The Comparative Guide to American Hospitals

Volume 1

2/15

Fourth Edition

The Comparative Guide to American Hospitals

Volume 1: Eastern Region

4,834 Hospitals with Key Personnel and 67 Quality Measures Relating to Heart Attack, Heart Failure, Pneumonia, Stroke, Blood Clots, Childhood Asthma, Emergency Room Care, Surgical Care, Preventative Care, Medical Imaging and Patient Experience

---

A SEDGWICK PRESS Book

Grey House Publishing

PUBLISHER: Leslie Mackenzie
SENIOR EDITOR: David Garoogian
EDITORIAL DIRECTOR: Laura Mars
PRODUCTION MANAGER: Kristen Thatcher
MARKETING DIRECTOR: Jessica Moody

A Sedgewick Press Book
Grey House Publishing, Inc.
4919 Route 22
Amenia, NY 12501
518.789.8700
FAX 845.373.6390
www.greyhouse.com
e-mail: books @greyhouse.com

Fourth Edition

Printed in Canada

Comparative guide to American hospitals. Vol. 1, Eastern region; [ed. David Garoogian]. — 4th ed. (2014)

4 v. ; cm.

Includes index.
"4,834 Hospitals with Key Personnel and 67 Quality Measures Relating to Heart Attack, Heart Failure, Pneumonia, Stroke, Blood Clots, Childhood Asthma, Emergency Room Care, Surgical Care, Preventative Care, Medical Imaging and Patient Experience."

1. Hospitals—United States—Directories. 2. Hospitals—United States—Periodicals. 3. Hospitals—Ratings—United States—Statistics—Periodicals. 4. Myocardial infarction—Hospitals—United States—Directories. 5. Heart failure—Hospitals—United States—Directories. 6. Pneumonia—Hospitals—United States—Directories. I. Garoogian, David.

RA977 .C66
610/.025

4-Volume Set	ISBN: 978-1-61925-457-2
Volume 1	**ISBN: 978-1-61925-458-9**
Volume 2	ISBN: 978-1-61925-459-6
Volume 3	ISBN: 978-1-61925-460-2
Volume 4	ISBN: 978-1-61925-461-9

Table of Contents

Introduction

This is the fourth edition of *The Comparative Guide to American Hospitals*. It reports on how 4,834 hospitals—**141 more than last edition**—in America measure up when caring for patients with a number of specific conditions. The third edition reported on **Heart Attacks, Heart Failure, Pneumonia, Childhood Asthma, Surgical Care, Use of Medical Imaging**, and **Patients' Hospital Experiences**. This fourth edition includes new data on **Blood Clot Prevention and Treatment, Emergency Room Care, Preventative Care, Stroke,** and **Medicare Spending**. Also new are appendices on **Surgical Complication Rates** and **Best Hospitals by Category**.

This work is based on a Federal study (Hospital Compare) in which short-term acute care and critical access hospitals around the country voluntarily report on quality measures to receive an incentive payment established by the Medicare Prescription Drug, Improvement and Modernization Act of 2003. Each hospital in this edition is rated on 67 recognized quality measures—**18 more than last edition**—and is compared to both state and national averages.

In *The Comparative Guide to American Hospitals,* the data is organized, sorted and ranked by our editors. It is this organization and ranking that makes *The Comparative Guide to American Hospitals* a unique and valuable tool to the health care consumer. Data is presented in such a way as to inform and educate the user, who can then put the facts into a meaningful context as hospitals are evaluated state by state.

Due to the increased data, and the regional use of such data, this edition is again comprised of four regional volumes—**Eastern, Southern, Central** and **Western**. In addition to comprehensive **hospital rankings and profiles** for all states in the region, each volume includes four Appendices with additional information.

In addition to the data from Hospital Compare, each hospital profile in *The Comparative Guide to American Hospitals* is comprised of value-added data from Grey House's *Directory of Hospital Personnel*. This critical contact data includes fax numbers, web sites, email addresses, and number of beds plus 24,458 key contact names—**783 more names than last edition.** In addition, each state chapter includes **State Hospital Rankings**.

Section One: State Hospital Rankings & State Profiles

The first section of each regional volume of *The Comparative Guide to American Hospitals* is arranged alphabetically by state. Each state chapter starts with a ranking section, unique to Grey House, that ranks hospitals in that state on how often they meet each of the 67 accepted quality protocols. The quality measures ranked in *The Comparative Guide to American Hospitals* are based on accepted, effective treatments supported by the Centers for Medicare & Medical Services of the US Department of Health & Human Services and the Hospital Quality Alliance (HQA)—a public/private collaboration established to promote on hospital quality of care. HQA represents consumers, hospitals, doctors, employers, accrediting organizations and Federal agencies.

Following the ranking section, hospital profiles are listed first by city, then alpha within city. Profiles include name, address, phone, fax, web site, hospital type and ownership, number of beds, and whether the hospital provides emergency services. Further, each profile includes an average of five key medical contacts—representing not only the facility's top administration but also the physicians specifically responsible for the care of heart, pneumonia, and asthma patients, as well as surgical care. Again, these data points are unique to *The Comparative Guide to American Hospitals*, and complete the picture for health care consumers searching for quality care.

The remainder of each hospital profile examines the 67 quality measures in detail, comparing the hospital's score with both the state and national average: These measures include:

- **Timely and Effective Care:**
    - **Blood Clot Prevention and Treatment** ***(NEW)*** measures include anticoagulation overlap therapy, ICU venous thromboembolism prophylaxis, incidence of potentially preventable VTE, UFH with dosages/platelet count monitoring, venous thromboembolism prophylaxis, and warfarin therapy discharge instructions
    - **Chest Pain/Possible Heart Attack Care** measures include aspirin at arrival, median time to ECG, median time to transfer, and fibrinolytic medication timing
    - **Children's Asthma Care** measures include receiving systemic corticosteroids, receiving home management plan, and receiving reliever medication
    - **Emergency Department** ***(NEW)*** measures include admittance decision time, head CT results within 45 minutes of arrival, patients who left ER before being seen, time from ER arrival to admittance, time from ER arrival to discharge, time spent in ER before being evaluated, and time to pain medications for long-bone fractures
    - **Heart Attack Care** measures include aspirin given at discharge, statin prescribed at discharge, fibrinolytic medication timing, and percutaneous coronary intervention within 90 minutes of arrival
    - **Heart Failure Care** measures include angiotensin converting enzyme inhibitor or angiotensin receptor blocker for left ventricular systolic dysfunction, discharge instructions given, and evaluation of left ventricular systolic function
    - **Pneumonia Care** measures include appropriate initial antibiotic, and blood culture timing
    - **Pregnancy and Delivery Care** ***(NEW)*** measures include newborn deliveries scheduled early
    - **Preventive Care** ***(NEW)*** measures include immunization for influenza and immunization for pneumonia
    - **Stroke Care** ***(NEW)*** measures include anticoagulation therapy for atrial fibrillation, antithrombotic therapy timing, assessed for rehabilitation, discharged on antithrombotic therapy, discharged on statin medication, thrombolytic therapy timing, venous thromboembolism prophylaxis, and written stroke educational materials given
    - **Surgical Care** measures include appropriate venous thromboembolism prophylaxis within 24 hours, appropriate beta blocker usage, controlled postoperative blood glucose, perioperative temperature management ***(NEW)***, prophylactic antibiotic timing, prophylactic antibiotic selection, prophylactic antibiotic stopped, and urinary catheter removal
- **Medicare Spending** ***(NEW)*** measures include Medicare spending per beneficiary
- **Use of Medical Imaging** measures include MRI for low back pain, cardiac imaging stress test before surgery ***(NEW)***, follow-up mammogram/ultrasound, combination brain/sinus CT scan ***(NEW)***, combination abdominal CT scan, and combination chest CT scan.
- **Survey of Patients' Hospital Experiences**
  HCAHPS (Hospital Consumer Assessment of Healthcare Providers and Systems) is a national, standardized survey of hospital patients. HCAHPS (pronounced "H-caps") was created to publicly report the patient's perspective of hospital care. The survey asks a random sample of recently discharged patients about important aspects of their hospital experience. The HCAHPS results allow consumers to make fair and objective comparisons between hospitals, and of individual hospitals to state and national benchmarks, on ten important measures of patients' perspectives of care:
    - How do patients rate the hospital overall?
    - How often did doctors communicate well with patients?
    - How often did nurses communicate well with patients?
    - How often did patients receive help quickly from hospital staff?
    - How often did staff explain about medicines before giving them to patients?
    - How often was patients' pain well controlled?
    - How often was the area around patients' rooms kept quiet at night?
    - How often were the patients' rooms and bathrooms kept clean?
    - Were patients given information about what to do during their recovery at home?
    - Would patients recommend the hospital to friends and family?

Section Two: Appendixes & Index

The second section of *The Comparative Guide to American Hospitals* includes:

- **Appendix A: 30-Day Death (Mortality) Rates** Unique to Grey House, this section takes data and organize it in a helpful, informative way for the reader. It lists hospitals nationwide that are "better" or "worse" than the national average, plus a State and National Summary of Hospital Mortality Rates.
- **Appendix B: 30-Day Readmission Rates** lists hospitals nationwide that are "better" or "worse" than the national average, plus a State and National Summary of Hospital Readmission Rates.
- **Appendix C: Surgical Complication Rates** lists hospitals nationwide that are "better" or "worse" than the national average, plus a State and National Summary of Hospital Readmission Rates. Surgical complications covered include:
  - A Wound That Splits Open After Surgery on the Abdomen or Pelvis
  - Accidental Cuts and Tears From Medical Treatment
  - Collapsed Lung Due to Medical Treatment
  - Deaths Among Patients With Serious Treatable Complications After Surgery
  - Rate of Complications for Hip/Knee Replacement Patients
  - Serious Blood Clots After Surgery
  - Serious Complications
- **Appendix D: Best Hospitals by Selected Category** lists best hospitals nationwide based on their average scores in 11 categories. The categories are:
  - Blood Clot Prevention and Treatment
  - Children's Asthma Care
  - Emergency Department Care
  - Heart Care
  - Pneumonia Care
  - Preventative Care
  - Stroke Care
  - Surgical Care
  - Patient's Hospital Experiences
  - Use of Medical Imaging
  - Lowest Medicare Spending per Beneficiary
- **Appendix E: Glossary** provides a list of 87 medical terms to make the best use possible of the data in this edition.
- **Regional Hospital Profile Index** lists hospitals included in each regional volume alphabetically, including city and state.
- **National Hospital Profile Index** lists all hospitals nationwide alphabetically, including volume number, city and state. Appears in Volume 4 only.

This completely revised fourth edition of *The Comparative Guide to American Hospitals* is a valuable guide for the entire medical community, with more hospitals, more criteria measures and more key executives than the last edition. It offers an indispensable snapshot of how hospitals measure up, not only to established "best practices," but also to each other.

We welcome your comments to this edition.

User's Guide

What is the *Comparative Guide to American Hospitals*?

The *Comparative Guide to American Hospitals* (CGAH) is based on a Federal study (Hospital Compare) in which short-term acute care and critical access hospitals around the country voluntarily report on quality measures to receive an incentive payment established by the Medicare Prescription Drug, Improvement and Modernization Act of 2003. Each hospital in this edition is rated on 67 recognized quality measures and is compared to both state and national averages. The measures are grouped into four major categories: Timely and Effective Care; Survey of Patients' Experiences; Use of Medical Imaging; and Medicare Spending Per Beneficiary.

Timely and Effective Care Measures (aka "Process of Care" Measures)

Process of care measures reported under the Hospital Inpatient Quality Reporting (IQR) and Outpatient Quality Reporting (OQR) programs show: 1) The percentage of hospital patients who receive treatments known to get the best results for certain common, serious medical conditions or surgical procedures; 2) How quickly hospitals treat patients who come to the hospital with certain medical emergencies. The measures only apply to patients for whom the recommended treatment would be appropriate. By law, any measures reported on the Hospital Compare website must reflect accepted standards of care, based on current scientific evidence. The measures are regularly reviewed and revised to ensure that they are up-to-date, and new measures and types of conditions and treatments are added over time. Process of care measures include:

- Blood Clot Prevention and Treatment
- Chest Pain/Possible Heart Attack Care
- Children's Asthma Care
- Emergency Department Care
- Heart Attack Care
- Heart Failure Care
- Pneumonia Care
- Pregnancy and Delivery Care
- Preventative Care
- Stroke Care
- Surgical Care Improvment Project

Where the Information Comes From

Measures of timely and effective care come from the data that hospitals get from medical records of their eligible patients, following standards for abstracting and reporting the information. Data submissions include auditing procedures and edit checks to assess whether data submitted are consistent with CMS's defined specifications. In addition, CMS validates the data submitted to provide assurance that the hospital, or its designated agent, can accurately abstract patient medical records and accurately submit data.

What Patients the Measures Apply To

The measures of timely and effective care apply to any adult patients treated at hospitals participating in the IQR and OQR programs for whom the recommended treatments would be appropriate, including Medicare patients, Medicare managed care patients, and non-Medicare patients. Hospitals with a large number of discharges may provide data from a sample of eligible Medicare and non-Medicare patients, based CMS sampling rules.

Risk Adjustment

The measures of timely and effective care do not require risk adjustment, because patients for whom the recommended treatment would not be appropriate are not included in the calculations.

Significance Testing

CMS does not perform tests of statistical significance in reporting the measures of timely and effective care. However, the smaller the sample size, the greater the difference in rates must be in order for that difference to be statistically meaningful. Large differences between individual hospitals' rates may be significant, but small differences between hospitals are usually not significant.

Reporting Period

These 50 measures are based on a reporting period of October 1, 2012 through September 30, 2013 except for the following: Emergency Department Care—Percentage of Patients Who Left the Emergency Department Before Being Seen—January 1, 2012 through December 31, 2012; Preventative Care—Patients Assessed and Given Influenza Vaccination—October 1, 2012 through March 31, 2013; All eight Stroke Care measures—January 1, 2013 through September 30, 2013; All six Blood Clot Prevention and Treatment measures—January 1, 2013 through September 30, 2013.

Survey of Patients' Experiences

The Centers for Medicare & Medicaid Services (CMS), along with the Agency for Healthcare Research and Quality (AHRQ), developed the HCAHPS (Hospital Consumer Assessment of Healthcare Providers and Systems) Survey, also known as Hospital CAHPS®, to provide a standardized survey instrument and data collection methodology for measuring patients' perspectives on hospital care. The HCAHPS Survey is administered to a random sample of patients continuously throughout the year. CMS cleans, adjusts and analyzes the data, then publicly reports the results.

Which Patients are Included
The HCAHPS survey is administered to a random sample of adult patients across medical conditions between 48 hours and six weeks after discharge; the survey is not restricted to Medicare beneficiaries.

Where the Information Comes From
All short-term, acute care, non-specialty hospitals are invited to participate in the HCAHPS Survey. Over 4,000 hospitals participate in HCAHPS. The goal is for each hospital to get at least 300 completed patient surveys per year. In general, the more patients that respond to the survey, the more the results shown on this website will reflect the experiences of all the patients who used that hospital. HCAHPS survey data must be collected by organizations that are trained by the federal government in HCAHPS data collection procedures. Data submitted to the HCAHPS data warehouse is cleaned, adjusted and analyzed by CMS, which calculates hospitals' HCAHPS scores and publicly reports them on the Hospital Compare website.

Adjusting Rates
Preparing the data for public reporting includes taking certain factors into account to ensure fair comparisons among hospitals. For example, the mix of patients can differ from one hospital to the next, and these differences in the patient mix can affect a hospital's HCAHPS results. Patient-mix adjustment takes these differences into account so that the survey results reported on this website are what would be expected for each hospital if all hospitals had a similar mix of patients.

Reporting Period
These 10 measures are based on a reporting period of October 1, 2012 through September 30, 2013.

Use of Medical Imaging

The six measures on the use of medical imaging show how often a hospital provides specific imaging tests for Medicare beneficiaries under circumstances where they may not be medically appropriate. Lower percentages suggest more efficient use of medical imaging. The purpose of reporting these measures is to reduce unnecessary exposure to contrast materials and/or radiation, to ensure adherence to evidence-based medicine and practice guidelines, and to prevent wasteful use of Medicare resources. The measures only apply to Medicare patients treated in hospital outpatient departments. It does not include tests performed in other ambulatory care settings or hospital inpatient settings.

What Patients are Included
Outpatient imaging efficiency measures apply only to Medicare beneficiaries enrolled in Original Medicare who were treated as outpatients in hospital facilities reimbursed through the Outpatient Prospective Payment System (OPPS). They do not include Medicare managed care patients, non-Medicare patients, or patients who were admitted to the hospital as inpatients.

Where the Information Comes From
CMS calculates imaging efficiency measures using data from claims that hospitals and physicians submit for Medicare beneficiaries enrolled in Original Medicare. The data are calculated only for hospitals paid through the Outpatient Prospective Payment System (OPPS). The measures are part of the Hospital Outpatient Quality Reporting Program (OQR).

Risk Adjustment
Outpatient imaging efficiency measures are not risk adjusted. However, measures specifications do not include cases where there were clear medical reasons for performing the tests.

Significance Testing
CMS does not perform tests of statistical significance in reporting the outpatient imaging efficiency measures. Large differences between hospitals' percentages may be significant, but small differences usually are not.

Reporting Period
These six measures are based on a reporting period of July 1, 2012 through June 30, 2013.

Medicare Spending per Beneficiary

The Medicare Spending per Beneficiary (MSPB) measure assesses Medicare Part A and Part B payments for services provided to a Medicare beneficiary during a spending-per-beneficiary episode that spans from three days prior to an inpatient hospital admission through 30 days after discharge. The payments included in this measure are price-standardized and risk-adjusted. Price standardization removes sources of variation that are due to geographic payment differences such as wage index and geographic practice cost differences, as well as indirect medical education (IME) or disproportionate share hospital (DSH) payments. Risk adjustment accounts for variation due to patient health status.

By measuring cost of care through this measure, CMS hopes to increase the transparency of care for consumers and recognize hospitals that are involved in the provision of high-quality care at lower cost to Medicare.

Reporting Period
This measure is based on a reporting period of January 1, 2012 through December 31, 2012.

Sample Entry

The listing below illustrates the kind of information that is or might be included in a Hospital Profile. Each numbered item of information is described in the paragraphs following the example.

1 ▶ **Cleveland Clinic**
9500 Euclid Avenue — Phone: 216-444-2200
Cleveland, OH 44195 — Fax: 216-445-7758
URL: www.clevelandclinic.org
Type: Acute Care Hospitals — Emergency Services: Yes
Ownership: Voluntary non-profit - Private — Beds: 1,113

2 ▶ **Key Personnel:**
CEO/President. . . . . Delos M Cosgrove, MD
Chief of Medical Staff . . . . Marc Harrison, MD
Infection Control. . . . . David L Longworth, MD
Operating Room. . . . . Allan Siperstein, MD
Pediatric Ambulatory Care . . . . . . Robert Wyllie, MD
Quality Assurance . . . . J Michael Henderson, MD
Radiology. . . . . Gregory P Borkowski, MD

3 ▶ Measure	Cases	This Hosp.	State Avg.	U.S. Avg.
4 ▶ **Blood Clot Prevention and Treatment**				
Anticoagulation Overlap Therapy[2]	400	98%	93%	93%
ICU Venous Thromboembolism Prophylaxis[2]	84	98%	93%	92%
Incidence of Potentially Preventable VTE[2]	168	2%	6%	10%
UFH with Dosages/Platelet Monitoring[2]	444	100%	98%	97%
Venous Thromboembolism Prophylaxis[2]	347	96%	88%	85%
Warfarin Therapy Discharge Instructions[2]	237	89%	79%	75%
5 ▶ **Chest Pain/Possible Heart Attack Care**				
Aspirin Given Within 24 Hours of Arrival	190	96%	97%	96%
Fibrinolytic Meds Within 30 Min. of Arrival[7]	-	-	44%	58%
Median Time to ECG (minutes)	197	6	6	7
Median Time to Transfer (minutes)[1]	-	-	58	60
6 ▶ **Children's Asthma Care**				
Received Home Management Plan of Care	74	99%	85%	88%
Received Reliever Medication	75	100%	100%	100%
Received Systemic Corticosteroids	74	100%	100%	100%
7 ▶ **Emergency Department**				
Admittance Decision Time (minutes)[2]	227	102	90	98%
Head CT Results Within 45 Min. of Arrival	11	91%	63%	57%
Patients Who Left ER Before Being Seen	82,229	2%	2%	2%
Time from ER Arrival to Admit. (minutes)[2]	228	304	265	274
Time from ER Arrival to Discharge (minutes)	294	131	128	134
Time in ER Before Being Evaluated (minutes)	417	11	22	26
Time to Pain Meds for Fractures (minutes)	194	46	54	57
8 ▶ **Heart Attack Care**				
Aspirin Given at Discharge	868	100%	99%	99%
Fibrinolytic Meds Within 30 Min. of Arrival[7]	-	-	80%	54%
PCI Within 90 Minutes of Arrival	13	92%	97%	96%
Statin Prescribed at Discharge	834	100%	98%	98%
9 ▶ **Heart Failure Care**				
ACE Inhibitor or ARB for LVSD[2]	287	99%	97%	97%
Discharge Instructions Given[2]	712	94%	96%	94%
Evaluation of LVS Function[2]	858	100%	100%	99%
10 ▶ **Medicare Spending**				
Medicare Hospital Spending per Patient	-	0.99	1.01	0.98
11 ▶ **Pneumonia Care**				
Appropriate Initial Antibiotic Given	84	94%	96%	95%
Blood Culture Timing	176	95%	98%	98%
12 ▶ **Pregnancy and Delivery Care**				
Newborn Deliveries Scheduled Early[1]	-	-	5%	6%
13 ▶ **Preventive Care**				
Immunization for Influenza[2]	577	96%	93%	90%
Immunization for Pneumonia[2]	747	95%	94%	92%
14 ▶ **Stroke Care**				
Anticoagulation Therapy for Atrial Fibrillation[2]	34	100%	95%	95%
Antithrombotic Therapy Timing[2]	180	96%	98%	98%
Assessed for Rehabilitation[2]	333	98%	98%	97%
Discharged on Antithrombotic Therapy[2]	221	100%	99%	99%
Discharged on Statin Medication[2]	152	99%	95%	94%
Thrombolytic Therapy Timing[1,2]	-	-	65%	66%
Venous Thromboembolism Prophylaxis[2]	349	100%	95%	94%
Written Stroke Educational Materials Given[2]	125	98%	92%	88%
15 ▶ **Surgical Care Improvement Project**				
Appropriate Beta Blocker Usage[2]	356	99%	98%	98%
Appropriate VTP Within 24 Hours[2]	447	99%	98%	98%
Controlled Postoperative Blood Glucose[2]	253	96%	97%	97%
Perioperative Temperature Management[2]	625	100%	100%	100%
Prophylactic Antibiotic Selection[2]	570	99%	99%	99%
Prophylactic Antibiotic Selection (Outpatient)	1,080	100%	98%	98%
Prophylactic Antibiotic Stopped[2]	554	97%	98%	98%
Prophylactic Antibiotic Timing[2]	570	99%	99%	99%
Prophylactic Antibiotic Timing (Outpatient)	563	97%	97%	98%
Urinary Catheter Removal[2]	381	98%	97%	97%
16 ▶ **Survey of Patients' Hospital Experiences**				
Area Around Room 'Always' Quiet at Night	300+	57%	58%	61%
Doctors 'Always' Communicated Well	300+	82%	80%	82%
Home Recovery Information Given	300+	90%	87%	85%
Hospital Given 9 or 10 on 10 Point Scale	300+	84%	72%	71%
Meds 'Always' Explained Before Given	300+	66%	64%	64%
Nurses 'Always' Communicated Well	300+	83%	81%	79%
Pain 'Always' Well Controlled	300+	72%	71%	71%
Room and Bathroom 'Always' Clean	300+	78%	75%	73%
Timely Help 'Always' Received	300+	68%	70%	68%
Would Definitely Recommend Hospital	300+	87%	71%	71%
17 ▶ **Use of Medical Imaging**				
Cardiac Imaging Stress Test before Surgery	4,179	6.7%	5.4%	5.3%
Combination Abdominal CT Scan	5,813	13.0%	7.1%	10.5%
Combination Brain/Sinus CT Scan	2,131	1.7%	2.8%	2.7%
Combination Chest CT Scan	6,539	0.1%	1.7%	2.7%
Follow-up Mammogram/Ultrasound	9,962	9.3%	8.7%	8.8%
Lumbar Spine MRI for Low Back Pain	661	31.9%	34.7%	37.2%

1▶ Hospital Name and Record Header: hospital name; street address; phone; fax; e-mail; URL; hospital type; ownership; emergency services (Yes/No); and number of beds.

2▶ Key Personnel: includes the names of key personnel primarily related to the conditions covered in this publication.

3▶ Hospital Compare Data: each profile contains data covering 67 measures contained in the Centers for Medicare & Medicaid Services Hospital Compare database. There are five columns:

Measure: the 67 quality measures reported.

There are 14 possible footnotes:

(1) The number of cases/patients is too few to report
This footnote is applied: when the number of cases/patients does not meet the required minimum amount for public reporting; when the number of cases/patients is too small to reliably tell how well a hospital is performing; and/or to protect personal health information.

(2) Data submitted were based on a sample of cases/patients
This footnote indicates that a hospital chose to submit data for a random sample of its cases/patients while following specific rules for how to select the patients.

(3) Results are based on a shorter time period than required
This footnote indicates that the hospital's results were based on data from less than the maximum possible time period generally used to collect data for a measure. See Reporting Periods for more information.

(4) Data suppressed by CMS (Centers for Medicare and Medicaid Services) for one or more quarters
The results for these measures were excluded for various reasons, such as data inaccuracies.

(5) Results are not available for this reporting period
This footnote is applied when the hospital does not have data to report.

(6) Fewer than 100 patients completed the HCAHPS survey.
This footnote is applied when the number of completed surveys the hospital or its vendor provided to CMS is less than 100. Use these scores with caution, as the number of surveys may be too low to reliably assess hospital performance.

(7) No cases met the criteria for this measure
This footnote is applied when a hospital did not have any cases meet the inclusion criteria for a measure.

(8) The lower limit of the confidence interval cannot be calculated
The lower limit of the confidence interval cannot be calculated if the number of observed infections equals zero.

(9) No data are available from the state/territory for this reporting period
This footnote is applied when: too few hospitals in a state/territory had data available; or no data was reported for this state/territory.

(10) The scores shown reflect fewer than 50 completed surveys.
This footnote is applied when the number of completed surveys the hospital or its vendor provided to CMS is less than 50. Use these scores with caution, as the number of surveys may be too low to reliably assess hospital performance.

(11) There were discrepancies in the data collection process
This footnote is applied when there have been deviations from data collection protocols. CMS is working to correct this situation.

(12) This measure does not apply to this hospital for this reporting period
This footnote is applied when: there were zero device days or procedures; the hospital does not have ICU locations; the hospital is a new member of the registry and didn't have an opportunity to submit any cases; or the hospital does not report this voluntary measure.

(13) Results cannot be calculated for this reporting period
This footnote is applied when: the number of predicted infections is less than 1; the number of observed MRSA or Clostridium difficile infections present on admission (community-onset prevalence) was above a pre-determined cut-point.

(14) The results for this state are combined with nearby states to protect confidentiality
This footnote is applied when a state has fewer than 10 hospitals in order to protect confidentiality. Results are combined as follows: 1) the District of Columbia and Delaware are combined; 2) Alaska and Washington are combined; 3) North Dakota and South Dakota are combined; and 4) New Hampshire and Vermont are combined. Hospitals located in Maryland and U.S. territories are excluded from the measure calculation.

Cases: the size of the data sample (number of patients) for each hospital and quality measure. In addition, the notation "0" is applied when a hospital provided care to patients with a condition, such as pneumonia, but the cases that the hospital submitted did not meet the specific criteria for being included in the calculation of the measure.

This Hospital: the performance rate that the hospital achieved for each quality measure. This value is expressed as a percentage of the sample size that was measured. The performance rate is calculated by dividing the numerator by the denominator. The denominator is the sum of all eligible cases (as defined in the measure specifications) submitted to the QIO Clinical Data Warehouse for the reporting period. The numerator is the sum of all eligible cases submitted for the same reporting period where the recommended care was provided.

State Average: the average rate for all hospitals reporting data in the state the hospital is located in.

U.S. Average: the average rate for all hospitals reporting nationwide.

Note: Beginning in December 2010, state and national averages for the process of care measures are calculated by summing the cases in the state or nation that "passed" the measure (Numerator) and dividing that sum by the number of cases in the state or national Denominator. For the national and state averages, a simple average was constructed where the numerator was the sum of all non-excluded hospitals' scores and the denominator was the total number of hospitals, each calculated at either the national or individual state level. For the process and survey measures, the national and state averages are calculated before excluding suppressed rates and are not recalculated using only published rates as was done prior to September 2009. Acute Care-VA Medical Centers are not included in the calculation of the national and state comparison rates.

The children's asthma care national and state averages are calculated differently. The average rate for all healthcare organizations in the nation that provide results for a measure. The average rate is calculated by dividing the total number of patients who had the recommended care provided for a measure by the total number of patients who met the inclusion and exclusion criteria for that measure in the nation for the timeframe being reported.

4▶ Blood Clot Prevention and Treatment

The measures listed below show how well hospitals are providing recommended care known to prevent or treat blood clots and how often blood clots occur that could have been prevented.

Anticoagulation Overlap Therapy

Patients with blood clots who got the recommended treatment, which includes using two different blood thinner medicines at the same time.
Patients who develop blood clots in their veins (also called venous thromboembolism, or VTE) need to get treatment that can break up the clots quickly and prevent others from forming. The recommended treatment is to first give a blood thinner that can get into the bloodstream quickly through an IV or injection (heparin), then give a slower-acting oral blood thinner medicine (warfarin), and continue giving both blood thinners for 5 days or until it is safe for the patient to transition off of the IV blood thinner and use only the oral blood thinner medicine. This measure shows the percentage of hospital patients who had a confirmed diagnosis of blood clot at hospital admission or during their hospital stay, and received both medicines for at least 5 days, or were discharged from the hospital on both kinds of medicine, unless their blood work showed they no longer needed it. *Higher percentages are better.*

ICU Venous Thromboembolism Prophylaxis

Patients who got treatment to prevent blood clots on the day of or day after being admitted to the intensive care unit (ICU).
Patients in the Intensive Care Unit (ICU) are at increased risk for developing blood clots in their veins (venous thromboembolism, or VTE), because they are in bed for a long period of time. These clots can break off and travel to other parts of the body, causing serious harm. Hospitals can prevent blood clots by routinely evaluating all patients for their risk of developing blood clots and using appropriate prevention and treatment procedures. Prevention can include compression stockings, blood thinners, and/or other medicines. This measure shows the percentage of ICU patients who received treatment to prevent blood clots: on the day of or day after arrival at the hospital; or on the day of or day after transfer to the ICU; or on the day of or day after having surgery. Patients who did not receive treatment may also be included in this measure, if they had paperwork in their chart to explain why. Reasons for not receiving treatment may include having a massive wound, actively bleeding, or having an allergy to blood thinners. *Higher percentages are better.*

Incidence of Potentially Preventable VTE
Patients who developed a blood clot while in the hospital who did not get treatment that could have prevented it. Because hospital patients often have to stay in bed for long periods of time, all patients admitted to the hospital are at increased risk of developing blood clots in their veins (also called venous thromboembolism or VTE) that can break off and travel to other parts of the body, like the heart, brain, or lung. Hospitals can prevent blood clots by routinely evaluating patients for their risk of developing blood clots and using appropriate prevention and treatment procedures. Prevention can include compression stockings, blood thinners, and/or other medicines. This measure shows the percentage of patients who developed blood clots while in the hospital who did not receive preventative treatment beforehand. *Lower percentages are better.*

UFH with Dosages/Platelet Monitoring
Patients with blood clots who were treated with an intravenous blood thinner, and then were checked to determine if the blood thinner was putting the patient at an increased risk of bleeding.
Patients who have been diagnosed with a blood clot (also called venous thromboembolism, or VTE) are usually treated with a blood thinner such as IV heparin. Some patients may be prescribed a type of IV heparin called unfractionated heparin (UFH). Unfractionated heparin carries a higher risk of increased bleeding than a different type of IV heparin (called low molecular weight heparin). Risk for bleeding increases because blood thinners increase the time it takes your blood to clot. The most common signs of increased bleeding include unusual bruising, nosebleeds, and bleeding gums. Because of their higher risk of bleeding, patients getting unfractionated heparin should be given regular blood tests to determine if they are at an increased risk of bleeding from getting the medication. This measure shows the percentage of patients who developed a blood clot at admission or during their hospital stay, treated with unfractionated IV heparin who had their blood checked using recommended procedures. *Higher percentages are better.*

Venous Thromboembolism Prophylaxis
Patients who got treatment to prevent blood clots on the day of or day after hospital admission or surgery. Because hospital patients often have to stay in bed for long periods of time, all patients admitted to the hospital are at increased risk of developing blood clots in their veins (also called venous thromboembolism, or VTE) that can break off and travel to other parts of the body, like the heart, brain, or lung. Hospitals can prevent blood clots by routinely evaluating patients for their risk of developing blood clots and using appropriate prevention and treatment procedures. Prevention can include compression stockings, blood thinners, and/or other medicines. This measure shows the percentage of patients who received treatment to prevent blood clots: on the day of or day after arrival at the hospital; or on the day of or day after having surgery. Patients who did not receive treatment may also be included in this measure, if they had paperwork in their chart to explain why. Reasons for not receiving treatment may include having a massive wound, actively bleeding, or having an allergy to blood thinners. *Higher percentages are better.*

Warfarin Therapy Discharge Instructions
Patients with blood clots who were discharged on a blood thinner medicine and received written instructions about that medicine.
Patients who develop blood clots (also called venous thromboembolism or VTE) will usually be given blood thinner medicines to take when they leave the hospital. Educating patients about how to take the medicine and its possible side effects can help prevent problems that could bring them back to the hospital. Before leaving the hospital, patients with a blood clot, who are taking a blood thinner medicine, and their caregiver should receive information about the following topics: Compliance (how to follow medication instructions); Diet (how to eat a healthy diet and avoid foods that interfere with blood thinners); Monitoring their blood thinner medicine; Adverse drug reactions (difficulty breathing, vomiting, nausea); When to call your health care provider (dizziness or weakness, a fall, bright red bleeding). This measure shows the percentage of patients diagnosed with a blood clot (either at admission or during their hospital stay) discharged from the hospital on blood thinners (anticoagulants or anticoagulant therapy or warfarin therapy) who received written educational instructions at hospital discharge. *Higher percentages are better.*

5▶ Chest Pain/Possible Heart Attack Care

Scientific evidence shows that the following measures represent the best practices for the treatment of chest pain/possible heart attack.

Aspirin Given Within 24 Hours of Arrival
Outpatients with chest pain or possible heart attack who got aspirin within 24 hours of arrival.
Blood clots can cause heart attacks. For many patients having a heart attack, taking aspirin soon after symptoms of a heart attack begin may help break up a clot and make the heart attack less severe. If patients have not taken aspirin themselves before going to the hospital, they should get aspirin when they arrive. Standards for care say that patients should get aspirin within 24 hours of arriving at the hospital. This measure tells what percent of patients got aspirin within this time period. *Higher percentages are better.*

Fibrinolytic Meds Within 30 Minutes of Arrival
Outpatients with chest pain or possible heart attack who got drugs to break up blood clots within 30 minutes of arrival.
Blood clots can cause heart attacks. Certain patients having a heart attack should get a "clot busting" drug to help break up the blood clots and improve blood flow to the heart. Standards for care say that a clot busting drug should be given within 30 minutes of arrival at the hospital. This measure tells the percent of patients who were given a clot busting drug within this time period. *Higher percentages are better.*

Average Time to ECG (minutes)
Average number of minutes before outpatients with chest pain or possible heart attack got an ECG.
"ECG" (sometimes called EKG) stands for electrocardiogram. An ECG is a test that can help doctors know whether patients are having a heart attack. Standards of care say that patients with chest pain or a possible heart attack should have an ECG upon arrival, preferably within 10 minutes. This measure shows the average number of minutes it takes before patients had an ECG (calculated as an arithmetic median). Sometimes patients get an ECG done before they get to the hospital (for example, by the ambulance staff). This is counted as "0 minutes." *Lower numbers are better.*

Average Time to Transfer (minutes)
Average number of minutes before outpatients with chest pain or possible heart attack who needed specialized care were transferred to another hospital.
If a hospital does not have the facilities to provide specialized heart attack care, it transfers patients with possible heart attack to another hospital that can give them this care. This measure shows how long it takes, on average, for hospitals to identify patients who need specialized heart attack care the hospital cannot provide and begin their transfer to another hospital. Specifically, it shows the average (arithmetic median) number of minutes it takes from the time patients arrive in the emergency department until they are transported to a different hospital. *Lower numbers are better.*

6▶ Children's Asthma Care

Scientific evidence shows that the following measures represent best practices for treating children with asthma.

Received Home Management Plan of Care
Children and their caregivers who received a home management plan of care document while hospitalized for asthma.
This measure shows the percentage of children with asthma and their caregivers who were given a home management plan of care document while hospitalized. Because asthma is a chronic condition, controlling a child's asthma symptoms at home will help reduce the risk of further attacks. Knowledge about the disease and its treatment is the key to good asthma control. Asthma that is not managed effectively may lead to more visits to the hospital. Medications can help prevent asthma symptoms and attacks from starting in the first place and can reduce how often attacks happen and severity of the attacks. It is important for children with asthma and their caregivers to know how to prevent asthma symptoms and attacks before they happen. The home management plan of care helps children with asthma and their caregivers develop a plan to manage the child's asthma symptoms and to know when to take action. It should address all of the following: arrangements for follow-up care; environmental control and control of other triggers; method and timing of rescue actions; use of controller medications; use of reliever medications. *Higher percentages are better.*

Received Reliever Medication
Children who received reliever medication while hospitalized for asthma.
National guidelines for treating children with asthma recommend using relievers in the severe phase and gradually cutting down the dosage of medications to provide control of asthma symptoms. Although there are guidelines for medication therapy for children with asthma, there is evidence that these guidelines are not being consistently followed. Using the appropriate medications will lower the risk of severe illness and/or death. This measure shows the percentage of children with asthma who were given reliever medication (like albuterol) while hospitalized. Relievers are medications that relax the bands of muscle surrounding the airways and make breathing easier. *Higher percentages are better.*

Received Systemic Corticosteroids
Children who received systemic corticosteroid medication (oral and IV medication that reduces inflammation and controls symptoms) while hospitalized for asthma.
Oral or IV steroid medications control severe asthma well. That is why they are important for hospital care. Unfortunately, they can cause serious side effects when used long-term. That is why they are mainly used for severe episodes or chronic severe asthma, which cannot be controlled with other medications (like inhaled or oral bronchodilators and anti-inflammatory medications). This measure shows the percentage of children with asthma who were given oral or IV steroid medications while hospitalized. These medications work in the body as a whole,

rather than just on the lungs. They help reduce inflammation and control allergic reactions. *Higher percentages are better.*

7▶ Emergency Department Care

Timely and effective care in hospital emergency departments is essential for good patient outcomes. Delays before receiving care in the emergency department can reduce the quality of care and increase risks and discomfort for patients with serious illnesses or injuries. Waiting times at different hospitals can vary widely, depending on the number of patients seen, staffing levels, efficiency, admitting procedures, or the availability of inpatient beds.

Admittance Decision Time (minutes)
For patients who had to be admitted to the hospital as an inpatient, average time patients spent in the emergency department, after the doctor decided to admit them as an inpatient before leaving the emergency department for their inpatient room.
Delays in transferring emergency department patients to an inpatient unit may be a sign that there's not enough staff or there's poor coordination among hospital departments. Long delays can also create more stress for patients and families. This measure shows the average (arithmetic median) time patients spent in the emergency department—from the time the doctor decided to admit them to the time they left the emergency department for an inpatient bed. *Lower numbers are better.*

Head CT Results Within 45 Minutes of Arrival
Percentage of patients who came to the emergency department with stroke symptoms who received brain scan results within 45 minutes of arrival.
People who suffer from strokes need to receive treatment immediately to lessen the amount of brain damage that occurs with any stroke. A scan of the brain must be taken to determine the type and severity of the stroke before treatment can be provided. Long waits may be a sign that the emergency department is understaffed or overcrowded and can lead to delayed diagnosis and treatment and may lead to further brain damage. Standards of care say that patients with stroke symptoms should receive brain scan results (to diagnose whether and how severely a stroke occurred) within 45 minutes of arriving at the emergency department. This measure shows the percentage of emergency department patients with stroke symptoms who received brain scan results within that time period. *Lower numbers are better.*

Patients Who Left ER Before Being Seen
Percentage of patients who left the emergency department before being seen.
Hospital emergency departments that have high percentages of patients who leave without being seen may not have the staff or resources to provide timely and effective emergency room care. Patients who leave the emergency department without being seen may be seriously ill, putting themselves at higher risk for poor health outcomes. This measure shows the percentage of all individuals who signed into an emergency department but left before being evaluated by a healthcare professional. *Lower numbers are better.*

Time from ER Arrival to Admittance (minutes)
For patients who had to be admitted to the hospital as an inpatient, average time patients spent in the emergency department, before they were admitted to the hospital as an inpatient.
Long stays in an emergency department before a patient is admitted may be a sign that the emergency department is understaffed or overcrowded. This may result in delays in treatment or lower quality care. This measure shows the average (arithmetic median) time patients spent in the emergency department—from the time they arrived to the time they left the emergency department for an inpatient bed. This number only includes patients who were admitted to the hospital as an inpatient. It does not include those people who went home. *Lower numbers are better.*

Time from ER Arrival to Discharge (minutes)
Average time patients spent in the emergency department before being sent home.
Long stays in the emergency department before a patient is sent home may be a sign that the emergency department is understaffed or overcrowded. This may result in delays in treatment, increased suffering for those who wait, and unpleasant treatment environments. This measure shows the average (arithmetic median) time in minutes that patients spent in the emergency department—from the time they arrived to the time they were sent home. It does not include patients who were later admitted to the hospital as inpatients, admitted for observation, transferred to another acute care hospital, or who left without being seen by a licensed provider. *Lower numbers are better.*

Time in ER Before Being Evaluated (minutes)
Average time patients spent in the emergency department before they were seen by a healthcare professional.
Delays in being seen by a healthcare provider may be a sign that the emergency department is understaffed or overcrowded. This may result in delays in treatment, lower quality care, and more stress for patients and families. For patients who were later sent home, this measure shows the average (arithmetic median) time in minutes

spent in the emergency department—from the time they arrived until the time they were seen by a healthcare professional. It does not include patients who were admitted to the hospital, who died in the emergency department, or who left without being seen. *Lower numbers are better.*

Time to Pain Meds for Fractures (minutes)
Average time patients who came to the emergency department with broken bones had to wait before receiving pain medication.
Long waits before a patient is treated may be a sign that the emergency department is understaffed or overcrowded. For patients with broken bones, long waits without pain medication cause unnecessary suffering. For all patients 2 years and older who came to the emergency department with a broken arm or leg, this shows the average (arithmetic median) time they waited before receiving pain medication. *Lower numbers are better.*

8 ▸ Heart Attack Care

Scientific evidence shows that the following measures represent the best practices for the treatment of heart attack.

Aspirin Given at Discharge
Heart attack patients given aspirin at discharge.
Blood clots can block blood vessels. Aspirin can help prevent blood clots from forming or help dissolve blood clots that have formed. Following a heart attack, continued use of aspirin may help reduce the risk of another heart attack. Aspirin can have side effects like stomach inflammation, bleeding, or allergic reactions. Talk to your health care provider before using aspirin on a regular basis to make sure it's safe for you. This measure shows what percentage of patients were given aspirin upon leaving the hospital. *Higher percentages are better.*

Fibrinolytic Meds Within 30 Minutes of Arrival
Heart attack patients given fibrinolytic medication within 30 minutes of arrival.
The heart is a muscle that gets oxygen through blood vessels. Sometimes blood clots can block these blood vessels and the heart can't get enough oxygen. This can cause a heart attack. Fibrinolytic drugs are medicines that can help dissolve blood clots in blood vessels and improve blood flow to your heart. Standards for care say that patients should get them within 30 minutes of arrival at the hospital. This measure shows what percentage of patients got fibrinolytic drugs within this time period. *Higher percentages are better.*

PCI Within 90 Minutes of Arrival
Heart attack patients given PCI within 90 minutes of arrival.
The heart is a muscle that gets oxygen through blood vessels. Sometimes blood clots can block these blood vessels, and the heart cannot get enough oxygen. This can cause a heart attack. Percutaneous coronary interventions (PCI) are procedures that are among the most effective ways to open blocked blood vessels and help prevent further heart muscle damage. A PCI is performed by a doctor to open the blockage and increase blood flow in blocked blood vessels. Improving blood flow to your heart as quickly as possible lessens the damage to your heart muscle, and it also can increase your chances of surviving a heart attack. There are three procedures commonly described by the term PCI. These procedures all involve a catheter (a flexible tube) that is inserted, often through your leg, and guided through the blood vessels to the blockage. The three procedures are: angioplasty—a balloon is inflated to open the blood vessel; stenting—a small wire tube called a stent is placed in the blood vessel to hold it open; atherectomy—a blade or laser cuts through and removes the blockage. Standards for care say that patients should receive a PCI within 90 minutes of arriving at the hospital. This measure shows what percentage of patients got a PCI within this time period. *Higher percentages are better.*

Statin Prescribed at Discharge
Heart attack patients given a prescription for a statin at discharge.
Statins are drugs used to lower cholesterol. Cholesterol is a fat (also called a lipid) that your body needs to work properly. Cholesterol levels that are too high can increase your chance of getting heart disease, stroke, and other problems. For patients who have had one or more heart attacks and have high cholesterol, taking statins can lower the chance that they'll have another heart attack or die. This measure shows the percent of patients who had a heart attack who got a prescription for a statin upon leaving the hospital. Patients who shouldn't take statins aren't included in this measure. *Higher numbers are better.*

9 ▸ Heart Failure Care

Scientific evidence shows that the following measures represent the best practices for the treatment of heart failure.

ACE Inhibitor or ARB for LVSD
Heart failure patients given ACE inhibitor or ARB for left ventricular systolic dysfunction (LVSD).
ACE (angiotensin converting enzyme) inhibitors and ARBs (angiotensin receptor blockers) are medicines used to treat patients with heart failure and are particularly beneficial in those patients with decreased function of the left side of the heart. Early treatment with ACE inhibitors and ARBs in patients who have heart failure symptoms or decreased heart function after a heart attack can also reduce their risk of death from future heart attacks. ACE

inhibitors and ARBs work by limiting the effects of a hormone that narrows blood vessels, and may thus lower blood pressure and reduce the work the heart has to perform. Since the ways in which these two kinds of drugs work are different, your doctor will decide which drug is most appropriate for you. Standards for care say that if patients have a heart attack and/or heart failure, they should get a prescription for ACE inhibitors or ARBs if they have decreased heart function before leaving the hospital. *Higher percentages are better.*

Discharge Instructions Given
Heart failure patients given discharge instructions.
Heart failure is a chronic condition. It results in symptoms such as shortness of breath, dizziness, and fatigue. Before you leave the hospital, the staff at the hospital should provide you with information to help you manage the symptoms after you get home. The information should include your information about: activity level (what you can and can't do); diet (what you should, and shouldn't eat or drink); medications; your follow-up appointment; watching your daily weight; and what to do if your symptoms get worse. *Higher percentages are better.*

Evaluation of LVS Function
Heart failure patients given an evaluation of left ventricular systolic (LVS) function.
The proper treatment for heart failure depends on what area of your heart is affected. An important test is to check how your heart is pumping, called an "evaluation of the left ventricular systolic function." It can tell your health care provider whether the left side of your heart is pumping properly. Other ways to check on how your heart is pumping include: your medical history; a physical examination; listening to your heart sounds; and other tests as ordered by a physician (like an ECG (electrocardiogram), chest x-ray, blood work, and an echocardiogram) *Higher percentages are better.*

10 ▶ Medicare Spending

The Medicare Hospital Spending per Patient measure shows whether Medicare spends more, less, or about the same on an episode of care for a Medicare patient treated in a specific hospital compared to how much Medicare spends on an episode of care across all hospitals nationally. This measure includes any Medicare Part A and Part B payments made for services provided to a patient during an episode of care, which includes the 3 days prior to the hospital stay, during the stay, and during the 30 days after discharge from the hospital. This result is a ratio calculated by dividing the amount Medicare spends per patient for an episode of care initiated at this hospital by the median (or middle) amount Medicare spent per episode of care nationally.

- A ratio equal to the national average means that Medicare spends ABOUT THE SAME per patient for an episode of care initiated at this hospital as it does per episode of care across all hospitals nationally.
- A ratio that is more than the national average means that Medicare spends MORE per patient for an episode of care initiated at this hospital than it does per episode of care across all hospitals nationally.
- A ratio that is less than the national average means that Medicare spends LESS per patient for an episode of care initiated at this hospital than it does per episode of care across all hospitals nationally.

11 ▶ Pneumonia Care

Scientific evidence shows that the following measures represent the best practices for the treatment of community-acquired pneumonia.

Appropriate Initial Antibiotic Given
Pneumonia patients given the most appropriate initial antibiotic(s).
Pneumonia is a lung infection that is usually caused by bacteria or a virus. If pneumonia is caused by bacteria, hospitals will treat the infection with antibiotics. Different bacteria are treated with different antibiotics. *Higher percentages are better.*

Blood Culture Timing
Pneumonia patients whose initial emergency room blood culture was performed prior to the administration of the first hospital dose of antibiotics.
Different types of bacteria can cause pneumonia. A blood culture is a test that can help your health care provider identify which bacteria may have caused your pneumonia, and which antibiotic should be prescribed. A blood culture is not always needed, but for patients who are first seen in the hospital emergency department, it is important for the accuracy of the test that a blood culture be conducted before any antibiotics are started. It is also important to start antibiotics as soon as possible. *Higher percentages are better.*

12▶ Pregnancy and Delivery Care

Newborn Deliveries Scheduled Early
Percent of newborns whose deliveries were scheduled too early (1-3 weeks early), when a scheduled delivery was not medically necessary.
Guidelines developed by doctors and researchers say it's best to wait until the 39th completed week of pregnancy to deliver your baby because important fetal development takes place in your baby's brain and lungs during the last few weeks of pregnancy. Sometimes women go into early labor on their own, and early deliveries can't be prevented. Sometimes, doctors decide that inducing labor or delivering a baby early by C-section (called "elective delivery") is in the best interest of the mother and the baby. In these cases, early deliveries are medically necessary. However, doctors may also decide to induce labor or deliver babies by C-section early as a convenience to themselves or their patient. This practice is not recommended. Hospitals should work with doctors and patients to avoid early elective deliveries when they are not medically necessary. This measure shows the percent of pregnancy women who had elective deliveries 1-3 weeks early (either vaginally or by C-section) who early deliveries were not medically necessary. Higher numbers may indicate that hospitals aren't doing enough to discourage this unsafe practice. *Lower percentages are better.*

13▶ Preventive Care

Hospitals and other healthcare providers play a crucial role in promoting, providing and educating patients about preventive services and screenings and maintaining the health of their communities. Many diseases are preventable through immunizations, screenings, treatment, and lifestyle changes. The information below shows how well the hospitals you selected are providing preventive services.

Immunization for Influenza
Patients assessed and given influenza vaccination.
Influenza, or the "flu," is a respiratory illness that is caused by flu viruses and easily spread from person to person. There are over 200,000 hospitalizations from the flu on average every year. An average of 36,000 Americans die annually due to the flu and its complications. The best way to prevent the flu is to get a flu shot each year during the fall season. Because flu viruses change from year to year, it is important to get a flu shot each year. *Higher percentages are better.*

Immunization for Pneumonia
Patients assessed and given pneumonia vaccination.
Pneumonia is an infection of the lungs that is caused by bacteria or a virus and can spread from person to person. A cold or flu that gets worse can turn into pneumonia. Although antibiotics such as penicillin were once very effective at treating pneumonia, the disease has mutated (changed) so these treatments are not as effective. The best way to prevent pneumonia is to get a flu shot each year (as flu often leads to pneumonia) and frequently washing your hands. Those who are more at risk of getting pneumonia, such as young children, people over the age of 65, people with a chronic illness (such as heart or lung disease or diabetes), or people who have had pneumonia before, should get the pneumonia vaccine. Ask your doctor when the best time to be vaccinated is for you. *Higher percentages are better.*

14▶ Stroke Care

Scientific evidence shows that the following measures show some of the standards of stroke care that hospitals should follow, for adults who have had a stroke.

Anticoagulation Therapy for Atrial Fibrillation
Ischemic stroke patients with a type of irregular heartbeat who were given a prescription for a blood thinner at discharge.
Patients admitted with an ischemic stroke who have an irregular heartbeat (also called atrial fibrillation or atrial flutter) are at greater risk of having another stroke. Research suggests that medicine that thins the blood (called an anticoagulant) reduces the chance of another stroke in these patients. This measure shows the percentage of patients admitted with ischemic stroke and an irregular heartbeat (atrial fibrillation/atrial flutter) who were prescribed an anticoagulant before they were discharged from the hospital. *Higher percentages are better.*

Antithrombotic Therapy Timing
Ischemic stroke patients who received medicine known to prevent complications caused by blood clots within 2 days of arriving at the hospital.
Ischemic stroke patients should get medicine known to reduce death, disability and the risk of another stroke (known as Antithrombotic Therapy) while in the hospital. Research shows that hospitals should start this medicine within 2 days of arriving at the hospital to prevent and treat clots and reduce the risk of complications from the stroke. Serious complications caused by strokes include changes in thinking and memory; muscle, joint, and nerve problems; or difficulty swallowing or eating; or blood clots. This measure shows the percentage of patients

admitted with an ischemic stroke who got antithrombotic therapy started within 2 days of arriving at the hospital. *Higher percentages are better.*

Assessed for Rehabilitation

Ischemic or hemorrhagic stroke patients who were evaluated for rehabilitation services.

Many ischemic stroke or hemorrhagic stroke patients will experience moderate or severe disability, including problems with physical, speech and mental functions. Stroke rehabilitation can help patients relearn those lost skills and regain independence. Once the stroke symptoms and related problems are under control, the hospital appropriate health care professionals should review the status of the patient and begin rehabilitation as soon as possible. Appropriate health care professionals include physicians, physical therapists, occupational therapists, speech and language therapists, and/or neuropsychologist. The earlier the patient starts rehabilitation, the better the recovery process. Patients who need stroke rehabilitation may begin while they are still at the hospital and continue in a rehabilitation setting that is right for the patient. These options include inpatient rehabilitation units (either stand-alone or part of a hospital/clinic), outpatient units (usually part of a hospital/clinic), nursing home, or home-based programs. This measure shows the percentage of patients admitted with an ischemic stroke or a hemorrhagic stroke who were evaluated for their need for rehabilitation services. *Higher percentages are better.*

Discharged on Antithrombotic Therapy

Ischemic stroke patients who received a prescription for medicine known to prevent complications caused by blood clots before discharge.

Patients admitted with an ischemic stroke are at risk for developing complications like another stroke even after discharge. These patients should get a prescription at discharge for a blood thinner that prevents complications like another stroke (called Antithrombotic Therapy.) Serious complications caused by strokes include changes in thinking and memory; muscle, joint, and nerve problems; or difficulty swallowing or eating; or blood clots. This measure shows the percentage of patients who were admitted with an ischemic stroke who were given a prescription for an antithrombotic before they were discharged from the hospital. *Higher percentages are better.*

Discharged on Statin Medication

Ischemic stroke patients needing medicine to lower cholesterol, who were given a prescription for this medicine before discharge.

Cholesterol is a fat (also called a lipid) that the body needs to work properly. Levels of bad cholesterol (LDL) that are too high can increase the chance of stroke, heart disease, and other problems. Medicines called statins can help lower LDL cholesterol levels. In patients with ischemic stroke who have high cholesterol, taking statins can help lower the chance of another stroke. This measure shows the percentage of patients admitted with an ischemic stroke who got a prescription for a statin before they were discharged from the hospital. Patients who shouldn't take statins are not included in this measure. *Higher percentages are better.*

Thrombolytic Therapy Timing

Ischemic stroke patients who got medicine to break up a blood clot within 3 hours after symptoms started.

Patients with ischemic stroke should get medicine called tissue plasminogen activator, or t-PA, to break up a blood clot within 3 hours after their symptoms start. T-PA is a kind of thrombolytic therapy. Research shows that hospitals that give t-PA within 3 hours after symptoms start can limit the damage and disability caused by an ischemic stroke. This measure shows the percentage of patients admitted with ischemic stroke who arrived in the emergency department (ED) within 2 hours of the onset of their symptoms and who got t-PA within three hours after the onset of their symptoms. *Higher percentages are better.*

Venous Thromboembolism Prophylaxis

Ischemic or hemorrhagic stroke patients who received treatment to keep blood clots from forming anywhere in the body within 2 days of arriving at the hospital.

Patients admitted to the hospital with ischemic stroke or hemorrhagic stroke are at increased risk of developing new blood clots in their veins that break off and travel to other parts of the body, like the brain or lung (also called venous thromboembolism). Research shows that hospitals should begin treatment to prevent new blood clots on the day of or day after these patients are arrived at the hospital. Treatment can include medicine, medical devices, or tightly fitting stockings designed to keep blood from clotting. This measure shows the percentage of patients admitted with an ischemic stroke or hemorrhagic stroke who either received treatment to prevent blood clots on the day of or day after arrival at the hospital or had paperwork in their chart to explain why they had not received this treatment. *Higher percentages are better.*

Written Stroke Educational Materials Given

Ischemic or hemorrhagic stroke patients or caregivers who received written educational materials about stroke care and prevention during the hospital stay.

Educating patients with ischemic stroke and hemorrhagic stroke and their caregivers about stroke care and prevention helps patients live healthier lives and reduces health care costs. During the hospital stay, hospital staff should give stroke patients and caregivers written information on: how to activate the hospital emergency system; the importance of doing follow-up after being released from the hospital; medicines prescribed at discharge;

what increases the chance of stroke; warning signs and symptoms of stroke. This measure shows the percentage of patients with an ischemic stroke or a hemorrhagic stroke or their caregivers who received written information about these topics during their hospital stay. *Higher percentages are better.*

15▶ Surgical Care Improvement Project

Scientific evidence shows that the following measures represent the best practices for preventing complications after certain surgeries: colon surgery, hip replacement, knee replacement, abdominal and vaginal hysterectomy, cardiac surgery- including coronary artery bypass grafts (CABG), and vascular surgery.

Appropriate Beta Blocker Usage
Surgery patients who were taking heart drugs called beta blockers before coming to the hospital, who were kept on the beta blockers during the period just before and after their surgery.
It is often standard procedure to stop taking usual medications for a while before and after surgery. But if patients who have been taking beta blockers suddenly stop taking them, they can have heart problems such as a fast heartbeat. For these patients, staying on beta blockers before and after surgery makes it less likely that they will have heart problems. This measure shows the percentage of patients who remained on beta blockers within this time period. *Higher percentages are better.*

Appropriate VTP Within 24 Hours
Patients who got treatment (venous thromboembolism prevention) at the right time (within 24 hours before or after their surgery) to help prevent blood clots after certain types of surgery.
Many factors influence a surgery patient's risk of developing a blood clot, including the type of surgery. When patients stay still for a long time after some types of surgery, they are more likely to develop a blood clot in the veins of the legs, thighs, or pelvis. A blood clot slows down the flow of blood, causing swelling, redness, and pain. A blood clot can also break off and travel to other parts of the body. If the blood clot gets into the lung, it is a serious problem that can sometimes cause death. Doctors can order treatments including blood-thinning medications, elastic support stockings, or mechanical air stockings that help with blood flow in the legs. These treatments need to be started at the right time, which is typically during the period that begins 24 hours before surgery and ends 24 hours after surgery. This measure shows the percentage of patients who received these treatments this time period. *Higher percentages are better.*

Controlled Postoperative Blood Glucose
Heart surgery patients whose blood sugar (blood glucose) is kept under good control in the days right after surgery.
Even if heart surgery patients do not have diabetes, keeping blood sugar under good control (200 mg/dL or less) after surgery lowers the risk of infection and other problems. This measure shows the percentage of patients who had their blood sugar kept under good control in the days right after surgery. *Higher percentages are better.*

Perioperative Temperature Management
Patients having surgery who were actively warmed in the operating room or whose body temperature was near normal by the end of surgery.
Hospitals can prevent surgical wound infections and other complications by keeping the patient's body temperature near normal during surgery. Medical research has shown that patients whose body temperatures drop during surgery have a greater risk of infection and their wounds may not heal as quickly. Standards of care say that patients should have their body temperature normal or near normal during the time period 30 minutes before the end of surgery to 15 minutes after anesthesia ended. This measure shows the percent of patients whose body temperature was normal or near normal within this time period. *Higher percentages are better.*

Prophylactic Antibiotic Selection
Surgery patients who were given the right kind of antibiotic to help prevent infection.
Surgical wound infections can be prevented. Medical research has shown that certain antibiotics work better to prevent wound infections for certain types of surgery. This measure shows the percentage of surgery patients who were given the right antibiotic during surgery. *Higher percentages are better.*

Prophylactic Antibiotic Selection (Outpatient)
Outpatients having surgery who got the right kind of antibiotic.
Hospitals can prevent surgical wound infections. Medical research has shown that certain antibiotics work better to prevent wound infections for certain types of surgery. Hospital staff should make sure patients get the antibiotic that works best for their type of surgery. This measure shows the percentage of patients who got the right antibiotic during surgery. *Higher percentages are better.*

Prophylactic Antibiotic Stopped
Surgery patients whose preventive antibiotics were stopped at the right time (within 24 hours after surgery).
Antibiotics are often given to patients before surgery to prevent infection. Taking these antibiotics for more than 24 hours after routine surgery is usually not necessary. Continuing the medication longer than necessary can in-

crease the risk of side effects such as stomach aches and serious types of diarrhea. Also, when antibiotics are used for too long, patients can develop resistance to them and the antibiotics won't work as well. This measure shows the percentage of patients who stopped getting preventive antibiotics within this time period. *Higher percentages are better.*

Prophylactic Antibiotic Timing
Surgery patients who were given an antibiotic at the right time (within one hour before surgery) to help prevent infection.
Surgical wound infections can be prevented. Medical research shows that surgery patients who get antibiotics within the hour before their surgery are less likely to get wound infections. Getting an antibiotic earlier, or after surgery begins, is not as effective. Hospital staff should make sure surgery patients get antibiotics at the right time. This measure shows the percentage of patients who got an antibiotic to prevent infection in this time period. *Higher percentages are better.*

Prophylactic Antibiotic Timing (Outpatient)
Outpatients having surgery who got an antibiotic at the right time (within one hour before surgery).
Hospitals can prevent surgical wound infections. Standards for care say that surgery patients who get antibiotics within an hour of their surgery are less likely to get wound infections. Getting an antibiotic earlier, or after surgery begins, is not as effective. This measure shows the percentage of patients who got an antibiotic in this time period. *Higher percentages are better.*

Urinary Catheter Removal
Surgery patients whose urinary catheters were removed on the first or second day after surgery.
Sometimes surgical patients need to have a urinary catheter, or thin tube, inserted into their bladder to help drain the urine. Catheters are usually attached to a bag that collects the urine. Surgery patients can develop infections when urinary catheters are left in place too long after surgery. Standards of care say that most surgery patients should have their urinary catheters removed within 2 days after surgery to help prevent infection. This measure shows the percent of surgery patients whose urinary catheters were removed on the first or second day after surgery. *Higher percentages are better.*

16▶ Survey of Patients' Hospital Experiences

The HCAHPS (Hospital Consumer Assessment of Healthcare Providers and Systems) Survey, also known as the CAHPS® Hospital Survey or Hospital CAHPS®, is a standardized survey instrument and data collection methodology that has been in use since 2006 to measure patients' perspectives of hospital care. A partnership of public and private organizations led by the Federal government, specifically the Centers for Medicare & Medicaid Services (CMS) and the Agency for Healthcare Research and Quality (AHRQ), created HCAHPS (pronounced "H-caps") to publicly report the patient's perspective of hospital care. The HCAHPS results posted on Hospital Compare allow consumers to make fair and objective comparisons between hospitals and with state and national averages, on important measures of patients' perspectives of care. For more on HCAHPS information, please visit the official HCAHPS website: www.hcahpsonline.org

The HCAHPS survey asks patients to give feedback about topics for which they are the best source of information. The survey asks patients to answer questions about their experiences in the hospital. To make sure the HCAHPS survey data is meaningful; patients only answer questions about topics with which they have experience. The HCAHPS survey asks patients to answer questions related to ten topics. The topics and questions are listed in the table below. Answers shown in italics are included in this publication.

Measure as it Appears in CGAH	HCAHPS Topic Text	HCAHPS Answer Description
Would Definitely Recommend Hospital	How do patients rate the hospital overall?	*Patients who gave a rating of 9 or 10 (high)*
		Patients who gave a rating of 7 or 8 (medium)
		Patients who gave a rating of 6 or lower (low)
Doctors 'Always' Communicated Well	How often did doctors communicate well with patients?	*Doctors always communicated well*
		Doctors usually communicated well
		Doctors sometimes or never communicated well
Nurses 'Always' Communicated Well	How often did nurses communicate well with patients?	*Nurses always communicated well*
		Nurses usually communicated well
		Nurses sometimes or never communicated well
Timely Help 'Always' Received	How often did patients receive help quickly from hospital staff?	*Patients always received help as soon as they wanted*
		Patients usually received help as soon as they wanted
		Patients sometimes or never received help as soon as they wanted

Measure as it Appears in CGAH	HCAHPS Topic Text	HCAHPS Answer Description
Meds 'Always' Explained Before Given	How often did staff explain about medicines before giving them to patients?	*Staff always explained*
		Staff usually explained
		Staff sometimes or never explained
Pain 'Always' Well Controlled	How often was patients' pain well controlled?	*Pain was always well controlled*
		Pain was usually well controlled
		Pain was sometimes or never well controlled
Area Around Room 'Always' Quiet at Night	How often was the area around patients' rooms kept quiet at night?	*Always quiet at night*
		Usually quiet at night
		Sometimes or never quiet at night
Room and Bathroom 'Always' Clean	How often were the patients' rooms and bathrooms kept clean?	*Room was always clean*
		Room was usually clean
		Room was sometimes or never clean
Home Recovery Information Given	Were patients given information about what to do during their recovery at home?	*YES, staff did give patients this information*
		NO, staff did not give patients this information
Would Definitely Recommend Hospital	Would patients recommend the hospital to friends and family?	*YES, patients would definitely recommend the hospital*
		YES, patients would probably recommend the hospital
		NO, patients would not recommend the hospital (they probably would not or definitely would not recommend it)

17 ▶ Use of Medical Imaging

"Medical imaging" tests create images of various parts of the body to screen for or diagnose medical conditions. Examples of medical imaging include CT scans, MRIs, and mammograms.

Cardiac Imaging Stress Test before Surgery

Outpatients who got cardiac imaging stress tests before low-risk outpatient surgery.
A cardiac stress test measures the heart's ability to respond when it is stressed, and can be useful in evaluating a patient's surgical risk. Experts agree, however, that these tests are not necessary before most low-risk outpatient surgical procedures, such as colonoscopies, cataract surgery, biopsies, or endoscopies (using an instrument to look inside the body) because these procedures put very little stress on the heart. Patients with certain risk factors that increase the likelihood of having complications are not included in the measure. This measure shows the percentage of all cardiac stress tests done in a hospital outpatient imaging department (using echocardiograms, CT scans, and MRIs) for Medicare patients who were going to have certain low-risk outpatient surgical procedures. Hospital outpatient imaging departments that have higher percentages on this measure may be giving people more tests than they need. *Hospitals that are rated well will have lower percentages.* If a percentage is high, it may mean that the facility is doing unnecessary cardiac imaging before some low-risk surgeries.

Combination Abdominal CT Scan

Outpatient CT scans of the abdomen that were "combination" (double) scans.
A CT scan (also called a CAT scan) uses multiple X-rays to produce detailed pictures of the inside of the body (bones, organs, and other body parts). For some, a substance called "contrast" is put into the patient's body before the scan begins, which help make parts of the body stand out more clearly. Contrast can be either swallowed or injected into a vein. Risks of contrast include possible harm to the kidneys or allergic reactions. Contrast shouldn't be used if it isn't needed. "Combination" CT scan means that the patient gets two CT scans—one scan without contrast, followed by a second scan with contrast. Standards of quality care say that most patients who are getting a CT scan of the chest should be given a single CT scan rather than a "combination" CT scan. Although combination CT scans are appropriate for some parts of the body and for some medical conditions, combination scans are usually not appropriate for the chest. The range for these measures is from 0% to 100%. For hospitals with higher percentages, it may mean that the facility is routinely giving patients combination CT scans of the chest or abdomen when a single scan is all they need. Giving patients two scans when they only need one needlessly doubles their exposure to radiation: Radiation exposure from a single CT scan of the chest is about 350 times higher than for an ordinary chest X-ray. For combination CT scans, radiation exposure is 700 times higher than for a chest X-ray because the patient is given two scans. For a combination CT scan, radiation exposure is 22 times higher than for an X-ray of the abdomen because the patient is given two scans. Radiation exposure from a single CT scan of the abdomen is about 11 times higher than for an ordinary X-ray of the abdomen. When contrast is used, there are risks that can include possible harm to the kidneys or allergic reactions (especially if the contrast is injected). To avoid unnecessary risk, contrast should be used only when it is needed. If you need to have a CT scan of the chest or abdomen, feel free to ask your doctor these questions to determine

what's best for your medical condition: Do you need a single scan—either with or without contrast—or is a combination scan necessary? Is using contrast appropriate for your medical condition? *Hospitals that are rated well will have lower percentages.* If a percentage is high, it may mean that the facility is doing unnecessary double/combination scans.

Combination Brain/Sinus CT Scan
Outpatients with brain CT scans who got a sinus CT scan at the same time.
Brain CTs and sinus CTs can be important tools for diagnosing problems that may be causing severe headaches or chronic sinus infections, but they also expose patients to high levels of radiation. Brain CT scans cover large parts of the sinuses, so ordering both tests may be unnecessary. For patients with chronic sinusitis, a sinus CT is usually done first before deciding if a brain CT is also needed. Experts do not recommend doing both tests at once, unless patients have head injuries or tumors. Hospital outpatient imaging departments that have higher percentages on this measure may be giving people more tests than they need, exposing them to too much radiation. This measure shows the percentage of brain CT scans done in a hospital outpatient imaging department where a sinus CT scan was done at the same time on the same Medicare patient. It does not count cases where doctors had questions about complications due to injuries, cancer, or serious infections. *Hospitals that are rated well will have lower percentages.* If a percentage is high, it may mean that the facility is doing unnecessary scans.

Combination Chest CT Scan
Outpatient CT scans of the chest that were "combination" (double) scans.
A CT scan (also called a CAT scan) uses multiple X-rays to produce detailed pictures of the inside of the body (bones, organs, and other body parts). For some, a substance called "contrast" is put into the patient's body before the scan begins, which help make parts of the body stand out more clearly. Contrast can be either swallowed or injected into a vein. Risks of contrast include possible harm to the kidneys or allergic reactions. Contrast shouldn't be used if it isn't needed. "Combination" CT scan means that the patient gets two CT scans—one scan without contrast, followed by a second scan with contrast. Standards of quality care say that most patients who are getting a CT scan of the chest should be given a single CT scan rather than a "combination" CT scan. Although combination CT scans are appropriate for some parts of the body and for some medical conditions, combination scans are usually not appropriate for the chest. The range for these measures is from 0% to 100%. For hospitals with higher percentages, it may mean that the facility is routinely giving patients combination CT scans of the chest or abdomen when a single scan is all they need. Giving patients two scans when they only need one needlessly doubles their exposure to radiation. Radiation exposure from a single CT scan of the chest is about 350 times higher than for an ordinary chest X-ray. For combination CT scans, radiation exposure is 700 times higher than for a chest X-ray because the patient is given two scans. For a combination CT scan, radiation exposure is 22 times higher than for an X-ray of the abdomen because the patient is given two scans. Radiation exposure from a single CT scan of the abdomen is about 11 times higher than for an ordinary X-ray of the abdomen. When contrast is used, there are risks that can include possible harm to the kidneys or allergic reactions (especially if the contrast is injected). To avoid unnecessary risk, contrast should be used only when it is needed. If you need to have a CT scan of the chest or abdomen, feel free to ask your doctor these questions to determine what's best for your medical condition: Do you need a single scan - either with or without contrast - or is a combination scan necessary? Is using contrast appropriate for your medical condition? *Hospitals that are rated well will have lower percentages.* If a percentage is high, it may mean that the facility is doing unnecessary double/combination scans.

Follow-up Mammogram/Ultrasound
Outpatients who had a follow-up mammogram, ultrasound, or MRI of the breast within 45 days after a screening mammogram.
A screening mammogram is an X-ray of the breast to check for possible breast cancer before it can be detected by women or health care professionals. Although mammography is a good test, it is not perfect. Some women who do not have breast cancer will have an abnormal mammogram (even though they are cancer free), and some women with breast cancer will have a normal screening mammogram (their cancer is missed). Some women may be asked to come back for follow-up testing if there are signs of possible breast cancer. A follow-up visit usually means having more tests (mammograms, an ultrasound, and/or an MRI of the breast). The numbers of women asked to follow-up varies widely among mammography facilities in the United States. There are many reasons for differences in follow-up rates including poor technique (blurry X-rays that need to be repeated), a lack of skill or experience interpreting the screening mammograms, medical history of the woman undergoing screening, and whether a woman is being screened for the first time or has previously undergone mammography screening. The follow-up rates reported here for mammography facilities include follow-up exams performed on the same day as screening mammograms, as well as those performed up to 45 days later. Medical evidence suggests that there may be a problem if a facility has either a very low or very high rate of follow-ups. *Although values for a very low follow-up rate have not been established, a follow-up rate near zero may indicate a facility that misses signs of cancer. Follow-up rates around 9% are typical. Research has established that a follow-up rate above 14% is not appropriate, and may indicate a facility doing unnecessary follow up.* If you have a screening

mammogram and you are called back for additional testing, ask your doctor why and what this additional testing means in your case for how he or she makes an accurate diagnosis.

Lumbar Spine MRI for Low Back Pain

Outpatients with low back pain who had an MRI without trying recommended treatments first, such as physical therapy.

An MRI (magnetic resonance imaging) is a test that uses a powerful magnetic field and a computer to produce detailed pictures of the inside of the body (bones, organs, and other body parts). Although MRI scans can be helpful for diagnosing low back pain, they can also be used too much. Low back pain can improve or go away within six weeks and an MRI may not be needed. Standards of care say that most patients with low back pain should start with treatment such as physical therapy or chiropractic care, and have an MRI only if the treatment doesn't help. Finding out whether treatment helps or not before having an MRI can be a safe and effective way to avoid unnecessary stress, risk, or cost of doing an MRI. For patients with certain conditions, getting an MRI right away is appropriate care. Patients with these conditions are not included in this measure. If you have low back pain, you, your doctor, and the medical imaging facility staff can talk about the best time to do an MRI if you need one. Since MRIs use magnets rather than x-rays, there is no radiation risk. However, because the magnets attract some kinds of metal, it's important for the technician to know if there are any metal objects or implants inside your body, such as pacemakers, artificial joints, screws, stents, plates, or staples. Metal objects can pose serious risk to you during the MRI and interfere with the test. For some MRIs, a substance called "contrast" is injected before the test to make parts of the body stand out more clearly on the images. Risks of contrast include possible harm to the kidneys or allergic reactions. Contrast shouldn't be used if it isn't needed. Having the test can be stressful for some people. Patients must hold still for about 15 to 45 minutes while lying on a table that moves inside a large scanning machine. While images are being taken, the machine makes loud noises. *Hospitals that are rated well will have lower percentages.* If a percentage is high, it may mean that the facility is doing unnecessary MRIs for low back pain.

Blood Clot Prevention and Treatment

Anticoagulation Overlap Therapy

Hospital Name	City	Rate	Cases
Rockville General Hospital[2]	Rockville	100%	47
Danbury Hospital[2]	Danbury	99%	110
Lawrence & Memorial Hospital[2]	New London	99%	70
Middlesex Hospital[2]	Middletown	99%	83
Norwalk Hospital Association[2]	Norwalk	99%	73
Bristol Hospital[2]	Bristol	98%	54
Greenwich Hospital Association[2]	Greenwich	96%	52
Hartford Hospital[2]	Hartford	96%	280
William W Backus Hospital[2]	Norwich	96%	100
The Hospital of Central Connecticut[2]	New Britain	95%	95
Manchester Memorial Hospital[2]	Manchester	95%	75
Waterbury Hospital[2]	Waterbury	95%	77
Griffin Hospital[2]	Derby	94%	35
John Dempsey Hospital[2]	Farmington	94%	53
Yale-New Haven Hospital[2]	New Haven	94%	319
Saint Francis Hospital & Medical Center[2]	Hartford	92%	227
Stamford Hospital[2]	Stamford	91%	80
Windham Comm Mem Hosp & Hatch Hosp[2]	Willimantic	91%	32
Charlotte Hungerford Hospital[2]	Torrington	88%	43
Bridgeport Hospital[2]	Bridgeport	79%	107
Midstate Medical Center[2]	Meriden	78%	73
Johnson Memorial Hospital[2]	Stafford Springs	72%	25
Saint Marys Hospital[2]	Waterbury	72%	65
Saint Vincent's Medical Center[2]	Bridgeport	64%	156

ICU Venous Thromboembolism Prophylaxis

Hospital Name	City	Rate	Cases
Bridgeport Hospital[2]	Bridgeport	100%	53
Danbury Hospital[2]	Danbury	100%	50
The Hospital of Central Connecticut[2]	New Britain	100%	54
William W Backus Hospital[2]	Norwich	100%	31
Greenwich Hospital Association[2]	Greenwich	98%	40
Midstate Medical Center[2]	Meriden	97%	37
Saint Francis Hospital & Medical Center[2]	Hartford	97%	64
Stamford Hospital[2]	Stamford	97%	59
Waterbury Hospital[2]	Waterbury	97%	65
Manchester Memorial Hospital[2]	Manchester	96%	93
Middlesex Hospital[2]	Middletown	96%	25
Day Kimball Hospital[2]	Putnam	95%	37
Griffin Hospital[2]	Derby	95%	84
Windham Comm Mem Hosp & Hatch Hosp[2]	Willimantic	95%	42
Bristol Hospital[2]	Bristol	92%	63
Hartford Hospital[2]	Hartford	92%	63
Milford Hospital[2]	Milford	92%	53
Saint Marys Hospital[2]	Waterbury	92%	51
Sharon Hospital[2]	Sharon	92%	95
John Dempsey Hospital[2]	Farmington	91%	58
Rockville General Hospital[2]	Rockville	91%	86
Yale-New Haven Hospital[2]	New Haven	89%	28
Saint Vincent's Medical Center[2]	Bridgeport	86%	49
Lawrence & Memorial Hospital[2]	New London	83%	84
Johnson Memorial Hospital[2]	Stafford Springs	77%	60
Charlotte Hungerford Hospital[2]	Torrington	76%	54

Incidence of Potentially Preventable VTE

Hospital Name	City	Rate	Cases
Danbury Hospital[2]	Danbury	0%	30
Yale-New Haven Hospital[2]	New Haven	4%	122
Bridgeport Hospital[2]	Bridgeport	6%	36
Hartford Hospital[2]	Hartford	7%	92
Saint Francis Hospital & Medical Center[2]	Hartford	11%	44
Saint Vincent's Medical Center[2]	Bridgeport	12%	32
John Dempsey Hospital[2]	Farmington	20%	25

UFH with Dosages/Platelet Count Monitoring

Hospital Name	City	Rate	Cases
Charlotte Hungerford Hospital[2]	Torrington	100%	36
Danbury Hospital[2]	Danbury	100%	35
Greenwich Hospital Association[2]	Greenwich	100%	26
Griffin Hospital[2]	Derby	100%	37
John Dempsey Hospital[2]	Farmington	100%	40
Lawrence & Memorial Hospital[2]	New London	100%	75
Manchester Memorial Hospital[2]	Manchester	100%	65
Middlesex Hospital[2]	Middletown	100%	49
Midstate Medical Center[2]	Meriden	100%	85
Rockville General Hospital[2]	Rockville	100%	42
Saint Francis Hospital & Medical Center[2]	Hartford	100%	226
William W Backus Hospital[2]	Norwich	100%	100
Waterbury Hospital[2]	Waterbury	99%	87
Bridgeport Hospital[2]	Bridgeport	98%	85
Hartford Hospital[2]	Hartford	98%	234
Norwalk Hospital Association[2]	Norwalk	98%	82
Stamford Hospital[2]	Stamford	95%	44
Yale-New Haven Hospital[2]	New Haven	94%	355
The Hospital of Central Connecticut[2]	New Britain	89%	47
Saint Marys Hospital[2]	Waterbury	85%	68
Saint Vincent's Medical Center[2]	Bridgeport	62%	126

Venous Thromboembolism Prophylaxis

Hospital Name	City	Rate	Cases
William W Backus Hospital[2]	Norwich	98%	369
Day Kimball Hospital[2]	Putnam	97%	267
The Hospital of Central Connecticut[2]	New Britain	97%	367
New Milford Hospital[2]	New Milford	97%	175
Bristol Hospital[2]	Bristol	95%	391
Griffin Hospital[2]	Derby	95%	376
Middlesex Hospital[2]	Middletown	95%	351
Norwalk Hospital Association[2]	Norwalk	95%	353
Stamford Hospital[2]	Stamford	95%	373
Waterbury Hospital[2]	Waterbury	95%	354
Masonic Home & Hospital	Wallingford	94%	293
Windham Comm Mem Hosp & Hatch Hosp[2]	Willimantic	94%	377
Bridgeport Hospital[2]	Bridgeport	93%	319
Hartford Hospital[2]	Hartford	91%	376
Milford Hospital[2]	Milford	91%	246
Danbury Hospital[2]	Danbury	90%	362
Yale-New Haven Hospital[2]	New Haven	90%	348
Rockville General Hospital[2]	Rockville	89%	248
John Dempsey Hospital[2]	Farmington	88%	292
Manchester Memorial Hospital[2]	Manchester	87%	317
Sharon Hospital[2]	Sharon	87%	134
Saint Marys Hospital[2]	Waterbury	85%	377
Midstate Medical Center[2]	Meriden	84%	419
Greenwich Hospital Association[2]	Greenwich	83%	322
Saint Francis Hospital & Medical Center[2]	Hartford	83%	402
Hebrew Home & Hospital	West Hartford	80%	84
Saint Vincent's Medical Center[2]	Bridgeport	80%	354
Lawrence & Memorial Hospital[2]	New London	74%	349
Johnson Memorial Hospital[2]	Stafford Springs	70%	276
Charlotte Hungerford Hospital[2]	Torrington	67%	369

Warfarin Therapy Discharge Instructions

Hospital Name	City	Rate	Cases
Saint Vincent's Medical Center[2]	Bridgeport	92%	102
Midstate Medical Center[2]	Meriden	91%	47
William W Backus Hospital[2]	Norwich	84%	77
The Hospital of Central Connecticut[2]	New Britain	83%	63
Middlesex Hospital[2]	Middletown	80%	54
Hartford Hospital[2]	Hartford	78%	179
Bristol Hospital[2]	Bristol	74%	38
Yale-New Haven Hospital[2]	New Haven	73%	205
Norwalk Hospital Association[2]	Norwalk	66%	47
Danbury Hospital[2]	Danbury	65%	77
Lawrence & Memorial Hospital[2]	New London	64%	44
Saint Francis Hospital & Medical Center[2]	Hartford	60%	139
Bridgeport Hospital[2]	Bridgeport	59%	63
Waterbury Hospital[2]	Waterbury	58%	38
Rockville General Hospital[2]	Rockville	52%	29
Manchester Memorial Hospital[2]	Manchester	37%	52
Saint Marys Hospital[2]	Waterbury	20%	44
Stamford Hospital[2]	Stamford	12%	57
Greenwich Hospital Association[2]	Greenwich	11%	35
John Dempsey Hospital[2]	Farmington	0%	32

Chest Pain/Possible Heart Attack Care

Aspirin Given Within 24 Hours of Arrival

Hospital Name	City	Rate	Cases
Middlesex Hospital	Middletown	100%	216
Sharon Hospital	Sharon	100%	50
Windham Comm Mem Hosp & Hatch Hosp	Willimantic	100%	39
Charlotte Hungerford Hospital	Torrington	99%	99
Bristol Hospital	Bristol	98%	54
New Milford Hospital	New Milford	98%	44
Rockville General Hospital	Rockville	98%	49
William W Backus Hospital	Norwich	98%	158
Griffin Hospital	Derby	97%	31
Midstate Medical Center	Meriden	97%	72
Day Kimball Hospital	Putnam	96%	100
Manchester Memorial Hospital	Manchester	96%	79
Johnson Memorial Hospital	Stafford Springs	91%	58

Average Time to ECG (minutes)

Hospital Name	City	Min.	Cases
Johnson Memorial Hospital	Stafford Springs	5	61
Rockville General Hospital	Rockville	5	52
William W Backus Hospital	Norwich	5	166
Charlotte Hungerford Hospital	Torrington	6	102
Day Kimball Hospital	Putnam	6	104
Griffin Hospital	Derby	7	32
Manchester Memorial Hospital	Manchester	7	79
New Milford Hospital	New Milford	7	43
Middlesex Hospital	Middletown	8	224
Midstate Medical Center	Meriden	8	76
Sharon Hospital	Sharon	8	52
Windham Comm Mem Hosp & Hatch Hosp	Willimantic	9	39
Bristol Hospital	Bristol	14	58

Average Time to Transfer (minutes)

Hospital Name	City	Min.	Cases
Middlesex Hospital	Middletown	51	51
William W Backus Hospital	Norwich	65	39

Children's Asthma Care

Received Home Management Plan of Care

Hospital Name	City	Rate	Cases
Connecticut Childrens Medical Center	Hartford	79%	267
Yale-New Haven Hospital[2]	New Haven	63%	316

Received Reliever Medication

Hospital Name	City	Rate	Cases
Connecticut Childrens Medical Center	Hartford	100%	267
Yale-New Haven Hospital[2]	New Haven	100%	317

Received Systemic Corticosteroids

Hospital Name	City	Rate	Cases
Connecticut Childrens Medical Center	Hartford	99%	267
Yale-New Haven Hospital[2]	New Haven	99%	316

Emergency Department

Admittance Decision Time (minutes)

Hospital Name	City	Min.	Cases
New Milford Hospital[2]	New Milford	57	428
Bristol Hospital[2]	Bristol	97	855
Yale-New Haven Hospital[2]	New Haven	100	316
Danbury Hospital[2]	Danbury	102	701
Norwalk Hospital Association[2]	Norwalk	104	698
Middlesex Hospital[2]	Middletown	117	808
Stamford Hospital[2]	Stamford	119	683
Griffin Hospital[2]	Derby	123	809
Lawrence & Memorial Hospital[2]	New London	130	589
Saint Marys Hospital[2]	Waterbury	135	650
Greenwich Hospital Association[2]	Greenwich	136	514
Milford Hospital[2]	Milford	137	525
Windham Comm Mem Hosp & Hatch Hosp[2]	Willimantic	138	589
Johnson Memorial Hospital[2]	Stafford Springs	146	402
Day Kimball Hospital[2]	Putnam	147	459
Charlotte Hungerford Hospital[2]	Torrington	148	864
Sharon Hospital[2]	Sharon	148	382
The Hospital of Central Connecticut[2]	New Britain	174	784
Midstate Medical Center[2]	Meriden	176	778
Hartford Hospital[2]	Hartford	180	616
John Dempsey Hospital[2]	Farmington	180	608
Saint Vincent's Medical Center[2]	Bridgeport	182	754
Waterbury Hospital[2]	Waterbury	190	787
Rockville General Hospital[2]	Rockville	192	518
Bridgeport Hospital[2]	Bridgeport	206	574
Saint Francis Hospital & Medical Center[2]	Hartford	215	646
William W Backus Hospital[2]	Norwich	220	768
Manchester Memorial Hospital[2]	Manchester	223	661

Head CT Results Within 45 Minutes of Arrival

Hospital Name	City	Rate	Cases
Middlesex Hospital	Middletown	77%	35

Patients Who Left ER Before Being Seen

Hospital Name	City	Rate	Cases
Charlotte Hungerford Hospital	Torrington	0%	41924
Greenwich Hospital Association	Greenwich	0%	43855
Johnson Memorial Hospital	Stafford Springs	0%	21007
New Milford Hospital	New Milford	0%	18213
Windham Comm Mem Hosp & Hatch Hosp	Willimantic	0%	36170
Bristol Hospital	Bristol	1%	39227
Danbury Hospital	Danbury	1%	70172
Day Kimball Hospital	Putnam	1%	27397
Griffin Hospital	Derby	1%	41113
The Hospital of Central Connecticut	New Britain	1%	110519
John Dempsey Hospital	Farmington	1%	29563
Lawrence & Memorial Hospital	New London	1%	78594
Middlesex Hospital	Middletown	1%	92456
Midstate Medical Center	Meriden	1%	60676
Milford Hospital	Milford	1%	24683
Norwalk Hospital Association	Norwalk	1%	50170
Rockville General Hospital	Rockville	1%	25311
Saint Vincent's Medical Center	Bridgeport	1%	82490
Sharon Hospital	Sharon	1%	15694
Stamford Hospital	Stamford	1%	51054
William W Backus Hospital	Norwich	1%	71056
Manchester Memorial Hospital	Manchester	2%	46449

NOTE: Hospital profiles are in alphabetical order by state, then city, then hospital within the city; Rankings exclude hospitals with less than 25 cases except for patient surveys which excludes hospitals with less than 100 cases; (a) 100-299 cases; (1) The number of cases/patients is too few to report; (2) Data submitted were based on a sample of cases/patients; (3) Results are based on a shorter time period than required; (4) Data suppressed by CMS for one or more quarters; (5) Results are not available for this reporting period; (6) Fewer than 100 patients completed the HCAHPS survey; (7) No cases met the criteria for this measure; (8) The lower limit of the confidence interval cannot be calculated if the number of observed infections equals zero; (9) No data are available from the state/territory for this reporting period; (10) The scores shown reflect fewer than 50 completed surveys; (11) There were discrepancies in the data collection process; (12) This measure does not apply to this hospital for this reporting period; (13) Results cannot be calculated for this reporting period; (14) The results for this state are combined with nearby states to protect confidentiality; Please refer to the User's Guide for a full explanation of data.

Hospital Name	City	Rate	Cases
Bridgeport Hospital	Bridgeport	3%	80689
Saint Francis Hospital & Medical Center	Hartford	3%	82584
Saint Marys Hospital	Waterbury	3%	71160
Hartford Hospital	Hartford	4%	100912
Waterbury Hospital	Waterbury	4%	56513
Yale-New Haven Hospital	New Haven	4%	151578

Time from ER Arrival to Being Admitted (minutes)

Hospital Name	City	Min.	Cases
New Milford Hospital[2]	New Milford	235	427
Windham Comm Mem Hosp & Hatch Hosp[2]	Willimantic	261	598
Bristol Hospital[2]	Bristol	276	862
Greenwich Hospital Association[2]	Greenwich	276	516
Middlesex Hospital[2]	Middletown	284	808
Danbury Hospital[2]	Danbury	286	701
Norwalk Hospital Association[2]	Norwalk	289	716
Sharon Hospital[2]	Sharon	296	389
Stamford Hospital[2]	Stamford	297	688
Yale-New Haven Hospital[2]	New Haven	301	331
William W Backus Hospital[2]	Norwich	309	773
The Hospital of Central Connecticut[2]	New Britain	316	786
Griffin Hospital[2]	Derby	317	816
Milford Hospital[2]	Milford	321	542
Johnson Memorial Hospital[2]	Stafford Springs	327	402
Day Kimball Hospital[2]	Putnam	338	465
John Dempsey Hospital[2]	Farmington	349	608
Charlotte Hungerford Hospital[2]	Torrington	355	864
Saint Vincent's Medical Center[2]	Bridgeport	384	772
Midstate Medical Center[2]	Meriden	392	778
Saint Marys Hospital[2]	Waterbury	400	710
Lawrence & Memorial Hospital[2]	New London	405	663
Rockville General Hospital[2]	Rockville	406	518
Waterbury Hospital[2]	Waterbury	422	858
Bridgeport Hospital[2]	Bridgeport	438	588
Saint Francis Hospital & Medical Center[2]	Hartford	452	661
Manchester Memorial Hospital[2]	Manchester	462	661
Hartford Hospital[2]	Hartford	494	627

Time from ER Arrival to Discharge (minutes)

Hospital Name	City	Min.	Cases
New Milford Hospital	New Milford	79	351
Windham Comm Mem Hosp & Hatch Hosp	Willimantic	90	406
The Hospital of Central Connecticut	New Britain	93	405
Sharon Hospital	Sharon	97	397
Charlotte Hungerford Hospital	Torrington	98	348
Middlesex Hospital	Middletown	105	593
Bristol Hospital	Bristol	113	467
William W Backus Hospital	Norwich	114	383
Johnson Memorial Hospital	Stafford Springs	118	364
Midstate Medical Center	Meriden	118	404
Lawrence & Memorial Hospital	New London	119	379
Day Kimball Hospital	Putnam	121	392
Danbury Hospital	Danbury	130	348
Griffin Hospital	Derby	130	376
Greenwich Hospital Association	Greenwich	133	344
Rockville General Hospital	Rockville	135	343
Manchester Memorial Hospital	Manchester	147	330
Saint Marys Hospital	Waterbury	148	376
Milford Hospital	Milford	150	404
Saint Vincent's Medical Center	Bridgeport	150	329
Norwalk Hospital Association	Norwalk	156	509
John Dempsey Hospital	Farmington	159	361
Stamford Hospital	Stamford	164	369
Waterbury Hospital	Waterbury	178	384
Bridgeport Hospital	Bridgeport	182	342
Saint Francis Hospital & Medical Center	Hartford	188	411
Yale-New Haven Hospital	New Haven	190	310
Hartford Hospital	Hartford	256	375

Time in ER Before Being Evaluated (minutes)

Hospital Name	City	Min.	Cases
Stamford Hospital	Stamford	14	419
Windham Comm Mem Hosp & Hatch Hosp	Willimantic	14	441
Johnson Memorial Hospital	Stafford Springs	17	418
Bristol Hospital	Bristol	18	503
Day Kimball Hospital	Putnam	18	444
Charlotte Hungerford Hospital	Torrington	20	387
New Milford Hospital	New Milford	20	355
The Hospital of Central Connecticut	New Britain	21	444
William W Backus Hospital	Norwich	23	420
Middlesex Hospital	Middletown	25	421
Sharon Hospital	Sharon	25	424
John Dempsey Hospital	Farmington	26	384
Danbury Hospital	Danbury	27	383
Saint Francis Hospital & Medical Center	Hartford	27	477
Milford Hospital	Milford	28	421
Saint Vincent's Medical Center	Bridgeport	28	381
Greenwich Hospital Association	Greenwich	31	383
Norwalk Hospital Association	Norwalk	32	546
Griffin Hospital	Derby	33	418
Saint Marys Hospital	Waterbury	36	309
Midstate Medical Center	Meriden	40	214
Lawrence & Memorial Hospital	New London	44	98
Yale-New Haven Hospital	New Haven	45	353
Rockville General Hospital	Rockville	59	244
Waterbury Hospital	Waterbury	67	417
Manchester Memorial Hospital	Manchester	74	267
Bridgeport Hospital	Bridgeport	79	301
Hartford Hospital	Hartford	94	399

Time to Pain Meds for Bone Fractures (minutes)

Hospital Name	City	Min.	Cases
Windham Comm Mem Hosp & Hatch Hosp	Willimantic	38	45
Charlotte Hungerford Hospital	Torrington	42	102
Rockville General Hospital	Rockville	43	68
Johnson Memorial Hospital	Stafford Springs	44	145
Middlesex Hospital	Middletown	44	80
Day Kimball Hospital	Putnam	45	69
William W Backus Hospital	Norwich	46	176
Midstate Medical Center	Meriden	47	144
New Milford Hospital	New Milford	47	93
John Dempsey Hospital	Farmington	48	72
Sharon Hospital	Sharon	50	92
Yale-New Haven Hospital	New Haven	50	224
Lawrence & Memorial Hospital	New London	51	172
Milford Hospital	Milford	52	62
Greenwich Hospital Association	Greenwich	53	157
Norwalk Hospital Association	Norwalk	54	178
Bristol Hospital	Bristol	56	91
Stamford Hospital	Stamford	56	153
The Hospital of Central Connecticut	New Britain	58	118
Saint Vincent's Medical Center	Bridgeport	64	81
Danbury Hospital	Danbury	65	209
Saint Francis Hospital & Medical Center	Hartford	69	77
Bridgeport Hospital	Bridgeport	70	56
Griffin Hospital	Derby	71	87
Manchester Memorial Hospital	Manchester	72	85
Saint Marys Hospital	Waterbury	80	244
Hartford Hospital	Hartford	82	110
Waterbury Hospital	Waterbury	92	132

Heart Attack Care

Aspirin Given at Discharge

Hospital Name	City	Rate	Cases
Danbury Hospital	Danbury	100%	344
Day Kimball Hospital	Putnam	100%	36
Griffin Hospital	Derby	100%	25
Hartford Hospital	Hartford	100%	913
The Hospital of Central Connecticut	New Britain	100%	171
John Dempsey Hospital	Farmington	100%	145
Middlesex Hospital	Middletown	100%	50
Midstate Medical Center	Meriden	100%	48
Saint Francis Hospital & Medical Center	Hartford	100%	537
Saint Marys Hospital	Waterbury	100%	176
Saint Vincent's Medical Center	Bridgeport	100%	415
West Haven VA Medical Center	West Haven	100%	28
Lawrence & Memorial Hospital	New London	99%	156
Norwalk Hospital Association	Norwalk	99%	76
Stamford Hospital	Stamford	99%	165
Yale-New Haven Hospital[2]	New Haven	99%	277
Bridgeport Hospital[2]	Bridgeport	98%	248
Greenwich Hospital Association[2]	Greenwich	98%	53
Waterbury Hospital	Waterbury	98%	201
Bristol Hospital	Bristol	97%	32
Charlotte Hungerford Hospital	Torrington	97%	30
William W Backus Hospital	Norwich	97%	36

PCI Within 90 Minutes of Arrival

Hospital Name	City	Rate	Cases
Danbury Hospital	Danbury	100%	66
Greenwich Hospital Association[2]	Greenwich	100%	29
Norwalk Hospital Association	Norwalk	100%	35
Stamford Hospital	Stamford	100%	41
Hartford Hospital	Hartford	98%	92
The Hospital of Central Connecticut	New Britain	97%	36
Yale-New Haven Hospital[2]	New Haven	97%	33
Saint Marys Hospital	Waterbury	96%	55
Bridgeport Hospital[2]	Bridgeport	94%	31
Saint Vincent's Medical Center	Bridgeport	94%	52
Waterbury Hospital	Waterbury	94%	47
Saint Francis Hospital & Medical Center	Hartford	93%	72
Lawrence & Memorial Hospital	New London	90%	60

Statin Prescribed at Discharge

Hospital Name	City	Rate	Cases
Bristol Hospital	Bristol	100%	34
Greenwich Hospital Association[2]	Greenwich	100%	56
John Dempsey Hospital	Farmington	100%	146
Norwalk Hospital Association	Norwalk	100%	78
Saint Francis Hospital & Medical Center	Hartford	100%	523
Saint Marys Hospital	Waterbury	100%	172
Saint Vincent's Medical Center	Bridgeport	100%	418
Sharon Hospital	Sharon	100%	25
West Haven VA Medical Center	West Haven	100%	29
Hartford Hospital	Hartford	99%	902
Stamford Hospital	Stamford	99%	164
Waterbury Hospital	Waterbury	99%	192
Bridgeport Hospital[2]	Bridgeport	98%	252
Danbury Hospital	Danbury	98%	340
Middlesex Hospital	Middletown	98%	43
Yale-New Haven Hospital[2]	New Haven	98%	274
Lawrence & Memorial Hospital	New London	97%	151
Griffin Hospital	Derby	96%	26
The Hospital of Central Connecticut	New Britain	95%	174
William W Backus Hospital	Norwich	94%	36
Midstate Medical Center	Meriden	92%	53
Day Kimball Hospital	Putnam	90%	31
Charlotte Hungerford Hospital	Torrington	81%	32
Manchester Memorial Hospital	Manchester	77%	26

Heart Failure Care

ACE Inhibitor or ARB for LVSD

Hospital Name	City	Rate	Cases
Griffin Hospital	Derby	100%	32
John Dempsey Hospital	Farmington	100%	48
Manchester Memorial Hospital	Manchester	100%	49
Saint Francis Hospital & Medical Center[2]	Hartford	100%	97
Saint Marys Hospital	Waterbury	100%	75
Saint Vincent's Medical Center	Bridgeport	100%	159
William W Backus Hospital	Norwich	100%	34
Danbury Hospital[2]	Danbury	99%	76
Stamford Hospital	Stamford	98%	123
Milford Hospital	Milford	97%	34
West Haven VA Medical Center	West Haven	97%	29
Greenwich Hospital Association[2]	Greenwich	96%	77
Middlesex Hospital	Middletown	96%	103
Midstate Medical Center	Meriden	96%	74
Rockville General Hospital	Rockville	96%	26
Hartford Hospital	Hartford	94%	272
Norwalk Hospital Association[2]	Norwalk	94%	51
Waterbury Hospital[2]	Waterbury	94%	84
Bridgeport Hospital[2]	Bridgeport	92%	59
The Hospital of Central Connecticut[2]	New Britain	92%	60
Yale-New Haven Hospital[2]	New Haven	91%	77
Lawrence & Memorial Hospital[2]	New London	89%	53
Bristol Hospital	Bristol	85%	41
Charlotte Hungerford Hospital	Torrington	82%	39

Discharge Instructions Given

Hospital Name	City	Rate	Cases
Day Kimball Hospital	Putnam	100%	55
Griffin Hospital	Derby	100%	119
John Dempsey Hospital	Farmington	100%	151
Saint Marys Hospital	Waterbury	99%	162
Saint Vincent's Medical Center	Bridgeport	99%	341
West Haven VA Medical Center	West Haven	99%	141
Greenwich Hospital Association[2]	Greenwich	98%	179
Stamford Hospital	Stamford	98%	211
William W Backus Hospital	Norwich	98%	161
Milford Hospital	Milford	97%	95
Sharon Hospital	Sharon	97%	35
Bridgeport Hospital[2]	Bridgeport	96%	177
Waterbury Hospital[2]	Waterbury	94%	181
Manchester Memorial Hospital	Manchester	93%	134
Windham Comm Mem Hosp & Hatch Hosp	Willimantic	93%	71
Bristol Hospital	Bristol	92%	96
Yale-New Haven Hospital[2]	New Haven	92%	243
Danbury Hospital[2]	Danbury	91%	218
Norwalk Hospital Association[2]	Norwalk	91%	188
Middlesex Hospital	Middletown	90%	261
Rockville General Hospital	Rockville	90%	79
Saint Francis Hospital & Medical Center[2]	Hartford	90%	208
Hartford Hospital	Hartford	89%	669
New Milford Hospital	New Milford	88%	32
The Hospital of Central Connecticut[2]	New Britain	87%	218
Midstate Medical Center	Meriden	87%	190
Lawrence & Memorial Hospital[2]	New London	86%	205
Charlotte Hungerford Hospital	Torrington	84%	100
Johnson Memorial Hospital	Stafford Springs	79%	61

Evaluation of LVS Function

Hospital Name	City	Rate	Cases
Danbury Hospital[2]	Danbury	100%	323
Day Kimball Hospital	Putnam	100%	89
Greenwich Hospital Association[2]	Greenwich	100%	245
Griffin Hospital	Derby	100%	175

NOTE: Hospital profiles are in alphabetical order by state, then city, then hospital within the city; Rankings exclude hospitals with less than 25 cases except for patient surveys which excludes hospitals with less than 100 cases; (a) 100-299 cases; (1) The number of cases/patients is too few to report; (2) Data submitted were based on a sample of cases/patients; (3) Results are based on a shorter time period than required; (4) Data suppressed by CMS for one or more quarters; (5) Results are not available for this reporting period; (6) Fewer than 100 patients completed the HCAHPS survey; (7) No cases met the criteria for this measure; (8) The lower limit of the confidence interval cannot be calculated if the number of observed infections equals zero; (9) No data are available from the state/territory for this reporting period; (10) The scores shown reflect fewer than 50 completed surveys; (11) There were discrepancies in the data collection process; (12) This measure does not apply to this hospital for this reporting period; (13) Results cannot be calculated for this reporting period; (14) The results for this state are combined with nearby states to protect confidentiality; Please refer to the User's Guide for a full explanation of data.

Hospital Name	City	Rate	Cases
Hartford Hospital	Hartford	100%	934
The Hospital of Central Connecticut[2]	New Britain	100%	333
John Dempsey Hospital	Farmington	100%	200
Johnson Memorial Hospital	Stafford Springs	100%	108
Lawrence & Memorial Hospital[2]	New London	100%	308
Manchester Memorial Hospital	Manchester	100%	202
Middlesex Hospital	Middletown	100%	402
Midstate Medical Center	Meriden	100%	307
New Milford Hospital	New Milford	100%	51
Norwalk Hospital Association[2]	Norwalk	100%	256
Saint Francis Hospital & Medical Center[2]	Hartford	100%	305
Saint Marys Hospital	Waterbury	100%	268
Saint Vincent's Medical Center	Bridgeport	100%	515
Stamford Hospital	Stamford	100%	308
Waterbury Hospital[2]	Waterbury	100%	304
William W Backus Hospital	Norwich	100%	234
Windham Comm Mem Hosp & Hatch Hosp	Willimantic	100%	109
Yale-New Haven Hospital[2]	New Haven	100%	341
Bridgeport Hospital[2]	Bridgeport	99%	262
Bristol Hospital	Bristol	99%	166
Milford Hospital	Milford	99%	150
West Haven VA Medical Center	West Haven	99%	163
Charlotte Hungerford Hospital	Torrington	98%	165
Sharon Hospital	Sharon	98%	57
Rockville General Hospital	Rockville	97%	113
Masonic Home & Hospital	Wallingford	74%	27

Medicare Spending

Medicare Spending per Patient (ratio)

Hospital Name	City	Ratio	Cases
Hebrew Home & Hospital	West Hartford	0.85	-
Sharon Hospital	Sharon	0.93	-
Windham Comm Mem Hosp & Hatch Hosp	Willimantic	0.96	-
The Hospital of Central Connecticut	New Britain	0.98	-
Middlesex Hospital	Middletown	0.98	-
Hartford Hospital	Hartford	0.99	-
Norwalk Hospital Association	Norwalk	0.99	-
John Dempsey Hospital	Farmington	1.00	-
Waterbury Hospital	Waterbury	1.00	-
Charlotte Hungerford Hospital	Torrington	1.01	-
Greenwich Hospital Association	Greenwich	1.01	-
Griffin Hospital	Derby	1.01	-
Midstate Medical Center	Meriden	1.01	-
Milford Hospital	Milford	1.01	-
Saint Marys Hospital	Waterbury	1.01	-
Yale-New Haven Hospital	New Haven	1.01	-
Lawrence & Memorial Hospital	New London	1.02	-
Danbury Hospital	Danbury	1.03	-
Day Kimball Hospital	Putnam	1.04	-
Saint Francis Hospital & Medical Center	Hartford	1.04	-
William W Backus Hospital	Norwich	1.04	-
Bridgeport Hospital	Bridgeport	1.05	-
Stamford Hospital	Stamford	1.05	-
Johnson Memorial Hospital	Stafford Springs	1.06	-
Saint Vincent's Medical Center	Bridgeport	1.06	-
Bristol Hospital	Bristol	1.07	-
Manchester Memorial Hospital	Manchester	1.07	-
Masonic Home & Hospital	Wallingford	1.07	-
Rockville General Hospital	Rockville	1.07	-
New Milford Hospital	New Milford	1.08	-

Pneumonia Care

Appropriate Initial Antibiotic Given

Hospital Name	City	Rate	Cases
The Hospital of Central Connecticut[2]	New Britain	100%	94
John Dempsey Hospital[2]	Farmington	100%	58
Milford Hospital[2]	Milford	100%	95
Norwalk Hospital Association[2]	Norwalk	100%	90
Sharon Hospital	Sharon	100%	38
Day Kimball Hospital	Putnam	99%	90
Griffin Hospital	Derby	99%	156
Johnson Memorial Hospital	Stafford Springs	99%	77
Saint Marys Hospital[2]	Waterbury	99%	83
William W Backus Hospital[2]	Norwich	99%	100
Yale-New Haven Hospital[2]	New Haven	99%	73
Middlesex Hospital	Middletown	98%	179
New Milford Hospital	New Milford	98%	63
Waterbury Hospital[2]	Waterbury	98%	105
Danbury Hospital[2]	Danbury	97%	115
Greenwich Hospital Association[2]	Greenwich	97%	74
Hartford Hospital	Hartford	97%	307
Rockville General Hospital[2]	Rockville	97%	102
Saint Vincent's Medical Center	Bridgeport	97%	219
Stamford Hospital	Stamford	97%	172
West Haven VA Medical Center	West Haven	97%	36
Charlotte Hungerford Hospital	Torrington	95%	110
Saint Francis Hospital & Medical Center[2]	Hartford	95%	74
Manchester Memorial Hospital[2]	Manchester	94%	100
Windham Comm Mem Hosp & Hatch Hosp	Willimantic	94%	87
Bristol Hospital	Bristol	93%	112
Midstate Medical Center[2]	Meriden	93%	113
Bridgeport Hospital[2]	Bridgeport	90%	73
Lawrence & Memorial Hospital[2]	New London	88%	80

Blood Culture Timing

Hospital Name	City	Rate	Cases
Norwalk Hospital Association[2]	Norwalk	100%	170
Waterbury Hospital[2]	Waterbury	100%	207
Day Kimball Hospital	Putnam	99%	157
Greenwich Hospital Association[2]	Greenwich	99%	125
The Hospital of Central Connecticut[2]	New Britain	99%	208
Rockville General Hospital[2]	Rockville	99%	181
Stamford Hospital	Stamford	99%	273
West Haven VA Medical Center	West Haven	99%	69
William W Backus Hospital[2]	Norwich	99%	73
Griffin Hospital	Derby	98%	231
Hartford Hospital	Hartford	98%	676
Manchester Memorial Hospital[2]	Manchester	98%	204
Middlesex Hospital	Middletown	98%	330
Saint Francis Hospital & Medical Center[2]	Hartford	98%	185
Saint Marys Hospital[2]	Waterbury	98%	180
Saint Vincent's Medical Center	Bridgeport	98%	379
Sharon Hospital	Sharon	98%	97
Windham Comm Mem Hosp & Hatch Hosp	Willimantic	98%	123
Johnson Memorial Hospital	Stafford Springs	97%	123
John Dempsey Hospital[2]	Farmington	96%	138
Midstate Medical Center[2]	Meriden	96%	200
Bristol Hospital	Bristol	95%	154
Charlotte Hungerford Hospital	Torrington	95%	157
Danbury Hospital[2]	Danbury	95%	65
Milford Hospital[2]	Milford	95%	159
Yale-New Haven Hospital[2]	New Haven	95%	203
Lawrence & Memorial Hospital[2]	New London	94%	125
New Milford Hospital	New Milford	93%	44
Bridgeport Hospital[2]	Bridgeport	92%	119

Pregnancy and Delivery Care

Newborns whose Deliveries were Scheduled Early

Hospital Name	City	Rate	Cases
Danbury Hospital[2]	Danbury	0%	30
Day Kimball Hospital[2]	Putnam	0%	25
The Hospital of Central Connecticut[2]	New Britain	0%	39
Norwalk Hospital Association[2]	Norwalk	0%	27
Saint Francis Hospital & Medical Center[2]	Hartford	0%	49
Sharon Hospital	Sharon	0%	34
Stamford Hospital[2]	Stamford	0%	35
William W Backus Hospital[2]	Norwich	0%	31
John Dempsey Hospital[2]	Farmington	1%	122
Middlesex Hospital[2]	Middletown	2%	61
Hartford Hospital[2]	Hartford	3%	64
Lawrence & Memorial Hospital[2]	New London	4%	28
Manchester Memorial Hospital	Manchester	4%	84
Griffin Hospital[2]	Derby	6%	32
Midstate Medical Center[2]	Meriden	6%	108
Windham Comm Mem Hosp & Hatch Hosp	Willimantic	8%	26
Waterbury Hospital[2]	Waterbury	9%	32
Bridgeport Hospital[2]	Bridgeport	10%	48
Yale-New Haven Hospital[2]	New Haven	10%	92
Charlotte Hungerford Hospital[2]	Torrington	11%	37
Saint Marys Hospital[2]	Waterbury	11%	47
Greenwich Hospital Association[2]	Greenwich	13%	30
Bristol Hospital[2]	Bristol	14%	36
Johnson Memorial Hospital[2]	Stafford Springs	19%	26

Preventive Care

Immunization for Influenza

Hospital Name	City	Rate	Cases
Griffin Hospital[2]	Derby	99%	551
John Dempsey Hospital[2]	Farmington	99%	550
Danbury Hospital[2]	Danbury	97%	517
Middlesex Hospital[2]	Middletown	97%	543
Norwalk Hospital Association[2]	Norwalk	97%	527
Saint Vincent's Medical Center[2]	Bridgeport	97%	556
The Hospital of Central Connecticut[2]	New Britain	96%	549
Windham Comm Mem Hosp & Hatch Hosp[2]	Willimantic	96%	400
Johnson Memorial Hospital[2]	Stafford Springs	95%	317
Stamford Hospital[2]	Stamford	95%	524
Manchester Memorial Hospital[2]	Manchester	94%	489
Milford Hospital[2]	Milford	94%	334
New Milford Hospital[2]	New Milford	94%	311
Midstate Medical Center[2]	Meriden	93%	552
Rockville General Hospital[2]	Rockville	92%	290
Waterbury Hospital[2]	Waterbury	92%	597
Bridgeport Hospital[2]	Bridgeport	91%	511
Saint Francis Hospital & Medical Center[2]	Hartford	91%	579
Sharon Hospital[2]	Sharon	91%	290
Lawrence & Memorial Hospital[2]	New London	90%	523
William W Backus Hospital[2]	Norwich	88%	562
Day Kimball Hospital[2]	Putnam	85%	414
Hartford Hospital[2]	Hartford	85%	554
Hebrew Home & Hospital	West Hartford	85%	87
Saint Marys Hospital[2]	Waterbury	85%	572
Bristol Hospital[2]	Bristol	82%	587
Charlotte Hungerford Hospital[2]	Torrington	81%	561
Masonic Home & Hospital	Wallingford	73%	251
Greenwich Hospital Association[2]	Greenwich	65%	470
Yale-New Haven Hospital[2]	New Haven	65%	539

Immunization for Pneumonia

Hospital Name	City	Rate	Cases
Danbury Hospital[2]	Danbury	99%	641
Griffin Hospital[2]	Derby	99%	725
Saint Vincent's Medical Center[2]	Bridgeport	98%	737
Johnson Memorial Hospital[2]	Stafford Springs	97%	421
Middlesex Hospital[2]	Middletown	97%	778
Milford Hospital[2]	Milford	97%	499
Stamford Hospital[2]	Stamford	97%	575
Windham Comm Mem Hosp & Hatch Hosp[2]	Willimantic	97%	536
New Milford Hospital[2]	New Milford	96%	427
Norwalk Hospital Association[2]	Norwalk	96%	632
Hebrew Home & Hospital	West Hartford	95%	131
Midstate Medical Center[2]	Meriden	95%	762
Saint Francis Hospital & Medical Center[2]	Hartford	95%	770
Waterbury Hospital[2]	Waterbury	95%	786
The Hospital of Central Connecticut[2]	New Britain	94%	717
William W Backus Hospital[2]	Norwich	94%	736
Day Kimball Hospital[2]	Putnam	93%	469
Sharon Hospital[2]	Sharon	92%	374
Bridgeport Hospital[2]	Bridgeport	91%	564
John Dempsey Hospital[2]	Farmington	91%	636
Manchester Memorial Hospital[2]	Manchester	91%	596
Rockville General Hospital[2]	Rockville	91%	448
Lawrence & Memorial Hospital[2]	New London	89%	675
Hartford Hospital[2]	Hartford	86%	693
Bristol Hospital[2]	Bristol	82%	757
Saint Marys Hospital[2]	Waterbury	82%	737
Masonic Home & Hospital	Wallingford	80%	412
Charlotte Hungerford Hospital[2]	Torrington	75%	787
Greenwich Hospital Association[2]	Greenwich	72%	500
Yale-New Haven Hospital[2]	New Haven	68%	549

Stroke Care

Anticoagulation Therapy for Atrial Fibrillation

Hospital Name	City	Rate	Cases
Hartford Hospital	Hartford	100%	74
Middlesex Hospital	Middletown	100%	26
Saint Francis Hospital & Medical Center	Hartford	90%	50

Antithrombotic Therapy Timing

Hospital Name	City	Rate	Cases
Bridgeport Hospital[2]	Bridgeport	100%	87
Bristol Hospital	Bristol	100%	38
Day Kimball Hospital	Putnam	100%	32
Greenwich Hospital Association[2]	Greenwich	100%	73
The Hospital of Central Connecticut	New Britain	100%	137
Manchester Memorial Hospital	Manchester	100%	45
Middlesex Hospital	Middletown	100%	124
Midstate Medical Center	Meriden	100%	94
Norwalk Hospital Association	Norwalk	100%	113
Rockville General Hospital	Rockville	100%	33
Saint Marys Hospital	Waterbury	100%	120
Windham Comm Mem Hosp & Hatch Hosp	Willimantic	100%	30
Yale-New Haven Hospital[2]	New Haven	100%	96
Hartford Hospital	Hartford	99%	236
Lawrence & Memorial Hospital	New London	99%	137
Stamford Hospital	Stamford	99%	102
Waterbury Hospital	Waterbury	99%	83
John Dempsey Hospital	Farmington	98%	44
William W Backus Hospital	Norwich	98%	116
Danbury Hospital	Danbury	97%	139
Griffin Hospital	Derby	97%	69
Saint Francis Hospital & Medical Center	Hartford	97%	264
Saint Vincent's Medical Center	Bridgeport	97%	136
Charlotte Hungerford Hospital	Torrington	95%	44

Assessed for Rehabilitation

Hospital Name	City	Rate	Cases
Day Kimball Hospital	Putnam	100%	30
Greenwich Hospital Association[2]	Greenwich	100%	84
Griffin Hospital	Derby	100%	74
Hartford Hospital	Hartford	100%	445
The Hospital of Central Connecticut	New Britain	100%	169
Middlesex Hospital	Middletown	100%	137

NOTE: Hospital profiles are in alphabetical order by state, then city, then hospital within the city; Rankings exclude hospitals with less than 25 cases except for patient surveys which excludes hospitals with less than 100 cases; (a) 100-299 cases; (1) The number of cases/patients is too few to report; (2) Data submitted were based on a sample of cases/patients; (3) Results are based on a shorter time period than required; (4) Data suppressed by CMS for one or more quarters; (5) Results are not available for this reporting period; (6) Fewer than 100 patients completed the HCAHPS survey; (7) No cases met the criteria for this measure; (8) The lower limit of the confidence interval cannot be calculated if the number of observed infections equals zero; (9) No data are available from the state/territory for this reporting period; (10) The scores shown reflect fewer than 50 completed surveys; (11) There were discrepancies in the data collection process; (12) This measure does not apply to this hospital for this reporting period; (13) Results cannot be calculated for this reporting period; (14) The results for this state are combined with nearby states to protect confidentiality; Please refer to the User's Guide for a full explanation of data.

Hospital Name	City	Rate	Cases
Milford Hospital	Milford	100%	27
Saint Marys Hospital	Waterbury	100%	123
Stamford Hospital	Stamford	100%	124
William W Backus Hospital	Norwich	100%	122
Yale-New Haven Hospital[2]	New Haven	100%	125
Bridgeport Hospital[2]	Bridgeport	99%	99
Midstate Medical Center	Meriden	99%	106
Saint Francis Hospital & Medical Center	Hartford	98%	338
Saint Vincent's Medical Center	Bridgeport	98%	175
Waterbury Hospital	Waterbury	98%	88
Bristol Hospital	Bristol	97%	39
John Dempsey Hospital	Farmington	97%	71
Lawrence & Memorial Hospital	New London	97%	150
Norwalk Hospital Association	Norwalk	97%	132
Danbury Hospital	Danbury	96%	180
Rockville General Hospital	Rockville	94%	32
Windham Comm Mem Hosp & Hatch Hosp	Willimantic	94%	34
Charlotte Hungerford Hospital	Torrington	92%	40
Manchester Memorial Hospital	Manchester	86%	42

Discharged on Antithrombotic Therapy

Hospital Name	City	Rate	Cases
Bristol Hospital	Bristol	100%	37
Charlotte Hungerford Hospital	Torrington	100%	39
Danbury Hospital	Danbury	100%	152
Day Kimball Hospital	Putnam	100%	29
John Dempsey Hospital	Farmington	100%	65
Manchester Memorial Hospital	Manchester	100%	41
Middlesex Hospital	Middletown	100%	133
Midstate Medical Center	Meriden	100%	101
Norwalk Hospital Association	Norwalk	100%	112
Rockville General Hospital	Rockville	100%	32
Saint Francis Hospital & Medical Center	Hartford	100%	277
Stamford Hospital	Stamford	100%	113
Waterbury Hospital	Waterbury	100%	79
William W Backus Hospital	Norwich	100%	119
Yale-New Haven Hospital[2]	New Haven	100%	100
Greenwich Hospital Association[2]	Greenwich	99%	68
Griffin Hospital	Derby	99%	67
Hartford Hospital	Hartford	99%	330
The Hospital of Central Connecticut	New Britain	99%	156
Lawrence & Memorial Hospital	New London	99%	135
Saint Vincent's Medical Center	Bridgeport	99%	155
Saint Marys Hospital	Waterbury	98%	112
Windham Comm Mem Hosp & Hatch Hosp	Willimantic	97%	32
Bridgeport Hospital[2]	Bridgeport	96%	89

Discharged on Statin Medication

Hospital Name	City	Rate	Cases
Waterbury Hospital	Waterbury	100%	62
Midstate Medical Center	Meriden	99%	79
Greenwich Hospital Association[2]	Greenwich	98%	58
John Dempsey Hospital	Farmington	98%	48
Middlesex Hospital	Middletown	98%	97
Stamford Hospital	Stamford	98%	93
Hartford Hospital	Hartford	97%	232
Norwalk Hospital Association	Norwalk	97%	88
Danbury Hospital	Danbury	96%	118
The Hospital of Central Connecticut	New Britain	96%	115
Yale-New Haven Hospital[2]	New Haven	96%	73
Saint Francis Hospital & Medical Center	Hartford	95%	212
Saint Vincent's Medical Center	Bridgeport	95%	127
William W Backus Hospital	Norwich	95%	87
Lawrence & Memorial Hospital	New London	94%	105
Saint Marys Hospital	Waterbury	94%	99
Rockville General Hospital	Rockville	93%	27
Day Kimball Hospital	Putnam	92%	25
Griffin Hospital	Derby	91%	56
Manchester Memorial Hospital	Manchester	91%	35
Bridgeport Hospital[2]	Bridgeport	90%	72
Bristol Hospital	Bristol	88%	34
Charlotte Hungerford Hospital	Torrington	76%	33

Thrombolytic Therapy Timing

Hospital Name	City	Rate	Cases
Hartford Hospital	Hartford	95%	37
Saint Francis Hospital & Medical Center	Hartford	50%	32

Venous Thromboembolism (VTE) Prophylaxis

Hospital Name	City	Rate	Cases
Griffin Hospital	Derby	100%	80
Waterbury Hospital	Waterbury	100%	100
Bridgeport Hospital[2]	Bridgeport	99%	110
Hartford Hospital	Hartford	99%	466
The Hospital of Central Connecticut	New Britain	99%	162
Midstate Medical Center	Meriden	99%	110
Stamford Hospital	Stamford	99%	127
Danbury Hospital	Danbury	98%	183
Greenwich Hospital Association[2]	Greenwich	98%	90

Hospital Name	City	Rate	Cases
William W Backus Hospital	Norwich	98%	123
Middlesex Hospital	Middletown	97%	139
Windham Comm Mem Hosp & Hatch Hosp	Willimantic	97%	31
Yale-New Haven Hospital[2]	New Haven	97%	125
Norwalk Hospital Association	Norwalk	96%	136
Bristol Hospital	Bristol	95%	41
Milford Hospital	Milford	94%	31
Lawrence & Memorial Hospital	New London	93%	161
Saint Francis Hospital & Medical Center	Hartford	92%	372
Day Kimball Hospital	Putnam	91%	34
Saint Marys Hospital	Waterbury	90%	134
Saint Vincent's Medical Center	Bridgeport	90%	167
Rockville General Hospital	Rockville	87%	30
John Dempsey Hospital	Farmington	80%	59
Manchester Memorial Hospital	Manchester	78%	40
Charlotte Hungerford Hospital	Torrington	73%	48

Written Stroke Educational Materials Given

Hospital Name	City	Rate	Cases
Griffin Hospital	Derby	100%	30
Midstate Medical Center	Meriden	100%	49
The Hospital of Central Connecticut	New Britain	99%	83
Danbury Hospital	Danbury	95%	82
Middlesex Hospital	Middletown	94%	81
Lawrence & Memorial Hospital	New London	93%	67
Stamford Hospital	Stamford	93%	56
William W Backus Hospital	Norwich	93%	60
Hartford Hospital	Hartford	92%	217
Greenwich Hospital Association[2]	Greenwich	91%	44
Bridgeport Hospital[2]	Bridgeport	90%	42
Saint Vincent's Medical Center	Bridgeport	89%	73
Norwalk Hospital Association	Norwalk	88%	60
Waterbury Hospital	Waterbury	84%	38
Saint Marys Hospital	Waterbury	66%	53
Yale-New Haven Hospital[2]	New Haven	58%	62
Manchester Memorial Hospital	Manchester	39%	31
Saint Francis Hospital & Medical Center	Hartford	25%	107
John Dempsey Hospital	Farmington	22%	41

Surgical Care Improvement Project

Appropriate Beta Blocker Usage

Hospital Name	City	Rate	Cases
Day Kimball Hospital	Putnam	100%	98
Greenwich Hospital Association[2]	Greenwich	100%	82
John Dempsey Hospital[2]	Farmington	100%	105
West Haven VA Medical Center[2]	West Haven	100%	149
Yale-New Haven Hospital[2]	New Haven	100%	244
Griffin Hospital	Derby	99%	77
Lawrence & Memorial Hospital[2]	New London	99%	133
Middlesex Hospital	Middletown	99%	359
Milford Hospital[2]	Milford	99%	123
Saint Francis Hospital & Medical Center[2]	Hartford	99%	282
Saint Marys Hospital[2]	Waterbury	99%	152
William W Backus Hospital[2]	Norwich	99%	142
Bridgeport Hospital[2]	Bridgeport	98%	161
Danbury Hospital[2]	Danbury	98%	288
Hartford Hospital[2]	Hartford	98%	320
The Hospital of Central Connecticut[2]	New Britain	98%	168
Midstate Medical Center[2]	Meriden	98%	208
New Milford Hospital	New Milford	98%	58
Norwalk Hospital Association[2]	Norwalk	98%	105
Saint Vincent's Medical Center[2]	Bridgeport	98%	200
Waterbury Hospital[2]	Waterbury	98%	183
Manchester Memorial Hospital[2]	Manchester	97%	146
Windham Comm Mem Hosp & Hatch Hosp	Willimantic	96%	27
Charlotte Hungerford Hospital	Torrington	95%	108
Stamford Hospital	Stamford	95%	192
Bristol Hospital	Bristol	88%	50
Johnson Memorial Hospital	Stafford Springs	85%	48

Appropriate VTP Within 24 Hours

Hospital Name	City	Rate	Cases
Hartford Hospital[2]	Hartford	100%	529
John Dempsey Hospital[2]	Farmington	100%	270
Saint Marys Hospital[2]	Waterbury	100%	334
Saint Vincent's Medical Center[2]	Bridgeport	100%	274
Yale-New Haven Hospital[2]	New Haven	100%	398
Bridgeport Hospital[2]	Bridgeport	99%	274
Charlotte Hungerford Hospital	Torrington	99%	278
Danbury Hospital[2]	Danbury	99%	509
Day Kimball Hospital	Putnam	99%	302
Griffin Hospital	Derby	99%	246
The Hospital of Central Connecticut[2]	New Britain	99%	412
Manchester Memorial Hospital[2]	Manchester	99%	401
Middlesex Hospital	Middletown	99%	995
Midstate Medical Center[2]	Meriden	99%	611
Milford Hospital[2]	Milford	99%	429
Stamford Hospital	Stamford	99%	546

Hospital Name	City	Rate	Cases
West Haven VA Medical Center[2]	West Haven	99%	175
Lawrence & Memorial Hospital[2]	New London	98%	363
New Milford Hospital	New Milford	98%	174
Norwalk Hospital Association[2]	Norwalk	98%	365
Saint Francis Hospital & Medical Center[2]	Hartford	98%	514
Waterbury Hospital[2]	Waterbury	98%	454
William W Backus Hospital[2]	Norwich	98%	413
Bristol Hospital	Bristol	97%	155
Greenwich Hospital Association[2]	Greenwich	97%	271
Windham Comm Mem Hosp & Hatch Hosp	Willimantic	97%	105
Johnson Memorial Hospital	Stafford Springs	95%	113
Rockville General Hospital	Rockville	94%	48
Sharon Hospital	Sharon	92%	96

Controlled Postoperative Blood Glucose

Hospital Name	City	Rate	Cases
Danbury Hospital[2]	Danbury	99%	139
Saint Marys Hospital[2]	Waterbury	99%	76
Saint Vincent's Medical Center[2]	Bridgeport	99%	113
Saint Francis Hospital & Medical Center[2]	Hartford	98%	172
Stamford Hospital	Stamford	98%	63
John Dempsey Hospital[2]	Farmington	97%	59
Bridgeport Hospital[2]	Bridgeport	95%	77
Waterbury Hospital[2]	Waterbury	94%	103
Yale-New Haven Hospital[2]	New Haven	94%	116
Hartford Hospital[2]	Hartford	90%	152
West Haven VA Medical Center[2]	West Haven	87%	77

Perioperative Temperature Management

Hospital Name	City	Rate	Cases
Danbury Hospital[2]	Danbury	100%	604
Day Kimball Hospital	Putnam	100%	334
Greenwich Hospital Association[2]	Greenwich	100%	318
Griffin Hospital	Derby	100%	282
Hartford Hospital[2]	Hartford	100%	804
The Hospital of Central Connecticut[2]	New Britain	100%	473
John Dempsey Hospital[2]	Farmington	100%	304
Manchester Memorial Hospital[2]	Manchester	100%	443
Middlesex Hospital	Middletown	100%	1131
Midstate Medical Center[2]	Meriden	100%	691
Milford Hospital[2]	Milford	100%	468
New Milford Hospital	New Milford	100%	192
Norwalk Hospital Association[2]	Norwalk	100%	423
Rockville General Hospital	Rockville	100%	67
Saint Marys Hospital[2]	Waterbury	100%	452
Saint Vincent's Medical Center[2]	Bridgeport	100%	350
Stamford Hospital	Stamford	100%	643
West Haven VA Medical Center[2]	West Haven	100%	213
William W Backus Hospital[2]	Norwich	100%	480
Windham Comm Mem Hosp & Hatch Hosp	Willimantic	100%	124
Bridgeport Hospital[2]	Bridgeport	99%	370
Johnson Memorial Hospital	Stafford Springs	99%	139
Saint Francis Hospital & Medical Center[2]	Hartford	99%	695
Waterbury Hospital[2]	Waterbury	99%	511
Bristol Hospital	Bristol	98%	215
Lawrence & Memorial Hospital[2]	New London	98%	450
Charlotte Hungerford Hospital	Torrington	97%	358
Yale-New Haven Hospital[2]	New Haven	96%	567
Sharon Hospital	Sharon	95%	109

Prophylactic Antibiotic Selection

Hospital Name	City	Rate	Cases
Danbury Hospital[2]	Danbury	100%	507
Day Kimball Hospital	Putnam	100%	243
Griffin Hospital	Derby	100%	161
Hartford Hospital[2]	Hartford	100%	578
John Dempsey Hospital[2]	Farmington	100%	242
Manchester Memorial Hospital[2]	Manchester	100%	268
Milford Hospital[2]	Milford	100%	334
Rockville General Hospital	Rockville	100%	26
Sharon Hospital	Sharon	100%	76
Stamford Hospital	Stamford	100%	378
West Haven VA Medical Center	West Haven	100%	174
William W Backus Hospital[2]	Norwich	100%	305
Bridgeport Hospital[2]	Bridgeport	99%	312
Charlotte Hungerford Hospital	Torrington	99%	224
Middlesex Hospital	Middletown	99%	760
New Milford Hospital	New Milford	99%	153
Norwalk Hospital Association[2]	Norwalk	99%	255
Saint Francis Hospital & Medical Center[2]	Hartford	99%	619
Saint Marys Hospital[2]	Waterbury	99%	355
Saint Vincent's Medical Center[2]	Bridgeport	99%	332
Waterbury Hospital[2]	Waterbury	99%	416
Windham Comm Mem Hosp & Hatch Hosp	Willimantic	99%	69
Yale-New Haven Hospital[2]	New Haven	99%	393
Greenwich Hospital Association[2]	Greenwich	98%	184
The Hospital of Central Connecticut[2]	New Britain	98%	284
Midstate Medical Center[2]	Meriden	98%	457
Lawrence & Memorial Hospital[2]	New London	97%	294
Bristol Hospital	Bristol	96%	114

NOTE: Hospital profiles are in alphabetical order by state, then city, then hospital within the city; Rankings exclude hospitals with less than 25 cases except for patient surveys which excludes hospitals with less than 100 cases; (a) 100-299 cases; (1) The number of cases/patients is too few to report; (2) Data submitted were based on a sample of cases/patients; (3) Results are based on a shorter time period than required; (4) Data suppressed by CMS for one or more quarters; (5) Results are not available for this reporting period; (6) Fewer than 100 patients completed the HCAHPS survey; (7) No cases met the criteria for this measure; (8) The lower limit of the confidence interval cannot be calculated if the number of observed infections equals zero; (9) No data are available from the state/territory for this reporting period; (10) The scores shown reflect fewer than 50 completed surveys; (11) There were discrepancies in the data collection process; (12) This measure does not apply to this hospital for this reporting period; (13) Results cannot be calculated for this reporting period; (14) The results for this state are combined with nearby states to protect confidentiality; Please refer to the User's Guide for a full explanation of data.

Johnson Memorial Hospital	Stafford Springs	96%	91

Prophylactic Antibiotic Selection (Outpatient)

Hospital Name	City	Rate	Cases
Day Kimball Hospital	Putnam	100%	42
Griffin Hospital	Derby	100%	34
Johnson Memorial Hospital	Stafford Springs	100%	53
Rockville General Hospital	Rockville	100%	80
William W Backus Hospital	Norwich	100%	202
Windham Comm Mem Hosp & Hatch Hosp	Willimantic	100%	33
Charlotte Hungerford Hospital	Torrington	99%	259
Danbury Hospital	Danbury	99%	557
Hartford Hospital	Hartford	99%	749
Manchester Memorial Hospital	Manchester	99%	259
Greenwich Hospital Association	Greenwich	98%	303
The Hospital of Central Connecticut	New Britain	98%	388
John Dempsey Hospital	Farmington	98%	301
Lawrence & Memorial Hospital	New London	98%	165
Middlesex Hospital	Middletown	98%	111
Saint Francis Hospital & Medical Center	Hartford	98%	688
Saint Marys Hospital	Waterbury	98%	367
Saint Vincent's Medical Center	Bridgeport	98%	240
Stamford Hospital	Stamford	98%	445
Waterbury Hospital	Waterbury	98%	207
Bridgeport Hospital	Bridgeport	97%	363
Bristol Hospital	Bristol	97%	118
Midstate Medical Center	Meriden	97%	176
Norwalk Hospital Association	Norwalk	97%	333
New Milford Hospital	New Milford	94%	72
Sharon Hospital	Sharon	88%	33
Yale-New Haven Hospital	New Haven	85%	500

Prophylactic Antibiotic Stopped

Hospital Name	City	Rate	Cases
The Hospital of Central Connecticut[2]	New Britain	100%	278
Manchester Memorial Hospital[2]	Manchester	100%	258
New Milford Hospital[2]	New Milford	100%	152
William W Backus Hospital[2]	Norwich	100%	302
Griffin Hospital	Derby	99%	154
John Dempsey Hospital[2]	Farmington	99%	236
Lawrence & Memorial Hospital[2]	New London	99%	291
Midstate Medical Center[2]	Meriden	99%	444
Milford Hospital[2]	Milford	99%	326
Norwalk Hospital Association[2]	Norwalk	99%	246
Saint Vincent's Medical Center[2]	Bridgeport	99%	312
Yale-New Haven Hospital[2]	New Haven	99%	365
Bridgeport Hospital[2]	Bridgeport	98%	292
Danbury Hospital[2]	Danbury	98%	487
Middlesex Hospital	Middletown	98%	750
Saint Francis Hospital & Medical Center[2]	Hartford	98%	601
Saint Marys Hospital[2]	Waterbury	98%	342
Stamford Hospital	Stamford	98%	365
Waterbury Hospital[2]	Waterbury	98%	407
West Haven VA Medical Center	West Haven	98%	161
Hartford Hospital[2]	Hartford	97%	559
Day Kimball Hospital	Putnam	96%	234
Johnson Memorial Hospital	Stafford Springs	95%	88
Sharon Hospital	Sharon	95%	73
Greenwich Hospital Association[2]	Greenwich	94%	182
Bristol Hospital	Bristol	93%	104
Charlotte Hungerford Hospital	Torrington	91%	215
Windham Comm Mem Hosp & Hatch Hosp	Willimantic	91%	67

Prophylactic Antibiotic Timing

Hospital Name	City	Rate	Cases
Danbury Hospital[2]	Danbury	100%	508
Day Kimball Hospital	Putnam	100%	243
Rockville General Hospital	Rockville	100%	26
Stamford Hospital	Stamford	100%	378
William W Backus Hospital[2]	Norwich	100%	305
Bridgeport Hospital[2]	Bridgeport	99%	313
Greenwich Hospital Association[2]	Greenwich	99%	185
Griffin Hospital	Derby	99%	161
John Dempsey Hospital[2]	Farmington	99%	244
Johnson Memorial Hospital	Stafford Springs	99%	91
Manchester Memorial Hospital[2]	Manchester	99%	268
New Milford Hospital	New Milford	99%	153
Saint Francis Hospital & Medical Center[2]	Hartford	99%	619
Saint Marys Hospital[2]	Waterbury	99%	355
Sharon Hospital	Sharon	99%	76
Waterbury Hospital[2]	Waterbury	99%	416
West Haven VA Medical Center	West Haven	99%	176
Hartford Hospital[2]	Hartford	98%	579
The Hospital of Central Connecticut[2]	New Britain	98%	285
Lawrence & Memorial Hospital[2]	New London	98%	294
Middlesex Hospital	Middletown	98%	762
Norwalk Hospital Association[2]	Norwalk	98%	255
Saint Vincent's Medical Center[2]	Bridgeport	98%	332
Bristol Hospital	Bristol	97%	114
Midstate Medical Center[2]	Meriden	97%	458
Milford Hospital[2]	Milford	97%	334
Windham Comm Mem Hosp & Hatch Hosp	Willimantic	97%	69
Yale-New Haven Hospital[2]	New Haven	97%	395
Charlotte Hungerford Hospital	Torrington	96%	224

Prophylactic Antibiotic Timing (Outpatient)

Hospital Name	City	Rate	Cases
Day Kimball Hospital	Putnam	100%	42
Johnson Memorial Hospital	Stafford Springs	100%	53
New Milford Hospital	New Milford	100%	72
Rockville General Hospital	Rockville	100%	80
Windham Comm Mem Hosp & Hatch Hosp	Willimantic	100%	33
Danbury Hospital	Danbury	99%	539
Manchester Memorial Hospital	Manchester	99%	259
Norwalk Hospital Association	Norwalk	99%	334
Stamford Hospital	Stamford	99%	439
William W Backus Hospital	Norwich	99%	202
Bridgeport Hospital	Bridgeport	98%	362
Greenwich Hospital Association	Greenwich	98%	307
Saint Marys Hospital	Waterbury	98%	367
Saint Vincent's Medical Center	Bridgeport	98%	242
Charlotte Hungerford Hospital	Torrington	97%	108
Griffin Hospital	Derby	97%	32
John Dempsey Hospital	Farmington	97%	306
Saint Francis Hospital & Medical Center	Hartford	97%	676
Waterbury Hospital	Waterbury	97%	209
Bristol Hospital	Bristol	96%	120
The Hospital of Central Connecticut	New Britain	96%	393
Lawrence & Memorial Hospital	New London	96%	167
Midstate Medical Center	Meriden	96%	178
Hartford Hospital	Hartford	95%	759
Yale-New Haven Hospital	New Haven	95%	508
Middlesex Hospital	Middletown	94%	115
Sharon Hospital	Sharon	89%	35

Urinary Catheter Removal

Hospital Name	City	Rate	Cases
Griffin Hospital	Derby	100%	163
John Dempsey Hospital[2]	Farmington	100%	232
Milford Hospital[2]	Milford	100%	391
Saint Francis Hospital & Medical Center[2]	Hartford	100%	331
West Haven VA Medical Center[2]	West Haven	100%	107
Saint Marys Hospital[2]	Waterbury	99%	177
Stamford Hospital	Stamford	99%	243
The Hospital of Central Connecticut[2]	New Britain	98%	327
Manchester Memorial Hospital[2]	Manchester	98%	130
Middlesex Hospital	Middletown	98%	834
Midstate Medical Center[2]	Meriden	98%	494
Saint Vincent's Medical Center[2]	Bridgeport	98%	313
William W Backus Hospital[2]	Norwich	98%	282
Danbury Hospital[2]	Danbury	97%	464
Hartford Hospital[2]	Hartford	97%	483
Rockville General Hospital	Rockville	97%	36
Waterbury Hospital[2]	Waterbury	97%	298
Windham Comm Mem Hosp & Hatch Hosp	Willimantic	97%	87
Bridgeport Hospital[2]	Bridgeport	96%	290
Day Kimball Hospital	Putnam	96%	53
Greenwich Hospital Association[2]	Greenwich	96%	98
Lawrence & Memorial Hospital[2]	New London	96%	255
Norwalk Hospital Association[2]	Norwalk	96%	97
Yale-New Haven Hospital[2]	New Haven	96%	392
Sharon Hospital	Sharon	95%	65
Charlotte Hungerford Hospital	Torrington	93%	98
Bristol Hospital	Bristol	89%	103
Johnson Memorial Hospital	Stafford Springs	89%	100
New Milford Hospital	New Milford	73%	30

Survey of Patients' Hospital Experiences

Area Around Room 'Always' Quiet at Night

Hospital Name	City	Rate	Cases
Midstate Medical Center	Meriden	62%	300+
Stamford Hospital	Stamford	60%	300+
New Milford Hospital	New Milford	59%	300+
Johnson Memorial Hospital	Stafford Springs	58%	300+
Milford Hospital	Milford	58%	300+
Greenwich Hospital Association	Greenwich	57%	300+
Middlesex Hospital	Middletown	57%	300+
Griffin Hospital	Derby	56%	300+
Saint Marys Hospital	Waterbury	56%	300+
Saint Vincent's Medical Center	Bridgeport	56%	300+
Sharon Hospital	Sharon	56%	300+
Saint Francis Hospital & Medical Center	Hartford	54%	300+
Bristol Hospital	Bristol	53%	300+
Norwalk Hospital Association	Norwalk	53%	300+
Waterbury Hospital	Waterbury	52%	300+
Lawrence & Memorial Hospital	New London	51%	300+
Manchester Memorial Hospital	Manchester	51%	300+
Yale-New Haven Hospital	New Haven	51%	300+
Danbury Hospital	Danbury	49%	300+
Day Kimball Hospital	Putnam	49%	300+
Rockville General Hospital	Rockville	48%	300+
The Hospital of Central Connecticut	New Britain	47%	300+
Windham Comm Mem Hosp & Hatch Hosp	Willimantic	47%	300+
William W Backus Hospital	Norwich	46%	300+
Bridgeport Hospital	Bridgeport	45%	300+
Charlotte Hungerford Hospital	Torrington	45%	300+
Hartford Hospital	Hartford	45%	300+
John Dempsey Hospital	Farmington	44%	300+

Doctors 'Always' Communicated Well

Hospital Name	City	Rate	Cases
Sharon Hospital	Sharon	83%	300+
Day Kimball Hospital	Putnam	82%	300+
Greenwich Hospital Association	Greenwich	82%	300+
Milford Hospital	Milford	82%	300+
New Milford Hospital	New Milford	82%	300+
Stamford Hospital	Stamford	82%	300+
Midstate Medical Center	Meriden	81%	300+
Norwalk Hospital Association	Norwalk	81%	300+
Windham Comm Mem Hosp & Hatch Hosp	Willimantic	81%	300+
Bridgeport Hospital	Bridgeport	80%	300+
Hartford Hospital	Hartford	80%	300+
The Hospital of Central Connecticut	New Britain	80%	300+
John Dempsey Hospital	Farmington	80%	300+
Middlesex Hospital	Middletown	80%	300+
Johnson Memorial Hospital	Stafford Springs	79%	300+
Lawrence & Memorial Hospital	New London	79%	300+
Saint Francis Hospital & Medical Center	Hartford	79%	300+
Saint Vincent's Medical Center	Bridgeport	79%	300+
William W Backus Hospital	Norwich	79%	300+
Yale-New Haven Hospital	New Haven	79%	300+
Bristol Hospital	Bristol	78%	300+
Danbury Hospital	Danbury	78%	300+
Griffin Hospital	Derby	78%	300+
Saint Marys Hospital	Waterbury	78%	300+
Waterbury Hospital	Waterbury	78%	300+
Charlotte Hungerford Hospital	Torrington	77%	300+
Manchester Memorial Hospital	Manchester	76%	300+
Rockville General Hospital	Rockville	73%	300+

Home Recovery Information Given

Hospital Name	City	Rate	Cases
Charlotte Hungerford Hospital	Torrington	89%	300+
Griffin Hospital	Derby	89%	300+
Bristol Hospital	Bristol	88%	300+
Day Kimball Hospital	Putnam	88%	300+
Hartford Hospital	Hartford	88%	300+
John Dempsey Hospital	Farmington	87%	300+
New Milford Hospital	New Milford	87%	300+
Waterbury Hospital	Waterbury	87%	300+
Windham Comm Mem Hosp & Hatch Hosp	Willimantic	87%	300+
Middlesex Hospital	Middletown	86%	300+
Rockville General Hospital	Rockville	86%	300+
Saint Marys Hospital	Waterbury	86%	300+
The Hospital of Central Connecticut	New Britain	85%	300+
Johnson Memorial Hospital	Stafford Springs	85%	300+
Midstate Medical Center	Meriden	85%	300+
Milford Hospital	Milford	85%	300+
Norwalk Hospital Association	Norwalk	85%	300+
Saint Francis Hospital & Medical Center	Hartford	85%	300+
Sharon Hospital	Sharon	85%	300+
Yale-New Haven Hospital	New Haven	85%	300+
Stamford Hospital	Stamford	83%	300+
Bridgeport Hospital	Bridgeport	82%	300+
Greenwich Hospital Association	Greenwich	82%	300+
Manchester Memorial Hospital	Manchester	82%	300+
Lawrence & Memorial Hospital	New London	81%	300+
Saint Vincent's Medical Center	Bridgeport	81%	300+
William W Backus Hospital	Norwich	81%	300+
Danbury Hospital	Danbury	80%	300+

Hospital Given 9 or 10 on 10 Point Scale

Hospital Name	City	Rate	Cases
Greenwich Hospital Association	Greenwich	83%	300+
Middlesex Hospital	Middletown	76%	300+
Griffin Hospital	Derby	75%	300+
Midstate Medical Center	Meriden	72%	300+
Milford Hospital	Milford	72%	300+
Day Kimball Hospital	Putnam	71%	300+
Stamford Hospital	Stamford	71%	300+
Yale-New Haven Hospital	New Haven	71%	300+
Norwalk Hospital Association	Norwalk	70%	300+
Saint Vincent's Medical Center	Bridgeport	70%	300+
New Milford Hospital	New Milford	69%	300+
Saint Francis Hospital & Medical Center	Hartford	69%	300+
Danbury Hospital	Danbury	68%	300+
John Dempsey Hospital	Farmington	68%	300+
Bristol Hospital	Bristol	67%	300+

NOTE: Hospital profiles are in alphabetical order by state, then city, then hospital within the city; Rankings exclude hospitals with less than 25 cases except for patient surveys which excludes hospitals with less than 100 cases; (a) 100-299 cases; (1) The number of cases/patients is too few to report; (2) Data submitted were based on a sample of cases/patients; (3) Results are based on a shorter time period than required; (4) Data suppressed by CMS for one or more quarters; (5) Results are not available for this reporting period; (6) Fewer than 100 patients completed the HCAHPS survey; (7) No cases met the criteria for this measure; (8) The lower limit of the confidence interval cannot be calculated if the number of observed infections equals zero; (9) No data are available from the state/territory for this reporting period; (10) The scores shown reflect fewer than 50 completed surveys; (11) There were discrepancies in the data collection process; (12) This measure does not apply to this hospital for this reporting period; (13) Results cannot be calculated for this reporting period; (14) The results for this state are combined with nearby states to protect confidentiality; Please refer to the User's Guide for a full explanation of data.

Hospital Name	City	Rate	Cases
Saint Marys Hospital	Waterbury	67%	300+
Sharon Hospital	Sharon	67%	300+
Bridgeport Hospital	Bridgeport	66%	300+
Hartford Hospital	Hartford	66%	300+
The Hospital of Central Connecticut	New Britain	65%	300+
William W Backus Hospital	Norwich	64%	300+
Charlotte Hungerford Hospital	Torrington	63%	300+
Johnson Memorial Hospital	Stafford Springs	63%	300+
Windham Comm Mem Hosp & Hatch Hosp	Willimantic	63%	300+
Manchester Memorial Hospital	Manchester	62%	300+
Waterbury Hospital	Waterbury	62%	300+
Lawrence & Memorial Hospital	New London	61%	300+
Rockville General Hospital	Rockville	58%	300+

Meds 'Always' Explained Before Given

Hospital Name	City	Rate	Cases
Day Kimball Hospital	Putnam	65%	300+
Griffin Hospital	Derby	65%	300+
Johnson Memorial Hospital	Stafford Springs	65%	300+
Milford Hospital	Milford	65%	300+
Sharon Hospital	Sharon	65%	300+
Greenwich Hospital Association	Greenwich	64%	300+
John Dempsey Hospital	Farmington	64%	300+
Midstate Medical Center	Meriden	64%	300+
Windham Comm Mem Hosp & Hatch Hosp	Willimantic	64%	300+
Bristol Hospital	Bristol	63%	300+
Charlotte Hungerford Hospital	Torrington	63%	300+
Middlesex Hospital	Middletown	63%	300+
Rockville General Hospital	Rockville	63%	300+
Stamford Hospital	Stamford	62%	300+
William W Backus Hospital	Norwich	62%	300+
Hartford Hospital	Hartford	61%	300+
The Hospital of Central Connecticut	New Britain	61%	300+
Saint Marys Hospital	Waterbury	61%	300+
Bridgeport Hospital	Bridgeport	60%	300+
New Milford Hospital	New Milford	60%	300+
Norwalk Hospital Association	Norwalk	60%	300+
Saint Francis Hospital & Medical Center	Hartford	60%	300+
Yale-New Haven Hospital	New Haven	60%	300+
Danbury Hospital	Danbury	59%	300+
Waterbury Hospital	Waterbury	59%	300+
Manchester Memorial Hospital	Manchester	58%	300+
Lawrence & Memorial Hospital	New London	57%	300+
Saint Vincent's Medical Center	Bridgeport	56%	300+

Nurses 'Always' Communicated Well

Hospital Name	City	Rate	Cases
Bristol Hospital	Bristol	82%	300+
Day Kimball Hospital	Putnam	82%	300+
Midstate Medical Center	Meriden	82%	300+
Sharon Hospital	Sharon	82%	300+
Bridgeport Hospital	Bridgeport	81%	300+
Greenwich Hospital Association	Greenwich	81%	300+
Johnson Memorial Hospital	Stafford Springs	81%	300+
Middlesex Hospital	Middletown	81%	300+
Stamford Hospital	Stamford	81%	300+
Milford Hospital	Milford	80%	300+
William W Backus Hospital	Norwich	80%	300+
Yale-New Haven Hospital	New Haven	80%	300+
Charlotte Hungerford Hospital	Torrington	79%	300+
Griffin Hospital	Derby	79%	300+
John Dempsey Hospital	Farmington	79%	300+
Hartford Hospital	Hartford	78%	300+
Lawrence & Memorial Hospital	New London	78%	300+
Windham Comm Mem Hosp & Hatch Hosp	Willimantic	78%	300+
Danbury Hospital	Danbury	77%	300+
The Hospital of Central Connecticut	New Britain	77%	300+
Manchester Memorial Hospital	Manchester	77%	300+
New Milford Hospital	New Milford	77%	300+
Norwalk Hospital Association	Norwalk	77%	300+
Saint Francis Hospital & Medical Center	Hartford	77%	300+
Saint Marys Hospital	Waterbury	77%	300+
Saint Vincent's Medical Center	Bridgeport	77%	300+
Waterbury Hospital	Waterbury	76%	300+
Rockville General Hospital	Rockville	75%	300+

Pain 'Always' Well Controlled

Hospital Name	City	Rate	Cases
Greenwich Hospital Association	Greenwich	77%	300+
Bristol Hospital	Bristol	75%	300+
Day Kimball Hospital	Putnam	75%	300+
Johnson Memorial Hospital	Stafford Springs	74%	300+
Stamford Hospital	Stamford	74%	300+
Bridgeport Hospital	Bridgeport	73%	300+
Windham Comm Mem Hosp & Hatch Hosp	Willimantic	73%	300+
Charlotte Hungerford Hospital	Torrington	72%	300+
Milford Hospital	Milford	72%	300+
Sharon Hospital	Sharon	72%	300+
William W Backus Hospital	Norwich	72%	300+
Middlesex Hospital	Middletown	71%	300+

Hospital Name	City	Rate	Cases
Midstate Medical Center	Meriden	71%	300+
Norwalk Hospital Association	Norwalk	71%	300+
Manchester Memorial Hospital	Manchester	70%	300+
Danbury Hospital	Danbury	69%	300+
Griffin Hospital	Derby	69%	300+
The Hospital of Central Connecticut	New Britain	69%	300+
Saint Vincent's Medical Center	Bridgeport	69%	300+
Hartford Hospital	Hartford	68%	300+
John Dempsey Hospital	Farmington	68%	300+
Lawrence & Memorial Hospital	New London	68%	300+
New Milford Hospital	New Milford	68%	300+
Saint Francis Hospital & Medical Center	Hartford	68%	300+
Saint Marys Hospital	Waterbury	68%	300+
Waterbury Hospital	Waterbury	68%	300+
Rockville General Hospital	Rockville	67%	300+
Yale-New Haven Hospital	New Haven	67%	300+

Room and Bathroom 'Always' Clean

Hospital Name	City	Rate	Cases
Milford Hospital	Milford	82%	300+
Greenwich Hospital Association	Greenwich	80%	300+
Sharon Hospital	Sharon	78%	300+
Griffin Hospital	Derby	77%	300+
Middlesex Hospital	Middletown	77%	300+
Midstate Medical Center	Meriden	77%	300+
Day Kimball Hospital	Putnam	76%	300+
The Hospital of Central Connecticut	New Britain	76%	300+
Johnson Memorial Hospital	Stafford Springs	75%	300+
Charlotte Hungerford Hospital	Torrington	73%	300+
Stamford Hospital	Stamford	73%	300+
Danbury Hospital	Danbury	72%	300+
Saint Francis Hospital & Medical Center	Hartford	72%	300+
Saint Marys Hospital	Waterbury	72%	300+
Bristol Hospital	Bristol	71%	300+
New Milford Hospital	New Milford	71%	300+
Norwalk Hospital Association	Norwalk	71%	300+
William W Backus Hospital	Norwich	71%	300+
Saint Vincent's Medical Center	Bridgeport	70%	300+
Windham Comm Mem Hosp & Hatch Hosp	Willimantic	70%	300+
Lawrence & Memorial Hospital	New London	69%	300+
Yale-New Haven Hospital	New Haven	68%	300+
Bridgeport Hospital	Bridgeport	67%	300+
John Dempsey Hospital	Farmington	67%	300+
Rockville General Hospital	Rockville	67%	300+
Waterbury Hospital	Waterbury	67%	300+
Hartford Hospital	Hartford	66%	300+
Manchester Memorial Hospital	Manchester	63%	300+

Timely Help 'Always' Received

Hospital Name	City	Rate	Cases
Greenwich Hospital Association	Greenwich	71%	300+
Middlesex Hospital	Middletown	71%	300+
Milford Hospital	Milford	71%	300+
Day Kimball Hospital	Putnam	70%	300+
Johnson Memorial Hospital	Stafford Springs	70%	300+
Midstate Medical Center	Meriden	70%	300+
Bristol Hospital	Bristol	67%	300+
Griffin Hospital	Derby	67%	300+
Charlotte Hungerford Hospital	Torrington	66%	300+
William W Backus Hospital	Norwich	66%	300+
Windham Comm Mem Hosp & Hatch Hosp	Willimantic	66%	300+
Bridgeport Hospital	Bridgeport	65%	300+
Yale-New Haven Hospital	New Haven	65%	300+
New Milford Hospital	New Milford	64%	300+
Sharon Hospital	Sharon	64%	300+
Stamford Hospital	Stamford	64%	300+
The Hospital of Central Connecticut	New Britain	63%	300+
Norwalk Hospital Association	Norwalk	63%	300+
Lawrence & Memorial Hospital	New London	62%	300+
Rockville General Hospital	Rockville	61%	300+
Saint Marys Hospital	Waterbury	61%	300+
Danbury Hospital	Danbury	60%	300+
Saint Francis Hospital & Medical Center	Hartford	60%	300+
Saint Vincent's Medical Center	Bridgeport	60%	300+
John Dempsey Hospital	Farmington	59%	300+
Manchester Memorial Hospital	Manchester	58%	300+
Waterbury Hospital	Waterbury	58%	300+
Hartford Hospital	Hartford	57%	300+

Would Definitely Recommend Hospital

Hospital Name	City	Rate	Cases
Greenwich Hospital Association	Greenwich	85%	300+
Middlesex Hospital	Middletown	78%	300+
Saint Vincent's Medical Center	Bridgeport	78%	300+
Stamford Hospital	Stamford	77%	300+
Griffin Hospital	Derby	76%	300+
Midstate Medical Center	Meriden	76%	300+
Norwalk Hospital Association	Norwalk	76%	300+
Saint Francis Hospital & Medical Center	Hartford	76%	300+
Yale-New Haven Hospital	New Haven	76%	300+

Hospital Name	City	Rate	Cases
Bridgeport Hospital	Bridgeport	75%	300+
John Dempsey Hospital	Farmington	74%	300+
New Milford Hospital	New Milford	74%	300+
Danbury Hospital	Danbury	73%	300+
Hartford Hospital	Hartford	73%	300+
Milford Hospital	Milford	73%	300+
Saint Marys Hospital	Waterbury	71%	300+
Sharon Hospital	Sharon	70%	300+
Day Kimball Hospital	Putnam	69%	300+
William W Backus Hospital	Norwich	69%	300+
Bristol Hospital	Bristol	68%	300+
The Hospital of Central Connecticut	New Britain	68%	300+
Lawrence & Memorial Hospital	New London	67%	300+
Waterbury Hospital	Waterbury	67%	300+
Johnson Memorial Hospital	Stafford Springs	66%	300+
Manchester Memorial Hospital	Manchester	66%	300+
Windham Comm Mem Hosp & Hatch Hosp	Willimantic	65%	300+
Rockville General Hospital	Rockville	63%	300+
Charlotte Hungerford Hospital	Torrington	60%	300+

Use of Medical Imaging

Cardiac Imaging Stress Test before OP Surgery

Hospital Name	City	Rate	Cases
New Milford Hospital	New Milford	2.0%	151
Manchester Memorial Hospital	Manchester	2.1%	243
Sharon Hospital	Sharon	2.8%	254
John Dempsey Hospital	Farmington	3.0%	331
Rockville General Hospital	Rockville	3.2%	124
Saint Marys Hospital	Waterbury	3.5%	317
Day Kimball Hospital	Putnam	3.6%	443
Danbury Hospital	Danbury	3.8%	1280
Norwalk Hospital Association	Norwalk	3.9%	154
The Hospital of Central Connecticut	New Britain	4.0%	176
Milford Hospital	Milford	4.1%	97
William W Backus Hospital	Norwich	4.2%	522
Lawrence & Memorial Hospital	New London	4.4%	724
Saint Francis Hospital & Medical Center	Hartford	4.4%	613
Windham Comm Mem Hosp & Hatch Hosp	Willimantic	4.5%	268
Bridgeport Hospital	Bridgeport	4.6%	1536
Yale-New Haven Hospital	New Haven	4.6%	1075
Hartford Hospital	Hartford	5.1%	784
Johnson Memorial Hospital	Stafford Springs	5.1%	99
Charlotte Hungerford Hospital	Torrington	5.4%	280
Saint Vincent's Medical Center	Bridgeport	5.4%	1594
Waterbury Hospital	Waterbury	5.5%	924
Stamford Hospital	Stamford	5.7%	653
Bristol Hospital	Bristol	6.3%	317
Greenwich Hospital Association	Greenwich	6.8%	443
Midstate Medical Center	Meriden	9.3%	118

Combination Abdominal CT Scan

Hospital Name	City	Rate	Cases
Griffin Hospital	Derby	1.1%	525
William W Backus Hospital	Norwich	1.1%	1397
Bristol Hospital	Bristol	1.4%	629
Hartford Hospital	Hartford	2.0%	636
Johnson Memorial Hospital	Stafford Springs	2.1%	388
Saint Francis Hospital & Medical Center	Hartford	2.3%	1412
Stamford Hospital	Stamford	2.3%	1484
Waterbury Hospital	Waterbury	2.8%	751
Danbury Hospital	Danbury	2.9%	1255
Manchester Memorial Hospital	Manchester	3.0%	943
Saint Marys Hospital	Waterbury	3.2%	760
Day Kimball Hospital	Putnam	3.6%	494
Windham Comm Mem Hosp & Hatch Hosp	Willimantic	3.7%	589
Rockville General Hospital	Rockville	3.9%	565
Lawrence & Memorial Hospital	New London	4.1%	1357
Sharon Hospital	Sharon	4.2%	312
Charlotte Hungerford Hospital	Torrington	4.9%	714
The Hospital of Central Connecticut	New Britain	4.9%	1432
Greenwich Hospital Association	Greenwich	5.1%	952
Midstate Medical Center	Meriden	5.7%	791
Milford Hospital	Milford	6.2%	353
Middlesex Hospital	Middletown	6.3%	1986
Yale-New Haven Hospital	New Haven	6.3%	3992
New Milford Hospital	New Milford	7.9%	433
Norwalk Hospital Association	Norwalk	9.4%	1484
John Dempsey Hospital	Farmington	12.0%	692
Bridgeport Hospital	Bridgeport	13.4%	396
Saint Vincent's Medical Center	Bridgeport	14.5%	830

Combination Brain/Sinus CT Scan

Hospital Name	City	Rate	Cases
Bristol Hospital	Bristol	0.7%	420
Johnson Memorial Hospital	Stafford Springs	1.2%	334
Middlesex Hospital	Middletown	1.2%	1181
Charlotte Hungerford Hospital	Torrington	1.3%	540
Yale-New Haven Hospital	New Haven	1.3%	2620

NOTE: Hospital profiles are in alphabetical order by state, then city, then hospital within the city; Rankings exclude hospitals with less than 25 cases except for patient surveys which excludes hospitals with less than 100 cases; (a) 100-299 cases; (1) The number of cases/patients is too few to report; (2) Data submitted were based on a sample of cases/patients; (3) Results are based on a shorter time period than required; (4) Data suppressed by CMS for one or more quarters; (5) Results are not available for this reporting period; (6) Fewer than 100 patients completed the HCAHPS survey; (7) No cases met the criteria for this measure; (8) The lower limit of the confidence interval cannot be calculated if the number of observed infections equals zero; (9) No data are available from the state/territory for this reporting period; (10) The scores shown reflect fewer than 50 completed surveys; (11) There were discrepancies in the data collection process; (12) This measure does not apply to this hospital for this reporting period; (13) Results cannot be calculated for this reporting period; (14) The results for this state are combined with nearby states to protect confidentiality; Please refer to the User's Guide for a full explanation of data.

Danbury Hospital	Danbury	1.4%	983
Hartford Hospital	Hartford	1.4%	910
John Dempsey Hospital	Farmington	1.8%	595
Day Kimball Hospital	Putnam	1.9%	479
Manchester Memorial Hospital	Manchester	1.9%	616
Lawrence & Memorial Hospital	New London	2.1%	1077
Saint Marys Hospital	Waterbury	2.1%	812
Waterbury Hospital	Waterbury	2.1%	780
The Hospital of Central Connecticut	New Britain	2.2%	1235
Midstate Medical Center	Meriden	2.2%	757
Norwalk Hospital Association	Norwalk	2.2%	963
William W Backus Hospital	Norwich	2.2%	999
Saint Francis Hospital & Medical Center	Hartford	2.6%	962
Saint Vincent's Medical Center	Bridgeport	3.5%	1013
Greenwich Hospital Association	Greenwich	3.6%	1039
Stamford Hospital	Stamford	4.1%	1139
Milford Hospital	Milford	5.8%	395

Combination Chest CT Scan

Hospital Name	City	Rate	Cases
Griffin Hospital	Derby	0.0%	477
John Dempsey Hospital	Farmington	0.0%	609
Johnson Memorial Hospital	Stafford Springs	0.0%	254
Lawrence & Memorial Hospital	New London	0.0%	1091
Midstate Medical Center	Meriden	0.0%	427
Milford Hospital	Milford	0.0%	119
Saint Marys Hospital	Waterbury	0.0%	463
Sharon Hospital	Sharon	0.0%	300
William W Backus Hospital	Norwich	0.0%	1335
Middlesex Hospital	Middletown	0.1%	1166
Manchester Memorial Hospital	Manchester	0.2%	879
Rockville General Hospital	Rockville	0.2%	516
Saint Francis Hospital & Medical Center	Hartford	0.2%	1061
Waterbury Hospital	Waterbury	0.2%	544
Bristol Hospital	Bristol	0.3%	386
Day Kimball Hospital	Putnam	0.3%	361
Greenwich Hospital Association	Greenwich	0.3%	698
Saint Vincent's Medical Center	Bridgeport	0.3%	400
Stamford Hospital	Stamford	0.4%	926
Yale-New Haven Hospital	New Haven	0.4%	4488
Hartford Hospital	Hartford	0.5%	213
Danbury Hospital	Danbury	0.6%	1251
The Hospital of Central Connecticut	New Britain	0.6%	713
New Milford Hospital	New Milford	0.9%	319
Norwalk Hospital Association	Norwalk	1.1%	1095
Charlotte Hungerford Hospital	Torrington	1.9%	319
Bridgeport Hospital	Bridgeport	12.2%	131
Windham Comm Mem Hosp & Hatch Hosp	Willimantic	22.0%	513

Follow-up Mammogram/Ultrasound

A follow-up rate near zero may indicate missed cancer; a rate higher than 14% may mean there is unnecessary follow up.

Hospital Name	City	Rate	Cases
Lawrence & Memorial Hospital	New London	8.1%	3186
Rockville General Hospital	Rockville	8.8%	1815
Day Kimball Hospital	Putnam	9.9%	1578
William W Backus Hospital	Norwich	10.0%	2355
Windham Comm Mem Hosp & Hatch Hosp	Willimantic	10.8%	1269
Saint Francis Hospital & Medical Center	Hartford	12.2%	1577
Johnson Memorial Hospital	Stafford Springs	12.8%	452
Manchester Memorial Hospital	Manchester	13.2%	441
Yale-New Haven Hospital	New Haven	13.5%	5446
The Hospital of Central Connecticut	New Britain	13.6%	2611
Bristol Hospital	Bristol	13.9%	209
Midstate Medical Center	Meriden	14.3%	872
John Dempsey Hospital	Farmington	14.4%	968
Sharon Hospital	Sharon	15.9%	889
Saint Marys Hospital	Waterbury	17.3%	508
Hartford Hospital	Hartford	17.5%	229
Waterbury Hospital	Waterbury	19.6%	199
Charlotte Hungerford Hospital	Torrington	20.6%	2097
Greenwich Hospital Association	Greenwich	21.8%	1910
Bridgeport Hospital	Bridgeport	23.2%	99
Middlesex Hospital	Middletown	24.3%	2723
New Milford Hospital	New Milford	26.2%	718
Griffin Hospital	Derby	28.2%	998
Danbury Hospital	Danbury	28.4%	1495
Saint Vincent's Medical Center	Bridgeport	32.2%	326
Norwalk Hospital Association	Norwalk	35.8%	3436
Stamford Hospital	Stamford	45.1%	2964

Lumbar Spine MRI for Low Back Pain

Hospital Name	City	Rate	Cases
Sharon Hospital	Sharon	22.1%	68
Manchester Memorial Hospital	Manchester	27.4%	73
John Dempsey Hospital	Farmington	28.7%	164
Midstate Medical Center	Meriden	29.9%	107
Danbury Hospital	Danbury	30.4%	161
Middlesex Hospital	Middletown	30.6%	206
Norwalk Hospital Association	Norwalk	32.0%	231
Griffin Hospital	Derby	32.1%	109
New Milford Hospital	New Milford	32.3%	93
The Hospital of Central Connecticut	New Britain	32.8%	119
Lawrence & Memorial Hospital	New London	33.3%	270
Stamford Hospital	Stamford	33.3%	117
Yale-New Haven Hospital	New Haven	34.4%	285
Bristol Hospital	Bristol	35.6%	73
Rockville General Hospital	Rockville	36.0%	89
William W Backus Hospital	Norwich	36.4%	294
Saint Francis Hospital & Medical Center	Hartford	38.8%	170
Greenwich Hospital Association	Greenwich	40.2%	179
Windham Comm Mem Hosp & Hatch Hosp	Willimantic	45.2%	93
Day Kimball Hospital	Putnam	45.8%	72

NOTE: Hospital profiles are in alphabetical order by state, then city, then hospital within the city; Rankings exclude hospitals with less than 25 cases except for patient surveys which excludes hospitals with less than 100 cases; (a) 100-299 cases; (1) The number of cases/patients is too few to report; (2) Data submitted were based on a sample of cases/patients; (3) Results are based on a shorter time period than required; (4) Data suppressed by CMS for one or more quarters; (5) Results are not available for this reporting period; (6) Fewer than 100 patients completed the HCAHPS survey; (7) No cases met the criteria for this measure; (8) The lower limit of the confidence interval cannot be calculated if the number of observed infections equals zero; (9) No data are available from the state/territory for this reporting period; (10) The scores shown reflect fewer than 50 completed surveys; (11) There were discrepancies in the data collection process; (12) This measure does not apply to this hospital for this reporting period; (13) Results cannot be calculated for this reporting period; (14) The results for this state are combined with nearby states to protect confidentiality; Please refer to the User's Guide for a full explanation of data.

Bridgeport Hospital

267 Grant Street
Bridgeport, CT 06610
Phone: 203-384-3000
Fax: 203-384-3943
E-mail: kawise@bpthosp.org
URL: www.bridgeporthospital.com
Type: Acute Care Hospitals
Emergency Services: Yes
Ownership: Voluntary non-profit - Private
Beds: 425

Key Personnel:

Infection Control. . . . . David Baker, MD
Operating Room. . . . . Karin Hooper, RN
CEO/President. . . . . William Jennings
Radiology. . . . . Alan D Kaye
Pediatric In-Patient Care . . . . Thomas Kennedy, MD
Quality Assurance . . . . Michael Liebowitz
Chief of Medical Staff . . . . Constantine Manthous, MD

Measure	Cases	This Hosp.	State Avg.	U.S. Avg.
Blood Clot Prevention and Treatment				
Anticoagulation Overlap Therapy[2]	107	79%	91%	93%
ICU Venous Thromboembolism Prophylaxis[2]	53	100%	93%	92%
Incidence of Potentially Preventable VTE[2]	36	6%	6%	10%
UFH with Dosages/Platelet Monitoring[2]	85	98%	95%	97%
Venous Thromboembolism Prophylaxis[2]	319	93%	89%	85%
Warfarin Therapy Discharge Instructions[2]	63	59%	64%	75%
Chest Pain/Possible Heart Attack Care				
Aspirin Given Within 24 Hours of Arrival[5]	-	-	98%	96%
Fibrinolytic Meds Within 30 Min. of Arrival[5]	-	-	33%	58%
Average Time to ECG (minutes)[5]	-	-	7	7
Average Time to Transfer (minutes)[5]	-	-	61	60
Children's Asthma Care				
Received Home Management Plan of Care	-	-	-	88%
Received Reliever Medication	-	-	-	100%
Received Systemic Corticosteroids	-	-	-	100%
Emergency Department				
Admittance Decision Time (minutes)[2]	574	206	147	98
Head CT Results Within 45 Min. of Arrival[1,3]	-	-	70%	57%
Patients Who Left ER Before Being Seen	80,689	3%	2%	2%
Time from ER Arrival to Admit. (minutes)[2]	588	438	338	274
Time from ER Arrival to Discharge (minutes)	342	182	131	134
Time in ER Before Being Evaluated (minutes)	301	79	28	26
Time to Pain Meds for Fractures (minutes)	56	70	55	57
Heart Attack Care				
Aspirin Given at Discharge[2]	248	98%	99%	99%
Fibrinolytic Meds Within 30 Min. of Arrival[2,7]	-	-	50%	54%
PCI Within 90 Minutes of Arrival[2]	31	94%	96%	96%
Statin Prescribed at Discharge[2]	252	98%	98%	98%
Heart Failure Care				
ACE Inhibitor or ARB for LVSD[2]	59	92%	96%	97%
Discharge Instructions Given[2]	177	96%	93%	94%
Evaluation of LVS Function[2]	262	99%	100%	99%
Medicare Spending				
Medicare Spending per Patient (ratio)	-	1.05	1.02	0.98
Pneumonia Care				
Appropriate Initial Antibiotic Given[2]	73	90%	97%	95%
Blood Culture Timing[2]	119	92%	97%	98%
Pregnancy and Delivery Care				
Newborn Deliveries Scheduled Early[2]	48	10%	5%	6%
Preventive Care				
Immunization for Influenza[2]	511	91%	90%	90%
Immunization for Pneumonia[2]	564	91%	91%	92%
Stroke Care				
Anticoagulation Therapy for Atrial Fibrillation[2]	12	83%	96%	95%
Antithrombotic Therapy Timing[2]	87	100%	99%	98%
Assessed for Rehabilitation[2]	99	99%	98%	97%
Discharged on Antithrombotic Therapy[2]	89	96%	99%	99%
Discharged on Statin Medication[2]	72	90%	95%	94%
Thrombolytic Therapy Timing[2]	13	92%	71%	66%
Venous Thromboembolism Prophylaxis[2]	110	99%	95%	94%
Written Stroke Educational Materials Given[2]	42	90%	80%	88%
Surgical Care Improvement Project				
Appropriate Beta Blocker Usage[2]	161	98%	98%	98%
Appropriate VTP Within 24 Hours[2]	274	99%	99%	98%
Controlled Postoperative Blood Glucose[2]	77	95%	96%	97%
Perioperative Temperature Management[2]	370	99%	99%	100%
Prophylactic Antibiotic Selection[2]	312	99%	99%	99%
Prophylactic Antibiotic Selection (Outpatient)	363	97%	97%	98%
Prophylactic Antibiotic Stopped[2]	292	98%	98%	98%
Prophylactic Antibiotic Timing[2]	313	99%	98%	99%
Prophylactic Antibiotic Timing (Outpatient)	362	98%	97%	98%
Urinary Catheter Removal[2]	290	96%	97%	97%
Survey of Patients' Hospital Experiences				
Area Around Room 'Always' Quiet at Night	300+	45%	52%	61%
Doctors 'Always' Communicated Well	300+	80%	80%	82%
Home Recovery Information Given	300+	82%	85%	85%
Hospital Given 9 or 10 on 10 Point Scale	300+	66%	68%	71%
Meds 'Always' Explained Before Given	300+	60%	62%	64%
Nurses 'Always' Communicated Well	300+	81%	78%	79%
Pain 'Always' Well Controlled	300+	73%	71%	71%
Room and Bathroom 'Always' Clean	300+	67%	71%	73%
Timely Help 'Always' Received	300+	65%	64%	68%
Would Definitely Recommend Hospital	300+	75%	71%	71%
Use of Medical Imaging				
Cardiac Imaging Stress Test before Surgery	1,536	4.6%	4.7%	5.3%
Combination Abdominal CT Scan	396	13.4%	5%	10.5%
Combination Brain/Sinus CT Scan[1]	-	-	2.3%	2.7%
Combination Chest CT Scan	131	12.2%	0.9%	2.7%
Follow-up Mammogram/Ultrasound	99	23.2%	19.5%	8.8%
Lumbar Spine MRI for Low Back Pain[1]	-	-	34.3%	37.2%

Saint Vincent's Medical Center

2800 Main St
Bridgeport, CT 06606
Phone: 203-576-5551
Fax: 203-576-5733
E-mail: info@svhs-ct.org
URL: www.stvincents.org
Type: Acute Care Hospitals
Emergency Services: Yes
Ownership: Voluntary non-profit - Church
Beds: 391

Key Personnel:

Quality Assurance . . . . Evelyn Gowel
Infection Control. . . . . Grace Kim, MD
Cardiac Laboratory. . . . . Edward Kosinski, MD
CEO/President. . . . . Stuart G. Marcus, MD, FACS
Operating Room. . . . . Nancy Newton
Radiology. . . . . Robert Russo, MD
Chief of Medical Staff . . . . Lawrence Schek, MD, FACC
Pediatric In-Patient Care . . . . Roy Schutzengel, MD

Measure	Cases	This Hosp.	State Avg.	U.S. Avg.
Blood Clot Prevention and Treatment				
Anticoagulation Overlap Therapy[2]	156	64%	91%	93%
ICU Venous Thromboembolism Prophylaxis[2]	49	86%	93%	92%
Incidence of Potentially Preventable VTE[2]	32	12%	6%	10%
UFH with Dosages/Platelet Monitoring[2]	126	62%	95%	97%
Venous Thromboembolism Prophylaxis[2]	354	80%	89%	85%
Warfarin Therapy Discharge Instructions[2]	102	92%	64%	75%
Chest Pain/Possible Heart Attack Care				
Aspirin Given Within 24 Hours of Arrival[3,7]	-	-	98%	96%
Fibrinolytic Meds Within 30 Min. of Arrival[5]	-	-	33%	58%
Average Time to ECG (minutes)[3,7]	-	-	7	7
Average Time to Transfer (minutes)[5]	-	-	61	60
Children's Asthma Care				
Received Home Management Plan of Care	-	-	-	88%
Received Reliever Medication	-	-	-	100%
Received Systemic Corticosteroids	-	-	-	100%
Emergency Department				
Admittance Decision Time (minutes)[2]	754	182	147	98
Head CT Results Within 45 Min. of Arrival[1]	-	-	70%	57%
Patients Who Left ER Before Being Seen	82,490	1%	2%	2%
Time from ER Arrival to Admit. (minutes)[2]	772	384	338	274
Time from ER Arrival to Discharge (minutes)	329	150	131	134
Time in ER Before Being Evaluated (minutes)	381	28	28	26
Time to Pain Meds for Fractures (minutes)	81	64	55	57
Heart Attack Care				
Aspirin Given at Discharge	415	100%	99%	99%
Fibrinolytic Meds Within 30 Min. of Arrival[7]	-	-	50%	54%
PCI Within 90 Minutes of Arrival	52	94%	96%	96%
Statin Prescribed at Discharge	418	100%	98%	98%
Heart Failure Care				
ACE Inhibitor or ARB for LVSD	159	100%	96%	97%
Discharge Instructions Given	341	99%	93%	94%
Evaluation of LVS Function	515	100%	100%	99%
Medicare Spending				
Medicare Spending per Patient (ratio)	-	1.06	1.02	0.98
Pneumonia Care				
Appropriate Initial Antibiotic Given	219	97%	97%	95%
Blood Culture Timing	379	98%	97%	98%
Pregnancy and Delivery Care				
Newborn Deliveries Scheduled Early[2]	21	0%	5%	6%
Preventive Care				
Immunization for Influenza[2]	556	97%	90%	90%
Immunization for Pneumonia[2]	737	98%	91%	92%
Stroke Care				
Anticoagulation Therapy for Atrial Fibrillation	22	95%	96%	95%
Antithrombotic Therapy Timing	136	97%	99%	98%
Assessed for Rehabilitation	175	98%	98%	97%
Discharged on Antithrombotic Therapy	155	99%	99%	99%
Discharged on Statin Medication	127	95%	95%	94%
Thrombolytic Therapy Timing[1]	-	-	71%	66%
Venous Thromboembolism Prophylaxis	167	90%	95%	94%
Written Stroke Educational Materials Given	73	89%	80%	88%
Surgical Care Improvement Project				
Appropriate Beta Blocker Usage[2]	200	98%	98%	98%
Appropriate VTP Within 24 Hours[2]	274	100%	99%	98%
Controlled Postoperative Blood Glucose[2]	113	99%	96%	97%
Perioperative Temperature Management[2]	350	100%	99%	100%
Prophylactic Antibiotic Selection[2]	332	99%	99%	99%
Prophylactic Antibiotic Selection (Outpatient)	240	98%	97%	98%
Prophylactic Antibiotic Stopped[2]	312	99%	98%	98%
Prophylactic Antibiotic Timing[2]	332	98%	98%	99%
Prophylactic Antibiotic Timing (Outpatient)	242	98%	97%	98%
Urinary Catheter Removal[2]	313	98%	97%	97%
Survey of Patients' Hospital Experiences				
Area Around Room 'Always' Quiet at Night	300+	56%	52%	61%
Doctors 'Always' Communicated Well	300+	79%	80%	82%
Home Recovery Information Given	300+	81%	85%	85%
Hospital Given 9 or 10 on 10 Point Scale	300+	70%	68%	71%
Meds 'Always' Explained Before Given	300+	56%	62%	64%
Nurses 'Always' Communicated Well	300+	77%	78%	79%
Pain 'Always' Well Controlled	300+	69%	71%	71%
Room and Bathroom 'Always' Clean	300+	70%	71%	73%
Timely Help 'Always' Received	300+	60%	64%	68%
Would Definitely Recommend Hospital	300+	78%	71%	71%
Use of Medical Imaging				
Cardiac Imaging Stress Test before Surgery	1,594	5.4%	4.7%	5.3%
Combination Abdominal CT Scan	830	14.5%	5%	10.5%
Combination Brain/Sinus CT Scan	1,013	3.5%	2.3%	2.7%
Combination Chest CT Scan	400	0.3%	0.9%	2.7%
Follow-up Mammogram/Ultrasound	326	32.2%	19.5%	8.8%
Lumbar Spine MRI for Low Back Pain[1]	-	-	34.3%	37.2%

Bristol Hospital

Brewster Rd
Bristol, CT 06010
Phone: 860-585-3000
Fax: 860-585-3058
E-mail: info@bristolhospital.org
URL: www.bristolhospital.org
Type: Acute Care Hospitals
Emergency Services: Yes
Ownership: Voluntary non-profit - Private
Beds: 152

Key Personnel:

Radiology. . . . . Carlos M Badiola, MD
Operating Room. . . . . Ara D Bagdasarian
CEO/President. . . . . Kurt A. Barwis, FACHE
Pediatric In-Patient Care . . . . Delbert Hodder, MD
Patient Relations . . . . Sheila Kempf, RN, PhD
Quality Assurance . . . . Karen Poole, RN
Chief of Medical Staff . . . . Kenneth Rhee, MD

Measure	Cases	This Hosp.	State Avg.	U.S. Avg.
Blood Clot Prevention and Treatment				
Anticoagulation Overlap Therapy[2]	54	98%	91%	93%
ICU Venous Thromboembolism Prophylaxis[2]	63	92%	93%	92%
Incidence of Potentially Preventable VTE[1,2]	-	-	6%	10%
UFH with Dosages/Platelet Monitoring[2]	24	100%	95%	97%
Venous Thromboembolism Prophylaxis[2]	391	95%	89%	85%
Warfarin Therapy Discharge Instructions[2]	38	74%	64%	75%
Chest Pain/Possible Heart Attack Care				
Aspirin Given Within 24 Hours of Arrival	54	98%	98%	96%

NOTE: Hospital profiles are in alphabetical order by state, then city, then hospital within the city; Rankings exclude hospitals with less than 25 cases except for patient surveys which excludes hospitals with less than 100 cases; (a) 100-299 cases; (1) The number of cases/patients is too few to report; (2) Data submitted were based on a sample of cases/patients; (3) Results are based on a shorter time period than required; (4) Data suppressed by CMS for one or more quarters; (5) Results are not available for this reporting period; (6) Fewer than 100 patients completed the HCAHPS survey; (7) No cases met the criteria for this measure; (8) The lower limit of the confidence interval cannot be calculated if the number of observed infections equals zero; (9) No data are available from the state/territory for this reporting period; (10) The scores shown reflect fewer than 50 completed surveys; (11) There were discrepancies in the data collection process; (12) This measure does not apply to this hospital for this reporting period; (13) Results cannot be calculated for this reporting period; (14) The results for this state are combined with nearby states to protect confidentiality; Please refer to the User's Guide for a full explanation of data.

Measure	Cases	This Hosp.	State Avg.	U.S. Avg.
Fibrinolytic Meds Within 30 Min. of Arrival[7]	-	-	33%	58%
Average Time to ECG (minutes)	58	14	7	7
Average Time to Transfer (minutes)	14	68	61	60
Children's Asthma Care				
Received Home Management Plan of Care	-	-	-	88%
Received Reliever Medication	-	-	-	100%
Received Systemic Corticosteroids	-	-	-	100%
Emergency Department				
Admittance Decision Time (minutes)[2]	855	97	147	98
Head CT Results Within 45 Min. of Arrival[1]	-	-	70%	57%
Patients Who Left ER Before Being Seen	39,227	1%	2%	2%
Time from ER Arrival to Admit. (minutes)[2]	862	276	338	274
Time from ER Arrival to Discharge (minutes)	467	113	131	134
Time in ER Before Being Evaluated (minutes)	503	18	28	26
Time to Pain Meds for Fractures (minutes)	91	56	55	57
Heart Attack Care				
Aspirin Given at Discharge	32	97%	99%	99%
Fibrinolytic Meds Within 30 Min. of Arrival[7]	-	-	50%	54%
PCI Within 90 Minutes of Arrival[7]	-	-	96%	96%
Statin Prescribed at Discharge	34	100%	98%	98%
Heart Failure Care				
ACE Inhibitor or ARB for LVSD	41	85%	96%	97%
Discharge Instructions Given	96	92%	93%	94%
Evaluation of LVS Function	166	99%	100%	99%
Medicare Spending				
Medicare Spending per Patient (ratio)	-	1.07	1.02	0.98
Pneumonia Care				
Appropriate Initial Antibiotic Given	112	93%	97%	95%
Blood Culture Timing	154	95%	97%	98%
Pregnancy and Delivery Care				
Newborn Deliveries Scheduled Early[2]	36	14%	5%	6%
Preventive Care				
Immunization for Influenza[2]	587	82%	90%	90%
Immunization for Pneumonia[2]	757	82%	91%	92%
Stroke Care				
Anticoagulation Therapy for Atrial Fibrillation[1]	-	-	96%	95%
Antithrombotic Therapy Timing	38	100%	99%	98%
Assessed for Rehabilitation	39	97%	98%	97%
Discharged on Antithrombotic Therapy	37	100%	99%	99%
Discharged on Statin Medication	34	88%	95%	94%
Thrombolytic Therapy Timing[1]	-	-	71%	66%
Venous Thromboembolism Prophylaxis	41	95%	95%	94%
Written Stroke Educational Materials Given	19	84%	80%	88%
Surgical Care Improvement Project				
Appropriate Beta Blocker Usage	50	88%	98%	98%
Appropriate VTP Within 24 Hours	155	97%	99%	98%
Controlled Postoperative Blood Glucose[7]	-	-	96%	97%
Perioperative Temperature Management	215	98%	99%	100%
Prophylactic Antibiotic Selection	114	96%	99%	99%
Prophylactic Antibiotic Selection (Outpatient)	118	97%	97%	98%
Prophylactic Antibiotic Stopped	104	93%	98%	98%
Prophylactic Antibiotic Timing	114	97%	98%	99%
Prophylactic Antibiotic Timing (Outpatient)	120	96%	97%	98%
Urinary Catheter Removal	103	89%	97%	97%
Survey of Patients' Hospital Experiences				
Area Around Room 'Always' Quiet at Night	300+	53%	52%	61%
Doctors 'Always' Communicated Well	300+	78%	80%	82%
Home Recovery Information Given	300+	88%	85%	85%
Hospital Given 9 or 10 on 10 Point Scale	300+	67%	68%	71%
Meds 'Always' Explained Before Given	300+	63%	62%	64%
Nurses 'Always' Communicated Well	300+	82%	78%	79%
Pain 'Always' Well Controlled	300+	75%	71%	71%
Room and Bathroom 'Always' Clean	300+	71%	71%	73%
Timely Help 'Always' Received	300+	67%	64%	68%
Would Definitely Recommend Hospital	300+	68%	71%	71%
Use of Medical Imaging				
Cardiac Imaging Stress Test before Surgery	317	6.3%	4.7%	5.3%
Combination Abdominal CT Scan	629	1.4%	5%	10.5%
Combination Brain/Sinus CT Scan	420	0.7%	2.3%	2.7%
Combination Chest CT Scan	386	0.3%	0.9%	2.7%
Follow-up Mammogram/Ultrasound	209	13.9%	19.5%	8.8%
Lumbar Spine MRI for Low Back Pain	73	35.6%	34.3%	37.2%

Danbury Hospital

24 Hospital Ave
Danbury, CT 06810
URL: www.danburyhospital.com
Phone: 203-797-7000
Fax: 203-797-7776
Type: Acute Care Hospitals
Emergency Services: Yes
Ownership: Voluntary non-profit - Private
Beds: 371

Key Personnel:

Pediatric In-Patient Care . . . . Raul Arguello, MD
Chairman/CEO . . . . James Kennedy
Chief of Medical Staff. . . . . Matthew Miller, MD
CEO/President. . . . . John M. Murphy, MD
Quality Assurance . . . . Dawn Myles, RN
Radiology. . . . . Fatejeet S. Sandhu, MD
Operating Room. . . . . Joanne Thompson, RN
Infection Control. . . . . Barbara Welch

Measure	Cases	This Hosp.	State Avg.	U.S. Avg.
Blood Clot Prevention and Treatment				
Anticoagulation Overlap Therapy[2]	110	99%	91%	93%
ICU Venous Thromboembolism Prophylaxis[2]	50	100%	93%	92%
Incidence of Potentially Preventable VTE[2]	30	0%	6%	10%
UFH with Dosages/Platelet Monitoring[2]	35	100%	95%	97%
Venous Thromboembolism Prophylaxis[2]	362	90%	89%	85%
Warfarin Therapy Discharge Instructions[2]	77	65%	64%	75%
Chest Pain/Possible Heart Attack Care				
Aspirin Given Within 24 Hours of Arrival[5]	-	-	98%	96%
Fibrinolytic Meds Within 30 Min. of Arrival[5]	-	-	33%	58%
Average Time to ECG (minutes)[5]	-	-	7	7
Average Time to Transfer (minutes)[5]	-	-	61	60
Children's Asthma Care				
Received Home Management Plan of Care	-	-	-	88%
Received Reliever Medication	-	-	-	100%
Received Systemic Corticosteroids	-	-	-	100%
Emergency Department				
Admittance Decision Time (minutes)[2]	701	102	147	98
Head CT Results Within 45 Min. of Arrival[1]	-	-	70%	57%
Patients Who Left ER Before Being Seen	70,172	1%	2%	2%
Time from ER Arrival to Admit. (minutes)[2]	701	286	338	274
Time from ER Arrival to Discharge (minutes)	348	130	131	134
Time in ER Before Being Evaluated (minutes)	383	27	28	26
Time to Pain Meds for Fractures (minutes)	209	65	55	57
Heart Attack Care				
Aspirin Given at Discharge	344	100%	99%	99%
Fibrinolytic Meds Within 30 Min. of Arrival[7]	-	-	50%	54%
PCI Within 90 Minutes of Arrival	66	100%	96%	96%
Statin Prescribed at Discharge	340	98%	98%	98%
Heart Failure Care				
ACE Inhibitor or ARB for LVSD[2]	76	99%	96%	97%
Discharge Instructions Given[2]	218	91%	93%	94%
Evaluation of LVS Function[2]	323	100%	100%	99%
Medicare Spending				
Medicare Spending per Patient (ratio)	-	1.03	1.02	0.98
Pneumonia Care				
Appropriate Initial Antibiotic Given[2]	115	97%	97%	95%
Blood Culture Timing[2]	65	95%	97%	98%
Pregnancy and Delivery Care				
Newborn Deliveries Scheduled Early[2]	30	0%	5%	6%
Preventive Care				
Immunization for Influenza[2]	517	97%	90%	90%
Immunization for Pneumonia[2]	641	99%	91%	92%
Stroke Care				
Anticoagulation Therapy for Atrial Fibrillation	20	100%	96%	95%
Antithrombotic Therapy Timing	139	97%	99%	98%
Assessed for Rehabilitation	180	96%	98%	97%
Discharged on Antithrombotic Therapy	152	100%	99%	99%
Discharged on Statin Medication	118	96%	95%	94%
Thrombolytic Therapy Timing	14	86%	71%	66%
Venous Thromboembolism Prophylaxis	183	98%	95%	94%
Written Stroke Educational Materials Given	82	95%	80%	88%
Surgical Care Improvement Project				
Appropriate Beta Blocker Usage[2]	288	98%	98%	98%
Appropriate VTP Within 24 Hours[2]	509	99%	99%	98%
Controlled Postoperative Blood Glucose[2]	139	99%	96%	97%
Perioperative Temperature Management[2]	604	100%	99%	100%
Prophylactic Antibiotic Selection[2]	507	100%	99%	99%
Prophylactic Antibiotic Selection (Outpatient)	557	99%	97%	98%
Prophylactic Antibiotic Stopped[2]	487	98%	98%	98%
Prophylactic Antibiotic Timing[2]	508	100%	98%	99%
Prophylactic Antibiotic Timing (Outpatient)	539	99%	97%	98%
Urinary Catheter Removal[2]	464	97%	97%	97%
Survey of Patients' Hospital Experiences				
Area Around Room 'Always' Quiet at Night	300+	49%	52%	61%
Doctors 'Always' Communicated Well	300+	78%	80%	82%
Home Recovery Information Given	300+	80%	85%	85%
Hospital Given 9 or 10 on 10 Point Scale	300+	68%	68%	71%
Meds 'Always' Explained Before Given	300+	59%	62%	64%
Nurses 'Always' Communicated Well	300+	77%	78%	79%
Pain 'Always' Well Controlled	300+	69%	71%	71%
Room and Bathroom 'Always' Clean	300+	72%	71%	73%
Timely Help 'Always' Received	300+	60%	64%	68%
Would Definitely Recommend Hospital	300+	73%	71%	71%
Use of Medical Imaging				
Cardiac Imaging Stress Test before Surgery	1,280	3.8%	4.7%	5.3%
Combination Abdominal CT Scan	1,255	2.9%	5%	10.5%
Combination Brain/Sinus CT Scan	983	1.4%	2.3%	2.7%
Combination Chest CT Scan	1,251	0.6%	0.9%	2.7%
Follow-up Mammogram/Ultrasound	1,495	28.4%	19.5%	8.8%
Lumbar Spine MRI for Low Back Pain	161	30.4%	34.3%	37.2%

Griffin Hospital

130 Division St
Derby, CT 06418
E-mail: griffin@griffinhealth.org
URL: www.griffinhealth.org
Phone: 203-732-7500
Fax: 203-732-7569
Type: Acute Care Hospitals
Emergency Services: Yes
Ownership: Voluntary non-profit - Other
Beds: 119

Key Personnel:

Chairman/CEO . . . . Joseph Andreana
Coronary Care . . . . Mary Ann Bertini
CEO/President. . . . . Patrick Charmel
Radiology. . . . . Christine Cooper
Quality Assurance . . . . Linda Evanko
Chief of Medical Staff. . . . . Kenneth Schwartz
Operating Room. . . . . Kim Viadero, RN
Pediatric In-Patient Care . . . . Anthony Wayne, MD

Measure	Cases	This Hosp.	State Avg.	U.S. Avg.
Blood Clot Prevention and Treatment				
Anticoagulation Overlap Therapy[2]	35	94%	91%	93%
ICU Venous Thromboembolism Prophylaxis[2]	84	95%	93%	92%
Incidence of Potentially Preventable VTE[1,2]	-	-	6%	10%
UFH with Dosages/Platelet Monitoring[2]	37	100%	95%	97%
Venous Thromboembolism Prophylaxis[2]	376	95%	89%	85%
Warfarin Therapy Discharge Instructions[2]	24	96%	64%	75%
Chest Pain/Possible Heart Attack Care				
Aspirin Given Within 24 Hours of Arrival	31	97%	98%	96%
Fibrinolytic Meds Within 30 Min. of Arrival[7]	-	-	33%	58%
Average Time to ECG (minutes)	32	7	7	7
Average Time to Transfer (minutes)	13	67	61	60
Children's Asthma Care				
Received Home Management Plan of Care	-	-	-	88%
Received Reliever Medication	-	-	-	100%
Received Systemic Corticosteroids	-	-	-	100%
Emergency Department				
Admittance Decision Time (minutes)[2]	809	123	147	98
Head CT Results Within 45 Min. of Arrival[7]	-	-	70%	57%
Patients Who Left ER Before Being Seen	41,113	1%	2%	2%
Time from ER Arrival to Admit. (minutes)[2]	816	317	338	274
Time from ER Arrival to Discharge (minutes)	376	130	131	134
Time in ER Before Being Evaluated (minutes)	418	33	28	26
Time to Pain Meds for Fractures (minutes)	87	71	55	57
Heart Attack Care				
Aspirin Given at Discharge	25	100%	99%	99%
Fibrinolytic Meds Within 30 Min. of Arrival[7]	-	-	50%	54%
PCI Within 90 Minutes of Arrival[7]	-	-	96%	96%
Statin Prescribed at Discharge	26	96%	98%	98%
Heart Failure Care				
ACE Inhibitor or ARB for LVSD	32	100%	96%	97%
Discharge Instructions Given	119	100%	93%	94%
Evaluation of LVS Function	175	100%	100%	99%

NOTE: Hospital profiles are in alphabetical order by state, then city, then hospital within the city; Rankings exclude hospitals with less than 25 cases except for patient surveys which excludes hospitals with less than 100 cases; (a) 100-299 cases; (1) The number of cases/patients is too few to report; (2) Data submitted were based on a sample of cases/patients; (3) Results are based on a shorter time period than required; (4) Data suppressed by CMS for one or more quarters; (5) Results are not available for this reporting period; (6) Fewer than 100 patients completed the HCAHPS survey; (7) No cases met the criteria for this measure; (8) The lower limit of the confidence interval cannot be calculated if the number of observed infections equals zero; (9) No data are available from the state/territory for this reporting period; (10) The scores shown reflect fewer than 50 completed surveys; (11) There were discrepancies in the data collection process; (12) This measure does not apply to this hospital for this reporting period; (13) Results cannot be calculated for this reporting period; (14) The results for this state are combined with nearby states to protect confidentiality; Please refer to the User's Guide for a full explanation of data.

Measure	Cases	This Hosp.	State Avg.	U.S. Avg.
Medicare Spending				
Medicare Spending per Patient (ratio)	-	1.01	1.02	0.98
Pneumonia Care				
Appropriate Initial Antibiotic Given	156	99%	97%	95%
Blood Culture Timing	231	98%	97%	98%
Pregnancy and Delivery Care				
Newborn Deliveries Scheduled Early[2]	32	6%	5%	6%
Preventive Care				
Immunization for Influenza[2]	551	99%	90%	90%
Immunization for Pneumonia[2]	725	99%	91%	92%
Stroke Care				
Anticoagulation Therapy for Atrial Fibrillation	16	88%	96%	95%
Antithrombotic Therapy Timing	69	97%	99%	98%
Assessed for Rehabilitation	74	100%	98%	97%
Discharged on Antithrombotic Therapy	67	99%	99%	99%
Discharged on Statin Medication	56	91%	95%	94%
Thrombolytic Therapy Timing[1]	-	-	71%	66%
Venous Thromboembolism Prophylaxis	80	100%	95%	94%
Written Stroke Educational Materials Given	30	100%	80%	88%
Surgical Care Improvement Project				
Appropriate Beta Blocker Usage	77	99%	98%	98%
Appropriate VTP Within 24 Hours	246	99%	99%	98%
Controlled Postoperative Blood Glucose[7]	-	-	96%	97%
Perioperative Temperature Management	282	100%	99%	100%
Prophylactic Antibiotic Selection	161	100%	99%	99%
Prophylactic Antibiotic Selection (Outpatient)	34	100%	97%	98%
Prophylactic Antibiotic Stopped	154	99%	98%	98%
Prophylactic Antibiotic Timing	161	99%	98%	99%
Prophylactic Antibiotic Timing (Outpatient)	32	97%	97%	98%
Urinary Catheter Removal	163	100%	97%	97%
Survey of Patients' Hospital Experiences				
Area Around Room 'Always' Quiet at Night	300+	56%	52%	61%
Doctors 'Always' Communicated Well	300+	78%	80%	82%
Home Recovery Information Given	300+	89%	85%	85%
Hospital Given 9 or 10 on 10 Point Scale	300+	75%	68%	71%
Meds 'Always' Explained Before Given	300+	65%	62%	64%
Nurses 'Always' Communicated Well	300+	79%	78%	79%
Pain 'Always' Well Controlled	300+	69%	71%	71%
Room and Bathroom 'Always' Clean	300+	77%	71%	73%
Timely Help 'Always' Received	300+	67%	64%	68%
Would Definitely Recommend Hospital	300+	76%	71%	71%
Use of Medical Imaging				
Cardiac Imaging Stress Test before Surgery[1]	-	-	4.7%	5.3%
Combination Abdominal CT Scan	525	1.1%	5%	10.5%
Combination Brain/Sinus CT Scan[1]	-	-	2.3%	2.7%
Combination Chest CT Scan	477	0.0%	0.9%	2.7%
Follow-up Mammogram/Ultrasound	998	28.2%	19.5%	8.8%
Lumbar Spine MRI for Low Back Pain	109	32.1%	34.3%	37.2%

John Dempsey Hospital

263 Farmington Ave
Farmington, CT 06032
Phone: 860-679-1145
Fax: 860-679-4515
E-mail: ccda@up.uchc.edu
URL: www.uconnhealth.orgorwww.uchc.edu
Type: Acute Care Hospitals
Emergency Services: Yes
Ownership: Government - Local
Beds: 204

Key Personnel:
CEO . . . . Carolle Andrews
Operating Room. . . . . Bruce Brenner
Radiology. . . . . XLawrence J Briggs
Chief of Medical Staff. . . . . Bruce Carlson
Ambulatory Care . . . . Marianne Dess-Santoro
Infection Control. . . . . Nancy Dupont
Quality Assurance . . . . Barry Kels, MD
Cardiac Laboratory. . . . . Dr Bruce Liang

Measure	Cases	This Hosp.	State Avg.	U.S. Avg.
Blood Clot Prevention and Treatment				
Anticoagulation Overlap Therapy[2]	53	94%	91%	93%
ICU Venous Thromboembolism Prophylaxis[2]	58	91%	93%	92%
Incidence of Potentially Preventable VTE[2]	25	20%	6%	10%
UFH with Dosages/Platelet Monitoring[2]	40	100%	95%	97%
Venous Thromboembolism Prophylaxis[2]	292	88%	89%	85%
Warfarin Therapy Discharge Instructions[2]	32	0%	64%	75%
Chest Pain/Possible Heart Attack Care				
Aspirin Given Within 24 Hours of Arrival[5]	-	-	98%	96%
Fibrinolytic Meds Within 30 Min. of Arrival[5]	-	-	33%	58%
Average Time to ECG (minutes)[5]	-	-	7	7
Average Time to Transfer (minutes)[5]	-	-	61	60
Children's Asthma Care				
Received Home Management Plan of Care	-	-	-	88%
Received Reliever Medication	-	-	-	100%
Received Systemic Corticosteroids	-	-	-	100%
Emergency Department				
Admittance Decision Time (minutes)[2]	608	180	147	98
Head CT Results Within 45 Min. of Arrival[1]	-	-	70%	57%
Patients Who Left ER Before Being Seen	29,563	1%	2%	2%
Time from ER Arrival to Admit. (minutes)[2]	608	349	338	274
Time from ER Arrival to Discharge (minutes)	361	159	131	134
Time in ER Before Being Evaluated (minutes)	384	26	28	26
Time to Pain Meds for Fractures (minutes)	72	48	55	57
Heart Attack Care				
Aspirin Given at Discharge	145	100%	99%	99%
Fibrinolytic Meds Within 30 Min. of Arrival[7]	-	-	50%	54%
PCI Within 90 Minutes of Arrival	23	91%	96%	96%
Statin Prescribed at Discharge	146	100%	98%	98%
Heart Failure Care				
ACE Inhibitor or ARB for LVSD	48	100%	96%	97%
Discharge Instructions Given	151	100%	93%	94%
Evaluation of LVS Function	200	100%	100%	99%
Medicare Spending				
Medicare Spending per Patient (ratio)	-	1.00	1.02	0.98
Pneumonia Care				
Appropriate Initial Antibiotic Given[2]	58	100%	97%	95%
Blood Culture Timing[2]	138	96%	97%	98%
Pregnancy and Delivery Care				
Newborn Deliveries Scheduled Early[2]	122	1%	5%	6%
Preventive Care				
Immunization for Influenza[2]	550	99%	90%	90%
Immunization for Pneumonia[2]	636	91%	91%	92%
Stroke Care				
Anticoagulation Therapy for Atrial Fibrillation[1]	-	-	96%	95%
Antithrombotic Therapy Timing	44	98%	99%	98%
Assessed for Rehabilitation	71	97%	98%	97%
Discharged on Antithrombotic Therapy	65	100%	99%	99%
Discharged on Statin Medication	48	98%	95%	94%
Thrombolytic Therapy Timing[1]	-	-	71%	66%
Venous Thromboembolism Prophylaxis	59	80%	95%	94%
Written Stroke Educational Materials Given	41	22%	80%	88%
Surgical Care Improvement Project				
Appropriate Beta Blocker Usage[2]	105	100%	98%	98%
Appropriate VTP Within 24 Hours[2]	270	100%	99%	98%
Controlled Postoperative Blood Glucose[2]	59	97%	96%	97%
Perioperative Temperature Management[2]	304	100%	99%	100%
Prophylactic Antibiotic Selection[2]	242	100%	99%	99%
Prophylactic Antibiotic Selection (Outpatient)	301	98%	97%	98%
Prophylactic Antibiotic Stopped[2]	236	99%	98%	98%
Prophylactic Antibiotic Timing[2]	244	99%	98%	99%
Prophylactic Antibiotic Timing (Outpatient)	306	97%	97%	98%
Urinary Catheter Removal[2]	232	100%	97%	97%
Survey of Patients' Hospital Experiences				
Area Around Room 'Always' Quiet at Night	300+	44%	52%	61%
Doctors 'Always' Communicated Well	300+	80%	80%	82%
Home Recovery Information Given	300+	87%	85%	85%
Hospital Given 9 or 10 on 10 Point Scale	300+	68%	68%	71%
Meds 'Always' Explained Before Given	300+	64%	62%	64%
Nurses 'Always' Communicated Well	300+	79%	78%	79%
Pain 'Always' Well Controlled	300+	68%	71%	71%
Room and Bathroom 'Always' Clean	300+	67%	71%	73%
Timely Help 'Always' Received	300+	59%	64%	68%
Would Definitely Recommend Hospital	300+	74%	71%	71%
Use of Medical Imaging				
Cardiac Imaging Stress Test before Surgery	331	3.0%	4.7%	5.3%
Combination Abdominal CT Scan	692	12.0%	5%	10.5%
Combination Brain/Sinus CT Scan	595	1.8%	2.3%	2.7%
Combination Chest CT Scan	609	0.0%	0.9%	2.7%
Follow-up Mammogram/Ultrasound	968	14.4%	19.5%	8.8%
Lumbar Spine MRI for Low Back Pain	164	28.7%	34.3%	37.2%

Greenwich Hospital Association

5 Perryridge Rd
Greenwich, CT 06830
Phone: 203-863-3000
Fax: 203-863-4604
E-mail: robin1@greenhosp
URL: www.greenhosp.org
Type: Acute Care Hospitals
Emergency Services: Yes
Ownership: Voluntary non-profit - Private
Beds: 174

Key Personnel:
Infection Control. . . . . Lillian Burns
CEO/President. . . . . Frank A Corvino
Quality Assurance . . . . Barbara Hughes
Pediatric Ambulatory Care . . . . . . Arnold B Korval, MD
Administrator . . . . Marc Kosak
Operating Room. . . . . Philip J McWhorter
Radiology. . . . . David J Mullen, MD
Chief of Medical Staff. . . . . Frederick E Siefert, MD

Measure	Cases	This Hosp.	State Avg.	U.S. Avg.
Blood Clot Prevention and Treatment				
Anticoagulation Overlap Therapy[2]	52	96%	91%	93%
ICU Venous Thromboembolism Prophylaxis[2]	40	98%	93%	92%
Incidence of Potentially Preventable VTE[1,2]	-	-	6%	10%
UFH with Dosages/Platelet Monitoring[2]	26	100%	95%	97%
Venous Thromboembolism Prophylaxis[2]	322	83%	89%	85%
Warfarin Therapy Discharge Instructions[2]	35	11%	64%	75%
Chest Pain/Possible Heart Attack Care				
Aspirin Given Within 24 Hours of Arrival[5]	-	-	98%	96%
Fibrinolytic Meds Within 30 Min. of Arrival[5]	-	-	33%	58%
Average Time to ECG (minutes)[5]	-	-	7	7
Average Time to Transfer (minutes)[5]	-	-	61	60
Children's Asthma Care				
Received Home Management Plan of Care	-	-	-	88%
Received Reliever Medication	-	-	-	100%
Received Systemic Corticosteroids	-	-	-	100%
Emergency Department				
Admittance Decision Time (minutes)[2]	514	136	147	98
Head CT Results Within 45 Min. of Arrival[1,3]	-	-	70%	57%
Patients Who Left ER Before Being Seen	43,855	0%	2%	2%
Time from ER Arrival to Admit. (minutes)[2]	516	276	338	274
Time from ER Arrival to Discharge (minutes)	344	133	131	134
Time in ER Before Being Evaluated (minutes)	383	31	28	26
Time to Pain Meds for Fractures (minutes)	157	53	55	57
Heart Attack Care				
Aspirin Given at Discharge[2]	53	98%	99%	99%
Fibrinolytic Meds Within 30 Min. of Arrival[2,7]	-	-	50%	54%
PCI Within 90 Minutes of Arrival[2]	29	100%	96%	96%
Statin Prescribed at Discharge[2]	56	100%	98%	98%
Heart Failure Care				
ACE Inhibitor or ARB for LVSD[2]	77	96%	96%	97%
Discharge Instructions Given[2]	179	98%	93%	94%
Evaluation of LVS Function[2]	245	100%	100%	99%
Medicare Spending				
Medicare Spending per Patient (ratio)	-	1.01	1.02	0.98
Pneumonia Care				
Appropriate Initial Antibiotic Given[2]	74	97%	97%	95%
Blood Culture Timing[2]	125	99%	97%	98%
Pregnancy and Delivery Care				
Newborn Deliveries Scheduled Early[2]	30	13%	5%	6%
Preventive Care				
Immunization for Influenza[2]	470	65%	90%	90%
Immunization for Pneumonia[2]	500	72%	91%	92%
Stroke Care				
Anticoagulation Therapy for Atrial Fibrillation[2]	11	100%	96%	95%
Antithrombotic Therapy Timing[2]	73	100%	99%	98%
Assessed for Rehabilitation[2]	84	100%	98%	97%
Discharged on Antithrombotic Therapy[2]	68	99%	99%	99%
Discharged on Statin Medication[2]	58	98%	95%	94%
Thrombolytic Therapy Timing[1,2]	-	-	71%	66%
Venous Thromboembolism Prophylaxis[2]	90	98%	95%	94%
Written Stroke Educational Materials Given[2]	44	91%	80%	88%
Surgical Care Improvement Project				
Appropriate Beta Blocker Usage[2]	82	100%	98%	98%
Appropriate VTP Within 24 Hours[2]	271	97%	99%	98%

NOTE: Hospital profiles are in alphabetical order by state, then city, then hospital within the city; Rankings exclude hospitals with less than 25 cases except for patient surveys which excludes hospitals with less than 100 cases; (a) 100-299 cases; (1) The number of cases/patients is too few to report; (2) Data submitted were based on a sample of cases/patients; (3) Results are based on a shorter time period than required; (4) Data suppressed by CMS for one or more quarters; (5) Results are not available for this reporting period; (6) Fewer than 100 patients completed the HCAHPS survey; (7) No cases met the criteria for this measure; (8) The lower limit of the confidence interval cannot be calculated if the number of observed infections equals zero; (9) No data are available from the state/territory for this reporting period; (10) The scores shown reflect fewer than 50 completed surveys; (11) There were discrepancies in the data collection process; (12) This measure does not apply to this hospital for this reporting period; (13) Results cannot be calculated for this reporting period; (14) The results for this state are combined with nearby states to protect confidentiality; Please refer to the User's Guide for a full explanation of data.

Measure	Cases	This Hosp.	State Avg.	U.S. Avg.
Controlled Postoperative Blood Glucose[2,7]	-	-	96%	97%
Perioperative Temperature Management[2]	318	100%	99%	100%
Prophylactic Antibiotic Selection[2]	184	98%	99%	99%
Prophylactic Antibiotic Selection (Outpatient)	303	98%	97%	98%
Prophylactic Antibiotic Stopped[2]	182	94%	98%	98%
Prophylactic Antibiotic Timing[2]	185	99%	98%	99%
Prophylactic Antibiotic Timing (Outpatient)	307	98%	97%	98%
Urinary Catheter Removal[2]	98	96%	97%	97%
Survey of Patients' Hospital Experiences				
Area Around Room 'Always' Quiet at Night	300+	57%	52%	61%
Doctors 'Always' Communicated Well	300+	82%	80%	82%
Home Recovery Information Given	300+	82%	85%	85%
Hospital Given 9 or 10 on 10 Point Scale	300+	83%	68%	71%
Meds 'Always' Explained Before Given	300+	64%	62%	64%
Nurses 'Always' Communicated Well	300+	81%	78%	79%
Pain 'Always' Well Controlled	300+	77%	71%	71%
Room and Bathroom 'Always' Clean	300+	80%	71%	73%
Timely Help 'Always' Received	300+	71%	64%	68%
Would Definitely Recommend Hospital	300+	85%	71%	71%
Use of Medical Imaging				
Cardiac Imaging Stress Test before Surgery	443	6.8%	4.7%	5.3%
Combination Abdominal CT Scan	952	5.1%	5%	10.5%
Combination Brain/Sinus CT Scan	1,039	3.6%	2.3%	2.7%
Combination Chest CT Scan	698	0.3%	0.9%	2.7%
Follow-up Mammogram/Ultrasound	1,910	21.8%	19.5%	8.8%
Lumbar Spine MRI for Low Back Pain	179	40.2%	34.3%	37.2%

Connecticut Childrens Medical Center

282 Washington Street Phone: 860-545-9000
Hartford, CT 06106 Fax: 860-545-8560
URL: www.ccmckids.org
Type: Childrens Emergency Services: Yes
Ownership: Voluntary non-profit - Private Beds: 135

Key Personnel:

Pediatric Ambulatory Care . . . . . . Carol Benjamin
Chief of Medical Staff. . . . . Paul H Dworkin, MD
CEO/President. . . . . Martin J Gavin
Quality Assurance . . . . Elizabeth Gnu
Radiology. . . . . Diane Jay
Cardiac Laboratory. . . . . Harris Lepold, MD
Infection Control. . . . . Jennifer Martin
Pediatric In-Patient Care . . . . Susan Maxwell

Measure	Cases	This Hosp.	State Avg.	U.S. Avg.
Blood Clot Prevention and Treatment				
Anticoagulation Overlap Therapy[5]	-	-	91%	93%
ICU Venous Thromboembolism Prophylaxis[5]	-	-	93%	92%
Incidence of Potentially Preventable VTE[5]	-	-	6%	10%
UFH with Dosages/Platelet Monitoring[5]	-	-	95%	97%
Venous Thromboembolism Prophylaxis[5]	-	-	89%	85%
Warfarin Therapy Discharge Instructions[5]	-	-	64%	75%
Chest Pain/Possible Heart Attack Care				
Aspirin Given Within 24 Hours of Arrival	-	-	98%	96%
Fibrinolytic Meds Within 30 Min. of Arrival	-	-	33%	58%
Average Time to ECG (minutes)	-	-	7	7
Average Time to Transfer (minutes)	-	-	61	60
Children's Asthma Care				
Received Home Management Plan of Care	267	79%	-	88%
Received Reliever Medication	267	100%	-	100%
Received Systemic Corticosteroids	267	99%	-	100%
Emergency Department				
Admittance Decision Time (minutes)[5]	-	-	147	98
Head CT Results Within 45 Min. of Arrival	-	-	70%	57%
Patients Who Left ER Before Being Seen	-	-	2%	2%
Time from ER Arrival to Admit. (minutes)[5]	-	-	338	274
Time from ER Arrival to Discharge (minutes)	-	-	131	134
Time in ER Before Being Evaluated (minutes)	-	-	28	26
Time to Pain Meds for Fractures (minutes)	-	-	55	57
Heart Attack Care				
Aspirin Given at Discharge[5]	-	-	99%	99%
Fibrinolytic Meds Within 30 Min. of Arrival[5]	-	-	50%	54%
PCI Within 90 Minutes of Arrival[5]	-	-	96%	96%
Statin Prescribed at Discharge[5]	-	-	98%	98%
Heart Failure Care				
ACE Inhibitor or ARB for LVSD[5]	-	-	96%	97%
Discharge Instructions Given[5]	-	-	93%	94%
Evaluation of LVS Function[5]	-	-	100%	99%
Medicare Spending				
Medicare Spending per Patient (ratio)	-	-	1.02	0.98
Pneumonia Care				
Appropriate Initial Antibiotic Given[5]	-	-	97%	95%
Blood Culture Timing[5]	-	-	97%	98%
Pregnancy and Delivery Care				
Newborn Deliveries Scheduled Early[5]	-	-	5%	6%
Preventive Care				
Immunization for Influenza[5]	-	-	90%	90%
Immunization for Pneumonia[5]	-	-	91%	92%
Stroke Care				
Anticoagulation Therapy for Atrial Fibrillation[5]	-	-	96%	95%
Antithrombotic Therapy Timing[5]	-	-	99%	98%
Assessed for Rehabilitation[5]	-	-	98%	97%
Discharged on Antithrombotic Therapy[5]	-	-	99%	99%
Discharged on Statin Medication[5]	-	-	95%	94%
Thrombolytic Therapy Timing[5]	-	-	71%	66%
Venous Thromboembolism Prophylaxis[5]	-	-	95%	94%
Written Stroke Educational Materials Given[5]	-	-	80%	88%
Surgical Care Improvement Project				
Appropriate Beta Blocker Usage[5]	-	-	98%	98%
Appropriate VTP Within 24 Hours[5]	-	-	99%	98%
Controlled Postoperative Blood Glucose[5]	-	-	96%	97%
Perioperative Temperature Management[5]	-	-	99%	100%
Prophylactic Antibiotic Selection[5]	-	-	99%	99%
Prophylactic Antibiotic Selection (Outpatient)	-	-	97%	98%
Prophylactic Antibiotic Stopped[5]	-	-	98%	98%
Prophylactic Antibiotic Timing[5]	-	-	98%	99%
Prophylactic Antibiotic Timing (Outpatient)	-	-	97%	98%
Urinary Catheter Removal[5]	-	-	97%	97%
Survey of Patients' Hospital Experiences				
Area Around Room 'Always' Quiet at Night[5]	-	-	52%	61%
Doctors 'Always' Communicated Well[5]	-	-	80%	82%
Home Recovery Information Given[5]	-	-	85%	85%
Hospital Given 9 or 10 on 10 Point Scale[5]	-	-	68%	71%
Meds 'Always' Explained Before Given[5]	-	-	62%	64%
Nurses 'Always' Communicated Well[5]	-	-	78%	79%
Pain 'Always' Well Controlled[5]	-	-	71%	71%
Room and Bathroom 'Always' Clean[5]	-	-	71%	73%
Timely Help 'Always' Received[5]	-	-	64%	68%
Would Definitely Recommend Hospital[5]	-	-	71%	71%
Use of Medical Imaging				
Cardiac Imaging Stress Test before Surgery	-	-	4.7%	5.3%
Combination Abdominal CT Scan	-	-	5%	10.5%
Combination Brain/Sinus CT Scan	-	-	2.3%	2.7%
Combination Chest CT Scan	-	-	0.9%	2.7%
Follow-up Mammogram/Ultrasound	-	-	19.5%	8.8%
Lumbar Spine MRI for Low Back Pain	-	-	34.3%	37.2%

Hartford Hospital

80 Seymour Street Phone: 860-545-5000
Hartford, CT 06102 Fax: 860-545-5066
URL: www.harthosp.org
Type: Acute Care Hospitals Emergency Services: Yes
Ownership: Voluntary non-profit - Private Beds: 867

Key Personnel:

Pediatric In-Patient Care . . . . Leonard Banco
Infection Control. . . . . Brian Cooper, MD
Radiology. . . . . Stewart Markowitz, MD
CEO/President. . . . . Stuart K. Markowitz, MD, FACR
Chief of Medical Staff. . . . . Stacy Nerenstone, MD
Quality Assurance . . . . Allison Reynolds
Operating Room. . . . . Barbara Rodirick

Measure	Cases	This Hosp.	State Avg.	U.S. Avg.
Blood Clot Prevention and Treatment				
Anticoagulation Overlap Therapy[2]	280	96%	91%	93%
ICU Venous Thromboembolism Prophylaxis[2]	63	92%	93%	92%
Incidence of Potentially Preventable VTE[2]	92	7%	6%	10%
UFH with Dosages/Platelet Monitoring[2]	234	98%	95%	97%
Venous Thromboembolism Prophylaxis[2]	376	91%	89%	85%
Warfarin Therapy Discharge Instructions[2]	179	78%	64%	75%
Chest Pain/Possible Heart Attack Care				
Aspirin Given Within 24 Hours of Arrival[1,3]	-	-	98%	96%
Fibrinolytic Meds Within 30 Min. of Arrival[5]	-	-	33%	58%
Average Time to ECG (minutes)[1,3]	-	-	7	7
Average Time to Transfer (minutes)[5]	-	-	61	60
Children's Asthma Care				
Received Home Management Plan of Care	-	-	-	88%
Received Reliever Medication	-	-	-	100%
Received Systemic Corticosteroids	-	-	-	100%
Emergency Department				
Admittance Decision Time (minutes)[2]	616	180	147	98
Head CT Results Within 45 Min. of Arrival[1,3]	-	-	70%	57%
Patients Who Left ER Before Being Seen	>100k	4%	2%	2%
Time from ER Arrival to Admit. (minutes)[2]	627	494	338	274
Time from ER Arrival to Discharge (minutes)	375	256	131	134
Time in ER Before Being Evaluated (minutes)	399	94	28	26
Time to Pain Meds for Fractures (minutes)	110	82	55	57
Heart Attack Care				
Aspirin Given at Discharge	913	100%	99%	99%
Fibrinolytic Meds Within 30 Min. of Arrival[1]	-	-	50%	54%
PCI Within 90 Minutes of Arrival	92	98%	96%	96%
Statin Prescribed at Discharge	902	99%	98%	98%
Heart Failure Care				
ACE Inhibitor or ARB for LVSD	272	94%	96%	97%
Discharge Instructions Given	669	89%	93%	94%
Evaluation of LVS Function	934	100%	100%	99%
Medicare Spending				
Medicare Spending per Patient (ratio)	-	0.99	1.02	0.98
Pneumonia Care				
Appropriate Initial Antibiotic Given	307	97%	97%	95%
Blood Culture Timing	676	98%	97%	98%
Pregnancy and Delivery Care				
Newborn Deliveries Scheduled Early[2]	64	3%	5%	6%
Preventive Care				
Immunization for Influenza[2]	554	85%	90%	90%
Immunization for Pneumonia[2]	693	86%	91%	92%
Stroke Care				
Anticoagulation Therapy for Atrial Fibrillation	74	100%	96%	95%
Antithrombotic Therapy Timing	236	99%	99%	98%
Assessed for Rehabilitation	445	100%	98%	97%
Discharged on Antithrombotic Therapy	330	99%	99%	99%
Discharged on Statin Medication	232	97%	95%	94%
Thrombolytic Therapy Timing	37	95%	71%	66%
Venous Thromboembolism Prophylaxis	466	99%	95%	94%
Written Stroke Educational Materials Given	217	92%	80%	88%
Surgical Care Improvement Project				
Appropriate Beta Blocker Usage[2]	320	98%	98%	98%
Appropriate VTP Within 24 Hours[2]	529	100%	99%	98%
Controlled Postoperative Blood Glucose[2]	152	90%	96%	97%
Perioperative Temperature Management[2]	804	100%	99%	100%
Prophylactic Antibiotic Selection[2]	578	100%	99%	99%
Prophylactic Antibiotic Selection (Outpatient)	749	99%	97%	98%
Prophylactic Antibiotic Stopped[2]	559	97%	98%	98%
Prophylactic Antibiotic Timing[2]	579	98%	98%	99%
Prophylactic Antibiotic Timing (Outpatient)	759	95%	97%	98%
Urinary Catheter Removal[2]	483	97%	97%	97%
Survey of Patients' Hospital Experiences				
Area Around Room 'Always' Quiet at Night	300+	45%	52%	61%
Doctors 'Always' Communicated Well	300+	80%	80%	82%
Home Recovery Information Given	300+	88%	85%	85%
Hospital Given 9 or 10 on 10 Point Scale	300+	66%	68%	71%
Meds 'Always' Explained Before Given	300+	61%	62%	64%
Nurses 'Always' Communicated Well	300+	78%	78%	79%
Pain 'Always' Well Controlled	300+	68%	71%	71%
Room and Bathroom 'Always' Clean	300+	66%	71%	73%
Timely Help 'Always' Received	300+	57%	64%	68%
Would Definitely Recommend Hospital	300+	73%	71%	71%
Use of Medical Imaging				
Cardiac Imaging Stress Test before Surgery	784	5.1%	4.7%	5.3%
Combination Abdominal CT Scan	636	2.0%	5%	10.5%
Combination Brain/Sinus CT Scan	910	1.4%	2.3%	2.7%
Combination Chest CT Scan	213	0.5%	0.9%	2.7%
Follow-up Mammogram/Ultrasound	229	17.5%	19.5%	8.8%

NOTE: Hospital profiles are in alphabetical order by state, then city, then hospital within the city; Rankings exclude hospitals with less than 25 cases except for patient surveys which excludes hospitals with less than 100 cases; (a) 100-299 cases; (1) The number of cases/patients is too few to report; (2) Data submitted were based on a sample of cases/patients; (3) Results are based on a shorter time period than required; (4) Data suppressed by CMS for one or more quarters; (5) Results are not available for this reporting period; (6) Fewer than 100 patients completed the HCAHPS survey; (7) No cases met the criteria for this measure; (8) The lower limit of the confidence interval cannot be calculated if the number of observed infections equals zero; (9) No data are available from the state/territory for this reporting period; (10) The scores shown reflect fewer than 50 completed surveys; (11) There were discrepancies in the data collection process; (12) This measure does not apply to this hospital for this reporting period; (13) Results cannot be calculated for this reporting period; (14) The results for this state are combined with nearby states to protect confidentiality; Please refer to the User's Guide for a full explanation of data.

Lumbar Spine MRI for Low Back Pain[1]	-	-	34.3%	37.2%

Saint Francis Hospital & Medical Center

114 Woodland Street Phone: 860-714-4000
Hartford, CT 06105 Fax: 860-714-8048
E-mail: webmaster@stfranciscare.org
URL: www.saintfranciscare.com
Type: Acute Care Hospitals Emergency Services: Yes
Ownership: Voluntary non-profit - Church Beds: 617
Key Personnel:
Quality Assurance . . . . Nancy Budds
President/CEO . . . . Christopher M. Dadlez, FACHE
Emergency Room . . . . Judy Wiehl, RN

Measure	Cases	This Hosp.	State Avg.	U.S. Avg.
Blood Clot Prevention and Treatment				
Anticoagulation Overlap Therapy[2]	227	92%	91%	93%
ICU Venous Thromboembolism Prophylaxis[2]	64	97%	93%	92%
Incidence of Potentially Preventable VTE[2]	44	11%	6%	10%
UFH with Dosages/Platelet Monitoring[2]	226	100%	95%	97%
Venous Thromboembolism Prophylaxis[2]	402	83%	89%	85%
Warfarin Therapy Discharge Instructions[2]	139	60%	64%	75%
Chest Pain/Possible Heart Attack Care				
Aspirin Given Within 24 Hours of Arrival[5]	-	-	98%	96%
Fibrinolytic Meds Within 30 Min. of Arrival[5]	-	-	33%	58%
Average Time to ECG (minutes)[5]	-	-	7	7
Average Time to Transfer (minutes)[5]	-	-	61	60
Children's Asthma Care				
Received Home Management Plan of Care	-	-	-	88%
Received Reliever Medication	-	-	-	100%
Received Systemic Corticosteroids	-	-	-	100%
Emergency Department				
Admittance Decision Time (minutes)[2]	646	215	147	98
Head CT Results Within 45 Min. of Arrival[1]	-	-	70%	57%
Patients Who Left ER Before Being Seen	82,584	3%	2%	2%
Time from ER Arrival to Admit. (minutes)[2]	661	452	338	274
Time from ER Arrival to Discharge (minutes)	411	188	131	134
Time in ER Before Being Evaluated (minutes)	477	27	28	26
Time to Pain Meds for Fractures (minutes)	77	69	55	57
Heart Attack Care				
Aspirin Given at Discharge	537	100%	99%	99%
Fibrinolytic Meds Within 30 Min. of Arrival[7]	-	-	50%	54%
PCI Within 90 Minutes of Arrival	72	93%	96%	96%
Statin Prescribed at Discharge	523	100%	98%	98%
Heart Failure Care				
ACE Inhibitor or ARB for LVSD[2]	97	100%	96%	97%
Discharge Instructions Given[2]	208	90%	93%	94%
Evaluation of LVS Function[2]	305	100%	100%	99%
Medicare Spending				
Medicare Spending per Patient (ratio)	-	1.04	1.02	0.98
Pneumonia Care				
Appropriate Initial Antibiotic Given[2]	74	95%	97%	95%
Blood Culture Timing[2]	185	98%	97%	98%
Pregnancy and Delivery Care				
Newborn Deliveries Scheduled Early[2]	49	0%	5%	6%
Preventive Care				
Immunization for Influenza[2]	579	91%	90%	90%
Immunization for Pneumonia[2]	770	95%	91%	92%
Stroke Care				
Anticoagulation Therapy for Atrial Fibrillation	50	90%	96%	95%
Antithrombotic Therapy Timing	264	97%	99%	98%
Assessed for Rehabilitation	338	98%	98%	97%
Discharged on Antithrombotic Therapy	277	100%	99%	99%
Discharged on Statin Medication	212	95%	95%	94%
Thrombolytic Therapy Timing	32	50%	71%	66%
Venous Thromboembolism Prophylaxis	372	92%	95%	94%
Written Stroke Educational Materials Given	107	25%	80%	88%
Surgical Care Improvement Project				
Appropriate Beta Blocker Usage[2]	282	99%	98%	98%
Appropriate VTP Within 24 Hours[2]	514	98%	99%	98%
Controlled Postoperative Blood Glucose[2]	172	98%	96%	97%
Perioperative Temperature Management[2]	695	99%	99%	100%
Prophylactic Antibiotic Selection[2]	619	99%	99%	99%
Prophylactic Antibiotic Selection (Outpatient)	688	98%	97%	98%
Prophylactic Antibiotic Stopped[2]	601	98%	98%	98%
Prophylactic Antibiotic Timing[2]	619	99%	98%	99%
Prophylactic Antibiotic Timing (Outpatient)	676	97%	97%	98%
Urinary Catheter Removal[2]	331	100%	97%	97%
Survey of Patients' Hospital Experiences				
Area Around Room 'Always' Quiet at Night	300+	54%	52%	61%
Doctors 'Always' Communicated Well	300+	79%	80%	82%
Home Recovery Information Given	300+	85%	85%	85%
Hospital Given 9 or 10 on 10 Point Scale	300+	69%	68%	71%
Meds 'Always' Explained Before Given	300+	60%	62%	64%
Nurses 'Always' Communicated Well	300+	77%	78%	79%
Pain 'Always' Well Controlled	300+	68%	71%	71%
Room and Bathroom 'Always' Clean	300+	72%	71%	73%
Timely Help 'Always' Received	300+	60%	64%	68%
Would Definitely Recommend Hospital	300+	76%	71%	71%
Use of Medical Imaging				
Cardiac Imaging Stress Test before Surgery	613	4.4%	4.7%	5.3%
Combination Abdominal CT Scan	1,412	2.3%	5%	10.5%
Combination Brain/Sinus CT Scan	962	2.6%	2.3%	2.7%
Combination Chest CT Scan	1,061	0.2%	0.9%	2.7%
Follow-up Mammogram/Ultrasound	1,577	12.2%	19.5%	8.8%
Lumbar Spine MRI for Low Back Pain	170	38.8%	34.3%	37.2%

Manchester Memorial Hospital

71 Haynes St Phone: 860-647-4780
Manchester, CT 06040 Fax: 860-533-3444
URL: www.echn.org
Type: Acute Care Hospitals Emergency Services: Yes
Ownership: Voluntary non-profit - Private Beds: 451
Key Personnel:
Emergency Room . . . . Robert F Carroll, MD
Cardiac Laboratory. . . . . Hazar Dahhan, MD
Radiology. . . . . Stephen Hauser
CEO/President. . . . . Peter J Karl
Pediatric In-Patient Care . . . . Jerome Lahman, MD
Quality Assurance . . . . Leona Mariani
Patient Relations . . . . Deborah A Parker, RN
Chief of Medical Staff. . . . . Joel J Reich

Measure	Cases	This Hosp.	State Avg.	U.S. Avg.
Blood Clot Prevention and Treatment				
Anticoagulation Overlap Therapy[2]	75	95%	91%	93%
ICU Venous Thromboembolism Prophylaxis[2]	93	96%	93%	92%
Incidence of Potentially Preventable VTE[2]	11	0%	6%	10%
UFH with Dosages/Platelet Monitoring[2]	65	100%	95%	97%
Venous Thromboembolism Prophylaxis[2]	317	87%	89%	85%
Warfarin Therapy Discharge Instructions[2]	52	37%	64%	75%
Chest Pain/Possible Heart Attack Care				
Aspirin Given Within 24 Hours of Arrival	79	96%	98%	96%
Fibrinolytic Meds Within 30 Min. of Arrival[1]	-	-	33%	58%
Average Time to ECG (minutes)	79	7	7	7
Average Time to Transfer (minutes)[1]	-	-	61	60
Children's Asthma Care				
Received Home Management Plan of Care	-	-	-	88%
Received Reliever Medication	-	-	-	100%
Received Systemic Corticosteroids	-	-	-	100%
Emergency Department				
Admittance Decision Time (minutes)[2]	661	223	147	98
Head CT Results Within 45 Min. of Arrival[1]	-	-	70%	57%
Patients Who Left ER Before Being Seen	46,449	2%	2%	2%
Time from ER Arrival to Admit. (minutes)[2]	661	462	338	274
Time from ER Arrival to Discharge (minutes)	330	147	131	134
Time in ER Before Being Evaluated (minutes)	267	74	28	26
Time to Pain Meds for Fractures (minutes)	85	72	55	57
Heart Attack Care				
Aspirin Given at Discharge	24	100%	99%	99%
Fibrinolytic Meds Within 30 Min. of Arrival[7]	-	-	50%	54%
PCI Within 90 Minutes of Arrival[7]	-	-	96%	96%
Statin Prescribed at Discharge	26	77%	98%	98%
Heart Failure Care				
ACE Inhibitor or ARB for LVSD	49	100%	96%	97%
Discharge Instructions Given	134	93%	93%	94%
Evaluation of LVS Function	202	100%	100%	99%
Medicare Spending				
Medicare Spending per Patient (ratio)	-	1.07	1.02	0.98
Pneumonia Care				
Appropriate Initial Antibiotic Given[2]	100	94%	97%	95%
Blood Culture Timing[2]	204	98%	97%	98%
Pregnancy and Delivery Care				
Newborn Deliveries Scheduled Early	84	4%	5%	6%
Preventive Care				
Immunization for Influenza[2]	489	94%	90%	90%
Immunization for Pneumonia[2]	596	91%	91%	92%
Stroke Care				
Anticoagulation Therapy for Atrial Fibrillation[1]	-	-	96%	95%
Antithrombotic Therapy Timing	45	100%	99%	98%
Assessed for Rehabilitation	42	86%	98%	97%
Discharged on Antithrombotic Therapy	41	100%	99%	99%
Discharged on Statin Medication	35	91%	95%	94%
Thrombolytic Therapy Timing[1]	-	-	71%	66%
Venous Thromboembolism Prophylaxis	40	78%	95%	94%
Written Stroke Educational Materials Given	31	39%	80%	88%
Surgical Care Improvement Project				
Appropriate Beta Blocker Usage[2]	146	97%	98%	98%
Appropriate VTP Within 24 Hours[2]	401	99%	99%	98%
Controlled Postoperative Blood Glucose[2,7]	-	-	96%	97%
Perioperative Temperature Management[2]	443	100%	99%	100%
Prophylactic Antibiotic Selection[2]	268	100%	99%	99%
Prophylactic Antibiotic Selection (Outpatient)	259	99%	97%	98%
Prophylactic Antibiotic Stopped[2]	258	100%	98%	98%
Prophylactic Antibiotic Timing[2]	268	99%	98%	99%
Prophylactic Antibiotic Timing (Outpatient)	259	99%	97%	98%
Urinary Catheter Removal[2]	130	98%	97%	97%
Survey of Patients' Hospital Experiences				
Area Around Room 'Always' Quiet at Night	300+	51%	52%	61%
Doctors 'Always' Communicated Well	300+	76%	80%	82%
Home Recovery Information Given	300+	82%	85%	85%
Hospital Given 9 or 10 on 10 Point Scale	300+	62%	68%	71%
Meds 'Always' Explained Before Given	300+	58%	62%	64%
Nurses 'Always' Communicated Well	300+	77%	78%	79%
Pain 'Always' Well Controlled	300+	70%	71%	71%
Room and Bathroom 'Always' Clean	300+	63%	71%	73%
Timely Help 'Always' Received	300+	58%	64%	68%
Would Definitely Recommend Hospital	300+	66%	71%	71%
Use of Medical Imaging				
Cardiac Imaging Stress Test before Surgery	243	2.1%	4.7%	5.3%
Combination Abdominal CT Scan	943	3.0%	5%	10.5%
Combination Brain/Sinus CT Scan	616	1.9%	2.3%	2.7%
Combination Chest CT Scan	879	0.2%	0.9%	2.7%
Follow-up Mammogram/Ultrasound	441	13.2%	19.5%	8.8%
Lumbar Spine MRI for Low Back Pain	73	27.4%	34.3%	37.2%

Midstate Medical Center

435 Lewis Ave Phone: 203-694-8200
Meriden, CT 06450 Fax: 203-694-7601
URL: www.midstatemedical.org
Type: Acute Care Hospitals Emergency Services: Yes
Ownership: Voluntary non-profit - Private Beds: 130
Key Personnel:
Pediatric In-Patient Care . . . . Luis Alonso, MD
Coronary Care . . . . Lynn Amarante, RN
Infection Control. . . . . Julia Chiarizio, RN
Quality Assurance . . . . Elizabeth Desanto
CEO/President. . . . . Lucille Janatka
Chief of Medical Staff . . . . Harold Kaplan, MD
Radiology. . . . . Allen Kratzer, MD
Operating Room. . . . . Peg Sherwood, RN

Measure	Cases	This Hosp.	State Avg.	U.S. Avg.
Blood Clot Prevention and Treatment				
Anticoagulation Overlap Therapy[2]	73	78%	91%	93%
ICU Venous Thromboembolism Prophylaxis[2]	37	97%	93%	92%
Incidence of Potentially Preventable VTE[1,2]	-	-	6%	10%
UFH with Dosages/Platelet Monitoring[2]	85	100%	95%	97%
Venous Thromboembolism Prophylaxis[2]	419	84%	89%	85%
Warfarin Therapy Discharge Instructions[2]	47	91%	64%	75%
Chest Pain/Possible Heart Attack Care				
Aspirin Given Within 24 Hours of Arrival	72	97%	98%	96%
Fibrinolytic Meds Within 30 Min. of Arrival[7]	-	-	33%	58%
Average Time to ECG (minutes)	76	8	7	7

NOTE: Hospital profiles are in alphabetical order by state, then city, then hospital within the city; Rankings exclude hospitals with less than 25 cases except for patient surveys which excludes hospitals with less than 100 cases; (a) 100-299 cases; (1) The number of cases/patients is too few to report; (2) Data submitted were based on a sample of cases/patients; (3) Results are based on a shorter time period than required; (4) Data suppressed by CMS for one or more quarters; (5) Results are not available for this reporting period; (6) Fewer than 100 patients completed the HCAHPS survey; (7) No cases met the criteria for this measure; (8) The lower limit of the confidence interval cannot be calculated if the number of observed infections equals zero; (9) No data are available from the state/territory for this reporting period; (10) The scores shown reflect fewer than 50 completed surveys; (11) There were discrepancies in the data collection process; (12) This measure does not apply to this hospital for this reporting period; (13) Results cannot be calculated for this reporting period; (14) The results for this state are combined with nearby states to protect confidentiality; Please refer to the User's Guide for a full explanation of data.

Measure	Cases	This Hosp.	State Avg.	U.S. Avg.
Average Time to Transfer (minutes)	19	88	61	60
Children's Asthma Care				
Received Home Management Plan of Care	-	-	-	88%
Received Reliever Medication	-	-	-	100%
Received Systemic Corticosteroids	-	-	-	100%
Emergency Department				
Admittance Decision Time (minutes)[2]	778	176	147	98
Head CT Results Within 45 Min. of Arrival[1]	-	-	70%	57%
Patients Who Left ER Before Being Seen	60,676	1%	2%	2%
Time from ER Arrival to Admit. (minutes)[2]	778	392	338	274
Time from ER Arrival to Discharge (minutes)	404	118	131	134
Time in ER Before Being Evaluated (minutes)	214	40	28	26
Time to Pain Meds for Fractures (minutes)	144	47	55	57
Heart Attack Care				
Aspirin Given at Discharge	48	100%	99%	99%
Fibrinolytic Meds Within 30 Min. of Arrival[7]	-	-	50%	54%
PCI Within 90 Minutes of Arrival[7]	-	-	96%	96%
Statin Prescribed at Discharge	53	92%	98%	98%
Heart Failure Care				
ACE Inhibitor or ARB for LVSD	74	96%	96%	97%
Discharge Instructions Given	190	87%	93%	94%
Evaluation of LVS Function	307	100%	100%	99%
Medicare Spending				
Medicare Spending per Patient (ratio)	-	1.01	1.02	0.98
Pneumonia Care				
Appropriate Initial Antibiotic Given[2]	113	93%	97%	95%
Blood Culture Timing[2]	200	96%	97%	98%
Pregnancy and Delivery Care				
Newborn Deliveries Scheduled Early[2]	108	6%	5%	6%
Preventive Care				
Immunization for Influenza[2]	552	93%	90%	90%
Immunization for Pneumonia[2]	762	95%	91%	92%
Stroke Care				
Anticoagulation Therapy for Atrial Fibrillation	15	93%	96%	95%
Antithrombotic Therapy Timing	94	100%	99%	98%
Assessed for Rehabilitation	106	99%	98%	97%
Discharged on Antithrombotic Therapy	101	100%	99%	99%
Discharged on Statin Medication	79	99%	95%	94%
Thrombolytic Therapy Timing[1]	-	-	71%	66%
Venous Thromboembolism Prophylaxis	110	99%	95%	94%
Written Stroke Educational Materials Given	49	100%	80%	88%
Surgical Care Improvement Project				
Appropriate Beta Blocker Usage[2]	208	98%	98%	98%
Appropriate VTP Within 24 Hours[2]	611	99%	99%	98%
Controlled Postoperative Blood Glucose[2,7]	-	-	96%	97%
Perioperative Temperature Management[2]	691	100%	99%	100%
Prophylactic Antibiotic Selection[2]	457	98%	99%	99%
Prophylactic Antibiotic Selection (Outpatient)	176	97%	97%	98%
Prophylactic Antibiotic Stopped[2]	444	99%	98%	98%
Prophylactic Antibiotic Timing[2]	458	97%	98%	99%
Prophylactic Antibiotic Timing (Outpatient)	178	96%	97%	98%
Urinary Catheter Removal[2]	494	98%	97%	97%
Survey of Patients' Hospital Experiences				
Area Around Room 'Always' Quiet at Night	300+	62%	52%	61%
Doctors 'Always' Communicated Well	300+	81%	80%	82%
Home Recovery Information Given	300+	85%	85%	85%
Hospital Given 9 or 10 on 10 Point Scale	300+	72%	68%	71%
Meds 'Always' Explained Before Given	300+	64%	62%	64%
Nurses 'Always' Communicated Well	300+	82%	78%	79%
Pain 'Always' Well Controlled	300+	71%	71%	71%
Room and Bathroom 'Always' Clean	300+	77%	71%	73%
Timely Help 'Always' Received	300+	70%	64%	68%
Would Definitely Recommend Hospital	300+	76%	71%	71%
Use of Medical Imaging				
Cardiac Imaging Stress Test before Surgery	118	9.3%	4.7%	5.3%
Combination Abdominal CT Scan	791	5.7%	5%	10.5%
Combination Brain/Sinus CT Scan	757	2.2%	2.3%	2.7%
Combination Chest CT Scan	427	0.0%	0.9%	2.7%
Follow-up Mammogram/Ultrasound	872	14.3%	19.5%	8.8%
Lumbar Spine MRI for Low Back Pain	107	29.9%	34.3%	37.2%

Middlesex Hospital

28 Crescent St
Middletown, CT 06457
URL: www.midhosp.org
Phone: 860-344-6000
Fax: 860-344-6568
Type: Acute Care Hospitals
Emergency Services: Yes
Ownership: Voluntary non-profit - Private
Beds: 193

Key Personnel:
Pediatric In-Patient Care . . . . Joseph Flanagan, MD
Radiology. . . . . Diana M Hull, Jr, MD
CEO/President. . . . . Robert G Kiely
Cardiac Laboratory. . . . . Arthur V McDowell, MD
Chief of Medical Staff. . . . . Arthur V McDowell
Emergency Room . . . . Jacquelyn Nelson, RN
Quality Assurance . . . . Cathleen O'Hara

Measure	Cases	This Hosp.	State Avg.	U.S. Avg.
Blood Clot Prevention and Treatment				
Anticoagulation Overlap Therapy[2]	83	99%	91%	93%
ICU Venous Thromboembolism Prophylaxis[2]	25	96%	93%	92%
Incidence of Potentially Preventable VTE[2]	16	6%	6%	10%
UFH with Dosages/Platelet Monitoring[2]	49	100%	95%	97%
Venous Thromboembolism Prophylaxis[2]	351	95%	89%	85%
Warfarin Therapy Discharge Instructions[2]	54	80%	64%	75%
Chest Pain/Possible Heart Attack Care				
Aspirin Given Within 24 Hours of Arrival	216	100%	98%	96%
Fibrinolytic Meds Within 30 Min. of Arrival[7]	-	-	33%	58%
Average Time to ECG (minutes)	224	8	7	7
Average Time to Transfer (minutes)	51	51	61	60
Children's Asthma Care				
Received Home Management Plan of Care	-	-	-	88%
Received Reliever Medication	-	-	-	100%
Received Systemic Corticosteroids	-	-	-	100%
Emergency Department				
Admittance Decision Time (minutes)[2]	808	117	147	98
Head CT Results Within 45 Min. of Arrival	35	77%	70%	57%
Patients Who Left ER Before Being Seen	92,456	1%	2%	2%
Time from ER Arrival to Admit. (minutes)[2]	808	284	338	274
Time from ER Arrival to Discharge (minutes)	593	105	131	134
Time in ER Before Being Evaluated (minutes)	421	25	28	26
Time to Pain Meds for Fractures (minutes)	80	44	55	57
Heart Attack Care				
Aspirin Given at Discharge	50	100%	99%	99%
Fibrinolytic Meds Within 30 Min. of Arrival[7]	-	-	50%	54%
PCI Within 90 Minutes of Arrival[7]	-	-	96%	96%
Statin Prescribed at Discharge	43	98%	98%	98%
Heart Failure Care				
ACE Inhibitor or ARB for LVSD	103	96%	96%	97%
Discharge Instructions Given	261	90%	93%	94%
Evaluation of LVS Function	402	100%	100%	99%
Medicare Spending				
Medicare Spending per Patient (ratio)	-	0.98	1.02	0.98
Pneumonia Care				
Appropriate Initial Antibiotic Given	179	98%	97%	95%
Blood Culture Timing	330	98%	97%	98%
Pregnancy and Delivery Care				
Newborn Deliveries Scheduled Early[2]	61	2%	5%	6%
Preventive Care				
Immunization for Influenza[2]	543	97%	90%	90%
Immunization for Pneumonia[2]	778	97%	91%	92%
Stroke Care				
Anticoagulation Therapy for Atrial Fibrillation	26	100%	96%	95%
Antithrombotic Therapy Timing	124	100%	99%	98%
Assessed for Rehabilitation	137	100%	98%	97%
Discharged on Antithrombotic Therapy	133	100%	99%	99%
Discharged on Statin Medication	97	98%	95%	94%
Thrombolytic Therapy Timing[1]	-	-	71%	66%
Venous Thromboembolism Prophylaxis	139	97%	95%	94%
Written Stroke Educational Materials Given	81	94%	80%	88%
Surgical Care Improvement Project				
Appropriate Beta Blocker Usage	359	99%	98%	98%
Appropriate VTP Within 24 Hours	995	99%	99%	98%
Controlled Postoperative Blood Glucose[7]	-	-	96%	97%
Perioperative Temperature Management	1,131	100%	99%	100%
Prophylactic Antibiotic Selection	760	99%	99%	99%
Prophylactic Antibiotic Selection (Outpatient)	111	98%	97%	98%
Prophylactic Antibiotic Stopped	750	98%	98%	98%
Prophylactic Antibiotic Timing	762	98%	98%	99%
Prophylactic Antibiotic Timing (Outpatient)	115	94%	97%	98%
Urinary Catheter Removal	834	98%	97%	97%
Survey of Patients' Hospital Experiences				
Area Around Room 'Always' Quiet at Night	300+	57%	52%	61%
Doctors 'Always' Communicated Well	300+	80%	80%	82%
Home Recovery Information Given	300+	86%	85%	85%
Hospital Given 9 or 10 on 10 Point Scale	300+	76%	68%	71%
Meds 'Always' Explained Before Given	300+	63%	62%	64%
Nurses 'Always' Communicated Well	300+	81%	78%	79%
Pain 'Always' Well Controlled	300+	71%	71%	71%
Room and Bathroom 'Always' Clean	300+	77%	71%	73%
Timely Help 'Always' Received	300+	71%	64%	68%
Would Definitely Recommend Hospital	300+	78%	71%	71%
Use of Medical Imaging				
Cardiac Imaging Stress Test before Surgery[7]	-	-	4.7%	5.3%
Combination Abdominal CT Scan	1,986	6.3%	5%	10.5%
Combination Brain/Sinus CT Scan	1,181	1.2%	2.3%	2.7%
Combination Chest CT Scan	1,166	0.1%	0.9%	2.7%
Follow-up Mammogram/Ultrasound	2,723	24.3%	19.5%	8.8%
Lumbar Spine MRI for Low Back Pain	206	30.6%	34.3%	37.2%

Milford Hospital

300 Seaside Avenue
Milford, CT 06460
URL: www.milfordhospital.org
Phone: 203-876-4000
Type: Acute Care Hospitals
Emergency Services: Yes
Ownership: Voluntary non-profit - Private
Beds: 106

Key Personnel:
Radiology. . . . . Vito Errico, MD
Operating Room. . . . . Rosemarie Esposito
Quality Assurance . . . . Lloyd Friedman, MD
Anesthesiology. . . . . Yair Grinberg, MD
Pediatric Ambulatory Care . . . . . . Jeffrey Gruskay, MD
Pediatric In-Patient Care . . . . Jeffrey Gruskay, MD
President/CEO. . . . . Joseph Pelaccia
Chief of Medical Staff. . . . . Nitai Riegler, MD

Measure	Cases	This Hosp.	State Avg.	U.S. Avg.
Blood Clot Prevention and Treatment				
Anticoagulation Overlap Therapy[2]	18	100%	91%	93%
ICU Venous Thromboembolism Prophylaxis[2]	53	92%	93%	92%
Incidence of Potentially Preventable VTE[1,2]	-	-	6%	10%
UFH with Dosages/Platelet Monitoring[2]	19	100%	95%	97%
Venous Thromboembolism Prophylaxis[2]	246	91%	89%	85%
Warfarin Therapy Discharge Instructions[1,2]	-	-	64%	75%
Chest Pain/Possible Heart Attack Care				
Aspirin Given Within 24 Hours of Arrival	12	100%	98%	96%
Fibrinolytic Meds Within 30 Min. of Arrival[7]	-	-	33%	58%
Average Time to ECG (minutes)	11	7	7	7
Average Time to Transfer (minutes)[1]	-	-	61	60
Children's Asthma Care				
Received Home Management Plan of Care	-	-	-	88%
Received Reliever Medication	-	-	-	100%
Received Systemic Corticosteroids	-	-	-	100%
Emergency Department				
Admittance Decision Time (minutes)[2]	525	137	147	98
Head CT Results Within 45 Min. of Arrival[1]	-	-	70%	57%
Patients Who Left ER Before Being Seen	24,683	1%	2%	2%
Time from ER Arrival to Admit. (minutes)[2]	542	321	338	274
Time from ER Arrival to Discharge (minutes)	404	150	131	134
Time in ER Before Being Evaluated (minutes)	421	28	28	26
Time to Pain Meds for Fractures (minutes)	62	52	55	57
Heart Attack Care				
Aspirin Given at Discharge[1]	-	-	99%	99%
Fibrinolytic Meds Within 30 Min. of Arrival[7]	-	-	50%	54%
PCI Within 90 Minutes of Arrival[7]	-	-	96%	96%
Statin Prescribed at Discharge[1]	-	-	98%	98%
Heart Failure Care				
ACE Inhibitor or ARB for LVSD	34	97%	96%	97%
Discharge Instructions Given	95	97%	93%	94%
Evaluation of LVS Function	150	99%	100%	99%
Medicare Spending				
Medicare Spending per Patient (ratio)	-	1.01	1.02	0.98

NOTE: Hospital profiles are in alphabetical order by state, then city, then hospital within the city; Rankings exclude hospitals with less than 25 cases except for patient surveys which excludes hospitals with less than 100 cases; (a) 100-299 cases; (1) The number of cases/patients is too few to report; (2) Data submitted were based on a sample of cases/patients; (3) Results are based on a shorter time period than required; (4) Data suppressed by CMS for one or more quarters; (5) Results are not available for this reporting period; (6) Fewer than 100 patients completed the HCAHPS survey; (7) No cases met the criteria for this measure; (8) The lower limit of the confidence interval cannot be calculated if the number of observed infections equals zero; (9) No data are available from the state/territory for this reporting period; (10) The scores shown reflect fewer than 50 completed surveys; (11) There were discrepancies in the data collection process; (12) This measure does not apply to this hospital for this reporting period; (13) Results cannot be calculated for this reporting period; (14) The results for this state are combined with nearby states to protect confidentiality; Please refer to the User's Guide for a full explanation of data.

Pneumonia Care				
Appropriate Initial Antibiotic Given[2]	95	100%	97%	95%
Blood Culture Timing[2]	159	95%	97%	98%
Pregnancy and Delivery Care				
Newborn Deliveries Scheduled Early[1,2]	-	-	5%	6%
Preventive Care				
Immunization for Influenza[2]	334	94%	90%	90%
Immunization for Pneumonia[2]	499	97%	91%	92%
Stroke Care				
Anticoagulation Therapy for Atrial Fibrillation[1]	-	-	96%	95%
Antithrombotic Therapy Timing	19	100%	99%	98%
Assessed for Rehabilitation	27	100%	98%	97%
Discharged on Antithrombotic Therapy	24	100%	99%	99%
Discharged on Statin Medication	20	90%	95%	94%
Thrombolytic Therapy Timing[1]	-	-	71%	66%
Venous Thromboembolism Prophylaxis	31	94%	95%	94%
Written Stroke Educational Materials Given	12	58%	80%	88%
Surgical Care Improvement Project				
Appropriate Beta Blocker Usage[2]	123	99%	98%	98%
Appropriate VTP Within 24 Hours[2]	429	99%	99%	98%
Controlled Postoperative Blood Glucose[2,7]	-	-	96%	97%
Perioperative Temperature Management[2]	468	100%	99%	100%
Prophylactic Antibiotic Selection[2]	334	100%	99%	99%
Prophylactic Antibiotic Selection (Outpatient)	20	95%	97%	98%
Prophylactic Antibiotic Stopped[2]	326	99%	98%	98%
Prophylactic Antibiotic Timing[2]	334	97%	98%	99%
Prophylactic Antibiotic Timing (Outpatient)	20	100%	97%	98%
Urinary Catheter Removal[2]	391	100%	97%	97%
Survey of Patients' Hospital Experiences				
Area Around Room 'Always' Quiet at Night	300+	58%	52%	61%
Doctors 'Always' Communicated Well	300+	82%	80%	82%
Home Recovery Information Given	300+	85%	85%	85%
Hospital Given 9 or 10 on 10 Point Scale	300+	72%	68%	71%
Meds 'Always' Explained Before Given	300+	65%	62%	64%
Nurses 'Always' Communicated Well	300+	80%	78%	79%
Pain 'Always' Well Controlled	300+	72%	71%	71%
Room and Bathroom 'Always' Clean	300+	82%	71%	73%
Timely Help 'Always' Received	300+	71%	64%	68%
Would Definitely Recommend Hospital	300+	73%	71%	71%
Use of Medical Imaging				
Cardiac Imaging Stress Test before Surgery	97	4.1%	4.7%	5.3%
Combination Abdominal CT Scan	353	6.2%	5%	10.5%
Combination Brain/Sinus CT Scan	395	5.8%	2.3%	2.7%
Combination Chest CT Scan	119	0.0%	0.9%	2.7%
Follow-up Mammogram/Ultrasound[1]	-	-	19.5%	8.8%
Lumbar Spine MRI for Low Back Pain[1]	-	-	34.3%	37.2%

The Hospital of Central Connecticut

100 Grand Street Phone: 860-224-5011
New Britain, CT 06050 Fax: 860-224-5779
E-mail: moreinfo@thocc.org
URL: www.thocc.org
Type: Acute Care Hospitals Emergency Services: Yes
Ownership: Voluntary non-profit - Other Beds: 330

Key Personnel:

Chief of Medical Staff.......... James L Bernene, MD
Intensive Care Unit........... Paula Bowley, RN
Infection Control............. Diane Dowling, RN
Emergency Room ....Jeffrey Finkelstein, MD
Patient Relations .... Elaine Greene
Radiology.................. Stephen Grund, MD
Quality Assurance .... Elizabeth Schuff
CEO/President............... Laurence Tanner

Measure	Cases	This Hosp.	State Avg.	U.S. Avg.
Blood Clot Prevention and Treatment				
Anticoagulation Overlap Therapy[2]	95	95%	91%	93%
ICU Venous Thromboembolism Prophylaxis[2]	54	100%	93%	92%
Incidence of Potentially Preventable VTE[2]	14	0%	6%	10%
UFH with Dosages/Platelet Monitoring[2]	47	89%	95%	97%
Venous Thromboembolism Prophylaxis[2]	367	97%	89%	85%
Warfarin Therapy Discharge Instructions[2]	63	83%	64%	75%
Chest Pain/Possible Heart Attack Care				
Aspirin Given Within 24 Hours of Arrival	14	93%	98%	96%
Fibrinolytic Meds Within 30 Min. of Arrival[7]	-	-	33%	58%
Average Time to ECG (minutes)	14	9	7	7
Average Time to Transfer (minutes)[7]	-	-	61	60
Children's Asthma Care				
Received Home Management Plan of Care	-	-	-	88%
Received Reliever Medication	-	-	-	100%
Received Systemic Corticosteroids	-	-	-	100%
Emergency Department				
Admittance Decision Time (minutes)[2]	784	174	147	98
Head CT Results Within 45 Min. of Arrival[1]	-	-	70%	57%
Patients Who Left ER Before Being Seen	>100k	1%	2%	2%
Time from ER Arrival to Admit. (minutes)[2]	786	316	338	274
Time from ER Arrival to Discharge (minutes)	405	93	131	134
Time in ER Before Being Evaluated (minutes)	444	21	28	26
Time to Pain Meds for Fractures (minutes)	118	58	55	57
Heart Attack Care				
Aspirin Given at Discharge	171	100%	99%	99%
Fibrinolytic Meds Within 30 Min. of Arrival[7]	-	-	50%	54%
PCI Within 90 Minutes of Arrival	36	97%	96%	96%
Statin Prescribed at Discharge	174	95%	98%	98%
Heart Failure Care				
ACE Inhibitor or ARB for LVSD[2]	60	92%	96%	97%
Discharge Instructions Given[2]	218	87%	93%	94%
Evaluation of LVS Function[2]	333	100%	100%	99%
Medicare Spending				
Medicare Spending per Patient (ratio)	-	0.98	1.02	0.98
Pneumonia Care				
Appropriate Initial Antibiotic Given[2]	94	100%	97%	95%
Blood Culture Timing[2]	208	99%	97%	98%
Pregnancy and Delivery Care				
Newborn Deliveries Scheduled Early[2]	39	0%	5%	6%
Preventive Care				
Immunization for Influenza[2]	549	96%	90%	90%
Immunization for Pneumonia[2]	717	94%	91%	92%
Stroke Care				
Anticoagulation Therapy for Atrial Fibrillation	23	96%	96%	95%
Antithrombotic Therapy Timing	137	100%	99%	98%
Assessed for Rehabilitation	169	100%	98%	97%
Discharged on Antithrombotic Therapy	156	99%	99%	99%
Discharged on Statin Medication	115	96%	95%	94%
Thrombolytic Therapy Timing[1]	-	-	71%	66%
Venous Thromboembolism Prophylaxis	162	99%	95%	94%
Written Stroke Educational Materials Given	83	99%	80%	88%
Surgical Care Improvement Project				
Appropriate Beta Blocker Usage[2]	168	98%	98%	98%
Appropriate VTP Within 24 Hours[2]	412	99%	99%	98%
Controlled Postoperative Blood Glucose[2,7]	-	-	96%	97%
Perioperative Temperature Management[2]	473	100%	99%	100%
Prophylactic Antibiotic Selection[2]	284	98%	99%	99%
Prophylactic Antibiotic Selection (Outpatient)	388	98%	97%	98%
Prophylactic Antibiotic Stopped[2]	278	100%	98%	98%
Prophylactic Antibiotic Timing[2]	285	98%	98%	99%
Prophylactic Antibiotic Timing (Outpatient)	393	96%	97%	98%
Urinary Catheter Removal[2]	327	98%	97%	97%
Survey of Patients' Hospital Experiences				
Area Around Room 'Always' Quiet at Night	300+	47%	52%	61%
Doctors 'Always' Communicated Well	300+	80%	80%	82%
Home Recovery Information Given	300+	85%	85%	85%
Hospital Given 9 or 10 on 10 Point Scale	300+	65%	68%	71%
Meds 'Always' Explained Before Given	300+	61%	62%	64%
Nurses 'Always' Communicated Well	300+	77%	78%	79%
Pain 'Always' Well Controlled	300+	69%	71%	71%
Room and Bathroom 'Always' Clean	300+	76%	71%	73%
Timely Help 'Always' Received	300+	63%	64%	68%
Would Definitely Recommend Hospital	300+	68%	71%	71%
Use of Medical Imaging				
Cardiac Imaging Stress Test before Surgery	176	4.0%	4.7%	5.3%
Combination Abdominal CT Scan	1,432	4.9%	5%	10.5%
Combination Brain/Sinus CT Scan	1,235	2.2%	2.3%	2.7%
Combination Chest CT Scan	713	0.6%	0.9%	2.7%
Follow-up Mammogram/Ultrasound	2,611	13.6%	19.5%	8.8%
Lumbar Spine MRI for Low Back Pain	119	32.8%	34.3%	37.2%

Yale-New Haven Hospital

20 York St Phone: 203-688-4242
New Haven, CT 06504 Fax: 203-688-3203
URL: www.ynhh.org
Type: Acute Care Hospitals Emergency Services: Yes
Ownership: Voluntary non-profit - Private Beds: 944

Key Personnel:

CEO .... Marna P Borgstrom
President .... Alan H. Friedman, MD
Radiology.................. Peter M. Glazer, MD
Chief of Medical Staff .... Peter N Herbert, MD
Anesthesiology............... Roberta L. Hines, MD
Pediatrics.................. George Lister, MD
Surgery .... Robert Udelsman, MD

Measure	Cases	This Hosp.	State Avg.	U.S. Avg.
Blood Clot Prevention and Treatment				
Anticoagulation Overlap Therapy[2]	319	94%	91%	93%
ICU Venous Thromboembolism Prophylaxis[2]	28	89%	93%	92%
Incidence of Potentially Preventable VTE[2]	122	4%	6%	10%
UFH with Dosages/Platelet Monitoring[2]	355	94%	95%	97%
Venous Thromboembolism Prophylaxis[2]	348	90%	89%	85%
Warfarin Therapy Discharge Instructions[2]	205	73%	64%	75%
Chest Pain/Possible Heart Attack Care				
Aspirin Given Within 24 Hours of Arrival[5]	-	-	98%	96%
Fibrinolytic Meds Within 30 Min. of Arrival[5]	-	-	33%	58%
Average Time to ECG (minutes)[5]	-	-	7	7
Average Time to Transfer (minutes)[5]	-	-	61	60
Children's Asthma Care				
Received Home Management Plan of Care[2]	316	63%	-	88%
Received Reliever Medication[2]	317	100%	-	100%
Received Systemic Corticosteroids[2]	316	99%	-	100%
Emergency Department				
Admittance Decision Time (minutes)[2]	316	100	147	98
Head CT Results Within 45 Min. of Arrival[5]	-	-	70%	57%
Patients Who Left ER Before Being Seen	>100k	4%	2%	2%
Time from ER Arrival to Admit. (minutes)[2]	331	301	338	274
Time from ER Arrival to Discharge (minutes)	310	190	131	134
Time in ER Before Being Evaluated (minutes)	353	45	28	26
Time to Pain Meds for Fractures (minutes)	224	50	55	57
Heart Attack Care				
Aspirin Given at Discharge[2]	277	99%	99%	99%
Fibrinolytic Meds Within 30 Min. of Arrival[2,7]	-	-	50%	54%
PCI Within 90 Minutes of Arrival[2]	33	97%	96%	96%
Statin Prescribed at Discharge[2]	274	98%	98%	98%
Heart Failure Care				
ACE Inhibitor or ARB for LVSD[2]	77	91%	96%	97%
Discharge Instructions Given[2]	243	92%	93%	94%
Evaluation of LVS Function[2]	341	100%	100%	99%
Medicare Spending				
Medicare Spending per Patient (ratio)	-	1.01	1.02	0.98
Pneumonia Care				
Appropriate Initial Antibiotic Given[2]	73	99%	97%	95%
Blood Culture Timing[2]	203	95%	97%	98%
Pregnancy and Delivery Care				
Newborn Deliveries Scheduled Early[2]	92	10%	5%	6%
Preventive Care				
Immunization for Influenza[2]	539	65%	90%	90%
Immunization for Pneumonia[2]	549	68%	91%	92%
Stroke Care				
Anticoagulation Therapy for Atrial Fibrillation[1,2]	-	-	96%	95%
Antithrombotic Therapy Timing[2]	96	100%	99%	98%
Assessed for Rehabilitation[2]	125	100%	98%	97%
Discharged on Antithrombotic Therapy[2]	100	100%	99%	99%
Discharged on Statin Medication[2]	73	96%	95%	94%
Thrombolytic Therapy Timing[1,2]	-	-	71%	66%
Venous Thromboembolism Prophylaxis[2]	125	97%	95%	94%
Written Stroke Educational Materials Given[2]	62	58%	80%	88%
Surgical Care Improvement Project				
Appropriate Beta Blocker Usage[2]	244	100%	98%	98%
Appropriate VTP Within 24 Hours[2]	398	100%	99%	98%
Controlled Postoperative Blood Glucose[2]	116	94%	96%	97%
Perioperative Temperature Management[2]	567	96%	99%	100%
Prophylactic Antibiotic Selection[2]	393	99%	99%	99%
Prophylactic Antibiotic Selection (Outpatient)	500	85%	97%	98%

NOTE: Hospital profiles are in alphabetical order by state, then city, then hospital within the city; Rankings exclude hospitals with less than 25 cases except for patient surveys which excludes hospitals with less than 100 cases; (a) 100-299 cases; (1) The number of cases/patients is too few to report; (2) Data submitted were based on a sample of cases/patients; (3) Results are based on a shorter time period than required; (4) Data suppressed by CMS for one or more quarters; (5) Results are not available for this reporting period; (6) Fewer than 100 patients completed the HCAHPS survey; (7) No cases met the criteria for this measure; (8) The lower limit of the confidence interval cannot be calculated if the number of observed infections equals zero; (9) No data are available from the state/territory for this reporting period; (10) The scores shown reflect fewer than 50 completed surveys; (11) There were discrepancies in the data collection process; (12) This measure does not apply to this hospital for this reporting period; (13) Results cannot be calculated for this reporting period; (14) The results for this state are combined with nearby states to protect confidentiality; Please refer to the User's Guide for a full explanation of data.

Measure	Cases	This Hosp.	State Avg.	U.S. Avg.
Prophylactic Antibiotic Stopped[2]	365	99%	98%	98%
Prophylactic Antibiotic Timing[2]	395	97%	98%	99%
Prophylactic Antibiotic Timing (Outpatient)	508	95%	97%	98%
Urinary Catheter Removal[2]	392	96%	97%	97%
Survey of Patients' Hospital Experiences				
Area Around Room 'Always' Quiet at Night	300+	51%	52%	61%
Doctors 'Always' Communicated Well	300+	79%	80%	82%
Home Recovery Information Given	300+	85%	85%	85%
Hospital Given 9 or 10 on 10 Point Scale	300+	71%	68%	71%
Meds 'Always' Explained Before Given	300+	60%	62%	64%
Nurses 'Always' Communicated Well	300+	80%	78%	79%
Pain 'Always' Well Controlled	300+	67%	71%	71%
Room and Bathroom 'Always' Clean	300+	68%	71%	73%
Timely Help 'Always' Received	300+	65%	64%	68%
Would Definitely Recommend Hospital	300+	76%	71%	71%
Use of Medical Imaging				
Cardiac Imaging Stress Test before Surgery	1,075	4.6%	4.7%	5.3%
Combination Abdominal CT Scan	3,992	6.3%	5%	10.5%
Combination Brain/Sinus CT Scan	2,620	1.3%	2.3%	2.7%
Combination Chest CT Scan	4,488	0.4%	0.9%	2.7%
Follow-up Mammogram/Ultrasound	5,446	13.5%	19.5%	8.8%
Lumbar Spine MRI for Low Back Pain	285	34.4%	34.3%	37.2%

Lawrence & Memorial Hospital

365 Montauk Ave
New London, CT 06320
Phone: 860-442-0711
Fax: 860-444-3717
E-mail: kanthony@lmhosp.org
URL: www.lmhospital.org
Type: Acute Care Hospitals
Emergency Services: Yes
Ownership: Voluntary non-profit - Private
Beds: 350

Key Personnel:
Operating Room. . . . . Joe Aldred
Radiology. . . . . Donna Blakley
Ambulatory Care . . . . Anthony Coppola, MD
CEO/President. . . . . Bruce D Cummings
Pediatric In-Patient Care . . . . Bernard N Giserman, MD
Emergency Room . . . . Ronnie Hanrahan, RN
Cardiac Laboratory. . . . . Gerry Mulholland
Quality Assurance . . . . Sherry Strammiello

Measure	Cases	This Hosp.	State Avg.	U.S. Avg.
Blood Clot Prevention and Treatment				
Anticoagulation Overlap Therapy[2]	70	99%	91%	93%
ICU Venous Thromboembolism Prophylaxis[2]	84	83%	93%	92%
Incidence of Potentially Preventable VTE[2]	14	7%	6%	10%
UFH with Dosages/Platelet Monitoring[2]	75	100%	95%	97%
Venous Thromboembolism Prophylaxis[2]	349	74%	89%	85%
Warfarin Therapy Discharge Instructions[2]	44	64%	64%	75%
Chest Pain/Possible Heart Attack Care				
Aspirin Given Within 24 Hours of Arrival	13	92%	98%	96%
Fibrinolytic Meds Within 30 Min. of Arrival[3,7]	-	-	33%	58%
Average Time to ECG (minutes)	13	5	7	7
Average Time to Transfer (minutes)[3,7]	-	-	61	60
Children's Asthma Care				
Received Home Management Plan of Care	-	-	-	88%
Received Reliever Medication	-	-	-	100%
Received Systemic Corticosteroids	-	-	-	100%
Emergency Department				
Admittance Decision Time (minutes)[2]	589	130	147	98
Head CT Results Within 45 Min. of Arrival	15	60%	70%	57%
Patients Who Left ER Before Being Seen	78,594	1%	2%	2%
Time from ER Arrival to Admit. (minutes)[2]	663	405	338	274
Time from ER Arrival to Discharge (minutes)	379	119	131	134
Time in ER Before Being Evaluated (minutes)	98	44	28	26
Time to Pain Meds for Fractures (minutes)	172	51	55	57
Heart Attack Care				
Aspirin Given at Discharge	156	99%	99%	99%
Fibrinolytic Meds Within 30 Min. of Arrival[7]	-	-	50%	54%
PCI Within 90 Minutes of Arrival	60	90%	96%	96%
Statin Prescribed at Discharge	151	97%	98%	98%
Heart Failure Care				
ACE Inhibitor or ARB for LVSD[2]	53	89%	96%	97%
Discharge Instructions Given[2]	205	86%	93%	94%
Evaluation of LVS Function[2]	308	100%	100%	99%
Medicare Spending				
Medicare Spending per Patient (ratio)	-	1.02	1.02	0.98
Pneumonia Care				
Appropriate Initial Antibiotic Given[2]	80	88%	97%	95%
Blood Culture Timing[2]	125	94%	97%	98%
Pregnancy and Delivery Care				
Newborn Deliveries Scheduled Early[2]	28	4%	5%	6%
Preventive Care				
Immunization for Influenza[2]	523	90%	90%	90%
Immunization for Pneumonia[2]	675	89%	91%	92%
Stroke Care				
Anticoagulation Therapy for Atrial Fibrillation	21	100%	96%	95%
Antithrombotic Therapy Timing	137	99%	99%	98%
Assessed for Rehabilitation	150	97%	98%	97%
Discharged on Antithrombotic Therapy	135	99%	99%	99%
Discharged on Statin Medication	105	94%	95%	94%
Thrombolytic Therapy Timing	16	88%	71%	66%
Venous Thromboembolism Prophylaxis	161	93%	95%	94%
Written Stroke Educational Materials Given	67	93%	80%	88%
Surgical Care Improvement Project				
Appropriate Beta Blocker Usage[2]	133	99%	98%	98%
Appropriate VTP Within 24 Hours[2]	363	98%	99%	98%
Controlled Postoperative Blood Glucose[2,7]	-	-	96%	97%
Perioperative Temperature Management[2]	450	98%	99%	100%
Prophylactic Antibiotic Selection[2]	294	97%	99%	99%
Prophylactic Antibiotic Selection (Outpatient)	165	98%	97%	98%
Prophylactic Antibiotic Stopped[2]	291	99%	98%	98%
Prophylactic Antibiotic Timing[2]	294	98%	98%	99%
Prophylactic Antibiotic Timing (Outpatient)	167	96%	97%	98%
Urinary Catheter Removal[2]	255	96%	97%	97%
Survey of Patients' Hospital Experiences				
Area Around Room 'Always' Quiet at Night	300+	51%	52%	61%
Doctors 'Always' Communicated Well	300+	79%	80%	82%
Home Recovery Information Given	300+	81%	85%	85%
Hospital Given 9 or 10 on 10 Point Scale	300+	61%	68%	71%
Meds 'Always' Explained Before Given	300+	57%	62%	64%
Nurses 'Always' Communicated Well	300+	78%	78%	79%
Pain 'Always' Well Controlled	300+	68%	71%	71%
Room and Bathroom 'Always' Clean	300+	69%	71%	73%
Timely Help 'Always' Received	300+	62%	64%	68%
Would Definitely Recommend Hospital	300+	67%	71%	71%
Use of Medical Imaging				
Cardiac Imaging Stress Test before Surgery	724	4.4%	4.7%	5.3%
Combination Abdominal CT Scan	1,357	4.1%	5%	10.5%
Combination Brain/Sinus CT Scan	1,077	2.1%	2.3%	2.7%
Combination Chest CT Scan	1,091	0.0%	0.9%	2.7%
Follow-up Mammogram/Ultrasound	3,186	8.1%	19.5%	8.8%
Lumbar Spine MRI for Low Back Pain	270	33.3%	34.3%	37.2%

New Milford Hospital

21 Elm St
New Milford, CT 06776
Phone: 860-355-2611
Fax: 860-210-7422
URL: www.newmilfordhospital.org
Type: Acute Care Hospitals
Emergency Services: Yes
Ownership: Voluntary non-profit - Private
Beds: 85

Key Personnel:
Operating Room. . . . . Courtney E Chambers, RN
Radiology. . . . . Andrea Q Crowley, MD
Pediatric Ambulatory Care . . . . . . Evan Hack, MD
Pediatric In-Patient Care . . . . Evan Hack, MD
Chief of Medical Staff . . . . Thomas Koobatian, MD
CEO/President. . . . . Richard E Pugh
Quality Assurance . . . . Linda Vryhof
Infection Control. . . . . Brenda Warren, RN

Measure	Cases	This Hosp.	State Avg.	U.S. Avg.
Blood Clot Prevention and Treatment				
Anticoagulation Overlap Therapy[2]	11	100%	91%	93%
ICU Venous Thromboembolism Prophylaxis[2]	24	96%	93%	92%
Incidence of Potentially Preventable VTE[1,2]	-	-	6%	10%
UFH with Dosages/Platelet Monitoring[1,2]	-	-	95%	97%
Venous Thromboembolism Prophylaxis[2]	175	97%	89%	85%
Warfarin Therapy Discharge Instructions[1,2]	-	-	64%	75%
Chest Pain/Possible Heart Attack Care				
Aspirin Given Within 24 Hours of Arrival	44	98%	98%	96%
Fibrinolytic Meds Within 30 Min. of Arrival[7]	-	-	33%	58%
Average Time to ECG (minutes)	43	7	7	7
Average Time to Transfer (minutes)	16	48	61	60
Children's Asthma Care				
Received Home Management Plan of Care	-	-	-	88%
Received Reliever Medication	-	-	-	100%
Received Systemic Corticosteroids	-	-	-	100%
Emergency Department				
Admittance Decision Time (minutes)[2]	428	57	147	98
Head CT Results Within 45 Min. of Arrival[1]	-	-	70%	57%
Patients Who Left ER Before Being Seen	18,213	0%	2%	2%
Time from ER Arrival to Admit. (minutes)[2]	427	235	338	274
Time from ER Arrival to Discharge (minutes)	351	79	131	134
Time in ER Before Being Evaluated (minutes)	355	20	28	26
Time to Pain Meds for Fractures (minutes)	93	47	55	57
Heart Attack Care				
Aspirin Given at Discharge[1]	-	-	99%	99%
Fibrinolytic Meds Within 30 Min. of Arrival[7]	-	-	50%	54%
PCI Within 90 Minutes of Arrival[7]	-	-	96%	96%
Statin Prescribed at Discharge[1]	-	-	98%	98%
Heart Failure Care				
ACE Inhibitor or ARB for LVSD	11	100%	96%	97%
Discharge Instructions Given	32	88%	93%	94%
Evaluation of LVS Function	51	100%	100%	99%
Medicare Spending				
Medicare Spending per Patient (ratio)	-	1.08	1.02	0.98
Pneumonia Care				
Appropriate Initial Antibiotic Given	63	98%	97%	95%
Blood Culture Timing	44	93%	97%	98%
Pregnancy and Delivery Care				
Newborn Deliveries Scheduled Early[1]	-	-	5%	6%
Preventive Care				
Immunization for Influenza[2]	311	94%	90%	90%
Immunization for Pneumonia[2]	427	96%	91%	92%
Stroke Care				
Anticoagulation Therapy for Atrial Fibrillation[1]	-	-	96%	95%
Antithrombotic Therapy Timing	20	100%	99%	98%
Assessed for Rehabilitation	20	100%	98%	97%
Discharged on Antithrombotic Therapy	18	100%	99%	99%
Discharged on Statin Medication	15	73%	95%	94%
Thrombolytic Therapy Timing[1]	-	-	71%	66%
Venous Thromboembolism Prophylaxis	21	90%	95%	94%
Written Stroke Educational Materials Given[1]	-	-	80%	88%
Surgical Care Improvement Project				
Appropriate Beta Blocker Usage	58	98%	98%	98%
Appropriate VTP Within 24 Hours	174	98%	99%	98%
Controlled Postoperative Blood Glucose[7]	-	-	96%	97%
Perioperative Temperature Management	192	100%	99%	100%
Prophylactic Antibiotic Selection	153	99%	99%	99%
Prophylactic Antibiotic Selection (Outpatient)	72	94%	97%	98%
Prophylactic Antibiotic Stopped	152	100%	98%	98%
Prophylactic Antibiotic Timing	153	99%	98%	99%
Prophylactic Antibiotic Timing (Outpatient)	72	100%	97%	98%
Urinary Catheter Removal	30	73%	97%	97%
Survey of Patients' Hospital Experiences				
Area Around Room 'Always' Quiet at Night	300+	59%	52%	61%
Doctors 'Always' Communicated Well	300+	82%	80%	82%
Home Recovery Information Given	300+	87%	85%	85%
Hospital Given 9 or 10 on 10 Point Scale	300+	69%	68%	71%
Meds 'Always' Explained Before Given	300+	60%	62%	64%
Nurses 'Always' Communicated Well	300+	77%	78%	79%
Pain 'Always' Well Controlled	300+	68%	71%	71%
Room and Bathroom 'Always' Clean	300+	71%	71%	73%
Timely Help 'Always' Received	300+	64%	64%	68%
Would Definitely Recommend Hospital	300+	74%	71%	71%
Use of Medical Imaging				
Cardiac Imaging Stress Test before Surgery	151	2.0%	4.7%	5.3%
Combination Abdominal CT Scan	433	7.9%	5%	10.5%
Combination Brain/Sinus CT Scan[1]	-	-	2.3%	2.7%
Combination Chest CT Scan	319	0.9%	0.9%	2.7%
Follow-up Mammogram/Ultrasound	718	26.2%	19.5%	8.8%
Lumbar Spine MRI for Low Back Pain	93	32.3%	34.3%	37.2%

NOTE: Hospital profiles are in alphabetical order by state, then city, then hospital within the city; Rankings exclude hospitals with less than 25 cases except for patient surveys which excludes hospitals with less than 100 cases; (a) 100-299 cases; (1) The number of cases/patients is too few to report; (2) Data submitted were based on a sample of cases/patients; (3) Results are based on a shorter time period than required; (4) Data suppressed by CMS for one or more quarters; (5) Results are not available for this reporting period; (6) Fewer than 100 patients completed the HCAHPS survey; (7) No cases met the criteria for this measure; (8) The lower limit of the confidence interval cannot be calculated if the number of observed infections equals zero; (9) No data are available from the state/territory for this reporting period; (10) The scores shown reflect fewer than 50 completed surveys; (11) There were discrepancies in the data collection process; (12) This measure does not apply to this hospital for this reporting period; (13) Results cannot be calculated for this reporting period; (14) The results for this state are combined with nearby states to protect confidentiality; Please refer to the User's Guide for a full explanation of data.

Norwalk Hospital Association

24 Stevens Street Phone: 203-852-2000
Norwalk, CT 06856 Fax: 203-855-3987
E-mail: hr@norwalkhealth.org
URL: www.norwalkhosp.org
Type: Acute Care Hospitals Emergency Services: Yes
Ownership: Voluntary non-profit - Private Beds: 328

Key Personnel:
Chief of Medical Staff. . . . . Thomas Ayoub, MD
Coronary Care . . . . Debbie Bailey
Quality Assurance . . . . Claire Davis, RN
CEO/President. . . . . Daniel DeBarba Jr.
Infection Control. . . . . Erin Fitzgerald
Radiology. . . . . Alan Richman, MD
Pediatric Ambulatory Care . . . . . . Vicki Smetak, MD
Pediatric In-Patient Care . . . . Vicki Smetak, MD

Measure	Cases	This Hosp.	State Avg.	U.S. Avg.
Blood Clot Prevention and Treatment				
Anticoagulation Overlap Therapy[2]	73	99%	91%	93%
ICU Venous Thromboembolism Prophylaxis[2]	23	100%	93%	92%
Incidence of Potentially Preventable VTE[2]	17	0%	6%	10%
UFH with Dosages/Platelet Monitoring[2]	82	98%	95%	97%
Venous Thromboembolism Prophylaxis[2]	353	95%	89%	85%
Warfarin Therapy Discharge Instructions[2]	47	66%	64%	75%
Chest Pain/Possible Heart Attack Care				
Aspirin Given Within 24 Hours of Arrival	16	94%	98%	96%
Fibrinolytic Meds Within 30 Min. of Arrival[3,7]	-	-	33%	58%
Average Time to ECG (minutes)	16	0	7	7
Average Time to Transfer (minutes)[3,7]	-	-	61	60
Children's Asthma Care				
Received Home Management Plan of Care	-	-	-	88%
Received Reliever Medication	-	-	-	100%
Received Systemic Corticosteroids	-	-	-	100%
Emergency Department				
Admittance Decision Time (minutes)[2]	698	104	147	98
Head CT Results Within 45 Min. of Arrival[1]	-	-	70%	57%
Patients Who Left ER Before Being Seen	50,170	1%	2%	2%
Time from ER Arrival to Admit. (minutes)[2]	716	289	338	274
Time from ER Arrival to Discharge (minutes)	509	156	131	134
Time in ER Before Being Evaluated (minutes)	546	32	28	26
Time to Pain Meds for Fractures (minutes)	178	54	55	57
Heart Attack Care				
Aspirin Given at Discharge	76	99%	99%	99%
Fibrinolytic Meds Within 30 Min. of Arrival[7]	-	-	50%	54%
PCI Within 90 Minutes of Arrival	35	100%	96%	96%
Statin Prescribed at Discharge	78	100%	98%	98%
Heart Failure Care				
ACE Inhibitor or ARB for LVSD[2]	51	94%	96%	97%
Discharge Instructions Given[2]	188	91%	93%	94%
Evaluation of LVS Function[2]	256	100%	100%	99%
Medicare Spending				
Medicare Spending per Patient (ratio)	-	0.99	1.02	0.98
Pneumonia Care				
Appropriate Initial Antibiotic Given[2]	90	100%	97%	95%
Blood Culture Timing[2]	170	100%	97%	98%
Pregnancy and Delivery Care				
Newborn Deliveries Scheduled Early[2]	27	0%	5%	6%
Preventive Care				
Immunization for Influenza[2]	527	97%	90%	90%
Immunization for Pneumonia[2]	632	96%	91%	92%
Stroke Care				
Anticoagulation Therapy for Atrial Fibrillation	22	100%	96%	95%
Antithrombotic Therapy Timing	113	100%	99%	98%
Assessed for Rehabilitation	132	97%	98%	97%
Discharged on Antithrombotic Therapy	112	100%	99%	99%
Discharged on Statin Medication	88	97%	95%	94%
Thrombolytic Therapy Timing[1]	-	-	71%	66%
Venous Thromboembolism Prophylaxis	136	96%	95%	94%
Written Stroke Educational Materials Given	60	88%	80%	88%
Surgical Care Improvement Project				
Appropriate Beta Blocker Usage[2]	105	98%	98%	98%
Appropriate VTP Within 24 Hours[2]	365	98%	99%	98%
Controlled Postoperative Blood Glucose[2,7]	-	-	96%	97%
Perioperative Temperature Management[2]	423	100%	99%	100%
Prophylactic Antibiotic Selection[2]	255	99%	99%	99%
Prophylactic Antibiotic Selection (Outpatient)	333	97%	97%	98%
Prophylactic Antibiotic Stopped[2]	246	99%	98%	98%
Prophylactic Antibiotic Timing[2]	255	98%	98%	99%
Prophylactic Antibiotic Timing (Outpatient)	334	99%	97%	98%
Urinary Catheter Removal[2]	97	96%	97%	97%
Survey of Patients' Hospital Experiences				
Area Around Room 'Always' Quiet at Night	300+	53%	52%	61%
Doctors 'Always' Communicated Well	300+	81%	80%	82%
Home Recovery Information Given	300+	85%	85%	85%
Hospital Given 9 or 10 on 10 Point Scale	300+	70%	68%	71%
Meds 'Always' Explained Before Given	300+	60%	62%	64%
Nurses 'Always' Communicated Well	300+	77%	78%	79%
Pain 'Always' Well Controlled	300+	71%	71%	71%
Room and Bathroom 'Always' Clean	300+	71%	71%	73%
Timely Help 'Always' Received	300+	63%	64%	68%
Would Definitely Recommend Hospital	300+	76%	71%	71%
Use of Medical Imaging				
Cardiac Imaging Stress Test before Surgery	154	3.9%	4.7%	5.3%
Combination Abdominal CT Scan	1,484	9.4%	5%	10.5%
Combination Brain/Sinus CT Scan	963	2.2%	2.3%	2.7%
Combination Chest CT Scan	1,095	1.1%	0.9%	2.7%
Follow-up Mammogram/Ultrasound	3,436	35.8%	19.5%	8.8%
Lumbar Spine MRI for Low Back Pain	231	32.0%	34.3%	37.2%

William W Backus Hospital

326 Washington St Phone: 860-889-8331
Norwich, CT 06360 Fax: 860-823-6329
E-mail: smawhiney@wwbh.org
URL: www.backushospital.org
Type: Acute Care Hospitals Emergency Services: Yes
Ownership: Voluntary non-profit - Other Beds: 20

Key Personnel:
Emergency Room . . . . Susan Davis, RN
Quality Assurance . . . . Joseph Hughes
Radiology. . . . . Herb Lustberg, MD
Pediatric Ambulatory Care . . . . . . Ravi Prakash, MD
Chief of Medical Staff. . . . . Peter Shea, MD
CEO/President. . . . . Dave Whitehead

Measure	Cases	This Hosp.	State Avg.	U.S. Avg.
Blood Clot Prevention and Treatment				
Anticoagulation Overlap Therapy[2]	100	96%	91%	93%
ICU Venous Thromboembolism Prophylaxis[2]	31	100%	93%	92%
Incidence of Potentially Preventable VTE[2]	19	0%	6%	10%
UFH with Dosages/Platelet Monitoring[2]	100	100%	95%	97%
Venous Thromboembolism Prophylaxis[2]	369	98%	89%	85%
Warfarin Therapy Discharge Instructions[2]	77	84%	64%	75%
Chest Pain/Possible Heart Attack Care				
Aspirin Given Within 24 Hours of Arrival	158	98%	98%	96%
Fibrinolytic Meds Within 30 Min. of Arrival[7]	-	-	33%	58%
Average Time to ECG (minutes)	166	5	7	7
Average Time to Transfer (minutes)	39	65	61	60
Children's Asthma Care				
Received Home Management Plan of Care	-	-	-	88%
Received Reliever Medication	-	-	-	100%
Received Systemic Corticosteroids	-	-	-	100%
Emergency Department				
Admittance Decision Time (minutes)[2]	768	220	147	98
Head CT Results Within 45 Min. of Arrival	13	92%	70%	57%
Patients Who Left ER Before Being Seen	71,056	1%	2%	2%
Time from ER Arrival to Admit. (minutes)[2]	773	309	338	274
Time from ER Arrival to Discharge (minutes)	383	114	131	134
Time in ER Before Being Evaluated (minutes)	420	23	28	26
Time to Pain Meds for Fractures (minutes)	176	46	55	57
Heart Attack Care				
Aspirin Given at Discharge	36	97%	99%	99%
Fibrinolytic Meds Within 30 Min. of Arrival[7]	-	-	50%	54%
PCI Within 90 Minutes of Arrival[7]	-	-	96%	96%
Statin Prescribed at Discharge	36	94%	98%	98%
Heart Failure Care				
ACE Inhibitor or ARB for LVSD	34	100%	96%	97%
Discharge Instructions Given	161	98%	93%	94%
Evaluation of LVS Function	234	100%	100%	99%
Medicare Spending				
Medicare Spending per Patient (ratio)	-	1.04	1.02	0.98
Pneumonia Care				
Appropriate Initial Antibiotic Given[2]	100	99%	97%	95%
Blood Culture Timing[2]	73	99%	97%	98%
Pregnancy and Delivery Care				
Newborn Deliveries Scheduled Early[2]	31	0%	5%	6%
Preventive Care				
Immunization for Influenza[2]	562	88%	90%	90%
Immunization for Pneumonia[2]	736	94%	91%	92%
Stroke Care				
Anticoagulation Therapy for Atrial Fibrillation	18	94%	96%	95%
Antithrombotic Therapy Timing	116	98%	99%	98%
Assessed for Rehabilitation	122	100%	98%	97%
Discharged on Antithrombotic Therapy	119	100%	99%	99%
Discharged on Statin Medication	87	95%	95%	94%
Thrombolytic Therapy Timing[1]	-	-	71%	66%
Venous Thromboembolism Prophylaxis	123	98%	95%	94%
Written Stroke Educational Materials Given	60	93%	80%	88%
Surgical Care Improvement Project				
Appropriate Beta Blocker Usage[2]	142	99%	98%	98%
Appropriate VTP Within 24 Hours[2]	413	98%	99%	98%
Controlled Postoperative Blood Glucose[2,7]	-	-	96%	97%
Perioperative Temperature Management[2]	480	100%	99%	100%
Prophylactic Antibiotic Selection[2]	305	100%	99%	99%
Prophylactic Antibiotic Selection (Outpatient)	202	100%	97%	98%
Prophylactic Antibiotic Stopped[2]	302	100%	98%	98%
Prophylactic Antibiotic Timing[2]	305	100%	98%	99%
Prophylactic Antibiotic Timing (Outpatient)	202	99%	97%	98%
Urinary Catheter Removal[2]	282	98%	97%	97%
Survey of Patients' Hospital Experiences				
Area Around Room 'Always' Quiet at Night	300+	46%	52%	61%
Doctors 'Always' Communicated Well	300+	79%	80%	82%
Home Recovery Information Given	300+	81%	85%	85%
Hospital Given 9 or 10 on 10 Point Scale	300+	64%	68%	71%
Meds 'Always' Explained Before Given	300+	62%	62%	64%
Nurses 'Always' Communicated Well	300+	80%	78%	79%
Pain 'Always' Well Controlled	300+	72%	71%	71%
Room and Bathroom 'Always' Clean	300+	71%	71%	73%
Timely Help 'Always' Received	300+	66%	64%	68%
Would Definitely Recommend Hospital	300+	69%	71%	71%
Use of Medical Imaging				
Cardiac Imaging Stress Test before Surgery	522	4.2%	4.7%	5.3%
Combination Abdominal CT Scan	1,397	1.1%	5%	10.5%
Combination Brain/Sinus CT Scan	999	2.2%	2.3%	2.7%
Combination Chest CT Scan	1,335	0.0%	0.9%	2.7%
Follow-up Mammogram/Ultrasound	2,355	10.0%	19.5%	8.8%
Lumbar Spine MRI for Low Back Pain	294	36.4%	34.3%	37.2%

Day Kimball Hospital

320 Pomfret Street Phone: 860-928-6541
Putnam, CT 06260 Fax: 860-963-6375
E-mail: ilisee@daykimball.org
URL: www.daykimball.org
Type: Acute Care Hospitals Emergency Services: Yes
Ownership: Voluntary non-profit - Private Beds: 103

Key Personnel:
Emergency Room . . . . Joel S Bogner
Patient Relations . . . . Sandra Bucci
Chief of Medical Staff. . . . . John Day
Intensive Care Unit. . . . . John Modica, MD
Quality Assurance . . . . Elaine Noren
Anesthesiology. . . . . Steven Schimmel, MD
President/CEO. . . . . Robert Smanik, FACHE
Infection Control. . . . . Douglas Waite, MD

Measure	Cases	This Hosp.	State Avg.	U.S. Avg.
Blood Clot Prevention and Treatment				
Anticoagulation Overlap Therapy[2]	21	100%	91%	93%
ICU Venous Thromboembolism Prophylaxis[2]	37	95%	93%	92%
Incidence of Potentially Preventable VTE[2,7]	-	-	6%	10%
UFH with Dosages/Platelet Monitoring[1,2]	-	-	95%	97%
Venous Thromboembolism Prophylaxis[2]	267	97%	89%	85%
Warfarin Therapy Discharge Instructions[2]	16	100%	64%	75%
Chest Pain/Possible Heart Attack Care				
Aspirin Given Within 24 Hours of Arrival	100	96%	98%	96%

NOTE: Hospital profiles are in alphabetical order by state, then city, then hospital within the city; Rankings exclude hospitals with less than 25 cases except for patient surveys which excludes hospitals with less than 100 cases; (a) 100-299 cases; (1) The number of cases/patients is too few to report; (2) Data submitted were based on a sample of cases/patients; (3) Results are based on a shorter time period than required; (4) Data suppressed by CMS for one or more quarters; (5) Results are not available for this reporting period; (6) Fewer than 100 patients completed the HCAHPS survey; (7) No cases met the criteria for this measure; (8) The lower limit of the confidence interval cannot be calculated if the number of observed infections equals zero; (9) No data are available from the state/territory for this reporting period; (10) The scores shown reflect fewer than 50 completed surveys; (11) There were discrepancies in the data collection process; (12) This measure does not apply to this hospital for this reporting period; (13) Results cannot be calculated for this reporting period; (14) The results for this state are combined with nearby states to protect confidentiality; Please refer to the User's Guide for a full explanation of data.

Measure	Cases	This Hosp.	State Avg.	U.S. Avg.
Fibrinolytic Meds Within 30 Min. of Arrival[7]	-	-	33%	58%
Average Time to ECG (minutes)	104	6	7	7
Average Time to Transfer (minutes)[1]	-	-	61	60
Children's Asthma Care				
Received Home Management Plan of Care	-	-	-	88%
Received Reliever Medication	-	-	-	100%
Received Systemic Corticosteroids	-	-	-	100%
Emergency Department				
Admittance Decision Time (minutes)[2]	459	147	147	98
Head CT Results Within 45 Min. of Arrival	22	68%	70%	57%
Patients Who Left ER Before Being Seen	27,397	1%	2%	2%
Time from ER Arrival to Admit. (minutes)[2]	465	338	338	274
Time from ER Arrival to Discharge (minutes)	392	121	131	134
Time in ER Before Being Evaluated (minutes)	444	18	28	26
Time to Pain Meds for Fractures (minutes)	69	45	55	57
Heart Attack Care				
Aspirin Given at Discharge	36	100%	99%	99%
Fibrinolytic Meds Within 30 Min. of Arrival[7]	-	-	50%	54%
PCI Within 90 Minutes of Arrival[7]	-	-	96%	96%
Statin Prescribed at Discharge	31	90%	98%	98%
Heart Failure Care				
ACE Inhibitor or ARB for LVSD	24	100%	96%	97%
Discharge Instructions Given	55	100%	93%	94%
Evaluation of LVS Function	89	100%	100%	99%
Medicare Spending				
Medicare Spending per Patient (ratio)	-	1.04	1.02	0.98
Pneumonia Care				
Appropriate Initial Antibiotic Given	90	99%	97%	95%
Blood Culture Timing	157	99%	97%	98%
Pregnancy and Delivery Care				
Newborn Deliveries Scheduled Early[2]	25	0%	5%	6%
Preventive Care				
Immunization for Influenza[2]	414	85%	90%	90%
Immunization for Pneumonia[2]	469	93%	91%	92%
Stroke Care				
Anticoagulation Therapy for Atrial Fibrillation[1]	-	-	96%	95%
Antithrombotic Therapy Timing	32	100%	99%	98%
Assessed for Rehabilitation	30	100%	98%	97%
Discharged on Antithrombotic Therapy	29	100%	99%	99%
Discharged on Statin Medication	25	92%	95%	94%
Thrombolytic Therapy Timing[1]	-	-	71%	66%
Venous Thromboembolism Prophylaxis	34	91%	95%	94%
Written Stroke Educational Materials Given	16	81%	80%	88%
Surgical Care Improvement Project				
Appropriate Beta Blocker Usage	98	100%	98%	98%
Appropriate VTP Within 24 Hours	302	99%	99%	98%
Controlled Postoperative Blood Glucose[7]	-	-	96%	97%
Perioperative Temperature Management	334	100%	99%	100%
Prophylactic Antibiotic Selection	243	100%	99%	99%
Prophylactic Antibiotic Selection (Outpatient)	42	100%	97%	98%
Prophylactic Antibiotic Stopped	234	96%	98%	98%
Prophylactic Antibiotic Timing	243	100%	98%	99%
Prophylactic Antibiotic Timing (Outpatient)	42	100%	97%	98%
Urinary Catheter Removal	53	96%	97%	97%
Survey of Patients' Hospital Experiences				
Area Around Room 'Always' Quiet at Night	300+	49%	52%	61%
Doctors 'Always' Communicated Well	300+	82%	80%	82%
Home Recovery Information Given	300+	88%	85%	85%
Hospital Given 9 or 10 on 10 Point Scale	300+	71%	68%	71%
Meds 'Always' Explained Before Given	300+	65%	62%	64%
Nurses 'Always' Communicated Well	300+	82%	78%	79%
Pain 'Always' Well Controlled	300+	75%	71%	71%
Room and Bathroom 'Always' Clean	300+	76%	71%	73%
Timely Help 'Always' Received	300+	70%	64%	68%
Would Definitely Recommend Hospital	300+	69%	71%	71%
Use of Medical Imaging				
Cardiac Imaging Stress Test before Surgery	443	3.6%	4.7%	5.3%
Combination Abdominal CT Scan	494	3.6%	5%	10.5%
Combination Brain/Sinus CT Scan	479	1.9%	2.3%	2.7%
Combination Chest CT Scan	361	0.3%	0.9%	2.7%
Follow-up Mammogram/Ultrasound	1,578	9.9%	19.5%	8.8%
Lumbar Spine MRI for Low Back Pain	72	45.8%	34.3%	37.2%

Rockville General Hospital

31 Union St
Rockville, CT 06066
E-mail: info@echn.org
URL: www.echn.org
Phone: 860-872-5160
Fax: 860-875-5336
Type: Acute Care Hospitals
Ownership: Voluntary non-profit - Other
Emergency Services: Yes
Beds: 102

Key Personnel:
Quality Assurance . . . . Leona Crosskey
President/CEO. . . . . Peter J Karl
Operating Room. . . . . Judy Montgomery
Chief of Medical Staff . . . . Deborah A Parker, RN
Chief of Medical Staff . . . . Joel J Reich
Coronary Care . . . . Richard Slutsky

Measure	Cases	This Hosp.	State Avg.	U.S. Avg.
Blood Clot Prevention and Treatment				
Anticoagulation Overlap Therapy[2]	47	100%	91%	93%
ICU Venous Thromboembolism Prophylaxis[2]	86	91%	93%	92%
Incidence of Potentially Preventable VTE[1,2]	-	-	6%	10%
UFH with Dosages/Platelet Monitoring[2]	42	100%	95%	97%
Venous Thromboembolism Prophylaxis[2]	248	89%	89%	85%
Warfarin Therapy Discharge Instructions[2]	29	52%	64%	75%
Chest Pain/Possible Heart Attack Care				
Aspirin Given Within 24 Hours of Arrival	49	98%	98%	96%
Fibrinolytic Meds Within 30 Min. of Arrival[1]	-	-	33%	58%
Average Time to ECG (minutes)	52	5	7	7
Average Time to Transfer (minutes)[1]	-	-	61	60
Children's Asthma Care				
Received Home Management Plan of Care	-	-	-	88%
Received Reliever Medication	-	-	-	100%
Received Systemic Corticosteroids	-	-	-	100%
Emergency Department				
Admittance Decision Time (minutes)[2]	518	192	147	98
Head CT Results Within 45 Min. of Arrival[1]	-	-	70%	57%
Patients Who Left ER Before Being Seen	25,311	1%	2%	2%
Time from ER Arrival to Admit. (minutes)[2]	518	406	338	274
Time from ER Arrival to Discharge (minutes)	343	135	131	134
Time in ER Before Being Evaluated (minutes)	244	59	28	26
Time to Pain Meds for Fractures (minutes)	68	43	55	57
Heart Attack Care				
Aspirin Given at Discharge[1]	-	-	99%	99%
Fibrinolytic Meds Within 30 Min. of Arrival[7]	-	-	50%	54%
PCI Within 90 Minutes of Arrival[7]	-	-	96%	96%
Statin Prescribed at Discharge[1]	-	-	98%	98%
Heart Failure Care				
ACE Inhibitor or ARB for LVSD	26	96%	96%	97%
Discharge Instructions Given	79	90%	93%	94%
Evaluation of LVS Function	113	97%	100%	99%
Medicare Spending				
Medicare Spending per Patient (ratio)	-	1.07	1.02	0.98
Pneumonia Care				
Appropriate Initial Antibiotic Given[2]	102	97%	97%	95%
Blood Culture Timing[2]	181	99%	97%	98%
Pregnancy and Delivery Care				
Newborn Deliveries Scheduled Early[7]	-	-	5%	6%
Preventive Care				
Immunization for Influenza[2]	290	92%	90%	90%
Immunization for Pneumonia[2]	448	91%	91%	92%
Stroke Care				
Anticoagulation Therapy for Atrial Fibrillation[1]	-	-	96%	95%
Antithrombotic Therapy Timing	33	100%	99%	98%
Assessed for Rehabilitation	32	94%	98%	97%
Discharged on Antithrombotic Therapy	32	100%	99%	99%
Discharged on Statin Medication	27	93%	95%	94%
Thrombolytic Therapy Timing[7]	-	-	71%	66%
Venous Thromboembolism Prophylaxis	30	87%	95%	94%
Written Stroke Educational Materials Given	20	55%	80%	88%
Surgical Care Improvement Project				
Appropriate Beta Blocker Usage	18	94%	98%	98%
Appropriate VTP Within 24 Hours	48	94%	99%	98%
Controlled Postoperative Blood Glucose[7]	-	-	96%	97%
Perioperative Temperature Management	67	100%	99%	100%
Prophylactic Antibiotic Selection	26	100%	99%	99%
Prophylactic Antibiotic Selection (Outpatient)	80	100%	97%	98%
Prophylactic Antibiotic Stopped	23	100%	98%	98%
Prophylactic Antibiotic Timing	26	100%	98%	99%
Prophylactic Antibiotic Timing (Outpatient)	80	100%	97%	98%
Urinary Catheter Removal	36	97%	97%	97%
Survey of Patients' Hospital Experiences				
Area Around Room 'Always' Quiet at Night	300+	48%	52%	61%
Doctors 'Always' Communicated Well	300+	73%	80%	82%
Home Recovery Information Given	300+	86%	85%	85%
Hospital Given 9 or 10 on 10 Point Scale	300+	58%	68%	71%
Meds 'Always' Explained Before Given	300+	63%	62%	64%
Nurses 'Always' Communicated Well	300+	75%	78%	79%
Pain 'Always' Well Controlled	300+	67%	71%	71%
Room and Bathroom 'Always' Clean	300+	67%	71%	73%
Timely Help 'Always' Received	300+	61%	64%	68%
Would Definitely Recommend Hospital	300+	63%	71%	71%
Use of Medical Imaging				
Cardiac Imaging Stress Test before Surgery	124	3.2%	4.7%	5.3%
Combination Abdominal CT Scan	565	3.9%	5%	10.5%
Combination Brain/Sinus CT Scan[1]	-	-	2.3%	2.7%
Combination Chest CT Scan	516	0.2%	0.9%	2.7%
Follow-up Mammogram/Ultrasound	1,815	8.8%	19.5%	8.8%
Lumbar Spine MRI for Low Back Pain	89	36.0%	34.3%	37.2%

Sharon Hospital

50 Hospital Hill Road, PO Box 789
Sharon, CT 06069
E-mail: info@sharonhospital.com
URL: www.sharonhospital.com
Phone: 860-364-4228
Fax: 860-364-4470
Type: Acute Care Hospitals
Ownership: Proprietary
Emergency Services: Yes
Beds: 25

Key Personnel:
Radiology. . . . . Joseph C Antonio
Operating Room. . . . . Patricia Carson
Pediatric In-Patient Care . . . . Virginia L Gray-Carke
Pediatric Ambulatory Care . . . . . . Susan Jessen
Infection Control. . . . . Diana Kelly
CEO/President. . . . . Kimberly Lumia
Cardiac Laboratory. . . . . Lee S Marcu
Chief of Medical Staff . . . . Michael D Parker, MD

Measure	Cases	This Hosp.	State Avg.	U.S. Avg.
Blood Clot Prevention and Treatment				
Anticoagulation Overlap Therapy[2]	14	100%	91%	93%
ICU Venous Thromboembolism Prophylaxis[2]	95	92%	93%	92%
Incidence of Potentially Preventable VTE[1,2]	-	-	6%	10%
UFH with Dosages/Platelet Monitoring[1,2]	-	-	95%	97%
Venous Thromboembolism Prophylaxis[2]	134	87%	89%	85%
Warfarin Therapy Discharge Instructions[1,2]	-	-	64%	75%
Chest Pain/Possible Heart Attack Care				
Aspirin Given Within 24 Hours of Arrival	50	100%	98%	96%
Fibrinolytic Meds Within 30 Min. of Arrival[1]	-	-	33%	58%
Average Time to ECG (minutes)	52	8	7	7
Average Time to Transfer (minutes)[7]	-	-	61	60
Children's Asthma Care				
Received Home Management Plan of Care	-	-	-	88%
Received Reliever Medication	-	-	-	100%
Received Systemic Corticosteroids	-	-	-	100%
Emergency Department				
Admittance Decision Time (minutes)[2]	382	148	147	98
Head CT Results Within 45 Min. of Arrival[1]	-	-	70%	57%
Patients Who Left ER Before Being Seen	15,694	1%	2%	2%
Time from ER Arrival to Admit. (minutes)[2]	389	296	338	274
Time from ER Arrival to Discharge (minutes)	397	97	131	134
Time in ER Before Being Evaluated (minutes)	424	25	28	26
Time to Pain Meds for Fractures (minutes)	92	50	55	57
Heart Attack Care				
Aspirin Given at Discharge	20	95%	99%	99%
Fibrinolytic Meds Within 30 Min. of Arrival[1]	-	-	50%	54%
PCI Within 90 Minutes of Arrival[7]	-	-	96%	96%
Statin Prescribed at Discharge	25	100%	98%	98%
Heart Failure Care				
ACE Inhibitor or ARB for LVSD[1]	-	-	96%	97%
Discharge Instructions Given	35	97%	93%	94%
Evaluation of LVS Function	57	98%	100%	99%
Medicare Spending				

NOTE: Hospital profiles are in alphabetical order by state, then city, then hospital within the city; Rankings exclude hospitals with less than 25 cases except for patient surveys which excludes hospitals with less than 100 cases; (a) 100-299 cases; (1) The number of cases/patients is too few to report; (2) Data submitted were based on a sample of cases/patients; (3) Results are based on a shorter time period than required; (4) Data suppressed by CMS for one or more quarters; (5) Results are not available for this reporting period; (6) Fewer than 100 patients completed the HCAHPS survey; (7) No cases met the criteria for this measure; (8) The lower limit of the confidence interval cannot be calculated if the number of observed infections equals zero; (9) No data are available from the state/territory for this reporting period; (10) The scores shown reflect fewer than 50 completed surveys; (11) There were discrepancies in the data collection process; (12) This measure does not apply to this hospital for this reporting period; (13) Results cannot be calculated for this reporting period; (14) The results for this state are combined with nearby states to protect confidentiality; Please refer to the User's Guide for a full explanation of data.

Measure	Cases	This Hosp.	State Avg.	U.S. Avg.
Medicare Spending per Patient (ratio)	-	0.93	1.02	0.98
Pneumonia Care				
Appropriate Initial Antibiotic Given	38	100%	97%	95%
Blood Culture Timing	97	98%	97%	98%
Pregnancy and Delivery Care				
Newborn Deliveries Scheduled Early	34	0%	5%	6%
Preventive Care				
Immunization for Influenza[2]	290	91%	90%	90%
Immunization for Pneumonia[2]	374	92%	91%	92%
Stroke Care				
Anticoagulation Therapy for Atrial Fibrillation[1]	-	-	96%	95%
Antithrombotic Therapy Timing	14	100%	99%	98%
Assessed for Rehabilitation	17	94%	98%	97%
Discharged on Antithrombotic Therapy	16	100%	99%	99%
Discharged on Statin Medication	13	100%	95%	94%
Thrombolytic Therapy Timing[1]	-	-	71%	66%
Venous Thromboembolism Prophylaxis	15	87%	95%	94%
Written Stroke Educational Materials Given[1]	-	-	80%	88%
Surgical Care Improvement Project				
Appropriate Beta Blocker Usage	24	96%	98%	98%
Appropriate VTP Within 24 Hours	96	92%	99%	98%
Controlled Postoperative Blood Glucose[7]	-	-	96%	97%
Perioperative Temperature Management	109	95%	99%	100%
Prophylactic Antibiotic Selection	76	100%	99%	99%
Prophylactic Antibiotic Selection (Outpatient)	33	88%	97%	98%
Prophylactic Antibiotic Stopped	73	95%	98%	98%
Prophylactic Antibiotic Timing	76	99%	98%	99%
Prophylactic Antibiotic Timing (Outpatient)	35	89%	97%	98%
Urinary Catheter Removal	65	95%	97%	97%
Survey of Patients' Hospital Experiences				
Area Around Room 'Always' Quiet at Night	300+	56%	52%	61%
Doctors 'Always' Communicated Well	300+	83%	80%	82%
Home Recovery Information Given	300+	85%	85%	85%
Hospital Given 9 or 10 on 10 Point Scale	300+	67%	68%	71%
Meds 'Always' Explained Before Given	300+	65%	62%	64%
Nurses 'Always' Communicated Well	300+	82%	78%	79%
Pain 'Always' Well Controlled	300+	72%	71%	71%
Room and Bathroom 'Always' Clean	300+	78%	71%	73%
Timely Help 'Always' Received	300+	64%	64%	68%
Would Definitely Recommend Hospital	300+	70%	71%	71%
Use of Medical Imaging				
Cardiac Imaging Stress Test before Surgery	254	2.8%	4.7%	5.3%
Combination Abdominal CT Scan	312	4.2%	5%	10.5%
Combination Brain/Sinus CT Scan[1]	-	-	2.3%	2.7%
Combination Chest CT Scan	300	0.0%	0.9%	2.7%
Follow-up Mammogram/Ultrasound	889	15.9%	19.5%	8.8%
Lumbar Spine MRI for Low Back Pain	68	22.1%	34.3%	37.2%

Johnson Memorial Hospital

201 Chestnut Hill Rd
Stafford Springs, CT 06076
Phone: 860-684-4251
Fax: 860-684-8459
URL: www.johnsonhealthnetwork.com
Type: Acute Care Hospitals
Emergency Services: Yes
Ownership: Voluntary non-profit - Private
Beds: 89

Key Personnel:

Quality Assurance . . . . Debra Abel
Radiology. . . . . Richard Buck
Operating Room. . . . . Stephanie Kelley, RN
CEO/President. . . . . Alfred A Lerz
Cardiac Laboratory. . . . . James Lietz
Chief of Medical Staff. . . . . Nicholas Salerno, MD

Measure	Cases	This Hosp.	State Avg.	U.S. Avg.
Blood Clot Prevention and Treatment				
Anticoagulation Overlap Therapy[2]	25	72%	91%	93%
ICU Venous Thromboembolism Prophylaxis[2]	60	77%	93%	92%
Incidence of Potentially Preventable VTE[1,2]	-	-	6%	10%
UFH with Dosages/Platelet Monitoring[2]	21	95%	95%	97%
Venous Thromboembolism Prophylaxis[2]	276	70%	89%	85%
Warfarin Therapy Discharge Instructions[2]	19	5%	64%	75%
Chest Pain/Possible Heart Attack Care				
Aspirin Given Within 24 Hours of Arrival	58	91%	98%	96%
Fibrinolytic Meds Within 30 Min. of Arrival[1]	-	-	33%	58%
Average Time to ECG (minutes)	61	5	7	7
Average Time to Transfer (minutes)[1]	-	-	61	60
Children's Asthma Care				
Received Home Management Plan of Care	-	-	-	88%
Received Reliever Medication	-	-	-	100%
Received Systemic Corticosteroids	-	-	-	100%
Emergency Department				
Admittance Decision Time (minutes)[2]	402	146	147	98
Head CT Results Within 45 Min. of Arrival[1]	-	-	70%	57%
Patients Who Left ER Before Being Seen	21,007	0%	2%	2%
Time from ER Arrival to Admit. (minutes)[2]	402	327	338	274
Time from ER Arrival to Discharge (minutes)	364	118	131	134
Time in ER Before Being Evaluated (minutes)	418	17	28	26
Time to Pain Meds for Fractures (minutes)	145	44	55	57
Heart Attack Care				
Aspirin Given at Discharge[1]	-	-	99%	99%
Fibrinolytic Meds Within 30 Min. of Arrival[7]	-	-	50%	54%
PCI Within 90 Minutes of Arrival[7]	-	-	96%	96%
Statin Prescribed at Discharge[1]	-	-	98%	98%
Heart Failure Care				
ACE Inhibitor or ARB for LVSD	16	88%	96%	97%
Discharge Instructions Given	61	79%	93%	94%
Evaluation of LVS Function	108	100%	100%	99%
Medicare Spending				
Medicare Spending per Patient (ratio)	-	1.06	1.02	0.98
Pneumonia Care				
Appropriate Initial Antibiotic Given	77	99%	97%	95%
Blood Culture Timing	123	97%	97%	98%
Pregnancy and Delivery Care				
Newborn Deliveries Scheduled Early[2]	26	19%	5%	6%
Preventive Care				
Immunization for Influenza[2]	317	95%	90%	90%
Immunization for Pneumonia[2]	421	97%	91%	92%
Stroke Care				
Anticoagulation Therapy for Atrial Fibrillation[1]	-	-	96%	95%
Antithrombotic Therapy Timing	12	100%	99%	98%
Assessed for Rehabilitation[1]	-	-	98%	97%
Discharged on Antithrombotic Therapy[1]	-	-	99%	99%
Discharged on Statin Medication[1]	-	-	95%	94%
Thrombolytic Therapy Timing[7]	-	-	71%	66%
Venous Thromboembolism Prophylaxis	13	69%	95%	94%
Written Stroke Educational Materials Given[1]	-	-	80%	88%
Surgical Care Improvement Project				
Appropriate Beta Blocker Usage	48	85%	98%	98%
Appropriate VTP Within 24 Hours	113	95%	99%	98%
Controlled Postoperative Blood Glucose[7]	-	-	96%	97%
Perioperative Temperature Management	139	99%	99%	100%
Prophylactic Antibiotic Selection	91	96%	99%	99%
Prophylactic Antibiotic Selection (Outpatient)	53	100%	97%	98%
Prophylactic Antibiotic Stopped	88	95%	98%	98%
Prophylactic Antibiotic Timing	91	99%	98%	99%
Prophylactic Antibiotic Timing (Outpatient)	53	100%	97%	98%
Urinary Catheter Removal	100	89%	97%	97%
Survey of Patients' Hospital Experiences				
Area Around Room 'Always' Quiet at Night	300+	58%	52%	61%
Doctors 'Always' Communicated Well	300+	79%	80%	82%
Home Recovery Information Given	300+	85%	85%	85%
Hospital Given 9 or 10 on 10 Point Scale	300+	63%	68%	71%
Meds 'Always' Explained Before Given	300+	65%	62%	64%
Nurses 'Always' Communicated Well	300+	81%	78%	79%
Pain 'Always' Well Controlled	300+	74%	71%	71%
Room and Bathroom 'Always' Clean	300+	75%	71%	73%
Timely Help 'Always' Received	300+	70%	64%	68%
Would Definitely Recommend Hospital	300+	66%	71%	71%
Use of Medical Imaging				
Cardiac Imaging Stress Test before Surgery	99	5.1%	4.7%	5.3%
Combination Abdominal CT Scan	388	2.1%	5%	10.5%
Combination Brain/Sinus CT Scan	334	1.2%	2.3%	2.7%
Combination Chest CT Scan	254	0.0%	0.9%	2.7%
Follow-up Mammogram/Ultrasound	452	12.8%	19.5%	8.8%
Lumbar Spine MRI for Low Back Pain[1]	-	-	34.3%	37.2%

Stamford Hospital

30 Shelburne Road
Stamford, CT 06904
Phone: 203-276-1000
Fax: 203-325-7223
E-mail: cmurphy@stamhealth.org
URL: www.stamhealth.org
Type: Acute Care Hospitals
Emergency Services: Yes
Ownership: Voluntary non-profit - Private
Beds: 305

Key Personnel:

Infection Control. . . . . Diane Baranowsky
CEO/President. . . . . Brian G Grissler
Chief of Medical Staff . . . . Sharon Kiely, MD
Radiology. . . . . James J McSweeney, MD
Pediatric Ambulatory Care . . . . . . Michael N Suchenski, MD
Quality Assurance . . . . Eva Winjarska
Operating Room. . . . . Beth Wolff, RN

Measure	Cases	This Hosp.	State Avg.	U.S. Avg.
Blood Clot Prevention and Treatment				
Anticoagulation Overlap Therapy[2]	80	91%	91%	93%
ICU Venous Thromboembolism Prophylaxis[2]	59	97%	93%	92%
Incidence of Potentially Preventable VTE[2]	18	6%	6%	10%
UFH with Dosages/Platelet Monitoring[2]	44	95%	95%	97%
Venous Thromboembolism Prophylaxis[2]	373	95%	89%	85%
Warfarin Therapy Discharge Instructions[2]	57	12%	64%	75%
Chest Pain/Possible Heart Attack Care				
Aspirin Given Within 24 Hours of Arrival[5]	-	-	98%	96%
Fibrinolytic Meds Within 30 Min. of Arrival[5]	-	-	33%	58%
Average Time to ECG (minutes)[5]	-	-	7	7
Average Time to Transfer (minutes)[5]	-	-	61	60
Children's Asthma Care				
Received Home Management Plan of Care	-	-	-	88%
Received Reliever Medication	-	-	-	100%
Received Systemic Corticosteroids	-	-	-	100%
Emergency Department				
Admittance Decision Time (minutes)[2]	683	119	147	98
Head CT Results Within 45 Min. of Arrival	11	55%	70%	57%
Patients Who Left ER Before Being Seen	51,054	1%	2%	2%
Time from ER Arrival to Admit. (minutes)[2]	688	297	338	274
Time from ER Arrival to Discharge (minutes)	369	164	131	134
Time in ER Before Being Evaluated (minutes)	419	14	28	26
Time to Pain Meds for Fractures (minutes)	153	56	55	57
Heart Attack Care				
Aspirin Given at Discharge	165	99%	99%	99%
Fibrinolytic Meds Within 30 Min. of Arrival[7]	-	-	50%	54%
PCI Within 90 Minutes of Arrival	41	100%	96%	96%
Statin Prescribed at Discharge	164	99%	98%	98%
Heart Failure Care				
ACE Inhibitor or ARB for LVSD	123	98%	96%	97%
Discharge Instructions Given	211	98%	93%	94%
Evaluation of LVS Function	308	100%	100%	99%
Medicare Spending				
Medicare Spending per Patient (ratio)	-	1.05	1.02	0.98
Pneumonia Care				
Appropriate Initial Antibiotic Given	172	97%	97%	95%
Blood Culture Timing	273	99%	97%	98%
Pregnancy and Delivery Care				
Newborn Deliveries Scheduled Early[2]	35	0%	5%	6%
Preventive Care				
Immunization for Influenza[2]	524	95%	90%	90%
Immunization for Pneumonia[2]	575	97%	91%	92%
Stroke Care				
Anticoagulation Therapy for Atrial Fibrillation	17	100%	96%	95%
Antithrombotic Therapy Timing	102	99%	99%	98%
Assessed for Rehabilitation	124	100%	98%	97%
Discharged on Antithrombotic Therapy	113	100%	99%	99%
Discharged on Statin Medication	93	98%	95%	94%
Thrombolytic Therapy Timing[1]	-	-	71%	66%
Venous Thromboembolism Prophylaxis	127	99%	95%	94%
Written Stroke Educational Materials Given	56	93%	80%	88%
Surgical Care Improvement Project				
Appropriate Beta Blocker Usage	192	95%	98%	98%
Appropriate VTP Within 24 Hours	546	99%	99%	98%
Controlled Postoperative Blood Glucose	63	98%	96%	97%
Perioperative Temperature Management	643	100%	99%	100%
Prophylactic Antibiotic Selection	378	100%	99%	99%

NOTE: Hospital profiles are in alphabetical order by state, then city, then hospital within the city; Rankings exclude hospitals with less than 25 cases except for patient surveys which excludes hospitals with less than 100 cases; (a) 100-299 cases; (1) The number of cases/patients is too few to report; (2) Data submitted were based on a sample of cases/patients; (3) Results are based on a shorter time period than required; (4) Data suppressed by CMS for one or more quarters; (5) Results are not available for this reporting period; (6) Fewer than 100 patients completed the HCAHPS survey; (7) No cases met the criteria for this measure; (8) The lower limit of the confidence interval cannot be calculated if the number of observed infections equals zero; (9) No data are available from the state/territory for this reporting period; (10) The scores shown reflect fewer than 50 completed surveys; (11) There were discrepancies in the data collection process; (12) This measure does not apply to this hospital for this reporting period; (13) Results cannot be calculated for this reporting period; (14) The results for this state are combined with nearby states to protect confidentiality; Please refer to the User's Guide for a full explanation of data.

Prophylactic Antibiotic Selection (Outpatient)	445	98%	97%	98%
Prophylactic Antibiotic Stopped	365	98%	98%	98%
Prophylactic Antibiotic Timing	378	100%	98%	99%
Prophylactic Antibiotic Timing (Outpatient)	439	99%	97%	98%
Urinary Catheter Removal	243	99%	97%	97%
Survey of Patients' Hospital Experiences				
Area Around Room 'Always' Quiet at Night	300+	60%	52%	61%
Doctors 'Always' Communicated Well	300+	82%	80%	82%
Home Recovery Information Given	300+	83%	85%	85%
Hospital Given 9 or 10 on 10 Point Scale	300+	71%	68%	71%
Meds 'Always' Explained Before Given	300+	62%	62%	64%
Nurses 'Always' Communicated Well	300+	81%	78%	79%
Pain 'Always' Well Controlled	300+	74%	71%	71%
Room and Bathroom 'Always' Clean	300+	73%	71%	73%
Timely Help 'Always' Received	300+	64%	64%	68%
Would Definitely Recommend Hospital	300+	77%	71%	71%
Use of Medical Imaging				
Cardiac Imaging Stress Test before Surgery	653	5.7%	4.7%	5.3%
Combination Abdominal CT Scan	1,484	2.3%	5%	10.5%
Combination Brain/Sinus CT Scan	1,139	4.1%	2.3%	2.7%
Combination Chest CT Scan	926	0.4%	0.9%	2.7%
Follow-up Mammogram/Ultrasound	2,964	45.1%	19.5%	8.8%
Lumbar Spine MRI for Low Back Pain	117	33.3%	34.3%	37.2%

Charlotte Hungerford Hospital

540 Litchfield St
Torrington, CT 06790
Phone: 860-496-6666
Fax: 860-482-8627
URL: www.charlottesweb.hungerford.org
Type: Acute Care Hospitals
Emergency Services: Yes
Ownership: Voluntary non-profit - Private
Beds: 109

Key Personnel:
Emergency Room . . . . Peter Bull
Radiology. . . . . Herman Coleman, MD
Quality Assurance . . . . Donna Feinstein
Operating Room. . . . . Timothy Gostkowski
Patient Relations . . . . Marty Mancuso
President/CEO. . . . . Daniel J McIntyre
Infection Control. . . . . Joseph O'Geen
Chief of Medical Staff. . . . . Mark Prete, MD

Measure	Cases	This Hosp.	State Avg.	U.S. Avg.
Blood Clot Prevention and Treatment				
Anticoagulation Overlap Therapy[2]	43	88%	91%	93%
ICU Venous Thromboembolism Prophylaxis[2]	54	76%	93%	92%
Incidence of Potentially Preventable VTE[1,2]	-	-	6%	10%
UFH with Dosages/Platelet Monitoring[2]	36	100%	95%	97%
Venous Thromboembolism Prophylaxis[2]	369	67%	89%	85%
Warfarin Therapy Discharge Instructions[2]	20	95%	64%	75%
Chest Pain/Possible Heart Attack Care				
Aspirin Given Within 24 Hours of Arrival	99	99%	98%	96%
Fibrinolytic Meds Within 30 Min. of Arrival[7]	-	-	33%	58%
Average Time to ECG (minutes)	102	6	7	7
Average Time to Transfer (minutes)[1]	-	-	61	60
Children's Asthma Care				
Received Home Management Plan of Care	-	-	-	88%
Received Reliever Medication	-	-	-	100%
Received Systemic Corticosteroids	-	-	-	100%
Emergency Department				
Admittance Decision Time (minutes)[2]	864	148	147	98
Head CT Results Within 45 Min. of Arrival	15	53%	70%	57%
Patients Who Left ER Before Being Seen	41,924	0%	2%	2%
Time from ER Arrival to Admit. (minutes)[2]	864	355	338	274
Time from ER Arrival to Discharge (minutes)	348	98	131	134
Time in ER Before Being Evaluated (minutes)	387	20	28	26
Time to Pain Meds for Fractures (minutes)	102	42	55	57
Heart Attack Care				
Aspirin Given at Discharge	30	97%	99%	99%
Fibrinolytic Meds Within 30 Min. of Arrival[7]	-	-	50%	54%
PCI Within 90 Minutes of Arrival[7]	-	-	96%	96%
Statin Prescribed at Discharge	32	81%	98%	98%
Heart Failure Care				
ACE Inhibitor or ARB for LVSD	39	82%	96%	97%
Discharge Instructions Given	100	84%	93%	94%
Evaluation of LVS Function	165	98%	100%	99%
Medicare Spending				
Medicare Spending per Patient (ratio)	-	1.01	1.02	0.98
Pneumonia Care				
Appropriate Initial Antibiotic Given	110	95%	97%	95%
Blood Culture Timing	157	95%	97%	98%
Pregnancy and Delivery Care				
Newborn Deliveries Scheduled Early[2]	37	11%	5%	6%
Preventive Care				
Immunization for Influenza[2]	561	81%	90%	90%
Immunization for Pneumonia[2]	787	75%	91%	92%
Stroke Care				
Anticoagulation Therapy for Atrial Fibrillation[1]	-	-	96%	95%
Antithrombotic Therapy Timing	44	95%	99%	98%
Assessed for Rehabilitation	40	92%	98%	97%
Discharged on Antithrombotic Therapy	39	100%	99%	99%
Discharged on Statin Medication	33	76%	95%	94%
Thrombolytic Therapy Timing[1]	-	-	71%	66%
Venous Thromboembolism Prophylaxis	48	73%	95%	94%
Written Stroke Educational Materials Given	16	88%	80%	88%
Surgical Care Improvement Project				
Appropriate Beta Blocker Usage	108	95%	98%	98%
Appropriate VTP Within 24 Hours	278	99%	99%	98%
Controlled Postoperative Blood Glucose[7]	-	-	96%	97%
Perioperative Temperature Management	358	97%	99%	100%
Prophylactic Antibiotic Selection	224	99%	99%	99%
Prophylactic Antibiotic Selection (Outpatient)	259	99%	97%	98%
Prophylactic Antibiotic Stopped	215	91%	98%	98%
Prophylactic Antibiotic Timing	224	96%	98%	99%
Prophylactic Antibiotic Timing (Outpatient)	108	97%	97%	98%
Urinary Catheter Removal	98	93%	97%	97%
Survey of Patients' Hospital Experiences				
Area Around Room 'Always' Quiet at Night	300+	45%	52%	61%
Doctors 'Always' Communicated Well	300+	77%	80%	82%
Home Recovery Information Given	300+	89%	85%	85%
Hospital Given 9 or 10 on 10 Point Scale	300+	63%	68%	71%
Meds 'Always' Explained Before Given	300+	63%	62%	64%
Nurses 'Always' Communicated Well	300+	79%	78%	79%
Pain 'Always' Well Controlled	300+	72%	71%	71%
Room and Bathroom 'Always' Clean	300+	73%	71%	73%
Timely Help 'Always' Received	300+	66%	64%	68%
Would Definitely Recommend Hospital	300+	60%	71%	71%
Use of Medical Imaging				
Cardiac Imaging Stress Test before Surgery	280	5.4%	4.7%	5.3%
Combination Abdominal CT Scan	714	4.9%	5%	10.5%
Combination Brain/Sinus CT Scan	540	1.3%	2.3%	2.7%
Combination Chest CT Scan	319	1.9%	0.9%	2.7%
Follow-up Mammogram/Ultrasound	2,097	20.6%	19.5%	8.8%
Lumbar Spine MRI for Low Back Pain[1]	-	-	34.3%	37.2%

Masonic Home & Hospital

22 Masonic Ave
Wallingford, CT 06492
Phone: 203-679-5900
Fax: 203-679-5038
E-mail: info@masonicare.org
URL: www.masonicare.org
Type: Acute Care Hospitals
Emergency Services: No
Ownership: Voluntary non-profit - Private
Beds: 548

Key Personnel:
Radiology. . . . . Jean Desrosiers
Ambulatory Care . . . . Carol Herbert, RN
Quality Assurance . . . . Tracey Lemay
CEO/President. . . . . Stephen B. McPherson
Infection Control. . . . . Irene Morris, RN
Chief of Medical Staff. . . . . Ronald Schwartz, MD

Measure	Cases	This Hosp.	State Avg.	U.S. Avg.
Blood Clot Prevention and Treatment				
Anticoagulation Overlap Therapy[7]	-	-	91%	93%
ICU Venous Thromboembolism Prophylaxis[7]	-	-	93%	92%
Incidence of Potentially Preventable VTE[7]	-	-	6%	10%
UFH with Dosages/Platelet Monitoring[7]	-	-	95%	97%
Venous Thromboembolism Prophylaxis	293	94%	89%	85%
Warfarin Therapy Discharge Instructions[7]	-	-	64%	75%
Chest Pain/Possible Heart Attack Care				
Aspirin Given Within 24 Hours of Arrival[5]	-	-	98%	96%
Fibrinolytic Meds Within 30 Min. of Arrival[5]	-	-	33%	58%
Average Time to ECG (minutes)[5]	-	-	7	7
Average Time to Transfer (minutes)[5]	-	-	61	60
Children's Asthma Care				
Received Home Management Plan of Care	-	-	-	88%
Received Reliever Medication	-	-	-	100%
Received Systemic Corticosteroids	-	-	-	100%
Emergency Department				
Admittance Decision Time (minutes)[7]	-	-	147	98
Head CT Results Within 45 Min. of Arrival[5]	-	-	70%	57%
Patients Who Left ER Before Being Seen[5]	-	-	2%	2%
Time from ER Arrival to Admit. (minutes)[7]	-	-	338	274
Time from ER Arrival to Discharge (minutes)[5]	-	-	131	134
Time in ER Before Being Evaluated (minutes)[5]	-	-	28	26
Time to Pain Meds for Fractures (minutes)[5]	-	-	55	57
Heart Attack Care				
Aspirin Given at Discharge[1]	-	-	99%	99%
Fibrinolytic Meds Within 30 Min. of Arrival[7]	-	-	50%	54%
PCI Within 90 Minutes of Arrival[7]	-	-	96%	96%
Statin Prescribed at Discharge[1]	-	-	98%	98%
Heart Failure Care				
ACE Inhibitor or ARB for LVSD[1]	-	-	96%	97%
Discharge Instructions Given[1]	-	-	93%	94%
Evaluation of LVS Function	27	74%	100%	99%
Medicare Spending				
Medicare Spending per Patient (ratio)	-	1.07	1.02	0.98
Pneumonia Care				
Appropriate Initial Antibiotic Given	17	53%	97%	95%
Blood Culture Timing[1]	-	-	97%	98%
Pregnancy and Delivery Care				
Newborn Deliveries Scheduled Early[7]	-	-	5%	6%
Preventive Care				
Immunization for Influenza	251	73%	90%	90%
Immunization for Pneumonia	412	80%	91%	92%
Stroke Care				
Anticoagulation Therapy for Atrial Fibrillation[5]	-	-	96%	95%
Antithrombotic Therapy Timing[5]	-	-	99%	98%
Assessed for Rehabilitation[5]	-	-	98%	97%
Discharged on Antithrombotic Therapy[5]	-	-	99%	99%
Discharged on Statin Medication[5]	-	-	95%	94%
Thrombolytic Therapy Timing[5]	-	-	71%	66%
Venous Thromboembolism Prophylaxis[5]	-	-	95%	94%
Written Stroke Educational Materials Given[5]	-	-	80%	88%
Surgical Care Improvement Project				
Appropriate Beta Blocker Usage[5]	-	-	98%	98%
Appropriate VTP Within 24 Hours[5]	-	-	99%	98%
Controlled Postoperative Blood Glucose[5]	-	-	96%	97%
Perioperative Temperature Management[5]	-	-	99%	100%
Prophylactic Antibiotic Selection[5]	-	-	99%	99%
Prophylactic Antibiotic Selection (Outpatient)[5]	-	-	97%	98%
Prophylactic Antibiotic Stopped[5]	-	-	98%	98%
Prophylactic Antibiotic Timing[5]	-	-	98%	99%
Prophylactic Antibiotic Timing (Outpatient)[5]	-	-	97%	98%
Urinary Catheter Removal[5]	-	-	97%	97%
Survey of Patients' Hospital Experiences				
Area Around Room 'Always' Quiet at Night[10]	<100	49%	52%	61%
Doctors 'Always' Communicated Well[10]	<100	73%	80%	82%
Home Recovery Information Given[10]	<100	88%	85%	85%
Hospital Given 9 or 10 on 10 Point Scale[10]	<100	75%	68%	71%
Meds 'Always' Explained Before Given[10]	<100	64%	62%	64%
Nurses 'Always' Communicated Well[10]	<100	73%	78%	79%
Pain 'Always' Well Controlled[10]	<100	71%	71%	71%
Room and Bathroom 'Always' Clean[10]	<100	71%	71%	73%
Timely Help 'Always' Received[10]	<100	64%	64%	68%
Would Definitely Recommend Hospital[10]	<100	70%	71%	71%
Use of Medical Imaging				
Cardiac Imaging Stress Test before Surgery[7]	-	-	4.7%	5.3%
Combination Abdominal CT Scan[7]	-	-	5%	10.5%
Combination Brain/Sinus CT Scan[7]	-	-	2.3%	2.7%
Combination Chest CT Scan[7]	-	-	0.9%	2.7%
Follow-up Mammogram/Ultrasound[7]	-	-	19.5%	8.8%
Lumbar Spine MRI for Low Back Pain[7]	-	-	34.3%	37.2%

NOTE: Hospital profiles are in alphabetical order by state, then city, then hospital within the city; Rankings exclude hospitals with less than 25 cases except for patient surveys which excludes hospitals with less than 100 cases; (a) 100-299 cases; (1) The number of cases/patients is too few to report; (2) Data submitted were based on a sample of cases/patients; (3) Results are based on a shorter time period than required; (4) Data suppressed by CMS for one or more quarters; (5) Results are not available for this reporting period; (6) Fewer than 100 patients completed the HCAHPS survey; (7) No cases met the criteria for this measure; (8) The lower limit of the confidence interval cannot be calculated if the number of observed infections equals zero; (9) No data are available from the state/territory for this reporting period; (10) The scores shown reflect fewer than 50 completed surveys; (11) There were discrepancies in the data collection process; (12) This measure does not apply to this hospital for this reporting period; (13) Results cannot be calculated for this reporting period; (14) The results for this state are combined with nearby states to protect confidentiality; Please refer to the User's Guide for a full explanation of data.

Saint Marys Hospital

56 Franklin St Phone: 203-574-6000
Waterbury, CT 06706 Fax: 203-709-7753
URL: www.stmh.org
Type: Acute Care Hospitals Emergency Services: Yes
Ownership: Voluntary non-profit - Other Beds: 347

Key Personnel:

Operating Room. . . . . Pat Clement
Emergency Room . . . . Dr Fisher
Pediatric Ambulatory Care . . . . . . M Alex Geertsmand
Pediatric In-Patient Care . . . . M Alex Geertsmand
Radiology. . . . . Robert Lehman, MD
Chairman/CEO . . . . Robert Mazaika
Chief of Medical Staff. . . . . Steven E. Schneider, MD, MBA
CEO/President. . . . . Chad W. Wable, FACHE

Measure	Cases	This Hosp.	State Avg.	U.S. Avg.
Blood Clot Prevention and Treatment				
Anticoagulation Overlap Therapy[2]	65	72%	91%	93%
ICU Venous Thromboembolism Prophylaxis[2]	51	92%	93%	92%
Incidence of Potentially Preventable VTE[2]	12	0%	6%	10%
UFH with Dosages/Platelet Monitoring[2]	68	85%	95%	97%
Venous Thromboembolism Prophylaxis[2]	377	85%	89%	85%
Warfarin Therapy Discharge Instructions[2]	44	20%	64%	75%
Chest Pain/Possible Heart Attack Care				
Aspirin Given Within 24 Hours of Arrival[5]	-	-	98%	96%
Fibrinolytic Meds Within 30 Min. of Arrival[5]	-	-	33%	58%
Average Time to ECG (minutes)[5]	-	-	7	7
Average Time to Transfer (minutes)[5]	-	-	61	60
Children's Asthma Care				
Received Home Management Plan of Care	-	-	-	88%
Received Reliever Medication	-	-	-	100%
Received Systemic Corticosteroids	-	-	-	100%
Emergency Department				
Admittance Decision Time (minutes)[2]	650	135	147	98
Head CT Results Within 45 Min. of Arrival[1]	-	-	70%	57%
Patients Who Left ER Before Being Seen	71,160	3%	2%	2%
Time from ER Arrival to Admit. (minutes)[2]	710	400	338	274
Time from ER Arrival to Discharge (minutes)	376	148	131	134
Time in ER Before Being Evaluated (minutes)	309	36	28	26
Time to Pain Meds for Fractures (minutes)	244	80	55	57
Heart Attack Care				
Aspirin Given at Discharge	176	100%	99%	99%
Fibrinolytic Meds Within 30 Min. of Arrival[7]	-	-	50%	54%
PCI Within 90 Minutes of Arrival	55	96%	96%	96%
Statin Prescribed at Discharge	172	100%	98%	98%
Heart Failure Care				
ACE Inhibitor or ARB for LVSD	75	100%	96%	97%
Discharge Instructions Given	162	99%	93%	94%
Evaluation of LVS Function	268	100%	100%	99%
Medicare Spending				
Medicare Spending per Patient (ratio)	-	1.01	1.02	0.98
Pneumonia Care				
Appropriate Initial Antibiotic Given[2]	83	99%	97%	95%
Blood Culture Timing[2]	180	98%	97%	98%
Pregnancy and Delivery Care				
Newborn Deliveries Scheduled Early[2]	47	11%	5%	6%
Preventive Care				
Immunization for Influenza[2]	572	85%	90%	90%
Immunization for Pneumonia[2]	737	82%	91%	92%
Stroke Care				
Anticoagulation Therapy for Atrial Fibrillation	18	100%	96%	95%
Antithrombotic Therapy Timing	120	100%	99%	98%
Assessed for Rehabilitation	123	100%	98%	97%
Discharged on Antithrombotic Therapy	112	98%	99%	99%
Discharged on Statin Medication	99	94%	95%	94%
Thrombolytic Therapy Timing	11	36%	71%	66%
Venous Thromboembolism Prophylaxis	134	90%	95%	94%
Written Stroke Educational Materials Given	53	66%	80%	88%
Surgical Care Improvement Project				
Appropriate Beta Blocker Usage[2]	152	99%	98%	98%
Appropriate VTP Within 24 Hours[2]	334	100%	99%	98%
Controlled Postoperative Blood Glucose[2]	76	99%	96%	97%
Perioperative Temperature Management[2]	452	100%	99%	100%
Prophylactic Antibiotic Selection[2]	355	99%	99%	99%
Prophylactic Antibiotic Selection (Outpatient)	367	98%	97%	98%
Prophylactic Antibiotic Stopped[2]	342	98%	98%	98%
Prophylactic Antibiotic Timing[2]	355	99%	98%	99%
Prophylactic Antibiotic Timing (Outpatient)	367	98%	97%	98%
Urinary Catheter Removal[2]	177	99%	97%	97%
Survey of Patients' Hospital Experiences				
Area Around Room 'Always' Quiet at Night	300+	56%	52%	61%
Doctors 'Always' Communicated Well	300+	78%	80%	82%
Home Recovery Information Given	300+	86%	85%	85%
Hospital Given 9 or 10 on 10 Point Scale	300+	67%	68%	71%
Meds 'Always' Explained Before Given	300+	61%	62%	64%
Nurses 'Always' Communicated Well	300+	77%	78%	79%
Pain 'Always' Well Controlled	300+	68%	71%	71%
Room and Bathroom 'Always' Clean	300+	72%	71%	73%
Timely Help 'Always' Received	300+	61%	64%	68%
Would Definitely Recommend Hospital	300+	71%	71%	71%
Use of Medical Imaging				
Cardiac Imaging Stress Test before Surgery	317	3.5%	4.7%	5.3%
Combination Abdominal CT Scan	760	3.2%	5%	10.5%
Combination Brain/Sinus CT Scan	812	2.1%	2.3%	2.7%
Combination Chest CT Scan	463	0.0%	0.9%	2.7%
Follow-up Mammogram/Ultrasound	508	17.3%	19.5%	8.8%
Lumbar Spine MRI for Low Back Pain[1]	-	-	34.3%	37.2%

Waterbury Hospital

64 Robbins St Phone: 203-573-6000
Waterbury, CT 06721 Fax: 203-573-7325
URL: www.waterburyhospital.org
Type: Acute Care Hospitals Emergency Services: Yes
Ownership: Voluntary non-profit - Private Beds: 357

Key Personnel:

Radiology. . . . . John DeLeon, MD
Chief of Medical Staff. . . . . Steve Eisen, MD
Emergency Room . . . . Kreig Middleman, MD
Anesthesiology. . . . . Neil Peterson, MD
Operating Room. . . . . Ellen Polokoff
Quality Assurance . . . . John Porter
CEO/President. . . . . John H Tobin
Infection Control. . . . . Maria Villaneuava

Measure	Cases	This Hosp.	State Avg.	U.S. Avg.
Blood Clot Prevention and Treatment				
Anticoagulation Overlap Therapy[2]	77	95%	91%	93%
ICU Venous Thromboembolism Prophylaxis[2]	65	97%	93%	92%
Incidence of Potentially Preventable VTE[2]	24	4%	6%	10%
UFH with Dosages/Platelet Monitoring[2]	87	99%	95%	97%
Venous Thromboembolism Prophylaxis[2]	354	95%	89%	85%
Warfarin Therapy Discharge Instructions[2]	38	58%	64%	75%
Chest Pain/Possible Heart Attack Care				
Aspirin Given Within 24 Hours of Arrival[5]	-	-	98%	96%
Fibrinolytic Meds Within 30 Min. of Arrival[5]	-	-	33%	58%
Average Time to ECG (minutes)[5]	-	-	7	7
Average Time to Transfer (minutes)[5]	-	-	61	60
Children's Asthma Care				
Received Home Management Plan of Care	-	-	-	88%
Received Reliever Medication	-	-	-	100%
Received Systemic Corticosteroids	-	-	-	100%
Emergency Department				
Admittance Decision Time (minutes)[2]	787	190	147	98
Head CT Results Within 45 Min. of Arrival	11	73%	70%	57%
Patients Who Left ER Before Being Seen	56,513	4%	2%	2%
Time from ER Arrival to Admit. (minutes)[2]	858	422	338	274
Time from ER Arrival to Discharge (minutes)	384	178	131	134
Time in ER Before Being Evaluated (minutes)	417	67	28	26
Time to Pain Meds for Fractures (minutes)	132	92	55	57
Heart Attack Care				
Aspirin Given at Discharge	201	98%	99%	99%
Fibrinolytic Meds Within 30 Min. of Arrival[7]	-	-	50%	54%
PCI Within 90 Minutes of Arrival	47	94%	96%	96%
Statin Prescribed at Discharge	192	99%	98%	98%
Heart Failure Care				
ACE Inhibitor or ARB for LVSD[2]	84	94%	96%	97%
Discharge Instructions Given[2]	181	94%	93%	94%
Evaluation of LVS Function[2]	304	100%	100%	99%
Medicare Spending				
Medicare Spending per Patient (ratio)	-	1.00	1.02	0.98
Pneumonia Care				
Appropriate Initial Antibiotic Given[2]	105	98%	97%	95%
Blood Culture Timing[2]	207	100%	97%	98%
Pregnancy and Delivery Care				
Newborn Deliveries Scheduled Early[2]	32	9%	5%	6%
Preventive Care				
Immunization for Influenza[2]	597	92%	90%	90%
Immunization for Pneumonia[2]	786	95%	91%	92%
Stroke Care				
Anticoagulation Therapy for Atrial Fibrillation	12	100%	96%	95%
Antithrombotic Therapy Timing	83	99%	99%	98%
Assessed for Rehabilitation	88	98%	98%	97%
Discharged on Antithrombotic Therapy	79	100%	99%	99%
Discharged on Statin Medication	62	100%	95%	94%
Thrombolytic Therapy Timing[1]	-	-	71%	66%
Venous Thromboembolism Prophylaxis	100	100%	95%	94%
Written Stroke Educational Materials Given	38	84%	80%	88%
Surgical Care Improvement Project				
Appropriate Beta Blocker Usage[2]	183	98%	98%	98%
Appropriate VTP Within 24 Hours[2]	454	98%	99%	98%
Controlled Postoperative Blood Glucose[2]	103	94%	96%	97%
Perioperative Temperature Management[2]	511	99%	99%	100%
Prophylactic Antibiotic Selection[2]	416	99%	99%	99%
Prophylactic Antibiotic Selection (Outpatient)	207	98%	97%	98%
Prophylactic Antibiotic Stopped[2]	407	98%	98%	98%
Prophylactic Antibiotic Timing[2]	416	99%	98%	99%
Prophylactic Antibiotic Timing (Outpatient)	209	97%	97%	98%
Urinary Catheter Removal[2]	298	97%	97%	97%
Survey of Patients' Hospital Experiences				
Area Around Room 'Always' Quiet at Night	300+	52%	52%	61%
Doctors 'Always' Communicated Well	300+	78%	80%	82%
Home Recovery Information Given	300+	87%	85%	85%
Hospital Given 9 or 10 on 10 Point Scale	300+	62%	68%	71%
Meds 'Always' Explained Before Given	300+	59%	62%	64%
Nurses 'Always' Communicated Well	300+	76%	78%	79%
Pain 'Always' Well Controlled	300+	68%	71%	71%
Room and Bathroom 'Always' Clean	300+	67%	71%	73%
Timely Help 'Always' Received	300+	58%	64%	68%
Would Definitely Recommend Hospital	300+	67%	71%	71%
Use of Medical Imaging				
Cardiac Imaging Stress Test before Surgery	924	5.5%	4.7%	5.3%
Combination Abdominal CT Scan	751	2.8%	5%	10.5%
Combination Brain/Sinus CT Scan	780	2.1%	2.3%	2.7%
Combination Chest CT Scan	544	0.2%	0.9%	2.7%
Follow-up Mammogram/Ultrasound	199	19.6%	19.5%	8.8%
Lumbar Spine MRI for Low Back Pain[1]	-	-	34.3%	37.2%

Hebrew Home & Hospital

1 Abrahms Boulevard Phone: 860-523-3800
West Hartford, CT 06117 Fax: 860-523-3949
E-mail: info@hebrewhealthcare.org
URL: www.hebrewhealthcare.org
Type: Acute Care Hospitals Emergency Services: No
Ownership: Voluntary non-profit - Private Beds: 334

Key Personnel:

CEO/President. . . . . Bonnie Gauthier
Infection Control. . . . . Barbara Joy, RN
Quality Assurance . . . . Linda McDonnell
Chief of Medical Staff. . . . . Kathy Mon, MD
Patient Relations . . . . Jennifer Terray

Measure	Cases	This Hosp.	State Avg.	U.S. Avg.
Blood Clot Prevention and Treatment				
Anticoagulation Overlap Therapy[7]	-	-	91%	93%
ICU Venous Thromboembolism Prophylaxis[7]	-	-	93%	92%
Incidence of Potentially Preventable VTE[7]	-	-	6%	10%
UFH with Dosages/Platelet Monitoring[7]	-	-	95%	97%
Venous Thromboembolism Prophylaxis	84	80%	89%	85%
Warfarin Therapy Discharge Instructions[7]	-	-	64%	75%
Chest Pain/Possible Heart Attack Care				
Aspirin Given Within 24 Hours of Arrival[5]	-	-	98%	96%
Fibrinolytic Meds Within 30 Min. of Arrival[5]	-	-	33%	58%
Average Time to ECG (minutes)[5]	-	-	7	7
Average Time to Transfer (minutes)[5]	-	-	61	60

NOTE: Hospital profiles are in alphabetical order by state, then city, then hospital within the city; Rankings exclude hospitals with less than 25 cases except for patient surveys which excludes hospitals with less than 100 cases; (a) 100-299 cases; (1) The number of cases/patients is too few to report; (2) Data submitted were based on a sample of cases/patients; (3) Results are based on a shorter time period than required; (4) Data suppressed by CMS for one or more quarters; (5) Results are not available for this reporting period; (6) Fewer than 100 patients completed the HCAHPS survey; (7) No cases met the criteria for this measure; (8) The lower limit of the confidence interval cannot be calculated if the number of observed infections equals zero; (9) No data are available from the state/territory for this reporting period; (10) The scores shown reflect fewer than 50 completed surveys; (11) There were discrepancies in the data collection process; (12) This measure does not apply to this hospital for this reporting period; (13) Results cannot be calculated for this reporting period; (14) The results for this state are combined with nearby states to protect confidentiality; Please refer to the User's Guide for a full explanation of data.

Measure	Cases	This Hosp.	State Avg.	U.S. Avg.
Children's Asthma Care				
Received Home Management Plan of Care	-	-	-	88%
Received Reliever Medication	-	-	-	100%
Received Systemic Corticosteroids	-	-	-	100%
Emergency Department				
Admittance Decision Time (minutes)[7]	-	-	147	98
Head CT Results Within 45 Min. of Arrival[5]	-	-	70%	57%
Patients Who Left ER Before Being Seen[5]	-	-	2%	2%
Time from ER Arrival to Admit. (minutes)[7]	-	-	338	274
Time from ER Arrival to Discharge (minutes)[5]	-	-	131	134
Time in ER Before Being Evaluated (minutes)[5]	-	-	28	26
Time to Pain Meds for Fractures (minutes)[5]	-	-	55	57
Heart Attack Care				
Aspirin Given at Discharge[5]	-	-	99%	99%
Fibrinolytic Meds Within 30 Min. of Arrival[5]	-	-	50%	54%
PCI Within 90 Minutes of Arrival[5]	-	-	96%	96%
Statin Prescribed at Discharge[5]	-	-	98%	98%
Heart Failure Care				
ACE Inhibitor or ARB for LVSD[5]	-	-	96%	97%
Discharge Instructions Given[5]	-	-	93%	94%
Evaluation of LVS Function[5]	-	-	100%	99%
Medicare Spending				
Medicare Spending per Patient (ratio)	-	0.85	1.02	0.98
Pneumonia Care				
Appropriate Initial Antibiotic Given[1,3]	-	-	97%	95%
Blood Culture Timing[3,7]	-	-	97%	98%
Pregnancy and Delivery Care				
Newborn Deliveries Scheduled Early[7]	-	-	5%	6%
Preventive Care				
Immunization for Influenza	87	85%	90%	90%
Immunization for Pneumonia	131	95%	91%	92%
Stroke Care				
Anticoagulation Therapy for Atrial Fibrillation[5]	-	-	96%	95%
Antithrombotic Therapy Timing[5]	-	-	99%	98%
Assessed for Rehabilitation[5]	-	-	98%	97%
Discharged on Antithrombotic Therapy[5]	-	-	99%	99%
Discharged on Statin Medication[5]	-	-	95%	94%
Thrombolytic Therapy Timing[5]	-	-	71%	66%
Venous Thromboembolism Prophylaxis[5]	-	-	95%	94%
Written Stroke Educational Materials Given[5]	-	-	80%	88%
Surgical Care Improvement Project				
Appropriate Beta Blocker Usage[5]	-	-	98%	98%
Appropriate VTP Within 24 Hours[5]	-	-	99%	98%
Controlled Postoperative Blood Glucose[5]	-	-	96%	97%
Perioperative Temperature Management[5]	-	-	99%	100%
Prophylactic Antibiotic Selection[5]	-	-	99%	99%
Prophylactic Antibiotic Selection (Outpatient)[5]	-	-	97%	98%
Prophylactic Antibiotic Stopped[5]	-	-	98%	98%
Prophylactic Antibiotic Timing[5]	-	-	98%	99%
Prophylactic Antibiotic Timing (Outpatient)[5]	-	-	97%	98%
Urinary Catheter Removal[5]	-	-	97%	97%
Survey of Patients' Hospital Experiences				
Area Around Room 'Always' Quiet at Night[10]	<100	-	52%	61%
Doctors 'Always' Communicated Well[10]	<100	100%	80%	82%
Home Recovery Information Given[10]	<100	82%	85%	85%
Hospital Given 9 or 10 on 10 Point Scale[10]	<100	55%	68%	71%
Meds 'Always' Explained Before Given[10]	<100	-	62%	64%
Nurses 'Always' Communicated Well[10]	<100	55%	78%	79%
Pain 'Always' Well Controlled[10]	<100	-	71%	71%
Room and Bathroom 'Always' Clean[10]	<100	52%	71%	73%
Timely Help 'Always' Received[10]	<100	-	64%	68%
Would Definitely Recommend Hospital[10]	<100	54%	71%	71%
Use of Medical Imaging				
Cardiac Imaging Stress Test before Surgery[7]	-	-	4.7%	5.3%
Combination Abdominal CT Scan[7]	-	-	5%	10.5%
Combination Brain/Sinus CT Scan[7]	-	-	2.3%	2.7%
Combination Chest CT Scan[7]	-	-	0.9%	2.7%
Follow-up Mammogram/Ultrasound[7]	-	-	19.5%	8.8%
Lumbar Spine MRI for Low Back Pain[7]	-	-	34.3%	37.2%

West Haven VA Medical Center

950 Campbell Avenue
West Haven, CT 06516
URL: www.visn1.med.va.gov/vact
Type: Acute Care - VA
Ownership: Government Federal

Phone: 203-932-5711
Fax: 203-937-3868
Emergency Services: No
Beds: 191

Key Personnel:
Operating Room. . . . . Cindy Christensen
Chief of Medical Staff. . . . . Michael H Ebert, MD
Quality Assurance . . . . Catherine Grabowski
CEO/President. . . . . Roger L Johnson
Pediatric In-Patient Care . . . . Margaret Veazey, RN, MSN

Measure	Cases	This Hosp.	State Avg.	U.S. Avg.
Blood Clot Prevention and Treatment				
Anticoagulation Overlap Therapy	-	-	91%	93%
ICU Venous Thromboembolism Prophylaxis	-	-	93%	92%
Incidence of Potentially Preventable VTE	-	-	6%	10%
UFH with Dosages/Platelet Monitoring	-	-	95%	97%
Venous Thromboembolism Prophylaxis	-	-	89%	85%
Warfarin Therapy Discharge Instructions	-	-	64%	75%
Chest Pain/Possible Heart Attack Care				
Aspirin Given Within 24 Hours of Arrival	-	-	98%	96%
Fibrinolytic Meds Within 30 Min. of Arrival	-	-	33%	58%
Average Time to ECG (minutes)	-	-	7	7
Average Time to Transfer (minutes)	-	-	61	60
Children's Asthma Care				
Received Home Management Plan of Care	-	-	-	88%
Received Reliever Medication	-	-	-	100%
Received Systemic Corticosteroids	-	-	-	100%
Emergency Department				
Admittance Decision Time (minutes)	-	-	147	98
Head CT Results Within 45 Min. of Arrival	-	-	70%	57%
Patients Who Left ER Before Being Seen	-	-	2%	2%
Time from ER Arrival to Admit. (minutes)	-	-	338	274
Time from ER Arrival to Discharge (minutes)	-	-	131	134
Time in ER Before Being Evaluated (minutes)	-	-	28	26
Time to Pain Meds for Fractures (minutes)	-	-	55	57
Heart Attack Care				
Aspirin Given at Discharge	28	100%	99%	99%
Fibrinolytic Meds Within 30 Min. of Arrival[5]	-	-	50%	54%
PCI Within 90 Minutes of Arrival[1]	-	-	96%	96%
Statin Prescribed at Discharge	29	100%	98%	98%
Heart Failure Care				
ACE Inhibitor or ARB for LVSD	29	97%	96%	97%
Discharge Instructions Given	141	99%	93%	94%
Evaluation of LVS Function	163	99%	100%	99%
Medicare Spending				
Medicare Spending per Patient (ratio)	-	-	1.02	0.98
Pneumonia Care				
Appropriate Initial Antibiotic Given	36	97%	97%	95%
Blood Culture Timing	69	99%	97%	98%
Pregnancy and Delivery Care				
Newborn Deliveries Scheduled Early	-	-	5%	6%
Preventive Care				
Immunization for Influenza[5]	-	-	90%	90%
Immunization for Pneumonia[5]	-	-	91%	92%
Stroke Care				
Anticoagulation Therapy for Atrial Fibrillation	-	-	96%	95%
Antithrombotic Therapy Timing	-	-	99%	98%
Assessed for Rehabilitation	-	-	98%	97%
Discharged on Antithrombotic Therapy	-	-	99%	99%
Discharged on Statin Medication	-	-	95%	94%
Thrombolytic Therapy Timing	-	-	71%	66%
Venous Thromboembolism Prophylaxis	-	-	95%	94%
Written Stroke Educational Materials Given	-	-	80%	88%
Surgical Care Improvement Project				
Appropriate Beta Blocker Usage[2]	149	100%	98%	98%
Appropriate VTP Within 24 Hours[2]	175	99%	99%	98%
Controlled Postoperative Blood Glucose[2]	77	87%	96%	97%
Perioperative Temperature Management[2]	213	100%	99%	100%
Prophylactic Antibiotic Selection	174	100%	99%	99%
Prophylactic Antibiotic Selection (Outpatient)	-	-	97%	98%
Prophylactic Antibiotic Stopped	161	98%	98%	98%
Prophylactic Antibiotic Timing	176	99%	98%	99%
Prophylactic Antibiotic Timing (Outpatient)	-	-	97%	98%
Urinary Catheter Removal[2]	107	100%	97%	97%
Survey of Patients' Hospital Experiences				
Area Around Room 'Always' Quiet at Night	-	-	52%	61%
Doctors 'Always' Communicated Well	-	-	80%	82%
Home Recovery Information Given	-	-	85%	85%
Hospital Given 9 or 10 on 10 Point Scale	-	-	68%	71%
Meds 'Always' Explained Before Given	-	-	62%	64%
Nurses 'Always' Communicated Well	-	-	78%	79%
Pain 'Always' Well Controlled	-	-	71%	71%
Room and Bathroom 'Always' Clean	-	-	71%	73%
Timely Help 'Always' Received	-	-	64%	68%
Would Definitely Recommend Hospital	-	-	71%	71%
Use of Medical Imaging				
Cardiac Imaging Stress Test before Surgery	-	-	4.7%	5.3%
Combination Abdominal CT Scan	-	-	5%	10.5%
Combination Brain/Sinus CT Scan	-	-	2.3%	2.7%
Combination Chest CT Scan	-	-	0.9%	2.7%
Follow-up Mammogram/Ultrasound	-	-	19.5%	8.8%
Lumbar Spine MRI for Low Back Pain	-	-	34.3%	37.2%

Windham Community Memorial Hospital & Hatch Hospital

112 Mansfield Ave
Willimantic, CT 06226
E-mail: info@windhamhospital.org
URL: www.wcmh.org
Type: Acute Care Hospitals
Ownership: Voluntary non-profit - Private

Phone: 860-456-9116
Fax: 860-456-6838
Emergency Services: Yes
Beds: 130

Key Personnel:
Radiology. . . . . Bruce Arose, MD
Pediatric Ambulatory Care . . . . . . Thomas Gorin
Pediatric In-Patient Care . . . . Thomas Gorin
Quality Assurance . . . . Annette Hansell
Chief of Medical Staff. . . . . Nadia Nashid, MD
Operating Room. . . . . Francis Siracusa
CEO/President. . . . . David A. Whitehead

Measure	Cases	This Hosp.	State Avg.	U.S. Avg.
Blood Clot Prevention and Treatment				
Anticoagulation Overlap Therapy[2]	32	91%	91%	93%
ICU Venous Thromboembolism Prophylaxis[2]	42	95%	93%	92%
Incidence of Potentially Preventable VTE[1,2]	-	-	6%	10%
UFH with Dosages/Platelet Monitoring[2]	12	50%	95%	97%
Venous Thromboembolism Prophylaxis[2]	377	94%	89%	85%
Warfarin Therapy Discharge Instructions[2]	22	9%	64%	75%
Chest Pain/Possible Heart Attack Care				
Aspirin Given Within 24 Hours of Arrival	39	100%	98%	96%
Fibrinolytic Meds Within 30 Min. of Arrival[1]	-	-	33%	58%
Average Time to ECG (minutes)	39	9	7	7
Average Time to Transfer (minutes)[1]	-	-	61	60
Children's Asthma Care				
Received Home Management Plan of Care	-	-	-	88%
Received Reliever Medication	-	-	-	100%
Received Systemic Corticosteroids	-	-	-	100%
Emergency Department				
Admittance Decision Time (minutes)[2]	589	138	147	98
Head CT Results Within 45 Min. of Arrival	16	69%	70%	57%
Patients Who Left ER Before Being Seen	36,170	0%	2%	2%
Time from ER Arrival to Admit. (minutes)[2]	598	261	338	274
Time from ER Arrival to Discharge (minutes)	406	90	131	134
Time in ER Before Being Evaluated (minutes)	441	14	28	26
Time to Pain Meds for Fractures (minutes)	45	38	55	57
Heart Attack Care				
Aspirin Given at Discharge	16	88%	99%	99%
Fibrinolytic Meds Within 30 Min. of Arrival[7]	-	-	50%	54%
PCI Within 90 Minutes of Arrival[7]	-	-	96%	96%
Statin Prescribed at Discharge	16	100%	98%	98%
Heart Failure Care				
ACE Inhibitor or ARB for LVSD	22	95%	96%	97%
Discharge Instructions Given	71	93%	93%	94%
Evaluation of LVS Function	109	100%	100%	99%
Medicare Spending				
Medicare Spending per Patient (ratio)	-	0.96	1.02	0.98

NOTE: Hospital profiles are in alphabetical order by state, then city, then hospital within the city; Rankings exclude hospitals with less than 25 cases except for patient surveys which excludes hospitals with less than 100 cases; (a) 100-299 cases; (1) The number of cases/patients is too few to report; (2) Data submitted were based on a sample of cases/patients; (3) Results are based on a shorter time period than required; (4) Data suppressed by CMS for one or more quarters; (5) Results are not available for this reporting period; (6) Fewer than 100 patients completed the HCAHPS survey; (7) No cases met the criteria for this measure; (8) The lower limit of the confidence interval cannot be calculated if the number of observed infections equals zero; (9) No data are available from the state/territory for this reporting period; (10) The scores shown reflect fewer than 50 completed surveys; (11) There were discrepancies in the data collection process; (12) This measure does not apply to this hospital for this reporting period; (13) Results cannot be calculated for this reporting period; (14) The results for this state are combined with nearby states to protect confidentiality; Please refer to the User's Guide for a full explanation of data.

Pneumonia Care				
Appropriate Initial Antibiotic Given	87	94%	97%	95%
Blood Culture Timing	123	98%	97%	98%
Pregnancy and Delivery Care				
Newborn Deliveries Scheduled Early	26	8%	5%	6%
Preventive Care				
Immunization for Influenza[2]	400	96%	90%	90%
Immunization for Pneumonia[2]	536	97%	91%	92%
Stroke Care				
Anticoagulation Therapy for Atrial Fibrillation	11	91%	96%	95%
Antithrombotic Therapy Timing	30	100%	99%	98%
Assessed for Rehabilitation	34	94%	98%	97%
Discharged on Antithrombotic Therapy	32	97%	99%	99%
Discharged on Statin Medication	23	100%	95%	94%
Thrombolytic Therapy Timing[1]	-	-	71%	66%
Venous Thromboembolism Prophylaxis	31	97%	95%	94%
Written Stroke Educational Materials Given	16	81%	80%	88%
Surgical Care Improvement Project				
Appropriate Beta Blocker Usage	27	96%	98%	98%
Appropriate VTP Within 24 Hours	105	97%	99%	98%
Controlled Postoperative Blood Glucose[7]	-	-	96%	97%
Perioperative Temperature Management	124	100%	99%	100%
Prophylactic Antibiotic Selection	69	99%	99%	99%
Prophylactic Antibiotic Selection (Outpatient)	33	100%	97%	98%
Prophylactic Antibiotic Stopped	67	91%	98%	98%
Prophylactic Antibiotic Timing	69	97%	98%	99%
Prophylactic Antibiotic Timing (Outpatient)	33	100%	97%	98%
Urinary Catheter Removal	87	97%	97%	97%
Survey of Patients' Hospital Experiences				
Area Around Room 'Always' Quiet at Night	300+	47%	52%	61%
Doctors 'Always' Communicated Well	300+	81%	80%	82%
Home Recovery Information Given	300+	87%	85%	85%
Hospital Given 9 or 10 on 10 Point Scale	300+	63%	68%	71%
Meds 'Always' Explained Before Given	300+	64%	62%	64%
Nurses 'Always' Communicated Well	300+	78%	78%	79%
Pain 'Always' Well Controlled	300+	73%	71%	71%
Room and Bathroom 'Always' Clean	300+	70%	71%	73%
Timely Help 'Always' Received	300+	66%	64%	68%
Would Definitely Recommend Hospital	300+	65%	71%	71%
Use of Medical Imaging				
Cardiac Imaging Stress Test before Surgery	268	4.5%	4.7%	5.3%
Combination Abdominal CT Scan	589	3.7%	5%	10.5%
Combination Brain/Sinus CT Scan[1]	-	-	2.3%	2.7%
Combination Chest CT Scan	513	22.0%	0.9%	2.7%
Follow-up Mammogram/Ultrasound	1,269	10.8%	19.5%	8.8%
Lumbar Spine MRI for Low Back Pain	93	45.2%	34.3%	37.2%

NOTE: Hospital profiles are in alphabetical order by state, then city, then hospital within the city; Rankings exclude hospitals with less than 25 cases except for patient surveys which excludes hospitals with less than 100 cases; (a) 100-299 cases; (1) The number of cases/patients is too few to report; (2) Data submitted were based on a sample of cases/patients; (3) Results are based on a shorter time period than required; (4) Data suppressed by CMS for one or more quarters; (5) Results are not available for this reporting period; (6) Fewer than 100 patients completed the HCAHPS survey; (7) No cases met the criteria for this measure; (8) The lower limit of the confidence interval cannot be calculated if the number of observed infections equals zero; (9) No data are available from the state/territory for this reporting period; (10) The scores shown reflect fewer than 50 completed surveys; (11) There were discrepancies in the data collection process; (12) This measure does not apply to this hospital for this reporting period; (13) Results cannot be calculated for this reporting period; (14) The results for this state are combined with nearby states to protect confidentiality; Please refer to the User's Guide for a full explanation of data.

Blood Clot Prevention and Treatment

Anticoagulation Overlap Therapy

Hospital Name	City	Rate	Cases
Saint Francis Hospital[2]	Wilmington	96%	25
Bayhealth - Milford Memorial Hospital[2]	Milford	95%	38
Beebe Medical Center[2]	Lewes	89%	87
Bayhealth - Kent General Hospital[2]	Dover	88%	101
Christiana Care Health Services[2]	Newark	86%	182

ICU Venous Thromboembolism Prophylaxis

Hospital Name	City	Rate	Cases
Christiana Care Health Services[2]	Newark	98%	48
Saint Francis Hospital[2]	Wilmington	96%	78
Bayhealth - Kent General Hospital[2]	Dover	95%	63
Nanticoke Memorial Hospital[2]	Seaford	95%	56
Beebe Medical Center[2]	Lewes	86%	59
Bayhealth - Milford Memorial Hospital[2]	Milford	83%	69

Incidence of Potentially Preventable VTE

Hospital Name	City	Rate	Cases
Christiana Care Health Services[2]	Newark	7%	90

UFH with Dosages/Platelet Count Monitoring

Hospital Name	City	Rate	Cases
Beebe Medical Center[2]	Lewes	98%	47
Bayhealth - Kent General Hospital[2]	Dover	96%	54
Christiana Care Health Services[2]	Newark	70%	105

Venous Thromboembolism Prophylaxis

Hospital Name	City	Rate	Cases
Christiana Care Health Services[2]	Newark	92%	370
Bayhealth - Milford Memorial Hospital[2]	Milford	91%	374
Bayhealth - Kent General Hospital[2]	Dover	87%	389
Saint Francis Hospital[2]	Wilmington	83%	364
Nanticoke Memorial Hospital[2]	Seaford	81%	390
Beebe Medical Center[2]	Lewes	68%	392

Warfarin Therapy Discharge Instructions

Hospital Name	City	Rate	Cases
Beebe Medical Center[2]	Lewes	42%	72
Bayhealth - Milford Memorial Hospital[2]	Milford	31%	29
Bayhealth - Kent General Hospital[2]	Dover	21%	71
Christiana Care Health Services[2]	Newark	15%	119

Chest Pain/Possible Heart Attack Care

Aspirin Given Within 24 Hours of Arrival

Hospital Name	City	Rate	Cases
Bayhealth - Milford Memorial Hospital	Milford	100%	25

Average Time to ECG (minutes)

Hospital Name	City	Min.	Cases
Bayhealth - Milford Memorial Hospital	Milford	6	26

Children's Asthma Care

No hospitals met the 25 case threshold.

Emergency Department

Admittance Decision Time (minutes)

Hospital Name	City	Min.	Cases
Nanticoke Memorial Hospital[2]	Seaford	130	719
Christiana Care Health Services[2]	Newark	156	182
Saint Francis Hospital[2]	Wilmington	166	644
Beebe Medical Center[2]	Lewes	201	717
Bayhealth - Milford Memorial Hospital[2]	Milford	236	669
Bayhealth - Kent General Hospital[2]	Dover	262	682

Head CT Results Within 45 Minutes of Arrival

Hospital Name	City	Rate	Cases
Beebe Medical Center	Lewes	72%	32

Patients Who Left ER Before Being Seen

Hospital Name	City	Rate	Cases
Beebe Medical Center	Lewes	0%	47316
Nanticoke Memorial Hospital	Seaford	2%	38433
Saint Francis Hospital	Wilmington	3%	35936
Bayhealth - Milford Memorial Hospital	Milford	4%	26013
Christiana Care Health Services	Newark	4%	173702
Bayhealth - Kent General Hospital	Dover	6%	44307

Time from ER Arrival to Being Admitted (minutes)

Hospital Name	City	Min.	Cases
Nanticoke Memorial Hospital[2]	Seaford	304	721
Saint Francis Hospital[2]	Wilmington	341	683
Beebe Medical Center[2]	Lewes	394	717
Bayhealth - Milford Memorial Hospital[2]	Milford	404	672
Christiana Care Health Services[2]	Newark	420	182
Bayhealth - Kent General Hospital[2]	Dover	455	685

Time from ER Arrival to Discharge (minutes)

Hospital Name	City	Min.	Cases
Saint Francis Hospital	Wilmington	112	380
Bayhealth - Milford Memorial Hospital	Milford	144	391
Nanticoke Memorial Hospital	Seaford	145	333
Beebe Medical Center	Lewes	148	367
Christiana Care Health Services[3]	Newark	185	171
Bayhealth - Kent General Hospital	Dover	213	385

Time in ER Before Being Evaluated (minutes)

Hospital Name	City	Min.	Cases
Beebe Medical Center	Lewes	29	399
Nanticoke Memorial Hospital	Seaford	34	381
Bayhealth - Milford Memorial Hospital	Milford	36	409
Saint Francis Hospital	Wilmington	40	401
Bayhealth - Kent General Hospital	Dover	44	413
Christiana Care Health Services	Newark	65	371

Time to Pain Meds for Bone Fractures (minutes)

Hospital Name	City	Min.	Cases
Beebe Medical Center	Lewes	67	131
Bayhealth - Kent General Hospital	Dover	68	164
Nanticoke Memorial Hospital	Seaford	69	103
Christiana Care Health Services	Newark	75	149
Bayhealth - Milford Memorial Hospital	Milford	86	47
Saint Francis Hospital	Wilmington	93	28

Heart Attack Care

Aspirin Given at Discharge

Hospital Name	City	Rate	Cases
Bayhealth - Kent General Hospital[2]	Dover	100%	280
Bayhealth - Milford Memorial Hospital	Milford	100%	26
Beebe Medical Center	Lewes	100%	215
Christiana Care Health Services	Newark	100%	738
Nanticoke Memorial Hospital	Seaford	99%	91
Saint Francis Hospital	Wilmington	99%	121

PCI Within 90 Minutes of Arrival

Hospital Name	City	Rate	Cases
Beebe Medical Center	Lewes	100%	26
Bayhealth - Kent General Hospital[2]	Dover	97%	34
Christiana Care Health Services	Newark	95%	153

Statin Prescribed at Discharge

Hospital Name	City	Rate	Cases
Bayhealth - Kent General Hospital[2]	Dover	100%	278
Bayhealth - Milford Memorial Hospital	Milford	100%	26
Christiana Care Health Services	Newark	100%	730
Nanticoke Memorial Hospital	Seaford	99%	97
Beebe Medical Center	Lewes	98%	210
Saint Francis Hospital	Wilmington	97%	112

Heart Failure Care

ACE Inhibitor or ARB for LVSD

Hospital Name	City	Rate	Cases
Bayhealth - Kent General Hospital[2]	Dover	100%	118
Saint Francis Hospital	Wilmington	100%	72
Wilmington VA Medical Center	Wilmington	100%	25
Bayhealth - Milford Memorial Hospital	Milford	99%	68
Nanticoke Memorial Hospital	Seaford	99%	67
Beebe Medical Center	Lewes	98%	92
Christiana Care Health Services[2]	Newark	97%	256

Discharge Instructions Given

Hospital Name	City	Rate	Cases
Wilmington VA Medical Center	Wilmington	100%	67
Saint Francis Hospital	Wilmington	99%	132
Beebe Medical Center	Lewes	97%	258
Bayhealth - Kent General Hospital[2]	Dover	96%	259
Bayhealth - Milford Memorial Hospital	Milford	95%	156
Christiana Care Health Services[2]	Newark	95%	686
Nanticoke Memorial Hospital	Seaford	95%	209

Evaluation of LVS Function

Hospital Name	City	Rate	Cases
Bayhealth - Kent General Hospital[2]	Dover	100%	310
Bayhealth - Milford Memorial Hospital	Milford	100%	193
Beebe Medical Center	Lewes	100%	329
Christiana Care Health Services[2]	Newark	100%	798
Nanticoke Memorial Hospital	Seaford	100%	299
Saint Francis Hospital	Wilmington	100%	149
Wilmington VA Medical Center	Wilmington	100%	72

Medicare Spending

Medicare Spending per Patient (ratio)

Hospital Name	City	Ratio	Cases
Bayhealth - Milford Memorial Hospital	Milford	0.97	-
Beebe Medical Center	Lewes	0.99	-
Nanticoke Memorial Hospital	Seaford	0.99	-
Christiana Care Health Services	Newark	1.00	-
Saint Francis Hospital	Wilmington	1.02	-
Bayhealth - Kent General Hospital	Dover	1.03	-

Pneumonia Care

Appropriate Initial Antibiotic Given

Hospital Name	City	Rate	Cases
Nanticoke Memorial Hospital	Seaford	100%	154
Bayhealth - Kent General Hospital[2]	Dover	99%	74
Beebe Medical Center	Lewes	99%	239
Saint Francis Hospital	Wilmington	98%	91
Christiana Care Health Services[2]	Newark	94%	277
Bayhealth - Milford Memorial Hospital[2]	Milford	93%	76

Blood Culture Timing

Hospital Name	City	Rate	Cases
Wilmington VA Medical Center	Wilmington	100%	35
Bayhealth - Kent General Hospital[2]	Dover	99%	151
Bayhealth - Milford Memorial Hospital[2]	Milford	99%	145
Beebe Medical Center	Lewes	99%	259
Saint Francis Hospital	Wilmington	99%	135
Christiana Care Health Services[2]	Newark	95%	353
Nanticoke Memorial Hospital	Seaford	95%	164

Pregnancy and Delivery Care

Newborns whose Deliveries were Scheduled Early

Hospital Name	City	Rate	Cases
Bayhealth - Milford Memorial Hospital	Milford	0%	25
Bayhealth - Kent General Hospital	Dover	1%	141
Christiana Care Health Services[2]	Newark	1%	368
Saint Francis Hospital	Wilmington	1%	74
Nanticoke Memorial Hospital[2]	Seaford	7%	27
Beebe Medical Center	Lewes	12%	65

Preventive Care

Immunization for Influenza

Hospital Name	City	Rate	Cases
Bayhealth - Milford Memorial Hospital[2]	Milford	99%	432
Bayhealth - Kent General Hospital[2]	Dover	98%	539
Wilmington VA Medical Center[2,3]	Wilmington	98%	144
Beebe Medical Center[2]	Lewes	97%	554
Saint Francis Hospital[2]	Wilmington	96%	539
Christiana Care Health Services[2]	Newark	91%	620
Nanticoke Memorial Hospital[2]	Seaford	91%	485

Immunization for Pneumonia

Hospital Name	City	Rate	Cases
Bayhealth - Milford Memorial Hospital[2]	Milford	99%	596
Beebe Medical Center[2]	Lewes	99%	785
Bayhealth - Kent General Hospital[2]	Dover	98%	658
Wilmington VA Medical Center[2,3]	Wilmington	97%	336
Saint Francis Hospital[2]	Wilmington	96%	568
Christiana Care Health Services[2]	Newark	93%	543
Nanticoke Memorial Hospital[2]	Seaford	86%	625

Stroke Care

Anticoagulation Therapy for Atrial Fibrillation

Hospital Name	City	Rate	Cases
Beebe Medical Center	Lewes	95%	38
Christiana Care Health Services[2]	Newark	92%	39

Antithrombotic Therapy Timing

Hospital Name	City	Rate	Cases
Nanticoke Memorial Hospital[2]	Seaford	99%	68
Bayhealth - Milford Memorial Hospital	Milford	98%	60

NOTE: Hospital profiles are in alphabetical order by state, then city, then hospital within the city; Rankings exclude hospitals with less than 25 cases except for patient surveys which excludes hospitals with less than 100 cases; (a) 100-299 cases; (1) The number of cases/patients is too few to report; (2) Data submitted were based on a sample of cases/patients; (3) Results are based on a shorter time period than required; (4) Data suppressed by CMS for one or more quarters; (5) Results are not available for this reporting period; (6) Fewer than 100 patients completed the HCAHPS survey; (7) No cases met the criteria for this measure; (8) The lower limit of the confidence interval cannot be calculated if the number of observed infections equals zero; (9) No data are available from the state/territory for this reporting period; (10) The scores shown reflect fewer than 50 completed surveys; (11) There were discrepancies in the data collection process; (12) This measure does not apply to this hospital for this reporting period; (13) Results cannot be calculated for this reporting period; (14) The results for this state are combined with nearby states to protect confidentiality; Please refer to the User's Guide for a full explanation of data.

Hospital Name	City	Rate	Cases
Saint Francis Hospital	Wilmington	97%	58
Bayhealth - Kent General Hospital	Dover	96%	139
Beebe Medical Center	Lewes	96%	139
Christiana Care Health Services[2]	Newark	94%	269

Assessed for Rehabilitation

Hospital Name	City	Rate	Cases
Christiana Care Health Services[2]	Newark	100%	384
Saint Francis Hospital	Wilmington	100%	59
Bayhealth - Kent General Hospital	Dover	99%	158
Bayhealth - Milford Memorial Hospital	Milford	99%	67
Nanticoke Memorial Hospital[2]	Seaford	96%	67
Beebe Medical Center	Lewes	93%	180

Discharged on Antithrombotic Therapy

Hospital Name	City	Rate	Cases
Nanticoke Memorial Hospital[2]	Seaford	100%	66
Saint Francis Hospital	Wilmington	100%	56
Bayhealth - Kent General Hospital	Dover	99%	139
Christiana Care Health Services[2]	Newark	99%	317
Beebe Medical Center	Lewes	97%	177
Bayhealth - Milford Memorial Hospital	Milford	94%	66

Discharged on Statin Medication

Hospital Name	City	Rate	Cases
Nanticoke Memorial Hospital[2]	Seaford	98%	59
Saint Francis Hospital	Wilmington	98%	46
Bayhealth - Kent General Hospital	Dover	97%	112
Christiana Care Health Services[2]	Newark	95%	256
Bayhealth - Milford Memorial Hospital	Milford	94%	47
Beebe Medical Center	Lewes	89%	144

Thrombolytic Therapy Timing

Hospital Name	City	Rate	Cases
Christiana Care Health Services[2]	Newark	97%	31

Venous Thromboembolism (VTE) Prophylaxis

Hospital Name	City	Rate	Cases
Beebe Medical Center	Lewes	97%	142
Christiana Care Health Services[2]	Newark	95%	393
Saint Francis Hospital	Wilmington	95%	62
Nanticoke Memorial Hospital[2]	Seaford	94%	67
Bayhealth - Kent General Hospital	Dover	84%	166
Bayhealth - Milford Memorial Hospital	Milford	78%	64

Written Stroke Educational Materials Given

Hospital Name	City	Rate	Cases
Saint Francis Hospital	Wilmington	100%	30
Bayhealth - Milford Memorial Hospital	Milford	97%	38
Bayhealth - Kent General Hospital	Dover	96%	80
Nanticoke Memorial Hospital[2]	Seaford	92%	37
Christiana Care Health Services[2]	Newark	86%	215
Beebe Medical Center	Lewes	75%	114

Surgical Care Improvement Project

Appropriate Beta Blocker Usage

Hospital Name	City	Rate	Cases
Bayhealth - Milford Memorial Hospital[2]	Milford	100%	58
Beebe Medical Center	Lewes	100%	532
Nanticoke Memorial Hospital[2]	Seaford	100%	64
Wilmington VA Medical Center[2]	Wilmington	100%	25
Christiana Care Health Services[2]	Newark	99%	381
Bayhealth - Kent General Hospital[2]	Dover	98%	242
Saint Francis Hospital	Wilmington	91%	70

Appropriate VTP Within 24 Hours

Hospital Name	City	Rate	Cases
Bayhealth - Milford Memorial Hospital[2]	Milford	100%	156
Beebe Medical Center	Lewes	100%	973
Wilmington VA Medical Center[2]	Wilmington	100%	53
Bayhealth - Kent General Hospital[2]	Dover	99%	421
Christiana Care Health Services[2]	Newark	99%	680
Nanticoke Memorial Hospital[2]	Seaford	96%	183
Saint Francis Hospital	Wilmington	95%	220

Controlled Postoperative Blood Glucose

Hospital Name	City	Rate	Cases
Bayhealth - Kent General Hospital[2]	Dover	100%	115
Christiana Care Health Services[2]	Newark	99%	203
Saint Francis Hospital	Wilmington	96%	27
Beebe Medical Center	Lewes	95%	123

Perioperative Temperature Management

Hospital Name	City	Rate	Cases
Bayhealth - Kent General Hospital[2]	Dover	100%	486
Bayhealth - Milford Memorial Hospital[2]	Milford	100%	177
Beebe Medical Center	Lewes	100%	1097
Christiana Care Health Services[2]	Newark	100%	889
Nanticoke Memorial Hospital[2]	Seaford	100%	211
Saint Francis Hospital	Wilmington	100%	265
Wilmington VA Medical Center[2]	Wilmington	100%	73

Prophylactic Antibiotic Selection

Hospital Name	City	Rate	Cases
Bayhealth - Kent General Hospital[2]	Dover	100%	424
Beebe Medical Center	Lewes	100%	925
Christiana Care Health Services[2]	Newark	100%	711
Nanticoke Memorial Hospital[2]	Seaford	100%	116
Bayhealth - Milford Memorial Hospital[2]	Milford	99%	112
Saint Francis Hospital	Wilmington	99%	168

Prophylactic Antibiotic Selection (Outpatient)

Hospital Name	City	Rate	Cases
Nanticoke Memorial Hospital	Seaford	100%	61
Saint Francis Hospital	Wilmington	100%	204
Christiana Care Health Services	Newark	99%	866
Bayhealth - Kent General Hospital	Dover	98%	174
Beebe Medical Center	Lewes	98%	405

Prophylactic Antibiotic Stopped

Hospital Name	City	Rate	Cases
Bayhealth - Milford Memorial Hospital[2]	Milford	100%	110
Christiana Care Health Services[2]	Newark	100%	700
Bayhealth - Kent General Hospital[2]	Dover	99%	405
Beebe Medical Center	Lewes	99%	920
Nanticoke Memorial Hospital[2]	Seaford	96%	113
Saint Francis Hospital	Wilmington	96%	159

Prophylactic Antibiotic Timing

Hospital Name	City	Rate	Cases
Beebe Medical Center	Lewes	100%	927
Bayhealth - Kent General Hospital[2]	Dover	99%	424
Christiana Care Health Services[2]	Newark	99%	712
Nanticoke Memorial Hospital[2]	Seaford	99%	116
Saint Francis Hospital	Wilmington	99%	168
Bayhealth - Milford Memorial Hospital[2]	Milford	98%	112

Prophylactic Antibiotic Timing (Outpatient)

Hospital Name	City	Rate	Cases
Beebe Medical Center	Lewes	100%	396
Saint Francis Hospital	Wilmington	100%	205
Bayhealth - Kent General Hospital	Dover	98%	176
Christiana Care Health Services	Newark	98%	855
Nanticoke Memorial Hospital	Seaford	90%	67

Urinary Catheter Removal

Hospital Name	City	Rate	Cases
Bayhealth - Milford Memorial Hospital[2]	Milford	100%	105
Beebe Medical Center	Lewes	100%	989
Wilmington VA Medical Center[2]	Wilmington	100%	41
Christiana Care Health Services[2]	Newark	99%	566
Bayhealth - Kent General Hospital[2]	Dover	98%	368
Saint Francis Hospital	Wilmington	95%	130
Nanticoke Memorial Hospital[2]	Seaford	93%	138

Survey of Patients' Hospital Experiences

Area Around Room 'Always' Quiet at Night

Hospital Name	City	Rate	Cases
Saint Francis Hospital	Wilmington	61%	300+
Bayhealth - Kent General Hospital	Dover	53%	300+
Beebe Medical Center	Lewes	51%	300+
Christiana Care Health Services[11]	Newark	51%	300+
Nanticoke Memorial Hospital	Seaford	50%	300+
Bayhealth - Milford Memorial Hospital	Milford	48%	300+

Doctors 'Always' Communicated Well

Hospital Name	City	Rate	Cases
Nanticoke Memorial Hospital	Seaford	82%	300+
Beebe Medical Center	Lewes	80%	300+
Christiana Care Health Services[11]	Newark	79%	300+
Bayhealth - Kent General Hospital	Dover	76%	300+
Bayhealth - Milford Memorial Hospital	Milford	76%	300+
Saint Francis Hospital	Wilmington	76%	300+

Home Recovery Information Given

Hospital Name	City	Rate	Cases
Nanticoke Memorial Hospital	Seaford	88%	300+
Bayhealth - Milford Memorial Hospital	Milford	86%	300+
Christiana Care Health Services[11]	Newark	86%	300+
Bayhealth - Kent General Hospital	Dover	84%	300+
Beebe Medical Center	Lewes	83%	300+
Saint Francis Hospital	Wilmington	81%	300+

Hospital Given 9 or 10 on 10 Point Scale

Hospital Name	City	Rate	Cases
Christiana Care Health Services[11]	Newark	72%	300+
Nanticoke Memorial Hospital	Seaford	70%	300+
Beebe Medical Center	Lewes	67%	300+
Bayhealth - Kent General Hospital	Dover	66%	300+
Saint Francis Hospital	Wilmington	65%	300+
Bayhealth - Milford Memorial Hospital	Milford	61%	300+

Meds 'Always' Explained Before Given

Hospital Name	City	Rate	Cases
Beebe Medical Center	Lewes	69%	300+
Nanticoke Memorial Hospital	Seaford	65%	300+
Christiana Care Health Services[11]	Newark	64%	300+
Bayhealth - Kent General Hospital	Dover	61%	300+
Bayhealth - Milford Memorial Hospital	Milford	61%	300+
Saint Francis Hospital	Wilmington	61%	300+

Nurses 'Always' Communicated Well

Hospital Name	City	Rate	Cases
Beebe Medical Center	Lewes	82%	300+
Nanticoke Memorial Hospital	Seaford	82%	300+
Bayhealth - Kent General Hospital	Dover	80%	300+
Christiana Care Health Services[11]	Newark	80%	300+
Bayhealth - Milford Memorial Hospital	Milford	76%	300+
Saint Francis Hospital	Wilmington	75%	300+

Pain 'Always' Well Controlled

Hospital Name	City	Rate	Cases
Beebe Medical Center	Lewes	73%	300+
Christiana Care Health Services[11]	Newark	71%	300+
Bayhealth - Milford Memorial Hospital	Milford	70%	300+
Nanticoke Memorial Hospital	Seaford	70%	300+
Saint Francis Hospital	Wilmington	70%	300+
Bayhealth - Kent General Hospital	Dover	69%	300+

Room and Bathroom 'Always' Clean

Hospital Name	City	Rate	Cases
Bayhealth - Kent General Hospital	Dover	72%	300+
Bayhealth - Milford Memorial Hospital	Milford	72%	300+
Nanticoke Memorial Hospital	Seaford	72%	300+
Beebe Medical Center	Lewes	71%	300+
Christiana Care Health Services[11]	Newark	71%	300+
Saint Francis Hospital	Wilmington	64%	300+

Timely Help 'Always' Received

Hospital Name	City	Rate	Cases
Beebe Medical Center	Lewes	70%	300+
Christiana Care Health Services[11]	Newark	70%	300+
Bayhealth - Kent General Hospital	Dover	66%	300+
Nanticoke Memorial Hospital	Seaford	66%	300+
Bayhealth - Milford Memorial Hospital	Milford	63%	300+
Saint Francis Hospital	Wilmington	63%	300+

Would Definitely Recommend Hospital

Hospital Name	City	Rate	Cases
Christiana Care Health Services[11]	Newark	76%	300+
Beebe Medical Center	Lewes	72%	300+
Bayhealth - Kent General Hospital	Dover	67%	300+
Nanticoke Memorial Hospital	Seaford	67%	300+
Saint Francis Hospital	Wilmington	66%	300+
Bayhealth - Milford Memorial Hospital	Milford	60%	300+

Use of Medical Imaging

Cardiac Imaging Stress Test before OP Surgery

Hospital Name	City	Rate	Cases
Beebe Medical Center	Lewes	3.2%	466
Bayhealth - Kent General Hospital	Dover	3.9%	726
Christiana Care Health Services	Newark	4.1%	1884
Nanticoke Memorial Hospital	Seaford	4.3%	300
Saint Francis Hospital	Wilmington	5.1%	137
Bayhealth - Milford Memorial Hospital	Milford	5.2%	675

Combination Abdominal CT Scan

Hospital Name	City	Rate	Cases
Saint Francis Hospital	Wilmington	2.1%	438
Nanticoke Memorial Hospital	Seaford	3.4%	893
Christiana Care Health Services	Newark	5.5%	4639
Beebe Medical Center	Lewes	5.8%	2673
Bayhealth - Milford Memorial Hospital	Milford	7.0%	848
Bayhealth - Kent General Hospital	Dover	8.7%	2211

NOTE: Hospital profiles are in alphabetical order by state, then city, then hospital within the city; Rankings exclude hospitals with less than 25 cases except for patient surveys which excludes hospitals with less than 100 cases; (a) 100-299 cases; (1) The number of cases/patients is too few to report; (2) Data submitted were based on a sample of cases/patients; (3) Results are based on a shorter time period than required; (4) Data suppressed by CMS for one or more quarters; (5) Results are not available for this reporting period; (6) Fewer than 100 patients completed the HCAHPS survey; (7) No cases met the criteria for this measure; (8) The lower limit of the confidence interval cannot be calculated if the number of observed infections equals zero; (9) No data are available from the state/territory for this reporting period; (10) The scores shown reflect fewer than 50 completed surveys; (11) There were discrepancies in the data collection process; (12) This measure does not apply to this hospital for this reporting period; (13) Results cannot be calculated for this reporting period; (14) The results for this state are combined with nearby states to protect confidentiality; Please refer to the User's Guide for a full explanation of data.

Combination Brain/Sinus CT Scan

Hospital Name	City	Rate	Cases
Christiana Care Health Services	Newark	0.0%	3024
Beebe Medical Center	Lewes	2.3%	1768
Nanticoke Memorial Hospital	Seaford	3.8%	807
Bayhealth - Milford Memorial Hospital	Milford	4.7%	619
Saint Francis Hospital	Wilmington	5.3%	550
Bayhealth - Kent General Hospital	Dover	5.7%	1603

Combination Chest CT Scan

Hospital Name	City	Rate	Cases
Nanticoke Memorial Hospital	Seaford	0.0%	618
Bayhealth - Kent General Hospital	Dover	0.1%	1519
Christiana Care Health Services	Newark	0.5%	4234
Saint Francis Hospital	Wilmington	1.3%	228
Bayhealth - Milford Memorial Hospital	Milford	1.4%	627
Beebe Medical Center	Lewes	1.5%	1966

Follow-up Mammogram/Ultrasound

A follow-up rate near zero may indicate missed cancer; a rate higher than 14% may mean there is unnecessary follow up.

Hospital Name	City	Rate	Cases
Saint Francis Hospital	Wilmington	3.6%	948
Beebe Medical Center	Lewes	6.0%	3793
Nanticoke Memorial Hospital	Seaford	8.6%	1506
Christiana Care Health Services	Newark	8.9%	4580
Bayhealth - Milford Memorial Hospital	Milford	12.9%	1216
Bayhealth - Kent General Hospital	Dover	13.7%	2978

Lumbar Spine MRI for Low Back Pain

Hospital Name	City	Rate	Cases
Bayhealth - Milford Memorial Hospital	Milford	23.4%	64
Bayhealth - Kent General Hospital	Dover	27.0%	148
Christiana Care Health Services	Newark	31.0%	583
Beebe Medical Center	Lewes	36.3%	234
Saint Francis Hospital	Wilmington	40.4%	47

NOTE: Hospital profiles are in alphabetical order by state, then city, then hospital within the city; Rankings exclude hospitals with less than 25 cases except for patient surveys which excludes hospitals with less than 100 cases; (a) 100-299 cases; (1) The number of cases/patients is too few to report; (2) Data submitted were based on a sample of cases/patients; (3) Results are based on a shorter time period than required; (4) Data suppressed by CMS for one or more quarters; (5) Results are not available for this reporting period; (6) Fewer than 100 patients completed the HCAHPS survey; (7) No cases met the criteria for this measure; (8) The lower limit of the confidence interval cannot be calculated if the number of observed infections equals zero; (9) No data are available from the state/territory for this reporting period; (10) The scores shown reflect fewer than 50 completed surveys; (11) There were discrepancies in the data collection process; (12) This measure does not apply to this hospital for this reporting period; (13) Results cannot be calculated for this reporting period; (14) The results for this state are combined with nearby states to protect confidentiality; Please refer to the User's Guide for a full explanation of data.

Bayhealth - Kent General Hospital

640 S State Street — Phone: 302-744-7001
Dover, DE 19901 — Fax: 302-735-3227
URL: www.bayhealth.org/about/kent.asp
Type: Acute Care Hospitals — Emergency Services: Yes
Ownership: Voluntary non-profit - Private — Beds: 231

Key Personnel:
Quality Assurance . . . . Joann Davis
Emergency Room . . . . Craig Hochstein, MD
CEO/President. . . . . Dennis E Klima
Patient Relations . . . . Cathy Marketto
Anesthesiology. . . . . Brian McCarthy
Ambulatory Care . . . . Al Pilong
Operating Room. . . . . Chris Price
Chief of Medical Staff. . . . . William Rosenfeld

Measure	Cases	This Hosp.	State Avg.	U.S. Avg.
Blood Clot Prevention and Treatment				
Anticoagulation Overlap Therapy[2]	101	88%	88%	93%
ICU Venous Thromboembolism Prophylaxis[2]	63	95%	92%	92%
Incidence of Potentially Preventable VTE[2]	14	0%	8%	10%
UFH with Dosages/Platelet Monitoring[2]	54	96%	84%	97%
Venous Thromboembolism Prophylaxis[2]	389	87%	83%	85%
Warfarin Therapy Discharge Instructions[2]	71	21%	27%	75%
Chest Pain/Possible Heart Attack Care				
Aspirin Given Within 24 Hours of Arrival	22	91%	95%	96%
Fibrinolytic Meds Within 30 Min. of Arrival[3,7]	-	-	-	58%
Average Time to ECG (minutes)	23	11	7	7
Average Time to Transfer (minutes)[3,7]	-	-	120	60
Children's Asthma Care				
Received Home Management Plan of Care	-	-	-	88%
Received Reliever Medication	-	-	-	100%
Received Systemic Corticosteroids	-	-	-	100%
Emergency Department				
Admittance Decision Time (minutes)[2]	682	262	190	98
Head CT Results Within 45 Min. of Arrival[1]	-	-	59%	57%
Patients Who Left ER Before Being Seen	44,307	6%	3%	2%
Time from ER Arrival to Admit. (minutes)[2]	685	455	374	274
Time from ER Arrival to Discharge (minutes)	385	213	153	134
Time in ER Before Being Evaluated (minutes)	413	44	40	26
Time to Pain Meds for Fractures (minutes)	164	68	72	57
Heart Attack Care				
Aspirin Given at Discharge[2]	280	100%	100%	99%
Fibrinolytic Meds Within 30 Min. of Arrival[2,7]	-	-	-	54%
PCI Within 90 Minutes of Arrival[2]	34	97%	97%	96%
Statin Prescribed at Discharge[2]	278	100%	99%	98%
Heart Failure Care				
ACE Inhibitor or ARB for LVSD[2]	118	100%	98%	97%
Discharge Instructions Given[2]	259	96%	96%	94%
Evaluation of LVS Function[2]	310	100%	100%	99%
Medicare Spending				
Medicare Spending per Patient (ratio)	-	1.03	1	0.98
Pneumonia Care				
Appropriate Initial Antibiotic Given[2]	74	99%	97%	95%
Blood Culture Timing[2]	151	99%	98%	98%
Pregnancy and Delivery Care				
Newborn Deliveries Scheduled Early	141	1%	2%	6%
Preventive Care				
Immunization for Influenza[2]	539	98%	95%	90%
Immunization for Pneumonia[2]	658	98%	96%	92%
Stroke Care				
Anticoagulation Therapy for Atrial Fibrillation	18	89%	92%	95%
Antithrombotic Therapy Timing	139	96%	96%	98%
Assessed for Rehabilitation	158	99%	98%	97%
Discharged on Antithrombotic Therapy	139	99%	98%	99%
Discharged on Statin Medication	112	97%	95%	94%
Thrombolytic Therapy Timing[1]	-	-	75%	66%
Venous Thromboembolism Prophylaxis	166	84%	92%	94%
Written Stroke Educational Materials Given	80	96%	87%	88%
Surgical Care Improvement Project				
Appropriate Beta Blocker Usage[2]	242	98%	99%	98%
Appropriate VTP Within 24 Hours[2]	421	99%	99%	98%
Controlled Postoperative Blood Glucose[2]	115	100%	98%	97%
Perioperative Temperature Management[2]	486	100%	100%	100%
Prophylactic Antibiotic Selection[2]	424	100%	100%	99%
Prophylactic Antibiotic Selection (Outpatient)	174	98%	99%	98%
Prophylactic Antibiotic Stopped[2]	405	99%	99%	98%
Prophylactic Antibiotic Timing[2]	424	99%	99%	99%
Prophylactic Antibiotic Timing (Outpatient)	176	98%	98%	98%
Urinary Catheter Removal[2]	368	98%	99%	97%
Survey of Patients' Hospital Experiences				
Area Around Room 'Always' Quiet at Night	300+	53%	52%	61%
Doctors 'Always' Communicated Well	300+	76%	78%	82%
Home Recovery Information Given	300+	84%	85%	85%
Hospital Given 9 or 10 on 10 Point Scale	300+	66%	67%	71%
Meds 'Always' Explained Before Given	300+	61%	64%	64%
Nurses 'Always' Communicated Well	300+	80%	79%	79%
Pain 'Always' Well Controlled	300+	69%	71%	71%
Room and Bathroom 'Always' Clean	300+	72%	70%	73%
Timely Help 'Always' Received	300+	66%	66%	68%
Would Definitely Recommend Hospital	300+	67%	68%	71%
Use of Medical Imaging				
Cardiac Imaging Stress Test before Surgery	726	3.9%	4.2%	5.3%
Combination Abdominal CT Scan	2,211	8.7%	6%	10.5%
Combination Brain/Sinus CT Scan	1,603	5.7%	2.7%	2.7%
Combination Chest CT Scan	1,519	0.1%	0.7%	2.7%
Follow-up Mammogram/Ultrasound	2,978	13.7%	9.1%	8.8%
Lumbar Spine MRI for Low Back Pain	148	27.0%	31.2%	37.2%

Beebe Medical Center

424 Savannah Rd — Phone: 302-645-3300
Lewes, DE 19958 — Fax: 302-645-3585
E-mail: khalen@bbmc.org
URL: www.beebemed.org
Type: Acute Care Hospitals — Emergency Services: Yes
Ownership: Voluntary non-profit - Private — Beds: 138

Key Personnel:
Radiology. . . . . Frances Esposito, MD
CEO/President. . . . . Jeffrey M Fried, FACHE
Operating Room. . . . . Perry Jeffrey
Pediatric Ambulatory Care . . . . . . Sautosh Reddy, MD
Pediatric In-Patient Care . . . . Sautosh Reddy, MD
Quality Assurance . . . . Barbara Reick
Chief of Medical Staff. . . . . Andrejs Strauss, MD
Patient Relations . . . . Ellen Tolbert

Measure	Cases	This Hosp.	State Avg.	U.S. Avg.
Blood Clot Prevention and Treatment				
Anticoagulation Overlap Therapy[2]	87	89%	88%	93%
ICU Venous Thromboembolism Prophylaxis[2]	59	86%	92%	92%
Incidence of Potentially Preventable VTE[1,2]	-	-	8%	10%
UFH with Dosages/Platelet Monitoring[2]	47	98%	84%	97%
Venous Thromboembolism Prophylaxis[2]	392	68%	83%	85%
Warfarin Therapy Discharge Instructions[2]	72	42%	27%	75%
Chest Pain/Possible Heart Attack Care				
Aspirin Given Within 24 Hours of Arrival[1,3]	-	-	95%	96%
Fibrinolytic Meds Within 30 Min. of Arrival[3,7]	-	-	-	58%
Average Time to ECG (minutes)[1,3]	-	-	7	7
Average Time to Transfer (minutes)[3,7]	-	-	120	60
Children's Asthma Care				
Received Home Management Plan of Care	-	-	-	88%
Received Reliever Medication	-	-	-	100%
Received Systemic Corticosteroids	-	-	-	100%
Emergency Department				
Admittance Decision Time (minutes)[2]	717	201	190	98
Head CT Results Within 45 Min. of Arrival	32	72%	59%	57%
Patients Who Left ER Before Being Seen	47,316	0%	3%	2%
Time from ER Arrival to Admit. (minutes)[2]	717	394	374	274
Time from ER Arrival to Discharge (minutes)	367	148	153	134
Time in ER Before Being Evaluated (minutes)	399	29	40	26
Time to Pain Meds for Fractures (minutes)	131	67	72	57
Heart Attack Care				
Aspirin Given at Discharge	215	100%	100%	99%
Fibrinolytic Meds Within 30 Min. of Arrival[7]	-	-	-	54%
PCI Within 90 Minutes of Arrival	26	100%	97%	96%
Statin Prescribed at Discharge	210	98%	99%	98%
Heart Failure Care				
ACE Inhibitor or ARB for LVSD	92	98%	98%	97%
Discharge Instructions Given	258	97%	96%	94%
Evaluation of LVS Function	329	100%	100%	99%
Medicare Spending				
Medicare Spending per Patient (ratio)	-	0.99	1	0.98
Pneumonia Care				
Appropriate Initial Antibiotic Given	239	99%	97%	95%
Blood Culture Timing	259	99%	98%	98%
Pregnancy and Delivery Care				
Newborn Deliveries Scheduled Early	65	12%	2%	6%
Preventive Care				
Immunization for Influenza[2]	554	97%	95%	90%
Immunization for Pneumonia[2]	785	99%	96%	92%
Stroke Care				
Anticoagulation Therapy for Atrial Fibrillation	38	95%	92%	95%
Antithrombotic Therapy Timing	139	96%	96%	98%
Assessed for Rehabilitation	180	93%	98%	97%
Discharged on Antithrombotic Therapy	177	97%	98%	99%
Discharged on Statin Medication	144	89%	95%	94%
Thrombolytic Therapy Timing[1]	-	-	75%	66%
Venous Thromboembolism Prophylaxis	142	97%	92%	94%
Written Stroke Educational Materials Given	114	75%	87%	88%
Surgical Care Improvement Project				
Appropriate Beta Blocker Usage	532	100%	99%	98%
Appropriate VTP Within 24 Hours	973	100%	99%	98%
Controlled Postoperative Blood Glucose	123	95%	98%	97%
Perioperative Temperature Management	1,097	100%	100%	100%
Prophylactic Antibiotic Selection	925	100%	100%	99%
Prophylactic Antibiotic Selection (Outpatient)	405	98%	99%	98%
Prophylactic Antibiotic Stopped	920	99%	99%	98%
Prophylactic Antibiotic Timing	927	100%	99%	99%
Prophylactic Antibiotic Timing (Outpatient)	396	100%	98%	98%
Urinary Catheter Removal	989	100%	99%	97%
Survey of Patients' Hospital Experiences				
Area Around Room 'Always' Quiet at Night	300+	51%	52%	61%
Doctors 'Always' Communicated Well	300+	80%	78%	82%
Home Recovery Information Given	300+	83%	85%	85%
Hospital Given 9 or 10 on 10 Point Scale	300+	67%	67%	71%
Meds 'Always' Explained Before Given	300+	69%	64%	64%
Nurses 'Always' Communicated Well	300+	82%	79%	79%
Pain 'Always' Well Controlled	300+	73%	71%	71%
Room and Bathroom 'Always' Clean	300+	71%	70%	73%
Timely Help 'Always' Received	300+	70%	66%	68%
Would Definitely Recommend Hospital	300+	72%	68%	71%
Use of Medical Imaging				
Cardiac Imaging Stress Test before Surgery	466	3.2%	4.2%	5.3%
Combination Abdominal CT Scan	2,673	5.8%	6%	10.5%
Combination Brain/Sinus CT Scan	1,768	2.3%	2.7%	2.7%
Combination Chest CT Scan	1,966	1.5%	0.7%	2.7%
Follow-up Mammogram/Ultrasound	3,793	6.0%	9.1%	8.8%
Lumbar Spine MRI for Low Back Pain	234	36.3%	31.2%	37.2%

Bayhealth - Milford Memorial Hospital

21 West Clarke Avenue — Phone: 302-422-3311
Milford, DE 19963
Type: Acute Care Hospitals — Emergency Services: Yes
Ownership: Proprietary

Measure	Cases	This Hosp.	State Avg.	U.S. Avg.
Blood Clot Prevention and Treatment				
Anticoagulation Overlap Therapy[2]	38	95%	88%	93%
ICU Venous Thromboembolism Prophylaxis[2]	69	83%	92%	92%
Incidence of Potentially Preventable VTE[1,2]	-	-	8%	10%
UFH with Dosages/Platelet Monitoring[2]	19	95%	84%	97%
Venous Thromboembolism Prophylaxis[2]	374	91%	83%	85%
Warfarin Therapy Discharge Instructions[2]	29	31%	27%	75%
Chest Pain/Possible Heart Attack Care				
Aspirin Given Within 24 Hours of Arrival	25	100%	95%	96%
Fibrinolytic Meds Within 30 Min. of Arrival[7]	-	-	-	58%
Average Time to ECG (minutes)	26	6	7	7
Average Time to Transfer (minutes)	12	120	120	60
Children's Asthma Care				
Received Home Management Plan of Care	-	-	-	88%
Received Reliever Medication	-	-	-	100%
Received Systemic Corticosteroids	-	-	-	100%
Emergency Department				

NOTE: Hospital profiles are in alphabetical order by state, then city, then hospital within the city; Rankings exclude hospitals with less than 25 cases except for patient surveys which excludes hospitals with less than 100 cases; (a) 100-299 cases; (1) The number of cases/patients is too few to report; (2) Data submitted were based on a sample of cases/patients; (3) Results are based on a shorter time period than required; (4) Data suppressed by CMS for one or more quarters; (5) Results are not available for this reporting period; (6) Fewer than 100 patients completed the HCAHPS survey; (7) No cases met the criteria for this measure; (8) The lower limit of the confidence interval cannot be calculated if the number of observed infections equals zero; (9) No data are available from the state/territory for this reporting period; (10) The scores shown reflect fewer than 50 completed surveys; (11) There were discrepancies in the data collection process; (12) This measure does not apply to this hospital for this reporting period; (13) Results cannot be calculated for this reporting period; (14) The results for this state are combined with nearby states to protect confidentiality; Please refer to the User's Guide for a full explanation of data.

Measure	Cases	This Hosp.	State Avg.	U.S. Avg.
Admittance Decision Time (minutes)[2]	669	236	190	98
Head CT Results Within 45 Min. of Arrival[1]	-	-	59%	57%
Patients Who Left ER Before Being Seen	26,013	4%	3%	2%
Time from ER Arrival to Admit. (minutes)[2]	672	404	374	274
Time from ER Arrival to Discharge (minutes)	391	144	153	134
Time in ER Before Being Evaluated (minutes)	409	36	40	26
Time to Pain Meds for Fractures (minutes)	47	86	72	57
Heart Attack Care				
Aspirin Given at Discharge	26	100%	100%	99%
Fibrinolytic Meds Within 30 Min. of Arrival[7]	-	-	-	54%
PCI Within 90 Minutes of Arrival[3,7]	-	-	97%	96%
Statin Prescribed at Discharge	26	100%	99%	98%
Heart Failure Care				
ACE Inhibitor or ARB for LVSD	68	99%	98%	97%
Discharge Instructions Given	156	95%	96%	94%
Evaluation of LVS Function	193	100%	100%	99%
Medicare Spending				
Medicare Spending per Patient (ratio)	-	0.97	1	0.98
Pneumonia Care				
Appropriate Initial Antibiotic Given[2]	76	93%	97%	95%
Blood Culture Timing[2]	145	99%	98%	98%
Pregnancy and Delivery Care				
Newborn Deliveries Scheduled Early	25	0%	2%	6%
Preventive Care				
Immunization for Influenza[2]	432	99%	95%	90%
Immunization for Pneumonia[2]	596	99%	96%	92%
Stroke Care				
Anticoagulation Therapy for Atrial Fibrillation	12	75%	92%	95%
Antithrombotic Therapy Timing	60	98%	96%	98%
Assessed for Rehabilitation	67	99%	98%	97%
Discharged on Antithrombotic Therapy	66	94%	98%	99%
Discharged on Statin Medication	47	94%	95%	94%
Thrombolytic Therapy Timing[1]	-	-	75%	66%
Venous Thromboembolism Prophylaxis	64	78%	92%	94%
Written Stroke Educational Materials Given	38	97%	87%	88%
Surgical Care Improvement Project				
Appropriate Beta Blocker Usage[2]	58	100%	99%	98%
Appropriate VTP Within 24 Hours[2]	156	100%	99%	98%
Controlled Postoperative Blood Glucose[2,3]	-	-	98%	97%
Perioperative Temperature Management[2]	177	100%	100%	100%
Prophylactic Antibiotic Selection[2]	112	99%	100%	99%
Prophylactic Antibiotic Selection (Outpatient)	23	87%	99%	98%
Prophylactic Antibiotic Stopped[2]	110	100%	99%	98%
Prophylactic Antibiotic Timing[2]	112	98%	99%	99%
Prophylactic Antibiotic Timing (Outpatient)	22	91%	98%	98%
Urinary Catheter Removal[2]	105	100%	99%	97%
Survey of Patients' Hospital Experiences				
Area Around Room 'Always' Quiet at Night	300+	48%	52%	61%
Doctors 'Always' Communicated Well	300+	76%	78%	82%
Home Recovery Information Given	300+	86%	85%	85%
Hospital Given 9 or 10 on 10 Point Scale	300+	61%	67%	71%
Meds 'Always' Explained Before Given	300+	61%	64%	64%
Nurses 'Always' Communicated Well	300+	76%	79%	79%
Pain 'Always' Well Controlled	300+	70%	71%	71%
Room and Bathroom 'Always' Clean	300+	72%	70%	73%
Timely Help 'Always' Received	300+	63%	66%	68%
Would Definitely Recommend Hospital	300+	60%	68%	71%
Use of Medical Imaging				
Cardiac Imaging Stress Test before Surgery	675	5.2%	4.2%	5.3%
Combination Abdominal CT Scan	848	7.0%	6%	10.5%
Combination Brain/Sinus CT Scan	619	4.7%	2.7%	2.7%
Combination Chest CT Scan	627	1.4%	0.7%	2.7%
Follow-up Mammogram/Ultrasound	1,216	12.9%	9.1%	8.8%
Lumbar Spine MRI for Low Back Pain	64	23.4%	31.2%	37.2%

Christiana Care Health Services

4755 Ogletown - Stanton Road
Newark, DE 19718
Phone: 302-733-1000
Fax: 302-428-5790
URL: www.christianacare.org
Type: Acute Care Hospitals
Emergency Services: Yes
Ownership: Voluntary non-profit - Private
Beds: 250
Key Personnel:
CEO .... Steve Daugherty
Chief of Medical Staff .... Michael D. Thomsberry, MD, MBA, CPE

Measure	Cases	This Hosp.	State Avg.	U.S. Avg.
Blood Clot Prevention and Treatment				
Anticoagulation Overlap Therapy[2]	182	86%	88%	93%
ICU Venous Thromboembolism Prophylaxis[2]	48	98%	92%	92%
Incidence of Potentially Preventable VTE[2]	90	7%	8%	10%
UFH with Dosages/Platelet Monitoring[2]	105	70%	84%	97%
Venous Thromboembolism Prophylaxis[2]	370	92%	83%	85%
Warfarin Therapy Discharge Instructions[2]	119	15%	27%	75%
Chest Pain/Possible Heart Attack Care				
Aspirin Given Within 24 Hours of Arrival[5]	-	-	95%	96%
Fibrinolytic Meds Within 30 Min. of Arrival[5]	-	-	-	58%
Average Time to ECG (minutes)[5]	-	-	7	7
Average Time to Transfer (minutes)[5]	-	-	120	60
Children's Asthma Care				
Received Home Management Plan of Care	-	-	-	88%
Received Reliever Medication	-	-	-	100%
Received Systemic Corticosteroids	-	-	-	100%
Emergency Department				
Admittance Decision Time (minutes)[2]	182	156	190	98
Head CT Results Within 45 Min. of Arrival[1]	-	-	59%	57%
Patients Who Left ER Before Being Seen	>100k	4%	3%	2%
Time from ER Arrival to Admit. (minutes)[2]	182	420	374	274
Time from ER Arrival to Discharge (minutes)[3]	171	185	153	134
Time in ER Before Being Evaluated (minutes)	371	65	40	26
Time to Pain Meds for Fractures (minutes)	149	75	72	57
Heart Attack Care				
Aspirin Given at Discharge	738	100%	100%	99%
Fibrinolytic Meds Within 30 Min. of Arrival[7]	-	-	-	54%
PCI Within 90 Minutes of Arrival	153	95%	97%	96%
Statin Prescribed at Discharge	730	100%	99%	98%
Heart Failure Care				
ACE Inhibitor or ARB for LVSD[2]	256	97%	98%	97%
Discharge Instructions Given[2]	686	95%	96%	94%
Evaluation of LVS Function[2]	798	100%	100%	99%
Medicare Spending				
Medicare Spending per Patient (ratio)	-	1.00	1	0.98
Pneumonia Care				
Appropriate Initial Antibiotic Given[2]	277	94%	97%	95%
Blood Culture Timing[2]	353	95%	98%	98%
Pregnancy and Delivery Care				
Newborn Deliveries Scheduled Early[2]	368	1%	2%	6%
Preventive Care				
Immunization for Influenza[2]	620	91%	95%	90%
Immunization for Pneumonia[2]	543	93%	96%	92%
Stroke Care				
Anticoagulation Therapy for Atrial Fibrillation[2]	39	92%	92%	95%
Antithrombotic Therapy Timing[2]	269	94%	96%	98%
Assessed for Rehabilitation[2]	384	100%	98%	97%
Discharged on Antithrombotic Therapy[2]	317	99%	98%	99%
Discharged on Statin Medication[2]	256	95%	95%	94%
Thrombolytic Therapy Timing[2]	31	97%	75%	66%
Venous Thromboembolism Prophylaxis[2]	393	95%	92%	94%
Written Stroke Educational Materials Given[2]	215	86%	87%	88%
Surgical Care Improvement Project				
Appropriate Beta Blocker Usage[2]	381	99%	99%	98%
Appropriate VTP Within 24 Hours[2]	680	99%	99%	98%
Controlled Postoperative Blood Glucose[2]	203	99%	98%	97%
Perioperative Temperature Management[2]	889	100%	100%	100%
Prophylactic Antibiotic Selection[2]	711	100%	100%	99%
Prophylactic Antibiotic Selection (Outpatient)	866	99%	99%	98%
Prophylactic Antibiotic Stopped[2]	700	100%	99%	98%
Prophylactic Antibiotic Timing[2]	712	99%	99%	99%
Prophylactic Antibiotic Timing (Outpatient)	855	98%	98%	98%
Urinary Catheter Removal[2]	566	99%	99%	97%
Survey of Patients' Hospital Experiences				
Area Around Room 'Always' Quiet at Night[11]	300+	51%	52%	61%
Doctors 'Always' Communicated Well[11]	300+	79%	78%	82%
Home Recovery Information Given[11]	300+	86%	85%	85%
Hospital Given 9 or 10 on 10 Point Scale[11]	300+	72%	67%	71%
Meds 'Always' Explained Before Given[11]	300+	64%	64%	64%
Nurses 'Always' Communicated Well[11]	300+	80%	79%	79%
Pain 'Always' Well Controlled[11]	300+	71%	71%	71%
Room and Bathroom 'Always' Clean[11]	300+	71%	70%	73%
Timely Help 'Always' Received[11]	300+	70%	66%	68%
Would Definitely Recommend Hospital[11]	300+	76%	68%	71%
Use of Medical Imaging				
Cardiac Imaging Stress Test before Surgery	1,884	4.1%	4.2%	5.3%
Combination Abdominal CT Scan	4,639	5.5%	6%	10.5%
Combination Brain/Sinus CT Scan	3,024	0.0%	2.7%	2.7%
Combination Chest CT Scan	4,234	0.5%	0.7%	2.7%
Follow-up Mammogram/Ultrasound	4,580	8.9%	9.1%	8.8%
Lumbar Spine MRI for Low Back Pain	583	31.0%	31.2%	37.2%

Nanticoke Memorial Hospital

801 Middleford Rd
Seaford, DE 19973
Phone: 302-629-6611
Fax: 302-629-4758
E-mail: nhshr@ce.net
URL: www.nanticoke.org
Type: Acute Care Hospitals
Emergency Services: Yes
Ownership: Voluntary non-profit - Private
Beds: 140
Key Personnel:
Operating Room............. Stephen D Carey
Radiology.................. Warren Cohen, MD
Pediatric Ambulatory Care ...... Patrick Jarvie, MD
Pediatric In-Patient Care .... Patrick Jarvie, MD
Emergency Room .... Yvonne O'Brien
Chairman/CEO .... Kent T. Peterson
CEO/President............... Steven A. Rose
Quality Assurance .... Barbara Young

Measure	Cases	This Hosp.	State Avg.	U.S. Avg.
Blood Clot Prevention and Treatment				
Anticoagulation Overlap Therapy[2]	20	85%	88%	93%
ICU Venous Thromboembolism Prophylaxis[2]	56	95%	92%	92%
Incidence of Potentially Preventable VTE[1,2]	-	-	8%	10%
UFH with Dosages/Platelet Monitoring[1,2]	-	-	84%	97%
Venous Thromboembolism Prophylaxis[2]	390	81%	83%	85%
Warfarin Therapy Discharge Instructions[2]	14	43%	27%	75%
Chest Pain/Possible Heart Attack Care				
Aspirin Given Within 24 Hours of Arrival[1]	-	-	95%	96%
Fibrinolytic Meds Within 30 Min. of Arrival[3,7]	-	-	-	58%
Average Time to ECG (minutes)[1]	-	-	7	7
Average Time to Transfer (minutes)[3,7]	-	-	120	60
Children's Asthma Care				
Received Home Management Plan of Care	-	-	-	88%
Received Reliever Medication	-	-	-	100%
Received Systemic Corticosteroids	-	-	-	100%
Emergency Department				
Admittance Decision Time (minutes)[2]	719	130	190	98
Head CT Results Within 45 Min. of Arrival	13	77%	59%	57%
Patients Who Left ER Before Being Seen	38,433	2%	3%	2%
Time from ER Arrival to Admit. (minutes)[2]	721	304	374	274
Time from ER Arrival to Discharge (minutes)	333	145	153	134
Time in ER Before Being Evaluated (minutes)	381	34	40	26
Time to Pain Meds for Fractures (minutes)	103	69	72	57
Heart Attack Care				
Aspirin Given at Discharge	91	99%	100%	99%
Fibrinolytic Meds Within 30 Min. of Arrival[7]	-	-	-	54%
PCI Within 90 Minutes of Arrival	22	100%	97%	96%
Statin Prescribed at Discharge	97	99%	99%	98%
Heart Failure Care				
ACE Inhibitor or ARB for LVSD	67	99%	98%	97%
Discharge Instructions Given	209	95%	96%	94%
Evaluation of LVS Function	299	100%	100%	99%
Medicare Spending				
Medicare Spending per Patient (ratio)	-	0.99	1	0.98
Pneumonia Care				
Appropriate Initial Antibiotic Given	154	100%	97%	95%
Blood Culture Timing	164	95%	98%	98%
Pregnancy and Delivery Care				
Newborn Deliveries Scheduled Early[2]	27	7%	2%	6%
Preventive Care				
Immunization for Influenza[2]	485	91%	95%	90%
Immunization for Pneumonia[2]	625	86%	96%	92%
Stroke Care				

NOTE: Hospital profiles are in alphabetical order by state, then city, then hospital within the city; Rankings exclude hospitals with less than 25 cases except for patient surveys which excludes hospitals with less than 100 cases; (a) 100-299 cases; (1) The number of cases/patients is too few to report; (2) Data submitted were based on a sample of cases/patients; (3) Results are based on a shorter time period than required; (4) Data suppressed by CMS for one or more quarters; (5) Results are not available for this reporting period; (6) Fewer than 100 patients completed the HCAHPS survey; (7) No cases met the criteria for this measure; (8) The lower limit of the confidence interval cannot be calculated if the number of observed infections equals zero; (9) No data are available from the state/territory for this reporting period; (10) The scores shown reflect fewer than 50 completed surveys; (11) There were discrepancies in the data collection process; (12) This measure does not apply to this hospital for this reporting period; (13) Results cannot be calculated for this reporting period; (14) The results for this state are combined with nearby states to protect confidentiality; Please refer to the User's Guide for a full explanation of data.

Anticoagulation Therapy for Atrial Fibrillation[2]	12	100%	92%	95%
Antithrombotic Therapy Timing[2]	68	99%	96%	98%
Assessed for Rehabilitation[2]	67	96%	98%	97%
Discharged on Antithrombotic Therapy[2]	66	100%	98%	99%
Discharged on Statin Medication[2]	59	98%	95%	94%
Thrombolytic Therapy Timing[1,2]	-	-	75%	66%
Venous Thromboembolism Prophylaxis[2]	67	94%	92%	94%
Written Stroke Educational Materials Given[2]	37	92%	87%	88%
Surgical Care Improvement Project				
Appropriate Beta Blocker Usage[2]	64	100%	99%	98%
Appropriate VTP Within 24 Hours[2]	183	96%	99%	98%
Controlled Postoperative Blood Glucose[2,7]	-	-	98%	97%
Perioperative Temperature Management[2]	211	100%	100%	100%
Prophylactic Antibiotic Selection[2]	116	100%	100%	99%
Prophylactic Antibiotic Selection (Outpatient)	61	100%	99%	98%
Prophylactic Antibiotic Stopped[2]	113	96%	99%	98%
Prophylactic Antibiotic Timing[2]	116	99%	99%	99%
Prophylactic Antibiotic Timing (Outpatient)	67	90%	98%	98%
Urinary Catheter Removal[2]	138	93%	99%	97%
Survey of Patients' Hospital Experiences				
Area Around Room 'Always' Quiet at Night	300+	50%	52%	61%
Doctors 'Always' Communicated Well	300+	82%	78%	82%
Home Recovery Information Given	300+	88%	85%	85%
Hospital Given 9 or 10 on 10 Point Scale	300+	70%	67%	71%
Meds 'Always' Explained Before Given	300+	65%	64%	64%
Nurses 'Always' Communicated Well	300+	82%	79%	79%
Pain 'Always' Well Controlled	300+	70%	71%	71%
Room and Bathroom 'Always' Clean	300+	72%	70%	73%
Timely Help 'Always' Received	300+	66%	66%	68%
Would Definitely Recommend Hospital	300+	67%	68%	71%
Use of Medical Imaging				
Cardiac Imaging Stress Test before Surgery	300	4.3%	4.2%	5.3%
Combination Abdominal CT Scan	893	3.4%	6%	10.5%
Combination Brain/Sinus CT Scan	807	3.8%	2.7%	2.7%
Combination Chest CT Scan	618	0.0%	0.7%	2.7%
Follow-up Mammogram/Ultrasound	1,506	8.6%	9.1%	8.8%
Lumbar Spine MRI for Low Back Pain[1]	-	-	31.2%	37.2%

Saint Francis Hospital

7th & Clayton Sts
Wilmington, DE 19805
Phone: 302-421-4100
URL: www.stfrancishealthcare.org
Type: Acute Care Hospitals
Emergency Services: Yes
Ownership: Voluntary non-profit - Private
Beds: 330

Key Personnel:
CEO/President. . . . . Clarence Laliberty

Measure	Cases	This Hosp.	State Avg.	U.S. Avg.
Blood Clot Prevention and Treatment				
Anticoagulation Overlap Therapy[2]	25	96%	88%	93%
ICU Venous Thromboembolism Prophylaxis[2]	78	96%	92%	92%
Incidence of Potentially Preventable VTE[1,2]	-	-	8%	10%
UFH with Dosages/Platelet Monitoring[1,2]	-	-	84%	97%
Venous Thromboembolism Prophylaxis[2]	364	83%	83%	85%
Warfarin Therapy Discharge Instructions[1,2]	-	-	27%	75%
Chest Pain/Possible Heart Attack Care				
Aspirin Given Within 24 Hours of Arrival[1,3]	-	-	95%	96%
Fibrinolytic Meds Within 30 Min. of Arrival[3,7]	-	-	-	58%
Average Time to ECG (minutes)[1,3]	-	-	7	7
Average Time to Transfer (minutes)[3,7]	-	-	120	60
Children's Asthma Care				
Received Home Management Plan of Care	-	-	-	88%
Received Reliever Medication	-	-	-	100%
Received Systemic Corticosteroids	-	-	-	100%
Emergency Department				
Admittance Decision Time (minutes)[2]	644	166	190	98
Head CT Results Within 45 Min. of Arrival[1]	-	-	59%	57%
Patients Who Left ER Before Being Seen	35,936	3%	3%	2%
Time from ER Arrival to Admit. (minutes)[2]	683	341	374	274
Time from ER Arrival to Discharge (minutes)	380	112	153	134
Time in ER Before Being Evaluated (minutes)	401	40	40	26
Time to Pain Meds for Fractures (minutes)	28	93	72	57
Heart Attack Care				
Aspirin Given at Discharge	121	99%	100%	99%
Fibrinolytic Meds Within 30 Min. of Arrival[7]	-	-	-	54%
PCI Within 90 Minutes of Arrival	21	100%	97%	96%
Statin Prescribed at Discharge	112	97%	99%	98%
Heart Failure Care				
ACE Inhibitor or ARB for LVSD	72	100%	98%	97%
Discharge Instructions Given	132	99%	96%	94%
Evaluation of LVS Function	149	100%	100%	99%
Medicare Spending				
Medicare Spending per Patient (ratio)	-	1.02	1	0.98
Pneumonia Care				
Appropriate Initial Antibiotic Given	91	98%	97%	95%
Blood Culture Timing	135	99%	98%	98%
Pregnancy and Delivery Care				
Newborn Deliveries Scheduled Early	74	1%	2%	6%
Preventive Care				
Immunization for Influenza[2]	539	96%	95%	90%
Immunization for Pneumonia[2]	568	96%	96%	92%
Stroke Care				
Anticoagulation Therapy for Atrial Fibrillation[1]	-	-	92%	95%
Antithrombotic Therapy Timing	58	97%	96%	98%
Assessed for Rehabilitation	59	100%	98%	97%
Discharged on Antithrombotic Therapy	56	100%	98%	99%
Discharged on Statin Medication	46	98%	95%	94%
Thrombolytic Therapy Timing[1]	-	-	75%	66%
Venous Thromboembolism Prophylaxis	62	95%	92%	94%
Written Stroke Educational Materials Given	30	100%	87%	88%
Surgical Care Improvement Project				
Appropriate Beta Blocker Usage	70	91%	99%	98%
Appropriate VTP Within 24 Hours	220	95%	99%	98%
Controlled Postoperative Blood Glucose	27	96%	98%	97%
Perioperative Temperature Management	265	100%	100%	100%
Prophylactic Antibiotic Selection	168	99%	100%	99%
Prophylactic Antibiotic Selection (Outpatient)	204	100%	99%	98%
Prophylactic Antibiotic Stopped	159	96%	99%	98%
Prophylactic Antibiotic Timing	168	99%	99%	99%
Prophylactic Antibiotic Timing (Outpatient)	205	100%	98%	98%
Urinary Catheter Removal	130	95%	99%	97%
Survey of Patients' Hospital Experiences				
Area Around Room 'Always' Quiet at Night	300+	61%	52%	61%
Doctors 'Always' Communicated Well	300+	76%	78%	82%
Home Recovery Information Given	300+	81%	85%	85%
Hospital Given 9 or 10 on 10 Point Scale	300+	65%	67%	71%
Meds 'Always' Explained Before Given	300+	61%	64%	64%
Nurses 'Always' Communicated Well	300+	75%	79%	79%
Pain 'Always' Well Controlled	300+	70%	71%	71%
Room and Bathroom 'Always' Clean	300+	64%	70%	73%
Timely Help 'Always' Received	300+	63%	66%	68%
Would Definitely Recommend Hospital	300+	66%	68%	71%
Use of Medical Imaging				
Cardiac Imaging Stress Test before Surgery	137	5.1%	4.2%	5.3%
Combination Abdominal CT Scan	438	2.1%	6%	10.5%
Combination Brain/Sinus CT Scan	550	5.3%	2.7%	2.7%
Combination Chest CT Scan	228	1.3%	0.7%	2.7%
Follow-up Mammogram/Ultrasound	948	3.6%	9.1%	8.8%
Lumbar Spine MRI for Low Back Pain	47	40.4%	31.2%	37.2%

Wilmington VA Medical Center

1601 Kirkwood Highway
Wilmington, DE 19805
Phone: 302-994-2511
Fax: 302-633-5591
URL: www.va.gov/wilmington
Type: Acute Care - VA
Emergency Services: No
Ownership: Government Federal
Beds: 120

Key Personnel:
Chief of Medical Staff. . . . . Robert M Boucher, MD
CEO/President. . . . . Charles M Dorman
Quality Assurance . . . . Melinda Haebel
Operating Room. . . . . Jeanne Long
Infection Control. . . . . Ted Martynowicz, DO
Cardiac Laboratory. . . . . Gaddum Reddy, MD

Measure	Cases	This Hosp.	State Avg.	U.S. Avg.
Blood Clot Prevention and Treatment				
Anticoagulation Overlap Therapy	-	-	88%	93%
ICU Venous Thromboembolism Prophylaxis	-	-	92%	92%
Incidence of Potentially Preventable VTE	-	-	8%	10%
UFH with Dosages/Platelet Monitoring	-	-	84%	97%
Venous Thromboembolism Prophylaxis	-	-	83%	85%
Warfarin Therapy Discharge Instructions	-	-	27%	75%
Chest Pain/Possible Heart Attack Care				
Aspirin Given Within 24 Hours of Arrival	-	-	95%	96%
Fibrinolytic Meds Within 30 Min. of Arrival	-	-	-	58%
Average Time to ECG (minutes)	-	-	7	7
Average Time to Transfer (minutes)	-	-	120	60
Children's Asthma Care				
Received Home Management Plan of Care	-	-	-	88%
Received Reliever Medication	-	-	-	100%
Received Systemic Corticosteroids	-	-	-	100%
Emergency Department				
Admittance Decision Time (minutes)	-	-	190	98
Head CT Results Within 45 Min. of Arrival	-	-	59%	57%
Patients Who Left ER Before Being Seen	-	-	3%	2%
Time from ER Arrival to Admit. (minutes)	-	-	374	274
Time from ER Arrival to Discharge (minutes)	-	-	153	134
Time in ER Before Being Evaluated (minutes)	-	-	40	26
Time to Pain Meds for Fractures (minutes)	-	-	72	57
Heart Attack Care				
Aspirin Given at Discharge[5]	-	-	100%	99%
Fibrinolytic Meds Within 30 Min. of Arrival[5]	-	-	-	54%
PCI Within 90 Minutes of Arrival[5]	-	-	97%	96%
Statin Prescribed at Discharge[5]	-	-	99%	98%
Heart Failure Care				
ACE Inhibitor or ARB for LVSD	25	100%	98%	97%
Discharge Instructions Given	67	100%	96%	94%
Evaluation of LVS Function	72	100%	100%	99%
Medicare Spending				
Medicare Spending per Patient (ratio)	-	-	1	0.98
Pneumonia Care				
Appropriate Initial Antibiotic Given[1]	21	100%	97%	95%
Blood Culture Timing	35	100%	98%	98%
Pregnancy and Delivery Care				
Newborn Deliveries Scheduled Early	-	-	2%	6%
Preventive Care				
Immunization for Influenza[2,3]	144	98%	95%	90%
Immunization for Pneumonia[2,3]	336	97%	96%	92%
Stroke Care				
Anticoagulation Therapy for Atrial Fibrillation	-	-	92%	95%
Antithrombotic Therapy Timing	-	-	96%	98%
Assessed for Rehabilitation	-	-	98%	97%
Discharged on Antithrombotic Therapy	-	-	98%	99%
Discharged on Statin Medication	-	-	95%	94%
Thrombolytic Therapy Timing	-	-	75%	66%
Venous Thromboembolism Prophylaxis	-	-	92%	94%
Written Stroke Educational Materials Given	-	-	87%	88%
Surgical Care Improvement Project				
Appropriate Beta Blocker Usage[2]	25	100%	99%	98%
Appropriate VTP Within 24 Hours[2]	53	100%	99%	98%
Controlled Postoperative Blood Glucose[5]	-	-	98%	97%
Perioperative Temperature Management[2]	73	100%	100%	100%
Prophylactic Antibiotic Selection[1]	14	100%	100%	99%
Prophylactic Antibiotic Selection (Outpatient)	-	-	99%	98%
Prophylactic Antibiotic Stopped[1]	14	100%	99%	98%
Prophylactic Antibiotic Timing[1]	14	100%	99%	99%
Prophylactic Antibiotic Timing (Outpatient)	-	-	98%	98%
Urinary Catheter Removal[2]	41	100%	99%	97%
Survey of Patients' Hospital Experiences				
Area Around Room 'Always' Quiet at Night	-	-	52%	61%
Doctors 'Always' Communicated Well	-	-	78%	82%
Home Recovery Information Given	-	-	85%	85%
Hospital Given 9 or 10 on 10 Point Scale	-	-	67%	71%
Meds 'Always' Explained Before Given	-	-	64%	64%
Nurses 'Always' Communicated Well	-	-	79%	79%
Pain 'Always' Well Controlled	-	-	71%	71%
Room and Bathroom 'Always' Clean	-	-	70%	73%
Timely Help 'Always' Received	-	-	66%	68%
Would Definitely Recommend Hospital	-	-	68%	71%
Use of Medical Imaging				
Cardiac Imaging Stress Test before Surgery	-	-	4.2%	5.3%

NOTE: Hospital profiles are in alphabetical order by state, then city, then hospital within the city; Rankings exclude hospitals with less than 25 cases except for patient surveys which excludes hospitals with less than 100 cases; (a) 100-299 cases; (1) The number of cases/patients is too few to report; (2) Data submitted were based on a sample of cases/patients; (3) Results are based on a shorter time period than required; (4) Data suppressed by CMS for one or more quarters; (5) Results are not available for this reporting period; (6) Fewer than 100 patients completed the HCAHPS survey; (7) No cases met the criteria for this measure; (8) The lower limit of the confidence interval cannot be calculated if the number of observed infections equals zero; (9) No data are available from the state/territory for this reporting period; (10) The scores shown reflect fewer than 50 completed surveys; (11) There were discrepancies in the data collection process; (12) This measure does not apply to this hospital for this reporting period; (13) Results cannot be calculated for this reporting period; (14) The results for this state are combined with nearby states to protect confidentiality; Please refer to the User's Guide for a full explanation of data.

Combination Abdominal CT Scan	-	-	6%	10.5%
Combination Brain/Sinus CT Scan	-	-	2.7%	2.7%
Combination Chest CT Scan	-	-	0.7%	2.7%
Follow-up Mammogram/Ultrasound	-	-	9.1%	8.8%
Lumbar Spine MRI for Low Back Pain	-	-	31.2%	37.2%

NOTE: Hospital profiles are in alphabetical order by state, then city, then hospital within the city; Rankings exclude hospitals with less than 25 cases except for patient surveys which excludes hospitals with less than 100 cases; (a) 100-299 cases; (1) The number of cases/patients is too few to report; (2) Data submitted were based on a sample of cases/patients; (3) Results are based on a shorter time period than required; (4) Data suppressed by CMS for one or more quarters; (5) Results are not available for this reporting period; (6) Fewer than 100 patients completed the HCAHPS survey; (7) No cases met the criteria for this measure; (8) The lower limit of the confidence interval cannot be calculated if the number of observed infections equals zero; (9) No data are available from the state/territory for this reporting period; (10) The scores shown reflect fewer than 50 completed surveys; (11) There were discrepancies in the data collection process; (12) This measure does not apply to this hospital for this reporting period; (13) Results cannot be calculated for this reporting period; (14) The results for this state are combined with nearby states to protect confidentiality; Please refer to the User's Guide for a full explanation of data.

Blood Clot Prevention and Treatment

Anticoagulation Overlap Therapy

Hospital Name	City	Rate	Cases
Sibley Memorial Hospital[2]	Washington	100%	26
Medstar Georgetown University Hospital[2]	Washington	97%	87
Medstar Washington Hospital Center[2]	Washington	97%	297
George Washington Univ Hospital[2]	Washington	95%	106
Howard University Hospital[2]	Washington	89%	66
Providence Hospital[2]	Washington	85%	82

ICU Venous Thromboembolism Prophylaxis

Hospital Name	City	Rate	Cases
George Washington Univ Hospital[2]	Washington	98%	87
Howard University Hospital[2]	Washington	98%	89
Medstar Georgetown University Hospital[2]	Washington	97%	86
Medstar Washington Hospital Center[2]	Washington	97%	97
Sibley Memorial Hospital[2]	Washington	97%	39
Providence Hospital[2]	Washington	92%	62
United Medical Center[2]	Washington	91%	87

Incidence of Potentially Preventable VTE

Hospital Name	City	Rate	Cases
Medstar Washington Hospital Center[2]	Washington	2%	118
Medstar Georgetown University Hospital[2]	Washington	7%	72
George Washington Univ Hospital[2]	Washington	10%	29

UFH with Dosages/Platelet Count Monitoring

Hospital Name	City	Rate	Cases
George Washington Univ Hospital[2]	Washington	100%	69
Medstar Georgetown University Hospital[2]	Washington	100%	82
Medstar Washington Hospital Center[2]	Washington	100%	133

Venous Thromboembolism Prophylaxis

Hospital Name	City	Rate	Cases
George Washington Univ Hospital[2]	Washington	92%	308
Medstar Washington Hospital Center[2]	Washington	90%	355
Howard University Hospital[2]	Washington	89%	254
Sibley Memorial Hospital[2]	Washington	87%	260
Medstar Georgetown University Hospital[2]	Washington	86%	302
Providence Hospital[2]	Washington	72%	360
United Medical Center[2]	Washington	65%	403

Warfarin Therapy Discharge Instructions

Hospital Name	City	Rate	Cases
Medstar Washington Hospital Center[2]	Washington	99%	207
George Washington Univ Hospital[2]	Washington	81%	84
Medstar Georgetown University Hospital[2]	Washington	58%	64
Howard University Hospital[2]	Washington	21%	48
Providence Hospital[2]	Washington	9%	56

Chest Pain/Possible Heart Attack Care

Aspirin Given Within 24 Hours of Arrival

Hospital Name	City	Rate	Cases
Sibley Memorial Hospital	Washington	100%	33
United Medical Center	Washington	89%	36

Average Time to ECG (minutes)

Hospital Name	City	Min.	Cases
Sibley Memorial Hospital	Washington	12	34
United Medical Center	Washington	32	36

Children's Asthma Care

Received Home Management Plan of Care

Hospital Name	City	Rate	Cases
Medstar Georgetown University Hospital[2]	Washington	90%	78
Children's Hospital NMC[2]	Washington	89%	375

Received Reliever Medication

Hospital Name	City	Rate	Cases
Children's Hospital NMC[2]	Washington	100%	375
Medstar Georgetown University Hospital	Washington	100%	79

Received Systemic Corticosteroids

Hospital Name	City	Rate	Cases
Children's Hospital NMC[2]	Washington	100%	374
Medstar Georgetown University Hospital	Washington	100%	79

Emergency Department

Admittance Decision Time (minutes)

Hospital Name	City	Min.	Cases
Sibley Memorial Hospital[2]	Washington	122	320
Medstar Georgetown University Hospital[2]	Washington	136	112
Howard University Hospital[2]	Washington	170	203
United Medical Center[2]	Washington	245	198
George Washington Univ Hospital[2]	Washington	250	388
Medstar Washington Hospital Center[2]	Washington	263	514
Providence Hospital[2]	Washington	290	527

Patients Who Left ER Before Being Seen

Hospital Name	City	Rate	Cases
Sibley Memorial Hospital	Washington	0%	34093
George Washington Univ Hospital	Washington	2%	74886
Medstar Georgetown University Hospital	Washington	2%	36823
Medstar Washington Hospital Center	Washington	2%	91968
Howard University Hospital	Washington	3%	59608
Providence Hospital	Washington	4%	49937
United Medical Center	Washington	6%	26110

Time from ER Arrival to Being Admitted (minutes)

Hospital Name	City	Min.	Cases
Sibley Memorial Hospital[2]	Washington	292	320
Medstar Georgetown University Hospital[2]	Washington	332	115
Howard University Hospital[2]	Washington	399	234
George Washington Univ Hospital[2]	Washington	470	393
Medstar Washington Hospital Center[2]	Washington	544	547
United Medical Center[2]	Washington	559	199
Providence Hospital[2]	Washington	614	529

Time from ER Arrival to Discharge (minutes)

Hospital Name	City	Min.	Cases
Sibley Memorial Hospital	Washington	123	556
Medstar Georgetown University Hospital	Washington	163	329
United Medical Center	Washington	173	333
Howard University Hospital	Washington	206	330
George Washington Univ Hospital	Washington	215	370
Medstar Washington Hospital Center	Washington	226	389
Providence Hospital	Washington	318	311

Time in ER Before Being Evaluated (minutes)

Hospital Name	City	Min.	Cases
Sibley Memorial Hospital	Washington	13	561
Medstar Georgetown University Hospital	Washington	35	373
George Washington Univ Hospital	Washington	48	418
Providence Hospital	Washington	75	369
Medstar Washington Hospital Center	Washington	88	414
Howard University Hospital	Washington	98	316
United Medical Center	Washington	102	436

Time to Pain Meds for Bone Fractures (minutes)

Hospital Name	City	Min.	Cases
Sibley Memorial Hospital	Washington	50	94
Medstar Georgetown University Hospital	Washington	64	74
George Washington Univ Hospital	Washington	78	195
Medstar Washington Hospital Center	Washington	89	105
Howard University Hospital	Washington	108	70
United Medical Center	Washington	118	96

Heart Attack Care

Aspirin Given at Discharge

Hospital Name	City	Rate	Cases
Providence Hospital	Washington	100%	41
Washington DC VA Medical Center	Washington	100%	54
George Washington Univ Hospital	Washington	98%	173
Medstar Washington Hospital Center[2]	Washington	98%	322
Howard University Hospital	Washington	96%	49
United Medical Center	Washington	81%	31

PCI Within 90 Minutes of Arrival

Hospital Name	City	Rate	Cases
George Washington Univ Hospital	Washington	96%	45

Statin Prescribed at Discharge

Hospital Name	City	Rate	Cases
Washington DC VA Medical Center	Washington	100%	51
George Washington Univ Hospital	Washington	99%	170
Medstar Washington Hospital Center[2]	Washington	99%	302
Howard University Hospital	Washington	94%	49
Providence Hospital	Washington	89%	37

Heart Failure Care

ACE Inhibitor or ARB for LVSD

Hospital Name	City	Rate	Cases
Medstar Georgetown University Hospital	Washington	100%	33
Sibley Memorial Hospital	Washington	100%	25
George Washington Univ Hospital[2]	Washington	98%	113
Washington DC VA Medical Center	Washington	98%	129
Medstar Washington Hospital Center[2]	Washington	97%	195
Howard University Hospital[2]	Washington	96%	109
Providence Hospital	Washington	89%	179
United Medical Center[2]	Washington	75%	122

Discharge Instructions Given

Hospital Name	City	Rate	Cases
George Washington Univ Hospital[2]	Washington	100%	311
Sibley Memorial Hospital	Washington	100%	61
Medstar Washington Hospital Center[2]	Washington	97%	383
Washington DC VA Medical Center	Washington	94%	185
Medstar Georgetown University Hospital	Washington	93%	70
Providence Hospital	Washington	90%	392
Howard University Hospital[2]	Washington	77%	220
United Medical Center[2]	Washington	55%	249

Evaluation of LVS Function

Hospital Name	City	Rate	Cases
George Washington Univ Hospital[2]	Washington	100%	336
Medstar Georgetown University Hospital	Washington	100%	91
Medstar Washington Hospital Center[2]	Washington	100%	418
Sibley Memorial Hospital	Washington	100%	85
Howard University Hospital[2]	Washington	99%	235
Washington DC VA Medical Center	Washington	99%	214
Providence Hospital	Washington	96%	481
United Medical Center[2]	Washington	92%	306

Medicare Spending

Medicare Spending per Patient (ratio)

Hospital Name	City	Ratio	Cases
Howard University Hospital	Washington	0.90	-
Sibley Memorial Hospital	Washington	0.97	-
George Washington Univ Hospital	Washington	0.99	-
Medstar Washington Hospital Center	Washington	0.99	-
Providence Hospital	Washington	0.99	-
Medstar Georgetown University Hospital	Washington	1.03	-
United Medical Center	Washington	1.05	-

Pneumonia Care

Appropriate Initial Antibiotic Given

Hospital Name	City	Rate	Cases
Sibley Memorial Hospital[2]	Washington	100%	76
George Washington Univ Hospital[2]	Washington	98%	82
Washington DC VA Medical Center	Washington	98%	42
Medstar Georgetown University Hospital[2]	Washington	97%	30
Medstar Washington Hospital Center[2]	Washington	96%	144
Howard University Hospital[2]	Washington	95%	43
United Medical Center[2]	Washington	91%	57
Providence Hospital	Washington	79%	102

Blood Culture Timing

Hospital Name	City	Rate	Cases
Sibley Memorial Hospital[2]	Washington	100%	140
Howard University Hospital[2]	Washington	96%	101
Medstar Washington Hospital Center[2]	Washington	96%	108
Medstar Georgetown University Hospital[2]	Washington	95%	63
Washington DC VA Medical Center	Washington	95%	85
George Washington Univ Hospital[2]	Washington	93%	130
Providence Hospital	Washington	87%	128
United Medical Center[2]	Washington	86%	114

Pregnancy and Delivery Care

Newborns whose Deliveries were Scheduled Early

Hospital Name	City	Rate	Cases
Howard University Hospital[2]	Washington	0%	30
Medstar Washington Hospital Center[2]	Washington	1%	108
Providence Hospital[2]	Washington	2%	46
United Medical Center[2]	Washington	10%	41
George Washington Univ Hospital[2]	Washington	12%	40
Sibley Memorial Hospital[2]	Washington	13%	61

Preventive Care

Immunization for Influenza

Hospital Name	City	Rate	Cases
Medstar Georgetown University Hospital[2]	Washington	97%	520
Sibley Memorial Hospital[2]	Washington	97%	453
Medstar Washington Hospital Center[2]	Washington	96%	556
Howard University Hospital[2]	Washington	91%	543
Providence Hospital[2]	Washington	81%	510
United Medical Center[2]	Washington	65%	443
George Washington Univ Hospital[2]	Washington	57%	546

NOTE: Hospital profiles are in alphabetical order by state, then city, then hospital within the city; Rankings exclude hospitals with less than 25 cases except for patient surveys which excludes hospitals with less than 100 cases; (a) 100-299 cases; (1) The number of cases/patients is too few to report; (2) Data submitted were based on a sample of cases/patients; (3) Results are based on a shorter time period than required; (4) Data suppressed by CMS for one or more quarters; (5) Results are not available for this reporting period; (6) Fewer than 100 patients completed the HCAHPS survey; (7) No cases met the criteria for this measure; (8) The lower limit of the confidence interval cannot be calculated if the number of observed infections equals zero; (9) No data are available from the state/territory for this reporting period; (10) The scores shown reflect fewer than 50 completed surveys; (11) There were discrepancies in the data collection process; (12) This measure does not apply to this hospital for this reporting period; (13) Results cannot be calculated for this reporting period; (14) The results for this state are combined with nearby states to protect confidentiality; Please refer to the User's Guide for a full explanation of data.

Immunization for Pneumonia

Hospital Name	City	Rate	Cases
Medstar Washington Hospital Center[2]	Washington	96%	714
Howard University Hospital[2]	Washington	95%	559
Medstar Georgetown University Hospital[2]	Washington	95%	485
Sibley Memorial Hospital[2]	Washington	94%	381
Providence Hospital[2]	Washington	81%	603
United Medical Center[2]	Washington	74%	589
George Washington Univ Hospital[2]	Washington	64%	534

Stroke Care

Antithrombotic Therapy Timing

Hospital Name	City	Rate	Cases
George Washington Univ Hospital[2]	Washington	99%	85
Howard University Hospital	Washington	99%	72
Providence Hospital	Washington	99%	127
Medstar Washington Hospital Center[2]	Washington	98%	100
Sibley Memorial Hospital	Washington	98%	51
Medstar Georgetown University Hospital	Washington	86%	80
United Medical Center	Washington	83%	30

Assessed for Rehabilitation

Hospital Name	City	Rate	Cases
George Washington Univ Hospital[2]	Washington	99%	128
Medstar Georgetown University Hospital	Washington	99%	181
Medstar Washington Hospital Center[2]	Washington	99%	147
Sibley Memorial Hospital	Washington	98%	62
Howard University Hospital	Washington	97%	72
Providence Hospital	Washington	95%	130
United Medical Center	Washington	77%	31

Discharged on Antithrombotic Therapy

Hospital Name	City	Rate	Cases
George Washington Univ Hospital[2]	Washington	100%	102
Sibley Memorial Hospital	Washington	100%	54
United Medical Center	Washington	100%	30
Howard University Hospital	Washington	98%	65
Medstar Georgetown University Hospital	Washington	98%	98
Medstar Washington Hospital Center[2]	Washington	98%	113
Providence Hospital	Washington	98%	113

Discharged on Statin Medication

Hospital Name	City	Rate	Cases
George Washington Univ Hospital[2]	Washington	100%	75
Howard University Hospital	Washington	100%	49
Sibley Memorial Hospital	Washington	100%	44
Medstar Georgetown University Hospital	Washington	97%	71
Medstar Washington Hospital Center[2]	Washington	95%	104
Providence Hospital	Washington	94%	86

Thrombolytic Therapy Timing

Hospital Name	City	Rate	Cases
George Washington Univ Hospital[2]	Washington	26%	31

Venous Thromboembolism (VTE) Prophylaxis

Hospital Name	City	Rate	Cases
Medstar Georgetown University Hospital	Washington	99%	211
Sibley Memorial Hospital	Washington	98%	60
George Washington Univ Hospital[2]	Washington	97%	137
Medstar Washington Hospital Center[2]	Washington	97%	148
Howard University Hospital	Washington	96%	77
Providence Hospital	Washington	92%	144
United Medical Center	Washington	64%	33

Written Stroke Educational Materials Given

Hospital Name	City	Rate	Cases
Medstar Georgetown University Hospital	Washington	99%	72
Providence Hospital	Washington	98%	62
Sibley Memorial Hospital	Washington	97%	34
Medstar Washington Hospital Center[2]	Washington	93%	61
Howard University Hospital	Washington	88%	49
George Washington Univ Hospital[2]	Washington	86%	92

Surgical Care Improvement Project

Appropriate Beta Blocker Usage

Hospital Name	City	Rate	Cases
George Washington Univ Hospital[2]	Washington	99%	185
Washington DC VA Medical Center[2]	Washington	98%	84
Medstar Georgetown University Hospital[2]	Washington	97%	78
Sibley Memorial Hospital[2]	Washington	97%	218
Medstar Washington Hospital Center[2]	Washington	95%	212
Howard University Hospital[2]	Washington	94%	34
Providence Hospital[2]	Washington	83%	107

Appropriate VTP Within 24 Hours

Hospital Name	City	Rate	Cases
George Washington Univ Hospital[2]	Washington	100%	366
Medstar Georgetown University Hospital[2]	Washington	98%	330
Medstar Washington Hospital Center[2]	Washington	98%	461
Sibley Memorial Hospital[2]	Washington	97%	1030
Howard University Hospital[2]	Washington	94%	187
Washington DC VA Medical Center[2]	Washington	91%	120
Providence Hospital[2]	Washington	84%	430
United Medical Center	Washington	83%	72

Controlled Postoperative Blood Glucose

Hospital Name	City	Rate	Cases
Medstar Washington Hospital Center[2]	Washington	95%	196
Washington DC VA Medical Center[2]	Washington	95%	92
George Washington Univ Hospital[2]	Washington	94%	81

Perioperative Temperature Management

Hospital Name	City	Rate	Cases
George Washington Univ Hospital[2]	Washington	100%	538
Medstar Georgetown University Hospital[2]	Washington	100%	380
Providence Hospital[2]	Washington	100%	490
Sibley Memorial Hospital[2]	Washington	99%	1113
Medstar Washington Hospital Center[2]	Washington	98%	612
Washington DC VA Medical Center[2]	Washington	98%	234
Howard University Hospital[2]	Washington	97%	232
United Medical Center	Washington	93%	88

Prophylactic Antibiotic Selection

Hospital Name	City	Rate	Cases
Medstar Washington Hospital Center[2]	Washington	100%	567
Washington DC VA Medical Center	Washington	100%	127
George Washington Univ Hospital[2]	Washington	99%	358
Medstar Georgetown University Hospital[2]	Washington	99%	218
Sibley Memorial Hospital[2]	Washington	99%	783
Howard University Hospital[2]	Washington	97%	144
Providence Hospital[2]	Washington	97%	316
United Medical Center	Washington	79%	29

Prophylactic Antibiotic Selection (Outpatient)

Hospital Name	City	Rate	Cases
Providence Hospital	Washington	99%	168
Medstar Georgetown University Hospital	Washington	98%	301
Medstar Washington Hospital Center	Washington	98%	695
George Washington Univ Hospital	Washington	96%	368
Sibley Memorial Hospital	Washington	92%	288
Howard University Hospital	Washington	85%	52

Prophylactic Antibiotic Stopped

Hospital Name	City	Rate	Cases
Sibley Memorial Hospital[2]	Washington	98%	775
Medstar Georgetown University Hospital[2]	Washington	97%	209
Medstar Washington Hospital Center[2]	Washington	97%	560
Washington DC VA Medical Center	Washington	96%	125
George Washington Univ Hospital[2]	Washington	93%	332
Howard University Hospital[2]	Washington	92%	132
Providence Hospital[2]	Washington	92%	310
United Medical Center	Washington	89%	28

Prophylactic Antibiotic Timing

Hospital Name	City	Rate	Cases
George Washington Univ Hospital[2]	Washington	99%	358
Medstar Washington Hospital Center[2]	Washington	99%	571
Sibley Memorial Hospital[2]	Washington	98%	786
Washington DC VA Medical Center	Washington	98%	127
Medstar Georgetown University Hospital[2]	Washington	97%	216
Providence Hospital[2]	Washington	96%	316
Howard University Hospital[2]	Washington	95%	144
United Medical Center	Washington	90%	29

Prophylactic Antibiotic Timing (Outpatient)

Hospital Name	City	Rate	Cases
George Washington Univ Hospital	Washington	98%	369
Medstar Washington Hospital Center	Washington	98%	684
Sibley Memorial Hospital	Washington	96%	291
Medstar Georgetown University Hospital	Washington	95%	303
Howard University Hospital	Washington	85%	39
Providence Hospital	Washington	71%	208

Urinary Catheter Removal

Hospital Name	City	Rate	Cases
George Washington Univ Hospital[2]	Washington	100%	381
Sibley Memorial Hospital[2]	Washington	99%	798
Washington DC VA Medical Center[2]	Washington	98%	123
Medstar Georgetown University Hospital[2]	Washington	97%	229
Medstar Washington Hospital Center[2]	Washington	95%	488
Howard University Hospital[2]	Washington	93%	123
Providence Hospital[2]	Washington	89%	327
United Medical Center	Washington	57%	46

Survey of Patients' Hospital Experiences

Area Around Room 'Always' Quiet at Night

Hospital Name	City	Rate	Cases
Howard University Hospital	Washington	67%	300+
Providence Hospital	Washington	62%	300+
Medstar Georgetown University Hospital	Washington	54%	300+
George Washington Univ Hospital	Washington	53%	300+
United Medical Center	Washington	51%	300+
Sibley Memorial Hospital	Washington	50%	300+
Medstar Washington Hospital Center	Washington	49%	300+

Doctors 'Always' Communicated Well

Hospital Name	City	Rate	Cases
Providence Hospital	Washington	80%	300+
Sibley Memorial Hospital	Washington	79%	300+
Howard University Hospital	Washington	78%	300+
Medstar Georgetown University Hospital	Washington	78%	300+
Medstar Washington Hospital Center	Washington	77%	300+
George Washington Univ Hospital	Washington	75%	300+
United Medical Center	Washington	72%	300+

Home Recovery Information Given

Hospital Name	City	Rate	Cases
Medstar Georgetown University Hospital	Washington	88%	300+
Medstar Washington Hospital Center	Washington	85%	300+
George Washington Univ Hospital	Washington	81%	300+
Providence Hospital	Washington	78%	300+
Howard University Hospital	Washington	76%	300+
Sibley Memorial Hospital	Washington	75%	300+
United Medical Center	Washington	62%	300+

Hospital Given 9 or 10 on 10 Point Scale

Hospital Name	City	Rate	Cases
Medstar Georgetown University Hospital	Washington	69%	300+
Medstar Washington Hospital Center	Washington	69%	300+
Providence Hospital	Washington	64%	300+
George Washington Univ Hospital	Washington	63%	300+
Sibley Memorial Hospital	Washington	62%	300+
Howard University Hospital	Washington	54%	300+
United Medical Center	Washington	38%	300+

Meds 'Always' Explained Before Given

Hospital Name	City	Rate	Cases
Medstar Georgetown University Hospital	Washington	58%	300+
Medstar Washington Hospital Center	Washington	58%	300+
Howard University Hospital	Washington	57%	300+
Sibley Memorial Hospital	Washington	57%	300+
Providence Hospital	Washington	55%	300+
George Washington Univ Hospital	Washington	54%	300+
United Medical Center	Washington	44%	300+

Nurses 'Always' Communicated Well

Hospital Name	City	Rate	Cases
Medstar Georgetown University Hospital	Washington	77%	300+
Medstar Washington Hospital Center	Washington	72%	300+
Providence Hospital	Washington	72%	300+
George Washington Univ Hospital	Washington	70%	300+
Howard University Hospital	Washington	69%	300+
Sibley Memorial Hospital	Washington	69%	300+
United Medical Center	Washington	62%	300+

Pain 'Always' Well Controlled

Hospital Name	City	Rate	Cases
Medstar Georgetown University Hospital	Washington	69%	300+
Sibley Memorial Hospital	Washington	69%	300+
Providence Hospital	Washington	65%	300+
George Washington Univ Hospital	Washington	63%	300+
Howard University Hospital	Washington	63%	300+
Medstar Washington Hospital Center	Washington	62%	300+
United Medical Center	Washington	58%	300+

Room and Bathroom 'Always' Clean

Hospital Name	City	Rate	Cases
Sibley Memorial Hospital	Washington	68%	300+
Providence Hospital	Washington	67%	300+
Howard University Hospital	Washington	63%	300+
George Washington Univ Hospital	Washington	60%	300+
Medstar Georgetown University Hospital	Washington	59%	300+
Medstar Washington Hospital Center	Washington	56%	300+
United Medical Center	Washington	53%	300+

NOTE: Hospital profiles are in alphabetical order by state, then city, then hospital within the city; Rankings exclude hospitals with less than 25 cases except for patient surveys which excludes hospitals with less than 100 cases; (a) 100-299 cases; (1) The number of cases/patients is too few to report; (2) Data submitted were based on a sample of cases/patients; (3) Results are based on a shorter time period than required; (4) Data suppressed by CMS for one or more quarters; (5) Results are not available for this reporting period; (6) Fewer than 100 patients completed the HCAHPS survey; (7) No cases met the criteria for this measure; (8) The lower limit of the confidence interval cannot be calculated if the number of observed infections equals zero; (9) No data are available from the state/territory for this reporting period; (10) The scores shown reflect fewer than 50 completed surveys; (11) There were discrepancies in the data collection process; (12) This measure does not apply to this hospital for this reporting period; (13) Results cannot be calculated for this reporting period; (14) The results for this state are combined with nearby states to protect confidentiality; Please refer to the User's Guide for a full explanation of data.

Timely Help 'Always' Received

Hospital Name	City	Rate	Cases
Providence Hospital	Washington	59%	300+
Medstar Georgetown University Hospital	Washington	57%	300+
Sibley Memorial Hospital	Washington	57%	300+
Howard University Hospital	Washington	55%	300+
George Washington Univ Hospital	Washington	53%	300+
Medstar Washington Hospital Center	Washington	53%	300+
United Medical Center	Washington	49%	300+

Would Definitely Recommend Hospital

Hospital Name	City	Rate	Cases
Medstar Georgetown University Hospital	Washington	76%	300+
Medstar Washington Hospital Center	Washington	72%	300+
Sibley Memorial Hospital	Washington	70%	300+
George Washington Univ Hospital	Washington	68%	300+
Providence Hospital	Washington	62%	300+
Howard University Hospital	Washington	56%	300+
United Medical Center	Washington	30%	300+

Use of Medical Imaging

Cardiac Imaging Stress Test before OP Surgery

Hospital Name	City	Rate	Cases
Providence Hospital	Washington	1.3%	75
George Washington Univ Hospital	Washington	5.3%	133
Sibley Memorial Hospital	Washington	5.4%	56
Medstar Washington Hospital Center	Washington	5.6%	539
Howard University Hospital	Washington	5.9%	102
Medstar Georgetown University Hospital	Washington	9.1%	285

Combination Abdominal CT Scan

Hospital Name	City	Rate	Cases
Medstar Washington Hospital Center	Washington	0.8%	2098
Sibley Memorial Hospital	Washington	2.2%	1096
United Medical Center	Washington	6.2%	195
Howard University Hospital	Washington	7.1%	439
Medstar Georgetown University Hospital	Washington	7.9%	1382
Providence Hospital	Washington	7.9%	822
George Washington Univ Hospital	Washington	8.0%	1102

Combination Brain/Sinus CT Scan

Hospital Name	City	Rate	Cases
Medstar Georgetown University Hospital	Washington	1.0%	394
Medstar Washington Hospital Center	Washington	3.2%	979
Providence Hospital	Washington	4.0%	757
United Medical Center	Washington	4.1%	413
Sibley Memorial Hospital	Washington	4.7%	615
Howard University Hospital	Washington	6.0%	448
George Washington Univ Hospital	Washington	7.1%	687

Combination Chest CT Scan

Hospital Name	City	Rate	Cases
Sibley Memorial Hospital	Washington	0.0%	694
United Medical Center	Washington	0.0%	135
Medstar Georgetown University Hospital	Washington	0.4%	1652
Medstar Washington Hospital Center	Washington	0.5%	1758
George Washington Univ Hospital	Washington	1.0%	691
Howard University Hospital	Washington	2.3%	219
Providence Hospital	Washington	3.5%	395

Follow-up Mammogram/Ultrasound

A follow-up rate near zero may indicate missed cancer; a rate higher than 14% may mean there is unnecessary follow up.

Hospital Name	City	Rate	Cases
Providence Hospital	Washington	3.4%	2055
Medstar Washington Hospital Center	Washington	6.7%	2554
Sibley Memorial Hospital	Washington	7.8%	2158
Howard University Hospital	Washington	8.7%	723
George Washington Univ Hospital	Washington	8.8%	739
United Medical Center	Washington	9.4%	395
Medstar Georgetown University Hospital	Washington	10.5%	891

Lumbar Spine MRI for Low Back Pain

Hospital Name	City	Rate	Cases
Medstar Washington Hospital Center	Washington	32.3%	201
Sibley Memorial Hospital	Washington	33.3%	183
George Washington Univ Hospital	Washington	33.8%	142
United Medical Center	Washington	34.8%	46
Medstar Georgetown University Hospital	Washington	35.1%	74
Providence Hospital	Washington	35.9%	142

NOTE: Hospital profiles are in alphabetical order by state, then city, then hospital within the city; Rankings exclude hospitals with less than 25 cases except for patient surveys which excludes hospitals with less than 100 cases; (a) 100-299 cases; (1) The number of cases/patients is too few to report; (2) Data submitted were based on a sample of cases/patients; (3) Results are based on a shorter time period than required; (4) Data suppressed by CMS for one or more quarters; (5) Results are not available for this reporting period; (6) Fewer than 100 patients completed the HCAHPS survey; (7) No cases met the criteria for this measure; (8) The lower limit of the confidence interval cannot be calculated if the number of observed infections equals zero; (9) No data are available from the state/territory for this reporting period; (10) The scores shown reflect fewer than 50 completed surveys; (11) There were discrepancies in the data collection process; (12) This measure does not apply to this hospital for this reporting period; (13) Results cannot be calculated for this reporting period; (14) The results for this state are combined with nearby states to protect confidentiality; Please refer to the User's Guide for a full explanation of data.

Children's Hospital NMC

111 Michigan Ave, NW Phone: 202-476-5000
Washington, DC 20010 Fax: 202-884-5987
URL: www.dcchildrens.com
Type: Childrens Emergency Services: Yes
Ownership: Voluntary non-profit - Private Beds: 279

Key Personnel:
Emergency Room . . . . James Chamberland, MD
Radiology. . . . . David Kushner, MD
Cardiac Laboratory. . . . . Gerard Robert Martin, MD
CEO/President. . . . . Kurt Newman, MD
Operating Room. . . . . Kurt D Newman, MD
Patient Relations . . . . Nellie Robinson, RN, MS
Pediatric In-Patient Care . . . . . . Peter Scheidt, MD
Chief of Medical Staff. . . . . David Wessel, MD

Measure	Cases	This Hosp.	State Avg.	U.S. Avg.
Blood Clot Prevention and Treatment				
Anticoagulation Overlap Therapy[5]	-	-	94%	93%
ICU Venous Thromboembolism Prophylaxis[5]	-	-	96%	92%
Incidence of Potentially Preventable VTE[5]	-	-	6%	10%
UFH with Dosages/Platelet Monitoring[5]	-	-	99%	97%
Venous Thromboembolism Prophylaxis[5]	-	-	82%	85%
Warfarin Therapy Discharge Instructions[5]	-	-	68%	75%
Chest Pain/Possible Heart Attack Care				
Aspirin Given Within 24 Hours of Arrival	-	-	95%	96%
Fibrinolytic Meds Within 30 Min. of Arrival	-	-	-	58%
Average Time to ECG (minutes)	-	-	19	7
Average Time to Transfer (minutes)	-	-	79	60
Children's Asthma Care				
Received Home Management Plan of Care[2]	375	89%	-	88%
Received Reliever Medication[2]	375	100%	-	100%
Received Systemic Corticosteroids[2]	374	100%	-	100%
Emergency Department				
Admittance Decision Time (minutes)[5]	-	-	226	98
Head CT Results Within 45 Min. of Arrival	-	-	18%	57%
Patients Who Left ER Before Being Seen	-	-	3%	2%
Time from ER Arrival to Admit. (minutes)[5]	-	-	479	274
Time from ER Arrival to Discharge (minutes)	-	-	186	134
Time in ER Before Being Evaluated (minutes)	-	-	53	26
Time to Pain Meds for Fractures (minutes)	-	-	80	57
Heart Attack Care				
Aspirin Given at Discharge[5]	-	-	97%	99%
Fibrinolytic Meds Within 30 Min. of Arrival[5]	-	-	-	54%
PCI Within 90 Minutes of Arrival[5]	-	-	88%	96%
Statin Prescribed at Discharge[5]	-	-	97%	98%
Heart Failure Care				
ACE Inhibitor or ARB for LVSD[5]	-	-	92%	97%
Discharge Instructions Given[5]	-	-	87%	94%
Evaluation of LVS Function[5]	-	-	98%	99%
Medicare Spending				
Medicare Spending per Patient (ratio)	-	-	1	0.98
Pneumonia Care				
Appropriate Initial Antibiotic Given[5]	-	-	93%	95%
Blood Culture Timing[5]	-	-	93%	98%
Pregnancy and Delivery Care				
Newborn Deliveries Scheduled Early[5]	-	-	6%	6%
Preventive Care				
Immunization for Influenza[5]	-	-	84%	90%
Immunization for Pneumonia[5]	-	-	85%	92%
Stroke Care				
Anticoagulation Therapy for Atrial Fibrillation[5]	-	-	94%	95%
Antithrombotic Therapy Timing[5]	-	-	96%	98%
Assessed for Rehabilitation[5]	-	-	97%	97%
Discharged on Antithrombotic Therapy[5]	-	-	99%	99%
Discharged on Statin Medication[5]	-	-	96%	94%
Thrombolytic Therapy Timing[5]	-	-	40%	66%
Venous Thromboembolism Prophylaxis[5]	-	-	95%	94%
Written Stroke Educational Materials Given[5]	-	-	90%	88%
Surgical Care Improvement Project				
Appropriate Beta Blocker Usage[5]	-	-	95%	98%
Appropriate VTP Within 24 Hours[5]	-	-	95%	98%
Controlled Postoperative Blood Glucose[5]	-	-	94%	97%
Perioperative Temperature Management[5]	-	-	99%	100%
Prophylactic Antibiotic Selection[5]	-	-	99%	99%
Prophylactic Antibiotic Selection (Outpatient)	-	-	97%	98%
Prophylactic Antibiotic Stopped[5]	-	-	96%	98%
Prophylactic Antibiotic Timing[5]	-	-	98%	99%
Prophylactic Antibiotic Timing (Outpatient)	-	-	94%	98%
Urinary Catheter Removal[5]	-	-	96%	97%
Survey of Patients' Hospital Experiences				
Area Around Room 'Always' Quiet at Night[5]	-	-	55%	61%
Doctors 'Always' Communicated Well[5]	-	-	77%	82%
Home Recovery Information Given[5]	-	-	78%	85%
Hospital Given 9 or 10 on 10 Point Scale[5]	-	-	60%	71%
Meds 'Always' Explained Before Given[5]	-	-	55%	64%
Nurses 'Always' Communicated Well[5]	-	-	70%	79%
Pain 'Always' Well Controlled[5]	-	-	64%	71%
Room and Bathroom 'Always' Clean[5]	-	-	61%	73%
Timely Help 'Always' Received[5]	-	-	55%	68%
Would Definitely Recommend Hospital[5]	-	-	62%	71%
Use of Medical Imaging				
Cardiac Imaging Stress Test before Surgery	-	-	6.2%	5.3%
Combination Abdominal CT Scan	-	-	4.8%	10.5%
Combination Brain/Sinus CT Scan	-	-	4.4%	2.7%
Combination Chest CT Scan	-	-	0.7%	2.7%
Follow-up Mammogram/Ultrasound	-	-	7%	8.8%
Lumbar Spine MRI for Low Back Pain	-	-	33.8%	37.2%

George Washington Univ Hospital

900 23rd Saint Nw Phone: 202-716-4605
Washington, DC 20037 Fax: 202-715-5206
URL: www.gwhospital.com
Type: Acute Care Hospitals Emergency Services: Yes
Ownership: Proprietary Beds: 371

Key Personnel:
Radiology. . . . . Mark Lerner
Chief of Medical Staff. . . . . Gary Little, MD
Quality Assurance . . . . Melanie Sage
Infection Control. . . . . Rita Smith, RN
Operating Room. . . . . Elizabeth White, RN
CEO/President. . . . . Barry A. Wolfman

Measure	Cases	This Hosp.	State Avg.	U.S. Avg.
Blood Clot Prevention and Treatment				
Anticoagulation Overlap Therapy[2]	106	95%	94%	93%
ICU Venous Thromboembolism Prophylaxis[2]	87	98%	96%	92%
Incidence of Potentially Preventable VTE[2]	29	10%	6%	10%
UFH with Dosages/Platelet Monitoring[2]	69	100%	99%	97%
Venous Thromboembolism Prophylaxis[2]	308	92%	82%	85%
Warfarin Therapy Discharge Instructions[2]	84	81%	68%	75%
Chest Pain/Possible Heart Attack Care				
Aspirin Given Within 24 Hours of Arrival[1,3]	-	-	95%	96%
Fibrinolytic Meds Within 30 Min. of Arrival[5]	-	-	-	58%
Average Time to ECG (minutes)[1,3]	-	-	19	7
Average Time to Transfer (minutes)[5]	-	-	79	60
Children's Asthma Care				
Received Home Management Plan of Care	-	-	-	88%
Received Reliever Medication	-	-	-	100%
Received Systemic Corticosteroids	-	-	-	100%
Emergency Department				
Admittance Decision Time (minutes)[2]	388	250	226	98
Head CT Results Within 45 Min. of Arrival[3,7]	-	-	18%	57%
Patients Who Left ER Before Being Seen	74,886	2%	3%	2%
Time from ER Arrival to Admit. (minutes)[2]	393	470	479	274
Time from ER Arrival to Discharge (minutes)	370	215	186	134
Time in ER Before Being Evaluated (minutes)	418	48	53	26
Time to Pain Meds for Fractures (minutes)	195	78	80	57
Heart Attack Care				
Aspirin Given at Discharge	173	98%	97%	99%
Fibrinolytic Meds Within 30 Min. of Arrival[7]	-	-	-	54%
PCI Within 90 Minutes of Arrival	45	96%	88%	96%
Statin Prescribed at Discharge	170	99%	97%	98%
Heart Failure Care				
ACE Inhibitor or ARB for LVSD[2]	113	98%	92%	97%
Discharge Instructions Given[2]	311	100%	87%	94%
Evaluation of LVS Function[2]	336	100%	98%	99%
Medicare Spending				
Medicare Spending per Patient (ratio)	-	0.99	1	0.98
Pneumonia Care				
Appropriate Initial Antibiotic Given[2]	82	98%	93%	95%
Blood Culture Timing[2]	130	93%	93%	98%
Pregnancy and Delivery Care				
Newborn Deliveries Scheduled Early[2]	40	12%	6%	6%
Preventive Care				
Immunization for Influenza[2]	546	57%	84%	90%
Immunization for Pneumonia[2]	534	64%	85%	92%
Stroke Care				
Anticoagulation Therapy for Atrial Fibrillation[2]	15	100%	94%	95%
Antithrombotic Therapy Timing[2]	85	99%	96%	98%
Assessed for Rehabilitation[2]	128	99%	97%	97%
Discharged on Antithrombotic Therapy[2]	102	100%	99%	99%
Discharged on Statin Medication[2]	75	100%	96%	94%
Thrombolytic Therapy Timing[2]	31	26%	40%	66%
Venous Thromboembolism Prophylaxis[2]	137	97%	95%	94%
Written Stroke Educational Materials Given[2]	92	86%	90%	88%
Surgical Care Improvement Project				
Appropriate Beta Blocker Usage[2]	185	99%	95%	98%
Appropriate VTP Within 24 Hours[2]	366	100%	95%	98%
Controlled Postoperative Blood Glucose[2]	81	94%	94%	97%
Perioperative Temperature Management[2]	538	100%	99%	100%
Prophylactic Antibiotic Selection[2]	358	99%	99%	99%
Prophylactic Antibiotic Selection (Outpatient)	368	96%	97%	98%
Prophylactic Antibiotic Stopped[2]	332	93%	96%	98%
Prophylactic Antibiotic Timing[2]	358	99%	98%	99%
Prophylactic Antibiotic Timing (Outpatient)	369	98%	94%	98%
Urinary Catheter Removal[2]	381	100%	96%	97%
Survey of Patients' Hospital Experiences				
Area Around Room 'Always' Quiet at Night	300+	53%	55%	61%
Doctors 'Always' Communicated Well	300+	75%	77%	82%
Home Recovery Information Given	300+	81%	78%	85%
Hospital Given 9 or 10 on 10 Point Scale	300+	63%	60%	71%
Meds 'Always' Explained Before Given	300+	54%	55%	64%
Nurses 'Always' Communicated Well	300+	70%	70%	79%
Pain 'Always' Well Controlled	300+	63%	64%	71%
Room and Bathroom 'Always' Clean	300+	60%	61%	73%
Timely Help 'Always' Received	300+	53%	55%	68%
Would Definitely Recommend Hospital	300+	68%	62%	71%
Use of Medical Imaging				
Cardiac Imaging Stress Test before Surgery	133	5.3%	6.2%	5.3%
Combination Abdominal CT Scan	1,102	8.0%	4.8%	10.5%
Combination Brain/Sinus CT Scan	687	7.1%	4.4%	2.7%
Combination Chest CT Scan	691	1.0%	0.7%	2.7%
Follow-up Mammogram/Ultrasound	739	8.8%	7%	8.8%
Lumbar Spine MRI for Low Back Pain	142	33.8%	33.8%	37.2%

Howard University Hospital

2041 Georgia Ave Nw Phone: 202-745-6100
Washington, DC 20060 Fax: 202-745-3731
URL: www.huhosp.org
Type: Acute Care Hospitals Emergency Services: Yes
Ownership: Voluntary non-profit - Other Beds: 482

Key Personnel:
Quality Assurance . . . . Norma Bent
Operating Room. . . . . Clive O Callender, MD FACS
Radiology. . . . . Andre J. Duerinckx, MD, PhD
Infection Control. . . . . John I McNeil, MD
CEO/President. . . . . H Patrick Swygert
Chief of Medical Staff. . . . . Alvin Thomas, MD
Cardiac Laboratory. . . . . Deborah Williams, MD
Pediatric In-Patient Care . . . . . . Michael A. Young, M.D., F.A.B.M.,

Measure	Cases	This Hosp.	State Avg.	U.S. Avg.
Blood Clot Prevention and Treatment				
Anticoagulation Overlap Therapy[2]	66	89%	94%	93%
ICU Venous Thromboembolism Prophylaxis[2]	89	98%	96%	92%
Incidence of Potentially Preventable VTE[2]	15	7%	6%	10%
UFH with Dosages/Platelet Monitoring[2]	22	91%	99%	97%
Venous Thromboembolism Prophylaxis[2]	254	89%	82%	85%
Warfarin Therapy Discharge Instructions[2]	48	21%	68%	75%
Chest Pain/Possible Heart Attack Care				
Aspirin Given Within 24 Hours of Arrival[1,3]	-	-	95%	96%
Fibrinolytic Meds Within 30 Min. of Arrival[5]	-	-	-	58%
Average Time to ECG (minutes)[1,3]	-	-	19	7
Average Time to Transfer (minutes)[5]	-	-	79	60

NOTE: Hospital profiles are in alphabetical order by state, then city, then hospital within the city; Rankings exclude hospitals with less than 25 cases except for patient surveys which excludes hospitals with less than 100 cases; (a) 100-299 cases; (1) The number of cases/patients is too few to report; (2) Data submitted were based on a sample of cases/patients; (3) Results are based on a shorter time period than required; (4) Data suppressed by CMS for one or more quarters; (5) Results are not available for this reporting period; (6) Fewer than 100 patients completed the HCAHPS survey; (7) No cases met the criteria for this measure; (8) The lower limit of the confidence interval cannot be calculated if the number of observed infections equals zero; (9) No data are available from the state/territory for this reporting period; (10) The scores shown reflect fewer than 50 completed surveys; (11) There were discrepancies in the data collection process; (12) This measure does not apply to this hospital for this reporting period; (13) Results cannot be calculated for this reporting period; (14) The results for this state are combined with nearby states to protect confidentiality; Please refer to the User's Guide for a full explanation of data.

Measure	Cases	This Hosp.	State Avg.	U.S. Avg.
Children's Asthma Care				
Received Home Management Plan of Care	14	71%	-	88%
Received Reliever Medication	14	100%	-	100%
Received Systemic Corticosteroids	14	86%	-	100%
Emergency Department				
Admittance Decision Time (minutes)[2]	203	170	226	98
Head CT Results Within 45 Min. of Arrival[1,3]	-	-	18%	57%
Patients Who Left ER Before Being Seen	59,608	3%	3%	2%
Time from ER Arrival to Admit. (minutes)[2]	234	399	479	274
Time from ER Arrival to Discharge (minutes)	330	206	186	134
Time in ER Before Being Evaluated (minutes)	316	98	53	26
Time to Pain Meds for Fractures (minutes)	70	108	80	57
Heart Attack Care				
Aspirin Given at Discharge	49	96%	97%	99%
Fibrinolytic Meds Within 30 Min. of Arrival[7]	-	-	-	54%
PCI Within 90 Minutes of Arrival[1]	-	-	88%	96%
Statin Prescribed at Discharge	49	94%	97%	98%
Heart Failure Care				
ACE Inhibitor or ARB for LVSD[2]	109	96%	92%	97%
Discharge Instructions Given[2]	220	77%	87%	94%
Evaluation of LVS Function[2]	235	99%	98%	99%
Medicare Spending				
Medicare Spending per Patient (ratio)	-	0.90	1	0.98
Pneumonia Care				
Appropriate Initial Antibiotic Given[2]	43	95%	93%	95%
Blood Culture Timing[2]	101	96%	93%	98%
Pregnancy and Delivery Care				
Newborn Deliveries Scheduled Early[2]	30	0%	6%	6%
Preventive Care				
Immunization for Influenza[2]	543	91%	84%	90%
Immunization for Pneumonia[2]	559	95%	85%	92%
Stroke Care				
Anticoagulation Therapy for Atrial Fibrillation[1]	-	-	94%	95%
Antithrombotic Therapy Timing	72	99%	96%	98%
Assessed for Rehabilitation	72	97%	97%	97%
Discharged on Antithrombotic Therapy	65	98%	99%	99%
Discharged on Statin Medication	49	100%	96%	94%
Thrombolytic Therapy Timing[1]	-	-	40%	66%
Venous Thromboembolism Prophylaxis	77	96%	95%	94%
Written Stroke Educational Materials Given	49	88%	90%	88%
Surgical Care Improvement Project				
Appropriate Beta Blocker Usage[2]	34	94%	95%	98%
Appropriate VTP Within 24 Hours[2]	187	94%	95%	98%
Controlled Postoperative Blood Glucose[2]	17	82%	94%	97%
Perioperative Temperature Management[2]	232	97%	99%	100%
Prophylactic Antibiotic Selection[2]	144	97%	99%	99%
Prophylactic Antibiotic Selection (Outpatient)	52	85%	97%	98%
Prophylactic Antibiotic Stopped[2]	132	92%	96%	98%
Prophylactic Antibiotic Timing[2]	144	95%	98%	99%
Prophylactic Antibiotic Timing (Outpatient)	39	85%	94%	98%
Urinary Catheter Removal[2]	123	93%	96%	97%
Survey of Patients' Hospital Experiences				
Area Around Room 'Always' Quiet at Night	300+	67%	55%	61%
Doctors 'Always' Communicated Well	300+	78%	77%	82%
Home Recovery Information Given	300+	76%	78%	85%
Hospital Given 9 or 10 on 10 Point Scale	300+	54%	60%	71%
Meds 'Always' Explained Before Given	300+	57%	55%	64%
Nurses 'Always' Communicated Well	300+	69%	70%	79%
Pain 'Always' Well Controlled	300+	63%	64%	71%
Room and Bathroom 'Always' Clean	300+	63%	61%	73%
Timely Help 'Always' Received	300+	55%	55%	68%
Would Definitely Recommend Hospital	300+	56%	62%	71%
Use of Medical Imaging				
Cardiac Imaging Stress Test before Surgery	102	5.9%	6.2%	5.3%
Combination Abdominal CT Scan	439	7.1%	4.8%	10.5%
Combination Brain/Sinus CT Scan	448	6.0%	4.4%	2.7%
Combination Chest CT Scan	219	2.3%	0.7%	2.7%
Follow-up Mammogram/Ultrasound	723	8.7%	7%	8.8%
Lumbar Spine MRI for Low Back Pain[1]	-	-	33.8%	37.2%

Medstar Georgetown University Hospital

3800 Reservoir Rd
Washington, DC 20007
Phone: 202-784-3000
Fax: 202-444-2875
URL: www.georgetownuniversityhospital.org
Type: Acute Care Hospitals
Emergency Services: Yes
Ownership: Voluntary non-profit - Private
Beds: 381

Key Personnel:
Chief of Medical Staff. . . . . Lisa M. Boyle, MD
CEO/President. . . . . Richard L. Goldberg, MD

Measure	Cases	This Hosp.	State Avg.	U.S. Avg.
Blood Clot Prevention and Treatment				
Anticoagulation Overlap Therapy[2]	87	97%	94%	93%
ICU Venous Thromboembolism Prophylaxis[2]	86	97%	96%	92%
Incidence of Potentially Preventable VTE[2]	72	7%	6%	10%
UFH with Dosages/Platelet Monitoring[2]	82	100%	99%	97%
Venous Thromboembolism Prophylaxis[2]	302	86%	82%	85%
Warfarin Therapy Discharge Instructions[2]	64	58%	68%	75%
Chest Pain/Possible Heart Attack Care				
Aspirin Given Within 24 Hours of Arrival	22	95%	95%	96%
Fibrinolytic Meds Within 30 Min. of Arrival[7]	-	-	-	58%
Average Time to ECG (minutes)	22	10	19	7
Average Time to Transfer (minutes)[1]	-	-	79	60
Children's Asthma Care				
Received Home Management Plan of Care[2]	78	90%	-	88%
Received Reliever Medication	79	100%	-	100%
Received Systemic Corticosteroids	79	100%	-	100%
Emergency Department				
Admittance Decision Time (minutes)[2]	112	136	226	98
Head CT Results Within 45 Min. of Arrival[1,3]	-	-	18%	57%
Patients Who Left ER Before Being Seen	36,823	2%	3%	2%
Time from ER Arrival to Admit. (minutes)[2]	115	332	479	274
Time from ER Arrival to Discharge (minutes)	329	163	186	134
Time in ER Before Being Evaluated (minutes)	373	35	53	26
Time to Pain Meds for Fractures (minutes)	74	64	80	57
Heart Attack Care				
Aspirin Given at Discharge	12	100%	97%	99%
Fibrinolytic Meds Within 30 Min. of Arrival[7]	-	-	-	54%
PCI Within 90 Minutes of Arrival[7]	-	-	88%	96%
Statin Prescribed at Discharge	12	100%	97%	98%
Heart Failure Care				
ACE Inhibitor or ARB for LVSD	33	100%	92%	97%
Discharge Instructions Given	70	93%	87%	94%
Evaluation of LVS Function	91	100%	98%	99%
Medicare Spending				
Medicare Spending per Patient (ratio)	-	1.03	1	0.98
Pneumonia Care				
Appropriate Initial Antibiotic Given[2]	30	97%	93%	95%
Blood Culture Timing[2]	63	95%	93%	98%
Pregnancy and Delivery Care				
Newborn Deliveries Scheduled Early[2]	13	0%	6%	6%
Preventive Care				
Immunization for Influenza[2]	520	97%	84%	90%
Immunization for Pneumonia[2]	485	95%	85%	92%
Stroke Care				
Anticoagulation Therapy for Atrial Fibrillation	19	95%	94%	95%
Antithrombotic Therapy Timing	80	86%	96%	98%
Assessed for Rehabilitation	181	99%	97%	97%
Discharged on Antithrombotic Therapy	98	98%	99%	99%
Discharged on Statin Medication	71	97%	96%	94%
Thrombolytic Therapy Timing[1]	-	-	40%	66%
Venous Thromboembolism Prophylaxis	211	99%	95%	94%
Written Stroke Educational Materials Given	72	99%	90%	88%
Surgical Care Improvement Project				
Appropriate Beta Blocker Usage[2]	78	97%	95%	98%
Appropriate VTP Within 24 Hours[2]	330	98%	95%	98%
Controlled Postoperative Blood Glucose[2,7]	-	-	94%	97%
Perioperative Temperature Management[2]	380	100%	99%	100%
Prophylactic Antibiotic Selection[2]	218	99%	99%	99%
Prophylactic Antibiotic Selection (Outpatient)	301	98%	97%	98%
Prophylactic Antibiotic Stopped[2]	209	97%	96%	98%
Prophylactic Antibiotic Timing[2]	216	97%	98%	99%
Prophylactic Antibiotic Timing (Outpatient)	303	95%	94%	98%
Urinary Catheter Removal[2]	229	97%	96%	97%
Survey of Patients' Hospital Experiences				
Area Around Room 'Always' Quiet at Night	300+	54%	55%	61%
Doctors 'Always' Communicated Well	300+	78%	77%	82%
Home Recovery Information Given	300+	88%	78%	85%
Hospital Given 9 or 10 on 10 Point Scale	300+	69%	60%	71%
Meds 'Always' Explained Before Given	300+	58%	55%	64%
Nurses 'Always' Communicated Well	300+	77%	70%	79%
Pain 'Always' Well Controlled	300+	69%	64%	71%
Room and Bathroom 'Always' Clean	300+	59%	61%	73%
Timely Help 'Always' Received	300+	57%	55%	68%
Would Definitely Recommend Hospital	300+	76%	62%	71%
Use of Medical Imaging				
Cardiac Imaging Stress Test before Surgery	285	9.1%	6.2%	5.3%
Combination Abdominal CT Scan	1,382	7.9%	4.8%	10.5%
Combination Brain/Sinus CT Scan	394	1.0%	4.4%	2.7%
Combination Chest CT Scan	1,652	0.4%	0.7%	2.7%
Follow-up Mammogram/Ultrasound	891	10.5%	7%	8.8%
Lumbar Spine MRI for Low Back Pain	74	35.1%	33.8%	37.2%

Medstar Washington Hospital Center

110 Irving Saint Nw
Washington, DC 20010
Phone: 202-877-7000
Fax: 202-877-3299
URL: www.whcenter.org
Type: Acute Care Hospitals
Emergency Services: Yes
Ownership: Voluntary non-profit - Other
Beds: 926

Key Personnel:
Cardiac Laboratory. . . . . Maureen Clancy
Infection Control. . . . . Nancy Donegan
Radiology. . . . . James S. Jelinek, MD, FACR
Chief of Medical Staff. . . . . Janis M Orlowski, MD
Coronary Care. . . . . Julio Panza, MD
Anesthesiology. . . . . Stephen D. Parker, MD, MBA
Operating Room. . . . . John J Ricotta, MD, FACS
CEO/President. . . . . John Sullivan

Measure	Cases	This Hosp.	State Avg.	U.S. Avg.
Blood Clot Prevention and Treatment				
Anticoagulation Overlap Therapy[2]	297	97%	94%	93%
ICU Venous Thromboembolism Prophylaxis[2]	97	97%	96%	92%
Incidence of Potentially Preventable VTE[2]	118	2%	6%	10%
UFH with Dosages/Platelet Monitoring[2]	133	100%	99%	97%
Venous Thromboembolism Prophylaxis[2]	355	90%	82%	85%
Warfarin Therapy Discharge Instructions[2]	207	99%	68%	75%
Chest Pain/Possible Heart Attack Care				
Aspirin Given Within 24 Hours of Arrival[5]	-	-	95%	96%
Fibrinolytic Meds Within 30 Min. of Arrival[5]	-	-	-	58%
Average Time to ECG (minutes)[5]	-	-	19	7
Average Time to Transfer (minutes)[5]	-	-	79	60
Children's Asthma Care				
Received Home Management Plan of Care	-	-	-	88%
Received Reliever Medication	-	-	-	100%
Received Systemic Corticosteroids	-	-	-	100%
Emergency Department				
Admittance Decision Time (minutes)[2]	514	263	226	98
Head CT Results Within 45 Min. of Arrival[3,7]	-	-	18%	57%
Patients Who Left ER Before Being Seen	91,968	2%	3%	2%
Time from ER Arrival to Admit. (minutes)[2]	547	544	479	274
Time from ER Arrival to Discharge (minutes)	389	226	186	134
Time in ER Before Being Evaluated (minutes)	414	88	53	26
Time to Pain Meds for Fractures (minutes)	105	89	80	57
Heart Attack Care				
Aspirin Given at Discharge[2]	322	98%	97%	99%
Fibrinolytic Meds Within 30 Min. of Arrival[2,7]	-	-	-	54%
PCI Within 90 Minutes of Arrival[1,2]	-	-	88%	96%
Statin Prescribed at Discharge[2]	302	99%	97%	98%
Heart Failure Care				
ACE Inhibitor or ARB for LVSD[2]	195	97%	92%	97%
Discharge Instructions Given[2]	383	97%	87%	94%
Evaluation of LVS Function[2]	418	100%	98%	99%
Medicare Spending				
Medicare Spending per Patient (ratio)	-	0.99	1	0.98
Pneumonia Care				
Appropriate Initial Antibiotic Given[2]	144	96%	93%	95%
Blood Culture Timing[2]	108	96%	93%	98%
Pregnancy and Delivery Care				

NOTE: Hospital profiles are in alphabetical order by state, then city, then hospital within the city; Rankings exclude hospitals with less than 25 cases except for patient surveys which excludes hospitals with less than 100 cases; (a) 100-299 cases; (1) The number of cases/patients is too few to report; (2) Data submitted were based on a sample of cases/patients; (3) Results are based on a shorter time period than required; (4) Data suppressed by CMS for one or more quarters; (5) Results are not available for this reporting period; (6) Fewer than 100 patients completed the HCAHPS survey; (7) No cases met the criteria for this measure; (8) The lower limit of the confidence interval cannot be calculated if the number of observed infections equals zero; (9) No data are available from the state/territory for this reporting period; (10) The scores shown reflect fewer than 50 completed surveys; (11) There were discrepancies in the data collection process; (12) This measure does not apply to this hospital for this reporting period; (13) Results cannot be calculated for this reporting period; (14) The results for this state are combined with nearby states to protect confidentiality; Please refer to the User's Guide for a full explanation of data.

Newborn Deliveries Scheduled Early[2]	108	1%	6%	6%
Preventive Care				
Immunization for Influenza[2]	556	96%	84%	90%
Immunization for Pneumonia[2]	714	96%	85%	92%
Stroke Care				
Anticoagulation Therapy for Atrial Fibrillation[2]	21	90%	94%	95%
Antithrombotic Therapy Timing[2]	100	98%	96%	98%
Assessed for Rehabilitation[2]	147	99%	97%	97%
Discharged on Antithrombotic Therapy[2]	113	98%	99%	99%
Discharged on Statin Medication[2]	104	95%	96%	94%
Thrombolytic Therapy Timing[1,2]	-	-	40%	66%
Venous Thromboembolism Prophylaxis[2]	148	97%	95%	94%
Written Stroke Educational Materials Given[2]	61	93%	90%	88%
Surgical Care Improvement Project				
Appropriate Beta Blocker Usage[2]	212	95%	95%	98%
Appropriate VTP Within 24 Hours[2]	461	98%	95%	98%
Controlled Postoperative Blood Glucose[2]	196	95%	94%	97%
Perioperative Temperature Management[2]	612	98%	99%	100%
Prophylactic Antibiotic Selection[2]	567	100%	99%	99%
Prophylactic Antibiotic Selection (Outpatient)	695	98%	97%	98%
Prophylactic Antibiotic Stopped[2]	560	97%	96%	98%
Prophylactic Antibiotic Timing[2]	571	99%	98%	99%
Prophylactic Antibiotic Timing (Outpatient)	684	98%	94%	98%
Urinary Catheter Removal[2]	488	95%	96%	97%
Survey of Patients' Hospital Experiences				
Area Around Room 'Always' Quiet at Night	300+	49%	55%	61%
Doctors 'Always' Communicated Well	300+	77%	77%	82%
Home Recovery Information Given	300+	85%	78%	85%
Hospital Given 9 or 10 on 10 Point Scale	300+	69%	60%	71%
Meds 'Always' Explained Before Given	300+	58%	55%	64%
Nurses 'Always' Communicated Well	300+	72%	70%	79%
Pain 'Always' Well Controlled	300+	62%	64%	71%
Room and Bathroom 'Always' Clean	300+	56%	61%	73%
Timely Help 'Always' Received	300+	53%	55%	68%
Would Definitely Recommend Hospital	300+	72%	62%	71%
Use of Medical Imaging				
Cardiac Imaging Stress Test before Surgery	539	5.6%	6.2%	5.3%
Combination Abdominal CT Scan	2,098	0.8%	4.8%	10.5%
Combination Brain/Sinus CT Scan	979	3.2%	4.4%	2.7%
Combination Chest CT Scan	1,758	0.5%	0.7%	2.7%
Follow-up Mammogram/Ultrasound	2,554	6.7%	7%	8.8%
Lumbar Spine MRI for Low Back Pain	201	32.3%	33.8%	37.2%

Providence Hospital

1150 Varnum Saint Ne
Washington, DC 20017
Phone: 202-269-7000
Fax: 202-269-7160
URL: www.provhosp.org
Type: Acute Care Hospitals
Emergency Services: Yes
Ownership: Voluntary non-profit - Private
Beds: 240

Key Personnel:
Intensive Care Unit. . . . . Byron Atkinson, RN
Operating Room. . . . . Willie C Blair
Radiology. . . . . Joel Bruce Bowers, RN
Quality Assurance . . . . Deborah Gill
CEO/President. . . . . Sister Carol Keehan
Infection Control. . . . . John Morrissey, MD
Pediatric In-Patient Care . . . . Jolan Rhodes, MD
Chief of Medical Staff. . . . . Robert Simmons

Measure	Cases	This Hosp.	State Avg.	U.S. Avg.
Blood Clot Prevention and Treatment				
Anticoagulation Overlap Therapy[2]	82	85%	94%	93%
ICU Venous Thromboembolism Prophylaxis[2]	62	92%	96%	92%
Incidence of Potentially Preventable VTE[2]	17	24%	6%	10%
UFH with Dosages/Platelet Monitoring[1,2]	-	-	99%	97%
Venous Thromboembolism Prophylaxis[2]	360	72%	82%	85%
Warfarin Therapy Discharge Instructions[2]	56	9%	68%	75%
Chest Pain/Possible Heart Attack Care				
Aspirin Given Within 24 Hours of Arrival	15	100%	95%	96%
Fibrinolytic Meds Within 30 Min. of Arrival[7]	-	-	-	58%
Average Time to ECG (minutes)	15	89	19	7
Average Time to Transfer (minutes)[1]	-	-	79	60
Children's Asthma Care				
Received Home Management Plan of Care	-	-	-	88%
Received Reliever Medication	-	-	-	100%
Received Systemic Corticosteroids	-	-	-	100%
Emergency Department				
Admittance Decision Time (minutes)[2]	527	290	226	98
Head CT Results Within 45 Min. of Arrival[1]	-	-	18%	57%
Patients Who Left ER Before Being Seen	49,937	4%	3%	2%
Time from ER Arrival to Admit. (minutes)[2]	529	614	479	274
Time from ER Arrival to Discharge (minutes)	311	318	186	134
Time in ER Before Being Evaluated (minutes)	369	75	53	26
Time to Pain Meds for Fractures (minutes)	14	120	80	57
Heart Attack Care				
Aspirin Given at Discharge	41	100%	97%	99%
Fibrinolytic Meds Within 30 Min. of Arrival[7]	-	-	-	54%
PCI Within 90 Minutes of Arrival[7]	-	-	88%	96%
Statin Prescribed at Discharge	37	89%	97%	98%
Heart Failure Care				
ACE Inhibitor or ARB for LVSD	179	89%	92%	97%
Discharge Instructions Given	392	90%	87%	94%
Evaluation of LVS Function	481	96%	98%	99%
Medicare Spending				
Medicare Spending per Patient (ratio)	-	0.99	1	0.98
Pneumonia Care				
Appropriate Initial Antibiotic Given	102	79%	93%	95%
Blood Culture Timing	128	87%	93%	98%
Pregnancy and Delivery Care				
Newborn Deliveries Scheduled Early[2]	46	2%	6%	6%
Preventive Care				
Immunization for Influenza[2]	510	81%	84%	90%
Immunization for Pneumonia[2]	603	81%	85%	92%
Stroke Care				
Anticoagulation Therapy for Atrial Fibrillation	14	86%	94%	95%
Antithrombotic Therapy Timing	127	99%	96%	98%
Assessed for Rehabilitation	130	95%	97%	97%
Discharged on Antithrombotic Therapy	113	98%	99%	99%
Discharged on Statin Medication	86	94%	96%	94%
Thrombolytic Therapy Timing[1]	-	-	40%	66%
Venous Thromboembolism Prophylaxis	144	92%	95%	94%
Written Stroke Educational Materials Given	62	98%	90%	88%
Surgical Care Improvement Project				
Appropriate Beta Blocker Usage[2]	107	83%	95%	98%
Appropriate VTP Within 24 Hours[2]	430	84%	95%	98%
Controlled Postoperative Blood Glucose[2,7]	-	-	94%	97%
Perioperative Temperature Management[2]	490	100%	99%	100%
Prophylactic Antibiotic Selection[2]	316	97%	99%	99%
Prophylactic Antibiotic Selection (Outpatient)	168	99%	97%	98%
Prophylactic Antibiotic Stopped[2]	310	92%	96%	98%
Prophylactic Antibiotic Timing[2]	316	96%	98%	99%
Prophylactic Antibiotic Timing (Outpatient)	208	71%	94%	98%
Urinary Catheter Removal[2]	327	89%	96%	97%
Survey of Patients' Hospital Experiences				
Area Around Room 'Always' Quiet at Night	300+	62%	55%	61%
Doctors 'Always' Communicated Well	300+	80%	77%	82%
Home Recovery Information Given	300+	78%	78%	85%
Hospital Given 9 or 10 on 10 Point Scale	300+	64%	60%	71%
Meds 'Always' Explained Before Given	300+	55%	55%	64%
Nurses 'Always' Communicated Well	300+	72%	70%	79%
Pain 'Always' Well Controlled	300+	65%	64%	71%
Room and Bathroom 'Always' Clean	300+	67%	61%	73%
Timely Help 'Always' Received	300+	59%	55%	68%
Would Definitely Recommend Hospital	300+	62%	62%	71%
Use of Medical Imaging				
Cardiac Imaging Stress Test before Surgery	75	1.3%	6.2%	5.3%
Combination Abdominal CT Scan	822	7.9%	4.8%	10.5%
Combination Brain/Sinus CT Scan	757	4.0%	4.4%	2.7%
Combination Chest CT Scan	395	3.5%	0.7%	2.7%
Follow-up Mammogram/Ultrasound	2,055	3.4%	7%	8.8%
Lumbar Spine MRI for Low Back Pain	142	35.9%	33.8%	37.2%

Sibley Memorial Hospital

5255 Loughboro Rd Nw
Washington, DC 20016
Phone: 202-537-4680
Fax: 202-364-8405
URL: www.sibley.org
Type: Acute Care Hospitals
Emergency Services: Yes
Ownership: Voluntary non-profit - Other
Beds: 328

Key Personnel:
CEO/President. . . . . Richard O. Davis, Ph.D.
Operating Room. . . . . Cindy Lee, RN
Chief of Medical Staff. . . . . Lawrence D. Ramunno
Patient Relations . . . . Joan Vincent, RN

Measure	Cases	This Hosp.	State Avg.	U.S. Avg.
Blood Clot Prevention and Treatment				
Anticoagulation Overlap Therapy[2]	26	100%	94%	93%
ICU Venous Thromboembolism Prophylaxis[2]	39	97%	96%	92%
Incidence of Potentially Preventable VTE[1,2]	-	-	6%	10%
UFH with Dosages/Platelet Monitoring[1,2]	-	-	99%	97%
Venous Thromboembolism Prophylaxis[2]	260	87%	82%	85%
Warfarin Therapy Discharge Instructions[2]	12	42%	68%	75%
Chest Pain/Possible Heart Attack Care				
Aspirin Given Within 24 Hours of Arrival	33	100%	95%	96%
Fibrinolytic Meds Within 30 Min. of Arrival[7]	-	-	-	58%
Average Time to ECG (minutes)	34	12	19	7
Average Time to Transfer (minutes)	11	105	79	60
Children's Asthma Care				
Received Home Management Plan of Care	-	-	-	88%
Received Reliever Medication	-	-	-	100%
Received Systemic Corticosteroids	-	-	-	100%
Emergency Department				
Admittance Decision Time (minutes)[2]	320	122	226	98
Head CT Results Within 45 Min. of Arrival[1]	-	-	18%	57%
Patients Who Left ER Before Being Seen	34,093	0%	3%	2%
Time from ER Arrival to Admit. (minutes)[2]	320	292	479	274
Time from ER Arrival to Discharge (minutes)	556	123	186	134
Time in ER Before Being Evaluated (minutes)	561	13	53	26
Time to Pain Meds for Fractures (minutes)	94	50	80	57
Heart Attack Care				
Aspirin Given at Discharge[2]	18	100%	97%	99%
Fibrinolytic Meds Within 30 Min. of Arrival[2,7]	-	-	-	54%
PCI Within 90 Minutes of Arrival[2,7]	-	-	88%	96%
Statin Prescribed at Discharge[2]	14	100%	97%	98%
Heart Failure Care				
ACE Inhibitor or ARB for LVSD	25	100%	92%	97%
Discharge Instructions Given	61	100%	87%	94%
Evaluation of LVS Function	85	100%	98%	99%
Medicare Spending				
Medicare Spending per Patient (ratio)	-	0.97	1	0.98
Pneumonia Care				
Appropriate Initial Antibiotic Given[2]	76	100%	93%	95%
Blood Culture Timing[2]	140	100%	93%	98%
Pregnancy and Delivery Care				
Newborn Deliveries Scheduled Early[2]	61	13%	6%	6%
Preventive Care				
Immunization for Influenza[2]	453	97%	84%	90%
Immunization for Pneumonia[2]	381	94%	85%	92%
Stroke Care				
Anticoagulation Therapy for Atrial Fibrillation	14	100%	94%	95%
Antithrombotic Therapy Timing	51	98%	96%	98%
Assessed for Rehabilitation	62	98%	97%	97%
Discharged on Antithrombotic Therapy	54	100%	99%	99%
Discharged on Statin Medication	44	100%	96%	94%
Thrombolytic Therapy Timing[1]	-	-	40%	66%
Venous Thromboembolism Prophylaxis	60	98%	95%	94%
Written Stroke Educational Materials Given	34	97%	90%	88%
Surgical Care Improvement Project				
Appropriate Beta Blocker Usage[2]	218	97%	95%	98%
Appropriate VTP Within 24 Hours[2]	1,030	97%	95%	98%
Controlled Postoperative Blood Glucose[2,7]	-	-	94%	97%
Perioperative Temperature Management[2]	1,113	99%	99%	100%
Prophylactic Antibiotic Selection[2]	783	99%	99%	99%
Prophylactic Antibiotic Selection (Outpatient)	288	92%	97%	98%
Prophylactic Antibiotic Stopped[2]	775	98%	96%	98%
Prophylactic Antibiotic Timing[2]	786	98%	98%	99%

NOTE: Hospital profiles are in alphabetical order by state, then city, then hospital within the city; Rankings exclude hospitals with less than 25 cases except for patient surveys which excludes hospitals with less than 100 cases; (a) 100-299 cases; (1) The number of cases/patients is too few to report; (2) Data submitted were based on a sample of cases/patients; (3) Results are based on a shorter time period than required; (4) Data suppressed by CMS for one or more quarters; (5) Results are not available for this reporting period; (6) Fewer than 100 patients completed the HCAHPS survey; (7) No cases met the criteria for this measure; (8) The lower limit of the confidence interval cannot be calculated if the number of observed infections equals zero; (9) No data are available from the state/territory for this reporting period; (10) The scores shown reflect fewer than 50 completed surveys; (11) There were discrepancies in the data collection process; (12) This measure does not apply to this hospital for this reporting period; (13) Results cannot be calculated for this reporting period; (14) The results for this state are combined with nearby states to protect confidentiality; Please refer to the User's Guide for a full explanation of data.

Measure	Cases	This Hosp.	State Avg.	U.S. Avg.
Prophylactic Antibiotic Timing (Outpatient)	291	96%	94%	98%
Urinary Catheter Removal[2]	798	99%	96%	97%
Survey of Patients' Hospital Experiences				
Area Around Room 'Always' Quiet at Night	300+	50%	55%	61%
Doctors 'Always' Communicated Well	300+	79%	77%	82%
Home Recovery Information Given	300+	75%	78%	85%
Hospital Given 9 or 10 on 10 Point Scale	300+	62%	60%	71%
Meds 'Always' Explained Before Given	300+	57%	55%	64%
Nurses 'Always' Communicated Well	300+	69%	70%	79%
Pain 'Always' Well Controlled	300+	69%	64%	71%
Room and Bathroom 'Always' Clean	300+	68%	61%	73%
Timely Help 'Always' Received	300+	57%	55%	68%
Would Definitely Recommend Hospital	300+	70%	62%	71%
Use of Medical Imaging				
Cardiac Imaging Stress Test before Surgery	56	5.4%	6.2%	5.3%
Combination Abdominal CT Scan	1,096	2.2%	4.8%	10.5%
Combination Brain/Sinus CT Scan	615	4.7%	4.4%	2.7%
Combination Chest CT Scan	694	0.0%	0.7%	2.7%
Follow-up Mammogram/Ultrasound	2,158	7.8%	7%	8.8%
Lumbar Spine MRI for Low Back Pain	183	33.3%	33.8%	37.2%

United Medical Center

1310 Southern Avenue Se
Washington, DC 20032
Phone: 202-574-6611
Fax: 202-574-6110
URL: www.greatersoutheastorg.verizonsupersite.com/home
Type: Acute Care Hospitals
Emergency Services: Yes
Ownership: Proprietary
Beds: 450

Key Personnel:
Pediatric In-Patient Care . . . . Gail Crossman, RN
Chief of Medical Staff . . . . Gilbert Daniel, MD
Operating Room. . . . . Ester Espartero, RN
Chairman/CEO . . . . Charles Hudson, Jr
Quality Assurance . . . . Paula Johnson
Pediatric Ambulatory Care . . . . . . Marilyn McPherson-Corde, MD
CEO/President. . . . . David Small
Radiology. . . . . Raymond Tu, MD

Measure	Cases	This Hosp.	State Avg.	U.S. Avg.
Blood Clot Prevention and Treatment				
Anticoagulation Overlap Therapy[2]	21	81%	94%	93%
ICU Venous Thromboembolism Prophylaxis[2]	87	91%	96%	92%
Incidence of Potentially Preventable VTE[1,2]	-	-	6%	10%
UFH with Dosages/Platelet Monitoring[1,2]	-	-	99%	97%
Venous Thromboembolism Prophylaxis[2]	403	65%	82%	85%
Warfarin Therapy Discharge Instructions[2]	16	0%	68%	75%
Chest Pain/Possible Heart Attack Care				
Aspirin Given Within 24 Hours of Arrival	36	89%	95%	96%
Fibrinolytic Meds Within 30 Min. of Arrival[7]	-	-	-	58%
Average Time to ECG (minutes)	36	32	19	7
Average Time to Transfer (minutes)[1]	-	-	79	60
Children's Asthma Care				
Received Home Management Plan of Care	-	-	-	88%
Received Reliever Medication	-	-	-	100%
Received Systemic Corticosteroids	-	-	-	100%
Emergency Department				
Admittance Decision Time (minutes)[2]	198	245	226	98
Head CT Results Within 45 Min. of Arrival[1]	-	-	18%	57%
Patients Who Left ER Before Being Seen	26,110	6%	3%	2%
Time from ER Arrival to Admit. (minutes)[2]	199	559	479	274
Time from ER Arrival to Discharge (minutes)	333	173	186	134
Time in ER Before Being Evaluated (minutes)	436	102	53	26
Time to Pain Meds for Fractures (minutes)	96	118	80	57
Heart Attack Care				
Aspirin Given at Discharge	31	81%	97%	99%
Fibrinolytic Meds Within 30 Min. of Arrival[7]	-	-	-	54%
PCI Within 90 Minutes of Arrival[7]	-	-	88%	96%
Statin Prescribed at Discharge	24	67%	97%	98%
Heart Failure Care				
ACE Inhibitor or ARB for LVSD[2]	122	75%	92%	97%
Discharge Instructions Given[2]	249	55%	87%	94%
Evaluation of LVS Function[2]	306	92%	98%	99%
Medicare Spending				
Medicare Spending per Patient (ratio)	-	1.05	1	0.98
Pneumonia Care				
Appropriate Initial Antibiotic Given[2]	57	91%	93%	95%
Blood Culture Timing[2]	114	86%	93%	98%
Pregnancy and Delivery Care				
Newborn Deliveries Scheduled Early[2]	41	10%	6%	6%
Preventive Care				
Immunization for Influenza[2]	443	65%	84%	90%
Immunization for Pneumonia[2]	589	74%	85%	92%
Stroke Care				
Anticoagulation Therapy for Atrial Fibrillation[1]	-	-	94%	95%
Antithrombotic Therapy Timing	30	83%	96%	98%
Assessed for Rehabilitation	31	77%	97%	97%
Discharged on Antithrombotic Therapy	30	100%	99%	99%
Discharged on Statin Medication	23	78%	96%	94%
Thrombolytic Therapy Timing[7]	-	-	40%	66%
Venous Thromboembolism Prophylaxis	33	64%	95%	94%
Written Stroke Educational Materials Given	13	0%	90%	88%
Surgical Care Improvement Project				
Appropriate Beta Blocker Usage	15	73%	95%	98%
Appropriate VTP Within 24 Hours	72	83%	95%	98%
Controlled Postoperative Blood Glucose[7]	-	-	94%	97%
Perioperative Temperature Management	88	93%	99%	100%
Prophylactic Antibiotic Selection	29	79%	99%	99%
Prophylactic Antibiotic Selection (Outpatient)	17	100%	97%	98%
Prophylactic Antibiotic Stopped	28	89%	96%	98%
Prophylactic Antibiotic Timing	29	90%	98%	99%
Prophylactic Antibiotic Timing (Outpatient)	20	85%	94%	98%
Urinary Catheter Removal	46	57%	96%	97%
Survey of Patients' Hospital Experiences				
Area Around Room 'Always' Quiet at Night	300+	51%	55%	61%
Doctors 'Always' Communicated Well	300+	72%	77%	82%
Home Recovery Information Given	300+	62%	78%	85%
Hospital Given 9 or 10 on 10 Point Scale	300+	38%	60%	71%
Meds 'Always' Explained Before Given	300+	44%	55%	64%
Nurses 'Always' Communicated Well	300+	62%	70%	79%
Pain 'Always' Well Controlled	300+	58%	64%	71%
Room and Bathroom 'Always' Clean	300+	53%	61%	73%
Timely Help 'Always' Received	300+	49%	55%	68%
Would Definitely Recommend Hospital	300+	30%	62%	71%
Use of Medical Imaging				
Cardiac Imaging Stress Test before Surgery[1]	-	-	6.2%	5.3%
Combination Abdominal CT Scan	195	6.2%	4.8%	10.5%
Combination Brain/Sinus CT Scan	413	4.1%	4.4%	2.7%
Combination Chest CT Scan	135	0.0%	0.7%	2.7%
Follow-up Mammogram/Ultrasound	395	9.4%	7%	8.8%
Lumbar Spine MRI for Low Back Pain	46	34.8%	33.8%	37.2%

Washington DC VA Medical Center

50 Irving Street NW
Washington, DC 20422
Phone: 202-745-8000
Fax: 202-745-8530
URL: www.washington.va.gov
Type: Acute Care - VA
Emergency Services: No
Ownership: Government Federal
Beds: 291

Key Personnel:
Radiology. . . . . Klemens H. Barth, MD
Quality Assurance . . . . Cathy Delligatti
Chief of Medical Staff . . . . Ross D. Fletcher, MD
CEO/President. . . . . Sanford M Garfunkel
Infection Control. . . . . Fred Gordin
Patient Relations . . . . Terry Koss
Operating Room. . . . . Charles Shuner
Surgery . . . . Jon White, MD

Measure	Cases	This Hosp.	State Avg.	U.S. Avg.
Blood Clot Prevention and Treatment				
Anticoagulation Overlap Therapy	-	-	94%	93%
ICU Venous Thromboembolism Prophylaxis	-	-	96%	92%
Incidence of Potentially Preventable VTE	-	-	6%	10%
UFH with Dosages/Platelet Monitoring	-	-	99%	97%
Venous Thromboembolism Prophylaxis	-	-	82%	85%
Warfarin Therapy Discharge Instructions	-	-	68%	75%
Chest Pain/Possible Heart Attack Care				
Aspirin Given Within 24 Hours of Arrival	-	-	95%	96%
Fibrinolytic Meds Within 30 Min. of Arrival	-	-	-	58%
Average Time to ECG (minutes)	-	-	19	7
Average Time to Transfer (minutes)	-	-	79	60
Children's Asthma Care				
Received Home Management Plan of Care	-	-	-	88%
Received Reliever Medication	-	-	-	100%
Received Systemic Corticosteroids	-	-	-	100%
Emergency Department				
Admittance Decision Time (minutes)	-	-	226	98
Head CT Results Within 45 Min. of Arrival	-	-	18%	57%
Patients Who Left ER Before Being Seen	-	-	3%	2%
Time from ER Arrival to Admit. (minutes)	-	-	479	274
Time from ER Arrival to Discharge (minutes)	-	-	186	134
Time in ER Before Being Evaluated (minutes)	-	-	53	26
Time to Pain Meds for Fractures (minutes)	-	-	80	57
Heart Attack Care				
Aspirin Given at Discharge	54	100%	97%	99%
Fibrinolytic Meds Within 30 Min. of Arrival[5]	-	-	-	54%
PCI Within 90 Minutes of Arrival[1]	-	-	88%	96%
Statin Prescribed at Discharge	51	100%	97%	98%
Heart Failure Care				
ACE Inhibitor or ARB for LVSD	129	98%	92%	97%
Discharge Instructions Given	185	94%	87%	94%
Evaluation of LVS Function	214	99%	98%	99%
Medicare Spending				
Medicare Spending per Patient (ratio)	-	-	1	0.98
Pneumonia Care				
Appropriate Initial Antibiotic Given	42	98%	93%	95%
Blood Culture Timing	85	95%	93%	98%
Pregnancy and Delivery Care				
Newborn Deliveries Scheduled Early	-	-	6%	6%
Preventive Care				
Immunization for Influenza[5]	-	-	84%	90%
Immunization for Pneumonia[5]	-	-	85%	92%
Stroke Care				
Anticoagulation Therapy for Atrial Fibrillation	-	-	94%	95%
Antithrombotic Therapy Timing	-	-	96%	98%
Assessed for Rehabilitation	-	-	97%	97%
Discharged on Antithrombotic Therapy	-	-	99%	99%
Discharged on Statin Medication	-	-	96%	94%
Thrombolytic Therapy Timing	-	-	40%	66%
Venous Thromboembolism Prophylaxis	-	-	95%	94%
Written Stroke Educational Materials Given	-	-	90%	88%
Surgical Care Improvement Project				
Appropriate Beta Blocker Usage[2]	84	98%	95%	98%
Appropriate VTP Within 24 Hours[2]	120	91%	95%	98%
Controlled Postoperative Blood Glucose[2]	92	95%	94%	97%
Perioperative Temperature Management[2]	234	98%	99%	100%
Prophylactic Antibiotic Selection	127	100%	99%	99%
Prophylactic Antibiotic Selection (Outpatient)	-	-	97%	98%
Prophylactic Antibiotic Stopped	125	96%	96%	98%
Prophylactic Antibiotic Timing	127	98%	98%	99%
Prophylactic Antibiotic Timing (Outpatient)	-	-	94%	98%
Urinary Catheter Removal[2]	123	98%	96%	97%
Survey of Patients' Hospital Experiences				
Area Around Room 'Always' Quiet at Night	-	-	55%	61%
Doctors 'Always' Communicated Well	-	-	77%	82%
Home Recovery Information Given	-	-	78%	85%
Hospital Given 9 or 10 on 10 Point Scale	-	-	60%	71%
Meds 'Always' Explained Before Given	-	-	55%	64%
Nurses 'Always' Communicated Well	-	-	70%	79%
Pain 'Always' Well Controlled	-	-	64%	71%
Room and Bathroom 'Always' Clean	-	-	61%	73%
Timely Help 'Always' Received	-	-	55%	68%
Would Definitely Recommend Hospital	-	-	62%	71%
Use of Medical Imaging				
Cardiac Imaging Stress Test before Surgery	-	-	6.2%	5.3%
Combination Abdominal CT Scan	-	-	4.8%	10.5%
Combination Brain/Sinus CT Scan	-	-	4.4%	2.7%
Combination Chest CT Scan	-	-	0.7%	2.7%
Follow-up Mammogram/Ultrasound	-	-	7%	8.8%
Lumbar Spine MRI for Low Back Pain	-	-	33.8%	37.2%

NOTE: Hospital profiles are in alphabetical order by state, then city, then hospital within the city; Rankings exclude hospitals with less than 25 cases except for patient surveys which excludes hospitals with less than 100 cases; (a) 100-299 cases; (1) The number of cases/patients is too few to report; (2) Data submitted were based on a sample of cases/patients; (3) Results are based on a shorter time period than required; (4) Data suppressed by CMS for one or more quarters; (5) Results are not available for this reporting period; (6) Fewer than 100 patients completed the HCAHPS survey; (7) No cases met the criteria for this measure; (8) The lower limit of the confidence interval cannot be calculated if the number of observed infections equals zero; (9) No data are available from the state/territory for this reporting period; (10) The scores shown reflect fewer than 50 completed surveys; (11) There were discrepancies in the data collection process; (12) This measure does not apply to this hospital for this reporting period; (13) Results cannot be calculated for this reporting period; (14) The results for this state are combined with nearby states to protect confidentiality; Please refer to the User's Guide for a full explanation of data.

Blood Clot Prevention and Treatment

Anticoagulation Overlap Therapy

Hospital Name	City	Rate	Cases
Saint Elizabeth Florence[2]	Florence	100%	60
Saint Elizabeth Ft Thomas[2]	Fort Thomas	100%	51
Saint Elizabeth Medical Center[2]	Lakeside Park	100%	134
Twin Lakes Regional Medical Center[2]	Leitchfield	100%	26
University of Kentucky Hospital[2]	Lexington	99%	166
Baptist Health Lexington[2]	Lexington	98%	87
Saint Joseph Hospital[2]	Lexington	98%	127
The Medical Center at Bowling Green[2]	Bowling Green	97%	110
Saint Joseph London[2]	London	97%	29
Baptist Health Louisville[2]	Louisville	96%	188
Baptist Health Madisonville[2]	Madisonville	96%	53
Baptist Health Richmond[2]	Richmond	96%	26
Saint Joseph East[2]	Lexington	96%	27
Baptist Health Paducah[2]	Paducah	95%	75
Pikeville Medical Center[2]	Pikeville	95%	55
Methodist Hospital[2]	Henderson	93%	29
Ephraim Mcdowell Regional Medical Center[2]	Danville	92%	53
King's Daughters' Medical Center[2]	Ashland	92%	106
Baptist Health Corbin[2]	Corbin	91%	33
Jewish Hospital & Saint Mary's Healthcare[2]	Louisville	91%	206
T J Samson Community Hospital[2]	Glasgow	91%	33
Norton Hospitals[2]	Louisville	88%	327
Lake Cumberland Regional Hospital[2]	Somerset	86%	59
Highlands Regional Medical Center[2]	Prestonsburg	84%	31
Jennie Stuart Medical Center[2]	Hopkinsville	84%	55
Owensboro Health Regional Hospital[2]	Owensboro	83%	104
University of Louisville Hospital[2]	Louisville	77%	65
Lourdes Hospital[2]	Paducah	75%	36
Hardin Memorial Hospital[2]	Elizabethtown	60%	83

ICU Venous Thromboembolism Prophylaxis

Hospital Name	City	Rate	Cases
Greenview Regional Hospital[2]	Bowling Green	100%	65
Kentucky River Medical Center[2]	Jackson	100%	53
King's Daughters' Medical Center[2]	Ashland	100%	57
Parkway Regional Hospital[2]	Fulton	100%	109
Three Rivers Medical Center[2]	Louisa	100%	78
Baptist Health Richmond[2]	Richmond	99%	102
Frankfort Regional Medical Center[2]	Frankfort	99%	90
Jackson Purchase Medical Center[2]	Mayfield	99%	89
Saint Elizabeth Ft Thomas[2]	Fort Thomas	99%	83
Baptist Health Louisville[2]	Louisville	98%	64
Hazard ARH Regional Medical Center[2]	Hazard	98%	82
Saint Elizabeth Florence[2]	Florence	98%	88
Saint Elizabeth Medical Center[2]	Lakeside Park	98%	82
Saint Joseph London[2]	London	98%	118
Georgetown Community Hospital[2]	Georgetown	97%	37
Clark Regional Medical Center[2]	Winchester	96%	73
Williamson ARH Hospital[2]	S Williamson	96%	49
Baptist Health Lagrange[2]	La Grange	95%	64
Lake Cumberland Regional Hospital[2]	Somerset	95%	91
Pikeville Medical Center[2]	Pikeville	95%	85
Taylor Regional Hospital[2]	Campbellsville	95%	59
University of Kentucky Hospital[2]	Lexington	95%	103
Baptist Health Lexington[2]	Lexington	94%	116
Baptist Health Paducah[2]	Paducah	94%	114
Jewish Hospital & Saint Mary's Healthcare[2]	Louisville	94%	139
The Medical Center at Bowling Green[2]	Bowling Green	94%	86
Our Lady of Bellefonte Hospital[2]	Ashland	94%	33
Spring View Hospital[2]	Lebanon	94%	31
Twin Lakes Regional Medical Center[2]	Leitchfield	94%	53
Logan Memorial Hospital[2]	Russellville	93%	28
Whitesburg ARH Hospital[2]	Whitesburg	91%	74
Baptist Health Corbin[2]	Corbin	90%	79
Memorial Hospital[2]	Manchester	90%	60
Flaget Memorial Hospital[2]	Bardstown	89%	27
Saint Claire Regional Medical Center[2]	Morehead	89%	142
Jennie Stuart Medical Center[2]	Hopkinsville	88%	89
Methodist Hospital[2]	Henderson	87%	68
Saint Joseph East[2]	Lexington	85%	74
University of Louisville Hospital[2]	Louisville	85%	129
Baptist Health Madisonville[2]	Madisonville	83%	107
Norton Hospitals[2]	Louisville	83%	129
Jewish Hospital - Shelbyville[2]	Shelbyville	82%	51
Harlan Appalachian Reg Healthcare Hosp[2]	Harlan	80%	70
Paul B Hall Regional Medical Center[2]	Paintsville	80%	83
T J Samson Community Hospital[2]	Glasgow	78%	81
Muhlenberg Community Hospital[2]	Greenville	77%	62
Owensboro Health Regional Hospital[2]	Owensboro	76%	101
Lourdes Hospital[2]	Paducah	75%	122
Hardin Memorial Hospital[2]	Elizabethtown	73%	73
Fleming County Hospital[2]	Flemingsburg	72%	117
Saint Joseph Hospital[2]	Lexington	72%	128
Saint Joseph Mount Sterling	Mount Sterling	72%	161
Murray - Calloway County Hospital[2]	Murray	70%	57
Clinton County Hospital[2]	Albany	68%	31
Middlesboro Appalachian Reg Healthcare[2]	Middlesboro	67%	54
Meadowview Regional Medical Center[2]	Maysville	60%	96
Marshall County Hospital	Benton	59%	133
Pineville Community Hospital[2]	Pineville	58%	67
Highlands Regional Medical Center[2]	Prestonsburg	53%	83
Ephraim Mcdowell Regional Medical Center[2]	Danville	46%	74

Incidence of Potentially Preventable VTE

Hospital Name	City	Rate	Cases
Baptist Health Louisville[2]	Louisville	2%	43
University of Kentucky Hospital[2]	Lexington	3%	78
University of Louisville Hospital[2]	Louisville	4%	53
Norton Hospitals[2]	Louisville	19%	85
Jewish Hospital & Saint Mary's Healthcare[2]	Louisville	22%	46

UFH with Dosages/Platelet Count Monitoring

Hospital Name	City	Rate	Cases
Baptist Health Corbin[2]	Corbin	100%	25
Baptist Health Lexington[2]	Lexington	100%	62
Baptist Health Louisville[2]	Louisville	100%	83
Baptist Health Madisonville[2]	Madisonville	100%	29
Ephraim Mcdowell Regional Medical Center[2]	Danville	100%	45
Jewish Hospital & Saint Mary's Healthcare[2]	Louisville	100%	123
King's Daughters' Medical Center[2]	Ashland	100%	68
The Medical Center at Bowling Green[2]	Bowling Green	100%	69
Owensboro Health Regional Hospital[2]	Owensboro	100%	31
Pikeville Medical Center[2]	Pikeville	100%	44
Saint Elizabeth Florence[2]	Florence	100%	64
Saint Elizabeth Ft Thomas[2]	Fort Thomas	100%	57
Saint Joseph Hospital[2]	Lexington	100%	60
University of Kentucky Hospital[2]	Lexington	100%	124
Saint Elizabeth Medical Center[2]	Lakeside Park	99%	169
Norton Hospitals[2]	Louisville	98%	182
T J Samson Community Hospital[2]	Glasgow	96%	27
University of Louisville Hospital[2]	Louisville	94%	51
Saint Joseph East[2]	Lexington	93%	28
Hardin Memorial Hospital[2]	Elizabethtown	53%	36

Venous Thromboembolism Prophylaxis

Hospital Name	City	Rate	Cases
Frankfort Regional Medical Center[2]	Frankfort	100%	328
Kentucky River Medical Center[2]	Jackson	100%	299
Baptist Health Richmond[2]	Richmond	99%	160
Bourbon Community Hospital[2]	Paris	99%	115
Greenview Regional Hospital[2]	Bowling Green	99%	327
Parkway Regional Hospital[2]	Fulton	99%	237
Three Rivers Medical Center[2]	Louisa	98%	234
Clark Regional Medical Center[2]	Winchester	97%	138
Georgetown Community Hospital[2]	Georgetown	97%	171
Harrison Memorial Hospital[2]	Cynthiana	97%	173
Saint Elizabeth Ft Thomas[2]	Fort Thomas	97%	406
Saint Elizabeth Florence[2]	Florence	96%	391
Saint Elizabeth Medical Center[2]	Lakeside Park	96%	364
Saint Elizabeth Grant[2]	Williamstown	95%	111
Saint Joseph London[2]	London	95%	346
Pikeville Medical Center[2]	Pikeville	94%	373
Williamson ARH Hospital[2]	S Williamson	94%	265
Baptist Health Lagrange[2]	La Grange	93%	195
Baptist Health Louisville[2]	Louisville	93%	328
Methodist Hospital[2]	Henderson	93%	377
King's Daughters' Medical Center[2]	Ashland	92%	353
Logan Memorial Hospital[2]	Russellville	92%	169
The Medical Center at Bowling Green[2]	Bowling Green	92%	366
Lake Cumberland Regional Hospital[2]	Somerset	90%	363
Saint Claire Regional Medical Center[2]	Morehead	89%	286
Spring View Hospital[2]	Lebanon	89%	123
Memorial Hospital[2]	Manchester	88%	208
Monroe County Medical Center[2]	Tompkinsville	87%	247
Taylor Regional Hospital[2]	Campbellsville	87%	218
University of Kentucky Hospital[2]	Lexington	87%	279
Baptist Health Paducah[2]	Paducah	86%	329
Harlan Appalachian Reg Healthcare Hosp[2]	Harlan	86%	354
Jackson Purchase Medical Center[2]	Mayfield	86%	310
Twin Lakes Regional Medical Center[2]	Leitchfield	86%	236
Westlake Regional Hospital[2]	Columbia	85%	229
Middlesboro Appalachian Reg Healthcare[2]	Middlesboro	84%	210
Baptist Health Lexington[2]	Lexington	83%	330
Whitesburg ARH Hospital[2]	Whitesburg	83%	324
Hazard ARH Regional Medical Center[2]	Hazard	81%	371
Bluegrass Community Hospital[2,3]	Versailles	80%	35
Jennie Stuart Medical Center[2]	Hopkinsville	80%	326
Muhlenberg Community Hospital[2]	Greenville	80%	126
Ephraim Mcdowell Regional Medical Center[2]	Danville	79%	521
Our Lady of Bellefonte Hospital[2]	Ashland	79%	329
Flaget Memorial Hospital[2]	Bardstown	77%	180
Jewish Hospital & Saint Mary's Healthcare[2]	Louisville	77%	472
Hardin Memorial Hospital[2]	Elizabethtown	75%	338
Lourdes Hospital[2]	Paducah	75%	269
Saint Joseph East[2]	Lexington	74%	349
Norton Hospitals[2]	Louisville	71%	418
Baptist Health Madisonville[2]	Madisonville	70%	337
Saint Joseph Mount Sterling	Mount Sterling	68%	732
University of Louisville Hospital[2]	Louisville	68%	220
Baptist Health Corbin[2]	Corbin	67%	283
Rockcastle County Hospital[2]	Mount Vernon	67%	110
Saint Joseph Hospital[2]	Lexington	67%	413
Paul B Hall Regional Medical Center[2]	Paintsville	66%	254
Jewish Hospital - Shelbyville[2]	Shelbyville	64%	165
T J Samson Community Hospital[2]	Glasgow	64%	353
Carroll County Memorial Hospital[3]	Carrollton	63%	263
Meadowview Regional Medical Center[2]	Maysville	61%	181
Fleming County Hospital[2]	Flemingsburg	60%	141
Murray - Calloway County Hospital[2]	Murray	56%	317
Owensboro Health Regional Hospital[2]	Owensboro	52%	343
Clinton County Hospital[2]	Albany	50%	163
Trigg County Hospital	Cadiz	47%	64
Crittenden Health System[2]	Marion	45%	112
Pineville Community Hospital[2]	Pineville	44%	209
Highlands Regional Medical Center[2]	Prestonsburg	38%	339
Cumberland County Hospital[2]	Burkesville	14%	336

Warfarin Therapy Discharge Instructions

Hospital Name	City	Rate	Cases
Ephraim Mcdowell Regional Medical Center[2]	Danville	100%	41
Pikeville Medical Center[2]	Pikeville	100%	40
Saint Elizabeth Florence[2]	Florence	100%	47
T J Samson Community Hospital[2]	Glasgow	100%	31
Saint Elizabeth Medical Center[2]	Lakeside Park	98%	104
Baptist Health Lexington[2]	Lexington	97%	66
Baptist Health Paducah[2]	Paducah	96%	47
Baptist Health Madisonville[2]	Madisonville	95%	42
The Medical Center at Bowling Green[2]	Bowling Green	95%	76
Saint Elizabeth Ft Thomas[2]	Fort Thomas	95%	43
Lourdes Hospital[2]	Paducah	93%	29
University of Kentucky Hospital[2]	Lexington	90%	126
Jennie Stuart Medical Center[2]	Hopkinsville	88%	34
Baptist Health Louisville[2]	Louisville	86%	133
Lake Cumberland Regional Hospital[2]	Somerset	86%	42
King's Daughters' Medical Center[2]	Ashland	78%	85
Owensboro Health Regional Hospital[2]	Owensboro	75%	71
Norton Hospitals[2]	Louisville	46%	213
University of Louisville Hospital[2]	Louisville	35%	43
Jewish Hospital & Saint Mary's Healthcare[2]	Louisville	34%	157
Saint Joseph Hospital[2]	Lexington	17%	89
Hardin Memorial Hospital[2]	Elizabethtown	7%	71

Chest Pain/Possible Heart Attack Care

Aspirin Given Within 24 Hours of Arrival

Hospital Name	City	Rate	Cases
Baptist Health Corbin	Corbin	100%	110
Baptist Health Lagrange	La Grange	100%	48
Clark Regional Medical Center	Winchester	100%	36
Flaget Memorial Hospital	Bardstown	100%	196
Fleming County Hospital	Flemingsburg	100%	49
Greenview Regional Hospital	Bowling Green	100%	27
Harlan Appalachian Reg Healthcare Hosp	Harlan	100%	81
Harrison Memorial Hospital	Cynthiana	100%	65
Highlands Regional Medical Center	Prestonsburg	100%	66
Kentucky River Medical Center	Jackson	100%	64
Parkway Regional Hospital	Fulton	100%	42
Saint Elizabeth Florence	Florence	100%	34
Saint Elizabeth Ft Thomas	Fort Thomas	100%	25
Three Rivers Medical Center	Louisa	100%	75
Frankfort Regional Medical Center	Frankfort	99%	128
Middlesboro Appalachian Reg Healthcare	Middlesboro	99%	77
Taylor Regional Hospital	Campbellsville	99%	75
Twin Lakes Regional Medical Center	Leitchfield	99%	83
Bourbon Community Hospital	Paris	98%	61
Georgetown Community Hospital	Georgetown	98%	118
Methodist Hospital	Henderson	98%	65
Muhlenberg Community Hospital	Greenville	98%	108
Russell County Hospital	Russell Springs	98%	59
Murray - Calloway County Hospital	Murray	97%	72
Pineville Community Hospital	Pineville	97%	31
Saint Elizabeth Grant	Williamstown	97%	61
Westlake Regional Hospital	Columbia	97%	34
Jewish Hospital & Saint Mary's Healthcare	Louisville	96%	156
Logan Memorial Hospital	Russellville	96%	122
Rockcastle County Hospital	Mount Vernon	96%	55
Spring View Hospital	Lebanon	96%	52
Jennie Stuart Medical Center	Hopkinsville	95%	164
Jewish Hospital - Shelbyville	Shelbyville	95%	39
Memorial Hospital	Manchester	94%	66
Paul B Hall Regional Medical Center	Paintsville	94%	81
Baptist Health Richmond	Richmond	93%	43
Clinton County Hospital	Albany	93%	28
Monroe County Medical Center	Tompkinsville	93%	44
Saint Joseph Mount Sterling	Mount Sterling	93%	104
Jackson Purchase Medical Center	Mayfield	92%	25

NOTE: Hospital profiles are in alphabetical order by state, then city, then hospital within the city; Rankings exclude hospitals with less than 25 cases except for patient surveys which excludes hospitals with less than 100 cases; (a) 100-299 cases; (1) The number of cases/patients is too few to report; (2) Data submitted were based on a sample of cases/patients; (3) Results are based on a shorter time period than required; (4) Data suppressed by CMS for one or more quarters; (5) Results are not available for this reporting period; (6) Fewer than 100 patients completed the HCAHPS survey; (7) No cases met the criteria for this measure; (8) The lower limit of the confidence interval cannot be calculated if the number of observed infections equals zero; (9) No data are available from the state/territory for this reporting period; (10) The scores shown reflect fewer than 50 completed surveys; (11) There were discrepancies in the data collection process; (12) This measure does not apply to this hospital for this reporting period; (13) Results cannot be calculated for this reporting period; (14) The results for this state are combined with nearby states to protect confidentiality; Please refer to the User's Guide for a full explanation of data.

Our Lady of Bellefonte Hospital	Ashland	88%	33
Marshall County Hospital[3]	Benton	86%	58
Casey County Hospital	Liberty	84%	44

Average Time to ECG (minutes)

Hospital Name	City	Min.	Cases
Baptist Health Richmond	Richmond	2	43
Clark Regional Medical Center	Winchester	2	39
Paul B Hall Regional Medical Center	Paintsville	2	88
Baptist Health Lagrange	La Grange	3	50
Kentucky River Medical Center	Jackson	3	65
Methodist Hospital	Henderson	3	66
Parkway Regional Hospital	Fulton	3	46
Rockcastle County Hospital	Mount Vernon	3	55
Three Rivers Medical Center	Louisa	3	78
Clinton County Hospital	Albany	4	28
Jackson Purchase Medical Center	Mayfield	4	26
Jewish Hospital & Saint Mary's Healthcare	Louisville	4	159
Jewish Hospital - Shelbyville	Shelbyville	4	39
Logan Memorial Hospital	Russellville	4	130
Muhlenberg Community Hospital	Greenville	4	114
Baptist Health Corbin	Corbin	5	111
Frankfort Regional Medical Center	Frankfort	5	126
Marshall County Hospital[3]	Benton	5	61
Middlesboro Appalachian Reg Healthcare	Middlesboro	5	82
Bourbon Community Hospital	Paris	6	63
Saint Elizabeth Grant	Williamstown	6	65
Saint Joseph Mount Sterling	Mount Sterling	6	113
Georgetown Community Hospital	Georgetown	7	124
Harlan Appalachian Reg Healthcare Hosp	Harlan	7	82
Monroe County Medical Center	Tompkinsville	7	43
Pineville Community Hospital	Pineville	7	31
Taylor Regional Hospital	Campbellsville	7	75
Casey County Hospital	Liberty	8	47
Flaget Memorial Hospital	Bardstown	8	199
Fleming County Hospital	Flemingsburg	8	52
Greenview Regional Hospital	Bowling Green	8	29
Harrison Memorial Hospital	Cynthiana	8	68
Spring View Hospital	Lebanon	8	52
Westlake Regional Hospital	Columbia	8	32
Twin Lakes Regional Medical Center	Leitchfield	9	85
Highlands Regional Medical Center	Prestonsburg	10	66
Memorial Hospital	Manchester	10	70
Murray - Calloway County Hospital	Murray	10	74
Russell County Hospital	Russell Springs	10	64
Jennie Stuart Medical Center	Hopkinsville	11	174
Saint Elizabeth Ft Thomas	Fort Thomas	11	25
Saint Elizabeth Florence	Florence	16	35
Our Lady of Bellefonte Hospital	Ashland	18	34

Average Time to Transfer (minutes)

Hospital Name	City	Min.	Cases
Frankfort Regional Medical Center	Frankfort	34	44
Three Rivers Medical Center	Louisa	40	25
Baptist Health Corbin	Corbin	61	38
Jennie Stuart Medical Center	Hopkinsville	78	26
Middlesboro Appalachian Reg Healthcare	Middlesboro	91	26

Children's Asthma Care

Received Home Management Plan of Care

Hospital Name	City	Rate	Cases
University of Kentucky Hospital	Lexington	98%	131
Norton Hospitals	Louisville	88%	596

Received Reliever Medication

Hospital Name	City	Rate	Cases
Norton Hospitals	Louisville	100%	596
University of Kentucky Hospital	Lexington	100%	131

Received Systemic Corticosteroids

Hospital Name	City	Rate	Cases
Norton Hospitals	Louisville	100%	597
University of Kentucky Hospital	Lexington	100%	127

Emergency Department

Admittance Decision Time (minutes)

Hospital Name	City	Min.	Cases
Crittenden Health System	Marion	35	324
Harrison Memorial Hospital[2]	Cynthiana	37	245
Monroe County Medical Center[2]	Tompkinsville	41	209
Whitesburg ARH Hospital[2]	Whitesburg	42	345
Parkway Regional Hospital[2]	Fulton	44	347
Bluegrass Community Hospital[2]	Versailles	46	175
Rockcastle County Hospital[2]	Mount Vernon	47	432
Ephraim Mcdowell Fort Logan Hospital[2]	Stanford	48	176
Spring View Hospital[2]	Lebanon	49	244
Bourbon Community Hospital[2]	Paris	50	478
Logan Memorial Hospital[2]	Russellville	50	361
Marshall County Hospital[2]	Benton	50	294
Baptist Health Lagrange[2]	La Grange	51	243
Muhlenberg Community Hospital[2]	Greenville	56	383
University of Louisville Hospital[2]	Louisville	57	539
Pikeville Medical Center[2]	Pikeville	58	361
Methodist Hospital[2]	Henderson	59	411
Taylor Regional Hospital[2]	Campbellsville	59	253
Baptist Health Richmond[2]	Richmond	60	321
Clinton County Hospital[2]	Albany	60	181
Owensboro Health Regional Hospital[2]	Owensboro	60	664
Saint Elizabeth Grant	Williamstown	60	223
Twin Lakes Regional Medical Center[2]	Leitchfield	61	310
Baptist Health Lexington[2]	Lexington	63	282
Frankfort Regional Medical Center[2]	Frankfort	63	503
Saint Joseph Martin[2]	Martin	64	375
Carroll County Memorial Hospital[2]	Carrollton	65	416
Jackson Purchase Medical Center[2]	Mayfield	65	488
Pineville Community Hospital[2]	Pineville	65	270
Saint Claire Regional Medical Center[2]	Morehead	65	405
Westlake Regional Hospital[2]	Columbia	65	355
Saint Joseph Mount Sterling	Mount Sterling	66	905
Middlesboro Appalachian Reg Healthcare[2]	Middlesboro	70	333
Murray - Calloway County Hospital[2]	Murray	70	359
Our Lady of Bellefonte Hospital[2]	Ashland	70	233
Williamson ARH Hospital[2]	S Williamson	72	378
Memorial Hospital[2]	Manchester	75	319
Paul B Hall Regional Medical Center[2]	Paintsville	75	426
Fleming County Hospital[2]	Flemingsburg	76	360
Georgetown Community Hospital[2]	Georgetown	76	243
Breckinridge Memorial Hospital	Hardinsburg	77	317
Clark Regional Medical Center[2]	Winchester	78	322
Ephraim Mcdowell Regional Medical Center[2]	Danville	80	781
Lake Cumberland Regional Hospital[2]	Somerset	80	348
The Medical Center at Bowling Green[2]	Bowling Green	80	264
Highlands Regional Medical Center[2]	Prestonsburg	81	391
Harlan Appalachian Reg Healthcare Hosp[2]	Harlan	82	541
Jennie Stuart Medical Center[2]	Hopkinsville	83	437
Lourdes Hospital[2]	Paducah	84	599
Flaget Memorial Hospital[2]	Bardstown	85	223
Meadowview Regional Medical Center[2]	Maysville	87	275
Saint Elizabeth Florence[2]	Florence	87	933
Three Rivers Medical Center[2]	Louisa	89	471
Baptist Health Louisville[2]	Louisville	91	446
T J Samson Community Hospital[2]	Glasgow	92	415
Baptist Health Corbin[2]	Corbin	94	451
Saint Elizabeth Ft Thomas[2]	Fort Thomas	94	960
Jewish Hospital - Shelbyville[2]	Shelbyville	95	382
Kentucky River Medical Center[2]	Jackson	100	516
King's Daughters' Medical Center[2]	Ashland	100	425
Baptist Health Madisonville[2]	Madisonville	102	609
Saint Elizabeth Medical Center[2]	Lakeside Park	104	528
Norton Hospitals[2]	Louisville	109	752
Baptist Health Paducah[2]	Paducah	110	511
Greenview Regional Hospital[2]	Bowling Green	110	506
Saint Joseph East[2]	Lexington	110	269
Saint Joseph London[2]	London	115	489
Hazard ARH Regional Medical Center[2]	Hazard	139	344
Hardin Memorial Hospital[2]	Elizabethtown	146	624
Saint Joseph Hospital[2]	Lexington	153	525
Jewish Hospital & Saint Mary's Healthcare[2]	Louisville	160	600
University of Kentucky Hospital[2]	Lexington	200	426

Head CT Results Within 45 Minutes of Arrival

Hospital Name	City	Rate	Cases
Baptist Health Madisonville	Madisonville	74%	27
Norton Hospitals	Louisville	69%	29
Frankfort Regional Medical Center	Frankfort	59%	27
Jewish Hospital & Saint Mary's Healthcare	Louisville	44%	27

Patients Who Left ER Before Being Seen

Hospital Name	City	Rate	Cases
Bourbon Community Hospital	Paris	0%	11573
Cumberland County Hospital	Burkesville	0%	6346
Ephraim Mcdowell Fort Logan Hospital	Stanford	0%	11895
Ephraim Mcdowell Regional Medical Center	Danville	0%	28550
Harrison Memorial Hospital	Cynthiana	0%	13676
Jackson Purchase Medical Center	Mayfield	0%	26073
Lake Cumberland Regional Hospital	Somerset	0%	40867
Livingston Hospital & Healthcare Services	Salem	0%	4651
Meadowview Regional Medical Center	Maysville	0%	19842
Methodist Hospital Union County	Morganfield	0%	8236
Morgan County ARH Hospital	West Liberty	0%	7653
Nicholas County Hospital	Carlisle	0%	3683
Pikeville Medical Center	Pikeville	0%	46114
Saint Elizabeth Florence	Florence	0%	50116
Saint Elizabeth Ft Thomas	Fort Thomas	0%	37132
Saint Elizabeth Grant	Williamstown	0%	18212
Saint Elizabeth Medical Center	Lakeside Park	0%	102802
Three Rivers Medical Center	Louisa	0%	18313
Baptist Health Corbin	Corbin	1%	40921
Baptist Health Richmond	Richmond	1%	30172
Bluegrass Community Hospital	Versailles	1%	9154
Caldwell Medical Center	Princeton	1%	11030
Carroll County Memorial Hospital	Carrollton	1%	10748
Clark Regional Medical Center	Winchester	1%	25209
Crittenden Health System	Marion	1%	4421
Fleming County Hospital	Flemingsburg	1%	9042
Georgetown Community Hospital	Georgetown	1%	22045
Greenview Regional Hospital	Bowling Green	1%	31297
Harlan Appalachian Reg Healthcare Hosp	Harlan	1%	21393
Hazard ARH Regional Medical Center	Hazard	1%	24382
Jane Todd Crawford Hospital	Greensburg	1%	5849
King's Daughters' Medical Center	Ashland	1%	73652
Lourdes Hospital	Paducah	1%	31746
Marcum & Wallace Memorial Hospital	Irvine	1%	14039
Marshall County Hospital	Benton	1%	8737
Mary Breckinridge ARH Hospital	Hyden	1%	9127
Methodist Hospital	Henderson	1%	28518
Monroe County Medical Center	Tompkinsville	1%	8177
Ohio County Hospital	Hartford	1%	15188
Parkway Regional Hospital	Fulton	1%	6093
Paul B Hall Regional Medical Center	Paintsville	1%	16252
Russell County Hospital	Russell Springs	1%	11762
Saint Claire Regional Medical Center	Morehead	1%	28534
Saint Joseph East	Lexington	1%	38568
Saint Joseph London	London	1%	48455
Spring View Hospital	Lebanon	1%	14821
T J Samson Community Hospital	Glasgow	1%	34624
Taylor Regional Hospital	Campbellsville	1%	20070
Trigg County Hospital	Cadiz	1%	3064
Westlake Regional Hospital	Columbia	1%	8755
Baptist Health Lagrange	La Grange	2%	15173
Baptist Health Louisville	Louisville	2%	53736
Casey County Hospital	Liberty	2%	6319
Frankfort Regional Medical Center	Frankfort	2%	31031
Highlands Regional Medical Center	Prestonsburg	2%	26413
Jennie Stuart Medical Center	Hopkinsville	2%	35087
Jewish Hospital & Saint Mary's Healthcare	Louisville	2%	169374
Jewish Hospital - Shelbyville	Shelbyville	2%	19313
Kentucky River Medical Center	Jackson	2%	21615
Knox County Hospital	Barbourville	2%	14264
Logan Memorial Hospital	Russellville	2%	13793
McDowell ARH Hospital	Mc Dowell	2%	9298
Middlesboro Appalachian Reg Healthcare	Middlesboro	2%	21813
Muhlenberg Community Hospital	Greenville	2%	20208
Murray - Calloway County Hospital	Murray	2%	18279
Norton Hospitals	Louisville	2%	210165
Our Lady of Bellefonte Hospital	Ashland	2%	26726
Rockcastle County Hospital	Mount Vernon	2%	11564
Saint Joseph Berea	Berea	2%	21825
Saint Joseph Hospital	Lexington	2%	42286
Twin Lakes Regional Medical Center	Leitchfield	2%	21834
University of Kentucky Hospital	Lexington	2%	91208
University of Louisville Hospital	Louisville	2%	43473
Wayne County Hospital	Monticello	2%	11230
Whitesburg ARH Hospital	Whitesburg	2%	37622
Williamson ARH Hospital	S Williamson	2%	17767
Baptist Health Madisonville	Madisonville	3%	30205
Hardin Memorial Hospital	Elizabethtown	3%	58521
Saint Joseph Martin	Martin	3%	15133
Baptist Health Lexington	Lexington	4%	32797
Baptist Health Paducah	Paducah	4%	37443
Breckinridge Memorial Hospital	Hardinsburg	4%	8537
Clinton County Hospital	Albany	4%	6322
The Medical Center at Bowling Green	Bowling Green	4%	47343
The Medical Center at Franklin	Franklin	4%	11489
The Medical Center at Scottsville	Scottsville	4%	8935
Owensboro Health Regional Hospital	Owensboro	4%	64812
Pineville Community Hospital	Pineville	4%	10828
Flaget Memorial Hospital	Bardstown	5%	21861
Memorial Hospital	Manchester	5%	18200
Saint Joseph Mount Sterling	Mount Sterling	5%	24509

Time from ER Arrival to Being Admitted (minutes)

Hospital Name	City	Min.	Cases
Trigg County Hospital[2,3]	Cadiz	115	49
Crittenden Health System	Marion	141	358
Monroe County Medical Center[2]	Tompkinsville	149	300
Saint Elizabeth Grant	Williamstown	169	223
Kentucky River Medical Center[2]	Jackson	170	517
Twin Lakes Regional Medical Center[2]	Leitchfield	175	310
Parkway Regional Hospital[2]	Fulton	180	348
Carroll County Memorial Hospital[2]	Carrollton	181	434
Logan Memorial Hospital[2]	Russellville	181	362
Bourbon Community Hospital[2]	Paris	187	478
Ephraim Mcdowell Fort Logan Hospital[2]	Stanford	188	184
Rockcastle County Hospital[2]	Mount Vernon	188	450
Methodist Hospital[2]	Henderson	194	458
Clinton County Hospital[2]	Albany	195	189

NOTE: Hospital profiles are in alphabetical order by state, then city, then hospital within the city; Rankings exclude hospitals with less than 25 cases except for patient surveys which excludes hospitals with less than 100 cases; (a) 100-299 cases; (1) The number of cases/patients is too few to report; (2) Data submitted were based on a sample of cases/patients; (3) Results are based on a shorter time period than required; (4) Data suppressed by CMS for one or more quarters; (5) Results are not available for this reporting period; (6) Fewer than 100 patients completed the HCAHPS survey; (7) No cases met the criteria for this measure; (8) The lower limit of the confidence interval cannot be calculated if the number of observed infections equals zero; (9) No data are available from the state/territory for this reporting period; (10) The scores shown reflect fewer than 50 completed surveys; (11) There were discrepancies in the data collection process; (12) This measure does not apply to this hospital for this reporting period; (13) Results cannot be calculated for this reporting period; (14) The results for this state are combined with nearby states to protect confidentiality; Please refer to the User's Guide for a full explanation of data.

Harrison Memorial Hospital[2]	Cynthiana	199	245
Middlesboro Appalachian Reg Healthcare[2]	Middlesboro	199	333
Marshall County Hospital[2]	Benton	200	339
Jackson Purchase Medical Center[2]	Mayfield	201	492
Bluegrass Community Hospital[2]	Versailles	204	175
Saint Claire Regional Medical Center[2]	Morehead	207	590
Taylor Regional Hospital[2]	Campbellsville	210	254
Lake Cumberland Regional Hospital[2]	Somerset	214	450
Whitesburg ARH Hospital[2]	Whitesburg	214	356
Pikeville Medical Center[2]	Pikeville	215	460
King's Daughters' Medical Center[2]	Ashland	218	426
Harlan Appalachian Reg Healthcare Hosp[2]	Harlan	219	569
Owensboro Health Regional Hospital[2]	Owensboro	220	669
Ephraim Mcdowell Regional Medical Center[2]	Danville	222	832
Westlake Regional Hospital[2]	Columbia	222	385
Fleming County Hospital[2]	Flemingsburg	225	362
Pineville Community Hospital[2]	Pineville	225	452
Baptist Health Lagrange[2]	La Grange	227	243
Georgetown Community Hospital[2]	Georgetown	228	243
Muhlenberg Community Hospital[2]	Greenville	228	437
Williamson ARH Hospital[2]	S Williamson	230	385
Saint Joseph Martin[2]	Martin	233	379
Baptist Health Richmond[2]	Richmond	234	347
Breckinridge Memorial Hospital	Hardinsburg	235	341
Three Rivers Medical Center[2]	Louisa	235	471
Frankfort Regional Medical Center[2]	Frankfort	236	503
Lourdes Hospital[2]	Paducah	236	618
Hazard ARH Regional Medical Center[2]	Hazard	244	346
Murray - Calloway County Hospital[2]	Murray	244	366
Spring View Hospital[2]	Lebanon	244	244
Baptist Health Lexington[2]	Lexington	246	282
Baptist Health Madisonville[2]	Madisonville	248	616
Greenview Regional Hospital[2]	Bowling Green	248	506
Memorial Hospital[2]	Manchester	250	370
Saint Elizabeth Florence[2]	Florence	250	933
Saint Elizabeth Ft Thomas[2]	Fort Thomas	254	961
Baptist Health Corbin[2]	Corbin	255	451
Meadowview Regional Medical Center[2]	Maysville	255	275
Saint Elizabeth Medical Center[2]	Lakeside Park	255	531
The Medical Center at Bowling Green[2]	Bowling Green	256	392
T J Samson Community Hospital[2]	Glasgow	256	460
Saint Joseph Mount Sterling	Mount Sterling	257	1053
Jennie Stuart Medical Center[2]	Hopkinsville	259	514
Paul B Hall Regional Medical Center[2]	Paintsville	262	426
Our Lady of Bellefonte Hospital[2]	Ashland	265	233
Highlands Regional Medical Center[2]	Prestonsburg	266	392
Flaget Memorial Hospital[2]	Bardstown	275	252
Baptist Health Louisville[2]	Louisville	280	493
Saint Joseph London[2]	London	280	518
Clark Regional Medical Center[2]	Winchester	285	324
Jewish Hospital - Shelbyville[2]	Shelbyville	285	406
Norton Hospitals[2]	Louisville	290	771
Saint Joseph East[2]	Lexington	292	281
Baptist Health Paducah[2]	Paducah	312	513
Hardin Memorial Hospital[2]	Elizabethtown	339	624
Jewish Hospital & Saint Mary's Healthcare[2]	Louisville	348	627
Saint Joseph Hospital[2]	Lexington	360	544
University of Louisville Hospital[2]	Louisville	368	559
University of Kentucky Hospital[2]	Lexington	444	435

Time from ER Arrival to Discharge (minutes)

Hospital Name	City	Min.	Cases
Crittenden Health System	Marion	68	381
Saint Elizabeth Grant	Williamstown	76	381
Jackson Purchase Medical Center	Mayfield	82	441
Bourbon Community Hospital	Paris	83	374
Kentucky River Medical Center	Jackson	84	358
Monroe County Medical Center	Tompkinsville	84	428
Marshall County Hospital[3]	Benton	89	705
Rockcastle County Hospital	Mount Vernon	91	373
Parkway Regional Hospital	Fulton	93	375
Twin Lakes Regional Medical Center	Leitchfield	94	374
Clinton County Hospital	Albany	95	439
Meadowview Regional Medical Center	Maysville	96	384
Harrison Memorial Hospital	Cynthiana	99	371
Trigg County Hospital	Cadiz	100	468
Logan Memorial Hospital	Russellville	102	420
Baptist Health Richmond	Richmond	104	486
Georgetown Community Hospital	Georgetown	109	425
Middlesboro Appalachian Reg Healthcare	Middlesboro	109	408
Westlake Regional Hospital	Columbia	109	535
Saint Elizabeth Medical Center	Lakeside Park	111	768
Saint Joseph Martin[3]	Martin	114	174
Methodist Hospital	Henderson	117	323
Taylor Regional Hospital	Campbellsville	117	394
Ephraim Mcdowell Regional Medical Center	Danville	118	660
Williamson ARH Hospital	S Williamson	118	408
Lourdes Hospital	Paducah	120	399
T J Samson Community Hospital	Glasgow	120	424
King's Daughters' Medical Center	Ashland	123	323
Saint Elizabeth Ft Thomas	Fort Thomas	123	379
Three Rivers Medical Center	Louisa	124	397
Spring View Hospital	Lebanon	125	409
Harlan Appalachian Reg Healthcare Hosp	Harlan	126	405
Fleming County Hospital	Flemingsburg	127	323
Greenview Regional Hospital	Bowling Green	127	478
Saint Elizabeth Florence	Florence	127	384
Paul B Hall Regional Medical Center	Paintsville	128	812
Muhlenberg Community Hospital	Greenville	129	376
Jewish Hospital & Saint Mary's Healthcare	Louisville	132	550
Pineville Community Hospital	Pineville	132	387
Pikeville Medical Center	Pikeville	133	463
Saint Joseph East	Lexington	134	374
Hazard ARH Regional Medical Center	Hazard	135	313
Murray - Calloway County Hospital	Murray	135	390
Owensboro Health Regional Hospital	Owensboro	135	307
Saint Joseph London	London	137	361
Saint Claire Regional Medical Center	Morehead	138	369
Saint Joseph Mount Sterling	Mount Sterling	139	369
Lake Cumberland Regional Hospital	Somerset	140	477
Clark Regional Medical Center	Winchester	143	397
Frankfort Regional Medical Center	Frankfort	143	435
Baptist Health Lagrange	La Grange	146	384
Jewish Hospital - Shelbyville	Shelbyville	149	399
Memorial Hospital	Manchester	149	347
Baptist Health Madisonville	Madisonville	150	369
Jennie Stuart Medical Center	Hopkinsville	150	350
Whitesburg ARH Hospital	Whitesburg	153	397
Baptist Health Corbin	Corbin	154	365
Saint Joseph Hospital	Lexington	154	368
Norton Hospitals	Louisville	162	1633
The Medical Center at Bowling Green	Bowling Green	170	375
Highlands Regional Medical Center	Prestonsburg	182	398
Our Lady of Bellefonte Hospital	Ashland	185	390
Hardin Memorial Hospital	Elizabethtown	189	390
Flaget Memorial Hospital	Bardstown	191	365
Baptist Health Lexington	Lexington	192	430
University of Kentucky Hospital	Lexington	200	349
Baptist Health Louisville	Louisville	218	350
Baptist Health Paducah	Paducah	220	353
University of Louisville Hospital	Louisville	240	318

Time in ER Before Being Evaluated (minutes)

Hospital Name	City	Min.	Cases
Hazard ARH Regional Medical Center	Hazard	8	421
Bourbon Community Hospital	Paris	11	406
Ephraim Mcdowell Regional Medical Center	Danville	11	686
Fleming County Hospital	Flemingsburg	11	361
Saint Elizabeth Grant	Williamstown	11	420
Harrison Memorial Hospital	Cynthiana	12	405
Kentucky River Medical Center	Jackson	12	418
Crittenden Health System	Marion	13	448
Georgetown Community Hospital	Georgetown	14	467
King's Daughters' Medical Center	Ashland	14	406
Baptist Health Corbin	Corbin	15	402
Greenview Regional Hospital	Bowling Green	15	502
Meadowview Regional Medical Center	Maysville	15	406
Rockcastle County Hospital	Mount Vernon	15	410
Trigg County Hospital	Cadiz	15	567
Clinton County Hospital	Albany	16	423
Jackson Purchase Medical Center	Mayfield	16	462
Parkway Regional Hospital	Fulton	16	423
Saint Elizabeth Medical Center	Lakeside Park	16	843
Twin Lakes Regional Medical Center	Leitchfield	17	397
Baptist Health Richmond	Richmond	18	561
Owensboro Health Regional Hospital	Owensboro	18	430
Pikeville Medical Center	Pikeville	18	486
Saint Joseph Martin[3]	Martin	18	192
Three Rivers Medical Center	Louisa	18	421
Lourdes Hospital	Paducah	19	415
Westlake Regional Hospital	Columbia	19	544
Frankfort Regional Medical Center	Frankfort	20	513
Lake Cumberland Regional Hospital	Somerset	20	504
Marshall County Hospital[3]	Benton	20	666
Saint Elizabeth Florence	Florence	20	421
Spring View Hospital	Lebanon	20	443
Clark Regional Medical Center	Winchester	21	463
Saint Elizabeth Ft Thomas	Fort Thomas	21	422
Taylor Regional Hospital	Campbellsville	21	442
Logan Memorial Hospital	Russellville	22	435
Saint Joseph London	London	22	390
Saint Claire Regional Medical Center	Morehead	23	245
Monroe County Medical Center	Tompkinsville	24	485
Jewish Hospital - Shelbyville	Shelbyville	26	406
University of Kentucky Hospital	Lexington	27	369
Baptist Health Lexington	Lexington	28	444
Murray - Calloway County Hospital	Murray	28	406
Saint Joseph East	Lexington	28	383
Middlesboro Appalachian Reg Healthcare	Middlesboro	29	439
Pineville Community Hospital	Pineville	29	417
Harlan Appalachian Reg Healthcare Hosp	Harlan	30	442
Williamson ARH Hospital	S Williamson	30	422
Baptist Health Madisonville	Madisonville	32	339
Jewish Hospital & Saint Mary's Healthcare	Louisville	32	610
T J Samson Community Hospital	Glasgow	33	336
Baptist Health Lagrange	La Grange	34	406
Saint Joseph Hospital	Lexington	34	384
Methodist Hospital	Henderson	35	334
Norton Hospitals	Louisville	35	1526
Paul B Hall Regional Medical Center	Paintsville	35	897
Jennie Stuart Medical Center	Hopkinsville	36	388
Muhlenberg Community Hospital	Greenville	40	391
Our Lady of Bellefonte Hospital	Ashland	40	151
Saint Joseph Mount Sterling	Mount Sterling	40	404
Flaget Memorial Hospital	Bardstown	42	415
Baptist Health Paducah	Paducah	46	406
Whitesburg ARH Hospital	Whitesburg	48	422
Baptist Health Louisville	Louisville	49	405
The Medical Center at Bowling Green	Bowling Green	50	399
Memorial Hospital	Manchester	50	275
Highlands Regional Medical Center	Prestonsburg	52	273
Hardin Memorial Hospital	Elizabethtown	58	405
University of Louisville Hospital	Louisville	66	337

Time to Pain Meds for Bone Fractures (minutes)

Hospital Name	City	Min.	Cases
Norton Hospitals	Louisville	26	446
Saint Elizabeth Grant	Williamstown	30	59
Georgetown Community Hospital	Georgetown	32	75
Clinton County Hospital	Albany	38	33
Ephraim Mcdowell Regional Medical Center	Danville	38	124
Greenview Regional Hospital	Bowling Green	38	139
Saint Joseph Martin[3]	Martin	38	46
Saint Elizabeth Medical Center	Lakeside Park	39	232
Frankfort Regional Medical Center	Frankfort	41	153
Lake Cumberland Regional Hospital	Somerset	42	158
Rockcastle County Hospital	Mount Vernon	42	26
Westlake Regional Hospital	Columbia	42	30
Clark Regional Medical Center	Winchester	44	97
Meadowview Regional Medical Center	Maysville	45	95
Saint Joseph London	London	46	176
Baptist Health Richmond	Richmond	47	100
Hazard ARH Regional Medical Center	Hazard	47	85
King's Daughters' Medical Center	Ashland	47	139
Lourdes Hospital	Paducah	48	102
Saint Elizabeth Ft Thomas	Fort Thomas	49	77
Bourbon Community Hospital	Paris	50	30
Saint Elizabeth Florence	Florence	51	143
Spring View Hospital	Lebanon	51	41
Jackson Purchase Medical Center	Mayfield	52	66
Jewish Hospital & Saint Mary's Healthcare	Louisville	53	296
Memorial Hospital	Manchester	54	59
Saint Joseph Hospital	Lexington	54	173
Harlan Appalachian Reg Healthcare Hosp	Harlan	55	65
Paul B Hall Regional Medical Center	Paintsville	55	66
Saint Joseph East	Lexington	55	136
Twin Lakes Regional Medical Center	Leitchfield	55	94
Baptist Health Corbin	Corbin	56	89
Fleming County Hospital	Flemingsburg	56	43
Owensboro Health Regional Hospital	Owensboro	56	285
Harrison Memorial Hospital	Cynthiana	57	48
Pineville Community Hospital	Pineville	57	37
Marshall County Hospital[3]	Benton	59	40
Pikeville Medical Center	Pikeville	59	219
T J Samson Community Hospital	Glasgow	62	138
Williamson ARH Hospital	S Williamson	63	83
Taylor Regional Hospital	Campbellsville	64	56
Logan Memorial Hospital	Russellville	66	30
Three Rivers Medical Center	Louisa	66	74
Baptist Health Madisonville	Madisonville	68	90
Baptist Health Lexington	Lexington	69	95
Methodist Hospital	Henderson	70	89
Middlesboro Appalachian Reg Healthcare	Middlesboro	70	84
Murray - Calloway County Hospital	Murray	70	81
Jewish Hospital - Shelbyville	Shelbyville	71	60
Kentucky River Medical Center	Jackson	73	81
The Medical Center at Bowling Green	Bowling Green	73	143
Highlands Regional Medical Center	Prestonsburg	74	82
Saint Claire Regional Medical Center	Morehead	74	83
University of Kentucky Hospital	Lexington	74	356
Whitesburg ARH Hospital	Whitesburg	74	88
Jennie Stuart Medical Center	Hopkinsville	75	102
Muhlenberg Community Hospital	Greenville	75	67
Baptist Health Louisville	Louisville	77	101
Baptist Health Paducah	Paducah	79	105
University of Louisville Hospital	Louisville	82	52
Our Lady of Bellefonte Hospital	Ashland	86	81
Saint Joseph Mount Sterling	Mount Sterling	87	130
Hardin Memorial Hospital	Elizabethtown	88	152
Flaget Memorial Hospital	Bardstown	89	133

NOTE: Hospital profiles are in alphabetical order by state, then city, then hospital within the city; Rankings exclude hospitals with less than 25 cases except for patient surveys which excludes hospitals with less than 100 cases; (a) 100-299 cases; (1) The number of cases/patients is too few to report; (2) Data submitted were based on a sample of cases/patients; (3) Results are based on a shorter time period than required; (4) Data suppressed by CMS for one or more quarters; (5) Results are not available for this reporting period; (6) Fewer than 100 patients completed the HCAHPS survey; (7) No cases met the criteria for this measure; (8) The lower limit of the confidence interval cannot be calculated if the number of observed infections equals zero; (9) No data are available from the state/territory for this reporting period; (10) The scores shown reflect fewer than 50 completed surveys; (11) There were discrepancies in the data collection process; (12) This measure does not apply to this hospital for this reporting period; (13) Results cannot be calculated for this reporting period; (14) The results for this state are combined with nearby states to protect confidentiality; Please refer to the User's Guide for a full explanation of data.

Heart Attack Care

Aspirin Given at Discharge

Hospital Name	City	Rate	Cases
Baptist Health Lexington	Lexington	100%	627
Baptist Health Louisville	Louisville	100%	500
Baptist Health Madisonville	Madisonville	100%	299
Baptist Health Paducah[2]	Paducah	100%	356
Baptist Health Richmond	Richmond	100%	37
Clark Regional Medical Center	Winchester	100%	30
Greenview Regional Hospital	Bowling Green	100%	30
Jewish Hospital & Saint Mary's Healthcare[2]	Louisville	100%	470
King's Daughters' Medical Center[2]	Ashland	100%	296
Lake Cumberland Regional Hospital[2]	Somerset	100%	253
Lexington VA Medical Center	Lexington	100%	74
Owensboro Health Regional Hospital	Owensboro	100%	371
Pikeville Medical Center	Pikeville	100%	340
Saint Claire Regional Medical Center	Morehead	100%	133
Saint Elizabeth Florence	Florence	100%	64
Saint Elizabeth Ft Thomas	Fort Thomas	100%	55
Saint Elizabeth Medical Center[2]	Lakeside Park	100%	327
Saint Joseph East	Lexington	100%	134
Saint Joseph Hospital[2]	Lexington	100%	354
Saint Joseph London	London	100%	345
University of Kentucky Hospital	Lexington	100%	355
University of Louisville Hospital	Louisville	100%	156
Ephraim Mcdowell Regional Medical Center	Danville	99%	174
Hardin Memorial Hospital	Elizabethtown	99%	235
Lourdes Hospital	Paducah	99%	169
Meadowview Regional Medical Center	Maysville	99%	117
Norton Hospitals	Louisville	99%	916
Hazard ARH Regional Medical Center	Hazard	97%	179
Louisville VA Medical Center	Louisville	97%	60
The Medical Center at Bowling Green	Bowling Green	97%	705
T J Samson Community Hospital	Glasgow	95%	207
Our Lady of Bellefonte Hospital	Ashland	94%	48

PCI Within 90 Minutes of Arrival

Hospital Name	City	Rate	Cases
Baptist Health Madisonville	Madisonville	100%	50
Hardin Memorial Hospital	Elizabethtown	100%	31
King's Daughters' Medical Center[2]	Ashland	100%	30
Lourdes Hospital	Paducah	100%	38
Norton Hospitals	Louisville	100%	87
Owensboro Health Regional Hospital	Owensboro	100%	57
Pikeville Medical Center	Pikeville	100%	32
Saint Joseph Hospital[2]	Lexington	100%	27
Baptist Health Lexington	Lexington	99%	72
Baptist Health Louisville	Louisville	98%	122
Baptist Health Paducah[2]	Paducah	98%	41
Saint Elizabeth Medical Center[2]	Lakeside Park	98%	43
Lake Cumberland Regional Hospital[2]	Somerset	96%	45
Meadowview Regional Medical Center	Maysville	96%	27
The Medical Center at Bowling Green	Bowling Green	95%	43
Ephraim Mcdowell Regional Medical Center	Danville	94%	32
Jewish Hospital & Saint Mary's Healthcare[2]	Louisville	94%	31
University of Kentucky Hospital	Lexington	93%	41
Saint Joseph London	London	92%	38
Saint Claire Regional Medical Center	Morehead	90%	31

Statin Prescribed at Discharge

Hospital Name	City	Rate	Cases
Baptist Health Lexington	Lexington	100%	613
Baptist Health Paducah[2]	Paducah	100%	342
Baptist Health Richmond	Richmond	100%	38
Greenview Regional Hospital	Bowling Green	100%	26
King's Daughters' Medical Center[2]	Ashland	100%	276
Louisville VA Medical Center	Louisville	100%	57
Lourdes Hospital	Paducah	100%	152
Pikeville Medical Center	Pikeville	100%	342
Saint Elizabeth Ft Thomas	Fort Thomas	100%	51
Saint Elizabeth Medical Center[2]	Lakeside Park	100%	312
Saint Joseph Hospital[2]	Lexington	100%	344
Saint Joseph London	London	100%	331
University of Kentucky Hospital	Lexington	100%	325
University of Louisville Hospital	Louisville	100%	151
Baptist Health Louisville	Louisville	99%	461
Ephraim Mcdowell Regional Medical Center	Danville	99%	166
Hardin Memorial Hospital	Elizabethtown	99%	223
Norton Hospitals	Louisville	99%	868
Owensboro Health Regional Hospital	Owensboro	99%	373
Saint Joseph East	Lexington	99%	135
Baptist Health Madisonville	Madisonville	98%	279
Saint Claire Regional Medical Center	Morehead	98%	128
Saint Elizabeth Florence	Florence	98%	59
Clark Regional Medical Center	Winchester	97%	29
Lake Cumberland Regional Hospital[2]	Somerset	97%	247
Jewish Hospital & Saint Mary's Healthcare[2]	Louisville	96%	446
Lexington VA Medical Center	Lexington	96%	76
Hazard ARH Regional Medical Center	Hazard	95%	173
Our Lady of Bellefonte Hospital	Ashland	94%	48
The Medical Center at Bowling Green	Bowling Green	88%	695
T J Samson Community Hospital	Glasgow	88%	195
Meadowview Regional Medical Center	Maysville	87%	103

Heart Failure Care

ACE Inhibitor or ARB for LVSD

Hospital Name	City	Rate	Cases
Baptist Health Corbin	Corbin	100%	46
Baptist Health Lagrange	La Grange	100%	25
Baptist Health Louisville	Louisville	100%	142
Baptist Health Paducah[2]	Paducah	100%	99
Ephraim Mcdowell Regional Medical Center	Danville	100%	71
Frankfort Regional Medical Center	Frankfort	100%	34
Jennie Stuart Medical Center	Hopkinsville	100%	36
Lourdes Hospital	Paducah	100%	99
Pikeville Medical Center	Pikeville	100%	90
Saint Claire Regional Medical Center	Morehead	100%	41
Saint Elizabeth Florence[2]	Florence	100%	59
Saint Elizabeth Ft Thomas[2]	Fort Thomas	100%	54
Saint Elizabeth Medical Center[2]	Lakeside Park	100%	83
Saint Joseph London	London	100%	86
University of Kentucky Hospital	Lexington	100%	211
Louisville VA Medical Center	Louisville	99%	95
University of Louisville Hospital	Louisville	99%	116
Baptist Health Lexington	Lexington	98%	116
Baptist Health Madisonville	Madisonville	98%	96
Norton Hospitals	Louisville	98%	339
Owensboro Health Regional Hospital	Owensboro	98%	193
Saint Joseph East	Lexington	98%	44
King's Daughters' Medical Center[2]	Ashland	97%	74
Saint Joseph Hospital[2]	Lexington	97%	89
Jackson Purchase Medical Center	Mayfield	96%	27
Hardin Memorial Hospital	Elizabethtown	95%	133
Lake Cumberland Regional Hospital[2]	Somerset	95%	79
Lexington VA Medical Center	Lexington	95%	65
Our Lady of Bellefonte Hospital	Ashland	95%	56
Memorial Hospital	Manchester	93%	28
Hazard ARH Regional Medical Center	Hazard	91%	54
T J Samson Community Hospital	Glasgow	90%	60
Methodist Hospital	Henderson	88%	49
Jewish Hospital & Saint Mary's Healthcare[2]	Louisville	86%	170
Whitesburg ARH Hospital	Whitesburg	85%	26
Middlesboro Appalachian Reg Healthcare	Middlesboro	82%	28
The Medical Center at Bowling Green	Bowling Green	78%	154

Discharge Instructions Given

Hospital Name	City	Rate	Cases
Baptist Health Richmond	Richmond	100%	47
Greenview Regional Hospital	Bowling Green	100%	57
Harrison Memorial Hospital	Cynthiana	100%	32
Jackson Purchase Medical Center	Mayfield	100%	63
King's Daughters' Medical Center[2]	Ashland	100%	261
Logan Memorial Hospital	Russellville	100%	29
McDowell ARH Hospital	Mc Dowell	100%	39
Memorial Hospital	Manchester	100%	132
Paul B Hall Regional Medical Center	Paintsville	100%	33
Pikeville Medical Center	Pikeville	100%	334
Rockcastle County Hospital	Mount Vernon	100%	29
Saint Elizabeth Florence[2]	Florence	100%	220
Saint Elizabeth Ft Thomas[2]	Fort Thomas	100%	189
Saint Elizabeth Medical Center[2]	Lakeside Park	100%	258
Spring View Hospital	Lebanon	100%	35
Three Rivers Medical Center	Louisa	100%	91
University of Kentucky Hospital	Lexington	100%	418
University of Louisville Hospital	Louisville	100%	210
Lexington VA Medical Center	Lexington	99%	196
Owensboro Health Regional Hospital	Owensboro	99%	443
Frankfort Regional Medical Center	Frankfort	98%	134
Harlan Appalachian Reg Healthcare Hosp	Harlan	98%	126
Highlands Regional Medical Center	Prestonsburg	98%	99
Kentucky River Medical Center	Jackson	97%	58
The Medical Center at Franklin	Franklin	97%	31
Baptist Health Corbin	Corbin	96%	149
Baptist Health Lagrange	La Grange	96%	71
Baptist Health Lexington	Lexington	96%	339
Flaget Memorial Hospital	Bardstown	96%	57
Fleming County Hospital	Flemingsburg	96%	57
Baptist Health Paducah[2]	Paducah	95%	240
Clark Regional Medical Center	Winchester	95%	42
Georgetown Community Hospital	Georgetown	95%	44
Jennie Stuart Medical Center	Hopkinsville	95%	59
Marshall County Hospital	Benton	95%	38
Norton Hospitals	Louisville	95%	1000
Saint Claire Regional Medical Center	Morehead	95%	126
Baptist Health Louisville	Louisville	94%	538
Lourdes Hospital	Paducah	94%	208
Whitesburg ARH Hospital	Whitesburg	94%	134
Marcum & Wallace Memorial Hospital[2]	Irvine	93%	28
Ephraim Mcdowell Regional Medical Center	Danville	92%	179
Hardin Memorial Hospital	Elizabethtown	92%	436
Louisville VA Medical Center	Louisville	92%	235
Williamson ARH Hospital	S Williamson	92%	91
Baptist Health Madisonville	Madisonville	91%	190
Saint Joseph London	London	91%	270
Saint Joseph Mount Sterling	Mount Sterling	91%	32
Lake Cumberland Regional Hospital[2]	Somerset	90%	214
The Medical Center at Bowling Green	Bowling Green	90%	455
Methodist Hospital	Henderson	90%	131
Twin Lakes Regional Medical Center	Leitchfield	90%	61
Hazard ARH Regional Medical Center	Hazard	89%	202
Middlesboro Appalachian Reg Healthcare	Middlesboro	89%	87
Cumberland County Hospital	Burkesville	88%	33
Meadowview Regional Medical Center	Maysville	88%	95
Pineville Community Hospital	Pineville	87%	112
T J Samson Community Hospital	Glasgow	87%	143
Knox County Hospital	Barbourville	86%	42
Monroe County Medical Center	Tompkinsville	86%	64
Crittenden Health System	Marion	85%	26
Our Lady of Bellefonte Hospital	Ashland	85%	207
Saint Joseph Martin	Martin	84%	25
Taylor Regional Hospital	Campbellsville	84%	45
Muhlenberg Community Hospital	Greenville	82%	38
Saint Joseph East	Lexington	81%	114
Ohio County Hospital	Hartford	79%	34
Clinton County Hospital	Albany	77%	30
Jewish Hospital & Saint Mary's Healthcare[2]	Louisville	73%	433
Saint Joseph Hospital[2]	Lexington	71%	276
Jewish Hospital - Shelbyville	Shelbyville	63%	70
Murray - Calloway County Hospital	Murray	41%	87

Evaluation of LVS Function

Hospital Name	City	Rate	Cases
Baptist Health Corbin	Corbin	100%	191
Baptist Health Lagrange	La Grange	100%	83
Baptist Health Lexington	Lexington	100%	410
Baptist Health Louisville	Louisville	100%	762
Baptist Health Madisonville	Madisonville	100%	241
Baptist Health Paducah[2]	Paducah	100%	295
Baptist Health Richmond	Richmond	100%	51
Bourbon Community Hospital	Paris	100%	30
Clark Regional Medical Center	Winchester	100%	51
Clinton County Hospital	Albany	100%	39
Flaget Memorial Hospital	Bardstown	100%	74
Frankfort Regional Medical Center	Frankfort	100%	160
Georgetown Community Hospital	Georgetown	100%	53
Greenview Regional Hospital	Bowling Green	100%	90
Hardin Memorial Hospital	Elizabethtown	100%	551
Harlan Appalachian Reg Healthcare Hosp	Harlan	100%	150
Harrison Memorial Hospital	Cynthiana	100%	36
Jackson Purchase Medical Center	Mayfield	100%	100
Jewish Hospital & Saint Mary's Healthcare[2]	Louisville	100%	538
Kentucky River Medical Center	Jackson	100%	73
King's Daughters' Medical Center[2]	Ashland	100%	299
Lake Cumberland Regional Hospital[2]	Somerset	100%	258
Lexington VA Medical Center	Lexington	100%	216
Logan Memorial Hospital	Russellville	100%	45
Louisville VA Medical Center	Louisville	100%	269
Lourdes Hospital	Paducah	100%	249
Mary Breckinridge ARH Hospital	Hyden	100%	39
McDowell ARH Hospital	Mc Dowell	100%	42
Middlesboro Appalachian Reg Healthcare	Middlesboro	100%	119
Muhlenberg Community Hospital	Greenville	100%	47
Norton Hospitals	Louisville	100%	1359
Owensboro Health Regional Hospital	Owensboro	100%	549
Parkway Regional Hospital	Fulton	100%	35
Paul B Hall Regional Medical Center	Paintsville	100%	46
Pikeville Medical Center	Pikeville	100%	369
Rockcastle County Hospital	Mount Vernon	100%	44
Saint Claire Regional Medical Center	Morehead	100%	163
Saint Elizabeth Florence[2]	Florence	100%	271
Saint Elizabeth Ft Thomas[2]	Fort Thomas	100%	243
Saint Elizabeth Medical Center[2]	Lakeside Park	100%	316
Saint Joseph Berea	Berea	100%	25
Saint Joseph East	Lexington	100%	140
Saint Joseph Hospital[2]	Lexington	100%	338
Saint Joseph London	London	100%	310
Saint Joseph Mount Sterling	Mount Sterling	100%	44
Taylor Regional Hospital	Campbellsville	100%	61
Three Rivers Medical Center	Louisa	100%	103
University of Kentucky Hospital	Lexington	100%	479
University of Louisville Hospital	Louisville	100%	232
Ephraim Mcdowell Regional Medical Center	Danville	99%	233
Fleming County Hospital	Flemingsburg	99%	67
Highlands Regional Medical Center	Prestonsburg	99%	116
Jewish Hospital - Shelbyville	Shelbyville	99%	85
Memorial Hospital	Manchester	99%	152
Methodist Hospital	Henderson	99%	165
Our Lady of Bellefonte Hospital	Ashland	99%	243
T J Samson Community Hospital	Glasgow	99%	186

NOTE: Hospital profiles are in alphabetical order by state, then city, then hospital within the city; Rankings exclude hospitals with less than 25 cases except for patient surveys which excludes hospitals with less than 100 cases; (a) 100-299 cases; (1) The number of cases/patients is too few to report; (2) Data submitted were based on a sample of cases/patients; (3) Results are based on a shorter time period than required; (4) Data suppressed by CMS for one or more quarters; (5) Results are not available for this reporting period; (6) Fewer than 100 patients completed the HCAHPS survey; (7) No cases met the criteria for this measure; (8) The lower limit of the confidence interval cannot be calculated if the number of observed infections equals zero; (9) No data are available from the state/territory for this reporting period; (10) The scores shown reflect fewer than 50 completed surveys; (11) There were discrepancies in the data collection process; (12) This measure does not apply to this hospital for this reporting period; (13) Results cannot be calculated for this reporting period; (14) The results for this state are combined with nearby states to protect confidentiality; Please refer to the User's Guide for a full explanation of data.

Twin Lakes Regional Medical Center	Leitchfield	99%	77
Hazard ARH Regional Medical Center	Hazard	98%	238
Meadowview Regional Medical Center	Maysville	98%	121
Williamson ARH Hospital	S Williamson	98%	107
Crittenden Health System	Marion	97%	39
Jennie Stuart Medical Center	Hopkinsville	97%	76
Marcum & Wallace Memorial Hospital[2]	Irvine	97%	33
Marshall County Hospital	Benton	96%	55
Monroe County Medical Center	Tompkinsville	96%	76
The Medical Center at Franklin	Franklin	95%	42
Ohio County Hospital	Hartford	95%	41
The Medical Center at Bowling Green	Bowling Green	94%	561
Carroll County Memorial Hospital	Carrollton	93%	30
Pineville Community Hospital	Pineville	93%	128
Saint Joseph Martin	Martin	93%	29
Whitesburg ARH Hospital	Whitesburg	88%	157
Murray - Calloway County Hospital	Murray	85%	99
Spring View Hospital	Lebanon	85%	62
Livingston Hospital & Healthcare Services	Salem	66%	29
Knox County Hospital	Barbourville	65%	46
Westlake Regional Hospital	Columbia	62%	32
Cumberland County Hospital	Burkesville	40%	40
Jane Todd Crawford Hospital	Greensburg	36%	42
Casey County Hospital	Liberty	11%	36

Medicare Spending

Medicare Spending per Patient (ratio)

Hospital Name	City	Ratio	Cases
Paul B Hall Regional Medical Center	Paintsville	0.84	-
Pineville Community Hospital	Pineville	0.85	-
Bourbon Community Hospital	Paris	0.86	-
Clark Regional Medical Center	Winchester	0.88	-
Muhlenberg Community Hospital	Greenville	0.89	-
Three Rivers Medical Center	Louisa	0.89	-
Flaget Memorial Hospital	Bardstown	0.90	-
Saint Joseph London	London	0.92	-
Spring View Hospital	Lebanon	0.92	-
Williamson ARH Hospital	S Williamson	0.92	-
Baptist Health Paducah	Paducah	0.93	-
Middlesboro Appalachian Reg Healthcare	Middlesboro	0.93	-
Pikeville Medical Center	Pikeville	0.93	-
Harrison Memorial Hospital	Cynthiana	0.94	-
Lourdes Hospital	Paducah	0.94	-
Memorial Hospital	Manchester	0.94	-
Monroe County Medical Center	Tompkinsville	0.94	-
Owensboro Health Regional Hospital	Owensboro	0.94	-
Baptist Health Lagrange	La Grange	0.95	-
Baptist Health Madisonville	Madisonville	0.95	-
Kentucky River Medical Center	Jackson	0.95	-
Our Lady of Bellefonte Hospital	Ashland	0.95	-
Rockcastle County Hospital	Mount Vernon	0.95	-
Twin Lakes Regional Medical Center	Leitchfield	0.95	-
Ephraim Mcdowell Regional Medical Center	Danville	0.96	-
Georgetown Community Hospital	Georgetown	0.96	-
Whitesburg ARH Hospital	Whitesburg	0.96	-
Hardin Memorial Hospital	Elizabethtown	0.97	-
Highlands Regional Medical Center	Prestonsburg	0.97	-
King's Daughters' Medical Center	Ashland	0.97	-
Murray - Calloway County Hospital	Murray	0.97	-
Saint Joseph East	Lexington	0.97	-
Saint Joseph Hospital	Lexington	0.97	-
Baptist Health Corbin	Corbin	0.98	-
Baptist Health Louisville	Louisville	0.98	-
Crittenden Health System	Marion	0.98	-
Jackson Purchase Medical Center	Mayfield	0.98	-
Jennie Stuart Medical Center	Hopkinsville	0.98	-
Lake Cumberland Regional Hospital	Somerset	0.98	-
Meadowview Regional Medical Center	Maysville	0.98	-
Saint Elizabeth Ft Thomas	Fort Thomas	0.98	-
Westlake Regional Hospital	Columbia	0.98	-
Saint Claire Regional Medical Center	Morehead	0.99	-
Fleming County Hospital	Flemingsburg	1.00	-
Harlan Appalachian Reg Healthcare Hosp	Harlan	1.00	-
Jewish Hospital & Saint Mary's Healthcare	Louisville	1.00	-
Saint Joseph Mount Sterling	Mount Sterling	1.00	-
T J Samson Community Hospital	Glasgow	1.00	-
University of Kentucky Hospital	Lexington	1.00	-
Methodist Hospital	Henderson	1.01	-
Norton Hospitals	Louisville	1.01	-
Frankfort Regional Medical Center	Frankfort	1.02	-
Hazard ARH Regional Medical Center	Hazard	1.02	-
Jewish Hospital - Shelbyville	Shelbyville	1.02	-
Parkway Regional Hospital	Fulton	1.02	-
Saint Elizabeth Medical Center	Lakeside Park	1.02	-
Taylor Regional Hospital	Campbellsville	1.02	-
University of Louisville Hospital	Louisville	1.02	-
Baptist Health Lexington	Lexington	1.03	-
Baptist Health Richmond	Richmond	1.03	-
Greenview Regional Hospital	Bowling Green	1.03	-
Logan Memorial Hospital	Russellville	1.03	-
Clinton County Hospital	Albany	1.04	-
The Medical Center at Bowling Green	Bowling Green	1.05	-
Saint Elizabeth Florence	Florence	1.06	-

Pneumonia Care

Appropriate Initial Antibiotic Given

Hospital Name	City	Rate	Cases
Carroll County Memorial Hospital	Carrollton	100%	28
Frankfort Regional Medical Center	Frankfort	100%	88
Mary Breckinridge ARH Hospital	Hyden	100%	38
Morgan County ARH Hospital	West Liberty	100%	51
Parkway Regional Hospital	Fulton	100%	53
Saint Elizabeth Medical Center[2]	Lakeside Park	100%	60
Three Rivers Medical Center	Louisa	100%	72
University of Kentucky Hospital	Lexington	100%	135
University of Louisville Hospital	Louisville	100%	53
Wayne County Hospital	Monticello	100%	48
Baptist Health Lexington	Lexington	99%	171
Baptist Health Paducah[2]	Paducah	99%	149
Fleming County Hospital	Flemingsburg	99%	115
Greenview Regional Hospital	Bowling Green	99%	71
King's Daughters' Medical Center[2]	Ashland	99%	85
Paul B Hall Regional Medical Center	Paintsville	99%	72
Pikeville Medical Center	Pikeville	99%	237
Saint Elizabeth Ft Thomas[2]	Fort Thomas	99%	72
Baptist Health Corbin	Corbin	98%	165
Baptist Health Lagrange	La Grange	98%	65
Baptist Health Richmond	Richmond	98%	82
Harrison Memorial Hospital	Cynthiana	98%	125
Kentucky River Medical Center	Jackson	98%	41
Logan Memorial Hospital	Russellville	98%	93
Lourdes Hospital	Paducah	98%	176
McDowell ARH Hospital	Mc Dowell	98%	47
Baptist Health Louisville	Louisville	97%	397
Baptist Health Madisonville	Madisonville	97%	115
Ephraim Mcdowell Regional Medical Center	Danville	97%	124
Harlan Appalachian Reg Healthcare Hosp	Harlan	97%	124
Louisville VA Medical Center	Louisville	97%	58
Meadowview Regional Medical Center	Maysville	97%	71
Owensboro Health Regional Hospital	Owensboro	97%	274
Rockcastle County Hospital	Mount Vernon	97%	33
Saint Elizabeth Florence[2]	Florence	97%	79
Saint Joseph Berea	Berea	97%	63
Ephraim Mcdowell Fort Logan Hospital	Stanford	96%	25
Flaget Memorial Hospital	Bardstown	96%	111
Jennie Stuart Medical Center	Hopkinsville	96%	158
Lake Cumberland Regional Hospital[2]	Somerset	96%	93
Memorial Hospital	Manchester	96%	223
Norton Hospitals	Louisville	96%	564
Saint Joseph East	Lexington	96%	96
Saint Joseph Martin	Martin	96%	46
Georgetown Community Hospital	Georgetown	95%	79
Methodist Hospital	Henderson	95%	141
Saint Joseph Hospital[2]	Lexington	95%	102
Twin Lakes Regional Medical Center	Leitchfield	95%	96
Whitesburg ARH Hospital	Whitesburg	95%	130
Clark Regional Medical Center	Winchester	94%	103
Hardin Memorial Hospital[2]	Elizabethtown	94%	79
Marcum & Wallace Memorial Hospital	Irvine	94%	31
Middlesboro Appalachian Reg Healthcare	Middlesboro	94%	93
Our Lady of Bellefonte Hospital	Ashland	94%	194
Saint Claire Regional Medical Center	Morehead	94%	117
Spring View Hospital	Lebanon	94%	109
Taylor Regional Hospital	Campbellsville	94%	88
Highlands Regional Medical Center	Prestonsburg	93%	107
Lexington VA Medical Center	Lexington	93%	67
Saint Joseph London	London	93%	135
T J Samson Community Hospital[2]	Glasgow	93%	85
Jackson Purchase Medical Center	Mayfield	92%	131
Jewish Hospital & Saint Mary's Healthcare[2]	Louisville	92%	145
Saint Joseph Mount Sterling	Mount Sterling	92%	128
Williamson ARH Hospital	S Williamson	92%	96
Methodist Hospital Union County	Morganfield	91%	46
Jewish Hospital - Shelbyville	Shelbyville	90%	59
The Medical Center at Bowling Green	Bowling Green	89%	174
Bourbon Community Hospital	Paris	88%	41
Russell County Hospital	Russell Springs	88%	60
Hazard ARH Regional Medical Center[2]	Hazard	87%	69
The Medical Center at Franklin	Franklin	87%	55
Muhlenberg Community Hospital	Greenville	85%	80
Jane Todd Crawford Hospital	Greensburg	84%	25
Ohio County Hospital	Hartford	83%	54
Clinton County Hospital	Albany	82%	72
Westlake Regional Hospital	Columbia	82%	60
Monroe County Medical Center	Tompkinsville	80%	50
Murray - Calloway County Hospital	Murray	80%	116
Marshall County Hospital	Benton	78%	45
Pineville Community Hospital	Pineville	76%	68
Caldwell Medical Center	Princeton	74%	27
Trigg County Hospital[2]	Cadiz	73%	26
Crittenden Health System	Marion	71%	45
Casey County Hospital	Liberty	70%	40
Knox County Hospital	Barbourville	69%	51
Cumberland County Hospital	Burkesville	56%	39

Blood Culture Timing

Hospital Name	City	Rate	Cases
Baptist Health Lagrange	La Grange	100%	112
Baptist Health Lexington	Lexington	100%	266
Baptist Health Madisonville	Madisonville	100%	169
Crittenden Health System	Marion	100%	35
Ephraim Mcdowell Fort Logan Hospital	Stanford	100%	43
Frankfort Regional Medical Center	Frankfort	100%	153
Harlan Appalachian Reg Healthcare Hosp	Harlan	100%	215
Jackson Purchase Medical Center	Mayfield	100%	215
Kentucky River Medical Center	Jackson	100%	60
Lake Cumberland Regional Hospital[2]	Somerset	100%	135
Lourdes Hospital	Paducah	100%	163
Methodist Hospital	Henderson	100%	154
Owensboro Health Regional Hospital	Owensboro	100%	378
Parkway Regional Hospital	Fulton	100%	57
Paul B Hall Regional Medical Center	Paintsville	100%	161
Pikeville Medical Center	Pikeville	100%	444
Saint Elizabeth Florence[2]	Florence	100%	111
Saint Joseph Berea	Berea	100%	68
Saint Joseph East	Lexington	100%	133
Three Rivers Medical Center	Louisa	100%	103
Wayne County Hospital	Monticello	100%	57
Baptist Health Corbin	Corbin	99%	286
Baptist Health Louisville	Louisville	99%	571
Baptist Health Paducah[2]	Paducah	99%	234
Ephraim Mcdowell Regional Medical Center	Danville	99%	263
Flaget Memorial Hospital	Bardstown	99%	156
Greenview Regional Hospital	Bowling Green	99%	111
Harrison Memorial Hospital	Cynthiana	99%	182
King's Daughters' Medical Center[2]	Ashland	99%	67
Logan Memorial Hospital	Russellville	99%	76
Mary Breckinridge ARH Hospital	Hyden	99%	67
Meadowview Regional Medical Center	Maysville	99%	116
Saint Elizabeth Ft Thomas[2]	Fort Thomas	99%	96
Saint Elizabeth Medical Center[2]	Lakeside Park	99%	87
Saint Joseph Hospital[2]	Lexington	99%	140
Spring View Hospital	Lebanon	99%	138
T J Samson Community Hospital[2]	Glasgow	99%	144
University of Kentucky Hospital	Lexington	99%	354
Baptist Health Richmond	Richmond	98%	147
Clark Regional Medical Center	Winchester	98%	144
Fleming County Hospital	Flemingsburg	98%	107
Georgetown Community Hospital	Georgetown	98%	104
Jennie Stuart Medical Center	Hopkinsville	98%	268
McDowell ARH Hospital	Mc Dowell	98%	65
Middlesboro Appalachian Reg Healthcare	Middlesboro	98%	115
Muhlenberg Community Hospital	Greenville	98%	91
Norton Hospitals	Louisville	98%	1063
Saint Joseph London	London	98%	189
Taylor Regional Hospital	Campbellsville	98%	81
Whitesburg ARH Hospital	Whitesburg	98%	125
Jewish Hospital & Saint Mary's Healthcare[2]	Louisville	97%	266
Lexington VA Medical Center	Lexington	97%	206
Louisville VA Medical Center	Louisville	97%	112
The Medical Center at Bowling Green	Bowling Green	97%	207
Memorial Hospital	Manchester	97%	278
Rockcastle County Hospital	Mount Vernon	97%	29
Saint Claire Regional Medical Center	Morehead	97%	237
Saint Joseph Mount Sterling	Mount Sterling	97%	182
University of Louisville Hospital	Louisville	97%	131
Williamson ARH Hospital	S Williamson	97%	100
Bourbon Community Hospital	Paris	96%	51
The James B Haggin Memorial Hospital	Harrodsburg	96%	50
Jewish Hospital - Shelbyville	Shelbyville	96%	123
Marshall County Hospital	Benton	96%	50
The Medical Center at Franklin	Franklin	96%	26
Pineville Community Hospital	Pineville	96%	91
Saint Joseph Martin	Martin	96%	52
Twin Lakes Regional Medical Center	Leitchfield	96%	162
Carroll County Memorial Hospital	Carrollton	95%	38
Hazard ARH Regional Medical Center[2]	Hazard	95%	81
Highlands Regional Medical Center	Prestonsburg	95%	140
Morgan County ARH Hospital	West Liberty	95%	65
Ohio County Hospital	Hartford	95%	55
Our Lady of Bellefonte Hospital	Ashland	95%	366
Hardin Memorial Hospital[2]	Elizabethtown	94%	108
Marcum & Wallace Memorial Hospital	Irvine	94%	31
Murray - Calloway County Hospital	Murray	93%	118
Westlake Regional Hospital	Columbia	91%	82
Knox County Hospital	Barbourville	90%	49
Caldwell Medical Center	Princeton	89%	37
Methodist Hospital Union County	Morganfield	82%	39
Monroe County Medical Center	Tompkinsville	80%	64

NOTE: Hospital profiles are in alphabetical order by state, then city, then hospital within the city; Rankings exclude hospitals with less than 25 cases except for patient surveys which excludes hospitals with less than 100 cases; (a) 100-299 cases; (1) The number of cases/patients is too few to report; (2) Data submitted were based on a sample of cases/patients; (3) Results are based on a shorter time period than required; (4) Data suppressed by CMS for one or more quarters; (5) Results are not available for this reporting period; (6) Fewer than 100 patients completed the HCAHPS survey; (7) No cases met the criteria for this measure; (8) The lower limit of the confidence interval cannot be calculated if the number of observed infections equals zero; (9) No data are available from the state/territory for this reporting period; (10) The scores shown reflect fewer than 50 completed surveys; (11) There were discrepancies in the data collection process; (12) This measure does not apply to this hospital for this reporting period; (13) Results cannot be calculated for this reporting period; (14) The results for this state are combined with nearby states to protect confidentiality; Please refer to the User's Guide for a full explanation of data.

Russell County Hospital	Russell Springs	77%	64

Pregnancy and Delivery Care

Newborns whose Deliveries were Scheduled Early

Hospital Name	City	Rate	Cases
Jewish Hospital & Saint Mary's Healthcare[4]	Louisville	-	90
Saint Elizabeth Medical Center[2]	Lakeside Park	0%	240
Baptist Health Lexington[2]	Lexington	1%	86
Baptist Health Louisville	Louisville	2%	264
Baptist Health Richmond[2]	Richmond	2%	63
Frankfort Regional Medical Center[2]	Frankfort	3%	30
Harrison Memorial Hospital[2]	Cynthiana	3%	31
King's Daughters' Medical Center[2]	Ashland	3%	32
Lourdes Hospital	Paducah	3%	30
Owensboro Health Regional Hospital[2]	Owensboro	3%	185
Pikeville Medical Center[2]	Pikeville	3%	39
Baptist Health Lagrange[2]	La Grange	4%	47
Ephraim Mcdowell Regional Medical Center	Danville	4%	46
Lake Cumberland Regional Hospital[2]	Somerset	4%	27
Saint Joseph East[2]	Lexington	6%	50
Saint Joseph Mount Sterling	Mount Sterling	6%	31
Spring View Hospital[2]	Lebanon	6%	31
Whitesburg ARH Hospital[2]	Whitesburg	7%	119
University of Louisville Hospital[2]	Louisville	8%	40
Norton Hospitals[2]	Louisville	9%	692
Twin Lakes Regional Medical Center	Leitchfield	9%	35
Saint Claire Regional Medical Center	Morehead	10%	40
Jackson Purchase Medical Center[2]	Mayfield	12%	42
Baptist Health Corbin[2]	Corbin	14%	36
Highlands Regional Medical Center	Prestonsburg	14%	101
The Medical Center at Bowling Green	Bowling Green	14%	284
Methodist Hospital[2]	Henderson	14%	69
Hardin Memorial Hospital[2]	Elizabethtown	16%	55
T J Samson Community Hospital[2]	Glasgow	16%	31
Taylor Regional Hospital	Campbellsville	18%	34
Hazard ARH Regional Medical Center[2]	Hazard	19%	47
Murray - Calloway County Hospital	Murray	26%	65
Jennie Stuart Medical Center	Hopkinsville	45%	168

Preventive Care

Immunization for Influenza

Hospital Name	City	Rate	Cases
Kentucky River Medical Center[2]	Jackson	100%	320
Parkway Regional Hospital[2]	Fulton	100%	305
Saint Elizabeth Florence[2]	Florence	100%	642
Saint Elizabeth Ft Thomas[2]	Fort Thomas	100%	597
Saint Elizabeth Grant	Williamstown	100%	160
Saint Elizabeth Medical Center[2]	Lakeside Park	100%	549
Baptist Health Lagrange[2]	La Grange	99%	288
Baptist Health Richmond[2]	Richmond	99%	375
Bourbon Community Hospital[2]	Paris	99%	285
Ephraim Mcdowell Regional Medical Center[2]	Danville	99%	832
Greenview Regional Hospital[2]	Bowling Green	99%	434
Harrison Memorial Hospital[2]	Cynthiana	99%	254
Lake Cumberland Regional Hospital[2]	Somerset	99%	520
Logan Memorial Hospital[2]	Russellville	99%	291
Three Rivers Medical Center[2]	Louisa	99%	310
Baptist Health Paducah[2]	Paducah	98%	535
Bluegrass Community Hospital[2]	Versailles	98%	159
Ephraim Mcdowell Fort Logan Hospital[2]	Stanford	98%	284
Georgetown Community Hospital[2]	Georgetown	98%	259
Jennie Stuart Medical Center[2]	Hopkinsville	98%	544
University of Kentucky Hospital[2]	Lexington	98%	523
Baptist Health Lexington[2]	Lexington	97%	499
Baptist Health Louisville[2]	Louisville	97%	534
Baptist Health Madisonville[2]	Madisonville	97%	522
Frankfort Regional Medical Center[2]	Frankfort	97%	435
Jackson Purchase Medical Center[2]	Mayfield	97%	382
King's Daughters' Medical Center[2]	Ashland	97%	598
Paul B Hall Regional Medical Center[2]	Paintsville	97%	415
Williamson ARH Hospital[2]	S Williamson	97%	318
Clark Regional Medical Center[2]	Winchester	96%	331
Clinton County Hospital[2]	Albany	96%	331
Fleming County Hospital[2]	Flemingsburg	96%	285
Saint Joseph Mount Sterling	Mount Sterling	96%	992
Spring View Hospital[2]	Lebanon	96%	258
T J Samson Community Hospital[2]	Glasgow	96%	495
Baptist Health Corbin[2]	Corbin	95%	520
Muhlenberg Community Hospital[2]	Greenville	95%	273
Saint Joseph East[2]	Lexington	95%	498
Saint Joseph London[2]	London	95%	523
Twin Lakes Regional Medical Center[2]	Leitchfield	95%	291
Marshall County Hospital[2]	Benton	94%	437
Saint Joseph Hospital[2]	Lexington	94%	606
Carroll County Memorial Hospital	Carrollton	93%	334
Hardin Memorial Hospital[2]	Elizabethtown	93%	525
Meadowview Regional Medical Center[2]	Maysville	93%	304
Norton Hospitals[2]	Louisville	93%	985
Pikeville Medical Center[2]	Pikeville	93%	561
Jewish Hospital & Saint Mary's Healthcare[2]	Louisville	92%	643
Pineville Community Hospital[2]	Pineville	92%	283
Flaget Memorial Hospital[2]	Bardstown	91%	301
Middlesboro Appalachian Reg Healthcare[2]	Middlesboro	91%	277
Our Lady of Bellefonte Hospital[2]	Ashland	91%	631
Saint Claire Regional Medical Center[2]	Morehead	91%	454
Lourdes Hospital[2]	Paducah	90%	596
The Medical Center at Bowling Green[2]	Bowling Green	90%	554
Cumberland County Hospital	Burkesville	89%	378
Harlan Appalachian Reg Healthcare Hosp[2]	Harlan	89%	414
Taylor Regional Hospital[2]	Campbellsville	89%	321
Crittenden Health System	Marion	88%	417
Rockcastle County Hospital[2]	Mount Vernon	88%	299
Memorial Hospital[2]	Manchester	85%	306
Methodist Hospital[2]	Henderson	85%	489
Saint Joseph Martin[2]	Martin	85%	288
Owensboro Health Regional Hospital[2]	Owensboro	83%	584
University of Louisville Hospital[2]	Louisville	82%	535
Jewish Hospital - Shelbyville[2]	Shelbyville	76%	286
Hazard ARH Regional Medical Center[2]	Hazard	75%	611
Monroe County Medical Center[2]	Tompkinsville	75%	317
Westlake Regional Hospital[2]	Columbia	75%	326
Whitesburg ARH Hospital[2]	Whitesburg	70%	398
Highlands Regional Medical Center[2]	Prestonsburg	67%	454
Trigg County Hospital[3]	Cadiz	65%	34
Murray - Calloway County Hospital[2]	Murray	51%	426

Immunization for Pneumonia

Hospital Name	City	Rate	Cases
Baptist Health Richmond[2]	Richmond	100%	407
Clinton County Hospital[2]	Albany	100%	470
Harrison Memorial Hospital[2]	Cynthiana	100%	324
Kentucky River Medical Center[2]	Jackson	100%	420
King's Daughters' Medical Center[2]	Ashland	100%	825
Lake Cumberland Regional Hospital[2]	Somerset	100%	625
Parkway Regional Hospital[2]	Fulton	100%	362
Saint Elizabeth Florence[2]	Florence	100%	911
Saint Elizabeth Ft Thomas[2]	Fort Thomas	100%	905
Saint Elizabeth Grant	Williamstown	100%	241
Saint Elizabeth Medical Center[2]	Lakeside Park	100%	676
Baptist Health Lagrange[2]	La Grange	99%	307
Baptist Health Paducah[2]	Paducah	99%	682
Bourbon Community Hospital[2]	Paris	99%	421
Ephraim Mcdowell Regional Medical Center[2]	Danville	99%	1128
Frankfort Regional Medical Center[2]	Frankfort	99%	549
Greenview Regional Hospital[2]	Bowling Green	99%	660
Paul B Hall Regional Medical Center[2]	Paintsville	99%	554
Saint Joseph Mount Sterling	Mount Sterling	99%	1268
Three Rivers Medical Center[2]	Louisa	99%	380
Clark Regional Medical Center[2]	Winchester	98%	352
Ephraim Mcdowell Fort Logan Hospital[2]	Stanford	98%	207
Logan Memorial Hospital[2]	Russellville	98%	476
Meadowview Regional Medical Center[2]	Maysville	98%	358
Saint Joseph London[2]	London	98%	621
Baptist Health Corbin[2]	Corbin	97%	550
Baptist Health Madisonville[2]	Madisonville	97%	694
Fleming County Hospital[2]	Flemingsburg	97%	486
Jennie Stuart Medical Center[2]	Hopkinsville	97%	623
Spring View Hospital[2]	Lebanon	97%	278
Williamson ARH Hospital[2]	S Williamson	97%	436
Baptist Health Lexington[2]	Lexington	96%	583
Memorial Hospital[2]	Manchester	96%	367
Muhlenberg Community Hospital[2]	Greenville	96%	435
T J Samson Community Hospital[2]	Glasgow	96%	570
Baptist Health Louisville[2]	Louisville	95%	673
Bluegrass Community Hospital[2]	Versailles	95%	233
Carroll County Memorial Hospital	Carrollton	95%	487
Crittenden Health System	Marion	95%	589
Georgetown Community Hospital[2]	Georgetown	95%	318
Harlan Appalachian Reg Healthcare Hosp[2]	Harlan	95%	539
Lourdes Hospital[2]	Paducah	95%	877
Marshall County Hospital[2]	Benton	95%	653
Pikeville Medical Center[2]	Pikeville	95%	709
Taylor Regional Hospital[2]	Campbellsville	95%	413
Flaget Memorial Hospital[2]	Bardstown	94%	390
Hardin Memorial Hospital[2]	Elizabethtown	94%	664
Jackson Purchase Medical Center[2]	Mayfield	94%	557
Middlesboro Appalachian Reg Healthcare[2]	Middlesboro	94%	337
Pineville Community Hospital[2]	Pineville	94%	330
Rockcastle County Hospital[2]	Mount Vernon	94%	465
Saint Joseph Hospital[2]	Lexington	94%	929
Cumberland County Hospital[2]	Burkesville	93%	579
Jewish Hospital - Shelbyville[2]	Shelbyville	93%	471
Methodist Hospital[2]	Henderson	93%	545
Saint Claire Regional Medical Center[2]	Morehead	93%	576
Saint Joseph Martin[2]	Martin	93%	411
Jewish Hospital & Saint Mary's Healthcare[2]	Louisville	92%	1208
Norton Hospitals[2]	Louisville	92%	1029
Saint Joseph East[2]	Lexington	92%	422
Twin Lakes Regional Medical Center[2]	Leitchfield	91%	385
The Medical Center at Bowling Green[2]	Bowling Green	89%	669
Our Lady of Bellefonte Hospital[2]	Ashland	89%	820
Owensboro Health Regional Hospital[2]	Owensboro	87%	767
University of Kentucky Hospital[2]	Lexington	87%	483
Whitesburg ARH Hospital[2]	Whitesburg	83%	463
Westlake Regional Hospital[2]	Columbia	82%	441
University of Louisville Hospital[2]	Louisville	81%	457
Hazard ARH Regional Medical Center[2]	Hazard	75%	864
Monroe County Medical Center[2]	Tompkinsville	75%	460
Highlands Regional Medical Center[2]	Prestonsburg	74%	496
Trigg County Hospital[2,3]	Cadiz	72%	79
Murray - Calloway County Hospital[2]	Murray	62%	507

Stroke Care

Anticoagulation Therapy for Atrial Fibrillation

Hospital Name	City	Rate	Cases
Baptist Health Louisville	Louisville	100%	56
Owensboro Health Regional Hospital	Owensboro	100%	26
University of Kentucky Hospital	Lexington	100%	70
University of Louisville Hospital	Louisville	98%	55
Baptist Health Paducah[2]	Paducah	97%	31
Jewish Hospital & Saint Mary's Healthcare[2]	Louisville	97%	31
Baptist Health Lexington	Lexington	96%	49
Norton Hospitals	Louisville	95%	57
Hardin Memorial Hospital	Elizabethtown	93%	30
The Medical Center at Bowling Green	Bowling Green	93%	30

Antithrombotic Therapy Timing

Hospital Name	City	Rate	Cases
Greenview Regional Hospital	Bowling Green	100%	41
Jennie Stuart Medical Center	Hopkinsville	100%	78
King's Daughters' Medical Center[2]	Ashland	100%	91
Lake Cumberland Regional Hospital[2]	Somerset	100%	97
Pikeville Medical Center	Pikeville	100%	105
Saint Claire Regional Medical Center	Morehead	100%	27
Twin Lakes Regional Medical Center	Leitchfield	100%	27
Baptist Health Lexington	Lexington	99%	252
Baptist Health Louisville	Louisville	99%	297
Baptist Health Paducah[2]	Paducah	99%	154
Norton Hospitals	Louisville	99%	360
Owensboro Health Regional Hospital	Owensboro	99%	211
Saint Elizabeth Florence[2]	Florence	99%	75
Saint Joseph Hospital[2]	Lexington	99%	103
University of Kentucky Hospital	Lexington	99%	391
Baptist Health Madisonville[2]	Madisonville	98%	65
Lourdes Hospital	Paducah	98%	98
Methodist Hospital[2]	Henderson	98%	41
Our Lady of Bellefonte Hospital	Ashland	98%	51
Saint Joseph London[2]	London	98%	49
University of Louisville Hospital	Louisville	98%	248
Baptist Health Corbin	Corbin	97%	33
Ephraim Mcdowell Regional Medical Center	Danville	97%	31
Hardin Memorial Hospital	Elizabethtown	97%	144
Saint Elizabeth Medical Center[2]	Lakeside Park	97%	100
Jewish Hospital & Saint Mary's Healthcare[2]	Louisville	96%	177
Saint Elizabeth Ft Thomas[2]	Fort Thomas	96%	70
Whitesburg ARH Hospital	Whitesburg	96%	28
The Medical Center at Bowling Green	Bowling Green	95%	251
Hazard ARH Regional Medical Center	Hazard	94%	53
Murray - Calloway County Hospital	Murray	94%	35
Jackson Purchase Medical Center	Mayfield	93%	28
Monroe County Medical Center	Tompkinsville	72%	36

Assessed for Rehabilitation

Hospital Name	City	Rate	Cases
Baptist Health Paducah[2]	Paducah	100%	182
Jewish Hospital & Saint Mary's Healthcare[2]	Louisville	100%	207
Pikeville Medical Center	Pikeville	100%	137
Saint Elizabeth Florence[2]	Florence	100%	98
Saint Elizabeth Ft Thomas[2]	Fort Thomas	100%	81
University of Kentucky Hospital	Lexington	100%	627
University of Louisville Hospital	Louisville	100%	423
Lake Cumberland Regional Hospital[2]	Somerset	99%	113
Saint Elizabeth Medical Center[2]	Lakeside Park	99%	127
Baptist Health Louisville	Louisville	98%	358
Greenview Regional Hospital	Bowling Green	98%	46
Hardin Memorial Hospital	Elizabethtown	98%	162
Norton Hospitals	Louisville	98%	499
Owensboro Health Regional Hospital	Owensboro	98%	238
Saint Joseph London[2]	London	98%	47
Baptist Health Lexington	Lexington	97%	332
Baptist Health Madisonville[2]	Madisonville	97%	70
King's Daughters' Medical Center[2]	Ashland	96%	100
Our Lady of Bellefonte Hospital	Ashland	96%	57
Twin Lakes Regional Medical Center	Leitchfield	96%	25
The Medical Center at Bowling Green	Bowling Green	95%	288
Ephraim Mcdowell Regional Medical Center	Danville	93%	30
Jackson Purchase Medical Center	Mayfield	93%	27

NOTE: Hospital profiles are in alphabetical order by state, then city, then hospital within the city; Rankings exclude hospitals with less than 25 cases except for patient surveys which excludes hospitals with less than 100 cases; (a) 100-299 cases; (1) The number of cases/patients is too few to report; (2) Data submitted were based on a sample of cases/patients; (3) Results are based on a shorter time period than required; (4) Data suppressed by CMS for one or more quarters; (5) Results are not available for this reporting period; (6) Fewer than 100 patients completed the HCAHPS survey; (7) No cases met the criteria for this measure; (8) The lower limit of the confidence interval cannot be calculated if the number of observed infections equals zero; (9) No data are available from the state/territory for this reporting period; (10) The scores shown reflect fewer than 50 completed surveys; (11) There were discrepancies in the data collection process; (12) This measure does not apply to this hospital for this reporting period; (13) Results cannot be calculated for this reporting period; (14) The results for this state are combined with nearby states to protect confidentiality; Please refer to the User's Guide for a full explanation of data.

Hospital Name	City	Rate	Cases
Saint Joseph Hospital[2]	Lexington	93%	120
Methodist Hospital[2]	Henderson	92%	37
Whitesburg ARH Hospital	Whitesburg	92%	26
Saint Claire Regional Medical Center	Morehead	90%	30
Lourdes Hospital	Paducah	86%	103
Fleming County Hospital	Flemingsburg	85%	26
Monroe County Medical Center	Tompkinsville	81%	31
Murray - Calloway County Hospital	Murray	80%	40
Baptist Health Corbin	Corbin	76%	34
Jennie Stuart Medical Center	Hopkinsville	74%	72
Hazard ARH Regional Medical Center	Hazard	71%	49

Discharged on Antithrombotic Therapy

Hospital Name	City	Rate	Cases
Baptist Health Corbin	Corbin	100%	30
Baptist Health Lexington	Lexington	100%	299
Baptist Health Louisville	Louisville	100%	320
Baptist Health Madisonville[2]	Madisonville	100%	67
Baptist Health Paducah[2]	Paducah	100%	165
Ephraim Mcdowell Regional Medical Center	Danville	100%	30
Greenview Regional Hospital	Bowling Green	100%	40
Jackson Purchase Medical Center	Mayfield	100%	25
Lake Cumberland Regional Hospital[2]	Somerset	100%	103
Norton Hospitals	Louisville	100%	402
Pikeville Medical Center	Pikeville	100%	125
Saint Elizabeth Florence[2]	Florence	100%	93
Saint Elizabeth Ft Thomas[2]	Fort Thomas	100%	77
Saint Elizabeth Medical Center[2]	Lakeside Park	100%	115
Saint Joseph London[2]	London	100%	47
University of Kentucky Hospital	Lexington	100%	507
University of Louisville Hospital	Louisville	100%	329
Jennie Stuart Medical Center	Hopkinsville	99%	69
Jewish Hospital & Saint Mary's Healthcare[2]	Louisville	99%	199
The Medical Center at Bowling Green	Bowling Green	99%	267
Saint Joseph Hospital[2]	Lexington	99%	109
Hardin Memorial Hospital	Elizabethtown	97%	152
King's Daughters' Medical Center[2]	Ashland	97%	94
Lourdes Hospital	Paducah	97%	100
Methodist Hospital[2]	Henderson	97%	35
Saint Claire Regional Medical Center	Morehead	97%	29
Our Lady of Bellefonte Hospital	Ashland	96%	57
Owensboro Health Regional Hospital	Owensboro	96%	218
Twin Lakes Regional Medical Center	Leitchfield	96%	25
Hazard ARH Regional Medical Center	Hazard	94%	48
Whitesburg ARH Hospital	Whitesburg	92%	25
Murray - Calloway County Hospital	Murray	89%	37
Monroe County Medical Center	Tompkinsville	58%	31

Discharged on Statin Medication

Hospital Name	City	Rate	Cases
Greenview Regional Hospital	Bowling Green	100%	27
Jewish Hospital & Saint Mary's Healthcare[2]	Louisville	100%	154
Lake Cumberland Regional Hospital[2]	Somerset	100%	84
Pikeville Medical Center	Pikeville	100%	102
Saint Elizabeth Florence[2]	Florence	100%	75
Saint Elizabeth Ft Thomas[2]	Fort Thomas	100%	56
Saint Joseph London[2]	London	100%	37
University of Kentucky Hospital	Lexington	100%	352
Baptist Health Lexington	Lexington	99%	238
Baptist Health Paducah[2]	Paducah	99%	117
Baptist Health Louisville	Louisville	98%	241
Saint Elizabeth Medical Center[2]	Lakeside Park	98%	86
University of Louisville Hospital	Louisville	98%	243
Baptist Health Madisonville[2]	Madisonville	96%	56
King's Daughters' Medical Center[2]	Ashland	96%	81
Owensboro Health Regional Hospital	Owensboro	95%	178
Norton Hospitals	Louisville	94%	321
Saint Joseph Hospital[2]	Lexington	93%	88
The Medical Center at Bowling Green	Bowling Green	92%	213
Our Lady of Bellefonte Hospital	Ashland	89%	37
Murray - Calloway County Hospital	Murray	84%	31
Saint Claire Regional Medical Center	Morehead	84%	25
Hardin Memorial Hospital	Elizabethtown	80%	123
Jennie Stuart Medical Center	Hopkinsville	80%	54
Lourdes Hospital	Paducah	76%	78
Hazard ARH Regional Medical Center	Hazard	75%	36
Methodist Hospital[2]	Henderson	72%	32
Monroe County Medical Center	Tompkinsville	35%	31

Thrombolytic Therapy Timing

Hospital Name	City	Rate	Cases
University of Kentucky Hospital	Lexington	100%	28
Baptist Health Louisville	Louisville	86%	29
Hardin Memorial Hospital	Elizabethtown	15%	27

Venous Thromboembolism (VTE) Prophylaxis

Hospital Name	City	Rate	Cases
Greenview Regional Hospital	Bowling Green	100%	50
Lake Cumberland Regional Hospital[2]	Somerset	100%	119
Saint Elizabeth Florence[2]	Florence	100%	92
Saint Elizabeth Ft Thomas[2]	Fort Thomas	100%	81
Saint Elizabeth Medical Center[2]	Lakeside Park	100%	132
Baptist Health Paducah[2]	Paducah	99%	187
Pikeville Medical Center	Pikeville	99%	125
University of Kentucky Hospital	Lexington	99%	590
University of Louisville Hospital	Louisville	99%	418
Our Lady of Bellefonte Hospital	Ashland	98%	52
Saint Joseph London[2]	London	98%	45
The Medical Center at Bowling Green	Bowling Green	97%	296
Baptist Health Louisville	Louisville	95%	378
Norton Hospitals	Louisville	95%	497
Owensboro Health Regional Hospital	Owensboro	94%	242
Baptist Health Lexington	Lexington	93%	330
Jackson Purchase Medical Center	Mayfield	93%	28
King's Daughters' Medical Center[2]	Ashland	93%	96
Jewish Hospital & Saint Mary's Healthcare[2]	Louisville	91%	202
Jennie Stuart Medical Center	Hopkinsville	89%	73
Lourdes Hospital	Paducah	89%	106
Twin Lakes Regional Medical Center	Leitchfield	89%	27
Hardin Memorial Hospital	Elizabethtown	85%	150
Ephraim Mcdowell Regional Medical Center	Danville	84%	32
Monroe County Medical Center	Tompkinsville	84%	37
Whitesburg ARH Hospital	Whitesburg	83%	30
Saint Joseph Hospital[2]	Lexington	82%	119
Methodist Hospital[2]	Henderson	80%	41
Baptist Health Corbin	Corbin	79%	34
Baptist Health Madisonville[2]	Madisonville	79%	68
Hazard ARH Regional Medical Center	Hazard	67%	51
Fleming County Hospital	Flemingsburg	64%	25
Murray - Calloway County Hospital	Murray	55%	40

Written Stroke Educational Materials Given

Hospital Name	City	Rate	Cases
Lourdes Hospital	Paducah	100%	64
Pikeville Medical Center	Pikeville	100%	88
Saint Elizabeth Ft Thomas[2]	Fort Thomas	100%	46
Saint Elizabeth Medical Center[2]	Lakeside Park	100%	68
University of Kentucky Hospital	Lexington	99%	348
Saint Elizabeth Florence[2]	Florence	98%	49
Our Lady of Bellefonte Hospital	Ashland	97%	37
Baptist Health Paducah[2]	Paducah	96%	109
King's Daughters' Medical Center[2]	Ashland	95%	61
University of Louisville Hospital	Louisville	93%	241
Baptist Health Lexington	Lexington	92%	199
Baptist Health Louisville	Louisville	92%	195
Lake Cumberland Regional Hospital[2]	Somerset	89%	65
The Medical Center at Bowling Green	Bowling Green	89%	174
Owensboro Health Regional Hospital	Owensboro	89%	141
Norton Hospitals	Louisville	88%	269
Hardin Memorial Hospital	Elizabethtown	87%	93
Saint Joseph London[2]	London	76%	33
Jewish Hospital & Saint Mary's Healthcare[2]	Louisville	73%	122
Baptist Health Madisonville[2]	Madisonville	58%	38
Jennie Stuart Medical Center	Hopkinsville	36%	39
Saint Joseph Hospital[2]	Lexington	22%	73
Hazard ARH Regional Medical Center	Hazard	3%	29

Surgical Care Improvement Project

Appropriate Beta Blocker Usage

Hospital Name	City	Rate	Cases
Baptist Health Corbin	Corbin	100%	93
Frankfort Regional Medical Center	Frankfort	100%	53
Greenview Regional Hospital	Bowling Green	100%	244
Lourdes Hospital[2]	Paducah	100%	486
Meadowview Regional Medical Center	Maysville	100%	40
Pikeville Medical Center	Pikeville	100%	381
Saint Elizabeth Florence	Florence	100%	66
Taylor Regional Hospital	Campbellsville	100%	53
Twin Lakes Regional Medical Center	Leitchfield	100%	34
University of Kentucky Hospital[2]	Lexington	100%	233
University of Louisville Hospital[2]	Louisville	100%	77
Baptist Health Lexington	Lexington	99%	692
Baptist Health Louisville	Louisville	99%	1372
Baptist Health Paducah[2]	Paducah	99%	339
Ephraim Mcdowell Regional Medical Center	Danville	99%	140
King's Daughters' Medical Center[2]	Ashland	99%	301
Saint Elizabeth Medical Center[2]	Lakeside Park	99%	270
Saint Joseph London	London	99%	161
Baptist Health Lagrange	La Grange	98%	53
Baptist Health Madisonville[2]	Madisonville	98%	188
Baptist Health Richmond	Richmond	98%	63
Clark Regional Medical Center	Winchester	98%	40
Methodist Hospital[2]	Henderson	98%	56
Owensboro Health Regional Hospital[2]	Owensboro	98%	370
Saint Claire Regional Medical Center[2]	Morehead	98%	51
Flaget Memorial Hospital[2]	Bardstown	97%	75
Jewish Hospital & Saint Mary's Healthcare[2]	Louisville	97%	343
Lake Cumberland Regional Hospital[2]	Somerset	97%	169
Saint Joseph East	Lexington	97%	216
The Medical Center at Bowling Green	Bowling Green	96%	489
Murray - Calloway County Hospital	Murray	96%	161
Norton Hospitals[2]	Louisville	96%	1287
Saint Joseph Hospital[2]	Lexington	96%	367
Our Lady of Bellefonte Hospital	Ashland	95%	200
Saint Elizabeth Ft Thomas	Fort Thomas	95%	39
Hazard ARH Regional Medical Center	Hazard	94%	116
Jewish Hospital - Shelbyville	Shelbyville	94%	34
Lexington VA Medical Center[2]	Lexington	94%	93
T J Samson Community Hospital[2]	Glasgow	94%	109
Jennie Stuart Medical Center	Hopkinsville	93%	102
Saint Joseph Mount Sterling	Mount Sterling	93%	91
Hardin Memorial Hospital[2]	Elizabethtown	92%	137
Louisville VA Medical Center[2]	Louisville	90%	58
Spring View Hospital	Lebanon	89%	27

Appropriate VTP Within 24 Hours

Hospital Name	City	Rate	Cases
Baptist Health Lexington	Lexington	100%	1274
Bluegrass Community Hospital	Versailles	100%	37
Fleming County Hospital	Flemingsburg	100%	25
Frankfort Regional Medical Center	Frankfort	100%	175
Harlan Appalachian Reg Healthcare Hosp	Harlan	100%	51
Harrison Memorial Hospital	Cynthiana	100%	44
Jewish Hospital - Shelbyville	Shelbyville	100%	69
Kentucky River Medical Center	Jackson	100%	27
King's Daughters' Medical Center[2]	Ashland	100%	345
Parkway Regional Hospital	Fulton	100%	47
Paul B Hall Regional Medical Center	Paintsville	100%	28
Pikeville Medical Center	Pikeville	100%	814
Saint Elizabeth Florence	Florence	100%	158
Saint Elizabeth Ft Thomas	Fort Thomas	100%	129
Saint Elizabeth Medical Center[2]	Lakeside Park	100%	434
Three Rivers Medical Center	Louisa	100%	29
University of Kentucky Hospital[2]	Lexington	100%	405
Baptist Health Corbin	Corbin	99%	199
Baptist Health Louisville	Louisville	99%	3101
Baptist Health Madisonville[2]	Madisonville	99%	388
Baptist Health Paducah[2]	Paducah	99%	704
Baptist Health Richmond	Richmond	99%	187
Clark Regional Medical Center	Winchester	99%	136
Flaget Memorial Hospital[2]	Bardstown	99%	282
Greenview Regional Hospital	Bowling Green	99%	621
Hardin Memorial Hospital[2]	Elizabethtown	99%	355
Jennie Stuart Medical Center	Hopkinsville	99%	323
Lake Cumberland Regional Hospital[2]	Somerset	99%	305
Lexington VA Medical Center[2]	Lexington	99%	202
Lourdes Hospital[2]	Paducah	99%	908
Saint Claire Regional Medical Center[2]	Morehead	99%	143
Spring View Hospital	Lebanon	99%	123
Taylor Regional Hospital	Campbellsville	99%	178
Baptist Health Lagrange	La Grange	98%	192
Hazard ARH Regional Medical Center	Hazard	98%	243
Louisville VA Medical Center[2]	Louisville	98%	143
Meadowview Regional Medical Center	Maysville	98%	133
Murray - Calloway County Hospital	Murray	98%	458
Saint Joseph London	London	98%	270
Saint Joseph Mount Sterling	Mount Sterling	98%	251
Twin Lakes Regional Medical Center	Leitchfield	98%	135
Ephraim Mcdowell Regional Medical Center	Danville	97%	336
Highlands Regional Medical Center	Prestonsburg	97%	101
Muhlenberg Community Hospital	Greenville	97%	63
Owensboro Health Regional Hospital[2]	Owensboro	97%	699
The Medical Center at Bowling Green	Bowling Green	96%	664
Norton Hospitals[2]	Louisville	96%	2563
Our Lady of Bellefonte Hospital	Ashland	96%	582
Saint Joseph East	Lexington	96%	637
Saint Joseph Hospital[2]	Lexington	96%	423
University of Louisville Hospital[2]	Louisville	96%	267
Jewish Hospital & Saint Mary's Healthcare[2]	Louisville	95%	496
T J Samson Community Hospital[2]	Glasgow	95%	263
Georgetown Community Hospital	Georgetown	94%	50
Saint Joseph Berea	Berea	94%	36
Methodist Hospital[2]	Henderson	93%	175
Whitesburg ARH Hospital	Whitesburg	93%	75
Williamson ARH Hospital	S Williamson	92%	37
Jackson Purchase Medical Center	Mayfield	87%	62
Pineville Community Hospital	Pineville	76%	29

Controlled Postoperative Blood Glucose

Hospital Name	City	Rate	Cases
Hazard ARH Regional Medical Center	Hazard	100%	37
Lake Cumberland Regional Hospital[2]	Somerset	100%	45
Owensboro Health Regional Hospital[2]	Owensboro	100%	190
Pikeville Medical Center	Pikeville	100%	125
Saint Elizabeth Medical Center[2]	Lakeside Park	100%	163
Baptist Health Louisville	Louisville	99%	331
King's Daughters' Medical Center[2]	Ashland	99%	124
Baptist Health Paducah[2]	Paducah	98%	124

NOTE: Hospital profiles are in alphabetical order by state, then city, then hospital within the city; Rankings exclude hospitals with less than 25 cases except for patient surveys which excludes hospitals with less than 100 cases; (a) 100-299 cases; (1) The number of cases/patients is too few to report; (2) Data submitted were based on a sample of cases/patients; (3) Results are based on a shorter time period than required; (4) Data suppressed by CMS for one or more quarters; (5) Results are not available for this reporting period; (6) Fewer than 100 patients completed the HCAHPS survey; (7) No cases met the criteria for this measure; (8) The lower limit of the confidence interval cannot be calculated if the number of observed infections equals zero; (9) No data are available from the state/territory for this reporting period; (10) The scores shown reflect fewer than 50 completed surveys; (11) There were discrepancies in the data collection process; (12) This measure does not apply to this hospital for this reporting period; (13) Results cannot be calculated for this reporting period; (14) The results for this state are combined with nearby states to protect confidentiality; Please refer to the User's Guide for a full explanation of data.

Hospital Name	City	Rate	Cases
Norton Hospitals[2]	Louisville	97%	413
Saint Joseph Hospital[2]	Lexington	97%	236
Baptist Health Lexington	Lexington	96%	411
Saint Joseph London	London	96%	52
University of Kentucky Hospital[2]	Lexington	96%	115
Jewish Hospital & Saint Mary's Healthcare[2]	Louisville	94%	159
Baptist Health Madisonville[2]	Madisonville	93%	90
Lourdes Hospital[2]	Paducah	93%	165
The Medical Center at Bowling Green	Bowling Green	88%	309

Perioperative Temperature Management

Hospital Name	City	Rate	Cases
Baptist Health Corbin	Corbin	100%	215
Baptist Health Lagrange	La Grange	100%	205
Baptist Health Lexington	Lexington	100%	1540
Baptist Health Louisville	Louisville	100%	3496
Baptist Health Madisonville[2]	Madisonville	100%	474
Baptist Health Paducah[2]	Paducah	100%	803
Baptist Health Richmond	Richmond	100%	229
Bluegrass Community Hospital	Versailles	100%	38
Clark Regional Medical Center	Winchester	100%	158
Ephraim Mcdowell Regional Medical Center	Danville	100%	406
Flaget Memorial Hospital[2]	Bardstown	100%	296
Fleming County Hospital	Flemingsburg	100%	26
Frankfort Regional Medical Center	Frankfort	100%	200
Georgetown Community Hospital	Georgetown	100%	52
Greenview Regional Hospital	Bowling Green	100%	694
Hardin Memorial Hospital[2]	Elizabethtown	100%	443
Harlan Appalachian Reg Healthcare Hosp	Harlan	100%	77
Harrison Memorial Hospital	Cynthiana	100%	53
Hazard ARH Regional Medical Center	Hazard	100%	270
Jackson Purchase Medical Center	Mayfield	100%	66
Jennie Stuart Medical Center	Hopkinsville	100%	400
Jewish Hospital & Saint Mary's Healthcare[2]	Louisville	100%	653
Jewish Hospital - Shelbyville	Shelbyville	100%	79
Kentucky River Medical Center	Jackson	100%	36
King's Daughters' Medical Center[2]	Ashland	100%	496
Lake Cumberland Regional Hospital[2]	Somerset	100%	382
Lourdes Hospital[2]	Paducah	100%	1122
Meadowview Regional Medical Center	Maysville	100%	137
Methodist Hospital[2]	Henderson	100%	200
Muhlenberg Community Hospital	Greenville	100%	69
Murray - Calloway County Hospital	Murray	100%	505
Our Lady of Bellefonte Hospital	Ashland	100%	609
Owensboro Health Regional Hospital[2]	Owensboro	100%	993
Parkway Regional Hospital	Fulton	100%	47
Paul B Hall Regional Medical Center	Paintsville	100%	31
Pikeville Medical Center	Pikeville	100%	898
Pineville Community Hospital	Pineville	100%	30
Saint Claire Regional Medical Center[2]	Morehead	100%	204
Saint Elizabeth Florence	Florence	100%	200
Saint Elizabeth Ft Thomas	Fort Thomas	100%	170
Saint Elizabeth Medical Center[2]	Lakeside Park	100%	548
Saint Joseph Berea	Berea	100%	39
Saint Joseph East	Lexington	100%	733
Saint Joseph Hospital[2]	Lexington	100%	643
Saint Joseph London	London	100%	317
Saint Joseph Mount Sterling	Mount Sterling	100%	270
Spring View Hospital	Lebanon	100%	144
T J Samson Community Hospital[2]	Glasgow	100%	306
Taylor Regional Hospital	Campbellsville	100%	186
Three Rivers Medical Center	Louisa	100%	35
Twin Lakes Regional Medical Center	Leitchfield	100%	145
University of Kentucky Hospital[2]	Lexington	100%	541
University of Louisville Hospital[2]	Louisville	100%	321
Whitesburg ARH Hospital	Whitesburg	100%	86
Williamson ARH Hospital	S Williamson	100%	44
Highlands Regional Medical Center	Prestonsburg	99%	121
Louisville VA Medical Center[2]	Louisville	99%	173
The Medical Center at Bowling Green	Bowling Green	99%	870
Norton Hospitals[2]	Louisville	99%	3538
Lexington VA Medical Center[2]	Lexington	98%	233

Prophylactic Antibiotic Selection

Hospital Name	City	Rate	Cases
Baptist Health Corbin	Corbin	100%	100
Baptist Health Lexington	Lexington	100%	1266
Bluegrass Community Hospital	Versailles	100%	35
Clark Regional Medical Center	Winchester	100%	126
Flaget Memorial Hospital[2]	Bardstown	100%	232
Georgetown Community Hospital	Georgetown	100%	25
Greenview Regional Hospital	Bowling Green	100%	549
Harlan Appalachian Reg Healthcare Hosp	Harlan	100%	51
Hazard ARH Regional Medical Center	Hazard	100%	197
Jackson Purchase Medical Center	Mayfield	100%	39
Jennie Stuart Medical Center	Hopkinsville	100%	300
King's Daughters' Medical Center[2]	Ashland	100%	407
Lourdes Hospital[2]	Paducah	100%	1033
Meadowview Regional Medical Center	Maysville	100%	116
Our Lady of Bellefonte Hospital	Ashland	100%	441
Parkway Regional Hospital	Fulton	100%	40
Pikeville Medical Center	Pikeville	100%	734
Saint Elizabeth Florence	Florence	100%	71
Saint Elizabeth Ft Thomas	Fort Thomas	100%	56
Saint Elizabeth Medical Center[2]	Lakeside Park	100%	501
Saint Joseph Berea	Berea	100%	27
Saint Joseph East	Lexington	100%	525
Saint Joseph Mount Sterling	Mount Sterling	100%	240
T J Samson Community Hospital[2]	Glasgow	100%	200
Baptist Health Lagrange	La Grange	99%	139
Baptist Health Louisville	Louisville	99%	2553
Baptist Health Madisonville[2]	Madisonville	99%	393
Baptist Health Paducah[2]	Paducah	99%	571
Baptist Health Richmond	Richmond	99%	168
Ephraim Mcdowell Regional Medical Center	Danville	99%	298
Frankfort Regional Medical Center	Frankfort	99%	124
Hardin Memorial Hospital[2]	Elizabethtown	99%	281
Jewish Hospital & Saint Mary's Healthcare[2]	Louisville	99%	551
Lexington VA Medical Center	Lexington	99%	126
The Medical Center at Bowling Green	Bowling Green	99%	743
Murray - Calloway County Hospital	Murray	99%	376
Norton Hospitals[2]	Louisville	99%	2681
Owensboro Health Regional Hospital[2]	Owensboro	99%	775
Saint Joseph London	London	99%	271
University of Kentucky Hospital[2]	Lexington	99%	424
University of Louisville Hospital[2]	Louisville	99%	191
Highlands Regional Medical Center	Prestonsburg	98%	94
Jewish Hospital - Shelbyville	Shelbyville	98%	49
Lake Cumberland Regional Hospital[2]	Somerset	98%	232
Muhlenberg Community Hospital	Greenville	98%	42
Saint Joseph Hospital[2]	Lexington	98%	515
Spring View Hospital	Lebanon	98%	119
Taylor Regional Hospital	Campbellsville	98%	122
Twin Lakes Regional Medical Center	Leitchfield	98%	96
Harrison Memorial Hospital	Cynthiana	97%	31
Louisville VA Medical Center	Louisville	97%	79
Whitesburg ARH Hospital	Whitesburg	96%	54
Methodist Hospital[2]	Henderson	95%	126
Saint Claire Regional Medical Center[2]	Morehead	93%	104

Prophylactic Antibiotic Selection (Outpatient)

Hospital Name	City	Rate	Cases
Baptist Health Corbin	Corbin	100%	267
Baptist Health Richmond	Richmond	100%	159
Frankfort Regional Medical Center	Frankfort	100%	134
Greenview Regional Hospital	Bowling Green	100%	125
Harlan Appalachian Reg Healthcare Hosp	Harlan	100%	37
Jennie Stuart Medical Center	Hopkinsville	100%	67
Lake Cumberland Regional Hospital	Somerset	100%	374
Middlesboro Appalachian Reg Healthcare	Middlesboro	100%	30
Saint Elizabeth Medical Center	Lakeside Park	100%	628
Spring View Hospital	Lebanon	100%	31
Twin Lakes Regional Medical Center	Leitchfield	100%	31
Baptist Health Lexington	Lexington	99%	1872
Baptist Health Louisville	Louisville	99%	1276
Baptist Health Paducah	Paducah	99%	604
Hardin Memorial Hospital	Elizabethtown	99%	463
Jackson Purchase Medical Center	Mayfield	99%	76
Jewish Hospital & Saint Mary's Healthcare	Louisville	99%	629
Kentucky River Medical Center	Jackson	99%	75
Saint Elizabeth Florence	Florence	99%	118
Saint Elizabeth Ft Thomas	Fort Thomas	99%	114
Baptist Health Madisonville	Madisonville	98%	184
Harrison Memorial Hospital	Cynthiana	98%	42
King's Daughters' Medical Center	Ashland	98%	637
Lourdes Hospital	Paducah	98%	204
Saint Joseph Hospital	Lexington	98%	800
Saint Joseph London	London	98%	234
Georgetown Community Hospital	Georgetown	97%	144
Hazard ARH Regional Medical Center	Hazard	97%	111
The Medical Center at Bowling Green	Bowling Green	97%	466
Norton Hospitals	Louisville	97%	1300
Saint Joseph East	Lexington	97%	421
Three Rivers Medical Center	Louisa	97%	33
Whitesburg ARH Hospital	Whitesburg	97%	138
Baptist Health Lagrange	La Grange	96%	77
Meadowview Regional Medical Center	Maysville	96%	115
Our Lady of Bellefonte Hospital	Ashland	96%	196
Owensboro Health Regional Hospital	Owensboro	96%	694
T J Samson Community Hospital	Glasgow	96%	192
University of Louisville Hospital	Louisville	96%	264
Ephraim Mcdowell Regional Medical Center	Danville	95%	234
Pikeville Medical Center	Pikeville	95%	204
University of Kentucky Hospital	Lexington	95%	611
Highlands Regional Medical Center	Prestonsburg	93%	89
Saint Claire Regional Medical Center	Morehead	93%	114
Saint Joseph Mount Sterling	Mount Sterling	93%	29
Taylor Regional Hospital	Campbellsville	90%	40
Methodist Hospital	Henderson	89%	128
Logan Memorial Hospital	Russellville	88%	25
Murray - Calloway County Hospital	Murray	87%	160
Flaget Memorial Hospital	Bardstown	82%	38
Pineville Community Hospital	Pineville	10%	31

Prophylactic Antibiotic Stopped

Hospital Name	City	Rate	Cases
Baptist Health Richmond	Richmond	100%	153
Bluegrass Community Hospital	Versailles	100%	34
Ephraim Mcdowell Regional Medical Center	Danville	100%	294
Flaget Memorial Hospital[2]	Bardstown	100%	226
Harlan Appalachian Reg Healthcare Hosp	Harlan	100%	44
Harrison Memorial Hospital	Cynthiana	100%	28
Jewish Hospital - Shelbyville	Shelbyville	100%	44
Parkway Regional Hospital	Fulton	100%	40
Pikeville Medical Center	Pikeville	100%	703
Saint Elizabeth Florence	Florence	100%	65
Saint Elizabeth Ft Thomas	Fort Thomas	100%	51
Saint Elizabeth Medical Center[2]	Lakeside Park	100%	484
Baptist Health Corbin	Corbin	99%	96
Baptist Health Lagrange	La Grange	99%	137
Baptist Health Lexington	Lexington	99%	1230
Baptist Health Louisville	Louisville	99%	2503
Frankfort Regional Medical Center	Frankfort	99%	120
Greenview Regional Hospital	Bowling Green	99%	530
Hardin Memorial Hospital[2]	Elizabethtown	99%	269
King's Daughters' Medical Center[2]	Ashland	99%	392
Lourdes Hospital[2]	Paducah	99%	834
Owensboro Health Regional Hospital[2]	Owensboro	99%	770
Saint Joseph East	Lexington	99%	521
Saint Joseph Mount Sterling	Mount Sterling	99%	234
Taylor Regional Hospital	Campbellsville	99%	119
Twin Lakes Regional Medical Center	Leitchfield	99%	96
Baptist Health Madisonville[2]	Madisonville	98%	384
Baptist Health Paducah[2]	Paducah	98%	558
Clark Regional Medical Center	Winchester	98%	126
Hazard ARH Regional Medical Center	Hazard	98%	187
Lexington VA Medical Center	Lexington	98%	124
Meadowview Regional Medical Center	Maysville	98%	114
Muhlenberg Community Hospital	Greenville	98%	41
Murray - Calloway County Hospital	Murray	98%	374
Norton Hospitals[2]	Louisville	98%	2590
Our Lady of Bellefonte Hospital	Ashland	98%	425
Saint Joseph Hospital[2]	Lexington	98%	490
Saint Joseph London	London	98%	251
University of Kentucky Hospital[2]	Lexington	98%	411
Jennie Stuart Medical Center	Hopkinsville	97%	298
Jewish Hospital & Saint Mary's Healthcare[2]	Louisville	97%	525
Lake Cumberland Regional Hospital[2]	Somerset	97%	214
Louisville VA Medical Center	Louisville	97%	78
The Medical Center at Bowling Green	Bowling Green	97%	733
Spring View Hospital	Lebanon	97%	115
Saint Joseph Berea	Berea	96%	27
Jackson Purchase Medical Center	Mayfield	95%	37
T J Samson Community Hospital[2]	Glasgow	95%	192
Highlands Regional Medical Center	Prestonsburg	93%	88
University of Louisville Hospital[2]	Louisville	93%	188
Methodist Hospital[2]	Henderson	92%	123
Saint Claire Regional Medical Center[2]	Morehead	91%	100
Whitesburg ARH Hospital	Whitesburg	88%	43

Prophylactic Antibiotic Timing

Hospital Name	City	Rate	Cases
Baptist Health Corbin	Corbin	100%	101
Baptist Health Lagrange	La Grange	100%	139
Baptist Health Madisonville[2]	Madisonville	100%	393
Bluegrass Community Hospital	Versailles	100%	35
Flaget Memorial Hospital[2]	Bardstown	100%	232
Frankfort Regional Medical Center	Frankfort	100%	124
Georgetown Community Hospital	Georgetown	100%	25
Greenview Regional Hospital	Bowling Green	100%	549
Hardin Memorial Hospital[2]	Elizabethtown	100%	282
Harlan Appalachian Reg Healthcare Hosp	Harlan	100%	52
Harrison Memorial Hospital	Cynthiana	100%	31
Hazard ARH Regional Medical Center	Hazard	100%	197
Highlands Regional Medical Center	Prestonsburg	100%	95
Jackson Purchase Medical Center	Mayfield	100%	39
Meadowview Regional Medical Center	Maysville	100%	116
Muhlenberg Community Hospital	Greenville	100%	42
Parkway Regional Hospital	Fulton	100%	40
Pikeville Medical Center	Pikeville	100%	735
Saint Elizabeth Florence	Florence	100%	71
Saint Elizabeth Ft Thomas	Fort Thomas	100%	56
Saint Elizabeth Medical Center[2]	Lakeside Park	100%	501
Saint Joseph Berea	Berea	100%	27
Saint Joseph East	Lexington	100%	525
Saint Joseph London	London	100%	272
Twin Lakes Regional Medical Center	Leitchfield	100%	97
University of Kentucky Hospital[2]	Lexington	100%	426
Whitesburg ARH Hospital	Whitesburg	100%	54
Baptist Health Lexington	Lexington	99%	1268
Baptist Health Louisville	Louisville	99%	2553

NOTE: Hospital profiles are in alphabetical order by state, then city, then hospital within the city; Rankings exclude hospitals with less than 25 cases except for patient surveys which excludes hospitals with less than 100 cases; (a) 100-299 cases; (1) The number of cases/patients is too few to report; (2) Data submitted were based on a sample of cases/patients; (3) Results are based on a shorter time period than required; (4) Data suppressed by CMS for one or more quarters; (5) Results are not available for this reporting period; (6) Fewer than 100 patients completed the HCAHPS survey; (7) No cases met the criteria for this measure; (8) The lower limit of the confidence interval cannot be calculated if the number of observed infections equals zero; (9) No data are available from the state/territory for this reporting period; (10) The scores shown reflect fewer than 50 completed surveys; (11) There were discrepancies in the data collection process; (12) This measure does not apply to this hospital for this reporting period; (13) Results cannot be calculated for this reporting period; (14) The results for this state are combined with nearby states to protect confidentiality; Please refer to the User's Guide for a full explanation of data.

Hospital Name	City	Rate	Cases
Baptist Health Paducah[2]	Paducah	99%	572
Baptist Health Richmond	Richmond	99%	168
Ephraim Mcdowell Regional Medical Center	Danville	99%	299
Lake Cumberland Regional Hospital[2]	Somerset	99%	233
Lexington VA Medical Center	Lexington	99%	126
Lourdes Hospital[2]	Paducah	99%	1034
Murray - Calloway County Hospital	Murray	99%	376
Our Lady of Bellefonte Hospital	Ashland	99%	441
Owensboro Health Regional Hospital[2]	Owensboro	99%	777
Saint Joseph Hospital[2]	Lexington	99%	515
Taylor Regional Hospital	Campbellsville	99%	122
Clark Regional Medical Center	Winchester	98%	126
Jennie Stuart Medical Center	Hopkinsville	98%	301
Jewish Hospital - Shelbyville	Shelbyville	98%	49
The Medical Center at Bowling Green	Bowling Green	98%	745
Methodist Hospital[2]	Henderson	98%	126
Norton Hospitals[2]	Louisville	98%	2685
Saint Joseph Mount Sterling	Mount Sterling	98%	240
Jewish Hospital & Saint Mary's Healthcare[2]	Louisville	97%	553
King's Daughters' Medical Center[2]	Ashland	97%	407
Louisville VA Medical Center	Louisville	97%	79
Spring View Hospital	Lebanon	97%	119
T J Samson Community Hospital[2]	Glasgow	97%	200
University of Louisville Hospital[2]	Louisville	97%	192
Saint Claire Regional Medical Center[2]	Morehead	95%	105

Prophylactic Antibiotic Timing (Outpatient)

Hospital Name	City	Rate	Cases
Baptist Health Corbin	Corbin	100%	267
Baptist Health Lexington	Lexington	100%	1872
Baptist Health Madisonville	Madisonville	100%	184
Baptist Health Richmond	Richmond	100%	159
Georgetown Community Hospital	Georgetown	100%	144
Harlan Appalachian Reg Healthcare Hosp	Harlan	100%	37
Harrison Memorial Hospital	Cynthiana	100%	42
Highlands Regional Medical Center	Prestonsburg	100%	75
Kentucky River Medical Center	Jackson	100%	75
King's Daughters' Medical Center	Ashland	100%	554
Middlesboro Appalachian Reg Healthcare	Middlesboro	100%	30
Saint Elizabeth Florence	Florence	100%	118
Saint Elizabeth Ft Thomas	Fort Thomas	100%	114
Saint Elizabeth Medical Center	Lakeside Park	100%	629
Saint Joseph East	Lexington	100%	421
Saint Joseph London	London	100%	234
Taylor Regional Hospital	Campbellsville	100%	40
Twin Lakes Regional Medical Center	Leitchfield	100%	31
Baptist Health Louisville	Louisville	99%	1239
Baptist Health Paducah	Paducah	99%	606
Frankfort Regional Medical Center	Frankfort	99%	134
Hardin Memorial Hospital	Elizabethtown	99%	465
Lake Cumberland Regional Hospital	Somerset	99%	374
Lourdes Hospital	Paducah	99%	206
Murray - Calloway County Hospital	Murray	99%	161
Our Lady of Bellefonte Hospital	Ashland	99%	197
Greenview Regional Hospital	Bowling Green	98%	127
Jackson Purchase Medical Center	Mayfield	97%	75
Saint Claire Regional Medical Center	Morehead	97%	73
Saint Joseph Hospital	Lexington	97%	812
Spring View Hospital	Lebanon	97%	32
Three Rivers Medical Center	Louisa	97%	30
Baptist Health Lagrange	La Grange	96%	78
Jewish Hospital & Saint Mary's Healthcare	Louisville	96%	639
Meadowview Regional Medical Center	Maysville	96%	113
T J Samson Community Hospital	Glasgow	96%	195
Flaget Memorial Hospital	Bardstown	95%	39
Methodist Hospital	Henderson	95%	131
Norton Hospitals	Louisville	95%	1322
University of Louisville Hospital	Louisville	94%	269
Pikeville Medical Center	Pikeville	93%	218
University of Kentucky Hospital	Lexington	93%	644
Whitesburg ARH Hospital	Whitesburg	93%	138
Ephraim Mcdowell Regional Medical Center	Danville	92%	246
Saint Joseph Mount Sterling	Mount Sterling	92%	26
The Medical Center at Bowling Green	Bowling Green	91%	482
Hazard ARH Regional Medical Center	Hazard	88%	109
Jennie Stuart Medical Center	Hopkinsville	87%	69
Owensboro Health Regional Hospital	Owensboro	87%	747

Urinary Catheter Removal

Hospital Name	City	Rate	Cases
Baptist Health Corbin	Corbin	100%	101
Bluegrass Community Hospital	Versailles	100%	37
Clark Regional Medical Center	Winchester	100%	81
Ephraim Mcdowell Regional Medical Center	Danville	100%	220
Frankfort Regional Medical Center	Frankfort	100%	139
Greenview Regional Hospital	Bowling Green	100%	460
Harrison Memorial Hospital	Cynthiana	100%	33
Meadowview Regional Medical Center	Maysville	100%	118
Muhlenberg Community Hospital	Greenville	100%	34
Pikeville Medical Center	Pikeville	100%	556
Saint Elizabeth Florence	Florence	100%	105
Saint Elizabeth Ft Thomas	Fort Thomas	100%	76
Saint Elizabeth Medical Center[2]	Lakeside Park	100%	241
Saint Joseph Berea	Berea	100%	29
University of Kentucky Hospital[2]	Lexington	100%	262
Baptist Health Lexington	Lexington	99%	900
Baptist Health Madisonville[2]	Madisonville	99%	392
Baptist Health Richmond	Richmond	99%	86
Flaget Memorial Hospital[2]	Bardstown	99%	264
King's Daughters' Medical Center[2]	Ashland	99%	421
Murray - Calloway County Hospital	Murray	99%	448
Twin Lakes Regional Medical Center	Leitchfield	99%	83
Baptist Health Louisville	Louisville	98%	1169
Baptist Health Paducah[2]	Paducah	98%	602
Hazard ARH Regional Medical Center	Hazard	98%	237
Our Lady of Bellefonte Hospital	Ashland	98%	454
Owensboro Health Regional Hospital[2]	Owensboro	98%	472
Parkway Regional Hospital	Fulton	98%	43
Saint Joseph London	London	98%	252
Saint Joseph Mount Sterling	Mount Sterling	98%	230
T J Samson Community Hospital[2]	Glasgow	98%	210
Baptist Health Lagrange	La Grange	97%	35
Georgetown Community Hospital	Georgetown	97%	32
Lake Cumberland Regional Hospital[2]	Somerset	97%	248
Lourdes Hospital[2]	Paducah	97%	643
Taylor Regional Hospital	Campbellsville	97%	88
The Medical Center at Bowling Green	Bowling Green	96%	762
Saint Claire Regional Medical Center[2]	Morehead	96%	117
Saint Joseph East	Lexington	96%	351
Highlands Regional Medical Center	Prestonsburg	95%	62
Jackson Purchase Medical Center	Mayfield	95%	38
Jennie Stuart Medical Center	Hopkinsville	95%	272
Norton Hospitals[2]	Louisville	95%	1864
Jewish Hospital & Saint Mary's Healthcare[2]	Louisville	94%	453
Lexington VA Medical Center[2]	Lexington	94%	49
Methodist Hospital[2]	Henderson	94%	108
Jewish Hospital - Shelbyville	Shelbyville	93%	55
Louisville VA Medical Center[2]	Louisville	93%	120
Hardin Memorial Hospital[2]	Elizabethtown	90%	292
Spring View Hospital	Lebanon	90%	70
University of Louisville Hospital[2]	Louisville	90%	162
Saint Joseph Hospital[2]	Lexington	88%	466

Survey of Patients' Hospital Experiences

Area Around Room 'Always' Quiet at Night

Hospital Name	City	Rate	Cases
Westlake Regional Hospital	Columbia	93%	(a)
Casey County Hospital	Liberty	79%	(a)
Clinton County Hospital	Albany	78%	300+
Parkway Regional Hospital	Fulton	78%	(a)
Monroe County Medical Center	Tompkinsville	75%	300+
Methodist Hospital Union County	Morganfield	73%	(a)
Logan Memorial Hospital	Russellville	72%	300+
Rockcastle County Hospital	Mount Vernon	72%	(a)
Fleming County Hospital	Flemingsburg	71%	300+
Saint Joseph Berea	Berea	70%	(a)
Wayne County Hospital	Monticello	70%	(a)
McDowell ARH Hospital	Mc Dowell	69%	(a)
Our Lady of Bellefonte Hospital	Ashland	69%	300+
Whitesburg ARH Hospital	Whitesburg	69%	300+
Middlesboro Appalachian Reg Healthcare	Middlesboro	68%	300+
Murray - Calloway County Hospital	Murray	68%	300+
Pikeville Medical Center	Pikeville	68%	300+
Saint Joseph London	London	68%	300+
Saint Joseph Mount Sterling	Mount Sterling	68%	300+
Three Rivers Medical Center	Louisa	68%	300+
Bourbon Community Hospital	Paris	67%	(a)
Methodist Hospital	Henderson	67%	300+
Ohio County Hospital	Hartford	67%	(a)
Clark Regional Medical Center	Winchester	66%	300+
Jewish Hospital - Shelbyville	Shelbyville	66%	(a)
Pineville Community Hospital	Pineville	66%	300+
T J Samson Community Hospital	Glasgow	66%	300+
Baptist Health Paducah	Paducah	65%	300+
Kentucky River Medical Center	Jackson	65%	300+
Marcum & Wallace Memorial Hospital	Irvine	65%	(a)
Saint Joseph East	Lexington	65%	300+
Williamson ARH Hospital	S Williamson	65%	300+
Greenview Regional Hospital	Bowling Green	64%	300+
King's Daughters' Medical Center	Ashland	64%	300+
The Medical Center at Bowling Green[11]	Bowling Green	64%	300+
Russell County Hospital	Russell Springs	64%	(a)
Flaget Memorial Hospital	Bardstown	63%	(a)
Harrison Memorial Hospital	Cynthiana	63%	300+
Paul B Hall Regional Medical Center	Paintsville	63%	(a)
Baptist Health Louisville	Louisville	62%	300+
Ephraim Mcdowell Fort Logan Hospital	Stanford	62%	(a)
Ephraim Mcdowell Regional Medical Center	Danville	62%	300+
Memorial Hospital[11]	Manchester	62%	(a)
University of Kentucky Hospital	Lexington	62%	300+
Georgetown Community Hospital	Georgetown	61%	300+
Harlan Appalachian Reg Healthcare Hosp	Harlan	61%	300+
Highlands Regional Medical Center	Prestonsburg	61%	300+
Muhlenberg Community Hospital	Greenville	61%	(a)
Saint Elizabeth Medical Center	Lakeside Park	61%	300+
Saint Joseph Hospital	Lexington	61%	300+
Spring View Hospital	Lebanon	61%	300+
Hazard ARH Regional Medical Center	Hazard	60%	300+
Jackson Purchase Medical Center	Mayfield	60%	300+
Owensboro Health Regional Hospital	Owensboro	60%	300+
Taylor Regional Hospital	Campbellsville	60%	300+
Twin Lakes Regional Medical Center	Leitchfield	60%	300+
Baptist Health Corbin	Corbin	59%	300+
Crittenden Health System	Marion	59%	(a)
Lake Cumberland Regional Hospital	Somerset	59%	300+
Saint Elizabeth Florence	Florence	59%	300+
Baptist Health Lagrange	La Grange	58%	300+
Baptist Health Richmond	Richmond	58%	300+
Frankfort Regional Medical Center	Frankfort	58%	300+
Jewish Hospital & Saint Mary's Healthcare	Louisville	58%	300+
Lourdes Hospital	Paducah	58%	300+
Saint Joseph Martin	Martin	57%	(a)
Baptist Health Lexington	Lexington	56%	300+
Jane Todd Crawford Hospital	Greensburg	56%	(a)
Meadowview Regional Medical Center	Maysville	56%	300+
Norton Hospitals	Louisville	56%	300+
Saint Claire Regional Medical Center	Morehead	56%	300+
Baptist Health Madisonville	Madisonville	54%	300+
Saint Elizabeth Ft Thomas	Fort Thomas	54%	300+
Jennie Stuart Medical Center	Hopkinsville	53%	300+
University of Louisville Hospital	Louisville	53%	300+
Hardin Memorial Hospital	Elizabethtown	51%	300+

Doctors 'Always' Communicated Well

Hospital Name	City	Rate	Cases
Westlake Regional Hospital	Columbia	100%	(a)
Casey County Hospital	Liberty	96%	(a)
Clinton County Hospital	Albany	96%	300+
Jane Todd Crawford Hospital	Greensburg	96%	(a)
Wayne County Hospital	Monticello	93%	(a)
Russell County Hospital	Russell Springs	91%	(a)
Marcum & Wallace Memorial Hospital	Irvine	90%	(a)
McDowell ARH Hospital	Mc Dowell	90%	(a)
Rockcastle County Hospital	Mount Vernon	90%	(a)
Middlesboro Appalachian Reg Healthcare	Middlesboro	89%	300+
Pikeville Medical Center	Pikeville	89%	300+
Georgetown Community Hospital	Georgetown	88%	300+
Harrison Memorial Hospital	Cynthiana	88%	300+
Logan Memorial Hospital	Russellville	88%	300+
Ohio County Hospital	Hartford	88%	(a)
Parkway Regional Hospital	Fulton	88%	(a)
Pineville Community Hospital	Pineville	88%	300+
Saint Joseph Berea	Berea	88%	(a)
Monroe County Medical Center	Tompkinsville	87%	300+
Murray - Calloway County Hospital	Murray	87%	300+
Saint Joseph Martin	Martin	87%	(a)
Three Rivers Medical Center	Louisa	87%	300+
Whitesburg ARH Hospital	Whitesburg	87%	300+
Crittenden Health System	Marion	86%	(a)
Fleming County Hospital	Flemingsburg	86%	300+
Hazard ARH Regional Medical Center	Hazard	86%	300+
Highlands Regional Medical Center	Prestonsburg	86%	300+
Methodist Hospital	Henderson	86%	300+
Williamson ARH Hospital	S Williamson	86%	300+
Methodist Hospital Union County	Morganfield	85%	(a)
Saint Claire Regional Medical Center	Morehead	85%	300+
T J Samson Community Hospital	Glasgow	85%	300+
Taylor Regional Hospital	Campbellsville	85%	300+
Baptist Health Corbin	Corbin	84%	300+
Our Lady of Bellefonte Hospital	Ashland	84%	300+
Clark Regional Medical Center	Winchester	83%	300+
Flaget Memorial Hospital	Bardstown	83%	(a)
Kentucky River Medical Center	Jackson	83%	300+
Muhlenberg Community Hospital	Greenville	83%	(a)
Paul B Hall Regional Medical Center	Paintsville	83%	(a)
Saint Joseph London	London	83%	300+
Twin Lakes Regional Medical Center	Leitchfield	83%	300+
Baptist Health Lexington	Lexington	82%	300+
Baptist Health Louisville	Louisville	82%	300+
Bourbon Community Hospital	Paris	82%	(a)
Ephraim Mcdowell Regional Medical Center	Danville	82%	300+
Greenview Regional Hospital	Bowling Green	82%	300+
Hardin Memorial Hospital	Elizabethtown	82%	300+
Jackson Purchase Medical Center	Mayfield	82%	300+
King's Daughters' Medical Center	Ashland	82%	300+
Saint Joseph Mount Sterling	Mount Sterling	82%	300+
Spring View Hospital	Lebanon	82%	300+
Baptist Health Lagrange	La Grange	81%	300+
Baptist Health Paducah	Paducah	81%	300+
Ephraim Mcdowell Fort Logan Hospital	Stanford	81%	(a)

NOTE: Hospital profiles are in alphabetical order by state, then city, then hospital within the city; Rankings exclude hospitals with less than 25 cases except for patient surveys which excludes hospitals with less than 100 cases; (a) 100-299 cases; (1) The number of cases/patients is too few to report; (2) Data submitted were based on a sample of cases/patients; (3) Results are based on a shorter time period than required; (4) Data suppressed by CMS for one or more quarters; (5) Results are not available for this reporting period; (6) Fewer than 100 patients completed the HCAHPS survey; (7) No cases met the criteria for this measure; (8) The lower limit of the confidence interval cannot be calculated if the number of observed infections equals zero; (9) No data are available from the state/territory for this reporting period; (10) The scores shown reflect fewer than 50 completed surveys; (11) There were discrepancies in the data collection process; (12) This measure does not apply to this hospital for this reporting period; (13) Results cannot be calculated for this reporting period; (14) The results for this state are combined with nearby states to protect confidentiality; Please refer to the User's Guide for a full explanation of data.

Frankfort Regional Medical Center	Frankfort	81%	300+
Lourdes Hospital	Paducah	81%	300+
Memorial Hospital[11]	Manchester	81%	(a)
Owensboro Health Regional Hospital	Owensboro	81%	300+
Baptist Health Madisonville	Madisonville	80%	300+
Harlan Appalachian Reg Healthcare Hosp	Harlan	80%	300+
Jewish Hospital - Shelbyville	Shelbyville	80%	(a)
Lake Cumberland Regional Hospital	Somerset	80%	300+
The Medical Center at Bowling Green[11]	Bowling Green	80%	300+
Saint Elizabeth Medical Center	Lakeside Park	80%	300+
Saint Joseph East	Lexington	80%	300+
Baptist Health Richmond	Richmond	79%	300+
Meadowview Regional Medical Center	Maysville	79%	300+
Saint Joseph Hospital	Lexington	79%	300+
University of Kentucky Hospital	Lexington	79%	300+
Jewish Hospital & Saint Mary's Healthcare	Louisville	78%	300+
Norton Hospitals	Louisville	78%	300+
Saint Elizabeth Ft Thomas	Fort Thomas	78%	300+
University of Louisville Hospital	Louisville	78%	300+
Jennie Stuart Medical Center	Hopkinsville	77%	300+
Saint Elizabeth Florence	Florence	77%	300+

Home Recovery Information Given

Hospital Name	City	Rate	Cases
Westlake Regional Hospital	Columbia	100%	(a)
Wayne County Hospital	Monticello	92%	(a)
Casey County Hospital	Liberty	91%	(a)
Pikeville Medical Center	Pikeville	90%	300+
Baptist Health Lexington	Lexington	89%	300+
Baptist Health Louisville	Louisville	89%	300+
Fleming County Hospital	Flemingsburg	89%	300+
Saint Claire Regional Medical Center	Morehead	89%	300+
Saint Elizabeth Ft Thomas	Fort Thomas	89%	300+
Saint Joseph Berea	Berea	89%	(a)
Saint Joseph Mount Sterling	Mount Sterling	89%	300+
Flaget Memorial Hospital	Bardstown	88%	(a)
Saint Elizabeth Medical Center	Lakeside Park	88%	300+
Saint Joseph East	Lexington	88%	300+
Georgetown Community Hospital	Georgetown	87%	300+
Greenview Regional Hospital	Bowling Green	87%	300+
Jane Todd Crawford Hospital	Greensburg	87%	(a)
Logan Memorial Hospital	Russellville	87%	300+
Marcum & Wallace Memorial Hospital	Irvine	87%	(a)
McDowell ARH Hospital	Mc Dowell	87%	(a)
The Medical Center at Bowling Green[11]	Bowling Green	87%	300+
Our Lady of Bellefonte Hospital	Ashland	87%	300+
Owensboro Health Regional Hospital	Owensboro	87%	300+
Saint Elizabeth Florence	Florence	87%	300+
Saint Joseph Hospital	Lexington	87%	300+
Three Rivers Medical Center	Louisa	87%	300+
Whitesburg ARH Hospital	Whitesburg	87%	300+
Baptist Health Lagrange	La Grange	86%	300+
Baptist Health Paducah	Paducah	86%	300+
Baptist Health Richmond	Richmond	86%	300+
Clark Regional Medical Center	Winchester	86%	300+
Jewish Hospital - Shelbyville	Shelbyville	86%	(a)
Middlesboro Appalachian Reg Healthcare	Middlesboro	86%	300+
Murray - Calloway County Hospital	Murray	86%	300+
Rockcastle County Hospital	Mount Vernon	86%	(a)
University of Kentucky Hospital	Lexington	86%	300+
Bourbon Community Hospital	Paris	85%	(a)
Frankfort Regional Medical Center	Frankfort	85%	300+
Harrison Memorial Hospital	Cynthiana	85%	300+
Meadowview Regional Medical Center	Maysville	85%	300+
Memorial Hospital[11]	Manchester	85%	(a)
Norton Hospitals	Louisville	85%	300+
Ohio County Hospital	Hartford	85%	(a)
Saint Joseph London	London	85%	300+
Taylor Regional Hospital	Campbellsville	85%	300+
Baptist Health Corbin	Corbin	84%	300+
Baptist Health Madisonville	Madisonville	84%	300+
Clinton County Hospital	Albany	84%	300+
Jackson Purchase Medical Center	Mayfield	84%	300+
Jennie Stuart Medical Center	Hopkinsville	84%	300+
Jewish Hospital & Saint Mary's Healthcare	Louisville	84%	300+
Parkway Regional Hospital	Fulton	84%	(a)
Pineville Community Hospital	Pineville	84%	300+
University of Louisville Hospital	Louisville	84%	300+
Ephraim Mcdowell Fort Logan Hospital	Stanford	83%	(a)
Hardin Memorial Hospital	Elizabethtown	83%	300+
Hazard ARH Regional Medical Center	Hazard	83%	300+
Highlands Regional Medical Center	Prestonsburg	83%	300+
Kentucky River Medical Center	Jackson	83%	300+
Lake Cumberland Regional Hospital	Somerset	83%	300+
Lourdes Hospital	Paducah	83%	300+
Muhlenberg Community Hospital	Greenville	83%	(a)
Williamson ARH Hospital	S Williamson	83%	300+
Harlan Appalachian Reg Healthcare Hosp	Harlan	82%	300+
Saint Joseph Martin	Martin	82%	(a)
Spring View Hospital	Lebanon	82%	300+
T J Samson Community Hospital	Glasgow	82%	300+
Ephraim Mcdowell Regional Medical Center	Danville	81%	300+
Methodist Hospital Union County	Morganfield	81%	(a)
Russell County Hospital	Russell Springs	81%	(a)
King's Daughters' Medical Center	Ashland	80%	300+
Methodist Hospital	Henderson	80%	300+
Monroe County Medical Center	Tompkinsville	80%	300+
Paul B Hall Regional Medical Center	Paintsville	80%	(a)
Crittenden Health System	Marion	78%	(a)
Twin Lakes Regional Medical Center	Leitchfield	77%	300+

Hospital Given 9 or 10 on 10 Point Scale

Hospital Name	City	Rate	Cases
Westlake Regional Hospital	Columbia	91%	(a)
Clinton County Hospital	Albany	86%	300+
Casey County Hospital	Liberty	82%	(a)
Baptist Health Louisville	Louisville	81%	300+
Rockcastle County Hospital	Mount Vernon	81%	(a)
Harrison Memorial Hospital	Cynthiana	80%	300+
Pikeville Medical Center	Pikeville	80%	300+
Marcum & Wallace Memorial Hospital	Irvine	79%	(a)
McDowell ARH Hospital	Mc Dowell	79%	(a)
Wayne County Hospital	Monticello	79%	(a)
Saint Joseph London	London	78%	300+
Flaget Memorial Hospital	Bardstown	77%	(a)
Our Lady of Bellefonte Hospital	Ashland	77%	300+
Saint Joseph Berea	Berea	77%	(a)
Saint Joseph Martin	Martin	77%	(a)
Baptist Health Lagrange	La Grange	76%	300+
Baptist Health Lexington	Lexington	76%	300+
Saint Joseph Mount Sterling	Mount Sterling	76%	300+
Baptist Health Paducah	Paducah	75%	300+
Fleming County Hospital	Flemingsburg	75%	300+
Pineville Community Hospital	Pineville	75%	300+
Saint Elizabeth Medical Center	Lakeside Park	75%	300+
Clark Regional Medical Center	Winchester	74%	300+
Greenview Regional Hospital	Bowling Green	74%	300+
Russell County Hospital	Russell Springs	74%	(a)
Ephraim Mcdowell Fort Logan Hospital	Stanford	73%	(a)
Jackson Purchase Medical Center	Mayfield	73%	300+
Saint Claire Regional Medical Center	Morehead	73%	300+
Williamson ARH Hospital	S Williamson	73%	300+
Kentucky River Medical Center	Jackson	72%	300+
Lourdes Hospital	Paducah	72%	300+
Owensboro Health Regional Hospital	Owensboro	72%	300+
University of Kentucky Hospital	Lexington	72%	300+
King's Daughters' Medical Center	Ashland	71%	300+
The Medical Center at Bowling Green[11]	Bowling Green	71%	300+
Methodist Hospital	Henderson	71%	300+
Murray - Calloway County Hospital	Murray	71%	300+
Saint Joseph East	Lexington	71%	300+
Twin Lakes Regional Medical Center	Leitchfield	71%	300+
University of Louisville Hospital	Louisville	71%	300+
Logan Memorial Hospital	Russellville	70%	300+
Parkway Regional Hospital	Fulton	70%	(a)
Saint Joseph Hospital	Lexington	70%	300+
T J Samson Community Hospital	Glasgow	70%	300+
Baptist Health Corbin	Corbin	69%	300+
Georgetown Community Hospital	Georgetown	69%	300+
Middlesboro Appalachian Reg Healthcare	Middlesboro	69%	300+
Saint Elizabeth Ft Thomas	Fort Thomas	69%	300+
Whitesburg ARH Hospital	Whitesburg	69%	300+
Ephraim Mcdowell Regional Medical Center	Danville	68%	300+
Methodist Hospital Union County	Morganfield	68%	(a)
Monroe County Medical Center	Tompkinsville	68%	300+
Norton Hospitals	Louisville	68%	300+
Spring View Hospital	Lebanon	68%	300+
Taylor Regional Hospital	Campbellsville	68%	300+
Three Rivers Medical Center	Louisa	68%	300+
Baptist Health Richmond	Richmond	67%	300+
Bourbon Community Hospital	Paris	67%	(a)
Hazard ARH Regional Medical Center	Hazard	67%	300+
Ohio County Hospital	Hartford	67%	(a)
Saint Elizabeth Florence	Florence	67%	300+
Jewish Hospital & Saint Mary's Healthcare	Louisville	66%	300+
Jewish Hospital - Shelbyville	Shelbyville	66%	(a)
Muhlenberg Community Hospital	Greenville	66%	(a)
Crittenden Health System	Marion	65%	(a)
Frankfort Regional Medical Center	Frankfort	65%	300+
Hardin Memorial Hospital	Elizabethtown	65%	300+
Harlan Appalachian Reg Healthcare Hosp	Harlan	65%	300+
Memorial Hospital[11]	Manchester	65%	(a)
Baptist Health Madisonville	Madisonville	64%	300+
Jane Todd Crawford Hospital	Greensburg	64%	(a)
Meadowview Regional Medical Center	Maysville	63%	300+
Highlands Regional Medical Center	Prestonsburg	62%	300+
Lake Cumberland Regional Hospital	Somerset	61%	300+
Paul B Hall Regional Medical Center	Paintsville	61%	(a)
Jennie Stuart Medical Center	Hopkinsville	58%	300+

Meds 'Always' Explained Before Given

Hospital Name	City	Rate	Cases
Westlake Regional Hospital	Columbia	99%	(a)
Rockcastle County Hospital	Mount Vernon	76%	(a)
Pikeville Medical Center	Pikeville	75%	300+
Saint Claire Regional Medical Center	Morehead	75%	300+
Ohio County Hospital	Hartford	74%	(a)
Saint Joseph Berea	Berea	74%	(a)
Wayne County Hospital	Monticello	73%	(a)
Clinton County Hospital	Albany	72%	300+
Marcum & Wallace Memorial Hospital	Irvine	71%	(a)
Russell County Hospital	Russell Springs	71%	(a)
Harrison Memorial Hospital	Cynthiana	70%	300+
Saint Joseph Martin	Martin	70%	(a)
Crittenden Health System	Marion	69%	(a)
Parkway Regional Hospital	Fulton	69%	(a)
Saint Joseph Mount Sterling	Mount Sterling	69%	300+
Three Rivers Medical Center	Louisa	69%	300+
Williamson ARH Hospital	S Williamson	69%	300+
Fleming County Hospital	Flemingsburg	68%	300+
Logan Memorial Hospital	Russellville	68%	300+
Saint Elizabeth Medical Center	Lakeside Park	68%	300+
Baptist Health Corbin	Corbin	67%	300+
Georgetown Community Hospital	Georgetown	67%	300+
Greenview Regional Hospital	Bowling Green	67%	300+
Jewish Hospital - Shelbyville	Shelbyville	67%	(a)
Middlesboro Appalachian Reg Healthcare	Middlesboro	67%	300+
Muhlenberg Community Hospital	Greenville	67%	(a)
Saint Joseph London	London	67%	300+
Baptist Health Louisville	Louisville	66%	300+
Bourbon Community Hospital	Paris	66%	(a)
Flaget Memorial Hospital	Bardstown	66%	(a)
Hardin Memorial Hospital	Elizabethtown	66%	300+
Memorial Hospital[11]	Manchester	66%	(a)
Our Lady of Bellefonte Hospital	Ashland	66%	300+
Saint Elizabeth Ft Thomas	Fort Thomas	66%	300+
Whitesburg ARH Hospital	Whitesburg	66%	300+
Baptist Health Lexington	Lexington	65%	300+
Clark Regional Medical Center	Winchester	65%	300+
Ephraim Mcdowell Fort Logan Hospital	Stanford	65%	(a)
Kentucky River Medical Center	Jackson	65%	300+
The Medical Center at Bowling Green[11]	Bowling Green	65%	300+
Methodist Hospital	Henderson	65%	300+
Monroe County Medical Center	Tompkinsville	65%	300+
University of Kentucky Hospital	Lexington	65%	300+
Baptist Health Lagrange	La Grange	64%	300+
Baptist Health Paducah	Paducah	64%	300+
Frankfort Regional Medical Center	Frankfort	64%	300+
Hazard ARH Regional Medical Center	Hazard	64%	300+
Meadowview Regional Medical Center	Maysville	64%	300+
Spring View Hospital	Lebanon	64%	300+
Ephraim Mcdowell Regional Medical Center	Danville	63%	300+
Highlands Regional Medical Center	Prestonsburg	63%	300+
Owensboro Health Regional Hospital	Owensboro	63%	300+
Paul B Hall Regional Medical Center	Paintsville	63%	(a)
Saint Elizabeth Florence	Florence	63%	300+
University of Louisville Hospital	Louisville	63%	300+
Harlan Appalachian Reg Healthcare Hosp	Harlan	62%	300+
Jennie Stuart Medical Center	Hopkinsville	62%	300+
McDowell ARH Hospital	Mc Dowell	62%	(a)
Murray - Calloway County Hospital	Murray	62%	300+
Saint Joseph East	Lexington	62%	300+
Saint Joseph Hospital	Lexington	62%	300+
Taylor Regional Hospital	Campbellsville	62%	300+
Casey County Hospital	Liberty	61%	(a)
King's Daughters' Medical Center	Ashland	61%	300+
Lourdes Hospital	Paducah	61%	300+
Norton Hospitals	Louisville	61%	300+
Twin Lakes Regional Medical Center	Leitchfield	61%	300+
Baptist Health Madisonville	Madisonville	60%	300+
Methodist Hospital Union County	Morganfield	60%	(a)
Jackson Purchase Medical Center	Mayfield	59%	300+
T J Samson Community Hospital	Glasgow	59%	300+
Baptist Health Richmond	Richmond	58%	300+
Jewish Hospital & Saint Mary's Healthcare	Louisville	58%	300+
Jane Todd Crawford Hospital	Greensburg	57%	(a)
Lake Cumberland Regional Hospital	Somerset	56%	300+
Pineville Community Hospital	Pineville	56%	300+

Nurses 'Always' Communicated Well

Hospital Name	City	Rate	Cases
Westlake Regional Hospital	Columbia	100%	(a)
Rockcastle County Hospital	Mount Vernon	89%	(a)
Clinton County Hospital	Albany	88%	300+
Marcum & Wallace Memorial Hospital	Irvine	88%	(a)
Russell County Hospital	Russell Springs	87%	(a)
Harrison Memorial Hospital	Cynthiana	86%	300+
Pikeville Medical Center	Pikeville	86%	300+
Wayne County Hospital	Monticello	86%	(a)
Saint Claire Regional Medical Center	Morehead	85%	300+

NOTE: Hospital profiles are in alphabetical order by state, then city, then hospital within the city; Rankings exclude hospitals with less than 25 cases except for patient surveys which excludes hospitals with less than 100 cases; (a) 100-299 cases; (1) The number of cases/patients is too few to report; (2) Data submitted were based on a sample of cases/patients; (3) Results are based on a shorter time period than required; (4) Data suppressed by CMS for one or more quarters; (5) Results are not available for this reporting period; (6) Fewer than 100 patients completed the HCAHPS survey; (7) No cases met the criteria for this measure; (8) The lower limit of the confidence interval cannot be calculated if the number of observed infections equals zero; (9) No data are available from the state/territory for this reporting period; (10) The scores shown reflect fewer than 50 completed surveys; (11) There were discrepancies in the data collection process; (12) This measure does not apply to this hospital for this reporting period; (13) Results cannot be calculated for this reporting period; (14) The results for this state are combined with nearby states to protect confidentiality; Please refer to the User's Guide for a full explanation of data.

Hospital Name	City	Rate	Cases
Casey County Hospital	Liberty	84%	(a)
McDowell ARH Hospital	Mc Dowell	84%	(a)
Methodist Hospital	Henderson	84%	300+
Saint Joseph Martin	Martin	84%	(a)
Baptist Health Lagrange	La Grange	83%	300+
Baptist Health Lexington	Lexington	83%	300+
Baptist Health Paducah	Paducah	83%	300+
Bourbon Community Hospital	Paris	83%	(a)
Kentucky River Medical Center	Jackson	83%	300+
Logan Memorial Hospital	Russellville	83%	300+
Memorial Hospital[11]	Manchester	83%	(a)
Our Lady of Bellefonte Hospital	Ashland	83%	300+
Saint Joseph Berea	Berea	83%	(a)
Crittenden Health System	Marion	82%	(a)
Saint Joseph London	London	82%	300+
T J Samson Community Hospital	Glasgow	82%	300+
Baptist Health Louisville	Louisville	81%	300+
Hardin Memorial Hospital	Elizabethtown	81%	300+
Monroe County Medical Center	Tompkinsville	81%	300+
Muhlenberg Community Hospital	Greenville	81%	(a)
Murray - Calloway County Hospital	Murray	81%	300+
Saint Elizabeth Medical Center	Lakeside Park	81%	300+
Saint Joseph Mount Sterling	Mount Sterling	81%	300+
Three Rivers Medical Center	Louisa	81%	300+
University of Kentucky Hospital	Lexington	81%	300+
Whitesburg ARH Hospital	Whitesburg	81%	300+
Williamson ARH Hospital	S Williamson	81%	300+
Ephraim Mcdowell Regional Medical Center	Danville	80%	300+
Flaget Memorial Hospital	Bardstown	80%	(a)
Fleming County Hospital	Flemingsburg	80%	300+
Georgetown Community Hospital	Georgetown	80%	300+
Methodist Hospital Union County	Morganfield	80%	(a)
Owensboro Health Regional Hospital	Owensboro	80%	300+
Parkway Regional Hospital	Fulton	80%	(a)
Pineville Community Hospital	Pineville	80%	300+
Taylor Regional Hospital	Campbellsville	80%	300+
Twin Lakes Regional Medical Center	Leitchfield	80%	300+
University of Louisville Hospital	Louisville	80%	300+
Ephraim Mcdowell Fort Logan Hospital	Stanford	79%	(a)
Greenview Regional Hospital	Bowling Green	79%	300+
Harlan Appalachian Reg Healthcare Hosp	Harlan	79%	300+
Highlands Regional Medical Center	Prestonsburg	79%	300+
Jane Todd Crawford Hospital	Greensburg	79%	(a)
Jewish Hospital - Shelbyville	Shelbyville	79%	(a)
King's Daughters' Medical Center	Ashland	79%	300+
Middlesboro Appalachian Reg Healthcare	Middlesboro	79%	300+
Ohio County Hospital	Hartford	79%	(a)
Saint Elizabeth Ft Thomas	Fort Thomas	79%	300+
Baptist Health Madisonville	Madisonville	78%	300+
Baptist Health Richmond	Richmond	78%	300+
Meadowview Regional Medical Center	Maysville	78%	300+
Saint Joseph East	Lexington	78%	300+
Baptist Health Corbin	Corbin	77%	300+
Hazard ARH Regional Medical Center	Hazard	77%	300+
Jackson Purchase Medical Center	Mayfield	77%	300+
Lourdes Hospital	Paducah	77%	300+
The Medical Center at Bowling Green[11]	Bowling Green	77%	300+
Norton Hospitals	Louisville	77%	300+
Paul B Hall Regional Medical Center	Paintsville	77%	(a)
Saint Joseph Hospital	Lexington	77%	300+
Spring View Hospital	Lebanon	77%	300+
Clark Regional Medical Center	Winchester	76%	300+
Frankfort Regional Medical Center	Frankfort	76%	300+
Saint Elizabeth Florence	Florence	76%	300+
Jennie Stuart Medical Center	Hopkinsville	74%	300+
Jewish Hospital & Saint Mary's Healthcare	Louisville	74%	300+
Lake Cumberland Regional Hospital	Somerset	74%	300+

Pain 'Always' Well Controlled

Hospital Name	City	Rate	Cases
Westlake Regional Hospital	Columbia	100%	(a)
Rockcastle County Hospital	Mount Vernon	83%	(a)
Russell County Hospital	Russell Springs	81%	(a)
Wayne County Hospital	Monticello	81%	(a)
Clinton County Hospital	Albany	80%	300+
Marcum & Wallace Memorial Hospital	Irvine	80%	(a)
Crittenden Health System	Marion	77%	(a)
McDowell ARH Hospital	Mc Dowell	77%	(a)
Pikeville Medical Center	Pikeville	77%	300+
Saint Joseph Mount Sterling	Mount Sterling	77%	300+
Baptist Health Lagrange	La Grange	76%	300+
Casey County Hospital	Liberty	76%	(a)
Harrison Memorial Hospital	Cynthiana	76%	300+
Baptist Health Lexington	Lexington	75%	300+
Methodist Hospital Union County	Morganfield	75%	(a)
Saint Joseph London	London	75%	300+
Baptist Health Louisville	Louisville	74%	300+
Kentucky River Medical Center	Jackson	74%	300+
Methodist Hospital	Henderson	74%	300+
Middlesboro Appalachian Reg Healthcare	Middlesboro	74%	300+
Our Lady of Bellefonte Hospital	Ashland	74%	300+
Parkway Regional Hospital	Fulton	74%	(a)
Baptist Health Corbin	Corbin	73%	300+
Baptist Health Paducah	Paducah	73%	300+
Flaget Memorial Hospital	Bardstown	73%	(a)
Fleming County Hospital	Flemingsburg	73%	300+
Saint Joseph Berea	Berea	73%	(a)
Three Rivers Medical Center	Louisa	73%	300+
Williamson ARH Hospital	S Williamson	73%	300+
Ephraim Mcdowell Regional Medical Center	Danville	72%	300+
Georgetown Community Hospital	Georgetown	72%	300+
Hardin Memorial Hospital	Elizabethtown	72%	300+
Harlan Appalachian Reg Healthcare Hosp	Harlan	72%	300+
Jane Todd Crawford Hospital	Greensburg	72%	(a)
Pineville Community Hospital	Pineville	72%	300+
Saint Claire Regional Medical Center	Morehead	72%	300+
University of Kentucky Hospital	Lexington	72%	300+
Bourbon Community Hospital	Paris	71%	(a)
Jewish Hospital - Shelbyville	Shelbyville	71%	(a)
Logan Memorial Hospital	Russellville	71%	300+
Muhlenberg Community Hospital	Greenville	71%	(a)
Murray - Calloway County Hospital	Murray	71%	300+
Saint Elizabeth Medical Center	Lakeside Park	71%	300+
Saint Joseph Martin	Martin	71%	(a)
Whitesburg ARH Hospital	Whitesburg	71%	300+
Greenview Regional Hospital	Bowling Green	70%	300+
Highlands Regional Medical Center	Prestonsburg	70%	300+
Jackson Purchase Medical Center	Mayfield	70%	300+
The Medical Center at Bowling Green[11]	Bowling Green	70%	300+
Norton Hospitals	Louisville	70%	300+
Saint Elizabeth Ft Thomas	Fort Thomas	70%	300+
Saint Joseph Hospital	Lexington	70%	300+
Baptist Health Madisonville	Madisonville	69%	300+
Hazard ARH Regional Medical Center	Hazard	69%	300+
Saint Elizabeth Florence	Florence	69%	300+
Spring View Hospital	Lebanon	69%	300+
Taylor Regional Hospital	Campbellsville	69%	300+
Frankfort Regional Medical Center	Frankfort	68%	300+
Jennie Stuart Medical Center	Hopkinsville	68%	300+
Lourdes Hospital	Paducah	68%	300+
Monroe County Medical Center	Tompkinsville	68%	300+
Owensboro Health Regional Hospital	Owensboro	68%	300+
Saint Joseph East	Lexington	68%	300+
T J Samson Community Hospital	Glasgow	68%	300+
Twin Lakes Regional Medical Center	Leitchfield	68%	300+
University of Louisville Hospital	Louisville	68%	300+
Baptist Health Richmond	Richmond	67%	300+
Clark Regional Medical Center	Winchester	67%	300+
King's Daughters' Medical Center	Ashland	67%	300+
Meadowview Regional Medical Center	Maysville	67%	300+
Memorial Hospital[11]	Manchester	67%	(a)
Ohio County Hospital	Hartford	67%	(a)
Jewish Hospital & Saint Mary's Healthcare	Louisville	66%	300+
Lake Cumberland Regional Hospital	Somerset	66%	300+
Paul B Hall Regional Medical Center	Paintsville	66%	(a)
Ephraim Mcdowell Fort Logan Hospital	Stanford	62%	(a)

Room and Bathroom 'Always' Clean

Hospital Name	City	Rate	Cases
Westlake Regional Hospital	Columbia	97%	(a)
Clinton County Hospital	Albany	92%	300+
Rockcastle County Hospital	Mount Vernon	88%	(a)
Russell County Hospital	Russell Springs	88%	(a)
Marcum & Wallace Memorial Hospital	Irvine	87%	(a)
Casey County Hospital	Liberty	85%	(a)
Saint Joseph Martin	Martin	84%	(a)
Harrison Memorial Hospital	Cynthiana	82%	300+
Pineville Community Hospital	Pineville	82%	300+
Three Rivers Medical Center	Louisa	82%	300+
Ephraim Mcdowell Fort Logan Hospital	Stanford	81%	(a)
T J Samson Community Hospital	Glasgow	81%	300+
Jane Todd Crawford Hospital	Greensburg	80%	(a)
Saint Joseph Berea	Berea	80%	(a)
Twin Lakes Regional Medical Center	Leitchfield	80%	300+
Wayne County Hospital	Monticello	80%	(a)
Logan Memorial Hospital	Russellville	79%	300+
Pikeville Medical Center	Pikeville	79%	300+
Saint Claire Regional Medical Center	Morehead	79%	300+
Saint Joseph Mount Sterling	Mount Sterling	79%	300+
Fleming County Hospital	Flemingsburg	78%	300+
Jewish Hospital - Shelbyville	Shelbyville	78%	(a)
McDowell ARH Hospital	Mc Dowell	78%	(a)
Monroe County Medical Center	Tompkinsville	78%	300+
Parkway Regional Hospital	Fulton	78%	(a)
Baptist Health Lexington	Lexington	77%	300+
Baptist Health Richmond	Richmond	77%	300+
Greenview Regional Hospital	Bowling Green	77%	300+
Memorial Hospital[11]	Manchester	77%	(a)
Methodist Hospital	Henderson	77%	300+
Whitesburg ARH Hospital	Whitesburg	77%	300+
Williamson ARH Hospital	S Williamson	77%	300+
Baptist Health Paducah	Paducah	76%	300+
Murray - Calloway County Hospital	Murray	76%	300+
Saint Joseph London	London	76%	300+
Taylor Regional Hospital	Campbellsville	76%	300+
Muhlenberg Community Hospital	Greenville	75%	(a)
Saint Elizabeth Ft Thomas	Fort Thomas	75%	300+
Ephraim Mcdowell Regional Medical Center	Danville	74%	300+
Harlan Appalachian Reg Healthcare Hosp	Harlan	74%	300+
Jackson Purchase Medical Center	Mayfield	74%	300+
Methodist Hospital Union County	Morganfield	74%	(a)
University of Kentucky Hospital	Lexington	74%	300+
Baptist Health Lagrange	La Grange	73%	300+
Kentucky River Medical Center	Jackson	73%	300+
Middlesboro Appalachian Reg Healthcare	Middlesboro	73%	300+
Hardin Memorial Hospital	Elizabethtown	72%	300+
Lourdes Hospital	Paducah	72%	300+
Our Lady of Bellefonte Hospital	Ashland	72%	300+
Bourbon Community Hospital	Paris	71%	(a)
Clark Regional Medical Center	Winchester	71%	300+
Jennie Stuart Medical Center	Hopkinsville	71%	300+
Baptist Health Corbin	Corbin	70%	300+
Baptist Health Madisonville	Madisonville	70%	300+
Meadowview Regional Medical Center	Maysville	70%	300+
The Medical Center at Bowling Green[11]	Bowling Green	70%	300+
Ohio County Hospital	Hartford	70%	(a)
Paul B Hall Regional Medical Center	Paintsville	70%	(a)
Spring View Hospital	Lebanon	70%	300+
Crittenden Health System	Marion	69%	(a)
Flaget Memorial Hospital	Bardstown	69%	(a)
Georgetown Community Hospital	Georgetown	69%	300+
Saint Elizabeth Medical Center	Lakeside Park	69%	300+
Baptist Health Louisville	Louisville	68%	300+
Hazard ARH Regional Medical Center	Hazard	68%	300+
Norton Hospitals	Louisville	68%	300+
Owensboro Health Regional Hospital	Owensboro	68%	300+
Saint Elizabeth Florence	Florence	68%	300+
Saint Joseph Hospital	Lexington	68%	300+
University of Louisville Hospital	Louisville	68%	300+
King's Daughters' Medical Center	Ashland	67%	300+
Lake Cumberland Regional Hospital	Somerset	67%	300+
Frankfort Regional Medical Center	Frankfort	66%	300+
Highlands Regional Medical Center	Prestonsburg	66%	300+
Saint Joseph East	Lexington	63%	300+
Jewish Hospital & Saint Mary's Healthcare	Louisville	61%	300+

Timely Help 'Always' Received

Hospital Name	City	Rate	Cases
Westlake Regional Hospital	Columbia	99%	(a)
Russell County Hospital	Russell Springs	80%	(a)
McDowell ARH Hospital	Mc Dowell	78%	(a)
Clinton County Hospital	Albany	77%	300+
Marcum & Wallace Memorial Hospital	Irvine	77%	(a)
Fleming County Hospital	Flemingsburg	75%	300+
Parkway Regional Hospital	Fulton	75%	(a)
Pineville Community Hospital	Pineville	75%	300+
Rockcastle County Hospital	Mount Vernon	75%	(a)
Saint Joseph Berea	Berea	75%	(a)
Saint Joseph London	London	75%	300+
Saint Joseph Martin	Martin	75%	(a)
Whitesburg ARH Hospital	Whitesburg	75%	300+
Williamson ARH Hospital	S Williamson	75%	300+
Pikeville Medical Center	Pikeville	74%	300+
Bourbon Community Hospital	Paris	73%	(a)
Kentucky River Medical Center	Jackson	73%	300+
Ephraim Mcdowell Fort Logan Hospital	Stanford	72%	(a)
Harrison Memorial Hospital	Cynthiana	72%	300+
Logan Memorial Hospital	Russellville	72%	300+
Memorial Hospital[11]	Manchester	72%	(a)
Middlesboro Appalachian Reg Healthcare	Middlesboro	72%	300+
T J Samson Community Hospital	Glasgow	72%	300+
Three Rivers Medical Center	Louisa	72%	300+
Murray - Calloway County Hospital	Murray	71%	300+
Saint Claire Regional Medical Center	Morehead	71%	300+
University of Kentucky Hospital	Lexington	71%	300+
Wayne County Hospital	Monticello	71%	(a)
Baptist Health Lagrange	La Grange	70%	300+
Methodist Hospital Union County	Morganfield	70%	(a)
Ohio County Hospital	Hartford	70%	(a)
Crittenden Health System	Marion	69%	(a)
Jane Todd Crawford Hospital	Greensburg	69%	(a)
Saint Joseph Mount Sterling	Mount Sterling	69%	300+
Baptist Health Madisonville	Madisonville	68%	300+
Baptist Health Paducah	Paducah	68%	300+
Harlan Appalachian Reg Healthcare Hosp	Harlan	68%	300+
King's Daughters' Medical Center	Ashland	68%	300+
Methodist Hospital	Henderson	68%	300+
Monroe County Medical Center	Tompkinsville	68%	300+
Our Lady of Bellefonte Hospital	Ashland	68%	300+
Twin Lakes Regional Medical Center	Leitchfield	68%	300+
Baptist Health Lexington	Lexington	67%	300+
Casey County Hospital	Liberty	67%	(a)
Baptist Health Louisville	Louisville	66%	300+

NOTE: Hospital profiles are in alphabetical order by state, then city, then hospital within the city; Rankings exclude hospitals with less than 25 cases except for patient surveys which excludes hospitals with less than 100 cases; (a) 100-299 cases; (1) The number of cases/patients is too few to report; (2) Data submitted were based on a sample of cases/patients; (3) Results are based on a shorter time period than required; (4) Data suppressed by CMS for one or more quarters; (5) Results are not available for this reporting period; (6) Fewer than 100 patients completed the HCAHPS survey; (7) No cases met the criteria for this measure; (8) The lower limit of the confidence interval cannot be calculated if the number of observed infections equals zero; (9) No data are available from the state/territory for this reporting period; (10) The scores shown reflect fewer than 50 completed surveys; (11) There were discrepancies in the data collection process; (12) This measure does not apply to this hospital for this reporting period; (13) Results cannot be calculated for this reporting period; (14) The results for this state are combined with nearby states to protect confidentiality; Please refer to the User's Guide for a full explanation of data.

Hospital Name	City	Rate	Cases
Ephraim Mcdowell Regional Medical Center	Danville	66%	300+
Saint Elizabeth Ft Thomas	Fort Thomas	66%	300+
Saint Elizabeth Medical Center	Lakeside Park	66%	300+
Spring View Hospital	Lebanon	66%	300+
Taylor Regional Hospital	Campbellsville	66%	300+
Clark Regional Medical Center	Winchester	65%	300+
Flaget Memorial Hospital	Bardstown	65%	(a)
Frankfort Regional Medical Center	Frankfort	65%	300+
Georgetown Community Hospital	Georgetown	65%	300+
Greenview Regional Hospital	Bowling Green	64%	300+
Saint Elizabeth Florence	Florence	64%	300+
University of Louisville Hospital	Louisville	64%	300+
Baptist Health Corbin	Corbin	63%	300+
Baptist Health Richmond	Richmond	63%	300+
Hazard ARH Regional Medical Center	Hazard	63%	300+
Jewish Hospital - Shelbyville	Shelbyville	63%	(a)
The Medical Center at Bowling Green[11]	Bowling Green	63%	300+
Muhlenberg Community Hospital	Greenville	63%	(a)
Norton Hospitals	Louisville	63%	300+
Owensboro Health Regional Hospital	Owensboro	63%	300+
Lake Cumberland Regional Hospital	Somerset	62%	300+
Saint Joseph Hospital	Lexington	62%	300+
Hardin Memorial Hospital	Elizabethtown	61%	300+
Highlands Regional Medical Center	Prestonsburg	61%	300+
Jennie Stuart Medical Center	Hopkinsville	61%	300+
Lourdes Hospital	Paducah	61%	300+
Meadowview Regional Medical Center	Maysville	61%	300+
Saint Joseph East	Lexington	61%	300+
Jackson Purchase Medical Center	Mayfield	60%	300+
Paul B Hall Regional Medical Center	Paintsville	60%	(a)
Jewish Hospital & Saint Mary's Healthcare	Louisville	55%	300+

Would Definitely Recommend Hospital

Hospital Name	City	Rate	Cases
Westlake Regional Hospital	Columbia	100%	(a)
Clinton County Hospital	Albany	86%	300+
Baptist Health Louisville	Louisville	84%	300+
Baptist Health Lexington	Lexington	82%	300+
Rockcastle County Hospital	Mount Vernon	82%	(a)
Saint Joseph Martin	Martin	82%	(a)
Pikeville Medical Center	Pikeville	81%	300+
Greenview Regional Hospital	Bowling Green	80%	300+
Our Lady of Bellefonte Hospital	Ashland	80%	300+
Casey County Hospital	Liberty	79%	(a)
Saint Joseph London	London	79%	300+
Baptist Health Paducah	Paducah	78%	300+
Marcum & Wallace Memorial Hospital	Irvine	78%	(a)
Saint Joseph Berea	Berea	78%	(a)
Harrison Memorial Hospital	Cynthiana	77%	300+
Saint Elizabeth Medical Center	Lakeside Park	77%	300+
Saint Joseph Mount Sterling	Mount Sterling	77%	300+
University of Kentucky Hospital	Lexington	77%	300+
Wayne County Hospital	Monticello	77%	(a)
McDowell ARH Hospital	Mc Dowell	76%	(a)
Saint Joseph East	Lexington	75%	300+
Williamson ARH Hospital	S Williamson	75%	300+
Baptist Health Lagrange	La Grange	74%	300+
Lourdes Hospital	Paducah	74%	300+
The Medical Center at Bowling Green[11]	Bowling Green	74%	300+
Saint Joseph Hospital	Lexington	74%	300+
Ephraim Mcdowell Fort Logan Hospital	Stanford	73%	(a)
Pineville Community Hospital	Pineville	73%	300+
University of Louisville Hospital	Louisville	73%	300+
King's Daughters' Medical Center	Ashland	72%	300+
Logan Memorial Hospital	Russellville	72%	300+
Owensboro Health Regional Hospital	Owensboro	72%	300+
Flaget Memorial Hospital	Bardstown	71%	(a)
Fleming County Hospital	Flemingsburg	71%	300+
Georgetown Community Hospital	Georgetown	71%	300+
Russell County Hospital	Russell Springs	71%	(a)
Clark Regional Medical Center	Winchester	70%	300+
Murray - Calloway County Hospital	Murray	70%	300+
Norton Hospitals	Louisville	70%	300+
Parkway Regional Hospital	Fulton	70%	(a)
Saint Claire Regional Medical Center	Morehead	70%	300+
Taylor Regional Hospital	Campbellsville	70%	300+
Whitesburg ARH Hospital	Whitesburg	70%	300+
Methodist Hospital	Henderson	69%	300+
Three Rivers Medical Center	Louisa	69%	300+
Baptist Health Corbin	Corbin	68%	300+
Crittenden Health System	Marion	68%	(a)
Hardin Memorial Hospital	Elizabethtown	68%	300+
Jackson Purchase Medical Center	Mayfield	68%	300+
Kentucky River Medical Center	Jackson	68%	300+
Methodist Hospital Union County	Morganfield	68%	(a)
T J Samson Community Hospital	Glasgow	68%	300+
Ephraim Mcdowell Regional Medical Center	Danville	67%	300+
Jane Todd Crawford Hospital	Greensburg	67%	(a)
Jewish Hospital & Saint Mary's Healthcare	Louisville	67%	300+
Ohio County Hospital	Hartford	67%	(a)
Saint Elizabeth Florence	Florence	67%	300+
Saint Elizabeth Ft Thomas	Fort Thomas	67%	300+
Twin Lakes Regional Medical Center	Leitchfield	67%	300+
Jewish Hospital - Shelbyville	Shelbyville	66%	(a)
Memorial Hospital[11]	Manchester	66%	(a)
Muhlenberg Community Hospital	Greenville	66%	(a)
Hazard ARH Regional Medical Center	Hazard	65%	300+
Middlesboro Appalachian Reg Healthcare	Middlesboro	65%	300+
Monroe County Medical Center	Tompkinsville	64%	300+
Spring View Hospital	Lebanon	64%	300+
Baptist Health Richmond	Richmond	63%	300+
Paul B Hall Regional Medical Center	Paintsville	63%	(a)
Baptist Health Madisonville	Madisonville	62%	300+
Frankfort Regional Medical Center	Frankfort	62%	300+
Harlan Appalachian Reg Healthcare Hosp	Harlan	62%	300+
Highlands Regional Medical Center	Prestonsburg	62%	300+
Lake Cumberland Regional Hospital	Somerset	60%	300+
Meadowview Regional Medical Center	Maysville	59%	300+
Bourbon Community Hospital	Paris	57%	(a)
Jennie Stuart Medical Center	Hopkinsville	55%	300+

Use of Medical Imaging

Cardiac Imaging Stress Test before OP Surgery

Hospital Name	City	Rate	Cases
Rockcastle County Hospital	Mount Vernon	0.6%	155
Kentucky River Medical Center	Jackson	1.7%	59
Frankfort Regional Medical Center	Frankfort	1.9%	53
Monroe County Medical Center	Tompkinsville	2.1%	192
Three Rivers Medical Center	Louisa	2.5%	161
Williamson ARH Hospital	S Williamson	2.6%	76
Saint Joseph East	Lexington	2.9%	70
Saint Joseph Mount Sterling	Mount Sterling	2.9%	174
Meadowview Regional Medical Center	Maysville	3.0%	404
Saint Elizabeth Grant	Williamstown	3.0%	203
Bourbon Community Hospital	Paris	3.3%	151
Paul B Hall Regional Medical Center	Paintsville	3.3%	90
Clark Regional Medical Center	Winchester	3.4%	116
Pikeville Medical Center	Pikeville	3.7%	673
Carroll County Memorial Hospital	Carrollton	3.8%	80
Middlesboro Appalachian Reg Healthcare	Middlesboro	3.8%	52
Russell County Hospital	Russell Springs	3.8%	133
Georgetown Community Hospital	Georgetown	3.9%	103
Baptist Health Lagrange	La Grange	4.0%	223
Saint Joseph Hospital	Lexington	4.0%	904
Saint Elizabeth Ft Thomas	Fort Thomas	4.2%	167
Saint Elizabeth Medical Center	Lakeside Park	4.2%	1904
Saint Joseph London	London	4.2%	1107
T J Samson Community Hospital	Glasgow	4.3%	326
Jewish Hospital - Shelbyville	Shelbyville	4.6%	197
Saint Claire Regional Medical Center	Morehead	4.6%	434
Spring View Hospital	Lebanon	4.6%	174
Caldwell Medical Center	Princeton	4.7%	148
Ephraim Mcdowell Regional Medical Center	Danville	4.7%	444
Norton Hospitals	Louisville	4.7%	2731
Pineville Community Hospital	Pineville	4.8%	83
Saint Elizabeth Florence	Florence	5.0%	179
Saint Joseph Berea	Berea	5.0%	200
Whitesburg ARH Hospital	Whitesburg	5.1%	59
Baptist Health Corbin	Corbin	5.2%	1062
Harrison Memorial Hospital	Cynthiana	5.3%	94
Baptist Health Richmond	Richmond	5.4%	205
Fleming County Hospital	Flemingsburg	5.4%	149
Marcum & Wallace Memorial Hospital	Irvine	5.4%	92
Taylor Regional Hospital	Campbellsville	5.4%	112
Jewish Hospital & Saint Mary's Healthcare	Louisville	5.5%	1448
Baptist Health Lexington	Lexington	5.6%	929
King's Daughters' Medical Center	Ashland	5.9%	2034
Our Lady of Bellefonte Hospital	Ashland	6.2%	612
Lake Cumberland Regional Hospital	Somerset	6.3%	239
Logan Memorial Hospital	Russellville	6.3%	79
Lourdes Hospital	Paducah	6.3%	1134
Murray - Calloway County Hospital	Murray	6.3%	253
Owensboro Health Regional Hospital	Owensboro	6.3%	971
University of Louisville Hospital	Louisville	6.6%	182
Twin Lakes Regional Medical Center	Leitchfield	6.7%	210
Baptist Health Louisville	Louisville	6.8%	1420
Greenview Regional Hospital	Bowling Green	6.8%	118
Methodist Hospital	Henderson	6.8%	222
Baptist Health Madisonville	Madisonville	7.2%	208
Highlands Regional Medical Center	Prestonsburg	7.2%	223
Harlan Appalachian Reg Healthcare Hosp	Harlan	7.4%	68
University of Kentucky Hospital	Lexington	7.7%	363
Baptist Health Paducah	Paducah	8.0%	1055
Hardin Memorial Hospital	Elizabethtown	8.7%	288
The Medical Center at Bowling Green	Bowling Green	9.2%	163

Combination Abdominal CT Scan

Hospital Name	City	Rate	Cases
Baptist Health Lagrange	La Grange	1.4%	370
Saint Claire Regional Medical Center	Morehead	1.4%	716
Wayne County Hospital	Monticello	1.8%	325
Williamson ARH Hospital	S Williamson	1.8%	170
Hazard ARH Regional Medical Center	Hazard	2.2%	408
Saint Joseph Martin	Martin	2.5%	239
Trigg County Hospital	Cadiz	2.5%	121
Carroll County Memorial Hospital	Carrollton	2.6%	153
Saint Joseph East	Lexington	2.7%	412
Georgetown Community Hospital	Georgetown	2.8%	317
Flaget Memorial Hospital	Bardstown	2.9%	593
Kentucky River Medical Center	Jackson	2.9%	345
Morgan County ARH Hospital	West Liberty	3.0%	132
University of Kentucky Hospital	Lexington	3.0%	1972
Frankfort Regional Medical Center	Frankfort	3.1%	486
Baptist Health Louisville	Louisville	3.2%	3701
Crittenden Health System	Marion	3.2%	158
Saint Elizabeth Florence	Florence	3.2%	677
Saint Elizabeth Ft Thomas	Fort Thomas	3.2%	600
Saint Joseph Hospital	Lexington	3.2%	771
The Medical Center at Scottsville	Scottsville	3.3%	181
Three Rivers Medical Center	Louisa	3.3%	241
Saint Elizabeth Grant	Williamstown	3.5%	347
Saint Elizabeth Medical Center	Lakeside Park	3.5%	1749
Mary Breckinridge ARH Hospital	Hyden	3.7%	163
Jewish Hospital - Shelbyville	Shelbyville	4.0%	430
McDowell ARH Hospital	Mc Dowell	4.3%	185
Saint Joseph Berea	Berea	4.3%	468
Baptist Health Lexington	Lexington	4.4%	1694
Parkway Regional Hospital	Fulton	4.6%	131
Jennie Stuart Medical Center	Hopkinsville	4.7%	847
Harrison Memorial Hospital	Cynthiana	5.0%	359
Baptist Health Madisonville	Madisonville	5.2%	705
University of Louisville Hospital	Louisville	5.4%	1151
Saint Joseph London	London	5.6%	1041
Jewish Hospital & Saint Mary's Healthcare	Louisville	5.8%	3511
Logan Memorial Hospital	Russellville	5.8%	329
Memorial Hospital	Manchester	5.8%	330
Ephraim Mcdowell Fort Logan Hospital	Stanford	6.3%	190
The James B Haggin Memorial Hospital	Harrodsburg	6.3%	224
Twin Lakes Regional Medical Center	Leitchfield	6.3%	332
Whitesburg ARH Hospital	Whitesburg	6.4%	280
Caldwell Medical Center	Princeton	6.6%	258
Baptist Health Richmond	Richmond	6.7%	639
Monroe County Medical Center	Tompkinsville	7.5%	212
Ohio County Hospital	Hartford	7.5%	308
Casey County Hospital	Liberty	7.7%	182
Methodist Hospital Union County	Morganfield	7.8%	128
Our Lady of Bellefonte Hospital	Ashland	7.9%	1124
Lourdes Hospital	Paducah	8.1%	1307
Hardin Memorial Hospital	Elizabethtown	8.2%	2219
Baptist Health Corbin	Corbin	8.4%	1080
Saint Joseph Mount Sterling	Mount Sterling	9.6%	554
The Medical Center at Bowling Green	Bowling Green	9.9%	816
Marcum & Wallace Memorial Hospital	Irvine	10.5%	334
The Medical Center at Franklin	Franklin	10.6%	216
Baptist Health Paducah	Paducah	11.4%	1476
Murray - Calloway County Hospital	Murray	11.4%	590
Norton Hospitals	Louisville	11.4%	4201
Marshall County Hospital	Benton	11.8%	287
Lake Cumberland Regional Hospital	Somerset	12.0%	1307
Paul B Hall Regional Medical Center	Paintsville	12.4%	510
Spring View Hospital	Lebanon	12.7%	299
Bluegrass Community Hospital	Versailles	12.8%	125
Cumberland County Hospital	Burkesville	12.9%	85
Knox County Hospital	Barbourville	13.3%	240
Bourbon Community Hospital	Paris	14.3%	196
Westlake Regional Hospital	Columbia	14.4%	209
King's Daughters' Medical Center	Ashland	14.7%	2232
T J Samson Community Hospital	Glasgow	15.2%	876
Methodist Hospital	Henderson	16.9%	516
Muhlenberg Community Hospital	Greenville	16.9%	255
Pikeville Medical Center	Pikeville	17.5%	1409
Taylor Regional Hospital	Campbellsville	17.7%	651
Clark Regional Medical Center	Winchester	18.0%	483
Ephraim Mcdowell Regional Medical Center	Danville	18.4%	841
Clinton County Hospital	Albany	19.0%	189
Greenview Regional Hospital	Bowling Green	19.2%	681
Middlesboro Appalachian Reg Healthcare	Middlesboro	19.8%	383
Rockcastle County Hospital	Mount Vernon	22.7%	282
Jackson Purchase Medical Center	Mayfield	26.2%	413
Pineville Community Hospital	Pineville	31.5%	375
Harlan Appalachian Reg Healthcare Hosp	Harlan	32.3%	362
Owensboro Health Regional Hospital	Owensboro	32.7%	1919
Highlands Regional Medical Center	Prestonsburg	33.8%	1097
Breckinridge Memorial Hospital	Hardinsburg	34.8%	256
Jane Todd Crawford Hospital	Greensburg	35.0%	180
Nicholas County Hospital	Carlisle	35.3%	51
Livingston Hospital & Healthcare Services	Salem	43.9%	187
Caverna Memorial Hospital	Horse Cave	47.7%	149
Meadowview Regional Medical Center	Maysville	49.8%	237
Russell County Hospital	Russell Springs	51.2%	287
Fleming County Hospital	Flemingsburg	53.8%	197

NOTE: Hospital profiles are in alphabetical order by state, then city, then hospital within the city; Rankings exclude hospitals with less than 25 cases except for patient surveys which excludes hospitals with less than 100 cases; (a) 100-299 cases; (1) The number of cases/patients is too few to report; (2) Data submitted were based on a sample of cases/patients; (3) Results are based on a shorter time period than required; (4) Data suppressed by CMS for one or more quarters; (5) Results are not available for this reporting period; (6) Fewer than 100 patients completed the HCAHPS survey; (7) No cases met the criteria for this measure; (8) The lower limit of the confidence interval cannot be calculated if the number of observed infections equals zero; (9) No data are available from the state/territory for this reporting period; (10) The scores shown reflect fewer than 50 completed surveys; (11) There were discrepancies in the data collection process; (12) This measure does not apply to this hospital for this reporting period; (13) Results cannot be calculated for this reporting period; (14) The results for this state are combined with nearby states to protect confidentiality; Please refer to the User's Guide for a full explanation of data.

Combination Brain/Sinus CT Scan

Hospital Name	City	Rate	Cases
Morgan County ARH Hospital	West Liberty	0.0%	201
Saint Joseph Martin	Martin	0.0%	246
Saint Elizabeth Grant	Williamstown	0.4%	239
Saint Elizabeth Medical Center	Lakeside Park	0.6%	1262
Caverna Memorial Hospital	Horse Cave	0.7%	137
Fleming County Hospital	Flemingsburg	0.8%	239
Carroll County Memorial Hospital	Carrollton	0.9%	226
Caldwell Medical Center	Princeton	1.1%	281
Frankfort Regional Medical Center	Frankfort	1.1%	561
Wayne County Hospital	Monticello	1.1%	285
Saint Elizabeth Florence	Florence	1.3%	593
Marcum & Wallace Memorial Hospital	Irvine	1.4%	356
Saint Joseph London	London	1.4%	919
Jewish Hospital - Shelbyville	Shelbyville	1.5%	395
King's Daughters' Medical Center	Ashland	1.6%	1219
Baptist Health Louisville	Louisville	2.0%	2332
Our Lady of Bellefonte Hospital	Ashland	2.0%	711
Ephraim Mcdowell Regional Medical Center	Danville	2.1%	678
Jennie Stuart Medical Center	Hopkinsville	2.3%	792
Baptist Health Madisonville	Madisonville	2.5%	690
Norton Hospitals	Louisville	2.5%	3420
Saint Elizabeth Ft Thomas	Fort Thomas	2.5%	513
Lake Cumberland Regional Hospital	Somerset	2.6%	862
Lourdes Hospital	Paducah	2.6%	947
T J Samson Community Hospital	Glasgow	2.6%	681
Baptist Health Lexington	Lexington	2.8%	956
Baptist Health Corbin	Corbin	3.0%	944
Owensboro Health Regional Hospital	Owensboro	3.1%	1534
Hardin Memorial Hospital	Elizabethtown	3.3%	1392
Highlands Regional Medical Center	Prestonsburg	3.5%	770
The Medical Center at Bowling Green	Bowling Green	3.5%	973
Saint Joseph Hospital	Lexington	3.6%	1021
University of Louisville Hospital	Louisville	3.6%	728
Baptist Health Paducah	Paducah	3.8%	1303
Jewish Hospital & Saint Mary's Healthcare	Louisville	3.9%	2773
Pikeville Medical Center	Pikeville	3.9%	1111
Saint Claire Regional Medical Center	Morehead	4.0%	652
Methodist Hospital	Henderson	4.1%	540
Middlesboro Appalachian Reg Healthcare	Middlesboro	4.1%	469
Taylor Regional Hospital	Campbellsville	4.2%	622
Flaget Memorial Hospital	Bardstown	4.3%	552
Harlan Appalachian Reg Healthcare Hosp	Harlan	4.5%	359
Kentucky River Medical Center	Jackson	4.8%	353
Meadowview Regional Medical Center	Maysville	4.9%	226
University of Kentucky Hospital	Lexington	5.3%	854
Saint Joseph Mount Sterling	Mount Sterling	5.5%	618
Clinton County Hospital	Albany	5.8%	191
Paul B Hall Regional Medical Center	Paintsville	5.9%	490
Murray - Calloway County Hospital	Murray	6.0%	521
Three Rivers Medical Center	Louisa	6.2%	321
Crittenden Health System	Marion	6.6%	106
Harrison Memorial Hospital	Cynthiana	7.4%	282
Bourbon Community Hospital	Paris	7.5%	201
Saint Joseph East	Lexington	8.3%	324

Combination Chest CT Scan

Hospital Name	City	Rate	Cases
Baptist Health Lagrange	La Grange	0.0%	242
Baptist Health Louisville	Louisville	0.0%	3075
Ephraim Mcdowell Regional Medical Center	Danville	0.0%	399
Hardin Memorial Hospital	Elizabethtown	0.0%	1639
Jackson Purchase Medical Center	Mayfield	0.0%	262
Jennie Stuart Medical Center	Hopkinsville	0.0%	443
Jewish Hospital - Shelbyville	Shelbyville	0.0%	374
Logan Memorial Hospital	Russellville	0.0%	111
Morgan County ARH Hospital	West Liberty	0.0%	53
Ohio County Hospital	Hartford	0.0%	133
Parkway Regional Hospital	Fulton	0.0%	85
Saint Elizabeth Grant	Williamstown	0.0%	204
Three Rivers Medical Center	Louisa	0.0%	150
Trigg County Hospital	Cadiz	0.0%	47
University of Kentucky Hospital	Lexington	0.0%	2354
University of Louisville Hospital	Louisville	0.0%	1493
Jewish Hospital & Saint Mary's Healthcare	Louisville	0.1%	2705
Saint Elizabeth Medical Center	Lakeside Park	0.2%	922
Flaget Memorial Hospital	Bardstown	0.3%	327
Meadowview Regional Medical Center	Maysville	0.4%	231
Saint Elizabeth Florence	Florence	0.4%	263
Saint Joseph Mount Sterling	Mount Sterling	0.4%	233
Harrison Memorial Hospital	Cynthiana	0.5%	187
Baptist Health Madisonville	Madisonville	0.6%	356
Frankfort Regional Medical Center	Frankfort	0.6%	158
Marshall County Hospital	Benton	0.6%	174
Williamson ARH Hospital	S Williamson	0.6%	170
Spring View Hospital	Lebanon	0.7%	146
Twin Lakes Regional Medical Center	Leitchfield	0.7%	293
Greenview Regional Hospital	Bowling Green	0.8%	133
Norton Hospitals	Louisville	0.9%	2881
Saint Elizabeth Ft Thomas	Fort Thomas	1.0%	293
Baptist Health Lexington	Lexington	1.1%	1416
Casey County Hospital	Liberty	1.2%	83
Carroll County Memorial Hospital	Carrollton	1.3%	79
Saint Joseph Martin	Martin	1.4%	140
Georgetown Community Hospital	Georgetown	1.5%	132
Bluegrass Community Hospital	Versailles	1.6%	61
The Medical Center at Scottsville	Scottsville	1.7%	58
Owensboro Health Regional Hospital	Owensboro	1.8%	1751
Baptist Health Corbin	Corbin	1.9%	535
Baptist Health Richmond	Richmond	1.9%	316
Breckinridge Memorial Hospital	Hardinsburg	2.0%	197
Fleming County Hospital	Flemingsburg	2.0%	148
Saint Claire Regional Medical Center	Morehead	2.0%	405
Caverna Memorial Hospital	Horse Cave	2.2%	89
Mary Breckinridge ARH Hospital	Hyden	2.4%	82
Muhlenberg Community Hospital	Greenville	2.4%	84
Bourbon Community Hospital	Paris	2.7%	111
Methodist Hospital Union County	Morganfield	2.7%	74
The Medical Center at Bowling Green	Bowling Green	3.0%	371
Monroe County Medical Center	Tompkinsville	3.5%	115
Saint Joseph Hospital	Lexington	3.5%	172
Crittenden Health System	Marion	3.6%	84
Whitesburg ARH Hospital	Whitesburg	4.2%	96
Saint Joseph Berea	Berea	4.3%	301
Saint Joseph East	Lexington	4.3%	94
Wayne County Hospital	Monticello	4.4%	114
The James B Haggin Memorial Hospital	Harrodsburg	4.5%	111
Knox County Hospital	Barbourville	5.9%	102
Hazard ARH Regional Medical Center	Hazard	6.1%	180
Saint Joseph London	London	6.3%	510
Methodist Hospital	Henderson	6.4%	295
Lake Cumberland Regional Hospital	Somerset	6.8%	755
King's Daughters' Medical Center	Ashland	7.6%	2052
Baptist Health Paducah	Paducah	7.7%	970
Murray - Calloway County Hospital	Murray	7.7%	350
Caldwell Medical Center	Princeton	8.2%	85
Our Lady of Bellefonte Hospital	Ashland	8.8%	611
Memorial Hospital	Manchester	9.0%	178
Lourdes Hospital	Paducah	9.5%	651
The Medical Center at Franklin	Franklin	10.0%	90
T J Samson Community Hospital	Glasgow	10.1%	642
Kentucky River Medical Center	Jackson	10.4%	96
Ephraim Mcdowell Fort Logan Hospital	Stanford	11.3%	71
McDowell ARH Hospital	Mc Dowell	11.7%	77
Marcum & Wallace Memorial Hospital	Irvine	11.9%	176
Jane Todd Crawford Hospital	Greensburg	12.2%	98
Taylor Regional Hospital	Campbellsville	13.8%	399
Russell County Hospital	Russell Springs	17.3%	191
Highlands Regional Medical Center	Prestonsburg	17.5%	492
Westlake Regional Hospital	Columbia	18.9%	90
Clinton County Hospital	Albany	19.6%	112
Clark Regional Medical Center	Winchester	22.0%	205
Paul B Hall Regional Medical Center	Paintsville	22.6%	212
Rockcastle County Hospital	Mount Vernon	23.4%	128
Middlesboro Appalachian Reg Healthcare	Middlesboro	25.0%	136
Pineville Community Hospital	Pineville	29.3%	157
Harlan Appalachian Reg Healthcare Hosp	Harlan	30.0%	170
Livingston Hospital & Healthcare Services	Salem	31.0%	58
Cumberland County Hospital	Burkesville	32.0%	50
Pikeville Medical Center	Pikeville	32.3%	1031

Follow-up Mammogram/Ultrasound

A follow-up rate near zero may indicate missed cancer; a rate higher than 14% may mean there is unnecessary follow up.

Hospital Name	City	Rate	Cases
Saint Joseph Hospital	Lexington	2.3%	844
Methodist Hospital Union County	Morganfield	2.5%	238
Caldwell Medical Center	Princeton	2.7%	444
Murray - Calloway County Hospital	Murray	3.2%	1091
Breckinridge Memorial Hospital	Hardinsburg	3.3%	335
Frankfort Regional Medical Center	Frankfort	3.6%	750
The Medical Center at Franklin	Franklin	3.6%	169
Muhlenberg Community Hospital	Greenville	3.7%	270
Georgetown Community Hospital	Georgetown	3.9%	409
Carroll County Memorial Hospital	Carrollton	4.0%	149
Crittenden Health System	Marion	4.1%	121
Kentucky River Medical Center	Jackson	4.1%	193
Rockcastle County Hospital	Mount Vernon	4.1%	341
Baptist Health Lagrange	La Grange	4.4%	662
T J Samson Community Hospital	Glasgow	4.5%	1257
Marshall County Hospital	Benton	4.6%	304
Livingston Hospital & Healthcare Services	Salem	4.8%	145
Knox County Hospital	Barbourville	4.9%	143
Ohio County Hospital	Hartford	5.0%	382
Saint Elizabeth Grant	Williamstown	5.2%	346
Twin Lakes Regional Medical Center	Leitchfield	5.2%	524
Memorial Hospital	Manchester	5.3%	208
Whitesburg ARH Hospital	Whitesburg	5.4%	240
Caverna Memorial Hospital	Horse Cave	5.6%	231
Marcum & Wallace Memorial Hospital	Irvine	5.6%	356
Saint Joseph Mount Sterling	Mount Sterling	5.6%	429
Spring View Hospital	Lebanon	5.7%	542
Russell County Hospital	Russell Springs	5.8%	292
Saint Elizabeth Medical Center	Lakeside Park	5.8%	3234
Saint Joseph East	Lexington	5.9%	1280
King's Daughters' Medical Center	Ashland	6.1%	2619
Baptist Health Louisville	Louisville	6.2%	3287
Jennie Stuart Medical Center	Hopkinsville	6.3%	1375
Pineville Community Hospital	Pineville	6.3%	349
Saint Joseph Berea	Berea	6.4%	359
Bourbon Community Hospital	Paris	6.7%	341
Clinton County Hospital	Albany	6.8%	265
Morgan County ARH Hospital	West Liberty	6.8%	103
Pikeville Medical Center	Pikeville	6.8%	1318
Saint Elizabeth Ft Thomas	Fort Thomas	6.8%	969
Saint Elizabeth Florence	Florence	6.9%	918
Highlands Regional Medical Center	Prestonsburg	7.0%	845
Jewish Hospital & Saint Mary's Healthcare	Louisville	7.1%	3899
Owensboro Health Regional Hospital	Owensboro	7.1%	4000
Trigg County Hospital	Cadiz	7.3%	286
Casey County Hospital	Liberty	7.5%	67
Baptist Health Corbin	Corbin	7.7%	1106
Jane Todd Crawford Hospital	Greensburg	7.7%	208
Methodist Hospital	Henderson	7.8%	670
Jewish Hospital - Shelbyville	Shelbyville	7.9%	722
Taylor Regional Hospital	Campbellsville	7.9%	995
Westlake Regional Hospital	Columbia	8.4%	119
Jackson Purchase Medical Center	Mayfield	8.5%	574
Our Lady of Bellefonte Hospital	Ashland	8.5%	1347
Ephraim Mcdowell Fort Logan Hospital	Stanford	8.7%	275
Bluegrass Community Hospital	Versailles	8.9%	235
McDowell ARH Hospital	Mc Dowell	9.0%	122
University of Louisville Hospital	Louisville	9.1%	1696
Wayne County Hospital	Monticello	9.1%	276
The Medical Center at Bowling Green	Bowling Green	9.7%	1658
Ephraim Mcdowell Regional Medical Center	Danville	9.8%	1460
Hardin Memorial Hospital	Elizabethtown	9.8%	2953
Meadowview Regional Medical Center	Maysville	9.9%	583
Baptist Health Lexington	Lexington	10.0%	3423
The Medical Center at Scottsville	Scottsville	10.0%	130
Logan Memorial Hospital	Russellville	10.3%	546
Norton Hospitals	Louisville	10.5%	4455
Saint Joseph Martin	Martin	10.5%	229
Parkway Regional Hospital	Fulton	10.6%	227
University of Kentucky Hospital	Lexington	10.7%	345
The James B Haggin Memorial Hospital	Harrodsburg	10.8%	251
Saint Claire Regional Medical Center	Morehead	10.9%	728
Flaget Memorial Hospital	Bardstown	11.3%	635
Greenview Regional Hospital	Bowling Green	11.5%	330
Baptist Health Paducah	Paducah	11.6%	1419
Lake Cumberland Regional Hospital	Somerset	12.1%	1258
Three Rivers Medical Center	Louisa	12.5%	160
Harlan Appalachian Reg Healthcare Hosp	Harlan	12.9%	317
Baptist Health Richmond	Richmond	13.7%	871
Clark Regional Medical Center	Winchester	13.8%	674
Mary Breckinridge ARH Hospital	Hyden	13.8%	87
Saint Joseph London	London	13.8%	509
Fleming County Hospital	Flemingsburg	14.0%	299
Middlesboro Appalachian Reg Healthcare	Middlesboro	14.7%	272
Harrison Memorial Hospital	Cynthiana	15.1%	372
Lourdes Hospital	Paducah	16.5%	1905
Monroe County Medical Center	Tompkinsville	17.9%	117
Williamson ARH Hospital	S Williamson	19.6%	168
Paul B Hall Regional Medical Center	Paintsville	31.1%	244

Lumbar Spine MRI for Low Back Pain

Hospital Name	City	Rate	Cases
Kentucky River Medical Center	Jackson	20.0%	80
Saint Elizabeth Ft Thomas	Fort Thomas	26.5%	83
Whitesburg ARH Hospital	Whitesburg	30.4%	92
Murray - Calloway County Hospital	Murray	31.0%	87
Baptist Health Madisonville	Madisonville	31.5%	89
Saint Joseph London	London	31.6%	76
Taylor Regional Hospital	Campbellsville	31.9%	119
Flaget Memorial Hospital	Bardstown	33.6%	134
T J Samson Community Hospital	Glasgow	34.3%	99
Three Rivers Medical Center	Louisa	34.6%	52
Hardin Memorial Hospital	Elizabethtown	34.7%	349
Meadowview Regional Medical Center	Maysville	35.4%	65
Norton Hospitals	Louisville	35.5%	833
Baptist Health Louisville	Louisville	35.7%	428
The Medical Center at Bowling Green	Bowling Green	36.5%	244
Baptist Health Lexington	Lexington	36.7%	218
King's Daughters' Medical Center	Ashland	36.9%	590
Middlesboro Appalachian Reg Healthcare	Middlesboro	36.9%	65
Saint Elizabeth Florence	Florence	37.0%	92
Lourdes Hospital	Paducah	37.3%	169
Pikeville Medical Center	Pikeville	37.3%	367
Highlands Regional Medical Center	Prestonsburg	37.5%	160
Saint Joseph Berea	Berea	38.1%	42
Muhlenberg Community Hospital	Greenville	38.2%	55

NOTE: Hospital profiles are in alphabetical order by state, then city, then hospital within the city; Rankings exclude hospitals with less than 25 cases except for patient surveys which excludes hospitals with less than 100 cases; (a) 100-299 cases; (1) The number of cases/patients is too few to report; (2) Data submitted were based on a sample of cases/patients; (3) Results are based on a shorter time period than required; (4) Data suppressed by CMS for one or more quarters; (5) Results are not available for this reporting period; (6) Fewer than 100 patients completed the HCAHPS survey; (7) No cases met the criteria for this measure; (8) The lower limit of the confidence interval cannot be calculated if the number of observed infections equals zero; (9) No data are available from the state/territory for this reporting period; (10) The scores shown reflect fewer than 50 completed surveys; (11) There were discrepancies in the data collection process; (12) This measure does not apply to this hospital for this reporting period; (13) Results cannot be calculated for this reporting period; (14) The results for this state are combined with nearby states to protect confidentiality; Please refer to the User's Guide for a full explanation of data.

University of Louisville Hospital	Louisville	38.4%	73
Jewish Hospital - Shelbyville	Shelbyville	38.6%	70
University of Kentucky Hospital	Lexington	38.6%	101
Owensboro Health Regional Hospital	Owensboro	38.8%	387
Ephraim Mcdowell Regional Medical Center	Danville	39.2%	283
Harlan Appalachian Reg Healthcare Hosp	Harlan	39.6%	96
Baptist Health Paducah	Paducah	39.7%	297
Our Lady of Bellefonte Hospital	Ashland	40.2%	251
Pineville Community Hospital	Pineville	40.2%	82
Paul B Hall Regional Medical Center	Paintsville	40.5%	42
Saint Elizabeth Grant	Williamstown	40.6%	96
Clark Regional Medical Center	Winchester	40.7%	59
Methodist Hospital	Henderson	41.3%	92
Saint Elizabeth Medical Center	Lakeside Park	41.5%	528
Jennie Stuart Medical Center	Hopkinsville	41.7%	96
Jewish Hospital & Saint Mary's Healthcare	Louisville	41.7%	540
Caldwell Medical Center	Princeton	42.6%	54
Twin Lakes Regional Medical Center	Leitchfield	42.9%	70
Saint Joseph Hospital	Lexington	43.5%	62
Rockcastle County Hospital	Mount Vernon	44.0%	50
Frankfort Regional Medical Center	Frankfort	44.3%	61
Logan Memorial Hospital	Russellville	44.3%	61
Spring View Hospital	Lebanon	44.3%	88
Baptist Health Corbin	Corbin	44.7%	179
Williamson ARH Hospital	S Williamson	45.1%	71
Memorial Hospital	Manchester	45.6%	79
Saint Claire Regional Medical Center	Morehead	46.7%	107
Greenview Regional Hospital	Bowling Green	47.8%	69
Saint Joseph Mount Sterling	Mount Sterling	48.9%	88
Lake Cumberland Regional Hospital	Somerset	49.7%	187
Baptist Health Richmond	Richmond	51.5%	66
Marcum & Wallace Memorial Hospital	Irvine	51.6%	62
McDowell ARH Hospital	Mc Dowell	55.0%	40
The James B Haggin Memorial Hospital	Harrodsburg	55.6%	45

NOTE: Hospital profiles are in alphabetical order by state, then city, then hospital within the city; Rankings exclude hospitals with less than 25 cases except for patient surveys which excludes hospitals with less than 100 cases; (a) 100-299 cases; (1) The number of cases/patients is too few to report; (2) Data submitted were based on a sample of cases/patients; (3) Results are based on a shorter time period than required; (4) Data suppressed by CMS for one or more quarters; (5) Results are not available for this reporting period; (6) Fewer than 100 patients completed the HCAHPS survey; (7) No cases met the criteria for this measure; (8) The lower limit of the confidence interval cannot be calculated if the number of observed infections equals zero; (9) No data are available from the state/territory for this reporting period; (10) The scores shown reflect fewer than 50 completed surveys; (11) There were discrepancies in the data collection process; (12) This measure does not apply to this hospital for this reporting period; (13) Results cannot be calculated for this reporting period; (14) The results for this state are combined with nearby states to protect confidentiality; Please refer to the User's Guide for a full explanation of data.

Clinton County Hospital

723 Burkesville Road
Albany, KY 42602
E-mail: info@clintoncountyhospital.com
URL: www.clintoncountyhospital.com
Type: Acute Care Hospitals
Ownership: Proprietary
Phone: 606-387-6421
Fax: 606-387-8550
Emergency Services: Yes
Beds: 42

Key Personnel:
Intensive Care Unit. . . . . Janice Beard
Emergency Room . . . . Tamara Collins
Operating Room. . . . . Tracy Cross
CEO/President. . . . . Randel A Flowers, PhD
Chief of Medical Staff . . . . Vicki Latham
Quality Assurance . . . . Pat Sewell
Radiology. . . . . Jai Singh
Infection Control. . . . . Linda Steele

Measure	Cases	This Hosp.	State Avg.	U.S. Avg.
Blood Clot Prevention and Treatment				
Anticoagulation Overlap Therapy[1,2]	-	-	90%	93%
ICU Venous Thromboembolism Prophylaxis[2]	31	68%	86%	92%
Incidence of Potentially Preventable VTE[1,2]	-	-	13%	10%
UFH with Dosages/Platelet Monitoring[1,2]	-	-	98%	97%
Venous Thromboembolism Prophylaxis[2]	163	50%	80%	85%
Warfarin Therapy Discharge Instructions[1,2]	-	-	72%	75%
Chest Pain/Possible Heart Attack Care				
Aspirin Given Within 24 Hours of Arrival	28	93%	97%	96%
Fibrinolytic Meds Within 30 Min. of Arrival[1,3]	-	-	63%	58%
Average Time to ECG (minutes)	28	4	6	7
Average Time to Transfer (minutes)[1,3]	-	-	61	60
Children's Asthma Care				
Received Home Management Plan of Care	-	-	-	88%
Received Reliever Medication	-	-	-	100%
Received Systemic Corticosteroids	-	-	-	100%
Emergency Department				
Admittance Decision Time (minutes)[2]	181	60	78	98
Head CT Results Within 45 Min. of Arrival[1]	-	-	55%	57%
Patients Who Left ER Before Being Seen	6,322	4%	2%	2%
Time from ER Arrival to Admit. (minutes)[2]	189	195	238	274
Time from ER Arrival to Discharge (minutes)	439	95	126	134
Time in ER Before Being Evaluated (minutes)	423	16	23	26
Time to Pain Meds for Fractures (minutes)	33	38	56	57
Heart Attack Care				
Aspirin Given at Discharge[1]	-	-	99%	99%
Fibrinolytic Meds Within 30 Min. of Arrival[7]	-	-	-	54%
PCI Within 90 Minutes of Arrival[7]	-	-	97%	96%
Statin Prescribed at Discharge[1]	-	-	97%	98%
Heart Failure Care				
ACE Inhibitor or ARB for LVSD	13	46%	95%	97%
Discharge Instructions Given	30	77%	92%	94%
Evaluation of LVS Function	39	100%	98%	99%
Medicare Spending				
Medicare Spending per Patient (ratio)	-	1.04	0.97	0.98
Pneumonia Care				
Appropriate Initial Antibiotic Given	72	82%	94%	95%
Blood Culture Timing	24	92%	98%	98%
Pregnancy and Delivery Care				
Newborn Deliveries Scheduled Early[7]	-	-	9%	6%
Preventive Care				
Immunization for Influenza[2]	331	96%	92%	90%
Immunization for Pneumonia[2]	470	100%	94%	92%
Stroke Care				
Anticoagulation Therapy for Atrial Fibrillation[1]	-	-	95%	95%
Antithrombotic Therapy Timing	15	93%	97%	98%
Assessed for Rehabilitation	13	85%	97%	97%
Discharged on Antithrombotic Therapy	13	85%	98%	99%
Discharged on Statin Medication[1]	-	-	93%	94%
Thrombolytic Therapy Timing[1]	-	-	59%	66%
Venous Thromboembolism Prophylaxis	16	75%	93%	94%
Written Stroke Educational Materials Given[1]	-	-	86%	88%
Surgical Care Improvement Project				
Appropriate Beta Blocker Usage[1,3]	-	-	98%	98%
Appropriate VTP Within 24 Hours[1,3]	-	-	98%	98%
Controlled Postoperative Blood Glucose[3,7]	-	-	96%	97%
Perioperative Temperature Management[1,3]	-	-	100%	100%
Prophylactic Antibiotic Selection[1,3]	-	-	99%	99%
Prophylactic Antibiotic Selection (Outpatient)[1,3]	-	-	97%	98%
Prophylactic Antibiotic Stopped[1,3]	-	-	98%	98%
Prophylactic Antibiotic Timing[1,3]	-	-	99%	99%
Prophylactic Antibiotic Timing (Outpatient)[1,3]	-	-	97%	98%
Urinary Catheter Removal[3,7]	-	-	97%	97%
Survey of Patients' Hospital Experiences				
Area Around Room 'Always' Quiet at Night	300+	78%	64%	61%
Doctors 'Always' Communicated Well	300+	96%	84%	82%
Home Recovery Information Given	300+	84%	86%	85%
Hospital Given 9 or 10 on 10 Point Scale	300+	86%	72%	71%
Meds 'Always' Explained Before Given	300+	72%	66%	64%
Nurses 'Always' Communicated Well	300+	88%	81%	79%
Pain 'Always' Well Controlled	300+	80%	73%	71%
Room and Bathroom 'Always' Clean	300+	92%	75%	73%
Timely Help 'Always' Received	300+	77%	69%	68%
Would Definitely Recommend Hospital	300+	86%	71%	71%
Use of Medical Imaging				
Cardiac Imaging Stress Test before Surgery[7]	-	-	5.3%	5.3%
Combination Abdominal CT Scan	189	19.0%	10.7%	10.5%
Combination Brain/Sinus CT Scan	191	5.8%	3.1%	2.7%
Combination Chest CT Scan	112	19.6%	4.3%	2.7%
Follow-up Mammogram/Ultrasound	265	6.8%	8.3%	8.8%
Lumbar Spine MRI for Low Back Pain[7]	-	-	38.9%	37.2%

King's Daughters' Medical Center

2201 Lexington Avenue
Ashland, KY 41101
URL: www.kdmc.com
Type: Acute Care Hospitals
Ownership: Voluntary non-profit - Private
Phone: 606-408-4000
Fax: 606-327-4805
Emergency Services: Yes
Beds: 341

Key Personnel:
Infection Control. . . . . Lea Acord
Chief of Medical Staff. . . . . Philip W Fioret
Radiology. . . . . Chun Kim, MD
Quality Assurance . . . . Sheryl Mahaney
Pediatric Ambulatory Care . . . . . . John Roger Potter, MD
Pediatric In-Patient Care . . . . John Roger Potter, MD
CEO/President. . . . . Kristie Whitlatch

Measure	Cases	This Hosp.	State Avg.	U.S. Avg.
Blood Clot Prevention and Treatment				
Anticoagulation Overlap Therapy[2]	106	92%	90%	93%
ICU Venous Thromboembolism Prophylaxis[2]	57	100%	86%	92%
Incidence of Potentially Preventable VTE[1,2]	-	-	13%	10%
UFH with Dosages/Platelet Monitoring[2]	68	100%	98%	97%
Venous Thromboembolism Prophylaxis[2]	353	92%	80%	85%
Warfarin Therapy Discharge Instructions[2]	85	78%	72%	75%
Chest Pain/Possible Heart Attack Care				
Aspirin Given Within 24 Hours of Arrival[1,3]	-	-	97%	96%
Fibrinolytic Meds Within 30 Min. of Arrival[5]	-	-	63%	58%
Average Time to ECG (minutes)[1,3]	-	-	6	7
Average Time to Transfer (minutes)[5]	-	-	61	60
Children's Asthma Care				
Received Home Management Plan of Care	-	-	-	88%
Received Reliever Medication	-	-	-	100%
Received Systemic Corticosteroids	-	-	-	100%
Emergency Department				
Admittance Decision Time (minutes)[2]	425	100	78	98
Head CT Results Within 45 Min. of Arrival[1]	-	-	55%	57%
Patients Who Left ER Before Being Seen	73,652	1%	2%	2%
Time from ER Arrival to Admit. (minutes)[2]	426	218	238	274
Time from ER Arrival to Discharge (minutes)	323	123	126	134
Time in ER Before Being Evaluated (minutes)	406	14	23	26
Time to Pain Meds for Fractures (minutes)	139	47	56	57
Heart Attack Care				
Aspirin Given at Discharge[2]	296	100%	99%	99%
Fibrinolytic Meds Within 30 Min. of Arrival[2,7]	-	-	-	54%
PCI Within 90 Minutes of Arrival[2]	30	100%	97%	96%
Statin Prescribed at Discharge[2]	276	100%	97%	98%
Heart Failure Care				
ACE Inhibitor or ARB for LVSD[2]	74	97%	95%	97%
Discharge Instructions Given[2]	261	100%	92%	94%
Evaluation of LVS Function[2]	299	100%	98%	99%
Medicare Spending				
Medicare Spending per Patient (ratio)	-	0.97	0.97	0.98
Pneumonia Care				
Appropriate Initial Antibiotic Given[2]	85	99%	94%	95%
Blood Culture Timing[2]	67	99%	98%	98%
Pregnancy and Delivery Care				
Newborn Deliveries Scheduled Early[2]	32	3%	9%	6%
Preventive Care				
Immunization for Influenza[2]	598	97%	92%	90%
Immunization for Pneumonia[2]	825	100%	94%	92%
Stroke Care				
Anticoagulation Therapy for Atrial Fibrillation[2]	22	91%	95%	95%
Antithrombotic Therapy Timing[2]	91	100%	97%	98%
Assessed for Rehabilitation[2]	100	96%	97%	97%
Discharged on Antithrombotic Therapy[2]	94	97%	98%	99%
Discharged on Statin Medication[2]	81	96%	93%	94%
Thrombolytic Therapy Timing[1,2]	-	-	59%	66%
Venous Thromboembolism Prophylaxis[2]	96	93%	93%	94%
Written Stroke Educational Materials Given[2]	61	95%	86%	88%
Surgical Care Improvement Project				
Appropriate Beta Blocker Usage[2]	301	99%	98%	98%
Appropriate VTP Within 24 Hours[2]	345	100%	98%	98%
Controlled Postoperative Blood Glucose[2]	124	99%	96%	97%
Perioperative Temperature Management[2]	496	100%	100%	100%
Prophylactic Antibiotic Selection[2]	407	100%	99%	99%
Prophylactic Antibiotic Selection (Outpatient)	637	98%	97%	98%
Prophylactic Antibiotic Stopped[2]	392	99%	98%	98%
Prophylactic Antibiotic Timing[2]	407	97%	99%	99%
Prophylactic Antibiotic Timing (Outpatient)	554	100%	97%	98%
Urinary Catheter Removal[2]	421	99%	97%	97%
Survey of Patients' Hospital Experiences				
Area Around Room 'Always' Quiet at Night	300+	64%	64%	61%
Doctors 'Always' Communicated Well	300+	82%	84%	82%
Home Recovery Information Given	300+	80%	86%	85%
Hospital Given 9 or 10 on 10 Point Scale	300+	71%	72%	71%
Meds 'Always' Explained Before Given	300+	61%	66%	64%
Nurses 'Always' Communicated Well	300+	79%	81%	79%
Pain 'Always' Well Controlled	300+	67%	73%	71%
Room and Bathroom 'Always' Clean	300+	67%	75%	73%
Timely Help 'Always' Received	300+	68%	69%	68%
Would Definitely Recommend Hospital	300+	72%	71%	71%
Use of Medical Imaging				
Cardiac Imaging Stress Test before Surgery	2,034	5.9%	5.3%	5.3%
Combination Abdominal CT Scan	2,232	14.7%	10.7%	10.5%
Combination Brain/Sinus CT Scan	1,219	1.6%	3.1%	2.7%
Combination Chest CT Scan	2,052	7.6%	4.3%	2.7%
Follow-up Mammogram/Ultrasound	2,619	6.1%	8.3%	8.8%
Lumbar Spine MRI for Low Back Pain	590	36.9%	38.9%	37.2%

Our Lady of Bellefonte Hospital

1000 Saint Christopher Drive
Ashland, KY 41101
URL: www.olbh.com
Type: Acute Care Hospitals
Ownership: Voluntary non-profit - Private
Phone: 606-833-3600
Fax: 606-833-3593
Emergency Services: Yes
Beds: 214

Key Personnel:
Chief of Medical Staff. . . . . Eugene DeGiorgio, MD
CEO/President. . . . . Mark Gordon

Measure	Cases	This Hosp.	State Avg.	U.S. Avg.
Blood Clot Prevention and Treatment				
Anticoagulation Overlap Therapy[2]	24	50%	90%	93%
ICU Venous Thromboembolism Prophylaxis[2]	33	94%	86%	92%
Incidence of Potentially Preventable VTE[1,2]	-	-	13%	10%
UFH with Dosages/Platelet Monitoring[1,2]	-	-	98%	97%
Venous Thromboembolism Prophylaxis[2]	329	79%	80%	85%
Warfarin Therapy Discharge Instructions[2]	18	61%	72%	75%
Chest Pain/Possible Heart Attack Care				
Aspirin Given Within 24 Hours of Arrival	33	88%	97%	96%
Fibrinolytic Meds Within 30 Min. of Arrival[7]	-	-	63%	58%
Average Time to ECG (minutes)	34	18	6	7
Average Time to Transfer (minutes)[7]	-	-	61	60
Children's Asthma Care				
Received Home Management Plan of Care	-	-	-	88%
Received Reliever Medication	-	-	-	100%

NOTE: Hospital profiles are in alphabetical order by state, then city, then hospital within the city; Rankings exclude hospitals with less than 25 cases except for patient surveys which excludes hospitals with less than 100 cases; (a) 100-299 cases; (1) The number of cases/patients is too few to report; (2) Data submitted were based on a sample of cases/patients; (3) Results are based on a shorter time period than required; (4) Data suppressed by CMS for one or more quarters; (5) Results are not available for this reporting period; (6) Fewer than 100 patients completed the HCAHPS survey; (7) No cases met the criteria for this measure; (8) The lower limit of the confidence interval cannot be calculated if the number of observed infections equals zero; (9) No data are available from the state/territory for this reporting period; (10) The scores shown reflect fewer than 50 completed surveys; (11) There were discrepancies in the data collection process; (12) This measure does not apply to this hospital for this reporting period; (13) Results cannot be calculated for this reporting period; (14) The results for this state are combined with nearby states to protect confidentiality; Please refer to the User's Guide for a full explanation of data.

Measure	Cases	This Hosp.	State Avg.	U.S. Avg.
Received Systemic Corticosteroids	-	-	-	100%
Emergency Department				
Admittance Decision Time (minutes)[2]	233	70	78	98
Head CT Results Within 45 Min. of Arrival[1]	-	-	55%	57%
Patients Who Left ER Before Being Seen	26,726	2%	2%	2%
Time from ER Arrival to Admit. (minutes)[2]	233	265	238	274
Time from ER Arrival to Discharge (minutes)	390	185	126	134
Time in ER Before Being Evaluated (minutes)	151	40	23	26
Time to Pain Meds for Fractures (minutes)	81	86	56	57
Heart Attack Care				
Aspirin Given at Discharge	48	94%	99%	99%
Fibrinolytic Meds Within 30 Min. of Arrival[7]	-	-	-	54%
PCI Within 90 Minutes of Arrival[7]	-	-	97%	96%
Statin Prescribed at Discharge	48	94%	97%	98%
Heart Failure Care				
ACE Inhibitor or ARB for LVSD	56	95%	95%	97%
Discharge Instructions Given	207	85%	92%	94%
Evaluation of LVS Function	243	99%	98%	99%
Medicare Spending				
Medicare Spending per Patient (ratio)	-	0.95	0.97	0.98
Pneumonia Care				
Appropriate Initial Antibiotic Given	194	94%	94%	95%
Blood Culture Timing	366	95%	98%	98%
Pregnancy and Delivery Care				
Newborn Deliveries Scheduled Early[7]	-	-	9%	6%
Preventive Care				
Immunization for Influenza[2]	631	91%	92%	90%
Immunization for Pneumonia[2]	820	89%	94%	92%
Stroke Care				
Anticoagulation Therapy for Atrial Fibrillation[1]	-	-	95%	95%
Antithrombotic Therapy Timing	51	98%	97%	98%
Assessed for Rehabilitation	57	96%	97%	97%
Discharged on Antithrombotic Therapy	57	96%	98%	99%
Discharged on Statin Medication	37	89%	93%	94%
Thrombolytic Therapy Timing[7]	-	-	59%	66%
Venous Thromboembolism Prophylaxis	52	98%	93%	94%
Written Stroke Educational Materials Given	37	97%	86%	88%
Surgical Care Improvement Project				
Appropriate Beta Blocker Usage	200	95%	98%	98%
Appropriate VTP Within 24 Hours	582	96%	98%	98%
Controlled Postoperative Blood Glucose[7]	-	-	96%	97%
Perioperative Temperature Management	609	100%	100%	100%
Prophylactic Antibiotic Selection	441	100%	99%	99%
Prophylactic Antibiotic Selection (Outpatient)	196	96%	97%	98%
Prophylactic Antibiotic Stopped	425	98%	98%	98%
Prophylactic Antibiotic Timing	441	99%	99%	99%
Prophylactic Antibiotic Timing (Outpatient)	197	99%	97%	98%
Urinary Catheter Removal	454	98%	97%	97%
Survey of Patients' Hospital Experiences				
Area Around Room 'Always' Quiet at Night	300+	69%	64%	61%
Doctors 'Always' Communicated Well	300+	84%	84%	82%
Home Recovery Information Given	300+	87%	86%	85%
Hospital Given 9 or 10 on 10 Point Scale	300+	77%	72%	71%
Meds 'Always' Explained Before Given	300+	66%	66%	64%
Nurses 'Always' Communicated Well	300+	83%	81%	79%
Pain 'Always' Well Controlled	300+	74%	73%	71%
Room and Bathroom 'Always' Clean	300+	72%	75%	73%
Timely Help 'Always' Received	300+	68%	69%	68%
Would Definitely Recommend Hospital	300+	80%	71%	71%
Use of Medical Imaging				
Cardiac Imaging Stress Test before Surgery	612	6.2%	5.3%	5.3%
Combination Abdominal CT Scan	1,124	7.9%	10.7%	10.5%
Combination Brain/Sinus CT Scan	711	2.0%	3.1%	2.7%
Combination Chest CT Scan	611	8.8%	4.3%	2.7%
Follow-up Mammogram/Ultrasound	1,347	8.5%	8.3%	8.8%
Lumbar Spine MRI for Low Back Pain	251	40.2%	38.9%	37.2%

Knox County Hospital

80 Hospital Drive
Barbourville, KY 40906
E-mail: webmaster@knoxcohospital.com
URL: www.knoxcohospital.com
Type: Critical Access Hospitals
Ownership: Government - Local

Phone: 606-546-4175
Fax: 606-545-5511
Emergency Services: Yes
Beds: 58

Key Personnel:
CEO/President. . . . . Ray Canady
Quality Assurance . . . . Rita Hammons
Radiology. . . . . Mike Standifer

Measure	Cases	This Hosp.	State Avg.	U.S. Avg.
Blood Clot Prevention and Treatment				
Anticoagulation Overlap Therapy[5]	-	-	90%	93%
ICU Venous Thromboembolism Prophylaxis[5]	-	-	86%	92%
Incidence of Potentially Preventable VTE[5]	-	-	13%	10%
UFH with Dosages/Platelet Monitoring[5]	-	-	98%	97%
Venous Thromboembolism Prophylaxis[5]	-	-	80%	85%
Warfarin Therapy Discharge Instructions[5]	-	-	72%	75%
Chest Pain/Possible Heart Attack Care				
Aspirin Given Within 24 Hours of Arrival[5]	-	-	97%	96%
Fibrinolytic Meds Within 30 Min. of Arrival[5]	-	-	63%	58%
Average Time to ECG (minutes)[5]	-	-	6	7
Average Time to Transfer (minutes)[5]	-	-	61	60
Children's Asthma Care				
Received Home Management Plan of Care	-	-	-	88%
Received Reliever Medication	-	-	-	100%
Received Systemic Corticosteroids	-	-	-	100%
Emergency Department				
Admittance Decision Time (minutes)[5]	-	-	78	98
Head CT Results Within 45 Min. of Arrival[5]	-	-	55%	57%
Patients Who Left ER Before Being Seen	14,264	2%	2%	2%
Time from ER Arrival to Admit. (minutes)[5]	-	-	238	274
Time from ER Arrival to Discharge (minutes)[5]	-	-	126	134
Time in ER Before Being Evaluated (minutes)[5]	-	-	23	26
Time to Pain Meds for Fractures (minutes)[5]	-	-	56	57
Heart Attack Care				
Aspirin Given at Discharge[1]	-	-	99%	99%
Fibrinolytic Meds Within 30 Min. of Arrival[7]	-	-	-	54%
PCI Within 90 Minutes of Arrival[7]	-	-	97%	96%
Statin Prescribed at Discharge[1]	-	-	97%	98%
Heart Failure Care				
ACE Inhibitor or ARB for LVSD[1]	-	-	95%	97%
Discharge Instructions Given	42	86%	92%	94%
Evaluation of LVS Function	46	65%	98%	99%
Medicare Spending				
Medicare Spending per Patient (ratio)	-	-	0.97	0.98
Pneumonia Care				
Appropriate Initial Antibiotic Given	51	69%	94%	95%
Blood Culture Timing	49	90%	98%	98%
Pregnancy and Delivery Care				
Newborn Deliveries Scheduled Early[5]	-	-	9%	6%
Preventive Care				
Immunization for Influenza[5]	-	-	92%	90%
Immunization for Pneumonia[5]	-	-	94%	92%
Stroke Care				
Anticoagulation Therapy for Atrial Fibrillation[5]	-	-	95%	95%
Antithrombotic Therapy Timing[5]	-	-	97%	98%
Assessed for Rehabilitation[5]	-	-	97%	97%
Discharged on Antithrombotic Therapy[5]	-	-	98%	99%
Discharged on Statin Medication[5]	-	-	93%	94%
Thrombolytic Therapy Timing[5]	-	-	59%	66%
Venous Thromboembolism Prophylaxis[5]	-	-	93%	94%
Written Stroke Educational Materials Given[5]	-	-	86%	88%
Surgical Care Improvement Project				
Appropriate Beta Blocker Usage[5]	-	-	98%	98%
Appropriate VTP Within 24 Hours[5]	-	-	98%	98%
Controlled Postoperative Blood Glucose[5]	-	-	96%	97%
Perioperative Temperature Management[5]	-	-	100%	100%
Prophylactic Antibiotic Selection[5]	-	-	99%	99%
Prophylactic Antibiotic Selection (Outpatient)[5]	-	-	97%	98%
Prophylactic Antibiotic Stopped[5]	-	-	98%	98%
Prophylactic Antibiotic Timing[5]	-	-	99%	99%
Prophylactic Antibiotic Timing (Outpatient)[5]	-	-	97%	98%
Urinary Catheter Removal[5]	-	-	97%	97%
Survey of Patients' Hospital Experiences				
Area Around Room 'Always' Quiet at Night[5]	-	-	64%	61%
Doctors 'Always' Communicated Well[5]	-	-	84%	82%
Home Recovery Information Given[5]	-	-	86%	85%
Hospital Given 9 or 10 on 10 Point Scale[5]	-	-	72%	71%
Meds 'Always' Explained Before Given[5]	-	-	66%	64%
Nurses 'Always' Communicated Well[5]	-	-	81%	79%
Pain 'Always' Well Controlled[5]	-	-	73%	71%
Room and Bathroom 'Always' Clean[5]	-	-	75%	73%
Timely Help 'Always' Received[5]	-	-	69%	68%
Would Definitely Recommend Hospital[5]	-	-	71%	71%
Use of Medical Imaging				
Cardiac Imaging Stress Test before Surgery[1]	-	-	5.3%	5.3%
Combination Abdominal CT Scan	240	13.3%	10.7%	10.5%
Combination Brain/Sinus CT Scan[1]	-	-	3.1%	2.7%
Combination Chest CT Scan	102	5.9%	4.3%	2.7%
Follow-up Mammogram/Ultrasound	143	4.9%	8.3%	8.8%
Lumbar Spine MRI for Low Back Pain[7]	-	-	38.9%	37.2%

Flaget Memorial Hospital

4305 New Shepherdsville Road
Bardstown, KY 40004
URL: www.flaget.com
Type: Acute Care Hospitals
Ownership: Voluntary non-profit - Private

Phone: 502-350-5000
Fax: 502-350-5036
Emergency Services: Yes
Beds: 52

Key Personnel:
Chief of Medical Staff . . . . Mark Abraham, MD
Quality Assurance . . . . Cheri Davidson
CEO/President. . . . . Bruce Klotkarh
Emergency Room . . . . Clara Powell, RN

Measure	Cases	This Hosp.	State Avg.	U.S. Avg.
Blood Clot Prevention and Treatment				
Anticoagulation Overlap Therapy[2]	11	91%	90%	93%
ICU Venous Thromboembolism Prophylaxis[2]	27	89%	86%	92%
Incidence of Potentially Preventable VTE[2,7]	-	-	13%	10%
UFH with Dosages/Platelet Monitoring[1,2]	-	-	98%	97%
Venous Thromboembolism Prophylaxis[2]	180	77%	80%	85%
Warfarin Therapy Discharge Instructions[1,2]	-	-	72%	75%
Chest Pain/Possible Heart Attack Care				
Aspirin Given Within 24 Hours of Arrival	196	100%	97%	96%
Fibrinolytic Meds Within 30 Min. of Arrival	19	68%	63%	58%
Average Time to ECG (minutes)	199	8	6	7
Average Time to Transfer (minutes)[1]	-	-	61	60
Children's Asthma Care				
Received Home Management Plan of Care	-	-	-	88%
Received Reliever Medication	-	-	-	100%
Received Systemic Corticosteroids	-	-	-	100%
Emergency Department				
Admittance Decision Time (minutes)[2]	223	85	78	98
Head CT Results Within 45 Min. of Arrival	16	25%	55%	57%
Patients Who Left ER Before Being Seen	21,861	5%	2%	2%
Time from ER Arrival to Admit. (minutes)[2]	252	275	238	274
Time from ER Arrival to Discharge (minutes)	365	191	126	134
Time in ER Before Being Evaluated (minutes)	415	42	23	26
Time to Pain Meds for Fractures (minutes)	133	89	56	57
Heart Attack Care				
Aspirin Given at Discharge[1]	-	-	99%	99%
Fibrinolytic Meds Within 30 Min. of Arrival[7]	-	-	-	54%
PCI Within 90 Minutes of Arrival[7]	-	-	97%	96%
Statin Prescribed at Discharge[1]	-	-	97%	98%
Heart Failure Care				
ACE Inhibitor or ARB for LVSD	19	89%	95%	97%
Discharge Instructions Given	57	96%	92%	94%
Evaluation of LVS Function	74	100%	98%	99%
Medicare Spending				
Medicare Spending per Patient (ratio)	-	0.90	0.97	0.98
Pneumonia Care				
Appropriate Initial Antibiotic Given	111	96%	94%	95%
Blood Culture Timing	156	99%	98%	98%
Pregnancy and Delivery Care				
Newborn Deliveries Scheduled Early[2]	19	0%	9%	6%

NOTE: Hospital profiles are in alphabetical order by state, then city, then hospital within the city; Rankings exclude hospitals with less than 25 cases except for patient surveys which excludes hospitals with less than 100 cases; (a) 100-299 cases; (1) The number of cases/patients is too few to report; (2) Data submitted were based on a sample of cases/patients; (3) Results are based on a shorter time period than required; (4) Data suppressed by CMS for one or more quarters; (5) Results are not available for this reporting period; (6) Fewer than 100 patients completed the HCAHPS survey; (7) No cases met the criteria for this measure; (8) The lower limit of the confidence interval cannot be calculated if the number of observed infections equals zero; (9) No data are available from the state/territory for this reporting period; (10) The scores shown reflect fewer than 50 completed surveys; (11) There were discrepancies in the data collection process; (12) This measure does not apply to this hospital for this reporting period; (13) Results cannot be calculated for this reporting period; (14) The results for this state are combined with nearby states to protect confidentiality; Please refer to the User's Guide for a full explanation of data.

Measure	Cases	This Hosp.	State Avg.	U.S. Avg.
Preventive Care				
Immunization for Influenza[2]	301	91%	92%	90%
Immunization for Pneumonia[2]	390	94%	94%	92%
Stroke Care				
Anticoagulation Therapy for Atrial Fibrillation[2,7]	-	-	95%	95%
Antithrombotic Therapy Timing[1,2]	-	-	97%	98%
Assessed for Rehabilitation[2]	12	100%	97%	97%
Discharged on Antithrombotic Therapy[2]	12	92%	98%	99%
Discharged on Statin Medication[2]	11	82%	93%	94%
Thrombolytic Therapy Timing[1,2]	-	-	59%	66%
Venous Thromboembolism Prophylaxis[1,2]	-	-	93%	94%
Written Stroke Educational Materials Given[1,2]	-	-	86%	88%
Surgical Care Improvement Project				
Appropriate Beta Blocker Usage[2]	75	97%	98%	98%
Appropriate VTP Within 24 Hours[2]	282	99%	98%	98%
Controlled Postoperative Blood Glucose[2,7]	-	-	96%	97%
Perioperative Temperature Management[2]	296	100%	100%	100%
Prophylactic Antibiotic Selection[2]	232	100%	99%	99%
Prophylactic Antibiotic Selection (Outpatient)	38	82%	97%	98%
Prophylactic Antibiotic Stopped[2]	226	100%	98%	98%
Prophylactic Antibiotic Timing[2]	232	100%	99%	99%
Prophylactic Antibiotic Timing (Outpatient)	39	95%	97%	98%
Urinary Catheter Removal[2]	264	99%	97%	97%
Survey of Patients' Hospital Experiences				
Area Around Room 'Always' Quiet at Night	(a)	63%	64%	61%
Doctors 'Always' Communicated Well	(a)	83%	84%	82%
Home Recovery Information Given	(a)	88%	86%	85%
Hospital Given 9 or 10 on 10 Point Scale	(a)	77%	72%	71%
Meds 'Always' Explained Before Given	(a)	66%	66%	64%
Nurses 'Always' Communicated Well	(a)	80%	81%	79%
Pain 'Always' Well Controlled	(a)	73%	73%	71%
Room and Bathroom 'Always' Clean	(a)	69%	75%	73%
Timely Help 'Always' Received	(a)	65%	69%	68%
Would Definitely Recommend Hospital	(a)	71%	71%	71%
Use of Medical Imaging				
Cardiac Imaging Stress Test before Surgery[1]	-	-	5.3%	5.3%
Combination Abdominal CT Scan	593	2.9%	10.7%	10.5%
Combination Brain/Sinus CT Scan	552	4.3%	3.1%	2.7%
Combination Chest CT Scan	327	0.3%	4.3%	2.7%
Follow-up Mammogram/Ultrasound	635	11.3%	8.3%	8.8%
Lumbar Spine MRI for Low Back Pain	134	33.6%	38.9%	37.2%

Marshall County Hospital

615 Old Symsonia Road
Benton, KY 42025
Phone: 270-527-4800
Fax: 270-527-4853
Type: Critical Access Hospitals
Emergency Services: Yes
Ownership: Govt - Hospital Dist/Auth
Beds: 80

Key Personnel:

Operating Room. . . . . Robert Beale
Coronary Care . . . . Lisa Bowlin
Intensive Care Unit. . . . . Lisa Bowlin
Quality Assurance . . . . Lisa Bowlin
CEO/President. . . . . Kathy Long
Chief of Medical Staff . . . . Glen Van Loon, MD
Infection Control. . . . . Mary Jo Myers
Emergency Room . . . . Sharon Sirls

Measure	Cases	This Hosp.	State Avg.	U.S. Avg.
Blood Clot Prevention and Treatment				
Anticoagulation Overlap Therapy[1]	-	-	90%	93%
ICU Venous Thromboembolism Prophylaxis	133	59%	86%	92%
Incidence of Potentially Preventable VTE[7]	-	-	13%	10%
UFH with Dosages/Platelet Monitoring[7]	-	-	98%	97%
Venous Thromboembolism Prophylaxis	15	13%	80%	85%
Warfarin Therapy Discharge Instructions[1]	-	-	72%	75%
Chest Pain/Possible Heart Attack Care				
Aspirin Given Within 24 Hours of Arrival[3]	58	86%	97%	96%
Fibrinolytic Meds Within 30 Min. of Arrival[1,3]	-	-	63%	58%
Average Time to ECG (minutes)[3]	61	5	6	7
Average Time to Transfer (minutes)[1,3]	-	-	61	60
Children's Asthma Care				
Received Home Management Plan of Care	-	-	-	88%
Received Reliever Medication	-	-	-	100%
Received Systemic Corticosteroids	-	-	-	100%
Emergency Department				
Admittance Decision Time (minutes)[2]	294	50	78	98
Head CT Results Within 45 Min. of Arrival[1,3]	-	-	55%	57%
Patients Who Left ER Before Being Seen	8,737	1%	2%	2%
Time from ER Arrival to Admit. (minutes)[2]	339	200	238	274
Time from ER Arrival to Discharge (minutes)[3]	705	89	126	134
Time in ER Before Being Evaluated (minutes)[3]	666	20	23	26
Time to Pain Meds for Fractures (minutes)[3]	40	59	56	57
Heart Attack Care				
Aspirin Given at Discharge[5]	-	-	99%	99%
Fibrinolytic Meds Within 30 Min. of Arrival[5]	-	-	-	54%
PCI Within 90 Minutes of Arrival[5]	-	-	97%	96%
Statin Prescribed at Discharge[5]	-	-	97%	98%
Heart Failure Care				
ACE Inhibitor or ARB for LVSD	16	81%	95%	97%
Discharge Instructions Given	38	95%	92%	94%
Evaluation of LVS Function	55	96%	98%	99%
Medicare Spending				
Medicare Spending per Patient (ratio)	-	-	0.97	0.98
Pneumonia Care				
Appropriate Initial Antibiotic Given	45	78%	94%	95%
Blood Culture Timing	50	96%	98%	98%
Pregnancy and Delivery Care				
Newborn Deliveries Scheduled Early[5]	-	-	9%	6%
Preventive Care				
Immunization for Influenza[2]	437	94%	92%	90%
Immunization for Pneumonia[2]	653	95%	94%	92%
Stroke Care				
Anticoagulation Therapy for Atrial Fibrillation[3,7]	-	-	95%	95%
Antithrombotic Therapy Timing[3,7]	-	-	97%	98%
Assessed for Rehabilitation[1,3]	-	-	97%	97%
Discharged on Antithrombotic Therapy[3,7]	-	-	98%	99%
Discharged on Statin Medication[3,7]	-	-	93%	94%
Thrombolytic Therapy Timing[3,7]	-	-	59%	66%
Venous Thromboembolism Prophylaxis[1,3]	-	-	93%	94%
Written Stroke Educational Materials Given[1,3]	-	-	86%	88%
Surgical Care Improvement Project				
Appropriate Beta Blocker Usage[3,7]	-	-	98%	98%
Appropriate VTP Within 24 Hours[1]	-	-	98%	98%
Controlled Postoperative Blood Glucose[3,7]	-	-	96%	97%
Perioperative Temperature Management[1]	-	-	100%	100%
Prophylactic Antibiotic Selection[1]	-	-	99%	99%
Prophylactic Antibiotic Selection (Outpatient)[5]	-	-	97%	98%
Prophylactic Antibiotic Stopped[1]	-	-	98%	98%
Prophylactic Antibiotic Timing[1]	-	-	99%	99%
Prophylactic Antibiotic Timing (Outpatient)[5]	-	-	97%	98%
Urinary Catheter Removal[1]	-	-	97%	97%
Survey of Patients' Hospital Experiences				
Area Around Room 'Always' Quiet at Night[5]	-	-	64%	61%
Doctors 'Always' Communicated Well[5]	-	-	84%	82%
Home Recovery Information Given[5]	-	-	86%	85%
Hospital Given 9 or 10 on 10 Point Scale[5]	-	-	72%	71%
Meds 'Always' Explained Before Given[5]	-	-	66%	64%
Nurses 'Always' Communicated Well[5]	-	-	81%	79%
Pain 'Always' Well Controlled[5]	-	-	73%	71%
Room and Bathroom 'Always' Clean[5]	-	-	75%	73%
Timely Help 'Always' Received[5]	-	-	69%	68%
Would Definitely Recommend Hospital[5]	-	-	71%	71%
Use of Medical Imaging				
Cardiac Imaging Stress Test before Surgery[1]	-	-	5.3%	5.3%
Combination Abdominal CT Scan	287	11.8%	10.7%	10.5%
Combination Brain/Sinus CT Scan[1]	-	-	3.1%	2.7%
Combination Chest CT Scan	174	0.6%	4.3%	2.7%
Follow-up Mammogram/Ultrasound	304	4.6%	8.3%	8.8%
Lumbar Spine MRI for Low Back Pain[7]	-	-	38.9%	37.2%

Saint Joseph Berea

305 Estill Street
Berea, KY 40403
Phone: 859-986-6500
Fax: 859-986-6768
E-mail: info@bereahospital.org
URL: www.bereahospital.org
Type: Critical Access Hospitals
Emergency Services: Yes
Ownership: Voluntary non-profit - Private
Beds: 48

Key Personnel:

Chief of Medical Staff . . . . Saves Desai, MD
CEO/President. . . . . Greg Gerard
Patient Relations . . . . Katie Heckman
Intensive Care Unit. . . . . Mary Kemper
Operating Room. . . . . Kent Kessler
Quality Assurance . . . . Darlene Matekovich
Emergency Room . . . . John Mullins, MD
Infection Control. . . . . Helen Rice

Measure	Cases	This Hosp.	State Avg.	U.S. Avg.
Blood Clot Prevention and Treatment				
Anticoagulation Overlap Therapy[5]	-	-	90%	93%
ICU Venous Thromboembolism Prophylaxis[5]	-	-	86%	92%
Incidence of Potentially Preventable VTE[5]	-	-	13%	10%
UFH with Dosages/Platelet Monitoring[5]	-	-	98%	97%
Venous Thromboembolism Prophylaxis[5]	-	-	80%	85%
Warfarin Therapy Discharge Instructions[5]	-	-	72%	75%
Chest Pain/Possible Heart Attack Care				
Aspirin Given Within 24 Hours of Arrival[5]	-	-	97%	96%
Fibrinolytic Meds Within 30 Min. of Arrival[5]	-	-	63%	58%
Average Time to ECG (minutes)[5]	-	-	6	7
Average Time to Transfer (minutes)[5]	-	-	61	60
Children's Asthma Care				
Received Home Management Plan of Care	-	-	-	88%
Received Reliever Medication	-	-	-	100%
Received Systemic Corticosteroids	-	-	-	100%
Emergency Department				
Admittance Decision Time (minutes)[5]	-	-	78	98
Head CT Results Within 45 Min. of Arrival[5]	-	-	55%	57%
Patients Who Left ER Before Being Seen	21,825	2%	2%	2%
Time from ER Arrival to Admit. (minutes)[5]	-	-	238	274
Time from ER Arrival to Discharge (minutes)[5]	-	-	126	134
Time in ER Before Being Evaluated (minutes)[5]	-	-	23	26
Time to Pain Meds for Fractures (minutes)[5]	-	-	56	57
Heart Attack Care				
Aspirin Given at Discharge[1]	-	-	99%	99%
Fibrinolytic Meds Within 30 Min. of Arrival[7]	-	-	-	54%
PCI Within 90 Minutes of Arrival[7]	-	-	97%	96%
Statin Prescribed at Discharge	11	100%	97%	98%
Heart Failure Care				
ACE Inhibitor or ARB for LVSD[1]	-	-	95%	97%
Discharge Instructions Given	19	100%	92%	94%
Evaluation of LVS Function	25	100%	98%	99%
Medicare Spending				
Medicare Spending per Patient (ratio)	-	-	0.97	0.98
Pneumonia Care				
Appropriate Initial Antibiotic Given	63	97%	94%	95%
Blood Culture Timing	68	100%	98%	98%
Pregnancy and Delivery Care				
Newborn Deliveries Scheduled Early[5]	-	-	9%	6%
Preventive Care				
Immunization for Influenza[5]	-	-	92%	90%
Immunization for Pneumonia[5]	-	-	94%	92%
Stroke Care				
Anticoagulation Therapy for Atrial Fibrillation[5]	-	-	95%	95%
Antithrombotic Therapy Timing[5]	-	-	97%	98%
Assessed for Rehabilitation[5]	-	-	97%	97%
Discharged on Antithrombotic Therapy[5]	-	-	98%	99%
Discharged on Statin Medication[5]	-	-	93%	94%
Thrombolytic Therapy Timing[5]	-	-	59%	66%
Venous Thromboembolism Prophylaxis[5]	-	-	93%	94%
Written Stroke Educational Materials Given[5]	-	-	86%	88%
Surgical Care Improvement Project				
Appropriate Beta Blocker Usage	14	100%	98%	98%
Appropriate VTP Within 24 Hours	36	94%	98%	98%
Controlled Postoperative Blood Glucose[7]	-	-	96%	97%
Perioperative Temperature Management	39	100%	100%	100%
Prophylactic Antibiotic Selection	27	100%	99%	99%
Prophylactic Antibiotic Selection (Outpatient)[5]	-	-	97%	98%
Prophylactic Antibiotic Stopped	27	96%	98%	98%
Prophylactic Antibiotic Timing	27	100%	99%	99%
Prophylactic Antibiotic Timing (Outpatient)[5]	-	-	97%	98%
Urinary Catheter Removal	29	100%	97%	97%
Survey of Patients' Hospital Experiences				
Area Around Room 'Always' Quiet at Night	(a)	70%	64%	61%

NOTE: Hospital profiles are in alphabetical order by state, then city, then hospital within the city; Rankings exclude hospitals with less than 25 cases except for patient surveys which excludes hospitals with less than 100 cases; (a) 100-299 cases; (1) The number of cases/patients is too few to report; (2) Data submitted were based on a sample of cases/patients; (3) Results are based on a shorter time period than required; (4) Data suppressed by CMS for one or more quarters; (5) Results are not available for this reporting period; (6) Fewer than 100 patients completed the HCAHPS survey; (7) No cases met the criteria for this measure; (8) The lower limit of the confidence interval cannot be calculated if the number of observed infections equals zero; (9) No data are available from the state/territory for this reporting period; (10) The scores shown reflect fewer than 50 completed surveys; (11) There were discrepancies in the data collection process; (12) This measure does not apply to this hospital for this reporting period; (13) Results cannot be calculated for this reporting period; (14) The results for this state are combined with nearby states to protect confidentiality; Please refer to the User's Guide for a full explanation of data.

Measure	Cases	This Hosp.	State Avg.	U.S. Avg.
Doctors 'Always' Communicated Well	(a)	88%	84%	82%
Home Recovery Information Given	(a)	89%	86%	85%
Hospital Given 9 or 10 on 10 Point Scale	(a)	77%	72%	71%
Meds 'Always' Explained Before Given	(a)	74%	66%	64%
Nurses 'Always' Communicated Well	(a)	83%	81%	79%
Pain 'Always' Well Controlled	(a)	73%	73%	71%
Room and Bathroom 'Always' Clean	(a)	80%	75%	73%
Timely Help 'Always' Received	(a)	75%	69%	68%
Would Definitely Recommend Hospital	(a)	78%	71%	71%
Use of Medical Imaging				
Cardiac Imaging Stress Test before Surgery	200	5.0%	5.3%	5.3%
Combination Abdominal CT Scan	468	4.3%	10.7%	10.5%
Combination Brain/Sinus CT Scan[1]	-	-	3.1%	2.7%
Combination Chest CT Scan	301	4.3%	4.3%	2.7%
Follow-up Mammogram/Ultrasound	359	6.4%	8.3%	8.8%
Lumbar Spine MRI for Low Back Pain	42	38.1%	38.9%	37.2%

Greenview Regional Hospital

1801 Ashley Circle
Bowling Green, KY 42104
Phone: 270-793-1000
URL: www.greenviewhospital.com
Type: Acute Care Hospitals
Emergency Services: Yes
Ownership: Proprietary
Beds: 211
Key Personnel:
CEO . . . . Mark Marsh

Measure	Cases	This Hosp.	State Avg.	U.S. Avg.
Blood Clot Prevention and Treatment				
Anticoagulation Overlap Therapy[2]	23	100%	90%	93%
ICU Venous Thromboembolism Prophylaxis[2]	65	100%	86%	92%
Incidence of Potentially Preventable VTE[1,2]	-	-	13%	10%
UFH with Dosages/Platelet Monitoring[1,2]	-	-	98%	97%
Venous Thromboembolism Prophylaxis[2]	327	99%	80%	85%
Warfarin Therapy Discharge Instructions[2]	19	100%	72%	75%
Chest Pain/Possible Heart Attack Care				
Aspirin Given Within 24 Hours of Arrival	27	100%	97%	96%
Fibrinolytic Meds Within 30 Min. of Arrival[7]	-	-	63%	58%
Average Time to ECG (minutes)	29	8	6	7
Average Time to Transfer (minutes)[1]	-	-	61	60
Children's Asthma Care				
Received Home Management Plan of Care	-	-	-	88%
Received Reliever Medication	-	-	-	100%
Received Systemic Corticosteroids	-	-	-	100%
Emergency Department				
Admittance Decision Time (minutes)[2]	506	110	78	98
Head CT Results Within 45 Min. of Arrival[1]	-	-	55%	57%
Patients Who Left ER Before Being Seen	31,297	1%	2%	2%
Time from ER Arrival to Admit. (minutes)[2]	506	248	238	274
Time from ER Arrival to Discharge (minutes)	478	127	126	134
Time in ER Before Being Evaluated (minutes)	502	15	23	26
Time to Pain Meds for Fractures (minutes)	139	38	56	57
Heart Attack Care				
Aspirin Given at Discharge	30	100%	99%	99%
Fibrinolytic Meds Within 30 Min. of Arrival[7]	-	-	-	54%
PCI Within 90 Minutes of Arrival[1]	-	-	97%	96%
Statin Prescribed at Discharge	26	100%	97%	98%
Heart Failure Care				
ACE Inhibitor or ARB for LVSD	16	100%	95%	97%
Discharge Instructions Given	57	100%	92%	94%
Evaluation of LVS Function	90	100%	98%	99%
Medicare Spending				
Medicare Spending per Patient (ratio)	-	1.03	0.97	0.98
Pneumonia Care				
Appropriate Initial Antibiotic Given	71	99%	94%	95%
Blood Culture Timing	111	99%	98%	98%
Pregnancy and Delivery Care				
Newborn Deliveries Scheduled Early[2,7]	-	-	9%	6%
Preventive Care				
Immunization for Influenza[2]	434	99%	92%	90%
Immunization for Pneumonia[2]	660	99%	94%	92%
Stroke Care				
Anticoagulation Therapy for Atrial Fibrillation[1]	-	-	95%	95%
Antithrombotic Therapy Timing	41	100%	97%	98%
Assessed for Rehabilitation	46	98%	97%	97%
Discharged on Antithrombotic Therapy	40	100%	98%	99%
Discharged on Statin Medication	27	100%	93%	94%
Thrombolytic Therapy Timing[1]	-	-	59%	66%
Venous Thromboembolism Prophylaxis	50	100%	93%	94%
Written Stroke Educational Materials Given	16	94%	86%	88%
Surgical Care Improvement Project				
Appropriate Beta Blocker Usage	244	100%	98%	98%
Appropriate VTP Within 24 Hours	621	99%	98%	98%
Controlled Postoperative Blood Glucose[7]	-	-	96%	97%
Perioperative Temperature Management	694	100%	100%	100%
Prophylactic Antibiotic Selection	549	100%	99%	99%
Prophylactic Antibiotic Selection (Outpatient)	125	100%	97%	98%
Prophylactic Antibiotic Stopped	530	99%	98%	98%
Prophylactic Antibiotic Timing	549	100%	99%	99%
Prophylactic Antibiotic Timing (Outpatient)	127	98%	97%	98%
Urinary Catheter Removal	460	100%	97%	97%
Survey of Patients' Hospital Experiences				
Area Around Room 'Always' Quiet at Night	300+	64%	64%	61%
Doctors 'Always' Communicated Well	300+	82%	84%	82%
Home Recovery Information Given	300+	87%	86%	85%
Hospital Given 9 or 10 on 10 Point Scale	300+	74%	72%	71%
Meds 'Always' Explained Before Given	300+	67%	66%	64%
Nurses 'Always' Communicated Well	300+	79%	81%	79%
Pain 'Always' Well Controlled	300+	70%	73%	71%
Room and Bathroom 'Always' Clean	300+	77%	75%	73%
Timely Help 'Always' Received	300+	64%	69%	68%
Would Definitely Recommend Hospital	300+	80%	71%	71%
Use of Medical Imaging				
Cardiac Imaging Stress Test before Surgery	118	6.8%	5.3%	5.3%
Combination Abdominal CT Scan	681	19.2%	10.7%	10.5%
Combination Brain/Sinus CT Scan[1]	-	-	3.1%	2.7%
Combination Chest CT Scan	133	0.8%	4.3%	2.7%
Follow-up Mammogram/Ultrasound	330	11.5%	8.3%	8.8%
Lumbar Spine MRI for Low Back Pain	69	47.8%	38.9%	37.2%

The Medical Center at Bowling Green

250 Park Street
Bowling Green, KY 42101
Phone: 270-745-1000
Fax: 270-745-1253
E-mail: skwebb@mcbg.org
URL: www.mcbg.org
Type: Acute Care Hospitals
Emergency Services: Yes
Ownership: Voluntary non-profit - Private
Beds: 330
Key Personnel:
Radiology. . . . . Ken Bartholomew, MD
Hemotology Center . . . . Sandy Durrance, RN
Pediatric Ambulatory Care . . . . . . Zahid Fraser, MD
Pediatric In-Patient Care . . . . Zahid Fraser, MD
Quality Assurance . . . . Gerri Glenn
CEO/President. . . . . Connie D. Smith, MD
Intensive Care Unit. . . . . Barbara Wolfe, RN

Measure	Cases	This Hosp.	State Avg.	U.S. Avg.
Blood Clot Prevention and Treatment				
Anticoagulation Overlap Therapy[2]	110	97%	90%	93%
ICU Venous Thromboembolism Prophylaxis[2]	86	94%	86%	92%
Incidence of Potentially Preventable VTE[1,2]	-	-	13%	10%
UFH with Dosages/Platelet Monitoring[2]	69	100%	98%	97%
Venous Thromboembolism Prophylaxis[2]	366	92%	80%	85%
Warfarin Therapy Discharge Instructions[2]	76	95%	72%	75%
Chest Pain/Possible Heart Attack Care				
Aspirin Given Within 24 Hours of Arrival[1,3]	-	-	97%	96%
Fibrinolytic Meds Within 30 Min. of Arrival[5]	-	-	63%	58%
Average Time to ECG (minutes)[1,3]	-	-	6	7
Average Time to Transfer (minutes)[5]	-	-	61	60
Children's Asthma Care				
Received Home Management Plan of Care	-	-	-	88%
Received Reliever Medication	-	-	-	100%
Received Systemic Corticosteroids	-	-	-	100%
Emergency Department				
Admittance Decision Time (minutes)[2]	264	80	78	98
Head CT Results Within 45 Min. of Arrival[1]	-	-	55%	57%
Patients Who Left ER Before Being Seen	47,343	4%	2%	2%
Time from ER Arrival to Admit. (minutes)[2]	392	256	238	274
Time from ER Arrival to Discharge (minutes)	375	170	126	134
Time in ER Before Being Evaluated (minutes)	399	50	23	26
Time to Pain Meds for Fractures (minutes)	143	73	56	57
Heart Attack Care				
Aspirin Given at Discharge	705	97%	99%	99%
Fibrinolytic Meds Within 30 Min. of Arrival[7]	-	-	-	54%
PCI Within 90 Minutes of Arrival	43	95%	97%	96%
Statin Prescribed at Discharge	695	88%	97%	98%
Heart Failure Care				
ACE Inhibitor or ARB for LVSD	154	78%	95%	97%
Discharge Instructions Given	455	90%	92%	94%
Evaluation of LVS Function	561	94%	98%	99%
Medicare Spending				
Medicare Spending per Patient (ratio)	-	1.05	0.97	0.98
Pneumonia Care				
Appropriate Initial Antibiotic Given	174	89%	94%	95%
Blood Culture Timing	207	97%	98%	98%
Pregnancy and Delivery Care				
Newborn Deliveries Scheduled Early	284	14%	9%	6%
Preventive Care				
Immunization for Influenza[2]	554	90%	92%	90%
Immunization for Pneumonia[2]	669	89%	94%	92%
Stroke Care				
Anticoagulation Therapy for Atrial Fibrillation	30	93%	95%	95%
Antithrombotic Therapy Timing	251	95%	97%	98%
Assessed for Rehabilitation	288	95%	97%	97%
Discharged on Antithrombotic Therapy	267	99%	98%	99%
Discharged on Statin Medication	213	92%	93%	94%
Thrombolytic Therapy Timing	20	45%	59%	66%
Venous Thromboembolism Prophylaxis	296	97%	93%	94%
Written Stroke Educational Materials Given	174	89%	86%	88%
Surgical Care Improvement Project				
Appropriate Beta Blocker Usage	489	96%	98%	98%
Appropriate VTP Within 24 Hours	664	96%	98%	98%
Controlled Postoperative Blood Glucose	309	88%	96%	97%
Perioperative Temperature Management	870	99%	100%	100%
Prophylactic Antibiotic Selection	743	99%	99%	99%
Prophylactic Antibiotic Selection (Outpatient)	466	97%	97%	98%
Prophylactic Antibiotic Stopped	733	97%	98%	98%
Prophylactic Antibiotic Timing	745	98%	99%	99%
Prophylactic Antibiotic Timing (Outpatient)	482	91%	97%	98%
Urinary Catheter Removal	762	96%	97%	97%
Survey of Patients' Hospital Experiences				
Area Around Room 'Always' Quiet at Night[11]	300+	64%	64%	61%
Doctors 'Always' Communicated Well[11]	300+	80%	84%	82%
Home Recovery Information Given[11]	300+	87%	86%	85%
Hospital Given 9 or 10 on 10 Point Scale[11]	300+	71%	72%	71%
Meds 'Always' Explained Before Given[11]	300+	65%	66%	64%
Nurses 'Always' Communicated Well[11]	300+	77%	81%	79%
Pain 'Always' Well Controlled[11]	300+	70%	73%	71%
Room and Bathroom 'Always' Clean[11]	300+	70%	75%	73%
Timely Help 'Always' Received[11]	300+	63%	69%	68%
Would Definitely Recommend Hospital[11]	300+	74%	71%	71%
Use of Medical Imaging				
Cardiac Imaging Stress Test before Surgery	163	9.2%	5.3%	5.3%
Combination Abdominal CT Scan	816	9.9%	10.7%	10.5%
Combination Brain/Sinus CT Scan	973	3.5%	3.1%	2.7%
Combination Chest CT Scan	371	3.0%	4.3%	2.7%
Follow-up Mammogram/Ultrasound	1,658	9.7%	8.3%	8.8%
Lumbar Spine MRI for Low Back Pain	244	36.5%	38.9%	37.2%

Cumberland County Hospital

299 Glasgow Road
Burkesville, KY 42717
Phone: 270-864-2511
Fax: 270-864-1307
E-mail: administration@cchospital.org
URL: www.cumberlandhospital.org
Type: Critical Access Hospitals
Emergency Services: Yes
Ownership: Voluntary non-profit - Other
Beds: 31
Key Personnel:
CEO/President. . . . . Edward J Sanford

Measure	Cases	This Hosp.	State Avg.	U.S. Avg.
Blood Clot Prevention and Treatment				
Anticoagulation Overlap Therapy[1,2]	-	-	90%	93%
ICU Venous Thromboembolism Prophylaxis[1,2]	-	-	86%	92%
Incidence of Potentially Preventable VTE[2,7]	-	-	13%	10%

NOTE: Hospital profiles are in alphabetical order by state, then city, then hospital within the city; Rankings exclude hospitals with less than 25 cases except for patient surveys which excludes hospitals with less than 100 cases; (a) 100-299 cases; (1) The number of cases/patients is too few to report; (2) Data submitted were based on a sample of cases/patients; (3) Results are based on a shorter time period than required; (4) Data suppressed by CMS for one or more quarters; (5) Results are not available for this reporting period; (6) Fewer than 100 patients completed the HCAHPS survey; (7) No cases met the criteria for this measure; (8) The lower limit of the confidence interval cannot be calculated if the number of observed infections equals zero; (9) No data are available from the state/territory for this reporting period; (10) The scores shown reflect fewer than 50 completed surveys; (11) There were discrepancies in the data collection process; (12) This measure does not apply to this hospital for this reporting period; (13) Results cannot be calculated for this reporting period; (14) The results for this state are combined with nearby states to protect confidentiality; Please refer to the User's Guide for a full explanation of data.

Measure	Cases	This Hosp.	State Avg.	U.S. Avg.
UFH with Dosages/Platelet Monitoring[1,2]	-	-	98%	97%
Venous Thromboembolism Prophylaxis[2]	336	14%	80%	85%
Warfarin Therapy Discharge Instructions[1,2]	-	-	72%	75%
Chest Pain/Possible Heart Attack Care				
Aspirin Given Within 24 Hours of Arrival	15	93%	97%	96%
Fibrinolytic Meds Within 30 Min. of Arrival[1]	-	-	63%	58%
Average Time to ECG (minutes)	16	5	6	7
Average Time to Transfer (minutes)[1]	-	-	61	60
Children's Asthma Care				
Received Home Management Plan of Care	-	-	-	88%
Received Reliever Medication	-	-	-	100%
Received Systemic Corticosteroids	-	-	-	100%
Emergency Department				
Admittance Decision Time (minutes)[5]	-	-	78	98
Head CT Results Within 45 Min. of Arrival[1,3]	-	-	55%	57%
Patients Who Left ER Before Being Seen	6,346	0%	2%	2%
Time from ER Arrival to Admit. (minutes)[5]	-	-	238	274
Time from ER Arrival to Discharge (minutes)[5]	-	-	126	134
Time in ER Before Being Evaluated (minutes)[5]	-	-	23	26
Time to Pain Meds for Fractures (minutes)[5]	-	-	56	57
Heart Attack Care				
Aspirin Given at Discharge[1]	-	-	99%	99%
Fibrinolytic Meds Within 30 Min. of Arrival[7]	-	-	-	54%
PCI Within 90 Minutes of Arrival[7]	-	-	97%	96%
Statin Prescribed at Discharge[1]	-	-	97%	98%
Heart Failure Care				
ACE Inhibitor or ARB for LVSD[1]	-	-	95%	97%
Discharge Instructions Given	33	88%	92%	94%
Evaluation of LVS Function	40	40%	98%	99%
Medicare Spending				
Medicare Spending per Patient (ratio)	-	-	0.97	0.98
Pneumonia Care				
Appropriate Initial Antibiotic Given	39	56%	94%	95%
Blood Culture Timing	23	96%	98%	98%
Pregnancy and Delivery Care				
Newborn Deliveries Scheduled Early[5]	-	-	9%	6%
Preventive Care				
Immunization for Influenza	378	89%	92%	90%
Immunization for Pneumonia[2]	579	93%	94%	92%
Stroke Care				
Anticoagulation Therapy for Atrial Fibrillation[3,7]	-	-	95%	95%
Antithrombotic Therapy Timing[1,3]	-	-	97%	98%
Assessed for Rehabilitation[1,3]	-	-	97%	97%
Discharged on Antithrombotic Therapy[1,3]	-	-	98%	99%
Discharged on Statin Medication[1,3]	-	-	93%	94%
Thrombolytic Therapy Timing[1,3]	-	-	59%	66%
Venous Thromboembolism Prophylaxis[1,3]	-	-	93%	94%
Written Stroke Educational Materials Given[1,3]	-	-	86%	88%
Surgical Care Improvement Project				
Appropriate Beta Blocker Usage[5]	-	-	98%	98%
Appropriate VTP Within 24 Hours[5]	-	-	98%	98%
Controlled Postoperative Blood Glucose[5]	-	-	96%	97%
Perioperative Temperature Management[5]	-	-	100%	100%
Prophylactic Antibiotic Selection[5]	-	-	99%	99%
Prophylactic Antibiotic Selection (Outpatient)[5]	-	-	97%	98%
Prophylactic Antibiotic Stopped[5]	-	-	98%	98%
Prophylactic Antibiotic Timing[5]	-	-	99%	99%
Prophylactic Antibiotic Timing (Outpatient)[5]	-	-	97%	98%
Urinary Catheter Removal[5]	-	-	97%	97%
Survey of Patients' Hospital Experiences				
Area Around Room 'Always' Quiet at Night[5]	-	-	64%	61%
Doctors 'Always' Communicated Well[5]	-	-	84%	82%
Home Recovery Information Given[5]	-	-	86%	85%
Hospital Given 9 or 10 on 10 Point Scale[5]	-	-	72%	71%
Meds 'Always' Explained Before Given[5]	-	-	66%	64%
Nurses 'Always' Communicated Well[5]	-	-	81%	79%
Pain 'Always' Well Controlled[5]	-	-	73%	71%
Room and Bathroom 'Always' Clean[5]	-	-	75%	73%
Timely Help 'Always' Received[5]	-	-	69%	68%
Would Definitely Recommend Hospital[5]	-	-	71%	71%
Use of Medical Imaging				
Cardiac Imaging Stress Test before Surgery[1]	-	-	5.3%	5.3%
Combination Abdominal CT Scan	85	12.9%	10.7%	10.5%
Combination Brain/Sinus CT Scan[1]	-	-	3.1%	2.7%
Combination Chest CT Scan	50	32.0%	4.3%	2.7%
Follow-up Mammogram/Ultrasound[7]	-	-	8.3%	8.8%
Lumbar Spine MRI for Low Back Pain[7]	-	-	38.9%	37.2%

Trigg County Hospital

254 Main Street
Cadiz, KY 42211
Phone: 270-522-3215
Fax: 270-522-6974
URL: www.trigghospital.org
Type: Critical Access Hospitals
Emergency Services: Yes
Ownership: Government - Local
Beds: 25

Key Personnel:

CEO/President. . . . . Alisa Coleman
Radiology. . . . . Jill Cunningham
Chief of Medical Staff. . . . . Stuart Harris, MD
Cardiac Laboratory. . . . . George Howe
Infection Control. . . . . Susanna May
Operating Room. . . . . Susanna May
Patient Relations . . . . Nicole Reamer
Emergency Room . . . . Frieda Wood

Measure	Cases	This Hosp.	State Avg.	U.S. Avg.
Blood Clot Prevention and Treatment				
Anticoagulation Overlap Therapy[7]	-	-	90%	93%
ICU Venous Thromboembolism Prophylaxis[7]	-	-	86%	92%
Incidence of Potentially Preventable VTE[7]	-	-	13%	10%
UFH with Dosages/Platelet Monitoring[7]	-	-	98%	97%
Venous Thromboembolism Prophylaxis	64	47%	80%	85%
Warfarin Therapy Discharge Instructions[7]	-	-	72%	75%
Chest Pain/Possible Heart Attack Care				
Aspirin Given Within 24 Hours of Arrival[1,3]	-	-	97%	96%
Fibrinolytic Meds Within 30 Min. of Arrival[3,7]	-	-	63%	58%
Average Time to ECG (minutes)[3]	11	7	6	7
Average Time to Transfer (minutes)[3,7]	-	-	61	60
Children's Asthma Care				
Received Home Management Plan of Care	-	-	-	88%
Received Reliever Medication	-	-	-	100%
Received Systemic Corticosteroids	-	-	-	100%
Emergency Department				
Admittance Decision Time (minutes)[2,3]	13	35	78	98
Head CT Results Within 45 Min. of Arrival[1,3]	-	-	55%	57%
Patients Who Left ER Before Being Seen	3,064	1%	2%	2%
Time from ER Arrival to Admit. (minutes)[2,3]	49	115	238	274
Time from ER Arrival to Discharge (minutes)	468	100	126	134
Time in ER Before Being Evaluated (minutes)	567	15	23	26
Time to Pain Meds for Fractures (minutes)[1,3]	-	-	56	57
Heart Attack Care				
Aspirin Given at Discharge[5]	-	-	99%	99%
Fibrinolytic Meds Within 30 Min. of Arrival[5]	-	-	-	54%
PCI Within 90 Minutes of Arrival[5]	-	-	97%	96%
Statin Prescribed at Discharge[5]	-	-	97%	98%
Heart Failure Care				
ACE Inhibitor or ARB for LVSD[3,7]	-	-	95%	97%
Discharge Instructions Given[3,7]	-	-	92%	94%
Evaluation of LVS Function[1,3]	-	-	98%	99%
Medicare Spending				
Medicare Spending per Patient (ratio)	-	-	0.97	0.98
Pneumonia Care				
Appropriate Initial Antibiotic Given[2]	26	73%	94%	95%
Blood Culture Timing[2]	17	94%	98%	98%
Pregnancy and Delivery Care				
Newborn Deliveries Scheduled Early[5]	-	-	9%	6%
Preventive Care				
Immunization for Influenza[3]	34	65%	92%	90%
Immunization for Pneumonia[2,3]	79	72%	94%	92%
Stroke Care				
Anticoagulation Therapy for Atrial Fibrillation[3,7]	-	-	95%	95%
Antithrombotic Therapy Timing[1,3]	-	-	97%	98%
Assessed for Rehabilitation[3,7]	-	-	97%	97%
Discharged on Antithrombotic Therapy[3,7]	-	-	98%	99%
Discharged on Statin Medication[3,7]	-	-	93%	94%
Thrombolytic Therapy Timing[3,7]	-	-	59%	66%
Venous Thromboembolism Prophylaxis[1,3]	-	-	93%	94%
Written Stroke Educational Materials Given[3,7]	-	-	86%	88%
Surgical Care Improvement Project				
Appropriate Beta Blocker Usage[5]	-	-	98%	98%
Appropriate VTP Within 24 Hours[5]	-	-	98%	98%
Controlled Postoperative Blood Glucose[5]	-	-	96%	97%
Perioperative Temperature Management[5]	-	-	100%	100%
Prophylactic Antibiotic Selection[5]	-	-	99%	99%
Prophylactic Antibiotic Selection (Outpatient)[5]	-	-	97%	98%
Prophylactic Antibiotic Stopped[5]	-	-	98%	98%
Prophylactic Antibiotic Timing[5]	-	-	99%	99%
Prophylactic Antibiotic Timing (Outpatient)[5]	-	-	97%	98%
Urinary Catheter Removal[5]	-	-	97%	97%
Survey of Patients' Hospital Experiences				
Area Around Room 'Always' Quiet at Night[10]	<100	72%	64%	61%
Doctors 'Always' Communicated Well[10]	<100	84%	84%	82%
Home Recovery Information Given[10]	<100	86%	86%	85%
Hospital Given 9 or 10 on 10 Point Scale[10]	<100	64%	72%	71%
Meds 'Always' Explained Before Given[10]	<100	64%	66%	64%
Nurses 'Always' Communicated Well[10]	<100	84%	81%	79%
Pain 'Always' Well Controlled[10]	<100	85%	73%	71%
Room and Bathroom 'Always' Clean[10]	<100	72%	75%	73%
Timely Help 'Always' Received[10]	<100	73%	69%	68%
Would Definitely Recommend Hospital[10]	<100	58%	71%	71%
Use of Medical Imaging				
Cardiac Imaging Stress Test before Surgery[7]	-	-	5.3%	5.3%
Combination Abdominal CT Scan	121	2.5%	10.7%	10.5%
Combination Brain/Sinus CT Scan[1]	-	-	3.1%	2.7%
Combination Chest CT Scan	47	0.0%	4.3%	2.7%
Follow-up Mammogram/Ultrasound	286	7.3%	8.3%	8.8%
Lumbar Spine MRI for Low Back Pain[1]	-	-	38.9%	37.2%

Taylor Regional Hospital

1700 Old Lebanon Road
Campbellsville, KY 42718
Phone: 270-465-3561
Fax: 270-789-5875
URL: www.tchosp.org
Type: Acute Care Hospitals
Emergency Services: Yes
Ownership: Govt - Hospital Dist/Auth
Beds: 90

Key Personnel:

Cardiology. . . . . Krishnan Challappa, M.D.
Anesthesiology. . . . . Gary Fraiz
Emergency Room . . . . Jennifer L Friend
Radiology. . . . . Cynthia Hart, MD
Anesthesiology. . . . . Paul Johnson, DO
Pulmonology . . . . Robert Karman
Radiology. . . . . Curtis Manning
CEO/President. . . . . Jane Wheatley

Measure	Cases	This Hosp.	State Avg.	U.S. Avg.
Blood Clot Prevention and Treatment				
Anticoagulation Overlap Therapy[2]	13	100%	90%	93%
ICU Venous Thromboembolism Prophylaxis[2]	59	95%	86%	92%
Incidence of Potentially Preventable VTE[1,2]	-	-	13%	10%
UFH with Dosages/Platelet Monitoring[2]	12	67%	98%	97%
Venous Thromboembolism Prophylaxis[2]	218	87%	80%	85%
Warfarin Therapy Discharge Instructions[1,2]	-	-	72%	75%
Chest Pain/Possible Heart Attack Care				
Aspirin Given Within 24 Hours of Arrival	75	99%	97%	96%
Fibrinolytic Meds Within 30 Min. of Arrival	16	81%	63%	58%
Average Time to ECG (minutes)	75	7	6	7
Average Time to Transfer (minutes)[1]	-	-	61	60
Children's Asthma Care				
Received Home Management Plan of Care	-	-	-	88%
Received Reliever Medication	-	-	-	100%
Received Systemic Corticosteroids	-	-	-	100%
Emergency Department				
Admittance Decision Time (minutes)[2]	253	59	78	98
Head CT Results Within 45 Min. of Arrival	13	62%	55%	57%
Patients Who Left ER Before Being Seen	20,070	1%	2%	2%
Time from ER Arrival to Admit. (minutes)[2]	254	210	238	274
Time from ER Arrival to Discharge (minutes)	394	117	126	134
Time in ER Before Being Evaluated (minutes)	442	21	23	26
Time to Pain Meds for Fractures (minutes)	56	64	56	57
Heart Attack Care				
Aspirin Given at Discharge	11	100%	99%	99%
Fibrinolytic Meds Within 30 Min. of Arrival[7]	-	-	-	54%
PCI Within 90 Minutes of Arrival[7]	-	-	97%	96%

NOTE: Hospital profiles are in alphabetical order by state, then city, then hospital within the city; Rankings exclude hospitals with less than 25 cases except for patient surveys which excludes hospitals with less than 100 cases; (a) 100-299 cases; (1) The number of cases/patients is too few to report; (2) Data submitted were based on a sample of cases/patients; (3) Results are based on a shorter time period than required; (4) Data suppressed by CMS for one or more quarters; (5) Results are not available for this reporting period; (6) Fewer than 100 patients completed the HCAHPS survey; (7) No cases met the criteria for this measure; (8) The lower limit of the confidence interval cannot be calculated if the number of observed infections equals zero; (9) No data are available from the state/territory for this reporting period; (10) The scores shown reflect fewer than 50 completed surveys; (11) There were discrepancies in the data collection process; (12) This measure does not apply to this hospital for this reporting period; (13) Results cannot be calculated for this reporting period; (14) The results for this state are combined with nearby states to protect confidentiality; Please refer to the User's Guide for a full explanation of data.

Measure	Cases	This Hosp.	State Avg.	U.S. Avg.
Statin Prescribed at Discharge	11	73%	97%	98%
Heart Failure Care				
ACE Inhibitor or ARB for LVSD	13	85%	95%	97%
Discharge Instructions Given	45	84%	92%	94%
Evaluation of LVS Function	61	100%	98%	99%
Medicare Spending				
Medicare Spending per Patient (ratio)	-	1.02	0.97	0.98
Pneumonia Care				
Appropriate Initial Antibiotic Given	88	94%	94%	95%
Blood Culture Timing	81	98%	98%	98%
Pregnancy and Delivery Care				
Newborn Deliveries Scheduled Early	34	18%	9%	6%
Preventive Care				
Immunization for Influenza[2]	321	89%	92%	90%
Immunization for Pneumonia[2]	413	95%	94%	92%
Stroke Care				
Anticoagulation Therapy for Atrial Fibrillation[7]	-	-	95%	95%
Antithrombotic Therapy Timing[1]	-	-	97%	98%
Assessed for Rehabilitation[1]	-	-	97%	97%
Discharged on Antithrombotic Therapy[1]	-	-	98%	99%
Discharged on Statin Medication[1]	-	-	93%	94%
Thrombolytic Therapy Timing[1]	-	-	59%	66%
Venous Thromboembolism Prophylaxis[1]	-	-	93%	94%
Written Stroke Educational Materials Given[7]	-	-	86%	88%
Surgical Care Improvement Project				
Appropriate Beta Blocker Usage	53	100%	98%	98%
Appropriate VTP Within 24 Hours	178	99%	98%	98%
Controlled Postoperative Blood Glucose[7]	-	-	96%	97%
Perioperative Temperature Management	186	100%	100%	100%
Prophylactic Antibiotic Selection	122	98%	99%	99%
Prophylactic Antibiotic Selection (Outpatient)	40	90%	97%	98%
Prophylactic Antibiotic Stopped	119	99%	98%	98%
Prophylactic Antibiotic Timing	122	99%	99%	99%
Prophylactic Antibiotic Timing (Outpatient)	40	100%	97%	98%
Urinary Catheter Removal	88	97%	97%	97%
Survey of Patients' Hospital Experiences				
Area Around Room 'Always' Quiet at Night	300+	60%	64%	61%
Doctors 'Always' Communicated Well	300+	85%	84%	82%
Home Recovery Information Given	300+	85%	86%	85%
Hospital Given 9 or 10 on 10 Point Scale	300+	68%	72%	71%
Meds 'Always' Explained Before Given	300+	62%	66%	64%
Nurses 'Always' Communicated Well	300+	80%	81%	79%
Pain 'Always' Well Controlled	300+	69%	73%	71%
Room and Bathroom 'Always' Clean	300+	76%	75%	73%
Timely Help 'Always' Received	300+	66%	69%	68%
Would Definitely Recommend Hospital	300+	70%	71%	71%
Use of Medical Imaging				
Cardiac Imaging Stress Test before Surgery	112	5.4%	5.3%	5.3%
Combination Abdominal CT Scan	651	17.7%	10.7%	10.5%
Combination Brain/Sinus CT Scan	622	4.2%	3.1%	2.7%
Combination Chest CT Scan	399	13.8%	4.3%	2.7%
Follow-up Mammogram/Ultrasound	995	7.9%	8.3%	8.8%
Lumbar Spine MRI for Low Back Pain	119	31.9%	38.9%	37.2%

Nicholas County Hospital

2325 Concrete Road
Carlisle, KY 40311
Phone: 859-289-7181
Fax: 859-289-7510
URL: www.johnsonmathers.org
Type: Critical Access Hospitals
Emergency Services: Yes
Ownership: Voluntary non-profit - Other
Beds: 18

Key Personnel:
Chief of Medical Staff.......... Stephen Besson, MD
Infection Control.............. Mendy Courtney, RN
Radiology.................... Otis Davis
CEO/President............... Doris Ecton
Emergency Room .... Carolyn Pope, RN

Measure	Cases	This Hosp.	State Avg.	U.S. Avg.
Blood Clot Prevention and Treatment				
Anticoagulation Overlap Therapy[5]	-	-	90%	93%
ICU Venous Thromboembolism Prophylaxis[5]	-	-	86%	92%
Incidence of Potentially Preventable VTE[5]	-	-	13%	10%
UFH with Dosages/Platelet Monitoring[5]	-	-	98%	97%
Venous Thromboembolism Prophylaxis[5]	-	-	80%	85%
Warfarin Therapy Discharge Instructions[5]	-	-	72%	75%
Chest Pain/Possible Heart Attack Care				
Aspirin Given Within 24 Hours of Arrival[1,3]	-	-	97%	96%
Fibrinolytic Meds Within 30 Min. of Arrival[3,7]	-	-	63%	58%
Average Time to ECG (minutes)[1,3]	-	-	6	7
Average Time to Transfer (minutes)[1,3]	-	-	61	60
Children's Asthma Care				
Received Home Management Plan of Care	-	-	-	88%
Received Reliever Medication	-	-	-	100%
Received Systemic Corticosteroids	-	-	-	100%
Emergency Department				
Admittance Decision Time (minutes)[5]	-	-	78	98
Head CT Results Within 45 Min. of Arrival[1,3]	-	-	55%	57%
Patients Who Left ER Before Being Seen	3,683	0%	2%	2%
Time from ER Arrival to Admit. (minutes)[5]	-	-	238	274
Time from ER Arrival to Discharge (minutes)[5]	-	-	126	134
Time in ER Before Being Evaluated (minutes)[5]	-	-	23	26
Time to Pain Meds for Fractures (minutes)[5]	-	-	56	57
Heart Attack Care				
Aspirin Given at Discharge[5]	-	-	99%	99%
Fibrinolytic Meds Within 30 Min. of Arrival[5]	-	-	-	54%
PCI Within 90 Minutes of Arrival[5]	-	-	97%	96%
Statin Prescribed at Discharge[5]	-	-	97%	98%
Heart Failure Care				
ACE Inhibitor or ARB for LVSD[1,3]	-	-	95%	97%
Discharge Instructions Given[1,3]	-	-	92%	94%
Evaluation of LVS Function[1,3]	-	-	98%	99%
Medicare Spending				
Medicare Spending per Patient (ratio)	-	-	0.97	0.98
Pneumonia Care				
Appropriate Initial Antibiotic Given	23	52%	94%	95%
Blood Culture Timing	18	89%	98%	98%
Pregnancy and Delivery Care				
Newborn Deliveries Scheduled Early[5]	-	-	9%	6%
Preventive Care				
Immunization for Influenza[5]	-	-	92%	90%
Immunization for Pneumonia[5]	-	-	94%	92%
Stroke Care				
Anticoagulation Therapy for Atrial Fibrillation[5]	-	-	95%	95%
Antithrombotic Therapy Timing[5]	-	-	97%	98%
Assessed for Rehabilitation[5]	-	-	97%	97%
Discharged on Antithrombotic Therapy[5]	-	-	98%	99%
Discharged on Statin Medication[5]	-	-	93%	94%
Thrombolytic Therapy Timing[5]	-	-	59%	66%
Venous Thromboembolism Prophylaxis[5]	-	-	93%	94%
Written Stroke Educational Materials Given[5]	-	-	86%	88%
Surgical Care Improvement Project				
Appropriate Beta Blocker Usage[5]	-	-	98%	98%
Appropriate VTP Within 24 Hours[5]	-	-	98%	98%
Controlled Postoperative Blood Glucose[5]	-	-	96%	97%
Perioperative Temperature Management[5]	-	-	100%	100%
Prophylactic Antibiotic Selection[5]	-	-	99%	99%
Prophylactic Antibiotic Selection (Outpatient)[5]	-	-	97%	98%
Prophylactic Antibiotic Stopped[5]	-	-	98%	98%
Prophylactic Antibiotic Timing[5]	-	-	99%	99%
Prophylactic Antibiotic Timing (Outpatient)[5]	-	-	97%	98%
Urinary Catheter Removal[5]	-	-	97%	97%
Survey of Patients' Hospital Experiences				
Area Around Room 'Always' Quiet at Night[5]	-	-	64%	61%
Doctors 'Always' Communicated Well[5]	-	-	84%	82%
Home Recovery Information Given[5]	-	-	86%	85%
Hospital Given 9 or 10 on 10 Point Scale[5]	-	-	72%	71%
Meds 'Always' Explained Before Given[5]	-	-	66%	64%
Nurses 'Always' Communicated Well[5]	-	-	81%	79%
Pain 'Always' Well Controlled[5]	-	-	73%	71%
Room and Bathroom 'Always' Clean[5]	-	-	75%	73%
Timely Help 'Always' Received[5]	-	-	69%	68%
Would Definitely Recommend Hospital[5]	-	-	71%	71%
Use of Medical Imaging				
Cardiac Imaging Stress Test before Surgery[7]	-	-	5.3%	5.3%
Combination Abdominal CT Scan	51	35.3%	10.7%	10.5%
Combination Brain/Sinus CT Scan[1]	-	-	3.1%	2.7%
Combination Chest CT Scan[1]	-	-	4.3%	2.7%
Follow-up Mammogram/Ultrasound[1]	-	-	8.3%	8.8%
Lumbar Spine MRI for Low Back Pain[7]	-	-	38.9%	37.2%

Carroll County Memorial Hospital

309 Eleventh Street
Carrollton, KY 41008
Phone: 502-732-4321
Fax: 502-732-3292
E-mail: mabel.burkhardt@nortonhealthcare.org
URL: www.ccmhosp.com
Type: Critical Access Hospitals
Emergency Services: Yes
Ownership: Voluntary non-profit - Private
Beds: 49

Key Personnel:
Intensive Care Unit............ Rhonda Clark
CEO/President................ Kim Dees
Operating Room.............. Trudy Gould
Chief of Medical Staff.......... Hari Nagaraj
Administrator .... Jeff Tindle, MHA
Emergency Room .... Allen Young

Measure	Cases	This Hosp.	State Avg.	U.S. Avg.
Blood Clot Prevention and Treatment				
Anticoagulation Overlap Therapy[1,3]	-	-	90%	93%
ICU Venous Thromboembolism Prophylaxis[3,7]	-	-	86%	92%
Incidence of Potentially Preventable VTE[3,7]	-	-	13%	10%
UFH with Dosages/Platelet Monitoring[3,7]	-	-	98%	97%
Venous Thromboembolism Prophylaxis[3]	263	63%	80%	85%
Warfarin Therapy Discharge Instructions[1,3]	-	-	72%	75%
Chest Pain/Possible Heart Attack Care				
Aspirin Given Within 24 Hours of Arrival[5]	-	-	97%	96%
Fibrinolytic Meds Within 30 Min. of Arrival[5]	-	-	63%	58%
Average Time to ECG (minutes)[5]	-	-	6	7
Average Time to Transfer (minutes)[5]	-	-	61	60
Children's Asthma Care				
Received Home Management Plan of Care	-	-	-	88%
Received Reliever Medication	-	-	-	100%
Received Systemic Corticosteroids	-	-	-	100%
Emergency Department				
Admittance Decision Time (minutes)[2]	416	65	78	98
Head CT Results Within 45 Min. of Arrival[5]	-	-	55%	57%
Patients Who Left ER Before Being Seen	10,748	1%	2%	2%
Time from ER Arrival to Admit. (minutes)[2]	434	181	238	274
Time from ER Arrival to Discharge (minutes)[5]	-	-	126	134
Time in ER Before Being Evaluated (minutes)[5]	-	-	23	26
Time to Pain Meds for Fractures (minutes)[5]	-	-	56	57
Heart Attack Care				
Aspirin Given at Discharge[1,3]	-	-	99%	99%
Fibrinolytic Meds Within 30 Min. of Arrival[3,7]	-	-	-	54%
PCI Within 90 Minutes of Arrival[3,7]	-	-	97%	96%
Statin Prescribed at Discharge[1,3]	-	-	97%	98%
Heart Failure Care				
ACE Inhibitor or ARB for LVSD[1]	-	-	95%	97%
Discharge Instructions Given	20	90%	92%	94%
Evaluation of LVS Function	30	93%	98%	99%
Medicare Spending				
Medicare Spending per Patient (ratio)	-	-	0.97	0.98
Pneumonia Care				
Appropriate Initial Antibiotic Given	28	100%	94%	95%
Blood Culture Timing	38	95%	98%	98%
Pregnancy and Delivery Care				
Newborn Deliveries Scheduled Early[5]	-	-	9%	6%
Preventive Care				
Immunization for Influenza	334	93%	92%	90%
Immunization for Pneumonia	487	95%	94%	92%
Stroke Care				
Anticoagulation Therapy for Atrial Fibrillation[1,3]	-	-	95%	95%
Antithrombotic Therapy Timing[1,3]	-	-	97%	98%
Assessed for Rehabilitation[1,3]	-	-	97%	97%
Discharged on Antithrombotic Therapy[1,3]	-	-	98%	99%
Discharged on Statin Medication[1,3]	-	-	93%	94%
Thrombolytic Therapy Timing[1,3]	-	-	59%	66%
Venous Thromboembolism Prophylaxis[1,3]	-	-	93%	94%
Written Stroke Educational Materials Given[1,3]	-	-	86%	88%
Surgical Care Improvement Project				
Appropriate Beta Blocker Usage[5]	-	-	98%	98%
Appropriate VTP Within 24 Hours[5]	-	-	98%	98%

NOTE: Hospital profiles are in alphabetical order by state, then city, then hospital within the city; Rankings exclude hospitals with less than 25 cases except for patient surveys which excludes hospitals with less than 100 cases; (a) 100-299 cases; (1) The number of cases/patients is too few to report; (2) Data submitted were based on a sample of cases/patients; (3) Results are based on a shorter time period than required; (4) Data suppressed by CMS for one or more quarters; (5) Results are not available for this reporting period; (6) Fewer than 100 patients completed the HCAHPS survey; (7) No cases met the criteria for this measure; (8) The lower limit of the confidence interval cannot be calculated if the number of observed infections equals zero; (9) No data are available from the state/territory for this reporting period; (10) The scores shown reflect fewer than 50 completed surveys; (11) There were discrepancies in the data collection process; (12) This measure does not apply to this hospital for this reporting period; (13) Results cannot be calculated for this reporting period; (14) The results for this state are combined with nearby states to protect confidentiality; Please refer to the User's Guide for a full explanation of data.

Measure	Cases	This Hosp.	State Avg.	U.S. Avg.
Controlled Postoperative Blood Glucose[5]	-	-	96%	97%
Perioperative Temperature Management[5]	-	-	100%	100%
Prophylactic Antibiotic Selection[5]	-	-	99%	99%
Prophylactic Antibiotic Selection (Outpatient)[5]	-	-	97%	98%
Prophylactic Antibiotic Stopped[5]	-	-	98%	98%
Prophylactic Antibiotic Timing[5]	-	-	99%	99%
Prophylactic Antibiotic Timing (Outpatient)[5]	-	-	97%	98%
Urinary Catheter Removal[5]	-	-	97%	97%
Survey of Patients' Hospital Experiences				
Area Around Room 'Always' Quiet at Night[5]	-	-	64%	61%
Doctors 'Always' Communicated Well[5]	-	-	84%	82%
Home Recovery Information Given[5]	-	-	86%	85%
Hospital Given 9 or 10 on 10 Point Scale[5]	-	-	72%	71%
Meds 'Always' Explained Before Given[5]	-	-	66%	64%
Nurses 'Always' Communicated Well[5]	-	-	81%	79%
Pain 'Always' Well Controlled[5]	-	-	73%	71%
Room and Bathroom 'Always' Clean[5]	-	-	75%	73%
Timely Help 'Always' Received[5]	-	-	69%	68%
Would Definitely Recommend Hospital[5]	-	-	71%	71%
Use of Medical Imaging				
Cardiac Imaging Stress Test before Surgery	80	3.8%	5.3%	5.3%
Combination Abdominal CT Scan	153	2.6%	10.7%	10.5%
Combination Brain/Sinus CT Scan	226	0.9%	3.1%	2.7%
Combination Chest CT Scan	79	1.3%	4.3%	2.7%
Follow-up Mammogram/Ultrasound	149	4.0%	8.3%	8.8%
Lumbar Spine MRI for Low Back Pain[1]	-	-	38.9%	37.2%

Westlake Regional Hospital

901 Westlake Drive
Columbia, KY 42728
Phone: 270-384-4753
Fax: 270-384-3742
URL: www.westlake-healthcare.org
Type: Acute Care Hospitals
Emergency Services: Yes
Ownership: Govt - Hospital Dist/Auth
Beds: 80

Key Personnel:

Emergency Room . . . . Celia Downey
Intensive Care Unit. . . . . Celia Downey
Operating Room. . . . . Kathy Hadley
Quality Assurance . . . . Jim Hagan
Chief of Medical Staff. . . . . Gary Partin, MD
Infection Control. . . . . Sharon Watson
Anesthesiology. . . . . Tom Wimmer

Measure	Cases	This Hosp.	State Avg.	U.S. Avg.
Blood Clot Prevention and Treatment				
Anticoagulation Overlap Therapy[1,2]	-	-	90%	93%
ICU Venous Thromboembolism Prophylaxis[2]	13	85%	86%	92%
Incidence of Potentially Preventable VTE[2,7]	-	-	13%	10%
UFH with Dosages/Platelet Monitoring[1,2]	-	-	98%	97%
Venous Thromboembolism Prophylaxis[2]	229	85%	80%	85%
Warfarin Therapy Discharge Instructions[1,2]	-	-	72%	75%
Chest Pain/Possible Heart Attack Care				
Aspirin Given Within 24 Hours of Arrival	34	97%	97%	96%
Fibrinolytic Meds Within 30 Min. of Arrival[1]	-	-	63%	58%
Average Time to ECG (minutes)	32	8	6	7
Average Time to Transfer (minutes)[1]	-	-	61	60
Children's Asthma Care				
Received Home Management Plan of Care	-	-	-	88%
Received Reliever Medication	-	-	-	100%
Received Systemic Corticosteroids	-	-	-	100%
Emergency Department				
Admittance Decision Time (minutes)[2]	355	65	78	98
Head CT Results Within 45 Min. of Arrival[1]	-	-	55%	57%
Patients Who Left ER Before Being Seen	8,755	1%	2%	2%
Time from ER Arrival to Admit. (minutes)[2]	385	222	238	274
Time from ER Arrival to Discharge (minutes)	535	109	126	134
Time in ER Before Being Evaluated (minutes)	544	19	23	26
Time to Pain Meds for Fractures (minutes)	30	42	56	57
Heart Attack Care				
Aspirin Given at Discharge[1]	-	-	99%	99%
Fibrinolytic Meds Within 30 Min. of Arrival[7]	-	-	-	54%
PCI Within 90 Minutes of Arrival[7]	-	-	97%	96%
Statin Prescribed at Discharge[1]	-	-	97%	98%
Heart Failure Care				
ACE Inhibitor or ARB for LVSD[1]	-	-	95%	97%
Discharge Instructions Given	19	100%	92%	94%
Evaluation of LVS Function	32	62%	98%	99%
Medicare Spending				
Medicare Spending per Patient (ratio)	-	0.98	0.97	0.98
Pneumonia Care				
Appropriate Initial Antibiotic Given	60	82%	94%	95%
Blood Culture Timing	82	91%	98%	98%
Pregnancy and Delivery Care				
Newborn Deliveries Scheduled Early[7]	-	-	9%	6%
Preventive Care				
Immunization for Influenza[2]	326	75%	92%	90%
Immunization for Pneumonia[2]	441	82%	94%	92%
Stroke Care				
Anticoagulation Therapy for Atrial Fibrillation[1]	-	-	95%	95%
Antithrombotic Therapy Timing[1]	-	-	97%	98%
Assessed for Rehabilitation[1]	-	-	97%	97%
Discharged on Antithrombotic Therapy[1]	-	-	98%	99%
Discharged on Statin Medication[1]	-	-	93%	94%
Thrombolytic Therapy Timing[1]	-	-	59%	66%
Venous Thromboembolism Prophylaxis[1]	-	-	93%	94%
Written Stroke Educational Materials Given[7]	-	-	86%	88%
Surgical Care Improvement Project				
Appropriate Beta Blocker Usage[3,7]	-	-	98%	98%
Appropriate VTP Within 24 Hours[1,3]	-	-	98%	98%
Controlled Postoperative Blood Glucose[3,7]	-	-	96%	97%
Perioperative Temperature Management[1,3]	-	-	100%	100%
Prophylactic Antibiotic Selection[1,3]	-	-	99%	99%
Prophylactic Antibiotic Selection (Outpatient)[1,3]	-	-	97%	98%
Prophylactic Antibiotic Stopped[1,3]	-	-	98%	98%
Prophylactic Antibiotic Timing[1,3]	-	-	99%	99%
Prophylactic Antibiotic Timing (Outpatient)[1,3]	-	-	97%	98%
Urinary Catheter Removal[1,3]	-	-	97%	97%
Survey of Patients' Hospital Experiences				
Area Around Room 'Always' Quiet at Night	(a)	93%	64%	61%
Doctors 'Always' Communicated Well	(a)	100%	84%	82%
Home Recovery Information Given	(a)	100%	86%	85%
Hospital Given 9 or 10 on 10 Point Scale	(a)	91%	72%	71%
Meds 'Always' Explained Before Given	(a)	99%	66%	64%
Nurses 'Always' Communicated Well	(a)	100%	81%	79%
Pain 'Always' Well Controlled	(a)	100%	73%	71%
Room and Bathroom 'Always' Clean	(a)	97%	75%	73%
Timely Help 'Always' Received	(a)	99%	69%	68%
Would Definitely Recommend Hospital	(a)	100%	71%	71%
Use of Medical Imaging				
Cardiac Imaging Stress Test before Surgery[1]	-	-	5.3%	5.3%
Combination Abdominal CT Scan	209	14.4%	10.7%	10.5%
Combination Brain/Sinus CT Scan[1]	-	-	3.1%	2.7%
Combination Chest CT Scan	90	18.9%	4.3%	2.7%
Follow-up Mammogram/Ultrasound	119	8.4%	8.3%	8.8%
Lumbar Spine MRI for Low Back Pain[1]	-	-	38.9%	37.2%

Baptist Health Corbin

One Trillium Way
Corbin, KY 40701
Phone: 606-528-1212
Fax: 606-528-9996
URL: www.baptistregional.com
Type: Acute Care Hospitals
Emergency Services: Yes
Ownership: Voluntary non-profit - Private
Beds: 240

Key Personnel:

Infection Control. . . . . Elizabeth Bryant
Intensive Care Unit. . . . . Donna Carroll
Radiology. . . . . William Daniel, II
Chief of Medical Staff . . . . Ross Halbleib
CEO/President. . . . . John Henson
Operating Room. . . . . George Liu
Quality Assurance . . . . Theresa Sidebottom

Measure	Cases	This Hosp.	State Avg.	U.S. Avg.
Blood Clot Prevention and Treatment				
Anticoagulation Overlap Therapy[2]	33	91%	90%	93%
ICU Venous Thromboembolism Prophylaxis[2]	79	90%	86%	92%
Incidence of Potentially Preventable VTE[1,2]	-	-	13%	10%
UFH with Dosages/Platelet Monitoring[2]	25	100%	98%	97%
Venous Thromboembolism Prophylaxis[2]	283	67%	80%	85%
Warfarin Therapy Discharge Instructions[2]	19	63%	72%	75%
Chest Pain/Possible Heart Attack Care				
Aspirin Given Within 24 Hours of Arrival	110	100%	97%	96%
Fibrinolytic Meds Within 30 Min. of Arrival[7]	-	-	63%	58%
Average Time to ECG (minutes)	111	5	6	7
Average Time to Transfer (minutes)	38	61	61	60
Children's Asthma Care				
Received Home Management Plan of Care	-	-	-	88%
Received Reliever Medication	-	-	-	100%
Received Systemic Corticosteroids	-	-	-	100%
Emergency Department				
Admittance Decision Time (minutes)[2]	451	94	78	98
Head CT Results Within 45 Min. of Arrival	20	40%	55%	57%
Patients Who Left ER Before Being Seen	40,921	1%	2%	2%
Time from ER Arrival to Admit. (minutes)[2]	451	255	238	274
Time from ER Arrival to Discharge (minutes)	365	154	126	134
Time in ER Before Being Evaluated (minutes)	402	15	23	26
Time to Pain Meds for Fractures (minutes)	89	56	56	57
Heart Attack Care				
Aspirin Given at Discharge	15	100%	99%	99%
Fibrinolytic Meds Within 30 Min. of Arrival[7]	-	-	-	54%
PCI Within 90 Minutes of Arrival[7]	-	-	97%	96%
Statin Prescribed at Discharge	11	100%	97%	98%
Heart Failure Care				
ACE Inhibitor or ARB for LVSD	46	100%	95%	97%
Discharge Instructions Given	149	96%	92%	94%
Evaluation of LVS Function	191	100%	98%	99%
Medicare Spending				
Medicare Spending per Patient (ratio)	-	0.98	0.97	0.98
Pneumonia Care				
Appropriate Initial Antibiotic Given	165	98%	94%	95%
Blood Culture Timing	286	99%	98%	98%
Pregnancy and Delivery Care				
Newborn Deliveries Scheduled Early[2]	36	14%	9%	6%
Preventive Care				
Immunization for Influenza[2]	520	95%	92%	90%
Immunization for Pneumonia[2]	550	97%	94%	92%
Stroke Care				
Anticoagulation Therapy for Atrial Fibrillation[1]	-	-	95%	95%
Antithrombotic Therapy Timing	33	97%	97%	98%
Assessed for Rehabilitation	34	76%	97%	97%
Discharged on Antithrombotic Therapy	30	100%	98%	99%
Discharged on Statin Medication	23	78%	93%	94%
Thrombolytic Therapy Timing[1]	-	-	59%	66%
Venous Thromboembolism Prophylaxis	34	79%	93%	94%
Written Stroke Educational Materials Given	20	80%	86%	88%
Surgical Care Improvement Project				
Appropriate Beta Blocker Usage	93	100%	98%	98%
Appropriate VTP Within 24 Hours	199	99%	98%	98%
Controlled Postoperative Blood Glucose[7]	-	-	96%	97%
Perioperative Temperature Management	215	100%	100%	100%
Prophylactic Antibiotic Selection	100	100%	99%	99%
Prophylactic Antibiotic Selection (Outpatient)	267	100%	97%	98%
Prophylactic Antibiotic Stopped	96	99%	98%	98%
Prophylactic Antibiotic Timing	101	100%	99%	99%
Prophylactic Antibiotic Timing (Outpatient)	267	100%	97%	98%
Urinary Catheter Removal	101	100%	97%	97%
Survey of Patients' Hospital Experiences				
Area Around Room 'Always' Quiet at Night	300+	59%	64%	61%
Doctors 'Always' Communicated Well	300+	84%	84%	82%
Home Recovery Information Given	300+	84%	86%	85%
Hospital Given 9 or 10 on 10 Point Scale	300+	69%	72%	71%
Meds 'Always' Explained Before Given	300+	67%	66%	64%
Nurses 'Always' Communicated Well	300+	77%	81%	79%
Pain 'Always' Well Controlled	300+	73%	73%	71%
Room and Bathroom 'Always' Clean	300+	70%	75%	73%
Timely Help 'Always' Received	300+	63%	69%	68%
Would Definitely Recommend Hospital	300+	68%	71%	71%
Use of Medical Imaging				
Cardiac Imaging Stress Test before Surgery	1,062	5.2%	5.3%	5.3%
Combination Abdominal CT Scan	1,080	8.4%	10.7%	10.5%
Combination Brain/Sinus CT Scan	944	3.0%	3.1%	2.7%
Combination Chest CT Scan	535	1.9%	4.3%	2.7%
Follow-up Mammogram/Ultrasound	1,106	7.7%	8.3%	8.8%
Lumbar Spine MRI for Low Back Pain	179	44.7%	38.9%	37.2%

NOTE: Hospital profiles are in alphabetical order by state, then city, then hospital within the city; Rankings exclude hospitals with less than 25 cases except for patient surveys which excludes hospitals with less than 100 cases; (a) 100-299 cases; (1) The number of cases/patients is too few to report; (2) Data submitted were based on a sample of cases/patients; (3) Results are based on a shorter time period than required; (4) Data suppressed by CMS for one or more quarters; (5) Results are not available for this reporting period; (6) Fewer than 100 patients completed the HCAHPS survey; (7) No cases met the criteria for this measure; (8) The lower limit of the confidence interval cannot be calculated if the number of observed infections equals zero; (9) No data are available from the state/territory for this reporting period; (10) The scores shown reflect fewer than 50 completed surveys; (11) There were discrepancies in the data collection process; (12) This measure does not apply to this hospital for this reporting period; (13) Results cannot be calculated for this reporting period; (14) The results for this state are combined with nearby states to protect confidentiality; Please refer to the User's Guide for a full explanation of data.

Harrison Memorial Hospital

1210 Ky Hwy 36 E
Cynthiana, KY 41031
Phone: 859-234-2300
Fax: 859-235-3699
URL: www.harrisonmemhosp.com
Type: Acute Care Hospitals
Emergency Services: Yes
Ownership: Voluntary non-profit - Other
Beds: 99

Key Personnel:
Radiology. Douglas C Crutcher
Chief of Medical Staff. . . . . David French
Emergency Room . . . . M Gainey

Measure	Cases	This Hosp.	State Avg.	U.S. Avg.
Blood Clot Prevention and Treatment				
Anticoagulation Overlap Therapy[2]	14	93%	90%	93%
ICU Venous Thromboembolism Prophylaxis[1,2]	-	-	86%	92%
Incidence of Potentially Preventable VTE[1,2]	-	-	13%	10%
UFH with Dosages/Platelet Monitoring[1,2]	-	-	98%	97%
Venous Thromboembolism Prophylaxis[2]	173	97%	80%	85%
Warfarin Therapy Discharge Instructions[1,2]	-	-	72%	75%
Chest Pain/Possible Heart Attack Care				
Aspirin Given Within 24 Hours of Arrival	65	100%	97%	96%
Fibrinolytic Meds Within 30 Min. of Arrival[1]	-	-	63%	58%
Average Time to ECG (minutes)	68	8	6	7
Average Time to Transfer (minutes)[1]	-	-	61	60
Children's Asthma Care				
Received Home Management Plan of Care	-	-	-	88%
Received Reliever Medication	-	-	-	100%
Received Systemic Corticosteroids	-	-	-	100%
Emergency Department				
Admittance Decision Time (minutes)[2]	245	37	78	98
Head CT Results Within 45 Min. of Arrival[1]	-	-	55%	57%
Patients Who Left ER Before Being Seen	13,676	0%	2%	2%
Time from ER Arrival to Admit. (minutes)[2]	245	199	238	274
Time from ER Arrival to Discharge (minutes)	371	99	126	134
Time in ER Before Being Evaluated (minutes)	405	12	23	26
Time to Pain Meds for Fractures (minutes)	48	57	56	57
Heart Attack Care				
Aspirin Given at Discharge[1]	-	-	99%	99%
Fibrinolytic Meds Within 30 Min. of Arrival[7]	-	-	-	54%
PCI Within 90 Minutes of Arrival[7]	-	-	97%	96%
Statin Prescribed at Discharge[1]	-	-	97%	98%
Heart Failure Care				
ACE Inhibitor or ARB for LVSD[1]	-	-	95%	97%
Discharge Instructions Given	32	100%	92%	94%
Evaluation of LVS Function	36	100%	98%	99%
Medicare Spending				
Medicare Spending per Patient (ratio)	-	0.94	0.97	0.98
Pneumonia Care				
Appropriate Initial Antibiotic Given	125	98%	94%	95%
Blood Culture Timing	182	99%	98%	98%
Pregnancy and Delivery Care				
Newborn Deliveries Scheduled Early[2]	31	3%	9%	6%
Preventive Care				
Immunization for Influenza[2]	254	99%	92%	90%
Immunization for Pneumonia[2]	324	100%	94%	92%
Stroke Care				
Anticoagulation Therapy for Atrial Fibrillation[7]	-	-	95%	95%
Antithrombotic Therapy Timing[1]	-	-	97%	98%
Assessed for Rehabilitation[1]	-	-	97%	97%
Discharged on Antithrombotic Therapy[1]	-	-	98%	99%
Discharged on Statin Medication[1]	-	-	93%	94%
Thrombolytic Therapy Timing[7]	-	-	59%	66%
Venous Thromboembolism Prophylaxis[1]	-	-	93%	94%
Written Stroke Educational Materials Given[1]	-	-	86%	88%
Surgical Care Improvement Project				
Appropriate Beta Blocker Usage	23	96%	98%	98%
Appropriate VTP Within 24 Hours	44	100%	98%	98%
Controlled Postoperative Blood Glucose[7]	-	-	96%	97%
Perioperative Temperature Management	53	100%	100%	100%
Prophylactic Antibiotic Selection	31	97%	99%	99%
Prophylactic Antibiotic Selection (Outpatient)	42	98%	97%	98%
Prophylactic Antibiotic Stopped	28	100%	98%	98%
Prophylactic Antibiotic Timing	31	100%	99%	99%
Prophylactic Antibiotic Timing (Outpatient)	42	100%	97%	98%
Urinary Catheter Removal	33	100%	97%	97%
Survey of Patients' Hospital Experiences				
Area Around Room 'Always' Quiet at Night	300+	63%	64%	61%
Doctors 'Always' Communicated Well	300+	88%	84%	82%
Home Recovery Information Given	300+	85%	86%	85%
Hospital Given 9 or 10 on 10 Point Scale	300+	80%	72%	71%
Meds 'Always' Explained Before Given	300+	70%	66%	64%
Nurses 'Always' Communicated Well	300+	86%	81%	79%
Pain 'Always' Well Controlled	300+	76%	73%	71%
Room and Bathroom 'Always' Clean	300+	82%	75%	73%
Timely Help 'Always' Received	300+	72%	69%	68%
Would Definitely Recommend Hospital	300+	77%	71%	71%
Use of Medical Imaging				
Cardiac Imaging Stress Test before Surgery	94	5.3%	5.3%	5.3%
Combination Abdominal CT Scan	359	5.0%	10.7%	10.5%
Combination Brain/Sinus CT Scan	282	7.4%	3.1%	2.7%
Combination Chest CT Scan	187	0.5%	4.3%	2.7%
Follow-up Mammogram/Ultrasound	372	15.1%	8.3%	8.8%
Lumbar Spine MRI for Low Back Pain[1]	-	-	38.9%	37.2%

Ephraim Mcdowell Regional Medical Center

217 South Third Street
Danville, KY 40422
Phone: 859-239-2409
Fax: 859-239-6960
E-mail: marketing@emhealth.org
URL: www.emrmc.com
Type: Acute Care Hospitals
Emergency Services: Yes
Ownership: Voluntary non-profit - Other
Beds: 177

Key Personnel:
Chief of Medical Staff. . . . . William P Baas
Quality Assurance . . . . Nancy Brooks
Coronary Care. . . . . Beth Carter
Operating Room. . . . . Paul DeLuca
Infection Control. . . . . Ginger Elliot
Pediatric Ambulatory Care . . . . . . Russel Goodwin, MD
Radiology. . . . . Shawn D Grant, MD
CEO/President. . . . . Clark Taylor

Measure	Cases	This Hosp.	State Avg.	U.S. Avg.
Blood Clot Prevention and Treatment				
Anticoagulation Overlap Therapy[2]	53	92%	90%	93%
ICU Venous Thromboembolism Prophylaxis[2]	74	46%	86%	92%
Incidence of Potentially Preventable VTE[2]	16	6%	13%	10%
UFH with Dosages/Platelet Monitoring[2]	45	100%	98%	97%
Venous Thromboembolism Prophylaxis[2]	521	79%	80%	85%
Warfarin Therapy Discharge Instructions[2]	41	100%	72%	75%
Chest Pain/Possible Heart Attack Care				
Aspirin Given Within 24 Hours of Arrival	12	100%	97%	96%
Fibrinolytic Meds Within 30 Min. of Arrival[7]	-	-	63%	58%
Average Time to ECG (minutes)	12	8	6	7
Average Time to Transfer (minutes)[1]	-	-	61	60
Children's Asthma Care				
Received Home Management Plan of Care	-	-	-	88%
Received Reliever Medication	-	-	-	100%
Received Systemic Corticosteroids	-	-	-	100%
Emergency Department				
Admittance Decision Time (minutes)[2]	781	80	78	98
Head CT Results Within 45 Min. of Arrival	18	39%	55%	57%
Patients Who Left ER Before Being Seen	28,550	0%	2%	2%
Time from ER Arrival to Admit. (minutes)[2]	832	222	238	274
Time from ER Arrival to Discharge (minutes)	660	118	126	134
Time in ER Before Being Evaluated (minutes)	686	11	23	26
Time to Pain Meds for Fractures (minutes)	124	38	56	57
Heart Attack Care				
Aspirin Given at Discharge	174	99%	99%	99%
Fibrinolytic Meds Within 30 Min. of Arrival[7]	-	-	-	54%
PCI Within 90 Minutes of Arrival	32	94%	97%	96%
Statin Prescribed at Discharge	166	99%	97%	98%
Heart Failure Care				
ACE Inhibitor or ARB for LVSD	71	100%	95%	97%
Discharge Instructions Given	179	92%	92%	94%
Evaluation of LVS Function	233	99%	98%	99%
Medicare Spending				
Medicare Spending per Patient (ratio)	-	0.96	0.97	0.98
Pneumonia Care				
Appropriate Initial Antibiotic Given	124	97%	94%	95%
Blood Culture Timing	263	99%	98%	98%
Pregnancy and Delivery Care				
Newborn Deliveries Scheduled Early	46	4%	9%	6%
Preventive Care				
Immunization for Influenza[2]	832	99%	92%	90%
Immunization for Pneumonia[2]	1,128	99%	94%	92%
Stroke Care				
Anticoagulation Therapy for Atrial Fibrillation[1]	-	-	95%	95%
Antithrombotic Therapy Timing	31	97%	97%	98%
Assessed for Rehabilitation	30	93%	97%	97%
Discharged on Antithrombotic Therapy	30	100%	98%	99%
Discharged on Statin Medication	22	95%	93%	94%
Thrombolytic Therapy Timing[1]	-	-	59%	66%
Venous Thromboembolism Prophylaxis	32	84%	93%	94%
Written Stroke Educational Materials Given	18	100%	86%	88%
Surgical Care Improvement Project				
Appropriate Beta Blocker Usage	140	99%	98%	98%
Appropriate VTP Within 24 Hours	336	97%	98%	98%
Controlled Postoperative Blood Glucose[7]	-	-	96%	97%
Perioperative Temperature Management	406	100%	100%	100%
Prophylactic Antibiotic Selection	298	99%	99%	99%
Prophylactic Antibiotic Selection (Outpatient)	234	95%	97%	98%
Prophylactic Antibiotic Stopped	294	100%	98%	98%
Prophylactic Antibiotic Timing	299	99%	99%	99%
Prophylactic Antibiotic Timing (Outpatient)	246	92%	97%	98%
Urinary Catheter Removal	220	100%	97%	97%
Survey of Patients' Hospital Experiences				
Area Around Room 'Always' Quiet at Night	300+	62%	64%	61%
Doctors 'Always' Communicated Well	300+	82%	84%	82%
Home Recovery Information Given	300+	81%	86%	85%
Hospital Given 9 or 10 on 10 Point Scale	300+	68%	72%	71%
Meds 'Always' Explained Before Given	300+	63%	66%	64%
Nurses 'Always' Communicated Well	300+	80%	81%	79%
Pain 'Always' Well Controlled	300+	72%	73%	71%
Room and Bathroom 'Always' Clean	300+	74%	75%	73%
Timely Help 'Always' Received	300+	66%	69%	68%
Would Definitely Recommend Hospital	300+	67%	71%	71%
Use of Medical Imaging				
Cardiac Imaging Stress Test before Surgery	444	4.7%	5.3%	5.3%
Combination Abdominal CT Scan	841	18.4%	10.7%	10.5%
Combination Brain/Sinus CT Scan	678	2.1%	3.1%	2.7%
Combination Chest CT Scan	399	0.0%	4.3%	2.7%
Follow-up Mammogram/Ultrasound	1,460	9.8%	8.3%	8.8%
Lumbar Spine MRI for Low Back Pain	283	39.2%	38.9%	37.2%

Hardin Memorial Hospital

913 North Dixie Avenue
Elizabethtown, KY 42701
Phone: 270-737-1212
Fax: 270-706-5125
URL: www.hmh.net
Type: Acute Care Hospitals
Emergency Services: Yes
Ownership: Government - Local
Beds: 300

Key Personnel:
Operating Room. . . . . Denise Adams
Quality Assurance . . . . Vivian Bishoff
CEO/President. . . . . David Gray
Infection Control. . . . . Jo Ellen Mackey
Radiology. . . . . Michael Oliff, MD
Pediatric Ambulatory Care . . . . . . Robert Padgett, MD
Pediatric In-Patient Care . . . . Robert Padgett, MD
Chief of Medical Staff. . . . . Cora Veza

Measure	Cases	This Hosp.	State Avg.	U.S. Avg.
Blood Clot Prevention and Treatment				
Anticoagulation Overlap Therapy[2]	83	60%	90%	93%
ICU Venous Thromboembolism Prophylaxis[2]	73	73%	86%	92%
Incidence of Potentially Preventable VTE[1,2]	-	-	13%	10%
UFH with Dosages/Platelet Monitoring[2]	36	53%	98%	97%
Venous Thromboembolism Prophylaxis[2]	338	75%	80%	85%
Warfarin Therapy Discharge Instructions[2]	71	7%	72%	75%
Chest Pain/Possible Heart Attack Care				
Aspirin Given Within 24 Hours of Arrival[1]	-	-	97%	96%
Fibrinolytic Meds Within 30 Min. of Arrival[3,7]	-	-	63%	58%
Average Time to ECG (minutes)[1]	-	-	6	7
Average Time to Transfer (minutes)[3,7]	-	-	61	60
Children's Asthma Care				

NOTE: Hospital profiles are in alphabetical order by state, then city, then hospital within the city; Rankings exclude hospitals with less than 25 cases except for patient surveys which excludes hospitals with less than 100 cases; (a) 100-299 cases; (1) The number of cases/patients is too few to report; (2) Data submitted were based on a sample of cases/patients; (3) Results are based on a shorter time period than required; (4) Data suppressed by CMS for one or more quarters; (5) Results are not available for this reporting period; (6) Fewer than 100 patients completed the HCAHPS survey; (7) No cases met the criteria for this measure; (8) The lower limit of the confidence interval cannot be calculated if the number of observed infections equals zero; (9) No data are available from the state/territory for this reporting period; (10) The scores shown reflect fewer than 50 completed surveys; (11) There were discrepancies in the data collection process; (12) This measure does not apply to this hospital for this reporting period; (13) Results cannot be calculated for this reporting period; (14) The results for this state are combined with nearby states to protect confidentiality; Please refer to the User's Guide for a full explanation of data.

Measure	Cases	This Hosp.	State Avg.	U.S. Avg.
Received Home Management Plan of Care	-	-	-	88%
Received Reliever Medication	-	-	-	100%
Received Systemic Corticosteroids	-	-	-	100%
Emergency Department				
Admittance Decision Time (minutes)[2]	624	146	78	98
Head CT Results Within 45 Min. of Arrival	17	53%	55%	57%
Patients Who Left ER Before Being Seen	58,521	3%	2%	2%
Time from ER Arrival to Admit. (minutes)[2]	624	339	238	274
Time from ER Arrival to Discharge (minutes)	390	189	126	134
Time in ER Before Being Evaluated (minutes)	405	58	23	26
Time to Pain Meds for Fractures (minutes)	152	88	56	57
Heart Attack Care				
Aspirin Given at Discharge	235	99%	99%	99%
Fibrinolytic Meds Within 30 Min. of Arrival[7]	-	-	-	54%
PCI Within 90 Minutes of Arrival	31	100%	97%	96%
Statin Prescribed at Discharge	223	99%	97%	98%
Heart Failure Care				
ACE Inhibitor or ARB for LVSD	133	95%	95%	97%
Discharge Instructions Given	436	92%	92%	94%
Evaluation of LVS Function	551	100%	98%	99%
Medicare Spending				
Medicare Spending per Patient (ratio)	-	0.97	0.97	0.98
Pneumonia Care				
Appropriate Initial Antibiotic Given[2]	79	94%	94%	95%
Blood Culture Timing[2]	108	94%	98%	98%
Pregnancy and Delivery Care				
Newborn Deliveries Scheduled Early[2]	55	16%	9%	6%
Preventive Care				
Immunization for Influenza[2]	525	93%	92%	90%
Immunization for Pneumonia[2]	664	94%	94%	92%
Stroke Care				
Anticoagulation Therapy for Atrial Fibrillation	30	93%	95%	95%
Antithrombotic Therapy Timing	144	97%	97%	98%
Assessed for Rehabilitation	162	98%	97%	97%
Discharged on Antithrombotic Therapy	152	97%	98%	99%
Discharged on Statin Medication	123	80%	93%	94%
Thrombolytic Therapy Timing	27	15%	59%	66%
Venous Thromboembolism Prophylaxis	150	85%	93%	94%
Written Stroke Educational Materials Given	93	87%	86%	88%
Surgical Care Improvement Project				
Appropriate Beta Blocker Usage[2]	137	92%	98%	98%
Appropriate VTP Within 24 Hours[2]	355	99%	98%	98%
Controlled Postoperative Blood Glucose[2,7]	-	-	96%	97%
Perioperative Temperature Management[2]	443	100%	100%	100%
Prophylactic Antibiotic Selection[2]	281	99%	99%	99%
Prophylactic Antibiotic Selection (Outpatient)	463	99%	97%	98%
Prophylactic Antibiotic Stopped[2]	269	99%	98%	98%
Prophylactic Antibiotic Timing[2]	282	100%	99%	99%
Prophylactic Antibiotic Timing (Outpatient)	465	99%	97%	98%
Urinary Catheter Removal[2]	292	90%	97%	97%
Survey of Patients' Hospital Experiences				
Area Around Room 'Always' Quiet at Night	300+	51%	64%	61%
Doctors 'Always' Communicated Well	300+	82%	84%	82%
Home Recovery Information Given	300+	83%	86%	85%
Hospital Given 9 or 10 on 10 Point Scale	300+	65%	72%	71%
Meds 'Always' Explained Before Given	300+	66%	66%	64%
Nurses 'Always' Communicated Well	300+	81%	81%	79%
Pain 'Always' Well Controlled	300+	72%	73%	71%
Room and Bathroom 'Always' Clean	300+	72%	75%	73%
Timely Help 'Always' Received	300+	61%	69%	68%
Would Definitely Recommend Hospital	300+	68%	71%	71%
Use of Medical Imaging				
Cardiac Imaging Stress Test before Surgery	288	8.7%	5.3%	5.3%
Combination Abdominal CT Scan	2,219	8.2%	10.7%	10.5%
Combination Brain/Sinus CT Scan	1,392	3.3%	3.1%	2.7%
Combination Chest CT Scan	1,639	0.0%	4.3%	2.7%
Follow-up Mammogram/Ultrasound	2,953	9.8%	8.3%	8.8%
Lumbar Spine MRI for Low Back Pain	349	34.7%	38.9%	37.2%

Fleming County Hospital

55 Foundation Drive
Flemingsburg, KY 41041
URL: www.flemingcountyhospital.org
Phone: 606-849-2351
Fax: 606-849-5005
Type: Acute Care Hospitals
Ownership: Voluntary non-profit - Other
Emergency Services: Yes
Beds: 52

Key Personnel:
CEO/President. . . . . Mark Armstrong
Emergency Room . . . . Roland Benton
Infection Control. . . . . Jeanne Conley, RN
Chief of Medical Staff . . . . Samuel W Gehring, MD
Quality Assurance . . . . Marsha Gorman
Radiology. . . . . Richard S Hartman, RT
Operating Room. . . . . Theresa Huber, RN
Intensive Care Unit. . . . . Helen McKay, RN

Measure	Cases	This Hosp.	State Avg.	U.S. Avg.
Blood Clot Prevention and Treatment				
Anticoagulation Overlap Therapy[1,2]	-	-	90%	93%
ICU Venous Thromboembolism Prophylaxis[2]	117	72%	86%	92%
Incidence of Potentially Preventable VTE[1,2]	-	-	13%	10%
UFH with Dosages/Platelet Monitoring[1,2]	-	-	98%	97%
Venous Thromboembolism Prophylaxis[2]	141	60%	80%	85%
Warfarin Therapy Discharge Instructions[1,2]	-	-	72%	75%
Chest Pain/Possible Heart Attack Care				
Aspirin Given Within 24 Hours of Arrival	49	100%	97%	96%
Fibrinolytic Meds Within 30 Min. of Arrival[7]	-	-	63%	58%
Average Time to ECG (minutes)	52	8	6	7
Average Time to Transfer (minutes)	12	70	61	60
Children's Asthma Care				
Received Home Management Plan of Care	-	-	-	88%
Received Reliever Medication	-	-	-	100%
Received Systemic Corticosteroids	-	-	-	100%
Emergency Department				
Admittance Decision Time (minutes)[2]	360	76	78	98
Head CT Results Within 45 Min. of Arrival[1]	-	-	55%	57%
Patients Who Left ER Before Being Seen	9,042	1%	2%	2%
Time from ER Arrival to Admit. (minutes)[2]	362	225	238	274
Time from ER Arrival to Discharge (minutes)	323	127	126	134
Time in ER Before Being Evaluated (minutes)	361	11	23	26
Time to Pain Meds for Fractures (minutes)	43	56	56	57
Heart Attack Care				
Aspirin Given at Discharge[1]	-	-	99%	99%
Fibrinolytic Meds Within 30 Min. of Arrival[7]	-	-	-	54%
PCI Within 90 Minutes of Arrival[7]	-	-	97%	96%
Statin Prescribed at Discharge[1]	-	-	97%	98%
Heart Failure Care				
ACE Inhibitor or ARB for LVSD[1]	-	-	95%	97%
Discharge Instructions Given	57	96%	92%	94%
Evaluation of LVS Function	67	99%	98%	99%
Medicare Spending				
Medicare Spending per Patient (ratio)	-	1.00	0.97	0.98
Pneumonia Care				
Appropriate Initial Antibiotic Given	115	99%	94%	95%
Blood Culture Timing	107	98%	98%	98%
Pregnancy and Delivery Care				
Newborn Deliveries Scheduled Early[7]	-	-	9%	6%
Preventive Care				
Immunization for Influenza[2]	285	96%	92%	90%
Immunization for Pneumonia[2]	486	97%	94%	92%
Stroke Care				
Anticoagulation Therapy for Atrial Fibrillation[1]	-	-	95%	95%
Antithrombotic Therapy Timing	24	88%	97%	98%
Assessed for Rehabilitation	26	85%	97%	97%
Discharged on Antithrombotic Therapy	23	83%	98%	99%
Discharged on Statin Medication	18	72%	93%	94%
Thrombolytic Therapy Timing[1]	-	-	59%	66%
Venous Thromboembolism Prophylaxis	25	64%	93%	94%
Written Stroke Educational Materials Given	13	69%	86%	88%
Surgical Care Improvement Project				
Appropriate Beta Blocker Usage[1]	-	-	98%	98%
Appropriate VTP Within 24 Hours	25	100%	98%	98%
Controlled Postoperative Blood Glucose[7]	-	-	96%	97%
Perioperative Temperature Management	26	100%	100%	100%
Prophylactic Antibiotic Selection	17	100%	99%	99%
Prophylactic Antibiotic Selection (Outpatient)	16	88%	97%	98%
Prophylactic Antibiotic Stopped	17	100%	98%	98%
Prophylactic Antibiotic Timing	17	94%	99%	99%
Prophylactic Antibiotic Timing (Outpatient)	16	100%	97%	98%
Urinary Catheter Removal	21	100%	97%	97%
Survey of Patients' Hospital Experiences				
Area Around Room 'Always' Quiet at Night	300+	71%	64%	61%
Doctors 'Always' Communicated Well	300+	86%	84%	82%
Home Recovery Information Given	300+	89%	86%	85%
Hospital Given 9 or 10 on 10 Point Scale	300+	75%	72%	71%
Meds 'Always' Explained Before Given	300+	68%	66%	64%
Nurses 'Always' Communicated Well	300+	80%	81%	79%
Pain 'Always' Well Controlled	300+	73%	73%	71%
Room and Bathroom 'Always' Clean	300+	78%	75%	73%
Timely Help 'Always' Received	300+	75%	69%	68%
Would Definitely Recommend Hospital	300+	71%	71%	71%
Use of Medical Imaging				
Cardiac Imaging Stress Test before Surgery	149	5.4%	5.3%	5.3%
Combination Abdominal CT Scan	197	53.8%	10.7%	10.5%
Combination Brain/Sinus CT Scan	239	0.8%	3.1%	2.7%
Combination Chest CT Scan	148	2.0%	4.3%	2.7%
Follow-up Mammogram/Ultrasound	299	14.0%	8.3%	8.8%
Lumbar Spine MRI for Low Back Pain[1]	-	-	38.9%	37.2%

Saint Elizabeth Florence

4900 Houston Road
Florence, KY 41042
URL: www.stlukehospitals.com
Phone: 859-212-5220
Fax: 859-212-5221
Type: Acute Care Hospitals
Ownership: Voluntary non-profit - Private
Emergency Services: Yes
Beds: 177

Key Personnel:
Operating Room. . . . . Beth Ackerson
Radiology. . . . . Carol Milburn, MD
Pediatric Ambulatory Care . . . . . . Ted Pappas, MD
Pediatric In-Patient Care . . . . . . Ted Pappas, MD
Quality Assurance . . . . Ron Reeser
CEO/President. . . . . Daniel M Vinson

Measure	Cases	This Hosp.	State Avg.	U.S. Avg.
Blood Clot Prevention and Treatment				
Anticoagulation Overlap Therapy[2]	60	100%	90%	93%
ICU Venous Thromboembolism Prophylaxis[2]	88	98%	86%	92%
Incidence of Potentially Preventable VTE[1,2]	-	-	13%	10%
UFH with Dosages/Platelet Monitoring[2]	64	100%	98%	97%
Venous Thromboembolism Prophylaxis[2]	391	96%	80%	85%
Warfarin Therapy Discharge Instructions[2]	47	100%	72%	75%
Chest Pain/Possible Heart Attack Care				
Aspirin Given Within 24 Hours of Arrival	34	100%	97%	96%
Fibrinolytic Meds Within 30 Min. of Arrival[7]	-	-	63%	58%
Average Time to ECG (minutes)	35	16	6	7
Average Time to Transfer (minutes)	14	58	61	60
Children's Asthma Care				
Received Home Management Plan of Care	-	-	-	88%
Received Reliever Medication	-	-	-	100%
Received Systemic Corticosteroids	-	-	-	100%
Emergency Department				
Admittance Decision Time (minutes)[2]	933	87	78	98
Head CT Results Within 45 Min. of Arrival[1]	-	-	55%	57%
Patients Who Left ER Before Being Seen	50,116	0%	2%	2%
Time from ER Arrival to Admit. (minutes)[2]	933	250	238	274
Time from ER Arrival to Discharge (minutes)	384	127	126	134
Time in ER Before Being Evaluated (minutes)	421	20	23	26
Time to Pain Meds for Fractures (minutes)	143	51	56	57
Heart Attack Care				
Aspirin Given at Discharge	64	100%	99%	99%
Fibrinolytic Meds Within 30 Min. of Arrival[7]	-	-	-	54%
PCI Within 90 Minutes of Arrival[7]	-	-	97%	96%
Statin Prescribed at Discharge	59	98%	97%	98%
Heart Failure Care				
ACE Inhibitor or ARB for LVSD[2]	59	100%	95%	97%
Discharge Instructions Given[2]	220	100%	92%	94%
Evaluation of LVS Function[2]	271	100%	98%	99%
Medicare Spending				
Medicare Spending per Patient (ratio)	-	1.06	0.97	0.98
Pneumonia Care				

NOTE: Hospital profiles are in alphabetical order by state, then city, then hospital within the city; Rankings exclude hospitals with less than 25 cases except for patient surveys which excludes hospitals with less than 100 cases; (a) 100-299 cases; (1) The number of cases/patients is too few to report; (2) Data submitted were based on a sample of cases/patients; (3) Results are based on a shorter time period than required; (4) Data suppressed by CMS for one or more quarters; (5) Results are not available for this reporting period; (6) Fewer than 100 patients completed the HCAHPS survey; (7) No cases met the criteria for this measure; (8) The lower limit of the confidence interval cannot be calculated if the number of observed infections equals zero; (9) No data are available from the state/territory for this reporting period; (10) The scores shown reflect fewer than 50 completed surveys; (11) There were discrepancies in the data collection process; (12) This measure does not apply to this hospital for this reporting period; (13) Results cannot be calculated for this reporting period; (14) The results for this state are combined with nearby states to protect confidentiality; Please refer to the User's Guide for a full explanation of data.

Appropriate Initial Antibiotic Given[2]	79	97%	94%	95%
Blood Culture Timing[2]	111	100%	98%	98%
Pregnancy and Delivery Care				
Newborn Deliveries Scheduled Early[7]	-	-	9%	6%
Preventive Care				
Immunization for Influenza[2]	642	100%	92%	90%
Immunization for Pneumonia[2]	911	100%	94%	92%
Stroke Care				
Anticoagulation Therapy for Atrial Fibrillation[1,2]	-	-	95%	95%
Antithrombotic Therapy Timing[2]	75	99%	97%	98%
Assessed for Rehabilitation[2]	98	100%	97%	97%
Discharged on Antithrombotic Therapy[2]	93	100%	98%	99%
Discharged on Statin Medication[2]	75	100%	93%	94%
Thrombolytic Therapy Timing[1,2]	-	-	59%	66%
Venous Thromboembolism Prophylaxis[2]	92	100%	93%	94%
Written Stroke Educational Materials Given[2]	49	98%	86%	88%
Surgical Care Improvement Project				
Appropriate Beta Blocker Usage	66	100%	98%	98%
Appropriate VTP Within 24 Hours	158	100%	98%	98%
Controlled Postoperative Blood Glucose[7]	-	-	96%	97%
Perioperative Temperature Management	200	100%	100%	100%
Prophylactic Antibiotic Selection	71	100%	99%	99%
Prophylactic Antibiotic Selection (Outpatient)	118	99%	97%	98%
Prophylactic Antibiotic Stopped	65	100%	98%	98%
Prophylactic Antibiotic Timing	71	100%	99%	99%
Prophylactic Antibiotic Timing (Outpatient)	118	100%	97%	98%
Urinary Catheter Removal	105	100%	97%	97%
Survey of Patients' Hospital Experiences				
Area Around Room 'Always' Quiet at Night	300+	59%	64%	61%
Doctors 'Always' Communicated Well	300+	77%	84%	82%
Home Recovery Information Given	300+	87%	86%	85%
Hospital Given 9 or 10 on 10 Point Scale	300+	67%	72%	71%
Meds 'Always' Explained Before Given	300+	63%	66%	64%
Nurses 'Always' Communicated Well	300+	76%	81%	79%
Pain 'Always' Well Controlled	300+	69%	73%	71%
Room and Bathroom 'Always' Clean	300+	68%	75%	73%
Timely Help 'Always' Received	300+	64%	69%	68%
Would Definitely Recommend Hospital	300+	67%	71%	71%
Use of Medical Imaging				
Cardiac Imaging Stress Test before Surgery	179	5.0%	5.3%	5.3%
Combination Abdominal CT Scan	677	3.2%	10.7%	10.5%
Combination Brain/Sinus CT Scan	593	1.3%	3.1%	2.7%
Combination Chest CT Scan	263	0.4%	4.3%	2.7%
Follow-up Mammogram/Ultrasound	918	6.9%	8.3%	8.8%
Lumbar Spine MRI for Low Back Pain	92	37.0%	38.9%	37.2%

Saint Elizabeth Ft Thomas

85 North Grand Avenue Phone: 859-572-3100
Fort Thomas, KY 41075 Fax: 859-572-3895
E-mail: lmw@chhs-nkey.org
URL: www.cardinalhill.org
Type: Acute Care Hospitals Emergency Services: Yes
Ownership: Voluntary non-profit - Private Beds: 33
Key Personnel:
CEO/President. . . . . Kerry Gillihan
Chief of Medical Staff. . . . . Patrica Miles

Measure	Cases	This Hosp.	State Avg.	U.S. Avg.
Blood Clot Prevention and Treatment				
Anticoagulation Overlap Therapy[2]	51	100%	90%	93%
ICU Venous Thromboembolism Prophylaxis[2]	83	99%	86%	92%
Incidence of Potentially Preventable VTE[1,2]	-	-	13%	10%
UFH with Dosages/Platelet Monitoring[2]	57	100%	98%	97%
Venous Thromboembolism Prophylaxis[2]	406	97%	80%	85%
Warfarin Therapy Discharge Instructions[2]	43	95%	72%	75%
Chest Pain/Possible Heart Attack Care				
Aspirin Given Within 24 Hours of Arrival	25	100%	97%	96%
Fibrinolytic Meds Within 30 Min. of Arrival[7]	-	-	63%	58%
Average Time to ECG (minutes)	25	11	6	7
Average Time to Transfer (minutes)	11	54	61	60
Children's Asthma Care				
Received Home Management Plan of Care	-	-	-	88%
Received Reliever Medication	-	-	-	100%
Received Systemic Corticosteroids	-	-	-	100%
Emergency Department				
Admittance Decision Time (minutes)[2]	960	94	78	98
Head CT Results Within 45 Min. of Arrival[1]	-	-	55%	57%
Patients Who Left ER Before Being Seen	37,132	0%	2%	2%
Time from ER Arrival to Admit. (minutes)[2]	961	254	238	274
Time from ER Arrival to Discharge (minutes)	379	123	126	134
Time in ER Before Being Evaluated (minutes)	422	21	23	26
Time to Pain Meds for Fractures (minutes)	77	49	56	57
Heart Attack Care				
Aspirin Given at Discharge	55	100%	99%	99%
Fibrinolytic Meds Within 30 Min. of Arrival[7]	-	-	-	54%
PCI Within 90 Minutes of Arrival[7]	-	-	97%	96%
Statin Prescribed at Discharge	51	100%	97%	98%
Heart Failure Care				
ACE Inhibitor or ARB for LVSD[2]	54	100%	95%	97%
Discharge Instructions Given[2]	189	100%	92%	94%
Evaluation of LVS Function[2]	243	100%	98%	99%
Medicare Spending				
Medicare Spending per Patient (ratio)	-	0.98	0.97	0.98
Pneumonia Care				
Appropriate Initial Antibiotic Given[2]	72	99%	94%	95%
Blood Culture Timing[2]	96	99%	98%	98%
Pregnancy and Delivery Care				
Newborn Deliveries Scheduled Early[7]	-	-	9%	6%
Preventive Care				
Immunization for Influenza[2]	597	100%	92%	90%
Immunization for Pneumonia[2]	905	100%	94%	92%
Stroke Care				
Anticoagulation Therapy for Atrial Fibrillation[1,2]	-	-	95%	95%
Antithrombotic Therapy Timing[2]	70	96%	97%	98%
Assessed for Rehabilitation[2]	81	100%	97%	97%
Discharged on Antithrombotic Therapy[2]	77	100%	98%	99%
Discharged on Statin Medication[2]	56	100%	93%	94%
Thrombolytic Therapy Timing[1,2]	-	-	59%	66%
Venous Thromboembolism Prophylaxis[2]	81	100%	93%	94%
Written Stroke Educational Materials Given[2]	46	100%	86%	88%
Surgical Care Improvement Project				
Appropriate Beta Blocker Usage	39	95%	98%	98%
Appropriate VTP Within 24 Hours	129	100%	98%	98%
Controlled Postoperative Blood Glucose[7]	-	-	96%	97%
Perioperative Temperature Management	170	100%	100%	100%
Prophylactic Antibiotic Selection	56	100%	99%	99%
Prophylactic Antibiotic Selection (Outpatient)	114	99%	97%	98%
Prophylactic Antibiotic Stopped	51	100%	98%	98%
Prophylactic Antibiotic Timing	56	100%	99%	99%
Prophylactic Antibiotic Timing (Outpatient)	114	100%	97%	98%
Urinary Catheter Removal	76	100%	97%	97%
Survey of Patients' Hospital Experiences				
Area Around Room 'Always' Quiet at Night	300+	54%	64%	61%
Doctors 'Always' Communicated Well	300+	78%	84%	82%
Home Recovery Information Given	300+	89%	86%	85%
Hospital Given 9 or 10 on 10 Point Scale	300+	69%	72%	71%
Meds 'Always' Explained Before Given	300+	66%	66%	64%
Nurses 'Always' Communicated Well	300+	79%	81%	79%
Pain 'Always' Well Controlled	300+	70%	73%	71%
Room and Bathroom 'Always' Clean	300+	75%	75%	73%
Timely Help 'Always' Received	300+	66%	69%	68%
Would Definitely Recommend Hospital	300+	67%	71%	71%
Use of Medical Imaging				
Cardiac Imaging Stress Test before Surgery	167	4.2%	5.3%	5.3%
Combination Abdominal CT Scan	600	3.2%	10.7%	10.5%
Combination Brain/Sinus CT Scan	513	2.5%	3.1%	2.7%
Combination Chest CT Scan	293	1.0%	4.3%	2.7%
Follow-up Mammogram/Ultrasound	969	6.8%	8.3%	8.8%
Lumbar Spine MRI for Low Back Pain	83	26.5%	38.9%	37.2%

Frankfort Regional Medical Center

299 Kings Daughters Drive Phone: 502-875-5240
Frankfort, KY 40601 Fax: 502-226-7936
URL: www.frankfortregional.com
Type: Acute Care Hospitals Emergency Services: Yes
Ownership: Proprietary Beds: 173
Key Personnel:
Emergency Room . . . . Timothy K Anderson
Chief of Medical Staff. . . . . Allen Haddix, MD
Operating Room. . . . . Becky Jernigan
CEO/President. . . . . Michael Mayo
Quality Assurance . . . . Pam Melton
Infection Control. . . . . Emily Mills
Patient Relations . . . . Karen Muzzillo
Cardiac Laboratory. . . . . Dave Sebastian

Measure	Cases	This Hosp.	State Avg.	U.S. Avg.
Blood Clot Prevention and Treatment				
Anticoagulation Overlap Therapy[2]	17	94%	90%	93%
ICU Venous Thromboembolism Prophylaxis[2]	90	99%	86%	92%
Incidence of Potentially Preventable VTE[1,2]	-	-	13%	10%
UFH with Dosages/Platelet Monitoring[1,2]	-	-	98%	97%
Venous Thromboembolism Prophylaxis[2]	328	100%	80%	85%
Warfarin Therapy Discharge Instructions[2]	13	100%	72%	75%
Chest Pain/Possible Heart Attack Care				
Aspirin Given Within 24 Hours of Arrival	128	99%	97%	96%
Fibrinolytic Meds Within 30 Min. of Arrival[1]	-	-	63%	58%
Average Time to ECG (minutes)	126	5	6	7
Average Time to Transfer (minutes)	44	34	61	60
Children's Asthma Care				
Received Home Management Plan of Care	-	-	-	88%
Received Reliever Medication	-	-	-	100%
Received Systemic Corticosteroids	-	-	-	100%
Emergency Department				
Admittance Decision Time (minutes)[2]	503	63	78	98
Head CT Results Within 45 Min. of Arrival	27	59%	55%	57%
Patients Who Left ER Before Being Seen	31,031	2%	2%	2%
Time from ER Arrival to Admit. (minutes)[2]	503	236	238	274
Time from ER Arrival to Discharge (minutes)	435	143	126	134
Time in ER Before Being Evaluated (minutes)	513	20	23	26
Time to Pain Meds for Fractures (minutes)	153	41	56	57
Heart Attack Care				
Aspirin Given at Discharge	14	100%	99%	99%
Fibrinolytic Meds Within 30 Min. of Arrival[7]	-	-	-	54%
PCI Within 90 Minutes of Arrival[7]	-	-	97%	96%
Statin Prescribed at Discharge	13	100%	97%	98%
Heart Failure Care				
ACE Inhibitor or ARB for LVSD	34	100%	95%	97%
Discharge Instructions Given	134	98%	92%	94%
Evaluation of LVS Function	160	100%	98%	99%
Medicare Spending				
Medicare Spending per Patient (ratio)	-	1.02	0.97	0.98
Pneumonia Care				
Appropriate Initial Antibiotic Given	88	100%	94%	95%
Blood Culture Timing	153	100%	98%	98%
Pregnancy and Delivery Care				
Newborn Deliveries Scheduled Early[2]	30	3%	9%	6%
Preventive Care				
Immunization for Influenza[2]	435	97%	92%	90%
Immunization for Pneumonia[2]	549	99%	94%	92%
Stroke Care				
Anticoagulation Therapy for Atrial Fibrillation[1,2]	-	-	95%	95%
Antithrombotic Therapy Timing[2]	19	89%	97%	98%
Assessed for Rehabilitation[2]	18	100%	97%	97%
Discharged on Antithrombotic Therapy[2]	18	100%	98%	99%
Discharged on Statin Medication[1,2]	-	-	93%	94%
Thrombolytic Therapy Timing[2,7]	-	-	59%	66%
Venous Thromboembolism Prophylaxis[2]	19	100%	93%	94%
Written Stroke Educational Materials Given[1,2]	-	-	86%	88%
Surgical Care Improvement Project				
Appropriate Beta Blocker Usage	53	100%	98%	98%
Appropriate VTP Within 24 Hours	175	100%	98%	98%
Controlled Postoperative Blood Glucose[7]	-	-	96%	97%
Perioperative Temperature Management	200	100%	100%	100%
Prophylactic Antibiotic Selection	124	99%	99%	99%
Prophylactic Antibiotic Selection (Outpatient)	134	100%	97%	98%
Prophylactic Antibiotic Stopped	120	99%	98%	98%
Prophylactic Antibiotic Timing	124	100%	99%	99%
Prophylactic Antibiotic Timing (Outpatient)	134	99%	97%	98%
Urinary Catheter Removal	139	100%	97%	97%
Survey of Patients' Hospital Experiences				
Area Around Room 'Always' Quiet at Night	300+	58%	64%	61%

NOTE: Hospital profiles are in alphabetical order by state, then city, then hospital within the city; Rankings exclude hospitals with less than 25 cases except for patient surveys which excludes hospitals with less than 100 cases; (a) 100-299 cases; (1) The number of cases/patients is too few to report; (2) Data submitted were based on a sample of cases/patients; (3) Results are based on a shorter time period than required; (4) Data suppressed by CMS for one or more quarters; (5) Results are not available for this reporting period; (6) Fewer than 100 patients completed the HCAHPS survey; (7) No cases met the criteria for this measure; (8) The lower limit of the confidence interval cannot be calculated if the number of observed infections equals zero; (9) No data are available from the state/territory for this reporting period; (10) The scores shown reflect fewer than 50 completed surveys; (11) There were discrepancies in the data collection process; (12) This measure does not apply to this hospital for this reporting period; (13) Results cannot be calculated for this reporting period; (14) The results for this state are combined with nearby states to protect confidentiality; Please refer to the User's Guide for a full explanation of data.

Measure	Cases	This Hosp.	State Avg.	U.S. Avg.
Doctors 'Always' Communicated Well	300+	81%	84%	82%
Home Recovery Information Given	300+	85%	86%	85%
Hospital Given 9 or 10 on 10 Point Scale	300+	65%	72%	71%
Meds 'Always' Explained Before Given	300+	64%	66%	64%
Nurses 'Always' Communicated Well	300+	76%	81%	79%
Pain 'Always' Well Controlled	300+	68%	73%	71%
Room and Bathroom 'Always' Clean	300+	66%	75%	73%
Timely Help 'Always' Received	300+	65%	69%	68%
Would Definitely Recommend Hospital	300+	62%	71%	71%
Use of Medical Imaging				
Cardiac Imaging Stress Test before Surgery	53	1.9%	5.3%	5.3%
Combination Abdominal CT Scan	486	3.1%	10.7%	10.5%
Combination Brain/Sinus CT Scan	561	1.1%	3.1%	2.7%
Combination Chest CT Scan	158	0.6%	4.3%	2.7%
Follow-up Mammogram/Ultrasound	750	3.6%	8.3%	8.8%
Lumbar Spine MRI for Low Back Pain	61	44.3%	38.9%	37.2%

The Medical Center at Franklin

1100 Brookhaven Road Phone: 270-598-4800
Franklin, KY 42135
URL: www.mcfrk.org
Type: Critical Access Hospitals Emergency Services: Yes
Ownership: Voluntary non-profit - Private Beds: 25
Key Personnel:
CEO/President. . . . . John C Desmarais

Measure	Cases	This Hosp.	State Avg.	U.S. Avg.
Blood Clot Prevention and Treatment				
Anticoagulation Overlap Therapy[5]	-	-	90%	93%
ICU Venous Thromboembolism Prophylaxis[5]	-	-	86%	92%
Incidence of Potentially Preventable VTE[5]	-	-	13%	10%
UFH with Dosages/Platelet Monitoring[5]	-	-	98%	97%
Venous Thromboembolism Prophylaxis[5]	-	-	80%	85%
Warfarin Therapy Discharge Instructions[5]	-	-	72%	75%
Chest Pain/Possible Heart Attack Care				
Aspirin Given Within 24 Hours of Arrival[5]	-	-	97%	96%
Fibrinolytic Meds Within 30 Min. of Arrival[5]	-	-	63%	58%
Average Time to ECG (minutes)[5]	-	-	6	7
Average Time to Transfer (minutes)[5]	-	-	61	60
Children's Asthma Care				
Received Home Management Plan of Care	-	-	-	88%
Received Reliever Medication	-	-	-	100%
Received Systemic Corticosteroids	-	-	-	100%
Emergency Department				
Admittance Decision Time (minutes)[5]	-	-	78	98
Head CT Results Within 45 Min. of Arrival[5]	-	-	55%	57%
Patients Who Left ER Before Being Seen	11,489	4%	2%	2%
Time from ER Arrival to Admit. (minutes)[5]	-	-	238	274
Time from ER Arrival to Discharge (minutes)[5]	-	-	126	134
Time in ER Before Being Evaluated (minutes)[5]	-	-	23	26
Time to Pain Meds for Fractures (minutes)[5]	-	-	56	57
Heart Attack Care				
Aspirin Given at Discharge[1,3]	-	-	99%	99%
Fibrinolytic Meds Within 30 Min. of Arrival[3,7]	-	-	-	54%
PCI Within 90 Minutes of Arrival[3,7]	-	-	97%	96%
Statin Prescribed at Discharge[3,7]	-	-	97%	98%
Heart Failure Care				
ACE Inhibitor or ARB for LVSD[1]	-	-	95%	97%
Discharge Instructions Given	31	97%	92%	94%
Evaluation of LVS Function	42	95%	98%	99%
Medicare Spending				
Medicare Spending per Patient (ratio)	-	-	0.97	0.98
Pneumonia Care				
Appropriate Initial Antibiotic Given	55	87%	94%	95%
Blood Culture Timing	26	96%	98%	98%
Pregnancy and Delivery Care				
Newborn Deliveries Scheduled Early[5]	-	-	9%	6%
Preventive Care				
Immunization for Influenza[5]	-	-	92%	90%
Immunization for Pneumonia[5]	-	-	94%	92%
Stroke Care				
Anticoagulation Therapy for Atrial Fibrillation[5]	-	-	95%	95%
Antithrombotic Therapy Timing[5]	-	-	97%	98%
Assessed for Rehabilitation[5]	-	-	97%	97%
Discharged on Antithrombotic Therapy[5]	-	-	98%	99%
Discharged on Statin Medication[5]	-	-	93%	94%
Thrombolytic Therapy Timing[5]	-	-	59%	66%
Venous Thromboembolism Prophylaxis[5]	-	-	93%	94%
Written Stroke Educational Materials Given[5]	-	-	86%	88%
Surgical Care Improvement Project				
Appropriate Beta Blocker Usage[5]	-	-	98%	98%
Appropriate VTP Within 24 Hours[5]	-	-	98%	98%
Controlled Postoperative Blood Glucose[5]	-	-	96%	97%
Perioperative Temperature Management[5]	-	-	100%	100%
Prophylactic Antibiotic Selection[5]	-	-	99%	99%
Prophylactic Antibiotic Selection (Outpatient)[5]	-	-	97%	98%
Prophylactic Antibiotic Stopped[5]	-	-	98%	98%
Prophylactic Antibiotic Timing[5]	-	-	99%	99%
Prophylactic Antibiotic Timing (Outpatient)[5]	-	-	97%	98%
Urinary Catheter Removal[5]	-	-	97%	97%
Survey of Patients' Hospital Experiences				
Area Around Room 'Always' Quiet at Night[5]	-	-	64%	61%
Doctors 'Always' Communicated Well[5]	-	-	84%	82%
Home Recovery Information Given[5]	-	-	86%	85%
Hospital Given 9 or 10 on 10 Point Scale[5]	-	-	72%	71%
Meds 'Always' Explained Before Given[5]	-	-	66%	64%
Nurses 'Always' Communicated Well[5]	-	-	81%	79%
Pain 'Always' Well Controlled[5]	-	-	73%	71%
Room and Bathroom 'Always' Clean[5]	-	-	75%	73%
Timely Help 'Always' Received[5]	-	-	69%	68%
Would Definitely Recommend Hospital[5]	-	-	71%	71%
Use of Medical Imaging				
Cardiac Imaging Stress Test before Surgery[1]	-	-	5.3%	5.3%
Combination Abdominal CT Scan	216	10.6%	10.7%	10.5%
Combination Brain/Sinus CT Scan[1]	-	-	3.1%	2.7%
Combination Chest CT Scan	90	10.0%	4.3%	2.7%
Follow-up Mammogram/Ultrasound	169	3.6%	8.3%	8.8%
Lumbar Spine MRI for Low Back Pain[1]	-	-	38.9%	37.2%

Parkway Regional Hospital

2000 Holiday Lane Phone: 270-472-2522
Fulton, KY 42041 Fax: 270-472-2438
URL: www.parkwayregionalhospital.com
Type: Acute Care Hospitals Emergency Services: Yes
Ownership: Proprietary Beds: 70
Key Personnel:
CEO/President. . . . . Michael Patterson

Measure	Cases	This Hosp.	State Avg.	U.S. Avg.
Blood Clot Prevention and Treatment				
Anticoagulation Overlap Therapy[1,2]	-	-	90%	93%
ICU Venous Thromboembolism Prophylaxis[2]	109	100%	86%	92%
Incidence of Potentially Preventable VTE[2,7]	-	-	13%	10%
UFH with Dosages/Platelet Monitoring[2,7]	-	-	98%	97%
Venous Thromboembolism Prophylaxis[2]	237	99%	80%	85%
Warfarin Therapy Discharge Instructions[1,2]	-	-	72%	75%
Chest Pain/Possible Heart Attack Care				
Aspirin Given Within 24 Hours of Arrival	42	100%	97%	96%
Fibrinolytic Meds Within 30 Min. of Arrival[1]	-	-	63%	58%
Average Time to ECG (minutes)	46	3	6	7
Average Time to Transfer (minutes)[1]	-	-	61	60
Children's Asthma Care				
Received Home Management Plan of Care	-	-	-	88%
Received Reliever Medication	-	-	-	100%
Received Systemic Corticosteroids	-	-	-	100%
Emergency Department				
Admittance Decision Time (minutes)[2]	347	44	78	98
Head CT Results Within 45 Min. of Arrival[1,3]	-	-	55%	57%
Patients Who Left ER Before Being Seen	6,093	1%	2%	2%
Time from ER Arrival to Admit. (minutes)[2]	348	180	238	274
Time from ER Arrival to Discharge (minutes)	375	93	126	134
Time in ER Before Being Evaluated (minutes)	423	16	23	26
Time to Pain Meds for Fractures (minutes)	23	72	56	57
Heart Attack Care				
Aspirin Given at Discharge[1]	-	-	99%	99%
Fibrinolytic Meds Within 30 Min. of Arrival[7]	-	-	-	54%
PCI Within 90 Minutes of Arrival[7]	-	-	97%	96%
Statin Prescribed at Discharge[1]	-	-	97%	98%
Heart Failure Care				
ACE Inhibitor or ARB for LVSD[1]	-	-	95%	97%
Discharge Instructions Given	23	100%	92%	94%
Evaluation of LVS Function	35	100%	98%	99%
Medicare Spending				
Medicare Spending per Patient (ratio)	-	1.02	0.97	0.98
Pneumonia Care				
Appropriate Initial Antibiotic Given	53	100%	94%	95%
Blood Culture Timing	57	100%	98%	98%
Pregnancy and Delivery Care				
Newborn Deliveries Scheduled Early[2,7]	-	-	9%	6%
Preventive Care				
Immunization for Influenza[2]	305	100%	92%	90%
Immunization for Pneumonia[2]	362	100%	94%	92%
Stroke Care				
Anticoagulation Therapy for Atrial Fibrillation[7]	-	-	95%	95%
Antithrombotic Therapy Timing[1]	-	-	97%	98%
Assessed for Rehabilitation[1]	-	-	97%	97%
Discharged on Antithrombotic Therapy[1]	-	-	98%	99%
Discharged on Statin Medication[1]	-	-	93%	94%
Thrombolytic Therapy Timing[1]	-	-	59%	66%
Venous Thromboembolism Prophylaxis[1]	-	-	93%	94%
Written Stroke Educational Materials Given[1]	-	-	86%	88%
Surgical Care Improvement Project				
Appropriate Beta Blocker Usage[1]	-	-	98%	98%
Appropriate VTP Within 24 Hours	47	100%	98%	98%
Controlled Postoperative Blood Glucose[7]	-	-	96%	97%
Perioperative Temperature Management	47	100%	100%	100%
Prophylactic Antibiotic Selection	40	100%	99%	99%
Prophylactic Antibiotic Selection (Outpatient)[1,3]	-	-	97%	98%
Prophylactic Antibiotic Stopped	40	100%	98%	98%
Prophylactic Antibiotic Timing	40	100%	99%	99%
Prophylactic Antibiotic Timing (Outpatient)[1,3]	-	-	97%	98%
Urinary Catheter Removal	43	98%	97%	97%
Survey of Patients' Hospital Experiences				
Area Around Room 'Always' Quiet at Night	(a)	78%	64%	61%
Doctors 'Always' Communicated Well	(a)	88%	84%	82%
Home Recovery Information Given	(a)	84%	86%	85%
Hospital Given 9 or 10 on 10 Point Scale	(a)	70%	72%	71%
Meds 'Always' Explained Before Given	(a)	69%	66%	64%
Nurses 'Always' Communicated Well	(a)	80%	81%	79%
Pain 'Always' Well Controlled	(a)	74%	73%	71%
Room and Bathroom 'Always' Clean	(a)	78%	75%	73%
Timely Help 'Always' Received	(a)	75%	69%	68%
Would Definitely Recommend Hospital	(a)	70%	71%	71%
Use of Medical Imaging				
Cardiac Imaging Stress Test before Surgery[1]	-	-	5.3%	5.3%
Combination Abdominal CT Scan	131	4.6%	10.7%	10.5%
Combination Brain/Sinus CT Scan[1]	-	-	3.1%	2.7%
Combination Chest CT Scan	85	0.0%	4.3%	2.7%
Follow-up Mammogram/Ultrasound	227	10.6%	8.3%	8.8%
Lumbar Spine MRI for Low Back Pain[1]	-	-	38.9%	37.2%

Georgetown Community Hospital

1140 Lexington Road Phone: 502-868-1100
Georgetown, KY 40324 Fax: 502-868-5607
URL: www.georgetowncommunityhospital.com
Type: Acute Care Hospitals Emergency Services: Yes
Ownership: Proprietary Beds: 75
Key Personnel:
Chief of Medical Staff. . . . . Kelly Burguss
CEO . . . . William Haugh
Emergency Room . . . . Philip Wagner

Measure	Cases	This Hosp.	State Avg.	U.S. Avg.
Blood Clot Prevention and Treatment				
Anticoagulation Overlap Therapy[2]	13	92%	90%	93%
ICU Venous Thromboembolism Prophylaxis[2]	37	97%	86%	92%
Incidence of Potentially Preventable VTE[1,2]	-	-	13%	10%
UFH with Dosages/Platelet Monitoring[1,2]	-	-	98%	97%
Venous Thromboembolism Prophylaxis[2]	171	97%	80%	85%
Warfarin Therapy Discharge Instructions[2]	12	100%	72%	75%
Chest Pain/Possible Heart Attack Care				
Aspirin Given Within 24 Hours of Arrival	118	98%	97%	96%

NOTE: Hospital profiles are in alphabetical order by state, then city, then hospital within the city; Rankings exclude hospitals with less than 25 cases except for patient surveys which excludes hospitals with less than 100 cases; (a) 100-299 cases; (1) The number of cases/patients is too few to report; (2) Data submitted were based on a sample of cases/patients; (3) Results are based on a shorter time period than required; (4) Data suppressed by CMS for one or more quarters; (5) Results are not available for this reporting period; (6) Fewer than 100 patients completed the HCAHPS survey; (7) No cases met the criteria for this measure; (8) The lower limit of the confidence interval cannot be calculated if the number of observed infections equals zero; (9) No data are available from the state/territory for this reporting period; (10) The scores shown reflect fewer than 50 completed surveys; (11) There were discrepancies in the data collection process; (12) This measure does not apply to this hospital for this reporting period; (13) Results cannot be calculated for this reporting period; (14) The results for this state are combined with nearby states to protect confidentiality; Please refer to the User's Guide for a full explanation of data.

Fibrinolytic Meds Within 30 Min. of Arrival[7]	-	-	63%	58%
Average Time to ECG (minutes)	124	7	6	7
Average Time to Transfer (minutes)[1]	-	-	61	60
Children's Asthma Care				
Received Home Management Plan of Care	-	-	-	88%
Received Reliever Medication	-	-	-	100%
Received Systemic Corticosteroids	-	-	-	100%
Emergency Department				
Admittance Decision Time (minutes)[2]	243	76	78	98
Head CT Results Within 45 Min. of Arrival[1]	-	-	55%	57%
Patients Who Left ER Before Being Seen	22,045	1%	2%	2%
Time from ER Arrival to Admit. (minutes)[2]	243	228	238	274
Time from ER Arrival to Discharge (minutes)	425	109	126	134
Time in ER Before Being Evaluated (minutes)	467	14	23	26
Time to Pain Meds for Fractures (minutes)	75	32	56	57
Heart Attack Care				
Aspirin Given at Discharge[1,3]	-	-	99%	99%
Fibrinolytic Meds Within 30 Min. of Arrival[3,7]	-	-	-	54%
PCI Within 90 Minutes of Arrival[3,7]	-	-	97%	96%
Statin Prescribed at Discharge[1,3]	-	-	97%	98%
Heart Failure Care				
ACE Inhibitor or ARB for LVSD	13	85%	95%	97%
Discharge Instructions Given	44	95%	92%	94%
Evaluation of LVS Function	53	100%	98%	99%
Medicare Spending				
Medicare Spending per Patient (ratio)	-	0.96	0.97	0.98
Pneumonia Care				
Appropriate Initial Antibiotic Given	79	95%	94%	95%
Blood Culture Timing	104	98%	98%	98%
Pregnancy and Delivery Care				
Newborn Deliveries Scheduled Early[2]	11	0%	9%	6%
Preventive Care				
Immunization for Influenza[2]	259	98%	92%	90%
Immunization for Pneumonia[2]	318	95%	94%	92%
Stroke Care				
Anticoagulation Therapy for Atrial Fibrillation[1]	-	-	95%	95%
Antithrombotic Therapy Timing	16	100%	97%	98%
Assessed for Rehabilitation	17	100%	97%	97%
Discharged on Antithrombotic Therapy	17	100%	98%	99%
Discharged on Statin Medication	15	93%	93%	94%
Thrombolytic Therapy Timing[7]	-	-	59%	66%
Venous Thromboembolism Prophylaxis	16	88%	93%	94%
Written Stroke Educational Materials Given[1]	-	-	86%	88%
Surgical Care Improvement Project				
Appropriate Beta Blocker Usage	20	90%	98%	98%
Appropriate VTP Within 24 Hours	50	94%	98%	98%
Controlled Postoperative Blood Glucose[7]	-	-	96%	97%
Perioperative Temperature Management	52	100%	100%	100%
Prophylactic Antibiotic Selection	25	100%	99%	99%
Prophylactic Antibiotic Selection (Outpatient)	144	97%	97%	98%
Prophylactic Antibiotic Stopped	23	100%	98%	98%
Prophylactic Antibiotic Timing	25	100%	99%	99%
Prophylactic Antibiotic Timing (Outpatient)	144	100%	97%	98%
Urinary Catheter Removal	32	97%	97%	97%
Survey of Patients' Hospital Experiences				
Area Around Room 'Always' Quiet at Night	300+	61%	64%	61%
Doctors 'Always' Communicated Well	300+	88%	84%	82%
Home Recovery Information Given	300+	87%	86%	85%
Hospital Given 9 or 10 on 10 Point Scale	300+	69%	72%	71%
Meds 'Always' Explained Before Given	300+	67%	66%	64%
Nurses 'Always' Communicated Well	300+	80%	81%	79%
Pain 'Always' Well Controlled	300+	72%	73%	71%
Room and Bathroom 'Always' Clean	300+	69%	75%	73%
Timely Help 'Always' Received	300+	65%	69%	68%
Would Definitely Recommend Hospital	300+	71%	71%	71%
Use of Medical Imaging				
Cardiac Imaging Stress Test before Surgery	103	3.9%	5.3%	5.3%
Combination Abdominal CT Scan	317	2.8%	10.7%	10.5%
Combination Brain/Sinus CT Scan[1]	-	-	3.1%	2.7%
Combination Chest CT Scan	132	1.5%	4.3%	2.7%
Follow-up Mammogram/Ultrasound	409	3.9%	8.3%	8.8%
Lumbar Spine MRI for Low Back Pain[1]	-	-	38.9%	37.2%

T J Samson Community Hospital

1301 North Race Street
Glasgow, KY 42141
E-mail: tjsamson@tjsamson.org
URL: www.tjsamson.org
Phone: 270-651-4159
Fax: 270-651-4848

Type: Acute Care Hospitals
Ownership: Voluntary non-profit - Other
Emergency Services: Yes
Beds: 196

Key Personnel:
Coronary Care . . . . Barbara Buss, RN
Infection Control. . . . . Millie Delk
Pediatric Ambulatory Care . . . . . . Melissa Dennison, MD
Pediatric In-Patient Care . . . . Melissa Dennison, MD
Chief of Medical Staff. . . . . Jeffery Sabolovic, MD
Radiology. . . . . Michael Shadowe
Quality Assurance . . . . Melanie Watson
CEO . . . . Bud Wethington

Measure	Cases	This Hosp.	State Avg.	U.S. Avg.
Blood Clot Prevention and Treatment				
Anticoagulation Overlap Therapy[2]	33	91%	90%	93%
ICU Venous Thromboembolism Prophylaxis[2]	81	78%	86%	92%
Incidence of Potentially Preventable VTE[1,2]	-	-	13%	10%
UFH with Dosages/Platelet Monitoring[2]	27	96%	98%	97%
Venous Thromboembolism Prophylaxis[2]	353	64%	80%	85%
Warfarin Therapy Discharge Instructions[2]	31	100%	72%	75%
Chest Pain/Possible Heart Attack Care				
Aspirin Given Within 24 Hours of Arrival[3]	16	94%	97%	96%
Fibrinolytic Meds Within 30 Min. of Arrival[3,7]	-	-	63%	58%
Average Time to ECG (minutes)[3]	15	15	6	7
Average Time to Transfer (minutes)[3,7]	-	-	61	60
Children's Asthma Care				
Received Home Management Plan of Care	-	-	-	88%
Received Reliever Medication	-	-	-	100%
Received Systemic Corticosteroids	-	-	-	100%
Emergency Department				
Admittance Decision Time (minutes)[2]	415	92	78	98
Head CT Results Within 45 Min. of Arrival	22	23%	55%	57%
Patients Who Left ER Before Being Seen	34,624	1%	2%	2%
Time from ER Arrival to Admit. (minutes)[2]	460	256	238	274
Time from ER Arrival to Discharge (minutes)	424	120	126	134
Time in ER Before Being Evaluated (minutes)	336	33	23	26
Time to Pain Meds for Fractures (minutes)	138	62	56	57
Heart Attack Care				
Aspirin Given at Discharge	207	95%	99%	99%
Fibrinolytic Meds Within 30 Min. of Arrival[7]	-	-	-	54%
PCI Within 90 Minutes of Arrival	24	83%	97%	96%
Statin Prescribed at Discharge	195	88%	97%	98%
Heart Failure Care				
ACE Inhibitor or ARB for LVSD	60	90%	95%	97%
Discharge Instructions Given	143	87%	92%	94%
Evaluation of LVS Function	186	99%	98%	99%
Medicare Spending				
Medicare Spending per Patient (ratio)	-	1.00	0.97	0.98
Pneumonia Care				
Appropriate Initial Antibiotic Given[2]	85	93%	94%	95%
Blood Culture Timing[2]	144	99%	98%	98%
Pregnancy and Delivery Care				
Newborn Deliveries Scheduled Early[2]	31	16%	9%	6%
Preventive Care				
Immunization for Influenza[2]	495	96%	92%	90%
Immunization for Pneumonia[2]	570	96%	94%	92%
Stroke Care				
Anticoagulation Therapy for Atrial Fibrillation[1]	-	-	95%	95%
Antithrombotic Therapy Timing[1]	-	-	97%	98%
Assessed for Rehabilitation[1]	-	-	97%	97%
Discharged on Antithrombotic Therapy[1]	-	-	98%	99%
Discharged on Statin Medication[1]	-	-	93%	94%
Thrombolytic Therapy Timing[1]	-	-	59%	66%
Venous Thromboembolism Prophylaxis[1]	-	-	93%	94%
Written Stroke Educational Materials Given[1]	-	-	86%	88%
Surgical Care Improvement Project				
Appropriate Beta Blocker Usage[2]	109	94%	98%	98%
Appropriate VTP Within 24 Hours[2]	263	95%	98%	98%
Controlled Postoperative Blood Glucose[2,7]	-	-	96%	97%
Perioperative Temperature Management[2]	306	100%	100%	100%
Prophylactic Antibiotic Selection[2]	200	100%	99%	99%
Prophylactic Antibiotic Selection (Outpatient)	192	96%	97%	98%
Prophylactic Antibiotic Stopped[2]	192	95%	98%	98%
Prophylactic Antibiotic Timing[2]	200	97%	99%	99%
Prophylactic Antibiotic Timing (Outpatient)	195	96%	97%	98%
Urinary Catheter Removal[2]	210	98%	97%	97%
Survey of Patients' Hospital Experiences				
Area Around Room 'Always' Quiet at Night	300+	66%	64%	61%
Doctors 'Always' Communicated Well	300+	85%	84%	82%
Home Recovery Information Given	300+	82%	86%	85%
Hospital Given 9 or 10 on 10 Point Scale	300+	70%	72%	71%
Meds 'Always' Explained Before Given	300+	59%	66%	64%
Nurses 'Always' Communicated Well	300+	82%	81%	79%
Pain 'Always' Well Controlled	300+	68%	73%	71%
Room and Bathroom 'Always' Clean	300+	81%	75%	73%
Timely Help 'Always' Received	300+	72%	69%	68%
Would Definitely Recommend Hospital	300+	68%	71%	71%
Use of Medical Imaging				
Cardiac Imaging Stress Test before Surgery	326	4.3%	5.3%	5.3%
Combination Abdominal CT Scan	876	15.2%	10.7%	10.5%
Combination Brain/Sinus CT Scan	681	2.6%	3.1%	2.7%
Combination Chest CT Scan	642	10.1%	4.3%	2.7%
Follow-up Mammogram/Ultrasound	1,257	4.5%	8.3%	8.8%
Lumbar Spine MRI for Low Back Pain	99	34.3%	38.9%	37.2%

Jane Todd Crawford Hospital

202-206 Milby Street
Greensburg, KY 42743
E-mail: jtodd@kih.net
Phone: 270-932-4211
Fax: 270-932-3504

Type: Critical Access Hospitals
Ownership: Voluntary non-profit - Private
Emergency Services: Yes
Beds: 64

Key Personnel:
CEO/President. . . . . Rex A Tungate

Measure	Cases	This Hosp.	State Avg.	U.S. Avg.
Blood Clot Prevention and Treatment				
Anticoagulation Overlap Therapy[5]	-	-	90%	93%
ICU Venous Thromboembolism Prophylaxis[5]	-	-	86%	92%
Incidence of Potentially Preventable VTE[5]	-	-	13%	10%
UFH with Dosages/Platelet Monitoring[5]	-	-	98%	97%
Venous Thromboembolism Prophylaxis[5]	-	-	80%	85%
Warfarin Therapy Discharge Instructions[5]	-	-	72%	75%
Chest Pain/Possible Heart Attack Care				
Aspirin Given Within 24 Hours of Arrival	11	73%	97%	96%
Fibrinolytic Meds Within 30 Min. of Arrival[1,3]	-	-	63%	58%
Average Time to ECG (minutes)	11	2	6	7
Average Time to Transfer (minutes)[1,3]	-	-	61	60
Children's Asthma Care				
Received Home Management Plan of Care	-	-	-	88%
Received Reliever Medication	-	-	-	100%
Received Systemic Corticosteroids	-	-	-	100%
Emergency Department				
Admittance Decision Time (minutes)[5]	-	-	78	98
Head CT Results Within 45 Min. of Arrival[5]	-	-	55%	57%
Patients Who Left ER Before Being Seen	5,849	1%	2%	2%
Time from ER Arrival to Admit. (minutes)[5]	-	-	238	274
Time from ER Arrival to Discharge (minutes)[5]	-	-	126	134
Time in ER Before Being Evaluated (minutes)[5]	-	-	23	26
Time to Pain Meds for Fractures (minutes)[5]	-	-	56	57
Heart Attack Care				
Aspirin Given at Discharge[1,3]	-	-	99%	99%
Fibrinolytic Meds Within 30 Min. of Arrival[3,7]	-	-	-	54%
PCI Within 90 Minutes of Arrival[3,7]	-	-	97%	96%
Statin Prescribed at Discharge[1,3]	-	-	97%	98%
Heart Failure Care				
ACE Inhibitor or ARB for LVSD[7]	-	-	95%	97%
Discharge Instructions Given	24	100%	92%	94%
Evaluation of LVS Function	42	36%	98%	99%
Medicare Spending				
Medicare Spending per Patient (ratio)	-	-	0.97	0.98
Pneumonia Care				
Appropriate Initial Antibiotic Given	25	84%	94%	95%
Blood Culture Timing[1]	-	-	98%	98%
Pregnancy and Delivery Care				

NOTE: Hospital profiles are in alphabetical order by state, then city, then hospital within the city; Rankings exclude hospitals with less than 25 cases except for patient surveys which excludes hospitals with less than 100 cases; (a) 100-299 cases; (1) The number of cases/patients is too few to report; (2) Data submitted were based on a sample of cases/patients; (3) Results are based on a shorter time period than required; (4) Data suppressed by CMS for one or more quarters; (5) Results are not available for this reporting period; (6) Fewer than 100 patients completed the HCAHPS survey; (7) No cases met the criteria for this measure; (8) The lower limit of the confidence interval cannot be calculated if the number of observed infections equals zero; (9) No data are available from the state/territory for this reporting period; (10) The scores shown reflect fewer than 50 completed surveys; (11) There were discrepancies in the data collection process; (12) This measure does not apply to this hospital for this reporting period; (13) Results cannot be calculated for this reporting period; (14) The results for this state are combined with nearby states to protect confidentiality; Please refer to the User's Guide for a full explanation of data.

Measure	Cases	This Hosp.	State Avg.	U.S. Avg.
Newborn Deliveries Scheduled Early[5]	-	-	9%	6%
Preventive Care				
Immunization for Influenza[5]	-	-	92%	90%
Immunization for Pneumonia[5]	-	-	94%	92%
Stroke Care				
Anticoagulation Therapy for Atrial Fibrillation[5]	-	-	95%	95%
Antithrombotic Therapy Timing[5]	-	-	97%	98%
Assessed for Rehabilitation[5]	-	-	97%	97%
Discharged on Antithrombotic Therapy[5]	-	-	98%	99%
Discharged on Statin Medication[5]	-	-	93%	94%
Thrombolytic Therapy Timing[5]	-	-	59%	66%
Venous Thromboembolism Prophylaxis[5]	-	-	93%	94%
Written Stroke Educational Materials Given[5]	-	-	86%	88%
Surgical Care Improvement Project				
Appropriate Beta Blocker Usage[5]	-	-	98%	98%
Appropriate VTP Within 24 Hours[5]	-	-	98%	98%
Controlled Postoperative Blood Glucose[5]	-	-	96%	97%
Perioperative Temperature Management[5]	-	-	100%	100%
Prophylactic Antibiotic Selection[5]	-	-	99%	99%
Prophylactic Antibiotic Selection (Outpatient)[5]	-	-	97%	98%
Prophylactic Antibiotic Stopped[5]	-	-	98%	98%
Prophylactic Antibiotic Timing[5]	-	-	99%	99%
Prophylactic Antibiotic Timing (Outpatient)[5]	-	-	97%	98%
Urinary Catheter Removal[5]	-	-	97%	97%
Survey of Patients' Hospital Experiences				
Area Around Room 'Always' Quiet at Night	(a)	56%	64%	61%
Doctors 'Always' Communicated Well	(a)	96%	84%	82%
Home Recovery Information Given	(a)	87%	86%	85%
Hospital Given 9 or 10 on 10 Point Scale	(a)	64%	72%	71%
Meds 'Always' Explained Before Given	(a)	57%	66%	64%
Nurses 'Always' Communicated Well	(a)	79%	81%	79%
Pain 'Always' Well Controlled	(a)	72%	73%	71%
Room and Bathroom 'Always' Clean	(a)	80%	75%	73%
Timely Help 'Always' Received	(a)	69%	69%	68%
Would Definitely Recommend Hospital	(a)	67%	71%	71%
Use of Medical Imaging				
Cardiac Imaging Stress Test before Surgery[7]	-	-	5.3%	5.3%
Combination Abdominal CT Scan	180	35.0%	10.7%	10.5%
Combination Brain/Sinus CT Scan[1]	-	-	3.1%	2.7%
Combination Chest CT Scan	98	12.2%	4.3%	2.7%
Follow-up Mammogram/Ultrasound	208	7.7%	8.3%	8.8%
Lumbar Spine MRI for Low Back Pain[7]	-	-	38.9%	37.2%

Muhlenberg Community Hospital

440 Hopkinsville Street
Greenville, KY 42345
URL: www.mchky.org
Type: Acute Care Hospitals
Ownership: Voluntary non-profit - Private

Phone: 270-338-8000
Fax: 270-338-8278
Emergency Services: Yes
Beds: 135

Key Personnel:

Pediatric Ambulatory Care . . . . . . Karla Davis
Pediatric In-Patient Care . . . . Karla Davis
CEO/President. . . . . Lloyd K Ford, JR
Infection Control. . . . . Beckie Penrod
Chief of Medical Staff . . . . Brad Sparks, MD
Operating Room. . . . . Fara Stewart
Coronary Care . . . . Kim Vender
Quality Assurance . . . . Michele Vincent

Measure	Cases	This Hosp.	State Avg.	U.S. Avg.
Blood Clot Prevention and Treatment				
Anticoagulation Overlap Therapy[1,2]	-	-	90%	93%
ICU Venous Thromboembolism Prophylaxis[2]	62	77%	86%	92%
Incidence of Potentially Preventable VTE[1,2]	-	-	13%	10%
UFH with Dosages/Platelet Monitoring[1,2]	-	-	98%	97%
Venous Thromboembolism Prophylaxis[2]	126	80%	80%	85%
Warfarin Therapy Discharge Instructions[1,2]	-	-	72%	75%
Chest Pain/Possible Heart Attack Care				
Aspirin Given Within 24 Hours of Arrival	108	98%	97%	96%
Fibrinolytic Meds Within 30 Min. of Arrival[1]	-	-	63%	58%
Average Time to ECG (minutes)	114	4	6	7
Average Time to Transfer (minutes)[1]	-	-	61	60
Children's Asthma Care				
Received Home Management Plan of Care	-	-	-	88%
Received Reliever Medication	-	-	-	100%
Received Systemic Corticosteroids	-	-	-	100%
Emergency Department				
Admittance Decision Time (minutes)[2]	383	56	78	98
Head CT Results Within 45 Min. of Arrival	11	0%	55%	57%
Patients Who Left ER Before Being Seen	20,208	2%	2%	2%
Time from ER Arrival to Admit. (minutes)[2]	437	228	238	274
Time from ER Arrival to Discharge (minutes)	376	129	126	134
Time in ER Before Being Evaluated (minutes)	391	40	23	26
Time to Pain Meds for Fractures (minutes)	67	75	56	57
Heart Attack Care				
Aspirin Given at Discharge[1]	-	-	99%	99%
Fibrinolytic Meds Within 30 Min. of Arrival[7]	-	-	-	54%
PCI Within 90 Minutes of Arrival[7]	-	-	97%	96%
Statin Prescribed at Discharge[1]	-	-	97%	98%
Heart Failure Care				
ACE Inhibitor or ARB for LVSD	12	92%	95%	97%
Discharge Instructions Given	38	82%	92%	94%
Evaluation of LVS Function	47	100%	98%	99%
Medicare Spending				
Medicare Spending per Patient (ratio)	-	0.89	0.97	0.98
Pneumonia Care				
Appropriate Initial Antibiotic Given	80	85%	94%	95%
Blood Culture Timing	91	98%	98%	98%
Pregnancy and Delivery Care				
Newborn Deliveries Scheduled Early[2,7]	-	-	9%	6%
Preventive Care				
Immunization for Influenza[2]	273	95%	92%	90%
Immunization for Pneumonia[2]	435	96%	94%	92%
Stroke Care				
Anticoagulation Therapy for Atrial Fibrillation[3,7]	-	-	95%	95%
Antithrombotic Therapy Timing[1,3]	-	-	97%	98%
Assessed for Rehabilitation[3,7]	-	-	97%	97%
Discharged on Antithrombotic Therapy[3,7]	-	-	98%	99%
Discharged on Statin Medication[3,7]	-	-	93%	94%
Thrombolytic Therapy Timing[3,7]	-	-	59%	66%
Venous Thromboembolism Prophylaxis[3,7]	-	-	93%	94%
Written Stroke Educational Materials Given[3,7]	-	-	86%	88%
Surgical Care Improvement Project				
Appropriate Beta Blocker Usage	24	88%	98%	98%
Appropriate VTP Within 24 Hours	63	97%	98%	98%
Controlled Postoperative Blood Glucose[7]	-	-	96%	97%
Perioperative Temperature Management	69	100%	100%	100%
Prophylactic Antibiotic Selection	42	98%	99%	99%
Prophylactic Antibiotic Selection (Outpatient)[1,3]	-	-	97%	98%
Prophylactic Antibiotic Stopped	41	98%	98%	98%
Prophylactic Antibiotic Timing	42	100%	99%	99%
Prophylactic Antibiotic Timing (Outpatient)[1,3]	-	-	97%	98%
Urinary Catheter Removal	34	100%	97%	97%
Survey of Patients' Hospital Experiences				
Area Around Room 'Always' Quiet at Night	(a)	61%	64%	61%
Doctors 'Always' Communicated Well	(a)	83%	84%	82%
Home Recovery Information Given	(a)	83%	86%	85%
Hospital Given 9 or 10 on 10 Point Scale	(a)	66%	72%	71%
Meds 'Always' Explained Before Given	(a)	67%	66%	64%
Nurses 'Always' Communicated Well	(a)	81%	81%	79%
Pain 'Always' Well Controlled	(a)	71%	73%	71%
Room and Bathroom 'Always' Clean	(a)	75%	75%	73%
Timely Help 'Always' Received	(a)	63%	69%	68%
Would Definitely Recommend Hospital	(a)	66%	71%	71%
Use of Medical Imaging				
Cardiac Imaging Stress Test before Surgery[1]	-	-	5.3%	5.3%
Combination Abdominal CT Scan	255	16.9%	10.7%	10.5%
Combination Brain/Sinus CT Scan[1]	-	-	3.1%	2.7%
Combination Chest CT Scan	84	2.4%	4.3%	2.7%
Follow-up Mammogram/Ultrasound	270	3.7%	8.3%	8.8%
Lumbar Spine MRI for Low Back Pain	55	38.2%	38.9%	37.2%

Breckinridge Memorial Hospital

1011 Old Highway 60
Hardinsburg, KY 40143
E-mail: info@breckhealth.org
URL: www.breckhealth.org
Type: Critical Access Hospitals
Ownership: Government - Local

Phone: 270-756-7000
Fax: 270-756-6510
Emergency Services: Yes
Beds: 45

Key Personnel:

Chief of Medical Staff . . . . Robert Chambliss, MD
CEO/President. . . . . Michael Cooper
Operating Room. . . . . Amy Mingus
Quality Assurance . . . . Ricky Moore
Emergency Room . . . . Patty White

Measure	Cases	This Hosp.	State Avg.	U.S. Avg.
Blood Clot Prevention and Treatment				
Anticoagulation Overlap Therapy[5]	-	-	90%	93%
ICU Venous Thromboembolism Prophylaxis[5]	-	-	86%	92%
Incidence of Potentially Preventable VTE[5]	-	-	13%	10%
UFH with Dosages/Platelet Monitoring[5]	-	-	98%	97%
Venous Thromboembolism Prophylaxis[5]	-	-	80%	85%
Warfarin Therapy Discharge Instructions[5]	-	-	72%	75%
Chest Pain/Possible Heart Attack Care				
Aspirin Given Within 24 Hours of Arrival[5]	-	-	97%	96%
Fibrinolytic Meds Within 30 Min. of Arrival[5]	-	-	63%	58%
Average Time to ECG (minutes)[5]	-	-	6	7
Average Time to Transfer (minutes)[5]	-	-	61	60
Children's Asthma Care				
Received Home Management Plan of Care	-	-	-	88%
Received Reliever Medication	-	-	-	100%
Received Systemic Corticosteroids	-	-	-	100%
Emergency Department				
Admittance Decision Time (minutes)	317	77	78	98
Head CT Results Within 45 Min. of Arrival[5]	-	-	55%	57%
Patients Who Left ER Before Being Seen	8,537	4%	2%	2%
Time from ER Arrival to Admit. (minutes)	341	235	238	274
Time from ER Arrival to Discharge (minutes)[5]	-	-	126	134
Time in ER Before Being Evaluated (minutes)[5]	-	-	23	26
Time to Pain Meds for Fractures (minutes)[5]	-	-	56	57
Heart Attack Care				
Aspirin Given at Discharge[5]	-	-	99%	99%
Fibrinolytic Meds Within 30 Min. of Arrival[5]	-	-	-	54%
PCI Within 90 Minutes of Arrival[5]	-	-	97%	96%
Statin Prescribed at Discharge[5]	-	-	97%	98%
Heart Failure Care				
ACE Inhibitor or ARB for LVSD[7]	-	-	95%	97%
Discharge Instructions Given[1]	-	-	92%	94%
Evaluation of LVS Function[1]	-	-	98%	99%
Medicare Spending				
Medicare Spending per Patient (ratio)	-	-	0.97	0.98
Pneumonia Care				
Appropriate Initial Antibiotic Given	13	54%	94%	95%
Blood Culture Timing	14	86%	98%	98%
Pregnancy and Delivery Care				
Newborn Deliveries Scheduled Early[5]	-	-	9%	6%
Preventive Care				
Immunization for Influenza[5]	-	-	92%	90%
Immunization for Pneumonia[5]	-	-	94%	92%
Stroke Care				
Anticoagulation Therapy for Atrial Fibrillation[5]	-	-	95%	95%
Antithrombotic Therapy Timing[5]	-	-	97%	98%
Assessed for Rehabilitation[5]	-	-	97%	97%
Discharged on Antithrombotic Therapy[5]	-	-	98%	99%
Discharged on Statin Medication[5]	-	-	93%	94%
Thrombolytic Therapy Timing[5]	-	-	59%	66%
Venous Thromboembolism Prophylaxis[5]	-	-	93%	94%
Written Stroke Educational Materials Given[5]	-	-	86%	88%
Surgical Care Improvement Project				
Appropriate Beta Blocker Usage[5]	-	-	98%	98%
Appropriate VTP Within 24 Hours[5]	-	-	98%	98%
Controlled Postoperative Blood Glucose[5]	-	-	96%	97%
Perioperative Temperature Management[5]	-	-	100%	100%
Prophylactic Antibiotic Selection[5]	-	-	99%	99%
Prophylactic Antibiotic Selection (Outpatient)[5]	-	-	97%	98%
Prophylactic Antibiotic Stopped[5]	-	-	98%	98%

NOTE: Hospital profiles are in alphabetical order by state, then city, then hospital within the city; Rankings exclude hospitals with less than 25 cases except for patient surveys which excludes hospitals with less than 100 cases; (a) 100-299 cases; (1) The number of cases/patients is too few to report; (2) Data submitted were based on a sample of cases/patients; (3) Results are based on a shorter time period than required; (4) Data suppressed by CMS for one or more quarters; (5) Results are not available for this reporting period; (6) Fewer than 100 patients completed the HCAHPS survey; (7) No cases met the criteria for this measure; (8) The lower limit of the confidence interval cannot be calculated if the number of observed infections equals zero; (9) No data are available from the state/territory for this reporting period; (10) The scores shown reflect fewer than 50 completed surveys; (11) There were discrepancies in the data collection process; (12) This measure does not apply to this hospital for this reporting period; (13) Results cannot be calculated for this reporting period; (14) The results for this state are combined with nearby states to protect confidentiality; Please refer to the User's Guide for a full explanation of data.

Measure	Cases	This Hosp.	State Avg.	U.S. Avg.
Prophylactic Antibiotic Timing[5]	-	-	99%	99%
Prophylactic Antibiotic Timing (Outpatient)[5]	-	-	97%	98%
Urinary Catheter Removal[5]	-	-	97%	97%
Survey of Patients' Hospital Experiences				
Area Around Room 'Always' Quiet at Night[5]	-	-	64%	61%
Doctors 'Always' Communicated Well[5]	-	-	84%	82%
Home Recovery Information Given[5]	-	-	86%	85%
Hospital Given 9 or 10 on 10 Point Scale[5]	-	-	72%	71%
Meds 'Always' Explained Before Given[5]	-	-	66%	64%
Nurses 'Always' Communicated Well[5]	-	-	81%	79%
Pain 'Always' Well Controlled[5]	-	-	73%	71%
Room and Bathroom 'Always' Clean[5]	-	-	75%	73%
Timely Help 'Always' Received[5]	-	-	69%	68%
Would Definitely Recommend Hospital[5]	-	-	71%	71%
Use of Medical Imaging				
Cardiac Imaging Stress Test before Surgery[7]	-	-	5.3%	5.3%
Combination Abdominal CT Scan	256	34.8%	10.7%	10.5%
Combination Brain/Sinus CT Scan[1]	-	-	3.1%	2.7%
Combination Chest CT Scan	197	2.0%	4.3%	2.7%
Follow-up Mammogram/Ultrasound	335	3.3%	8.3%	8.8%
Lumbar Spine MRI for Low Back Pain[1]	-	-	38.9%	37.2%

Harlan Appalachian Regional Healthcare Hospital

81 Ball Park Road Phone: 606-573-8100
Harlan, KY 40831 Fax: 606-573-8200
URL: www.arh.org
Type: Acute Care Hospitals Emergency Services: Yes
Ownership: Voluntary non-profit - Other Beds: 150

Key Personnel:
Chief of Medical Staff.......... Amir Ahmad, MD
Cardiac Laboratory............ Johnnie Bargo
Quality Assurance .... Russ Barker
CEO/President............... Jerry W Haynes
Emergency Room .... Donna Middleton, RN
Radiology.................... Gregory Y Tiu

Measure	Cases	This Hosp.	State Avg.	U.S. Avg.
Blood Clot Prevention and Treatment				
Anticoagulation Overlap Therapy[1,2]	-	-	90%	93%
ICU Venous Thromboembolism Prophylaxis[2]	70	80%	86%	92%
Incidence of Potentially Preventable VTE[2,7]	-	-	13%	10%
UFH with Dosages/Platelet Monitoring[1,2]	-	-	98%	97%
Venous Thromboembolism Prophylaxis[2]	354	86%	80%	85%
Warfarin Therapy Discharge Instructions[1,2]	-	-	72%	75%
Chest Pain/Possible Heart Attack Care				
Aspirin Given Within 24 Hours of Arrival	81	100%	97%	96%
Fibrinolytic Meds Within 30 Min. of Arrival[1]	-	-	63%	58%
Average Time to ECG (minutes)	82	7	6	7
Average Time to Transfer (minutes)[7]	-	-	61	60
Children's Asthma Care				
Received Home Management Plan of Care	-	-	-	88%
Received Reliever Medication	-	-	-	100%
Received Systemic Corticosteroids	-	-	-	100%
Emergency Department				
Admittance Decision Time (minutes)[2]	541	82	78	98
Head CT Results Within 45 Min. of Arrival[1]	-	-	55%	57%
Patients Who Left ER Before Being Seen	21,393	1%	2%	2%
Time from ER Arrival to Admit. (minutes)[2]	569	219	238	274
Time from ER Arrival to Discharge (minutes)	405	126	126	134
Time in ER Before Being Evaluated (minutes)	442	30	23	26
Time to Pain Meds for Fractures (minutes)	65	55	56	57
Heart Attack Care				
Aspirin Given at Discharge[1]	-	-	99%	99%
Fibrinolytic Meds Within 30 Min. of Arrival[7]	-	-	-	54%
PCI Within 90 Minutes of Arrival[7]	-	-	97%	96%
Statin Prescribed at Discharge[1]	-	-	97%	98%
Heart Failure Care				
ACE Inhibitor or ARB for LVSD	23	100%	95%	97%
Discharge Instructions Given	126	98%	92%	94%
Evaluation of LVS Function	150	100%	98%	99%
Medicare Spending				
Medicare Spending per Patient (ratio)	-	1.00	0.97	0.98
Pneumonia Care				
Appropriate Initial Antibiotic Given	124	97%	94%	95%
Blood Culture Timing	215	100%	98%	98%
Pregnancy and Delivery Care				
Newborn Deliveries Scheduled Early	19	5%	9%	6%
Preventive Care				
Immunization for Influenza[2]	414	89%	92%	90%
Immunization for Pneumonia[2]	539	95%	94%	92%
Stroke Care				
Anticoagulation Therapy for Atrial Fibrillation[1]	-	-	95%	95%
Antithrombotic Therapy Timing	19	84%	97%	98%
Assessed for Rehabilitation	17	100%	97%	97%
Discharged on Antithrombotic Therapy	15	93%	98%	99%
Discharged on Statin Medication	11	82%	93%	94%
Thrombolytic Therapy Timing[7]	-	-	59%	66%
Venous Thromboembolism Prophylaxis	18	89%	93%	94%
Written Stroke Educational Materials Given[1]	-	-	86%	88%
Surgical Care Improvement Project				
Appropriate Beta Blocker Usage	12	100%	98%	98%
Appropriate VTP Within 24 Hours	51	100%	98%	98%
Controlled Postoperative Blood Glucose[7]	-	-	96%	97%
Perioperative Temperature Management	77	100%	100%	100%
Prophylactic Antibiotic Selection	51	100%	99%	99%
Prophylactic Antibiotic Selection (Outpatient)	37	100%	97%	98%
Prophylactic Antibiotic Stopped	44	100%	98%	98%
Prophylactic Antibiotic Timing	52	100%	99%	99%
Prophylactic Antibiotic Timing (Outpatient)	37	100%	97%	98%
Urinary Catheter Removal[1]	-	-	97%	97%
Survey of Patients' Hospital Experiences				
Area Around Room 'Always' Quiet at Night	300+	61%	64%	61%
Doctors 'Always' Communicated Well	300+	80%	84%	82%
Home Recovery Information Given	300+	82%	86%	85%
Hospital Given 9 or 10 on 10 Point Scale	300+	65%	72%	71%
Meds 'Always' Explained Before Given	300+	62%	66%	64%
Nurses 'Always' Communicated Well	300+	79%	81%	79%
Pain 'Always' Well Controlled	300+	72%	73%	71%
Room and Bathroom 'Always' Clean	300+	74%	75%	73%
Timely Help 'Always' Received	300+	68%	69%	68%
Would Definitely Recommend Hospital	300+	62%	71%	71%
Use of Medical Imaging				
Cardiac Imaging Stress Test before Surgery	68	7.4%	5.3%	5.3%
Combination Abdominal CT Scan	362	32.3%	10.7%	10.5%
Combination Brain/Sinus CT Scan	359	4.5%	3.1%	2.7%
Combination Chest CT Scan	170	30.0%	4.3%	2.7%
Follow-up Mammogram/Ultrasound	317	12.9%	8.3%	8.8%
Lumbar Spine MRI for Low Back Pain	96	39.6%	38.9%	37.2%

The James B Haggin Memorial Hospital

464 Linden Avenue Phone: 859-734-5441
Harrodsburg, KY 40330 Fax: 859-734-5563
Type: Critical Access Hospitals Emergency Services: Yes
Ownership: Voluntary non-profit - Other Beds: 59

Key Personnel:
Anesthesiology............... Anjum Bux, MD
Chief of Medical Staff.......... Nick G. Dedman, MD
Radiology.................... Danny Hall, MD
Pediatrics.................... Pamela G. Johnson, MD
Surgery...................... John H. Lacy, MD
CEO/President............... Victoria L. Reed, DHA, FACHE
Cardiology................... David Sihau, MD

Measure	Cases	This Hosp.	State Avg.	U.S. Avg.
Blood Clot Prevention and Treatment				
Anticoagulation Overlap Therapy[5]	-	-	90%	93%
ICU Venous Thromboembolism Prophylaxis[5]	-	-	86%	92%
Incidence of Potentially Preventable VTE[5]	-	-	13%	10%
UFH with Dosages/Platelet Monitoring[5]	-	-	98%	97%
Venous Thromboembolism Prophylaxis[5]	-	-	80%	85%
Warfarin Therapy Discharge Instructions[5]	-	-	72%	75%
Chest Pain/Possible Heart Attack Care				
Aspirin Given Within 24 Hours of Arrival[5]	-	-	97%	96%
Fibrinolytic Meds Within 30 Min. of Arrival[5]	-	-	63%	58%
Average Time to ECG (minutes)[5]	-	-	6	7
Average Time to Transfer (minutes)[5]	-	-	61	60
Children's Asthma Care				
Received Home Management Plan of Care	-	-	-	88%
Received Reliever Medication	-	-	-	100%
Received Systemic Corticosteroids	-	-	-	100%
Emergency Department				
Admittance Decision Time (minutes)[5]	-	-	78	98
Head CT Results Within 45 Min. of Arrival[5]	-	-	55%	57%
Patients Who Left ER Before Being Seen[5]	-	-	2%	2%
Time from ER Arrival to Admit. (minutes)[5]	-	-	238	274
Time from ER Arrival to Discharge (minutes)[5]	-	-	126	134
Time in ER Before Being Evaluated (minutes)[5]	-	-	23	26
Time to Pain Meds for Fractures (minutes)[5]	-	-	56	57
Heart Attack Care				
Aspirin Given at Discharge[5]	-	-	99%	99%
Fibrinolytic Meds Within 30 Min. of Arrival[5]	-	-	-	54%
PCI Within 90 Minutes of Arrival[5]	-	-	97%	96%
Statin Prescribed at Discharge[5]	-	-	97%	98%
Heart Failure Care				
ACE Inhibitor or ARB for LVSD[1]	-	-	95%	97%
Discharge Instructions Given[1]	-	-	92%	94%
Evaluation of LVS Function[1]	-	-	98%	99%
Medicare Spending				
Medicare Spending per Patient (ratio)	-	-	0.97	0.98
Pneumonia Care				
Appropriate Initial Antibiotic Given	22	64%	94%	95%
Blood Culture Timing	50	96%	98%	98%
Pregnancy and Delivery Care				
Newborn Deliveries Scheduled Early[5]	-	-	9%	6%
Preventive Care				
Immunization for Influenza[5]	-	-	92%	90%
Immunization for Pneumonia[5]	-	-	94%	92%
Stroke Care				
Anticoagulation Therapy for Atrial Fibrillation[5]	-	-	95%	95%
Antithrombotic Therapy Timing[5]	-	-	97%	98%
Assessed for Rehabilitation[5]	-	-	97%	97%
Discharged on Antithrombotic Therapy[5]	-	-	98%	99%
Discharged on Statin Medication[5]	-	-	93%	94%
Thrombolytic Therapy Timing[5]	-	-	59%	66%
Venous Thromboembolism Prophylaxis[5]	-	-	93%	94%
Written Stroke Educational Materials Given[5]	-	-	86%	88%
Surgical Care Improvement Project				
Appropriate Beta Blocker Usage[1,3]	-	-	98%	98%
Appropriate VTP Within 24 Hours[1,3]	-	-	98%	98%
Controlled Postoperative Blood Glucose[3,7]	-	-	96%	97%
Perioperative Temperature Management[1,3]	-	-	100%	100%
Prophylactic Antibiotic Selection[1,3]	-	-	99%	99%
Prophylactic Antibiotic Selection (Outpatient)[5]	-	-	97%	98%
Prophylactic Antibiotic Stopped[1,3]	-	-	98%	98%
Prophylactic Antibiotic Timing[1,3]	-	-	99%	99%
Prophylactic Antibiotic Timing (Outpatient)[5]	-	-	97%	98%
Urinary Catheter Removal[1,3]	-	-	97%	97%
Survey of Patients' Hospital Experiences				
Area Around Room 'Always' Quiet at Night[5]	-	-	64%	61%
Doctors 'Always' Communicated Well[5]	-	-	84%	82%
Home Recovery Information Given[5]	-	-	86%	85%
Hospital Given 9 or 10 on 10 Point Scale[5]	-	-	72%	71%
Meds 'Always' Explained Before Given[5]	-	-	66%	64%
Nurses 'Always' Communicated Well[5]	-	-	81%	79%
Pain 'Always' Well Controlled[5]	-	-	73%	71%
Room and Bathroom 'Always' Clean[5]	-	-	75%	73%
Timely Help 'Always' Received[5]	-	-	69%	68%
Would Definitely Recommend Hospital[5]	-	-	71%	71%
Use of Medical Imaging				
Cardiac Imaging Stress Test before Surgery[7]	-	-	5.3%	5.3%
Combination Abdominal CT Scan	224	6.3%	10.7%	10.5%
Combination Brain/Sinus CT Scan[1]	-	-	3.1%	2.7%
Combination Chest CT Scan	111	4.5%	4.3%	2.7%
Follow-up Mammogram/Ultrasound	251	10.8%	8.3%	8.8%
Lumbar Spine MRI for Low Back Pain	45	55.6%	38.9%	37.2%

Ohio County Hospital

1211 Old Main Street Phone: 270-298-7411
Hartford, KY 42347 Fax: 270-298-3758
URL: www.ohiocountyhospital.com
Type: Critical Access Hospitals Emergency Services: Yes
Ownership: Proprietary Beds: 68

Key Personnel:
Radiology.................... Bruce Bu

NOTE: Hospital profiles are in alphabetical order by state, then city, then hospital within the city; Rankings exclude hospitals with less than 25 cases except for patient surveys which excludes hospitals with less than 100 cases; (a) 100-299 cases; (1) The number of cases/patients is too few to report; (2) Data submitted were based on a sample of cases/patients; (3) Results are based on a shorter time period than required; (4) Data suppressed by CMS for one or more quarters; (5) Results are not available for this reporting period; (6) Fewer than 100 patients completed the HCAHPS survey; (7) No cases met the criteria for this measure; (8) The lower limit of the confidence interval cannot be calculated if the number of observed infections equals zero; (9) No data are available from the state/territory for this reporting period; (10) The scores shown reflect fewer than 50 completed surveys; (11) There were discrepancies in the data collection process; (12) This measure does not apply to this hospital for this reporting period; (13) Results cannot be calculated for this reporting period; (14) The results for this state are combined with nearby states to protect confidentiality; Please refer to the User's Guide for a full explanation of data.

Patient Relations . . . . Brenda Newcom, RN
CEO/President. . . . . Blaine Pieper
Chief of Medical Staff. . . . . Leticia Tuker

Measure	Cases	This Hosp.	State Avg.	U.S. Avg.
Blood Clot Prevention and Treatment				
Anticoagulation Overlap Therapy[5]	-	-	90%	93%
ICU Venous Thromboembolism Prophylaxis[5]	-	-	86%	92%
Incidence of Potentially Preventable VTE[5]	-	-	13%	10%
UFH with Dosages/Platelet Monitoring[5]	-	-	98%	97%
Venous Thromboembolism Prophylaxis[5]	-	-	80%	85%
Warfarin Therapy Discharge Instructions[5]	-	-	72%	75%
Chest Pain/Possible Heart Attack Care				
Aspirin Given Within 24 Hours of Arrival[5]	-	-	97%	96%
Fibrinolytic Meds Within 30 Min. of Arrival[5]	-	-	63%	58%
Average Time to ECG (minutes)[5]	-	-	6	7
Average Time to Transfer (minutes)[5]	-	-	61	60
Children's Asthma Care				
Received Home Management Plan of Care	-	-	-	88%
Received Reliever Medication	-	-	-	100%
Received Systemic Corticosteroids	-	-	-	100%
Emergency Department				
Admittance Decision Time (minutes)[5]	-	-	78	98
Head CT Results Within 45 Min. of Arrival[5]	-	-	55%	57%
Patients Who Left ER Before Being Seen	15,188	1%	2%	2%
Time from ER Arrival to Admit. (minutes)[5]	-	-	238	274
Time from ER Arrival to Discharge (minutes)[5]	-	-	126	134
Time in ER Before Being Evaluated (minutes)[5]	-	-	23	26
Time to Pain Meds for Fractures (minutes)[5]	-	-	56	57
Heart Attack Care				
Aspirin Given at Discharge[1,3]	-	-	99%	99%
Fibrinolytic Meds Within 30 Min. of Arrival[3,7]	-	-	-	54%
PCI Within 90 Minutes of Arrival[3,7]	-	-	97%	96%
Statin Prescribed at Discharge[1,3]	-	-	97%	98%
Heart Failure Care				
ACE Inhibitor or ARB for LVSD	15	80%	95%	97%
Discharge Instructions Given	34	79%	92%	94%
Evaluation of LVS Function	41	95%	98%	99%
Medicare Spending				
Medicare Spending per Patient (ratio)	-	-	0.97	0.98
Pneumonia Care				
Appropriate Initial Antibiotic Given	54	83%	94%	95%
Blood Culture Timing	55	95%	98%	98%
Pregnancy and Delivery Care				
Newborn Deliveries Scheduled Early[5]	-	-	9%	6%
Preventive Care				
Immunization for Influenza[5]	-	-	92%	90%
Immunization for Pneumonia[5]	-	-	94%	92%
Stroke Care				
Anticoagulation Therapy for Atrial Fibrillation[5]	-	-	95%	95%
Antithrombotic Therapy Timing[5]	-	-	97%	98%
Assessed for Rehabilitation[5]	-	-	97%	97%
Discharged on Antithrombotic Therapy[5]	-	-	98%	99%
Discharged on Statin Medication[5]	-	-	93%	94%
Thrombolytic Therapy Timing[5]	-	-	59%	66%
Venous Thromboembolism Prophylaxis[5]	-	-	93%	94%
Written Stroke Educational Materials Given[5]	-	-	86%	88%
Surgical Care Improvement Project				
Appropriate Beta Blocker Usage[1]	-	-	98%	98%
Appropriate VTP Within 24 Hours	17	82%	98%	98%
Controlled Postoperative Blood Glucose[7]	-	-	96%	97%
Perioperative Temperature Management	18	89%	100%	100%
Prophylactic Antibiotic Selection[1]	-	-	99%	99%
Prophylactic Antibiotic Selection (Outpatient)[5]	-	-	97%	98%
Prophylactic Antibiotic Stopped[1]	-	-	98%	98%
Prophylactic Antibiotic Timing[1]	-	-	99%	99%
Prophylactic Antibiotic Timing (Outpatient)[5]	-	-	97%	98%
Urinary Catheter Removal	11	73%	97%	97%
Survey of Patients' Hospital Experiences				
Area Around Room 'Always' Quiet at Night	(a)	67%	64%	61%
Doctors 'Always' Communicated Well	(a)	88%	84%	82%
Home Recovery Information Given	(a)	85%	86%	85%
Hospital Given 9 or 10 on 10 Point Scale	(a)	67%	72%	71%
Meds 'Always' Explained Before Given	(a)	74%	66%	64%
Nurses 'Always' Communicated Well	(a)	79%	81%	79%
Pain 'Always' Well Controlled	(a)	67%	73%	71%
Room and Bathroom 'Always' Clean	(a)	70%	75%	73%
Timely Help 'Always' Received	(a)	70%	69%	68%
Would Definitely Recommend Hospital	(a)	67%	71%	71%
Use of Medical Imaging				
Cardiac Imaging Stress Test before Surgery[1]	-	-	5.3%	5.3%
Combination Abdominal CT Scan	308	7.5%	10.7%	10.5%
Combination Brain/Sinus CT Scan[1]	-	-	3.1%	2.7%
Combination Chest CT Scan	133	0.0%	4.3%	2.7%
Follow-up Mammogram/Ultrasound	382	5.0%	8.3%	8.8%
Lumbar Spine MRI for Low Back Pain[1]	-	-	38.9%	37.2%

Hazard ARH Regional Medical Center

100 Medical Center Drive — Phone: 606-439-6600
Hazard, KY 41701 — Fax: 606-439-6682
E-mail: afugate@arh.org
URL: www.arh.org/hazard
Type: Acute Care Hospitals — Emergency Services: Yes
Ownership: Voluntary non-profit - Private — Beds: 308
Key Personnel:
Intensive Care Unit. . . . . Wanda Combs, RN
Emergency Room . . . . Lisa Hall
Radiology. . . . . Doug Morgan, RT
Chief of Medical Staff. . . . . Dr. Syamala Reddy
CEO/President. . . . . Dan Stone
Infection Control. . . . . Tonda Young

Measure	Cases	This Hosp.	State Avg.	U.S. Avg.
Blood Clot Prevention and Treatment				
Anticoagulation Overlap Therapy[1,2]	-	-	90%	93%
ICU Venous Thromboembolism Prophylaxis[2]	82	98%	86%	92%
Incidence of Potentially Preventable VTE[2]	12	8%	13%	10%
UFH with Dosages/Platelet Monitoring[2]	18	100%	98%	97%
Venous Thromboembolism Prophylaxis[2]	371	81%	80%	85%
Warfarin Therapy Discharge Instructions[1,2]	-	-	72%	75%
Chest Pain/Possible Heart Attack Care				
Aspirin Given Within 24 Hours of Arrival[1]	-	-	97%	96%
Fibrinolytic Meds Within 30 Min. of Arrival[3,7]	-	-	63%	58%
Average Time to ECG (minutes)[1]	-	-	6	7
Average Time to Transfer (minutes)[3,7]	-	-	61	60
Children's Asthma Care				
Received Home Management Plan of Care	-	-	-	88%
Received Reliever Medication	-	-	-	100%
Received Systemic Corticosteroids	-	-	-	100%
Emergency Department				
Admittance Decision Time (minutes)[2]	344	139	78	98
Head CT Results Within 45 Min. of Arrival[1]	-	-	55%	57%
Patients Who Left ER Before Being Seen	24,382	1%	2%	2%
Time from ER Arrival to Admit. (minutes)[2]	346	244	238	274
Time from ER Arrival to Discharge (minutes)	313	135	126	134
Time in ER Before Being Evaluated (minutes)	421	8	23	26
Time to Pain Meds for Fractures (minutes)	85	47	56	57
Heart Attack Care				
Aspirin Given at Discharge	179	97%	99%	99%
Fibrinolytic Meds Within 30 Min. of Arrival[7]	-	-	-	54%
PCI Within 90 Minutes of Arrival	21	90%	97%	96%
Statin Prescribed at Discharge	173	95%	97%	98%
Heart Failure Care				
ACE Inhibitor or ARB for LVSD	54	91%	95%	97%
Discharge Instructions Given	202	89%	92%	94%
Evaluation of LVS Function	238	98%	98%	99%
Medicare Spending				
Medicare Spending per Patient (ratio)	-	1.02	0.97	0.98
Pneumonia Care				
Appropriate Initial Antibiotic Given[2]	69	87%	94%	95%
Blood Culture Timing[2]	81	95%	98%	98%
Pregnancy and Delivery Care				
Newborn Deliveries Scheduled Early[2]	47	19%	9%	6%
Preventive Care				
Immunization for Influenza[2]	611	75%	92%	90%
Immunization for Pneumonia[2]	864	75%	94%	92%
Stroke Care				
Anticoagulation Therapy for Atrial Fibrillation[1]	-	-	95%	95%
Antithrombotic Therapy Timing	53	94%	97%	98%
Assessed for Rehabilitation	49	71%	97%	97%
Discharged on Antithrombotic Therapy	48	94%	98%	99%
Discharged on Statin Medication	36	75%	93%	94%
Thrombolytic Therapy Timing[1]	-	-	59%	66%
Venous Thromboembolism Prophylaxis	51	67%	93%	94%
Written Stroke Educational Materials Given	29	3%	86%	88%
Surgical Care Improvement Project				
Appropriate Beta Blocker Usage	116	94%	98%	98%
Appropriate VTP Within 24 Hours	243	98%	98%	98%
Controlled Postoperative Blood Glucose	37	100%	96%	97%
Perioperative Temperature Management	270	100%	100%	100%
Prophylactic Antibiotic Selection	197	100%	99%	99%
Prophylactic Antibiotic Selection (Outpatient)	111	97%	97%	98%
Prophylactic Antibiotic Stopped	187	98%	98%	98%
Prophylactic Antibiotic Timing	197	100%	99%	99%
Prophylactic Antibiotic Timing (Outpatient)	109	88%	97%	98%
Urinary Catheter Removal	237	98%	97%	97%
Survey of Patients' Hospital Experiences				
Area Around Room 'Always' Quiet at Night	300+	60%	64%	61%
Doctors 'Always' Communicated Well	300+	86%	84%	82%
Home Recovery Information Given	300+	83%	86%	85%
Hospital Given 9 or 10 on 10 Point Scale	300+	67%	72%	71%
Meds 'Always' Explained Before Given	300+	64%	66%	64%
Nurses 'Always' Communicated Well	300+	77%	81%	79%
Pain 'Always' Well Controlled	300+	69%	73%	71%
Room and Bathroom 'Always' Clean	300+	68%	75%	73%
Timely Help 'Always' Received	300+	63%	69%	68%
Would Definitely Recommend Hospital	300+	65%	71%	71%
Use of Medical Imaging				
Cardiac Imaging Stress Test before Surgery[1]	-	-	5.3%	5.3%
Combination Abdominal CT Scan	408	2.2%	10.7%	10.5%
Combination Brain/Sinus CT Scan[1]	-	-	3.1%	2.7%
Combination Chest CT Scan	180	6.1%	4.3%	2.7%
Follow-up Mammogram/Ultrasound[7]	-	-	8.3%	8.8%
Lumbar Spine MRI for Low Back Pain[1]	-	-	38.9%	37.2%

Methodist Hospital

1305 N Elm St — Phone: 270-827-7700
Henderson, KY 42420 — Fax: 270-827-7129
E-mail: info@methodisthospital.net
URL: www.methodisthospital.net
Type: Acute Care Hospitals — Emergency Services: Yes
Ownership: Voluntary non-profit - Church — Beds: 197
Key Personnel:
Emergency Room . . . . Salim Akrabawi, RN
Pediatric In-Patient Care . . . . Rita Barron
Coronary Care. . . . . Brenda Dossett
Radiology. . . . . Anthony Perkins
Patient Relations . . . . Bill Schwartz
Chief of Medical Staff. . . . . Mohit K Sheth, MD
Cardiac Laboratory. . . . . Sandy Shuler
Intensive Care Unit. . . . . Beverly Skaggs

Measure	Cases	This Hosp.	State Avg.	U.S. Avg.
Blood Clot Prevention and Treatment				
Anticoagulation Overlap Therapy[2]	29	93%	90%	93%
ICU Venous Thromboembolism Prophylaxis[2]	68	87%	86%	92%
Incidence of Potentially Preventable VTE[1,2]	-	-	13%	10%
UFH with Dosages/Platelet Monitoring[1,2]	-	-	98%	97%
Venous Thromboembolism Prophylaxis[2]	377	93%	80%	85%
Warfarin Therapy Discharge Instructions[2]	20	100%	72%	75%
Chest Pain/Possible Heart Attack Care				
Aspirin Given Within 24 Hours of Arrival	65	98%	97%	96%
Fibrinolytic Meds Within 30 Min. of Arrival[1]	-	-	63%	58%
Average Time to ECG (minutes)	66	3	6	7
Average Time to Transfer (minutes)	15	53	61	60
Children's Asthma Care				
Received Home Management Plan of Care	-	-	-	88%
Received Reliever Medication	-	-	-	100%
Received Systemic Corticosteroids	-	-	-	100%
Emergency Department				
Admittance Decision Time (minutes)[2]	411	59	78	98
Head CT Results Within 45 Min. of Arrival	12	50%	55%	57%
Patients Who Left ER Before Being Seen	28,518	1%	2%	2%

NOTE: Hospital profiles are in alphabetical order by state, then city, then hospital within the city; Rankings exclude hospitals with less than 25 cases except for patient surveys which excludes hospitals with less than 100 cases; (a) 100-299 cases; (1) The number of cases/patients is too few to report; (2) Data submitted were based on a sample of cases/patients; (3) Results are based on a shorter time period than required; (4) Data suppressed by CMS for one or more quarters; (5) Results are not available for this reporting period; (6) Fewer than 100 patients completed the HCAHPS survey; (7) No cases met the criteria for this measure; (8) The lower limit of the confidence interval cannot be calculated if the number of observed infections equals zero; (9) No data are available from the state/territory for this reporting period; (10) The scores shown reflect fewer than 50 completed surveys; (11) There were discrepancies in the data collection process; (12) This measure does not apply to this hospital for this reporting period; (13) Results cannot be calculated for this reporting period; (14) The results for this state are combined with nearby states to protect confidentiality; Please refer to the User's Guide for a full explanation of data.

Measure	Cases	This Hosp.	State Avg.	U.S. Avg.
Time from ER Arrival to Admit. (minutes)[2]	458	194	238	274
Time from ER Arrival to Discharge (minutes)	323	117	126	134
Time in ER Before Being Evaluated (minutes)	334	35	23	26
Time to Pain Meds for Fractures (minutes)	89	70	56	57
Heart Attack Care				
Aspirin Given at Discharge	12	92%	99%	99%
Fibrinolytic Meds Within 30 Min. of Arrival[7]	-	-	-	54%
PCI Within 90 Minutes of Arrival[7]	-	-	97%	96%
Statin Prescribed at Discharge	12	83%	97%	98%
Heart Failure Care				
ACE Inhibitor or ARB for LVSD	49	88%	95%	97%
Discharge Instructions Given	131	90%	92%	94%
Evaluation of LVS Function	165	99%	98%	99%
Medicare Spending				
Medicare Spending per Patient (ratio)	-	1.01	0.97	0.98
Pneumonia Care				
Appropriate Initial Antibiotic Given	141	95%	94%	95%
Blood Culture Timing	154	100%	98%	98%
Pregnancy and Delivery Care				
Newborn Deliveries Scheduled Early[2]	69	14%	9%	6%
Preventive Care				
Immunization for Influenza[2]	489	85%	92%	90%
Immunization for Pneumonia[2]	545	93%	94%	92%
Stroke Care				
Anticoagulation Therapy for Atrial Fibrillation[1,2]	-	-	95%	95%
Antithrombotic Therapy Timing[2]	41	98%	97%	98%
Assessed for Rehabilitation[2]	37	92%	97%	97%
Discharged on Antithrombotic Therapy[2]	35	97%	98%	99%
Discharged on Statin Medication[2]	32	72%	93%	94%
Thrombolytic Therapy Timing[1,2]	-	-	59%	66%
Venous Thromboembolism Prophylaxis[2]	41	80%	93%	94%
Written Stroke Educational Materials Given[2]	20	90%	86%	88%
Surgical Care Improvement Project				
Appropriate Beta Blocker Usage[2]	56	98%	98%	98%
Appropriate VTP Within 24 Hours[2]	175	93%	98%	98%
Controlled Postoperative Blood Glucose[2,7]	-	-	96%	97%
Perioperative Temperature Management[2]	200	100%	100%	100%
Prophylactic Antibiotic Selection[2]	126	95%	99%	99%
Prophylactic Antibiotic Selection (Outpatient)	128	89%	97%	98%
Prophylactic Antibiotic Stopped[2]	123	92%	98%	98%
Prophylactic Antibiotic Timing[2]	126	98%	99%	99%
Prophylactic Antibiotic Timing (Outpatient)	131	95%	97%	98%
Urinary Catheter Removal[2]	108	94%	97%	97%
Survey of Patients' Hospital Experiences				
Area Around Room 'Always' Quiet at Night	300+	67%	64%	61%
Doctors 'Always' Communicated Well	300+	86%	84%	82%
Home Recovery Information Given	300+	80%	86%	85%
Hospital Given 9 or 10 on 10 Point Scale	300+	71%	72%	71%
Meds 'Always' Explained Before Given	300+	65%	66%	64%
Nurses 'Always' Communicated Well	300+	84%	81%	79%
Pain 'Always' Well Controlled	300+	74%	73%	71%
Room and Bathroom 'Always' Clean	300+	77%	75%	73%
Timely Help 'Always' Received	300+	68%	69%	68%
Would Definitely Recommend Hospital	300+	69%	71%	71%
Use of Medical Imaging				
Cardiac Imaging Stress Test before Surgery	222	6.8%	5.3%	5.3%
Combination Abdominal CT Scan	516	16.9%	10.7%	10.5%
Combination Brain/Sinus CT Scan	540	4.1%	3.1%	2.7%
Combination Chest CT Scan	295	6.4%	4.3%	2.7%
Follow-up Mammogram/Ultrasound	670	7.8%	8.3%	8.8%
Lumbar Spine MRI for Low Back Pain	92	41.3%	38.9%	37.2%

Jennie Stuart Medical Center

320 West 18th Street
Hopkinsville, KY 42240
Phone: 270-887-0100
Fax: 270-887-0254
URL: www.jsmc.org
Type: Acute Care Hospitals
Emergency Services: Yes
Ownership: Voluntary non-profit - Private
Beds: 194

Key Personnel:
Chief of Medical Staff.......... Travis Calhoun
Radiology.................... Michael Clark
Operating Room............... J Giannini
Pediatric Ambulatory Care...... Ronald Howard
Pediatric In-Patient Care....... Ronald Howard
Infection Control.............. Betty Jones
President/CEO................ Eric Lee
Quality Assurance............ Eric Lee

Measure	Cases	This Hosp.	State Avg.	U.S. Avg.
Blood Clot Prevention and Treatment				
Anticoagulation Overlap Therapy[2]	55	84%	90%	93%
ICU Venous Thromboembolism Prophylaxis[2]	89	88%	86%	92%
Incidence of Potentially Preventable VTE[1,2]	-	-	13%	10%
UFH with Dosages/Platelet Monitoring[1,2]	-	-	98%	97%
Venous Thromboembolism Prophylaxis[2]	326	80%	80%	85%
Warfarin Therapy Discharge Instructions[2]	34	88%	72%	75%
Chest Pain/Possible Heart Attack Care				
Aspirin Given Within 24 Hours of Arrival	164	95%	97%	96%
Fibrinolytic Meds Within 30 Min. of Arrival[1]	-	-	63%	58%
Average Time to ECG (minutes)	174	11	6	7
Average Time to Transfer (minutes)	26	78	61	60
Children's Asthma Care				
Received Home Management Plan of Care	-	-	-	88%
Received Reliever Medication	-	-	-	100%
Received Systemic Corticosteroids	-	-	-	100%
Emergency Department				
Admittance Decision Time (minutes)[2]	437	83	78	98
Head CT Results Within 45 Min. of Arrival	22	36%	55%	57%
Patients Who Left ER Before Being Seen	35,087	2%	2%	2%
Time from ER Arrival to Admit. (minutes)[2]	514	259	238	274
Time from ER Arrival to Discharge (minutes)	350	150	126	134
Time in ER Before Being Evaluated (minutes)	388	36	23	26
Time to Pain Meds for Fractures (minutes)	102	75	56	57
Heart Attack Care				
Aspirin Given at Discharge	11	91%	99%	99%
Fibrinolytic Meds Within 30 Min. of Arrival[7]	-	-	-	54%
PCI Within 90 Minutes of Arrival[7]	-	-	97%	96%
Statin Prescribed at Discharge[1]	-	-	97%	98%
Heart Failure Care				
ACE Inhibitor or ARB for LVSD	36	100%	95%	97%
Discharge Instructions Given	59	95%	92%	94%
Evaluation of LVS Function	76	97%	98%	99%
Medicare Spending				
Medicare Spending per Patient (ratio)	-	0.98	0.97	0.98
Pneumonia Care				
Appropriate Initial Antibiotic Given	158	96%	94%	95%
Blood Culture Timing	268	98%	98%	98%
Pregnancy and Delivery Care				
Newborn Deliveries Scheduled Early	168	45%	9%	6%
Preventive Care				
Immunization for Influenza[2]	544	98%	92%	90%
Immunization for Pneumonia[2]	623	97%	94%	92%
Stroke Care				
Anticoagulation Therapy for Atrial Fibrillation[1]	-	-	95%	95%
Antithrombotic Therapy Timing	78	100%	97%	98%
Assessed for Rehabilitation	72	74%	97%	97%
Discharged on Antithrombotic Therapy	69	99%	98%	99%
Discharged on Statin Medication	54	80%	93%	94%
Thrombolytic Therapy Timing[1]	-	-	59%	66%
Venous Thromboembolism Prophylaxis	73	89%	93%	94%
Written Stroke Educational Materials Given	39	36%	86%	88%
Surgical Care Improvement Project				
Appropriate Beta Blocker Usage	102	93%	98%	98%
Appropriate VTP Within 24 Hours	323	99%	98%	98%
Controlled Postoperative Blood Glucose[7]	-	-	96%	97%
Perioperative Temperature Management	400	100%	100%	100%
Prophylactic Antibiotic Selection	300	100%	99%	99%
Prophylactic Antibiotic Selection (Outpatient)	67	100%	97%	98%
Prophylactic Antibiotic Stopped	298	97%	98%	98%
Prophylactic Antibiotic Timing	301	98%	99%	99%
Prophylactic Antibiotic Timing (Outpatient)	69	87%	97%	98%
Urinary Catheter Removal	272	95%	97%	97%
Survey of Patients' Hospital Experiences				
Area Around Room 'Always' Quiet at Night	300+	53%	64%	61%
Doctors 'Always' Communicated Well	300+	77%	84%	82%
Home Recovery Information Given	300+	84%	86%	85%
Hospital Given 9 or 10 on 10 Point Scale	300+	58%	72%	71%
Meds 'Always' Explained Before Given	300+	62%	66%	64%
Nurses 'Always' Communicated Well	300+	74%	81%	79%
Pain 'Always' Well Controlled	300+	68%	73%	71%
Room and Bathroom 'Always' Clean	300+	71%	75%	73%
Timely Help 'Always' Received	300+	61%	69%	68%
Would Definitely Recommend Hospital	300+	55%	71%	71%
Use of Medical Imaging				
Cardiac Imaging Stress Test before Surgery[1]	-	-	5.3%	5.3%
Combination Abdominal CT Scan	847	4.7%	10.7%	10.5%
Combination Brain/Sinus CT Scan	792	2.3%	3.1%	2.7%
Combination Chest CT Scan	443	0.0%	4.3%	2.7%
Follow-up Mammogram/Ultrasound	1,375	6.3%	8.3%	8.8%
Lumbar Spine MRI for Low Back Pain	96	41.7%	38.9%	37.2%

Caverna Memorial Hospital

1501 South Dixie Street
Horse Cave, KY 42749
Phone: 270-786-2191
Fax: 270-786-1557
URL: www.cavernahospital.com
Type: Critical Access Hospitals
Emergency Services: Yes
Ownership: Voluntary non-profit - Private
Beds: 25

Key Personnel:
Radiology.................. Jannice Aaron, MD
CEO/President............... Alan Alexander
Chief of Medical Staff.......... David N Catlett
Cardiology.................. Krishnan K. Challapa, MD
Pulmonology................ Michael Zachek, MD

Measure	Cases	This Hosp.	State Avg.	U.S. Avg.
Blood Clot Prevention and Treatment				
Anticoagulation Overlap Therapy[5]	-	-	90%	93%
ICU Venous Thromboembolism Prophylaxis[5]	-	-	86%	92%
Incidence of Potentially Preventable VTE[5]	-	-	13%	10%
UFH with Dosages/Platelet Monitoring[5]	-	-	98%	97%
Venous Thromboembolism Prophylaxis[5]	-	-	80%	85%
Warfarin Therapy Discharge Instructions[5]	-	-	72%	75%
Chest Pain/Possible Heart Attack Care				
Aspirin Given Within 24 Hours of Arrival[5]	-	-	97%	96%
Fibrinolytic Meds Within 30 Min. of Arrival[5]	-	-	63%	58%
Average Time to ECG (minutes)[5]	-	-	6	7
Average Time to Transfer (minutes)[5]	-	-	61	60
Children's Asthma Care				
Received Home Management Plan of Care	-	-	-	88%
Received Reliever Medication	-	-	-	100%
Received Systemic Corticosteroids	-	-	-	100%
Emergency Department				
Admittance Decision Time (minutes)[2,3]	23	75	78	98
Head CT Results Within 45 Min. of Arrival[5]	-	-	55%	57%
Patients Who Left ER Before Being Seen[5]	-	-	2%	2%
Time from ER Arrival to Admit. (minutes)[2,3]	23	260	238	274
Time from ER Arrival to Discharge (minutes)[5]	-	-	126	134
Time in ER Before Being Evaluated (minutes)[5]	-	-	23	26
Time to Pain Meds for Fractures (minutes)[5]	-	-	56	57
Heart Attack Care				
Aspirin Given at Discharge[5]	-	-	99%	99%
Fibrinolytic Meds Within 30 Min. of Arrival[5]	-	-	-	54%
PCI Within 90 Minutes of Arrival[5]	-	-	97%	96%
Statin Prescribed at Discharge[5]	-	-	97%	98%
Heart Failure Care				
ACE Inhibitor or ARB for LVSD[1,2]	-	-	95%	97%
Discharge Instructions Given[1,2]	-	-	92%	94%
Evaluation of LVS Function[2,3]	21	33%	98%	99%
Medicare Spending				
Medicare Spending per Patient (ratio)	-	-	0.97	0.98
Pneumonia Care				
Appropriate Initial Antibiotic Given[2,3]	12	58%	94%	95%
Blood Culture Timing[1,2]	-	-	98%	98%
Pregnancy and Delivery Care				
Newborn Deliveries Scheduled Early[5]	-	-	9%	6%
Preventive Care				
Immunization for Influenza[5]	-	-	92%	90%
Immunization for Pneumonia[5]	-	-	94%	92%
Stroke Care				
Anticoagulation Therapy for Atrial Fibrillation[5]	-	-	95%	95%
Antithrombotic Therapy Timing[5]	-	-	97%	98%
Assessed for Rehabilitation[5]	-	-	97%	97%
Discharged on Antithrombotic Therapy[5]	-	-	98%	99%

NOTE: Hospital profiles are in alphabetical order by state, then city, then hospital within the city; Rankings exclude hospitals with less than 25 cases except for patient surveys which excludes hospitals with less than 100 cases; (a) 100-299 cases; (1) The number of cases/patients is too few to report; (2) Data submitted were based on a sample of cases/patients; (3) Results are based on a shorter time period than required; (4) Data suppressed by CMS for one or more quarters; (5) Results are not available for this reporting period; (6) Fewer than 100 patients completed the HCAHPS survey; (7) No cases met the criteria for this measure; (8) The lower limit of the confidence interval cannot be calculated if the number of observed infections equals zero; (9) No data are available from the state/territory for this reporting period; (10) The scores shown reflect fewer than 50 completed surveys; (11) There were discrepancies in the data collection process; (12) This measure does not apply to this hospital for this reporting period; (13) Results cannot be calculated for this reporting period; (14) The results for this state are combined with nearby states to protect confidentiality; Please refer to the User's Guide for a full explanation of data.

Discharged on Statin Medication[5]	-	-	93%	94%
Thrombolytic Therapy Timing[5]	-	-	59%	66%
Venous Thromboembolism Prophylaxis[5]	-	-	93%	94%
Written Stroke Educational Materials Given[5]	-	-	86%	88%
Surgical Care Improvement Project				
Appropriate Beta Blocker Usage[5]	-	-	98%	98%
Appropriate VTP Within 24 Hours[5]	-	-	98%	98%
Controlled Postoperative Blood Glucose[5]	-	-	96%	97%
Perioperative Temperature Management[5]	-	-	100%	100%
Prophylactic Antibiotic Selection[5]	-	-	99%	99%
Prophylactic Antibiotic Selection (Outpatient)[5]	-	-	97%	98%
Prophylactic Antibiotic Stopped[5]	-	-	98%	98%
Prophylactic Antibiotic Timing[5]	-	-	99%	99%
Prophylactic Antibiotic Timing (Outpatient)[5]	-	-	97%	98%
Urinary Catheter Removal[5]	-	-	97%	97%
Survey of Patients' Hospital Experiences				
Area Around Room 'Always' Quiet at Night[5]	-	-	64%	61%
Doctors 'Always' Communicated Well[5]	-	-	84%	82%
Home Recovery Information Given[5]	-	-	86%	85%
Hospital Given 9 or 10 on 10 Point Scale[5]	-	-	72%	71%
Meds 'Always' Explained Before Given[5]	-	-	66%	64%
Nurses 'Always' Communicated Well[5]	-	-	81%	79%
Pain 'Always' Well Controlled[5]	-	-	73%	71%
Room and Bathroom 'Always' Clean[5]	-	-	75%	73%
Timely Help 'Always' Received[5]	-	-	69%	68%
Would Definitely Recommend Hospital[5]	-	-	71%	71%
Use of Medical Imaging				
Cardiac Imaging Stress Test before Surgery[7]	-	-	5.3%	5.3%
Combination Abdominal CT Scan	149	47.7%	10.7%	10.5%
Combination Brain/Sinus CT Scan	137	0.7%	3.1%	2.7%
Combination Chest CT Scan	89	2.2%	4.3%	2.7%
Follow-up Mammogram/Ultrasound	231	5.6%	8.3%	8.8%
Lumbar Spine MRI for Low Back Pain[1]	-	-	38.9%	37.2%

Mary Breckinridge ARH Hospital

130 Kate Ireland Drive | Phone: 606-672-2901
Hyden, KY 41749 | Fax: 606-672-3626
Type: Critical Access Hospitals | Emergency Services: Yes
Ownership: Voluntary non-profit - Private | Beds: 40

Key Personnel:
Quality Assurance .... Betty Helen Couch
Operating Room.............. Linda Craft
CEO/President............... William Hall
Emergency Room .... Edith Hensley
Infection Control............. Mona Howard
Chief of Medical Staff.......... Roy Varghese, MD

Measure	Cases	This Hosp.	State Avg.	U.S. Avg.
Blood Clot Prevention and Treatment				
Anticoagulation Overlap Therapy[5]	-	-	90%	93%
ICU Venous Thromboembolism Prophylaxis[5]	-	-	86%	92%
Incidence of Potentially Preventable VTE[5]	-	-	13%	10%
UFH with Dosages/Platelet Monitoring[5]	-	-	98%	97%
Venous Thromboembolism Prophylaxis[5]	-	-	80%	85%
Warfarin Therapy Discharge Instructions[5]	-	-	72%	75%
Chest Pain/Possible Heart Attack Care				
Aspirin Given Within 24 Hours of Arrival[5]	-	-	97%	96%
Fibrinolytic Meds Within 30 Min. of Arrival[5]	-	-	63%	58%
Average Time to ECG (minutes)[5]	-	-	6	7
Average Time to Transfer (minutes)[5]	-	-	61	60
Children's Asthma Care				
Received Home Management Plan of Care	-	-	-	88%
Received Reliever Medication	-	-	-	100%
Received Systemic Corticosteroids	-	-	-	100%
Emergency Department				
Admittance Decision Time (minutes)[5]	-	-	78	98
Head CT Results Within 45 Min. of Arrival[5]	-	-	55%	57%
Patients Who Left ER Before Being Seen	9,127	1%	2%	2%
Time from ER Arrival to Admit. (minutes)[5]	-	-	238	274
Time from ER Arrival to Discharge (minutes)[5]	-	-	126	134
Time in ER Before Being Evaluated (minutes)[5]	-	-	23	26
Time to Pain Meds for Fractures (minutes)[5]	-	-	56	57
Heart Attack Care				
Aspirin Given at Discharge[5]	-	-	99%	99%
Fibrinolytic Meds Within 30 Min. of Arrival[5]	-	-	-	54%
PCI Within 90 Minutes of Arrival[5]	-	-	97%	96%
Statin Prescribed at Discharge[5]	-	-	97%	98%
Heart Failure Care				
ACE Inhibitor or ARB for LVSD[1]	-	-	95%	97%
Discharge Instructions Given	22	100%	92%	94%
Evaluation of LVS Function	39	100%	98%	99%
Medicare Spending				
Medicare Spending per Patient (ratio)	-	-	0.97	0.98
Pneumonia Care				
Appropriate Initial Antibiotic Given	38	100%	94%	95%
Blood Culture Timing	67	99%	98%	98%
Pregnancy and Delivery Care				
Newborn Deliveries Scheduled Early[5]	-	-	9%	6%
Preventive Care				
Immunization for Influenza[5]	-	-	92%	90%
Immunization for Pneumonia[5]	-	-	94%	92%
Stroke Care				
Anticoagulation Therapy for Atrial Fibrillation[5]	-	-	95%	95%
Antithrombotic Therapy Timing[5]	-	-	97%	98%
Assessed for Rehabilitation[5]	-	-	97%	97%
Discharged on Antithrombotic Therapy[5]	-	-	98%	99%
Discharged on Statin Medication[5]	-	-	93%	94%
Thrombolytic Therapy Timing[5]	-	-	59%	66%
Venous Thromboembolism Prophylaxis[5]	-	-	93%	94%
Written Stroke Educational Materials Given[5]	-	-	86%	88%
Surgical Care Improvement Project				
Appropriate Beta Blocker Usage[5]	-	-	98%	98%
Appropriate VTP Within 24 Hours[5]	-	-	98%	98%
Controlled Postoperative Blood Glucose[5]	-	-	96%	97%
Perioperative Temperature Management[5]	-	-	100%	100%
Prophylactic Antibiotic Selection[5]	-	-	99%	99%
Prophylactic Antibiotic Selection (Outpatient)[5]	-	-	97%	98%
Prophylactic Antibiotic Stopped[5]	-	-	98%	98%
Prophylactic Antibiotic Timing[5]	-	-	99%	99%
Prophylactic Antibiotic Timing (Outpatient)[5]	-	-	97%	98%
Urinary Catheter Removal[5]	-	-	97%	97%
Survey of Patients' Hospital Experiences				
Area Around Room 'Always' Quiet at Night[5]	-	-	64%	61%
Doctors 'Always' Communicated Well[5]	-	-	84%	82%
Home Recovery Information Given[5]	-	-	86%	85%
Hospital Given 9 or 10 on 10 Point Scale[5]	-	-	72%	71%
Meds 'Always' Explained Before Given[5]	-	-	66%	64%
Nurses 'Always' Communicated Well[5]	-	-	81%	79%
Pain 'Always' Well Controlled[5]	-	-	73%	71%
Room and Bathroom 'Always' Clean[5]	-	-	75%	73%
Timely Help 'Always' Received[5]	-	-	69%	68%
Would Definitely Recommend Hospital[5]	-	-	71%	71%
Use of Medical Imaging				
Cardiac Imaging Stress Test before Surgery[7]	-	-	5.3%	5.3%
Combination Abdominal CT Scan	163	3.7%	10.7%	10.5%
Combination Brain/Sinus CT Scan[1]	-	-	3.1%	2.7%
Combination Chest CT Scan	82	2.4%	4.3%	2.7%
Follow-up Mammogram/Ultrasound	87	13.8%	8.3%	8.8%
Lumbar Spine MRI for Low Back Pain[1]	-	-	38.9%	37.2%

Marcum & Wallace Memorial Hospital

60 Mercy Court | Phone: 606-723-2115
Irvine, KY 40336 | Fax: 606-723-6549
Type: Critical Access Hospitals | Emergency Services: Yes
Ownership: Voluntary non-profit - Private | Beds: 26

Key Personnel:
Quality Assurance .... Susan Ftarling
Emergency Room .... Jenith Smith
CEO .... Susan Starling

Measure	Cases	This Hosp.	State Avg.	U.S. Avg.
Blood Clot Prevention and Treatment				
Anticoagulation Overlap Therapy[5]	-	-	90%	93%
ICU Venous Thromboembolism Prophylaxis[5]	-	-	86%	92%
Incidence of Potentially Preventable VTE[5]	-	-	13%	10%
UFH with Dosages/Platelet Monitoring[5]	-	-	98%	97%
Venous Thromboembolism Prophylaxis[5]	-	-	80%	85%
Warfarin Therapy Discharge Instructions[5]	-	-	72%	75%
Chest Pain/Possible Heart Attack Care				
Aspirin Given Within 24 Hours of Arrival[5]	-	-	97%	96%
Fibrinolytic Meds Within 30 Min. of Arrival[5]	-	-	63%	58%
Average Time to ECG (minutes)[5]	-	-	6	7
Average Time to Transfer (minutes)[5]	-	-	61	60
Children's Asthma Care				
Received Home Management Plan of Care	-	-	-	88%
Received Reliever Medication	-	-	-	100%
Received Systemic Corticosteroids	-	-	-	100%
Emergency Department				
Admittance Decision Time (minutes)[5]	-	-	78	98
Head CT Results Within 45 Min. of Arrival[5]	-	-	55%	57%
Patients Who Left ER Before Being Seen	14,039	1%	2%	2%
Time from ER Arrival to Admit. (minutes)[5]	-	-	238	274
Time from ER Arrival to Discharge (minutes)[5]	-	-	126	134
Time in ER Before Being Evaluated (minutes)[5]	-	-	23	26
Time to Pain Meds for Fractures (minutes)[5]	-	-	56	57
Heart Attack Care				
Aspirin Given at Discharge[5]	-	-	99%	99%
Fibrinolytic Meds Within 30 Min. of Arrival[5]	-	-	-	54%
PCI Within 90 Minutes of Arrival[5]	-	-	97%	96%
Statin Prescribed at Discharge[5]	-	-	97%	98%
Heart Failure Care				
ACE Inhibitor or ARB for LVSD[1,2]	-	-	95%	97%
Discharge Instructions Given[2]	28	93%	92%	94%
Evaluation of LVS Function[2]	33	97%	98%	99%
Medicare Spending				
Medicare Spending per Patient (ratio)	-	-	0.97	0.98
Pneumonia Care				
Appropriate Initial Antibiotic Given	31	94%	94%	95%
Blood Culture Timing	31	94%	98%	98%
Pregnancy and Delivery Care				
Newborn Deliveries Scheduled Early[5]	-	-	9%	6%
Preventive Care				
Immunization for Influenza[5]	-	-	92%	90%
Immunization for Pneumonia[5]	-	-	94%	92%
Stroke Care				
Anticoagulation Therapy for Atrial Fibrillation[5]	-	-	95%	95%
Antithrombotic Therapy Timing[5]	-	-	97%	98%
Assessed for Rehabilitation[5]	-	-	97%	97%
Discharged on Antithrombotic Therapy[5]	-	-	98%	99%
Discharged on Statin Medication[5]	-	-	93%	94%
Thrombolytic Therapy Timing[5]	-	-	59%	66%
Venous Thromboembolism Prophylaxis[5]	-	-	93%	94%
Written Stroke Educational Materials Given[5]	-	-	86%	88%
Surgical Care Improvement Project				
Appropriate Beta Blocker Usage[5]	-	-	98%	98%
Appropriate VTP Within 24 Hours[5]	-	-	98%	98%
Controlled Postoperative Blood Glucose[5]	-	-	96%	97%
Perioperative Temperature Management[5]	-	-	100%	100%
Prophylactic Antibiotic Selection[5]	-	-	99%	99%
Prophylactic Antibiotic Selection (Outpatient)[5]	-	-	97%	98%
Prophylactic Antibiotic Stopped[5]	-	-	98%	98%
Prophylactic Antibiotic Timing[5]	-	-	99%	99%
Prophylactic Antibiotic Timing (Outpatient)[5]	-	-	97%	98%
Urinary Catheter Removal[5]	-	-	97%	97%
Survey of Patients' Hospital Experiences				
Area Around Room 'Always' Quiet at Night	(a)	65%	64%	61%
Doctors 'Always' Communicated Well	(a)	90%	84%	82%
Home Recovery Information Given	(a)	87%	86%	85%
Hospital Given 9 or 10 on 10 Point Scale	(a)	79%	72%	71%
Meds 'Always' Explained Before Given	(a)	71%	66%	64%
Nurses 'Always' Communicated Well	(a)	88%	81%	79%
Pain 'Always' Well Controlled	(a)	80%	73%	71%
Room and Bathroom 'Always' Clean	(a)	87%	75%	73%
Timely Help 'Always' Received	(a)	77%	69%	68%
Would Definitely Recommend Hospital	(a)	78%	71%	71%
Use of Medical Imaging				
Cardiac Imaging Stress Test before Surgery	92	5.4%	5.3%	5.3%
Combination Abdominal CT Scan	334	10.5%	10.7%	10.5%
Combination Brain/Sinus CT Scan	356	1.4%	3.1%	2.7%
Combination Chest CT Scan	176	11.9%	4.3%	2.7%

NOTE: Hospital profiles are in alphabetical order by state, then city, then hospital within the city; Rankings exclude hospitals with less than 25 cases except for patient surveys which excludes hospitals with less than 100 cases; (a) 100-299 cases; (1) The number of cases/patients is too few to report; (2) Data submitted were based on a sample of cases/patients; (3) Results are based on a shorter time period than required; (4) Data suppressed by CMS for one or more quarters; (5) Results are not available for this reporting period; (6) Fewer than 100 patients completed the HCAHPS survey; (7) No cases met the criteria for this measure; (8) The lower limit of the confidence interval cannot be calculated if the number of observed infections equals zero; (9) No data are available from the state/territory for this reporting period; (10) The scores shown reflect fewer than 50 completed surveys; (11) There were discrepancies in the data collection process; (12) This measure does not apply to this hospital for this reporting period; (13) Results cannot be calculated for this reporting period; (14) The results for this state are combined with nearby states to protect confidentiality; Please refer to the User's Guide for a full explanation of data.

Follow-up Mammogram/Ultrasound	356	5.6%	8.3%	8.8%
Lumbar Spine MRI for Low Back Pain	62	51.6%	38.9%	37.2%

Kentucky River Medical Center

540 Jett Drive Phone: 606-666-6000
Jackson, KY 41339 Fax: 606-666-6107
URL: www.kentuckyrivermc.com
Type: Acute Care Hospitals Emergency Services: Yes
Ownership: Voluntary non-profit - Other Beds: 55
Key Personnel:
Quality Assurance .... Carolyn S Lipp

Measure	Cases	This Hosp.	State Avg.	U.S. Avg.
Blood Clot Prevention and Treatment				
Anticoagulation Overlap Therapy[1,2]	-	-	90%	93%
ICU Venous Thromboembolism Prophylaxis[2]	53	100%	86%	92%
Incidence of Potentially Preventable VTE[2,7]	-	-	13%	10%
UFH with Dosages/Platelet Monitoring[1,2]	-	-	98%	97%
Venous Thromboembolism Prophylaxis[2]	299	100%	80%	85%
Warfarin Therapy Discharge Instructions[1,2]	-	-	72%	75%
Chest Pain/Possible Heart Attack Care				
Aspirin Given Within 24 Hours of Arrival	64	100%	97%	96%
Fibrinolytic Meds Within 30 Min. of Arrival[1]	-	-	63%	58%
Average Time to ECG (minutes)	65	3	6	7
Average Time to Transfer (minutes)[1]	-	-	61	60
Children's Asthma Care				
Received Home Management Plan of Care	-	-	-	88%
Received Reliever Medication	-	-	-	100%
Received Systemic Corticosteroids	-	-	-	100%
Emergency Department				
Admittance Decision Time (minutes)[2]	516	100	78	98
Head CT Results Within 45 Min. of Arrival[1]	-	-	55%	57%
Patients Who Left ER Before Being Seen	21,615	2%	2%	2%
Time from ER Arrival to Admit. (minutes)[2]	517	170	238	274
Time from ER Arrival to Discharge (minutes)	358	84	126	134
Time in ER Before Being Evaluated (minutes)	418	12	23	26
Time to Pain Meds for Fractures (minutes)	81	73	56	57
Heart Attack Care				
Aspirin Given at Discharge[1]	-	-	99%	99%
Fibrinolytic Meds Within 30 Min. of Arrival[7]	-	-	-	54%
PCI Within 90 Minutes of Arrival[7]	-	-	97%	96%
Statin Prescribed at Discharge[1]	-	-	97%	98%
Heart Failure Care				
ACE Inhibitor or ARB for LVSD	18	100%	95%	97%
Discharge Instructions Given	58	97%	92%	94%
Evaluation of LVS Function	73	100%	98%	99%
Medicare Spending				
Medicare Spending per Patient (ratio)	-	0.95	0.97	0.98
Pneumonia Care				
Appropriate Initial Antibiotic Given	41	98%	94%	95%
Blood Culture Timing	60	100%	98%	98%
Pregnancy and Delivery Care				
Newborn Deliveries Scheduled Early[2,7]	-	-	9%	6%
Preventive Care				
Immunization for Influenza[2]	320	100%	92%	90%
Immunization for Pneumonia[2]	420	100%	94%	92%
Stroke Care				
Anticoagulation Therapy for Atrial Fibrillation[7]	-	-	95%	95%
Antithrombotic Therapy Timing[1]	-	-	97%	98%
Assessed for Rehabilitation[1]	-	-	97%	97%
Discharged on Antithrombotic Therapy[1]	-	-	98%	99%
Discharged on Statin Medication[1]	-	-	93%	94%
Thrombolytic Therapy Timing[7]	-	-	59%	66%
Venous Thromboembolism Prophylaxis[1]	-	-	93%	94%
Written Stroke Educational Materials Given[1]	-	-	86%	88%
Surgical Care Improvement Project				
Appropriate Beta Blocker Usage[1]	-	-	98%	98%
Appropriate VTP Within 24 Hours	27	100%	98%	98%
Controlled Postoperative Blood Glucose[7]	-	-	96%	97%
Perioperative Temperature Management	36	100%	100%	100%
Prophylactic Antibiotic Selection	18	94%	99%	99%
Prophylactic Antibiotic Selection (Outpatient)	75	99%	97%	98%
Prophylactic Antibiotic Stopped	18	89%	98%	98%
Prophylactic Antibiotic Timing	18	100%	99%	99%
Prophylactic Antibiotic Timing (Outpatient)	75	100%	97%	98%
Urinary Catheter Removal	14	100%	97%	97%
Survey of Patients' Hospital Experiences				
Area Around Room 'Always' Quiet at Night	300+	65%	64%	61%
Doctors 'Always' Communicated Well	300+	83%	84%	82%
Home Recovery Information Given	300+	83%	86%	85%
Hospital Given 9 or 10 on 10 Point Scale	300+	72%	72%	71%
Meds 'Always' Explained Before Given	300+	65%	66%	64%
Nurses 'Always' Communicated Well	300+	83%	81%	79%
Pain 'Always' Well Controlled	300+	74%	73%	71%
Room and Bathroom 'Always' Clean	300+	73%	75%	73%
Timely Help 'Always' Received	300+	73%	69%	68%
Would Definitely Recommend Hospital	300+	68%	71%	71%
Use of Medical Imaging				
Cardiac Imaging Stress Test before Surgery	59	1.7%	5.3%	5.3%
Combination Abdominal CT Scan	345	2.9%	10.7%	10.5%
Combination Brain/Sinus CT Scan	353	4.8%	3.1%	2.7%
Combination Chest CT Scan	96	10.4%	4.3%	2.7%
Follow-up Mammogram/Ultrasound	193	4.1%	8.3%	8.8%
Lumbar Spine MRI for Low Back Pain	80	20.0%	38.9%	37.2%

Baptist Health Lagrange

1025 New Moody Lane Phone: 502-222-5388
La Grange, KY 40031 Fax: 502-222-3411
URL: www.baptistnortheast.com
Type: Acute Care Hospitals Emergency Services: Yes
Ownership: Voluntary non-profit - Private Beds: 120
Key Personnel:
Quality Assurance .... Toby Bilbro
Infection Control............. Marilyn Czape
Cardiac Laboratory............ Maureen Holmes
Coronary Care .... Lynn Rigon
Operating Room............... Barbara Ritchie
Radiology................... Rommi Wadlington
Chief of Medical Staff.......... Richardzabeth Waggen, MD

Measure	Cases	This Hosp.	State Avg.	U.S. Avg.
Blood Clot Prevention and Treatment				
Anticoagulation Overlap Therapy[2]	11	91%	90%	93%
ICU Venous Thromboembolism Prophylaxis[2]	64	95%	86%	92%
Incidence of Potentially Preventable VTE[2,7]	-	-	13%	10%
UFH with Dosages/Platelet Monitoring[1,2]	-	-	98%	97%
Venous Thromboembolism Prophylaxis[2]	195	93%	80%	85%
Warfarin Therapy Discharge Instructions[1,2]	-	-	72%	75%
Chest Pain/Possible Heart Attack Care				
Aspirin Given Within 24 Hours of Arrival	48	100%	97%	96%
Fibrinolytic Meds Within 30 Min. of Arrival[7]	-	-	63%	58%
Average Time to ECG (minutes)	50	3	6	7
Average Time to Transfer (minutes)[1]	-	-	61	60
Children's Asthma Care				
Received Home Management Plan of Care	-	-	-	88%
Received Reliever Medication	-	-	-	100%
Received Systemic Corticosteroids	-	-	-	100%
Emergency Department				
Admittance Decision Time (minutes)[2]	243	51	78	98
Head CT Results Within 45 Min. of Arrival[1]	-	-	55%	57%
Patients Who Left ER Before Being Seen	15,173	2%	2%	2%
Time from ER Arrival to Admit. (minutes)[2]	243	227	238	274
Time from ER Arrival to Discharge (minutes)	384	146	126	134
Time in ER Before Being Evaluated (minutes)	406	34	23	26
Time to Pain Meds for Fractures (minutes)	19	68	56	57
Heart Attack Care				
Aspirin Given at Discharge[1]	-	-	99%	99%
Fibrinolytic Meds Within 30 Min. of Arrival[7]	-	-	-	54%
PCI Within 90 Minutes of Arrival[7]	-	-	97%	96%
Statin Prescribed at Discharge[1]	-	-	97%	98%
Heart Failure Care				
ACE Inhibitor or ARB for LVSD	25	100%	95%	97%
Discharge Instructions Given	71	96%	92%	94%
Evaluation of LVS Function	83	100%	98%	99%
Medicare Spending				
Medicare Spending per Patient (ratio)	-	0.95	0.97	0.98
Pneumonia Care				
Appropriate Initial Antibiotic Given	65	98%	94%	95%
Blood Culture Timing	112	100%	98%	98%
Pregnancy and Delivery Care				
Newborn Deliveries Scheduled Early[2]	47	4%	9%	6%
Preventive Care				
Immunization for Influenza[2]	288	99%	92%	90%
Immunization for Pneumonia[2]	307	99%	94%	92%
Stroke Care				
Anticoagulation Therapy for Atrial Fibrillation[7]	-	-	95%	95%
Antithrombotic Therapy Timing	17	100%	97%	98%
Assessed for Rehabilitation	23	100%	97%	97%
Discharged on Antithrombotic Therapy	23	100%	98%	99%
Discharged on Statin Medication	20	90%	93%	94%
Thrombolytic Therapy Timing[1]	-	-	59%	66%
Venous Thromboembolism Prophylaxis	23	100%	93%	94%
Written Stroke Educational Materials Given	14	100%	86%	88%
Surgical Care Improvement Project				
Appropriate Beta Blocker Usage	53	98%	98%	98%
Appropriate VTP Within 24 Hours	192	98%	98%	98%
Controlled Postoperative Blood Glucose[7]	-	-	96%	97%
Perioperative Temperature Management	205	100%	100%	100%
Prophylactic Antibiotic Selection	139	99%	99%	99%
Prophylactic Antibiotic Selection (Outpatient)	77	96%	97%	98%
Prophylactic Antibiotic Stopped	137	99%	98%	98%
Prophylactic Antibiotic Timing	139	100%	99%	99%
Prophylactic Antibiotic Timing (Outpatient)	78	96%	97%	98%
Urinary Catheter Removal	35	97%	97%	97%
Survey of Patients' Hospital Experiences				
Area Around Room 'Always' Quiet at Night	300+	58%	64%	61%
Doctors 'Always' Communicated Well	300+	81%	84%	82%
Home Recovery Information Given	300+	86%	86%	85%
Hospital Given 9 or 10 on 10 Point Scale	300+	76%	72%	71%
Meds 'Always' Explained Before Given	300+	64%	66%	64%
Nurses 'Always' Communicated Well	300+	83%	81%	79%
Pain 'Always' Well Controlled	300+	76%	73%	71%
Room and Bathroom 'Always' Clean	300+	73%	75%	73%
Timely Help 'Always' Received	300+	70%	69%	68%
Would Definitely Recommend Hospital	300+	74%	71%	71%
Use of Medical Imaging				
Cardiac Imaging Stress Test before Surgery	223	4.0%	5.3%	5.3%
Combination Abdominal CT Scan	370	1.4%	10.7%	10.5%
Combination Brain/Sinus CT Scan[1]	-	-	3.1%	2.7%
Combination Chest CT Scan	242	0.0%	4.3%	2.7%
Follow-up Mammogram/Ultrasound	662	4.4%	8.3%	8.8%
Lumbar Spine MRI for Low Back Pain[1]	-	-	38.9%	37.2%

Saint Elizabeth Medical Center

1 Medical Village Drive Phone: 859-292-2000
Lakeside Park, KY 41017 Fax: 859-301-5178
E-mail: contact@stelizabeth.com
URL: www.stelizabeth.com
Type: Acute Care Hospitals Emergency Services: Yes
Ownership: Voluntary non-profit - Church Beds: 684
Key Personnel:
Infection Control.............. Patty Burns
Quality Assurance .... Lisa Frey
Pediatric In-Patient Care .... Mary Garamy, RN
Radiology.................... Lloyd Gill
CEO/President................ Joseph W Gross
Operating Room............... Sue Sansone, RN
Chief of Medical Staff.......... Phillip B Schworer, MD

Measure	Cases	This Hosp.	State Avg.	U.S. Avg.
Blood Clot Prevention and Treatment				
Anticoagulation Overlap Therapy[2]	134	100%	90%	93%
ICU Venous Thromboembolism Prophylaxis[2]	82	98%	86%	92%
Incidence of Potentially Preventable VTE[2]	21	24%	13%	10%
UFH with Dosages/Platelet Monitoring[2]	169	99%	98%	97%
Venous Thromboembolism Prophylaxis[2]	364	96%	80%	85%
Warfarin Therapy Discharge Instructions[2]	104	98%	72%	75%
Chest Pain/Possible Heart Attack Care				
Aspirin Given Within 24 Hours of Arrival	19	95%	97%	96%
Fibrinolytic Meds Within 30 Min. of Arrival[3,7]	-	-	63%	58%
Average Time to ECG (minutes)	22	14	6	7
Average Time to Transfer (minutes)[3,7]	-	-	61	60
Children's Asthma Care				
Received Home Management Plan of Care	-	-	-	88%

NOTE: Hospital profiles are in alphabetical order by state, then city, then hospital within the city; Rankings exclude hospitals with less than 25 cases except for patient surveys which excludes hospitals with less than 100 cases; (a) 100-299 cases; (1) The number of cases/patients is too few to report; (2) Data submitted were based on a sample of cases/patients; (3) Results are based on a shorter time period than required; (4) Data suppressed by CMS for one or more quarters; (5) Results are not available for this reporting period; (6) Fewer than 100 patients completed the HCAHPS survey; (7) No cases met the criteria for this measure; (8) The lower limit of the confidence interval cannot be calculated if the number of observed infections equals zero; (9) No data are available from the state/territory for this reporting period; (10) The scores shown reflect fewer than 50 completed surveys; (11) There were discrepancies in the data collection process; (12) This measure does not apply to this hospital for this reporting period; (13) Results cannot be calculated for this reporting period; (14) The results for this state are combined with nearby states to protect confidentiality; Please refer to the User's Guide for a full explanation of data.

Measure	Cases	This Hosp.	State Avg.	U.S. Avg.
Received Reliever Medication	-	-	-	100%
Received Systemic Corticosteroids	-	-	-	100%
Emergency Department				
Admittance Decision Time (minutes)[2]	528	104	78	98
Head CT Results Within 45 Min. of Arrival[1]	-	-	55%	57%
Patients Who Left ER Before Being Seen	>100k	0%	2%	2%
Time from ER Arrival to Admit. (minutes)[2]	531	255	238	274
Time from ER Arrival to Discharge (minutes)	768	111	126	134
Time in ER Before Being Evaluated (minutes)	843	16	23	26
Time to Pain Meds for Fractures (minutes)	232	39	56	57
Heart Attack Care				
Aspirin Given at Discharge[2]	327	100%	99%	99%
Fibrinolytic Meds Within 30 Min. of Arrival[2,7]	-	-	-	54%
PCI Within 90 Minutes of Arrival[2]	43	98%	97%	96%
Statin Prescribed at Discharge[2]	312	100%	97%	98%
Heart Failure Care				
ACE Inhibitor or ARB for LVSD[2]	83	100%	95%	97%
Discharge Instructions Given[2]	258	100%	92%	94%
Evaluation of LVS Function[2]	316	100%	98%	99%
Medicare Spending				
Medicare Spending per Patient (ratio)	-	1.02	0.97	0.98
Pneumonia Care				
Appropriate Initial Antibiotic Given[2]	60	100%	94%	95%
Blood Culture Timing[2]	87	99%	98%	98%
Pregnancy and Delivery Care				
Newborn Deliveries Scheduled Early[2]	240	0%	9%	6%
Preventive Care				
Immunization for Influenza[2]	549	100%	92%	90%
Immunization for Pneumonia[2]	676	100%	94%	92%
Stroke Care				
Anticoagulation Therapy for Atrial Fibrillation[2]	16	100%	95%	95%
Antithrombotic Therapy Timing[2]	100	97%	97%	98%
Assessed for Rehabilitation[2]	127	99%	97%	97%
Discharged on Antithrombotic Therapy[2]	115	100%	98%	99%
Discharged on Statin Medication[2]	86	98%	93%	94%
Thrombolytic Therapy Timing[1,2]	-	-	59%	66%
Venous Thromboembolism Prophylaxis[2]	132	100%	93%	94%
Written Stroke Educational Materials Given[2]	68	100%	86%	88%
Surgical Care Improvement Project				
Appropriate Beta Blocker Usage[2]	270	99%	98%	98%
Appropriate VTP Within 24 Hours[2]	434	100%	98%	98%
Controlled Postoperative Blood Glucose[2]	163	100%	96%	97%
Perioperative Temperature Management[2]	548	100%	100%	100%
Prophylactic Antibiotic Selection[2]	501	100%	99%	99%
Prophylactic Antibiotic Selection (Outpatient)	628	100%	97%	98%
Prophylactic Antibiotic Stopped[2]	484	100%	98%	98%
Prophylactic Antibiotic Timing[2]	501	100%	99%	99%
Prophylactic Antibiotic Timing (Outpatient)	629	100%	97%	98%
Urinary Catheter Removal[2]	241	100%	97%	97%
Survey of Patients' Hospital Experiences				
Area Around Room 'Always' Quiet at Night	300+	61%	64%	61%
Doctors 'Always' Communicated Well	300+	80%	84%	82%
Home Recovery Information Given	300+	88%	86%	85%
Hospital Given 9 or 10 on 10 Point Scale	300+	75%	72%	71%
Meds 'Always' Explained Before Given	300+	68%	66%	64%
Nurses 'Always' Communicated Well	300+	81%	81%	79%
Pain 'Always' Well Controlled	300+	71%	73%	71%
Room and Bathroom 'Always' Clean	300+	69%	75%	73%
Timely Help 'Always' Received	300+	66%	69%	68%
Would Definitely Recommend Hospital	300+	77%	71%	71%
Use of Medical Imaging				
Cardiac Imaging Stress Test before Surgery	1,904	4.2%	5.3%	5.3%
Combination Abdominal CT Scan	1,749	3.5%	10.7%	10.5%
Combination Brain/Sinus CT Scan	1,262	0.6%	3.1%	2.7%
Combination Chest CT Scan	922	0.2%	4.3%	2.7%
Follow-up Mammogram/Ultrasound	3,234	5.8%	8.3%	8.8%
Lumbar Spine MRI for Low Back Pain	528	41.5%	38.9%	37.2%

Spring View Hospital

320 Loretto Road — Phone: 270-692-5145
Lebanon, KY 40033 — Fax: 270-692-5155
Type: Acute Care Hospitals — Emergency Services: Yes
Ownership: Proprietary — Beds: 113

Measure	Cases	This Hosp.	State Avg.	U.S. Avg.
Blood Clot Prevention and Treatment				
Anticoagulation Overlap Therapy[1,2]	-	-	90%	93%
ICU Venous Thromboembolism Prophylaxis[2]	31	94%	86%	92%
Incidence of Potentially Preventable VTE[2,7]	-	-	13%	10%
UFH with Dosages/Platelet Monitoring[1,2]	-	-	98%	97%
Venous Thromboembolism Prophylaxis[2]	123	89%	80%	85%
Warfarin Therapy Discharge Instructions[1,2]	-	-	72%	75%
Chest Pain/Possible Heart Attack Care				
Aspirin Given Within 24 Hours of Arrival	52	96%	97%	96%
Fibrinolytic Meds Within 30 Min. of Arrival[1]	-	-	63%	58%
Average Time to ECG (minutes)	52	8	6	7
Average Time to Transfer (minutes)[1]	-	-	61	60
Children's Asthma Care				
Received Home Management Plan of Care	-	-	-	88%
Received Reliever Medication	-	-	-	100%
Received Systemic Corticosteroids	-	-	-	100%
Emergency Department				
Admittance Decision Time (minutes)[2]	244	49	78	98
Head CT Results Within 45 Min. of Arrival	13	54%	55%	57%
Patients Who Left ER Before Being Seen	14,821	1%	2%	2%
Time from ER Arrival to Admit. (minutes)[2]	244	244	238	274
Time from ER Arrival to Discharge (minutes)	409	125	126	134
Time in ER Before Being Evaluated (minutes)	443	20	23	26
Time to Pain Meds for Fractures (minutes)	41	51	56	57
Heart Attack Care				
Aspirin Given at Discharge[1,3]	-	-	99%	99%
Fibrinolytic Meds Within 30 Min. of Arrival[3,7]	-	-	-	54%
PCI Within 90 Minutes of Arrival[3,7]	-	-	97%	96%
Statin Prescribed at Discharge[1,3]	-	-	97%	98%
Heart Failure Care				
ACE Inhibitor or ARB for LVSD[1]	-	-	95%	97%
Discharge Instructions Given	35	100%	92%	94%
Evaluation of LVS Function	62	85%	98%	99%
Medicare Spending				
Medicare Spending per Patient (ratio)	-	0.92	0.97	0.98
Pneumonia Care				
Appropriate Initial Antibiotic Given	109	94%	94%	95%
Blood Culture Timing	138	99%	98%	98%
Pregnancy and Delivery Care				
Newborn Deliveries Scheduled Early[2]	31	6%	9%	6%
Preventive Care				
Immunization for Influenza[2]	258	96%	92%	90%
Immunization for Pneumonia[2]	278	97%	94%	92%
Stroke Care				
Anticoagulation Therapy for Atrial Fibrillation[7]	-	-	95%	95%
Antithrombotic Therapy Timing[1]	-	-	97%	98%
Assessed for Rehabilitation[1]	-	-	97%	97%
Discharged on Antithrombotic Therapy[1]	-	-	98%	99%
Discharged on Statin Medication[1]	-	-	93%	94%
Thrombolytic Therapy Timing[7]	-	-	59%	66%
Venous Thromboembolism Prophylaxis[1]	-	-	93%	94%
Written Stroke Educational Materials Given[7]	-	-	86%	88%
Surgical Care Improvement Project				
Appropriate Beta Blocker Usage	27	89%	98%	98%
Appropriate VTP Within 24 Hours	123	99%	98%	98%
Controlled Postoperative Blood Glucose[7]	-	-	96%	97%
Perioperative Temperature Management	144	100%	100%	100%
Prophylactic Antibiotic Selection	119	98%	99%	99%
Prophylactic Antibiotic Selection (Outpatient)	31	100%	97%	98%
Prophylactic Antibiotic Stopped	115	97%	98%	98%
Prophylactic Antibiotic Timing	119	97%	99%	99%
Prophylactic Antibiotic Timing (Outpatient)	32	97%	97%	98%
Urinary Catheter Removal	70	90%	97%	97%
Survey of Patients' Hospital Experiences				
Area Around Room 'Always' Quiet at Night	300+	61%	64%	61%
Doctors 'Always' Communicated Well	300+	82%	84%	82%
Home Recovery Information Given	300+	82%	86%	85%
Hospital Given 9 or 10 on 10 Point Scale	300+	68%	72%	71%
Meds 'Always' Explained Before Given	300+	64%	66%	64%
Nurses 'Always' Communicated Well	300+	77%	81%	79%
Pain 'Always' Well Controlled	300+	69%	73%	71%
Room and Bathroom 'Always' Clean	300+	70%	75%	73%
Timely Help 'Always' Received	300+	66%	69%	68%
Would Definitely Recommend Hospital	300+	64%	71%	71%
Use of Medical Imaging				
Cardiac Imaging Stress Test before Surgery	174	4.6%	5.3%	5.3%
Combination Abdominal CT Scan	299	12.7%	10.7%	10.5%
Combination Brain/Sinus CT Scan[1]	-	-	3.1%	2.7%
Combination Chest CT Scan	146	0.7%	4.3%	2.7%
Follow-up Mammogram/Ultrasound	542	5.7%	8.3%	8.8%
Lumbar Spine MRI for Low Back Pain	88	44.3%	38.9%	37.2%

Twin Lakes Regional Medical Center

910 Wallace Avenue — Phone: 270-259-9400
Leitchfield, KY 42754 — Fax: 270-259-9524
URL: www.tlrmc.com
Type: Acute Care Hospitals — Emergency Services: Yes
Ownership: Voluntary non-profit - Other — Beds: 75

Key Personnel:
Radiology. . . . . Kenneth Dennison
CEO/President. . . . . Stephen L Meredith

Measure	Cases	This Hosp.	State Avg.	U.S. Avg.
Blood Clot Prevention and Treatment				
Anticoagulation Overlap Therapy[2]	26	100%	90%	93%
ICU Venous Thromboembolism Prophylaxis[2]	53	94%	86%	92%
Incidence of Potentially Preventable VTE[1,2]	-	-	13%	10%
UFH with Dosages/Platelet Monitoring[1,2]	-	-	98%	97%
Venous Thromboembolism Prophylaxis[2]	236	86%	80%	85%
Warfarin Therapy Discharge Instructions[2]	17	100%	72%	75%
Chest Pain/Possible Heart Attack Care				
Aspirin Given Within 24 Hours of Arrival	83	99%	97%	96%
Fibrinolytic Meds Within 30 Min. of Arrival	11	91%	63%	58%
Average Time to ECG (minutes)	85	9	6	7
Average Time to Transfer (minutes)[1]	-	-	61	60
Children's Asthma Care				
Received Home Management Plan of Care	-	-	-	88%
Received Reliever Medication	-	-	-	100%
Received Systemic Corticosteroids	-	-	-	100%
Emergency Department				
Admittance Decision Time (minutes)[2]	310	61	78	98
Head CT Results Within 45 Min. of Arrival[1]	-	-	55%	57%
Patients Who Left ER Before Being Seen	21,834	2%	2%	2%
Time from ER Arrival to Admit. (minutes)[2]	310	175	238	274
Time from ER Arrival to Discharge (minutes)	374	94	126	134
Time in ER Before Being Evaluated (minutes)	397	17	23	26
Time to Pain Meds for Fractures (minutes)	94	55	56	57
Heart Attack Care				
Aspirin Given at Discharge[1]	-	-	99%	99%
Fibrinolytic Meds Within 30 Min. of Arrival[7]	-	-	-	54%
PCI Within 90 Minutes of Arrival[7]	-	-	97%	96%
Statin Prescribed at Discharge[1]	-	-	97%	98%
Heart Failure Care				
ACE Inhibitor or ARB for LVSD	12	100%	95%	97%
Discharge Instructions Given	61	90%	92%	94%
Evaluation of LVS Function	77	99%	98%	99%
Medicare Spending				
Medicare Spending per Patient (ratio)	-	0.95	0.97	0.98
Pneumonia Care				
Appropriate Initial Antibiotic Given	96	95%	94%	95%
Blood Culture Timing	162	96%	98%	98%
Pregnancy and Delivery Care				
Newborn Deliveries Scheduled Early	35	9%	9%	6%
Preventive Care				
Immunization for Influenza[2]	291	95%	92%	90%
Immunization for Pneumonia[2]	385	91%	94%	92%
Stroke Care				
Anticoagulation Therapy for Atrial Fibrillation[1]	-	-	95%	95%
Antithrombotic Therapy Timing	27	100%	97%	98%
Assessed for Rehabilitation	25	96%	97%	97%

NOTE: Hospital profiles are in alphabetical order by state, then city, then hospital within the city; Rankings exclude hospitals with less than 25 cases except for patient surveys which excludes hospitals with less than 100 cases; (a) 100-299 cases; (1) The number of cases/patients is too few to report; (2) Data submitted were based on a sample of cases/patients; (3) Results are based on a shorter time period than required; (4) Data suppressed by CMS for one or more quarters; (5) Results are not available for this reporting period; (6) Fewer than 100 patients completed the HCAHPS survey; (7) No cases met the criteria for this measure; (8) The lower limit of the confidence interval cannot be calculated if the number of observed infections equals zero; (9) No data are available from the state/territory for this reporting period; (10) The scores shown reflect fewer than 50 completed surveys; (11) There were discrepancies in the data collection process; (12) This measure does not apply to this hospital for this reporting period; (13) Results cannot be calculated for this reporting period; (14) The results for this state are combined with nearby states to protect confidentiality; Please refer to the User's Guide for a full explanation of data.

Measure	Cases	This Hosp.	State Avg.	U.S. Avg.
Discharged on Antithrombotic Therapy	25	96%	98%	99%
Discharged on Statin Medication	20	90%	93%	94%
Thrombolytic Therapy Timing[1]	-	-	59%	66%
Venous Thromboembolism Prophylaxis	27	89%	93%	94%
Written Stroke Educational Materials Given	13	77%	86%	88%
Surgical Care Improvement Project				
Appropriate Beta Blocker Usage	34	100%	98%	98%
Appropriate VTP Within 24 Hours	135	98%	98%	98%
Controlled Postoperative Blood Glucose[7]	-	-	96%	97%
Perioperative Temperature Management	145	100%	100%	100%
Prophylactic Antibiotic Selection	96	98%	99%	99%
Prophylactic Antibiotic Selection (Outpatient)	31	100%	97%	98%
Prophylactic Antibiotic Stopped	96	99%	98%	98%
Prophylactic Antibiotic Timing	97	100%	99%	99%
Prophylactic Antibiotic Timing (Outpatient)	31	100%	97%	98%
Urinary Catheter Removal	83	99%	97%	97%
Survey of Patients' Hospital Experiences				
Area Around Room 'Always' Quiet at Night	300+	60%	64%	61%
Doctors 'Always' Communicated Well	300+	83%	84%	82%
Home Recovery Information Given	300+	77%	86%	85%
Hospital Given 9 or 10 on 10 Point Scale	300+	71%	72%	71%
Meds 'Always' Explained Before Given	300+	61%	66%	64%
Nurses 'Always' Communicated Well	300+	80%	81%	79%
Pain 'Always' Well Controlled	300+	68%	73%	71%
Room and Bathroom 'Always' Clean	300+	80%	75%	73%
Timely Help 'Always' Received	300+	68%	69%	68%
Would Definitely Recommend Hospital	300+	67%	71%	71%
Use of Medical Imaging				
Cardiac Imaging Stress Test before Surgery	210	6.7%	5.3%	5.3%
Combination Abdominal CT Scan	332	6.3%	10.7%	10.5%
Combination Brain/Sinus CT Scan[1]	-	-	3.1%	2.7%
Combination Chest CT Scan	293	0.7%	4.3%	2.7%
Follow-up Mammogram/Ultrasound	524	5.2%	8.3%	8.8%
Lumbar Spine MRI for Low Back Pain	70	42.9%	38.9%	37.2%

Baptist Health Lexington

1740 Nicholasville Road
Lexington, KY 40503
Phone: 859-260-6104
Fax: 859-260-6117
URL: www.centralbap.com
Type: Acute Care Hospitals
Emergency Services: Yes
Ownership: Voluntary non-profit - Other
Beds: 383

Key Personnel:
Infection Control. . . . . Dee Anderson, RN
Pediatric In-Patient Care . . . . Carole Bales
Operating Room. . . . . Kathleen Blair
Radiology. . . . . Bill Broaddis
Quality Assurance . . . . Lynn Kolokowski
Coronary Care. . . . . Norma Lake
CEO/President. . . . . William G Sisson
Chief of Medical Staff. . . . . Jon Voss, MD

Measure	Cases	This Hosp.	State Avg.	U.S. Avg.
Blood Clot Prevention and Treatment				
Anticoagulation Overlap Therapy[2]	87	98%	90%	93%
ICU Venous Thromboembolism Prophylaxis[2]	116	94%	86%	92%
Incidence of Potentially Preventable VTE[1,2]	-	-	13%	10%
UFH with Dosages/Platelet Monitoring[2]	62	100%	98%	97%
Venous Thromboembolism Prophylaxis[2]	330	83%	80%	85%
Warfarin Therapy Discharge Instructions[2]	66	97%	72%	75%
Chest Pain/Possible Heart Attack Care				
Aspirin Given Within 24 Hours of Arrival[3,7]	-	-	97%	96%
Fibrinolytic Meds Within 30 Min. of Arrival[5]	-	-	63%	58%
Average Time to ECG (minutes)[3,7]	-	-	6	7
Average Time to Transfer (minutes)[5]	-	-	61	60
Children's Asthma Care				
Received Home Management Plan of Care	-	-	-	88%
Received Reliever Medication	-	-	-	100%
Received Systemic Corticosteroids	-	-	-	100%
Emergency Department				
Admittance Decision Time (minutes)[2]	282	63	78	98
Head CT Results Within 45 Min. of Arrival[1]	-	-	55%	57%
Patients Who Left ER Before Being Seen	32,797	4%	2%	2%
Time from ER Arrival to Admit. (minutes)[2]	282	246	238	274
Time from ER Arrival to Discharge (minutes)	430	192	126	134
Time in ER Before Being Evaluated (minutes)	444	28	23	26
Time to Pain Meds for Fractures (minutes)	95	69	56	57
Heart Attack Care				
Aspirin Given at Discharge	627	100%	99%	99%
Fibrinolytic Meds Within 30 Min. of Arrival[7]	-	-	-	54%
PCI Within 90 Minutes of Arrival	72	99%	97%	96%
Statin Prescribed at Discharge	613	100%	97%	98%
Heart Failure Care				
ACE Inhibitor or ARB for LVSD	116	98%	95%	97%
Discharge Instructions Given	339	96%	92%	94%
Evaluation of LVS Function	410	100%	98%	99%
Medicare Spending				
Medicare Spending per Patient (ratio)	-	1.03	0.97	0.98
Pneumonia Care				
Appropriate Initial Antibiotic Given	171	99%	94%	95%
Blood Culture Timing	266	100%	98%	98%
Pregnancy and Delivery Care				
Newborn Deliveries Scheduled Early[2]	86	1%	9%	6%
Preventive Care				
Immunization for Influenza[2]	499	97%	92%	90%
Immunization for Pneumonia[2]	583	96%	94%	92%
Stroke Care				
Anticoagulation Therapy for Atrial Fibrillation	49	96%	95%	95%
Antithrombotic Therapy Timing	252	99%	97%	98%
Assessed for Rehabilitation	332	97%	97%	97%
Discharged on Antithrombotic Therapy	299	100%	98%	99%
Discharged on Statin Medication	238	99%	93%	94%
Thrombolytic Therapy Timing	22	91%	59%	66%
Venous Thromboembolism Prophylaxis	330	93%	93%	94%
Written Stroke Educational Materials Given	199	92%	86%	88%
Surgical Care Improvement Project				
Appropriate Beta Blocker Usage	692	99%	98%	98%
Appropriate VTP Within 24 Hours	1,274	100%	98%	98%
Controlled Postoperative Blood Glucose	411	96%	96%	97%
Perioperative Temperature Management	1,540	100%	100%	100%
Prophylactic Antibiotic Selection	1,266	100%	99%	99%
Prophylactic Antibiotic Selection (Outpatient)	1,872	99%	97%	98%
Prophylactic Antibiotic Stopped	1,230	99%	98%	98%
Prophylactic Antibiotic Timing	1,268	99%	99%	99%
Prophylactic Antibiotic Timing (Outpatient)	1,872	100%	97%	98%
Urinary Catheter Removal	900	99%	97%	97%
Survey of Patients' Hospital Experiences				
Area Around Room 'Always' Quiet at Night	300+	56%	64%	61%
Doctors 'Always' Communicated Well	300+	82%	84%	82%
Home Recovery Information Given	300+	89%	86%	85%
Hospital Given 9 or 10 on 10 Point Scale	300+	76%	72%	71%
Meds 'Always' Explained Before Given	300+	65%	66%	64%
Nurses 'Always' Communicated Well	300+	83%	81%	79%
Pain 'Always' Well Controlled	300+	75%	73%	71%
Room and Bathroom 'Always' Clean	300+	77%	75%	73%
Timely Help 'Always' Received	300+	67%	69%	68%
Would Definitely Recommend Hospital	300+	82%	71%	71%
Use of Medical Imaging				
Cardiac Imaging Stress Test before Surgery	929	5.6%	5.3%	5.3%
Combination Abdominal CT Scan	1,694	4.4%	10.7%	10.5%
Combination Brain/Sinus CT Scan	956	2.8%	3.1%	2.7%
Combination Chest CT Scan	1,416	1.1%	4.3%	2.7%
Follow-up Mammogram/Ultrasound	3,423	10.0%	8.3%	8.8%
Lumbar Spine MRI for Low Back Pain	218	36.7%	38.9%	37.2%

Lexington VA Medical Center

1101 Veterans Drive
Lexington, KY 40502
Phone: 859-233-4511
Fax: 859-281-4911
URL: www.lexington.va.gov
Type: Acute Care - VA
Emergency Services: No
Ownership: Government Federal
Beds: 99

Key Personnel:
Quality Assurance . . . . Linda Cranfill
Ambulatory Care . . . . James Flueck, MD
Chief of Medical Staff. . . . . Emma Metcalf, MD
Anesthesiology. . . . . Daniel Reese, MD
Patient Relations . . . . Melinda Washburn, RN, MSN

Measure	Cases	This Hosp.	State Avg.	U.S. Avg.
Blood Clot Prevention and Treatment				
Anticoagulation Overlap Therapy	-	-	90%	93%
ICU Venous Thromboembolism Prophylaxis	-	-	86%	92%
Incidence of Potentially Preventable VTE	-	-	13%	10%
UFH with Dosages/Platelet Monitoring	-	-	98%	97%
Venous Thromboembolism Prophylaxis	-	-	80%	85%
Warfarin Therapy Discharge Instructions	-	-	72%	75%
Chest Pain/Possible Heart Attack Care				
Aspirin Given Within 24 Hours of Arrival	-	-	97%	96%
Fibrinolytic Meds Within 30 Min. of Arrival	-	-	63%	58%
Average Time to ECG (minutes)	-	-	6	7
Average Time to Transfer (minutes)	-	-	61	60
Children's Asthma Care				
Received Home Management Plan of Care	-	-	-	88%
Received Reliever Medication	-	-	-	100%
Received Systemic Corticosteroids	-	-	-	100%
Emergency Department				
Admittance Decision Time (minutes)	-	-	78	98
Head CT Results Within 45 Min. of Arrival	-	-	55%	57%
Patients Who Left ER Before Being Seen	-	-	2%	2%
Time from ER Arrival to Admit. (minutes)	-	-	238	274
Time from ER Arrival to Discharge (minutes)	-	-	126	134
Time in ER Before Being Evaluated (minutes)	-	-	23	26
Time to Pain Meds for Fractures (minutes)	-	-	56	57
Heart Attack Care				
Aspirin Given at Discharge	74	100%	99%	99%
Fibrinolytic Meds Within 30 Min. of Arrival[5]	-	-	-	54%
PCI Within 90 Minutes of Arrival[1]	-	-	97%	96%
Statin Prescribed at Discharge	76	96%	97%	98%
Heart Failure Care				
ACE Inhibitor or ARB for LVSD	65	95%	95%	97%
Discharge Instructions Given	196	99%	92%	94%
Evaluation of LVS Function	216	100%	98%	99%
Medicare Spending				
Medicare Spending per Patient (ratio)	-	-	0.97	0.98
Pneumonia Care				
Appropriate Initial Antibiotic Given	67	93%	94%	95%
Blood Culture Timing	206	97%	98%	98%
Pregnancy and Delivery Care				
Newborn Deliveries Scheduled Early	-	-	9%	6%
Preventive Care				
Immunization for Influenza[5]	-	-	92%	90%
Immunization for Pneumonia[5]	-	-	94%	92%
Stroke Care				
Anticoagulation Therapy for Atrial Fibrillation	-	-	95%	95%
Antithrombotic Therapy Timing	-	-	97%	98%
Assessed for Rehabilitation	-	-	97%	97%
Discharged on Antithrombotic Therapy	-	-	98%	99%
Discharged on Statin Medication	-	-	93%	94%
Thrombolytic Therapy Timing	-	-	59%	66%
Venous Thromboembolism Prophylaxis	-	-	93%	94%
Written Stroke Educational Materials Given	-	-	86%	88%
Surgical Care Improvement Project				
Appropriate Beta Blocker Usage[2]	93	94%	98%	98%
Appropriate VTP Within 24 Hours[2]	202	99%	98%	98%
Controlled Postoperative Blood Glucose[5]	-	-	96%	97%
Perioperative Temperature Management[2]	233	98%	100%	100%
Prophylactic Antibiotic Selection	126	99%	99%	99%
Prophylactic Antibiotic Selection (Outpatient)	-	-	97%	98%
Prophylactic Antibiotic Stopped	124	98%	98%	98%
Prophylactic Antibiotic Timing	126	99%	99%	99%
Prophylactic Antibiotic Timing (Outpatient)	-	-	97%	98%
Urinary Catheter Removal[2]	49	94%	97%	97%
Survey of Patients' Hospital Experiences				
Area Around Room 'Always' Quiet at Night	-	-	64%	61%
Doctors 'Always' Communicated Well	-	-	84%	82%
Home Recovery Information Given	-	-	86%	85%
Hospital Given 9 or 10 on 10 Point Scale	-	-	72%	71%
Meds 'Always' Explained Before Given	-	-	66%	64%
Nurses 'Always' Communicated Well	-	-	81%	79%
Pain 'Always' Well Controlled	-	-	73%	71%
Room and Bathroom 'Always' Clean	-	-	75%	73%
Timely Help 'Always' Received	-	-	69%	68%
Would Definitely Recommend Hospital	-	-	71%	71%

NOTE: Hospital profiles are in alphabetical order by state, then city, then hospital within the city; Rankings exclude hospitals with less than 25 cases except for patient surveys which excludes hospitals with less than 100 cases; (a) 100-299 cases; (1) The number of cases/patients is too few to report; (2) Data submitted were based on a sample of cases/patients; (3) Results are based on a shorter time period than required; (4) Data suppressed by CMS for one or more quarters; (5) Results are not available for this reporting period; (6) Fewer than 100 patients completed the HCAHPS survey; (7) No cases met the criteria for this measure; (8) The lower limit of the confidence interval cannot be calculated if the number of observed infections equals zero; (9) No data are available from the state/territory for this reporting period; (10) The scores shown reflect fewer than 50 completed surveys; (11) There were discrepancies in the data collection process; (12) This measure does not apply to this hospital for this reporting period; (13) Results cannot be calculated for this reporting period; (14) The results for this state are combined with nearby states to protect confidentiality; Please refer to the User's Guide for a full explanation of data.

Measure	Cases	This Hosp.	State Avg.	U.S. Avg.
Use of Medical Imaging				
Cardiac Imaging Stress Test before Surgery	-	-	5.3%	5.3%
Combination Abdominal CT Scan	-	-	10.7%	10.5%
Combination Brain/Sinus CT Scan	-	-	3.1%	2.7%
Combination Chest CT Scan	-	-	4.3%	2.7%
Follow-up Mammogram/Ultrasound	-	-	8.3%	8.8%
Lumbar Spine MRI for Low Back Pain	-	-	38.9%	37.2%

Saint Joseph East

150 North Eagle Creek Drive
Lexington, KY 40509
URL: www.sjhlex.org
Phone: 859-967-5000
Fax: 859-967-5766
Type: Acute Care Hospitals
Emergency Services: Yes
Ownership: Voluntary non-profit - Church
Beds: 174

Key Personnel:
CEO/President. . . . . Gene Woods

Measure	Cases	This Hosp.	State Avg.	U.S. Avg.
Blood Clot Prevention and Treatment				
Anticoagulation Overlap Therapy[2]	27	96%	90%	93%
ICU Venous Thromboembolism Prophylaxis[2]	74	85%	86%	92%
Incidence of Potentially Preventable VTE[1,2]	-	-	13%	10%
UFH with Dosages/Platelet Monitoring[2]	28	93%	98%	97%
Venous Thromboembolism Prophylaxis[2]	349	74%	80%	85%
Warfarin Therapy Discharge Instructions[2]	23	22%	72%	75%
Chest Pain/Possible Heart Attack Care				
Aspirin Given Within 24 Hours of Arrival[1,3]	-	-	97%	96%
Fibrinolytic Meds Within 30 Min. of Arrival[5]	-	-	63%	58%
Average Time to ECG (minutes)[1,3]	-	-	6	7
Average Time to Transfer (minutes)[5]	-	-	61	60
Children's Asthma Care				
Received Home Management Plan of Care	-	-	-	88%
Received Reliever Medication	-	-	-	100%
Received Systemic Corticosteroids	-	-	-	100%
Emergency Department				
Admittance Decision Time (minutes)[2]	269	110	78	98
Head CT Results Within 45 Min. of Arrival[1]	-	-	55%	57%
Patients Who Left ER Before Being Seen	38,568	1%	2%	2%
Time from ER Arrival to Admit. (minutes)[2]	281	292	238	274
Time from ER Arrival to Discharge (minutes)	374	134	126	134
Time in ER Before Being Evaluated (minutes)	383	28	23	26
Time to Pain Meds for Fractures (minutes)	136	55	56	57
Heart Attack Care				
Aspirin Given at Discharge	134	100%	99%	99%
Fibrinolytic Meds Within 30 Min. of Arrival[7]	-	-	-	54%
PCI Within 90 Minutes of Arrival	18	67%	97%	96%
Statin Prescribed at Discharge	135	99%	97%	98%
Heart Failure Care				
ACE Inhibitor or ARB for LVSD	44	98%	95%	97%
Discharge Instructions Given	114	81%	92%	94%
Evaluation of LVS Function	140	100%	98%	99%
Medicare Spending				
Medicare Spending per Patient (ratio)	-	0.97	0.97	0.98
Pneumonia Care				
Appropriate Initial Antibiotic Given	96	96%	94%	95%
Blood Culture Timing	133	100%	98%	98%
Pregnancy and Delivery Care				
Newborn Deliveries Scheduled Early[2]	50	6%	9%	6%
Preventive Care				
Immunization for Influenza[2]	498	95%	92%	90%
Immunization for Pneumonia[2]	422	92%	94%	92%
Stroke Care				
Anticoagulation Therapy for Atrial Fibrillation[1,2]	-	-	95%	95%
Antithrombotic Therapy Timing[2]	17	100%	97%	98%
Assessed for Rehabilitation[2]	22	95%	97%	97%
Discharged on Antithrombotic Therapy[2]	22	100%	98%	99%
Discharged on Statin Medication[2]	15	93%	93%	94%
Thrombolytic Therapy Timing[2,7]	-	-	59%	66%
Venous Thromboembolism Prophylaxis[2]	17	76%	93%	94%
Written Stroke Educational Materials Given[2]	20	15%	86%	88%
Surgical Care Improvement Project				
Appropriate Beta Blocker Usage	216	97%	98%	98%
Appropriate VTP Within 24 Hours	637	96%	98%	98%
Controlled Postoperative Blood Glucose[7]	-	-	96%	97%
Perioperative Temperature Management	733	100%	100%	100%
Prophylactic Antibiotic Selection	525	100%	99%	99%
Prophylactic Antibiotic Selection (Outpatient)	421	97%	97%	98%
Prophylactic Antibiotic Stopped	521	99%	98%	98%
Prophylactic Antibiotic Timing	525	100%	99%	99%
Prophylactic Antibiotic Timing (Outpatient)	421	100%	97%	98%
Urinary Catheter Removal	351	96%	97%	97%
Survey of Patients' Hospital Experiences				
Area Around Room 'Always' Quiet at Night	300+	65%	64%	61%
Doctors 'Always' Communicated Well	300+	80%	84%	82%
Home Recovery Information Given	300+	88%	86%	85%
Hospital Given 9 or 10 on 10 Point Scale	300+	71%	72%	71%
Meds 'Always' Explained Before Given	300+	62%	66%	64%
Nurses 'Always' Communicated Well	300+	78%	81%	79%
Pain 'Always' Well Controlled	300+	68%	73%	71%
Room and Bathroom 'Always' Clean	300+	63%	75%	73%
Timely Help 'Always' Received	300+	61%	69%	68%
Would Definitely Recommend Hospital	300+	75%	71%	71%
Use of Medical Imaging				
Cardiac Imaging Stress Test before Surgery	70	2.9%	5.3%	5.3%
Combination Abdominal CT Scan	412	2.7%	10.7%	10.5%
Combination Brain/Sinus CT Scan	324	8.3%	3.1%	2.7%
Combination Chest CT Scan	94	4.3%	4.3%	2.7%
Follow-up Mammogram/Ultrasound	1,280	5.9%	8.3%	8.8%
Lumbar Spine MRI for Low Back Pain[1]	-	-	38.9%	37.2%

Saint Joseph Hospital

One Saint Joseph Drive
Lexington, KY 40504
URL: www.sjhlex.org
Phone: 859-313-1000
Fax: 859-260-6117
Type: Acute Care Hospitals
Emergency Services: Yes
Ownership: Voluntary non-profit - Church
Beds: 468

Key Personnel:
Operating Room. . . . . Judy Behnhardy
Anesthesiology. . . . . Wayne Graff, MD
Chief of Medical Staff . . . . Dennis B Kelly, MD
Emergency Room . . . . Barry Parsley, MD
Radiology. . . . . Chris Riley, MD
Quality Assurance . . . . Cherri Tichenor
Pediatric Ambulatory Care . . . . . Walter Yates, MD
Pediatric In-Patient Care . . . . Walter Yates, MD

Measure	Cases	This Hosp.	State Avg.	U.S. Avg.
Blood Clot Prevention and Treatment				
Anticoagulation Overlap Therapy[2]	127	98%	90%	93%
ICU Venous Thromboembolism Prophylaxis[2]	128	72%	86%	92%
Incidence of Potentially Preventable VTE[2]	22	9%	13%	10%
UFH with Dosages/Platelet Monitoring[2]	60	100%	98%	97%
Venous Thromboembolism Prophylaxis[2]	413	67%	80%	85%
Warfarin Therapy Discharge Instructions[2]	89	17%	72%	75%
Chest Pain/Possible Heart Attack Care				
Aspirin Given Within 24 Hours of Arrival	14	93%	97%	96%
Fibrinolytic Meds Within 30 Min. of Arrival[3,7]	-	-	63%	58%
Average Time to ECG (minutes)	14	10	6	7
Average Time to Transfer (minutes)[1,3]	-	-	61	60
Children's Asthma Care				
Received Home Management Plan of Care	-	-	-	88%
Received Reliever Medication	-	-	-	100%
Received Systemic Corticosteroids	-	-	-	100%
Emergency Department				
Admittance Decision Time (minutes)[2]	525	153	78	98
Head CT Results Within 45 Min. of Arrival[1]	-	-	55%	57%
Patients Who Left ER Before Being Seen	42,286	2%	2%	2%
Time from ER Arrival to Admit. (minutes)[2]	544	360	238	274
Time from ER Arrival to Discharge (minutes)	368	154	126	134
Time in ER Before Being Evaluated (minutes)	384	34	23	26
Time to Pain Meds for Fractures (minutes)	173	54	56	57
Heart Attack Care				
Aspirin Given at Discharge[2]	354	100%	99%	99%
Fibrinolytic Meds Within 30 Min. of Arrival[2,7]	-	-	-	54%
PCI Within 90 Minutes of Arrival[2]	27	100%	97%	96%
Statin Prescribed at Discharge[2]	344	100%	97%	98%
Heart Failure Care				
ACE Inhibitor or ARB for LVSD[2]	89	97%	95%	97%
Discharge Instructions Given[2]	276	71%	92%	94%
Evaluation of LVS Function[2]	338	100%	98%	99%
Medicare Spending				
Medicare Spending per Patient (ratio)	-	0.97	0.97	0.98
Pneumonia Care				
Appropriate Initial Antibiotic Given[2]	102	95%	94%	95%
Blood Culture Timing[2]	140	99%	98%	98%
Pregnancy and Delivery Care				
Newborn Deliveries Scheduled Early[2,7]	-	-	9%	6%
Preventive Care				
Immunization for Influenza[2]	606	94%	92%	90%
Immunization for Pneumonia[2]	929	94%	94%	92%
Stroke Care				
Anticoagulation Therapy for Atrial Fibrillation[1,2]	-	-	95%	95%
Antithrombotic Therapy Timing[2]	103	99%	97%	98%
Assessed for Rehabilitation[2]	120	93%	97%	97%
Discharged on Antithrombotic Therapy[2]	109	99%	98%	99%
Discharged on Statin Medication[2]	88	93%	93%	94%
Thrombolytic Therapy Timing[1,2]	-	-	59%	66%
Venous Thromboembolism Prophylaxis[2]	119	82%	93%	94%
Written Stroke Educational Materials Given[2]	73	22%	86%	88%
Surgical Care Improvement Project				
Appropriate Beta Blocker Usage[2]	367	96%	98%	98%
Appropriate VTP Within 24 Hours[2]	423	96%	98%	98%
Controlled Postoperative Blood Glucose[2]	236	97%	96%	97%
Perioperative Temperature Management[2]	643	100%	100%	100%
Prophylactic Antibiotic Selection[2]	515	98%	99%	99%
Prophylactic Antibiotic Selection (Outpatient)	800	98%	97%	98%
Prophylactic Antibiotic Stopped[2]	490	98%	98%	98%
Prophylactic Antibiotic Timing[2]	515	99%	99%	99%
Prophylactic Antibiotic Timing (Outpatient)	812	97%	97%	98%
Urinary Catheter Removal[2]	466	88%	97%	97%
Survey of Patients' Hospital Experiences				
Area Around Room 'Always' Quiet at Night	300+	61%	64%	61%
Doctors 'Always' Communicated Well	300+	79%	84%	82%
Home Recovery Information Given	300+	87%	86%	85%
Hospital Given 9 or 10 on 10 Point Scale	300+	70%	72%	71%
Meds 'Always' Explained Before Given	300+	62%	66%	64%
Nurses 'Always' Communicated Well	300+	77%	81%	79%
Pain 'Always' Well Controlled	300+	70%	73%	71%
Room and Bathroom 'Always' Clean	300+	68%	75%	73%
Timely Help 'Always' Received	300+	62%	69%	68%
Would Definitely Recommend Hospital	300+	74%	71%	71%
Use of Medical Imaging				
Cardiac Imaging Stress Test before Surgery	904	4.0%	5.3%	5.3%
Combination Abdominal CT Scan	771	3.2%	10.7%	10.5%
Combination Brain/Sinus CT Scan	1,021	3.6%	3.1%	2.7%
Combination Chest CT Scan	172	3.5%	4.3%	2.7%
Follow-up Mammogram/Ultrasound	844	2.3%	8.3%	8.8%
Lumbar Spine MRI for Low Back Pain	62	43.5%	38.9%	37.2%

University of Kentucky Hospital

800 Rose Street
Lexington, KY 40536
URL: www.uhealthcare.uky.edu
Phone: 859-323-5000
Fax: 859-323-2044
Type: Acute Care Hospitals
Emergency Services: Yes
Ownership: Government - State
Beds: 473

Key Personnel:
Quality Assurance . . . . Jennifer Blakeley
Infection Control. . . . . Martin Evans, MD
Radiology. . . . . Todd Hickey
Chief of Medical Staff . . . . Courtney Higdon
Pediatric In-Patient Care . . . . Sherry Holmes, RN
Operating Room. . . . . Patricia Seabolt, RN
Coronary Care . . . . Ann Wiard, RN

Measure	Cases	This Hosp.	State Avg.	U.S. Avg.
Blood Clot Prevention and Treatment				
Anticoagulation Overlap Therapy[2]	166	99%	90%	93%
ICU Venous Thromboembolism Prophylaxis[2]	103	95%	86%	92%
Incidence of Potentially Preventable VTE[2]	78	3%	13%	10%
UFH with Dosages/Platelet Monitoring[2]	124	100%	98%	97%
Venous Thromboembolism Prophylaxis[2]	279	87%	80%	85%
Warfarin Therapy Discharge Instructions[2]	126	90%	72%	75%
Chest Pain/Possible Heart Attack Care				
Aspirin Given Within 24 Hours of Arrival[5]	-	-	97%	96%

NOTE: Hospital profiles are in alphabetical order by state, then city, then hospital within the city; Rankings exclude hospitals with less than 25 cases except for patient surveys which excludes hospitals with less than 100 cases; (a) 100-299 cases; (1) The number of cases/patients is too few to report; (2) Data submitted were based on a sample of cases/patients; (3) Results are based on a shorter time period than required; (4) Data suppressed by CMS for one or more quarters; (5) Results are not available for this reporting period; (6) Fewer than 100 patients completed the HCAHPS survey; (7) No cases met the criteria for this measure; (8) The lower limit of the confidence interval cannot be calculated if the number of observed infections equals zero; (9) No data are available from the state/territory for this reporting period; (10) The scores shown reflect fewer than 50 completed surveys; (11) There were discrepancies in the data collection process; (12) This measure does not apply to this hospital for this reporting period; (13) Results cannot be calculated for this reporting period; (14) The results for this state are combined with nearby states to protect confidentiality; Please refer to the User's Guide for a full explanation of data.

Measure	Cases	This Hosp.	State Avg.	U.S. Avg.
Fibrinolytic Meds Within 30 Min. of Arrival[5]	-	-	63%	58%
Average Time to ECG (minutes)[5]	-	-	6	7
Average Time to Transfer (minutes)[5]	-	-	61	60
Children's Asthma Care				
Received Home Management Plan of Care	131	98%	-	88%
Received Reliever Medication	131	100%	-	100%
Received Systemic Corticosteroids	127	100%	-	100%
Emergency Department				
Admittance Decision Time (minutes)[2]	426	200	78	98
Head CT Results Within 45 Min. of Arrival[1]	-	-	55%	57%
Patients Who Left ER Before Being Seen	91,208	2%	2%	2%
Time from ER Arrival to Admit. (minutes)[2]	435	444	238	274
Time from ER Arrival to Discharge (minutes)	349	200	126	134
Time in ER Before Being Evaluated (minutes)	369	27	23	26
Time to Pain Meds for Fractures (minutes)	356	74	56	57
Heart Attack Care				
Aspirin Given at Discharge	355	100%	99%	99%
Fibrinolytic Meds Within 30 Min. of Arrival[7]	-	-	-	54%
PCI Within 90 Minutes of Arrival	41	93%	97%	96%
Statin Prescribed at Discharge	325	100%	97%	98%
Heart Failure Care				
ACE Inhibitor or ARB for LVSD	211	100%	95%	97%
Discharge Instructions Given	418	100%	92%	94%
Evaluation of LVS Function	479	100%	98%	99%
Medicare Spending				
Medicare Spending per Patient (ratio)	-	1.00	0.97	0.98
Pneumonia Care				
Appropriate Initial Antibiotic Given	135	100%	94%	95%
Blood Culture Timing	354	99%	98%	98%
Pregnancy and Delivery Care				
Newborn Deliveries Scheduled Early[2]	24	0%	9%	6%
Preventive Care				
Immunization for Influenza[2]	523	98%	92%	90%
Immunization for Pneumonia[2]	483	87%	94%	92%
Stroke Care				
Anticoagulation Therapy for Atrial Fibrillation	70	100%	95%	95%
Antithrombotic Therapy Timing	391	99%	97%	98%
Assessed for Rehabilitation	627	100%	97%	97%
Discharged on Antithrombotic Therapy	507	100%	98%	99%
Discharged on Statin Medication	352	100%	93%	94%
Thrombolytic Therapy Timing	28	100%	59%	66%
Venous Thromboembolism Prophylaxis	590	99%	93%	94%
Written Stroke Educational Materials Given	348	99%	86%	88%
Surgical Care Improvement Project				
Appropriate Beta Blocker Usage[2]	233	100%	98%	98%
Appropriate VTP Within 24 Hours[2]	405	100%	98%	98%
Controlled Postoperative Blood Glucose[2]	115	96%	96%	97%
Perioperative Temperature Management[2]	541	100%	100%	100%
Prophylactic Antibiotic Selection[2]	424	99%	99%	99%
Prophylactic Antibiotic Selection (Outpatient)	611	95%	97%	98%
Prophylactic Antibiotic Stopped[2]	411	98%	98%	98%
Prophylactic Antibiotic Timing[2]	426	100%	99%	99%
Prophylactic Antibiotic Timing (Outpatient)	644	93%	97%	98%
Urinary Catheter Removal[2]	262	100%	97%	97%
Survey of Patients' Hospital Experiences				
Area Around Room 'Always' Quiet at Night	300+	62%	64%	61%
Doctors 'Always' Communicated Well	300+	79%	84%	82%
Home Recovery Information Given	300+	86%	86%	85%
Hospital Given 9 or 10 on 10 Point Scale	300+	72%	72%	71%
Meds 'Always' Explained Before Given	300+	65%	66%	64%
Nurses 'Always' Communicated Well	300+	81%	81%	79%
Pain 'Always' Well Controlled	300+	72%	73%	71%
Room and Bathroom 'Always' Clean	300+	74%	75%	73%
Timely Help 'Always' Received	300+	71%	69%	68%
Would Definitely Recommend Hospital	300+	77%	71%	71%
Use of Medical Imaging				
Cardiac Imaging Stress Test before Surgery	363	7.7%	5.3%	5.3%
Combination Abdominal CT Scan	1,972	3.0%	10.7%	10.5%
Combination Brain/Sinus CT Scan	854	5.3%	3.1%	2.7%
Combination Chest CT Scan	2,354	0.0%	4.3%	2.7%
Follow-up Mammogram/Ultrasound	345	10.7%	8.3%	8.8%
Lumbar Spine MRI for Low Back Pain	101	38.6%	38.9%	37.2%

Casey County Hospital

187 Wolford Avenue — Phone: 606-787-6275
Liberty, KY 42539 — Fax: 606-787-9717
Type: Critical Access Hospitals — Emergency Services: Yes
Ownership: Govt - Hospital Dist/Auth — Beds: 24
Key Personnel:
Emergency Room . . . . Linda Mackey
CEO/President. . . . . Rusty Tungate

Measure	Cases	This Hosp.	State Avg.	U.S. Avg.
Blood Clot Prevention and Treatment				
Anticoagulation Overlap Therapy[5]	-	-	90%	93%
ICU Venous Thromboembolism Prophylaxis[5]	-	-	86%	92%
Incidence of Potentially Preventable VTE[5]	-	-	13%	10%
UFH with Dosages/Platelet Monitoring[5]	-	-	98%	97%
Venous Thromboembolism Prophylaxis[5]	-	-	80%	85%
Warfarin Therapy Discharge Instructions[5]	-	-	72%	75%
Chest Pain/Possible Heart Attack Care				
Aspirin Given Within 24 Hours of Arrival	44	84%	97%	96%
Fibrinolytic Meds Within 30 Min. of Arrival[1]	-	-	63%	58%
Average Time to ECG (minutes)	47	8	6	7
Average Time to Transfer (minutes)[1]	-	-	61	60
Children's Asthma Care				
Received Home Management Plan of Care	-	-	-	88%
Received Reliever Medication	-	-	-	100%
Received Systemic Corticosteroids	-	-	-	100%
Emergency Department				
Admittance Decision Time (minutes)[5]	-	-	78	98
Head CT Results Within 45 Min. of Arrival[5]	-	-	55%	57%
Patients Who Left ER Before Being Seen	6,319	2%	2%	2%
Time from ER Arrival to Admit. (minutes)[5]	-	-	238	274
Time from ER Arrival to Discharge (minutes)[5]	-	-	126	134
Time in ER Before Being Evaluated (minutes)[5]	-	-	23	26
Time to Pain Meds for Fractures (minutes)[5]	-	-	56	57
Heart Attack Care				
Aspirin Given at Discharge[3,7]	-	-	99%	99%
Fibrinolytic Meds Within 30 Min. of Arrival[3,7]	-	-	-	54%
PCI Within 90 Minutes of Arrival[3,7]	-	-	97%	96%
Statin Prescribed at Discharge[3,7]	-	-	97%	98%
Heart Failure Care				
ACE Inhibitor or ARB for LVSD[1]	-	-	95%	97%
Discharge Instructions Given	22	100%	92%	94%
Evaluation of LVS Function	36	11%	98%	99%
Medicare Spending				
Medicare Spending per Patient (ratio)	-	-	0.97	0.98
Pneumonia Care				
Appropriate Initial Antibiotic Given	40	70%	94%	95%
Blood Culture Timing[7]	-	-	98%	98%
Pregnancy and Delivery Care				
Newborn Deliveries Scheduled Early[5]	-	-	9%	6%
Preventive Care				
Immunization for Influenza[5]	-	-	92%	90%
Immunization for Pneumonia[5]	-	-	94%	92%
Stroke Care				
Anticoagulation Therapy for Atrial Fibrillation[5]	-	-	95%	95%
Antithrombotic Therapy Timing[5]	-	-	97%	98%
Assessed for Rehabilitation[5]	-	-	97%	97%
Discharged on Antithrombotic Therapy[5]	-	-	98%	99%
Discharged on Statin Medication[5]	-	-	93%	94%
Thrombolytic Therapy Timing[5]	-	-	59%	66%
Venous Thromboembolism Prophylaxis[5]	-	-	93%	94%
Written Stroke Educational Materials Given[5]	-	-	86%	88%
Surgical Care Improvement Project				
Appropriate Beta Blocker Usage[5]	-	-	98%	98%
Appropriate VTP Within 24 Hours[5]	-	-	98%	98%
Controlled Postoperative Blood Glucose[5]	-	-	96%	97%
Perioperative Temperature Management[5]	-	-	100%	100%
Prophylactic Antibiotic Selection[5]	-	-	99%	99%
Prophylactic Antibiotic Selection (Outpatient)[5]	-	-	97%	98%
Prophylactic Antibiotic Stopped[5]	-	-	98%	98%
Prophylactic Antibiotic Timing[5]	-	-	99%	99%
Prophylactic Antibiotic Timing (Outpatient)[5]	-	-	97%	98%
Urinary Catheter Removal[5]	-	-	97%	97%
Survey of Patients' Hospital Experiences				
Area Around Room 'Always' Quiet at Night	(a)	79%	64%	61%
Doctors 'Always' Communicated Well	(a)	96%	84%	82%
Home Recovery Information Given	(a)	91%	86%	85%
Hospital Given 9 or 10 on 10 Point Scale	(a)	82%	72%	71%
Meds 'Always' Explained Before Given	(a)	61%	66%	64%
Nurses 'Always' Communicated Well	(a)	84%	81%	79%
Pain 'Always' Well Controlled	(a)	76%	73%	71%
Room and Bathroom 'Always' Clean	(a)	85%	75%	73%
Timely Help 'Always' Received	(a)	67%	69%	68%
Would Definitely Recommend Hospital	(a)	79%	71%	71%
Use of Medical Imaging				
Cardiac Imaging Stress Test before Surgery[7]	-	-	5.3%	5.3%
Combination Abdominal CT Scan	182	7.7%	10.7%	10.5%
Combination Brain/Sinus CT Scan[1]	-	-	3.1%	2.7%
Combination Chest CT Scan	83	1.2%	4.3%	2.7%
Follow-up Mammogram/Ultrasound	67	7.5%	8.3%	8.8%
Lumbar Spine MRI for Low Back Pain[7]	-	-	38.9%	37.2%

Saint Joseph London

1001 Saint Joseph Lane — Phone: 606-330-6000
London, KY 40741
URL: www.sjhlex.org
Type: Acute Care Hospitals — Emergency Services: Yes
Ownership: Voluntary non-profit - Private

Measure	Cases	This Hosp.	State Avg.	U.S. Avg.
Blood Clot Prevention and Treatment				
Anticoagulation Overlap Therapy[2]	29	97%	90%	93%
ICU Venous Thromboembolism Prophylaxis[2]	118	98%	86%	92%
Incidence of Potentially Preventable VTE[1,2]	-	-	13%	10%
UFH with Dosages/Platelet Monitoring[2]	17	100%	98%	97%
Venous Thromboembolism Prophylaxis[2]	346	95%	80%	85%
Warfarin Therapy Discharge Instructions[2]	23	91%	72%	75%
Chest Pain/Possible Heart Attack Care				
Aspirin Given Within 24 Hours of Arrival	12	92%	97%	96%
Fibrinolytic Meds Within 30 Min. of Arrival[1,3]	-	-	63%	58%
Average Time to ECG (minutes)	13	6	6	7
Average Time to Transfer (minutes)[1,3]	-	-	61	60
Children's Asthma Care				
Received Home Management Plan of Care	-	-	-	88%
Received Reliever Medication	-	-	-	100%
Received Systemic Corticosteroids	-	-	-	100%
Emergency Department				
Admittance Decision Time (minutes)[2]	489	115	78	98
Head CT Results Within 45 Min. of Arrival	12	67%	55%	57%
Patients Who Left ER Before Being Seen	48,455	1%	2%	2%
Time from ER Arrival to Admit. (minutes)[2]	518	280	238	274
Time from ER Arrival to Discharge (minutes)	361	137	126	134
Time in ER Before Being Evaluated (minutes)	390	22	23	26
Time to Pain Meds for Fractures (minutes)	176	46	56	57
Heart Attack Care				
Aspirin Given at Discharge	345	100%	99%	99%
Fibrinolytic Meds Within 30 Min. of Arrival[7]	-	-	-	54%
PCI Within 90 Minutes of Arrival	38	92%	97%	96%
Statin Prescribed at Discharge	331	100%	97%	98%
Heart Failure Care				
ACE Inhibitor or ARB for LVSD	86	100%	95%	97%
Discharge Instructions Given	270	91%	92%	94%
Evaluation of LVS Function	310	100%	98%	99%
Medicare Spending				
Medicare Spending per Patient (ratio)	-	0.92	0.97	0.98
Pneumonia Care				
Appropriate Initial Antibiotic Given	135	93%	94%	95%
Blood Culture Timing	189	98%	98%	98%
Pregnancy and Delivery Care				
Newborn Deliveries Scheduled Early[2]	12	8%	9%	6%
Preventive Care				
Immunization for Influenza[2]	523	95%	92%	90%
Immunization for Pneumonia[2]	621	98%	94%	92%
Stroke Care				
Anticoagulation Therapy for Atrial Fibrillation[1,2]	-	-	95%	95%
Antithrombotic Therapy Timing[2]	49	98%	97%	98%
Assessed for Rehabilitation[2]	47	98%	97%	97%

NOTE: Hospital profiles are in alphabetical order by state, then city, then hospital within the city; Rankings exclude hospitals with less than 25 cases except for patient surveys which excludes hospitals with less than 100 cases; (a) 100-299 cases; (1) The number of cases/patients is too few to report; (2) Data submitted were based on a sample of cases/patients; (3) Results are based on a shorter time period than required; (4) Data suppressed by CMS for one or more quarters; (5) Results are not available for this reporting period; (6) Fewer than 100 patients completed the HCAHPS survey; (7) No cases met the criteria for this measure; (8) The lower limit of the confidence interval cannot be calculated if the number of observed infections equals zero; (9) No data are available from the state/territory for this reporting period; (10) The scores shown reflect fewer than 50 completed surveys; (11) There were discrepancies in the data collection process; (12) This measure does not apply to this hospital for this reporting period; (13) Results cannot be calculated for this reporting period; (14) The results for this state are combined with nearby states to protect confidentiality; Please refer to the User's Guide for a full explanation of data.

Measure	Cases	This Hosp.	State Avg.	U.S. Avg.
Discharged on Antithrombotic Therapy[2]	47	100%	98%	99%
Discharged on Statin Medication[2]	37	100%	93%	94%
Thrombolytic Therapy Timing[1,2]	-	-	59%	66%
Venous Thromboembolism Prophylaxis[2]	45	98%	93%	94%
Written Stroke Educational Materials Given[2]	33	76%	86%	88%
Surgical Care Improvement Project				
Appropriate Beta Blocker Usage	161	99%	98%	98%
Appropriate VTP Within 24 Hours	270	98%	98%	98%
Controlled Postoperative Blood Glucose	52	96%	96%	97%
Perioperative Temperature Management	317	100%	100%	100%
Prophylactic Antibiotic Selection	271	99%	99%	99%
Prophylactic Antibiotic Selection (Outpatient)	234	98%	97%	98%
Prophylactic Antibiotic Stopped	251	98%	98%	98%
Prophylactic Antibiotic Timing	272	100%	99%	99%
Prophylactic Antibiotic Timing (Outpatient)	234	100%	97%	98%
Urinary Catheter Removal	252	98%	97%	97%
Survey of Patients' Hospital Experiences				
Area Around Room 'Always' Quiet at Night	300+	68%	64%	61%
Doctors 'Always' Communicated Well	300+	83%	84%	82%
Home Recovery Information Given	300+	85%	86%	85%
Hospital Given 9 or 10 on 10 Point Scale	300+	78%	72%	71%
Meds 'Always' Explained Before Given	300+	67%	66%	64%
Nurses 'Always' Communicated Well	300+	82%	81%	79%
Pain 'Always' Well Controlled	300+	75%	73%	71%
Room and Bathroom 'Always' Clean	300+	76%	75%	73%
Timely Help 'Always' Received	300+	75%	69%	68%
Would Definitely Recommend Hospital	300+	79%	71%	71%
Use of Medical Imaging				
Cardiac Imaging Stress Test before Surgery	1,107	4.2%	5.3%	5.3%
Combination Abdominal CT Scan	1,041	5.6%	10.7%	10.5%
Combination Brain/Sinus CT Scan	919	1.4%	3.1%	2.7%
Combination Chest CT Scan	510	6.3%	4.3%	2.7%
Follow-up Mammogram/Ultrasound	509	13.8%	8.3%	8.8%
Lumbar Spine MRI for Low Back Pain	76	31.6%	38.9%	37.2%

Three Rivers Medical Center

2485 Highway 644
Louisa, KY 41230
Phone: 606-638-9451
Fax: 606-638-9494
URL: www.threeriversmedicalcenter.com
Type: Acute Care Hospitals
Ownership: Proprietary
Emergency Services: Yes
Beds: 90

Key Personnel:
Radiology. . . . . Paul V Akers
Chief of Medical Staff. . . . . Lee Balaklaw
Cardiac Laboratory. . . . . Joe Bevans
CEO/President. . . . . Greg Kiser
Emergency Room . . . . Dian Ratcliff
Operating Room. . . . . Barbara Robinson, MD
Quality Assurance . . . . Betty Slone

Measure	Cases	This Hosp.	State Avg.	U.S. Avg.
Blood Clot Prevention and Treatment				
Anticoagulation Overlap Therapy[2]	16	100%	90%	93%
ICU Venous Thromboembolism Prophylaxis[2]	78	100%	86%	92%
Incidence of Potentially Preventable VTE[2,7]	-	-	13%	10%
UFH with Dosages/Platelet Monitoring[2,7]	-	-	98%	97%
Venous Thromboembolism Prophylaxis[2]	234	98%	80%	85%
Warfarin Therapy Discharge Instructions[2]	16	100%	72%	75%
Chest Pain/Possible Heart Attack Care				
Aspirin Given Within 24 Hours of Arrival	75	100%	97%	96%
Fibrinolytic Meds Within 30 Min. of Arrival[1]	-	-	63%	58%
Average Time to ECG (minutes)	78	3	6	7
Average Time to Transfer (minutes)	25	40	61	60
Children's Asthma Care				
Received Home Management Plan of Care	-	-	-	88%
Received Reliever Medication	-	-	-	100%
Received Systemic Corticosteroids	-	-	-	100%
Emergency Department				
Admittance Decision Time (minutes)[2]	471	89	78	98
Head CT Results Within 45 Min. of Arrival[1]	-	-	55%	57%
Patients Who Left ER Before Being Seen	18,313	0%	2%	2%
Time from ER Arrival to Admit. (minutes)[2]	471	235	238	274
Time from ER Arrival to Discharge (minutes)	397	124	126	134
Time in ER Before Being Evaluated (minutes)	421	18	23	26
Time to Pain Meds for Fractures (minutes)	74	66	56	57
Heart Attack Care				
Aspirin Given at Discharge[1]	-	-	99%	99%
Fibrinolytic Meds Within 30 Min. of Arrival[7]	-	-	-	54%
PCI Within 90 Minutes of Arrival[7]	-	-	97%	96%
Statin Prescribed at Discharge[1]	-	-	97%	98%
Heart Failure Care				
ACE Inhibitor or ARB for LVSD	18	100%	95%	97%
Discharge Instructions Given	91	100%	92%	94%
Evaluation of LVS Function	103	100%	98%	99%
Medicare Spending				
Medicare Spending per Patient (ratio)	-	0.89	0.97	0.98
Pneumonia Care				
Appropriate Initial Antibiotic Given	72	100%	94%	95%
Blood Culture Timing	103	100%	98%	98%
Pregnancy and Delivery Care				
Newborn Deliveries Scheduled Early[1,2]	-	-	9%	6%
Preventive Care				
Immunization for Influenza[2]	310	99%	92%	90%
Immunization for Pneumonia[2]	380	99%	94%	92%
Stroke Care				
Anticoagulation Therapy for Atrial Fibrillation[1]	-	-	95%	95%
Antithrombotic Therapy Timing	13	92%	97%	98%
Assessed for Rehabilitation[1]	-	-	97%	97%
Discharged on Antithrombotic Therapy[1]	-	-	98%	99%
Discharged on Statin Medication[1]	-	-	93%	94%
Thrombolytic Therapy Timing[1]	-	-	59%	66%
Venous Thromboembolism Prophylaxis	12	92%	93%	94%
Written Stroke Educational Materials Given[1]	-	-	86%	88%
Surgical Care Improvement Project				
Appropriate Beta Blocker Usage[1]	-	-	98%	98%
Appropriate VTP Within 24 Hours	29	100%	98%	98%
Controlled Postoperative Blood Glucose[7]	-	-	96%	97%
Perioperative Temperature Management	35	100%	100%	100%
Prophylactic Antibiotic Selection	22	91%	99%	99%
Prophylactic Antibiotic Selection (Outpatient)	33	97%	97%	98%
Prophylactic Antibiotic Stopped	21	100%	98%	98%
Prophylactic Antibiotic Timing	22	100%	99%	99%
Prophylactic Antibiotic Timing (Outpatient)	30	97%	97%	98%
Urinary Catheter Removal[1]	-	-	97%	97%
Survey of Patients' Hospital Experiences				
Area Around Room 'Always' Quiet at Night	300+	68%	64%	61%
Doctors 'Always' Communicated Well	300+	87%	84%	82%
Home Recovery Information Given	300+	87%	86%	85%
Hospital Given 9 or 10 on 10 Point Scale	300+	68%	72%	71%
Meds 'Always' Explained Before Given	300+	69%	66%	64%
Nurses 'Always' Communicated Well	300+	81%	81%	79%
Pain 'Always' Well Controlled	300+	73%	73%	71%
Room and Bathroom 'Always' Clean	300+	82%	75%	73%
Timely Help 'Always' Received	300+	72%	69%	68%
Would Definitely Recommend Hospital	300+	69%	71%	71%
Use of Medical Imaging				
Cardiac Imaging Stress Test before Surgery	161	2.5%	5.3%	5.3%
Combination Abdominal CT Scan	241	3.3%	10.7%	10.5%
Combination Brain/Sinus CT Scan	321	6.2%	3.1%	2.7%
Combination Chest CT Scan	150	0.0%	4.3%	2.7%
Follow-up Mammogram/Ultrasound	160	12.5%	8.3%	8.8%
Lumbar Spine MRI for Low Back Pain	52	34.6%	38.9%	37.2%

Baptist Health Louisville

4000 Kresge Way
Louisville, KY 40207
Phone: 502-897-8100
Fax: 502-897-8020
E-mail: bheinfocenter@bhsi.com
URL: www.baptisteast.com
Type: Acute Care Hospitals
Ownership: Voluntary non-profit - Private
Emergency Services: Yes
Beds: 519

Key Personnel:
Infection Control. . . . . Connie Baker
Intensive Care Unit. . . . . Paul Battes
Hemotology Center . . . . Denise Carroll
Radiology. . . . . Robert Elliott, MD
CEO/President. . . . . David Gray

Measure	Cases	This Hosp.	State Avg.	U.S. Avg.
Blood Clot Prevention and Treatment				
Anticoagulation Overlap Therapy[2]	188	96%	90%	93%
ICU Venous Thromboembolism Prophylaxis[2]	64	98%	86%	92%
Incidence of Potentially Preventable VTE[2]	43	2%	13%	10%
UFH with Dosages/Platelet Monitoring[2]	83	100%	98%	97%
Venous Thromboembolism Prophylaxis[2]	328	93%	80%	85%
Warfarin Therapy Discharge Instructions[2]	133	86%	72%	75%
Chest Pain/Possible Heart Attack Care				
Aspirin Given Within 24 Hours of Arrival[1,3]	-	-	97%	96%
Fibrinolytic Meds Within 30 Min. of Arrival[5]	-	-	63%	58%
Average Time to ECG (minutes)[1,3]	-	-	6	7
Average Time to Transfer (minutes)[5]	-	-	61	60
Children's Asthma Care				
Received Home Management Plan of Care	-	-	-	88%
Received Reliever Medication	-	-	-	100%
Received Systemic Corticosteroids	-	-	-	100%
Emergency Department				
Admittance Decision Time (minutes)[2]	446	91	78	98
Head CT Results Within 45 Min. of Arrival[1]	-	-	55%	57%
Patients Who Left ER Before Being Seen	53,736	2%	2%	2%
Time from ER Arrival to Admit. (minutes)[2]	493	280	238	274
Time from ER Arrival to Discharge (minutes)	350	218	126	134
Time in ER Before Being Evaluated (minutes)	405	49	23	26
Time to Pain Meds for Fractures (minutes)	101	77	56	57
Heart Attack Care				
Aspirin Given at Discharge	500	100%	99%	99%
Fibrinolytic Meds Within 30 Min. of Arrival[7]	-	-	-	54%
PCI Within 90 Minutes of Arrival	122	98%	97%	96%
Statin Prescribed at Discharge	461	99%	97%	98%
Heart Failure Care				
ACE Inhibitor or ARB for LVSD	142	100%	95%	97%
Discharge Instructions Given	538	94%	92%	94%
Evaluation of LVS Function	762	100%	98%	99%
Medicare Spending				
Medicare Spending per Patient (ratio)	-	0.98	0.97	0.98
Pneumonia Care				
Appropriate Initial Antibiotic Given	397	97%	94%	95%
Blood Culture Timing	571	99%	98%	98%
Pregnancy and Delivery Care				
Newborn Deliveries Scheduled Early	264	2%	9%	6%
Preventive Care				
Immunization for Influenza[2]	534	97%	92%	90%
Immunization for Pneumonia[2]	673	95%	94%	92%
Stroke Care				
Anticoagulation Therapy for Atrial Fibrillation	56	100%	95%	95%
Antithrombotic Therapy Timing	297	99%	97%	98%
Assessed for Rehabilitation	358	98%	97%	97%
Discharged on Antithrombotic Therapy	320	100%	98%	99%
Discharged on Statin Medication	241	98%	93%	94%
Thrombolytic Therapy Timing	29	86%	59%	66%
Venous Thromboembolism Prophylaxis	378	95%	93%	94%
Written Stroke Educational Materials Given	195	92%	86%	88%
Surgical Care Improvement Project				
Appropriate Beta Blocker Usage	1,372	99%	98%	98%
Appropriate VTP Within 24 Hours	3,101	99%	98%	98%
Controlled Postoperative Blood Glucose	331	99%	96%	97%
Perioperative Temperature Management	3,496	100%	100%	100%
Prophylactic Antibiotic Selection	2,553	99%	99%	99%
Prophylactic Antibiotic Selection (Outpatient)	1,276	99%	97%	98%
Prophylactic Antibiotic Stopped	2,503	99%	98%	98%
Prophylactic Antibiotic Timing	2,553	99%	99%	99%
Prophylactic Antibiotic Timing (Outpatient)	1,239	99%	97%	98%
Urinary Catheter Removal	1,169	98%	97%	97%
Survey of Patients' Hospital Experiences				
Area Around Room 'Always' Quiet at Night	300+	62%	64%	61%
Doctors 'Always' Communicated Well	300+	82%	84%	82%
Home Recovery Information Given	300+	89%	86%	85%
Hospital Given 9 or 10 on 10 Point Scale	300+	81%	72%	71%
Meds 'Always' Explained Before Given	300+	66%	66%	64%
Nurses 'Always' Communicated Well	300+	81%	81%	79%
Pain 'Always' Well Controlled	300+	74%	73%	71%
Room and Bathroom 'Always' Clean	300+	68%	75%	73%
Timely Help 'Always' Received	300+	66%	69%	68%
Would Definitely Recommend Hospital	300+	84%	71%	71%

NOTE: Hospital profiles are in alphabetical order by state, then city, then hospital within the city; Rankings exclude hospitals with less than 25 cases except for patient surveys which excludes hospitals with less than 100 cases; (a) 100-299 cases; (1) The number of cases/patients is too few to report; (2) Data submitted were based on a sample of cases/patients; (3) Results are based on a shorter time period than required; (4) Data suppressed by CMS for one or more quarters; (5) Results are not available for this reporting period; (6) Fewer than 100 patients completed the HCAHPS survey; (7) No cases met the criteria for this measure; (8) The lower limit of the confidence interval cannot be calculated if the number of observed infections equals zero; (9) No data are available from the state/territory for this reporting period; (10) The scores shown reflect fewer than 50 completed surveys; (11) There were discrepancies in the data collection process; (12) This measure does not apply to this hospital for this reporting period; (13) Results cannot be calculated for this reporting period; (14) The results for this state are combined with nearby states to protect confidentiality; Please refer to the User's Guide for a full explanation of data.

Use of Medical Imaging				
Cardiac Imaging Stress Test before Surgery	1,420	6.8%	5.3%	5.3%
Combination Abdominal CT Scan	3,701	3.2%	10.7%	10.5%
Combination Brain/Sinus CT Scan	2,332	2.0%	3.1%	2.7%
Combination Chest CT Scan	3,075	0.0%	4.3%	2.7%
Follow-up Mammogram/Ultrasound	3,287	6.2%	8.3%	8.8%
Lumbar Spine MRI for Low Back Pain	428	35.7%	38.9%	37.2%

Jewish Hospital & Saint Mary's Healthcare

200 Abraham Flexner Way Phone: 502-587-4011
Louisville, KY 40202
URL: www.jhhs.org
Type: Acute Care Hospitals Emergency Services: Yes
Ownership: Voluntary non-profit - Private

Key Personnel:

Anesthesiology. . . . . Atul Barry, MD
Operating Room. . . . . Lisa Jackson
Emergency Room . . . . Tom Neal
Ambulatory Care . . . . Luis R Scheker, MD
CEO/President. . . . . Robert L Shircliff
Chief of Medical Staff. . . . . Lynn T Simon, MDMBACHE

Measure	Cases	This Hosp.	State Avg.	U.S. Avg.
Blood Clot Prevention and Treatment				
Anticoagulation Overlap Therapy[2]	206	91%	90%	93%
ICU Venous Thromboembolism Prophylaxis[2]	139	94%	86%	92%
Incidence of Potentially Preventable VTE[2]	46	22%	13%	10%
UFH with Dosages/Platelet Monitoring[2]	123	100%	98%	97%
Venous Thromboembolism Prophylaxis[2]	472	77%	80%	85%
Warfarin Therapy Discharge Instructions[2]	157	34%	72%	75%
Chest Pain/Possible Heart Attack Care				
Aspirin Given Within 24 Hours of Arrival	156	96%	97%	96%
Fibrinolytic Meds Within 30 Min. of Arrival[7]	-	-	63%	58%
Average Time to ECG (minutes)	159	4	6	7
Average Time to Transfer (minutes)[1]	-	-	61	60
Children's Asthma Care				
Received Home Management Plan of Care	-	-	-	88%
Received Reliever Medication	-	-	-	100%
Received Systemic Corticosteroids	-	-	-	100%
Emergency Department				
Admittance Decision Time (minutes)[2]	600	160	78	98
Head CT Results Within 45 Min. of Arrival	27	44%	55%	57%
Patients Who Left ER Before Being Seen	>100k	2%	2%	2%
Time from ER Arrival to Admit. (minutes)[2]	627	348	238	274
Time from ER Arrival to Discharge (minutes)	550	132	126	134
Time in ER Before Being Evaluated (minutes)	610	32	23	26
Time to Pain Meds for Fractures (minutes)	296	53	56	57
Heart Attack Care				
Aspirin Given at Discharge[2]	470	100%	99%	99%
Fibrinolytic Meds Within 30 Min. of Arrival[2,7]	-	-	-	54%
PCI Within 90 Minutes of Arrival[2]	31	94%	97%	96%
Statin Prescribed at Discharge[2]	446	96%	97%	98%
Heart Failure Care				
ACE Inhibitor or ARB for LVSD[2]	170	86%	95%	97%
Discharge Instructions Given[2]	433	73%	92%	94%
Evaluation of LVS Function[2]	538	100%	98%	99%
Medicare Spending				
Medicare Spending per Patient (ratio)	-	1.00	0.97	0.98
Pneumonia Care				
Appropriate Initial Antibiotic Given[2]	145	92%	94%	95%
Blood Culture Timing[2]	266	97%	98%	98%
Pregnancy and Delivery Care				
Newborn Deliveries Scheduled Early[4]	-	-	9%	6%
Preventive Care				
Immunization for Influenza[2]	643	92%	92%	90%
Immunization for Pneumonia[2]	1,208	92%	94%	92%
Stroke Care				
Anticoagulation Therapy for Atrial Fibrillation[2]	31	97%	95%	95%
Antithrombotic Therapy Timing[2]	177	96%	97%	98%
Assessed for Rehabilitation[2]	207	100%	97%	97%
Discharged on Antithrombotic Therapy[2]	199	99%	98%	99%
Discharged on Statin Medication[2]	154	100%	93%	94%
Thrombolytic Therapy Timing[1,2]	-	-	59%	66%
Venous Thromboembolism Prophylaxis[2]	202	91%	93%	94%
Written Stroke Educational Materials Given[2]	122	73%	86%	88%
Surgical Care Improvement Project				
Appropriate Beta Blocker Usage[2]	343	97%	98%	98%
Appropriate VTP Within 24 Hours[2]	496	95%	98%	98%
Controlled Postoperative Blood Glucose[2]	159	94%	96%	97%
Perioperative Temperature Management[2]	653	100%	100%	100%
Prophylactic Antibiotic Selection[2]	551	99%	99%	99%
Prophylactic Antibiotic Selection (Outpatient)	629	99%	97%	98%
Prophylactic Antibiotic Stopped[2]	525	97%	98%	98%
Prophylactic Antibiotic Timing[2]	553	97%	99%	99%
Prophylactic Antibiotic Timing (Outpatient)	639	96%	97%	98%
Urinary Catheter Removal[2]	453	94%	97%	97%
Survey of Patients' Hospital Experiences				
Area Around Room 'Always' Quiet at Night	300+	58%	64%	61%
Doctors 'Always' Communicated Well	300+	78%	84%	82%
Home Recovery Information Given	300+	84%	86%	85%
Hospital Given 9 or 10 on 10 Point Scale	300+	66%	72%	71%
Meds 'Always' Explained Before Given	300+	58%	66%	64%
Nurses 'Always' Communicated Well	300+	74%	81%	79%
Pain 'Always' Well Controlled	300+	66%	73%	71%
Room and Bathroom 'Always' Clean	300+	61%	75%	73%
Timely Help 'Always' Received	300+	55%	69%	68%
Would Definitely Recommend Hospital	300+	67%	71%	71%
Use of Medical Imaging				
Cardiac Imaging Stress Test before Surgery	1,448	5.5%	5.3%	5.3%
Combination Abdominal CT Scan	3,511	5.8%	10.7%	10.5%
Combination Brain/Sinus CT Scan	2,773	3.9%	3.1%	2.7%
Combination Chest CT Scan	2,705	0.1%	4.3%	2.7%
Follow-up Mammogram/Ultrasound	3,899	7.1%	8.3%	8.8%
Lumbar Spine MRI for Low Back Pain	540	41.7%	38.9%	37.2%

Louisville VA Medical Center

800 Zorn Avenue Phone: 502-287-4000
Louisville, KY 40206 Fax: 502-287-6225
E-mail: sander.larry-j@lousville.va.gov
URL: www.va.gov/603louisville
Type: Acute Care - VA Emergency Services: No
Ownership: Government Federal Beds: 168

Key Personnel:

Emergency Room . . . . Ruby Leverson
Infection Control. . . . . Alberta Mozee, RN
Patient Relations . . . . Kathleen Rajoevich, RN
Chief of Medical Staff. . . . . Lisa Vuocolo, MD
Quality Assurance . . . . Verena Wheatley

Measure	Cases	This Hosp.	State Avg.	U.S. Avg.
Blood Clot Prevention and Treatment				
Anticoagulation Overlap Therapy	-	-	90%	93%
ICU Venous Thromboembolism Prophylaxis	-	-	86%	92%
Incidence of Potentially Preventable VTE	-	-	13%	10%
UFH with Dosages/Platelet Monitoring	-	-	98%	97%
Venous Thromboembolism Prophylaxis	-	-	80%	85%
Warfarin Therapy Discharge Instructions	-	-	72%	75%
Chest Pain/Possible Heart Attack Care				
Aspirin Given Within 24 Hours of Arrival	-	-	97%	96%
Fibrinolytic Meds Within 30 Min. of Arrival	-	-	63%	58%
Average Time to ECG (minutes)	-	-	6	7
Average Time to Transfer (minutes)	-	-	61	60
Children's Asthma Care				
Received Home Management Plan of Care	-	-	-	88%
Received Reliever Medication	-	-	-	100%
Received Systemic Corticosteroids	-	-	-	100%
Emergency Department				
Admittance Decision Time (minutes)	-	-	78	98
Head CT Results Within 45 Min. of Arrival	-	-	55%	57%
Patients Who Left ER Before Being Seen	-	-	2%	2%
Time from ER Arrival to Admit. (minutes)	-	-	238	274
Time from ER Arrival to Discharge (minutes)	-	-	126	134
Time in ER Before Being Evaluated (minutes)	-	-	23	26
Time to Pain Meds for Fractures (minutes)	-	-	56	57
Heart Attack Care				
Aspirin Given at Discharge	60	97%	99%	99%
Fibrinolytic Meds Within 30 Min. of Arrival[5]	-	-	-	54%
PCI Within 90 Minutes of Arrival[1]	-	-	97%	96%
Statin Prescribed at Discharge	57	100%	97%	98%
Heart Failure Care				
ACE Inhibitor or ARB for LVSD	95	99%	95%	97%
Discharge Instructions Given	235	92%	92%	94%
Evaluation of LVS Function	269	100%	98%	99%
Medicare Spending				
Medicare Spending per Patient (ratio)	-	-	0.97	0.98
Pneumonia Care				
Appropriate Initial Antibiotic Given	58	97%	94%	95%
Blood Culture Timing	112	97%	98%	98%
Pregnancy and Delivery Care				
Newborn Deliveries Scheduled Early	-	-	9%	6%
Preventive Care				
Immunization for Influenza[5]	-	-	92%	90%
Immunization for Pneumonia[5]	-	-	94%	92%
Stroke Care				
Anticoagulation Therapy for Atrial Fibrillation	-	-	95%	95%
Antithrombotic Therapy Timing	-	-	97%	98%
Assessed for Rehabilitation	-	-	97%	97%
Discharged on Antithrombotic Therapy	-	-	98%	99%
Discharged on Statin Medication	-	-	93%	94%
Thrombolytic Therapy Timing	-	-	59%	66%
Venous Thromboembolism Prophylaxis	-	-	93%	94%
Written Stroke Educational Materials Given	-	-	86%	88%
Surgical Care Improvement Project				
Appropriate Beta Blocker Usage[2]	58	90%	98%	98%
Appropriate VTP Within 24 Hours[2]	143	98%	98%	98%
Controlled Postoperative Blood Glucose[5]	-	-	96%	97%
Perioperative Temperature Management[2]	173	99%	100%	100%
Prophylactic Antibiotic Selection	79	97%	99%	99%
Prophylactic Antibiotic Selection (Outpatient)	-	-	97%	98%
Prophylactic Antibiotic Stopped	78	97%	98%	98%
Prophylactic Antibiotic Timing	79	97%	99%	99%
Prophylactic Antibiotic Timing (Outpatient)	-	-	97%	98%
Urinary Catheter Removal[2]	120	93%	97%	97%
Survey of Patients' Hospital Experiences				
Area Around Room 'Always' Quiet at Night	-	-	64%	61%
Doctors 'Always' Communicated Well	-	-	84%	82%
Home Recovery Information Given	-	-	86%	85%
Hospital Given 9 or 10 on 10 Point Scale	-	-	72%	71%
Meds 'Always' Explained Before Given	-	-	66%	64%
Nurses 'Always' Communicated Well	-	-	81%	79%
Pain 'Always' Well Controlled	-	-	73%	71%
Room and Bathroom 'Always' Clean	-	-	75%	73%
Timely Help 'Always' Received	-	-	69%	68%
Would Definitely Recommend Hospital	-	-	71%	71%
Use of Medical Imaging				
Cardiac Imaging Stress Test before Surgery	-	-	5.3%	5.3%
Combination Abdominal CT Scan	-	-	10.7%	10.5%
Combination Brain/Sinus CT Scan	-	-	3.1%	2.7%
Combination Chest CT Scan	-	-	4.3%	2.7%
Follow-up Mammogram/Ultrasound	-	-	8.3%	8.8%
Lumbar Spine MRI for Low Back Pain	-	-	38.9%	37.2%

Norton Hospitals

200 East Chestnut Street Phone: 502-629-6560
Louisville, KY 40202
URL: www.nortonhealthcare.com
Type: Acute Care Hospitals Emergency Services: Yes
Ownership: Voluntary non-profit - Private

Key Personnel:

President . . . . Russell F. Cox
CEO . . . . Stephen A. Williams

Measure	Cases	This Hosp.	State Avg.	U.S. Avg.
Blood Clot Prevention and Treatment				
Anticoagulation Overlap Therapy[2]	327	88%	90%	93%
ICU Venous Thromboembolism Prophylaxis[2]	129	83%	86%	92%
Incidence of Potentially Preventable VTE[2]	85	19%	13%	10%
UFH with Dosages/Platelet Monitoring[2]	182	98%	98%	97%
Venous Thromboembolism Prophylaxis[2]	418	71%	80%	85%
Warfarin Therapy Discharge Instructions[2]	213	46%	72%	75%
Chest Pain/Possible Heart Attack Care				
Aspirin Given Within 24 Hours of Arrival	23	96%	97%	96%
Fibrinolytic Meds Within 30 Min. of Arrival[7]	-	-	63%	58%
Average Time to ECG (minutes)	23	6	6	7

NOTE: Hospital profiles are in alphabetical order by state, then city, then hospital within the city; Rankings exclude hospitals with less than 25 cases except for patient surveys which excludes hospitals with less than 100 cases; (a) 100-299 cases; (1) The number of cases/patients is too few to report; (2) Data submitted were based on a sample of cases/patients; (3) Results are based on a shorter time period than required; (4) Data suppressed by CMS for one or more quarters; (5) Results are not available for this reporting period; (6) Fewer than 100 patients completed the HCAHPS survey; (7) No cases met the criteria for this measure; (8) The lower limit of the confidence interval cannot be calculated if the number of observed infections equals zero; (9) No data are available from the state/territory for this reporting period; (10) The scores shown reflect fewer than 50 completed surveys; (11) There were discrepancies in the data collection process; (12) This measure does not apply to this hospital for this reporting period; (13) Results cannot be calculated for this reporting period; (14) The results for this state are combined with nearby states to protect confidentiality; Please refer to the User's Guide for a full explanation of data.

Measure	Cases	This Hosp.	State Avg.	U.S. Avg.
Average Time to Transfer (minutes)	11	51	61	60
Children's Asthma Care				
Received Home Management Plan of Care	596	88%	-	88%
Received Reliever Medication	596	100%	-	100%
Received Systemic Corticosteroids	597	100%	-	100%
Emergency Department				
Admittance Decision Time (minutes)[2]	752	109	78	98
Head CT Results Within 45 Min. of Arrival	29	69%	55%	57%
Patients Who Left ER Before Being Seen	>100k	2%	2%	2%
Time from ER Arrival to Admit. (minutes)[2]	771	290	238	274
Time from ER Arrival to Discharge (minutes)	1,633	162	126	134
Time in ER Before Being Evaluated (minutes)	1,526	35	23	26
Time to Pain Meds for Fractures (minutes)	446	26	56	57
Heart Attack Care				
Aspirin Given at Discharge	916	99%	99%	99%
Fibrinolytic Meds Within 30 Min. of Arrival[7]	-	-	-	54%
PCI Within 90 Minutes of Arrival	87	100%	97%	96%
Statin Prescribed at Discharge	868	99%	97%	98%
Heart Failure Care				
ACE Inhibitor or ARB for LVSD	339	98%	95%	97%
Discharge Instructions Given	1,000	95%	92%	94%
Evaluation of LVS Function	1,359	100%	98%	99%
Medicare Spending				
Medicare Spending per Patient (ratio)	-	1.01	0.97	0.98
Pneumonia Care				
Appropriate Initial Antibiotic Given	564	96%	94%	95%
Blood Culture Timing	1,063	98%	98%	98%
Pregnancy and Delivery Care				
Newborn Deliveries Scheduled Early[2]	692	9%	9%	6%
Preventive Care				
Immunization for Influenza[2]	985	93%	92%	90%
Immunization for Pneumonia[2]	1,029	92%	94%	92%
Stroke Care				
Anticoagulation Therapy for Atrial Fibrillation	57	95%	95%	95%
Antithrombotic Therapy Timing	360	99%	97%	98%
Assessed for Rehabilitation	499	98%	97%	97%
Discharged on Antithrombotic Therapy	402	100%	98%	99%
Discharged on Statin Medication	321	94%	93%	94%
Thrombolytic Therapy Timing	22	86%	59%	66%
Venous Thromboembolism Prophylaxis	497	95%	93%	94%
Written Stroke Educational Materials Given	269	88%	86%	88%
Surgical Care Improvement Project				
Appropriate Beta Blocker Usage[2]	1,287	96%	98%	98%
Appropriate VTP Within 24 Hours[2]	2,563	96%	98%	98%
Controlled Postoperative Blood Glucose[2]	413	97%	96%	97%
Perioperative Temperature Management[2]	3,538	99%	100%	100%
Prophylactic Antibiotic Selection[2]	2,681	99%	99%	99%
Prophylactic Antibiotic Selection (Outpatient)	1,300	97%	97%	98%
Prophylactic Antibiotic Stopped[2]	2,590	98%	98%	98%
Prophylactic Antibiotic Timing[2]	2,685	98%	99%	99%
Prophylactic Antibiotic Timing (Outpatient)	1,322	95%	97%	98%
Urinary Catheter Removal[2]	1,864	95%	97%	97%
Survey of Patients' Hospital Experiences				
Area Around Room 'Always' Quiet at Night	300+	56%	64%	61%
Doctors 'Always' Communicated Well	300+	78%	84%	82%
Home Recovery Information Given	300+	85%	86%	85%
Hospital Given 9 or 10 on 10 Point Scale	300+	68%	72%	71%
Meds 'Always' Explained Before Given	300+	61%	66%	64%
Nurses 'Always' Communicated Well	300+	77%	81%	79%
Pain 'Always' Well Controlled	300+	70%	73%	71%
Room and Bathroom 'Always' Clean	300+	68%	75%	73%
Timely Help 'Always' Received	300+	63%	69%	68%
Would Definitely Recommend Hospital	300+	70%	71%	71%
Use of Medical Imaging				
Cardiac Imaging Stress Test before Surgery	2,731	4.7%	5.3%	5.3%
Combination Abdominal CT Scan	4,201	11.4%	10.7%	10.5%
Combination Brain/Sinus CT Scan	3,420	2.5%	3.1%	2.7%
Combination Chest CT Scan	2,881	0.9%	4.3%	2.7%
Follow-up Mammogram/Ultrasound	4,455	10.5%	8.3%	8.8%
Lumbar Spine MRI for Low Back Pain	833	35.5%	38.9%	37.2%

University of Louisville Hospital

530 South Jackson Street — Phone: 502-562-3000
Louisville, KY 40202 — Fax: 502-562-3593
URL: www.uoflhealthcare.org
Type: Acute Care Hospitals — Emergency Services: Yes
Ownership: Voluntary non-profit - Private — Beds: 404

Key Personnel:
CEO/President. . . . . Ken Marshall
Operating Room. . . . . Patty Melvin
Chief of Medical Staff . . . . Mark Pfeifer, MD
Anesthesiology. . . . . Anupama Wadhwa

Measure	Cases	This Hosp.	State Avg.	U.S. Avg.
Blood Clot Prevention and Treatment				
Anticoagulation Overlap Therapy[2]	65	77%	90%	93%
ICU Venous Thromboembolism Prophylaxis[2]	129	85%	86%	92%
Incidence of Potentially Preventable VTE[2]	53	4%	13%	10%
UFH with Dosages/Platelet Monitoring[2]	51	94%	98%	97%
Venous Thromboembolism Prophylaxis[2]	220	68%	80%	85%
Warfarin Therapy Discharge Instructions[2]	43	35%	72%	75%
Chest Pain/Possible Heart Attack Care				
Aspirin Given Within 24 Hours of Arrival[1,3]	-	-	97%	96%
Fibrinolytic Meds Within 30 Min. of Arrival[3,7]	-	-	63%	58%
Average Time to ECG (minutes)[1,3]	-	-	6	7
Average Time to Transfer (minutes)[1,3]	-	-	61	60
Children's Asthma Care				
Received Home Management Plan of Care	-	-	-	88%
Received Reliever Medication	-	-	-	100%
Received Systemic Corticosteroids	-	-	-	100%
Emergency Department				
Admittance Decision Time (minutes)[2]	539	57	78	98
Head CT Results Within 45 Min. of Arrival[5]	-	-	55%	57%
Patients Who Left ER Before Being Seen	43,473	2%	2%	2%
Time from ER Arrival to Admit. (minutes)[2]	559	368	238	274
Time from ER Arrival to Discharge (minutes)	318	240	126	134
Time in ER Before Being Evaluated (minutes)	337	66	23	26
Time to Pain Meds for Fractures (minutes)	52	82	56	57
Heart Attack Care				
Aspirin Given at Discharge	156	100%	99%	99%
Fibrinolytic Meds Within 30 Min. of Arrival[7]	-	-	-	54%
PCI Within 90 Minutes of Arrival	15	100%	97%	96%
Statin Prescribed at Discharge	151	100%	97%	98%
Heart Failure Care				
ACE Inhibitor or ARB for LVSD	116	99%	95%	97%
Discharge Instructions Given	210	100%	92%	94%
Evaluation of LVS Function	232	100%	98%	99%
Medicare Spending				
Medicare Spending per Patient (ratio)	-	1.02	0.97	0.98
Pneumonia Care				
Appropriate Initial Antibiotic Given	53	100%	94%	95%
Blood Culture Timing	131	97%	98%	98%
Pregnancy and Delivery Care				
Newborn Deliveries Scheduled Early[2]	40	8%	9%	6%
Preventive Care				
Immunization for Influenza[2]	535	82%	92%	90%
Immunization for Pneumonia[2]	457	81%	94%	92%
Stroke Care				
Anticoagulation Therapy for Atrial Fibrillation	55	98%	95%	95%
Antithrombotic Therapy Timing	248	98%	97%	98%
Assessed for Rehabilitation	423	100%	97%	97%
Discharged on Antithrombotic Therapy	329	100%	98%	99%
Discharged on Statin Medication	243	98%	93%	94%
Thrombolytic Therapy Timing	24	92%	59%	66%
Venous Thromboembolism Prophylaxis	418	99%	93%	94%
Written Stroke Educational Materials Given	241	93%	86%	88%
Surgical Care Improvement Project				
Appropriate Beta Blocker Usage[2]	77	100%	98%	98%
Appropriate VTP Within 24 Hours[2]	267	96%	98%	98%
Controlled Postoperative Blood Glucose[1,2]	-	-	96%	97%
Perioperative Temperature Management[2]	321	100%	100%	100%
Prophylactic Antibiotic Selection[2]	191	99%	99%	99%
Prophylactic Antibiotic Selection (Outpatient)	264	96%	97%	98%
Prophylactic Antibiotic Stopped[2]	188	93%	98%	98%
Prophylactic Antibiotic Timing[2]	192	97%	99%	99%
Prophylactic Antibiotic Timing (Outpatient)	269	94%	97%	98%
Urinary Catheter Removal[2]	162	90%	97%	97%
Survey of Patients' Hospital Experiences				
Area Around Room 'Always' Quiet at Night	300+	53%	64%	61%
Doctors 'Always' Communicated Well	300+	78%	84%	82%
Home Recovery Information Given	300+	84%	86%	85%
Hospital Given 9 or 10 on 10 Point Scale	300+	71%	72%	71%
Meds 'Always' Explained Before Given	300+	63%	66%	64%
Nurses 'Always' Communicated Well	300+	80%	81%	79%
Pain 'Always' Well Controlled	300+	68%	73%	71%
Room and Bathroom 'Always' Clean	300+	68%	75%	73%
Timely Help 'Always' Received	300+	64%	69%	68%
Would Definitely Recommend Hospital	300+	73%	71%	71%
Use of Medical Imaging				
Cardiac Imaging Stress Test before Surgery	182	6.6%	5.3%	5.3%
Combination Abdominal CT Scan	1,151	5.4%	10.7%	10.5%
Combination Brain/Sinus CT Scan	728	3.6%	3.1%	2.7%
Combination Chest CT Scan	1,493	0.0%	4.3%	2.7%
Follow-up Mammogram/Ultrasound	1,696	9.1%	8.3%	8.8%
Lumbar Spine MRI for Low Back Pain	73	38.4%	38.9%	37.2%

Baptist Health Madisonville

900 Hospital Drive — Phone: 270-825-5100
Madisonville, KY 42431 — Fax: 270-825-6650
E-mail: info@trover.org
URL: www.troverfoundation.org
Type: Acute Care Hospitals — Emergency Services: Yes
Ownership: Voluntary non-profit - Private — Beds: 410

Key Personnel:
CEO/President. . . . . Bobby Dampier
Radiology. . . . . Kavita Erickson
Chairman/CEO . . . . Allen Rudd

Measure	Cases	This Hosp.	State Avg.	U.S. Avg.
Blood Clot Prevention and Treatment				
Anticoagulation Overlap Therapy[2]	53	96%	90%	93%
ICU Venous Thromboembolism Prophylaxis[2]	107	83%	86%	92%
Incidence of Potentially Preventable VTE[1,2]	-	-	13%	10%
UFH with Dosages/Platelet Monitoring[2]	29	100%	98%	97%
Venous Thromboembolism Prophylaxis[2]	337	70%	80%	85%
Warfarin Therapy Discharge Instructions[2]	42	95%	72%	75%
Chest Pain/Possible Heart Attack Care				
Aspirin Given Within 24 Hours of Arrival[3,7]	-	-	97%	96%
Fibrinolytic Meds Within 30 Min. of Arrival[5]	-	-	63%	58%
Average Time to ECG (minutes)[1,3]	-	-	6	7
Average Time to Transfer (minutes)[5]	-	-	61	60
Children's Asthma Care				
Received Home Management Plan of Care	-	-	-	88%
Received Reliever Medication	-	-	-	100%
Received Systemic Corticosteroids	-	-	-	100%
Emergency Department				
Admittance Decision Time (minutes)[2]	609	102	78	98
Head CT Results Within 45 Min. of Arrival	27	74%	55%	57%
Patients Who Left ER Before Being Seen	30,205	3%	2%	2%
Time from ER Arrival to Admit. (minutes)[2]	616	248	238	274
Time from ER Arrival to Discharge (minutes)	369	150	126	134
Time in ER Before Being Evaluated (minutes)	339	32	23	26
Time to Pain Meds for Fractures (minutes)	90	68	56	57
Heart Attack Care				
Aspirin Given at Discharge	299	100%	99%	99%
Fibrinolytic Meds Within 30 Min. of Arrival[7]	-	-	-	54%
PCI Within 90 Minutes of Arrival	50	100%	97%	96%
Statin Prescribed at Discharge	279	98%	97%	98%
Heart Failure Care				
ACE Inhibitor or ARB for LVSD	96	98%	95%	97%
Discharge Instructions Given	190	91%	92%	94%
Evaluation of LVS Function	241	100%	98%	99%
Medicare Spending				
Medicare Spending per Patient (ratio)	-	0.95	0.97	0.98
Pneumonia Care				
Appropriate Initial Antibiotic Given	115	97%	94%	95%
Blood Culture Timing	169	100%	98%	98%
Pregnancy and Delivery Care				
Newborn Deliveries Scheduled Early[2]	15	0%	9%	6%

NOTE: Hospital profiles are in alphabetical order by state, then city, then hospital within the city; Rankings exclude hospitals with less than 25 cases except for patient surveys which excludes hospitals with less than 100 cases; (a) 100-299 cases; (1) The number of cases/patients is too few to report; (2) Data submitted were based on a sample of cases/patients; (3) Results are based on a shorter time period than required; (4) Data suppressed by CMS for one or more quarters; (5) Results are not available for this reporting period; (6) Fewer than 100 patients completed the HCAHPS survey; (7) No cases met the criteria for this measure; (8) The lower limit of the confidence interval cannot be calculated if the number of observed infections equals zero; (9) No data are available from the state/territory for this reporting period; (10) The scores shown reflect fewer than 50 completed surveys; (11) There were discrepancies in the data collection process; (12) This measure does not apply to this hospital for this reporting period; (13) Results cannot be calculated for this reporting period; (14) The results for this state are combined with nearby states to protect confidentiality; Please refer to the User's Guide for a full explanation of data.

Measure	Cases	This Hosp.	State Avg.	U.S. Avg.
Preventive Care				
Immunization for Influenza[2]	522	97%	92%	90%
Immunization for Pneumonia[2]	694	97%	94%	92%
Stroke Care				
Anticoagulation Therapy for Atrial Fibrillation[1,2]	-	-	95%	95%
Antithrombotic Therapy Timing[2]	65	98%	97%	98%
Assessed for Rehabilitation[2]	70	97%	97%	97%
Discharged on Antithrombotic Therapy[2]	67	100%	98%	99%
Discharged on Statin Medication[2]	56	96%	93%	94%
Thrombolytic Therapy Timing[1,2]	-	-	59%	66%
Venous Thromboembolism Prophylaxis[2]	68	79%	93%	94%
Written Stroke Educational Materials Given[2]	38	58%	86%	88%
Surgical Care Improvement Project				
Appropriate Beta Blocker Usage[2]	188	98%	98%	98%
Appropriate VTP Within 24 Hours[2]	388	99%	98%	98%
Controlled Postoperative Blood Glucose[2]	90	93%	96%	97%
Perioperative Temperature Management[2]	474	100%	100%	100%
Prophylactic Antibiotic Selection[2]	393	99%	99%	99%
Prophylactic Antibiotic Selection (Outpatient)	184	98%	97%	98%
Prophylactic Antibiotic Stopped[2]	384	98%	98%	98%
Prophylactic Antibiotic Timing[2]	393	100%	99%	99%
Prophylactic Antibiotic Timing (Outpatient)	184	100%	97%	98%
Urinary Catheter Removal[2]	392	99%	97%	97%
Survey of Patients' Hospital Experiences				
Area Around Room 'Always' Quiet at Night	300+	54%	64%	61%
Doctors 'Always' Communicated Well	300+	80%	84%	82%
Home Recovery Information Given	300+	84%	86%	85%
Hospital Given 9 or 10 on 10 Point Scale	300+	64%	72%	71%
Meds 'Always' Explained Before Given	300+	60%	66%	64%
Nurses 'Always' Communicated Well	300+	78%	81%	79%
Pain 'Always' Well Controlled	300+	69%	73%	71%
Room and Bathroom 'Always' Clean	300+	70%	75%	73%
Timely Help 'Always' Received	300+	68%	69%	68%
Would Definitely Recommend Hospital	300+	62%	71%	71%
Use of Medical Imaging				
Cardiac Imaging Stress Test before Surgery	208	7.2%	5.3%	5.3%
Combination Abdominal CT Scan	705	5.2%	10.7%	10.5%
Combination Brain/Sinus CT Scan	690	2.5%	3.1%	2.7%
Combination Chest CT Scan	356	0.6%	4.3%	2.7%
Follow-up Mammogram/Ultrasound[7]	-	-	8.3%	8.8%
Lumbar Spine MRI for Low Back Pain	89	31.5%	38.9%	37.2%

Memorial Hospital

210 Marie Langdon Drive
Manchester, KY 40962
Phone: 606-598-5104
Fax: 606-598-7008
E-mail: rosann.may@ahss.org
URL: www.manchestermemorial.com
Type: Acute Care Hospitals
Emergency Services: Yes
Ownership: Voluntary non-profit - Church
Beds: 63

Key Personnel:

Emergency Room .... Kathy Campbell
Quality Assurance .... Melissa Culver
Chief of Medical Staff.......... Kishore Javhav
CEO/President............... Erika Skula, MBA

Measure	Cases	This Hosp.	State Avg.	U.S. Avg.
Blood Clot Prevention and Treatment				
Anticoagulation Overlap Therapy[1,2]	-	-	90%	93%
ICU Venous Thromboembolism Prophylaxis[2]	60	90%	86%	92%
Incidence of Potentially Preventable VTE[2,7]	-	-	13%	10%
UFH with Dosages/Platelet Monitoring[1,2]	-	-	98%	97%
Venous Thromboembolism Prophylaxis[2]	208	88%	80%	85%
Warfarin Therapy Discharge Instructions[1,2]	-	-	72%	75%
Chest Pain/Possible Heart Attack Care				
Aspirin Given Within 24 Hours of Arrival	66	94%	97%	96%
Fibrinolytic Meds Within 30 Min. of Arrival[7]	-	-	63%	58%
Average Time to ECG (minutes)	70	10	6	7
Average Time to Transfer (minutes)[1]	-	-	61	60
Children's Asthma Care				
Received Home Management Plan of Care	-	-	-	88%
Received Reliever Medication	-	-	-	100%
Received Systemic Corticosteroids	-	-	-	100%
Emergency Department				
Admittance Decision Time (minutes)[2]	319	75	78	98
Head CT Results Within 45 Min. of Arrival[1]	-	-	55%	57%
Patients Who Left ER Before Being Seen	18,200	5%	2%	2%
Time from ER Arrival to Admit. (minutes)[2]	370	250	238	274
Time from ER Arrival to Discharge (minutes)	347	149	126	134
Time in ER Before Being Evaluated (minutes)	275	50	23	26
Time to Pain Meds for Fractures (minutes)	59	54	56	57
Heart Attack Care				
Aspirin Given at Discharge[1]	-	-	99%	99%
Fibrinolytic Meds Within 30 Min. of Arrival[7]	-	-	-	54%
PCI Within 90 Minutes of Arrival[7]	-	-	97%	96%
Statin Prescribed at Discharge[1]	-	-	97%	98%
Heart Failure Care				
ACE Inhibitor or ARB for LVSD	28	93%	95%	97%
Discharge Instructions Given	132	100%	92%	94%
Evaluation of LVS Function	152	99%	98%	99%
Medicare Spending				
Medicare Spending per Patient (ratio)	-	0.94	0.97	0.98
Pneumonia Care				
Appropriate Initial Antibiotic Given	223	96%	94%	95%
Blood Culture Timing	278	97%	98%	98%
Pregnancy and Delivery Care				
Newborn Deliveries Scheduled Early[2]	16	0%	9%	6%
Preventive Care				
Immunization for Influenza[2]	306	85%	92%	90%
Immunization for Pneumonia[2]	367	96%	94%	92%
Stroke Care				
Anticoagulation Therapy for Atrial Fibrillation[7]	-	-	95%	95%
Antithrombotic Therapy Timing[1]	-	-	97%	98%
Assessed for Rehabilitation[1]	-	-	97%	97%
Discharged on Antithrombotic Therapy[1]	-	-	98%	99%
Discharged on Statin Medication[1]	-	-	93%	94%
Thrombolytic Therapy Timing[7]	-	-	59%	66%
Venous Thromboembolism Prophylaxis[1]	-	-	93%	94%
Written Stroke Educational Materials Given[1]	-	-	86%	88%
Surgical Care Improvement Project				
Appropriate Beta Blocker Usage[1]	-	-	98%	98%
Appropriate VTP Within 24 Hours	13	100%	98%	98%
Controlled Postoperative Blood Glucose[7]	-	-	96%	97%
Perioperative Temperature Management	15	100%	100%	100%
Prophylactic Antibiotic Selection[1]	-	-	99%	99%
Prophylactic Antibiotic Selection (Outpatient)	15	100%	97%	98%
Prophylactic Antibiotic Stopped[1]	-	-	98%	98%
Prophylactic Antibiotic Timing[1]	-	-	99%	99%
Prophylactic Antibiotic Timing (Outpatient)	15	100%	97%	98%
Urinary Catheter Removal[7]	-	-	97%	97%
Survey of Patients' Hospital Experiences				
Area Around Room 'Always' Quiet at Night[11]	(a)	62%	64%	61%
Doctors 'Always' Communicated Well[11]	(a)	81%	84%	82%
Home Recovery Information Given[11]	(a)	85%	86%	85%
Hospital Given 9 or 10 on 10 Point Scale[11]	(a)	65%	72%	71%
Meds 'Always' Explained Before Given[11]	(a)	66%	66%	64%
Nurses 'Always' Communicated Well[11]	(a)	83%	81%	79%
Pain 'Always' Well Controlled[11]	(a)	67%	73%	71%
Room and Bathroom 'Always' Clean[11]	(a)	77%	75%	73%
Timely Help 'Always' Received[11]	(a)	72%	69%	68%
Would Definitely Recommend Hospital[11]	(a)	66%	71%	71%
Use of Medical Imaging				
Cardiac Imaging Stress Test before Surgery[1]	-	-	5.3%	5.3%
Combination Abdominal CT Scan	330	5.8%	10.7%	10.5%
Combination Brain/Sinus CT Scan[1]	-	-	3.1%	2.7%
Combination Chest CT Scan	178	9.0%	4.3%	2.7%
Follow-up Mammogram/Ultrasound	208	5.3%	8.3%	8.8%
Lumbar Spine MRI for Low Back Pain	79	45.6%	38.9%	37.2%

Crittenden Health System

520 West Gum Street
Marion, KY 42064
Phone: 270-965-5281
Fax: 270-965-1061
URL: www.crittenden-health.org
Type: Acute Care Hospitals
Emergency Services: Yes
Ownership: Proprietary
Beds: 50

Key Personnel:

CEO/President............... Jim Cristenson
Chairman/CEO .... Caroline Kieffer
Radiology.................... Carl Watkins

Measure	Cases	This Hosp.	State Avg.	U.S. Avg.
Blood Clot Prevention and Treatment				
Anticoagulation Overlap Therapy[1,2]	-	-	90%	93%
ICU Venous Thromboembolism Prophylaxis[2]	24	67%	86%	92%
Incidence of Potentially Preventable VTE[1,2]	-	-	13%	10%
UFH with Dosages/Platelet Monitoring[2,7]	-	-	98%	97%
Venous Thromboembolism Prophylaxis[2]	112	45%	80%	85%
Warfarin Therapy Discharge Instructions[1,2]	-	-	72%	75%
Chest Pain/Possible Heart Attack Care				
Aspirin Given Within 24 Hours of Arrival	12	92%	97%	96%
Fibrinolytic Meds Within 30 Min. of Arrival[1]	-	-	63%	58%
Average Time to ECG (minutes)	13	3	6	7
Average Time to Transfer (minutes)[1]	-	-	61	60
Children's Asthma Care				
Received Home Management Plan of Care	-	-	-	88%
Received Reliever Medication	-	-	-	100%
Received Systemic Corticosteroids	-	-	-	100%
Emergency Department				
Admittance Decision Time (minutes)	324	35	78	98
Head CT Results Within 45 Min. of Arrival[7]	-	-	55%	57%
Patients Who Left ER Before Being Seen	4,421	1%	2%	2%
Time from ER Arrival to Admit. (minutes)	358	141	238	274
Time from ER Arrival to Discharge (minutes)	381	68	126	134
Time in ER Before Being Evaluated (minutes)	448	13	23	26
Time to Pain Meds for Fractures (minutes)	17	63	56	57
Heart Attack Care				
Aspirin Given at Discharge[1,3]	-	-	99%	99%
Fibrinolytic Meds Within 30 Min. of Arrival[3,7]	-	-	-	54%
PCI Within 90 Minutes of Arrival[3,7]	-	-	97%	96%
Statin Prescribed at Discharge[1,3]	-	-	97%	98%
Heart Failure Care				
ACE Inhibitor or ARB for LVSD[1]	-	-	95%	97%
Discharge Instructions Given	26	85%	92%	94%
Evaluation of LVS Function	39	97%	98%	99%
Medicare Spending				
Medicare Spending per Patient (ratio)	-	0.98	0.97	0.98
Pneumonia Care				
Appropriate Initial Antibiotic Given	45	71%	94%	95%
Blood Culture Timing	35	100%	98%	98%
Pregnancy and Delivery Care				
Newborn Deliveries Scheduled Early[7]	-	-	9%	6%
Preventive Care				
Immunization for Influenza	417	88%	92%	90%
Immunization for Pneumonia	589	95%	94%	92%
Stroke Care				
Anticoagulation Therapy for Atrial Fibrillation[1]	-	-	95%	95%
Antithrombotic Therapy Timing[1]	-	-	97%	98%
Assessed for Rehabilitation[1]	-	-	97%	97%
Discharged on Antithrombotic Therapy[1]	-	-	98%	99%
Discharged on Statin Medication[1]	-	-	93%	94%
Thrombolytic Therapy Timing[1]	-	-	59%	66%
Venous Thromboembolism Prophylaxis[1]	-	-	93%	94%
Written Stroke Educational Materials Given[1]	-	-	86%	88%
Surgical Care Improvement Project				
Appropriate Beta Blocker Usage[3,7]	-	-	98%	98%
Appropriate VTP Within 24 Hours[1,3]	-	-	98%	98%
Controlled Postoperative Blood Glucose[3,7]	-	-	96%	97%
Perioperative Temperature Management[1,3]	-	-	100%	100%
Prophylactic Antibiotic Selection[3,7]	-	-	99%	99%
Prophylactic Antibiotic Selection (Outpatient)[1,3]	-	-	97%	98%
Prophylactic Antibiotic Stopped[3,7]	-	-	98%	98%
Prophylactic Antibiotic Timing[3,7]	-	-	99%	99%
Prophylactic Antibiotic Timing (Outpatient)[1,3]	-	-	97%	98%
Urinary Catheter Removal[1,3]	-	-	97%	97%
Survey of Patients' Hospital Experiences				
Area Around Room 'Always' Quiet at Night	(a)	59%	64%	61%
Doctors 'Always' Communicated Well	(a)	86%	84%	82%
Home Recovery Information Given	(a)	78%	86%	85%
Hospital Given 9 or 10 on 10 Point Scale	(a)	65%	72%	71%
Meds 'Always' Explained Before Given	(a)	69%	66%	64%
Nurses 'Always' Communicated Well	(a)	82%	81%	79%
Pain 'Always' Well Controlled	(a)	77%	73%	71%

NOTE: Hospital profiles are in alphabetical order by state, then city, then hospital within the city; Rankings exclude hospitals with less than 25 cases except for patient surveys which excludes hospitals with less than 100 cases; (a) 100-299 cases; (1) The number of cases/patients is too few to report; (2) Data submitted were based on a sample of cases/patients; (3) Results are based on a shorter time period than required; (4) Data suppressed by CMS for one or more quarters; (5) Results are not available for this reporting period; (6) Fewer than 100 patients completed the HCAHPS survey; (7) No cases met the criteria for this measure; (8) The lower limit of the confidence interval cannot be calculated if the number of observed infections equals zero; (9) No data are available from the state/territory for this reporting period; (10) The scores shown reflect fewer than 50 completed surveys; (11) There were discrepancies in the data collection process; (12) This measure does not apply to this hospital for this reporting period; (13) Results cannot be calculated for this reporting period; (14) The results for this state are combined with nearby states to protect confidentiality; Please refer to the User's Guide for a full explanation of data.

Measure	Cases	This Hosp.	State Avg.	U.S. Avg.
Room and Bathroom 'Always' Clean	(a)	69%	75%	73%
Timely Help 'Always' Received	(a)	69%	69%	68%
Would Definitely Recommend Hospital	(a)	68%	71%	71%
Use of Medical Imaging				
Cardiac Imaging Stress Test before Surgery[1]	-	-	5.3%	5.3%
Combination Abdominal CT Scan	158	3.2%	10.7%	10.5%
Combination Brain/Sinus CT Scan	106	6.6%	3.1%	2.7%
Combination Chest CT Scan	84	3.6%	4.3%	2.7%
Follow-up Mammogram/Ultrasound	121	4.1%	8.3%	8.8%
Lumbar Spine MRI for Low Back Pain[1]	-	-	38.9%	37.2%

Saint Joseph Martin

11203 Main Street Phone: 606-285-6401
Martin, KY 41649
URL: www.catholichealth.net
Type: Critical Access Hospitals Emergency Services: Yes
Ownership: Voluntary non-profit - Private Beds: 25

Key Personnel:
Operating Room. . . . . Danita Hampton, RN BSN
Pediatric In-Patient Care . . . . Mary Little, RN BSN
Infection Control. . . . . Mary Martin, RN, CIC
Quality Assurance . . . . Olive Martin, MT
Anesthesiology. . . . . William Montgomery, CRNA
Emergency Room . . . . Ronald Ross, RN BSN
CEO/President. . . . . Kathy Stumbo

Measure	Cases	This Hosp.	State Avg.	U.S. Avg.
Blood Clot Prevention and Treatment				
Anticoagulation Overlap Therapy[5]	-	-	90%	93%
ICU Venous Thromboembolism Prophylaxis[5]	-	-	86%	92%
Incidence of Potentially Preventable VTE[5]	-	-	13%	10%
UFH with Dosages/Platelet Monitoring[5]	-	-	98%	97%
Venous Thromboembolism Prophylaxis[5]	-	-	80%	85%
Warfarin Therapy Discharge Instructions[5]	-	-	72%	75%
Chest Pain/Possible Heart Attack Care				
Aspirin Given Within 24 Hours of Arrival[3]	11	100%	97%	96%
Fibrinolytic Meds Within 30 Min. of Arrival[1,3]	-	-	63%	58%
Average Time to ECG (minutes)[3]	12	10	6	7
Average Time to Transfer (minutes)[3,7]	-	-	61	60
Children's Asthma Care				
Received Home Management Plan of Care	-	-	-	88%
Received Reliever Medication	-	-	-	100%
Received Systemic Corticosteroids	-	-	-	100%
Emergency Department				
Admittance Decision Time (minutes)[2]	375	64	78	98
Head CT Results Within 45 Min. of Arrival[5]	-	-	55%	57%
Patients Who Left ER Before Being Seen	15,133	3%	2%	2%
Time from ER Arrival to Admit. (minutes)[2]	379	233	238	274
Time from ER Arrival to Discharge (minutes)[3]	174	114	126	134
Time in ER Before Being Evaluated (minutes)[3]	192	18	23	26
Time to Pain Meds for Fractures (minutes)[3]	46	38	56	57
Heart Attack Care				
Aspirin Given at Discharge[5]	-	-	99%	99%
Fibrinolytic Meds Within 30 Min. of Arrival[5]	-	-	-	54%
PCI Within 90 Minutes of Arrival[5]	-	-	97%	96%
Statin Prescribed at Discharge[5]	-	-	97%	98%
Heart Failure Care				
ACE Inhibitor or ARB for LVSD[1]	-	-	95%	97%
Discharge Instructions Given	25	84%	92%	94%
Evaluation of LVS Function	29	93%	98%	99%
Medicare Spending				
Medicare Spending per Patient (ratio)	-	-	0.97	0.98
Pneumonia Care				
Appropriate Initial Antibiotic Given	46	96%	94%	95%
Blood Culture Timing	52	96%	98%	98%
Pregnancy and Delivery Care				
Newborn Deliveries Scheduled Early[5]	-	-	9%	6%
Preventive Care				
Immunization for Influenza[2]	288	85%	92%	90%
Immunization for Pneumonia[2]	411	93%	94%	92%
Stroke Care				
Anticoagulation Therapy for Atrial Fibrillation[5]	-	-	95%	95%
Antithrombotic Therapy Timing[5]	-	-	97%	98%
Assessed for Rehabilitation[5]	-	-	97%	97%
Discharged on Antithrombotic Therapy[5]	-	-	98%	99%
Discharged on Statin Medication[5]	-	-	93%	94%
Thrombolytic Therapy Timing[5]	-	-	59%	66%
Venous Thromboembolism Prophylaxis[5]	-	-	93%	94%
Written Stroke Educational Materials Given[5]	-	-	86%	88%
Surgical Care Improvement Project				
Appropriate Beta Blocker Usage[5]	-	-	98%	98%
Appropriate VTP Within 24 Hours[5]	-	-	98%	98%
Controlled Postoperative Blood Glucose[5]	-	-	96%	97%
Perioperative Temperature Management[5]	-	-	100%	100%
Prophylactic Antibiotic Selection[5]	-	-	99%	99%
Prophylactic Antibiotic Selection (Outpatient)[5]	-	-	97%	98%
Prophylactic Antibiotic Stopped[5]	-	-	98%	98%
Prophylactic Antibiotic Timing[5]	-	-	99%	99%
Prophylactic Antibiotic Timing (Outpatient)[5]	-	-	97%	98%
Urinary Catheter Removal[5]	-	-	97%	97%
Survey of Patients' Hospital Experiences				
Area Around Room 'Always' Quiet at Night	(a)	57%	64%	61%
Doctors 'Always' Communicated Well	(a)	87%	84%	82%
Home Recovery Information Given	(a)	82%	86%	85%
Hospital Given 9 or 10 on 10 Point Scale	(a)	77%	72%	71%
Meds 'Always' Explained Before Given	(a)	70%	66%	64%
Nurses 'Always' Communicated Well	(a)	84%	81%	79%
Pain 'Always' Well Controlled	(a)	71%	73%	71%
Room and Bathroom 'Always' Clean	(a)	84%	75%	73%
Timely Help 'Always' Received	(a)	75%	69%	68%
Would Definitely Recommend Hospital	(a)	82%	71%	71%
Use of Medical Imaging				
Cardiac Imaging Stress Test before Surgery[1]	-	-	5.3%	5.3%
Combination Abdominal CT Scan	239	2.5%	10.7%	10.5%
Combination Brain/Sinus CT Scan	246	0.0%	3.1%	2.7%
Combination Chest CT Scan	140	1.4%	4.3%	2.7%
Follow-up Mammogram/Ultrasound	229	10.5%	8.3%	8.8%
Lumbar Spine MRI for Low Back Pain[1]	-	-	38.9%	37.2%

Jackson Purchase Medical Center

1099 Medical Center Circle Phone: 270-251-4500
Mayfield, KY 42066 Fax: 270-251-4507
URL: www.jacksonpurchase.com
Type: Acute Care Hospitals Emergency Services: Yes
Ownership: Govt - Hospital Dist/Auth Beds: 107

Key Personnel:
Infection Control. . . . . Ronnica Adams, RD, LD
CEO . . . . David Anderson
Radiology. . . . . John J Beasley, RT(R)
Intensive Care Unit. . . . . Julia Grove
Quality Assurance . . . . Denise Hawks
Operating Room. . . . . Edward McWhirt, RN, BSN
Emergency Room . . . . Della Thurston, RN
Chief of Medical Staff. . . . . David Zetter, MD

Measure	Cases	This Hosp.	State Avg.	U.S. Avg.
Blood Clot Prevention and Treatment				
Anticoagulation Overlap Therapy[2]	24	88%	90%	93%
ICU Venous Thromboembolism Prophylaxis[2]	89	99%	86%	92%
Incidence of Potentially Preventable VTE[1,2]	-	-	13%	10%
UFH with Dosages/Platelet Monitoring[2,7]	-	-	98%	97%
Venous Thromboembolism Prophylaxis[2]	310	86%	80%	85%
Warfarin Therapy Discharge Instructions[2]	11	91%	72%	75%
Chest Pain/Possible Heart Attack Care				
Aspirin Given Within 24 Hours of Arrival	25	92%	97%	96%
Fibrinolytic Meds Within 30 Min. of Arrival[7]	-	-	63%	58%
Average Time to ECG (minutes)	26	4	6	7
Average Time to Transfer (minutes)[1]	-	-	61	60
Children's Asthma Care				
Received Home Management Plan of Care	-	-	-	88%
Received Reliever Medication	-	-	-	100%
Received Systemic Corticosteroids	-	-	-	100%
Emergency Department				
Admittance Decision Time (minutes)[2]	488	65	78	98
Head CT Results Within 45 Min. of Arrival[1]	-	-	55%	57%
Patients Who Left ER Before Being Seen	26,073	0%	2%	2%
Time from ER Arrival to Admit. (minutes)[2]	492	201	238	274
Time from ER Arrival to Discharge (minutes)	441	82	126	134
Time in ER Before Being Evaluated (minutes)	462	16	23	26
Time to Pain Meds for Fractures (minutes)	66	52	56	57
Heart Attack Care				
Aspirin Given at Discharge	17	94%	99%	99%
Fibrinolytic Meds Within 30 Min. of Arrival[7]	-	-	-	54%
PCI Within 90 Minutes of Arrival[7]	-	-	97%	96%
Statin Prescribed at Discharge	14	93%	97%	98%
Heart Failure Care				
ACE Inhibitor or ARB for LVSD	27	96%	95%	97%
Discharge Instructions Given	63	100%	92%	94%
Evaluation of LVS Function	100	100%	98%	99%
Medicare Spending				
Medicare Spending per Patient (ratio)	-	0.98	0.97	0.98
Pneumonia Care				
Appropriate Initial Antibiotic Given	131	92%	94%	95%
Blood Culture Timing	215	100%	98%	98%
Pregnancy and Delivery Care				
Newborn Deliveries Scheduled Early[2]	42	12%	9%	6%
Preventive Care				
Immunization for Influenza[2]	382	97%	92%	90%
Immunization for Pneumonia[2]	557	94%	94%	92%
Stroke Care				
Anticoagulation Therapy for Atrial Fibrillation[1]	-	-	95%	95%
Antithrombotic Therapy Timing	28	93%	97%	98%
Assessed for Rehabilitation	27	93%	97%	97%
Discharged on Antithrombotic Therapy	25	100%	98%	99%
Discharged on Statin Medication	24	88%	93%	94%
Thrombolytic Therapy Timing[1]	-	-	59%	66%
Venous Thromboembolism Prophylaxis	28	93%	93%	94%
Written Stroke Educational Materials Given	15	100%	86%	88%
Surgical Care Improvement Project				
Appropriate Beta Blocker Usage	23	87%	98%	98%
Appropriate VTP Within 24 Hours	62	87%	98%	98%
Controlled Postoperative Blood Glucose[7]	-	-	96%	97%
Perioperative Temperature Management	66	100%	100%	100%
Prophylactic Antibiotic Selection	39	100%	99%	99%
Prophylactic Antibiotic Selection (Outpatient)	76	99%	97%	98%
Prophylactic Antibiotic Stopped	37	95%	98%	98%
Prophylactic Antibiotic Timing	39	100%	99%	99%
Prophylactic Antibiotic Timing (Outpatient)	75	97%	97%	98%
Urinary Catheter Removal	38	95%	97%	97%
Survey of Patients' Hospital Experiences				
Area Around Room 'Always' Quiet at Night	300+	60%	64%	61%
Doctors 'Always' Communicated Well	300+	82%	84%	82%
Home Recovery Information Given	300+	84%	86%	85%
Hospital Given 9 or 10 on 10 Point Scale	300+	73%	72%	71%
Meds 'Always' Explained Before Given	300+	59%	66%	64%
Nurses 'Always' Communicated Well	300+	77%	81%	79%
Pain 'Always' Well Controlled	300+	70%	73%	71%
Room and Bathroom 'Always' Clean	300+	74%	75%	73%
Timely Help 'Always' Received	300+	60%	69%	68%
Would Definitely Recommend Hospital	300+	68%	71%	71%
Use of Medical Imaging				
Cardiac Imaging Stress Test before Surgery[1]	-	-	5.3%	5.3%
Combination Abdominal CT Scan	413	26.2%	10.7%	10.5%
Combination Brain/Sinus CT Scan[1]	-	-	3.1%	2.7%
Combination Chest CT Scan	262	0.0%	4.3%	2.7%
Follow-up Mammogram/Ultrasound	574	8.5%	8.3%	8.8%
Lumbar Spine MRI for Low Back Pain[1]	-	-	38.9%	37.2%

Meadowview Regional Medical Center

989 Medical Park Drive Phone: 606-759-5311
Maysville, KY 41056 Fax: 606-759-5616
URL: www.meadowviewregional.com
Type: Acute Care Hospitals Emergency Services: Yes
Ownership: Proprietary Beds: 101

Key Personnel:
Quality Assurance . . . . Pam Brant, RN
Emergency Room . . . . June Fultz
Intensive Care Unit. . . . . June Fultz
Radiology. . . . . Richard Hartman
Chief of Medical Staff. . . . . Rick Hartman
CEO . . . . Robert Parker
Infection Control. . . . . Clare Vetter

Measure	Cases	This Hosp.	State Avg.	U.S. Avg.
Blood Clot Prevention and Treatment				

NOTE: Hospital profiles are in alphabetical order by state, then city, then hospital within the city; Rankings exclude hospitals with less than 25 cases except for patient surveys which excludes hospitals with less than 100 cases; (a) 100-299 cases; (1) The number of cases/patients is too few to report; (2) Data submitted were based on a sample of cases/patients; (3) Results are based on a shorter time period than required; (4) Data suppressed by CMS for one or more quarters; (5) Results are not available for this reporting period; (6) Fewer than 100 patients completed the HCAHPS survey; (7) No cases met the criteria for this measure; (8) The lower limit of the confidence interval cannot be calculated if the number of observed infections equals zero; (9) No data are available from the state/territory for this reporting period; (10) The scores shown reflect fewer than 50 completed surveys; (11) There were discrepancies in the data collection process; (12) This measure does not apply to this hospital for this reporting period; (13) Results cannot be calculated for this reporting period; (14) The results for this state are combined with nearby states to protect confidentiality; Please refer to the User's Guide for a full explanation of data.

Measure	Cases	This Hosp.	State Avg.	U.S. Avg.
Anticoagulation Overlap Therapy[2]	11	82%	90%	93%
ICU Venous Thromboembolism Prophylaxis[2]	96	60%	86%	92%
Incidence of Potentially Preventable VTE[1,2]	-	-	13%	10%
UFH with Dosages/Platelet Monitoring[1,2]	-	-	98%	97%
Venous Thromboembolism Prophylaxis[2]	181	61%	80%	85%
Warfarin Therapy Discharge Instructions[1,2]	-	-	72%	75%
Chest Pain/Possible Heart Attack Care				
Aspirin Given Within 24 Hours of Arrival	14	100%	97%	96%
Fibrinolytic Meds Within 30 Min. of Arrival[3,7]	-	-	63%	58%
Average Time to ECG (minutes)	17	2	6	7
Average Time to Transfer (minutes)[1,3]	-	-	61	60
Children's Asthma Care				
Received Home Management Plan of Care	-	-	-	88%
Received Reliever Medication	-	-	-	100%
Received Systemic Corticosteroids	-	-	-	100%
Emergency Department				
Admittance Decision Time (minutes)[2]	275	87	78	98
Head CT Results Within 45 Min. of Arrival[1]	-	-	55%	57%
Patients Who Left ER Before Being Seen	19,842	0%	2%	2%
Time from ER Arrival to Admit. (minutes)[2]	275	255	238	274
Time from ER Arrival to Discharge (minutes)	384	96	126	134
Time in ER Before Being Evaluated (minutes)	406	15	23	26
Time to Pain Meds for Fractures (minutes)	95	45	56	57
Heart Attack Care				
Aspirin Given at Discharge	117	99%	99%	99%
Fibrinolytic Meds Within 30 Min. of Arrival[7]	-	-	-	54%
PCI Within 90 Minutes of Arrival	27	96%	97%	96%
Statin Prescribed at Discharge	103	87%	97%	98%
Heart Failure Care				
ACE Inhibitor or ARB for LVSD	20	95%	95%	97%
Discharge Instructions Given	95	88%	92%	94%
Evaluation of LVS Function	121	98%	98%	99%
Medicare Spending				
Medicare Spending per Patient (ratio)	-	0.98	0.97	0.98
Pneumonia Care				
Appropriate Initial Antibiotic Given	71	97%	94%	95%
Blood Culture Timing	116	99%	98%	98%
Pregnancy and Delivery Care				
Newborn Deliveries Scheduled Early[1,2]	-	-	9%	6%
Preventive Care				
Immunization for Influenza[2]	304	93%	92%	90%
Immunization for Pneumonia[2]	358	98%	94%	92%
Stroke Care				
Anticoagulation Therapy for Atrial Fibrillation[1]	-	-	95%	95%
Antithrombotic Therapy Timing	18	89%	97%	98%
Assessed for Rehabilitation	18	89%	97%	97%
Discharged on Antithrombotic Therapy	18	94%	98%	99%
Discharged on Statin Medication	15	73%	93%	94%
Thrombolytic Therapy Timing[1]	-	-	59%	66%
Venous Thromboembolism Prophylaxis	19	58%	93%	94%
Written Stroke Educational Materials Given[1]	-	-	86%	88%
Surgical Care Improvement Project				
Appropriate Beta Blocker Usage	40	100%	98%	98%
Appropriate VTP Within 24 Hours	133	98%	98%	98%
Controlled Postoperative Blood Glucose[7]	-	-	96%	97%
Perioperative Temperature Management	137	100%	100%	100%
Prophylactic Antibiotic Selection	116	100%	99%	99%
Prophylactic Antibiotic Selection (Outpatient)	115	96%	97%	98%
Prophylactic Antibiotic Stopped	114	98%	98%	98%
Prophylactic Antibiotic Timing	116	100%	99%	99%
Prophylactic Antibiotic Timing (Outpatient)	113	96%	97%	98%
Urinary Catheter Removal	118	100%	97%	97%
Survey of Patients' Hospital Experiences				
Area Around Room 'Always' Quiet at Night	300+	56%	64%	61%
Doctors 'Always' Communicated Well	300+	79%	84%	82%
Home Recovery Information Given	300+	85%	86%	85%
Hospital Given 9 or 10 on 10 Point Scale	300+	63%	72%	71%
Meds 'Always' Explained Before Given	300+	64%	66%	64%
Nurses 'Always' Communicated Well	300+	78%	81%	79%
Pain 'Always' Well Controlled	300+	67%	73%	71%
Room and Bathroom 'Always' Clean	300+	70%	75%	73%
Timely Help 'Always' Received	300+	61%	69%	68%
Would Definitely Recommend Hospital	300+	59%	71%	71%
Use of Medical Imaging				
Cardiac Imaging Stress Test before Surgery	404	3.0%	5.3%	5.3%
Combination Abdominal CT Scan	237	49.8%	10.7%	10.5%
Combination Brain/Sinus CT Scan	226	4.9%	3.1%	2.7%
Combination Chest CT Scan	231	0.4%	4.3%	2.7%
Follow-up Mammogram/Ultrasound	583	9.9%	8.3%	8.8%
Lumbar Spine MRI for Low Back Pain	65	35.4%	38.9%	37.2%

McDowell ARH Hospital

9879 Kentucky Route 122
Mc Dowell, KY 41647
Phone: 606-377-3400
Fax: 606-377-3433
E-mail: mcdowellarh@arh.org
URL: www.arh.org/mcdowell
Type: Critical Access Hospitals
Emergency Services: Yes
Ownership: Voluntary non-profit - Private
Beds: 25

Key Personnel:
Operating Room. . . . . Josephine Akers
CEO . . . . Russ Barker
Radiology. . . . . Dhirenkumar I Desai, MD
Quality Assurance . . . . Jeff Frazier
Chief of Medical Staff. . . . . Dr. Bradley Moore
Pediatric In-Patient Care . . . . Vivian Ong, MD
Emergency Room . . . . Francisco G Rivera, MD
Anesthesiology. . . . . Kerry Slona, CRNA

Measure	Cases	This Hosp.	State Avg.	U.S. Avg.
Blood Clot Prevention and Treatment				
Anticoagulation Overlap Therapy[5]	-	-	90%	93%
ICU Venous Thromboembolism Prophylaxis[5]	-	-	86%	92%
Incidence of Potentially Preventable VTE[5]	-	-	13%	10%
UFH with Dosages/Platelet Monitoring[5]	-	-	98%	97%
Venous Thromboembolism Prophylaxis[5]	-	-	80%	85%
Warfarin Therapy Discharge Instructions[5]	-	-	72%	75%
Chest Pain/Possible Heart Attack Care				
Aspirin Given Within 24 Hours of Arrival[5]	-	-	97%	96%
Fibrinolytic Meds Within 30 Min. of Arrival[5]	-	-	63%	58%
Average Time to ECG (minutes)[5]	-	-	6	7
Average Time to Transfer (minutes)[5]	-	-	61	60
Children's Asthma Care				
Received Home Management Plan of Care	-	-	-	88%
Received Reliever Medication	-	-	-	100%
Received Systemic Corticosteroids	-	-	-	100%
Emergency Department				
Admittance Decision Time (minutes)[5]	-	-	78	98
Head CT Results Within 45 Min. of Arrival[5]	-	-	55%	57%
Patients Who Left ER Before Being Seen	9,298	2%	2%	2%
Time from ER Arrival to Admit. (minutes)[5]	-	-	238	274
Time from ER Arrival to Discharge (minutes)[5]	-	-	126	134
Time in ER Before Being Evaluated (minutes)[5]	-	-	23	26
Time to Pain Meds for Fractures (minutes)[5]	-	-	56	57
Heart Attack Care				
Aspirin Given at Discharge[3,7]	-	-	99%	99%
Fibrinolytic Meds Within 30 Min. of Arrival[3,7]	-	-	-	54%
PCI Within 90 Minutes of Arrival[3,7]	-	-	97%	96%
Statin Prescribed at Discharge[3,7]	-	-	97%	98%
Heart Failure Care				
ACE Inhibitor or ARB for LVSD	11	100%	95%	97%
Discharge Instructions Given	39	100%	92%	94%
Evaluation of LVS Function	42	100%	98%	99%
Medicare Spending				
Medicare Spending per Patient (ratio)	-	-	0.97	0.98
Pneumonia Care				
Appropriate Initial Antibiotic Given	47	98%	94%	95%
Blood Culture Timing	65	98%	98%	98%
Pregnancy and Delivery Care				
Newborn Deliveries Scheduled Early[5]	-	-	9%	6%
Preventive Care				
Immunization for Influenza[5]	-	-	92%	90%
Immunization for Pneumonia[5]	-	-	94%	92%
Stroke Care				
Anticoagulation Therapy for Atrial Fibrillation[5]	-	-	95%	95%
Antithrombotic Therapy Timing[5]	-	-	97%	98%
Assessed for Rehabilitation[5]	-	-	97%	97%
Discharged on Antithrombotic Therapy[5]	-	-	98%	99%
Discharged on Statin Medication[5]	-	-	93%	94%
Thrombolytic Therapy Timing[5]	-	-	59%	66%
Venous Thromboembolism Prophylaxis[5]	-	-	93%	94%
Written Stroke Educational Materials Given[5]	-	-	86%	88%
Surgical Care Improvement Project				
Appropriate Beta Blocker Usage[5]	-	-	98%	98%
Appropriate VTP Within 24 Hours[5]	-	-	98%	98%
Controlled Postoperative Blood Glucose[5]	-	-	96%	97%
Perioperative Temperature Management[5]	-	-	100%	100%
Prophylactic Antibiotic Selection[5]	-	-	99%	99%
Prophylactic Antibiotic Selection (Outpatient)[5]	-	-	97%	98%
Prophylactic Antibiotic Stopped[5]	-	-	98%	98%
Prophylactic Antibiotic Timing[5]	-	-	99%	99%
Prophylactic Antibiotic Timing (Outpatient)[5]	-	-	97%	98%
Urinary Catheter Removal[5]	-	-	97%	97%
Survey of Patients' Hospital Experiences				
Area Around Room 'Always' Quiet at Night	(a)	69%	64%	61%
Doctors 'Always' Communicated Well	(a)	90%	84%	82%
Home Recovery Information Given	(a)	87%	86%	85%
Hospital Given 9 or 10 on 10 Point Scale	(a)	79%	72%	71%
Meds 'Always' Explained Before Given	(a)	62%	66%	64%
Nurses 'Always' Communicated Well	(a)	84%	81%	79%
Pain 'Always' Well Controlled	(a)	77%	73%	71%
Room and Bathroom 'Always' Clean	(a)	78%	75%	73%
Timely Help 'Always' Received	(a)	78%	69%	68%
Would Definitely Recommend Hospital	(a)	76%	71%	71%
Use of Medical Imaging				
Cardiac Imaging Stress Test before Surgery[7]	-	-	5.3%	5.3%
Combination Abdominal CT Scan	185	4.3%	10.7%	10.5%
Combination Brain/Sinus CT Scan[1]	-	-	3.1%	2.7%
Combination Chest CT Scan	77	11.7%	4.3%	2.7%
Follow-up Mammogram/Ultrasound	122	9.0%	8.3%	8.8%
Lumbar Spine MRI for Low Back Pain	40	55.0%	38.9%	37.2%

Middlesboro Appalachian Regional Healthcare Hospital

3600 West Cumberland Avenue
Middlesboro, KY 40965
Phone: 606-242-1101
Fax: 606-248-3903
URL: www.arh.org/middlesboro
Type: Acute Care Hospitals
Emergency Services: Yes
Ownership: Voluntary non-profit - Private
Beds: 96

Key Personnel:
Operating Room. . . . . Charles Crumley, RN
Quality Assurance . . . . Lisa Dooley
CEO/President. . . . . Jerry W Haynes
Chief of Medical Staff . . . . Vicente Kaw, MD
Pediatric Ambulatory Care . . . . . . Houshang Khorram, MD
Pediatric In-Patient Care . . . . . . Houshang Khorram, MD
Infection Control. . . . . Shirley Lovell
Radiology. . . . . Ashok R Patel, MD

Measure	Cases	This Hosp.	State Avg.	U.S. Avg.
Blood Clot Prevention and Treatment				
Anticoagulation Overlap Therapy[1,2]	-	-	90%	93%
ICU Venous Thromboembolism Prophylaxis[2]	54	67%	86%	92%
Incidence of Potentially Preventable VTE[2,7]	-	-	13%	10%
UFH with Dosages/Platelet Monitoring[2,7]	-	-	98%	97%
Venous Thromboembolism Prophylaxis[2]	210	84%	80%	85%
Warfarin Therapy Discharge Instructions[1,2]	-	-	72%	75%
Chest Pain/Possible Heart Attack Care				
Aspirin Given Within 24 Hours of Arrival	77	99%	97%	96%
Fibrinolytic Meds Within 30 Min. of Arrival[1]	-	-	63%	58%
Average Time to ECG (minutes)	82	5	6	7
Average Time to Transfer (minutes)	26	91	61	60
Children's Asthma Care				
Received Home Management Plan of Care	-	-	-	88%
Received Reliever Medication	-	-	-	100%
Received Systemic Corticosteroids	-	-	-	100%
Emergency Department				
Admittance Decision Time (minutes)[2]	333	70	78	98
Head CT Results Within 45 Min. of Arrival	11	18%	55%	57%
Patients Who Left ER Before Being Seen	21,813	2%	2%	2%
Time from ER Arrival to Admit. (minutes)[2]	333	199	238	274
Time from ER Arrival to Discharge (minutes)	408	109	126	134
Time in ER Before Being Evaluated (minutes)	439	29	23	26

NOTE: Hospital profiles are in alphabetical order by state, then city, then hospital within the city; Rankings exclude hospitals with less than 25 cases except for patient surveys which excludes hospitals with less than 100 cases; (a) 100-299 cases; (1) The number of cases/patients is too few to report; (2) Data submitted were based on a sample of cases/patients; (3) Results are based on a shorter time period than required; (4) Data suppressed by CMS for one or more quarters; (5) Results are not available for this reporting period; (6) Fewer than 100 patients completed the HCAHPS survey; (7) No cases met the criteria for this measure; (8) The lower limit of the confidence interval cannot be calculated if the number of observed infections equals zero; (9) No data are available from the state/territory for this reporting period; (10) The scores shown reflect fewer than 50 completed surveys; (11) There were discrepancies in the data collection process; (12) This measure does not apply to this hospital for this reporting period; (13) Results cannot be calculated for this reporting period; (14) The results for this state are combined with nearby states to protect confidentiality; Please refer to the User's Guide for a full explanation of data.

Measure	Cases	This Hosp.	State Avg.	U.S. Avg.
Time to Pain Meds for Fractures (minutes)	84	70	56	57
Heart Attack Care				
Aspirin Given at Discharge[1]	-	-	99%	99%
Fibrinolytic Meds Within 30 Min. of Arrival[7]	-	-	-	54%
PCI Within 90 Minutes of Arrival[7]	-	-	97%	96%
Statin Prescribed at Discharge[1]	-	-	97%	98%
Heart Failure Care				
ACE Inhibitor or ARB for LVSD	28	82%	95%	97%
Discharge Instructions Given	87	89%	92%	94%
Evaluation of LVS Function	119	100%	98%	99%
Medicare Spending				
Medicare Spending per Patient (ratio)	-	0.93	0.97	0.98
Pneumonia Care				
Appropriate Initial Antibiotic Given	93	94%	94%	95%
Blood Culture Timing	115	98%	98%	98%
Pregnancy and Delivery Care				
Newborn Deliveries Scheduled Early[2]	17	18%	9%	6%
Preventive Care				
Immunization for Influenza[2]	277	91%	92%	90%
Immunization for Pneumonia[2]	337	94%	94%	92%
Stroke Care				
Anticoagulation Therapy for Atrial Fibrillation[1]	-	-	95%	95%
Antithrombotic Therapy Timing[1]	-	-	97%	98%
Assessed for Rehabilitation	11	100%	97%	97%
Discharged on Antithrombotic Therapy[1]	-	-	98%	99%
Discharged on Statin Medication[1]	-	-	93%	94%
Thrombolytic Therapy Timing[1]	-	-	59%	66%
Venous Thromboembolism Prophylaxis	11	45%	93%	94%
Written Stroke Educational Materials Given[1]	-	-	86%	88%
Surgical Care Improvement Project				
Appropriate Beta Blocker Usage[1]	-	-	98%	98%
Appropriate VTP Within 24 Hours	16	94%	98%	98%
Controlled Postoperative Blood Glucose[7]	-	-	96%	97%
Perioperative Temperature Management	21	100%	100%	100%
Prophylactic Antibiotic Selection	11	100%	99%	99%
Prophylactic Antibiotic Selection (Outpatient)	30	100%	97%	98%
Prophylactic Antibiotic Stopped[1]	-	-	98%	98%
Prophylactic Antibiotic Timing	11	100%	99%	99%
Prophylactic Antibiotic Timing (Outpatient)	30	100%	97%	98%
Urinary Catheter Removal[1]	-	-	97%	97%
Survey of Patients' Hospital Experiences				
Area Around Room 'Always' Quiet at Night	300+	68%	64%	61%
Doctors 'Always' Communicated Well	300+	89%	84%	82%
Home Recovery Information Given	300+	86%	86%	85%
Hospital Given 9 or 10 on 10 Point Scale	300+	69%	72%	71%
Meds 'Always' Explained Before Given	300+	67%	66%	64%
Nurses 'Always' Communicated Well	300+	79%	81%	79%
Pain 'Always' Well Controlled	300+	74%	73%	71%
Room and Bathroom 'Always' Clean	300+	73%	75%	73%
Timely Help 'Always' Received	300+	72%	69%	68%
Would Definitely Recommend Hospital	300+	65%	71%	71%
Use of Medical Imaging				
Cardiac Imaging Stress Test before Surgery	52	3.8%	5.3%	5.3%
Combination Abdominal CT Scan	383	19.8%	10.7%	10.5%
Combination Brain/Sinus CT Scan	469	4.1%	3.1%	2.7%
Combination Chest CT Scan	136	25.0%	4.3%	2.7%
Follow-up Mammogram/Ultrasound	272	14.7%	8.3%	8.8%
Lumbar Spine MRI for Low Back Pain	65	36.9%	38.9%	37.2%

Wayne County Hospital

166 Hospital Street
Monticello, KY 42633
Phone: 606-348-9343
Fax: 606-348-5796
E-mail: wchospital@kih.net
URL: www.waynehospital.org
Type: Critical Access Hospitals
Emergency Services: Yes
Ownership: Voluntary non-profit - Other
Beds: 30

Key Personnel:
Emergency Room . . . . Patricia Brenson
Chief of Medical Staff . . . . Walter Koscrenski
CEO . . . . Daren L. Relph, PS-CCP

Measure	Cases	This Hosp.	State Avg.	U.S. Avg.
Blood Clot Prevention and Treatment				
Anticoagulation Overlap Therapy[5]	-	-	90%	93%
ICU Venous Thromboembolism Prophylaxis[5]	-	-	86%	92%
Incidence of Potentially Preventable VTE[5]	-	-	13%	10%
UFH with Dosages/Platelet Monitoring[5]	-	-	98%	97%
Venous Thromboembolism Prophylaxis[5]	-	-	80%	85%
Warfarin Therapy Discharge Instructions[5]	-	-	72%	75%
Chest Pain/Possible Heart Attack Care				
Aspirin Given Within 24 Hours of Arrival[5]	-	-	97%	96%
Fibrinolytic Meds Within 30 Min. of Arrival[5]	-	-	63%	58%
Average Time to ECG (minutes)[5]	-	-	6	7
Average Time to Transfer (minutes)[5]	-	-	61	60
Children's Asthma Care				
Received Home Management Plan of Care	-	-	-	88%
Received Reliever Medication	-	-	-	100%
Received Systemic Corticosteroids	-	-	-	100%
Emergency Department				
Admittance Decision Time (minutes)[5]	-	-	78	98
Head CT Results Within 45 Min. of Arrival[5]	-	-	55%	57%
Patients Who Left ER Before Being Seen	11,230	2%	2%	2%
Time from ER Arrival to Admit. (minutes)[5]	-	-	238	274
Time from ER Arrival to Discharge (minutes)[5]	-	-	126	134
Time in ER Before Being Evaluated (minutes)[5]	-	-	23	26
Time to Pain Meds for Fractures (minutes)[5]	-	-	56	57
Heart Attack Care				
Aspirin Given at Discharge[3,7]	-	-	99%	99%
Fibrinolytic Meds Within 30 Min. of Arrival[3,7]	-	-	-	54%
PCI Within 90 Minutes of Arrival[3,7]	-	-	97%	96%
Statin Prescribed at Discharge[3,7]	-	-	97%	98%
Heart Failure Care				
ACE Inhibitor or ARB for LVSD[1,2]	-	-	95%	97%
Discharge Instructions Given[2]	15	100%	92%	94%
Evaluation of LVS Function[2]	17	100%	98%	99%
Medicare Spending				
Medicare Spending per Patient (ratio)	-	-	0.97	0.98
Pneumonia Care				
Appropriate Initial Antibiotic Given	48	100%	94%	95%
Blood Culture Timing	57	100%	98%	98%
Pregnancy and Delivery Care				
Newborn Deliveries Scheduled Early[5]	-	-	9%	6%
Preventive Care				
Immunization for Influenza[5]	-	-	92%	90%
Immunization for Pneumonia[5]	-	-	94%	92%
Stroke Care				
Anticoagulation Therapy for Atrial Fibrillation[5]	-	-	95%	95%
Antithrombotic Therapy Timing[5]	-	-	97%	98%
Assessed for Rehabilitation[5]	-	-	97%	97%
Discharged on Antithrombotic Therapy[5]	-	-	98%	99%
Discharged on Statin Medication[5]	-	-	93%	94%
Thrombolytic Therapy Timing[5]	-	-	59%	66%
Venous Thromboembolism Prophylaxis[5]	-	-	93%	94%
Written Stroke Educational Materials Given[5]	-	-	86%	88%
Surgical Care Improvement Project				
Appropriate Beta Blocker Usage[5]	-	-	98%	98%
Appropriate VTP Within 24 Hours[5]	-	-	98%	98%
Controlled Postoperative Blood Glucose[5]	-	-	96%	97%
Perioperative Temperature Management[5]	-	-	100%	100%
Prophylactic Antibiotic Selection[5]	-	-	99%	99%
Prophylactic Antibiotic Selection (Outpatient)[5]	-	-	97%	98%
Prophylactic Antibiotic Stopped[5]	-	-	98%	98%
Prophylactic Antibiotic Timing[5]	-	-	99%	99%
Prophylactic Antibiotic Timing (Outpatient)[5]	-	-	97%	98%
Urinary Catheter Removal[5]	-	-	97%	97%
Survey of Patients' Hospital Experiences				
Area Around Room 'Always' Quiet at Night	(a)	70%	64%	61%
Doctors 'Always' Communicated Well	(a)	93%	84%	82%
Home Recovery Information Given	(a)	92%	86%	85%
Hospital Given 9 or 10 on 10 Point Scale	(a)	79%	72%	71%
Meds 'Always' Explained Before Given	(a)	73%	66%	64%
Nurses 'Always' Communicated Well	(a)	86%	81%	79%
Pain 'Always' Well Controlled	(a)	81%	73%	71%
Room and Bathroom 'Always' Clean	(a)	80%	75%	73%
Timely Help 'Always' Received	(a)	71%	69%	68%
Would Definitely Recommend Hospital	(a)	77%	71%	71%
Use of Medical Imaging				
Cardiac Imaging Stress Test before Surgery[7]	-	-	5.3%	5.3%
Combination Abdominal CT Scan	325	1.8%	10.7%	10.5%
Combination Brain/Sinus CT Scan	285	1.1%	3.1%	2.7%
Combination Chest CT Scan	114	4.4%	4.3%	2.7%
Follow-up Mammogram/Ultrasound	276	9.1%	8.3%	8.8%
Lumbar Spine MRI for Low Back Pain[1]	-	-	38.9%	37.2%

Saint Claire Regional Medical Center

222 Medical Circle
Morehead, KY 40351
Phone: 606-783-6500
Fax: 606-783-6503
E-mail: mjneff@st-claire.org
URL: www.st-claire.org
Type: Acute Care Hospitals
Emergency Services: Yes
Ownership: Government - Federal
Beds: 159

Key Personnel:
Operating Room. . . . . Lisa Amburgey
Radiology. . . . . Charles Butler
Quality Assurance . . . . Linda Fultz
Infection Control. . . . . Charlette Kinney
Cardiac Laboratory. . . . . Charlotte Lewis
Pediatric In-Patient Care . . . . Nancy Maggard
Chief of Medical Staff . . . . Will Mehlan, MD
CEO/President. . . . . Mark J Neff

Measure	Cases	This Hosp.	State Avg.	U.S. Avg.
Blood Clot Prevention and Treatment				
Anticoagulation Overlap Therapy[2]	22	73%	90%	93%
ICU Venous Thromboembolism Prophylaxis[2]	142	89%	86%	92%
Incidence of Potentially Preventable VTE[1,2]	-	-	13%	10%
UFH with Dosages/Platelet Monitoring[2]	15	100%	98%	97%
Venous Thromboembolism Prophylaxis[2]	286	89%	80%	85%
Warfarin Therapy Discharge Instructions[2]	19	100%	72%	75%
Chest Pain/Possible Heart Attack Care				
Aspirin Given Within 24 Hours of Arrival	24	96%	97%	96%
Fibrinolytic Meds Within 30 Min. of Arrival[3,7]	-	-	63%	58%
Average Time to ECG (minutes)	24	6	6	7
Average Time to Transfer (minutes)[1,3]	-	-	61	60
Children's Asthma Care				
Received Home Management Plan of Care[1]	-	-	-	88%
Received Reliever Medication[1]	-	-	-	100%
Received Systemic Corticosteroids[1]	-	-	-	100%
Emergency Department				
Admittance Decision Time (minutes)[2]	405	65	78	98
Head CT Results Within 45 Min. of Arrival	18	61%	55%	57%
Patients Who Left ER Before Being Seen	28,534	1%	2%	2%
Time from ER Arrival to Admit. (minutes)[2]	590	207	238	274
Time from ER Arrival to Discharge (minutes)	369	138	126	134
Time in ER Before Being Evaluated (minutes)	245	23	23	26
Time to Pain Meds for Fractures (minutes)	83	74	56	57
Heart Attack Care				
Aspirin Given at Discharge	133	100%	99%	99%
Fibrinolytic Meds Within 30 Min. of Arrival[7]	-	-	-	54%
PCI Within 90 Minutes of Arrival	31	90%	97%	96%
Statin Prescribed at Discharge	128	98%	97%	98%
Heart Failure Care				
ACE Inhibitor or ARB for LVSD	41	100%	95%	97%
Discharge Instructions Given	126	95%	92%	94%
Evaluation of LVS Function	163	100%	98%	99%
Medicare Spending				
Medicare Spending per Patient (ratio)	-	0.99	0.97	0.98
Pneumonia Care				
Appropriate Initial Antibiotic Given	117	94%	94%	95%
Blood Culture Timing	237	97%	98%	98%
Pregnancy and Delivery Care				
Newborn Deliveries Scheduled Early	40	10%	9%	6%
Preventive Care				
Immunization for Influenza[2]	454	91%	92%	90%
Immunization for Pneumonia[2]	576	93%	94%	92%
Stroke Care				
Anticoagulation Therapy for Atrial Fibrillation[1]	-	-	95%	95%
Antithrombotic Therapy Timing	27	100%	97%	98%
Assessed for Rehabilitation	30	90%	97%	97%
Discharged on Antithrombotic Therapy	29	97%	98%	99%
Discharged on Statin Medication	25	84%	93%	94%

NOTE: Hospital profiles are in alphabetical order by state, then city, then hospital within the city; Rankings exclude hospitals with less than 25 cases except for patient surveys which excludes hospitals with less than 100 cases; (a) 100-299 cases; (1) The number of cases/patients is too few to report; (2) Data submitted were based on a sample of cases/patients; (3) Results are based on a shorter time period than required; (4) Data suppressed by CMS for one or more quarters; (5) Results are not available for this reporting period; (6) Fewer than 100 patients completed the HCAHPS survey; (7) No cases met the criteria for this measure; (8) The lower limit of the confidence interval cannot be calculated if the number of observed infections equals zero; (9) No data are available from the state/territory for this reporting period; (10) The scores shown reflect fewer than 50 completed surveys; (11) There were discrepancies in the data collection process; (12) This measure does not apply to this hospital for this reporting period; (13) Results cannot be calculated for this reporting period; (14) The results for this state are combined with nearby states to protect confidentiality; Please refer to the User's Guide for a full explanation of data.

Thrombolytic Therapy Timing[1]	-	-	59%	66%
Venous Thromboembolism Prophylaxis	20	85%	93%	94%
Written Stroke Educational Materials Given	17	76%	86%	88%
Surgical Care Improvement Project				
Appropriate Beta Blocker Usage[2]	51	98%	98%	98%
Appropriate VTP Within 24 Hours[2]	143	99%	98%	98%
Controlled Postoperative Blood Glucose[2,7]	-	-	96%	97%
Perioperative Temperature Management[2]	204	100%	100%	100%
Prophylactic Antibiotic Selection[2]	104	93%	99%	99%
Prophylactic Antibiotic Selection (Outpatient)	114	93%	97%	98%
Prophylactic Antibiotic Stopped[2]	100	91%	98%	98%
Prophylactic Antibiotic Timing[2]	105	95%	99%	99%
Prophylactic Antibiotic Timing (Outpatient)	73	97%	97%	98%
Urinary Catheter Removal[2]	117	96%	97%	97%
Survey of Patients' Hospital Experiences				
Area Around Room 'Always' Quiet at Night	300+	56%	64%	61%
Doctors 'Always' Communicated Well	300+	85%	84%	82%
Home Recovery Information Given	300+	89%	86%	85%
Hospital Given 9 or 10 on 10 Point Scale	300+	73%	72%	71%
Meds 'Always' Explained Before Given	300+	75%	66%	64%
Nurses 'Always' Communicated Well	300+	85%	81%	79%
Pain 'Always' Well Controlled	300+	72%	73%	71%
Room and Bathroom 'Always' Clean	300+	79%	75%	73%
Timely Help 'Always' Received	300+	71%	69%	68%
Would Definitely Recommend Hospital	300+	70%	71%	71%
Use of Medical Imaging				
Cardiac Imaging Stress Test before Surgery	434	4.6%	5.3%	5.3%
Combination Abdominal CT Scan	716	1.4%	10.7%	10.5%
Combination Brain/Sinus CT Scan	652	4.0%	3.1%	2.7%
Combination Chest CT Scan	405	2.0%	4.3%	2.7%
Follow-up Mammogram/Ultrasound	728	10.9%	8.3%	8.8%
Lumbar Spine MRI for Low Back Pain	107	46.7%	38.9%	37.2%

Methodist Hospital Union County

4604 Us Highway 60 West
Morganfield, KY 42437
Phone: 270-389-3030
Fax: 270-389-5059
E-mail: pdonahue@methodisthospital.net
URL: www.methodisthospitaluc.net
Type: Critical Access Hospitals
Emergency Services: Yes
Ownership: Voluntary non-profit - Church
Beds: 25

Key Personnel:
Emergency Room . . . . William Clapp, MD
Coronary Care . . . . Peggy Creighton, RN
Pediatric In-Patient Care . . . . Peggy Creighton, RN
Chief of Medical Staff . . . . William Guyette, MD
Radiology . . . . William Guyette, MD
Operating Room . . . . Vinod Joni, MD
Infection Control . . . . Marie White, RN
Quality Assurance . . . . Marie Whits, RN

Measure	Cases	This Hosp.	State Avg.	U.S. Avg.
Blood Clot Prevention and Treatment				
Anticoagulation Overlap Therapy[5]	-	-	90%	93%
ICU Venous Thromboembolism Prophylaxis[5]	-	-	86%	92%
Incidence of Potentially Preventable VTE[5]	-	-	13%	10%
UFH with Dosages/Platelet Monitoring[5]	-	-	98%	97%
Venous Thromboembolism Prophylaxis[5]	-	-	80%	85%
Warfarin Therapy Discharge Instructions[5]	-	-	72%	75%
Chest Pain/Possible Heart Attack Care				
Aspirin Given Within 24 Hours of Arrival[5]	-	-	97%	96%
Fibrinolytic Meds Within 30 Min. of Arrival[5]	-	-	63%	58%
Average Time to ECG (minutes)[5]	-	-	6	7
Average Time to Transfer (minutes)[5]	-	-	61	60
Children's Asthma Care				
Received Home Management Plan of Care	-	-	-	88%
Received Reliever Medication	-	-	-	100%
Received Systemic Corticosteroids	-	-	-	100%
Emergency Department				
Admittance Decision Time (minutes)[5]	-	-	78	98
Head CT Results Within 45 Min. of Arrival[5]	-	-	55%	57%
Patients Who Left ER Before Being Seen	8,236	0%	2%	2%
Time from ER Arrival to Admit. (minutes)[5]	-	-	238	274
Time from ER Arrival to Discharge (minutes)[5]	-	-	126	134
Time in ER Before Being Evaluated (minutes)[5]	-	-	23	26
Time to Pain Meds for Fractures (minutes)[5]	-	-	56	57
Heart Attack Care				
Aspirin Given at Discharge[5]	-	-	99%	99%
Fibrinolytic Meds Within 30 Min. of Arrival[5]	-	-	-	54%
PCI Within 90 Minutes of Arrival[5]	-	-	97%	96%
Statin Prescribed at Discharge[5]	-	-	97%	98%
Heart Failure Care				
ACE Inhibitor or ARB for LVSD[1]	-	-	95%	97%
Discharge Instructions Given	16	100%	92%	94%
Evaluation of LVS Function	21	95%	98%	99%
Medicare Spending				
Medicare Spending per Patient (ratio)	-	-	0.97	0.98
Pneumonia Care				
Appropriate Initial Antibiotic Given	46	91%	94%	95%
Blood Culture Timing	39	82%	98%	98%
Pregnancy and Delivery Care				
Newborn Deliveries Scheduled Early[3,7]	-	-	9%	6%
Preventive Care				
Immunization for Influenza[5]	-	-	92%	90%
Immunization for Pneumonia[5]	-	-	94%	92%
Stroke Care				
Anticoagulation Therapy for Atrial Fibrillation[5]	-	-	95%	95%
Antithrombotic Therapy Timing[5]	-	-	97%	98%
Assessed for Rehabilitation[5]	-	-	97%	97%
Discharged on Antithrombotic Therapy[5]	-	-	98%	99%
Discharged on Statin Medication[5]	-	-	93%	94%
Thrombolytic Therapy Timing[5]	-	-	59%	66%
Venous Thromboembolism Prophylaxis[5]	-	-	93%	94%
Written Stroke Educational Materials Given[5]	-	-	86%	88%
Surgical Care Improvement Project				
Appropriate Beta Blocker Usage[5]	-	-	98%	98%
Appropriate VTP Within 24 Hours[5]	-	-	98%	98%
Controlled Postoperative Blood Glucose[5]	-	-	96%	97%
Perioperative Temperature Management[5]	-	-	100%	100%
Prophylactic Antibiotic Selection[5]	-	-	99%	99%
Prophylactic Antibiotic Selection (Outpatient)[5]	-	-	97%	98%
Prophylactic Antibiotic Stopped[5]	-	-	98%	98%
Prophylactic Antibiotic Timing[5]	-	-	99%	99%
Prophylactic Antibiotic Timing (Outpatient)[5]	-	-	97%	98%
Urinary Catheter Removal[5]	-	-	97%	97%
Survey of Patients' Hospital Experiences				
Area Around Room 'Always' Quiet at Night	(a)	73%	64%	61%
Doctors 'Always' Communicated Well	(a)	85%	84%	82%
Home Recovery Information Given	(a)	81%	86%	85%
Hospital Given 9 or 10 on 10 Point Scale	(a)	68%	72%	71%
Meds 'Always' Explained Before Given	(a)	60%	66%	64%
Nurses 'Always' Communicated Well	(a)	80%	81%	79%
Pain 'Always' Well Controlled	(a)	75%	73%	71%
Room and Bathroom 'Always' Clean	(a)	74%	75%	73%
Timely Help 'Always' Received	(a)	70%	69%	68%
Would Definitely Recommend Hospital	(a)	68%	71%	71%
Use of Medical Imaging				
Cardiac Imaging Stress Test before Surgery[7]	-	-	5.3%	5.3%
Combination Abdominal CT Scan	128	7.8%	10.7%	10.5%
Combination Brain/Sinus CT Scan[1]	-	-	3.1%	2.7%
Combination Chest CT Scan	74	2.7%	4.3%	2.7%
Follow-up Mammogram/Ultrasound	238	2.5%	8.3%	8.8%
Lumbar Spine MRI for Low Back Pain[7]	-	-	38.9%	37.2%

Saint Joseph Mount Sterling

225 Falcon Drive
Mount Sterling, KY 40353
Phone: 859-498-1220
Fax: 859-498-5155
URL: www.marychiles.org
Type: Acute Care Hospitals
Emergency Services: Yes
Ownership: Voluntary non-profit - Private
Beds: 63

Key Personnel:
Operating Room . . . . Sheila Barnes, RN
Radiology . . . . Tim Damron
Pediatric In-Patient Care . . . . Rick Hall, MD
Patient Relations . . . . Tammye Hood, RN
Chief of Medical Staff . . . . John Merryman, MD
Infection Control . . . . Lisa Ray, RN
CEO/President . . . . Patrick A Romano, JR
Surgery . . . . Dr. Ryan Sutherland, MD

Measure	Cases	This Hosp.	State Avg.	U.S. Avg.
Blood Clot Prevention and Treatment				
Anticoagulation Overlap Therapy	20	90%	90%	93%
ICU Venous Thromboembolism Prophylaxis	161	72%	86%	92%
Incidence of Potentially Preventable VTE[1]	-	-	13%	10%
UFH with Dosages/Platelet Monitoring[1]	-	-	98%	97%
Venous Thromboembolism Prophylaxis	732	68%	80%	85%
Warfarin Therapy Discharge Instructions	13	92%	72%	75%
Chest Pain/Possible Heart Attack Care				
Aspirin Given Within 24 Hours of Arrival	104	93%	97%	96%
Fibrinolytic Meds Within 30 Min. of Arrival[1]	-	-	63%	58%
Average Time to ECG (minutes)	113	6	6	7
Average Time to Transfer (minutes)[1]	-	-	61	60
Children's Asthma Care				
Received Home Management Plan of Care	-	-	-	88%
Received Reliever Medication	-	-	-	100%
Received Systemic Corticosteroids	-	-	-	100%
Emergency Department				
Admittance Decision Time (minutes)	905	66	78	98
Head CT Results Within 45 Min. of Arrival[1]	-	-	55%	57%
Patients Who Left ER Before Being Seen	24,509	5%	2%	2%
Time from ER Arrival to Admit. (minutes)	1,053	257	238	274
Time from ER Arrival to Discharge (minutes)	369	139	126	134
Time in ER Before Being Evaluated (minutes)	404	40	23	26
Time to Pain Meds for Fractures (minutes)	130	87	56	57
Heart Attack Care				
Aspirin Given at Discharge[1]	-	-	99%	99%
Fibrinolytic Meds Within 30 Min. of Arrival[7]	-	-	-	54%
PCI Within 90 Minutes of Arrival[7]	-	-	97%	96%
Statin Prescribed at Discharge[1]	-	-	97%	98%
Heart Failure Care				
ACE Inhibitor or ARB for LVSD	11	100%	95%	97%
Discharge Instructions Given	32	91%	92%	94%
Evaluation of LVS Function	44	100%	98%	99%
Medicare Spending				
Medicare Spending per Patient (ratio)	-	1.00	0.97	0.98
Pneumonia Care				
Appropriate Initial Antibiotic Given	128	92%	94%	95%
Blood Culture Timing	182	97%	98%	98%
Pregnancy and Delivery Care				
Newborn Deliveries Scheduled Early	31	6%	9%	6%
Preventive Care				
Immunization for Influenza	992	96%	92%	90%
Immunization for Pneumonia	1,268	99%	94%	92%
Stroke Care				
Anticoagulation Therapy for Atrial Fibrillation[1]	-	-	95%	95%
Antithrombotic Therapy Timing	14	93%	97%	98%
Assessed for Rehabilitation	11	100%	97%	97%
Discharged on Antithrombotic Therapy[1]	-	-	98%	99%
Discharged on Statin Medication[1]	-	-	93%	94%
Thrombolytic Therapy Timing[1]	-	-	59%	66%
Venous Thromboembolism Prophylaxis	13	77%	93%	94%
Written Stroke Educational Materials Given[1]	-	-	86%	88%
Surgical Care Improvement Project				
Appropriate Beta Blocker Usage	91	93%	98%	98%
Appropriate VTP Within 24 Hours	251	98%	98%	98%
Controlled Postoperative Blood Glucose[7]	-	-	96%	97%
Perioperative Temperature Management	270	100%	100%	100%
Prophylactic Antibiotic Selection	240	100%	99%	99%
Prophylactic Antibiotic Selection (Outpatient)	29	93%	97%	98%
Prophylactic Antibiotic Stopped	234	99%	98%	98%
Prophylactic Antibiotic Timing	240	98%	99%	99%
Prophylactic Antibiotic Timing (Outpatient)	26	92%	97%	98%
Urinary Catheter Removal	230	98%	97%	97%
Survey of Patients' Hospital Experiences				
Area Around Room 'Always' Quiet at Night	300+	68%	64%	61%
Doctors 'Always' Communicated Well	300+	82%	84%	82%
Home Recovery Information Given	300+	89%	86%	85%
Hospital Given 9 or 10 on 10 Point Scale	300+	76%	72%	71%
Meds 'Always' Explained Before Given	300+	69%	66%	64%
Nurses 'Always' Communicated Well	300+	81%	81%	79%
Pain 'Always' Well Controlled	300+	77%	73%	71%
Room and Bathroom 'Always' Clean	300+	79%	75%	73%

NOTE: Hospital profiles are in alphabetical order by state, then city, then hospital within the city; Rankings exclude hospitals with less than 25 cases except for patient surveys which excludes hospitals with less than 100 cases; (a) 100-299 cases; (1) The number of cases/patients is too few to report; (2) Data submitted were based on a sample of cases/patients; (3) Results are based on a shorter time period than required; (4) Data suppressed by CMS for one or more quarters; (5) Results are not available for this reporting period; (6) Fewer than 100 patients completed the HCAHPS survey; (7) No cases met the criteria for this measure; (8) The lower limit of the confidence interval cannot be calculated if the number of observed infections equals zero; (9) No data are available from the state/territory for this reporting period; (10) The scores shown reflect fewer than 50 completed surveys; (11) There were discrepancies in the data collection process; (12) This measure does not apply to this hospital for this reporting period; (13) Results cannot be calculated for this reporting period; (14) The results for this state are combined with nearby states to protect confidentiality; Please refer to the User's Guide for a full explanation of data.

Timely Help 'Always' Received	300+	69%	69%	68%
Would Definitely Recommend Hospital	300+	77%	71%	71%
Use of Medical Imaging				
Cardiac Imaging Stress Test before Surgery	174	2.9%	5.3%	5.3%
Combination Abdominal CT Scan	554	9.6%	10.7%	10.5%
Combination Brain/Sinus CT Scan	618	5.5%	3.1%	2.7%
Combination Chest CT Scan	233	0.4%	4.3%	2.7%
Follow-up Mammogram/Ultrasound	429	5.6%	8.3%	8.8%
Lumbar Spine MRI for Low Back Pain	88	48.9%	38.9%	37.2%

Rockcastle County Hospital

145 Newcomb Avenue
Mount Vernon, KY 40456
Phone: 606-256-2195
Fax: 606-256-3232
URL: www.rockcastlehospital.com
Type: Acute Care Hospitals
Emergency Services: Yes
Ownership: Voluntary non-profit - Private
Beds: 86

Key Personnel:
Chief of Medical Staff.......... Jon Arvin
Infection Control............. Traci Bullens
Quality Assurance .... Stephen Estes
CEO/President............... Stephen A Estes
Radiology.................. Eduard Gomez
Operating Room............. Christian Knecht
Emergency Room .... William P McElwain, MD
Anesthesiology............... Tiffany Patrick

Measure	Cases	This Hosp.	State Avg.	U.S. Avg.
Blood Clot Prevention and Treatment				
Anticoagulation Overlap Therapy[1,2]	-	-	90%	93%
ICU Venous Thromboembolism Prophylaxis[2,7]	-	-	86%	92%
Incidence of Potentially Preventable VTE[2,7]	-	-	13%	10%
UFH with Dosages/Platelet Monitoring[2,7]	-	-	98%	97%
Venous Thromboembolism Prophylaxis[2]	110	67%	80%	85%
Warfarin Therapy Discharge Instructions[1,2]	-	-	72%	75%
Chest Pain/Possible Heart Attack Care				
Aspirin Given Within 24 Hours of Arrival	55	96%	97%	96%
Fibrinolytic Meds Within 30 Min. of Arrival[7]	-	-	63%	58%
Average Time to ECG (minutes)	55	3	6	7
Average Time to Transfer (minutes)[1]	-	-	61	60
Children's Asthma Care				
Received Home Management Plan of Care	-	-	-	88%
Received Reliever Medication	-	-	-	100%
Received Systemic Corticosteroids	-	-	-	100%
Emergency Department				
Admittance Decision Time (minutes)[2]	432	47	78	98
Head CT Results Within 45 Min. of Arrival[1]	-	-	55%	57%
Patients Who Left ER Before Being Seen	11,564	2%	2%	2%
Time from ER Arrival to Admit. (minutes)[2]	450	188	238	274
Time from ER Arrival to Discharge (minutes)	373	91	126	134
Time in ER Before Being Evaluated (minutes)	410	15	23	26
Time to Pain Meds for Fractures (minutes)	26	42	56	57
Heart Attack Care				
Aspirin Given at Discharge[1]	-	-	99%	99%
Fibrinolytic Meds Within 30 Min. of Arrival[7]	-	-	-	54%
PCI Within 90 Minutes of Arrival[7]	-	-	97%	96%
Statin Prescribed at Discharge[1]	-	-	97%	98%
Heart Failure Care				
ACE Inhibitor or ARB for LVSD[1]	-	-	95%	97%
Discharge Instructions Given	29	100%	92%	94%
Evaluation of LVS Function	44	100%	98%	99%
Medicare Spending				
Medicare Spending per Patient (ratio)	-	0.95	0.97	0.98
Pneumonia Care				
Appropriate Initial Antibiotic Given	33	97%	94%	95%
Blood Culture Timing	29	97%	98%	98%
Pregnancy and Delivery Care				
Newborn Deliveries Scheduled Early[7]	-	-	9%	6%
Preventive Care				
Immunization for Influenza[2]	299	88%	92%	90%
Immunization for Pneumonia[2]	465	94%	94%	92%
Stroke Care				
Anticoagulation Therapy for Atrial Fibrillation[7]	-	-	95%	95%
Antithrombotic Therapy Timing[1]	-	-	97%	98%
Assessed for Rehabilitation[1]	-	-	97%	97%
Discharged on Antithrombotic Therapy[1]	-	-	98%	99%
Discharged on Statin Medication[1]	-	-	93%	94%
Thrombolytic Therapy Timing[7]	-	-	59%	66%
Venous Thromboembolism Prophylaxis[1]	-	-	93%	94%
Written Stroke Educational Materials Given[1]	-	-	86%	88%
Surgical Care Improvement Project				
Appropriate Beta Blocker Usage[5]	-	-	98%	98%
Appropriate VTP Within 24 Hours[5]	-	-	98%	98%
Controlled Postoperative Blood Glucose[5]	-	-	96%	97%
Perioperative Temperature Management[5]	-	-	100%	100%
Prophylactic Antibiotic Selection[5]	-	-	99%	99%
Prophylactic Antibiotic Selection (Outpatient)[1,3]	-	-	97%	98%
Prophylactic Antibiotic Stopped[5]	-	-	98%	98%
Prophylactic Antibiotic Timing[5]	-	-	99%	99%
Prophylactic Antibiotic Timing (Outpatient)[1,3]	-	-	97%	98%
Urinary Catheter Removal[5]	-	-	97%	97%
Survey of Patients' Hospital Experiences				
Area Around Room 'Always' Quiet at Night	(a)	72%	64%	61%
Doctors 'Always' Communicated Well	(a)	90%	84%	82%
Home Recovery Information Given	(a)	86%	86%	85%
Hospital Given 9 or 10 on 10 Point Scale	(a)	81%	72%	71%
Meds 'Always' Explained Before Given	(a)	76%	66%	64%
Nurses 'Always' Communicated Well	(a)	89%	81%	79%
Pain 'Always' Well Controlled	(a)	83%	73%	71%
Room and Bathroom 'Always' Clean	(a)	88%	75%	73%
Timely Help 'Always' Received	(a)	75%	69%	68%
Would Definitely Recommend Hospital	(a)	82%	71%	71%
Use of Medical Imaging				
Cardiac Imaging Stress Test before Surgery	155	0.6%	5.3%	5.3%
Combination Abdominal CT Scan	282	22.7%	10.7%	10.5%
Combination Brain/Sinus CT Scan[1]	-	-	3.1%	2.7%
Combination Chest CT Scan	128	23.4%	4.3%	2.7%
Follow-up Mammogram/Ultrasound	341	4.1%	8.3%	8.8%
Lumbar Spine MRI for Low Back Pain	50	44.0%	38.9%	37.2%

Murray - Calloway County Hospital

803 Poplar Street
Murray, KY 42071
Phone: 270-762-1100
Fax: 270-767-3600
E-mail: info@murrayhospital.org
URL: www.murrayhospital.org
Type: Acute Care Hospitals
Emergency Services: Yes
Ownership: Voluntary non-profit - Other
Beds: 366

Key Personnel:
Chief of Medical Staff.......... Dr Richard Crouch, MD
Emergency Room .... Jerry Edwards, MD
Operating Room............. Mary Hension, RN
Intensive Care Unit............ Jeanne Mathis, RN
Radiology.................. Felipe Patino
CEO/President............... Jerry Penner III
Patient Relations .... Allen Peters
Infection Control............. Lisa Ray, RN

Measure	Cases	This Hosp.	State Avg.	U.S. Avg.
Blood Clot Prevention and Treatment				
Anticoagulation Overlap Therapy[1,2]	-	-	90%	93%
ICU Venous Thromboembolism Prophylaxis[2]	57	70%	86%	92%
Incidence of Potentially Preventable VTE[1,2]	-	-	13%	10%
UFH with Dosages/Platelet Monitoring[1,2]	-	-	98%	97%
Venous Thromboembolism Prophylaxis[2]	317	56%	80%	85%
Warfarin Therapy Discharge Instructions[1,2]	-	-	72%	75%
Chest Pain/Possible Heart Attack Care				
Aspirin Given Within 24 Hours of Arrival	72	97%	97%	96%
Fibrinolytic Meds Within 30 Min. of Arrival[7]	-	-	63%	58%
Average Time to ECG (minutes)	74	10	6	7
Average Time to Transfer (minutes)[1]	-	-	61	60
Children's Asthma Care				
Received Home Management Plan of Care	-	-	-	88%
Received Reliever Medication	-	-	-	100%
Received Systemic Corticosteroids	-	-	-	100%
Emergency Department				
Admittance Decision Time (minutes)[2]	359	70	78	98
Head CT Results Within 45 Min. of Arrival	18	33%	55%	57%
Patients Who Left ER Before Being Seen	18,279	2%	2%	2%
Time from ER Arrival to Admit. (minutes)[2]	366	244	238	274
Time from ER Arrival to Discharge (minutes)	390	135	126	134
Time in ER Before Being Evaluated (minutes)	406	28	23	26
Time to Pain Meds for Fractures (minutes)	81	70	56	57
Heart Attack Care				
Aspirin Given at Discharge	14	86%	99%	99%
Fibrinolytic Meds Within 30 Min. of Arrival[7]	-	-	-	54%
PCI Within 90 Minutes of Arrival[7]	-	-	97%	96%
Statin Prescribed at Discharge	15	47%	97%	98%
Heart Failure Care				
ACE Inhibitor or ARB for LVSD	23	61%	95%	97%
Discharge Instructions Given	87	41%	92%	94%
Evaluation of LVS Function	99	85%	98%	99%
Medicare Spending				
Medicare Spending per Patient (ratio)	-	0.97	0.97	0.98
Pneumonia Care				
Appropriate Initial Antibiotic Given	116	80%	94%	95%
Blood Culture Timing	118	93%	98%	98%
Pregnancy and Delivery Care				
Newborn Deliveries Scheduled Early	65	26%	9%	6%
Preventive Care				
Immunization for Influenza[2]	426	51%	92%	90%
Immunization for Pneumonia[2]	507	62%	94%	92%
Stroke Care				
Anticoagulation Therapy for Atrial Fibrillation[1]	-	-	95%	95%
Antithrombotic Therapy Timing	35	94%	97%	98%
Assessed for Rehabilitation	40	80%	97%	97%
Discharged on Antithrombotic Therapy	37	89%	98%	99%
Discharged on Statin Medication	31	84%	93%	94%
Thrombolytic Therapy Timing	13	0%	59%	66%
Venous Thromboembolism Prophylaxis	40	55%	93%	94%
Written Stroke Educational Materials Given	22	45%	86%	88%
Surgical Care Improvement Project				
Appropriate Beta Blocker Usage	161	96%	98%	98%
Appropriate VTP Within 24 Hours	458	98%	98%	98%
Controlled Postoperative Blood Glucose[7]	-	-	96%	97%
Perioperative Temperature Management	505	100%	100%	100%
Prophylactic Antibiotic Selection	376	99%	99%	99%
Prophylactic Antibiotic Selection (Outpatient)	160	87%	97%	98%
Prophylactic Antibiotic Stopped	374	98%	98%	98%
Prophylactic Antibiotic Timing	376	99%	99%	99%
Prophylactic Antibiotic Timing (Outpatient)	161	99%	97%	98%
Urinary Catheter Removal	448	99%	97%	97%
Survey of Patients' Hospital Experiences				
Area Around Room 'Always' Quiet at Night	300+	68%	64%	61%
Doctors 'Always' Communicated Well	300+	87%	84%	82%
Home Recovery Information Given	300+	86%	86%	85%
Hospital Given 9 or 10 on 10 Point Scale	300+	71%	72%	71%
Meds 'Always' Explained Before Given	300+	62%	66%	64%
Nurses 'Always' Communicated Well	300+	81%	81%	79%
Pain 'Always' Well Controlled	300+	71%	73%	71%
Room and Bathroom 'Always' Clean	300+	76%	75%	73%
Timely Help 'Always' Received	300+	71%	69%	68%
Would Definitely Recommend Hospital	300+	70%	71%	71%
Use of Medical Imaging				
Cardiac Imaging Stress Test before Surgery	253	6.3%	5.3%	5.3%
Combination Abdominal CT Scan	590	11.4%	10.7%	10.5%
Combination Brain/Sinus CT Scan	521	6.0%	3.1%	2.7%
Combination Chest CT Scan	350	7.7%	4.3%	2.7%
Follow-up Mammogram/Ultrasound	1,091	3.2%	8.3%	8.8%
Lumbar Spine MRI for Low Back Pain	87	31.0%	38.9%	37.2%

Owensboro Health Regional Hospital

1201 Pleasant Valley Road
Owensboro, KY 42303
Phone: 270-688-2000
Fax: 270-685-7195
URL: www.omhs.org
Type: Acute Care Hospitals
Emergency Services: Yes
Ownership: Voluntary non-profit - Private
Beds: 447

Key Personnel:
Cardiac Laboratory............ Liz Belt
Quality Assurance .... Pam Cox
Emergency Room .... Debbie Eoch
Operating Room............. Marti Gaw
Chief of Medical Staff.......... R. Wathen Medley, MD
CEO/President............... Philip Patterson, FACHE
Radiology.................. Donna Ross
Surgery.................... Michael Scherm, MD

NOTE: Hospital profiles are in alphabetical order by state, then city, then hospital within the city; Rankings exclude hospitals with less than 25 cases except for patient surveys which excludes hospitals with less than 100 cases; (a) 100-299 cases; (1) The number of cases/patients is too few to report; (2) Data submitted were based on a sample of cases/patients; (3) Results are based on a shorter time period than required; (4) Data suppressed by CMS for one or more quarters; (5) Results are not available for this reporting period; (6) Fewer than 100 patients completed the HCAHPS survey; (7) No cases met the criteria for this measure; (8) The lower limit of the confidence interval cannot be calculated if the number of observed infections equals zero; (9) No data are available from the state/territory for this reporting period; (10) The scores shown reflect fewer than 50 completed surveys; (11) There were discrepancies in the data collection process; (12) This measure does not apply to this hospital for this reporting period; (13) Results cannot be calculated for this reporting period; (14) The results for this state are combined with nearby states to protect confidentiality; Please refer to the User's Guide for a full explanation of data.

Measure	Cases	This Hosp.	State Avg.	U.S. Avg.
Blood Clot Prevention and Treatment				
Anticoagulation Overlap Therapy[2]	104	83%	90%	93%
ICU Venous Thromboembolism Prophylaxis[2]	101	76%	86%	92%
Incidence of Potentially Preventable VTE[2]	16	31%	13%	10%
UFH with Dosages/Platelet Monitoring[2]	31	100%	98%	97%
Venous Thromboembolism Prophylaxis[2]	343	52%	80%	85%
Warfarin Therapy Discharge Instructions[2]	71	75%	72%	75%
Chest Pain/Possible Heart Attack Care				
Aspirin Given Within 24 Hours of Arrival[5]	-	-	97%	96%
Fibrinolytic Meds Within 30 Min. of Arrival[5]	-	-	63%	58%
Average Time to ECG (minutes)[5]	-	-	6	7
Average Time to Transfer (minutes)[5]	-	-	61	60
Children's Asthma Care				
Received Home Management Plan of Care	-	-	-	88%
Received Reliever Medication	-	-	-	100%
Received Systemic Corticosteroids	-	-	-	100%
Emergency Department				
Admittance Decision Time (minutes)[2]	664	60	78	98
Head CT Results Within 45 Min. of Arrival[1]	-	-	55%	57%
Patients Who Left ER Before Being Seen	64,812	4%	2%	2%
Time from ER Arrival to Admit. (minutes)[2]	669	220	238	274
Time from ER Arrival to Discharge (minutes)	307	135	126	134
Time in ER Before Being Evaluated (minutes)	430	18	23	26
Time to Pain Meds for Fractures (minutes)	285	56	56	57
Heart Attack Care				
Aspirin Given at Discharge	371	100%	99%	99%
Fibrinolytic Meds Within 30 Min. of Arrival[7]	-	-	-	54%
PCI Within 90 Minutes of Arrival	57	100%	97%	96%
Statin Prescribed at Discharge	373	99%	97%	98%
Heart Failure Care				
ACE Inhibitor or ARB for LVSD	193	98%	95%	97%
Discharge Instructions Given	443	99%	92%	94%
Evaluation of LVS Function	549	100%	98%	99%
Medicare Spending				
Medicare Spending per Patient (ratio)	-	0.94	0.97	0.98
Pneumonia Care				
Appropriate Initial Antibiotic Given	274	97%	94%	95%
Blood Culture Timing	378	100%	98%	98%
Pregnancy and Delivery Care				
Newborn Deliveries Scheduled Early[2]	185	3%	9%	6%
Preventive Care				
Immunization for Influenza[2]	584	83%	92%	90%
Immunization for Pneumonia[2]	767	87%	94%	92%
Stroke Care				
Anticoagulation Therapy for Atrial Fibrillation	26	100%	95%	95%
Antithrombotic Therapy Timing	211	99%	97%	98%
Assessed for Rehabilitation	238	98%	97%	97%
Discharged on Antithrombotic Therapy	218	96%	98%	99%
Discharged on Statin Medication	178	95%	93%	94%
Thrombolytic Therapy Timing	14	71%	59%	66%
Venous Thromboembolism Prophylaxis	242	94%	93%	94%
Written Stroke Educational Materials Given	141	89%	86%	88%
Surgical Care Improvement Project				
Appropriate Beta Blocker Usage[2]	370	98%	98%	98%
Appropriate VTP Within 24 Hours[2]	699	97%	98%	98%
Controlled Postoperative Blood Glucose[2]	190	100%	96%	97%
Perioperative Temperature Management[2]	993	100%	100%	100%
Prophylactic Antibiotic Selection[2]	775	99%	99%	99%
Prophylactic Antibiotic Selection (Outpatient)	694	96%	97%	98%
Prophylactic Antibiotic Stopped[2]	770	99%	98%	98%
Prophylactic Antibiotic Timing[2]	777	99%	99%	99%
Prophylactic Antibiotic Timing (Outpatient)	747	87%	97%	98%
Urinary Catheter Removal[2]	472	98%	97%	97%
Survey of Patients' Hospital Experiences				
Area Around Room 'Always' Quiet at Night	300+	60%	64%	61%
Doctors 'Always' Communicated Well	300+	81%	84%	82%
Home Recovery Information Given	300+	87%	86%	85%
Hospital Given 9 or 10 on 10 Point Scale	300+	72%	72%	71%
Meds 'Always' Explained Before Given	300+	63%	66%	64%
Nurses 'Always' Communicated Well	300+	80%	81%	79%
Pain 'Always' Well Controlled	300+	68%	73%	71%
Room and Bathroom 'Always' Clean	300+	68%	75%	73%
Timely Help 'Always' Received	300+	63%	69%	68%
Would Definitely Recommend Hospital	300+	72%	71%	71%
Use of Medical Imaging				
Cardiac Imaging Stress Test before Surgery	971	6.3%	5.3%	5.3%
Combination Abdominal CT Scan	1,919	32.7%	10.7%	10.5%
Combination Brain/Sinus CT Scan	1,534	3.1%	3.1%	2.7%
Combination Chest CT Scan	1,751	1.8%	4.3%	2.7%
Follow-up Mammogram/Ultrasound	4,000	7.1%	8.3%	8.8%
Lumbar Spine MRI for Low Back Pain	387	38.8%	38.9%	37.2%

New Horizons Medical Center

330 Roland Avenue Phone: 502-484-4656
Owenton, KY 40359
URL: www.newhorizonsmedicalcenter.org
Type: Critical Access Hospitals Emergency Services: Yes
Ownership: Proprietary
Key Personnel:
CEO/President. . . . . Bernard T Poe

Measure	Cases	This Hosp.	State Avg.	U.S. Avg.
Blood Clot Prevention and Treatment				
Anticoagulation Overlap Therapy[5]	-	-	90%	93%
ICU Venous Thromboembolism Prophylaxis[5]	-	-	86%	92%
Incidence of Potentially Preventable VTE[5]	-	-	13%	10%
UFH with Dosages/Platelet Monitoring[5]	-	-	98%	97%
Venous Thromboembolism Prophylaxis[5]	-	-	80%	85%
Warfarin Therapy Discharge Instructions[5]	-	-	72%	75%
Chest Pain/Possible Heart Attack Care				
Aspirin Given Within 24 Hours of Arrival	-	-	97%	96%
Fibrinolytic Meds Within 30 Min. of Arrival	-	-	63%	58%
Average Time to ECG (minutes)	-	-	6	7
Average Time to Transfer (minutes)	-	-	61	60
Children's Asthma Care				
Received Home Management Plan of Care	-	-	-	88%
Received Reliever Medication	-	-	-	100%
Received Systemic Corticosteroids	-	-	-	100%
Emergency Department				
Admittance Decision Time (minutes)[5]	-	-	78	98
Head CT Results Within 45 Min. of Arrival	-	-	55%	57%
Patients Who Left ER Before Being Seen	-	-	2%	2%
Time from ER Arrival to Admit. (minutes)[5]	-	-	238	274
Time from ER Arrival to Discharge (minutes)	-	-	126	134
Time in ER Before Being Evaluated (minutes)	-	-	23	26
Time to Pain Meds for Fractures (minutes)	-	-	56	57
Heart Attack Care				
Aspirin Given at Discharge[5]	-	-	99%	99%
Fibrinolytic Meds Within 30 Min. of Arrival[5]	-	-	-	54%
PCI Within 90 Minutes of Arrival[5]	-	-	97%	96%
Statin Prescribed at Discharge[5]	-	-	97%	98%
Heart Failure Care				
ACE Inhibitor or ARB for LVSD[1]	-	-	95%	97%
Discharge Instructions Given	12	92%	92%	94%
Evaluation of LVS Function	12	67%	98%	99%
Medicare Spending				
Medicare Spending per Patient (ratio)	-	-	0.97	0.98
Pneumonia Care				
Appropriate Initial Antibiotic Given	21	81%	94%	95%
Blood Culture Timing	20	95%	98%	98%
Pregnancy and Delivery Care				
Newborn Deliveries Scheduled Early[5]	-	-	9%	6%
Preventive Care				
Immunization for Influenza[5]	-	-	92%	90%
Immunization for Pneumonia[5]	-	-	94%	92%
Stroke Care				
Anticoagulation Therapy for Atrial Fibrillation[5]	-	-	95%	95%
Antithrombotic Therapy Timing[5]	-	-	97%	98%
Assessed for Rehabilitation[5]	-	-	97%	97%
Discharged on Antithrombotic Therapy[5]	-	-	98%	99%
Discharged on Statin Medication[5]	-	-	93%	94%
Thrombolytic Therapy Timing[5]	-	-	59%	66%
Venous Thromboembolism Prophylaxis[5]	-	-	93%	94%
Written Stroke Educational Materials Given[5]	-	-	86%	88%
Surgical Care Improvement Project				
Appropriate Beta Blocker Usage[5]	-	-	98%	98%
Appropriate VTP Within 24 Hours[5]	-	-	98%	98%
Controlled Postoperative Blood Glucose[5]	-	-	96%	97%
Perioperative Temperature Management[5]	-	-	100%	100%
Prophylactic Antibiotic Selection[5]	-	-	99%	99%
Prophylactic Antibiotic Selection (Outpatient)	-	-	97%	98%
Prophylactic Antibiotic Stopped[5]	-	-	98%	98%
Prophylactic Antibiotic Timing[5]	-	-	99%	99%
Prophylactic Antibiotic Timing (Outpatient)	-	-	97%	98%
Urinary Catheter Removal[5]	-	-	97%	97%
Survey of Patients' Hospital Experiences				
Area Around Room 'Always' Quiet at Night[5]	-	-	64%	61%
Doctors 'Always' Communicated Well[5]	-	-	84%	82%
Home Recovery Information Given[5]	-	-	86%	85%
Hospital Given 9 or 10 on 10 Point Scale[5]	-	-	72%	71%
Meds 'Always' Explained Before Given[5]	-	-	66%	64%
Nurses 'Always' Communicated Well[5]	-	-	81%	79%
Pain 'Always' Well Controlled[5]	-	-	73%	71%
Room and Bathroom 'Always' Clean[5]	-	-	75%	73%
Timely Help 'Always' Received[5]	-	-	69%	68%
Would Definitely Recommend Hospital[5]	-	-	71%	71%
Use of Medical Imaging				
Cardiac Imaging Stress Test before Surgery	-	-	5.3%	5.3%
Combination Abdominal CT Scan	-	-	10.7%	10.5%
Combination Brain/Sinus CT Scan	-	-	3.1%	2.7%
Combination Chest CT Scan	-	-	4.3%	2.7%
Follow-up Mammogram/Ultrasound	-	-	8.3%	8.8%
Lumbar Spine MRI for Low Back Pain	-	-	38.9%	37.2%

Baptist Health Paducah

2501 Kentucky Avenue Phone: 270-575-2100
Paducah, KY 42003 Fax: 270-575-2217
URL: www.westernbaptist.com
Type: Acute Care Hospitals Emergency Services: Yes
Ownership: Voluntary non-profit - Church Beds: 349
Key Personnel:
Pediatric Ambulatory Care . . . . . . Glenda Channey, MD
Pediatric In-Patient Care . . . . Glenda Channey, MD
Quality Assurance . . . . Meri Curtis
Operating Room. . . . . Ted Henderson
Infection Control. . . . . Chris Nutty
Radiology. . . . . Bob Seely
Chief of Medical Staff . . . . Eric Shields, MD
CEO/President. . . . . Scott Ware

Measure	Cases	This Hosp.	State Avg.	U.S. Avg.
Blood Clot Prevention and Treatment				
Anticoagulation Overlap Therapy[2]	75	95%	90%	93%
ICU Venous Thromboembolism Prophylaxis[2]	114	94%	86%	92%
Incidence of Potentially Preventable VTE[2]	14	7%	13%	10%
UFH with Dosages/Platelet Monitoring[1,2]	-	-	98%	97%
Venous Thromboembolism Prophylaxis[2]	329	86%	80%	85%
Warfarin Therapy Discharge Instructions[2]	47	96%	72%	75%
Chest Pain/Possible Heart Attack Care				
Aspirin Given Within 24 Hours of Arrival[1,3]	-	-	97%	96%
Fibrinolytic Meds Within 30 Min. of Arrival[5]	-	-	63%	58%
Average Time to ECG (minutes)[1,3]	-	-	6	7
Average Time to Transfer (minutes)[5]	-	-	61	60
Children's Asthma Care				
Received Home Management Plan of Care	-	-	-	88%
Received Reliever Medication	-	-	-	100%
Received Systemic Corticosteroids	-	-	-	100%
Emergency Department				
Admittance Decision Time (minutes)[2]	511	110	78	98
Head CT Results Within 45 Min. of Arrival[1]	-	-	55%	57%
Patients Who Left ER Before Being Seen	37,443	4%	2%	2%
Time from ER Arrival to Admit. (minutes)[2]	513	312	238	274
Time from ER Arrival to Discharge (minutes)	353	220	126	134
Time in ER Before Being Evaluated (minutes)	406	46	23	26
Time to Pain Meds for Fractures (minutes)	105	79	56	57
Heart Attack Care				
Aspirin Given at Discharge[2]	356	100%	99%	99%
Fibrinolytic Meds Within 30 Min. of Arrival[2,7]	-	-	-	54%
PCI Within 90 Minutes of Arrival[2]	41	98%	97%	96%
Statin Prescribed at Discharge[2]	342	100%	97%	98%

NOTE: Hospital profiles are in alphabetical order by state, then city, then hospital within the city; Rankings exclude hospitals with less than 25 cases except for patient surveys which excludes hospitals with less than 100 cases; (a) 100-299 cases; (1) The number of cases/patients is too few to report; (2) Data submitted were based on a sample of cases/patients; (3) Results are based on a shorter time period than required; (4) Data suppressed by CMS for one or more quarters; (5) Results are not available for this reporting period; (6) Fewer than 100 patients completed the HCAHPS survey; (7) No cases met the criteria for this measure; (8) The lower limit of the confidence interval cannot be calculated if the number of observed infections equals zero; (9) No data are available from the state/territory for this reporting period; (10) The scores shown reflect fewer than 50 completed surveys; (11) There were discrepancies in the data collection process; (12) This measure does not apply to this hospital for this reporting period; (13) Results cannot be calculated for this reporting period; (14) The results for this state are combined with nearby states to protect confidentiality; Please refer to the User's Guide for a full explanation of data.

Heart Failure Care				
ACE Inhibitor or ARB for LVSD[2]	99	100%	95%	97%
Discharge Instructions Given[2]	240	95%	92%	94%
Evaluation of LVS Function[2]	295	100%	98%	99%
Medicare Spending				
Medicare Spending per Patient (ratio)	-	0.93	0.97	0.98
Pneumonia Care				
Appropriate Initial Antibiotic Given[2]	149	99%	94%	95%
Blood Culture Timing[2]	234	99%	98%	98%
Pregnancy and Delivery Care				
Newborn Deliveries Scheduled Early[2]	22	5%	9%	6%
Preventive Care				
Immunization for Influenza[2]	535	98%	92%	90%
Immunization for Pneumonia[2]	682	99%	94%	92%
Stroke Care				
Anticoagulation Therapy for Atrial Fibrillation[2]	31	97%	95%	95%
Antithrombotic Therapy Timing[2]	154	99%	97%	98%
Assessed for Rehabilitation[2]	182	100%	97%	97%
Discharged on Antithrombotic Therapy[2]	165	100%	98%	99%
Discharged on Statin Medication[2]	117	99%	93%	94%
Thrombolytic Therapy Timing[1,2]	-	-	59%	66%
Venous Thromboembolism Prophylaxis[2]	187	99%	93%	94%
Written Stroke Educational Materials Given[2]	109	96%	86%	88%
Surgical Care Improvement Project				
Appropriate Beta Blocker Usage[2]	339	99%	98%	98%
Appropriate VTP Within 24 Hours[2]	704	99%	98%	98%
Controlled Postoperative Blood Glucose[2]	124	98%	96%	97%
Perioperative Temperature Management[2]	803	100%	100%	100%
Prophylactic Antibiotic Selection[2]	571	99%	99%	99%
Prophylactic Antibiotic Selection (Outpatient)	604	99%	97%	98%
Prophylactic Antibiotic Stopped[2]	558	98%	98%	98%
Prophylactic Antibiotic Timing[2]	572	99%	99%	99%
Prophylactic Antibiotic Timing (Outpatient)	606	99%	97%	98%
Urinary Catheter Removal[2]	602	98%	97%	97%
Survey of Patients' Hospital Experiences				
Area Around Room 'Always' Quiet at Night	300+	65%	64%	61%
Doctors 'Always' Communicated Well	300+	81%	84%	82%
Home Recovery Information Given	300+	86%	86%	85%
Hospital Given 9 or 10 on 10 Point Scale	300+	75%	72%	71%
Meds 'Always' Explained Before Given	300+	64%	66%	64%
Nurses 'Always' Communicated Well	300+	83%	81%	79%
Pain 'Always' Well Controlled	300+	73%	73%	71%
Room and Bathroom 'Always' Clean	300+	76%	75%	73%
Timely Help 'Always' Received	300+	68%	69%	68%
Would Definitely Recommend Hospital	300+	78%	71%	71%
Use of Medical Imaging				
Cardiac Imaging Stress Test before Surgery	1,055	8.0%	5.3%	5.3%
Combination Abdominal CT Scan	1,476	11.4%	10.7%	10.5%
Combination Brain/Sinus CT Scan	1,303	3.8%	3.1%	2.7%
Combination Chest CT Scan	970	7.7%	4.3%	2.7%
Follow-up Mammogram/Ultrasound	1,419	11.6%	8.3%	8.8%
Lumbar Spine MRI for Low Back Pain	297	39.7%	38.9%	37.2%

Lourdes Hospital

1530 Lone Oak Road
Paducah, KY 42003
URL: www.ehealthconnection.com
Type: Acute Care Hospitals
Ownership: Voluntary non-profit - Church

Phone: 270-444-2444
Fax: 270-444-2980
Emergency Services: Yes
Beds: 389

Key Personnel:
Radiology.................. William E Adams, MD
Emergency Room .... Philip E Anderson
Operating Room.............. Jason David Banister
Anesthesiology............... Blane Graw, MD
CEO/President.............. Steven Grinnell
Chief of Medical Staff.......... Daniel Howard
Quality Assurance .... Jan Kincer

Measure	Cases	This Hosp.	State Avg.	U.S. Avg.
Blood Clot Prevention and Treatment				
Anticoagulation Overlap Therapy[2]	36	75%	90%	93%
ICU Venous Thromboembolism Prophylaxis[2]	122	75%	86%	92%
Incidence of Potentially Preventable VTE[1,2]	-	-	13%	10%
UFH with Dosages/Platelet Monitoring[2,7]	-	-	98%	97%
Venous Thromboembolism Prophylaxis[2]	269	75%	80%	85%
Warfarin Therapy Discharge Instructions[2]	29	93%	72%	75%
Chest Pain/Possible Heart Attack Care				
Aspirin Given Within 24 Hours of Arrival[5]	-	-	97%	96%
Fibrinolytic Meds Within 30 Min. of Arrival[5]	-	-	63%	58%
Average Time to ECG (minutes)[5]	-	-	6	7
Average Time to Transfer (minutes)[5]	-	-	61	60
Children's Asthma Care				
Received Home Management Plan of Care	-	-	-	88%
Received Reliever Medication	-	-	-	100%
Received Systemic Corticosteroids	-	-	-	100%
Emergency Department				
Admittance Decision Time (minutes)[2]	599	84	78	98
Head CT Results Within 45 Min. of Arrival[1,3]	-	-	55%	57%
Patients Who Left ER Before Being Seen	31,746	1%	2%	2%
Time from ER Arrival to Admit. (minutes)[2]	618	236	238	274
Time from ER Arrival to Discharge (minutes)	399	120	126	134
Time in ER Before Being Evaluated (minutes)	415	19	23	26
Time to Pain Meds for Fractures (minutes)	102	48	56	57
Heart Attack Care				
Aspirin Given at Discharge	169	99%	99%	99%
Fibrinolytic Meds Within 30 Min. of Arrival[7]	-	-	-	54%
PCI Within 90 Minutes of Arrival	38	100%	97%	96%
Statin Prescribed at Discharge	152	100%	97%	98%
Heart Failure Care				
ACE Inhibitor or ARB for LVSD	99	100%	95%	97%
Discharge Instructions Given	208	94%	92%	94%
Evaluation of LVS Function	249	100%	98%	99%
Medicare Spending				
Medicare Spending per Patient (ratio)	-	0.94	0.97	0.98
Pneumonia Care				
Appropriate Initial Antibiotic Given	176	98%	94%	95%
Blood Culture Timing	163	100%	98%	98%
Pregnancy and Delivery Care				
Newborn Deliveries Scheduled Early	30	3%	9%	6%
Preventive Care				
Immunization for Influenza[2]	596	90%	92%	90%
Immunization for Pneumonia[2]	877	95%	94%	92%
Stroke Care				
Anticoagulation Therapy for Atrial Fibrillation[1]	-	-	95%	95%
Antithrombotic Therapy Timing	98	98%	97%	98%
Assessed for Rehabilitation	103	86%	97%	97%
Discharged on Antithrombotic Therapy	100	97%	98%	99%
Discharged on Statin Medication	78	76%	93%	94%
Thrombolytic Therapy Timing[1]	-	-	59%	66%
Venous Thromboembolism Prophylaxis	106	89%	93%	94%
Written Stroke Educational Materials Given	64	100%	86%	88%
Surgical Care Improvement Project				
Appropriate Beta Blocker Usage[2]	486	100%	98%	98%
Appropriate VTP Within 24 Hours[2]	908	99%	98%	98%
Controlled Postoperative Blood Glucose[2]	165	93%	96%	97%
Perioperative Temperature Management[2]	1,122	100%	100%	100%
Prophylactic Antibiotic Selection[2]	1,033	100%	99%	99%
Prophylactic Antibiotic Selection (Outpatient)	204	98%	97%	98%
Prophylactic Antibiotic Stopped[2]	834	99%	98%	98%
Prophylactic Antibiotic Timing[2]	1,034	99%	99%	99%
Prophylactic Antibiotic Timing (Outpatient)	206	99%	97%	98%
Urinary Catheter Removal[2]	643	97%	97%	97%
Survey of Patients' Hospital Experiences				
Area Around Room 'Always' Quiet at Night	300+	58%	64%	61%
Doctors 'Always' Communicated Well	300+	81%	84%	82%
Home Recovery Information Given	300+	83%	86%	85%
Hospital Given 9 or 10 on 10 Point Scale	300+	72%	72%	71%
Meds 'Always' Explained Before Given	300+	61%	66%	64%
Nurses 'Always' Communicated Well	300+	77%	81%	79%
Pain 'Always' Well Controlled	300+	68%	73%	71%
Room and Bathroom 'Always' Clean	300+	72%	75%	73%
Timely Help 'Always' Received	300+	61%	69%	68%
Would Definitely Recommend Hospital	300+	74%	71%	71%
Use of Medical Imaging				
Cardiac Imaging Stress Test before Surgery	1,134	6.3%	5.3%	5.3%
Combination Abdominal CT Scan	1,307	8.1%	10.7%	10.5%
Combination Brain/Sinus CT Scan	947	2.6%	3.1%	2.7%
Combination Chest CT Scan	651	9.5%	4.3%	2.7%
Follow-up Mammogram/Ultrasound	1,905	16.5%	8.3%	8.8%
Lumbar Spine MRI for Low Back Pain	169	37.3%	38.9%	37.2%

Paul B Hall Regional Medical Center

625 James S Trimble Boulevard
Paintsville, KY 41240
URL: www.pbhrmc.com
Type: Acute Care Hospitals
Ownership: Proprietary

Phone: 606-789-3511
Fax: 606-789-6486
Emergency Services: Yes
Beds: 72

Key Personnel:
Operating Room.............. JoAnn Allen
Radiology.................. Jon E Anderson
Emergency Room .... Willard C Arnold
Intensive Care Unit............ Patricia Foley
CEO/President.............. Deborah L Trimble

Measure	Cases	This Hosp.	State Avg.	U.S. Avg.
Blood Clot Prevention and Treatment				
Anticoagulation Overlap Therapy[2]	11	100%	90%	93%
ICU Venous Thromboembolism Prophylaxis[2]	83	80%	86%	92%
Incidence of Potentially Preventable VTE[2,7]	-	-	13%	10%
UFH with Dosages/Platelet Monitoring[1,2]	-	-	98%	97%
Venous Thromboembolism Prophylaxis[2]	254	66%	80%	85%
Warfarin Therapy Discharge Instructions[1,2]	-	-	72%	75%
Chest Pain/Possible Heart Attack Care				
Aspirin Given Within 24 Hours of Arrival	81	94%	97%	96%
Fibrinolytic Meds Within 30 Min. of Arrival[1]	-	-	63%	58%
Average Time to ECG (minutes)	88	2	6	7
Average Time to Transfer (minutes)[1]	-	-	61	60
Children's Asthma Care				
Received Home Management Plan of Care	-	-	-	88%
Received Reliever Medication	-	-	-	100%
Received Systemic Corticosteroids	-	-	-	100%
Emergency Department				
Admittance Decision Time (minutes)[2]	426	75	78	98
Head CT Results Within 45 Min. of Arrival	16	81%	55%	57%
Patients Who Left ER Before Being Seen	16,252	1%	2%	2%
Time from ER Arrival to Admit. (minutes)[2]	426	262	238	274
Time from ER Arrival to Discharge (minutes)	812	128	126	134
Time in ER Before Being Evaluated (minutes)	897	35	23	26
Time to Pain Meds for Fractures (minutes)	66	55	56	57
Heart Attack Care				
Aspirin Given at Discharge[1]	-	-	99%	99%
Fibrinolytic Meds Within 30 Min. of Arrival[7]	-	-	-	54%
PCI Within 90 Minutes of Arrival[7]	-	-	97%	96%
Statin Prescribed at Discharge[1]	-	-	97%	98%
Heart Failure Care				
ACE Inhibitor or ARB for LVSD[1]	-	-	95%	97%
Discharge Instructions Given	33	100%	92%	94%
Evaluation of LVS Function	46	100%	98%	99%
Medicare Spending				
Medicare Spending per Patient (ratio)	-	0.84	0.97	0.98
Pneumonia Care				
Appropriate Initial Antibiotic Given	72	99%	94%	95%
Blood Culture Timing	161	100%	98%	98%
Pregnancy and Delivery Care				
Newborn Deliveries Scheduled Early[1]	-	-	9%	6%
Preventive Care				
Immunization for Influenza[2]	415	97%	92%	90%
Immunization for Pneumonia[2]	554	99%	94%	92%
Stroke Care				
Anticoagulation Therapy for Atrial Fibrillation[1]	-	-	95%	95%
Antithrombotic Therapy Timing	13	100%	97%	98%
Assessed for Rehabilitation	12	100%	97%	97%
Discharged on Antithrombotic Therapy	12	100%	98%	99%
Discharged on Statin Medication[1]	-	-	93%	94%
Thrombolytic Therapy Timing[1]	-	-	59%	66%
Venous Thromboembolism Prophylaxis	13	85%	93%	94%
Written Stroke Educational Materials Given[1]	-	-	86%	88%
Surgical Care Improvement Project				
Appropriate Beta Blocker Usage	13	100%	98%	98%
Appropriate VTP Within 24 Hours	28	100%	98%	98%
Controlled Postoperative Blood Glucose[7]	-	-	96%	97%
Perioperative Temperature Management	31	100%	100%	100%

NOTE: Hospital profiles are in alphabetical order by state, then city, then hospital within the city; Rankings exclude hospitals with less than 25 cases except for patient surveys which excludes hospitals with less than 100 cases; (a) 100-299 cases; (1) The number of cases/patients is too few to report; (2) Data submitted were based on a sample of cases/patients; (3) Results are based on a shorter time period than required; (4) Data suppressed by CMS for one or more quarters; (5) Results are not available for this reporting period; (6) Fewer than 100 patients completed the HCAHPS survey; (7) No cases met the criteria for this measure; (8) The lower limit of the confidence interval cannot be calculated if the number of observed infections equals zero; (9) No data are available from the state/territory for this reporting period; (10) The scores shown reflect fewer than 50 completed surveys; (11) There were discrepancies in the data collection process; (12) This measure does not apply to this hospital for this reporting period; (13) Results cannot be calculated for this reporting period; (14) The results for this state are combined with nearby states to protect confidentiality; Please refer to the User's Guide for a full explanation of data.

Measure	Cases	This Hosp.	State Avg.	U.S. Avg.
Prophylactic Antibiotic Selection[1]	-	-	99%	99%
Prophylactic Antibiotic Selection (Outpatient)	14	100%	97%	98%
Prophylactic Antibiotic Stopped[1]	-	-	98%	98%
Prophylactic Antibiotic Timing[1]	-	-	99%	99%
Prophylactic Antibiotic Timing (Outpatient)	15	93%	97%	98%
Urinary Catheter Removal[1]	-	-	97%	97%
Survey of Patients' Hospital Experiences				
Area Around Room 'Always' Quiet at Night	(a)	63%	64%	61%
Doctors 'Always' Communicated Well	(a)	83%	84%	82%
Home Recovery Information Given	(a)	80%	86%	85%
Hospital Given 9 or 10 on 10 Point Scale	(a)	61%	72%	71%
Meds 'Always' Explained Before Given	(a)	63%	66%	64%
Nurses 'Always' Communicated Well	(a)	77%	81%	79%
Pain 'Always' Well Controlled	(a)	66%	73%	71%
Room and Bathroom 'Always' Clean	(a)	70%	75%	73%
Timely Help 'Always' Received	(a)	60%	69%	68%
Would Definitely Recommend Hospital	(a)	63%	71%	71%
Use of Medical Imaging				
Cardiac Imaging Stress Test before Surgery	90	3.3%	5.3%	5.3%
Combination Abdominal CT Scan	510	12.4%	10.7%	10.5%
Combination Brain/Sinus CT Scan	490	5.9%	3.1%	2.7%
Combination Chest CT Scan	212	22.6%	4.3%	2.7%
Follow-up Mammogram/Ultrasound	244	31.1%	8.3%	8.8%
Lumbar Spine MRI for Low Back Pain	42	40.5%	38.9%	37.2%

Bourbon Community Hospital

9 Linville Drive
Paris, KY 40361
Phone: 859-987-3600
Fax: 859-987-1003
URL: www.bourbonhospital.com
Type: Acute Care Hospitals
Emergency Services: Yes
Ownership: Proprietary
Beds: 58

Key Personnel:
Chief of Medical Staff.......... Charles Allran
Radiology.................. Jerry Anderson
Emergency Room .... Robert Biddle, MD
Intensive Care Unit............ Donna Davis, RN
Infection Control.............. Marsha Haney, RN
CEO/President............... Joe Koch
Quality Assurance .... Jennie Rockidge, RN
Operating Room.............. C Schulstad, RN

Measure	Cases	This Hosp.	State Avg.	U.S. Avg.
Blood Clot Prevention and Treatment				
Anticoagulation Overlap Therapy[1,2]	-	-	90%	93%
ICU Venous Thromboembolism Prophylaxis[2]	22	95%	86%	92%
Incidence of Potentially Preventable VTE[2,7]	-	-	13%	10%
UFH with Dosages/Platelet Monitoring[1,2]	-	-	98%	97%
Venous Thromboembolism Prophylaxis[2]	115	99%	80%	85%
Warfarin Therapy Discharge Instructions[1,2]	-	-	72%	75%
Chest Pain/Possible Heart Attack Care				
Aspirin Given Within 24 Hours of Arrival	61	98%	97%	96%
Fibrinolytic Meds Within 30 Min. of Arrival[7]	-	-	63%	58%
Average Time to ECG (minutes)	63	6	6	7
Average Time to Transfer (minutes)[1]	-	-	61	60
Children's Asthma Care				
Received Home Management Plan of Care	-	-	-	88%
Received Reliever Medication	-	-	-	100%
Received Systemic Corticosteroids	-	-	-	100%
Emergency Department				
Admittance Decision Time (minutes)[2]	478	50	78	98
Head CT Results Within 45 Min. of Arrival[1]	-	-	55%	57%
Patients Who Left ER Before Being Seen	11,573	0%	2%	2%
Time from ER Arrival to Admit. (minutes)[2]	478	187	238	274
Time from ER Arrival to Discharge (minutes)	374	83	126	134
Time in ER Before Being Evaluated (minutes)	406	11	23	26
Time to Pain Meds for Fractures (minutes)	30	50	56	57
Heart Attack Care				
Aspirin Given at Discharge[7]	-	-	99%	99%
Fibrinolytic Meds Within 30 Min. of Arrival[7]	-	-	-	54%
PCI Within 90 Minutes of Arrival[7]	-	-	97%	96%
Statin Prescribed at Discharge[7]	-	-	97%	98%
Heart Failure Care				
ACE Inhibitor or ARB for LVSD[1]	-	-	95%	97%
Discharge Instructions Given	23	100%	92%	94%
Evaluation of LVS Function	30	100%	98%	99%
Medicare Spending				
Medicare Spending per Patient (ratio)	-	0.86	0.97	0.98
Pneumonia Care				
Appropriate Initial Antibiotic Given	41	88%	94%	95%
Blood Culture Timing	51	96%	98%	98%
Pregnancy and Delivery Care				
Newborn Deliveries Scheduled Early[2,7]	-	-	9%	6%
Preventive Care				
Immunization for Influenza[2]	285	99%	92%	90%
Immunization for Pneumonia[2]	421	99%	94%	92%
Stroke Care				
Anticoagulation Therapy for Atrial Fibrillation[3,7]	-	-	95%	95%
Antithrombotic Therapy Timing[1,3]	-	-	97%	98%
Assessed for Rehabilitation[1,3]	-	-	97%	97%
Discharged on Antithrombotic Therapy[1,3]	-	-	98%	99%
Discharged on Statin Medication[1,3]	-	-	93%	94%
Thrombolytic Therapy Timing[3,7]	-	-	59%	66%
Venous Thromboembolism Prophylaxis[1,3]	-	-	93%	94%
Written Stroke Educational Materials Given[3,7]	-	-	86%	88%
Surgical Care Improvement Project				
Appropriate Beta Blocker Usage[1]	-	-	98%	98%
Appropriate VTP Within 24 Hours[1]	-	-	98%	98%
Controlled Postoperative Blood Glucose[7]	-	-	96%	97%
Perioperative Temperature Management[1]	-	-	100%	100%
Prophylactic Antibiotic Selection[1]	-	-	99%	99%
Prophylactic Antibiotic Selection (Outpatient)	11	91%	97%	98%
Prophylactic Antibiotic Stopped[1]	-	-	98%	98%
Prophylactic Antibiotic Timing[1]	-	-	99%	99%
Prophylactic Antibiotic Timing (Outpatient)	11	100%	97%	98%
Urinary Catheter Removal[1]	-	-	97%	97%
Survey of Patients' Hospital Experiences				
Area Around Room 'Always' Quiet at Night	(a)	67%	64%	61%
Doctors 'Always' Communicated Well	(a)	82%	84%	82%
Home Recovery Information Given	(a)	85%	86%	85%
Hospital Given 9 or 10 on 10 Point Scale	(a)	67%	72%	71%
Meds 'Always' Explained Before Given	(a)	66%	66%	64%
Nurses 'Always' Communicated Well	(a)	83%	81%	79%
Pain 'Always' Well Controlled	(a)	71%	73%	71%
Room and Bathroom 'Always' Clean	(a)	71%	75%	73%
Timely Help 'Always' Received	(a)	73%	69%	68%
Would Definitely Recommend Hospital	(a)	57%	71%	71%
Use of Medical Imaging				
Cardiac Imaging Stress Test before Surgery	151	3.3%	5.3%	5.3%
Combination Abdominal CT Scan	196	14.3%	10.7%	10.5%
Combination Brain/Sinus CT Scan	201	7.5%	3.1%	2.7%
Combination Chest CT Scan	111	2.7%	4.3%	2.7%
Follow-up Mammogram/Ultrasound	341	6.7%	8.3%	8.8%
Lumbar Spine MRI for Low Back Pain[1]	-	-	38.9%	37.2%

Pikeville Medical Center

911 Bypass Road
Pikeville, KY 41501
Phone: 606-218-3500
Fax: 606-437-4996
URL: www.pikevillehospital.org
Type: Acute Care Hospitals
Emergency Services: Yes
Ownership: Voluntary non-profit - Private
Beds: 221

Key Personnel:
Pediatric In-Patient Care .... Sheila Belcher
Quality Assurance .... Mary Combs
Radiology.................. Dennis H Halbert
Chief of Medical Staff.......... William M Johnson
CEO/President............... Walter E May
Pediatric Ambulatory Care ...... Willena Moore
Operating Room.............. Ernestine Mullins
Patient Relations .... Patty Thompson

Measure	Cases	This Hosp.	State Avg.	U.S. Avg.
Blood Clot Prevention and Treatment				
Anticoagulation Overlap Therapy[2]	55	95%	90%	93%
ICU Venous Thromboembolism Prophylaxis[2]	85	95%	86%	92%
Incidence of Potentially Preventable VTE[2]	12	8%	13%	10%
UFH with Dosages/Platelet Monitoring[2]	44	100%	98%	97%
Venous Thromboembolism Prophylaxis[2]	373	94%	80%	85%
Warfarin Therapy Discharge Instructions[2]	40	100%	72%	75%
Chest Pain/Possible Heart Attack Care				
Aspirin Given Within 24 Hours of Arrival[1,3]	-	-	97%	96%
Fibrinolytic Meds Within 30 Min. of Arrival[5]	-	-	63%	58%
Average Time to ECG (minutes)[1,3]	-	-	6	7
Average Time to Transfer (minutes)[5]	-	-	61	60
Children's Asthma Care				
Received Home Management Plan of Care	-	-	-	88%
Received Reliever Medication	-	-	-	100%
Received Systemic Corticosteroids	-	-	-	100%
Emergency Department				
Admittance Decision Time (minutes)[2]	361	58	78	98
Head CT Results Within 45 Min. of Arrival[1]	-	-	55%	57%
Patients Who Left ER Before Being Seen	46,114	0%	2%	2%
Time from ER Arrival to Admit. (minutes)[2]	460	215	238	274
Time from ER Arrival to Discharge (minutes)	463	133	126	134
Time in ER Before Being Evaluated (minutes)	486	18	23	26
Time to Pain Meds for Fractures (minutes)	219	59	56	57
Heart Attack Care				
Aspirin Given at Discharge	340	100%	99%	99%
Fibrinolytic Meds Within 30 Min. of Arrival[1]	-	-	-	54%
PCI Within 90 Minutes of Arrival	32	100%	97%	96%
Statin Prescribed at Discharge	342	100%	97%	98%
Heart Failure Care				
ACE Inhibitor or ARB for LVSD	90	100%	95%	97%
Discharge Instructions Given	334	100%	92%	94%
Evaluation of LVS Function	369	100%	98%	99%
Medicare Spending				
Medicare Spending per Patient (ratio)	-	0.93	0.97	0.98
Pneumonia Care				
Appropriate Initial Antibiotic Given	237	99%	94%	95%
Blood Culture Timing	444	100%	98%	98%
Pregnancy and Delivery Care				
Newborn Deliveries Scheduled Early[2]	39	3%	9%	6%
Preventive Care				
Immunization for Influenza[2]	561	93%	92%	90%
Immunization for Pneumonia[2]	709	95%	94%	92%
Stroke Care				
Anticoagulation Therapy for Atrial Fibrillation	12	100%	95%	95%
Antithrombotic Therapy Timing	105	100%	97%	98%
Assessed for Rehabilitation	137	100%	97%	97%
Discharged on Antithrombotic Therapy	125	100%	98%	99%
Discharged on Statin Medication	102	100%	93%	94%
Thrombolytic Therapy Timing[1]	-	-	59%	66%
Venous Thromboembolism Prophylaxis	125	99%	93%	94%
Written Stroke Educational Materials Given	88	100%	86%	88%
Surgical Care Improvement Project				
Appropriate Beta Blocker Usage	381	100%	98%	98%
Appropriate VTP Within 24 Hours	814	100%	98%	98%
Controlled Postoperative Blood Glucose	125	100%	96%	97%
Perioperative Temperature Management	898	100%	100%	100%
Prophylactic Antibiotic Selection	734	100%	99%	99%
Prophylactic Antibiotic Selection (Outpatient)	204	95%	97%	98%
Prophylactic Antibiotic Stopped	703	100%	98%	98%
Prophylactic Antibiotic Timing	735	100%	99%	99%
Prophylactic Antibiotic Timing (Outpatient)	218	93%	97%	98%
Urinary Catheter Removal	556	100%	97%	97%
Survey of Patients' Hospital Experiences				
Area Around Room 'Always' Quiet at Night	300+	68%	64%	61%
Doctors 'Always' Communicated Well	300+	89%	84%	82%
Home Recovery Information Given	300+	90%	86%	85%
Hospital Given 9 or 10 on 10 Point Scale	300+	80%	72%	71%
Meds 'Always' Explained Before Given	300+	75%	66%	64%
Nurses 'Always' Communicated Well	300+	86%	81%	79%
Pain 'Always' Well Controlled	300+	77%	73%	71%
Room and Bathroom 'Always' Clean	300+	79%	75%	73%
Timely Help 'Always' Received	300+	74%	69%	68%
Would Definitely Recommend Hospital	300+	81%	71%	71%
Use of Medical Imaging				
Cardiac Imaging Stress Test before Surgery	673	3.7%	5.3%	5.3%
Combination Abdominal CT Scan	1,409	17.5%	10.7%	10.5%
Combination Brain/Sinus CT Scan	1,111	3.9%	3.1%	2.7%
Combination Chest CT Scan	1,031	32.3%	4.3%	2.7%
Follow-up Mammogram/Ultrasound	1,318	6.8%	8.3%	8.8%
Lumbar Spine MRI for Low Back Pain	367	37.3%	38.9%	37.2%

NOTE: Hospital profiles are in alphabetical order by state, then city, then hospital within the city; Rankings exclude hospitals with less than 25 cases except for patient surveys which excludes hospitals with less than 100 cases; (a) 100-299 cases; (1) The number of cases/patients is too few to report; (2) Data submitted were based on a sample of cases/patients; (3) Results are based on a shorter time period than required; (4) Data suppressed by CMS for one or more quarters; (5) Results are not available for this reporting period; (6) Fewer than 100 patients completed the HCAHPS survey; (7) No cases met the criteria for this measure; (8) The lower limit of the confidence interval cannot be calculated if the number of observed infections equals zero; (9) No data are available from the state/territory for this reporting period; (10) The scores shown reflect fewer than 50 completed surveys; (11) There were discrepancies in the data collection process; (12) This measure does not apply to this hospital for this reporting period; (13) Results cannot be calculated for this reporting period; (14) The results for this state are combined with nearby states to protect confidentiality; Please refer to the User's Guide for a full explanation of data.

Pineville Community Hospital

850 Riverview Avenue
Pineville, KY 40977
Phone: 606-337-3051
Fax: 606-337-4284
URL: www.pinevillehospital.com
Type: Acute Care Hospitals
Emergency Services: Yes
Ownership: Voluntary non-profit - Other
Beds: 150

Key Personnel:
Anesthesiology. . . . . Shannon Cheech, CRNA
Emergency Room . . . . Nora Ciford
Operating Room. . . . . Scott Emerick
Quality Assurance . . . . Brooke Jones

Measure	Cases	This Hosp.	State Avg.	U.S. Avg.
Blood Clot Prevention and Treatment				
Anticoagulation Overlap Therapy[1,2]	-	-	90%	93%
ICU Venous Thromboembolism Prophylaxis[2]	67	58%	86%	92%
Incidence of Potentially Preventable VTE[1,2]	-	-	13%	10%
UFH with Dosages/Platelet Monitoring[2,7]	-	-	98%	97%
Venous Thromboembolism Prophylaxis[2]	209	44%	80%	85%
Warfarin Therapy Discharge Instructions[1,2]	-	-	72%	75%
Chest Pain/Possible Heart Attack Care				
Aspirin Given Within 24 Hours of Arrival	31	97%	97%	96%
Fibrinolytic Meds Within 30 Min. of Arrival[1]	-	-	63%	58%
Average Time to ECG (minutes)	31	7	6	7
Average Time to Transfer (minutes)[1]	-	-	61	60
Children's Asthma Care				
Received Home Management Plan of Care	-	-	-	88%
Received Reliever Medication	-	-	-	100%
Received Systemic Corticosteroids	-	-	-	100%
Emergency Department				
Admittance Decision Time (minutes)[2]	270	65	78	98
Head CT Results Within 45 Min. of Arrival[1]	-	-	55%	57%
Patients Who Left ER Before Being Seen	10,828	4%	2%	2%
Time from ER Arrival to Admit. (minutes)[2]	452	225	238	274
Time from ER Arrival to Discharge (minutes)	387	132	126	134
Time in ER Before Being Evaluated (minutes)	417	29	23	26
Time to Pain Meds for Fractures (minutes)	37	57	56	57
Heart Attack Care				
Aspirin Given at Discharge[1,3]	-	-	99%	99%
Fibrinolytic Meds Within 30 Min. of Arrival[3,7]	-	-	-	54%
PCI Within 90 Minutes of Arrival[3,7]	-	-	97%	96%
Statin Prescribed at Discharge[1,3]	-	-	97%	98%
Heart Failure Care				
ACE Inhibitor or ARB for LVSD	22	91%	95%	97%
Discharge Instructions Given	112	87%	92%	94%
Evaluation of LVS Function	128	93%	98%	99%
Medicare Spending				
Medicare Spending per Patient (ratio)	-	0.85	0.97	0.98
Pneumonia Care				
Appropriate Initial Antibiotic Given	68	76%	94%	95%
Blood Culture Timing	91	96%	98%	98%
Pregnancy and Delivery Care				
Newborn Deliveries Scheduled Early[7]	-	-	9%	6%
Preventive Care				
Immunization for Influenza[2]	283	92%	92%	90%
Immunization for Pneumonia[2]	330	94%	94%	92%
Stroke Care				
Anticoagulation Therapy for Atrial Fibrillation[1,3]	-	-	95%	95%
Antithrombotic Therapy Timing[1,3]	-	-	97%	98%
Assessed for Rehabilitation[1,3]	-	-	97%	97%
Discharged on Antithrombotic Therapy[1,3]	-	-	98%	99%
Discharged on Statin Medication[1,3]	-	-	93%	94%
Thrombolytic Therapy Timing[1,3]	-	-	59%	66%
Venous Thromboembolism Prophylaxis[1,3]	-	-	93%	94%
Written Stroke Educational Materials Given[1,3]	-	-	86%	88%
Surgical Care Improvement Project				
Appropriate Beta Blocker Usage[1]	-	-	98%	98%
Appropriate VTP Within 24 Hours	29	76%	98%	98%
Controlled Postoperative Blood Glucose[7]	-	-	96%	97%
Perioperative Temperature Management	30	100%	100%	100%
Prophylactic Antibiotic Selection	21	76%	99%	99%
Prophylactic Antibiotic Selection (Outpatient)	31	10%	97%	98%
Prophylactic Antibiotic Stopped	21	57%	98%	98%
Prophylactic Antibiotic Timing	21	81%	99%	99%
Prophylactic Antibiotic Timing (Outpatient)[1]	-	-	97%	98%
Urinary Catheter Removal	13	69%	97%	97%
Survey of Patients' Hospital Experiences				
Area Around Room 'Always' Quiet at Night	300+	66%	64%	61%
Doctors 'Always' Communicated Well	300+	88%	84%	82%
Home Recovery Information Given	300+	84%	86%	85%
Hospital Given 9 or 10 on 10 Point Scale	300+	75%	72%	71%
Meds 'Always' Explained Before Given	300+	56%	66%	64%
Nurses 'Always' Communicated Well	300+	80%	81%	79%
Pain 'Always' Well Controlled	300+	72%	73%	71%
Room and Bathroom 'Always' Clean	300+	82%	75%	73%
Timely Help 'Always' Received	300+	75%	69%	68%
Would Definitely Recommend Hospital	300+	73%	71%	71%
Use of Medical Imaging				
Cardiac Imaging Stress Test before Surgery	83	4.8%	5.3%	5.3%
Combination Abdominal CT Scan	375	31.5%	10.7%	10.5%
Combination Brain/Sinus CT Scan[1]	-	-	3.1%	2.7%
Combination Chest CT Scan	157	29.3%	4.3%	2.7%
Follow-up Mammogram/Ultrasound	349	6.3%	8.3%	8.8%
Lumbar Spine MRI for Low Back Pain	82	40.2%	38.9%	37.2%

Highlands Regional Medical Center

5000 Kentucky Route 321
Prestonsburg, KY 41653
Phone: 606-886-8511
Fax: 606-886-7534
E-mail: info@hrmc.org
URL: www.hrmc.org
Type: Acute Care Hospitals
Emergency Services: Yes
Ownership: Proprietary
Beds: 184

Key Personnel:
Operating Room. . . . . Faruque Ahmed
Intensive Care Unit. . . . . Sharon Dingus
Quality Assurance . . . . Eunice Hull
Infection Control. . . . . Norcie Jervis
Anesthesiology. . . . . Jonathan Korshin
Emergency Room . . . . Dena Patton
Chief of Medical Staff. . . . . Sujatha Reddy

Measure	Cases	This Hosp.	State Avg.	U.S. Avg.
Blood Clot Prevention and Treatment				
Anticoagulation Overlap Therapy[2]	31	84%	90%	93%
ICU Venous Thromboembolism Prophylaxis[2]	83	53%	86%	92%
Incidence of Potentially Preventable VTE[2]	11	45%	13%	10%
UFH with Dosages/Platelet Monitoring[1,2]	-	-	98%	97%
Venous Thromboembolism Prophylaxis[2]	339	38%	80%	85%
Warfarin Therapy Discharge Instructions[2]	24	29%	72%	75%
Chest Pain/Possible Heart Attack Care				
Aspirin Given Within 24 Hours of Arrival	66	100%	97%	96%
Fibrinolytic Meds Within 30 Min. of Arrival[7]	-	-	63%	58%
Average Time to ECG (minutes)	66	10	6	7
Average Time to Transfer (minutes)[1]	-	-	61	60
Children's Asthma Care				
Received Home Management Plan of Care	-	-	-	88%
Received Reliever Medication	-	-	-	100%
Received Systemic Corticosteroids	-	-	-	100%
Emergency Department				
Admittance Decision Time (minutes)[2]	391	81	78	98
Head CT Results Within 45 Min. of Arrival	14	36%	55%	57%
Patients Who Left ER Before Being Seen	26,413	2%	2%	2%
Time from ER Arrival to Admit. (minutes)[2]	392	266	238	274
Time from ER Arrival to Discharge (minutes)	398	182	126	134
Time in ER Before Being Evaluated (minutes)	273	52	23	26
Time to Pain Meds for Fractures (minutes)	82	74	56	57
Heart Attack Care				
Aspirin Given at Discharge	23	100%	99%	99%
Fibrinolytic Meds Within 30 Min. of Arrival[7]	-	-	-	54%
PCI Within 90 Minutes of Arrival[7]	-	-	97%	96%
Statin Prescribed at Discharge	14	57%	97%	98%
Heart Failure Care				
ACE Inhibitor or ARB for LVSD	19	95%	95%	97%
Discharge Instructions Given	99	98%	92%	94%
Evaluation of LVS Function	116	99%	98%	99%
Medicare Spending				
Medicare Spending per Patient (ratio)	-	0.97	0.97	0.98
Pneumonia Care				
Appropriate Initial Antibiotic Given	107	93%	94%	95%
Blood Culture Timing	140	95%	98%	98%
Pregnancy and Delivery Care				
Newborn Deliveries Scheduled Early	101	14%	9%	6%
Preventive Care				
Immunization for Influenza[2]	454	67%	92%	90%
Immunization for Pneumonia[2]	496	74%	94%	92%
Stroke Care				
Anticoagulation Therapy for Atrial Fibrillation[1]	-	-	95%	95%
Antithrombotic Therapy Timing	18	94%	97%	98%
Assessed for Rehabilitation	15	67%	97%	97%
Discharged on Antithrombotic Therapy	15	93%	98%	99%
Discharged on Statin Medication	15	60%	93%	94%
Thrombolytic Therapy Timing[1]	-	-	59%	66%
Venous Thromboembolism Prophylaxis	18	50%	93%	94%
Written Stroke Educational Materials Given	13	69%	86%	88%
Surgical Care Improvement Project				
Appropriate Beta Blocker Usage	21	95%	98%	98%
Appropriate VTP Within 24 Hours	101	97%	98%	98%
Controlled Postoperative Blood Glucose[7]	-	-	96%	97%
Perioperative Temperature Management	121	99%	100%	100%
Prophylactic Antibiotic Selection	94	98%	99%	99%
Prophylactic Antibiotic Selection (Outpatient)	89	93%	97%	98%
Prophylactic Antibiotic Stopped	88	93%	98%	98%
Prophylactic Antibiotic Timing	95	100%	99%	99%
Prophylactic Antibiotic Timing (Outpatient)	75	100%	97%	98%
Urinary Catheter Removal	62	95%	97%	97%
Survey of Patients' Hospital Experiences				
Area Around Room 'Always' Quiet at Night	300+	61%	64%	61%
Doctors 'Always' Communicated Well	300+	86%	84%	82%
Home Recovery Information Given	300+	83%	86%	85%
Hospital Given 9 or 10 on 10 Point Scale	300+	62%	72%	71%
Meds 'Always' Explained Before Given	300+	63%	66%	64%
Nurses 'Always' Communicated Well	300+	79%	81%	79%
Pain 'Always' Well Controlled	300+	70%	73%	71%
Room and Bathroom 'Always' Clean	300+	66%	75%	73%
Timely Help 'Always' Received	300+	61%	69%	68%
Would Definitely Recommend Hospital	300+	62%	71%	71%
Use of Medical Imaging				
Cardiac Imaging Stress Test before Surgery	223	7.2%	5.3%	5.3%
Combination Abdominal CT Scan	1,097	33.8%	10.7%	10.5%
Combination Brain/Sinus CT Scan	770	3.5%	3.1%	2.7%
Combination Chest CT Scan	492	17.5%	4.3%	2.7%
Follow-up Mammogram/Ultrasound	845	7.0%	8.3%	8.8%
Lumbar Spine MRI for Low Back Pain	160	37.5%	38.9%	37.2%

Caldwell Medical Center

100 Medical Center Drive
Princeton, KY 42445
Phone: 270-365-0300
Fax: 270-365-6694
E-mail: info@caldwellhosp.org
URL: www.caldwellhosp.org
Type: Critical Access Hospitals
Emergency Services: Yes
Ownership: Govt - Hospital Dist/Auth
Beds: 25

Key Personnel:
CEO . . . . Charles Lovell
Infection Control. . . . . Tonya Magowan
Operating Room. . . . . Tammy Mcconnel
Radiology. . . . . Sandy Stephans

Measure	Cases	This Hosp.	State Avg.	U.S. Avg.
Blood Clot Prevention and Treatment				
Anticoagulation Overlap Therapy[5]	-	-	90%	93%
ICU Venous Thromboembolism Prophylaxis[5]	-	-	86%	92%
Incidence of Potentially Preventable VTE[5]	-	-	13%	10%
UFH with Dosages/Platelet Monitoring[5]	-	-	98%	97%
Venous Thromboembolism Prophylaxis[5]	-	-	80%	85%
Warfarin Therapy Discharge Instructions[5]	-	-	72%	75%
Chest Pain/Possible Heart Attack Care				
Aspirin Given Within 24 Hours of Arrival[5]	-	-	97%	96%
Fibrinolytic Meds Within 30 Min. of Arrival[5]	-	-	63%	58%
Average Time to ECG (minutes)[5]	-	-	6	7
Average Time to Transfer (minutes)[5]	-	-	61	60
Children's Asthma Care				
Received Home Management Plan of Care	-	-	-	88%
Received Reliever Medication	-	-	-	100%

NOTE: Hospital profiles are in alphabetical order by state, then city, then hospital within the city; Rankings exclude hospitals with less than 25 cases except for patient surveys which excludes hospitals with less than 100 cases; (a) 100-299 cases; (1) The number of cases/patients is too few to report; (2) Data submitted were based on a sample of cases/patients; (3) Results are based on a shorter time period than required; (4) Data suppressed by CMS for one or more quarters; (5) Results are not available for this reporting period; (6) Fewer than 100 patients completed the HCAHPS survey; (7) No cases met the criteria for this measure; (8) The lower limit of the confidence interval cannot be calculated if the number of observed infections equals zero; (9) No data are available from the state/territory for this reporting period; (10) The scores shown reflect fewer than 50 completed surveys; (11) There were discrepancies in the data collection process; (12) This measure does not apply to this hospital for this reporting period; (13) Results cannot be calculated for this reporting period; (14) The results for this state are combined with nearby states to protect confidentiality; Please refer to the User's Guide for a full explanation of data.

Measure	Cases	This Hosp.	State Avg.	U.S. Avg.
Received Systemic Corticosteroids	-	-	-	100%
Emergency Department				
Admittance Decision Time (minutes)[5]	-	-	78	98
Head CT Results Within 45 Min. of Arrival[5]	-	-	55%	57%
Patients Who Left ER Before Being Seen	11,030	1%	2%	2%
Time from ER Arrival to Admit. (minutes)[5]	-	-	238	274
Time from ER Arrival to Discharge (minutes)[5]	-	-	126	134
Time in ER Before Being Evaluated (minutes)[5]	-	-	23	26
Time to Pain Meds for Fractures (minutes)[5]	-	-	56	57
Heart Attack Care				
Aspirin Given at Discharge[5]	-	-	99%	99%
Fibrinolytic Meds Within 30 Min. of Arrival[5]	-	-	-	54%
PCI Within 90 Minutes of Arrival[5]	-	-	97%	96%
Statin Prescribed at Discharge[5]	-	-	97%	98%
Heart Failure Care				
ACE Inhibitor or ARB for LVSD[1]	-	-	95%	97%
Discharge Instructions Given[1]	-	-	92%	94%
Evaluation of LVS Function[1]	-	-	98%	99%
Medicare Spending				
Medicare Spending per Patient (ratio)	-	-	0.97	0.98
Pneumonia Care				
Appropriate Initial Antibiotic Given	27	74%	94%	95%
Blood Culture Timing	37	89%	98%	98%
Pregnancy and Delivery Care				
Newborn Deliveries Scheduled Early[5]	-	-	9%	6%
Preventive Care				
Immunization for Influenza[5]	-	-	92%	90%
Immunization for Pneumonia[5]	-	-	94%	92%
Stroke Care				
Anticoagulation Therapy for Atrial Fibrillation[5]	-	-	95%	95%
Antithrombotic Therapy Timing[5]	-	-	97%	98%
Assessed for Rehabilitation[5]	-	-	97%	97%
Discharged on Antithrombotic Therapy[5]	-	-	98%	99%
Discharged on Statin Medication[5]	-	-	93%	94%
Thrombolytic Therapy Timing[5]	-	-	59%	66%
Venous Thromboembolism Prophylaxis[5]	-	-	93%	94%
Written Stroke Educational Materials Given[5]	-	-	86%	88%
Surgical Care Improvement Project				
Appropriate Beta Blocker Usage[5]	-	-	98%	98%
Appropriate VTP Within 24 Hours[5]	-	-	98%	98%
Controlled Postoperative Blood Glucose[5]	-	-	96%	97%
Perioperative Temperature Management[5]	-	-	100%	100%
Prophylactic Antibiotic Selection[5]	-	-	99%	99%
Prophylactic Antibiotic Selection (Outpatient)[5]	-	-	97%	98%
Prophylactic Antibiotic Stopped[5]	-	-	98%	98%
Prophylactic Antibiotic Timing[5]	-	-	99%	99%
Prophylactic Antibiotic Timing (Outpatient)[5]	-	-	97%	98%
Urinary Catheter Removal[5]	-	-	97%	97%
Survey of Patients' Hospital Experiences				
Area Around Room 'Always' Quiet at Night[5]	-	-	64%	61%
Doctors 'Always' Communicated Well[5]	-	-	84%	82%
Home Recovery Information Given[5]	-	-	86%	85%
Hospital Given 9 or 10 on 10 Point Scale[5]	-	-	72%	71%
Meds 'Always' Explained Before Given[5]	-	-	66%	64%
Nurses 'Always' Communicated Well[5]	-	-	81%	79%
Pain 'Always' Well Controlled[5]	-	-	73%	71%
Room and Bathroom 'Always' Clean[5]	-	-	75%	73%
Timely Help 'Always' Received[5]	-	-	69%	68%
Would Definitely Recommend Hospital[5]	-	-	71%	71%
Use of Medical Imaging				
Cardiac Imaging Stress Test before Surgery	148	4.7%	5.3%	5.3%
Combination Abdominal CT Scan	258	6.6%	10.7%	10.5%
Combination Brain/Sinus CT Scan	281	1.1%	3.1%	2.7%
Combination Chest CT Scan	85	8.2%	4.3%	2.7%
Follow-up Mammogram/Ultrasound	444	2.7%	8.3%	8.8%
Lumbar Spine MRI for Low Back Pain	54	42.6%	38.9%	37.2%

Baptist Health Richmond

801 Eastern Bypass | Phone: 859-623-3131
Richmond, KY 40475 | Fax: 859-625-3535
URL: www.pattieaclay.org
Type: Acute Care Hospitals | Emergency Services: Yes
Ownership: Voluntary non-profit - Private | Beds: 105

Key Personnel:
Chief of Medical Staff . . . . Patricia Barnwell
Emergency Room . . . . Pat Cornelison, RN
Operating Room. . . . . S Fritz, RN
President . . . . C. Todd Jones, MHA
Cardiac Laboratory. . . . . Shelia Powell, RN
Quality Assurance . . . . Janie Rosanbalm, RN

Measure	Cases	This Hosp.	State Avg.	U.S. Avg.
Blood Clot Prevention and Treatment				
Anticoagulation Overlap Therapy[2]	26	96%	90%	93%
ICU Venous Thromboembolism Prophylaxis[2]	102	99%	86%	92%
Incidence of Potentially Preventable VTE[1,2]	-	-	13%	10%
UFH with Dosages/Platelet Monitoring[2]	12	100%	98%	97%
Venous Thromboembolism Prophylaxis[2]	160	99%	80%	85%
Warfarin Therapy Discharge Instructions[2]	20	100%	72%	75%
Chest Pain/Possible Heart Attack Care				
Aspirin Given Within 24 Hours of Arrival	43	93%	97%	96%
Fibrinolytic Meds Within 30 Min. of Arrival[7]	-	-	63%	58%
Average Time to ECG (minutes)	43	2	6	7
Average Time to Transfer (minutes)[1]	-	-	61	60
Children's Asthma Care				
Received Home Management Plan of Care	-	-	-	88%
Received Reliever Medication	-	-	-	100%
Received Systemic Corticosteroids	-	-	-	100%
Emergency Department				
Admittance Decision Time (minutes)[2]	321	60	78	98
Head CT Results Within 45 Min. of Arrival	13	100%	55%	57%
Patients Who Left ER Before Being Seen	30,172	1%	2%	2%
Time from ER Arrival to Admit. (minutes)[2]	347	234	238	274
Time from ER Arrival to Discharge (minutes)	486	104	126	134
Time in ER Before Being Evaluated (minutes)	561	18	23	26
Time to Pain Meds for Fractures (minutes)	100	47	56	57
Heart Attack Care				
Aspirin Given at Discharge	37	100%	99%	99%
Fibrinolytic Meds Within 30 Min. of Arrival[7]	-	-	-	54%
PCI Within 90 Minutes of Arrival[1]	-	-	97%	96%
Statin Prescribed at Discharge	38	100%	97%	98%
Heart Failure Care				
ACE Inhibitor or ARB for LVSD	24	100%	95%	97%
Discharge Instructions Given	47	100%	92%	94%
Evaluation of LVS Function	51	100%	98%	99%
Medicare Spending				
Medicare Spending per Patient (ratio)	-	1.03	0.97	0.98
Pneumonia Care				
Appropriate Initial Antibiotic Given	82	98%	94%	95%
Blood Culture Timing	147	98%	98%	98%
Pregnancy and Delivery Care				
Newborn Deliveries Scheduled Early[2]	63	2%	9%	6%
Preventive Care				
Immunization for Influenza[2]	375	99%	92%	90%
Immunization for Pneumonia[2]	407	100%	94%	92%
Stroke Care				
Anticoagulation Therapy for Atrial Fibrillation[1]	-	-	95%	95%
Antithrombotic Therapy Timing[1]	-	-	97%	98%
Assessed for Rehabilitation[1]	-	-	97%	97%
Discharged on Antithrombotic Therapy[1]	-	-	98%	99%
Discharged on Statin Medication[1]	-	-	93%	94%
Thrombolytic Therapy Timing[7]	-	-	59%	66%
Venous Thromboembolism Prophylaxis[1]	-	-	93%	94%
Written Stroke Educational Materials Given[1]	-	-	86%	88%
Surgical Care Improvement Project				
Appropriate Beta Blocker Usage	63	98%	98%	98%
Appropriate VTP Within 24 Hours	187	99%	98%	98%
Controlled Postoperative Blood Glucose[7]	-	-	96%	97%
Perioperative Temperature Management	229	100%	100%	100%
Prophylactic Antibiotic Selection	168	99%	99%	99%
Prophylactic Antibiotic Selection (Outpatient)	159	100%	97%	98%
Prophylactic Antibiotic Stopped	153	100%	98%	98%
Prophylactic Antibiotic Timing	168	99%	99%	99%
Prophylactic Antibiotic Timing (Outpatient)	159	100%	97%	98%
Urinary Catheter Removal	86	99%	97%	97%
Survey of Patients' Hospital Experiences				
Area Around Room 'Always' Quiet at Night	300+	58%	64%	61%
Doctors 'Always' Communicated Well	300+	79%	84%	82%
Home Recovery Information Given	300+	86%	86%	85%
Hospital Given 9 or 10 on 10 Point Scale	300+	67%	72%	71%
Meds 'Always' Explained Before Given	300+	58%	66%	64%
Nurses 'Always' Communicated Well	300+	78%	81%	79%
Pain 'Always' Well Controlled	300+	67%	73%	71%
Room and Bathroom 'Always' Clean	300+	77%	75%	73%
Timely Help 'Always' Received	300+	63%	69%	68%
Would Definitely Recommend Hospital	300+	63%	71%	71%
Use of Medical Imaging				
Cardiac Imaging Stress Test before Surgery	205	5.4%	5.3%	5.3%
Combination Abdominal CT Scan	639	6.7%	10.7%	10.5%
Combination Brain/Sinus CT Scan[1]	-	-	3.1%	2.7%
Combination Chest CT Scan	316	1.9%	4.3%	2.7%
Follow-up Mammogram/Ultrasound	871	13.7%	8.3%	8.8%
Lumbar Spine MRI for Low Back Pain	66	51.5%	38.9%	37.2%

Russell County Hospital

153 Dowell Road | Phone: 270-866-4141
Russell Springs, KY 42642 | Fax: 270-866-2136
URL: www.russellcohospital.org
Type: Critical Access Hospitals | Emergency Services: Yes
Ownership: Government - Local | Beds: 45

Key Personnel:
Chairman/CEO . . . . Charles Blankenship
CEO/President. . . . . Gary Delsorge
Operating Room. . . . . Vijay Jain, MD
CEO . . . . Robert Ramey
Emergency Room . . . . Paula Roy, MD
Radiology. . . . . Jerry Westerfield, MD

Measure	Cases	This Hosp.	State Avg.	U.S. Avg.
Blood Clot Prevention and Treatment				
Anticoagulation Overlap Therapy[5]	-	-	90%	93%
ICU Venous Thromboembolism Prophylaxis[5]	-	-	86%	92%
Incidence of Potentially Preventable VTE[5]	-	-	13%	10%
UFH with Dosages/Platelet Monitoring[5]	-	-	98%	97%
Venous Thromboembolism Prophylaxis[5]	-	-	80%	85%
Warfarin Therapy Discharge Instructions[5]	-	-	72%	75%
Chest Pain/Possible Heart Attack Care				
Aspirin Given Within 24 Hours of Arrival	59	98%	97%	96%
Fibrinolytic Meds Within 30 Min. of Arrival[1]	-	-	63%	58%
Average Time to ECG (minutes)	64	10	6	7
Average Time to Transfer (minutes)[1]	-	-	61	60
Children's Asthma Care				
Received Home Management Plan of Care	-	-	-	88%
Received Reliever Medication	-	-	-	100%
Received Systemic Corticosteroids	-	-	-	100%
Emergency Department				
Admittance Decision Time (minutes)[5]	-	-	78	98
Head CT Results Within 45 Min. of Arrival[5]	-	-	55%	57%
Patients Who Left ER Before Being Seen	11,762	1%	2%	2%
Time from ER Arrival to Admit. (minutes)[5]	-	-	238	274
Time from ER Arrival to Discharge (minutes)[5]	-	-	126	134
Time in ER Before Being Evaluated (minutes)[5]	-	-	23	26
Time to Pain Meds for Fractures (minutes)[5]	-	-	56	57
Heart Attack Care				
Aspirin Given at Discharge[1,3]	-	-	99%	99%
Fibrinolytic Meds Within 30 Min. of Arrival[3,7]	-	-	-	54%
PCI Within 90 Minutes of Arrival[3,7]	-	-	97%	96%
Statin Prescribed at Discharge[1,3]	-	-	97%	98%
Heart Failure Care				
ACE Inhibitor or ARB for LVSD[1]	-	-	95%	97%
Discharge Instructions Given[1]	-	-	92%	94%
Evaluation of LVS Function	13	100%	98%	99%
Medicare Spending				
Medicare Spending per Patient (ratio)	-	-	0.97	0.98
Pneumonia Care				
Appropriate Initial Antibiotic Given	60	88%	94%	95%
Blood Culture Timing	64	77%	98%	98%

NOTE: Hospital profiles are in alphabetical order by state, then city, then hospital within the city; Rankings exclude hospitals with less than 25 cases except for patient surveys which excludes hospitals with less than 100 cases; (a) 100-299 cases; (1) The number of cases/patients is too few to report; (2) Data submitted were based on a sample of cases/patients; (3) Results are based on a shorter time period than required; (4) Data suppressed by CMS for one or more quarters; (5) Results are not available for this reporting period; (6) Fewer than 100 patients completed the HCAHPS survey; (7) No cases met the criteria for this measure; (8) The lower limit of the confidence interval cannot be calculated if the number of observed infections equals zero; (9) No data are available from the state/territory for this reporting period; (10) The scores shown reflect fewer than 50 completed surveys; (11) There were discrepancies in the data collection process; (12) This measure does not apply to this hospital for this reporting period; (13) Results cannot be calculated for this reporting period; (14) The results for this state are combined with nearby states to protect confidentiality; Please refer to the User's Guide for a full explanation of data.

Measure	Cases	This Hosp.	State Avg.	U.S. Avg.
Pregnancy and Delivery Care				
Newborn Deliveries Scheduled Early[5]	-	-	9%	6%
Preventive Care				
Immunization for Influenza[5]	-	-	92%	90%
Immunization for Pneumonia[5]	-	-	94%	92%
Stroke Care				
Anticoagulation Therapy for Atrial Fibrillation[5]	-	-	95%	95%
Antithrombotic Therapy Timing[5]	-	-	97%	98%
Assessed for Rehabilitation[5]	-	-	97%	97%
Discharged on Antithrombotic Therapy[5]	-	-	98%	99%
Discharged on Statin Medication[5]	-	-	93%	94%
Thrombolytic Therapy Timing[5]	-	-	59%	66%
Venous Thromboembolism Prophylaxis[5]	-	-	93%	94%
Written Stroke Educational Materials Given[5]	-	-	86%	88%
Surgical Care Improvement Project				
Appropriate Beta Blocker Usage[5]	-	-	98%	98%
Appropriate VTP Within 24 Hours[5]	-	-	98%	98%
Controlled Postoperative Blood Glucose[5]	-	-	96%	97%
Perioperative Temperature Management[5]	-	-	100%	100%
Prophylactic Antibiotic Selection[5]	-	-	99%	99%
Prophylactic Antibiotic Selection (Outpatient)[5]	-	-	97%	98%
Prophylactic Antibiotic Stopped[5]	-	-	98%	98%
Prophylactic Antibiotic Timing[5]	-	-	99%	99%
Prophylactic Antibiotic Timing (Outpatient)[5]	-	-	97%	98%
Urinary Catheter Removal[5]	-	-	97%	97%
Survey of Patients' Hospital Experiences				
Area Around Room 'Always' Quiet at Night	(a)	64%	64%	61%
Doctors 'Always' Communicated Well	(a)	91%	84%	82%
Home Recovery Information Given	(a)	81%	86%	85%
Hospital Given 9 or 10 on 10 Point Scale	(a)	74%	72%	71%
Meds 'Always' Explained Before Given	(a)	71%	66%	64%
Nurses 'Always' Communicated Well	(a)	87%	81%	79%
Pain 'Always' Well Controlled	(a)	81%	73%	71%
Room and Bathroom 'Always' Clean	(a)	88%	75%	73%
Timely Help 'Always' Received	(a)	80%	69%	68%
Would Definitely Recommend Hospital	(a)	71%	71%	71%
Use of Medical Imaging				
Cardiac Imaging Stress Test before Surgery	133	3.8%	5.3%	5.3%
Combination Abdominal CT Scan	287	51.2%	10.7%	10.5%
Combination Brain/Sinus CT Scan[1]	-	-	3.1%	2.7%
Combination Chest CT Scan	191	17.3%	4.3%	2.7%
Follow-up Mammogram/Ultrasound	292	5.8%	8.3%	8.8%
Lumbar Spine MRI for Low Back Pain[1]	-	-	38.9%	37.2%

Logan Memorial Hospital

1625 Nashville Street
Russellville, KY 42276
Phone: 270-726-4011
Fax: 270-726-7465
URL: www.loganmemorial.com
Type: Acute Care Hospitals
Emergency Services: Yes
Ownership: Proprietary
Beds: 100

Key Personnel:
Chief of Medical Staff.......... Muhammad Ahmad, MD
CEO .... Jim Bills
Cardiac Laboratory............ Shirley Blick
Operating Room............... Adam Ellis
Quality Assurance .... June Massingille
Infection Control.............. Joyce Noe
Radiology.................... Todd Talmadge

Measure	Cases	This Hosp.	State Avg.	U.S. Avg.
Blood Clot Prevention and Treatment				
Anticoagulation Overlap Therapy[1,2]	-	-	90%	93%
ICU Venous Thromboembolism Prophylaxis[2]	28	93%	86%	92%
Incidence of Potentially Preventable VTE[1,2]	-	-	13%	10%
UFH with Dosages/Platelet Monitoring[1,2]	-	-	98%	97%
Venous Thromboembolism Prophylaxis[2]	169	92%	80%	85%
Warfarin Therapy Discharge Instructions[1,2]	-	-	72%	75%
Chest Pain/Possible Heart Attack Care				
Aspirin Given Within 24 Hours of Arrival	122	96%	97%	96%
Fibrinolytic Meds Within 30 Min. of Arrival[1]	-	-	63%	58%
Average Time to ECG (minutes)	130	4	6	7
Average Time to Transfer (minutes)[1]	-	-	61	60
Children's Asthma Care				
Received Home Management Plan of Care	-	-	-	88%
Received Reliever Medication	-	-	-	100%
Received Systemic Corticosteroids	-	-	-	100%
Emergency Department				
Admittance Decision Time (minutes)[2]	361	50	78	98
Head CT Results Within 45 Min. of Arrival[1]	-	-	55%	57%
Patients Who Left ER Before Being Seen	13,793	2%	2%	2%
Time from ER Arrival to Admit. (minutes)[2]	362	181	238	274
Time from ER Arrival to Discharge (minutes)	420	102	126	134
Time in ER Before Being Evaluated (minutes)	435	22	23	26
Time to Pain Meds for Fractures (minutes)	30	66	56	57
Heart Attack Care				
Aspirin Given at Discharge[1]	-	-	99%	99%
Fibrinolytic Meds Within 30 Min. of Arrival[7]	-	-	-	54%
PCI Within 90 Minutes of Arrival[7]	-	-	97%	96%
Statin Prescribed at Discharge[1]	-	-	97%	98%
Heart Failure Care				
ACE Inhibitor or ARB for LVSD[1]	-	-	95%	97%
Discharge Instructions Given	29	100%	92%	94%
Evaluation of LVS Function	45	100%	98%	99%
Medicare Spending				
Medicare Spending per Patient (ratio)	-	1.03	0.97	0.98
Pneumonia Care				
Appropriate Initial Antibiotic Given	93	98%	94%	95%
Blood Culture Timing	76	99%	98%	98%
Pregnancy and Delivery Care				
Newborn Deliveries Scheduled Early[2,7]	-	-	9%	6%
Preventive Care				
Immunization for Influenza[2]	291	99%	92%	90%
Immunization for Pneumonia[2]	476	98%	94%	92%
Stroke Care				
Anticoagulation Therapy for Atrial Fibrillation[1]	-	-	95%	95%
Antithrombotic Therapy Timing[1]	-	-	97%	98%
Assessed for Rehabilitation[1]	-	-	97%	97%
Discharged on Antithrombotic Therapy[1]	-	-	98%	99%
Discharged on Statin Medication[1]	-	-	93%	94%
Thrombolytic Therapy Timing[7]	-	-	59%	66%
Venous Thromboembolism Prophylaxis[1]	-	-	93%	94%
Written Stroke Educational Materials Given[1]	-	-	86%	88%
Surgical Care Improvement Project				
Appropriate Beta Blocker Usage[1]	-	-	98%	98%
Appropriate VTP Within 24 Hours	13	100%	98%	98%
Controlled Postoperative Blood Glucose[7]	-	-	96%	97%
Perioperative Temperature Management	15	100%	100%	100%
Prophylactic Antibiotic Selection[1]	-	-	99%	99%
Prophylactic Antibiotic Selection (Outpatient)	25	88%	97%	98%
Prophylactic Antibiotic Stopped[1]	-	-	98%	98%
Prophylactic Antibiotic Timing[1]	-	-	99%	99%
Prophylactic Antibiotic Timing (Outpatient)	24	92%	97%	98%
Urinary Catheter Removal[1]	-	-	97%	97%
Survey of Patients' Hospital Experiences				
Area Around Room 'Always' Quiet at Night	300+	72%	64%	61%
Doctors 'Always' Communicated Well	300+	88%	84%	82%
Home Recovery Information Given	300+	87%	86%	85%
Hospital Given 9 or 10 on 10 Point Scale	300+	70%	72%	71%
Meds 'Always' Explained Before Given	300+	68%	66%	64%
Nurses 'Always' Communicated Well	300+	83%	81%	79%
Pain 'Always' Well Controlled	300+	71%	73%	71%
Room and Bathroom 'Always' Clean	300+	79%	75%	73%
Timely Help 'Always' Received	300+	72%	69%	68%
Would Definitely Recommend Hospital	300+	72%	71%	71%
Use of Medical Imaging				
Cardiac Imaging Stress Test before Surgery	79	6.3%	5.3%	5.3%
Combination Abdominal CT Scan	329	5.8%	10.7%	10.5%
Combination Brain/Sinus CT Scan[1]	-	-	3.1%	2.7%
Combination Chest CT Scan	111	0.0%	4.3%	2.7%
Follow-up Mammogram/Ultrasound	546	10.3%	8.3%	8.8%
Lumbar Spine MRI for Low Back Pain	61	44.3%	38.9%	37.2%

Livingston Hospital & Healthcare Services

131 Hospital Drive
Salem, KY 42078
Phone: 270-988-2299
Fax: 270-988-3900
URL: www.lhhs.org
Type: Critical Access Hospitals
Emergency Services: Yes
Ownership: Proprietary
Beds: 25

Key Personnel:
CEO .... Mark Edward
Quality Assurance .... Pat Fletcher
Radiology.................... William Guyette

Measure	Cases	This Hosp.	State Avg.	U.S. Avg.
Blood Clot Prevention and Treatment				
Anticoagulation Overlap Therapy[5]	-	-	90%	93%
ICU Venous Thromboembolism Prophylaxis[5]	-	-	86%	92%
Incidence of Potentially Preventable VTE[5]	-	-	13%	10%
UFH with Dosages/Platelet Monitoring[5]	-	-	98%	97%
Venous Thromboembolism Prophylaxis[5]	-	-	80%	85%
Warfarin Therapy Discharge Instructions[5]	-	-	72%	75%
Chest Pain/Possible Heart Attack Care				
Aspirin Given Within 24 Hours of Arrival[5]	-	-	97%	96%
Fibrinolytic Meds Within 30 Min. of Arrival[5]	-	-	63%	58%
Average Time to ECG (minutes)[5]	-	-	6	7
Average Time to Transfer (minutes)[5]	-	-	61	60
Children's Asthma Care				
Received Home Management Plan of Care	-	-	-	88%
Received Reliever Medication	-	-	-	100%
Received Systemic Corticosteroids	-	-	-	100%
Emergency Department				
Admittance Decision Time (minutes)[5]	-	-	78	98
Head CT Results Within 45 Min. of Arrival[5]	-	-	55%	57%
Patients Who Left ER Before Being Seen	4,651	0%	2%	2%
Time from ER Arrival to Admit. (minutes)[5]	-	-	238	274
Time from ER Arrival to Discharge (minutes)[5]	-	-	126	134
Time in ER Before Being Evaluated (minutes)[5]	-	-	23	26
Time to Pain Meds for Fractures (minutes)[5]	-	-	56	57
Heart Attack Care				
Aspirin Given at Discharge[5]	-	-	99%	99%
Fibrinolytic Meds Within 30 Min. of Arrival[5]	-	-	-	54%
PCI Within 90 Minutes of Arrival[5]	-	-	97%	96%
Statin Prescribed at Discharge[5]	-	-	97%	98%
Heart Failure Care				
ACE Inhibitor or ARB for LVSD[1]	-	-	95%	97%
Discharge Instructions Given	13	92%	92%	94%
Evaluation of LVS Function	29	66%	98%	99%
Medicare Spending				
Medicare Spending per Patient (ratio)		-	0.97	0.98
Pneumonia Care				
Appropriate Initial Antibiotic Given	15	100%	94%	95%
Blood Culture Timing[1]	-	-	98%	98%
Pregnancy and Delivery Care				
Newborn Deliveries Scheduled Early[5]	-	-	9%	6%
Preventive Care				
Immunization for Influenza[5]	-	-	92%	90%
Immunization for Pneumonia[5]	-	-	94%	92%
Stroke Care				
Anticoagulation Therapy for Atrial Fibrillation[5]	-	-	95%	95%
Antithrombotic Therapy Timing[5]	-	-	97%	98%
Assessed for Rehabilitation[5]	-	-	97%	97%
Discharged on Antithrombotic Therapy[5]	-	-	98%	99%
Discharged on Statin Medication[5]	-	-	93%	94%
Thrombolytic Therapy Timing[5]	-	-	59%	66%
Venous Thromboembolism Prophylaxis[5]	-	-	93%	94%
Written Stroke Educational Materials Given[5]	-	-	86%	88%
Surgical Care Improvement Project				
Appropriate Beta Blocker Usage[5]	-	-	98%	98%
Appropriate VTP Within 24 Hours[5]	-	-	98%	98%
Controlled Postoperative Blood Glucose[5]	-	-	96%	97%
Perioperative Temperature Management[5]	-	-	100%	100%
Prophylactic Antibiotic Selection[5]	-	-	99%	99%
Prophylactic Antibiotic Selection (Outpatient)[5]	-	-	97%	98%
Prophylactic Antibiotic Stopped[5]	-	-	98%	98%
Prophylactic Antibiotic Timing[5]	-	-	99%	99%
Prophylactic Antibiotic Timing (Outpatient)[5]	-	-	97%	98%

NOTE: Hospital profiles are in alphabetical order by state, then city, then hospital within the city; Rankings exclude hospitals with less than 25 cases except for patient surveys which excludes hospitals with less than 100 cases; (a) 100-299 cases; (1) The number of cases/patients is too few to report; (2) Data submitted were based on a sample of cases/patients; (3) Results are based on a shorter time period than required; (4) Data suppressed by CMS for one or more quarters; (5) Results are not available for this reporting period; (6) Fewer than 100 patients completed the HCAHPS survey; (7) No cases met the criteria for this measure; (8) The lower limit of the confidence interval cannot be calculated if the number of observed infections equals zero; (9) No data are available from the state/territory for this reporting period; (10) The scores shown reflect fewer than 50 completed surveys; (11) There were discrepancies in the data collection process; (12) This measure does not apply to this hospital for this reporting period; (13) Results cannot be calculated for this reporting period; (14) The results for this state are combined with nearby states to protect confidentiality; Please refer to the User's Guide for a full explanation of data.

Measure	Cases	This Hosp.	State Avg.	U.S. Avg.
Urinary Catheter Removal[5]	-	-	97%	97%
Survey of Patients' Hospital Experiences				
Area Around Room 'Always' Quiet at Night[5]	-	-	64%	61%
Doctors 'Always' Communicated Well[5]	-	-	84%	82%
Home Recovery Information Given[5]	-	-	86%	85%
Hospital Given 9 or 10 on 10 Point Scale[5]	-	-	72%	71%
Meds 'Always' Explained Before Given[5]	-	-	66%	64%
Nurses 'Always' Communicated Well[5]	-	-	81%	79%
Pain 'Always' Well Controlled[5]	-	-	73%	71%
Room and Bathroom 'Always' Clean[5]	-	-	75%	73%
Timely Help 'Always' Received[5]	-	-	69%	68%
Would Definitely Recommend Hospital[5]	-	-	71%	71%
Use of Medical Imaging				
Cardiac Imaging Stress Test before Surgery[1]	-	-	5.3%	5.3%
Combination Abdominal CT Scan	187	43.9%	10.7%	10.5%
Combination Brain/Sinus CT Scan[1]	-	-	3.1%	2.7%
Combination Chest CT Scan	58	31.0%	4.3%	2.7%
Follow-up Mammogram/Ultrasound	145	4.8%	8.3%	8.8%
Lumbar Spine MRI for Low Back Pain[1]	-	-	38.9%	37.2%

The Medical Center at Scottsville

456 Burnley Road
Scottsville, KY 42164
Type: Critical Access Hospitals
Ownership: Voluntary non-profit - Private
Phone: 270-622-2800
Fax: 270-622-2208
Emergency Services: Yes
Beds: 157

Measure	Cases	This Hosp.	State Avg.	U.S. Avg.
Blood Clot Prevention and Treatment				
Anticoagulation Overlap Therapy[5]	-	-	90%	93%
ICU Venous Thromboembolism Prophylaxis[5]	-	-	86%	92%
Incidence of Potentially Preventable VTE[5]	-	-	13%	10%
UFH with Dosages/Platelet Monitoring[5]	-	-	98%	97%
Venous Thromboembolism Prophylaxis[5]	-	-	80%	85%
Warfarin Therapy Discharge Instructions[5]	-	-	72%	75%
Chest Pain/Possible Heart Attack Care				
Aspirin Given Within 24 Hours of Arrival[5]	-	-	97%	96%
Fibrinolytic Meds Within 30 Min. of Arrival[5]	-	-	63%	58%
Average Time to ECG (minutes)[5]	-	-	6	7
Average Time to Transfer (minutes)[5]	-	-	61	60
Children's Asthma Care				
Received Home Management Plan of Care	-	-	-	88%
Received Reliever Medication	-	-	-	100%
Received Systemic Corticosteroids	-	-	-	100%
Emergency Department				
Admittance Decision Time (minutes)[5]	-	-	78	98
Head CT Results Within 45 Min. of Arrival[5]	-	-	55%	57%
Patients Who Left ER Before Being Seen	8,935	4%	2%	2%
Time from ER Arrival to Admit. (minutes)[5]	-	-	238	274
Time from ER Arrival to Discharge (minutes)[5]	-	-	126	134
Time in ER Before Being Evaluated (minutes)[5]	-	-	23	26
Time to Pain Meds for Fractures (minutes)[5]	-	-	56	57
Heart Attack Care				
Aspirin Given at Discharge[5]	-	-	99%	99%
Fibrinolytic Meds Within 30 Min. of Arrival[5]	-	-	-	54%
PCI Within 90 Minutes of Arrival[5]	-	-	97%	96%
Statin Prescribed at Discharge[5]	-	-	97%	98%
Heart Failure Care				
ACE Inhibitor or ARB for LVSD[1]	-	-	95%	97%
Discharge Instructions Given[1]	-	-	92%	94%
Evaluation of LVS Function	13	85%	98%	99%
Medicare Spending				
Medicare Spending per Patient (ratio)	-	-	0.97	0.98
Pneumonia Care				
Appropriate Initial Antibiotic Given[2]	23	100%	94%	95%
Blood Culture Timing[2]	21	95%	98%	98%
Pregnancy and Delivery Care				
Newborn Deliveries Scheduled Early[5]	-	-	9%	6%
Preventive Care				
Immunization for Influenza[5]	-	-	92%	90%
Immunization for Pneumonia[5]	-	-	94%	92%
Stroke Care				
Anticoagulation Therapy for Atrial Fibrillation[5]	-	-	95%	95%
Antithrombotic Therapy Timing[5]	-	-	97%	98%
Assessed for Rehabilitation[5]	-	-	97%	97%
Discharged on Antithrombotic Therapy[5]	-	-	98%	99%
Discharged on Statin Medication[5]	-	-	93%	94%
Thrombolytic Therapy Timing[5]	-	-	59%	66%
Venous Thromboembolism Prophylaxis[5]	-	-	93%	94%
Written Stroke Educational Materials Given[5]	-	-	86%	88%
Surgical Care Improvement Project				
Appropriate Beta Blocker Usage[5]	-	-	98%	98%
Appropriate VTP Within 24 Hours[5]	-	-	98%	98%
Controlled Postoperative Blood Glucose[5]	-	-	96%	97%
Perioperative Temperature Management[5]	-	-	100%	100%
Prophylactic Antibiotic Selection[5]	-	-	99%	99%
Prophylactic Antibiotic Selection (Outpatient)[5]	-	-	97%	98%
Prophylactic Antibiotic Stopped[5]	-	-	98%	98%
Prophylactic Antibiotic Timing[5]	-	-	99%	99%
Prophylactic Antibiotic Timing (Outpatient)[5]	-	-	97%	98%
Urinary Catheter Removal[5]	-	-	97%	97%
Survey of Patients' Hospital Experiences				
Area Around Room 'Always' Quiet at Night[5]	-	-	64%	61%
Doctors 'Always' Communicated Well[5]	-	-	84%	82%
Home Recovery Information Given[5]	-	-	86%	85%
Hospital Given 9 or 10 on 10 Point Scale[5]	-	-	72%	71%
Meds 'Always' Explained Before Given[5]	-	-	66%	64%
Nurses 'Always' Communicated Well[5]	-	-	81%	79%
Pain 'Always' Well Controlled[5]	-	-	73%	71%
Room and Bathroom 'Always' Clean[5]	-	-	75%	73%
Timely Help 'Always' Received[5]	-	-	69%	68%
Would Definitely Recommend Hospital[5]	-	-	71%	71%
Use of Medical Imaging				
Cardiac Imaging Stress Test before Surgery[7]	-	-	5.3%	5.3%
Combination Abdominal CT Scan	181	3.3%	10.7%	10.5%
Combination Brain/Sinus CT Scan[1]	-	-	3.1%	2.7%
Combination Chest CT Scan	58	1.7%	4.3%	2.7%
Follow-up Mammogram/Ultrasound	130	10.0%	8.3%	8.8%
Lumbar Spine MRI for Low Back Pain[1]	-	-	38.9%	37.2%

Jewish Hospital - Shelbyville

727 Hospital Drive
Shelbyville, KY 40065
Type: Acute Care Hospitals
Ownership: Voluntary non-profit - Private
Phone: 502-647-4300
Emergency Services: Yes

Measure	Cases	This Hosp.	State Avg.	U.S. Avg.
Blood Clot Prevention and Treatment				
Anticoagulation Overlap Therapy[2]	19	89%	90%	93%
ICU Venous Thromboembolism Prophylaxis[2]	51	82%	86%	92%
Incidence of Potentially Preventable VTE[1,2]	-	-	13%	10%
UFH with Dosages/Platelet Monitoring[1,2]	-	-	98%	97%
Venous Thromboembolism Prophylaxis[2]	165	64%	80%	85%
Warfarin Therapy Discharge Instructions[2]	15	0%	72%	75%
Chest Pain/Possible Heart Attack Care				
Aspirin Given Within 24 Hours of Arrival	39	95%	97%	96%
Fibrinolytic Meds Within 30 Min. of Arrival[1]	-	-	63%	58%
Average Time to ECG (minutes)	39	4	6	7
Average Time to Transfer (minutes)[1]	-	-	61	60
Children's Asthma Care				
Received Home Management Plan of Care	-	-	-	88%
Received Reliever Medication	-	-	-	100%
Received Systemic Corticosteroids	-	-	-	100%
Emergency Department				
Admittance Decision Time (minutes)[2]	382	95	78	98
Head CT Results Within 45 Min. of Arrival[1]	-	-	55%	57%
Patients Who Left ER Before Being Seen	19,313	2%	2%	2%
Time from ER Arrival to Admit. (minutes)[2]	406	285	238	274
Time from ER Arrival to Discharge (minutes)	399	149	126	134
Time in ER Before Being Evaluated (minutes)	406	26	23	26
Time to Pain Meds for Fractures (minutes)	60	71	56	57
Heart Attack Care				
Aspirin Given at Discharge[1]	-	-	99%	99%
Fibrinolytic Meds Within 30 Min. of Arrival[7]	-	-	-	54%
PCI Within 90 Minutes of Arrival[7]	-	-	97%	96%
Statin Prescribed at Discharge[1]	-	-	97%	98%
Heart Failure Care				
ACE Inhibitor or ARB for LVSD	20	55%	95%	97%
Discharge Instructions Given	70	63%	92%	94%
Evaluation of LVS Function	85	99%	98%	99%
Medicare Spending				
Medicare Spending per Patient (ratio)	-	1.02	0.97	0.98
Pneumonia Care				
Appropriate Initial Antibiotic Given	59	90%	94%	95%
Blood Culture Timing	123	96%	98%	98%
Pregnancy and Delivery Care				
Newborn Deliveries Scheduled Early[7]	-	-	9%	6%
Preventive Care				
Immunization for Influenza[2]	286	76%	92%	90%
Immunization for Pneumonia[2]	471	93%	94%	92%
Stroke Care				
Anticoagulation Therapy for Atrial Fibrillation[3,7]	-	-	95%	95%
Antithrombotic Therapy Timing[1,3]	-	-	97%	98%
Assessed for Rehabilitation[3,7]	-	-	97%	97%
Discharged on Antithrombotic Therapy[3,7]	-	-	98%	99%
Discharged on Statin Medication[3,7]	-	-	93%	94%
Thrombolytic Therapy Timing[3,7]	-	-	59%	66%
Venous Thromboembolism Prophylaxis[1,3]	-	-	93%	94%
Written Stroke Educational Materials Given[3,7]	-	-	86%	88%
Surgical Care Improvement Project				
Appropriate Beta Blocker Usage	34	94%	98%	98%
Appropriate VTP Within 24 Hours	69	100%	98%	98%
Controlled Postoperative Blood Glucose[7]	-	-	96%	97%
Perioperative Temperature Management	79	100%	100%	100%
Prophylactic Antibiotic Selection	49	98%	99%	99%
Prophylactic Antibiotic Selection (Outpatient)	14	93%	97%	98%
Prophylactic Antibiotic Stopped	44	100%	98%	98%
Prophylactic Antibiotic Timing	49	98%	99%	99%
Prophylactic Antibiotic Timing (Outpatient)	17	53%	97%	98%
Urinary Catheter Removal	55	93%	97%	97%
Survey of Patients' Hospital Experiences				
Area Around Room 'Always' Quiet at Night	(a)	66%	64%	61%
Doctors 'Always' Communicated Well	(a)	80%	84%	82%
Home Recovery Information Given	(a)	86%	86%	85%
Hospital Given 9 or 10 on 10 Point Scale	(a)	66%	72%	71%
Meds 'Always' Explained Before Given	(a)	67%	66%	64%
Nurses 'Always' Communicated Well	(a)	79%	81%	79%
Pain 'Always' Well Controlled	(a)	71%	73%	71%
Room and Bathroom 'Always' Clean	(a)	78%	75%	73%
Timely Help 'Always' Received	(a)	63%	69%	68%
Would Definitely Recommend Hospital	(a)	66%	71%	71%
Use of Medical Imaging				
Cardiac Imaging Stress Test before Surgery	197	4.6%	5.3%	5.3%
Combination Abdominal CT Scan	430	4.0%	10.7%	10.5%
Combination Brain/Sinus CT Scan	395	1.5%	3.1%	2.7%
Combination Chest CT Scan	374	0.0%	4.3%	2.7%
Follow-up Mammogram/Ultrasound	722	7.9%	8.3%	8.8%
Lumbar Spine MRI for Low Back Pain	70	38.6%	38.9%	37.2%

Lake Cumberland Regional Hospital

305 Langdon Street
Somerset, KY 42502
URL: www.lakecumberlandhospital.com
Type: Acute Care Hospitals
Ownership: Proprietary
Phone: 606-679-7441
Fax: 606-678-9919
Emergency Services: Yes
Beds: 234

Key Personnel:

Radiology. . . . . William M Baker
Quality Assurance . . . . Pat Brinson
Intensive Care Unit. . . . . Dottie Campbell, RN
Chief of Medical Staff . . . . Michael Citalo
Operating Room. . . . . Lindae Cook
Infection Control. . . . . Judy Kaen, RN
Emergency Room . . . . Mel Medroso, MD
CEO/President. . . . . Jeff Seraphine

Measure	Cases	This Hosp.	State Avg.	U.S. Avg.
Blood Clot Prevention and Treatment				
Anticoagulation Overlap Therapy[2]	59	86%	90%	93%
ICU Venous Thromboembolism Prophylaxis[2]	91	95%	86%	92%
Incidence of Potentially Preventable VTE[2]	11	9%	13%	10%
UFH with Dosages/Platelet Monitoring[2]	15	87%	98%	97%
Venous Thromboembolism Prophylaxis[2]	363	90%	80%	85%

NOTE: Hospital profiles are in alphabetical order by state, then city, then hospital within the city; Rankings exclude hospitals with less than 25 cases except for patient surveys which excludes hospitals with less than 100 cases; (a) 100-299 cases; (1) The number of cases/patients is too few to report; (2) Data submitted were based on a sample of cases/patients; (3) Results are based on a shorter time period than required; (4) Data suppressed by CMS for one or more quarters; (5) Results are not available for this reporting period; (6) Fewer than 100 patients completed the HCAHPS survey; (7) No cases met the criteria for this measure; (8) The lower limit of the confidence interval cannot be calculated if the number of observed infections equals zero; (9) No data are available from the state/territory for this reporting period; (10) The scores shown reflect fewer than 50 completed surveys; (11) There were discrepancies in the data collection process; (12) This measure does not apply to this hospital for this reporting period; (13) Results cannot be calculated for this reporting period; (14) The results for this state are combined with nearby states to protect confidentiality; Please refer to the User's Guide for a full explanation of data.

Measure	Cases	This Hosp.	State Avg.	U.S. Avg.
Warfarin Therapy Discharge Instructions[2]	42	86%	72%	75%
Chest Pain/Possible Heart Attack Care				
Aspirin Given Within 24 Hours of Arrival	16	88%	97%	96%
Fibrinolytic Meds Within 30 Min. of Arrival[3,7]	-	-	63%	58%
Average Time to ECG (minutes)	17	8	6	7
Average Time to Transfer (minutes)[3,7]	-	-	61	60
Children's Asthma Care				
Received Home Management Plan of Care	-	-	-	88%
Received Reliever Medication	-	-	-	100%
Received Systemic Corticosteroids	-	-	-	100%
Emergency Department				
Admittance Decision Time (minutes)[2]	348	80	78	98
Head CT Results Within 45 Min. of Arrival	12	100%	55%	57%
Patients Who Left ER Before Being Seen	40,867	0%	2%	2%
Time from ER Arrival to Admit. (minutes)[2]	450	214	238	274
Time from ER Arrival to Discharge (minutes)	477	140	126	134
Time in ER Before Being Evaluated (minutes)	504	20	23	26
Time to Pain Meds for Fractures (minutes)	158	42	56	57
Heart Attack Care				
Aspirin Given at Discharge[2]	253	100%	99%	99%
Fibrinolytic Meds Within 30 Min. of Arrival[2,7]	-	-	-	54%
PCI Within 90 Minutes of Arrival[2]	45	96%	97%	96%
Statin Prescribed at Discharge[2]	247	97%	97%	98%
Heart Failure Care				
ACE Inhibitor or ARB for LVSD[2]	79	95%	95%	97%
Discharge Instructions Given[2]	214	90%	92%	94%
Evaluation of LVS Function[2]	258	100%	98%	99%
Medicare Spending				
Medicare Spending per Patient (ratio)	-	0.98	0.97	0.98
Pneumonia Care				
Appropriate Initial Antibiotic Given[2]	93	96%	94%	95%
Blood Culture Timing[2]	135	100%	98%	98%
Pregnancy and Delivery Care				
Newborn Deliveries Scheduled Early[2]	27	4%	9%	6%
Preventive Care				
Immunization for Influenza[2]	520	99%	92%	90%
Immunization for Pneumonia[2]	625	100%	94%	92%
Stroke Care				
Anticoagulation Therapy for Atrial Fibrillation[2]	15	100%	95%	95%
Antithrombotic Therapy Timing[2]	97	100%	97%	98%
Assessed for Rehabilitation[2]	113	99%	97%	97%
Discharged on Antithrombotic Therapy[2]	103	100%	98%	99%
Discharged on Statin Medication[2]	84	100%	93%	94%
Thrombolytic Therapy Timing[1,2]	-	-	59%	66%
Venous Thromboembolism Prophylaxis[2]	119	100%	93%	94%
Written Stroke Educational Materials Given[2]	65	89%	86%	88%
Surgical Care Improvement Project				
Appropriate Beta Blocker Usage[2]	169	97%	98%	98%
Appropriate VTP Within 24 Hours[2]	305	99%	98%	98%
Controlled Postoperative Blood Glucose[2]	45	100%	96%	97%
Perioperative Temperature Management[2]	382	100%	100%	100%
Prophylactic Antibiotic Selection[2]	232	98%	99%	99%
Prophylactic Antibiotic Selection (Outpatient)	374	100%	97%	98%
Prophylactic Antibiotic Stopped[2]	214	97%	98%	98%
Prophylactic Antibiotic Timing[2]	233	99%	99%	99%
Prophylactic Antibiotic Timing (Outpatient)	374	99%	97%	98%
Urinary Catheter Removal[2]	248	97%	97%	97%
Survey of Patients' Hospital Experiences				
Area Around Room 'Always' Quiet at Night	300+	59%	64%	61%
Doctors 'Always' Communicated Well	300+	80%	84%	82%
Home Recovery Information Given	300+	83%	86%	85%
Hospital Given 9 or 10 on 10 Point Scale	300+	61%	72%	71%
Meds 'Always' Explained Before Given	300+	56%	66%	64%
Nurses 'Always' Communicated Well	300+	74%	81%	79%
Pain 'Always' Well Controlled	300+	66%	73%	71%
Room and Bathroom 'Always' Clean	300+	67%	75%	73%
Timely Help 'Always' Received	300+	62%	69%	68%
Would Definitely Recommend Hospital	300+	60%	71%	71%
Use of Medical Imaging				
Cardiac Imaging Stress Test before Surgery	239	6.3%	5.3%	5.3%
Combination Abdominal CT Scan	1,307	12.0%	10.7%	10.5%
Combination Brain/Sinus CT Scan	862	2.6%	3.1%	2.7%
Combination Chest CT Scan	755	6.8%	4.3%	2.7%
Follow-up Mammogram/Ultrasound	1,258	12.1%	8.3%	8.8%
Lumbar Spine MRI for Low Back Pain	187	49.7%	38.9%	37.2%

Williamson ARH Hospital

260 Hospital Drive
South Williamson, KY 41503
Phone: 606-237-1700
Fax: 606-237-1701
URL: www.arh.org
Type: Acute Care Hospitals
Emergency Services: Yes
Ownership: Proprietary
Beds: 113

Key Personnel:
CEO/President. . . . . Wes Dangerfield
Radiology. . . . . Jagadishwar Dev, MD
Infection Control. . . . . Sheila Hall, RN
Pediatric Ambulatory Care . . . . . . Charles Johnson, MD
Pediatric In-Patient Care . . . . Charles Johnson, MD
Chief of Medical Staff. . . . . Mansoor Mahmood, MD
Quality Assurance . . . . Karen Reed
Coronary Care. . . . . Elizabeth Smith, RN

Measure	Cases	This Hosp.	State Avg.	U.S. Avg.
Blood Clot Prevention and Treatment				
Anticoagulation Overlap Therapy[2]	14	100%	90%	93%
ICU Venous Thromboembolism Prophylaxis[2]	49	96%	86%	92%
Incidence of Potentially Preventable VTE[1,2]	-	-	13%	10%
UFH with Dosages/Platelet Monitoring[1,2]	-	-	98%	97%
Venous Thromboembolism Prophylaxis[2]	265	94%	80%	85%
Warfarin Therapy Discharge Instructions[2]	11	100%	72%	75%
Chest Pain/Possible Heart Attack Care				
Aspirin Given Within 24 Hours of Arrival	21	90%	97%	96%
Fibrinolytic Meds Within 30 Min. of Arrival[1]	-	-	63%	58%
Average Time to ECG (minutes)	22	4	6	7
Average Time to Transfer (minutes)[1]	-	-	61	60
Children's Asthma Care				
Received Home Management Plan of Care	-	-	-	88%
Received Reliever Medication	-	-	-	100%
Received Systemic Corticosteroids	-	-	-	100%
Emergency Department				
Admittance Decision Time (minutes)[2]	378	72	78	98
Head CT Results Within 45 Min. of Arrival[1,3]	-	-	55%	57%
Patients Who Left ER Before Being Seen	17,767	2%	2%	2%
Time from ER Arrival to Admit. (minutes)[2]	385	230	238	274
Time from ER Arrival to Discharge (minutes)	408	118	126	134
Time in ER Before Being Evaluated (minutes)	422	30	23	26
Time to Pain Meds for Fractures (minutes)	83	63	56	57
Heart Attack Care				
Aspirin Given at Discharge[7]	-	-	99%	99%
Fibrinolytic Meds Within 30 Min. of Arrival[7]	-	-	-	54%
PCI Within 90 Minutes of Arrival[7]	-	-	97%	96%
Statin Prescribed at Discharge[1]	-	-	97%	98%
Heart Failure Care				
ACE Inhibitor or ARB for LVSD	19	95%	95%	97%
Discharge Instructions Given	91	92%	92%	94%
Evaluation of LVS Function	107	98%	98%	99%
Medicare Spending				
Medicare Spending per Patient (ratio)	-	0.92	0.97	0.98
Pneumonia Care				
Appropriate Initial Antibiotic Given	96	92%	94%	95%
Blood Culture Timing	100	97%	98%	98%
Pregnancy and Delivery Care				
Newborn Deliveries Scheduled Early[2]	11	27%	9%	6%
Preventive Care				
Immunization for Influenza[2]	318	97%	92%	90%
Immunization for Pneumonia[2]	436	97%	94%	92%
Stroke Care				
Anticoagulation Therapy for Atrial Fibrillation[1]	-	-	95%	95%
Antithrombotic Therapy Timing[1]	-	-	97%	98%
Assessed for Rehabilitation[1]	-	-	97%	97%
Discharged on Antithrombotic Therapy[1]	-	-	98%	99%
Discharged on Statin Medication[1]	-	-	93%	94%
Thrombolytic Therapy Timing[7]	-	-	59%	66%
Venous Thromboembolism Prophylaxis[1]	-	-	93%	94%
Written Stroke Educational Materials Given[1]	-	-	86%	88%
Surgical Care Improvement Project				
Appropriate Beta Blocker Usage[1]	-	-	98%	98%
Appropriate VTP Within 24 Hours	37	92%	98%	98%
Controlled Postoperative Blood Glucose[7]	-	-	96%	97%
Perioperative Temperature Management	44	100%	100%	100%
Prophylactic Antibiotic Selection	15	100%	99%	99%
Prophylactic Antibiotic Selection (Outpatient)	12	92%	97%	98%
Prophylactic Antibiotic Stopped	13	92%	98%	98%
Prophylactic Antibiotic Timing	15	100%	99%	99%
Prophylactic Antibiotic Timing (Outpatient)[1]	-	-	97%	98%
Urinary Catheter Removal	14	100%	97%	97%
Survey of Patients' Hospital Experiences				
Area Around Room 'Always' Quiet at Night	300+	65%	64%	61%
Doctors 'Always' Communicated Well	300+	86%	84%	82%
Home Recovery Information Given	300+	83%	86%	85%
Hospital Given 9 or 10 on 10 Point Scale	300+	73%	72%	71%
Meds 'Always' Explained Before Given	300+	69%	66%	64%
Nurses 'Always' Communicated Well	300+	81%	81%	79%
Pain 'Always' Well Controlled	300+	73%	73%	71%
Room and Bathroom 'Always' Clean	300+	77%	75%	73%
Timely Help 'Always' Received	300+	75%	69%	68%
Would Definitely Recommend Hospital	300+	75%	71%	71%
Use of Medical Imaging				
Cardiac Imaging Stress Test before Surgery	76	2.6%	5.3%	5.3%
Combination Abdominal CT Scan	170	1.8%	10.7%	10.5%
Combination Brain/Sinus CT Scan[1]	-	-	3.1%	2.7%
Combination Chest CT Scan	170	0.6%	4.3%	2.7%
Follow-up Mammogram/Ultrasound	168	19.6%	8.3%	8.8%
Lumbar Spine MRI for Low Back Pain	71	45.1%	38.9%	37.2%

Ephraim Mcdowell Fort Logan Hospital

110 Metker Trail
Stanford, KY 40484
Phone: 606-365-4600
Fax: 606-365-7900
E-mail: flh@searnet.com
URL: www.emhealth.org
Type: Critical Access Hospitals
Emergency Services: Yes
Ownership: Voluntary non-profit - Private
Beds: 25

Key Personnel:
CEO/President. . . . . Vicki A Darnell
Radiology. . . . . Shawn D Grant
Chief of Medical Staff . . . . Narea James, MD
Emergency Room . . . . Paula Ledford, DON
Infection Control. . . . . Mary Lou Lynn, RN
Anesthesiology. . . . . Balazs Makaj, MD

Measure	Cases	This Hosp.	State Avg.	U.S. Avg.
Blood Clot Prevention and Treatment				
Anticoagulation Overlap Therapy[5]	-	-	90%	93%
ICU Venous Thromboembolism Prophylaxis[5]	-	-	86%	92%
Incidence of Potentially Preventable VTE[5]	-	-	13%	10%
UFH with Dosages/Platelet Monitoring[5]	-	-	98%	97%
Venous Thromboembolism Prophylaxis[5]	-	-	80%	85%
Warfarin Therapy Discharge Instructions[5]	-	-	72%	75%
Chest Pain/Possible Heart Attack Care				
Aspirin Given Within 24 Hours of Arrival[5]	-	-	97%	96%
Fibrinolytic Meds Within 30 Min. of Arrival[5]	-	-	63%	58%
Average Time to ECG (minutes)[5]	-	-	6	7
Average Time to Transfer (minutes)[5]	-	-	61	60
Children's Asthma Care				
Received Home Management Plan of Care	-	-	-	88%
Received Reliever Medication	-	-	-	100%
Received Systemic Corticosteroids	-	-	-	100%
Emergency Department				
Admittance Decision Time (minutes)[2]	176	48	78	98
Head CT Results Within 45 Min. of Arrival[5]	-	-	55%	57%
Patients Who Left ER Before Being Seen	11,895	0%	2%	2%
Time from ER Arrival to Admit. (minutes)[2]	184	188	238	274
Time from ER Arrival to Discharge (minutes)[5]	-	-	126	134
Time in ER Before Being Evaluated (minutes)[5]	-	-	23	26
Time to Pain Meds for Fractures (minutes)[5]	-	-	56	57
Heart Attack Care				
Aspirin Given at Discharge[1,3]	-	-	99%	99%
Fibrinolytic Meds Within 30 Min. of Arrival[3,7]	-	-	-	54%
PCI Within 90 Minutes of Arrival[3,7]	-	-	97%	96%
Statin Prescribed at Discharge[3,7]	-	-	97%	98%
Heart Failure Care				
ACE Inhibitor or ARB for LVSD[1]	-	-	95%	97%

NOTE: Hospital profiles are in alphabetical order by state, then city, then hospital within the city; Rankings exclude hospitals with less than 25 cases except for patient surveys which excludes hospitals with less than 100 cases; (a) 100-299 cases; (1) The number of cases/patients is too few to report; (2) Data submitted were based on a sample of cases/patients; (3) Results are based on a shorter time period than required; (4) Data suppressed by CMS for one or more quarters; (5) Results are not available for this reporting period; (6) Fewer than 100 patients completed the HCAHPS survey; (7) No cases met the criteria for this measure; (8) The lower limit of the confidence interval cannot be calculated if the number of observed infections equals zero; (9) No data are available from the state/territory for this reporting period; (10) The scores shown reflect fewer than 50 completed surveys; (11) There were discrepancies in the data collection process; (12) This measure does not apply to this hospital for this reporting period; (13) Results cannot be calculated for this reporting period; (14) The results for this state are combined with nearby states to protect confidentiality; Please refer to the User's Guide for a full explanation of data.

Measure	Cases	This Hosp.	State Avg.	U.S. Avg.
Discharge Instructions Given[1]	-	-	92%	94%
Evaluation of LVS Function[1]	-	-	98%	99%
Medicare Spending				
Medicare Spending per Patient (ratio)	-	-	0.97	0.98
Pneumonia Care				
Appropriate Initial Antibiotic Given	25	96%	94%	95%
Blood Culture Timing	43	100%	98%	98%
Pregnancy and Delivery Care				
Newborn Deliveries Scheduled Early[5]	-	-	9%	6%
Preventive Care				
Immunization for Influenza[2]	284	98%	92%	90%
Immunization for Pneumonia[2]	207	98%	94%	92%
Stroke Care				
Anticoagulation Therapy for Atrial Fibrillation[5]	-	-	95%	95%
Antithrombotic Therapy Timing[5]	-	-	97%	98%
Assessed for Rehabilitation[5]	-	-	97%	97%
Discharged on Antithrombotic Therapy[5]	-	-	98%	99%
Discharged on Statin Medication[5]	-	-	93%	94%
Thrombolytic Therapy Timing[5]	-	-	59%	66%
Venous Thromboembolism Prophylaxis[5]	-	-	93%	94%
Written Stroke Educational Materials Given[5]	-	-	86%	88%
Surgical Care Improvement Project				
Appropriate Beta Blocker Usage[3,7]	-	-	98%	98%
Appropriate VTP Within 24 Hours[1,3]	-	-	98%	98%
Controlled Postoperative Blood Glucose[3,7]	-	-	96%	97%
Perioperative Temperature Management[1,3]	-	-	100%	100%
Prophylactic Antibiotic Selection[1,3]	-	-	99%	99%
Prophylactic Antibiotic Selection (Outpatient)[5]	-	-	97%	98%
Prophylactic Antibiotic Stopped[1,3]	-	-	98%	98%
Prophylactic Antibiotic Timing[1,3]	-	-	99%	99%
Prophylactic Antibiotic Timing (Outpatient)[5]	-	-	97%	98%
Urinary Catheter Removal[3,7]	-	-	97%	97%
Survey of Patients' Hospital Experiences				
Area Around Room 'Always' Quiet at Night	(a)	62%	64%	61%
Doctors 'Always' Communicated Well	(a)	81%	84%	82%
Home Recovery Information Given	(a)	83%	86%	85%
Hospital Given 9 or 10 on 10 Point Scale	(a)	73%	72%	71%
Meds 'Always' Explained Before Given	(a)	65%	66%	64%
Nurses 'Always' Communicated Well	(a)	79%	81%	79%
Pain 'Always' Well Controlled	(a)	62%	73%	71%
Room and Bathroom 'Always' Clean	(a)	81%	75%	73%
Timely Help 'Always' Received	(a)	72%	69%	68%
Would Definitely Recommend Hospital	(a)	73%	71%	71%
Use of Medical Imaging				
Cardiac Imaging Stress Test before Surgery[7]	-	-	5.3%	5.3%
Combination Abdominal CT Scan	190	6.3%	10.7%	10.5%
Combination Brain/Sinus CT Scan[1]	-	-	3.1%	2.7%
Combination Chest CT Scan	71	11.3%	4.3%	2.7%
Follow-up Mammogram/Ultrasound	275	8.7%	8.3%	8.8%
Lumbar Spine MRI for Low Back Pain[1]	-	-	38.9%	37.2%

Monroe County Medical Center

529 Capp Harlan Road
Tompkinsville, KY 42167
URL: www.mcmccares.com
Phone: 270-487-9231
Fax: 270-487-5784
Type: Acute Care Hospitals
Ownership: Voluntary non-profit - Private
Emergency Services: Yes
Beds: 49

Key Personnel:
Emergency Room . . . . Moujahed Achtar
Radiology. . . . . Joseph J Brennan
President . . . . Greg Crabtree, D.M.D.
Infection Control. . . . . Lisa Davis, RN
Chief of Medical Staff. . . . . Kimberly Eakle Hume
Quality Assurance . . . . Dana Hammer
CEO . . . . Vicky McFall
CEO/President. . . . . Vicky McFall

Measure	Cases	This Hosp.	State Avg.	U.S. Avg.
Blood Clot Prevention and Treatment				
Anticoagulation Overlap Therapy[2]	15	47%	90%	93%
ICU Venous Thromboembolism Prophylaxis[2,7]	-	-	86%	92%
Incidence of Potentially Preventable VTE[2,7]	-	-	13%	10%
UFH with Dosages/Platelet Monitoring[1,2]	-	-	98%	97%
Venous Thromboembolism Prophylaxis[2]	247	87%	80%	85%
Warfarin Therapy Discharge Instructions[2]	13	62%	72%	75%
Chest Pain/Possible Heart Attack Care				
Aspirin Given Within 24 Hours of Arrival	44	93%	97%	96%
Fibrinolytic Meds Within 30 Min. of Arrival[1]	-	-	63%	58%
Average Time to ECG (minutes)	43	7	6	7
Average Time to Transfer (minutes)[1]	-	-	61	60
Children's Asthma Care				
Received Home Management Plan of Care	-	-	-	88%
Received Reliever Medication	-	-	-	100%
Received Systemic Corticosteroids	-	-	-	100%
Emergency Department				
Admittance Decision Time (minutes)[2]	209	41	78	98
Head CT Results Within 45 Min. of Arrival[1]	-	-	55%	57%
Patients Who Left ER Before Being Seen	8,177	1%	2%	2%
Time from ER Arrival to Admit. (minutes)[2]	300	149	238	274
Time from ER Arrival to Discharge (minutes)	428	84	126	134
Time in ER Before Being Evaluated (minutes)	485	24	23	26
Time to Pain Meds for Fractures (minutes)	18	75	56	57
Heart Attack Care				
Aspirin Given at Discharge[1]	-	-	99%	99%
Fibrinolytic Meds Within 30 Min. of Arrival[7]	-	-	-	54%
PCI Within 90 Minutes of Arrival[7]	-	-	97%	96%
Statin Prescribed at Discharge[1]	-	-	97%	98%
Heart Failure Care				
ACE Inhibitor or ARB for LVSD	12	67%	95%	97%
Discharge Instructions Given	64	86%	92%	94%
Evaluation of LVS Function	76	96%	98%	99%
Medicare Spending				
Medicare Spending per Patient (ratio)		0.94	0.97	0.98
Pneumonia Care				
Appropriate Initial Antibiotic Given	50	80%	94%	95%
Blood Culture Timing	64	80%	98%	98%
Pregnancy and Delivery Care				
Newborn Deliveries Scheduled Early[7]	-	-	9%	6%
Preventive Care				
Immunization for Influenza[2]	317	75%	92%	90%
Immunization for Pneumonia[2]	460	75%	94%	92%
Stroke Care				
Anticoagulation Therapy for Atrial Fibrillation[1]	-	-	95%	95%
Antithrombotic Therapy Timing	36	72%	97%	98%
Assessed for Rehabilitation	31	81%	97%	97%
Discharged on Antithrombotic Therapy	31	58%	98%	99%
Discharged on Statin Medication	31	35%	93%	94%
Thrombolytic Therapy Timing[7]	-	-	59%	66%
Venous Thromboembolism Prophylaxis	37	84%	93%	94%
Written Stroke Educational Materials Given	16	69%	86%	88%
Surgical Care Improvement Project				
Appropriate Beta Blocker Usage[5]	-	-	98%	98%
Appropriate VTP Within 24 Hours[5]	-	-	98%	98%
Controlled Postoperative Blood Glucose[5]	-	-	96%	97%
Perioperative Temperature Management[5]	-	-	100%	100%
Prophylactic Antibiotic Selection[5]	-	-	99%	99%
Prophylactic Antibiotic Selection (Outpatient)[5]	-	-	97%	98%
Prophylactic Antibiotic Stopped[5]	-	-	98%	98%
Prophylactic Antibiotic Timing[5]	-	-	99%	99%
Prophylactic Antibiotic Timing (Outpatient)[5]	-	-	97%	98%
Urinary Catheter Removal[5]	-	-	97%	97%
Survey of Patients' Hospital Experiences				
Area Around Room 'Always' Quiet at Night	300+	75%	64%	61%
Doctors 'Always' Communicated Well	300+	87%	84%	82%
Home Recovery Information Given	300+	80%	86%	85%
Hospital Given 9 or 10 on 10 Point Scale	300+	68%	72%	71%
Meds 'Always' Explained Before Given	300+	65%	66%	64%
Nurses 'Always' Communicated Well	300+	81%	81%	79%
Pain 'Always' Well Controlled	300+	68%	73%	71%
Room and Bathroom 'Always' Clean	300+	78%	75%	73%
Timely Help 'Always' Received	300+	68%	69%	68%
Would Definitely Recommend Hospital	300+	64%	71%	71%
Use of Medical Imaging				
Cardiac Imaging Stress Test before Surgery	192	2.1%	5.3%	5.3%
Combination Abdominal CT Scan	212	7.5%	10.7%	10.5%
Combination Brain/Sinus CT Scan[1]	-	-	3.1%	2.7%
Combination Chest CT Scan	115	3.5%	4.3%	2.7%
Follow-up Mammogram/Ultrasound	117	17.9%	8.3%	8.8%
Lumbar Spine MRI for Low Back Pain[1]	-	-	38.9%	37.2%

Bluegrass Community Hospital

360 Amsden Avenue
Versailles, KY 40383
Phone: 859-879-2300
Fax: 859-873-1016
Type: Critical Access Hospitals
Ownership: Proprietary
Emergency Services: Yes
Beds: 73

Key Personnel:
Infection Control. . . . . Tina Cairell
Chief of Medical Staff. . . . . W Foley
Intensive Care Unit. . . . . Dale Goodin, MD
CEO . . . . Tommy Haggard
Quality Assurance . . . . Barbara Kauppi
Pediatric Ambulatory Care . . . . . . C Rener
Pediatric In-Patient Care . . . . C Rener
Operating Room. . . . . Sherri Taylor, RN

Measure	Cases	This Hosp.	State Avg.	U.S. Avg.
Blood Clot Prevention and Treatment				
Anticoagulation Overlap Therapy[1,2]	-	-	90%	93%
ICU Venous Thromboembolism Prophylaxis[1,2]	-	-	86%	92%
Incidence of Potentially Preventable VTE[2,3]	-	-	13%	10%
UFH with Dosages/Platelet Monitoring[2,3]	-	-	98%	97%
Venous Thromboembolism Prophylaxis[2,3]	35	80%	80%	85%
Warfarin Therapy Discharge Instructions[1,2]	-	-	72%	75%
Chest Pain/Possible Heart Attack Care				
Aspirin Given Within 24 Hours of Arrival[5]	-	-	97%	96%
Fibrinolytic Meds Within 30 Min. of Arrival[5]	-	-	63%	58%
Average Time to ECG (minutes)[5]	-	-	6	7
Average Time to Transfer (minutes)[5]	-	-	61	60
Children's Asthma Care				
Received Home Management Plan of Care	-	-	-	88%
Received Reliever Medication	-	-	-	100%
Received Systemic Corticosteroids	-	-	-	100%
Emergency Department				
Admittance Decision Time (minutes)[2]	175	46	78	98
Head CT Results Within 45 Min. of Arrival[5]	-	-	55%	57%
Patients Who Left ER Before Being Seen	9,154	1%	2%	2%
Time from ER Arrival to Admit. (minutes)[2]	175	204	238	274
Time from ER Arrival to Discharge (minutes)[5]	-	-	126	134
Time in ER Before Being Evaluated (minutes)[5]	-	-	23	26
Time to Pain Meds for Fractures (minutes)[5]	-	-	56	57
Heart Attack Care				
Aspirin Given at Discharge[5]	-	-	99%	99%
Fibrinolytic Meds Within 30 Min. of Arrival[5]	-	-	-	54%
PCI Within 90 Minutes of Arrival[5]	-	-	97%	96%
Statin Prescribed at Discharge[5]	-	-	97%	98%
Heart Failure Care				
ACE Inhibitor or ARB for LVSD[1]	-	-	95%	97%
Discharge Instructions Given[1]	-	-	92%	94%
Evaluation of LVS Function	14	100%	98%	99%
Medicare Spending				
Medicare Spending per Patient (ratio)	-	-	0.97	0.98
Pneumonia Care				
Appropriate Initial Antibiotic Given	12	100%	94%	95%
Blood Culture Timing	13	100%	98%	98%
Pregnancy and Delivery Care				
Newborn Deliveries Scheduled Early[2,7]	-	-	9%	6%
Preventive Care				
Immunization for Influenza[2]	159	98%	92%	90%
Immunization for Pneumonia[2]	233	95%	94%	92%
Stroke Care				
Anticoagulation Therapy for Atrial Fibrillation[5]	-	-	95%	95%
Antithrombotic Therapy Timing[5]	-	-	97%	98%
Assessed for Rehabilitation[5]	-	-	97%	97%
Discharged on Antithrombotic Therapy[5]	-	-	98%	99%
Discharged on Statin Medication[5]	-	-	93%	94%
Thrombolytic Therapy Timing[5]	-	-	59%	66%
Venous Thromboembolism Prophylaxis[5]	-	-	93%	94%
Written Stroke Educational Materials Given[5]	-	-	86%	88%
Surgical Care Improvement Project				
Appropriate Beta Blocker Usage	11	100%	98%	98%
Appropriate VTP Within 24 Hours	37	100%	98%	98%
Controlled Postoperative Blood Glucose[7]	-	-	96%	97%

NOTE: Hospital profiles are in alphabetical order by state, then city, then hospital within the city; Rankings exclude hospitals with less than 25 cases except for patient surveys which excludes hospitals with less than 100 cases; (a) 100-299 cases; (1) The number of cases/patients is too few to report; (2) Data submitted were based on a sample of cases/patients; (3) Results are based on a shorter time period than required; (4) Data suppressed by CMS for one or more quarters; (5) Results are not available for this reporting period; (6) Fewer than 100 patients completed the HCAHPS survey; (7) No cases met the criteria for this measure; (8) The lower limit of the confidence interval cannot be calculated if the number of observed infections equals zero; (9) No data are available from the state/territory for this reporting period; (10) The scores shown reflect fewer than 50 completed surveys; (11) There were discrepancies in the data collection process; (12) This measure does not apply to this hospital for this reporting period; (13) Results cannot be calculated for this reporting period; (14) The results for this state are combined with nearby states to protect confidentiality; Please refer to the User's Guide for a full explanation of data.

Measure	Cases	This Hosp.	State Avg.	U.S. Avg.
Perioperative Temperature Management	38	100%	100%	100%
Prophylactic Antibiotic Selection	35	100%	99%	99%
Prophylactic Antibiotic Selection (Outpatient)[5]	-	-	97%	98%
Prophylactic Antibiotic Stopped	34	100%	98%	98%
Prophylactic Antibiotic Timing	35	100%	99%	99%
Prophylactic Antibiotic Timing (Outpatient)[5]	-	-	97%	98%
Urinary Catheter Removal	37	100%	97%	97%
Survey of Patients' Hospital Experiences				
Area Around Room 'Always' Quiet at Night[6]	<100	73%	64%	61%
Doctors 'Always' Communicated Well[6]	<100	84%	84%	82%
Home Recovery Information Given[6]	<100	89%	86%	85%
Hospital Given 9 or 10 on 10 Point Scale[6]	<100	76%	72%	71%
Meds 'Always' Explained Before Given[6]	<100	81%	66%	64%
Nurses 'Always' Communicated Well[6]	<100	82%	81%	79%
Pain 'Always' Well Controlled[6]	<100	77%	73%	71%
Room and Bathroom 'Always' Clean[6]	<100	68%	75%	73%
Timely Help 'Always' Received[6]	<100	76%	69%	68%
Would Definitely Recommend Hospital[6]	<100	67%	71%	71%
Use of Medical Imaging				
Cardiac Imaging Stress Test before Surgery[1]	-	-	5.3%	5.3%
Combination Abdominal CT Scan	125	12.8%	10.7%	10.5%
Combination Brain/Sinus CT Scan[1]	-	-	3.1%	2.7%
Combination Chest CT Scan	61	1.6%	4.3%	2.7%
Follow-up Mammogram/Ultrasound	235	8.9%	8.3%	8.8%
Lumbar Spine MRI for Low Back Pain[1]	-	-	38.9%	37.2%

Morgan County ARH Hospital

476 Liberty Road Phone: 606-743-3186
West Liberty, KY 41472 Fax: 606-743-9604
URL: www.arh.org/morgan
Type: Critical Access Hospitals Emergency Services: Yes
Ownership: Voluntary non-profit - Private Beds: 50

Key Personnel:
Chief of Medical Staff.......... James D. Frederick, MD
CEO/President.............. Timothy A Hatfield
Infection Control.............. Patricia Lewis, RN
Quality Assurance .... Dolores Luke
Emergency Room .... Gail Perry, RN

Measure	Cases	This Hosp.	State Avg.	U.S. Avg.
Blood Clot Prevention and Treatment				
Anticoagulation Overlap Therapy[5]	-	-	90%	93%
ICU Venous Thromboembolism Prophylaxis[5]	-	-	86%	92%
Incidence of Potentially Preventable VTE[5]	-	-	13%	10%
UFH with Dosages/Platelet Monitoring[5]	-	-	98%	97%
Venous Thromboembolism Prophylaxis[5]	-	-	80%	85%
Warfarin Therapy Discharge Instructions[5]	-	-	72%	75%
Chest Pain/Possible Heart Attack Care				
Aspirin Given Within 24 Hours of Arrival[5]	-	-	97%	96%
Fibrinolytic Meds Within 30 Min. of Arrival[5]	-	-	63%	58%
Average Time to ECG (minutes)[5]	-	-	6	7
Average Time to Transfer (minutes)[5]	-	-	61	60
Children's Asthma Care				
Received Home Management Plan of Care	-	-	-	88%
Received Reliever Medication	-	-	-	100%
Received Systemic Corticosteroids	-	-	-	100%
Emergency Department				
Admittance Decision Time (minutes)[5]	-	-	78	98
Head CT Results Within 45 Min. of Arrival[5]	-	-	55%	57%
Patients Who Left ER Before Being Seen	7,653	0%	2%	2%
Time from ER Arrival to Admit. (minutes)[5]	-	-	238	274
Time from ER Arrival to Discharge (minutes)[5]	-	-	126	134
Time in ER Before Being Evaluated (minutes)[5]	-	-	23	26
Time to Pain Meds for Fractures (minutes)[5]	-	-	56	57
Heart Attack Care				
Aspirin Given at Discharge[3,7]	-	-	99%	99%
Fibrinolytic Meds Within 30 Min. of Arrival[3,7]	-	-	-	54%
PCI Within 90 Minutes of Arrival[3,7]	-	-	97%	96%
Statin Prescribed at Discharge[3,7]	-	-	97%	98%
Heart Failure Care				
ACE Inhibitor or ARB for LVSD[1]	-	-	95%	97%
Discharge Instructions Given	14	93%	92%	94%
Evaluation of LVS Function	20	90%	98%	99%
Medicare Spending				
Medicare Spending per Patient (ratio)	-	-	0.97	0.98
Pneumonia Care				
Appropriate Initial Antibiotic Given	51	100%	94%	95%
Blood Culture Timing	65	95%	98%	98%
Pregnancy and Delivery Care				
Newborn Deliveries Scheduled Early[5]	-	-	9%	6%
Preventive Care				
Immunization for Influenza[5]	-	-	92%	90%
Immunization for Pneumonia[5]	-	-	94%	92%
Stroke Care				
Anticoagulation Therapy for Atrial Fibrillation[5]	-	-	95%	95%
Antithrombotic Therapy Timing[5]	-	-	97%	98%
Assessed for Rehabilitation[5]	-	-	97%	97%
Discharged on Antithrombotic Therapy[5]	-	-	98%	99%
Discharged on Statin Medication[5]	-	-	93%	94%
Thrombolytic Therapy Timing[5]	-	-	59%	66%
Venous Thromboembolism Prophylaxis[5]	-	-	93%	94%
Written Stroke Educational Materials Given[5]	-	-	86%	88%
Surgical Care Improvement Project				
Appropriate Beta Blocker Usage[5]	-	-	98%	98%
Appropriate VTP Within 24 Hours[5]	-	-	98%	98%
Controlled Postoperative Blood Glucose[5]	-	-	96%	97%
Perioperative Temperature Management[5]	-	-	100%	100%
Prophylactic Antibiotic Selection[5]	-	-	99%	99%
Prophylactic Antibiotic Selection (Outpatient)[5]	-	-	97%	98%
Prophylactic Antibiotic Stopped[5]	-	-	98%	98%
Prophylactic Antibiotic Timing[5]	-	-	99%	99%
Prophylactic Antibiotic Timing (Outpatient)[5]	-	-	97%	98%
Urinary Catheter Removal[5]	-	-	97%	97%
Survey of Patients' Hospital Experiences				
Area Around Room 'Always' Quiet at Night[6]	<100	85%	64%	61%
Doctors 'Always' Communicated Well[6]	<100	93%	84%	82%
Home Recovery Information Given[6]	<100	97%	86%	85%
Hospital Given 9 or 10 on 10 Point Scale[6]	<100	79%	72%	71%
Meds 'Always' Explained Before Given[6]	<100	85%	66%	64%
Nurses 'Always' Communicated Well[6]	<100	90%	81%	79%
Pain 'Always' Well Controlled[6]	<100	86%	73%	71%
Room and Bathroom 'Always' Clean[6]	<100	95%	75%	73%
Timely Help 'Always' Received[6]	<100	80%	69%	68%
Would Definitely Recommend Hospital[6]	<100	83%	71%	71%
Use of Medical Imaging				
Cardiac Imaging Stress Test before Surgery[7]	-	-	5.3%	5.3%
Combination Abdominal CT Scan	132	3.0%	10.7%	10.5%
Combination Brain/Sinus CT Scan	201	0.0%	3.1%	2.7%
Combination Chest CT Scan	53	0.0%	4.3%	2.7%
Follow-up Mammogram/Ultrasound	103	6.8%	8.3%	8.8%
Lumbar Spine MRI for Low Back Pain[1]	-	-	38.9%	37.2%

Whitesburg ARH Hospital

240 Hospital Road Phone: 606-633-3500
Whitesburg, KY 41858 Fax: 606-633-3652
URL: www.arh.org/whitesburg
Type: Acute Care Hospitals Emergency Services: Yes
Ownership: Voluntary non-profit - Other Beds: 82

Key Personnel:
Radiology.................. John J Beasley
Patient Relations .... Heather Burton
Operating Room............. Charles Crumley
CEO/President.............. Jerry W Haynes
Infection Control............. Glenda Helton
Coronary Care.............. Teresa Hogg
Quality Assurance .... Gail McConnell
Chief of Medical Staff.......... PS Chandra Shekar, MD

Measure	Cases	This Hosp.	State Avg.	U.S. Avg.
Blood Clot Prevention and Treatment				
Anticoagulation Overlap Therapy[2]	22	68%	90%	93%
ICU Venous Thromboembolism Prophylaxis[2]	74	91%	86%	92%
Incidence of Potentially Preventable VTE[1,2]	-	-	13%	10%
UFH with Dosages/Platelet Monitoring[1,2]	-	-	98%	97%
Venous Thromboembolism Prophylaxis[2]	324	83%	80%	85%
Warfarin Therapy Discharge Instructions[2]	12	100%	72%	75%
Chest Pain/Possible Heart Attack Care				
Aspirin Given Within 24 Hours of Arrival	21	100%	97%	96%
Fibrinolytic Meds Within 30 Min. of Arrival[1,3]	-	-	63%	58%
Average Time to ECG (minutes)	22	6	6	7
Average Time to Transfer (minutes)[1,3]	-	-	61	60
Children's Asthma Care				
Received Home Management Plan of Care	-	-	-	88%
Received Reliever Medication	-	-	-	100%
Received Systemic Corticosteroids	-	-	-	100%
Emergency Department				
Admittance Decision Time (minutes)[2]	345	42	78	98
Head CT Results Within 45 Min. of Arrival[1]	-	-	55%	57%
Patients Who Left ER Before Being Seen	37,622	2%	2%	2%
Time from ER Arrival to Admit. (minutes)[2]	356	214	238	274
Time from ER Arrival to Discharge (minutes)	397	153	126	134
Time in ER Before Being Evaluated (minutes)	422	48	23	26
Time to Pain Meds for Fractures (minutes)	88	74	56	57
Heart Attack Care				
Aspirin Given at Discharge[1]	-	-	99%	99%
Fibrinolytic Meds Within 30 Min. of Arrival[7]	-	-	-	54%
PCI Within 90 Minutes of Arrival[7]	-	-	97%	96%
Statin Prescribed at Discharge[1]	-	-	97%	98%
Heart Failure Care				
ACE Inhibitor or ARB for LVSD	26	85%	95%	97%
Discharge Instructions Given	134	94%	92%	94%
Evaluation of LVS Function	157	88%	98%	99%
Medicare Spending				
Medicare Spending per Patient (ratio)	-	0.96	0.97	0.98
Pneumonia Care				
Appropriate Initial Antibiotic Given	130	95%	94%	95%
Blood Culture Timing	125	98%	98%	98%
Pregnancy and Delivery Care				
Newborn Deliveries Scheduled Early[2]	119	7%	9%	6%
Preventive Care				
Immunization for Influenza[2]	398	70%	92%	90%
Immunization for Pneumonia[2]	463	83%	94%	92%
Stroke Care				
Anticoagulation Therapy for Atrial Fibrillation[1]	-	-	95%	95%
Antithrombotic Therapy Timing	28	96%	97%	98%
Assessed for Rehabilitation	26	92%	97%	97%
Discharged on Antithrombotic Therapy	25	92%	98%	99%
Discharged on Statin Medication	24	75%	93%	94%
Thrombolytic Therapy Timing[1]	-	-	59%	66%
Venous Thromboembolism Prophylaxis	30	83%	93%	94%
Written Stroke Educational Materials Given	17	59%	86%	88%
Surgical Care Improvement Project				
Appropriate Beta Blocker Usage	20	90%	98%	98%
Appropriate VTP Within 24 Hours	75	93%	98%	98%
Controlled Postoperative Blood Glucose[7]	-	-	96%	97%
Perioperative Temperature Management	86	100%	100%	100%
Prophylactic Antibiotic Selection	54	96%	99%	99%
Prophylactic Antibiotic Selection (Outpatient)	138	97%	97%	98%
Prophylactic Antibiotic Stopped	43	88%	98%	98%
Prophylactic Antibiotic Timing	54	100%	99%	99%
Prophylactic Antibiotic Timing (Outpatient)	138	93%	97%	98%
Urinary Catheter Removal	16	100%	97%	97%
Survey of Patients' Hospital Experiences				
Area Around Room 'Always' Quiet at Night	300+	69%	64%	61%
Doctors 'Always' Communicated Well	300+	87%	84%	82%
Home Recovery Information Given	300+	87%	86%	85%
Hospital Given 9 or 10 on 10 Point Scale	300+	69%	72%	71%
Meds 'Always' Explained Before Given	300+	66%	66%	64%
Nurses 'Always' Communicated Well	300+	81%	81%	79%
Pain 'Always' Well Controlled	300+	71%	73%	71%
Room and Bathroom 'Always' Clean	300+	77%	75%	73%
Timely Help 'Always' Received	300+	75%	69%	68%
Would Definitely Recommend Hospital	300+	70%	71%	71%
Use of Medical Imaging				
Cardiac Imaging Stress Test before Surgery	59	5.1%	5.3%	5.3%
Combination Abdominal CT Scan	280	6.4%	10.7%	10.5%
Combination Brain/Sinus CT Scan[1]	-	-	3.1%	2.7%
Combination Chest CT Scan	96	4.2%	4.3%	2.7%
Follow-up Mammogram/Ultrasound	240	5.4%	8.3%	8.8%
Lumbar Spine MRI for Low Back Pain	92	30.4%	38.9%	37.2%

NOTE: Hospital profiles are in alphabetical order by state, then city, then hospital within the city; Rankings exclude hospitals with less than 25 cases except for patient surveys which excludes hospitals with less than 100 cases; (a) 100-299 cases; (1) The number of cases/patients is too few to report; (2) Data submitted were based on a sample of cases/patients; (3) Results are based on a shorter time period than required; (4) Data suppressed by CMS for one or more quarters; (5) Results are not available for this reporting period; (6) Fewer than 100 patients completed the HCAHPS survey; (7) No cases met the criteria for this measure; (8) The lower limit of the confidence interval cannot be calculated if the number of observed infections equals zero; (9) No data are available from the state/territory for this reporting period; (10) The scores shown reflect fewer than 50 completed surveys; (11) There were discrepancies in the data collection process; (12) This measure does not apply to this hospital for this reporting period; (13) Results cannot be calculated for this reporting period; (14) The results for this state are combined with nearby states to protect confidentiality; Please refer to the User's Guide for a full explanation of data.

Saint Elizabeth Grant

238 Barnes Road Phone: 859-824-8240
Williamstown, KY 41097 Fax: 859-824-8118
URL: www.stelizabeth.com
Type: Critical Access Hospitals Emergency Services: Yes
Ownership: Voluntary non-profit - Church Beds: 30
Key Personnel:
CEO/President. . . . . Joseph Gross
Chief of Medical Staff. . . . . LeRoy Kendall, MD

Measure	Cases	This Hosp.	State Avg.	U.S. Avg.
Blood Clot Prevention and Treatment				
Anticoagulation Overlap Therapy[1,2]	-	-	90%	93%
ICU Venous Thromboembolism Prophylaxis[2,7]	-	-	86%	92%
Incidence of Potentially Preventable VTE[2,7]	-	-	13%	10%
UFH with Dosages/Platelet Monitoring[2,7]	-	-	98%	97%
Venous Thromboembolism Prophylaxis[2]	111	95%	80%	85%
Warfarin Therapy Discharge Instructions[1,2]	-	-	72%	75%
Chest Pain/Possible Heart Attack Care				
Aspirin Given Within 24 Hours of Arrival	61	97%	97%	96%
Fibrinolytic Meds Within 30 Min. of Arrival[7]	-	-	63%	58%
Average Time to ECG (minutes)	65	6	6	7
Average Time to Transfer (minutes)[1]	-	-	61	60
Children's Asthma Care				
Received Home Management Plan of Care	-	-	-	88%
Received Reliever Medication	-	-	-	100%
Received Systemic Corticosteroids	-	-	-	100%
Emergency Department				
Admittance Decision Time (minutes)	223	60	78	98
Head CT Results Within 45 Min. of Arrival[1]	-	-	55%	57%
Patients Who Left ER Before Being Seen	18,212	0%	2%	2%
Time from ER Arrival to Admit. (minutes)	223	169	238	274
Time from ER Arrival to Discharge (minutes)	381	76	126	134
Time in ER Before Being Evaluated (minutes)	420	11	23	26
Time to Pain Meds for Fractures (minutes)	59	30	56	57
Heart Attack Care				
Aspirin Given at Discharge[5]	-	-	99%	99%
Fibrinolytic Meds Within 30 Min. of Arrival[5]	-	-	-	54%
PCI Within 90 Minutes of Arrival[5]	-	-	97%	96%
Statin Prescribed at Discharge[5]	-	-	97%	98%
Heart Failure Care				
ACE Inhibitor or ARB for LVSD[1]	-	-	95%	97%
Discharge Instructions Given[1]	-	-	92%	94%
Evaluation of LVS Function[1]	-	-	98%	99%
Medicare Spending				
Medicare Spending per Patient (ratio)	-	-	0.97	0.98
Pneumonia Care				
Appropriate Initial Antibiotic Given	13	85%	94%	95%
Blood Culture Timing[1]	-	-	98%	98%
Pregnancy and Delivery Care				
Newborn Deliveries Scheduled Early[7]	-	-	9%	6%
Preventive Care				
Immunization for Influenza	160	100%	92%	90%
Immunization for Pneumonia	241	100%	94%	92%
Stroke Care				
Anticoagulation Therapy for Atrial Fibrillation[3,7]	-	-	95%	95%
Antithrombotic Therapy Timing[3,7]	-	-	97%	98%
Assessed for Rehabilitation[1,3]	-	-	97%	97%
Discharged on Antithrombotic Therapy[3,7]	-	-	98%	99%
Discharged on Statin Medication[3,7]	-	-	93%	94%
Thrombolytic Therapy Timing[3,7]	-	-	59%	66%
Venous Thromboembolism Prophylaxis[1,3]	-	-	93%	94%
Written Stroke Educational Materials Given[1,3]	-	-	86%	88%
Surgical Care Improvement Project				
Appropriate Beta Blocker Usage[5]	-	-	98%	98%
Appropriate VTP Within 24 Hours[5]	-	-	98%	98%
Controlled Postoperative Blood Glucose[5]	-	-	96%	97%
Perioperative Temperature Management[5]	-	-	100%	100%
Prophylactic Antibiotic Selection[5]	-	-	99%	99%
Prophylactic Antibiotic Selection (Outpatient)[5]	-	-	97%	98%
Prophylactic Antibiotic Stopped[5]	-	-	98%	98%
Prophylactic Antibiotic Timing[5]	-	-	99%	99%
Prophylactic Antibiotic Timing (Outpatient)[5]	-	-	97%	98%
Urinary Catheter Removal[5]	-	-	97%	97%
Survey of Patients' Hospital Experiences				
Area Around Room 'Always' Quiet at Night[6]	<100	73%	64%	61%
Doctors 'Always' Communicated Well[6]	<100	93%	84%	82%
Home Recovery Information Given[6]	<100	91%	86%	85%
Hospital Given 9 or 10 on 10 Point Scale[6]	<100	85%	72%	71%
Meds 'Always' Explained Before Given[6]	<100	73%	66%	64%
Nurses 'Always' Communicated Well[6]	<100	89%	81%	79%
Pain 'Always' Well Controlled[6]	<100	80%	73%	71%
Room and Bathroom 'Always' Clean[6]	<100	84%	75%	73%
Timely Help 'Always' Received[6]	<100	85%	69%	68%
Would Definitely Recommend Hospital[6]	<100	85%	71%	71%
Use of Medical Imaging				
Cardiac Imaging Stress Test before Surgery	203	3.0%	5.3%	5.3%
Combination Abdominal CT Scan	347	3.5%	10.7%	10.5%
Combination Brain/Sinus CT Scan	239	0.4%	3.1%	2.7%
Combination Chest CT Scan	204	0.0%	4.3%	2.7%
Follow-up Mammogram/Ultrasound	346	5.2%	8.3%	8.8%
Lumbar Spine MRI for Low Back Pain	96	40.6%	38.9%	37.2%

Clark Regional Medical Center

175 Hospital Drive Phone: 859-737-8559
Winchester, KY 40391 Fax: 859-744-6408
URL: www.clarkregional.org
Type: Acute Care Hospitals Emergency Services: Yes
Ownership: Proprietary Beds: 100
Key Personnel:
Chief of Medical Staff. . . . . Richard Chamberlin, MD
Radiology. . . . . William Cooper
CEO . . . . Cherie Sibley

Measure	Cases	This Hosp.	State Avg.	U.S. Avg.
Blood Clot Prevention and Treatment				
Anticoagulation Overlap Therapy[1,2]	-	-	90%	93%
ICU Venous Thromboembolism Prophylaxis[2]	73	96%	86%	92%
Incidence of Potentially Preventable VTE[1,2]	-	-	13%	10%
UFH with Dosages/Platelet Monitoring[1,2]	-	-	98%	97%
Venous Thromboembolism Prophylaxis[2]	138	97%	80%	85%
Warfarin Therapy Discharge Instructions[1,2]	-	-	72%	75%
Chest Pain/Possible Heart Attack Care				
Aspirin Given Within 24 Hours of Arrival	36	100%	97%	96%
Fibrinolytic Meds Within 30 Min. of Arrival[7]	-	-	63%	58%
Average Time to ECG (minutes)	39	2	6	7
Average Time to Transfer (minutes)[1]	-	-	61	60
Children's Asthma Care				
Received Home Management Plan of Care	-	-	-	88%
Received Reliever Medication	-	-	-	100%
Received Systemic Corticosteroids	-	-	-	100%
Emergency Department				
Admittance Decision Time (minutes)[2]	322	78	78	98
Head CT Results Within 45 Min. of Arrival[1]	-	-	55%	57%
Patients Who Left ER Before Being Seen	25,209	1%	2%	2%
Time from ER Arrival to Admit. (minutes)[2]	324	285	238	274
Time from ER Arrival to Discharge (minutes)	397	143	126	134
Time in ER Before Being Evaluated (minutes)	463	21	23	26
Time to Pain Meds for Fractures (minutes)	97	44	56	57
Heart Attack Care				
Aspirin Given at Discharge	30	100%	99%	99%
Fibrinolytic Meds Within 30 Min. of Arrival[7]	-	-	-	54%
PCI Within 90 Minutes of Arrival[7]	-	-	97%	96%
Statin Prescribed at Discharge	29	97%	97%	98%
Heart Failure Care				
ACE Inhibitor or ARB for LVSD	14	86%	95%	97%
Discharge Instructions Given	42	95%	92%	94%
Evaluation of LVS Function	51	100%	98%	99%
Medicare Spending				
Medicare Spending per Patient (ratio)	-	0.88	0.97	0.98
Pneumonia Care				
Appropriate Initial Antibiotic Given	103	94%	94%	95%
Blood Culture Timing	144	98%	98%	98%
Pregnancy and Delivery Care				
Newborn Deliveries Scheduled Early[2]	14	0%	9%	6%
Preventive Care				
Immunization for Influenza[2]	331	96%	92%	90%
Immunization for Pneumonia[2]	352	98%	94%	92%
Stroke Care				
Anticoagulation Therapy for Atrial Fibrillation[7]	-	-	95%	95%
Antithrombotic Therapy Timing	13	100%	97%	98%
Assessed for Rehabilitation	15	100%	97%	97%
Discharged on Antithrombotic Therapy	13	100%	98%	99%
Discharged on Statin Medication[1]	-	-	93%	94%
Thrombolytic Therapy Timing[1]	-	-	59%	66%
Venous Thromboembolism Prophylaxis	13	92%	93%	94%
Written Stroke Educational Materials Given[1]	-	-	86%	88%
Surgical Care Improvement Project				
Appropriate Beta Blocker Usage	40	98%	98%	98%
Appropriate VTP Within 24 Hours	136	99%	98%	98%
Controlled Postoperative Blood Glucose[7]	-	-	96%	97%
Perioperative Temperature Management	158	100%	100%	100%
Prophylactic Antibiotic Selection	126	100%	99%	99%
Prophylactic Antibiotic Selection (Outpatient)	12	83%	97%	98%
Prophylactic Antibiotic Stopped	126	98%	98%	98%
Prophylactic Antibiotic Timing	126	98%	99%	99%
Prophylactic Antibiotic Timing (Outpatient)	14	79%	97%	98%
Urinary Catheter Removal	81	100%	97%	97%
Survey of Patients' Hospital Experiences				
Area Around Room 'Always' Quiet at Night	300+	66%	64%	61%
Doctors 'Always' Communicated Well	300+	83%	84%	82%
Home Recovery Information Given	300+	86%	86%	85%
Hospital Given 9 or 10 on 10 Point Scale	300+	74%	72%	71%
Meds 'Always' Explained Before Given	300+	65%	66%	64%
Nurses 'Always' Communicated Well	300+	76%	81%	79%
Pain 'Always' Well Controlled	300+	67%	73%	71%
Room and Bathroom 'Always' Clean	300+	71%	75%	73%
Timely Help 'Always' Received	300+	65%	69%	68%
Would Definitely Recommend Hospital	300+	70%	71%	71%
Use of Medical Imaging				
Cardiac Imaging Stress Test before Surgery	116	3.4%	5.3%	5.3%
Combination Abdominal CT Scan	483	18.0%	10.7%	10.5%
Combination Brain/Sinus CT Scan[1]	-	-	3.1%	2.7%
Combination Chest CT Scan	205	22.0%	4.3%	2.7%
Follow-up Mammogram/Ultrasound	674	13.8%	8.3%	8.8%
Lumbar Spine MRI for Low Back Pain	59	40.7%	38.9%	37.2%

NOTE: Hospital profiles are in alphabetical order by state, then city, then hospital within the city; Rankings exclude hospitals with less than 25 cases except for patient surveys which excludes hospitals with less than 100 cases; (a) 100-299 cases; (1) The number of cases/patients is too few to report; (2) Data submitted were based on a sample of cases/patients; (3) Results are based on a shorter time period than required; (4) Data suppressed by CMS for one or more quarters; (5) Results are not available for this reporting period; (6) Fewer than 100 patients completed the HCAHPS survey; (7) No cases met the criteria for this measure; (8) The lower limit of the confidence interval cannot be calculated if the number of observed infections equals zero; (9) No data are available from the state/territory for this reporting period; (10) The scores shown reflect fewer than 50 completed surveys; (11) There were discrepancies in the data collection process; (12) This measure does not apply to this hospital for this reporting period; (13) Results cannot be calculated for this reporting period; (14) The results for this state are combined with nearby states to protect confidentiality; Please refer to the User's Guide for a full explanation of data.

Blood Clot Prevention and Treatment

Anticoagulation Overlap Therapy

Hospital Name	City	Rate	Cases
Eastern Maine Medical Center[2]	Bangor	100%	79
Mid Coast Hospital[2]	Brunswick	100%	34
Saint Joseph Hospital[2]	Bangor	100%	31
Southern Maine Medical Center[2]	Biddeford	100%	54
York Hospital[2]	York	100%	25
Maine Medical Center[2]	Portland	99%	157
Mainegeneral Medical Center[2]	Augusta	99%	73
Mercy Hospital[2]	Portland	97%	34
Central Maine Medical Center[2]	Lewiston	94%	71

ICU Venous Thromboembolism Prophylaxis

Hospital Name	City	Rate	Cases
Franklin Memorial Hospital[2]	Farmington	100%	42
Inland Hospital[2]	Waterville	100%	47
Maine Medical Center[2]	Portland	100%	50
Central Maine Medical Center[2]	Lewiston	98%	90
Maine Coast Memorial Hospital[2]	Ellsworth	98%	55
Mid Coast Hospital[2]	Brunswick	98%	109
Cary Medical Center[2]	Caribou	97%	35
York Hospital[2]	York	97%	62
Henrietta D Goodall Hospital[2]	Sanford	96%	57
Mainegeneral Medical Center[2]	Augusta	96%	93
Parkview Adventist Medical Center[2]	Brunswick	96%	91
Southern Maine Medical Center[2]	Biddeford	96%	52
Eastern Maine Medical Center[2]	Bangor	95%	104
Saint Joseph Hospital[2]	Bangor	95%	43
The Aroostook Medical Center[2]	Presque Isle	94%	101
Redington Fairview General Hospital[2]	Skowhegan	92%	36
Saint Marys Regional Medical Center[2]	Lewiston	90%	41
Miles Memorial Hospital[2]	Damariscotta	89%	94

Incidence of Potentially Preventable VTE

Hospital Name	City	Rate	Cases
Maine Medical Center[2]	Portland	2%	49

UFH with Dosages/Platelet Count Monitoring

Hospital Name	City	Rate	Cases
Eastern Maine Medical Center[2]	Bangor	100%	87
Maine Medical Center[2]	Portland	100%	174
Mainegeneral Medical Center[2]	Augusta	100%	50
Saint Joseph Hospital[2]	Bangor	100%	32

Venous Thromboembolism Prophylaxis

Hospital Name	City	Rate	Cases
Franklin Memorial Hospital[2]	Farmington	100%	219
Inland Hospital[2]	Waterville	99%	98
Northern Maine Medical Center[2]	Fort Kent	99%	97
Redington Fairview General Hospital[2]	Skowhegan	99%	136
Maine Coast Memorial Hospital[2]	Ellsworth	98%	156
Maine Medical Center[2]	Portland	98%	340
Penobscot Valley Hospital[2,3]	Lincoln	98%	62
Calais Regional Hospital	Calais	97%	317
Parkview Adventist Medical Center[2]	Brunswick	97%	248
Henrietta D Goodall Hospital[2]	Sanford	96%	137
Mercy Hospital[2]	Portland	96%	294
Saint Joseph Hospital[2]	Bangor	96%	363
York Hospital[2]	York	96%	251
The Aroostook Medical Center[2]	Presque Isle	95%	362
Penobscot Bay Medical Center[2]	Rockport	95%	274
Saint Marys Regional Medical Center[2]	Lewiston	94%	250
Eastern Maine Medical Center[2]	Bangor	93%	309
Central Maine Medical Center[2]	Lewiston	92%	325
Southern Maine Medical Center[2]	Biddeford	92%	326
Mid Coast Hospital[2]	Brunswick	91%	296
Mainegeneral Medical Center[2]	Augusta	90%	330
Miles Memorial Hospital[2]	Damariscotta	89%	113
Cary Medical Center[2]	Caribou	84%	139

Warfarin Therapy Discharge Instructions

Hospital Name	City	Rate	Cases
Mainegeneral Medical Center[2]	Augusta	100%	56
Eastern Maine Medical Center[2]	Bangor	97%	58
Mid Coast Hospital[2]	Brunswick	84%	31
Southern Maine Medical Center[2]	Biddeford	83%	42
Maine Medical Center[2]	Portland	73%	114
Central Maine Medical Center[2]	Lewiston	63%	57

Chest Pain/Possible Heart Attack Care

Aspirin Given Within 24 Hours of Arrival

Hospital Name	City	Rate	Cases
The Aroostook Medical Center	Presque Isle	100%	38
Henrietta D Goodall Hospital	Sanford	100%	84
Houlton Regional Hospital	Houlton	100%	36
Maine Coast Memorial Hospital	Ellsworth	100%	36
Mainegeneral Medical Center	Augusta	100%	120
Mid Coast Hospital	Brunswick	100%	41
Miles Memorial Hospital	Damariscotta	100%	71
Saint Marys Regional Medical Center	Lewiston	100%	28
Southern Maine Medical Center	Biddeford	100%	92
Stephens Memorial Hospital	Norway	100%	36
Calais Regional Hospital	Calais	98%	66
Inland Hospital	Waterville	98%	50
Penobscot Bay Medical Center	Rockport	98%	53
Franklin Memorial Hospital	Farmington	97%	35
Redington Fairview General Hospital	Skowhegan	97%	64

Fibrinolytic Meds Within 30 Minutes of Arrival

Hospital Name	City	Rate	Cases
Mainegeneral Medical Center	Augusta	97%	35

Average Time to ECG (minutes)

Hospital Name	City	Min.	Cases
Mid Coast Hospital	Brunswick	0	41
Calais Regional Hospital	Calais	3	66
Stephens Memorial Hospital	Norway	3	39
Houlton Regional Hospital	Houlton	4	38
Southern Maine Medical Center	Biddeford	4	92
Inland Hospital	Waterville	5	51
The Aroostook Medical Center	Presque Isle	6	38
Henrietta D Goodall Hospital	Sanford	6	86
Mainegeneral Medical Center	Augusta	6	123
Miles Memorial Hospital	Damariscotta	6	74
Penobscot Valley Hospital	Lincoln	6	25
Franklin Memorial Hospital	Farmington	7	32
Penobscot Bay Medical Center	Rockport	7	54
Saint Marys Regional Medical Center	Lewiston	9	28
Maine Coast Memorial Hospital	Ellsworth	10	38
Redington Fairview General Hospital	Skowhegan	12	71

Average Time to Transfer (minutes)

Hospital Name	City	Min.	Cases
Southern Maine Medical Center	Biddeford	30	33

Children's Asthma Care

No hospitals met the 25 case threshold.

Emergency Department

Admittance Decision Time (minutes)

Hospital Name	City	Min.	Cases
Stephens Memorial Hospital[2]	Norway	53	387
Northern Maine Medical Center[2]	Fort Kent	58	316
York Hospital[2]	York	66	422
Southern Maine Medical Center[2]	Biddeford	70	738
Cary Medical Center[2]	Caribou	71	398
Penobscot Valley Hospital[2]	Lincoln	80	444
Redington Fairview General Hospital[2]	Skowhegan	98	442
Parkview Adventist Medical Center[2]	Brunswick	104	314
Central Maine Medical Center[2]	Lewiston	105	613
Maine Medical Center[2]	Portland	107	464
Inland Hospital[2]	Waterville	109	355
Franklin Memorial Hospital[2]	Farmington	114	415
Mid Coast Hospital[2]	Brunswick	116	588
Penobscot Bay Medical Center[2]	Rockport	121	458
Saint Joseph Hospital[2]	Bangor	122	620
Saint Marys Regional Medical Center[2]	Lewiston	142	371
Maine Coast Memorial Hospital[2]	Ellsworth	145	353
Mainegeneral Medical Center[2]	Augusta	145	732
Mount Desert Island Hospital[2,3]	Bar Harbor	145	285
Mercy Hospital[2]	Portland	147	453
Miles Memorial Hospital[2]	Damariscotta	147	252
The Aroostook Medical Center[2]	Presque Isle	150	326
Henrietta D Goodall Hospital[2]	Sanford	164	435
Eastern Maine Medical Center[2]	Bangor	228	90

Head CT Results Within 45 Minutes of Arrival

Hospital Name	City	Rate	Cases
Maine Medical Center	Portland	11%	27

Patients Who Left ER Before Being Seen

Hospital Name	City	Rate	Cases
Maine Coast Memorial Hospital	Ellsworth	0%	18058
Mount Desert Island Hospital	Bar Harbor	0%	6287
Northern Maine Medical Center	Fort Kent	0%	6579
Parkview Adventist Medical Center	Brunswick	0%	9390
Saint Andrews Hospital	Boothbay Hrbr	0%	4632
York Hospital	York	0%	29027
Cary Medical Center	Caribou	1%	18711
Franklin Memorial Hospital	Farmington	1%	16598
Henrietta D Goodall Hospital	Sanford	1%	21644
Mainegeneral Medical Center	Augusta	1%	60234
Mercy Hospital	Portland	1%	27579
Mid Coast Hospital	Brunswick	1%	24140
Miles Memorial Hospital	Damariscotta	1%	12331
Penobscot Bay Medical Center	Rockport	1%	23770
Saint Joseph Hospital	Bangor	1%	25013
Saint Marys Regional Medical Center	Lewiston	1%	34187
Stephens Memorial Hospital	Norway	1%	18568
The Aroostook Medical Center	Presque Isle	2%	14942
Central Maine Medical Center	Lewiston	2%	46841
Eastern Maine Medical Center	Bangor	2%	40349
Inland Hospital	Waterville	2%	14744
Maine Medical Center	Portland	2%	66049
Southern Maine Medical Center	Biddeford	2%	41548

Time from ER Arrival to Being Admitted (minutes)

Hospital Name	City	Min.	Cases
Northern Maine Medical Center[2]	Fort Kent	202	331
Parkview Adventist Medical Center[2]	Brunswick	222	504
York Hospital[2]	York	224	442
Penobscot Valley Hospital[2]	Lincoln	233	451
Stephens Memorial Hospital[2]	Norway	236	423
Cary Medical Center[2]	Caribou	253	400
The Aroostook Medical Center[2]	Presque Isle	254	334
Franklin Memorial Hospital[2]	Farmington	263	415
Mount Desert Island Hospital[2,3]	Bar Harbor	268	285
Maine Coast Memorial Hospital[2]	Ellsworth	280	361
Mid Coast Hospital[2]	Brunswick	283	588
Penobscot Bay Medical Center[2]	Rockport	288	458
Central Maine Medical Center[2]	Lewiston	291	634
Redington Fairview General Hospital[2]	Skowhegan	295	442
Inland Hospital[2]	Waterville	300	360
Miles Memorial Hospital[2]	Damariscotta	303	386
Henrietta D Goodall Hospital[2]	Sanford	318	445
Mainegeneral Medical Center[2]	Augusta	322	759
Southern Maine Medical Center[2]	Biddeford	322	756
Saint Joseph Hospital[2]	Bangor	324	620
Maine Medical Center[2]	Portland	342	486
Saint Marys Regional Medical Center[2]	Lewiston	354	374
Eastern Maine Medical Center[2]	Bangor	376	289
Mercy Hospital[2]	Portland	407	470

Time from ER Arrival to Discharge (minutes)

Hospital Name	City	Min.	Cases
York Hospital	York	86	369
Penobscot Valley Hospital[3]	Lincoln	89	231
Cary Medical Center	Caribou	96	368
Northern Maine Medical Center	Fort Kent	101	368
Franklin Memorial Hospital	Farmington	102	453
Parkview Adventist Medical Center	Brunswick	104	369
Stephens Memorial Hospital	Norway	109	376
Inland Hospital	Waterville	110	382
Miles Memorial Hospital	Damariscotta	110	353
The Aroostook Medical Center	Presque Isle	111	400
Henrietta D Goodall Hospital	Sanford	111	372
Penobscot Bay Medical Center	Rockport	111	382
Saint Marys Regional Medical Center	Lewiston	113	368
Maine Coast Memorial Hospital	Ellsworth	115	393
Mid Coast Hospital	Brunswick	120	374
Mount Desert Island Hospital[3]	Bar Harbor	126	138
Redington Fairview General Hospital	Skowhegan	128	393
Mainegeneral Medical Center	Augusta	132	398
Southern Maine Medical Center	Biddeford	146	329
Central Maine Medical Center	Lewiston	158	371
Mercy Hospital	Portland	160	350
Saint Joseph Hospital	Bangor	164	363
Eastern Maine Medical Center	Bangor	176	344
Maine Medical Center	Portland	236	360

Time in ER Before Being Evaluated (minutes)

Hospital Name	City	Min.	Cases
York Hospital	York	14	406
Penobscot Bay Medical Center	Rockport	18	408
Henrietta D Goodall Hospital	Sanford	20	408
Parkview Adventist Medical Center	Brunswick	21	395
Saint Marys Regional Medical Center	Lewiston	21	416
Miles Memorial Hospital	Damariscotta	24	292
Stephens Memorial Hospital	Norway	24	404
Saint Joseph Hospital	Bangor	25	401
Franklin Memorial Hospital	Farmington	26	477
Mount Desert Island Hospital[3]	Bar Harbor	26	145
Northern Maine Medical Center	Fort Kent	26	404
Penobscot Valley Hospital[3]	Lincoln	27	250
Inland Hospital	Waterville	30	328
Mercy Hospital	Portland	30	330
Cary Medical Center	Caribou	31	378
Maine Coast Memorial Hospital	Ellsworth	31	306
The Aroostook Medical Center	Presque Isle	32	292
Mainegeneral Medical Center	Augusta	33	415
Maine Medical Center	Portland	36	411

NOTE: Hospital profiles are in alphabetical order by state, then city, then hospital within the city; Rankings exclude hospitals with less than 25 cases except for patient surveys which excludes hospitals with less than 100 cases; (a) 100-299 cases; (1) The number of cases/patients is too few to report; (2) Data submitted were based on a sample of cases/patients; (3) Results are based on a shorter time period than required; (4) Data suppressed by CMS for one or more quarters; (5) Results are not available for this reporting period; (6) Fewer than 100 patients completed the HCAHPS survey; (7) No cases met the criteria for this measure; (8) The lower limit of the confidence interval cannot be calculated if the number of observed infections equals zero; (9) No data are available from the state/territory for this reporting period; (10) The scores shown reflect fewer than 50 completed surveys; (11) There were discrepancies in the data collection process; (12) This measure does not apply to this hospital for this reporting period; (13) Results cannot be calculated for this reporting period; (14) The results for this state are combined with nearby states to protect confidentiality; Please refer to the User's Guide for a full explanation of data.

Mid Coast Hospital	Brunswick	37	174
Eastern Maine Medical Center	Bangor	44	244
Redington Fairview General Hospital	Skowhegan	44	435
Central Maine Medical Center	Lewiston	45	415
Southern Maine Medical Center	Biddeford	50	262

Time to Pain Meds for Bone Fractures (minutes)

Hospital Name	City	Min.	Cases
Penobscot Bay Medical Center	Rockport	26	68
Mainegeneral Medical Center	Augusta	31	111
Henrietta D Goodall Hospital	Sanford	34	46
York Hospital	York	35	60
Parkview Adventist Medical Center	Brunswick	36	42
Franklin Memorial Hospital	Farmington	40	83
Inland Hospital	Waterville	42	43
Miles Memorial Hospital	Damariscotta	42	32
The Aroostook Medical Center	Presque Isle	48	60
Maine Coast Memorial Hospital	Ellsworth	49	51
Saint Marys Regional Medical Center	Lewiston	49	54
Cary Medical Center	Caribou	52	34
Mercy Hospital	Portland	55	65
Southern Maine Medical Center	Biddeford	55	99
Maine Medical Center	Portland	57	291
Mid Coast Hospital	Brunswick	62	62
Redington Fairview General Hospital	Skowhegan	64	84
Saint Joseph Hospital	Bangor	65	107
Eastern Maine Medical Center	Bangor	67	169
Penobscot Valley Hospital	Lincoln	77	25
Central Maine Medical Center	Lewiston	85	123

Heart Attack Care

Aspirin Given at Discharge

Hospital Name	City	Rate	Cases
The Aroostook Medical Center	Presque Isle	100%	41
Central Maine Medical Center[2]	Lewiston	100%	329
Eastern Maine Medical Center	Bangor	100%	1002
Maine Medical Center	Portland	100%	1138
Mid Coast Hospital	Brunswick	100%	30
Saint Joseph Hospital	Bangor	100%	36
Saint Marys Regional Medical Center	Lewiston	100%	26
Southern Maine Medical Center	Biddeford	100%	60
York Hospital	York	100%	63
Mainegeneral Medical Center	Augusta	99%	91
Maine Coast Memorial Hospital	Ellsworth	98%	62

PCI Within 90 Minutes of Arrival

Hospital Name	City	Rate	Cases
Maine Medical Center	Portland	97%	77
Central Maine Medical Center[2]	Lewiston	96%	50
Eastern Maine Medical Center	Bangor	96%	25

Statin Prescribed at Discharge

Hospital Name	City	Rate	Cases
The Aroostook Medical Center	Presque Isle	100%	35
Eastern Maine Medical Center	Bangor	100%	953
Maine Coast Memorial Hospital	Ellsworth	100%	58
Mainegeneral Medical Center	Augusta	100%	84
Saint Marys Regional Medical Center	Lewiston	100%	27
York Hospital	York	100%	62
Central Maine Medical Center[2]	Lewiston	99%	323
Maine Medical Center	Portland	99%	1108
Saint Joseph Hospital	Bangor	97%	34
Southern Maine Medical Center	Biddeford	97%	59

Heart Failure Care

ACE Inhibitor or ARB for LVSD

Hospital Name	City	Rate	Cases
The Aroostook Medical Center	Presque Isle	100%	32
Central Maine Medical Center	Lewiston	100%	64
Eastern Maine Medical Center	Bangor	100%	88
Mainegeneral Medical Center	Augusta	100%	48
Mid Coast Hospital	Brunswick	100%	29
Southern Maine Medical Center	Biddeford	100%	29
York Hospital	York	100%	25
Maine Medical Center	Portland	99%	109
Saint Joseph Hospital	Bangor	93%	27

Discharge Instructions Given

Hospital Name	City	Rate	Cases
Central Maine Medical Center	Lewiston	100%	201
Inland Hospital	Waterville	100%	35
Mainegeneral Medical Center	Augusta	100%	180
Mid Coast Hospital	Brunswick	100%	106
Miles Memorial Hospital[2]	Damariscotta	100%	49
Northern Maine Medical Center	Fort Kent	100%	28
Penobscot Bay Medical Center	Rockport	100%	55
The Aroostook Medical Center	Presque Isle	99%	83
Eastern Maine Medical Center	Bangor	99%	375
Saint Joseph Hospital	Bangor	99%	110
Cary Medical Center	Caribou	98%	65
Franklin Memorial Hospital	Farmington	98%	64
Maine Coast Memorial Hospital	Ellsworth	98%	43
Redington Fairview General Hospital	Skowhegan	98%	49
Saint Marys Regional Medical Center	Lewiston	98%	47
Houlton Regional Hospital	Houlton	97%	32
Maine Medical Center	Portland	97%	424
Parkview Adventist Medical Center	Brunswick	97%	29
Southern Maine Medical Center	Biddeford	97%	158
Sebasticook Valley Hospital	Pittsfield	96%	28
York Hospital	York	95%	117
Mercy Hospital	Portland	93%	82
Stephens Memorial Hospital	Norway	93%	30
Togus VA Medical Center	Augusta	87%	68
Henrietta D Goodall Hospital	Sanford	84%	57

Evaluation of LVS Function

Hospital Name	City	Rate	Cases
The Aroostook Medical Center	Presque Isle	100%	100
Bridgton Hospital	Bridgton	100%	30
Calais Regional Hospital	Calais	100%	27
Cary Medical Center	Caribou	100%	86
Central Maine Medical Center	Lewiston	100%	265
Eastern Maine Medical Center	Bangor	100%	444
Franklin Memorial Hospital	Farmington	100%	83
Henrietta D Goodall Hospital	Sanford	100%	95
Houlton Regional Hospital	Houlton	100%	47
Inland Hospital	Waterville	100%	48
Maine Coast Memorial Hospital	Ellsworth	100%	57
Maine Medical Center	Portland	100%	593
Mainegeneral Medical Center	Augusta	100%	227
Mayo Regional Hospital	Dover Foxcroft	100%	29
Mercy Hospital	Portland	100%	112
Mid Coast Hospital	Brunswick	100%	124
Miles Memorial Hospital[2]	Damariscotta	100%	81
Mount Desert Island Hospital	Bar Harbor	100%	25
Northern Maine Medical Center	Fort Kent	100%	46
Parkview Adventist Medical Center	Brunswick	100%	34
Penobscot Bay Medical Center	Rockport	100%	70
Penobscot Valley Hospital	Lincoln	100%	38
Redington Fairview General Hospital	Skowhegan	100%	78
Rumford Hospital	Rumford	100%	35
Saint Joseph Hospital	Bangor	100%	152
Saint Marys Regional Medical Center	Lewiston	100%	74
Sebasticook Valley Hospital	Pittsfield	100%	29
Southern Maine Medical Center	Biddeford	100%	206
Stephens Memorial Hospital	Norway	100%	41
Waldo County General Hospital	Belfast	100%	25
Togus VA Medical Center	Augusta	99%	83
York Hospital	York	99%	143

Medicare Spending

Medicare Spending per Patient (ratio)

Hospital Name	City	Ratio	Cases
The Aroostook Medical Center	Presque Isle	0.86	-
Northern Maine Medical Center	Fort Kent	0.87	-
Franklin Memorial Hospital	Farmington	0.88	-
Cary Medical Center	Caribou	0.89	-
Parkview Adventist Medical Center	Brunswick	0.91	-
Maine Coast Memorial Hospital	Ellsworth	0.94	-
Penobscot Bay Medical Center	Rockport	0.94	-
Henrietta D Goodall Hospital	Sanford	0.95	-
Mid Coast Hospital	Brunswick	0.95	-
Saint Joseph Hospital	Bangor	0.96	-
Central Maine Medical Center	Lewiston	0.97	-
Saint Marys Regional Medical Center	Lewiston	0.97	-
York Hospital	York	0.97	-
Inland Hospital	Waterville	0.98	-
Mainegeneral Medical Center	Augusta	0.98	-
Southern Maine Medical Center	Biddeford	0.98	-
Eastern Maine Medical Center	Bangor	0.99	-
Maine Medical Center	Portland	0.99	-
Miles Memorial Hospital	Damariscotta	0.99	-
Mercy Hospital	Portland	1.00	-

Pneumonia Care

Appropriate Initial Antibiotic Given

Hospital Name	City	Rate	Cases
Bridgton Hospital	Bridgton	100%	29
Down East Community Hospital	Machias	100%	51
Franklin Memorial Hospital	Farmington	100%	55
Maine Medical Center	Portland	100%	120
Penobscot Valley Hospital[2]	Lincoln	100%	46
Sebasticook Valley Hospital	Pittsfield	100%	27
Togus VA Medical Center	Augusta	100%	30
Henrietta D Goodall Hospital	Sanford	99%	76
Mainegeneral Medical Center	Augusta	99%	255
Saint Marys Regional Medical Center	Lewiston	99%	77
Cary Medical Center	Caribou	98%	45
Central Maine Medical Center[2]	Lewiston	98%	111
Eastern Maine Medical Center	Bangor	98%	119
Maine Coast Memorial Hospital	Ellsworth	98%	55
Redington Fairview General Hospital	Skowhegan	98%	83
Southern Maine Medical Center	Biddeford	98%	122
Stephens Memorial Hospital[2]	Norway	98%	55
Calais Regional Hospital	Calais	97%	29
Houlton Regional Hospital	Houlton	97%	33
Mercy Hospital	Portland	97%	112
Waldo County General Hospital	Belfast	97%	35
The Aroostook Medical Center	Presque Isle	96%	46
Mid Coast Hospital[2]	Brunswick	96%	107
Penobscot Bay Medical Center	Rockport	96%	77
Saint Joseph Hospital	Bangor	96%	151
York Hospital	York	96%	67
Mayo Regional Hospital	Dover Foxcroft	94%	34
Inland Hospital[2]	Waterville	93%	30
Miles Memorial Hospital	Damariscotta	93%	27
Parkview Adventist Medical Center	Brunswick	93%	30

Blood Culture Timing

Hospital Name	City	Rate	Cases
The Aroostook Medical Center	Presque Isle	100%	106
Calais Regional Hospital	Calais	100%	53
Down East Community Hospital	Machias	100%	59
Maine Coast Memorial Hospital	Ellsworth	100%	99
Mayo Regional Hospital	Dover Foxcroft	100%	54
Mercy Hospital	Portland	100%	144
Mount Desert Island Hospital	Bar Harbor	100%	28
Rumford Hospital	Rumford	100%	28
Southern Maine Medical Center	Biddeford	100%	86
Togus VA Medical Center	Augusta	100%	39
Waldo County General Hospital	Belfast	100%	50
Cary Medical Center	Caribou	99%	75
Maine Medical Center	Portland	99%	215
Eastern Maine Medical Center	Bangor	98%	261
Henrietta D Goodall Hospital	Sanford	98%	138
Houlton Regional Hospital	Houlton	98%	62
Inland Hospital[2]	Waterville	98%	46
Mainegeneral Medical Center	Augusta	98%	312
Miles Memorial Hospital	Damariscotta	98%	55
Northern Maine Medical Center	Fort Kent	98%	49
Penobscot Bay Medical Center	Rockport	98%	121
Stephens Memorial Hospital[2]	Norway	98%	94
York Hospital	York	98%	132
Bridgton Hospital	Bridgton	97%	36
Millinocket Regional Hospital	Millinocket	97%	32
Saint Joseph Hospital	Bangor	97%	247
Sebasticook Valley Hospital	Pittsfield	97%	29
Franklin Memorial Hospital	Farmington	96%	75
Saint Marys Regional Medical Center	Lewiston	96%	93
Redington Fairview General Hospital	Skowhegan	95%	110
Central Maine Medical Center[2]	Lewiston	94%	82
Mid Coast Hospital[2]	Brunswick	94%	83

Pregnancy and Delivery Care

Newborns whose Deliveries were Scheduled Early

Hospital Name	City	Rate	Cases
Inland Hospital	Waterville	0%	40
Maine Coast Memorial Hospital	Ellsworth	0%	39
Mainegeneral Medical Center	Augusta	0%	46
Saint Marys Regional Medical Center	Lewiston	0%	33
Southern Maine Medical Center	Biddeford	0%	71
Central Maine Medical Center	Lewiston	2%	50
Maine Medical Center	Portland	2%	121
Mercy Hospital	Portland	2%	40
Mid Coast Hospital	Brunswick	3%	36
Eastern Maine Medical Center	Bangor	5%	98

Preventive Care

Immunization for Influenza

Hospital Name	City	Rate	Cases
Franklin Memorial Hospital[2]	Farmington	100%	274
Mount Desert Island Hospital[2,3]	Bar Harbor	100%	131
Northern Maine Medical Center[2]	Fort Kent	100%	289
Henrietta D Goodall Hospital[2]	Sanford	99%	267
York Hospital[2]	York	99%	304
The Aroostook Medical Center[2]	Presque Isle	98%	294
Calais Regional Hospital	Calais	98%	306
Maine Coast Memorial Hospital[2]	Ellsworth	98%	289
Redington Fairview General Hospital[2]	Skowhegan	98%	285
Inland Hospital[2]	Waterville	97%	289

NOTE: Hospital profiles are in alphabetical order by state, then city, then hospital within the city; Rankings exclude hospitals with less than 25 cases except for patient surveys which excludes hospitals with less than 100 cases; (a) 100-299 cases; (1) The number of cases/patients is too few to report; (2) Data submitted were based on a sample of cases/patients; (3) Results are based on a shorter time period than required; (4) Data suppressed by CMS for one or more quarters; (5) Results are not available for this reporting period; (6) Fewer than 100 patients completed the HCAHPS survey; (7) No cases met the criteria for this measure; (8) The lower limit of the confidence interval cannot be calculated if the number of observed infections equals zero; (9) No data are available from the state/territory for this reporting period; (10) The scores shown reflect fewer than 50 completed surveys; (11) There were discrepancies in the data collection process; (12) This measure does not apply to this hospital for this reporting period; (13) Results cannot be calculated for this reporting period; (14) The results for this state are combined with nearby states to protect confidentiality; Please refer to the User's Guide for a full explanation of data.

Hospital Name	City	Rate	Cases
Parkview Adventist Medical Center[2]	Brunswick	97%	308
Stephens Memorial Hospital[2]	Norway	97%	304
Cary Medical Center[2]	Caribou	96%	283
Miles Memorial Hospital[2]	Damariscotta	96%	295
Southern Maine Medical Center[2]	Biddeford	96%	509
Saint Joseph Hospital[2]	Bangor	95%	384
Mainegeneral Medical Center[2]	Augusta	94%	519
Penobscot Valley Hospital[2]	Lincoln	93%	276
Central Maine Medical Center[2]	Lewiston	92%	585
Mercy Hospital[2]	Portland	92%	539
Togus VA Medical Center[2,3]	Augusta	90%	143
Saint Marys Regional Medical Center[2]	Lewiston	89%	474
Eastern Maine Medical Center[2]	Bangor	85%	553
Maine Medical Center[2]	Portland	85%	552
Penobscot Bay Medical Center[2]	Rockport	82%	299
Mid Coast Hospital[2]	Brunswick	76%	416

Immunization for Pneumonia

Hospital Name	City	Rate	Cases
Henrietta D Goodall Hospital[2]	Sanford	100%	383
Mount Desert Island Hospital[2,3]	Bar Harbor	100%	253
Northern Maine Medical Center[2]	Fort Kent	100%	356
The Aroostook Medical Center[2]	Presque Isle	99%	405
Calais Regional Hospital	Calais	99%	425
Franklin Memorial Hospital[2]	Farmington	99%	347
Inland Hospital[2]	Waterville	99%	327
Maine Coast Memorial Hospital[2]	Ellsworth	99%	386
Penobscot Valley Hospital[2]	Lincoln	99%	406
York Hospital[2]	York	99%	412
Miles Memorial Hospital[2]	Damariscotta	98%	444
Parkview Adventist Medical Center[2]	Brunswick	98%	485
Redington Fairview General Hospital[2]	Skowhegan	98%	391
Stephens Memorial Hospital[2]	Norway	98%	444
Cary Medical Center[2]	Caribou	97%	382
Mainegeneral Medical Center[2]	Augusta	97%	680
Eastern Maine Medical Center[2]	Bangor	95%	674
Saint Joseph Hospital[2]	Bangor	95%	631
Saint Marys Regional Medical Center[2]	Lewiston	94%	477
Southern Maine Medical Center[2]	Biddeford	94%	727
Togus VA Medical Center[2,3]	Augusta	93%	317
Mercy Hospital[2]	Portland	92%	680
Central Maine Medical Center[2]	Lewiston	89%	798
Penobscot Bay Medical Center[2]	Rockport	84%	418
Maine Medical Center[2]	Portland	81%	625
Mid Coast Hospital[2]	Brunswick	79%	531

Stroke Care

Anticoagulation Therapy for Atrial Fibrillation

Hospital Name	City	Rate	Cases
Eastern Maine Medical Center	Bangor	100%	26
Maine Medical Center	Portland	94%	33

Antithrombotic Therapy Timing

Hospital Name	City	Rate	Cases
Henrietta D Goodall Hospital	Sanford	100%	27
Maine Coast Memorial Hospital	Ellsworth	100%	26
Mainegeneral Medical Center	Augusta	100%	77
Northern Maine Medical Center	Fort Kent	100%	26
Penobscot Bay Medical Center	Rockport	100%	54
Redington Fairview General Hospital	Skowhegan	100%	26
Saint Joseph Hospital	Bangor	100%	42
Saint Marys Regional Medical Center	Lewiston	100%	32
Southern Maine Medical Center	Biddeford	100%	79
York Hospital	York	100%	38
Eastern Maine Medical Center	Bangor	99%	162
Central Maine Medical Center	Lewiston	98%	91
Mid Coast Hospital	Brunswick	98%	54
Maine Medical Center	Portland	97%	157

Assessed for Rehabilitation

Hospital Name	City	Rate	Cases
Maine Coast Memorial Hospital	Ellsworth	100%	36
Mainegeneral Medical Center	Augusta	100%	87
Mid Coast Hospital	Brunswick	100%	54
Saint Joseph Hospital	Bangor	100%	40
Saint Marys Regional Medical Center	Lewiston	100%	34
Eastern Maine Medical Center	Bangor	99%	234
Southern Maine Medical Center	Biddeford	99%	91
Central Maine Medical Center	Lewiston	98%	123
York Hospital	York	98%	40
Penobscot Bay Medical Center	Rockport	97%	70
Henrietta D Goodall Hospital	Sanford	96%	26
Maine Medical Center	Portland	96%	259

Discharged on Antithrombotic Therapy

Hospital Name	City	Rate	Cases
Central Maine Medical Center	Lewiston	100%	106
Eastern Maine Medical Center	Bangor	100%	192
Henrietta D Goodall Hospital	Sanford	100%	26
Maine Coast Memorial Hospital	Ellsworth	100%	34
Maine Medical Center	Portland	100%	192
Mainegeneral Medical Center	Augusta	100%	81
Mid Coast Hospital	Brunswick	100%	53
Penobscot Bay Medical Center	Rockport	100%	69
Saint Joseph Hospital	Bangor	100%	37
Southern Maine Medical Center	Biddeford	100%	83
York Hospital	York	100%	39
Saint Marys Regional Medical Center	Lewiston	97%	31

Discharged on Statin Medication

Hospital Name	City	Rate	Cases
Southern Maine Medical Center	Biddeford	100%	69
York Hospital	York	100%	27
Eastern Maine Medical Center	Bangor	99%	151
Mid Coast Hospital	Brunswick	98%	44
Penobscot Bay Medical Center	Rockport	98%	52
Central Maine Medical Center	Lewiston	97%	79
Saint Joseph Hospital	Bangor	97%	32
Maine Medical Center	Portland	96%	157
Mainegeneral Medical Center	Augusta	94%	69

Thrombolytic Therapy Timing

Hospital Name	City	Rate	Cases
Maine Medical Center	Portland	18%	94

Venous Thromboembolism (VTE) Prophylaxis

Hospital Name	City	Rate	Cases
Northern Maine Medical Center	Fort Kent	100%	27
Saint Marys Regional Medical Center	Lewiston	100%	34
Eastern Maine Medical Center	Bangor	99%	244
Mainegeneral Medical Center	Augusta	98%	87
Mid Coast Hospital	Brunswick	98%	55
Central Maine Medical Center	Lewiston	97%	113
Maine Coast Memorial Hospital	Ellsworth	97%	33
Henrietta D Goodall Hospital	Sanford	96%	27
Southern Maine Medical Center	Biddeford	96%	89
York Hospital	York	95%	38
Saint Joseph Hospital	Bangor	93%	45
Maine Medical Center	Portland	92%	268
Penobscot Bay Medical Center	Rockport	91%	66
Mercy Hospital	Portland	89%	28

Written Stroke Educational Materials Given

Hospital Name	City	Rate	Cases
Mainegeneral Medical Center	Augusta	100%	37
Penobscot Bay Medical Center	Rockport	97%	36
Eastern Maine Medical Center	Bangor	95%	100
Central Maine Medical Center	Lewiston	93%	69
Southern Maine Medical Center	Biddeford	80%	40
Maine Medical Center	Portland	66%	115

Surgical Care Improvement Project

Appropriate Beta Blocker Usage

Hospital Name	City	Rate	Cases
Cary Medical Center[2]	Caribou	100%	59
Eastern Maine Medical Center[2]	Bangor	100%	575
Henrietta D Goodall Hospital	Sanford	100%	51
Inland Hospital[2]	Waterville	100%	32
Maine Medical Center[2]	Portland	100%	305
Miles Memorial Hospital	Damariscotta	100%	42
Millinocket Regional Hospital	Millinocket	100%	31
Saint Marys Regional Medical Center[2]	Lewiston	100%	139
Southern Maine Medical Center	Biddeford	100%	143
Stephens Memorial Hospital[2]	Norway	100%	30
Togus VA Medical Center[2]	Augusta	100%	31
Waldo County General Hospital	Belfast	100%	32
Mainegeneral Medical Center[2]	Augusta	99%	183
Mercy Hospital[2]	Portland	99%	187
Saint Joseph Hospital[2]	Bangor	99%	128
The Aroostook Medical Center	Presque Isle	98%	51
Central Maine Medical Center[2]	Lewiston	98%	246
Maine Coast Memorial Hospital	Ellsworth	98%	64
Mid Coast Hospital	Brunswick	98%	59
York Hospital[2]	York	98%	83
Franklin Memorial Hospital	Farmington	97%	29
Penobscot Bay Medical Center	Rockport	97%	76
Mayo Regional Hospital[2]	Dover Foxcroft	96%	26

Appropriate VTP Within 24 Hours

Hospital Name	City	Rate	Cases
The Aroostook Medical Center	Presque Isle	100%	95
Cary Medical Center[2]	Caribou	100%	152
Down East Community Hospital	Machias	100%	33
Eastern Maine Medical Center[2]	Bangor	100%	763
Franklin Memorial Hospital	Farmington	100%	120
Maine Medical Center[2]	Portland	100%	437
Miles Memorial Hospital	Damariscotta	100%	111
Millinocket Regional Hospital	Millinocket	100%	56
Mount Desert Island Hospital	Bar Harbor	100%	32
Parkview Adventist Medical Center[3]	Brunswick	100%	51
Penobscot Bay Medical Center	Rockport	100%	204
Redington Fairview General Hospital	Skowhegan	100%	58
Saint Marys Regional Medical Center[2]	Lewiston	100%	445
Southern Maine Medical Center	Biddeford	100%	370
Central Maine Medical Center[2]	Lewiston	99%	336
Henrietta D Goodall Hospital	Sanford	99%	156
Inland Hospital[2]	Waterville	99%	76
Maine Coast Memorial Hospital	Ellsworth	99%	178
Mainegeneral Medical Center[2]	Augusta	99%	519
Mayo Regional Hospital[2]	Dover Foxcroft	99%	91
Mercy Hospital[2]	Portland	99%	548
Saint Joseph Hospital[2]	Bangor	99%	422
York Hospital[2]	York	99%	237
Blue Hill Memorial Hospital	Blue Hill	98%	44
Calais Regional Hospital	Calais	98%	52
Stephens Memorial Hospital[2]	Norway	98%	100
Waldo County General Hospital	Belfast	98%	120
Mid Coast Hospital	Brunswick	94%	235
Togus VA Medical Center[2]	Augusta	94%	139

Controlled Postoperative Blood Glucose

Hospital Name	City	Rate	Cases
Central Maine Medical Center[2]	Lewiston	99%	108
Maine Medical Center[2]	Portland	99%	198
Eastern Maine Medical Center[2]	Bangor	98%	305

Perioperative Temperature Management

Hospital Name	City	Rate	Cases
The Aroostook Medical Center	Presque Isle	100%	122
Blue Hill Memorial Hospital	Blue Hill	100%	50
Calais Regional Hospital	Calais	100%	58
Cary Medical Center[2]	Caribou	100%	155
Central Maine Medical Center[2]	Lewiston	100%	590
Down East Community Hospital	Machias	100%	28
Eastern Maine Medical Center[2]	Bangor	100%	1011
Franklin Memorial Hospital	Farmington	100%	128
Inland Hospital[2]	Waterville	100%	118
Maine Coast Memorial Hospital	Ellsworth	100%	206
Mainegeneral Medical Center[2]	Augusta	100%	611
Mayo Regional Hospital[2]	Dover Foxcroft	100%	102
Mercy Hospital[2]	Portland	100%	618
Mid Coast Hospital	Brunswick	100%	246
Miles Memorial Hospital	Damariscotta	100%	131
Millinocket Regional Hospital	Millinocket	100%	60
Mount Desert Island Hospital	Bar Harbor	100%	36
Parkview Adventist Medical Center[3]	Brunswick	100%	60
Penobscot Bay Medical Center	Rockport	100%	237
Redington Fairview General Hospital	Skowhegan	100%	61
Saint Marys Regional Medical Center[2]	Lewiston	100%	478
Southern Maine Medical Center	Biddeford	100%	435
Stephens Memorial Hospital[2]	Norway	100%	113
Waldo County General Hospital	Belfast	100%	138
York Hospital[2]	York	100%	281
Henrietta D Goodall Hospital	Sanford	99%	168
Maine Medical Center[2]	Portland	99%	700
Saint Joseph Hospital[2]	Bangor	99%	452
Togus VA Medical Center[2]	Augusta	98%	149

Prophylactic Antibiotic Selection

Hospital Name	City	Rate	Cases
Blue Hill Memorial Hospital	Blue Hill	100%	45
Cary Medical Center[2]	Caribou	100%	133
Down East Community Hospital	Machias	100%	29
Eastern Maine Medical Center[2]	Bangor	100%	1029
Franklin Memorial Hospital	Farmington	100%	75
Maine Coast Memorial Hospital	Ellsworth	100%	135
Maine Medical Center[2]	Portland	100%	640
Mayo Regional Hospital[2]	Dover Foxcroft	100%	92
Mercy Hospital[2]	Portland	100%	471
Millinocket Regional Hospital	Millinocket	100%	48
Parkview Adventist Medical Center[3]	Brunswick	100%	39
Redington Fairview General Hospital	Skowhegan	100%	45
Saint Marys Regional Medical Center[2]	Lewiston	100%	319
Southern Maine Medical Center	Biddeford	100%	301
Stephens Memorial Hospital[2]	Norway	100%	76
Togus VA Medical Center	Augusta	100%	117
Waldo County General Hospital	Belfast	100%	97
The Aroostook Medical Center	Presque Isle	99%	79
Henrietta D Goodall Hospital	Sanford	99%	145
Inland Hospital[2]	Waterville	99%	90
Mainegeneral Medical Center[2]	Augusta	99%	419
Mid Coast Hospital	Brunswick	99%	176
Miles Memorial Hospital	Damariscotta	99%	104
Penobscot Bay Medical Center	Rockport	99%	174

NOTE: Hospital profiles are in alphabetical order by state, then city, then hospital within the city; Rankings exclude hospitals with less than 25 cases except for patient surveys which excludes hospitals with less than 100 cases; (a) 100-299 cases; (1) The number of cases/patients is too few to report; (2) Data submitted were based on a sample of cases/patients; (3) Results are based on a shorter time period than required; (4) Data suppressed by CMS for one or more quarters; (5) Results are not available for this reporting period; (6) Fewer than 100 patients completed the HCAHPS survey; (7) No cases met the criteria for this measure; (8) The lower limit of the confidence interval cannot be calculated if the number of observed infections equals zero; (9) No data are available from the state/territory for this reporting period; (10) The scores shown reflect fewer than 50 completed surveys; (11) There were discrepancies in the data collection process; (12) This measure does not apply to this hospital for this reporting period; (13) Results cannot be calculated for this reporting period; (14) The results for this state are combined with nearby states to protect confidentiality; Please refer to the User's Guide for a full explanation of data.

Hospital Name	City	Rate	Cases
Saint Joseph Hospital[2]	Bangor	99%	349
York Hospital[2]	York	99%	182
Calais Regional Hospital	Calais	98%	53
Central Maine Medical Center[2]	Lewiston	98%	464

Prophylactic Antibiotic Selection (Outpatient)

Hospital Name	City	Rate	Cases
Cary Medical Center	Caribou	100%	114
Franklin Memorial Hospital	Farmington	100%	33
Inland Hospital	Waterville	100%	208
Saint Joseph Hospital	Bangor	100%	278
The Aroostook Medical Center	Presque Isle	99%	139
Maine Coast Memorial Hospital	Ellsworth	99%	84
Mercy Hospital	Portland	99%	580
Mid Coast Hospital	Brunswick	99%	88
York Hospital	York	99%	109
Eastern Maine Medical Center	Bangor	98%	965
Maine Medical Center	Portland	98%	972
Mainegeneral Medical Center	Augusta	98%	380
Stephens Memorial Hospital	Norway	98%	44
Central Maine Medical Center	Lewiston	97%	460
Penobscot Bay Medical Center	Rockport	97%	71
Saint Marys Regional Medical Center	Lewiston	93%	169

Prophylactic Antibiotic Stopped

Hospital Name	City	Rate	Cases
The Aroostook Medical Center	Presque Isle	100%	77
Calais Regional Hospital	Calais	100%	52
Eastern Maine Medical Center[2]	Bangor	100%	996
Inland Hospital[2]	Waterville	100%	88
Maine Coast Memorial Hospital	Ellsworth	100%	131
Mainegeneral Medical Center[2]	Augusta	100%	407
Mayo Regional Hospital[2]	Dover Foxcroft	100%	90
Mercy Hospital[2]	Portland	100%	464
Millinocket Regional Hospital	Millinocket	100%	48
Parkview Adventist Medical Center[3]	Brunswick	100%	39
Southern Maine Medical Center	Biddeford	100%	300
York Hospital[2]	York	100%	180
Central Maine Medical Center[2]	Lewiston	99%	452
Franklin Memorial Hospital	Farmington	99%	71
Mid Coast Hospital	Brunswick	99%	173
Saint Joseph Hospital[2]	Bangor	99%	348
Saint Marys Regional Medical Center[2]	Lewiston	99%	307
Stephens Memorial Hospital[2]	Norway	99%	75
Blue Hill Memorial Hospital	Blue Hill	98%	45
Cary Medical Center[2]	Caribou	98%	131
Henrietta D Goodall Hospital	Sanford	98%	144
Maine Medical Center[2]	Portland	98%	637
Penobscot Bay Medical Center	Rockport	98%	172
Redington Fairview General Hospital	Skowhegan	98%	43
Down East Community Hospital	Machias	97%	29
Miles Memorial Hospital	Damariscotta	97%	102
Togus VA Medical Center	Augusta	97%	115
Waldo County General Hospital	Belfast	96%	94

Prophylactic Antibiotic Timing

Hospital Name	City	Rate	Cases
Calais Regional Hospital	Calais	100%	53
Cary Medical Center[2]	Caribou	100%	133
Down East Community Hospital	Machias	100%	29
Eastern Maine Medical Center[2]	Bangor	100%	1032
Franklin Memorial Hospital	Farmington	100%	75
Inland Hospital[2]	Waterville	100%	90
Maine Coast Memorial Hospital	Ellsworth	100%	135
Mainegeneral Medical Center[2]	Augusta	100%	419
Mayo Regional Hospital[2]	Dover Foxcroft	100%	92
Mid Coast Hospital	Brunswick	100%	176
Parkview Adventist Medical Center[3]	Brunswick	100%	39
Redington Fairview General Hospital	Skowhegan	100%	45
Saint Joseph Hospital[2]	Bangor	100%	350
Southern Maine Medical Center	Biddeford	100%	301
Stephens Memorial Hospital[2]	Norway	100%	76
The Aroostook Medical Center	Presque Isle	99%	79
Central Maine Medical Center[2]	Lewiston	99%	465
Henrietta D Goodall Hospital	Sanford	99%	145
Mercy Hospital[2]	Portland	99%	471
Penobscot Bay Medical Center	Rockport	99%	174
Saint Marys Regional Medical Center[2]	Lewiston	99%	319
Waldo County General Hospital	Belfast	99%	97
York Hospital[2]	York	99%	182
Blue Hill Memorial Hospital	Blue Hill	98%	45
Millinocket Regional Hospital	Millinocket	98%	48
Maine Medical Center[2]	Portland	97%	639
Togus VA Medical Center	Augusta	97%	117
Miles Memorial Hospital	Damariscotta	95%	104

Prophylactic Antibiotic Timing (Outpatient)

Hospital Name	City	Rate	Cases
Franklin Memorial Hospital	Farmington	100%	32
Mercy Hospital	Portland	100%	562
Saint Joseph Hospital	Bangor	100%	279
Stephens Memorial Hospital	Norway	100%	44
The Aroostook Medical Center	Presque Isle	99%	98
Inland Hospital	Waterville	99%	210
Mainegeneral Medical Center	Augusta	99%	326
Central Maine Medical Center	Lewiston	98%	389
York Hospital	York	98%	97
Cary Medical Center	Caribou	96%	27
Eastern Maine Medical Center	Bangor	96%	877
Penobscot Bay Medical Center	Rockport	96%	46
Mid Coast Hospital	Brunswick	94%	84
Maine Medical Center	Portland	93%	1005
Maine Coast Memorial Hospital	Ellsworth	90%	31
Saint Marys Regional Medical Center	Lewiston	88%	118

Urinary Catheter Removal

Hospital Name	City	Rate	Cases
The Aroostook Medical Center	Presque Isle	100%	81
Cary Medical Center[2]	Caribou	100%	131
Eastern Maine Medical Center[2]	Bangor	100%	492
Franklin Memorial Hospital	Farmington	100%	64
Inland Hospital[2]	Waterville	100%	74
Maine Coast Memorial Hospital	Ellsworth	100%	47
Maine Medical Center[2]	Portland	100%	417
Mayo Regional Hospital[2]	Dover Foxcroft	100%	85
Mount Desert Island Hospital	Bar Harbor	100%	31
Parkview Adventist Medical Center[3]	Brunswick	100%	43
Saint Joseph Hospital[2]	Bangor	100%	106
Saint Marys Regional Medical Center[2]	Lewiston	100%	157
Southern Maine Medical Center	Biddeford	100%	265
Henrietta D Goodall Hospital	Sanford	99%	99
York Hospital[2]	York	99%	172
Miles Memorial Hospital	Damariscotta	98%	91
Millinocket Regional Hospital	Millinocket	98%	59
Penobscot Bay Medical Center	Rockport	98%	125
Redington Fairview General Hospital	Skowhegan	98%	47
Mainegeneral Medical Center[2]	Augusta	97%	322
Mercy Hospital[2]	Portland	97%	488
Mid Coast Hospital	Brunswick	97%	96
Stephens Memorial Hospital[2]	Norway	97%	87
Waldo County General Hospital	Belfast	97%	102
Central Maine Medical Center[2]	Lewiston	94%	248

Survey of Patients' Hospital Experiences

Area Around Room 'Always' Quiet at Night

Hospital Name	City	Rate	Cases
Mount Desert Island Hospital	Bar Harbor	71%	(a)
Mercy Hospital	Portland	70%	300+
Blue Hill Memorial Hospital	Blue Hill	68%	(a)
Stephens Memorial Hospital	Norway	67%	(a)
Millinocket Regional Hospital	Millinocket	65%	(a)
Rumford Hospital	Rumford	65%	(a)
York Hospital	York	65%	300+
Inland Hospital	Waterville	64%	(a)
Redington Fairview General Hospital	Skowhegan	64%	300+
Cary Medical Center	Caribou	61%	300+
Mayo Regional Hospital	Dover Foxcroft	61%	(a)
Saint Joseph Hospital	Bangor	61%	300+
Bridgton Hospital	Bridgton	60%	(a)
Calais Regional Hospital	Calais	60%	(a)
Down East Community Hospital	Machias	60%	(a)
Henrietta D Goodall Hospital	Sanford	60%	(a)
Sebasticook Valley Hospital	Pittsfield	60%	(a)
Northern Maine Medical Center	Fort Kent	59%	(a)
Parkview Adventist Medical Center	Brunswick	59%	(a)
Penobscot Valley Hospital	Lincoln	59%	(a)
Miles Memorial Hospital	Damariscotta	58%	300+
Penobscot Bay Medical Center	Rockport	58%	300+
Saint Marys Regional Medical Center	Lewiston	58%	300+
Maine Coast Memorial Hospital	Ellsworth	57%	300+
Central Maine Medical Center	Lewiston	55%	300+
Maine Medical Center	Portland	55%	300+
Houlton Regional Hospital	Houlton	54%	(a)
Waldo County General Hospital	Belfast	52%	(a)
Mid Coast Hospital	Brunswick	51%	300+
Mainegeneral Medical Center	Augusta	48%	300+
The Aroostook Medical Center	Presque Isle	47%	300+
Franklin Memorial Hospital	Farmington	47%	(a)
Southern Maine Medical Center	Biddeford	46%	300+
Eastern Maine Medical Center	Bangor	45%	300+

Doctors 'Always' Communicated Well

Hospital Name	City	Rate	Cases
Mount Desert Island Hospital	Bar Harbor	92%	(a)
Parkview Adventist Medical Center	Brunswick	92%	(a)
Millinocket Regional Hospital	Millinocket	89%	(a)
York Hospital	York	89%	300+
Houlton Regional Hospital	Houlton	87%	(a)
Calais Regional Hospital	Calais	86%	(a)
Down East Community Hospital	Machias	86%	(a)
Northern Maine Medical Center	Fort Kent	86%	(a)
Redington Fairview General Hospital	Skowhegan	86%	300+
Cary Medical Center	Caribou	84%	300+
Maine Coast Memorial Hospital	Ellsworth	84%	300+
Mayo Regional Hospital	Dover Foxcroft	84%	(a)
Mercy Hospital	Portland	84%	300+
Mid Coast Hospital	Brunswick	84%	300+
Miles Memorial Hospital	Damariscotta	84%	300+
Saint Joseph Hospital	Bangor	84%	300+
Stephens Memorial Hospital	Norway	84%	(a)
Blue Hill Memorial Hospital	Blue Hill	83%	(a)
Inland Hospital	Waterville	83%	(a)
Penobscot Valley Hospital	Lincoln	83%	(a)
Saint Marys Regional Medical Center	Lewiston	83%	300+
Penobscot Bay Medical Center	Rockport	82%	300+
Bridgton Hospital	Bridgton	81%	(a)
Franklin Memorial Hospital	Farmington	81%	(a)
Maine Medical Center	Portland	81%	300+
Mainegeneral Medical Center	Augusta	81%	300+
Henrietta D Goodall Hospital	Sanford	80%	(a)
Rumford Hospital	Rumford	80%	(a)
Southern Maine Medical Center	Biddeford	80%	300+
Central Maine Medical Center	Lewiston	79%	300+
Eastern Maine Medical Center	Bangor	79%	300+
Waldo County General Hospital	Belfast	79%	(a)
The Aroostook Medical Center	Presque Isle	75%	300+
Sebasticook Valley Hospital	Pittsfield	71%	(a)

Home Recovery Information Given

Hospital Name	City	Rate	Cases
Mount Desert Island Hospital	Bar Harbor	96%	(a)
Bridgton Hospital	Bridgton	95%	(a)
Parkview Adventist Medical Center	Brunswick	95%	(a)
Blue Hill Memorial Hospital	Blue Hill	94%	(a)
Mercy Hospital	Portland	93%	300+
Stephens Memorial Hospital	Norway	93%	(a)
Saint Joseph Hospital	Bangor	92%	300+
Inland Hospital	Waterville	91%	(a)
Mayo Regional Hospital	Dover Foxcroft	91%	(a)
Redington Fairview General Hospital	Skowhegan	91%	300+
Cary Medical Center	Caribou	90%	300+
Central Maine Medical Center	Lewiston	90%	300+
Maine Coast Memorial Hospital	Ellsworth	90%	300+
Millinocket Regional Hospital	Millinocket	90%	(a)
York Hospital	York	90%	300+
Calais Regional Hospital	Calais	89%	(a)
Mid Coast Hospital	Brunswick	89%	300+
Sebasticook Valley Hospital	Pittsfield	89%	(a)
Waldo County General Hospital	Belfast	89%	(a)
Eastern Maine Medical Center	Bangor	88%	300+
Franklin Memorial Hospital	Farmington	88%	(a)
Maine Medical Center	Portland	88%	300+
Mainegeneral Medical Center	Augusta	88%	300+
Miles Memorial Hospital	Damariscotta	88%	300+
Penobscot Bay Medical Center	Rockport	88%	300+
Rumford Hospital	Rumford	88%	(a)
Houlton Regional Hospital	Houlton	87%	(a)
Penobscot Valley Hospital	Lincoln	87%	(a)
The Aroostook Medical Center	Presque Isle	86%	300+
Henrietta D Goodall Hospital	Sanford	86%	(a)
Saint Marys Regional Medical Center	Lewiston	86%	300+
Southern Maine Medical Center	Biddeford	86%	300+
Down East Community Hospital	Machias	85%	(a)
Northern Maine Medical Center	Fort Kent	85%	(a)

Hospital Given 9 or 10 on 10 Point Scale

Hospital Name	City	Rate	Cases
Mount Desert Island Hospital	Bar Harbor	88%	(a)
Millinocket Regional Hospital	Millinocket	84%	(a)
York Hospital	York	84%	300+
Parkview Adventist Medical Center	Brunswick	82%	(a)
Blue Hill Memorial Hospital	Blue Hill	81%	(a)
Mercy Hospital	Portland	79%	300+
Miles Memorial Hospital	Damariscotta	79%	300+
Calais Regional Hospital	Calais	77%	(a)
Cary Medical Center	Caribou	77%	300+
Mid Coast Hospital	Brunswick	77%	300+
Redington Fairview General Hospital	Skowhegan	77%	300+
Saint Joseph Hospital	Bangor	77%	300+
Maine Medical Center	Portland	76%	300+
Inland Hospital	Waterville	75%	(a)
Maine Coast Memorial Hospital	Ellsworth	75%	300+
Mayo Regional Hospital	Dover Foxcroft	75%	(a)
Rumford Hospital	Rumford	75%	(a)
Saint Marys Regional Medical Center	Lewiston	75%	300+
Waldo County General Hospital	Belfast	74%	(a)
Central Maine Medical Center	Lewiston	73%	300+

NOTE: Hospital profiles are in alphabetical order by state, then city, then hospital within the city; Rankings exclude hospitals with less than 25 cases except for patient surveys which excludes hospitals with less than 100 cases; (a) 100-299 cases; (1) The number of cases/patients is too few to report; (2) Data submitted were based on a sample of cases/patients; (3) Results are based on a shorter time period than required; (4) Data suppressed by CMS for one or more quarters; (5) Results are not available for this reporting period; (6) Fewer than 100 patients completed the HCAHPS survey; (7) No cases met the criteria for this measure; (8) The lower limit of the confidence interval cannot be calculated if the number of observed infections equals zero; (9) No data are available from the state/territory for this reporting period; (10) The scores shown reflect fewer than 50 completed surveys; (11) There were discrepancies in the data collection process; (12) This measure does not apply to this hospital for this reporting period; (13) Results cannot be calculated for this reporting period; (14) The results for this state are combined with nearby states to protect confidentiality; Please refer to the User's Guide for a full explanation of data.

Hospital Name	City	Rate	Cases
Penobscot Valley Hospital	Lincoln	73%	(a)
Stephens Memorial Hospital	Norway	73%	(a)
Bridgton Hospital	Bridgton	72%	(a)
Eastern Maine Medical Center	Bangor	70%	300+
The Aroostook Medical Center	Presque Isle	69%	300+
Franklin Memorial Hospital	Farmington	69%	(a)
Houlton Regional Hospital	Houlton	69%	(a)
Northern Maine Medical Center	Fort Kent	69%	(a)
Southern Maine Medical Center	Biddeford	68%	300+
Down East Community Hospital	Machias	67%	(a)
Penobscot Bay Medical Center	Rockport	67%	300+
Sebasticook Valley Hospital	Pittsfield	65%	(a)
Mainegeneral Medical Center	Augusta	64%	300+
Henrietta D Goodall Hospital	Sanford	62%	(a)

Meds 'Always' Explained Before Given

Hospital Name	City	Rate	Cases
Millinocket Regional Hospital	Millinocket	79%	(a)
Blue Hill Memorial Hospital	Blue Hill	78%	(a)
Mayo Regional Hospital	Dover Foxcroft	77%	(a)
Bridgton Hospital	Bridgton	76%	(a)
Mount Desert Island Hospital	Bar Harbor	76%	(a)
Parkview Adventist Medical Center	Brunswick	74%	(a)
Houlton Regional Hospital	Houlton	73%	(a)
Stephens Memorial Hospital	Norway	73%	(a)
York Hospital	York	73%	300+
Calais Regional Hospital	Calais	72%	(a)
Down East Community Hospital	Machias	72%	(a)
Redington Fairview General Hospital	Skowhegan	72%	300+
Cary Medical Center	Caribou	71%	300+
Miles Memorial Hospital	Damariscotta	70%	300+
Northern Maine Medical Center	Fort Kent	70%	(a)
Franklin Memorial Hospital	Farmington	69%	(a)
Maine Coast Memorial Hospital	Ellsworth	69%	300+
Central Maine Medical Center	Lewiston	68%	300+
Inland Hospital	Waterville	68%	(a)
Saint Joseph Hospital	Bangor	68%	300+
Saint Marys Regional Medical Center	Lewiston	68%	300+
Mid Coast Hospital	Brunswick	67%	300+
Mainegeneral Medical Center	Augusta	66%	300+
Mercy Hospital	Portland	66%	300+
Maine Medical Center	Portland	65%	300+
Eastern Maine Medical Center	Bangor	64%	300+
Penobscot Bay Medical Center	Rockport	64%	300+
Penobscot Valley Hospital	Lincoln	64%	(a)
Rumford Hospital	Rumford	64%	(a)
Sebasticook Valley Hospital	Pittsfield	64%	(a)
The Aroostook Medical Center	Presque Isle	63%	300+
Henrietta D Goodall Hospital	Sanford	63%	(a)
Southern Maine Medical Center	Biddeford	62%	300+
Waldo County General Hospital	Belfast	61%	(a)

Nurses 'Always' Communicated Well

Hospital Name	City	Rate	Cases
Millinocket Regional Hospital	Millinocket	91%	(a)
Mount Desert Island Hospital	Bar Harbor	91%	(a)
York Hospital	York	88%	300+
Blue Hill Memorial Hospital	Blue Hill	87%	(a)
Cary Medical Center	Caribou	85%	300+
Northern Maine Medical Center	Fort Kent	85%	(a)
Redington Fairview General Hospital	Skowhegan	85%	300+
Calais Regional Hospital	Calais	84%	(a)
Houlton Regional Hospital	Houlton	84%	(a)
Mayo Regional Hospital	Dover Foxcroft	84%	(a)
Miles Memorial Hospital	Damariscotta	84%	300+
Stephens Memorial Hospital	Norway	84%	(a)
Down East Community Hospital	Machias	83%	(a)
Inland Hospital	Waterville	83%	(a)
Maine Coast Memorial Hospital	Ellsworth	82%	300+
Mercy Hospital	Portland	82%	300+
Parkview Adventist Medical Center	Brunswick	82%	(a)
Saint Marys Regional Medical Center	Lewiston	82%	300+
Central Maine Medical Center	Lewiston	81%	300+
Penobscot Valley Hospital	Lincoln	81%	(a)
Rumford Hospital	Rumford	81%	(a)
Saint Joseph Hospital	Bangor	81%	300+
Bridgton Hospital	Bridgton	80%	(a)
Eastern Maine Medical Center	Bangor	80%	300+
Franklin Memorial Hospital	Farmington	80%	(a)
Maine Medical Center	Portland	80%	300+
Mainegeneral Medical Center	Augusta	80%	300+
Waldo County General Hospital	Belfast	80%	(a)
Mid Coast Hospital	Brunswick	79%	300+
Sebasticook Valley Hospital	Pittsfield	79%	(a)
Penobscot Bay Medical Center	Rockport	78%	300+
Southern Maine Medical Center	Biddeford	77%	300+
The Aroostook Medical Center	Presque Isle	75%	300+
Henrietta D Goodall Hospital	Sanford	72%	(a)

Pain 'Always' Well Controlled

Hospital Name	City	Rate	Cases
Calais Regional Hospital	Calais	86%	(a)
Mount Desert Island Hospital	Bar Harbor	84%	(a)
Millinocket Regional Hospital	Millinocket	81%	(a)
Blue Hill Memorial Hospital	Blue Hill	78%	(a)
Cary Medical Center	Caribou	78%	300+
York Hospital	York	76%	300+
Maine Coast Memorial Hospital	Ellsworth	75%	300+
Parkview Adventist Medical Center	Brunswick	75%	(a)
Bridgton Hospital	Bridgton	74%	(a)
Down East Community Hospital	Machias	74%	(a)
Mayo Regional Hospital	Dover Foxcroft	74%	(a)
Maine Medical Center	Portland	73%	300+
Mid Coast Hospital	Brunswick	73%	300+
Saint Joseph Hospital	Bangor	73%	300+
Waldo County General Hospital	Belfast	73%	(a)
Houlton Regional Hospital	Houlton	72%	(a)
Inland Hospital	Waterville	72%	(a)
Mercy Hospital	Portland	72%	300+
Stephens Memorial Hospital	Norway	72%	(a)
Central Maine Medical Center	Lewiston	71%	300+
Sebasticook Valley Hospital	Pittsfield	71%	(a)
Franklin Memorial Hospital	Farmington	70%	(a)
Miles Memorial Hospital	Damariscotta	70%	300+
Penobscot Bay Medical Center	Rockport	70%	300+
Redington Fairview General Hospital	Skowhegan	70%	300+
Eastern Maine Medical Center	Bangor	69%	300+
Rumford Hospital	Rumford	69%	(a)
Southern Maine Medical Center	Biddeford	69%	300+
The Aroostook Medical Center	Presque Isle	68%	300+
Mainegeneral Medical Center	Augusta	68%	300+
Northern Maine Medical Center	Fort Kent	68%	(a)
Saint Marys Regional Medical Center	Lewiston	68%	300+
Penobscot Valley Hospital	Lincoln	67%	(a)
Henrietta D Goodall Hospital	Sanford	64%	(a)

Room and Bathroom 'Always' Clean

Hospital Name	City	Rate	Cases
Blue Hill Memorial Hospital	Blue Hill	93%	(a)
Mayo Regional Hospital	Dover Foxcroft	90%	(a)
Millinocket Regional Hospital	Millinocket	90%	(a)
Maine Coast Memorial Hospital	Ellsworth	86%	300+
Calais Regional Hospital	Calais	85%	(a)
Inland Hospital	Waterville	85%	(a)
Mount Desert Island Hospital	Bar Harbor	85%	(a)
Parkview Adventist Medical Center	Brunswick	85%	(a)
Penobscot Valley Hospital	Lincoln	84%	(a)
Redington Fairview General Hospital	Skowhegan	84%	300+
Saint Marys Regional Medical Center	Lewiston	82%	300+
Stephens Memorial Hospital	Norway	82%	(a)
York Hospital	York	82%	300+
Bridgton Hospital	Bridgton	81%	(a)
Rumford Hospital	Rumford	81%	(a)
The Aroostook Medical Center	Presque Isle	80%	300+
Franklin Memorial Hospital	Farmington	80%	(a)
Northern Maine Medical Center	Fort Kent	80%	(a)
Houlton Regional Hospital	Houlton	79%	(a)
Waldo County General Hospital	Belfast	79%	(a)
Down East Community Hospital	Machias	78%	(a)
Saint Joseph Hospital	Bangor	78%	300+
Central Maine Medical Center	Lewiston	76%	300+
Eastern Maine Medical Center	Bangor	76%	300+
Mainegeneral Medical Center	Augusta	76%	300+
Mid Coast Hospital	Brunswick	76%	300+
Miles Memorial Hospital	Damariscotta	75%	300+
Maine Medical Center	Portland	74%	300+
Cary Medical Center	Caribou	73%	300+
Henrietta D Goodall Hospital	Sanford	73%	(a)
Mercy Hospital	Portland	73%	300+
Penobscot Bay Medical Center	Rockport	72%	300+
Sebasticook Valley Hospital	Pittsfield	70%	(a)
Southern Maine Medical Center	Biddeford	66%	300+

Timely Help 'Always' Received

Hospital Name	City	Rate	Cases
Millinocket Regional Hospital	Millinocket	85%	(a)
Mount Desert Island Hospital	Bar Harbor	85%	(a)
Cary Medical Center	Caribou	82%	300+
Calais Regional Hospital	Calais	79%	(a)
Blue Hill Memorial Hospital	Blue Hill	78%	(a)
Houlton Regional Hospital	Houlton	77%	(a)
Inland Hospital	Waterville	76%	(a)
Northern Maine Medical Center	Fort Kent	75%	(a)
York Hospital	York	75%	300+
Mayo Regional Hospital	Dover Foxcroft	74%	(a)
Miles Memorial Hospital	Damariscotta	74%	300+
Parkview Adventist Medical Center	Brunswick	74%	(a)
Stephens Memorial Hospital	Norway	74%	(a)
Down East Community Hospital	Machias	73%	(a)
Redington Fairview General Hospital	Skowhegan	73%	300+
Sebasticook Valley Hospital	Pittsfield	73%	(a)
Maine Coast Memorial Hospital	Ellsworth	72%	300+
Bridgton Hospital	Bridgton	71%	(a)
Mid Coast Hospital	Brunswick	71%	300+
Waldo County General Hospital	Belfast	71%	(a)
Mercy Hospital	Portland	69%	300+
Penobscot Bay Medical Center	Rockport	69%	300+
Saint Marys Regional Medical Center	Lewiston	69%	300+
Franklin Memorial Hospital	Farmington	68%	(a)
Penobscot Valley Hospital	Lincoln	68%	(a)
Rumford Hospital	Rumford	68%	(a)
Saint Joseph Hospital	Bangor	68%	300+
Central Maine Medical Center	Lewiston	67%	300+
Henrietta D Goodall Hospital	Sanford	66%	(a)
The Aroostook Medical Center	Presque Isle	65%	300+
Maine Medical Center	Portland	65%	300+
Mainegeneral Medical Center	Augusta	65%	300+
Eastern Maine Medical Center	Bangor	64%	300+
Southern Maine Medical Center	Biddeford	60%	300+

Would Definitely Recommend Hospital

Hospital Name	City	Rate	Cases
Mount Desert Island Hospital	Bar Harbor	91%	(a)
York Hospital	York	89%	300+
Mercy Hospital	Portland	84%	300+
Mid Coast Hospital	Brunswick	84%	300+
Parkview Adventist Medical Center	Brunswick	84%	(a)
Inland Hospital	Waterville	83%	(a)
Millinocket Regional Hospital	Millinocket	83%	(a)
Saint Joseph Hospital	Bangor	83%	300+
Cary Medical Center	Caribou	81%	300+
Saint Marys Regional Medical Center	Lewiston	81%	300+
Bridgton Hospital	Bridgton	80%	(a)
Maine Coast Memorial Hospital	Ellsworth	80%	300+
Miles Memorial Hospital	Damariscotta	80%	300+
Blue Hill Memorial Hospital	Blue Hill	79%	(a)
Calais Regional Hospital	Calais	79%	(a)
Maine Medical Center	Portland	79%	300+
Redington Fairview General Hospital	Skowhegan	79%	300+
Central Maine Medical Center	Lewiston	77%	300+
Eastern Maine Medical Center	Bangor	75%	300+
Stephens Memorial Hospital	Norway	75%	(a)
Waldo County General Hospital	Belfast	75%	(a)
Mayo Regional Hospital	Dover Foxcroft	73%	(a)
Rumford Hospital	Rumford	73%	(a)
Penobscot Valley Hospital	Lincoln	72%	(a)
Northern Maine Medical Center	Fort Kent	71%	(a)
Sebasticook Valley Hospital	Pittsfield	71%	(a)
Southern Maine Medical Center	Biddeford	70%	300+
Franklin Memorial Hospital	Farmington	68%	(a)
The Aroostook Medical Center	Presque Isle	67%	300+
Down East Community Hospital	Machias	67%	(a)
Houlton Regional Hospital	Houlton	67%	(a)
Mainegeneral Medical Center	Augusta	67%	300+
Penobscot Bay Medical Center	Rockport	66%	300+
Henrietta D Goodall Hospital	Sanford	64%	(a)

Use of Medical Imaging

Cardiac Imaging Stress Test before OP Surgery

Hospital Name	City	Rate	Cases
Redington Fairview General Hospital	Skowhegan	1.8%	165
Penobscot Bay Medical Center	Rockport	2.3%	266
Cary Medical Center	Caribou	2.7%	182
Mid Coast Hospital	Brunswick	2.9%	278
Miles Memorial Hospital	Damariscotta	3.2%	125
Southern Maine Medical Center	Biddeford	3.5%	462
Houlton Regional Hospital	Houlton	3.8%	106
The Aroostook Medical Center	Presque Isle	4.0%	302
Maine Coast Memorial Hospital	Ellsworth	4.1%	169
Henrietta D Goodall Hospital	Sanford	4.3%	139
Maine Medical Center	Portland	4.4%	1816
Mainegeneral Medical Center	Augusta	4.8%	520
Saint Joseph Hospital	Bangor	4.8%	248
Franklin Memorial Hospital	Farmington	4.9%	144
Parkview Adventist Medical Center	Brunswick	4.9%	81
Central Maine Medical Center	Lewiston	5.0%	704
Eastern Maine Medical Center	Bangor	5.0%	686
Sebasticook Valley Hospital	Pittsfield	5.2%	229
Bridgton Hospital	Bridgton	5.7%	70
Northern Maine Medical Center	Fort Kent	6.0%	116
Millinocket Regional Hospital	Millinocket	6.2%	130
Inland Hospital	Waterville	6.7%	282
Saint Marys Regional Medical Center	Lewiston	6.9%	174
Stephens Memorial Hospital	Norway	7.0%	86
York Hospital	York	7.3%	683
Mercy Hospital	Portland	7.4%	163
Rumford Hospital	Rumford	7.4%	68

NOTE: Hospital profiles are in alphabetical order by state, then city, then hospital within the city; Rankings exclude hospitals with less than 25 cases except for patient surveys which excludes hospitals with less than 100 cases; (a) 100-299 cases; (1) The number of cases/patients is too few to report; (2) Data submitted were based on a sample of cases/patients; (3) Results are based on a shorter time period than required; (4) Data suppressed by CMS for one or more quarters; (5) Results are not available for this reporting period; (6) Fewer than 100 patients completed the HCAHPS survey; (7) No cases met the criteria for this measure; (8) The lower limit of the confidence interval cannot be calculated if the number of observed infections equals zero; (9) No data are available from the state/territory for this reporting period; (10) The scores shown reflect fewer than 50 completed surveys; (11) There were discrepancies in the data collection process; (12) This measure does not apply to this hospital for this reporting period; (13) Results cannot be calculated for this reporting period; (14) The results for this state are combined with nearby states to protect confidentiality; Please refer to the User's Guide for a full explanation of data.

Penobscot Valley Hospital	Lincoln	10.6%	104

Combination Abdominal CT Scan

Hospital Name	City	Rate	Cases
Inland Hospital	Waterville	1.9%	314
Saint Andrews Hospital	Boothbay Hrbr	1.9%	106
Eastern Maine Medical Center	Bangor	2.0%	1475
Houlton Regional Hospital	Houlton	2.7%	415
Rumford Hospital	Rumford	2.7%	264
Bridgton Hospital	Bridgton	2.8%	398
Mainegeneral Medical Center	Augusta	2.9%	1268
Maine Medical Center	Portland	3.2%	1833
Penobscot Valley Hospital	Lincoln	3.2%	186
Calais Regional Hospital	Calais	3.4%	268
Miles Memorial Hospital	Damariscotta	3.4%	324
Millinocket Regional Hospital	Millinocket	3.9%	152
Henrietta D Goodall Hospital	Sanford	4.0%	427
Saint Joseph Hospital	Bangor	4.0%	631
Down East Community Hospital	Machias	4.3%	304
Penobscot Bay Medical Center	Rockport	4.3%	506
Sebasticook Valley Hospital	Pittsfield	4.5%	290
Maine Coast Memorial Hospital	Ellsworth	4.6%	435
Stephens Memorial Hospital	Norway	4.6%	459
Saint Marys Regional Medical Center	Lewiston	4.9%	697
Mid Coast Hospital	Brunswick	5.1%	666
Central Maine Medical Center	Lewiston	5.3%	943
Southern Maine Medical Center	Biddeford	5.4%	988
Parkview Adventist Medical Center	Brunswick	6.1%	230
Mount Desert Island Hospital	Bar Harbor	6.3%	206
Cary Medical Center	Caribou	6.7%	478
Redington Fairview General Hospital	Skowhegan	7.8%	526
Mercy Hospital	Portland	8.2%	671
York Hospital	York	8.7%	700
Franklin Memorial Hospital	Farmington	11.7%	412
The Aroostook Medical Center	Presque Isle	16.8%	537
Northern Maine Medical Center	Fort Kent	29.6%	297

Combination Brain/Sinus CT Scan

Hospital Name	City	Rate	Cases
Sebasticook Valley Hospital	Pittsfield	0.0%	245
Inland Hospital	Waterville	0.4%	232
Penobscot Valley Hospital	Lincoln	0.5%	185
Redington Fairview General Hospital	Skowhegan	0.5%	621
Penobscot Bay Medical Center	Rockport	0.7%	421
Mainegeneral Medical Center	Augusta	0.8%	972
Maine Medical Center	Portland	1.0%	1253
Mid Coast Hospital	Brunswick	1.2%	502
Saint Marys Regional Medical Center	Lewiston	1.5%	525
York Hospital	York	1.5%	467
Stephens Memorial Hospital	Norway	1.6%	381
Southern Maine Medical Center	Biddeford	2.0%	939
Eastern Maine Medical Center	Bangor	2.4%	637
Mercy Hospital	Portland	2.4%	506
Central Maine Medical Center	Lewiston	2.5%	603

Combination Chest CT Scan

Hospital Name	City	Rate	Cases
Down East Community Hospital	Machias	0.0%	128
Eastern Maine Medical Center	Bangor	0.0%	1563
Inland Hospital	Waterville	0.0%	137
Mainegeneral Medical Center	Augusta	0.0%	963
Mid Coast Hospital	Brunswick	0.0%	580
Millinocket Regional Hospital	Millinocket	0.0%	89
Mount Desert Island Hospital	Bar Harbor	0.0%	93
Rumford Hospital	Rumford	0.0%	164
Saint Joseph Hospital	Bangor	0.0%	366
Sebasticook Valley Hospital	Pittsfield	0.0%	102
Southern Maine Medical Center	Biddeford	0.0%	663
Central Maine Medical Center	Lewiston	0.1%	794
Cary Medical Center	Caribou	0.2%	403
Saint Marys Regional Medical Center	Lewiston	0.2%	473
York Hospital	York	0.2%	463
Henrietta D Goodall Hospital	Sanford	0.3%	286
Mercy Hospital	Portland	0.3%	372
Houlton Regional Hospital	Houlton	0.4%	224
Bridgton Hospital	Bridgton	0.5%	196
Penobscot Bay Medical Center	Rockport	0.5%	439
Miles Memorial Hospital	Damariscotta	0.6%	156
Maine Medical Center	Portland	0.8%	1685
Penobscot Valley Hospital	Lincoln	1.1%	88
Maine Coast Memorial Hospital	Ellsworth	1.2%	173
Redington Fairview General Hospital	Skowhegan	1.2%	253
Saint Andrews Hospital	Boothbay Hrbr	1.9%	53
Parkview Adventist Medical Center	Brunswick	2.1%	143
Calais Regional Hospital	Calais	2.2%	139
Stephens Memorial Hospital	Norway	2.4%	332
Franklin Memorial Hospital	Farmington	2.6%	230
Northern Maine Medical Center	Fort Kent	4.9%	288
The Aroostook Medical Center	Presque Isle	5.1%	410

Follow-up Mammogram/Ultrasound

A follow-up rate near zero may indicate missed cancer; a rate higher than 14% may mean there is unnecessary follow up.

Hospital Name	City	Rate	Cases
Inland Hospital	Waterville	4.1%	703
Maine Coast Memorial Hospital	Ellsworth	4.3%	834
Sebasticook Valley Hospital	Pittsfield	4.8%	725
Rumford Hospital	Rumford	4.9%	492
Eastern Maine Medical Center	Bangor	5.0%	1452
Saint Andrews Hospital	Boothbay Hrbr	5.3%	169
Bridgton Hospital	Bridgton	5.4%	698
Mainegeneral Medical Center	Augusta	5.5%	3153
Mount Desert Island Hospital	Bar Harbor	5.7%	351
Southern Maine Medical Center	Biddeford	6.2%	1986
Central Maine Medical Center	Lewiston	6.4%	1949
Saint Joseph Hospital	Bangor	6.5%	2794
Miles Memorial Hospital	Damariscotta	7.1%	663
Redington Fairview General Hospital	Skowhegan	7.1%	829
Mid Coast Hospital	Brunswick	7.3%	1133
Stephens Memorial Hospital	Norway	7.4%	1113
Saint Marys Regional Medical Center	Lewiston	7.5%	1166
Penobscot Valley Hospital	Lincoln	7.8%	348
York Hospital	York	7.9%	1980
Down East Community Hospital	Machias	8.0%	477
The Aroostook Medical Center	Presque Isle	8.1%	1339
Franklin Memorial Hospital	Farmington	8.2%	1128
Mercy Hospital	Portland	9.2%	2010
Calais Regional Hospital	Calais	9.3%	398
Houlton Regional Hospital	Houlton	9.5%	462
Northern Maine Medical Center	Fort Kent	9.6%	757
Maine Medical Center	Portland	10.5%	2066
Parkview Adventist Medical Center	Brunswick	11.3%	627
Millinocket Regional Hospital	Millinocket	13.4%	426
Cary Medical Center	Caribou	13.8%	809
Henrietta D Goodall Hospital	Sanford	14.9%	964

Lumbar Spine MRI for Low Back Pain

Hospital Name	City	Rate	Cases
York Hospital	York	28.4%	74
Inland Hospital	Waterville	30.6%	62
Mercy Hospital	Portland	33.1%	130
Mid Coast Hospital	Brunswick	34.0%	150
Maine Medical Center	Portland	34.2%	152
Saint Joseph Hospital	Bangor	34.2%	199
Cary Medical Center	Caribou	34.6%	78
Franklin Memorial Hospital	Farmington	35.5%	124
Henrietta D Goodall Hospital	Sanford	36.5%	96
Saint Marys Regional Medical Center	Lewiston	36.5%	126
Southern Maine Medical Center	Biddeford	37.0%	127
Eastern Maine Medical Center	Bangor	37.5%	341
Bridgton Hospital	Bridgton	37.7%	53
Miles Memorial Hospital	Damariscotta	39.3%	61
Maine Coast Memorial Hospital	Ellsworth	39.5%	81
Sebasticook Valley Hospital	Pittsfield	41.5%	65
Northern Maine Medical Center	Fort Kent	44.7%	76
Stephens Memorial Hospital	Norway	53.2%	94

NOTE: Hospital profiles are in alphabetical order by state, then city, then hospital within the city; Rankings exclude hospitals with less than 25 cases except for patient surveys which excludes hospitals with less than 100 cases; (a) 100-299 cases; (1) The number of cases/patients is too few to report; (2) Data submitted were based on a sample of cases/patients; (3) Results are based on a shorter time period than required; (4) Data suppressed by CMS for one or more quarters; (5) Results are not available for this reporting period; (6) Fewer than 100 patients completed the HCAHPS survey; (7) No cases met the criteria for this measure; (8) The lower limit of the confidence interval cannot be calculated if the number of observed infections equals zero; (9) No data are available from the state/territory for this reporting period; (10) The scores shown reflect fewer than 50 completed surveys; (11) There were discrepancies in the data collection process; (12) This measure does not apply to this hospital for this reporting period; (13) Results cannot be calculated for this reporting period; (14) The results for this state are combined with nearby states to protect confidentiality; Please refer to the User's Guide for a full explanation of data.

Mainegeneral Medical Center

35 Medical Center Parkway Phone: 207-872-1000
Augusta, ME 04330 Fax: 207-872-4665
URL: www.mainegeneral.org
Type: Acute Care Hospitals Emergency Services: Yes
Ownership: Voluntary non-profit - Other Beds: 246
Key Personnel:
CEO/President. . . . . Scott B Bullock
Radiology. . . . . Paul D Gagliardi
Chief of Medical Staff. . . . . Thomas J Keating

Measure	Cases	This Hosp.	State Avg.	U.S. Avg.
Blood Clot Prevention and Treatment				
Anticoagulation Overlap Therapy[2]	73	99%	98%	93%
ICU Venous Thromboembolism Prophylaxis[2]	93	96%	96%	92%
Incidence of Potentially Preventable VTE[1,2]	-	-	2%	10%
UFH with Dosages/Platelet Monitoring[2]	50	100%	100%	97%
Venous Thromboembolism Prophylaxis[2]	330	90%	95%	85%
Warfarin Therapy Discharge Instructions[2]	56	100%	84%	75%
Chest Pain/Possible Heart Attack Care				
Aspirin Given Within 24 Hours of Arrival	120	100%	99%	96%
Fibrinolytic Meds Within 30 Min. of Arrival	35	97%	86%	58%
Average Time to ECG (minutes)	123	6	6	7
Average Time to Transfer (minutes)[7]	-	-	49	60
Children's Asthma Care				
Received Home Management Plan of Care	-	-	-	88%
Received Reliever Medication	-	-	-	100%
Received Systemic Corticosteroids	-	-	-	100%
Emergency Department				
Admittance Decision Time (minutes)[2]	732	145	110	98
Head CT Results Within 45 Min. of Arrival	18	50%	44%	57%
Patients Who Left ER Before Being Seen	60,234	1%	1%	2%
Time from ER Arrival to Admit. (minutes)[2]	759	322	288	274
Time from ER Arrival to Discharge (minutes)	398	132	122	134
Time in ER Before Being Evaluated (minutes)	415	33	28	26
Time to Pain Meds for Fractures (minutes)	111	31	52	57
Heart Attack Care				
Aspirin Given at Discharge	91	99%	100%	99%
Fibrinolytic Meds Within 30 Min. of Arrival[7]	-	-	50%	54%
PCI Within 90 Minutes of Arrival[7]	-	-	96%	96%
Statin Prescribed at Discharge	84	100%	99%	98%
Heart Failure Care				
ACE Inhibitor or ARB for LVSD	48	100%	99%	97%
Discharge Instructions Given	180	100%	98%	94%
Evaluation of LVS Function	227	100%	100%	99%
Medicare Spending				
Medicare Spending per Patient (ratio)	-	0.98	0.95	0.98
Pneumonia Care				
Appropriate Initial Antibiotic Given	255	99%	98%	95%
Blood Culture Timing	312	98%	98%	98%
Pregnancy and Delivery Care				
Newborn Deliveries Scheduled Early	46	0%	2%	6%
Preventive Care				
Immunization for Influenza[2]	519	94%	93%	90%
Immunization for Pneumonia[2]	680	97%	94%	92%
Stroke Care				
Anticoagulation Therapy for Atrial Fibrillation	18	100%	98%	95%
Antithrombotic Therapy Timing	77	100%	99%	98%
Assessed for Rehabilitation	87	100%	98%	97%
Discharged on Antithrombotic Therapy	81	100%	100%	99%
Discharged on Statin Medication	69	94%	97%	94%
Thrombolytic Therapy Timing[1]	-	-	29%	66%
Venous Thromboembolism Prophylaxis	87	98%	96%	94%
Written Stroke Educational Materials Given	37	100%	86%	88%
Surgical Care Improvement Project				
Appropriate Beta Blocker Usage[2]	183	99%	99%	98%
Appropriate VTP Within 24 Hours[2]	519	99%	99%	98%
Controlled Postoperative Blood Glucose[2,7]	-	-	99%	97%
Perioperative Temperature Management[2]	611	100%	100%	100%
Prophylactic Antibiotic Selection[2]	419	99%	99%	99%
Prophylactic Antibiotic Selection (Outpatient)	380	98%	98%	98%
Prophylactic Antibiotic Stopped[2]	407	100%	99%	98%
Prophylactic Antibiotic Timing[2]	419	100%	99%	99%
Prophylactic Antibiotic Timing (Outpatient)	326	99%	96%	98%
Urinary Catheter Removal[2]	322	97%	99%	97%
Survey of Patients' Hospital Experiences				
Area Around Room 'Always' Quiet at Night	300+	48%	59%	61%
Doctors 'Always' Communicated Well	300+	81%	83%	82%
Home Recovery Information Given	300+	88%	90%	85%
Hospital Given 9 or 10 on 10 Point Scale	300+	64%	74%	71%
Meds 'Always' Explained Before Given	300+	66%	69%	64%
Nurses 'Always' Communicated Well	300+	80%	82%	79%
Pain 'Always' Well Controlled	300+	68%	73%	71%
Room and Bathroom 'Always' Clean	300+	76%	80%	73%
Timely Help 'Always' Received	300+	65%	72%	68%
Would Definitely Recommend Hospital	300+	67%	77%	71%
Use of Medical Imaging				
Cardiac Imaging Stress Test before Surgery	520	4.8%	4.8%	5.3%
Combination Abdominal CT Scan	1,268	2.9%	5.2%	10.5%
Combination Brain/Sinus CT Scan	972	0.8%	1.7%	2.7%
Combination Chest CT Scan	963	0.0%	0.7%	2.7%
Follow-up Mammogram/Ultrasound	3,153	5.5%	7.7%	8.8%
Lumbar Spine MRI for Low Back Pain[1]	-	-	37.5%	37.2%

Togus VA Medical Center

1 VA Center Phone: 207-623-8411
Augusta, ME 04330
URL: www.maine.va.gov
Type: Acute Care - VA Emergency Services: No
Ownership: Government Federal Beds: 67

Measure	Cases	This Hosp.	State Avg.	U.S. Avg.
Blood Clot Prevention and Treatment				
Anticoagulation Overlap Therapy	-	-	98%	93%
ICU Venous Thromboembolism Prophylaxis	-	-	96%	92%
Incidence of Potentially Preventable VTE	-	-	2%	10%
UFH with Dosages/Platelet Monitoring	-	-	100%	97%
Venous Thromboembolism Prophylaxis	-	-	95%	85%
Warfarin Therapy Discharge Instructions	-	-	84%	75%
Chest Pain/Possible Heart Attack Care				
Aspirin Given Within 24 Hours of Arrival	-	-	99%	96%
Fibrinolytic Meds Within 30 Min. of Arrival	-	-	86%	58%
Average Time to ECG (minutes)	-	-	6	7
Average Time to Transfer (minutes)	-	-	49	60
Children's Asthma Care				
Received Home Management Plan of Care	-	-	-	88%
Received Reliever Medication	-	-	-	100%
Received Systemic Corticosteroids	-	-	-	100%
Emergency Department				
Admittance Decision Time (minutes)	-	-	110	98
Head CT Results Within 45 Min. of Arrival	-	-	44%	57%
Patients Who Left ER Before Being Seen	-	-	1%	2%
Time from ER Arrival to Admit. (minutes)	-	-	288	274
Time from ER Arrival to Discharge (minutes)	-	-	122	134
Time in ER Before Being Evaluated (minutes)	-	-	28	26
Time to Pain Meds for Fractures (minutes)	-	-	52	57
Heart Attack Care				
Aspirin Given at Discharge[5]	-	-	100%	99%
Fibrinolytic Meds Within 30 Min. of Arrival[5]	-	-	50%	54%
PCI Within 90 Minutes of Arrival[5]	-	-	96%	96%
Statin Prescribed at Discharge[5]	-	-	99%	98%
Heart Failure Care				
ACE Inhibitor or ARB for LVSD[1]	24	71%	99%	97%
Discharge Instructions Given	68	87%	98%	94%
Evaluation of LVS Function	83	99%	100%	99%
Medicare Spending				
Medicare Spending per Patient (ratio)	-	-	0.95	0.98
Pneumonia Care				
Appropriate Initial Antibiotic Given	30	100%	98%	95%
Blood Culture Timing	39	100%	98%	98%
Pregnancy and Delivery Care				
Newborn Deliveries Scheduled Early	-	-	2%	6%
Preventive Care				
Immunization for Influenza[2,3]	143	90%	93%	90%
Immunization for Pneumonia[2,3]	317	93%	94%	92%
Stroke Care				
Anticoagulation Therapy for Atrial Fibrillation	-	-	98%	95%
Antithrombotic Therapy Timing	-	-	99%	98%
Assessed for Rehabilitation	-	-	98%	97%
Discharged on Antithrombotic Therapy	-	-	100%	99%
Discharged on Statin Medication	-	-	97%	94%
Thrombolytic Therapy Timing	-	-	29%	66%
Venous Thromboembolism Prophylaxis	-	-	96%	94%
Written Stroke Educational Materials Given	-	-	86%	88%
Surgical Care Improvement Project				
Appropriate Beta Blocker Usage[2]	31	100%	99%	98%
Appropriate VTP Within 24 Hours[2]	139	94%	99%	98%
Controlled Postoperative Blood Glucose[5]	-	-	99%	97%
Perioperative Temperature Management[2]	149	98%	100%	100%
Prophylactic Antibiotic Selection	117	100%	99%	99%
Prophylactic Antibiotic Selection (Outpatient)	-	-	98%	98%
Prophylactic Antibiotic Stopped	115	97%	99%	98%
Prophylactic Antibiotic Timing	117	97%	99%	99%
Prophylactic Antibiotic Timing (Outpatient)	-	-	96%	98%
Urinary Catheter Removal[1,2]	19	79%	99%	97%
Survey of Patients' Hospital Experiences				
Area Around Room 'Always' Quiet at Night	-	-	59%	61%
Doctors 'Always' Communicated Well	-	-	83%	82%
Home Recovery Information Given	-	-	90%	85%
Hospital Given 9 or 10 on 10 Point Scale	-	-	74%	71%
Meds 'Always' Explained Before Given	-	-	69%	64%
Nurses 'Always' Communicated Well	-	-	82%	79%
Pain 'Always' Well Controlled	-	-	73%	71%
Room and Bathroom 'Always' Clean	-	-	80%	73%
Timely Help 'Always' Received	-	-	72%	68%
Would Definitely Recommend Hospital	-	-	77%	71%
Use of Medical Imaging				
Cardiac Imaging Stress Test before Surgery	-	-	4.8%	5.3%
Combination Abdominal CT Scan	-	-	5.2%	10.5%
Combination Brain/Sinus CT Scan	-	-	1.7%	2.7%
Combination Chest CT Scan	-	-	0.7%	2.7%
Follow-up Mammogram/Ultrasound	-	-	7.7%	8.8%
Lumbar Spine MRI for Low Back Pain	-	-	37.5%	37.2%

Eastern Maine Medical Center

489 State St, PO Box 404 Phone: 207-973-7000
Bangor, ME 04401 Fax: 207-973-7865
URL: www.emh.org
Type: Acute Care Hospitals Emergency Services: Yes
Ownership: Voluntary non-profit - Private Beds: 441
Key Personnel:
CEO/President. . . . . Deborah Carey Johnson, RN
Chief of Medical Staff. . . . . James A Raczek, MD

Measure	Cases	This Hosp.	State Avg.	U.S. Avg.
Blood Clot Prevention and Treatment				
Anticoagulation Overlap Therapy[2]	79	100%	98%	93%
ICU Venous Thromboembolism Prophylaxis[2]	104	95%	96%	92%
Incidence of Potentially Preventable VTE[2]	24	4%	2%	10%
UFH with Dosages/Platelet Monitoring[2]	87	100%	100%	97%
Venous Thromboembolism Prophylaxis[2]	309	93%	95%	85%
Warfarin Therapy Discharge Instructions[2]	58	97%	84%	75%
Chest Pain/Possible Heart Attack Care				
Aspirin Given Within 24 Hours of Arrival[1,3]	-	-	99%	96%
Fibrinolytic Meds Within 30 Min. of Arrival[5]	-	-	86%	58%
Average Time to ECG (minutes)[1,3]	-	-	6	7
Average Time to Transfer (minutes)[5]	-	-	49	60
Children's Asthma Care				
Received Home Management Plan of Care	-	-	-	88%
Received Reliever Medication	-	-	-	100%
Received Systemic Corticosteroids	-	-	-	100%
Emergency Department				
Admittance Decision Time (minutes)[2]	90	228	110	98
Head CT Results Within 45 Min. of Arrival[1]	-	-	44%	57%
Patients Who Left ER Before Being Seen	40,349	2%	1%	2%
Time from ER Arrival to Admit. (minutes)[2]	289	376	288	274
Time from ER Arrival to Discharge (minutes)	344	176	122	134
Time in ER Before Being Evaluated (minutes)	244	44	28	26
Time to Pain Meds for Fractures (minutes)	169	67	52	57
Heart Attack Care				
Aspirin Given at Discharge	1,002	100%	100%	99%

NOTE: Hospital profiles are in alphabetical order by state, then city, then hospital within the city; Rankings exclude hospitals with less than 25 cases except for patient surveys which excludes hospitals with less than 100 cases; (a) 100-299 cases; (1) The number of cases/patients is too few to report; (2) Data submitted were based on a sample of cases/patients; (3) Results are based on a shorter time period than required; (4) Data suppressed by CMS for one or more quarters; (5) Results are not available for this reporting period; (6) Fewer than 100 patients completed the HCAHPS survey; (7) No cases met the criteria for this measure; (8) The lower limit of the confidence interval cannot be calculated if the number of observed infections equals zero; (9) No data are available from the state/territory for this reporting period; (10) The scores shown reflect fewer than 50 completed surveys; (11) There were discrepancies in the data collection process; (12) This measure does not apply to this hospital for this reporting period; (13) Results cannot be calculated for this reporting period; (14) The results for this state are combined with nearby states to protect confidentiality; Please refer to the User's Guide for a full explanation of data.

Measure	Cases	This Hosp.	State Avg.	U.S. Avg.
Fibrinolytic Meds Within 30 Min. of Arrival[1]	-	-	50%	54%
PCI Within 90 Minutes of Arrival	25	96%	96%	96%
Statin Prescribed at Discharge	953	100%	99%	98%
Heart Failure Care				
ACE Inhibitor or ARB for LVSD	88	100%	99%	97%
Discharge Instructions Given	375	99%	98%	94%
Evaluation of LVS Function	444	100%	100%	99%
Medicare Spending				
Medicare Spending per Patient (ratio)	-	0.99	0.95	0.98
Pneumonia Care				
Appropriate Initial Antibiotic Given	119	98%	98%	95%
Blood Culture Timing	261	98%	98%	98%
Pregnancy and Delivery Care				
Newborn Deliveries Scheduled Early	98	5%	2%	6%
Preventive Care				
Immunization for Influenza[2]	553	85%	93%	90%
Immunization for Pneumonia[2]	674	95%	94%	92%
Stroke Care				
Anticoagulation Therapy for Atrial Fibrillation	26	100%	98%	95%
Antithrombotic Therapy Timing	162	99%	99%	98%
Assessed for Rehabilitation	234	99%	98%	97%
Discharged on Antithrombotic Therapy	192	100%	100%	99%
Discharged on Statin Medication	151	99%	97%	94%
Thrombolytic Therapy Timing[1]	-	-	29%	66%
Venous Thromboembolism Prophylaxis	244	99%	96%	94%
Written Stroke Educational Materials Given	100	95%	86%	88%
Surgical Care Improvement Project				
Appropriate Beta Blocker Usage[2]	575	100%	99%	98%
Appropriate VTP Within 24 Hours[2]	763	100%	99%	98%
Controlled Postoperative Blood Glucose[2]	305	98%	99%	97%
Perioperative Temperature Management[2]	1,011	100%	100%	100%
Prophylactic Antibiotic Selection[2]	1,029	100%	99%	99%
Prophylactic Antibiotic Selection (Outpatient)	965	98%	98%	98%
Prophylactic Antibiotic Stopped[2]	996	100%	99%	98%
Prophylactic Antibiotic Timing[2]	1,032	100%	99%	99%
Prophylactic Antibiotic Timing (Outpatient)	877	96%	96%	98%
Urinary Catheter Removal[2]	492	100%	99%	97%
Survey of Patients' Hospital Experiences				
Area Around Room 'Always' Quiet at Night	300+	45%	59%	61%
Doctors 'Always' Communicated Well	300+	79%	83%	82%
Home Recovery Information Given	300+	88%	90%	85%
Hospital Given 9 or 10 on 10 Point Scale	300+	70%	74%	71%
Meds 'Always' Explained Before Given	300+	64%	69%	64%
Nurses 'Always' Communicated Well	300+	80%	82%	79%
Pain 'Always' Well Controlled	300+	69%	73%	71%
Room and Bathroom 'Always' Clean	300+	76%	80%	73%
Timely Help 'Always' Received	300+	64%	72%	68%
Would Definitely Recommend Hospital	300+	75%	77%	71%
Use of Medical Imaging				
Cardiac Imaging Stress Test before Surgery	686	5.0%	4.8%	5.3%
Combination Abdominal CT Scan	1,475	2.0%	5.2%	10.5%
Combination Brain/Sinus CT Scan	637	2.4%	1.7%	2.7%
Combination Chest CT Scan	1,563	0.0%	0.7%	2.7%
Follow-up Mammogram/Ultrasound	1,452	5.0%	7.7%	8.8%
Lumbar Spine MRI for Low Back Pain	341	37.5%	37.5%	37.2%

Saint Joseph Hospital

360 Broadway
Bangor, ME 04401
Phone: 207-262-1000
Fax: 207-262-1922
URL: www.stjoeshealing.com
Type: Acute Care Hospitals
Emergency Services: Yes
Ownership: Voluntary non-profit - Church
Beds: 100

Key Personnel:
Radiology.................. David Ahola
CEO/President.............. Sister Mary Norberta, CSSF
Chief of Medical Staff.......... David Renedo, MD
Patient Relations .... Dianne Swandal, BSN

Measure	Cases	This Hosp.	State Avg.	U.S. Avg.
Blood Clot Prevention and Treatment				
Anticoagulation Overlap Therapy[2]	31	100%	98%	93%
ICU Venous Thromboembolism Prophylaxis[2]	43	95%	96%	92%
Incidence of Potentially Preventable VTE[1,2]	-	-	2%	10%
UFH with Dosages/Platelet Monitoring[2]	32	100%	100%	97%
Venous Thromboembolism Prophylaxis[2]	363	96%	95%	85%
Warfarin Therapy Discharge Instructions[2]	21	100%	84%	75%
Chest Pain/Possible Heart Attack Care				
Aspirin Given Within 24 Hours of Arrival	19	100%	99%	96%
Fibrinolytic Meds Within 30 Min. of Arrival[7]	-	-	86%	58%
Average Time to ECG (minutes)	19	9	6	7
Average Time to Transfer (minutes)[1]	-	-	49	60
Children's Asthma Care				
Received Home Management Plan of Care	-	-	-	88%
Received Reliever Medication	-	-	-	100%
Received Systemic Corticosteroids	-	-	-	100%
Emergency Department				
Admittance Decision Time (minutes)[2]	620	122	110	98
Head CT Results Within 45 Min. of Arrival[1]	-	-	44%	57%
Patients Who Left ER Before Being Seen	25,013	1%	1%	2%
Time from ER Arrival to Admit. (minutes)[2]	620	324	288	274
Time from ER Arrival to Discharge (minutes)	363	164	122	134
Time in ER Before Being Evaluated (minutes)	401	25	28	26
Time to Pain Meds for Fractures (minutes)	107	65	52	57
Heart Attack Care				
Aspirin Given at Discharge	36	100%	100%	99%
Fibrinolytic Meds Within 30 Min. of Arrival[7]	-	-	50%	54%
PCI Within 90 Minutes of Arrival[7]	-	-	96%	96%
Statin Prescribed at Discharge	34	97%	99%	98%
Heart Failure Care				
ACE Inhibitor or ARB for LVSD	27	93%	99%	97%
Discharge Instructions Given	110	99%	98%	94%
Evaluation of LVS Function	152	100%	100%	99%
Medicare Spending				
Medicare Spending per Patient (ratio)	-	0.96	0.95	0.98
Pneumonia Care				
Appropriate Initial Antibiotic Given	151	96%	98%	95%
Blood Culture Timing	247	97%	98%	98%
Pregnancy and Delivery Care				
Newborn Deliveries Scheduled Early[7]	-	-	2%	6%
Preventive Care				
Immunization for Influenza[2]	384	95%	93%	90%
Immunization for Pneumonia[2]	631	95%	94%	92%
Stroke Care				
Anticoagulation Therapy for Atrial Fibrillation[1]	-	-	98%	95%
Antithrombotic Therapy Timing	42	100%	99%	98%
Assessed for Rehabilitation	40	100%	98%	97%
Discharged on Antithrombotic Therapy	37	100%	100%	99%
Discharged on Statin Medication	32	97%	97%	94%
Thrombolytic Therapy Timing[1]	-	-	29%	66%
Venous Thromboembolism Prophylaxis	45	93%	96%	94%
Written Stroke Educational Materials Given	17	94%	86%	88%
Surgical Care Improvement Project				
Appropriate Beta Blocker Usage[2]	128	99%	99%	98%
Appropriate VTP Within 24 Hours[2]	422	99%	99%	98%
Controlled Postoperative Blood Glucose[2,7]	-	-	99%	97%
Perioperative Temperature Management[2]	452	99%	100%	100%
Prophylactic Antibiotic Selection[2]	349	99%	99%	99%
Prophylactic Antibiotic Selection (Outpatient)	278	100%	98%	98%
Prophylactic Antibiotic Stopped[2]	348	99%	99%	98%
Prophylactic Antibiotic Timing[2]	350	100%	99%	99%
Prophylactic Antibiotic Timing (Outpatient)	279	100%	96%	98%
Urinary Catheter Removal[2]	106	100%	99%	97%
Survey of Patients' Hospital Experiences				
Area Around Room 'Always' Quiet at Night	300+	61%	59%	61%
Doctors 'Always' Communicated Well	300+	84%	83%	82%
Home Recovery Information Given	300+	92%	90%	85%
Hospital Given 9 or 10 on 10 Point Scale	300+	77%	74%	71%
Meds 'Always' Explained Before Given	300+	68%	69%	64%
Nurses 'Always' Communicated Well	300+	81%	82%	79%
Pain 'Always' Well Controlled	300+	73%	73%	71%
Room and Bathroom 'Always' Clean	300+	78%	80%	73%
Timely Help 'Always' Received	300+	68%	72%	68%
Would Definitely Recommend Hospital	300+	83%	77%	71%
Use of Medical Imaging				
Cardiac Imaging Stress Test before Surgery	248	4.8%	4.8%	5.3%
Combination Abdominal CT Scan	631	4.0%	5.2%	10.5%
Combination Brain/Sinus CT Scan[1]	-	-	1.7%	2.7%
Combination Chest CT Scan	366	0.0%	0.7%	2.7%
Follow-up Mammogram/Ultrasound	2,794	6.5%	7.7%	8.8%
Lumbar Spine MRI for Low Back Pain	199	34.2%	37.5%	37.2%

Mount Desert Island Hospital

10 Wayman Lane, PO Box 8
Bar Harbor, ME 04609
Phone: 207-288-5081
Fax: 207-288-5874
E-mail: crdev@mdihospital.org
URL: www.mdihospital.com
Type: Critical Access Hospitals
Emergency Services: Yes
Ownership: Voluntary non-profit - Private
Beds: 49

Key Personnel:
Chief of Medical Staff.......... John M Benson, MD
CEO/President.............. Arthur J Blank
Emergency Room .... Michael Lewin, MD
Chairman/CEO .... Vincent C. Messer, PhD
Quality Assurance .... Jean Wolf

Measure	Cases	This Hosp.	State Avg.	U.S. Avg.
Blood Clot Prevention and Treatment				
Anticoagulation Overlap Therapy[1]	-	-	98%	93%
ICU Venous Thromboembolism Prophylaxis[7]	-	-	96%	92%
Incidence of Potentially Preventable VTE[7]	-	-	2%	10%
UFH with Dosages/Platelet Monitoring[1]	-	-	100%	97%
Venous Thromboembolism Prophylaxis[7]	-	-	95%	85%
Warfarin Therapy Discharge Instructions[1]	-	-	84%	75%
Chest Pain/Possible Heart Attack Care				
Aspirin Given Within 24 Hours of Arrival[1,3]	-	-	99%	96%
Fibrinolytic Meds Within 30 Min. of Arrival[1,3]	-	-	86%	58%
Average Time to ECG (minutes)[1,3]	-	-	6	7
Average Time to Transfer (minutes)[3,7]	-	-	49	60
Children's Asthma Care				
Received Home Management Plan of Care	-	-	-	88%
Received Reliever Medication	-	-	-	100%
Received Systemic Corticosteroids	-	-	-	100%
Emergency Department				
Admittance Decision Time (minutes)[2,3]	285	145	110	98
Head CT Results Within 45 Min. of Arrival[1,3]	-	-	44%	57%
Patients Who Left ER Before Being Seen	6,287	0%	1%	2%
Time from ER Arrival to Admit. (minutes)[2,3]	285	268	288	274
Time from ER Arrival to Discharge (minutes)[3]	138	126	122	134
Time in ER Before Being Evaluated (minutes)[3]	145	26	28	26
Time to Pain Meds for Fractures (minutes)[5]	-	-	52	57
Heart Attack Care				
Aspirin Given at Discharge[1]	-	-	100%	99%
Fibrinolytic Meds Within 30 Min. of Arrival[7]	-	-	50%	54%
PCI Within 90 Minutes of Arrival[7]	-	-	96%	96%
Statin Prescribed at Discharge[1]	-	-	99%	98%
Heart Failure Care				
ACE Inhibitor or ARB for LVSD[1]	-	-	99%	97%
Discharge Instructions Given	13	100%	98%	94%
Evaluation of LVS Function	25	100%	100%	99%
Medicare Spending				
Medicare Spending per Patient (ratio)	-	-	0.95	0.98
Pneumonia Care				
Appropriate Initial Antibiotic Given	18	100%	98%	95%
Blood Culture Timing	28	100%	98%	98%
Pregnancy and Delivery Care				
Newborn Deliveries Scheduled Early[1,3]	-	-	2%	6%
Preventive Care				
Immunization for Influenza[2,3]	131	100%	93%	90%
Immunization for Pneumonia[2,3]	253	100%	94%	92%
Stroke Care				
Anticoagulation Therapy for Atrial Fibrillation[1]	-	-	98%	95%
Antithrombotic Therapy Timing[1]	-	-	99%	98%
Assessed for Rehabilitation[1]	-	-	98%	97%
Discharged on Antithrombotic Therapy[1]	-	-	100%	99%
Discharged on Statin Medication[1]	-	-	97%	94%
Thrombolytic Therapy Timing[7]	-	-	29%	66%
Venous Thromboembolism Prophylaxis[1]	-	-	96%	94%
Written Stroke Educational Materials Given[1]	-	-	86%	88%
Surgical Care Improvement Project				
Appropriate Beta Blocker Usage[1]	-	-	99%	98%
Appropriate VTP Within 24 Hours	32	100%	99%	98%

NOTE: Hospital profiles are in alphabetical order by state, then city, then hospital within the city; Rankings exclude hospitals with less than 25 cases except for patient surveys which excludes hospitals with less than 100 cases; (a) 100-299 cases; (1) The number of cases/patients is too few to report; (2) Data submitted were based on a sample of cases/patients; (3) Results are based on a shorter time period than required; (4) Data suppressed by CMS for one or more quarters; (5) Results are not available for this reporting period; (6) Fewer than 100 patients completed the HCAHPS survey; (7) No cases met the criteria for this measure; (8) The lower limit of the confidence interval cannot be calculated if the number of observed infections equals zero; (9) No data are available from the state/territory for this reporting period; (10) The scores shown reflect fewer than 50 completed surveys; (11) There were discrepancies in the data collection process; (12) This measure does not apply to this hospital for this reporting period; (13) Results cannot be calculated for this reporting period; (14) The results for this state are combined with nearby states to protect confidentiality; Please refer to the User's Guide for a full explanation of data.

Controlled Postoperative Blood Glucose[7]	-	-	99%	97%
Perioperative Temperature Management	36	100%	100%	100%
Prophylactic Antibiotic Selection	24	100%	99%	99%
Prophylactic Antibiotic Selection (Outpatient)[1,3]	-	-	98%	98%
Prophylactic Antibiotic Stopped	24	100%	99%	98%
Prophylactic Antibiotic Timing	24	100%	99%	99%
Prophylactic Antibiotic Timing (Outpatient)[1,3]	-	-	96%	98%
Urinary Catheter Removal	31	100%	99%	97%
Survey of Patients' Hospital Experiences				
Area Around Room 'Always' Quiet at Night	(a)	71%	59%	61%
Doctors 'Always' Communicated Well	(a)	92%	83%	82%
Home Recovery Information Given	(a)	96%	90%	85%
Hospital Given 9 or 10 on 10 Point Scale	(a)	88%	74%	71%
Meds 'Always' Explained Before Given	(a)	76%	69%	64%
Nurses 'Always' Communicated Well	(a)	91%	82%	79%
Pain 'Always' Well Controlled	(a)	84%	73%	71%
Room and Bathroom 'Always' Clean	(a)	85%	80%	73%
Timely Help 'Always' Received	(a)	85%	72%	68%
Would Definitely Recommend Hospital	(a)	91%	77%	71%
Use of Medical Imaging				
Cardiac Imaging Stress Test before Surgery[1]	-	-	4.8%	5.3%
Combination Abdominal CT Scan	206	6.3%	5.2%	10.5%
Combination Brain/Sinus CT Scan[1]	-	-	1.7%	2.7%
Combination Chest CT Scan	93	0.0%	0.7%	2.7%
Follow-up Mammogram/Ultrasound	351	5.7%	7.7%	8.8%
Lumbar Spine MRI for Low Back Pain[1]	-	-	37.5%	37.2%

Waldo County General Hospital

PO Box 287
Belfast, ME 04915
Phone: 207-338-2500
Fax: 207-338-9382
E-mail: inquires@wchi.com
URL: www.wchi.com
Type: Critical Access Hospitals
Emergency Services: Yes
Ownership: Voluntary non-profit - Private
Beds: 25

Key Personnel:
CEO/President. . . . . Mark Biscone
Emergency Room . . . . Camille C Canova
Radiology. . . . . John P Gay

Measure	Cases	This Hosp.	State Avg.	U.S. Avg.
Blood Clot Prevention and Treatment				
Anticoagulation Overlap Therapy[5]	-	-	98%	93%
ICU Venous Thromboembolism Prophylaxis[5]	-	-	96%	92%
Incidence of Potentially Preventable VTE[5]	-	-	2%	10%
UFH with Dosages/Platelet Monitoring[5]	-	-	100%	97%
Venous Thromboembolism Prophylaxis[5]	-	-	95%	85%
Warfarin Therapy Discharge Instructions[5]	-	-	84%	75%
Chest Pain/Possible Heart Attack Care				
Aspirin Given Within 24 Hours of Arrival	-	-	99%	96%
Fibrinolytic Meds Within 30 Min. of Arrival	-	-	86%	58%
Average Time to ECG (minutes)	-	-	6	7
Average Time to Transfer (minutes)	-	-	49	60
Children's Asthma Care				
Received Home Management Plan of Care	-	-	-	88%
Received Reliever Medication	-	-	-	100%
Received Systemic Corticosteroids	-	-	-	100%
Emergency Department				
Admittance Decision Time (minutes)[5]	-	-	110	98
Head CT Results Within 45 Min. of Arrival	-	-	44%	57%
Patients Who Left ER Before Being Seen	-	-	1%	2%
Time from ER Arrival to Admit. (minutes)[5]	-	-	288	274
Time from ER Arrival to Discharge (minutes)	-	-	122	134
Time in ER Before Being Evaluated (minutes)	-	-	28	26
Time to Pain Meds for Fractures (minutes)	-	-	52	57
Heart Attack Care				
Aspirin Given at Discharge	17	94%	100%	99%
Fibrinolytic Meds Within 30 Min. of Arrival[7]	-	-	50%	54%
PCI Within 90 Minutes of Arrival[3,7]	-	-	96%	96%
Statin Prescribed at Discharge	16	100%	99%	98%
Heart Failure Care				
ACE Inhibitor or ARB for LVSD[1]	-	-	99%	97%
Discharge Instructions Given	17	100%	98%	94%
Evaluation of LVS Function	25	100%	100%	99%
Medicare Spending				
Medicare Spending per Patient (ratio)	-	-	0.95	0.98
Pneumonia Care				
Appropriate Initial Antibiotic Given	35	97%	98%	95%
Blood Culture Timing	50	100%	98%	98%
Pregnancy and Delivery Care				
Newborn Deliveries Scheduled Early[2]	17	0%	2%	6%
Preventive Care				
Immunization for Influenza[5]	-	-	93%	90%
Immunization for Pneumonia[5]	-	-	94%	92%
Stroke Care				
Anticoagulation Therapy for Atrial Fibrillation[5]	-	-	98%	95%
Antithrombotic Therapy Timing[5]	-	-	99%	98%
Assessed for Rehabilitation[5]	-	-	98%	97%
Discharged on Antithrombotic Therapy[5]	-	-	100%	99%
Discharged on Statin Medication[5]	-	-	97%	94%
Thrombolytic Therapy Timing[5]	-	-	29%	66%
Venous Thromboembolism Prophylaxis[5]	-	-	96%	94%
Written Stroke Educational Materials Given[5]	-	-	86%	88%
Surgical Care Improvement Project				
Appropriate Beta Blocker Usage	32	100%	99%	98%
Appropriate VTP Within 24 Hours	120	98%	99%	98%
Controlled Postoperative Blood Glucose[3,7]	-	-	99%	97%
Perioperative Temperature Management	138	100%	100%	100%
Prophylactic Antibiotic Selection	97	100%	99%	99%
Prophylactic Antibiotic Selection (Outpatient)	-	-	98%	98%
Prophylactic Antibiotic Stopped	94	96%	99%	98%
Prophylactic Antibiotic Timing	97	99%	99%	99%
Prophylactic Antibiotic Timing (Outpatient)	-	-	96%	98%
Urinary Catheter Removal	102	97%	99%	97%
Survey of Patients' Hospital Experiences				
Area Around Room 'Always' Quiet at Night	(a)	52%	59%	61%
Doctors 'Always' Communicated Well	(a)	79%	83%	82%
Home Recovery Information Given	(a)	89%	90%	85%
Hospital Given 9 or 10 on 10 Point Scale	(a)	74%	74%	71%
Meds 'Always' Explained Before Given	(a)	61%	69%	64%
Nurses 'Always' Communicated Well	(a)	80%	82%	79%
Pain 'Always' Well Controlled	(a)	73%	73%	71%
Room and Bathroom 'Always' Clean	(a)	79%	80%	73%
Timely Help 'Always' Received	(a)	71%	72%	68%
Would Definitely Recommend Hospital	(a)	75%	77%	71%
Use of Medical Imaging				
Cardiac Imaging Stress Test before Surgery	-	-	4.8%	5.3%
Combination Abdominal CT Scan	-	-	5.2%	10.5%
Combination Brain/Sinus CT Scan	-	-	1.7%	2.7%
Combination Chest CT Scan	-	-	0.7%	2.7%
Follow-up Mammogram/Ultrasound	-	-	7.7%	8.8%
Lumbar Spine MRI for Low Back Pain	-	-	37.5%	37.2%

Southern Maine Medical Center

1 Medical Center Drive
Biddeford, ME 04005
Phone: 207-283-7000
Fax: 207-283-7020
E-mail: info@smmc.org
URL: www.smmc.org
Type: Acute Care Hospitals
Emergency Services: Yes
Ownership: Voluntary non-profit - Private
Beds: 150

Key Personnel:
Chief of Medical Staff. . . . . Michael Albaum, MD
Operating Room. . . . . Toni Clark, RN
Radiology. . . . . Stephen M Madigan
Quality Assurance . . . . Melissa McClay
CEO/President. . . . . Ed McGeachey
Emergency Room . . . . Gina Quinn-Skillings, MD
Coronary Care. . . . . Kathy Viger, RN

Measure	Cases	This Hosp.	State Avg.	U.S. Avg.
Blood Clot Prevention and Treatment				
Anticoagulation Overlap Therapy[2]	54	100%	98%	93%
ICU Venous Thromboembolism Prophylaxis[2]	52	96%	96%	92%
Incidence of Potentially Preventable VTE[1,2]	-	-	2%	10%
UFH with Dosages/Platelet Monitoring[2]	19	100%	100%	97%
Venous Thromboembolism Prophylaxis[2]	326	92%	95%	85%
Warfarin Therapy Discharge Instructions[2]	42	83%	84%	75%
Chest Pain/Possible Heart Attack Care				
Aspirin Given Within 24 Hours of Arrival	92	100%	99%	96%
Fibrinolytic Meds Within 30 Min. of Arrival[7]	-	-	86%	58%
Average Time to ECG (minutes)	92	4	6	7
Average Time to Transfer (minutes)	33	30	49	60
Children's Asthma Care				
Received Home Management Plan of Care	-	-	-	88%
Received Reliever Medication	-	-	-	100%
Received Systemic Corticosteroids	-	-	-	100%
Emergency Department				
Admittance Decision Time (minutes)[2]	738	70	110	98
Head CT Results Within 45 Min. of Arrival	12	8%	44%	57%
Patients Who Left ER Before Being Seen	41,548	2%	1%	2%
Time from ER Arrival to Admit. (minutes)[2]	756	322	288	274
Time from ER Arrival to Discharge (minutes)	329	146	122	134
Time in ER Before Being Evaluated (minutes)	262	50	28	26
Time to Pain Meds for Fractures (minutes)	99	55	52	57
Heart Attack Care				
Aspirin Given at Discharge	60	100%	100%	99%
Fibrinolytic Meds Within 30 Min. of Arrival[7]	-	-	50%	54%
PCI Within 90 Minutes of Arrival[7]	-	-	96%	96%
Statin Prescribed at Discharge	59	97%	99%	98%
Heart Failure Care				
ACE Inhibitor or ARB for LVSD	29	100%	99%	97%
Discharge Instructions Given	158	97%	98%	94%
Evaluation of LVS Function	206	100%	100%	99%
Medicare Spending				
Medicare Spending per Patient (ratio)	-	0.98	0.95	0.98
Pneumonia Care				
Appropriate Initial Antibiotic Given	122	98%	98%	95%
Blood Culture Timing	86	100%	98%	98%
Pregnancy and Delivery Care				
Newborn Deliveries Scheduled Early	71	0%	2%	6%
Preventive Care				
Immunization for Influenza[2]	509	96%	93%	90%
Immunization for Pneumonia[2]	727	94%	94%	92%
Stroke Care				
Anticoagulation Therapy for Atrial Fibrillation	14	100%	98%	95%
Antithrombotic Therapy Timing	79	100%	99%	98%
Assessed for Rehabilitation	91	99%	98%	97%
Discharged on Antithrombotic Therapy	83	100%	100%	99%
Discharged on Statin Medication	69	100%	97%	94%
Thrombolytic Therapy Timing[1]	-	-	29%	66%
Venous Thromboembolism Prophylaxis	89	96%	96%	94%
Written Stroke Educational Materials Given	40	80%	86%	88%
Surgical Care Improvement Project				
Appropriate Beta Blocker Usage	143	100%	99%	98%
Appropriate VTP Within 24 Hours	370	100%	99%	98%
Controlled Postoperative Blood Glucose[7]	-	-	99%	97%
Perioperative Temperature Management	435	100%	100%	100%
Prophylactic Antibiotic Selection	301	100%	99%	99%
Prophylactic Antibiotic Selection (Outpatient)	17	100%	98%	98%
Prophylactic Antibiotic Stopped	300	100%	99%	98%
Prophylactic Antibiotic Timing	301	100%	99%	99%
Prophylactic Antibiotic Timing (Outpatient)	17	94%	96%	98%
Urinary Catheter Removal	265	100%	99%	97%
Survey of Patients' Hospital Experiences				
Area Around Room 'Always' Quiet at Night	300+	46%	59%	61%
Doctors 'Always' Communicated Well	300+	80%	83%	82%
Home Recovery Information Given	300+	86%	90%	85%
Hospital Given 9 or 10 on 10 Point Scale	300+	68%	74%	71%
Meds 'Always' Explained Before Given	300+	62%	69%	64%
Nurses 'Always' Communicated Well	300+	77%	82%	79%
Pain 'Always' Well Controlled	300+	69%	73%	71%
Room and Bathroom 'Always' Clean	300+	66%	80%	73%
Timely Help 'Always' Received	300+	60%	72%	68%
Would Definitely Recommend Hospital	300+	70%	77%	71%
Use of Medical Imaging				
Cardiac Imaging Stress Test before Surgery	462	3.5%	4.8%	5.3%
Combination Abdominal CT Scan	988	5.4%	5.2%	10.5%
Combination Brain/Sinus CT Scan	939	2.0%	1.7%	2.7%
Combination Chest CT Scan	663	0.0%	0.7%	2.7%
Follow-up Mammogram/Ultrasound	1,986	6.2%	7.7%	8.8%
Lumbar Spine MRI for Low Back Pain	127	37.0%	37.5%	37.2%

NOTE: Hospital profiles are in alphabetical order by state, then city, then hospital within the city; Rankings exclude hospitals with less than 25 cases except for patient surveys which excludes hospitals with less than 100 cases; (a) 100-299 cases; (1) The number of cases/patients is too few to report; (2) Data submitted were based on a sample of cases/patients; (3) Results are based on a shorter time period than required; (4) Data suppressed by CMS for one or more quarters; (5) Results are not available for this reporting period; (6) Fewer than 100 patients completed the HCAHPS survey; (7) No cases met the criteria for this measure; (8) The lower limit of the confidence interval cannot be calculated if the number of observed infections equals zero; (9) No data are available from the state/territory for this reporting period; (10) The scores shown reflect fewer than 50 completed surveys; (11) There were discrepancies in the data collection process; (12) This measure does not apply to this hospital for this reporting period; (13) Results cannot be calculated for this reporting period; (14) The results for this state are combined with nearby states to protect confidentiality; Please refer to the User's Guide for a full explanation of data.

Blue Hill Memorial Hospital

57 Water Street
Blue Hill, ME 04614
Phone: 207-374-2836
Fax: 207-374-5368
URL: www.bhmh.org/default.html
Type: Critical Access Hospitals
Emergency Services: Yes
Ownership: Voluntary non-profit - Private
Beds: 25

Key Personnel:
Chief of Medical Staff. . . . . Robert Baroody
President/CEO. . . . . John Ronan, FACHE
Radiology. . . . . Richard Seger

Measure	Cases	This Hosp.	State Avg.	U.S. Avg.
Blood Clot Prevention and Treatment				
Anticoagulation Overlap Therapy[5]	-	-	98%	93%
ICU Venous Thromboembolism Prophylaxis[5]	-	-	96%	92%
Incidence of Potentially Preventable VTE[5]	-	-	2%	10%
UFH with Dosages/Platelet Monitoring[5]	-	-	100%	97%
Venous Thromboembolism Prophylaxis[5]	-	-	95%	85%
Warfarin Therapy Discharge Instructions[5]	-	-	84%	75%
Chest Pain/Possible Heart Attack Care				
Aspirin Given Within 24 Hours of Arrival	-	-	99%	96%
Fibrinolytic Meds Within 30 Min. of Arrival	-	-	86%	58%
Average Time to ECG (minutes)	-	-	6	7
Average Time to Transfer (minutes)	-	-	49	60
Children's Asthma Care				
Received Home Management Plan of Care	-	-	-	88%
Received Reliever Medication	-	-	-	100%
Received Systemic Corticosteroids	-	-	-	100%
Emergency Department				
Admittance Decision Time (minutes)[5]	-	-	110	98
Head CT Results Within 45 Min. of Arrival	-	-	44%	57%
Patients Who Left ER Before Being Seen	-	-	1%	2%
Time from ER Arrival to Admit. (minutes)[5]	-	-	288	274
Time from ER Arrival to Discharge (minutes)	-	-	122	134
Time in ER Before Being Evaluated (minutes)	-	-	28	26
Time to Pain Meds for Fractures (minutes)	-	-	52	57
Heart Attack Care				
Aspirin Given at Discharge[1]	-	-	100%	99%
Fibrinolytic Meds Within 30 Min. of Arrival[7]	-	-	50%	54%
PCI Within 90 Minutes of Arrival[3,7]	-	-	96%	96%
Statin Prescribed at Discharge[1]	-	-	99%	98%
Heart Failure Care				
ACE Inhibitor or ARB for LVSD[1]	-	-	99%	97%
Discharge Instructions Given[1]	-	-	98%	94%
Evaluation of LVS Function	15	100%	100%	99%
Medicare Spending				
Medicare Spending per Patient (ratio)	-	-	0.95	0.98
Pneumonia Care				
Appropriate Initial Antibiotic Given	15	100%	98%	95%
Blood Culture Timing	19	100%	98%	98%
Pregnancy and Delivery Care				
Newborn Deliveries Scheduled Early[5]	-	-	2%	6%
Preventive Care				
Immunization for Influenza[5]	-	-	93%	90%
Immunization for Pneumonia[5]	-	-	94%	92%
Stroke Care				
Anticoagulation Therapy for Atrial Fibrillation[5]	-	-	98%	95%
Antithrombotic Therapy Timing[5]	-	-	99%	98%
Assessed for Rehabilitation[5]	-	-	98%	97%
Discharged on Antithrombotic Therapy[5]	-	-	100%	99%
Discharged on Statin Medication[5]	-	-	97%	94%
Thrombolytic Therapy Timing[5]	-	-	29%	66%
Venous Thromboembolism Prophylaxis[5]	-	-	96%	94%
Written Stroke Educational Materials Given[5]	-	-	86%	88%
Surgical Care Improvement Project				
Appropriate Beta Blocker Usage	12	100%	99%	98%
Appropriate VTP Within 24 Hours	44	98%	99%	98%
Controlled Postoperative Blood Glucose[3,7]	-	-	99%	97%
Perioperative Temperature Management	50	100%	100%	100%
Prophylactic Antibiotic Selection	45	100%	99%	99%
Prophylactic Antibiotic Selection (Outpatient)	-	-	98%	98%
Prophylactic Antibiotic Stopped	45	98%	99%	98%
Prophylactic Antibiotic Timing	45	98%	99%	99%
Prophylactic Antibiotic Timing (Outpatient)	-	-	96%	98%
Urinary Catheter Removal[1]	-	-	99%	97%
Survey of Patients' Hospital Experiences				
Area Around Room 'Always' Quiet at Night	(a)	68%	59%	61%
Doctors 'Always' Communicated Well	(a)	83%	83%	82%
Home Recovery Information Given	(a)	94%	90%	85%
Hospital Given 9 or 10 on 10 Point Scale	(a)	81%	74%	71%
Meds 'Always' Explained Before Given	(a)	78%	69%	64%
Nurses 'Always' Communicated Well	(a)	87%	82%	79%
Pain 'Always' Well Controlled	(a)	78%	73%	71%
Room and Bathroom 'Always' Clean	(a)	93%	80%	73%
Timely Help 'Always' Received	(a)	78%	72%	68%
Would Definitely Recommend Hospital	(a)	79%	77%	71%
Use of Medical Imaging				
Cardiac Imaging Stress Test before Surgery	-	-	4.8%	5.3%
Combination Abdominal CT Scan	-	-	5.2%	10.5%
Combination Brain/Sinus CT Scan	-	-	1.7%	2.7%
Combination Chest CT Scan	-	-	0.7%	2.7%
Follow-up Mammogram/Ultrasound	-	-	7.7%	8.8%
Lumbar Spine MRI for Low Back Pain	-	-	37.5%	37.2%

Saint Andrews Hospital

6 Saint Andrews Lane
Boothbay Harbor, ME 04538
Phone: 207-633-2121
Fax: 207-633-5173
E-mail: mpinkham@standrewshealthcare.org
URL: www.standrewshealthcare.org
Type: Critical Access Hospitals
Emergency Services: Yes
Ownership: Voluntary non-profit - Private
Beds: 15

Key Personnel:
CEO/President. . . . . James W Donovan
Radiology. . . . . Bernadette V Jakomin, MD
Chief of Medical Staff. . . . . Jana Kazalski, DO
Emergency Room . . . . Matthew Sleeth, MD
Infection Control. . . . . Joan Taylor
Quality Assurance . . . . Charles White

Measure	Cases	This Hosp.	State Avg.	U.S. Avg.
Blood Clot Prevention and Treatment				
Anticoagulation Overlap Therapy[5]	-	-	98%	93%
ICU Venous Thromboembolism Prophylaxis[5]	-	-	96%	92%
Incidence of Potentially Preventable VTE[5]	-	-	2%	10%
UFH with Dosages/Platelet Monitoring[5]	-	-	100%	97%
Venous Thromboembolism Prophylaxis[5]	-	-	95%	85%
Warfarin Therapy Discharge Instructions[5]	-	-	84%	75%
Chest Pain/Possible Heart Attack Care				
Aspirin Given Within 24 Hours of Arrival[5]	-	-	99%	96%
Fibrinolytic Meds Within 30 Min. of Arrival[5]	-	-	86%	58%
Average Time to ECG (minutes)[5]	-	-	6	7
Average Time to Transfer (minutes)[5]	-	-	49	60
Children's Asthma Care				
Received Home Management Plan of Care	-	-	-	88%
Received Reliever Medication	-	-	-	100%
Received Systemic Corticosteroids	-	-	-	100%
Emergency Department				
Admittance Decision Time (minutes)[5]	-	-	110	98
Head CT Results Within 45 Min. of Arrival[5]	-	-	44%	57%
Patients Who Left ER Before Being Seen	4,632	0%	1%	2%
Time from ER Arrival to Admit. (minutes)[5]	-	-	288	274
Time from ER Arrival to Discharge (minutes)[5]	-	-	122	134
Time in ER Before Being Evaluated (minutes)[5]	-	-	28	26
Time to Pain Meds for Fractures (minutes)[5]	-	-	52	57
Heart Attack Care				
Aspirin Given at Discharge[5]	-	-	100%	99%
Fibrinolytic Meds Within 30 Min. of Arrival[5]	-	-	50%	54%
PCI Within 90 Minutes of Arrival[5]	-	-	96%	96%
Statin Prescribed at Discharge[5]	-	-	99%	98%
Heart Failure Care				
ACE Inhibitor or ARB for LVSD[5]	-	-	99%	97%
Discharge Instructions Given[5]	-	-	98%	94%
Evaluation of LVS Function[5]	-	-	100%	99%
Medicare Spending				
Medicare Spending per Patient (ratio)	-	-	0.95	0.98
Pneumonia Care				
Appropriate Initial Antibiotic Given[5]	-	-	98%	95%
Blood Culture Timing[5]	-	-	98%	98%
Pregnancy and Delivery Care				
Newborn Deliveries Scheduled Early[7]	-	-	2%	6%
Preventive Care				
Immunization for Influenza[5]	-	-	93%	90%
Immunization for Pneumonia[5]	-	-	94%	92%
Stroke Care				
Anticoagulation Therapy for Atrial Fibrillation[5]	-	-	98%	95%
Antithrombotic Therapy Timing[5]	-	-	99%	98%
Assessed for Rehabilitation[5]	-	-	98%	97%
Discharged on Antithrombotic Therapy[5]	-	-	100%	99%
Discharged on Statin Medication[5]	-	-	97%	94%
Thrombolytic Therapy Timing[5]	-	-	29%	66%
Venous Thromboembolism Prophylaxis[5]	-	-	96%	94%
Written Stroke Educational Materials Given[5]	-	-	86%	88%
Surgical Care Improvement Project				
Appropriate Beta Blocker Usage[5]	-	-	99%	98%
Appropriate VTP Within 24 Hours[5]	-	-	99%	98%
Controlled Postoperative Blood Glucose[5]	-	-	99%	97%
Perioperative Temperature Management[5]	-	-	100%	100%
Prophylactic Antibiotic Selection[5]	-	-	99%	99%
Prophylactic Antibiotic Selection (Outpatient)[5]	-	-	98%	98%
Prophylactic Antibiotic Stopped[5]	-	-	99%	98%
Prophylactic Antibiotic Timing[5]	-	-	99%	99%
Prophylactic Antibiotic Timing (Outpatient)[5]	-	-	96%	98%
Urinary Catheter Removal[5]	-	-	99%	97%
Survey of Patients' Hospital Experiences				
Area Around Room 'Always' Quiet at Night[5]	-	-	59%	61%
Doctors 'Always' Communicated Well[5]	-	-	83%	82%
Home Recovery Information Given[5]	-	-	90%	85%
Hospital Given 9 or 10 on 10 Point Scale[5]	-	-	74%	71%
Meds 'Always' Explained Before Given[5]	-	-	69%	64%
Nurses 'Always' Communicated Well[5]	-	-	82%	79%
Pain 'Always' Well Controlled[5]	-	-	73%	71%
Room and Bathroom 'Always' Clean[5]	-	-	80%	73%
Timely Help 'Always' Received[5]	-	-	72%	68%
Would Definitely Recommend Hospital[5]	-	-	77%	71%
Use of Medical Imaging				
Cardiac Imaging Stress Test before Surgery[7]	-	-	4.8%	5.3%
Combination Abdominal CT Scan	106	1.9%	5.2%	10.5%
Combination Brain/Sinus CT Scan[1]	-	-	1.7%	2.7%
Combination Chest CT Scan	53	1.9%	0.7%	2.7%
Follow-up Mammogram/Ultrasound	169	5.3%	7.7%	8.8%
Lumbar Spine MRI for Low Back Pain[7]	-	-	37.5%	37.2%

Bridgton Hospital

10 Hospital Drive
Bridgton, ME 04009
Phone: 207-647-6000
Fax: 207-647-4209
E-mail: dubay@bh.com
URL: www.bridgtonhospital.com
Type: Critical Access Hospitals
Emergency Services: Yes
Ownership: Voluntary non-profit - Private
Beds: 40

Key Personnel:
Infection Control. . . . . Marcia Elliott, RN
Operating Room. . . . . Genise Knowlton, RN
Chief of Medical Staff. . . . . Henry Roy, III, MD
Pediatric Ambulatory Care . . . . . . Wenda L Saunders, MD
Pediatric In-Patient Care . . . . Wenda L Saunders, MD
Quality Assurance . . . . Kathy Wohlenberg

Measure	Cases	This Hosp.	State Avg.	U.S. Avg.
Blood Clot Prevention and Treatment				
Anticoagulation Overlap Therapy[5]	-	-	98%	93%
ICU Venous Thromboembolism Prophylaxis[5]	-	-	96%	92%
Incidence of Potentially Preventable VTE[5]	-	-	2%	10%
UFH with Dosages/Platelet Monitoring[5]	-	-	100%	97%
Venous Thromboembolism Prophylaxis[5]	-	-	95%	85%
Warfarin Therapy Discharge Instructions[5]	-	-	84%	75%
Chest Pain/Possible Heart Attack Care				
Aspirin Given Within 24 Hours of Arrival[5]	-	-	99%	96%
Fibrinolytic Meds Within 30 Min. of Arrival[5]	-	-	86%	58%
Average Time to ECG (minutes)[5]	-	-	6	7
Average Time to Transfer (minutes)[5]	-	-	49	60
Children's Asthma Care				
Received Home Management Plan of Care	-	-	-	88%
Received Reliever Medication	-	-	-	100%
Received Systemic Corticosteroids	-	-	-	100%

NOTE: Hospital profiles are in alphabetical order by state, then city, then hospital within the city; Rankings exclude hospitals with less than 25 cases except for patient surveys which excludes hospitals with less than 100 cases; (a) 100-299 cases; (1) The number of cases/patients is too few to report; (2) Data submitted were based on a sample of cases/patients; (3) Results are based on a shorter time period than required; (4) Data suppressed by CMS for one or more quarters; (5) Results are not available for this reporting period; (6) Fewer than 100 patients completed the HCAHPS survey; (7) No cases met the criteria for this measure; (8) The lower limit of the confidence interval cannot be calculated if the number of observed infections equals zero; (9) No data are available from the state/territory for this reporting period; (10) The scores shown reflect fewer than 50 completed surveys; (11) There were discrepancies in the data collection process; (12) This measure does not apply to this hospital for this reporting period; (13) Results cannot be calculated for this reporting period; (14) The results for this state are combined with nearby states to protect confidentiality; Please refer to the User's Guide for a full explanation of data.

Measure	Cases	This Hosp.	State Avg.	U.S. Avg.
Emergency Department				
Admittance Decision Time (minutes)[5]	-	-	110	98
Head CT Results Within 45 Min. of Arrival[5]	-	-	44%	57%
Patients Who Left ER Before Being Seen[5]	-	-	1%	2%
Time from ER Arrival to Admit. (minutes)[5]	-	-	288	274
Time from ER Arrival to Discharge (minutes)[5]	-	-	122	134
Time in ER Before Being Evaluated (minutes)[5]	-	-	28	26
Time to Pain Meds for Fractures (minutes)[5]	-	-	52	57
Heart Attack Care				
Aspirin Given at Discharge[5]	-	-	100%	99%
Fibrinolytic Meds Within 30 Min. of Arrival[5]	-	-	50%	54%
PCI Within 90 Minutes of Arrival[5]	-	-	96%	96%
Statin Prescribed at Discharge[5]	-	-	99%	98%
Heart Failure Care				
ACE Inhibitor or ARB for LVSD[1]	-	-	99%	97%
Discharge Instructions Given	23	96%	98%	94%
Evaluation of LVS Function	30	100%	100%	99%
Medicare Spending				
Medicare Spending per Patient (ratio)	-	-	0.95	0.98
Pneumonia Care				
Appropriate Initial Antibiotic Given	29	100%	98%	95%
Blood Culture Timing	36	97%	98%	98%
Pregnancy and Delivery Care				
Newborn Deliveries Scheduled Early[5]	-	-	2%	6%
Preventive Care				
Immunization for Influenza[5]	-	-	93%	90%
Immunization for Pneumonia[5]	-	-	94%	92%
Stroke Care				
Anticoagulation Therapy for Atrial Fibrillation[5]	-	-	98%	95%
Antithrombotic Therapy Timing[5]	-	-	99%	98%
Assessed for Rehabilitation[5]	-	-	98%	97%
Discharged on Antithrombotic Therapy[5]	-	-	100%	99%
Discharged on Statin Medication[5]	-	-	97%	94%
Thrombolytic Therapy Timing[5]	-	-	29%	66%
Venous Thromboembolism Prophylaxis[5]	-	-	96%	94%
Written Stroke Educational Materials Given[5]	-	-	86%	88%
Surgical Care Improvement Project				
Appropriate Beta Blocker Usage[1,3]	-	-	99%	98%
Appropriate VTP Within 24 Hours[3]	16	94%	99%	98%
Controlled Postoperative Blood Glucose[3,7]	-	-	99%	97%
Perioperative Temperature Management[3]	17	100%	100%	100%
Prophylactic Antibiotic Selection[1,3]	-	-	99%	99%
Prophylactic Antibiotic Selection (Outpatient)[5]	-	-	98%	98%
Prophylactic Antibiotic Stopped[1,3]	-	-	99%	98%
Prophylactic Antibiotic Timing[1,3]	-	-	99%	99%
Prophylactic Antibiotic Timing (Outpatient)[5]	-	-	96%	98%
Urinary Catheter Removal[3]	11	91%	99%	97%
Survey of Patients' Hospital Experiences				
Area Around Room 'Always' Quiet at Night	(a)	60%	59%	61%
Doctors 'Always' Communicated Well	(a)	81%	83%	82%
Home Recovery Information Given	(a)	95%	90%	85%
Hospital Given 9 or 10 on 10 Point Scale	(a)	72%	74%	71%
Meds 'Always' Explained Before Given	(a)	76%	69%	64%
Nurses 'Always' Communicated Well	(a)	80%	82%	79%
Pain 'Always' Well Controlled	(a)	74%	73%	71%
Room and Bathroom 'Always' Clean	(a)	81%	80%	73%
Timely Help 'Always' Received	(a)	71%	72%	68%
Would Definitely Recommend Hospital	(a)	80%	77%	71%
Use of Medical Imaging				
Cardiac Imaging Stress Test before Surgery	70	5.7%	4.8%	5.3%
Combination Abdominal CT Scan	398	2.8%	5.2%	10.5%
Combination Brain/Sinus CT Scan[1]	-	-	1.7%	2.7%
Combination Chest CT Scan	196	0.5%	0.7%	2.7%
Follow-up Mammogram/Ultrasound	698	5.4%	7.7%	8.8%
Lumbar Spine MRI for Low Back Pain	53	37.7%	37.5%	37.2%

Mid Coast Hospital

123 Medical Center Drive
Brunswick, ME 04011
Phone: 207-729-0181
Fax: 207-373-6744
URL: www.midcoasthealth.com
Type: Acute Care Hospitals
Emergency Services: Yes
Ownership: Voluntary non-profit - Private
Beds: 104

Key Personnel:

Radiology. . . . . John J Chomyn
Emergency Room . . . . Marlene Cormier
Quality Assurance . . . . George Hunter
Infection Control. . . . . Lorna MacKinnon, RN
Chief of Medical Staff . . . . Scott Mills, MD
CEO/President. . . . . Herbert Paris
Intensive Care Unit. . . . . Brian Viele

Measure	Cases	This Hosp.	State Avg.	U.S. Avg.
Blood Clot Prevention and Treatment				
Anticoagulation Overlap Therapy[2]	34	100%	98%	93%
ICU Venous Thromboembolism Prophylaxis[2]	109	98%	96%	92%
Incidence of Potentially Preventable VTE[2,7]	-	-	2%	10%
UFH with Dosages/Platelet Monitoring[1,2]	-	-	100%	97%
Venous Thromboembolism Prophylaxis[2]	296	91%	95%	85%
Warfarin Therapy Discharge Instructions[2]	31	84%	84%	75%
Chest Pain/Possible Heart Attack Care				
Aspirin Given Within 24 Hours of Arrival	41	100%	99%	96%
Fibrinolytic Meds Within 30 Min. of Arrival	11	100%	86%	58%
Average Time to ECG (minutes)	41	0	6	7
Average Time to Transfer (minutes)[7]	-	-	49	60
Children's Asthma Care				
Received Home Management Plan of Care	-	-	-	88%
Received Reliever Medication	-	-	-	100%
Received Systemic Corticosteroids	-	-	-	100%
Emergency Department				
Admittance Decision Time (minutes)[2]	588	116	110	98
Head CT Results Within 45 Min. of Arrival[1]	-	-	44%	57%
Patients Who Left ER Before Being Seen	24,140	1%	1%	2%
Time from ER Arrival to Admit. (minutes)[2]	588	283	288	274
Time from ER Arrival to Discharge (minutes)	374	120	122	134
Time in ER Before Being Evaluated (minutes)	174	37	28	26
Time to Pain Meds for Fractures (minutes)	62	62	52	57
Heart Attack Care				
Aspirin Given at Discharge	30	100%	100%	99%
Fibrinolytic Meds Within 30 Min. of Arrival[7]	-	-	50%	54%
PCI Within 90 Minutes of Arrival[7]	-	-	96%	96%
Statin Prescribed at Discharge	24	100%	99%	98%
Heart Failure Care				
ACE Inhibitor or ARB for LVSD	29	100%	99%	97%
Discharge Instructions Given	106	100%	98%	94%
Evaluation of LVS Function	124	100%	100%	99%
Medicare Spending				
Medicare Spending per Patient (ratio)	-	0.95	0.95	0.98
Pneumonia Care				
Appropriate Initial Antibiotic Given[2]	107	96%	98%	95%
Blood Culture Timing[2]	83	94%	98%	98%
Pregnancy and Delivery Care				
Newborn Deliveries Scheduled Early	36	3%	2%	6%
Preventive Care				
Immunization for Influenza[2]	416	76%	93%	90%
Immunization for Pneumonia[2]	531	79%	94%	92%
Stroke Care				
Anticoagulation Therapy for Atrial Fibrillation[1]	-	-	98%	95%
Antithrombotic Therapy Timing	54	98%	99%	98%
Assessed for Rehabilitation	54	100%	98%	97%
Discharged on Antithrombotic Therapy	53	100%	100%	99%
Discharged on Statin Medication	44	98%	97%	94%
Thrombolytic Therapy Timing[7]	-	-	29%	66%
Venous Thromboembolism Prophylaxis	55	98%	96%	94%
Written Stroke Educational Materials Given	23	96%	86%	88%
Surgical Care Improvement Project				
Appropriate Beta Blocker Usage	59	98%	99%	98%
Appropriate VTP Within 24 Hours	235	94%	99%	98%
Controlled Postoperative Blood Glucose[7]	-	-	99%	97%
Perioperative Temperature Management	246	100%	100%	100%
Prophylactic Antibiotic Selection	176	99%	99%	99%
Prophylactic Antibiotic Selection (Outpatient)	88	99%	98%	98%
Prophylactic Antibiotic Stopped	173	99%	99%	98%
Prophylactic Antibiotic Timing	176	100%	99%	99%
Prophylactic Antibiotic Timing (Outpatient)	84	94%	96%	98%
Urinary Catheter Removal	96	97%	99%	97%
Survey of Patients' Hospital Experiences				
Area Around Room 'Always' Quiet at Night	300+	51%	59%	61%
Doctors 'Always' Communicated Well	300+	84%	83%	82%
Home Recovery Information Given	300+	89%	90%	85%
Hospital Given 9 or 10 on 10 Point Scale	300+	77%	74%	71%
Meds 'Always' Explained Before Given	300+	67%	69%	64%
Nurses 'Always' Communicated Well	300+	79%	82%	79%
Pain 'Always' Well Controlled	300+	73%	73%	71%
Room and Bathroom 'Always' Clean	300+	76%	80%	73%
Timely Help 'Always' Received	300+	71%	72%	68%
Would Definitely Recommend Hospital	300+	84%	77%	71%
Use of Medical Imaging				
Cardiac Imaging Stress Test before Surgery	278	2.9%	4.8%	5.3%
Combination Abdominal CT Scan	666	5.1%	5.2%	10.5%
Combination Brain/Sinus CT Scan	502	1.2%	1.7%	2.7%
Combination Chest CT Scan	580	0.0%	0.7%	2.7%
Follow-up Mammogram/Ultrasound	1,133	7.3%	7.7%	8.8%
Lumbar Spine MRI for Low Back Pain	150	34.0%	37.5%	37.2%

Parkview Adventist Medical Center

329 Main St
Brunswick, ME 04011
Phone: 207-373-2000
Fax: 207-373-2161
URL: www.parkviewamc.org
Type: Acute Care Hospitals
Emergency Services: Yes
Ownership: Voluntary non-profit - Church
Beds: 55

Key Personnel:

Emergency Room . . . . Charles Armstrong
Hemotology Center . . . . Trudi Chase
Anesthesiology. . . . . J. Scott Ewert
Radiology. . . . . Keith Fleming
Cardiology . . . . Patrick Lawrence
CEO/President. . . . . Ted Lewis
Pediatric In-Patient Care . . . . Larry Losey, MD
Pediatric Ambulatory Care . . . . . . Lawrence Losey, MD

Measure	Cases	This Hosp.	State Avg.	U.S. Avg.
Blood Clot Prevention and Treatment				
Anticoagulation Overlap Therapy[1,2]	-	-	98%	93%
ICU Venous Thromboembolism Prophylaxis[2]	91	96%	96%	92%
Incidence of Potentially Preventable VTE[1,2]	-	-	2%	10%
UFH with Dosages/Platelet Monitoring[1,2]	-	-	100%	97%
Venous Thromboembolism Prophylaxis[2]	248	97%	95%	85%
Warfarin Therapy Discharge Instructions[1,2]	-	-	84%	75%
Chest Pain/Possible Heart Attack Care				
Aspirin Given Within 24 Hours of Arrival	20	100%	99%	96%
Fibrinolytic Meds Within 30 Min. of Arrival[7]	-	-	86%	58%
Average Time to ECG (minutes)	20	8	6	7
Average Time to Transfer (minutes)[1]	-	-	49	60
Children's Asthma Care				
Received Home Management Plan of Care	-	-	-	88%
Received Reliever Medication	-	-	-	100%
Received Systemic Corticosteroids	-	-	-	100%
Emergency Department				
Admittance Decision Time (minutes)[2]	314	104	110	98
Head CT Results Within 45 Min. of Arrival[1]	-	-	44%	57%
Patients Who Left ER Before Being Seen	9,390	0%	1%	2%
Time from ER Arrival to Admit. (minutes)[2]	504	222	288	274
Time from ER Arrival to Discharge (minutes)	369	104	122	134
Time in ER Before Being Evaluated (minutes)	395	21	28	26
Time to Pain Meds for Fractures (minutes)	42	36	52	57
Heart Attack Care				
Aspirin Given at Discharge[1]	-	-	100%	99%
Fibrinolytic Meds Within 30 Min. of Arrival[7]	-	-	50%	54%
PCI Within 90 Minutes of Arrival[7]	-	-	96%	96%
Statin Prescribed at Discharge[1]	-	-	99%	98%
Heart Failure Care				
ACE Inhibitor or ARB for LVSD[1]	-	-	99%	97%
Discharge Instructions Given	29	97%	98%	94%
Evaluation of LVS Function	34	100%	100%	99%
Medicare Spending				
Medicare Spending per Patient (ratio)	-	0.91	0.95	0.98
Pneumonia Care				
Appropriate Initial Antibiotic Given	30	93%	98%	95%
Blood Culture Timing	20	95%	98%	98%
Pregnancy and Delivery Care				
Newborn Deliveries Scheduled Early[7]	-	-	2%	6%
Preventive Care				
Immunization for Influenza[2]	308	97%	93%	90%

NOTE: Hospital profiles are in alphabetical order by state, then city, then hospital within the city; Rankings exclude hospitals with less than 25 cases except for patient surveys which excludes hospitals with less than 100 cases; (a) 100-299 cases; (1) The number of cases/patients is too few to report; (2) Data submitted were based on a sample of cases/patients; (3) Results are based on a shorter time period than required; (4) Data suppressed by CMS for one or more quarters; (5) Results are not available for this reporting period; (6) Fewer than 100 patients completed the HCAHPS survey; (7) No cases met the criteria for this measure; (8) The lower limit of the confidence interval cannot be calculated if the number of observed infections equals zero; (9) No data are available from the state/territory for this reporting period; (10) The scores shown reflect fewer than 50 completed surveys; (11) There were discrepancies in the data collection process; (12) This measure does not apply to this hospital for this reporting period; (13) Results cannot be calculated for this reporting period; (14) The results for this state are combined with nearby states to protect confidentiality; Please refer to the User's Guide for a full explanation of data.

Measure	Cases	This Hosp.	State Avg.	U.S. Avg.
Immunization for Pneumonia[2]	485	98%	94%	92%
Stroke Care				
Anticoagulation Therapy for Atrial Fibrillation[1]	-	-	98%	95%
Antithrombotic Therapy Timing[1]	-	-	99%	98%
Assessed for Rehabilitation[1]	-	-	98%	97%
Discharged on Antithrombotic Therapy[1]	-	-	100%	99%
Discharged on Statin Medication[1]	-	-	97%	94%
Thrombolytic Therapy Timing[7]	-	-	29%	66%
Venous Thromboembolism Prophylaxis[1]	-	-	96%	94%
Written Stroke Educational Materials Given[1]	-	-	86%	88%
Surgical Care Improvement Project				
Appropriate Beta Blocker Usage[3]	20	100%	99%	98%
Appropriate VTP Within 24 Hours[3]	51	100%	99%	98%
Controlled Postoperative Blood Glucose[3,7]	-	-	99%	97%
Perioperative Temperature Management[3]	60	100%	100%	100%
Prophylactic Antibiotic Selection[3]	39	100%	99%	99%
Prophylactic Antibiotic Selection (Outpatient)	13	85%	98%	98%
Prophylactic Antibiotic Stopped[3]	39	100%	99%	98%
Prophylactic Antibiotic Timing[3]	39	100%	99%	99%
Prophylactic Antibiotic Timing (Outpatient)[1]	-	-	96%	98%
Urinary Catheter Removal[3]	43	100%	99%	97%
Survey of Patients' Hospital Experiences				
Area Around Room 'Always' Quiet at Night	(a)	59%	59%	61%
Doctors 'Always' Communicated Well	(a)	92%	83%	82%
Home Recovery Information Given	(a)	95%	90%	85%
Hospital Given 9 or 10 on 10 Point Scale	(a)	82%	74%	71%
Meds 'Always' Explained Before Given	(a)	74%	69%	64%
Nurses 'Always' Communicated Well	(a)	82%	82%	79%
Pain 'Always' Well Controlled	(a)	75%	73%	71%
Room and Bathroom 'Always' Clean	(a)	85%	80%	73%
Timely Help 'Always' Received	(a)	74%	72%	68%
Would Definitely Recommend Hospital	(a)	84%	77%	71%
Use of Medical Imaging				
Cardiac Imaging Stress Test before Surgery	81	4.9%	4.8%	5.3%
Combination Abdominal CT Scan	230	6.1%	5.2%	10.5%
Combination Brain/Sinus CT Scan[1]	-	-	1.7%	2.7%
Combination Chest CT Scan	143	2.1%	0.7%	2.7%
Follow-up Mammogram/Ultrasound	627	11.3%	7.7%	8.8%
Lumbar Spine MRI for Low Back Pain[1]	-	-	37.5%	37.2%

Calais Regional Hospital

24 Hospital Lane
Calais, ME 04619
Phone: 207-454-7521
Fax: 207-454-3616
URL: www.calaishospital.com
Type: Critical Access Hospitals
Emergency Services: Yes
Ownership: Voluntary non-profit - Private
Beds: 49

Key Personnel:
Radiology. . . . . Edward Barrera, MD
Emergency Room . . . . Cressey Brazier, MD
Operating Room. . . . . Robert Chagrasulis, RN
CEO/President. . . . . Ray H Davis, Jr
Infection Control. . . . . Stacey Doten
Quality Assurance . . . . Stacey Doten
Intensive Care Unit. . . . . Barbara Wheaton, RN
Chief of Medical Staff. . . . . Peter S Wilkinson, DO

Measure	Cases	This Hosp.	State Avg.	U.S. Avg.
Blood Clot Prevention and Treatment				
Anticoagulation Overlap Therapy[1]	-	-	98%	93%
ICU Venous Thromboembolism Prophylaxis[7]	-	-	96%	92%
Incidence of Potentially Preventable VTE[7]	-	-	2%	10%
UFH with Dosages/Platelet Monitoring[1]	-	-	100%	97%
Venous Thromboembolism Prophylaxis	317	97%	95%	85%
Warfarin Therapy Discharge Instructions[1]	-	-	84%	75%
Chest Pain/Possible Heart Attack Care				
Aspirin Given Within 24 Hours of Arrival	66	98%	99%	96%
Fibrinolytic Meds Within 30 Min. of Arrival[1]	-	-	86%	58%
Average Time to ECG (minutes)	66	3	6	7
Average Time to Transfer (minutes)[7]	-	-	49	60
Children's Asthma Care				
Received Home Management Plan of Care	-	-	-	88%
Received Reliever Medication	-	-	-	100%
Received Systemic Corticosteroids	-	-	-	100%
Emergency Department				
Admittance Decision Time (minutes)[5]	-	-	110	98
Head CT Results Within 45 Min. of Arrival[1]	-	-	44%	57%
Patients Who Left ER Before Being Seen[5]	-	-	1%	2%
Time from ER Arrival to Admit. (minutes)[5]	-	-	288	274
Time from ER Arrival to Discharge (minutes)[5]	-	-	122	134
Time in ER Before Being Evaluated (minutes)[5]	-	-	28	26
Time to Pain Meds for Fractures (minutes)	22	38	52	57
Heart Attack Care				
Aspirin Given at Discharge	14	100%	100%	99%
Fibrinolytic Meds Within 30 Min. of Arrival[7]	-	-	50%	54%
PCI Within 90 Minutes of Arrival[3,7]	-	-	96%	96%
Statin Prescribed at Discharge[1]	-	-	99%	98%
Heart Failure Care				
ACE Inhibitor or ARB for LVSD[1]	-	-	99%	97%
Discharge Instructions Given	21	100%	98%	94%
Evaluation of LVS Function	27	100%	100%	99%
Medicare Spending				
Medicare Spending per Patient (ratio)	-	-	0.95	0.98
Pneumonia Care				
Appropriate Initial Antibiotic Given	29	97%	98%	95%
Blood Culture Timing	53	100%	98%	98%
Pregnancy and Delivery Care				
Newborn Deliveries Scheduled Early[5]	-	-	2%	6%
Preventive Care				
Immunization for Influenza	306	98%	93%	90%
Immunization for Pneumonia	425	99%	94%	92%
Stroke Care				
Anticoagulation Therapy for Atrial Fibrillation[5]	-	-	98%	95%
Antithrombotic Therapy Timing[5]	-	-	99%	98%
Assessed for Rehabilitation[5]	-	-	98%	97%
Discharged on Antithrombotic Therapy[5]	-	-	100%	99%
Discharged on Statin Medication[5]	-	-	97%	94%
Thrombolytic Therapy Timing[5]	-	-	29%	66%
Venous Thromboembolism Prophylaxis[5]	-	-	96%	94%
Written Stroke Educational Materials Given[5]	-	-	86%	88%
Surgical Care Improvement Project				
Appropriate Beta Blocker Usage	16	94%	99%	98%
Appropriate VTP Within 24 Hours	52	98%	99%	98%
Controlled Postoperative Blood Glucose[3,7]	-	-	99%	97%
Perioperative Temperature Management	58	100%	100%	100%
Prophylactic Antibiotic Selection	53	98%	99%	99%
Prophylactic Antibiotic Selection (Outpatient)[1,3]	-	-	98%	98%
Prophylactic Antibiotic Stopped	52	100%	99%	98%
Prophylactic Antibiotic Timing	53	100%	99%	99%
Prophylactic Antibiotic Timing (Outpatient)[1,3]	-	-	96%	98%
Urinary Catheter Removal	17	100%	99%	97%
Survey of Patients' Hospital Experiences				
Area Around Room 'Always' Quiet at Night	(a)	60%	59%	61%
Doctors 'Always' Communicated Well	(a)	86%	83%	82%
Home Recovery Information Given	(a)	89%	90%	85%
Hospital Given 9 or 10 on 10 Point Scale	(a)	77%	74%	71%
Meds 'Always' Explained Before Given	(a)	72%	69%	64%
Nurses 'Always' Communicated Well	(a)	84%	82%	79%
Pain 'Always' Well Controlled	(a)	86%	73%	71%
Room and Bathroom 'Always' Clean	(a)	85%	80%	73%
Timely Help 'Always' Received	(a)	79%	72%	68%
Would Definitely Recommend Hospital	(a)	79%	77%	71%
Use of Medical Imaging				
Cardiac Imaging Stress Test before Surgery[1]	-	-	4.8%	5.3%
Combination Abdominal CT Scan	268	3.4%	5.2%	10.5%
Combination Brain/Sinus CT Scan[1]	-	-	1.7%	2.7%
Combination Chest CT Scan	139	2.2%	0.7%	2.7%
Follow-up Mammogram/Ultrasound	398	9.3%	7.7%	8.8%
Lumbar Spine MRI for Low Back Pain[1]	-	-	37.5%	37.2%

Cary Medical Center

163 Van Buren Rd, Suite 1
Caribou, ME 04736
Phone: 207-498-3111
Fax: 207-496-2631
E-mail: mfreeman@cary.carymed.org
URL: www.carymedicalcenter.org
Type: Acute Care Hospitals
Emergency Services: Yes
Ownership: Government - Local
Beds: 65

Key Personnel:
Chief of Medical Staff. . . . . Krista Burchill
Cardiac Laboratory. . . . . Gus Cains
Intensive Care Unit. . . . . Jackie Deboe
CEO/President. . . . . Kris Doody, RN
Emergency Room . . . . Daniel Harrigan, MD
Quality Assurance . . . . Darlene Higgins
Radiology. . . . . John Stewart

Measure	Cases	This Hosp.	State Avg.	U.S. Avg.
Blood Clot Prevention and Treatment				
Anticoagulation Overlap Therapy[2]	14	79%	98%	93%
ICU Venous Thromboembolism Prophylaxis[2]	35	97%	96%	92%
Incidence of Potentially Preventable VTE[1,2]	-	-	2%	10%
UFH with Dosages/Platelet Monitoring[1,2]	-	-	100%	97%
Venous Thromboembolism Prophylaxis[2]	139	84%	95%	85%
Warfarin Therapy Discharge Instructions[2]	11	91%	84%	75%
Chest Pain/Possible Heart Attack Care				
Aspirin Given Within 24 Hours of Arrival[1,3]	-	-	99%	96%
Fibrinolytic Meds Within 30 Min. of Arrival[1,3]	-	-	86%	58%
Average Time to ECG (minutes)[1,3]	-	-	6	7
Average Time to Transfer (minutes)[3,7]	-	-	49	60
Children's Asthma Care				
Received Home Management Plan of Care	-	-	-	88%
Received Reliever Medication	-	-	-	100%
Received Systemic Corticosteroids	-	-	-	100%
Emergency Department				
Admittance Decision Time (minutes)[2]	398	71	110	98
Head CT Results Within 45 Min. of Arrival[3,7]	-	-	44%	57%
Patients Who Left ER Before Being Seen	18,711	1%	1%	2%
Time from ER Arrival to Admit. (minutes)[2]	400	253	288	274
Time from ER Arrival to Discharge (minutes)	368	96	122	134
Time in ER Before Being Evaluated (minutes)	378	31	28	26
Time to Pain Meds for Fractures (minutes)	34	52	52	57
Heart Attack Care				
Aspirin Given at Discharge	14	100%	100%	99%
Fibrinolytic Meds Within 30 Min. of Arrival[7]	-	-	50%	54%
PCI Within 90 Minutes of Arrival[7]	-	-	96%	96%
Statin Prescribed at Discharge	15	100%	99%	98%
Heart Failure Care				
ACE Inhibitor or ARB for LVSD	19	100%	99%	97%
Discharge Instructions Given	65	98%	98%	94%
Evaluation of LVS Function	86	100%	100%	99%
Medicare Spending				
Medicare Spending per Patient (ratio)	-	0.89	0.95	0.98
Pneumonia Care				
Appropriate Initial Antibiotic Given	45	98%	98%	95%
Blood Culture Timing	75	99%	98%	98%
Pregnancy and Delivery Care				
Newborn Deliveries Scheduled Early	12	0%	2%	6%
Preventive Care				
Immunization for Influenza[2]	283	96%	93%	90%
Immunization for Pneumonia[2]	382	97%	94%	92%
Stroke Care				
Anticoagulation Therapy for Atrial Fibrillation[7]	-	-	98%	95%
Antithrombotic Therapy Timing	12	92%	99%	98%
Assessed for Rehabilitation	12	100%	98%	97%
Discharged on Antithrombotic Therapy	11	100%	100%	99%
Discharged on Statin Medication[1]	-	-	97%	94%
Thrombolytic Therapy Timing[1]	-	-	29%	66%
Venous Thromboembolism Prophylaxis	13	100%	96%	94%
Written Stroke Educational Materials Given[1]	-	-	86%	88%
Surgical Care Improvement Project				
Appropriate Beta Blocker Usage[2]	59	100%	99%	98%
Appropriate VTP Within 24 Hours[2]	152	100%	99%	98%
Controlled Postoperative Blood Glucose[2,7]	-	-	99%	97%
Perioperative Temperature Management[2]	155	100%	100%	100%
Prophylactic Antibiotic Selection[2]	133	100%	99%	99%
Prophylactic Antibiotic Selection (Outpatient)	114	100%	98%	98%
Prophylactic Antibiotic Stopped[2]	131	98%	99%	98%
Prophylactic Antibiotic Timing[2]	133	100%	99%	99%
Prophylactic Antibiotic Timing (Outpatient)	27	96%	96%	98%
Urinary Catheter Removal[2]	131	100%	99%	97%
Survey of Patients' Hospital Experiences				
Area Around Room 'Always' Quiet at Night	300+	61%	59%	61%
Doctors 'Always' Communicated Well	300+	84%	83%	82%

NOTE: Hospital profiles are in alphabetical order by state, then city, then hospital within the city; Rankings exclude hospitals with less than 25 cases except for patient surveys which excludes hospitals with less than 100 cases; (a) 100-299 cases; (1) The number of cases/patients is too few to report; (2) Data submitted were based on a sample of cases/patients; (3) Results are based on a shorter time period than required; (4) Data suppressed by CMS for one or more quarters; (5) Results are not available for this reporting period; (6) Fewer than 100 patients completed the HCAHPS survey; (7) No cases met the criteria for this measure; (8) The lower limit of the confidence interval cannot be calculated if the number of observed infections equals zero; (9) No data are available from the state/territory for this reporting period; (10) The scores shown reflect fewer than 50 completed surveys; (11) There were discrepancies in the data collection process; (12) This measure does not apply to this hospital for this reporting period; (13) Results cannot be calculated for this reporting period; (14) The results for this state are combined with nearby states to protect confidentiality; Please refer to the User's Guide for a full explanation of data.

Measure	Cases	This Hosp.	State Avg.	U.S. Avg.
Home Recovery Information Given	300+	90%	90%	85%
Hospital Given 9 or 10 on 10 Point Scale	300+	77%	74%	71%
Meds 'Always' Explained Before Given	300+	71%	69%	64%
Nurses 'Always' Communicated Well	300+	85%	82%	79%
Pain 'Always' Well Controlled	300+	78%	73%	71%
Room and Bathroom 'Always' Clean	300+	73%	80%	73%
Timely Help 'Always' Received	300+	82%	72%	68%
Would Definitely Recommend Hospital	300+	81%	77%	71%
Use of Medical Imaging				
Cardiac Imaging Stress Test before Surgery	182	2.7%	4.8%	5.3%
Combination Abdominal CT Scan	478	6.7%	5.2%	10.5%
Combination Brain/Sinus CT Scan[1]	-	-	1.7%	2.7%
Combination Chest CT Scan	403	0.2%	0.7%	2.7%
Follow-up Mammogram/Ultrasound	809	13.8%	7.7%	8.8%
Lumbar Spine MRI for Low Back Pain	78	34.6%	37.5%	37.2%

Miles Memorial Hospital

35 Miles Street
Damariscotta, ME 04543
Phone: 207-563-1234
Fax: 207-563-4710
E-mail: info@mileshealthcare.org
URL: www.mileshealthcare.org
Type: Acute Care Hospitals
Emergency Services: Yes
Ownership: Voluntary non-profit - Private
Beds: 35

Key Personnel:
Patient Relations . . . . Vicky Bell
Emergency Room . . . . Janet Fowle
Chief of Medical Staff. . . . . Timothy Goltz
Anesthesiology. . . . . Russ Maek, MD
CEO/President. . . . . Judith C Tarr

Measure	Cases	This Hosp.	State Avg.	U.S. Avg.
Blood Clot Prevention and Treatment				
Anticoagulation Overlap Therapy[1,2]	-	-	98%	93%
ICU Venous Thromboembolism Prophylaxis[2]	94	89%	96%	92%
Incidence of Potentially Preventable VTE[2,7]	-	-	2%	10%
UFH with Dosages/Platelet Monitoring[1,2]	-	-	100%	97%
Venous Thromboembolism Prophylaxis[2]	113	89%	95%	85%
Warfarin Therapy Discharge Instructions[1,2]	-	-	84%	75%
Chest Pain/Possible Heart Attack Care				
Aspirin Given Within 24 Hours of Arrival	71	100%	99%	96%
Fibrinolytic Meds Within 30 Min. of Arrival[1]	-	-	86%	58%
Average Time to ECG (minutes)	74	6	6	7
Average Time to Transfer (minutes)[7]	-	-	49	60
Children's Asthma Care				
Received Home Management Plan of Care	-	-	-	88%
Received Reliever Medication	-	-	-	100%
Received Systemic Corticosteroids	-	-	-	100%
Emergency Department				
Admittance Decision Time (minutes)[2]	252	147	110	98
Head CT Results Within 45 Min. of Arrival[1]	-	-	44%	57%
Patients Who Left ER Before Being Seen	12,331	1%	1%	2%
Time from ER Arrival to Admit. (minutes)[2]	386	303	288	274
Time from ER Arrival to Discharge (minutes)	353	110	122	134
Time in ER Before Being Evaluated (minutes)	292	24	28	26
Time to Pain Meds for Fractures (minutes)	32	42	52	57
Heart Attack Care				
Aspirin Given at Discharge[7]	-	-	100%	99%
Fibrinolytic Meds Within 30 Min. of Arrival[7]	-	-	50%	54%
PCI Within 90 Minutes of Arrival[7]	-	-	96%	96%
Statin Prescribed at Discharge[7]	-	-	99%	98%
Heart Failure Care				
ACE Inhibitor or ARB for LVSD[1,2]	-	-	99%	97%
Discharge Instructions Given[2]	49	100%	98%	94%
Evaluation of LVS Function[2]	81	100%	100%	99%
Medicare Spending				
Medicare Spending per Patient (ratio)	-	0.99	0.95	0.98
Pneumonia Care				
Appropriate Initial Antibiotic Given	27	93%	98%	95%
Blood Culture Timing	55	98%	98%	98%
Pregnancy and Delivery Care				
Newborn Deliveries Scheduled Early[1]	-	-	2%	6%
Preventive Care				
Immunization for Influenza[2]	295	96%	93%	90%
Immunization for Pneumonia[2]	444	98%	94%	92%
Stroke Care				
Anticoagulation Therapy for Atrial Fibrillation[1]	-	-	98%	95%
Antithrombotic Therapy Timing	20	100%	99%	98%
Assessed for Rehabilitation	22	95%	98%	97%
Discharged on Antithrombotic Therapy	22	100%	100%	99%
Discharged on Statin Medication	16	100%	97%	94%
Thrombolytic Therapy Timing[1]	-	-	29%	66%
Venous Thromboembolism Prophylaxis	20	90%	96%	94%
Written Stroke Educational Materials Given	16	94%	86%	88%
Surgical Care Improvement Project				
Appropriate Beta Blocker Usage	42	100%	99%	98%
Appropriate VTP Within 24 Hours	111	100%	99%	98%
Controlled Postoperative Blood Glucose[7]	-	-	99%	97%
Perioperative Temperature Management	131	100%	100%	100%
Prophylactic Antibiotic Selection	104	99%	99%	99%
Prophylactic Antibiotic Selection (Outpatient)[1]	-	-	98%	98%
Prophylactic Antibiotic Stopped	102	97%	99%	98%
Prophylactic Antibiotic Timing	104	95%	99%	99%
Prophylactic Antibiotic Timing (Outpatient)[1]	-	-	96%	98%
Urinary Catheter Removal	91	98%	99%	97%
Survey of Patients' Hospital Experiences				
Area Around Room 'Always' Quiet at Night	300+	58%	59%	61%
Doctors 'Always' Communicated Well	300+	84%	83%	82%
Home Recovery Information Given	300+	88%	90%	85%
Hospital Given 9 or 10 on 10 Point Scale	300+	79%	74%	71%
Meds 'Always' Explained Before Given	300+	70%	69%	64%
Nurses 'Always' Communicated Well	300+	84%	82%	79%
Pain 'Always' Well Controlled	300+	70%	73%	71%
Room and Bathroom 'Always' Clean	300+	75%	80%	73%
Timely Help 'Always' Received	300+	74%	72%	68%
Would Definitely Recommend Hospital	300+	80%	77%	71%
Use of Medical Imaging				
Cardiac Imaging Stress Test before Surgery	125	3.2%	4.8%	5.3%
Combination Abdominal CT Scan	324	3.4%	5.2%	10.5%
Combination Brain/Sinus CT Scan[1]	-	-	1.7%	2.7%
Combination Chest CT Scan	156	0.6%	0.7%	2.7%
Follow-up Mammogram/Ultrasound	663	7.1%	7.7%	8.8%
Lumbar Spine MRI for Low Back Pain	61	39.3%	37.5%	37.2%

Mayo Regional Hospital

897 West Main Street
Dover Foxcroft, ME 04426
Phone: 207-564-4251
Fax: 207-564-4356
E-mail: tlizotte@mayohospital.com
URL: www.mayohospital.com
Type: Critical Access Hospitals
Emergency Services: Yes
Ownership: Govt - Hospital Dist/Auth
Beds: 25

Key Personnel:
Radiology. . . . . Joan Lovell
Chief of Medical Staff. . . . . Thomas Murray, MD
Infection Control. . . . . Kristy Pratley, RN
Quality Assurance . . . . Cheryl Roberts
CEO . . . . Marie Vienneau
Operating Room. . . . . Linda Zimmerman

Measure	Cases	This Hosp.	State Avg.	U.S. Avg.
Blood Clot Prevention and Treatment				
Anticoagulation Overlap Therapy[5]	-	-	98%	93%
ICU Venous Thromboembolism Prophylaxis[5]	-	-	96%	92%
Incidence of Potentially Preventable VTE[5]	-	-	2%	10%
UFH with Dosages/Platelet Monitoring[5]	-	-	100%	97%
Venous Thromboembolism Prophylaxis[5]	-	-	95%	85%
Warfarin Therapy Discharge Instructions[5]	-	-	84%	75%
Chest Pain/Possible Heart Attack Care				
Aspirin Given Within 24 Hours of Arrival	-	-	99%	96%
Fibrinolytic Meds Within 30 Min. of Arrival	-	-	86%	58%
Average Time to ECG (minutes)	-	-	6	7
Average Time to Transfer (minutes)	-	-	49	60
Children's Asthma Care				
Received Home Management Plan of Care	-	-	-	88%
Received Reliever Medication	-	-	-	100%
Received Systemic Corticosteroids	-	-	-	100%
Emergency Department				
Admittance Decision Time (minutes)[5]	-	-	110	98
Head CT Results Within 45 Min. of Arrival	-	-	44%	57%
Patients Who Left ER Before Being Seen	-	-	1%	2%
Time from ER Arrival to Admit. (minutes)[5]	-	-	288	274
Time from ER Arrival to Discharge (minutes)	-	-	122	134
Time in ER Before Being Evaluated (minutes)	-	-	28	26
Time to Pain Meds for Fractures (minutes)	-	-	52	57
Heart Attack Care				
Aspirin Given at Discharge[1]	-	-	100%	99%
Fibrinolytic Meds Within 30 Min. of Arrival[7]	-	-	50%	54%
PCI Within 90 Minutes of Arrival[7]	-	-	96%	96%
Statin Prescribed at Discharge[1]	-	-	99%	98%
Heart Failure Care				
ACE Inhibitor or ARB for LVSD[1]	-	-	99%	97%
Discharge Instructions Given	19	100%	98%	94%
Evaluation of LVS Function	29	100%	100%	99%
Medicare Spending				
Medicare Spending per Patient (ratio)	-	-	0.95	0.98
Pneumonia Care				
Appropriate Initial Antibiotic Given	34	94%	98%	95%
Blood Culture Timing	54	100%	98%	98%
Pregnancy and Delivery Care				
Newborn Deliveries Scheduled Early[5]	-	-	2%	6%
Preventive Care				
Immunization for Influenza[5]	-	-	93%	90%
Immunization for Pneumonia[5]	-	-	94%	92%
Stroke Care				
Anticoagulation Therapy for Atrial Fibrillation[5]	-	-	98%	95%
Antithrombotic Therapy Timing[5]	-	-	99%	98%
Assessed for Rehabilitation[5]	-	-	98%	97%
Discharged on Antithrombotic Therapy[5]	-	-	100%	99%
Discharged on Statin Medication[5]	-	-	97%	94%
Thrombolytic Therapy Timing[5]	-	-	29%	66%
Venous Thromboembolism Prophylaxis[5]	-	-	96%	94%
Written Stroke Educational Materials Given[5]	-	-	86%	88%
Surgical Care Improvement Project				
Appropriate Beta Blocker Usage[2]	26	96%	99%	98%
Appropriate VTP Within 24 Hours[2]	91	99%	99%	98%
Controlled Postoperative Blood Glucose[2,7]	-	-	99%	97%
Perioperative Temperature Management[2]	102	100%	100%	100%
Prophylactic Antibiotic Selection[2]	92	100%	99%	99%
Prophylactic Antibiotic Selection (Outpatient)	-	-	98%	98%
Prophylactic Antibiotic Stopped[2]	90	100%	99%	98%
Prophylactic Antibiotic Timing[2]	92	100%	99%	99%
Prophylactic Antibiotic Timing (Outpatient)	-	-	96%	98%
Urinary Catheter Removal[2]	85	100%	99%	97%
Survey of Patients' Hospital Experiences				
Area Around Room 'Always' Quiet at Night	(a)	61%	59%	61%
Doctors 'Always' Communicated Well	(a)	84%	83%	82%
Home Recovery Information Given	(a)	91%	90%	85%
Hospital Given 9 or 10 on 10 Point Scale	(a)	75%	74%	71%
Meds 'Always' Explained Before Given	(a)	77%	69%	64%
Nurses 'Always' Communicated Well	(a)	84%	82%	79%
Pain 'Always' Well Controlled	(a)	74%	73%	71%
Room and Bathroom 'Always' Clean	(a)	90%	80%	73%
Timely Help 'Always' Received	(a)	74%	72%	68%
Would Definitely Recommend Hospital	(a)	73%	77%	71%
Use of Medical Imaging				
Cardiac Imaging Stress Test before Surgery	-	-	4.8%	5.3%
Combination Abdominal CT Scan	-	-	5.2%	10.5%
Combination Brain/Sinus CT Scan	-	-	1.7%	2.7%
Combination Chest CT Scan	-	-	0.7%	2.7%
Follow-up Mammogram/Ultrasound	-	-	7.7%	8.8%
Lumbar Spine MRI for Low Back Pain	-	-	37.5%	37.2%

Maine Coast Memorial Hospital

50 Union Street
Ellsworth, ME 04605
Phone: 207-667-5311
Fax: 207-664-5305
E-mail: dbunker@mainehospital.org
URL: www.mainehospital.org
Type: Acute Care Hospitals
Emergency Services: Yes
Ownership: Voluntary non-profit - Other
Beds: 64

Key Personnel:
Emergency Room . . . . Kenneth Christian, MD
Chief of Medical Staff. . . . . Peter Ossanna, MD
CEO/President. . . . . Charlie D. Therrien

Measure	Cases	This Hosp.	State Avg.	U.S. Avg.

NOTE: Hospital profiles are in alphabetical order by state, then city, then hospital within the city; Rankings exclude hospitals with less than 25 cases except for patient surveys which excludes hospitals with less than 100 cases; (a) 100-299 cases; (1) The number of cases/patients is too few to report; (2) Data submitted were based on a sample of cases/patients; (3) Results are based on a shorter time period than required; (4) Data suppressed by CMS for one or more quarters; (5) Results are not available for this reporting period; (6) Fewer than 100 patients completed the HCAHPS survey; (7) No cases met the criteria for this measure; (8) The lower limit of the confidence interval cannot be calculated if the number of observed infections equals zero; (9) No data are available from the state/territory for this reporting period; (10) The scores shown reflect fewer than 50 completed surveys; (11) There were discrepancies in the data collection process; (12) This measure does not apply to this hospital for this reporting period; (13) Results cannot be calculated for this reporting period; (14) The results for this state are combined with nearby states to protect confidentiality; Please refer to the User's Guide for a full explanation of data.

Blood Clot Prevention and Treatment				
Anticoagulation Overlap Therapy[2]	11	91%	98%	93%
ICU Venous Thromboembolism Prophylaxis[2]	55	98%	96%	92%
Incidence of Potentially Preventable VTE[1,2]	-	-	2%	10%
UFH with Dosages/Platelet Monitoring[1,2]	-	-	100%	97%
Venous Thromboembolism Prophylaxis[2]	156	98%	95%	85%
Warfarin Therapy Discharge Instructions[2]	11	82%	84%	75%
Chest Pain/Possible Heart Attack Care				
Aspirin Given Within 24 Hours of Arrival	36	100%	99%	96%
Fibrinolytic Meds Within 30 Min. of Arrival[1]	-	-	86%	58%
Average Time to ECG (minutes)	38	10	6	7
Average Time to Transfer (minutes)[7]	-	-	49	60
Children's Asthma Care				
Received Home Management Plan of Care	-	-	-	88%
Received Reliever Medication	-	-	-	100%
Received Systemic Corticosteroids	-	-	-	100%
Emergency Department				
Admittance Decision Time (minutes)[2]	353	145	110	98
Head CT Results Within 45 Min. of Arrival[1]	-	-	44%	57%
Patients Who Left ER Before Being Seen	18,058	0%	1%	2%
Time from ER Arrival to Admit. (minutes)[2]	361	280	288	274
Time from ER Arrival to Discharge (minutes)	393	115	122	134
Time in ER Before Being Evaluated (minutes)	306	31	28	26
Time to Pain Meds for Fractures (minutes)	51	49	52	57
Heart Attack Care				
Aspirin Given at Discharge	62	98%	100%	99%
Fibrinolytic Meds Within 30 Min. of Arrival[7]	-	-	50%	54%
PCI Within 90 Minutes of Arrival[7]	-	-	96%	96%
Statin Prescribed at Discharge	58	100%	99%	98%
Heart Failure Care				
ACE Inhibitor or ARB for LVSD[1]	-	-	99%	97%
Discharge Instructions Given	43	98%	98%	94%
Evaluation of LVS Function	57	100%	100%	99%
Medicare Spending				
Medicare Spending per Patient (ratio)	-	0.94	0.95	0.98
Pneumonia Care				
Appropriate Initial Antibiotic Given	55	98%	98%	95%
Blood Culture Timing	99	100%	98%	98%
Pregnancy and Delivery Care				
Newborn Deliveries Scheduled Early	39	0%	2%	6%
Preventive Care				
Immunization for Influenza[2]	289	98%	93%	90%
Immunization for Pneumonia[2]	386	99%	94%	92%
Stroke Care				
Anticoagulation Therapy for Atrial Fibrillation[1]	-	-	98%	95%
Antithrombotic Therapy Timing	26	100%	99%	98%
Assessed for Rehabilitation	36	100%	98%	97%
Discharged on Antithrombotic Therapy	34	100%	100%	99%
Discharged on Statin Medication	24	92%	97%	94%
Thrombolytic Therapy Timing[1]	-	-	29%	66%
Venous Thromboembolism Prophylaxis	33	97%	96%	94%
Written Stroke Educational Materials Given	18	56%	86%	88%
Surgical Care Improvement Project				
Appropriate Beta Blocker Usage	64	98%	99%	98%
Appropriate VTP Within 24 Hours	178	99%	99%	98%
Controlled Postoperative Blood Glucose[7]	-	-	99%	97%
Perioperative Temperature Management	206	100%	100%	100%
Prophylactic Antibiotic Selection	135	100%	99%	99%
Prophylactic Antibiotic Selection (Outpatient)	84	99%	98%	98%
Prophylactic Antibiotic Stopped	131	100%	99%	98%
Prophylactic Antibiotic Timing	135	100%	99%	99%
Prophylactic Antibiotic Timing (Outpatient)	31	90%	96%	98%
Urinary Catheter Removal	47	100%	99%	97%
Survey of Patients' Hospital Experiences				
Area Around Room 'Always' Quiet at Night	300+	57%	59%	61%
Doctors 'Always' Communicated Well	300+	84%	83%	82%
Home Recovery Information Given	300+	90%	90%	85%
Hospital Given 9 or 10 on 10 Point Scale	300+	75%	74%	71%
Meds 'Always' Explained Before Given	300+	69%	69%	64%
Nurses 'Always' Communicated Well	300+	82%	82%	79%
Pain 'Always' Well Controlled	300+	75%	73%	71%
Room and Bathroom 'Always' Clean	300+	86%	80%	73%
Timely Help 'Always' Received	300+	72%	72%	68%
Would Definitely Recommend Hospital	300+	80%	77%	71%
Use of Medical Imaging				
Cardiac Imaging Stress Test before Surgery	169	4.1%	4.8%	5.3%
Combination Abdominal CT Scan	435	4.6%	5.2%	10.5%
Combination Brain/Sinus CT Scan[1]	-	-	1.7%	2.7%
Combination Chest CT Scan	173	1.2%	0.7%	2.7%
Follow-up Mammogram/Ultrasound	834	4.3%	7.7%	8.8%
Lumbar Spine MRI for Low Back Pain	81	39.5%	37.5%	37.2%

Franklin Memorial Hospital

111 Franklin Health Commons
Farmington, ME 04938
Phone: 207-778-6031
Fax: 207-779-2548
E-mail: batt@fchn.org
URL: www.fchn.org
Type: Acute Care Hospitals
Emergency Services: Yes
Ownership: Voluntary non-profit - Private
Beds: 70

Key Personnel:
CEO/President. . . . . Rebecca Arsenault
Cardiac Laboratory. . . . . Joel Chandler
Quality Assurance . . . . Mary Drake
Chief of Medical Staff . . . . Rodrick Prior, MD
Emergency Room . . . . Steven Zanella

Measure	Cases	This Hosp.	State Avg.	U.S. Avg.
Blood Clot Prevention and Treatment				
Anticoagulation Overlap Therapy[2]	17	100%	98%	93%
ICU Venous Thromboembolism Prophylaxis[2]	42	100%	96%	92%
Incidence of Potentially Preventable VTE[2,7]	-	-	2%	10%
UFH with Dosages/Platelet Monitoring[1,2]	-	-	100%	97%
Venous Thromboembolism Prophylaxis[2]	219	100%	95%	85%
Warfarin Therapy Discharge Instructions[2]	14	93%	84%	75%
Chest Pain/Possible Heart Attack Care				
Aspirin Given Within 24 Hours of Arrival	35	97%	99%	96%
Fibrinolytic Meds Within 30 Min. of Arrival[1]	-	-	86%	58%
Average Time to ECG (minutes)	32	7	6	7
Average Time to Transfer (minutes)[1]	-	-	49	60
Children's Asthma Care				
Received Home Management Plan of Care	-	-	-	88%
Received Reliever Medication	-	-	-	100%
Received Systemic Corticosteroids	-	-	-	100%
Emergency Department				
Admittance Decision Time (minutes)[2]	415	114	110	98
Head CT Results Within 45 Min. of Arrival[1]	-	-	44%	57%
Patients Who Left ER Before Being Seen	16,598	1%	1%	2%
Time from ER Arrival to Admit. (minutes)[2]	415	263	288	274
Time from ER Arrival to Discharge (minutes)	453	102	122	134
Time in ER Before Being Evaluated (minutes)	477	26	28	26
Time to Pain Meds for Fractures (minutes)	83	40	52	57
Heart Attack Care				
Aspirin Given at Discharge	13	100%	100%	99%
Fibrinolytic Meds Within 30 Min. of Arrival[7]	-	-	50%	54%
PCI Within 90 Minutes of Arrival[7]	-	-	96%	96%
Statin Prescribed at Discharge	14	93%	99%	98%
Heart Failure Care				
ACE Inhibitor or ARB for LVSD	19	95%	99%	97%
Discharge Instructions Given	64	98%	98%	94%
Evaluation of LVS Function	83	100%	100%	99%
Medicare Spending				
Medicare Spending per Patient (ratio)	-	0.88	0.95	0.98
Pneumonia Care				
Appropriate Initial Antibiotic Given	55	100%	98%	95%
Blood Culture Timing	75	96%	98%	98%
Pregnancy and Delivery Care				
Newborn Deliveries Scheduled Early[1]	-	-	2%	6%
Preventive Care				
Immunization for Influenza[2]	274	100%	93%	90%
Immunization for Pneumonia[2]	347	99%	94%	92%
Stroke Care				
Anticoagulation Therapy for Atrial Fibrillation[1]	-	-	98%	95%
Antithrombotic Therapy Timing	15	93%	99%	98%
Assessed for Rehabilitation	15	100%	98%	97%
Discharged on Antithrombotic Therapy	14	100%	100%	99%
Discharged on Statin Medication	13	92%	97%	94%
Thrombolytic Therapy Timing[1]	-	-	29%	66%
Venous Thromboembolism Prophylaxis	14	100%	96%	94%
Written Stroke Educational Materials Given	11	91%	86%	88%
Surgical Care Improvement Project				
Appropriate Beta Blocker Usage	29	97%	99%	98%
Appropriate VTP Within 24 Hours	120	100%	99%	98%
Controlled Postoperative Blood Glucose[7]	-	-	99%	97%
Perioperative Temperature Management	128	100%	100%	100%
Prophylactic Antibiotic Selection	75	100%	99%	99%
Prophylactic Antibiotic Selection (Outpatient)	33	100%	98%	98%
Prophylactic Antibiotic Stopped	71	99%	99%	98%
Prophylactic Antibiotic Timing	75	100%	99%	99%
Prophylactic Antibiotic Timing (Outpatient)	32	100%	96%	98%
Urinary Catheter Removal	64	100%	99%	97%
Survey of Patients' Hospital Experiences				
Area Around Room 'Always' Quiet at Night	(a)	47%	59%	61%
Doctors 'Always' Communicated Well	(a)	81%	83%	82%
Home Recovery Information Given	(a)	88%	90%	85%
Hospital Given 9 or 10 on 10 Point Scale	(a)	69%	74%	71%
Meds 'Always' Explained Before Given	(a)	69%	69%	64%
Nurses 'Always' Communicated Well	(a)	80%	82%	79%
Pain 'Always' Well Controlled	(a)	70%	73%	71%
Room and Bathroom 'Always' Clean	(a)	80%	80%	73%
Timely Help 'Always' Received	(a)	68%	72%	68%
Would Definitely Recommend Hospital	(a)	68%	77%	71%
Use of Medical Imaging				
Cardiac Imaging Stress Test before Surgery	144	4.9%	4.8%	5.3%
Combination Abdominal CT Scan	412	11.7%	5.2%	10.5%
Combination Brain/Sinus CT Scan[1]	-	-	1.7%	2.7%
Combination Chest CT Scan	230	2.6%	0.7%	2.7%
Follow-up Mammogram/Ultrasound	1,128	8.2%	7.7%	8.8%
Lumbar Spine MRI for Low Back Pain	124	35.5%	37.5%	37.2%

Northern Maine Medical Center

194 E Main Street
Fort Kent, ME 04743
Phone: 207-834-3195
Fax: 207-834-2202
E-mail: robin.damboise@nmmc.org
URL: www.nmmc.org
Type: Acute Care Hospitals
Emergency Services: Yes
Ownership: Voluntary non-profit - Private
Beds: 52

Key Personnel:
Radiology. . . . . Baharak Bagheri, MD
CEO/President. . . . . Martin B Bernstein
Operating Room. . . . . Jill Daigle
Quality Assurance . . . . Sue Devoe
President . . . . Norman Fournier, MD
Chief of Medical Staff . . . . Guy Raymond, MD
Infection Control. . . . . Tina Soucy
Cardiac Laboratory. . . . . Don Thersault

Measure	Cases	This Hosp.	State Avg.	U.S. Avg.
Blood Clot Prevention and Treatment				
Anticoagulation Overlap Therapy[2,7]	-	-	98%	93%
ICU Venous Thromboembolism Prophylaxis[2]	23	96%	96%	92%
Incidence of Potentially Preventable VTE[1,2]	-	-	2%	10%
UFH with Dosages/Platelet Monitoring[2,7]	-	-	100%	97%
Venous Thromboembolism Prophylaxis[2]	97	99%	95%	85%
Warfarin Therapy Discharge Instructions[2,7]	-	-	84%	75%
Chest Pain/Possible Heart Attack Care				
Aspirin Given Within 24 Hours of Arrival	15	100%	99%	96%
Fibrinolytic Meds Within 30 Min. of Arrival[1]	-	-	86%	58%
Average Time to ECG (minutes)	15	0	6	7
Average Time to Transfer (minutes)[7]	-	-	49	60
Children's Asthma Care				
Received Home Management Plan of Care	-	-	-	88%
Received Reliever Medication	-	-	-	100%
Received Systemic Corticosteroids	-	-	-	100%
Emergency Department				
Admittance Decision Time (minutes)[2]	316	58	110	98
Head CT Results Within 45 Min. of Arrival[1]	-	-	44%	57%
Patients Who Left ER Before Being Seen	6,579	0%	1%	2%
Time from ER Arrival to Admit. (minutes)[2]	331	202	288	274
Time from ER Arrival to Discharge (minutes)	368	101	122	134
Time in ER Before Being Evaluated (minutes)	404	26	28	26
Time to Pain Meds for Fractures (minutes)	22	32	52	57
Heart Attack Care				

NOTE: Hospital profiles are in alphabetical order by state, then city, then hospital within the city; Rankings exclude hospitals with less than 25 cases except for patient surveys which excludes hospitals with less than 100 cases; (a) 100-299 cases; (1) The number of cases/patients is too few to report; (2) Data submitted were based on a sample of cases/patients; (3) Results are based on a shorter time period than required; (4) Data suppressed by CMS for one or more quarters; (5) Results are not available for this reporting period; (6) Fewer than 100 patients completed the HCAHPS survey; (7) No cases met the criteria for this measure; (8) The lower limit of the confidence interval cannot be calculated if the number of observed infections equals zero; (9) No data are available from the state/territory for this reporting period; (10) The scores shown reflect fewer than 50 completed surveys; (11) There were discrepancies in the data collection process; (12) This measure does not apply to this hospital for this reporting period; (13) Results cannot be calculated for this reporting period; (14) The results for this state are combined with nearby states to protect confidentiality; Please refer to the User's Guide for a full explanation of data.

Measure	Cases	This Hosp.	State Avg.	U.S. Avg.
Aspirin Given at Discharge[1]	-	-	100%	99%
Fibrinolytic Meds Within 30 Min. of Arrival[7]	-	-	50%	54%
PCI Within 90 Minutes of Arrival[7]	-	-	96%	96%
Statin Prescribed at Discharge[1]	-	-	99%	98%
Heart Failure Care				
ACE Inhibitor or ARB for LVSD	17	100%	99%	97%
Discharge Instructions Given	28	100%	98%	94%
Evaluation of LVS Function	46	100%	100%	99%
Medicare Spending				
Medicare Spending per Patient (ratio)	-	0.87	0.95	0.98
Pneumonia Care				
Appropriate Initial Antibiotic Given	23	100%	98%	95%
Blood Culture Timing	49	98%	98%	98%
Pregnancy and Delivery Care				
Newborn Deliveries Scheduled Early[1]	-	-	2%	6%
Preventive Care				
Immunization for Influenza[2]	289	100%	93%	90%
Immunization for Pneumonia[2]	356	100%	94%	92%
Stroke Care				
Anticoagulation Therapy for Atrial Fibrillation[1]	-	-	98%	95%
Antithrombotic Therapy Timing	26	100%	99%	98%
Assessed for Rehabilitation	24	100%	98%	97%
Discharged on Antithrombotic Therapy	24	100%	100%	99%
Discharged on Statin Medication	23	96%	97%	94%
Thrombolytic Therapy Timing[7]	-	-	29%	66%
Venous Thromboembolism Prophylaxis	27	100%	96%	94%
Written Stroke Educational Materials Given[1]	-	-	86%	88%
Surgical Care Improvement Project				
Appropriate Beta Blocker Usage[1,3]	-	-	99%	98%
Appropriate VTP Within 24 Hours[3]	12	92%	99%	98%
Controlled Postoperative Blood Glucose[3,7]	-	-	99%	97%
Perioperative Temperature Management[3]	14	100%	100%	100%
Prophylactic Antibiotic Selection[1,3]	-	-	99%	99%
Prophylactic Antibiotic Selection (Outpatient)[1]	-	-	98%	98%
Prophylactic Antibiotic Stopped[1,3]	-	-	99%	98%
Prophylactic Antibiotic Timing[1,3]	-	-	99%	99%
Prophylactic Antibiotic Timing (Outpatient)[1]	-	-	96%	98%
Urinary Catheter Removal[3]	11	91%	99%	97%
Survey of Patients' Hospital Experiences				
Area Around Room 'Always' Quiet at Night	(a)	59%	59%	61%
Doctors 'Always' Communicated Well	(a)	86%	83%	82%
Home Recovery Information Given	(a)	85%	90%	85%
Hospital Given 9 or 10 on 10 Point Scale	(a)	69%	74%	71%
Meds 'Always' Explained Before Given	(a)	70%	69%	64%
Nurses 'Always' Communicated Well	(a)	85%	82%	79%
Pain 'Always' Well Controlled	(a)	68%	73%	71%
Room and Bathroom 'Always' Clean	(a)	80%	80%	73%
Timely Help 'Always' Received	(a)	75%	72%	68%
Would Definitely Recommend Hospital	(a)	71%	77%	71%
Use of Medical Imaging				
Cardiac Imaging Stress Test before Surgery	116	6.0%	4.8%	5.3%
Combination Abdominal CT Scan	297	29.6%	5.2%	10.5%
Combination Brain/Sinus CT Scan[1]	-	-	1.7%	2.7%
Combination Chest CT Scan	288	4.9%	0.7%	2.7%
Follow-up Mammogram/Ultrasound	757	9.6%	7.7%	8.8%
Lumbar Spine MRI for Low Back Pain	76	44.7%	37.5%	37.2%

Charles A Dean Memorial Hospital

Pritham Avenue PO Box 1129 Phone: 207-695-5200
Greenville, ME 04441 Fax: 207-695-2329
URL: www.cadean.org/default.htm
Type: Critical Access Hospitals Emergency Services: Yes
Ownership: Voluntary non-profit - Private Beds: 14

Key Personnel:
Patient Relations . . . . Dan Blue
CEO/President. . . . . Geno Murray

Measure	Cases	This Hosp.	State Avg.	U.S. Avg.
Blood Clot Prevention and Treatment				
Anticoagulation Overlap Therapy[5]	-	-	98%	93%
ICU Venous Thromboembolism Prophylaxis[5]	-	-	96%	92%
Incidence of Potentially Preventable VTE[5]	-	-	2%	10%
UFH with Dosages/Platelet Monitoring[5]	-	-	100%	97%
Venous Thromboembolism Prophylaxis[5]	-	-	95%	85%
Warfarin Therapy Discharge Instructions[5]	-	-	84%	75%
Chest Pain/Possible Heart Attack Care				
Aspirin Given Within 24 Hours of Arrival	-	-	99%	96%
Fibrinolytic Meds Within 30 Min. of Arrival	-	-	86%	58%
Average Time to ECG (minutes)	-	-	6	7
Average Time to Transfer (minutes)	-	-	49	60
Children's Asthma Care				
Received Home Management Plan of Care	-	-	-	88%
Received Reliever Medication	-	-	-	100%
Received Systemic Corticosteroids	-	-	-	100%
Emergency Department				
Admittance Decision Time (minutes)[5]	-	-	110	98
Head CT Results Within 45 Min. of Arrival	-	-	44%	57%
Patients Who Left ER Before Being Seen	-	-	1%	2%
Time from ER Arrival to Admit. (minutes)[5]	-	-	288	274
Time from ER Arrival to Discharge (minutes)	-	-	122	134
Time in ER Before Being Evaluated (minutes)	-	-	28	26
Time to Pain Meds for Fractures (minutes)	-	-	52	57
Heart Attack Care				
Aspirin Given at Discharge[3,7]	-	-	100%	99%
Fibrinolytic Meds Within 30 Min. of Arrival[3,7]	-	-	50%	54%
PCI Within 90 Minutes of Arrival[3,7]	-	-	96%	96%
Statin Prescribed at Discharge[3,7]	-	-	99%	98%
Heart Failure Care				
ACE Inhibitor or ARB for LVSD[1,3]	-	-	99%	97%
Discharge Instructions Given[1,3]	-	-	98%	94%
Evaluation of LVS Function[1,3]	-	-	100%	99%
Medicare Spending				
Medicare Spending per Patient (ratio)	-	-	0.95	0.98
Pneumonia Care				
Appropriate Initial Antibiotic Given[7]	-	-	98%	95%
Blood Culture Timing[7]	-	-	98%	98%
Pregnancy and Delivery Care				
Newborn Deliveries Scheduled Early[5]	-	-	2%	6%
Preventive Care				
Immunization for Influenza[5]	-	-	93%	90%
Immunization for Pneumonia[5]	-	-	94%	92%
Stroke Care				
Anticoagulation Therapy for Atrial Fibrillation[5]	-	-	98%	95%
Antithrombotic Therapy Timing[5]	-	-	99%	98%
Assessed for Rehabilitation[5]	-	-	98%	97%
Discharged on Antithrombotic Therapy[5]	-	-	100%	99%
Discharged on Statin Medication[5]	-	-	97%	94%
Thrombolytic Therapy Timing[5]	-	-	29%	66%
Venous Thromboembolism Prophylaxis[5]	-	-	96%	94%
Written Stroke Educational Materials Given[5]	-	-	86%	88%
Surgical Care Improvement Project				
Appropriate Beta Blocker Usage[5]	-	-	99%	98%
Appropriate VTP Within 24 Hours[5]	-	-	99%	98%
Controlled Postoperative Blood Glucose[5]	-	-	99%	97%
Perioperative Temperature Management[5]	-	-	100%	100%
Prophylactic Antibiotic Selection[5]	-	-	99%	99%
Prophylactic Antibiotic Selection (Outpatient)	-	-	98%	98%
Prophylactic Antibiotic Stopped[5]	-	-	99%	98%
Prophylactic Antibiotic Timing[5]	-	-	99%	99%
Prophylactic Antibiotic Timing (Outpatient)	-	-	96%	98%
Urinary Catheter Removal[5]	-	-	99%	97%
Survey of Patients' Hospital Experiences				
Area Around Room 'Always' Quiet at Night[6]	<100	60%	59%	61%
Doctors 'Always' Communicated Well[6]	<100	92%	83%	82%
Home Recovery Information Given[6]	<100	95%	90%	85%
Hospital Given 9 or 10 on 10 Point Scale[6]	<100	86%	74%	71%
Meds 'Always' Explained Before Given[6]	<100	78%	69%	64%
Nurses 'Always' Communicated Well[6]	<100	88%	82%	79%
Pain 'Always' Well Controlled[6]	<100	84%	73%	71%
Room and Bathroom 'Always' Clean[6]	<100	81%	80%	73%
Timely Help 'Always' Received[6]	<100	79%	72%	68%
Would Definitely Recommend Hospital[6]	<100	88%	77%	71%
Use of Medical Imaging				
Cardiac Imaging Stress Test before Surgery	-	-	4.8%	5.3%
Combination Abdominal CT Scan	-	-	5.2%	10.5%
Combination Brain/Sinus CT Scan	-	-	1.7%	2.7%
Combination Chest CT Scan	-	-	0.7%	2.7%
Follow-up Mammogram/Ultrasound	-	-	7.7%	8.8%
Lumbar Spine MRI for Low Back Pain	-	-	37.5%	37.2%

Houlton Regional Hospital

20 Hartford Street Phone: 207-532-2900
Houlton, ME 04730 Fax: 207-532-4755
E-mail: info@houltonregional.org
URL: www.houlton.net/hrh
Type: Critical Access Hospitals Emergency Services: Yes
Ownership: Voluntary non-profit - Private Beds: 91

Key Personnel:
Chief of Medical Staff . . . . Philip Mc Farnei, MD
CEO/President. . . . . Thomas J Moakler

Measure	Cases	This Hosp.	State Avg.	U.S. Avg.
Blood Clot Prevention and Treatment				
Anticoagulation Overlap Therapy[5]	-	-	98%	93%
ICU Venous Thromboembolism Prophylaxis[5]	-	-	96%	92%
Incidence of Potentially Preventable VTE[5]	-	-	2%	10%
UFH with Dosages/Platelet Monitoring[5]	-	-	100%	97%
Venous Thromboembolism Prophylaxis[5]	-	-	95%	85%
Warfarin Therapy Discharge Instructions[5]	-	-	84%	75%
Chest Pain/Possible Heart Attack Care				
Aspirin Given Within 24 Hours of Arrival	36	100%	99%	96%
Fibrinolytic Meds Within 30 Min. of Arrival[1]	-	-	86%	58%
Average Time to ECG (minutes)	38	4	6	7
Average Time to Transfer (minutes)[1]	-	-	49	60
Children's Asthma Care				
Received Home Management Plan of Care	-	-	-	88%
Received Reliever Medication	-	-	-	100%
Received Systemic Corticosteroids	-	-	-	100%
Emergency Department				
Admittance Decision Time (minutes)[5]	-	-	110	98
Head CT Results Within 45 Min. of Arrival[5]	-	-	44%	57%
Patients Who Left ER Before Being Seen[5]	-	-	1%	2%
Time from ER Arrival to Admit. (minutes)[5]	-	-	288	274
Time from ER Arrival to Discharge (minutes)[5]	-	-	122	134
Time in ER Before Being Evaluated (minutes)[5]	-	-	28	26
Time to Pain Meds for Fractures (minutes)[5]	-	-	52	57
Heart Attack Care				
Aspirin Given at Discharge[1]	-	-	100%	99%
Fibrinolytic Meds Within 30 Min. of Arrival[7]	-	-	50%	54%
PCI Within 90 Minutes of Arrival[7]	-	-	96%	96%
Statin Prescribed at Discharge[1]	-	-	99%	98%
Heart Failure Care				
ACE Inhibitor or ARB for LVSD[1]	-	-	99%	97%
Discharge Instructions Given	32	97%	98%	94%
Evaluation of LVS Function	47	100%	100%	99%
Medicare Spending				
Medicare Spending per Patient (ratio)	-	-	0.95	0.98
Pneumonia Care				
Appropriate Initial Antibiotic Given	33	97%	98%	95%
Blood Culture Timing	62	98%	98%	98%
Pregnancy and Delivery Care				
Newborn Deliveries Scheduled Early[5]	-	-	2%	6%
Preventive Care				
Immunization for Influenza[5]	-	-	93%	90%
Immunization for Pneumonia[5]	-	-	94%	92%
Stroke Care				
Anticoagulation Therapy for Atrial Fibrillation[5]	-	-	98%	95%
Antithrombotic Therapy Timing[5]	-	-	99%	98%
Assessed for Rehabilitation[5]	-	-	98%	97%
Discharged on Antithrombotic Therapy[5]	-	-	100%	99%
Discharged on Statin Medication[5]	-	-	97%	94%
Thrombolytic Therapy Timing[5]	-	-	29%	66%
Venous Thromboembolism Prophylaxis[5]	-	-	96%	94%
Written Stroke Educational Materials Given[5]	-	-	86%	88%
Surgical Care Improvement Project				
Appropriate Beta Blocker Usage[1,3]	-	-	99%	98%
Appropriate VTP Within 24 Hours[3]	13	100%	99%	98%
Controlled Postoperative Blood Glucose[3,7]	-	-	99%	97%
Perioperative Temperature Management[3]	13	100%	100%	100%
Prophylactic Antibiotic Selection[1,3]	-	-	99%	99%

NOTE: Hospital profiles are in alphabetical order by state, then city, then hospital within the city; Rankings exclude hospitals with less than 25 cases except for patient surveys which excludes hospitals with less than 100 cases; (a) 100-299 cases; (1) The number of cases/patients is too few to report; (2) Data submitted were based on a sample of cases/patients; (3) Results are based on a shorter time period than required; (4) Data suppressed by CMS for one or more quarters; (5) Results are not available for this reporting period; (6) Fewer than 100 patients completed the HCAHPS survey; (7) No cases met the criteria for this measure; (8) The lower limit of the confidence interval cannot be calculated if the number of observed infections equals zero; (9) No data are available from the state/territory for this reporting period; (10) The scores shown reflect fewer than 50 completed surveys; (11) There were discrepancies in the data collection process; (12) This measure does not apply to this hospital for this reporting period; (13) Results cannot be calculated for this reporting period; (14) The results for this state are combined with nearby states to protect confidentiality; Please refer to the User's Guide for a full explanation of data.

Measure	Cases	This Hosp.	State Avg.	U.S. Avg.
Prophylactic Antibiotic Selection (Outpatient)	24	96%	98%	98%
Prophylactic Antibiotic Stopped[1,3]	-	-	99%	98%
Prophylactic Antibiotic Timing[1,3]	-	-	99%	99%
Prophylactic Antibiotic Timing (Outpatient)	13	92%	96%	98%
Urinary Catheter Removal[1,3]	-	-	99%	97%
Survey of Patients' Hospital Experiences				
Area Around Room 'Always' Quiet at Night	(a)	54%	59%	61%
Doctors 'Always' Communicated Well	(a)	87%	83%	82%
Home Recovery Information Given	(a)	87%	90%	85%
Hospital Given 9 or 10 on 10 Point Scale	(a)	69%	74%	71%
Meds 'Always' Explained Before Given	(a)	73%	69%	64%
Nurses 'Always' Communicated Well	(a)	84%	82%	79%
Pain 'Always' Well Controlled	(a)	72%	73%	71%
Room and Bathroom 'Always' Clean	(a)	79%	80%	73%
Timely Help 'Always' Received	(a)	77%	72%	68%
Would Definitely Recommend Hospital	(a)	67%	77%	71%
Use of Medical Imaging				
Cardiac Imaging Stress Test before Surgery	106	3.8%	4.8%	5.3%
Combination Abdominal CT Scan	415	2.7%	5.2%	10.5%
Combination Brain/Sinus CT Scan[1]	-	-	1.7%	2.7%
Combination Chest CT Scan	224	0.4%	0.7%	2.7%
Follow-up Mammogram/Ultrasound	462	9.5%	7.7%	8.8%
Lumbar Spine MRI for Low Back Pain[1]	-	-	37.5%	37.2%

Central Maine Medical Center

300 Main Street Phone: 207-795-0111
Lewiston, ME 04240 Fax: 207-795-5687
E-mail: cmmc@cmmc.org
URL: www.cmmc.org
Type: Acute Care Hospitals Emergency Services: Yes
Ownership: Voluntary non-profit - Private Beds: 250

Key Personnel:
CEO/President. . . . . Peter Chalke
Emergency Room . . . . John Fields, RN
Cardiac Laboratory. . . . . Susan Horton
Pediatric Ambulatory Care . . . . . . Stephen Jacobs, MD
Pediatric In-Patient Care . . . . Stephen Jacobs, MD
Quality Assurance . . . . Sharon King
Radiology. . . . . Barry Kutzen, MD
Chief of Medical Staff. . . . . Lanny Oliver

Measure	Cases	This Hosp.	State Avg.	U.S. Avg.
Blood Clot Prevention and Treatment				
Anticoagulation Overlap Therapy[2]	71	94%	98%	93%
ICU Venous Thromboembolism Prophylaxis[2]	90	98%	96%	92%
Incidence of Potentially Preventable VTE[1,2]	-	-	2%	10%
UFH with Dosages/Platelet Monitoring[2]	24	100%	100%	97%
Venous Thromboembolism Prophylaxis[2]	325	92%	95%	85%
Warfarin Therapy Discharge Instructions[2]	57	63%	84%	75%
Chest Pain/Possible Heart Attack Care				
Aspirin Given Within 24 Hours of Arrival[1,3]	-	-	99%	96%
Fibrinolytic Meds Within 30 Min. of Arrival[5]	-	-	86%	58%
Average Time to ECG (minutes)[3,7]	-	-	6	7
Average Time to Transfer (minutes)[5]	-	-	49	60
Children's Asthma Care				
Received Home Management Plan of Care	-	-	-	88%
Received Reliever Medication	-	-	-	100%
Received Systemic Corticosteroids	-	-	-	100%
Emergency Department				
Admittance Decision Time (minutes)[2]	613	105	110	98
Head CT Results Within 45 Min. of Arrival[1]	-	-	44%	57%
Patients Who Left ER Before Being Seen	46,841	2%	1%	2%
Time from ER Arrival to Admit. (minutes)[2]	634	291	288	274
Time from ER Arrival to Discharge (minutes)	371	158	122	134
Time in ER Before Being Evaluated (minutes)	415	45	28	26
Time to Pain Meds for Fractures (minutes)	123	85	52	57
Heart Attack Care				
Aspirin Given at Discharge[2]	329	100%	100%	99%
Fibrinolytic Meds Within 30 Min. of Arrival[2,7]	-	-	50%	54%
PCI Within 90 Minutes of Arrival[2]	50	96%	96%	96%
Statin Prescribed at Discharge[2]	323	99%	99%	98%
Heart Failure Care				
ACE Inhibitor or ARB for LVSD	64	100%	99%	97%
Discharge Instructions Given	201	100%	98%	94%
Evaluation of LVS Function	265	100%	100%	99%
Medicare Spending				
Medicare Spending per Patient (ratio)	-	0.97	0.95	0.98
Pneumonia Care				
Appropriate Initial Antibiotic Given[2]	111	98%	98%	95%
Blood Culture Timing[2]	82	94%	98%	98%
Pregnancy and Delivery Care				
Newborn Deliveries Scheduled Early	50	2%	2%	6%
Preventive Care				
Immunization for Influenza[2]	585	92%	93%	90%
Immunization for Pneumonia[2]	798	89%	94%	92%
Stroke Care				
Anticoagulation Therapy for Atrial Fibrillation[1]	-	-	98%	95%
Antithrombotic Therapy Timing	91	98%	99%	98%
Assessed for Rehabilitation	123	98%	98%	97%
Discharged on Antithrombotic Therapy	106	100%	100%	99%
Discharged on Statin Medication	79	97%	97%	94%
Thrombolytic Therapy Timing[1]	-	-	29%	66%
Venous Thromboembolism Prophylaxis	113	97%	96%	94%
Written Stroke Educational Materials Given	69	93%	86%	88%
Surgical Care Improvement Project				
Appropriate Beta Blocker Usage[2]	246	98%	99%	98%
Appropriate VTP Within 24 Hours[2]	336	99%	99%	98%
Controlled Postoperative Blood Glucose[2]	108	99%	99%	97%
Perioperative Temperature Management[2]	590	100%	100%	100%
Prophylactic Antibiotic Selection[2]	464	98%	99%	99%
Prophylactic Antibiotic Selection (Outpatient)	460	97%	98%	98%
Prophylactic Antibiotic Stopped[2]	452	99%	99%	98%
Prophylactic Antibiotic Timing[2]	465	99%	99%	99%
Prophylactic Antibiotic Timing (Outpatient)	389	98%	96%	98%
Urinary Catheter Removal[2]	248	94%	99%	97%
Survey of Patients' Hospital Experiences				
Area Around Room 'Always' Quiet at Night	300+	55%	59%	61%
Doctors 'Always' Communicated Well	300+	79%	83%	82%
Home Recovery Information Given	300+	90%	90%	85%
Hospital Given 9 or 10 on 10 Point Scale	300+	73%	74%	71%
Meds 'Always' Explained Before Given	300+	68%	69%	64%
Nurses 'Always' Communicated Well	300+	81%	82%	79%
Pain 'Always' Well Controlled	300+	71%	73%	71%
Room and Bathroom 'Always' Clean	300+	76%	80%	73%
Timely Help 'Always' Received	300+	67%	72%	68%
Would Definitely Recommend Hospital	300+	77%	77%	71%
Use of Medical Imaging				
Cardiac Imaging Stress Test before Surgery	704	5.0%	4.8%	5.3%
Combination Abdominal CT Scan	943	5.3%	5.2%	10.5%
Combination Brain/Sinus CT Scan	603	2.5%	1.7%	2.7%
Combination Chest CT Scan	794	0.1%	0.7%	2.7%
Follow-up Mammogram/Ultrasound	1,949	6.4%	7.7%	8.8%
Lumbar Spine MRI for Low Back Pain[7]	-	-	37.5%	37.2%

Saint Marys Regional Medical Center

Campus Avenue - PO Box 291 Phone: 207-777-8100
Lewiston, ME 04240 Fax: 207-777-8800
URL: www.stmarysmaine.com
Type: Acute Care Hospitals Emergency Services: Yes
Ownership: Voluntary non-profit - Private Beds: 233

Key Personnel:
Chief of Medical Staff. . . . . Peter Beeckel
Quality Assurance . . . . Kathleen Bremer
Radiology. . . . . Cindy Brousseau
CEO/President. . . . . James Cassidy
Operating Room. . . . . Justin Clark
Pediatric Ambulatory Care . . . . . . Linda Glass, MD
Pediatric In-Patient Care . . . . Linda Glass, MD
Infection Control. . . . . Diane Theriault, RN

Measure	Cases	This Hosp.	State Avg.	U.S. Avg.
Blood Clot Prevention and Treatment				
Anticoagulation Overlap Therapy[2]	24	100%	98%	93%
ICU Venous Thromboembolism Prophylaxis[2]	41	90%	96%	92%
Incidence of Potentially Preventable VTE[1,2]	-	-	2%	10%
UFH with Dosages/Platelet Monitoring[1,2]	-	-	100%	97%
Venous Thromboembolism Prophylaxis[2]	250	94%	95%	85%
Warfarin Therapy Discharge Instructions[2]	17	100%	84%	75%
Chest Pain/Possible Heart Attack Care				
Aspirin Given Within 24 Hours of Arrival	28	100%	99%	96%
Fibrinolytic Meds Within 30 Min. of Arrival[7]	-	-	86%	58%
Average Time to ECG (minutes)	28	9	6	7
Average Time to Transfer (minutes)[1]	-	-	49	60
Children's Asthma Care				
Received Home Management Plan of Care	-	-	-	88%
Received Reliever Medication	-	-	-	100%
Received Systemic Corticosteroids	-	-	-	100%
Emergency Department				
Admittance Decision Time (minutes)[2]	371	142	110	98
Head CT Results Within 45 Min. of Arrival[1]	-	-	44%	57%
Patients Who Left ER Before Being Seen	34,187	1%	1%	2%
Time from ER Arrival to Admit. (minutes)[2]	374	354	288	274
Time from ER Arrival to Discharge (minutes)	368	113	122	134
Time in ER Before Being Evaluated (minutes)	416	21	28	26
Time to Pain Meds for Fractures (minutes)	54	49	52	57
Heart Attack Care				
Aspirin Given at Discharge	26	100%	100%	99%
Fibrinolytic Meds Within 30 Min. of Arrival[7]	-	-	50%	54%
PCI Within 90 Minutes of Arrival[7]	-	-	96%	96%
Statin Prescribed at Discharge	27	100%	99%	98%
Heart Failure Care				
ACE Inhibitor or ARB for LVSD	14	100%	99%	97%
Discharge Instructions Given	47	98%	98%	94%
Evaluation of LVS Function	74	100%	100%	99%
Medicare Spending				
Medicare Spending per Patient (ratio)	-	0.97	0.95	0.98
Pneumonia Care				
Appropriate Initial Antibiotic Given	77	99%	98%	95%
Blood Culture Timing	93	96%	98%	98%
Pregnancy and Delivery Care				
Newborn Deliveries Scheduled Early	33	0%	2%	6%
Preventive Care				
Immunization for Influenza[2]	474	89%	93%	90%
Immunization for Pneumonia[2]	477	94%	94%	92%
Stroke Care				
Anticoagulation Therapy for Atrial Fibrillation	13	100%	98%	95%
Antithrombotic Therapy Timing	32	100%	99%	98%
Assessed for Rehabilitation	34	100%	98%	97%
Discharged on Antithrombotic Therapy	31	97%	100%	99%
Discharged on Statin Medication	23	100%	97%	94%
Thrombolytic Therapy Timing	13	8%	29%	66%
Venous Thromboembolism Prophylaxis	34	100%	96%	94%
Written Stroke Educational Materials Given[1]	-	-	86%	88%
Surgical Care Improvement Project				
Appropriate Beta Blocker Usage[2]	139	100%	99%	98%
Appropriate VTP Within 24 Hours[2]	445	100%	99%	98%
Controlled Postoperative Blood Glucose[2,7]	-	-	99%	97%
Perioperative Temperature Management[2]	478	100%	100%	100%
Prophylactic Antibiotic Selection[2]	319	100%	99%	99%
Prophylactic Antibiotic Selection (Outpatient)	169	93%	98%	98%
Prophylactic Antibiotic Stopped[2]	307	99%	99%	98%
Prophylactic Antibiotic Timing[2]	319	99%	99%	99%
Prophylactic Antibiotic Timing (Outpatient)	118	88%	96%	98%
Urinary Catheter Removal[2]	157	100%	99%	97%
Survey of Patients' Hospital Experiences				
Area Around Room 'Always' Quiet at Night	300+	58%	59%	61%
Doctors 'Always' Communicated Well	300+	83%	83%	82%
Home Recovery Information Given	300+	86%	90%	85%
Hospital Given 9 or 10 on 10 Point Scale	300+	75%	74%	71%
Meds 'Always' Explained Before Given	300+	68%	69%	64%
Nurses 'Always' Communicated Well	300+	82%	82%	79%
Pain 'Always' Well Controlled	300+	68%	73%	71%
Room and Bathroom 'Always' Clean	300+	82%	80%	73%
Timely Help 'Always' Received	300+	69%	72%	68%
Would Definitely Recommend Hospital	300+	81%	77%	71%
Use of Medical Imaging				
Cardiac Imaging Stress Test before Surgery	174	6.9%	4.8%	5.3%
Combination Abdominal CT Scan	697	4.9%	5.2%	10.5%
Combination Brain/Sinus CT Scan	525	1.5%	1.7%	2.7%
Combination Chest CT Scan	473	0.2%	0.7%	2.7%
Follow-up Mammogram/Ultrasound	1,166	7.5%	7.7%	8.8%
Lumbar Spine MRI for Low Back Pain	126	36.5%	37.5%	37.2%

NOTE: Hospital profiles are in alphabetical order by state, then city, then hospital within the city; Rankings exclude hospitals with less than 25 cases except for patient surveys which excludes hospitals with less than 100 cases; (a) 100-299 cases; (1) The number of cases/patients is too few to report; (2) Data submitted were based on a sample of cases/patients; (3) Results are based on a shorter time period than required; (4) Data suppressed by CMS for one or more quarters; (5) Results are not available for this reporting period; (6) Fewer than 100 patients completed the HCAHPS survey; (7) No cases met the criteria for this measure; (8) The lower limit of the confidence interval cannot be calculated if the number of observed infections equals zero; (9) No data are available from the state/territory for this reporting period; (10) The scores shown reflect fewer than 50 completed surveys; (11) There were discrepancies in the data collection process; (12) This measure does not apply to this hospital for this reporting period; (13) Results cannot be calculated for this reporting period; (14) The results for this state are combined with nearby states to protect confidentiality; Please refer to the User's Guide for a full explanation of data.

Penobscot Valley Hospital

7 Transalpine Road, PO Box 368 | Phone: 207-794-3321
Lincoln, ME 04457 | Fax: 207-794-6490
E-mail: info@pvhhealthcare.org
URL: www.pvhhealthcare.org
Type: Critical Access Hospitals | Emergency Services: Yes
Ownership: Voluntary non-profit - Private | Beds: 25

Key Personnel:
Surgery . . . . Glenn Deyo, MD
Emergency Room . . . . David Ettinger
Quality Assurance . . . . Penelope Kneeland
Pediatrics. . . . . Patricia Noble
CEO/President. . . . . Ronald Victory

Measure	Cases	This Hosp.	State Avg.	U.S. Avg.
Blood Clot Prevention and Treatment				
Anticoagulation Overlap Therapy[2,3]	-	-	98%	93%
ICU Venous Thromboembolism Prophylaxis[1,2]	-	-	96%	92%
Incidence of Potentially Preventable VTE[2,3]	-	-	2%	10%
UFH with Dosages/Platelet Monitoring[2,3]	-	-	100%	97%
Venous Thromboembolism Prophylaxis[2,3]	62	98%	95%	85%
Warfarin Therapy Discharge Instructions[2,3]	-	-	84%	75%
Chest Pain/Possible Heart Attack Care				
Aspirin Given Within 24 Hours of Arrival	24	96%	99%	96%
Fibrinolytic Meds Within 30 Min. of Arrival[1]	-	-	86%	58%
Average Time to ECG (minutes)	25	6	6	7
Average Time to Transfer (minutes)[1]	-	-	49	60
Children's Asthma Care				
Received Home Management Plan of Care	-	-	-	88%
Received Reliever Medication	-	-	-	100%
Received Systemic Corticosteroids	-	-	-	100%
Emergency Department				
Admittance Decision Time (minutes)[2]	444	80	110	98
Head CT Results Within 45 Min. of Arrival[1]	-	-	44%	57%
Patients Who Left ER Before Being Seen[5]	-	-	1%	2%
Time from ER Arrival to Admit. (minutes)[2]	451	233	288	274
Time from ER Arrival to Discharge (minutes)[3]	231	89	122	134
Time in ER Before Being Evaluated (minutes)[3]	250	27	28	26
Time to Pain Meds for Fractures (minutes)	25	77	52	57
Heart Attack Care				
Aspirin Given at Discharge[1,2]	-	-	100%	99%
Fibrinolytic Meds Within 30 Min. of Arrival[2,7]	-	-	50%	54%
PCI Within 90 Minutes of Arrival[2,7]	-	-	96%	96%
Statin Prescribed at Discharge[1,2]	-	-	99%	98%
Heart Failure Care				
ACE Inhibitor or ARB for LVSD[1]	-	-	99%	97%
Discharge Instructions Given	24	96%	98%	94%
Evaluation of LVS Function	38	100%	100%	99%
Medicare Spending				
Medicare Spending per Patient (ratio)	-	-	0.95	0.98
Pneumonia Care				
Appropriate Initial Antibiotic Given[2]	46	100%	98%	95%
Blood Culture Timing[2]	23	96%	98%	98%
Pregnancy and Delivery Care				
Newborn Deliveries Scheduled Early[5]	-	-	2%	6%
Preventive Care				
Immunization for Influenza[2]	276	93%	93%	90%
Immunization for Pneumonia[2]	406	99%	94%	92%
Stroke Care				
Anticoagulation Therapy for Atrial Fibrillation[7]	-	-	98%	95%
Antithrombotic Therapy Timing	14	100%	99%	98%
Assessed for Rehabilitation	14	100%	98%	97%
Discharged on Antithrombotic Therapy	13	100%	100%	99%
Discharged on Statin Medication	13	100%	97%	94%
Thrombolytic Therapy Timing[7]	-	-	29%	66%
Venous Thromboembolism Prophylaxis	15	93%	96%	94%
Written Stroke Educational Materials Given[1]	-	-	86%	88%
Surgical Care Improvement Project				
Appropriate Beta Blocker Usage[1]	-	-	99%	98%
Appropriate VTP Within 24 Hours	13	100%	99%	98%
Controlled Postoperative Blood Glucose[7]	-	-	99%	97%
Perioperative Temperature Management	15	100%	100%	100%
Prophylactic Antibiotic Selection[1]	-	-	99%	99%
Prophylactic Antibiotic Selection (Outpatient)[3,7]	-	-	98%	98%
Prophylactic Antibiotic Stopped[1]	-	-	99%	98%
Prophylactic Antibiotic Timing[1]	-	-	99%	99%
Prophylactic Antibiotic Timing (Outpatient)[3,7]	-	-	96%	98%
Urinary Catheter Removal	13	100%	99%	97%
Survey of Patients' Hospital Experiences				
Area Around Room 'Always' Quiet at Night	(a)	59%	59%	61%
Doctors 'Always' Communicated Well	(a)	83%	83%	82%
Home Recovery Information Given	(a)	87%	90%	85%
Hospital Given 9 or 10 on 10 Point Scale	(a)	73%	74%	71%
Meds 'Always' Explained Before Given	(a)	64%	69%	64%
Nurses 'Always' Communicated Well	(a)	81%	82%	79%
Pain 'Always' Well Controlled	(a)	67%	73%	71%
Room and Bathroom 'Always' Clean	(a)	84%	80%	73%
Timely Help 'Always' Received	(a)	68%	72%	68%
Would Definitely Recommend Hospital	(a)	72%	77%	71%
Use of Medical Imaging				
Cardiac Imaging Stress Test before Surgery	104	10.6%	4.8%	5.3%
Combination Abdominal CT Scan	186	3.2%	5.2%	10.5%
Combination Brain/Sinus CT Scan	185	0.5%	1.7%	2.7%
Combination Chest CT Scan	88	1.1%	0.7%	2.7%
Follow-up Mammogram/Ultrasound	348	7.8%	7.7%	8.8%
Lumbar Spine MRI for Low Back Pain[1]	-	-	37.5%	37.2%

Down East Community Hospital

11 Hospital Drive | Phone: 207-255-3356
Machias, ME 04654 | Fax: 207-255-0427
E-mail: mjgripp@dech.org
URL: www.dech.org
Type: Critical Access Hospitals | Emergency Services: Yes
Ownership: Voluntary non-profit - Private | Beds: 36

Key Personnel:
Infection Control. . . . . Bart Brizee, RN
Patient Relations . . . . Vicki Brown
Operating Room. . . . . Jane Foshay, RN, CRNFA
President/CEO. . . . . Ralph Gabarro, FACHE
Quality Assurance . . . . Sue Jones-Burr
Radiology. . . . . Karen Krigman, MD
Emergency Room . . . . Kristzina Morin, DO
Chief of Medical Staff. . . . . David Rioux, DO

Measure	Cases	This Hosp.	State Avg.	U.S. Avg.
Blood Clot Prevention and Treatment				
Anticoagulation Overlap Therapy[5]	-	-	98%	93%
ICU Venous Thromboembolism Prophylaxis[5]	-	-	96%	92%
Incidence of Potentially Preventable VTE[5]	-	-	2%	10%
UFH with Dosages/Platelet Monitoring[5]	-	-	100%	97%
Venous Thromboembolism Prophylaxis[5]	-	-	95%	85%
Warfarin Therapy Discharge Instructions[5]	-	-	84%	75%
Chest Pain/Possible Heart Attack Care				
Aspirin Given Within 24 Hours of Arrival[5]	-	-	99%	96%
Fibrinolytic Meds Within 30 Min. of Arrival[5]	-	-	86%	58%
Average Time to ECG (minutes)[5]	-	-	6	7
Average Time to Transfer (minutes)[5]	-	-	49	60
Children's Asthma Care				
Received Home Management Plan of Care	-	-	-	88%
Received Reliever Medication	-	-	-	100%
Received Systemic Corticosteroids	-	-	-	100%
Emergency Department				
Admittance Decision Time (minutes)[5]	-	-	110	98
Head CT Results Within 45 Min. of Arrival[5]	-	-	44%	57%
Patients Who Left ER Before Being Seen[5]	-	-	1%	2%
Time from ER Arrival to Admit. (minutes)[5]	-	-	288	274
Time from ER Arrival to Discharge (minutes)[5]	-	-	122	134
Time in ER Before Being Evaluated (minutes)[5]	-	-	28	26
Time to Pain Meds for Fractures (minutes)[5]	-	-	52	57
Heart Attack Care				
Aspirin Given at Discharge	12	100%	100%	99%
Fibrinolytic Meds Within 30 Min. of Arrival[7]	-	-	50%	54%
PCI Within 90 Minutes of Arrival[7]	-	-	96%	96%
Statin Prescribed at Discharge	11	100%	99%	98%
Heart Failure Care				
ACE Inhibitor or ARB for LVSD[1]	-	-	99%	97%
Discharge Instructions Given	15	100%	98%	94%
Evaluation of LVS Function	19	100%	100%	99%
Medicare Spending				
Medicare Spending per Patient (ratio)	-	-	0.95	0.98
Pneumonia Care				
Appropriate Initial Antibiotic Given	51	100%	98%	95%
Blood Culture Timing	59	100%	98%	98%
Pregnancy and Delivery Care				
Newborn Deliveries Scheduled Early[5]	-	-	2%	6%
Preventive Care				
Immunization for Influenza[5]	-	-	93%	90%
Immunization for Pneumonia[3,7]	-	-	94%	92%
Stroke Care				
Anticoagulation Therapy for Atrial Fibrillation[5]	-	-	98%	95%
Antithrombotic Therapy Timing[5]	-	-	99%	98%
Assessed for Rehabilitation[5]	-	-	98%	97%
Discharged on Antithrombotic Therapy[5]	-	-	100%	99%
Discharged on Statin Medication[5]	-	-	97%	94%
Thrombolytic Therapy Timing[5]	-	-	29%	66%
Venous Thromboembolism Prophylaxis[5]	-	-	96%	94%
Written Stroke Educational Materials Given[5]	-	-	86%	88%
Surgical Care Improvement Project				
Appropriate Beta Blocker Usage[1]	-	-	99%	98%
Appropriate VTP Within 24 Hours	33	100%	99%	98%
Controlled Postoperative Blood Glucose[7]	-	-	99%	97%
Perioperative Temperature Management	28	100%	100%	100%
Prophylactic Antibiotic Selection	29	100%	99%	99%
Prophylactic Antibiotic Selection (Outpatient)[5]	-	-	98%	98%
Prophylactic Antibiotic Stopped	29	97%	99%	98%
Prophylactic Antibiotic Timing	29	100%	99%	99%
Prophylactic Antibiotic Timing (Outpatient)[5]	-	-	96%	98%
Urinary Catheter Removal	23	100%	99%	97%
Survey of Patients' Hospital Experiences				
Area Around Room 'Always' Quiet at Night	(a)	60%	59%	61%
Doctors 'Always' Communicated Well	(a)	86%	83%	82%
Home Recovery Information Given	(a)	85%	90%	85%
Hospital Given 9 or 10 on 10 Point Scale	(a)	67%	74%	71%
Meds 'Always' Explained Before Given	(a)	72%	69%	64%
Nurses 'Always' Communicated Well	(a)	83%	82%	79%
Pain 'Always' Well Controlled	(a)	74%	73%	71%
Room and Bathroom 'Always' Clean	(a)	78%	80%	73%
Timely Help 'Always' Received	(a)	73%	72%	68%
Would Definitely Recommend Hospital	(a)	67%	77%	71%
Use of Medical Imaging				
Cardiac Imaging Stress Test before Surgery[1]	-	-	4.8%	5.3%
Combination Abdominal CT Scan	304	4.3%	5.2%	10.5%
Combination Brain/Sinus CT Scan[1]	-	-	1.7%	2.7%
Combination Chest CT Scan	128	0.0%	0.7%	2.7%
Follow-up Mammogram/Ultrasound	477	8.0%	7.7%	8.8%
Lumbar Spine MRI for Low Back Pain[1]	-	-	37.5%	37.2%

Millinocket Regional Hospital

200 Somerset Street | Phone: 207-723-5161
Millinocket, ME 04462 | Fax: 207-723-4913
URL: www.mrhme.org
Type: Critical Access Hospitals | Emergency Services: Yes
Ownership: Voluntary non-profit - Private | Beds: 42

Key Personnel:
Radiology. . . . . John Connolly, MD
Cardiology . . . . Kathleen Harper, DO
Chief of Medical Staff. . . . . Daniel Herbert, MD
Surgery . . . . Mark Kowalski, MD
Quality Assurance . . . . Mary Marter, RN
Emergency Room . . . . Stephanie Thompson, RN
CEO/President. . . . . Marie Vienneau

Measure	Cases	This Hosp.	State Avg.	U.S. Avg.
Blood Clot Prevention and Treatment				
Anticoagulation Overlap Therapy[5]	-	-	98%	93%
ICU Venous Thromboembolism Prophylaxis[5]	-	-	96%	92%
Incidence of Potentially Preventable VTE[5]	-	-	2%	10%
UFH with Dosages/Platelet Monitoring[5]	-	-	100%	97%
Venous Thromboembolism Prophylaxis[5]	-	-	95%	85%
Warfarin Therapy Discharge Instructions[5]	-	-	84%	75%
Chest Pain/Possible Heart Attack Care				
Aspirin Given Within 24 Hours of Arrival[5]	-	-	99%	96%
Fibrinolytic Meds Within 30 Min. of Arrival[5]	-	-	86%	58%
Average Time to ECG (minutes)[5]	-	-	6	7
Average Time to Transfer (minutes)[5]	-	-	49	60

NOTE: *Hospital profiles are in alphabetical order by state, then city, then hospital within the city; Rankings exclude hospitals with less than 25 cases except for patient surveys which excludes hospitals with less than 100 cases; (a) 100-299 cases; (1) The number of cases/patients is too few to report; (2) Data submitted were based on a sample of cases/patients; (3) Results are based on a shorter time period than required; (4) Data suppressed by CMS for one or more quarters; (5) Results are not available for this reporting period; (6) Fewer than 100 patients completed the HCAHPS survey; (7) No cases met the criteria for this measure; (8) The lower limit of the confidence interval cannot be calculated if the number of observed infections equals zero; (9) No data are available from the state/territory for this reporting period; (10) The scores shown reflect fewer than 50 completed surveys; (11) There were discrepancies in the data collection process; (12) This measure does not apply to this hospital for this reporting period; (13) Results cannot be calculated for this reporting period; (14) The results for this state are combined with nearby states to protect confidentiality; Please refer to the User's Guide for a full explanation of data.*

Measure	Cases	This Hosp.	State Avg.	U.S. Avg.
Children's Asthma Care				
Received Home Management Plan of Care	-	-	-	88%
Received Reliever Medication	-	-	-	100%
Received Systemic Corticosteroids	-	-	-	100%
Emergency Department				
Admittance Decision Time (minutes)[5]	-	-	110	98
Head CT Results Within 45 Min. of Arrival[5]	-	-	44%	57%
Patients Who Left ER Before Being Seen[5]	-	-	1%	2%
Time from ER Arrival to Admit. (minutes)[5]	-	-	288	274
Time from ER Arrival to Discharge (minutes)[5]	-	-	122	134
Time in ER Before Being Evaluated (minutes)[5]	-	-	28	26
Time to Pain Meds for Fractures (minutes)[5]	-	-	52	57
Heart Attack Care				
Aspirin Given at Discharge[1,3]	-	-	100%	99%
Fibrinolytic Meds Within 30 Min. of Arrival[3,7]	-	-	50%	54%
PCI Within 90 Minutes of Arrival[3,7]	-	-	96%	96%
Statin Prescribed at Discharge[1,3]	-	-	99%	98%
Heart Failure Care				
ACE Inhibitor or ARB for LVSD[1]	-	-	99%	97%
Discharge Instructions Given	20	100%	98%	94%
Evaluation of LVS Function	23	96%	100%	99%
Medicare Spending				
Medicare Spending per Patient (ratio)	-	-	0.95	0.98
Pneumonia Care				
Appropriate Initial Antibiotic Given	17	100%	98%	95%
Blood Culture Timing	32	97%	98%	98%
Pregnancy and Delivery Care				
Newborn Deliveries Scheduled Early[5]	-	-	2%	6%
Preventive Care				
Immunization for Influenza[5]	-	-	93%	90%
Immunization for Pneumonia[5]	-	-	94%	92%
Stroke Care				
Anticoagulation Therapy for Atrial Fibrillation[5]	-	-	98%	95%
Antithrombotic Therapy Timing[5]	-	-	99%	98%
Assessed for Rehabilitation[5]	-	-	98%	97%
Discharged on Antithrombotic Therapy[5]	-	-	100%	99%
Discharged on Statin Medication[5]	-	-	97%	94%
Thrombolytic Therapy Timing[5]	-	-	29%	66%
Venous Thromboembolism Prophylaxis[5]	-	-	96%	94%
Written Stroke Educational Materials Given[5]	-	-	86%	88%
Surgical Care Improvement Project				
Appropriate Beta Blocker Usage	31	100%	99%	98%
Appropriate VTP Within 24 Hours	56	100%	99%	98%
Controlled Postoperative Blood Glucose[7]	-	-	99%	97%
Perioperative Temperature Management	60	100%	100%	100%
Prophylactic Antibiotic Selection	48	100%	99%	99%
Prophylactic Antibiotic Selection (Outpatient)[5]	-	-	98%	98%
Prophylactic Antibiotic Stopped	48	100%	99%	98%
Prophylactic Antibiotic Timing	48	98%	99%	99%
Prophylactic Antibiotic Timing (Outpatient)[5]	-	-	96%	98%
Urinary Catheter Removal	59	98%	99%	97%
Survey of Patients' Hospital Experiences				
Area Around Room 'Always' Quiet at Night	(a)	65%	59%	61%
Doctors 'Always' Communicated Well	(a)	89%	83%	82%
Home Recovery Information Given	(a)	90%	90%	85%
Hospital Given 9 or 10 on 10 Point Scale	(a)	84%	74%	71%
Meds 'Always' Explained Before Given	(a)	79%	69%	64%
Nurses 'Always' Communicated Well	(a)	91%	82%	79%
Pain 'Always' Well Controlled	(a)	81%	73%	71%
Room and Bathroom 'Always' Clean	(a)	90%	80%	73%
Timely Help 'Always' Received	(a)	85%	72%	68%
Would Definitely Recommend Hospital	(a)	83%	77%	71%
Use of Medical Imaging				
Cardiac Imaging Stress Test before Surgery	130	6.2%	4.8%	5.3%
Combination Abdominal CT Scan	152	3.9%	5.2%	10.5%
Combination Brain/Sinus CT Scan[1]	-	-	1.7%	2.7%
Combination Chest CT Scan	89	0.0%	0.7%	2.7%
Follow-up Mammogram/Ultrasound	426	13.4%	7.7%	8.8%
Lumbar Spine MRI for Low Back Pain[1]	-	-	37.5%	37.2%

Stephens Memorial Hospital

181 Main Street
Norway, ME 04268
Phone: 207-743-5933
Type: Critical Access Hospitals
Emergency Services: Yes
Ownership: Voluntary non-profit - Private

Measure	Cases	This Hosp.	State Avg.	U.S. Avg.
Blood Clot Prevention and Treatment				
Anticoagulation Overlap Therapy[5]	-	-	98%	93%
ICU Venous Thromboembolism Prophylaxis[5]	-	-	96%	92%
Incidence of Potentially Preventable VTE[5]	-	-	2%	10%
UFH with Dosages/Platelet Monitoring[5]	-	-	100%	97%
Venous Thromboembolism Prophylaxis[5]	-	-	95%	85%
Warfarin Therapy Discharge Instructions[5]	-	-	84%	75%
Chest Pain/Possible Heart Attack Care				
Aspirin Given Within 24 Hours of Arrival	36	100%	99%	96%
Fibrinolytic Meds Within 30 Min. of Arrival[1]	-	-	86%	58%
Average Time to ECG (minutes)	39	3	6	7
Average Time to Transfer (minutes)[1]	-	-	49	60
Children's Asthma Care				
Received Home Management Plan of Care	-	-	-	88%
Received Reliever Medication	-	-	-	100%
Received Systemic Corticosteroids	-	-	-	100%
Emergency Department				
Admittance Decision Time (minutes)[2]	387	53	110	98
Head CT Results Within 45 Min. of Arrival[5]	-	-	44%	57%
Patients Who Left ER Before Being Seen	18,568	1%	1%	2%
Time from ER Arrival to Admit. (minutes)[2]	423	236	288	274
Time from ER Arrival to Discharge (minutes)	376	109	122	134
Time in ER Before Being Evaluated (minutes)	404	24	28	26
Time to Pain Meds for Fractures (minutes)[5]	-	-	52	57
Heart Attack Care				
Aspirin Given at Discharge[1]	-	-	100%	99%
Fibrinolytic Meds Within 30 Min. of Arrival[7]	-	-	50%	54%
PCI Within 90 Minutes of Arrival[7]	-	-	96%	96%
Statin Prescribed at Discharge	11	82%	99%	98%
Heart Failure Care				
ACE Inhibitor or ARB for LVSD	12	100%	99%	97%
Discharge Instructions Given	30	93%	98%	94%
Evaluation of LVS Function	41	100%	100%	99%
Medicare Spending				
Medicare Spending per Patient (ratio)	-	-	0.95	0.98
Pneumonia Care				
Appropriate Initial Antibiotic Given[2]	55	98%	98%	95%
Blood Culture Timing[2]	94	98%	98%	98%
Pregnancy and Delivery Care				
Newborn Deliveries Scheduled Early	13	0%	2%	6%
Preventive Care				
Immunization for Influenza[2]	304	97%	93%	90%
Immunization for Pneumonia[2]	444	98%	94%	92%
Stroke Care				
Anticoagulation Therapy for Atrial Fibrillation[5]	-	-	98%	95%
Antithrombotic Therapy Timing[5]	-	-	99%	98%
Assessed for Rehabilitation[5]	-	-	98%	97%
Discharged on Antithrombotic Therapy[5]	-	-	100%	99%
Discharged on Statin Medication[5]	-	-	97%	94%
Thrombolytic Therapy Timing[5]	-	-	29%	66%
Venous Thromboembolism Prophylaxis[5]	-	-	96%	94%
Written Stroke Educational Materials Given[5]	-	-	86%	88%
Surgical Care Improvement Project				
Appropriate Beta Blocker Usage[2]	30	100%	99%	98%
Appropriate VTP Within 24 Hours[2]	100	98%	99%	98%
Controlled Postoperative Blood Glucose[2,7]	-	-	99%	97%
Perioperative Temperature Management[2]	113	100%	100%	100%
Prophylactic Antibiotic Selection[2]	76	100%	99%	99%
Prophylactic Antibiotic Selection (Outpatient)	44	98%	98%	98%
Prophylactic Antibiotic Stopped[2]	75	99%	99%	98%
Prophylactic Antibiotic Timing[2]	76	100%	99%	99%
Prophylactic Antibiotic Timing (Outpatient)	44	100%	96%	98%
Urinary Catheter Removal[2]	87	97%	99%	97%
Survey of Patients' Hospital Experiences				
Area Around Room 'Always' Quiet at Night	(a)	67%	59%	61%
Doctors 'Always' Communicated Well	(a)	84%	83%	82%
Home Recovery Information Given	(a)	93%	90%	85%
Hospital Given 9 or 10 on 10 Point Scale	(a)	73%	74%	71%
Meds 'Always' Explained Before Given	(a)	73%	69%	64%
Nurses 'Always' Communicated Well	(a)	84%	82%	79%
Pain 'Always' Well Controlled	(a)	72%	73%	71%
Room and Bathroom 'Always' Clean	(a)	82%	80%	73%
Timely Help 'Always' Received	(a)	74%	72%	68%
Would Definitely Recommend Hospital	(a)	75%	77%	71%
Use of Medical Imaging				
Cardiac Imaging Stress Test before Surgery	86	7.0%	4.8%	5.3%
Combination Abdominal CT Scan	459	4.6%	5.2%	10.5%
Combination Brain/Sinus CT Scan	381	1.6%	1.7%	2.7%
Combination Chest CT Scan	332	2.4%	0.7%	2.7%
Follow-up Mammogram/Ultrasound	1,113	7.4%	7.7%	8.8%
Lumbar Spine MRI for Low Back Pain	94	53.2%	37.5%	37.2%

Sebasticook Valley Hospital

447 North Main Street
Pittsfield, ME 04967
Phone: 207-487-5141
Fax: 207-487-3204
URL: www.sebasticookhospital.org
Type: Critical Access Hospitals
Emergency Services: Yes
Ownership: Voluntary non-profit - Private
Beds: 25

Key Personnel:
Quality Assurance . . . . Sharon King
Chief of Medical Staff . . . . Mohammad Niayesh, MD, FACS
Administrator . . . . Michael Peterson, FACHE
CEO/President. . . . . Terri Vieira

Measure	Cases	This Hosp.	State Avg.	U.S. Avg.
Blood Clot Prevention and Treatment				
Anticoagulation Overlap Therapy[5]	-	-	98%	93%
ICU Venous Thromboembolism Prophylaxis[5]	-	-	96%	92%
Incidence of Potentially Preventable VTE[5]	-	-	2%	10%
UFH with Dosages/Platelet Monitoring[5]	-	-	100%	97%
Venous Thromboembolism Prophylaxis[5]	-	-	95%	85%
Warfarin Therapy Discharge Instructions[5]	-	-	84%	75%
Chest Pain/Possible Heart Attack Care				
Aspirin Given Within 24 Hours of Arrival[3]	14	100%	99%	96%
Fibrinolytic Meds Within 30 Min. of Arrival[1,3]	-	-	86%	58%
Average Time to ECG (minutes)[3]	14	12	6	7
Average Time to Transfer (minutes)[3,7]	-	-	49	60
Children's Asthma Care				
Received Home Management Plan of Care	-	-	-	88%
Received Reliever Medication	-	-	-	100%
Received Systemic Corticosteroids	-	-	-	100%
Emergency Department				
Admittance Decision Time (minutes)[5]	-	-	110	98
Head CT Results Within 45 Min. of Arrival[5]	-	-	44%	57%
Patients Who Left ER Before Being Seen[5]	-	-	1%	2%
Time from ER Arrival to Admit. (minutes)[5]	-	-	288	274
Time from ER Arrival to Discharge (minutes)[5]	-	-	122	134
Time in ER Before Being Evaluated (minutes)[5]	-	-	28	26
Time to Pain Meds for Fractures (minutes)[5]	-	-	52	57
Heart Attack Care				
Aspirin Given at Discharge[1]	-	-	100%	99%
Fibrinolytic Meds Within 30 Min. of Arrival[7]	-	-	50%	54%
PCI Within 90 Minutes of Arrival[7]	-	-	96%	96%
Statin Prescribed at Discharge[1]	-	-	99%	98%
Heart Failure Care				
ACE Inhibitor or ARB for LVSD[1]	-	-	99%	97%
Discharge Instructions Given	28	96%	98%	94%
Evaluation of LVS Function	29	100%	100%	99%
Medicare Spending				
Medicare Spending per Patient (ratio)	-	-	0.95	0.98
Pneumonia Care				
Appropriate Initial Antibiotic Given	27	100%	98%	95%
Blood Culture Timing	29	97%	98%	98%
Pregnancy and Delivery Care				
Newborn Deliveries Scheduled Early[5]	-	-	2%	6%
Preventive Care				
Immunization for Influenza[5]	-	-	93%	90%
Immunization for Pneumonia[5]	-	-	94%	92%
Stroke Care				
Anticoagulation Therapy for Atrial Fibrillation[5]	-	-	98%	95%

NOTE: Hospital profiles are in alphabetical order by state, then city, then hospital within the city; Rankings exclude hospitals with less than 25 cases except for patient surveys which excludes hospitals with less than 100 cases; (a) 100-299 cases; (1) The number of cases/patients is too few to report; (2) Data submitted were based on a sample of cases/patients; (3) Results are based on a shorter time period than required; (4) Data suppressed by CMS for one or more quarters; (5) Results are not available for this reporting period; (6) Fewer than 100 patients completed the HCAHPS survey; (7) No cases met the criteria for this measure; (8) The lower limit of the confidence interval cannot be calculated if the number of observed infections equals zero; (9) No data are available from the state/territory for this reporting period; (10) The scores shown reflect fewer than 50 completed surveys; (11) There were discrepancies in the data collection process; (12) This measure does not apply to this hospital for this reporting period; (13) Results cannot be calculated for this reporting period; (14) The results for this state are combined with nearby states to protect confidentiality; Please refer to the User's Guide for a full explanation of data.

Measure	Cases	This Hosp.	State Avg.	U.S. Avg.
Antithrombotic Therapy Timing[5]	-	-	99%	98%
Assessed for Rehabilitation[5]	-	-	98%	97%
Discharged on Antithrombotic Therapy[5]	-	-	100%	99%
Discharged on Statin Medication[5]	-	-	97%	94%
Thrombolytic Therapy Timing[5]	-	-	29%	66%
Venous Thromboembolism Prophylaxis[5]	-	-	96%	94%
Written Stroke Educational Materials Given[5]	-	-	86%	88%
Surgical Care Improvement Project				
Appropriate Beta Blocker Usage[1]	-	-	99%	98%
Appropriate VTP Within 24 Hours	21	100%	99%	98%
Controlled Postoperative Blood Glucose[7]	-	-	99%	97%
Perioperative Temperature Management	23	100%	100%	100%
Prophylactic Antibiotic Selection	15	100%	99%	99%
Prophylactic Antibiotic Selection (Outpatient)[5]	-	-	98%	98%
Prophylactic Antibiotic Stopped	15	100%	99%	98%
Prophylactic Antibiotic Timing	15	100%	99%	99%
Prophylactic Antibiotic Timing (Outpatient)[5]	-	-	96%	98%
Urinary Catheter Removal	14	100%	99%	97%
Survey of Patients' Hospital Experiences				
Area Around Room 'Always' Quiet at Night	(a)	60%	59%	61%
Doctors 'Always' Communicated Well	(a)	71%	83%	82%
Home Recovery Information Given	(a)	89%	90%	85%
Hospital Given 9 or 10 on 10 Point Scale	(a)	65%	74%	71%
Meds 'Always' Explained Before Given	(a)	64%	69%	64%
Nurses 'Always' Communicated Well	(a)	79%	82%	79%
Pain 'Always' Well Controlled	(a)	71%	73%	71%
Room and Bathroom 'Always' Clean	(a)	70%	80%	73%
Timely Help 'Always' Received	(a)	73%	72%	68%
Would Definitely Recommend Hospital	(a)	71%	77%	71%
Use of Medical Imaging				
Cardiac Imaging Stress Test before Surgery	229	5.2%	4.8%	5.3%
Combination Abdominal CT Scan	290	4.5%	5.2%	10.5%
Combination Brain/Sinus CT Scan	245	0.0%	1.7%	2.7%
Combination Chest CT Scan	102	0.0%	0.7%	2.7%
Follow-up Mammogram/Ultrasound	725	4.8%	7.7%	8.8%
Lumbar Spine MRI for Low Back Pain	65	41.5%	37.5%	37.2%

Maine Medical Center

22 Bramhall St
Portland, ME 04102
Phone: 207-662-0111
Fax: 207-871-6212
URL: www.mmc.org
Type: Acute Care Hospitals
Emergency Services: Yes
Ownership: Voluntary non-profit - Private
Beds: 605
Key Personnel:
Operating Room............. Karen Dumond
CEO/President............... Richard W. Peterson, FACHE
Chief of Medical Staff.......... James H. Zeitlin, MD, MPH

Measure	Cases	This Hosp.	State Avg.	U.S. Avg.
Blood Clot Prevention and Treatment				
Anticoagulation Overlap Therapy[2]	157	99%	98%	93%
ICU Venous Thromboembolism Prophylaxis[2]	50	100%	96%	92%
Incidence of Potentially Preventable VTE[2]	49	2%	2%	10%
UFH with Dosages/Platelet Monitoring[2]	174	100%	100%	97%
Venous Thromboembolism Prophylaxis[2]	340	98%	95%	85%
Warfarin Therapy Discharge Instructions[2]	114	73%	84%	75%
Chest Pain/Possible Heart Attack Care				
Aspirin Given Within 24 Hours of Arrival[3,7]	-	-	99%	96%
Fibrinolytic Meds Within 30 Min. of Arrival[5]	-	-	86%	58%
Average Time to ECG (minutes)[3,7]	-	-	6	7
Average Time to Transfer (minutes)[5]	-	-	49	60
Children's Asthma Care				
Received Home Management Plan of Care	-	-	-	88%
Received Reliever Medication	-	-	-	100%
Received Systemic Corticosteroids	-	-	-	100%
Emergency Department				
Admittance Decision Time (minutes)[2]	464	107	110	98
Head CT Results Within 45 Min. of Arrival	27	11%	44%	57%
Patients Who Left ER Before Being Seen	66,049	2%	1%	2%
Time from ER Arrival to Admit. (minutes)[2]	486	342	288	274
Time from ER Arrival to Discharge (minutes)	360	236	122	134
Time in ER Before Being Evaluated (minutes)	411	36	28	26
Time to Pain Meds for Fractures (minutes)	291	57	52	57
Heart Attack Care				
Aspirin Given at Discharge	1,138	100%	100%	99%
Fibrinolytic Meds Within 30 Min. of Arrival[7]	-	-	50%	54%
PCI Within 90 Minutes of Arrival	77	97%	96%	96%
Statin Prescribed at Discharge	1,108	99%	99%	98%
Heart Failure Care				
ACE Inhibitor or ARB for LVSD	109	99%	99%	97%
Discharge Instructions Given	424	97%	98%	94%
Evaluation of LVS Function	593	100%	100%	99%
Medicare Spending				
Medicare Spending per Patient (ratio)	-	0.99	0.95	0.98
Pneumonia Care				
Appropriate Initial Antibiotic Given	120	100%	98%	95%
Blood Culture Timing	215	99%	98%	98%
Pregnancy and Delivery Care				
Newborn Deliveries Scheduled Early	121	2%	2%	6%
Preventive Care				
Immunization for Influenza[2]	552	85%	93%	90%
Immunization for Pneumonia[2]	625	81%	94%	92%
Stroke Care				
Anticoagulation Therapy for Atrial Fibrillation	33	94%	98%	95%
Antithrombotic Therapy Timing	157	97%	99%	98%
Assessed for Rehabilitation	259	96%	98%	97%
Discharged on Antithrombotic Therapy	192	100%	100%	99%
Discharged on Statin Medication	157	96%	97%	94%
Thrombolytic Therapy Timing	94	18%	29%	66%
Venous Thromboembolism Prophylaxis	268	92%	96%	94%
Written Stroke Educational Materials Given	115	66%	86%	88%
Surgical Care Improvement Project				
Appropriate Beta Blocker Usage[2]	305	100%	99%	98%
Appropriate VTP Within 24 Hours[2]	437	100%	99%	98%
Controlled Postoperative Blood Glucose[2]	198	99%	99%	97%
Perioperative Temperature Management[2]	700	99%	100%	100%
Prophylactic Antibiotic Selection[2]	640	100%	99%	99%
Prophylactic Antibiotic Selection (Outpatient)	972	98%	98%	98%
Prophylactic Antibiotic Stopped[2]	637	98%	99%	98%
Prophylactic Antibiotic Timing[2]	639	97%	99%	99%
Prophylactic Antibiotic Timing (Outpatient)	1,005	93%	96%	98%
Urinary Catheter Removal[2]	417	100%	99%	97%
Survey of Patients' Hospital Experiences				
Area Around Room 'Always' Quiet at Night	300+	55%	59%	61%
Doctors 'Always' Communicated Well	300+	81%	83%	82%
Home Recovery Information Given	300+	88%	90%	85%
Hospital Given 9 or 10 on 10 Point Scale	300+	76%	74%	71%
Meds 'Always' Explained Before Given	300+	65%	69%	64%
Nurses 'Always' Communicated Well	300+	80%	82%	79%
Pain 'Always' Well Controlled	300+	73%	73%	71%
Room and Bathroom 'Always' Clean	300+	74%	80%	73%
Timely Help 'Always' Received	300+	65%	72%	68%
Would Definitely Recommend Hospital	300+	79%	77%	71%
Use of Medical Imaging				
Cardiac Imaging Stress Test before Surgery	1,816	4.4%	4.8%	5.3%
Combination Abdominal CT Scan	1,833	3.2%	5.2%	10.5%
Combination Brain/Sinus CT Scan	1,253	1.0%	1.7%	2.7%
Combination Chest CT Scan	1,685	0.8%	0.7%	2.7%
Follow-up Mammogram/Ultrasound	2,066	10.5%	7.7%	8.8%
Lumbar Spine MRI for Low Back Pain	152	34.2%	37.5%	37.2%

Mercy Hospital

144 State Street
Portland, ME 04101
Phone: 207-879-3000
Fax: 207-879-3666
URL: www.mercyhospital.com
Type: Acute Care Hospitals
Emergency Services: Yes
Ownership: Voluntary non-profit - Church
Key Personnel:
Emergency Room .... Rebecca Bloch
Patient Relations .... Jill Berry Bowen, RN, CHE
Radiology.................. Greatorex David
Chief of Medical Staff......... Stephen Sears, MD
CEO/President.............. Eileen F Skinner

Measure	Cases	This Hosp.	State Avg.	U.S. Avg.
Blood Clot Prevention and Treatment				
Anticoagulation Overlap Therapy[2]	34	97%	98%	93%
ICU Venous Thromboembolism Prophylaxis[1,2]	-	-	96%	92%
Incidence of Potentially Preventable VTE[1,2]	-	-	2%	10%
UFH with Dosages/Platelet Monitoring[2]	19	100%	100%	97%
Venous Thromboembolism Prophylaxis[2]	294	96%	95%	85%
Warfarin Therapy Discharge Instructions[2]	20	55%	84%	75%
Chest Pain/Possible Heart Attack Care				
Aspirin Given Within 24 Hours of Arrival[1]	-	-	99%	96%
Fibrinolytic Meds Within 30 Min. of Arrival[7]	-	-	86%	58%
Average Time to ECG (minutes)[1]	-	-	6	7
Average Time to Transfer (minutes)[1]	-	-	49	60
Children's Asthma Care				
Received Home Management Plan of Care	-	-	-	88%
Received Reliever Medication	-	-	-	100%
Received Systemic Corticosteroids	-	-	-	100%
Emergency Department				
Admittance Decision Time (minutes)[2]	453	147	110	98
Head CT Results Within 45 Min. of Arrival[1]	-	-	44%	57%
Patients Who Left ER Before Being Seen	27,579	1%	1%	2%
Time from ER Arrival to Admit. (minutes)[2]	470	407	288	274
Time from ER Arrival to Discharge (minutes)	350	160	122	134
Time in ER Before Being Evaluated (minutes)	330	30	28	26
Time to Pain Meds for Fractures (minutes)	65	55	52	57
Heart Attack Care				
Aspirin Given at Discharge	22	100%	100%	99%
Fibrinolytic Meds Within 30 Min. of Arrival[7]	-	-	50%	54%
PCI Within 90 Minutes of Arrival[7]	-	-	96%	96%
Statin Prescribed at Discharge	20	100%	99%	98%
Heart Failure Care				
ACE Inhibitor or ARB for LVSD	14	100%	99%	97%
Discharge Instructions Given	82	93%	98%	94%
Evaluation of LVS Function	112	100%	100%	99%
Medicare Spending				
Medicare Spending per Patient (ratio)	-	1.00	0.95	0.98
Pneumonia Care				
Appropriate Initial Antibiotic Given	112	97%	98%	95%
Blood Culture Timing	144	100%	98%	98%
Pregnancy and Delivery Care				
Newborn Deliveries Scheduled Early	40	2%	2%	6%
Preventive Care				
Immunization for Influenza[2]	539	92%	93%	90%
Immunization for Pneumonia[2]	680	92%	94%	92%
Stroke Care				
Anticoagulation Therapy for Atrial Fibrillation[1]	-	-	98%	95%
Antithrombotic Therapy Timing	22	100%	99%	98%
Assessed for Rehabilitation	18	100%	98%	97%
Discharged on Antithrombotic Therapy	16	94%	100%	99%
Discharged on Statin Medication	13	100%	97%	94%
Thrombolytic Therapy Timing[1]	-	-	29%	66%
Venous Thromboembolism Prophylaxis	28	89%	96%	94%
Written Stroke Educational Materials Given[1]	-	-	86%	88%
Surgical Care Improvement Project				
Appropriate Beta Blocker Usage[2]	187	99%	99%	98%
Appropriate VTP Within 24 Hours[2]	548	99%	99%	98%
Controlled Postoperative Blood Glucose[2,7]	-	-	99%	97%
Perioperative Temperature Management[2]	618	100%	100%	100%
Prophylactic Antibiotic Selection[2]	471	100%	99%	99%
Prophylactic Antibiotic Selection (Outpatient)	580	99%	98%	98%
Prophylactic Antibiotic Stopped[2]	464	100%	99%	98%
Prophylactic Antibiotic Timing[2]	471	99%	99%	99%
Prophylactic Antibiotic Timing (Outpatient)	562	100%	96%	98%
Urinary Catheter Removal[2]	488	97%	99%	97%
Survey of Patients' Hospital Experiences				
Area Around Room 'Always' Quiet at Night	300+	70%	59%	61%
Doctors 'Always' Communicated Well	300+	84%	83%	82%
Home Recovery Information Given	300+	93%	90%	85%
Hospital Given 9 or 10 on 10 Point Scale	300+	79%	74%	71%
Meds 'Always' Explained Before Given	300+	66%	69%	64%
Nurses 'Always' Communicated Well	300+	82%	82%	79%
Pain 'Always' Well Controlled	300+	72%	73%	71%
Room and Bathroom 'Always' Clean	300+	73%	80%	73%
Timely Help 'Always' Received	300+	69%	72%	68%
Would Definitely Recommend Hospital	300+	84%	77%	71%
Use of Medical Imaging				

NOTE: Hospital profiles are in alphabetical order by state, then city, then hospital within the city; Rankings exclude hospitals with less than 25 cases except for patient surveys which excludes hospitals with less than 100 cases; (a) 100-299 cases; (1) The number of cases/patients is too few to report; (2) Data submitted were based on a sample of cases/patients; (3) Results are based on a shorter time period than required; (4) Data suppressed by CMS for one or more quarters; (5) Results are not available for this reporting period; (6) Fewer than 100 patients completed the HCAHPS survey; (7) No cases met the criteria for this measure; (8) The lower limit of the confidence interval cannot be calculated if the number of observed infections equals zero; (9) No data are available from the state/territory for this reporting period; (10) The scores shown reflect fewer than 50 completed surveys; (11) There were discrepancies in the data collection process; (12) This measure does not apply to this hospital for this reporting period; (13) Results cannot be calculated for this reporting period; (14) The results for this state are combined with nearby states to protect confidentiality; Please refer to the User's Guide for a full explanation of data.

Measure	Cases	This Hosp.	State Avg.	U.S. Avg.
Cardiac Imaging Stress Test before Surgery	163	7.4%	4.8%	5.3%
Combination Abdominal CT Scan	671	8.2%	5.2%	10.5%
Combination Brain/Sinus CT Scan	506	2.4%	1.7%	2.7%
Combination Chest CT Scan	372	0.3%	0.7%	2.7%
Follow-up Mammogram/Ultrasound	2,010	9.2%	7.7%	8.8%
Lumbar Spine MRI for Low Back Pain	130	33.1%	37.5%	37.2%

The Aroostook Medical Center

140 Academy Saint - PO Box 151
Presque Isle, ME 04769
Phone: 207-768-4000
Fax: 207-768-4226
URL: www.tamc.org
Type: Acute Care Hospitals
Emergency Services: Yes
Ownership: Voluntary non-profit - Private
Beds: 177

Key Personnel:

Chief of Medical Staff.......... Lawrence Crystal
Emergency Room .... Sharon Lesbear
CEO/President............... David A Peterson
Quality Assurance .... Stephen A Poitras

Measure	Cases	This Hosp.	State Avg.	U.S. Avg.
Blood Clot Prevention and Treatment				
Anticoagulation Overlap Therapy[1,2]	-	-	98%	93%
ICU Venous Thromboembolism Prophylaxis[2]	101	94%	96%	92%
Incidence of Potentially Preventable VTE[1,2]	-	-	2%	10%
UFH with Dosages/Platelet Monitoring[1,2]	-	-	100%	97%
Venous Thromboembolism Prophylaxis[2]	362	95%	95%	85%
Warfarin Therapy Discharge Instructions[2]	11	100%	84%	75%
Chest Pain/Possible Heart Attack Care				
Aspirin Given Within 24 Hours of Arrival	38	100%	99%	96%
Fibrinolytic Meds Within 30 Min. of Arrival	12	67%	86%	58%
Average Time to ECG (minutes)	38	6	6	7
Average Time to Transfer (minutes)[7]	-	-	49	60
Children's Asthma Care				
Received Home Management Plan of Care	-	-	-	88%
Received Reliever Medication	-	-	-	100%
Received Systemic Corticosteroids	-	-	-	100%
Emergency Department				
Admittance Decision Time (minutes)[2]	326	150	110	98
Head CT Results Within 45 Min. of Arrival[1]	-	-	44%	57%
Patients Who Left ER Before Being Seen	14,942	2%	1%	2%
Time from ER Arrival to Admit. (minutes)[2]	334	254	288	274
Time from ER Arrival to Discharge (minutes)	400	111	122	134
Time in ER Before Being Evaluated (minutes)	292	32	28	26
Time to Pain Meds for Fractures (minutes)	60	48	52	57
Heart Attack Care				
Aspirin Given at Discharge	41	100%	100%	99%
Fibrinolytic Meds Within 30 Min. of Arrival[1]	-	-	50%	54%
PCI Within 90 Minutes of Arrival[7]	-	-	96%	96%
Statin Prescribed at Discharge	35	100%	99%	98%
Heart Failure Care				
ACE Inhibitor or ARB for LVSD	32	100%	99%	97%
Discharge Instructions Given	83	99%	98%	94%
Evaluation of LVS Function	100	100%	100%	99%
Medicare Spending				
Medicare Spending per Patient (ratio)	-	0.86	0.95	0.98
Pneumonia Care				
Appropriate Initial Antibiotic Given	46	96%	98%	95%
Blood Culture Timing	106	100%	98%	98%
Pregnancy and Delivery Care				
Newborn Deliveries Scheduled Early[1]	-	-	2%	6%
Preventive Care				
Immunization for Influenza[2]	294	98%	93%	90%
Immunization for Pneumonia[2]	405	99%	94%	92%
Stroke Care				
Anticoagulation Therapy for Atrial Fibrillation[1]	-	-	98%	95%
Antithrombotic Therapy Timing	14	100%	99%	98%
Assessed for Rehabilitation	14	100%	98%	97%
Discharged on Antithrombotic Therapy	14	100%	100%	99%
Discharged on Statin Medication	12	92%	97%	94%
Thrombolytic Therapy Timing[1]	-	-	29%	66%
Venous Thromboembolism Prophylaxis	15	100%	96%	94%
Written Stroke Educational Materials Given[1]	-	-	86%	88%
Surgical Care Improvement Project				
Appropriate Beta Blocker Usage	51	98%	99%	98%
Appropriate VTP Within 24 Hours	95	100%	99%	98%
Controlled Postoperative Blood Glucose[7]	-	-	99%	97%
Perioperative Temperature Management	122	100%	100%	100%
Prophylactic Antibiotic Selection	79	99%	99%	99%
Prophylactic Antibiotic Selection (Outpatient)	139	99%	98%	98%
Prophylactic Antibiotic Stopped	77	100%	99%	98%
Prophylactic Antibiotic Timing	79	99%	99%	99%
Prophylactic Antibiotic Timing (Outpatient)	98	99%	96%	98%
Urinary Catheter Removal	81	100%	99%	97%
Survey of Patients' Hospital Experiences				
Area Around Room 'Always' Quiet at Night	300+	47%	59%	61%
Doctors 'Always' Communicated Well	300+	75%	83%	82%
Home Recovery Information Given	300+	86%	90%	85%
Hospital Given 9 or 10 on 10 Point Scale	300+	69%	74%	71%
Meds 'Always' Explained Before Given	300+	63%	69%	64%
Nurses 'Always' Communicated Well	300+	75%	82%	79%
Pain 'Always' Well Controlled	300+	68%	73%	71%
Room and Bathroom 'Always' Clean	300+	80%	80%	73%
Timely Help 'Always' Received	300+	65%	72%	68%
Would Definitely Recommend Hospital	300+	67%	77%	71%
Use of Medical Imaging				
Cardiac Imaging Stress Test before Surgery	302	4.0%	4.8%	5.3%
Combination Abdominal CT Scan	537	16.8%	5.2%	10.5%
Combination Brain/Sinus CT Scan[1]	-	-	1.7%	2.7%
Combination Chest CT Scan	410	5.1%	0.7%	2.7%
Follow-up Mammogram/Ultrasound	1,339	8.1%	7.7%	8.8%
Lumbar Spine MRI for Low Back Pain[1]	-	-	37.5%	37.2%

Penobscot Bay Medical Center

6 Glen Cove Drive
Rockport, ME 04856
Phone: 207-596-8000
Fax: 207-593-6710
URL: www.nehealth.org
Type: Acute Care Hospitals
Emergency Services: Yes
Ownership: Voluntary non-profit - Private
Beds: 106

Key Personnel:

Radiology.................... Charles A Crans, Jr
CEO/President............... Roy Hitthing

Measure	Cases	This Hosp.	State Avg.	U.S. Avg.
Blood Clot Prevention and Treatment				
Anticoagulation Overlap Therapy[2]	15	100%	98%	93%
ICU Venous Thromboembolism Prophylaxis[2]	14	93%	96%	92%
Incidence of Potentially Preventable VTE[1,2]	-	-	2%	10%
UFH with Dosages/Platelet Monitoring[1,2]	-	-	100%	97%
Venous Thromboembolism Prophylaxis[2]	274	95%	95%	85%
Warfarin Therapy Discharge Instructions[2]	14	93%	84%	75%
Chest Pain/Possible Heart Attack Care				
Aspirin Given Within 24 Hours of Arrival	53	98%	99%	96%
Fibrinolytic Meds Within 30 Min. of Arrival	15	73%	86%	58%
Average Time to ECG (minutes)	54	7	6	7
Average Time to Transfer (minutes)[7]	-	-	49	60
Children's Asthma Care				
Received Home Management Plan of Care	-	-	-	88%
Received Reliever Medication	-	-	-	100%
Received Systemic Corticosteroids	-	-	-	100%
Emergency Department				
Admittance Decision Time (minutes)[2]	458	121	110	98
Head CT Results Within 45 Min. of Arrival[1]	-	-	44%	57%
Patients Who Left ER Before Being Seen	23,770	1%	1%	2%
Time from ER Arrival to Admit. (minutes)[2]	458	288	288	274
Time from ER Arrival to Discharge (minutes)	382	111	122	134
Time in ER Before Being Evaluated (minutes)	408	18	28	26
Time to Pain Meds for Fractures (minutes)	68	26	52	57
Heart Attack Care				
Aspirin Given at Discharge	23	96%	100%	99%
Fibrinolytic Meds Within 30 Min. of Arrival[7]	-	-	50%	54%
PCI Within 90 Minutes of Arrival[7]	-	-	96%	96%
Statin Prescribed at Discharge	24	88%	99%	98%
Heart Failure Care				
ACE Inhibitor or ARB for LVSD	14	100%	99%	97%
Discharge Instructions Given	55	100%	98%	94%
Evaluation of LVS Function	70	100%	100%	99%
Medicare Spending				
Medicare Spending per Patient (ratio)	-	0.94	0.95	0.98
Pneumonia Care				
Appropriate Initial Antibiotic Given	77	96%	98%	95%
Blood Culture Timing	121	98%	98%	98%
Pregnancy and Delivery Care				
Newborn Deliveries Scheduled Early	21	0%	2%	6%
Preventive Care				
Immunization for Influenza[2]	299	82%	93%	90%
Immunization for Pneumonia[2]	418	84%	94%	92%
Stroke Care				
Anticoagulation Therapy for Atrial Fibrillation[1]	-	-	98%	95%
Antithrombotic Therapy Timing	54	100%	99%	98%
Assessed for Rehabilitation	70	97%	98%	97%
Discharged on Antithrombotic Therapy	69	100%	100%	99%
Discharged on Statin Medication	52	98%	97%	94%
Thrombolytic Therapy Timing[1]	-	-	29%	66%
Venous Thromboembolism Prophylaxis	66	91%	96%	94%
Written Stroke Educational Materials Given	36	97%	86%	88%
Surgical Care Improvement Project				
Appropriate Beta Blocker Usage	76	97%	99%	98%
Appropriate VTP Within 24 Hours	204	100%	99%	98%
Controlled Postoperative Blood Glucose[7]	-	-	99%	97%
Perioperative Temperature Management	237	100%	100%	100%
Prophylactic Antibiotic Selection	174	99%	99%	99%
Prophylactic Antibiotic Selection (Outpatient)	71	97%	98%	98%
Prophylactic Antibiotic Stopped	172	98%	99%	98%
Prophylactic Antibiotic Timing	174	99%	99%	99%
Prophylactic Antibiotic Timing (Outpatient)	46	96%	96%	98%
Urinary Catheter Removal	125	98%	99%	97%
Survey of Patients' Hospital Experiences				
Area Around Room 'Always' Quiet at Night	300+	58%	59%	61%
Doctors 'Always' Communicated Well	300+	82%	83%	82%
Home Recovery Information Given	300+	88%	90%	85%
Hospital Given 9 or 10 on 10 Point Scale	300+	67%	74%	71%
Meds 'Always' Explained Before Given	300+	64%	69%	64%
Nurses 'Always' Communicated Well	300+	78%	82%	79%
Pain 'Always' Well Controlled	300+	70%	73%	71%
Room and Bathroom 'Always' Clean	300+	72%	80%	73%
Timely Help 'Always' Received	300+	69%	72%	68%
Would Definitely Recommend Hospital	300+	66%	77%	71%
Use of Medical Imaging				
Cardiac Imaging Stress Test before Surgery	266	2.3%	4.8%	5.3%
Combination Abdominal CT Scan	506	4.3%	5.2%	10.5%
Combination Brain/Sinus CT Scan	421	0.7%	1.7%	2.7%
Combination Chest CT Scan	439	0.5%	0.7%	2.7%
Follow-up Mammogram/Ultrasound[7]	-	-	7.7%	8.8%
Lumbar Spine MRI for Low Back Pain[1]	-	-	37.5%	37.2%

Rumford Hospital

420 Franklin Street
Rumford, ME 04276
Phone: 207-369-1000
Fax: 207-369-0834
URL: www.rumfordhospital.org
Type: Critical Access Hospitals
Emergency Services: Yes
Ownership: Voluntary non-profit - Private
Beds: 49

Key Personnel:

Radiology.................... John J Bennett
CEO/President............... John Welsh

Measure	Cases	This Hosp.	State Avg.	U.S. Avg.
Blood Clot Prevention and Treatment				
Anticoagulation Overlap Therapy[5]	-	-	98%	93%
ICU Venous Thromboembolism Prophylaxis[5]	-	-	96%	92%
Incidence of Potentially Preventable VTE[5]	-	-	2%	10%
UFH with Dosages/Platelet Monitoring[5]	-	-	100%	97%
Venous Thromboembolism Prophylaxis[5]	-	-	95%	85%
Warfarin Therapy Discharge Instructions[5]	-	-	84%	75%
Chest Pain/Possible Heart Attack Care				
Aspirin Given Within 24 Hours of Arrival[5]	-	-	99%	96%
Fibrinolytic Meds Within 30 Min. of Arrival[5]	-	-	86%	58%
Average Time to ECG (minutes)[5]	-	-	6	7
Average Time to Transfer (minutes)[5]	-	-	49	60
Children's Asthma Care				
Received Home Management Plan of Care	-	-	-	88%
Received Reliever Medication	-	-	-	100%
Received Systemic Corticosteroids	-	-	-	100%

NOTE: Hospital profiles are in alphabetical order by state, then city, then hospital within the city; Rankings exclude hospitals with less than 25 cases except for patient surveys which excludes hospitals with less than 100 cases; (a) 100-299 cases; (1) The number of cases/patients is too few to report; (2) Data submitted were based on a sample of cases/patients; (3) Results are based on a shorter time period than required; (4) Data suppressed by CMS for one or more quarters; (5) Results are not available for this reporting period; (6) Fewer than 100 patients completed the HCAHPS survey; (7) No cases met the criteria for this measure; (8) The lower limit of the confidence interval cannot be calculated if the number of observed infections equals zero; (9) No data are available from the state/territory for this reporting period; (10) The scores shown reflect fewer than 50 completed surveys; (11) There were discrepancies in the data collection process; (12) This measure does not apply to this hospital for this reporting period; (13) Results cannot be calculated for this reporting period; (14) The results for this state are combined with nearby states to protect confidentiality; Please refer to the User's Guide for a full explanation of data.

Measure	Cases	This Hosp.	State Avg.	U.S. Avg.
Emergency Department				
Admittance Decision Time (minutes)[5]	-	-	110	98
Head CT Results Within 45 Min. of Arrival[5]	-	-	44%	57%
Patients Who Left ER Before Being Seen[5]	-	-	1%	2%
Time from ER Arrival to Admit. (minutes)[5]	-	-	288	274
Time from ER Arrival to Discharge (minutes)[5]	-	-	122	134
Time in ER Before Being Evaluated (minutes)[5]	-	-	28	26
Time to Pain Meds for Fractures (minutes)[5]	-	-	52	57
Heart Attack Care				
Aspirin Given at Discharge[5]	-	-	100%	99%
Fibrinolytic Meds Within 30 Min. of Arrival[5]	-	-	50%	54%
PCI Within 90 Minutes of Arrival[5]	-	-	96%	96%
Statin Prescribed at Discharge[5]	-	-	99%	98%
Heart Failure Care				
ACE Inhibitor or ARB for LVSD[1]	-	-	99%	97%
Discharge Instructions Given	22	100%	98%	94%
Evaluation of LVS Function	35	100%	100%	99%
Medicare Spending				
Medicare Spending per Patient (ratio)	-	-	0.95	0.98
Pneumonia Care				
Appropriate Initial Antibiotic Given	21	100%	98%	95%
Blood Culture Timing	28	100%	98%	98%
Pregnancy and Delivery Care				
Newborn Deliveries Scheduled Early[5]	-	-	2%	6%
Preventive Care				
Immunization for Influenza[5]	-	-	93%	90%
Immunization for Pneumonia[5]	-	-	94%	92%
Stroke Care				
Anticoagulation Therapy for Atrial Fibrillation[5]	-	-	98%	95%
Antithrombotic Therapy Timing[5]	-	-	99%	98%
Assessed for Rehabilitation[5]	-	-	98%	97%
Discharged on Antithrombotic Therapy[5]	-	-	100%	99%
Discharged on Statin Medication[5]	-	-	97%	94%
Thrombolytic Therapy Timing[5]	-	-	29%	66%
Venous Thromboembolism Prophylaxis[5]	-	-	96%	94%
Written Stroke Educational Materials Given[5]	-	-	86%	88%
Surgical Care Improvement Project				
Appropriate Beta Blocker Usage[1,3]	-	-	99%	98%
Appropriate VTP Within 24 Hours[1,3]	-	-	99%	98%
Controlled Postoperative Blood Glucose[3,7]	-	-	99%	97%
Perioperative Temperature Management[1,3]	-	-	100%	100%
Prophylactic Antibiotic Selection[1,3]	-	-	99%	99%
Prophylactic Antibiotic Selection (Outpatient)[5]	-	-	98%	98%
Prophylactic Antibiotic Stopped[1,3]	-	-	99%	98%
Prophylactic Antibiotic Timing[1,3]	-	-	99%	99%
Prophylactic Antibiotic Timing (Outpatient)[5]	-	-	96%	98%
Urinary Catheter Removal[1,3]	-	-	99%	97%
Survey of Patients' Hospital Experiences				
Area Around Room 'Always' Quiet at Night	(a)	65%	59%	61%
Doctors 'Always' Communicated Well	(a)	80%	83%	82%
Home Recovery Information Given	(a)	88%	90%	85%
Hospital Given 9 or 10 on 10 Point Scale	(a)	75%	74%	71%
Meds 'Always' Explained Before Given	(a)	64%	69%	64%
Nurses 'Always' Communicated Well	(a)	81%	82%	79%
Pain 'Always' Well Controlled	(a)	69%	73%	71%
Room and Bathroom 'Always' Clean	(a)	81%	80%	73%
Timely Help 'Always' Received	(a)	68%	72%	68%
Would Definitely Recommend Hospital	(a)	73%	77%	71%
Use of Medical Imaging				
Cardiac Imaging Stress Test before Surgery	68	7.4%	4.8%	5.3%
Combination Abdominal CT Scan	264	2.7%	5.2%	10.5%
Combination Brain/Sinus CT Scan[1]	-	-	1.7%	2.7%
Combination Chest CT Scan	164	0.0%	0.7%	2.7%
Follow-up Mammogram/Ultrasound	492	4.9%	7.7%	8.8%
Lumbar Spine MRI for Low Back Pain[7]	-	-	37.5%	37.2%

Henrietta D Goodall Hospital

25 June Street
Sanford, ME 04073
Phone: 207-324-4310
Fax: 207-490-7328
E-mail: mfroning@goodallhospital.org
URL: www.goodallhospital.org
Type: Acute Care Hospitals
Emergency Services: Yes
Ownership: Voluntary non-profit - Private
Beds: 137

Key Personnel:
Emergency Room . . . . John Bartley, MD
Radiology. . . . . Edward M Cruz
Operating Room. . . . . Ken Gillis
Patient Relations . . . . Lorraine D Masure
Chief of Medical Staff . . . . Mark A Rautenberg
Quality Assurance . . . . Eliot Sanantagosl
CEO/President. . . . . Darlene Stromstad
Anesthesiology. . . . . Leonid I Temkin, MD

Measure	Cases	This Hosp.	State Avg.	U.S. Avg.
Blood Clot Prevention and Treatment				
Anticoagulation Overlap Therapy[2]	20	95%	98%	93%
ICU Venous Thromboembolism Prophylaxis[2]	57	96%	96%	92%
Incidence of Potentially Preventable VTE[1,2]	-	-	2%	10%
UFH with Dosages/Platelet Monitoring[1,2]	-	-	100%	97%
Venous Thromboembolism Prophylaxis[2]	137	96%	95%	85%
Warfarin Therapy Discharge Instructions[2]	16	75%	84%	75%
Chest Pain/Possible Heart Attack Care				
Aspirin Given Within 24 Hours of Arrival	84	100%	99%	96%
Fibrinolytic Meds Within 30 Min. of Arrival	17	76%	86%	58%
Average Time to ECG (minutes)	86	6	6	7
Average Time to Transfer (minutes)[7]	-	-	49	60
Children's Asthma Care				
Received Home Management Plan of Care	-	-	-	88%
Received Reliever Medication	-	-	-	100%
Received Systemic Corticosteroids	-	-	-	100%
Emergency Department				
Admittance Decision Time (minutes)[2]	435	164	110	98
Head CT Results Within 45 Min. of Arrival[1]	-	-	44%	57%
Patients Who Left ER Before Being Seen	21,644	1%	1%	2%
Time from ER Arrival to Admit. (minutes)[2]	445	318	288	274
Time from ER Arrival to Discharge (minutes)	372	111	122	134
Time in ER Before Being Evaluated (minutes)	408	20	28	26
Time to Pain Meds for Fractures (minutes)	46	34	52	57
Heart Attack Care				
Aspirin Given at Discharge	13	100%	100%	99%
Fibrinolytic Meds Within 30 Min. of Arrival[7]	-	-	50%	54%
PCI Within 90 Minutes of Arrival[7]	-	-	96%	96%
Statin Prescribed at Discharge	12	100%	99%	98%
Heart Failure Care				
ACE Inhibitor or ARB for LVSD[1]	-	-	99%	97%
Discharge Instructions Given	57	84%	98%	94%
Evaluation of LVS Function	95	100%	100%	99%
Medicare Spending				
Medicare Spending per Patient (ratio)	-	0.95	0.95	0.98
Pneumonia Care				
Appropriate Initial Antibiotic Given	76	99%	98%	95%
Blood Culture Timing	138	98%	98%	98%
Pregnancy and Delivery Care				
Newborn Deliveries Scheduled Early	14	7%	2%	6%
Preventive Care				
Immunization for Influenza[2]	267	99%	93%	90%
Immunization for Pneumonia[2]	383	100%	94%	92%
Stroke Care				
Anticoagulation Therapy for Atrial Fibrillation[1]	-	-	98%	95%
Antithrombotic Therapy Timing	27	100%	99%	98%
Assessed for Rehabilitation	26	96%	98%	97%
Discharged on Antithrombotic Therapy	26	100%	100%	99%
Discharged on Statin Medication	24	100%	97%	94%
Thrombolytic Therapy Timing[7]	-	-	29%	66%
Venous Thromboembolism Prophylaxis	27	96%	96%	94%
Written Stroke Educational Materials Given	12	58%	86%	88%
Surgical Care Improvement Project				
Appropriate Beta Blocker Usage	51	100%	99%	98%
Appropriate VTP Within 24 Hours	156	99%	99%	98%
Controlled Postoperative Blood Glucose[7]	-	-	99%	97%
Perioperative Temperature Management	168	99%	100%	100%
Prophylactic Antibiotic Selection	145	99%	99%	99%
Prophylactic Antibiotic Selection (Outpatient)	18	100%	98%	98%
Prophylactic Antibiotic Stopped	144	98%	99%	98%
Prophylactic Antibiotic Timing	145	99%	99%	99%
Prophylactic Antibiotic Timing (Outpatient)	18	100%	96%	98%
Urinary Catheter Removal	99	99%	99%	97%
Survey of Patients' Hospital Experiences				
Area Around Room 'Always' Quiet at Night	(a)	60%	59%	61%
Doctors 'Always' Communicated Well	(a)	80%	83%	82%
Home Recovery Information Given	(a)	86%	90%	85%
Hospital Given 9 or 10 on 10 Point Scale	(a)	62%	74%	71%
Meds 'Always' Explained Before Given	(a)	63%	69%	64%
Nurses 'Always' Communicated Well	(a)	72%	82%	79%
Pain 'Always' Well Controlled	(a)	64%	73%	71%
Room and Bathroom 'Always' Clean	(a)	73%	80%	73%
Timely Help 'Always' Received	(a)	66%	72%	68%
Would Definitely Recommend Hospital	(a)	64%	77%	71%
Use of Medical Imaging				
Cardiac Imaging Stress Test before Surgery	139	4.3%	4.8%	5.3%
Combination Abdominal CT Scan	427	4.0%	5.2%	10.5%
Combination Brain/Sinus CT Scan[1]	-	-	1.7%	2.7%
Combination Chest CT Scan	286	0.3%	0.7%	2.7%
Follow-up Mammogram/Ultrasound	964	14.9%	7.7%	8.8%
Lumbar Spine MRI for Low Back Pain	96	36.5%	37.5%	37.2%

Redington Fairview General Hospital

46 Fairview Ave
Skowhegan, ME 04976
Phone: 207-474-5121
Fax: 207-474-5121
E-mail: info@rfgh.net
URL: www.rfgh.net
Type: Critical Access Hospitals
Emergency Services: Yes
Ownership: Voluntary non-profit - Other
Beds: 65

Key Personnel:
Radiology. . . . . Anthony Van Dyck, MD
Quality Assurance . . . . Alma Fournier, RN
Chief of Medical Staff . . . . Roger Renfrew, MD
Pediatric Ambulatory Care . . . . . . Ruby Rodriguez
Pediatric In-Patient Care . . . . Ruby Rodriguez
Infection Control. . . . . Peg Shore
Intensive Care Unit. . . . . Sandy Whiting
CEO/President. . . . . Richard Willett

Measure	Cases	This Hosp.	State Avg.	U.S. Avg.
Blood Clot Prevention and Treatment				
Anticoagulation Overlap Therapy[1,2]	-	-	98%	93%
ICU Venous Thromboembolism Prophylaxis[2]	36	92%	96%	92%
Incidence of Potentially Preventable VTE[1,2]	-	-	2%	10%
UFH with Dosages/Platelet Monitoring[1,2]	-	-	100%	97%
Venous Thromboembolism Prophylaxis[2]	136	99%	95%	85%
Warfarin Therapy Discharge Instructions[1,2]	-	-	84%	75%
Chest Pain/Possible Heart Attack Care				
Aspirin Given Within 24 Hours of Arrival	64	97%	99%	96%
Fibrinolytic Meds Within 30 Min. of Arrival	12	75%	86%	58%
Average Time to ECG (minutes)	71	12	6	7
Average Time to Transfer (minutes)[7]	-	-	49	60
Children's Asthma Care				
Received Home Management Plan of Care	-	-	-	88%
Received Reliever Medication	-	-	-	100%
Received Systemic Corticosteroids	-	-	-	100%
Emergency Department				
Admittance Decision Time (minutes)[2]	442	98	110	98
Head CT Results Within 45 Min. of Arrival	12	42%	44%	57%
Patients Who Left ER Before Being Seen[5]	-	-	1%	2%
Time from ER Arrival to Admit. (minutes)[2]	442	295	288	274
Time from ER Arrival to Discharge (minutes)	393	128	122	134
Time in ER Before Being Evaluated (minutes)	435	44	28	26
Time to Pain Meds for Fractures (minutes)	84	64	52	57
Heart Attack Care				
Aspirin Given at Discharge	18	100%	100%	99%
Fibrinolytic Meds Within 30 Min. of Arrival[7]	-	-	50%	54%
PCI Within 90 Minutes of Arrival[7]	-	-	96%	96%
Statin Prescribed at Discharge	19	100%	99%	98%
Heart Failure Care				
ACE Inhibitor or ARB for LVSD	14	100%	99%	97%
Discharge Instructions Given	49	98%	98%	94%

NOTE: Hospital profiles are in alphabetical order by state, then city, then hospital within the city; Rankings exclude hospitals with less than 25 cases except for patient surveys which excludes hospitals with less than 100 cases; (a) 100-299 cases; (1) The number of cases/patients is too few to report; (2) Data submitted were based on a sample of cases/patients; (3) Results are based on a shorter time period than required; (4) Data suppressed by CMS for one or more quarters; (5) Results are not available for this reporting period; (6) Fewer than 100 patients completed the HCAHPS survey; (7) No cases met the criteria for this measure; (8) The lower limit of the confidence interval cannot be calculated if the number of observed infections equals zero; (9) No data are available from the state/territory for this reporting period; (10) The scores shown reflect fewer than 50 completed surveys; (11) There were discrepancies in the data collection process; (12) This measure does not apply to this hospital for this reporting period; (13) Results cannot be calculated for this reporting period; (14) The results for this state are combined with nearby states to protect confidentiality; Please refer to the User's Guide for a full explanation of data.

Measure	Cases	This Hosp.	State Avg.	U.S. Avg.
Evaluation of LVS Function	78	100%	100%	99%
Medicare Spending				
Medicare Spending per Patient (ratio)	-	-	0.95	0.98
Pneumonia Care				
Appropriate Initial Antibiotic Given	83	98%	98%	95%
Blood Culture Timing	110	95%	98%	98%
Pregnancy and Delivery Care				
Newborn Deliveries Scheduled Early[1,3]	-	-	2%	6%
Preventive Care				
Immunization for Influenza[2]	285	98%	93%	90%
Immunization for Pneumonia[2]	391	98%	94%	92%
Stroke Care				
Anticoagulation Therapy for Atrial Fibrillation[1]	-	-	98%	95%
Antithrombotic Therapy Timing	26	100%	99%	98%
Assessed for Rehabilitation	24	100%	98%	97%
Discharged on Antithrombotic Therapy	21	100%	100%	99%
Discharged on Statin Medication	13	100%	97%	94%
Thrombolytic Therapy Timing[1]	-	-	29%	66%
Venous Thromboembolism Prophylaxis	24	100%	96%	94%
Written Stroke Educational Materials Given	12	75%	86%	88%
Surgical Care Improvement Project				
Appropriate Beta Blocker Usage	15	100%	99%	98%
Appropriate VTP Within 24 Hours	58	100%	99%	98%
Controlled Postoperative Blood Glucose[7]	-	-	99%	97%
Perioperative Temperature Management	61	100%	100%	100%
Prophylactic Antibiotic Selection	45	100%	99%	99%
Prophylactic Antibiotic Selection (Outpatient)[1]	-	-	98%	98%
Prophylactic Antibiotic Stopped	43	98%	99%	98%
Prophylactic Antibiotic Timing	45	100%	99%	99%
Prophylactic Antibiotic Timing (Outpatient)[1]	-	-	96%	98%
Urinary Catheter Removal	47	98%	99%	97%
Survey of Patients' Hospital Experiences				
Area Around Room 'Always' Quiet at Night	300+	64%	59%	61%
Doctors 'Always' Communicated Well	300+	86%	83%	82%
Home Recovery Information Given	300+	91%	90%	85%
Hospital Given 9 or 10 on 10 Point Scale	300+	77%	74%	71%
Meds 'Always' Explained Before Given	300+	72%	69%	64%
Nurses 'Always' Communicated Well	300+	85%	82%	79%
Pain 'Always' Well Controlled	300+	70%	73%	71%
Room and Bathroom 'Always' Clean	300+	84%	80%	73%
Timely Help 'Always' Received	300+	73%	72%	68%
Would Definitely Recommend Hospital	300+	79%	77%	71%
Use of Medical Imaging				
Cardiac Imaging Stress Test before Surgery	165	1.8%	4.8%	5.3%
Combination Abdominal CT Scan	526	7.8%	5.2%	10.5%
Combination Brain/Sinus CT Scan	621	0.5%	1.7%	2.7%
Combination Chest CT Scan	253	1.2%	0.7%	2.7%
Follow-up Mammogram/Ultrasound	829	7.1%	7.7%	8.8%
Lumbar Spine MRI for Low Back Pain[7]	-	-	37.5%	37.2%

Inland Hospital

200 Kennedy Memorial Drive
Waterville, ME 04901
Phone: 207-861-3012
URL: www.inlandhospital.org
Type: Acute Care Hospitals
Emergency Services: Yes
Ownership: Voluntary non-profit - Private
Beds: 78
Key Personnel:
Radiology. Hugh R Caggiano
CEO/President. . . . . John Dalton
Chief of Medical Staff. . . . . Michael Palumbo

Measure	Cases	This Hosp.	State Avg.	U.S. Avg.
Blood Clot Prevention and Treatment				
Anticoagulation Overlap Therapy[1,2]	-	-	98%	93%
ICU Venous Thromboembolism Prophylaxis[2]	47	100%	96%	92%
Incidence of Potentially Preventable VTE[2,7]	-	-	2%	10%
UFH with Dosages/Platelet Monitoring[1,2]	-	-	100%	97%
Venous Thromboembolism Prophylaxis[2]	98	99%	95%	85%
Warfarin Therapy Discharge Instructions[1,2]	-	-	84%	75%
Chest Pain/Possible Heart Attack Care				
Aspirin Given Within 24 Hours of Arrival	50	98%	99%	96%
Fibrinolytic Meds Within 30 Min. of Arrival[1]	-	-	86%	58%
Average Time to ECG (minutes)	51	5	6	7
Average Time to Transfer (minutes)[1]	-	-	49	60
Children's Asthma Care				
Received Home Management Plan of Care	-	-	-	88%
Received Reliever Medication	-	-	-	100%
Received Systemic Corticosteroids	-	-	-	100%
Emergency Department				
Admittance Decision Time (minutes)[2]	355	109	110	98
Head CT Results Within 45 Min. of Arrival[1]	-	-	44%	57%
Patients Who Left ER Before Being Seen	14,744	2%	1%	2%
Time from ER Arrival to Admit. (minutes)[2]	360	300	288	274
Time from ER Arrival to Discharge (minutes)	382	110	122	134
Time in ER Before Being Evaluated (minutes)	328	30	28	26
Time to Pain Meds for Fractures (minutes)	43	42	52	57
Heart Attack Care				
Aspirin Given at Discharge[1]	-	-	100%	99%
Fibrinolytic Meds Within 30 Min. of Arrival[7]	-	-	50%	54%
PCI Within 90 Minutes of Arrival[7]	-	-	96%	96%
Statin Prescribed at Discharge	11	91%	99%	98%
Heart Failure Care				
ACE Inhibitor or ARB for LVSD	16	100%	99%	97%
Discharge Instructions Given	35	100%	98%	94%
Evaluation of LVS Function	48	100%	100%	99%
Medicare Spending				
Medicare Spending per Patient (ratio)	-	0.98	0.95	0.98
Pneumonia Care				
Appropriate Initial Antibiotic Given[2]	30	93%	98%	95%
Blood Culture Timing[2]	46	98%	98%	98%
Pregnancy and Delivery Care				
Newborn Deliveries Scheduled Early	40	0%	2%	6%
Preventive Care				
Immunization for Influenza[2]	289	97%	93%	90%
Immunization for Pneumonia[2]	327	99%	94%	92%
Stroke Care				
Anticoagulation Therapy for Atrial Fibrillation[1,2]	-	-	98%	95%
Antithrombotic Therapy Timing[2]	14	100%	99%	98%
Assessed for Rehabilitation[2]	18	100%	98%	97%
Discharged on Antithrombotic Therapy[2]	17	94%	100%	99%
Discharged on Statin Medication[2]	13	92%	97%	94%
Thrombolytic Therapy Timing[2,7]	-	-	29%	66%
Venous Thromboembolism Prophylaxis[2]	16	100%	96%	94%
Written Stroke Educational Materials Given[1,2]	-	-	86%	88%
Surgical Care Improvement Project				
Appropriate Beta Blocker Usage[2]	32	100%	99%	98%
Appropriate VTP Within 24 Hours[2]	76	99%	99%	98%
Controlled Postoperative Blood Glucose[2,7]	-	-	99%	97%
Perioperative Temperature Management[2]	118	100%	100%	100%
Prophylactic Antibiotic Selection[2]	90	99%	99%	99%
Prophylactic Antibiotic Selection (Outpatient)	208	100%	98%	98%
Prophylactic Antibiotic Stopped[2]	88	100%	99%	98%
Prophylactic Antibiotic Timing[2]	90	100%	99%	99%
Prophylactic Antibiotic Timing (Outpatient)	210	99%	96%	98%
Urinary Catheter Removal[2]	74	100%	99%	97%
Survey of Patients' Hospital Experiences				
Area Around Room 'Always' Quiet at Night	(a)	64%	59%	61%
Doctors 'Always' Communicated Well	(a)	83%	83%	82%
Home Recovery Information Given	(a)	91%	90%	85%
Hospital Given 9 or 10 on 10 Point Scale	(a)	75%	74%	71%
Meds 'Always' Explained Before Given	(a)	68%	69%	64%
Nurses 'Always' Communicated Well	(a)	83%	82%	79%
Pain 'Always' Well Controlled	(a)	72%	73%	71%
Room and Bathroom 'Always' Clean	(a)	85%	80%	73%
Timely Help 'Always' Received	(a)	76%	72%	68%
Would Definitely Recommend Hospital	(a)	83%	77%	71%
Use of Medical Imaging				
Cardiac Imaging Stress Test before Surgery	282	6.7%	4.8%	5.3%
Combination Abdominal CT Scan	314	1.9%	5.2%	10.5%
Combination Brain/Sinus CT Scan	232	0.4%	1.7%	2.7%
Combination Chest CT Scan	137	0.0%	0.7%	2.7%
Follow-up Mammogram/Ultrasound	703	4.1%	7.7%	8.8%
Lumbar Spine MRI for Low Back Pain	62	30.6%	37.5%	37.2%

York Hospital

15 Hospital Drive
York, ME 03909
Phone: 207-363-4321
Fax: 207-363-3858
E-mail: cr@yorkhospital.com
URL: www.yorkhospital.com
Type: Acute Care Hospitals
Emergency Services: Yes
Ownership: Voluntary non-profit - Private
Beds: 79
Key Personnel:
Radiology. Edward Michael Cruz
Coronary Care . . . . Larry Pedrovich
Infection Control. . . . . Shirley Peverly
Quality Assurance . . . . Eliot Smith, MD
Emergency Room . . . . Elliot Smith, MD

Measure	Cases	This Hosp.	State Avg.	U.S. Avg.
Blood Clot Prevention and Treatment				
Anticoagulation Overlap Therapy[2]	25	100%	98%	93%
ICU Venous Thromboembolism Prophylaxis[2]	62	97%	96%	92%
Incidence of Potentially Preventable VTE[1,2]	-	-	2%	10%
UFH with Dosages/Platelet Monitoring[1,2]	-	-	100%	97%
Venous Thromboembolism Prophylaxis[2]	251	96%	95%	85%
Warfarin Therapy Discharge Instructions[2]	24	100%	84%	75%
Chest Pain/Possible Heart Attack Care				
Aspirin Given Within 24 Hours of Arrival[1,3]	-	-	99%	96%
Fibrinolytic Meds Within 30 Min. of Arrival[3,7]	-	-	86%	58%
Average Time to ECG (minutes)[1,3]	-	-	6	7
Average Time to Transfer (minutes)[3,7]	-	-	49	60
Children's Asthma Care				
Received Home Management Plan of Care	-	-	-	88%
Received Reliever Medication	-	-	-	100%
Received Systemic Corticosteroids	-	-	-	100%
Emergency Department				
Admittance Decision Time (minutes)[2]	422	66	110	98
Head CT Results Within 45 Min. of Arrival[1]	-	-	44%	57%
Patients Who Left ER Before Being Seen	29,027	0%	1%	2%
Time from ER Arrival to Admit. (minutes)[2]	442	224	288	274
Time from ER Arrival to Discharge (minutes)	369	86	122	134
Time in ER Before Being Evaluated (minutes)	406	14	28	26
Time to Pain Meds for Fractures (minutes)	60	35	52	57
Heart Attack Care				
Aspirin Given at Discharge	63	100%	100%	99%
Fibrinolytic Meds Within 30 Min. of Arrival[7]	-	-	50%	54%
PCI Within 90 Minutes of Arrival[1]	-	-	96%	96%
Statin Prescribed at Discharge	62	100%	99%	98%
Heart Failure Care				
ACE Inhibitor or ARB for LVSD	25	100%	99%	97%
Discharge Instructions Given	117	95%	98%	94%
Evaluation of LVS Function	143	99%	100%	99%
Medicare Spending				
Medicare Spending per Patient (ratio)	-	0.97	0.95	0.98
Pneumonia Care				
Appropriate Initial Antibiotic Given	67	96%	98%	95%
Blood Culture Timing	132	98%	98%	98%
Pregnancy and Delivery Care				
Newborn Deliveries Scheduled Early[2]	24	0%	2%	6%
Preventive Care				
Immunization for Influenza[2]	304	99%	93%	90%
Immunization for Pneumonia[2]	412	99%	94%	92%
Stroke Care				
Anticoagulation Therapy for Atrial Fibrillation	11	100%	98%	95%
Antithrombotic Therapy Timing	38	100%	99%	98%
Assessed for Rehabilitation	40	98%	98%	97%
Discharged on Antithrombotic Therapy	39	100%	100%	99%
Discharged on Statin Medication	27	100%	97%	94%
Thrombolytic Therapy Timing[1]	-	-	29%	66%
Venous Thromboembolism Prophylaxis	38	95%	96%	94%
Written Stroke Educational Materials Given	23	96%	86%	88%
Surgical Care Improvement Project				
Appropriate Beta Blocker Usage[2]	83	98%	99%	98%
Appropriate VTP Within 24 Hours[2]	237	99%	99%	98%
Controlled Postoperative Blood Glucose[2,7]	-	-	99%	97%
Perioperative Temperature Management[2]	281	100%	100%	100%
Prophylactic Antibiotic Selection[2]	182	99%	99%	99%
Prophylactic Antibiotic Selection (Outpatient)	109	99%	98%	98%
Prophylactic Antibiotic Stopped[2]	180	100%	99%	98%

NOTE: Hospital profiles are in alphabetical order by state, then city, then hospital within the city; Rankings exclude hospitals with less than 25 cases except for patient surveys which excludes hospitals with less than 100 cases; (a) 100-299 cases; (1) The number of cases/patients is too few to report; (2) Data submitted were based on a sample of cases/patients; (3) Results are based on a shorter time period than required; (4) Data suppressed by CMS for one or more quarters; (5) Results are not available for this reporting period; (6) Fewer than 100 patients completed the HCAHPS survey; (7) No cases met the criteria for this measure; (8) The lower limit of the confidence interval cannot be calculated if the number of observed infections equals zero; (9) No data are available from the state/territory for this reporting period; (10) The scores shown reflect fewer than 50 completed surveys; (11) There were discrepancies in the data collection process; (12) This measure does not apply to this hospital for this reporting period; (13) Results cannot be calculated for this reporting period; (14) The results for this state are combined with nearby states to protect confidentiality; Please refer to the User's Guide for a full explanation of data.

Prophylactic Antibiotic Timing[2]	182	99%	99%	99%
Prophylactic Antibiotic Timing (Outpatient)	97	98%	96%	98%
Urinary Catheter Removal[2]	172	99%	99%	97%
Survey of Patients' Hospital Experiences				
Area Around Room 'Always' Quiet at Night	300+	65%	59%	61%
Doctors 'Always' Communicated Well	300+	89%	83%	82%
Home Recovery Information Given	300+	90%	90%	85%
Hospital Given 9 or 10 on 10 Point Scale	300+	84%	74%	71%
Meds 'Always' Explained Before Given	300+	73%	69%	64%
Nurses 'Always' Communicated Well	300+	88%	82%	79%
Pain 'Always' Well Controlled	300+	76%	73%	71%
Room and Bathroom 'Always' Clean	300+	82%	80%	73%
Timely Help 'Always' Received	300+	75%	72%	68%
Would Definitely Recommend Hospital	300+	89%	77%	71%
Use of Medical Imaging				
Cardiac Imaging Stress Test before Surgery	683	7.3%	4.8%	5.3%
Combination Abdominal CT Scan	700	8.7%	5.2%	10.5%
Combination Brain/Sinus CT Scan	467	1.5%	1.7%	2.7%
Combination Chest CT Scan	463	0.2%	0.7%	2.7%
Follow-up Mammogram/Ultrasound	1,980	7.9%	7.7%	8.8%
Lumbar Spine MRI for Low Back Pain	74	28.4%	37.5%	37.2%

NOTE: Hospital profiles are in alphabetical order by state, then city, then hospital within the city; Rankings exclude hospitals with less than 25 cases except for patient surveys which excludes hospitals with less than 100 cases; (a) 100-299 cases; (1) The number of cases/patients is too few to report; (2) Data submitted were based on a sample of cases/patients; (3) Results are based on a shorter time period than required; (4) Data suppressed by CMS for one or more quarters; (5) Results are not available for this reporting period; (6) Fewer than 100 patients completed the HCAHPS survey; (7) No cases met the criteria for this measure; (8) The lower limit of the confidence interval cannot be calculated if the number of observed infections equals zero; (9) No data are available from the state/territory for this reporting period; (10) The scores shown reflect fewer than 50 completed surveys; (11) There were discrepancies in the data collection process; (12) This measure does not apply to this hospital for this reporting period; (13) Results cannot be calculated for this reporting period; (14) The results for this state are combined with nearby states to protect confidentiality; Please refer to the User's Guide for a full explanation of data.

Blood Clot Prevention and Treatment

Anticoagulation Overlap Therapy

Hospital Name	City	Rate	Cases
Calvert Memorial Hospital[2]	Prince Frederick	100%	48
Doctors' Community Hospital[2]	Lanham	100%	100
Univ of MD Shore Med Ctr at Easton[2,3]	Easton	100%	36
Johns Hopkins Bayview Medical Center[2]	Baltimore	99%	107
Mercy Medical Center[2]	Baltimore	99%	108
Northwest Hospital Center[2]	Randallstown	99%	95
University of Maryland Medical Center[2]	Baltimore	99%	194
Medstar Good Samaritan Hospital[2]	Baltimore	98%	103
Medstar Montgomery Medical Center[2]	Olney	98%	63
Saint Agnes Hospital[2]	Baltimore	98%	147
Shady Grove Adventist Hospital[2]	Rockville	98%	82
Sinai Hospital of Baltimore[2]	Baltimore	98%	132
Suburban Hospital[2]	Bethesda	98%	84
Univ of MD Charles Reg Med Ctr[2]	La Plata	98%	89
Univ of MD St Joseph Med Ctr[2,3]	Towson	98%	62
Atlantic General Hospital[2]	Berlin	97%	30
Frederick Memorial Hospital[2]	Frederick	97%	146
Greater Baltimore Medical Center[2,3]	Baltimore	97%	73
Carroll Hospital Center[2]	Westminster	96%	93
Fort Washington Hospital[2]	Fort Washington	96%	26
Peninsula Regional Medical Center[2]	Salisbury	96%	138
Univ of MD Balto Washington Med Ctr[2,3]	Glen Burnie	95%	129
Medstar Southern Maryland Hospital Center[2]	Clinton	94%	99
Anne Arundel Medical Center[2]	Annapolis	93%	167
Meritus Medical Center	Hagerstown	93%	154
Upper Chesapeake Medical Center[2]	Bel Air	93%	86
Washington Adventist Hospital[2]	Takoma Park	93%	73
Medstar Saint Mary's Hospital[2]	Leonardtown	92%	53
Medstar Franklin Square Medical Center[2]	Baltimore	89%	123
Prince Georges Hospital Center[2]	Cheverly	89%	89
Howard County General Hospital[2]	Columbia	86%	152
Laurel Regional Medical Center[2]	Laurel	83%	42
Medstar Harbor Hospital[2]	Baltimore	74%	65
Medstar Union Memorial Hospital[2]	Baltimore	73%	88

ICU Venous Thromboembolism Prophylaxis

Hospital Name	City	Rate	Cases
Carroll Hospital Center[2]	Westminster	100%	87
Doctors' Community Hospital[2]	Lanham	100%	60
Mercy Medical Center[2]	Baltimore	100%	71
Saint Agnes Hospital[2]	Baltimore	100%	39
Union Hospital of Cecil County	Elkton	100%	120
Univ of MD Shore Med Ctr-Chestertown[2]	Chestertown	100%	45
Frederick Memorial Hospital[2]	Frederick	98%	49
Medstar Good Samaritan Hospital[2]	Baltimore	98%	40
Sinai Hospital of Baltimore[2]	Baltimore	98%	57
Univ of MD Med Ctr Midtown Campus[2,3]	Baltimore	98%	51
Fort Washington Hospital[2]	Fort Washington	97%	33
Peninsula Regional Medical Center[2]	Salisbury	97%	131
Prince Georges Hospital Center[2]	Cheverly	97%	176
Suburban Hospital[2]	Bethesda	97%	75
Univ of MD Charles Reg Med Ctr[2]	La Plata	97%	69
Anne Arundel Medical Center[2]	Annapolis	96%	49
Medstar Harbor Hospital[2]	Baltimore	96%	92
Meritus Medical Center	Hagerstown	96%	1148
Univ of MD Balto Washington Med Ctr[2,3]	Glen Burnie	96%	57
University of Maryland Medical Center[2]	Baltimore	96%	101
Washington Adventist Hospital[2]	Takoma Park	96%	80
Medstar Montgomery Medical Center[2]	Olney	95%	40
Univ of MD St Joseph Med Ctr[2,3]	Towson	95%	42
Harford Memorial Hospital[2]	Havre De Grace	94%	34
Medstar Saint Mary's Hospital[2]	Leonardtown	93%	42
Upper Chesapeake Medical Center[2]	Bel Air	92%	37
Howard County General Hospital[2]	Columbia	91%	35
Laurel Regional Medical Center[2]	Laurel	91%	96
Medstar Southern Maryland Hospital Center[2]	Clinton	87%	52
Medstar Franklin Square Medical Center[2]	Baltimore	85%	52
Atlantic General Hospital[2]	Berlin	84%	50
Garrett County Memorial Hospital	Oakland	82%	129
Medstar Union Memorial Hospital[2]	Baltimore	82%	56
Bon Secours Hospital[2]	Baltimore	68%	40
Johns Hopkins Bayview Medical Center[2]	Baltimore	67%	127

Incidence of Potentially Preventable VTE

Hospital Name	City	Rate	Cases
Doctors' Community Hospital[2]	Lanham	0%	34
Sinai Hospital of Baltimore[2]	Baltimore	0%	38
University of Maryland Medical Center[2]	Baltimore	1%	113
Shady Grove Adventist Hospital[2]	Rockville	2%	52
Medstar Good Samaritan Hospital[2]	Baltimore	3%	35
Prince Georges Hospital Center[2]	Cheverly	3%	33
Univ of MD Balto Washington Med Ctr[2,3]	Glen Burnie	4%	27
Johns Hopkins Bayview Medical Center[2]	Baltimore	5%	42
Suburban Hospital[2]	Bethesda	5%	38
Anne Arundel Medical Center[2]	Annapolis	10%	41
Howard County General Hospital[2]	Columbia	11%	28
Mercy Medical Center[2]	Baltimore	12%	40
Medstar Union Memorial Hospital[2]	Baltimore	14%	44

UFH with Dosages/Platelet Count Monitoring

Hospital Name	City	Rate	Cases
Anne Arundel Medical Center[2]	Annapolis	100%	35
Carroll Hospital Center[2]	Westminster	100%	84
Doctors' Community Hospital[2]	Lanham	100%	37
Frederick Memorial Hospital[2]	Frederick	100%	180
Greater Baltimore Medical Center[2,3]	Baltimore	100%	39
Howard County General Hospital[2]	Columbia	100%	163
Johns Hopkins Bayview Medical Center[2]	Baltimore	100%	97
Medstar Franklin Square Medical Center[2]	Baltimore	100%	61
Medstar Southern Maryland Hospital Center[2]	Clinton	100%	27
Northwest Hospital Center[2]	Randallstown	100%	38
Peninsula Regional Medical Center[2]	Salisbury	100%	33
Sinai Hospital of Baltimore[2]	Baltimore	100%	86
Univ of MD Balto Washington Med Ctr[2,3]	Glen Burnie	100%	70
Univ of MD Charles Reg Med Ctr[2]	La Plata	100%	35
Univ of MD St Joseph Med Ctr[2,3]	Towson	100%	38
Upper Chesapeake Medical Center[2]	Bel Air	100%	79
Medstar Good Samaritan Hospital[2]	Baltimore	99%	86
Mercy Medical Center[2]	Baltimore	99%	100
Saint Agnes Hospital[2]	Baltimore	99%	118
Meritus Medical Center	Hagerstown	98%	140
Prince Georges Hospital Center[2]	Cheverly	97%	37
University of Maryland Medical Center[2]	Baltimore	95%	202
Medstar Union Memorial Hospital[2]	Baltimore	94%	83
Washington Adventist Hospital[2]	Takoma Park	92%	25
Medstar Harbor Hospital[2]	Baltimore	42%	53

Venous Thromboembolism Prophylaxis

Hospital Name	City	Rate	Cases
Doctors' Community Hospital[2]	Lanham	100%	389
Univ of MD Balto Washington Med Ctr[2,3]	Glen Burnie	99%	209
Calvert Memorial Hospital[2]	Prince Frederick	98%	348
Greater Baltimore Medical Center[2,3]	Baltimore	98%	223
Saint Agnes Hospital[2]	Baltimore	98%	391
Sinai Hospital of Baltimore[2]	Baltimore	98%	536
Mercy Medical Center[2]	Baltimore	97%	259
Carroll Hospital Center[2]	Westminster	96%	277
Harford Memorial Hospital[2]	Havre De Grace	96%	280
Medstar Montgomery Medical Center[2]	Olney	96%	409
Union Hospital of Cecil County	Elkton	96%	645
Northwest Hospital Center[2]	Randallstown	95%	421
Peninsula Regional Medical Center[2]	Salisbury	95%	265
Shady Grove Adventist Hospital[2]	Rockville	95%	362
Univ of MD Shore Med Ctr-Chestertown[2]	Chestertown	94%	239
Univ of MD Shore Med Ctr at Easton[2,3]	Easton	94%	232
Fort Washington Hospital[2]	Fort Washington	93%	230
Meritus Medical Center	Hagerstown	93%	5414
Univ of MD Charles Reg Med Ctr[2]	La Plata	93%	385
Upper Chesapeake Medical Center[2]	Bel Air	93%	368
Prince Georges Hospital Center[2]	Cheverly	91%	281
Frederick Memorial Hospital[2]	Frederick	89%	319
University of Maryland Medical Center[2]	Baltimore	89%	278
Anne Arundel Medical Center[2]	Annapolis	87%	287
Univ of MD Med Ctr Midtown Campus[2,3]	Baltimore	87%	146
Laurel Regional Medical Center[2]	Laurel	86%	322
Johns Hopkins Bayview Medical Center[2]	Baltimore	85%	304
Medstar Harbor Hospital[2]	Baltimore	85%	304
Suburban Hospital[2]	Bethesda	85%	249
Washington Adventist Hospital[2]	Takoma Park	84%	286
Medstar Good Samaritan Hospital[2]	Baltimore	83%	369
Medstar Southern Maryland Hospital Center[2]	Clinton	81%	335
Univ of MD St Joseph Med Ctr[2,3]	Towson	81%	171
Medstar Union Memorial Hospital[2]	Baltimore	80%	271
Medstar Franklin Square Medical Center[2]	Baltimore	79%	351
Howard County General Hospital[2]	Columbia	74%	358
Medstar Saint Mary's Hospital[2]	Leonardtown	73%	314
Garrett County Memorial Hospital	Oakland	72%	655
Atlantic General Hospital[2]	Berlin	70%	254
Bon Secours Hospital[2]	Baltimore	68%	259

Warfarin Therapy Discharge Instructions

Hospital Name	City	Rate	Cases
Doctors' Community Hospital[2]	Lanham	100%	73
Carroll Hospital Center[2]	Westminster	99%	78
Peninsula Regional Medical Center[2]	Salisbury	99%	88
Univ of MD Balto Washington Med Ctr[2,3]	Glen Burnie	99%	83
Shady Grove Adventist Hospital[2]	Rockville	98%	41
Medstar Good Samaritan Hospital[2]	Baltimore	97%	62
Univ of MD Charles Reg Med Ctr[2]	La Plata	97%	74
Upper Chesapeake Medical Center[2]	Bel Air	97%	62
Calvert Memorial Hospital[2]	Prince Frederick	96%	48
Medstar Montgomery Medical Center[2]	Olney	96%	50
Sinai Hospital of Baltimore[2]	Baltimore	95%	88
Howard County General Hospital[2]	Columbia	94%	129
Greater Baltimore Medical Center[2,3]	Baltimore	92%	40
Meritus Medical Center	Hagerstown	92%	119
University of Maryland Medical Center[2]	Baltimore	92%	113
Medstar Saint Mary's Hospital[2]	Leonardtown	86%	37
Northwest Hospital Center[2]	Randallstown	82%	67
Prince Georges Hospital Center[2]	Cheverly	75%	65
Medstar Union Memorial Hospital[2]	Baltimore	73%	63
Johns Hopkins Bayview Medical Center[2]	Baltimore	72%	67
Frederick Memorial Hospital[2]	Frederick	70%	107
Mercy Medical Center[2]	Baltimore	68%	75
Suburban Hospital[2]	Bethesda	66%	47
Univ of MD St Joseph Med Ctr[2,3]	Towson	64%	45
Saint Agnes Hospital[2]	Baltimore	61%	102
Laurel Regional Medical Center[2]	Laurel	59%	32
Anne Arundel Medical Center[2]	Annapolis	53%	118
Washington Adventist Hospital[2]	Takoma Park	53%	47
Medstar Harbor Hospital[2]	Baltimore	44%	50
Medstar Southern Maryland Hospital Center[2]	Clinton	39%	67
Medstar Franklin Square Medical Center[2]	Baltimore	15%	102

Chest Pain/Possible Heart Attack Care

No hospitals met the 25 case threshold.

Children's Asthma Care

Received Home Management Plan of Care

Hospital Name	City	Rate	Cases
Univ of MD Balto Washington Med Ctr	Glen Burnie	94%	48

Received Reliever Medication

Hospital Name	City	Rate	Cases
Carroll Hospital Center	Westminster	100%	26
Univ of MD Balto Washington Med Ctr	Glen Burnie	100%	50

Received Systemic Corticosteroids

Hospital Name	City	Rate	Cases
Carroll Hospital Center	Westminster	100%	26
Univ of MD Balto Washington Med Ctr	Glen Burnie	100%	50

Emergency Department

Admittance Decision Time (minutes)

Hospital Name	City	Min.	Cases
Edward Mccready Memorial Hospital	Crisfield	40	152
Garrett County Memorial Hospital	Oakland	55	1209
Univ of MD Shore Med Ctr-Chestertown[2]	Chestertown	62	550
Atlantic General Hospital[2]	Berlin	64	510
Fort Washington Hospital[2]	Fort Washington	85	413
Union Hospital of Cecil County	Elkton	96	1184
Carroll Hospital Center[2]	Westminster	99	780
Peninsula Regional Medical Center[2]	Salisbury	102	598
Univ of MD St Joseph Med Ctr[2,3]	Towson	108	230
Univ of MD Shore Med Ctr at Easton[2]	Easton	109	825
Frederick Memorial Hospital[2]	Frederick	110	675
Upper Chesapeake Medical Center[2]	Bel Air	110	612
Univ of MD Charles Reg Med Ctr[2]	La Plata	113	1060
Sinai Hospital of Baltimore[2]	Baltimore	115	719
Harford Memorial Hospital[2]	Havre De Grace	116	391
Medstar Saint Mary's Hospital[2]	Leonardtown	121	600
Medstar Union Memorial Hospital[2]	Baltimore	126	447
Univ of MD Med Ctr Midtown Campus[2]	Baltimore	127	240
Greater Baltimore Medical Center[2,3]	Baltimore	133	227
Medstar Montgomery Medical Center[2]	Olney	136	768
Medstar Good Samaritan Hospital[2]	Baltimore	141	525
Northwest Hospital Center[2]	Randallstown	141	1137
Holy Cross Hospital[2]	Silver Spring	142	420
Saint Agnes Hospital[2]	Baltimore	144	814
Medstar Harbor Hospital[2]	Baltimore	145	396
Medstar Franklin Square Medical Center[2]	Baltimore	150	588
Howard County General Hospital[2,3]	Columbia	160	402
Shady Grove Adventist Hospital[2]	Rockville	164	499
Laurel Regional Medical Center[2]	Laurel	168	660
Medstar Southern Maryland Hospital Center[2,3]	Clinton	168	793
Bon Secours Hospital[2]	Baltimore	174	120
Univ of MD Balto Washington Med Ctr[2]	Glen Burnie	183	1245
Calvert Memorial Hospital[2]	Prince Frederick	187	717
Meritus Medical Center[2]	Hagerstown	192	5070
Doctors' Community Hospital[2]	Lanham	193	903
Washington Adventist Hospital[2]	Takoma Park	197	554
Suburban Hospital[2]	Bethesda	211	654
Johns Hopkins Bayview Medical Center[2]	Baltimore	215	619
Anne Arundel Medical Center[2]	Annapolis	272	742
Prince Georges Hospital Center[2]	Cheverly	301	457
University of Maryland Medical Center[2]	Baltimore	336	283

Patients Who Left ER Before Being Seen

Hospital Name	City	Rate	Cases
Northwest Hospital Center	Randallstown	3%	64917

NOTE: Hospital profiles are in alphabetical order by state, then city, then hospital within the city; Rankings exclude hospitals with less than 25 cases except for patient surveys which excludes hospitals with less than 100 cases; (a) 100-299 cases; (1) The number of cases/patients is too few to report; (2) Data submitted were based on a sample of cases/patients; (3) Results are based on a shorter time period than required; (4) Data suppressed by CMS for one or more quarters; (5) Results are not available for this reporting period; (6) Fewer than 100 patients completed the HCAHPS survey; (7) No cases met the criteria for this measure; (8) The lower limit of the confidence interval cannot be calculated if the number of observed infections equals zero; (9) No data are available from the state/territory for this reporting period; (10) The scores shown reflect fewer than 50 completed surveys; (11) There were discrepancies in the data collection process; (12) This measure does not apply to this hospital for this reporting period; (13) Results cannot be calculated for this reporting period; (14) The results for this state are combined with nearby states to protect confidentiality; Please refer to the User's Guide for a full explanation of data.

Time from ER Arrival to Being Admitted (minutes)

Hospital Name	City	Min.	Cases
Edward Mccready Memorial Hospital	Crisfield	192	152
Atlantic General Hospital[2]	Berlin	207	510
Garrett County Memorial Hospital	Oakland	215	1211
Fort Washington Hospital[2]	Fort Washington	256	453
Peninsula Regional Medical Center[2]	Salisbury	271	600
Medstar Montgomery Medical Center[2]	Olney	288	787
Univ of MD Shore Med Ctr-Chestertown[2]	Chestertown	300	553
Carroll Hospital Center[2]	Westminster	306	780
Union Hospital of Cecil County	Elkton	307	1187
Medstar Saint Mary's Hospital[2]	Leonardtown	313	604
Univ of MD Charles Reg Med Ctr[2]	La Plata	313	1061
Medstar Union Memorial Hospital[2]	Baltimore	320	523
Medstar Harbor Hospital[2]	Baltimore	325	407
Univ of MD St Joseph Med Ctr[2,3]	Towson	327	247
Harford Memorial Hospital[2]	Havre De Grace	336	518
Greater Baltimore Medical Center[2,3]	Baltimore	346	229
Frederick Memorial Hospital[2]	Frederick	349	694
Univ of MD Shore Med Ctr at Easton[2]	Easton	353	862
Meritus Medical Center[2]	Hagerstown	362	5144
Sinai Hospital of Baltimore[2]	Baltimore	370	719
Upper Chesapeake Medical Center[2]	Bel Air	372	714
Univ of MD Med Ctr Midtown Campus[2]	Baltimore	377	367
Medstar Franklin Square Medical Center[2]	Baltimore	378	628
Medstar Southern Maryland Hospital Center[2,3]	Clinton	384	801
Northwest Hospital Center[2]	Randallstown	384	1138
Univ of MD Balto Washington Med Ctr[2]	Glen Burnie	386	1248
Holy Cross Hospital[2]	Silver Spring	400	421
Shady Grove Adventist Hospital[2]	Rockville	402	500
Medstar Good Samaritan Hospital[2]	Baltimore	405	552
Suburban Hospital[2]	Bethesda	410	679
Johns Hopkins Bayview Medical Center[2]	Baltimore	411	619
Saint Agnes Hospital[2]	Baltimore	414	816
Bon Secours Hospital[2]	Baltimore	415	155
Washington Adventist Hospital[2]	Takoma Park	427	560
Calvert Memorial Hospital[2]	Prince Frederick	428	717
Laurel Regional Medical Center[2]	Laurel	430	661
Howard County General Hospital[2,3]	Columbia	462	416
Doctors' Community Hospital[2]	Lanham	492	933
Anne Arundel Medical Center[2]	Annapolis	494	745
Prince Georges Hospital Center[2]	Cheverly	550	509
University of Maryland Medical Center[2]	Baltimore	639	327

Heart Attack Care

Aspirin Given at Discharge

Hospital Name	City	Rate	Cases
Anne Arundel Medical Center	Annapolis	100%	240
Calvert Memorial Hospital	Prince Frederick	100%	28
Carroll Hospital Center	Westminster	100%	96
Frederick Memorial Hospital	Frederick	100%	216
Holy Cross Hospital	Silver Spring	100%	92
Johns Hopkins Bayview Medical Center	Baltimore	100%	227
Northwest Hospital Center	Randallstown	100%	51
Peninsula Regional Medical Center	Salisbury	100%	479
Prince Georges Hospital Center[2]	Cheverly	100%	144
Saint Agnes Hospital	Baltimore	100%	215
Shady Grove Adventist Hospital	Rockville	100%	202
Suburban Hospital	Bethesda	100%	238
Univ of MD Balto Washington Med Ctr	Glen Burnie	100%	222
University of Maryland Medical Center	Baltimore	100%	489
Upper Chesapeake Medical Center	Bel Air	100%	150
VA Maryland Healthcare System - Baltimore	Baltimore	100%	45
Washington Adventist Hospital	Takoma Park	100%	364
Western Maryland Regional Medical Center	Cumberland	100%	274
The Johns Hopkins Hospital	Baltimore	99%	523
Sinai Hospital of Baltimore	Baltimore	99%	389
Univ of MD St Joseph Med Ctr[2,3]	Towson	99%	139
Howard County General Hospital	Columbia	98%	83
Medstar Franklin Square Medical Center	Baltimore	98%	167
Medstar Harbor Hospital	Baltimore	98%	51
Medstar Union Memorial Hospital	Baltimore	98%	516
Meritus Medical Center	Hagerstown	98%	124
Univ of MD Shore Med Ctr at Easton	Easton	98%	45
Medstar Southern Maryland Hospital Center[3]	Clinton	97%	153
Laurel Regional Medical Center	Laurel	96%	27
Medstar Good Samaritan Hospital	Baltimore	93%	72

PCI Within 90 Minutes of Arrival

Hospital Name	City	Rate	Cases
Frederick Memorial Hospital	Frederick	100%	88
Holy Cross Hospital	Silver Spring	100%	47
Meritus Medical Center	Hagerstown	100%	54
Shady Grove Adventist Hospital	Rockville	100%	68
Upper Chesapeake Medical Center	Bel Air	100%	83
Univ of MD Balto Washington Med Ctr	Glen Burnie	97%	87
Washington Adventist Hospital	Takoma Park	97%	31
Saint Agnes Hospital	Baltimore	96%	74
Johns Hopkins Bayview Medical Center	Baltimore	95%	38
Sinai Hospital of Baltimore	Baltimore	95%	56
Anne Arundel Medical Center	Annapolis	94%	89
Carroll Hospital Center	Westminster	94%	51
Medstar Southern Maryland Hospital Center[3]	Clinton	93%	42
Peninsula Regional Medical Center	Salisbury	93%	70
Suburban Hospital	Bethesda	92%	39
Howard County General Hospital	Columbia	90%	58
Western Maryland Regional Medical Center	Cumberland	85%	40
Medstar Franklin Square Medical Center	Baltimore	83%	69
Medstar Union Memorial Hospital	Baltimore	83%	29
Prince Georges Hospital Center[2]	Cheverly	56%	25

Statin Prescribed at Discharge

Hospital Name	City	Rate	Cases
Calvert Memorial Hospital	Prince Frederick	100%	30
Carroll Hospital Center	Westminster	100%	95
Frederick Memorial Hospital	Frederick	100%	208
Holy Cross Hospital	Silver Spring	100%	93
Howard County General Hospital	Columbia	100%	85
Johns Hopkins Bayview Medical Center	Baltimore	100%	220
Peninsula Regional Medical Center	Salisbury	100%	476
Shady Grove Adventist Hospital	Rockville	100%	205
Suburban Hospital	Bethesda	100%	220
Univ of MD Balto Washington Med Ctr	Glen Burnie	100%	218
University of Maryland Medical Center	Baltimore	100%	481
Upper Chesapeake Medical Center	Bel Air	100%	146
Washington Adventist Hospital	Takoma Park	100%	356
The Johns Hopkins Hospital	Baltimore	99%	505
Medstar Franklin Square Medical Center	Baltimore	99%	168
Medstar Good Samaritan Hospital	Baltimore	99%	69
Saint Agnes Hospital	Baltimore	99%	209
Univ of MD St Joseph Med Ctr[2,3]	Towson	99%	131
Anne Arundel Medical Center	Annapolis	98%	240
Medstar Harbor Hospital	Baltimore	98%	51
Sinai Hospital of Baltimore	Baltimore	98%	370
VA Maryland Healthcare System - Baltimore	Baltimore	98%	48
Western Maryland Regional Medical Center	Cumberland	98%	245
Meritus Medical Center	Hagerstown	97%	117
Prince Georges Hospital Center[2]	Cheverly	97%	143
Medstar Union Memorial Hospital	Baltimore	94%	475
Northwest Hospital Center	Randallstown	94%	53
Laurel Regional Medical Center	Laurel	93%	28
Medstar Southern Maryland Hospital Center[3]	Clinton	93%	149
Univ of MD Shore Med Ctr at Easton	Easton	92%	40

Heart Failure Care

ACE Inhibitor or ARB for LVSD

Hospital Name	City	Rate	Cases
Calvert Memorial Hospital	Prince Frederick	100%	36
Carroll Hospital Center[2]	Westminster	100%	52
Doctors' Community Hospital	Lanham	100%	114
Frederick Memorial Hospital	Frederick	100%	102
Holy Cross Hospital[2]	Silver Spring	100%	141
The Johns Hopkins Hospital[2]	Baltimore	100%	160
Laurel Regional Medical Center	Laurel	100%	47
Medstar Montgomery Medical Center	Olney	100%	54
Saint Agnes Hospital	Baltimore	100%	191
Shady Grove Adventist Hospital	Rockville	100%	122
Sinai Hospital of Baltimore	Baltimore	100%	248
Suburban Hospital[2]	Bethesda	100%	114
Univ of MD Balto Washington Med Ctr	Glen Burnie	100%	169
Univ of MD Charles Reg Med Ctr	La Plata	100%	59
Univ of MD Med Ctr Midtown Campus	Baltimore	100%	48
Upper Chesapeake Medical Center	Bel Air	100%	62
Northwest Hospital Center	Randallstown	99%	156
University of Maryland Medical Center	Baltimore	99%	198
Univ of MD Shore Med Ctr at Easton[2]	Easton	99%	138
Fort Washington Hospital	Fort Washington	98%	49
Greater Baltimore Medical Center[3]	Baltimore	98%	45
Medstar Saint Mary's Hospital[2]	Leonardtown	98%	46
Peninsula Regional Medical Center	Salisbury	98%	170
Univ of MD St Joseph Med Ctr[2,3]	Towson	98%	41
Western Maryland Regional Medical Center	Cumberland	98%	103
Medstar Good Samaritan Hospital	Baltimore	97%	212
Meritus Medical Center	Hagerstown	97%	61
VA Maryland Healthcare System - Baltimore	Baltimore	97%	117
Washington Adventist Hospital	Takoma Park	97%	146
Anne Arundel Medical Center	Annapolis	96%	181
Howard County General Hospital[2]	Columbia	96%	79
Johns Hopkins Bayview Medical Center	Baltimore	96%	240
Medstar Union Memorial Hospital	Baltimore	96%	187
Prince Georges Hospital Center[2]	Cheverly	96%	113
Univ of MD Shore Med Ctr-Chestertown	Chestertown	96%	28
Medstar Franklin Square Medical Center	Baltimore	93%	168
Medstar Harbor Hospital	Baltimore	92%	103
Bon Secours Hospital	Baltimore	90%	59
Mercy Medical Center	Baltimore	89%	123
Atlantic General Hospital	Berlin	88%	26
Medstar Southern Maryland Hospital Center[3]	Clinton	85%	166

Discharge Instructions Given

Hospital Name	City	Rate	Cases
Calvert Memorial Hospital	Prince Frederick	100%	245
Greater Baltimore Medical Center[3]	Baltimore	100%	164
Peninsula Regional Medical Center	Salisbury	100%	465
Shady Grove Adventist Hospital	Rockville	100%	232
Union Hospital of Cecil County	Elkton	100%	57
Univ of MD Med Ctr Midtown Campus	Baltimore	100%	108
Univ of MD Shore Med Ctr-Chestertown	Chestertown	100%	75
Carroll Hospital Center[2]	Westminster	99%	180
Fort Washington Hospital	Fort Washington	99%	118
The Johns Hopkins Hospital[2]	Baltimore	99%	385
Univ of MD Charles Reg Med Ctr	La Plata	99%	213
Upper Chesapeake Medical Center	Bel Air	99%	254
Anne Arundel Medical Center	Annapolis	98%	490
Doctors' Community Hospital	Lanham	98%	291
Harford Memorial Hospital	Havre De Grace	98%	124
Univ of MD St Joseph Med Ctr[2,3]	Towson	98%	107
Laurel Regional Medical Center	Laurel	97%	116
Johns Hopkins Bayview Medical Center	Baltimore	96%	535
Medstar Montgomery Medical Center	Olney	96%	123
Medstar Saint Mary's Hospital[2]	Leonardtown	96%	179
Univ of MD Shore Med Ctr at Easton[2]	Easton	96%	338
Holy Cross Hospital[2]	Silver Spring	95%	317
Howard County General Hospital[2]	Columbia	95%	250
Sinai Hospital of Baltimore	Baltimore	95%	575
Univ of MD Balto Washington Med Ctr	Glen Burnie	95%	553
Garrett County Memorial Hospital	Oakland	94%	69
Medstar Harbor Hospital	Baltimore	94%	243
Meritus Medical Center	Hagerstown	94%	250
Northwest Hospital Center	Randallstown	94%	353
Saint Agnes Hospital	Baltimore	94%	491
University of Maryland Medical Center	Baltimore	94%	332
VA Maryland Healthcare System - Baltimore	Baltimore	94%	222
Frederick Memorial Hospital	Frederick	93%	325
Mercy Medical Center	Baltimore	93%	238
Washington Adventist Hospital	Takoma Park	93%	239
Medstar Good Samaritan Hospital	Baltimore	92%	481
Medstar Union Memorial Hospital	Baltimore	89%	448
Bon Secours Hospital	Baltimore	88%	179
Western Maryland Regional Medical Center	Cumberland	88%	208
Suburban Hospital[2]	Bethesda	83%	233
Atlantic General Hospital	Berlin	82%	110
Prince Georges Hospital Center[2]	Cheverly	82%	276
Medstar Franklin Square Medical Center	Baltimore	74%	566
Medstar Southern Maryland Hospital Center[3]	Clinton	62%	454

Evaluation of LVS Function

Hospital Name	City	Rate	Cases
Bon Secours Hospital	Baltimore	100%	199
Calvert Memorial Hospital	Prince Frederick	100%	242
Carroll Hospital Center[2]	Westminster	100%	220
Doctors' Community Hospital	Lanham	100%	339
Frederick Memorial Hospital	Frederick	100%	430
Garrett County Memorial Hospital	Oakland	100%	77
Harford Memorial Hospital	Havre De Grace	100%	151
Holy Cross Hospital[2]	Silver Spring	100%	407
The Johns Hopkins Hospital[2]	Baltimore	100%	431
Medstar Good Samaritan Hospital	Baltimore	100%	673
Medstar Montgomery Medical Center	Olney	100%	177
Medstar Saint Mary's Hospital[2]	Leonardtown	100%	215
Mercy Medical Center	Baltimore	100%	274
Meritus Medical Center	Hagerstown	100%	310
Northwest Hospital Center	Randallstown	100%	458
Peninsula Regional Medical Center	Salisbury	100%	611
Saint Agnes Hospital	Baltimore	100%	592
Shady Grove Adventist Hospital	Rockville	100%	317
Union Hospital of Cecil County	Elkton	100%	78
Univ of MD Balto Washington Med Ctr	Glen Burnie	100%	627
Univ of MD Charles Reg Med Ctr	La Plata	100%	260
University of Maryland Medical Center	Baltimore	100%	391
Univ of MD Med Ctr Midtown Campus	Baltimore	100%	138
Univ of MD St Joseph Med Ctr[2,3]	Towson	100%	132
Univ of MD Shore Med Ctr-Chestertown	Chestertown	100%	93
Univ of MD Shore Med Ctr at Easton[2]	Easton	100%	417
Upper Chesapeake Medical Center	Bel Air	100%	330
VA Maryland Healthcare System - Baltimore	Baltimore	100%	235
Washington Adventist Hospital	Takoma Park	100%	315
Western Maryland Regional Medical Center	Cumberland	100%	269
Anne Arundel Medical Center	Annapolis	99%	596
Fort Washington Hospital	Fort Washington	99%	138
Greater Baltimore Medical Center[3]	Baltimore	99%	242
Howard County General Hospital[2]	Columbia	99%	304
Johns Hopkins Bayview Medical Center	Baltimore	99%	658
Laurel Regional Medical Center	Laurel	99%	144
Medstar Franklin Square Medical Center	Baltimore	99%	726
Prince Georges Hospital Center[2]	Cheverly	99%	295
Sinai Hospital of Baltimore	Baltimore	99%	691

NOTE: Hospital profiles are in alphabetical order by state, then city, then hospital within the city; Rankings exclude hospitals with less than 25 cases except for patient surveys which excludes hospitals with less than 100 cases; (a) 100-299 cases; (1) The number of cases/patients is too few to report; (2) Data submitted were based on a sample of cases/patients; (3) Results are based on a shorter time period than required; (4) Data suppressed by CMS for one or more quarters; (5) Results are not available for this reporting period; (6) Fewer than 100 patients completed the HCAHPS survey; (7) No cases met the criteria for this measure; (8) The lower limit of the confidence interval cannot be calculated if the number of observed infections equals zero; (9) No data are available from the state/territory for this reporting period; (10) The scores shown reflect fewer than 50 completed surveys; (11) There were discrepancies in the data collection process; (12) This measure does not apply to this hospital for this reporting period; (13) Results cannot be calculated for this reporting period; (14) The results for this state are combined with nearby states to protect confidentiality; Please refer to the User's Guide for a full explanation of data.

Hospital Name	City	Rate	Cases
Suburban Hospital[2]	Bethesda	99%	333
Medstar Harbor Hospital	Baltimore	98%	291
Atlantic General Hospital	Berlin	96%	148
Medstar Southern Maryland Hospital Center[3]	Clinton	96%	498
Medstar Union Memorial Hospital	Baltimore	95%	506

Medicare Spending

Data was not available for this measure.

Pneumonia Care

Appropriate Initial Antibiotic Given

Hospital Name	City	Rate	Cases
Fort Washington Hospital	Fort Washington	100%	46
The Johns Hopkins Hospital[2]	Baltimore	100%	41
Medstar Saint Mary's Hospital[2]	Leonardtown	100%	77
Saint Agnes Hospital[2]	Baltimore	100%	59
Univ of MD Charles Reg Med Ctr[2]	La Plata	100%	98
University of Maryland Medical Center	Baltimore	100%	46
Univ of MD Med Ctr Midtown Campus	Baltimore	100%	42
Frederick Memorial Hospital	Frederick	99%	269
Greater Baltimore Medical Center[3]	Baltimore	99%	103
Harford Memorial Hospital	Havre De Grace	99%	121
Holy Cross Hospital[2]	Silver Spring	99%	165
Medstar Montgomery Medical Center	Olney	99%	159
Sinai Hospital of Baltimore	Baltimore	99%	132
Suburban Hospital[2]	Bethesda	99%	113
Washington Adventist Hospital	Takoma Park	99%	76
Atlantic General Hospital	Berlin	98%	128
Doctors' Community Hospital	Lanham	98%	307
Garrett County Memorial Hospital	Oakland	98%	42
Northwest Hospital Center[2]	Randallstown	98%	129
Union Hospital of Cecil County	Elkton	98%	124
Univ of MD Balto Washington Med Ctr	Glen Burnie	98%	418
Univ of MD Shore Med Ctr-Chestertown	Chestertown	98%	41
Bon Secours Hospital	Baltimore	97%	93
Howard County General Hospital[2]	Columbia	97%	77
Johns Hopkins Bayview Medical Center	Baltimore	97%	169
Medstar Harbor Hospital	Baltimore	97%	156
Shady Grove Adventist Hospital[2]	Rockville	97%	196
Carroll Hospital Center[2]	Westminster	96%	99
Laurel Regional Medical Center	Laurel	96%	101
Medstar Franklin Square Medical Center	Baltimore	96%	346
Medstar Union Memorial Hospital	Baltimore	96%	98
Upper Chesapeake Medical Center	Bel Air	96%	248
VA Maryland Healthcare System - Baltimore	Baltimore	96%	55
Western Maryland Regional Medical Center	Cumberland	96%	180
Anne Arundel Medical Center	Annapolis	95%	284
Calvert Memorial Hospital	Prince Frederick	95%	168
Medstar Good Samaritan Hospital	Baltimore	95%	169
Peninsula Regional Medical Center	Salisbury	95%	294
Univ of MD St Joseph Med Ctr[2,3]	Towson	95%	37
Medstar Southern Maryland Hospital Center[2,3]	Clinton	94%	62
Prince Georges Hospital Center[2]	Cheverly	94%	69
Univ of MD Shore Med Ctr at Easton	Easton	94%	157
Meritus Medical Center	Hagerstown	93%	437
Mercy Medical Center	Baltimore	92%	89

Blood Culture Timing

Hospital Name	City	Rate	Cases
Calvert Memorial Hospital	Prince Frederick	100%	216
Harford Memorial Hospital	Havre De Grace	100%	201
The Johns Hopkins Hospital[2]	Baltimore	100%	42
Shady Grove Adventist Hospital[2]	Rockville	100%	220
University of Maryland Medical Center	Baltimore	100%	99
Upper Chesapeake Medical Center	Bel Air	100%	437
Atlantic General Hospital	Berlin	99%	164
Bon Secours Hospital	Baltimore	99%	170
Frederick Memorial Hospital	Frederick	99%	285
Holy Cross Hospital[2]	Silver Spring	99%	262
Medstar Montgomery Medical Center	Olney	99%	205
Medstar Union Memorial Hospital	Baltimore	99%	166
Suburban Hospital[2]	Bethesda	99%	192
Univ of MD Charles Reg Med Ctr[2]	La Plata	99%	155
Univ of MD Med Ctr Midtown Campus	Baltimore	99%	145
Washington Adventist Hospital	Takoma Park	99%	143
Carroll Hospital Center[2]	Westminster	98%	165
Garrett County Memorial Hospital	Oakland	98%	44
Howard County General Hospital[2]	Columbia	98%	139
Johns Hopkins Bayview Medical Center	Baltimore	98%	98
Medstar Saint Mary's Hospital[2]	Leonardtown	98%	130
Northwest Hospital Center[2]	Randallstown	98%	218
Sinai Hospital of Baltimore	Baltimore	98%	320
Univ of MD Balto Washington Med Ctr	Glen Burnie	98%	280
Anne Arundel Medical Center	Annapolis	97%	463
Doctors' Community Hospital	Lanham	97%	505
Greater Baltimore Medical Center[3]	Baltimore	97%	149
Peninsula Regional Medical Center	Salisbury	97%	451
Union Hospital of Cecil County	Elkton	97%	227
VA Maryland Healthcare System - Baltimore	Baltimore	97%	120
Western Maryland Regional Medical Center	Cumberland	97%	355
Meritus Medical Center	Hagerstown	96%	741
Univ of MD Shore Med Ctr at Easton	Easton	96%	186
Fort Washington Hospital	Fort Washington	95%	75
Medstar Harbor Hospital	Baltimore	94%	292
Prince Georges Hospital Center[2]	Cheverly	94%	126
Saint Agnes Hospital[2]	Baltimore	94%	214
Univ of MD St Joseph Med Ctr[2,3]	Towson	94%	62
Medstar Good Samaritan Hospital	Baltimore	92%	351
Mercy Medical Center	Baltimore	92%	105
Laurel Regional Medical Center	Laurel	91%	158
Univ of MD Shore Med Ctr-Chestertown	Chestertown	91%	67
Medstar Franklin Square Medical Center	Baltimore	89%	369
Medstar Southern Maryland Hospital Center[2,3]	Clinton	82%	50

Pregnancy and Delivery Care

No hospitals met the 25 case threshold.

Preventive Care

Immunization for Influenza

Hospital Name	City	Rate	Cases
Doctors' Community Hospital[2]	Lanham	100%	597
Univ of MD Shore Med Ctr-Chestertown[2]	Chestertown	100%	319
Northwest Hospital Center[2]	Randallstown	99%	597
Harford Memorial Hospital[2]	Havre De Grace	98%	485
Holy Cross Hospital[2]	Silver Spring	98%	484
Medstar Montgomery Medical Center[2]	Olney	98%	648
Medstar Saint Mary's Hospital[2]	Leonardtown	98%	547
Univ of MD Med Ctr Midtown Campus[2]	Baltimore	98%	579
Anne Arundel Medical Center[2]	Annapolis	97%	819
Howard County General Hospital[2,3]	Columbia	97%	243
Meritus Medical Center[2]	Hagerstown	97%	7246
Union Hospital of Cecil County	Elkton	97%	782
Univ of MD Charles Reg Med Ctr[2]	La Plata	97%	611
Upper Chesapeake Medical Center[2]	Bel Air	97%	521
Garrett County Memorial Hospital	Oakland	96%	937
Laurel Regional Medical Center[2]	Laurel	96%	459
Medstar Good Samaritan Hospital[2]	Baltimore	96%	591
Univ of MD Shore Med Ctr at Easton[2]	Easton	96%	529
Washington Adventist Hospital[2]	Takoma Park	96%	509
Carroll Hospital Center[2]	Westminster	95%	553
Fort Washington Hospital[2]	Fort Washington	95%	289
Saint Agnes Hospital[2]	Baltimore	95%	551
Suburban Hospital[2]	Bethesda	95%	589
Frederick Memorial Hospital[2]	Frederick	94%	511
Johns Hopkins Bayview Medical Center[2]	Baltimore	94%	536
Medstar Franklin Square Medical Center[2]	Baltimore	94%	574
Sinai Hospital of Baltimore[2]	Baltimore	94%	691
Calvert Memorial Hospital[2]	Prince Frederick	93%	553
Atlantic General Hospital[2]	Berlin	92%	302
University of Maryland Medical Center[2]	Baltimore	91%	807
Greater Baltimore Medical Center[2,3]	Baltimore	89%	271
Peninsula Regional Medical Center[2]	Salisbury	89%	533
Univ of MD Balto Washington Med Ctr[2]	Glen Burnie	89%	824
Medstar Harbor Hospital[2]	Baltimore	87%	513
Prince Georges Hospital Center[2]	Cheverly	87%	479
Medstar Union Memorial Hospital[2]	Baltimore	86%	496
Medstar Southern Maryland Hospital Center[2,3]	Clinton	84%	304
Shady Grove Adventist Hospital[2]	Rockville	83%	463
Bon Secours Hospital[2]	Baltimore	74%	592
Edward Mccready Memorial Hospital	Crisfield	52%	79

Immunization for Pneumonia

Hospital Name	City	Rate	Cases
Doctors' Community Hospital[2]	Lanham	99%	780
Harford Memorial Hospital[2]	Havre De Grace	99%	582
Medstar Saint Mary's Hospital[2]	Leonardtown	99%	640
Northwest Hospital Center[2]	Randallstown	99%	911
Union Hospital of Cecil County	Elkton	99%	1122
Univ of MD Med Ctr Midtown Campus[2]	Baltimore	99%	695
Upper Chesapeake Medical Center[2]	Bel Air	99%	664
Suburban Hospital[2]	Bethesda	98%	799
Univ of MD Shore Med Ctr-Chestertown[2]	Chestertown	98%	499
Calvert Memorial Hospital[2]	Prince Frederick	97%	585
Garrett County Memorial Hospital	Oakland	97%	1082
Holy Cross Hospital[2]	Silver Spring	97%	452
Howard County General Hospital[2,3]	Columbia	97%	388
Johns Hopkins Bayview Medical Center[2]	Baltimore	97%	683
Anne Arundel Medical Center[2]	Annapolis	96%	830
Carroll Hospital Center[2]	Westminster	96%	733
Meritus Medical Center[2]	Hagerstown	96%	5069
Medstar Montgomery Medical Center[2]	Olney	95%	753
Sinai Hospital of Baltimore[2]	Baltimore	95%	844
Univ of MD Charles Reg Med Ctr[2]	La Plata	95%	762
Univ of MD St Joseph Med Ctr[2,3]	Towson	95%	320
Univ of MD Shore Med Ctr at Easton[2]	Easton	95%	694
Medstar Good Samaritan Hospital[2]	Baltimore	94%	918
Washington Adventist Hospital[2]	Takoma Park	94%	551
Fort Washington Hospital[2]	Fort Washington	93%	417
Univ of MD Balto Washington Med Ctr[2]	Glen Burnie	93%	1112
Greater Baltimore Medical Center[2,3]	Baltimore	92%	275
Medstar Union Memorial Hospital[2]	Baltimore	92%	753
Saint Agnes Hospital[2]	Baltimore	92%	720
University of Maryland Medical Center[2]	Baltimore	92%	722
Medstar Franklin Square Medical Center[2]	Baltimore	91%	713
Medstar Southern Maryland Hospital Center[2,3]	Clinton	91%	654
Laurel Regional Medical Center[2]	Laurel	90%	512
Medstar Harbor Hospital[2]	Baltimore	89%	639
Frederick Memorial Hospital[2]	Frederick	88%	606
Peninsula Regional Medical Center[2]	Salisbury	88%	669
Atlantic General Hospital[2]	Berlin	87%	500
Prince Georges Hospital Center[2]	Cheverly	82%	456
Bon Secours Hospital[2]	Baltimore	80%	690
Shady Grove Adventist Hospital[2]	Rockville	70%	424
Edward Mccready Memorial Hospital[3]	Crisfield	35%	109

Stroke Care

Antithrombotic Therapy Timing

Hospital Name	City	Rate	Cases
Laurel Regional Medical Center	Laurel	97%	36
Medstar Union Memorial Hospital	Baltimore	97%	59
Prince Georges Hospital Center	Cheverly	96%	92

Assessed for Rehabilitation

Hospital Name	City	Rate	Cases
Prince Georges Hospital Center	Cheverly	98%	91
Medstar Union Memorial Hospital	Baltimore	97%	60
Laurel Regional Medical Center	Laurel	91%	43

Discharged on Antithrombotic Therapy

Hospital Name	City	Rate	Cases
Prince Georges Hospital Center	Cheverly	98%	85
Laurel Regional Medical Center	Laurel	95%	39
Medstar Union Memorial Hospital	Baltimore	95%	59

Discharged on Statin Medication

Hospital Name	City	Rate	Cases
Medstar Union Memorial Hospital	Baltimore	100%	50
Laurel Regional Medical Center	Laurel	97%	37
Prince Georges Hospital Center	Cheverly	95%	76

Venous Thromboembolism (VTE) Prophylaxis

Hospital Name	City	Rate	Cases
Laurel Regional Medical Center	Laurel	93%	41
Prince Georges Hospital Center	Cheverly	89%	103
Medstar Union Memorial Hospital	Baltimore	87%	61

Written Stroke Educational Materials Given

Hospital Name	City	Rate	Cases
Medstar Union Memorial Hospital	Baltimore	100%	34
Prince Georges Hospital Center	Cheverly	63%	54

Surgical Care Improvement Project

Appropriate Beta Blocker Usage

Hospital Name	City	Rate	Cases
Calvert Memorial Hospital	Prince Frederick	100%	61
Garrett County Memorial Hospital	Oakland	100%	71
Harford Memorial Hospital	Havre De Grace	100%	32
Holy Cross Hospital[2]	Silver Spring	100%	159
Saint Agnes Hospital[2]	Baltimore	100%	117
Union Hospital of Cecil County	Elkton	100%	105
Univ of MD Med Ctr Midtown Campus	Baltimore	100%	30
Upper Chesapeake Medical Center[2]	Bel Air	100%	223
Frederick Memorial Hospital[2]	Frederick	99%	262
The Johns Hopkins Hospital[2]	Baltimore	99%	345
Mercy Medical Center[2]	Baltimore	99%	349
Suburban Hospital[2]	Bethesda	99%	449
Univ of MD Balto Washington Med Ctr[2]	Glen Burnie	99%	306
Washington Adventist Hospital	Takoma Park	99%	253
Western Maryland Regional Medical Center	Cumberland	99%	357
Atlantic General Hospital	Berlin	98%	92
Carroll Hospital Center[2]	Westminster	98%	112
Doctors' Community Hospital[2]	Lanham	98%	121
Greater Baltimore Medical Center[3]	Baltimore	98%	152
Medstar Montgomery Medical Center	Olney	98%	128
Medstar Saint Mary's Hospital[2]	Leonardtown	98%	61
Sinai Hospital of Baltimore[2]	Baltimore	98%	378
Univ of MD St Joseph Med Ctr[2,3]	Towson	98%	97
Fort Washington Hospital	Fort Washington	97%	30
Howard County General Hospital[2]	Columbia	97%	101
Laurel Regional Medical Center	Laurel	97%	36
Medstar Franklin Square Medical Center[2]	Baltimore	97%	347
Medstar Union Memorial Hospital[2]	Baltimore	97%	313
Shady Grove Adventist Hospital	Rockville	97%	236

NOTE: Hospital profiles are in alphabetical order by state, then city, then hospital within the city; Rankings exclude hospitals with less than 25 cases except for patient surveys which excludes hospitals with less than 100 cases; (a) 100-299 cases; (1) The number of cases/patients is too few to report; (2) Data submitted were based on a sample of cases/patients; (3) Results are based on a shorter time period than required; (4) Data suppressed by CMS for one or more quarters; (5) Results are not available for this reporting period; (6) Fewer than 100 patients completed the HCAHPS survey; (7) No cases met the criteria for this measure; (8) The lower limit of the confidence interval cannot be calculated if the number of observed infections equals zero; (9) No data are available from the state/territory for this reporting period; (10) The scores shown reflect fewer than 50 completed surveys; (11) There were discrepancies in the data collection process; (12) This measure does not apply to this hospital for this reporting period; (13) Results cannot be calculated for this reporting period; (14) The results for this state are combined with nearby states to protect confidentiality; Please refer to the User's Guide for a full explanation of data.

University of Maryland Medical Center[2]	Baltimore	97%	612
Univ of MD Shore Med Ctr-Chestertown	Chestertown	97%	29
VA Maryland Healthcare System - Baltimore[2]	Baltimore	97%	59
Peninsula Regional Medical Center[2]	Salisbury	96%	210
Univ of MD Charles Reg Med Ctr[2]	La Plata	96%	102
Univ of MD Shore Med Ctr at Easton	Easton	96%	216
Johns Hopkins Bayview Medical Center[2]	Baltimore	95%	209
Meritus Medical Center	Hagerstown	95%	378
Anne Arundel Medical Center[2]	Annapolis	94%	248
Northwest Hospital Center	Randallstown	94%	86
Medstar Good Samaritan Hospital	Baltimore	93%	272
Medstar Harbor Hospital[2]	Baltimore	90%	168
Medstar Southern Maryland Hospital Center[2,3]	Clinton	90%	120
Prince Georges Hospital Center[2]	Cheverly	83%	30

Appropriate VTP Within 24 Hours

Hospital Name	City	Rate	Cases
Bon Secours Hospital	Baltimore	100%	60
Calvert Memorial Hospital	Prince Frederick	100%	183
Harford Memorial Hospital	Havre De Grace	100%	106
Holy Cross Hospital[2]	Silver Spring	100%	618
Mercy Medical Center[2]	Baltimore	100%	1310
Saint Agnes Hospital[2]	Baltimore	100%	376
Carroll Hospital Center[2]	Westminster	99%	395
Doctors' Community Hospital[2]	Lanham	99%	410
Fort Washington Hospital	Fort Washington	99%	134
Frederick Memorial Hospital[2]	Frederick	99%	751
The Johns Hopkins Hospital[2]	Baltimore	99%	343
Medstar Montgomery Medical Center	Olney	99%	401
Meritus Medical Center	Hagerstown	99%	1072
Shady Grove Adventist Hospital	Rockville	99%	853
Union Hospital of Cecil County	Elkton	99%	282
Univ of MD Balto Washington Med Ctr[2]	Glen Burnie	99%	726
Univ of MD Charles Reg Med Ctr[2]	La Plata	99%	330
Upper Chesapeake Medical Center[2]	Bel Air	99%	599
Western Maryland Regional Medical Center	Cumberland	99%	653
Greater Baltimore Medical Center[3]	Baltimore	98%	531
Howard County General Hospital[2]	Columbia	98%	367
Johns Hopkins Bayview Medical Center[2]	Baltimore	98%	601
Medstar Good Samaritan Hospital	Baltimore	98%	815
Medstar Saint Mary's Hospital[2]	Leonardtown	98%	240
Sinai Hospital of Baltimore[2]	Baltimore	98%	648
Suburban Hospital[2]	Bethesda	98%	1311
Univ of MD St Joseph Med Ctr[2,3]	Towson	98%	127
Washington Adventist Hospital	Takoma Park	98%	217
Atlantic General Hospital	Berlin	97%	259
Medstar Franklin Square Medical Center[2]	Baltimore	97%	661
Medstar Harbor Hospital[2]	Baltimore	97%	523
Medstar Southern Maryland Hospital Center[2,3]	Clinton	97%	378
Medstar Union Memorial Hospital[2]	Baltimore	97%	609
Northwest Hospital Center	Randallstown	97%	253
Peninsula Regional Medical Center[2]	Salisbury	97%	308
Univ of MD Med Ctr Midtown Campus	Baltimore	97%	107
Univ of MD Shore Med Ctr-Chestertown	Chestertown	97%	87
Univ of MD Shore Med Ctr at Easton	Easton	97%	565
Anne Arundel Medical Center[2]	Annapolis	96%	786
Garrett County Memorial Hospital	Oakland	95%	209
Laurel Regional Medical Center	Laurel	94%	99
University of Maryland Medical Center[2]	Baltimore	94%	806
VA Maryland Healthcare System - Baltimore[2]	Baltimore	88%	151
Prince Georges Hospital Center[2]	Cheverly	84%	154

Controlled Postoperative Blood Glucose

Hospital Name	City	Rate	Cases
Washington Adventist Hospital	Takoma Park	100%	278
Sinai Hospital of Baltimore[2]	Baltimore	99%	267
Western Maryland Regional Medical Center	Cumberland	98%	171
Peninsula Regional Medical Center[2]	Salisbury	97%	135
The Johns Hopkins Hospital[2]	Baltimore	96%	391
Suburban Hospital[2]	Bethesda	96%	171
University of Maryland Medical Center[2]	Baltimore	95%	562
Medstar Union Memorial Hospital[2]	Baltimore	91%	163
Univ of MD St Joseph Med Ctr[2,3]	Towson	90%	63

Perioperative Temperature Management

Hospital Name	City	Rate	Cases
Atlantic General Hospital	Berlin	100%	279
Bon Secours Hospital	Baltimore	100%	64
Calvert Memorial Hospital	Prince Frederick	100%	231
Carroll Hospital Center[2]	Westminster	100%	559
Doctors' Community Hospital[2]	Lanham	100%	460
Fort Washington Hospital	Fort Washington	100%	141
Frederick Memorial Hospital[2]	Frederick	100%	873
Garrett County Memorial Hospital	Oakland	100%	214
Greater Baltimore Medical Center[3]	Baltimore	100%	668
Harford Memorial Hospital	Havre De Grace	100%	118
Holy Cross Hospital[2]	Silver Spring	100%	715
Howard County General Hospital[2]	Columbia	100%	415
Johns Hopkins Bayview Medical Center[2]	Baltimore	100%	704
The Johns Hopkins Hospital[2]	Baltimore	100%	485
Laurel Regional Medical Center	Laurel	100%	143
Medstar Franklin Square Medical Center[2]	Baltimore	100%	923
Medstar Good Samaritan Hospital	Baltimore	100%	902
Medstar Montgomery Medical Center	Olney	100%	452
Medstar Saint Mary's Hospital[2]	Leonardtown	100%	294
Medstar Southern Maryland Hospital Center[2,3]	Clinton	100%	466
Mercy Medical Center[2]	Baltimore	100%	1532
Meritus Medical Center	Hagerstown	100%	1184
Northwest Hospital Center	Randallstown	100%	300
Peninsula Regional Medical Center[2]	Salisbury	100%	397
Saint Agnes Hospital[2]	Baltimore	100%	463
Shady Grove Adventist Hospital	Rockville	100%	977
Sinai Hospital of Baltimore[2]	Baltimore	100%	755
Suburban Hospital[2]	Bethesda	100%	1399
Univ of MD Balto Washington Med Ctr[2]	Glen Burnie	100%	914
Univ of MD Charles Reg Med Ctr[2]	La Plata	100%	357
University of Maryland Medical Center[2]	Baltimore	100%	1076
Univ of MD Med Ctr Midtown Campus	Baltimore	100%	122
Univ of MD Shore Med Ctr at Easton	Easton	100%	668
Upper Chesapeake Medical Center[2]	Bel Air	100%	703
Washington Adventist Hospital	Takoma Park	100%	289
Western Maryland Regional Medical Center	Cumberland	100%	799
Union Hospital of Cecil County	Elkton	99%	312
Univ of MD St Joseph Med Ctr[2,3]	Towson	99%	181
Univ of MD Shore Med Ctr-Chestertown	Chestertown	99%	105
Anne Arundel Medical Center[2]	Annapolis	98%	1008
Medstar Harbor Hospital[2]	Baltimore	98%	610
VA Maryland Healthcare System - Baltimore[2]	Baltimore	98%	181
Medstar Union Memorial Hospital[2]	Baltimore	97%	810
Prince Georges Hospital Center[2]	Cheverly	97%	192

Prophylactic Antibiotic Selection

Hospital Name	City	Rate	Cases
Bon Secours Hospital	Baltimore	100%	28
Doctors' Community Hospital[2]	Lanham	100%	305
Fort Washington Hospital	Fort Washington	100%	95
Harford Memorial Hospital	Havre De Grace	100%	74
Holy Cross Hospital[2]	Silver Spring	100%	394
Medstar Saint Mary's Hospital[2]	Leonardtown	100%	242
Meritus Medical Center	Hagerstown	100%	758
Shady Grove Adventist Hospital	Rockville	100%	650
Univ of MD Balto Washington Med Ctr[2]	Glen Burnie	100%	656
Univ of MD Charles Reg Med Ctr[2]	La Plata	100%	232
Univ of MD Med Ctr Midtown Campus	Baltimore	100%	52
Univ of MD St Joseph Med Ctr[2,3]	Towson	100%	170
VA Maryland Healthcare System - Baltimore	Baltimore	100%	67
Washington Adventist Hospital	Takoma Park	100%	427
Western Maryland Regional Medical Center	Cumberland	100%	703
Calvert Memorial Hospital	Prince Frederick	99%	179
Carroll Hospital Center[2]	Westminster	99%	377
Frederick Memorial Hospital[2]	Frederick	99%	675
Greater Baltimore Medical Center[3]	Baltimore	99%	401
Johns Hopkins Bayview Medical Center[2]	Baltimore	99%	530
The Johns Hopkins Hospital[2]	Baltimore	99%	572
Medstar Harbor Hospital[2]	Baltimore	99%	462
Medstar Montgomery Medical Center	Olney	99%	305
Medstar Southern Maryland Hospital Center[2,3]	Clinton	99%	312
Mercy Medical Center[2]	Baltimore	99%	1326
Peninsula Regional Medical Center[2]	Salisbury	99%	410
Saint Agnes Hospital[2]	Baltimore	99%	284
Suburban Hospital[2]	Bethesda	99%	1345
Univ of MD Shore Med Ctr-Chestertown	Chestertown	99%	70
Univ of MD Shore Med Ctr at Easton	Easton	99%	498
Upper Chesapeake Medical Center[2]	Bel Air	99%	469
Garrett County Memorial Hospital	Oakland	98%	167
Medstar Good Samaritan Hospital	Baltimore	98%	661
Medstar Union Memorial Hospital[2]	Baltimore	98%	663
Northwest Hospital Center	Randallstown	98%	176
Sinai Hospital of Baltimore[2]	Baltimore	98%	708
Union Hospital of Cecil County	Elkton	98%	184
University of Maryland Medical Center[2]	Baltimore	98%	1036
Anne Arundel Medical Center[2]	Annapolis	97%	676
Atlantic General Hospital	Berlin	97%	179
Howard County General Hospital[2]	Columbia	97%	262
Laurel Regional Medical Center	Laurel	97%	76
Medstar Franklin Square Medical Center[2]	Baltimore	96%	621
Prince Georges Hospital Center[2]	Cheverly	83%	82

Prophylactic Antibiotic Selection (Outpatient)

Hospital Name	City	Rate	Cases
Holy Cross Hospital	Silver Spring	98%	719

Prophylactic Antibiotic Stopped

Hospital Name	City	Rate	Cases
Bon Secours Hospital	Baltimore	100%	27
Harford Memorial Hospital	Havre De Grace	100%	73
The Johns Hopkins Hospital[2]	Baltimore	100%	561
Northwest Hospital Center	Randallstown	100%	164
Univ of MD Balto Washington Med Ctr[2]	Glen Burnie	100%	637
Univ of MD Med Ctr Midtown Campus	Baltimore	100%	51
Upper Chesapeake Medical Center[2]	Bel Air	100%	464
Western Maryland Regional Medical Center	Cumberland	100%	694
Frederick Memorial Hospital[2]	Frederick	99%	655
Holy Cross Hospital[2]	Silver Spring	99%	373
Saint Agnes Hospital[2]	Baltimore	99%	273
Sinai Hospital of Baltimore[2]	Baltimore	99%	667
Suburban Hospital[2]	Bethesda	99%	1336
Univ of MD Charles Reg Med Ctr[2]	La Plata	99%	213
Univ of MD St Joseph Med Ctr[2,3]	Towson	99%	164
Univ of MD Shore Med Ctr-Chestertown	Chestertown	99%	70
Washington Adventist Hospital	Takoma Park	99%	424
Anne Arundel Medical Center[2]	Annapolis	98%	667
Calvert Memorial Hospital	Prince Frederick	98%	166
Doctors' Community Hospital[2]	Lanham	98%	287
Fort Washington Hospital	Fort Washington	98%	93
Howard County General Hospital[2]	Columbia	98%	256
Johns Hopkins Bayview Medical Center[2]	Baltimore	98%	519
Medstar Montgomery Medical Center	Olney	98%	285
Mercy Medical Center[2]	Baltimore	98%	1315
Meritus Medical Center	Hagerstown	98%	740
Shady Grove Adventist Hospital	Rockville	98%	632
Union Hospital of Cecil County	Elkton	98%	177
Carroll Hospital Center[2]	Westminster	97%	372
Medstar Franklin Square Medical Center[2]	Baltimore	97%	605
Medstar Good Samaritan Hospital	Baltimore	97%	638
Medstar Saint Mary's Hospital[2]	Leonardtown	97%	238
Peninsula Regional Medical Center[2]	Salisbury	97%	401
University of Maryland Medical Center[2]	Baltimore	97%	972
Univ of MD Shore Med Ctr at Easton	Easton	97%	490
Atlantic General Hospital	Berlin	96%	177
Garrett County Memorial Hospital	Oakland	96%	163
Greater Baltimore Medical Center[3]	Baltimore	96%	391
Laurel Regional Medical Center	Laurel	96%	73
Medstar Union Memorial Hospital[2]	Baltimore	96%	655
Medstar Harbor Hospital[2]	Baltimore	94%	451
Medstar Southern Maryland Hospital Center[2,3]	Clinton	94%	306
VA Maryland Healthcare System - Baltimore	Baltimore	94%	66
Prince Georges Hospital Center[2]	Cheverly	90%	77

Prophylactic Antibiotic Timing

Hospital Name	City	Rate	Cases
Atlantic General Hospital	Berlin	100%	179
Bon Secours Hospital	Baltimore	100%	28
Fort Washington Hospital	Fort Washington	100%	95
Frederick Memorial Hospital[2]	Frederick	100%	675
Laurel Regional Medical Center	Laurel	100%	76
Medstar Saint Mary's Hospital[2]	Leonardtown	100%	242
Saint Agnes Hospital[2]	Baltimore	100%	285
Univ of MD Balto Washington Med Ctr[2]	Glen Burnie	100%	656
Univ of MD Charles Reg Med Ctr[2]	La Plata	100%	232
Western Maryland Regional Medical Center	Cumberland	100%	703
Garrett County Memorial Hospital	Oakland	99%	167
Harford Memorial Hospital	Havre De Grace	99%	74
Holy Cross Hospital[2]	Silver Spring	99%	393
Howard County General Hospital[2]	Columbia	99%	262
Medstar Montgomery Medical Center	Olney	99%	305
Medstar Southern Maryland Hospital Center[2,3]	Clinton	99%	312
Northwest Hospital Center	Randallstown	99%	176
Shady Grove Adventist Hospital	Rockville	99%	651
Sinai Hospital of Baltimore[2]	Baltimore	99%	709
Union Hospital of Cecil County	Elkton	99%	184
University of Maryland Medical Center[2]	Baltimore	99%	1040
Univ of MD St Joseph Med Ctr[2,3]	Towson	99%	172
Univ of MD Shore Med Ctr at Easton	Easton	99%	499
Upper Chesapeake Medical Center[2]	Bel Air	99%	469
Washington Adventist Hospital	Takoma Park	99%	427
Anne Arundel Medical Center[2]	Annapolis	98%	675
Calvert Memorial Hospital	Prince Frederick	98%	179
Carroll Hospital Center[2]	Westminster	98%	377
Doctors' Community Hospital[2]	Lanham	98%	306
Johns Hopkins Bayview Medical Center[2]	Baltimore	98%	530
The Johns Hopkins Hospital[2]	Baltimore	98%	574
Medstar Franklin Square Medical Center[2]	Baltimore	98%	622
Medstar Good Samaritan Hospital	Baltimore	98%	661
Mercy Medical Center[2]	Baltimore	98%	1327
Meritus Medical Center	Hagerstown	98%	759
Peninsula Regional Medical Center[2]	Salisbury	98%	411
Suburban Hospital[2]	Bethesda	98%	1346
Univ of MD Med Ctr Midtown Campus	Baltimore	98%	52
Medstar Harbor Hospital[2]	Baltimore	97%	462
VA Maryland Healthcare System - Baltimore	Baltimore	96%	68
Greater Baltimore Medical Center[3]	Baltimore	94%	401
Univ of MD Shore Med Ctr-Chestertown	Chestertown	94%	70
Prince Georges Hospital Center[2]	Cheverly	89%	83
Medstar Union Memorial Hospital[2]	Baltimore	72%	770

Prophylactic Antibiotic Timing (Outpatient)

Hospital Name	City	Rate	Cases
Holy Cross Hospital	Silver Spring	98%	724

NOTE: Hospital profiles are in alphabetical order by state, then city, then hospital within the city; Rankings exclude hospitals with less than 25 cases except for patient surveys which excludes hospitals with less than 100 cases; (a) 100-299 cases; (1) The number of cases/patients is too few to report; (2) Data submitted were based on a sample of cases/patients; (3) Results are based on a shorter time period than required; (4) Data suppressed by CMS for one or more quarters; (5) Results are not available for this reporting period; (6) Fewer than 100 patients completed the HCAHPS survey; (7) No cases met the criteria for this measure; (8) The lower limit of the confidence interval cannot be calculated if the number of observed infections equals zero; (9) No data are available from the state/territory for this reporting period; (10) The scores shown reflect fewer than 50 completed surveys; (11) There were discrepancies in the data collection process; (12) This measure does not apply to this hospital for this reporting period; (13) Results cannot be calculated for this reporting period; (14) The results for this state are combined with nearby states to protect confidentiality; Please refer to the User's Guide for a full explanation of data.

Urinary Catheter Removal

Hospital Name	City	Rate	Cases
Bon Secours Hospital	Baltimore	100%	30
Calvert Memorial Hospital	Prince Frederick	100%	137
Fort Washington Hospital	Fort Washington	100%	34
Frederick Memorial Hospital[2]	Frederick	100%	638
Harford Memorial Hospital	Havre De Grace	100%	97
Holy Cross Hospital[2]	Silver Spring	100%	296
Medstar Montgomery Medical Center	Olney	100%	318
Mercy Medical Center[2]	Baltimore	100%	1119
Shady Grove Adventist Hospital	Rockville	100%	744
Sinai Hospital of Baltimore[2]	Baltimore	100%	603
Univ of MD Balto Washington Med Ctr[2]	Glen Burnie	100%	350
Univ of MD Med Ctr Midtown Campus	Baltimore	100%	65
Washington Adventist Hospital	Takoma Park	100%	428
Carroll Hospital Center[2]	Westminster	99%	278
Doctors' Community Hospital[2]	Lanham	99%	274
Medstar Saint Mary's Hospital[2]	Leonardtown	99%	228
Peninsula Regional Medical Center[2]	Salisbury	99%	318
Suburban Hospital[2]	Bethesda	99%	906
Univ of MD Charles Reg Med Ctr[2]	La Plata	99%	278
University of Maryland Medical Center[2]	Baltimore	99%	966
Upper Chesapeake Medical Center[2]	Bel Air	99%	390
Western Maryland Regional Medical Center	Cumberland	99%	158
Johns Hopkins Bayview Medical Center[2]	Baltimore	98%	511
The Johns Hopkins Hospital[2]	Baltimore	98%	346
Medstar Franklin Square Medical Center[2]	Baltimore	98%	578
Union Hospital of Cecil County	Elkton	98%	241
Howard County General Hospital[2]	Columbia	97%	269
Medstar Good Samaritan Hospital	Baltimore	97%	750
Saint Agnes Hospital[2]	Baltimore	97%	353
Univ of MD Shore Med Ctr-Chestertown	Chestertown	97%	65
Univ of MD Shore Med Ctr at Easton	Easton	97%	477
Anne Arundel Medical Center[2]	Annapolis	96%	661
Garrett County Memorial Hospital	Oakland	96%	161
Greater Baltimore Medical Center[3]	Baltimore	96%	365
Laurel Regional Medical Center	Laurel	95%	77
Medstar Harbor Hospital[2]	Baltimore	95%	377
Meritus Medical Center	Hagerstown	95%	455
Univ of MD St Joseph Med Ctr[2,3]	Towson	95%	106
VA Maryland Healthcare System - Baltimore[2]	Baltimore	95%	101
Atlantic General Hospital	Berlin	94%	249
Northwest Hospital Center	Randallstown	92%	146
Prince Georges Hospital Center[2]	Cheverly	92%	116
Medstar Union Memorial Hospital[2]	Baltimore	90%	248
Medstar Southern Maryland Hospital Center[2,3]	Clinton	89%	133

Survey of Patients' Hospital Experiences

Area Around Room 'Always' Quiet at Night

Hospital Name	City	Rate	Cases
Mercy Medical Center	Baltimore	68%	300+
The Johns Hopkins Hospital	Baltimore	66%	300+
Doctors' Community Hospital	Lanham	64%	300+
Medstar Union Memorial Hospital	Baltimore	64%	300+
Medstar Saint Mary's Hospital	Leonardtown	63%	300+
Anne Arundel Medical Center	Annapolis	62%	300+
Bon Secours Hospital	Baltimore	62%	300+
Univ of MD Med Ctr Midtown Campus	Baltimore	62%	300+
Medstar Good Samaritan Hospital	Baltimore	61%	300+
Medstar Harbor Hospital	Baltimore	61%	300+
Frederick Memorial Hospital	Frederick	60%	300+
Western Maryland Regional Medical Center	Cumberland	60%	300+
Prince Georges Hospital Center	Cheverly	59%	300+
Saint Agnes Hospital	Baltimore	59%	300+
Holy Cross Hospital	Silver Spring	58%	300+
Sinai Hospital of Baltimore	Baltimore	58%	300+
Univ of MD Shore Med Ctr-Chestertown	Chestertown	58%	300+
Upper Chesapeake Medical Center	Bel Air	57%	300+
Harford Memorial Hospital	Havre De Grace	56%	300+
Laurel Regional Medical Center	Laurel	56%	300+
Meritus Medical Center	Hagerstown	56%	300+
Univ of MD Balto Washington Med Ctr	Glen Burnie	56%	300+
Carroll Hospital Center	Westminster	55%	300+
Univ of MD Shore Med Ctr at Easton	Easton	55%	300+
Howard County General Hospital	Columbia	54%	300+
Washington Adventist Hospital	Takoma Park	54%	300+
Atlantic General Hospital	Berlin	53%	300+
Calvert Memorial Hospital	Prince Frederick	53%	300+
Fort Washington Hospital	Fort Washington	53%	(a)
Garrett County Memorial Hospital	Oakland	53%	300+
Greater Baltimore Medical Center	Baltimore	53%	300+
Medstar Montgomery Medical Center	Olney	53%	(a)
Northwest Hospital Center	Randallstown	53%	300+
Univ of MD Charles Reg Med Ctr	La Plata	53%	300+
University of Maryland Medical Center	Baltimore	53%	300+
Suburban Hospital	Bethesda	52%	300+
Medstar Franklin Square Medical Center	Baltimore	51%	300+
Peninsula Regional Medical Center	Salisbury	51%	300+
Shady Grove Adventist Hospital	Rockville	51%	300+
Union Hospital of Cecil County	Elkton	51%	300+
Johns Hopkins Bayview Medical Center	Baltimore	50%	300+

Doctors 'Always' Communicated Well

Hospital Name	City	Rate	Cases
Garrett County Memorial Hospital	Oakland	84%	300+
Mercy Medical Center	Baltimore	84%	300+
Univ of MD Shore Med Ctr-Chestertown	Chestertown	82%	300+
Univ of MD Shore Med Ctr at Easton	Easton	82%	300+
The Johns Hopkins Hospital	Baltimore	81%	300+
University of Maryland Medical Center	Baltimore	81%	300+
Anne Arundel Medical Center	Annapolis	80%	300+
Atlantic General Hospital	Berlin	80%	300+
Medstar Good Samaritan Hospital	Baltimore	80%	300+
Medstar Harbor Hospital	Baltimore	80%	300+
Medstar Union Memorial Hospital	Baltimore	80%	300+
Western Maryland Regional Medical Center	Cumberland	80%	300+
Carroll Hospital Center	Westminster	79%	300+
Harford Memorial Hospital	Havre De Grace	79%	300+
Johns Hopkins Bayview Medical Center	Baltimore	79%	300+
Medstar Saint Mary's Hospital	Leonardtown	79%	300+
Calvert Memorial Hospital	Prince Frederick	78%	300+
Doctors' Community Hospital	Lanham	78%	300+
Greater Baltimore Medical Center	Baltimore	78%	300+
Medstar Franklin Square Medical Center	Baltimore	78%	300+
Saint Agnes Hospital	Baltimore	78%	300+
Univ of MD Balto Washington Med Ctr	Glen Burnie	78%	300+
Frederick Memorial Hospital	Frederick	77%	300+
Peninsula Regional Medical Center	Salisbury	77%	300+
Shady Grove Adventist Hospital	Rockville	77%	300+
Suburban Hospital	Bethesda	77%	300+
Union Hospital of Cecil County	Elkton	77%	300+
Univ of MD Charles Reg Med Ctr	La Plata	77%	300+
Upper Chesapeake Medical Center	Bel Air	77%	300+
Washington Adventist Hospital	Takoma Park	77%	300+
Bon Secours Hospital	Baltimore	76%	300+
Northwest Hospital Center	Randallstown	76%	300+
Sinai Hospital of Baltimore	Baltimore	76%	300+
Univ of MD Med Ctr Midtown Campus	Baltimore	76%	300+
Fort Washington Hospital	Fort Washington	75%	(a)
Holy Cross Hospital	Silver Spring	75%	300+
Meritus Medical Center	Hagerstown	75%	300+
Howard County General Hospital	Columbia	74%	300+
Medstar Montgomery Medical Center	Olney	74%	(a)
Prince Georges Hospital Center	Cheverly	73%	300+
Laurel Regional Medical Center	Laurel	69%	300+

Home Recovery Information Given

Hospital Name	City	Rate	Cases
Medstar Saint Mary's Hospital	Leonardtown	90%	300+
Union Hospital of Cecil County	Elkton	90%	300+
Western Maryland Regional Medical Center	Cumberland	90%	300+
Atlantic General Hospital	Berlin	89%	300+
Mercy Medical Center	Baltimore	89%	300+
Anne Arundel Medical Center	Annapolis	88%	300+
Johns Hopkins Bayview Medical Center	Baltimore	88%	300+
Medstar Franklin Square Medical Center	Baltimore	88%	300+
University of Maryland Medical Center	Baltimore	88%	300+
Univ of MD Shore Med Ctr-Chestertown	Chestertown	88%	300+
Frederick Memorial Hospital	Frederick	87%	300+
The Johns Hopkins Hospital	Baltimore	87%	300+
Medstar Union Memorial Hospital	Baltimore	87%	300+
Carroll Hospital Center	Westminster	86%	300+
Garrett County Memorial Hospital	Oakland	86%	300+
Medstar Good Samaritan Hospital	Baltimore	86%	300+
Peninsula Regional Medical Center	Salisbury	86%	300+
Univ of MD Balto Washington Med Ctr	Glen Burnie	86%	300+
Calvert Memorial Hospital	Prince Frederick	85%	300+
Medstar Harbor Hospital	Baltimore	85%	300+
Medstar Montgomery Medical Center	Olney	85%	(a)
Univ of MD Shore Med Ctr at Easton	Easton	85%	300+
Doctors' Community Hospital	Lanham	84%	300+
Harford Memorial Hospital	Havre De Grace	84%	300+
Meritus Medical Center	Hagerstown	84%	300+
Shady Grove Adventist Hospital	Rockville	84%	300+
Univ of MD Med Ctr Midtown Campus	Baltimore	83%	300+
Upper Chesapeake Medical Center	Bel Air	83%	300+
Washington Adventist Hospital	Takoma Park	83%	300+
Greater Baltimore Medical Center	Baltimore	82%	300+
Northwest Hospital Center	Randallstown	82%	300+
Saint Agnes Hospital	Baltimore	82%	300+
Sinai Hospital of Baltimore	Baltimore	82%	300+
Univ of MD Charles Reg Med Ctr	La Plata	82%	300+
Holy Cross Hospital	Silver Spring	80%	300+
Howard County General Hospital	Columbia	80%	300+
Suburban Hospital	Bethesda	80%	300+
Bon Secours Hospital	Baltimore	79%	300+
Prince Georges Hospital Center	Cheverly	79%	300+
Laurel Regional Medical Center	Laurel	78%	300+
Fort Washington Hospital	Fort Washington	77%	(a)

Hospital Given 9 or 10 on 10 Point Scale

Hospital Name	City	Rate	Cases
The Johns Hopkins Hospital	Baltimore	83%	300+
Anne Arundel Medical Center	Annapolis	78%	300+
Mercy Medical Center	Baltimore	76%	300+
Atlantic General Hospital	Berlin	75%	300+
Carroll Hospital Center	Westminster	73%	300+
Medstar Saint Mary's Hospital	Leonardtown	73%	300+
Greater Baltimore Medical Center	Baltimore	72%	300+
Medstar Harbor Hospital	Baltimore	72%	300+
Medstar Union Memorial Hospital	Baltimore	72%	300+
Garrett County Memorial Hospital	Oakland	71%	300+
Medstar Franklin Square Medical Center	Baltimore	71%	300+
Suburban Hospital	Bethesda	69%	300+
University of Maryland Medical Center	Baltimore	69%	300+
Frederick Memorial Hospital	Frederick	68%	300+
Doctors' Community Hospital	Lanham	67%	300+
Peninsula Regional Medical Center	Salisbury	67%	300+
Sinai Hospital of Baltimore	Baltimore	67%	300+
Univ of MD Balto Washington Med Ctr	Glen Burnie	67%	300+
Howard County General Hospital	Columbia	66%	300+
Medstar Good Samaritan Hospital	Baltimore	66%	300+
Meritus Medical Center	Hagerstown	66%	300+
Harford Memorial Hospital	Havre De Grace	65%	300+
Western Maryland Regional Medical Center	Cumberland	65%	300+
Holy Cross Hospital	Silver Spring	64%	300+
Johns Hopkins Bayview Medical Center	Baltimore	64%	300+
Medstar Montgomery Medical Center	Olney	64%	(a)
Univ of MD Shore Med Ctr at Easton	Easton	64%	300+
Upper Chesapeake Medical Center	Bel Air	64%	300+
Calvert Memorial Hospital	Prince Frederick	63%	300+
Washington Adventist Hospital	Takoma Park	63%	300+
Saint Agnes Hospital	Baltimore	62%	300+
Northwest Hospital Center	Randallstown	61%	300+
Univ of MD Shore Med Ctr-Chestertown	Chestertown	60%	300+
Union Hospital of Cecil County	Elkton	59%	300+
Univ of MD Charles Reg Med Ctr	La Plata	59%	300+
Shady Grove Adventist Hospital	Rockville	55%	300+
Univ of MD Med Ctr Midtown Campus	Baltimore	52%	300+
Bon Secours Hospital	Baltimore	48%	300+
Fort Washington Hospital	Fort Washington	48%	(a)
Laurel Regional Medical Center	Laurel	48%	300+
Prince Georges Hospital Center	Cheverly	48%	300+

Meds 'Always' Explained Before Given

Hospital Name	City	Rate	Cases
Carroll Hospital Center	Westminster	65%	300+
The Johns Hopkins Hospital	Baltimore	65%	300+
Anne Arundel Medical Center	Annapolis	64%	300+
Harford Memorial Hospital	Havre De Grace	64%	300+
Mercy Medical Center	Baltimore	64%	300+
University of Maryland Medical Center	Baltimore	64%	300+
Atlantic General Hospital	Berlin	63%	300+
Garrett County Memorial Hospital	Oakland	63%	300+
Medstar Franklin Square Medical Center	Baltimore	63%	300+
Western Maryland Regional Medical Center	Cumberland	63%	300+
Medstar Saint Mary's Hospital	Leonardtown	62%	300+
Johns Hopkins Bayview Medical Center	Baltimore	61%	300+
Univ of MD Shore Med Ctr at Easton	Easton	61%	300+
Upper Chesapeake Medical Center	Bel Air	61%	300+
Doctors' Community Hospital	Lanham	60%	300+
Frederick Memorial Hospital	Frederick	60%	300+
Medstar Harbor Hospital	Baltimore	60%	300+
Univ of MD Balto Washington Med Ctr	Glen Burnie	60%	300+
Medstar Union Memorial Hospital	Baltimore	59%	300+
Northwest Hospital Center	Randallstown	59%	300+
Suburban Hospital	Bethesda	59%	300+
Calvert Memorial Hospital	Prince Frederick	58%	300+
Peninsula Regional Medical Center	Salisbury	58%	300+
Sinai Hospital of Baltimore	Baltimore	58%	300+
Univ of MD Shore Med Ctr-Chestertown	Chestertown	58%	300+
Bon Secours Hospital	Baltimore	57%	300+
Medstar Good Samaritan Hospital	Baltimore	57%	300+
Meritus Medical Center	Hagerstown	56%	300+
Union Hospital of Cecil County	Elkton	56%	300+
Univ of MD Charles Reg Med Ctr	La Plata	56%	300+
Greater Baltimore Medical Center	Baltimore	55%	300+
Medstar Montgomery Medical Center	Olney	55%	(a)
Saint Agnes Hospital	Baltimore	55%	300+
Washington Adventist Hospital	Takoma Park	55%	300+
Holy Cross Hospital	Silver Spring	54%	300+
Howard County General Hospital	Columbia	53%	300+
Prince Georges Hospital Center	Cheverly	52%	300+
Univ of MD Med Ctr Midtown Campus	Baltimore	52%	300+
Laurel Regional Medical Center	Laurel	51%	300+
Fort Washington Hospital	Fort Washington	50%	(a)
Shady Grove Adventist Hospital	Rockville	50%	300+

NOTE: Hospital profiles are in alphabetical order by state, then city, then hospital within the city; Rankings exclude hospitals with less than 25 cases except for patient surveys which excludes hospitals with less than 100 cases; (a) 100-299 cases; (1) The number of cases/patients is too few to report; (2) Data submitted were based on a sample of cases/patients; (3) Results are based on a shorter time period than required; (4) Data suppressed by CMS for one or more quarters; (5) Results are not available for this reporting period; (6) Fewer than 100 patients completed the HCAHPS survey; (7) No cases met the criteria for this measure; (8) The lower limit of the confidence interval cannot be calculated if the number of observed infections equals zero; (9) No data are available from the state/territory for this reporting period; (10) The scores shown reflect fewer than 50 completed surveys; (11) There were discrepancies in the data collection process; (12) This measure does not apply to this hospital for this reporting period; (13) Results cannot be calculated for this reporting period; (14) The results for this state are combined with nearby states to protect confidentiality; Please refer to the User's Guide for a full explanation of data.

Nurses 'Always' Communicated Well

Hospital Name	City	Rate	Cases
Carroll Hospital Center	Westminster	82%	300+
The Johns Hopkins Hospital	Baltimore	82%	300+
Atlantic General Hospital	Berlin	81%	300+
Mercy Medical Center	Baltimore	81%	300+
Anne Arundel Medical Center	Annapolis	80%	300+
Garrett County Memorial Hospital	Oakland	80%	300+
Frederick Memorial Hospital	Frederick	79%	300+
Harford Memorial Hospital	Havre De Grace	79%	300+
Medstar Saint Mary's Hospital	Leonardtown	79%	300+
Univ of MD Shore Med Ctr at Easton	Easton	79%	300+
Medstar Franklin Square Medical Center	Baltimore	78%	300+
Medstar Union Memorial Hospital	Baltimore	78%	300+
Upper Chesapeake Medical Center	Bel Air	78%	300+
Western Maryland Regional Medical Center	Cumberland	78%	300+
Medstar Good Samaritan Hospital	Baltimore	77%	300+
Medstar Harbor Hospital	Baltimore	77%	300+
Univ of MD Shore Med Ctr-Chestertown	Chestertown	77%	300+
Johns Hopkins Bayview Medical Center	Baltimore	76%	300+
Univ of MD Balto Washington Med Ctr	Glen Burnie	76%	300+
University of Maryland Medical Center	Baltimore	76%	300+
Doctors' Community Hospital	Lanham	75%	300+
Meritus Medical Center	Hagerstown	75%	300+
Northwest Hospital Center	Randallstown	75%	300+
Peninsula Regional Medical Center	Salisbury	75%	300+
Sinai Hospital of Baltimore	Baltimore	75%	300+
Calvert Memorial Hospital	Prince Frederick	74%	300+
Howard County General Hospital	Columbia	73%	300+
Suburban Hospital	Bethesda	73%	300+
Union Hospital of Cecil County	Elkton	73%	300+
Greater Baltimore Medical Center	Baltimore	72%	300+
Saint Agnes Hospital	Baltimore	72%	300+
Washington Adventist Hospital	Takoma Park	72%	300+
Holy Cross Hospital	Silver Spring	71%	300+
Univ of MD Charles Reg Med Ctr	La Plata	71%	300+
Medstar Montgomery Medical Center	Olney	70%	(a)
Univ of MD Med Ctr Midtown Campus	Baltimore	70%	300+
Bon Secours Hospital	Baltimore	68%	300+
Fort Washington Hospital	Fort Washington	67%	(a)
Shady Grove Adventist Hospital	Rockville	67%	300+
Laurel Regional Medical Center	Laurel	66%	300+
Prince Georges Hospital Center	Cheverly	63%	300+

Room and Bathroom 'Always' Clean

Hospital Name	City	Rate	Cases
Garrett County Memorial Hospital	Oakland	76%	300+
Medstar Saint Mary's Hospital	Leonardtown	74%	300+
Mercy Medical Center	Baltimore	74%	300+
Doctors' Community Hospital	Lanham	72%	300+
Frederick Memorial Hospital	Frederick	72%	300+
Anne Arundel Medical Center	Annapolis	71%	300+
Atlantic General Hospital	Berlin	71%	300+
Harford Memorial Hospital	Havre De Grace	71%	300+
Carroll Hospital Center	Westminster	70%	300+
The Johns Hopkins Hospital	Baltimore	70%	300+
Western Maryland Regional Medical Center	Cumberland	70%	300+
Meritus Medical Center	Hagerstown	68%	300+
Medstar Harbor Hospital	Baltimore	67%	300+
Upper Chesapeake Medical Center	Bel Air	67%	300+
Sinai Hospital of Baltimore	Baltimore	66%	300+
Univ of MD Balto Washington Med Ctr	Glen Burnie	66%	300+
Univ of MD Charles Reg Med Ctr	La Plata	66%	300+
Univ of MD Shore Med Ctr-Chestertown	Chestertown	66%	300+
Medstar Good Samaritan Hospital	Baltimore	65%	300+
Medstar Union Memorial Hospital	Baltimore	65%	300+
Peninsula Regional Medical Center	Salisbury	65%	300+
Univ of MD Shore Med Ctr at Easton	Easton	65%	300+
Bon Secours Hospital	Baltimore	64%	300+
Calvert Memorial Hospital	Prince Frederick	64%	300+
Suburban Hospital	Bethesda	64%	300+
Medstar Montgomery Medical Center	Olney	63%	(a)
Howard County General Hospital	Columbia	62%	300+
Union Hospital of Cecil County	Elkton	62%	300+
University of Maryland Medical Center	Baltimore	61%	300+
Prince Georges Hospital Center	Cheverly	60%	300+
Washington Adventist Hospital	Takoma Park	59%	300+
Holy Cross Hospital	Silver Spring	58%	300+
Medstar Franklin Square Medical Center	Baltimore	58%	300+
Northwest Hospital Center	Randallstown	58%	300+
Saint Agnes Hospital	Baltimore	58%	300+
Univ of MD Med Ctr Midtown Campus	Baltimore	58%	300+
Johns Hopkins Bayview Medical Center	Baltimore	57%	300+
Greater Baltimore Medical Center	Baltimore	56%	300+
Fort Washington Hospital	Fort Washington	54%	(a)
Shady Grove Adventist Hospital	Rockville	54%	300+
Laurel Regional Medical Center	Laurel	53%	300+

Would Definitely Recommend Hospital

Hospital Name	City	Rate	Cases
The Johns Hopkins Hospital	Baltimore	86%	300+
Anne Arundel Medical Center	Annapolis	81%	300+
Mercy Medical Center	Baltimore	80%	300+
Greater Baltimore Medical Center	Baltimore	76%	300+
Medstar Union Memorial Hospital	Baltimore	75%	300+
Suburban Hospital	Bethesda	74%	300+
University of Maryland Medical Center	Baltimore	74%	300+
Atlantic General Hospital	Berlin	73%	300+
Carroll Hospital Center	Westminster	73%	300+
Medstar Saint Mary's Hospital	Leonardtown	72%	300+
Howard County General Hospital	Columbia	71%	300+
Medstar Franklin Square Medical Center	Baltimore	71%	300+
Medstar Montgomery Medical Center	Olney	71%	(a)
Garrett County Memorial Hospital	Oakland	70%	300+
Medstar Good Samaritan Hospital	Baltimore	70%	300+
Peninsula Regional Medical Center	Salisbury	70%	300+
Sinai Hospital of Baltimore	Baltimore	70%	300+
Holy Cross Hospital	Silver Spring	69%	300+
Medstar Harbor Hospital	Baltimore	69%	300+
Univ of MD Balto Washington Med Ctr	Glen Burnie	69%	300+
Doctors' Community Hospital	Lanham	68%	300+
Frederick Memorial Hospital	Frederick	67%	300+
Washington Adventist Hospital	Takoma Park	67%	300+
Harford Memorial Hospital	Havre De Grace	66%	300+
Johns Hopkins Bayview Medical Center	Baltimore	66%	300+
Univ of MD Shore Med Ctr at Easton	Easton	66%	300+
Upper Chesapeake Medical Center	Bel Air	66%	300+
Saint Agnes Hospital	Baltimore	65%	300+
Meritus Medical Center	Hagerstown	64%	300+
Western Maryland Regional Medical Center	Cumberland	63%	300+
Northwest Hospital Center	Randallstown	62%	300+
Union Hospital of Cecil County	Elkton	62%	300+
Calvert Memorial Hospital	Prince Frederick	61%	300+
Shady Grove Adventist Hospital	Rockville	60%	300+
Univ of MD Charles Reg Med Ctr	La Plata	60%	300+
Univ of MD Shore Med Ctr-Chestertown	Chestertown	56%	300+
Univ of MD Med Ctr Midtown Campus	Baltimore	54%	300+
Fort Washington Hospital	Fort Washington	52%	(a)
Laurel Regional Medical Center	Laurel	49%	300+
Prince Georges Hospital Center	Cheverly	47%	300+
Bon Secours Hospital	Baltimore	43%	300+

Pain 'Always' Well Controlled

Hospital Name	City	Rate	Cases
Anne Arundel Medical Center	Annapolis	74%	300+
Atlantic General Hospital	Berlin	73%	300+
Medstar Harbor Hospital	Baltimore	72%	300+
Mercy Medical Center	Baltimore	72%	300+
Frederick Memorial Hospital	Frederick	71%	300+
Garrett County Memorial Hospital	Oakland	71%	300+
Harford Memorial Hospital	Havre De Grace	71%	300+
Carroll Hospital Center	Westminster	70%	300+
The Johns Hopkins Hospital	Baltimore	70%	300+
Medstar Franklin Square Medical Center	Baltimore	70%	300+
Medstar Saint Mary's Hospital	Leonardtown	70%	300+
Medstar Union Memorial Hospital	Baltimore	70%	300+
Univ of MD Shore Med Ctr at Easton	Easton	70%	300+
Univ of MD Balto Washington Med Ctr	Glen Burnie	69%	300+
University of Maryland Medical Center	Baltimore	69%	300+
Western Maryland Regional Medical Center	Cumberland	69%	300+
Medstar Good Samaritan Hospital	Baltimore	68%	300+
Meritus Medical Center	Hagerstown	68%	300+
Sinai Hospital of Baltimore	Baltimore	68%	300+
Univ of MD Shore Med Ctr-Chestertown	Chestertown	68%	300+
Doctors' Community Hospital	Lanham	67%	300+
Howard County General Hospital	Columbia	67%	300+
Upper Chesapeake Medical Center	Bel Air	67%	300+
Greater Baltimore Medical Center	Baltimore	65%	300+
Holy Cross Hospital	Silver Spring	65%	300+
Johns Hopkins Bayview Medical Center	Baltimore	65%	300+
Laurel Regional Medical Center	Laurel	65%	300+
Peninsula Regional Medical Center	Salisbury	65%	300+
Saint Agnes Hospital	Baltimore	65%	300+
Washington Adventist Hospital	Takoma Park	65%	300+
Calvert Memorial Hospital	Prince Frederick	64%	300+
Suburban Hospital	Bethesda	64%	300+
Univ of MD Charles Reg Med Ctr	La Plata	64%	300+
Northwest Hospital Center	Randallstown	63%	300+
Bon Secours Hospital	Baltimore	61%	300+
Prince Georges Hospital Center	Cheverly	60%	300+
Union Hospital of Cecil County	Elkton	60%	300+
Univ of MD Med Ctr Midtown Campus	Baltimore	60%	300+
Fort Washington Hospital	Fort Washington	59%	(a)
Medstar Montgomery Medical Center	Olney	59%	(a)
Shady Grove Adventist Hospital	Rockville	58%	300+

Timely Help 'Always' Received

Hospital Name	City	Rate	Cases
Garrett County Memorial Hospital	Oakland	72%	300+
Carroll Hospital Center	Westminster	70%	300+
Univ of MD Shore Med Ctr-Chestertown	Chestertown	70%	300+
Atlantic General Hospital	Berlin	69%	300+
Univ of MD Shore Med Ctr at Easton	Easton	67%	300+
Anne Arundel Medical Center	Annapolis	66%	300+
Medstar Union Memorial Hospital	Baltimore	66%	300+
Mercy Medical Center	Baltimore	65%	300+
Medstar Harbor Hospital	Baltimore	64%	300+
The Johns Hopkins Hospital	Baltimore	63%	300+
Medstar Saint Mary's Hospital	Leonardtown	63%	300+
Western Maryland Regional Medical Center	Cumberland	63%	300+
Frederick Memorial Hospital	Frederick	62%	300+
Harford Memorial Hospital	Havre De Grace	62%	300+
Peninsula Regional Medical Center	Salisbury	61%	300+
Calvert Memorial Hospital	Prince Frederick	59%	300+
Sinai Hospital of Baltimore	Baltimore	59%	300+
Union Hospital of Cecil County	Elkton	59%	300+
Univ of MD Balto Washington Med Ctr	Glen Burnie	59%	300+
University of Maryland Medical Center	Baltimore	59%	300+
Upper Chesapeake Medical Center	Bel Air	59%	300+
Doctors' Community Hospital	Lanham	58%	300+
Johns Hopkins Bayview Medical Center	Baltimore	58%	300+
Howard County General Hospital	Columbia	57%	300+
Meritus Medical Center	Hagerstown	57%	300+
Medstar Franklin Square Medical Center	Baltimore	55%	300+
Medstar Good Samaritan Hospital	Baltimore	55%	300+
Univ of MD Charles Reg Med Ctr	La Plata	55%	300+
Washington Adventist Hospital	Takoma Park	55%	300+
Greater Baltimore Medical Center	Baltimore	54%	300+
Univ of MD Med Ctr Midtown Campus	Baltimore	54%	300+
Holy Cross Hospital	Silver Spring	53%	300+
Medstar Montgomery Medical Center	Olney	53%	(a)
Saint Agnes Hospital	Baltimore	53%	300+
Fort Washington Hospital	Fort Washington	51%	(a)
Laurel Regional Medical Center	Laurel	51%	300+
Northwest Hospital Center	Randallstown	51%	300+
Suburban Hospital	Bethesda	50%	300+
Bon Secours Hospital	Baltimore	46%	300+
Prince Georges Hospital Center	Cheverly	43%	300+
Shady Grove Adventist Hospital	Rockville	43%	300+

Use of Medical Imaging

Cardiac Imaging Stress Test before OP Surgery

Hospital Name	City	Rate	Cases
Medstar Saint Mary's Hospital	Leonardtown	0.0%	68
Atlantic General Hospital	Berlin	3.0%	164
Upper Chesapeake Medical Center	Bel Air	3.8%	968
Washington Adventist Hospital	Takoma Park	4.2%	96
Laurel Regional Medical Center	Laurel	4.3%	115
Medstar Union Memorial Hospital	Baltimore	4.5%	445
Union Hospital of Cecil County	Elkton	4.5%	267
Peninsula Regional Medical Center	Salisbury	4.8%	248
Western Maryland Regional Medical Center	Cumberland	5.1%	415
Medstar Franklin Square Medical Center	Baltimore	5.2%	734
Shady Grove Adventist Hospital	Rockville	5.3%	113
The Johns Hopkins Hospital	Baltimore	5.4%	483
Carroll Hospital Center	Westminster	5.5%	293
Univ of MD Shore Med Ctr at Easton	Easton	5.7%	193
Anne Arundel Medical Center	Annapolis	5.8%	364
Johns Hopkins Bayview Medical Center	Baltimore	6.3%	459
Univ of MD Balto Washington Med Ctr	Glen Burnie	6.3%	541
Garrett County Memorial Hospital	Oakland	6.6%	167
Saint Agnes Hospital	Baltimore	6.6%	588
Sinai Hospital of Baltimore	Baltimore	6.6%	363
Howard County General Hospital	Columbia	7.0%	314
Medstar Good Samaritan Hospital	Baltimore	7.3%	467
Medstar Harbor Hospital	Baltimore	7.3%	317
Medstar Southern Maryland Hospital Center	Clinton	7.4%	122
Harford Memorial Hospital	Havre De Grace	7.5%	374
Calvert Memorial Hospital	Prince Frederick	7.7%	455
Mercy Medical Center	Baltimore	8.0%	535
Bon Secours Hospital	Baltimore	8.1%	124
Univ of MD Med Ctr Midtown Campus	Baltimore	8.5%	141
Medstar Montgomery Medical Center	Olney	8.6%	93
Northwest Hospital Center	Randallstown	8.7%	104
University of Maryland Medical Center	Baltimore	8.8%	400
Univ of MD St Joseph Med Ctr	Towson	9.3%	269
Greater Baltimore Medical Center	Baltimore	13.1%	359

Combination Abdominal CT Scan

Hospital Name	City	Rate	Cases
Medstar Franklin Square Medical Center	Baltimore	0.1%	1228
Carroll Hospital Center	Westminster	0.4%	818
Calvert Memorial Hospital	Prince Frederick	0.5%	384
Medstar Montgomery Medical Center	Olney	0.5%	568

NOTE: Hospital profiles are in alphabetical order by state, then city, then hospital within the city; Rankings exclude hospitals with less than 25 cases except for patient surveys which excludes hospitals with less than 100 cases; (a) 100-299 cases; (1) The number of cases/patients is too few to report; (2) Data submitted were based on a sample of cases/patients; (3) Results are based on a shorter time period than required; (4) Data suppressed by CMS for one or more quarters; (5) Results are not available for this reporting period; (6) Fewer than 100 patients completed the HCAHPS survey; (7) No cases met the criteria for this measure; (8) The lower limit of the confidence interval cannot be calculated if the number of observed infections equals zero; (9) No data are available from the state/territory for this reporting period; (10) The scores shown reflect fewer than 50 completed surveys; (11) There were discrepancies in the data collection process; (12) This measure does not apply to this hospital for this reporting period; (13) Results cannot be calculated for this reporting period; (14) The results for this state are combined with nearby states to protect confidentiality; Please refer to the User's Guide for a full explanation of data.

Doctors' Community Hospital	Lanham	0.7%	568
Meritus Medical Center	Hagerstown	0.7%	1218
Shady Grove Adventist Hospital	Rockville	0.7%	547
Univ of MD Balto Washington Med Ctr	Glen Burnie	0.7%	1066
Medstar Southern Maryland Hospital Center	Clinton	1.2%	256
Anne Arundel Medical Center	Annapolis	1.3%	1004
Edward Mccready Memorial Hospital	Crisfield	1.3%	158
Bon Secours Hospital	Baltimore	1.5%	205
Holy Cross Hospital	Silver Spring	1.5%	543
Prince Georges Hospital Center	Cheverly	1.5%	269
Fort Washington Hospital	Fort Washington	1.7%	401
Northwest Hospital Center	Randallstown	1.8%	798
The Johns Hopkins Hospital	Baltimore	2.0%	2882
Laurel Regional Medical Center	Laurel	2.0%	294
Univ of MD Charles Reg Med Ctr	La Plata	2.0%	689
University of Maryland Medical Center	Baltimore	2.1%	1107
Saint Agnes Hospital	Baltimore	2.3%	908
Medstar Good Samaritan Hospital	Baltimore	2.6%	760
Peninsula Regional Medical Center	Salisbury	2.6%	1824
Medstar Saint Mary's Hospital	Leonardtown	3.0%	951
Upper Chesapeake Medical Center	Bel Air	3.3%	1290
Howard County General Hospital	Columbia	3.6%	692
Univ of MD Med Ctr Midtown Campus	Baltimore	3.8%	212
Medstar Harbor Hospital	Baltimore	3.9%	409
Medstar Union Memorial Hospital	Baltimore	3.9%	697
Sinai Hospital of Baltimore	Baltimore	3.9%	916
Washington Adventist Hospital	Takoma Park	4.0%	351
Univ of MD St Joseph Med Ctr	Towson	4.5%	333
Univ of MD Shore Med Ctr-Chestertown	Chestertown	4.8%	560
Frederick Memorial Hospital	Frederick	5.3%	879
Western Maryland Regional Medical Center	Cumberland	5.7%	1158
Univ of MD Shore Med Ctr at Easton	Easton	6.1%	1061
Garrett County Memorial Hospital	Oakland	6.5%	522
Greater Baltimore Medical Center	Baltimore	6.5%	1020
Suburban Hospital	Bethesda	7.0%	842
Union Hospital of Cecil County	Elkton	7.0%	972
Harford Memorial Hospital	Havre De Grace	7.4%	814
Johns Hopkins Bayview Medical Center	Baltimore	8.5%	1100
Atlantic General Hospital	Berlin	9.3%	1332
Mercy Medical Center	Baltimore	13.8%	1139

Combination Brain/Sinus CT Scan

Hospital Name	City	Rate	Cases
Medstar Franklin Square Medical Center	Baltimore	0.7%	1753
Medstar Southern Maryland Hospital Center	Clinton	0.9%	466
Union Hospital of Cecil County	Elkton	1.9%	648
Fort Washington Hospital	Fort Washington	2.1%	605
Univ of MD Shore Med Ctr-Chestertown	Chestertown	2.1%	435
Medstar Saint Mary's Hospital	Leonardtown	2.4%	826
Medstar Union Memorial Hospital	Baltimore	2.4%	582
Peninsula Regional Medical Center	Salisbury	2.4%	1815
Meritus Medical Center	Hagerstown	2.8%	1468
Frederick Memorial Hospital	Frederick	3.3%	1221
Univ of MD Shore Med Ctr at Easton	Easton	3.3%	1439
Univ of MD Charles Reg Med Ctr	La Plata	3.6%	831
Shady Grove Adventist Hospital	Rockville	3.8%	973
Harford Memorial Hospital	Havre De Grace	3.9%	813
Sinai Hospital of Baltimore	Baltimore	3.9%	1190
Anne Arundel Medical Center	Annapolis	4.0%	1290
Laurel Regional Medical Center	Laurel	4.0%	445
Medstar Good Samaritan Hospital	Baltimore	4.0%	1133
University of Maryland Medical Center	Baltimore	4.3%	554
Atlantic General Hospital	Berlin	4.4%	1058
Garrett County Memorial Hospital	Oakland	4.4%	436
Univ of MD Balto Washington Med Ctr	Glen Burnie	4.9%	1790
Greater Baltimore Medical Center	Baltimore	5.0%	973
Northwest Hospital Center	Randallstown	5.1%	1161
Upper Chesapeake Medical Center	Bel Air	5.1%	1555
Western Maryland Regional Medical Center	Cumberland	5.1%	1190
Saint Agnes Hospital	Baltimore	5.3%	1306
Howard County General Hospital	Columbia	5.9%	1243
Holy Cross Hospital	Silver Spring	6.0%	1168
The Johns Hopkins Hospital	Baltimore	6.0%	736
Johns Hopkins Bayview Medical Center	Baltimore	6.1%	838
Carroll Hospital Center	Westminster	6.6%	1466
Prince Georges Hospital Center	Cheverly	6.7%	388
Suburban Hospital	Bethesda	6.8%	1160
Univ of MD Med Ctr Midtown Campus	Baltimore	7.8%	244
Bon Secours Hospital	Baltimore	8.0%	299
Medstar Montgomery Medical Center	Olney	10.3%	918

Combination Chest CT Scan

Hospital Name	City	Rate	Cases
Bon Secours Hospital	Baltimore	0.0%	109
Calvert Memorial Hospital	Prince Frederick	0.0%	175
Carroll Hospital Center	Westminster	0.0%	131
Fort Washington Hospital	Fort Washington	0.0%	64
Garrett County Memorial Hospital	Oakland	0.0%	247
Holy Cross Hospital	Silver Spring	0.0%	282
Medstar Good Samaritan Hospital	Baltimore	0.0%	438
Medstar Harbor Hospital	Baltimore	0.0%	255
Medstar Montgomery Medical Center	Olney	0.0%	258
Peninsula Regional Medical Center	Salisbury	0.0%	1160
Shady Grove Adventist Hospital	Rockville	0.0%	102
Univ of MD Balto Washington Med Ctr	Glen Burnie	0.0%	401
Univ of MD Med Ctr Midtown Campus	Baltimore	0.0%	113
The Johns Hopkins Hospital	Baltimore	0.1%	4928
Mercy Medical Center	Baltimore	0.2%	832
Northwest Hospital Center	Randallstown	0.2%	483
University of Maryland Medical Center	Baltimore	0.2%	1267
Univ of MD Shore Med Ctr at Easton	Easton	0.2%	438
Atlantic General Hospital	Berlin	0.3%	868
Medstar Franklin Square Medical Center	Baltimore	0.3%	290
Meritus Medical Center	Hagerstown	0.3%	287
Upper Chesapeake Medical Center	Bel Air	0.4%	828
Anne Arundel Medical Center	Annapolis	0.5%	191
Doctors' Community Hospital	Lanham	0.5%	220
Western Maryland Regional Medical Center	Cumberland	0.5%	783
Medstar Union Memorial Hospital	Baltimore	0.7%	614
Edward Mccready Memorial Hospital	Crisfield	0.9%	111
Laurel Regional Medical Center	Laurel	1.0%	101
Union Hospital of Cecil County	Elkton	1.0%	691
Harford Memorial Hospital	Havre De Grace	1.1%	471
Univ of MD Charles Reg Med Ctr	La Plata	1.1%	268
Saint Agnes Hospital	Baltimore	1.2%	727
Medstar Saint Mary's Hospital	Leonardtown	1.3%	540
Medstar Southern Maryland Hospital Center	Clinton	1.6%	63
Prince Georges Hospital Center	Cheverly	1.6%	129
Univ of MD Shore Med Ctr-Chestertown	Chestertown	1.8%	275
Sinai Hospital of Baltimore	Baltimore	2.2%	648
Suburban Hospital	Bethesda	2.2%	358
Univ of MD St Joseph Med Ctr	Towson	2.2%	92
Washington Adventist Hospital	Takoma Park	3.1%	128
Frederick Memorial Hospital	Frederick	4.1%	246
Howard County General Hospital	Columbia	4.2%	521
Johns Hopkins Bayview Medical Center	Baltimore	4.4%	1241
Greater Baltimore Medical Center	Baltimore	8.1%	493

Follow-up Mammogram/Ultrasound

A follow-up rate near zero may indicate missed cancer; a rate higher than 14% may mean there is unnecessary follow up.

Hospital Name	City	Rate	Cases
The Johns Hopkins Hospital	Baltimore	2.7%	1055
Northwest Hospital Center	Randallstown	3.6%	1012
Univ of MD Med Ctr Midtown Campus	Baltimore	5.2%	212
Medstar Saint Mary's Hospital	Leonardtown	6.2%	577
Saint Agnes Hospital	Baltimore	6.6%	243
Atlantic General Hospital	Berlin	7.0%	1985
Sinai Hospital of Baltimore	Baltimore	7.2%	514
Harford Memorial Hospital	Havre De Grace	7.4%	591
Holy Cross Hospital	Silver Spring	7.9%	151
Prince Georges Hospital Center	Cheverly	7.9%	101
Univ of MD Shore Med Ctr-Chestertown	Chestertown	8.0%	879
University of Maryland Medical Center	Baltimore	9.1%	1054
Peninsula Regional Medical Center	Salisbury	9.4%	1383
Union Hospital of Cecil County	Elkton	9.4%	1228
Medstar Good Samaritan Hospital	Baltimore	9.7%	858
Univ of MD Charles Reg Med Ctr	La Plata	9.8%	305
Washington Adventist Hospital	Takoma Park	10.4%	260
Medstar Union Memorial Hospital	Baltimore	10.5%	1040
Univ of MD Shore Med Ctr at Easton	Easton	10.7%	917
Medstar Harbor Hospital	Baltimore	11.2%	456
Upper Chesapeake Medical Center	Bel Air	11.5%	480
Howard County General Hospital	Columbia	13.3%	105
Bon Secours Hospital	Baltimore	13.5%	126
Fort Washington Hospital	Fort Washington	13.9%	158
Johns Hopkins Bayview Medical Center	Baltimore	16.3%	264
Mercy Medical Center	Baltimore	18.3%	1530
Edward Mccready Memorial Hospital	Crisfield	67.8%	307

Lumbar Spine MRI for Low Back Pain

Hospital Name	City	Rate	Cases
Medstar Union Memorial Hospital	Baltimore	26.3%	95
The Johns Hopkins Hospital	Baltimore	26.6%	139
Medstar Saint Mary's Hospital	Leonardtown	32.1%	140
Atlantic General Hospital	Berlin	34.5%	113
Mercy Medical Center	Baltimore	34.5%	139
Harford Memorial Hospital	Havre De Grace	37.0%	100
Sinai Hospital of Baltimore	Baltimore	38.7%	62
Western Maryland Regional Medical Center	Cumberland	38.7%	155
Medstar Harbor Hospital	Baltimore	38.9%	54
Upper Chesapeake Medical Center	Bel Air	40.2%	87
Johns Hopkins Bayview Medical Center	Baltimore	40.9%	44
Univ of MD Shore Med Ctr at Easton	Easton	40.9%	132
Union Hospital of Cecil County	Elkton	42.7%	82
Univ of MD Shore Med Ctr-Chestertown	Chestertown	43.1%	51
Northwest Hospital Center	Randallstown	44.4%	36
Medstar Good Samaritan Hospital	Baltimore	46.6%	131
Peninsula Regional Medical Center	Salisbury	60.6%	94

NOTE: Hospital profiles are in alphabetical order by state, then city, then hospital within the city; Rankings exclude hospitals with less than 25 cases except for patient surveys which excludes hospitals with less than 100 cases; (a) 100-299 cases; (1) The number of cases/patients is too few to report; (2) Data submitted were based on a sample of cases/patients; (3) Results are based on a shorter time period than required; (4) Data suppressed by CMS for one or more quarters; (5) Results are not available for this reporting period; (6) Fewer than 100 patients completed the HCAHPS survey; (7) No cases met the criteria for this measure; (8) The lower limit of the confidence interval cannot be calculated if the number of observed infections equals zero; (9) No data are available from the state/territory for this reporting period; (10) The scores shown reflect fewer than 50 completed surveys; (11) There were discrepancies in the data collection process; (12) This measure does not apply to this hospital for this reporting period; (13) Results cannot be calculated for this reporting period; (14) The results for this state are combined with nearby states to protect confidentiality; Please refer to the User's Guide for a full explanation of data.

Anne Arundel Medical Center

2001 Medical Parkway
Annapolis, MD 21401
URL: www.aahs.org
Type: Acute Care Hospitals
Ownership: Voluntary non-profit - Private
Phone: 443-481-1307
Fax: 443-481-4707
Emergency Services: Yes
Beds: 316

Key Personnel:
CEO/President. . . . . Victoria W. Bayless
Infection Control. . . . . Mary Clance, MD
Quality Assurance . . . . Shirley J Knelly
Operating Room. . . . . Sue Patton, RN
Pediatric In-Patient Care . . . . Karen Peddicord, PhD
Chief of Medical Staff. . . . . Mitchell Schwartz, MD

Measure	Cases	This Hosp.	State Avg.	U.S. Avg.
Blood Clot Prevention and Treatment				
Anticoagulation Overlap Therapy[2]	167	93%	94%	93%
ICU Venous Thromboembolism Prophylaxis[2]	49	96%	94%	92%
Incidence of Potentially Preventable VTE[2]	41	10%	7%	10%
UFH with Dosages/Platelet Monitoring[2]	35	100%	97%	97%
Venous Thromboembolism Prophylaxis[2]	287	87%	90%	85%
Warfarin Therapy Discharge Instructions[2]	118	53%	78%	75%
Chest Pain/Possible Heart Attack Care				
Aspirin Given Within 24 Hours of Arrival[5]	-	-	100%	96%
Fibrinolytic Meds Within 30 Min. of Arrival[5]	-	-	-	58%
Average Time to ECG (minutes)[5]	-	-	6	7
Average Time to Transfer (minutes)[5]	-	-	32	60
Children's Asthma Care				
Received Home Management Plan of Care	-	-	-	88%
Received Reliever Medication	-	-	-	100%
Received Systemic Corticosteroids	-	-	-	100%
Emergency Department				
Admittance Decision Time (minutes)[2]	742	272	143	98
Head CT Results Within 45 Min. of Arrival[5]	-	-	-	57%
Patients Who Left ER Before Being Seen[5]	-	-	3%	2%
Time from ER Arrival to Admit. (minutes)[2]	745	494	357	274
Time from ER Arrival to Discharge (minutes)[5]	-	-	-	134
Time in ER Before Being Evaluated (minutes)[5]	-	-	-	26
Time to Pain Meds for Fractures (minutes)[5]	-	-	-	57
Heart Attack Care				
Aspirin Given at Discharge	240	100%	99%	99%
Fibrinolytic Meds Within 30 Min. of Arrival[7]	-	-	-	54%
PCI Within 90 Minutes of Arrival	89	94%	93%	96%
Statin Prescribed at Discharge	240	98%	98%	98%
Heart Failure Care				
ACE Inhibitor or ARB for LVSD	181	96%	97%	97%
Discharge Instructions Given	490	98%	93%	94%
Evaluation of LVS Function	596	99%	99%	99%
Medicare Spending				
Medicare Spending per Patient (ratio)	-	-	-	0.98
Pneumonia Care				
Appropriate Initial Antibiotic Given	284	95%	97%	95%
Blood Culture Timing	463	97%	97%	98%
Pregnancy and Delivery Care				
Newborn Deliveries Scheduled Early[5]	-	-	-	6%
Preventive Care				
Immunization for Influenza[2]	819	97%	94%	90%
Immunization for Pneumonia[2]	830	96%	94%	92%
Stroke Care				
Anticoagulation Therapy for Atrial Fibrillation[5]	-	-	95%	95%
Antithrombotic Therapy Timing[5]	-	-	95%	98%
Assessed for Rehabilitation[5]	-	-	96%	97%
Discharged on Antithrombotic Therapy[5]	-	-	95%	99%
Discharged on Statin Medication[5]	-	-	97%	94%
Thrombolytic Therapy Timing[5]	-	-	-	66%
Venous Thromboembolism Prophylaxis[5]	-	-	89%	94%
Written Stroke Educational Materials Given[5]	-	-	77%	88%
Surgical Care Improvement Project				
Appropriate Beta Blocker Usage[2]	248	94%	97%	98%
Appropriate VTP Within 24 Hours[2]	786	96%	98%	98%
Controlled Postoperative Blood Glucose[2,7]	-	-	96%	97%
Perioperative Temperature Management[2]	1,008	98%	100%	100%
Prophylactic Antibiotic Selection[2]	676	97%	99%	99%
Prophylactic Antibiotic Selection (Outpatient)[5]	-	-	98%	98%
Prophylactic Antibiotic Stopped[2]	667	98%	98%	98%
Prophylactic Antibiotic Timing[2]	675	98%	97%	99%
Prophylactic Antibiotic Timing (Outpatient)[5]	-	-	98%	98%
Urinary Catheter Removal[2]	661	96%	98%	97%
Survey of Patients' Hospital Experiences				
Area Around Room 'Always' Quiet at Night	300+	62%	57%	61%
Doctors 'Always' Communicated Well	300+	80%	78%	82%
Home Recovery Information Given	300+	88%	85%	85%
Hospital Given 9 or 10 on 10 Point Scale	300+	78%	65%	71%
Meds 'Always' Explained Before Given	300+	64%	58%	64%
Nurses 'Always' Communicated Well	300+	80%	75%	79%
Pain 'Always' Well Controlled	300+	74%	67%	71%
Room and Bathroom 'Always' Clean	300+	71%	64%	73%
Timely Help 'Always' Received	300+	66%	58%	68%
Would Definitely Recommend Hospital	300+	81%	67%	71%
Use of Medical Imaging				
Cardiac Imaging Stress Test before Surgery	364	5.8%	6.4%	5.3%
Combination Abdominal CT Scan	1,004	1.3%	3.8%	10.5%
Combination Brain/Sinus CT Scan	1,290	4.0%	4.3%	2.7%
Combination Chest CT Scan	191	0.5%	1%	2.7%
Follow-up Mammogram/Ultrasound[7]	-	-	10.2%	8.8%
Lumbar Spine MRI for Low Back Pain[1]	-	-	38.2%	37.2%

Bon Secours Hospital

2000 W Baltimore Street
Baltimore, MD 21223
URL: www.bonsecours.org/baltimore
Type: Acute Care Hospitals
Ownership: Voluntary non-profit - Private
Phone: 410-362-3000
Fax: 410-442-1082
Emergency Services: Yes
Beds: 208

Key Personnel:
Radiology. . . . . Adolfo M Alonso, MD
Chief of Medical Staff. . . . . Efem Imoke, MD
CEO . . . . Dr Samuel L Ross, FACHE
Quality Assurance . . . . William Law, MD
Patient Relations . . . . Jean Phaire
Ambulatory Care . . . . Reed Winston, MD

Measure	Cases	This Hosp.	State Avg.	U.S. Avg.
Blood Clot Prevention and Treatment				
Anticoagulation Overlap Therapy[2]	19	74%	94%	93%
ICU Venous Thromboembolism Prophylaxis[2]	40	68%	94%	92%
Incidence of Potentially Preventable VTE[1,2]	-	-	7%	10%
UFH with Dosages/Platelet Monitoring[1,2]	-	-	97%	97%
Venous Thromboembolism Prophylaxis[2]	259	68%	90%	85%
Warfarin Therapy Discharge Instructions[2]	16	6%	78%	75%
Chest Pain/Possible Heart Attack Care				
Aspirin Given Within 24 Hours of Arrival[5]	-	-	100%	96%
Fibrinolytic Meds Within 30 Min. of Arrival[5]	-	-	-	58%
Average Time to ECG (minutes)[5]	-	-	6	7
Average Time to Transfer (minutes)[5]	-	-	32	60
Children's Asthma Care				
Received Home Management Plan of Care	-	-	-	88%
Received Reliever Medication	-	-	-	100%
Received Systemic Corticosteroids	-	-	-	100%
Emergency Department				
Admittance Decision Time (minutes)[2]	120	174	143	98
Head CT Results Within 45 Min. of Arrival[5]	-	-	-	57%
Patients Who Left ER Before Being Seen[5]	-	-	3%	2%
Time from ER Arrival to Admit. (minutes)[2]	155	415	357	274
Time from ER Arrival to Discharge (minutes)[5]	-	-	-	134
Time in ER Before Being Evaluated (minutes)[5]	-	-	-	26
Time to Pain Meds for Fractures (minutes)[5]	-	-	-	57
Heart Attack Care				
Aspirin Given at Discharge[1,3]	-	-	99%	99%
Fibrinolytic Meds Within 30 Min. of Arrival[3,7]	-	-	-	54%
PCI Within 90 Minutes of Arrival[3,7]	-	-	93%	96%
Statin Prescribed at Discharge[1,3]	-	-	98%	98%
Heart Failure Care				
ACE Inhibitor or ARB for LVSD	59	90%	97%	97%
Discharge Instructions Given	179	88%	93%	94%
Evaluation of LVS Function	199	100%	99%	99%
Medicare Spending				
Medicare Spending per Patient (ratio)	-	-	-	0.98
Pneumonia Care				
Appropriate Initial Antibiotic Given	93	97%	97%	95%
Blood Culture Timing	170	99%	97%	98%
Pregnancy and Delivery Care				
Newborn Deliveries Scheduled Early[5]	-	-	-	6%
Preventive Care				
Immunization for Influenza[2]	592	74%	94%	90%
Immunization for Pneumonia[2]	690	80%	94%	92%
Stroke Care				
Anticoagulation Therapy for Atrial Fibrillation[5]	-	-	95%	95%
Antithrombotic Therapy Timing[5]	-	-	95%	98%
Assessed for Rehabilitation[5]	-	-	96%	97%
Discharged on Antithrombotic Therapy[5]	-	-	95%	99%
Discharged on Statin Medication[5]	-	-	97%	94%
Thrombolytic Therapy Timing[5]	-	-	-	66%
Venous Thromboembolism Prophylaxis[5]	-	-	89%	94%
Written Stroke Educational Materials Given[5]	-	-	77%	88%
Surgical Care Improvement Project				
Appropriate Beta Blocker Usage	20	100%	97%	98%
Appropriate VTP Within 24 Hours	60	100%	98%	98%
Controlled Postoperative Blood Glucose[7]	-	-	96%	97%
Perioperative Temperature Management	64	100%	100%	100%
Prophylactic Antibiotic Selection	28	100%	99%	99%
Prophylactic Antibiotic Selection (Outpatient)[5]	-	-	98%	98%
Prophylactic Antibiotic Stopped	27	100%	98%	98%
Prophylactic Antibiotic Timing	28	100%	97%	99%
Prophylactic Antibiotic Timing (Outpatient)[5]	-	-	98%	98%
Urinary Catheter Removal	30	100%	98%	97%
Survey of Patients' Hospital Experiences				
Area Around Room 'Always' Quiet at Night	300+	62%	57%	61%
Doctors 'Always' Communicated Well	300+	76%	78%	82%
Home Recovery Information Given	300+	79%	85%	85%
Hospital Given 9 or 10 on 10 Point Scale	300+	48%	65%	71%
Meds 'Always' Explained Before Given	300+	57%	58%	64%
Nurses 'Always' Communicated Well	300+	68%	75%	79%
Pain 'Always' Well Controlled	300+	61%	67%	71%
Room and Bathroom 'Always' Clean	300+	64%	64%	73%
Timely Help 'Always' Received	300+	46%	58%	68%
Would Definitely Recommend Hospital	300+	43%	67%	71%
Use of Medical Imaging				
Cardiac Imaging Stress Test before Surgery	124	8.1%	6.4%	5.3%
Combination Abdominal CT Scan	205	1.5%	3.8%	10.5%
Combination Brain/Sinus CT Scan	299	8.0%	4.3%	2.7%
Combination Chest CT Scan	109	0.0%	1%	2.7%
Follow-up Mammogram/Ultrasound	126	13.5%	10.2%	8.8%
Lumbar Spine MRI for Low Back Pain[1]	-	-	38.2%	37.2%

Greater Baltimore Medical Center

6701 North Charles Street
Baltimore, MD 21204
URL: www.gbmc.org
Type: Acute Care Hospitals
Ownership: Voluntary non-profit - Private
Phone: 443-849-2000
Fax: 410-828-3024
Emergency Services: Yes
Beds: 372

Key Personnel:
Operating Room. . . . . Dale Buchbinder, MD
CEO/President. . . . . John B. Chessare, MD
Pediatric Ambulatory Care . . . . . . Timothy F Doran, MD
Quality Assurance . . . . Paul Masser
Hemotology Center . . . . Laurie Mead
Radiology. . . . . H Alexander Munitz, MD
Chief of Medical Staff. . . . . John Saunders, Jr., MD
Emergency Room . . . . Jeffrey Sternlicht, MD

Measure	Cases	This Hosp.	State Avg.	U.S. Avg.
Blood Clot Prevention and Treatment				
Anticoagulation Overlap Therapy[2,3]	73	97%	94%	93%
ICU Venous Thromboembolism Prophylaxis[2,3]	17	100%	94%	92%
Incidence of Potentially Preventable VTE[1,2]	-	-	7%	10%
UFH with Dosages/Platelet Monitoring[2,3]	39	100%	97%	97%
Venous Thromboembolism Prophylaxis[2,3]	223	98%	90%	85%
Warfarin Therapy Discharge Instructions[2,3]	40	92%	78%	75%
Chest Pain/Possible Heart Attack Care				
Aspirin Given Within 24 Hours of Arrival[5]	-	-	100%	96%
Fibrinolytic Meds Within 30 Min. of Arrival[5]	-	-	-	58%
Average Time to ECG (minutes)[5]	-	-	6	7
Average Time to Transfer (minutes)[5]	-	-	32	60
Children's Asthma Care				
Received Home Management Plan of Care	-	-	-	88%

NOTE: Hospital profiles are in alphabetical order by state, then city, then hospital within the city; Rankings exclude hospitals with less than 25 cases except for patient surveys which excludes hospitals with less than 100 cases; (a) 100-299 cases; (1) The number of cases/patients is too few to report; (2) Data submitted were based on a sample of cases/patients; (3) Results are based on a shorter time period than required; (4) Data suppressed by CMS for one or more quarters; (5) Results are not available for this reporting period; (6) Fewer than 100 patients completed the HCAHPS survey; (7) No cases met the criteria for this measure; (8) The lower limit of the confidence interval cannot be calculated if the number of observed infections equals zero; (9) No data are available from the state/territory for this reporting period; (10) The scores shown reflect fewer than 50 completed surveys; (11) There were discrepancies in the data collection process; (12) This measure does not apply to this hospital for this reporting period; (13) Results cannot be calculated for this reporting period; (14) The results for this state are combined with nearby states to protect confidentiality; Please refer to the User's Guide for a full explanation of data.

Measure	Cases	This Hosp.	State Avg.	U.S. Avg.
Received Reliever Medication	-	-	-	100%
Received Systemic Corticosteroids	-	-	-	100%
Emergency Department				
Admittance Decision Time (minutes)[2,3]	227	133	143	98
Head CT Results Within 45 Min. of Arrival[5]	-	-	-	57%
Patients Who Left ER Before Being Seen[5]	-	-	3%	2%
Time from ER Arrival to Admit. (minutes)[2,3]	229	346	357	274
Time from ER Arrival to Discharge (minutes)[5]	-	-	-	134
Time in ER Before Being Evaluated (minutes)[5]	-	-	-	26
Time to Pain Meds for Fractures (minutes)[5]	-	-	-	57
Heart Attack Care				
Aspirin Given at Discharge[1,3]	-	-	99%	99%
Fibrinolytic Meds Within 30 Min. of Arrival[3,7]	-	-	-	54%
PCI Within 90 Minutes of Arrival[3,7]	-	-	93%	96%
Statin Prescribed at Discharge[1,3]	-	-	98%	98%
Heart Failure Care				
ACE Inhibitor or ARB for LVSD[3]	45	98%	97%	97%
Discharge Instructions Given[3]	164	100%	93%	94%
Evaluation of LVS Function[3]	242	99%	99%	99%
Medicare Spending				
Medicare Spending per Patient (ratio)	-	-	-	0.98
Pneumonia Care				
Appropriate Initial Antibiotic Given[3]	103	99%	97%	95%
Blood Culture Timing[3]	149	97%	97%	98%
Pregnancy and Delivery Care				
Newborn Deliveries Scheduled Early[5]	-	-	-	6%
Preventive Care				
Immunization for Influenza[2,3]	271	89%	94%	90%
Immunization for Pneumonia[2,3]	275	92%	94%	92%
Stroke Care				
Anticoagulation Therapy for Atrial Fibrillation[5]	-	-	95%	95%
Antithrombotic Therapy Timing[5]	-	-	95%	98%
Assessed for Rehabilitation[5]	-	-	96%	97%
Discharged on Antithrombotic Therapy[5]	-	-	95%	99%
Discharged on Statin Medication[5]	-	-	97%	94%
Thrombolytic Therapy Timing[5]	-	-	-	66%
Venous Thromboembolism Prophylaxis[5]	-	-	89%	94%
Written Stroke Educational Materials Given[5]	-	-	77%	88%
Surgical Care Improvement Project				
Appropriate Beta Blocker Usage[3]	152	98%	97%	98%
Appropriate VTP Within 24 Hours[3]	531	98%	98%	98%
Controlled Postoperative Blood Glucose[3,7]	-	-	96%	97%
Perioperative Temperature Management[3]	668	100%	100%	100%
Prophylactic Antibiotic Selection[3]	401	99%	99%	99%
Prophylactic Antibiotic Selection (Outpatient)[5]	-	-	98%	98%
Prophylactic Antibiotic Stopped[3]	391	96%	98%	98%
Prophylactic Antibiotic Timing[3]	401	94%	97%	99%
Prophylactic Antibiotic Timing (Outpatient)[5]	-	-	98%	98%
Urinary Catheter Removal[3]	365	96%	98%	97%
Survey of Patients' Hospital Experiences				
Area Around Room 'Always' Quiet at Night	300+	53%	57%	61%
Doctors 'Always' Communicated Well	300+	78%	78%	82%
Home Recovery Information Given	300+	82%	85%	85%
Hospital Given 9 or 10 on 10 Point Scale	300+	72%	65%	71%
Meds 'Always' Explained Before Given	300+	55%	58%	64%
Nurses 'Always' Communicated Well	300+	72%	75%	79%
Pain 'Always' Well Controlled	300+	65%	67%	71%
Room and Bathroom 'Always' Clean	300+	56%	64%	73%
Timely Help 'Always' Received	300+	54%	58%	68%
Would Definitely Recommend Hospital	300+	76%	67%	71%
Use of Medical Imaging				
Cardiac Imaging Stress Test before Surgery	359	13.1%	6.4%	5.3%
Combination Abdominal CT Scan	1,020	6.5%	3.8%	10.5%
Combination Brain/Sinus CT Scan	973	5.0%	4.3%	2.7%
Combination Chest CT Scan	493	8.1%	1%	2.7%
Follow-up Mammogram/Ultrasound[7]	-	-	10.2%	8.8%
Lumbar Spine MRI for Low Back Pain[1]	-	-	38.2%	37.2%

Johns Hopkins Bayview Medical Center

4940 Eastern Avenue
Baltimore, MD 21224
Phone: 410-550-0123
Fax: 410-550-0184
URL: www.hopkinsbayview.org
Type: Acute Care Hospitals
Emergency Services: Yes
Ownership: Voluntary non-profit - Private
Beds: 565

Key Personnel:
CEO/President. . . . . Richard G. Bennett, MD
Radiology. . . . . Mark Bohlman, MD
Pediatric Ambulatory Care . . . . . . Mike Crocetti, MD
Coronary Care . . . . Robert Gibson, MD
Pediatric In-Patient Care . . . . Archie Golden, MD
Chief of Medical Staff . . . . David Hellmann, MD
Infection Control . . . . Jeanne LeClair
Operating Room. . . . . Thomas Magnuson, MD

Measure	Cases	This Hosp.	State Avg.	U.S. Avg.
Blood Clot Prevention and Treatment				
Anticoagulation Overlap Therapy[2]	107	99%	94%	93%
ICU Venous Thromboembolism Prophylaxis[2]	127	67%	94%	92%
Incidence of Potentially Preventable VTE[2]	42	5%	7%	10%
UFH with Dosages/Platelet Monitoring[2]	97	100%	97%	97%
Venous Thromboembolism Prophylaxis[2]	304	85%	90%	85%
Warfarin Therapy Discharge Instructions[2]	67	72%	78%	75%
Chest Pain/Possible Heart Attack Care				
Aspirin Given Within 24 Hours of Arrival[5]	-	-	100%	96%
Fibrinolytic Meds Within 30 Min. of Arrival[5]	-	-	-	58%
Average Time to ECG (minutes)[5]	-	-	6	7
Average Time to Transfer (minutes)[5]	-	-	32	60
Children's Asthma Care				
Received Home Management Plan of Care	-	-	-	88%
Received Reliever Medication	-	-	-	100%
Received Systemic Corticosteroids	-	-	-	100%
Emergency Department				
Admittance Decision Time (minutes)[2]	619	215	143	98
Head CT Results Within 45 Min. of Arrival[5]	-	-	-	57%
Patients Who Left ER Before Being Seen[5]	-	-	3%	2%
Time from ER Arrival to Admit. (minutes)[2]	619	411	357	274
Time from ER Arrival to Discharge (minutes)[5]	-	-	-	134
Time in ER Before Being Evaluated (minutes)[5]	-	-	-	26
Time to Pain Meds for Fractures (minutes)[5]	-	-	-	57
Heart Attack Care				
Aspirin Given at Discharge	227	100%	99%	99%
Fibrinolytic Meds Within 30 Min. of Arrival[7]	-	-	-	54%
PCI Within 90 Minutes of Arrival	38	95%	93%	96%
Statin Prescribed at Discharge	220	100%	98%	98%
Heart Failure Care				
ACE Inhibitor or ARB for LVSD	240	96%	97%	97%
Discharge Instructions Given	535	96%	93%	94%
Evaluation of LVS Function	658	99%	99%	99%
Medicare Spending				
Medicare Spending per Patient (ratio)	-	-	-	0.98
Pneumonia Care				
Appropriate Initial Antibiotic Given	169	97%	97%	95%
Blood Culture Timing	98	98%	97%	98%
Pregnancy and Delivery Care				
Newborn Deliveries Scheduled Early[5]	-	-	-	6%
Preventive Care				
Immunization for Influenza[2]	536	94%	94%	90%
Immunization for Pneumonia[2]	683	97%	94%	92%
Stroke Care				
Anticoagulation Therapy for Atrial Fibrillation[5]	-	-	95%	95%
Antithrombotic Therapy Timing[5]	-	-	95%	98%
Assessed for Rehabilitation[5]	-	-	96%	97%
Discharged on Antithrombotic Therapy[5]	-	-	95%	99%
Discharged on Statin Medication[5]	-	-	97%	94%
Thrombolytic Therapy Timing[5]	-	-	-	66%
Venous Thromboembolism Prophylaxis[5]	-	-	89%	94%
Written Stroke Educational Materials Given[5]	-	-	77%	88%
Surgical Care Improvement Project				
Appropriate Beta Blocker Usage[2]	209	95%	97%	98%
Appropriate VTP Within 24 Hours[2]	601	98%	98%	98%
Controlled Postoperative Blood Glucose[2,7]	-	-	96%	97%
Perioperative Temperature Management[2]	704	100%	100%	100%
Prophylactic Antibiotic Selection[2]	530	99%	99%	99%
Prophylactic Antibiotic Selection (Outpatient)[5]	-	-	98%	98%
Prophylactic Antibiotic Stopped[2]	519	98%	98%	98%
Prophylactic Antibiotic Timing[2]	530	98%	97%	99%
Prophylactic Antibiotic Timing (Outpatient)[5]	-	-	98%	98%
Urinary Catheter Removal[2]	511	98%	98%	97%
Survey of Patients' Hospital Experiences				
Area Around Room 'Always' Quiet at Night	300+	50%	57%	61%
Doctors 'Always' Communicated Well	300+	79%	78%	82%
Home Recovery Information Given	300+	88%	85%	85%
Hospital Given 9 or 10 on 10 Point Scale	300+	64%	65%	71%
Meds 'Always' Explained Before Given	300+	61%	58%	64%
Nurses 'Always' Communicated Well	300+	76%	75%	79%
Pain 'Always' Well Controlled	300+	65%	67%	71%
Room and Bathroom 'Always' Clean	300+	57%	64%	73%
Timely Help 'Always' Received	300+	58%	58%	68%
Would Definitely Recommend Hospital	300+	66%	67%	71%
Use of Medical Imaging				
Cardiac Imaging Stress Test before Surgery	459	6.3%	6.4%	5.3%
Combination Abdominal CT Scan	1,100	8.5%	3.8%	10.5%
Combination Brain/Sinus CT Scan	838	6.1%	4.3%	2.7%
Combination Chest CT Scan	1,241	4.4%	1%	2.7%
Follow-up Mammogram/Ultrasound	264	16.3%	10.2%	8.8%
Lumbar Spine MRI for Low Back Pain	44	40.9%	38.2%	37.2%

The Johns Hopkins Hospital

600 North Wolfe Street
Baltimore, MD 21287
Phone: 410-955-9540
Fax: 410-955-0890
E-mail: drichma@jhmi.edu
URL: www.jhmi.edu
Type: Acute Care Hospitals
Emergency Services: Yes
Ownership: Voluntary non-profit - Private
Beds: 1,036

Key Personnel:
Chief of Medical Staff. . . . . Edward Benz, MD
Pediatric Ambulatory Care . . . . . . George Dover, MD
Pediatric In-Patient Care . . . . George Dover, MD
Infection Control. . . . . John Froggatt, III, DP
Quality Assurance . . . . Rick Kidwell
Anesthesiology. . . . . Dr. Daniel Nyhan
CEO/President. . . . . Ronald R Peterson, MD
Radiology. . . . . George Saba

Measure	Cases	This Hosp.	State Avg.	U.S. Avg.
Blood Clot Prevention and Treatment				
Anticoagulation Overlap Therapy[5]	-	-	94%	93%
ICU Venous Thromboembolism Prophylaxis[5]	-	-	94%	92%
Incidence of Potentially Preventable VTE[5]	-	-	7%	10%
UFH with Dosages/Platelet Monitoring[5]	-	-	97%	97%
Venous Thromboembolism Prophylaxis[5]	-	-	90%	85%
Warfarin Therapy Discharge Instructions[5]	-	-	78%	75%
Chest Pain/Possible Heart Attack Care				
Aspirin Given Within 24 Hours of Arrival[5]	-	-	100%	96%
Fibrinolytic Meds Within 30 Min. of Arrival[5]	-	-	-	58%
Average Time to ECG (minutes)[5]	-	-	6	7
Average Time to Transfer (minutes)[5]	-	-	32	60
Children's Asthma Care				
Received Home Management Plan of Care	-	-	-	88%
Received Reliever Medication	-	-	-	100%
Received Systemic Corticosteroids	-	-	-	100%
Emergency Department				
Admittance Decision Time (minutes)[5]	-	-	143	98
Head CT Results Within 45 Min. of Arrival[5]	-	-	-	57%
Patients Who Left ER Before Being Seen[5]	-	-	3%	2%
Time from ER Arrival to Admit. (minutes)[5]	-	-	357	274
Time from ER Arrival to Discharge (minutes)[5]	-	-	-	134
Time in ER Before Being Evaluated (minutes)[5]	-	-	-	26
Time to Pain Meds for Fractures (minutes)[5]	-	-	-	57
Heart Attack Care				
Aspirin Given at Discharge	523	99%	99%	99%
Fibrinolytic Meds Within 30 Min. of Arrival[7]	-	-	-	54%
PCI Within 90 Minutes of Arrival	11	82%	93%	96%
Statin Prescribed at Discharge	505	99%	98%	98%
Heart Failure Care				
ACE Inhibitor or ARB for LVSD[2]	160	100%	97%	97%
Discharge Instructions Given[2]	385	99%	93%	94%
Evaluation of LVS Function[2]	431	100%	99%	99%

NOTE: Hospital profiles are in alphabetical order by state, then city, then hospital within the city; Rankings exclude hospitals with less than 25 cases except for patient surveys which excludes hospitals with less than 100 cases; (a) 100-299 cases; (1) The number of cases/patients is too few to report; (2) Data submitted were based on a sample of cases/patients; (3) Results are based on a shorter time period than required; (4) Data suppressed by CMS for one or more quarters; (5) Results are not available for this reporting period; (6) Fewer than 100 patients completed the HCAHPS survey; (7) No cases met the criteria for this measure; (8) The lower limit of the confidence interval cannot be calculated if the number of observed infections equals zero; (9) No data are available from the state/territory for this reporting period; (10) The scores shown reflect fewer than 50 completed surveys; (11) There were discrepancies in the data collection process; (12) This measure does not apply to this hospital for this reporting period; (13) Results cannot be calculated for this reporting period; (14) The results for this state are combined with nearby states to protect confidentiality; Please refer to the User's Guide for a full explanation of data.

Measure	Cases	This Hosp.	State Avg.	U.S. Avg.
Medicare Spending				
Medicare Spending per Patient (ratio)	-	-	-	0.98
Pneumonia Care				
Appropriate Initial Antibiotic Given[2]	41	100%	97%	95%
Blood Culture Timing[2]	42	100%	97%	98%
Pregnancy and Delivery Care				
Newborn Deliveries Scheduled Early[5]	-	-	-	6%
Preventive Care				
Immunization for Influenza[5]	-	-	94%	90%
Immunization for Pneumonia[5]	-	-	94%	92%
Stroke Care				
Anticoagulation Therapy for Atrial Fibrillation[5]	-	-	95%	95%
Antithrombotic Therapy Timing[5]	-	-	95%	98%
Assessed for Rehabilitation[5]	-	-	96%	97%
Discharged on Antithrombotic Therapy[5]	-	-	95%	99%
Discharged on Statin Medication[5]	-	-	97%	94%
Thrombolytic Therapy Timing[5]	-	-	-	66%
Venous Thromboembolism Prophylaxis[5]	-	-	89%	94%
Written Stroke Educational Materials Given[5]	-	-	77%	88%
Surgical Care Improvement Project				
Appropriate Beta Blocker Usage[2]	345	99%	97%	98%
Appropriate VTP Within 24 Hours[2]	343	99%	98%	98%
Controlled Postoperative Blood Glucose[2]	391	96%	96%	97%
Perioperative Temperature Management[2]	485	100%	100%	100%
Prophylactic Antibiotic Selection[2]	572	99%	99%	99%
Prophylactic Antibiotic Selection (Outpatient)[5]	-	-	98%	98%
Prophylactic Antibiotic Stopped[2]	561	100%	98%	98%
Prophylactic Antibiotic Timing[2]	574	98%	97%	99%
Prophylactic Antibiotic Timing (Outpatient)[5]	-	-	98%	98%
Urinary Catheter Removal[2]	346	98%	98%	97%
Survey of Patients' Hospital Experiences				
Area Around Room 'Always' Quiet at Night	300+	66%	57%	61%
Doctors 'Always' Communicated Well	300+	81%	78%	82%
Home Recovery Information Given	300+	87%	85%	85%
Hospital Given 9 or 10 on 10 Point Scale	300+	83%	65%	71%
Meds 'Always' Explained Before Given	300+	65%	58%	64%
Nurses 'Always' Communicated Well	300+	82%	75%	79%
Pain 'Always' Well Controlled	300+	70%	67%	71%
Room and Bathroom 'Always' Clean	300+	70%	64%	73%
Timely Help 'Always' Received	300+	63%	58%	68%
Would Definitely Recommend Hospital	300+	86%	67%	71%
Use of Medical Imaging				
Cardiac Imaging Stress Test before Surgery	483	5.4%	6.4%	5.3%
Combination Abdominal CT Scan	2,882	2.0%	3.8%	10.5%
Combination Brain/Sinus CT Scan	736	6.0%	4.3%	2.7%
Combination Chest CT Scan	4,928	0.1%	1%	2.7%
Follow-up Mammogram/Ultrasound	1,055	2.7%	10.2%	8.8%
Lumbar Spine MRI for Low Back Pain	139	26.6%	38.2%	37.2%

Medstar Franklin Square Medical Center

9000 Franklin Square Drive
Baltimore, MD 21237
URL: www.franklinsquare.org
Type: Acute Care Hospitals
Ownership: Voluntary non-profit - Private
Phone: 443-777-7850
Fax: 443-777-7904
Emergency Services: Yes
Beds: 380

Key Personnel:
Radiology. . . . . Blair Andrew
Pediatric Ambulatory Care . . . . . . Scott Krugman, MD
Operating Room. . . . . Beth Leilich, RN
CEO/President. . . . . Samuel E. Moskowitz, FACHE
Emergency Room . . . . Michael Pipkin, MD
Surgery . . . . Bridget Schall
Chief of Medical Staff. . . . . Anthony Sclama, MD
Quality Assurance . . . . Jacqueline Spielman

Measure	Cases	This Hosp.	State Avg.	U.S. Avg.
Blood Clot Prevention and Treatment				
Anticoagulation Overlap Therapy[2]	123	89%	94%	93%
ICU Venous Thromboembolism Prophylaxis[2]	52	85%	94%	92%
Incidence of Potentially Preventable VTE[2]	19	11%	7%	10%
UFH with Dosages/Platelet Monitoring[2]	61	100%	97%	97%
Venous Thromboembolism Prophylaxis[2]	351	79%	90%	85%
Warfarin Therapy Discharge Instructions[2]	102	15%	78%	75%
Chest Pain/Possible Heart Attack Care				
Aspirin Given Within 24 Hours of Arrival[5]	-	-	100%	96%
Fibrinolytic Meds Within 30 Min. of Arrival[5]	-	-	-	58%
Average Time to ECG (minutes)[5]	-	-	6	7
Average Time to Transfer (minutes)[5]	-	-	32	60
Children's Asthma Care				
Received Home Management Plan of Care	-	-	-	88%
Received Reliever Medication	-	-	-	100%
Received Systemic Corticosteroids	-	-	-	100%
Emergency Department				
Admittance Decision Time (minutes)[2]	588	150	143	98
Head CT Results Within 45 Min. of Arrival[5]	-	-	-	57%
Patients Who Left ER Before Being Seen[5]	-	-	3%	2%
Time from ER Arrival to Admit. (minutes)[2]	628	378	357	274
Time from ER Arrival to Discharge (minutes)[5]	-	-	-	134
Time in ER Before Being Evaluated (minutes)[5]	-	-	-	26
Time to Pain Meds for Fractures (minutes)[5]	-	-	-	57
Heart Attack Care				
Aspirin Given at Discharge	167	98%	99%	99%
Fibrinolytic Meds Within 30 Min. of Arrival[7]	-	-	-	54%
PCI Within 90 Minutes of Arrival	69	83%	93%	96%
Statin Prescribed at Discharge	168	99%	98%	98%
Heart Failure Care				
ACE Inhibitor or ARB for LVSD	168	93%	97%	97%
Discharge Instructions Given	566	74%	93%	94%
Evaluation of LVS Function	726	99%	99%	99%
Medicare Spending				
Medicare Spending per Patient (ratio)	-	-	-	0.98
Pneumonia Care				
Appropriate Initial Antibiotic Given	346	96%	97%	95%
Blood Culture Timing	369	89%	97%	98%
Pregnancy and Delivery Care				
Newborn Deliveries Scheduled Early[5]	-	-	-	6%
Preventive Care				
Immunization for Influenza[2]	574	94%	94%	90%
Immunization for Pneumonia[2]	713	91%	94%	92%
Stroke Care				
Anticoagulation Therapy for Atrial Fibrillation[5]	-	-	95%	95%
Antithrombotic Therapy Timing[5]	-	-	95%	98%
Assessed for Rehabilitation[5]	-	-	96%	97%
Discharged on Antithrombotic Therapy[5]	-	-	95%	99%
Discharged on Statin Medication[5]	-	-	97%	94%
Thrombolytic Therapy Timing[5]	-	-	-	66%
Venous Thromboembolism Prophylaxis[5]	-	-	89%	94%
Written Stroke Educational Materials Given[5]	-	-	77%	88%
Surgical Care Improvement Project				
Appropriate Beta Blocker Usage[2]	347	97%	97%	98%
Appropriate VTP Within 24 Hours[2]	661	97%	98%	98%
Controlled Postoperative Blood Glucose[2,7]	-	-	96%	97%
Perioperative Temperature Management[2]	923	100%	100%	100%
Prophylactic Antibiotic Selection[2]	621	96%	99%	99%
Prophylactic Antibiotic Selection (Outpatient)[5]	-	-	98%	98%
Prophylactic Antibiotic Stopped[2]	605	97%	98%	98%
Prophylactic Antibiotic Timing[2]	622	98%	97%	99%
Prophylactic Antibiotic Timing (Outpatient)[5]	-	-	98%	98%
Urinary Catheter Removal[2]	578	98%	98%	97%
Survey of Patients' Hospital Experiences				
Area Around Room 'Always' Quiet at Night	300+	51%	57%	61%
Doctors 'Always' Communicated Well	300+	78%	78%	82%
Home Recovery Information Given	300+	88%	85%	85%
Hospital Given 9 or 10 on 10 Point Scale	300+	71%	65%	71%
Meds 'Always' Explained Before Given	300+	63%	58%	64%
Nurses 'Always' Communicated Well	300+	78%	75%	79%
Pain 'Always' Well Controlled	300+	70%	67%	71%
Room and Bathroom 'Always' Clean	300+	58%	64%	73%
Timely Help 'Always' Received	300+	55%	58%	68%
Would Definitely Recommend Hospital	300+	71%	67%	71%
Use of Medical Imaging				
Cardiac Imaging Stress Test before Surgery	734	5.2%	6.4%	5.3%
Combination Abdominal CT Scan	1,228	0.1%	3.8%	10.5%
Combination Brain/Sinus CT Scan	1,753	0.7%	4.3%	2.7%
Combination Chest CT Scan	290	0.3%	1%	2.7%
Follow-up Mammogram/Ultrasound[7]	-	-	10.2%	8.8%
Lumbar Spine MRI for Low Back Pain[1]	-	-	38.2%	37.2%

Medstar Good Samaritan Hospital

5601 Loch Raven Boulevard
Baltimore, MD 21239
URL: www.goodsam-md.org
Type: Acute Care Hospitals
Ownership: Voluntary non-profit - Other
Phone: 443-444-3902
Fax: 410-532-5929
Emergency Services: Yes
Beds: 317

Key Personnel:
Cardiac Laboratory. . . . . Linda Hawes, RN
CEO/President. . . . . Jeffrey Matton
Emergency Room . . . . Kevin Scruggs, MD
Anesthesiology. . . . . Michael Sendak, MD
Quality Assurance . . . . Ken Walsch
Operating Room. . . . . Jeremy Weiner, MD
Chief of Medical Staff . . . . David Weisman, DO
Radiology. . . . . Allan Weksberg, MD

Measure	Cases	This Hosp.	State Avg.	U.S. Avg.
Blood Clot Prevention and Treatment				
Anticoagulation Overlap Therapy[2]	103	98%	94%	93%
ICU Venous Thromboembolism Prophylaxis[2]	40	98%	94%	92%
Incidence of Potentially Preventable VTE[2]	35	3%	7%	10%
UFH with Dosages/Platelet Monitoring[2]	86	99%	97%	97%
Venous Thromboembolism Prophylaxis[2]	369	83%	90%	85%
Warfarin Therapy Discharge Instructions[2]	62	97%	78%	75%
Chest Pain/Possible Heart Attack Care				
Aspirin Given Within 24 Hours of Arrival[5]	-	-	100%	96%
Fibrinolytic Meds Within 30 Min. of Arrival[5]	-	-	-	58%
Average Time to ECG (minutes)[5]	-	-	6	7
Average Time to Transfer (minutes)[5]	-	-	32	60
Children's Asthma Care				
Received Home Management Plan of Care	-	-	-	88%
Received Reliever Medication	-	-	-	100%
Received Systemic Corticosteroids	-	-	-	100%
Emergency Department				
Admittance Decision Time (minutes)[2]	525	141	143	98
Head CT Results Within 45 Min. of Arrival[5]	-	-	-	57%
Patients Who Left ER Before Being Seen[5]	-	-	3%	2%
Time from ER Arrival to Admit. (minutes)[2]	552	405	357	274
Time from ER Arrival to Discharge (minutes)[5]	-	-	-	134
Time in ER Before Being Evaluated (minutes)[5]	-	-	-	26
Time to Pain Meds for Fractures (minutes)[5]	-	-	-	57
Heart Attack Care				
Aspirin Given at Discharge	72	93%	99%	99%
Fibrinolytic Meds Within 30 Min. of Arrival[7]	-	-	-	54%
PCI Within 90 Minutes of Arrival[7]	-	-	93%	96%
Statin Prescribed at Discharge	69	99%	98%	98%
Heart Failure Care				
ACE Inhibitor or ARB for LVSD	212	97%	97%	97%
Discharge Instructions Given	481	92%	93%	94%
Evaluation of LVS Function	673	100%	99%	99%
Medicare Spending				
Medicare Spending per Patient (ratio)	-	-	-	0.98
Pneumonia Care				
Appropriate Initial Antibiotic Given	169	95%	97%	95%
Blood Culture Timing	351	92%	97%	98%
Pregnancy and Delivery Care				
Newborn Deliveries Scheduled Early[5]	-	-	-	6%
Preventive Care				
Immunization for Influenza[2]	591	96%	94%	90%
Immunization for Pneumonia[2]	918	94%	94%	92%
Stroke Care				
Anticoagulation Therapy for Atrial Fibrillation[5]	-	-	95%	95%
Antithrombotic Therapy Timing[5]	-	-	95%	98%
Assessed for Rehabilitation[5]	-	-	96%	97%
Discharged on Antithrombotic Therapy[5]	-	-	95%	99%
Discharged on Statin Medication[5]	-	-	97%	94%
Thrombolytic Therapy Timing[5]	-	-	-	66%
Venous Thromboembolism Prophylaxis[5]	-	-	89%	94%
Written Stroke Educational Materials Given[5]	-	-	77%	88%
Surgical Care Improvement Project				
Appropriate Beta Blocker Usage	272	93%	97%	98%
Appropriate VTP Within 24 Hours	815	98%	98%	98%
Controlled Postoperative Blood Glucose[7]	-	-	96%	97%
Perioperative Temperature Management	902	100%	100%	100%
Prophylactic Antibiotic Selection	661	98%	99%	99%

NOTE: Hospital profiles are in alphabetical order by state, then city, then hospital within the city; Rankings exclude hospitals with less than 25 cases except for patient surveys which excludes hospitals with less than 100 cases; (a) 100-299 cases; (1) The number of cases/patients is too few to report; (2) Data submitted were based on a sample of cases/patients; (3) Results are based on a shorter time period than required; (4) Data suppressed by CMS for one or more quarters; (5) Results are not available for this reporting period; (6) Fewer than 100 patients completed the HCAHPS survey; (7) No cases met the criteria for this measure; (8) The lower limit of the confidence interval cannot be calculated if the number of observed infections equals zero; (9) No data are available from the state/territory for this reporting period; (10) The scores shown reflect fewer than 50 completed surveys; (11) There were discrepancies in the data collection process; (12) This measure does not apply to this hospital for this reporting period; (13) Results cannot be calculated for this reporting period; (14) The results for this state are combined with nearby states to protect confidentiality; Please refer to the User's Guide for a full explanation of data.

Measure	Cases	This Hosp.	State Avg.	U.S. Avg.
Prophylactic Antibiotic Selection (Outpatient)[5]	-	-	98%	98%
Prophylactic Antibiotic Stopped	638	97%	98%	98%
Prophylactic Antibiotic Timing	661	98%	97%	99%
Prophylactic Antibiotic Timing (Outpatient)[5]	-	-	98%	98%
Urinary Catheter Removal	750	97%	98%	97%
Survey of Patients' Hospital Experiences				
Area Around Room 'Always' Quiet at Night	300+	61%	57%	61%
Doctors 'Always' Communicated Well	300+	80%	78%	82%
Home Recovery Information Given	300+	86%	85%	85%
Hospital Given 9 or 10 on 10 Point Scale	300+	66%	65%	71%
Meds 'Always' Explained Before Given	300+	57%	58%	64%
Nurses 'Always' Communicated Well	300+	77%	75%	79%
Pain 'Always' Well Controlled	300+	68%	67%	71%
Room and Bathroom 'Always' Clean	300+	65%	64%	73%
Timely Help 'Always' Received	300+	55%	58%	68%
Would Definitely Recommend Hospital	300+	70%	67%	71%
Use of Medical Imaging				
Cardiac Imaging Stress Test before Surgery	467	7.3%	6.4%	5.3%
Combination Abdominal CT Scan	760	2.6%	3.8%	10.5%
Combination Brain/Sinus CT Scan	1,133	4.0%	4.3%	2.7%
Combination Chest CT Scan	438	0.0%	1%	2.7%
Follow-up Mammogram/Ultrasound	858	9.7%	10.2%	8.8%
Lumbar Spine MRI for Low Back Pain	131	46.6%	38.2%	37.2%

Medstar Harbor Hospital

3001 South Hanover Street
Baltimore, MD 21225
Phone: 410-350-3201
Fax: 410-350-2052
URL: www.harborhospital.org
Type: Acute Care Hospitals
Emergency Services: Yes
Ownership: Voluntary non-profit - Private
Beds: 182

Key Personnel:
Operating Room. . . . . Ashok Agrawal, RN
Pediatric In-Patient Care . . . . Shahid Aziz, MD
Anesthesiology. . . . . Allan Birenberg, MD
Ambulatory Care . . . . Joel N Bryan
Radiology. . . . . Mohsen Gharib
Emergency Room . . . . Tammy Kile, MD
President . . . . Dennis W. Pullin, FACHE
Quality Assurance . . . . Christine Swearingen

Measure	Cases	This Hosp.	State Avg.	U.S. Avg.
Blood Clot Prevention and Treatment				
Anticoagulation Overlap Therapy[2]	65	74%	94%	93%
ICU Venous Thromboembolism Prophylaxis[2]	92	96%	94%	92%
Incidence of Potentially Preventable VTE[2]	14	29%	7%	10%
UFH with Dosages/Platelet Monitoring[2]	53	42%	97%	97%
Venous Thromboembolism Prophylaxis[2]	304	85%	90%	85%
Warfarin Therapy Discharge Instructions[2]	50	44%	78%	75%
Chest Pain/Possible Heart Attack Care				
Aspirin Given Within 24 Hours of Arrival[5]	-	-	100%	96%
Fibrinolytic Meds Within 30 Min. of Arrival[5]	-	-	-	58%
Average Time to ECG (minutes)[5]	-	-	6	7
Average Time to Transfer (minutes)[5]	-	-	32	60
Children's Asthma Care				
Received Home Management Plan of Care	-	-	-	88%
Received Reliever Medication	-	-	-	100%
Received Systemic Corticosteroids	-	-	-	100%
Emergency Department				
Admittance Decision Time (minutes)[2]	396	145	143	98
Head CT Results Within 45 Min. of Arrival[5]	-	-	-	57%
Patients Who Left ER Before Being Seen[5]	-	-	3%	2%
Time from ER Arrival to Admit. (minutes)[2]	407	325	357	274
Time from ER Arrival to Discharge (minutes)[5]	-	-	-	134
Time in ER Before Being Evaluated (minutes)[5]	-	-	-	26
Time to Pain Meds for Fractures (minutes)[5]	-	-	-	57
Heart Attack Care				
Aspirin Given at Discharge	51	98%	99%	99%
Fibrinolytic Meds Within 30 Min. of Arrival[7]	-	-	-	54%
PCI Within 90 Minutes of Arrival[7]	-	-	93%	96%
Statin Prescribed at Discharge	51	98%	98%	98%
Heart Failure Care				
ACE Inhibitor or ARB for LVSD	103	92%	97%	97%
Discharge Instructions Given	243	94%	93%	94%
Evaluation of LVS Function	291	98%	99%	99%
Medicare Spending				
Medicare Spending per Patient (ratio)	-	-	-	0.98
Pneumonia Care				
Appropriate Initial Antibiotic Given	156	97%	97%	95%
Blood Culture Timing	292	94%	97%	98%
Pregnancy and Delivery Care				
Newborn Deliveries Scheduled Early[5]	-	-	-	6%
Preventive Care				
Immunization for Influenza[2]	513	87%	94%	90%
Immunization for Pneumonia[2]	639	89%	94%	92%
Stroke Care				
Anticoagulation Therapy for Atrial Fibrillation[5]	-	-	95%	95%
Antithrombotic Therapy Timing[5]	-	-	95%	98%
Assessed for Rehabilitation[5]	-	-	96%	97%
Discharged on Antithrombotic Therapy[5]	-	-	95%	99%
Discharged on Statin Medication[5]	-	-	97%	94%
Thrombolytic Therapy Timing[5]	-	-	-	66%
Venous Thromboembolism Prophylaxis[5]	-	-	89%	94%
Written Stroke Educational Materials Given[5]	-	-	77%	88%
Surgical Care Improvement Project				
Appropriate Beta Blocker Usage[2]	168	90%	97%	98%
Appropriate VTP Within 24 Hours[2]	523	97%	98%	98%
Controlled Postoperative Blood Glucose[2,7]	-	-	96%	97%
Perioperative Temperature Management[2]	610	98%	100%	100%
Prophylactic Antibiotic Selection[2]	462	99%	99%	99%
Prophylactic Antibiotic Selection (Outpatient)[5]	-	-	98%	98%
Prophylactic Antibiotic Stopped[2]	451	94%	98%	98%
Prophylactic Antibiotic Timing[2]	462	97%	97%	99%
Prophylactic Antibiotic Timing (Outpatient)[5]	-	-	98%	98%
Urinary Catheter Removal[2]	377	95%	98%	97%
Survey of Patients' Hospital Experiences				
Area Around Room 'Always' Quiet at Night	300+	61%	57%	61%
Doctors 'Always' Communicated Well	300+	80%	78%	82%
Home Recovery Information Given	300+	85%	85%	85%
Hospital Given 9 or 10 on 10 Point Scale	300+	72%	65%	71%
Meds 'Always' Explained Before Given	300+	60%	58%	64%
Nurses 'Always' Communicated Well	300+	77%	75%	79%
Pain 'Always' Well Controlled	300+	72%	67%	71%
Room and Bathroom 'Always' Clean	300+	67%	64%	73%
Timely Help 'Always' Received	300+	64%	58%	68%
Would Definitely Recommend Hospital	300+	69%	67%	71%
Use of Medical Imaging				
Cardiac Imaging Stress Test before Surgery	317	7.3%	6.4%	5.3%
Combination Abdominal CT Scan	409	3.9%	3.8%	10.5%
Combination Brain/Sinus CT Scan[1]	-	-	4.3%	2.7%
Combination Chest CT Scan	255	0.0%	1%	2.7%
Follow-up Mammogram/Ultrasound	456	11.2%	10.2%	8.8%
Lumbar Spine MRI for Low Back Pain	54	38.9%	38.2%	37.2%

Medstar Union Memorial Hospital

201 East University Parkway
Baltimore, MD 21218
Phone: 410-554-2227
Fax: 410-554-2652
URL: www.unionmemorial.org
Type: Acute Care Hospitals
Emergency Services: Yes
Ownership: Voluntary non-profit - Other
Beds: 249

Key Personnel:
CEO/President. . . . . Bradley S. Chambers
Infection Control. . . . . Barbara Elau
Chief of Medical Staff. . . . . Robert Ferguson, MD
Quality Assurance . . . . Anne Flood
Pediatric Ambulatory Care . . . . . . Jay Gopal, MD
Operating Room. . . . . Kathy Mucei
Radiology. . . . . Carlton Sexton
Chair/CEO . . . . Christopher G. Wunder

Measure	Cases	This Hosp.	State Avg.	U.S. Avg.
Blood Clot Prevention and Treatment				
Anticoagulation Overlap Therapy[2]	88	73%	94%	93%
ICU Venous Thromboembolism Prophylaxis[2]	56	82%	94%	92%
Incidence of Potentially Preventable VTE[2]	44	14%	7%	10%
UFH with Dosages/Platelet Monitoring[2]	83	94%	97%	97%
Venous Thromboembolism Prophylaxis[2]	271	80%	90%	85%
Warfarin Therapy Discharge Instructions[2]	63	73%	78%	75%
Chest Pain/Possible Heart Attack Care				
Aspirin Given Within 24 Hours of Arrival[5]	-	-	100%	96%
Fibrinolytic Meds Within 30 Min. of Arrival[5]	-	-	-	58%
Average Time to ECG (minutes)[5]	-	-	6	7
Average Time to Transfer (minutes)[5]	-	-	32	60
Children's Asthma Care				
Received Home Management Plan of Care	-	-	-	88%
Received Reliever Medication	-	-	-	100%
Received Systemic Corticosteroids	-	-	-	100%
Emergency Department				
Admittance Decision Time (minutes)[2]	447	126	143	98
Head CT Results Within 45 Min. of Arrival[5]	-	-	-	57%
Patients Who Left ER Before Being Seen[5]	-	-	3%	2%
Time from ER Arrival to Admit. (minutes)[2]	523	320	357	274
Time from ER Arrival to Discharge (minutes)[5]	-	-	-	134
Time in ER Before Being Evaluated (minutes)[5]	-	-	-	26
Time to Pain Meds for Fractures (minutes)[5]	-	-	-	57
Heart Attack Care				
Aspirin Given at Discharge	516	98%	99%	99%
Fibrinolytic Meds Within 30 Min. of Arrival[7]	-	-	-	54%
PCI Within 90 Minutes of Arrival	29	83%	93%	96%
Statin Prescribed at Discharge	475	94%	98%	98%
Heart Failure Care				
ACE Inhibitor or ARB for LVSD	187	96%	97%	97%
Discharge Instructions Given	448	89%	93%	94%
Evaluation of LVS Function	506	95%	99%	99%
Medicare Spending				
Medicare Spending per Patient (ratio)	-	-	-	0.98
Pneumonia Care				
Appropriate Initial Antibiotic Given	98	96%	97%	95%
Blood Culture Timing	166	99%	97%	98%
Pregnancy and Delivery Care				
Newborn Deliveries Scheduled Early[5]	-	-	-	6%
Preventive Care				
Immunization for Influenza[2]	496	86%	94%	90%
Immunization for Pneumonia[2]	753	92%	94%	92%
Stroke Care				
Anticoagulation Therapy for Atrial Fibrillation[1]	-	-	95%	95%
Antithrombotic Therapy Timing	59	97%	95%	98%
Assessed for Rehabilitation	60	97%	96%	97%
Discharged on Antithrombotic Therapy	59	95%	95%	99%
Discharged on Statin Medication	50	100%	97%	94%
Thrombolytic Therapy Timing[1]	-	-	-	66%
Venous Thromboembolism Prophylaxis	61	87%	89%	94%
Written Stroke Educational Materials Given	34	100%	77%	88%
Surgical Care Improvement Project				
Appropriate Beta Blocker Usage[2]	313	97%	97%	98%
Appropriate VTP Within 24 Hours[2]	609	97%	98%	98%
Controlled Postoperative Blood Glucose[2]	163	91%	96%	97%
Perioperative Temperature Management[2]	810	97%	100%	100%
Prophylactic Antibiotic Selection[2]	663	98%	99%	99%
Prophylactic Antibiotic Selection (Outpatient)[5]	-	-	98%	98%
Prophylactic Antibiotic Stopped[2]	655	96%	98%	98%
Prophylactic Antibiotic Timing[2]	770	72%	97%	99%
Prophylactic Antibiotic Timing (Outpatient)[5]	-	-	98%	98%
Urinary Catheter Removal[2]	248	90%	98%	97%
Survey of Patients' Hospital Experiences				
Area Around Room 'Always' Quiet at Night	300+	64%	57%	61%
Doctors 'Always' Communicated Well	300+	80%	78%	82%
Home Recovery Information Given	300+	87%	85%	85%
Hospital Given 9 or 10 on 10 Point Scale	300+	72%	65%	71%
Meds 'Always' Explained Before Given	300+	59%	58%	64%
Nurses 'Always' Communicated Well	300+	78%	75%	79%
Pain 'Always' Well Controlled	300+	70%	67%	71%
Room and Bathroom 'Always' Clean	300+	65%	64%	73%
Timely Help 'Always' Received	300+	66%	58%	68%
Would Definitely Recommend Hospital	300+	75%	67%	71%
Use of Medical Imaging				
Cardiac Imaging Stress Test before Surgery	445	4.5%	6.4%	5.3%
Combination Abdominal CT Scan	697	3.9%	3.8%	10.5%
Combination Brain/Sinus CT Scan	582	2.4%	4.3%	2.7%
Combination Chest CT Scan	614	0.7%	1%	2.7%
Follow-up Mammogram/Ultrasound	1,040	10.5%	10.2%	8.8%
Lumbar Spine MRI for Low Back Pain	95	26.3%	38.2%	37.2%

NOTE: Hospital profiles are in alphabetical order by state, then city, then hospital within the city; Rankings exclude hospitals with less than 25 cases except for patient surveys which excludes hospitals with less than 100 cases; (a) 100-299 cases; (1) The number of cases/patients is too few to report; (2) Data submitted were based on a sample of cases/patients; (3) Results are based on a shorter time period than required; (4) Data suppressed by CMS for one or more quarters; (5) Results are not available for this reporting period; (6) Fewer than 100 patients completed the HCAHPS survey; (7) No cases met the criteria for this measure; (8) The lower limit of the confidence interval cannot be calculated if the number of observed infections equals zero; (9) No data are available from the state/territory for this reporting period; (10) The scores shown reflect fewer than 50 completed surveys; (11) There were discrepancies in the data collection process; (12) This measure does not apply to this hospital for this reporting period; (13) Results cannot be calculated for this reporting period; (14) The results for this state are combined with nearby states to protect confidentiality; Please refer to the User's Guide for a full explanation of data.

Mercy Medical Center

301 Saint Paul Place
Baltimore, MD 21202
Phone: 410-332-9237
URL: www.mdmercy.com
Type: Acute Care Hospitals
Emergency Services: Yes
Ownership: Voluntary non-profit - Church

Key Personnel:
CEO/President. . . . . Thomas Mullen

Measure	Cases	This Hosp.	State Avg.	U.S. Avg.
Blood Clot Prevention and Treatment				
Anticoagulation Overlap Therapy[2]	108	99%	94%	93%
ICU Venous Thromboembolism Prophylaxis[2]	71	100%	94%	92%
Incidence of Potentially Preventable VTE[2]	40	12%	7%	10%
UFH with Dosages/Platelet Monitoring[2]	100	99%	97%	97%
Venous Thromboembolism Prophylaxis[2]	259	97%	90%	85%
Warfarin Therapy Discharge Instructions[2]	75	68%	78%	75%
Chest Pain/Possible Heart Attack Care				
Aspirin Given Within 24 Hours of Arrival[5]	-	-	100%	96%
Fibrinolytic Meds Within 30 Min. of Arrival[5]	-	-	-	58%
Average Time to ECG (minutes)[5]	-	-	6	7
Average Time to Transfer (minutes)[5]	-	-	32	60
Children's Asthma Care				
Received Home Management Plan of Care	-	-	-	88%
Received Reliever Medication	-	-	-	100%
Received Systemic Corticosteroids	-	-	-	100%
Emergency Department				
Admittance Decision Time (minutes)[5]	-	-	143	98
Head CT Results Within 45 Min. of Arrival[5]	-	-	-	57%
Patients Who Left ER Before Being Seen[5]	-	-	3%	2%
Time from ER Arrival to Admit. (minutes)[5]	-	-	357	274
Time from ER Arrival to Discharge (minutes)[5]	-	-	-	134
Time in ER Before Being Evaluated (minutes)[5]	-	-	-	26
Time to Pain Meds for Fractures (minutes)[5]	-	-	-	57
Heart Attack Care				
Aspirin Given at Discharge	16	100%	99%	99%
Fibrinolytic Meds Within 30 Min. of Arrival[7]	-	-	-	54%
PCI Within 90 Minutes of Arrival[7]	-	-	93%	96%
Statin Prescribed at Discharge	17	100%	98%	98%
Heart Failure Care				
ACE Inhibitor or ARB for LVSD	123	89%	97%	97%
Discharge Instructions Given	238	93%	93%	94%
Evaluation of LVS Function	274	100%	99%	99%
Medicare Spending				
Medicare Spending per Patient (ratio)	-	-	-	0.98
Pneumonia Care				
Appropriate Initial Antibiotic Given	89	92%	97%	95%
Blood Culture Timing	105	92%	97%	98%
Pregnancy and Delivery Care				
Newborn Deliveries Scheduled Early[5]	-	-	-	6%
Preventive Care				
Immunization for Influenza[5]	-	-	94%	90%
Immunization for Pneumonia[5]	-	-	94%	92%
Stroke Care				
Anticoagulation Therapy for Atrial Fibrillation[5]	-	-	95%	95%
Antithrombotic Therapy Timing[5]	-	-	95%	98%
Assessed for Rehabilitation[5]	-	-	96%	97%
Discharged on Antithrombotic Therapy[5]	-	-	95%	99%
Discharged on Statin Medication[5]	-	-	97%	94%
Thrombolytic Therapy Timing[5]	-	-	-	66%
Venous Thromboembolism Prophylaxis[5]	-	-	89%	94%
Written Stroke Educational Materials Given[5]	-	-	77%	88%
Surgical Care Improvement Project				
Appropriate Beta Blocker Usage[2]	349	99%	97%	98%
Appropriate VTP Within 24 Hours[2]	1,310	100%	98%	98%
Controlled Postoperative Blood Glucose[2,7]	-	-	96%	97%
Perioperative Temperature Management[2]	1,532	100%	100%	100%
Prophylactic Antibiotic Selection[2]	1,326	99%	99%	99%
Prophylactic Antibiotic Selection (Outpatient)[5]	-	-	98%	98%
Prophylactic Antibiotic Stopped[2]	1,315	98%	98%	98%
Prophylactic Antibiotic Timing[2]	1,327	98%	97%	99%
Prophylactic Antibiotic Timing (Outpatient)[5]	-	-	98%	98%
Urinary Catheter Removal[2]	1,119	100%	98%	97%
Survey of Patients' Hospital Experiences				
Area Around Room 'Always' Quiet at Night	300+	68%	57%	61%
Doctors 'Always' Communicated Well	300+	84%	78%	82%
Home Recovery Information Given	300+	89%	85%	85%
Hospital Given 9 or 10 on 10 Point Scale	300+	76%	65%	71%
Meds 'Always' Explained Before Given	300+	64%	58%	64%
Nurses 'Always' Communicated Well	300+	81%	75%	79%
Pain 'Always' Well Controlled	300+	72%	67%	71%
Room and Bathroom 'Always' Clean	300+	74%	64%	73%
Timely Help 'Always' Received	300+	65%	58%	68%
Would Definitely Recommend Hospital	300+	80%	67%	71%
Use of Medical Imaging				
Cardiac Imaging Stress Test before Surgery	535	8.0%	6.4%	5.3%
Combination Abdominal CT Scan	1,139	13.8%	3.8%	10.5%
Combination Brain/Sinus CT Scan[1]	-	-	4.3%	2.7%
Combination Chest CT Scan	832	0.2%	1%	2.7%
Follow-up Mammogram/Ultrasound	1,530	18.3%	10.2%	8.8%
Lumbar Spine MRI for Low Back Pain	139	34.5%	38.2%	37.2%

Saint Agnes Hospital

900 Caton Avenue
Baltimore, MD 21229
Phone: 410-368-2101
Fax: 410-368-3536
E-mail: info@stagnes.org
URL: www.stagnes.org
Type: Acute Care Hospitals
Emergency Services: Yes
Ownership: Voluntary non-profit - Church
Beds: 323

Key Personnel:
Pediatric In-Patient Care . . . . Michael Burke, MD
Patient Relations . . . . Yolanda Copeland
Operating Room. . . . . Dorothy James
Chief of Medical Staff. . . . . Adrian Long, MD
Quality Assurance . . . . Mike Moriarty, MD
CEO/President. . . . . Bonnie Phipps
Emergency Room . . . . Kevin Scruggs
Radiology. . . . . Robert Stroud, MD

Measure	Cases	This Hosp.	State Avg.	U.S. Avg.
Blood Clot Prevention and Treatment				
Anticoagulation Overlap Therapy[2]	147	98%	94%	93%
ICU Venous Thromboembolism Prophylaxis[2]	39	100%	94%	92%
Incidence of Potentially Preventable VTE[1,2]	-	-	7%	10%
UFH with Dosages/Platelet Monitoring[2]	118	99%	97%	97%
Venous Thromboembolism Prophylaxis[2]	391	98%	90%	85%
Warfarin Therapy Discharge Instructions[2]	102	61%	78%	75%
Chest Pain/Possible Heart Attack Care				
Aspirin Given Within 24 Hours of Arrival[5]	-	-	100%	96%
Fibrinolytic Meds Within 30 Min. of Arrival[5]	-	-	-	58%
Average Time to ECG (minutes)[5]	-	-	6	7
Average Time to Transfer (minutes)[5]	-	-	32	60
Children's Asthma Care				
Received Home Management Plan of Care	-	-	-	88%
Received Reliever Medication	-	-	-	100%
Received Systemic Corticosteroids	-	-	-	100%
Emergency Department				
Admittance Decision Time (minutes)[2]	814	144	143	98
Head CT Results Within 45 Min. of Arrival[5]	-	-	-	57%
Patients Who Left ER Before Being Seen[5]	-	-	3%	2%
Time from ER Arrival to Admit. (minutes)[2]	816	414	357	274
Time from ER Arrival to Discharge (minutes)[5]	-	-	-	134
Time in ER Before Being Evaluated (minutes)[5]	-	-	-	26
Time to Pain Meds for Fractures (minutes)[5]	-	-	-	57
Heart Attack Care				
Aspirin Given at Discharge	215	100%	99%	99%
Fibrinolytic Meds Within 30 Min. of Arrival[7]	-	-	-	54%
PCI Within 90 Minutes of Arrival	74	96%	93%	96%
Statin Prescribed at Discharge	209	99%	98%	98%
Heart Failure Care				
ACE Inhibitor or ARB for LVSD	191	100%	97%	97%
Discharge Instructions Given	491	94%	93%	94%
Evaluation of LVS Function	592	100%	99%	99%
Medicare Spending				
Medicare Spending per Patient (ratio)	-	-	-	0.98
Pneumonia Care				
Appropriate Initial Antibiotic Given[2]	59	100%	97%	95%
Blood Culture Timing[2]	214	94%	97%	98%
Pregnancy and Delivery Care				
Newborn Deliveries Scheduled Early[5]	-	-	-	6%
Preventive Care				
Immunization for Influenza[2]	551	95%	94%	90%
Immunization for Pneumonia[2]	720	92%	94%	92%
Stroke Care				
Anticoagulation Therapy for Atrial Fibrillation[5]	-	-	95%	95%
Antithrombotic Therapy Timing[5]	-	-	95%	98%
Assessed for Rehabilitation[5]	-	-	96%	97%
Discharged on Antithrombotic Therapy[5]	-	-	95%	99%
Discharged on Statin Medication[5]	-	-	97%	94%
Thrombolytic Therapy Timing[5]	-	-	-	66%
Venous Thromboembolism Prophylaxis[5]	-	-	89%	94%
Written Stroke Educational Materials Given[5]	-	-	77%	88%
Surgical Care Improvement Project				
Appropriate Beta Blocker Usage[2]	117	100%	97%	98%
Appropriate VTP Within 24 Hours[2]	376	100%	98%	98%
Controlled Postoperative Blood Glucose[2,7]	-	-	96%	97%
Perioperative Temperature Management[2]	463	100%	100%	100%
Prophylactic Antibiotic Selection[2]	284	99%	99%	99%
Prophylactic Antibiotic Selection (Outpatient)[5]	-	-	98%	98%
Prophylactic Antibiotic Stopped[2]	273	99%	98%	98%
Prophylactic Antibiotic Timing[2]	285	100%	97%	99%
Prophylactic Antibiotic Timing (Outpatient)[5]	-	-	98%	98%
Urinary Catheter Removal[2]	353	97%	98%	97%
Survey of Patients' Hospital Experiences				
Area Around Room 'Always' Quiet at Night	300+	59%	57%	61%
Doctors 'Always' Communicated Well	300+	78%	78%	82%
Home Recovery Information Given	300+	82%	85%	85%
Hospital Given 9 or 10 on 10 Point Scale	300+	62%	65%	71%
Meds 'Always' Explained Before Given	300+	55%	58%	64%
Nurses 'Always' Communicated Well	300+	72%	75%	79%
Pain 'Always' Well Controlled	300+	65%	67%	71%
Room and Bathroom 'Always' Clean	300+	58%	64%	73%
Timely Help 'Always' Received	300+	53%	58%	68%
Would Definitely Recommend Hospital	300+	65%	67%	71%
Use of Medical Imaging				
Cardiac Imaging Stress Test before Surgery	588	6.6%	6.4%	5.3%
Combination Abdominal CT Scan	908	2.3%	3.8%	10.5%
Combination Brain/Sinus CT Scan	1,306	5.3%	4.3%	2.7%
Combination Chest CT Scan	727	1.2%	1%	2.7%
Follow-up Mammogram/Ultrasound	243	6.6%	10.2%	8.8%
Lumbar Spine MRI for Low Back Pain[1]	-	-	38.2%	37.2%

Sinai Hospital of Baltimore

2401 West Belvedere Avenue
Baltimore, MD 21215
Phone: 410-601-5131
Fax: 410-601-9055
URL: www.sinai-balt.com
Type: Acute Care Hospitals
Emergency Services: Yes
Ownership: Voluntary non-profit - Other
Beds: 467

Key Personnel:
Coronary Care . . . . Valerie Allen
Infection Control. . . . . Katleen Arias
Chief of Medical Staff. . . . . Lorrie Liang, MD
Radiology. . . . . Noah I Lightman, MD
Quality Assurance . . . . Sheila McClahahan
CEO/President. . . . . Amy Perry
Pediatric Ambulatory Care . . . . . . Joseph M Wiley, MD
Pediatric In-Patient Care . . . . Joseph M Wiley, MD

Measure	Cases	This Hosp.	State Avg.	U.S. Avg.
Blood Clot Prevention and Treatment				
Anticoagulation Overlap Therapy[2]	132	98%	94%	93%
ICU Venous Thromboembolism Prophylaxis[2]	57	98%	94%	92%
Incidence of Potentially Preventable VTE[2]	38	0%	7%	10%
UFH with Dosages/Platelet Monitoring[2]	86	100%	97%	97%
Venous Thromboembolism Prophylaxis[2]	536	98%	90%	85%
Warfarin Therapy Discharge Instructions[2]	88	95%	78%	75%
Chest Pain/Possible Heart Attack Care				
Aspirin Given Within 24 Hours of Arrival[5]	-	-	100%	96%
Fibrinolytic Meds Within 30 Min. of Arrival[5]	-	-	-	58%
Average Time to ECG (minutes)[5]	-	-	6	7
Average Time to Transfer (minutes)[5]	-	-	32	60
Children's Asthma Care				
Received Home Management Plan of Care	-	-	-	88%
Received Reliever Medication	-	-	-	100%

NOTE: Hospital profiles are in alphabetical order by state, then city, then hospital within the city; Rankings exclude hospitals with less than 25 cases except for patient surveys which excludes hospitals with less than 100 cases; (a) 100-299 cases; (1) The number of cases/patients is too few to report; (2) Data submitted were based on a sample of cases/patients; (3) Results are based on a shorter time period than required; (4) Data suppressed by CMS for one or more quarters; (5) Results are not available for this reporting period; (6) Fewer than 100 patients completed the HCAHPS survey; (7) No cases met the criteria for this measure; (8) The lower limit of the confidence interval cannot be calculated if the number of observed infections equals zero; (9) No data are available from the state/territory for this reporting period; (10) The scores shown reflect fewer than 50 completed surveys; (11) There were discrepancies in the data collection process; (12) This measure does not apply to this hospital for this reporting period; (13) Results cannot be calculated for this reporting period; (14) The results for this state are combined with nearby states to protect confidentiality; Please refer to the User's Guide for a full explanation of data.

Measure	Cases	This Hosp.	State Avg.	U.S. Avg.
Received Systemic Corticosteroids	-	-	-	100%
Emergency Department				
Admittance Decision Time (minutes)[2]	719	115	143	98
Head CT Results Within 45 Min. of Arrival[5]	-	-	-	57%
Patients Who Left ER Before Being Seen[5]	-	-	3%	2%
Time from ER Arrival to Admit. (minutes)[2]	719	370	357	274
Time from ER Arrival to Discharge (minutes)[5]	-	-	-	134
Time in ER Before Being Evaluated (minutes)[5]	-	-	-	26
Time to Pain Meds for Fractures (minutes)[5]	-	-	-	57
Heart Attack Care				
Aspirin Given at Discharge	389	99%	99%	99%
Fibrinolytic Meds Within 30 Min. of Arrival[7]	-	-	-	54%
PCI Within 90 Minutes of Arrival	56	95%	93%	96%
Statin Prescribed at Discharge	370	98%	98%	98%
Heart Failure Care				
ACE Inhibitor or ARB for LVSD	248	100%	97%	97%
Discharge Instructions Given	575	95%	93%	94%
Evaluation of LVS Function	691	99%	99%	99%
Medicare Spending				
Medicare Spending per Patient (ratio)	-	-	-	0.98
Pneumonia Care				
Appropriate Initial Antibiotic Given	132	99%	97%	95%
Blood Culture Timing	320	98%	97%	98%
Pregnancy and Delivery Care				
Newborn Deliveries Scheduled Early[5]	-	-	-	6%
Preventive Care				
Immunization for Influenza[2]	691	94%	94%	90%
Immunization for Pneumonia[2]	844	95%	94%	92%
Stroke Care				
Anticoagulation Therapy for Atrial Fibrillation[5]	-	-	95%	95%
Antithrombotic Therapy Timing[5]	-	-	95%	98%
Assessed for Rehabilitation[5]	-	-	96%	97%
Discharged on Antithrombotic Therapy[5]	-	-	95%	99%
Discharged on Statin Medication[5]	-	-	97%	94%
Thrombolytic Therapy Timing[5]	-	-	-	66%
Venous Thromboembolism Prophylaxis[5]	-	-	89%	94%
Written Stroke Educational Materials Given[5]	-	-	77%	88%
Surgical Care Improvement Project				
Appropriate Beta Blocker Usage[2]	378	98%	97%	98%
Appropriate VTP Within 24 Hours[2]	648	98%	98%	98%
Controlled Postoperative Blood Glucose[2]	267	99%	96%	97%
Perioperative Temperature Management[2]	755	100%	100%	100%
Prophylactic Antibiotic Selection[2]	708	98%	99%	99%
Prophylactic Antibiotic Selection (Outpatient)[5]	-	-	98%	98%
Prophylactic Antibiotic Stopped[2]	667	99%	98%	98%
Prophylactic Antibiotic Timing[2]	709	99%	97%	99%
Prophylactic Antibiotic Timing (Outpatient)[5]	-	-	98%	98%
Urinary Catheter Removal[2]	603	100%	98%	97%
Survey of Patients' Hospital Experiences				
Area Around Room 'Always' Quiet at Night	300+	58%	57%	61%
Doctors 'Always' Communicated Well	300+	76%	78%	82%
Home Recovery Information Given	300+	82%	85%	85%
Hospital Given 9 or 10 on 10 Point Scale	300+	67%	65%	71%
Meds 'Always' Explained Before Given	300+	58%	58%	64%
Nurses 'Always' Communicated Well	300+	75%	75%	79%
Pain 'Always' Well Controlled	300+	68%	67%	71%
Room and Bathroom 'Always' Clean	300+	66%	64%	73%
Timely Help 'Always' Received	300+	59%	58%	68%
Would Definitely Recommend Hospital	300+	70%	67%	71%
Use of Medical Imaging				
Cardiac Imaging Stress Test before Surgery	363	6.6%	6.4%	5.3%
Combination Abdominal CT Scan	916	3.9%	3.8%	10.5%
Combination Brain/Sinus CT Scan	1,190	3.9%	4.3%	2.7%
Combination Chest CT Scan	648	2.2%	1%	2.7%
Follow-up Mammogram/Ultrasound	514	7.2%	10.2%	8.8%
Lumbar Spine MRI for Low Back Pain	62	38.7%	38.2%	37.2%

University of Maryland Medical Center

22 South Greene Street
Baltimore, MD 21201
URL: www.umm.edu
Type: Acute Care Hospitals
Ownership: Voluntary non-profit - Private
Phone: 410-328-8667
Fax: 410-328-8664
Emergency Services: Yes
Beds: 650

Key Personnel:

Emergency Room . . . . Robert Barish, MD
Pediatric Ambulatory Care . . . . . . Michael Berman, MD
Pediatric In-Patient Care . . . . Michael Berman, MD
Quality Assurance . . . . Josephine Goode-Johnson
Chief of Medical Staff . . . . Jonathan E. Gottlieb, MD
Infection Control. . . . . Joan Hebden
CEO/President. . . . . Jeffrey A. Rivest, MD
Radiology. . . . . Philip A Templeton, MD

Measure	Cases	This Hosp.	State Avg.	U.S. Avg.
Blood Clot Prevention and Treatment				
Anticoagulation Overlap Therapy[2]	194	99%	94%	93%
ICU Venous Thromboembolism Prophylaxis[2]	101	96%	94%	92%
Incidence of Potentially Preventable VTE[2]	113	1%	7%	10%
UFH with Dosages/Platelet Monitoring[2]	202	95%	97%	97%
Venous Thromboembolism Prophylaxis[2]	278	89%	90%	85%
Warfarin Therapy Discharge Instructions[2]	113	92%	78%	75%
Chest Pain/Possible Heart Attack Care				
Aspirin Given Within 24 Hours of Arrival[5]	-	-	100%	96%
Fibrinolytic Meds Within 30 Min. of Arrival[5]	-	-	-	58%
Average Time to ECG (minutes)[5]	-	-	6	7
Average Time to Transfer (minutes)[5]	-	-	32	60
Children's Asthma Care				
Received Home Management Plan of Care	-	-	-	88%
Received Reliever Medication	-	-	-	100%
Received Systemic Corticosteroids	-	-	-	100%
Emergency Department				
Admittance Decision Time (minutes)[2]	283	336	143	98
Head CT Results Within 45 Min. of Arrival[5]	-	-	-	57%
Patients Who Left ER Before Being Seen[5]	-	-	3%	2%
Time from ER Arrival to Admit. (minutes)[2]	327	639	357	274
Time from ER Arrival to Discharge (minutes)[5]	-	-	-	134
Time in ER Before Being Evaluated (minutes)[5]	-	-	-	26
Time to Pain Meds for Fractures (minutes)[5]	-	-	-	57
Heart Attack Care				
Aspirin Given at Discharge	489	100%	99%	99%
Fibrinolytic Meds Within 30 Min. of Arrival[7]	-	-	-	54%
PCI Within 90 Minutes of Arrival	16	81%	93%	96%
Statin Prescribed at Discharge	481	100%	98%	98%
Heart Failure Care				
ACE Inhibitor or ARB for LVSD	198	99%	97%	97%
Discharge Instructions Given	332	94%	93%	94%
Evaluation of LVS Function	391	100%	99%	99%
Medicare Spending				
Medicare Spending per Patient (ratio)	-	-	-	0.98
Pneumonia Care				
Appropriate Initial Antibiotic Given	46	100%	97%	95%
Blood Culture Timing	99	100%	97%	98%
Pregnancy and Delivery Care				
Newborn Deliveries Scheduled Early[5]	-	-	-	6%
Preventive Care				
Immunization for Influenza[2]	807	91%	94%	90%
Immunization for Pneumonia[2]	722	92%	94%	92%
Stroke Care				
Anticoagulation Therapy for Atrial Fibrillation[5]	-	-	95%	95%
Antithrombotic Therapy Timing[5]	-	-	95%	98%
Assessed for Rehabilitation[5]	-	-	96%	97%
Discharged on Antithrombotic Therapy[5]	-	-	95%	99%
Discharged on Statin Medication[5]	-	-	97%	94%
Thrombolytic Therapy Timing[5]	-	-	-	66%
Venous Thromboembolism Prophylaxis[5]	-	-	89%	94%
Written Stroke Educational Materials Given[5]	-	-	77%	88%
Surgical Care Improvement Project				
Appropriate Beta Blocker Usage[2]	612	97%	97%	98%
Appropriate VTP Within 24 Hours[2]	806	94%	98%	98%
Controlled Postoperative Blood Glucose[2]	562	95%	96%	97%
Perioperative Temperature Management[2]	1,076	100%	100%	100%
Prophylactic Antibiotic Selection[2]	1,036	98%	99%	99%
Prophylactic Antibiotic Selection (Outpatient)[5]	-	-	98%	98%
Prophylactic Antibiotic Stopped[2]	972	97%	98%	98%
Prophylactic Antibiotic Timing[2]	1,040	99%	97%	99%
Prophylactic Antibiotic Timing (Outpatient)[5]	-	-	98%	98%
Urinary Catheter Removal[2]	966	99%	98%	97%
Survey of Patients' Hospital Experiences				
Area Around Room 'Always' Quiet at Night	300+	53%	57%	61%
Doctors 'Always' Communicated Well	300+	81%	78%	82%
Home Recovery Information Given	300+	88%	85%	85%
Hospital Given 9 or 10 on 10 Point Scale	300+	69%	65%	71%
Meds 'Always' Explained Before Given	300+	64%	58%	64%
Nurses 'Always' Communicated Well	300+	76%	75%	79%
Pain 'Always' Well Controlled	300+	69%	67%	71%
Room and Bathroom 'Always' Clean	300+	61%	64%	73%
Timely Help 'Always' Received	300+	59%	58%	68%
Would Definitely Recommend Hospital	300+	74%	67%	71%
Use of Medical Imaging				
Cardiac Imaging Stress Test before Surgery	400	8.8%	6.4%	5.3%
Combination Abdominal CT Scan	1,107	2.1%	3.8%	10.5%
Combination Brain/Sinus CT Scan	554	4.3%	4.3%	2.7%
Combination Chest CT Scan	1,267	0.2%	1%	2.7%
Follow-up Mammogram/Ultrasound	1,054	9.1%	10.2%	8.8%
Lumbar Spine MRI for Low Back Pain[1]	-	-	38.2%	37.2%

University of Maryland Medical Center Midtown Campus

827 Linden Avenue
Baltimore, MD 21201
URL: www.marylandgeneral.org
Type: Acute Care Hospitals
Ownership: Voluntary non-profit - Other
Phone: 410-225-8996
Fax: 410-669-8368
Emergency Services: Yes
Beds: 238

Key Personnel:

Chief of Medical Staff. . . . . William Anthony, MD
Pediatric In-Patient Care . . . . Mario Gonzalez
CEO/President. . . . . Sylvia Smith Johnson
Ambulatory Care . . . . Brian Krebs
Emergency Room . . . . Rhamin Ligon, MD
Operating Room. . . . . Jeanne Queen, RN

Measure	Cases	This Hosp.	State Avg.	U.S. Avg.
Blood Clot Prevention and Treatment				
Anticoagulation Overlap Therapy[2,3]	24	100%	94%	93%
ICU Venous Thromboembolism Prophylaxis[2,3]	51	98%	94%	92%
Incidence of Potentially Preventable VTE[1,2]	-	-	7%	10%
UFH with Dosages/Platelet Monitoring[2,3]	12	100%	97%	97%
Venous Thromboembolism Prophylaxis[2,3]	146	87%	90%	85%
Warfarin Therapy Discharge Instructions[2,3]	14	86%	78%	75%
Chest Pain/Possible Heart Attack Care				
Aspirin Given Within 24 Hours of Arrival[5]	-	-	100%	96%
Fibrinolytic Meds Within 30 Min. of Arrival[5]	-	-	-	58%
Average Time to ECG (minutes)[5]	-	-	6	7
Average Time to Transfer (minutes)[5]	-	-	32	60
Children's Asthma Care				
Received Home Management Plan of Care	-	-	-	88%
Received Reliever Medication	-	-	-	100%
Received Systemic Corticosteroids	-	-	-	100%
Emergency Department				
Admittance Decision Time (minutes)[2]	240	127	143	98
Head CT Results Within 45 Min. of Arrival[5]	-	-	-	57%
Patients Who Left ER Before Being Seen[5]	-	-	3%	2%
Time from ER Arrival to Admit. (minutes)[2]	367	377	357	274
Time from ER Arrival to Discharge (minutes)[5]	-	-	-	134
Time in ER Before Being Evaluated (minutes)[5]	-	-	-	26
Time to Pain Meds for Fractures (minutes)[5]	-	-	-	57
Heart Attack Care				
Aspirin Given at Discharge[1]	-	-	99%	99%
Fibrinolytic Meds Within 30 Min. of Arrival[7]	-	-	-	54%
PCI Within 90 Minutes of Arrival[7]	-	-	93%	96%
Statin Prescribed at Discharge[1]	-	-	98%	98%
Heart Failure Care				
ACE Inhibitor or ARB for LVSD	48	100%	97%	97%
Discharge Instructions Given	108	100%	93%	94%
Evaluation of LVS Function	138	100%	99%	99%
Medicare Spending				
Medicare Spending per Patient (ratio)	-	-	-	0.98

NOTE: Hospital profiles are in alphabetical order by state, then city, then hospital within the city; Rankings exclude hospitals with less than 25 cases except for patient surveys which excludes hospitals with less than 100 cases; (a) 100-299 cases; (1) The number of cases/patients is too few to report; (2) Data submitted were based on a sample of cases/patients; (3) Results are based on a shorter time period than required; (4) Data suppressed by CMS for one or more quarters; (5) Results are not available for this reporting period; (6) Fewer than 100 patients completed the HCAHPS survey; (7) No cases met the criteria for this measure; (8) The lower limit of the confidence interval cannot be calculated if the number of observed infections equals zero; (9) No data are available from the state/territory for this reporting period; (10) The scores shown reflect fewer than 50 completed surveys; (11) There were discrepancies in the data collection process; (12) This measure does not apply to this hospital for this reporting period; (13) Results cannot be calculated for this reporting period; (14) The results for this state are combined with nearby states to protect confidentiality; Please refer to the User's Guide for a full explanation of data.

Measure	Cases	This Hosp.	State Avg.	U.S. Avg.
Pneumonia Care				
Appropriate Initial Antibiotic Given	42	100%	97%	95%
Blood Culture Timing	145	99%	97%	98%
Pregnancy and Delivery Care				
Newborn Deliveries Scheduled Early[5]	-	-	-	6%
Preventive Care				
Immunization for Influenza[2]	579	98%	94%	90%
Immunization for Pneumonia[2]	695	99%	94%	92%
Stroke Care				
Anticoagulation Therapy for Atrial Fibrillation[5]	-	-	95%	95%
Antithrombotic Therapy Timing[5]	-	-	95%	98%
Assessed for Rehabilitation[5]	-	-	96%	97%
Discharged on Antithrombotic Therapy[5]	-	-	95%	99%
Discharged on Statin Medication[5]	-	-	97%	94%
Thrombolytic Therapy Timing[5]	-	-	-	66%
Venous Thromboembolism Prophylaxis[5]	-	-	89%	94%
Written Stroke Educational Materials Given[5]	-	-	77%	88%
Surgical Care Improvement Project				
Appropriate Beta Blocker Usage	30	100%	97%	98%
Appropriate VTP Within 24 Hours	107	97%	98%	98%
Controlled Postoperative Blood Glucose[7]	-	-	96%	97%
Perioperative Temperature Management	122	100%	100%	100%
Prophylactic Antibiotic Selection	52	100%	99%	99%
Prophylactic Antibiotic Selection (Outpatient)[5]	-	-	98%	98%
Prophylactic Antibiotic Stopped	51	100%	98%	98%
Prophylactic Antibiotic Timing	52	98%	97%	99%
Prophylactic Antibiotic Timing (Outpatient)[5]	-	-	98%	98%
Urinary Catheter Removal	65	100%	98%	97%
Survey of Patients' Hospital Experiences				
Area Around Room 'Always' Quiet at Night	300+	62%	57%	61%
Doctors 'Always' Communicated Well	300+	76%	78%	82%
Home Recovery Information Given	300+	83%	85%	85%
Hospital Given 9 or 10 on 10 Point Scale	300+	52%	65%	71%
Meds 'Always' Explained Before Given	300+	52%	58%	64%
Nurses 'Always' Communicated Well	300+	70%	75%	79%
Pain 'Always' Well Controlled	300+	60%	67%	71%
Room and Bathroom 'Always' Clean	300+	58%	64%	73%
Timely Help 'Always' Received	300+	54%	58%	68%
Would Definitely Recommend Hospital	300+	54%	67%	71%
Use of Medical Imaging				
Cardiac Imaging Stress Test before Surgery	141	8.5%	6.4%	5.3%
Combination Abdominal CT Scan	212	3.8%	3.8%	10.5%
Combination Brain/Sinus CT Scan	244	7.8%	4.3%	2.7%
Combination Chest CT Scan	113	0.0%	1%	2.7%
Follow-up Mammogram/Ultrasound	212	5.2%	10.2%	8.8%
Lumbar Spine MRI for Low Back Pain[1]	-	-	38.2%	37.2%

University of Maryland Rehabilitation & Orthopaedic Institute

2200 Kernan Drive
Baltimore, MD 21207
Phone: 410-448-6701
Type: Acute Care Hospitals
Emergency Services: No
Ownership: Voluntary non-profit - Other

Measure	Cases	This Hosp.	State Avg.	U.S. Avg.
Blood Clot Prevention and Treatment				
Anticoagulation Overlap Therapy	-	-	94%	93%
ICU Venous Thromboembolism Prophylaxis	-	-	94%	92%
Incidence of Potentially Preventable VTE	-	-	7%	10%
UFH with Dosages/Platelet Monitoring	-	-	97%	97%
Venous Thromboembolism Prophylaxis	-	-	90%	85%
Warfarin Therapy Discharge Instructions	-	-	78%	75%
Chest Pain/Possible Heart Attack Care				
Aspirin Given Within 24 Hours of Arrival[5]	-	-	100%	96%
Fibrinolytic Meds Within 30 Min. of Arrival[5]	-	-	-	58%
Average Time to ECG (minutes)[5]	-	-	6	7
Average Time to Transfer (minutes)[5]	-	-	32	60
Children's Asthma Care				
Received Home Management Plan of Care	-	-	-	88%
Received Reliever Medication	-	-	-	100%
Received Systemic Corticosteroids	-	-	-	100%
Emergency Department				
Admittance Decision Time (minutes)	-	-	143	98
Head CT Results Within 45 Min. of Arrival[5]	-	-	-	57%
Patients Who Left ER Before Being Seen[5]	-	-	3%	2%
Time from ER Arrival to Admit. (minutes)	-	-	357	274
Time from ER Arrival to Discharge (minutes)[5]	-	-	-	134
Time in ER Before Being Evaluated (minutes)[5]	-	-	-	26
Time to Pain Meds for Fractures (minutes)[5]	-	-	-	57
Heart Attack Care				
Aspirin Given at Discharge	-	-	99%	99%
Fibrinolytic Meds Within 30 Min. of Arrival	-	-	-	54%
PCI Within 90 Minutes of Arrival	-	-	93%	96%
Statin Prescribed at Discharge	-	-	98%	98%
Heart Failure Care				
ACE Inhibitor or ARB for LVSD	-	-	97%	97%
Discharge Instructions Given	-	-	93%	94%
Evaluation of LVS Function	-	-	99%	99%
Medicare Spending				
Medicare Spending per Patient (ratio)	-	-	-	0.98
Pneumonia Care				
Appropriate Initial Antibiotic Given	-	-	97%	95%
Blood Culture Timing	-	-	97%	98%
Pregnancy and Delivery Care				
Newborn Deliveries Scheduled Early	-	-	-	6%
Preventive Care				
Immunization for Influenza	-	-	94%	90%
Immunization for Pneumonia	-	-	94%	92%
Stroke Care				
Anticoagulation Therapy for Atrial Fibrillation	-	-	95%	95%
Antithrombotic Therapy Timing	-	-	95%	98%
Assessed for Rehabilitation	-	-	96%	97%
Discharged on Antithrombotic Therapy	-	-	95%	99%
Discharged on Statin Medication	-	-	97%	94%
Thrombolytic Therapy Timing	-	-	-	66%
Venous Thromboembolism Prophylaxis	-	-	89%	94%
Written Stroke Educational Materials Given	-	-	77%	88%
Surgical Care Improvement Project				
Appropriate Beta Blocker Usage	-	-	97%	98%
Appropriate VTP Within 24 Hours	-	-	98%	98%
Controlled Postoperative Blood Glucose	-	-	96%	97%
Perioperative Temperature Management	-	-	100%	100%
Prophylactic Antibiotic Selection	-	-	99%	99%
Prophylactic Antibiotic Selection (Outpatient)[5]	-	-	98%	98%
Prophylactic Antibiotic Stopped	-	-	98%	98%
Prophylactic Antibiotic Timing	-	-	97%	99%
Prophylactic Antibiotic Timing (Outpatient)[5]	-	-	98%	98%
Urinary Catheter Removal	-	-	98%	97%
Survey of Patients' Hospital Experiences				
Area Around Room 'Always' Quiet at Night	-	-	57%	61%
Doctors 'Always' Communicated Well	-	-	78%	82%
Home Recovery Information Given	-	-	85%	85%
Hospital Given 9 or 10 on 10 Point Scale	-	-	65%	71%
Meds 'Always' Explained Before Given	-	-	58%	64%
Nurses 'Always' Communicated Well	-	-	75%	79%
Pain 'Always' Well Controlled	-	-	67%	71%
Room and Bathroom 'Always' Clean	-	-	64%	73%
Timely Help 'Always' Received	-	-	58%	68%
Would Definitely Recommend Hospital	-	-	67%	71%
Use of Medical Imaging				
Cardiac Imaging Stress Test before Surgery[7]	-	-	6.4%	5.3%
Combination Abdominal CT Scan[1]	-	-	3.8%	10.5%
Combination Brain/Sinus CT Scan[7]	-	-	4.3%	2.7%
Combination Chest CT Scan[7]	-	-	1%	2.7%
Follow-up Mammogram/Ultrasound[7]	-	-	10.2%	8.8%
Lumbar Spine MRI for Low Back Pain[7]	-	-	38.2%	37.2%

VA Maryland Healthcare System - Baltimore

10 North Greene Street
Baltimore, MD 21201
Phone: 410-605-7016
URL: www.maryland.va.gov
Type: Acute Care - VA
Emergency Services: No
Ownership: Government Federal
Beds: 137

Measure	Cases	This Hosp.	State Avg.	U.S. Avg.
Blood Clot Prevention and Treatment				
Anticoagulation Overlap Therapy	-	-	94%	93%
ICU Venous Thromboembolism Prophylaxis	-	-	94%	92%
Incidence of Potentially Preventable VTE	-	-	7%	10%
UFH with Dosages/Platelet Monitoring	-	-	97%	97%
Venous Thromboembolism Prophylaxis	-	-	90%	85%
Warfarin Therapy Discharge Instructions	-	-	78%	75%
Chest Pain/Possible Heart Attack Care				
Aspirin Given Within 24 Hours of Arrival	-	-	100%	96%
Fibrinolytic Meds Within 30 Min. of Arrival	-	-	-	58%
Average Time to ECG (minutes)	-	-	6	7
Average Time to Transfer (minutes)	-	-	32	60
Children's Asthma Care				
Received Home Management Plan of Care	-	-	-	88%
Received Reliever Medication	-	-	-	100%
Received Systemic Corticosteroids	-	-	-	100%
Emergency Department				
Admittance Decision Time (minutes)	-	-	143	98
Head CT Results Within 45 Min. of Arrival	-	-	-	57%
Patients Who Left ER Before Being Seen	-	-	3%	2%
Time from ER Arrival to Admit. (minutes)	-	-	357	274
Time from ER Arrival to Discharge (minutes)	-	-	-	134
Time in ER Before Being Evaluated (minutes)	-	-	-	26
Time to Pain Meds for Fractures (minutes)	-	-	-	57
Heart Attack Care				
Aspirin Given at Discharge	45	100%	99%	99%
Fibrinolytic Meds Within 30 Min. of Arrival[5]	-	-	-	54%
PCI Within 90 Minutes of Arrival[1]	-	-	93%	96%
Statin Prescribed at Discharge	48	98%	98%	98%
Heart Failure Care				
ACE Inhibitor or ARB for LVSD	117	97%	97%	97%
Discharge Instructions Given	222	94%	93%	94%
Evaluation of LVS Function	235	100%	99%	99%
Medicare Spending				
Medicare Spending per Patient (ratio)	-	-	-	0.98
Pneumonia Care				
Appropriate Initial Antibiotic Given	55	96%	97%	95%
Blood Culture Timing	120	97%	97%	98%
Pregnancy and Delivery Care				
Newborn Deliveries Scheduled Early	-	-	-	6%
Preventive Care				
Immunization for Influenza[5]	-	-	94%	90%
Immunization for Pneumonia[5]	-	-	94%	92%
Stroke Care				
Anticoagulation Therapy for Atrial Fibrillation	-	-	95%	95%
Antithrombotic Therapy Timing	-	-	95%	98%
Assessed for Rehabilitation	-	-	96%	97%
Discharged on Antithrombotic Therapy	-	-	95%	99%
Discharged on Statin Medication	-	-	97%	94%
Thrombolytic Therapy Timing	-	-	-	66%
Venous Thromboembolism Prophylaxis	-	-	89%	94%
Written Stroke Educational Materials Given	-	-	77%	88%
Surgical Care Improvement Project				
Appropriate Beta Blocker Usage[2]	59	97%	97%	98%
Appropriate VTP Within 24 Hours[2]	151	88%	98%	98%
Controlled Postoperative Blood Glucose[5]	-	-	96%	97%
Perioperative Temperature Management[2]	181	98%	100%	100%
Prophylactic Antibiotic Selection	67	100%	99%	99%
Prophylactic Antibiotic Selection (Outpatient)	-	-	98%	98%
Prophylactic Antibiotic Stopped	66	94%	98%	98%
Prophylactic Antibiotic Timing	68	96%	97%	99%
Prophylactic Antibiotic Timing (Outpatient)	-	-	98%	98%
Urinary Catheter Removal[2]	101	95%	98%	97%
Survey of Patients' Hospital Experiences				
Area Around Room 'Always' Quiet at Night	-	-	57%	61%
Doctors 'Always' Communicated Well	-	-	78%	82%
Home Recovery Information Given	-	-	85%	85%
Hospital Given 9 or 10 on 10 Point Scale	-	-	65%	71%
Meds 'Always' Explained Before Given	-	-	58%	64%
Nurses 'Always' Communicated Well	-	-	75%	79%
Pain 'Always' Well Controlled	-	-	67%	71%
Room and Bathroom 'Always' Clean	-	-	64%	73%
Timely Help 'Always' Received	-	-	58%	68%

NOTE: Hospital profiles are in alphabetical order by state, then city, then hospital within the city; Rankings exclude hospitals with less than 25 cases except for patient surveys which excludes hospitals with less than 100 cases; (a) 100-299 cases; (1) The number of cases/patients is too few to report; (2) Data submitted were based on a sample of cases/patients; (3) Results are based on a shorter time period than required; (4) Data suppressed by CMS for one or more quarters; (5) Results are not available for this reporting period; (6) Fewer than 100 patients completed the HCAHPS survey; (7) No cases met the criteria for this measure; (8) The lower limit of the confidence interval cannot be calculated if the number of observed infections equals zero; (9) No data are available from the state/territory for this reporting period; (10) The scores shown reflect fewer than 50 completed surveys; (11) There were discrepancies in the data collection process; (12) This measure does not apply to this hospital for this reporting period; (13) Results cannot be calculated for this reporting period; (14) The results for this state are combined with nearby states to protect confidentiality; Please refer to the User's Guide for a full explanation of data.

Measure	Cases	This Hosp.	State Avg.	U.S. Avg.
Would Definitely Recommend Hospital	-	-	67%	71%
Use of Medical Imaging				
Cardiac Imaging Stress Test before Surgery	-	-	6.4%	5.3%
Combination Abdominal CT Scan	-	-	3.8%	10.5%
Combination Brain/Sinus CT Scan	-	-	4.3%	2.7%
Combination Chest CT Scan	-	-	1%	2.7%
Follow-up Mammogram/Ultrasound	-	-	10.2%	8.8%
Lumbar Spine MRI for Low Back Pain	-	-	38.2%	37.2%

Upper Chesapeake Medical Center

500 Upper Chesapeake Drive — Phone: 443-643-3303
Bel Air, MD 21014 — Fax: 443-643-4210
URL: www.uchs.org
Type: Acute Care Hospitals — Emergency Services: Yes
Ownership: Voluntary non-profit - Other — Beds: 143

Key Personnel:
Pediatric In-Patient Care .... Marianne Fridberg, MD
Quality Assurance .... Jane Gordon
Operating Room.............. Robert Hoofnagle
Emergency Room .... Charlotte Meck
Radiology.................. Brian Monroe, MD
CEO/President.............. Lyle Ernest Sheldon, FACHE
Intensive Care Unit........... Antoinette Spevetz, MD
Chief of Medical Staff.......... Peggy Vaughan, MD

Measure	Cases	This Hosp.	State Avg.	U.S. Avg.
Blood Clot Prevention and Treatment				
Anticoagulation Overlap Therapy[2]	86	93%	94%	93%
ICU Venous Thromboembolism Prophylaxis[2]	37	92%	94%	92%
Incidence of Potentially Preventable VTE[1,2]	-	-	7%	10%
UFH with Dosages/Platelet Monitoring[2]	79	100%	97%	97%
Venous Thromboembolism Prophylaxis[2]	368	93%	90%	85%
Warfarin Therapy Discharge Instructions[2]	62	97%	78%	75%
Chest Pain/Possible Heart Attack Care				
Aspirin Given Within 24 Hours of Arrival[5]	-	-	100%	96%
Fibrinolytic Meds Within 30 Min. of Arrival[5]	-	-	-	58%
Average Time to ECG (minutes)[5]	-	-	6	7
Average Time to Transfer (minutes)[5]	-	-	32	60
Children's Asthma Care				
Received Home Management Plan of Care	-	-	-	88%
Received Reliever Medication	-	-	-	100%
Received Systemic Corticosteroids	-	-	-	100%
Emergency Department				
Admittance Decision Time (minutes)[2]	612	110	143	98
Head CT Results Within 45 Min. of Arrival[5]	-	-	-	57%
Patients Who Left ER Before Being Seen[5]	-	-	3%	2%
Time from ER Arrival to Admit. (minutes)[2]	714	372	357	274
Time from ER Arrival to Discharge (minutes)[5]	-	-	-	134
Time in ER Before Being Evaluated (minutes)[5]	-	-	-	26
Time to Pain Meds for Fractures (minutes)[5]	-	-	-	57
Heart Attack Care				
Aspirin Given at Discharge	150	100%	99%	99%
Fibrinolytic Meds Within 30 Min. of Arrival[7]	-	-	-	54%
PCI Within 90 Minutes of Arrival	83	100%	93%	96%
Statin Prescribed at Discharge	146	100%	98%	98%
Heart Failure Care				
ACE Inhibitor or ARB for LVSD	62	100%	97%	97%
Discharge Instructions Given	254	99%	93%	94%
Evaluation of LVS Function	330	100%	99%	99%
Medicare Spending				
Medicare Spending per Patient (ratio)	-	-	-	0.98
Pneumonia Care				
Appropriate Initial Antibiotic Given	248	96%	97%	95%
Blood Culture Timing	437	100%	97%	98%
Pregnancy and Delivery Care				
Newborn Deliveries Scheduled Early[5]	-	-	-	6%
Preventive Care				
Immunization for Influenza[2]	521	97%	94%	90%
Immunization for Pneumonia[2]	664	99%	94%	92%
Stroke Care				
Anticoagulation Therapy for Atrial Fibrillation[5]	-	-	95%	95%
Antithrombotic Therapy Timing[5]	-	-	95%	98%
Assessed for Rehabilitation[5]	-	-	96%	97%
Discharged on Antithrombotic Therapy[5]	-	-	95%	99%
Discharged on Statin Medication[5]	-	-	97%	94%
Thrombolytic Therapy Timing[5]	-	-	-	66%
Venous Thromboembolism Prophylaxis[5]	-	-	89%	94%
Written Stroke Educational Materials Given[5]	-	-	77%	88%
Surgical Care Improvement Project				
Appropriate Beta Blocker Usage[2]	223	100%	97%	98%
Appropriate VTP Within 24 Hours[2]	599	99%	98%	98%
Controlled Postoperative Blood Glucose[2,7]	-	-	96%	97%
Perioperative Temperature Management[2]	703	100%	100%	100%
Prophylactic Antibiotic Selection[2]	469	99%	99%	99%
Prophylactic Antibiotic Selection (Outpatient)[5]	-	-	98%	98%
Prophylactic Antibiotic Stopped[2]	464	100%	98%	98%
Prophylactic Antibiotic Timing[2]	469	99%	97%	99%
Prophylactic Antibiotic Timing (Outpatient)[5]	-	-	98%	98%
Urinary Catheter Removal[2]	390	99%	98%	97%
Survey of Patients' Hospital Experiences				
Area Around Room 'Always' Quiet at Night	300+	57%	57%	61%
Doctors 'Always' Communicated Well	300+	77%	78%	82%
Home Recovery Information Given	300+	83%	85%	85%
Hospital Given 9 or 10 on 10 Point Scale	300+	64%	65%	71%
Meds 'Always' Explained Before Given	300+	61%	58%	64%
Nurses 'Always' Communicated Well	300+	78%	75%	79%
Pain 'Always' Well Controlled	300+	67%	67%	71%
Room and Bathroom 'Always' Clean	300+	67%	64%	73%
Timely Help 'Always' Received	300+	59%	58%	68%
Would Definitely Recommend Hospital	300+	66%	67%	71%
Use of Medical Imaging				
Cardiac Imaging Stress Test before Surgery	968	3.8%	6.4%	5.3%
Combination Abdominal CT Scan	1,290	3.3%	3.8%	10.5%
Combination Brain/Sinus CT Scan	1,555	5.1%	4.3%	2.7%
Combination Chest CT Scan	828	0.4%	1%	2.7%
Follow-up Mammogram/Ultrasound	480	11.5%	10.2%	8.8%
Lumbar Spine MRI for Low Back Pain	87	40.2%	38.2%	37.2%

Atlantic General Hospital

9733 Healthway Drive — Phone: 410-641-9601
Berlin, MD 21811 — Fax: 410-641-9670
E-mail: agh@atlanticgeneral.org
URL: www.atlanticgeneral.org
Type: Acute Care Hospitals — Emergency Services: Yes
Ownership: Voluntary non-profit - Private — Beds: 62

Key Personnel:
Chair/CEO.................. John H. Burbage, Jr.
Chief of Medical Staff.......... Edwin Castaneda
Radiology.................. Simmi Chawla
CEO/President.............. Michael Franklin, FACHE
Infection Control............. Michaelann Frate, RN
Quality Assurance .... Charles Gizora
Coronary Care.............. Scott Rose
Operating Room.............. Shirley Spirk

Measure	Cases	This Hosp.	State Avg.	U.S. Avg.
Blood Clot Prevention and Treatment				
Anticoagulation Overlap Therapy[2]	30	97%	94%	93%
ICU Venous Thromboembolism Prophylaxis[2]	50	84%	94%	92%
Incidence of Potentially Preventable VTE[1,2]	-	-	7%	10%
UFH with Dosages/Platelet Monitoring[1,2]	-	-	97%	97%
Venous Thromboembolism Prophylaxis[2]	254	70%	90%	85%
Warfarin Therapy Discharge Instructions[2]	18	94%	78%	75%
Chest Pain/Possible Heart Attack Care				
Aspirin Given Within 24 Hours of Arrival[5]	-	-	100%	96%
Fibrinolytic Meds Within 30 Min. of Arrival[5]	-	-	-	58%
Average Time to ECG (minutes)[5]	-	-	6	7
Average Time to Transfer (minutes)[5]	-	-	32	60
Children's Asthma Care				
Received Home Management Plan of Care	-	-	-	88%
Received Reliever Medication	-	-	-	100%
Received Systemic Corticosteroids	-	-	-	100%
Emergency Department				
Admittance Decision Time (minutes)[2]	510	64	143	98
Head CT Results Within 45 Min. of Arrival[5]	-	-	-	57%
Patients Who Left ER Before Being Seen[5]	-	-	3%	2%
Time from ER Arrival to Admit. (minutes)[2]	510	207	357	274
Time from ER Arrival to Discharge (minutes)[5]	-	-	-	134
Time in ER Before Being Evaluated (minutes)[5]	-	-	-	26
Time to Pain Meds for Fractures (minutes)[5]	-	-	-	57
Heart Attack Care				
Aspirin Given at Discharge[1]	-	-	99%	99%
Fibrinolytic Meds Within 30 Min. of Arrival[3,7]	-	-	-	54%
PCI Within 90 Minutes of Arrival[3,7]	-	-	93%	96%
Statin Prescribed at Discharge[1]	-	-	98%	98%
Heart Failure Care				
ACE Inhibitor or ARB for LVSD	26	88%	97%	97%
Discharge Instructions Given	110	82%	93%	94%
Evaluation of LVS Function	148	96%	99%	99%
Medicare Spending				
Medicare Spending per Patient (ratio)	-	-	-	0.98
Pneumonia Care				
Appropriate Initial Antibiotic Given	128	98%	97%	95%
Blood Culture Timing	164	99%	97%	98%
Pregnancy and Delivery Care				
Newborn Deliveries Scheduled Early[5]	-	-	-	6%
Preventive Care				
Immunization for Influenza[2]	302	92%	94%	90%
Immunization for Pneumonia[2]	500	87%	94%	92%
Stroke Care				
Anticoagulation Therapy for Atrial Fibrillation[5]	-	-	95%	95%
Antithrombotic Therapy Timing[5]	-	-	95%	98%
Assessed for Rehabilitation[5]	-	-	96%	97%
Discharged on Antithrombotic Therapy[5]	-	-	95%	99%
Discharged on Statin Medication[5]	-	-	97%	94%
Thrombolytic Therapy Timing[5]	-	-	-	66%
Venous Thromboembolism Prophylaxis[5]	-	-	89%	94%
Written Stroke Educational Materials Given[5]	-	-	77%	88%
Surgical Care Improvement Project				
Appropriate Beta Blocker Usage	92	98%	97%	98%
Appropriate VTP Within 24 Hours	259	97%	98%	98%
Controlled Postoperative Blood Glucose[7]	-	-	96%	97%
Perioperative Temperature Management	279	100%	100%	100%
Prophylactic Antibiotic Selection	179	97%	99%	99%
Prophylactic Antibiotic Selection (Outpatient)[5]	-	-	98%	98%
Prophylactic Antibiotic Stopped	177	96%	98%	98%
Prophylactic Antibiotic Timing	179	100%	97%	99%
Prophylactic Antibiotic Timing (Outpatient)[5]	-	-	98%	98%
Urinary Catheter Removal	249	94%	98%	97%
Survey of Patients' Hospital Experiences				
Area Around Room 'Always' Quiet at Night	300+	53%	57%	61%
Doctors 'Always' Communicated Well	300+	80%	78%	82%
Home Recovery Information Given	300+	89%	85%	85%
Hospital Given 9 or 10 on 10 Point Scale	300+	75%	65%	71%
Meds 'Always' Explained Before Given	300+	63%	58%	64%
Nurses 'Always' Communicated Well	300+	81%	75%	79%
Pain 'Always' Well Controlled	300+	73%	67%	71%
Room and Bathroom 'Always' Clean	300+	71%	64%	73%
Timely Help 'Always' Received	300+	69%	58%	68%
Would Definitely Recommend Hospital	300+	73%	67%	71%
Use of Medical Imaging				
Cardiac Imaging Stress Test before Surgery	164	3.0%	6.4%	5.3%
Combination Abdominal CT Scan	1,332	9.3%	3.8%	10.5%
Combination Brain/Sinus CT Scan	1,058	4.4%	4.3%	2.7%
Combination Chest CT Scan	868	0.3%	1%	2.7%
Follow-up Mammogram/Ultrasound	1,985	7.0%	10.2%	8.8%
Lumbar Spine MRI for Low Back Pain	113	34.5%	38.2%	37.2%

Suburban Hospital

8600 Old Georgetown Road — Phone: 301-896-2576
Bethesda, MD 20814 — Fax: 301-897-1339
URL: www.suburbanhospital.org
Type: Acute Care Hospitals — Emergency Services: Yes
Ownership: Voluntary non-profit - Private — Beds: 366

Key Personnel:
Radiology.................. Stephan Cisternino, MD
Infection Control............. Fred Gill, MD
CEO/President.............. Gene E. Green, MD, MBA
Anesthesiology.............. Steven Hopper, MD
Quality Assurance .... Mary Monen
Chief of Medical Staff.......... Dr Eugene Passamani
Emergency Room .... Robert J Rothstein, MD
Patient Relations .... Jacky Schultz

Measure	Cases	This Hosp.	State Avg.	U.S. Avg.

NOTE: Hospital profiles are in alphabetical order by state, then city, then hospital within the city; Rankings exclude hospitals with less than 25 cases except for patient surveys which excludes hospitals with less than 100 cases; (a) 100-299 cases; (1) The number of cases/patients is too few to report; (2) Data submitted were based on a sample of cases/patients; (3) Results are based on a shorter time period than required; (4) Data suppressed by CMS for one or more quarters; (5) Results are not available for this reporting period; (6) Fewer than 100 patients completed the HCAHPS survey; (7) No cases met the criteria for this measure; (8) The lower limit of the confidence interval cannot be calculated if the number of observed infections equals zero; (9) No data are available from the state/territory for this reporting period; (10) The scores shown reflect fewer than 50 completed surveys; (11) There were discrepancies in the data collection process; (12) This measure does not apply to this hospital for this reporting period; (13) Results cannot be calculated for this reporting period; (14) The results for this state are combined with nearby states to protect confidentiality; Please refer to the User's Guide for a full explanation of data.

Measure	Cases	This Hosp.	State Avg.	U.S. Avg.
Blood Clot Prevention and Treatment				
Anticoagulation Overlap Therapy[2]	84	98%	94%	93%
ICU Venous Thromboembolism Prophylaxis[2]	75	97%	94%	92%
Incidence of Potentially Preventable VTE[2]	38	5%	7%	10%
UFH with Dosages/Platelet Monitoring[2]	24	100%	97%	97%
Venous Thromboembolism Prophylaxis[2]	249	85%	90%	85%
Warfarin Therapy Discharge Instructions[2]	47	66%	78%	75%
Chest Pain/Possible Heart Attack Care				
Aspirin Given Within 24 Hours of Arrival[5]	-	-	100%	96%
Fibrinolytic Meds Within 30 Min. of Arrival[5]	-	-	-	58%
Average Time to ECG (minutes)[5]	-	-	6	7
Average Time to Transfer (minutes)[5]	-	-	32	60
Children's Asthma Care				
Received Home Management Plan of Care	-	-	-	88%
Received Reliever Medication	-	-	-	100%
Received Systemic Corticosteroids	-	-	-	100%
Emergency Department				
Admittance Decision Time (minutes)[2]	654	211	143	98
Head CT Results Within 45 Min. of Arrival[5]	-	-	-	57%
Patients Who Left ER Before Being Seen[5]	-	-	3%	2%
Time from ER Arrival to Admit. (minutes)[2]	679	410	357	274
Time from ER Arrival to Discharge (minutes)[5]	-	-	-	134
Time in ER Before Being Evaluated (minutes)[5]	-	-	-	26
Time to Pain Meds for Fractures (minutes)[5]	-	-	-	57
Heart Attack Care				
Aspirin Given at Discharge	238	100%	99%	99%
Fibrinolytic Meds Within 30 Min. of Arrival[7]	-	-	-	54%
PCI Within 90 Minutes of Arrival	39	92%	93%	96%
Statin Prescribed at Discharge	220	100%	98%	98%
Heart Failure Care				
ACE Inhibitor or ARB for LVSD[2]	114	100%	97%	97%
Discharge Instructions Given[2]	233	83%	93%	94%
Evaluation of LVS Function[2]	333	99%	99%	99%
Medicare Spending				
Medicare Spending per Patient (ratio)	-	-	-	0.98
Pneumonia Care				
Appropriate Initial Antibiotic Given[2]	113	99%	97%	95%
Blood Culture Timing[2]	192	99%	97%	98%
Pregnancy and Delivery Care				
Newborn Deliveries Scheduled Early[5]	-	-	-	6%
Preventive Care				
Immunization for Influenza[2]	589	95%	94%	90%
Immunization for Pneumonia[2]	799	98%	94%	92%
Stroke Care				
Anticoagulation Therapy for Atrial Fibrillation[5]	-	-	95%	95%
Antithrombotic Therapy Timing[5]	-	-	95%	98%
Assessed for Rehabilitation[5]	-	-	96%	97%
Discharged on Antithrombotic Therapy[5]	-	-	95%	99%
Discharged on Statin Medication[5]	-	-	97%	94%
Thrombolytic Therapy Timing[5]	-	-	-	66%
Venous Thromboembolism Prophylaxis[5]	-	-	89%	94%
Written Stroke Educational Materials Given[5]	-	-	77%	88%
Surgical Care Improvement Project				
Appropriate Beta Blocker Usage[2]	449	99%	97%	98%
Appropriate VTP Within 24 Hours[2]	1,311	98%	98%	98%
Controlled Postoperative Blood Glucose[2]	171	96%	96%	97%
Perioperative Temperature Management[2]	1,399	100%	100%	100%
Prophylactic Antibiotic Selection[2]	1,345	99%	99%	99%
Prophylactic Antibiotic Selection (Outpatient)[5]	-	-	98%	98%
Prophylactic Antibiotic Stopped[2]	1,336	99%	98%	98%
Prophylactic Antibiotic Timing[2]	1,346	98%	97%	99%
Prophylactic Antibiotic Timing (Outpatient)[5]	-	-	98%	98%
Urinary Catheter Removal[2]	906	99%	98%	97%
Survey of Patients' Hospital Experiences				
Area Around Room 'Always' Quiet at Night	300+	52%	57%	61%
Doctors 'Always' Communicated Well	300+	77%	78%	82%
Home Recovery Information Given	300+	80%	85%	85%
Hospital Given 9 or 10 on 10 Point Scale	300+	69%	65%	71%
Meds 'Always' Explained Before Given	300+	59%	58%	64%
Nurses 'Always' Communicated Well	300+	73%	75%	79%
Pain 'Always' Well Controlled	300+	64%	67%	71%
Room and Bathroom 'Always' Clean	300+	64%	64%	73%
Timely Help 'Always' Received	300+	50%	58%	68%
Would Definitely Recommend Hospital	300+	74%	67%	71%
Use of Medical Imaging				
Cardiac Imaging Stress Test before Surgery[1]	-	-	6.4%	5.3%
Combination Abdominal CT Scan	842	7.0%	3.8%	10.5%
Combination Brain/Sinus CT Scan	1,160	6.8%	4.3%	2.7%
Combination Chest CT Scan	358	2.2%	1%	2.7%
Follow-up Mammogram/Ultrasound[7]	-	-	10.2%	8.8%
Lumbar Spine MRI for Low Back Pain[1]	-	-	38.2%	37.2%

University of Maryland Shore Medical Center at Chestertown

100 Brown Street
Chestertown, MD 21620
Phone: 410-778-7668
Type: Acute Care Hospitals
Emergency Services: Yes
Ownership: Voluntary non-profit - Private

Key Personnel:
Radiology. . . . . Brian Monroe, M.D
Anesthesiology. . . . . Rodger Oursler, M.D
CEO/President. . . . . Lyle E. Sheldon, FACHE

Measure	Cases	This Hosp.	State Avg.	U.S. Avg.
Blood Clot Prevention and Treatment				
Anticoagulation Overlap Therapy[2]	17	76%	94%	93%
ICU Venous Thromboembolism Prophylaxis[2]	45	100%	94%	92%
Incidence of Potentially Preventable VTE[1,2]	-	-	7%	10%
UFH with Dosages/Platelet Monitoring[1,2]	-	-	97%	97%
Venous Thromboembolism Prophylaxis[2]	239	94%	90%	85%
Warfarin Therapy Discharge Instructions[1,2]	-	-	78%	75%
Chest Pain/Possible Heart Attack Care				
Aspirin Given Within 24 Hours of Arrival[5]	-	-	100%	96%
Fibrinolytic Meds Within 30 Min. of Arrival[5]	-	-	-	58%
Average Time to ECG (minutes)[5]	-	-	6	7
Average Time to Transfer (minutes)[5]	-	-	32	60
Children's Asthma Care				
Received Home Management Plan of Care	-	-	-	88%
Received Reliever Medication	-	-	-	100%
Received Systemic Corticosteroids	-	-	-	100%
Emergency Department				
Admittance Decision Time (minutes)[2]	550	62	143	98
Head CT Results Within 45 Min. of Arrival[5]	-	-	-	57%
Patients Who Left ER Before Being Seen[5]	-	-	3%	2%
Time from ER Arrival to Admit. (minutes)[2]	553	300	357	274
Time from ER Arrival to Discharge (minutes)[5]	-	-	-	134
Time in ER Before Being Evaluated (minutes)[5]	-	-	-	26
Time to Pain Meds for Fractures (minutes)[5]	-	-	-	57
Heart Attack Care				
Aspirin Given at Discharge[1]	-	-	99%	99%
Fibrinolytic Meds Within 30 Min. of Arrival[1]	-	-	-	54%
PCI Within 90 Minutes of Arrival[7]	-	-	93%	96%
Statin Prescribed at Discharge[1]	-	-	98%	98%
Heart Failure Care				
ACE Inhibitor or ARB for LVSD	28	96%	97%	97%
Discharge Instructions Given	75	100%	93%	94%
Evaluation of LVS Function	93	100%	99%	99%
Medicare Spending				
Medicare Spending per Patient (ratio)	-	-	-	0.98
Pneumonia Care				
Appropriate Initial Antibiotic Given	41	98%	97%	95%
Blood Culture Timing	67	91%	97%	98%
Pregnancy and Delivery Care				
Newborn Deliveries Scheduled Early[5]	-	-	-	6%
Preventive Care				
Immunization for Influenza[2]	319	100%	94%	90%
Immunization for Pneumonia[2]	499	98%	94%	92%
Stroke Care				
Anticoagulation Therapy for Atrial Fibrillation[5]	-	-	95%	95%
Antithrombotic Therapy Timing[5]	-	-	95%	98%
Assessed for Rehabilitation[5]	-	-	96%	97%
Discharged on Antithrombotic Therapy[5]	-	-	95%	99%
Discharged on Statin Medication[5]	-	-	97%	94%
Thrombolytic Therapy Timing[5]	-	-	-	66%
Venous Thromboembolism Prophylaxis[5]	-	-	89%	94%
Written Stroke Educational Materials Given[5]	-	-	77%	88%
Surgical Care Improvement Project				
Appropriate Beta Blocker Usage	29	97%	97%	98%
Appropriate VTP Within 24 Hours	87	97%	98%	98%
Controlled Postoperative Blood Glucose[7]	-	-	96%	97%
Perioperative Temperature Management	105	99%	100%	100%
Prophylactic Antibiotic Selection	70	99%	99%	99%
Prophylactic Antibiotic Selection (Outpatient)[5]	-	-	98%	98%
Prophylactic Antibiotic Stopped	70	99%	98%	98%
Prophylactic Antibiotic Timing	70	94%	97%	99%
Prophylactic Antibiotic Timing (Outpatient)[5]	-	-	98%	98%
Urinary Catheter Removal	65	97%	98%	97%
Survey of Patients' Hospital Experiences				
Area Around Room 'Always' Quiet at Night	300+	58%	57%	61%
Doctors 'Always' Communicated Well	300+	82%	78%	82%
Home Recovery Information Given	300+	88%	85%	85%
Hospital Given 9 or 10 on 10 Point Scale	300+	60%	65%	71%
Meds 'Always' Explained Before Given	300+	58%	58%	64%
Nurses 'Always' Communicated Well	300+	77%	75%	79%
Pain 'Always' Well Controlled	300+	68%	67%	71%
Room and Bathroom 'Always' Clean	300+	66%	64%	73%
Timely Help 'Always' Received	300+	70%	58%	68%
Would Definitely Recommend Hospital	300+	56%	67%	71%
Use of Medical Imaging				
Cardiac Imaging Stress Test before Surgery[1]	-	-	6.4%	5.3%
Combination Abdominal CT Scan	560	4.8%	3.8%	10.5%
Combination Brain/Sinus CT Scan	435	2.1%	4.3%	2.7%
Combination Chest CT Scan	275	1.8%	1%	2.7%
Follow-up Mammogram/Ultrasound	879	8.0%	10.2%	8.8%
Lumbar Spine MRI for Low Back Pain	51	43.1%	38.2%	37.2%

Prince Georges Hospital Center

3001 Hospital Drive
Cheverly, MD 20785
Phone: 301-618-2000
Fax: 301-618-2547
URL: www.princegeorgeshospital.org
Type: Acute Care Hospitals
Emergency Services: Yes
Ownership: Voluntary non-profit - Private
Beds: 290

Key Personnel:
Radiology. . . . . David Blanton, MD
Infection Control. . . . . Jackie Cohran
Pediatric Ambulatory Care . . . . . . Frederick Corder, MD
Pediatric In-Patient Care . . . . Frederick Corder, MD
CEO/President. . . . . G T Dunlop Ecker
Quality Assurance . . . . Brigid Krizek
Chief of Medical Staff. . . . . Shirley Morgan

Measure	Cases	This Hosp.	State Avg.	U.S. Avg.
Blood Clot Prevention and Treatment				
Anticoagulation Overlap Therapy[2]	89	89%	94%	93%
ICU Venous Thromboembolism Prophylaxis[2]	176	97%	94%	92%
Incidence of Potentially Preventable VTE[2]	33	3%	7%	10%
UFH with Dosages/Platelet Monitoring[2]	37	97%	97%	97%
Venous Thromboembolism Prophylaxis[2]	281	91%	90%	85%
Warfarin Therapy Discharge Instructions[2]	65	75%	78%	75%
Chest Pain/Possible Heart Attack Care				
Aspirin Given Within 24 Hours of Arrival[5]	-	-	100%	96%
Fibrinolytic Meds Within 30 Min. of Arrival[5]	-	-	-	58%
Average Time to ECG (minutes)[5]	-	-	6	7
Average Time to Transfer (minutes)[5]	-	-	32	60
Children's Asthma Care				
Received Home Management Plan of Care[1]	-	-	-	88%
Received Reliever Medication[1]	-	-	-	100%
Received Systemic Corticosteroids[1]	-	-	-	100%
Emergency Department				
Admittance Decision Time (minutes)[2]	457	301	143	98
Head CT Results Within 45 Min. of Arrival[5]	-	-	-	57%
Patients Who Left ER Before Being Seen[5]	-	-	3%	2%
Time from ER Arrival to Admit. (minutes)[2]	509	550	357	274
Time from ER Arrival to Discharge (minutes)[5]	-	-	-	134
Time in ER Before Being Evaluated (minutes)[5]	-	-	-	26
Time to Pain Meds for Fractures (minutes)[5]	-	-	-	57
Heart Attack Care				
Aspirin Given at Discharge[2]	144	100%	99%	99%
Fibrinolytic Meds Within 30 Min. of Arrival[2,7]	-	-	-	54%
PCI Within 90 Minutes of Arrival[2]	25	56%	93%	96%
Statin Prescribed at Discharge[2]	143	97%	98%	98%

NOTE: Hospital profiles are in alphabetical order by state, then city, then hospital within the city; Rankings exclude hospitals with less than 25 cases except for patient surveys which excludes hospitals with less than 100 cases; (a) 100-299 cases; (1) The number of cases/patients is too few to report; (2) Data submitted were based on a sample of cases/patients; (3) Results are based on a shorter time period than required; (4) Data suppressed by CMS for one or more quarters; (5) Results are not available for this reporting period; (6) Fewer than 100 patients completed the HCAHPS survey; (7) No cases met the criteria for this measure; (8) The lower limit of the confidence interval cannot be calculated if the number of observed infections equals zero; (9) No data are available from the state/territory for this reporting period; (10) The scores shown reflect fewer than 50 completed surveys; (11) There were discrepancies in the data collection process; (12) This measure does not apply to this hospital for this reporting period; (13) Results cannot be calculated for this reporting period; (14) The results for this state are combined with nearby states to protect confidentiality; Please refer to the User's Guide for a full explanation of data.

Measure	Cases	This Hosp.	State Avg.	U.S. Avg.
Heart Failure Care				
ACE Inhibitor or ARB for LVSD[2]	113	96%	97%	97%
Discharge Instructions Given[2]	276	82%	93%	94%
Evaluation of LVS Function[2]	295	99%	99%	99%
Medicare Spending				
Medicare Spending per Patient (ratio)	-	-	-	0.98
Pneumonia Care				
Appropriate Initial Antibiotic Given[2]	69	94%	97%	95%
Blood Culture Timing[2]	126	94%	97%	98%
Pregnancy and Delivery Care				
Newborn Deliveries Scheduled Early[5]	-	-	-	6%
Preventive Care				
Immunization for Influenza[2]	479	87%	94%	90%
Immunization for Pneumonia[2]	456	82%	94%	92%
Stroke Care				
Anticoagulation Therapy for Atrial Fibrillation[1]	-	-	95%	95%
Antithrombotic Therapy Timing	92	96%	95%	98%
Assessed for Rehabilitation	91	98%	96%	97%
Discharged on Antithrombotic Therapy	85	98%	95%	99%
Discharged on Statin Medication	76	95%	97%	94%
Thrombolytic Therapy Timing[1]	-	-	-	66%
Venous Thromboembolism Prophylaxis	103	89%	89%	94%
Written Stroke Educational Materials Given	54	63%	77%	88%
Surgical Care Improvement Project				
Appropriate Beta Blocker Usage[2]	30	83%	97%	98%
Appropriate VTP Within 24 Hours[2]	154	84%	98%	98%
Controlled Postoperative Blood Glucose[1,2]	-	-	96%	97%
Perioperative Temperature Management[2]	192	97%	100%	100%
Prophylactic Antibiotic Selection[2]	82	83%	99%	99%
Prophylactic Antibiotic Selection (Outpatient)[5]	-	-	98%	98%
Prophylactic Antibiotic Stopped[2]	77	90%	98%	98%
Prophylactic Antibiotic Timing[2]	83	89%	97%	99%
Prophylactic Antibiotic Timing (Outpatient)[5]	-	-	98%	98%
Urinary Catheter Removal[2]	116	92%	98%	97%
Survey of Patients' Hospital Experiences				
Area Around Room 'Always' Quiet at Night	300+	59%	57%	61%
Doctors 'Always' Communicated Well	300+	73%	78%	82%
Home Recovery Information Given	300+	79%	85%	85%
Hospital Given 9 or 10 on 10 Point Scale	300+	48%	65%	71%
Meds 'Always' Explained Before Given	300+	52%	58%	64%
Nurses 'Always' Communicated Well	300+	63%	75%	79%
Pain 'Always' Well Controlled	300+	60%	67%	71%
Room and Bathroom 'Always' Clean	300+	60%	64%	73%
Timely Help 'Always' Received	300+	43%	58%	68%
Would Definitely Recommend Hospital	300+	47%	67%	71%
Use of Medical Imaging				
Cardiac Imaging Stress Test before Surgery[1]	-	-	6.4%	5.3%
Combination Abdominal CT Scan	269	1.5%	3.8%	10.5%
Combination Brain/Sinus CT Scan	388	6.7%	4.3%	2.7%
Combination Chest CT Scan	129	1.6%	1%	2.7%
Follow-up Mammogram/Ultrasound	101	7.9%	10.2%	8.8%
Lumbar Spine MRI for Low Back Pain[1]	-	-	38.2%	37.2%

Medstar Southern Maryland Hospital Center

7503 Surratts Road
Clinton, MD 20735
Phone: 301-868-8000
URL: www.medstarhealth.org
Type: Acute Care Hospitals
Emergency Services: Yes
Ownership: Voluntary non-profit - Private

Measure	Cases	This Hosp.	State Avg.	U.S. Avg.
Blood Clot Prevention and Treatment				
Anticoagulation Overlap Therapy[2]	99	94%	94%	93%
ICU Venous Thromboembolism Prophylaxis[2]	52	87%	94%	92%
Incidence of Potentially Preventable VTE[1,2]	-	-	7%	10%
UFH with Dosages/Platelet Monitoring[2]	27	100%	97%	97%
Venous Thromboembolism Prophylaxis[2]	335	81%	90%	85%
Warfarin Therapy Discharge Instructions[2]	67	39%	78%	75%
Chest Pain/Possible Heart Attack Care				
Aspirin Given Within 24 Hours of Arrival[5]	-	-	100%	96%
Fibrinolytic Meds Within 30 Min. of Arrival[5]	-	-	-	58%
Average Time to ECG (minutes)[5]	-	-	6	7
Average Time to Transfer (minutes)[5]	-	-	32	60
Children's Asthma Care				
Received Home Management Plan of Care	-	-	-	88%
Received Reliever Medication	-	-	-	100%
Received Systemic Corticosteroids	-	-	-	100%
Emergency Department				
Admittance Decision Time (minutes)[2,3]	793	168	143	98
Head CT Results Within 45 Min. of Arrival[5]	-	-	-	57%
Patients Who Left ER Before Being Seen[5]	-	-	3%	2%
Time from ER Arrival to Admit. (minutes)[2,3]	801	384	357	274
Time from ER Arrival to Discharge (minutes)[5]	-	-	-	134
Time in ER Before Being Evaluated (minutes)[5]	-	-	-	26
Time to Pain Meds for Fractures (minutes)[5]	-	-	-	57
Heart Attack Care				
Aspirin Given at Discharge[3]	153	97%	99%	99%
Fibrinolytic Meds Within 30 Min. of Arrival[3,7]	-	-	-	54%
PCI Within 90 Minutes of Arrival[3]	42	93%	93%	96%
Statin Prescribed at Discharge[3]	149	93%	98%	98%
Heart Failure Care				
ACE Inhibitor or ARB for LVSD[3]	166	85%	97%	97%
Discharge Instructions Given[3]	454	62%	93%	94%
Evaluation of LVS Function[3]	498	96%	99%	99%
Medicare Spending				
Medicare Spending per Patient (ratio)	-	-	-	0.98
Pneumonia Care				
Appropriate Initial Antibiotic Given[2,3]	62	94%	97%	95%
Blood Culture Timing[2,3]	50	82%	97%	98%
Pregnancy and Delivery Care				
Newborn Deliveries Scheduled Early[5]	-	-	-	6%
Preventive Care				
Immunization for Influenza[2,3]	304	84%	94%	90%
Immunization for Pneumonia[2,3]	654	91%	94%	92%
Stroke Care				
Anticoagulation Therapy for Atrial Fibrillation[5]	-	-	95%	95%
Antithrombotic Therapy Timing[5]	-	-	95%	98%
Assessed for Rehabilitation[5]	-	-	96%	97%
Discharged on Antithrombotic Therapy[5]	-	-	95%	99%
Discharged on Statin Medication[5]	-	-	97%	94%
Thrombolytic Therapy Timing[5]	-	-	-	66%
Venous Thromboembolism Prophylaxis[5]	-	-	89%	94%
Written Stroke Educational Materials Given[5]	-	-	77%	88%
Surgical Care Improvement Project				
Appropriate Beta Blocker Usage[2,3]	120	90%	97%	98%
Appropriate VTP Within 24 Hours[2,3]	378	97%	98%	98%
Controlled Postoperative Blood Glucose[2,3]	-	-	96%	97%
Perioperative Temperature Management[2,3]	466	100%	100%	100%
Prophylactic Antibiotic Selection[2,3]	312	99%	99%	99%
Prophylactic Antibiotic Selection (Outpatient)[5]	-	-	98%	98%
Prophylactic Antibiotic Stopped[2,3]	306	94%	98%	98%
Prophylactic Antibiotic Timing[2,3]	312	99%	97%	99%
Prophylactic Antibiotic Timing (Outpatient)[5]	-	-	98%	98%
Urinary Catheter Removal[2,3]	133	89%	98%	97%
Survey of Patients' Hospital Experiences				
Area Around Room 'Always' Quiet at Night[5]	-	-	57%	61%
Doctors 'Always' Communicated Well[5]	-	-	78%	82%
Home Recovery Information Given[5]	-	-	85%	85%
Hospital Given 9 or 10 on 10 Point Scale[5]	-	-	65%	71%
Meds 'Always' Explained Before Given[5]	-	-	58%	64%
Nurses 'Always' Communicated Well[5]	-	-	75%	79%
Pain 'Always' Well Controlled[5]	-	-	67%	71%
Room and Bathroom 'Always' Clean[5]	-	-	64%	73%
Timely Help 'Always' Received[5]	-	-	58%	68%
Would Definitely Recommend Hospital[5]	-	-	67%	71%
Use of Medical Imaging				
Cardiac Imaging Stress Test before Surgery	122	7.4%	6.4%	5.3%
Combination Abdominal CT Scan	256	1.2%	3.8%	10.5%
Combination Brain/Sinus CT Scan	466	0.9%	4.3%	2.7%
Combination Chest CT Scan	63	1.6%	1%	2.7%
Follow-up Mammogram/Ultrasound[7]	-	-	10.2%	8.8%
Lumbar Spine MRI for Low Back Pain[1]	-	-	38.2%	37.2%

Howard County General Hospital

5755 Cedar Lane
Columbia, MD 21044
Phone: 410-740-7890
Fax: 410-740-7610
URL: www.hcgh.org
Type: Acute Care Hospitals
Emergency Services: Yes
Ownership: Voluntary non-profit - Private
Beds: 208

Key Personnel:
Operating Room. . . . . Francine Black
Quality Assurance . . . . Judy Brown
Radiology. . . . . John Dunn
Chief of Medical Staff . . . . Jonathan Fish, MD

Measure	Cases	This Hosp.	State Avg.	U.S. Avg.
Blood Clot Prevention and Treatment				
Anticoagulation Overlap Therapy[2]	152	86%	94%	93%
ICU Venous Thromboembolism Prophylaxis[2]	35	91%	94%	92%
Incidence of Potentially Preventable VTE[2]	28	11%	7%	10%
UFH with Dosages/Platelet Monitoring[2]	163	100%	97%	97%
Venous Thromboembolism Prophylaxis[2]	358	74%	90%	85%
Warfarin Therapy Discharge Instructions[2]	129	94%	78%	75%
Chest Pain/Possible Heart Attack Care				
Aspirin Given Within 24 Hours of Arrival[5]	-	-	100%	96%
Fibrinolytic Meds Within 30 Min. of Arrival[5]	-	-	-	58%
Average Time to ECG (minutes)[5]	-	-	6	7
Average Time to Transfer (minutes)[5]	-	-	32	60
Children's Asthma Care				
Received Home Management Plan of Care	-	-	-	88%
Received Reliever Medication	-	-	-	100%
Received Systemic Corticosteroids	-	-	-	100%
Emergency Department				
Admittance Decision Time (minutes)[2,3]	402	160	143	98
Head CT Results Within 45 Min. of Arrival[5]	-	-	-	57%
Patients Who Left ER Before Being Seen[5]	-	-	3%	2%
Time from ER Arrival to Admit. (minutes)[2,3]	416	462	357	274
Time from ER Arrival to Discharge (minutes)[5]	-	-	-	134
Time in ER Before Being Evaluated (minutes)[5]	-	-	-	26
Time to Pain Meds for Fractures (minutes)[5]	-	-	-	57
Heart Attack Care				
Aspirin Given at Discharge	83	98%	99%	99%
Fibrinolytic Meds Within 30 Min. of Arrival[7]	-	-	-	54%
PCI Within 90 Minutes of Arrival	58	90%	93%	96%
Statin Prescribed at Discharge	85	100%	98%	98%
Heart Failure Care				
ACE Inhibitor or ARB for LVSD[2]	79	96%	97%	97%
Discharge Instructions Given[2]	250	95%	93%	94%
Evaluation of LVS Function[2]	304	99%	99%	99%
Medicare Spending				
Medicare Spending per Patient (ratio)	-	-	-	0.98
Pneumonia Care				
Appropriate Initial Antibiotic Given[2]	77	97%	97%	95%
Blood Culture Timing[2]	139	98%	97%	98%
Pregnancy and Delivery Care				
Newborn Deliveries Scheduled Early[5]	-	-	-	6%
Preventive Care				
Immunization for Influenza[2,3]	243	97%	94%	90%
Immunization for Pneumonia[2,3]	388	97%	94%	92%
Stroke Care				
Anticoagulation Therapy for Atrial Fibrillation[5]	-	-	95%	95%
Antithrombotic Therapy Timing[5]	-	-	95%	98%
Assessed for Rehabilitation[5]	-	-	96%	97%
Discharged on Antithrombotic Therapy[5]	-	-	95%	99%
Discharged on Statin Medication[5]	-	-	97%	94%
Thrombolytic Therapy Timing[5]	-	-	-	66%
Venous Thromboembolism Prophylaxis[5]	-	-	89%	94%
Written Stroke Educational Materials Given[5]	-	-	77%	88%
Surgical Care Improvement Project				
Appropriate Beta Blocker Usage[2]	101	97%	97%	98%
Appropriate VTP Within 24 Hours[2]	367	98%	98%	98%
Controlled Postoperative Blood Glucose[2,7]	-	-	96%	97%
Perioperative Temperature Management[2]	415	100%	100%	100%
Prophylactic Antibiotic Selection[2]	262	97%	99%	99%
Prophylactic Antibiotic Selection (Outpatient)[5]	-	-	98%	98%
Prophylactic Antibiotic Stopped[2]	256	98%	98%	98%
Prophylactic Antibiotic Timing[2]	262	99%	97%	99%

NOTE: Hospital profiles are in alphabetical order by state, then city, then hospital within the city; Rankings exclude hospitals with less than 25 cases except for patient surveys which excludes hospitals with less than 100 cases; (a) 100-299 cases; (1) The number of cases/patients is too few to report; (2) Data submitted were based on a sample of cases/patients; (3) Results are based on a shorter time period than required; (4) Data suppressed by CMS for one or more quarters; (5) Results are not available for this reporting period; (6) Fewer than 100 patients completed the HCAHPS survey; (7) No cases met the criteria for this measure; (8) The lower limit of the confidence interval cannot be calculated if the number of observed infections equals zero; (9) No data are available from the state/territory for this reporting period; (10) The scores shown reflect fewer than 50 completed surveys; (11) There were discrepancies in the data collection process; (12) This measure does not apply to this hospital for this reporting period; (13) Results cannot be calculated for this reporting period; (14) The results for this state are combined with nearby states to protect confidentiality; Please refer to the User's Guide for a full explanation of data.

Prophylactic Antibiotic Timing (Outpatient)[5]	-	-	98%	98%
Urinary Catheter Removal[2]	269	97%	98%	97%
Survey of Patients' Hospital Experiences				
Area Around Room 'Always' Quiet at Night	300+	54%	57%	61%
Doctors 'Always' Communicated Well	300+	74%	78%	82%
Home Recovery Information Given	300+	80%	85%	85%
Hospital Given 9 or 10 on 10 Point Scale	300+	66%	65%	71%
Meds 'Always' Explained Before Given	300+	53%	58%	64%
Nurses 'Always' Communicated Well	300+	73%	75%	79%
Pain 'Always' Well Controlled	300+	67%	67%	71%
Room and Bathroom 'Always' Clean	300+	62%	64%	73%
Timely Help 'Always' Received	300+	57%	58%	68%
Would Definitely Recommend Hospital	300+	71%	67%	71%
Use of Medical Imaging				
Cardiac Imaging Stress Test before Surgery	314	7.0%	6.4%	5.3%
Combination Abdominal CT Scan	692	3.6%	3.8%	10.5%
Combination Brain/Sinus CT Scan	1,243	5.9%	4.3%	2.7%
Combination Chest CT Scan	521	4.2%	1%	2.7%
Follow-up Mammogram/Ultrasound	105	13.3%	10.2%	8.8%
Lumbar Spine MRI for Low Back Pain[1]	-	-	38.2%	37.2%

Edward Mccready Memorial Hospital

201 Hall Highway
Crisfield, MD 21817
Phone: 410-726-9496
Fax: 410-968-3005
E-mail: mccreadyhospital@aol.com
Type: Acute Care Hospitals
Emergency Services: Yes
Ownership: Voluntary non-profit - Private
Beds: 104

Key Personnel:

Chief of Medical Staff.......... Michael Atkins
Radiology.................... Mary Lynne Everett
CEO .... Joy A. Strand

Measure	Cases	This Hosp.	State Avg.	U.S. Avg.
Blood Clot Prevention and Treatment				
Anticoagulation Overlap Therapy[1,3]	-	-	94%	93%
ICU Venous Thromboembolism Prophylaxis[3,7]	-	-	94%	92%
Incidence of Potentially Preventable VTE[3,7]	-	-	7%	10%
UFH with Dosages/Platelet Monitoring[3,7]	-	-	97%	97%
Venous Thromboembolism Prophylaxis[1,3]	-	-	90%	85%
Warfarin Therapy Discharge Instructions[3,7]	-	-	78%	75%
Chest Pain/Possible Heart Attack Care				
Aspirin Given Within 24 Hours of Arrival[5]	-	-	100%	96%
Fibrinolytic Meds Within 30 Min. of Arrival[5]	-	-	-	58%
Average Time to ECG (minutes)[5]	-	-	6	7
Average Time to Transfer (minutes)[5]	-	-	32	60
Children's Asthma Care				
Received Home Management Plan of Care	-	-	-	88%
Received Reliever Medication	-	-	-	100%
Received Systemic Corticosteroids	-	-	-	100%
Emergency Department				
Admittance Decision Time (minutes)	152	40	143	98
Head CT Results Within 45 Min. of Arrival[5]	-	-	-	57%
Patients Who Left ER Before Being Seen[5]	-	-	3%	2%
Time from ER Arrival to Admit. (minutes)	152	192	357	274
Time from ER Arrival to Discharge (minutes)[5]	-	-	-	134
Time in ER Before Being Evaluated (minutes)[5]	-	-	-	26
Time to Pain Meds for Fractures (minutes)[5]	-	-	-	57
Heart Attack Care				
Aspirin Given at Discharge[1,3]	-	-	99%	99%
Fibrinolytic Meds Within 30 Min. of Arrival[3,7]	-	-	-	54%
PCI Within 90 Minutes of Arrival[3,7]	-	-	93%	96%
Statin Prescribed at Discharge[1,3]	-	-	98%	98%
Heart Failure Care				
ACE Inhibitor or ARB for LVSD[3]	11	82%	97%	97%
Discharge Instructions Given[3]	14	93%	93%	94%
Evaluation of LVS Function[3]	23	83%	99%	99%
Medicare Spending				
Medicare Spending per Patient (ratio)	-	-	-	0.98
Pneumonia Care				
Appropriate Initial Antibiotic Given[1,3]	-	-	97%	95%
Blood Culture Timing[3]	11	91%	97%	98%
Pregnancy and Delivery Care				
Newborn Deliveries Scheduled Early[5]	-	-	-	6%
Preventive Care				
Immunization for Influenza	79	52%	94%	90%
Immunization for Pneumonia[3]	109	35%	94%	92%
Stroke Care				
Anticoagulation Therapy for Atrial Fibrillation[3,7]	-	-	95%	95%
Antithrombotic Therapy Timing[1,3]	-	-	95%	98%
Assessed for Rehabilitation[1,3]	-	-	96%	97%
Discharged on Antithrombotic Therapy[1,3]	-	-	95%	99%
Discharged on Statin Medication[1,3]	-	-	97%	94%
Thrombolytic Therapy Timing[1,3]	-	-	-	66%
Venous Thromboembolism Prophylaxis[1,3]	-	-	89%	94%
Written Stroke Educational Materials Given[1,3]	-	-	77%	88%
Surgical Care Improvement Project				
Appropriate Beta Blocker Usage[5]	-	-	97%	98%
Appropriate VTP Within 24 Hours[5]	-	-	98%	98%
Controlled Postoperative Blood Glucose[5]	-	-	96%	97%
Perioperative Temperature Management[5]	-	-	100%	100%
Prophylactic Antibiotic Selection[5]	-	-	99%	99%
Prophylactic Antibiotic Selection (Outpatient)[5]	-	-	98%	98%
Prophylactic Antibiotic Stopped[5]	-	-	98%	98%
Prophylactic Antibiotic Timing[5]	-	-	97%	99%
Prophylactic Antibiotic Timing (Outpatient)[5]	-	-	98%	98%
Urinary Catheter Removal[5]	-	-	98%	97%
Survey of Patients' Hospital Experiences				
Area Around Room 'Always' Quiet at Night[5]	-	-	57%	61%
Doctors 'Always' Communicated Well[5]	-	-	78%	82%
Home Recovery Information Given[5]	-	-	85%	85%
Hospital Given 9 or 10 on 10 Point Scale[5]	-	-	65%	71%
Meds 'Always' Explained Before Given[5]	-	-	58%	64%
Nurses 'Always' Communicated Well[5]	-	-	75%	79%
Pain 'Always' Well Controlled[5]	-	-	67%	71%
Room and Bathroom 'Always' Clean[5]	-	-	64%	73%
Timely Help 'Always' Received[5]	-	-	58%	68%
Would Definitely Recommend Hospital[5]	-	-	67%	71%
Use of Medical Imaging				
Cardiac Imaging Stress Test before Surgery[1]	-	-	6.4%	5.3%
Combination Abdominal CT Scan	158	1.3%	3.8%	10.5%
Combination Brain/Sinus CT Scan[1]	-	-	4.3%	2.7%
Combination Chest CT Scan	111	0.9%	1%	2.7%
Follow-up Mammogram/Ultrasound	307	67.8%	10.2%	8.8%
Lumbar Spine MRI for Low Back Pain[1]	-	-	38.2%	37.2%

Western Maryland Regional Medical Center

12500 Willowbrook Road
Cumberland, MD 21502
Phone: 240-964-8001
URL: www.wmhs.com
Type: Acute Care Hospitals
Emergency Services: Yes
Ownership: Voluntary non-profit - Private
Beds: 275

Measure	Cases	This Hosp.	State Avg.	U.S. Avg.
Blood Clot Prevention and Treatment				
Anticoagulation Overlap Therapy[5]	-	-	94%	93%
ICU Venous Thromboembolism Prophylaxis[5]	-	-	94%	92%
Incidence of Potentially Preventable VTE[5]	-	-	7%	10%
UFH with Dosages/Platelet Monitoring[5]	-	-	97%	97%
Venous Thromboembolism Prophylaxis[5]	-	-	90%	85%
Warfarin Therapy Discharge Instructions[5]	-	-	78%	75%
Chest Pain/Possible Heart Attack Care				
Aspirin Given Within 24 Hours of Arrival[5]	-	-	100%	96%
Fibrinolytic Meds Within 30 Min. of Arrival[5]	-	-	-	58%
Average Time to ECG (minutes)[5]	-	-	6	7
Average Time to Transfer (minutes)[5]	-	-	32	60
Children's Asthma Care				
Received Home Management Plan of Care	-	-	-	88%
Received Reliever Medication	-	-	-	100%
Received Systemic Corticosteroids	-	-	-	100%
Emergency Department				
Admittance Decision Time (minutes)[5]	-	-	143	98
Head CT Results Within 45 Min. of Arrival[5]	-	-	-	57%
Patients Who Left ER Before Being Seen[5]	-	-	3%	2%
Time from ER Arrival to Admit. (minutes)[5]	-	-	357	274
Time from ER Arrival to Discharge (minutes)[5]	-	-	-	134
Time in ER Before Being Evaluated (minutes)[5]	-	-	-	26
Time to Pain Meds for Fractures (minutes)[5]	-	-	-	57
Heart Attack Care				
Aspirin Given at Discharge	274	100%	99%	99%
Fibrinolytic Meds Within 30 Min. of Arrival[7]	-	-	-	54%
PCI Within 90 Minutes of Arrival	40	85%	93%	96%
Statin Prescribed at Discharge	245	98%	98%	98%
Heart Failure Care				
ACE Inhibitor or ARB for LVSD	103	98%	97%	97%
Discharge Instructions Given	208	88%	93%	94%
Evaluation of LVS Function	269	100%	99%	99%
Medicare Spending				
Medicare Spending per Patient (ratio)	-	-	-	0.98
Pneumonia Care				
Appropriate Initial Antibiotic Given	180	96%	97%	95%
Blood Culture Timing	355	97%	97%	98%
Pregnancy and Delivery Care				
Newborn Deliveries Scheduled Early[5]	-	-	-	6%
Preventive Care				
Immunization for Influenza[5]	-	-	94%	90%
Immunization for Pneumonia[5]	-	-	94%	92%
Stroke Care				
Anticoagulation Therapy for Atrial Fibrillation[5]	-	-	95%	95%
Antithrombotic Therapy Timing[5]	-	-	95%	98%
Assessed for Rehabilitation[5]	-	-	96%	97%
Discharged on Antithrombotic Therapy[5]	-	-	95%	99%
Discharged on Statin Medication[5]	-	-	97%	94%
Thrombolytic Therapy Timing[5]	-	-	-	66%
Venous Thromboembolism Prophylaxis[5]	-	-	89%	94%
Written Stroke Educational Materials Given[5]	-	-	77%	88%
Surgical Care Improvement Project				
Appropriate Beta Blocker Usage	357	99%	97%	98%
Appropriate VTP Within 24 Hours	653	99%	98%	98%
Controlled Postoperative Blood Glucose	171	98%	96%	97%
Perioperative Temperature Management	799	100%	100%	100%
Prophylactic Antibiotic Selection	703	100%	99%	99%
Prophylactic Antibiotic Selection (Outpatient)[5]	-	-	98%	98%
Prophylactic Antibiotic Stopped	694	100%	98%	98%
Prophylactic Antibiotic Timing	703	100%	97%	99%
Prophylactic Antibiotic Timing (Outpatient)[5]	-	-	98%	98%
Urinary Catheter Removal	158	99%	98%	97%
Survey of Patients' Hospital Experiences				
Area Around Room 'Always' Quiet at Night	300+	60%	57%	61%
Doctors 'Always' Communicated Well	300+	80%	78%	82%
Home Recovery Information Given	300+	90%	85%	85%
Hospital Given 9 or 10 on 10 Point Scale	300+	65%	65%	71%
Meds 'Always' Explained Before Given	300+	63%	58%	64%
Nurses 'Always' Communicated Well	300+	78%	75%	79%
Pain 'Always' Well Controlled	300+	69%	67%	71%
Room and Bathroom 'Always' Clean	300+	70%	64%	73%
Timely Help 'Always' Received	300+	63%	58%	68%
Would Definitely Recommend Hospital	300+	63%	67%	71%
Use of Medical Imaging				
Cardiac Imaging Stress Test before Surgery	415	5.1%	6.4%	5.3%
Combination Abdominal CT Scan	1,158	5.7%	3.8%	10.5%
Combination Brain/Sinus CT Scan	1,190	5.1%	4.3%	2.7%
Combination Chest CT Scan	783	0.5%	1%	2.7%
Follow-up Mammogram/Ultrasound[1]	-	-	10.2%	8.8%
Lumbar Spine MRI for Low Back Pain	155	38.7%	38.2%	37.2%

University of Maryland Shore Medical Center at Easton

219 South Washington Street
Easton, MD 21601
Phone: 410-822-1000
Fax: 410-740-8603
URL: www.shorehealth.org
Type: Acute Care Hospitals
Emergency Services: Yes
Ownership: Voluntary non-profit - Private
Beds: 250

Key Personnel:

Radiology.................... Stephen Brigham
Chief of Medical Staff.......... John Condit, MD
Pediatric Ambulatory Care ...... Brian Corden
Pediatric In-Patient Care .... Brian Corden
Quality Assurance .... Jeanne Lusby
CEO/President............... Joseph Ross

Measure	Cases	This Hosp.	State Avg.	U.S. Avg.
Blood Clot Prevention and Treatment				

NOTE: Hospital profiles are in alphabetical order by state, then city, then hospital within the city; Rankings exclude hospitals with less than 25 cases except for patient surveys which excludes hospitals with less than 100 cases; (a) 100-299 cases; (1) The number of cases/patients is too few to report; (2) Data submitted were based on a sample of cases/patients; (3) Results are based on a shorter time period than required; (4) Data suppressed by CMS for one or more quarters; (5) Results are not available for this reporting period; (6) Fewer than 100 patients completed the HCAHPS survey; (7) No cases met the criteria for this measure; (8) The lower limit of the confidence interval cannot be calculated if the number of observed infections equals zero; (9) No data are available from the state/territory for this reporting period; (10) The scores shown reflect fewer than 50 completed surveys; (11) There were discrepancies in the data collection process; (12) This measure does not apply to this hospital for this reporting period; (13) Results cannot be calculated for this reporting period; (14) The results for this state are combined with nearby states to protect confidentiality; Please refer to the User's Guide for a full explanation of data.

Measure	Cases	This Hosp.	State Avg.	U.S. Avg.
Anticoagulation Overlap Therapy[2,3]	36	100%	94%	93%
ICU Venous Thromboembolism Prophylaxis[2,3]	19	95%	94%	92%
Incidence of Potentially Preventable VTE[1,2]	-	-	7%	10%
UFH with Dosages/Platelet Monitoring[1,2]	-	-	97%	97%
Venous Thromboembolism Prophylaxis[2,3]	232	94%	90%	85%
Warfarin Therapy Discharge Instructions[2,3]	24	92%	78%	75%
Chest Pain/Possible Heart Attack Care				
Aspirin Given Within 24 Hours of Arrival[5]	-	-	100%	96%
Fibrinolytic Meds Within 30 Min. of Arrival[5]	-	-	-	58%
Average Time to ECG (minutes)[5]	-	-	6	7
Average Time to Transfer (minutes)[5]	-	-	32	60
Children's Asthma Care				
Received Home Management Plan of Care	-	-	-	88%
Received Reliever Medication	-	-	-	100%
Received Systemic Corticosteroids	-	-	-	100%
Emergency Department				
Admittance Decision Time (minutes)[2]	825	109	143	98
Head CT Results Within 45 Min. of Arrival[5]	-	-	-	57%
Patients Who Left ER Before Being Seen[5]	-	-	3%	2%
Time from ER Arrival to Admit. (minutes)[2]	862	353	357	274
Time from ER Arrival to Discharge (minutes)[5]	-	-	-	134
Time in ER Before Being Evaluated (minutes)[5]	-	-	-	26
Time to Pain Meds for Fractures (minutes)[5]	-	-	-	57
Heart Attack Care				
Aspirin Given at Discharge	45	98%	99%	99%
Fibrinolytic Meds Within 30 Min. of Arrival[7]	-	-	-	54%
PCI Within 90 Minutes of Arrival[3,7]	-	-	93%	96%
Statin Prescribed at Discharge	40	92%	98%	98%
Heart Failure Care				
ACE Inhibitor or ARB for LVSD[2]	138	99%	97%	97%
Discharge Instructions Given[2]	338	96%	93%	94%
Evaluation of LVS Function[2]	417	100%	99%	99%
Medicare Spending				
Medicare Spending per Patient (ratio)	-	-	-	0.98
Pneumonia Care				
Appropriate Initial Antibiotic Given	157	94%	97%	95%
Blood Culture Timing	186	96%	97%	98%
Pregnancy and Delivery Care				
Newborn Deliveries Scheduled Early[5]	-	-	-	6%
Preventive Care				
Immunization for Influenza[2]	529	96%	94%	90%
Immunization for Pneumonia[2]	694	95%	94%	92%
Stroke Care				
Anticoagulation Therapy for Atrial Fibrillation[5]	-	-	95%	95%
Antithrombotic Therapy Timing[5]	-	-	95%	98%
Assessed for Rehabilitation[5]	-	-	96%	97%
Discharged on Antithrombotic Therapy[5]	-	-	95%	99%
Discharged on Statin Medication[5]	-	-	97%	94%
Thrombolytic Therapy Timing[5]	-	-	-	66%
Venous Thromboembolism Prophylaxis[5]	-	-	89%	94%
Written Stroke Educational Materials Given[5]	-	-	77%	88%
Surgical Care Improvement Project				
Appropriate Beta Blocker Usage	216	96%	97%	98%
Appropriate VTP Within 24 Hours	565	97%	98%	98%
Controlled Postoperative Blood Glucose[7]	-	-	96%	97%
Perioperative Temperature Management	668	100%	100%	100%
Prophylactic Antibiotic Selection	498	99%	99%	99%
Prophylactic Antibiotic Selection (Outpatient)[5]	-	-	98%	98%
Prophylactic Antibiotic Stopped	490	97%	98%	98%
Prophylactic Antibiotic Timing	499	99%	97%	99%
Prophylactic Antibiotic Timing (Outpatient)[5]	-	-	98%	98%
Urinary Catheter Removal	477	97%	98%	97%
Survey of Patients' Hospital Experiences				
Area Around Room 'Always' Quiet at Night	300+	55%	57%	61%
Doctors 'Always' Communicated Well	300+	82%	78%	82%
Home Recovery Information Given	300+	85%	85%	85%
Hospital Given 9 or 10 on 10 Point Scale	300+	64%	65%	71%
Meds 'Always' Explained Before Given	300+	61%	58%	64%
Nurses 'Always' Communicated Well	300+	79%	75%	79%
Pain 'Always' Well Controlled	300+	70%	67%	71%
Room and Bathroom 'Always' Clean	300+	65%	64%	73%
Timely Help 'Always' Received	300+	67%	58%	68%
Would Definitely Recommend Hospital	300+	66%	67%	71%
Use of Medical Imaging				
Cardiac Imaging Stress Test before Surgery	193	5.7%	6.4%	5.3%
Combination Abdominal CT Scan	1,061	6.1%	3.8%	10.5%
Combination Brain/Sinus CT Scan	1,439	3.3%	4.3%	2.7%
Combination Chest CT Scan	438	0.2%	1%	2.7%
Follow-up Mammogram/Ultrasound	917	10.7%	10.2%	8.8%
Lumbar Spine MRI for Low Back Pain	132	40.9%	38.2%	37.2%

Union Hospital of Cecil County

106 Bow Street
Elkton, MD 21921
Phone: 410-392-7009
Fax: 410-392-9486
URL: www.uhcc.com
Type: Acute Care Hospitals
Emergency Services: Yes
Ownership: Voluntary non-profit - Private
Beds: 116

Key Personnel:

Quality Assurance . . . . Michelle Adams
Chief of Medical Staff . . . . Paticia Clark
Pulmonology . . . . Theodora Fynn, MD
Radiology . . . . Constance Gerassimak
CEO/President . . . . Kenneth S Lewis, MD
Infection Control . . . . Helen Paxton
Emergency Room . . . . Jeffrey Tiongson, MD

Measure	Cases	This Hosp.	State Avg.	U.S. Avg.
Blood Clot Prevention and Treatment				
Anticoagulation Overlap Therapy	22	100%	94%	93%
ICU Venous Thromboembolism Prophylaxis	120	100%	94%	92%
Incidence of Potentially Preventable VTE[1]	-	-	7%	10%
UFH with Dosages/Platelet Monitoring	16	100%	97%	97%
Venous Thromboembolism Prophylaxis	645	96%	90%	85%
Warfarin Therapy Discharge Instructions	16	81%	78%	75%
Chest Pain/Possible Heart Attack Care				
Aspirin Given Within 24 Hours of Arrival[5]	-	-	100%	96%
Fibrinolytic Meds Within 30 Min. of Arrival[5]	-	-	-	58%
Average Time to ECG (minutes)[5]	-	-	6	7
Average Time to Transfer (minutes)[5]	-	-	32	60
Children's Asthma Care				
Received Home Management Plan of Care	-	-	-	88%
Received Reliever Medication	-	-	-	100%
Received Systemic Corticosteroids	-	-	-	100%
Emergency Department				
Admittance Decision Time (minutes)	1,184	96	143	98
Head CT Results Within 45 Min. of Arrival[5]	-	-	-	57%
Patients Who Left ER Before Being Seen[5]	-	-	3%	2%
Time from ER Arrival to Admit. (minutes)	1,187	307	357	274
Time from ER Arrival to Discharge (minutes)[5]	-	-	-	134
Time in ER Before Being Evaluated (minutes)[5]	-	-	-	26
Time to Pain Meds for Fractures (minutes)[5]	-	-	-	57
Heart Attack Care				
Aspirin Given at Discharge	20	100%	99%	99%
Fibrinolytic Meds Within 30 Min. of Arrival[7]	-	-	-	54%
PCI Within 90 Minutes of Arrival[7]	-	-	93%	96%
Statin Prescribed at Discharge	17	100%	98%	98%
Heart Failure Care				
ACE Inhibitor or ARB for LVSD	16	100%	97%	97%
Discharge Instructions Given	57	100%	93%	94%
Evaluation of LVS Function	78	100%	99%	99%
Medicare Spending				
Medicare Spending per Patient (ratio)	-	-	-	0.98
Pneumonia Care				
Appropriate Initial Antibiotic Given	124	98%	97%	95%
Blood Culture Timing	227	97%	97%	98%
Pregnancy and Delivery Care				
Newborn Deliveries Scheduled Early[5]	-	-	-	6%
Preventive Care				
Immunization for Influenza	782	97%	94%	90%
Immunization for Pneumonia	1,122	99%	94%	92%
Stroke Care				
Anticoagulation Therapy for Atrial Fibrillation[5]	-	-	95%	95%
Antithrombotic Therapy Timing[5]	-	-	95%	98%
Assessed for Rehabilitation[5]	-	-	96%	97%
Discharged on Antithrombotic Therapy[5]	-	-	95%	99%
Discharged on Statin Medication[5]	-	-	97%	94%
Thrombolytic Therapy Timing[5]	-	-	-	66%
Venous Thromboembolism Prophylaxis[5]	-	-	89%	94%
Written Stroke Educational Materials Given[5]	-	-	77%	88%
Surgical Care Improvement Project				
Appropriate Beta Blocker Usage	105	100%	97%	98%
Appropriate VTP Within 24 Hours	282	99%	98%	98%
Controlled Postoperative Blood Glucose[7]	-	-	96%	97%
Perioperative Temperature Management	312	99%	100%	100%
Prophylactic Antibiotic Selection	184	98%	99%	99%
Prophylactic Antibiotic Selection (Outpatient)[5]	-	-	98%	98%
Prophylactic Antibiotic Stopped	177	98%	98%	98%
Prophylactic Antibiotic Timing	184	99%	97%	99%
Prophylactic Antibiotic Timing (Outpatient)[5]	-	-	98%	98%
Urinary Catheter Removal	241	98%	98%	97%
Survey of Patients' Hospital Experiences				
Area Around Room 'Always' Quiet at Night	300+	51%	57%	61%
Doctors 'Always' Communicated Well	300+	77%	78%	82%
Home Recovery Information Given	300+	90%	85%	85%
Hospital Given 9 or 10 on 10 Point Scale	300+	59%	65%	71%
Meds 'Always' Explained Before Given	300+	56%	58%	64%
Nurses 'Always' Communicated Well	300+	73%	75%	79%
Pain 'Always' Well Controlled	300+	60%	67%	71%
Room and Bathroom 'Always' Clean	300+	62%	64%	73%
Timely Help 'Always' Received	300+	59%	58%	68%
Would Definitely Recommend Hospital	300+	62%	67%	71%
Use of Medical Imaging				
Cardiac Imaging Stress Test before Surgery	267	4.5%	6.4%	5.3%
Combination Abdominal CT Scan	972	7.0%	3.8%	10.5%
Combination Brain/Sinus CT Scan	648	1.9%	4.3%	2.7%
Combination Chest CT Scan	691	1.0%	1%	2.7%
Follow-up Mammogram/Ultrasound	1,228	9.4%	10.2%	8.8%
Lumbar Spine MRI for Low Back Pain	82	42.7%	38.2%	37.2%

Fort Washington Hospital

11711 Livingston Road
Fort Washington, MD 20744
Phone: 301-292-7000
Fax: 301-203-2216
URL: www.fortwashington.org
Type: Acute Care Hospitals
Emergency Services: Yes
Ownership: Voluntary non-profit - Other
Beds: 43

Key Personnel:

Chief of Medical Staff . . . . Samir Azer, MD
Radiology . . . . Vimla Bhooshan
Emergency Room . . . . Patrick Daly, MD
CEO/President . . . . Verna S. Meacham, CEO
Intensive Care Unit . . . . Amir Mirza-Alikhani, MD
Operating Room . . . . Socorro Obedoza
Infection Control . . . . Carmen Resusseccion, RN
Anesthesiology . . . . Christopher Smith, MD

Measure	Cases	This Hosp.	State Avg.	U.S. Avg.
Blood Clot Prevention and Treatment				
Anticoagulation Overlap Therapy[2]	26	96%	94%	93%
ICU Venous Thromboembolism Prophylaxis[2]	33	97%	94%	92%
Incidence of Potentially Preventable VTE[1,2]	-	-	7%	10%
UFH with Dosages/Platelet Monitoring[1,2]	-	-	97%	97%
Venous Thromboembolism Prophylaxis[2]	230	93%	90%	85%
Warfarin Therapy Discharge Instructions[2]	23	87%	78%	75%
Chest Pain/Possible Heart Attack Care				
Aspirin Given Within 24 Hours of Arrival[5]	-	-	100%	96%
Fibrinolytic Meds Within 30 Min. of Arrival[5]	-	-	-	58%
Average Time to ECG (minutes)[5]	-	-	6	7
Average Time to Transfer (minutes)[5]	-	-	32	60
Children's Asthma Care				
Received Home Management Plan of Care	-	-	-	88%
Received Reliever Medication	-	-	-	100%
Received Systemic Corticosteroids	-	-	-	100%
Emergency Department				
Admittance Decision Time (minutes)[2]	413	85	143	98
Head CT Results Within 45 Min. of Arrival[5]	-	-	-	57%
Patients Who Left ER Before Being Seen[5]	-	-	3%	2%
Time from ER Arrival to Admit. (minutes)[2]	453	256	357	274
Time from ER Arrival to Discharge (minutes)[5]	-	-	-	134
Time in ER Before Being Evaluated (minutes)[5]	-	-	-	26
Time to Pain Meds for Fractures (minutes)[5]	-	-	-	57
Heart Attack Care				
Aspirin Given at Discharge[1]	-	-	99%	99%

NOTE: Hospital profiles are in alphabetical order by state, then city, then hospital within the city; Rankings exclude hospitals with less than 25 cases except for patient surveys which excludes hospitals with less than 100 cases; (a) 100-299 cases; (1) The number of cases/patients is too few to report; (2) Data submitted were based on a sample of cases/patients; (3) Results are based on a shorter time period than required; (4) Data suppressed by CMS for one or more quarters; (5) Results are not available for this reporting period; (6) Fewer than 100 patients completed the HCAHPS survey; (7) No cases met the criteria for this measure; (8) The lower limit of the confidence interval cannot be calculated if the number of observed infections equals zero; (9) No data are available from the state/territory for this reporting period; (10) The scores shown reflect fewer than 50 completed surveys; (11) There were discrepancies in the data collection process; (12) This measure does not apply to this hospital for this reporting period; (13) Results cannot be calculated for this reporting period; (14) The results for this state are combined with nearby states to protect confidentiality; Please refer to the User's Guide for a full explanation of data.

Measure	Cases	This Hosp.	State Avg.	U.S. Avg.
Fibrinolytic Meds Within 30 Min. of Arrival[7]	-	-	-	54%
PCI Within 90 Minutes of Arrival[3,7]	-	-	93%	96%
Statin Prescribed at Discharge[1]	-	-	98%	98%
Heart Failure Care				
ACE Inhibitor or ARB for LVSD	49	98%	97%	97%
Discharge Instructions Given	118	99%	93%	94%
Evaluation of LVS Function	138	99%	99%	99%
Medicare Spending				
Medicare Spending per Patient (ratio)	-	-	-	0.98
Pneumonia Care				
Appropriate Initial Antibiotic Given	46	100%	97%	95%
Blood Culture Timing	75	95%	97%	98%
Pregnancy and Delivery Care				
Newborn Deliveries Scheduled Early[5]	-	-	-	6%
Preventive Care				
Immunization for Influenza[2]	289	95%	94%	90%
Immunization for Pneumonia[2]	417	93%	94%	92%
Stroke Care				
Anticoagulation Therapy for Atrial Fibrillation[5]	-	-	95%	95%
Antithrombotic Therapy Timing[5]	-	-	95%	98%
Assessed for Rehabilitation[5]	-	-	96%	97%
Discharged on Antithrombotic Therapy[5]	-	-	95%	99%
Discharged on Statin Medication[5]	-	-	97%	94%
Thrombolytic Therapy Timing[5]	-	-	-	66%
Venous Thromboembolism Prophylaxis[5]	-	-	89%	94%
Written Stroke Educational Materials Given[5]	-	-	77%	88%
Surgical Care Improvement Project				
Appropriate Beta Blocker Usage	30	97%	97%	98%
Appropriate VTP Within 24 Hours	134	99%	98%	98%
Controlled Postoperative Blood Glucose[3,7]	-	-	96%	97%
Perioperative Temperature Management	141	100%	100%	100%
Prophylactic Antibiotic Selection	95	100%	99%	99%
Prophylactic Antibiotic Selection (Outpatient)[5]	-	-	98%	98%
Prophylactic Antibiotic Stopped	93	98%	98%	98%
Prophylactic Antibiotic Timing	95	100%	97%	99%
Prophylactic Antibiotic Timing (Outpatient)[5]	-	-	98%	98%
Urinary Catheter Removal	34	100%	98%	97%
Survey of Patients' Hospital Experiences				
Area Around Room 'Always' Quiet at Night	(a)	53%	57%	61%
Doctors 'Always' Communicated Well	(a)	75%	78%	82%
Home Recovery Information Given	(a)	77%	85%	85%
Hospital Given 9 or 10 on 10 Point Scale	(a)	48%	65%	71%
Meds 'Always' Explained Before Given	(a)	50%	58%	64%
Nurses 'Always' Communicated Well	(a)	67%	75%	79%
Pain 'Always' Well Controlled	(a)	59%	67%	71%
Room and Bathroom 'Always' Clean	(a)	54%	64%	73%
Timely Help 'Always' Received	(a)	51%	58%	68%
Would Definitely Recommend Hospital	(a)	52%	67%	71%
Use of Medical Imaging				
Cardiac Imaging Stress Test before Surgery[1]	-	-	6.4%	5.3%
Combination Abdominal CT Scan	401	1.7%	3.8%	10.5%
Combination Brain/Sinus CT Scan	605	2.1%	4.3%	2.7%
Combination Chest CT Scan	64	0.0%	1%	2.7%
Follow-up Mammogram/Ultrasound	158	13.9%	10.2%	8.8%
Lumbar Spine MRI for Low Back Pain[7]	-	-	38.2%	37.2%

Frederick Memorial Hospital

400 West Seventh St — Phone: 240-566-3300
Frederick, MD 21701 — Fax: 301-698-3292
URL: www.fmh.org
Type: Acute Care Hospitals — Emergency Services: Yes
Ownership: Voluntary non-profit - Private — Beds: 253

Key Personnel:
Chief of Medical Staff.......... Gene Ashe
Emergency Room .... Laila Beaulieu
Radiology.................. Tom Bonnor
President/CEO.............. Thomas A Kleinhanzl
Pediatric In-Patient Care .... James Lee
Cardiac Laboratory........... Michael Levangie
Quality Assurance .... Craig Rosendale
Operating Room............. Katherine Smith, RN

Measure	Cases	This Hosp.	State Avg.	U.S. Avg.
Blood Clot Prevention and Treatment				
Anticoagulation Overlap Therapy[2]	146	97%	94%	93%
ICU Venous Thromboembolism Prophylaxis[2]	49	98%	94%	92%
Incidence of Potentially Preventable VTE[2]	21	5%	7%	10%
UFH with Dosages/Platelet Monitoring[2]	180	100%	97%	97%
Venous Thromboembolism Prophylaxis[2]	319	89%	90%	85%
Warfarin Therapy Discharge Instructions[2]	107	70%	78%	75%
Chest Pain/Possible Heart Attack Care				
Aspirin Given Within 24 Hours of Arrival[5]	-	-	100%	96%
Fibrinolytic Meds Within 30 Min. of Arrival[5]	-	-	-	58%
Average Time to ECG (minutes)[5]	-	-	6	7
Average Time to Transfer (minutes)[5]	-	-	32	60
Children's Asthma Care				
Received Home Management Plan of Care	-	-	-	88%
Received Reliever Medication	-	-	-	100%
Received Systemic Corticosteroids	-	-	-	100%
Emergency Department				
Admittance Decision Time (minutes)[2]	675	110	143	98
Head CT Results Within 45 Min. of Arrival[5]	-	-	-	57%
Patients Who Left ER Before Being Seen[5]	-	-	3%	2%
Time from ER Arrival to Admit. (minutes)[2]	694	349	357	274
Time from ER Arrival to Discharge (minutes)[5]	-	-	-	134
Time in ER Before Being Evaluated (minutes)[5]	-	-	-	26
Time to Pain Meds for Fractures (minutes)[5]	-	-	-	57
Heart Attack Care				
Aspirin Given at Discharge	216	100%	99%	99%
Fibrinolytic Meds Within 30 Min. of Arrival[7]	-	-	-	54%
PCI Within 90 Minutes of Arrival	88	100%	93%	96%
Statin Prescribed at Discharge	208	100%	98%	98%
Heart Failure Care				
ACE Inhibitor or ARB for LVSD	102	100%	97%	97%
Discharge Instructions Given	325	93%	93%	94%
Evaluation of LVS Function	430	100%	99%	99%
Medicare Spending				
Medicare Spending per Patient (ratio)	-	-	-	0.98
Pneumonia Care				
Appropriate Initial Antibiotic Given	269	99%	97%	95%
Blood Culture Timing	285	99%	97%	98%
Pregnancy and Delivery Care				
Newborn Deliveries Scheduled Early[5]	-	-	-	6%
Preventive Care				
Immunization for Influenza[2]	511	94%	94%	90%
Immunization for Pneumonia[2]	606	88%	94%	92%
Stroke Care				
Anticoagulation Therapy for Atrial Fibrillation[5]	-	-	95%	95%
Antithrombotic Therapy Timing[5]	-	-	95%	98%
Assessed for Rehabilitation[5]	-	-	96%	97%
Discharged on Antithrombotic Therapy[5]	-	-	95%	99%
Discharged on Statin Medication[5]	-	-	97%	94%
Thrombolytic Therapy Timing[5]	-	-	-	66%
Venous Thromboembolism Prophylaxis[5]	-	-	89%	94%
Written Stroke Educational Materials Given[5]	-	-	77%	88%
Surgical Care Improvement Project				
Appropriate Beta Blocker Usage[2]	262	99%	97%	98%
Appropriate VTP Within 24 Hours[2]	751	99%	98%	98%
Controlled Postoperative Blood Glucose[2,7]	-	-	96%	97%
Perioperative Temperature Management[2]	873	100%	100%	100%
Prophylactic Antibiotic Selection[2]	675	99%	99%	99%
Prophylactic Antibiotic Selection (Outpatient)[5]	-	-	98%	98%
Prophylactic Antibiotic Stopped[2]	655	99%	98%	98%
Prophylactic Antibiotic Timing[2]	675	100%	97%	99%
Prophylactic Antibiotic Timing (Outpatient)[5]	-	-	98%	98%
Urinary Catheter Removal[2]	638	100%	98%	97%
Survey of Patients' Hospital Experiences				
Area Around Room 'Always' Quiet at Night	300+	60%	57%	61%
Doctors 'Always' Communicated Well	300+	77%	78%	82%
Home Recovery Information Given	300+	87%	85%	85%
Hospital Given 9 or 10 on 10 Point Scale	300+	68%	65%	71%
Meds 'Always' Explained Before Given	300+	60%	58%	64%
Nurses 'Always' Communicated Well	300+	79%	75%	79%
Pain 'Always' Well Controlled	300+	71%	67%	71%
Room and Bathroom 'Always' Clean	300+	72%	64%	73%
Timely Help 'Always' Received	300+	62%	58%	68%
Would Definitely Recommend Hospital	300+	67%	67%	71%
Use of Medical Imaging				
Cardiac Imaging Stress Test before Surgery[7]	-	-	6.4%	5.3%
Combination Abdominal CT Scan	879	5.3%	3.8%	10.5%
Combination Brain/Sinus CT Scan	1,221	3.3%	4.3%	2.7%
Combination Chest CT Scan	246	4.1%	1%	2.7%
Follow-up Mammogram/Ultrasound[7]	-	-	10.2%	8.8%
Lumbar Spine MRI for Low Back Pain[1]	-	-	38.2%	37.2%

University of MD Balto Washington Medical Center

301 Hospital Drive — Phone: 410-595-1967
Glen Burnie, MD 21061 — Fax: 410-595-1958
URL: www.bwmc.umms.org
Type: Acute Care Hospitals — Emergency Services: Yes
Ownership: Voluntary non-profit - Other — Beds: 286

Key Personnel:
Radiology.................. James Cary
Quality Assurance .... Lynda Dabrowski
Infection Control............. Donna Lemmert
Chief of Medical Staff.......... Lawrence Linder, MD, FACEP
Operating Room............. Joyce Myers, RN
CEO/President............... Karen E. Olscamp
Emergency Room .... Carol Ann Sperry, RN
Pediatric Ambulatory Care ...... Eric Sundel, MD

Measure	Cases	This Hosp.	State Avg.	U.S. Avg.
Blood Clot Prevention and Treatment				
Anticoagulation Overlap Therapy[2,3]	129	95%	94%	93%
ICU Venous Thromboembolism Prophylaxis[2,3]	57	96%	94%	92%
Incidence of Potentially Preventable VTE[2,3]	27	4%	7%	10%
UFH with Dosages/Platelet Monitoring[2,3]	70	100%	97%	97%
Venous Thromboembolism Prophylaxis[2,3]	209	99%	90%	85%
Warfarin Therapy Discharge Instructions[2,3]	83	99%	78%	75%
Chest Pain/Possible Heart Attack Care				
Aspirin Given Within 24 Hours of Arrival[5]	-	-	100%	96%
Fibrinolytic Meds Within 30 Min. of Arrival[5]	-	-	-	58%
Average Time to ECG (minutes)[5]	-	-	6	7
Average Time to Transfer (minutes)[5]	-	-	32	60
Children's Asthma Care				
Received Home Management Plan of Care	48	94%	-	88%
Received Reliever Medication	50	100%	-	100%
Received Systemic Corticosteroids	50	100%	-	100%
Emergency Department				
Admittance Decision Time (minutes)[2]	1,245	183	143	98
Head CT Results Within 45 Min. of Arrival[5]	-	-	-	57%
Patients Who Left ER Before Being Seen[5]	-	-	3%	2%
Time from ER Arrival to Admit. (minutes)[2]	1,248	386	357	274
Time from ER Arrival to Discharge (minutes)[5]	-	-	-	134
Time in ER Before Being Evaluated (minutes)[5]	-	-	-	26
Time to Pain Meds for Fractures (minutes)[5]	-	-	-	57
Heart Attack Care				
Aspirin Given at Discharge	222	100%	99%	99%
Fibrinolytic Meds Within 30 Min. of Arrival[7]	-	-	-	54%
PCI Within 90 Minutes of Arrival	87	97%	93%	96%
Statin Prescribed at Discharge	218	100%	98%	98%
Heart Failure Care				
ACE Inhibitor or ARB for LVSD	169	100%	97%	97%
Discharge Instructions Given	553	95%	93%	94%
Evaluation of LVS Function	627	100%	99%	99%
Medicare Spending				
Medicare Spending per Patient (ratio)	-	-	-	0.98
Pneumonia Care				
Appropriate Initial Antibiotic Given	418	98%	97%	95%
Blood Culture Timing	280	98%	97%	98%
Pregnancy and Delivery Care				
Newborn Deliveries Scheduled Early[5]	-	-	-	6%
Preventive Care				
Immunization for Influenza[2]	824	89%	94%	90%
Immunization for Pneumonia[2]	1,112	93%	94%	92%
Stroke Care				
Anticoagulation Therapy for Atrial Fibrillation[5]	-	-	95%	95%
Antithrombotic Therapy Timing[5]	-	-	95%	98%
Assessed for Rehabilitation[5]	-	-	96%	97%
Discharged on Antithrombotic Therapy[5]	-	-	95%	99%
Discharged on Statin Medication[5]	-	-	97%	94%
Thrombolytic Therapy Timing[5]	-	-	-	66%

NOTE: Hospital profiles are in alphabetical order by state, then city, then hospital within the city; Rankings exclude hospitals with less than 25 cases except for patient surveys which excludes hospitals with less than 100 cases; (a) 100-299 cases; (1) The number of cases/patients is too few to report; (2) Data submitted were based on a sample of cases/patients; (3) Results are based on a shorter time period than required; (4) Data suppressed by CMS for one or more quarters; (5) Results are not available for this reporting period; (6) Fewer than 100 patients completed the HCAHPS survey; (7) No cases met the criteria for this measure; (8) The lower limit of the confidence interval cannot be calculated if the number of observed infections equals zero; (9) No data are available from the state/territory for this reporting period; (10) The scores shown reflect fewer than 50 completed surveys; (11) There were discrepancies in the data collection process; (12) This measure does not apply to this hospital for this reporting period; (13) Results cannot be calculated for this reporting period; (14) The results for this state are combined with nearby states to protect confidentiality; Please refer to the User's Guide for a full explanation of data.

Venous Thromboembolism Prophylaxis[5]	-	-	89%	94%
Written Stroke Educational Materials Given[5]	-	-	77%	88%
Surgical Care Improvement Project				
Appropriate Beta Blocker Usage[2]	306	99%	97%	98%
Appropriate VTP Within 24 Hours[2]	726	99%	98%	98%
Controlled Postoperative Blood Glucose[2,3]	-	-	96%	97%
Perioperative Temperature Management[2]	914	100%	100%	100%
Prophylactic Antibiotic Selection[2]	656	100%	99%	99%
Prophylactic Antibiotic Selection (Outpatient)[5]	-	-	98%	98%
Prophylactic Antibiotic Stopped[2]	637	100%	98%	98%
Prophylactic Antibiotic Timing[2]	656	100%	97%	99%
Prophylactic Antibiotic Timing (Outpatient)[5]	-	-	98%	98%
Urinary Catheter Removal[2]	350	100%	98%	97%
Survey of Patients' Hospital Experiences				
Area Around Room 'Always' Quiet at Night	300+	56%	57%	61%
Doctors 'Always' Communicated Well	300+	78%	78%	82%
Home Recovery Information Given	300+	86%	85%	85%
Hospital Given 9 or 10 on 10 Point Scale	300+	67%	65%	71%
Meds 'Always' Explained Before Given	300+	60%	58%	64%
Nurses 'Always' Communicated Well	300+	76%	75%	79%
Pain 'Always' Well Controlled	300+	69%	67%	71%
Room and Bathroom 'Always' Clean	300+	66%	64%	73%
Timely Help 'Always' Received	300+	59%	58%	68%
Would Definitely Recommend Hospital	300+	69%	67%	71%
Use of Medical Imaging				
Cardiac Imaging Stress Test before Surgery	541	6.3%	6.4%	5.3%
Combination Abdominal CT Scan	1,066	0.7%	3.8%	10.5%
Combination Brain/Sinus CT Scan	1,790	4.9%	4.3%	2.7%
Combination Chest CT Scan	401	0.0%	1%	2.7%
Follow-up Mammogram/Ultrasound[7]	-	-	10.2%	8.8%
Lumbar Spine MRI for Low Back Pain[1]	-	-	38.2%	37.2%

Meritus Medical Center

11116 Medical Campus Road Phone: 240-313-9500
Hagerstown, MD 21742
URL: www.meritushealth.com
Type: Acute Care Hospitals Emergency Services: Yes
Ownership: Voluntary non-profit - Private Beds: 341

Key Personnel:
Chief of Medical Staff. . . . . Heather Lorenzo, MD
President/CEO. . . . . Joseph P Ross

Measure	Cases	This Hosp.	State Avg.	U.S. Avg.
Blood Clot Prevention and Treatment				
Anticoagulation Overlap Therapy	154	93%	94%	93%
ICU Venous Thromboembolism Prophylaxis	1,148	96%	94%	92%
Incidence of Potentially Preventable VTE	19	5%	7%	10%
UFH with Dosages/Platelet Monitoring	140	98%	97%	97%
Venous Thromboembolism Prophylaxis	5,414	93%	90%	85%
Warfarin Therapy Discharge Instructions	119	92%	78%	75%
Chest Pain/Possible Heart Attack Care				
Aspirin Given Within 24 Hours of Arrival[5]	-	-	100%	96%
Fibrinolytic Meds Within 30 Min. of Arrival[5]	-	-	-	58%
Average Time to ECG (minutes)[5]	-	-	6	7
Average Time to Transfer (minutes)[5]	-	-	32	60
Children's Asthma Care				
Received Home Management Plan of Care	-	-	-	88%
Received Reliever Medication	-	-	-	100%
Received Systemic Corticosteroids	-	-	-	100%
Emergency Department				
Admittance Decision Time (minutes)[2]	5,070	192	143	98
Head CT Results Within 45 Min. of Arrival[5]	-	-	-	57%
Patients Who Left ER Before Being Seen[5]	-	-	3%	2%
Time from ER Arrival to Admit. (minutes)[2]	5,144	362	357	274
Time from ER Arrival to Discharge (minutes)[5]	-	-	-	134
Time in ER Before Being Evaluated (minutes)[5]	-	-	-	26
Time to Pain Meds for Fractures (minutes)[5]	-	-	-	57
Heart Attack Care				
Aspirin Given at Discharge	124	98%	99%	99%
Fibrinolytic Meds Within 30 Min. of Arrival[7]	-	-	-	54%
PCI Within 90 Minutes of Arrival	54	100%	93%	96%
Statin Prescribed at Discharge	117	97%	98%	98%
Heart Failure Care				
ACE Inhibitor or ARB for LVSD	61	97%	97%	97%
Discharge Instructions Given	250	94%	93%	94%
Evaluation of LVS Function	310	100%	99%	99%
Medicare Spending				
Medicare Spending per Patient (ratio)	-	-	-	0.98
Pneumonia Care				
Appropriate Initial Antibiotic Given	437	93%	97%	95%
Blood Culture Timing	741	96%	97%	98%
Pregnancy and Delivery Care				
Newborn Deliveries Scheduled Early[5]	-	-	-	6%
Preventive Care				
Immunization for Influenza[2]	7,246	97%	94%	90%
Immunization for Pneumonia[2]	5,069	96%	94%	92%
Stroke Care				
Anticoagulation Therapy for Atrial Fibrillation[5]	-	-	95%	95%
Antithrombotic Therapy Timing[5]	-	-	95%	98%
Assessed for Rehabilitation[5]	-	-	96%	97%
Discharged on Antithrombotic Therapy[5]	-	-	95%	99%
Discharged on Statin Medication[5]	-	-	97%	94%
Thrombolytic Therapy Timing[5]	-	-	-	66%
Venous Thromboembolism Prophylaxis[5]	-	-	89%	94%
Written Stroke Educational Materials Given[5]	-	-	77%	88%
Surgical Care Improvement Project				
Appropriate Beta Blocker Usage	378	95%	97%	98%
Appropriate VTP Within 24 Hours	1,072	99%	98%	98%
Controlled Postoperative Blood Glucose[7]	-	-	96%	97%
Perioperative Temperature Management	1,184	100%	100%	100%
Prophylactic Antibiotic Selection	758	100%	99%	99%
Prophylactic Antibiotic Selection (Outpatient)[5]	-	-	98%	98%
Prophylactic Antibiotic Stopped	740	98%	98%	98%
Prophylactic Antibiotic Timing	759	98%	97%	99%
Prophylactic Antibiotic Timing (Outpatient)[5]	-	-	98%	98%
Urinary Catheter Removal	455	95%	98%	97%
Survey of Patients' Hospital Experiences				
Area Around Room 'Always' Quiet at Night	300+	56%	57%	61%
Doctors 'Always' Communicated Well	300+	75%	78%	82%
Home Recovery Information Given	300+	84%	85%	85%
Hospital Given 9 or 10 on 10 Point Scale	300+	66%	65%	71%
Meds 'Always' Explained Before Given	300+	56%	58%	64%
Nurses 'Always' Communicated Well	300+	75%	75%	79%
Pain 'Always' Well Controlled	300+	68%	67%	71%
Room and Bathroom 'Always' Clean	300+	68%	64%	73%
Timely Help 'Always' Received	300+	57%	58%	68%
Would Definitely Recommend Hospital	300+	64%	67%	71%
Use of Medical Imaging				
Cardiac Imaging Stress Test before Surgery[1]	-	-	6.4%	5.3%
Combination Abdominal CT Scan	1,218	0.7%	3.8%	10.5%
Combination Brain/Sinus CT Scan	1,468	2.8%	4.3%	2.7%
Combination Chest CT Scan	287	0.3%	1%	2.7%
Follow-up Mammogram/Ultrasound[7]	-	-	10.2%	8.8%
Lumbar Spine MRI for Low Back Pain[1]	-	-	38.2%	37.2%

Harford Memorial Hospital

501 South Union Avenue Phone: 443-643-3303
Havre De Grace, MD 21078 Fax: 443-643-3404
URL: www.uchs.org
Type: Acute Care Hospitals Emergency Services: Yes
Ownership: Voluntary non-profit - Private Beds: 102

Key Personnel:
Emergency Room . . . . Fermin Barrueto, MD
Surgery . . . . Mark Gonze, MD
Pediatrics. . . . . Paul Lomonico, MD
Radiology. . . . . Brain Monroe, MD
Anesthesiology. . . . . Rodger Oursler, MD
President . . . . Angela Poppe Ries, MD
President/CEO. . . . . Lyle Ernest Sheldon, FACHE
Chief of Medical Staff. . . . . Peggy Vaughan

Measure	Cases	This Hosp.	State Avg.	U.S. Avg.
Blood Clot Prevention and Treatment				
Anticoagulation Overlap Therapy[2]	20	80%	94%	93%
ICU Venous Thromboembolism Prophylaxis[2]	34	94%	94%	92%
Incidence of Potentially Preventable VTE[1,2]	-	-	7%	10%
UFH with Dosages/Platelet Monitoring[2]	18	100%	97%	97%
Venous Thromboembolism Prophylaxis[2]	280	96%	90%	85%
Warfarin Therapy Discharge Instructions[2]	14	79%	78%	75%
Chest Pain/Possible Heart Attack Care				
Aspirin Given Within 24 Hours of Arrival[5]	-	-	100%	96%
Fibrinolytic Meds Within 30 Min. of Arrival[5]	-	-	-	58%
Average Time to ECG (minutes)[5]	-	-	6	7
Average Time to Transfer (minutes)[5]	-	-	32	60
Children's Asthma Care				
Received Home Management Plan of Care	-	-	-	88%
Received Reliever Medication	-	-	-	100%
Received Systemic Corticosteroids	-	-	-	100%
Emergency Department				
Admittance Decision Time (minutes)[2]	391	116	143	98
Head CT Results Within 45 Min. of Arrival[5]	-	-	-	57%
Patients Who Left ER Before Being Seen[5]	-	-	3%	2%
Time from ER Arrival to Admit. (minutes)[2]	518	336	357	274
Time from ER Arrival to Discharge (minutes)[5]	-	-	-	134
Time in ER Before Being Evaluated (minutes)[5]	-	-	-	26
Time to Pain Meds for Fractures (minutes)[5]	-	-	-	57
Heart Attack Care				
Aspirin Given at Discharge	20	100%	99%	99%
Fibrinolytic Meds Within 30 Min. of Arrival[7]	-	-	-	54%
PCI Within 90 Minutes of Arrival[3,7]	-	-	93%	96%
Statin Prescribed at Discharge	15	100%	98%	98%
Heart Failure Care				
ACE Inhibitor or ARB for LVSD	23	100%	97%	97%
Discharge Instructions Given	124	98%	93%	94%
Evaluation of LVS Function	151	100%	99%	99%
Medicare Spending				
Medicare Spending per Patient (ratio)	-	-	-	0.98
Pneumonia Care				
Appropriate Initial Antibiotic Given	121	99%	97%	95%
Blood Culture Timing	201	100%	97%	98%
Pregnancy and Delivery Care				
Newborn Deliveries Scheduled Early[5]	-	-	-	6%
Preventive Care				
Immunization for Influenza[2]	485	98%	94%	90%
Immunization for Pneumonia[2]	582	99%	94%	92%
Stroke Care				
Anticoagulation Therapy for Atrial Fibrillation[5]	-	-	95%	95%
Antithrombotic Therapy Timing[5]	-	-	95%	98%
Assessed for Rehabilitation[5]	-	-	96%	97%
Discharged on Antithrombotic Therapy[5]	-	-	95%	99%
Discharged on Statin Medication[5]	-	-	97%	94%
Thrombolytic Therapy Timing[5]	-	-	-	66%
Venous Thromboembolism Prophylaxis[5]	-	-	89%	94%
Written Stroke Educational Materials Given[5]	-	-	77%	88%
Surgical Care Improvement Project				
Appropriate Beta Blocker Usage	32	100%	97%	98%
Appropriate VTP Within 24 Hours	106	100%	98%	98%
Controlled Postoperative Blood Glucose[7]	-	-	96%	97%
Perioperative Temperature Management	118	100%	100%	100%
Prophylactic Antibiotic Selection	74	100%	99%	99%
Prophylactic Antibiotic Selection (Outpatient)[5]	-	-	98%	98%
Prophylactic Antibiotic Stopped	73	100%	98%	98%
Prophylactic Antibiotic Timing	74	99%	97%	99%
Prophylactic Antibiotic Timing (Outpatient)[5]	-	-	98%	98%
Urinary Catheter Removal	97	100%	98%	97%
Survey of Patients' Hospital Experiences				
Area Around Room 'Always' Quiet at Night	300+	56%	57%	61%
Doctors 'Always' Communicated Well	300+	79%	78%	82%
Home Recovery Information Given	300+	84%	85%	85%
Hospital Given 9 or 10 on 10 Point Scale	300+	65%	65%	71%
Meds 'Always' Explained Before Given	300+	64%	58%	64%
Nurses 'Always' Communicated Well	300+	79%	75%	79%
Pain 'Always' Well Controlled	300+	71%	67%	71%
Room and Bathroom 'Always' Clean	300+	71%	64%	73%
Timely Help 'Always' Received	300+	62%	58%	68%
Would Definitely Recommend Hospital	300+	66%	67%	71%
Use of Medical Imaging				
Cardiac Imaging Stress Test before Surgery	374	7.5%	6.4%	5.3%
Combination Abdominal CT Scan	814	7.4%	3.8%	10.5%
Combination Brain/Sinus CT Scan	813	3.9%	4.3%	2.7%
Combination Chest CT Scan	471	1.1%	1%	2.7%

NOTE: Hospital profiles are in alphabetical order by state, then city, then hospital within the city; Rankings exclude hospitals with less than 25 cases except for patient surveys which excludes hospitals with less than 100 cases; (a) 100-299 cases; (1) The number of cases/patients is too few to report; (2) Data submitted were based on a sample of cases/patients; (3) Results are based on a shorter time period than required; (4) Data suppressed by CMS for one or more quarters; (5) Results are not available for this reporting period; (6) Fewer than 100 patients completed the HCAHPS survey; (7) No cases met the criteria for this measure; (8) The lower limit of the confidence interval cannot be calculated if the number of observed infections equals zero; (9) No data are available from the state/territory for this reporting period; (10) The scores shown reflect fewer than 50 completed surveys; (11) There were discrepancies in the data collection process; (12) This measure does not apply to this hospital for this reporting period; (13) Results cannot be calculated for this reporting period; (14) The results for this state are combined with nearby states to protect confidentiality; Please refer to the User's Guide for a full explanation of data.

Follow-up Mammogram/Ultrasound	591	7.4%	10.2%	8.8%
Lumbar Spine MRI for Low Back Pain	100	37.0%	38.2%	37.2%

University of Maryland Charles Regional Medical Center

5 Garrett Avenue Phone: 301-609-4265
La Plata, MD 20646 Fax: 301-609-4191
E-mail: civistatoday@civista.org
URL: www.civista.org
Type: Acute Care Hospitals Emergency Services: Yes
Ownership: Voluntary non-profit - Private Beds: 116

Key Personnel:
Radiology. Edward Druy
Infection Control. . . . . James Dunn
Quality Assurance . . . . Florence Moran
Chief of Medical Staff. . . . . Seetaramayya Nagula, MD
Intensive Care Unit. . . . . Dana Smith
Emergency Room . . . . Stephen M Smith
CEO/President. . . . . Christine Stefanides

Measure	Cases	This Hosp.	State Avg.	U.S. Avg.
Blood Clot Prevention and Treatment				
Anticoagulation Overlap Therapy[2]	89	98%	94%	93%
ICU Venous Thromboembolism Prophylaxis[2]	69	97%	94%	92%
Incidence of Potentially Preventable VTE[2]	13	8%	7%	10%
UFH with Dosages/Platelet Monitoring[2]	35	100%	97%	97%
Venous Thromboembolism Prophylaxis[2]	385	93%	90%	85%
Warfarin Therapy Discharge Instructions[2]	74	97%	78%	75%
Chest Pain/Possible Heart Attack Care				
Aspirin Given Within 24 Hours of Arrival[5]	-	-	100%	96%
Fibrinolytic Meds Within 30 Min. of Arrival[5]	-	-	-	58%
Average Time to ECG (minutes)[5]	-	-	6	7
Average Time to Transfer (minutes)[5]	-	-	32	60
Children's Asthma Care				
Received Home Management Plan of Care	-	-	-	88%
Received Reliever Medication	-	-	-	100%
Received Systemic Corticosteroids	-	-	-	100%
Emergency Department				
Admittance Decision Time (minutes)[2]	1,060	113	143	98
Head CT Results Within 45 Min. of Arrival[5]	-	-	-	57%
Patients Who Left ER Before Being Seen[5]	-	-	3%	2%
Time from ER Arrival to Admit. (minutes)[2]	1,061	313	357	274
Time from ER Arrival to Discharge (minutes)[5]	-	-	-	134
Time in ER Before Being Evaluated (minutes)[5]	-	-	-	26
Time to Pain Meds for Fractures (minutes)[5]	-	-	-	57
Heart Attack Care				
Aspirin Given at Discharge[1]	-	-	99%	99%
Fibrinolytic Meds Within 30 Min. of Arrival[7]	-	-	-	54%
PCI Within 90 Minutes of Arrival[3,7]	-	-	93%	96%
Statin Prescribed at Discharge[1]	-	-	98%	98%
Heart Failure Care				
ACE Inhibitor or ARB for LVSD	59	100%	97%	97%
Discharge Instructions Given	213	99%	93%	94%
Evaluation of LVS Function	260	100%	99%	99%
Medicare Spending				
Medicare Spending per Patient (ratio)	-	-	-	0.98
Pneumonia Care				
Appropriate Initial Antibiotic Given[2]	98	100%	97%	95%
Blood Culture Timing[2]	155	99%	97%	98%
Pregnancy and Delivery Care				
Newborn Deliveries Scheduled Early[5]	-	-	-	6%
Preventive Care				
Immunization for Influenza[2]	611	97%	94%	90%
Immunization for Pneumonia[2]	762	95%	94%	92%
Stroke Care				
Anticoagulation Therapy for Atrial Fibrillation[5]	-	-	95%	95%
Antithrombotic Therapy Timing[5]	-	-	95%	98%
Assessed for Rehabilitation[5]	-	-	96%	97%
Discharged on Antithrombotic Therapy[5]	-	-	95%	99%
Discharged on Statin Medication[5]	-	-	97%	94%
Thrombolytic Therapy Timing[5]	-	-	-	66%
Venous Thromboembolism Prophylaxis[5]	-	-	89%	94%
Written Stroke Educational Materials Given[5]	-	-	77%	88%
Surgical Care Improvement Project				
Appropriate Beta Blocker Usage[2]	102	96%	97%	98%
Appropriate VTP Within 24 Hours[2]	330	99%	98%	98%
Controlled Postoperative Blood Glucose[2,7]	-	-	96%	97%
Perioperative Temperature Management[2]	357	100%	100%	100%
Prophylactic Antibiotic Selection[2]	232	100%	99%	99%
Prophylactic Antibiotic Selection (Outpatient)[5]	-	-	98%	98%
Prophylactic Antibiotic Stopped[2]	213	99%	98%	98%
Prophylactic Antibiotic Timing[2]	232	100%	97%	99%
Prophylactic Antibiotic Timing (Outpatient)[5]	-	-	98%	98%
Urinary Catheter Removal[2]	278	99%	98%	97%
Survey of Patients' Hospital Experiences				
Area Around Room 'Always' Quiet at Night	300+	53%	57%	61%
Doctors 'Always' Communicated Well	300+	77%	78%	82%
Home Recovery Information Given	300+	82%	85%	85%
Hospital Given 9 or 10 on 10 Point Scale	300+	59%	65%	71%
Meds 'Always' Explained Before Given	300+	56%	58%	64%
Nurses 'Always' Communicated Well	300+	71%	75%	79%
Pain 'Always' Well Controlled	300+	64%	67%	71%
Room and Bathroom 'Always' Clean	300+	66%	64%	73%
Timely Help 'Always' Received	300+	55%	58%	68%
Would Definitely Recommend Hospital	300+	60%	67%	71%
Use of Medical Imaging				
Cardiac Imaging Stress Test before Surgery[1]	-	-	6.4%	5.3%
Combination Abdominal CT Scan	689	2.0%	3.8%	10.5%
Combination Brain/Sinus CT Scan	831	3.6%	4.3%	2.7%
Combination Chest CT Scan	268	1.1%	1%	2.7%
Follow-up Mammogram/Ultrasound	305	9.8%	10.2%	8.8%
Lumbar Spine MRI for Low Back Pain[1]	-	-	38.2%	37.2%

Doctors' Community Hospital

8118 Good Luck Road Phone: 301-552-8085
Lanham, MD 20706 Fax: 301-552-7937
URL: www.dchweb.org
Type: Acute Care Hospitals Emergency Services: Yes
Ownership: Proprietary Beds: 250

Key Personnel:
Pediatric In-Patient Care . . . . Paula L. Bruening
CEO . . . . Philip Down
Emergency Room . . . . Nancy Haupt, RN
Chief of Medical Staff. . . . . Gabriel Jaffe, MD
Radiology. Louis Kirschner, MD
Quality Assurance . . . . Peg Kostopoulos
Cardiac Laboratory. . . . . Cecily Ludka

Measure	Cases	This Hosp.	State Avg.	U.S. Avg.
Blood Clot Prevention and Treatment				
Anticoagulation Overlap Therapy[2]	100	100%	94%	93%
ICU Venous Thromboembolism Prophylaxis[2]	60	100%	94%	92%
Incidence of Potentially Preventable VTE[2]	34	0%	7%	10%
UFH with Dosages/Platelet Monitoring[2]	37	100%	97%	97%
Venous Thromboembolism Prophylaxis[2]	389	100%	90%	85%
Warfarin Therapy Discharge Instructions[2]	73	100%	78%	75%
Chest Pain/Possible Heart Attack Care				
Aspirin Given Within 24 Hours of Arrival[5]	-	-	100%	96%
Fibrinolytic Meds Within 30 Min. of Arrival[5]	-	-	-	58%
Average Time to ECG (minutes)[5]	-	-	6	7
Average Time to Transfer (minutes)[5]	-	-	32	60
Children's Asthma Care				
Received Home Management Plan of Care	-	-	-	88%
Received Reliever Medication	-	-	-	100%
Received Systemic Corticosteroids	-	-	-	100%
Emergency Department				
Admittance Decision Time (minutes)[2]	903	193	143	98
Head CT Results Within 45 Min. of Arrival[5]	-	-	-	57%
Patients Who Left ER Before Being Seen[5]	-	-	3%	2%
Time from ER Arrival to Admit. (minutes)[2]	933	492	357	274
Time from ER Arrival to Discharge (minutes)[5]	-	-	-	134
Time in ER Before Being Evaluated (minutes)[5]	-	-	-	26
Time to Pain Meds for Fractures (minutes)[5]	-	-	-	57
Heart Attack Care				
Aspirin Given at Discharge	15	100%	99%	99%
Fibrinolytic Meds Within 30 Min. of Arrival[7]	-	-	-	54%
PCI Within 90 Minutes of Arrival[7]	-	-	93%	96%
Statin Prescribed at Discharge	11	100%	98%	98%
Heart Failure Care				
ACE Inhibitor or ARB for LVSD	114	100%	97%	97%
Discharge Instructions Given	291	98%	93%	94%
Evaluation of LVS Function	339	100%	99%	99%
Medicare Spending				
Medicare Spending per Patient (ratio)	-	-	-	0.98
Pneumonia Care				
Appropriate Initial Antibiotic Given	307	98%	97%	95%
Blood Culture Timing	505	97%	97%	98%
Pregnancy and Delivery Care				
Newborn Deliveries Scheduled Early[5]	-	-	-	6%
Preventive Care				
Immunization for Influenza[2]	597	100%	94%	90%
Immunization for Pneumonia[2]	780	99%	94%	92%
Stroke Care				
Anticoagulation Therapy for Atrial Fibrillation[5]	-	-	95%	95%
Antithrombotic Therapy Timing[5]	-	-	95%	98%
Assessed for Rehabilitation[5]	-	-	96%	97%
Discharged on Antithrombotic Therapy[5]	-	-	95%	99%
Discharged on Statin Medication[5]	-	-	97%	94%
Thrombolytic Therapy Timing[5]	-	-	-	66%
Venous Thromboembolism Prophylaxis[5]	-	-	89%	94%
Written Stroke Educational Materials Given[5]	-	-	77%	88%
Surgical Care Improvement Project				
Appropriate Beta Blocker Usage[2]	121	98%	97%	98%
Appropriate VTP Within 24 Hours[2]	410	99%	98%	98%
Controlled Postoperative Blood Glucose[2,7]	-	-	96%	97%
Perioperative Temperature Management[2]	460	100%	100%	100%
Prophylactic Antibiotic Selection[2]	305	100%	99%	99%
Prophylactic Antibiotic Selection (Outpatient)[5]	-	-	98%	98%
Prophylactic Antibiotic Stopped[2]	287	98%	98%	98%
Prophylactic Antibiotic Timing[2]	306	98%	97%	99%
Prophylactic Antibiotic Timing (Outpatient)[5]	-	-	98%	98%
Urinary Catheter Removal[2]	274	99%	98%	97%
Survey of Patients' Hospital Experiences				
Area Around Room 'Always' Quiet at Night	300+	64%	57%	61%
Doctors 'Always' Communicated Well	300+	78%	78%	82%
Home Recovery Information Given	300+	84%	85%	85%
Hospital Given 9 or 10 on 10 Point Scale	300+	67%	65%	71%
Meds 'Always' Explained Before Given	300+	60%	58%	64%
Nurses 'Always' Communicated Well	300+	75%	75%	79%
Pain 'Always' Well Controlled	300+	67%	67%	71%
Room and Bathroom 'Always' Clean	300+	72%	64%	73%
Timely Help 'Always' Received	300+	58%	58%	68%
Would Definitely Recommend Hospital	300+	68%	67%	71%
Use of Medical Imaging				
Cardiac Imaging Stress Test before Surgery[1]	-	-	6.4%	5.3%
Combination Abdominal CT Scan	568	0.7%	3.8%	10.5%
Combination Brain/Sinus CT Scan[1]	-	-	4.3%	2.7%
Combination Chest CT Scan	220	0.5%	1%	2.7%
Follow-up Mammogram/Ultrasound[7]	-	-	10.2%	8.8%
Lumbar Spine MRI for Low Back Pain[1]	-	-	38.2%	37.2%

Laurel Regional Medical Center

7300 Van Dusen Road Phone: 301-725-4300
Laurel, MD 20707 Fax: 301-497-7953
URL: www.laurelregionalhospital.org
Type: Acute Care Hospitals Emergency Services: Yes
Ownership: Voluntary non-profit - Private Beds: 146

Key Personnel:
Radiology. Meghal Antani
Emergency Room . . . . Gerald Apollon
Chief of Medical Staff. . . . . Neil Meade
Anesthesiology. . . . . Jon Newsome, MD
Patient Relations . . . . Suzy Novotny
CEO/President. . . . . Douglas Shepherd
Infection Control. . . . . Barbara Thieman

Measure	Cases	This Hosp.	State Avg.	U.S. Avg.
Blood Clot Prevention and Treatment				
Anticoagulation Overlap Therapy[2]	42	83%	94%	93%
ICU Venous Thromboembolism Prophylaxis[2]	96	91%	94%	92%
Incidence of Potentially Preventable VTE[1,2]	-	-	7%	10%
UFH with Dosages/Platelet Monitoring[2]	15	100%	97%	97%
Venous Thromboembolism Prophylaxis[2]	322	86%	90%	85%
Warfarin Therapy Discharge Instructions[2]	32	59%	78%	75%
Chest Pain/Possible Heart Attack Care				

NOTE: Hospital profiles are in alphabetical order by state, then city, then hospital within the city; Rankings exclude hospitals with less than 25 cases except for patient surveys which excludes hospitals with less than 100 cases; (a) 100-299 cases; (1) The number of cases/patients is too few to report; (2) Data submitted were based on a sample of cases/patients; (3) Results are based on a shorter time period than required; (4) Data suppressed by CMS for one or more quarters; (5) Results are not available for this reporting period; (6) Fewer than 100 patients completed the HCAHPS survey; (7) No cases met the criteria for this measure; (8) The lower limit of the confidence interval cannot be calculated if the number of observed infections equals zero; (9) No data are available from the state/territory for this reporting period; (10) The scores shown reflect fewer than 50 completed surveys; (11) There were discrepancies in the data collection process; (12) This measure does not apply to this hospital for this reporting period; (13) Results cannot be calculated for this reporting period; (14) The results for this state are combined with nearby states to protect confidentiality; Please refer to the User's Guide for a full explanation of data.

Measure	Cases	This Hosp.	State Avg.	U.S. Avg.
Aspirin Given Within 24 Hours of Arrival[5]	-	-	100%	96%
Fibrinolytic Meds Within 30 Min. of Arrival[5]	-	-	-	58%
Average Time to ECG (minutes)[5]	-	-	6	7
Average Time to Transfer (minutes)[5]	-	-	32	60
Children's Asthma Care				
Received Home Management Plan of Care	-	-	-	88%
Received Reliever Medication	-	-	-	100%
Received Systemic Corticosteroids	-	-	-	100%
Emergency Department				
Admittance Decision Time (minutes)[2]	660	168	143	98
Head CT Results Within 45 Min. of Arrival[5]	-	-	-	57%
Patients Who Left ER Before Being Seen[5]	-	-	3%	2%
Time from ER Arrival to Admit. (minutes)[2]	661	430	357	274
Time from ER Arrival to Discharge (minutes)[5]	-	-	-	134
Time in ER Before Being Evaluated (minutes)[5]	-	-	-	26
Time to Pain Meds for Fractures (minutes)[5]	-	-	-	57
Heart Attack Care				
Aspirin Given at Discharge	27	96%	99%	99%
Fibrinolytic Meds Within 30 Min. of Arrival[7]	-	-	-	54%
PCI Within 90 Minutes of Arrival[7]	-	-	93%	96%
Statin Prescribed at Discharge	28	93%	98%	98%
Heart Failure Care				
ACE Inhibitor or ARB for LVSD	47	100%	97%	97%
Discharge Instructions Given	116	97%	93%	94%
Evaluation of LVS Function	144	99%	99%	99%
Medicare Spending				
Medicare Spending per Patient (ratio)	-	-	-	0.98
Pneumonia Care				
Appropriate Initial Antibiotic Given	101	96%	97%	95%
Blood Culture Timing	158	91%	97%	98%
Pregnancy and Delivery Care				
Newborn Deliveries Scheduled Early[5]	-	-	-	6%
Preventive Care				
Immunization for Influenza[2]	459	96%	94%	90%
Immunization for Pneumonia[2]	512	90%	94%	92%
Stroke Care				
Anticoagulation Therapy for Atrial Fibrillation[1]	-	-	95%	95%
Antithrombotic Therapy Timing	36	97%	95%	98%
Assessed for Rehabilitation	43	91%	96%	97%
Discharged on Antithrombotic Therapy	39	95%	95%	99%
Discharged on Statin Medication	37	97%	97%	94%
Thrombolytic Therapy Timing[1]	-	-	-	66%
Venous Thromboembolism Prophylaxis	41	93%	89%	94%
Written Stroke Educational Materials Given	23	83%	77%	88%
Surgical Care Improvement Project				
Appropriate Beta Blocker Usage	36	97%	97%	98%
Appropriate VTP Within 24 Hours	99	94%	98%	98%
Controlled Postoperative Blood Glucose[7]	-	-	96%	97%
Perioperative Temperature Management	143	100%	100%	100%
Prophylactic Antibiotic Selection	76	97%	99%	99%
Prophylactic Antibiotic Selection (Outpatient)[5]	-	-	98%	98%
Prophylactic Antibiotic Stopped	73	96%	98%	98%
Prophylactic Antibiotic Timing	76	100%	97%	99%
Prophylactic Antibiotic Timing (Outpatient)[5]	-	-	98%	98%
Urinary Catheter Removal	77	95%	98%	97%
Survey of Patients' Hospital Experiences				
Area Around Room 'Always' Quiet at Night	300+	56%	57%	61%
Doctors 'Always' Communicated Well	300+	69%	78%	82%
Home Recovery Information Given	300+	78%	85%	85%
Hospital Given 9 or 10 on 10 Point Scale	300+	48%	65%	71%
Meds 'Always' Explained Before Given	300+	51%	58%	64%
Nurses 'Always' Communicated Well	300+	66%	75%	79%
Pain 'Always' Well Controlled	300+	65%	67%	71%
Room and Bathroom 'Always' Clean	300+	53%	64%	73%
Timely Help 'Always' Received	300+	51%	58%	68%
Would Definitely Recommend Hospital	300+	49%	67%	71%
Use of Medical Imaging				
Cardiac Imaging Stress Test before Surgery	115	4.3%	6.4%	5.3%
Combination Abdominal CT Scan	294	2.0%	3.8%	10.5%
Combination Brain/Sinus CT Scan	445	4.0%	4.3%	2.7%
Combination Chest CT Scan	101	1.0%	1%	2.7%
Follow-up Mammogram/Ultrasound[1]	-	-	10.2%	8.8%
Lumbar Spine MRI for Low Back Pain[1]	-	-	38.2%	37.2%

Medstar Saint Mary's Hospital

25500 Point Lookout Road
Leonardtown, MD 20650
URL: www.smhwecare.com
Type: Acute Care Hospitals
Ownership: Voluntary non-profit - Private
Phone: 301-475-6001
Fax: 301-475-5388
Emergency Services: Yes
Beds: 110

Key Personnel:
Emergency Room . . . . Eveline Ane
Chief of Medical Staff. . . . . Cindy Daly, MD
Radiology. . . . . Bolivia Davis
President . . . . Christine R. Wray, FACHE

Measure	Cases	This Hosp.	State Avg.	U.S. Avg.
Blood Clot Prevention and Treatment				
Anticoagulation Overlap Therapy[2]	53	92%	94%	93%
ICU Venous Thromboembolism Prophylaxis[2]	42	93%	94%	92%
Incidence of Potentially Preventable VTE[1,2]	-	-	7%	10%
UFH with Dosages/Platelet Monitoring[1,2]	-	-	97%	97%
Venous Thromboembolism Prophylaxis[2]	314	73%	90%	85%
Warfarin Therapy Discharge Instructions[2]	37	86%	78%	75%
Chest Pain/Possible Heart Attack Care				
Aspirin Given Within 24 Hours of Arrival[5]	-	-	100%	96%
Fibrinolytic Meds Within 30 Min. of Arrival[5]	-	-	-	58%
Average Time to ECG (minutes)[5]	-	-	6	7
Average Time to Transfer (minutes)[5]	-	-	32	60
Children's Asthma Care				
Received Home Management Plan of Care	-	-	-	88%
Received Reliever Medication	-	-	-	100%
Received Systemic Corticosteroids	-	-	-	100%
Emergency Department				
Admittance Decision Time (minutes)[2]	600	121	143	98
Head CT Results Within 45 Min. of Arrival[5]	-	-	-	57%
Patients Who Left ER Before Being Seen[5]	-	-	3%	2%
Time from ER Arrival to Admit. (minutes)[2]	604	313	357	274
Time from ER Arrival to Discharge (minutes)[5]	-	-	-	134
Time in ER Before Being Evaluated (minutes)[5]	-	-	-	26
Time to Pain Meds for Fractures (minutes)[5]	-	-	-	57
Heart Attack Care				
Aspirin Given at Discharge	21	100%	99%	99%
Fibrinolytic Meds Within 30 Min. of Arrival[7]	-	-	-	54%
PCI Within 90 Minutes of Arrival[7]	-	-	93%	96%
Statin Prescribed at Discharge	16	100%	98%	98%
Heart Failure Care				
ACE Inhibitor or ARB for LVSD[2]	46	98%	97%	97%
Discharge Instructions Given[2]	179	96%	93%	94%
Evaluation of LVS Function[2]	215	100%	99%	99%
Medicare Spending				
Medicare Spending per Patient (ratio)	-	-	-	0.98
Pneumonia Care				
Appropriate Initial Antibiotic Given[2]	77	100%	97%	95%
Blood Culture Timing[2]	130	98%	97%	98%
Pregnancy and Delivery Care				
Newborn Deliveries Scheduled Early[5]	-	-	-	6%
Preventive Care				
Immunization for Influenza[2]	547	98%	94%	90%
Immunization for Pneumonia[2]	640	99%	94%	92%
Stroke Care				
Anticoagulation Therapy for Atrial Fibrillation[5]	-	-	95%	95%
Antithrombotic Therapy Timing[5]	-	-	95%	98%
Assessed for Rehabilitation[5]	-	-	96%	97%
Discharged on Antithrombotic Therapy[5]	-	-	95%	99%
Discharged on Statin Medication[5]	-	-	97%	94%
Thrombolytic Therapy Timing[5]	-	-	-	66%
Venous Thromboembolism Prophylaxis[5]	-	-	89%	94%
Written Stroke Educational Materials Given[5]	-	-	77%	88%
Surgical Care Improvement Project				
Appropriate Beta Blocker Usage[2]	61	98%	97%	98%
Appropriate VTP Within 24 Hours[2]	240	98%	98%	98%
Controlled Postoperative Blood Glucose[2,7]	-	-	96%	97%
Perioperative Temperature Management[2]	294	100%	100%	100%
Prophylactic Antibiotic Selection[2]	242	100%	99%	99%
Prophylactic Antibiotic Selection (Outpatient)[5]	-	-	98%	98%
Prophylactic Antibiotic Stopped[2]	238	97%	98%	98%
Prophylactic Antibiotic Timing[2]	242	100%	97%	99%
Prophylactic Antibiotic Timing (Outpatient)[5]	-	-	98%	98%
Urinary Catheter Removal[2]	228	99%	98%	97%
Survey of Patients' Hospital Experiences				
Area Around Room 'Always' Quiet at Night	300+	63%	57%	61%
Doctors 'Always' Communicated Well	300+	79%	78%	82%
Home Recovery Information Given	300+	90%	85%	85%
Hospital Given 9 or 10 on 10 Point Scale	300+	73%	65%	71%
Meds 'Always' Explained Before Given	300+	62%	58%	64%
Nurses 'Always' Communicated Well	300+	79%	75%	79%
Pain 'Always' Well Controlled	300+	70%	67%	71%
Room and Bathroom 'Always' Clean	300+	74%	64%	73%
Timely Help 'Always' Received	300+	63%	58%	68%
Would Definitely Recommend Hospital	300+	72%	67%	71%
Use of Medical Imaging				
Cardiac Imaging Stress Test before Surgery	68	0.0%	6.4%	5.3%
Combination Abdominal CT Scan	951	3.0%	3.8%	10.5%
Combination Brain/Sinus CT Scan	826	2.4%	4.3%	2.7%
Combination Chest CT Scan	540	1.3%	1%	2.7%
Follow-up Mammogram/Ultrasound	577	6.2%	10.2%	8.8%
Lumbar Spine MRI for Low Back Pain	140	32.1%	38.2%	37.2%

Garrett County Memorial Hospital

251 North Fourth Street
Oakland, MD 21550
URL: www.gcmh.com
Type: Acute Care Hospitals
Ownership: Voluntary non-profit - Private
Phone: 301-533-4173
Fax: 301-533-4328
Emergency Services: Yes
Beds: 76

Key Personnel:
CEO/President. . . . . Donald P Battista
Radiology. . . . . James K Benjamin
Infection Control. . . . . Linda Danjou, RN
Operating Room. . . . . Elaine Geroski, RN
Coronary Care . . . . Dale Hair, RN
Chief of Medical Staff . . . . Richard Perry, MD

Measure	Cases	This Hosp.	State Avg.	U.S. Avg.
Blood Clot Prevention and Treatment				
Anticoagulation Overlap Therapy	12	75%	94%	93%
ICU Venous Thromboembolism Prophylaxis	129	82%	94%	92%
Incidence of Potentially Preventable VTE[1]	-	-	7%	10%
UFH with Dosages/Platelet Monitoring[1]	-	-	97%	97%
Venous Thromboembolism Prophylaxis	655	72%	90%	85%
Warfarin Therapy Discharge Instructions[1]	-	-	78%	75%
Chest Pain/Possible Heart Attack Care				
Aspirin Given Within 24 Hours of Arrival[5]	-	-	100%	96%
Fibrinolytic Meds Within 30 Min. of Arrival[5]	-	-	-	58%
Average Time to ECG (minutes)[5]	-	-	6	7
Average Time to Transfer (minutes)[5]	-	-	32	60
Children's Asthma Care				
Received Home Management Plan of Care	-	-	-	88%
Received Reliever Medication	-	-	-	100%
Received Systemic Corticosteroids	-	-	-	100%
Emergency Department				
Admittance Decision Time (minutes)	1,209	55	143	98
Head CT Results Within 45 Min. of Arrival[5]	-	-	-	57%
Patients Who Left ER Before Being Seen[5]	-	-	3%	2%
Time from ER Arrival to Admit. (minutes)	1,211	215	357	274
Time from ER Arrival to Discharge (minutes)[5]	-	-	-	134
Time in ER Before Being Evaluated (minutes)[5]	-	-	-	26
Time to Pain Meds for Fractures (minutes)[5]	-	-	-	57
Heart Attack Care				
Aspirin Given at Discharge	14	86%	99%	99%
Fibrinolytic Meds Within 30 Min. of Arrival[7]	-	-	-	54%
PCI Within 90 Minutes of Arrival[7]	-	-	93%	96%
Statin Prescribed at Discharge	13	62%	98%	98%
Heart Failure Care				
ACE Inhibitor or ARB for LVSD	21	100%	97%	97%
Discharge Instructions Given	69	94%	93%	94%
Evaluation of LVS Function	77	100%	99%	99%
Medicare Spending				
Medicare Spending per Patient (ratio)	-	-	-	0.98
Pneumonia Care				
Appropriate Initial Antibiotic Given	42	98%	97%	95%

NOTE: Hospital profiles are in alphabetical order by state, then city, then hospital within the city; Rankings exclude hospitals with less than 25 cases except for patient surveys which excludes hospitals with less than 100 cases; (a) 100-299 cases; (1) The number of cases/patients is too few to report; (2) Data submitted were based on a sample of cases/patients; (3) Results are based on a shorter time period than required; (4) Data suppressed by CMS for one or more quarters; (5) Results are not available for this reporting period; (6) Fewer than 100 patients completed the HCAHPS survey; (7) No cases met the criteria for this measure; (8) The lower limit of the confidence interval cannot be calculated if the number of observed infections equals zero; (9) No data are available from the state/territory for this reporting period; (10) The scores shown reflect fewer than 50 completed surveys; (11) There were discrepancies in the data collection process; (12) This measure does not apply to this hospital for this reporting period; (13) Results cannot be calculated for this reporting period; (14) The results for this state are combined with nearby states to protect confidentiality; Please refer to the User's Guide for a full explanation of data.

Measure	Cases	This Hosp.	State Avg.	U.S. Avg.
Blood Culture Timing	44	98%	97%	98%
Pregnancy and Delivery Care				
Newborn Deliveries Scheduled Early[5]	-	-	-	6%
Preventive Care				
Immunization for Influenza	937	96%	94%	90%
Immunization for Pneumonia	1,082	97%	94%	92%
Stroke Care				
Anticoagulation Therapy for Atrial Fibrillation[5]	-	-	95%	95%
Antithrombotic Therapy Timing[5]	-	-	95%	98%
Assessed for Rehabilitation[5]	-	-	96%	97%
Discharged on Antithrombotic Therapy[5]	-	-	95%	99%
Discharged on Statin Medication[5]	-	-	97%	94%
Thrombolytic Therapy Timing[5]	-	-	-	66%
Venous Thromboembolism Prophylaxis[5]	-	-	89%	94%
Written Stroke Educational Materials Given[5]	-	-	77%	88%
Surgical Care Improvement Project				
Appropriate Beta Blocker Usage	71	100%	97%	98%
Appropriate VTP Within 24 Hours	209	95%	98%	98%
Controlled Postoperative Blood Glucose[7]	-	-	96%	97%
Perioperative Temperature Management	214	100%	100%	100%
Prophylactic Antibiotic Selection	167	98%	99%	99%
Prophylactic Antibiotic Selection (Outpatient)[5]	-	-	98%	98%
Prophylactic Antibiotic Stopped	163	96%	98%	98%
Prophylactic Antibiotic Timing	167	99%	97%	99%
Prophylactic Antibiotic Timing (Outpatient)[5]	-	-	98%	98%
Urinary Catheter Removal	161	96%	98%	97%
Survey of Patients' Hospital Experiences				
Area Around Room 'Always' Quiet at Night	300+	53%	57%	61%
Doctors 'Always' Communicated Well	300+	84%	78%	82%
Home Recovery Information Given	300+	86%	85%	85%
Hospital Given 9 or 10 on 10 Point Scale	300+	71%	65%	71%
Meds 'Always' Explained Before Given	300+	63%	58%	64%
Nurses 'Always' Communicated Well	300+	80%	75%	79%
Pain 'Always' Well Controlled	300+	71%	67%	71%
Room and Bathroom 'Always' Clean	300+	76%	64%	73%
Timely Help 'Always' Received	300+	72%	58%	68%
Would Definitely Recommend Hospital	300+	70%	67%	71%
Use of Medical Imaging				
Cardiac Imaging Stress Test before Surgery	167	6.6%	6.4%	5.3%
Combination Abdominal CT Scan	522	6.5%	3.8%	10.5%
Combination Brain/Sinus CT Scan	436	4.4%	4.3%	2.7%
Combination Chest CT Scan	247	0.0%	1%	2.7%
Follow-up Mammogram/Ultrasound[7]	-	-	10.2%	8.8%
Lumbar Spine MRI for Low Back Pain[7]	-	-	38.2%	37.2%

Medstar Montgomery Medical Center

18101 Prince Philip Drive
Olney, MD 20832
URL: www.montgomerygeneral.com
Type: Acute Care Hospitals
Ownership: Voluntary non-profit - Private

Phone: 301-774-8882
Fax: 301-774-7389
Emergency Services: Yes
Beds: 244

Key Personnel:
Quality Assurance .... Nancy Barlow
Emergency Room .... Andy Divine
Operating Room.............. Rene Gelber
Pediatric Ambulatory Care ...... Sheila Ideerda, MD
Pediatric In-Patient Care .... Sheila Ideerda, MD
Chief of Medical Staff.......... Roger F Leonard, MD
CEO/President................ Peter W Monge

Measure	Cases	This Hosp.	State Avg.	U.S. Avg.
Blood Clot Prevention and Treatment				
Anticoagulation Overlap Therapy[2]	63	98%	94%	93%
ICU Venous Thromboembolism Prophylaxis[2]	40	95%	94%	92%
Incidence of Potentially Preventable VTE[2]	11	0%	7%	10%
UFH with Dosages/Platelet Monitoring[1,2]	-	-	97%	97%
Venous Thromboembolism Prophylaxis[2]	409	96%	90%	85%
Warfarin Therapy Discharge Instructions[2]	50	96%	78%	75%
Chest Pain/Possible Heart Attack Care				
Aspirin Given Within 24 Hours of Arrival[5]	-	-	100%	96%
Fibrinolytic Meds Within 30 Min. of Arrival[5]	-	-	-	58%
Average Time to ECG (minutes)[5]	-	-	6	7
Average Time to Transfer (minutes)[5]	-	-	32	60
Children's Asthma Care				
Received Home Management Plan of Care	-	-	-	88%
Received Reliever Medication	-	-	-	100%
Received Systemic Corticosteroids	-	-	-	100%
Emergency Department				
Admittance Decision Time (minutes)[2]	768	136	143	98
Head CT Results Within 45 Min. of Arrival[5]	-	-	-	57%
Patients Who Left ER Before Being Seen[5]	-	-	3%	2%
Time from ER Arrival to Admit. (minutes)[2]	787	288	357	274
Time from ER Arrival to Discharge (minutes)[5]	-	-	-	134
Time in ER Before Being Evaluated (minutes)[5]	-	-	-	26
Time to Pain Meds for Fractures (minutes)[5]	-	-	-	57
Heart Attack Care				
Aspirin Given at Discharge	21	100%	99%	99%
Fibrinolytic Meds Within 30 Min. of Arrival[7]	-	-	-	54%
PCI Within 90 Minutes of Arrival[7]	-	-	93%	96%
Statin Prescribed at Discharge	21	100%	98%	98%
Heart Failure Care				
ACE Inhibitor or ARB for LVSD	54	100%	97%	97%
Discharge Instructions Given	123	96%	93%	94%
Evaluation of LVS Function	177	100%	99%	99%
Medicare Spending				
Medicare Spending per Patient (ratio)	-	-	-	0.98
Pneumonia Care				
Appropriate Initial Antibiotic Given	159	99%	97%	95%
Blood Culture Timing	205	99%	97%	98%
Pregnancy and Delivery Care				
Newborn Deliveries Scheduled Early[5]	-	-	-	6%
Preventive Care				
Immunization for Influenza[2]	648	98%	94%	90%
Immunization for Pneumonia[2]	753	95%	94%	92%
Stroke Care				
Anticoagulation Therapy for Atrial Fibrillation[5]	-	-	95%	95%
Antithrombotic Therapy Timing[5]	-	-	95%	98%
Assessed for Rehabilitation[5]	-	-	96%	97%
Discharged on Antithrombotic Therapy[5]	-	-	95%	99%
Discharged on Statin Medication[5]	-	-	97%	94%
Thrombolytic Therapy Timing[5]	-	-	-	66%
Venous Thromboembolism Prophylaxis[5]	-	-	89%	94%
Written Stroke Educational Materials Given[5]	-	-	77%	88%
Surgical Care Improvement Project				
Appropriate Beta Blocker Usage	128	98%	97%	98%
Appropriate VTP Within 24 Hours	401	99%	98%	98%
Controlled Postoperative Blood Glucose[7]	-	-	96%	97%
Perioperative Temperature Management	452	100%	100%	100%
Prophylactic Antibiotic Selection	305	99%	99%	99%
Prophylactic Antibiotic Selection (Outpatient)[5]	-	-	98%	98%
Prophylactic Antibiotic Stopped	285	98%	98%	98%
Prophylactic Antibiotic Timing	305	99%	97%	99%
Prophylactic Antibiotic Timing (Outpatient)[5]	-	-	98%	98%
Urinary Catheter Removal	318	100%	98%	97%
Survey of Patients' Hospital Experiences				
Area Around Room 'Always' Quiet at Night	(a)	53%	57%	61%
Doctors 'Always' Communicated Well	(a)	74%	78%	82%
Home Recovery Information Given	(a)	85%	85%	85%
Hospital Given 9 or 10 on 10 Point Scale	(a)	64%	65%	71%
Meds 'Always' Explained Before Given	(a)	55%	58%	64%
Nurses 'Always' Communicated Well	(a)	70%	75%	79%
Pain 'Always' Well Controlled	(a)	59%	67%	71%
Room and Bathroom 'Always' Clean	(a)	63%	64%	73%
Timely Help 'Always' Received	(a)	53%	58%	68%
Would Definitely Recommend Hospital	(a)	71%	67%	71%
Use of Medical Imaging				
Cardiac Imaging Stress Test before Surgery	93	8.6%	6.4%	5.3%
Combination Abdominal CT Scan	568	0.5%	3.8%	10.5%
Combination Brain/Sinus CT Scan	918	10.3%	4.3%	2.7%
Combination Chest CT Scan	258	0.0%	1%	2.7%
Follow-up Mammogram/Ultrasound[7]	-	-	10.2%	8.8%
Lumbar Spine MRI for Low Back Pain[1]	-	-	38.2%	37.2%

Calvert Memorial Hospital

100 Hospital Road
Prince Frederick, MD 20678
URL: www.calverthospital.com
Type: Acute Care Hospitals
Ownership: Voluntary non-profit - Other

Phone: 410-535-8239
Fax: 410-535-4125
Emergency Services: Yes
Beds: 88

Key Personnel:
Quality Assurance .... Susan Dohony
Intensive Care Unit............ Annie Lockhart
Patient Relations .... Mattie Lowery
Chief of Medical Staff.......... Robert Schlager, MD
Infection Control.............. Judith Sturgis
Operating Room............... Gretchen West
CEO/President................ James J Xinis
Radiology.................... Guillermo Zambrano

Measure	Cases	This Hosp.	State Avg.	U.S. Avg.
Blood Clot Prevention and Treatment				
Anticoagulation Overlap Therapy[2]	48	100%	94%	93%
ICU Venous Thromboembolism Prophylaxis[2]	21	100%	94%	92%
Incidence of Potentially Preventable VTE[1,2]	-	-	7%	10%
UFH with Dosages/Platelet Monitoring[1,2]	-	-	97%	97%
Venous Thromboembolism Prophylaxis[2]	348	98%	90%	85%
Warfarin Therapy Discharge Instructions[2]	48	96%	78%	75%
Chest Pain/Possible Heart Attack Care				
Aspirin Given Within 24 Hours of Arrival[5]	-	-	100%	96%
Fibrinolytic Meds Within 30 Min. of Arrival[5]	-	-	-	58%
Average Time to ECG (minutes)[5]	-	-	6	7
Average Time to Transfer (minutes)[5]	-	-	32	60
Children's Asthma Care				
Received Home Management Plan of Care	-	-	-	88%
Received Reliever Medication	-	-	-	100%
Received Systemic Corticosteroids	-	-	-	100%
Emergency Department				
Admittance Decision Time (minutes)[2]	717	187	143	98
Head CT Results Within 45 Min. of Arrival[5]	-	-	-	57%
Patients Who Left ER Before Being Seen[5]	-	-	3%	2%
Time from ER Arrival to Admit. (minutes)[2]	717	428	357	274
Time from ER Arrival to Discharge (minutes)[5]	-	-	-	134
Time in ER Before Being Evaluated (minutes)[5]	-	-	-	26
Time to Pain Meds for Fractures (minutes)[5]	-	-	-	57
Heart Attack Care				
Aspirin Given at Discharge	28	100%	99%	99%
Fibrinolytic Meds Within 30 Min. of Arrival[7]	-	-	-	54%
PCI Within 90 Minutes of Arrival[3,7]	-	-	93%	96%
Statin Prescribed at Discharge	30	100%	98%	98%
Heart Failure Care				
ACE Inhibitor or ARB for LVSD	36	100%	97%	97%
Discharge Instructions Given	245	100%	93%	94%
Evaluation of LVS Function	242	100%	99%	99%
Medicare Spending				
Medicare Spending per Patient (ratio)	-	-	-	0.98
Pneumonia Care				
Appropriate Initial Antibiotic Given	168	95%	97%	95%
Blood Culture Timing	216	100%	97%	98%
Pregnancy and Delivery Care				
Newborn Deliveries Scheduled Early[5]	-	-	-	6%
Preventive Care				
Immunization for Influenza[2]	553	93%	94%	90%
Immunization for Pneumonia[2]	585	97%	94%	92%
Stroke Care				
Anticoagulation Therapy for Atrial Fibrillation[5]	-	-	95%	95%
Antithrombotic Therapy Timing[5]	-	-	95%	98%
Assessed for Rehabilitation[5]	-	-	96%	97%
Discharged on Antithrombotic Therapy[5]	-	-	95%	99%
Discharged on Statin Medication[5]	-	-	97%	94%
Thrombolytic Therapy Timing[5]	-	-	-	66%
Venous Thromboembolism Prophylaxis[5]	-	-	89%	94%
Written Stroke Educational Materials Given[5]	-	-	77%	88%
Surgical Care Improvement Project				
Appropriate Beta Blocker Usage	61	100%	97%	98%
Appropriate VTP Within 24 Hours	183	100%	98%	98%
Controlled Postoperative Blood Glucose[7]	-	-	96%	97%
Perioperative Temperature Management	231	100%	100%	100%
Prophylactic Antibiotic Selection	179	99%	99%	99%

NOTE: Hospital profiles are in alphabetical order by state, then city, then hospital within the city; Rankings exclude hospitals with less than 25 cases except for patient surveys which excludes hospitals with less than 100 cases; (a) 100-299 cases; (1) The number of cases/patients is too few to report; (2) Data submitted were based on a sample of cases/patients; (3) Results are based on a shorter time period than required; (4) Data suppressed by CMS for one or more quarters; (5) Results are not available for this reporting period; (6) Fewer than 100 patients completed the HCAHPS survey; (7) No cases met the criteria for this measure; (8) The lower limit of the confidence interval cannot be calculated if the number of observed infections equals zero; (9) No data are available from the state/territory for this reporting period; (10) The scores shown reflect fewer than 50 completed surveys; (11) There were discrepancies in the data collection process; (12) This measure does not apply to this hospital for this reporting period; (13) Results cannot be calculated for this reporting period; (14) The results for this state are combined with nearby states to protect confidentiality; Please refer to the User's Guide for a full explanation of data.

Measure	Cases	This Hosp.	State Avg.	U.S. Avg.
Prophylactic Antibiotic Selection (Outpatient)[5]	-	-	98%	98%
Prophylactic Antibiotic Stopped	166	98%	98%	98%
Prophylactic Antibiotic Timing	179	98%	97%	99%
Prophylactic Antibiotic Timing (Outpatient)[5]	-	-	98%	98%
Urinary Catheter Removal	137	100%	98%	97%
Survey of Patients' Hospital Experiences				
Area Around Room 'Always' Quiet at Night	300+	53%	57%	61%
Doctors 'Always' Communicated Well	300+	78%	78%	82%
Home Recovery Information Given	300+	85%	85%	85%
Hospital Given 9 or 10 on 10 Point Scale	300+	63%	65%	71%
Meds 'Always' Explained Before Given	300+	58%	58%	64%
Nurses 'Always' Communicated Well	300+	74%	75%	79%
Pain 'Always' Well Controlled	300+	64%	67%	71%
Room and Bathroom 'Always' Clean	300+	64%	64%	73%
Timely Help 'Always' Received	300+	59%	58%	68%
Would Definitely Recommend Hospital	300+	61%	67%	71%
Use of Medical Imaging				
Cardiac Imaging Stress Test before Surgery	455	7.7%	6.4%	5.3%
Combination Abdominal CT Scan	384	0.5%	3.8%	10.5%
Combination Brain/Sinus CT Scan[1]	-	-	4.3%	2.7%
Combination Chest CT Scan	175	0.0%	1%	2.7%
Follow-up Mammogram/Ultrasound[7]	-	-	10.2%	8.8%
Lumbar Spine MRI for Low Back Pain[1]	-	-	38.2%	37.2%

Northwest Hospital Center

5401 Old Court Road
Randallstown, MD 21133
Phone: 410-521-5995
Fax: 410-521-7269
URL: www.lifebridgehealth.org
Type: Acute Care Hospitals
Emergency Services: Yes
Ownership: Voluntary non-profit - Private
Beds: 240

Key Personnel:

Radiology. . . . . George Allen
Quality Assurance . . . . Candy Hamner
Patient Relations . . . . Sue Jalbert
CEO/President. . . . . Dave Krajewski
Intensive Care Unit. . . . . Christopher Lee, RN
Anesthesiology. . . . . Charles Leve, MD
Emergency Room . . . . Deborah Macy

Measure	Cases	This Hosp.	State Avg.	U.S. Avg.
Blood Clot Prevention and Treatment				
Anticoagulation Overlap Therapy[2]	95	99%	94%	93%
ICU Venous Thromboembolism Prophylaxis[2]	22	95%	94%	92%
Incidence of Potentially Preventable VTE[1,2]	-	-	7%	10%
UFH with Dosages/Platelet Monitoring[2]	38	100%	97%	97%
Venous Thromboembolism Prophylaxis[2]	421	95%	90%	85%
Warfarin Therapy Discharge Instructions[2]	67	82%	78%	75%
Chest Pain/Possible Heart Attack Care				
Aspirin Given Within 24 Hours of Arrival[5]	-	-	100%	96%
Fibrinolytic Meds Within 30 Min. of Arrival[5]	-	-	-	58%
Average Time to ECG (minutes)[5]	-	-	6	7
Average Time to Transfer (minutes)[5]	-	-	32	60
Children's Asthma Care				
Received Home Management Plan of Care	-	-	-	88%
Received Reliever Medication	-	-	-	100%
Received Systemic Corticosteroids	-	-	-	100%
Emergency Department				
Admittance Decision Time (minutes)[2]	1,137	141	143	98
Head CT Results Within 45 Min. of Arrival[5]	-	-	-	57%
Patients Who Left ER Before Being Seen	64,917	3%	3%	2%
Time from ER Arrival to Admit. (minutes)[2]	1,138	384	357	274
Time from ER Arrival to Discharge (minutes)[5]	-	-	-	134
Time in ER Before Being Evaluated (minutes)[5]	-	-	-	26
Time to Pain Meds for Fractures (minutes)[5]	-	-	-	57
Heart Attack Care				
Aspirin Given at Discharge	51	100%	99%	99%
Fibrinolytic Meds Within 30 Min. of Arrival[7]	-	-	-	54%
PCI Within 90 Minutes of Arrival[3,7]	-	-	93%	96%
Statin Prescribed at Discharge	53	94%	98%	98%
Heart Failure Care				
ACE Inhibitor or ARB for LVSD	156	99%	97%	97%
Discharge Instructions Given	353	94%	93%	94%
Evaluation of LVS Function	458	100%	99%	99%
Medicare Spending				
Medicare Spending per Patient (ratio)	-	-	-	0.98
Pneumonia Care				
Appropriate Initial Antibiotic Given[2]	129	98%	97%	95%
Blood Culture Timing[2]	218	98%	97%	98%
Pregnancy and Delivery Care				
Newborn Deliveries Scheduled Early[3,7]	-	-	-	6%
Preventive Care				
Immunization for Influenza[2]	597	99%	94%	90%
Immunization for Pneumonia[2]	911	99%	94%	92%
Stroke Care				
Anticoagulation Therapy for Atrial Fibrillation[5]	-	-	95%	95%
Antithrombotic Therapy Timing[5]	-	-	95%	98%
Assessed for Rehabilitation[5]	-	-	96%	97%
Discharged on Antithrombotic Therapy[5]	-	-	95%	99%
Discharged on Statin Medication[5]	-	-	97%	94%
Thrombolytic Therapy Timing[5]	-	-	-	66%
Venous Thromboembolism Prophylaxis[5]	-	-	89%	94%
Written Stroke Educational Materials Given[5]	-	-	77%	88%
Surgical Care Improvement Project				
Appropriate Beta Blocker Usage	86	94%	97%	98%
Appropriate VTP Within 24 Hours	253	97%	98%	98%
Controlled Postoperative Blood Glucose[7]	-	-	96%	97%
Perioperative Temperature Management	300	100%	100%	100%
Prophylactic Antibiotic Selection	176	98%	99%	99%
Prophylactic Antibiotic Selection (Outpatient)[5]	-	-	98%	98%
Prophylactic Antibiotic Stopped	164	100%	98%	98%
Prophylactic Antibiotic Timing	176	99%	97%	99%
Prophylactic Antibiotic Timing (Outpatient)[5]	-	-	98%	98%
Urinary Catheter Removal	146	92%	98%	97%
Survey of Patients' Hospital Experiences				
Area Around Room 'Always' Quiet at Night	300+	53%	57%	61%
Doctors 'Always' Communicated Well	300+	76%	78%	82%
Home Recovery Information Given	300+	82%	85%	85%
Hospital Given 9 or 10 on 10 Point Scale	300+	61%	65%	71%
Meds 'Always' Explained Before Given	300+	59%	58%	64%
Nurses 'Always' Communicated Well	300+	75%	75%	79%
Pain 'Always' Well Controlled	300+	63%	67%	71%
Room and Bathroom 'Always' Clean	300+	58%	64%	73%
Timely Help 'Always' Received	300+	51%	58%	68%
Would Definitely Recommend Hospital	300+	62%	67%	71%
Use of Medical Imaging				
Cardiac Imaging Stress Test before Surgery	104	8.7%	6.4%	5.3%
Combination Abdominal CT Scan	798	1.8%	3.8%	10.5%
Combination Brain/Sinus CT Scan	1,161	5.1%	4.3%	2.7%
Combination Chest CT Scan	483	0.2%	1%	2.7%
Follow-up Mammogram/Ultrasound	1,012	3.6%	10.2%	8.8%
Lumbar Spine MRI for Low Back Pain	36	44.4%	38.2%	37.2%

Shady Grove Adventist Hospital

9901 Medical Center Drive
Rockville, MD 20850
Phone: 240-826-6517
Fax: 301-315-3043
URL: www.adventisthealthcare.com/sgah
Type: Acute Care Hospitals
Emergency Services: Yes
Ownership: Voluntary non-profit - Church
Beds: 268

Key Personnel:

Chair/CEO . . . . Terry Forde
CEO/President. . . . . John Sackett
Chief of Medical Staff. . . . . Kevin Smothers, MD

Measure	Cases	This Hosp.	State Avg.	U.S. Avg.
Blood Clot Prevention and Treatment				
Anticoagulation Overlap Therapy[2]	82	98%	94%	93%
ICU Venous Thromboembolism Prophylaxis[2]	12	100%	94%	92%
Incidence of Potentially Preventable VTE[2]	52	2%	7%	10%
UFH with Dosages/Platelet Monitoring[2]	19	100%	97%	97%
Venous Thromboembolism Prophylaxis[2]	362	95%	90%	85%
Warfarin Therapy Discharge Instructions[2]	41	98%	78%	75%
Chest Pain/Possible Heart Attack Care				
Aspirin Given Within 24 Hours of Arrival[5]	-	-	100%	96%
Fibrinolytic Meds Within 30 Min. of Arrival[5]	-	-	-	58%
Average Time to ECG (minutes)[5]	-	-	6	7
Average Time to Transfer (minutes)[5]	-	-	32	60
Children's Asthma Care				
Received Home Management Plan of Care	-	-	-	88%
Received Reliever Medication	-	-	-	100%
Received Systemic Corticosteroids	-	-	-	100%
Emergency Department				
Admittance Decision Time (minutes)[2]	499	164	143	98
Head CT Results Within 45 Min. of Arrival[5]	-	-	-	57%
Patients Who Left ER Before Being Seen[5]	-	-	3%	2%
Time from ER Arrival to Admit. (minutes)[2]	500	402	357	274
Time from ER Arrival to Discharge (minutes)[5]	-	-	-	134
Time in ER Before Being Evaluated (minutes)[5]	-	-	-	26
Time to Pain Meds for Fractures (minutes)[5]	-	-	-	57
Heart Attack Care				
Aspirin Given at Discharge	202	100%	99%	99%
Fibrinolytic Meds Within 30 Min. of Arrival[7]	-	-	-	54%
PCI Within 90 Minutes of Arrival	68	100%	93%	96%
Statin Prescribed at Discharge	205	100%	98%	98%
Heart Failure Care				
ACE Inhibitor or ARB for LVSD	122	100%	97%	97%
Discharge Instructions Given	232	100%	93%	94%
Evaluation of LVS Function	317	100%	99%	99%
Medicare Spending				
Medicare Spending per Patient (ratio)	-	-	-	0.98
Pneumonia Care				
Appropriate Initial Antibiotic Given[2]	196	97%	97%	95%
Blood Culture Timing[2]	220	100%	97%	98%
Pregnancy and Delivery Care				
Newborn Deliveries Scheduled Early[5]	-	-	-	6%
Preventive Care				
Immunization for Influenza[2]	463	83%	94%	90%
Immunization for Pneumonia[2]	424	70%	94%	92%
Stroke Care				
Anticoagulation Therapy for Atrial Fibrillation[5]	-	-	95%	95%
Antithrombotic Therapy Timing[5]	-	-	95%	98%
Assessed for Rehabilitation[5]	-	-	96%	97%
Discharged on Antithrombotic Therapy[5]	-	-	95%	99%
Discharged on Statin Medication[5]	-	-	97%	94%
Thrombolytic Therapy Timing[5]	-	-	-	66%
Venous Thromboembolism Prophylaxis[5]	-	-	89%	94%
Written Stroke Educational Materials Given[5]	-	-	77%	88%
Surgical Care Improvement Project				
Appropriate Beta Blocker Usage	236	97%	97%	98%
Appropriate VTP Within 24 Hours	853	99%	98%	98%
Controlled Postoperative Blood Glucose[7]	-	-	96%	97%
Perioperative Temperature Management	977	100%	100%	100%
Prophylactic Antibiotic Selection	650	100%	99%	99%
Prophylactic Antibiotic Selection (Outpatient)[5]	-	-	98%	98%
Prophylactic Antibiotic Stopped	632	98%	98%	98%
Prophylactic Antibiotic Timing	651	99%	97%	99%
Prophylactic Antibiotic Timing (Outpatient)[5]	-	-	98%	98%
Urinary Catheter Removal	744	100%	98%	97%
Survey of Patients' Hospital Experiences				
Area Around Room 'Always' Quiet at Night	300+	51%	57%	61%
Doctors 'Always' Communicated Well	300+	77%	78%	82%
Home Recovery Information Given	300+	84%	85%	85%
Hospital Given 9 or 10 on 10 Point Scale	300+	55%	65%	71%
Meds 'Always' Explained Before Given	300+	50%	58%	64%
Nurses 'Always' Communicated Well	300+	67%	75%	79%
Pain 'Always' Well Controlled	300+	58%	67%	71%
Room and Bathroom 'Always' Clean	300+	54%	64%	73%
Timely Help 'Always' Received	300+	43%	58%	68%
Would Definitely Recommend Hospital	300+	60%	67%	71%
Use of Medical Imaging				
Cardiac Imaging Stress Test before Surgery	113	5.3%	6.4%	5.3%
Combination Abdominal CT Scan	547	0.7%	3.8%	10.5%
Combination Brain/Sinus CT Scan	973	3.8%	4.3%	2.7%
Combination Chest CT Scan	102	0.0%	1%	2.7%
Follow-up Mammogram/Ultrasound[1]	-	-	10.2%	8.8%
Lumbar Spine MRI for Low Back Pain[1]	-	-	38.2%	37.2%

NOTE: Hospital profiles are in alphabetical order by state, then city, then hospital within the city; Rankings exclude hospitals with less than 25 cases except for patient surveys which excludes hospitals with less than 100 cases; (a) 100-299 cases; (1) The number of cases/patients is too few to report; (2) Data submitted were based on a sample of cases/patients; (3) Results are based on a shorter time period than required; (4) Data suppressed by CMS for one or more quarters; (5) Results are not available for this reporting period; (6) Fewer than 100 patients completed the HCAHPS survey; (7) No cases met the criteria for this measure; (8) The lower limit of the confidence interval cannot be calculated if the number of observed infections equals zero; (9) No data are available from the state/territory for this reporting period; (10) The scores shown reflect fewer than 50 completed surveys; (11) There were discrepancies in the data collection process; (12) This measure does not apply to this hospital for this reporting period; (13) Results cannot be calculated for this reporting period; (14) The results for this state are combined with nearby states to protect confidentiality; Please refer to the User's Guide for a full explanation of data.

Peninsula Regional Medical Center

100 East Carroll Avenue | Phone: 410-543-7111
Salisbury, MD 21801 | Fax: 410-543-7179
URL: www.peninsula.org
Type: Acute Care Hospitals | Emergency Services: Yes
Ownership: Voluntary non-profit - Private | Beds: 362

Key Personnel:
Coronary Care . . . . Mary Beth D'Amico
Pediatric Ambulatory Care . . . . . . Andras Kovacs, MD
Chief of Medical Staff . . . . Thomas P Lawrence, MD
Chairman/CEO . . . . William McCain
Quality Assurance . . . . Susan McDonald
Radiology. . . . . Mary Lou Melhorn
Infection Control . . . . Karen Mihalik, RN
CEO/President. . . . . Peggy Naleppa

Measure	Cases	This Hosp.	State Avg.	U.S. Avg.
Blood Clot Prevention and Treatment				
Anticoagulation Overlap Therapy[2]	138	96%	94%	93%
ICU Venous Thromboembolism Prophylaxis[2]	131	97%	94%	92%
Incidence of Potentially Preventable VTE[1,2]	-	-	7%	10%
UFH with Dosages/Platelet Monitoring[2]	33	100%	97%	97%
Venous Thromboembolism Prophylaxis[2]	265	95%	90%	85%
Warfarin Therapy Discharge Instructions[2]	88	99%	78%	75%
Chest Pain/Possible Heart Attack Care				
Aspirin Given Within 24 Hours of Arrival[5]	-	-	100%	96%
Fibrinolytic Meds Within 30 Min. of Arrival[5]	-	-	-	58%
Average Time to ECG (minutes)[5]	-	-	6	7
Average Time to Transfer (minutes)[5]	-	-	32	60
Children's Asthma Care				
Received Home Management Plan of Care	-	-	-	88%
Received Reliever Medication	-	-	-	100%
Received Systemic Corticosteroids	-	-	-	100%
Emergency Department				
Admittance Decision Time (minutes)[2]	598	102	143	98
Head CT Results Within 45 Min. of Arrival[5]	-	-	-	57%
Patients Who Left ER Before Being Seen[5]	-	-	3%	2%
Time from ER Arrival to Admit. (minutes)[2]	600	271	357	274
Time from ER Arrival to Discharge (minutes)[5]	-	-	-	134
Time in ER Before Being Evaluated (minutes)[5]	-	-	-	26
Time to Pain Meds for Fractures (minutes)[5]	-	-	-	57
Heart Attack Care				
Aspirin Given at Discharge	479	100%	99%	99%
Fibrinolytic Meds Within 30 Min. of Arrival[7]	-	-	-	54%
PCI Within 90 Minutes of Arrival	70	93%	93%	96%
Statin Prescribed at Discharge	476	100%	98%	98%
Heart Failure Care				
ACE Inhibitor or ARB for LVSD	170	98%	97%	97%
Discharge Instructions Given	465	100%	93%	94%
Evaluation of LVS Function	611	100%	99%	99%
Medicare Spending				
Medicare Spending per Patient (ratio)	-	-	-	0.98
Pneumonia Care				
Appropriate Initial Antibiotic Given	294	95%	97%	95%
Blood Culture Timing	451	97%	97%	98%
Pregnancy and Delivery Care				
Newborn Deliveries Scheduled Early[5]	-	-	-	6%
Preventive Care				
Immunization for Influenza[2]	533	89%	94%	90%
Immunization for Pneumonia[2]	669	88%	94%	92%
Stroke Care				
Anticoagulation Therapy for Atrial Fibrillation[5]	-	-	95%	95%
Antithrombotic Therapy Timing[5]	-	-	95%	98%
Assessed for Rehabilitation[5]	-	-	96%	97%
Discharged on Antithrombotic Therapy[5]	-	-	95%	99%
Discharged on Statin Medication[5]	-	-	97%	94%
Thrombolytic Therapy Timing[5]	-	-	-	66%
Venous Thromboembolism Prophylaxis[5]	-	-	89%	94%
Written Stroke Educational Materials Given[5]	-	-	77%	88%
Surgical Care Improvement Project				
Appropriate Beta Blocker Usage[2]	210	96%	97%	98%
Appropriate VTP Within 24 Hours[2]	308	97%	98%	98%
Controlled Postoperative Blood Glucose[2]	135	97%	96%	97%
Perioperative Temperature Management[2]	397	100%	100%	100%
Prophylactic Antibiotic Selection[2]	410	99%	99%	99%
Prophylactic Antibiotic Selection (Outpatient)[5]	-	-	98%	98%
Prophylactic Antibiotic Stopped[2]	401	97%	98%	98%
Prophylactic Antibiotic Timing[2]	411	98%	97%	99%
Prophylactic Antibiotic Timing (Outpatient)[5]	-	-	98%	98%
Urinary Catheter Removal[2]	318	99%	98%	97%
Survey of Patients' Hospital Experiences				
Area Around Room 'Always' Quiet at Night	300+	51%	57%	61%
Doctors 'Always' Communicated Well	300+	77%	78%	82%
Home Recovery Information Given	300+	86%	85%	85%
Hospital Given 9 or 10 on 10 Point Scale	300+	67%	65%	71%
Meds 'Always' Explained Before Given	300+	58%	58%	64%
Nurses 'Always' Communicated Well	300+	75%	75%	79%
Pain 'Always' Well Controlled	300+	65%	67%	71%
Room and Bathroom 'Always' Clean	300+	65%	64%	73%
Timely Help 'Always' Received	300+	61%	58%	68%
Would Definitely Recommend Hospital	300+	70%	67%	71%
Use of Medical Imaging				
Cardiac Imaging Stress Test before Surgery	248	4.8%	6.4%	5.3%
Combination Abdominal CT Scan	1,824	2.6%	3.8%	10.5%
Combination Brain/Sinus CT Scan	1,815	2.4%	4.3%	2.7%
Combination Chest CT Scan	1,160	0.0%	1%	2.7%
Follow-up Mammogram/Ultrasound	1,383	9.4%	10.2%	8.8%
Lumbar Spine MRI for Low Back Pain	94	60.6%	38.2%	37.2%

Holy Cross Hospital

1500 Forest Glen Road | Phone: 301-754-7000
Silver Spring, MD 20910 | Fax: 301-754-7031
URL: www.holycrosshealth.org
Type: Acute Care Hospitals | Emergency Services: Yes
Ownership: Voluntary non-profit - Church | Beds: 443

Key Personnel:
Intensive Care Unit. . . . . Crystal Beckford, RN
Pediatric In-Patient Care . . . . Jane Chase
Chief of Medical Staff. . . . . Blair M. Eig, MD
Infection Control. . . . . Mary Mohla
Emergency Room . . . . Laurence Oufiero, MD
CEO/President. . . . . Kevin J. Sexton
Quality Assurance . . . . Carolyn Simonsen
Radiology. . . . . Robert Zimmermann, MD

Measure	Cases	This Hosp.	State Avg.	U.S. Avg.
Blood Clot Prevention and Treatment				
Anticoagulation Overlap Therapy[5]	-	-	94%	93%
ICU Venous Thromboembolism Prophylaxis[5]	-	-	94%	92%
Incidence of Potentially Preventable VTE[5]	-	-	7%	10%
UFH with Dosages/Platelet Monitoring[5]	-	-	97%	97%
Venous Thromboembolism Prophylaxis[5]	-	-	90%	85%
Warfarin Therapy Discharge Instructions[5]	-	-	78%	75%
Chest Pain/Possible Heart Attack Care				
Aspirin Given Within 24 Hours of Arrival[3]	16	100%	100%	96%
Fibrinolytic Meds Within 30 Min. of Arrival[3,7]	-	-	-	58%
Average Time to ECG (minutes)[3]	17	6	6	7
Average Time to Transfer (minutes)[1,3]	-	-	32	60
Children's Asthma Care				
Received Home Management Plan of Care	-	-	-	88%
Received Reliever Medication	-	-	-	100%
Received Systemic Corticosteroids	-	-	-	100%
Emergency Department				
Admittance Decision Time (minutes)[2]	420	142	143	98
Head CT Results Within 45 Min. of Arrival[5]	-	-	-	57%
Patients Who Left ER Before Being Seen[5]	-	-	3%	2%
Time from ER Arrival to Admit. (minutes)[2]	421	400	357	274
Time from ER Arrival to Discharge (minutes)[5]	-	-	-	134
Time in ER Before Being Evaluated (minutes)[5]	-	-	-	26
Time to Pain Meds for Fractures (minutes)[5]	-	-	-	57
Heart Attack Care				
Aspirin Given at Discharge	92	100%	99%	99%
Fibrinolytic Meds Within 30 Min. of Arrival[7]	-	-	-	54%
PCI Within 90 Minutes of Arrival	47	100%	93%	96%
Statin Prescribed at Discharge	93	100%	98%	98%
Heart Failure Care				
ACE Inhibitor or ARB for LVSD[2]	141	100%	97%	97%
Discharge Instructions Given[2]	317	95%	93%	94%
Evaluation of LVS Function[2]	407	100%	99%	99%
Medicare Spending				
Medicare Spending per Patient (ratio)	-	-	-	0.98
Pneumonia Care				
Appropriate Initial Antibiotic Given[2]	165	99%	97%	95%
Blood Culture Timing[2]	262	99%	97%	98%
Pregnancy and Delivery Care				
Newborn Deliveries Scheduled Early[5]	-	-	-	6%
Preventive Care				
Immunization for Influenza[2]	484	98%	94%	90%
Immunization for Pneumonia[2]	452	97%	94%	92%
Stroke Care				
Anticoagulation Therapy for Atrial Fibrillation[5]	-	-	95%	95%
Antithrombotic Therapy Timing[5]	-	-	95%	98%
Assessed for Rehabilitation[5]	-	-	96%	97%
Discharged on Antithrombotic Therapy[5]	-	-	95%	99%
Discharged on Statin Medication[5]	-	-	97%	94%
Thrombolytic Therapy Timing[5]	-	-	-	66%
Venous Thromboembolism Prophylaxis[5]	-	-	89%	94%
Written Stroke Educational Materials Given[5]	-	-	77%	88%
Surgical Care Improvement Project				
Appropriate Beta Blocker Usage[2]	159	100%	97%	98%
Appropriate VTP Within 24 Hours[2]	618	100%	98%	98%
Controlled Postoperative Blood Glucose[2,7]	-	-	96%	97%
Perioperative Temperature Management[2]	715	100%	100%	100%
Prophylactic Antibiotic Selection[2]	394	100%	99%	99%
Prophylactic Antibiotic Selection (Outpatient)	719	98%	98%	98%
Prophylactic Antibiotic Stopped[2]	373	99%	98%	98%
Prophylactic Antibiotic Timing[2]	393	99%	97%	99%
Prophylactic Antibiotic Timing (Outpatient)	724	98%	98%	98%
Urinary Catheter Removal[2]	296	100%	98%	97%
Survey of Patients' Hospital Experiences				
Area Around Room 'Always' Quiet at Night	300+	58%	57%	61%
Doctors 'Always' Communicated Well	300+	75%	78%	82%
Home Recovery Information Given	300+	80%	85%	85%
Hospital Given 9 or 10 on 10 Point Scale	300+	64%	65%	71%
Meds 'Always' Explained Before Given	300+	54%	58%	64%
Nurses 'Always' Communicated Well	300+	71%	75%	79%
Pain 'Always' Well Controlled	300+	65%	67%	71%
Room and Bathroom 'Always' Clean	300+	58%	64%	73%
Timely Help 'Always' Received	300+	53%	58%	68%
Would Definitely Recommend Hospital	300+	69%	67%	71%
Use of Medical Imaging				
Cardiac Imaging Stress Test before Surgery[1]	-	-	6.4%	5.3%
Combination Abdominal CT Scan	543	1.5%	3.8%	10.5%
Combination Brain/Sinus CT Scan	1,168	6.0%	4.3%	2.7%
Combination Chest CT Scan	282	0.0%	1%	2.7%
Follow-up Mammogram/Ultrasound	151	7.9%	10.2%	8.8%
Lumbar Spine MRI for Low Back Pain[1]	-	-	38.2%	37.2%

Washington Adventist Hospital

7600 Carroll Avenue | Phone: 301-891-5651
Takoma Park, MD 20912
URL: www.adventisthealthcare.com/wah
Type: Acute Care Hospitals | Emergency Services: Yes
Ownership: Voluntary non-profit - Private | Beds: 252

Key Personnel:
Cardiology . . . . David M. Brill, MD
CEO/President. . . . . Terry Forde
Chief of Medical Staff . . . . Randall Wagner, MD

Measure	Cases	This Hosp.	State Avg.	U.S. Avg.
Blood Clot Prevention and Treatment				
Anticoagulation Overlap Therapy[2]	73	93%	94%	93%
ICU Venous Thromboembolism Prophylaxis[2]	80	96%	94%	92%
Incidence of Potentially Preventable VTE[1,2]	-	-	7%	10%
UFH with Dosages/Platelet Monitoring[2]	25	92%	97%	97%
Venous Thromboembolism Prophylaxis[2]	286	84%	90%	85%
Warfarin Therapy Discharge Instructions[2]	47	53%	78%	75%
Chest Pain/Possible Heart Attack Care				
Aspirin Given Within 24 Hours of Arrival[5]	-	-	100%	96%
Fibrinolytic Meds Within 30 Min. of Arrival[5]	-	-	-	58%
Average Time to ECG (minutes)[5]	-	-	6	7
Average Time to Transfer (minutes)[5]	-	-	32	60
Children's Asthma Care				
Received Home Management Plan of Care	-	-	-	88%

NOTE: Hospital profiles are in alphabetical order by state, then city, then hospital within the city; Rankings exclude hospitals with less than 25 cases except for patient surveys which excludes hospitals with less than 100 cases; (a) 100-299 cases; (1) The number of cases/patients is too few to report; (2) Data submitted were based on a sample of cases/patients; (3) Results are based on a shorter time period than required; (4) Data suppressed by CMS for one or more quarters; (5) Results are not available for this reporting period; (6) Fewer than 100 patients completed the HCAHPS survey; (7) No cases met the criteria for this measure; (8) The lower limit of the confidence interval cannot be calculated if the number of observed infections equals zero; (9) No data are available from the state/territory for this reporting period; (10) The scores shown reflect fewer than 50 completed surveys; (11) There were discrepancies in the data collection process; (12) This measure does not apply to this hospital for this reporting period; (13) Results cannot be calculated for this reporting period; (14) The results for this state are combined with nearby states to protect confidentiality; Please refer to the User's Guide for a full explanation of data.

Measure	Cases	This Hosp.	State Avg.	U.S. Avg.
Received Reliever Medication	-	-	-	100%
Received Systemic Corticosteroids	-	-	-	100%
Emergency Department				
Admittance Decision Time (minutes)[2]	554	197	143	98
Head CT Results Within 45 Min. of Arrival[5]	-	-	-	57%
Patients Who Left ER Before Being Seen[5]	-	-	3%	2%
Time from ER Arrival to Admit. (minutes)[2]	560	427	357	274
Time from ER Arrival to Discharge (minutes)[5]	-	-	-	134
Time in ER Before Being Evaluated (minutes)[5]	-	-	-	26
Time to Pain Meds for Fractures (minutes)[5]	-	-	-	57
Heart Attack Care				
Aspirin Given at Discharge	364	100%	99%	99%
Fibrinolytic Meds Within 30 Min. of Arrival[7]	-	-	-	54%
PCI Within 90 Minutes of Arrival	31	97%	93%	96%
Statin Prescribed at Discharge	356	100%	98%	98%
Heart Failure Care				
ACE Inhibitor or ARB for LVSD	146	97%	97%	97%
Discharge Instructions Given	239	93%	93%	94%
Evaluation of LVS Function	315	100%	99%	99%
Medicare Spending				
Medicare Spending per Patient (ratio)	-	-	-	0.98
Pneumonia Care				
Appropriate Initial Antibiotic Given	76	99%	97%	95%
Blood Culture Timing	143	99%	97%	98%
Pregnancy and Delivery Care				
Newborn Deliveries Scheduled Early[5]	-	-	-	6%
Preventive Care				
Immunization for Influenza[2]	509	96%	94%	90%
Immunization for Pneumonia[2]	551	94%	94%	92%
Stroke Care				
Anticoagulation Therapy for Atrial Fibrillation[5]	-	-	95%	95%
Antithrombotic Therapy Timing[5]	-	-	95%	98%
Assessed for Rehabilitation[5]	-	-	96%	97%
Discharged on Antithrombotic Therapy[5]	-	-	95%	99%
Discharged on Statin Medication[5]	-	-	97%	94%
Thrombolytic Therapy Timing[5]	-	-	-	66%
Venous Thromboembolism Prophylaxis[5]	-	-	89%	94%
Written Stroke Educational Materials Given[5]	-	-	77%	88%
Surgical Care Improvement Project				
Appropriate Beta Blocker Usage	253	99%	97%	98%
Appropriate VTP Within 24 Hours	217	98%	98%	98%
Controlled Postoperative Blood Glucose	278	100%	96%	97%
Perioperative Temperature Management	289	100%	100%	100%
Prophylactic Antibiotic Selection	427	100%	99%	99%
Prophylactic Antibiotic Selection (Outpatient)[5]	-	-	98%	98%
Prophylactic Antibiotic Stopped	424	99%	98%	98%
Prophylactic Antibiotic Timing	427	99%	97%	99%
Prophylactic Antibiotic Timing (Outpatient)[5]	-	-	98%	98%
Urinary Catheter Removal	428	100%	98%	97%
Survey of Patients' Hospital Experiences				
Area Around Room 'Always' Quiet at Night	300+	54%	57%	61%
Doctors 'Always' Communicated Well	300+	77%	78%	82%
Home Recovery Information Given	300+	83%	85%	85%
Hospital Given 9 or 10 on 10 Point Scale	300+	63%	65%	71%
Meds 'Always' Explained Before Given	300+	55%	58%	64%
Nurses 'Always' Communicated Well	300+	72%	75%	79%
Pain 'Always' Well Controlled	300+	65%	67%	71%
Room and Bathroom 'Always' Clean	300+	59%	64%	73%
Timely Help 'Always' Received	300+	55%	58%	68%
Would Definitely Recommend Hospital	300+	67%	67%	71%
Use of Medical Imaging				
Cardiac Imaging Stress Test before Surgery	96	4.2%	6.4%	5.3%
Combination Abdominal CT Scan	351	4.0%	3.8%	10.5%
Combination Brain/Sinus CT Scan[1]	-	-	4.3%	2.7%
Combination Chest CT Scan	128	3.1%	1%	2.7%
Follow-up Mammogram/Ultrasound	260	10.4%	10.2%	8.8%
Lumbar Spine MRI for Low Back Pain[1]	-	-	38.2%	37.2%

University of Maryland Saint Joseph Medical Center

7601 Osler Drive
Towson, MD 21204
Phone: 410-337-1000
Type: Acute Care Hospitals
Emergency Services: Yes
Ownership: Voluntary non-profit - Private

Measure	Cases	This Hosp.	State Avg.	U.S. Avg.
Blood Clot Prevention and Treatment				
Anticoagulation Overlap Therapy[2,3]	62	98%	94%	93%
ICU Venous Thromboembolism Prophylaxis[2,3]	42	95%	94%	92%
Incidence of Potentially Preventable VTE[1,2]	-	-	7%	10%
UFH with Dosages/Platelet Monitoring[2,3]	38	100%	97%	97%
Venous Thromboembolism Prophylaxis[2,3]	171	81%	90%	85%
Warfarin Therapy Discharge Instructions[2,3]	45	64%	78%	75%
Chest Pain/Possible Heart Attack Care				
Aspirin Given Within 24 Hours of Arrival[5]	-	-	100%	96%
Fibrinolytic Meds Within 30 Min. of Arrival[5]	-	-	-	58%
Average Time to ECG (minutes)[5]	-	-	6	7
Average Time to Transfer (minutes)[5]	-	-	32	60
Children's Asthma Care				
Received Home Management Plan of Care	-	-	-	88%
Received Reliever Medication	-	-	-	100%
Received Systemic Corticosteroids	-	-	-	100%
Emergency Department				
Admittance Decision Time (minutes)[2,3]	230	108	143	98
Head CT Results Within 45 Min. of Arrival[5]	-	-	-	57%
Patients Who Left ER Before Being Seen[5]	-	-	3%	2%
Time from ER Arrival to Admit. (minutes)[2,3]	247	327	357	274
Time from ER Arrival to Discharge (minutes)[5]	-	-	-	134
Time in ER Before Being Evaluated (minutes)[5]	-	-	-	26
Time to Pain Meds for Fractures (minutes)[5]	-	-	-	57
Heart Attack Care				
Aspirin Given at Discharge[2,3]	139	99%	99%	99%
Fibrinolytic Meds Within 30 Min. of Arrival[2,3]	-	-	-	54%
PCI Within 90 Minutes of Arrival[2,3]	19	89%	93%	96%
Statin Prescribed at Discharge[2,3]	131	99%	98%	98%
Heart Failure Care				
ACE Inhibitor or ARB for LVSD[2,3]	41	98%	97%	97%
Discharge Instructions Given[2,3]	107	98%	93%	94%
Evaluation of LVS Function[2,3]	132	100%	99%	99%
Medicare Spending				
Medicare Spending per Patient (ratio)	-	-	-	0.98
Pneumonia Care				
Appropriate Initial Antibiotic Given[2,3]	37	95%	97%	95%
Blood Culture Timing[2,3]	62	94%	97%	98%
Pregnancy and Delivery Care				
Newborn Deliveries Scheduled Early[5]	-	-	-	6%
Preventive Care				
Immunization for Influenza[5]	-	-	94%	90%
Immunization for Pneumonia[2,3]	320	95%	94%	92%
Stroke Care				
Anticoagulation Therapy for Atrial Fibrillation[5]	-	-	95%	95%
Antithrombotic Therapy Timing[5]	-	-	95%	98%
Assessed for Rehabilitation[5]	-	-	96%	97%
Discharged on Antithrombotic Therapy[5]	-	-	95%	99%
Discharged on Statin Medication[5]	-	-	97%	94%
Thrombolytic Therapy Timing[5]	-	-	-	66%
Venous Thromboembolism Prophylaxis[5]	-	-	89%	94%
Written Stroke Educational Materials Given[5]	-	-	77%	88%
Surgical Care Improvement Project				
Appropriate Beta Blocker Usage[2,3]	97	98%	97%	98%
Appropriate VTP Within 24 Hours[2,3]	127	98%	98%	98%
Controlled Postoperative Blood Glucose[2,3]	63	90%	96%	97%
Perioperative Temperature Management[2,3]	181	99%	100%	100%
Prophylactic Antibiotic Selection[2,3]	170	100%	99%	99%
Prophylactic Antibiotic Selection (Outpatient)[5]	-	-	98%	98%
Prophylactic Antibiotic Stopped[2,3]	164	99%	98%	98%
Prophylactic Antibiotic Timing[2,3]	172	99%	97%	99%
Prophylactic Antibiotic Timing (Outpatient)[5]	-	-	98%	98%
Urinary Catheter Removal[2,3]	106	95%	98%	97%
Survey of Patients' Hospital Experiences				
Area Around Room 'Always' Quiet at Night[5]	-	-	57%	61%
Doctors 'Always' Communicated Well[5]	-	-	78%	82%
Home Recovery Information Given[5]	-	-	85%	85%
Hospital Given 9 or 10 on 10 Point Scale[5]	-	-	65%	71%
Meds 'Always' Explained Before Given[5]	-	-	58%	64%
Nurses 'Always' Communicated Well[5]	-	-	75%	79%
Pain 'Always' Well Controlled[5]	-	-	67%	71%
Room and Bathroom 'Always' Clean[5]	-	-	64%	73%
Timely Help 'Always' Received[5]	-	-	58%	68%
Would Definitely Recommend Hospital[5]	-	-	67%	71%
Use of Medical Imaging				
Cardiac Imaging Stress Test before Surgery	269	9.3%	6.4%	5.3%
Combination Abdominal CT Scan	333	4.5%	3.8%	10.5%
Combination Brain/Sinus CT Scan[1]	-	-	4.3%	2.7%
Combination Chest CT Scan	92	2.2%	1%	2.7%
Follow-up Mammogram/Ultrasound[7]	-	-	10.2%	8.8%
Lumbar Spine MRI for Low Back Pain[1]	-	-	38.2%	37.2%

Carroll Hospital Center

200 Memorial Ave
Westminster, MD 21157
Phone: 410-848-3000
Fax: 410-871-6325
E-mail: info@carrollhospitalcenter.org
URL: www.carrollhospitalcenter.org
Type: Acute Care Hospitals
Emergency Services: Yes
Ownership: Voluntary non-profit - Private
Beds: 200

Key Personnel:

Radiology. . . . . Sandy D'Arrigo
Pediatric In-Patient Care . . . . Linda Grogan
Quality Assurance . . . . Mary Ann Kowalczyk
Chief of Medical Staff . . . . Mark Olszyk, MD, MBA, CPE, F
Operating Room. . . . . Kate Painter
Patient Relations . . . . Leslie Simmons
President/CEO. . . . . Leslie Simmons, RN, FACHE
Operating Room. . . . . Robert White, MBA, MHA, FACHE

Measure	Cases	This Hosp.	State Avg.	U.S. Avg.
Blood Clot Prevention and Treatment				
Anticoagulation Overlap Therapy[2]	93	96%	94%	93%
ICU Venous Thromboembolism Prophylaxis[2]	87	100%	94%	92%
Incidence of Potentially Preventable VTE[1,2]	-	-	7%	10%
UFH with Dosages/Platelet Monitoring[2]	84	100%	97%	97%
Venous Thromboembolism Prophylaxis[2]	277	96%	90%	85%
Warfarin Therapy Discharge Instructions[2]	78	99%	78%	75%
Chest Pain/Possible Heart Attack Care				
Aspirin Given Within 24 Hours of Arrival[5]	-	-	100%	96%
Fibrinolytic Meds Within 30 Min. of Arrival[5]	-	-	-	58%
Average Time to ECG (minutes)[5]	-	-	6	7
Average Time to Transfer (minutes)[5]	-	-	32	60
Children's Asthma Care				
Received Home Management Plan of Care	24	88%	-	88%
Received Reliever Medication	26	100%	-	100%
Received Systemic Corticosteroids	26	100%	-	100%
Emergency Department				
Admittance Decision Time (minutes)[2]	780	99	143	98
Head CT Results Within 45 Min. of Arrival[5]	-	-	-	57%
Patients Who Left ER Before Being Seen[5]	-	-	3%	2%
Time from ER Arrival to Admit. (minutes)[2]	780	306	357	274
Time from ER Arrival to Discharge (minutes)[5]	-	-	-	134
Time in ER Before Being Evaluated (minutes)[5]	-	-	-	26
Time to Pain Meds for Fractures (minutes)[5]	-	-	-	57
Heart Attack Care				
Aspirin Given at Discharge	96	100%	99%	99%
Fibrinolytic Meds Within 30 Min. of Arrival[7]	-	-	-	54%
PCI Within 90 Minutes of Arrival	51	94%	93%	96%
Statin Prescribed at Discharge	95	100%	98%	98%
Heart Failure Care				
ACE Inhibitor or ARB for LVSD[2]	52	100%	97%	97%
Discharge Instructions Given[2]	180	99%	93%	94%
Evaluation of LVS Function[2]	220	100%	99%	99%
Medicare Spending				
Medicare Spending per Patient (ratio)	-	-	-	0.98
Pneumonia Care				
Appropriate Initial Antibiotic Given[2]	99	96%	97%	95%
Blood Culture Timing[2]	165	98%	97%	98%
Pregnancy and Delivery Care				
Newborn Deliveries Scheduled Early[5]	-	-	-	6%
Preventive Care				

NOTE: Hospital profiles are in alphabetical order by state, then city, then hospital within the city; Rankings exclude hospitals with less than 25 cases except for patient surveys which excludes hospitals with less than 100 cases; (a) 100-299 cases; (1) The number of cases/patients is too few to report; (2) Data submitted were based on a sample of cases/patients; (3) Results are based on a shorter time period than required; (4) Data suppressed by CMS for one or more quarters; (5) Results are not available for this reporting period; (6) Fewer than 100 patients completed the HCAHPS survey; (7) No cases met the criteria for this measure; (8) The lower limit of the confidence interval cannot be calculated if the number of observed infections equals zero; (9) No data are available from the state/territory for this reporting period; (10) The scores shown reflect fewer than 50 completed surveys; (11) There were discrepancies in the data collection process; (12) This measure does not apply to this hospital for this reporting period; (13) Results cannot be calculated for this reporting period; (14) The results for this state are combined with nearby states to protect confidentiality; Please refer to the User's Guide for a full explanation of data.

Immunization for Influenza[2]	553	95%	94%	90%
Immunization for Pneumonia[2]	733	96%	94%	92%
Stroke Care				
Anticoagulation Therapy for Atrial Fibrillation[5]	-	-	95%	95%
Antithrombotic Therapy Timing[5]	-	-	95%	98%
Assessed for Rehabilitation[5]	-	-	96%	97%
Discharged on Antithrombotic Therapy[5]	-	-	95%	99%
Discharged on Statin Medication[5]	-	-	97%	94%
Thrombolytic Therapy Timing[5]	-	-	-	66%
Venous Thromboembolism Prophylaxis[5]	-	-	89%	94%
Written Stroke Educational Materials Given[5]	-	-	77%	88%
Surgical Care Improvement Project				
Appropriate Beta Blocker Usage[2]	112	98%	97%	98%
Appropriate VTP Within 24 Hours[2]	395	99%	98%	98%
Controlled Postoperative Blood Glucose[2,7]	-	-	96%	97%
Perioperative Temperature Management[2]	559	100%	100%	100%
Prophylactic Antibiotic Selection[2]	377	99%	99%	99%
Prophylactic Antibiotic Selection (Outpatient)[5]	-	-	98%	98%
Prophylactic Antibiotic Stopped[2]	372	97%	98%	98%
Prophylactic Antibiotic Timing[2]	377	98%	97%	99%
Prophylactic Antibiotic Timing (Outpatient)[5]	-	-	98%	98%
Urinary Catheter Removal[2]	278	99%	98%	97%
Survey of Patients' Hospital Experiences				
Area Around Room 'Always' Quiet at Night	300+	55%	57%	61%
Doctors 'Always' Communicated Well	300+	79%	78%	82%
Home Recovery Information Given	300+	86%	85%	85%
Hospital Given 9 or 10 on 10 Point Scale	300+	73%	65%	71%
Meds 'Always' Explained Before Given	300+	65%	58%	64%
Nurses 'Always' Communicated Well	300+	82%	75%	79%
Pain 'Always' Well Controlled	300+	70%	67%	71%
Room and Bathroom 'Always' Clean	300+	70%	64%	73%
Timely Help 'Always' Received	300+	70%	58%	68%
Would Definitely Recommend Hospital	300+	73%	67%	71%
Use of Medical Imaging				
Cardiac Imaging Stress Test before Surgery	293	5.5%	6.4%	5.3%
Combination Abdominal CT Scan	818	0.4%	3.8%	10.5%
Combination Brain/Sinus CT Scan	1,466	6.6%	4.3%	2.7%
Combination Chest CT Scan	131	0.0%	1%	2.7%
Follow-up Mammogram/Ultrasound[7]	-	-	10.2%	8.8%
Lumbar Spine MRI for Low Back Pain[1]	-	-	38.2%	37.2%

NOTE: Hospital profiles are in alphabetical order by state, then city, then hospital within the city; Rankings exclude hospitals with less than 25 cases except for patient surveys which excludes hospitals with less than 100 cases; (a) 100-299 cases; (1) The number of cases/patients is too few to report; (2) Data submitted were based on a sample of cases/patients; (3) Results are based on a shorter time period than required; (4) Data suppressed by CMS for one or more quarters; (5) Results are not available for this reporting period; (6) Fewer than 100 patients completed the HCAHPS survey; (7) No cases met the criteria for this measure; (8) The lower limit of the confidence interval cannot be calculated if the number of observed infections equals zero; (9) No data are available from the state/territory for this reporting period; (10) The scores shown reflect fewer than 50 completed surveys; (11) There were discrepancies in the data collection process; (12) This measure does not apply to this hospital for this reporting period; (13) Results cannot be calculated for this reporting period; (14) The results for this state are combined with nearby states to protect confidentiality; Please refer to the User's Guide for a full explanation of data.

Blood Clot Prevention and Treatment

Anticoagulation Overlap Therapy

Hospital Name	City	Rate	Cases
Beth Israel Deaconess Hospital - Milton[2]	Milton	100%	41
Boston Medical Center Corporation[2]	Boston	100%	93
Brigham & Women's Faulkner Hospital[2]	Boston	100%	27
Cambridge Health Alliance[2]	Cambridge	100%	61
The Cooley Dickinson Hospital[2]	Northampton	100%	39
Emerson Hospital[2]	W Concord	100%	46
Massachusetts General Hospital[2]	Boston	100%	224
Metrowest Medical Center[2]	Framingham	100%	45
Mount Auburn Hospital[2]	Cambridge	100%	55
Newton - Wellesley Hospital[2]	Newton	100%	52
Saint Elizabeth's Medical Center[2]	Brighton	100%	53
South Shore Hospital[2]	S Weymouth	100%	158
Umass Memorial Medical Center[2]	Worcester	100%	236
Winchester Hospital[2]	Winchester	100%	67
Beverly Hospital Corporation[2]	Beverly	99%	88
Good Samaritan Medical Center[2]	Brockton	99%	101
Lahey Hosp & Med Ctr-Burlington[2]	Burlington	99%	165
Saint Vincent Hospital[2]	Worcester	99%	131
Signature Healthcare Brockton Hospital[2]	Brockton	99%	74
Anna Jaques Hospital[2]	Newburyport	98%	40
Berkshire Medical Center[2]	Pittsfield	98%	50
Milford Regional Medical Center[2]	Milford	98%	50
Morton Hospital[2]	Taunton	98%	45
Southcoast Hospital Group[2]	Fall River	98%	255
Sturdy Memorial Hospital[2]	Attleboro	98%	56
Brigham & Women's Hospital[2]	Boston	97%	179
Hallmark Health System[2]	Melrose	97%	69
Lowell General Hospital[2]	Lowell	97%	58
Saint Anne's Hospital[2]	Fall River	97%	62
Baystate Medical Center[2]	Springfield	96%	189
Cape Cod Hospital[2]	Hyannis	96%	123
Holy Family Hospital[2]	Methuen	96%	67
Tufts Medical Center[2]	Boston	96%	94
Beth Israel Deaconess Medical Center[2]	Boston	95%	177
Falmouth Hospital[2]	Falmouth	95%	43
Holyoke Medical Center[2]	Holyoke	95%	42
North Shore Medical Center[2]	Salem	93%	112
Mercy Medical Center[2]	Springfield	92%	79
Healthalliance Hospitals[2]	Leominster	91%	53
Jordan Hospital[2]	Plymouth	90%	60
Saints Medical Center[2]	Lowell	89%	27
Merrimack Valley Hospital[2]	Haverhill	88%	25
Norwood Hospital[2]	Norwood	87%	85
Lawrence General Hospital[2]	Lawrence	84%	49
Heywood Hospital[2]	Gardner	73%	26

ICU Venous Thromboembolism Prophylaxis

Hospital Name	City	Rate	Cases
Berkshire Medical Center[2]	Pittsfield	100%	73
Cape Cod Hospital[2]	Hyannis	100%	42
The Cooley Dickinson Hospital[2]	Northampton	100%	37
Falmouth Hospital[2]	Falmouth	100%	65
Healthalliance Hospitals[2]	Leominster	100%	111
Lahey Hosp & Med Ctr-Burlington[2]	Burlington	100%	69
Nashoba Valley Medical Center[2]	Ayer	100%	38
Sturdy Memorial Hospital[2]	Attleboro	100%	71
Wing Memorial Hospital & Medical Center[2]	Palmer	100%	38
Massachusetts General Hospital[2]	Boston	99%	79
Metrowest Medical Center[2]	Framingham	99%	71
Signature Healthcare Brockton Hospital[2]	Brockton	99%	71
Umass Memorial Medical Center[2]	Worcester	99%	121
Milford Regional Medical Center[2]	Milford	98%	56
Baystate Medical Center[2]	Springfield	97%	75
Beth Israel Deaconess Medical Center[2]	Boston	97%	103
Saint Vincent Hospital[2]	Worcester	97%	78
Good Samaritan Medical Center[2]	Brockton	96%	52
Saint Anne's Hospital[2]	Fall River	96%	68
South Shore Hospital[2]	S Weymouth	96%	73
Anna Jaques Hospital[2]	Newburyport	95%	41
Brigham & Women's Hospital[2]	Boston	95%	56
Carney Hospital[2]	Boston	95%	64
Jordan Hospital[2]	Plymouth	95%	58
North Adams Regional Hospital[2]	North Adams	94%	104
Beth Israel Deaconess Hospital - Needham[2]	Needham	93%	54
Emerson Hospital[2]	W Concord	93%	69
Holyoke Medical Center[2]	Holyoke	93%	44
Marlborough Hospital[2]	Marlborough	93%	74
Mount Auburn Hospital[2]	Cambridge	93%	91
Norwood Hospital[2]	Norwood	93%	30
Heywood Hospital[2]	Gardner	92%	40
Morton Hospital[2]	Taunton	92%	63
Newton - Wellesley Hospital[2]	Newton	92%	62
Beverly Hospital Corporation[2]	Beverly	91%	44
Tufts Medical Center[2]	Boston	91%	206
Southcoast Hospital Group[2]	Fall River	90%	63
Baystate Franklin Medical Center[2]	Greenfield	89%	37
Cambridge Health Alliance[2]	Cambridge	89%	62
Hallmark Health System[2]	Melrose	89%	37
Saint Elizabeth's Medical Center[2]	Brighton	89%	83
Beth Israel Deaconess Hospital - Milton[2]	Milton	88%	65
Boston Medical Center Corporation[2]	Boston	87%	85
Merrimack Valley Hospital[2]	Haverhill	84%	55
Winchester Hospital[2]	Winchester	81%	27
Holy Family Hospital[2]	Methuen	79%	85
Saints Medical Center[2]	Lowell	77%	31
Harrington Memorial Hospital[2]	Southbridge	73%	52
Lawrence General Hospital[2]	Lawrence	73%	67
North Shore Medical Center[2]	Salem	62%	74

Incidence of Potentially Preventable VTE

Hospital Name	City	Rate	Cases
Umass Memorial Medical Center[2]	Worcester	0%	58
Beth Israel Deaconess Medical Center[2]	Boston	2%	57
Brigham & Women's Hospital[2]	Boston	2%	81
Lahey Hosp & Med Ctr-Burlington[2]	Burlington	3%	58
Saint Vincent Hospital[2]	Worcester	3%	37
Massachusetts General Hospital[2]	Boston	4%	111
Boston Medical Center Corporation[2]	Boston	7%	41
Baystate Medical Center[2]	Springfield	8%	62
South Shore Hospital[2]	S Weymouth	9%	33
Tufts Medical Center[2]	Boston	9%	45
Southcoast Hospital Group[2]	Fall River	15%	34

UFH with Dosages/Platelet Count Monitoring

Hospital Name	City	Rate	Cases
Baystate Medical Center[2]	Springfield	100%	145
Berkshire Medical Center[2]	Pittsfield	100%	41
Beverly Hospital Corporation[2]	Beverly	100%	39
Brigham & Women's Hospital[2]	Boston	100%	240
Cambridge Health Alliance[2]	Cambridge	100%	55
Good Samaritan Medical Center[2]	Brockton	100%	47
Holy Family Hospital[2]	Methuen	100%	34
Lahey Hosp & Med Ctr-Burlington[2]	Burlington	100%	132
Lawrence General Hospital[2]	Lawrence	100%	34
Mercy Medical Center[2]	Springfield	100%	46
Metrowest Medical Center[2]	Framingham	100%	28
Mount Auburn Hospital[2]	Cambridge	100%	49
North Shore Medical Center[2]	Salem	100%	73
Saint Anne's Hospital[2]	Fall River	100%	28
Saint Vincent Hospital[2]	Worcester	100%	94
Signature Healthcare Brockton Hospital[2]	Brockton	100%	36
South Shore Hospital[2]	S Weymouth	100%	82
Southcoast Hospital Group[2]	Fall River	100%	206
Sturdy Memorial Hospital[2]	Attleboro	100%	46
Tufts Medical Center[2]	Boston	100%	97
Winchester Hospital[2]	Winchester	100%	34
Norwood Hospital[2]	Norwood	99%	81
Umass Memorial Medical Center[2]	Worcester	99%	156
Saint Elizabeth's Medical Center[2]	Brighton	98%	58
Lowell General Hospital[2]	Lowell	96%	27
Cape Cod Hospital[2]	Hyannis	95%	99
Boston Medical Center Corporation[2]	Boston	93%	67
Massachusetts General Hospital[2]	Boston	92%	232
Beth Israel Deaconess Medical Center[2]	Boston	0%	199

Venous Thromboembolism Prophylaxis

Hospital Name	City	Rate	Cases
The Cooley Dickinson Hospital[2]	Northampton	100%	369
New England Baptist Hospital[2]	Boston	100%	106
Berkshire Medical Center[2]	Pittsfield	99%	333
Falmouth Hospital[2]	Falmouth	99%	307
Sturdy Memorial Hospital[2]	Attleboro	99%	349
Noble Hospital[2]	Westfield	98%	266
Brigham & Women's Faulkner Hospital[2]	Boston	97%	286
North Adams Regional Hospital[2]	North Adams	97%	112
Wing Memorial Hospital & Medical Center[2]	Palmer	97%	239
Baystate Mary Lane Hospital[2]	Ware	96%	112
Beth Israel Deaconess Hospital - Needham[2]	Needham	96%	168
Saint Vincent Hospital[2]	Worcester	96%	348
Holyoke Medical Center[2]	Holyoke	95%	389
Massachusetts General Hospital[2]	Boston	95%	341
Norwood Hospital[2]	Norwood	95%	352
Beth Israel Deaconess Medical Center[2]	Boston	94%	326
Mercy Medical Center[2]	Springfield	94%	377
South Shore Hospital[2]	S Weymouth	94%	396
Jordan Hospital[2]	Plymouth	93%	322
Lowell General Hospital[2]	Lowell	93%	341
Metrowest Medical Center[2]	Framingham	93%	302
Nashoba Valley Medical Center[2]	Ayer	93%	174
Baystate Medical Center[2]	Springfield	92%	376
Boston Medical Center Corporation[2]	Boston	92%	359
Massachusetts Eye & Ear Infirmary[2]	Boston	92%	160
Signature Healthcare Brockton Hospital[2]	Brockton	92%	344
Emerson Hospital[2]	W Concord	91%	240
Heywood Hospital[2]	Gardner	91%	319
Umass Memorial Medical Center[2]	Worcester	91%	311
Baystate Franklin Medical Center[2]	Greenfield	90%	227
Cape Cod Hospital[2]	Hyannis	90%	355
Lahey Hosp & Med Ctr-Burlington[2]	Burlington	90%	351
Milford Regional Medical Center[2]	Milford	90%	365
Good Samaritan Medical Center[2]	Brockton	89%	351
Mount Auburn Hospital[2]	Cambridge	89%	348
Newton - Wellesley Hospital[2]	Newton	89%	305
Cambridge Health Alliance[2]	Cambridge	88%	313
Healthalliance Hospitals[2]	Leominster	88%	444
Carney Hospital[2]	Boston	87%	305
Brigham & Women's Hospital[2]	Boston	86%	347
Harrington Memorial Hospital[2]	Southbridge	85%	290
Morton Hospital[2]	Taunton	84%	324
Southcoast Hospital Group[2]	Fall River	84%	369
Beverly Hospital Corporation[2]	Beverly	83%	279
Quincy Medical Center[2]	Quincy	83%	365
Anna Jaques Hospital[2]	Newburyport	79%	323
Beth Israel Deaconess Hospital - Milton[2]	Milton	79%	341
Marlborough Hospital[2]	Marlborough	79%	210
Winchester Hospital[2]	Winchester	79%	375
Lawrence General Hospital[2]	Lawrence	78%	369
Saint Elizabeth's Medical Center[2]	Brighton	78%	269
Tufts Medical Center[2]	Boston	76%	288
Saint Anne's Hospital[2]	Fall River	74%	348
Merrimack Valley Hospital[2]	Haverhill	73%	259
North Shore Medical Center[2]	Salem	73%	372
Saints Medical Center[2]	Lowell	73%	407
Holy Family Hospital[2]	Methuen	72%	287
Hallmark Health System[2]	Melrose	65%	297
Clinton Hospital Association[2]	Clinton	64%	97
Nantucket Cottage Hospital[2]	Nantucket	26%	136

Warfarin Therapy Discharge Instructions

Hospital Name	City	Rate	Cases
Beth Israel Deaconess Hospital - Milton[2]	Milton	100%	27
Saint Anne's Hospital[2]	Fall River	100%	46
Winchester Hospital[2]	Winchester	100%	43
Brigham & Women's Hospital[2]	Boston	99%	114
Berkshire Medical Center[2]	Pittsfield	98%	41
Hallmark Health System[2]	Melrose	98%	53
Holy Family Hospital[2]	Methuen	98%	41
Good Samaritan Medical Center[2]	Brockton	97%	79
Southcoast Hospital Group[2]	Fall River	96%	184
Norwood Hospital[2]	Norwood	95%	75
Saint Elizabeth's Medical Center[2]	Brighton	95%	41
Emerson Hospital[2]	W Concord	94%	33
North Shore Medical Center[2]	Salem	93%	82
The Cooley Dickinson Hospital[2]	Northampton	92%	26
South Shore Hospital[2]	S Weymouth	92%	115
Sturdy Memorial Hospital[2]	Attleboro	92%	38
Jordan Hospital[2]	Plymouth	90%	41
Massachusetts General Hospital[2]	Boston	90%	143
Morton Hospital[2]	Taunton	86%	37
Newton - Wellesley Hospital[2]	Newton	85%	48
Cambridge Health Alliance[2]	Cambridge	82%	49
Cape Cod Hospital[2]	Hyannis	82%	77
Baystate Medical Center[2]	Springfield	80%	141
Milford Regional Medical Center[2]	Milford	79%	34
Anna Jaques Hospital[2]	Newburyport	76%	29
Umass Memorial Medical Center[2]	Worcester	76%	160
Mercy Medical Center[2]	Springfield	75%	60
Metrowest Medical Center[2]	Framingham	72%	29
Lahey Hosp & Med Ctr-Burlington[2]	Burlington	71%	112
Saint Vincent Hospital[2]	Worcester	69%	87
Signature Healthcare Brockton Hospital[2]	Brockton	69%	52
Lowell General Hospital[2]	Lowell	59%	37
Beverly Hospital Corporation[2]	Beverly	55%	62
Beth Israel Deaconess Medical Center[2]	Boston	47%	109
Lawrence General Hospital[2]	Lawrence	39%	33
Boston Medical Center Corporation[2]	Boston	34%	71
Falmouth Hospital[2]	Falmouth	34%	29
Healthalliance Hospitals[2]	Leominster	8%	38
Mount Auburn Hospital[2]	Cambridge	2%	44
Tufts Medical Center[2]	Boston	1%	69

Chest Pain/Possible Heart Attack Care

Aspirin Given Within 24 Hours of Arrival

Hospital Name	City	Rate	Cases
Anna Jaques Hospital	Newburyport	100%	64
Baystate Franklin Medical Center	Greenfield	100%	48
Baystate Mary Lane Hospital	Ware	100%	33
Berkshire Medical Center	Pittsfield	100%	93
Beth Israel Deaconess Hospital - Needham	Needham	100%	61
Beverly Hospital Corporation	Beverly	100%	68
Brigham & Women's Faulkner Hospital	Boston	100%	49
Cambridge Health Alliance	Cambridge	100%	85
Carney Hospital	Boston	100%	41
The Cooley Dickinson Hospital	Northampton	100%	90
Metrowest Medical Center	Framingham	100%	33

NOTE: Hospital profiles are in alphabetical order by state, then city, then hospital within the city; Rankings exclude hospitals with less than 25 cases except for patient surveys which excludes hospitals with less than 100 cases; (a) 100-299 cases; (1) The number of cases/patients is too few to report; (2) Data submitted were based on a sample of cases/patients; (3) Results are based on a shorter time period than required; (4) Data suppressed by CMS for one or more quarters; (5) Results are not available for this reporting period; (6) Fewer than 100 patients completed the HCAHPS survey; (7) No cases met the criteria for this measure; (8) The lower limit of the confidence interval cannot be calculated if the number of observed infections equals zero; (9) No data are available from the state/territory for this reporting period; (10) The scores shown reflect fewer than 50 completed surveys; (11) There were discrepancies in the data collection process; (12) This measure does not apply to this hospital for this reporting period; (13) Results cannot be calculated for this reporting period; (14) The results for this state are combined with nearby states to protect confidentiality; Please refer to the User's Guide for a full explanation of data.

Nashoba Valley Medical Center	Ayer	100%	36
Newton - Wellesley Hospital	Newton	100%	112
Noble Hospital	Westfield	100%	50
Signature Healthcare Brockton Hospital	Brockton	100%	25
Winchester Hospital	Winchester	100%	99
Beth Israel Deaconess Hospital - Milton	Milton	99%	74
Healthalliance Hospitals	Leominster	99%	173
Milford Regional Medical Center	Milford	99%	70
Jordan Hospital	Plymouth	98%	82
Mercy Medical Center	Springfield	98%	55
Morton Hospital	Taunton	98%	63
North Adams Regional Hospital	North Adams	98%	58
Southcoast Hospital Group	Fall River	98%	150
Sturdy Memorial Hospital	Attleboro	98%	125
Emerson Hospital	W Concord	97%	34
Good Samaritan Medical Center	Brockton	97%	29
Hallmark Health System	Melrose	97%	71
Holyoke Medical Center	Holyoke	97%	59
Marlborough Hospital	Marlborough	97%	58
Quincy Medical Center	Quincy	97%	62
South Shore Hospital	S Weymouth	96%	28
Norwood Hospital	Norwood	94%	66
Saints Medical Center	Lowell	94%	36
Harrington Memorial Hospital	Southbridge	93%	88
Lawrence General Hospital	Lawrence	93%	28
Wing Memorial Hospital & Medical Center	Palmer	93%	57
Heywood Hospital	Gardner	91%	139
Holy Family Hospital	Methuen	89%	28
Nantucket Cottage Hospital	Nantucket	87%	31

Fibrinolytic Meds Within 30 Minutes of Arrival

Hospital Name	City	Rate	Cases
Berkshire Medical Center	Pittsfield	72%	25

Average Time to ECG (minutes)

Hospital Name	City	Min.	Cases
Norwood Hospital	Norwood	0	68
Good Samaritan Medical Center	Brockton	1	33
Metrowest Medical Center	Framingham	1	35
Quincy Medical Center	Quincy	4	63
Signature Healthcare Brockton Hospital	Brockton	4	29
Anna Jaques Hospital	Newburyport	5	67
Brigham & Women's Faulkner Hospital	Boston	5	47
The Cooley Dickinson Hospital	Northampton	5	93
Harrington Memorial Hospital	Southbridge	5	99
Holyoke Medical Center	Holyoke	5	60
Milford Regional Medical Center	Milford	5	70
Newton - Wellesley Hospital	Newton	5	114
Berkshire Medical Center	Pittsfield	6	95
Marlborough Hospital	Marlborough	6	61
Mercy Medical Center	Springfield	6	57
Morton Hospital	Taunton	6	65
Nashoba Valley Medical Center	Ayer	6	36
Beverly Hospital Corporation	Beverly	7	72
Noble Hospital	Westfield	7	51
North Adams Regional Hospital	North Adams	7	63
Saints Medical Center	Lowell	7	35
Southcoast Hospital Group	Fall River	7	157
Baystate Franklin Medical Center	Greenfield	8	48
Holy Family Hospital	Methuen	8	33
South Shore Hospital	S Weymouth	8	29
Wing Memorial Hospital & Medical Center	Palmer	8	55
Cambridge Health Alliance	Cambridge	9	90
Healthalliance Hospitals	Leominster	9	174
Heywood Hospital	Gardner	9	145
Baystate Mary Lane Hospital	Ware	10	35
Beth Israel Deaconess Hospital - Needham	Needham	10	62
Emerson Hospital	W Concord	10	34
Hallmark Health System	Melrose	10	72
Jordan Hospital	Plymouth	10	87
Nantucket Cottage Hospital	Nantucket	10	30
Beth Israel Deaconess Hospital - Milton	Milton	11	75
Sturdy Memorial Hospital	Attleboro	11	126
Lawrence General Hospital	Lawrence	12	30
Winchester Hospital	Winchester	12	101
Carney Hospital	Boston	14	40

Average Time to Transfer (minutes)

Hospital Name	City	Min.	Cases
Southcoast Hospital Group	Fall River	54	50
Winchester Hospital	Winchester	75	31

Children's Asthma Care

Received Home Management Plan of Care

Hospital Name	City	Rate	Cases
Baystate Medical Center	Springfield	95%	109
Boston Children's Hospital[2]	Boston	62%	332

Received Reliever Medication

Hospital Name	City	Rate	Cases
Baystate Medical Center	Springfield	100%	109
Boston Children's Hospital[2]	Boston	100%	332

Received Systemic Corticosteroids

Hospital Name	City	Rate	Cases
Baystate Medical Center	Springfield	100%	109
Boston Children's Hospital[2]	Boston	100%	332

Emergency Department

Admittance Decision Time (minutes)

Hospital Name	City	Min.	Cases
Clinton Hospital Association[2]	Clinton	40	243
Nantucket Cottage Hospital[2]	Nantucket	44	148
Noble Hospital[2]	Westfield	48	723
Nashoba Valley Medical Center[2]	Ayer	52	422
Wing Memorial Hospital & Medical Center[2]	Palmer	55	336
Berkshire Medical Center[2]	Pittsfield	58	798
Baystate Mary Lane Hospital[2]	Ware	65	322
North Adams Regional Hospital[2]	North Adams	69	333
Fairview Hospital[2]	Great Barrington	73	391
Beth Israel Deaconess Hospital - Milton[2]	Milton	75	942
The Cooley Dickinson Hospital[2]	Northampton	80	825
Harrington Memorial Hospital[2]	Southbridge	80	565
Lahey Hosp & Med Ctr-Burlington[2]	Burlington	84	534
Brigham & Women's Faulkner Hospital[2]	Boston	86	638
Healthalliance Hospitals[2]	Leominster	92	579
Cambridge Health Alliance[2]	Cambridge	94	716
Sturdy Memorial Hospital[2]	Attleboro	96	630
Hallmark Health System[2]	Melrose	97	785
Merrimack Valley Hospital[2]	Haverhill	97	383
Anna Jaques Hospital[2]	Newburyport	98	664
Baystate Franklin Medical Center[2]	Greenfield	100	430
Saint Anne's Hospital[2]	Fall River	100	793
Beth Israel Deaconess Hospital - Needham[2]	Needham	104	384
Morton Hospital[2]	Taunton	105	687
Brigham & Women's Hospital[2]	Boston	108	327
Winchester Hospital[2]	Winchester	111	649
Carney Hospital[2]	Boston	113	653
Southcoast Hospital Group[2]	Fall River	113	694
Metrowest Medical Center[2]	Framingham	115	833
Milford Regional Medical Center[2]	Milford	116	810
Good Samaritan Medical Center[2]	Brockton	119	904
Newton - Wellesley Hospital[2]	Newton	123	393
Mount Auburn Hospital[2]	Cambridge	127	480
Emerson Hospital[2]	W Concord	132	394
Heywood Hospital[2]	Gardner	132	430
Lowell General Hospital[2]	Lowell	136	606
Beth Israel Deaconess Medical Center[2]	Boston	138	568
Mercy Medical Center[2]	Springfield	140	795
Quincy Medical Center[2]	Quincy	141	803
Holy Family Hospital[2]	Methuen	147	674
Norwood Hospital[2]	Norwood	148	920
Tufts Medical Center[2]	Boston	148	362
Beverly Hospital Corporation[2]	Beverly	150	520
Marlborough Hospital[2]	Marlborough	150	306
Saint Vincent Hospital[2]	Worcester	150	775
Holyoke Medical Center[2]	Holyoke	153	1859
Signature Healthcare Brockton Hospital[2]	Brockton	160	488
Baystate Medical Center[2]	Springfield	163	578
Cape Cod Hospital[2]	Hyannis	172	915
Saint Elizabeth's Medical Center[2]	Brighton	173	402
Lawrence General Hospital[2]	Lawrence	175	671
North Shore Medical Center[2]	Salem	175	563
Boston Medical Center Corporation[2]	Boston	178	654
Umass Memorial Medical Center[2]	Worcester	180	171
Massachusetts General Hospital[2]	Boston	184	520
Saints Medical Center[2]	Lowell	185	775
Jordan Hospital[2]	Plymouth	203	792
Falmouth Hospital[2]	Falmouth	217	843
South Shore Hospital[2]	S Weymouth	327	750

Head CT Results Within 45 Minutes of Arrival

Hospital Name	City	Rate	Cases
Good Samaritan Medical Center	Brockton	92%	25
The Cooley Dickinson Hospital	Northampton	86%	29
Southcoast Hospital Group	Fall River	78%	88
Lawrence General Hospital	Lawrence	63%	27

Patients Who Left ER Before Being Seen

Hospital Name	City	Rate	Cases
Beth Israel Deaconess Hospital - Milton	Milton	0%	25715
Beth Israel Deaconess Hospital - Needham	Needham	0%	14842
Cambridge Health Alliance	Cambridge	0%	96953
Morton Hospital	Taunton	0%	47019
Anna Jaques Hospital	Newburyport	1%	32473
Baystate Mary Lane Hospital	Ware	1%	15597
Beth Israel Deaconess Medical Center	Boston	1%	55526
Brigham & Women's Hospital	Boston	1%	61276
Cape Cod Hospital	Hyannis	1%	91260
Carney Hospital	Boston	1%	30214
Hallmark Health System	Melrose	1%	60962
Harrington Memorial Hospital	Southbridge	1%	38075
Jordan Hospital	Plymouth	1%	51042
Massachusetts Eye & Ear Infirmary	Boston	1%	19642
Metrowest Medical Center	Framingham	1%	66959
Milford Regional Medical Center	Milford	1%	56534
Nantucket Cottage Hospital	Nantucket	1%	11291
Nashoba Valley Medical Center	Ayer	1%	13332
Newton - Wellesley Hospital	Newton	1%	61170
Noble Hospital	Westfield	1%	29285
Norwood Hospital	Norwood	1%	44114
Saint Elizabeth's Medical Center	Brighton	1%	37175
Saint Vincent Hospital	Worcester	1%	68808
South Shore Hospital	S Weymouth	1%	85353
Sturdy Memorial Hospital	Attleboro	1%	50822
Tufts Medical Center	Boston	1%	41763
Winchester Hospital	Winchester	1%	51242
Baystate Franklin Medical Center	Greenfield	2%	27831
Beverly Hospital Corporation	Beverly	2%	64420
Brigham & Women's Faulkner Hospital	Boston	2%	25840
Clinton Hospital Association	Clinton	2%	13486
The Cooley Dickinson Hospital	Northampton	2%	36658
Emerson Hospital	W Concord	2%	27072
Heywood Hospital	Gardner	2%	24635
Holy Family Hospital	Methuen	2%	46468
Lahey Hosp & Med Ctr-Burlington	Burlington	2%	54931
Marlborough Hospital	Marlborough	2%	27245
Massachusetts General Hospital	Boston	2%	99942
Mount Auburn Hospital	Cambridge	2%	37343
Saints Medical Center	Lowell	2%	44627
Signature Healthcare Brockton Hospital	Brockton	2%	62520
Southcoast Hospital Group	Fall River	2%	191494
Umass Memorial Medical Center	Worcester	2%	145622
Wing Memorial Hospital & Medical Center	Palmer	2%	24613
Berkshire Medical Center	Pittsfield	3%	56805
Good Samaritan Medical Center	Brockton	3%	55682
Holyoke Medical Center	Holyoke	3%	46193
Lawrence General Hospital	Lawrence	3%	72995
North Adams Regional Hospital	North Adams	3%	21443
North Shore Medical Center	Salem	3%	78078
Quincy Medical Center	Quincy	3%	31423
Saint Anne's Hospital	Fall River	3%	41460
Boston Medical Center Corporation	Boston	4%	130258
Healthalliance Hospitals	Leominster	4%	45012
Lowell General Hospital	Lowell	4%	55796
Mercy Medical Center	Springfield	4%	76434
Merrimack Valley Hospital	Haverhill	6%	19554
Baystate Medical Center	Springfield	7%	110349
Falmouth Hospital	Falmouth	9%	3869

Time from ER Arrival to Being Admitted (minutes)

Hospital Name	City	Min.	Cases
Nashoba Valley Medical Center[2]	Ayer	213	438
Clinton Hospital Association[2]	Clinton	215	295
Wing Memorial Hospital & Medical Center[2]	Palmer	220	379
Baystate Mary Lane Hospital[2]	Ware	231	485
Noble Hospital[2]	Westfield	235	757
Harrington Memorial Hospital[2]	Southbridge	236	566
Beth Israel Deaconess Hospital - Milton[2]	Milton	247	947
Sturdy Memorial Hospital[2]	Attleboro	262	634
Berkshire Medical Center[2]	Pittsfield	265	801
Carney Hospital[2]	Boston	275	658
Hallmark Health System[2]	Melrose	277	785
Healthalliance Hospitals[2]	Leominster	281	595
Brigham & Women's Faulkner Hospital[2]	Boston	283	638
Cambridge Health Alliance[2]	Cambridge	283	725
Anna Jaques Hospital[2]	Newburyport	292	667
Baystate Franklin Medical Center[2]	Greenfield	292	480
Southcoast Hospital Group[2]	Fall River	293	720
Beth Israel Deaconess Hospital - Needham[2]	Needham	294	414
Emerson Hospital[2]	W Concord	294	400
The Cooley Dickinson Hospital[2]	Northampton	296	826
Fairview Hospital[2]	Great Barrington	298	426
Mount Auburn Hospital[2]	Cambridge	300	484
Morton Hospital[2]	Taunton	301	739
Boston Medical Center Corporation[2]	Boston	302	654
Newton - Wellesley Hospital[2]	Newton	302	404
North Adams Regional Hospital[2]	North Adams	304	335
Saint Anne's Hospital[2]	Fall River	305	799
Winchester Hospital[2]	Winchester	307	657
Metrowest Medical Center[2]	Framingham	309	835
Beverly Hospital Corporation[2]	Beverly	310	522
Brigham & Women's Hospital[2]	Boston	311	338
Nantucket Cottage Hospital[2]	Nantucket	312	148
Milford Regional Medical Center[2]	Milford	316	810
Quincy Medical Center[2]	Quincy	320	805

NOTE: Hospital profiles are in alphabetical order by state, then city, then hospital within the city; Rankings exclude hospitals with less than 25 cases except for patient surveys which excludes hospitals with less than 100 cases; (a) 100-299 cases; (1) The number of cases/patients is too few to report; (2) Data submitted were based on a sample of cases/patients; (3) Results are based on a shorter time period than required; (4) Data suppressed by CMS for one or more quarters; (5) Results are not available for this reporting period; (6) Fewer than 100 patients completed the HCAHPS survey; (7) No cases met the criteria for this measure; (8) The lower limit of the confidence interval cannot be calculated if the number of observed infections equals zero; (9) No data are available from the state/territory for this reporting period; (10) The scores shown reflect fewer than 50 completed surveys; (11) There were discrepancies in the data collection process; (12) This measure does not apply to this hospital for this reporting period; (13) Results cannot be calculated for this reporting period; (14) The results for this state are combined with nearby states to protect confidentiality; Please refer to the User's Guide for a full explanation of data.

Hospital Name	City	Min.	Cases
Holyoke Medical Center[2]	Holyoke	322	1859
Lahey Hosp & Med Ctr-Burlington[2]	Burlington	323	587
Beth Israel Deaconess Medical Center[2]	Boston	325	571
Saint Elizabeth's Medical Center[2]	Brighton	331	403
Cape Cod Hospital[2]	Hyannis	337	915
Signature Healthcare Brockton Hospital[2]	Brockton	337	488
Holy Family Hospital[2]	Methuen	338	682
Lawrence General Hospital[2]	Lawrence	338	675
Norwood Hospital[2]	Norwood	339	927
Good Samaritan Medical Center[2]	Brockton	340	908
North Shore Medical Center[2]	Salem	346	563
Tufts Medical Center[2]	Boston	348	362
Mercy Medical Center[2]	Springfield	352	795
Heywood Hospital[2]	Gardner	360	430
Saints Medical Center[2]	Lowell	366	792
Marlborough Hospital[2]	Marlborough	370	388
Merrimack Valley Hospital[2]	Haverhill	374	453
Saint Vincent Hospital[2]	Worcester	376	775
Lowell General Hospital[2]	Lowell	378	621
Falmouth Hospital[2]	Falmouth	394	844
Umass Memorial Medical Center[2]	Worcester	394	592
Baystate Medical Center[2]	Springfield	396	589
Massachusetts General Hospital[2]	Boston	408	523
Jordan Hospital[2]	Plymouth	446	792
South Shore Hospital[2]	S Weymouth	577	754

Time from ER Arrival to Discharge (minutes)

Hospital Name	City	Min.	Cases
Baystate Mary Lane Hospital	Ware	90	369
Harrington Memorial Hospital	Southbridge	99	359
Cambridge Health Alliance	Cambridge	100	414
Wing Memorial Hospital & Medical Center	Palmer	102	314
Nantucket Cottage Hospital	Nantucket	104	363
Noble Hospital	Westfield	107	542
Clinton Hospital Association	Clinton	110	344
Falmouth Hospital	Falmouth	120	368
Nashoba Valley Medical Center	Ayer	120	361
Massachusetts Eye & Ear Infirmary	Boston	123	189
North Adams Regional Hospital	North Adams	128	436
Sturdy Memorial Hospital	Attleboro	128	348
Cape Cod Hospital	Hyannis	129	396
Emerson Hospital	W Concord	130	351
Southcoast Hospital Group	Fall River	133	324
Anna Jaques Hospital	Newburyport	135	367
Lawrence General Hospital	Lawrence	138	419
Baystate Franklin Medical Center	Greenfield	139	375
Beth Israel Deaconess Hospital - Milton	Milton	142	371
Hallmark Health System	Melrose	142	334
Beth Israel Deaconess Hospital - Needham	Needham	145	358
Lahey Hosp & Med Ctr-Burlington	Burlington	145	351
North Shore Medical Center	Salem	145	344
Carney Hospital	Boston	146	359
Beverly Hospital Corporation	Beverly	147	396
Metrowest Medical Center	Framingham	148	375
Saint Elizabeth's Medical Center	Brighton	148	367
Newton - Wellesley Hospital	Newton	149	337
Morton Hospital	Taunton	150	349
Holyoke Medical Center	Holyoke	153	391
Milford Regional Medical Center	Milford	154	385
Saints Medical Center	Lowell	154	380
Mount Auburn Hospital	Cambridge	159	325
Saint Vincent Hospital	Worcester	159	404
Berkshire Medical Center	Pittsfield	160	385
Signature Healthcare Brockton Hospital	Brockton	161	290
Brigham & Women's Faulkner Hospital	Boston	162	252
Quincy Medical Center	Quincy	164	388
Tufts Medical Center	Boston	164	354
Marlborough Hospital	Marlborough	167	267
Saint Anne's Hospital	Fall River	167	344
Healthalliance Hospitals	Leominster	168	324
Mercy Medical Center	Springfield	169	384
Norwood Hospital	Norwood	172	369
The Cooley Dickinson Hospital	Northampton	173	357
Jordan Hospital	Plymouth	178	358
Umass Memorial Medical Center	Worcester	179	325
Winchester Hospital	Winchester	179	318
Brigham & Women's Hospital	Boston	180	306
South Shore Hospital	S Weymouth	182	376
Boston Medical Center Corporation	Boston	186	341
Holy Family Hospital	Methuen	186	381
Lowell General Hospital	Lowell	192	389
Massachusetts General Hospital	Boston	210	278
Good Samaritan Medical Center	Brockton	212	339
Heywood Hospital	Gardner	212	344
Merrimack Valley Hospital	Haverhill	226	343
Beth Israel Deaconess Medical Center	Boston	242	1716
Baystate Medical Center	Springfield	252	378

Time in ER Before Being Evaluated (minutes)

Hospital Name	City	Min.	Cases
Harrington Memorial Hospital	Southbridge	4	403
Massachusetts General Hospital	Boston	9	395
Cape Cod Hospital	Hyannis	10	434
Cambridge Health Alliance	Cambridge	13	457
Sturdy Memorial Hospital	Attleboro	14	408
Baystate Mary Lane Hospital	Ware	17	279
Falmouth Hospital	Falmouth	18	417
Beth Israel Deaconess Hospital - Needham	Needham	21	406
Brigham & Women's Hospital	Boston	21	326
Nashoba Valley Medical Center	Ayer	22	386
Quincy Medical Center	Quincy	22	388
Nantucket Cottage Hospital	Nantucket	23	384
Milford Regional Medical Center	Milford	24	428
Noble Hospital	Westfield	24	494
Clinton Hospital Association	Clinton	25	379
Carney Hospital	Boston	29	384
Norwood Hospital	Norwood	29	361
Saint Vincent Hospital	Worcester	29	437
Brigham & Women's Faulkner Hospital	Boston	32	384
Morton Hospital	Taunton	32	389
North Adams Regional Hospital	North Adams	32	492
Metrowest Medical Center	Framingham	33	423
Tufts Medical Center	Boston	34	401
Wing Memorial Hospital & Medical Center	Palmer	36	338
Beth Israel Deaconess Hospital - Milton	Milton	39	416
Hallmark Health System	Melrose	39	382
North Shore Medical Center	Salem	39	383
Saint Elizabeth's Medical Center	Brighton	39	370
Anna Jaques Hospital	Newburyport	42	408
Beth Israel Deaconess Medical Center	Boston	42	1406
Jordan Hospital	Plymouth	42	408
Signature Healthcare Brockton Hospital	Brockton	42	398
South Shore Hospital	S Weymouth	42	408
Boston Medical Center Corporation	Boston	44	376
Emerson Hospital	W Concord	44	374
Winchester Hospital	Winchester	44	342
Berkshire Medical Center	Pittsfield	45	383
Umass Memorial Medical Center	Worcester	45	336
Holyoke Medical Center	Holyoke	46	441
Southcoast Hospital Group	Fall River	46	319
Beverly Hospital Corporation	Beverly	47	479
Heywood Hospital	Gardner	47	398
Lahey Hosp & Med Ctr-Burlington	Burlington	47	353
Mount Auburn Hospital	Cambridge	48	425
Baystate Franklin Medical Center	Greenfield	50	320
The Cooley Dickinson Hospital	Northampton	50	400
Saints Medical Center	Lowell	54	270
Holy Family Hospital	Methuen	60	353
Saint Anne's Hospital	Fall River	61	393
Healthalliance Hospitals	Leominster	65	193
Marlborough Hospital	Marlborough	65	295
Good Samaritan Medical Center	Brockton	66	352
Merrimack Valley Hospital	Haverhill	66	296
Mercy Medical Center	Springfield	70	410
Massachusetts Eye & Ear Infirmary	Boston	73	311
Lawrence General Hospital	Lawrence	75	423
Lowell General Hospital	Lowell	79	428
Baystate Medical Center	Springfield	91	261

Time to Pain Meds for Bone Fractures (minutes)

Hospital Name	City	Min.	Cases
North Shore Medical Center	Salem	28	173
Metrowest Medical Center	Framingham	37	156
Cape Cod Hospital	Hyannis	38	225
Harrington Memorial Hospital	Southbridge	38	121
Brigham & Women's Hospital	Boston	43	50
Nashoba Valley Medical Center	Ayer	43	46
Cambridge Health Alliance	Cambridge	44	110
Beth Israel Deaconess Hospital - Needham	Needham	45	54
Signature Healthcare Brockton Hospital	Brockton	45	115
Tufts Medical Center	Boston	47	63
Carney Hospital	Boston	50	31
Marlborough Hospital	Marlborough	50	77
Nantucket Cottage Hospital	Nantucket	50	46
The Cooley Dickinson Hospital	Northampton	52	121
Noble Hospital	Westfield	52	75
Brigham & Women's Faulkner Hospital	Boston	53	35
Baystate Mary Lane Hospital	Ware	54	59
Hallmark Health System	Melrose	54	99
Mount Auburn Hospital	Cambridge	54	72
Southcoast Hospital Group	Fall River	55	242
Umass Memorial Medical Center	Worcester	55	341
Clinton Hospital Association	Clinton	56	38
Baystate Medical Center	Springfield	58	274
Anna Jaques Hospital	Newburyport	59	123
Newton - Wellesley Hospital	Newton	59	189
Norwood Hospital	Norwood	59	125
Winchester Hospital	Winchester	59	169
North Adams Regional Hospital	North Adams	60	29
Lawrence General Hospital	Lawrence	61	161
Beverly Hospital Corporation	Beverly	62	270
Saint Vincent Hospital	Worcester	63	239
South Shore Hospital	S Weymouth	63	423
Baystate Franklin Medical Center	Greenfield	65	77
Beth Israel Deaconess Hospital - Milton	Milton	66	58
Holy Family Hospital	Methuen	66	82
Mercy Medical Center	Springfield	66	170
Massachusetts General Hospital	Boston	67	105
Milford Regional Medical Center	Milford	67	214
Morton Hospital	Taunton	68	67
Heywood Hospital	Gardner	69	78
Wing Memorial Hospital & Medical Center	Palmer	69	55
Lahey Hosp & Med Ctr-Burlington	Burlington	70	69
Quincy Medical Center	Quincy	71	71
Boston Medical Center Corporation	Boston	72	149
Healthalliance Hospitals	Leominster	73	149
Jordan Hospital	Plymouth	76	62
Saint Anne's Hospital	Fall River	76	51
Saints Medical Center	Lowell	76	65
Sturdy Memorial Hospital	Attleboro	76	68
Emerson Hospital	W Concord	77	35
Falmouth Hospital	Falmouth	77	117
Good Samaritan Medical Center	Brockton	77	102
Berkshire Medical Center	Pittsfield	78	124
Saint Elizabeth's Medical Center	Brighton	78	43
Beth Israel Deaconess Medical Center	Boston	79	43
Holyoke Medical Center	Holyoke	79	78
Lowell General Hospital	Lowell	82	162
Merrimack Valley Hospital	Haverhill	113	46

Heart Attack Care

Aspirin Given at Discharge

Hospital Name	City	Rate	Cases
Baystate Medical Center	Springfield	100%	1051
Berkshire Medical Center	Pittsfield	100%	49
Beth Israel Deaconess Medical Center	Boston	100%	558
Beverly Hospital Corporation	Beverly	100%	139
Boston Medical Center Corporation	Boston	100%	352
Brigham & Women's Hospital	Boston	100%	495
Cape Cod Hospital[2]	Hyannis	100%	299
The Cooley Dickinson Hospital	Northampton	100%	26
Good Samaritan Medical Center	Brockton	100%	154
Hallmark Health System	Melrose	100%	88
Healthalliance Hospitals	Leominster	100%	41
Holy Family Hospital	Methuen	100%	90
Holyoke Medical Center	Holyoke	100%	27
Lowell General Hospital[2]	Lowell	100%	238
Mercy Medical Center	Springfield	100%	55
Merrimack Valley Hospital	Haverhill	100%	25
Mount Auburn Hospital	Cambridge	100%	213
North Shore Medical Center	Salem	100%	245
Norwood Hospital	Norwood	100%	89
Saint Anne's Hospital	Fall River	100%	26
Saint Vincent Hospital	Worcester	100%	303
Saints Medical Center	Lowell	100%	25
Signature Healthcare Brockton Hospital	Brockton	100%	149
South Shore Hospital	S Weymouth	100%	305
Tufts Medical Center	Boston	100%	364
Umass Memorial Medical Center[2]	Worcester	100%	332
VA Boston Healthcare Sys-Jamaica Plain	Jamaica Plain	100%	29
Winchester Hospital[2]	Winchester	100%	25
Lahey Hosp & Med Ctr-Burlington	Burlington	99%	575
Massachusetts General Hospital	Boston	99%	676
Metrowest Medical Center	Framingham	99%	99
Saint Elizabeth's Medical Center	Brighton	99%	335
Southcoast Hospital Group[2]	Fall River	99%	628
Jordan Hospital	Plymouth	98%	43
Lawrence General Hospital	Lawrence	98%	159
Morton Hospital	Taunton	97%	33
Cambridge Health Alliance	Cambridge	96%	25
Harrington Memorial Hospital	Southbridge	96%	26
Milford Regional Medical Center	Milford	94%	52
Heywood Hospital	Gardner	93%	43
Anna Jaques Hospital	Newburyport	92%	25

PCI Within 90 Minutes of Arrival

Hospital Name	City	Rate	Cases
Metrowest Medical Center	Framingham	100%	44
Mount Auburn Hospital	Cambridge	100%	25
Saint Vincent Hospital	Worcester	100%	47
South Shore Hospital	S Weymouth	99%	108
Brigham & Women's Hospital	Boston	98%	51
Lahey Hosp & Med Ctr-Burlington	Burlington	98%	64
Lowell General Hospital[2]	Lowell	98%	63
Signature Healthcare Brockton Hospital	Brockton	98%	57
Southcoast Hospital Group[2]	Fall River	98%	64
Beth Israel Deaconess Medical Center	Boston	97%	32

NOTE: Hospital profiles are in alphabetical order by state, then city, then hospital within the city; Rankings exclude hospitals with less than 25 cases except for patient surveys which excludes hospitals with less than 100 cases; (a) 100-299 cases; (1) The number of cases/patients is too few to report; (2) Data submitted were based on a sample of cases/patients; (3) Results are based on a shorter time period than required; (4) Data suppressed by CMS for one or more quarters; (5) Results are not available for this reporting period; (6) Fewer than 100 patients completed the HCAHPS survey; (7) No cases met the criteria for this measure; (8) The lower limit of the confidence interval cannot be calculated if the number of observed infections equals zero; (9) No data are available from the state/territory for this reporting period; (10) The scores shown reflect fewer than 50 completed surveys; (11) There were discrepancies in the data collection process; (12) This measure does not apply to this hospital for this reporting period; (13) Results cannot be calculated for this reporting period; (14) The results for this state are combined with nearby states to protect confidentiality; Please refer to the User's Guide for a full explanation of data.

Hospital Name	City	Rate	Cases
Beverly Hospital Corporation	Beverly	97%	37
Lawrence General Hospital	Lawrence	97%	31
Cape Cod Hospital[2]	Hyannis	96%	57
Massachusetts General Hospital	Boston	96%	49
Norwood Hospital	Norwood	96%	45
Baystate Medical Center	Springfield	95%	112
North Shore Medical Center	Salem	95%	61
Good Samaritan Medical Center	Brockton	93%	42
Umass Memorial Medical Center[2]	Worcester	91%	79
Boston Medical Center Corporation	Boston	90%	31
Holy Family Hospital	Methuen	89%	35

Statin Prescribed at Discharge

Hospital Name	City	Rate	Cases
Baystate Medical Center	Springfield	100%	1041
Berkshire Medical Center	Pittsfield	100%	49
Beth Israel Deaconess Medical Center	Boston	100%	558
Beverly Hospital Corporation	Beverly	100%	121
Brigham & Women's Hospital	Boston	100%	480
Hallmark Health System	Melrose	100%	85
Healthalliance Hospitals	Leominster	100%	38
Holy Family Hospital	Methuen	100%	85
Lowell General Hospital[2]	Lowell	100%	242
Mercy Medical Center	Springfield	100%	54
Metrowest Medical Center	Framingham	100%	95
Mount Auburn Hospital	Cambridge	100%	205
North Shore Medical Center	Salem	100%	242
Saint Vincent Hospital	Worcester	100%	299
South Shore Hospital	S Weymouth	100%	294
Tufts Medical Center	Boston	100%	355
Umass Memorial Medical Center[2]	Worcester	100%	335
VA Boston Healthcare Sys-Jamaica Plain	Jamaica Plain	100%	31
Lahey Hosp & Med Ctr-Burlington	Burlington	99%	565
Massachusetts General Hospital	Boston	99%	658
Signature Healthcare Brockton Hospital	Brockton	99%	158
Boston Medical Center Corporation	Boston	98%	343
Cape Cod Hospital[2]	Hyannis	98%	277
Norwood Hospital	Norwood	98%	86
Southcoast Hospital Group[2]	Fall River	98%	603
Good Samaritan Medical Center	Brockton	97%	147
Saint Elizabeth's Medical Center	Brighton	97%	326
Cambridge Health Alliance	Cambridge	96%	26
Harrington Memorial Hospital	Southbridge	96%	26
Holyoke Medical Center	Holyoke	96%	28
Lawrence General Hospital	Lawrence	96%	145
Milford Regional Medical Center	Milford	96%	52
Saint Anne's Hospital	Fall River	96%	25
Winchester Hospital[2]	Winchester	96%	28
Jordan Hospital	Plymouth	95%	43
The Cooley Dickinson Hospital	Northampton	92%	25
Heywood Hospital	Gardner	90%	40
Falmouth Hospital	Falmouth	89%	28
Morton Hospital	Taunton	88%	33
Anna Jaques Hospital	Newburyport	84%	25

Heart Failure Care

ACE Inhibitor or ARB for LVSD

Hospital Name	City	Rate	Cases
Berkshire Medical Center	Pittsfield	100%	37
Beth Israel Deaconess Medical Center[2]	Boston	100%	104
Beverly Hospital Corporation	Beverly	100%	89
Brigham & Women's Faulkner Hospital	Boston	100%	26
Carney Hospital	Boston	100%	31
Newton - Wellesley Hospital[2]	Newton	100%	28
Signature Healthcare Brockton Hospital	Brockton	100%	50
South Shore Hospital	S Weymouth	100%	118
Baystate Medical Center	Springfield	99%	252
Brigham & Women's Hospital[2]	Boston	99%	88
Lowell General Hospital[2]	Lowell	99%	70
Mount Auburn Hospital	Cambridge	99%	82
North Shore Medical Center	Salem	99%	95
Saint Vincent Hospital	Worcester	99%	138
Tufts Medical Center	Boston	99%	159
The Cooley Dickinson Hospital	Northampton	98%	53
Harrington Memorial Hospital	Southbridge	98%	41
Metrowest Medical Center	Framingham	98%	59
Southcoast Hospital Group[2]	Fall River	98%	280
Sturdy Memorial Hospital	Attleboro	98%	51
Holyoke Medical Center	Holyoke	97%	34
Norwood Hospital	Norwood	97%	68
Quincy Medical Center	Quincy	97%	35
Umass Memorial Medical Center[2]	Worcester	97%	103
Mercy Medical Center	Springfield	96%	67
Massachusetts General Hospital[2]	Boston	95%	61
Cambridge Health Alliance	Cambridge	94%	47
Good Samaritan Medical Center	Brockton	94%	141
Healthalliance Hospitals[2]	Leominster	94%	52
Heywood Hospital	Gardner	94%	48
Lahey Hosp & Med Ctr-Burlington[2]	Burlington	94%	48
Winchester Hospital[2]	Winchester	94%	54
Boston Medical Center Corporation[2]	Boston	93%	95
Cape Cod Hospital[2]	Hyannis	93%	82
Holy Family Hospital	Methuen	92%	48
Saint Elizabeth's Medical Center	Brighton	92%	91
Saints Medical Center[2]	Lowell	92%	48
Jordan Hospital	Plymouth	91%	45
Anna Jaques Hospital	Newburyport	90%	31
Baystate Franklin Medical Center	Greenfield	90%	30
Saint Anne's Hospital	Fall River	90%	39
Milford Regional Medical Center	Milford	89%	65
Beth Israel Deaconess Hospital - Milton	Milton	88%	32
Lawrence General Hospital	Lawrence	88%	102
Morton Hospital	Taunton	88%	57
VA Boston Healthcare Sys-Jamaica Plain	Jamaica Plain	87%	93
Hallmark Health System[2]	Melrose	85%	46

Discharge Instructions Given

Hospital Name	City	Rate	Cases
Baystate Mary Lane Hospital	Ware	100%	35
Berkshire Medical Center	Pittsfield	100%	227
Beth Israel Deaconess Hospital - Milton	Milton	100%	158
Beth Israel Deaconess Medical Center[2]	Boston	100%	309
Brigham & Women's Faulkner Hospital	Boston	100%	126
Brigham & Women's Hospital[2]	Boston	100%	234
Lahey Hosp & Med Ctr-Burlington[2]	Burlington	100%	205
Martha's Vineyard Hospital	Oak Bluffs	100%	28
Mount Auburn Hospital	Cambridge	100%	202
Nashoba Valley Medical Center	Ayer	100%	54
Noble Hospital	Westfield	100%	92
North Adams Regional Hospital	North Adams	100%	63
Signature Healthcare Brockton Hospital	Brockton	100%	144
Sturdy Memorial Hospital	Attleboro	100%	127
Wing Memorial Hospital & Medical Center	Palmer	100%	83
Beth Israel Deaconess Hospital - Needham	Needham	99%	77
Boston Medical Center Corporation[2]	Boston	99%	270
Newton - Wellesley Hospital[2]	Newton	99%	144
Saint Vincent Hospital	Worcester	99%	432
VA Boston Healthcare Sys-Jamaica Plain	Jamaica Plain	99%	253
Anna Jaques Hospital	Newburyport	98%	143
Baystate Franklin Medical Center	Greenfield	98%	88
Baystate Medical Center	Springfield	98%	908
Carney Hospital	Boston	98%	83
Falmouth Hospital	Falmouth	98%	150
Tufts Medical Center	Boston	98%	287
Jordan Hospital	Plymouth	97%	175
Mercy Medical Center	Springfield	97%	200
South Shore Hospital	S Weymouth	97%	473
Beverly Hospital Corporation	Beverly	95%	275
Healthalliance Hospitals[2]	Leominster	95%	164
Holy Family Hospital	Methuen	95%	177
Metrowest Medical Center	Framingham	95%	244
Saint Anne's Hospital	Fall River	95%	168
Good Samaritan Medical Center	Brockton	94%	315
Holyoke Medical Center	Holyoke	94%	141
Lowell General Hospital[2]	Lowell	94%	239
North Shore Medical Center	Salem	94%	427
Saint Elizabeth's Medical Center	Brighton	94%	190
Southcoast Hospital Group[2]	Fall River	94%	734
Umass Memorial Medical Center[2]	Worcester	94%	218
Cape Cod Hospital[2]	Hyannis	93%	191
The Cooley Dickinson Hospital	Northampton	93%	140
Harrington Memorial Hospital	Southbridge	93%	119
Morton Hospital	Taunton	93%	148
Merrimack Valley Hospital	Haverhill	92%	72
Quincy Medical Center	Quincy	92%	110
Cambridge Health Alliance	Cambridge	91%	185
Massachusetts General Hospital[2]	Boston	91%	211
Milford Regional Medical Center	Milford	91%	184
Emerson Hospital	W Concord	90%	86
Hallmark Health System[2]	Melrose	90%	174
Heywood Hospital	Gardner	90%	121
Marlborough Hospital	Marlborough	88%	100
Saints Medical Center[2]	Lowell	84%	172
Norwood Hospital	Norwood	83%	202
Winchester Hospital[2]	Winchester	82%	187
Lawrence General Hospital	Lawrence	81%	304
Clinton Hospital Association	Clinton	79%	33

Evaluation of LVS Function

Hospital Name	City	Rate	Cases
Anna Jaques Hospital	Newburyport	100%	183
Baystate Franklin Medical Center	Greenfield	100%	122
Baystate Medical Center	Springfield	100%	1159
Berkshire Medical Center	Pittsfield	100%	299
Beth Israel Deaconess Hospital - Needham	Needham	100%	100
Beth Israel Deaconess Medical Center[2]	Boston	100%	407
Beverly Hospital Corporation	Beverly	100%	406
Boston Medical Center Corporation[2]	Boston	100%	309
Brigham & Women's Faulkner Hospital	Boston	100%	188
Brigham & Women's Hospital[2]	Boston	100%	286
Carney Hospital	Boston	100%	108
The Cooley Dickinson Hospital	Northampton	100%	187
Fairview Hospital	Great Barrington	100%	27
Falmouth Hospital	Falmouth	100%	221
Good Samaritan Medical Center	Brockton	100%	475
Hallmark Health System[2]	Melrose	100%	244
Healthalliance Hospitals[2]	Leominster	100%	226
Holyoke Medical Center	Holyoke	100%	210
Jordan Hospital	Plymouth	100%	244
Lahey Hosp & Med Ctr-Burlington[2]	Burlington	100%	278
Lawrence General Hospital	Lawrence	100%	418
Marlborough Hospital	Marlborough	100%	137
Martha's Vineyard Hospital	Oak Bluffs	100%	28
Massachusetts General Hospital[2]	Boston	100%	286
Mercy Medical Center	Springfield	100%	283
Merrimack Valley Hospital	Haverhill	100%	120
Milford Regional Medical Center	Milford	100%	274
Morton Hospital	Taunton	100%	227
Mount Auburn Hospital	Cambridge	100%	294
Nashoba Valley Medical Center	Ayer	100%	80
Newton - Wellesley Hospital[2]	Newton	100%	216
North Adams Regional Hospital	North Adams	100%	91
North Shore Medical Center	Salem	100%	598
Norwood Hospital	Norwood	100%	295
Saint Anne's Hospital	Fall River	100%	217
Saint Elizabeth's Medical Center	Brighton	100%	280
Saint Vincent Hospital	Worcester	100%	620
Signature Healthcare Brockton Hospital	Brockton	100%	190
South Shore Hospital	S Weymouth	100%	743
Southcoast Hospital Group[2]	Fall River	100%	1033
Sturdy Memorial Hospital	Attleboro	100%	182
Tufts Medical Center	Boston	100%	352
Umass Memorial Medical Center[2]	Worcester	100%	293
VA Boston Healthcare Sys-Jamaica Plain	Jamaica Plain	100%	299
Winchester Hospital[2]	Winchester	100%	245
Wing Memorial Hospital & Medical Center	Palmer	100%	114
Beth Israel Deaconess Hospital - Milton	Milton	99%	187
Cambridge Health Alliance	Cambridge	99%	237
Cape Cod Hospital[2]	Hyannis	99%	289
Emerson Hospital	W Concord	99%	137
Harrington Memorial Hospital	Southbridge	99%	159
Holy Family Hospital	Methuen	99%	241
Lowell General Hospital[2]	Lowell	99%	338
Metrowest Medical Center	Framingham	99%	365
Noble Hospital	Westfield	99%	119
Quincy Medical Center	Quincy	99%	144
Saints Medical Center[2]	Lowell	99%	245
Baystate Mary Lane Hospital	Ware	98%	43
Heywood Hospital	Gardner	98%	146
Clinton Hospital Association	Clinton	94%	35

Medicare Spending

Medicare Spending per Patient (ratio)

Hospital Name	City	Ratio	Cases
Nantucket Cottage Hospital	Nantucket	0.87	-
Adcare Hospital of Worcester	Worcester	0.91	-
Beth Israel Deaconess Hospital - Milton	Milton	0.96	-
Heywood Hospital	Gardner	0.97	-
Beth Israel Deaconess Hospital - Needham	Needham	0.98	-
Baystate Franklin Medical Center	Greenfield	0.99	-
Lowell General Hospital	Lowell	0.99	-
Berkshire Medical Center	Pittsfield	1.00	-
Falmouth Hospital	Falmouth	1.00	-
Harrington Memorial Hospital	Southbridge	1.00	-
Holyoke Medical Center	Holyoke	1.00	-
Massachusetts Eye & Ear Infirmary	Boston	1.00	-
Brigham & Women's Hospital	Boston	1.01	-
Carney Hospital	Boston	1.01	-
Massachusetts General Hospital	Boston	1.01	-
New England Baptist Hospital	Boston	1.01	-
Newton - Wellesley Hospital	Newton	1.01	-
Norwood Hospital	Norwood	1.01	-
Saint Vincent Hospital	Worcester	1.01	-
Boston Medical Center Corporation	Boston	1.02	-
Lahey Hosp & Med Ctr-Burlington	Burlington	1.02	-
Saint Anne's Hospital	Fall River	1.02	-
Signature Healthcare Brockton Hospital	Brockton	1.02	-
Winchester Hospital	Winchester	1.02	-
Cape Cod Hospital	Hyannis	1.03	-
Metrowest Medical Center	Framingham	1.03	-
Milford Regional Medical Center	Milford	1.03	-
Baystate Medical Center	Springfield	1.04	-
Beth Israel Deaconess Medical Center	Boston	1.04	-
Beverly Hospital Corporation	Beverly	1.04	-
Brigham & Women's Faulkner Hospital	Boston	1.04	-
The Cooley Dickinson Hospital	Northampton	1.04	-
Emerson Hospital	W Concord	1.04	-
Jordan Hospital	Plymouth	1.04	-

NOTE: Hospital profiles are in alphabetical order by state, then city, then hospital within the city; Rankings exclude hospitals with less than 25 cases except for patient surveys which excludes hospitals with less than 100 cases; (a) 100-299 cases; (1) The number of cases/patients is too few to report; (2) Data submitted were based on a sample of cases/patients; (3) Results are based on a shorter time period than required; (4) Data suppressed by CMS for one or more quarters; (5) Results are not available for this reporting period; (6) Fewer than 100 patients completed the HCAHPS survey; (7) No cases met the criteria for this measure; (8) The lower limit of the confidence interval cannot be calculated if the number of observed infections equals zero; (9) No data are available from the state/territory for this reporting period; (10) The scores shown reflect fewer than 50 completed surveys; (11) There were discrepancies in the data collection process; (12) This measure does not apply to this hospital for this reporting period; (13) Results cannot be calculated for this reporting period; (14) The results for this state are combined with nearby states to protect confidentiality; Please refer to the User's Guide for a full explanation of data.

Hospital Name	City	Rate	Cases
Mercy Medical Center	Springfield	1.04	-
North Adams Regional Hospital	North Adams	1.04	-
North Shore Medical Center	Salem	1.04	-
Saints Medical Center	Lowell	1.04	-
Tufts Medical Center	Boston	1.04	-
Baystate Mary Lane Hospital	Ware	1.05	-
Healthalliance Hospitals	Leominster	1.05	-
Saint Elizabeth's Medical Center	Brighton	1.05	-
Cambridge Health Alliance	Cambridge	1.06	-
Good Samaritan Medical Center	Brockton	1.06	-
Mount Auburn Hospital	Cambridge	1.06	-
Southcoast Hospital Group	Fall River	1.06	-
Wing Memorial Hospital & Medical Center	Palmer	1.06	-
Marlborough Hospital	Marlborough	1.07	-
South Shore Hospital	S Weymouth	1.07	-
Anna Jaques Hospital	Newburyport	1.08	-
Noble Hospital	Westfield	1.08	-
Sturdy Memorial Hospital	Attleboro	1.08	-
Umass Memorial Medical Center	Worcester	1.08	-
Morton Hospital	Taunton	1.09	-
Quincy Medical Center	Quincy	1.09	-
Hallmark Health System	Melrose	1.10	-
Lawrence General Hospital	Lawrence	1.10	-
Clinton Hospital Association	Clinton	1.11	-
Holy Family Hospital	Methuen	1.11	-
Merrimack Valley Hospital	Haverhill	1.13	-
Nashoba Valley Medical Center	Ayer	1.13	-

Pneumonia Care

Appropriate Initial Antibiotic Given

Hospital Name	City	Rate	Cases
Berkshire Medical Center	Pittsfield	100%	178
Beth Israel Deaconess Hospital - Milton[2]	Milton	100%	121
Beth Israel Deaconess Hospital - Needham	Needham	100%	47
Beverly Hospital Corporation	Beverly	100%	293
Brigham & Women's Faulkner Hospital[2]	Boston	100%	80
Brigham & Women's Hospital[2]	Boston	100%	27
Carney Hospital	Boston	100%	58
Falmouth Hospital	Falmouth	100%	98
Lahey Hosp & Med Ctr-Burlington[2]	Burlington	100%	51
Mercy Medical Center	Springfield	100%	130
Noble Hospital	Westfield	100%	104
North Adams Regional Hospital	North Adams	100%	74
Signature Healthcare Brockton Hospital	Brockton	100%	138
Baystate Medical Center	Springfield	99%	268
The Cooley Dickinson Hospital	Northampton	99%	145
Holy Family Hospital	Methuen	99%	149
Merrimack Valley Hospital	Haverhill	99%	93
Metrowest Medical Center	Framingham	99%	181
Norwood Hospital	Norwood	99%	117
Saint Elizabeth's Medical Center	Brighton	99%	71
Boston Medical Center Corporation[2]	Boston	98%	82
Good Samaritan Medical Center	Brockton	98%	228
Hallmark Health System[2]	Melrose	98%	90
Healthalliance Hospitals[2]	Leominster	98%	83
Lawrence General Hospital	Lawrence	98%	153
Lowell General Hospital[2]	Lowell	98%	132
Nashoba Valley Medical Center	Ayer	98%	56
Saint Anne's Hospital	Fall River	98%	134
Saint Vincent Hospital	Worcester	98%	331
South Shore Hospital	S Weymouth	98%	341
Southcoast Hospital Group[2]	Fall River	98%	651
Sturdy Memorial Hospital	Attleboro	98%	105
Tufts Medical Center	Boston	98%	66
Harrington Memorial Hospital	Southbridge	97%	72
Holyoke Medical Center	Holyoke	97%	92
Jordan Hospital	Plymouth	97%	136
Martha's Vineyard Hospital	Oak Bluffs	97%	29
Mount Auburn Hospital	Cambridge	97%	213
North Shore Medical Center	Salem	97%	328
Umass Memorial Medical Center[2]	Worcester	97%	68
Winchester Hospital[2]	Winchester	97%	101
Anna Jaques Hospital	Newburyport	96%	123
Beth Israel Deaconess Medical Center[2]	Boston	96%	74
Cape Cod Hospital	Hyannis	96%	269
Emerson Hospital	W Concord	96%	107
Marlborough Hospital	Marlborough	96%	82
Wing Memorial Hospital & Medical Center	Palmer	96%	78
Baystate Franklin Medical Center	Greenfield	95%	87
Cambridge Health Alliance	Cambridge	95%	197
Fairview Hospital	Great Barrington	95%	38
Milford Regional Medical Center	Milford	95%	174
Morton Hospital	Taunton	94%	118
Quincy Medical Center	Quincy	94%	109
Baystate Mary Lane Hospital	Ware	92%	66
Massachusetts General Hospital[2]	Boston	92%	48
Newton - Wellesley Hospital[2]	Newton	92%	86
Heywood Hospital	Gardner	91%	105
VA Boston Healthcare Sys-Jamaica Plain	Jamaica Plain	90%	77
Saints Medical Center[2]	Lowell	89%	96

Blood Culture Timing

Hospital Name	City	Rate	Cases
Athol Memorial Hospital	Athol	100%	26
Berkshire Medical Center	Pittsfield	100%	355
Brigham & Women's Faulkner Hospital[2]	Boston	100%	65
Cape Cod Hospital	Hyannis	100%	426
Carney Hospital	Boston	100%	70
Fairview Hospital	Great Barrington	100%	65
Falmouth Hospital	Falmouth	100%	204
Massachusetts General Hospital[2]	Boston	100%	58
Mercy Medical Center	Springfield	100%	252
Metrowest Medical Center	Framingham	100%	215
Mount Auburn Hospital	Cambridge	100%	250
Nashoba Valley Medical Center	Ayer	100%	28
Noble Hospital	Westfield	100%	152
Signature Healthcare Brockton Hospital	Brockton	100%	105
Beverly Hospital Corporation	Beverly	99%	505
The Cooley Dickinson Hospital	Northampton	99%	198
Emerson Hospital	W Concord	99%	161
Good Samaritan Medical Center	Brockton	99%	185
Healthalliance Hospitals[2]	Leominster	99%	147
Heywood Hospital	Gardner	99%	183
Holy Family Hospital	Methuen	99%	146
Merrimack Valley Hospital	Haverhill	99%	83
Newton - Wellesley Hospital[2]	Newton	99%	147
Sturdy Memorial Hospital	Attleboro	99%	194
Anna Jaques Hospital	Newburyport	98%	180
Baystate Medical Center	Springfield	98%	436
Harrington Memorial Hospital	Southbridge	98%	121
Jordan Hospital	Plymouth	98%	212
Lahey Hosp & Med Ctr-Burlington[2]	Burlington	98%	88
Lowell General Hospital[2]	Lowell	98%	185
Morton Hospital	Taunton	98%	174
North Shore Medical Center	Salem	98%	450
Saint Anne's Hospital	Fall River	98%	139
Saint Vincent Hospital	Worcester	98%	617
Wing Memorial Hospital & Medical Center	Palmer	98%	158
Baystate Mary Lane Hospital	Ware	97%	73
Beth Israel Deaconess Medical Center[2]	Boston	97%	228
Brigham & Women's Hospital[2]	Boston	97%	64
Cambridge Health Alliance	Cambridge	97%	327
Clinton Hospital Association	Clinton	97%	32
Lawrence General Hospital	Lawrence	97%	258
Marlborough Hospital	Marlborough	97%	118
North Adams Regional Hospital	North Adams	97%	126
Quincy Medical Center	Quincy	97%	109
Saint Elizabeth's Medical Center	Brighton	97%	108
Southcoast Hospital Group[2]	Fall River	97%	901
Winchester Hospital[2]	Winchester	97%	148
Holyoke Medical Center	Holyoke	96%	194
Martha's Vineyard Hospital	Oak Bluffs	96%	56
Milford Regional Medical Center	Milford	96%	289
Saints Medical Center[2]	Lowell	96%	181
South Shore Hospital	S Weymouth	96%	185
Tufts Medical Center	Boston	96%	154
Beth Israel Deaconess Hospital - Milton[2]	Milton	95%	173
Hallmark Health System[2]	Melrose	95%	150
VA Boston Healthcare Sys-Jamaica Plain	Jamaica Plain	95%	131
Baystate Franklin Medical Center	Greenfield	94%	127
Boston Medical Center Corporation[2]	Boston	94%	102
Norwood Hospital	Norwood	92%	120
Umass Memorial Medical Center[2]	Worcester	88%	100
Beth Israel Deaconess Hospital - Needham	Needham	87%	82

Pregnancy and Delivery Care

Newborns whose Deliveries were Scheduled Early

Hospital Name	City	Rate	Cases
Anna Jaques Hospital[2]	Newburyport	0%	93
Berkshire Medical Center	Pittsfield	0%	42
Cape Cod Hospital	Hyannis	0%	41
Good Samaritan Medical Center	Brockton	0%	77
Holyoke Medical Center[2]	Holyoke	0%	25
Jordan Hospital	Plymouth	0%	28
Lawrence General Hospital[2]	Lawrence	0%	26
Metrowest Medical Center[2]	Framingham	0%	65
Milford Regional Medical Center	Milford	0%	92
Mount Auburn Hospital[2]	Cambridge	0%	38
Signature Healthcare Brockton Hospital	Brockton	0%	100
South Shore Hospital	S Weymouth	0%	465
Mercy Medical Center	Springfield	1%	103
Saint Vincent Hospital	Worcester	1%	143
Beth Israel Deaconess Medical Center	Boston	2%	321
Southcoast Hospital Group[2]	Fall River	2%	62
Umass Memorial Medical Center	Worcester	2%	248
Baystate Medical Center	Springfield	3%	297
Brigham & Women's Hospital[2]	Boston	3%	78
Cambridge Health Alliance[2]	Cambridge	3%	34
Falmouth Hospital	Falmouth	3%	29
Winchester Hospital[2]	Winchester	4%	28
Lowell General Hospital[2]	Lowell	5%	44
Heywood Hospital	Gardner	6%	36
Holy Family Hospital	Methuen	6%	87
Newton - Wellesley Hospital[2]	Newton	6%	53
Saint Elizabeth's Medical Center	Brighton	6%	47
Massachusetts General Hospital[2]	Boston	10%	31
Beverly Hospital Corporation[2]	Beverly	14%	44

Preventive Care

Immunization for Influenza

Hospital Name	City	Rate	Cases
Beth Israel Deaconess Hospital - Milton[2]	Milton	99%	520
Massachusetts General Hospital[2]	Boston	99%	540
Nashoba Valley Medical Center[2]	Ayer	99%	310
North Adams Regional Hospital[2]	North Adams	99%	294
Newton - Wellesley Hospital[2]	Newton	98%	455
Saint Vincent Hospital[2]	Worcester	98%	594
Brigham & Women's Faulkner Hospital[2]	Boston	97%	597
Mercy Medical Center[2]	Springfield	97%	558
North Shore Medical Center[2]	Salem	97%	538
Saint Anne's Hospital[2]	Fall River	97%	602
Sturdy Memorial Hospital[2]	Attleboro	97%	532
Winchester Hospital[2]	Winchester	97%	491
Anna Jaques Hospital[2]	Newburyport	96%	556
Baystate Franklin Medical Center[2]	Greenfield	96%	326
Beth Israel Deaconess Hospital - Needham[2]	Needham	96%	298
Beth Israel Deaconess Medical Center[2]	Boston	96%	658
Hallmark Health System[2]	Melrose	96%	541
Marlborough Hospital[2]	Marlborough	96%	397
Wing Memorial Hospital & Medical Center[2]	Palmer	96%	322
Metrowest Medical Center[2]	Framingham	95%	561
Southcoast Hospital Group[2]	Fall River	95%	545
Tufts Medical Center[2]	Boston	95%	542
Baystate Mary Lane Hospital[2]	Ware	94%	301
Berkshire Medical Center[2]	Pittsfield	94%	564
The Cooley Dickinson Hospital[2]	Northampton	94%	547
Good Samaritan Medical Center[2]	Brockton	94%	617
Holyoke Medical Center[2]	Holyoke	94%	589
Noble Hospital[2]	Westfield	94%	573
South Shore Hospital[2]	S Weymouth	94%	536
Fairview Hospital[2]	Great Barrington	93%	272
Heywood Hospital[2]	Gardner	93%	423
Jordan Hospital[2]	Plymouth	93%	518
Merrimack Valley Hospital[2]	Haverhill	93%	295
Quincy Medical Center[2]	Quincy	93%	590
Signature Healthcare Brockton Hospital[2]	Brockton	93%	549
Cambridge Health Alliance[2]	Cambridge	92%	507
Norwood Hospital[2]	Norwood	92%	575
Bedford VA Medical Center[2,3]	Bedford	91%	149
Brigham & Women's Hospital[2]	Boston	91%	494
Lahey Hosp & Med Ctr-Burlington[2]	Burlington	91%	585
Mount Auburn Hospital[2]	Cambridge	91%	526
Lawrence General Hospital[2]	Lawrence	90%	548
New England Baptist Hospital[2]	Boston	90%	621
Baystate Medical Center[2]	Springfield	89%	557
Falmouth Hospital[2]	Falmouth	89%	551
Harrington Memorial Hospital[2]	Southbridge	89%	352
Holy Family Hospital[2]	Methuen	88%	520
Saints Medical Center[2]	Lowell	88%	512
Boston Medical Center Corporation[2]	Boston	87%	599
Carney Hospital[2]	Boston	87%	485
Milford Regional Medical Center[2]	Milford	86%	547
Healthalliance Hospitals[2]	Leominster	85%	500
Umass Memorial Medical Center[2]	Worcester	85%	509
Cape Cod Hospital[2]	Hyannis	84%	581
Lowell General Hospital[2]	Lowell	84%	499
Northampton VA Medical Center[2,3]	Leeds	84%	146
Clinton Hospital Association[2]	Clinton	82%	285
Morton Hospital[2]	Taunton	81%	538
Emerson Hospital[2]	W Concord	80%	501
Nantucket Cottage Hospital	Nantucket	79%	62
Saint Elizabeth's Medical Center[2]	Brighton	76%	553
Beverly Hospital Corporation[2]	Beverly	69%	513
Adcare Hospital of Worcester[2]	Worcester	61%	568
Massachusetts Eye & Ear Infirmary[2]	Boston	54%	309

Immunization for Pneumonia

Hospital Name	City	Rate	Cases
Brigham & Women's Faulkner Hospital[2]	Boston	99%	749
Saint Vincent Hospital[2]	Worcester	99%	744
Anna Jaques Hospital[2]	Newburyport	98%	605
Noble Hospital[2]	Westfield	98%	663
North Adams Regional Hospital[2]	North Adams	98%	383
Sturdy Memorial Hospital[2]	Attleboro	98%	670
Baystate Franklin Medical Center[2]	Greenfield	96%	439
Baystate Mary Lane Hospital[2]	Ware	96%	452
The Cooley Dickinson Hospital[2]	Northampton	96%	713

NOTE: Hospital profiles are in alphabetical order by state, then city, then hospital within the city; Rankings exclude hospitals with less than 25 cases except for patient surveys which excludes hospitals with less than 100 cases; (a) 100-299 cases; (1) The number of cases/patients is too few to report; (2) Data submitted were based on a sample of cases/patients; (3) Results are based on a shorter time period than required; (4) Data suppressed by CMS for one or more quarters; (5) Results are not available for this reporting period; (6) Fewer than 100 patients completed the HCAHPS survey; (7) No cases met the criteria for this measure; (8) The lower limit of the confidence interval cannot be calculated if the number of observed infections equals zero; (9) No data are available from the state/territory for this reporting period; (10) The scores shown reflect fewer than 50 completed surveys; (11) There were discrepancies in the data collection process; (12) This measure does not apply to this hospital for this reporting period; (13) Results cannot be calculated for this reporting period; (14) The results for this state are combined with nearby states to protect confidentiality; Please refer to the User's Guide for a full explanation of data.

Holyoke Medical Center[2]	Holyoke	96%	1785
Metrowest Medical Center[2]	Framingham	96%	726
Nashoba Valley Medical Center[2]	Ayer	96%	434
Saint Anne's Hospital[2]	Fall River	96%	867
Carney Hospital[2]	Boston	95%	564
Hallmark Health System[2]	Melrose	95%	695
Jordan Hospital[2]	Plymouth	95%	700
Mercy Medical Center[2]	Springfield	95%	712
North Shore Medical Center[2]	Salem	95%	725
South Shore Hospital[2]	S Weymouth	95%	603
Baystate Medical Center[2]	Springfield	94%	651
Fairview Hospital[2]	Great Barrington	94%	335
Good Samaritan Medical Center[2]	Brockton	94%	774
Norwood Hospital[2]	Norwood	94%	754
Southcoast Hospital Group[2]	Fall River	94%	713
Tufts Medical Center[2]	Boston	94%	554
Wing Memorial Hospital & Medical Center[2]	Palmer	94%	439
Berkshire Medical Center[2]	Pittsfield	93%	772
Beth Israel Deaconess Hospital - Needham[2]	Needham	93%	465
Brigham & Women's Hospital[2]	Boston	93%	484
Morton Hospital[2]	Taunton	93%	738
Mount Auburn Hospital[2]	Cambridge	93%	586
Signature Healthcare Brockton Hospital[2]	Brockton	93%	626
Harrington Memorial Hospital[2]	Southbridge	92%	453
Marlborough Hospital[2]	Marlborough	92%	456
Massachusetts General Hospital[2]	Boston	92%	601
Winchester Hospital[2]	Winchester	92%	594
Falmouth Hospital[2]	Falmouth	91%	802
Lahey Hosp & Med Ctr-Burlington[2]	Burlington	91%	845
Newton - Wellesley Hospital[2]	Newton	91%	444
Holy Family Hospital[2]	Methuen	90%	651
Cambridge Health Alliance[2]	Cambridge	89%	566
Emerson Hospital[2]	W Concord	89%	468
Beth Israel Deaconess Hospital - Milton[2]	Milton	88%	771
Milford Regional Medical Center[2]	Milford	88%	720
Northampton VA Medical Center[2,3]	Leeds	88%	130
Quincy Medical Center[2]	Quincy	88%	709
Saints Medical Center[2]	Lowell	88%	736
Heywood Hospital[2]	Gardner	87%	516
Lawrence General Hospital[2]	Lawrence	87%	597
Lowell General Hospital[2]	Lowell	87%	534
Umass Memorial Medical Center[2]	Worcester	87%	572
Cape Cod Hospital[2]	Hyannis	86%	867
Healthalliance Hospitals[2]	Leominster	86%	666
Saint Elizabeth's Medical Center[2]	Brighton	86%	656
Merrimack Valley Hospital[2]	Haverhill	85%	436
New England Baptist Hospital[2]	Boston	84%	775
Boston Medical Center Corporation[2]	Boston	83%	605
Bedford VA Medical Center[2,3]	Bedford	81%	124
Beth Israel Deaconess Medical Center[2]	Boston	80%	721
Beverly Hospital Corporation[2]	Beverly	73%	580
Clinton Hospital Association[2]	Clinton	70%	482
Nantucket Cottage Hospital[2]	Nantucket	68%	117
Adcare Hospital of Worcester[2]	Worcester	54%	352
Massachusetts Eye & Ear Infirmary[2]	Boston	37%	268
Winchester Hospital[2]	Winchester	100%	37
Baystate Medical Center	Springfield	99%	275
Boston Medical Center Corporation	Boston	99%	144
Newton - Wellesley Hospital	Newton	99%	69
Norwood Hospital	Norwood	99%	75
Saint Vincent Hospital	Worcester	99%	154
South Shore Hospital	S Weymouth	99%	194
Baystate Franklin Medical Center	Greenfield	98%	40
Cambridge Health Alliance	Cambridge	98%	50
Falmouth Hospital	Falmouth	98%	61
Lawrence General Hospital	Lawrence	98%	83
Massachusetts General Hospital[2]	Boston	98%	85
Metrowest Medical Center	Framingham	98%	82
Morton Hospital	Taunton	98%	48
Tufts Medical Center	Boston	98%	97
Anna Jaques Hospital	Newburyport	97%	67
Hallmark Health System[2]	Melrose	97%	70
Holy Family Hospital	Methuen	97%	58
Jordan Hospital	Plymouth	97%	66
Milford Regional Medical Center	Milford	97%	71
Umass Memorial Medical Center[2]	Worcester	97%	63
Brigham & Women's Hospital[2]	Boston	96%	54
Good Samaritan Medical Center	Brockton	96%	95
Healthalliance Hospitals[2]	Leominster	96%	77
Mercy Medical Center	Springfield	96%	94
Saint Anne's Hospital	Fall River	96%	55
Lahey Hosp & Med Ctr-Burlington[2]	Burlington	95%	66
Quincy Medical Center	Quincy	95%	43
Saints Medical Center	Lowell	95%	60
Beth Israel Deaconess Medical Center[2]	Boston	94%	151
Lowell General Hospital[2]	Lowell	94%	101
Merrimack Valley Hospital	Haverhill	90%	29
Saint Elizabeth's Medical Center	Brighton	86%	59

Stroke Care

Anticoagulation Therapy for Atrial Fibrillation

Hospital Name	City	Rate	Cases
Berkshire Medical Center	Pittsfield	100%	31
Beverly Hospital Corporation	Beverly	100%	30
Boston Medical Center Corporation	Boston	100%	28
Cape Cod Hospital[2]	Hyannis	100%	25
Norwood Hospital	Norwood	100%	26
South Shore Hospital	S Weymouth	100%	32
Southcoast Hospital Group	Fall River	99%	73
Baystate Medical Center	Springfield	98%	45
Beth Israel Deaconess Medical Center[2]	Boston	98%	44
Saint Vincent Hospital	Worcester	97%	31

Antithrombotic Therapy Timing

Hospital Name	City	Rate	Cases
Berkshire Medical Center	Pittsfield	100%	96
Beth Israel Deaconess Hospital - Milton	Milton	100%	31
Beverly Hospital Corporation	Beverly	100%	119
Brigham & Women's Faulkner Hospital	Boston	100%	38
Cape Cod Hospital[2]	Hyannis	100%	103
Carney Hospital	Boston	100%	45
The Cooley Dickinson Hospital	Northampton	100%	36
Emerson Hospital	W Concord	100%	52
Harrington Memorial Hospital	Southbridge	100%	30
Holyoke Medical Center	Holyoke	100%	34
Marlborough Hospital	Marlborough	100%	25
Mount Auburn Hospital	Cambridge	100%	87
North Adams Regional Hospital	North Adams	100%	38
North Shore Medical Center[2]	Salem	100%	70
Signature Healthcare Brockton Hospital	Brockton	100%	65
Southcoast Hospital Group	Fall River	100%	344
Sturdy Memorial Hospital	Attleboro	100%	63

Assessed for Rehabilitation

Hospital Name	City	Rate	Cases
Baystate Medical Center	Springfield	100%	352
Berkshire Medical Center	Pittsfield	100%	136
Beth Israel Deaconess Hospital - Milton	Milton	100%	35
Boston Medical Center Corporation	Boston	100%	208
The Cooley Dickinson Hospital	Northampton	100%	44
Falmouth Hospital	Falmouth	100%	70
Newton - Wellesley Hospital	Newton	100%	97
North Adams Regional Hospital	North Adams	100%	38
Sturdy Memorial Hospital	Attleboro	100%	66
Winchester Hospital[2]	Winchester	100%	35
Wing Memorial Hospital & Medical Center	Palmer	100%	25
Saint Vincent Hospital	Worcester	99%	176
South Shore Hospital	S Weymouth	99%	221
Beverly Hospital Corporation	Beverly	98%	134
Brigham & Women's Faulkner Hospital	Boston	98%	40
Emerson Hospital	W Concord	98%	59
Mercy Medical Center	Springfield	98%	112
Saint Anne's Hospital	Fall River	98%	63
Southcoast Hospital Group	Fall River	98%	351
Anna Jaques Hospital	Newburyport	97%	68
Cape Cod Hospital[2]	Hyannis	97%	127
Harrington Memorial Hospital	Southbridge	97%	31
Holy Family Hospital	Methuen	97%	65
Marlborough Hospital	Marlborough	97%	31
Metrowest Medical Center	Framingham	97%	90
Signature Healthcare Brockton Hospital	Brockton	97%	73
Umass Memorial Medical Center[2]	Worcester	97%	103
Holyoke Medical Center	Holyoke	96%	57
Massachusetts General Hospital[2]	Boston	96%	144
Mount Auburn Hospital	Cambridge	96%	115
North Shore Medical Center[2]	Salem	96%	80
Lahey Hosp & Med Ctr-Burlington[2]	Burlington	95%	101
Milford Regional Medical Center	Milford	95%	75
Jordan Hospital	Plymouth	94%	64
Merrimack Valley Hospital	Haverhill	94%	31
Saint Elizabeth's Medical Center	Brighton	94%	77
Saints Medical Center	Lowell	94%	65
Baystate Franklin Medical Center	Greenfield	93%	42
Brigham & Women's Hospital[2]	Boston	93%	102
Carney Hospital	Boston	93%	43
Quincy Medical Center	Quincy	93%	42
Lowell General Hospital[2]	Lowell	92%	118
Tufts Medical Center	Boston	92%	192
Beth Israel Deaconess Medical Center[2]	Boston	91%	288
Good Samaritan Medical Center	Brockton	91%	91
Morton Hospital	Taunton	90%	52
Lawrence General Hospital	Lawrence	88%	91
Norwood Hospital	Norwood	88%	82
Cambridge Health Alliance	Cambridge	84%	50
Healthalliance Hospitals[2]	Leominster	82%	78
Hallmark Health System[2]	Melrose	79%	78

Discharged on Antithrombotic Therapy

Hospital Name	City	Rate	Cases
Anna Jaques Hospital	Newburyport	100%	67
Baystate Franklin Medical Center	Greenfield	100%	42
Baystate Medical Center	Springfield	100%	291
Berkshire Medical Center	Pittsfield	100%	130
Beverly Hospital Corporation	Beverly	100%	129
Brigham & Women's Faulkner Hospital	Boston	100%	35
Brigham & Women's Hospital[2]	Boston	100%	70
Carney Hospital	Boston	100%	41
The Cooley Dickinson Hospital	Northampton	100%	40
Emerson Hospital	W Concord	100%	55
Falmouth Hospital	Falmouth	100%	62
Healthalliance Hospitals[2]	Leominster	100%	74
Holyoke Medical Center	Holyoke	100%	55
Jordan Hospital	Plymouth	100%	62
Lahey Hosp & Med Ctr-Burlington[2]	Burlington	100%	78
Lawrence General Hospital	Lawrence	100%	83
Marlborough Hospital	Marlborough	100%	31
Massachusetts General Hospital[2]	Boston	100%	102
Mercy Medical Center	Springfield	100%	95
Metrowest Medical Center	Framingham	100%	86
Morton Hospital	Taunton	100%	51
Mount Auburn Hospital	Cambridge	100%	100
Newton - Wellesley Hospital	Newton	100%	91
North Adams Regional Hospital	North Adams	100%	37
North Shore Medical Center[2]	Salem	100%	77
Norwood Hospital	Norwood	100%	81
Saint Anne's Hospital	Fall River	100%	55
Saint Elizabeth's Medical Center	Brighton	100%	68
Saint Vincent Hospital	Worcester	100%	158
Saints Medical Center	Lowell	100%	62
Signature Healthcare Brockton Hospital	Brockton	100%	73
South Shore Hospital	S Weymouth	100%	198
Southcoast Hospital Group	Fall River	100%	327
Tufts Medical Center	Boston	100%	111
Winchester Hospital[2]	Winchester	100%	31
Wing Memorial Hospital & Medical Center	Palmer	100%	25
Beth Israel Deaconess Medical Center[2]	Boston	99%	193
Boston Medical Center Corporation	Boston	99%	170
Cape Cod Hospital[2]	Hyannis	99%	106
Hallmark Health System[2]	Melrose	99%	76
Lowell General Hospital[2]	Lowell	99%	109
Milford Regional Medical Center	Milford	99%	75
Umass Memorial Medical Center[2]	Worcester	99%	83
Good Samaritan Medical Center	Brockton	98%	88
Holy Family Hospital	Methuen	98%	59
Quincy Medical Center	Quincy	98%	41
Sturdy Memorial Hospital	Attleboro	98%	64
Beth Israel Deaconess Hospital - Milton	Milton	97%	33
Harrington Memorial Hospital	Southbridge	97%	30
Cambridge Health Alliance	Cambridge	94%	49
Merrimack Valley Hospital	Haverhill	90%	30

Discharged on Statin Medication

Hospital Name	City	Rate	Cases
Baystate Medical Center	Springfield	100%	223
Berkshire Medical Center	Pittsfield	100%	101
Brigham & Women's Faulkner Hospital	Boston	100%	32
Brigham & Women's Hospital[2]	Boston	100%	48
Falmouth Hospital	Falmouth	100%	50
Metrowest Medical Center	Framingham	100%	67
Milford Regional Medical Center	Milford	100%	61
Newton - Wellesley Hospital	Newton	100%	62
North Adams Regional Hospital	North Adams	100%	29
Quincy Medical Center	Quincy	100%	29
South Shore Hospital	S Weymouth	100%	174
Tufts Medical Center	Boston	100%	94
Boston Medical Center Corporation	Boston	99%	135
Lowell General Hospital[2]	Lowell	99%	87
Mercy Medical Center	Springfield	99%	73
Morton Hospital	Taunton	98%	45
North Shore Medical Center[2]	Salem	98%	62
Southcoast Hospital Group	Fall River	98%	266
Sturdy Memorial Hospital	Attleboro	98%	49
Baystate Franklin Medical Center	Greenfield	97%	32
Cape Cod Hospital[2]	Hyannis	97%	72
Holyoke Medical Center	Holyoke	97%	38
Massachusetts General Hospital[2]	Boston	97%	78
Norwood Hospital	Norwood	97%	70
Saint Vincent Hospital	Worcester	97%	114
Signature Healthcare Brockton Hospital	Brockton	97%	71
Umass Memorial Medical Center[2]	Worcester	97%	66
Harrington Memorial Hospital	Southbridge	96%	26
Beth Israel Deaconess Medical Center[2]	Boston	95%	148
Mount Auburn Hospital	Cambridge	95%	77
Carney Hospital	Boston	94%	31
Lahey Hosp & Med Ctr-Burlington[2]	Burlington	94%	63
Cambridge Health Alliance	Cambridge	93%	43
Hallmark Health System[2]	Melrose	93%	61

NOTE: Hospital profiles are in alphabetical order by state, then city, then hospital within the city; Rankings exclude hospitals with less than 25 cases except for patient surveys which excludes hospitals with less than 100 cases; (a) 100-299 cases; (1) The number of cases/patients is too few to report; (2) Data submitted were based on a sample of cases/patients; (3) Results are based on a shorter time period than required; (4) Data suppressed by CMS for one or more quarters; (5) Results are not available for this reporting period; (6) Fewer than 100 patients completed the HCAHPS survey; (7) No cases met the criteria for this measure; (8) The lower limit of the confidence interval cannot be calculated if the number of observed infections equals zero; (9) No data are available from the state/territory for this reporting period; (10) The scores shown reflect fewer than 50 completed surveys; (11) There were discrepancies in the data collection process; (12) This measure does not apply to this hospital for this reporting period; (13) Results cannot be calculated for this reporting period; (14) The results for this state are combined with nearby states to protect confidentiality; Please refer to the User's Guide for a full explanation of data.

Hospital Name	City	Rate	Cases
Saint Anne's Hospital	Fall River	93%	45
Good Samaritan Medical Center	Brockton	92%	80
Holy Family Hospital	Methuen	92%	48
Emerson Hospital	W Concord	91%	34
Jordan Hospital	Plymouth	91%	54
Saint Elizabeth's Medical Center	Brighton	90%	58
Beth Israel Deaconess Hospital - Milton	Milton	89%	28
Healthalliance Hospitals[2]	Leominster	89%	62
The Cooley Dickinson Hospital	Northampton	88%	33
Lawrence General Hospital	Lawrence	88%	58
Beverly Hospital Corporation	Beverly	84%	105
Winchester Hospital[2]	Winchester	84%	25
Anna Jaques Hospital	Newburyport	83%	60
Saints Medical Center	Lowell	82%	55

Thrombolytic Therapy Timing

Hospital Name	City	Rate	Cases
Baystate Medical Center	Springfield	50%	34

Venous Thromboembolism (VTE) Prophylaxis

Hospital Name	City	Rate	Cases
Berkshire Medical Center	Pittsfield	100%	113
Falmouth Hospital	Falmouth	100%	69
Newton - Wellesley Hospital	Newton	100%	94
North Adams Regional Hospital	North Adams	100%	38
North Shore Medical Center[2]	Salem	99%	78
Baystate Medical Center	Springfield	98%	368
Cape Cod Hospital[2]	Hyannis	98%	126
Lahey Hosp & Med Ctr-Burlington[2]	Burlington	98%	107
Saint Vincent Hospital	Worcester	98%	181
Sturdy Memorial Hospital	Attleboro	98%	65
Boston Medical Center Corporation	Boston	97%	212
Brigham & Women's Faulkner Hospital	Boston	97%	38
Harrington Memorial Hospital	Southbridge	97%	30
Mercy Medical Center	Springfield	97%	122
Holyoke Medical Center	Holyoke	96%	53
Southcoast Hospital Group	Fall River	96%	364
Tufts Medical Center	Boston	96%	200
Umass Memorial Medical Center[2]	Worcester	96%	101
Baystate Franklin Medical Center	Greenfield	95%	39
Beth Israel Deaconess Medical Center[2]	Boston	95%	294
Lowell General Hospital[2]	Lowell	95%	118
South Shore Hospital	S Weymouth	95%	202
Brigham & Women's Hospital[2]	Boston	94%	108
Massachusetts General Hospital[2]	Boston	94%	150
Milford Regional Medical Center	Milford	94%	71
Mount Auburn Hospital	Cambridge	94%	109
Metrowest Medical Center	Framingham	93%	88
Saint Elizabeth's Medical Center	Brighton	93%	75
Cambridge Health Alliance	Cambridge	92%	52
Norwood Hospital	Norwood	92%	87
Signature Healthcare Brockton Hospital	Brockton	92%	75
Carney Hospital	Boston	91%	45
Marlborough Hospital	Marlborough	91%	32
The Cooley Dickinson Hospital	Northampton	90%	42
Emerson Hospital	W Concord	90%	58
Beverly Hospital Corporation	Beverly	89%	143
Good Samaritan Medical Center	Brockton	89%	97
Holy Family Hospital	Methuen	89%	66
Saint Anne's Hospital	Fall River	89%	64
Anna Jaques Hospital	Newburyport	88%	67
Quincy Medical Center	Quincy	88%	48
Jordan Hospital	Plymouth	87%	69
Merrimack Valley Hospital	Haverhill	87%	30
Morton Hospital	Taunton	87%	52
Beth Israel Deaconess Hospital - Milton	Milton	84%	32
Hallmark Health System[2]	Melrose	82%	74
Healthalliance Hospitals[2]	Leominster	81%	80
Saints Medical Center	Lowell	80%	65
Lawrence General Hospital	Lawrence	79%	91
Winchester Hospital[2]	Winchester	78%	41

Written Stroke Educational Materials Given

Hospital Name	City	Rate	Cases
Brigham & Women's Faulkner Hospital	Boston	100%	27
Emerson Hospital	W Concord	100%	33
Falmouth Hospital	Falmouth	100%	31
Holyoke Medical Center	Holyoke	100%	26
Newton - Wellesley Hospital	Newton	100%	50
Boston Medical Center Corporation	Boston	99%	113
Good Samaritan Medical Center	Brockton	98%	49
Mercy Medical Center	Springfield	98%	52
North Shore Medical Center[2]	Salem	98%	40
Saint Vincent Hospital	Worcester	98%	87
Baystate Medical Center	Springfield	97%	181
Berkshire Medical Center	Pittsfield	97%	86
Morton Hospital	Taunton	97%	29
Saint Anne's Hospital	Fall River	97%	36
Jordan Hospital	Plymouth	96%	27
Signature Healthcare Brockton Hospital	Brockton	95%	40
Sturdy Memorial Hospital	Attleboro	95%	37
South Shore Hospital	S Weymouth	94%	106
Massachusetts General Hospital[2]	Boston	93%	76
Saints Medical Center	Lowell	93%	29
Norwood Hospital	Norwood	91%	47
Southcoast Hospital Group	Fall River	90%	163
Metrowest Medical Center	Framingham	87%	45
Milford Regional Medical Center	Milford	87%	38
Lowell General Hospital[2]	Lowell	86%	59
Beverly Hospital Corporation	Beverly	85%	65
Anna Jaques Hospital	Newburyport	82%	34
Saint Elizabeth's Medical Center	Brighton	77%	35
Umass Memorial Medical Center[2]	Worcester	76%	37
Hallmark Health System[2]	Melrose	74%	46
Cape Cod Hospital[2]	Hyannis	73%	56
Mount Auburn Hospital	Cambridge	70%	61
Lahey Hosp & Med Ctr-Burlington[2]	Burlington	65%	51
Cambridge Health Alliance	Cambridge	64%	33
Brigham & Women's Hospital[2]	Boston	55%	62
Beth Israel Deaconess Medical Center[2]	Boston	45%	136
Tufts Medical Center	Boston	22%	86
Lawrence General Hospital	Lawrence	19%	43
Healthalliance Hospitals[2]	Leominster	0%	44

Surgical Care Improvement Project

Appropriate Beta Blocker Usage

Hospital Name	City	Rate	Cases
Berkshire Medical Center	Pittsfield	100%	223
Beth Israel Deaconess Hospital - Milton[2]	Milton	100%	90
Beth Israel Deaconess Medical Center[2]	Boston	100%	481
Brigham & Women's Faulkner Hospital[2]	Boston	100%	60
Brigham & Women's Hospital[2]	Boston	100%	243
Carney Hospital	Boston	100%	48
Healthalliance Hospitals[2]	Leominster	100%	95
Holy Family Hospital[2]	Methuen	100%	200
Lahey Hosp & Med Ctr-Burlington[2]	Burlington	100%	255
Marlborough Hospital	Marlborough	100%	73
Massachusetts General Hospital[2]	Boston	100%	286
Merrimack Valley Hospital	Haverhill	100%	40
Nashoba Valley Medical Center	Ayer	100%	38
New England Baptist Hospital[2]	Boston	100%	322
Noble Hospital	Westfield	100%	30
North Shore Medical Center[2]	Salem	100%	203
Saint Anne's Hospital[2]	Fall River	100%	188
Anna Jaques Hospital	Newburyport	99%	88
Falmouth Hospital	Falmouth	99%	183
Metrowest Medical Center	Framingham	99%	170
Mount Auburn Hospital	Cambridge	99%	301
Norwood Hospital[2]	Norwood	99%	183
Quincy Medical Center	Quincy	99%	139
Southcoast Hospital Group[2]	Fall River	99%	560
Sturdy Memorial Hospital	Attleboro	99%	172
Tufts Medical Center[2]	Boston	99%	374
Umass Memorial Medical Center[2]	Worcester	99%	218
VA Boston Healthcare Sys-Jamaica Plain[2]	Jamaica Plain	99%	177
Baystate Medical Center[2]	Springfield	98%	243
Beverly Hospital Corporation	Beverly	98%	300
Boston Medical Center Corporation[2]	Boston	98%	270
Cape Cod Hospital[2]	Hyannis	98%	384
The Cooley Dickinson Hospital[2]	Northampton	98%	107
Holyoke Medical Center	Holyoke	98%	63
Lawrence General Hospital	Lawrence	98%	66
Lowell General Hospital[2]	Lowell	98%	256
Mercy Medical Center	Springfield	98%	220
Milford Regional Medical Center	Milford	98%	113
North Adams Regional Hospital	North Adams	98%	64
Saint Elizabeth's Medical Center[2]	Brighton	98%	390
Saint Vincent Hospital	Worcester	98%	534
Signature Healthcare Brockton Hospital	Brockton	98%	116
Good Samaritan Medical Center[2]	Brockton	97%	199
Hallmark Health System[2]	Melrose	97%	115
Heywood Hospital	Gardner	97%	77
Morton Hospital	Taunton	97%	137
Jordan Hospital	Plymouth	96%	219
Beth Israel Deaconess Hospital - Needham	Needham	95%	38
South Shore Hospital	S Weymouth	95%	324
Winchester Hospital[2]	Winchester	94%	124
Newton - Wellesley Hospital[2]	Newton	93%	76
Saints Medical Center	Lowell	93%	27
Cambridge Health Alliance[2]	Cambridge	92%	36
Baystate Franklin Medical Center[2]	Greenfield	91%	32
Emerson Hospital	W Concord	91%	121
Harrington Memorial Hospital	Southbridge	90%	52

Appropriate VTP Within 24 Hours

Hospital Name	City	Rate	Cases
Beth Israel Deaconess Hospital - Needham	Needham	100%	110
Beth Israel Deaconess Medical Center[2]	Boston	100%	878
Boston Medical Center Corporation[2]	Boston	100%	474
Brigham & Women's Hospital[2]	Boston	100%	425
Fairview Hospital	Great Barrington	100%	52
Lahey Hosp & Med Ctr-Burlington[2]	Burlington	100%	338
Mount Auburn Hospital	Cambridge	100%	528
Saint Vincent Hospital	Worcester	100%	1089
Signature Healthcare Brockton Hospital	Brockton	100%	311
Sturdy Memorial Hospital	Attleboro	100%	434
VA Boston Healthcare Sys-Jamaica Plain[2]	Jamaica Plain	100%	298
Baystate Medical Center[2]	Springfield	99%	404
Berkshire Medical Center	Pittsfield	99%	680
Beth Israel Deaconess Hospital - Milton[2]	Milton	99%	267
Beverly Hospital Corporation	Beverly	99%	926
Brigham & Women's Faulkner Hospital[2]	Boston	99%	251
Cambridge Health Alliance[2]	Cambridge	99%	156
Cape Cod Hospital[2]	Hyannis	99%	830
Carney Hospital	Boston	99%	140
The Cooley Dickinson Hospital[2]	Northampton	99%	452
Falmouth Hospital	Falmouth	99%	559
Good Samaritan Medical Center[2]	Brockton	99%	521
Hallmark Health System[2]	Melrose	99%	298
Heywood Hospital	Gardner	99%	242
Massachusetts General Hospital[2]	Boston	99%	460
Mercy Medical Center	Springfield	99%	702
Metrowest Medical Center	Framingham	99%	443
Newton - Wellesley Hospital[2]	Newton	99%	304
North Adams Regional Hospital	North Adams	99%	146
North Shore Medical Center[2]	Salem	99%	272
Saint Anne's Hospital[2]	Fall River	99%	405
Saint Elizabeth's Medical Center[2]	Brighton	99%	254
South Shore Hospital	S Weymouth	99%	881
Tufts Medical Center[2]	Boston	99%	387
Winchester Hospital[2]	Winchester	99%	293
Anna Jaques Hospital	Newburyport	98%	251
Jordan Hospital	Plymouth	98%	631
Lowell General Hospital[2]	Lowell	98%	635
Marlborough Hospital	Marlborough	98%	181
New England Baptist Hospital[2]	Boston	98%	1156
Norwood Hospital[2]	Norwood	98%	372
Quincy Medical Center	Quincy	98%	360
Southcoast Hospital Group[2]	Fall River	98%	1034
Umass Memorial Medical Center[2]	Worcester	98%	335
Emerson Hospital	W Concord	97%	446
Harrington Memorial Hospital	Southbridge	97%	146
Holy Family Hospital[2]	Methuen	97%	502
Merrimack Valley Hospital	Haverhill	97%	109
Morton Hospital	Taunton	97%	299
Saints Medical Center	Lowell	97%	74
Wing Memorial Hospital & Medical Center	Palmer	97%	38
Healthalliance Hospitals[2]	Leominster	96%	234
Milford Regional Medical Center	Milford	96%	356
Noble Hospital	Westfield	96%	83
Holyoke Medical Center	Holyoke	95%	183
Baystate Franklin Medical Center[2]	Greenfield	94%	122
Baystate Mary Lane Hospital	Ware	94%	47
Lawrence General Hospital	Lawrence	94%	230
Nashoba Valley Medical Center	Ayer	93%	72

Controlled Postoperative Blood Glucose

Hospital Name	City	Rate	Cases
Brigham & Women's Hospital[2]	Boston	99%	132
Mount Auburn Hospital	Cambridge	99%	161
Lahey Hosp & Med Ctr-Burlington[2]	Burlington	98%	131
Saint Vincent Hospital	Worcester	98%	159
Southcoast Hospital Group[2]	Fall River	98%	224
Umass Memorial Medical Center[2]	Worcester	98%	130
Boston Medical Center Corporation[2]	Boston	97%	163
North Shore Medical Center[2]	Salem	97%	117
Tufts Medical Center[2]	Boston	97%	287
VA Boston Healthcare Sys-Jamaica Plain[2]	Jamaica Plain	97%	180
Beth Israel Deaconess Medical Center[2]	Boston	96%	203
Cape Cod Hospital[2]	Hyannis	95%	130
Massachusetts General Hospital[2]	Boston	94%	145
Baystate Medical Center[2]	Springfield	93%	152
Saint Elizabeth's Medical Center[2]	Brighton	91%	336

Perioperative Temperature Management

Hospital Name	City	Rate	Cases
Anna Jaques Hospital	Newburyport	100%	294
Baystate Franklin Medical Center[2]	Greenfield	100%	153
Baystate Medical Center[2]	Springfield	100%	532
Berkshire Medical Center	Pittsfield	100%	781
Beth Israel Deaconess Hospital - Milton[2]	Milton	100%	317
Beth Israel Deaconess Hospital - Needham	Needham	100%	114
Beth Israel Deaconess Medical Center[2]	Boston	100%	1110
Beverly Hospital Corporation	Beverly	100%	1077
Boston Medical Center Corporation[2]	Boston	100%	610
Brigham & Women's Faulkner Hospital[2]	Boston	100%	289
Brigham & Women's Hospital[2]	Boston	100%	556
Cambridge Health Alliance[2]	Cambridge	100%	188
Cape Cod Hospital[2]	Hyannis	100%	956

NOTE: Hospital profiles are in alphabetical order by state, then city, then hospital within the city; Rankings exclude hospitals with less than 25 cases except for patient surveys which excludes hospitals with less than 100 cases; (a) 100-299 cases; (1) The number of cases/patients is too few to report; (2) Data submitted were based on a sample of cases/patients; (3) Results are based on a shorter time period than required; (4) Data suppressed by CMS for one or more quarters; (5) Results are not available for this reporting period; (6) Fewer than 100 patients completed the HCAHPS survey; (7) No cases met the criteria for this measure; (8) The lower limit of the confidence interval cannot be calculated if the number of observed infections equals zero; (9) No data are available from the state/territory for this reporting period; (10) The scores shown reflect fewer than 50 completed surveys; (11) There were discrepancies in the data collection process; (12) This measure does not apply to this hospital for this reporting period; (13) Results cannot be calculated for this reporting period; (14) The results for this state are combined with nearby states to protect confidentiality; Please refer to the User's Guide for a full explanation of data.

Hospital Name	City	Rate	Cases
Carney Hospital	Boston	100%	159
The Cooley Dickinson Hospital[2]	Northampton	100%	509
Emerson Hospital	W Concord	100%	500
Fairview Hospital	Great Barrington	100%	57
Falmouth Hospital	Falmouth	100%	642
Good Samaritan Medical Center[2]	Brockton	100%	693
Hallmark Health System[2]	Melrose	100%	343
Healthalliance Hospitals[2]	Leominster	100%	279
Heywood Hospital	Gardner	100%	266
Holy Family Hospital[2]	Methuen	100%	551
Jordan Hospital	Plymouth	100%	720
Lahey Hosp & Med Ctr-Burlington[2]	Burlington	100%	477
Lawrence General Hospital	Lawrence	100%	280
Lowell General Hospital[2]	Lowell	100%	755
Massachusetts General Hospital[2]	Boston	100%	628
Mercy Medical Center	Springfield	100%	857
Metrowest Medical Center	Framingham	100%	539
Milford Regional Medical Center	Milford	100%	394
Morton Hospital	Taunton	100%	355
Mount Auburn Hospital	Cambridge	100%	623
Nashoba Valley Medical Center	Ayer	100%	80
New England Baptist Hospital[2]	Boston	100%	1305
Newton - Wellesley Hospital[2]	Newton	100%	346
Noble Hospital	Westfield	100%	94
North Adams Regional Hospital	North Adams	100%	175
North Shore Medical Center[2]	Salem	100%	337
Norwood Hospital[2]	Norwood	100%	455
Quincy Medical Center	Quincy	100%	421
Saint Elizabeth's Medical Center[2]	Brighton	100%	432
Saint Vincent Hospital	Worcester	100%	1342
Saints Medical Center	Lowell	100%	78
Signature Healthcare Brockton Hospital	Brockton	100%	359
Southcoast Hospital Group[2]	Fall River	100%	1258
Sturdy Memorial Hospital	Attleboro	100%	529
Tufts Medical Center[2]	Boston	100%	543
Umass Memorial Medical Center[2]	Worcester	100%	470
Winchester Hospital[2]	Winchester	100%	385
Wing Memorial Hospital & Medical Center	Palmer	100%	43
Harrington Memorial Hospital	Southbridge	99%	164
Marlborough Hospital	Marlborough	99%	193
Merrimack Valley Hospital	Haverhill	99%	120
South Shore Hospital	S Weymouth	99%	994
VA Boston Healthcare Sys-Jamaica Plain[2]	Jamaica Plain	99%	364
Baystate Mary Lane Hospital	Ware	98%	55
Saint Anne's Hospital[2]	Fall River	98%	517
Holyoke Medical Center	Holyoke	97%	207

Prophylactic Antibiotic Selection

Hospital Name	City	Rate	Cases
Baystate Mary Lane Hospital	Ware	100%	35
Baystate Medical Center[2]	Springfield	100%	489
Berkshire Medical Center	Pittsfield	100%	478
Beth Israel Deaconess Hospital - Needham	Needham	100%	67
Beth Israel Deaconess Medical Center[2]	Boston	100%	750
Beverly Hospital Corporation	Beverly	100%	838
The Cooley Dickinson Hospital[2]	Northampton	100%	390
Fairview Hospital	Great Barrington	100%	39
Heywood Hospital	Gardner	100%	212
Lahey Hosp & Med Ctr-Burlington[2]	Burlington	100%	408
Marlborough Hospital	Marlborough	100%	163
Massachusetts General Hospital[2]	Boston	100%	473
Mercy Medical Center	Springfield	100%	423
Mount Auburn Hospital	Cambridge	100%	594
Newton - Wellesley Hospital[2]	Newton	100%	226
Noble Hospital	Westfield	100%	71
North Adams Regional Hospital	North Adams	100%	138
Norwood Hospital[2]	Norwood	100%	314
Saint Anne's Hospital[2]	Fall River	100%	432
Saints Medical Center	Lowell	100%	39
Signature Healthcare Brockton Hospital	Brockton	100%	249
Tufts Medical Center[2]	Boston	100%	628
VA Boston Healthcare Sys-Jamaica Plain	Jamaica Plain	100%	411
Beth Israel Deaconess Hospital - Milton[2]	Milton	99%	220
Boston Medical Center Corporation[2]	Boston	99%	543
Brigham & Women's Faulkner Hospital[2]	Boston	99%	153
Brigham & Women's Hospital[2]	Boston	99%	420
Cape Cod Hospital[2]	Hyannis	99%	863
Carney Hospital	Boston	99%	99
Falmouth Hospital	Falmouth	99%	512
Hallmark Health System[2]	Melrose	99%	239
Harrington Memorial Hospital	Southbridge	99%	121
Holy Family Hospital[2]	Methuen	99%	434
Holyoke Medical Center	Holyoke	99%	149
Jordan Hospital	Plymouth	99%	521
Lowell General Hospital[2]	Lowell	99%	562
Milford Regional Medical Center	Milford	99%	276
New England Baptist Hospital[2]	Boston	99%	1186
North Shore Medical Center[2]	Salem	99%	341
Quincy Medical Center	Quincy	99%	279
Saint Elizabeth's Medical Center[2]	Brighton	99%	567
Saint Vincent Hospital	Worcester	99%	986
South Shore Hospital	S Weymouth	99%	645
Southcoast Hospital Group[2]	Fall River	99%	951
Sturdy Memorial Hospital	Attleboro	99%	339
Umass Memorial Medical Center[2]	Worcester	99%	403
Anna Jaques Hospital	Newburyport	98%	213
Cambridge Health Alliance[2]	Cambridge	98%	100
Emerson Hospital	W Concord	98%	379
Good Samaritan Medical Center[2]	Brockton	98%	528
Merrimack Valley Hospital	Haverhill	98%	83
Metrowest Medical Center	Framingham	98%	287
Morton Hospital	Taunton	98%	256
Nashoba Valley Medical Center	Ayer	98%	60
Winchester Hospital[2]	Winchester	98%	252
Healthalliance Hospitals[2]	Leominster	97%	185
Lawrence General Hospital	Lawrence	97%	137
Baystate Franklin Medical Center[2]	Greenfield	96%	89

Prophylactic Antibiotic Selection (Outpatient)

Hospital Name	City	Rate	Cases
Carney Hospital	Boston	100%	32
Falmouth Hospital	Falmouth	100%	79
Hallmark Health System	Melrose	100%	83
Mount Auburn Hospital	Cambridge	100%	346
Quincy Medical Center	Quincy	100%	28
Saint Anne's Hospital	Fall River	100%	72
Signature Healthcare Brockton Hospital	Brockton	100%	42
Tufts Medical Center	Boston	100%	202
Wing Memorial Hospital & Medical Center	Palmer	100%	52
Anna Jaques Hospital	Newburyport	99%	101
Baystate Medical Center	Springfield	99%	627
Berkshire Medical Center	Pittsfield	99%	322
Beverly Hospital Corporation	Beverly	99%	256
Brigham & Women's Faulkner Hospital	Boston	99%	146
Cape Cod Hospital	Hyannis	99%	475
Emerson Hospital	W Concord	99%	160
Healthalliance Hospitals	Leominster	99%	105
Lahey Hosp & Med Ctr-Burlington	Burlington	99%	719
Mercy Medical Center	Springfield	99%	597
New England Baptist Hospital	Boston	99%	588
Newton - Wellesley Hospital	Newton	99%	513
Norwood Hospital	Norwood	99%	109
Saint Elizabeth's Medical Center	Brighton	99%	176
Beth Israel Deaconess Medical Center	Boston	98%	888
Boston Medical Center Corporation	Boston	98%	238
Brigham & Women's Hospital	Boston	98%	623
Cambridge Health Alliance	Cambridge	98%	184
Good Samaritan Medical Center	Brockton	98%	203
Lowell General Hospital	Lowell	98%	368
Massachusetts General Hospital	Boston	98%	609
Metrowest Medical Center	Framingham	98%	255
North Shore Medical Center	Salem	98%	467
Winchester Hospital	Winchester	98%	172
The Cooley Dickinson Hospital	Northampton	97%	167
Milford Regional Medical Center	Milford	97%	133
Morton Hospital	Taunton	97%	36
Saint Vincent Hospital	Worcester	97%	544
South Shore Hospital	S Weymouth	97%	317
Southcoast Hospital Group	Fall River	97%	921
Umass Memorial Medical Center	Worcester	97%	390
Holyoke Medical Center	Holyoke	96%	55
Lawrence General Hospital	Lawrence	96%	112
Beth Israel Deaconess Hospital - Needham	Needham	94%	47
Holy Family Hospital	Methuen	94%	105
Jordan Hospital	Plymouth	94%	145
Nashoba Valley Medical Center	Ayer	93%	59
Harrington Memorial Hospital	Southbridge	92%	65
Beth Israel Deaconess Hospital - Milton	Milton	89%	44
Heywood Hospital	Gardner	89%	133
Sturdy Memorial Hospital	Attleboro	82%	97

Prophylactic Antibiotic Stopped

Hospital Name	City	Rate	Cases
Anna Jaques Hospital	Newburyport	100%	209
Berkshire Medical Center	Pittsfield	100%	471
Beverly Hospital Corporation	Beverly	100%	821
Brigham & Women's Faulkner Hospital[2]	Boston	100%	153
Carney Hospital	Boston	100%	96
Fairview Hospital	Great Barrington	100%	39
Falmouth Hospital	Falmouth	100%	503
Hallmark Health System[2]	Melrose	100%	229
Metrowest Medical Center	Framingham	100%	278
Mount Auburn Hospital	Cambridge	100%	591
Newton - Wellesley Hospital[2]	Newton	100%	225
North Adams Regional Hospital	North Adams	100%	136
Saints Medical Center	Lowell	100%	39
Signature Healthcare Brockton Hospital	Brockton	100%	243
Sturdy Memorial Hospital	Attleboro	100%	318
Tufts Medical Center[2]	Boston	100%	614
VA Boston Healthcare Sys-Jamaica Plain	Jamaica Plain	100%	410
Winchester Hospital[2]	Winchester	100%	252
Baystate Medical Center[2]	Springfield	99%	475
Beth Israel Deaconess Medical Center[2]	Boston	99%	737
Cape Cod Hospital[2]	Hyannis	99%	847
The Cooley Dickinson Hospital[2]	Northampton	99%	389
Good Samaritan Medical Center[2]	Brockton	99%	516
Harrington Memorial Hospital	Southbridge	99%	116
Heywood Hospital	Gardner	99%	209
Holyoke Medical Center	Holyoke	99%	146
Jordan Hospital	Plymouth	99%	512
Lowell General Hospital[2]	Lowell	99%	549
Noble Hospital	Westfield	99%	70
Norwood Hospital[2]	Norwood	99%	307
Saint Anne's Hospital[2]	Fall River	99%	426
Saint Vincent Hospital	Worcester	99%	972
South Shore Hospital	S Weymouth	99%	641
Umass Memorial Medical Center[2]	Worcester	99%	392
Brigham & Women's Hospital[2]	Boston	98%	413
Emerson Hospital	W Concord	98%	370
Healthalliance Hospitals[2]	Leominster	98%	180
Holy Family Hospital[2]	Methuen	98%	424
Lahey Hosp & Med Ctr-Burlington[2]	Burlington	98%	392
Marlborough Hospital	Marlborough	98%	160
Milford Regional Medical Center	Milford	98%	265
New England Baptist Hospital[2]	Boston	98%	1185
North Shore Medical Center[2]	Salem	98%	334
Southcoast Hospital Group[2]	Fall River	98%	928
Baystate Mary Lane Hospital	Ware	97%	34
Beth Israel Deaconess Hospital - Milton[2]	Milton	97%	213
Boston Medical Center Corporation[2]	Boston	97%	517
Lawrence General Hospital	Lawrence	97%	133
Massachusetts General Hospital[2]	Boston	97%	458
Mercy Medical Center	Springfield	97%	400
Morton Hospital	Taunton	97%	250
Quincy Medical Center	Quincy	97%	274
Saint Elizabeth's Medical Center[2]	Brighton	96%	551
Beth Israel Deaconess Hospital - Needham	Needham	95%	61
Merrimack Valley Hospital	Haverhill	95%	82
Cambridge Health Alliance[2]	Cambridge	93%	99
Nashoba Valley Medical Center	Ayer	92%	60
Baystate Franklin Medical Center[2]	Greenfield	91%	88

Prophylactic Antibiotic Timing

Hospital Name	City	Rate	Cases
Anna Jaques Hospital	Newburyport	100%	213
Baystate Mary Lane Hospital	Ware	100%	35
Baystate Medical Center[2]	Springfield	100%	489
Beth Israel Deaconess Medical Center[2]	Boston	100%	750
Beverly Hospital Corporation	Beverly	100%	839
The Cooley Dickinson Hospital[2]	Northampton	100%	390
Fairview Hospital	Great Barrington	100%	39
Falmouth Hospital	Falmouth	100%	512
Holy Family Hospital[2]	Methuen	100%	435
Milford Regional Medical Center	Milford	100%	276
Morton Hospital	Taunton	100%	256
Newton - Wellesley Hospital[2]	Newton	100%	227
North Adams Regional Hospital	North Adams	100%	138
Quincy Medical Center	Quincy	100%	280
Saint Anne's Hospital[2]	Fall River	100%	433
Saints Medical Center	Lowell	100%	39
Signature Healthcare Brockton Hospital	Brockton	100%	249
VA Boston Healthcare Sys-Jamaica Plain	Jamaica Plain	100%	411
Berkshire Medical Center	Pittsfield	99%	478
Boston Medical Center Corporation[2]	Boston	99%	544
Brigham & Women's Hospital[2]	Boston	99%	422
Cape Cod Hospital[2]	Hyannis	99%	863
Good Samaritan Medical Center[2]	Brockton	99%	528
Hallmark Health System[2]	Melrose	99%	241
Heywood Hospital	Gardner	99%	213
Holyoke Medical Center	Holyoke	99%	150
Jordan Hospital	Plymouth	99%	521
Lahey Hosp & Med Ctr-Burlington[2]	Burlington	99%	408
Lowell General Hospital[2]	Lowell	99%	562
Massachusetts General Hospital[2]	Boston	99%	474
Mercy Medical Center	Springfield	99%	424
Merrimack Valley Hospital	Haverhill	99%	83
Metrowest Medical Center	Framingham	99%	287
Mount Auburn Hospital	Cambridge	99%	594
New England Baptist Hospital[2]	Boston	99%	1186
Noble Hospital	Westfield	99%	71
North Shore Medical Center[2]	Salem	99%	342
Norwood Hospital[2]	Norwood	99%	315
Saint Elizabeth's Medical Center[2]	Brighton	99%	569
South Shore Hospital	S Weymouth	99%	647
Southcoast Hospital Group[2]	Fall River	99%	953
Sturdy Memorial Hospital	Attleboro	99%	340
Umass Memorial Medical Center[2]	Worcester	99%	403
Winchester Hospital[2]	Winchester	99%	253
Cambridge Health Alliance[2]	Cambridge	98%	100
Carney Hospital	Boston	98%	99
Emerson Hospital	W Concord	98%	380
Healthalliance Hospitals[2]	Leominster	98%	185

NOTE: Hospital profiles are in alphabetical order by state, then city, then hospital within the city; Rankings exclude hospitals with less than 25 cases except for patient surveys which excludes hospitals with less than 100 cases; (a) 100-299 cases; (1) The number of cases/patients is too few to report; (2) Data submitted were based on a sample of cases/patients; (3) Results are based on a shorter time period than required; (4) Data suppressed by CMS for one or more quarters; (5) Results are not available for this reporting period; (6) Fewer than 100 patients completed the HCAHPS survey; (7) No cases met the criteria for this measure; (8) The lower limit of the confidence interval cannot be calculated if the number of observed infections equals zero; (9) No data are available from the state/territory for this reporting period; (10) The scores shown reflect fewer than 50 completed surveys; (11) There were discrepancies in the data collection process; (12) This measure does not apply to this hospital for this reporting period; (13) Results cannot be calculated for this reporting period; (14) The results for this state are combined with nearby states to protect confidentiality; Please refer to the User's Guide for a full explanation of data.

Hospital Name	City	Rate	Cases
Marlborough Hospital	Marlborough	98%	163
Nashoba Valley Medical Center	Ayer	98%	60
Saint Vincent Hospital	Worcester	98%	986
Tufts Medical Center[2]	Boston	98%	630
Baystate Franklin Medical Center[2]	Greenfield	97%	89
Brigham & Women's Faulkner Hospital[2]	Boston	97%	154
Harrington Memorial Hospital	Southbridge	97%	121
Beth Israel Deaconess Hospital - Milton[2]	Milton	96%	220
Beth Israel Deaconess Hospital - Needham	Needham	96%	67
Lawrence General Hospital	Lawrence	96%	137

Prophylactic Antibiotic Timing (Outpatient)

Hospital Name	City	Rate	Cases
Beth Israel Deaconess Hospital - Needham	Needham	100%	47
Brigham & Women's Faulkner Hospital	Boston	100%	145
Carney Hospital	Boston	100%	30
Holyoke Medical Center	Holyoke	100%	55
Mount Auburn Hospital	Cambridge	100%	347
Saint Anne's Hospital	Fall River	100%	71
Signature Healthcare Brockton Hospital	Brockton	100%	42
Tufts Medical Center	Boston	100%	108
Anna Jaques Hospital	Newburyport	99%	101
Baystate Medical Center	Springfield	99%	627
Berkshire Medical Center	Pittsfield	99%	246
Beverly Hospital Corporation	Beverly	99%	256
Cape Cod Hospital	Hyannis	99%	476
The Cooley Dickinson Hospital	Northampton	99%	167
Emerson Hospital	W Concord	99%	161
Falmouth Hospital	Falmouth	99%	79
Good Samaritan Medical Center	Brockton	99%	205
Lahey Hosp & Med Ctr-Burlington	Burlington	99%	427
Mercy Medical Center	Springfield	99%	597
Milford Regional Medical Center	Milford	99%	131
New England Baptist Hospital	Boston	99%	588
Newton - Wellesley Hospital	Newton	99%	514
Umass Memorial Medical Center	Worcester	99%	387
Beth Israel Deaconess Hospital - Milton	Milton	98%	44
Beth Israel Deaconess Medical Center	Boston	98%	845
Holy Family Hospital	Methuen	98%	105
Lowell General Hospital	Lowell	98%	374
North Shore Medical Center	Salem	98%	471
Norwood Hospital	Norwood	98%	109
South Shore Hospital	S Weymouth	98%	322
Southcoast Hospital Group	Fall River	98%	936
Brigham & Women's Hospital	Boston	97%	620
Cambridge Health Alliance	Cambridge	97%	67
Jordan Hospital	Plymouth	97%	147
Massachusetts General Hospital	Boston	97%	583
Metrowest Medical Center	Framingham	97%	257
Saint Vincent Hospital	Worcester	97%	546
Hallmark Health System	Melrose	96%	84
Quincy Medical Center	Quincy	96%	28
Winchester Hospital	Winchester	96%	175
Harrington Memorial Hospital	Southbridge	95%	65
Healthalliance Hospitals	Leominster	95%	101
Saint Elizabeth's Medical Center	Brighton	95%	178
Boston Medical Center Corporation	Boston	94%	243
Sturdy Memorial Hospital	Attleboro	94%	101
Morton Hospital	Taunton	92%	39
Lawrence General Hospital	Lawrence	90%	116
Nashoba Valley Medical Center	Ayer	89%	57
Heywood Hospital	Gardner	82%	94

Urinary Catheter Removal

Hospital Name	City	Rate	Cases
Anna Jaques Hospital	Newburyport	100%	194
Baystate Mary Lane Hospital	Ware	100%	43
Beth Israel Deaconess Hospital - Milton[2]	Milton	100%	231
Beth Israel Deaconess Medical Center[2]	Boston	100%	720
Brigham & Women's Faulkner Hospital[2]	Boston	100%	142
Falmouth Hospital	Falmouth	100%	463
Lahey Hosp & Med Ctr-Burlington[2]	Burlington	100%	209
Baystate Medical Center[2]	Springfield	99%	387
Berkshire Medical Center	Pittsfield	99%	295
The Cooley Dickinson Hospital[2]	Northampton	99%	387
Hallmark Health System[2]	Melrose	99%	185
Harrington Memorial Hospital	Southbridge	99%	135
Milford Regional Medical Center	Milford	99%	295
New England Baptist Hospital[2]	Boston	99%	723
Norwood Hospital[2]	Norwood	99%	255
Saint Anne's Hospital[2]	Fall River	99%	378
Saint Elizabeth's Medical Center[2]	Brighton	99%	454
Saint Vincent Hospital	Worcester	99%	966
Sturdy Memorial Hospital	Attleboro	99%	360
VA Boston Healthcare Sys-Jamaica Plain[2]	Jamaica Plain	99%	326
Winchester Hospital[2]	Winchester	99%	212
Beverly Hospital Corporation	Beverly	98%	846
Healthalliance Hospitals[2]	Leominster	98%	171
Holy Family Hospital[2]	Methuen	98%	396
Marlborough Hospital	Marlborough	98%	172
Mercy Medical Center	Springfield	98%	482
Metrowest Medical Center	Framingham	98%	245
Newton - Wellesley Hospital[2]	Newton	98%	95
Umass Memorial Medical Center[2]	Worcester	98%	298
Boston Medical Center Corporation[2]	Boston	97%	262
Brigham & Women's Hospital[2]	Boston	97%	330
Cape Cod Hospital[2]	Hyannis	97%	749
Massachusetts General Hospital[2]	Boston	97%	354
Signature Healthcare Brockton Hospital	Brockton	97%	77
South Shore Hospital	S Weymouth	97%	215
Southcoast Hospital Group[2]	Fall River	97%	782
Tufts Medical Center[2]	Boston	97%	495
Emerson Hospital	W Concord	96%	420
Lowell General Hospital[2]	Lowell	96%	456
Mount Auburn Hospital	Cambridge	96%	562
Beth Israel Deaconess Hospital - Needham	Needham	95%	80
Carney Hospital	Boston	95%	100
Quincy Medical Center	Quincy	95%	264
Morton Hospital	Taunton	94%	151
Noble Hospital	Westfield	94%	32
North Shore Medical Center[2]	Salem	94%	312
Nashoba Valley Medical Center	Ayer	93%	69
Cambridge Health Alliance[2]	Cambridge	92%	103
Jordan Hospital	Plymouth	92%	295
Baystate Franklin Medical Center[2]	Greenfield	91%	80
Good Samaritan Medical Center[2]	Brockton	90%	114
Merrimack Valley Hospital	Haverhill	90%	88
Heywood Hospital	Gardner	89%	189
Lawrence General Hospital	Lawrence	84%	173
Holyoke Medical Center	Holyoke	81%	62
Saints Medical Center	Lowell	76%	41

Survey of Patients' Hospital Experiences

Area Around Room 'Always' Quiet at Night

Hospital Name	City	Rate	Cases
Baystate Mary Lane Hospital	Ware	69%	300+
Athol Memorial Hospital	Athol	68%	(a)
Martha's Vineyard Hospital	Oak Bluffs	68%	(a)
Mount Auburn Hospital	Cambridge	66%	300+
Carney Hospital	Boston	63%	300+
Clinton Hospital Association	Clinton	61%	(a)
Brigham & Women's Faulkner Hospital	Boston	59%	300+
Fairview Hospital	Great Barrington	59%	(a)
Lowell General Hospital	Lowell	58%	300+
Baystate Franklin Medical Center	Greenfield	56%	300+
Beth Israel Deaconess Hospital - Milton	Milton	56%	300+
Brigham & Women's Hospital	Boston	56%	300+
Cambridge Health Alliance	Cambridge	56%	300+
Heywood Hospital	Gardner	56%	300+
Newton - Wellesley Hospital	Newton	56%	300+
Beth Israel Deaconess Hospital - Needham	Needham	55%	300+
The Cooley Dickinson Hospital	Northampton	55%	300+
Emerson Hospital	W Concord	55%	300+
South Shore Hospital	S Weymouth	55%	300+
Tufts Medical Center	Boston	55%	300+
Harrington Memorial Hospital	Southbridge	54%	300+
Nashoba Valley Medical Center	Ayer	54%	300+
North Adams Regional Hospital	North Adams	54%	300+
Saints Medical Center	Lowell	54%	300+
Wing Memorial Hospital & Medical Center	Palmer	54%	300+
Anna Jaques Hospital	Newburyport	53%	300+
Massachusetts General Hospital	Boston	53%	300+
Metrowest Medical Center[11]	Framingham	53%	300+
New England Baptist Hospital	Boston	53%	300+
Cape Cod Hospital	Hyannis	52%	300+
Healthalliance Hospitals	Leominster	52%	300+
Holyoke Medical Center	Holyoke	52%	300+
Lawrence General Hospital	Lawrence	52%	300+
Beth Israel Deaconess Medical Center	Boston	51%	300+
Hallmark Health System	Melrose	51%	300+
Merrimack Valley Hospital	Haverhill	50%	300+
Noble Hospital	Westfield	50%	300+
North Shore Medical Center	Salem	50%	300+
Saint Anne's Hospital	Fall River	50%	300+
Winchester Hospital[11]	Winchester	50%	300+
Baystate Medical Center	Springfield	49%	300+
Beverly Hospital Corporation	Beverly	49%	300+
Boston Medical Center Corporation	Boston	49%	300+
Holy Family Hospital	Methuen	49%	300+
Milford Regional Medical Center	Milford	49%	300+
Saint Elizabeth's Medical Center	Brighton	49%	300+
Sturdy Memorial Hospital	Attleboro	49%	300+
Berkshire Medical Center	Pittsfield	48%	300+
Lahey Hosp & Med Ctr-Burlington	Burlington	48%	300+
Saint Vincent Hospital[11]	Worcester	47%	300+
Southcoast Hospital Group	Fall River	47%	300+
Falmouth Hospital	Falmouth	46%	300+
Jordan Hospital	Plymouth	46%	300+
Umass Memorial Medical Center	Worcester	46%	300+
Morton Hospital	Taunton	45%	300+
Quincy Medical Center	Quincy	45%	300+
Good Samaritan Medical Center	Brockton	44%	300+
Mercy Medical Center	Springfield	44%	300+
Signature Healthcare Brockton Hospital	Brockton	44%	300+
Marlborough Hospital	Marlborough	41%	300+
Norwood Hospital	Norwood	41%	300+
Massachusetts Eye & Ear Infirmary	Boston	36%	300+

Doctors 'Always' Communicated Well

Hospital Name	City	Rate	Cases
Beth Israel Deaconess Hospital - Milton	Milton	85%	300+
Brigham & Women's Faulkner Hospital	Boston	85%	300+
New England Baptist Hospital	Boston	85%	300+
Baystate Mary Lane Hospital	Ware	84%	300+
Beth Israel Deaconess Hospital - Needham	Needham	84%	300+
Mount Auburn Hospital	Cambridge	84%	300+
Newton - Wellesley Hospital	Newton	84%	300+
Athol Memorial Hospital	Athol	83%	(a)
Fairview Hospital	Great Barrington	83%	(a)
Hallmark Health System	Melrose	83%	300+
Milford Regional Medical Center	Milford	83%	300+
Brigham & Women's Hospital	Boston	82%	300+
Clinton Hospital Association	Clinton	82%	(a)
Emerson Hospital	W Concord	82%	300+
Heywood Hospital	Gardner	82%	300+
Martha's Vineyard Hospital	Oak Bluffs	82%	(a)
South Shore Hospital	S Weymouth	82%	300+
Wing Memorial Hospital & Medical Center	Palmer	82%	300+
Cambridge Health Alliance	Cambridge	81%	300+
Lawrence General Hospital	Lawrence	81%	300+
Massachusetts General Hospital	Boston	81%	300+
Noble Hospital	Westfield	81%	300+
Winchester Hospital[11]	Winchester	81%	300+
Baystate Franklin Medical Center	Greenfield	80%	300+
Beth Israel Deaconess Medical Center	Boston	80%	300+
Cape Cod Hospital	Hyannis	80%	300+
Harrington Memorial Hospital	Southbridge	80%	300+
Healthalliance Hospitals	Leominster	80%	300+
Holyoke Medical Center	Holyoke	80%	300+
Lahey Hosp & Med Ctr-Burlington	Burlington	80%	300+
Lowell General Hospital	Lowell	80%	300+
Massachusetts Eye & Ear Infirmary	Boston	80%	300+
Saint Elizabeth's Medical Center	Brighton	80%	300+
Sturdy Memorial Hospital	Attleboro	80%	300+
Tufts Medical Center	Boston	80%	300+
Anna Jaques Hospital	Newburyport	79%	300+
Baystate Medical Center	Springfield	79%	300+
Boston Medical Center Corporation	Boston	79%	300+
Carney Hospital	Boston	79%	300+
Falmouth Hospital	Falmouth	79%	300+
Merrimack Valley Hospital	Haverhill	79%	300+
Metrowest Medical Center[11]	Framingham	79%	300+
North Adams Regional Hospital	North Adams	79%	300+
Saint Vincent Hospital[11]	Worcester	79%	300+
Saints Medical Center	Lowell	79%	300+
Southcoast Hospital Group	Fall River	79%	300+
Berkshire Medical Center	Pittsfield	78%	300+
Beverly Hospital Corporation	Beverly	78%	300+
Jordan Hospital	Plymouth	78%	300+
Marlborough Hospital	Marlborough	78%	300+
North Shore Medical Center	Salem	78%	300+
Norwood Hospital	Norwood	78%	300+
Signature Healthcare Brockton Hospital	Brockton	78%	300+
The Cooley Dickinson Hospital	Northampton	77%	300+
Holy Family Hospital	Methuen	77%	300+
Saint Anne's Hospital	Fall River	77%	300+
Umass Memorial Medical Center	Worcester	77%	300+
Morton Hospital	Taunton	76%	300+
Nashoba Valley Medical Center	Ayer	76%	300+
Mercy Medical Center	Springfield	75%	300+
Good Samaritan Medical Center	Brockton	74%	300+
Quincy Medical Center	Quincy	74%	300+

Home Recovery Information Given

Hospital Name	City	Rate	Cases
New England Baptist Hospital	Boston	95%	300+
Fairview Hospital	Great Barrington	92%	(a)
North Adams Regional Hospital	North Adams	92%	300+
Brigham & Women's Faulkner Hospital	Boston	91%	300+
Milford Regional Medical Center	Milford	91%	300+
Baystate Mary Lane Hospital	Ware	90%	300+
Massachusetts General Hospital	Boston	90%	300+
South Shore Hospital	S Weymouth	90%	300+
Tufts Medical Center	Boston	90%	300+
Brigham & Women's Hospital	Boston	89%	300+
Hallmark Health System	Melrose	89%	300+
Martha's Vineyard Hospital	Oak Bluffs	89%	(a)
Newton - Wellesley Hospital	Newton	89%	300+
Noble Hospital	Westfield	89%	300+

NOTE: Hospital profiles are in alphabetical order by state, then city, then hospital within the city; Rankings exclude hospitals with less than 25 cases except for patient surveys which excludes hospitals with less than 100 cases; (a) 100-299 cases; (1) The number of cases/patients is too few to report; (2) Data submitted were based on a sample of cases/patients; (3) Results are based on a shorter time period than required; (4) Data suppressed by CMS for one or more quarters; (5) Results are not available for this reporting period; (6) Fewer than 100 patients completed the HCAHPS survey; (7) No cases met the criteria for this measure; (8) The lower limit of the confidence interval cannot be calculated if the number of observed infections equals zero; (9) No data are available from the state/territory for this reporting period; (10) The scores shown reflect fewer than 50 completed surveys; (11) There were discrepancies in the data collection process; (12) This measure does not apply to this hospital for this reporting period; (13) Results cannot be calculated for this reporting period; (14) The results for this state are combined with nearby states to protect confidentiality; Please refer to the User's Guide for a full explanation of data.

Saint Vincent Hospital[11]	Worcester	89%	300+
Umass Memorial Medical Center	Worcester	89%	300+
Wing Memorial Hospital & Medical Center	Palmer	89%	300+
Baystate Franklin Medical Center	Greenfield	88%	300+
Baystate Medical Center	Springfield	88%	300+
Berkshire Medical Center	Pittsfield	88%	300+
Beth Israel Deaconess Hospital - Milton	Milton	88%	300+
Beth Israel Deaconess Medical Center	Boston	88%	300+
Holyoke Medical Center	Holyoke	88%	300+
Lahey Hosp & Med Ctr-Burlington	Burlington	88%	300+
Merrimack Valley Hospital	Haverhill	88%	300+
Metrowest Medical Center[11]	Framingham	88%	300+
Saint Anne's Hospital	Fall River	88%	300+
Southcoast Hospital Group	Fall River	88%	300+
Anna Jaques Hospital	Newburyport	87%	300+
Athol Memorial Hospital	Athol	87%	(a)
Beth Israel Deaconess Hospital - Needham	Needham	87%	300+
Cambridge Health Alliance	Cambridge	87%	300+
Clinton Hospital Association	Clinton	87%	(a)
Holy Family Hospital	Methuen	87%	300+
Mount Auburn Hospital	Cambridge	87%	300+
Signature Healthcare Brockton Hospital	Brockton	87%	300+
Sturdy Memorial Hospital	Attleboro	87%	300+
Winchester Hospital[11]	Winchester	87%	300+
Beverly Hospital Corporation	Beverly	86%	300+
Boston Medical Center Corporation	Boston	86%	300+
Falmouth Hospital	Falmouth	86%	300+
Healthalliance Hospitals	Leominster	86%	300+
Jordan Hospital	Plymouth	86%	300+
Lawrence General Hospital	Lawrence	86%	300+
North Shore Medical Center	Salem	86%	300+
Norwood Hospital	Norwood	86%	300+
Cape Cod Hospital	Hyannis	85%	300+
The Cooley Dickinson Hospital	Northampton	85%	300+
Emerson Hospital	W Concord	85%	300+
Harrington Memorial Hospital	Southbridge	85%	300+
Lowell General Hospital	Lowell	85%	300+
Mercy Medical Center	Springfield	85%	300+
Saint Elizabeth's Medical Center	Brighton	85%	300+
Saints Medical Center	Lowell	85%	300+
Good Samaritan Medical Center	Brockton	84%	300+
Heywood Hospital	Gardner	84%	300+
Marlborough Hospital	Marlborough	84%	300+
Quincy Medical Center	Quincy	84%	300+
Carney Hospital	Boston	83%	300+
Massachusetts Eye & Ear Infirmary	Boston	83%	300+
Morton Hospital	Taunton	83%	300+
Nashoba Valley Medical Center	Ayer	82%	300+

Hospital Given 9 or 10 on 10 Point Scale

Hospital Name	City	Rate	Cases
Fairview Hospital	Great Barrington	86%	(a)
New England Baptist Hospital	Boston	86%	300+
Brigham & Women's Hospital	Boston	82%	300+
Massachusetts General Hospital	Boston	81%	300+
Lahey Hosp & Med Ctr-Burlington	Burlington	79%	300+
Martha's Vineyard Hospital	Oak Bluffs	79%	(a)
Mount Auburn Hospital	Cambridge	78%	300+
Newton - Wellesley Hospital	Newton	78%	300+
Clinton Hospital Association	Clinton	77%	(a)
Milford Regional Medical Center	Milford	76%	300+
Winchester Hospital[11]	Winchester	76%	300+
Beth Israel Deaconess Medical Center	Boston	75%	300+
Cape Cod Hospital	Hyannis	75%	300+
Baystate Mary Lane Hospital	Ware	74%	300+
Brigham & Women's Faulkner Hospital	Boston	74%	300+
Wing Memorial Hospital & Medical Center	Palmer	74%	300+
Beth Israel Deaconess Hospital - Needham	Needham	73%	300+
The Cooley Dickinson Hospital	Northampton	72%	300+
Emerson Hospital	W Concord	72%	300+
Saint Vincent Hospital[11]	Worcester	72%	300+
South Shore Hospital	S Weymouth	72%	300+
Tufts Medical Center	Boston	72%	300+
Harrington Memorial Hospital	Southbridge	71%	300+
Heywood Hospital	Gardner	71%	300+
Lowell General Hospital	Lowell	71%	300+
Sturdy Memorial Hospital	Attleboro	71%	300+
Anna Jaques Hospital	Newburyport	70%	300+
Athol Memorial Hospital	Athol	70%	(a)
Beverly Hospital Corporation	Beverly	70%	300+
Holyoke Medical Center	Holyoke	70%	300+
Noble Hospital	Westfield	70%	300+
Baystate Medical Center	Springfield	69%	300+
Beth Israel Deaconess Hospital - Milton	Milton	69%	300+
Hallmark Health System	Melrose	69%	300+
North Shore Medical Center	Salem	69%	300+
Berkshire Medical Center	Pittsfield	68%	300+
Boston Medical Center Corporation	Boston	68%	300+
Falmouth Hospital	Falmouth	68%	300+
Massachusetts Eye & Ear Infirmary	Boston	68%	300+
Metrowest Medical Center[11]	Framingham	68%	300+

Healthalliance Hospitals	Leominster	67%	300+
Baystate Franklin Medical Center	Greenfield	66%	300+
Lawrence General Hospital	Lawrence	65%	300+
North Adams Regional Hospital	North Adams	65%	300+
Saints Medical Center	Lowell	65%	300+
Saint Anne's Hospital	Fall River	64%	300+
Saint Elizabeth's Medical Center	Brighton	64%	300+
Umass Memorial Medical Center	Worcester	64%	300+
Cambridge Health Alliance	Cambridge	63%	300+
Holy Family Hospital	Methuen	63%	300+
Mercy Medical Center	Springfield	63%	300+
Signature Healthcare Brockton Hospital	Brockton	63%	300+
Southcoast Hospital Group	Fall River	63%	300+
Jordan Hospital	Plymouth	61%	300+
Merrimack Valley Hospital	Haverhill	59%	300+
Good Samaritan Medical Center	Brockton	57%	300+
Marlborough Hospital	Marlborough	57%	300+
Carney Hospital	Boston	55%	300+
Nashoba Valley Medical Center	Ayer	55%	300+
Norwood Hospital	Norwood	54%	300+
Quincy Medical Center	Quincy	52%	300+
Morton Hospital	Taunton	50%	300+

Meds 'Always' Explained Before Given

Hospital Name	City	Rate	Cases
Fairview Hospital	Great Barrington	76%	(a)
Clinton Hospital Association	Clinton	73%	(a)
Athol Memorial Hospital	Athol	71%	(a)
Baystate Mary Lane Hospital	Ware	71%	300+
Martha's Vineyard Hospital	Oak Bluffs	70%	(a)
Brigham & Women's Faulkner Hospital	Boston	69%	300+
Milford Regional Medical Center	Milford	69%	300+
Beth Israel Deaconess Hospital - Milton	Milton	68%	300+
The Cooley Dickinson Hospital	Northampton	68%	300+
South Shore Hospital	S Weymouth	68%	300+
Winchester Hospital[11]	Winchester	68%	300+
Brigham & Women's Hospital	Boston	67%	300+
Harrington Memorial Hospital	Southbridge	67%	300+
Holyoke Medical Center	Holyoke	67%	300+
New England Baptist Hospital	Boston	67%	300+
Noble Hospital	Westfield	67%	300+
Signature Healthcare Brockton Hospital	Brockton	67%	300+
Tufts Medical Center	Boston	67%	300+
Wing Memorial Hospital & Medical Center	Palmer	67%	300+
Beth Israel Deaconess Medical Center	Boston	66%	300+
Sturdy Memorial Hospital	Attleboro	66%	300+
Boston Medical Center Corporation	Boston	65%	300+
Massachusetts General Hospital	Boston	65%	300+
Newton - Wellesley Hospital	Newton	65%	300+
North Adams Regional Hospital	North Adams	65%	300+
Beverly Hospital Corporation	Beverly	64%	300+
Cape Cod Hospital	Hyannis	64%	300+
Heywood Hospital	Gardner	64%	300+
Lawrence General Hospital	Lawrence	64%	300+
Lowell General Hospital	Lowell	64%	300+
Mount Auburn Hospital	Cambridge	64%	300+
Nashoba Valley Medical Center	Ayer	64%	300+
Anna Jaques Hospital	Newburyport	63%	300+
Hallmark Health System	Melrose	63%	300+
Lahey Hosp & Med Ctr-Burlington	Burlington	63%	300+
Marlborough Hospital	Marlborough	63%	300+
Saint Elizabeth's Medical Center	Brighton	63%	300+
Baystate Franklin Medical Center	Greenfield	62%	300+
Berkshire Medical Center	Pittsfield	62%	300+
Beth Israel Deaconess Hospital - Needham	Needham	62%	300+
Emerson Hospital	W Concord	62%	300+
Healthalliance Hospitals	Leominster	62%	300+
Metrowest Medical Center[11]	Framingham	62%	300+
Norwood Hospital	Norwood	62%	300+
Saint Vincent Hospital[11]	Worcester	62%	300+
Saints Medical Center	Lowell	62%	300+
Southcoast Hospital Group	Fall River	62%	300+
Baystate Medical Center	Springfield	61%	300+
Cambridge Health Alliance	Cambridge	61%	300+
Carney Hospital	Boston	61%	300+
Merrimack Valley Hospital	Haverhill	61%	300+
Falmouth Hospital	Falmouth	60%	300+
Saint Anne's Hospital	Fall River	60%	300+
Holy Family Hospital	Methuen	59%	300+
Jordan Hospital	Plymouth	59%	300+
North Shore Medical Center	Salem	59%	300+
Umass Memorial Medical Center	Worcester	58%	300+
Good Samaritan Medical Center	Brockton	57%	300+
Morton Hospital	Taunton	57%	300+
Quincy Medical Center	Quincy	56%	300+
Massachusetts Eye & Ear Infirmary	Boston	52%	300+
Mercy Medical Center	Springfield	52%	300+

Nurses 'Always' Communicated Well

Hospital Name	City	Rate	Cases
Fairview Hospital	Great Barrington	90%	(a)
New England Baptist Hospital	Boston	87%	300+
Baystate Mary Lane Hospital	Ware	85%	300+
Beth Israel Deaconess Hospital - Milton	Milton	84%	300+
Clinton Hospital Association	Clinton	84%	(a)
Martha's Vineyard Hospital	Oak Bluffs	84%	(a)
Anna Jaques Hospital	Newburyport	83%	300+
Athol Memorial Hospital	Athol	83%	(a)
Milford Regional Medical Center	Milford	83%	300+
Winchester Hospital[11]	Winchester	83%	300+
Brigham & Women's Faulkner Hospital	Boston	82%	300+
Hallmark Health System	Melrose	82%	300+
Lawrence General Hospital	Lawrence	82%	300+
Massachusetts General Hospital	Boston	82%	300+
Mount Auburn Hospital	Cambridge	82%	300+
South Shore Hospital	S Weymouth	82%	300+
Berkshire Medical Center	Pittsfield	81%	300+
Beverly Hospital Corporation	Beverly	81%	300+
Brigham & Women's Hospital	Boston	81%	300+
Emerson Hospital	W Concord	81%	300+
Harrington Memorial Hospital	Southbridge	81%	300+
Heywood Hospital	Gardner	81%	300+
Holyoke Medical Center	Holyoke	81%	300+
Lahey Hosp & Med Ctr-Burlington	Burlington	81%	300+
Newton - Wellesley Hospital	Newton	81%	300+
North Adams Regional Hospital	North Adams	81%	300+
Baystate Franklin Medical Center	Greenfield	80%	300+
Beth Israel Deaconess Hospital - Needham	Needham	80%	300+
Beth Israel Deaconess Medical Center	Boston	80%	300+
Lowell General Hospital	Lowell	80%	300+
Noble Hospital	Westfield	80%	300+
Sturdy Memorial Hospital	Attleboro	80%	300+
Tufts Medical Center	Boston	80%	300+
Cape Cod Hospital	Hyannis	79%	300+
Merrimack Valley Hospital	Haverhill	79%	300+
Metrowest Medical Center[11]	Framingham	79%	300+
Saints Medical Center	Lowell	79%	300+
Southcoast Hospital Group	Fall River	79%	300+
Wing Memorial Hospital & Medical Center	Palmer	79%	300+
The Cooley Dickinson Hospital	Northampton	78%	300+
Healthalliance Hospitals	Leominster	78%	300+
Saint Anne's Hospital	Fall River	78%	300+
Signature Healthcare Brockton Hospital	Brockton	78%	300+
Falmouth Hospital	Falmouth	77%	300+
Marlborough Hospital	Marlborough	77%	300+
North Shore Medical Center	Salem	77%	300+
Saint Vincent Hospital[11]	Worcester	77%	300+
Baystate Medical Center	Springfield	76%	300+
Cambridge Health Alliance	Cambridge	76%	300+
Carney Hospital	Boston	76%	300+
Holy Family Hospital	Methuen	76%	300+
Norwood Hospital	Norwood	76%	300+
Saint Elizabeth's Medical Center	Brighton	76%	300+
Jordan Hospital	Plymouth	75%	300+
Nashoba Valley Medical Center	Ayer	75%	300+
Good Samaritan Medical Center	Brockton	74%	300+
Umass Memorial Medical Center	Worcester	74%	300+
Boston Medical Center Corporation	Boston	73%	300+
Mercy Medical Center	Springfield	72%	300+
Morton Hospital	Taunton	72%	300+
Massachusetts Eye & Ear Infirmary	Boston	71%	300+
Quincy Medical Center	Quincy	71%	300+

Pain 'Always' Well Controlled

Hospital Name	City	Rate	Cases
Fairview Hospital	Great Barrington	82%	(a)
Martha's Vineyard Hospital	Oak Bluffs	78%	(a)
Baystate Mary Lane Hospital	Ware	76%	300+
Mount Auburn Hospital	Cambridge	76%	300+
Clinton Hospital Association	Clinton	75%	(a)
Emerson Hospital	W Concord	75%	300+
Hallmark Health System	Melrose	75%	300+
New England Baptist Hospital	Boston	75%	300+
North Adams Regional Hospital	North Adams	75%	300+
Anna Jaques Hospital	Newburyport	74%	300+
Milford Regional Medical Center	Milford	74%	300+
South Shore Hospital	S Weymouth	74%	300+
Brigham & Women's Faulkner Hospital	Boston	73%	300+
Harrington Memorial Hospital	Southbridge	73%	300+
Heywood Hospital	Gardner	73%	300+
Lahey Hosp & Med Ctr-Burlington	Burlington	73%	300+
Sturdy Memorial Hospital	Attleboro	73%	300+
Beverly Hospital Corporation	Beverly	72%	300+
Lawrence General Hospital	Lawrence	72%	300+
Lowell General Hospital	Lowell	72%	300+
Noble Hospital	Westfield	72%	300+
Signature Healthcare Brockton Hospital	Brockton	72%	300+
Beth Israel Deaconess Hospital - Milton	Milton	71%	300+

NOTE: Hospital profiles are in alphabetical order by state, then city, then hospital within the city; Rankings exclude hospitals with less than 25 cases except for patient surveys which excludes hospitals with less than 100 cases; (a) 100-299 cases; (1) The number of cases/patients is too few to report; (2) Data submitted were based on a sample of cases/patients; (3) Results are based on a shorter time period than required; (4) Data suppressed by CMS for one or more quarters; (5) Results are not available for this reporting period; (6) Fewer than 100 patients completed the HCAHPS survey; (7) No cases met the criteria for this measure; (8) The lower limit of the confidence interval cannot be calculated if the number of observed infections equals zero; (9) No data are available from the state/territory for this reporting period; (10) The scores shown reflect fewer than 50 completed surveys; (11) There were discrepancies in the data collection process; (12) This measure does not apply to this hospital for this reporting period; (13) Results cannot be calculated for this reporting period; (14) The results for this state are combined with nearby states to protect confidentiality; Please refer to the User's Guide for a full explanation of data.

Cape Cod Hospital	Hyannis	71%	300+
The Cooley Dickinson Hospital	Northampton	71%	300+
Massachusetts General Hospital	Boston	71%	300+
Newton - Wellesley Hospital	Newton	71%	300+
Southcoast Hospital Group	Fall River	71%	300+
Winchester Hospital[11]	Winchester	71%	300+
Athol Memorial Hospital	Athol	70%	(a)
Baystate Franklin Medical Center	Greenfield	70%	300+
Baystate Medical Center	Springfield	70%	300+
Berkshire Medical Center	Pittsfield	70%	300+
Beth Israel Deaconess Hospital - Needham	Needham	70%	300+
Falmouth Hospital	Falmouth	70%	300+
Healthalliance Hospitals	Leominster	70%	300+
Nashoba Valley Medical Center	Ayer	70%	300+
Saints Medical Center	Lowell	70%	300+
Tufts Medical Center	Boston	70%	300+
Beth Israel Deaconess Medical Center	Boston	69%	300+
Brigham & Women's Hospital	Boston	69%	300+
Holy Family Hospital	Methuen	69%	300+
Holyoke Medical Center	Holyoke	69%	300+
Jordan Hospital	Plymouth	69%	300+
Merrimack Valley Hospital	Haverhill	69%	300+
Metrowest Medical Center[11]	Framingham	69%	300+
North Shore Medical Center	Salem	69%	300+
Carney Hospital	Boston	68%	300+
Massachusetts Eye & Ear Infirmary	Boston	68%	300+
Morton Hospital	Taunton	68%	300+
Saint Anne's Hospital	Fall River	68%	300+
Saint Vincent Hospital[11]	Worcester	68%	300+
Cambridge Health Alliance	Cambridge	67%	300+
Norwood Hospital	Norwood	67%	300+
Saint Elizabeth's Medical Center	Brighton	67%	300+
Wing Memorial Hospital & Medical Center	Palmer	67%	300+
Good Samaritan Medical Center	Brockton	66%	300+
Umass Memorial Medical Center	Worcester	66%	300+
Marlborough Hospital	Marlborough	64%	300+
Mercy Medical Center	Springfield	64%	300+
Quincy Medical Center	Quincy	64%	300+
Boston Medical Center Corporation	Boston	63%	300+

Room and Bathroom 'Always' Clean

Hospital Name	City	Rate	Cases
Wing Memorial Hospital & Medical Center	Palmer	83%	300+
Clinton Hospital Association	Clinton	82%	(a)
New England Baptist Hospital	Boston	81%	300+
Athol Memorial Hospital	Athol	80%	(a)
Harrington Memorial Hospital	Southbridge	80%	300+
Baystate Mary Lane Hospital	Ware	79%	300+
Martha's Vineyard Hospital	Oak Bluffs	79%	(a)
Nashoba Valley Medical Center	Ayer	78%	300+
Newton - Wellesley Hospital	Newton	78%	300+
Sturdy Memorial Hospital	Attleboro	78%	300+
Fairview Hospital	Great Barrington	77%	(a)
Cape Cod Hospital	Hyannis	76%	300+
Mount Auburn Hospital	Cambridge	76%	300+
The Cooley Dickinson Hospital	Northampton	75%	300+
Heywood Hospital	Gardner	75%	300+
Holyoke Medical Center	Holyoke	75%	300+
North Adams Regional Hospital	North Adams	75%	300+
Saints Medical Center	Lowell	75%	300+
Brigham & Women's Faulkner Hospital	Boston	74%	300+
Massachusetts General Hospital	Boston	74%	300+
Noble Hospital	Westfield	74%	300+
Saint Anne's Hospital	Fall River	74%	300+
Anna Jaques Hospital	Newburyport	73%	300+
Beth Israel Deaconess Hospital - Milton	Milton	73%	300+
Falmouth Hospital	Falmouth	73%	300+
Lowell General Hospital	Lowell	73%	300+
Merrimack Valley Hospital	Haverhill	73%	300+
Berkshire Medical Center	Pittsfield	72%	300+
Hallmark Health System	Melrose	72%	300+
Healthalliance Hospitals	Leominster	72%	300+
Lahey Hosp & Med Ctr-Burlington	Burlington	72%	300+
Lawrence General Hospital	Lawrence	72%	300+
Milford Regional Medical Center	Milford	72%	300+
South Shore Hospital	S Weymouth	72%	300+
Southcoast Hospital Group	Fall River	72%	300+
Emerson Hospital	W Concord	71%	300+
Winchester Hospital[11]	Winchester	71%	300+
Beth Israel Deaconess Hospital - Needham	Needham	70%	300+
Beverly Hospital Corporation	Beverly	70%	300+
Cambridge Health Alliance	Cambridge	70%	300+
North Shore Medical Center	Salem	70%	300+
Norwood Hospital	Norwood	70%	300+
Saint Vincent Hospital[11]	Worcester	70%	300+
Baystate Franklin Medical Center	Greenfield	69%	300+
Carney Hospital	Boston	69%	300+
Tufts Medical Center	Boston	69%	300+
Beth Israel Deaconess Medical Center	Boston	68%	300+
Boston Medical Center Corporation	Boston	68%	300+
Marlborough Hospital	Marlborough	68%	300+
Metrowest Medical Center[11]	Framingham	68%	300+
Baystate Medical Center	Springfield	67%	300+
Brigham & Women's Hospital	Boston	67%	300+
Holy Family Hospital	Methuen	66%	300+
Mercy Medical Center	Springfield	66%	300+
Saint Elizabeth's Medical Center	Brighton	65%	300+
Umass Memorial Medical Center	Worcester	65%	300+
Massachusetts Eye & Ear Infirmary	Boston	64%	300+
Quincy Medical Center	Quincy	64%	300+
Jordan Hospital	Plymouth	62%	300+
Morton Hospital	Taunton	62%	300+
Signature Healthcare Brockton Hospital	Brockton	62%	300+
Good Samaritan Medical Center	Brockton	60%	300+

Timely Help 'Always' Received

Hospital Name	City	Rate	Cases
Fairview Hospital	Great Barrington	84%	(a)
Clinton Hospital Association	Clinton	82%	(a)
Martha's Vineyard Hospital	Oak Bluffs	79%	(a)
Athol Memorial Hospital	Athol	74%	(a)
Brigham & Women's Faulkner Hospital	Boston	74%	300+
Noble Hospital	Westfield	74%	300+
North Adams Regional Hospital	North Adams	73%	300+
Harrington Memorial Hospital	Southbridge	72%	300+
Mount Auburn Hospital	Cambridge	72%	300+
New England Baptist Hospital	Boston	72%	300+
Anna Jaques Hospital	Newburyport	71%	300+
Baystate Mary Lane Hospital	Ware	71%	300+
Hallmark Health System	Melrose	70%	300+
Winchester Hospital[11]	Winchester	70%	300+
Baystate Franklin Medical Center	Greenfield	69%	300+
Brigham & Women's Hospital	Boston	69%	300+
Milford Regional Medical Center	Milford	69%	300+
Emerson Hospital	W Concord	68%	300+
Saints Medical Center	Lowell	68%	300+
Signature Healthcare Brockton Hospital	Brockton	68%	300+
South Shore Hospital	S Weymouth	68%	300+
Newton - Wellesley Hospital	Newton	67%	300+
The Cooley Dickinson Hospital	Northampton	66%	300+
Lowell General Hospital	Lowell	66%	300+
Metrowest Medical Center[11]	Framingham	66%	300+
Beth Israel Deaconess Hospital - Milton	Milton	65%	300+
Heywood Hospital	Gardner	65%	300+
Holyoke Medical Center	Holyoke	65%	300+
Lawrence General Hospital	Lawrence	65%	300+
Massachusetts General Hospital	Boston	65%	300+
North Shore Medical Center	Salem	65%	300+
Saint Anne's Hospital	Fall River	65%	300+
Beverly Hospital Corporation	Beverly	64%	300+
Healthalliance Hospitals	Leominster	64%	300+
Lahey Hosp & Med Ctr-Burlington	Burlington	64%	300+
Merrimack Valley Hospital	Haverhill	64%	300+
Cape Cod Hospital	Hyannis	63%	300+
Marlborough Hospital	Marlborough	63%	300+
Saint Vincent Hospital[11]	Worcester	63%	300+
Sturdy Memorial Hospital	Attleboro	63%	300+
Tufts Medical Center	Boston	63%	300+
Wing Memorial Hospital & Medical Center	Palmer	63%	300+
Berkshire Medical Center	Pittsfield	62%	300+
Baystate Medical Center	Springfield	61%	300+
Beth Israel Deaconess Hospital - Needham	Needham	61%	300+
Carney Hospital	Boston	61%	300+
Falmouth Hospital	Falmouth	61%	300+
Holy Family Hospital	Methuen	61%	300+
Southcoast Hospital Group	Fall River	61%	300+
Beth Israel Deaconess Medical Center	Boston	60%	300+
Cambridge Health Alliance	Cambridge	60%	300+
Jordan Hospital	Plymouth	59%	300+
Massachusetts Eye & Ear Infirmary	Boston	59%	300+
Morton Hospital	Taunton	59%	300+
Quincy Medical Center	Quincy	59%	300+
Saint Elizabeth's Medical Center	Brighton	59%	300+
Boston Medical Center Corporation	Boston	58%	300+
Nashoba Valley Medical Center	Ayer	58%	300+
Norwood Hospital	Norwood	56%	300+
Mercy Medical Center	Springfield	55%	300+
Good Samaritan Medical Center	Brockton	54%	300+
Umass Memorial Medical Center	Worcester	54%	300+

Would Definitely Recommend Hospital

Hospital Name	City	Rate	Cases
New England Baptist Hospital	Boston	91%	300+
Fairview Hospital	Great Barrington	90%	(a)
Massachusetts General Hospital	Boston	90%	300+
Brigham & Women's Hospital	Boston	86%	300+
Mount Auburn Hospital	Cambridge	84%	300+
Newton - Wellesley Hospital	Newton	84%	300+
Clinton Hospital Association	Clinton	83%	(a)
Milford Regional Medical Center	Milford	82%	300+
Beth Israel Deaconess Hospital - Needham	Needham	81%	300+
Lahey Hosp & Med Ctr-Burlington	Burlington	81%	300+
Martha's Vineyard Hospital	Oak Bluffs	81%	(a)
Beth Israel Deaconess Medical Center	Boston	80%	300+
Winchester Hospital[11]	Winchester	80%	300+
Wing Memorial Hospital & Medical Center	Palmer	80%	300+
The Cooley Dickinson Hospital	Northampton	79%	300+
Brigham & Women's Faulkner Hospital	Boston	78%	300+
Cape Cod Hospital	Hyannis	78%	300+
Emerson Hospital	W Concord	78%	300+
Massachusetts Eye & Ear Infirmary	Boston	78%	300+
South Shore Hospital	S Weymouth	78%	300+
Heywood Hospital	Gardner	77%	300+
Lowell General Hospital	Lowell	77%	300+
Saint Vincent Hospital[11]	Worcester	77%	300+
Baystate Mary Lane Hospital	Ware	76%	300+
Tufts Medical Center	Boston	76%	300+
Baystate Medical Center	Springfield	75%	300+
Falmouth Hospital	Falmouth	75%	300+
Beth Israel Deaconess Hospital - Milton	Milton	74%	300+
Beverly Hospital Corporation	Beverly	74%	300+
Harrington Memorial Hospital	Southbridge	74%	300+
Lawrence General Hospital	Lawrence	74%	300+
Anna Jaques Hospital	Newburyport	73%	300+
Holyoke Medical Center	Holyoke	73%	300+
North Shore Medical Center	Salem	73%	300+
Sturdy Memorial Hospital	Attleboro	73%	300+
Hallmark Health System	Melrose	71%	300+
Metrowest Medical Center[11]	Framingham	71%	300+
Umass Memorial Medical Center	Worcester	71%	300+
Berkshire Medical Center	Pittsfield	70%	300+
Boston Medical Center Corporation	Boston	70%	300+
Athol Memorial Hospital	Athol	69%	(a)
Holy Family Hospital	Methuen	69%	300+
Noble Hospital	Westfield	69%	300+
Saint Elizabeth's Medical Center	Brighton	69%	300+
Baystate Franklin Medical Center	Greenfield	68%	300+
Jordan Hospital	Plymouth	68%	300+
Mercy Medical Center	Springfield	68%	300+
Saints Medical Center	Lowell	68%	300+
Healthalliance Hospitals	Leominster	67%	300+
North Adams Regional Hospital	North Adams	67%	300+
Saint Anne's Hospital	Fall River	67%	300+
Southcoast Hospital Group	Fall River	66%	300+
Marlborough Hospital	Marlborough	65%	300+
Signature Healthcare Brockton Hospital	Brockton	65%	300+
Cambridge Health Alliance	Cambridge	64%	300+
Good Samaritan Medical Center	Brockton	61%	300+
Nashoba Valley Medical Center	Ayer	61%	300+
Quincy Medical Center	Quincy	60%	300+
Carney Hospital	Boston	58%	300+
Norwood Hospital	Norwood	57%	300+
Merrimack Valley Hospital	Haverhill	56%	300+
Morton Hospital	Taunton	50%	300+

Use of Medical Imaging

Cardiac Imaging Stress Test before OP Surgery

Hospital Name	City	Rate	Cases
Holyoke Medical Center	Holyoke	1.7%	236
Milford Regional Medical Center	Milford	1.8%	275
Saint Vincent Hospital	Worcester	2.2%	589
North Adams Regional Hospital	North Adams	2.5%	119
Lowell General Hospital	Lowell	2.9%	171
Noble Hospital	Westfield	3.4%	89
New England Baptist Hospital	Boston	3.6%	84
Merrimack Valley Hospital	Haverhill	3.8%	78
Saints Medical Center	Lowell	3.8%	160
Good Samaritan Medical Center	Brockton	3.9%	439
The Cooley Dickinson Hospital	Northampton	4.0%	101
Emerson Hospital	W Concord	4.0%	202
Saint Elizabeth's Medical Center	Brighton	4.0%	323
Mercy Medical Center	Springfield	4.1%	537
Morton Hospital	Taunton	4.2%	333
Nashoba Valley Medical Center	Ayer	4.3%	211
Sturdy Memorial Hospital	Attleboro	4.3%	162
Boston Medical Center Corporation	Boston	4.5%	584
Lawrence General Hospital	Lawrence	4.5%	419
North Shore Medical Center	Salem	4.5%	799
Healthalliance Hospitals	Leominster	4.7%	255
Beverly Hospital Corporation	Beverly	5.0%	516
Cambridge Health Alliance	Cambridge	5.0%	262
Winchester Hospital	Winchester	5.0%	362
Massachusetts General Hospital	Boston	5.1%	2179
Berkshire Medical Center	Pittsfield	5.2%	616
Brigham & Women's Faulkner Hospital	Boston	5.2%	290
Harrington Memorial Hospital	Southbridge	5.2%	211
Southcoast Hospital Group	Fall River	5.3%	1165
Umass Memorial Medical Center	Worcester	5.3%	992
Beth Israel Deaconess Medical Center	Boston	5.4%	926
Newton - Wellesley Hospital	Newton	5.6%	486

NOTE: Hospital profiles are in alphabetical order by state, then city, then hospital within the city; Rankings exclude hospitals with less than 25 cases except for patient surveys which excludes hospitals with less than 100 cases; (a) 100-299 cases; (1) The number of cases/patients is too few to report; (2) Data submitted were based on a sample of cases/patients; (3) Results are based on a shorter time period than required; (4) Data suppressed by CMS for one or more quarters; (5) Results are not available for this reporting period; (6) Fewer than 100 patients completed the HCAHPS survey; (7) No cases met the criteria for this measure; (8) The lower limit of the confidence interval cannot be calculated if the number of observed infections equals zero; (9) No data are available from the state/territory for this reporting period; (10) The scores shown reflect fewer than 50 completed surveys; (11) There were discrepancies in the data collection process; (12) This measure does not apply to this hospital for this reporting period; (13) Results cannot be calculated for this reporting period; (14) The results for this state are combined with nearby states to protect confidentiality; Please refer to the User's Guide for a full explanation of data.

Norwood Hospital	Norwood	5.6%	354
Saint Anne's Hospital	Fall River	5.6%	161
Holy Family Hospital	Methuen	5.7%	476
South Shore Hospital	S Weymouth	5.7%	422
Baystate Medical Center	Springfield	5.8%	1093
Lahey Hosp & Med Ctr-Burlington	Burlington	5.8%	1714
Wing Memorial Hospital & Medical Center	Palmer	5.9%	118
Heywood Hospital	Gardner	6.0%	266
Signature Healthcare Brockton Hospital	Brockton	6.3%	252
Beth Israel Deaconess Hospital - Needham	Needham	6.4%	312
Metrowest Medical Center	Framingham	6.4%	187
Baystate Mary Lane Hospital	Ware	6.5%	62
Baystate Franklin Medical Center	Greenfield	6.7%	224
Carney Hospital	Boston	7.1%	154
Hallmark Health System	Melrose	7.1%	490
Mount Auburn Hospital	Cambridge	7.1%	434
Tufts Medical Center	Boston	7.1%	382
Marlborough Hospital	Marlborough	7.5%	214
Quincy Medical Center	Quincy	7.6%	118
Brigham & Women's Hospital	Boston	7.9%	951
Anna Jaques Hospital	Newburyport	8.5%	343
Beth Israel Deaconess Hospital - Milton	Milton	9.3%	193
Jordan Hospital	Plymouth	9.3%	205

Combination Abdominal CT Scan

Hospital Name	City	Rate	Cases
Saint Vincent Hospital	Worcester	1.1%	646
Healthalliance Hospitals	Leominster	1.8%	665
Noble Hospital	Westfield	1.9%	468
Baystate Medical Center	Springfield	2.1%	2020
Clinton Hospital Association	Clinton	2.5%	157
Heywood Hospital	Gardner	2.7%	482
South Shore Hospital	S Weymouth	2.7%	1455
Milford Regional Medical Center	Milford	2.8%	1126
Hallmark Health System	Melrose	2.9%	1453
Quincy Medical Center	Quincy	2.9%	648
Marlborough Hospital	Marlborough	3.0%	363
Wing Memorial Hospital & Medical Center	Palmer	3.0%	433
Falmouth Hospital	Falmouth	3.1%	950
Baystate Mary Lane Hospital	Ware	3.4%	267
Morton Hospital	Taunton	3.4%	827
Anna Jaques Hospital	Newburyport	3.5%	741
Holyoke Medical Center	Holyoke	3.5%	849
Beverly Hospital Corporation	Beverly	3.6%	1380
Nashoba Valley Medical Center	Ayer	3.6%	309
Jordan Hospital	Plymouth	3.7%	1294
Tufts Medical Center	Boston	3.7%	747
Brigham & Women's Faulkner Hospital	Boston	3.9%	925
Lowell General Hospital	Lowell	4.0%	1033
Massachusetts General Hospital	Boston	4.0%	5626
Emerson Hospital	W Concord	4.1%	678
The Cooley Dickinson Hospital	Northampton	4.4%	949
Signature Healthcare Brockton Hospital	Brockton	4.4%	839
Saints Medical Center	Lowell	4.5%	625
Berkshire Medical Center	Pittsfield	4.6%	1696
Southcoast Hospital Group	Fall River	4.6%	3382
Boston Medical Center Corporation	Boston	4.7%	1217
Norwood Hospital	Norwood	5.1%	875
North Adams Regional Hospital	North Adams	5.2%	594
Cambridge Health Alliance	Cambridge	5.3%	625
Mercy Medical Center	Springfield	5.4%	1240
Nantucket Cottage Hospital	Nantucket	5.4%	111
Harrington Memorial Hospital	Southbridge	5.5%	477
Saint Anne's Hospital	Fall River	5.5%	854
Good Samaritan Medical Center	Brockton	5.6%	1129
Merrimack Valley Hospital	Haverhill	5.8%	378
Winchester Hospital	Winchester	6.0%	1179
Sturdy Memorial Hospital	Attleboro	6.3%	860
Cape Cod Hospital	Hyannis	6.4%	2791
Baystate Franklin Medical Center	Greenfield	6.8%	584
New England Baptist Hospital	Boston	7.0%	201
Brigham & Women's Hospital	Boston	7.1%	2085
North Shore Medical Center	Salem	7.1%	1787
Beth Israel Deaconess Hospital - Milton	Milton	7.2%	553
Holy Family Hospital	Methuen	7.4%	890
Lawrence General Hospital	Lawrence	7.4%	942
Newton - Wellesley Hospital	Newton	7.4%	1168
Carney Hospital	Boston	8.1%	358
Umass Memorial Medical Center	Worcester	8.5%	1974
Saint Elizabeth's Medical Center	Brighton	11.2%	667
Metrowest Medical Center	Framingham	11.3%	797
Beth Israel Deaconess Hospital - Needham	Needham	11.7%	463
Lahey Hosp & Med Ctr-Burlington	Burlington	13.8%	2728
Mount Auburn Hospital	Cambridge	14.9%	881
Beth Israel Deaconess Medical Center	Boston	16.5%	2321

Combination Brain/Sinus CT Scan

Hospital Name	City	Rate	Cases
Massachusetts General Hospital	Boston	0.4%	1306
The Cooley Dickinson Hospital	Northampton	0.6%	657
Nashoba Valley Medical Center	Ayer	0.7%	280
Sturdy Memorial Hospital	Attleboro	0.8%	891
Beth Israel Deaconess Hospital - Needham	Needham	1.0%	495
South Shore Hospital	S Weymouth	1.0%	1535
Saint Elizabeth's Medical Center	Brighton	1.1%	369
Baystate Medical Center	Springfield	1.3%	1657
Newton - Wellesley Hospital	Newton	1.3%	1131
Brigham & Women's Hospital	Boston	1.4%	1110
Lowell General Hospital	Lowell	1.4%	775
Beverly Hospital Corporation	Beverly	1.5%	1218
Norwood Hospital	Norwood	1.5%	660
Healthalliance Hospitals	Leominster	1.6%	628
Milford Regional Medical Center	Milford	1.6%	920
Mount Auburn Hospital	Cambridge	1.6%	752
Beth Israel Deaconess Hospital - Milton	Milton	1.8%	553
Beth Israel Deaconess Medical Center	Boston	1.8%	1261
Emerson Hospital	W Concord	1.8%	665
Saint Anne's Hospital	Fall River	1.9%	587
Baystate Franklin Medical Center	Greenfield	2.0%	458
Lawrence General Hospital	Lawrence	2.0%	986
Holy Family Hospital	Methuen	2.1%	780
Wing Memorial Hospital & Medical Center	Palmer	2.1%	437
North Adams Regional Hospital	North Adams	2.2%	489
North Shore Medical Center	Salem	2.2%	1389
Umass Memorial Medical Center	Worcester	2.2%	1336
Lahey Hosp & Med Ctr-Burlington	Burlington	2.3%	1546
Mercy Medical Center	Springfield	2.3%	1223
Quincy Medical Center	Quincy	2.3%	694
Saints Medical Center	Lowell	2.4%	625
Morton Hospital	Taunton	2.5%	1037
Falmouth Hospital	Falmouth	2.6%	1087
Jordan Hospital	Plymouth	2.6%	1049
Anna Jaques Hospital	Newburyport	2.8%	676
Holyoke Medical Center	Holyoke	2.9%	920
Good Samaritan Medical Center	Brockton	3.0%	911
Signature Healthcare Brockton Hospital	Brockton	3.2%	742
Metrowest Medical Center	Framingham	3.3%	915
Cape Cod Hospital	Hyannis	3.4%	2095
Winchester Hospital	Winchester	3.4%	955
Boston Medical Center Corporation	Boston	3.5%	810
Southcoast Hospital Group	Fall River	3.5%	3527
Berkshire Medical Center	Pittsfield	4.0%	1002
Merrimack Valley Hospital	Haverhill	4.0%	494
Noble Hospital	Westfield	4.1%	467
Hallmark Health System	Melrose	5.9%	1617

Combination Chest CT Scan

Hospital Name	City	Rate	Cases
Baystate Medical Center	Springfield	0.0%	1600
Beth Israel Deaconess Hospital - Milton	Milton	0.0%	312
Brigham & Women's Faulkner Hospital	Boston	0.0%	908
Cambridge Health Alliance	Cambridge	0.0%	346
The Cooley Dickinson Hospital	Northampton	0.0%	668
Emerson Hospital	W Concord	0.0%	588
Harrington Memorial Hospital	Southbridge	0.0%	331
Healthalliance Hospitals	Leominster	0.0%	527
Heywood Hospital	Gardner	0.0%	329
Holyoke Medical Center	Holyoke	0.0%	269
Lahey Hosp & Med Ctr-Burlington	Burlington	0.0%	2982
Massachusetts Eye & Ear Infirmary	Boston	0.0%	520
Mercy Medical Center	Springfield	0.0%	610
Milford Regional Medical Center	Milford	0.0%	930
Mount Auburn Hospital	Cambridge	0.0%	760
Nantucket Cottage Hospital	Nantucket	0.0%	117
Nashoba Valley Medical Center	Ayer	0.0%	161
Newton - Wellesley Hospital	Newton	0.0%	1396
North Shore Medical Center	Salem	0.0%	1544
Saint Elizabeth's Medical Center	Brighton	0.0%	607
Saint Vincent Hospital	Worcester	0.0%	503
Signature Healthcare Brockton Hospital	Brockton	0.0%	519
Umass Memorial Medical Center	Worcester	0.0%	1946
Brigham & Women's Hospital	Boston	0.1%	4001
Good Samaritan Medical Center	Brockton	0.1%	957
Massachusetts General Hospital	Boston	0.1%	7673
Saint Anne's Hospital	Fall River	0.1%	763
Tufts Medical Center	Boston	0.1%	1040
Winchester Hospital	Winchester	0.1%	905
Anna Jaques Hospital	Newburyport	0.2%	632
Beth Israel Deaconess Medical Center	Boston	0.2%	2633
Beverly Hospital Corporation	Beverly	0.2%	1202
Lowell General Hospital	Lowell	0.2%	824
Norwood Hospital	Norwood	0.2%	606
Sturdy Memorial Hospital	Attleboro	0.2%	427
Beth Israel Deaconess Hospital - Needham	Needham	0.3%	315
Wing Memorial Hospital & Medical Center	Palmer	0.3%	327
Marlborough Hospital	Marlborough	0.4%	226
Noble Hospital	Westfield	0.4%	269
Baystate Franklin Medical Center	Greenfield	0.5%	373
Boston Medical Center Corporation	Boston	0.5%	1294
Carney Hospital	Boston	0.5%	220
Morton Hospital	Taunton	0.6%	619
Metrowest Medical Center	Framingham	0.7%	733
Baystate Mary Lane Hospital	Ware	0.8%	133
Quincy Medical Center	Quincy	0.8%	365
Falmouth Hospital	Falmouth	0.9%	545
Southcoast Hospital Group	Fall River	1.0%	2147
Cape Cod Hospital	Hyannis	1.3%	1919
Berkshire Medical Center	Pittsfield	1.7%	1693
North Adams Regional Hospital	North Adams	1.7%	418
Jordan Hospital	Plymouth	1.8%	930
New England Baptist Hospital	Boston	2.1%	241
Saints Medical Center	Lowell	2.1%	431
Hallmark Health System	Melrose	2.5%	1091
Holy Family Hospital	Methuen	2.8%	822
South Shore Hospital	S Weymouth	2.9%	1188
Lawrence General Hospital	Lawrence	3.7%	650
Merrimack Valley Hospital	Haverhill	4.3%	304

Follow-up Mammogram/Ultrasound

A follow-up rate near zero may indicate missed cancer; a rate higher than 14% may mean there is unnecessary follow up.

Hospital Name	City	Rate	Cases
Tufts Medical Center	Boston	2.2%	1191
Beth Israel Deaconess Hospital - Milton	Milton	4.1%	1042
Massachusetts General Hospital	Boston	4.7%	7641
Marlborough Hospital	Marlborough	4.8%	1043
North Shore Medical Center	Salem	5.3%	6493
North Adams Regional Hospital	North Adams	5.4%	1438
Signature Healthcare Brockton Hospital	Brockton	5.6%	1098
Carney Hospital	Boston	5.7%	922
Morton Hospital	Taunton	5.9%	2029
Nantucket Cottage Hospital	Nantucket	6.1%	179
Milford Regional Medical Center	Milford	6.2%	2107
Beth Israel Deaconess Hospital - Needham	Needham	6.3%	710
Boston Medical Center Corporation	Boston	6.3%	3118
Healthalliance Hospitals	Leominster	6.4%	1365
Beth Israel Deaconess Medical Center	Boston	6.5%	2825
Clinton Hospital Association	Clinton	6.5%	449
Brigham & Women's Hospital	Boston	6.6%	4414
Cambridge Health Alliance	Cambridge	7.0%	1385
The Cooley Dickinson Hospital	Northampton	7.0%	2142
Heywood Hospital	Gardner	7.0%	813
Wing Memorial Hospital & Medical Center	Palmer	7.0%	801
Saint Vincent Hospital	Worcester	7.2%	713
Harrington Memorial Hospital	Southbridge	7.3%	1210
Baystate Franklin Medical Center	Greenfield	7.4%	793
Beverly Hospital Corporation	Beverly	7.7%	3760
Jordan Hospital	Plymouth	7.7%	2798
Falmouth Hospital	Falmouth	7.8%	2742
Holyoke Medical Center	Holyoke	8.0%	1551
Saint Elizabeth's Medical Center	Brighton	8.0%	1396
South Shore Hospital	S Weymouth	8.1%	2940
Berkshire Medical Center	Pittsfield	8.2%	3648
Lowell General Hospital	Lowell	8.2%	1746
Anna Jaques Hospital	Newburyport	8.3%	2295
Saints Medical Center	Lowell	8.3%	1455
Sturdy Memorial Hospital	Attleboro	8.6%	2212
Brigham & Women's Faulkner Hospital	Boston	8.8%	6373
Winchester Hospital	Winchester	8.9%	2895
Lahey Hosp & Med Ctr-Burlington	Burlington	9.0%	6128
Mount Auburn Hospital	Cambridge	9.0%	2390
Baystate Medical Center	Springfield	9.4%	3832
Lawrence General Hospital	Lawrence	9.7%	920
Cape Cod Hospital	Hyannis	9.8%	4633
Southcoast Hospital Group	Fall River	9.9%	6855
Mercy Medical Center	Springfield	10.1%	2191
Newton - Wellesley Hospital	Newton	10.8%	3353
Quincy Medical Center	Quincy	11.2%	927
Merrimack Valley Hospital	Haverhill	11.3%	917
Good Samaritan Medical Center	Brockton	12.0%	2075
Holy Family Hospital	Methuen	12.0%	1118
Hallmark Health System	Melrose	12.3%	4248
Nashoba Valley Medical Center	Ayer	12.4%	354
Norwood Hospital	Norwood	12.5%	925
Noble Hospital	Westfield	12.7%	883
Baystate Mary Lane Hospital	Ware	13.2%	439
Saint Anne's Hospital	Fall River	15.4%	1355
Metrowest Medical Center	Framingham	15.7%	2681
Emerson Hospital	W Concord	16.4%	2208
Umass Memorial Medical Center	Worcester	21.2%	4331

Lumbar Spine MRI for Low Back Pain

Hospital Name	City	Rate	Cases
The Cooley Dickinson Hospital	Northampton	27.8%	216
Falmouth Hospital	Falmouth	28.1%	199
Massachusetts General Hospital	Boston	28.4%	264
Jordan Hospital	Plymouth	29.1%	172
Beth Israel Deaconess Medical Center	Boston	30.0%	207
North Shore Medical Center	Salem	30.7%	417
Morton Hospital	Taunton	30.9%	110
Beverly Hospital Corporation	Beverly	31.0%	271

NOTE: Hospital profiles are in alphabetical order by state, then city, then hospital within the city; Rankings exclude hospitals with less than 25 cases except for patient surveys which excludes hospitals with less than 100 cases; (a) 100-299 cases; (1) The number of cases/patients is too few to report; (2) Data submitted were based on a sample of cases/patients; (3) Results are based on a shorter time period than required; (4) Data suppressed by CMS for one or more quarters; (5) Results are not available for this reporting period; (6) Fewer than 100 patients completed the HCAHPS survey; (7) No cases met the criteria for this measure; (8) The lower limit of the confidence interval cannot be calculated if the number of observed infections equals zero; (9) No data are available from the state/territory for this reporting period; (10) The scores shown reflect fewer than 50 completed surveys; (11) There were discrepancies in the data collection process; (12) This measure does not apply to this hospital for this reporting period; (13) Results cannot be calculated for this reporting period; (14) The results for this state are combined with nearby states to protect confidentiality; Please refer to the User's Guide for a full explanation of data.

Winchester Hospital	Winchester	31.0%	126
Noble Hospital	Westfield	31.4%	51
South Shore Hospital	S Weymouth	32.4%	148
Boston Medical Center Corporation	Boston	32.5%	237
Brigham & Women's Hospital	Boston	32.8%	378
Sturdy Memorial Hospital	Attleboro	33.7%	187
Lahey Hosp & Med Ctr-Burlington	Burlington	34.0%	462
New England Baptist Hospital	Boston	34.0%	303
North Adams Regional Hospital	North Adams	34.1%	82
Southcoast Hospital Group	Fall River	34.1%	229
Cambridge Health Alliance	Cambridge	34.4%	93
Newton - Wellesley Hospital	Newton	35.1%	222
Holy Family Hospital	Methuen	35.4%	277
Signature Healthcare Brockton Hospital	Brockton	35.5%	155
Berkshire Medical Center	Pittsfield	36.7%	256
Cape Cod Hospital	Hyannis	37.8%	312
Holyoke Medical Center	Holyoke	38.0%	92
Good Samaritan Medical Center	Brockton	38.1%	181
Hallmark Health System	Melrose	38.2%	207
Saint Elizabeth's Medical Center	Brighton	38.3%	107
Milford Regional Medical Center	Milford	38.8%	134
Emerson Hospital	W Concord	39.2%	130
Baystate Medical Center	Springfield	39.6%	134
Quincy Medical Center	Quincy	40.8%	71
Mount Auburn Hospital	Cambridge	41.2%	182
Harrington Memorial Hospital	Southbridge	41.5%	82
Brigham & Women's Faulkner Hospital	Boston	41.9%	74
Saint Anne's Hospital	Fall River	42.3%	220
Heywood Hospital	Gardner	46.5%	99
Saint Vincent Hospital	Worcester	46.5%	71
Tufts Medical Center	Boston	47.2%	106
Beth Israel Deaconess Hospital - Needham	Needham	47.7%	65
Carney Hospital	Boston	49.1%	57
Beth Israel Deaconess Hospital - Milton	Milton	49.5%	93

NOTE: Hospital profiles are in alphabetical order by state, then city, then hospital within the city; Rankings exclude hospitals with less than 25 cases except for patient surveys which excludes hospitals with less than 100 cases; (a) 100-299 cases; (1) The number of cases/patients is too few to report; (2) Data submitted were based on a sample of cases/patients; (3) Results are based on a shorter time period than required; (4) Data suppressed by CMS for one or more quarters; (5) Results are not available for this reporting period; (6) Fewer than 100 patients completed the HCAHPS survey; (7) No cases met the criteria for this measure; (8) The lower limit of the confidence interval cannot be calculated if the number of observed infections equals zero; (9) No data are available from the state/territory for this reporting period; (10) The scores shown reflect fewer than 50 completed surveys; (11) There were discrepancies in the data collection process; (12) This measure does not apply to this hospital for this reporting period; (13) Results cannot be calculated for this reporting period; (14) The results for this state are combined with nearby states to protect confidentiality; Please refer to the User's Guide for a full explanation of data.

Athol Memorial Hospital

2033 Main Street Phone: 978-249-3511
Athol, MA 01331 Fax: 978-249-2651
URL: www.atholhospital.org
Type: Critical Access Hospitals Emergency Services: Yes
Ownership: Voluntary non-profit - Private Beds: 33

Key Personnel:
President/CEO. . . . . Win Brown
Chief of Medical Staff. . . . . Mohsen Noreldin, MD
Radiology. . . . . Paul Sabel
Emergency Room . . . . John Skrzypczak, MD

Measure	Cases	This Hosp.	State Avg.	U.S. Avg.
Blood Clot Prevention and Treatment				
Anticoagulation Overlap Therapy[5]	-	-	97%	93%
ICU Venous Thromboembolism Prophylaxis[5]	-	-	92%	92%
Incidence of Potentially Preventable VTE[5]	-	-	7%	10%
UFH with Dosages/Platelet Monitoring[5]	-	-	91%	97%
Venous Thromboembolism Prophylaxis[5]	-	-	87%	85%
Warfarin Therapy Discharge Instructions[5]	-	-	77%	75%
Chest Pain/Possible Heart Attack Care				
Aspirin Given Within 24 Hours of Arrival	-	-	97%	96%
Fibrinolytic Meds Within 30 Min. of Arrival	-	-	73%	58%
Average Time to ECG (minutes)	-	-	7	7
Average Time to Transfer (minutes)	-	-	55	60
Children's Asthma Care				
Received Home Management Plan of Care	-	-	-	88%
Received Reliever Medication	-	-	-	100%
Received Systemic Corticosteroids	-	-	-	100%
Emergency Department				
Admittance Decision Time (minutes)[5]	-	-	119	98
Head CT Results Within 45 Min. of Arrival	-	-	70%	57%
Patients Who Left ER Before Being Seen	-	-	2%	2%
Time from ER Arrival to Admit. (minutes)[5]	-	-	313	274
Time from ER Arrival to Discharge (minutes)	-	-	156	134
Time in ER Before Being Evaluated (minutes)	-	-	36	26
Time to Pain Meds for Fractures (minutes)	-	-	59	57
Heart Attack Care				
Aspirin Given at Discharge[1]	-	-	100%	99%
Fibrinolytic Meds Within 30 Min. of Arrival[7]	-	-	100%	54%
PCI Within 90 Minutes of Arrival[7]	-	-	96%	96%
Statin Prescribed at Discharge[1]	-	-	99%	98%
Heart Failure Care				
ACE Inhibitor or ARB for LVSD[1]	-	-	96%	97%
Discharge Instructions Given[1]	-	-	95%	94%
Evaluation of LVS Function	21	95%	100%	99%
Medicare Spending				
Medicare Spending per Patient (ratio)	-	-	1.03	0.98
Pneumonia Care				
Appropriate Initial Antibiotic Given	17	94%	97%	95%
Blood Culture Timing	26	100%	98%	98%
Pregnancy and Delivery Care				
Newborn Deliveries Scheduled Early[3,7]	-	-	2%	6%
Preventive Care				
Immunization for Influenza[5]	-	-	91%	90%
Immunization for Pneumonia[5]	-	-	91%	92%
Stroke Care				
Anticoagulation Therapy for Atrial Fibrillation[5]	-	-	97%	95%
Antithrombotic Therapy Timing[5]	-	-	98%	98%
Assessed for Rehabilitation[5]	-	-	96%	97%
Discharged on Antithrombotic Therapy[5]	-	-	100%	99%
Discharged on Statin Medication[5]	-	-	96%	94%
Thrombolytic Therapy Timing[5]	-	-	68%	66%
Venous Thromboembolism Prophylaxis[5]	-	-	94%	94%
Written Stroke Educational Materials Given[5]	-	-	82%	88%
Surgical Care Improvement Project				
Appropriate Beta Blocker Usage[1]	-	-	98%	98%
Appropriate VTP Within 24 Hours[1]	-	-	99%	98%
Controlled Postoperative Blood Glucose[7]	-	-	96%	97%
Perioperative Temperature Management[1]	-	-	100%	100%
Prophylactic Antibiotic Selection[1]	-	-	99%	99%
Prophylactic Antibiotic Selection (Outpatient)	-	-	98%	98%
Prophylactic Antibiotic Stopped[1]	-	-	99%	98%
Prophylactic Antibiotic Timing[1]	-	-	99%	99%
Prophylactic Antibiotic Timing (Outpatient)	-	-	98%	98%
Urinary Catheter Removal[1]	-	-	97%	97%
Survey of Patients' Hospital Experiences				
Area Around Room 'Always' Quiet at Night	(a)	68%	52%	61%
Doctors 'Always' Communicated Well	(a)	83%	80%	82%
Home Recovery Information Given	(a)	87%	87%	85%
Hospital Given 9 or 10 on 10 Point Scale	(a)	70%	69%	71%
Meds 'Always' Explained Before Given	(a)	71%	64%	64%
Nurses 'Always' Communicated Well	(a)	83%	79%	79%
Pain 'Always' Well Controlled	(a)	70%	71%	71%
Room and Bathroom 'Always' Clean	(a)	80%	72%	73%
Timely Help 'Always' Received	(a)	74%	66%	68%
Would Definitely Recommend Hospital	(a)	69%	73%	71%
Use of Medical Imaging				
Cardiac Imaging Stress Test before Surgery	-	-	5.4%	5.3%
Combination Abdominal CT Scan	-	-	6.3%	10.5%
Combination Brain/Sinus CT Scan	-	-	2.4%	2.7%
Combination Chest CT Scan	-	-	0.5%	2.7%
Follow-up Mammogram/Ultrasound	-	-	8.9%	8.8%
Lumbar Spine MRI for Low Back Pain	-	-	35.3%	37.2%

Sturdy Memorial Hospital

211 Park Street Phone: 508-222-5200
Attleboro, MA 02703 Fax: 508-236-7909
URL: www.sturdymemorial.org
Type: Acute Care Hospitals Emergency Services: Yes
Ownership: Voluntary non-profit - Other Beds: 138

Key Personnel:
Emergency Room . . . . Bruce Auerbach
Pediatric Ambulatory Care . . . . . . Heather Collupy
Pediatric In-Patient Care . . . . Heather Collupy
Radiology. . . . . Jay Daly, MD
Chief of Medical Staff. . . . . Daniel Pietro
CEO/President. . . . . Linda J Shyavitz
Quality Assurance . . . . Sharon Simmoneau

Measure	Cases	This Hosp.	State Avg.	U.S. Avg.
Blood Clot Prevention and Treatment				
Anticoagulation Overlap Therapy[2]	56	98%	97%	93%
ICU Venous Thromboembolism Prophylaxis[2]	71	100%	92%	92%
Incidence of Potentially Preventable VTE[1,2]	-	-	7%	10%
UFH with Dosages/Platelet Monitoring[2]	46	100%	91%	97%
Venous Thromboembolism Prophylaxis[2]	349	99%	87%	85%
Warfarin Therapy Discharge Instructions[2]	38	92%	77%	75%
Chest Pain/Possible Heart Attack Care				
Aspirin Given Within 24 Hours of Arrival	125	98%	97%	96%
Fibrinolytic Meds Within 30 Min. of Arrival[7]	-	-	73%	58%
Average Time to ECG (minutes)	126	11	7	7
Average Time to Transfer (minutes)	17	41	55	60
Children's Asthma Care				
Received Home Management Plan of Care	-	-	-	88%
Received Reliever Medication	-	-	-	100%
Received Systemic Corticosteroids	-	-	-	100%
Emergency Department				
Admittance Decision Time (minutes)[2]	630	96	119	98
Head CT Results Within 45 Min. of Arrival	14	50%	70%	57%
Patients Who Left ER Before Being Seen	50,822	1%	2%	2%
Time from ER Arrival to Admit. (minutes)[2]	634	262	313	274
Time from ER Arrival to Discharge (minutes)	348	128	156	134
Time in ER Before Being Evaluated (minutes)	408	14	36	26
Time to Pain Meds for Fractures (minutes)	68	76	59	57
Heart Attack Care				
Aspirin Given at Discharge	21	100%	100%	99%
Fibrinolytic Meds Within 30 Min. of Arrival[7]	-	-	100%	54%
PCI Within 90 Minutes of Arrival[7]	-	-	96%	96%
Statin Prescribed at Discharge	18	100%	99%	98%
Heart Failure Care				
ACE Inhibitor or ARB for LVSD	51	98%	96%	97%
Discharge Instructions Given	127	100%	95%	94%
Evaluation of LVS Function	182	100%	100%	99%
Medicare Spending				
Medicare Spending per Patient (ratio)	-	1.08	1.03	0.98
Pneumonia Care				
Appropriate Initial Antibiotic Given	105	98%	97%	95%
Blood Culture Timing	194	99%	98%	98%
Pregnancy and Delivery Care				
Newborn Deliveries Scheduled Early[2]	19	5%	2%	6%
Preventive Care				
Immunization for Influenza[2]	532	97%	91%	90%
Immunization for Pneumonia[2]	670	98%	91%	92%
Stroke Care				
Anticoagulation Therapy for Atrial Fibrillation	15	100%	97%	95%
Antithrombotic Therapy Timing	63	100%	98%	98%
Assessed for Rehabilitation	66	100%	96%	97%
Discharged on Antithrombotic Therapy	64	98%	100%	99%
Discharged on Statin Medication	49	98%	96%	94%
Thrombolytic Therapy Timing[1]	-	-	68%	66%
Venous Thromboembolism Prophylaxis	65	98%	94%	94%
Written Stroke Educational Materials Given	37	95%	82%	88%
Surgical Care Improvement Project				
Appropriate Beta Blocker Usage	172	99%	98%	98%
Appropriate VTP Within 24 Hours	434	100%	99%	98%
Controlled Postoperative Blood Glucose[7]	-	-	96%	97%
Perioperative Temperature Management	529	100%	100%	100%
Prophylactic Antibiotic Selection	339	99%	99%	99%
Prophylactic Antibiotic Selection (Outpatient)	97	82%	98%	98%
Prophylactic Antibiotic Stopped	318	100%	99%	98%
Prophylactic Antibiotic Timing	340	99%	99%	99%
Prophylactic Antibiotic Timing (Outpatient)	101	94%	98%	98%
Urinary Catheter Removal	360	99%	97%	97%
Survey of Patients' Hospital Experiences				
Area Around Room 'Always' Quiet at Night	300+	49%	52%	61%
Doctors 'Always' Communicated Well	300+	80%	80%	82%
Home Recovery Information Given	300+	87%	87%	85%
Hospital Given 9 or 10 on 10 Point Scale	300+	71%	69%	71%
Meds 'Always' Explained Before Given	300+	66%	64%	64%
Nurses 'Always' Communicated Well	300+	80%	79%	79%
Pain 'Always' Well Controlled	300+	73%	71%	71%
Room and Bathroom 'Always' Clean	300+	78%	72%	73%
Timely Help 'Always' Received	300+	63%	66%	68%
Would Definitely Recommend Hospital	300+	73%	73%	71%
Use of Medical Imaging				
Cardiac Imaging Stress Test before Surgery	162	4.3%	5.4%	5.3%
Combination Abdominal CT Scan	860	6.3%	6.3%	10.5%
Combination Brain/Sinus CT Scan	891	0.8%	2.4%	2.7%
Combination Chest CT Scan	427	0.2%	0.5%	2.7%
Follow-up Mammogram/Ultrasound	2,212	8.6%	8.9%	8.8%
Lumbar Spine MRI for Low Back Pain	187	33.7%	35.3%	37.2%

Nashoba Valley Medical Center

200 Groton Road Phone: 978-784-9000
Ayer, MA 01432 Fax: 978-784-9690
URL: www.nashobamed.com
Type: Acute Care Hospitals Emergency Services: Yes
Ownership: Proprietary Beds: 49

Key Personnel:
Radiology. . . . . Jerome M Auerbach
Chief of Medical Staff. . . . . Michelle Gordon
President . . . . Salvatore Perla
CEO/President. . . . . Steve Roach

Measure	Cases	This Hosp.	State Avg.	U.S. Avg.
Blood Clot Prevention and Treatment				
Anticoagulation Overlap Therapy[2]	13	92%	97%	93%
ICU Venous Thromboembolism Prophylaxis[2]	38	100%	92%	92%
Incidence of Potentially Preventable VTE[1,2]	-	-	7%	10%
UFH with Dosages/Platelet Monitoring[1,2]	-	-	91%	97%
Venous Thromboembolism Prophylaxis[2]	174	93%	87%	85%
Warfarin Therapy Discharge Instructions[1,2]	-	-	77%	75%
Chest Pain/Possible Heart Attack Care				
Aspirin Given Within 24 Hours of Arrival	36	100%	97%	96%
Fibrinolytic Meds Within 30 Min. of Arrival[7]	-	-	73%	58%
Average Time to ECG (minutes)	36	6	7	7
Average Time to Transfer (minutes)[1]	-	-	55	60
Children's Asthma Care				
Received Home Management Plan of Care	-	-	-	88%
Received Reliever Medication	-	-	-	100%
Received Systemic Corticosteroids	-	-	-	100%
Emergency Department				

NOTE: *Hospital profiles are in alphabetical order by state, then city, then hospital within the city; Rankings exclude hospitals with less than 25 cases except for patient surveys which excludes hospitals with less than 100 cases; (a) 100-299 cases; (1) The number of cases/patients is too few to report; (2) Data submitted were based on a sample of cases/patients; (3) Results are based on a shorter time period than required; (4) Data suppressed by CMS for one or more quarters; (5) Results are not available for this reporting period; (6) Fewer than 100 patients completed the HCAHPS survey; (7) No cases met the criteria for this measure; (8) The lower limit of the confidence interval cannot be calculated if the number of observed infections equals zero; (9) No data are available from the state/territory for this reporting period; (10) The scores shown reflect fewer than 50 completed surveys; (11) There were discrepancies in the data collection process; (12) This measure does not apply to this hospital for this reporting period; (13) Results cannot be calculated for this reporting period; (14) The results for this state are combined with nearby states to protect confidentiality; Please refer to the User's Guide for a full explanation of data.*

Admittance Decision Time (minutes)[2]	422	52	119	98
Head CT Results Within 45 Min. of Arrival[1]	-	-	70%	57%
Patients Who Left ER Before Being Seen	13,332	1%	2%	2%
Time from ER Arrival to Admit. (minutes)[2]	438	213	313	274
Time from ER Arrival to Discharge (minutes)	361	120	156	134
Time in ER Before Being Evaluated (minutes)	386	22	36	26
Time to Pain Meds for Fractures (minutes)	46	43	59	57
Heart Attack Care				
Aspirin Given at Discharge[1]	-	-	100%	99%
Fibrinolytic Meds Within 30 Min. of Arrival[7]	-	-	100%	54%
PCI Within 90 Minutes of Arrival[7]	-	-	96%	96%
Statin Prescribed at Discharge[1]	-	-	99%	98%
Heart Failure Care				
ACE Inhibitor or ARB for LVSD	24	100%	96%	97%
Discharge Instructions Given	54	100%	95%	94%
Evaluation of LVS Function	80	100%	100%	99%
Medicare Spending				
Medicare Spending per Patient (ratio)	-	1.13	1.03	0.98
Pneumonia Care				
Appropriate Initial Antibiotic Given	56	98%	97%	95%
Blood Culture Timing	28	100%	98%	98%
Pregnancy and Delivery Care				
Newborn Deliveries Scheduled Early[7]	-	-	2%	6%
Preventive Care				
Immunization for Influenza[2]	310	99%	91%	90%
Immunization for Pneumonia[2]	434	96%	91%	92%
Stroke Care				
Anticoagulation Therapy for Atrial Fibrillation[1]	-	-	97%	95%
Antithrombotic Therapy Timing	16	100%	98%	98%
Assessed for Rehabilitation	15	93%	96%	97%
Discharged on Antithrombotic Therapy	15	100%	100%	99%
Discharged on Statin Medication	13	100%	96%	94%
Thrombolytic Therapy Timing[7]	-	-	68%	66%
Venous Thromboembolism Prophylaxis	18	83%	94%	94%
Written Stroke Educational Materials Given[1]	-	-	82%	88%
Surgical Care Improvement Project				
Appropriate Beta Blocker Usage	38	100%	98%	98%
Appropriate VTP Within 24 Hours	72	93%	99%	98%
Controlled Postoperative Blood Glucose[7]	-	-	96%	97%
Perioperative Temperature Management	80	100%	100%	100%
Prophylactic Antibiotic Selection	60	98%	99%	99%
Prophylactic Antibiotic Selection (Outpatient)	59	93%	98%	98%
Prophylactic Antibiotic Stopped	60	92%	99%	98%
Prophylactic Antibiotic Timing	60	98%	99%	99%
Prophylactic Antibiotic Timing (Outpatient)	57	89%	98%	98%
Urinary Catheter Removal	69	93%	97%	97%
Survey of Patients' Hospital Experiences				
Area Around Room 'Always' Quiet at Night	300+	54%	52%	61%
Doctors 'Always' Communicated Well	300+	76%	80%	82%
Home Recovery Information Given	300+	82%	87%	85%
Hospital Given 9 or 10 on 10 Point Scale	300+	55%	69%	71%
Meds 'Always' Explained Before Given	300+	64%	64%	64%
Nurses 'Always' Communicated Well	300+	75%	79%	79%
Pain 'Always' Well Controlled	300+	70%	71%	71%
Room and Bathroom 'Always' Clean	300+	78%	72%	73%
Timely Help 'Always' Received	300+	58%	66%	68%
Would Definitely Recommend Hospital	300+	61%	73%	71%
Use of Medical Imaging				
Cardiac Imaging Stress Test before Surgery	211	4.3%	5.4%	5.3%
Combination Abdominal CT Scan	309	3.6%	6.3%	10.5%
Combination Brain/Sinus CT Scan	280	0.7%	2.4%	2.7%
Combination Chest CT Scan	161	0.0%	0.5%	2.7%
Follow-up Mammogram/Ultrasound	354	12.4%	8.9%	8.8%
Lumbar Spine MRI for Low Back Pain[1]	-	-	35.3%	37.2%

Bedford VA Medical Center

200 Springs Road
Bedford, MA 01730
Phone: 781-275-7500
Fax: 781-687-2101
URL: www.visn1.med.va.gov/bedford
Type: Acute Care - VA
Emergency Services: No
Ownership: Government Federal
Beds: 502
Key Personnel:
Chief of Medical Staff . . . . Gregory Binus, MD
Quality Assurance . . . . Michael Carey
CEO/President. . . . . Tammy A Follensbee
Infection Control. . . . . Gloria Jarnis
Patient Relations . . . . Karen Kubik
Radiology. . . . . Pat Sacco
Ambulatory Care . . . . James Schlosser, MD

Measure	Cases	This Hosp.	State Avg.	U.S. Avg.
Blood Clot Prevention and Treatment				
Anticoagulation Overlap Therapy	-	-	97%	93%
ICU Venous Thromboembolism Prophylaxis	-	-	92%	92%
Incidence of Potentially Preventable VTE	-	-	7%	10%
UFH with Dosages/Platelet Monitoring	-	-	91%	97%
Venous Thromboembolism Prophylaxis	-	-	87%	85%
Warfarin Therapy Discharge Instructions	-	-	77%	75%
Chest Pain/Possible Heart Attack Care				
Aspirin Given Within 24 Hours of Arrival	-	-	97%	96%
Fibrinolytic Meds Within 30 Min. of Arrival	-	-	73%	58%
Average Time to ECG (minutes)	-	-	7	7
Average Time to Transfer (minutes)	-	-	55	60
Children's Asthma Care				
Received Home Management Plan of Care	-	-	-	88%
Received Reliever Medication	-	-	-	100%
Received Systemic Corticosteroids	-	-	-	100%
Emergency Department				
Admittance Decision Time (minutes)	-	-	119	98
Head CT Results Within 45 Min. of Arrival	-	-	70%	57%
Patients Who Left ER Before Being Seen	-	-	2%	2%
Time from ER Arrival to Admit. (minutes)	-	-	313	274
Time from ER Arrival to Discharge (minutes)	-	-	156	134
Time in ER Before Being Evaluated (minutes)	-	-	36	26
Time to Pain Meds for Fractures (minutes)	-	-	59	57
Heart Attack Care				
Aspirin Given at Discharge[5]	-	-	100%	99%
Fibrinolytic Meds Within 30 Min. of Arrival[5]	-	-	100%	54%
PCI Within 90 Minutes of Arrival[5]	-	-	96%	96%
Statin Prescribed at Discharge[5]	-	-	99%	98%
Heart Failure Care				
ACE Inhibitor or ARB for LVSD[5]	-	-	96%	97%
Discharge Instructions Given[5]	-	-	95%	94%
Evaluation of LVS Function[5]	-	-	100%	99%
Medicare Spending				
Medicare Spending per Patient (ratio)	-	-	1.03	0.98
Pneumonia Care				
Appropriate Initial Antibiotic Given[5]	-	-	97%	95%
Blood Culture Timing[5]	-	-	98%	98%
Pregnancy and Delivery Care				
Newborn Deliveries Scheduled Early	-	-	2%	6%
Preventive Care				
Immunization for Influenza[2,3]	149	91%	91%	90%
Immunization for Pneumonia[2,3]	124	81%	91%	92%
Stroke Care				
Anticoagulation Therapy for Atrial Fibrillation	-	-	97%	95%
Antithrombotic Therapy Timing	-	-	98%	98%
Assessed for Rehabilitation	-	-	96%	97%
Discharged on Antithrombotic Therapy	-	-	100%	99%
Discharged on Statin Medication	-	-	96%	94%
Thrombolytic Therapy Timing	-	-	68%	66%
Venous Thromboembolism Prophylaxis	-	-	94%	94%
Written Stroke Educational Materials Given	-	-	82%	88%
Surgical Care Improvement Project				
Appropriate Beta Blocker Usage[5]	-	-	98%	98%
Appropriate VTP Within 24 Hours[5]	-	-	99%	98%
Controlled Postoperative Blood Glucose[5]	-	-	96%	97%
Perioperative Temperature Management[5]	-	-	100%	100%
Prophylactic Antibiotic Selection[5]	-	-	99%	99%
Prophylactic Antibiotic Selection (Outpatient)	-	-	98%	98%
Prophylactic Antibiotic Stopped[5]	-	-	99%	98%
Prophylactic Antibiotic Timing[5]	-	-	99%	99%
Prophylactic Antibiotic Timing (Outpatient)	-	-	98%	98%
Urinary Catheter Removal[5]	-	-	97%	97%
Survey of Patients' Hospital Experiences				
Area Around Room 'Always' Quiet at Night	-	-	52%	61%
Doctors 'Always' Communicated Well	-	-	80%	82%
Home Recovery Information Given	-	-	87%	85%
Hospital Given 9 or 10 on 10 Point Scale	-	-	69%	71%
Meds 'Always' Explained Before Given	-	-	64%	64%
Nurses 'Always' Communicated Well	-	-	79%	79%
Pain 'Always' Well Controlled	-	-	71%	71%
Room and Bathroom 'Always' Clean	-	-	72%	73%
Timely Help 'Always' Received	-	-	66%	68%
Would Definitely Recommend Hospital	-	-	73%	71%
Use of Medical Imaging				
Cardiac Imaging Stress Test before Surgery	-	-	5.4%	5.3%
Combination Abdominal CT Scan	-	-	6.3%	10.5%
Combination Brain/Sinus CT Scan	-	-	2.4%	2.7%
Combination Chest CT Scan	-	-	0.5%	2.7%
Follow-up Mammogram/Ultrasound	-	-	8.9%	8.8%
Lumbar Spine MRI for Low Back Pain	-	-	35.3%	37.2%

Beverly Hospital Corporation

85 Herrick Street
Beverly, MA 01915
Phone: 978-922-3000
Fax: 978-921-7025
URL: www.beverlyhospital.org
Type: Acute Care Hospitals
Emergency Services: Yes
Ownership: Voluntary non-profit - Private
Beds: 227
Key Personnel:
Radiology. . . . . Stephen A Barrand
CEO . . . . Denise Conroy
Chief of Medical Staff . . . . Peter H. Short, MD

Measure	Cases	This Hosp.	State Avg.	U.S. Avg.
Blood Clot Prevention and Treatment				
Anticoagulation Overlap Therapy[2]	88	99%	97%	93%
ICU Venous Thromboembolism Prophylaxis[2]	44	91%	92%	92%
Incidence of Potentially Preventable VTE[2]	11	36%	7%	10%
UFH with Dosages/Platelet Monitoring[2]	39	100%	91%	97%
Venous Thromboembolism Prophylaxis[2]	279	83%	87%	85%
Warfarin Therapy Discharge Instructions[2]	62	55%	77%	75%
Chest Pain/Possible Heart Attack Care				
Aspirin Given Within 24 Hours of Arrival	68	100%	97%	96%
Fibrinolytic Meds Within 30 Min. of Arrival[7]	-	-	73%	58%
Average Time to ECG (minutes)	72	7	7	7
Average Time to Transfer (minutes)	12	38	55	60
Children's Asthma Care				
Received Home Management Plan of Care	-	-	-	88%
Received Reliever Medication	-	-	-	100%
Received Systemic Corticosteroids	-	-	-	100%
Emergency Department				
Admittance Decision Time (minutes)[2]	520	150	119	98
Head CT Results Within 45 Min. of Arrival	15	67%	70%	57%
Patients Who Left ER Before Being Seen	64,420	2%	2%	2%
Time from ER Arrival to Admit. (minutes)[2]	522	310	313	274
Time from ER Arrival to Discharge (minutes)	396	147	156	134
Time in ER Before Being Evaluated (minutes)	479	47	36	26
Time to Pain Meds for Fractures (minutes)	270	62	59	57
Heart Attack Care				
Aspirin Given at Discharge	139	100%	100%	99%
Fibrinolytic Meds Within 30 Min. of Arrival[7]	-	-	100%	54%
PCI Within 90 Minutes of Arrival	37	97%	96%	96%
Statin Prescribed at Discharge	121	100%	99%	98%
Heart Failure Care				
ACE Inhibitor or ARB for LVSD	89	100%	96%	97%
Discharge Instructions Given	275	95%	95%	94%
Evaluation of LVS Function	406	100%	100%	99%
Medicare Spending				
Medicare Spending per Patient (ratio)	-	1.04	1.03	0.98
Pneumonia Care				
Appropriate Initial Antibiotic Given	293	100%	97%	95%
Blood Culture Timing	505	99%	98%	98%
Pregnancy and Delivery Care				
Newborn Deliveries Scheduled Early[2]	44	14%	2%	6%
Preventive Care				
Immunization for Influenza[2]	513	69%	91%	90%
Immunization for Pneumonia[2]	580	73%	91%	92%
Stroke Care				
Anticoagulation Therapy for Atrial Fibrillation	30	100%	97%	95%
Antithrombotic Therapy Timing	119	100%	98%	98%

NOTE: Hospital profiles are in alphabetical order by state, then city, then hospital within the city; Rankings exclude hospitals with less than 25 cases except for patient surveys which excludes hospitals with less than 100 cases; (a) 100-299 cases; (1) The number of cases/patients is too few to report; (2) Data submitted were based on a sample of cases/patients; (3) Results are based on a shorter time period than required; (4) Data suppressed by CMS for one or more quarters; (5) Results are not available for this reporting period; (6) Fewer than 100 patients completed the HCAHPS survey; (7) No cases met the criteria for this measure; (8) The lower limit of the confidence interval cannot be calculated if the number of observed infections equals zero; (9) No data are available from the state/territory for this reporting period; (10) The scores shown reflect fewer than 50 completed surveys; (11) There were discrepancies in the data collection process; (12) This measure does not apply to this hospital for this reporting period; (13) Results cannot be calculated for this reporting period; (14) The results for this state are combined with nearby states to protect confidentiality; Please refer to the User's Guide for a full explanation of data.

Measure	Cases	This Hosp.	State Avg.	U.S. Avg.
Assessed for Rehabilitation	134	98%	96%	97%
Discharged on Antithrombotic Therapy	129	100%	100%	99%
Discharged on Statin Medication	105	84%	96%	94%
Thrombolytic Therapy Timing	14	79%	68%	66%
Venous Thromboembolism Prophylaxis	143	89%	94%	94%
Written Stroke Educational Materials Given	65	85%	82%	88%
Surgical Care Improvement Project				
Appropriate Beta Blocker Usage	300	98%	98%	98%
Appropriate VTP Within 24 Hours	926	99%	99%	98%
Controlled Postoperative Blood Glucose[7]	-	-	96%	97%
Perioperative Temperature Management	1,077	100%	100%	100%
Prophylactic Antibiotic Selection	838	100%	99%	99%
Prophylactic Antibiotic Selection (Outpatient)	256	99%	98%	98%
Prophylactic Antibiotic Stopped	821	100%	99%	98%
Prophylactic Antibiotic Timing	839	100%	99%	99%
Prophylactic Antibiotic Timing (Outpatient)	256	99%	98%	98%
Urinary Catheter Removal	846	98%	97%	97%
Survey of Patients' Hospital Experiences				
Area Around Room 'Always' Quiet at Night	300+	49%	52%	61%
Doctors 'Always' Communicated Well	300+	78%	80%	82%
Home Recovery Information Given	300+	86%	87%	85%
Hospital Given 9 or 10 on 10 Point Scale	300+	70%	69%	71%
Meds 'Always' Explained Before Given	300+	64%	64%	64%
Nurses 'Always' Communicated Well	300+	81%	79%	79%
Pain 'Always' Well Controlled	300+	72%	71%	71%
Room and Bathroom 'Always' Clean	300+	70%	72%	73%
Timely Help 'Always' Received	300+	64%	66%	68%
Would Definitely Recommend Hospital	300+	74%	73%	71%
Use of Medical Imaging				
Cardiac Imaging Stress Test before Surgery	516	5.0%	5.4%	5.3%
Combination Abdominal CT Scan	1,380	3.6%	6.3%	10.5%
Combination Brain/Sinus CT Scan	1,218	1.5%	2.4%	2.7%
Combination Chest CT Scan	1,202	0.2%	0.5%	2.7%
Follow-up Mammogram/Ultrasound	3,760	7.7%	8.9%	8.8%
Lumbar Spine MRI for Low Back Pain	271	31.0%	35.3%	37.2%

Beth Israel Deaconess Medical Center

330 Brookline Avenue
Boston, MA 02215
Phone: 617-667-7000
Fax: 617-667-8155
URL: www.bidmc.harvard.edu
Type: Acute Care Hospitals
Emergency Services: Yes
Ownership: Voluntary non-profit - Private
Beds: 591

Key Personnel:

Hemotology Center . . . . Jerome Groopman, MD
Infection Control. . . . . AW Karchmer, MD
Radiology. . . . . Jonathan B. Kruskal, MD
Chief of Medical Staff. . . . . Robert Moellering, MD
Anesthesiology. . . . . Brett Simon, MD, PhD
CEO/President. . . . . Kevin Tabb, MD
Quality Assurance . . . . Beverly Waite, RN
Emergency Room . . . . Richard E. Wolfe

Measure	Cases	This Hosp.	State Avg.	U.S. Avg.
Blood Clot Prevention and Treatment				
Anticoagulation Overlap Therapy[2]	177	95%	97%	93%
ICU Venous Thromboembolism Prophylaxis[2]	103	97%	92%	92%
Incidence of Potentially Preventable VTE[2]	57	2%	7%	10%
UFH with Dosages/Platelet Monitoring[2]	199	0%	91%	97%
Venous Thromboembolism Prophylaxis[2]	326	94%	87%	85%
Warfarin Therapy Discharge Instructions[2]	109	47%	77%	75%
Chest Pain/Possible Heart Attack Care				
Aspirin Given Within 24 Hours of Arrival[5]	-	-	97%	96%
Fibrinolytic Meds Within 30 Min. of Arrival[5]	-	-	73%	58%
Average Time to ECG (minutes)[5]	-	-	7	7
Average Time to Transfer (minutes)[5]	-	-	55	60
Children's Asthma Care				
Received Home Management Plan of Care	-	-	-	88%
Received Reliever Medication	-	-	-	100%
Received Systemic Corticosteroids	-	-	-	100%
Emergency Department				
Admittance Decision Time (minutes)[2]	568	138	119	98
Head CT Results Within 45 Min. of Arrival[3,7]	-	-	70%	57%
Patients Who Left ER Before Being Seen	55,526	1%	2%	2%
Time from ER Arrival to Admit. (minutes)[2]	571	325	313	274
Time from ER Arrival to Discharge (minutes)	1,716	242	156	134
Time in ER Before Being Evaluated (minutes)	1,406	42	36	26
Time to Pain Meds for Fractures (minutes)	43	79	59	57
Heart Attack Care				
Aspirin Given at Discharge	558	100%	100%	99%
Fibrinolytic Meds Within 30 Min. of Arrival[7]	-	-	100%	54%
PCI Within 90 Minutes of Arrival	32	97%	96%	96%
Statin Prescribed at Discharge	558	100%	99%	98%
Heart Failure Care				
ACE Inhibitor or ARB for LVSD[2]	104	100%	96%	97%
Discharge Instructions Given[2]	309	100%	95%	94%
Evaluation of LVS Function[2]	407	100%	100%	99%
Medicare Spending				
Medicare Spending per Patient (ratio)	-	1.04	1.03	0.98
Pneumonia Care				
Appropriate Initial Antibiotic Given[2]	74	96%	97%	95%
Blood Culture Timing[2]	228	97%	98%	98%
Pregnancy and Delivery Care				
Newborn Deliveries Scheduled Early	321	2%	2%	6%
Preventive Care				
Immunization for Influenza[2]	658	96%	91%	90%
Immunization for Pneumonia[2]	721	80%	91%	92%
Stroke Care				
Anticoagulation Therapy for Atrial Fibrillation[2]	44	98%	97%	95%
Antithrombotic Therapy Timing[2]	151	94%	98%	98%
Assessed for Rehabilitation[2]	288	91%	96%	97%
Discharged on Antithrombotic Therapy[2]	193	99%	100%	99%
Discharged on Statin Medication[2]	148	95%	96%	94%
Thrombolytic Therapy Timing[1,2]	-	-	68%	66%
Venous Thromboembolism Prophylaxis[2]	294	95%	94%	94%
Written Stroke Educational Materials Given[2]	136	45%	82%	88%
Surgical Care Improvement Project				
Appropriate Beta Blocker Usage[2]	481	100%	98%	98%
Appropriate VTP Within 24 Hours[2]	878	100%	99%	98%
Controlled Postoperative Blood Glucose[2]	203	96%	96%	97%
Perioperative Temperature Management[2]	1,110	100%	100%	100%
Prophylactic Antibiotic Selection[2]	750	100%	99%	99%
Prophylactic Antibiotic Selection (Outpatient)	888	98%	98%	98%
Prophylactic Antibiotic Stopped[2]	737	99%	99%	98%
Prophylactic Antibiotic Timing[2]	750	100%	99%	99%
Prophylactic Antibiotic Timing (Outpatient)	845	98%	98%	98%
Urinary Catheter Removal[2]	720	100%	97%	97%
Survey of Patients' Hospital Experiences				
Area Around Room 'Always' Quiet at Night	300+	51%	52%	61%
Doctors 'Always' Communicated Well	300+	80%	80%	82%
Home Recovery Information Given	300+	88%	87%	85%
Hospital Given 9 or 10 on 10 Point Scale	300+	75%	69%	71%
Meds 'Always' Explained Before Given	300+	66%	64%	64%
Nurses 'Always' Communicated Well	300+	80%	79%	79%
Pain 'Always' Well Controlled	300+	69%	71%	71%
Room and Bathroom 'Always' Clean	300+	68%	72%	73%
Timely Help 'Always' Received	300+	60%	66%	68%
Would Definitely Recommend Hospital	300+	80%	73%	71%
Use of Medical Imaging				
Cardiac Imaging Stress Test before Surgery	926	5.4%	5.4%	5.3%
Combination Abdominal CT Scan	2,321	16.5%	6.3%	10.5%
Combination Brain/Sinus CT Scan	1,261	1.8%	2.4%	2.7%
Combination Chest CT Scan	2,633	0.2%	0.5%	2.7%
Follow-up Mammogram/Ultrasound	2,825	6.5%	8.9%	8.8%
Lumbar Spine MRI for Low Back Pain	207	30.0%	35.3%	37.2%

Boston Children's Hospital

300 Longwood Avenue
Boston, MA 02115
Phone: 617-735-6000
URL: www.childrenshospital.org
Type: Childrens
Emergency Services: Yes
Ownership: Voluntary non-profit - Private
Beds: 396

Key Personnel:

Emergency Room . . . . Richard G. Bachur, MD
President . . . . Sandra Fenwick
CEO . . . . Sandra L. Fenwick
Cardiology . . . . James Lock, PhD
Radiology. . . . . Richard L Robertson, Jr., MD
Surgery . . . . Robert C. Shamberger, MD
Infection Control. . . . . Michael Wessels, MD
Hemotology Center . . . . David A. Williams, MD

Measure	Cases	This Hosp.	State Avg.	U.S. Avg.
Blood Clot Prevention and Treatment				
Anticoagulation Overlap Therapy[5]	-	-	97%	93%
ICU Venous Thromboembolism Prophylaxis[5]	-	-	92%	92%
Incidence of Potentially Preventable VTE[5]	-	-	7%	10%
UFH with Dosages/Platelet Monitoring[5]	-	-	91%	97%
Venous Thromboembolism Prophylaxis[5]	-	-	87%	85%
Warfarin Therapy Discharge Instructions[5]	-	-	77%	75%
Chest Pain/Possible Heart Attack Care				
Aspirin Given Within 24 Hours of Arrival	-	-	97%	96%
Fibrinolytic Meds Within 30 Min. of Arrival	-	-	73%	58%
Average Time to ECG (minutes)	-	-	7	7
Average Time to Transfer (minutes)	-	-	55	60
Children's Asthma Care				
Received Home Management Plan of Care[2]	332	62%	-	88%
Received Reliever Medication[2]	332	100%	-	100%
Received Systemic Corticosteroids[2]	332	100%	-	100%
Emergency Department				
Admittance Decision Time (minutes)[5]	-	-	119	98
Head CT Results Within 45 Min. of Arrival	-	-	70%	57%
Patients Who Left ER Before Being Seen	-	-	2%	2%
Time from ER Arrival to Admit. (minutes)[5]	-	-	313	274
Time from ER Arrival to Discharge (minutes)	-	-	156	134
Time in ER Before Being Evaluated (minutes)	-	-	36	26
Time to Pain Meds for Fractures (minutes)	-	-	59	57
Heart Attack Care				
Aspirin Given at Discharge[5]	-	-	100%	99%
Fibrinolytic Meds Within 30 Min. of Arrival[5]	-	-	100%	54%
PCI Within 90 Minutes of Arrival[5]	-	-	96%	96%
Statin Prescribed at Discharge[5]	-	-	99%	98%
Heart Failure Care				
ACE Inhibitor or ARB for LVSD[5]	-	-	96%	97%
Discharge Instructions Given[5]	-	-	95%	94%
Evaluation of LVS Function[5]	-	-	100%	99%
Medicare Spending				
Medicare Spending per Patient (ratio)	-	-	1.03	0.98
Pneumonia Care				
Appropriate Initial Antibiotic Given[5]	-	-	97%	95%
Blood Culture Timing[5]	-	-	98%	98%
Pregnancy and Delivery Care				
Newborn Deliveries Scheduled Early[5]	-	-	2%	6%
Preventive Care				
Immunization for Influenza[5]	-	-	91%	90%
Immunization for Pneumonia[5]	-	-	91%	92%
Stroke Care				
Anticoagulation Therapy for Atrial Fibrillation[5]	-	-	97%	95%
Antithrombotic Therapy Timing[5]	-	-	98%	98%
Assessed for Rehabilitation[5]	-	-	96%	97%
Discharged on Antithrombotic Therapy[5]	-	-	100%	99%
Discharged on Statin Medication[5]	-	-	96%	94%
Thrombolytic Therapy Timing[5]	-	-	68%	66%
Venous Thromboembolism Prophylaxis[5]	-	-	94%	94%
Written Stroke Educational Materials Given[5]	-	-	82%	88%
Surgical Care Improvement Project				
Appropriate Beta Blocker Usage[5]	-	-	98%	98%
Appropriate VTP Within 24 Hours[5]	-	-	99%	98%
Controlled Postoperative Blood Glucose[5]	-	-	96%	97%
Perioperative Temperature Management[5]	-	-	100%	100%
Prophylactic Antibiotic Selection[5]	-	-	99%	99%
Prophylactic Antibiotic Selection (Outpatient)	-	-	98%	98%
Prophylactic Antibiotic Stopped[5]	-	-	99%	98%
Prophylactic Antibiotic Timing[5]	-	-	99%	99%
Prophylactic Antibiotic Timing (Outpatient)	-	-	98%	98%
Urinary Catheter Removal[5]	-	-	97%	97%
Survey of Patients' Hospital Experiences				
Area Around Room 'Always' Quiet at Night[5]	-	-	52%	61%
Doctors 'Always' Communicated Well[5]	-	-	80%	82%
Home Recovery Information Given[5]	-	-	87%	85%
Hospital Given 9 or 10 on 10 Point Scale[5]	-	-	69%	71%
Meds 'Always' Explained Before Given[5]	-	-	64%	64%
Nurses 'Always' Communicated Well[5]	-	-	79%	79%
Pain 'Always' Well Controlled[5]	-	-	71%	71%

NOTE: Hospital profiles are in alphabetical order by state, then city, then hospital within the city; Rankings exclude hospitals with less than 25 cases except for patient surveys which excludes hospitals with less than 100 cases; (a) 100-299 cases; (1) The number of cases/patients is too few to report; (2) Data submitted were based on a sample of cases/patients; (3) Results are based on a shorter time period than required; (4) Data suppressed by CMS for one or more quarters; (5) Results are not available for this reporting period; (6) Fewer than 100 patients completed the HCAHPS survey; (7) No cases met the criteria for this measure; (8) The lower limit of the confidence interval cannot be calculated if the number of observed infections equals zero; (9) No data are available from the state/territory for this reporting period; (10) The scores shown reflect fewer than 50 completed surveys; (11) There were discrepancies in the data collection process; (12) This measure does not apply to this hospital for this reporting period; (13) Results cannot be calculated for this reporting period; (14) The results for this state are combined with nearby states to protect confidentiality; Please refer to the User's Guide for a full explanation of data.

Measure	Cases	This Hosp.	State Avg.	U.S. Avg.
Room and Bathroom 'Always' Clean[5]	-	-	72%	73%
Timely Help 'Always' Received[5]	-	-	66%	68%
Would Definitely Recommend Hospital[5]	-	-	73%	71%
Use of Medical Imaging				
Cardiac Imaging Stress Test before Surgery	-	-	5.4%	5.3%
Combination Abdominal CT Scan	-	-	6.3%	10.5%
Combination Brain/Sinus CT Scan	-	-	2.4%	2.7%
Combination Chest CT Scan	-	-	0.5%	2.7%
Follow-up Mammogram/Ultrasound	-	-	8.9%	8.8%
Lumbar Spine MRI for Low Back Pain	-	-	35.3%	37.2%

Boston Medical Center Corporation

1 Boston Medical Center Place
Boston, MA 02118
Phone: 617-638-8000
Fax: 617-638-8538
URL: www.bmc.org
Type: Acute Care Hospitals
Emergency Services: Yes
Ownership: Voluntary non-profit - Private
Beds: 581

Key Personnel:
Coronary Care . . . . Peter Burke, MD
Chief of Medical Staff . . . . Ravin Davidoff, MBBCh
Pediatric Ambulatory Care . . . . . . Doug Hoffman, MD
Pediatric In-Patient Care . . . . Chi-Cheng Huang, MD
Cardiac Laboratory. . . . . Alice Jacobs, MD
Operating Room. . . . . Keith Lewis, MD
Radiology. . . . . Alexander Norbash, MD
CEO/President. . . . . Kate Walsh

Measure	Cases	This Hosp.	State Avg.	U.S. Avg.
Blood Clot Prevention and Treatment				
Anticoagulation Overlap Therapy[2]	93	100%	97%	93%
ICU Venous Thromboembolism Prophylaxis[2]	85	87%	92%	92%
Incidence of Potentially Preventable VTE[2]	41	7%	7%	10%
UFH with Dosages/Platelet Monitoring[2]	67	93%	91%	97%
Venous Thromboembolism Prophylaxis[2]	359	92%	87%	85%
Warfarin Therapy Discharge Instructions[2]	71	34%	77%	75%
Chest Pain/Possible Heart Attack Care				
Aspirin Given Within 24 Hours of Arrival[5]	-	-	97%	96%
Fibrinolytic Meds Within 30 Min. of Arrival[5]	-	-	73%	58%
Average Time to ECG (minutes)[5]	-	-	7	7
Average Time to Transfer (minutes)[5]	-	-	55	60
Children's Asthma Care				
Received Home Management Plan of Care	-	-	-	88%
Received Reliever Medication	-	-	-	100%
Received Systemic Corticosteroids	-	-	-	100%
Emergency Department				
Admittance Decision Time (minutes)[2]	654	178	119	98
Head CT Results Within 45 Min. of Arrival[7]	-	-	70%	57%
Patients Who Left ER Before Being Seen	>100k	4%	2%	2%
Time from ER Arrival to Admit. (minutes)[2]	654	302	313	274
Time from ER Arrival to Discharge (minutes)	341	186	156	134
Time in ER Before Being Evaluated (minutes)	376	44	36	26
Time to Pain Meds for Fractures (minutes)	149	72	59	57
Heart Attack Care				
Aspirin Given at Discharge	352	100%	100%	99%
Fibrinolytic Meds Within 30 Min. of Arrival[7]	-	-	100%	54%
PCI Within 90 Minutes of Arrival	31	90%	96%	96%
Statin Prescribed at Discharge	343	98%	99%	98%
Heart Failure Care				
ACE Inhibitor or ARB for LVSD[2]	95	93%	96%	97%
Discharge Instructions Given[2]	270	99%	95%	94%
Evaluation of LVS Function[2]	309	100%	100%	99%
Medicare Spending				
Medicare Spending per Patient (ratio)	-	1.02	1.03	0.98
Pneumonia Care				
Appropriate Initial Antibiotic Given[2]	82	98%	97%	95%
Blood Culture Timing[2]	102	94%	98%	98%
Pregnancy and Delivery Care				
Newborn Deliveries Scheduled Early[2]	23	4%	2%	6%
Preventive Care				
Immunization for Influenza[2]	599	87%	91%	90%
Immunization for Pneumonia[2]	605	83%	91%	92%
Stroke Care				
Anticoagulation Therapy for Atrial Fibrillation	28	100%	97%	95%
Antithrombotic Therapy Timing	144	99%	98%	98%
Assessed for Rehabilitation	208	100%	96%	97%
Discharged on Antithrombotic Therapy	170	99%	100%	99%
Discharged on Statin Medication	135	99%	96%	94%
Thrombolytic Therapy Timing	15	87%	68%	66%
Venous Thromboembolism Prophylaxis	212	97%	94%	94%
Written Stroke Educational Materials Given	113	99%	82%	88%
Surgical Care Improvement Project				
Appropriate Beta Blocker Usage[2]	270	98%	98%	98%
Appropriate VTP Within 24 Hours[2]	474	100%	99%	98%
Controlled Postoperative Blood Glucose[2]	163	97%	96%	97%
Perioperative Temperature Management[2]	610	100%	100%	100%
Prophylactic Antibiotic Selection[2]	543	99%	99%	99%
Prophylactic Antibiotic Selection (Outpatient)	238	98%	98%	98%
Prophylactic Antibiotic Stopped[2]	517	97%	99%	98%
Prophylactic Antibiotic Timing[2]	544	99%	99%	99%
Prophylactic Antibiotic Timing (Outpatient)	243	94%	98%	98%
Urinary Catheter Removal[2]	262	97%	97%	97%
Survey of Patients' Hospital Experiences				
Area Around Room 'Always' Quiet at Night	300+	49%	52%	61%
Doctors 'Always' Communicated Well	300+	79%	80%	82%
Home Recovery Information Given	300+	86%	87%	85%
Hospital Given 9 or 10 on 10 Point Scale	300+	68%	69%	71%
Meds 'Always' Explained Before Given	300+	65%	64%	64%
Nurses 'Always' Communicated Well	300+	73%	79%	79%
Pain 'Always' Well Controlled	300+	63%	71%	71%
Room and Bathroom 'Always' Clean	300+	68%	72%	73%
Timely Help 'Always' Received	300+	58%	66%	68%
Would Definitely Recommend Hospital	300+	70%	73%	71%
Use of Medical Imaging				
Cardiac Imaging Stress Test before Surgery	584	4.5%	5.4%	5.3%
Combination Abdominal CT Scan	1,217	4.7%	6.3%	10.5%
Combination Brain/Sinus CT Scan	810	3.5%	2.4%	2.7%
Combination Chest CT Scan	1,294	0.5%	0.5%	2.7%
Follow-up Mammogram/Ultrasound	3,118	6.3%	8.9%	8.8%
Lumbar Spine MRI for Low Back Pain	237	32.5%	35.3%	37.2%

Brigham & Women's Faulkner Hospital

1153 Centre Street
Boston, MA 02130
Phone: 617-983-7000
Fax: 617-524-8663
URL: www.brighamandwomensfaulkner.org
Type: Acute Care Hospitals
Emergency Services: Yes
Ownership: Voluntary non-profit - Private
Beds: 150

Key Personnel:
Radiology. . . . . Andrew N. Aikins, MD
Anesthesiology. . . . . James Gessner
Chief of Medical Staff . . . . Geoffrey Sherwood
Patient Relations . . . . Rosemarie Shortt
CEO/President. . . . . David J Trull
Emergency Room . . . . Ashley Yeats

Measure	Cases	This Hosp.	State Avg.	U.S. Avg.
Blood Clot Prevention and Treatment				
Anticoagulation Overlap Therapy[2]	27	100%	97%	93%
ICU Venous Thromboembolism Prophylaxis[2]	23	87%	92%	92%
Incidence of Potentially Preventable VTE[1,2]	-	-	7%	10%
UFH with Dosages/Platelet Monitoring[1,2]	-	-	91%	97%
Venous Thromboembolism Prophylaxis[2]	286	97%	87%	85%
Warfarin Therapy Discharge Instructions[2]	18	100%	77%	75%
Chest Pain/Possible Heart Attack Care				
Aspirin Given Within 24 Hours of Arrival	49	100%	97%	96%
Fibrinolytic Meds Within 30 Min. of Arrival[7]	-	-	73%	58%
Average Time to ECG (minutes)	47	5	7	7
Average Time to Transfer (minutes)[7]	-	-	55	60
Children's Asthma Care				
Received Home Management Plan of Care	-	-	-	88%
Received Reliever Medication	-	-	-	100%
Received Systemic Corticosteroids	-	-	-	100%
Emergency Department				
Admittance Decision Time (minutes)[2]	638	86	119	98
Head CT Results Within 45 Min. of Arrival	21	62%	70%	57%
Patients Who Left ER Before Being Seen	25,840	2%	2%	2%
Time from ER Arrival to Admit. (minutes)[2]	638	283	313	274
Time from ER Arrival to Discharge (minutes)	252	162	156	134
Time in ER Before Being Evaluated (minutes)	384	32	36	26
Time to Pain Meds for Fractures (minutes)	35	53	59	57
Heart Attack Care				
Aspirin Given at Discharge	20	100%	100%	99%
Fibrinolytic Meds Within 30 Min. of Arrival[7]	-	-	100%	54%
PCI Within 90 Minutes of Arrival[7]	-	-	96%	96%
Statin Prescribed at Discharge	22	100%	99%	98%
Heart Failure Care				
ACE Inhibitor or ARB for LVSD	26	100%	96%	97%
Discharge Instructions Given	126	100%	95%	94%
Evaluation of LVS Function	188	100%	100%	99%
Medicare Spending				
Medicare Spending per Patient (ratio)	-	1.04	1.03	0.98
Pneumonia Care				
Appropriate Initial Antibiotic Given[2]	80	100%	97%	95%
Blood Culture Timing[2]	65	100%	98%	98%
Pregnancy and Delivery Care				
Newborn Deliveries Scheduled Early[7]	-	-	2%	6%
Preventive Care				
Immunization for Influenza[2]	597	97%	91%	90%
Immunization for Pneumonia[2]	749	99%	91%	92%
Stroke Care				
Anticoagulation Therapy for Atrial Fibrillation[1]	-	-	97%	95%
Antithrombotic Therapy Timing	38	100%	98%	98%
Assessed for Rehabilitation	40	98%	96%	97%
Discharged on Antithrombotic Therapy	35	100%	100%	99%
Discharged on Statin Medication	32	100%	96%	94%
Thrombolytic Therapy Timing[1]	-	-	68%	66%
Venous Thromboembolism Prophylaxis	38	97%	94%	94%
Written Stroke Educational Materials Given	27	100%	82%	88%
Surgical Care Improvement Project				
Appropriate Beta Blocker Usage[2]	60	100%	98%	98%
Appropriate VTP Within 24 Hours[2]	251	99%	99%	98%
Controlled Postoperative Blood Glucose[2,7]	-	-	96%	97%
Perioperative Temperature Management[2]	289	100%	100%	100%
Prophylactic Antibiotic Selection[2]	153	99%	99%	99%
Prophylactic Antibiotic Selection (Outpatient)	146	99%	98%	98%
Prophylactic Antibiotic Stopped[2]	153	100%	99%	98%
Prophylactic Antibiotic Timing[2]	154	97%	99%	99%
Prophylactic Antibiotic Timing (Outpatient)	145	100%	98%	98%
Urinary Catheter Removal[2]	142	100%	97%	97%
Survey of Patients' Hospital Experiences				
Area Around Room 'Always' Quiet at Night	300+	59%	52%	61%
Doctors 'Always' Communicated Well	300+	85%	80%	82%
Home Recovery Information Given	300+	91%	87%	85%
Hospital Given 9 or 10 on 10 Point Scale	300+	74%	69%	71%
Meds 'Always' Explained Before Given	300+	69%	64%	64%
Nurses 'Always' Communicated Well	300+	82%	79%	79%
Pain 'Always' Well Controlled	300+	73%	71%	71%
Room and Bathroom 'Always' Clean	300+	74%	72%	73%
Timely Help 'Always' Received	300+	74%	66%	68%
Would Definitely Recommend Hospital	300+	78%	73%	71%
Use of Medical Imaging				
Cardiac Imaging Stress Test before Surgery	290	5.2%	5.4%	5.3%
Combination Abdominal CT Scan	925	3.9%	6.3%	10.5%
Combination Brain/Sinus CT Scan[1]	-	-	2.4%	2.7%
Combination Chest CT Scan	908	0.0%	0.5%	2.7%
Follow-up Mammogram/Ultrasound	6,373	8.8%	8.9%	8.8%
Lumbar Spine MRI for Low Back Pain	74	41.9%	35.3%	37.2%

Brigham & Women's Hospital

75 Francis Street
Boston, MA 02115
Phone: 617-732-5500
Fax: 617-582-6130
URL: www.brighamandwomens.org
Type: Acute Care Hospitals
Emergency Services: Yes
Ownership: Voluntary non-profit - Private
Beds: 725

Key Personnel:
Radiology. . . . . Piran Aliabadi
CEO/President. . . . . Gary Gottlieb, MD, MBA
President . . . . Elizabeth G. Nabel, MD
Anesthesiology. . . . . Charles Vacante, MD
Emergency Room . . . . Ron Walls, MD
Chief of Medical Staff . . . . Anthony Whittemore

Measure	Cases	This Hosp.	State Avg.	U.S. Avg.
Blood Clot Prevention and Treatment				
Anticoagulation Overlap Therapy[2]	179	97%	97%	93%
ICU Venous Thromboembolism Prophylaxis[2]	56	95%	92%	92%

NOTE: Hospital profiles are in alphabetical order by state, then city, then hospital within the city; Rankings exclude hospitals with less than 25 cases except for patient surveys which excludes hospitals with less than 100 cases; (a) 100-299 cases; (1) The number of cases/patients is too few to report; (2) Data submitted were based on a sample of cases/patients; (3) Results are based on a shorter time period than required; (4) Data suppressed by CMS for one or more quarters; (5) Results are not available for this reporting period; (6) Fewer than 100 patients completed the HCAHPS survey; (7) No cases met the criteria for this measure; (8) The lower limit of the confidence interval cannot be calculated if the number of observed infections equals zero; (9) No data are available from the state/territory for this reporting period; (10) The scores shown reflect fewer than 50 completed surveys; (11) There were discrepancies in the data collection process; (12) This measure does not apply to this hospital for this reporting period; (13) Results cannot be calculated for this reporting period; (14) The results for this state are combined with nearby states to protect confidentiality; Please refer to the User's Guide for a full explanation of data.

Measure	Cases	This Hosp.	State Avg.	U.S. Avg.
Incidence of Potentially Preventable VTE[2]	81	2%	7%	10%
UFH with Dosages/Platelet Monitoring[2]	240	100%	91%	97%
Venous Thromboembolism Prophylaxis[2]	347	86%	87%	85%
Warfarin Therapy Discharge Instructions[2]	114	99%	77%	75%
Chest Pain/Possible Heart Attack Care				
Aspirin Given Within 24 Hours of Arrival[1]	-	-	97%	96%
Fibrinolytic Meds Within 30 Min. of Arrival[5]	-	-	73%	58%
Average Time to ECG (minutes)[1]	-	-	7	7
Average Time to Transfer (minutes)[5]	-	-	55	60
Children's Asthma Care				
Received Home Management Plan of Care	-	-	-	88%
Received Reliever Medication	-	-	-	100%
Received Systemic Corticosteroids	-	-	-	100%
Emergency Department				
Admittance Decision Time (minutes)[2]	327	108	119	98
Head CT Results Within 45 Min. of Arrival[7]	-	-	70%	57%
Patients Who Left ER Before Being Seen	61,276	1%	2%	2%
Time from ER Arrival to Admit. (minutes)[2]	338	311	313	274
Time from ER Arrival to Discharge (minutes)	306	180	156	134
Time in ER Before Being Evaluated (minutes)	326	21	36	26
Time to Pain Meds for Fractures (minutes)	50	43	59	57
Heart Attack Care				
Aspirin Given at Discharge	495	100%	100%	99%
Fibrinolytic Meds Within 30 Min. of Arrival[7]	-	-	100%	54%
PCI Within 90 Minutes of Arrival	51	98%	96%	96%
Statin Prescribed at Discharge	480	100%	99%	98%
Heart Failure Care				
ACE Inhibitor or ARB for LVSD[2]	88	99%	96%	97%
Discharge Instructions Given[2]	234	100%	95%	94%
Evaluation of LVS Function[2]	286	100%	100%	99%
Medicare Spending				
Medicare Spending per Patient (ratio)	-	1.01	1.03	0.98
Pneumonia Care				
Appropriate Initial Antibiotic Given[2]	27	100%	97%	95%
Blood Culture Timing[2]	64	97%	98%	98%
Pregnancy and Delivery Care				
Newborn Deliveries Scheduled Early[2]	78	3%	2%	6%
Preventive Care				
Immunization for Influenza[2]	494	91%	91%	90%
Immunization for Pneumonia[2]	484	93%	91%	92%
Stroke Care				
Anticoagulation Therapy for Atrial Fibrillation[2]	18	94%	97%	95%
Antithrombotic Therapy Timing[2]	54	96%	98%	98%
Assessed for Rehabilitation[2]	102	93%	96%	97%
Discharged on Antithrombotic Therapy[2]	70	100%	100%	99%
Discharged on Statin Medication[2]	48	100%	96%	94%
Thrombolytic Therapy Timing[1,2]	-	-	68%	66%
Venous Thromboembolism Prophylaxis[2]	108	94%	94%	94%
Written Stroke Educational Materials Given[2]	62	55%	82%	88%
Surgical Care Improvement Project				
Appropriate Beta Blocker Usage[2]	243	100%	98%	98%
Appropriate VTP Within 24 Hours[2]	425	100%	99%	98%
Controlled Postoperative Blood Glucose[2]	132	99%	96%	97%
Perioperative Temperature Management[2]	556	100%	100%	100%
Prophylactic Antibiotic Selection[2]	420	99%	99%	99%
Prophylactic Antibiotic Selection (Outpatient)	623	98%	98%	98%
Prophylactic Antibiotic Stopped[2]	413	98%	99%	98%
Prophylactic Antibiotic Timing[2]	422	99%	99%	99%
Prophylactic Antibiotic Timing (Outpatient)	620	97%	98%	98%
Urinary Catheter Removal[2]	330	97%	97%	97%
Survey of Patients' Hospital Experiences				
Area Around Room 'Always' Quiet at Night	300+	56%	52%	61%
Doctors 'Always' Communicated Well	300+	82%	80%	82%
Home Recovery Information Given	300+	89%	87%	85%
Hospital Given 9 or 10 on 10 Point Scale	300+	82%	69%	71%
Meds 'Always' Explained Before Given	300+	67%	64%	64%
Nurses 'Always' Communicated Well	300+	81%	79%	79%
Pain 'Always' Well Controlled	300+	69%	71%	71%
Room and Bathroom 'Always' Clean	300+	67%	72%	73%
Timely Help 'Always' Received	300+	69%	66%	68%
Would Definitely Recommend Hospital	300+	86%	73%	71%
Use of Medical Imaging				
Cardiac Imaging Stress Test before Surgery	951	7.9%	5.4%	5.3%
Combination Abdominal CT Scan	2,085	7.1%	6.3%	10.5%
Combination Brain/Sinus CT Scan	1,110	1.4%	2.4%	2.7%
Combination Chest CT Scan	4,001	0.1%	0.5%	2.7%
Follow-up Mammogram/Ultrasound	4,414	6.6%	8.9%	8.8%
Lumbar Spine MRI for Low Back Pain	378	32.8%	35.3%	37.2%

Carney Hospital

2100 Dorchester Avenue
Boston, MA 02124
Phone: 617-506-2000
E-mail: chmail@cchcs.org
URL: www.caritascarney.org
Type: Acute Care Hospitals
Emergency Services: Yes
Ownership: Proprietary
Beds: 228

Key Personnel:

Infection Control. . . . . Philip Carling, MD
President . . . . Andy Davis
Radiology. . . . . Alexander L Feinstein, MD
Cardiac Laboratory. . . . . Francis Hubbard, MD
Pediatric Ambulatory Care . . . . . . Claudia Lavin, MD
Chief of Medical Staff. . . . . Gregory McSweeney
Operating Room. . . . . Cadet Nissage, RN
Quality Assurance . . . . Carol Torosian

Measure	Cases	This Hosp.	State Avg.	U.S. Avg.
Blood Clot Prevention and Treatment				
Anticoagulation Overlap Therapy[2]	15	100%	97%	93%
ICU Venous Thromboembolism Prophylaxis[2]	64	95%	92%	92%
Incidence of Potentially Preventable VTE[1,2]	-	-	7%	10%
UFH with Dosages/Platelet Monitoring[1,2]	-	-	91%	97%
Venous Thromboembolism Prophylaxis[2]	305	87%	87%	85%
Warfarin Therapy Discharge Instructions[2]	11	91%	77%	75%
Chest Pain/Possible Heart Attack Care				
Aspirin Given Within 24 Hours of Arrival	41	100%	97%	96%
Fibrinolytic Meds Within 30 Min. of Arrival[7]	-	-	73%	58%
Average Time to ECG (minutes)	40	14	7	7
Average Time to Transfer (minutes)[1]	-	-	55	60
Children's Asthma Care				
Received Home Management Plan of Care	-	-	-	88%
Received Reliever Medication	-	-	-	100%
Received Systemic Corticosteroids	-	-	-	100%
Emergency Department				
Admittance Decision Time (minutes)[2]	653	113	119	98
Head CT Results Within 45 Min. of Arrival[1]	-	-	70%	57%
Patients Who Left ER Before Being Seen	30,214	1%	2%	2%
Time from ER Arrival to Admit. (minutes)[2]	658	275	313	274
Time from ER Arrival to Discharge (minutes)	359	146	156	134
Time in ER Before Being Evaluated (minutes)	384	29	36	26
Time to Pain Meds for Fractures (minutes)	31	50	59	57
Heart Attack Care				
Aspirin Given at Discharge[1]	-	-	100%	99%
Fibrinolytic Meds Within 30 Min. of Arrival[7]	-	-	100%	54%
PCI Within 90 Minutes of Arrival[7]	-	-	96%	96%
Statin Prescribed at Discharge[1]	-	-	99%	98%
Heart Failure Care				
ACE Inhibitor or ARB for LVSD	31	100%	96%	97%
Discharge Instructions Given	83	98%	95%	94%
Evaluation of LVS Function	108	100%	100%	99%
Medicare Spending				
Medicare Spending per Patient (ratio)	-	1.01	1.03	0.98
Pneumonia Care				
Appropriate Initial Antibiotic Given	58	100%	97%	95%
Blood Culture Timing	70	100%	98%	98%
Pregnancy and Delivery Care				
Newborn Deliveries Scheduled Early[7]	-	-	2%	6%
Preventive Care				
Immunization for Influenza[2]	485	87%	91%	90%
Immunization for Pneumonia[2]	564	95%	91%	92%
Stroke Care				
Anticoagulation Therapy for Atrial Fibrillation[1]	-	-	97%	95%
Antithrombotic Therapy Timing	45	100%	98%	98%
Assessed for Rehabilitation	43	93%	96%	97%
Discharged on Antithrombotic Therapy	41	100%	100%	99%
Discharged on Statin Medication	31	94%	96%	94%
Thrombolytic Therapy Timing[1]	-	-	68%	66%
Venous Thromboembolism Prophylaxis	45	91%	94%	94%
Written Stroke Educational Materials Given	21	90%	82%	88%
Surgical Care Improvement Project				
Appropriate Beta Blocker Usage	48	100%	98%	98%
Appropriate VTP Within 24 Hours	140	99%	99%	98%
Controlled Postoperative Blood Glucose[7]	-	-	96%	97%
Perioperative Temperature Management	159	100%	100%	100%
Prophylactic Antibiotic Selection	99	99%	99%	99%
Prophylactic Antibiotic Selection (Outpatient)	32	100%	98%	98%
Prophylactic Antibiotic Stopped	96	100%	99%	98%
Prophylactic Antibiotic Timing	99	98%	99%	99%
Prophylactic Antibiotic Timing (Outpatient)	30	100%	98%	98%
Urinary Catheter Removal	100	95%	97%	97%
Survey of Patients' Hospital Experiences				
Area Around Room 'Always' Quiet at Night	300+	63%	52%	61%
Doctors 'Always' Communicated Well	300+	79%	80%	82%
Home Recovery Information Given	300+	83%	87%	85%
Hospital Given 9 or 10 on 10 Point Scale	300+	55%	69%	71%
Meds 'Always' Explained Before Given	300+	61%	64%	64%
Nurses 'Always' Communicated Well	300+	76%	79%	79%
Pain 'Always' Well Controlled	300+	68%	71%	71%
Room and Bathroom 'Always' Clean	300+	69%	72%	73%
Timely Help 'Always' Received	300+	61%	66%	68%
Would Definitely Recommend Hospital	300+	58%	73%	71%
Use of Medical Imaging				
Cardiac Imaging Stress Test before Surgery	154	7.1%	5.4%	5.3%
Combination Abdominal CT Scan	358	8.1%	6.3%	10.5%
Combination Brain/Sinus CT Scan[1]	-	-	2.4%	2.7%
Combination Chest CT Scan	220	0.5%	0.5%	2.7%
Follow-up Mammogram/Ultrasound	922	5.7%	8.9%	8.8%
Lumbar Spine MRI for Low Back Pain	57	49.1%	35.3%	37.2%

Dana - Farber Cancer Institute

450 Brookline Avenue
Boston, MA 02115
Phone: 617-632-3000
Fax: 617-667-9619
E-mail: dana-farbercontactus@dfci.harvard.edu
URL: www.dana-farber.org
Type: Acute Care Hospitals
Emergency Services: No
Ownership: Voluntary non-profit - Private
Beds: 57

Key Personnel:

CEO/President. . . . . Edward J Benz Jr, MD
Chief of Medical Staff. . . . . Craig A. Bunnell, MD, MBA, MPH
Hemotology Center . . . . James D Griffin, MD
Radiology. . . . . Jay R Harris, MD
Pediatric Ambulatory Care . . . . . . Stuart H Orkin, MD
Patient Relations . . . . Patricia Reid Ponte, RN

Measure	Cases	This Hosp.	State Avg.	U.S. Avg.
Blood Clot Prevention and Treatment				
Anticoagulation Overlap Therapy[5]	-	-	97%	93%
ICU Venous Thromboembolism Prophylaxis[5]	-	-	92%	92%
Incidence of Potentially Preventable VTE[5]	-	-	7%	10%
UFH with Dosages/Platelet Monitoring[5]	-	-	91%	97%
Venous Thromboembolism Prophylaxis[5]	-	-	87%	85%
Warfarin Therapy Discharge Instructions[5]	-	-	77%	75%
Chest Pain/Possible Heart Attack Care				
Aspirin Given Within 24 Hours of Arrival	-	-	97%	96%
Fibrinolytic Meds Within 30 Min. of Arrival	-	-	73%	58%
Average Time to ECG (minutes)	-	-	7	7
Average Time to Transfer (minutes)	-	-	55	60
Children's Asthma Care				
Received Home Management Plan of Care	-	-	-	88%
Received Reliever Medication	-	-	-	100%
Received Systemic Corticosteroids	-	-	-	100%
Emergency Department				
Admittance Decision Time (minutes)[5]	-	-	119	98
Head CT Results Within 45 Min. of Arrival	-	-	70%	57%
Patients Who Left ER Before Being Seen	-	-	2%	2%
Time from ER Arrival to Admit. (minutes)[5]	-	-	313	274
Time from ER Arrival to Discharge (minutes)	-	-	156	134
Time in ER Before Being Evaluated (minutes)	-	-	36	26
Time to Pain Meds for Fractures (minutes)	-	-	59	57
Heart Attack Care				
Aspirin Given at Discharge[5]	-	-	100%	99%
Fibrinolytic Meds Within 30 Min. of Arrival[5]	-	-	100%	54%

NOTE: Hospital profiles are in alphabetical order by state, then city, then hospital within the city; Rankings exclude hospitals with less than 25 cases except for patient surveys which excludes hospitals with less than 100 cases; (a) 100-299 cases; (1) The number of cases/patients is too few to report; (2) Data submitted were based on a sample of cases/patients; (3) Results are based on a shorter time period than required; (4) Data suppressed by CMS for one or more quarters; (5) Results are not available for this reporting period; (6) Fewer than 100 patients completed the HCAHPS survey; (7) No cases met the criteria for this measure; (8) The lower limit of the confidence interval cannot be calculated if the number of observed infections equals zero; (9) No data are available from the state/territory for this reporting period; (10) The scores shown reflect fewer than 50 completed surveys; (11) There were discrepancies in the data collection process; (12) This measure does not apply to this hospital for this reporting period; (13) Results cannot be calculated for this reporting period; (14) The results for this state are combined with nearby states to protect confidentiality; Please refer to the User's Guide for a full explanation of data.

Measure	Cases	This Hosp.	State Avg.	U.S. Avg.
PCI Within 90 Minutes of Arrival[5]	-	-	96%	96%
Statin Prescribed at Discharge[5]	-	-	99%	98%
Heart Failure Care				
ACE Inhibitor or ARB for LVSD[5]	-	-	96%	97%
Discharge Instructions Given[5]	-	-	95%	94%
Evaluation of LVS Function[5]	-	-	100%	99%
Medicare Spending				
Medicare Spending per Patient (ratio)	-	-	1.03	0.98
Pneumonia Care				
Appropriate Initial Antibiotic Given[1]	-	-	97%	95%
Blood Culture Timing	12	100%	98%	98%
Pregnancy and Delivery Care				
Newborn Deliveries Scheduled Early[3,7]	-	-	2%	6%
Preventive Care				
Immunization for Influenza[5]	-	-	91%	90%
Immunization for Pneumonia[5]	-	-	91%	92%
Stroke Care				
Anticoagulation Therapy for Atrial Fibrillation[5]	-	-	97%	95%
Antithrombotic Therapy Timing[5]	-	-	98%	98%
Assessed for Rehabilitation[5]	-	-	96%	97%
Discharged on Antithrombotic Therapy[5]	-	-	100%	99%
Discharged on Statin Medication[5]	-	-	96%	94%
Thrombolytic Therapy Timing[5]	-	-	68%	66%
Venous Thromboembolism Prophylaxis[5]	-	-	94%	94%
Written Stroke Educational Materials Given[5]	-	-	82%	88%
Surgical Care Improvement Project				
Appropriate Beta Blocker Usage[5]	-	-	98%	98%
Appropriate VTP Within 24 Hours[5]	-	-	99%	98%
Controlled Postoperative Blood Glucose[5]	-	-	96%	97%
Perioperative Temperature Management[5]	-	-	100%	100%
Prophylactic Antibiotic Selection[5]	-	-	99%	99%
Prophylactic Antibiotic Selection (Outpatient)	-	-	98%	98%
Prophylactic Antibiotic Stopped[5]	-	-	99%	98%
Prophylactic Antibiotic Timing[5]	-	-	99%	99%
Prophylactic Antibiotic Timing (Outpatient)	-	-	98%	98%
Urinary Catheter Removal[5]	-	-	97%	97%
Survey of Patients' Hospital Experiences				
Area Around Room 'Always' Quiet at Night[5]	-	-	52%	61%
Doctors 'Always' Communicated Well[5]	-	-	80%	82%
Home Recovery Information Given[5]	-	-	87%	85%
Hospital Given 9 or 10 on 10 Point Scale[5]	-	-	69%	71%
Meds 'Always' Explained Before Given[5]	-	-	64%	64%
Nurses 'Always' Communicated Well[5]	-	-	79%	79%
Pain 'Always' Well Controlled[5]	-	-	71%	71%
Room and Bathroom 'Always' Clean[5]	-	-	72%	73%
Timely Help 'Always' Received[5]	-	-	66%	68%
Would Definitely Recommend Hospital[5]	-	-	73%	71%
Use of Medical Imaging				
Cardiac Imaging Stress Test before Surgery	-	-	5.4%	5.3%
Combination Abdominal CT Scan	-	-	6.3%	10.5%
Combination Brain/Sinus CT Scan	-	-	2.4%	2.7%
Combination Chest CT Scan	-	-	0.5%	2.7%
Follow-up Mammogram/Ultrasound	-	-	8.9%	8.8%
Lumbar Spine MRI for Low Back Pain	-	-	35.3%	37.2%

Massachusetts Eye & Ear Infirmary

243 Charles Street
Boston, MA 02114
Phone: 617-523-7900
Fax: 617-573-3444
URL: www.meei.harvard.edu
Type: Acute Care Hospitals
Emergency Services: Yes
Ownership: Voluntary non-profit - Private
Beds: 42

Key Personnel:

Radiology. . . . . Paul Caruso
Patient Relations . . . . Carol Covell, RN
Chief of Medical Staff. . . . . Sunil Eappen, MD
CEO/President. . . . . John Fernandez
Emergency Room . . . . Matthew Gardiner, MD
Chairman/CEO . . . . Wycliffe Grousbeck
Anesthesiology. . . . . Salvatore Zasta, MD

Measure	Cases	This Hosp.	State Avg.	U.S. Avg.
Blood Clot Prevention and Treatment				
Anticoagulation Overlap Therapy[2,7]	-	-	97%	93%
ICU Venous Thromboembolism Prophylaxis[2,7]	-	-	92%	92%
Incidence of Potentially Preventable VTE[2,7]	-	-	7%	10%
UFH with Dosages/Platelet Monitoring[2,7]	-	-	91%	97%
Venous Thromboembolism Prophylaxis[2]	160	92%	87%	85%
Warfarin Therapy Discharge Instructions[2,7]	-	-	77%	75%
Chest Pain/Possible Heart Attack Care				
Aspirin Given Within 24 Hours of Arrival[5]	-	-	97%	96%
Fibrinolytic Meds Within 30 Min. of Arrival[5]	-	-	73%	58%
Average Time to ECG (minutes)[5]	-	-	7	7
Average Time to Transfer (minutes)[5]	-	-	55	60
Children's Asthma Care				
Received Home Management Plan of Care	-	-	-	88%
Received Reliever Medication	-	-	-	100%
Received Systemic Corticosteroids	-	-	-	100%
Emergency Department				
Admittance Decision Time (minutes)[1,2]	-	-	119	98
Head CT Results Within 45 Min. of Arrival[5]	-	-	70%	57%
Patients Who Left ER Before Being Seen	19,642	1%	2%	2%
Time from ER Arrival to Admit. (minutes)[1,2]	-	-	313	274
Time from ER Arrival to Discharge (minutes)	189	123	156	134
Time in ER Before Being Evaluated (minutes)	311	73	36	26
Time to Pain Meds for Fractures (minutes)[5]	-	-	59	57
Heart Attack Care				
Aspirin Given at Discharge[5]	-	-	100%	99%
Fibrinolytic Meds Within 30 Min. of Arrival[5]	-	-	100%	54%
PCI Within 90 Minutes of Arrival[5]	-	-	96%	96%
Statin Prescribed at Discharge[5]	-	-	99%	98%
Heart Failure Care				
ACE Inhibitor or ARB for LVSD[5]	-	-	96%	97%
Discharge Instructions Given[5]	-	-	95%	94%
Evaluation of LVS Function[5]	-	-	100%	99%
Medicare Spending				
Medicare Spending per Patient (ratio)	-	1.00	1.03	0.98
Pneumonia Care				
Appropriate Initial Antibiotic Given[5]	-	-	97%	95%
Blood Culture Timing[5]	-	-	98%	98%
Pregnancy and Delivery Care				
Newborn Deliveries Scheduled Early[7]	-	-	2%	6%
Preventive Care				
Immunization for Influenza[2]	309	54%	91%	90%
Immunization for Pneumonia[2]	268	37%	91%	92%
Stroke Care				
Anticoagulation Therapy for Atrial Fibrillation[5]	-	-	97%	95%
Antithrombotic Therapy Timing[5]	-	-	98%	98%
Assessed for Rehabilitation[5]	-	-	96%	97%
Discharged on Antithrombotic Therapy[5]	-	-	100%	99%
Discharged on Statin Medication[5]	-	-	96%	94%
Thrombolytic Therapy Timing[5]	-	-	68%	66%
Venous Thromboembolism Prophylaxis[5]	-	-	94%	94%
Written Stroke Educational Materials Given[5]	-	-	82%	88%
Surgical Care Improvement Project				
Appropriate Beta Blocker Usage[5]	-	-	98%	98%
Appropriate VTP Within 24 Hours[5]	-	-	99%	98%
Controlled Postoperative Blood Glucose[5]	-	-	96%	97%
Perioperative Temperature Management[5]	-	-	100%	100%
Prophylactic Antibiotic Selection[5]	-	-	99%	99%
Prophylactic Antibiotic Selection (Outpatient)[5]	-	-	98%	98%
Prophylactic Antibiotic Stopped[5]	-	-	99%	98%
Prophylactic Antibiotic Timing[5]	-	-	99%	99%
Prophylactic Antibiotic Timing (Outpatient)[5]	-	-	98%	98%
Urinary Catheter Removal[5]	-	-	97%	97%
Survey of Patients' Hospital Experiences				
Area Around Room 'Always' Quiet at Night	300+	36%	52%	61%
Doctors 'Always' Communicated Well	300+	80%	80%	82%
Home Recovery Information Given	300+	83%	87%	85%
Hospital Given 9 or 10 on 10 Point Scale	300+	68%	69%	71%
Meds 'Always' Explained Before Given	300+	52%	64%	64%
Nurses 'Always' Communicated Well	300+	71%	79%	79%
Pain 'Always' Well Controlled	300+	68%	71%	71%
Room and Bathroom 'Always' Clean	300+	64%	72%	73%
Timely Help 'Always' Received	300+	59%	66%	68%
Would Definitely Recommend Hospital	300+	78%	73%	71%
Use of Medical Imaging				
Cardiac Imaging Stress Test before Surgery[7]	-	-	5.4%	5.3%
Combination Abdominal CT Scan[1]	-	-	6.3%	10.5%
Combination Brain/Sinus CT Scan[1]	-	-	2.4%	2.7%
Combination Chest CT Scan	520	0.0%	0.5%	2.7%
Follow-up Mammogram/Ultrasound[7]	-	-	8.9%	8.8%
Lumbar Spine MRI for Low Back Pain[7]	-	-	35.3%	37.2%

Massachusetts General Hospital

55 Fruit Street
Boston, MA 02114
Phone: 617-726-2000
Fax: 617-724-7632
URL: www.massgeneral.org
Type: Acute Care Hospitals
Emergency Services: Yes
Ownership: Voluntary non-profit - Private
Beds: 868

Key Personnel:

Radiology. . . . . James A Brink, MD
Hemotology Center . . . . Zareh N Demirjian
President . . . . Peter L. Slavin, MD
Chair/CEO . . . . David Torchiana, MD
Pediatric In-Patient Care . . . . Joseph Vacanti, MD
Pediatrics. . . . . Joseph Vacanti, MD
Anesthesiology. . . . . Jeanine Wiener Kronish, MD

Measure	Cases	This Hosp.	State Avg.	U.S. Avg.
Blood Clot Prevention and Treatment				
Anticoagulation Overlap Therapy[2]	224	100%	97%	93%
ICU Venous Thromboembolism Prophylaxis[2]	79	99%	92%	92%
Incidence of Potentially Preventable VTE[2]	111	4%	7%	10%
UFH with Dosages/Platelet Monitoring[2]	232	92%	91%	97%
Venous Thromboembolism Prophylaxis[2]	341	95%	87%	85%
Warfarin Therapy Discharge Instructions[2]	143	90%	77%	75%
Chest Pain/Possible Heart Attack Care				
Aspirin Given Within 24 Hours of Arrival[1,3]	-	-	97%	96%
Fibrinolytic Meds Within 30 Min. of Arrival[3,7]	-	-	73%	58%
Average Time to ECG (minutes)[1,3]	-	-	7	7
Average Time to Transfer (minutes)[3,7]	-	-	55	60
Children's Asthma Care				
Received Home Management Plan of Care	-	-	-	88%
Received Reliever Medication	-	-	-	100%
Received Systemic Corticosteroids	-	-	-	100%
Emergency Department				
Admittance Decision Time (minutes)[2]	520	184	119	98
Head CT Results Within 45 Min. of Arrival[1]	-	-	70%	57%
Patients Who Left ER Before Being Seen	99,942	2%	2%	2%
Time from ER Arrival to Admit. (minutes)[2]	523	408	313	274
Time from ER Arrival to Discharge (minutes)	278	210	156	134
Time in ER Before Being Evaluated (minutes)	395	9	36	26
Time to Pain Meds for Fractures (minutes)	105	67	59	57
Heart Attack Care				
Aspirin Given at Discharge	676	99%	100%	99%
Fibrinolytic Meds Within 30 Min. of Arrival[7]	-	-	100%	54%
PCI Within 90 Minutes of Arrival	49	96%	96%	96%
Statin Prescribed at Discharge	658	99%	99%	98%
Heart Failure Care				
ACE Inhibitor or ARB for LVSD[2]	61	95%	96%	97%
Discharge Instructions Given[2]	211	91%	95%	94%
Evaluation of LVS Function[2]	286	100%	100%	99%
Medicare Spending				
Medicare Spending per Patient (ratio)	-	1.01	1.03	0.98
Pneumonia Care				
Appropriate Initial Antibiotic Given[2]	48	92%	97%	95%
Blood Culture Timing[2]	58	100%	98%	98%
Pregnancy and Delivery Care				
Newborn Deliveries Scheduled Early[2]	31	10%	2%	6%
Preventive Care				
Immunization for Influenza[2]	540	99%	91%	90%
Immunization for Pneumonia[2]	601	92%	91%	92%
Stroke Care				
Anticoagulation Therapy for Atrial Fibrillation[2]	14	86%	97%	95%
Antithrombotic Therapy Timing[2]	85	98%	98%	98%
Assessed for Rehabilitation[2]	144	96%	96%	97%
Discharged on Antithrombotic Therapy[2]	102	100%	100%	99%
Discharged on Statin Medication[2]	78	97%	96%	94%
Thrombolytic Therapy Timing[1,2]	-	-	68%	66%
Venous Thromboembolism Prophylaxis[2]	150	94%	94%	94%
Written Stroke Educational Materials Given[2]	76	93%	82%	88%
Surgical Care Improvement Project				

NOTE: Hospital profiles are in alphabetical order by state, then city, then hospital within the city; Rankings exclude hospitals with less than 25 cases except for patient surveys which excludes hospitals with less than 100 cases; (a) 100-299 cases; (1) The number of cases/patients is too few to report; (2) Data submitted were based on a sample of cases/patients; (3) Results are based on a shorter time period than required; (4) Data suppressed by CMS for one or more quarters; (5) Results are not available for this reporting period; (6) Fewer than 100 patients completed the HCAHPS survey; (7) No cases met the criteria for this measure; (8) The lower limit of the confidence interval cannot be calculated if the number of observed infections equals zero; (9) No data are available from the state/territory for this reporting period; (10) The scores shown reflect fewer than 50 completed surveys; (11) There were discrepancies in the data collection process; (12) This measure does not apply to this hospital for this reporting period; (13) Results cannot be calculated for this reporting period; (14) The results for this state are combined with nearby states to protect confidentiality; Please refer to the User's Guide for a full explanation of data.

Measure	Cases	This Hosp.	State Avg.	U.S. Avg.
Appropriate Beta Blocker Usage[2]	286	100%	98%	98%
Appropriate VTP Within 24 Hours[2]	460	99%	99%	98%
Controlled Postoperative Blood Glucose[2]	145	94%	96%	97%
Perioperative Temperature Management[2]	628	100%	100%	100%
Prophylactic Antibiotic Selection[2]	473	100%	99%	99%
Prophylactic Antibiotic Selection (Outpatient)	609	98%	98%	98%
Prophylactic Antibiotic Stopped[2]	458	97%	99%	98%
Prophylactic Antibiotic Timing[2]	474	99%	99%	99%
Prophylactic Antibiotic Timing (Outpatient)	583	97%	98%	98%
Urinary Catheter Removal[2]	354	97%	97%	97%
Survey of Patients' Hospital Experiences				
Area Around Room 'Always' Quiet at Night	300+	53%	52%	61%
Doctors 'Always' Communicated Well	300+	81%	80%	82%
Home Recovery Information Given	300+	90%	87%	85%
Hospital Given 9 or 10 on 10 Point Scale	300+	81%	69%	71%
Meds 'Always' Explained Before Given	300+	65%	64%	64%
Nurses 'Always' Communicated Well	300+	82%	79%	79%
Pain 'Always' Well Controlled	300+	71%	71%	71%
Room and Bathroom 'Always' Clean	300+	74%	72%	73%
Timely Help 'Always' Received	300+	65%	66%	68%
Would Definitely Recommend Hospital	300+	90%	73%	71%
Use of Medical Imaging				
Cardiac Imaging Stress Test before Surgery	2,179	5.1%	5.4%	5.3%
Combination Abdominal CT Scan	5,626	4.0%	6.3%	10.5%
Combination Brain/Sinus CT Scan	1,306	0.4%	2.4%	2.7%
Combination Chest CT Scan	7,673	0.1%	0.5%	2.7%
Follow-up Mammogram/Ultrasound	7,641	4.7%	8.9%	8.8%
Lumbar Spine MRI for Low Back Pain	264	28.4%	35.3%	37.2%

New England Baptist Hospital

125 Parker Hill Avenue
Boston, MA 02120
Phone: 617-754-5800
Fax: 617-754-5800
E-mail: nebhweb@caregroup.harvard.edu
URL: www.nebh.caregroup.org
Type: Acute Care Hospitals
Emergency Services: No
Ownership: Voluntary non-profit - Private
Beds: 141

Key Personnel:

Anesthesiology. . . . . Rueben Azocar
Pediatric In-Patient Care . . . . Marylou Buyse
Hemotology Center . . . . Elie Choufani
Chief of Medical Staff. . . . . James F Green
CEO/President. . . . . Trish Hannon, FACHE
Radiology. . . . . James R Hill, MD
Quality Assurance . . . . Marcella Malay
Operating Room. . . . . Pauline Robitaille, RN

Measure	Cases	This Hosp.	State Avg.	U.S. Avg.
Blood Clot Prevention and Treatment				
Anticoagulation Overlap Therapy[1,2]	-	-	97%	93%
ICU Venous Thromboembolism Prophylaxis[2]	12	100%	92%	92%
Incidence of Potentially Preventable VTE[1,2]	-	-	7%	10%
UFH with Dosages/Platelet Monitoring[1,2]	-	-	91%	97%
Venous Thromboembolism Prophylaxis[2]	106	100%	87%	85%
Warfarin Therapy Discharge Instructions[1,2]	-	-	77%	75%
Chest Pain/Possible Heart Attack Care				
Aspirin Given Within 24 Hours of Arrival[5]	-	-	97%	96%
Fibrinolytic Meds Within 30 Min. of Arrival[5]	-	-	73%	58%
Average Time to ECG (minutes)[5]	-	-	7	7
Average Time to Transfer (minutes)[5]	-	-	55	60
Children's Asthma Care				
Received Home Management Plan of Care	-	-	-	88%
Received Reliever Medication	-	-	-	100%
Received Systemic Corticosteroids	-	-	-	100%
Emergency Department				
Admittance Decision Time (minutes)[2,7]	-	-	119	98
Head CT Results Within 45 Min. of Arrival[5]	-	-	70%	57%
Patients Who Left ER Before Being Seen[5]	-	-	2%	2%
Time from ER Arrival to Admit. (minutes)[2,7]	-	-	313	274
Time from ER Arrival to Discharge (minutes)[5]	-	-	156	134
Time in ER Before Being Evaluated (minutes)[5]	-	-	36	26
Time to Pain Meds for Fractures (minutes)[5]	-	-	59	57
Heart Attack Care				
Aspirin Given at Discharge[3,7]	-	-	100%	99%
Fibrinolytic Meds Within 30 Min. of Arrival[3,7]	-	-	100%	54%
PCI Within 90 Minutes of Arrival[3,7]	-	-	96%	96%
Statin Prescribed at Discharge[3,7]	-	-	99%	98%
Heart Failure Care				
ACE Inhibitor or ARB for LVSD[1]	-	-	96%	97%
Discharge Instructions Given	15	100%	95%	94%
Evaluation of LVS Function	22	100%	100%	99%
Medicare Spending				
Medicare Spending per Patient (ratio)	-	1.01	1.03	0.98
Pneumonia Care				
Appropriate Initial Antibiotic Given	12	92%	97%	95%
Blood Culture Timing[1]	-	-	98%	98%
Pregnancy and Delivery Care				
Newborn Deliveries Scheduled Early[7]	-	-	2%	6%
Preventive Care				
Immunization for Influenza[2]	621	90%	91%	90%
Immunization for Pneumonia[2]	775	84%	91%	92%
Stroke Care				
Anticoagulation Therapy for Atrial Fibrillation[3,7]	-	-	97%	95%
Antithrombotic Therapy Timing[1,3]	-	-	98%	98%
Assessed for Rehabilitation[1,3]	-	-	96%	97%
Discharged on Antithrombotic Therapy[1,3]	-	-	100%	99%
Discharged on Statin Medication[1,3]	-	-	96%	94%
Thrombolytic Therapy Timing[3,7]	-	-	68%	66%
Venous Thromboembolism Prophylaxis[1,3]	-	-	94%	94%
Written Stroke Educational Materials Given[3,7]	-	-	82%	88%
Surgical Care Improvement Project				
Appropriate Beta Blocker Usage[2]	322	100%	98%	98%
Appropriate VTP Within 24 Hours[2]	1,156	98%	99%	98%
Controlled Postoperative Blood Glucose[2,7]	-	-	96%	97%
Perioperative Temperature Management[2]	1,305	100%	100%	100%
Prophylactic Antibiotic Selection[2]	1,186	99%	99%	99%
Prophylactic Antibiotic Selection (Outpatient)	588	99%	98%	98%
Prophylactic Antibiotic Stopped[2]	1,185	98%	99%	98%
Prophylactic Antibiotic Timing[2]	1,186	99%	99%	99%
Prophylactic Antibiotic Timing (Outpatient)	588	99%	98%	98%
Urinary Catheter Removal[2]	723	99%	97%	97%
Survey of Patients' Hospital Experiences				
Area Around Room 'Always' Quiet at Night	300+	53%	52%	61%
Doctors 'Always' Communicated Well	300+	85%	80%	82%
Home Recovery Information Given	300+	95%	87%	85%
Hospital Given 9 or 10 on 10 Point Scale	300+	86%	69%	71%
Meds 'Always' Explained Before Given	300+	67%	64%	64%
Nurses 'Always' Communicated Well	300+	87%	79%	79%
Pain 'Always' Well Controlled	300+	75%	71%	71%
Room and Bathroom 'Always' Clean	300+	81%	72%	73%
Timely Help 'Always' Received	300+	72%	66%	68%
Would Definitely Recommend Hospital	300+	91%	73%	71%
Use of Medical Imaging				
Cardiac Imaging Stress Test before Surgery	84	3.6%	5.4%	5.3%
Combination Abdominal CT Scan	201	7.0%	6.3%	10.5%
Combination Brain/Sinus CT Scan[1]	-	-	2.4%	2.7%
Combination Chest CT Scan	241	2.1%	0.5%	2.7%
Follow-up Mammogram/Ultrasound[7]	-	-	8.9%	8.8%
Lumbar Spine MRI for Low Back Pain	303	34.0%	35.3%	37.2%

Tufts Medical Center

800 Washington Street
Boston, MA 02111
Phone: 617-636-5000
Fax: 617-636-4658
URL: www.tuftsmedicalcenter.org
Type: Acute Care Hospitals
Emergency Services: Yes
Ownership: Voluntary non-profit - Private
Beds: 515

Key Personnel:

Emergency Room . . . . Brien Barnewolt, MD
Quality Assurance . . . . Susan Fletcher
Pediatric Ambulatory Care . . . . . . John Schreiber
Infection Control. . . . . David Syndeman, MD
Intensive Care Unit. . . . . Chris Veary, RN
CEO/President. . . . . Michael Wagner, MD
Chief of Medical Staff. . . . . Saul Weingart, MD, PhD
Radiology. . . . . Kent Yusel, MD

Measure	Cases	This Hosp.	State Avg.	U.S. Avg.
Blood Clot Prevention and Treatment				
Anticoagulation Overlap Therapy[2]	94	96%	97%	93%
ICU Venous Thromboembolism Prophylaxis[2]	206	91%	92%	92%
Incidence of Potentially Preventable VTE[2]	45	9%	7%	10%
UFH with Dosages/Platelet Monitoring[2]	97	100%	91%	97%
Venous Thromboembolism Prophylaxis[2]	288	76%	87%	85%
Warfarin Therapy Discharge Instructions[2]	69	1%	77%	75%
Chest Pain/Possible Heart Attack Care				
Aspirin Given Within 24 Hours of Arrival[5]	-	-	97%	96%
Fibrinolytic Meds Within 30 Min. of Arrival[5]	-	-	73%	58%
Average Time to ECG (minutes)[5]	-	-	7	7
Average Time to Transfer (minutes)[5]	-	-	55	60
Children's Asthma Care				
Received Home Management Plan of Care	-	-	-	88%
Received Reliever Medication	-	-	-	100%
Received Systemic Corticosteroids	-	-	-	100%
Emergency Department				
Admittance Decision Time (minutes)[2]	362	148	119	98
Head CT Results Within 45 Min. of Arrival[3,7]	-	-	70%	57%
Patients Who Left ER Before Being Seen	41,763	1%	2%	2%
Time from ER Arrival to Admit. (minutes)[2]	362	348	313	274
Time from ER Arrival to Discharge (minutes)	354	164	156	134
Time in ER Before Being Evaluated (minutes)	401	34	36	26
Time to Pain Meds for Fractures (minutes)	63	47	59	57
Heart Attack Care				
Aspirin Given at Discharge	364	100%	100%	99%
Fibrinolytic Meds Within 30 Min. of Arrival[7]	-	-	100%	54%
PCI Within 90 Minutes of Arrival	13	92%	96%	96%
Statin Prescribed at Discharge	355	100%	99%	98%
Heart Failure Care				
ACE Inhibitor or ARB for LVSD	159	99%	96%	97%
Discharge Instructions Given	287	98%	95%	94%
Evaluation of LVS Function	352	100%	100%	99%
Medicare Spending				
Medicare Spending per Patient (ratio)	-	1.04	1.03	0.98
Pneumonia Care				
Appropriate Initial Antibiotic Given	66	98%	97%	95%
Blood Culture Timing	154	96%	98%	98%
Pregnancy and Delivery Care				
Newborn Deliveries Scheduled Early[1,2]	-	-	2%	6%
Preventive Care				
Immunization for Influenza[2]	542	95%	91%	90%
Immunization for Pneumonia[2]	554	94%	91%	92%
Stroke Care				
Anticoagulation Therapy for Atrial Fibrillation	15	93%	97%	95%
Antithrombotic Therapy Timing	97	98%	98%	98%
Assessed for Rehabilitation	192	92%	96%	97%
Discharged on Antithrombotic Therapy	111	100%	100%	99%
Discharged on Statin Medication	94	100%	96%	94%
Thrombolytic Therapy Timing[1]	-	-	68%	66%
Venous Thromboembolism Prophylaxis	200	96%	94%	94%
Written Stroke Educational Materials Given	86	22%	82%	88%
Surgical Care Improvement Project				
Appropriate Beta Blocker Usage[2]	374	99%	98%	98%
Appropriate VTP Within 24 Hours[2]	387	99%	99%	98%
Controlled Postoperative Blood Glucose[2]	287	97%	96%	97%
Perioperative Temperature Management[2]	543	100%	100%	100%
Prophylactic Antibiotic Selection[2]	628	100%	99%	99%
Prophylactic Antibiotic Selection (Outpatient)	202	100%	98%	98%
Prophylactic Antibiotic Stopped[2]	614	100%	99%	98%
Prophylactic Antibiotic Timing[2]	630	98%	99%	99%
Prophylactic Antibiotic Timing (Outpatient)	108	100%	98%	98%
Urinary Catheter Removal[2]	495	97%	97%	97%
Survey of Patients' Hospital Experiences				
Area Around Room 'Always' Quiet at Night	300+	55%	52%	61%
Doctors 'Always' Communicated Well	300+	80%	80%	82%
Home Recovery Information Given	300+	90%	87%	85%
Hospital Given 9 or 10 on 10 Point Scale	300+	72%	69%	71%
Meds 'Always' Explained Before Given	300+	67%	64%	64%
Nurses 'Always' Communicated Well	300+	80%	79%	79%
Pain 'Always' Well Controlled	300+	70%	71%	71%
Room and Bathroom 'Always' Clean	300+	69%	72%	73%
Timely Help 'Always' Received	300+	63%	66%	68%
Would Definitely Recommend Hospital	300+	76%	73%	71%
Use of Medical Imaging				
Cardiac Imaging Stress Test before Surgery	382	7.1%	5.4%	5.3%

NOTE: Hospital profiles are in alphabetical order by state, then city, then hospital within the city; Rankings exclude hospitals with less than 25 cases except for patient surveys which excludes hospitals with less than 100 cases; (a) 100-299 cases; (1) The number of cases/patients is too few to report; (2) Data submitted were based on a sample of cases/patients; (3) Results are based on a shorter time period than required; (4) Data suppressed by CMS for one or more quarters; (5) Results are not available for this reporting period; (6) Fewer than 100 patients completed the HCAHPS survey; (7) No cases met the criteria for this measure; (8) The lower limit of the confidence interval cannot be calculated if the number of observed infections equals zero; (9) No data are available from the state/territory for this reporting period; (10) The scores shown reflect fewer than 50 completed surveys; (11) There were discrepancies in the data collection process; (12) This measure does not apply to this hospital for this reporting period; (13) Results cannot be calculated for this reporting period; (14) The results for this state are combined with nearby states to protect confidentiality; Please refer to the User's Guide for a full explanation of data.

Combination Abdominal CT Scan	747	3.7%	6.3%	10.5%
Combination Brain/Sinus CT Scan[1]	-	-	2.4%	2.7%
Combination Chest CT Scan	1,040	0.1%	0.5%	2.7%
Follow-up Mammogram/Ultrasound	1,191	2.2%	8.9%	8.8%
Lumbar Spine MRI for Low Back Pain	106	47.2%	35.3%	37.2%

Saint Elizabeth's Medical Center

736 Cambridge Street
Brighton, MA 02135
Phone: 617-789-3000
Fax: 617-789-2438
E-mail: semcmail@cchcs.org
URL: www.semc.org
Type: Acute Care Hospitals
Emergency Services: Yes
Ownership: Proprietary
Beds: 317

Key Personnel:
Infection Control. . . . . Christine Duffy, RN
CEO/President. . . . . Kevin Hannifan
Operating Room. . . . . Carol Hinar
Radiology. . . . . R Eugene Langevin, Jr, DM
Quality Assurance . . . . Barbara Lightizer
Chief of Medical Staff. . . . . John O Pastore, MD
Pediatric Ambulatory Care . . . . . . Ronald Pye, MD
Pediatric In-Patient Care . . . . Ronald Pye, MD

Measure	Cases	This Hosp.	State Avg.	U.S. Avg.
Blood Clot Prevention and Treatment				
Anticoagulation Overlap Therapy[2]	53	100%	97%	93%
ICU Venous Thromboembolism Prophylaxis[2]	83	89%	92%	92%
Incidence of Potentially Preventable VTE[1,2]	-	-	7%	10%
UFH with Dosages/Platelet Monitoring[2]	58	98%	91%	97%
Venous Thromboembolism Prophylaxis[2]	269	78%	87%	85%
Warfarin Therapy Discharge Instructions[2]	41	95%	77%	75%
Chest Pain/Possible Heart Attack Care				
Aspirin Given Within 24 Hours of Arrival[3,7]	-	-	97%	96%
Fibrinolytic Meds Within 30 Min. of Arrival[5]	-	-	73%	58%
Average Time to ECG (minutes)[3,7]	-	-	7	7
Average Time to Transfer (minutes)[5]	-	-	55	60
Children's Asthma Care				
Received Home Management Plan of Care	-	-	-	88%
Received Reliever Medication	-	-	-	100%
Received Systemic Corticosteroids	-	-	-	100%
Emergency Department				
Admittance Decision Time (minutes)[2]	402	173	119	98
Head CT Results Within 45 Min. of Arrival[1]	-	-	70%	57%
Patients Who Left ER Before Being Seen	37,175	1%	2%	2%
Time from ER Arrival to Admit. (minutes)[2]	403	331	313	274
Time from ER Arrival to Discharge (minutes)	367	148	156	134
Time in ER Before Being Evaluated (minutes)	370	39	36	26
Time to Pain Meds for Fractures (minutes)	43	78	59	57
Heart Attack Care				
Aspirin Given at Discharge	335	99%	100%	99%
Fibrinolytic Meds Within 30 Min. of Arrival[7]	-	-	100%	54%
PCI Within 90 Minutes of Arrival	19	84%	96%	96%
Statin Prescribed at Discharge	326	97%	99%	98%
Heart Failure Care				
ACE Inhibitor or ARB for LVSD	91	92%	96%	97%
Discharge Instructions Given	190	94%	95%	94%
Evaluation of LVS Function	280	100%	100%	99%
Medicare Spending				
Medicare Spending per Patient (ratio)	-	1.05	1.03	0.98
Pneumonia Care				
Appropriate Initial Antibiotic Given	71	99%	97%	95%
Blood Culture Timing	108	97%	98%	98%
Pregnancy and Delivery Care				
Newborn Deliveries Scheduled Early	47	6%	2%	6%
Preventive Care				
Immunization for Influenza[2]	553	76%	91%	90%
Immunization for Pneumonia[2]	656	86%	91%	92%
Stroke Care				
Anticoagulation Therapy for Atrial Fibrillation[1]	-	-	97%	95%
Antithrombotic Therapy Timing	59	86%	98%	98%
Assessed for Rehabilitation	77	94%	96%	97%
Discharged on Antithrombotic Therapy	68	100%	100%	99%
Discharged on Statin Medication	58	90%	96%	94%
Thrombolytic Therapy Timing[1]	-	-	68%	66%
Venous Thromboembolism Prophylaxis	75	93%	94%	94%
Written Stroke Educational Materials Given	35	77%	82%	88%
Surgical Care Improvement Project				
Appropriate Beta Blocker Usage[2]	390	98%	98%	98%
Appropriate VTP Within 24 Hours[2]	254	99%	99%	98%
Controlled Postoperative Blood Glucose[2]	336	91%	96%	97%
Perioperative Temperature Management[2]	432	100%	100%	100%
Prophylactic Antibiotic Selection[2]	567	99%	99%	99%
Prophylactic Antibiotic Selection (Outpatient)	176	99%	98%	98%
Prophylactic Antibiotic Stopped[2]	551	96%	99%	98%
Prophylactic Antibiotic Timing[2]	569	99%	99%	99%
Prophylactic Antibiotic Timing (Outpatient)	178	95%	98%	98%
Urinary Catheter Removal[2]	454	99%	97%	97%
Survey of Patients' Hospital Experiences				
Area Around Room 'Always' Quiet at Night	300+	49%	52%	61%
Doctors 'Always' Communicated Well	300+	80%	80%	82%
Home Recovery Information Given	300+	85%	87%	85%
Hospital Given 9 or 10 on 10 Point Scale	300+	64%	69%	71%
Meds 'Always' Explained Before Given	300+	63%	64%	64%
Nurses 'Always' Communicated Well	300+	76%	79%	79%
Pain 'Always' Well Controlled	300+	67%	71%	71%
Room and Bathroom 'Always' Clean	300+	65%	72%	73%
Timely Help 'Always' Received	300+	59%	66%	68%
Would Definitely Recommend Hospital	300+	69%	73%	71%
Use of Medical Imaging				
Cardiac Imaging Stress Test before Surgery	323	4.0%	5.4%	5.3%
Combination Abdominal CT Scan	667	11.2%	6.3%	10.5%
Combination Brain/Sinus CT Scan	369	1.1%	2.4%	2.7%
Combination Chest CT Scan	607	0.0%	0.5%	2.7%
Follow-up Mammogram/Ultrasound	1,396	8.0%	8.9%	8.8%
Lumbar Spine MRI for Low Back Pain	107	38.3%	35.3%	37.2%

Good Samaritan Medical Center

235 North Pearl Street
Brockton, MA 02301
Phone: 508-427-3000
URL: www.goodsamaritanmedical.org
Type: Acute Care Hospitals
Emergency Services: Yes
Ownership: Proprietary

Key Personnel:
President . . . . John A Jurczyk, FACHE

Measure	Cases	This Hosp.	State Avg.	U.S. Avg.
Blood Clot Prevention and Treatment				
Anticoagulation Overlap Therapy[2]	101	99%	97%	93%
ICU Venous Thromboembolism Prophylaxis[2]	52	96%	92%	92%
Incidence of Potentially Preventable VTE[1,2]	-	-	7%	10%
UFH with Dosages/Platelet Monitoring[2]	47	100%	91%	97%
Venous Thromboembolism Prophylaxis[2]	351	89%	87%	85%
Warfarin Therapy Discharge Instructions[2]	79	97%	77%	75%
Chest Pain/Possible Heart Attack Care				
Aspirin Given Within 24 Hours of Arrival	29	97%	97%	96%
Fibrinolytic Meds Within 30 Min. of Arrival[3,7]	-	-	73%	58%
Average Time to ECG (minutes)	33	1	7	7
Average Time to Transfer (minutes)[1,3]	-	-	55	60
Children's Asthma Care				
Received Home Management Plan of Care	-	-	-	88%
Received Reliever Medication	-	-	-	100%
Received Systemic Corticosteroids	-	-	-	100%
Emergency Department				
Admittance Decision Time (minutes)[2]	904	119	119	98
Head CT Results Within 45 Min. of Arrival	25	92%	70%	57%
Patients Who Left ER Before Being Seen	55,682	3%	2%	2%
Time from ER Arrival to Admit. (minutes)[2]	908	340	313	274
Time from ER Arrival to Discharge (minutes)	339	212	156	134
Time in ER Before Being Evaluated (minutes)	352	66	36	26
Time to Pain Meds for Fractures (minutes)	102	77	59	57
Heart Attack Care				
Aspirin Given at Discharge	154	100%	100%	99%
Fibrinolytic Meds Within 30 Min. of Arrival[7]	-	-	100%	54%
PCI Within 90 Minutes of Arrival	42	93%	96%	96%
Statin Prescribed at Discharge	147	97%	99%	98%
Heart Failure Care				
ACE Inhibitor or ARB for LVSD	141	94%	96%	97%
Discharge Instructions Given	315	94%	95%	94%
Evaluation of LVS Function	475	100%	100%	99%
Medicare Spending				
Medicare Spending per Patient (ratio)	-	1.06	1.03	0.98
Pneumonia Care				
Appropriate Initial Antibiotic Given	228	98%	97%	95%
Blood Culture Timing	185	99%	98%	98%
Pregnancy and Delivery Care				
Newborn Deliveries Scheduled Early	77	0%	2%	6%
Preventive Care				
Immunization for Influenza[2]	617	94%	91%	90%
Immunization for Pneumonia[2]	774	94%	91%	92%
Stroke Care				
Anticoagulation Therapy for Atrial Fibrillation	14	93%	97%	95%
Antithrombotic Therapy Timing	95	96%	98%	98%
Assessed for Rehabilitation	91	91%	96%	97%
Discharged on Antithrombotic Therapy	88	98%	100%	99%
Discharged on Statin Medication	80	92%	96%	94%
Thrombolytic Therapy Timing[1]	-	-	68%	66%
Venous Thromboembolism Prophylaxis	97	89%	94%	94%
Written Stroke Educational Materials Given	49	98%	82%	88%
Surgical Care Improvement Project				
Appropriate Beta Blocker Usage[2]	199	97%	98%	98%
Appropriate VTP Within 24 Hours[2]	521	99%	99%	98%
Controlled Postoperative Blood Glucose[2,7]	-	-	96%	97%
Perioperative Temperature Management[2]	693	100%	100%	100%
Prophylactic Antibiotic Selection[2]	528	98%	99%	99%
Prophylactic Antibiotic Selection (Outpatient)	203	98%	98%	98%
Prophylactic Antibiotic Stopped[2]	516	99%	99%	98%
Prophylactic Antibiotic Timing[2]	528	99%	99%	99%
Prophylactic Antibiotic Timing (Outpatient)	205	99%	98%	98%
Urinary Catheter Removal[2]	114	90%	97%	97%
Survey of Patients' Hospital Experiences				
Area Around Room 'Always' Quiet at Night	300+	44%	52%	61%
Doctors 'Always' Communicated Well	300+	74%	80%	82%
Home Recovery Information Given	300+	84%	87%	85%
Hospital Given 9 or 10 on 10 Point Scale	300+	57%	69%	71%
Meds 'Always' Explained Before Given	300+	57%	64%	64%
Nurses 'Always' Communicated Well	300+	74%	79%	79%
Pain 'Always' Well Controlled	300+	66%	71%	71%
Room and Bathroom 'Always' Clean	300+	60%	72%	73%
Timely Help 'Always' Received	300+	54%	66%	68%
Would Definitely Recommend Hospital	300+	61%	73%	71%
Use of Medical Imaging				
Cardiac Imaging Stress Test before Surgery	439	3.9%	5.4%	5.3%
Combination Abdominal CT Scan	1,129	5.6%	6.3%	10.5%
Combination Brain/Sinus CT Scan	911	3.0%	2.4%	2.7%
Combination Chest CT Scan	957	0.1%	0.5%	2.7%
Follow-up Mammogram/Ultrasound	2,075	12.0%	8.9%	8.8%
Lumbar Spine MRI for Low Back Pain	181	38.1%	35.3%	37.2%

Signature Healthcare Brockton Hospital

680 Center Street
Brockton, MA 02302
Phone: 508-941-7000
Fax: 508-941-6300
URL: www.brocktonhospital.com
Type: Acute Care Hospitals
Emergency Services: Yes
Ownership: Voluntary non-profit - Other
Beds: 245

Key Personnel:
CEO/President. . . . . Dr Goodman
Emergency Room . . . . Kate McMenon
Chief of Medical Staff. . . . . Burton J Polanski, MD

Measure	Cases	This Hosp.	State Avg.	U.S. Avg.
Blood Clot Prevention and Treatment				
Anticoagulation Overlap Therapy[2]	74	99%	97%	93%
ICU Venous Thromboembolism Prophylaxis[2]	71	99%	92%	92%
Incidence of Potentially Preventable VTE[1,2]	-	-	7%	10%
UFH with Dosages/Platelet Monitoring[2]	36	100%	91%	97%
Venous Thromboembolism Prophylaxis[2]	344	92%	87%	85%
Warfarin Therapy Discharge Instructions[2]	52	69%	77%	75%
Chest Pain/Possible Heart Attack Care				
Aspirin Given Within 24 Hours of Arrival	25	100%	97%	96%
Fibrinolytic Meds Within 30 Min. of Arrival[3,7]	-	-	73%	58%
Average Time to ECG (minutes)	29	4	7	7
Average Time to Transfer (minutes)[3,7]	-	-	55	60
Children's Asthma Care				

NOTE: Hospital profiles are in alphabetical order by state, then city, then hospital within the city; Rankings exclude hospitals with less than 25 cases except for patient surveys which excludes hospitals with less than 100 cases; (a) 100-299 cases; (1) The number of cases/patients is too few to report; (2) Data submitted were based on a sample of cases/patients; (3) Results are based on a shorter time period than required; (4) Data suppressed by CMS for one or more quarters; (5) Results are not available for this reporting period; (6) Fewer than 100 patients completed the HCAHPS survey; (7) No cases met the criteria for this measure; (8) The lower limit of the confidence interval cannot be calculated if the number of observed infections equals zero; (9) No data are available from the state/territory for this reporting period; (10) The scores shown reflect fewer than 50 completed surveys; (11) There were discrepancies in the data collection process; (12) This measure does not apply to this hospital for this reporting period; (13) Results cannot be calculated for this reporting period; (14) The results for this state are combined with nearby states to protect confidentiality; Please refer to the User's Guide for a full explanation of data.

Measure	Cases	This Hosp.	State Avg.	U.S. Avg.
Received Home Management Plan of Care	-	-	-	88%
Received Reliever Medication	-	-	-	100%
Received Systemic Corticosteroids	-	-	-	100%
Emergency Department				
Admittance Decision Time (minutes)[2]	488	160	119	98
Head CT Results Within 45 Min. of Arrival	12	58%	70%	57%
Patients Who Left ER Before Being Seen	62,520	2%	2%	2%
Time from ER Arrival to Admit. (minutes)[2]	488	337	313	274
Time from ER Arrival to Discharge (minutes)	290	161	156	134
Time in ER Before Being Evaluated (minutes)	398	42	36	26
Time to Pain Meds for Fractures (minutes)	115	45	59	57
Heart Attack Care				
Aspirin Given at Discharge	149	100%	100%	99%
Fibrinolytic Meds Within 30 Min. of Arrival[7]	-	-	100%	54%
PCI Within 90 Minutes of Arrival	57	98%	96%	96%
Statin Prescribed at Discharge	158	99%	99%	98%
Heart Failure Care				
ACE Inhibitor or ARB for LVSD	50	100%	96%	97%
Discharge Instructions Given	144	100%	95%	94%
Evaluation of LVS Function	190	100%	100%	99%
Medicare Spending				
Medicare Spending per Patient (ratio)	-	1.02	1.03	0.98
Pneumonia Care				
Appropriate Initial Antibiotic Given	138	100%	97%	95%
Blood Culture Timing	105	100%	98%	98%
Pregnancy and Delivery Care				
Newborn Deliveries Scheduled Early	100	0%	2%	6%
Preventive Care				
Immunization for Influenza[2]	549	93%	91%	90%
Immunization for Pneumonia[2]	626	93%	91%	92%
Stroke Care				
Anticoagulation Therapy for Atrial Fibrillation	11	100%	97%	95%
Antithrombotic Therapy Timing	65	100%	98%	98%
Assessed for Rehabilitation	73	97%	96%	97%
Discharged on Antithrombotic Therapy	73	100%	100%	99%
Discharged on Statin Medication	71	97%	96%	94%
Thrombolytic Therapy Timing	12	100%	68%	66%
Venous Thromboembolism Prophylaxis	75	92%	94%	94%
Written Stroke Educational Materials Given	40	95%	82%	88%
Surgical Care Improvement Project				
Appropriate Beta Blocker Usage	116	98%	98%	98%
Appropriate VTP Within 24 Hours	311	100%	99%	98%
Controlled Postoperative Blood Glucose[7]	-	-	96%	97%
Perioperative Temperature Management	359	100%	100%	100%
Prophylactic Antibiotic Selection	249	100%	99%	99%
Prophylactic Antibiotic Selection (Outpatient)	42	100%	98%	98%
Prophylactic Antibiotic Stopped	243	100%	99%	98%
Prophylactic Antibiotic Timing	249	100%	99%	99%
Prophylactic Antibiotic Timing (Outpatient)	42	100%	98%	98%
Urinary Catheter Removal	77	97%	97%	97%
Survey of Patients' Hospital Experiences				
Area Around Room 'Always' Quiet at Night	300+	44%	52%	61%
Doctors 'Always' Communicated Well	300+	78%	80%	82%
Home Recovery Information Given	300+	87%	87%	85%
Hospital Given 9 or 10 on 10 Point Scale	300+	63%	69%	71%
Meds 'Always' Explained Before Given	300+	67%	64%	64%
Nurses 'Always' Communicated Well	300+	78%	79%	79%
Pain 'Always' Well Controlled	300+	72%	71%	71%
Room and Bathroom 'Always' Clean	300+	62%	72%	73%
Timely Help 'Always' Received	300+	68%	66%	68%
Would Definitely Recommend Hospital	300+	65%	73%	71%
Use of Medical Imaging				
Cardiac Imaging Stress Test before Surgery	252	6.3%	5.4%	5.3%
Combination Abdominal CT Scan	839	4.4%	6.3%	10.5%
Combination Brain/Sinus CT Scan	742	3.2%	2.4%	2.7%
Combination Chest CT Scan	519	0.0%	0.5%	2.7%
Follow-up Mammogram/Ultrasound	1,098	5.6%	8.9%	8.8%
Lumbar Spine MRI for Low Back Pain	155	35.5%	35.3%	37.2%

Lahey Hospital & Medical Center - Burlington

41 & 45 Mall Road Phone: 781-744-5100
Burlington, MA 01803 Fax: 781-744-8920
URL: www.lahey.org
Type: Acute Care Hospitals Emergency Services: Yes
Ownership: Voluntary non-profit - Private Beds: 317

Key Personnel:

Emergency Room . . . . Jean Brown
Patient Relations . . . . Roger J Cameron
Radiology. . . . . Anna Chacko, MD
CEO/President. . . . . Joanne Conroy, MD
Anesthesiology. . . . . Micheal Entrup, MD
Quality Assurance . . . . Joseph M Healy, PhD
Operating Room. . . . . Roger L Jenkins, MD
Pediatric In-Patient Care . . . . Claire Wilson, MD

Measure	Cases	This Hosp.	State Avg.	U.S. Avg.
Blood Clot Prevention and Treatment				
Anticoagulation Overlap Therapy[2]	165	99%	97%	93%
ICU Venous Thromboembolism Prophylaxis[2]	69	100%	92%	92%
Incidence of Potentially Preventable VTE[2]	58	3%	7%	10%
UFH with Dosages/Platelet Monitoring[2]	132	100%	91%	97%
Venous Thromboembolism Prophylaxis[2]	351	90%	87%	85%
Warfarin Therapy Discharge Instructions[2]	112	71%	77%	75%
Chest Pain/Possible Heart Attack Care				
Aspirin Given Within 24 Hours of Arrival[5]	-	-	97%	96%
Fibrinolytic Meds Within 30 Min. of Arrival[5]	-	-	73%	58%
Average Time to ECG (minutes)[5]	-	-	7	7
Average Time to Transfer (minutes)[5]	-	-	55	60
Children's Asthma Care				
Received Home Management Plan of Care	-	-	-	88%
Received Reliever Medication	-	-	-	100%
Received Systemic Corticosteroids	-	-	-	100%
Emergency Department				
Admittance Decision Time (minutes)[2]	534	84	119	98
Head CT Results Within 45 Min. of Arrival[1,3]	-	-	70%	57%
Patients Who Left ER Before Being Seen	54,931	2%	2%	2%
Time from ER Arrival to Admit. (minutes)[2]	587	323	313	274
Time from ER Arrival to Discharge (minutes)	351	145	156	134
Time in ER Before Being Evaluated (minutes)	353	47	36	26
Time to Pain Meds for Fractures (minutes)	69	70	59	57
Heart Attack Care				
Aspirin Given at Discharge	575	99%	100%	99%
Fibrinolytic Meds Within 30 Min. of Arrival[7]	-	-	100%	54%
PCI Within 90 Minutes of Arrival	64	98%	96%	96%
Statin Prescribed at Discharge	565	99%	99%	98%
Heart Failure Care				
ACE Inhibitor or ARB for LVSD[2]	48	94%	96%	97%
Discharge Instructions Given[2]	205	100%	95%	94%
Evaluation of LVS Function[2]	278	100%	100%	99%
Medicare Spending				
Medicare Spending per Patient (ratio)	-	1.02	1.03	0.98
Pneumonia Care				
Appropriate Initial Antibiotic Given[2]	51	100%	97%	95%
Blood Culture Timing[2]	88	98%	98%	98%
Pregnancy and Delivery Care				
Newborn Deliveries Scheduled Early[7]	-	-	2%	6%
Preventive Care				
Immunization for Influenza[2]	585	91%	91%	90%
Immunization for Pneumonia[2]	845	91%	91%	92%
Stroke Care				
Anticoagulation Therapy for Atrial Fibrillation[2]	16	88%	97%	95%
Antithrombotic Therapy Timing[2]	66	95%	98%	98%
Assessed for Rehabilitation[2]	101	95%	96%	97%
Discharged on Antithrombotic Therapy[2]	78	100%	100%	99%
Discharged on Statin Medication[2]	63	94%	96%	94%
Thrombolytic Therapy Timing[1,2]	-	-	68%	66%
Venous Thromboembolism Prophylaxis[2]	107	98%	94%	94%
Written Stroke Educational Materials Given[2]	51	65%	82%	88%
Surgical Care Improvement Project				
Appropriate Beta Blocker Usage[2]	255	100%	98%	98%
Appropriate VTP Within 24 Hours[2]	338	100%	99%	98%
Controlled Postoperative Blood Glucose[2]	131	98%	96%	97%
Perioperative Temperature Management[2]	477	100%	100%	100%
Prophylactic Antibiotic Selection[2]	408	100%	99%	99%
Prophylactic Antibiotic Selection (Outpatient)	719	99%	98%	98%
Prophylactic Antibiotic Stopped[2]	392	98%	99%	98%
Prophylactic Antibiotic Timing[2]	408	99%	99%	99%
Prophylactic Antibiotic Timing (Outpatient)	427	99%	98%	98%
Urinary Catheter Removal[2]	209	100%	97%	97%
Survey of Patients' Hospital Experiences				
Area Around Room 'Always' Quiet at Night	300+	48%	52%	61%
Doctors 'Always' Communicated Well	300+	80%	80%	82%
Home Recovery Information Given	300+	88%	87%	85%
Hospital Given 9 or 10 on 10 Point Scale	300+	79%	69%	71%
Meds 'Always' Explained Before Given	300+	63%	64%	64%
Nurses 'Always' Communicated Well	300+	81%	79%	79%
Pain 'Always' Well Controlled	300+	73%	71%	71%
Room and Bathroom 'Always' Clean	300+	72%	72%	73%
Timely Help 'Always' Received	300+	64%	66%	68%
Would Definitely Recommend Hospital	300+	81%	73%	71%
Use of Medical Imaging				
Cardiac Imaging Stress Test before Surgery	1,714	5.8%	5.4%	5.3%
Combination Abdominal CT Scan	2,728	13.8%	6.3%	10.5%
Combination Brain/Sinus CT Scan	1,546	2.3%	2.4%	2.7%
Combination Chest CT Scan	2,982	0.0%	0.5%	2.7%
Follow-up Mammogram/Ultrasound	6,128	9.0%	8.9%	8.8%
Lumbar Spine MRI for Low Back Pain	462	34.0%	35.3%	37.2%

Cambridge Health Alliance

1493 Cambridge Street Phone: 617-665-2300
Cambridge, MA 02138 Fax: 617-665-3545
Type: Acute Care Hospitals Emergency Services: Yes
Ownership: Government - Local Beds: 270

Key Personnel:

Pediatrics. . . . . Greg Hagan, MD
Radiology. . . . . Carol Hulka, MD
Anesthesiology. . . . . Ron Minter, MD
Chief of Medical Staff . . . . Assaad Sayah, MD
Surgery . . . . Steven Schwaitzberg, MD
CEO/President. . . . . Patrick Wardell
Emergency Room . . . . Thomas Workman

Measure	Cases	This Hosp.	State Avg.	U.S. Avg.
Blood Clot Prevention and Treatment				
Anticoagulation Overlap Therapy[2]	61	100%	97%	93%
ICU Venous Thromboembolism Prophylaxis[2]	62	89%	92%	92%
Incidence of Potentially Preventable VTE[2]	20	5%	7%	10%
UFH with Dosages/Platelet Monitoring[2]	55	100%	91%	97%
Venous Thromboembolism Prophylaxis[2]	313	88%	87%	85%
Warfarin Therapy Discharge Instructions[2]	49	82%	77%	75%
Chest Pain/Possible Heart Attack Care				
Aspirin Given Within 24 Hours of Arrival	85	100%	97%	96%
Fibrinolytic Meds Within 30 Min. of Arrival[7]	-	-	73%	58%
Average Time to ECG (minutes)	90	9	7	7
Average Time to Transfer (minutes)	23	62	55	60
Children's Asthma Care				
Received Home Management Plan of Care	-	-	-	88%
Received Reliever Medication	-	-	-	100%
Received Systemic Corticosteroids	-	-	-	100%
Emergency Department				
Admittance Decision Time (minutes)[2]	716	94	119	98
Head CT Results Within 45 Min. of Arrival[1]	-	-	70%	57%
Patients Who Left ER Before Being Seen	96,953	0%	2%	2%
Time from ER Arrival to Admit. (minutes)[2]	725	283	313	274
Time from ER Arrival to Discharge (minutes)	414	100	156	134
Time in ER Before Being Evaluated (minutes)	457	13	36	26
Time to Pain Meds for Fractures (minutes)	110	44	59	57
Heart Attack Care				
Aspirin Given at Discharge	25	96%	100%	99%
Fibrinolytic Meds Within 30 Min. of Arrival[7]	-	-	100%	54%
PCI Within 90 Minutes of Arrival[7]	-	-	96%	96%
Statin Prescribed at Discharge	26	96%	99%	98%
Heart Failure Care				
ACE Inhibitor or ARB for LVSD	47	94%	96%	97%
Discharge Instructions Given	185	91%	95%	94%
Evaluation of LVS Function	237	99%	100%	99%
Medicare Spending				
Medicare Spending per Patient (ratio)	-	1.06	1.03	0.98
Pneumonia Care				

NOTE: Hospital profiles are in alphabetical order by state, then city, then hospital within the city; Rankings exclude hospitals with less than 25 cases except for patient surveys which excludes hospitals with less than 100 cases; (a) 100-299 cases; (1) The number of cases/patients is too few to report; (2) Data submitted were based on a sample of cases/patients; (3) Results are based on a shorter time period than required; (4) Data suppressed by CMS for one or more quarters; (5) Results are not available for this reporting period; (6) Fewer than 100 patients completed the HCAHPS survey; (7) No cases met the criteria for this measure; (8) The lower limit of the confidence interval cannot be calculated if the number of observed infections equals zero; (9) No data are available from the state/territory for this reporting period; (10) The scores shown reflect fewer than 50 completed surveys; (11) There were discrepancies in the data collection process; (12) This measure does not apply to this hospital for this reporting period; (13) Results cannot be calculated for this reporting period; (14) The results for this state are combined with nearby states to protect confidentiality; Please refer to the User's Guide for a full explanation of data.

Appropriate Initial Antibiotic Given	197	95%	97%	95%
Blood Culture Timing	327	97%	98%	98%
Pregnancy and Delivery Care				
Newborn Deliveries Scheduled Early[2]	34	3%	2%	6%
Preventive Care				
Immunization for Influenza[2]	507	92%	91%	90%
Immunization for Pneumonia[2]	566	89%	91%	92%
Stroke Care				
Anticoagulation Therapy for Atrial Fibrillation[1]	-	-	97%	95%
Antithrombotic Therapy Timing	50	98%	98%	98%
Assessed for Rehabilitation	50	84%	96%	97%
Discharged on Antithrombotic Therapy	49	94%	100%	99%
Discharged on Statin Medication	43	93%	96%	94%
Thrombolytic Therapy Timing[1]	-	-	68%	66%
Venous Thromboembolism Prophylaxis	52	92%	94%	94%
Written Stroke Educational Materials Given	33	64%	82%	88%
Surgical Care Improvement Project				
Appropriate Beta Blocker Usage[2]	36	92%	98%	98%
Appropriate VTP Within 24 Hours[2]	156	99%	99%	98%
Controlled Postoperative Blood Glucose[2,7]	-	-	96%	97%
Perioperative Temperature Management[2]	188	100%	100%	100%
Prophylactic Antibiotic Selection[2]	100	98%	99%	99%
Prophylactic Antibiotic Selection (Outpatient)	184	98%	98%	98%
Prophylactic Antibiotic Stopped[2]	99	93%	99%	98%
Prophylactic Antibiotic Timing[2]	100	98%	99%	99%
Prophylactic Antibiotic Timing (Outpatient)	67	97%	98%	98%
Urinary Catheter Removal[2]	103	92%	97%	97%
Survey of Patients' Hospital Experiences				
Area Around Room 'Always' Quiet at Night	300+	56%	52%	61%
Doctors 'Always' Communicated Well	300+	81%	80%	82%
Home Recovery Information Given	300+	87%	87%	85%
Hospital Given 9 or 10 on 10 Point Scale	300+	63%	69%	71%
Meds 'Always' Explained Before Given	300+	61%	64%	64%
Nurses 'Always' Communicated Well	300+	76%	79%	79%
Pain 'Always' Well Controlled	300+	67%	71%	71%
Room and Bathroom 'Always' Clean	300+	70%	72%	73%
Timely Help 'Always' Received	300+	60%	66%	68%
Would Definitely Recommend Hospital	300+	64%	73%	71%
Use of Medical Imaging				
Cardiac Imaging Stress Test before Surgery	262	5.0%	5.4%	5.3%
Combination Abdominal CT Scan	625	5.3%	6.3%	10.5%
Combination Brain/Sinus CT Scan[1]	-	-	2.4%	2.7%
Combination Chest CT Scan	346	0.0%	0.5%	2.7%
Follow-up Mammogram/Ultrasound	1,385	7.0%	8.9%	8.8%
Lumbar Spine MRI for Low Back Pain	93	34.4%	35.3%	37.2%

Mount Auburn Hospital

330 Mount Auburn Street
Cambridge, MA 02138
Phone: 617-492-3500
Fax: 617-499-5168
URL: www.mountauburnhospital.org
Type: Acute Care Hospitals
Emergency Services: Yes
Ownership: Voluntary non-profit - Private
Beds: 183

Key Personnel:

Operating Room. . . . . Frederick F Bartlett
CEO/President. . . . . Jeanette Clough
Radiology. . . . . Madeline S Crivello, MD
Emergency Room . . . . Jeanne Donvon
Cardiac Laboratory. . . . . Spanley Forwand, MD
Pediatric In-Patient Care . . . . . . David A Link
Quality Assurance . . . . Janet Long
Chief of Medical Staff. . . . . Ryan Sullivan, MD

Measure	Cases	This Hosp.	State Avg.	U.S. Avg.
Blood Clot Prevention and Treatment				
Anticoagulation Overlap Therapy[2]	55	100%	97%	93%
ICU Venous Thromboembolism Prophylaxis[2]	91	93%	92%	92%
Incidence of Potentially Preventable VTE[1,2]	-	-	7%	10%
UFH with Dosages/Platelet Monitoring[2]	49	100%	91%	97%
Venous Thromboembolism Prophylaxis[2]	348	89%	87%	85%
Warfarin Therapy Discharge Instructions[2]	44	2%	77%	75%
Chest Pain/Possible Heart Attack Care				
Aspirin Given Within 24 Hours of Arrival[5]	-	-	97%	96%
Fibrinolytic Meds Within 30 Min. of Arrival[5]	-	-	73%	58%
Average Time to ECG (minutes)[5]	-	-	7	7
Average Time to Transfer (minutes)[5]	-	-	55	60
Children's Asthma Care				
Received Home Management Plan of Care	-	-	-	88%
Received Reliever Medication	-	-	-	100%
Received Systemic Corticosteroids	-	-	-	100%
Emergency Department				
Admittance Decision Time (minutes)[2]	480	127	119	98
Head CT Results Within 45 Min. of Arrival[1,3]	-	-	70%	57%
Patients Who Left ER Before Being Seen	37,343	2%	2%	2%
Time from ER Arrival to Admit. (minutes)[2]	484	300	313	274
Time from ER Arrival to Discharge (minutes)	325	159	156	134
Time in ER Before Being Evaluated (minutes)	425	48	36	26
Time to Pain Meds for Fractures (minutes)	72	54	59	57
Heart Attack Care				
Aspirin Given at Discharge	213	100%	100%	99%
Fibrinolytic Meds Within 30 Min. of Arrival[7]	-	-	100%	54%
PCI Within 90 Minutes of Arrival	25	100%	96%	96%
Statin Prescribed at Discharge	205	100%	99%	98%
Heart Failure Care				
ACE Inhibitor or ARB for LVSD	82	99%	96%	97%
Discharge Instructions Given	202	100%	95%	94%
Evaluation of LVS Function	294	100%	100%	99%
Medicare Spending				
Medicare Spending per Patient (ratio)	-	1.06	1.03	0.98
Pneumonia Care				
Appropriate Initial Antibiotic Given	213	97%	97%	95%
Blood Culture Timing	250	100%	98%	98%
Pregnancy and Delivery Care				
Newborn Deliveries Scheduled Early[2]	38	0%	2%	6%
Preventive Care				
Immunization for Influenza[2]	526	91%	91%	90%
Immunization for Pneumonia[2]	586	93%	91%	92%
Stroke Care				
Anticoagulation Therapy for Atrial Fibrillation[1]	-	-	97%	95%
Antithrombotic Therapy Timing	87	100%	98%	98%
Assessed for Rehabilitation	115	96%	96%	97%
Discharged on Antithrombotic Therapy	100	100%	100%	99%
Discharged on Statin Medication	77	95%	96%	94%
Thrombolytic Therapy Timing[1]	-	-	68%	66%
Venous Thromboembolism Prophylaxis	109	94%	94%	94%
Written Stroke Educational Materials Given	61	70%	82%	88%
Surgical Care Improvement Project				
Appropriate Beta Blocker Usage	301	99%	98%	98%
Appropriate VTP Within 24 Hours	528	100%	99%	98%
Controlled Postoperative Blood Glucose	161	99%	96%	97%
Perioperative Temperature Management	623	100%	100%	100%
Prophylactic Antibiotic Selection	594	100%	99%	99%
Prophylactic Antibiotic Selection (Outpatient)	346	100%	98%	98%
Prophylactic Antibiotic Stopped	591	100%	99%	98%
Prophylactic Antibiotic Timing	594	99%	99%	99%
Prophylactic Antibiotic Timing (Outpatient)	347	100%	98%	98%
Urinary Catheter Removal	562	96%	97%	97%
Survey of Patients' Hospital Experiences				
Area Around Room 'Always' Quiet at Night	300+	66%	52%	61%
Doctors 'Always' Communicated Well	300+	84%	80%	82%
Home Recovery Information Given	300+	87%	87%	85%
Hospital Given 9 or 10 on 10 Point Scale	300+	78%	69%	71%
Meds 'Always' Explained Before Given	300+	64%	64%	64%
Nurses 'Always' Communicated Well	300+	82%	79%	79%
Pain 'Always' Well Controlled	300+	76%	71%	71%
Room and Bathroom 'Always' Clean	300+	76%	72%	73%
Timely Help 'Always' Received	300+	72%	66%	68%
Would Definitely Recommend Hospital	300+	84%	73%	71%
Use of Medical Imaging				
Cardiac Imaging Stress Test before Surgery	434	7.1%	5.4%	5.3%
Combination Abdominal CT Scan	881	14.9%	6.3%	10.5%
Combination Brain/Sinus CT Scan	752	1.6%	2.4%	2.7%
Combination Chest CT Scan	760	0.0%	0.5%	2.7%
Follow-up Mammogram/Ultrasound	2,390	9.0%	8.9%	8.8%
Lumbar Spine MRI for Low Back Pain	182	41.2%	35.3%	37.2%

Clinton Hospital Association

201 Highland Street
Clinton, MA 01510
Phone: 978-368-3000
Fax: 978-368-3766
URL: www.umassmemorial.org
Type: Acute Care Hospitals
Emergency Services: Yes
Ownership: Voluntary non-profit - Other
Beds: 781

Key Personnel:

CEO/President. . . . . Sheila Daly, RN, MS, CPHQ
Pediatric In-Patient Care . . . . Marianne Felice, MD
Radiology. . . . . JosephA Ferrucci, MD
Cardiac Laboratory. . . . . Daniel Fisher, MD, PhD
Chief of Medical Staff . . . . Cheryl Lapriore, MD
Infection Control. . . . . Lawrence Madoff, MD
Quality Assurance . . . . Karen Plainte, RN, MBA
Coronary Care . . . . Craig Smith, MD

Measure	Cases	This Hosp.	State Avg.	U.S. Avg.
Blood Clot Prevention and Treatment				
Anticoagulation Overlap Therapy[1,2]	-	-	97%	93%
ICU Venous Thromboembolism Prophylaxis[2,7]	-	-	92%	92%
Incidence of Potentially Preventable VTE[2,7]	-	-	7%	10%
UFH with Dosages/Platelet Monitoring[2,7]	-	-	91%	97%
Venous Thromboembolism Prophylaxis[2]	97	64%	87%	85%
Warfarin Therapy Discharge Instructions[2,7]	-	-	77%	75%
Chest Pain/Possible Heart Attack Care				
Aspirin Given Within 24 Hours of Arrival	24	100%	97%	96%
Fibrinolytic Meds Within 30 Min. of Arrival[7]	-	-	73%	58%
Average Time to ECG (minutes)	24	4	7	7
Average Time to Transfer (minutes)[1]	-	-	55	60
Children's Asthma Care				
Received Home Management Plan of Care	-	-	-	88%
Received Reliever Medication	-	-	-	100%
Received Systemic Corticosteroids	-	-	-	100%
Emergency Department				
Admittance Decision Time (minutes)[2]	243	40	119	98
Head CT Results Within 45 Min. of Arrival[1]	-	-	70%	57%
Patients Who Left ER Before Being Seen	13,486	2%	2%	2%
Time from ER Arrival to Admit. (minutes)[2]	295	215	313	274
Time from ER Arrival to Discharge (minutes)	344	110	156	134
Time in ER Before Being Evaluated (minutes)	379	25	36	26
Time to Pain Meds for Fractures (minutes)	38	56	59	57
Heart Attack Care				
Aspirin Given at Discharge[1,3]	-	-	100%	99%
Fibrinolytic Meds Within 30 Min. of Arrival[3,7]	-	-	100%	54%
PCI Within 90 Minutes of Arrival[3,7]	-	-	96%	96%
Statin Prescribed at Discharge[1,3]	-	-	99%	98%
Heart Failure Care				
ACE Inhibitor or ARB for LVSD[1]	-	-	96%	97%
Discharge Instructions Given	33	79%	95%	94%
Evaluation of LVS Function	35	94%	100%	99%
Medicare Spending				
Medicare Spending per Patient (ratio)	-	1.11	1.03	0.98
Pneumonia Care				
Appropriate Initial Antibiotic Given	24	92%	97%	95%
Blood Culture Timing	32	97%	98%	98%
Pregnancy and Delivery Care				
Newborn Deliveries Scheduled Early[7]	-	-	2%	6%
Preventive Care				
Immunization for Influenza[2]	285	82%	91%	90%
Immunization for Pneumonia[2]	482	70%	91%	92%
Stroke Care				
Anticoagulation Therapy for Atrial Fibrillation[3,7]	-	-	97%	95%
Antithrombotic Therapy Timing[1,3]	-	-	98%	98%
Assessed for Rehabilitation[1,3]	-	-	96%	97%
Discharged on Antithrombotic Therapy[1,3]	-	-	100%	99%
Discharged on Statin Medication[1,3]	-	-	96%	94%
Thrombolytic Therapy Timing[1,3]	-	-	68%	66%
Venous Thromboembolism Prophylaxis[1,3]	-	-	94%	94%
Written Stroke Educational Materials Given[3,7]	-	-	82%	88%
Surgical Care Improvement Project				
Appropriate Beta Blocker Usage[5]	-	-	98%	98%
Appropriate VTP Within 24 Hours[5]	-	-	99%	98%
Controlled Postoperative Blood Glucose[5]	-	-	96%	97%
Perioperative Temperature Management[5]	-	-	100%	100%
Prophylactic Antibiotic Selection[5]	-	-	99%	99%

NOTE: Hospital profiles are in alphabetical order by state, then city, then hospital within the city; Rankings exclude hospitals with less than 25 cases except for patient surveys which excludes hospitals with less than 100 cases; (a) 100-299 cases; (1) The number of cases/patients is too few to report; (2) Data submitted were based on a sample of cases/patients; (3) Results are based on a shorter time period than required; (4) Data suppressed by CMS for one or more quarters; (5) Results are not available for this reporting period; (6) Fewer than 100 patients completed the HCAHPS survey; (7) No cases met the criteria for this measure; (8) The lower limit of the confidence interval cannot be calculated if the number of observed infections equals zero; (9) No data are available from the state/territory for this reporting period; (10) The scores shown reflect fewer than 50 completed surveys; (11) There were discrepancies in the data collection process; (12) This measure does not apply to this hospital for this reporting period; (13) Results cannot be calculated for this reporting period; (14) The results for this state are combined with nearby states to protect confidentiality; Please refer to the User's Guide for a full explanation of data.

Measure	Cases	This Hosp.	State Avg.	U.S. Avg.
Prophylactic Antibiotic Selection (Outpatient)[5]	-	-	98%	98%
Prophylactic Antibiotic Stopped[5]	-	-	99%	98%
Prophylactic Antibiotic Timing[5]	-	-	99%	99%
Prophylactic Antibiotic Timing (Outpatient)[5]	-	-	98%	98%
Urinary Catheter Removal[5]	-	-	97%	97%
Survey of Patients' Hospital Experiences				
Area Around Room 'Always' Quiet at Night	(a)	61%	52%	61%
Doctors 'Always' Communicated Well	(a)	82%	80%	82%
Home Recovery Information Given	(a)	87%	87%	85%
Hospital Given 9 or 10 on 10 Point Scale	(a)	77%	69%	71%
Meds 'Always' Explained Before Given	(a)	73%	64%	64%
Nurses 'Always' Communicated Well	(a)	84%	79%	79%
Pain 'Always' Well Controlled	(a)	75%	71%	71%
Room and Bathroom 'Always' Clean	(a)	82%	72%	73%
Timely Help 'Always' Received	(a)	82%	66%	68%
Would Definitely Recommend Hospital	(a)	83%	73%	71%
Use of Medical Imaging				
Cardiac Imaging Stress Test before Surgery[1]	-	-	5.4%	5.3%
Combination Abdominal CT Scan	157	2.5%	6.3%	10.5%
Combination Brain/Sinus CT Scan[1]	-	-	2.4%	2.7%
Combination Chest CT Scan[1]	-	-	0.5%	2.7%
Follow-up Mammogram/Ultrasound	449	6.5%	8.9%	8.8%
Lumbar Spine MRI for Low Back Pain[7]	-	-	35.3%	37.2%

Saint Anne's Hospital

795 Middle Street
Fall River, MA 02721
Phone: 508-674-5600
Fax: 508-675-5647
E-mail: sahmail@cchcs.org
URL: www.saintanneshospital.org
Type: Acute Care Hospitals
Emergency Services: Yes
Ownership: Proprietary
Beds: 165

Key Personnel:
Quality Assurance . . . . Jane Benevides, RN
Pediatric Ambulatory Care . . . . . . Joan Benevides, RN
Radiology. . . . . Franklin A DePeters
Infection Control. . . . . Diane Gauvin, RN
Pediatric In-Patient Care . . . . Nellie Jacob
Chief of Medical Staff. . . . . Malcolm W MacDonald
CEO/President. . . . . Michael Metzler
Coronary Care . . . . Kristine Walker, RN

Measure	Cases	This Hosp.	State Avg.	U.S. Avg.
Blood Clot Prevention and Treatment				
Anticoagulation Overlap Therapy[2]	62	97%	97%	93%
ICU Venous Thromboembolism Prophylaxis[2]	68	96%	92%	92%
Incidence of Potentially Preventable VTE[2]	11	18%	7%	10%
UFH with Dosages/Platelet Monitoring[2]	28	100%	91%	97%
Venous Thromboembolism Prophylaxis[2]	348	74%	87%	85%
Warfarin Therapy Discharge Instructions[2]	46	100%	77%	75%
Chest Pain/Possible Heart Attack Care				
Aspirin Given Within 24 Hours of Arrival	14	100%	97%	96%
Fibrinolytic Meds Within 30 Min. of Arrival[7]	-	-	73%	58%
Average Time to ECG (minutes)	15	11	7	7
Average Time to Transfer (minutes)[1]	-	-	55	60
Children's Asthma Care				
Received Home Management Plan of Care	-	-	-	88%
Received Reliever Medication	-	-	-	100%
Received Systemic Corticosteroids	-	-	-	100%
Emergency Department				
Admittance Decision Time (minutes)[2]	793	100	119	98
Head CT Results Within 45 Min. of Arrival[1]	-	-	70%	57%
Patients Who Left ER Before Being Seen	41,460	3%	2%	2%
Time from ER Arrival to Admit. (minutes)[2]	799	305	313	274
Time from ER Arrival to Discharge (minutes)	344	167	156	134
Time in ER Before Being Evaluated (minutes)	393	61	36	26
Time to Pain Meds for Fractures (minutes)	51	76	59	57
Heart Attack Care				
Aspirin Given at Discharge	26	100%	100%	99%
Fibrinolytic Meds Within 30 Min. of Arrival[7]	-	-	100%	54%
PCI Within 90 Minutes of Arrival[7]	-	-	96%	96%
Statin Prescribed at Discharge	25	96%	99%	98%
Heart Failure Care				
ACE Inhibitor or ARB for LVSD	39	90%	96%	97%
Discharge Instructions Given	168	95%	95%	94%
Evaluation of LVS Function	217	100%	100%	99%
Medicare Spending				
Medicare Spending per Patient (ratio)	-	1.02	1.03	0.98
Pneumonia Care				
Appropriate Initial Antibiotic Given	134	98%	97%	95%
Blood Culture Timing	139	98%	98%	98%
Pregnancy and Delivery Care				
Newborn Deliveries Scheduled Early[7]	-	-	2%	6%
Preventive Care				
Immunization for Influenza[2]	602	97%	91%	90%
Immunization for Pneumonia[2]	867	96%	91%	92%
Stroke Care				
Anticoagulation Therapy for Atrial Fibrillation[1]	-	-	97%	95%
Antithrombotic Therapy Timing	55	96%	98%	98%
Assessed for Rehabilitation	63	98%	96%	97%
Discharged on Antithrombotic Therapy	55	100%	100%	99%
Discharged on Statin Medication	45	93%	96%	94%
Thrombolytic Therapy Timing[1]	-	-	68%	66%
Venous Thromboembolism Prophylaxis	64	89%	94%	94%
Written Stroke Educational Materials Given	36	97%	82%	88%
Surgical Care Improvement Project				
Appropriate Beta Blocker Usage[2]	188	100%	98%	98%
Appropriate VTP Within 24 Hours[2]	405	99%	99%	98%
Controlled Postoperative Blood Glucose[2,7]	-	-	96%	97%
Perioperative Temperature Management[2]	517	98%	100%	100%
Prophylactic Antibiotic Selection[2]	432	100%	99%	99%
Prophylactic Antibiotic Selection (Outpatient)	72	100%	98%	98%
Prophylactic Antibiotic Stopped[2]	426	99%	99%	98%
Prophylactic Antibiotic Timing[2]	433	100%	99%	99%
Prophylactic Antibiotic Timing (Outpatient)	71	100%	98%	98%
Urinary Catheter Removal[2]	378	99%	97%	97%
Survey of Patients' Hospital Experiences				
Area Around Room 'Always' Quiet at Night	300+	50%	52%	61%
Doctors 'Always' Communicated Well	300+	77%	80%	82%
Home Recovery Information Given	300+	88%	87%	85%
Hospital Given 9 or 10 on 10 Point Scale	300+	64%	69%	71%
Meds 'Always' Explained Before Given	300+	60%	64%	64%
Nurses 'Always' Communicated Well	300+	78%	79%	79%
Pain 'Always' Well Controlled	300+	68%	71%	71%
Room and Bathroom 'Always' Clean	300+	74%	72%	73%
Timely Help 'Always' Received	300+	65%	66%	68%
Would Definitely Recommend Hospital	300+	67%	73%	71%
Use of Medical Imaging				
Cardiac Imaging Stress Test before Surgery	161	5.6%	5.4%	5.3%
Combination Abdominal CT Scan	854	5.5%	6.3%	10.5%
Combination Brain/Sinus CT Scan	587	1.9%	2.4%	2.7%
Combination Chest CT Scan	763	0.1%	0.5%	2.7%
Follow-up Mammogram/Ultrasound	1,355	15.4%	8.9%	8.8%
Lumbar Spine MRI for Low Back Pain	220	42.3%	35.3%	37.2%

Southcoast Hospital Group

363 Highland Avenue
Fall River, MA 02720
Phone: 508-679-3131
Fax: 508-679-7144
URL: www.southcoast.org/charlton
Type: Acute Care Hospitals
Emergency Services: Yes
Ownership: Voluntary non-profit - Private
Beds: 362

Key Personnel:
CEO/President. . . . . John B Day
Chief of Medical Staff. . . . . Eugene McMahon, MD, MBA

Measure	Cases	This Hosp.	State Avg.	U.S. Avg.
Blood Clot Prevention and Treatment				
Anticoagulation Overlap Therapy[2]	255	98%	97%	93%
ICU Venous Thromboembolism Prophylaxis[2]	63	90%	92%	92%
Incidence of Potentially Preventable VTE[2]	34	15%	7%	10%
UFH with Dosages/Platelet Monitoring[2]	206	100%	91%	97%
Venous Thromboembolism Prophylaxis[2]	369	84%	87%	85%
Warfarin Therapy Discharge Instructions[2]	184	96%	77%	75%
Chest Pain/Possible Heart Attack Care				
Aspirin Given Within 24 Hours of Arrival	150	98%	97%	96%
Fibrinolytic Meds Within 30 Min. of Arrival[7]	-	-	73%	58%
Average Time to ECG (minutes)	157	7	7	7
Average Time to Transfer (minutes)	50	54	55	60
Children's Asthma Care				
Received Home Management Plan of Care	-	-	-	88%
Received Reliever Medication	-	-	-	100%
Received Systemic Corticosteroids	-	-	-	100%
Emergency Department				
Admittance Decision Time (minutes)[2]	694	113	119	98
Head CT Results Within 45 Min. of Arrival	88	78%	70%	57%
Patients Who Left ER Before Being Seen	>100k	2%	2%	2%
Time from ER Arrival to Admit. (minutes)[2]	720	293	313	274
Time from ER Arrival to Discharge (minutes)	324	133	156	134
Time in ER Before Being Evaluated (minutes)	319	46	36	26
Time to Pain Meds for Fractures (minutes)	242	55	59	57
Heart Attack Care				
Aspirin Given at Discharge[2]	628	99%	100%	99%
Fibrinolytic Meds Within 30 Min. of Arrival[2,7]	-	-	100%	54%
PCI Within 90 Minutes of Arrival[2]	64	98%	96%	96%
Statin Prescribed at Discharge[2]	603	98%	99%	98%
Heart Failure Care				
ACE Inhibitor or ARB for LVSD[2]	280	98%	96%	97%
Discharge Instructions Given[2]	734	94%	95%	94%
Evaluation of LVS Function[2]	1,033	100%	100%	99%
Medicare Spending				
Medicare Spending per Patient (ratio)	-	1.06	1.03	0.98
Pneumonia Care				
Appropriate Initial Antibiotic Given[2]	651	98%	97%	95%
Blood Culture Timing[2]	901	97%	98%	98%
Pregnancy and Delivery Care				
Newborn Deliveries Scheduled Early[2]	62	2%	2%	6%
Preventive Care				
Immunization for Influenza[2]	545	95%	91%	90%
Immunization for Pneumonia[2]	713	94%	91%	92%
Stroke Care				
Anticoagulation Therapy for Atrial Fibrillation	73	99%	97%	95%
Antithrombotic Therapy Timing	344	100%	98%	98%
Assessed for Rehabilitation	351	98%	96%	97%
Discharged on Antithrombotic Therapy	327	100%	100%	99%
Discharged on Statin Medication	266	98%	96%	94%
Thrombolytic Therapy Timing[1]	-	-	68%	66%
Venous Thromboembolism Prophylaxis	364	96%	94%	94%
Written Stroke Educational Materials Given	163	90%	82%	88%
Surgical Care Improvement Project				
Appropriate Beta Blocker Usage[2]	560	99%	98%	98%
Appropriate VTP Within 24 Hours[2]	1,034	98%	99%	98%
Controlled Postoperative Blood Glucose[2]	224	98%	96%	97%
Perioperative Temperature Management[2]	1,258	100%	100%	100%
Prophylactic Antibiotic Selection[2]	951	99%	99%	99%
Prophylactic Antibiotic Selection (Outpatient)	921	97%	98%	98%
Prophylactic Antibiotic Stopped[2]	928	98%	99%	98%
Prophylactic Antibiotic Timing[2]	953	99%	99%	99%
Prophylactic Antibiotic Timing (Outpatient)	936	98%	98%	98%
Urinary Catheter Removal[2]	782	97%	97%	97%
Survey of Patients' Hospital Experiences				
Area Around Room 'Always' Quiet at Night	300+	47%	52%	61%
Doctors 'Always' Communicated Well	300+	79%	80%	82%
Home Recovery Information Given	300+	88%	87%	85%
Hospital Given 9 or 10 on 10 Point Scale	300+	63%	69%	71%
Meds 'Always' Explained Before Given	300+	62%	64%	64%
Nurses 'Always' Communicated Well	300+	79%	79%	79%
Pain 'Always' Well Controlled	300+	71%	71%	71%
Room and Bathroom 'Always' Clean	300+	72%	72%	73%
Timely Help 'Always' Received	300+	61%	66%	68%
Would Definitely Recommend Hospital	300+	66%	73%	71%
Use of Medical Imaging				
Cardiac Imaging Stress Test before Surgery	1,165	5.3%	5.4%	5.3%
Combination Abdominal CT Scan	3,382	4.6%	6.3%	10.5%
Combination Brain/Sinus CT Scan	3,527	3.5%	2.4%	2.7%
Combination Chest CT Scan	2,147	1.0%	0.5%	2.7%
Follow-up Mammogram/Ultrasound	6,855	9.9%	8.9%	8.8%
Lumbar Spine MRI for Low Back Pain	229	34.1%	35.3%	37.2%

NOTE: Hospital profiles are in alphabetical order by state, then city, then hospital within the city; Rankings exclude hospitals with less than 25 cases except for patient surveys which excludes hospitals with less than 100 cases; (a) 100-299 cases; (1) The number of cases/patients is too few to report; (2) Data submitted were based on a sample of cases/patients; (3) Results are based on a shorter time period than required; (4) Data suppressed by CMS for one or more quarters; (5) Results are not available for this reporting period; (6) Fewer than 100 patients completed the HCAHPS survey; (7) No cases met the criteria for this measure; (8) The lower limit of the confidence interval cannot be calculated if the number of observed infections equals zero; (9) No data are available from the state/territory for this reporting period; (10) The scores shown reflect fewer than 50 completed surveys; (11) There were discrepancies in the data collection process; (12) This measure does not apply to this hospital for this reporting period; (13) Results cannot be calculated for this reporting period; (14) The results for this state are combined with nearby states to protect confidentiality; Please refer to the User's Guide for a full explanation of data.

Falmouth Hospital

67 & 100 Ter Heun Drive
Falmouth, MA 02540
URL: www.capecodhealth.com
Type: Acute Care Hospitals
Ownership: Voluntary non-profit - Private
Phone: 508-548-5300
Fax: 508-457-3857
Emergency Services: Yes
Beds: 95

Key Personnel:
Radiology. . . . . Kenneth L Caswell
Emergency Room . . . . Herbert Gray, MD
CEO/President. . . . . Susan Wing

Measure	Cases	This Hosp.	State Avg.	U.S. Avg.
Blood Clot Prevention and Treatment				
Anticoagulation Overlap Therapy[2]	43	95%	97%	93%
ICU Venous Thromboembolism Prophylaxis[2]	65	100%	92%	92%
Incidence of Potentially Preventable VTE[1,2]	-	-	7%	10%
UFH with Dosages/Platelet Monitoring[2]	12	100%	91%	97%
Venous Thromboembolism Prophylaxis[2]	307	99%	87%	85%
Warfarin Therapy Discharge Instructions[2]	29	34%	77%	75%
Chest Pain/Possible Heart Attack Care				
Aspirin Given Within 24 Hours of Arrival	17	94%	97%	96%
Fibrinolytic Meds Within 30 Min. of Arrival[7]	-	-	73%	58%
Average Time to ECG (minutes)	18	5	7	7
Average Time to Transfer (minutes)[7]	-	-	55	60
Children's Asthma Care				
Received Home Management Plan of Care	-	-	-	88%
Received Reliever Medication	-	-	-	100%
Received Systemic Corticosteroids	-	-	-	100%
Emergency Department				
Admittance Decision Time (minutes)[2]	843	217	119	98
Head CT Results Within 45 Min. of Arrival	22	64%	70%	57%
Patients Who Left ER Before Being Seen	3,869	9%	2%	2%
Time from ER Arrival to Admit. (minutes)[2]	844	394	313	274
Time from ER Arrival to Discharge (minutes)	368	120	156	134
Time in ER Before Being Evaluated (minutes)	417	18	36	26
Time to Pain Meds for Fractures (minutes)	117	77	59	57
Heart Attack Care				
Aspirin Given at Discharge	24	100%	100%	99%
Fibrinolytic Meds Within 30 Min. of Arrival[7]	-	-	100%	54%
PCI Within 90 Minutes of Arrival[7]	-	-	96%	96%
Statin Prescribed at Discharge	28	89%	99%	98%
Heart Failure Care				
ACE Inhibitor or ARB for LVSD	24	100%	96%	97%
Discharge Instructions Given	150	98%	95%	94%
Evaluation of LVS Function	221	100%	100%	99%
Medicare Spending				
Medicare Spending per Patient (ratio)	-	1.00	1.03	0.98
Pneumonia Care				
Appropriate Initial Antibiotic Given	98	100%	97%	95%
Blood Culture Timing	204	100%	98%	98%
Pregnancy and Delivery Care				
Newborn Deliveries Scheduled Early	29	3%	2%	6%
Preventive Care				
Immunization for Influenza[2]	551	89%	91%	90%
Immunization for Pneumonia[2]	802	91%	91%	92%
Stroke Care				
Anticoagulation Therapy for Atrial Fibrillation	16	100%	97%	95%
Antithrombotic Therapy Timing	61	98%	98%	98%
Assessed for Rehabilitation	70	100%	96%	97%
Discharged on Antithrombotic Therapy	62	100%	100%	99%
Discharged on Statin Medication	50	100%	96%	94%
Thrombolytic Therapy Timing[7]	-	-	68%	66%
Venous Thromboembolism Prophylaxis	69	100%	94%	94%
Written Stroke Educational Materials Given	31	100%	82%	88%
Surgical Care Improvement Project				
Appropriate Beta Blocker Usage	183	99%	98%	98%
Appropriate VTP Within 24 Hours	559	99%	99%	98%
Controlled Postoperative Blood Glucose[7]	-	-	96%	97%
Perioperative Temperature Management	642	100%	100%	100%
Prophylactic Antibiotic Selection	512	99%	99%	99%
Prophylactic Antibiotic Selection (Outpatient)	79	100%	98%	98%
Prophylactic Antibiotic Stopped	503	100%	99%	98%
Prophylactic Antibiotic Timing	512	100%	99%	99%
Prophylactic Antibiotic Timing (Outpatient)	79	99%	98%	98%
Urinary Catheter Removal	463	100%	97%	97%
Survey of Patients' Hospital Experiences				
Area Around Room 'Always' Quiet at Night	300+	46%	52%	61%
Doctors 'Always' Communicated Well	300+	79%	80%	82%
Home Recovery Information Given	300+	86%	87%	85%
Hospital Given 9 or 10 on 10 Point Scale	300+	68%	69%	71%
Meds 'Always' Explained Before Given	300+	60%	64%	64%
Nurses 'Always' Communicated Well	300+	77%	79%	79%
Pain 'Always' Well Controlled	300+	70%	71%	71%
Room and Bathroom 'Always' Clean	300+	73%	72%	73%
Timely Help 'Always' Received	300+	61%	66%	68%
Would Definitely Recommend Hospital	300+	75%	73%	71%
Use of Medical Imaging				
Cardiac Imaging Stress Test before Surgery[1]	-	-	5.4%	5.3%
Combination Abdominal CT Scan	950	3.1%	6.3%	10.5%
Combination Brain/Sinus CT Scan	1,087	2.6%	2.4%	2.7%
Combination Chest CT Scan	545	0.9%	0.5%	2.7%
Follow-up Mammogram/Ultrasound	2,742	7.8%	8.9%	8.8%
Lumbar Spine MRI for Low Back Pain	199	28.1%	35.3%	37.2%

Metrowest Medical Center

115 Lincoln Street
Framingham, MA 01701
E-mail: webmaster@mwmc.com
URL: www.mwmc.com
Type: Acute Care Hospitals
Ownership: Voluntary non-profit - Private
Phone: 508-383-1000
Fax: 508-383-1011
Emergency Services: Yes
Beds: 368

Key Personnel:
Radiology. . . . . Bill Buff, MD
Surgery . . . . Riad Cachecho, MD
CEO/President. . . . . Barbara Doyle, MHA, RN
Anesthesiology. . . . . Stephen Kapaon, MD
Cardiology . . . . George Kinzfogl, MD
Emergency Room . . . . Lisa Sotir, MD
Pediatrics. . . . . Jerry Wortzman, MD
Chief of Medical Staff. . . . . Jerry M. Wortzman, MD, MM

Measure	Cases	This Hosp.	State Avg.	U.S. Avg.
Blood Clot Prevention and Treatment				
Anticoagulation Overlap Therapy[2]	45	100%	97%	93%
ICU Venous Thromboembolism Prophylaxis[2]	71	99%	92%	92%
Incidence of Potentially Preventable VTE[1,2]	-	-	7%	10%
UFH with Dosages/Platelet Monitoring[2]	28	100%	91%	97%
Venous Thromboembolism Prophylaxis[2]	302	93%	87%	85%
Warfarin Therapy Discharge Instructions[2]	29	72%	77%	75%
Chest Pain/Possible Heart Attack Care				
Aspirin Given Within 24 Hours of Arrival	33	100%	97%	96%
Fibrinolytic Meds Within 30 Min. of Arrival[7]	-	-	73%	58%
Average Time to ECG (minutes)	35	1	7	7
Average Time to Transfer (minutes)[1]	-	-	55	60
Children's Asthma Care				
Received Home Management Plan of Care	-	-	-	88%
Received Reliever Medication	-	-	-	100%
Received Systemic Corticosteroids	-	-	-	100%
Emergency Department				
Admittance Decision Time (minutes)[2]	833	115	119	98
Head CT Results Within 45 Min. of Arrival	16	75%	70%	57%
Patients Who Left ER Before Being Seen	66,959	1%	2%	2%
Time from ER Arrival to Admit. (minutes)[2]	835	309	313	274
Time from ER Arrival to Discharge (minutes)	375	148	156	134
Time in ER Before Being Evaluated (minutes)	423	33	36	26
Time to Pain Meds for Fractures (minutes)	156	37	59	57
Heart Attack Care				
Aspirin Given at Discharge	99	99%	100%	99%
Fibrinolytic Meds Within 30 Min. of Arrival[7]	-	-	100%	54%
PCI Within 90 Minutes of Arrival	44	100%	96%	96%
Statin Prescribed at Discharge	95	100%	99%	98%
Heart Failure Care				
ACE Inhibitor or ARB for LVSD	59	98%	96%	97%
Discharge Instructions Given	244	95%	95%	94%
Evaluation of LVS Function	365	99%	100%	99%
Medicare Spending				
Medicare Spending per Patient (ratio)	-	1.03	1.03	0.98
Pneumonia Care				
Appropriate Initial Antibiotic Given	181	99%	97%	95%
Blood Culture Timing	215	100%	98%	98%
Pregnancy and Delivery Care				
Newborn Deliveries Scheduled Early[2]	65	0%	2%	6%
Preventive Care				
Immunization for Influenza[2]	561	95%	91%	90%
Immunization for Pneumonia[2]	726	96%	91%	92%
Stroke Care				
Anticoagulation Therapy for Atrial Fibrillation	17	94%	97%	95%
Antithrombotic Therapy Timing	82	98%	98%	98%
Assessed for Rehabilitation	90	97%	96%	97%
Discharged on Antithrombotic Therapy	86	100%	100%	99%
Discharged on Statin Medication	67	100%	96%	94%
Thrombolytic Therapy Timing	11	82%	68%	66%
Venous Thromboembolism Prophylaxis	88	93%	94%	94%
Written Stroke Educational Materials Given	45	87%	82%	88%
Surgical Care Improvement Project				
Appropriate Beta Blocker Usage	170	99%	98%	98%
Appropriate VTP Within 24 Hours	443	99%	99%	98%
Controlled Postoperative Blood Glucose[7]	-	-	96%	97%
Perioperative Temperature Management	539	100%	100%	100%
Prophylactic Antibiotic Selection	287	98%	99%	99%
Prophylactic Antibiotic Selection (Outpatient)	255	98%	98%	98%
Prophylactic Antibiotic Stopped	278	100%	99%	98%
Prophylactic Antibiotic Timing	287	99%	99%	99%
Prophylactic Antibiotic Timing (Outpatient)	257	97%	98%	98%
Urinary Catheter Removal	245	98%	97%	97%
Survey of Patients' Hospital Experiences				
Area Around Room 'Always' Quiet at Night[11]	300+	53%	52%	61%
Doctors 'Always' Communicated Well[11]	300+	79%	80%	82%
Home Recovery Information Given[11]	300+	88%	87%	85%
Hospital Given 9 or 10 on 10 Point Scale[11]	300+	68%	69%	71%
Meds 'Always' Explained Before Given[11]	300+	62%	64%	64%
Nurses 'Always' Communicated Well[11]	300+	79%	79%	79%
Pain 'Always' Well Controlled[11]	300+	69%	71%	71%
Room and Bathroom 'Always' Clean[11]	300+	68%	72%	73%
Timely Help 'Always' Received[11]	300+	66%	66%	68%
Would Definitely Recommend Hospital[11]	300+	71%	73%	71%
Use of Medical Imaging				
Cardiac Imaging Stress Test before Surgery	187	6.4%	5.4%	5.3%
Combination Abdominal CT Scan	797	11.3%	6.3%	10.5%
Combination Brain/Sinus CT Scan	915	3.3%	2.4%	2.7%
Combination Chest CT Scan	733	0.7%	0.5%	2.7%
Follow-up Mammogram/Ultrasound	2,681	15.7%	8.9%	8.8%
Lumbar Spine MRI for Low Back Pain[1]	-	-	35.3%	37.2%

Heywood Hospital

242 Green Street
Gardner, MA 01440
Type: Acute Care Hospitals
Ownership: Voluntary non-profit - Private
Phone: 978-632-3420
Fax: 978-630-6596
Emergency Services: Yes
Beds: 132

Key Personnel:
Chief of Medical Staff. . . . . Bruce K. Bertrand
CEO/President. . . . . Winfield S. Brown, MSB, MHA, FACHE
Emergency Room . . . . Kunle Fajana, MD
Chair/CEO. . . . . Kenneth J. Pierce

Measure	Cases	This Hosp.	State Avg.	U.S. Avg.
Blood Clot Prevention and Treatment				
Anticoagulation Overlap Therapy[2]	26	73%	97%	93%
ICU Venous Thromboembolism Prophylaxis[2]	40	92%	92%	92%
Incidence of Potentially Preventable VTE[1,2]	-	-	7%	10%
UFH with Dosages/Platelet Monitoring[1,2]	-	-	91%	97%
Venous Thromboembolism Prophylaxis[2]	319	91%	87%	85%
Warfarin Therapy Discharge Instructions[2]	21	81%	77%	75%
Chest Pain/Possible Heart Attack Care				
Aspirin Given Within 24 Hours of Arrival	139	91%	97%	96%
Fibrinolytic Meds Within 30 Min. of Arrival[7]	-	-	73%	58%
Average Time to ECG (minutes)	145	9	7	7
Average Time to Transfer (minutes)	11	54	55	60
Children's Asthma Care				
Received Home Management Plan of Care	-	-	-	88%
Received Reliever Medication	-	-	-	100%
Received Systemic Corticosteroids	-	-	-	100%

NOTE: Hospital profiles are in alphabetical order by state, then city, then hospital within the city; Rankings exclude hospitals with less than 25 cases except for patient surveys which excludes hospitals with less than 100 cases; (a) 100-299 cases; (1) The number of cases/patients is too few to report; (2) Data submitted were based on a sample of cases/patients; (3) Results are based on a shorter time period than required; (4) Data suppressed by CMS for one or more quarters; (5) Results are not available for this reporting period; (6) Fewer than 100 patients completed the HCAHPS survey; (7) No cases met the criteria for this measure; (8) The lower limit of the confidence interval cannot be calculated if the number of observed infections equals zero; (9) No data are available from the state/territory for this reporting period; (10) The scores shown reflect fewer than 50 completed surveys; (11) There were discrepancies in the data collection process; (12) This measure does not apply to this hospital for this reporting period; (13) Results cannot be calculated for this reporting period; (14) The results for this state are combined with nearby states to protect confidentiality; Please refer to the User's Guide for a full explanation of data.

Emergency Department				
Admittance Decision Time (minutes)[2]	430	132	119	98
Head CT Results Within 45 Min. of Arrival	20	45%	70%	57%
Patients Who Left ER Before Being Seen	24,635	2%	2%	2%
Time from ER Arrival to Admit. (minutes)[2]	430	360	313	274
Time from ER Arrival to Discharge (minutes)	344	212	156	134
Time in ER Before Being Evaluated (minutes)	398	47	36	26
Time to Pain Meds for Fractures (minutes)	78	69	59	57
Heart Attack Care				
Aspirin Given at Discharge	43	93%	100%	99%
Fibrinolytic Meds Within 30 Min. of Arrival[7]	-	-	100%	54%
PCI Within 90 Minutes of Arrival[7]	-	-	96%	96%
Statin Prescribed at Discharge	40	90%	99%	98%
Heart Failure Care				
ACE Inhibitor or ARB for LVSD	48	94%	96%	97%
Discharge Instructions Given	121	90%	95%	94%
Evaluation of LVS Function	146	98%	100%	99%
Medicare Spending				
Medicare Spending per Patient (ratio)	-	0.97	1.03	0.98
Pneumonia Care				
Appropriate Initial Antibiotic Given	105	91%	97%	95%
Blood Culture Timing	183	99%	98%	98%
Pregnancy and Delivery Care				
Newborn Deliveries Scheduled Early	36	6%	2%	6%
Preventive Care				
Immunization for Influenza[2]	423	93%	91%	90%
Immunization for Pneumonia[2]	516	87%	91%	92%
Stroke Care				
Anticoagulation Therapy for Atrial Fibrillation[1]	-	-	97%	95%
Antithrombotic Therapy Timing	20	100%	98%	98%
Assessed for Rehabilitation	18	94%	96%	97%
Discharged on Antithrombotic Therapy	18	100%	100%	99%
Discharged on Statin Medication	15	87%	96%	94%
Thrombolytic Therapy Timing[7]	-	-	68%	66%
Venous Thromboembolism Prophylaxis	21	95%	94%	94%
Written Stroke Educational Materials Given[1]	-	-	82%	88%
Surgical Care Improvement Project				
Appropriate Beta Blocker Usage	77	97%	98%	98%
Appropriate VTP Within 24 Hours	242	99%	99%	98%
Controlled Postoperative Blood Glucose[7]	-	-	96%	97%
Perioperative Temperature Management	266	100%	100%	100%
Prophylactic Antibiotic Selection	212	100%	99%	99%
Prophylactic Antibiotic Selection (Outpatient)	133	89%	98%	98%
Prophylactic Antibiotic Stopped	209	99%	99%	98%
Prophylactic Antibiotic Timing	213	99%	99%	99%
Prophylactic Antibiotic Timing (Outpatient)	94	82%	98%	98%
Urinary Catheter Removal	189	89%	97%	97%
Survey of Patients' Hospital Experiences				
Area Around Room 'Always' Quiet at Night	300+	56%	52%	61%
Doctors 'Always' Communicated Well	300+	82%	80%	82%
Home Recovery Information Given	300+	84%	87%	85%
Hospital Given 9 or 10 on 10 Point Scale	300+	71%	69%	71%
Meds 'Always' Explained Before Given	300+	64%	64%	64%
Nurses 'Always' Communicated Well	300+	81%	79%	79%
Pain 'Always' Well Controlled	300+	73%	71%	71%
Room and Bathroom 'Always' Clean	300+	75%	72%	73%
Timely Help 'Always' Received	300+	65%	66%	68%
Would Definitely Recommend Hospital	300+	77%	73%	71%
Use of Medical Imaging				
Cardiac Imaging Stress Test before Surgery	266	6.0%	5.4%	5.3%
Combination Abdominal CT Scan	482	2.7%	6.3%	10.5%
Combination Brain/Sinus CT Scan[1]	-	-	2.4%	2.7%
Combination Chest CT Scan	329	0.0%	0.5%	2.7%
Follow-up Mammogram/Ultrasound	813	7.0%	8.9%	8.8%
Lumbar Spine MRI for Low Back Pain	99	46.5%	35.3%	37.2%

Fairview Hospital

29 Lewis Avenue
Great Barrington, MA 01230
E-mail: bholcomb@bhsl.org
URL: www.berkshirehealthsystems.com
Type: Critical Access Hospitals
Ownership: Voluntary non-profit - Private
Phone: 413-528-0790
Fax: 413-528-0290
Emergency Services: Yes
Beds: 24

Key Personnel:
Cardiac Laboratory. . . . . Phillip Bhark
Chief of Medical Staff . . . . Brian Burke
CEO/President. . . . . Eugene Dellea
Radiology. . . . . Bob Dillon
Infection Control. . . . . Geraldine McQuoid
Quality Assurance . . . . Pavani Rangachari
Emergency Room . . . . Donna Sena
Operating Room. . . . . Donna Wichman

Measure	Cases	This Hosp.	State Avg.	U.S. Avg.
Blood Clot Prevention and Treatment				
Anticoagulation Overlap Therapy[5]	-	-	97%	93%
ICU Venous Thromboembolism Prophylaxis[5]	-	-	92%	92%
Incidence of Potentially Preventable VTE[5]	-	-	7%	10%
UFH with Dosages/Platelet Monitoring[5]	-	-	91%	97%
Venous Thromboembolism Prophylaxis[5]	-	-	87%	85%
Warfarin Therapy Discharge Instructions[5]	-	-	77%	75%
Chest Pain/Possible Heart Attack Care				
Aspirin Given Within 24 Hours of Arrival	-	-	97%	96%
Fibrinolytic Meds Within 30 Min. of Arrival	-	-	73%	58%
Average Time to ECG (minutes)	-	-	7	7
Average Time to Transfer (minutes)	-	-	55	60
Children's Asthma Care				
Received Home Management Plan of Care	-	-	-	88%
Received Reliever Medication	-	-	-	100%
Received Systemic Corticosteroids	-	-	-	100%
Emergency Department				
Admittance Decision Time (minutes)[2]	391	73	119	98
Head CT Results Within 45 Min. of Arrival	-	-	70%	57%
Patients Who Left ER Before Being Seen	-	-	2%	2%
Time from ER Arrival to Admit. (minutes)[2]	426	298	313	274
Time from ER Arrival to Discharge (minutes)	-	-	156	134
Time in ER Before Being Evaluated (minutes)	-	-	36	26
Time to Pain Meds for Fractures (minutes)	-	-	59	57
Heart Attack Care				
Aspirin Given at Discharge[1]	-	-	100%	99%
Fibrinolytic Meds Within 30 Min. of Arrival[7]	-	-	100%	54%
PCI Within 90 Minutes of Arrival[3,7]	-	-	96%	96%
Statin Prescribed at Discharge[1]	-	-	99%	98%
Heart Failure Care				
ACE Inhibitor or ARB for LVSD[1]	-	-	96%	97%
Discharge Instructions Given	20	95%	95%	94%
Evaluation of LVS Function	27	100%	100%	99%
Medicare Spending				
Medicare Spending per Patient (ratio)	-	-	1.03	0.98
Pneumonia Care				
Appropriate Initial Antibiotic Given	38	95%	97%	95%
Blood Culture Timing	65	100%	98%	98%
Pregnancy and Delivery Care				
Newborn Deliveries Scheduled Early[3]	12	0%	2%	6%
Preventive Care				
Immunization for Influenza[2]	272	93%	91%	90%
Immunization for Pneumonia[2]	335	94%	91%	92%
Stroke Care				
Anticoagulation Therapy for Atrial Fibrillation[5]	-	-	97%	95%
Antithrombotic Therapy Timing[5]	-	-	98%	98%
Assessed for Rehabilitation[5]	-	-	96%	97%
Discharged on Antithrombotic Therapy[5]	-	-	100%	99%
Discharged on Statin Medication[5]	-	-	96%	94%
Thrombolytic Therapy Timing[5]	-	-	68%	66%
Venous Thromboembolism Prophylaxis[5]	-	-	94%	94%
Written Stroke Educational Materials Given[5]	-	-	82%	88%
Surgical Care Improvement Project				
Appropriate Beta Blocker Usage	14	100%	98%	98%
Appropriate VTP Within 24 Hours	52	100%	99%	98%
Controlled Postoperative Blood Glucose[7]	-	-	96%	97%
Perioperative Temperature Management	57	100%	100%	100%
Prophylactic Antibiotic Selection	39	100%	99%	99%
Prophylactic Antibiotic Selection (Outpatient)	-	-	98%	98%
Prophylactic Antibiotic Stopped	39	100%	99%	98%
Prophylactic Antibiotic Timing	39	100%	99%	99%
Prophylactic Antibiotic Timing (Outpatient)	-	-	98%	98%
Urinary Catheter Removal	11	91%	97%	97%
Survey of Patients' Hospital Experiences				
Area Around Room 'Always' Quiet at Night	(a)	59%	52%	61%
Doctors 'Always' Communicated Well	(a)	83%	80%	82%
Home Recovery Information Given	(a)	92%	87%	85%
Hospital Given 9 or 10 on 10 Point Scale	(a)	86%	69%	71%
Meds 'Always' Explained Before Given	(a)	76%	64%	64%
Nurses 'Always' Communicated Well	(a)	90%	79%	79%
Pain 'Always' Well Controlled	(a)	82%	71%	71%
Room and Bathroom 'Always' Clean	(a)	77%	72%	73%
Timely Help 'Always' Received	(a)	84%	66%	68%
Would Definitely Recommend Hospital	(a)	90%	73%	71%
Use of Medical Imaging				
Cardiac Imaging Stress Test before Surgery	-	-	5.4%	5.3%
Combination Abdominal CT Scan	-	-	6.3%	10.5%
Combination Brain/Sinus CT Scan	-	-	2.4%	2.7%
Combination Chest CT Scan	-	-	0.5%	2.7%
Follow-up Mammogram/Ultrasound	-	-	8.9%	8.8%
Lumbar Spine MRI for Low Back Pain	-	-	35.3%	37.2%

Baystate Franklin Medical Center

164 High Street
Greenfield, MA 01301
URL: www.baystatehealth.com
Type: Acute Care Hospitals
Ownership: Voluntary non-profit - Private
Phone: 413-773-0211
Emergency Services: Yes
Beds: 93

Key Personnel:
CEO/President. . . . . Chuck Gijanto

Measure	Cases	This Hosp.	State Avg.	U.S. Avg.
Blood Clot Prevention and Treatment				
Anticoagulation Overlap Therapy[2]	14	100%	97%	93%
ICU Venous Thromboembolism Prophylaxis[2]	37	89%	92%	92%
Incidence of Potentially Preventable VTE[2,7]	-	-	7%	10%
UFH with Dosages/Platelet Monitoring[1,2]	-	-	91%	97%
Venous Thromboembolism Prophylaxis[2]	227	90%	87%	85%
Warfarin Therapy Discharge Instructions[2]	11	82%	77%	75%
Chest Pain/Possible Heart Attack Care				
Aspirin Given Within 24 Hours of Arrival	48	100%	97%	96%
Fibrinolytic Meds Within 30 Min. of Arrival[1]	-	-	73%	58%
Average Time to ECG (minutes)	48	8	7	7
Average Time to Transfer (minutes)[1]	-	-	55	60
Children's Asthma Care				
Received Home Management Plan of Care	-	-	-	88%
Received Reliever Medication	-	-	-	100%
Received Systemic Corticosteroids	-	-	-	100%
Emergency Department				
Admittance Decision Time (minutes)[2]	430	100	119	98
Head CT Results Within 45 Min. of Arrival[1]	-	-	70%	57%
Patients Who Left ER Before Being Seen	27,831	2%	2%	2%
Time from ER Arrival to Admit. (minutes)[2]	480	292	313	274
Time from ER Arrival to Discharge (minutes)	375	139	156	134
Time in ER Before Being Evaluated (minutes)	320	50	36	26
Time to Pain Meds for Fractures (minutes)	77	65	59	57
Heart Attack Care				
Aspirin Given at Discharge	15	93%	100%	99%
Fibrinolytic Meds Within 30 Min. of Arrival[7]	-	-	100%	54%
PCI Within 90 Minutes of Arrival[7]	-	-	96%	96%
Statin Prescribed at Discharge	14	100%	99%	98%
Heart Failure Care				
ACE Inhibitor or ARB for LVSD	30	90%	96%	97%
Discharge Instructions Given	88	98%	95%	94%
Evaluation of LVS Function	122	100%	100%	99%
Medicare Spending				
Medicare Spending per Patient (ratio)	-	0.99	1.03	0.98
Pneumonia Care				
Appropriate Initial Antibiotic Given	87	95%	97%	95%
Blood Culture Timing	127	94%	98%	98%
Pregnancy and Delivery Care				

NOTE: Hospital profiles are in alphabetical order by state, then city, then hospital within the city; Rankings exclude hospitals with less than 25 cases except for patient surveys which excludes hospitals with less than 100 cases; (a) 100-299 cases; (1) The number of cases/patients is too few to report; (2) Data submitted were based on a sample of cases/patients; (3) Results are based on a shorter time period than required; (4) Data suppressed by CMS for one or more quarters; (5) Results are not available for this reporting period; (6) Fewer than 100 patients completed the HCAHPS survey; (7) No cases met the criteria for this measure; (8) The lower limit of the confidence interval cannot be calculated if the number of observed infections equals zero; (9) No data are available from the state/territory for this reporting period; (10) The scores shown reflect fewer than 50 completed surveys; (11) There were discrepancies in the data collection process; (12) This measure does not apply to this hospital for this reporting period; (13) Results cannot be calculated for this reporting period; (14) The results for this state are combined with nearby states to protect confidentiality; Please refer to the User's Guide for a full explanation of data.

Measure	Cases	This Hosp.	State Avg.	U.S. Avg.
Newborn Deliveries Scheduled Early[2]	14	7%	2%	6%
Preventive Care				
Immunization for Influenza[2]	326	96%	91%	90%
Immunization for Pneumonia[2]	439	96%	91%	92%
Stroke Care				
Anticoagulation Therapy for Atrial Fibrillation[1]	-	-	97%	95%
Antithrombotic Therapy Timing	40	98%	98%	98%
Assessed for Rehabilitation	42	93%	96%	97%
Discharged on Antithrombotic Therapy	42	100%	100%	99%
Discharged on Statin Medication	32	97%	96%	94%
Thrombolytic Therapy Timing[7]	-	-	68%	66%
Venous Thromboembolism Prophylaxis	39	95%	94%	94%
Written Stroke Educational Materials Given	21	95%	82%	88%
Surgical Care Improvement Project				
Appropriate Beta Blocker Usage[2]	32	91%	98%	98%
Appropriate VTP Within 24 Hours[2]	122	94%	99%	98%
Controlled Postoperative Blood Glucose[2,7]	-	-	96%	97%
Perioperative Temperature Management[2]	153	100%	100%	100%
Prophylactic Antibiotic Selection[2]	89	96%	99%	99%
Prophylactic Antibiotic Selection (Outpatient)	17	100%	98%	98%
Prophylactic Antibiotic Stopped[2]	88	91%	99%	98%
Prophylactic Antibiotic Timing[2]	89	97%	99%	99%
Prophylactic Antibiotic Timing (Outpatient)	17	100%	98%	98%
Urinary Catheter Removal[2]	80	91%	97%	97%
Survey of Patients' Hospital Experiences				
Area Around Room 'Always' Quiet at Night	300+	56%	52%	61%
Doctors 'Always' Communicated Well	300+	80%	80%	82%
Home Recovery Information Given	300+	88%	87%	85%
Hospital Given 9 or 10 on 10 Point Scale	300+	66%	69%	71%
Meds 'Always' Explained Before Given	300+	62%	64%	64%
Nurses 'Always' Communicated Well	300+	80%	79%	79%
Pain 'Always' Well Controlled	300+	70%	71%	71%
Room and Bathroom 'Always' Clean	300+	69%	72%	73%
Timely Help 'Always' Received	300+	69%	66%	68%
Would Definitely Recommend Hospital	300+	68%	73%	71%
Use of Medical Imaging				
Cardiac Imaging Stress Test before Surgery	224	6.7%	5.4%	5.3%
Combination Abdominal CT Scan	584	6.8%	6.3%	10.5%
Combination Brain/Sinus CT Scan	458	2.0%	2.4%	2.7%
Combination Chest CT Scan	373	0.5%	0.5%	2.7%
Follow-up Mammogram/Ultrasound	793	7.4%	8.9%	8.8%
Lumbar Spine MRI for Low Back Pain[7]	-	-	35.3%	37.2%

Merrimack Valley Hospital

140 Lincoln Avenue Phone: 978-374-2000
Haverhill, MA 01830 Fax: 978-521-8138
E-mail: lester.schindel@merrimackvalleyhospital.com
URL: www.merrimackvalleyhospital.com

Type: Acute Care Hospitals Emergency Services: Yes
Ownership: Proprietary Beds: 108

Key Personnel:

Infection Control. . . . . Doris Bobryk-Rana, RN
President . . . . Michael G. Callum, MD
Radiology. . . . . Lawrence M Casha, MD
Operating Room. . . . . Cheryl Durkee, RN
President . . . . Mark Girard, MD, MBA
Chief of Medical Staff. . . . . George F Kwass, MD
Quality Assurance . . . . Gloria Swanbon
Chairman/CEO . . . . Ralph de la Torre, MD

Measure	Cases	This Hosp.	State Avg.	U.S. Avg.
Blood Clot Prevention and Treatment				
Anticoagulation Overlap Therapy[2]	25	88%	97%	93%
ICU Venous Thromboembolism Prophylaxis[2]	55	84%	92%	92%
Incidence of Potentially Preventable VTE[1,2]	-	-	7%	10%
UFH with Dosages/Platelet Monitoring[1,2]	-	-	91%	97%
Venous Thromboembolism Prophylaxis[2]	259	73%	87%	85%
Warfarin Therapy Discharge Instructions[2]	18	89%	77%	75%
Chest Pain/Possible Heart Attack Care				
Aspirin Given Within 24 Hours of Arrival	24	88%	97%	96%
Fibrinolytic Meds Within 30 Min. of Arrival[7]	-	-	73%	58%
Average Time to ECG (minutes)	24	9	7	7
Average Time to Transfer (minutes)	16	62	55	60
Children's Asthma Care				
Received Home Management Plan of Care	-	-	-	88%
Received Reliever Medication	-	-	-	100%
Received Systemic Corticosteroids	-	-	-	100%
Emergency Department				
Admittance Decision Time (minutes)[2]	383	97	119	98
Head CT Results Within 45 Min. of Arrival[1]	-	-	70%	57%
Patients Who Left ER Before Being Seen	19,554	6%	2%	2%
Time from ER Arrival to Admit. (minutes)[2]	453	374	313	274
Time from ER Arrival to Discharge (minutes)	343	226	156	134
Time in ER Before Being Evaluated (minutes)	296	66	36	26
Time to Pain Meds for Fractures (minutes)	46	113	59	57
Heart Attack Care				
Aspirin Given at Discharge	25	100%	100%	99%
Fibrinolytic Meds Within 30 Min. of Arrival[7]	-	-	100%	54%
PCI Within 90 Minutes of Arrival[7]	-	-	96%	96%
Statin Prescribed at Discharge	16	94%	99%	98%
Heart Failure Care				
ACE Inhibitor or ARB for LVSD	22	82%	96%	97%
Discharge Instructions Given	72	92%	95%	94%
Evaluation of LVS Function	120	100%	100%	99%
Medicare Spending				
Medicare Spending per Patient (ratio)	-	1.13	1.03	0.98
Pneumonia Care				
Appropriate Initial Antibiotic Given	93	99%	97%	95%
Blood Culture Timing	83	99%	98%	98%
Pregnancy and Delivery Care				
Newborn Deliveries Scheduled Early[7]	-	-	2%	6%
Preventive Care				
Immunization for Influenza[2]	295	93%	91%	90%
Immunization for Pneumonia[2]	436	85%	91%	92%
Stroke Care				
Anticoagulation Therapy for Atrial Fibrillation[1]	-	-	97%	95%
Antithrombotic Therapy Timing	29	90%	98%	98%
Assessed for Rehabilitation	31	94%	96%	97%
Discharged on Antithrombotic Therapy	30	90%	100%	99%
Discharged on Statin Medication	22	73%	96%	94%
Thrombolytic Therapy Timing[1]	-	-	68%	66%
Venous Thromboembolism Prophylaxis	30	87%	94%	94%
Written Stroke Educational Materials Given	18	94%	82%	88%
Surgical Care Improvement Project				
Appropriate Beta Blocker Usage	40	100%	98%	98%
Appropriate VTP Within 24 Hours	109	97%	99%	98%
Controlled Postoperative Blood Glucose[7]	-	-	96%	97%
Perioperative Temperature Management	120	99%	100%	100%
Prophylactic Antibiotic Selection	83	98%	99%	99%
Prophylactic Antibiotic Selection (Outpatient)	14	79%	98%	98%
Prophylactic Antibiotic Stopped	82	95%	99%	98%
Prophylactic Antibiotic Timing	83	99%	99%	99%
Prophylactic Antibiotic Timing (Outpatient)	14	93%	98%	98%
Urinary Catheter Removal	88	90%	97%	97%
Survey of Patients' Hospital Experiences				
Area Around Room 'Always' Quiet at Night	300+	50%	52%	61%
Doctors 'Always' Communicated Well	300+	79%	80%	82%
Home Recovery Information Given	300+	88%	87%	85%
Hospital Given 9 or 10 on 10 Point Scale	300+	59%	69%	71%
Meds 'Always' Explained Before Given	300+	61%	64%	64%
Nurses 'Always' Communicated Well	300+	79%	79%	79%
Pain 'Always' Well Controlled	300+	69%	71%	71%
Room and Bathroom 'Always' Clean	300+	73%	72%	73%
Timely Help 'Always' Received	300+	64%	66%	68%
Would Definitely Recommend Hospital	300+	56%	73%	71%
Use of Medical Imaging				
Cardiac Imaging Stress Test before Surgery	78	3.8%	5.4%	5.3%
Combination Abdominal CT Scan	378	5.8%	6.3%	10.5%
Combination Brain/Sinus CT Scan	494	4.0%	2.4%	2.7%
Combination Chest CT Scan	304	4.3%	0.5%	2.7%
Follow-up Mammogram/Ultrasound	917	11.3%	8.9%	8.8%
Lumbar Spine MRI for Low Back Pain[1]	-	-	35.3%	37.2%

Holyoke Medical Center

575 Beech Street Phone: 413-534-2500
Holyoke, MA 01040 Fax: 413-534-2664
URL: www.holyokehealth.com

Type: Acute Care Hospitals Emergency Services: Yes
Ownership: Voluntary non-profit - Private Beds: 202

Key Personnel:

Chief of Medical Staff. . . . . M Saleem Bajwa
Emergency Room . . . . Joseph Chang
Quality Assurance . . . . Clark Fenn
Operating Room. . . . . Brigid Glackin
Radiology. . . . . Won Park
CEO/President. . . . . Hank J Porten

Measure	Cases	This Hosp.	State Avg.	U.S. Avg.
Blood Clot Prevention and Treatment				
Anticoagulation Overlap Therapy[2]	42	95%	97%	93%
ICU Venous Thromboembolism Prophylaxis[2]	44	93%	92%	92%
Incidence of Potentially Preventable VTE[1,2]	-	-	7%	10%
UFH with Dosages/Platelet Monitoring[2]	16	100%	91%	97%
Venous Thromboembolism Prophylaxis[2]	389	95%	87%	85%
Warfarin Therapy Discharge Instructions[2]	24	92%	77%	75%
Chest Pain/Possible Heart Attack Care				
Aspirin Given Within 24 Hours of Arrival	59	97%	97%	96%
Fibrinolytic Meds Within 30 Min. of Arrival[7]	-	-	73%	58%
Average Time to ECG (minutes)	60	5	7	7
Average Time to Transfer (minutes)[1]	-	-	55	60
Children's Asthma Care				
Received Home Management Plan of Care	-	-	-	88%
Received Reliever Medication	-	-	-	100%
Received Systemic Corticosteroids	-	-	-	100%
Emergency Department				
Admittance Decision Time (minutes)[2]	1,859	153	119	98
Head CT Results Within 45 Min. of Arrival[1]	-	-	70%	57%
Patients Who Left ER Before Being Seen	46,193	3%	2%	2%
Time from ER Arrival to Admit. (minutes)[2]	1,859	322	313	274
Time from ER Arrival to Discharge (minutes)	391	153	156	134
Time in ER Before Being Evaluated (minutes)	441	46	36	26
Time to Pain Meds for Fractures (minutes)	78	79	59	57
Heart Attack Care				
Aspirin Given at Discharge	27	100%	100%	99%
Fibrinolytic Meds Within 30 Min. of Arrival[7]	-	-	100%	54%
PCI Within 90 Minutes of Arrival[7]	-	-	96%	96%
Statin Prescribed at Discharge	28	96%	99%	98%
Heart Failure Care				
ACE Inhibitor or ARB for LVSD	34	97%	96%	97%
Discharge Instructions Given	141	94%	95%	94%
Evaluation of LVS Function	210	100%	100%	99%
Medicare Spending				
Medicare Spending per Patient (ratio)	-	1.00	1.03	0.98
Pneumonia Care				
Appropriate Initial Antibiotic Given	92	97%	97%	95%
Blood Culture Timing	194	96%	98%	98%
Pregnancy and Delivery Care				
Newborn Deliveries Scheduled Early[2]	25	0%	2%	6%
Preventive Care				
Immunization for Influenza[2]	589	94%	91%	90%
Immunization for Pneumonia[2]	1,785	96%	91%	92%
Stroke Care				
Anticoagulation Therapy for Atrial Fibrillation	16	100%	97%	95%
Antithrombotic Therapy Timing	34	100%	98%	98%
Assessed for Rehabilitation	57	96%	96%	97%
Discharged on Antithrombotic Therapy	55	100%	100%	99%
Discharged on Statin Medication	38	97%	96%	94%
Thrombolytic Therapy Timing	18	100%	68%	66%
Venous Thromboembolism Prophylaxis	53	96%	94%	94%
Written Stroke Educational Materials Given	26	100%	82%	88%
Surgical Care Improvement Project				
Appropriate Beta Blocker Usage	63	98%	98%	98%
Appropriate VTP Within 24 Hours	183	95%	99%	98%
Controlled Postoperative Blood Glucose[7]	-	-	96%	97%
Perioperative Temperature Management	207	97%	100%	100%
Prophylactic Antibiotic Selection	149	99%	99%	99%
Prophylactic Antibiotic Selection (Outpatient)	55	96%	98%	98%
Prophylactic Antibiotic Stopped	146	99%	99%	98%

NOTE: Hospital profiles are in alphabetical order by state, then city, then hospital within the city; Rankings exclude hospitals with less than 25 cases except for patient surveys which excludes hospitals with less than 100 cases; (a) 100-299 cases; (1) The number of cases/patients is too few to report; (2) Data submitted were based on a sample of cases/patients; (3) Results are based on a shorter time period than required; (4) Data suppressed by CMS for one or more quarters; (5) Results are not available for this reporting period; (6) Fewer than 100 patients completed the HCAHPS survey; (7) No cases met the criteria for this measure; (8) The lower limit of the confidence interval cannot be calculated if the number of observed infections equals zero; (9) No data are available from the state/territory for this reporting period; (10) The scores shown reflect fewer than 50 completed surveys; (11) There were discrepancies in the data collection process; (12) This measure does not apply to this hospital for this reporting period; (13) Results cannot be calculated for this reporting period; (14) The results for this state are combined with nearby states to protect confidentiality; Please refer to the User's Guide for a full explanation of data.

Measure	Cases	This Hosp.	State Avg.	U.S. Avg.
Prophylactic Antibiotic Timing	150	99%	99%	99%
Prophylactic Antibiotic Timing (Outpatient)	55	100%	98%	98%
Urinary Catheter Removal	62	81%	97%	97%
Survey of Patients' Hospital Experiences				
Area Around Room 'Always' Quiet at Night	300+	52%	52%	61%
Doctors 'Always' Communicated Well	300+	80%	80%	82%
Home Recovery Information Given	300+	88%	87%	85%
Hospital Given 9 or 10 on 10 Point Scale	300+	70%	69%	71%
Meds 'Always' Explained Before Given	300+	67%	64%	64%
Nurses 'Always' Communicated Well	300+	81%	79%	79%
Pain 'Always' Well Controlled	300+	69%	71%	71%
Room and Bathroom 'Always' Clean	300+	75%	72%	73%
Timely Help 'Always' Received	300+	65%	66%	68%
Would Definitely Recommend Hospital	300+	73%	73%	71%
Use of Medical Imaging				
Cardiac Imaging Stress Test before Surgery	236	1.7%	5.4%	5.3%
Combination Abdominal CT Scan	849	3.5%	6.3%	10.5%
Combination Brain/Sinus CT Scan	920	2.9%	2.4%	2.7%
Combination Chest CT Scan	269	0.0%	0.5%	2.7%
Follow-up Mammogram/Ultrasound	1,551	8.0%	8.9%	8.8%
Lumbar Spine MRI for Low Back Pain	92	38.0%	35.3%	37.2%

Cape Cod Hospital

88 Lewis Bay Road
Hyannis, MA 02601
Phone: 508-771-1800
Fax: 508-790-7964
URL: www.capecodhealth.org
Type: Acute Care Hospitals
Emergency Services: Yes
Ownership: Voluntary non-profit - Private
Beds: 272

Key Personnel:

Pediatric Ambulatory Care . . . . . . Kenneth Colmer, MD
Pediatric In-Patient Care . . . . Kenneth Colmer, MD
Operating Room. . . . . Bonnie Finkle, RN
Chief of Medical Staff . . . . Donald A. Guadagnoli, MD
Emergency Room . . . . Dwayne Hendrick
Radiology. . . . . Gordan Kanzer, MD
CEO/President. . . . . Michael K. Lauf, MBA
Chairman/CEO . . . . William Zammer

Measure	Cases	This Hosp.	State Avg.	U.S. Avg.
Blood Clot Prevention and Treatment				
Anticoagulation Overlap Therapy[2]	123	96%	97%	93%
ICU Venous Thromboembolism Prophylaxis[2]	42	100%	92%	92%
Incidence of Potentially Preventable VTE[1,2]	-	-	7%	10%
UFH with Dosages/Platelet Monitoring[2]	99	95%	91%	97%
Venous Thromboembolism Prophylaxis[2]	355	90%	87%	85%
Warfarin Therapy Discharge Instructions[2]	77	82%	77%	75%
Chest Pain/Possible Heart Attack Care				
Aspirin Given Within 24 Hours of Arrival[1]	-	-	97%	96%
Fibrinolytic Meds Within 30 Min. of Arrival[3,7]	-	-	73%	58%
Average Time to ECG (minutes)[1]	-	-	7	7
Average Time to Transfer (minutes)[3,7]	-	-	55	60
Children's Asthma Care				
Received Home Management Plan of Care	-	-	-	88%
Received Reliever Medication	-	-	-	100%
Received Systemic Corticosteroids	-	-	-	100%
Emergency Department				
Admittance Decision Time (minutes)[2]	915	172	119	98
Head CT Results Within 45 Min. of Arrival	23	52%	70%	57%
Patients Who Left ER Before Being Seen	91,260	1%	2%	2%
Time from ER Arrival to Admit. (minutes)[2]	915	337	313	274
Time from ER Arrival to Discharge (minutes)	396	129	156	134
Time in ER Before Being Evaluated (minutes)	434	10	36	26
Time to Pain Meds for Fractures (minutes)	225	38	59	57
Heart Attack Care				
Aspirin Given at Discharge[2]	299	100%	100%	99%
Fibrinolytic Meds Within 30 Min. of Arrival[2,7]	-	-	100%	54%
PCI Within 90 Minutes of Arrival[2]	57	96%	96%	96%
Statin Prescribed at Discharge[2]	277	98%	99%	98%
Heart Failure Care				
ACE Inhibitor or ARB for LVSD[2]	82	93%	96%	97%
Discharge Instructions Given[2]	191	93%	95%	94%
Evaluation of LVS Function[2]	289	99%	100%	99%
Medicare Spending				
Medicare Spending per Patient (ratio)	-	1.03	1.03	0.98
Pneumonia Care				
Appropriate Initial Antibiotic Given	269	96%	97%	95%
Blood Culture Timing	426	100%	98%	98%
Pregnancy and Delivery Care				
Newborn Deliveries Scheduled Early	41	0%	2%	6%
Preventive Care				
Immunization for Influenza[2]	581	84%	91%	90%
Immunization for Pneumonia[2]	867	86%	91%	92%
Stroke Care				
Anticoagulation Therapy for Atrial Fibrillation[2]	25	100%	97%	95%
Antithrombotic Therapy Timing[2]	103	100%	98%	98%
Assessed for Rehabilitation[2]	127	97%	96%	97%
Discharged on Antithrombotic Therapy[2]	106	99%	100%	99%
Discharged on Statin Medication[2]	72	97%	96%	94%
Thrombolytic Therapy Timing[1,2]	-	-	68%	66%
Venous Thromboembolism Prophylaxis[2]	126	98%	94%	94%
Written Stroke Educational Materials Given[2]	56	73%	82%	88%
Surgical Care Improvement Project				
Appropriate Beta Blocker Usage[2]	384	98%	98%	98%
Appropriate VTP Within 24 Hours[2]	830	99%	99%	98%
Controlled Postoperative Blood Glucose[2]	130	95%	96%	97%
Perioperative Temperature Management[2]	956	100%	100%	100%
Prophylactic Antibiotic Selection[2]	863	99%	99%	99%
Prophylactic Antibiotic Selection (Outpatient)	475	99%	98%	98%
Prophylactic Antibiotic Stopped[2]	847	99%	99%	98%
Prophylactic Antibiotic Timing[2]	863	99%	99%	99%
Prophylactic Antibiotic Timing (Outpatient)	476	99%	98%	98%
Urinary Catheter Removal[2]	749	97%	97%	97%
Survey of Patients' Hospital Experiences				
Area Around Room 'Always' Quiet at Night	300+	52%	52%	61%
Doctors 'Always' Communicated Well	300+	80%	80%	82%
Home Recovery Information Given	300+	85%	87%	85%
Hospital Given 9 or 10 on 10 Point Scale	300+	75%	69%	71%
Meds 'Always' Explained Before Given	300+	64%	64%	64%
Nurses 'Always' Communicated Well	300+	79%	79%	79%
Pain 'Always' Well Controlled	300+	71%	71%	71%
Room and Bathroom 'Always' Clean	300+	76%	72%	73%
Timely Help 'Always' Received	300+	63%	66%	68%
Would Definitely Recommend Hospital	300+	78%	73%	71%
Use of Medical Imaging				
Cardiac Imaging Stress Test before Surgery[1]	-	-	5.4%	5.3%
Combination Abdominal CT Scan	2,791	6.4%	6.3%	10.5%
Combination Brain/Sinus CT Scan	2,095	3.4%	2.4%	2.7%
Combination Chest CT Scan	1,919	1.3%	0.5%	2.7%
Follow-up Mammogram/Ultrasound	4,633	9.8%	8.9%	8.8%
Lumbar Spine MRI for Low Back Pain	312	37.8%	35.3%	37.2%

VA Boston Healthcare System - Jamaica Plain

150 S. Huntington Avenue
Jamaica Plain, MA 02130
Phone: 617-232-9500
URL: www.vaww.visn1.med.va.gov/boston
Type: Acute Care - VA
Emergency Services: No
Ownership: Government Federal
Beds: 376

Key Personnel:

Quality Assurance . . . . Lynn Cannavho, RN
Chief of Medical Staff . . . . Michael E Charness, MD
Emergency Room . . . . Arthur Robins, MD

Measure	Cases	This Hosp.	State Avg.	U.S. Avg.
Blood Clot Prevention and Treatment				
Anticoagulation Overlap Therapy	-	-	97%	93%
ICU Venous Thromboembolism Prophylaxis	-	-	92%	92%
Incidence of Potentially Preventable VTE	-	-	7%	10%
UFH with Dosages/Platelet Monitoring	-	-	91%	97%
Venous Thromboembolism Prophylaxis	-	-	87%	85%
Warfarin Therapy Discharge Instructions	-	-	77%	75%
Chest Pain/Possible Heart Attack Care				
Aspirin Given Within 24 Hours of Arrival	-	-	97%	96%
Fibrinolytic Meds Within 30 Min. of Arrival	-	-	73%	58%
Average Time to ECG (minutes)	-	-	7	7
Average Time to Transfer (minutes)	-	-	55	60
Children's Asthma Care				
Received Home Management Plan of Care	-	-	-	88%
Received Reliever Medication	-	-	-	100%
Received Systemic Corticosteroids	-	-	-	100%
Emergency Department				
Admittance Decision Time (minutes)	-	-	119	98
Head CT Results Within 45 Min. of Arrival	-	-	70%	57%
Patients Who Left ER Before Being Seen	-	-	2%	2%
Time from ER Arrival to Admit. (minutes)	-	-	313	274
Time from ER Arrival to Discharge (minutes)	-	-	156	134
Time in ER Before Being Evaluated (minutes)	-	-	36	26
Time to Pain Meds for Fractures (minutes)	-	-	59	57
Heart Attack Care				
Aspirin Given at Discharge	29	100%	100%	99%
Fibrinolytic Meds Within 30 Min. of Arrival[5]	-	-	100%	54%
PCI Within 90 Minutes of Arrival[1]	-	-	96%	96%
Statin Prescribed at Discharge	31	100%	99%	98%
Heart Failure Care				
ACE Inhibitor or ARB for LVSD	93	87%	96%	97%
Discharge Instructions Given	253	99%	95%	94%
Evaluation of LVS Function	299	100%	100%	99%
Medicare Spending				
Medicare Spending per Patient (ratio)	-	-	1.03	0.98
Pneumonia Care				
Appropriate Initial Antibiotic Given	77	90%	97%	95%
Blood Culture Timing	131	95%	98%	98%
Pregnancy and Delivery Care				
Newborn Deliveries Scheduled Early	-	-	2%	6%
Preventive Care				
Immunization for Influenza[5]	-	-	91%	90%
Immunization for Pneumonia[5]	-	-	91%	92%
Stroke Care				
Anticoagulation Therapy for Atrial Fibrillation	-	-	97%	95%
Antithrombotic Therapy Timing	-	-	98%	98%
Assessed for Rehabilitation	-	-	96%	97%
Discharged on Antithrombotic Therapy	-	-	100%	99%
Discharged on Statin Medication	-	-	96%	94%
Thrombolytic Therapy Timing	-	-	68%	66%
Venous Thromboembolism Prophylaxis	-	-	94%	94%
Written Stroke Educational Materials Given	-	-	82%	88%
Surgical Care Improvement Project				
Appropriate Beta Blocker Usage[2]	177	99%	98%	98%
Appropriate VTP Within 24 Hours[2]	298	100%	99%	98%
Controlled Postoperative Blood Glucose[2]	180	97%	96%	97%
Perioperative Temperature Management[2]	364	99%	100%	100%
Prophylactic Antibiotic Selection	411	100%	99%	99%
Prophylactic Antibiotic Selection (Outpatient)	-	-	98%	98%
Prophylactic Antibiotic Stopped	410	100%	99%	98%
Prophylactic Antibiotic Timing	411	100%	99%	99%
Prophylactic Antibiotic Timing (Outpatient)	-	-	98%	98%
Urinary Catheter Removal[2]	326	99%	97%	97%
Survey of Patients' Hospital Experiences				
Area Around Room 'Always' Quiet at Night	-	-	52%	61%
Doctors 'Always' Communicated Well	-	-	80%	82%
Home Recovery Information Given	-	-	87%	85%
Hospital Given 9 or 10 on 10 Point Scale	-	-	69%	71%
Meds 'Always' Explained Before Given	-	-	64%	64%
Nurses 'Always' Communicated Well	-	-	79%	79%
Pain 'Always' Well Controlled	-	-	71%	71%
Room and Bathroom 'Always' Clean	-	-	72%	73%
Timely Help 'Always' Received	-	-	66%	68%
Would Definitely Recommend Hospital	-	-	73%	71%
Use of Medical Imaging				
Cardiac Imaging Stress Test before Surgery	-	-	5.4%	5.3%
Combination Abdominal CT Scan	-	-	6.3%	10.5%
Combination Brain/Sinus CT Scan	-	-	2.4%	2.7%
Combination Chest CT Scan	-	-	0.5%	2.7%
Follow-up Mammogram/Ultrasound	-	-	8.9%	8.8%
Lumbar Spine MRI for Low Back Pain	-	-	35.3%	37.2%

Lawrence General Hospital

One General Street
Lawrence, MA 01842
Phone: 978-683-4000
Fax: 978-946-8175
URL: www.lawrencegeneral.org
Type: Acute Care Hospitals
Emergency Services: Yes
Ownership: Voluntary non-profit - Private
Beds: 190

Key Personnel:

Chief of Medical Staff . . . . Brian Callahan

NOTE: Hospital profiles are in alphabetical order by state, then city, then hospital within the city; Rankings exclude hospitals with less than 25 cases except for patient surveys which excludes hospitals with less than 100 cases; (a) 100-299 cases; (1) The number of cases/patients is too few to report; (2) Data submitted were based on a sample of cases/patients; (3) Results are based on a shorter time period than required; (4) Data suppressed by CMS for one or more quarters; (5) Results are not available for this reporting period; (6) Fewer than 100 patients completed the HCAHPS survey; (7) No cases met the criteria for this measure; (8) The lower limit of the confidence interval cannot be calculated if the number of observed infections equals zero; (9) No data are available from the state/territory for this reporting period; (10) The scores shown reflect fewer than 50 completed surveys; (11) There were discrepancies in the data collection process; (12) This measure does not apply to this hospital for this reporting period; (13) Results cannot be calculated for this reporting period; (14) The results for this state are combined with nearby states to protect confidentiality; Please refer to the User's Guide for a full explanation of data.

Emergency Room .... Patrick Curran
Quality Assurance .... Theresa Dunn Sievers, MS, RN, CPHQ, C
Quality Assurance .... Janet Nelson
President/CEO............... Dianne J. Wilson

Measure	Cases	This Hosp.	State Avg.	U.S. Avg.
Blood Clot Prevention and Treatment				
Anticoagulation Overlap Therapy[2]	49	84%	97%	93%
ICU Venous Thromboembolism Prophylaxis[2]	67	73%	92%	92%
Incidence of Potentially Preventable VTE[1,2]	-	-	7%	10%
UFH with Dosages/Platelet Monitoring[2]	34	100%	91%	97%
Venous Thromboembolism Prophylaxis[2]	369	78%	87%	85%
Warfarin Therapy Discharge Instructions[2]	33	39%	77%	75%
Chest Pain/Possible Heart Attack Care				
Aspirin Given Within 24 Hours of Arrival	28	93%	97%	96%
Fibrinolytic Meds Within 30 Min. of Arrival[7]	-	-	73%	58%
Average Time to ECG (minutes)	30	12	7	7
Average Time to Transfer (minutes)[1]	-	-	55	60
Children's Asthma Care				
Received Home Management Plan of Care	-	-	-	88%
Received Reliever Medication	-	-	-	100%
Received Systemic Corticosteroids	-	-	-	100%
Emergency Department				
Admittance Decision Time (minutes)[2]	671	175	119	98
Head CT Results Within 45 Min. of Arrival	27	63%	70%	57%
Patients Who Left ER Before Being Seen	72,995	3%	2%	2%
Time from ER Arrival to Admit. (minutes)[2]	675	338	313	274
Time from ER Arrival to Discharge (minutes)	419	138	156	134
Time in ER Before Being Evaluated (minutes)	423	75	36	26
Time to Pain Meds for Fractures (minutes)	161	61	59	57
Heart Attack Care				
Aspirin Given at Discharge	159	98%	100%	99%
Fibrinolytic Meds Within 30 Min. of Arrival[7]	-	-	100%	54%
PCI Within 90 Minutes of Arrival	31	97%	96%	96%
Statin Prescribed at Discharge	145	96%	99%	98%
Heart Failure Care				
ACE Inhibitor or ARB for LVSD	102	88%	96%	97%
Discharge Instructions Given	304	81%	95%	94%
Evaluation of LVS Function	418	100%	100%	99%
Medicare Spending				
Medicare Spending per Patient (ratio)	-	1.10	1.03	0.98
Pneumonia Care				
Appropriate Initial Antibiotic Given	153	98%	97%	95%
Blood Culture Timing	258	97%	98%	98%
Pregnancy and Delivery Care				
Newborn Deliveries Scheduled Early[2]	26	0%	2%	6%
Preventive Care				
Immunization for Influenza[2]	548	90%	91%	90%
Immunization for Pneumonia[2]	597	87%	91%	92%
Stroke Care				
Anticoagulation Therapy for Atrial Fibrillation	21	100%	97%	95%
Antithrombotic Therapy Timing	83	98%	98%	98%
Assessed for Rehabilitation	91	88%	96%	97%
Discharged on Antithrombotic Therapy	83	100%	100%	99%
Discharged on Statin Medication	58	88%	96%	94%
Thrombolytic Therapy Timing[1]	-	-	68%	66%
Venous Thromboembolism Prophylaxis	91	79%	94%	94%
Written Stroke Educational Materials Given	43	19%	82%	88%
Surgical Care Improvement Project				
Appropriate Beta Blocker Usage	66	98%	98%	98%
Appropriate VTP Within 24 Hours	230	94%	99%	98%
Controlled Postoperative Blood Glucose[7]	-	-	96%	97%
Perioperative Temperature Management	280	100%	100%	100%
Prophylactic Antibiotic Selection	137	97%	99%	99%
Prophylactic Antibiotic Selection (Outpatient)	112	96%	98%	98%
Prophylactic Antibiotic Stopped	133	97%	99%	98%
Prophylactic Antibiotic Timing	137	96%	99%	99%
Prophylactic Antibiotic Timing (Outpatient)	116	90%	98%	98%
Urinary Catheter Removal	173	84%	97%	97%
Survey of Patients' Hospital Experiences				
Area Around Room 'Always' Quiet at Night	300+	52%	52%	61%
Doctors 'Always' Communicated Well	300+	81%	80%	82%
Home Recovery Information Given	300+	86%	87%	85%
Hospital Given 9 or 10 on 10 Point Scale	300+	65%	69%	71%
Meds 'Always' Explained Before Given	300+	64%	64%	64%
Nurses 'Always' Communicated Well	300+	82%	79%	79%
Pain 'Always' Well Controlled	300+	72%	71%	71%
Room and Bathroom 'Always' Clean	300+	72%	72%	73%
Timely Help 'Always' Received	300+	65%	66%	68%
Would Definitely Recommend Hospital	300+	74%	73%	71%
Use of Medical Imaging				
Cardiac Imaging Stress Test before Surgery	419	4.5%	5.4%	5.3%
Combination Abdominal CT Scan	942	7.4%	6.3%	10.5%
Combination Brain/Sinus CT Scan	986	2.0%	2.4%	2.7%
Combination Chest CT Scan	650	3.7%	0.5%	2.7%
Follow-up Mammogram/Ultrasound	920	9.7%	8.9%	8.8%
Lumbar Spine MRI for Low Back Pain[7]	-	-	35.3%	37.2%

Northampton VA Medical Center

421 N Main St
Leeds, MA 01053
Phone: 413-584-4040
Fax: 413-582-3040
E-mail: lastname.firstname@med.va.gov
URL: www.visn1.med.va.gov/northampton
Type: Acute Care - VA
Emergency Services: No
Ownership: Government Federal
Beds: 167

Key Personnel:
Infection Control.............. Don Braman
CEO/President............... Mary A Dowling
Chief of Medical Staff.......... George Fuller, MD
Quality Assurance .... Michael Walsh
Patient Relations .... Rosemary Westerman

Measure	Cases	This Hosp.	State Avg.	U.S. Avg.
Blood Clot Prevention and Treatment				
Anticoagulation Overlap Therapy	-	-	97%	93%
ICU Venous Thromboembolism Prophylaxis	-	-	92%	92%
Incidence of Potentially Preventable VTE	-	-	7%	10%
UFH with Dosages/Platelet Monitoring	-	-	91%	97%
Venous Thromboembolism Prophylaxis	-	-	87%	85%
Warfarin Therapy Discharge Instructions	-	-	77%	75%
Chest Pain/Possible Heart Attack Care				
Aspirin Given Within 24 Hours of Arrival	-	-	97%	96%
Fibrinolytic Meds Within 30 Min. of Arrival	-	-	73%	58%
Average Time to ECG (minutes)	-	-	7	7
Average Time to Transfer (minutes)	-	-	55	60
Children's Asthma Care				
Received Home Management Plan of Care	-	-	-	88%
Received Reliever Medication	-	-	-	100%
Received Systemic Corticosteroids	-	-	-	100%
Emergency Department				
Admittance Decision Time (minutes)	-	-	119	98
Head CT Results Within 45 Min. of Arrival	-	-	70%	57%
Patients Who Left ER Before Being Seen	-	-	2%	2%
Time from ER Arrival to Admit. (minutes)	-	-	313	274
Time from ER Arrival to Discharge (minutes)	-	-	156	134
Time in ER Before Being Evaluated (minutes)	-	-	36	26
Time to Pain Meds for Fractures (minutes)	-	-	59	57
Heart Attack Care				
Aspirin Given at Discharge[5]	-	-	100%	99%
Fibrinolytic Meds Within 30 Min. of Arrival[5]	-	-	100%	54%
PCI Within 90 Minutes of Arrival[5]	-	-	96%	96%
Statin Prescribed at Discharge[5]	-	-	99%	98%
Heart Failure Care				
ACE Inhibitor or ARB for LVSD[5]	-	-	96%	97%
Discharge Instructions Given[5]	-	-	95%	94%
Evaluation of LVS Function[5]	-	-	100%	99%
Medicare Spending				
Medicare Spending per Patient (ratio)	-	-	1.03	0.98
Pneumonia Care				
Appropriate Initial Antibiotic Given[5]	-	-	97%	95%
Blood Culture Timing[5]	-	-	98%	98%
Pregnancy and Delivery Care				
Newborn Deliveries Scheduled Early	-	-	2%	6%
Preventive Care				
Immunization for Influenza[2,3]	146	84%	91%	90%
Immunization for Pneumonia[2,3]	130	88%	91%	92%
Stroke Care				
Anticoagulation Therapy for Atrial Fibrillation	-	-	97%	95%
Antithrombotic Therapy Timing	-	-	98%	98%
Assessed for Rehabilitation	-	-	96%	97%
Discharged on Antithrombotic Therapy	-	-	100%	99%
Discharged on Statin Medication	-	-	96%	94%
Thrombolytic Therapy Timing	-	-	68%	66%
Venous Thromboembolism Prophylaxis	-	-	94%	94%
Written Stroke Educational Materials Given	-	-	82%	88%
Surgical Care Improvement Project				
Appropriate Beta Blocker Usage[5]	-	-	98%	98%
Appropriate VTP Within 24 Hours[5]	-	-	99%	98%
Controlled Postoperative Blood Glucose[5]	-	-	96%	97%
Perioperative Temperature Management[5]	-	-	100%	100%
Prophylactic Antibiotic Selection[5]	-	-	99%	99%
Prophylactic Antibiotic Selection (Outpatient)	-	-	98%	98%
Prophylactic Antibiotic Stopped[5]	-	-	99%	98%
Prophylactic Antibiotic Timing[5]	-	-	99%	99%
Prophylactic Antibiotic Timing (Outpatient)	-	-	98%	98%
Urinary Catheter Removal[5]	-	-	97%	97%
Survey of Patients' Hospital Experiences				
Area Around Room 'Always' Quiet at Night	-	-	52%	61%
Doctors 'Always' Communicated Well	-	-	80%	82%
Home Recovery Information Given	-	-	87%	85%
Hospital Given 9 or 10 on 10 Point Scale	-	-	69%	71%
Meds 'Always' Explained Before Given	-	-	64%	64%
Nurses 'Always' Communicated Well	-	-	79%	79%
Pain 'Always' Well Controlled	-	-	71%	71%
Room and Bathroom 'Always' Clean	-	-	72%	73%
Timely Help 'Always' Received	-	-	66%	68%
Would Definitely Recommend Hospital	-	-	73%	71%
Use of Medical Imaging				
Cardiac Imaging Stress Test before Surgery	-	-	5.4%	5.3%
Combination Abdominal CT Scan	-	-	6.3%	10.5%
Combination Brain/Sinus CT Scan	-	-	2.4%	2.7%
Combination Chest CT Scan	-	-	0.5%	2.7%
Follow-up Mammogram/Ultrasound	-	-	8.9%	8.8%
Lumbar Spine MRI for Low Back Pain	-	-	35.3%	37.2%

Healthalliance Hospitals

60 Hospital Road
Leominster, MA 01453
Phone: 978-466-2000
Fax: 978-466-2200
URL: www.healthalliance.com
Type: Acute Care Hospitals
Emergency Services: Yes
Ownership: Voluntary non-profit - Other
Beds: 154

Key Personnel:
Radiology.................. Daniel P Berman
Chair/CEO.................. Paul D'Onfro, Esq.
Operating Room............. Benjamin Grajales
Quality Assurance .... Cathy Hawke
Chief of Medical Staff.......... Daniel O'Leary, MD
CEO/President.............. Deborah Weymouth, FACHE

Measure	Cases	This Hosp.	State Avg.	U.S. Avg.
Blood Clot Prevention and Treatment				
Anticoagulation Overlap Therapy[2]	53	91%	97%	93%
ICU Venous Thromboembolism Prophylaxis[2]	111	100%	92%	92%
Incidence of Potentially Preventable VTE[1,2]	-	-	7%	10%
UFH with Dosages/Platelet Monitoring[1,2]	-	-	91%	97%
Venous Thromboembolism Prophylaxis[2]	444	88%	87%	85%
Warfarin Therapy Discharge Instructions[2]	38	8%	77%	75%
Chest Pain/Possible Heart Attack Care				
Aspirin Given Within 24 Hours of Arrival	173	99%	97%	96%
Fibrinolytic Meds Within 30 Min. of Arrival[7]	-	-	73%	58%
Average Time to ECG (minutes)	174	9	7	7
Average Time to Transfer (minutes)	18	45	55	60
Children's Asthma Care				
Received Home Management Plan of Care	-	-	-	88%
Received Reliever Medication	-	-	-	100%
Received Systemic Corticosteroids	-	-	-	100%
Emergency Department				
Admittance Decision Time (minutes)[2]	579	92	119	98
Head CT Results Within 45 Min. of Arrival	23	87%	70%	57%
Patients Who Left ER Before Being Seen	45,012	4%	2%	2%
Time from ER Arrival to Admit. (minutes)[2]	595	281	313	274
Time from ER Arrival to Discharge (minutes)	324	168	156	134

NOTE: Hospital profiles are in alphabetical order by state, then city, then hospital within the city; Rankings exclude hospitals with less than 25 cases except for patient surveys which excludes hospitals with less than 100 cases; (a) 100-299 cases; (1) The number of cases/patients is too few to report; (2) Data submitted were based on a sample of cases/patients; (3) Results are based on a shorter time period than required; (4) Data suppressed by CMS for one or more quarters; (5) Results are not available for this reporting period; (6) Fewer than 100 patients completed the HCAHPS survey; (7) No cases met the criteria for this measure; (8) The lower limit of the confidence interval cannot be calculated if the number of observed infections equals zero; (9) No data are available from the state/territory for this reporting period; (10) The scores shown reflect fewer than 50 completed surveys; (11) There were discrepancies in the data collection process; (12) This measure does not apply to this hospital for this reporting period; (13) Results cannot be calculated for this reporting period; (14) The results for this state are combined with nearby states to protect confidentiality; Please refer to the User's Guide for a full explanation of data.

Measure	Cases	This Hosp.	State Avg.	U.S. Avg.
Time in ER Before Being Evaluated (minutes)	193	65	36	26
Time to Pain Meds for Fractures (minutes)	149	73	59	57
Heart Attack Care				
Aspirin Given at Discharge	41	100%	100%	99%
Fibrinolytic Meds Within 30 Min. of Arrival[7]	-	-	100%	54%
PCI Within 90 Minutes of Arrival[7]	-	-	96%	96%
Statin Prescribed at Discharge	38	100%	99%	98%
Heart Failure Care				
ACE Inhibitor or ARB for LVSD[2]	52	94%	96%	97%
Discharge Instructions Given[2]	164	95%	95%	94%
Evaluation of LVS Function[2]	226	100%	100%	99%
Medicare Spending				
Medicare Spending per Patient (ratio)	-	1.05	1.03	0.98
Pneumonia Care				
Appropriate Initial Antibiotic Given[2]	83	98%	97%	95%
Blood Culture Timing[2]	147	99%	98%	98%
Pregnancy and Delivery Care				
Newborn Deliveries Scheduled Early[2]	21	5%	2%	6%
Preventive Care				
Immunization for Influenza[2]	500	85%	91%	90%
Immunization for Pneumonia[2]	666	86%	91%	92%
Stroke Care				
Anticoagulation Therapy for Atrial Fibrillation[2]	12	67%	97%	95%
Antithrombotic Therapy Timing[2]	77	96%	98%	98%
Assessed for Rehabilitation[2]	78	82%	96%	97%
Discharged on Antithrombotic Therapy[2]	74	100%	100%	99%
Discharged on Statin Medication[2]	62	89%	96%	94%
Thrombolytic Therapy Timing[1,2]	-	-	68%	66%
Venous Thromboembolism Prophylaxis[2]	80	81%	94%	94%
Written Stroke Educational Materials Given[2]	44	0%	82%	88%
Surgical Care Improvement Project				
Appropriate Beta Blocker Usage[2]	95	100%	98%	98%
Appropriate VTP Within 24 Hours[2]	234	96%	99%	98%
Controlled Postoperative Blood Glucose[2,7]	-	-	96%	97%
Perioperative Temperature Management[2]	279	100%	100%	100%
Prophylactic Antibiotic Selection[2]	185	97%	99%	99%
Prophylactic Antibiotic Selection (Outpatient)	105	99%	98%	98%
Prophylactic Antibiotic Stopped[2]	180	98%	99%	98%
Prophylactic Antibiotic Timing[2]	185	98%	99%	99%
Prophylactic Antibiotic Timing (Outpatient)	101	95%	98%	98%
Urinary Catheter Removal[2]	171	98%	97%	97%
Survey of Patients' Hospital Experiences				
Area Around Room 'Always' Quiet at Night	300+	52%	52%	61%
Doctors 'Always' Communicated Well	300+	80%	80%	82%
Home Recovery Information Given	300+	86%	87%	85%
Hospital Given 9 or 10 on 10 Point Scale	300+	67%	69%	71%
Meds 'Always' Explained Before Given	300+	62%	64%	64%
Nurses 'Always' Communicated Well	300+	78%	79%	79%
Pain 'Always' Well Controlled	300+	70%	71%	71%
Room and Bathroom 'Always' Clean	300+	72%	72%	73%
Timely Help 'Always' Received	300+	64%	66%	68%
Would Definitely Recommend Hospital	300+	67%	73%	71%
Use of Medical Imaging				
Cardiac Imaging Stress Test before Surgery	255	4.7%	5.4%	5.3%
Combination Abdominal CT Scan	665	1.8%	6.3%	10.5%
Combination Brain/Sinus CT Scan	628	1.6%	2.4%	2.7%
Combination Chest CT Scan	527	0.0%	0.5%	2.7%
Follow-up Mammogram/Ultrasound	1,365	6.4%	8.9%	8.8%
Lumbar Spine MRI for Low Back Pain[7]	-	-	35.3%	37.2%

Lowell General Hospital

295 Varnum Avenue
Lowell, MA 01854
URL: www.lowellgeneral.org
Phone: 978-937-6000
Fax: 978-452-4169
Type: Acute Care Hospitals
Ownership: Voluntary non-profit - Private
Emergency Services: Yes
Beds: 208

Key Personnel:
Radiology.................... Scott D Abel
CEO .... Normand E Deschene
Infection Control.............. Karen Kennet
Coronary Care................ Patricia Morse
Quality Assurance .... Gina O'Connor
Chief of Medical Staff.......... Wayne E Pasanen, MD
Pediatric Ambulatory Care ...... Michelle Saboliauskas
Operating Room............... Nicholas Spirito

Measure	Cases	This Hosp.	State Avg.	U.S. Avg.
Blood Clot Prevention and Treatment				
Anticoagulation Overlap Therapy[2]	58	97%	97%	93%
ICU Venous Thromboembolism Prophylaxis[2]	20	60%	92%	92%
Incidence of Potentially Preventable VTE[2]	12	0%	7%	10%
UFH with Dosages/Platelet Monitoring[2]	27	96%	91%	97%
Venous Thromboembolism Prophylaxis[2]	341	93%	87%	85%
Warfarin Therapy Discharge Instructions[2]	37	59%	77%	75%
Chest Pain/Possible Heart Attack Care				
Aspirin Given Within 24 Hours of Arrival[1]	-	-	97%	96%
Fibrinolytic Meds Within 30 Min. of Arrival[3,7]	-	-	73%	58%
Average Time to ECG (minutes)[1]	-	-	7	7
Average Time to Transfer (minutes)[3,7]	-	-	55	60
Children's Asthma Care				
Received Home Management Plan of Care	-	-	-	88%
Received Reliever Medication	-	-	-	100%
Received Systemic Corticosteroids	-	-	-	100%
Emergency Department				
Admittance Decision Time (minutes)[2]	606	136	119	98
Head CT Results Within 45 Min. of Arrival	12	92%	70%	57%
Patients Who Left ER Before Being Seen	55,796	4%	2%	2%
Time from ER Arrival to Admit. (minutes)[2]	621	378	313	274
Time from ER Arrival to Discharge (minutes)	389	192	156	134
Time in ER Before Being Evaluated (minutes)	428	79	36	26
Time to Pain Meds for Fractures (minutes)	162	82	59	57
Heart Attack Care				
Aspirin Given at Discharge[2]	238	100%	100%	99%
Fibrinolytic Meds Within 30 Min. of Arrival[2,7]	-	-	100%	54%
PCI Within 90 Minutes of Arrival[2]	63	98%	96%	96%
Statin Prescribed at Discharge[2]	242	100%	99%	98%
Heart Failure Care				
ACE Inhibitor or ARB for LVSD[2]	70	99%	96%	97%
Discharge Instructions Given[2]	239	94%	95%	94%
Evaluation of LVS Function[2]	338	99%	100%	99%
Medicare Spending				
Medicare Spending per Patient (ratio)	-	0.99	1.03	0.98
Pneumonia Care				
Appropriate Initial Antibiotic Given[2]	132	98%	97%	95%
Blood Culture Timing[2]	185	98%	98%	98%
Pregnancy and Delivery Care				
Newborn Deliveries Scheduled Early[2]	44	5%	2%	6%
Preventive Care				
Immunization for Influenza[2]	499	84%	91%	90%
Immunization for Pneumonia[2]	534	87%	91%	92%
Stroke Care				
Anticoagulation Therapy for Atrial Fibrillation[2]	16	88%	97%	95%
Antithrombotic Therapy Timing[2]	101	94%	98%	98%
Assessed for Rehabilitation[2]	118	92%	96%	97%
Discharged on Antithrombotic Therapy[2]	109	99%	100%	99%
Discharged on Statin Medication[2]	87	99%	96%	94%
Thrombolytic Therapy Timing[1,2]	-	-	68%	66%
Venous Thromboembolism Prophylaxis[2]	118	95%	94%	94%
Written Stroke Educational Materials Given[2]	59	86%	82%	88%
Surgical Care Improvement Project				
Appropriate Beta Blocker Usage[2]	256	98%	98%	98%
Appropriate VTP Within 24 Hours[2]	635	98%	99%	98%
Controlled Postoperative Blood Glucose[2,7]	-	-	96%	97%
Perioperative Temperature Management[2]	755	100%	100%	100%
Prophylactic Antibiotic Selection[2]	562	99%	99%	99%
Prophylactic Antibiotic Selection (Outpatient)	368	98%	98%	98%
Prophylactic Antibiotic Stopped[2]	549	99%	99%	98%
Prophylactic Antibiotic Timing[2]	562	99%	99%	99%
Prophylactic Antibiotic Timing (Outpatient)	374	98%	98%	98%
Urinary Catheter Removal[2]	456	96%	97%	97%
Survey of Patients' Hospital Experiences				
Area Around Room 'Always' Quiet at Night	300+	58%	52%	61%
Doctors 'Always' Communicated Well	300+	80%	80%	82%
Home Recovery Information Given	300+	85%	87%	85%
Hospital Given 9 or 10 on 10 Point Scale	300+	71%	69%	71%
Meds 'Always' Explained Before Given	300+	64%	64%	64%
Nurses 'Always' Communicated Well	300+	80%	79%	79%
Pain 'Always' Well Controlled	300+	72%	71%	71%
Room and Bathroom 'Always' Clean	300+	73%	72%	73%
Timely Help 'Always' Received	300+	66%	66%	68%
Would Definitely Recommend Hospital	300+	77%	73%	71%
Use of Medical Imaging				
Cardiac Imaging Stress Test before Surgery	171	2.9%	5.4%	5.3%
Combination Abdominal CT Scan	1,033	4.0%	6.3%	10.5%
Combination Brain/Sinus CT Scan	775	1.4%	2.4%	2.7%
Combination Chest CT Scan	824	0.2%	0.5%	2.7%
Follow-up Mammogram/Ultrasound	1,746	8.2%	8.9%	8.8%
Lumbar Spine MRI for Low Back Pain[1]	-	-	35.3%	37.2%

Saints Medical Center

1 Hospital Drive
Lowell, MA 01852
Phone: 978-458-1411
Fax: 978-458-8369
Type: Acute Care Hospitals
Ownership: Voluntary non-profit - Church
Emergency Services: Yes
Beds: 227

Key Personnel:
Operating Room............... Winnie Beaton
Quality Assurance .... Marjorie Boldt
Chief of Medical Staff.......... Peter S Connolly
President................... Billy Parish
Emergency Room .... Margrett Thibault
Radiology.................... Paul S Tower
Cardiac Laboratory............ Pammella Waksmonski

Measure	Cases	This Hosp.	State Avg.	U.S. Avg.
Blood Clot Prevention and Treatment				
Anticoagulation Overlap Therapy[2]	27	89%	97%	93%
ICU Venous Thromboembolism Prophylaxis[2]	31	77%	92%	92%
Incidence of Potentially Preventable VTE[1,2]	-	-	7%	10%
UFH with Dosages/Platelet Monitoring[2]	13	100%	91%	97%
Venous Thromboembolism Prophylaxis[2]	407	73%	87%	85%
Warfarin Therapy Discharge Instructions[2]	15	80%	77%	75%
Chest Pain/Possible Heart Attack Care				
Aspirin Given Within 24 Hours of Arrival	36	94%	97%	96%
Fibrinolytic Meds Within 30 Min. of Arrival[7]	-	-	73%	58%
Average Time to ECG (minutes)	35	7	7	7
Average Time to Transfer (minutes)	12	37	55	60
Children's Asthma Care				
Received Home Management Plan of Care	-	-	-	88%
Received Reliever Medication	-	-	-	100%
Received Systemic Corticosteroids	-	-	-	100%
Emergency Department				
Admittance Decision Time (minutes)[2]	775	185	119	98
Head CT Results Within 45 Min. of Arrival	11	36%	70%	57%
Patients Who Left ER Before Being Seen	44,627	2%	2%	2%
Time from ER Arrival to Admit. (minutes)[2]	792	366	313	274
Time from ER Arrival to Discharge (minutes)	380	154	156	134
Time in ER Before Being Evaluated (minutes)	270	54	36	26
Time to Pain Meds for Fractures (minutes)	65	76	59	57
Heart Attack Care				
Aspirin Given at Discharge	25	100%	100%	99%
Fibrinolytic Meds Within 30 Min. of Arrival[7]	-	-	100%	54%
PCI Within 90 Minutes of Arrival[7]	-	-	96%	96%
Statin Prescribed at Discharge	23	96%	99%	98%
Heart Failure Care				
ACE Inhibitor or ARB for LVSD[2]	48	92%	96%	97%
Discharge Instructions Given[2]	172	84%	95%	94%
Evaluation of LVS Function[2]	245	99%	100%	99%
Medicare Spending				
Medicare Spending per Patient (ratio)	-	1.04	1.03	0.98
Pneumonia Care				
Appropriate Initial Antibiotic Given[2]	96	89%	97%	95%
Blood Culture Timing[2]	181	96%	98%	98%
Pregnancy and Delivery Care				
Newborn Deliveries Scheduled Early[7]	-	-	2%	6%
Preventive Care				
Immunization for Influenza[2]	512	88%	91%	90%
Immunization for Pneumonia[2]	736	88%	91%	92%
Stroke Care				
Anticoagulation Therapy for Atrial Fibrillation[1]	-	-	97%	95%
Antithrombotic Therapy Timing	60	95%	98%	98%
Assessed for Rehabilitation	65	94%	96%	97%
Discharged on Antithrombotic Therapy	62	100%	100%	99%
Discharged on Statin Medication	55	82%	96%	94%

NOTE: Hospital profiles are in alphabetical order by state, then city, then hospital within the city; Rankings exclude hospitals with less than 25 cases except for patient surveys which excludes hospitals with less than 100 cases; (a) 100-299 cases; (1) The number of cases/patients is too few to report; (2) Data submitted were based on a sample of cases/patients; (3) Results are based on a shorter time period than required; (4) Data suppressed by CMS for one or more quarters; (5) Results are not available for this reporting period; (6) Fewer than 100 patients completed the HCAHPS survey; (7) No cases met the criteria for this measure; (8) The lower limit of the confidence interval cannot be calculated if the number of observed infections equals zero; (9) No data are available from the state/territory for this reporting period; (10) The scores shown reflect fewer than 50 completed surveys; (11) There were discrepancies in the data collection process; (12) This measure does not apply to this hospital for this reporting period; (13) Results cannot be calculated for this reporting period; (14) The results for this state are combined with nearby states to protect confidentiality; Please refer to the User's Guide for a full explanation of data.

Measure	Cases	This Hosp.	State Avg.	U.S. Avg.
Thrombolytic Therapy Timing[1]	-	-	68%	66%
Venous Thromboembolism Prophylaxis	65	80%	94%	94%
Written Stroke Educational Materials Given	29	93%	82%	88%
Surgical Care Improvement Project				
Appropriate Beta Blocker Usage	27	93%	98%	98%
Appropriate VTP Within 24 Hours	74	97%	99%	98%
Controlled Postoperative Blood Glucose[7]	-	-	96%	97%
Perioperative Temperature Management	78	100%	100%	100%
Prophylactic Antibiotic Selection	39	100%	99%	99%
Prophylactic Antibiotic Selection (Outpatient)	11	100%	98%	98%
Prophylactic Antibiotic Stopped	39	100%	99%	98%
Prophylactic Antibiotic Timing	39	100%	99%	99%
Prophylactic Antibiotic Timing (Outpatient)	11	91%	98%	98%
Urinary Catheter Removal	41	76%	97%	97%
Survey of Patients' Hospital Experiences				
Area Around Room 'Always' Quiet at Night	300+	54%	52%	61%
Doctors 'Always' Communicated Well	300+	79%	80%	82%
Home Recovery Information Given	300+	85%	87%	85%
Hospital Given 9 or 10 on 10 Point Scale	300+	65%	69%	71%
Meds 'Always' Explained Before Given	300+	62%	64%	64%
Nurses 'Always' Communicated Well	300+	79%	79%	79%
Pain 'Always' Well Controlled	300+	70%	71%	71%
Room and Bathroom 'Always' Clean	300+	75%	72%	73%
Timely Help 'Always' Received	300+	68%	66%	68%
Would Definitely Recommend Hospital	300+	68%	73%	71%
Use of Medical Imaging				
Cardiac Imaging Stress Test before Surgery	160	3.8%	5.4%	5.3%
Combination Abdominal CT Scan	625	4.5%	6.3%	10.5%
Combination Brain/Sinus CT Scan	625	2.4%	2.4%	2.7%
Combination Chest CT Scan	431	2.1%	0.5%	2.7%
Follow-up Mammogram/Ultrasound	1,455	8.3%	8.9%	8.8%
Lumbar Spine MRI for Low Back Pain[7]	-	-	35.3%	37.2%

Marlborough Hospital

157 Union Street
Marlborough, MA 01752
Phone: 508-481-5000
Fax: 508-485-9123
E-mail: gorfinkb@ummhc.org
Type: Acute Care Hospitals
Emergency Services: Yes
Ownership: Voluntary non-profit - Private
Beds: 104

Key Personnel:
Cardiac Laboratory............ Carlucci Daniel
Emergency Room .... Katharyn Kennedy, MD
Pediatric Ambulatory Care...... Ricardo Lewitus, MD
Chief of Medical Staff.......... Bhalchandra Parulkar, MD
CEO/President............... John Polanowicz
Quality Assurance .... Sue Scott
Operating Room............. Markian Stecyk, MD
Radiology.................. Mark Sykes, MD

Measure	Cases	This Hosp.	State Avg.	U.S. Avg.
Blood Clot Prevention and Treatment				
Anticoagulation Overlap Therapy[2]	17	100%	97%	93%
ICU Venous Thromboembolism Prophylaxis[2]	74	93%	92%	92%
Incidence of Potentially Preventable VTE[1,2]	-	-	7%	10%
UFH with Dosages/Platelet Monitoring[1,2]	-	-	91%	97%
Venous Thromboembolism Prophylaxis[2]	210	79%	87%	85%
Warfarin Therapy Discharge Instructions[2]	15	33%	77%	75%
Chest Pain/Possible Heart Attack Care				
Aspirin Given Within 24 Hours of Arrival	58	97%	97%	96%
Fibrinolytic Meds Within 30 Min. of Arrival[7]	-	-	73%	58%
Average Time to ECG (minutes)	61	6	7	7
Average Time to Transfer (minutes)[1]	-	-	55	60
Children's Asthma Care				
Received Home Management Plan of Care	-	-	-	88%
Received Reliever Medication	-	-	-	100%
Received Systemic Corticosteroids	-	-	-	100%
Emergency Department				
Admittance Decision Time (minutes)[2]	306	150	119	98
Head CT Results Within 45 Min. of Arrival[1]	-	-	70%	57%
Patients Who Left ER Before Being Seen	27,245	2%	2%	2%
Time from ER Arrival to Admit. (minutes)[2]	388	370	313	274
Time from ER Arrival to Discharge (minutes)	267	167	156	134
Time in ER Before Being Evaluated (minutes)	295	65	36	26
Time to Pain Meds for Fractures (minutes)	77	50	59	57
Heart Attack Care				
Aspirin Given at Discharge	14	100%	100%	99%
Fibrinolytic Meds Within 30 Min. of Arrival[7]	-	-	100%	54%
PCI Within 90 Minutes of Arrival[7]	-	-	96%	96%
Statin Prescribed at Discharge	14	93%	99%	98%
Heart Failure Care				
ACE Inhibitor or ARB for LVSD	22	100%	96%	97%
Discharge Instructions Given	100	88%	95%	94%
Evaluation of LVS Function	137	100%	100%	99%
Medicare Spending				
Medicare Spending per Patient (ratio)	-	1.07	1.03	0.98
Pneumonia Care				
Appropriate Initial Antibiotic Given	82	96%	97%	95%
Blood Culture Timing	118	97%	98%	98%
Pregnancy and Delivery Care				
Newborn Deliveries Scheduled Early[7]	-	-	2%	6%
Preventive Care				
Immunization for Influenza[2]	397	96%	91%	90%
Immunization for Pneumonia[2]	456	92%	91%	92%
Stroke Care				
Anticoagulation Therapy for Atrial Fibrillation[1]	-	-	97%	95%
Antithrombotic Therapy Timing	25	100%	98%	98%
Assessed for Rehabilitation	31	97%	96%	97%
Discharged on Antithrombotic Therapy	31	100%	100%	99%
Discharged on Statin Medication	22	100%	96%	94%
Thrombolytic Therapy Timing[1]	-	-	68%	66%
Venous Thromboembolism Prophylaxis	32	91%	94%	94%
Written Stroke Educational Materials Given	14	86%	82%	88%
Surgical Care Improvement Project				
Appropriate Beta Blocker Usage	73	100%	98%	98%
Appropriate VTP Within 24 Hours	181	98%	99%	98%
Controlled Postoperative Blood Glucose[7]	-	-	96%	97%
Perioperative Temperature Management	193	99%	100%	100%
Prophylactic Antibiotic Selection	163	100%	99%	99%
Prophylactic Antibiotic Selection (Outpatient)	24	100%	98%	98%
Prophylactic Antibiotic Stopped	160	98%	99%	98%
Prophylactic Antibiotic Timing	163	98%	99%	99%
Prophylactic Antibiotic Timing (Outpatient)	24	100%	98%	98%
Urinary Catheter Removal	172	98%	97%	97%
Survey of Patients' Hospital Experiences				
Area Around Room 'Always' Quiet at Night	300+	41%	52%	61%
Doctors 'Always' Communicated Well	300+	78%	80%	82%
Home Recovery Information Given	300+	84%	87%	85%
Hospital Given 9 or 10 on 10 Point Scale	300+	57%	69%	71%
Meds 'Always' Explained Before Given	300+	63%	64%	64%
Nurses 'Always' Communicated Well	300+	77%	79%	79%
Pain 'Always' Well Controlled	300+	64%	71%	71%
Room and Bathroom 'Always' Clean	300+	68%	72%	73%
Timely Help 'Always' Received	300+	63%	66%	68%
Would Definitely Recommend Hospital	300+	65%	73%	71%
Use of Medical Imaging				
Cardiac Imaging Stress Test before Surgery	214	7.5%	5.4%	5.3%
Combination Abdominal CT Scan	363	3.0%	6.3%	10.5%
Combination Brain/Sinus CT Scan[1]	-	-	2.4%	2.7%
Combination Chest CT Scan	226	0.4%	0.5%	2.7%
Follow-up Mammogram/Ultrasound	1,043	4.8%	8.9%	8.8%
Lumbar Spine MRI for Low Back Pain[7]	-	-	35.3%	37.2%

Hallmark Health System

585 Lebanon Street
Melrose, MA 02176
Phone: 781-979-3000
Fax: 781-979-3069
URL: www.hallmarkhealth.org
Type: Acute Care Hospitals
Emergency Services: Yes
Ownership: Voluntary non-profit - Private
Beds: 234

Key Personnel:
Pediatric In-Patient Care .... Karen Harvey-Wilkes, MD
Radiology.................. Eric Henrikson, MD
Anesthesiology............... Fathalla Mashali, MD
Emergency Room .... Joseph Pennacchio, MD
CEO/President............... Michael V Sack
Chief of Medical Staff.......... Mike Summerer, MD

Measure	Cases	This Hosp.	State Avg.	U.S. Avg.
Blood Clot Prevention and Treatment				
Anticoagulation Overlap Therapy[2]	69	97%	97%	93%
ICU Venous Thromboembolism Prophylaxis[2]	37	89%	92%	92%
Incidence of Potentially Preventable VTE[2]	15	0%	7%	10%
UFH with Dosages/Platelet Monitoring[2]	15	93%	91%	97%
Venous Thromboembolism Prophylaxis[2]	297	65%	87%	85%
Warfarin Therapy Discharge Instructions[2]	53	98%	77%	75%
Chest Pain/Possible Heart Attack Care				
Aspirin Given Within 24 Hours of Arrival	71	97%	97%	96%
Fibrinolytic Meds Within 30 Min. of Arrival[7]	-	-	73%	58%
Average Time to ECG (minutes)	72	10	7	7
Average Time to Transfer (minutes)	13	82	55	60
Children's Asthma Care				
Received Home Management Plan of Care	-	-	-	88%
Received Reliever Medication	-	-	-	100%
Received Systemic Corticosteroids	-	-	-	100%
Emergency Department				
Admittance Decision Time (minutes)[2]	785	97	119	98
Head CT Results Within 45 Min. of Arrival[1]	-	-	70%	57%
Patients Who Left ER Before Being Seen	60,962	1%	2%	2%
Time from ER Arrival to Admit. (minutes)[2]	785	277	313	274
Time from ER Arrival to Discharge (minutes)	334	142	156	134
Time in ER Before Being Evaluated (minutes)	382	39	36	26
Time to Pain Meds for Fractures (minutes)	99	54	59	57
Heart Attack Care				
Aspirin Given at Discharge	88	100%	100%	99%
Fibrinolytic Meds Within 30 Min. of Arrival[7]	-	-	100%	54%
PCI Within 90 Minutes of Arrival	23	96%	96%	96%
Statin Prescribed at Discharge	85	100%	99%	98%
Heart Failure Care				
ACE Inhibitor or ARB for LVSD[2]	46	85%	96%	97%
Discharge Instructions Given[2]	174	90%	95%	94%
Evaluation of LVS Function[2]	244	100%	100%	99%
Medicare Spending				
Medicare Spending per Patient (ratio)	-	1.10	1.03	0.98
Pneumonia Care				
Appropriate Initial Antibiotic Given[2]	90	98%	97%	95%
Blood Culture Timing[2]	150	95%	98%	98%
Pregnancy and Delivery Care				
Newborn Deliveries Scheduled Early[2]	21	0%	2%	6%
Preventive Care				
Immunization for Influenza[2]	541	96%	91%	90%
Immunization for Pneumonia[2]	695	95%	91%	92%
Stroke Care				
Anticoagulation Therapy for Atrial Fibrillation[2]	15	100%	97%	95%
Antithrombotic Therapy Timing[2]	70	97%	98%	98%
Assessed for Rehabilitation[2]	78	79%	96%	97%
Discharged on Antithrombotic Therapy[2]	76	99%	100%	99%
Discharged on Statin Medication[2]	61	93%	96%	94%
Thrombolytic Therapy Timing[1,2]	-	-	68%	66%
Venous Thromboembolism Prophylaxis[2]	74	82%	94%	94%
Written Stroke Educational Materials Given[2]	46	74%	82%	88%
Surgical Care Improvement Project				
Appropriate Beta Blocker Usage[2]	115	97%	98%	98%
Appropriate VTP Within 24 Hours[2]	298	99%	99%	98%
Controlled Postoperative Blood Glucose[2,7]	-	-	96%	97%
Perioperative Temperature Management[2]	343	100%	100%	100%
Prophylactic Antibiotic Selection[2]	239	99%	99%	99%
Prophylactic Antibiotic Selection (Outpatient)	83	100%	98%	98%
Prophylactic Antibiotic Stopped[2]	229	100%	99%	98%
Prophylactic Antibiotic Timing[2]	241	99%	99%	99%
Prophylactic Antibiotic Timing (Outpatient)	84	96%	98%	98%
Urinary Catheter Removal[2]	185	99%	97%	97%
Survey of Patients' Hospital Experiences				
Area Around Room 'Always' Quiet at Night	300+	51%	52%	61%
Doctors 'Always' Communicated Well	300+	83%	80%	82%
Home Recovery Information Given	300+	89%	87%	85%
Hospital Given 9 or 10 on 10 Point Scale	300+	69%	69%	71%
Meds 'Always' Explained Before Given	300+	63%	64%	64%
Nurses 'Always' Communicated Well	300+	82%	79%	79%
Pain 'Always' Well Controlled	300+	75%	71%	71%
Room and Bathroom 'Always' Clean	300+	72%	72%	73%
Timely Help 'Always' Received	300+	70%	66%	68%
Would Definitely Recommend Hospital	300+	71%	73%	71%
Use of Medical Imaging				

NOTE: Hospital profiles are in alphabetical order by state, then city, then hospital within the city; Rankings exclude hospitals with less than 25 cases except for patient surveys which excludes hospitals with less than 100 cases; (a) 100-299 cases; (1) The number of cases/patients is too few to report; (2) Data submitted were based on a sample of cases/patients; (3) Results are based on a shorter time period than required; (4) Data suppressed by CMS for one or more quarters; (5) Results are not available for this reporting period; (6) Fewer than 100 patients completed the HCAHPS survey; (7) No cases met the criteria for this measure; (8) The lower limit of the confidence interval cannot be calculated if the number of observed infections equals zero; (9) No data are available from the state/territory for this reporting period; (10) The scores shown reflect fewer than 50 completed surveys; (11) There were discrepancies in the data collection process; (12) This measure does not apply to this hospital for this reporting period; (13) Results cannot be calculated for this reporting period; (14) The results for this state are combined with nearby states to protect confidentiality; Please refer to the User's Guide for a full explanation of data.

Measure	Cases	This Hosp.	State Avg.	U.S. Avg.
Cardiac Imaging Stress Test before Surgery	490	7.1%	5.4%	5.3%
Combination Abdominal CT Scan	1,453	2.9%	6.3%	10.5%
Combination Brain/Sinus CT Scan	1,617	5.9%	2.4%	2.7%
Combination Chest CT Scan	1,091	2.5%	0.5%	2.7%
Follow-up Mammogram/Ultrasound	4,248	12.3%	8.9%	8.8%
Lumbar Spine MRI for Low Back Pain	207	38.2%	35.3%	37.2%

Holy Family Hospital

70 East Street
Methuen, MA 01844
Phone: 978-687-0156
Fax: 978-688-7689
E-mail: hfhmail@cchcs.org
URL: www.holyfamilyhosp.org
Type: Acute Care Hospitals
Emergency Services: Yes
Ownership: Proprietary
Beds: 271

Key Personnel:
Pediatric Ambulatory Care . . . . . . David Avila, DO
Pediatric In-Patient Care . . . . David Avila, DO
Quality Assurance . . . . Carolyn Candiello
Emergency Room . . . . Laurie Crawford, RN
Radiology. . . . . Robert C Hannon, MD
Chief of Medical Staff . . . . Sally A Hood, MD
CEO/President. . . . . Lester P Schindel

Measure	Cases	This Hosp.	State Avg.	U.S. Avg.
Blood Clot Prevention and Treatment				
Anticoagulation Overlap Therapy[2]	67	96%	97%	93%
ICU Venous Thromboembolism Prophylaxis[2]	85	79%	92%	92%
Incidence of Potentially Preventable VTE[2]	24	29%	7%	10%
UFH with Dosages/Platelet Monitoring[2]	34	100%	91%	97%
Venous Thromboembolism Prophylaxis[2]	287	72%	87%	85%
Warfarin Therapy Discharge Instructions[2]	41	98%	77%	75%
Chest Pain/Possible Heart Attack Care				
Aspirin Given Within 24 Hours of Arrival	28	89%	97%	96%
Fibrinolytic Meds Within 30 Min. of Arrival[3,7]	-	-	73%	58%
Average Time to ECG (minutes)	33	8	7	7
Average Time to Transfer (minutes)[1,3]	-	-	55	60
Children's Asthma Care				
Received Home Management Plan of Care	-	-	-	88%
Received Reliever Medication	-	-	-	100%
Received Systemic Corticosteroids	-	-	-	100%
Emergency Department				
Admittance Decision Time (minutes)[2]	674	147	119	98
Head CT Results Within 45 Min. of Arrival[1]	-	-	70%	57%
Patients Who Left ER Before Being Seen	46,468	2%	2%	2%
Time from ER Arrival to Admit. (minutes)[2]	682	338	313	274
Time from ER Arrival to Discharge (minutes)	381	186	156	134
Time in ER Before Being Evaluated (minutes)	353	60	36	26
Time to Pain Meds for Fractures (minutes)	82	66	59	57
Heart Attack Care				
Aspirin Given at Discharge	90	100%	100%	99%
Fibrinolytic Meds Within 30 Min. of Arrival[7]	-	-	100%	54%
PCI Within 90 Minutes of Arrival	35	89%	96%	96%
Statin Prescribed at Discharge	85	100%	99%	98%
Heart Failure Care				
ACE Inhibitor or ARB for LVSD	48	92%	96%	97%
Discharge Instructions Given	177	95%	95%	94%
Evaluation of LVS Function	241	99%	100%	99%
Medicare Spending				
Medicare Spending per Patient (ratio)	-	1.11	1.03	0.98
Pneumonia Care				
Appropriate Initial Antibiotic Given	149	99%	97%	95%
Blood Culture Timing	146	99%	98%	98%
Pregnancy and Delivery Care				
Newborn Deliveries Scheduled Early	87	6%	2%	6%
Preventive Care				
Immunization for Influenza[2]	520	88%	91%	90%
Immunization for Pneumonia[2]	651	90%	91%	92%
Stroke Care				
Anticoagulation Therapy for Atrial Fibrillation	14	93%	97%	95%
Antithrombotic Therapy Timing	58	97%	98%	98%
Assessed for Rehabilitation	65	97%	96%	97%
Discharged on Antithrombotic Therapy	59	98%	100%	99%
Discharged on Statin Medication	48	92%	96%	94%
Thrombolytic Therapy Timing[1]	-	-	68%	66%
Venous Thromboembolism Prophylaxis	66	89%	94%	94%
Written Stroke Educational Materials Given	23	100%	82%	88%
Surgical Care Improvement Project				
Appropriate Beta Blocker Usage[2]	200	100%	98%	98%
Appropriate VTP Within 24 Hours[2]	502	97%	99%	98%
Controlled Postoperative Blood Glucose[2,7]	-	-	96%	97%
Perioperative Temperature Management[2]	551	100%	100%	100%
Prophylactic Antibiotic Selection[2]	434	99%	99%	99%
Prophylactic Antibiotic Selection (Outpatient)	105	94%	98%	98%
Prophylactic Antibiotic Stopped[2]	424	98%	99%	98%
Prophylactic Antibiotic Timing[2]	435	100%	99%	99%
Prophylactic Antibiotic Timing (Outpatient)	105	98%	98%	98%
Urinary Catheter Removal[2]	396	98%	97%	97%
Survey of Patients' Hospital Experiences				
Area Around Room 'Always' Quiet at Night	300+	49%	52%	61%
Doctors 'Always' Communicated Well	300+	77%	80%	82%
Home Recovery Information Given	300+	87%	87%	85%
Hospital Given 9 or 10 on 10 Point Scale	300+	63%	69%	71%
Meds 'Always' Explained Before Given	300+	59%	64%	64%
Nurses 'Always' Communicated Well	300+	76%	79%	79%
Pain 'Always' Well Controlled	300+	69%	71%	71%
Room and Bathroom 'Always' Clean	300+	66%	72%	73%
Timely Help 'Always' Received	300+	61%	66%	68%
Would Definitely Recommend Hospital	300+	69%	73%	71%
Use of Medical Imaging				
Cardiac Imaging Stress Test before Surgery	476	5.7%	5.4%	5.3%
Combination Abdominal CT Scan	890	7.4%	6.3%	10.5%
Combination Brain/Sinus CT Scan	780	2.1%	2.4%	2.7%
Combination Chest CT Scan	822	2.8%	0.5%	2.7%
Follow-up Mammogram/Ultrasound	1,118	12.0%	8.9%	8.8%
Lumbar Spine MRI for Low Back Pain	277	35.4%	35.3%	37.2%

Milford Regional Medical Center

14 Prospect Street
Milford, MA 01757
Phone: 508-473-1190
Fax: 508-634-9124
URL: www.milfordregional.org
Type: Acute Care Hospitals
Emergency Services: Yes
Ownership: Voluntary non-profit - Other
Beds: 121

Key Personnel:
Emergency Room . . . . Donna Auger
Operating Room. . . . . Tom Cook, RN
Chief of Medical Staff. . . . . Albert A Crimaldi, MD
Infection Control. . . . . Kim Knox, RN
Quality Assurance . . . . Ann Northrop
CEO . . . . Francis M Saba
Intensive Care Unit. . . . . Mary Small
Cardiac Laboratory. . . . . Nancy Tomaso

Measure	Cases	This Hosp.	State Avg.	U.S. Avg.
Blood Clot Prevention and Treatment				
Anticoagulation Overlap Therapy[2]	50	98%	97%	93%
ICU Venous Thromboembolism Prophylaxis[2]	56	98%	92%	92%
Incidence of Potentially Preventable VTE[1,2]	-	-	7%	10%
UFH with Dosages/Platelet Monitoring[2]	18	100%	91%	97%
Venous Thromboembolism Prophylaxis[2]	365	90%	87%	85%
Warfarin Therapy Discharge Instructions[2]	34	79%	77%	75%
Chest Pain/Possible Heart Attack Care				
Aspirin Given Within 24 Hours of Arrival	70	99%	97%	96%
Fibrinolytic Meds Within 30 Min. of Arrival[7]	-	-	73%	58%
Average Time to ECG (minutes)	70	5	7	7
Average Time to Transfer (minutes)	19	60	55	60
Children's Asthma Care				
Received Home Management Plan of Care	-	-	-	88%
Received Reliever Medication	-	-	-	100%
Received Systemic Corticosteroids	-	-	-	100%
Emergency Department				
Admittance Decision Time (minutes)[2]	810	116	119	98
Head CT Results Within 45 Min. of Arrival	19	68%	70%	57%
Patients Who Left ER Before Being Seen	56,534	1%	2%	2%
Time from ER Arrival to Admit. (minutes)[2]	810	316	313	274
Time from ER Arrival to Discharge (minutes)	385	154	156	134
Time in ER Before Being Evaluated (minutes)	428	24	36	26
Time to Pain Meds for Fractures (minutes)	214	67	59	57
Heart Attack Care				
Aspirin Given at Discharge	52	94%	100%	99%
Fibrinolytic Meds Within 30 Min. of Arrival[7]	-	-	100%	54%
PCI Within 90 Minutes of Arrival[7]	-	-	96%	96%
Statin Prescribed at Discharge	52	96%	99%	98%
Heart Failure Care				
ACE Inhibitor or ARB for LVSD	65	89%	96%	97%
Discharge Instructions Given	184	91%	95%	94%
Evaluation of LVS Function	274	100%	100%	99%
Medicare Spending				
Medicare Spending per Patient (ratio)	-	1.03	1.03	0.98
Pneumonia Care				
Appropriate Initial Antibiotic Given	174	95%	97%	95%
Blood Culture Timing	289	96%	98%	98%
Pregnancy and Delivery Care				
Newborn Deliveries Scheduled Early	92	0%	2%	6%
Preventive Care				
Immunization for Influenza[2]	547	86%	91%	90%
Immunization for Pneumonia[2]	720	88%	91%	92%
Stroke Care				
Anticoagulation Therapy for Atrial Fibrillation	13	100%	97%	95%
Antithrombotic Therapy Timing	71	97%	98%	98%
Assessed for Rehabilitation	75	95%	96%	97%
Discharged on Antithrombotic Therapy	75	99%	100%	99%
Discharged on Statin Medication	61	100%	96%	94%
Thrombolytic Therapy Timing[1]	-	-	68%	66%
Venous Thromboembolism Prophylaxis	71	94%	94%	94%
Written Stroke Educational Materials Given	38	87%	82%	88%
Surgical Care Improvement Project				
Appropriate Beta Blocker Usage	113	98%	98%	98%
Appropriate VTP Within 24 Hours	356	96%	99%	98%
Controlled Postoperative Blood Glucose[7]	-	-	96%	97%
Perioperative Temperature Management	394	100%	100%	100%
Prophylactic Antibiotic Selection	276	99%	99%	99%
Prophylactic Antibiotic Selection (Outpatient)	133	97%	98%	98%
Prophylactic Antibiotic Stopped	265	98%	99%	98%
Prophylactic Antibiotic Timing	276	100%	99%	99%
Prophylactic Antibiotic Timing (Outpatient)	131	99%	98%	98%
Urinary Catheter Removal	295	99%	97%	97%
Survey of Patients' Hospital Experiences				
Area Around Room 'Always' Quiet at Night	300+	49%	52%	61%
Doctors 'Always' Communicated Well	300+	83%	80%	82%
Home Recovery Information Given	300+	91%	87%	85%
Hospital Given 9 or 10 on 10 Point Scale	300+	76%	69%	71%
Meds 'Always' Explained Before Given	300+	69%	64%	64%
Nurses 'Always' Communicated Well	300+	83%	79%	79%
Pain 'Always' Well Controlled	300+	74%	71%	71%
Room and Bathroom 'Always' Clean	300+	72%	72%	73%
Timely Help 'Always' Received	300+	69%	66%	68%
Would Definitely Recommend Hospital	300+	82%	73%	71%
Use of Medical Imaging				
Cardiac Imaging Stress Test before Surgery	275	1.8%	5.4%	5.3%
Combination Abdominal CT Scan	1,126	2.8%	6.3%	10.5%
Combination Brain/Sinus CT Scan	920	1.6%	2.4%	2.7%
Combination Chest CT Scan	930	0.0%	0.5%	2.7%
Follow-up Mammogram/Ultrasound	2,107	6.2%	8.9%	8.8%
Lumbar Spine MRI for Low Back Pain	134	38.8%	35.3%	37.2%

Beth Israel Deaconess Hospital - Milton

199 Reedsdale Road
Milton, MA 02186
Phone: 617-696-4600
Fax: 617-696-8323
E-mail: webmaster@miltonhospital.org
URL: www.miltonhosital.org
Type: Acute Care Hospitals
Emergency Services: Yes
Ownership: Government - Federal
Beds: 113

Key Personnel:
Surgery . . . . Elliot Chaikof, MD
Radiology. . . . . Jonathan B. Kruskal, MD
Patient Relations . . . . Cynthia Page
Chief of Medical Staff . . . . Joseph Raduazzo, MD
Anesthesiology. . . . . Brett Simon, MD, PhD
Intensive Care Unit. . . . . Deebble Sulo
President/CEO. . . . . Kevin Tabb, MD
Emergency Room . . . . Richard E. Wolfe, MD

Measure	Cases	This Hosp.	State Avg.	U.S. Avg.
Blood Clot Prevention and Treatment				
Anticoagulation Overlap Therapy[2]	41	100%	97%	93%

NOTE: Hospital profiles are in alphabetical order by state, then city, then hospital within the city; Rankings exclude hospitals with less than 25 cases except for patient surveys which excludes hospitals with less than 100 cases; (a) 100-299 cases; (1) The number of cases/patients is too few to report; (2) Data submitted were based on a sample of cases/patients; (3) Results are based on a shorter time period than required; (4) Data suppressed by CMS for one or more quarters; (5) Results are not available for this reporting period; (6) Fewer than 100 patients completed the HCAHPS survey; (7) No cases met the criteria for this measure; (8) The lower limit of the confidence interval cannot be calculated if the number of observed infections equals zero; (9) No data are available from the state/territory for this reporting period; (10) The scores shown reflect fewer than 50 completed surveys; (11) There were discrepancies in the data collection process; (12) This measure does not apply to this hospital for this reporting period; (13) Results cannot be calculated for this reporting period; (14) The results for this state are combined with nearby states to protect confidentiality; Please refer to the User's Guide for a full explanation of data.

Measure	Cases	This Hosp.	State Avg.	U.S. Avg.
ICU Venous Thromboembolism Prophylaxis[2]	65	88%	92%	92%
Incidence of Potentially Preventable VTE[1,2]	-	-	7%	10%
UFH with Dosages/Platelet Monitoring[2]	22	91%	91%	97%
Venous Thromboembolism Prophylaxis[2]	341	79%	87%	85%
Warfarin Therapy Discharge Instructions[2]	27	100%	77%	75%
Chest Pain/Possible Heart Attack Care				
Aspirin Given Within 24 Hours of Arrival	74	99%	97%	96%
Fibrinolytic Meds Within 30 Min. of Arrival[7]	-	-	73%	58%
Average Time to ECG (minutes)	75	11	7	7
Average Time to Transfer (minutes)	20	89	55	60
Children's Asthma Care				
Received Home Management Plan of Care	-	-	-	88%
Received Reliever Medication	-	-	-	100%
Received Systemic Corticosteroids	-	-	-	100%
Emergency Department				
Admittance Decision Time (minutes)[2]	942	75	119	98
Head CT Results Within 45 Min. of Arrival	11	73%	70%	57%
Patients Who Left ER Before Being Seen	25,715	0%	2%	2%
Time from ER Arrival to Admit. (minutes)[2]	947	247	313	274
Time from ER Arrival to Discharge (minutes)	371	142	156	134
Time in ER Before Being Evaluated (minutes)	416	39	36	26
Time to Pain Meds for Fractures (minutes)	58	66	59	57
Heart Attack Care				
Aspirin Given at Discharge	22	100%	100%	99%
Fibrinolytic Meds Within 30 Min. of Arrival[7]	-	-	100%	54%
PCI Within 90 Minutes of Arrival[7]	-	-	96%	96%
Statin Prescribed at Discharge	22	95%	99%	98%
Heart Failure Care				
ACE Inhibitor or ARB for LVSD	32	88%	96%	97%
Discharge Instructions Given	158	100%	95%	94%
Evaluation of LVS Function	187	99%	100%	99%
Medicare Spending				
Medicare Spending per Patient (ratio)	-	0.96	1.03	0.98
Pneumonia Care				
Appropriate Initial Antibiotic Given[2]	121	100%	97%	95%
Blood Culture Timing[2]	173	95%	98%	98%
Pregnancy and Delivery Care				
Newborn Deliveries Scheduled Early[7]	-	-	2%	6%
Preventive Care				
Immunization for Influenza[2]	520	99%	91%	90%
Immunization for Pneumonia[2]	771	88%	91%	92%
Stroke Care				
Anticoagulation Therapy for Atrial Fibrillation[1]	-	-	97%	95%
Antithrombotic Therapy Timing	31	100%	98%	98%
Assessed for Rehabilitation	35	100%	96%	97%
Discharged on Antithrombotic Therapy	33	97%	100%	99%
Discharged on Statin Medication	28	89%	96%	94%
Thrombolytic Therapy Timing[1]	-	-	68%	66%
Venous Thromboembolism Prophylaxis	32	84%	94%	94%
Written Stroke Educational Materials Given	23	100%	82%	88%
Surgical Care Improvement Project				
Appropriate Beta Blocker Usage[2]	90	100%	98%	98%
Appropriate VTP Within 24 Hours[2]	267	99%	99%	98%
Controlled Postoperative Blood Glucose[2,7]	-	-	96%	97%
Perioperative Temperature Management[2]	317	100%	100%	100%
Prophylactic Antibiotic Selection[2]	220	99%	99%	99%
Prophylactic Antibiotic Selection (Outpatient)	44	89%	98%	98%
Prophylactic Antibiotic Stopped[2]	213	97%	99%	98%
Prophylactic Antibiotic Timing[2]	220	96%	99%	99%
Prophylactic Antibiotic Timing (Outpatient)	44	98%	98%	98%
Urinary Catheter Removal[2]	231	100%	97%	97%
Survey of Patients' Hospital Experiences				
Area Around Room 'Always' Quiet at Night	300+	56%	52%	61%
Doctors 'Always' Communicated Well	300+	85%	80%	82%
Home Recovery Information Given	300+	88%	87%	85%
Hospital Given 9 or 10 on 10 Point Scale	300+	69%	69%	71%
Meds 'Always' Explained Before Given	300+	68%	64%	64%
Nurses 'Always' Communicated Well	300+	84%	79%	79%
Pain 'Always' Well Controlled	300+	71%	71%	71%
Room and Bathroom 'Always' Clean	300+	73%	72%	73%
Timely Help 'Always' Received	300+	65%	66%	68%
Would Definitely Recommend Hospital	300+	74%	73%	71%
Use of Medical Imaging				
Cardiac Imaging Stress Test before Surgery	193	9.3%	5.4%	5.3%
Combination Abdominal CT Scan	553	7.2%	6.3%	10.5%
Combination Brain/Sinus CT Scan	553	1.8%	2.4%	2.7%
Combination Chest CT Scan	312	0.0%	0.5%	2.7%
Follow-up Mammogram/Ultrasound	1,042	4.1%	8.9%	8.8%
Lumbar Spine MRI for Low Back Pain	93	49.5%	35.3%	37.2%

Nantucket Cottage Hospital

57 Prospect Street
Nantucket, MA 02554
Phone: 508-228-1200
Fax: 508-825-8249
E-mail: crdcontact@ackhosp.org
URL: www.nantuckethospital.org
Type: Acute Care Hospitals
Emergency Services: Yes
Ownership: Voluntary non-profit - Private
Beds: 19

Key Personnel:
Patient Relations . . . . Jane Bonvini, RN
Infection Control. . . . . Charlene Chadwick, RN
Quality Assurance . . . . Jan Ellsworth
CEO/President. . . . . Sylvia Getman
Chief of Medical Staff . . . . Timothy J Lepore, MD
Operating Room. . . . . Kevin Lurie, RN
Radiology. . . . . Oliver Pomeroy

Measure	Cases	This Hosp.	State Avg.	U.S. Avg.
Blood Clot Prevention and Treatment				
Anticoagulation Overlap Therapy[2,7]	-	-	97%	93%
ICU Venous Thromboembolism Prophylaxis[2,7]	-	-	92%	92%
Incidence of Potentially Preventable VTE[2,7]	-	-	7%	10%
UFH with Dosages/Platelet Monitoring[2,7]	-	-	91%	97%
Venous Thromboembolism Prophylaxis[2]	136	26%	87%	85%
Warfarin Therapy Discharge Instructions[2,7]	-	-	77%	75%
Chest Pain/Possible Heart Attack Care				
Aspirin Given Within 24 Hours of Arrival	31	87%	97%	96%
Fibrinolytic Meds Within 30 Min. of Arrival[1]	-	-	73%	58%
Average Time to ECG (minutes)	30	10	7	7
Average Time to Transfer (minutes)[1]	-	-	55	60
Children's Asthma Care				
Received Home Management Plan of Care	-	-	-	88%
Received Reliever Medication	-	-	-	100%
Received Systemic Corticosteroids	-	-	-	100%
Emergency Department				
Admittance Decision Time (minutes)[2]	148	44	119	98
Head CT Results Within 45 Min. of Arrival	12	25%	70%	57%
Patients Who Left ER Before Being Seen	11,291	1%	2%	2%
Time from ER Arrival to Admit. (minutes)[2]	148	312	313	274
Time from ER Arrival to Discharge (minutes)	363	104	156	134
Time in ER Before Being Evaluated (minutes)	384	23	36	26
Time to Pain Meds for Fractures (minutes)	46	50	59	57
Heart Attack Care				
Aspirin Given at Discharge[5]	-	-	100%	99%
Fibrinolytic Meds Within 30 Min. of Arrival[5]	-	-	100%	54%
PCI Within 90 Minutes of Arrival[5]	-	-	96%	96%
Statin Prescribed at Discharge[5]	-	-	99%	98%
Heart Failure Care				
ACE Inhibitor or ARB for LVSD[3,7]	-	-	96%	97%
Discharge Instructions Given[1,3]	-	-	95%	94%
Evaluation of LVS Function[1,3]	-	-	100%	99%
Medicare Spending				
Medicare Spending per Patient (ratio)	-	0.87	1.03	0.98
Pneumonia Care				
Appropriate Initial Antibiotic Given	15	60%	97%	95%
Blood Culture Timing[1]	-	-	98%	98%
Pregnancy and Delivery Care				
Newborn Deliveries Scheduled Early	15	0%	2%	6%
Preventive Care				
Immunization for Influenza	62	79%	91%	90%
Immunization for Pneumonia[2]	117	68%	91%	92%
Stroke Care				
Anticoagulation Therapy for Atrial Fibrillation[5]	-	-	97%	95%
Antithrombotic Therapy Timing[5]	-	-	98%	98%
Assessed for Rehabilitation[5]	-	-	96%	97%
Discharged on Antithrombotic Therapy[5]	-	-	100%	99%
Discharged on Statin Medication[5]	-	-	96%	94%
Thrombolytic Therapy Timing[5]	-	-	68%	66%
Venous Thromboembolism Prophylaxis[5]	-	-	94%	94%
Written Stroke Educational Materials Given[5]	-	-	82%	88%
Surgical Care Improvement Project				
Appropriate Beta Blocker Usage[5]	-	-	98%	98%
Appropriate VTP Within 24 Hours[5]	-	-	99%	98%
Controlled Postoperative Blood Glucose[5]	-	-	96%	97%
Perioperative Temperature Management[5]	-	-	100%	100%
Prophylactic Antibiotic Selection[5]	-	-	99%	99%
Prophylactic Antibiotic Selection (Outpatient)[5]	-	-	98%	98%
Prophylactic Antibiotic Stopped[5]	-	-	99%	98%
Prophylactic Antibiotic Timing[5]	-	-	99%	99%
Prophylactic Antibiotic Timing (Outpatient)[5]	-	-	98%	98%
Urinary Catheter Removal[5]	-	-	97%	97%
Survey of Patients' Hospital Experiences				
Area Around Room 'Always' Quiet at Night[6]	<100	54%	52%	61%
Doctors 'Always' Communicated Well[6]	<100	83%	80%	82%
Home Recovery Information Given[6]	<100	83%	87%	85%
Hospital Given 9 or 10 on 10 Point Scale[6]	<100	79%	69%	71%
Meds 'Always' Explained Before Given[6]	<100	60%	64%	64%
Nurses 'Always' Communicated Well[6]	<100	82%	79%	79%
Pain 'Always' Well Controlled[6]	<100	72%	71%	71%
Room and Bathroom 'Always' Clean[6]	<100	62%	72%	73%
Timely Help 'Always' Received[6]	<100	79%	66%	68%
Would Definitely Recommend Hospital[6]	<100	82%	73%	71%
Use of Medical Imaging				
Cardiac Imaging Stress Test before Surgery[7]	-	-	5.4%	5.3%
Combination Abdominal CT Scan	111	5.4%	6.3%	10.5%
Combination Brain/Sinus CT Scan[1]	-	-	2.4%	2.7%
Combination Chest CT Scan	117	0.0%	0.5%	2.7%
Follow-up Mammogram/Ultrasound	179	6.1%	8.9%	8.8%
Lumbar Spine MRI for Low Back Pain[1]	-	-	35.3%	37.2%

Beth Israel Deaconess Hospital - Needham

148 Chestnut Street
Needham, MA 02494
Phone: 781-453-3000
Fax: 781-453-5786
URL: www.caregroup.org
Type: Acute Care Hospitals
Emergency Services: Yes
Ownership: Government - Local
Beds: 58

Key Personnel:
Surgery . . . . Elliot Chaikof, MD
Chair/CEO . . . . Daniel Jick
Cardiac Laboratory. . . . . Joseph P Kannam, MD
Radiology. . . . . Jonathan B. Kruskal, MD
Anesthesiology. . . . . Brett Simon, MD, PhD
CEO/President. . . . . Kevin Tabb, MD
Emergency Room . . . . Richard E. Wolfe, MD

Measure	Cases	This Hosp.	State Avg.	U.S. Avg.
Blood Clot Prevention and Treatment				
Anticoagulation Overlap Therapy[2]	19	95%	97%	93%
ICU Venous Thromboembolism Prophylaxis[2]	54	93%	92%	92%
Incidence of Potentially Preventable VTE[2,7]	-	-	7%	10%
UFH with Dosages/Platelet Monitoring[1,2]	-	-	91%	97%
Venous Thromboembolism Prophylaxis[2]	168	96%	87%	85%
Warfarin Therapy Discharge Instructions[2]	17	35%	77%	75%
Chest Pain/Possible Heart Attack Care				
Aspirin Given Within 24 Hours of Arrival	61	100%	97%	96%
Fibrinolytic Meds Within 30 Min. of Arrival[7]	-	-	73%	58%
Average Time to ECG (minutes)	62	10	7	7
Average Time to Transfer (minutes)	13	59	55	60
Children's Asthma Care				
Received Home Management Plan of Care	-	-	-	88%
Received Reliever Medication	-	-	-	100%
Received Systemic Corticosteroids	-	-	-	100%
Emergency Department				
Admittance Decision Time (minutes)[2]	384	104	119	98
Head CT Results Within 45 Min. of Arrival	14	64%	70%	57%
Patients Who Left ER Before Being Seen	14,842	0%	2%	2%
Time from ER Arrival to Admit. (minutes)[2]	414	294	313	274
Time from ER Arrival to Discharge (minutes)	358	145	156	134
Time in ER Before Being Evaluated (minutes)	406	21	36	26
Time to Pain Meds for Fractures (minutes)	54	45	59	57
Heart Attack Care				
Aspirin Given at Discharge	14	100%	100%	99%
Fibrinolytic Meds Within 30 Min. of Arrival[7]	-	-	100%	54%

NOTE: Hospital profiles are in alphabetical order by state, then city, then hospital within the city; Rankings exclude hospitals with less than 25 cases except for patient surveys which excludes hospitals with less than 100 cases; (a) 100-299 cases; (1) The number of cases/patients is too few to report; (2) Data submitted were based on a sample of cases/patients; (3) Results are based on a shorter time period than required; (4) Data suppressed by CMS for one or more quarters; (5) Results are not available for this reporting period; (6) Fewer than 100 patients completed the HCAHPS survey; (7) No cases met the criteria for this measure; (8) The lower limit of the confidence interval cannot be calculated if the number of observed infections equals zero; (9) No data are available from the state/territory for this reporting period; (10) The scores shown reflect fewer than 50 completed surveys; (11) There were discrepancies in the data collection process; (12) This measure does not apply to this hospital for this reporting period; (13) Results cannot be calculated for this reporting period; (14) The results for this state are combined with nearby states to protect confidentiality; Please refer to the User's Guide for a full explanation of data.

Measure	Cases	This Hosp.	State Avg.	U.S. Avg.
PCI Within 90 Minutes of Arrival[7]	-	-	96%	96%
Statin Prescribed at Discharge	12	100%	99%	98%
Heart Failure Care				
ACE Inhibitor or ARB for LVSD	12	100%	96%	97%
Discharge Instructions Given	77	99%	95%	94%
Evaluation of LVS Function	100	100%	100%	99%
Medicare Spending				
Medicare Spending per Patient (ratio)	-	0.98	1.03	0.98
Pneumonia Care				
Appropriate Initial Antibiotic Given	47	100%	97%	95%
Blood Culture Timing	82	87%	98%	98%
Pregnancy and Delivery Care				
Newborn Deliveries Scheduled Early[7]	-	-	2%	6%
Preventive Care				
Immunization for Influenza[2]	298	96%	91%	90%
Immunization for Pneumonia[2]	465	93%	91%	92%
Stroke Care				
Anticoagulation Therapy for Atrial Fibrillation[1]	-	-	97%	95%
Antithrombotic Therapy Timing	20	100%	98%	98%
Assessed for Rehabilitation	21	100%	96%	97%
Discharged on Antithrombotic Therapy	20	100%	100%	99%
Discharged on Statin Medication	17	100%	96%	94%
Thrombolytic Therapy Timing[7]	-	-	68%	66%
Venous Thromboembolism Prophylaxis	17	100%	94%	94%
Written Stroke Educational Materials Given	11	100%	82%	88%
Surgical Care Improvement Project				
Appropriate Beta Blocker Usage	38	95%	98%	98%
Appropriate VTP Within 24 Hours	110	100%	99%	98%
Controlled Postoperative Blood Glucose[7]	-	-	96%	97%
Perioperative Temperature Management	114	100%	100%	100%
Prophylactic Antibiotic Selection	67	100%	99%	99%
Prophylactic Antibiotic Selection (Outpatient)	47	94%	98%	98%
Prophylactic Antibiotic Stopped	61	95%	99%	98%
Prophylactic Antibiotic Timing	67	96%	99%	99%
Prophylactic Antibiotic Timing (Outpatient)	47	100%	98%	98%
Urinary Catheter Removal	80	95%	97%	97%
Survey of Patients' Hospital Experiences				
Area Around Room 'Always' Quiet at Night	300+	55%	52%	61%
Doctors 'Always' Communicated Well	300+	84%	80%	82%
Home Recovery Information Given	300+	87%	87%	85%
Hospital Given 9 or 10 on 10 Point Scale	300+	73%	69%	71%
Meds 'Always' Explained Before Given	300+	62%	64%	64%
Nurses 'Always' Communicated Well	300+	80%	79%	79%
Pain 'Always' Well Controlled	300+	70%	71%	71%
Room and Bathroom 'Always' Clean	300+	70%	72%	73%
Timely Help 'Always' Received	300+	61%	66%	68%
Would Definitely Recommend Hospital	300+	81%	73%	71%
Use of Medical Imaging				
Cardiac Imaging Stress Test before Surgery	312	6.4%	5.4%	5.3%
Combination Abdominal CT Scan	463	11.7%	6.3%	10.5%
Combination Brain/Sinus CT Scan	495	1.0%	2.4%	2.7%
Combination Chest CT Scan	315	0.3%	0.5%	2.7%
Follow-up Mammogram/Ultrasound	710	6.3%	8.9%	8.8%
Lumbar Spine MRI for Low Back Pain	65	47.7%	35.3%	37.2%

Anna Jaques Hospital

25 Highland Avenue
Newburyport, MA 01950
URL: www.ajh.org
Type: Acute Care Hospitals
Ownership: Voluntary non-profit - Private
Phone: 978-463-1000
Fax: 978-463-1250
Emergency Services: Yes
Beds: 123

Key Personnel:
Radiology. . . . . Maximina Boutes, MD
Cardiac Laboratory. . . . . Jackie Carroll
Anesthesiology. . . . . Eduardo D'Agostino, MD
Chief of Medical Staff . . . . Gail B. Fayre, MD
Emergency Room . . . . Joe Hull, MD
Quality Assurance . . . . Kathy Lucy, RN
CEO/President. . . . . Delia O'Connor, FACHE
Hemotology Center . . . . Paul Spieler, MD

Measure	Cases	This Hosp.	State Avg.	U.S. Avg.
Blood Clot Prevention and Treatment				
Anticoagulation Overlap Therapy[2]	40	98%	97%	93%
ICU Venous Thromboembolism Prophylaxis[2]	41	95%	92%	92%
Incidence of Potentially Preventable VTE[1,2]	-	-	7%	10%
UFH with Dosages/Platelet Monitoring[2]	16	100%	91%	97%
Venous Thromboembolism Prophylaxis[2]	323	79%	87%	85%
Warfarin Therapy Discharge Instructions[2]	29	76%	77%	75%
Chest Pain/Possible Heart Attack Care				
Aspirin Given Within 24 Hours of Arrival	64	100%	97%	96%
Fibrinolytic Meds Within 30 Min. of Arrival[7]	-	-	73%	58%
Average Time to ECG (minutes)	67	5	7	7
Average Time to Transfer (minutes)	21	60	55	60
Children's Asthma Care				
Received Home Management Plan of Care	-	-	-	88%
Received Reliever Medication	-	-	-	100%
Received Systemic Corticosteroids	-	-	-	100%
Emergency Department				
Admittance Decision Time (minutes)[2]	664	98	119	98
Head CT Results Within 45 Min. of Arrival	17	82%	70%	57%
Patients Who Left ER Before Being Seen	32,473	1%	2%	2%
Time from ER Arrival to Admit. (minutes)[2]	667	292	313	274
Time from ER Arrival to Discharge (minutes)	367	135	156	134
Time in ER Before Being Evaluated (minutes)	408	42	36	26
Time to Pain Meds for Fractures (minutes)	123	59	59	57
Heart Attack Care				
Aspirin Given at Discharge	25	92%	100%	99%
Fibrinolytic Meds Within 30 Min. of Arrival[7]	-	-	100%	54%
PCI Within 90 Minutes of Arrival[7]	-	-	96%	96%
Statin Prescribed at Discharge	25	84%	99%	98%
Heart Failure Care				
ACE Inhibitor or ARB for LVSD	31	90%	96%	97%
Discharge Instructions Given	143	98%	95%	94%
Evaluation of LVS Function	183	100%	100%	99%
Medicare Spending				
Medicare Spending per Patient (ratio)	-	1.08	1.03	0.98
Pneumonia Care				
Appropriate Initial Antibiotic Given	123	96%	97%	95%
Blood Culture Timing	180	98%	98%	98%
Pregnancy and Delivery Care				
Newborn Deliveries Scheduled Early[2]	93	0%	2%	6%
Preventive Care				
Immunization for Influenza[2]	556	96%	91%	90%
Immunization for Pneumonia[2]	605	98%	91%	92%
Stroke Care				
Anticoagulation Therapy for Atrial Fibrillation[1]	-	-	97%	95%
Antithrombotic Therapy Timing	67	97%	98%	98%
Assessed for Rehabilitation	68	97%	96%	97%
Discharged on Antithrombotic Therapy	67	100%	100%	99%
Discharged on Statin Medication	60	83%	96%	94%
Thrombolytic Therapy Timing[1]	-	-	68%	66%
Venous Thromboembolism Prophylaxis	67	88%	94%	94%
Written Stroke Educational Materials Given	34	82%	82%	88%
Surgical Care Improvement Project				
Appropriate Beta Blocker Usage	88	99%	98%	98%
Appropriate VTP Within 24 Hours	251	98%	99%	98%
Controlled Postoperative Blood Glucose[7]	-	-	96%	97%
Perioperative Temperature Management	294	100%	100%	100%
Prophylactic Antibiotic Selection	213	98%	99%	99%
Prophylactic Antibiotic Selection (Outpatient)	101	99%	98%	98%
Prophylactic Antibiotic Stopped	209	100%	99%	98%
Prophylactic Antibiotic Timing	213	100%	99%	99%
Prophylactic Antibiotic Timing (Outpatient)	101	99%	98%	98%
Urinary Catheter Removal	194	100%	97%	97%
Survey of Patients' Hospital Experiences				
Area Around Room 'Always' Quiet at Night	300+	53%	52%	61%
Doctors 'Always' Communicated Well	300+	79%	80%	82%
Home Recovery Information Given	300+	87%	87%	85%
Hospital Given 9 or 10 on 10 Point Scale	300+	70%	69%	71%
Meds 'Always' Explained Before Given	300+	63%	64%	64%
Nurses 'Always' Communicated Well	300+	83%	79%	79%
Pain 'Always' Well Controlled	300+	74%	71%	71%
Room and Bathroom 'Always' Clean	300+	73%	72%	73%
Timely Help 'Always' Received	300+	71%	66%	68%
Would Definitely Recommend Hospital	300+	73%	73%	71%
Use of Medical Imaging				
Cardiac Imaging Stress Test before Surgery	343	8.5%	5.4%	5.3%
Combination Abdominal CT Scan	741	3.5%	6.3%	10.5%
Combination Brain/Sinus CT Scan	676	2.8%	2.4%	2.7%
Combination Chest CT Scan	632	0.2%	0.5%	2.7%
Follow-up Mammogram/Ultrasound	2,295	8.3%	8.9%	8.8%
Lumbar Spine MRI for Low Back Pain[7]	-	-	35.3%	37.2%

Newton - Wellesley Hospital

2014 Washington Street
Newton, MA 02462
URL: www.nwh.org
Type: Acute Care Hospitals
Ownership: Voluntary non-profit - Other
Phone: 617-243-6000
Fax: 617-243-6990
Emergency Services: Yes
Beds: 290

Key Personnel:
Pediatric Ambulatory Care . . . . Joel Bass, MD
Pediatric In-Patient Care . . . . Joel Bass, MD
Quality Assurance . . . . Marci Cass
Operating Room. . . . . Anna DaSilva, RN
Chief of Medical Staff. . . . . Laurence Friedman, MD
Infection Control. . . . . Sue MacDonald
Radiology. . . . . Steven Miller, MD
CEO/President. . . . . Kerry R. Watson

Measure	Cases	This Hosp.	State Avg.	U.S. Avg.
Blood Clot Prevention and Treatment				
Anticoagulation Overlap Therapy[2]	52	100%	97%	93%
ICU Venous Thromboembolism Prophylaxis[2]	62	92%	92%	92%
Incidence of Potentially Preventable VTE[2]	11	0%	7%	10%
UFH with Dosages/Platelet Monitoring[2]	20	100%	91%	97%
Venous Thromboembolism Prophylaxis[2]	305	89%	87%	85%
Warfarin Therapy Discharge Instructions[2]	48	85%	77%	75%
Chest Pain/Possible Heart Attack Care				
Aspirin Given Within 24 Hours of Arrival	112	100%	97%	96%
Fibrinolytic Meds Within 30 Min. of Arrival[7]	-	-	73%	58%
Average Time to ECG (minutes)	114	5	7	7
Average Time to Transfer (minutes)[7]	-	-	55	60
Children's Asthma Care				
Received Home Management Plan of Care	-	-	-	88%
Received Reliever Medication	-	-	-	100%
Received Systemic Corticosteroids	-	-	-	100%
Emergency Department				
Admittance Decision Time (minutes)[2]	393	123	119	98
Head CT Results Within 45 Min. of Arrival	22	73%	70%	57%
Patients Who Left ER Before Being Seen	61,170	1%	2%	2%
Time from ER Arrival to Admit. (minutes)[2]	404	302	313	274
Time from ER Arrival to Discharge (minutes)	337	149	156	134
Time in ER Before Being Evaluated (minutes)[1]	-	-	36	26
Time to Pain Meds for Fractures (minutes)	189	59	59	57
Heart Attack Care				
Aspirin Given at Discharge	24	100%	100%	99%
Fibrinolytic Meds Within 30 Min. of Arrival[7]	-	-	100%	54%
PCI Within 90 Minutes of Arrival[7]	-	-	96%	96%
Statin Prescribed at Discharge	23	100%	99%	98%
Heart Failure Care				
ACE Inhibitor or ARB for LVSD[2]	28	100%	96%	97%
Discharge Instructions Given[2]	144	99%	95%	94%
Evaluation of LVS Function[2]	216	100%	100%	99%
Medicare Spending				
Medicare Spending per Patient (ratio)	-	1.01	1.03	0.98
Pneumonia Care				
Appropriate Initial Antibiotic Given[2]	86	92%	97%	95%
Blood Culture Timing[2]	147	99%	98%	98%
Pregnancy and Delivery Care				
Newborn Deliveries Scheduled Early[2]	53	6%	2%	6%
Preventive Care				
Immunization for Influenza[2]	455	98%	91%	90%
Immunization for Pneumonia[2]	444	91%	91%	92%
Stroke Care				
Anticoagulation Therapy for Atrial Fibrillation	21	100%	97%	95%
Antithrombotic Therapy Timing	69	99%	98%	98%
Assessed for Rehabilitation	97	100%	96%	97%
Discharged on Antithrombotic Therapy	91	100%	100%	99%
Discharged on Statin Medication	62	100%	96%	94%
Thrombolytic Therapy Timing	14	100%	68%	66%
Venous Thromboembolism Prophylaxis	94	100%	94%	94%

NOTE: Hospital profiles are in alphabetical order by state, then city, then hospital within the city; Rankings exclude hospitals with less than 25 cases except for patient surveys which excludes hospitals with less than 100 cases; (a) 100-299 cases; (1) The number of cases/patients is too few to report; (2) Data submitted were based on a sample of cases/patients; (3) Results are based on a shorter time period than required; (4) Data suppressed by CMS for one or more quarters; (5) Results are not available for this reporting period; (6) Fewer than 100 patients completed the HCAHPS survey; (7) No cases met the criteria for this measure; (8) The lower limit of the confidence interval cannot be calculated if the number of observed infections equals zero; (9) No data are available from the state/territory for this reporting period; (10) The scores shown reflect fewer than 50 completed surveys; (11) There were discrepancies in the data collection process; (12) This measure does not apply to this hospital for this reporting period; (13) Results cannot be calculated for this reporting period; (14) The results for this state are combined with nearby states to protect confidentiality; Please refer to the User's Guide for a full explanation of data.

Measure	Cases	This Hosp.	State Avg.	U.S. Avg.
Written Stroke Educational Materials Given	50	100%	82%	88%
Surgical Care Improvement Project				
Appropriate Beta Blocker Usage[2]	76	93%	98%	98%
Appropriate VTP Within 24 Hours[2]	304	99%	99%	98%
Controlled Postoperative Blood Glucose[2,7]	-	-	96%	97%
Perioperative Temperature Management[2]	346	100%	100%	100%
Prophylactic Antibiotic Selection[2]	226	100%	99%	99%
Prophylactic Antibiotic Selection (Outpatient)	513	99%	98%	98%
Prophylactic Antibiotic Stopped[2]	225	100%	99%	98%
Prophylactic Antibiotic Timing[2]	227	100%	99%	99%
Prophylactic Antibiotic Timing (Outpatient)	514	99%	98%	98%
Urinary Catheter Removal[2]	95	98%	97%	97%
Survey of Patients' Hospital Experiences				
Area Around Room 'Always' Quiet at Night	300+	56%	52%	61%
Doctors 'Always' Communicated Well	300+	84%	80%	82%
Home Recovery Information Given	300+	89%	87%	85%
Hospital Given 9 or 10 on 10 Point Scale	300+	78%	69%	71%
Meds 'Always' Explained Before Given	300+	65%	64%	64%
Nurses 'Always' Communicated Well	300+	81%	79%	79%
Pain 'Always' Well Controlled	300+	71%	71%	71%
Room and Bathroom 'Always' Clean	300+	78%	72%	73%
Timely Help 'Always' Received	300+	67%	66%	68%
Would Definitely Recommend Hospital	300+	84%	73%	71%
Use of Medical Imaging				
Cardiac Imaging Stress Test before Surgery	486	5.6%	5.4%	5.3%
Combination Abdominal CT Scan	1,168	7.4%	6.3%	10.5%
Combination Brain/Sinus CT Scan	1,131	1.3%	2.4%	2.7%
Combination Chest CT Scan	1,396	0.0%	0.5%	2.7%
Follow-up Mammogram/Ultrasound	3,353	10.8%	8.9%	8.8%
Lumbar Spine MRI for Low Back Pain	222	35.1%	35.3%	37.2%

North Adams Regional Hospital

71 Hospital Avenue
North Adams, MA 01247
URL: www.nbhealth.org
Type: Acute Care Hospitals
Ownership: Voluntary non-profit - Private
Phone: 413-664-5000
Fax: 413-664-5028
Emergency Services: Yes
Beds: 134

Key Personnel:
Chief of Medical Staff . . . . Paul Donovan, MD
CEO/President . . . . Richard T Palmisano

Measure	Cases	This Hosp.	State Avg.	U.S. Avg.
Blood Clot Prevention and Treatment				
Anticoagulation Overlap Therapy[2]	13	100%	97%	93%
ICU Venous Thromboembolism Prophylaxis[2]	104	94%	92%	92%
Incidence of Potentially Preventable VTE[2,7]	-	-	7%	10%
UFH with Dosages/Platelet Monitoring[1,2]	-	-	91%	97%
Venous Thromboembolism Prophylaxis[2]	112	97%	87%	85%
Warfarin Therapy Discharge Instructions[1,2]	-	-	77%	75%
Chest Pain/Possible Heart Attack Care				
Aspirin Given Within 24 Hours of Arrival	58	98%	97%	96%
Fibrinolytic Meds Within 30 Min. of Arrival	14	79%	73%	58%
Average Time to ECG (minutes)	63	7	7	7
Average Time to Transfer (minutes)[7]	-	-	55	60
Children's Asthma Care				
Received Home Management Plan of Care	-	-	-	88%
Received Reliever Medication	-	-	-	100%
Received Systemic Corticosteroids	-	-	-	100%
Emergency Department				
Admittance Decision Time (minutes)[2]	333	69	119	98
Head CT Results Within 45 Min. of Arrival[1]	-	-	70%	57%
Patients Who Left ER Before Being Seen	21,443	3%	2%	2%
Time from ER Arrival to Admit. (minutes)[2]	335	304	313	274
Time from ER Arrival to Discharge (minutes)	436	128	156	134
Time in ER Before Being Evaluated (minutes)	492	32	36	26
Time to Pain Meds for Fractures (minutes)	29	60	59	57
Heart Attack Care				
Aspirin Given at Discharge	11	100%	100%	99%
Fibrinolytic Meds Within 30 Min. of Arrival[7]	-	-	100%	54%
PCI Within 90 Minutes of Arrival[7]	-	-	96%	96%
Statin Prescribed at Discharge	11	100%	99%	98%
Heart Failure Care				
ACE Inhibitor or ARB for LVSD	13	100%	96%	97%
Discharge Instructions Given	63	100%	95%	94%
Evaluation of LVS Function	91	100%	100%	99%
Medicare Spending				
Medicare Spending per Patient (ratio)	-	1.04	1.03	0.98
Pneumonia Care				
Appropriate Initial Antibiotic Given	74	100%	97%	95%
Blood Culture Timing	126	97%	98%	98%
Pregnancy and Delivery Care				
Newborn Deliveries Scheduled Early[1]	-	-	2%	6%
Preventive Care				
Immunization for Influenza[2]	294	99%	91%	90%
Immunization for Pneumonia[2]	383	98%	91%	92%
Stroke Care				
Anticoagulation Therapy for Atrial Fibrillation	11	100%	97%	95%
Antithrombotic Therapy Timing	38	100%	98%	98%
Assessed for Rehabilitation	38	100%	96%	97%
Discharged on Antithrombotic Therapy	37	100%	100%	99%
Discharged on Statin Medication	29	100%	96%	94%
Thrombolytic Therapy Timing[7]	-	-	68%	66%
Venous Thromboembolism Prophylaxis	38	100%	94%	94%
Written Stroke Educational Materials Given	14	100%	82%	88%
Surgical Care Improvement Project				
Appropriate Beta Blocker Usage	64	98%	98%	98%
Appropriate VTP Within 24 Hours	146	99%	99%	98%
Controlled Postoperative Blood Glucose[7]	-	-	96%	97%
Perioperative Temperature Management	175	100%	100%	100%
Prophylactic Antibiotic Selection	138	100%	99%	99%
Prophylactic Antibiotic Selection (Outpatient)	21	100%	98%	98%
Prophylactic Antibiotic Stopped	136	100%	99%	98%
Prophylactic Antibiotic Timing	138	100%	99%	99%
Prophylactic Antibiotic Timing (Outpatient)	22	95%	98%	98%
Urinary Catheter Removal	16	100%	97%	97%
Survey of Patients' Hospital Experiences				
Area Around Room 'Always' Quiet at Night	300+	54%	52%	61%
Doctors 'Always' Communicated Well	300+	79%	80%	82%
Home Recovery Information Given	300+	92%	87%	85%
Hospital Given 9 or 10 on 10 Point Scale	300+	65%	69%	71%
Meds 'Always' Explained Before Given	300+	65%	64%	64%
Nurses 'Always' Communicated Well	300+	81%	79%	79%
Pain 'Always' Well Controlled	300+	75%	71%	71%
Room and Bathroom 'Always' Clean	300+	75%	72%	73%
Timely Help 'Always' Received	300+	73%	66%	68%
Would Definitely Recommend Hospital	300+	67%	73%	71%
Use of Medical Imaging				
Cardiac Imaging Stress Test before Surgery	119	2.5%	5.4%	5.3%
Combination Abdominal CT Scan	594	5.2%	6.3%	10.5%
Combination Brain/Sinus CT Scan	489	2.2%	2.4%	2.7%
Combination Chest CT Scan	418	1.7%	0.5%	2.7%
Follow-up Mammogram/Ultrasound	1,438	5.4%	8.9%	8.8%
Lumbar Spine MRI for Low Back Pain	82	34.1%	35.3%	37.2%

The Cooley Dickinson Hospital

30 Locust Street
Northampton, MA 01060
URL: www.cooley-dickinson.org
Type: Acute Care Hospitals
Ownership: Voluntary non-profit - Private
Phone: 413-582-2000
Fax: 413-582-2951
Emergency Services: Yes
Beds: 125

Key Personnel:
Radiology . . . . George G Hartnell
Quality Assurance . . . . Joanne LaBelle
CEO/President . . . . Joanne Marqusee
Chair/CEO . . . . Matthew Pitoniak
Chief of Medical Staff . . . . Margaret Russo, MD

Measure	Cases	This Hosp.	State Avg.	U.S. Avg.
Blood Clot Prevention and Treatment				
Anticoagulation Overlap Therapy[2]	39	100%	97%	93%
ICU Venous Thromboembolism Prophylaxis[2]	37	100%	92%	92%
Incidence of Potentially Preventable VTE[1,2]	-	-	7%	10%
UFH with Dosages/Platelet Monitoring[1,2]	-	-	91%	97%
Venous Thromboembolism Prophylaxis[2]	369	100%	87%	85%
Warfarin Therapy Discharge Instructions[2]	26	92%	77%	75%
Chest Pain/Possible Heart Attack Care				
Aspirin Given Within 24 Hours of Arrival	90	100%	97%	96%
Fibrinolytic Meds Within 30 Min. of Arrival[1]	-	-	73%	58%
Average Time to ECG (minutes)	93	5	7	7
Average Time to Transfer (minutes)	22	30	55	60
Children's Asthma Care				
Received Home Management Plan of Care	-	-	-	88%
Received Reliever Medication	-	-	-	100%
Received Systemic Corticosteroids	-	-	-	100%
Emergency Department				
Admittance Decision Time (minutes)[2]	825	80	119	98
Head CT Results Within 45 Min. of Arrival	29	86%	70%	57%
Patients Who Left ER Before Being Seen	36,658	2%	2%	2%
Time from ER Arrival to Admit. (minutes)[2]	826	296	313	274
Time from ER Arrival to Discharge (minutes)	357	173	156	134
Time in ER Before Being Evaluated (minutes)	400	50	36	26
Time to Pain Meds for Fractures (minutes)	121	52	59	57
Heart Attack Care				
Aspirin Given at Discharge	26	100%	100%	99%
Fibrinolytic Meds Within 30 Min. of Arrival[7]	-	-	100%	54%
PCI Within 90 Minutes of Arrival[7]	-	-	96%	96%
Statin Prescribed at Discharge	25	92%	99%	98%
Heart Failure Care				
ACE Inhibitor or ARB for LVSD	53	98%	96%	97%
Discharge Instructions Given	140	93%	95%	94%
Evaluation of LVS Function	187	100%	100%	99%
Medicare Spending				
Medicare Spending per Patient (ratio)	-	1.04	1.03	0.98
Pneumonia Care				
Appropriate Initial Antibiotic Given	145	99%	97%	95%
Blood Culture Timing	198	99%	98%	98%
Pregnancy and Delivery Care				
Newborn Deliveries Scheduled Early[2]	17	0%	2%	6%
Preventive Care				
Immunization for Influenza[2]	547	94%	91%	90%
Immunization for Pneumonia[2]	713	96%	91%	92%
Stroke Care				
Anticoagulation Therapy for Atrial Fibrillation[1]	-	-	97%	95%
Antithrombotic Therapy Timing	36	100%	98%	98%
Assessed for Rehabilitation	44	100%	96%	97%
Discharged on Antithrombotic Therapy	40	100%	100%	99%
Discharged on Statin Medication	33	88%	96%	94%
Thrombolytic Therapy Timing[7]	-	-	68%	66%
Venous Thromboembolism Prophylaxis	42	90%	94%	94%
Written Stroke Educational Materials Given	19	100%	82%	88%
Surgical Care Improvement Project				
Appropriate Beta Blocker Usage[2]	107	98%	98%	98%
Appropriate VTP Within 24 Hours[2]	452	99%	99%	98%
Controlled Postoperative Blood Glucose[2,7]	-	-	96%	97%
Perioperative Temperature Management[2]	509	100%	100%	100%
Prophylactic Antibiotic Selection[2]	390	100%	99%	99%
Prophylactic Antibiotic Selection (Outpatient)	167	97%	98%	98%
Prophylactic Antibiotic Stopped[2]	389	99%	99%	98%
Prophylactic Antibiotic Timing[2]	390	100%	99%	99%
Prophylactic Antibiotic Timing (Outpatient)	167	99%	98%	98%
Urinary Catheter Removal[2]	387	99%	97%	97%
Survey of Patients' Hospital Experiences				
Area Around Room 'Always' Quiet at Night	300+	55%	52%	61%
Doctors 'Always' Communicated Well	300+	77%	80%	82%
Home Recovery Information Given	300+	85%	87%	85%
Hospital Given 9 or 10 on 10 Point Scale	300+	72%	69%	71%
Meds 'Always' Explained Before Given	300+	68%	64%	64%
Nurses 'Always' Communicated Well	300+	78%	79%	79%
Pain 'Always' Well Controlled	300+	71%	71%	71%
Room and Bathroom 'Always' Clean	300+	75%	72%	73%
Timely Help 'Always' Received	300+	66%	66%	68%
Would Definitely Recommend Hospital	300+	79%	73%	71%
Use of Medical Imaging				
Cardiac Imaging Stress Test before Surgery	101	4.0%	5.4%	5.3%
Combination Abdominal CT Scan	949	4.4%	6.3%	10.5%
Combination Brain/Sinus CT Scan	657	0.6%	2.4%	2.7%
Combination Chest CT Scan	668	0.0%	0.5%	2.7%
Follow-up Mammogram/Ultrasound	2,142	7.0%	8.9%	8.8%
Lumbar Spine MRI for Low Back Pain	216	27.8%	35.3%	37.2%

NOTE: Hospital profiles are in alphabetical order by state, then city, then hospital within the city; Rankings exclude hospitals with less than 25 cases except for patient surveys which excludes hospitals with less than 100 cases; (a) 100-299 cases; (1) The number of cases/patients is too few to report; (2) Data submitted were based on a sample of cases/patients; (3) Results are based on a shorter time period than required; (4) Data suppressed by CMS for one or more quarters; (5) Results are not available for this reporting period; (6) Fewer than 100 patients completed the HCAHPS survey; (7) No cases met the criteria for this measure; (8) The lower limit of the confidence interval cannot be calculated if the number of observed infections equals zero; (9) No data are available from the state/territory for this reporting period; (10) The scores shown reflect fewer than 50 completed surveys; (11) There were discrepancies in the data collection process; (12) This measure does not apply to this hospital for this reporting period; (13) Results cannot be calculated for this reporting period; (14) The results for this state are combined with nearby states to protect confidentiality; Please refer to the User's Guide for a full explanation of data.

Norwood Hospital

800 Washington Street
Norwood, MA 02062
Phone: 508-772-1000
Fax: 781-278-6820
URL: www.caritasnorwood.org
Type: Acute Care Hospitals
Emergency Services: Yes
Ownership: Proprietary
Beds: 265

Key Personnel:
Chief of Medical Staff. . . . . Michael Ginsburg, MD
CEO/President. . . . . Margaret Hanson
Cardiac Laboratory. . . . . John Kinch, MD
Radiology. . . . . Kevin Loughlin, MD
Quality Assurance . . . . Kathleen Turke
Pediatric Ambulatory Care . . . . . . Bruce Weinstock, MD

Measure	Cases	This Hosp.	State Avg.	U.S. Avg.
Blood Clot Prevention and Treatment				
Anticoagulation Overlap Therapy[2]	85	87%	97%	93%
ICU Venous Thromboembolism Prophylaxis[2]	30	93%	92%	92%
Incidence of Potentially Preventable VTE[1,2]	-	-	7%	10%
UFH with Dosages/Platelet Monitoring[2]	81	99%	91%	97%
Venous Thromboembolism Prophylaxis[2]	352	95%	87%	85%
Warfarin Therapy Discharge Instructions[2]	75	95%	77%	75%
Chest Pain/Possible Heart Attack Care				
Aspirin Given Within 24 Hours of Arrival	66	94%	97%	96%
Fibrinolytic Meds Within 30 Min. of Arrival[7]	-	-	73%	58%
Average Time to ECG (minutes)	68	0	7	7
Average Time to Transfer (minutes)[1]	-	-	55	60
Children's Asthma Care				
Received Home Management Plan of Care	-	-	-	88%
Received Reliever Medication	-	-	-	100%
Received Systemic Corticosteroids	-	-	-	100%
Emergency Department				
Admittance Decision Time (minutes)[2]	920	148	119	98
Head CT Results Within 45 Min. of Arrival	16	81%	70%	57%
Patients Who Left ER Before Being Seen	44,114	1%	2%	2%
Time from ER Arrival to Admit. (minutes)[2]	927	339	313	274
Time from ER Arrival to Discharge (minutes)	369	172	156	134
Time in ER Before Being Evaluated (minutes)	361	29	36	26
Time to Pain Meds for Fractures (minutes)	125	59	59	57
Heart Attack Care				
Aspirin Given at Discharge	89	100%	100%	99%
Fibrinolytic Meds Within 30 Min. of Arrival[7]	-	-	100%	54%
PCI Within 90 Minutes of Arrival	45	96%	96%	96%
Statin Prescribed at Discharge	86	98%	99%	98%
Heart Failure Care				
ACE Inhibitor or ARB for LVSD	68	97%	96%	97%
Discharge Instructions Given	202	83%	95%	94%
Evaluation of LVS Function	295	100%	100%	99%
Medicare Spending				
Medicare Spending per Patient (ratio)	-	1.01	1.03	0.98
Pneumonia Care				
Appropriate Initial Antibiotic Given	117	99%	97%	95%
Blood Culture Timing	120	92%	98%	98%
Pregnancy and Delivery Care				
Newborn Deliveries Scheduled Early	14	0%	2%	6%
Preventive Care				
Immunization for Influenza[2]	575	92%	91%	90%
Immunization for Pneumonia[2]	754	94%	91%	92%
Stroke Care				
Anticoagulation Therapy for Atrial Fibrillation	26	100%	97%	95%
Antithrombotic Therapy Timing	75	99%	98%	98%
Assessed for Rehabilitation	82	88%	96%	97%
Discharged on Antithrombotic Therapy	81	100%	100%	99%
Discharged on Statin Medication	70	97%	96%	94%
Thrombolytic Therapy Timing[1]	-	-	68%	66%
Venous Thromboembolism Prophylaxis	87	92%	94%	94%
Written Stroke Educational Materials Given	47	91%	82%	88%
Surgical Care Improvement Project				
Appropriate Beta Blocker Usage[2]	183	99%	98%	98%
Appropriate VTP Within 24 Hours[2]	372	98%	99%	98%
Controlled Postoperative Blood Glucose[2,7]	-	-	96%	97%
Perioperative Temperature Management[2]	455	100%	100%	100%
Prophylactic Antibiotic Selection[2]	314	100%	99%	99%
Prophylactic Antibiotic Selection (Outpatient)	109	99%	98%	98%
Prophylactic Antibiotic Stopped[2]	307	99%	99%	98%
Prophylactic Antibiotic Timing[2]	315	99%	99%	99%
Prophylactic Antibiotic Timing (Outpatient)	109	98%	98%	98%
Urinary Catheter Removal[2]	255	99%	97%	97%
Survey of Patients' Hospital Experiences				
Area Around Room 'Always' Quiet at Night	300+	41%	52%	61%
Doctors 'Always' Communicated Well	300+	78%	80%	82%
Home Recovery Information Given	300+	86%	87%	85%
Hospital Given 9 or 10 on 10 Point Scale	300+	54%	69%	71%
Meds 'Always' Explained Before Given	300+	62%	64%	64%
Nurses 'Always' Communicated Well	300+	76%	79%	79%
Pain 'Always' Well Controlled	300+	67%	71%	71%
Room and Bathroom 'Always' Clean	300+	70%	72%	73%
Timely Help 'Always' Received	300+	56%	66%	68%
Would Definitely Recommend Hospital	300+	57%	73%	71%
Use of Medical Imaging				
Cardiac Imaging Stress Test before Surgery	354	5.6%	5.4%	5.3%
Combination Abdominal CT Scan	875	5.1%	6.3%	10.5%
Combination Brain/Sinus CT Scan	660	1.5%	2.4%	2.7%
Combination Chest CT Scan	606	0.2%	0.5%	2.7%
Follow-up Mammogram/Ultrasound	925	12.5%	8.9%	8.8%
Lumbar Spine MRI for Low Back Pain[1]	-	-	35.3%	37.2%

Martha's Vineyard Hospital

One Hospital Road PO Box 1477
Oak Bluffs, MA 02557
Phone: 508-693-0410
Fax: 508-693-5971
URL: www.marthasvineyardhospital.com
Type: Critical Access Hospitals
Emergency Services: No
Ownership: Voluntary non-profit - Private
Beds: 32

Key Personnel:
Operating Room. . . . . Denise Fraser, MD
Pediatric In-Patient Care . . . . Michael Goldfein, MD
Cardiac Laboratory. . . . . Timothy Gurey, MD
Radiology. . . . . Stephen Miller, MD
Chief of Medical Staff. . . . . Pieter Pil, M.D., PhD
CEO/President. . . . . Timothy J. Walsh
Quality Assurance . . . . Dedie Wieler
Emergency Room . . . . Jeffrey Zack, MD

Measure	Cases	This Hosp.	State Avg.	U.S. Avg.
Blood Clot Prevention and Treatment				
Anticoagulation Overlap Therapy[5]	-	-	97%	93%
ICU Venous Thromboembolism Prophylaxis[5]	-	-	92%	92%
Incidence of Potentially Preventable VTE[5]	-	-	7%	10%
UFH with Dosages/Platelet Monitoring[5]	-	-	91%	97%
Venous Thromboembolism Prophylaxis[5]	-	-	87%	85%
Warfarin Therapy Discharge Instructions[5]	-	-	77%	75%
Chest Pain/Possible Heart Attack Care				
Aspirin Given Within 24 Hours of Arrival	-	-	97%	96%
Fibrinolytic Meds Within 30 Min. of Arrival	-	-	73%	58%
Average Time to ECG (minutes)	-	-	7	7
Average Time to Transfer (minutes)	-	-	55	60
Children's Asthma Care				
Received Home Management Plan of Care	-	-	-	88%
Received Reliever Medication	-	-	-	100%
Received Systemic Corticosteroids	-	-	-	100%
Emergency Department				
Admittance Decision Time (minutes)[5]	-	-	119	98
Head CT Results Within 45 Min. of Arrival	-	-	70%	57%
Patients Who Left ER Before Being Seen	-	-	2%	2%
Time from ER Arrival to Admit. (minutes)[5]	-	-	313	274
Time from ER Arrival to Discharge (minutes)	-	-	156	134
Time in ER Before Being Evaluated (minutes)	-	-	36	26
Time to Pain Meds for Fractures (minutes)	-	-	59	57
Heart Attack Care				
Aspirin Given at Discharge[5]	-	-	100%	99%
Fibrinolytic Meds Within 30 Min. of Arrival[5]	-	-	100%	54%
PCI Within 90 Minutes of Arrival[5]	-	-	96%	96%
Statin Prescribed at Discharge[5]	-	-	99%	98%
Heart Failure Care				
ACE Inhibitor or ARB for LVSD[1]	-	-	96%	97%
Discharge Instructions Given	28	100%	95%	94%
Evaluation of LVS Function	28	100%	100%	99%
Medicare Spending				
Medicare Spending per Patient (ratio)	-	-	1.03	0.98
Pneumonia Care				
Appropriate Initial Antibiotic Given	29	97%	97%	95%
Blood Culture Timing	56	96%	98%	98%
Pregnancy and Delivery Care				
Newborn Deliveries Scheduled Early[5]	-	-	2%	6%
Preventive Care				
Immunization for Influenza[5]	-	-	91%	90%
Immunization for Pneumonia[5]	-	-	91%	92%
Stroke Care				
Anticoagulation Therapy for Atrial Fibrillation[5]	-	-	97%	95%
Antithrombotic Therapy Timing[5]	-	-	98%	98%
Assessed for Rehabilitation[5]	-	-	96%	97%
Discharged on Antithrombotic Therapy[5]	-	-	100%	99%
Discharged on Statin Medication[5]	-	-	96%	94%
Thrombolytic Therapy Timing[5]	-	-	68%	66%
Venous Thromboembolism Prophylaxis[5]	-	-	94%	94%
Written Stroke Educational Materials Given[5]	-	-	82%	88%
Surgical Care Improvement Project				
Appropriate Beta Blocker Usage[5]	-	-	98%	98%
Appropriate VTP Within 24 Hours[5]	-	-	99%	98%
Controlled Postoperative Blood Glucose[5]	-	-	96%	97%
Perioperative Temperature Management[5]	-	-	100%	100%
Prophylactic Antibiotic Selection[5]	-	-	99%	99%
Prophylactic Antibiotic Selection (Outpatient)	-	-	98%	98%
Prophylactic Antibiotic Stopped[5]	-	-	99%	98%
Prophylactic Antibiotic Timing[5]	-	-	99%	99%
Prophylactic Antibiotic Timing (Outpatient)	-	-	98%	98%
Urinary Catheter Removal[5]	-	-	97%	97%
Survey of Patients' Hospital Experiences				
Area Around Room 'Always' Quiet at Night	(a)	68%	52%	61%
Doctors 'Always' Communicated Well	(a)	82%	80%	82%
Home Recovery Information Given	(a)	89%	87%	85%
Hospital Given 9 or 10 on 10 Point Scale	(a)	79%	69%	71%
Meds 'Always' Explained Before Given	(a)	70%	64%	64%
Nurses 'Always' Communicated Well	(a)	84%	79%	79%
Pain 'Always' Well Controlled	(a)	78%	71%	71%
Room and Bathroom 'Always' Clean	(a)	79%	72%	73%
Timely Help 'Always' Received	(a)	79%	66%	68%
Would Definitely Recommend Hospital	(a)	81%	73%	71%
Use of Medical Imaging				
Cardiac Imaging Stress Test before Surgery	-	-	5.4%	5.3%
Combination Abdominal CT Scan	-	-	6.3%	10.5%
Combination Brain/Sinus CT Scan	-	-	2.4%	2.7%
Combination Chest CT Scan	-	-	0.5%	2.7%
Follow-up Mammogram/Ultrasound	-	-	8.9%	8.8%
Lumbar Spine MRI for Low Back Pain	-	-	35.3%	37.2%

Wing Memorial Hospital & Medical Center

40 Wright Street
Palmer, MA 01069
Phone: 413-283-7651
Fax: 413-284-5117
URL: www.winghealth.org
Type: Acute Care Hospitals
Emergency Services: Yes
Ownership: Voluntary non-profit - Other
Beds: 74

Key Personnel:
CEO/President. . . . . Charles Cavagnaro III, MD
Patient Relations . . . . Maria Darasz
Operating Room. . . . . Sue Keenan, RN
Quality Assurance . . . . Ronald Krystofik
Radiology. . . . . Susaney C Londie
Chief of Medical Staff. . . . . David Maguire, MD
Emergency Room . . . . Lori Striplin, RN

Measure	Cases	This Hosp.	State Avg.	U.S. Avg.
Blood Clot Prevention and Treatment				
Anticoagulation Overlap Therapy[2]	15	100%	97%	93%
ICU Venous Thromboembolism Prophylaxis[2]	38	100%	92%	92%
Incidence of Potentially Preventable VTE[2,7]	-	-	7%	10%
UFH with Dosages/Platelet Monitoring[1,2]	-	-	91%	97%
Venous Thromboembolism Prophylaxis[2]	239	97%	87%	85%
Warfarin Therapy Discharge Instructions[2]	12	100%	77%	75%
Chest Pain/Possible Heart Attack Care				
Aspirin Given Within 24 Hours of Arrival	57	93%	97%	96%
Fibrinolytic Meds Within 30 Min. of Arrival[7]	-	-	73%	58%
Average Time to ECG (minutes)	55	8	7	7
Average Time to Transfer (minutes)	15	78	55	60
Children's Asthma Care				

NOTE: Hospital profiles are in alphabetical order by state, then city, then hospital within the city; Rankings exclude hospitals with less than 25 cases except for patient surveys which excludes hospitals with less than 100 cases; (a) 100-299 cases; (1) The number of cases/patients is too few to report; (2) Data submitted were based on a sample of cases/patients; (3) Results are based on a shorter time period than required; (4) Data suppressed by CMS for one or more quarters; (5) Results are not available for this reporting period; (6) Fewer than 100 patients completed the HCAHPS survey; (7) No cases met the criteria for this measure; (8) The lower limit of the confidence interval cannot be calculated if the number of observed infections equals zero; (9) No data are available from the state/territory for this reporting period; (10) The scores shown reflect fewer than 50 completed surveys; (11) There were discrepancies in the data collection process; (12) This measure does not apply to this hospital for this reporting period; (13) Results cannot be calculated for this reporting period; (14) The results for this state are combined with nearby states to protect confidentiality; Please refer to the User's Guide for a full explanation of data.

Measure	Cases	This Hosp.	State Avg.	U.S. Avg.
Received Home Management Plan of Care	-	-	-	88%
Received Reliever Medication	-	-	-	100%
Received Systemic Corticosteroids	-	-	-	100%
Emergency Department				
Admittance Decision Time (minutes)[2]	336	55	119	98
Head CT Results Within 45 Min. of Arrival	14	50%	70%	57%
Patients Who Left ER Before Being Seen	24,613	2%	2%	2%
Time from ER Arrival to Admit. (minutes)[2]	379	220	313	274
Time from ER Arrival to Discharge (minutes)	314	102	156	134
Time in ER Before Being Evaluated (minutes)	338	36	36	26
Time to Pain Meds for Fractures (minutes)	55	69	59	57
Heart Attack Care				
Aspirin Given at Discharge	16	100%	100%	99%
Fibrinolytic Meds Within 30 Min. of Arrival[7]	-	-	100%	54%
PCI Within 90 Minutes of Arrival[7]	-	-	96%	96%
Statin Prescribed at Discharge	17	94%	99%	98%
Heart Failure Care				
ACE Inhibitor or ARB for LVSD	17	100%	96%	97%
Discharge Instructions Given	83	100%	95%	94%
Evaluation of LVS Function	114	100%	100%	99%
Medicare Spending				
Medicare Spending per Patient (ratio)	-	1.06	1.03	0.98
Pneumonia Care				
Appropriate Initial Antibiotic Given	78	96%	97%	95%
Blood Culture Timing	158	98%	98%	98%
Pregnancy and Delivery Care				
Newborn Deliveries Scheduled Early[7]	-	-	2%	6%
Preventive Care				
Immunization for Influenza[2]	322	96%	91%	90%
Immunization for Pneumonia[2]	439	94%	91%	92%
Stroke Care				
Anticoagulation Therapy for Atrial Fibrillation[1]	-	-	97%	95%
Antithrombotic Therapy Timing	23	96%	98%	98%
Assessed for Rehabilitation	25	100%	96%	97%
Discharged on Antithrombotic Therapy	25	100%	100%	99%
Discharged on Statin Medication	22	100%	96%	94%
Thrombolytic Therapy Timing[7]	-	-	68%	66%
Venous Thromboembolism Prophylaxis	21	100%	94%	94%
Written Stroke Educational Materials Given	15	100%	82%	88%
Surgical Care Improvement Project				
Appropriate Beta Blocker Usage	12	100%	98%	98%
Appropriate VTP Within 24 Hours	38	97%	99%	98%
Controlled Postoperative Blood Glucose[7]	-	-	96%	97%
Perioperative Temperature Management	43	100%	100%	100%
Prophylactic Antibiotic Selection	23	100%	99%	99%
Prophylactic Antibiotic Selection (Outpatient)	52	100%	98%	98%
Prophylactic Antibiotic Stopped	21	100%	99%	98%
Prophylactic Antibiotic Timing	23	100%	99%	99%
Prophylactic Antibiotic Timing (Outpatient)	16	94%	98%	98%
Urinary Catheter Removal	12	100%	97%	97%
Survey of Patients' Hospital Experiences				
Area Around Room 'Always' Quiet at Night	300+	54%	52%	61%
Doctors 'Always' Communicated Well	300+	82%	80%	82%
Home Recovery Information Given	300+	89%	87%	85%
Hospital Given 9 or 10 on 10 Point Scale	300+	74%	69%	71%
Meds 'Always' Explained Before Given	300+	67%	64%	64%
Nurses 'Always' Communicated Well	300+	79%	79%	79%
Pain 'Always' Well Controlled	300+	67%	71%	71%
Room and Bathroom 'Always' Clean	300+	83%	72%	73%
Timely Help 'Always' Received	300+	63%	66%	68%
Would Definitely Recommend Hospital	300+	80%	73%	71%
Use of Medical Imaging				
Cardiac Imaging Stress Test before Surgery	118	5.9%	5.4%	5.3%
Combination Abdominal CT Scan	433	3.0%	6.3%	10.5%
Combination Brain/Sinus CT Scan	437	2.1%	2.4%	2.7%
Combination Chest CT Scan	327	0.3%	0.5%	2.7%
Follow-up Mammogram/Ultrasound	801	7.0%	8.9%	8.8%
Lumbar Spine MRI for Low Back Pain[7]	-	-	35.3%	37.2%

Berkshire Medical Center

725 North Street
Pittsfield, MA 01201
URL: www.berkshirehealthsystems.org
Type: Acute Care Hospitals
Ownership: Voluntary non-profit - Other

Phone: 413-447-2000
Fax: 413-447-2091
Emergency Services: Yes
Beds: 302

Key Personnel:
Radiology. . . . . Curtis Brasseur, DO
Pediatric In-Patient Care . . . . Michael Fabrizio, MD
Anesthesiology. . . . . Raymond Gary Sohl, MD
Emergency Room . . . . Ronald Hayden, MD
Chief of Medical Staff. . . . . John Kearns, MD
CEO/President. . . . . David E Phelps
Surgery . . . . Parvis Sadighi, MD
Operating Room. . . . . Diana Vallone, RN

Measure	Cases	This Hosp.	State Avg.	U.S. Avg.
Blood Clot Prevention and Treatment				
Anticoagulation Overlap Therapy[2]	50	98%	97%	93%
ICU Venous Thromboembolism Prophylaxis[2]	73	100%	92%	92%
Incidence of Potentially Preventable VTE[1,2]	-	-	7%	10%
UFH with Dosages/Platelet Monitoring[2]	41	100%	91%	97%
Venous Thromboembolism Prophylaxis[2]	333	99%	87%	85%
Warfarin Therapy Discharge Instructions[2]	41	98%	77%	75%
Chest Pain/Possible Heart Attack Care				
Aspirin Given Within 24 Hours of Arrival	93	100%	97%	96%
Fibrinolytic Meds Within 30 Min. of Arrival	25	72%	73%	58%
Average Time to ECG (minutes)	95	6	7	7
Average Time to Transfer (minutes)[7]	-	-	55	60
Children's Asthma Care				
Received Home Management Plan of Care	-	-	-	88%
Received Reliever Medication	-	-	-	100%
Received Systemic Corticosteroids	-	-	-	100%
Emergency Department				
Admittance Decision Time (minutes)[2]	798	58	119	98
Head CT Results Within 45 Min. of Arrival[1]	-	-	70%	57%
Patients Who Left ER Before Being Seen	56,805	3%	2%	2%
Time from ER Arrival to Admit. (minutes)[2]	801	265	313	274
Time from ER Arrival to Discharge (minutes)	385	160	156	134
Time in ER Before Being Evaluated (minutes)	383	45	36	26
Time to Pain Meds for Fractures (minutes)	124	78	59	57
Heart Attack Care				
Aspirin Given at Discharge	49	100%	100%	99%
Fibrinolytic Meds Within 30 Min. of Arrival[7]	-	-	100%	54%
PCI Within 90 Minutes of Arrival[7]	-	-	96%	96%
Statin Prescribed at Discharge	49	100%	99%	98%
Heart Failure Care				
ACE Inhibitor or ARB for LVSD	37	100%	96%	97%
Discharge Instructions Given	227	100%	95%	94%
Evaluation of LVS Function	299	100%	100%	99%
Medicare Spending				
Medicare Spending per Patient (ratio)	-	1.00	1.03	0.98
Pneumonia Care				
Appropriate Initial Antibiotic Given	178	100%	97%	95%
Blood Culture Timing	355	100%	98%	98%
Pregnancy and Delivery Care				
Newborn Deliveries Scheduled Early	42	0%	2%	6%
Preventive Care				
Immunization for Influenza[2]	564	94%	91%	90%
Immunization for Pneumonia[2]	772	93%	91%	92%
Stroke Care				
Anticoagulation Therapy for Atrial Fibrillation	31	100%	97%	95%
Antithrombotic Therapy Timing	96	100%	98%	98%
Assessed for Rehabilitation	136	100%	96%	97%
Discharged on Antithrombotic Therapy	130	100%	100%	99%
Discharged on Statin Medication	101	100%	96%	94%
Thrombolytic Therapy Timing[1]	-	-	68%	66%
Venous Thromboembolism Prophylaxis	113	100%	94%	94%
Written Stroke Educational Materials Given	86	97%	82%	88%
Surgical Care Improvement Project				
Appropriate Beta Blocker Usage	223	100%	98%	98%
Appropriate VTP Within 24 Hours	680	99%	99%	98%
Controlled Postoperative Blood Glucose[7]	-	-	96%	97%
Perioperative Temperature Management	781	100%	100%	100%
Prophylactic Antibiotic Selection	478	100%	99%	99%
Prophylactic Antibiotic Selection (Outpatient)	322	99%	98%	98%
Prophylactic Antibiotic Stopped	471	100%	99%	98%
Prophylactic Antibiotic Timing	478	99%	99%	99%
Prophylactic Antibiotic Timing (Outpatient)	246	99%	98%	98%
Urinary Catheter Removal	295	99%	97%	97%
Survey of Patients' Hospital Experiences				
Area Around Room 'Always' Quiet at Night	300+	48%	52%	61%
Doctors 'Always' Communicated Well	300+	78%	80%	82%
Home Recovery Information Given	300+	88%	87%	85%
Hospital Given 9 or 10 on 10 Point Scale	300+	68%	69%	71%
Meds 'Always' Explained Before Given	300+	62%	64%	64%
Nurses 'Always' Communicated Well	300+	81%	79%	79%
Pain 'Always' Well Controlled	300+	70%	71%	71%
Room and Bathroom 'Always' Clean	300+	72%	72%	73%
Timely Help 'Always' Received	300+	62%	66%	68%
Would Definitely Recommend Hospital	300+	70%	73%	71%
Use of Medical Imaging				
Cardiac Imaging Stress Test before Surgery	616	5.2%	5.4%	5.3%
Combination Abdominal CT Scan	1,696	4.6%	6.3%	10.5%
Combination Brain/Sinus CT Scan	1,002	4.0%	2.4%	2.7%
Combination Chest CT Scan	1,693	1.7%	0.5%	2.7%
Follow-up Mammogram/Ultrasound	3,648	8.2%	8.9%	8.8%
Lumbar Spine MRI for Low Back Pain	256	36.7%	35.3%	37.2%

Jordan Hospital

275 Sandwich Street
Plymouth, MA 02360
URL: www.jordanhospital.org
Type: Acute Care Hospitals
Ownership: Voluntary non-profit - Private

Phone: 508-746-2000
Fax: 508-830-1131
Emergency Services: Yes
Beds: 139

Key Personnel:
Emergency Room . . . . Erin Ackland, MD
Patient Relations . . . . Carrol Dillitlane
Chair/CEO . . . . Clark Hinkley
CEO/President. . . . . Peter J Holden
Chief of Medical Staff . . . . Harvey J Kowaloff, MD, MMM
Radiology. . . . . Stephen Trehu

Measure	Cases	This Hosp.	State Avg.	U.S. Avg.
Blood Clot Prevention and Treatment				
Anticoagulation Overlap Therapy[2]	60	90%	97%	93%
ICU Venous Thromboembolism Prophylaxis[2]	58	95%	92%	92%
Incidence of Potentially Preventable VTE[1,2]	-	-	7%	10%
UFH with Dosages/Platelet Monitoring[2]	19	100%	91%	97%
Venous Thromboembolism Prophylaxis[2]	322	93%	87%	85%
Warfarin Therapy Discharge Instructions[2]	41	90%	77%	75%
Chest Pain/Possible Heart Attack Care				
Aspirin Given Within 24 Hours of Arrival	82	98%	97%	96%
Fibrinolytic Meds Within 30 Min. of Arrival[7]	-	-	73%	58%
Average Time to ECG (minutes)	87	10	7	7
Average Time to Transfer (minutes)[1]	-	-	55	60
Children's Asthma Care				
Received Home Management Plan of Care	-	-	-	88%
Received Reliever Medication	-	-	-	100%
Received Systemic Corticosteroids	-	-	-	100%
Emergency Department				
Admittance Decision Time (minutes)[2]	792	203	119	98
Head CT Results Within 45 Min. of Arrival	21	67%	70%	57%
Patients Who Left ER Before Being Seen	51,042	1%	2%	2%
Time from ER Arrival to Admit. (minutes)[2]	792	446	313	274
Time from ER Arrival to Discharge (minutes)	358	178	156	134
Time in ER Before Being Evaluated (minutes)	408	42	36	26
Time to Pain Meds for Fractures (minutes)	62	76	59	57
Heart Attack Care				
Aspirin Given at Discharge	43	98%	100%	99%
Fibrinolytic Meds Within 30 Min. of Arrival[7]	-	-	100%	54%
PCI Within 90 Minutes of Arrival[7]	-	-	96%	96%
Statin Prescribed at Discharge	43	95%	99%	98%
Heart Failure Care				
ACE Inhibitor or ARB for LVSD	45	91%	96%	97%
Discharge Instructions Given	175	97%	95%	94%
Evaluation of LVS Function	244	100%	100%	99%
Medicare Spending				
Medicare Spending per Patient (ratio)	-	1.04	1.03	0.98
Pneumonia Care				

NOTE: Hospital profiles are in alphabetical order by state, then city, then hospital within the city; Rankings exclude hospitals with less than 25 cases except for patient surveys which excludes hospitals with less than 100 cases; (a) 100-299 cases; (1) The number of cases/patients is too few to report; (2) Data submitted were based on a sample of cases/patients; (3) Results are based on a shorter time period than required; (4) Data suppressed by CMS for one or more quarters; (5) Results are not available for this reporting period; (6) Fewer than 100 patients completed the HCAHPS survey; (7) No cases met the criteria for this measure; (8) The lower limit of the confidence interval cannot be calculated if the number of observed infections equals zero; (9) No data are available from the state/territory for this reporting period; (10) The scores shown reflect fewer than 50 completed surveys; (11) There were discrepancies in the data collection process; (12) This measure does not apply to this hospital for this reporting period; (13) Results cannot be calculated for this reporting period; (14) The results for this state are combined with nearby states to protect confidentiality; Please refer to the User's Guide for a full explanation of data.

Measure	Cases	This Hosp.	State Avg.	U.S. Avg.
Appropriate Initial Antibiotic Given	136	97%	97%	95%
Blood Culture Timing	212	98%	98%	98%
Pregnancy and Delivery Care				
Newborn Deliveries Scheduled Early	28	0%	2%	6%
Preventive Care				
Immunization for Influenza[2]	518	93%	91%	90%
Immunization for Pneumonia[2]	700	95%	91%	92%
Stroke Care				
Anticoagulation Therapy for Atrial Fibrillation[1]	-	-	97%	95%
Antithrombotic Therapy Timing	66	97%	98%	98%
Assessed for Rehabilitation	64	94%	96%	97%
Discharged on Antithrombotic Therapy	62	100%	100%	99%
Discharged on Statin Medication	54	91%	96%	94%
Thrombolytic Therapy Timing[1]	-	-	68%	66%
Venous Thromboembolism Prophylaxis	69	87%	94%	94%
Written Stroke Educational Materials Given	27	96%	82%	88%
Surgical Care Improvement Project				
Appropriate Beta Blocker Usage	219	96%	98%	98%
Appropriate VTP Within 24 Hours	631	98%	99%	98%
Controlled Postoperative Blood Glucose[7]	-	-	96%	97%
Perioperative Temperature Management	720	100%	100%	100%
Prophylactic Antibiotic Selection	521	99%	99%	99%
Prophylactic Antibiotic Selection (Outpatient)	145	94%	98%	98%
Prophylactic Antibiotic Stopped	512	99%	99%	98%
Prophylactic Antibiotic Timing	521	99%	99%	99%
Prophylactic Antibiotic Timing (Outpatient)	147	97%	98%	98%
Urinary Catheter Removal	295	92%	97%	97%
Survey of Patients' Hospital Experiences				
Area Around Room 'Always' Quiet at Night	300+	46%	52%	61%
Doctors 'Always' Communicated Well	300+	78%	80%	82%
Home Recovery Information Given	300+	86%	87%	85%
Hospital Given 9 or 10 on 10 Point Scale	300+	61%	69%	71%
Meds 'Always' Explained Before Given	300+	59%	64%	64%
Nurses 'Always' Communicated Well	300+	75%	79%	79%
Pain 'Always' Well Controlled	300+	69%	71%	71%
Room and Bathroom 'Always' Clean	300+	62%	72%	73%
Timely Help 'Always' Received	300+	59%	66%	68%
Would Definitely Recommend Hospital	300+	68%	73%	71%
Use of Medical Imaging				
Cardiac Imaging Stress Test before Surgery	205	9.3%	5.4%	5.3%
Combination Abdominal CT Scan	1,294	3.7%	6.3%	10.5%
Combination Brain/Sinus CT Scan	1,049	2.6%	2.4%	2.7%
Combination Chest CT Scan	930	1.8%	0.5%	2.7%
Follow-up Mammogram/Ultrasound	2,798	7.7%	8.9%	8.8%
Lumbar Spine MRI for Low Back Pain	172	29.1%	35.3%	37.2%

Quincy Medical Center

114 Whitwell Street
Quincy, MA 02169
URL: www.quincymc.org
Type: Acute Care Hospitals
Ownership: Proprietary
Phone: 617-773-6100
Fax: 617-376-4019
Emergency Services: Yes
Beds: 282

Key Personnel:
Quality Assurance .... Sandi Austin
CEO/President................ Donna Rubinate

Measure	Cases	This Hosp.	State Avg.	U.S. Avg.
Blood Clot Prevention and Treatment				
Anticoagulation Overlap Therapy[2]	18	89%	97%	93%
ICU Venous Thromboembolism Prophylaxis[2]	20	85%	92%	92%
Incidence of Potentially Preventable VTE[1,2]	-	-	7%	10%
UFH with Dosages/Platelet Monitoring[1,2]	-	-	91%	97%
Venous Thromboembolism Prophylaxis[2]	365	83%	87%	85%
Warfarin Therapy Discharge Instructions[2]	11	73%	77%	75%
Chest Pain/Possible Heart Attack Care				
Aspirin Given Within 24 Hours of Arrival	62	97%	97%	96%
Fibrinolytic Meds Within 30 Min. of Arrival[7]	-	-	73%	58%
Average Time to ECG (minutes)	63	4	7	7
Average Time to Transfer (minutes)	17	38	55	60
Children's Asthma Care				
Received Home Management Plan of Care	-	-	-	88%
Received Reliever Medication	-	-	-	100%
Received Systemic Corticosteroids	-	-	-	100%
Emergency Department				
Admittance Decision Time (minutes)[2]	803	141	119	98
Head CT Results Within 45 Min. of Arrival[1]	-	-	70%	57%
Patients Who Left ER Before Being Seen	31,423	3%	2%	2%
Time from ER Arrival to Admit. (minutes)[2]	805	320	313	274
Time from ER Arrival to Discharge (minutes)	388	164	156	134
Time in ER Before Being Evaluated (minutes)	388	22	36	26
Time to Pain Meds for Fractures (minutes)	71	71	59	57
Heart Attack Care				
Aspirin Given at Discharge	23	100%	100%	99%
Fibrinolytic Meds Within 30 Min. of Arrival[1]	-	-	100%	54%
PCI Within 90 Minutes of Arrival[7]	-	-	96%	96%
Statin Prescribed at Discharge	22	95%	99%	98%
Heart Failure Care				
ACE Inhibitor or ARB for LVSD	35	97%	96%	97%
Discharge Instructions Given	110	92%	95%	94%
Evaluation of LVS Function	144	99%	100%	99%
Medicare Spending				
Medicare Spending per Patient (ratio)	-	1.09	1.03	0.98
Pneumonia Care				
Appropriate Initial Antibiotic Given	109	94%	97%	95%
Blood Culture Timing	109	97%	98%	98%
Pregnancy and Delivery Care				
Newborn Deliveries Scheduled Early[7]	-	-	2%	6%
Preventive Care				
Immunization for Influenza[2]	590	93%	91%	90%
Immunization for Pneumonia[2]	709	88%	91%	92%
Stroke Care				
Anticoagulation Therapy for Atrial Fibrillation[1]	-	-	97%	95%
Antithrombotic Therapy Timing	43	95%	98%	98%
Assessed for Rehabilitation	42	93%	96%	97%
Discharged on Antithrombotic Therapy	41	98%	100%	99%
Discharged on Statin Medication	29	100%	96%	94%
Thrombolytic Therapy Timing[1]	-	-	68%	66%
Venous Thromboembolism Prophylaxis	48	88%	94%	94%
Written Stroke Educational Materials Given	22	91%	82%	88%
Surgical Care Improvement Project				
Appropriate Beta Blocker Usage	139	99%	98%	98%
Appropriate VTP Within 24 Hours	360	98%	99%	98%
Controlled Postoperative Blood Glucose[7]	-	-	96%	97%
Perioperative Temperature Management	421	100%	100%	100%
Prophylactic Antibiotic Selection	279	99%	99%	99%
Prophylactic Antibiotic Selection (Outpatient)	28	100%	98%	98%
Prophylactic Antibiotic Stopped	274	97%	99%	98%
Prophylactic Antibiotic Timing	280	100%	99%	99%
Prophylactic Antibiotic Timing (Outpatient)	28	96%	98%	98%
Urinary Catheter Removal	264	95%	97%	97%
Survey of Patients' Hospital Experiences				
Area Around Room 'Always' Quiet at Night	300+	45%	52%	61%
Doctors 'Always' Communicated Well	300+	74%	80%	82%
Home Recovery Information Given	300+	84%	87%	85%
Hospital Given 9 or 10 on 10 Point Scale	300+	52%	69%	71%
Meds 'Always' Explained Before Given	300+	56%	64%	64%
Nurses 'Always' Communicated Well	300+	71%	79%	79%
Pain 'Always' Well Controlled	300+	64%	71%	71%
Room and Bathroom 'Always' Clean	300+	64%	72%	73%
Timely Help 'Always' Received	300+	59%	66%	68%
Would Definitely Recommend Hospital	300+	60%	73%	71%
Use of Medical Imaging				
Cardiac Imaging Stress Test before Surgery	118	7.6%	5.4%	5.3%
Combination Abdominal CT Scan	648	2.9%	6.3%	10.5%
Combination Brain/Sinus CT Scan	694	2.3%	2.4%	2.7%
Combination Chest CT Scan	365	0.8%	0.5%	2.7%
Follow-up Mammogram/Ultrasound	927	11.2%	8.9%	8.8%
Lumbar Spine MRI for Low Back Pain	71	40.8%	35.3%	37.2%

North Shore Medical Center

81 Highland Avenue
Salem, MA 01970
URL: www.nsmc.partners.org
Type: Acute Care Hospitals
Ownership: Voluntary non-profit - Private
Phone: 978-741-1215
Fax: 978-744-9110
Emergency Services: Yes
Beds: 260

Key Personnel:
Emergency Room .... Everett Lyn, MD
Pediatrics.................. Mark H. Mandell, MD
Anesthesiology................ Johanna O'Connor, MD
Chief of Medical Staff.......... Mitchell S. Rein, MD
Cardiac Laboratory............ David J. Roberts, MD
CEO/President.............. Robert G. Rorton
Surgery .... Marc Rubin, MD
Radiology................... M. Christian Semine, MD

Measure	Cases	This Hosp.	State Avg.	U.S. Avg.
Blood Clot Prevention and Treatment				
Anticoagulation Overlap Therapy[2]	112	93%	97%	93%
ICU Venous Thromboembolism Prophylaxis[2]	74	62%	92%	92%
Incidence of Potentially Preventable VTE[2]	20	20%	7%	10%
UFH with Dosages/Platelet Monitoring[2]	73	100%	91%	97%
Venous Thromboembolism Prophylaxis[2]	372	73%	87%	85%
Warfarin Therapy Discharge Instructions[2]	82	93%	77%	75%
Chest Pain/Possible Heart Attack Care				
Aspirin Given Within 24 Hours of Arrival[1,3]	-	-	97%	96%
Fibrinolytic Meds Within 30 Min. of Arrival[3,7]	-	-	73%	58%
Average Time to ECG (minutes)[1,3]	-	-	7	7
Average Time to Transfer (minutes)[3,7]	-	-	55	60
Children's Asthma Care				
Received Home Management Plan of Care	-	-	-	88%
Received Reliever Medication	-	-	-	100%
Received Systemic Corticosteroids	-	-	-	100%
Emergency Department				
Admittance Decision Time (minutes)[2]	563	175	119	98
Head CT Results Within 45 Min. of Arrival	18	61%	70%	57%
Patients Who Left ER Before Being Seen	78,078	3%	2%	2%
Time from ER Arrival to Admit. (minutes)[2]	563	346	313	274
Time from ER Arrival to Discharge (minutes)	344	145	156	134
Time in ER Before Being Evaluated (minutes)	383	39	36	26
Time to Pain Meds for Fractures (minutes)	173	28	59	57
Heart Attack Care				
Aspirin Given at Discharge	245	100%	100%	99%
Fibrinolytic Meds Within 30 Min. of Arrival[7]	-	-	100%	54%
PCI Within 90 Minutes of Arrival	61	95%	96%	96%
Statin Prescribed at Discharge	242	100%	99%	98%
Heart Failure Care				
ACE Inhibitor or ARB for LVSD	95	99%	96%	97%
Discharge Instructions Given	427	94%	95%	94%
Evaluation of LVS Function	598	100%	100%	99%
Medicare Spending				
Medicare Spending per Patient (ratio)	-	1.04	1.03	0.98
Pneumonia Care				
Appropriate Initial Antibiotic Given	328	97%	97%	95%
Blood Culture Timing	450	98%	98%	98%
Pregnancy and Delivery Care				
Newborn Deliveries Scheduled Early[2]	18	0%	2%	6%
Preventive Care				
Immunization for Influenza[2]	538	97%	91%	90%
Immunization for Pneumonia[2]	725	95%	91%	92%
Stroke Care				
Anticoagulation Therapy for Atrial Fibrillation[2]	18	100%	97%	95%
Antithrombotic Therapy Timing[2]	70	100%	98%	98%
Assessed for Rehabilitation[2]	80	96%	96%	97%
Discharged on Antithrombotic Therapy[2]	77	100%	100%	99%
Discharged on Statin Medication[2]	62	98%	96%	94%
Thrombolytic Therapy Timing[2]	18	39%	68%	66%
Venous Thromboembolism Prophylaxis[2]	78	99%	94%	94%
Written Stroke Educational Materials Given[2]	40	98%	82%	88%
Surgical Care Improvement Project				
Appropriate Beta Blocker Usage[2]	203	100%	98%	98%
Appropriate VTP Within 24 Hours[2]	272	99%	99%	98%
Controlled Postoperative Blood Glucose[2]	117	97%	96%	97%
Perioperative Temperature Management[2]	337	100%	100%	100%
Prophylactic Antibiotic Selection[2]	341	99%	99%	99%
Prophylactic Antibiotic Selection (Outpatient)	467	98%	98%	98%
Prophylactic Antibiotic Stopped[2]	334	98%	99%	98%
Prophylactic Antibiotic Timing[2]	342	99%	99%	99%
Prophylactic Antibiotic Timing (Outpatient)	471	98%	98%	98%
Urinary Catheter Removal[2]	312	94%	97%	97%
Survey of Patients' Hospital Experiences				
Area Around Room 'Always' Quiet at Night	300+	50%	52%	61%
Doctors 'Always' Communicated Well	300+	78%	80%	82%

NOTE: Hospital profiles are in alphabetical order by state, then city, then hospital within the city; Rankings exclude hospitals with less than 25 cases except for patient surveys which excludes hospitals with less than 100 cases; (a) 100-299 cases; (1) The number of cases/patients is too few to report; (2) Data submitted were based on a sample of cases/patients; (3) Results are based on a shorter time period than required; (4) Data suppressed by CMS for one or more quarters; (5) Results are not available for this reporting period; (6) Fewer than 100 patients completed the HCAHPS survey; (7) No cases met the criteria for this measure; (8) The lower limit of the confidence interval cannot be calculated if the number of observed infections equals zero; (9) No data are available from the state/territory for this reporting period; (10) The scores shown reflect fewer than 50 completed surveys; (11) There were discrepancies in the data collection process; (12) This measure does not apply to this hospital for this reporting period; (13) Results cannot be calculated for this reporting period; (14) The results for this state are combined with nearby states to protect confidentiality; Please refer to the User's Guide for a full explanation of data.

Home Recovery Information Given	300+	86%	87%	85%
Hospital Given 9 or 10 on 10 Point Scale	300+	69%	69%	71%
Meds 'Always' Explained Before Given	300+	59%	64%	64%
Nurses 'Always' Communicated Well	300+	77%	79%	79%
Pain 'Always' Well Controlled	300+	69%	71%	71%
Room and Bathroom 'Always' Clean	300+	70%	72%	73%
Timely Help 'Always' Received	300+	65%	66%	68%
Would Definitely Recommend Hospital	300+	73%	73%	71%
Use of Medical Imaging				
Cardiac Imaging Stress Test before Surgery	799	4.5%	5.4%	5.3%
Combination Abdominal CT Scan	1,787	7.1%	6.3%	10.5%
Combination Brain/Sinus CT Scan	1,389	2.2%	2.4%	2.7%
Combination Chest CT Scan	1,544	0.0%	0.5%	2.7%
Follow-up Mammogram/Ultrasound	6,493	5.3%	8.9%	8.8%
Lumbar Spine MRI for Low Back Pain	417	30.7%	35.3%	37.2%

South Shore Hospital

55 Fogg Road
South Weymouth, MA 02190
Phone: 781-340-8000
Fax: 781-337-3768
URL: www.southshorehospital.org
Type: Acute Care Hospitals
Emergency Services: Yes
Ownership: Voluntary non-profit - Private
Beds: 303

Key Personnel:

CEO/President. . . . . Joseph Cahill
Anesthesiology. . . . . Mark Canning, MD
Radiology. . . . . Russell Kelley, MD
Chair/CEO . . . . Kenneth Kirkland
Surgery . . . . Frederick Millham, MD
Chief of Medical Staff . . . . John Stevenson, MD
Emergency Room . . . . Jason Tracy, MD
Pediatrics. . . . . Mark Waltzman, MD

Measure	Cases	This Hosp.	State Avg.	U.S. Avg.
Blood Clot Prevention and Treatment				
Anticoagulation Overlap Therapy[2]	158	100%	97%	93%
ICU Venous Thromboembolism Prophylaxis[2]	73	96%	92%	92%
Incidence of Potentially Preventable VTE[2]	33	9%	7%	10%
UFH with Dosages/Platelet Monitoring[2]	82	100%	91%	97%
Venous Thromboembolism Prophylaxis[2]	396	94%	87%	85%
Warfarin Therapy Discharge Instructions[2]	115	92%	77%	75%
Chest Pain/Possible Heart Attack Care				
Aspirin Given Within 24 Hours of Arrival	28	96%	97%	96%
Fibrinolytic Meds Within 30 Min. of Arrival[3,7]	-	-	73%	58%
Average Time to ECG (minutes)	29	8	7	7
Average Time to Transfer (minutes)[3,7]	-	-	55	60
Children's Asthma Care				
Received Home Management Plan of Care	-	-	-	88%
Received Reliever Medication	-	-	-	100%
Received Systemic Corticosteroids	-	-	-	100%
Emergency Department				
Admittance Decision Time (minutes)[2]	750	327	119	98
Head CT Results Within 45 Min. of Arrival	18	78%	70%	57%
Patients Who Left ER Before Being Seen	85,353	1%	2%	2%
Time from ER Arrival to Admit. (minutes)[2]	754	577	313	274
Time from ER Arrival to Discharge (minutes)	376	182	156	134
Time in ER Before Being Evaluated (minutes)	408	42	36	26
Time to Pain Meds for Fractures (minutes)	423	63	59	57
Heart Attack Care				
Aspirin Given at Discharge	305	100%	100%	99%
Fibrinolytic Meds Within 30 Min. of Arrival[7]	-	-	100%	54%
PCI Within 90 Minutes of Arrival	108	99%	96%	96%
Statin Prescribed at Discharge	294	100%	99%	98%
Heart Failure Care				
ACE Inhibitor or ARB for LVSD	118	100%	96%	97%
Discharge Instructions Given	473	97%	95%	94%
Evaluation of LVS Function	743	100%	100%	99%
Medicare Spending				
Medicare Spending per Patient (ratio)	-	1.07	1.03	0.98
Pneumonia Care				
Appropriate Initial Antibiotic Given	341	98%	97%	95%
Blood Culture Timing	185	96%	98%	98%
Pregnancy and Delivery Care				
Newborn Deliveries Scheduled Early	465	0%	2%	6%
Preventive Care				
Immunization for Influenza[2]	536	94%	91%	90%
Immunization for Pneumonia[2]	603	95%	91%	92%
Stroke Care				
Anticoagulation Therapy for Atrial Fibrillation	32	100%	97%	95%
Antithrombotic Therapy Timing	194	99%	98%	98%
Assessed for Rehabilitation	221	99%	96%	97%
Discharged on Antithrombotic Therapy	198	100%	100%	99%
Discharged on Statin Medication	174	100%	96%	94%
Thrombolytic Therapy Timing[1]	-	-	68%	66%
Venous Thromboembolism Prophylaxis	202	95%	94%	94%
Written Stroke Educational Materials Given	106	94%	82%	88%
Surgical Care Improvement Project				
Appropriate Beta Blocker Usage	324	95%	98%	98%
Appropriate VTP Within 24 Hours	881	99%	99%	98%
Controlled Postoperative Blood Glucose[7]	-	-	96%	97%
Perioperative Temperature Management	994	99%	100%	100%
Prophylactic Antibiotic Selection	645	99%	99%	99%
Prophylactic Antibiotic Selection (Outpatient)	317	97%	98%	98%
Prophylactic Antibiotic Stopped	641	99%	99%	98%
Prophylactic Antibiotic Timing	647	99%	99%	99%
Prophylactic Antibiotic Timing (Outpatient)	322	98%	98%	98%
Urinary Catheter Removal	215	97%	97%	97%
Survey of Patients' Hospital Experiences				
Area Around Room 'Always' Quiet at Night	300+	55%	52%	61%
Doctors 'Always' Communicated Well	300+	82%	80%	82%
Home Recovery Information Given	300+	90%	87%	85%
Hospital Given 9 or 10 on 10 Point Scale	300+	72%	69%	71%
Meds 'Always' Explained Before Given	300+	68%	64%	64%
Nurses 'Always' Communicated Well	300+	82%	79%	79%
Pain 'Always' Well Controlled	300+	74%	71%	71%
Room and Bathroom 'Always' Clean	300+	72%	72%	73%
Timely Help 'Always' Received	300+	68%	66%	68%
Would Definitely Recommend Hospital	300+	78%	73%	71%
Use of Medical Imaging				
Cardiac Imaging Stress Test before Surgery	422	5.7%	5.4%	5.3%
Combination Abdominal CT Scan	1,455	2.7%	6.3%	10.5%
Combination Brain/Sinus CT Scan	1,535	1.0%	2.4%	2.7%
Combination Chest CT Scan	1,188	2.9%	0.5%	2.7%
Follow-up Mammogram/Ultrasound	2,940	8.1%	8.9%	8.8%
Lumbar Spine MRI for Low Back Pain	148	32.4%	35.3%	37.2%

Harrington Memorial Hospital

100 South Street
Southbridge, MA 01550
Phone: 508-765-9771
Fax: 508-764-2486
E-mail: hr@harringtonhospital.org
URL: www.harringtonhospital.org
Type: Acute Care Hospitals
Emergency Services: Yes
Ownership: Voluntary non-profit - Private
Beds: 113

Key Personnel:

Pediatric In-Patient Care . . . . Ann Beaudry
Operating Room. . . . . Laura Fortin
Emergency Room . . . . Michael P Gaudet
Chief of Medical Staff . . . . Vladas Litani, MD
Quality Assurance . . . . Marlene Mach
President/CEO. . . . . Edward Moore
Intensive Care Unit. . . . . Marsha Woodard
Infection Control. . . . . Judith Zaido

Measure	Cases	This Hosp.	State Avg.	U.S. Avg.
Blood Clot Prevention and Treatment				
Anticoagulation Overlap Therapy[2]	13	69%	97%	93%
ICU Venous Thromboembolism Prophylaxis[2]	52	73%	92%	92%
Incidence of Potentially Preventable VTE[1,2]	-	-	7%	10%
UFH with Dosages/Platelet Monitoring[1,2]	-	-	91%	97%
Venous Thromboembolism Prophylaxis[2]	290	85%	87%	85%
Warfarin Therapy Discharge Instructions[2]	13	8%	77%	75%
Chest Pain/Possible Heart Attack Care				
Aspirin Given Within 24 Hours of Arrival	88	93%	97%	96%
Fibrinolytic Meds Within 30 Min. of Arrival[7]	-	-	73%	58%
Average Time to ECG (minutes)	99	5	7	7
Average Time to Transfer (minutes)	14	51	55	60
Children's Asthma Care				
Received Home Management Plan of Care	-	-	-	88%
Received Reliever Medication	-	-	-	100%
Received Systemic Corticosteroids	-	-	-	100%
Emergency Department				
Admittance Decision Time (minutes)[2]	565	80	119	98
Head CT Results Within 45 Min. of Arrival	13	46%	70%	57%
Patients Who Left ER Before Being Seen	38,075	1%	2%	2%
Time from ER Arrival to Admit. (minutes)[2]	566	236	313	274
Time from ER Arrival to Discharge (minutes)	359	99	156	134
Time in ER Before Being Evaluated (minutes)	403	4	36	26
Time to Pain Meds for Fractures (minutes)	121	38	59	57
Heart Attack Care				
Aspirin Given at Discharge	26	96%	100%	99%
Fibrinolytic Meds Within 30 Min. of Arrival[7]	-	-	100%	54%
PCI Within 90 Minutes of Arrival[7]	-	-	96%	96%
Statin Prescribed at Discharge	26	96%	99%	98%
Heart Failure Care				
ACE Inhibitor or ARB for LVSD	41	98%	96%	97%
Discharge Instructions Given	119	93%	95%	94%
Evaluation of LVS Function	159	99%	100%	99%
Medicare Spending				
Medicare Spending per Patient (ratio)	-	1.00	1.03	0.98
Pneumonia Care				
Appropriate Initial Antibiotic Given	72	97%	97%	95%
Blood Culture Timing	121	98%	98%	98%
Pregnancy and Delivery Care				
Newborn Deliveries Scheduled Early	17	0%	2%	6%
Preventive Care				
Immunization for Influenza[2]	352	89%	91%	90%
Immunization for Pneumonia[2]	453	92%	91%	92%
Stroke Care				
Anticoagulation Therapy for Atrial Fibrillation[1]	-	-	97%	95%
Antithrombotic Therapy Timing	30	100%	98%	98%
Assessed for Rehabilitation	31	97%	96%	97%
Discharged on Antithrombotic Therapy	30	97%	100%	99%
Discharged on Statin Medication	26	96%	96%	94%
Thrombolytic Therapy Timing[1]	-	-	68%	66%
Venous Thromboembolism Prophylaxis	30	97%	94%	94%
Written Stroke Educational Materials Given	20	100%	82%	88%
Surgical Care Improvement Project				
Appropriate Beta Blocker Usage	52	90%	98%	98%
Appropriate VTP Within 24 Hours	146	97%	99%	98%
Controlled Postoperative Blood Glucose[7]	-	-	96%	97%
Perioperative Temperature Management	164	99%	100%	100%
Prophylactic Antibiotic Selection	121	99%	99%	99%
Prophylactic Antibiotic Selection (Outpatient)	65	92%	98%	98%
Prophylactic Antibiotic Stopped	116	99%	99%	98%
Prophylactic Antibiotic Timing	121	97%	99%	99%
Prophylactic Antibiotic Timing (Outpatient)	65	95%	98%	98%
Urinary Catheter Removal	135	99%	97%	97%
Survey of Patients' Hospital Experiences				
Area Around Room 'Always' Quiet at Night	300+	54%	52%	61%
Doctors 'Always' Communicated Well	300+	80%	80%	82%
Home Recovery Information Given	300+	85%	87%	85%
Hospital Given 9 or 10 on 10 Point Scale	300+	71%	69%	71%
Meds 'Always' Explained Before Given	300+	67%	64%	64%
Nurses 'Always' Communicated Well	300+	81%	79%	79%
Pain 'Always' Well Controlled	300+	73%	71%	71%
Room and Bathroom 'Always' Clean	300+	80%	72%	73%
Timely Help 'Always' Received	300+	72%	66%	68%
Would Definitely Recommend Hospital	300+	74%	73%	71%
Use of Medical Imaging				
Cardiac Imaging Stress Test before Surgery	211	5.2%	5.4%	5.3%
Combination Abdominal CT Scan	477	5.5%	6.3%	10.5%
Combination Brain/Sinus CT Scan[1]	-	-	2.4%	2.7%
Combination Chest CT Scan	331	0.0%	0.5%	2.7%
Follow-up Mammogram/Ultrasound	1,210	7.3%	8.9%	8.8%
Lumbar Spine MRI for Low Back Pain	82	41.5%	35.3%	37.2%

Baystate Medical Center

759 Chestnut Street
Springfield, MA 01199
Phone: 413-794-0000
Fax: 413-794-3832
URL: www.baystatehealth.com
Type: Acute Care Hospitals
Emergency Services: Yes
Ownership: Voluntary non-profit - Private
Beds: 653

Key Personnel:

Quality Assurance . . . . Evan M Benjamin, MD
Chief of Medical Staff . . . . Martin Broder, MD

NOTE: Hospital profiles are in alphabetical order by state, then city, then hospital within the city; Rankings exclude hospitals with less than 25 cases except for patient surveys which excludes hospitals with less than 100 cases; (a) 100-299 cases; (1) The number of cases/patients is too few to report; (2) Data submitted were based on a sample of cases/patients; (3) Results are based on a shorter time period than required; (4) Data suppressed by CMS for one or more quarters; (5) Results are not available for this reporting period; (6) Fewer than 100 patients completed the HCAHPS survey; (7) No cases met the criteria for this measure; (8) The lower limit of the confidence interval cannot be calculated if the number of observed infections equals zero; (9) No data are available from the state/territory for this reporting period; (10) The scores shown reflect fewer than 50 completed surveys; (11) There were discrepancies in the data collection process; (12) This measure does not apply to this hospital for this reporting period; (13) Results cannot be calculated for this reporting period; (14) The results for this state are combined with nearby states to protect confidentiality; Please refer to the User's Guide for a full explanation of data.

Operating Room. . . . . Deborah A Provost
Pediatric Ambulatory Care . . . . . . Edward Reiter, MD
Pediatric In-Patient Care . . . . Edward Reiter, MD
Radiology. . . . . Eckert Sachsse, MD
Emergency Room . . . . John Santoro, MD
CEO/President. . . . . Mark R Tolosky

Measure	Cases	This Hosp.	State Avg.	U.S. Avg.
Blood Clot Prevention and Treatment				
Anticoagulation Overlap Therapy[2]	189	96%	97%	93%
ICU Venous Thromboembolism Prophylaxis[2]	75	97%	92%	92%
Incidence of Potentially Preventable VTE[2]	62	8%	7%	10%
UFH with Dosages/Platelet Monitoring[2]	145	100%	91%	97%
Venous Thromboembolism Prophylaxis[2]	376	92%	87%	85%
Warfarin Therapy Discharge Instructions[2]	141	80%	77%	75%
Chest Pain/Possible Heart Attack Care				
Aspirin Given Within 24 Hours of Arrival[1]	-	-	97%	96%
Fibrinolytic Meds Within 30 Min. of Arrival[3,7]	-	-	73%	58%
Average Time to ECG (minutes)[1]	-	-	7	7
Average Time to Transfer (minutes)[3,7]	-	-	55	60
Children's Asthma Care				
Received Home Management Plan of Care	109	95%	-	88%
Received Reliever Medication	109	100%	-	100%
Received Systemic Corticosteroids	109	100%	-	100%
Emergency Department				
Admittance Decision Time (minutes)[2]	578	163	119	98
Head CT Results Within 45 Min. of Arrival[1]	-	-	70%	57%
Patients Who Left ER Before Being Seen	>100k	7%	2%	2%
Time from ER Arrival to Admit. (minutes)[2]	589	396	313	274
Time from ER Arrival to Discharge (minutes)	378	252	156	134
Time in ER Before Being Evaluated (minutes)	261	91	36	26
Time to Pain Meds for Fractures (minutes)	274	58	59	57
Heart Attack Care				
Aspirin Given at Discharge	1,051	100%	100%	99%
Fibrinolytic Meds Within 30 Min. of Arrival[1]	-	-	100%	54%
PCI Within 90 Minutes of Arrival	112	95%	96%	96%
Statin Prescribed at Discharge	1,041	100%	99%	98%
Heart Failure Care				
ACE Inhibitor or ARB for LVSD	252	99%	96%	97%
Discharge Instructions Given	908	98%	95%	94%
Evaluation of LVS Function	1,159	100%	100%	99%
Medicare Spending				
Medicare Spending per Patient (ratio)	-	1.04	1.03	0.98
Pneumonia Care				
Appropriate Initial Antibiotic Given	268	99%	97%	95%
Blood Culture Timing	436	98%	98%	98%
Pregnancy and Delivery Care				
Newborn Deliveries Scheduled Early	297	3%	2%	6%
Preventive Care				
Immunization for Influenza[2]	557	89%	91%	90%
Immunization for Pneumonia[2]	651	94%	91%	92%
Stroke Care				
Anticoagulation Therapy for Atrial Fibrillation	45	98%	97%	95%
Antithrombotic Therapy Timing	275	99%	98%	98%
Assessed for Rehabilitation	352	100%	96%	97%
Discharged on Antithrombotic Therapy	291	100%	100%	99%
Discharged on Statin Medication	223	100%	96%	94%
Thrombolytic Therapy Timing	34	50%	68%	66%
Venous Thromboembolism Prophylaxis	368	98%	94%	94%
Written Stroke Educational Materials Given	181	97%	82%	88%
Surgical Care Improvement Project				
Appropriate Beta Blocker Usage[2]	243	98%	98%	98%
Appropriate VTP Within 24 Hours[2]	404	99%	99%	98%
Controlled Postoperative Blood Glucose[2]	152	93%	96%	97%
Perioperative Temperature Management[2]	532	100%	100%	100%
Prophylactic Antibiotic Selection[2]	489	100%	99%	99%
Prophylactic Antibiotic Selection (Outpatient)	627	99%	98%	98%
Prophylactic Antibiotic Stopped[2]	475	99%	99%	98%
Prophylactic Antibiotic Timing[2]	489	100%	99%	99%
Prophylactic Antibiotic Timing (Outpatient)	627	99%	98%	98%
Urinary Catheter Removal[2]	387	99%	97%	97%
Survey of Patients' Hospital Experiences				
Area Around Room 'Always' Quiet at Night	300+	49%	52%	61%
Doctors 'Always' Communicated Well	300+	79%	80%	82%
Home Recovery Information Given	300+	88%	87%	85%
Hospital Given 9 or 10 on 10 Point Scale	300+	69%	69%	71%
Meds 'Always' Explained Before Given	300+	61%	64%	64%
Nurses 'Always' Communicated Well	300+	76%	79%	79%
Pain 'Always' Well Controlled	300+	70%	71%	71%
Room and Bathroom 'Always' Clean	300+	67%	72%	73%
Timely Help 'Always' Received	300+	61%	66%	68%
Would Definitely Recommend Hospital	300+	75%	73%	71%
Use of Medical Imaging				
Cardiac Imaging Stress Test before Surgery	1,093	5.8%	5.4%	5.3%
Combination Abdominal CT Scan	2,020	2.1%	6.3%	10.5%
Combination Brain/Sinus CT Scan	1,657	1.3%	2.4%	2.7%
Combination Chest CT Scan	1,600	0.0%	0.5%	2.7%
Follow-up Mammogram/Ultrasound	3,832	9.4%	8.9%	8.8%
Lumbar Spine MRI for Low Back Pain	134	39.6%	35.3%	37.2%

Mercy Medical Center

271 Carew Street
Springfield, MA 01104
URL: www.mercycares.com
Type: Acute Care Hospitals
Ownership: Voluntary non-profit - Private
Phone: 413-748-9000
Fax: 413-748-9609
Emergency Services: Yes
Beds: 182

Key Personnel:
Radiology. . . . . Gregory Blackman
Chief of Medical Staff. . . . . P Henri Lamonthe
CEO/President. . . . . Vince J McCorkle

Measure	Cases	This Hosp.	State Avg.	U.S. Avg.
Blood Clot Prevention and Treatment				
Anticoagulation Overlap Therapy[2]	79	92%	97%	93%
ICU Venous Thromboembolism Prophylaxis[2]	14	100%	92%	92%
Incidence of Potentially Preventable VTE[2]	11	9%	7%	10%
UFH with Dosages/Platelet Monitoring[2]	46	100%	91%	97%
Venous Thromboembolism Prophylaxis[2]	377	94%	87%	85%
Warfarin Therapy Discharge Instructions[2]	60	75%	77%	75%
Chest Pain/Possible Heart Attack Care				
Aspirin Given Within 24 Hours of Arrival	55	98%	97%	96%
Fibrinolytic Meds Within 30 Min. of Arrival[7]	-	-	73%	58%
Average Time to ECG (minutes)	57	6	7	7
Average Time to Transfer (minutes)	15	53	55	60
Children's Asthma Care				
Received Home Management Plan of Care	-	-	-	88%
Received Reliever Medication	-	-	-	100%
Received Systemic Corticosteroids	-	-	-	100%
Emergency Department				
Admittance Decision Time (minutes)[2]	795	140	119	98
Head CT Results Within 45 Min. of Arrival[1]	-	-	70%	57%
Patients Who Left ER Before Being Seen	76,434	4%	2%	2%
Time from ER Arrival to Admit. (minutes)[2]	795	352	313	274
Time from ER Arrival to Discharge (minutes)	384	169	156	134
Time in ER Before Being Evaluated (minutes)	410	70	36	26
Time to Pain Meds for Fractures (minutes)	170	66	59	57
Heart Attack Care				
Aspirin Given at Discharge	55	100%	100%	99%
Fibrinolytic Meds Within 30 Min. of Arrival[7]	-	-	100%	54%
PCI Within 90 Minutes of Arrival[7]	-	-	96%	96%
Statin Prescribed at Discharge	54	100%	99%	98%
Heart Failure Care				
ACE Inhibitor or ARB for LVSD	67	96%	96%	97%
Discharge Instructions Given	200	97%	95%	94%
Evaluation of LVS Function	283	100%	100%	99%
Medicare Spending				
Medicare Spending per Patient (ratio)	-	1.04	1.03	0.98
Pneumonia Care				
Appropriate Initial Antibiotic Given	130	100%	97%	95%
Blood Culture Timing	252	100%	98%	98%
Pregnancy and Delivery Care				
Newborn Deliveries Scheduled Early	103	1%	2%	6%
Preventive Care				
Immunization for Influenza[2]	558	97%	91%	90%
Immunization for Pneumonia[2]	712	95%	91%	92%
Stroke Care				
Anticoagulation Therapy for Atrial Fibrillation	14	71%	97%	95%
Antithrombotic Therapy Timing	94	96%	98%	98%
Assessed for Rehabilitation	112	98%	96%	97%
Discharged on Antithrombotic Therapy	95	100%	100%	99%
Discharged on Statin Medication	73	99%	96%	94%
Thrombolytic Therapy Timing[1]	-	-	68%	66%
Venous Thromboembolism Prophylaxis	122	97%	94%	94%
Written Stroke Educational Materials Given	52	98%	82%	88%
Surgical Care Improvement Project				
Appropriate Beta Blocker Usage	220	98%	98%	98%
Appropriate VTP Within 24 Hours	702	99%	99%	98%
Controlled Postoperative Blood Glucose[7]	-	-	96%	97%
Perioperative Temperature Management	857	100%	100%	100%
Prophylactic Antibiotic Selection	423	100%	99%	99%
Prophylactic Antibiotic Selection (Outpatient)	597	99%	98%	98%
Prophylactic Antibiotic Stopped	400	97%	99%	98%
Prophylactic Antibiotic Timing	424	99%	99%	99%
Prophylactic Antibiotic Timing (Outpatient)	597	99%	98%	98%
Urinary Catheter Removal	482	98%	97%	97%
Survey of Patients' Hospital Experiences				
Area Around Room 'Always' Quiet at Night	300+	44%	52%	61%
Doctors 'Always' Communicated Well	300+	75%	80%	82%
Home Recovery Information Given	300+	85%	87%	85%
Hospital Given 9 or 10 on 10 Point Scale	300+	63%	69%	71%
Meds 'Always' Explained Before Given	300+	52%	64%	64%
Nurses 'Always' Communicated Well	300+	72%	79%	79%
Pain 'Always' Well Controlled	300+	64%	71%	71%
Room and Bathroom 'Always' Clean	300+	66%	72%	73%
Timely Help 'Always' Received	300+	55%	66%	68%
Would Definitely Recommend Hospital	300+	68%	73%	71%
Use of Medical Imaging				
Cardiac Imaging Stress Test before Surgery	537	4.1%	5.4%	5.3%
Combination Abdominal CT Scan	1,240	5.4%	6.3%	10.5%
Combination Brain/Sinus CT Scan	1,223	2.3%	2.4%	2.7%
Combination Chest CT Scan	610	0.0%	0.5%	2.7%
Follow-up Mammogram/Ultrasound	2,191	10.1%	8.9%	8.8%
Lumbar Spine MRI for Low Back Pain[7]	-	-	35.3%	37.2%

Morton Hospital

88 Washington Street
Taunton, MA 02780
URL: www.mortonhospital.org
Type: Acute Care Hospitals
Ownership: Proprietary
Phone: 508-828-7000
Fax: 508-824-6947
Emergency Services: Yes
Beds: 152

Key Personnel:
President . . . . Kim Bassett, RN, BSN, MBA
Intensive Care Unit. . . . . Donna Chase, RN
Radiology. . . . . Richard S Jennis
Infection Control. . . . . Marie Lebrun, RN
Anesthesiology. . . . . Bijan Naikai, MD
CEO/President. . . . . Thomas C Porter
Quality Assurance . . . . Richard J Slavick

Measure	Cases	This Hosp.	State Avg.	U.S. Avg.
Blood Clot Prevention and Treatment				
Anticoagulation Overlap Therapy[2]	45	98%	97%	93%
ICU Venous Thromboembolism Prophylaxis[2]	63	92%	92%	92%
Incidence of Potentially Preventable VTE[1,2]	-	-	7%	10%
UFH with Dosages/Platelet Monitoring[2]	24	96%	91%	97%
Venous Thromboembolism Prophylaxis[2]	324	84%	87%	85%
Warfarin Therapy Discharge Instructions[2]	37	86%	77%	75%
Chest Pain/Possible Heart Attack Care				
Aspirin Given Within 24 Hours of Arrival	63	98%	97%	96%
Fibrinolytic Meds Within 30 Min. of Arrival[7]	-	-	73%	58%
Average Time to ECG (minutes)	65	6	7	7
Average Time to Transfer (minutes)	11	82	55	60
Children's Asthma Care				
Received Home Management Plan of Care	-	-	-	88%
Received Reliever Medication	-	-	-	100%
Received Systemic Corticosteroids	-	-	-	100%
Emergency Department				
Admittance Decision Time (minutes)[2]	687	105	119	98
Head CT Results Within 45 Min. of Arrival	15	93%	70%	57%
Patients Who Left ER Before Being Seen	47,019	0%	2%	2%
Time from ER Arrival to Admit. (minutes)[2]	739	301	313	274
Time from ER Arrival to Discharge (minutes)	349	150	156	134
Time in ER Before Being Evaluated (minutes)	389	32	36	26

NOTE: Hospital profiles are in alphabetical order by state, then city, then hospital within the city; Rankings exclude hospitals with less than 25 cases except for patient surveys which excludes hospitals with less than 100 cases; (a) 100-299 cases; (1) The number of cases/patients is too few to report; (2) Data submitted were based on a sample of cases/patients; (3) Results are based on a shorter time period than required; (4) Data suppressed by CMS for one or more quarters; (5) Results are not available for this reporting period; (6) Fewer than 100 patients completed the HCAHPS survey; (7) No cases met the criteria for this measure; (8) The lower limit of the confidence interval cannot be calculated if the number of observed infections equals zero; (9) No data are available from the state/territory for this reporting period; (10) The scores shown reflect fewer than 50 completed surveys; (11) There were discrepancies in the data collection process; (12) This measure does not apply to this hospital for this reporting period; (13) Results cannot be calculated for this reporting period; (14) The results for this state are combined with nearby states to protect confidentiality; Please refer to the User's Guide for a full explanation of data.

Measure	Cases	This Hosp.	State Avg.	U.S. Avg.
Time to Pain Meds for Fractures (minutes)	67	68	59	57
Heart Attack Care				
Aspirin Given at Discharge	33	97%	100%	99%
Fibrinolytic Meds Within 30 Min. of Arrival[7]	-	-	100%	54%
PCI Within 90 Minutes of Arrival[7]	-	-	96%	96%
Statin Prescribed at Discharge	33	88%	99%	98%
Heart Failure Care				
ACE Inhibitor or ARB for LVSD	57	88%	96%	97%
Discharge Instructions Given	148	93%	95%	94%
Evaluation of LVS Function	227	100%	100%	99%
Medicare Spending				
Medicare Spending per Patient (ratio)	-	1.09	1.03	0.98
Pneumonia Care				
Appropriate Initial Antibiotic Given	118	94%	97%	95%
Blood Culture Timing	174	98%	98%	98%
Pregnancy and Delivery Care				
Newborn Deliveries Scheduled Early	15	0%	2%	6%
Preventive Care				
Immunization for Influenza[2]	538	81%	91%	90%
Immunization for Pneumonia[2]	738	93%	91%	92%
Stroke Care				
Anticoagulation Therapy for Atrial Fibrillation[1]	-	-	97%	95%
Antithrombotic Therapy Timing	48	98%	98%	98%
Assessed for Rehabilitation	52	90%	96%	97%
Discharged on Antithrombotic Therapy	51	100%	100%	99%
Discharged on Statin Medication	45	98%	96%	94%
Thrombolytic Therapy Timing[1]	-	-	68%	66%
Venous Thromboembolism Prophylaxis	52	87%	94%	94%
Written Stroke Educational Materials Given	29	97%	82%	88%
Surgical Care Improvement Project				
Appropriate Beta Blocker Usage	137	97%	98%	98%
Appropriate VTP Within 24 Hours	299	97%	99%	98%
Controlled Postoperative Blood Glucose[7]	-	-	96%	97%
Perioperative Temperature Management	355	100%	100%	100%
Prophylactic Antibiotic Selection	256	98%	99%	99%
Prophylactic Antibiotic Selection (Outpatient)	36	97%	98%	98%
Prophylactic Antibiotic Stopped	250	97%	99%	98%
Prophylactic Antibiotic Timing	256	100%	99%	99%
Prophylactic Antibiotic Timing (Outpatient)	39	92%	98%	98%
Urinary Catheter Removal	151	94%	97%	97%
Survey of Patients' Hospital Experiences				
Area Around Room 'Always' Quiet at Night	300+	45%	52%	61%
Doctors 'Always' Communicated Well	300+	76%	80%	82%
Home Recovery Information Given	300+	83%	87%	85%
Hospital Given 9 or 10 on 10 Point Scale	300+	50%	69%	71%
Meds 'Always' Explained Before Given	300+	57%	64%	64%
Nurses 'Always' Communicated Well	300+	72%	79%	79%
Pain 'Always' Well Controlled	300+	68%	71%	71%
Room and Bathroom 'Always' Clean	300+	62%	72%	73%
Timely Help 'Always' Received	300+	59%	66%	68%
Would Definitely Recommend Hospital	300+	50%	73%	71%
Use of Medical Imaging				
Cardiac Imaging Stress Test before Surgery	333	4.2%	5.4%	5.3%
Combination Abdominal CT Scan	827	3.4%	6.3%	10.5%
Combination Brain/Sinus CT Scan	1,037	2.5%	2.4%	2.7%
Combination Chest CT Scan	619	0.6%	0.5%	2.7%
Follow-up Mammogram/Ultrasound	2,029	5.9%	8.9%	8.8%
Lumbar Spine MRI for Low Back Pain	110	30.9%	35.3%	37.2%

Emerson Hospital

Old Road To 9 Acre Corner
W Concord, MA 01742
Phone: 978-369-1400
Fax: 978-287-3726
URL: www.emersonhospital.org
Type: Acute Care Hospitals
Emergency Services: Yes
Ownership: Voluntary non-profit - Private
Beds: 167

Key Personnel:

Chair/CEO . . . . Paul Birch
Radiology. . . . . Mark A Connaughton, MD
Operating Room. . . . . Diane Kalinowski
Chief of Medical Staff . . . . C. Gregory Martin, MD
CEO/President. . . . . Christine C Schuster
Pediatric In-Patient Care . . . . Marianne Sutton
Quality Assurance . . . . Regina Vurzynski
Emergency Room . . . . Alan Woodward

Measure	Cases	This Hosp.	State Avg.	U.S. Avg.
Blood Clot Prevention and Treatment				
Anticoagulation Overlap Therapy[2]	46	100%	97%	93%
ICU Venous Thromboembolism Prophylaxis[2]	69	93%	92%	92%
Incidence of Potentially Preventable VTE[2]	12	8%	7%	10%
UFH with Dosages/Platelet Monitoring[2]	20	100%	91%	97%
Venous Thromboembolism Prophylaxis[2]	240	91%	87%	85%
Warfarin Therapy Discharge Instructions[2]	33	94%	77%	75%
Chest Pain/Possible Heart Attack Care				
Aspirin Given Within 24 Hours of Arrival	34	97%	97%	96%
Fibrinolytic Meds Within 30 Min. of Arrival[7]	-	-	73%	58%
Average Time to ECG (minutes)	34	10	7	7
Average Time to Transfer (minutes)	13	45	55	60
Children's Asthma Care				
Received Home Management Plan of Care	-	-	-	88%
Received Reliever Medication	-	-	-	100%
Received Systemic Corticosteroids	-	-	-	100%
Emergency Department				
Admittance Decision Time (minutes)[2]	394	132	119	98
Head CT Results Within 45 Min. of Arrival[1]	-	-	70%	57%
Patients Who Left ER Before Being Seen	27,072	2%	2%	2%
Time from ER Arrival to Admit. (minutes)[2]	400	294	313	274
Time from ER Arrival to Discharge (minutes)	351	130	156	134
Time in ER Before Being Evaluated (minutes)	374	44	36	26
Time to Pain Meds for Fractures (minutes)	35	77	59	57
Heart Attack Care				
Aspirin Given at Discharge	19	100%	100%	99%
Fibrinolytic Meds Within 30 Min. of Arrival[7]	-	-	100%	54%
PCI Within 90 Minutes of Arrival[7]	-	-	96%	96%
Statin Prescribed at Discharge	18	100%	99%	98%
Heart Failure Care				
ACE Inhibitor or ARB for LVSD	20	100%	96%	97%
Discharge Instructions Given	86	90%	95%	94%
Evaluation of LVS Function	137	99%	100%	99%
Medicare Spending				
Medicare Spending per Patient (ratio)	-	1.04	1.03	0.98
Pneumonia Care				
Appropriate Initial Antibiotic Given	107	96%	97%	95%
Blood Culture Timing	161	99%	98%	98%
Pregnancy and Delivery Care				
Newborn Deliveries Scheduled Early[2]	12	8%	2%	6%
Preventive Care				
Immunization for Influenza[2]	501	80%	91%	90%
Immunization for Pneumonia[2]	468	89%	91%	92%
Stroke Care				
Anticoagulation Therapy for Atrial Fibrillation	13	92%	97%	95%
Antithrombotic Therapy Timing	52	100%	98%	98%
Assessed for Rehabilitation	59	98%	96%	97%
Discharged on Antithrombotic Therapy	55	100%	100%	99%
Discharged on Statin Medication	34	91%	96%	94%
Thrombolytic Therapy Timing[1]	-	-	68%	66%
Venous Thromboembolism Prophylaxis	58	90%	94%	94%
Written Stroke Educational Materials Given	33	100%	82%	88%
Surgical Care Improvement Project				
Appropriate Beta Blocker Usage	121	91%	98%	98%
Appropriate VTP Within 24 Hours	446	97%	99%	98%
Controlled Postoperative Blood Glucose[7]	-	-	96%	97%
Perioperative Temperature Management	500	100%	100%	100%
Prophylactic Antibiotic Selection	379	98%	99%	99%
Prophylactic Antibiotic Selection (Outpatient)	160	99%	98%	98%
Prophylactic Antibiotic Stopped	370	98%	99%	98%
Prophylactic Antibiotic Timing	380	98%	99%	99%
Prophylactic Antibiotic Timing (Outpatient)	161	99%	98%	98%
Urinary Catheter Removal	420	96%	97%	97%
Survey of Patients' Hospital Experiences				
Area Around Room 'Always' Quiet at Night	300+	55%	52%	61%
Doctors 'Always' Communicated Well	300+	82%	80%	82%
Home Recovery Information Given	300+	85%	87%	85%
Hospital Given 9 or 10 on 10 Point Scale	300+	72%	69%	71%
Meds 'Always' Explained Before Given	300+	62%	64%	64%
Nurses 'Always' Communicated Well	300+	81%	79%	79%
Pain 'Always' Well Controlled	300+	75%	71%	71%
Room and Bathroom 'Always' Clean	300+	71%	72%	73%
Timely Help 'Always' Received	300+	68%	66%	68%
Would Definitely Recommend Hospital	300+	78%	73%	71%
Use of Medical Imaging				
Cardiac Imaging Stress Test before Surgery	202	4.0%	5.4%	5.3%
Combination Abdominal CT Scan	678	4.1%	6.3%	10.5%
Combination Brain/Sinus CT Scan	665	1.8%	2.4%	2.7%
Combination Chest CT Scan	588	0.0%	0.5%	2.7%
Follow-up Mammogram/Ultrasound	2,208	16.4%	8.9%	8.8%
Lumbar Spine MRI for Low Back Pain	130	39.2%	35.3%	37.2%

Baystate Mary Lane Hospital

85 South Street
Ware, MA 01082
Phone: 413-967-6211
Fax: 413-967-2109
URL: www.baystatehealth.com
Type: Acute Care Hospitals
Emergency Services: Yes
Ownership: Voluntary non-profit - Private
Beds: 31

Key Personnel:

Quality Assurance . . . . Clare Burgess
Coronary Care . . . . Tina Frazier, RN
Chief of Medical Staff . . . . Richard Gerstein, MD
CEO/President. . . . . Mark A. Keroack, MD, MPH
Infection Control. . . . . Rosalie Rymarski, RN
Radiology. . . . . Eckart Sachsse
Pediatric Ambulatory Care . . . . . . Jeannette Tokarz, MD
Pediatric In-Patient Care . . . . Jeannette Tokarz, MD

Measure	Cases	This Hosp.	State Avg.	U.S. Avg.
Blood Clot Prevention and Treatment				
Anticoagulation Overlap Therapy[1,2]	-	-	97%	93%
ICU Venous Thromboembolism Prophylaxis[1,2]	-	-	92%	92%
Incidence of Potentially Preventable VTE[2,7]	-	-	7%	10%
UFH with Dosages/Platelet Monitoring[1,2]	-	-	91%	97%
Venous Thromboembolism Prophylaxis[2]	112	96%	87%	85%
Warfarin Therapy Discharge Instructions[1,2]	-	-	77%	75%
Chest Pain/Possible Heart Attack Care				
Aspirin Given Within 24 Hours of Arrival	33	100%	97%	96%
Fibrinolytic Meds Within 30 Min. of Arrival[1]	-	-	73%	58%
Average Time to ECG (minutes)	35	10	7	7
Average Time to Transfer (minutes)[1]	-	-	55	60
Children's Asthma Care				
Received Home Management Plan of Care	-	-	-	88%
Received Reliever Medication	-	-	-	100%
Received Systemic Corticosteroids	-	-	-	100%
Emergency Department				
Admittance Decision Time (minutes)[2]	322	65	119	98
Head CT Results Within 45 Min. of Arrival[1,3]	-	-	70%	57%
Patients Who Left ER Before Being Seen	15,597	1%	2%	2%
Time from ER Arrival to Admit. (minutes)[2]	485	231	313	274
Time from ER Arrival to Discharge (minutes)	369	90	156	134
Time in ER Before Being Evaluated (minutes)	279	17	36	26
Time to Pain Meds for Fractures (minutes)	59	54	59	57
Heart Attack Care				
Aspirin Given at Discharge[1]	-	-	100%	99%
Fibrinolytic Meds Within 30 Min. of Arrival[7]	-	-	100%	54%
PCI Within 90 Minutes of Arrival[7]	-	-	96%	96%
Statin Prescribed at Discharge	11	91%	99%	98%
Heart Failure Care				
ACE Inhibitor or ARB for LVSD	11	100%	96%	97%
Discharge Instructions Given	35	100%	95%	94%
Evaluation of LVS Function	43	98%	100%	99%
Medicare Spending				
Medicare Spending per Patient (ratio)	-	1.05	1.03	0.98
Pneumonia Care				
Appropriate Initial Antibiotic Given	66	92%	97%	95%
Blood Culture Timing	73	97%	98%	98%
Pregnancy and Delivery Care				
Newborn Deliveries Scheduled Early[7]	-	-	2%	6%
Preventive Care				
Immunization for Influenza[2]	301	94%	91%	90%
Immunization for Pneumonia[2]	452	96%	91%	92%
Stroke Care				
Anticoagulation Therapy for Atrial Fibrillation[1]	-	-	97%	95%
Antithrombotic Therapy Timing	12	100%	98%	98%
Assessed for Rehabilitation	11	91%	96%	97%

NOTE: Hospital profiles are in alphabetical order by state, then city, then hospital within the city; Rankings exclude hospitals with less than 25 cases except for patient surveys which excludes hospitals with less than 100 cases; (a) 100-299 cases; (1) The number of cases/patients is too few to report; (2) Data submitted were based on a sample of cases/patients; (3) Results are based on a shorter time period than required; (4) Data suppressed by CMS for one or more quarters; (5) Results are not available for this reporting period; (6) Fewer than 100 patients completed the HCAHPS survey; (7) No cases met the criteria for this measure; (8) The lower limit of the confidence interval cannot be calculated if the number of observed infections equals zero; (9) No data are available from the state/territory for this reporting period; (10) The scores shown reflect fewer than 50 completed surveys; (11) There were discrepancies in the data collection process; (12) This measure does not apply to this hospital for this reporting period; (13) Results cannot be calculated for this reporting period; (14) The results for this state are combined with nearby states to protect confidentiality; Please refer to the User's Guide for a full explanation of data.

Discharged on Antithrombotic Therapy	11	100%	100%	99%
Discharged on Statin Medication[1]	-	-	96%	94%
Thrombolytic Therapy Timing[1]	-	-	68%	66%
Venous Thromboembolism Prophylaxis	11	91%	94%	94%
Written Stroke Educational Materials Given[1]	-	-	82%	88%
Surgical Care Improvement Project				
Appropriate Beta Blocker Usage	13	100%	98%	98%
Appropriate VTP Within 24 Hours	47	94%	99%	98%
Controlled Postoperative Blood Glucose[7]	-	-	96%	97%
Perioperative Temperature Management	55	98%	100%	100%
Prophylactic Antibiotic Selection	35	100%	99%	99%
Prophylactic Antibiotic Selection (Outpatient)[1,3]	-	-	98%	98%
Prophylactic Antibiotic Stopped	34	97%	99%	98%
Prophylactic Antibiotic Timing	35	100%	99%	99%
Prophylactic Antibiotic Timing (Outpatient)[1,3]	-	-	98%	98%
Urinary Catheter Removal	43	100%	97%	97%
Survey of Patients' Hospital Experiences				
Area Around Room 'Always' Quiet at Night	300+	69%	52%	61%
Doctors 'Always' Communicated Well	300+	84%	80%	82%
Home Recovery Information Given	300+	90%	87%	85%
Hospital Given 9 or 10 on 10 Point Scale	300+	74%	69%	71%
Meds 'Always' Explained Before Given	300+	71%	64%	64%
Nurses 'Always' Communicated Well	300+	85%	79%	79%
Pain 'Always' Well Controlled	300+	76%	71%	71%
Room and Bathroom 'Always' Clean	300+	79%	72%	73%
Timely Help 'Always' Received	300+	71%	66%	68%
Would Definitely Recommend Hospital	300+	76%	73%	71%
Use of Medical Imaging				
Cardiac Imaging Stress Test before Surgery	62	6.5%	5.4%	5.3%
Combination Abdominal CT Scan	267	3.4%	6.3%	10.5%
Combination Brain/Sinus CT Scan[1]	-	-	2.4%	2.7%
Combination Chest CT Scan	133	0.8%	0.5%	2.7%
Follow-up Mammogram/Ultrasound	439	13.2%	8.9%	8.8%
Lumbar Spine MRI for Low Back Pain[7]	-	-	35.3%	37.2%

Noble Hospital

115 West Silver Street
Westfield, MA 01085
Phone: 413-568-2811
Fax: 413-562-5855
E-mail: hcote@noblehealth.org
URL: www.noblehospital.org
Type: Acute Care Hospitals
Emergency Services: Yes
Ownership: Government - Federal
Beds: 97

Key Personnel:
CEO/President. . . . . George Koller
Emergency Room . . . . David B Peterson
Chief of Medical Staff. . . . . Stanley Strzemeko

Measure	Cases	This Hosp.	State Avg.	U.S. Avg.
Blood Clot Prevention and Treatment				
Anticoagulation Overlap Therapy[2]	21	100%	97%	93%
ICU Venous Thromboembolism Prophylaxis[2]	22	100%	92%	92%
Incidence of Potentially Preventable VTE[2,7]	-	-	7%	10%
UFH with Dosages/Platelet Monitoring[1,2]	-	-	91%	97%
Venous Thromboembolism Prophylaxis[2]	266	98%	87%	85%
Warfarin Therapy Discharge Instructions[2]	19	100%	77%	75%
Chest Pain/Possible Heart Attack Care				
Aspirin Given Within 24 Hours of Arrival	50	100%	97%	96%
Fibrinolytic Meds Within 30 Min. of Arrival[7]	-	-	73%	58%
Average Time to ECG (minutes)	51	7	7	7
Average Time to Transfer (minutes)	11	28	55	60
Children's Asthma Care				
Received Home Management Plan of Care	-	-	-	88%
Received Reliever Medication	-	-	-	100%
Received Systemic Corticosteroids	-	-	-	100%
Emergency Department				
Admittance Decision Time (minutes)[2]	723	48	119	98
Head CT Results Within 45 Min. of Arrival	13	69%	70%	57%
Patients Who Left ER Before Being Seen	29,285	1%	2%	2%
Time from ER Arrival to Admit. (minutes)[2]	757	235	313	274
Time from ER Arrival to Discharge (minutes)	542	107	156	134
Time in ER Before Being Evaluated (minutes)	494	24	36	26
Time to Pain Meds for Fractures (minutes)	75	52	59	57
Heart Attack Care				
Aspirin Given at Discharge[1]	-	-	100%	99%
Fibrinolytic Meds Within 30 Min. of Arrival[7]	-	-	100%	54%
PCI Within 90 Minutes of Arrival[7]	-	-	96%	96%
Statin Prescribed at Discharge[1]	-	-	99%	98%
Heart Failure Care				
ACE Inhibitor or ARB for LVSD	11	100%	96%	97%
Discharge Instructions Given	92	100%	95%	94%
Evaluation of LVS Function	119	99%	100%	99%
Medicare Spending				
Medicare Spending per Patient (ratio)	-	1.08	1.03	0.98
Pneumonia Care				
Appropriate Initial Antibiotic Given	104	100%	97%	95%
Blood Culture Timing	152	100%	98%	98%
Pregnancy and Delivery Care				
Newborn Deliveries Scheduled Early[7]	-	-	2%	6%
Preventive Care				
Immunization for Influenza[2]	573	94%	91%	90%
Immunization for Pneumonia[2]	663	98%	91%	92%
Stroke Care				
Anticoagulation Therapy for Atrial Fibrillation[1]	-	-	97%	95%
Antithrombotic Therapy Timing	22	100%	98%	98%
Assessed for Rehabilitation	24	100%	96%	97%
Discharged on Antithrombotic Therapy	22	100%	100%	99%
Discharged on Statin Medication	18	94%	96%	94%
Thrombolytic Therapy Timing[7]	-	-	68%	66%
Venous Thromboembolism Prophylaxis	22	100%	94%	94%
Written Stroke Educational Materials Given	11	100%	82%	88%
Surgical Care Improvement Project				
Appropriate Beta Blocker Usage	30	100%	98%	98%
Appropriate VTP Within 24 Hours	83	96%	99%	98%
Controlled Postoperative Blood Glucose[7]	-	-	96%	97%
Perioperative Temperature Management	94	100%	100%	100%
Prophylactic Antibiotic Selection	71	100%	99%	99%
Prophylactic Antibiotic Selection (Outpatient)	18	94%	98%	98%
Prophylactic Antibiotic Stopped	70	99%	99%	98%
Prophylactic Antibiotic Timing	71	99%	99%	99%
Prophylactic Antibiotic Timing (Outpatient)	20	90%	98%	98%
Urinary Catheter Removal	32	94%	97%	97%
Survey of Patients' Hospital Experiences				
Area Around Room 'Always' Quiet at Night	300+	50%	52%	61%
Doctors 'Always' Communicated Well	300+	81%	80%	82%
Home Recovery Information Given	300+	89%	87%	85%
Hospital Given 9 or 10 on 10 Point Scale	300+	70%	69%	71%
Meds 'Always' Explained Before Given	300+	67%	64%	64%
Nurses 'Always' Communicated Well	300+	80%	79%	79%
Pain 'Always' Well Controlled	300+	72%	71%	71%
Room and Bathroom 'Always' Clean	300+	74%	72%	73%
Timely Help 'Always' Received	300+	74%	66%	68%
Would Definitely Recommend Hospital	300+	69%	73%	71%
Use of Medical Imaging				
Cardiac Imaging Stress Test before Surgery	89	3.4%	5.4%	5.3%
Combination Abdominal CT Scan	468	1.9%	6.3%	10.5%
Combination Brain/Sinus CT Scan	467	4.1%	2.4%	2.7%
Combination Chest CT Scan	269	0.4%	0.5%	2.7%
Follow-up Mammogram/Ultrasound	883	12.7%	8.9%	8.8%
Lumbar Spine MRI for Low Back Pain	51	31.4%	35.3%	37.2%

Winchester Hospital

41 Highland Avenue
Winchester, MA 01890
Phone: 781-729-9000
Fax: 781-756-2923
URL: www.winchesterhospital.org
Type: Acute Care Hospitals
Emergency Services: Yes
Ownership: Voluntary non-profit - Private
Beds: 200

Key Personnel:
Infection Control. . . . . Kay Deackoff, RN
Chief of Medical Staff. . . . . Donald J Deraska
Pediatric Ambulatory Care . . . . . . Martha McCarty, MD
Operating Room. . . . . Claire O'Brien
Cardiac Laboratory. . . . . Joseph Pappalardo
President/CEO. . . . . Kevin Smith
Quality Assurance . . . . Celeste Steele

Measure	Cases	This Hosp.	State Avg.	U.S. Avg.
Blood Clot Prevention and Treatment				
Anticoagulation Overlap Therapy[2]	67	100%	97%	93%
ICU Venous Thromboembolism Prophylaxis[2]	27	81%	92%	92%
Incidence of Potentially Preventable VTE[1,2]	-	-	7%	10%
UFH with Dosages/Platelet Monitoring[2]	34	100%	91%	97%
Venous Thromboembolism Prophylaxis[2]	375	79%	87%	85%
Warfarin Therapy Discharge Instructions[2]	43	100%	77%	75%
Chest Pain/Possible Heart Attack Care				
Aspirin Given Within 24 Hours of Arrival	99	100%	97%	96%
Fibrinolytic Meds Within 30 Min. of Arrival[7]	-	-	73%	58%
Average Time to ECG (minutes)	101	12	7	7
Average Time to Transfer (minutes)	31	75	55	60
Children's Asthma Care				
Received Home Management Plan of Care	-	-	-	88%
Received Reliever Medication	-	-	-	100%
Received Systemic Corticosteroids	-	-	-	100%
Emergency Department				
Admittance Decision Time (minutes)[2]	649	111	119	98
Head CT Results Within 45 Min. of Arrival	20	70%	70%	57%
Patients Who Left ER Before Being Seen	51,242	1%	2%	2%
Time from ER Arrival to Admit. (minutes)[2]	657	307	313	274
Time from ER Arrival to Discharge (minutes)	318	179	156	134
Time in ER Before Being Evaluated (minutes)	342	44	36	26
Time to Pain Meds for Fractures (minutes)	169	59	59	57
Heart Attack Care				
Aspirin Given at Discharge[2]	25	100%	100%	99%
Fibrinolytic Meds Within 30 Min. of Arrival[2,7]	-	-	100%	54%
PCI Within 90 Minutes of Arrival[2,7]	-	-	96%	96%
Statin Prescribed at Discharge[2]	28	96%	99%	98%
Heart Failure Care				
ACE Inhibitor or ARB for LVSD[2]	54	94%	96%	97%
Discharge Instructions Given[2]	187	82%	95%	94%
Evaluation of LVS Function[2]	245	100%	100%	99%
Medicare Spending				
Medicare Spending per Patient (ratio)	-	1.02	1.03	0.98
Pneumonia Care				
Appropriate Initial Antibiotic Given[2]	101	97%	97%	95%
Blood Culture Timing[2]	148	97%	98%	98%
Pregnancy and Delivery Care				
Newborn Deliveries Scheduled Early[2]	28	4%	2%	6%
Preventive Care				
Immunization for Influenza[2]	491	97%	91%	90%
Immunization for Pneumonia[2]	594	92%	91%	92%
Stroke Care				
Anticoagulation Therapy for Atrial Fibrillation[2]	11	91%	97%	95%
Antithrombotic Therapy Timing[2]	37	100%	98%	98%
Assessed for Rehabilitation[2]	35	100%	96%	97%
Discharged on Antithrombotic Therapy[2]	31	100%	100%	99%
Discharged on Statin Medication[2]	25	84%	96%	94%
Thrombolytic Therapy Timing[1,2]	-	-	68%	66%
Venous Thromboembolism Prophylaxis[2]	41	78%	94%	94%
Written Stroke Educational Materials Given[2]	14	64%	82%	88%
Surgical Care Improvement Project				
Appropriate Beta Blocker Usage[2]	124	94%	98%	98%
Appropriate VTP Within 24 Hours[2]	293	99%	99%	98%
Controlled Postoperative Blood Glucose[2,7]	-	-	96%	97%
Perioperative Temperature Management[2]	385	100%	100%	100%
Prophylactic Antibiotic Selection[2]	252	98%	99%	99%
Prophylactic Antibiotic Selection (Outpatient)	172	98%	98%	98%
Prophylactic Antibiotic Stopped[2]	252	100%	99%	98%
Prophylactic Antibiotic Timing[2]	253	99%	99%	99%
Prophylactic Antibiotic Timing (Outpatient)	175	96%	98%	98%
Urinary Catheter Removal[2]	212	99%	97%	97%
Survey of Patients' Hospital Experiences				
Area Around Room 'Always' Quiet at Night[11]	300+	50%	52%	61%
Doctors 'Always' Communicated Well[11]	300+	81%	80%	82%
Home Recovery Information Given[11]	300+	87%	87%	85%
Hospital Given 9 or 10 on 10 Point Scale[11]	300+	76%	69%	71%
Meds 'Always' Explained Before Given[11]	300+	68%	64%	64%
Nurses 'Always' Communicated Well[11]	300+	83%	79%	79%
Pain 'Always' Well Controlled[11]	300+	71%	71%	71%
Room and Bathroom 'Always' Clean[11]	300+	71%	72%	73%
Timely Help 'Always' Received[11]	300+	70%	66%	68%
Would Definitely Recommend Hospital[11]	300+	80%	73%	71%
Use of Medical Imaging				

NOTE: Hospital profiles are in alphabetical order by state, then city, then hospital within the city; Rankings exclude hospitals with less than 25 cases except for patient surveys which excludes hospitals with less than 100 cases; (a) 100-299 cases; (1) The number of cases/patients is too few to report; (2) Data submitted were based on a sample of cases/patients; (3) Results are based on a shorter time period than required; (4) Data suppressed by CMS for one or more quarters; (5) Results are not available for this reporting period; (6) Fewer than 100 patients completed the HCAHPS survey; (7) No cases met the criteria for this measure; (8) The lower limit of the confidence interval cannot be calculated if the number of observed infections equals zero; (9) No data are available from the state/territory for this reporting period; (10) The scores shown reflect fewer than 50 completed surveys; (11) There were discrepancies in the data collection process; (12) This measure does not apply to this hospital for this reporting period; (13) Results cannot be calculated for this reporting period; (14) The results for this state are combined with nearby states to protect confidentiality; Please refer to the User's Guide for a full explanation of data.

Cardiac Imaging Stress Test before Surgery	362	5.0%	5.4%	5.3%
Combination Abdominal CT Scan	1,179	6.0%	6.3%	10.5%
Combination Brain/Sinus CT Scan	955	3.4%	2.4%	2.7%
Combination Chest CT Scan	905	0.1%	0.5%	2.7%
Follow-up Mammogram/Ultrasound	2,895	8.9%	8.9%	8.8%
Lumbar Spine MRI for Low Back Pain	126	31.0%	35.3%	37.2%

Adcare Hospital of Worcester

107 Lincoln Street
Worcester, MA 01605
Phone: 508-799-9000
Fax: 508-753-3733
E-mail: info@adcare.com
URL: www.adcare.com
Type: Acute Care Hospitals
Emergency Services: No
Ownership: Voluntary non-profit - Church
Beds: 114

Key Personnel:
President . . . . Jeffrey W. Hillis
Quality Assurance . . . . Karole A Mesier
Operating Room. . . . . Petrice M. Muchowski, Sc.D
Chief of Medical Staff. . . . . Ronald F Pike, MD

Measure	Cases	This Hosp.	State Avg.	U.S. Avg.
Blood Clot Prevention and Treatment				
Anticoagulation Overlap Therapy[2,7]	-	-	97%	93%
ICU Venous Thromboembolism Prophylaxis[2,7]	-	-	92%	92%
Incidence of Potentially Preventable VTE[2,7]	-	-	7%	10%
UFH with Dosages/Platelet Monitoring[2,7]	-	-	91%	97%
Venous Thromboembolism Prophylaxis[2,7]	-	-	87%	85%
Warfarin Therapy Discharge Instructions[2,7]	-	-	77%	75%
Chest Pain/Possible Heart Attack Care				
Aspirin Given Within 24 Hours of Arrival[5]	-	-	97%	96%
Fibrinolytic Meds Within 30 Min. of Arrival[5]	-	-	73%	58%
Average Time to ECG (minutes)[5]	-	-	7	7
Average Time to Transfer (minutes)[5]	-	-	55	60
Children's Asthma Care				
Received Home Management Plan of Care	-	-	-	88%
Received Reliever Medication	-	-	-	100%
Received Systemic Corticosteroids	-	-	-	100%
Emergency Department				
Admittance Decision Time (minutes)[2,7]	-	-	119	98
Head CT Results Within 45 Min. of Arrival[5]	-	-	70%	57%
Patients Who Left ER Before Being Seen[5]	-	-	2%	2%
Time from ER Arrival to Admit. (minutes)[2,7]	-	-	313	274
Time from ER Arrival to Discharge (minutes)[5]	-	-	156	134
Time in ER Before Being Evaluated (minutes)[5]	-	-	36	26
Time to Pain Meds for Fractures (minutes)[5]	-	-	59	57
Heart Attack Care				
Aspirin Given at Discharge[5]	-	-	100%	99%
Fibrinolytic Meds Within 30 Min. of Arrival[5]	-	-	100%	54%
PCI Within 90 Minutes of Arrival[5]	-	-	96%	96%
Statin Prescribed at Discharge[5]	-	-	99%	98%
Heart Failure Care				
ACE Inhibitor or ARB for LVSD[5]	-	-	96%	97%
Discharge Instructions Given[5]	-	-	95%	94%
Evaluation of LVS Function[5]	-	-	100%	99%
Medicare Spending				
Medicare Spending per Patient (ratio)	-	0.91	1.03	0.98
Pneumonia Care				
Appropriate Initial Antibiotic Given[5]	-	-	97%	95%
Blood Culture Timing[5]	-	-	98%	98%
Pregnancy and Delivery Care				
Newborn Deliveries Scheduled Early[7]	-	-	2%	6%
Preventive Care				
Immunization for Influenza[2]	568	61%	91%	90%
Immunization for Pneumonia[2]	352	54%	91%	92%
Stroke Care				
Anticoagulation Therapy for Atrial Fibrillation[5]	-	-	97%	95%
Antithrombotic Therapy Timing[5]	-	-	98%	98%
Assessed for Rehabilitation[5]	-	-	96%	97%
Discharged on Antithrombotic Therapy[5]	-	-	100%	99%
Discharged on Statin Medication[5]	-	-	96%	94%
Thrombolytic Therapy Timing[5]	-	-	68%	66%
Venous Thromboembolism Prophylaxis[5]	-	-	94%	94%
Written Stroke Educational Materials Given[5]	-	-	82%	88%
Surgical Care Improvement Project				
Appropriate Beta Blocker Usage[5]	-	-	98%	98%
Appropriate VTP Within 24 Hours[5]	-	-	99%	98%
Controlled Postoperative Blood Glucose[5]	-	-	96%	97%
Perioperative Temperature Management[5]	-	-	100%	100%
Prophylactic Antibiotic Selection[5]	-	-	99%	99%
Prophylactic Antibiotic Selection (Outpatient)[5]	-	-	98%	98%
Prophylactic Antibiotic Stopped[5]	-	-	99%	98%
Prophylactic Antibiotic Timing[5]	-	-	99%	99%
Prophylactic Antibiotic Timing (Outpatient)[5]	-	-	98%	98%
Urinary Catheter Removal[5]	-	-	97%	97%
Survey of Patients' Hospital Experiences				
Area Around Room 'Always' Quiet at Night[1]	-	-	52%	61%
Doctors 'Always' Communicated Well[1]	-	-	80%	82%
Home Recovery Information Given[1]	-	-	87%	85%
Hospital Given 9 or 10 on 10 Point Scale[1]	-	-	69%	71%
Meds 'Always' Explained Before Given[1]	-	-	64%	64%
Nurses 'Always' Communicated Well[1]	-	-	79%	79%
Pain 'Always' Well Controlled[1]	-	-	71%	71%
Room and Bathroom 'Always' Clean[1]	-	-	72%	73%
Timely Help 'Always' Received[1]	-	-	66%	68%
Would Definitely Recommend Hospital[1]	-	-	73%	71%
Use of Medical Imaging				
Cardiac Imaging Stress Test before Surgery[7]	-	-	5.4%	5.3%
Combination Abdominal CT Scan[7]	-	-	6.3%	10.5%
Combination Brain/Sinus CT Scan[7]	-	-	2.4%	2.7%
Combination Chest CT Scan[7]	-	-	0.5%	2.7%
Follow-up Mammogram/Ultrasound[7]	-	-	8.9%	8.8%
Lumbar Spine MRI for Low Back Pain[7]	-	-	35.3%	37.2%

Saint Vincent Hospital

123 Summer Street
Worcester, MA 01608
Phone: 508-363-5000
Fax: 508-363-5387
E-mail: dennis.irish@tenethealth.com
URL: www.stvincenthospital.com
Type: Acute Care Hospitals
Emergency Services: Yes
Ownership: Proprietary
Beds: 349

Key Personnel:
Radiology. . . . . David Bader, MD
Emergency Room . . . . Michael Burns, MD
Pediatric Ambulatory Care . . . . . . William Horgan, OD, MD
Quality Assurance . . . . Jill Lyons, RN
CEO/President. . . . . Steven MacLauchlan
Cardiac Laboratory. . . . . Gordon Saperia
Anesthesiology. . . . . Akmal Wahid, MD
Chief of Medical Staff . . . . Douglas Waite, MD

Measure	Cases	This Hosp.	State Avg.	U.S. Avg.
Blood Clot Prevention and Treatment				
Anticoagulation Overlap Therapy[2]	131	99%	97%	93%
ICU Venous Thromboembolism Prophylaxis[2]	78	97%	92%	92%
Incidence of Potentially Preventable VTE[2]	37	3%	7%	10%
UFH with Dosages/Platelet Monitoring[2]	94	100%	91%	97%
Venous Thromboembolism Prophylaxis[2]	348	96%	87%	85%
Warfarin Therapy Discharge Instructions[2]	87	69%	77%	75%
Chest Pain/Possible Heart Attack Care				
Aspirin Given Within 24 Hours of Arrival[1]	-	-	97%	96%
Fibrinolytic Meds Within 30 Min. of Arrival[5]	-	-	73%	58%
Average Time to ECG (minutes)[1]	-	-	7	7
Average Time to Transfer (minutes)[5]	-	-	55	60
Children's Asthma Care				
Received Home Management Plan of Care	-	-	-	88%
Received Reliever Medication	-	-	-	100%
Received Systemic Corticosteroids	-	-	-	100%
Emergency Department				
Admittance Decision Time (minutes)[2]	775	150	119	98
Head CT Results Within 45 Min. of Arrival[1]	-	-	70%	57%
Patients Who Left ER Before Being Seen	68,808	1%	2%	2%
Time from ER Arrival to Admit. (minutes)[2]	775	376	313	274
Time from ER Arrival to Discharge (minutes)	404	159	156	134
Time in ER Before Being Evaluated (minutes)	437	29	36	26
Time to Pain Meds for Fractures (minutes)	239	63	59	57
Heart Attack Care				
Aspirin Given at Discharge	303	100%	100%	99%
Fibrinolytic Meds Within 30 Min. of Arrival[7]	-	-	100%	54%
PCI Within 90 Minutes of Arrival	47	100%	96%	96%
Statin Prescribed at Discharge	299	100%	99%	98%
Heart Failure Care				
ACE Inhibitor or ARB for LVSD	138	99%	96%	97%
Discharge Instructions Given	432	99%	95%	94%
Evaluation of LVS Function	620	100%	100%	99%
Medicare Spending				
Medicare Spending per Patient (ratio)	-	1.01	1.03	0.98
Pneumonia Care				
Appropriate Initial Antibiotic Given	331	98%	97%	95%
Blood Culture Timing	617	98%	98%	98%
Pregnancy and Delivery Care				
Newborn Deliveries Scheduled Early	143	1%	2%	6%
Preventive Care				
Immunization for Influenza[2]	594	98%	91%	90%
Immunization for Pneumonia[2]	744	99%	91%	92%
Stroke Care				
Anticoagulation Therapy for Atrial Fibrillation	31	97%	97%	95%
Antithrombotic Therapy Timing	154	99%	98%	98%
Assessed for Rehabilitation	176	99%	96%	97%
Discharged on Antithrombotic Therapy	158	100%	100%	99%
Discharged on Statin Medication	114	97%	96%	94%
Thrombolytic Therapy Timing[1]	-	-	68%	66%
Venous Thromboembolism Prophylaxis	181	98%	94%	94%
Written Stroke Educational Materials Given	87	98%	82%	88%
Surgical Care Improvement Project				
Appropriate Beta Blocker Usage	534	98%	98%	98%
Appropriate VTP Within 24 Hours	1,089	100%	99%	98%
Controlled Postoperative Blood Glucose	159	98%	96%	97%
Perioperative Temperature Management	1,342	100%	100%	100%
Prophylactic Antibiotic Selection	986	99%	99%	99%
Prophylactic Antibiotic Selection (Outpatient)	544	97%	98%	98%
Prophylactic Antibiotic Stopped	972	99%	99%	98%
Prophylactic Antibiotic Timing	986	98%	99%	99%
Prophylactic Antibiotic Timing (Outpatient)	546	97%	98%	98%
Urinary Catheter Removal	966	99%	97%	97%
Survey of Patients' Hospital Experiences				
Area Around Room 'Always' Quiet at Night[11]	300+	47%	52%	61%
Doctors 'Always' Communicated Well[11]	300+	79%	80%	82%
Home Recovery Information Given[11]	300+	89%	87%	85%
Hospital Given 9 or 10 on 10 Point Scale[11]	300+	72%	69%	71%
Meds 'Always' Explained Before Given[11]	300+	62%	64%	64%
Nurses 'Always' Communicated Well[11]	300+	77%	79%	79%
Pain 'Always' Well Controlled[11]	300+	68%	71%	71%
Room and Bathroom 'Always' Clean[11]	300+	70%	72%	73%
Timely Help 'Always' Received[11]	300+	63%	66%	68%
Would Definitely Recommend Hospital[11]	300+	77%	73%	71%
Use of Medical Imaging				
Cardiac Imaging Stress Test before Surgery	589	2.2%	5.4%	5.3%
Combination Abdominal CT Scan	646	1.1%	6.3%	10.5%
Combination Brain/Sinus CT Scan[1]	-	-	2.4%	2.7%
Combination Chest CT Scan	503	0.0%	0.5%	2.7%
Follow-up Mammogram/Ultrasound	713	7.2%	8.9%	8.8%
Lumbar Spine MRI for Low Back Pain	71	46.5%	35.3%	37.2%

Umass Memorial Medical Center

55 Lake Avenue North
Worcester, MA 01655
Phone: 508-334-1000
Fax: 508-856-5225
URL: www.umassmemorial.org
Type: Acute Care Hospitals
Emergency Services: Yes
Ownership: Voluntary non-profit - Private
Beds: 771

Key Personnel:
Operating Room. . . . . David Ayers, MD
Pediatric Ambulatory Care . . . . . . Marianne Felice, MD
Pediatric In-Patient Care . . . . Marianne Felice, MD
Radiology. . . . . Krishna Kandarpa, MD
CEO/President. . . . . John O'Brien
Cardiac Laboratory. . . . . Robert Phillips, MD
Chief of Medical Staff . . . . Stephen Tosi, MD

Measure	Cases	This Hosp.	State Avg.	U.S. Avg.
Blood Clot Prevention and Treatment				
Anticoagulation Overlap Therapy[2]	236	100%	97%	93%
ICU Venous Thromboembolism Prophylaxis[2]	121	99%	92%	92%
Incidence of Potentially Preventable VTE[2]	58	0%	7%	10%
UFH with Dosages/Platelet Monitoring[2]	156	99%	91%	97%
Venous Thromboembolism Prophylaxis[2]	311	91%	87%	85%

NOTE: Hospital profiles are in alphabetical order by state, then city, then hospital within the city; Rankings exclude hospitals with less than 25 cases except for patient surveys which excludes hospitals with less than 100 cases; (a) 100-299 cases; (1) The number of cases/patients is too few to report; (2) Data submitted were based on a sample of cases/patients; (3) Results are based on a shorter time period than required; (4) Data suppressed by CMS for one or more quarters; (5) Results are not available for this reporting period; (6) Fewer than 100 patients completed the HCAHPS survey; (7) No cases met the criteria for this measure; (8) The lower limit of the confidence interval cannot be calculated if the number of observed infections equals zero; (9) No data are available from the state/territory for this reporting period; (10) The scores shown reflect fewer than 50 completed surveys; (11) There were discrepancies in the data collection process; (12) This measure does not apply to this hospital for this reporting period; (13) Results cannot be calculated for this reporting period; (14) The results for this state are combined with nearby states to protect confidentiality; Please refer to the User's Guide for a full explanation of data.

Measure				
Warfarin Therapy Discharge Instructions[2]	160	76%	77%	75%
Chest Pain/Possible Heart Attack Care				
Aspirin Given Within 24 Hours of Arrival[1,3]	-	-	97%	96%
Fibrinolytic Meds Within 30 Min. of Arrival[3,7]	-	-	73%	58%
Average Time to ECG (minutes)[1,3]	-	-	7	7
Average Time to Transfer (minutes)[3,7]	-	-	55	60
Children's Asthma Care				
Received Home Management Plan of Care	-	-	-	88%
Received Reliever Medication	-	-	-	100%
Received Systemic Corticosteroids	-	-	-	100%
Emergency Department				
Admittance Decision Time (minutes)[2]	171	180	119	98
Head CT Results Within 45 Min. of Arrival[7]	-	-	70%	57%
Patients Who Left ER Before Being Seen	>100k	2%	2%	2%
Time from ER Arrival to Admit. (minutes)[2]	592	394	313	274
Time from ER Arrival to Discharge (minutes)	325	179	156	134
Time in ER Before Being Evaluated (minutes)	336	45	36	26
Time to Pain Meds for Fractures (minutes)	341	55	59	57
Heart Attack Care				
Aspirin Given at Discharge[2]	332	100%	100%	99%
Fibrinolytic Meds Within 30 Min. of Arrival[2,7]	-	-	100%	54%
PCI Within 90 Minutes of Arrival[2]	79	91%	96%	96%
Statin Prescribed at Discharge[2]	335	100%	99%	98%
Heart Failure Care				
ACE Inhibitor or ARB for LVSD[2]	103	97%	96%	97%
Discharge Instructions Given[2]	218	94%	95%	94%
Evaluation of LVS Function[2]	293	100%	100%	99%
Medicare Spending				
Medicare Spending per Patient (ratio)	-	1.08	1.03	0.98
Pneumonia Care				
Appropriate Initial Antibiotic Given[2]	68	97%	97%	95%
Blood Culture Timing[2]	100	88%	98%	98%
Pregnancy and Delivery Care				
Newborn Deliveries Scheduled Early	248	2%	2%	6%
Preventive Care				
Immunization for Influenza[2]	509	85%	91%	90%
Immunization for Pneumonia[2]	572	87%	91%	92%
Stroke Care				
Anticoagulation Therapy for Atrial Fibrillation[2]	16	100%	97%	95%
Antithrombotic Therapy Timing[2]	63	97%	98%	98%
Assessed for Rehabilitation[2]	103	97%	96%	97%
Discharged on Antithrombotic Therapy[2]	83	99%	100%	99%
Discharged on Statin Medication[2]	66	97%	96%	94%
Thrombolytic Therapy Timing[1,2]	-	-	68%	66%
Venous Thromboembolism Prophylaxis[2]	101	96%	94%	94%
Written Stroke Educational Materials Given[2]	37	76%	82%	88%
Surgical Care Improvement Project				
Appropriate Beta Blocker Usage[2]	218	99%	98%	98%
Appropriate VTP Within 24 Hours[2]	335	98%	99%	98%
Controlled Postoperative Blood Glucose[2]	130	98%	96%	97%
Perioperative Temperature Management[2]	470	100%	100%	100%
Prophylactic Antibiotic Selection[2]	403	99%	99%	99%
Prophylactic Antibiotic Selection (Outpatient)	390	97%	98%	98%
Prophylactic Antibiotic Stopped[2]	392	99%	99%	98%
Prophylactic Antibiotic Timing[2]	403	99%	99%	99%
Prophylactic Antibiotic Timing (Outpatient)	387	99%	98%	98%
Urinary Catheter Removal[2]	298	98%	97%	97%
Survey of Patients' Hospital Experiences				
Area Around Room 'Always' Quiet at Night	300+	46%	52%	61%
Doctors 'Always' Communicated Well	300+	77%	80%	82%
Home Recovery Information Given	300+	89%	87%	85%
Hospital Given 9 or 10 on 10 Point Scale	300+	64%	69%	71%
Meds 'Always' Explained Before Given	300+	58%	64%	64%
Nurses 'Always' Communicated Well	300+	74%	79%	79%
Pain 'Always' Well Controlled	300+	66%	71%	71%
Room and Bathroom 'Always' Clean	300+	65%	72%	73%
Timely Help 'Always' Received	300+	54%	66%	68%
Would Definitely Recommend Hospital	300+	71%	73%	71%
Use of Medical Imaging				
Cardiac Imaging Stress Test before Surgery	992	5.3%	5.4%	5.3%
Combination Abdominal CT Scan	1,974	8.5%	6.3%	10.5%
Combination Brain/Sinus CT Scan	1,336	2.2%	2.4%	2.7%
Combination Chest CT Scan	1,946	0.0%	0.5%	2.7%
Follow-up Mammogram/Ultrasound	4,331	21.2%	8.9%	8.8%
Lumbar Spine MRI for Low Back Pain[7]	-	-	35.3%	37.2%

NOTE: Hospital profiles are in alphabetical order by state, then city, then hospital within the city; Rankings exclude hospitals with less than 25 cases except for patient surveys which excludes hospitals with less than 100 cases; (a) 100-299 cases; (1) The number of cases/patients is too few to report; (2) Data submitted were based on a sample of cases/patients; (3) Results are based on a shorter time period than required; (4) Data suppressed by CMS for one or more quarters; (5) Results are not available for this reporting period; (6) Fewer than 100 patients completed the HCAHPS survey; (7) No cases met the criteria for this measure; (8) The lower limit of the confidence interval cannot be calculated if the number of observed infections equals zero; (9) No data are available from the state/territory for this reporting period; (10) The scores shown reflect fewer than 50 completed surveys; (11) There were discrepancies in the data collection process; (12) This measure does not apply to this hospital for this reporting period; (13) Results cannot be calculated for this reporting period; (14) The results for this state are combined with nearby states to protect confidentiality; Please refer to the User's Guide for a full explanation of data.

Blood Clot Prevention and Treatment

Anticoagulation Overlap Therapy

Hospital Name	City	Rate	Cases
Cheshire Medical Center[2]	Keene	100%	30
Concord Hospital[2]	Concord	100%	110
Frisbie Memorial Hospital[2]	Rochester	100%	29
Lakes Region General Hospital[2]	Laconia	100%	55
Parkland Medical Center[2]	Derry	100%	32
Portsmouth Regional Hospital[2]	Portsmouth	100%	26
Saint Joseph Hospital[2]	Nashua	100%	52
Wentworth - Douglass Hospital[2]	Dover	100%	49
Elliot Hospital[2]	Manchester	98%	51
Southern Nh Medical Center[2]	Nashua	98%	55
Catholic Medical Center[2]	Manchester	97%	92
Mary Hitchcock Memorial Hospital[2]	Lebanon	96%	81
Exeter Hospital[2]	Exeter	94%	36

ICU Venous Thromboembolism Prophylaxis

Hospital Name	City	Rate	Cases
Cheshire Medical Center[2]	Keene	100%	45
Parkland Medical Center[2]	Derry	100%	49
Portsmouth Regional Hospital[2]	Portsmouth	100%	91
Southern Nh Medical Center[2]	Nashua	100%	36
Mary Hitchcock Memorial Hospital[2]	Lebanon	98%	93
Catholic Medical Center[2]	Manchester	97%	62
Exeter Hospital[2]	Exeter	96%	48
Saint Joseph Hospital[2]	Nashua	96%	54
Frisbie Memorial Hospital[2]	Rochester	94%	51
Lakes Region General Hospital[2]	Laconia	93%	92
Wentworth - Douglass Hospital[2]	Dover	91%	67
Concord Hospital[2]	Concord	88%	50
Elliot Hospital[2]	Manchester	87%	47

Incidence of Potentially Preventable VTE

Hospital Name	City	Rate	Cases
Mary Hitchcock Memorial Hospital[2]	Lebanon	5%	39

UFH with Dosages/Platelet Count Monitoring

Hospital Name	City	Rate	Cases
Catholic Medical Center[2]	Manchester	100%	36
Concord Hospital[2]	Concord	100%	52
Lakes Region General Hospital[2]	Laconia	100%	46
Mary Hitchcock Memorial Hospital[2]	Lebanon	100%	73
Southern Nh Medical Center[2]	Nashua	100%	39
Wentworth - Douglass Hospital[2]	Dover	100%	44

Venous Thromboembolism Prophylaxis

Hospital Name	City	Rate	Cases
Portsmouth Regional Hospital[2]	Portsmouth	100%	311
Exeter Hospital[2]	Exeter	98%	333
Frisbie Memorial Hospital[2]	Rochester	98%	245
Parkland Medical Center[2]	Derry	98%	307
Valley Regional Hospital[2]	Claremont	98%	108
Wentworth - Douglass Hospital[2]	Dover	97%	372
Franklin Regional Hospital[2]	Franklin	94%	81
Mary Hitchcock Memorial Hospital[2]	Lebanon	91%	342
Concord Hospital[2]	Concord	90%	340
Southern Nh Medical Center[2]	Nashua	90%	344
Catholic Medical Center[2]	Manchester	89%	339
Cheshire Medical Center[2]	Keene	89%	233
Elliot Hospital[2]	Manchester	89%	330
Lakes Region General Hospital[2]	Laconia	89%	312
Saint Joseph Hospital[2]	Nashua	88%	314

Warfarin Therapy Discharge Instructions

Hospital Name	City	Rate	Cases
Cheshire Medical Center[2]	Keene	100%	25
Saint Joseph Hospital[2]	Nashua	100%	39
Wentworth - Douglass Hospital[2]	Dover	100%	37
Southern Nh Medical Center[2]	Nashua	94%	48
Concord Hospital[2]	Concord	88%	90
Catholic Medical Center[2]	Manchester	85%	67
Elliot Hospital[2]	Manchester	82%	38
Lakes Region General Hospital[2]	Laconia	61%	36
Exeter Hospital[2]	Exeter	31%	35
Mary Hitchcock Memorial Hospital[2]	Lebanon	7%	56

Chest Pain/Possible Heart Attack Care

Aspirin Given Within 24 Hours of Arrival

Hospital Name	City	Rate	Cases
Cheshire Medical Center	Keene	100%	89
Frisbie Memorial Hospital	Rochester	100%	41
Monadnock Community Hospital	Peterborough	100%	37
Speare Memorial Hospital	Plymouth	100%	56
Upper Connecticut Valley Hospital[3]	Colebrook	100%	27
Lakes Region General Hospital	Laconia	97%	99

Average Time to ECG (minutes)

Hospital Name	City	Min.	Cases
Cheshire Medical Center	Keene	7	93
Frisbie Memorial Hospital	Rochester	8	45
Speare Memorial Hospital	Plymouth	8	56
Upper Connecticut Valley Hospital[3]	Colebrook	9	26
Lakes Region General Hospital	Laconia	10	100
Monadnock Community Hospital	Peterborough	11	37

Children's Asthma Care

No hospitals met the 25 case threshold.

Emergency Department

Admittance Decision Time (minutes)

Hospital Name	City	Min.	Cases
Monadnock Community Hospital[2]	Peterborough	58	386
Parkland Medical Center[2]	Derry	69	659
Franklin Regional Hospital[2]	Franklin	70	296
Littleton Regional Healthcare[2]	Littleton	82	251
Speare Memorial Hospital[2]	Plymouth	84	400
Portsmouth Regional Hospital[2]	Portsmouth	90	665
Exeter Hospital[2]	Exeter	94	774
Lakes Region General Hospital[2]	Laconia	95	489
Saint Joseph Hospital[2]	Nashua	96	632
Frisbie Memorial Hospital[2]	Rochester	117	446
Elliot Hospital[2]	Manchester	133	445
Concord Hospital[2]	Concord	135	493
Wentworth - Douglass Hospital[2]	Dover	135	425
Southern Nh Medical Center[2]	Nashua	140	541
Catholic Medical Center[2]	Manchester	192	455
Cheshire Medical Center[2]	Keene	200	386
Mary Hitchcock Memorial Hospital[2]	Lebanon	247	284

Patients Who Left ER Before Being Seen

Hospital Name	City	Rate	Cases
Speare Memorial Hospital	Plymouth	0%	14526
Wentworth - Douglass Hospital	Dover	0%	40606
Frisbie Memorial Hospital	Rochester	1%	28975
Mary Hitchcock Memorial Hospital	Lebanon	1%	31543
Parkland Medical Center	Derry	1%	24321
Portsmouth Regional Hospital	Portsmouth	1%	25992
Saint Joseph Hospital	Nashua	1%	33159
Southern Nh Medical Center	Nashua	1%	44644
Catholic Medical Center	Manchester	2%	34503
Cheshire Medical Center	Keene	2%	27033
Concord Hospital	Concord	2%	46959
Elliot Hospital	Manchester	2%	53513
Exeter Hospital	Exeter	2%	31963
Franklin Regional Hospital	Franklin	2%	10936
Lakes Region General Hospital	Laconia	2%	21715

Time from ER Arrival to Being Admitted (minutes)

Hospital Name	City	Min.	Cases
Parkland Medical Center[2]	Derry	237	668
Saint Joseph Hospital[2]	Nashua	242	657
Alice Peck Day Memorial Hospital[2]	Lebanon	244	26
Portsmouth Regional Hospital[2]	Portsmouth	245	670
Speare Memorial Hospital[2]	Plymouth	256	407
Monadnock Community Hospital[2]	Peterborough	277	405
Franklin Regional Hospital[2]	Franklin	280	298
Wentworth - Douglass Hospital[2]	Dover	289	593
Concord Hospital[2]	Concord	302	505
Littleton Regional Healthcare[2]	Littleton	308	270
Southern Nh Medical Center[2]	Nashua	308	569
Elliot Hospital[2]	Manchester	309	482
Frisbie Memorial Hospital[2]	Rochester	313	446
Exeter Hospital[2]	Exeter	317	784
Catholic Medical Center[2]	Manchester	344	460
Lakes Region General Hospital[2]	Laconia	354	528
Cheshire Medical Center[2]	Keene	358	386
Mary Hitchcock Memorial Hospital[2]	Lebanon	370	286

Time from ER Arrival to Discharge (minutes)

Hospital Name	City	Min.	Cases
Franklin Regional Hospital	Franklin	100	372
Speare Memorial Hospital[3]	Plymouth	113	284
Saint Joseph Hospital	Nashua	115	358
Portsmouth Regional Hospital	Portsmouth	120	447
Parkland Medical Center	Derry	122	436
Wentworth - Douglass Hospital	Dover	123	363
Frisbie Memorial Hospital	Rochester	124	381
Cheshire Medical Center	Keene	131	372
Southern Nh Medical Center	Nashua	149	435
Catholic Medical Center	Manchester	163	322
Concord Hospital	Concord	170	277
Lakes Region General Hospital	Laconia	173	322
Mary Hitchcock Memorial Hospital	Lebanon	176	353
Exeter Hospital	Exeter	184	382
Elliot Hospital	Manchester	190	327

Time in ER Before Being Evaluated (minutes)

Hospital Name	City	Min.	Cases
Parkland Medical Center	Derry	13	491
Portsmouth Regional Hospital	Portsmouth	17	498
Wentworth - Douglass Hospital	Dover	21	372
Saint Joseph Hospital	Nashua	24	382
Speare Memorial Hospital[3]	Plymouth	26	287
Frisbie Memorial Hospital	Rochester	28	400
Franklin Regional Hospital	Franklin	30	406
Southern Nh Medical Center	Nashua	31	477
Elliot Hospital	Manchester	36	345
Mary Hitchcock Memorial Hospital	Lebanon	36	290
Cheshire Medical Center	Keene	38	407
Catholic Medical Center	Manchester	46	372
Concord Hospital	Concord	46	364
Lakes Region General Hospital	Laconia	48	344
Exeter Hospital	Exeter	90	313

Time to Pain Meds for Bone Fractures (minutes)

Hospital Name	City	Min.	Cases
Parkland Medical Center	Derry	36	71
Portsmouth Regional Hospital	Portsmouth	40	75
Wentworth - Douglass Hospital	Dover	40	97
Saint Joseph Hospital	Nashua	46	103
Concord Hospital	Concord	55	108
Elliot Hospital	Manchester	55	129
Franklin Regional Hospital	Franklin	55	31
Frisbie Memorial Hospital	Rochester	56	100
Cheshire Medical Center	Keene	58	65
Lakes Region General Hospital	Laconia	67	108
Southern Nh Medical Center	Nashua	73	146
Catholic Medical Center	Manchester	74	60
Mary Hitchcock Memorial Hospital	Lebanon	78	143
Exeter Hospital	Exeter	79	152

Heart Attack Care

Aspirin Given at Discharge

Hospital Name	City	Rate	Cases
Catholic Medical Center	Manchester	100%	477
Concord Hospital	Concord	100%	229
Elliot Hospital	Manchester	100%	121
Exeter Hospital	Exeter	100%	131
Parkland Medical Center	Derry	100%	75
Portsmouth Regional Hospital	Portsmouth	100%	298
Saint Joseph Hospital[2]	Nashua	100%	97
Southern Nh Medical Center	Nashua	100%	103
Wentworth - Douglass Hospital	Dover	100%	125
Mary Hitchcock Memorial Hospital[2]	Lebanon	99%	507

PCI Within 90 Minutes of Arrival

Hospital Name	City	Rate	Cases
Portsmouth Regional Hospital	Portsmouth	100%	26
Southern Nh Medical Center	Nashua	100%	30
Exeter Hospital	Exeter	97%	36
Catholic Medical Center	Manchester	96%	54
Concord Hospital	Concord	95%	65
Mary Hitchcock Memorial Hospital[2]	Lebanon	86%	36

Statin Prescribed at Discharge

Hospital Name	City	Rate	Cases
Catholic Medical Center	Manchester	100%	472
Concord Hospital	Concord	100%	221
Elliot Hospital	Manchester	100%	110
Mary Hitchcock Memorial Hospital[2]	Lebanon	100%	502
Parkland Medical Center	Derry	100%	74
Portsmouth Regional Hospital	Portsmouth	100%	285
Saint Joseph Hospital[2]	Nashua	100%	97
Exeter Hospital	Exeter	99%	119
Southern Nh Medical Center	Nashua	99%	101
Wentworth - Douglass Hospital	Dover	98%	124

Heart Failure Care

ACE Inhibitor or ARB for LVSD

Hospital Name	City	Rate	Cases
Catholic Medical Center[2]	Manchester	100%	86
Concord Hospital	Concord	100%	98
Elliot Hospital	Manchester	100%	47
Mary Hitchcock Memorial Hospital[2]	Lebanon	100%	67
Portsmouth Regional Hospital	Portsmouth	100%	45
Saint Joseph Hospital[2]	Nashua	100%	39
Southern Nh Medical Center	Nashua	100%	45

NOTE: Hospital profiles are in alphabetical order by state, then city, then hospital within the city; Rankings exclude hospitals with less than 25 cases except for patient surveys which excludes hospitals with less than 100 cases; (a) 100-299 cases; (1) The number of cases/patients is too few to report; (2) Data submitted were based on a sample of cases/patients; (3) Results are based on a shorter time period than required; (4) Data suppressed by CMS for one or more quarters; (5) Results are not available for this reporting period; (6) Fewer than 100 patients completed the HCAHPS survey; (7) No cases met the criteria for this measure; (8) The lower limit of the confidence interval cannot be calculated if the number of observed infections equals zero; (9) No data are available from the state/territory for this reporting period; (10) The scores shown reflect fewer than 50 completed surveys; (11) There were discrepancies in the data collection process; (12) This measure does not apply to this hospital for this reporting period; (13) Results cannot be calculated for this reporting period; (14) The results for this state are combined with nearby states to protect confidentiality; Please refer to the User's Guide for a full explanation of data.

Hospital Name	City	Rate	Cases
Wentworth - Douglass Hospital	Dover	98%	46
Lakes Region General Hospital[2]	Laconia	97%	34
Parkland Medical Center	Derry	97%	35
Exeter Hospital	Exeter	94%	47

Discharge Instructions Given

Hospital Name	City	Rate	Cases
Androscoggin Valley Hospital	Berlin	100%	32
Catholic Medical Center[2]	Manchester	100%	244
Cheshire Medical Center	Keene	100%	65
Exeter Hospital	Exeter	100%	141
Frisbie Memorial Hospital	Rochester	100%	98
The Memorial Hospital[2]	North Conway	100%	30
Portsmouth Regional Hospital	Portsmouth	100%	122
Southern Nh Medical Center	Nashua	100%	151
Speare Memorial Hospital	Plymouth	100%	27
Parkland Medical Center	Derry	99%	108
Saint Joseph Hospital[2]	Nashua	99%	137
Concord Hospital	Concord	98%	256
Elliot Hospital	Manchester	97%	175
Mary Hitchcock Memorial Hospital[2]	Lebanon	96%	242
Lakes Region General Hospital[2]	Laconia	90%	73
Wentworth - Douglass Hospital	Dover	86%	171

Evaluation of LVS Function

Hospital Name	City	Rate	Cases
Androscoggin Valley Hospital	Berlin	100%	37
Catholic Medical Center[2]	Manchester	100%	289
Cheshire Medical Center	Keene	100%	89
Concord Hospital	Concord	100%	334
Elliot Hospital	Manchester	100%	246
Exeter Hospital	Exeter	100%	198
Huggins Hospital	Wolfeboro	100%	34
Lakes Region General Hospital[2]	Laconia	100%	122
Mary Hitchcock Memorial Hospital[2]	Lebanon	100%	296
The Memorial Hospital[2]	North Conway	100%	42
Monadnock Community Hospital[2]	Peterborough	100%	44
Parkland Medical Center	Derry	100%	144
Portsmouth Regional Hospital	Portsmouth	100%	171
Saint Joseph Hospital[2]	Nashua	100%	176
Speare Memorial Hospital	Plymouth	100%	31
Wentworth - Douglass Hospital	Dover	100%	216
Southern Nh Medical Center	Nashua	99%	195
Frisbie Memorial Hospital	Rochester	98%	120
Valley Regional Hospital	Claremont	97%	29

Medicare Spending

Medicare Spending per Patient (ratio)

Hospital Name	City	Ratio	Cases
Cheshire Medical Center	Keene	0.99	-
Mary Hitchcock Memorial Hospital	Lebanon	0.99	-
Exeter Hospital	Exeter	1.00	-
Concord Hospital	Concord	1.01	-
Portsmouth Regional Hospital	Portsmouth	1.02	-
Saint Joseph Hospital	Nashua	1.02	-
Southern Nh Medical Center	Nashua	1.02	-
Lakes Region General Hospital	Laconia	1.03	-
Wentworth - Douglass Hospital	Dover	1.03	-
Catholic Medical Center	Manchester	1.04	-
Elliot Hospital	Manchester	1.05	-
Frisbie Memorial Hospital	Rochester	1.05	-
Parkland Medical Center	Derry	1.08	-

Pneumonia Care

Appropriate Initial Antibiotic Given

Hospital Name	City	Rate	Cases
Androscoggin Valley Hospital	Berlin	100%	26
Cheshire Medical Center[2]	Keene	100%	70
Huggins Hospital	Wolfeboro	100%	50
Littleton Regional Healthcare	Littleton	100%	32
Portsmouth Regional Hospital	Portsmouth	100%	57
Southern Nh Medical Center	Nashua	100%	159
Speare Memorial Hospital	Plymouth	100%	42
Elliot Hospital[2]	Manchester	99%	79
Parkland Medical Center	Derry	99%	86
Concord Hospital	Concord	98%	247
Exeter Hospital	Exeter	98%	111
Lakes Region General Hospital[2]	Laconia	97%	60
Valley Regional Hospital	Claremont	96%	46
Catholic Medical Center[2]	Manchester	95%	80
Frisbie Memorial Hospital	Rochester	95%	120
Mary Hitchcock Memorial Hospital[2]	Lebanon	95%	64
Wentworth - Douglass Hospital[2]	Dover	95%	100
The Memorial Hospital[2]	North Conway	94%	50
Saint Joseph Hospital[2]	Nashua	94%	82
Monadnock Community Hospital	Peterborough	89%	36
Franklin Regional Hospital[2]	Franklin	85%	27

Blood Culture Timing

Hospital Name	City	Rate	Cases
Franklin Regional Hospital[2]	Franklin	100%	39
Littleton Regional Healthcare	Littleton	100%	36
New London Hospital	New London	100%	31
Portsmouth Regional Hospital	Portsmouth	100%	105
Southern Nh Medical Center	Nashua	100%	245
Valley Regional Hospital	Claremont	100%	49
Cheshire Medical Center[2]	Keene	99%	136
Huggins Hospital	Wolfeboro	99%	70
The Memorial Hospital[2]	North Conway	99%	78
Monadnock Community Hospital	Peterborough	99%	75
Parkland Medical Center	Derry	99%	148
Speare Memorial Hospital	Plymouth	99%	71
Catholic Medical Center[2]	Manchester	98%	129
Concord Hospital	Concord	98%	259
Exeter Hospital	Exeter	98%	198
Lakes Region General Hospital[2]	Laconia	98%	98
Saint Joseph Hospital[2]	Nashua	98%	150
Elliot Hospital[2]	Manchester	97%	118
Wentworth - Douglass Hospital[2]	Dover	97%	182
Frisbie Memorial Hospital	Rochester	96%	130
Mary Hitchcock Memorial Hospital[2]	Lebanon	85%	94

Pregnancy and Delivery Care

Newborns whose Deliveries were Scheduled Early

Hospital Name	City	Rate	Cases
Elliot Hospital[2]	Manchester	0%	35
Frisbie Memorial Hospital	Rochester	0%	48
Lakes Region General Hospital	Laconia	0%	33
Wentworth - Douglass Hospital	Dover	5%	44
Exeter Hospital	Exeter	6%	32
Southern Nh Medical Center	Nashua	6%	63

Preventive Care

Immunization for Influenza

Hospital Name	City	Rate	Cases
Catholic Medical Center[2]	Manchester	99%	521
Elliot Hospital[2]	Manchester	99%	494
Cheshire Medical Center[2]	Keene	98%	299
Parkland Medical Center[2]	Derry	98%	421
Portsmouth Regional Hospital[2]	Portsmouth	98%	549
Speare Memorial Hospital[2]	Plymouth	98%	292
Wentworth - Douglass Hospital[2]	Dover	98%	533
Franklin Regional Hospital[2]	Franklin	97%	232
Frisbie Memorial Hospital[2]	Rochester	97%	337
Southern Nh Medical Center[2]	Nashua	96%	532
Saint Joseph Hospital[2]	Nashua	95%	494
Concord Hospital[2]	Concord	94%	519
Lakes Region General Hospital[2]	Laconia	94%	385
Monadnock Community Hospital[2]	Peterborough	92%	285
Littleton Regional Healthcare[2]	Littleton	89%	287
Exeter Hospital[2]	Exeter	88%	520
Mary Hitchcock Memorial Hospital[2]	Lebanon	87%	631

Immunization for Pneumonia

Hospital Name	City	Rate	Cases
Catholic Medical Center[2]	Manchester	100%	707
Franklin Regional Hospital[2]	Franklin	99%	357
Portsmouth Regional Hospital[2]	Portsmouth	99%	741
Cheshire Medical Center[2]	Keene	98%	371
Frisbie Memorial Hospital[2]	Rochester	98%	419
Parkland Medical Center[2]	Derry	97%	552
Speare Memorial Hospital[2]	Plymouth	97%	367
Lakes Region General Hospital[2]	Laconia	96%	561
Wentworth - Douglass Hospital[2]	Dover	96%	696
Elliot Hospital[2]	Manchester	95%	511
Monadnock Community Hospital[2]	Peterborough	95%	382
Exeter Hospital[2]	Exeter	94%	710
Saint Joseph Hospital[2]	Nashua	94%	637
Concord Hospital[2]	Concord	93%	639
Southern Nh Medical Center[2]	Nashua	90%	536
Littleton Regional Healthcare[2]	Littleton	88%	304
Mary Hitchcock Memorial Hospital[2]	Lebanon	87%	698
Alice Peck Day Memorial Hospital[2]	Lebanon	82%	44

Stroke Care

Anticoagulation Therapy for Atrial Fibrillation

Hospital Name	City	Rate	Cases
Mary Hitchcock Memorial Hospital[2]	Lebanon	95%	38

Antithrombotic Therapy Timing

Hospital Name	City	Rate	Cases
Catholic Medical Center	Manchester	100%	70
Cheshire Medical Center	Keene	100%	30
Exeter Hospital	Exeter	100%	44
Frisbie Memorial Hospital	Rochester	100%	36
Lakes Region General Hospital[2]	Laconia	100%	50
Mary Hitchcock Memorial Hospital[2]	Lebanon	100%	143
Parkland Medical Center[2]	Derry	100%	36
Portsmouth Regional Hospital	Portsmouth	100%	47
Saint Joseph Hospital[2]	Nashua	100%	57
Southern Nh Medical Center	Nashua	100%	60
Concord Hospital[2]	Concord	99%	80
Elliot Hospital	Manchester	99%	81
Wentworth - Douglass Hospital	Dover	93%	54

Assessed for Rehabilitation

Hospital Name	City	Rate	Cases
Cheshire Medical Center	Keene	100%	30
Frisbie Memorial Hospital	Rochester	100%	37
Portsmouth Regional Hospital	Portsmouth	100%	71
Southern Nh Medical Center	Nashua	100%	67
Wentworth - Douglass Hospital	Dover	100%	58
Parkland Medical Center[2]	Derry	98%	45
Concord Hospital[2]	Concord	97%	89
Elliot Hospital	Manchester	97%	114
Saint Joseph Hospital[2]	Nashua	97%	68
Exeter Hospital	Exeter	96%	46
Lakes Region General Hospital[2]	Laconia	94%	48
Mary Hitchcock Memorial Hospital[2]	Lebanon	94%	267
Catholic Medical Center	Manchester	92%	83

Discharged on Antithrombotic Therapy

Hospital Name	City	Rate	Cases
Catholic Medical Center	Manchester	100%	76
Cheshire Medical Center	Keene	100%	29
Concord Hospital[2]	Concord	100%	84
Exeter Hospital	Exeter	100%	42
Frisbie Memorial Hospital	Rochester	100%	35
Lakes Region General Hospital[2]	Laconia	100%	48
Parkland Medical Center[2]	Derry	100%	42
Portsmouth Regional Hospital	Portsmouth	100%	54
Saint Joseph Hospital[2]	Nashua	100%	64
Southern Nh Medical Center	Nashua	100%	62
Wentworth - Douglass Hospital	Dover	100%	53
Mary Hitchcock Memorial Hospital[2]	Lebanon	99%	187
Elliot Hospital	Manchester	98%	96

Discharged on Statin Medication

Hospital Name	City	Rate	Cases
Parkland Medical Center[2]	Derry	100%	35
Portsmouth Regional Hospital	Portsmouth	100%	47
Southern Nh Medical Center	Nashua	100%	51
Wentworth - Douglass Hospital	Dover	100%	41
Catholic Medical Center	Manchester	98%	65
Mary Hitchcock Memorial Hospital[2]	Lebanon	98%	149
Lakes Region General Hospital[2]	Laconia	97%	39
Elliot Hospital	Manchester	96%	73
Concord Hospital[2]	Concord	94%	65
Saint Joseph Hospital[2]	Nashua	91%	47
Exeter Hospital	Exeter	88%	32
Frisbie Memorial Hospital	Rochester	88%	26

Venous Thromboembolism (VTE) Prophylaxis

Hospital Name	City	Rate	Cases
Exeter Hospital	Exeter	100%	41
Parkland Medical Center[2]	Derry	100%	45
Portsmouth Regional Hospital	Portsmouth	100%	70
Southern Nh Medical Center	Nashua	98%	57
Wentworth - Douglass Hospital	Dover	98%	57
Saint Joseph Hospital[2]	Nashua	96%	68
Catholic Medical Center	Manchester	95%	74
Mary Hitchcock Memorial Hospital[2]	Lebanon	95%	283
Frisbie Memorial Hospital	Rochester	92%	39
Concord Hospital[2]	Concord	90%	84
Lakes Region General Hospital[2]	Laconia	89%	53
Elliot Hospital	Manchester	88%	97
Cheshire Medical Center	Keene	67%	30

Written Stroke Educational Materials Given

Hospital Name	City	Rate	Cases
Portsmouth Regional Hospital	Portsmouth	100%	35
Southern Nh Medical Center	Nashua	100%	36
Saint Joseph Hospital[2]	Nashua	93%	29
Mary Hitchcock Memorial Hospital[2]	Lebanon	87%	133
Wentworth - Douglass Hospital	Dover	83%	30
Concord Hospital[2]	Concord	78%	50
Catholic Medical Center	Manchester	74%	43
Elliot Hospital	Manchester	69%	51
Exeter Hospital	Exeter	4%	28

NOTE: Hospital profiles are in alphabetical order by state, then city, then hospital within the city; Rankings exclude hospitals with less than 25 cases except for patient surveys which excludes hospitals with less than 100 cases; (a) 100-299 cases; (1) The number of cases/patients is too few to report; (2) Data submitted were based on a sample of cases/patients; (3) Results are based on a shorter time period than required; (4) Data suppressed by CMS for one or more quarters; (5) Results are not available for this reporting period; (6) Fewer than 100 patients completed the HCAHPS survey; (7) No cases met the criteria for this measure; (8) The lower limit of the confidence interval cannot be calculated if the number of observed infections equals zero; (9) No data are available from the state/territory for this reporting period; (10) The scores shown reflect fewer than 50 completed surveys; (11) There were discrepancies in the data collection process; (12) This measure does not apply to this hospital for this reporting period; (13) Results cannot be calculated for this reporting period; (14) The results for this state are combined with nearby states to protect confidentiality; Please refer to the User's Guide for a full explanation of data.

Surgical Care Improvement Project

Appropriate Beta Blocker Usage

Hospital Name	City	Rate	Cases
Cheshire Medical Center	Keene	100%	69
Elliot Hospital[2]	Manchester	100%	78
Littleton Regional Healthcare[2]	Littleton	100%	48
Parkland Medical Center	Derry	100%	51
Portsmouth Regional Hospital[2]	Portsmouth	100%	265
Catholic Medical Center[2]	Manchester	99%	215
Lakes Region General Hospital[2]	Laconia	99%	148
Mary Hitchcock Memorial Hospital[2]	Lebanon	99%	307
Southern Nh Medical Center	Nashua	98%	128
Wentworth - Douglass Hospital[2]	Dover	98%	125
Concord Hospital[2]	Concord	97%	151
Saint Joseph Hospital[2]	Nashua	97%	69
Frisbie Memorial Hospital	Rochester	96%	90
Exeter Hospital	Exeter	95%	150

Appropriate VTP Within 24 Hours

Hospital Name	City	Rate	Cases
Androscoggin Valley Hospital	Berlin	100%	63
Frisbie Memorial Hospital	Rochester	100%	208
Huggins Hospital	Wolfeboro	100%	83
Littleton Regional Healthcare[2]	Littleton	100%	158
Mary Hitchcock Memorial Hospital[2]	Lebanon	100%	449
The Memorial Hospital	North Conway	100%	63
Monadnock Community Hospital	Peterborough	100%	58
Portsmouth Regional Hospital[2]	Portsmouth	100%	377
Speare Memorial Hospital	Plymouth	100%	64
Weeks Medical Center	Lancaster	100%	34
Concord Hospital[2]	Concord	99%	256
Elliot Hospital[2]	Manchester	99%	301
Parkland Medical Center	Derry	99%	112
Southern Nh Medical Center	Nashua	99%	436
Alice Peck Day Memorial Hospital[2]	Lebanon	98%	58
Exeter Hospital	Exeter	98%	392
Lakes Region General Hospital[2]	Laconia	98%	371
New London Hospital	New London	98%	42
Saint Joseph Hospital[2]	Nashua	98%	222
Catholic Medical Center[2]	Manchester	97%	230
Cheshire Medical Center	Keene	95%	230
Wentworth - Douglass Hospital[2]	Dover	94%	316

Controlled Postoperative Blood Glucose

Hospital Name	City	Rate	Cases
Catholic Medical Center[2]	Manchester	99%	130
Portsmouth Regional Hospital[2]	Portsmouth	99%	181
Concord Hospital[2]	Concord	97%	109
Mary Hitchcock Memorial Hospital[2]	Lebanon	96%	207

Perioperative Temperature Management

Hospital Name	City	Rate	Cases
Alice Peck Day Memorial Hospital[2]	Lebanon	100%	80
Androscoggin Valley Hospital	Berlin	100%	71
Catholic Medical Center[2]	Manchester	100%	418
Concord Hospital[2]	Concord	100%	345
Elliot Hospital[2]	Manchester	100%	376
Exeter Hospital	Exeter	100%	458
Frisbie Memorial Hospital	Rochester	100%	244
Huggins Hospital	Wolfeboro	100%	89
Lakes Region General Hospital[2]	Laconia	100%	455
Littleton Regional Healthcare[2]	Littleton	100%	187
Mary Hitchcock Memorial Hospital[2]	Lebanon	100%	656
The Memorial Hospital	North Conway	100%	66
Monadnock Community Hospital	Peterborough	100%	64
New London Hospital	New London	100%	69
Parkland Medical Center	Derry	100%	167
Portsmouth Regional Hospital[2]	Portsmouth	100%	435
Saint Joseph Hospital[2]	Nashua	100%	266
Southern Nh Medical Center	Nashua	100%	480
Speare Memorial Hospital	Plymouth	100%	72
Valley Regional Hospital	Claremont	100%	52
Weeks Medical Center	Lancaster	100%	36
Wentworth - Douglass Hospital[2]	Dover	100%	396
Cheshire Medical Center	Keene	99%	258

Prophylactic Antibiotic Selection

Hospital Name	City	Rate	Cases
Androscoggin Valley Hospital	Berlin	100%	62
Catholic Medical Center[2]	Manchester	100%	334
Cheshire Medical Center	Keene	100%	197
Frisbie Memorial Hospital	Rochester	100%	175
Huggins Hospital	Wolfeboro	100%	47
Lakes Region General Hospital[2]	Laconia	100%	272
The Memorial Hospital	North Conway	100%	45
Portsmouth Regional Hospital[2]	Portsmouth	100%	430
Southern Nh Medical Center	Nashua	100%	307
Speare Memorial Hospital	Plymouth	100%	48
Concord Hospital[2]	Concord	99%	326
Exeter Hospital	Exeter	99%	306
Littleton Regional Healthcare[2]	Littleton	99%	145
Mary Hitchcock Memorial Hospital[2]	Lebanon	99%	600
Wentworth - Douglass Hospital[2]	Dover	99%	276
Elliot Hospital[2]	Manchester	98%	254
Saint Joseph Hospital[2]	Nashua	98%	174
Alice Peck Day Memorial Hospital[2]	Lebanon	97%	70
Weeks Medical Center	Lancaster	97%	31
Monadnock Community Hospital	Peterborough	96%	55
Parkland Medical Center	Derry	95%	60
New London Hospital	New London	94%	31

Prophylactic Antibiotic Selection (Outpatient)

Hospital Name	City	Rate	Cases
Cheshire Medical Center	Keene	100%	116
Lakes Region General Hospital	Laconia	100%	148
New London Hospital	New London	100%	98
Portsmouth Regional Hospital	Portsmouth	100%	268
Southern Nh Medical Center	Nashua	100%	343
Concord Hospital	Concord	99%	421
Elliot Hospital	Manchester	99%	430
Mary Hitchcock Memorial Hospital	Lebanon	99%	668
Parkland Medical Center	Derry	99%	141
Wentworth - Douglass Hospital	Dover	99%	300
Catholic Medical Center	Manchester	98%	427
Exeter Hospital	Exeter	98%	100
Frisbie Memorial Hospital	Rochester	98%	120
Saint Joseph Hospital	Nashua	98%	116

Prophylactic Antibiotic Stopped

Hospital Name	City	Rate	Cases
Alice Peck Day Memorial Hospital[2]	Lebanon	100%	70
Exeter Hospital	Exeter	100%	302
Huggins Hospital	Wolfeboro	100%	47
Lakes Region General Hospital[2]	Laconia	100%	267
New London Hospital	New London	100%	31
Parkland Medical Center	Derry	100%	57
Portsmouth Regional Hospital[2]	Portsmouth	100%	411
Saint Joseph Hospital[2]	Nashua	100%	171
Androscoggin Valley Hospital	Berlin	98%	60
Catholic Medical Center[2]	Manchester	98%	325
Cheshire Medical Center	Keene	98%	196
Elliot Hospital[2]	Manchester	98%	247
Frisbie Memorial Hospital	Rochester	98%	175
Littleton Regional Healthcare[2]	Littleton	98%	144
The Memorial Hospital	North Conway	98%	44
Speare Memorial Hospital	Plymouth	98%	46
Wentworth - Douglass Hospital[2]	Dover	98%	273
Concord Hospital[2]	Concord	97%	320
Southern Nh Medical Center	Nashua	97%	300
Weeks Medical Center	Lancaster	97%	29
Mary Hitchcock Memorial Hospital[2]	Lebanon	95%	592
Monadnock Community Hospital	Peterborough	91%	54

Prophylactic Antibiotic Timing

Hospital Name	City	Rate	Cases
Androscoggin Valley Hospital	Berlin	100%	62
Monadnock Community Hospital	Peterborough	100%	55
New London Hospital	New London	100%	31
Portsmouth Regional Hospital[2]	Portsmouth	100%	430
Southern Nh Medical Center	Nashua	100%	307
Speare Memorial Hospital	Plymouth	100%	48
Weeks Medical Center	Lancaster	100%	31
Catholic Medical Center[2]	Manchester	99%	334
Cheshire Medical Center	Keene	99%	197
Concord Hospital[2]	Concord	99%	326
Elliot Hospital[2]	Manchester	99%	255
Exeter Hospital	Exeter	99%	306
Saint Joseph Hospital[2]	Nashua	99%	174
Wentworth - Douglass Hospital[2]	Dover	99%	276
Frisbie Memorial Hospital	Rochester	98%	175
Huggins Hospital	Wolfeboro	98%	47
Littleton Regional Healthcare[2]	Littleton	98%	145
Mary Hitchcock Memorial Hospital[2]	Lebanon	98%	601
The Memorial Hospital	North Conway	98%	45
Parkland Medical Center	Derry	97%	60
Lakes Region General Hospital[2]	Laconia	96%	272
Alice Peck Day Memorial Hospital[2]	Lebanon	93%	71

Prophylactic Antibiotic Timing (Outpatient)

Hospital Name	City	Rate	Cases
Catholic Medical Center	Manchester	100%	425
Frisbie Memorial Hospital	Rochester	100%	120
Portsmouth Regional Hospital	Portsmouth	100%	269
Cheshire Medical Center	Keene	99%	83
Concord Hospital	Concord	99%	410
New London Hospital	New London	99%	98
Parkland Medical Center	Derry	99%	85
Saint Joseph Hospital	Nashua	99%	116
Wentworth - Douglass Hospital	Dover	99%	300
Elliot Hospital	Manchester	98%	428
Southern Nh Medical Center	Nashua	98%	344
Lakes Region General Hospital	Laconia	97%	150
Exeter Hospital	Exeter	96%	101
Mary Hitchcock Memorial Hospital	Lebanon	96%	582

Urinary Catheter Removal

Hospital Name	City	Rate	Cases
Androscoggin Valley Hospital	Berlin	100%	52
Cheshire Medical Center	Keene	100%	186
Frisbie Memorial Hospital	Rochester	100%	177
Huggins Hospital	Wolfeboro	100%	61
Littleton Regional Healthcare[2]	Littleton	100%	126
The Memorial Hospital	North Conway	100%	38
New London Hospital	New London	100%	37
Parkland Medical Center	Derry	100%	89
Portsmouth Regional Hospital[2]	Portsmouth	100%	333
Southern Nh Medical Center	Nashua	100%	291
Speare Memorial Hospital	Plymouth	100%	55
Valley Regional Hospital	Claremont	100%	42
Weeks Medical Center	Lancaster	100%	31
Catholic Medical Center[2]	Manchester	99%	316
Concord Hospital[2]	Concord	99%	251
Saint Joseph Hospital[2]	Nashua	99%	95
Alice Peck Day Memorial Hospital[2]	Lebanon	98%	54
Elliot Hospital[2]	Manchester	98%	239
Lakes Region General Hospital[2]	Laconia	98%	309
Wentworth - Douglass Hospital[2]	Dover	98%	283
Exeter Hospital	Exeter	94%	139
Mary Hitchcock Memorial Hospital[2]	Lebanon	92%	501

Survey of Patients' Hospital Experiences

Area Around Room 'Always' Quiet at Night

Hospital Name	City	Rate	Cases
Frisbie Memorial Hospital	Rochester	73%	300+
Huggins Hospital	Wolfeboro	66%	(a)
Saint Joseph Hospital	Nashua	65%	300+
Valley Regional Hospital	Claremont	65%	(a)
Lakes Region General Hospital	Laconia	61%	300+
New London Hospital	New London	61%	(a)
Parkland Medical Center	Derry	61%	300+
Speare Memorial Hospital	Plymouth	60%	300+
Wentworth - Douglass Hospital	Dover	60%	300+
Monadnock Community Hospital	Peterborough	59%	300+
Portsmouth Regional Hospital	Portsmouth	59%	300+
Alice Peck Day Memorial Hospital	Lebanon	58%	300+
Exeter Hospital	Exeter	58%	300+
Littleton Regional Healthcare	Littleton	58%	(a)
Androscoggin Valley Hospital	Berlin	56%	(a)
Southern Nh Medical Center	Nashua	54%	300+
Catholic Medical Center	Manchester	53%	300+
Concord Hospital	Concord	52%	300+
Cheshire Medical Center	Keene	51%	300+
Elliot Hospital	Manchester	50%	300+
The Memorial Hospital	North Conway	49%	(a)
Mary Hitchcock Memorial Hospital	Lebanon	41%	300+

Doctors 'Always' Communicated Well

Hospital Name	City	Rate	Cases
Littleton Regional Healthcare	Littleton	87%	(a)
Speare Memorial Hospital	Plymouth	87%	300+
Valley Regional Hospital	Claremont	86%	(a)
Androscoggin Valley Hospital	Berlin	84%	(a)
Alice Peck Day Memorial Hospital	Lebanon	83%	300+
Cheshire Medical Center	Keene	83%	300+
Frisbie Memorial Hospital	Rochester	83%	300+
Monadnock Community Hospital	Peterborough	83%	300+
Wentworth - Douglass Hospital	Dover	83%	300+
Catholic Medical Center	Manchester	82%	300+
Exeter Hospital	Exeter	81%	300+
New London Hospital	New London	81%	(a)
Portsmouth Regional Hospital	Portsmouth	81%	300+
Elliot Hospital	Manchester	80%	300+
Mary Hitchcock Memorial Hospital	Lebanon	80%	300+
The Memorial Hospital	North Conway	80%	(a)
Concord Hospital	Concord	79%	300+
Southern Nh Medical Center	Nashua	79%	300+
Lakes Region General Hospital	Laconia	78%	300+
Parkland Medical Center	Derry	78%	300+
Saint Joseph Hospital	Nashua	78%	300+
Huggins Hospital	Wolfeboro	77%	(a)

Home Recovery Information Given

Hospital Name	City	Rate	Cases
Wentworth - Douglass Hospital	Dover	93%	300+
The Memorial Hospital	North Conway	92%	(a)

NOTE: Hospital profiles are in alphabetical order by state, then city, then hospital within the city; Rankings exclude hospitals with less than 25 cases except for patient surveys which excludes hospitals with less than 100 cases; (a) 100-299 cases; (1) The number of cases/patients is too few to report; (2) Data submitted were based on a sample of cases/patients; (3) Results are based on a shorter time period than required; (4) Data suppressed by CMS for one or more quarters; (5) Results are not available for this reporting period; (6) Fewer than 100 patients completed the HCAHPS survey; (7) No cases met the criteria for this measure; (8) The lower limit of the confidence interval cannot be calculated if the number of observed infections equals zero; (9) No data are available from the state/territory for this reporting period; (10) The scores shown reflect fewer than 50 completed surveys; (11) There were discrepancies in the data collection process; (12) This measure does not apply to this hospital for this reporting period; (13) Results cannot be calculated for this reporting period; (14) The results for this state are combined with nearby states to protect confidentiality; Please refer to the User's Guide for a full explanation of data.

Parkland Medical Center	Derry	92%	300+
Portsmouth Regional Hospital	Portsmouth	90%	300+
Southern Nh Medical Center	Nashua	90%	300+
Alice Peck Day Memorial Hospital	Lebanon	89%	300+
Cheshire Medical Center	Keene	89%	300+
Elliot Hospital	Manchester	89%	300+
Frisbie Memorial Hospital	Rochester	89%	300+
Mary Hitchcock Memorial Hospital	Lebanon	89%	300+
Monadnock Community Hospital	Peterborough	89%	300+
Exeter Hospital	Exeter	88%	300+
Lakes Region General Hospital	Laconia	88%	300+
Littleton Regional Healthcare	Littleton	88%	(a)
Speare Memorial Hospital	Plymouth	88%	300+
Androscoggin Valley Hospital	Berlin	87%	(a)
Catholic Medical Center	Manchester	87%	300+
Concord Hospital	Concord	87%	300+
Huggins Hospital	Wolfeboro	87%	(a)
Saint Joseph Hospital	Nashua	87%	300+
Valley Regional Hospital	Claremont	83%	(a)
New London Hospital	New London	81%	(a)

Hospital Given 9 or 10 on 10 Point Scale

Hospital Name	City	Rate	Cases
Exeter Hospital	Exeter	79%	300+
Wentworth - Douglass Hospital	Dover	78%	300+
Mary Hitchcock Memorial Hospital	Lebanon	77%	300+
Androscoggin Valley Hospital	Berlin	76%	(a)
Concord Hospital	Concord	76%	300+
Alice Peck Day Memorial Hospital	Lebanon	75%	300+
Monadnock Community Hospital	Peterborough	75%	300+
Southern Nh Medical Center	Nashua	74%	300+
Frisbie Memorial Hospital	Rochester	73%	300+
Saint Joseph Hospital	Nashua	73%	300+
Speare Memorial Hospital	Plymouth	73%	300+
Catholic Medical Center	Manchester	72%	300+
Cheshire Medical Center	Keene	71%	300+
Littleton Regional Healthcare	Littleton	71%	(a)
New London Hospital	New London	71%	(a)
Portsmouth Regional Hospital	Portsmouth	70%	300+
Elliot Hospital	Manchester	66%	300+
Parkland Medical Center	Derry	66%	300+
Valley Regional Hospital	Claremont	66%	(a)
Huggins Hospital	Wolfeboro	63%	(a)
Lakes Region General Hospital	Laconia	63%	300+
The Memorial Hospital	North Conway	61%	(a)

Meds 'Always' Explained Before Given

Hospital Name	City	Rate	Cases
Littleton Regional Healthcare	Littleton	73%	(a)
Speare Memorial Hospital	Plymouth	71%	300+
Wentworth - Douglass Hospital	Dover	71%	300+
Exeter Hospital	Exeter	70%	300+
Frisbie Memorial Hospital	Rochester	70%	300+
Alice Peck Day Memorial Hospital	Lebanon	68%	300+
Cheshire Medical Center	Keene	68%	300+
Androscoggin Valley Hospital	Berlin	67%	(a)
Concord Hospital	Concord	67%	300+
Monadnock Community Hospital	Peterborough	66%	300+
Parkland Medical Center	Derry	66%	300+
New London Hospital	New London	65%	(a)
Southern Nh Medical Center	Nashua	65%	300+
Catholic Medical Center	Manchester	64%	300+
Mary Hitchcock Memorial Hospital	Lebanon	64%	300+
Lakes Region General Hospital	Laconia	63%	300+
Portsmouth Regional Hospital	Portsmouth	63%	300+
Saint Joseph Hospital	Nashua	63%	300+
The Memorial Hospital	North Conway	62%	(a)
Valley Regional Hospital	Claremont	62%	(a)
Huggins Hospital	Wolfeboro	60%	(a)
Elliot Hospital	Manchester	58%	300+

Nurses 'Always' Communicated Well

Hospital Name	City	Rate	Cases
Monadnock Community Hospital	Peterborough	85%	300+
Speare Memorial Hospital	Plymouth	84%	300+
Androscoggin Valley Hospital	Berlin	83%	(a)
Cheshire Medical Center	Keene	83%	300+
Exeter Hospital	Exeter	83%	300+
Frisbie Memorial Hospital	Rochester	83%	300+
Valley Regional Hospital	Claremont	83%	(a)
Alice Peck Day Memorial Hospital	Lebanon	82%	300+
Concord Hospital	Concord	82%	300+
Saint Joseph Hospital	Nashua	82%	300+
Wentworth - Douglass Hospital	Dover	82%	300+
Catholic Medical Center	Manchester	81%	300+
Parkland Medical Center	Derry	80%	300+
Southern Nh Medical Center	Nashua	79%	300+
Mary Hitchcock Memorial Hospital	Lebanon	78%	300+
The Memorial Hospital	North Conway	78%	(a)
Portsmouth Regional Hospital	Portsmouth	78%	300+
Lakes Region General Hospital	Laconia	77%	300+
Littleton Regional Healthcare	Littleton	77%	(a)
New London Hospital	New London	77%	(a)
Huggins Hospital	Wolfeboro	76%	(a)
Elliot Hospital	Manchester	74%	300+

Pain 'Always' Well Controlled

Hospital Name	City	Rate	Cases
Androscoggin Valley Hospital	Berlin	78%	(a)
Speare Memorial Hospital	Plymouth	77%	300+
Frisbie Memorial Hospital	Rochester	76%	300+
Littleton Regional Healthcare	Littleton	76%	(a)
Exeter Hospital	Exeter	75%	300+
Monadnock Community Hospital	Peterborough	74%	300+
New London Hospital	New London	74%	(a)
Valley Regional Hospital	Claremont	74%	(a)
Cheshire Medical Center	Keene	73%	300+
Wentworth - Douglass Hospital	Dover	73%	300+
Concord Hospital	Concord	72%	300+
Lakes Region General Hospital	Laconia	72%	300+
Parkland Medical Center	Derry	72%	300+
Saint Joseph Hospital	Nashua	72%	300+
Southern Nh Medical Center	Nashua	72%	300+
Huggins Hospital	Wolfeboro	70%	(a)
Mary Hitchcock Memorial Hospital	Lebanon	70%	300+
The Memorial Hospital	North Conway	69%	(a)
Alice Peck Day Memorial Hospital	Lebanon	68%	300+
Catholic Medical Center	Manchester	68%	300+
Portsmouth Regional Hospital	Portsmouth	68%	300+
Elliot Hospital	Manchester	66%	300+

Room and Bathroom 'Always' Clean

Hospital Name	City	Rate	Cases
Speare Memorial Hospital	Plymouth	84%	300+
Wentworth - Douglass Hospital	Dover	83%	300+
Androscoggin Valley Hospital	Berlin	81%	(a)
New London Hospital	New London	81%	(a)
Frisbie Memorial Hospital	Rochester	80%	300+
Monadnock Community Hospital	Peterborough	80%	300+
Littleton Regional Healthcare	Littleton	79%	(a)
Parkland Medical Center	Derry	79%	300+
Huggins Hospital	Wolfeboro	78%	(a)
Cheshire Medical Center	Keene	77%	300+
Lakes Region General Hospital	Laconia	76%	300+
Saint Joseph Hospital	Nashua	75%	300+
Valley Regional Hospital	Claremont	75%	(a)
Southern Nh Medical Center	Nashua	74%	300+
Exeter Hospital	Exeter	73%	300+
The Memorial Hospital	North Conway	73%	(a)
Catholic Medical Center	Manchester	72%	300+
Alice Peck Day Memorial Hospital	Lebanon	71%	300+
Portsmouth Regional Hospital	Portsmouth	71%	300+
Elliot Hospital	Manchester	70%	300+
Concord Hospital	Concord	69%	300+
Mary Hitchcock Memorial Hospital	Lebanon	67%	300+

Timely Help 'Always' Received

Hospital Name	City	Rate	Cases
Monadnock Community Hospital	Peterborough	78%	300+
Speare Memorial Hospital	Plymouth	77%	300+
Frisbie Memorial Hospital	Rochester	76%	300+
Littleton Regional Healthcare	Littleton	76%	(a)
Huggins Hospital	Wolfeboro	75%	(a)
New London Hospital	New London	75%	(a)
Valley Regional Hospital	Claremont	74%	(a)
Alice Peck Day Memorial Hospital	Lebanon	72%	300+
Mary Hitchcock Memorial Hospital	Lebanon	72%	300+
Androscoggin Valley Hospital	Berlin	71%	(a)
Parkland Medical Center	Derry	70%	300+
Wentworth - Douglass Hospital	Dover	70%	300+
Catholic Medical Center	Manchester	69%	300+
Cheshire Medical Center	Keene	69%	300+
Exeter Hospital	Exeter	69%	300+
Lakes Region General Hospital	Laconia	69%	300+
Concord Hospital	Concord	68%	300+
Southern Nh Medical Center	Nashua	67%	300+
Saint Joseph Hospital	Nashua	65%	300+
The Memorial Hospital	North Conway	62%	(a)
Portsmouth Regional Hospital	Portsmouth	61%	300+
Elliot Hospital	Manchester	60%	300+

Would Definitely Recommend Hospital

Hospital Name	City	Rate	Cases
Wentworth - Douglass Hospital	Dover	84%	300+
Mary Hitchcock Memorial Hospital	Lebanon	83%	300+
Alice Peck Day Memorial Hospital	Lebanon	82%	300+
Concord Hospital	Concord	80%	300+
Monadnock Community Hospital	Peterborough	79%	300+
Catholic Medical Center	Manchester	78%	300+
Exeter Hospital	Exeter	78%	300+
Southern Nh Medical Center	Nashua	77%	300+
Androscoggin Valley Hospital	Berlin	76%	(a)
Saint Joseph Hospital	Nashua	76%	300+
Speare Memorial Hospital	Plymouth	76%	300+
Littleton Regional Healthcare	Littleton	75%	(a)
New London Hospital	New London	75%	(a)
Portsmouth Regional Hospital	Portsmouth	75%	300+
Valley Regional Hospital	Claremont	74%	(a)
Cheshire Medical Center	Keene	73%	300+
Frisbie Memorial Hospital	Rochester	72%	300+
Elliot Hospital	Manchester	71%	300+
Parkland Medical Center	Derry	69%	300+
Huggins Hospital	Wolfeboro	64%	(a)
Lakes Region General Hospital	Laconia	63%	300+
The Memorial Hospital	North Conway	62%	(a)

Use of Medical Imaging

Cardiac Imaging Stress Test before OP Surgery

Hospital Name	City	Rate	Cases
Parkland Medical Center	Derry	2.7%	258
Monadnock Community Hospital	Peterborough	3.1%	127
Concord Hospital	Concord	3.4%	712
Weeks Medical Center	Lancaster	3.4%	175
Speare Memorial Hospital	Plymouth	3.8%	158
New London Hospital	New London	4.1%	97
Mary Hitchcock Memorial Hospital	Lebanon	4.5%	1040
Catholic Medical Center	Manchester	4.6%	1142
Cheshire Medical Center	Keene	4.7%	379
Elliot Hospital	Manchester	5.0%	774
Southern Nh Medical Center	Nashua	5.0%	678
Lakes Region General Hospital	Laconia	5.3%	319
Exeter Hospital	Exeter	5.4%	534
Saint Joseph Hospital	Nashua	5.7%	438
Frisbie Memorial Hospital	Rochester	6.3%	269
Wentworth - Douglass Hospital	Dover	6.4%	468
Portsmouth Regional Hospital	Portsmouth	6.5%	339
Huggins Hospital	Wolfeboro	6.7%	119

Combination Abdominal CT Scan

Hospital Name	City	Rate	Cases
Franklin Regional Hospital	Franklin	1.2%	167
Catholic Medical Center	Manchester	1.3%	705
Cheshire Medical Center	Keene	1.3%	898
Mary Hitchcock Memorial Hospital	Lebanon	2.7%	1805
Frisbie Memorial Hospital	Rochester	3.7%	732
Valley Regional Hospital	Claremont	4.1%	171
Upper Connecticut Valley Hospital	Colebrook	4.2%	118
Speare Memorial Hospital	Plymouth	4.8%	312
Elliot Hospital	Manchester	4.9%	1088
Saint Joseph Hospital	Nashua	5.0%	741
Wentworth - Douglass Hospital	Dover	5.0%	1097
Concord Hospital	Concord	5.5%	836
Monadnock Community Hospital	Peterborough	5.8%	362
Huggins Hospital	Wolfeboro	6.3%	383
Lakes Region General Hospital	Laconia	6.3%	716
Parkland Medical Center	Derry	6.5%	321
New London Hospital	New London	7.8%	244
Southern Nh Medical Center	Nashua	8.5%	772
Portsmouth Regional Hospital	Portsmouth	9.3%	525
Exeter Hospital	Exeter	10.8%	781
Weeks Medical Center	Lancaster	35.8%	187

Combination Brain/Sinus CT Scan

Hospital Name	City	Rate	Cases
New London Hospital	New London	0.4%	243
Portsmouth Regional Hospital	Portsmouth	0.6%	530
Valley Regional Hospital	Claremont	0.8%	261
Saint Joseph Hospital	Nashua	0.9%	541
Mary Hitchcock Memorial Hospital	Lebanon	1.3%	629
Cheshire Medical Center	Keene	1.7%	599
Frisbie Memorial Hospital	Rochester	1.7%	578
Parkland Medical Center	Derry	2.2%	495
Catholic Medical Center	Manchester	2.4%	995
Southern Nh Medical Center	Nashua	2.4%	915
Concord Hospital	Concord	2.9%	957
Lakes Region General Hospital	Laconia	3.1%	737
Elliot Hospital	Manchester	3.3%	1099
Wentworth - Douglass Hospital	Dover	3.5%	779
Exeter Hospital	Exeter	3.7%	711

Combination Chest CT Scan

Hospital Name	City	Rate	Cases
Catholic Medical Center	Manchester	0.0%	397
Cheshire Medical Center	Keene	0.0%	800
Franklin Regional Hospital	Franklin	0.0%	93
Frisbie Memorial Hospital	Rochester	0.0%	666
Monadnock Community Hospital	Peterborough	0.0%	213

NOTE: Hospital profiles are in alphabetical order by state, then city, then hospital within the city; Rankings exclude hospitals with less than 25 cases except for patient surveys which excludes hospitals with less than 100 cases; (a) 100-299 cases; (1) The number of cases/patients is too few to report; (2) Data submitted were based on a sample of cases/patients; (3) Results are based on a shorter time period than required; (4) Data suppressed by CMS for one or more quarters; (5) Results are not available for this reporting period; (6) Fewer than 100 patients completed the HCAHPS survey; (7) No cases met the criteria for this measure; (8) The lower limit of the confidence interval cannot be calculated if the number of observed infections equals zero; (9) No data are available from the state/territory for this reporting period; (10) The scores shown reflect fewer than 50 completed surveys; (11) There were discrepancies in the data collection process; (12) This measure does not apply to this hospital for this reporting period; (13) Results cannot be calculated for this reporting period; (14) The results for this state are combined with nearby states to protect confidentiality; Please refer to the User's Guide for a full explanation of data.

Parkland Medical Center	Derry	0.0%	194
Portsmouth Regional Hospital	Portsmouth	0.0%	318
Saint Joseph Hospital	Nashua	0.0%	532
Speare Memorial Hospital	Plymouth	0.0%	130
Wentworth - Douglass Hospital	Dover	0.0%	1100
Elliot Hospital	Manchester	0.1%	727
Mary Hitchcock Memorial Hospital	Lebanon	0.1%	2351
Concord Hospital	Concord	0.2%	492
Lakes Region General Hospital	Laconia	0.2%	407
Southern Nh Medical Center	Nashua	0.6%	634
Exeter Hospital	Exeter	1.0%	670
Weeks Medical Center	Lancaster	1.8%	113
Huggins Hospital	Wolfeboro	2.4%	248
New London Hospital	New London	2.7%	112
Valley Regional Hospital	Claremont	3.8%	78
Upper Connecticut Valley Hospital	Colebrook	7.1%	70

Follow-up Mammogram/Ultrasound

A follow-up rate near zero may indicate missed cancer; a rate higher than 14% may mean there is unnecessary follow up.

Hospital Name	City	Rate	Cases
Weeks Medical Center	Lancaster	2.5%	278
Huggins Hospital	Wolfeboro	4.3%	678
Parkland Medical Center	Derry	4.5%	337
Cheshire Medical Center	Keene	4.9%	1737
Upper Connecticut Valley Hospital	Colebrook	4.9%	226
Exeter Hospital	Exeter	5.0%	2386
Concord Hospital	Concord	6.5%	1188
Southern Nh Medical Center	Nashua	8.1%	2382
Elliot Hospital	Manchester	8.4%	2501
Speare Memorial Hospital	Plymouth	8.6%	664
Franklin Regional Hospital	Franklin	8.7%	381
Lakes Region General Hospital	Laconia	8.9%	1945
Mary Hitchcock Memorial Hospital	Lebanon	9.4%	3149
Saint Joseph Hospital	Nashua	10.0%	2100
Catholic Medical Center	Manchester	10.2%	1622
Valley Regional Hospital	Claremont	10.4%	596
Monadnock Community Hospital	Peterborough	10.5%	849
New London Hospital	New London	10.6%	930
Portsmouth Regional Hospital	Portsmouth	13.0%	1878

Lumbar Spine MRI for Low Back Pain

Hospital Name	City	Rate	Cases
Portsmouth Regional Hospital	Portsmouth	23.9%	197
Wentworth - Douglass Hospital	Dover	28.8%	125
Catholic Medical Center	Manchester	30.3%	109
Elliot Hospital	Manchester	31.3%	265
Southern Nh Medical Center	Nashua	31.8%	151
Lakes Region General Hospital	Laconia	33.1%	154
Mary Hitchcock Memorial Hospital	Lebanon	33.2%	404
New London Hospital	New London	33.3%	48
Frisbie Memorial Hospital	Rochester	35.7%	112
Monadnock Community Hospital	Peterborough	36.0%	75
Exeter Hospital	Exeter	36.5%	200
Saint Joseph Hospital	Nashua	36.5%	115
Cheshire Medical Center	Keene	37.2%	148
Concord Hospital	Concord	38.5%	52
Speare Memorial Hospital	Plymouth	40.0%	50
Weeks Medical Center	Lancaster	42.9%	42
Huggins Hospital	Wolfeboro	48.0%	50

NOTE: Hospital profiles are in alphabetical order by state, then city, then hospital within the city; Rankings exclude hospitals with less than 25 cases except for patient surveys which excludes hospitals with less than 100 cases; (a) 100-299 cases; (1) The number of cases/patients is too few to report; (2) Data submitted were based on a sample of cases/patients; (3) Results are based on a shorter time period than required; (4) Data suppressed by CMS for one or more quarters; (5) Results are not available for this reporting period; (6) Fewer than 100 patients completed the HCAHPS survey; (7) No cases met the criteria for this measure; (8) The lower limit of the confidence interval cannot be calculated if the number of observed infections equals zero; (9) No data are available from the state/territory for this reporting period; (10) The scores shown reflect fewer than 50 completed surveys; (11) There were discrepancies in the data collection process; (12) This measure does not apply to this hospital for this reporting period; (13) Results cannot be calculated for this reporting period; (14) The results for this state are combined with nearby states to protect confidentiality; Please refer to the User's Guide for a full explanation of data.

Androscoggin Valley Hospital

59 Page Hill Road Phone: 603-752-2200
Berlin, NH 03570 Fax: 603-752-2376
E-mail: info@avhnh.com
URL: www.avhnh.com
Type: Critical Access Hospitals Emergency Services: Yes
Ownership: Voluntary non-profit - Private Beds: 92

Key Personnel:
Pediatric In-Patient Care .... Brenda Aubin, RN, BSN
Pediatric Ambulatory Care ...... Brian Beals, MD
Operating Room.............. Suzie Holland, RN
CEO/President.............. Russell G Keene
Infection Control............. Thomas Marallo, MT
Quality Assurance .... John McDowell, MD
Radiology................... Janet Sherman, RDMS, CT
Pulmonology .... Dr. Peggy M Simon

Measure	Cases	This Hosp.	State Avg.	U.S. Avg.
Blood Clot Prevention and Treatment				
Anticoagulation Overlap Therapy[5]	-	-	99%	93%
ICU Venous Thromboembolism Prophylaxis[5]	-	-	96%	92%
Incidence of Potentially Preventable VTE[5]	-	-	2%	10%
UFH with Dosages/Platelet Monitoring[5]	-	-	100%	97%
Venous Thromboembolism Prophylaxis[5]	-	-	93%	85%
Warfarin Therapy Discharge Instructions[5]	-	-	77%	75%
Chest Pain/Possible Heart Attack Care				
Aspirin Given Within 24 Hours of Arrival	-	-	99%	96%
Fibrinolytic Meds Within 30 Min. of Arrival	-	-	82%	58%
Average Time to ECG (minutes)	-	-	8	7
Average Time to Transfer (minutes)	-	-	52	60
Children's Asthma Care				
Received Home Management Plan of Care	-	-	-	88%
Received Reliever Medication	-	-	-	100%
Received Systemic Corticosteroids	-	-	-	100%
Emergency Department				
Admittance Decision Time (minutes)[5]	-	-	107	98
Head CT Results Within 45 Min. of Arrival	-	-	61%	57%
Patients Who Left ER Before Being Seen	-	-	1%	2%
Time from ER Arrival to Admit. (minutes)[5]	-	-	292	274
Time from ER Arrival to Discharge (minutes)	-	-	139	134
Time in ER Before Being Evaluated (minutes)	-	-	30	26
Time to Pain Meds for Fractures (minutes)	-	-	59	57
Heart Attack Care				
Aspirin Given at Discharge[1,3]	-	-	100%	99%
Fibrinolytic Meds Within 30 Min. of Arrival[3,7]	-	-	50%	54%
PCI Within 90 Minutes of Arrival[3,7]	-	-	95%	96%
Statin Prescribed at Discharge[3,7]	-	-	100%	98%
Heart Failure Care				
ACE Inhibitor or ARB for LVSD[1]	-	-	98%	97%
Discharge Instructions Given	32	100%	97%	94%
Evaluation of LVS Function	37	100%	100%	99%
Medicare Spending				
Medicare Spending per Patient (ratio)	-	-	1.01	0.98
Pneumonia Care				
Appropriate Initial Antibiotic Given	26	100%	97%	95%
Blood Culture Timing	15	100%	98%	98%
Pregnancy and Delivery Care				
Newborn Deliveries Scheduled Early[5]	-	-	2%	6%
Preventive Care				
Immunization for Influenza[5]	-	-	95%	90%
Immunization for Pneumonia[5]	-	-	95%	92%
Stroke Care				
Anticoagulation Therapy for Atrial Fibrillation[5]	-	-	96%	95%
Antithrombotic Therapy Timing[5]	-	-	99%	98%
Assessed for Rehabilitation[5]	-	-	96%	97%
Discharged on Antithrombotic Therapy[5]	-	-	100%	99%
Discharged on Statin Medication[5]	-	-	95%	94%
Thrombolytic Therapy Timing[5]	-	-	57%	66%
Venous Thromboembolism Prophylaxis[5]	-	-	94%	94%
Written Stroke Educational Materials Given[5]	-	-	76%	88%
Surgical Care Improvement Project				
Appropriate Beta Blocker Usage[5]	-	-	98%	98%
Appropriate VTP Within 24 Hours	63	100%	99%	98%
Controlled Postoperative Blood Glucose[3,7]	-	-	98%	97%
Perioperative Temperature Management	71	100%	100%	100%
Prophylactic Antibiotic Selection	62	100%	99%	99%
Prophylactic Antibiotic Selection (Outpatient)	-	-	99%	98%
Prophylactic Antibiotic Stopped	60	98%	98%	98%
Prophylactic Antibiotic Timing	62	100%	99%	99%
Prophylactic Antibiotic Timing (Outpatient)	-	-	98%	98%
Urinary Catheter Removal	52	100%	98%	97%
Survey of Patients' Hospital Experiences				
Area Around Room 'Always' Quiet at Night	(a)	56%	57%	61%
Doctors 'Always' Communicated Well	(a)	84%	81%	82%
Home Recovery Information Given	(a)	87%	88%	85%
Hospital Given 9 or 10 on 10 Point Scale	(a)	76%	71%	71%
Meds 'Always' Explained Before Given	(a)	67%	65%	64%
Nurses 'Always' Communicated Well	(a)	83%	80%	79%
Pain 'Always' Well Controlled	(a)	78%	72%	71%
Room and Bathroom 'Always' Clean	(a)	81%	76%	73%
Timely Help 'Always' Received	(a)	71%	70%	68%
Would Definitely Recommend Hospital	(a)	76%	74%	71%
Use of Medical Imaging				
Cardiac Imaging Stress Test before Surgery	-	-	4.7%	5.3%
Combination Abdominal CT Scan	-	-	5.6%	10.5%
Combination Brain/Sinus CT Scan	-	-	2.3%	2.7%
Combination Chest CT Scan	-	-	0.5%	2.7%
Follow-up Mammogram/Ultrasound	-	-	8.2%	8.8%
Lumbar Spine MRI for Low Back Pain	-	-	33.5%	37.2%

Valley Regional Hospital

243 Elm Street Phone: 603-542-7771
Claremont, NH 03743 Fax: 603-542-3403
URL: www.vrh.org
Type: Critical Access Hospitals Emergency Services: Yes
Ownership: Voluntary non-profit - Private Beds: 45

Key Personnel:
Chief of Medical Staff.......... Roy M Barnes
CEO/President.............. Claire Bowen
Quality Assurance .... Sandy Gee
Radiology................... Katherine F Gerke
Emergency Room .... Joseph Hagan, MD

Measure	Cases	This Hosp.	State Avg.	U.S. Avg.
Blood Clot Prevention and Treatment				
Anticoagulation Overlap Therapy[1,2]	-	-	99%	93%
ICU Venous Thromboembolism Prophylaxis[1,2]	-	-	96%	92%
Incidence of Potentially Preventable VTE[2,7]	-	-	2%	10%
UFH with Dosages/Platelet Monitoring[1,2]	-	-	100%	97%
Venous Thromboembolism Prophylaxis[2]	108	98%	93%	85%
Warfarin Therapy Discharge Instructions[1,2]	-	-	77%	75%
Chest Pain/Possible Heart Attack Care				
Aspirin Given Within 24 Hours of Arrival[5]	-	-	99%	96%
Fibrinolytic Meds Within 30 Min. of Arrival[5]	-	-	82%	58%
Average Time to ECG (minutes)[5]	-	-	8	7
Average Time to Transfer (minutes)[5]	-	-	52	60
Children's Asthma Care				
Received Home Management Plan of Care	-	-	-	88%
Received Reliever Medication	-	-	-	100%
Received Systemic Corticosteroids	-	-	-	100%
Emergency Department				
Admittance Decision Time (minutes)[5]	-	-	107	98
Head CT Results Within 45 Min. of Arrival[5]	-	-	61%	57%
Patients Who Left ER Before Being Seen[5]	-	-	1%	2%
Time from ER Arrival to Admit. (minutes)[5]	-	-	292	274
Time from ER Arrival to Discharge (minutes)[5]	-	-	139	134
Time in ER Before Being Evaluated (minutes)[5]	-	-	30	26
Time to Pain Meds for Fractures (minutes)[5]	-	-	59	57
Heart Attack Care				
Aspirin Given at Discharge[1]	-	-	100%	99%
Fibrinolytic Meds Within 30 Min. of Arrival[1]	-	-	50%	54%
PCI Within 90 Minutes of Arrival[7]	-	-	95%	96%
Statin Prescribed at Discharge[1]	-	-	100%	98%
Heart Failure Care				
ACE Inhibitor or ARB for LVSD[1]	-	-	98%	97%
Discharge Instructions Given	18	100%	97%	94%
Evaluation of LVS Function	29	97%	100%	99%
Medicare Spending				
Medicare Spending per Patient (ratio)	-	-	1.01	0.98
Pneumonia Care				
Appropriate Initial Antibiotic Given	46	96%	97%	95%
Blood Culture Timing	49	100%	98%	98%
Pregnancy and Delivery Care				
Newborn Deliveries Scheduled Early[3,7]	-	-	2%	6%
Preventive Care				
Immunization for Influenza[5]	-	-	95%	90%
Immunization for Pneumonia[5]	-	-	95%	92%
Stroke Care				
Anticoagulation Therapy for Atrial Fibrillation[1]	-	-	96%	95%
Antithrombotic Therapy Timing[1]	-	-	99%	98%
Assessed for Rehabilitation[1]	-	-	96%	97%
Discharged on Antithrombotic Therapy[1]	-	-	100%	99%
Discharged on Statin Medication[1]	-	-	95%	94%
Thrombolytic Therapy Timing[7]	-	-	57%	66%
Venous Thromboembolism Prophylaxis[1]	-	-	94%	94%
Written Stroke Educational Materials Given[1]	-	-	76%	88%
Surgical Care Improvement Project				
Appropriate Beta Blocker Usage	12	100%	98%	98%
Appropriate VTP Within 24 Hours[7]	-	-	99%	98%
Controlled Postoperative Blood Glucose[7]	-	-	98%	97%
Perioperative Temperature Management	52	100%	100%	100%
Prophylactic Antibiotic Selection[7]	-	-	99%	99%
Prophylactic Antibiotic Selection (Outpatient)	15	100%	99%	98%
Prophylactic Antibiotic Stopped[7]	-	-	98%	98%
Prophylactic Antibiotic Timing[7]	-	-	99%	99%
Prophylactic Antibiotic Timing (Outpatient)	15	100%	98%	98%
Urinary Catheter Removal	42	100%	98%	97%
Survey of Patients' Hospital Experiences				
Area Around Room 'Always' Quiet at Night	(a)	65%	57%	61%
Doctors 'Always' Communicated Well	(a)	86%	81%	82%
Home Recovery Information Given	(a)	83%	88%	85%
Hospital Given 9 or 10 on 10 Point Scale	(a)	66%	71%	71%
Meds 'Always' Explained Before Given	(a)	62%	65%	64%
Nurses 'Always' Communicated Well	(a)	83%	80%	79%
Pain 'Always' Well Controlled	(a)	74%	72%	71%
Room and Bathroom 'Always' Clean	(a)	75%	76%	73%
Timely Help 'Always' Received	(a)	74%	70%	68%
Would Definitely Recommend Hospital	(a)	74%	74%	71%
Use of Medical Imaging				
Cardiac Imaging Stress Test before Surgery[1]	-	-	4.7%	5.3%
Combination Abdominal CT Scan	171	4.1%	5.6%	10.5%
Combination Brain/Sinus CT Scan	261	0.8%	2.3%	2.7%
Combination Chest CT Scan	78	3.8%	0.5%	2.7%
Follow-up Mammogram/Ultrasound	596	10.4%	8.2%	8.8%
Lumbar Spine MRI for Low Back Pain[1]	-	-	33.5%	37.2%

Upper Connecticut Valley Hospital

181 Corliss Lane Phone: 603-237-4971
Colebrook, NH 03576 Fax: 603-237-4452
E-mail: ann.morrison@hitchcock.org
URL: www.dartmouth-hitchcock.org/ucvh
Type: Critical Access Hospitals Emergency Services: Yes
Ownership: Voluntary non-profit - Private Beds: 16

Key Personnel:
Infection Control............. Carol Bunnell, RN
Emergency Room .... Sharon Curtis, MD
Quality Assurance .... Irene Dodge
CEO/President.............. Louise A McCleery
Anesthesiology.............. Dan McClenahan, CRNA
Chief of Medical Staff.......... Robert Soucy

Measure	Cases	This Hosp.	State Avg.	U.S. Avg.
Blood Clot Prevention and Treatment				
Anticoagulation Overlap Therapy[5]	-	-	99%	93%
ICU Venous Thromboembolism Prophylaxis[5]	-	-	96%	92%
Incidence of Potentially Preventable VTE[5]	-	-	2%	10%
UFH with Dosages/Platelet Monitoring[5]	-	-	100%	97%
Venous Thromboembolism Prophylaxis[5]	-	-	93%	85%
Warfarin Therapy Discharge Instructions[5]	-	-	77%	75%
Chest Pain/Possible Heart Attack Care				
Aspirin Given Within 24 Hours of Arrival[3]	27	100%	99%	96%
Fibrinolytic Meds Within 30 Min. of Arrival[1,3]	-	-	82%	58%
Average Time to ECG (minutes)[3]	26	9	8	7
Average Time to Transfer (minutes)[3,7]	-	-	52	60

NOTE: Hospital profiles are in alphabetical order by state, then city, then hospital within the city; Rankings exclude hospitals with less than 25 cases except for patient surveys which excludes hospitals with less than 100 cases; (a) 100-299 cases; (1) The number of cases/patients is too few to report; (2) Data submitted were based on a sample of cases/patients; (3) Results are based on a shorter time period than required; (4) Data suppressed by CMS for one or more quarters; (5) Results are not available for this reporting period; (6) Fewer than 100 patients completed the HCAHPS survey; (7) No cases met the criteria for this measure; (8) The lower limit of the confidence interval cannot be calculated if the number of observed infections equals zero; (9) No data are available from the state/territory for this reporting period; (10) The scores shown reflect fewer than 50 completed surveys; (11) There were discrepancies in the data collection process; (12) This measure does not apply to this hospital for this reporting period; (13) Results cannot be calculated for this reporting period; (14) The results for this state are combined with nearby states to protect confidentiality; Please refer to the User's Guide for a full explanation of data.

Measure	Cases	This Hosp.	State Avg.	U.S. Avg.
Children's Asthma Care				
Received Home Management Plan of Care	-	-	-	88%
Received Reliever Medication	-	-	-	100%
Received Systemic Corticosteroids	-	-	-	100%
Emergency Department				
Admittance Decision Time (minutes)[5]	-	-	107	98
Head CT Results Within 45 Min. of Arrival[5]	-	-	61%	57%
Patients Who Left ER Before Being Seen[5]	-	-	1%	2%
Time from ER Arrival to Admit. (minutes)[5]	-	-	292	274
Time from ER Arrival to Discharge (minutes)[5]	-	-	139	134
Time in ER Before Being Evaluated (minutes)[5]	-	-	30	26
Time to Pain Meds for Fractures (minutes)[5]	-	-	59	57
Heart Attack Care				
Aspirin Given at Discharge[1]	-	-	100%	99%
Fibrinolytic Meds Within 30 Min. of Arrival[7]	-	-	50%	54%
PCI Within 90 Minutes of Arrival[7]	-	-	95%	96%
Statin Prescribed at Discharge[1]	-	-	100%	98%
Heart Failure Care				
ACE Inhibitor or ARB for LVSD[1]	-	-	98%	97%
Discharge Instructions Given	16	100%	97%	94%
Evaluation of LVS Function	17	88%	100%	99%
Medicare Spending				
Medicare Spending per Patient (ratio)	-	-	1.01	0.98
Pneumonia Care				
Appropriate Initial Antibiotic Given[1]	-	-	97%	95%
Blood Culture Timing[1]	-	-	98%	98%
Pregnancy and Delivery Care				
Newborn Deliveries Scheduled Early[5]	-	-	2%	6%
Preventive Care				
Immunization for Influenza[5]	-	-	95%	90%
Immunization for Pneumonia[5]	-	-	95%	92%
Stroke Care				
Anticoagulation Therapy for Atrial Fibrillation[5]	-	-	96%	95%
Antithrombotic Therapy Timing[5]	-	-	99%	98%
Assessed for Rehabilitation[5]	-	-	96%	97%
Discharged on Antithrombotic Therapy[5]	-	-	100%	99%
Discharged on Statin Medication[5]	-	-	95%	94%
Thrombolytic Therapy Timing[5]	-	-	57%	66%
Venous Thromboembolism Prophylaxis[5]	-	-	94%	94%
Written Stroke Educational Materials Given[5]	-	-	76%	88%
Surgical Care Improvement Project				
Appropriate Beta Blocker Usage[5]	-	-	98%	98%
Appropriate VTP Within 24 Hours[5]	-	-	99%	98%
Controlled Postoperative Blood Glucose[5]	-	-	98%	97%
Perioperative Temperature Management[5]	-	-	100%	100%
Prophylactic Antibiotic Selection[5]	-	-	99%	99%
Prophylactic Antibiotic Selection (Outpatient)[5]	-	-	99%	98%
Prophylactic Antibiotic Stopped[5]	-	-	98%	98%
Prophylactic Antibiotic Timing[5]	-	-	99%	99%
Prophylactic Antibiotic Timing (Outpatient)[5]	-	-	98%	98%
Urinary Catheter Removal[5]	-	-	98%	97%
Survey of Patients' Hospital Experiences				
Area Around Room 'Always' Quiet at Night[5]	-	-	57%	61%
Doctors 'Always' Communicated Well[5]	-	-	81%	82%
Home Recovery Information Given[5]	-	-	88%	85%
Hospital Given 9 or 10 on 10 Point Scale[5]	-	-	71%	71%
Meds 'Always' Explained Before Given[5]	-	-	65%	64%
Nurses 'Always' Communicated Well[5]	-	-	80%	79%
Pain 'Always' Well Controlled[5]	-	-	72%	71%
Room and Bathroom 'Always' Clean[5]	-	-	76%	73%
Timely Help 'Always' Received[5]	-	-	70%	68%
Would Definitely Recommend Hospital[5]	-	-	74%	71%
Use of Medical Imaging				
Cardiac Imaging Stress Test before Surgery[7]	-	-	4.7%	5.3%
Combination Abdominal CT Scan	118	4.2%	5.6%	10.5%
Combination Brain/Sinus CT Scan[1]	-	-	2.3%	2.7%
Combination Chest CT Scan	70	7.1%	0.5%	2.7%
Follow-up Mammogram/Ultrasound	226	4.9%	8.2%	8.8%
Lumbar Spine MRI for Low Back Pain[7]	-	-	33.5%	37.2%

Concord Hospital

250 Pleasant St
Concord, NH 03301
Phone: 603-225-2711
Fax: 603-228-7346
E-mail: karr@crhc.org
URL: www.concordhospital.org
Type: Acute Care Hospitals
Emergency Services: Yes
Ownership: Voluntary non-profit - Private
Beds: 295

Key Personnel:
Chief of Medical Staff. . . . . David F Green, MD
Quality Assurance . . . . Nancy Hacking
Emergency Room . . . . Leslie Mahoney
Operating Room. . . . . Noreen Nixon
CEO/President. . . . . Robert P. Steigmeyer
Radiology. . . . . Maureen Trombly

Measure	Cases	This Hosp.	State Avg.	U.S. Avg.
Blood Clot Prevention and Treatment				
Anticoagulation Overlap Therapy[2]	110	100%	99%	93%
ICU Venous Thromboembolism Prophylaxis[2]	50	88%	96%	92%
Incidence of Potentially Preventable VTE[1,2]	-	-	2%	10%
UFH with Dosages/Platelet Monitoring[2]	52	100%	100%	97%
Venous Thromboembolism Prophylaxis[2]	340	90%	93%	85%
Warfarin Therapy Discharge Instructions[2]	90	88%	77%	75%
Chest Pain/Possible Heart Attack Care				
Aspirin Given Within 24 Hours of Arrival[3,7]	-	-	99%	96%
Fibrinolytic Meds Within 30 Min. of Arrival[5]	-	-	82%	58%
Average Time to ECG (minutes)[3,7]	-	-	8	7
Average Time to Transfer (minutes)[5]	-	-	52	60
Children's Asthma Care				
Received Home Management Plan of Care	-	-	-	88%
Received Reliever Medication	-	-	-	100%
Received Systemic Corticosteroids	-	-	-	100%
Emergency Department				
Admittance Decision Time (minutes)[2]	493	135	107	98
Head CT Results Within 45 Min. of Arrival	19	79%	61%	57%
Patients Who Left ER Before Being Seen	46,959	2%	1%	2%
Time from ER Arrival to Admit. (minutes)[2]	505	302	292	274
Time from ER Arrival to Discharge (minutes)	277	170	139	134
Time in ER Before Being Evaluated (minutes)	364	46	30	26
Time to Pain Meds for Fractures (minutes)	108	55	59	57
Heart Attack Care				
Aspirin Given at Discharge	229	100%	100%	99%
Fibrinolytic Meds Within 30 Min. of Arrival[7]	-	-	50%	54%
PCI Within 90 Minutes of Arrival	65	95%	95%	96%
Statin Prescribed at Discharge	221	100%	100%	98%
Heart Failure Care				
ACE Inhibitor or ARB for LVSD	98	100%	98%	97%
Discharge Instructions Given	256	98%	97%	94%
Evaluation of LVS Function	334	100%	100%	99%
Medicare Spending				
Medicare Spending per Patient (ratio)	-	1.01	1.01	0.98
Pneumonia Care				
Appropriate Initial Antibiotic Given	247	98%	97%	95%
Blood Culture Timing	259	98%	98%	98%
Pregnancy and Delivery Care				
Newborn Deliveries Scheduled Early[2]	20	0%	2%	6%
Preventive Care				
Immunization for Influenza[2]	519	94%	95%	90%
Immunization for Pneumonia[2]	639	93%	95%	92%
Stroke Care				
Anticoagulation Therapy for Atrial Fibrillation[2]	16	100%	96%	95%
Antithrombotic Therapy Timing[2]	80	99%	99%	98%
Assessed for Rehabilitation[2]	89	97%	96%	97%
Discharged on Antithrombotic Therapy[2]	84	100%	100%	99%
Discharged on Statin Medication[2]	65	94%	95%	94%
Thrombolytic Therapy Timing[1,2]	-	-	57%	66%
Venous Thromboembolism Prophylaxis[2]	84	90%	94%	94%
Written Stroke Educational Materials Given[2]	50	78%	76%	88%
Surgical Care Improvement Project				
Appropriate Beta Blocker Usage[2]	151	97%	98%	98%
Appropriate VTP Within 24 Hours[2]	256	99%	99%	98%
Controlled Postoperative Blood Glucose[2]	109	97%	98%	97%
Perioperative Temperature Management[2]	345	100%	100%	100%
Prophylactic Antibiotic Selection[2]	326	99%	99%	99%
Prophylactic Antibiotic Selection (Outpatient)	421	99%	99%	98%
Prophylactic Antibiotic Stopped[2]	320	97%	98%	98%
Prophylactic Antibiotic Timing[2]	326	99%	99%	99%
Prophylactic Antibiotic Timing (Outpatient)	410	99%	98%	98%
Urinary Catheter Removal[2]	251	99%	98%	97%
Survey of Patients' Hospital Experiences				
Area Around Room 'Always' Quiet at Night	300+	52%	57%	61%
Doctors 'Always' Communicated Well	300+	79%	81%	82%
Home Recovery Information Given	300+	87%	88%	85%
Hospital Given 9 or 10 on 10 Point Scale	300+	76%	71%	71%
Meds 'Always' Explained Before Given	300+	67%	65%	64%
Nurses 'Always' Communicated Well	300+	82%	80%	79%
Pain 'Always' Well Controlled	300+	72%	72%	71%
Room and Bathroom 'Always' Clean	300+	69%	76%	73%
Timely Help 'Always' Received	300+	68%	70%	68%
Would Definitely Recommend Hospital	300+	80%	74%	71%
Use of Medical Imaging				
Cardiac Imaging Stress Test before Surgery	712	3.4%	4.7%	5.3%
Combination Abdominal CT Scan	836	5.5%	5.6%	10.5%
Combination Brain/Sinus CT Scan	957	2.9%	2.3%	2.7%
Combination Chest CT Scan	492	0.2%	0.5%	2.7%
Follow-up Mammogram/Ultrasound	1,188	6.5%	8.2%	8.8%
Lumbar Spine MRI for Low Back Pain	52	38.5%	33.5%	37.2%

Parkland Medical Center

1 Parkland Drive
Derry, NH 03038
Phone: 603-421-2100
Fax: 603-421-2111
URL: www.parklandmedicalcenter.com
Type: Acute Care Hospitals
Emergency Services: Yes
Ownership: Proprietary
Beds: 78

Key Personnel:
Cardiology . . . . Craig C Berry, MD
Cardiology . . . . Jeffery F Bleakley
Operating Room. . . . . Donald Colacchio, MD
CEO/President. . . . . Anne Jamieson
Pediatric In-Patient Care . . . . Christopher Peterson, MD
Quality Assurance . . . . Anne Sands

Measure	Cases	This Hosp.	State Avg.	U.S. Avg.
Blood Clot Prevention and Treatment				
Anticoagulation Overlap Therapy[2]	32	100%	99%	93%
ICU Venous Thromboembolism Prophylaxis[2]	49	100%	96%	92%
Incidence of Potentially Preventable VTE[1,2]	-	-	2%	10%
UFH with Dosages/Platelet Monitoring[2]	11	100%	100%	97%
Venous Thromboembolism Prophylaxis[2]	307	98%	93%	85%
Warfarin Therapy Discharge Instructions[2]	24	96%	77%	75%
Chest Pain/Possible Heart Attack Care				
Aspirin Given Within 24 Hours of Arrival[1,3]	-	-	99%	96%
Fibrinolytic Meds Within 30 Min. of Arrival[3,7]	-	-	82%	58%
Average Time to ECG (minutes)[1,3]	-	-	8	7
Average Time to Transfer (minutes)[1,3]	-	-	52	60
Children's Asthma Care				
Received Home Management Plan of Care	-	-	-	88%
Received Reliever Medication	-	-	-	100%
Received Systemic Corticosteroids	-	-	-	100%
Emergency Department				
Admittance Decision Time (minutes)[2]	659	69	107	98
Head CT Results Within 45 Min. of Arrival[1]	-	-	61%	57%
Patients Who Left ER Before Being Seen	24,321	1%	1%	2%
Time from ER Arrival to Admit. (minutes)[2]	668	237	292	274
Time from ER Arrival to Discharge (minutes)	436	122	139	134
Time in ER Before Being Evaluated (minutes)	491	13	30	26
Time to Pain Meds for Fractures (minutes)	71	36	59	57
Heart Attack Care				
Aspirin Given at Discharge	75	100%	100%	99%
Fibrinolytic Meds Within 30 Min. of Arrival[7]	-	-	50%	54%
PCI Within 90 Minutes of Arrival	15	100%	95%	96%
Statin Prescribed at Discharge	74	100%	100%	98%
Heart Failure Care				
ACE Inhibitor or ARB for LVSD	35	97%	98%	97%
Discharge Instructions Given	108	99%	97%	94%
Evaluation of LVS Function	144	100%	100%	99%
Medicare Spending				
Medicare Spending per Patient (ratio)	-	1.08	1.01	0.98
Pneumonia Care				
Appropriate Initial Antibiotic Given	86	99%	97%	95%

NOTE: Hospital profiles are in alphabetical order by state, then city, then hospital within the city; Rankings exclude hospitals with less than 25 cases except for patient surveys which excludes hospitals with less than 100 cases; (a) 100-299 cases; (1) The number of cases/patients is too few to report; (2) Data submitted were based on a sample of cases/patients; (3) Results are based on a shorter time period than required; (4) Data suppressed by CMS for one or more quarters; (5) Results are not available for this reporting period; (6) Fewer than 100 patients completed the HCAHPS survey; (7) No cases met the criteria for this measure; (8) The lower limit of the confidence interval cannot be calculated if the number of observed infections equals zero; (9) No data are available from the state/territory for this reporting period; (10) The scores shown reflect fewer than 50 completed surveys; (11) There were discrepancies in the data collection process; (12) This measure does not apply to this hospital for this reporting period; (13) Results cannot be calculated for this reporting period; (14) The results for this state are combined with nearby states to protect confidentiality; Please refer to the User's Guide for a full explanation of data.

Blood Culture Timing	148	99%	98%	98%
Pregnancy and Delivery Care				
Newborn Deliveries Scheduled Early[2]	15	0%	2%	6%
Preventive Care				
Immunization for Influenza[2]	421	98%	95%	90%
Immunization for Pneumonia[2]	552	97%	95%	92%
Stroke Care				
Anticoagulation Therapy for Atrial Fibrillation[1,2]	-	-	96%	95%
Antithrombotic Therapy Timing[2]	36	100%	99%	98%
Assessed for Rehabilitation[2]	45	98%	96%	97%
Discharged on Antithrombotic Therapy[2]	42	100%	100%	99%
Discharged on Statin Medication[2]	35	100%	95%	94%
Thrombolytic Therapy Timing[1,2]	-	-	57%	66%
Venous Thromboembolism Prophylaxis[2]	45	100%	94%	94%
Written Stroke Educational Materials Given[2]	22	100%	76%	88%
Surgical Care Improvement Project				
Appropriate Beta Blocker Usage	51	100%	98%	98%
Appropriate VTP Within 24 Hours	112	99%	99%	98%
Controlled Postoperative Blood Glucose[7]	-	-	98%	97%
Perioperative Temperature Management	167	100%	100%	100%
Prophylactic Antibiotic Selection	60	95%	99%	99%
Prophylactic Antibiotic Selection (Outpatient)	141	99%	99%	98%
Prophylactic Antibiotic Stopped	57	100%	98%	98%
Prophylactic Antibiotic Timing	60	97%	99%	99%
Prophylactic Antibiotic Timing (Outpatient)	85	99%	98%	98%
Urinary Catheter Removal	89	100%	98%	97%
Survey of Patients' Hospital Experiences				
Area Around Room 'Always' Quiet at Night	300+	61%	57%	61%
Doctors 'Always' Communicated Well	300+	78%	81%	82%
Home Recovery Information Given	300+	92%	88%	85%
Hospital Given 9 or 10 on 10 Point Scale	300+	66%	71%	71%
Meds 'Always' Explained Before Given	300+	66%	65%	64%
Nurses 'Always' Communicated Well	300+	80%	80%	79%
Pain 'Always' Well Controlled	300+	72%	72%	71%
Room and Bathroom 'Always' Clean	300+	79%	76%	73%
Timely Help 'Always' Received	300+	70%	70%	68%
Would Definitely Recommend Hospital	300+	69%	74%	71%
Use of Medical Imaging				
Cardiac Imaging Stress Test before Surgery	258	2.7%	4.7%	5.3%
Combination Abdominal CT Scan	321	6.5%	5.6%	10.5%
Combination Brain/Sinus CT Scan	495	2.2%	2.3%	2.7%
Combination Chest CT Scan	194	0.0%	0.5%	2.7%
Follow-up Mammogram/Ultrasound	337	4.5%	8.2%	8.8%
Lumbar Spine MRI for Low Back Pain[1]	-	-	33.5%	37.2%

Wentworth - Douglass Hospital

789 Central Ave
Dover, NH 03820
Phone: 603-740-2580
Fax: 603-740-2242
URL: www.wdhospital.com
Type: Acute Care Hospitals
Emergency Services: Yes
Ownership: Voluntary non-profit - Private
Beds: 178

Key Personnel:
Radiology. . . . . Bernard M Casey, MD
Emergency Room . . . . Owen MacCausland, MD
Chief of Medical Staff. . . . . James McKenna, MD
Anesthesiology. . . . . James Tobin, MD
Pediatric Ambulatory Care . . . . . . Andre Vanderzanden, MD
Pediatric In-Patient Care . . . . Andre Vanderzanden, MD

Measure	Cases	This Hosp.	State Avg.	U.S. Avg.
Blood Clot Prevention and Treatment				
Anticoagulation Overlap Therapy[2]	49	100%	99%	93%
ICU Venous Thromboembolism Prophylaxis[2]	67	91%	96%	92%
Incidence of Potentially Preventable VTE[1,2]	-	-	2%	10%
UFH with Dosages/Platelet Monitoring[2]	44	100%	100%	97%
Venous Thromboembolism Prophylaxis[2]	372	97%	93%	85%
Warfarin Therapy Discharge Instructions[2]	37	100%	77%	75%
Chest Pain/Possible Heart Attack Care				
Aspirin Given Within 24 Hours of Arrival[1,3]	-	-	99%	96%
Fibrinolytic Meds Within 30 Min. of Arrival[3,7]	-	-	82%	58%
Average Time to ECG (minutes)[1,3]	-	-	8	7
Average Time to Transfer (minutes)[3,7]	-	-	52	60
Children's Asthma Care				
Received Home Management Plan of Care	-	-	-	88%
Received Reliever Medication	-	-	-	100%
Received Systemic Corticosteroids	-	-	-	100%
Emergency Department				
Admittance Decision Time (minutes)[2]	425	135	107	98
Head CT Results Within 45 Min. of Arrival	18	67%	61%	57%
Patients Who Left ER Before Being Seen	40,606	0%	1%	2%
Time from ER Arrival to Admit. (minutes)[2]	593	289	292	274
Time from ER Arrival to Discharge (minutes)	363	123	139	134
Time in ER Before Being Evaluated (minutes)	372	21	30	26
Time to Pain Meds for Fractures (minutes)	97	40	59	57
Heart Attack Care				
Aspirin Given at Discharge	125	100%	100%	99%
Fibrinolytic Meds Within 30 Min. of Arrival[7]	-	-	50%	54%
PCI Within 90 Minutes of Arrival	22	95%	95%	96%
Statin Prescribed at Discharge	124	98%	100%	98%
Heart Failure Care				
ACE Inhibitor or ARB for LVSD	46	98%	98%	97%
Discharge Instructions Given	171	86%	97%	94%
Evaluation of LVS Function	216	100%	100%	99%
Medicare Spending				
Medicare Spending per Patient (ratio)	-	1.03	1.01	0.98
Pneumonia Care				
Appropriate Initial Antibiotic Given[2]	100	95%	97%	95%
Blood Culture Timing[2]	182	97%	98%	98%
Pregnancy and Delivery Care				
Newborn Deliveries Scheduled Early	44	5%	2%	6%
Preventive Care				
Immunization for Influenza[2]	533	98%	95%	90%
Immunization for Pneumonia[2]	696	96%	95%	92%
Stroke Care				
Anticoagulation Therapy for Atrial Fibrillation[1]	-	-	96%	95%
Antithrombotic Therapy Timing	54	93%	99%	98%
Assessed for Rehabilitation	58	100%	96%	97%
Discharged on Antithrombotic Therapy	53	100%	100%	99%
Discharged on Statin Medication	41	100%	95%	94%
Thrombolytic Therapy Timing[1]	-	-	57%	66%
Venous Thromboembolism Prophylaxis	57	98%	94%	94%
Written Stroke Educational Materials Given	30	83%	76%	88%
Surgical Care Improvement Project				
Appropriate Beta Blocker Usage[2]	125	98%	98%	98%
Appropriate VTP Within 24 Hours[2]	316	94%	99%	98%
Controlled Postoperative Blood Glucose[2,7]	-	-	98%	97%
Perioperative Temperature Management[2]	396	100%	100%	100%
Prophylactic Antibiotic Selection[2]	276	99%	99%	99%
Prophylactic Antibiotic Selection (Outpatient)	300	99%	99%	98%
Prophylactic Antibiotic Stopped[2]	273	98%	98%	98%
Prophylactic Antibiotic Timing[2]	276	99%	99%	99%
Prophylactic Antibiotic Timing (Outpatient)	300	99%	98%	98%
Urinary Catheter Removal[2]	283	98%	98%	97%
Survey of Patients' Hospital Experiences				
Area Around Room 'Always' Quiet at Night	300+	60%	57%	61%
Doctors 'Always' Communicated Well	300+	83%	81%	82%
Home Recovery Information Given	300+	93%	88%	85%
Hospital Given 9 or 10 on 10 Point Scale	300+	78%	71%	71%
Meds 'Always' Explained Before Given	300+	71%	65%	64%
Nurses 'Always' Communicated Well	300+	82%	80%	79%
Pain 'Always' Well Controlled	300+	73%	72%	71%
Room and Bathroom 'Always' Clean	300+	83%	76%	73%
Timely Help 'Always' Received	300+	70%	70%	68%
Would Definitely Recommend Hospital	300+	84%	74%	71%
Use of Medical Imaging				
Cardiac Imaging Stress Test before Surgery	468	6.4%	4.7%	5.3%
Combination Abdominal CT Scan	1,097	5.0%	5.6%	10.5%
Combination Brain/Sinus CT Scan	779	3.5%	2.3%	2.7%
Combination Chest CT Scan	1,100	0.0%	0.5%	2.7%
Follow-up Mammogram/Ultrasound[7]	-	-	8.2%	8.8%
Lumbar Spine MRI for Low Back Pain	125	28.8%	33.5%	37.2%

Exeter Hospital

5 Alumni Drive
Exeter, NH 03833
Phone: 603-778-7311
Fax: 603-778-6592
URL: www.exeterhospital.com
Type: Acute Care Hospitals
Emergency Services: Yes
Ownership: Voluntary non-profit - Private
Beds: 100

Key Personnel:
CEO/President. . . . . Kevin Callahan
Quality Assurance . . . . Lori Chabot
Emergency Room . . . . Mark Josephs, MD
Operating Room. . . . . Sheryl LaPlume
Pediatric In-Patient Care . . . . Steve Loh, MD
Pediatric Ambulatory Care . . . . . . Gregory Prazar, MD

Measure	Cases	This Hosp.	State Avg.	U.S. Avg.
Blood Clot Prevention and Treatment				
Anticoagulation Overlap Therapy[2]	36	94%	99%	93%
ICU Venous Thromboembolism Prophylaxis[2]	48	96%	96%	92%
Incidence of Potentially Preventable VTE[1,2]	-	-	2%	10%
UFH with Dosages/Platelet Monitoring[2]	15	93%	100%	97%
Venous Thromboembolism Prophylaxis[2]	333	98%	93%	85%
Warfarin Therapy Discharge Instructions[2]	35	31%	77%	75%
Chest Pain/Possible Heart Attack Care				
Aspirin Given Within 24 Hours of Arrival[1,3]	-	-	99%	96%
Fibrinolytic Meds Within 30 Min. of Arrival[5]	-	-	82%	58%
Average Time to ECG (minutes)[1,3]	-	-	8	7
Average Time to Transfer (minutes)[5]	-	-	52	60
Children's Asthma Care				
Received Home Management Plan of Care	-	-	-	88%
Received Reliever Medication	-	-	-	100%
Received Systemic Corticosteroids	-	-	-	100%
Emergency Department				
Admittance Decision Time (minutes)[2]	774	94	107	98
Head CT Results Within 45 Min. of Arrival	18	44%	61%	57%
Patients Who Left ER Before Being Seen	31,963	2%	1%	2%
Time from ER Arrival to Admit. (minutes)[2]	784	317	292	274
Time from ER Arrival to Discharge (minutes)	382	184	139	134
Time in ER Before Being Evaluated (minutes)	313	90	30	26
Time to Pain Meds for Fractures (minutes)	152	79	59	57
Heart Attack Care				
Aspirin Given at Discharge	131	100%	100%	99%
Fibrinolytic Meds Within 30 Min. of Arrival[7]	-	-	50%	54%
PCI Within 90 Minutes of Arrival	36	97%	95%	96%
Statin Prescribed at Discharge	119	99%	100%	98%
Heart Failure Care				
ACE Inhibitor or ARB for LVSD	47	94%	98%	97%
Discharge Instructions Given	141	100%	97%	94%
Evaluation of LVS Function	198	100%	100%	99%
Medicare Spending				
Medicare Spending per Patient (ratio)	-	1.00	1.01	0.98
Pneumonia Care				
Appropriate Initial Antibiotic Given	111	98%	97%	95%
Blood Culture Timing	198	98%	98%	98%
Pregnancy and Delivery Care				
Newborn Deliveries Scheduled Early	32	6%	2%	6%
Preventive Care				
Immunization for Influenza[2]	520	88%	95%	90%
Immunization for Pneumonia[2]	710	94%	95%	92%
Stroke Care				
Anticoagulation Therapy for Atrial Fibrillation[1]	-	-	96%	95%
Antithrombotic Therapy Timing	44	100%	99%	98%
Assessed for Rehabilitation	46	96%	96%	97%
Discharged on Antithrombotic Therapy	42	100%	100%	99%
Discharged on Statin Medication	32	88%	95%	94%
Thrombolytic Therapy Timing	17	0%	57%	66%
Venous Thromboembolism Prophylaxis	41	100%	94%	94%
Written Stroke Educational Materials Given	28	4%	76%	88%
Surgical Care Improvement Project				
Appropriate Beta Blocker Usage	150	95%	98%	98%
Appropriate VTP Within 24 Hours	392	98%	99%	98%
Controlled Postoperative Blood Glucose[7]	-	-	98%	97%
Perioperative Temperature Management	458	100%	100%	100%
Prophylactic Antibiotic Selection	306	99%	99%	99%
Prophylactic Antibiotic Selection (Outpatient)	100	98%	99%	98%
Prophylactic Antibiotic Stopped	302	100%	98%	98%

NOTE: Hospital profiles are in alphabetical order by state, then city, then hospital within the city; Rankings exclude hospitals with less than 25 cases except for patient surveys which excludes hospitals with less than 100 cases; (a) 100-299 cases; (1) The number of cases/patients is too few to report; (2) Data submitted were based on a sample of cases/patients; (3) Results are based on a shorter time period than required; (4) Data suppressed by CMS for one or more quarters; (5) Results are not available for this reporting period; (6) Fewer than 100 patients completed the HCAHPS survey; (7) No cases met the criteria for this measure; (8) The lower limit of the confidence interval cannot be calculated if the number of observed infections equals zero; (9) No data are available from the state/territory for this reporting period; (10) The scores shown reflect fewer than 50 completed surveys; (11) There were discrepancies in the data collection process; (12) This measure does not apply to this hospital for this reporting period; (13) Results cannot be calculated for this reporting period; (14) The results for this state are combined with nearby states to protect confidentiality; Please refer to the User's Guide for a full explanation of data.

Measure	Cases	This Hosp.	State Avg.	U.S. Avg.
Prophylactic Antibiotic Timing	306	99%	99%	99%
Prophylactic Antibiotic Timing (Outpatient)	101	96%	98%	98%
Urinary Catheter Removal	139	94%	98%	97%
Survey of Patients' Hospital Experiences				
Area Around Room 'Always' Quiet at Night	300+	58%	57%	61%
Doctors 'Always' Communicated Well	300+	81%	81%	82%
Home Recovery Information Given	300+	88%	88%	85%
Hospital Given 9 or 10 on 10 Point Scale	300+	79%	71%	71%
Meds 'Always' Explained Before Given	300+	70%	65%	64%
Nurses 'Always' Communicated Well	300+	83%	80%	79%
Pain 'Always' Well Controlled	300+	75%	72%	71%
Room and Bathroom 'Always' Clean	300+	73%	76%	73%
Timely Help 'Always' Received	300+	69%	70%	68%
Would Definitely Recommend Hospital	300+	78%	74%	71%
Use of Medical Imaging				
Cardiac Imaging Stress Test before Surgery	534	5.4%	4.7%	5.3%
Combination Abdominal CT Scan	781	10.8%	5.6%	10.5%
Combination Brain/Sinus CT Scan	711	3.7%	2.3%	2.7%
Combination Chest CT Scan	670	1.0%	0.5%	2.7%
Follow-up Mammogram/Ultrasound	2,386	5.0%	8.2%	8.8%
Lumbar Spine MRI for Low Back Pain	200	36.5%	33.5%	37.2%

Franklin Regional Hospital

15 Aiken Avenue
Franklin, NH 03235
Phone: 603-934-2060
Fax: 603-934-4616
E-mail: info@lrgh.org
URL: www.lrgh.org
Type: Critical Access Hospitals
Emergency Services: Yes
Ownership: Voluntary non-profit - Private
Beds: 25

Key Personnel:
Radiology. . . . . Robert C Andrews, MD
CEO/President. . . . . Tom Clearmont
Quality Assurance . . . . Kathy Fuller
Infection Control. . . . . Marcia Hansen
Operating Room. . . . . Virginia McCabe-Crum, RN
Intensive Care Unit. . . . . Marilyn Minichiello, RN
Emergency Room . . . . Paul Racicot, MD
Chief of Medical Staff. . . . . Peter Walkley

Measure	Cases	This Hosp.	State Avg.	U.S. Avg.
Blood Clot Prevention and Treatment				
Anticoagulation Overlap Therapy[1,2]	-	-	99%	93%
ICU Venous Thromboembolism Prophylaxis[2]	24	96%	96%	92%
Incidence of Potentially Preventable VTE[2,7]	-	-	2%	10%
UFH with Dosages/Platelet Monitoring[1,2]	-	-	100%	97%
Venous Thromboembolism Prophylaxis[2]	81	94%	93%	85%
Warfarin Therapy Discharge Instructions[1,2]	-	-	77%	75%
Chest Pain/Possible Heart Attack Care				
Aspirin Given Within 24 Hours of Arrival	17	100%	99%	96%
Fibrinolytic Meds Within 30 Min. of Arrival[7]	-	-	82%	58%
Average Time to ECG (minutes)	17	3	8	7
Average Time to Transfer (minutes)[1]	-	-	52	60
Children's Asthma Care				
Received Home Management Plan of Care	-	-	-	88%
Received Reliever Medication	-	-	-	100%
Received Systemic Corticosteroids	-	-	-	100%
Emergency Department				
Admittance Decision Time (minutes)[2]	296	70	107	98
Head CT Results Within 45 Min. of Arrival[1]	-	-	61%	57%
Patients Who Left ER Before Being Seen	10,936	2%	1%	2%
Time from ER Arrival to Admit. (minutes)[2]	298	280	292	274
Time from ER Arrival to Discharge (minutes)	372	100	139	134
Time in ER Before Being Evaluated (minutes)	406	30	30	26
Time to Pain Meds for Fractures (minutes)	31	55	59	57
Heart Attack Care				
Aspirin Given at Discharge[1,2]	-	-	100%	99%
Fibrinolytic Meds Within 30 Min. of Arrival[2,7]	-	-	50%	54%
PCI Within 90 Minutes of Arrival[2,7]	-	-	95%	96%
Statin Prescribed at Discharge[1,2]	-	-	100%	98%
Heart Failure Care				
ACE Inhibitor or ARB for LVSD[1,2]	-	-	98%	97%
Discharge Instructions Given[1,2]	-	-	97%	94%
Evaluation of LVS Function[2]	17	88%	100%	99%
Medicare Spending				
Medicare Spending per Patient (ratio)	-	-	1.01	0.98
Pneumonia Care				
Appropriate Initial Antibiotic Given[2]	27	85%	97%	95%
Blood Culture Timing[2]	39	100%	98%	98%
Pregnancy and Delivery Care				
Newborn Deliveries Scheduled Early[7]	-	-	2%	6%
Preventive Care				
Immunization for Influenza[2]	232	97%	95%	90%
Immunization for Pneumonia[2]	357	99%	95%	92%
Stroke Care				
Anticoagulation Therapy for Atrial Fibrillation[1,2]	-	-	96%	95%
Antithrombotic Therapy Timing[1,2]	-	-	99%	98%
Assessed for Rehabilitation[1,2]	-	-	96%	97%
Discharged on Antithrombotic Therapy[1,2]	-	-	100%	99%
Discharged on Statin Medication[1,2]	-	-	95%	94%
Thrombolytic Therapy Timing[1,2]	-	-	57%	66%
Venous Thromboembolism Prophylaxis[2]	13	100%	94%	94%
Written Stroke Educational Materials Given[1,2]	-	-	76%	88%
Surgical Care Improvement Project				
Appropriate Beta Blocker Usage[1,3]	-	-	98%	98%
Appropriate VTP Within 24 Hours[1,3]	-	-	99%	98%
Controlled Postoperative Blood Glucose[3,7]	-	-	98%	97%
Perioperative Temperature Management[1,3]	-	-	100%	100%
Prophylactic Antibiotic Selection[1,3]	-	-	99%	99%
Prophylactic Antibiotic Selection (Outpatient)[1,3]	-	-	99%	98%
Prophylactic Antibiotic Stopped[1,3]	-	-	98%	98%
Prophylactic Antibiotic Timing[1,3]	-	-	99%	99%
Prophylactic Antibiotic Timing (Outpatient)[1,3]	-	-	98%	98%
Urinary Catheter Removal[1,3]	-	-	98%	97%
Survey of Patients' Hospital Experiences				
Area Around Room 'Always' Quiet at Night[6]	<100	51%	57%	61%
Doctors 'Always' Communicated Well[6]	<100	66%	81%	82%
Home Recovery Information Given[6]	<100	86%	88%	85%
Hospital Given 9 or 10 on 10 Point Scale[6]	<100	58%	71%	71%
Meds 'Always' Explained Before Given[6]	<100	51%	65%	64%
Nurses 'Always' Communicated Well[6]	<100	73%	80%	79%
Pain 'Always' Well Controlled[6]	<100	72%	72%	71%
Room and Bathroom 'Always' Clean[6]	<100	80%	76%	73%
Timely Help 'Always' Received[6]	<100	57%	70%	68%
Would Definitely Recommend Hospital[6]	<100	56%	74%	71%
Use of Medical Imaging				
Cardiac Imaging Stress Test before Surgery[1]	-	-	4.7%	5.3%
Combination Abdominal CT Scan	167	1.2%	5.6%	10.5%
Combination Brain/Sinus CT Scan[1]	-	-	2.3%	2.7%
Combination Chest CT Scan	93	0.0%	0.5%	2.7%
Follow-up Mammogram/Ultrasound	381	8.7%	8.2%	8.8%
Lumbar Spine MRI for Low Back Pain[1]	-	-	33.5%	37.2%

Cheshire Medical Center

580 Court Street
Keene, NH 03431
Phone: 603-354-5400
Fax: 603-354-6519
URL: www.cheshire-med.com
Type: Acute Care Hospitals
Emergency Services: Yes
Ownership: Voluntary non-profit - Private
Beds: 169

Key Personnel:
Operating Room. . . . . James Bowden
Chief of Medical Staff. . . . . Don Caruso
CEO/President. . . . . Arthur Nichols
Emergency Room . . . . Cheryl Pinney
Coronary Care . . . . Carl Szot
Chair/CEO . . . . Gregg Tewksbury

Measure	Cases	This Hosp.	State Avg.	U.S. Avg.
Blood Clot Prevention and Treatment				
Anticoagulation Overlap Therapy[2]	30	100%	99%	93%
ICU Venous Thromboembolism Prophylaxis[2]	45	100%	96%	92%
Incidence of Potentially Preventable VTE[1,2]	-	-	2%	10%
UFH with Dosages/Platelet Monitoring[2]	15	100%	100%	97%
Venous Thromboembolism Prophylaxis[2]	233	89%	93%	85%
Warfarin Therapy Discharge Instructions[2]	25	100%	77%	75%
Chest Pain/Possible Heart Attack Care				
Aspirin Given Within 24 Hours of Arrival	89	100%	99%	96%
Fibrinolytic Meds Within 30 Min. of Arrival	12	92%	82%	58%
Average Time to ECG (minutes)	93	7	8	7
Average Time to Transfer (minutes)[7]	-	-	52	60
Children's Asthma Care				
Received Home Management Plan of Care	-	-	-	88%
Received Reliever Medication	-	-	-	100%
Received Systemic Corticosteroids	-	-	-	100%
Emergency Department				
Admittance Decision Time (minutes)[2]	386	200	107	98
Head CT Results Within 45 Min. of Arrival[1]	-	-	61%	57%
Patients Who Left ER Before Being Seen	27,033	2%	1%	2%
Time from ER Arrival to Admit. (minutes)[2]	386	358	292	274
Time from ER Arrival to Discharge (minutes)	372	131	139	134
Time in ER Before Being Evaluated (minutes)	407	38	30	26
Time to Pain Meds for Fractures (minutes)	65	58	59	57
Heart Attack Care				
Aspirin Given at Discharge	17	100%	100%	99%
Fibrinolytic Meds Within 30 Min. of Arrival[1]	-	-	50%	54%
PCI Within 90 Minutes of Arrival[7]	-	-	95%	96%
Statin Prescribed at Discharge	17	100%	100%	98%
Heart Failure Care				
ACE Inhibitor or ARB for LVSD	20	100%	98%	97%
Discharge Instructions Given	65	100%	97%	94%
Evaluation of LVS Function	89	100%	100%	99%
Medicare Spending				
Medicare Spending per Patient (ratio)	-	0.99	1.01	0.98
Pneumonia Care				
Appropriate Initial Antibiotic Given[2]	70	100%	97%	95%
Blood Culture Timing[2]	136	99%	98%	98%
Pregnancy and Delivery Care				
Newborn Deliveries Scheduled Early[1]	-	-	2%	6%
Preventive Care				
Immunization for Influenza[2]	299	98%	95%	90%
Immunization for Pneumonia[2]	371	98%	95%	92%
Stroke Care				
Anticoagulation Therapy for Atrial Fibrillation[1]	-	-	96%	95%
Antithrombotic Therapy Timing	30	100%	99%	98%
Assessed for Rehabilitation	30	100%	96%	97%
Discharged on Antithrombotic Therapy	29	100%	100%	99%
Discharged on Statin Medication	24	50%	95%	94%
Thrombolytic Therapy Timing[7]	-	-	57%	66%
Venous Thromboembolism Prophylaxis	30	67%	94%	94%
Written Stroke Educational Materials Given	11	73%	76%	88%
Surgical Care Improvement Project				
Appropriate Beta Blocker Usage	69	100%	98%	98%
Appropriate VTP Within 24 Hours	230	95%	99%	98%
Controlled Postoperative Blood Glucose[7]	-	-	98%	97%
Perioperative Temperature Management	258	99%	100%	100%
Prophylactic Antibiotic Selection	197	100%	99%	99%
Prophylactic Antibiotic Selection (Outpatient)	116	100%	99%	98%
Prophylactic Antibiotic Stopped	196	98%	98%	98%
Prophylactic Antibiotic Timing	197	99%	99%	99%
Prophylactic Antibiotic Timing (Outpatient)	83	99%	98%	98%
Urinary Catheter Removal	186	100%	98%	97%
Survey of Patients' Hospital Experiences				
Area Around Room 'Always' Quiet at Night	300+	51%	57%	61%
Doctors 'Always' Communicated Well	300+	83%	81%	82%
Home Recovery Information Given	300+	89%	88%	85%
Hospital Given 9 or 10 on 10 Point Scale	300+	71%	71%	71%
Meds 'Always' Explained Before Given	300+	68%	65%	64%
Nurses 'Always' Communicated Well	300+	83%	80%	79%
Pain 'Always' Well Controlled	300+	73%	72%	71%
Room and Bathroom 'Always' Clean	300+	77%	76%	73%
Timely Help 'Always' Received	300+	69%	70%	68%
Would Definitely Recommend Hospital	300+	73%	74%	71%
Use of Medical Imaging				
Cardiac Imaging Stress Test before Surgery	379	4.7%	4.7%	5.3%
Combination Abdominal CT Scan	898	1.3%	5.6%	10.5%
Combination Brain/Sinus CT Scan	599	1.7%	2.3%	2.7%
Combination Chest CT Scan	800	0.0%	0.5%	2.7%
Follow-up Mammogram/Ultrasound	1,737	4.9%	8.2%	8.8%
Lumbar Spine MRI for Low Back Pain	148	37.2%	33.5%	37.2%

NOTE: Hospital profiles are in alphabetical order by state, then city, then hospital within the city; Rankings exclude hospitals with less than 25 cases except for patient surveys which excludes hospitals with less than 100 cases; (a) 100-299 cases; (1) The number of cases/patients is too few to report; (2) Data submitted were based on a sample of cases/patients; (3) Results are based on a shorter time period than required; (4) Data suppressed by CMS for one or more quarters; (5) Results are not available for this reporting period; (6) Fewer than 100 patients completed the HCAHPS survey; (7) No cases met the criteria for this measure; (8) The lower limit of the confidence interval cannot be calculated if the number of observed infections equals zero; (9) No data are available from the state/territory for this reporting period; (10) The scores shown reflect fewer than 50 completed surveys; (11) There were discrepancies in the data collection process; (12) This measure does not apply to this hospital for this reporting period; (13) Results cannot be calculated for this reporting period; (14) The results for this state are combined with nearby states to protect confidentiality; Please refer to the User's Guide for a full explanation of data.

Lakes Region General Hospital

80 Highland St Phone: 603-524-3211
Laconia, NH 03246 Fax: 603-527-2887
URL: www.lrgh.org
Type: Acute Care Hospitals Emergency Services: Yes
Ownership: Voluntary non-profit - Private Beds: 143

Key Personnel:
Radiology. . . . . Robert C Andrews
Operating Room. . . . . Alan Awrich, RN
Emergency Room . . . . Andre Beauboeuf
Infection Control. . . . . Darlene Burrows, RN
CEO/President. . . . . Thomas Clairmont
Chairman/CEO . . . . Scott R Clarenbach
Chief of Medical Staff. . . . . Peter Doane, MD

Measure	Cases	This Hosp.	State Avg.	U.S. Avg.
Blood Clot Prevention and Treatment				
Anticoagulation Overlap Therapy[2]	55	100%	99%	93%
ICU Venous Thromboembolism Prophylaxis[2]	92	93%	96%	92%
Incidence of Potentially Preventable VTE[1,2]	-	-	2%	10%
UFH with Dosages/Platelet Monitoring[2]	46	100%	100%	97%
Venous Thromboembolism Prophylaxis[2]	312	89%	93%	85%
Warfarin Therapy Discharge Instructions[2]	36	61%	77%	75%
Chest Pain/Possible Heart Attack Care				
Aspirin Given Within 24 Hours of Arrival	99	97%	99%	96%
Fibrinolytic Meds Within 30 Min. of Arrival[1]	-	-	82%	58%
Average Time to ECG (minutes)	100	10	8	7
Average Time to Transfer (minutes)	17	42	52	60
Children's Asthma Care				
Received Home Management Plan of Care	-	-	-	88%
Received Reliever Medication	-	-	-	100%
Received Systemic Corticosteroids	-	-	-	100%
Emergency Department				
Admittance Decision Time (minutes)[2]	489	95	107	98
Head CT Results Within 45 Min. of Arrival[1]	-	-	61%	57%
Patients Who Left ER Before Being Seen	21,715	2%	1%	2%
Time from ER Arrival to Admit. (minutes)[2]	528	354	292	274
Time from ER Arrival to Discharge (minutes)	322	173	139	134
Time in ER Before Being Evaluated (minutes)	344	48	30	26
Time to Pain Meds for Fractures (minutes)	108	67	59	57
Heart Attack Care				
Aspirin Given at Discharge[1,2]	-	-	100%	99%
Fibrinolytic Meds Within 30 Min. of Arrival[2,7]	-	-	50%	54%
PCI Within 90 Minutes of Arrival[2,7]	-	-	95%	96%
Statin Prescribed at Discharge[1,2]	-	-	100%	98%
Heart Failure Care				
ACE Inhibitor or ARB for LVSD[2]	34	97%	98%	97%
Discharge Instructions Given[2]	73	90%	97%	94%
Evaluation of LVS Function[2]	122	100%	100%	99%
Medicare Spending				
Medicare Spending per Patient (ratio)	-	1.03	1.01	0.98
Pneumonia Care				
Appropriate Initial Antibiotic Given[2]	60	97%	97%	95%
Blood Culture Timing[2]	98	98%	98%	98%
Pregnancy and Delivery Care				
Newborn Deliveries Scheduled Early	33	0%	2%	6%
Preventive Care				
Immunization for Influenza[2]	385	94%	95%	90%
Immunization for Pneumonia[2]	561	96%	95%	92%
Stroke Care				
Anticoagulation Therapy for Atrial Fibrillation[1,2]	-	-	96%	95%
Antithrombotic Therapy Timing[2]	50	100%	99%	98%
Assessed for Rehabilitation[2]	48	94%	96%	97%
Discharged on Antithrombotic Therapy[2]	48	100%	100%	99%
Discharged on Statin Medication[2]	39	97%	95%	94%
Thrombolytic Therapy Timing[1,2]	-	-	57%	66%
Venous Thromboembolism Prophylaxis[2]	53	89%	94%	94%
Written Stroke Educational Materials Given[2]	23	13%	76%	88%
Surgical Care Improvement Project				
Appropriate Beta Blocker Usage[2]	148	99%	98%	98%
Appropriate VTP Within 24 Hours[2]	371	98%	99%	98%
Controlled Postoperative Blood Glucose[2,7]	-	-	98%	97%
Perioperative Temperature Management[2]	455	100%	100%	100%
Prophylactic Antibiotic Selection[2]	272	100%	99%	99%
Prophylactic Antibiotic Selection (Outpatient)	148	100%	99%	98%
Prophylactic Antibiotic Stopped[2]	267	100%	98%	98%
Prophylactic Antibiotic Timing[2]	272	96%	99%	99%
Prophylactic Antibiotic Timing (Outpatient)	150	97%	98%	98%
Urinary Catheter Removal[2]	309	98%	98%	97%
Survey of Patients' Hospital Experiences				
Area Around Room 'Always' Quiet at Night	300+	61%	57%	61%
Doctors 'Always' Communicated Well	300+	78%	81%	82%
Home Recovery Information Given	300+	88%	88%	85%
Hospital Given 9 or 10 on 10 Point Scale	300+	63%	71%	71%
Meds 'Always' Explained Before Given	300+	63%	65%	64%
Nurses 'Always' Communicated Well	300+	77%	80%	79%
Pain 'Always' Well Controlled	300+	72%	72%	71%
Room and Bathroom 'Always' Clean	300+	76%	76%	73%
Timely Help 'Always' Received	300+	69%	70%	68%
Would Definitely Recommend Hospital	300+	63%	74%	71%
Use of Medical Imaging				
Cardiac Imaging Stress Test before Surgery	319	5.3%	4.7%	5.3%
Combination Abdominal CT Scan	716	6.3%	5.6%	10.5%
Combination Brain/Sinus CT Scan	737	3.1%	2.3%	2.7%
Combination Chest CT Scan	407	0.2%	0.5%	2.7%
Follow-up Mammogram/Ultrasound	1,945	8.9%	8.2%	8.8%
Lumbar Spine MRI for Low Back Pain	154	33.1%	33.5%	37.2%

Weeks Medical Center

173 Middle Street Phone: 603-788-4911
Lancaster, NH 03584 Fax: 603-788-5027
URL: www.weeks.hitchcock.org
Type: Critical Access Hospitals Emergency Services: Yes
Ownership: Voluntary non-profit - Private Beds: 25

Key Personnel:
Emergency Room . . . . John Dege, MD
Intensive Care Unit. . . . . Chandre Engelbert
CEO/President. . . . . Scott W Howe
Chief of Medical Staff. . . . . Jeffrey Johnson, MD
Anesthesiology. . . . . Donna Walker, CNE
Radiology. . . . . Russel S Williams

Measure	Cases	This Hosp.	State Avg.	U.S. Avg.
Blood Clot Prevention and Treatment				
Anticoagulation Overlap Therapy[5]	-	-	99%	93%
ICU Venous Thromboembolism Prophylaxis[5]	-	-	96%	92%
Incidence of Potentially Preventable VTE[5]	-	-	2%	10%
UFH with Dosages/Platelet Monitoring[5]	-	-	100%	97%
Venous Thromboembolism Prophylaxis[5]	-	-	93%	85%
Warfarin Therapy Discharge Instructions[5]	-	-	77%	75%
Chest Pain/Possible Heart Attack Care				
Aspirin Given Within 24 Hours of Arrival[3]	17	100%	99%	96%
Fibrinolytic Meds Within 30 Min. of Arrival[1,3]	-	-	82%	58%
Average Time to ECG (minutes)[3]	17	9	8	7
Average Time to Transfer (minutes)[3,7]	-	-	52	60
Children's Asthma Care				
Received Home Management Plan of Care	-	-	-	88%
Received Reliever Medication	-	-	-	100%
Received Systemic Corticosteroids	-	-	-	100%
Emergency Department				
Admittance Decision Time (minutes)[5]	-	-	107	98
Head CT Results Within 45 Min. of Arrival[5]	-	-	61%	57%
Patients Who Left ER Before Being Seen[5]	-	-	1%	2%
Time from ER Arrival to Admit. (minutes)[5]	-	-	292	274
Time from ER Arrival to Discharge (minutes)[5]	-	-	139	134
Time in ER Before Being Evaluated (minutes)[5]	-	-	30	26
Time to Pain Meds for Fractures (minutes)[5]	-	-	59	57
Heart Attack Care				
Aspirin Given at Discharge	11	100%	100%	99%
Fibrinolytic Meds Within 30 Min. of Arrival[7]	-	-	50%	54%
PCI Within 90 Minutes of Arrival[7]	-	-	95%	96%
Statin Prescribed at Discharge[1]	-	-	100%	98%
Heart Failure Care				
ACE Inhibitor or ARB for LVSD[1]	-	-	98%	97%
Discharge Instructions Given[1]	-	-	97%	94%
Evaluation of LVS Function	16	100%	100%	99%
Medicare Spending				
Medicare Spending per Patient (ratio)	-	-	1.01	0.98
Pneumonia Care				
Appropriate Initial Antibiotic Given	18	100%	97%	95%
Blood Culture Timing	18	94%	98%	98%
Pregnancy and Delivery Care				
Newborn Deliveries Scheduled Early[5]	-	-	2%	6%
Preventive Care				
Immunization for Influenza[5]	-	-	95%	90%
Immunization for Pneumonia[5]	-	-	95%	92%
Stroke Care				
Anticoagulation Therapy for Atrial Fibrillation[5]	-	-	96%	95%
Antithrombotic Therapy Timing[5]	-	-	99%	98%
Assessed for Rehabilitation[5]	-	-	96%	97%
Discharged on Antithrombotic Therapy[5]	-	-	100%	99%
Discharged on Statin Medication[5]	-	-	95%	94%
Thrombolytic Therapy Timing[5]	-	-	57%	66%
Venous Thromboembolism Prophylaxis[5]	-	-	94%	94%
Written Stroke Educational Materials Given[5]	-	-	76%	88%
Surgical Care Improvement Project				
Appropriate Beta Blocker Usage[1]	-	-	98%	98%
Appropriate VTP Within 24 Hours	34	100%	99%	98%
Controlled Postoperative Blood Glucose[7]	-	-	98%	97%
Perioperative Temperature Management	36	100%	100%	100%
Prophylactic Antibiotic Selection	31	97%	99%	99%
Prophylactic Antibiotic Selection (Outpatient)[5]	-	-	99%	98%
Prophylactic Antibiotic Stopped	29	97%	98%	98%
Prophylactic Antibiotic Timing	31	100%	99%	99%
Prophylactic Antibiotic Timing (Outpatient)[5]	-	-	98%	98%
Urinary Catheter Removal	31	100%	98%	97%
Survey of Patients' Hospital Experiences				
Area Around Room 'Always' Quiet at Night[5]	-	-	57%	61%
Doctors 'Always' Communicated Well[5]	-	-	81%	82%
Home Recovery Information Given[5]	-	-	88%	85%
Hospital Given 9 or 10 on 10 Point Scale[5]	-	-	71%	71%
Meds 'Always' Explained Before Given[5]	-	-	65%	64%
Nurses 'Always' Communicated Well[5]	-	-	80%	79%
Pain 'Always' Well Controlled[5]	-	-	72%	71%
Room and Bathroom 'Always' Clean[5]	-	-	76%	73%
Timely Help 'Always' Received[5]	-	-	70%	68%
Would Definitely Recommend Hospital[5]	-	-	74%	71%
Use of Medical Imaging				
Cardiac Imaging Stress Test before Surgery	175	3.4%	4.7%	5.3%
Combination Abdominal CT Scan	187	35.8%	5.6%	10.5%
Combination Brain/Sinus CT Scan[1]	-	-	2.3%	2.7%
Combination Chest CT Scan	113	1.8%	0.5%	2.7%
Follow-up Mammogram/Ultrasound	278	2.5%	8.2%	8.8%
Lumbar Spine MRI for Low Back Pain	42	42.9%	33.5%	37.2%

Alice Peck Day Memorial Hospital

10 Alice Peck Day Drive Phone: 603-448-3121
Lebanon, NH 03766 Fax: 603-443-9620
Type: Critical Access Hospitals Emergency Services: Yes
Ownership: Voluntary non-profit - Private Beds: 82

Key Personnel:
CEO/President. . . . . Harry G Dorman III
Radiology. . . . . Katherine Gerke, RI
Infection Control. . . . . Thom Goodwin
Operating Room. . . . . David Kroner
Chief of Medical Staff. . . . . Brian Lombard
Quality Assurance . . . . Lora Smith
Pediatric Ambulatory Care . . . . . . Douglas Williamson, MD

Measure	Cases	This Hosp.	State Avg.	U.S. Avg.
Blood Clot Prevention and Treatment				
Anticoagulation Overlap Therapy[5]	-	-	99%	93%
ICU Venous Thromboembolism Prophylaxis[5]	-	-	96%	92%
Incidence of Potentially Preventable VTE[5]	-	-	2%	10%
UFH with Dosages/Platelet Monitoring[5]	-	-	100%	97%
Venous Thromboembolism Prophylaxis[5]	-	-	93%	85%
Warfarin Therapy Discharge Instructions[5]	-	-	77%	75%
Chest Pain/Possible Heart Attack Care				
Aspirin Given Within 24 Hours of Arrival	-	-	99%	96%
Fibrinolytic Meds Within 30 Min. of Arrival	-	-	82%	58%
Average Time to ECG (minutes)	-	-	8	7
Average Time to Transfer (minutes)	-	-	52	60
Children's Asthma Care				
Received Home Management Plan of Care	-	-	-	88%
Received Reliever Medication	-	-	-	100%

NOTE: Hospital profiles are in alphabetical order by state, then city, then hospital within the city; Rankings exclude hospitals with less than 25 cases except for patient surveys which excludes hospitals with less than 100 cases; (a) 100-299 cases; (1) The number of cases/patients is too few to report; (2) Data submitted were based on a sample of cases/patients; (3) Results are based on a shorter time period than required; (4) Data suppressed by CMS for one or more quarters; (5) Results are not available for this reporting period; (6) Fewer than 100 patients completed the HCAHPS survey; (7) No cases met the criteria for this measure; (8) The lower limit of the confidence interval cannot be calculated if the number of observed infections equals zero; (9) No data are available from the state/territory for this reporting period; (10) The scores shown reflect fewer than 50 completed surveys; (11) There were discrepancies in the data collection process; (12) This measure does not apply to this hospital for this reporting period; (13) Results cannot be calculated for this reporting period; (14) The results for this state are combined with nearby states to protect confidentiality; Please refer to the User's Guide for a full explanation of data.

Measure	Cases	This Hosp.	State Avg.	U.S. Avg.
Received Systemic Corticosteroids	-	-	-	100%
Emergency Department				
Admittance Decision Time (minutes)[2]	18	78	107	98
Head CT Results Within 45 Min. of Arrival	-	-	61%	57%
Patients Who Left ER Before Being Seen	-	-	1%	2%
Time from ER Arrival to Admit. (minutes)[2]	26	244	292	274
Time from ER Arrival to Discharge (minutes)	-	-	139	134
Time in ER Before Being Evaluated (minutes)	-	-	30	26
Time to Pain Meds for Fractures (minutes)	-	-	59	57
Heart Attack Care				
Aspirin Given at Discharge[1,3]	-	-	100%	99%
Fibrinolytic Meds Within 30 Min. of Arrival[3,7]	-	-	50%	54%
PCI Within 90 Minutes of Arrival[3,7]	-	-	95%	96%
Statin Prescribed at Discharge[1,3]	-	-	100%	98%
Heart Failure Care				
ACE Inhibitor or ARB for LVSD[1]	-	-	98%	97%
Discharge Instructions Given[1]	-	-	97%	94%
Evaluation of LVS Function[1]	-	-	100%	99%
Medicare Spending				
Medicare Spending per Patient (ratio)	-	-	1.01	0.98
Pneumonia Care				
Appropriate Initial Antibiotic Given	16	100%	97%	95%
Blood Culture Timing	14	93%	98%	98%
Pregnancy and Delivery Care				
Newborn Deliveries Scheduled Early[5]	-	-	2%	6%
Preventive Care				
Immunization for Influenza[2]	23	74%	95%	90%
Immunization for Pneumonia[2]	44	82%	95%	92%
Stroke Care				
Anticoagulation Therapy for Atrial Fibrillation[5]	-	-	96%	95%
Antithrombotic Therapy Timing[5]	-	-	99%	98%
Assessed for Rehabilitation[5]	-	-	96%	97%
Discharged on Antithrombotic Therapy[5]	-	-	100%	99%
Discharged on Statin Medication[5]	-	-	95%	94%
Thrombolytic Therapy Timing[5]	-	-	57%	66%
Venous Thromboembolism Prophylaxis[5]	-	-	94%	94%
Written Stroke Educational Materials Given[5]	-	-	76%	88%
Surgical Care Improvement Project				
Appropriate Beta Blocker Usage[2]	20	95%	98%	98%
Appropriate VTP Within 24 Hours[2]	58	98%	99%	98%
Controlled Postoperative Blood Glucose[2,7]	-	-	98%	97%
Perioperative Temperature Management[2]	80	100%	100%	100%
Prophylactic Antibiotic Selection[2]	70	97%	99%	99%
Prophylactic Antibiotic Selection (Outpatient)	-	-	99%	98%
Prophylactic Antibiotic Stopped[2]	70	100%	98%	98%
Prophylactic Antibiotic Timing[2]	71	93%	99%	99%
Prophylactic Antibiotic Timing (Outpatient)	-	-	98%	98%
Urinary Catheter Removal[2]	54	98%	98%	97%
Survey of Patients' Hospital Experiences				
Area Around Room 'Always' Quiet at Night	300+	58%	57%	61%
Doctors 'Always' Communicated Well	300+	83%	81%	82%
Home Recovery Information Given	300+	89%	88%	85%
Hospital Given 9 or 10 on 10 Point Scale	300+	75%	71%	71%
Meds 'Always' Explained Before Given	300+	68%	65%	64%
Nurses 'Always' Communicated Well	300+	82%	80%	79%
Pain 'Always' Well Controlled	300+	68%	72%	71%
Room and Bathroom 'Always' Clean	300+	71%	76%	73%
Timely Help 'Always' Received	300+	72%	70%	68%
Would Definitely Recommend Hospital	300+	82%	74%	71%
Use of Medical Imaging				
Cardiac Imaging Stress Test before Surgery	-	-	4.7%	5.3%
Combination Abdominal CT Scan	-	-	5.6%	10.5%
Combination Brain/Sinus CT Scan	-	-	2.3%	2.7%
Combination Chest CT Scan	-	-	0.5%	2.7%
Follow-up Mammogram/Ultrasound	-	-	8.2%	8.8%
Lumbar Spine MRI for Low Back Pain	-	-	33.5%	37.2%

Mary Hitchcock Memorial Hospital

1 Medical Center Drive
Lebanon, NH 03756
URL: www.dhmc.org
Phone: 603-650-5000
Fax: 603-653-1906
Type: Acute Care Hospitals
Emergency Services: Yes
Ownership: Voluntary non-profit - Other
Beds: 400

Key Personnel:
Radiology. . . . . Monte Clinton
Chief of Medical Staff. . . . . Thomas Colacchio, MD
Operating Room. . . . . Doug Heavisides
Pediatric In-Patient Care . . . . Aden Henry
Infection Control. . . . . Judy Ptak
Quality Assurance . . . . Sally Trombly
CEO/President. . . . . James W Varnum

Measure	Cases	This Hosp.	State Avg.	U.S. Avg.
Blood Clot Prevention and Treatment				
Anticoagulation Overlap Therapy[2]	81	96%	99%	93%
ICU Venous Thromboembolism Prophylaxis[2]	93	98%	96%	92%
Incidence of Potentially Preventable VTE[2]	39	5%	2%	10%
UFH with Dosages/Platelet Monitoring[2]	73	100%	100%	97%
Venous Thromboembolism Prophylaxis[2]	342	91%	93%	85%
Warfarin Therapy Discharge Instructions[2]	56	7%	77%	75%
Chest Pain/Possible Heart Attack Care				
Aspirin Given Within 24 Hours of Arrival[5]	-	-	99%	96%
Fibrinolytic Meds Within 30 Min. of Arrival[5]	-	-	82%	58%
Average Time to ECG (minutes)[5]	-	-	8	7
Average Time to Transfer (minutes)[5]	-	-	52	60
Children's Asthma Care				
Received Home Management Plan of Care	-	-	-	88%
Received Reliever Medication	-	-	-	100%
Received Systemic Corticosteroids	-	-	-	100%
Emergency Department				
Admittance Decision Time (minutes)[2]	284	247	107	98
Head CT Results Within 45 Min. of Arrival[5]	-	-	61%	57%
Patients Who Left ER Before Being Seen	31,543	1%	1%	2%
Time from ER Arrival to Admit. (minutes)[2]	286	370	292	274
Time from ER Arrival to Discharge (minutes)	353	176	139	134
Time in ER Before Being Evaluated (minutes)	290	36	30	26
Time to Pain Meds for Fractures (minutes)	143	78	59	57
Heart Attack Care				
Aspirin Given at Discharge[2]	507	99%	100%	99%
Fibrinolytic Meds Within 30 Min. of Arrival[2,7]	-	-	50%	54%
PCI Within 90 Minutes of Arrival[2]	36	86%	95%	96%
Statin Prescribed at Discharge[2]	502	100%	100%	98%
Heart Failure Care				
ACE Inhibitor or ARB for LVSD[2]	67	100%	98%	97%
Discharge Instructions Given[2]	242	96%	97%	94%
Evaluation of LVS Function[2]	296	100%	100%	99%
Medicare Spending				
Medicare Spending per Patient (ratio)	-	0.99	1.01	0.98
Pneumonia Care				
Appropriate Initial Antibiotic Given[2]	64	95%	97%	95%
Blood Culture Timing[2]	94	85%	98%	98%
Pregnancy and Delivery Care				
Newborn Deliveries Scheduled Early	19	0%	2%	6%
Preventive Care				
Immunization for Influenza[2]	631	87%	95%	90%
Immunization for Pneumonia[2]	698	87%	95%	92%
Stroke Care				
Anticoagulation Therapy for Atrial Fibrillation[2]	38	95%	96%	95%
Antithrombotic Therapy Timing[2]	143	100%	99%	98%
Assessed for Rehabilitation[2]	267	94%	96%	97%
Discharged on Antithrombotic Therapy[2]	187	99%	100%	99%
Discharged on Statin Medication[2]	149	98%	95%	94%
Thrombolytic Therapy Timing[2]	13	77%	57%	66%
Venous Thromboembolism Prophylaxis[2]	283	95%	94%	94%
Written Stroke Educational Materials Given[2]	133	87%	76%	88%
Surgical Care Improvement Project				
Appropriate Beta Blocker Usage[2]	307	99%	98%	98%
Appropriate VTP Within 24 Hours[2]	449	100%	99%	98%
Controlled Postoperative Blood Glucose[2]	207	96%	98%	97%
Perioperative Temperature Management[2]	656	100%	100%	100%
Prophylactic Antibiotic Selection[2]	600	99%	99%	99%
Prophylactic Antibiotic Selection (Outpatient)	668	99%	99%	98%
Prophylactic Antibiotic Stopped[2]	592	95%	98%	98%
Prophylactic Antibiotic Timing[2]	601	98%	99%	99%
Prophylactic Antibiotic Timing (Outpatient)	582	96%	98%	98%
Urinary Catheter Removal[2]	501	92%	98%	97%
Survey of Patients' Hospital Experiences				
Area Around Room 'Always' Quiet at Night	300+	41%	57%	61%
Doctors 'Always' Communicated Well	300+	80%	81%	82%
Home Recovery Information Given	300+	89%	88%	85%
Hospital Given 9 or 10 on 10 Point Scale	300+	77%	71%	71%
Meds 'Always' Explained Before Given	300+	64%	65%	64%
Nurses 'Always' Communicated Well	300+	78%	80%	79%
Pain 'Always' Well Controlled	300+	70%	72%	71%
Room and Bathroom 'Always' Clean	300+	67%	76%	73%
Timely Help 'Always' Received	300+	72%	70%	68%
Would Definitely Recommend Hospital	300+	83%	74%	71%
Use of Medical Imaging				
Cardiac Imaging Stress Test before Surgery	1,040	4.5%	4.7%	5.3%
Combination Abdominal CT Scan	1,805	2.7%	5.6%	10.5%
Combination Brain/Sinus CT Scan	629	1.3%	2.3%	2.7%
Combination Chest CT Scan	2,351	0.1%	0.5%	2.7%
Follow-up Mammogram/Ultrasound	3,149	9.4%	8.2%	8.8%
Lumbar Spine MRI for Low Back Pain	404	33.2%	33.5%	37.2%

Littleton Regional Healthcare

600 Saint Johnsbury Road
Littleton, NH 03561
URL: www.littletonhospital.org
Phone: 603-444-9000
Fax: 603-444-0443
Type: Critical Access Hospitals
Emergency Services: Yes
Ownership: Voluntary non-profit - Private

Key Personnel:
Operating Room. . . . . Jean Courteau
Emergency Room . . . . Edward Duffy, MD
Quality Assurance . . . . Linda Gilmore
Pediatric Ambulatory Care . . . . . . William Lakey, MD
Infection Control. . . . . Kris Major
Intensive Care Unit. . . . . Lois Peraino
CEO . . . . Warren West, FACHE
Chief of Medical Staff. . . . . Clare Wilmot

Measure	Cases	This Hosp.	State Avg.	U.S. Avg.
Blood Clot Prevention and Treatment				
Anticoagulation Overlap Therapy[5]	-	-	99%	93%
ICU Venous Thromboembolism Prophylaxis[5]	-	-	96%	92%
Incidence of Potentially Preventable VTE[5]	-	-	2%	10%
UFH with Dosages/Platelet Monitoring[5]	-	-	100%	97%
Venous Thromboembolism Prophylaxis[5]	-	-	93%	85%
Warfarin Therapy Discharge Instructions[5]	-	-	77%	75%
Chest Pain/Possible Heart Attack Care				
Aspirin Given Within 24 Hours of Arrival	-	-	99%	96%
Fibrinolytic Meds Within 30 Min. of Arrival	-	-	82%	58%
Average Time to ECG (minutes)	-	-	8	7
Average Time to Transfer (minutes)	-	-	52	60
Children's Asthma Care				
Received Home Management Plan of Care	-	-	-	88%
Received Reliever Medication	-	-	-	100%
Received Systemic Corticosteroids	-	-	-	100%
Emergency Department				
Admittance Decision Time (minutes)[2]	251	82	107	98
Head CT Results Within 45 Min. of Arrival	-	-	61%	57%
Patients Who Left ER Before Being Seen	-	-	1%	2%
Time from ER Arrival to Admit. (minutes)[2]	270	308	292	274
Time from ER Arrival to Discharge (minutes)	-	-	139	134
Time in ER Before Being Evaluated (minutes)	-	-	30	26
Time to Pain Meds for Fractures (minutes)	-	-	59	57
Heart Attack Care				
Aspirin Given at Discharge[1,3]	-	-	100%	99%
Fibrinolytic Meds Within 30 Min. of Arrival[3,7]	-	-	50%	54%
PCI Within 90 Minutes of Arrival[3,7]	-	-	95%	96%
Statin Prescribed at Discharge[1,3]	-	-	100%	98%
Heart Failure Care				
ACE Inhibitor or ARB for LVSD[1]	-	-	98%	97%
Discharge Instructions Given[1]	-	-	97%	94%
Evaluation of LVS Function	11	100%	100%	99%
Medicare Spending				
Medicare Spending per Patient (ratio)	-	-	1.01	0.98

NOTE: Hospital profiles are in alphabetical order by state, then city, then hospital within the city; Rankings exclude hospitals with less than 25 cases except for patient surveys which excludes hospitals with less than 100 cases; (a) 100-299 cases; (1) The number of cases/patients is too few to report; (2) Data submitted were based on a sample of cases/patients; (3) Results are based on a shorter time period than required; (4) Data suppressed by CMS for one or more quarters; (5) Results are not available for this reporting period; (6) Fewer than 100 patients completed the HCAHPS survey; (7) No cases met the criteria for this measure; (8) The lower limit of the confidence interval cannot be calculated if the number of observed infections equals zero; (9) No data are available from the state/territory for this reporting period; (10) The scores shown reflect fewer than 50 completed surveys; (11) There were discrepancies in the data collection process; (12) This measure does not apply to this hospital for this reporting period; (13) Results cannot be calculated for this reporting period; (14) The results for this state are combined with nearby states to protect confidentiality; Please refer to the User's Guide for a full explanation of data.

Measure	Cases	This Hosp.	State Avg.	U.S. Avg.
Pneumonia Care				
Appropriate Initial Antibiotic Given	32	100%	97%	95%
Blood Culture Timing	36	100%	98%	98%
Pregnancy and Delivery Care				
Newborn Deliveries Scheduled Early[5]	-	-	2%	6%
Preventive Care				
Immunization for Influenza[2]	287	89%	95%	90%
Immunization for Pneumonia[2]	304	88%	95%	92%
Stroke Care				
Anticoagulation Therapy for Atrial Fibrillation[5]	-	-	96%	95%
Antithrombotic Therapy Timing[5]	-	-	99%	98%
Assessed for Rehabilitation[5]	-	-	96%	97%
Discharged on Antithrombotic Therapy[5]	-	-	100%	99%
Discharged on Statin Medication[5]	-	-	95%	94%
Thrombolytic Therapy Timing[5]	-	-	57%	66%
Venous Thromboembolism Prophylaxis[5]	-	-	94%	94%
Written Stroke Educational Materials Given[5]	-	-	76%	88%
Surgical Care Improvement Project				
Appropriate Beta Blocker Usage[2]	48	100%	98%	98%
Appropriate VTP Within 24 Hours[2]	158	100%	99%	98%
Controlled Postoperative Blood Glucose[2,7]	-	-	98%	97%
Perioperative Temperature Management[2]	187	100%	100%	100%
Prophylactic Antibiotic Selection[2]	145	99%	99%	99%
Prophylactic Antibiotic Selection (Outpatient)	-	-	99%	98%
Prophylactic Antibiotic Stopped[2]	144	98%	98%	98%
Prophylactic Antibiotic Timing[2]	145	98%	99%	99%
Prophylactic Antibiotic Timing (Outpatient)	-	-	98%	98%
Urinary Catheter Removal[2]	126	100%	98%	97%
Survey of Patients' Hospital Experiences				
Area Around Room 'Always' Quiet at Night	(a)	58%	57%	61%
Doctors 'Always' Communicated Well	(a)	87%	81%	82%
Home Recovery Information Given	(a)	88%	88%	85%
Hospital Given 9 or 10 on 10 Point Scale	(a)	71%	71%	71%
Meds 'Always' Explained Before Given	(a)	73%	65%	64%
Nurses 'Always' Communicated Well	(a)	77%	80%	79%
Pain 'Always' Well Controlled	(a)	76%	72%	71%
Room and Bathroom 'Always' Clean	(a)	79%	76%	73%
Timely Help 'Always' Received	(a)	76%	70%	68%
Would Definitely Recommend Hospital	(a)	75%	74%	71%
Use of Medical Imaging				
Cardiac Imaging Stress Test before Surgery	-	-	4.7%	5.3%
Combination Abdominal CT Scan	-	-	5.6%	10.5%
Combination Brain/Sinus CT Scan	-	-	2.3%	2.7%
Combination Chest CT Scan	-	-	0.5%	2.7%
Follow-up Mammogram/Ultrasound	-	-	8.2%	8.8%
Lumbar Spine MRI for Low Back Pain	-	-	33.5%	37.2%

Catholic Medical Center

100 Mcgregor Street
Manchester, NH 03102
Phone: 603-668-3545
Fax: 603-668-5348
URL: www.catholicmedicalcenter.org
Type: Acute Care Hospitals
Emergency Services: Yes
Ownership: Voluntary non-profit - Private
Beds: 224

Key Personnel:
Chief of Medical Staff.......... Raef Fahmy, DPM
Cardiac Laboratory............ Louis A Fink, MD FACC
President.................... Connor J. Haugh, MD
Pediatric In-Patient Care .... Kevin Hodges, MD
Patient Relations .... Tina Legere
Quality Assurance .... Diane Rogier
Operating Room.............. Lisa Roux, MD FACS
Emergency Room .... Kathleen Zaffino, MD

Measure	Cases	This Hosp.	State Avg.	U.S. Avg.
Blood Clot Prevention and Treatment				
Anticoagulation Overlap Therapy[2]	92	97%	99%	93%
ICU Venous Thromboembolism Prophylaxis[2]	62	97%	96%	92%
Incidence of Potentially Preventable VTE[2]	23	0%	2%	10%
UFH with Dosages/Platelet Monitoring[2]	36	100%	100%	97%
Venous Thromboembolism Prophylaxis[2]	339	89%	93%	85%
Warfarin Therapy Discharge Instructions[2]	67	85%	77%	75%
Chest Pain/Possible Heart Attack Care				
Aspirin Given Within 24 Hours of Arrival[1,3]	-	-	99%	96%
Fibrinolytic Meds Within 30 Min. of Arrival[3,7]	-	-	82%	58%
Average Time to ECG (minutes)[1,3]	-	-	8	7
Average Time to Transfer (minutes)[3,7]	-	-	52	60
Children's Asthma Care				
Received Home Management Plan of Care	-	-	-	88%
Received Reliever Medication	-	-	-	100%
Received Systemic Corticosteroids	-	-	-	100%
Emergency Department				
Admittance Decision Time (minutes)[2]	455	192	107	98
Head CT Results Within 45 Min. of Arrival	19	63%	61%	57%
Patients Who Left ER Before Being Seen	34,503	2%	1%	2%
Time from ER Arrival to Admit. (minutes)[2]	460	344	292	274
Time from ER Arrival to Discharge (minutes)	322	163	139	134
Time in ER Before Being Evaluated (minutes)	372	46	30	26
Time to Pain Meds for Fractures (minutes)	60	74	59	57
Heart Attack Care				
Aspirin Given at Discharge	477	100%	100%	99%
Fibrinolytic Meds Within 30 Min. of Arrival[7]	-	-	50%	54%
PCI Within 90 Minutes of Arrival	54	96%	95%	96%
Statin Prescribed at Discharge	472	100%	100%	98%
Heart Failure Care				
ACE Inhibitor or ARB for LVSD[2]	86	100%	98%	97%
Discharge Instructions Given[2]	244	100%	97%	94%
Evaluation of LVS Function[2]	289	100%	100%	99%
Medicare Spending				
Medicare Spending per Patient (ratio)	-	1.04	1.01	0.98
Pneumonia Care				
Appropriate Initial Antibiotic Given[2]	80	95%	97%	95%
Blood Culture Timing[2]	129	98%	98%	98%
Pregnancy and Delivery Care				
Newborn Deliveries Scheduled Early[1,2]	-	-	2%	6%
Preventive Care				
Immunization for Influenza[2]	521	99%	95%	90%
Immunization for Pneumonia[2]	707	100%	95%	92%
Stroke Care				
Anticoagulation Therapy for Atrial Fibrillation	13	92%	96%	95%
Antithrombotic Therapy Timing	70	100%	99%	98%
Assessed for Rehabilitation	83	92%	96%	97%
Discharged on Antithrombotic Therapy	76	100%	100%	99%
Discharged on Statin Medication	65	98%	95%	94%
Thrombolytic Therapy Timing[7]	-	-	57%	66%
Venous Thromboembolism Prophylaxis	74	95%	94%	94%
Written Stroke Educational Materials Given	43	74%	76%	88%
Surgical Care Improvement Project				
Appropriate Beta Blocker Usage[2]	215	99%	98%	98%
Appropriate VTP Within 24 Hours[2]	230	97%	99%	98%
Controlled Postoperative Blood Glucose[2]	130	99%	98%	97%
Perioperative Temperature Management[2]	418	100%	100%	100%
Prophylactic Antibiotic Selection[2]	334	100%	99%	99%
Prophylactic Antibiotic Selection (Outpatient)	427	98%	99%	98%
Prophylactic Antibiotic Stopped[2]	325	98%	98%	98%
Prophylactic Antibiotic Timing[2]	334	99%	99%	99%
Prophylactic Antibiotic Timing (Outpatient)	425	100%	98%	98%
Urinary Catheter Removal[2]	316	99%	98%	97%
Survey of Patients' Hospital Experiences				
Area Around Room 'Always' Quiet at Night	300+	53%	57%	61%
Doctors 'Always' Communicated Well	300+	82%	81%	82%
Home Recovery Information Given	300+	87%	88%	85%
Hospital Given 9 or 10 on 10 Point Scale	300+	72%	71%	71%
Meds 'Always' Explained Before Given	300+	64%	65%	64%
Nurses 'Always' Communicated Well	300+	81%	80%	79%
Pain 'Always' Well Controlled	300+	68%	72%	71%
Room and Bathroom 'Always' Clean	300+	72%	76%	73%
Timely Help 'Always' Received	300+	69%	70%	68%
Would Definitely Recommend Hospital	300+	78%	74%	71%
Use of Medical Imaging				
Cardiac Imaging Stress Test before Surgery	1,142	4.6%	4.7%	5.3%
Combination Abdominal CT Scan	705	1.3%	5.6%	10.5%
Combination Brain/Sinus CT Scan	995	2.4%	2.3%	2.7%
Combination Chest CT Scan	397	0.0%	0.5%	2.7%
Follow-up Mammogram/Ultrasound	1,622	10.2%	8.2%	8.8%
Lumbar Spine MRI for Low Back Pain	109	30.3%	33.5%	37.2%

Elliot Hospital

1 Elliot Way
Manchester, NH 03103
Phone: 603-669-5300
Fax: 603-627-0561
URL: www.elliothospital.org
Type: Acute Care Hospitals
Emergency Services: Yes
Ownership: Voluntary non-profit - Private
Beds: 296

Key Personnel:
Infection Control............. Lynda Caine
Pediatric In-Patient Care .... Liz Castrogiovanni
Radiology.................. Richard Frechette
Cardiac Laboratory............ Laurie King
Quality Assurance .... MaryAnn McEntee
Chief of Medical Staff.......... Dr Mark Myers
CEO/President............... James T. Woodward
Operating Room.............. Laurie York

Measure	Cases	This Hosp.	State Avg.	U.S. Avg.
Blood Clot Prevention and Treatment				
Anticoagulation Overlap Therapy[2]	51	98%	99%	93%
ICU Venous Thromboembolism Prophylaxis[2]	47	87%	96%	92%
Incidence of Potentially Preventable VTE[1,2]	-	-	2%	10%
UFH with Dosages/Platelet Monitoring[2]	24	100%	100%	97%
Venous Thromboembolism Prophylaxis[2]	330	89%	93%	85%
Warfarin Therapy Discharge Instructions[2]	38	82%	77%	75%
Chest Pain/Possible Heart Attack Care				
Aspirin Given Within 24 Hours of Arrival[1]	-	-	99%	96%
Fibrinolytic Meds Within 30 Min. of Arrival[3,7]	-	-	82%	58%
Average Time to ECG (minutes)[1]	-	-	8	7
Average Time to Transfer (minutes)[1,3]	-	-	52	60
Children's Asthma Care				
Received Home Management Plan of Care	-	-	-	88%
Received Reliever Medication	-	-	-	100%
Received Systemic Corticosteroids	-	-	-	100%
Emergency Department				
Admittance Decision Time (minutes)[2]	445	133	107	98
Head CT Results Within 45 Min. of Arrival	11	45%	61%	57%
Patients Who Left ER Before Being Seen	53,513	2%	1%	2%
Time from ER Arrival to Admit. (minutes)[2]	482	309	292	274
Time from ER Arrival to Discharge (minutes)	327	190	139	134
Time in ER Before Being Evaluated (minutes)	345	36	30	26
Time to Pain Meds for Fractures (minutes)	129	55	59	57
Heart Attack Care				
Aspirin Given at Discharge	121	100%	100%	99%
Fibrinolytic Meds Within 30 Min. of Arrival[7]	-	-	50%	54%
PCI Within 90 Minutes of Arrival	20	75%	95%	96%
Statin Prescribed at Discharge	110	100%	100%	98%
Heart Failure Care				
ACE Inhibitor or ARB for LVSD	47	100%	98%	97%
Discharge Instructions Given	175	97%	97%	94%
Evaluation of LVS Function	246	100%	100%	99%
Medicare Spending				
Medicare Spending per Patient (ratio)	-	1.05	1.01	0.98
Pneumonia Care				
Appropriate Initial Antibiotic Given[2]	79	99%	97%	95%
Blood Culture Timing[2]	118	97%	98%	98%
Pregnancy and Delivery Care				
Newborn Deliveries Scheduled Early[2]	35	0%	2%	6%
Preventive Care				
Immunization for Influenza[2]	494	99%	95%	90%
Immunization for Pneumonia[2]	511	95%	95%	92%
Stroke Care				
Anticoagulation Therapy for Atrial Fibrillation	21	95%	96%	95%
Antithrombotic Therapy Timing	81	99%	99%	98%
Assessed for Rehabilitation	114	97%	96%	97%
Discharged on Antithrombotic Therapy	96	98%	100%	99%
Discharged on Statin Medication	73	96%	95%	94%
Thrombolytic Therapy Timing[1]	-	-	57%	66%
Venous Thromboembolism Prophylaxis	97	88%	94%	94%
Written Stroke Educational Materials Given	51	69%	76%	88%
Surgical Care Improvement Project				
Appropriate Beta Blocker Usage[2]	78	100%	98%	98%
Appropriate VTP Within 24 Hours[2]	301	99%	99%	98%
Controlled Postoperative Blood Glucose[2,7]	-	-	98%	97%
Perioperative Temperature Management[2]	376	100%	100%	100%
Prophylactic Antibiotic Selection[2]	254	98%	99%	99%

NOTE: Hospital profiles are in alphabetical order by state, then city, then hospital within the city; Rankings exclude hospitals with less than 25 cases except for patient surveys which excludes hospitals with less than 100 cases; (a) 100-299 cases; (1) The number of cases/patients is too few to report; (2) Data submitted were based on a sample of cases/patients; (3) Results are based on a shorter time period than required; (4) Data suppressed by CMS for one or more quarters; (5) Results are not available for this reporting period; (6) Fewer than 100 patients completed the HCAHPS survey; (7) No cases met the criteria for this measure; (8) The lower limit of the confidence interval cannot be calculated if the number of observed infections equals zero; (9) No data are available from the state/territory for this reporting period; (10) The scores shown reflect fewer than 50 completed surveys; (11) There were discrepancies in the data collection process; (12) This measure does not apply to this hospital for this reporting period; (13) Results cannot be calculated for this reporting period; (14) The results for this state are combined with nearby states to protect confidentiality; Please refer to the User's Guide for a full explanation of data.

Measure	Cases	This Hosp.	State Avg.	U.S. Avg.
Prophylactic Antibiotic Selection (Outpatient)	430	99%	99%	98%
Prophylactic Antibiotic Stopped[2]	247	98%	98%	98%
Prophylactic Antibiotic Timing[2]	255	99%	99%	99%
Prophylactic Antibiotic Timing (Outpatient)	428	98%	98%	98%
Urinary Catheter Removal[2]	239	98%	98%	97%
Survey of Patients' Hospital Experiences				
Area Around Room 'Always' Quiet at Night	300+	50%	57%	61%
Doctors 'Always' Communicated Well	300+	80%	81%	82%
Home Recovery Information Given	300+	89%	88%	85%
Hospital Given 9 or 10 on 10 Point Scale	300+	66%	71%	71%
Meds 'Always' Explained Before Given	300+	58%	65%	64%
Nurses 'Always' Communicated Well	300+	74%	80%	79%
Pain 'Always' Well Controlled	300+	66%	72%	71%
Room and Bathroom 'Always' Clean	300+	70%	76%	73%
Timely Help 'Always' Received	300+	60%	70%	68%
Would Definitely Recommend Hospital	300+	71%	74%	71%
Use of Medical Imaging				
Cardiac Imaging Stress Test before Surgery	774	5.0%	4.7%	5.3%
Combination Abdominal CT Scan	1,088	4.9%	5.6%	10.5%
Combination Brain/Sinus CT Scan	1,099	3.3%	2.3%	2.7%
Combination Chest CT Scan	727	0.1%	0.5%	2.7%
Follow-up Mammogram/Ultrasound	2,501	8.4%	8.2%	8.8%
Lumbar Spine MRI for Low Back Pain	265	31.3%	33.5%	37.2%

Saint Joseph Hospital

172 Kinsley St
Nashua, NH 03060
Phone: 603-882-3000
Fax: 603-889-1651
URL: www.stjosephhospital.com
Type: Acute Care Hospitals
Emergency Services: Yes
Ownership: Voluntary non-profit - Other
Beds: 208

Key Personnel:
CEO/President. . . . . Peter B Davis
Pediatric Ambulatory Care . . . . . . Ann Dobbins, MD
Pediatric In-Patient Care . . . . Ann Dobbins, MD
Quality Assurance . . . . Barbara Dotson
Chief of Medical Staff. . . . . John Posner, MD
Radiology. . . . . Don Wiess, MD

Measure	Cases	This Hosp.	State Avg.	U.S. Avg.
Blood Clot Prevention and Treatment				
Anticoagulation Overlap Therapy[2]	52	100%	99%	93%
ICU Venous Thromboembolism Prophylaxis[2]	54	96%	96%	92%
Incidence of Potentially Preventable VTE[2]	12	0%	2%	10%
UFH with Dosages/Platelet Monitoring[2]	15	100%	100%	97%
Venous Thromboembolism Prophylaxis[2]	314	88%	93%	85%
Warfarin Therapy Discharge Instructions[2]	39	100%	77%	75%
Chest Pain/Possible Heart Attack Care				
Aspirin Given Within 24 Hours of Arrival[1,3]	-	-	99%	96%
Fibrinolytic Meds Within 30 Min. of Arrival[3,7]	-	-	82%	58%
Average Time to ECG (minutes)[1,3]	-	-	8	7
Average Time to Transfer (minutes)[1,3]	-	-	52	60
Children's Asthma Care				
Received Home Management Plan of Care	-	-	-	88%
Received Reliever Medication	-	-	-	100%
Received Systemic Corticosteroids	-	-	-	100%
Emergency Department				
Admittance Decision Time (minutes)[2]	632	96	107	98
Head CT Results Within 45 Min. of Arrival[1]	-	-	61%	57%
Patients Who Left ER Before Being Seen	33,159	1%	1%	2%
Time from ER Arrival to Admit. (minutes)[2]	657	242	292	274
Time from ER Arrival to Discharge (minutes)	358	115	139	134
Time in ER Before Being Evaluated (minutes)	382	24	30	26
Time to Pain Meds for Fractures (minutes)	103	46	59	57
Heart Attack Care				
Aspirin Given at Discharge[2]	97	100%	100%	99%
Fibrinolytic Meds Within 30 Min. of Arrival[2,7]	-	-	50%	54%
PCI Within 90 Minutes of Arrival[2]	11	100%	95%	96%
Statin Prescribed at Discharge[2]	97	100%	100%	98%
Heart Failure Care				
ACE Inhibitor or ARB for LVSD[2]	39	100%	98%	97%
Discharge Instructions Given[2]	137	99%	97%	94%
Evaluation of LVS Function[2]	176	100%	100%	99%
Medicare Spending				
Medicare Spending per Patient (ratio)	-	1.02	1.01	0.98
Pneumonia Care				
Appropriate Initial Antibiotic Given[2]	82	94%	97%	95%
Blood Culture Timing[2]	150	98%	98%	98%
Pregnancy and Delivery Care				
Newborn Deliveries Scheduled Early[2]	14	0%	2%	6%
Preventive Care				
Immunization for Influenza[2]	494	95%	95%	90%
Immunization for Pneumonia[2]	637	94%	95%	92%
Stroke Care				
Anticoagulation Therapy for Atrial Fibrillation[2]	21	100%	96%	95%
Antithrombotic Therapy Timing[2]	57	100%	99%	98%
Assessed for Rehabilitation[2]	68	97%	96%	97%
Discharged on Antithrombotic Therapy[2]	64	100%	100%	99%
Discharged on Statin Medication[2]	47	91%	95%	94%
Thrombolytic Therapy Timing[1,2]	-	-	57%	66%
Venous Thromboembolism Prophylaxis[2]	68	96%	94%	94%
Written Stroke Educational Materials Given[2]	29	93%	76%	88%
Surgical Care Improvement Project				
Appropriate Beta Blocker Usage[2]	69	97%	98%	98%
Appropriate VTP Within 24 Hours[2]	222	98%	99%	98%
Controlled Postoperative Blood Glucose[2,7]	-	-	98%	97%
Perioperative Temperature Management[2]	266	100%	100%	100%
Prophylactic Antibiotic Selection[2]	174	98%	99%	99%
Prophylactic Antibiotic Selection (Outpatient)	116	98%	99%	98%
Prophylactic Antibiotic Stopped[2]	171	100%	98%	98%
Prophylactic Antibiotic Timing[2]	174	99%	99%	99%
Prophylactic Antibiotic Timing (Outpatient)	116	99%	98%	98%
Urinary Catheter Removal[2]	95	99%	98%	97%
Survey of Patients' Hospital Experiences				
Area Around Room 'Always' Quiet at Night	300+	65%	57%	61%
Doctors 'Always' Communicated Well	300+	78%	81%	82%
Home Recovery Information Given	300+	87%	88%	85%
Hospital Given 9 or 10 on 10 Point Scale	300+	73%	71%	71%
Meds 'Always' Explained Before Given	300+	63%	65%	64%
Nurses 'Always' Communicated Well	300+	82%	80%	79%
Pain 'Always' Well Controlled	300+	72%	72%	71%
Room and Bathroom 'Always' Clean	300+	75%	76%	73%
Timely Help 'Always' Received	300+	65%	70%	68%
Would Definitely Recommend Hospital	300+	76%	74%	71%
Use of Medical Imaging				
Cardiac Imaging Stress Test before Surgery	438	5.7%	4.7%	5.3%
Combination Abdominal CT Scan	741	5.0%	5.6%	10.5%
Combination Brain/Sinus CT Scan	541	0.9%	2.3%	2.7%
Combination Chest CT Scan	532	0.0%	0.5%	2.7%
Follow-up Mammogram/Ultrasound	2,100	10.0%	8.2%	8.8%
Lumbar Spine MRI for Low Back Pain	115	36.5%	33.5%	37.2%

Southern Nh Medical Center

8 Prospect Street
Nashua, NH 03060
Phone: 603-577-2000
URL: www.snhmc.org
Type: Acute Care Hospitals
Emergency Services: Yes
Ownership: Voluntary non-profit - Private
Beds: 188

Key Personnel:
Chief of Medical Staff. . . . . Sean W Fitzpatrick
CEO/President. . . . . Thomas E Wilhelmsen

Measure	Cases	This Hosp.	State Avg.	U.S. Avg.
Blood Clot Prevention and Treatment				
Anticoagulation Overlap Therapy[2]	55	98%	99%	93%
ICU Venous Thromboembolism Prophylaxis[2]	36	100%	96%	92%
Incidence of Potentially Preventable VTE[1,2]	-	-	2%	10%
UFH with Dosages/Platelet Monitoring[2]	39	100%	100%	97%
Venous Thromboembolism Prophylaxis[2]	344	90%	93%	85%
Warfarin Therapy Discharge Instructions[2]	48	94%	77%	75%
Chest Pain/Possible Heart Attack Care				
Aspirin Given Within 24 Hours of Arrival[1,3]	-	-	99%	96%
Fibrinolytic Meds Within 30 Min. of Arrival[3,7]	-	-	82%	58%
Average Time to ECG (minutes)[1,3]	-	-	8	7
Average Time to Transfer (minutes)[3,7]	-	-	52	60
Children's Asthma Care				
Received Home Management Plan of Care	-	-	-	88%
Received Reliever Medication	-	-	-	100%
Received Systemic Corticosteroids	-	-	-	100%
Emergency Department				
Admittance Decision Time (minutes)[2]	541	140	107	98
Head CT Results Within 45 Min. of Arrival[1]	-	-	61%	57%
Patients Who Left ER Before Being Seen	44,644	1%	1%	2%
Time from ER Arrival to Admit. (minutes)[2]	569	308	292	274
Time from ER Arrival to Discharge (minutes)	435	149	139	134
Time in ER Before Being Evaluated (minutes)	477	31	30	26
Time to Pain Meds for Fractures (minutes)	146	73	59	57
Heart Attack Care				
Aspirin Given at Discharge	103	100%	100%	99%
Fibrinolytic Meds Within 30 Min. of Arrival[7]	-	-	50%	54%
PCI Within 90 Minutes of Arrival	30	100%	95%	96%
Statin Prescribed at Discharge	101	99%	100%	98%
Heart Failure Care				
ACE Inhibitor or ARB for LVSD	45	100%	98%	97%
Discharge Instructions Given	151	100%	97%	94%
Evaluation of LVS Function	195	99%	100%	99%
Medicare Spending				
Medicare Spending per Patient (ratio)	-	1.02	1.01	0.98
Pneumonia Care				
Appropriate Initial Antibiotic Given	159	100%	97%	95%
Blood Culture Timing	245	100%	98%	98%
Pregnancy and Delivery Care				
Newborn Deliveries Scheduled Early	63	6%	2%	6%
Preventive Care				
Immunization for Influenza[2]	532	96%	95%	90%
Immunization for Pneumonia[2]	536	90%	95%	92%
Stroke Care				
Anticoagulation Therapy for Atrial Fibrillation	16	100%	96%	95%
Antithrombotic Therapy Timing	60	100%	99%	98%
Assessed for Rehabilitation	67	100%	96%	97%
Discharged on Antithrombotic Therapy	62	100%	100%	99%
Discharged on Statin Medication	51	100%	95%	94%
Thrombolytic Therapy Timing[7]	-	-	57%	66%
Venous Thromboembolism Prophylaxis	57	98%	94%	94%
Written Stroke Educational Materials Given	36	100%	76%	88%
Surgical Care Improvement Project				
Appropriate Beta Blocker Usage	128	98%	98%	98%
Appropriate VTP Within 24 Hours	436	99%	99%	98%
Controlled Postoperative Blood Glucose[7]	-	-	98%	97%
Perioperative Temperature Management	480	100%	100%	100%
Prophylactic Antibiotic Selection	307	100%	99%	99%
Prophylactic Antibiotic Selection (Outpatient)	343	100%	99%	98%
Prophylactic Antibiotic Stopped	300	97%	98%	98%
Prophylactic Antibiotic Timing	307	100%	99%	99%
Prophylactic Antibiotic Timing (Outpatient)	344	98%	98%	98%
Urinary Catheter Removal	291	100%	98%	97%
Survey of Patients' Hospital Experiences				
Area Around Room 'Always' Quiet at Night	300+	54%	57%	61%
Doctors 'Always' Communicated Well	300+	79%	81%	82%
Home Recovery Information Given	300+	90%	88%	85%
Hospital Given 9 or 10 on 10 Point Scale	300+	74%	71%	71%
Meds 'Always' Explained Before Given	300+	65%	65%	64%
Nurses 'Always' Communicated Well	300+	79%	80%	79%
Pain 'Always' Well Controlled	300+	72%	72%	71%
Room and Bathroom 'Always' Clean	300+	74%	76%	73%
Timely Help 'Always' Received	300+	67%	70%	68%
Would Definitely Recommend Hospital	300+	77%	74%	71%
Use of Medical Imaging				
Cardiac Imaging Stress Test before Surgery	678	5.0%	4.7%	5.3%
Combination Abdominal CT Scan	772	8.5%	5.6%	10.5%
Combination Brain/Sinus CT Scan	915	2.4%	2.3%	2.7%
Combination Chest CT Scan	634	0.6%	0.5%	2.7%
Follow-up Mammogram/Ultrasound	2,382	8.1%	8.2%	8.8%
Lumbar Spine MRI for Low Back Pain	151	31.8%	33.5%	37.2%

New London Hospital

273 County Road
New London, NH 03257
Phone: 603-526-2911
Fax: 603-526-2990
URL: www.newlondonhospital.org
Type: Critical Access Hospitals
Emergency Services: Yes
Ownership: Voluntary non-profit - Private
Beds: 25

Key Personnel:
Radiology. . . . . Katrina Acosta, MD
Infection Control. . . . . Jean Hughes Dowe

NOTE: Hospital profiles are in alphabetical order by state, then city, then hospital within the city; Rankings exclude hospitals with less than 25 cases except for patient surveys which excludes hospitals with less than 100 cases; (a) 100-299 cases; (1) The number of cases/patients is too few to report; (2) Data submitted were based on a sample of cases/patients; (3) Results are based on a shorter time period than required; (4) Data suppressed by CMS for one or more quarters; (5) Results are not available for this reporting period; (6) Fewer than 100 patients completed the HCAHPS survey; (7) No cases met the criteria for this measure; (8) The lower limit of the confidence interval cannot be calculated if the number of observed infections equals zero; (9) No data are available from the state/territory for this reporting period; (10) The scores shown reflect fewer than 50 completed surveys; (11) There were discrepancies in the data collection process; (12) This measure does not apply to this hospital for this reporting period; (13) Results cannot be calculated for this reporting period; (14) The results for this state are combined with nearby states to protect confidentiality; Please refer to the User's Guide for a full explanation of data.

Quality Assurance .... Kieran Kays
CEO/President................ Bruce King
Anesthesiology............... Bryant Matthew, CRNA
Operating Room.............. Patricia Miller, RN
Chief of Medical Staff.......... Douglas Moran, MD
Emergency Room .... Kent Wheeler

Measure	Cases	This Hosp.	State Avg.	U.S. Avg.
Blood Clot Prevention and Treatment				
Anticoagulation Overlap Therapy[5]	-	-	99%	93%
ICU Venous Thromboembolism Prophylaxis[5]	-	-	96%	92%
Incidence of Potentially Preventable VTE[5]	-	-	2%	10%
UFH with Dosages/Platelet Monitoring[5]	-	-	100%	97%
Venous Thromboembolism Prophylaxis[5]	-	-	93%	85%
Warfarin Therapy Discharge Instructions[5]	-	-	77%	75%
Chest Pain/Possible Heart Attack Care				
Aspirin Given Within 24 Hours of Arrival	17	100%	99%	96%
Fibrinolytic Meds Within 30 Min. of Arrival[7]	-	-	82%	58%
Average Time to ECG (minutes)	17	2	8	7
Average Time to Transfer (minutes)[1]	-	-	52	60
Children's Asthma Care				
Received Home Management Plan of Care	-	-	-	88%
Received Reliever Medication	-	-	-	100%
Received Systemic Corticosteroids	-	-	-	100%
Emergency Department				
Admittance Decision Time (minutes)[5]	-	-	107	98
Head CT Results Within 45 Min. of Arrival[5]	-	-	61%	57%
Patients Who Left ER Before Being Seen[5]	-	-	1%	2%
Time from ER Arrival to Admit. (minutes)[5]	-	-	292	274
Time from ER Arrival to Discharge (minutes)[5]	-	-	139	134
Time in ER Before Being Evaluated (minutes)[5]	-	-	30	26
Time to Pain Meds for Fractures (minutes)[5]	-	-	59	57
Heart Attack Care				
Aspirin Given at Discharge[1]	-	-	100%	99%
Fibrinolytic Meds Within 30 Min. of Arrival[3,7]	-	-	50%	54%
PCI Within 90 Minutes of Arrival[3,7]	-	-	95%	96%
Statin Prescribed at Discharge[1]	-	-	100%	98%
Heart Failure Care				
ACE Inhibitor or ARB for LVSD[1]	-	-	98%	97%
Discharge Instructions Given	13	62%	97%	94%
Evaluation of LVS Function	22	95%	100%	99%
Medicare Spending				
Medicare Spending per Patient (ratio)	-	-	1.01	0.98
Pneumonia Care				
Appropriate Initial Antibiotic Given	17	100%	97%	95%
Blood Culture Timing	31	100%	98%	98%
Pregnancy and Delivery Care				
Newborn Deliveries Scheduled Early[5]	-	-	2%	6%
Preventive Care				
Immunization for Influenza[5]	-	-	95%	90%
Immunization for Pneumonia[5]	-	-	95%	92%
Stroke Care				
Anticoagulation Therapy for Atrial Fibrillation[5]	-	-	96%	95%
Antithrombotic Therapy Timing[5]	-	-	99%	98%
Assessed for Rehabilitation[5]	-	-	96%	97%
Discharged on Antithrombotic Therapy[5]	-	-	100%	99%
Discharged on Statin Medication[5]	-	-	95%	94%
Thrombolytic Therapy Timing[5]	-	-	57%	66%
Venous Thromboembolism Prophylaxis[5]	-	-	94%	94%
Written Stroke Educational Materials Given[5]	-	-	76%	88%
Surgical Care Improvement Project				
Appropriate Beta Blocker Usage	22	95%	98%	98%
Appropriate VTP Within 24 Hours	42	98%	99%	98%
Controlled Postoperative Blood Glucose[7]	-	-	98%	97%
Perioperative Temperature Management	69	100%	100%	100%
Prophylactic Antibiotic Selection	31	94%	99%	99%
Prophylactic Antibiotic Selection (Outpatient)	98	100%	99%	98%
Prophylactic Antibiotic Stopped	31	100%	98%	98%
Prophylactic Antibiotic Timing	31	100%	99%	99%
Prophylactic Antibiotic Timing (Outpatient)	98	99%	98%	98%
Urinary Catheter Removal	37	100%	98%	97%
Survey of Patients' Hospital Experiences				
Area Around Room 'Always' Quiet at Night	(a)	61%	57%	61%
Doctors 'Always' Communicated Well	(a)	81%	81%	82%
Home Recovery Information Given	(a)	81%	88%	85%
Hospital Given 9 or 10 on 10 Point Scale	(a)	71%	71%	71%
Meds 'Always' Explained Before Given	(a)	65%	65%	64%
Nurses 'Always' Communicated Well	(a)	77%	80%	79%
Pain 'Always' Well Controlled	(a)	74%	72%	71%
Room and Bathroom 'Always' Clean	(a)	81%	76%	73%
Timely Help 'Always' Received	(a)	75%	70%	68%
Would Definitely Recommend Hospital	(a)	75%	74%	71%
Use of Medical Imaging				
Cardiac Imaging Stress Test before Surgery	97	4.1%	4.7%	5.3%
Combination Abdominal CT Scan	244	7.8%	5.6%	10.5%
Combination Brain/Sinus CT Scan	243	0.4%	2.3%	2.7%
Combination Chest CT Scan	112	2.7%	0.5%	2.7%
Follow-up Mammogram/Ultrasound	930	10.6%	8.2%	8.8%
Lumbar Spine MRI for Low Back Pain	48	33.3%	33.5%	37.2%

The Memorial Hospital

3073 White Mountain Highway
North Conway, NH 03860
Phone: 603-356-5461
Fax: 603-356-9121
Type: Critical Access Hospitals
Emergency Services: Yes
Ownership: Voluntary non-profit - Private
Beds: 35

Key Personnel:
Infection Control............ Andrea Murphy, RN
Quality Assurance .... Susan Perrault
CEO/President................ Gary Poquette
Chief of Medical Staff.......... Diane Snow
Radiology.................... Ray H VanWyngarden

Measure	Cases	This Hosp.	State Avg.	U.S. Avg.
Blood Clot Prevention and Treatment				
Anticoagulation Overlap Therapy[5]	-	-	99%	93%
ICU Venous Thromboembolism Prophylaxis[5]	-	-	96%	92%
Incidence of Potentially Preventable VTE[5]	-	-	2%	10%
UFH with Dosages/Platelet Monitoring[5]	-	-	100%	97%
Venous Thromboembolism Prophylaxis[5]	-	-	93%	85%
Warfarin Therapy Discharge Instructions[5]	-	-	77%	75%
Chest Pain/Possible Heart Attack Care				
Aspirin Given Within 24 Hours of Arrival	-	-	99%	96%
Fibrinolytic Meds Within 30 Min. of Arrival	-	-	82%	58%
Average Time to ECG (minutes)	-	-	8	7
Average Time to Transfer (minutes)	-	-	52	60
Children's Asthma Care				
Received Home Management Plan of Care	-	-	-	88%
Received Reliever Medication	-	-	-	100%
Received Systemic Corticosteroids	-	-	-	100%
Emergency Department				
Admittance Decision Time (minutes)[5]	-	-	107	98
Head CT Results Within 45 Min. of Arrival	-	-	61%	57%
Patients Who Left ER Before Being Seen	-	-	1%	2%
Time from ER Arrival to Admit. (minutes)[5]	-	-	292	274
Time from ER Arrival to Discharge (minutes)	-	-	139	134
Time in ER Before Being Evaluated (minutes)	-	-	30	26
Time to Pain Meds for Fractures (minutes)	-	-	59	57
Heart Attack Care				
Aspirin Given at Discharge[1]	-	-	100%	99%
Fibrinolytic Meds Within 30 Min. of Arrival[7]	-	-	50%	54%
PCI Within 90 Minutes of Arrival[7]	-	-	95%	96%
Statin Prescribed at Discharge[1]	-	-	100%	98%
Heart Failure Care				
ACE Inhibitor or ARB for LVSD[1,2]	-	-	98%	97%
Discharge Instructions Given[2]	30	100%	97%	94%
Evaluation of LVS Function[2]	42	100%	100%	99%
Medicare Spending				
Medicare Spending per Patient (ratio)	-	-	1.01	0.98
Pneumonia Care				
Appropriate Initial Antibiotic Given[2]	50	94%	97%	95%
Blood Culture Timing[2]	78	99%	98%	98%
Pregnancy and Delivery Care				
Newborn Deliveries Scheduled Early[5]	-	-	2%	6%
Preventive Care				
Immunization for Influenza[5]	-	-	95%	90%
Immunization for Pneumonia[5]	-	-	95%	92%
Stroke Care				
Anticoagulation Therapy for Atrial Fibrillation[5]	-	-	96%	95%
Antithrombotic Therapy Timing[5]	-	-	99%	98%
Assessed for Rehabilitation[5]	-	-	96%	97%
Discharged on Antithrombotic Therapy[5]	-	-	100%	99%
Discharged on Statin Medication[5]	-	-	95%	94%
Thrombolytic Therapy Timing[5]	-	-	57%	66%
Venous Thromboembolism Prophylaxis[5]	-	-	94%	94%
Written Stroke Educational Materials Given[5]	-	-	76%	88%
Surgical Care Improvement Project				
Appropriate Beta Blocker Usage[1]	-	-	98%	98%
Appropriate VTP Within 24 Hours	63	100%	99%	98%
Controlled Postoperative Blood Glucose[7]	-	-	98%	97%
Perioperative Temperature Management	66	100%	100%	100%
Prophylactic Antibiotic Selection	45	100%	99%	99%
Prophylactic Antibiotic Selection (Outpatient)	-	-	99%	98%
Prophylactic Antibiotic Stopped	44	98%	98%	98%
Prophylactic Antibiotic Timing	45	98%	99%	99%
Prophylactic Antibiotic Timing (Outpatient)	-	-	98%	98%
Urinary Catheter Removal	38	100%	98%	97%
Survey of Patients' Hospital Experiences				
Area Around Room 'Always' Quiet at Night	(a)	49%	57%	61%
Doctors 'Always' Communicated Well	(a)	80%	81%	82%
Home Recovery Information Given	(a)	92%	88%	85%
Hospital Given 9 or 10 on 10 Point Scale	(a)	61%	71%	71%
Meds 'Always' Explained Before Given	(a)	62%	65%	64%
Nurses 'Always' Communicated Well	(a)	78%	80%	79%
Pain 'Always' Well Controlled	(a)	69%	72%	71%
Room and Bathroom 'Always' Clean	(a)	73%	76%	73%
Timely Help 'Always' Received	(a)	62%	70%	68%
Would Definitely Recommend Hospital	(a)	62%	74%	71%
Use of Medical Imaging				
Cardiac Imaging Stress Test before Surgery	-	-	4.7%	5.3%
Combination Abdominal CT Scan	-	-	5.6%	10.5%
Combination Brain/Sinus CT Scan	-	-	2.3%	2.7%
Combination Chest CT Scan	-	-	0.5%	2.7%
Follow-up Mammogram/Ultrasound	-	-	8.2%	8.8%
Lumbar Spine MRI for Low Back Pain	-	-	33.5%	37.2%

Monadnock Community Hospital

452 Old Street Road
Peterborough, NH 03458
Phone: 603-924-7191
Fax: 603-924-9586
E-mail: info@monadnockhospital.org
URL: www.monadnockhospital.org
Type: Critical Access Hospitals
Emergency Services: Yes
Ownership: Proprietary
Beds: 62

Key Personnel:
Intensive Care Unit............ Dianne Bolton
Pediatric In-Patient Care .... Jeffrey Boxer, MD
Infection Control.............. Diana Clang
CEO/President................ Cynthia K. McGuire
Operating Room.............. Edwin S Menor, RN
Radiology.................... Bhojwani Rajesh, MD
Chief of Medical Staff.......... John Schlegelmilch, MD
Quality Assurance .... Margaret Viverito

Measure	Cases	This Hosp.	State Avg.	U.S. Avg.
Blood Clot Prevention and Treatment				
Anticoagulation Overlap Therapy[5]	-	-	99%	93%
ICU Venous Thromboembolism Prophylaxis[5]	-	-	96%	92%
Incidence of Potentially Preventable VTE[5]	-	-	2%	10%
UFH with Dosages/Platelet Monitoring[5]	-	-	100%	97%
Venous Thromboembolism Prophylaxis[5]	-	-	93%	85%
Warfarin Therapy Discharge Instructions[5]	-	-	77%	75%
Chest Pain/Possible Heart Attack Care				
Aspirin Given Within 24 Hours of Arrival	37	100%	99%	96%
Fibrinolytic Meds Within 30 Min. of Arrival[1]	-	-	82%	58%
Average Time to ECG (minutes)	37	11	8	7
Average Time to Transfer (minutes)[1]	-	-	52	60
Children's Asthma Care				
Received Home Management Plan of Care	-	-	-	88%
Received Reliever Medication	-	-	-	100%
Received Systemic Corticosteroids	-	-	-	100%
Emergency Department				
Admittance Decision Time (minutes)[2]	386	58	107	98
Head CT Results Within 45 Min. of Arrival[5]	-	-	61%	57%
Patients Who Left ER Before Being Seen[5]	-	-	1%	2%

NOTE: Hospital profiles are in alphabetical order by state, then city, then hospital within the city; Rankings exclude hospitals with less than 25 cases except for patient surveys which excludes hospitals with less than 100 cases; (a) 100-299 cases; (1) The number of cases/patients is too few to report; (2) Data submitted were based on a sample of cases/patients; (3) Results are based on a shorter time period than required; (4) Data suppressed by CMS for one or more quarters; (5) Results are not available for this reporting period; (6) Fewer than 100 patients completed the HCAHPS survey; (7) No cases met the criteria for this measure; (8) The lower limit of the confidence interval cannot be calculated if the number of observed infections equals zero; (9) No data are available from the state/territory for this reporting period; (10) The scores shown reflect fewer than 50 completed surveys; (11) There were discrepancies in the data collection process; (12) This measure does not apply to this hospital for this reporting period; (13) Results cannot be calculated for this reporting period; (14) The results for this state are combined with nearby states to protect confidentiality; Please refer to the User's Guide for a full explanation of data.

Measure	Cases	This Hosp.	State Avg.	U.S. Avg.
Time from ER Arrival to Admit. (minutes)[2]	405	277	292	274
Time from ER Arrival to Discharge (minutes)[5]	-	-	139	134
Time in ER Before Being Evaluated (minutes)[5]	-	-	30	26
Time to Pain Meds for Fractures (minutes)[5]	-	-	59	57
Heart Attack Care				
Aspirin Given at Discharge[1]	-	-	100%	99%
Fibrinolytic Meds Within 30 Min. of Arrival[7]	-	-	50%	54%
PCI Within 90 Minutes of Arrival[3,7]	-	-	95%	96%
Statin Prescribed at Discharge[1]	-	-	100%	98%
Heart Failure Care				
ACE Inhibitor or ARB for LVSD[1,2]	-	-	98%	97%
Discharge Instructions Given[2]	23	91%	97%	94%
Evaluation of LVS Function[2]	44	100%	100%	99%
Medicare Spending				
Medicare Spending per Patient (ratio)	-	-	1.01	0.98
Pneumonia Care				
Appropriate Initial Antibiotic Given	36	89%	97%	95%
Blood Culture Timing	75	99%	98%	98%
Pregnancy and Delivery Care				
Newborn Deliveries Scheduled Early[5]	-	-	2%	6%
Preventive Care				
Immunization for Influenza[2]	285	92%	95%	90%
Immunization for Pneumonia[2]	382	95%	95%	92%
Stroke Care				
Anticoagulation Therapy for Atrial Fibrillation[5]	-	-	96%	95%
Antithrombotic Therapy Timing[5]	-	-	99%	98%
Assessed for Rehabilitation[5]	-	-	96%	97%
Discharged on Antithrombotic Therapy[5]	-	-	100%	99%
Discharged on Statin Medication[5]	-	-	95%	94%
Thrombolytic Therapy Timing[5]	-	-	57%	66%
Venous Thromboembolism Prophylaxis[5]	-	-	94%	94%
Written Stroke Educational Materials Given[5]	-	-	76%	88%
Surgical Care Improvement Project				
Appropriate Beta Blocker Usage	21	100%	98%	98%
Appropriate VTP Within 24 Hours	58	100%	99%	98%
Controlled Postoperative Blood Glucose[3,7]	-	-	98%	97%
Perioperative Temperature Management	64	100%	100%	100%
Prophylactic Antibiotic Selection	55	96%	99%	99%
Prophylactic Antibiotic Selection (Outpatient)	19	95%	99%	98%
Prophylactic Antibiotic Stopped	54	91%	98%	98%
Prophylactic Antibiotic Timing	55	100%	99%	99%
Prophylactic Antibiotic Timing (Outpatient)	19	100%	98%	98%
Urinary Catheter Removal	14	86%	98%	97%
Survey of Patients' Hospital Experiences				
Area Around Room 'Always' Quiet at Night	300+	59%	57%	61%
Doctors 'Always' Communicated Well	300+	83%	81%	82%
Home Recovery Information Given	300+	89%	88%	85%
Hospital Given 9 or 10 on 10 Point Scale	300+	75%	71%	71%
Meds 'Always' Explained Before Given	300+	66%	65%	64%
Nurses 'Always' Communicated Well	300+	85%	80%	79%
Pain 'Always' Well Controlled	300+	74%	72%	71%
Room and Bathroom 'Always' Clean	300+	80%	76%	73%
Timely Help 'Always' Received	300+	78%	70%	68%
Would Definitely Recommend Hospital	300+	79%	74%	71%
Use of Medical Imaging				
Cardiac Imaging Stress Test before Surgery	127	3.1%	4.7%	5.3%
Combination Abdominal CT Scan	362	5.8%	5.6%	10.5%
Combination Brain/Sinus CT Scan[1]	-	-	2.3%	2.7%
Combination Chest CT Scan	213	0.0%	0.5%	2.7%
Follow-up Mammogram/Ultrasound	849	10.5%	8.2%	8.8%
Lumbar Spine MRI for Low Back Pain	75	36.0%	33.5%	37.2%

Speare Memorial Hospital

16 Hospital Road
Plymouth, NH 03264
Phone: 603-536-1120
Fax: 603-536-4828
URL: www.spearehospital.com
Type: Critical Access Hospitals
Emergency Services: Yes
Ownership: Voluntary non-profit - Private
Beds: 47

Key Personnel:

Radiology.................. Michael Beckerman
Operating Room............. John Bentwood
Chief of Medical Staff.......... Joseph Ebner
Quality Assurance .... Priscilla Farrell
Infection Control.............. Ann Graves
CEO/President................ Michelle McEwen, FACHE, CPA
Emergency Room .... Alex Medlacot
President .... Kevin Young

Measure	Cases	This Hosp.	State Avg.	U.S. Avg.
Blood Clot Prevention and Treatment				
Anticoagulation Overlap Therapy[5]	-	-	99%	93%
ICU Venous Thromboembolism Prophylaxis[5]	-	-	96%	92%
Incidence of Potentially Preventable VTE[5]	-	-	2%	10%
UFH with Dosages/Platelet Monitoring[5]	-	-	100%	97%
Venous Thromboembolism Prophylaxis[5]	-	-	93%	85%
Warfarin Therapy Discharge Instructions[5]	-	-	77%	75%
Chest Pain/Possible Heart Attack Care				
Aspirin Given Within 24 Hours of Arrival	56	100%	99%	96%
Fibrinolytic Meds Within 30 Min. of Arrival[1]	-	-	82%	58%
Average Time to ECG (minutes)	56	8	8	7
Average Time to Transfer (minutes)[7]	-	-	52	60
Children's Asthma Care				
Received Home Management Plan of Care	-	-	-	88%
Received Reliever Medication	-	-	-	100%
Received Systemic Corticosteroids	-	-	-	100%
Emergency Department				
Admittance Decision Time (minutes)[2]	400	84	107	98
Head CT Results Within 45 Min. of Arrival[5]	-	-	61%	57%
Patients Who Left ER Before Being Seen	14,526	0%	1%	2%
Time from ER Arrival to Admit. (minutes)[2]	407	256	292	274
Time from ER Arrival to Discharge (minutes)[3]	284	113	139	134
Time in ER Before Being Evaluated (minutes)[3]	287	26	30	26
Time to Pain Meds for Fractures (minutes)[5]	-	-	59	57
Heart Attack Care				
Aspirin Given at Discharge[3,7]	-	-	100%	99%
Fibrinolytic Meds Within 30 Min. of Arrival[3,7]	-	-	50%	54%
PCI Within 90 Minutes of Arrival[5]	-	-	95%	96%
Statin Prescribed at Discharge[3,7]	-	-	100%	98%
Heart Failure Care				
ACE Inhibitor or ARB for LVSD[1]	-	-	98%	97%
Discharge Instructions Given	27	100%	97%	94%
Evaluation of LVS Function	31	100%	100%	99%
Medicare Spending				
Medicare Spending per Patient (ratio)	-	-	1.01	0.98
Pneumonia Care				
Appropriate Initial Antibiotic Given	42	100%	97%	95%
Blood Culture Timing	71	99%	98%	98%
Pregnancy and Delivery Care				
Newborn Deliveries Scheduled Early	19	0%	2%	6%
Preventive Care				
Immunization for Influenza[2]	292	98%	95%	90%
Immunization for Pneumonia[2]	367	97%	95%	92%
Stroke Care				
Anticoagulation Therapy for Atrial Fibrillation[5]	-	-	96%	95%
Antithrombotic Therapy Timing[5]	-	-	99%	98%
Assessed for Rehabilitation[5]	-	-	96%	97%
Discharged on Antithrombotic Therapy[5]	-	-	100%	99%
Discharged on Statin Medication[5]	-	-	95%	94%
Thrombolytic Therapy Timing[5]	-	-	57%	66%
Venous Thromboembolism Prophylaxis[5]	-	-	94%	94%
Written Stroke Educational Materials Given[5]	-	-	76%	88%
Surgical Care Improvement Project				
Appropriate Beta Blocker Usage	17	100%	98%	98%
Appropriate VTP Within 24 Hours	64	100%	99%	98%
Controlled Postoperative Blood Glucose[3,7]	-	-	98%	97%
Perioperative Temperature Management	72	100%	100%	100%
Prophylactic Antibiotic Selection	48	100%	99%	99%
Prophylactic Antibiotic Selection (Outpatient)	22	100%	99%	98%
Prophylactic Antibiotic Stopped	46	98%	98%	98%
Prophylactic Antibiotic Timing	48	100%	99%	99%
Prophylactic Antibiotic Timing (Outpatient)	22	100%	98%	98%
Urinary Catheter Removal	55	100%	98%	97%
Survey of Patients' Hospital Experiences				
Area Around Room 'Always' Quiet at Night	300+	60%	57%	61%
Doctors 'Always' Communicated Well	300+	87%	81%	82%
Home Recovery Information Given	300+	88%	88%	85%
Hospital Given 9 or 10 on 10 Point Scale	300+	73%	71%	71%
Meds 'Always' Explained Before Given	300+	71%	65%	64%
Nurses 'Always' Communicated Well	300+	84%	80%	79%
Pain 'Always' Well Controlled	300+	77%	72%	71%
Room and Bathroom 'Always' Clean	300+	84%	76%	73%
Timely Help 'Always' Received	300+	77%	70%	68%
Would Definitely Recommend Hospital	300+	76%	74%	71%
Use of Medical Imaging				
Cardiac Imaging Stress Test before Surgery	158	3.8%	4.7%	5.3%
Combination Abdominal CT Scan	312	4.8%	5.6%	10.5%
Combination Brain/Sinus CT Scan[1]	-	-	2.3%	2.7%
Combination Chest CT Scan	130	0.0%	0.5%	2.7%
Follow-up Mammogram/Ultrasound	664	8.6%	8.2%	8.8%
Lumbar Spine MRI for Low Back Pain	50	40.0%	33.5%	37.2%

Portsmouth Regional Hospital

333 Borthwick Ave
Portsmouth, NH 03801
Phone: 603-436-5110
Fax: 603-433-5245
URL: www.portsmouthhospital.com
Type: Acute Care Hospitals
Emergency Services: Yes
Ownership: Proprietary
Beds: 209

Key Personnel:

CEO/President................ William Schurer
Chief of Medical Staff.......... Iva Schwartz, MD

Measure	Cases	This Hosp.	State Avg.	U.S. Avg.
Blood Clot Prevention and Treatment				
Anticoagulation Overlap Therapy[2]	26	100%	99%	93%
ICU Venous Thromboembolism Prophylaxis[2]	91	100%	96%	92%
Incidence of Potentially Preventable VTE[1,2]	-	-	2%	10%
UFH with Dosages/Platelet Monitoring[2]	16	100%	100%	97%
Venous Thromboembolism Prophylaxis[2]	311	100%	93%	85%
Warfarin Therapy Discharge Instructions[2]	19	100%	77%	75%
Chest Pain/Possible Heart Attack Care				
Aspirin Given Within 24 Hours of Arrival[1,3]	-	-	99%	96%
Fibrinolytic Meds Within 30 Min. of Arrival[5]	-	-	82%	58%
Average Time to ECG (minutes)[1,3]	-	-	8	7
Average Time to Transfer (minutes)[5]	-	-	52	60
Children's Asthma Care				
Received Home Management Plan of Care	-	-	-	88%
Received Reliever Medication	-	-	-	100%
Received Systemic Corticosteroids	-	-	-	100%
Emergency Department				
Admittance Decision Time (minutes)[2]	665	90	107	98
Head CT Results Within 45 Min. of Arrival[1]	-	-	61%	57%
Patients Who Left ER Before Being Seen	25,992	1%	1%	2%
Time from ER Arrival to Admit. (minutes)[2]	670	245	292	274
Time from ER Arrival to Discharge (minutes)	447	120	139	134
Time in ER Before Being Evaluated (minutes)	498	17	30	26
Time to Pain Meds for Fractures (minutes)	75	40	59	57
Heart Attack Care				
Aspirin Given at Discharge	298	100%	100%	99%
Fibrinolytic Meds Within 30 Min. of Arrival[7]	-	-	50%	54%
PCI Within 90 Minutes of Arrival	26	100%	95%	96%
Statin Prescribed at Discharge	285	100%	100%	98%
Heart Failure Care				
ACE Inhibitor or ARB for LVSD	45	100%	98%	97%
Discharge Instructions Given	122	100%	97%	94%
Evaluation of LVS Function	171	100%	100%	99%
Medicare Spending				
Medicare Spending per Patient (ratio)	-	1.02	1.01	0.98
Pneumonia Care				
Appropriate Initial Antibiotic Given	57	100%	97%	95%
Blood Culture Timing	105	100%	98%	98%
Pregnancy and Delivery Care				
Newborn Deliveries Scheduled Early[2]	23	4%	2%	6%
Preventive Care				
Immunization for Influenza[2]	549	98%	95%	90%
Immunization for Pneumonia[2]	741	99%	95%	92%
Stroke Care				
Anticoagulation Therapy for Atrial Fibrillation	15	100%	96%	95%
Antithrombotic Therapy Timing	47	100%	99%	98%
Assessed for Rehabilitation	71	100%	96%	97%
Discharged on Antithrombotic Therapy	54	100%	100%	99%
Discharged on Statin Medication	47	100%	95%	94%
Thrombolytic Therapy Timing[1]	-	-	57%	66%

NOTE: Hospital profiles are in alphabetical order by state, then city, then hospital within the city; Rankings exclude hospitals with less than 25 cases except for patient surveys which excludes hospitals with less than 100 cases; (a) 100-299 cases; (1) The number of cases/patients is too few to report; (2) Data submitted were based on a sample of cases/patients; (3) Results are based on a shorter time period than required; (4) Data suppressed by CMS for one or more quarters; (5) Results are not available for this reporting period; (6) Fewer than 100 patients completed the HCAHPS survey; (7) No cases met the criteria for this measure; (8) The lower limit of the confidence interval cannot be calculated if the number of observed infections equals zero; (9) No data are available from the state/territory for this reporting period; (10) The scores shown reflect fewer than 50 completed surveys; (11) There were discrepancies in the data collection process; (12) This measure does not apply to this hospital for this reporting period; (13) Results cannot be calculated for this reporting period; (14) The results for this state are combined with nearby states to protect confidentiality; Please refer to the User's Guide for a full explanation of data.

Measure	Cases	This Hosp.	State Avg.	U.S. Avg.
Venous Thromboembolism Prophylaxis	70	100%	94%	94%
Written Stroke Educational Materials Given	35	100%	76%	88%
Surgical Care Improvement Project				
Appropriate Beta Blocker Usage[2]	265	100%	98%	98%
Appropriate VTP Within 24 Hours[2]	377	100%	99%	98%
Controlled Postoperative Blood Glucose[2]	181	99%	98%	97%
Perioperative Temperature Management[2]	435	100%	100%	100%
Prophylactic Antibiotic Selection[2]	430	100%	99%	99%
Prophylactic Antibiotic Selection (Outpatient)	268	100%	99%	98%
Prophylactic Antibiotic Stopped[2]	411	100%	98%	98%
Prophylactic Antibiotic Timing[2]	430	100%	99%	99%
Prophylactic Antibiotic Timing (Outpatient)	269	100%	98%	98%
Urinary Catheter Removal[2]	333	100%	98%	97%
Survey of Patients' Hospital Experiences				
Area Around Room 'Always' Quiet at Night	300+	59%	57%	61%
Doctors 'Always' Communicated Well	300+	81%	81%	82%
Home Recovery Information Given	300+	90%	88%	85%
Hospital Given 9 or 10 on 10 Point Scale	300+	70%	71%	71%
Meds 'Always' Explained Before Given	300+	63%	65%	64%
Nurses 'Always' Communicated Well	300+	78%	80%	79%
Pain 'Always' Well Controlled	300+	68%	72%	71%
Room and Bathroom 'Always' Clean	300+	71%	76%	73%
Timely Help 'Always' Received	300+	61%	70%	68%
Would Definitely Recommend Hospital	300+	75%	74%	71%
Use of Medical Imaging				
Cardiac Imaging Stress Test before Surgery	339	6.5%	4.7%	5.3%
Combination Abdominal CT Scan	525	9.3%	5.6%	10.5%
Combination Brain/Sinus CT Scan	530	0.6%	2.3%	2.7%
Combination Chest CT Scan	318	0.0%	0.5%	2.7%
Follow-up Mammogram/Ultrasound	1,878	13.0%	8.2%	8.8%
Lumbar Spine MRI for Low Back Pain	197	23.9%	33.5%	37.2%

Frisbie Memorial Hospital

11 Whitehall Road
Rochester, NH 03867
E-mail: fmh3666@rscs.net
URL: www.frisbiehospital.com
Phone: 603-332-5211
Fax: 603-332-2699
Type: Acute Care Hospitals
Ownership: Voluntary non-profit - Private
Emergency Services: Yes
Beds: 122

Key Personnel:
Radiology. . . . . Albert Chang
Patient Relations . . . . Karen Dutcher
CEO/President. . . . . Alvin Felgar
Intensive Care Unit. . . . . Sally Gallot
Pediatric In-Patient Care . . . . Wallace Hubbard, MD
Quality Assurance . . . . Ellen Littlefield
Operating Room. . . . . Joseph Shields
Chief of Medical Staff . . . . Sara Stacey, MD

Measure	Cases	This Hosp.	State Avg.	U.S. Avg.
Blood Clot Prevention and Treatment				
Anticoagulation Overlap Therapy[2]	29	100%	99%	93%
ICU Venous Thromboembolism Prophylaxis[2]	51	94%	96%	92%
Incidence of Potentially Preventable VTE[1,2]	-	-	2%	10%
UFH with Dosages/Platelet Monitoring[2]	11	100%	100%	97%
Venous Thromboembolism Prophylaxis[2]	245	98%	93%	85%
Warfarin Therapy Discharge Instructions[2]	20	85%	77%	75%
Chest Pain/Possible Heart Attack Care				
Aspirin Given Within 24 Hours of Arrival	41	100%	99%	96%
Fibrinolytic Meds Within 30 Min. of Arrival[7]	-	-	82%	58%
Average Time to ECG (minutes)	45	8	8	7
Average Time to Transfer (minutes)[1]	-	-	52	60
Children's Asthma Care				
Received Home Management Plan of Care	-	-	-	88%
Received Reliever Medication	-	-	-	100%
Received Systemic Corticosteroids	-	-	-	100%
Emergency Department				
Admittance Decision Time (minutes)[2]	446	117	107	98
Head CT Results Within 45 Min. of Arrival[1,3]	-	-	61%	57%
Patients Who Left ER Before Being Seen	28,975	1%	1%	2%
Time from ER Arrival to Admit. (minutes)[2]	446	313	292	274
Time from ER Arrival to Discharge (minutes)	381	124	139	134
Time in ER Before Being Evaluated (minutes)	400	28	30	26
Time to Pain Meds for Fractures (minutes)	100	56	59	57
Heart Attack Care				
Aspirin Given at Discharge	14	100%	100%	99%
Fibrinolytic Meds Within 30 Min. of Arrival[7]	-	-	50%	54%
PCI Within 90 Minutes of Arrival[7]	-	-	95%	96%
Statin Prescribed at Discharge	12	100%	100%	98%
Heart Failure Care				
ACE Inhibitor or ARB for LVSD	17	100%	98%	97%
Discharge Instructions Given	98	100%	97%	94%
Evaluation of LVS Function	120	98%	100%	99%
Medicare Spending				
Medicare Spending per Patient (ratio)	-	1.05	1.01	0.98
Pneumonia Care				
Appropriate Initial Antibiotic Given	120	95%	97%	95%
Blood Culture Timing	130	96%	98%	98%
Pregnancy and Delivery Care				
Newborn Deliveries Scheduled Early	48	0%	2%	6%
Preventive Care				
Immunization for Influenza[2]	337	97%	95%	90%
Immunization for Pneumonia[2]	419	98%	95%	92%
Stroke Care				
Anticoagulation Therapy for Atrial Fibrillation[1]	-	-	96%	95%
Antithrombotic Therapy Timing	36	100%	99%	98%
Assessed for Rehabilitation	37	100%	96%	97%
Discharged on Antithrombotic Therapy	35	100%	100%	99%
Discharged on Statin Medication	26	88%	95%	94%
Thrombolytic Therapy Timing[1]	-	-	57%	66%
Venous Thromboembolism Prophylaxis	39	92%	94%	94%
Written Stroke Educational Materials Given	20	50%	76%	88%
Surgical Care Improvement Project				
Appropriate Beta Blocker Usage	90	96%	98%	98%
Appropriate VTP Within 24 Hours	208	100%	99%	98%
Controlled Postoperative Blood Glucose[7]	-	-	98%	97%
Perioperative Temperature Management	244	100%	100%	100%
Prophylactic Antibiotic Selection	175	100%	99%	99%
Prophylactic Antibiotic Selection (Outpatient)	120	98%	99%	98%
Prophylactic Antibiotic Stopped	175	98%	98%	98%
Prophylactic Antibiotic Timing	175	98%	99%	99%
Prophylactic Antibiotic Timing (Outpatient)	120	100%	98%	98%
Urinary Catheter Removal	177	100%	98%	97%
Survey of Patients' Hospital Experiences				
Area Around Room 'Always' Quiet at Night	300+	73%	57%	61%
Doctors 'Always' Communicated Well	300+	83%	81%	82%
Home Recovery Information Given	300+	89%	88%	85%
Hospital Given 9 or 10 on 10 Point Scale	300+	73%	71%	71%
Meds 'Always' Explained Before Given	300+	70%	65%	64%
Nurses 'Always' Communicated Well	300+	83%	80%	79%
Pain 'Always' Well Controlled	300+	76%	72%	71%
Room and Bathroom 'Always' Clean	300+	80%	76%	73%
Timely Help 'Always' Received	300+	76%	70%	68%
Would Definitely Recommend Hospital	300+	72%	74%	71%
Use of Medical Imaging				
Cardiac Imaging Stress Test before Surgery	269	6.3%	4.7%	5.3%
Combination Abdominal CT Scan	732	3.7%	5.6%	10.5%
Combination Brain/Sinus CT Scan	578	1.7%	2.3%	2.7%
Combination Chest CT Scan	666	0.0%	0.5%	2.7%
Follow-up Mammogram/Ultrasound[7]	-	-	8.2%	8.8%
Lumbar Spine MRI for Low Back Pain	112	35.7%	33.5%	37.2%

Huggins Hospital

240 South Main Street
Wolfeboro, NH 03894
E-mail: askhuggins@hugginshospital.org
URL: www.hugginshospital.org
Phone: 603-569-7500
Fax: 603-569-7509
Type: Critical Access Hospitals
Ownership: Voluntary non-profit - Private
Emergency Services: Yes
Beds: 55

Key Personnel:
Surgery . . . . Thomas M. Barton, MD
Chief of Medical Staff. . . . . John S. Boornazian, MD
Infection Control. . . . . Linda Brookes
CEO/President. . . . . Michael P. Connelly
Emergency Room . . . . Jim Copenhaver, MD
Pediatric In-Patient Care . . . . Harley W Heath, MD
Quality Assurance . . . . Rebecca Mason
Chairman/CEO . . . . Timothy Sullivan

Measure	Cases	This Hosp.	State Avg.	U.S. Avg.
Blood Clot Prevention and Treatment				
Anticoagulation Overlap Therapy[5]	-	-	99%	93%
ICU Venous Thromboembolism Prophylaxis[5]	-	-	96%	92%
Incidence of Potentially Preventable VTE[5]	-	-	2%	10%
UFH with Dosages/Platelet Monitoring[5]	-	-	100%	97%
Venous Thromboembolism Prophylaxis[5]	-	-	93%	85%
Warfarin Therapy Discharge Instructions[5]	-	-	77%	75%
Chest Pain/Possible Heart Attack Care				
Aspirin Given Within 24 Hours of Arrival[5]	-	-	99%	96%
Fibrinolytic Meds Within 30 Min. of Arrival[5]	-	-	82%	58%
Average Time to ECG (minutes)[5]	-	-	8	7
Average Time to Transfer (minutes)[5]	-	-	52	60
Children's Asthma Care				
Received Home Management Plan of Care	-	-	-	88%
Received Reliever Medication	-	-	-	100%
Received Systemic Corticosteroids	-	-	-	100%
Emergency Department				
Admittance Decision Time (minutes)[5]	-	-	107	98
Head CT Results Within 45 Min. of Arrival[5]	-	-	61%	57%
Patients Who Left ER Before Being Seen[5]	-	-	1%	2%
Time from ER Arrival to Admit. (minutes)[5]	-	-	292	274
Time from ER Arrival to Discharge (minutes)[5]	-	-	139	134
Time in ER Before Being Evaluated (minutes)[5]	-	-	30	26
Time to Pain Meds for Fractures (minutes)[5]	-	-	59	57
Heart Attack Care				
Aspirin Given at Discharge[1]	-	-	100%	99%
Fibrinolytic Meds Within 30 Min. of Arrival[7]	-	-	50%	54%
PCI Within 90 Minutes of Arrival[3,7]	-	-	95%	96%
Statin Prescribed at Discharge[1]	-	-	100%	98%
Heart Failure Care				
ACE Inhibitor or ARB for LVSD	17	100%	98%	97%
Discharge Instructions Given	21	100%	97%	94%
Evaluation of LVS Function	34	100%	100%	99%
Medicare Spending				
Medicare Spending per Patient (ratio)	-	-	1.01	0.98
Pneumonia Care				
Appropriate Initial Antibiotic Given	50	100%	97%	95%
Blood Culture Timing	70	99%	98%	98%
Pregnancy and Delivery Care				
Newborn Deliveries Scheduled Early[5]	-	-	2%	6%
Preventive Care				
Immunization for Influenza[5]	-	-	95%	90%
Immunization for Pneumonia[5]	-	-	95%	92%
Stroke Care				
Anticoagulation Therapy for Atrial Fibrillation[5]	-	-	96%	95%
Antithrombotic Therapy Timing[5]	-	-	99%	98%
Assessed for Rehabilitation[5]	-	-	96%	97%
Discharged on Antithrombotic Therapy[5]	-	-	100%	99%
Discharged on Statin Medication[5]	-	-	95%	94%
Thrombolytic Therapy Timing[5]	-	-	57%	66%
Venous Thromboembolism Prophylaxis[5]	-	-	94%	94%
Written Stroke Educational Materials Given[5]	-	-	76%	88%
Surgical Care Improvement Project				
Appropriate Beta Blocker Usage[1]	-	-	98%	98%
Appropriate VTP Within 24 Hours	83	100%	99%	98%
Controlled Postoperative Blood Glucose[3,7]	-	-	98%	97%
Perioperative Temperature Management	89	100%	100%	100%
Prophylactic Antibiotic Selection	47	100%	99%	99%
Prophylactic Antibiotic Selection (Outpatient)[5]	-	-	99%	98%
Prophylactic Antibiotic Stopped	47	100%	98%	98%
Prophylactic Antibiotic Timing	47	98%	99%	99%
Prophylactic Antibiotic Timing (Outpatient)[5]	-	-	98%	98%
Urinary Catheter Removal	61	100%	98%	97%
Survey of Patients' Hospital Experiences				
Area Around Room 'Always' Quiet at Night	(a)	66%	57%	61%
Doctors 'Always' Communicated Well	(a)	77%	81%	82%
Home Recovery Information Given	(a)	87%	88%	85%
Hospital Given 9 or 10 on 10 Point Scale	(a)	63%	71%	71%
Meds 'Always' Explained Before Given	(a)	60%	65%	64%
Nurses 'Always' Communicated Well	(a)	76%	80%	79%
Pain 'Always' Well Controlled	(a)	70%	72%	71%
Room and Bathroom 'Always' Clean	(a)	78%	76%	73%

NOTE: Hospital profiles are in alphabetical order by state, then city, then hospital within the city; Rankings exclude hospitals with less than 25 cases except for patient surveys which excludes hospitals with less than 100 cases; (a) 100-299 cases; (1) The number of cases/patients is too few to report; (2) Data submitted were based on a sample of cases/patients; (3) Results are based on a shorter time period than required; (4) Data suppressed by CMS for one or more quarters; (5) Results are not available for this reporting period; (6) Fewer than 100 patients completed the HCAHPS survey; (7) No cases met the criteria for this measure; (8) The lower limit of the confidence interval cannot be calculated if the number of observed infections equals zero; (9) No data are available from the state/territory for this reporting period; (10) The scores shown reflect fewer than 50 completed surveys; (11) There were discrepancies in the data collection process; (12) This measure does not apply to this hospital for this reporting period; (13) Results cannot be calculated for this reporting period; (14) The results for this state are combined with nearby states to protect confidentiality; Please refer to the User's Guide for a full explanation of data.

Timely Help 'Always' Received	(a)	75%	70%	68%
Would Definitely Recommend Hospital	(a)	64%	74%	71%
Use of Medical Imaging				
Cardiac Imaging Stress Test before Surgery	119	6.7%	4.7%	5.3%
Combination Abdominal CT Scan	383	6.3%	5.6%	10.5%
Combination Brain/Sinus CT Scan[1]	-	-	2.3%	2.7%
Combination Chest CT Scan	248	2.4%	0.5%	2.7%
Follow-up Mammogram/Ultrasound	678	4.3%	8.2%	8.8%
Lumbar Spine MRI for Low Back Pain	50	48.0%	33.5%	37.2%

Cottage Hospital

90 Swiftwater Rd
Woodsville, NH 03785
Phone: 603-747-9000
Fax: 603-747-3310
E-mail: myhospital@cottagehospital.org
URL: www.cottagehospital.org

Type: Critical Access Hospitals
Emergency Services: Yes
Ownership: Voluntary non-profit - Private
Beds: 25

Key Personnel:

Quality Assurance . . . . Laurie Hughes
Chief of Medical Staff . . . . Mealanie Lawrence, MD
Infection Control . . . . Mary Ruppert, RN
Radiology . . . . Marcy Rushford, RT
CEO/President . . . . Maria Ryan, PhD
Cardiac Laboratory . . . . Lori Taylor
Operating Room . . . . Patricia Thaver, RN

Measure	Cases	This Hosp.	State Avg.	U.S. Avg.
Blood Clot Prevention and Treatment				
Anticoagulation Overlap Therapy[5]	-	-	99%	93%
ICU Venous Thromboembolism Prophylaxis[5]	-	-	96%	92%
Incidence of Potentially Preventable VTE[5]	-	-	2%	10%
UFH with Dosages/Platelet Monitoring[5]	-	-	100%	97%
Venous Thromboembolism Prophylaxis[5]	-	-	93%	85%
Warfarin Therapy Discharge Instructions[5]	-	-	77%	75%
Chest Pain/Possible Heart Attack Care				
Aspirin Given Within 24 Hours of Arrival	-	-	99%	96%
Fibrinolytic Meds Within 30 Min. of Arrival	-	-	82%	58%
Average Time to ECG (minutes)	-	-	8	7
Average Time to Transfer (minutes)	-	-	52	60
Children's Asthma Care				
Received Home Management Plan of Care	-	-	-	88%
Received Reliever Medication	-	-	-	100%
Received Systemic Corticosteroids	-	-	-	100%
Emergency Department				
Admittance Decision Time (minutes)[5]	-	-	107	98
Head CT Results Within 45 Min. of Arrival	-	-	61%	57%
Patients Who Left ER Before Being Seen	-	-	1%	2%
Time from ER Arrival to Admit. (minutes)[5]	-	-	292	274
Time from ER Arrival to Discharge (minutes)	-	-	139	134
Time in ER Before Being Evaluated (minutes)	-	-	30	26
Time to Pain Meds for Fractures (minutes)	-	-	59	57
Heart Attack Care				
Aspirin Given at Discharge[1,3]	-	-	100%	99%
Fibrinolytic Meds Within 30 Min. of Arrival[3,7]	-	-	50%	54%
PCI Within 90 Minutes of Arrival[3,7]	-	-	95%	96%
Statin Prescribed at Discharge[1,3]	-	-	100%	98%
Heart Failure Care				
ACE Inhibitor or ARB for LVSD[3,7]	-	-	98%	97%
Discharge Instructions Given[1,3]	-	-	97%	94%
Evaluation of LVS Function[1,3]	-	-	100%	99%
Medicare Spending				
Medicare Spending per Patient (ratio)	-	-	1.01	0.98
Pneumonia Care				
Appropriate Initial Antibiotic Given[1,3]	-	-	97%	95%
Blood Culture Timing[3]	12	100%	98%	98%
Pregnancy and Delivery Care				
Newborn Deliveries Scheduled Early[5]	-	-	2%	6%
Preventive Care				
Immunization for Influenza[5]	-	-	95%	90%
Immunization for Pneumonia[5]	-	-	95%	92%
Stroke Care				
Anticoagulation Therapy for Atrial Fibrillation[5]	-	-	96%	95%
Antithrombotic Therapy Timing[5]	-	-	99%	98%
Assessed for Rehabilitation[5]	-	-	96%	97%
Discharged on Antithrombotic Therapy[5]	-	-	100%	99%
Discharged on Statin Medication[5]	-	-	95%	94%
Thrombolytic Therapy Timing[5]	-	-	57%	66%
Venous Thromboembolism Prophylaxis[5]	-	-	94%	94%
Written Stroke Educational Materials Given[5]	-	-	76%	88%
Surgical Care Improvement Project				
Appropriate Beta Blocker Usage[1,3]	-	-	98%	98%
Appropriate VTP Within 24 Hours[3]	22	100%	99%	98%
Controlled Postoperative Blood Glucose[3,7]	-	-	98%	97%
Perioperative Temperature Management[3]	23	100%	100%	100%
Prophylactic Antibiotic Selection[3]	14	100%	99%	99%
Prophylactic Antibiotic Selection (Outpatient)	-	-	99%	98%
Prophylactic Antibiotic Stopped[3]	14	100%	98%	98%
Prophylactic Antibiotic Timing[3]	14	93%	99%	99%
Prophylactic Antibiotic Timing (Outpatient)	-	-	98%	98%
Urinary Catheter Removal[3]	20	100%	98%	97%
Survey of Patients' Hospital Experiences				
Area Around Room 'Always' Quiet at Night[5]	-	-	57%	61%
Doctors 'Always' Communicated Well[5]	-	-	81%	82%
Home Recovery Information Given[5]	-	-	88%	85%
Hospital Given 9 or 10 on 10 Point Scale[5]	-	-	71%	71%
Meds 'Always' Explained Before Given[5]	-	-	65%	64%
Nurses 'Always' Communicated Well[5]	-	-	80%	79%
Pain 'Always' Well Controlled[5]	-	-	72%	71%
Room and Bathroom 'Always' Clean[5]	-	-	76%	73%
Timely Help 'Always' Received[5]	-	-	70%	68%
Would Definitely Recommend Hospital[5]	-	-	74%	71%
Use of Medical Imaging				
Cardiac Imaging Stress Test before Surgery	-	-	4.7%	5.3%
Combination Abdominal CT Scan	-	-	5.6%	10.5%
Combination Brain/Sinus CT Scan	-	-	2.3%	2.7%
Combination Chest CT Scan	-	-	0.5%	2.7%
Follow-up Mammogram/Ultrasound	-	-	8.2%	8.8%
Lumbar Spine MRI for Low Back Pain	-	-	33.5%	37.2%

NOTE: Hospital profiles are in alphabetical order by state, then city, then hospital within the city; Rankings exclude hospitals with less than 25 cases except for patient surveys which excludes hospitals with less than 100 cases; (a) 100-299 cases; (1) The number of cases/patients is too few to report; (2) Data submitted were based on a sample of cases/patients; (3) Results are based on a shorter time period than required; (4) Data suppressed by CMS for one or more quarters; (5) Results are not available for this reporting period; (6) Fewer than 100 patients completed the HCAHPS survey; (7) No cases met the criteria for this measure; (8) The lower limit of the confidence interval cannot be calculated if the number of observed infections equals zero; (9) No data are available from the state/territory for this reporting period; (10) The scores shown reflect fewer than 50 completed surveys; (11) There were discrepancies in the data collection process; (12) This measure does not apply to this hospital for this reporting period; (13) Results cannot be calculated for this reporting period; (14) The results for this state are combined with nearby states to protect confidentiality; Please refer to the User's Guide for a full explanation of data.

Blood Clot Prevention and Treatment

Anticoagulation Overlap Therapy

Hospital Name	City	Rate	Cases
Atlanticare Regional Medical Center[2]	Atlantic City	100%	250
Chilton Medical Center[2]	Pompton Plains	100%	80
Hackensack - Umc Mountainside[2]	Montclair	100%	61
Palisades Medical Center[2]	North Bergen	100%	36
Univ Med Ctr of Princeton-Plainsboro[2]	Plainsboro	100%	79
Robert Wood Johnson University Hospital[2]	New Brunswick	99%	155
Saint Francis Medical Center[2]	Trenton	98%	42
Overlook Medical Center[2]	Summit	97%	144
University Hospital[2]	Newark	97%	95
Inspira Medical Center Vineland[2]	Vineland	96%	78
Jersey Shore University Medical Center[2]	Neptune	96%	128
Capital Health Medical Center - Hopewell[2]	Pennington	95%	76
Englewood Hospital & Medical Center[2]	Englewood	95%	41
Saint Peter's University Hospital[2]	New Brunswick	95%	80
Virtua West Jersey Hospitals Berlin[2]	Berlin	95%	268
Capital Health System - Fuld Campus[2]	Trenton	94%	72
Inspira Medical Center Elmer[2]	Elmer	94%	51
Morristown Medical Center[2]	Morristown	94%	235
Newton Memorial Hospital[2]	Newton	94%	54
Ocean Medical Center[2]	Brick	94%	82
Trinitas Regional Medical Center[2]	Elizabeth	94%	84
Bayshore Community Hospital[2]	Holmdel	93%	57
Our Lady of Lourdes Medical Center[2]	Camden	93%	113
Saint Clare's Hospital[2]	Denville	93%	71
Virtua Mem Hosp of Burlington County[2]	Mount Holly	93%	146
Hackensack University Medical Center[2]	Hackensack	92%	241
Memorial Hospital of Salem County[2]	Salem	92%	39
Southern Ocean Medical Center[2]	Manahawkin	92%	63
Lourdes Med Ctr of Burlington County[2]	Willingboro	89%	66
Hunterdon Medical Center[2]	Flemington	88%	49
Saint Joseph's Regional Medical Center[2]	Paterson	88%	120
Cooper University Hospital[2]	Camden	87%	137
Holy Name Medical Center[2]	Teaneck	87%	97
Libertyhealth-Jersey City Med Ctr[2]	Jersey City	87%	89
Kennedy Univ Hosp-Stratford Div[2]	Stratford	86%	257
Community Medical Center[2]	Toms River	85%	198
Newark Beth Israel Medical Center[2]	Newark	85%	130
Somerset Medical Center[2]	Somerville	85%	122
Monmouth Medical Center - Southern Campus[2]	Lakewood	84%	43
Riverview Medical Center[2]	Red Bank	83%	52
Robert Wood Johnson Univ Hosp-Rahway[2]	Rahway	83%	48
Saint Barnabas Medical Center[2]	Livingston	83%	162
Centrastate Medical Center[2]	Freehold	81%	64
Raritan Bay Medical Center[2]	Perth Amboy	81%	103
Robert W Johnson Univ Hosp-Hamilton[2]	Hamilton	81%	98
Saint Mary's Hospital - Passaic[2]	Passaic	81%	47
Carepoint Health - Christ Hospital[2]	Jersey City	80%	54
Monmouth Medical Center[2]	Long Branch	78%	67
Cape Regional Medical Center[2]	Cape May CH	76%	63
Inspira Medical Center Woodbury[2]	Woodbury	76%	66
Saint Luke's Warren Hospital[2]	Phillipsburg	74%	61
Valley Hospital[2]	Ridgewood	73%	246
Shore Medical Center[2]	Somers Point	65%	71
Clara Maass Medical Center[2]	Belleville	64%	77
East Orange General Hospital[2]	East Orange	64%	59
JFK Med Ctr-A M Yelencsics Comm Hosp[2]	Edison	58%	164
Saint Michael's Medical Center[2]	Newark	52%	44

ICU Venous Thromboembolism Prophylaxis

Hospital Name	City	Rate	Cases
Carepoint Health-Bayonne Hosp Ctr[2]	Bayonne	100%	90
Chilton Medical Center[2]	Pompton Plains	100%	46
Englewood Hospital & Medical Center[2]	Englewood	100%	55
Jersey Shore University Medical Center[2]	Neptune	100%	69
Ocean Medical Center[2]	Brick	100%	49
Bayshore Community Hospital[2]	Holmdel	99%	92
Capital Health System - Fuld Campus[2]	Trenton	99%	148
Centrastate Medical Center[2]	Freehold	99%	67
Kennedy Univ Hosp-Stratford Div[2]	Stratford	99%	78
Saint Luke's Warren Hospital[2]	Phillipsburg	99%	88
Capital Health Medical Center - Hopewell[2]	Pennington	98%	99
Community Medical Center[2]	Toms River	98%	66
Overlook Medical Center[2]	Summit	98%	89
Robert W Johnson Univ Hosp-Hamilton[2]	Hamilton	98%	91
Saint Peter's University Hospital[2]	New Brunswick	98%	66
Atlanticare Regional Medical Center[2]	Atlantic City	97%	71
Carepoint Health - Christ Hospital[2]	Jersey City	97%	60
Deborah Heart & Lung Center[2]	Browns Mills	97%	183
Hackensack - Umc Mountainside[2]	Montclair	97%	64
Hunterdon Medical Center[2]	Flemington	97%	62
Inspira Medical Center Vineland[2]	Vineland	97%	113
Robert Wood Johnson University Hospital[2]	New Brunswick	97%	79
Saint Francis Medical Center[2]	Trenton	97%	118
Virtua Mem Hosp of Burlington County[2]	Mount Holly	97%	67
Monmouth Medical Center[2]	Long Branch	96%	67
Riverview Medical Center[2]	Red Bank	96%	74
Carepoint Health - Hoboken UMC[2]	Hoboken	95%	42
Inspira Medical Center Woodbury[2]	Woodbury	95%	61
Shore Medical Center[2]	Somers Point	95%	65
Trinitas Regional Medical Center[2]	Elizabeth	95%	86
Morristown Medical Center[2]	Morristown	94%	85
Saint Clare's Hospital[2]	Denville	94%	68
Southern Ocean Medical Center[2]	Manahawkin	94%	86
University Hospital[2]	Newark	94%	83
Valley Hospital[2]	Ridgewood	94%	64
Cape Regional Medical Center[2]	Cape May CH	93%	92
Saint Michael's Medical Center[2]	Newark	93%	91
Univ Med Ctr of Princeton-Plainsboro[2]	Plainsboro	93%	44
Cooper University Hospital[2]	Camden	92%	76
Holy Name Medical Center[2]	Teaneck	92%	38
Meadowlands Hospital Medical Center[2]	Secaucus	92%	75
Newton Memorial Hospital[2]	Newton	92%	78
Virtua West Jersey Hospitals Berlin[2]	Berlin	92%	51
Libertyhealth-Jersey City Med Ctr[2]	Jersey City	91%	109
Memorial Hospital of Salem County[2]	Salem	91%	105
Saint Barnabas Medical Center[2]	Livingston	91%	58
Saint Joseph's Regional Medical Center[2]	Paterson	91%	158
Palisades Medical Center[2]	North Bergen	90%	39
East Orange General Hospital[2]	East Orange	89%	65
Saint Mary's Hospital - Passaic[2]	Passaic	88%	86
Hackensack University Medical Center[2]	Hackensack	87%	54
Newark Beth Israel Medical Center[2]	Newark	87%	79
Robert Wood Johnson Univ Hosp-Rahway[2]	Rahway	86%	96
Lourdes Med Ctr of Burlington County[2]	Willingboro	85%	108
Our Lady of Lourdes Medical Center[2]	Camden	85%	114
Raritan Bay Medical Center[2]	Perth Amboy	85%	108
Monmouth Medical Center - Southern Campus[2]	Lakewood	84%	51
Clara Maass Medical Center[2]	Belleville	82%	61
Hackettstown Regional Medical Center[2]	Hackettstown	81%	52
Inspira Medical Center Elmer[2]	Elmer	78%	50
Somerset Medical Center[2]	Somerville	75%	60
JFK Med Ctr-A M Yelencsics Comm Hosp[2]	Edison	67%	73

Incidence of Potentially Preventable VTE

Hospital Name	City	Rate	Cases
Capital Health Medical Center - Hopewell[2]	Pennington	0%	28
Capital Health System - Fuld Campus[2]	Trenton	0%	46
Saint Peter's University Hospital[2]	New Brunswick	0%	32
Jersey Shore University Medical Center[2]	Neptune	3%	30
Overlook Medical Center[2]	Summit	3%	33
Virtua Mem Hosp of Burlington County[2]	Mount Holly	3%	32
Morristown Medical Center[2]	Morristown	4%	82
Robert Wood Johnson University Hospital[2]	New Brunswick	4%	57
Trinitas Regional Medical Center[2]	Elizabeth	4%	26
Cooper University Hospital[2]	Camden	5%	88
Kennedy Univ Hosp-Stratford Div[2]	Stratford	5%	57
Atlanticare Regional Medical Center[2]	Atlantic City	6%	64
Libertyhealth-Jersey City Med Ctr[2]	Jersey City	7%	42
Newark Beth Israel Medical Center[2]	Newark	7%	68
University Hospital[2]	Newark	7%	61
Holy Name Medical Center[2]	Teaneck	8%	61
Saint Barnabas Medical Center[2]	Livingston	8%	74
Hackensack University Medical Center[2]	Hackensack	10%	101
Virtua West Jersey Hospitals Berlin[2]	Berlin	11%	54
Valley Hospital[2]	Ridgewood	21%	72
Raritan Bay Medical Center[2]	Perth Amboy	22%	32
Monmouth Medical Center[2]	Long Branch	27%	26
Clara Maass Medical Center[2]	Belleville	33%	27
JFK Med Ctr-A M Yelencsics Comm Hosp[2]	Edison	33%	51

UFH with Dosages/Platelet Count Monitoring

Hospital Name	City	Rate	Cases
Atlanticare Regional Medical Center[2]	Atlantic City	100%	281
Bayshore Community Hospital[2]	Holmdel	100%	56
Cape Regional Medical Center[2]	Cape May CH	100%	66
Capital Health Medical Center - Hopewell[2]	Pennington	100%	89
Capital Health System - Fuld Campus[2]	Trenton	100%	75
Carepoint Health - Christ Hospital[2]	Jersey City	100%	40
Centrastate Medical Center[2]	Freehold	100%	68
Cooper University Hospital[2]	Camden	100%	154
Deborah Heart & Lung Center[2]	Browns Mills	100%	31
East Orange General Hospital[2]	East Orange	100%	28
Hackensack - Umc Mountainside[2]	Montclair	100%	34
Hackensack University Medical Center[2]	Hackensack	100%	240
Hackettstown Regional Medical Center[2]	Hackettstown	100%	29
Holy Name Medical Center[2]	Teaneck	100%	80
Inspira Medical Center Elmer[2]	Elmer	100%	50
Inspira Medical Center Woodbury[2]	Woodbury	100%	33
Jersey Shore University Medical Center[2]	Neptune	100%	131
Kennedy Univ Hosp-Stratford Div[2]	Stratford	100%	270
Libertyhealth-Jersey City Med Ctr[2]	Jersey City	100%	59
Lourdes Med Ctr of Burlington County[2]	Willingboro	100%	54
Morristown Medical Center[2]	Morristown	100%	248
Newark Beth Israel Medical Center[2]	Newark	100%	110
Ocean Medical Center[2]	Brick	100%	44
Our Lady of Lourdes Medical Center[2]	Camden	100%	120
Overlook Medical Center[2]	Summit	100%	80
Robert W Johnson Univ Hosp-Hamilton[2]	Hamilton	100%	104
Saint Francis Medical Center[2]	Trenton	100%	42
Saint Joseph's Regional Medical Center[2]	Paterson	100%	36
Saint Luke's Warren Hospital[2]	Phillipsburg	100%	38
Shore Medical Center[2]	Somers Point	100%	103
Somerset Medical Center[2]	Somerville	100%	130
Southern Ocean Medical Center[2]	Manahawkin	100%	44
Univ Med Ctr of Princeton-Plainsboro[2]	Plainsboro	100%	36
Community Medical Center[2]	Toms River	99%	101
Inspira Medical Center Vineland[2]	Vineland	99%	74
Saint Clare's Hospital[2]	Denville	99%	93
Saint Peter's University Hospital[2]	New Brunswick	99%	84
Monmouth Medical Center[2]	Long Branch	98%	50
Saint Mary's Hospital - Passaic[2]	Passaic	98%	56
Valley Hospital[2]	Ridgewood	98%	130
Raritan Bay Medical Center[2]	Perth Amboy	97%	79
Saint Barnabas Medical Center[2]	Livingston	97%	95
Trinitas Regional Medical Center[2]	Elizabeth	97%	31
University Hospital[2]	Newark	97%	89
Robert Wood Johnson Univ Hosp-Rahway[2]	Rahway	96%	27
JFK Med Ctr-A M Yelencsics Comm Hosp[2]	Edison	95%	133
Riverview Medical Center[2]	Red Bank	95%	39
Robert Wood Johnson University Hospital[2]	New Brunswick	95%	172
Hunterdon Medical Center[2]	Flemington	94%	34
Virtua West Jersey Hospitals Berlin[2]	Berlin	94%	232
Newton Memorial Hospital[2]	Newton	92%	25
Virtua Mem Hosp of Burlington County[2]	Mount Holly	92%	126

Venous Thromboembolism Prophylaxis

Hospital Name	City	Rate	Cases
Carepoint Health-Bayonne Hosp Ctr[2]	Bayonne	100%	429
Chilton Medical Center[2]	Pompton Plains	100%	404
Centrastate Medical Center[2]	Freehold	99%	449
Englewood Hospital & Medical Center[2]	Englewood	98%	363
Robert Wood Johnson University Hospital[2]	New Brunswick	98%	339
Saint Peter's University Hospital[2]	New Brunswick	98%	357
Saint Luke's Warren Hospital[2]	Phillipsburg	97%	390
Kennedy Univ Hosp-Stratford Div[2]	Stratford	96%	330
Capital Health Medical Center - Hopewell[2]	Pennington	94%	333
Capital Health System - Fuld Campus[2]	Trenton	94%	302
Inspira Medical Center Woodbury[2]	Woodbury	94%	391
Hunterdon Medical Center[2]	Flemington	93%	410
Inspira Medical Center Vineland[2]	Vineland	93%	379
Saint Francis Medical Center[2]	Trenton	92%	309
University Hospital[2]	Newark	92%	292
Bayshore Community Hospital[2]	Holmdel	91%	406
Ocean Medical Center[2]	Brick	91%	402
Virtua Mem Hosp of Burlington County[2]	Mount Holly	91%	414
Community Medical Center[2]	Toms River	90%	422
Memorial Hospital of Salem County[2]	Salem	90%	334
Newton Memorial Hospital[2]	Newton	90%	391
Jersey Shore University Medical Center[2]	Neptune	89%	384
Overlook Medical Center[2]	Summit	89%	340
Deborah Heart & Lung Center[2]	Browns Mills	88%	277
Univ Med Ctr of Princeton-Plainsboro[2]	Plainsboro	88%	340
Robert W Johnson Univ Hosp-Hamilton[2]	Hamilton	87%	312
Southern Ocean Medical Center[2]	Manahawkin	87%	395
Cooper University Hospital[2]	Camden	86%	302
Saint Joseph's Regional Medical Center[2]	Paterson	86%	731
Atlanticare Regional Medical Center[2]	Atlantic City	85%	331
Carepoint Health - Hoboken UMC[2]	Hoboken	85%	293
Shore Medical Center[2]	Somers Point	84%	373
Meadowlands Hospital Medical Center[2]	Secaucus	82%	212
Our Lady of Lourdes Medical Center[2]	Camden	82%	355
Carepoint Health - Christ Hospital[2]	Jersey City	81%	426
Monmouth Medical Center[2]	Long Branch	81%	367
Cape Regional Medical Center[2]	Cape May CH	80%	348
East Orange General Hospital[2]	East Orange	80%	425
Hackensack - Umc Mountainside[2]	Montclair	80%	366
Saint Clare's Hospital[2]	Denville	80%	348
Trinitas Regional Medical Center[2]	Elizabeth	80%	418
Virtua West Jersey Hospitals Berlin[2]	Berlin	80%	381
Hackettstown Regional Medical Center[2]	Hackettstown	77%	314
Holy Name Medical Center[2]	Teaneck	77%	433
Valley Hospital[2]	Ridgewood	77%	393
Morristown Medical Center[2]	Morristown	76%	344
Saint Barnabas Medical Center[2]	Livingston	76%	389
Saint Mary's Hospital - Passaic[2]	Passaic	76%	389
Inspira Medical Center Elmer[2]	Elmer	75%	319
Raritan Bay Medical Center[2]	Perth Amboy	75%	381
Bergen Regional Medical Center[2]	Paramus	72%	54
Libertyhealth-Jersey City Med Ctr[2]	Jersey City	72%	317
Clara Maass Medical Center[2]	Belleville	71%	408
Saint Michael's Medical Center[2]	Newark	71%	332
Palisades Medical Center[2]	North Bergen	70%	402
Hackensack University Medical Center[2]	Hackensack	69%	398
Monmouth Medical Center - Southern Campus[2]	Lakewood	68%	383
Newark Beth Israel Medical Center[2]	Newark	68%	437
Lourdes Med Ctr of Burlington County[2]	Willingboro	66%	301
Riverview Medical Center[2]	Red Bank	61%	375

NOTE: Hospital profiles are in alphabetical order by state, then city, then hospital within the city; Rankings exclude hospitals with less than 25 cases except for patient surveys which excludes hospitals with less than 100 cases; (a) 100-299 cases; (1) The number of cases/patients is too few to report; (2) Data submitted were based on a sample of cases/patients; (3) Results are based on a shorter time period than required; (4) Data suppressed by CMS for one or more quarters; (5) Results are not available for this reporting period; (6) Fewer than 100 patients completed the HCAHPS survey; (7) No cases met the criteria for this measure; (8) The lower limit of the confidence interval cannot be calculated if the number of observed infections equals zero; (9) No data are available from the state/territory for this reporting period; (10) The scores shown reflect fewer than 50 completed surveys; (11) There were discrepancies in the data collection process; (12) This measure does not apply to this hospital for this reporting period; (13) Results cannot be calculated for this reporting period; (14) The results for this state are combined with nearby states to protect confidentiality; Please refer to the User's Guide for a full explanation of data.

Hospital Name	City	Rate	Cases
Robert Wood Johnson Univ Hosp-Rahway[2]	Rahway	59%	407
Somerset Medical Center[2]	Somerville	56%	376
JFK Med Ctr-A M Yelencsics Comm Hosp[2]	Edison	45%	435

Warfarin Therapy Discharge Instructions

Hospital Name	City	Rate	Cases
Chilton Medical Center[2]	Pompton Plains	100%	49
Holy Name Medical Center[2]	Teaneck	100%	51
Inspira Medical Center Elmer[2]	Elmer	100%	40
Inspira Medical Center Woodbury[2]	Woodbury	100%	45
Newton Memorial Hospital[2]	Newton	100%	36
Riverview Medical Center[2]	Red Bank	100%	26
Robert Wood Johnson University Hospital[2]	New Brunswick	100%	91
Robert Wood Johnson Univ Hosp-Rahway[2]	Rahway	100%	26
Saint Francis Medical Center[2]	Trenton	100%	31
Saint Mary's Hospital - Passaic[2]	Passaic	100%	32
Saint Joseph's Regional Medical Center[2]	Paterson	98%	98
Bayshore Community Hospital[2]	Holmdel	97%	36
Hackensack - Umc Mountainside[2]	Montclair	97%	38
Monmouth Medical Center[2]	Long Branch	97%	36
Saint Clare's Hospital[2]	Denville	96%	46
Univ Med Ctr of Princeton-Plainsboro[2]	Plainsboro	94%	52
Hunterdon Medical Center[2]	Flemington	93%	29
Memorial Hospital of Salem County[2]	Salem	93%	27
Cooper University Hospital[2]	Camden	92%	93
Southern Ocean Medical Center[2]	Manahawkin	91%	35
Virtua West Jersey Hospitals Berlin[2]	Berlin	90%	185
Saint Peter's University Hospital[2]	New Brunswick	89%	55
Cape Regional Medical Center[2]	Cape May CH	88%	48
Community Medical Center[2]	Toms River	88%	107
Inspira Medical Center Vineland[2]	Vineland	86%	58
Capital Health Medical Center - Hopewell[2]	Pennington	85%	54
Overlook Medical Center[2]	Summit	84%	95
Saint Barnabas Medical Center[2]	Livingston	82%	97
Somerset Medical Center[2]	Somerville	82%	87
Ocean Medical Center[2]	Brick	81%	54
Trinitas Regional Medical Center[2]	Elizabeth	81%	53
Morristown Medical Center[2]	Morristown	80%	152
Our Lady of Lourdes Medical Center[2]	Camden	78%	73
Hackensack University Medical Center[2]	Hackensack	77%	128
Jersey Shore University Medical Center[2]	Neptune	77%	75
East Orange General Hospital[2]	East Orange	76%	33
Kennedy Univ Hosp-Stratford Div[2]	Stratford	76%	154
Atlanticare Regional Medical Center[2]	Atlantic City	74%	144
Carepoint Health - Christ Hospital[2]	Jersey City	74%	38
Capital Health System - Fuld Campus[2]	Trenton	72%	47
Newark Beth Israel Medical Center[2]	Newark	72%	80
Lourdes Med Ctr of Burlington County[2]	Willingboro	70%	47
Clara Maass Medical Center[2]	Belleville	62%	40
Saint Luke's Warren Hospital[2]	Phillipsburg	62%	39
Virtua Mem Hosp of Burlington County[2]	Mount Holly	60%	113
Libertyhealth-Jersey City Med Ctr[2]	Jersey City	56%	63
Raritan Bay Medical Center[2]	Perth Amboy	56%	64
Saint Michael's Medical Center[2]	Newark	56%	25
Shore Medical Center[2]	Somers Point	48%	44
University Hospital[2]	Newark	38%	58
JFK Med Ctr-A M Yelencsics Comm Hosp[2]	Edison	27%	81
Robert W Johnson Univ Hosp-Hamilton[2]	Hamilton	23%	62
Centrastate Medical Center[2]	Freehold	18%	38
Valley Hospital[2]	Ridgewood	17%	150

Chest Pain/Possible Heart Attack Care

Aspirin Given Within 24 Hours of Arrival

Hospital Name	City	Rate	Cases
Bayshore Community Hospital	Holmdel	100%	72
Centrastate Medical Center	Freehold	100%	117
Community Medical Center	Toms River	100%	33
Newton Memorial Hospital[3]	Newton	100%	32
Ocean Medical Center	Brick	100%	25
Saint Clare's Hospital	Denville	100%	26
Saint Luke's Warren Hospital	Phillipsburg	100%	43
Shore Medical Center	Somers Point	100%	59
Virtua Mem Hosp of Burlington County	Mount Holly	100%	28
Virtua West Jersey Hospitals Berlin	Berlin	100%	77
Cape Regional Medical Center	Cape May CH	99%	117
Inspira Medical Center Vineland	Vineland	99%	152
Kennedy Univ Hosp-Stratford Div	Stratford	99%	149
Inspira Medical Center Elmer	Elmer	98%	46
Lourdes Med Ctr of Burlington County	Willingboro	98%	661
Southern Ocean Medical Center	Manahawkin	98%	115
Memorial Hospital of Salem County	Salem	94%	32

Average Time to ECG (minutes)

Hospital Name	City	Min.	Cases
Centrastate Medical Center	Freehold	4	116
Saint Clare's Hospital	Denville	4	28
Virtua West Jersey Hospitals Berlin	Berlin	4	78
Inspira Medical Center Elmer	Elmer	5	47
Bayshore Community Hospital	Holmdel	6	70
Cape Regional Medical Center	Cape May CH	6	117
Inspira Medical Center Vineland	Vineland	6	154
Ocean Medical Center	Brick	6	27
Saint Luke's Warren Hospital	Phillipsburg	6	43
Lourdes Med Ctr of Burlington County	Willingboro	7	682
Memorial Hospital of Salem County	Salem	7	31
Virtua Mem Hosp of Burlington County	Mount Holly	7	29
Community Medical Center	Toms River	8	32
Kennedy Univ Hosp-Stratford Div	Stratford	8	149
Newton Memorial Hospital[3]	Newton	8	32
Southern Ocean Medical Center	Manahawkin	8	116
Shore Medical Center	Somers Point	11	59

Average Time to Transfer (minutes)

Hospital Name	City	Min.	Cases
Lourdes Med Ctr of Burlington County	Willingboro	66	30
Inspira Medical Center Vineland	Vineland	69	25
Southern Ocean Medical Center	Manahawkin	76	27
Shore Medical Center	Somers Point	80	31

Children's Asthma Care

Received Home Management Plan of Care

Hospital Name	City	Rate	Cases
Saint Peter's University Hospital	New Brunswick	97%	185

Received Reliever Medication

Hospital Name	City	Rate	Cases
Saint Peter's University Hospital	New Brunswick	100%	186

Received Systemic Corticosteroids

Hospital Name	City	Rate	Cases
Saint Peter's University Hospital	New Brunswick	100%	186

Emergency Department

Admittance Decision Time (minutes)

Hospital Name	City	Min.	Cases
Valley Hospital[2]	Ridgewood	71	747
Ocean Medical Center[2]	Brick	73	874
Saint Francis Medical Center[2]	Trenton	80	660
Carepoint Health - Christ Hospital[2]	Jersey City	82	674
Inspira Medical Center Woodbury[2]	Woodbury	82	932
Monmouth Medical Center - Southern Campus[2]	Lakewood	88	796
Univ Med Ctr of Princeton-Plainsboro[2]	Plainsboro	88	587
Saint Mary's Hospital - Passaic[2]	Passaic	90	471
Inspira Medical Center Elmer[2]	Elmer	94	528
Saint Joseph's Regional Medical Center[2]	Paterson	100	1719
Palisades Medical Center[2]	North Bergen	104	766
Robert W Johnson Univ Hosp-Hamilton[2]	Hamilton	110	777
Hackettstown Regional Medical Center[2]	Hackettstown	117	499
Inspira Medical Center Vineland[2]	Vineland	120	655
Riverview Medical Center[2]	Red Bank	121	755
Memorial Hospital of Salem County[2]	Salem	123	692
Saint Luke's Warren Hospital[2]	Phillipsburg	124	870
Bergen Regional Medical Center[2]	Paramus	129	132
Raritan Bay Medical Center[2]	Perth Amboy	130	802
Carepoint Health - Hoboken UMC[2]	Hoboken	133	550
Chilton Medical Center[2]	Pompton Plains	134	736
Jersey Shore University Medical Center[2]	Neptune	136	721
Southern Ocean Medical Center[2]	Manahawkin	136	978
Monmouth Medical Center[2]	Long Branch	139	369
Holy Name Medical Center[2]	Teaneck	142	782
Capital Health Medical Center - Hopewell[2]	Pennington	144	576
Meadowlands Hospital Medical Center[2]	Secaucus	144	532
Somerset Medical Center[2]	Somerville	144	810
Hackensack - Umc Mountainside[2]	Montclair	146	707
Bayshore Community Hospital[2]	Holmdel	148	1011
Hunterdon Medical Center[2]	Flemington	148	773
Virtua West Jersey Hospitals Berlin[2]	Berlin	148	611
Carepoint Health-Bayonne Hosp Ctr[2]	Bayonne	149	745
Overlook Medical Center[2]	Summit	149	465
Cape Regional Medical Center[2]	Cape May CH	152	969
Trinitas Regional Medical Center[2]	Elizabeth	153	652
Centrastate Medical Center[2]	Freehold	156	724
Saint Barnabas Medical Center[2]	Livingston	161	489
Community Medical Center[2]	Toms River	162	829
Robert Wood Johnson Univ Hosp-Rahway[2]	Rahway	163	1102
Saint Peter's University Hospital[2]	New Brunswick	164	454
Atlanticare Regional Medical Center[2]	Atlantic City	167	810
Shore Medical Center[2]	Somers Point	170	798
Lourdes Med Ctr of Burlington County[2]	Willingboro	181	1026
JFK Med Ctr-A M Yelencsics Comm Hosp[2]	Edison	187	585
Englewood Hospital & Medical Center[2]	Englewood	194	659
Libertyhealth-Jersey City Med Ctr[2]	Jersey City	198	581
Morristown Medical Center[2]	Morristown	198	491
Saint Clare's Hospital[2]	Denville	203	737
Saint Michael's Medical Center[2]	Newark	205	853
Virtua Mem Hosp of Burlington County[2]	Mount Holly	207	625
Kennedy Univ Hosp-Stratford Div[2]	Stratford	208	1005
Clara Maass Medical Center[2]	Belleville	227	233
Newton Memorial Hospital[2]	Newton	228	908
Capital Health System - Fuld Campus[2]	Trenton	233	877
University Hospital[2]	Newark	234	648
East Orange General Hospital[2]	East Orange	240	734
Cooper University Hospital[2]	Camden	242	620
Our Lady of Lourdes Medical Center[2]	Camden	254	678
Robert Wood Johnson University Hospital[2]	New Brunswick	260	622
Hackensack University Medical Center[2]	Hackensack	315	451
Newark Beth Israel Medical Center[2]	Newark	520	489

Head CT Results Within 45 Minutes of Arrival

Hospital Name	City	Rate	Cases
Inspira Medical Center Woodbury	Woodbury	91%	32
Inspira Medical Center Vineland	Vineland	80%	40
Cape Regional Medical Center	Cape May CH	79%	43
Ocean Medical Center	Brick	79%	29
Virtua West Jersey Hospitals Berlin	Berlin	70%	60
Lourdes Med Ctr of Burlington County	Willingboro	65%	43

Patients Who Left ER Before Being Seen

Hospital Name	City	Rate	Cases
Bayshore Community Hospital	Holmdel	0%	33080
Cape Regional Medical Center	Cape May CH	0%	47206
Chilton Medical Center	Pompton Plains	0%	49132
Monmouth Medical Center - Southern Campus	Lakewood	0%	24736
Morristown Medical Center	Morristown	0%	82239
Robert Wood Johnson University Hospital	New Brunswick	0%	96445
Saint Peter's University Hospital	New Brunswick	0%	66771
Shore Medical Center	Somers Point	0%	46714
Valley Hospital	Ridgewood	0%	76812
Virtua Mem Hosp of Burlington County	Mount Holly	0%	69134
Capital Health Medical Center - Hopewell	Pennington	1%	35117
Centrastate Medical Center	Freehold	1%	65888
Community Medical Center	Toms River	1%	95465
Englewood Hospital & Medical Center	Englewood	1%	47790
Hackensack - Umc Mountainside	Montclair	1%	40261
Hackensack University Medical Center	Hackensack	1%	125093
Hackettstown Regional Medical Center	Hackettstown	1%	21898
Holy Name Medical Center	Teaneck	1%	55879
Hunterdon Medical Center	Flemington	1%	34172
JFK Med Ctr-A M Yelencsics Comm Hosp	Edison	1%	32384
Lourdes Med Ctr of Burlington County	Willingboro	1%	68134
Meadowlands Hospital Medical Center	Secaucus	1%	20593
Memorial Hospital of Salem County	Salem	1%	21079
Monmouth Medical Center	Long Branch	1%	51193
Ocean Medical Center	Brick	1%	78458
Our Lady of Lourdes Medical Center	Camden	1%	59096
Overlook Medical Center	Summit	1%	92424
Palisades Medical Center	North Bergen	1%	39423
Robert W Johnson Univ Hosp-Hamilton	Hamilton	1%	56257
Robert Wood Johnson Univ Hosp-Rahway	Rahway	1%	31661
Saint Barnabas Medical Center	Livingston	1%	87741
Saint Clare's Hospital	Denville	1%	72338
Saint Luke's Warren Hospital	Phillipsburg	1%	30267
Saint Mary's Hospital - Passaic	Passaic	1%	33703
Saint Michael's Medical Center	Newark	1%	35619
Somerset Medical Center	Somerville	1%	54695
Virtua West Jersey Hospitals Berlin	Berlin	1%	148036
Atlanticare Regional Medical Center	Atlantic City	2%	136262
Bergen Regional Medical Center	Paramus	2%	16292
Carepoint Health-Bayonne Hosp Ctr	Bayonne	2%	28516
Carepoint Health - Christ Hospital	Jersey City	2%	48971
Carepoint Health - Hoboken UMC	Hoboken	2%	40186
Inspira Medical Center Woodbury	Woodbury	2%	59663
Kennedy Univ Hosp-Stratford Div	Stratford	2%	149457
Newton Memorial Hospital	Newton	2%	29174
Raritan Bay Medical Center	Perth Amboy	2%	48708
Riverview Medical Center	Red Bank	2%	42147
Saint Joseph's Regional Medical Center	Paterson	2%	166714
Clara Maass Medical Center	Belleville	3%	39658
Inspira Medical Center Elmer	Elmer	3%	22341
Jersey Shore University Medical Center	Neptune	3%	88610
Southern Ocean Medical Center	Manahawkin	3%	40455
Trinitas Regional Medical Center	Elizabeth	3%	70449
Univ Med Ctr of Princeton-Plainsboro	Plainsboro	3%	42162
Inspira Medical Center Vineland	Vineland	4%	92479
Libertyhealth-Jersey City Med Ctr	Jersey City	4%	86863
Saint Francis Medical Center	Trenton	4%	35589
Cooper University Hospital	Camden	5%	58126
Newark Beth Israel Medical Center	Newark	5%	44282
Capital Health System - Fuld Campus	Trenton	7%	61333
East Orange General Hospital	East Orange	8%	6794
University Hospital	Newark	9%	96588

NOTE: Hospital profiles are in alphabetical order by state, then city, then hospital within the city; Rankings exclude hospitals with less than 25 cases except for patient surveys which excludes hospitals with less than 100 cases; (a) 100-299 cases; (1) The number of cases/patients is too few to report; (2) Data submitted were based on a sample of cases/patients; (3) Results are based on a shorter time period than required; (4) Data suppressed by CMS for one or more quarters; (5) Results are not available for this reporting period; (6) Fewer than 100 patients completed the HCAHPS survey; (7) No cases met the criteria for this measure; (8) The lower limit of the confidence interval cannot be calculated if the number of observed infections equals zero; (9) No data are available from the state/territory for this reporting period; (10) The scores shown reflect fewer than 50 completed surveys; (11) There were discrepancies in the data collection process; (12) This measure does not apply to this hospital for this reporting period; (13) Results cannot be calculated for this reporting period; (14) The results for this state are combined with nearby states to protect confidentiality; Please refer to the User's Guide for a full explanation of data.

Time from ER Arrival to Being Admitted (minutes)

Hospital Name	City	Min.	Cases
Ocean Medical Center[2]	Brick	261	874
Saint Mary's Hospital - Passaic[2]	Passaic	270	632
Saint Luke's Warren Hospital[2]	Phillipsburg	271	937
Meadowlands Hospital Medical Center[2]	Secaucus	277	533
Memorial Hospital of Salem County[2]	Salem	283	696
Valley Hospital[2]	Ridgewood	283	747
Hackettstown Regional Medical Center[2]	Hackettstown	287	569
Saint Francis Medical Center[2]	Trenton	288	662
Cape Regional Medical Center[2]	Cape May CH	298	976
Univ Med Ctr of Princeton-Plainsboro[2]	Plainsboro	300	589
Inspira Medical Center Elmer[2]	Elmer	306	530
Monmouth Medical Center[2]	Long Branch	308	372
Saint Joseph's Regional Medical Center[2]	Paterson	314	1755
Hunterdon Medical Center[2]	Flemington	317	774
Shore Medical Center[2]	Somers Point	320	798
Hackensack - Umc Mountainside[2]	Montclair	322	711
Monmouth Medical Center - Southern Campus[2]	Lakewood	322	802
Bayshore Community Hospital[2]	Holmdel	324	1011
Chilton Medical Center[2]	Pompton Plains	327	739
Virtua West Jersey Hospitals Berlin[2]	Berlin	330	612
Carepoint Health-Bayonne Hosp Ctr[2]	Bayonne	332	749
Robert W Johnson Univ Hosp-Hamilton[2]	Hamilton	332	829
Holy Name Medical Center[2]	Teaneck	333	790
Virtua Mem Hosp of Burlington County[2]	Mount Holly	337	633
Carepoint Health - Christ Hospital[2]	Jersey City	339	709
Atlanticare Regional Medical Center[2]	Atlantic City	340	810
Palisades Medical Center[2]	North Bergen	340	766
Southern Ocean Medical Center[2]	Manahawkin	340	991
Inspira Medical Center Woodbury[2]	Woodbury	347	932
Carepoint Health - Hoboken UMC[2]	Hoboken	350	564
Jersey Shore University Medical Center[2]	Neptune	352	730
Inspira Medical Center Vineland[2]	Vineland	357	657
Saint Peter's University Hospital[2]	New Brunswick	357	455
Robert Wood Johnson Univ Hosp-Rahway[2]	Rahway	363	1194
Lourdes Med Ctr of Burlington County[2]	Willingboro	364	1028
Riverview Medical Center[2]	Red Bank	364	755
Bergen Regional Medical Center[2]	Paramus	368	132
Overlook Medical Center[2]	Summit	372	504
Centrastate Medical Center[2]	Freehold	376	729
Raritan Bay Medical Center[2]	Perth Amboy	376	802
Kennedy Univ Hosp-Stratford Div[2]	Stratford	377	1021
Saint Barnabas Medical Center[2]	Livingston	378	489
Englewood Hospital & Medical Center[2]	Englewood	392	659
Cooper University Hospital[2]	Camden	396	621
Morristown Medical Center[2]	Morristown	404	520
Saint Clare's Hospital[2]	Denville	404	780
Our Lady of Lourdes Medical Center[2]	Camden	407	678
Trinitas Regional Medical Center[2]	Elizabeth	410	655
Capital Health Medical Center - Hopewell[2]	Pennington	421	588
JFK Med Ctr-A M Yelencsics Comm Hosp[2]	Edison	434	588
Newton Memorial Hospital[2]	Newton	436	909
Somerset Medical Center[2]	Somerville	436	819
Community Medical Center[2]	Toms River	442	829
Saint Michael's Medical Center[2]	Newark	448	860
Robert Wood Johnson University Hospital[2]	New Brunswick	458	630
Hackensack University Medical Center[2]	Hackensack	477	472
Capital Health System - Fuld Campus[2]	Trenton	496	952
Libertyhealth-Jersey City Med Ctr[2]	Jersey City	508	736
East Orange General Hospital[2]	East Orange	520	735
Clara Maass Medical Center[2]	Belleville	522	233
University Hospital[2]	Newark	546	649
Newark Beth Israel Medical Center[2]	Newark	897	498

Time from ER Arrival to Discharge (minutes)

Hospital Name	City	Min.	Cases
Chilton Medical Center	Pompton Plains	92	385
Ocean Medical Center	Brick	94	390
Monmouth Medical Center - Southern Campus	Lakewood	96	382
Lourdes Med Ctr of Burlington County	Willingboro	108	372
Virtua West Jersey Hospitals Berlin	Berlin	118	401
Saint Clare's Hospital	Denville	120	434
Saint Luke's Warren Hospital	Phillipsburg	123	376
Virtua Mem Hosp of Burlington County	Mount Holly	124	362
Cape Regional Medical Center	Cape May CH	125	383
Meadowlands Hospital Medical Center	Secaucus	125	400
Hackettstown Regional Medical Center	Hackettstown	127	360
Robert Wood Johnson Univ Hosp-Rahway	Rahway	129	385
Raritan Bay Medical Center	Perth Amboy	130	366
Saint Peter's University Hospital	New Brunswick	132	409
Monmouth Medical Center	Long Branch	134	394
Shore Medical Center	Somers Point	134	402
Robert Wood Johnson University Hospital	New Brunswick	135	379
Inspira Medical Center Vineland	Vineland	138	948
Memorial Hospital of Salem County	Salem	139	364
Bayshore Community Hospital	Holmdel	141	365
Atlanticare Regional Medical Center	Atlantic City	142	395
Our Lady of Lourdes Medical Center	Camden	144	379
Carepoint Health - Christ Hospital	Jersey City	145	360
Saint Barnabas Medical Center	Livingston	145	375
Bergen Regional Medical Center	Paramus	147	235
Capital Health Medical Center - Hopewell	Pennington	147	423
Saint Francis Medical Center	Trenton	147	360
Carepoint Health - Hoboken UMC	Hoboken	148	293
Riverview Medical Center	Red Bank	149	386
Saint Joseph's Regional Medical Center	Paterson	150	780
Overlook Medical Center	Summit	151	403
Clara Maass Medical Center	Belleville	152	344
Holy Name Medical Center	Teaneck	153	382
Kennedy Univ Hosp-Stratford Div	Stratford	153	379
JFK Med Ctr-A M Yelencsics Comm Hosp	Edison	154	358
Saint Mary's Hospital - Passaic	Passaic	154	338
East Orange General Hospital	East Orange	155	309
Hackensack - Umc Mountainside	Montclair	155	441
Community Medical Center	Toms River	158	360
Univ Med Ctr of Princeton-Plainsboro	Plainsboro	158	392
Valley Hospital	Ridgewood	160	399
Somerset Medical Center	Somerville	161	406
Capital Health System - Fuld Campus	Trenton	162	383
Southern Ocean Medical Center	Manahawkin	162	372
Carepoint Health-Bayonne Hosp Ctr	Bayonne	164	401
Morristown Medical Center	Morristown	165	382
Robert W Johnson Univ Hosp-Hamilton	Hamilton	169	356
Centrastate Medical Center	Freehold	170	373
Jersey Shore University Medical Center	Neptune	170	389
Palisades Medical Center	North Bergen	170	316
Hackensack University Medical Center	Hackensack	174	341
Cooper University Hospital	Camden	175	331
Trinitas Regional Medical Center	Elizabeth	175	351
Englewood Hospital & Medical Center	Englewood	176	413
Inspira Medical Center Woodbury	Woodbury	176	390
Hunterdon Medical Center	Flemington	177	399
Inspira Medical Center Elmer	Elmer	181	2848
Libertyhealth-Jersey City Med Ctr	Jersey City	184	364
Newton Memorial Hospital	Newton	187	374
Newark Beth Israel Medical Center	Newark	189	398
Saint Michael's Medical Center	Newark	197	365
University Hospital	Newark	252	289

Time in ER Before Being Evaluated (minutes)

Hospital Name	City	Min.	Cases
Saint Barnabas Medical Center	Livingston	14	421
Our Lady of Lourdes Medical Center	Camden	17	435
Lourdes Med Ctr of Burlington County	Willingboro	18	426
Memorial Hospital of Salem County	Salem	18	422
Cape Regional Medical Center	Cape May CH	19	431
Kennedy Univ Hosp-Stratford Div	Stratford	19	428
Monmouth Medical Center - Southern Campus	Lakewood	19	397
Shore Medical Center	Somers Point	20	414
Ocean Medical Center	Brick	21	428
Bayshore Community Hospital	Holmdel	22	429
Chilton Medical Center	Pompton Plains	22	384
Atlanticare Regional Medical Center	Atlantic City	23	429
Meadowlands Hospital Medical Center	Secaucus	24	430
Monmouth Medical Center	Long Branch	24	342
Robert Wood Johnson University Hospital	New Brunswick	25	431
Valley Hospital	Ridgewood	25	433
Hackettstown Regional Medical Center	Hackettstown	26	383
Inspira Medical Center Vineland	Vineland	26	1037
Saint Francis Medical Center	Trenton	26	389
Univ Med Ctr of Princeton-Plainsboro	Plainsboro	27	427
Capital Health Medical Center - Hopewell	Pennington	28	432
Riverview Medical Center	Red Bank	29	428
Saint Clare's Hospital	Denville	29	466
Bergen Regional Medical Center	Paramus	30	401
Inspira Medical Center Elmer	Elmer	30	2981
Palisades Medical Center	North Bergen	30	381
Saint Joseph's Regional Medical Center	Paterson	30	884
Carepoint Health-Bayonne Hosp Ctr	Bayonne	31	444
Morristown Medical Center	Morristown	31	401
Newton Memorial Hospital	Newton	31	375
Carepoint Health - Christ Hospital	Jersey City	32	423
Inspira Medical Center Woodbury	Woodbury	32	429
Overlook Medical Center	Summit	32	387
Robert Wood Johnson Univ Hosp-Rahway	Rahway	32	408
Saint Peter's University Hospital	New Brunswick	32	432
Capital Health System - Fuld Campus	Trenton	33	432
Carepoint Health - Hoboken UMC	Hoboken	34	277
Holy Name Medical Center	Teaneck	34	427
JFK Med Ctr-A M Yelencsics Comm Hosp	Edison	34	422
Saint Luke's Warren Hospital	Phillipsburg	34	414
Saint Mary's Hospital - Passaic	Passaic	35	404
Southern Ocean Medical Center	Manahawkin	35	421
Englewood Hospital & Medical Center	Englewood	36	428
Libertyhealth-Jersey City Med Ctr	Jersey City	36	420
Somerset Medical Center	Somerville	37	396
Cooper University Hospital	Camden	39	400
Centrastate Medical Center	Freehold	40	384
Trinitas Regional Medical Center	Elizabeth	41	408
Hunterdon Medical Center	Flemington	43	411
Robert W Johnson Univ Hosp-Hamilton	Hamilton	43	375
Hackensack University Medical Center	Hackensack	44	376
Virtua West Jersey Hospitals Berlin	Berlin	44	381
Clara Maass Medical Center	Belleville	48	432
Community Medical Center	Toms River	50	424
East Orange General Hospital	East Orange	55	333
Jersey Shore University Medical Center	Neptune	55	430
Virtua Mem Hosp of Burlington County	Mount Holly	57	389
Hackensack - Umc Mountainside	Montclair	63	459
Raritan Bay Medical Center	Perth Amboy	69	405
Saint Michael's Medical Center	Newark	72	432
Newark Beth Israel Medical Center	Newark	75	430
University Hospital	Newark	90	327

Time to Pain Meds for Bone Fractures (minutes)

Hospital Name	City	Min.	Cases
Virtua West Jersey Hospitals Berlin	Berlin	33	282
Capital Health Medical Center - Hopewell	Pennington	39	136
Saint Barnabas Medical Center	Livingston	39	223
Shore Medical Center	Somers Point	42	85
JFK Med Ctr-A M Yelencsics Comm Hosp	Edison	44	237
Robert Wood Johnson University Hospital	New Brunswick	44	302
Valley Hospital	Ridgewood	45	249
Saint Luke's Warren Hospital	Phillipsburg	46	70
Bayshore Community Hospital	Holmdel	48	197
Riverview Medical Center	Red Bank	48	171
Robert W Johnson Univ Hosp-Hamilton	Hamilton	49	164
Meadowlands Hospital Medical Center	Secaucus	50	29
Ocean Medical Center	Brick	51	185
Robert Wood Johnson Univ Hosp-Rahway	Rahway	51	67
Centrastate Medical Center	Freehold	52	211
Lourdes Med Ctr of Burlington County	Willingboro	52	143
Monmouth Medical Center - Southern Campus	Lakewood	52	105
Morristown Medical Center	Morristown	52	247
Saint Clare's Hospital	Denville	52	198
Hunterdon Medical Center	Flemington	53	111
Our Lady of Lourdes Medical Center	Camden	53	69
Carepoint Health - Hoboken UMC	Hoboken	54	109
Univ Med Ctr of Princeton-Plainsboro	Plainsboro	55	124
Atlanticare Regional Medical Center	Atlantic City	56	180
Chilton Medical Center	Pompton Plains	56	32
Inspira Medical Center Vineland	Vineland	56	203
Saint Peter's University Hospital	New Brunswick	56	168
Somerset Medical Center	Somerville	56	138
Cape Regional Medical Center	Cape May CH	57	101
Carepoint Health-Bayonne Hosp Ctr	Bayonne	58	66
Newton Memorial Hospital	Newton	58	117
Saint Francis Medical Center	Trenton	58	88
Holy Name Medical Center	Teaneck	59	131
Saint Joseph's Regional Medical Center	Paterson	60	372
Hackensack University Medical Center	Hackensack	61	384
Inspira Medical Center Woodbury	Woodbury	62	132
Trinitas Regional Medical Center	Elizabeth	63	232
Overlook Medical Center	Summit	64	263
Kennedy Univ Hosp-Stratford Div	Stratford	65	310
Saint Mary's Hospital - Passaic	Passaic	67	92
Inspira Medical Center Elmer	Elmer	68	74
Jersey Shore University Medical Center	Neptune	68	221
Memorial Hospital of Salem County	Salem	68	82
Monmouth Medical Center	Long Branch	68	258
Southern Ocean Medical Center	Manahawkin	68	129
Virtua Mem Hosp of Burlington County	Mount Holly	68	148
Libertyhealth-Jersey City Med Ctr	Jersey City	69	120
Clara Maass Medical Center	Belleville	72	250
Hackensack - Umc Mountainside	Montclair	72	118
Raritan Bay Medical Center	Perth Amboy	72	151
Carepoint Health - Christ Hospital	Jersey City	73	92
Hackettstown Regional Medical Center	Hackettstown	76	98
Capital Health System - Fuld Campus	Trenton	78	65
Englewood Hospital & Medical Center	Englewood	79	182
Saint Michael's Medical Center	Newark	79	34
Community Medical Center	Toms River	82	162
Cooper University Hospital	Camden	83	174
Palisades Medical Center	North Bergen	84	84
Newark Beth Israel Medical Center	Newark	88	139
East Orange General Hospital	East Orange	95	39
University Hospital	Newark	115	179

Heart Attack Care

Aspirin Given at Discharge

Hospital Name	City	Rate	Cases
Atlanticare Regional Medical Center[2]	Atlantic City	100%	341
Bayshore Community Hospital	Holmdel	100%	47
Capital Health Medical Center - Hopewell	Pennington	100%	62
Carepoint Health-Bayonne Hosp Ctr	Bayonne	100%	156
Centrastate Medical Center[2]	Freehold	100%	30
Chilton Medical Center	Pompton Plains	100%	128
Clara Maass Medical Center[2]	Belleville	100%	203
Community Medical Center[2]	Toms River	100%	235

NOTE: Hospital profiles are in alphabetical order by state, then city, then hospital within the city; Rankings exclude hospitals with less than 25 cases except for patient surveys which excludes hospitals with less than 100 cases; (a) 100-299 cases; (1) The number of cases/patients is too few to report; (2) Data submitted were based on a sample of cases/patients; (3) Results are based on a shorter time period than required; (4) Data suppressed by CMS for one or more quarters; (5) Results are not available for this reporting period; (6) Fewer than 100 patients completed the HCAHPS survey; (7) No cases met the criteria for this measure; (8) The lower limit of the confidence interval cannot be calculated if the number of observed infections equals zero; (9) No data are available from the state/territory for this reporting period; (10) The scores shown reflect fewer than 50 completed surveys; (11) There were discrepancies in the data collection process; (12) This measure does not apply to this hospital for this reporting period; (13) Results cannot be calculated for this reporting period; (14) The results for this state are combined with nearby states to protect confidentiality; Please refer to the User's Guide for a full explanation of data.

Cooper University Hospital[2]	Camden	100%	277
Deborah Heart & Lung Center	Browns Mills	100%	337
Englewood Hospital & Medical Center	Englewood	100%	342
Hackensack University Medical Center	Hackensack	100%	603
Hackettstown Regional Medical Center	Hackettstown	100%	36
Holy Name Medical Center	Teaneck	100%	190
Hunterdon Medical Center	Flemington	100%	104
Inspira Medical Center Vineland	Vineland	100%	47
Inspira Medical Center Woodbury	Woodbury	100%	143
Jersey Shore University Medical Center	Neptune	100%	778
JFK Med Ctr-A M Yelencsics Comm Hosp	Edison	100%	265
Kennedy Univ Hosp-Stratford Div	Stratford	100%	117
Libertyhealth-Jersey City Med Ctr	Jersey City	100%	362
Monmouth Medical Center - Southern Campus	Lakewood	100%	57
Newark Beth Israel Medical Center[2]	Newark	100%	284
Our Lady of Lourdes Medical Center[2]	Camden	100%	341
Palisades Medical Center	North Bergen	100%	39
Riverview Medical Center	Red Bank	100%	155
Robert W Johnson Univ Hosp-Hamilton	Hamilton	100%	81
Robert Wood Johnson Univ Hosp-Rahway	Rahway	100%	68
Saint Barnabas Medical Center	Livingston	100%	241
Saint Mary's Hospital - Passaic	Passaic	100%	90
Saint Peter's University Hospital	New Brunswick	100%	79
University Hospital	Newark	100%	106
Valley Hospital[2]	Ridgewood	100%	307
Virtua Mem Hosp of Burlington County	Mount Holly	100%	160
Virtua West Jersey Hospitals Berlin	Berlin	100%	340
Hackensack - Umc Mountainside	Montclair	99%	84
Morristown Medical Center[2]	Morristown	99%	328
Ocean Medical Center	Brick	99%	135
Overlook Medical Center	Summit	99%	251
Robert Wood Johnson University Hospital	New Brunswick	99%	797
Saint Clare's Hospital	Denville	99%	137
Saint Francis Medical Center	Trenton	99%	291
Saint Joseph's Regional Medical Center	Paterson	99%	518
Trinitas Regional Medical Center	Elizabeth	99%	121
Carepoint Health - Christ Hospital	Jersey City	98%	96
Monmouth Medical Center	Long Branch	98%	53
Saint Michael's Medical Center	Newark	98%	162
Somerset Medical Center[2]	Somerville	98%	217
Univ Med Ctr of Princeton-Plainsboro	Plainsboro	98%	57
Shore Medical Center	Somers Point	97%	31
Raritan Bay Medical Center	Perth Amboy	95%	231
Newton Memorial Hospital	Newton	94%	36
East Orange General Hospital	East Orange	93%	54
Cape Regional Medical Center	Cape May CH	90%	29
Southern Ocean Medical Center	Manahawkin	89%	36

PCI Within 90 Minutes of Arrival

Hospital Name	City	Rate	Cases
Community Medical Center[2]	Toms River	100%	46
Hackensack - Umc Mountainside	Montclair	100%	28
Holy Name Medical Center	Teaneck	100%	35
Newark Beth Israel Medical Center[2]	Newark	100%	46
Overlook Medical Center	Summit	100%	44
Saint Clare's Hospital	Denville	100%	40
Saint Mary's Hospital - Passaic	Passaic	100%	25
Somerset Medical Center[2]	Somerville	100%	64
Inspira Medical Center Woodbury	Woodbury	99%	68
Jersey Shore University Medical Center	Neptune	98%	86
Robert Wood Johnson University Hospital	New Brunswick	98%	107
Valley Hospital[2]	Ridgewood	98%	44
Clara Maass Medical Center[2]	Belleville	97%	35
Hunterdon Medical Center	Flemington	97%	35
Saint Barnabas Medical Center	Livingston	97%	29
Carepoint Health - Christ Hospital	Jersey City	96%	25
Riverview Medical Center	Red Bank	96%	51
Robert Wood Johnson Univ Hosp-Rahway	Rahway	96%	25
Saint Joseph's Regional Medical Center	Paterson	96%	81
Atlanticare Regional Medical Center[2]	Atlantic City	95%	81
Chilton Medical Center	Pompton Plains	95%	57
Hackensack University Medical Center	Hackensack	95%	86
Ocean Medical Center	Brick	95%	40
JFK Med Ctr-A M Yelencsics Comm Hosp	Edison	94%	68
Virtua West Jersey Hospitals Berlin	Berlin	94%	51
Saint Francis Medical Center	Trenton	93%	28
Libertyhealth-Jersey City Med Ctr	Jersey City	92%	37
Englewood Hospital & Medical Center	Englewood	91%	33
Robert W Johnson Univ Hosp-Hamilton	Hamilton	91%	33
Morristown Medical Center[2]	Morristown	90%	29
Virtua Mem Hosp of Burlington County	Mount Holly	90%	39
Trinitas Regional Medical Center	Elizabeth	89%	27
Raritan Bay Medical Center	Perth Amboy	79%	43

Statin Prescribed at Discharge

Hospital Name	City	Rate	Cases
Atlanticare Regional Medical Center[2]	Atlantic City	100%	322
Bayshore Community Hospital	Holmdel	100%	42
Carepoint Health-Bayonne Hosp Ctr	Bayonne	100%	145
Centrastate Medical Center[2]	Freehold	100%	30
Chilton Medical Center	Pompton Plains	100%	136
Clara Maass Medical Center[2]	Belleville	100%	207
Community Medical Center[2]	Toms River	100%	206
Cooper University Hospital[2]	Camden	100%	274
Deborah Heart & Lung Center	Browns Mills	100%	326
Hackensack - Umc Mountainside	Montclair	100%	77
Hackensack University Medical Center	Hackensack	100%	602
Hackettstown Regional Medical Center	Hackettstown	100%	37
Holy Name Medical Center	Teaneck	100%	191
Hunterdon Medical Center	Flemington	100%	105
Inspira Medical Center Woodbury	Woodbury	100%	141
Jersey Shore University Medical Center	Neptune	100%	758
JFK Med Ctr-A M Yelencsics Comm Hosp	Edison	100%	261
Libertyhealth-Jersey City Med Ctr	Jersey City	100%	364
Monmouth Medical Center	Long Branch	100%	47
Newark Beth Israel Medical Center[2]	Newark	100%	274
Our Lady of Lourdes Medical Center[2]	Camden	100%	342
Riverview Medical Center	Red Bank	100%	150
Robert Wood Johnson University Hospital	New Brunswick	100%	759
Robert W Johnson Univ Hosp-Hamilton	Hamilton	100%	76
Robert Wood Johnson Univ Hosp-Rahway	Rahway	100%	66
Saint Barnabas Medical Center	Livingston	100%	233
Saint Francis Medical Center	Trenton	100%	281
Saint Mary's Hospital - Passaic	Passaic	100%	85
Saint Peter's University Hospital	New Brunswick	100%	83
University Hospital	Newark	100%	104
Valley Hospital[2]	Ridgewood	100%	311
Virtua Mem Hosp of Burlington County	Mount Holly	100%	152
Englewood Hospital & Medical Center	Englewood	99%	339
Kennedy Univ Hosp-Stratford Div	Stratford	99%	115
Virtua West Jersey Hospitals Berlin	Berlin	99%	333
Capital Health Medical Center - Hopewell	Pennington	98%	55
Monmouth Medical Center - Southern Campus	Lakewood	98%	57
Ocean Medical Center	Brick	98%	129
Overlook Medical Center	Summit	98%	250
Saint Clare's Hospital	Denville	98%	136
Saint Joseph's Regional Medical Center	Paterson	98%	507
Trinitas Regional Medical Center	Elizabeth	98%	123
Univ Med Ctr of Princeton-Plainsboro	Plainsboro	98%	53
Morristown Medical Center[2]	Morristown	97%	325
Saint Michael's Medical Center	Newark	97%	169
Somerset Medical Center[2]	Somerville	97%	206
Cape Regional Medical Center	Cape May CH	96%	28
East Orange General Hospital	East Orange	96%	48
Raritan Bay Medical Center	Perth Amboy	95%	244
Newton Memorial Hospital	Newton	94%	36
Southern Ocean Medical Center	Manahawkin	94%	33
Shore Medical Center	Somers Point	93%	30
Carepoint Health - Christ Hospital	Jersey City	92%	96
Inspira Medical Center Vineland	Vineland	92%	48
Palisades Medical Center	North Bergen	91%	35

Heart Failure Care

ACE Inhibitor or ARB for LVSD

Hospital Name	City	Rate	Cases
Atlanticare Regional Medical Center[2]	Atlantic City	100%	172
Bayshore Community Hospital	Holmdel	100%	48
Capital Health System - Fuld Campus	Trenton	100%	73
Carepoint Health-Bayonne Hosp Ctr[2]	Bayonne	100%	61
Carepoint Health - Hoboken UMC	Hoboken	100%	59
Centrastate Medical Center[2]	Freehold	100%	72
Chilton Medical Center	Pompton Plains	100%	77
Clara Maass Medical Center[2]	Belleville	100%	81
Community Medical Center[2]	Toms River	100%	78
Cooper University Hospital[2]	Camden	100%	120
Hackettstown Regional Medical Center	Hackettstown	100%	27
Holy Name Medical Center[2]	Teaneck	100%	61
Hunterdon Medical Center	Flemington	100%	43
Inspira Medical Center Woodbury	Woodbury	100%	94
Libertyhealth-Jersey City Med Ctr[2]	Jersey City	100%	140
Memorial Hospital of Salem County	Salem	100%	44
Monmouth Medical Center - Southern Campus	Lakewood	100%	69
Newark Beth Israel Medical Center[2]	Newark	100%	126
Our Lady of Lourdes Medical Center[2]	Camden	100%	86
Overlook Medical Center[2]	Summit	100%	92
Palisades Medical Center[2]	North Bergen	100%	51
Riverview Medical Center[2]	Red Bank	100%	41
Robert Wood Johnson Univ Hosp-Rahway	Rahway	100%	78
Saint Barnabas Medical Center[2]	Livingston	100%	77
Saint Francis Medical Center	Trenton	100%	67
Saint Mary's Hospital - Passaic[2]	Passaic	100%	95
Saint Peter's University Hospital	New Brunswick	100%	68
University Hospital	Newark	100%	181
Valley Hospital[2]	Ridgewood	100%	94
Virtua Mem Hosp of Burlington County	Mount Holly	100%	97
Virtua West Jersey Hospitals Berlin	Berlin	100%	153
Carepoint Health - Christ Hospital	Jersey City	99%	79
Deborah Heart & Lung Center	Browns Mills	99%	150
East Orange General Hospital[2]	East Orange	99%	73
Englewood Hospital & Medical Center	Englewood	99%	147
Hackensack - Umc Mountainside	Montclair	99%	94
Robert Wood Johnson University Hospital	New Brunswick	99%	321
Robert W Johnson Univ Hosp-Hamilton	Hamilton	99%	67
Saint Joseph's Regional Medical Center[2]	Paterson	99%	194
Capital Health Medical Center - Hopewell	Pennington	98%	49
Inspira Medical Center Vineland[2]	Vineland	98%	88
Jersey Shore University Medical Center[2]	Neptune	98%	103
Lourdes Med Ctr of Burlington County[2]	Willingboro	98%	44
Monmouth Medical Center[2]	Long Branch	98%	55
Newton Memorial Hospital	Newton	98%	48
Somerset Medical Center[2]	Somerville	98%	60
Hackensack University Medical Center	Hackensack	97%	261
JFK Med Ctr-A M Yelencsics Comm Hosp	Edison	97%	138
Saint Clare's Hospital	Denville	97%	95
Shore Medical Center[2]	Somers Point	97%	73
Southern Ocean Medical Center	Manahawkin	96%	55
Kennedy Univ Hosp-Stratford Div	Stratford	95%	155
Univ Med Ctr of Princeton-Plainsboro[2]	Plainsboro	95%	57
Raritan Bay Medical Center[2]	Perth Amboy	94%	125
VA New Jersey Health Care System	East Orange	94%	49
Saint Michael's Medical Center[2]	Newark	93%	151
Ocean Medical Center[2]	Brick	91%	70
Cape Regional Medical Center	Cape May CH	90%	69
Inspira Medical Center Elmer[2]	Elmer	86%	37
Morristown Medical Center[2]	Morristown	85%	131
Trinitas Regional Medical Center	Elizabeth	83%	157

Discharge Instructions Given

Hospital Name	City	Rate	Cases
Carepoint Health-Bayonne Hosp Ctr[2]	Bayonne	100%	168
Carepoint Health - Hoboken UMC	Hoboken	100%	98
Clara Maass Medical Center[2]	Belleville	100%	229
Community Medical Center[2]	Toms River	100%	192
Deborah Heart & Lung Center	Browns Mills	100%	333
Hackensack - Umc Mountainside	Montclair	100%	218
Hackettstown Regional Medical Center	Hackettstown	100%	117
Holy Name Medical Center[2]	Teaneck	100%	217
Inspira Medical Center Elmer[2]	Elmer	100%	114
Inspira Medical Center Vineland[2]	Vineland	100%	201
Inspira Medical Center Woodbury	Woodbury	100%	311
Libertyhealth-Jersey City Med Ctr[2]	Jersey City	100%	270
Meadowlands Hospital Medical Center	Secaucus	100%	41
Monmouth Medical Center[2]	Long Branch	100%	176
Monmouth Medical Center - Southern Campus	Lakewood	100%	173
Newark Beth Israel Medical Center[2]	Newark	100%	282
Overlook Medical Center[2]	Summit	100%	229
Riverview Medical Center[2]	Red Bank	100%	167
Saint Francis Medical Center	Trenton	100%	142
Saint Luke's Warren Hospital	Phillipsburg	100%	96
Saint Mary's Hospital - Passaic[2]	Passaic	100%	223
Somerset Medical Center[2]	Somerville	100%	210
University Hospital	Newark	100%	249
Atlanticare Regional Medical Center[2]	Atlantic City	99%	446
Cooper University Hospital[2]	Camden	99%	253
Jersey Shore University Medical Center[2]	Neptune	99%	213
Newton Memorial Hospital	Newton	99%	189
Palisades Medical Center[2]	North Bergen	99%	171
Robert Wood Johnson University Hospital	New Brunswick	99%	748
Saint Barnabas Medical Center[2]	Livingston	99%	248
Saint Michael's Medical Center[2]	Newark	99%	252
Saint Peter's University Hospital	New Brunswick	99%	213
Memorial Hospital of Salem County	Salem	98%	121
Our Lady of Lourdes Medical Center[2]	Camden	98%	262
Raritan Bay Medical Center[2]	Perth Amboy	98%	289
Robert Wood Johnson Univ Hosp-Rahway	Rahway	98%	176
Saint Clare's Hospital	Denville	98%	297
Virtua Mem Hosp of Burlington County	Mount Holly	98%	342
Bayshore Community Hospital	Holmdel	97%	178
Carepoint Health - Christ Hospital	Jersey City	97%	232
Chilton Medical Center	Pompton Plains	97%	199
Hackensack University Medical Center	Hackensack	97%	570
Kennedy Univ Hosp-Stratford Div	Stratford	97%	657
Morristown Medical Center[2]	Morristown	97%	217
Saint Joseph's Regional Medical Center[2]	Paterson	97%	480
Valley Hospital[2]	Ridgewood	97%	208
Capital Health System - Fuld Campus	Trenton	96%	141
Centrastate Medical Center[2]	Freehold	96%	182
Englewood Hospital & Medical Center	Englewood	96%	338
Southern Ocean Medical Center	Manahawkin	96%	158
Univ Med Ctr of Princeton-Plainsboro[2]	Plainsboro	96%	178
Virtua West Jersey Hospitals Berlin	Berlin	96%	531
Lourdes Med Ctr of Burlington County[2]	Willingboro	95%	164
Capital Health Medical Center - Hopewell	Pennington	94%	144
VA New Jersey Health Care System	East Orange	93%	68
Cape Regional Medical Center	Cape May CH	92%	184
Trinitas Regional Medical Center	Elizabeth	92%	342
Hunterdon Medical Center	Flemington	91%	120
Ocean Medical Center[2]	Brick	91%	181
Shore Medical Center[2]	Somers Point	91%	218
JFK Med Ctr-A M Yelencsics Comm Hosp	Edison	90%	348

NOTE: Hospital profiles are in alphabetical order by state, then city, then hospital within the city; Rankings exclude hospitals with less than 25 cases except for patient surveys which excludes hospitals with less than 100 cases; (a) 100-299 cases; (1) The number of cases/patients is too few to report; (2) Data submitted were based on a sample of cases/patients; (3) Results are based on a shorter time period than required; (4) Data suppressed by CMS for one or more quarters; (5) Results are not available for this reporting period; (6) Fewer than 100 patients completed the HCAHPS survey; (7) No cases met the criteria for this measure; (8) The lower limit of the confidence interval cannot be calculated if the number of observed infections equals zero; (9) No data are available from the state/territory for this reporting period; (10) The scores shown reflect fewer than 50 completed surveys; (11) There were discrepancies in the data collection process; (12) This measure does not apply to this hospital for this reporting period; (13) Results cannot be calculated for this reporting period; (14) The results for this state are combined with nearby states to protect confidentiality; Please refer to the User's Guide for a full explanation of data.

Hospital Name	City	Rate	Cases
Robert W Johnson Univ Hosp-Hamilton	Hamilton	89%	243
East Orange General Hospital[2]	East Orange	68%	169

Evaluation of LVS Function

Hospital Name	City	Rate	Cases
Atlanticare Regional Medical Center[2]	Atlantic City	100%	563
Bayshore Community Hospital	Holmdel	100%	270
Capital Health Medical Center - Hopewell	Pennington	100%	181
Capital Health System - Fuld Campus	Trenton	100%	187
Carepoint Health-Bayonne Hosp Ctr[2]	Bayonne	100%	264
Carepoint Health - Hoboken UMC	Hoboken	100%	144
Centrastate Medical Center[2]	Freehold	100%	293
Chilton Medical Center	Pompton Plains	100%	299
Clara Maass Medical Center[2]	Belleville	100%	309
Community Medical Center[2]	Toms River	100%	312
Cooper University Hospital[2]	Camden	100%	288
Deborah Heart & Lung Center	Browns Mills	100%	403
Hackensack - Umc Mountainside	Montclair	100%	333
Hackensack University Medical Center	Hackensack	100%	812
Hackettstown Regional Medical Center	Hackettstown	100%	188
Holy Name Medical Center[2]	Teaneck	100%	316
Inspira Medical Center Vineland[2]	Vineland	100%	261
Inspira Medical Center Woodbury	Woodbury	100%	383
Jersey Shore University Medical Center[2]	Neptune	100%	315
JFK Med Ctr-A M Yelencsics Comm Hosp	Edison	100%	546
Kennedy Univ Hosp-Stratford Div	Stratford	100%	899
Libertyhealth-Jersey City Med Ctr[2]	Jersey City	100%	335
Lourdes Med Ctr of Burlington County[2]	Willingboro	100%	205
Monmouth Medical Center[2]	Long Branch	100%	256
Monmouth Medical Center - Southern Campus	Lakewood	100%	322
Morristown Medical Center[2]	Morristown	100%	323
Newark Beth Israel Medical Center[2]	Newark	100%	339
Our Lady of Lourdes Medical Center[2]	Camden	100%	326
Overlook Medical Center[2]	Summit	100%	302
Riverview Medical Center[2]	Red Bank	100%	262
Robert Wood Johnson University Hospital	New Brunswick	100%	1040
Robert W Johnson Univ Hosp-Hamilton	Hamilton	100%	333
Robert Wood Johnson Univ Hosp-Rahway	Rahway	100%	308
Saint Barnabas Medical Center[2]	Livingston	100%	325
Saint Clare's Hospital	Denville	100%	464
Saint Francis Medical Center	Trenton	100%	186
Saint Joseph's Regional Medical Center[2]	Paterson	100%	658
Saint Luke's Warren Hospital	Phillipsburg	100%	142
Saint Mary's Hospital - Passaic[2]	Passaic	100%	315
Saint Peter's University Hospital	New Brunswick	100%	296
Somerset Medical Center[2]	Somerville	100%	308
Southern Ocean Medical Center	Manahawkin	100%	233
Trinitas Regional Medical Center	Elizabeth	100%	437
University Hospital	Newark	100%	288
Univ Med Ctr of Princeton-Plainsboro[2]	Plainsboro	100%	281
VA New Jersey Health Care System	East Orange	100%	73
Valley Hospital[2]	Ridgewood	100%	330
Virtua Mem Hosp of Burlington County	Mount Holly	100%	484
Virtua West Jersey Hospitals Berlin	Berlin	100%	746
Carepoint Health - Christ Hospital	Jersey City	99%	300
East Orange General Hospital[2]	East Orange	99%	244
Englewood Hospital & Medical Center	Englewood	99%	481
Hunterdon Medical Center	Flemington	99%	166
Inspira Medical Center Elmer[2]	Elmer	99%	135
Memorial Hospital of Salem County	Salem	99%	143
Newton Memorial Hospital	Newton	99%	270
Saint Michael's Medical Center[2]	Newark	99%	315
Shore Medical Center[2]	Somers Point	99%	269
Cape Regional Medical Center	Cape May CH	98%	238
Ocean Medical Center[2]	Brick	98%	292
Palisades Medical Center[2]	North Bergen	98%	259
Raritan Bay Medical Center[2]	Perth Amboy	98%	466
Meadowlands Hospital Medical Center	Secaucus	96%	46

Medicare Spending

Medicare Spending per Patient (ratio)

Hospital Name	City	Ratio	Cases
Cape Regional Medical Center	Cape May CH	0.98	-
Inspira Medical Center Elmer	Elmer	0.98	-
Newton Memorial Hospital	Newton	0.98	-
Shore Medical Center	Somers Point	0.98	-
Deborah Heart & Lung Center	Browns Mills	0.99	-
Hunterdon Medical Center	Flemington	1.02	-
Inspira Medical Center Woodbury	Woodbury	1.02	-
Kennedy Univ Hosp-Stratford Div	Stratford	1.02	-
Memorial Hospital of Salem County	Salem	1.02	-
Saint Luke's Warren Hospital	Phillipsburg	1.02	-
Virtua Mem Hosp of Burlington County	Mount Holly	1.02	-
Capital Health Medical Center - Hopewell	Pennington	1.03	-
Cooper University Hospital	Camden	1.03	-
Lourdes Med Ctr of Burlington County	Willingboro	1.03	-
Our Lady of Lourdes Medical Center	Camden	1.03	-
Southern Ocean Medical Center	Manahawkin	1.04	-
Virtua West Jersey Hospitals Berlin	Berlin	1.04	-
Inspira Medical Center Vineland	Vineland	1.05	-
Overlook Medical Center	Summit	1.05	-
Atlanticare Regional Medical Center	Atlantic City	1.06	-
Bergen Regional Medical Center	Paramus	1.06	-
Morristown Medical Center	Morristown	1.06	-
Riverview Medical Center	Red Bank	1.06	-
Saint Peter's University Hospital	New Brunswick	1.06	-
University Hospital	Newark	1.06	-
Bayshore Community Hospital	Holmdel	1.07	-
Capital Health System - Fuld Campus	Trenton	1.07	-
Centrastate Medical Center	Freehold	1.07	-
Englewood Hospital & Medical Center	Englewood	1.07	-
Hackettstown Regional Medical Center	Hackettstown	1.07	-
Palisades Medical Center	North Bergen	1.07	-
Raritan Bay Medical Center	Perth Amboy	1.07	-
Robert W Johnson Univ Hosp-Hamilton	Hamilton	1.07	-
Saint Clare's Hospital	Denville	1.07	-
Univ Med Ctr of Princeton-Plainsboro	Plainsboro	1.07	-
Community Medical Center	Toms River	1.08	-
Hackensack - Umc Mountainside	Montclair	1.08	-
Holy Name Medical Center	Teaneck	1.08	-
Jersey Shore University Medical Center	Neptune	1.08	-
Saint Barnabas Medical Center	Livingston	1.08	-
Chilton Medical Center	Pompton Plains	1.09	-
Robert Wood Johnson University Hospital	New Brunswick	1.09	-
Valley Hospital	Ridgewood	1.09	-
Monmouth Medical Center - Southern Campus	Lakewood	1.10	-
Ocean Medical Center	Brick	1.10	-
Carepoint Health - Christ Hospital	Jersey City	1.11	-
Carepoint Health - Hoboken UMC	Hoboken	1.11	-
Hackensack University Medical Center	Hackensack	1.11	-
Monmouth Medical Center	Long Branch	1.11	-
Saint Francis Medical Center	Trenton	1.11	-
Saint Joseph's Regional Medical Center	Paterson	1.11	-
Saint Mary's Hospital - Passaic	Passaic	1.11	-
Saint Michael's Medical Center	Newark	1.11	-
Libertyhealth-Jersey City Med Ctr	Jersey City	1.12	-
Newark Beth Israel Medical Center	Newark	1.12	-
Somerset Medical Center	Somerville	1.12	-
Carepoint Health-Bayonne Hosp Ctr	Bayonne	1.13	-
Clara Maass Medical Center	Belleville	1.13	-
Meadowlands Hospital Medical Center	Secaucus	1.13	-
Trinitas Regional Medical Center	Elizabeth	1.14	-
Robert Wood Johnson Univ Hosp-Rahway	Rahway	1.15	-
East Orange General Hospital	East Orange	1.17	-
JFK Med Ctr-A M Yelencsics Comm Hosp	Edison	1.17	-

Pneumonia Care

Appropriate Initial Antibiotic Given

Hospital Name	City	Rate	Cases
Carepoint Health-Bayonne Hosp Ctr[2]	Bayonne	100%	71
Cooper University Hospital[2]	Camden	100%	57
East Orange General Hospital[2]	East Orange	100%	52
Hackensack - Umc Mountainside	Montclair	100%	140
Hackettstown Regional Medical Center	Hackettstown	100%	107
Hunterdon Medical Center[2]	Flemington	100%	106
Inspira Medical Center Vineland[2]	Vineland	100%	48
Libertyhealth-Jersey City Med Ctr[2]	Jersey City	100%	94
Monmouth Medical Center - Southern Campus	Lakewood	100%	132
Our Lady of Lourdes Medical Center[2]	Camden	100%	82
Riverview Medical Center[2]	Red Bank	100%	123
Saint Barnabas Medical Center[2]	Livingston	100%	118
Saint Francis Medical Center	Trenton	100%	71
Somerset Medical Center[2]	Somerville	100%	80
University Hospital	Newark	100%	91
Bayshore Community Hospital[2]	Holmdel	99%	102
Carepoint Health - Hoboken UMC	Hoboken	99%	85
Centrastate Medical Center[2]	Freehold	99%	222
Chilton Medical Center[2]	Pompton Plains	99%	97
Englewood Hospital & Medical Center	Englewood	99%	122
Inspira Medical Center Woodbury	Woodbury	99%	197
Jersey Shore University Medical Center[2]	Neptune	99%	74
JFK Med Ctr-A M Yelencsics Comm Hosp	Edison	99%	238
Newark Beth Israel Medical Center[2]	Newark	99%	92
Robert Wood Johnson University Hospital	New Brunswick	99%	164
Valley Hospital[2]	Ridgewood	99%	88
Capital Health System - Fuld Campus	Trenton	98%	106
Clara Maass Medical Center[2]	Belleville	98%	125
Community Medical Center[2]	Toms River	98%	119
Kennedy Univ Hosp-Stratford Div	Stratford	98%	524
Lourdes Med Ctr of Burlington County[2]	Willingboro	98%	89
Memorial Hospital of Salem County	Salem	98%	60
Saint Mary's Hospital - Passaic[2]	Passaic	98%	112
Saint Peter's University Hospital[2]	New Brunswick	98%	129
Shore Medical Center[2]	Somers Point	98%	95
Univ Med Ctr of Princeton-Plainsboro[2]	Plainsboro	98%	92
Cape Regional Medical Center	Cape May CH	97%	206
Capital Health Medical Center - Hopewell	Pennington	97%	103
Inspira Medical Center Elmer[2]	Elmer	97%	60
Meadowlands Hospital Medical Center	Secaucus	97%	62
Monmouth Medical Center[2]	Long Branch	97%	88
Ocean Medical Center[2]	Brick	97%	115
Palisades Medical Center[2]	North Bergen	97%	92
Saint Luke's Warren Hospital	Phillipsburg	97%	118
Southern Ocean Medical Center	Manahawkin	97%	158
Virtua Mem Hosp of Burlington County	Mount Holly	97%	238
Virtua West Jersey Hospitals Berlin	Berlin	97%	497
Atlanticare Regional Medical Center[2]	Atlantic City	96%	238
Hackensack University Medical Center	Hackensack	96%	356
Newton Memorial Hospital[2]	Newton	96%	99
Overlook Medical Center[2]	Summit	96%	94
Robert Wood Johnson Univ Hosp-Rahway	Rahway	96%	95
Saint Clare's Hospital	Denville	96%	169
Saint Joseph's Regional Medical Center[2]	Paterson	96%	216
Trinitas Regional Medical Center[2]	Elizabeth	96%	54
Morristown Medical Center[2]	Morristown	95%	99
Raritan Bay Medical Center[2]	Perth Amboy	95%	173
Robert W Johnson Univ Hosp-Hamilton	Hamilton	95%	209
Saint Michael's Medical Center[2]	Newark	95%	76
Carepoint Health - Christ Hospital	Jersey City	93%	123
Holy Name Medical Center[2]	Teaneck	93%	134
Bergen Regional Medical Center	Paramus	84%	32
VA New Jersey Health Care System	East Orange	81%	31

Blood Culture Timing

Hospital Name	City	Rate	Cases
Cape Regional Medical Center	Cape May CH	100%	394
Capital Health Medical Center - Hopewell	Pennington	100%	216
Carepoint Health-Bayonne Hosp Ctr[2]	Bayonne	100%	133
Chilton Medical Center[2]	Pompton Plains	100%	166
Clara Maass Medical Center[2]	Belleville	100%	196
Hackensack - Umc Mountainside	Montclair	100%	252
Hackettstown Regional Medical Center	Hackettstown	100%	204
JFK Med Ctr-A M Yelencsics Comm Hosp	Edison	100%	545
Libertyhealth-Jersey City Med Ctr[2]	Jersey City	100%	206
Lourdes Med Ctr of Burlington County[2]	Willingboro	100%	164
Monmouth Medical Center[2]	Long Branch	100%	159
Monmouth Medical Center - Southern Campus	Lakewood	100%	221
Riverview Medical Center[2]	Red Bank	100%	198
Robert W Johnson Univ Hosp-Hamilton	Hamilton	100%	425
Saint Barnabas Medical Center[2]	Livingston	100%	96
Saint Francis Medical Center	Trenton	100%	121
Saint Mary's Hospital - Passaic[2]	Passaic	100%	182
Saint Peter's University Hospital[2]	New Brunswick	100%	289
Univ Med Ctr of Princeton-Plainsboro[2]	Plainsboro	100%	172
Virtua Mem Hosp of Burlington County	Mount Holly	100%	403
Virtua West Jersey Hospitals Berlin	Berlin	100%	956
Atlanticare Regional Medical Center[2]	Atlantic City	99%	447
Bayshore Community Hospital[2]	Holmdel	99%	157
Capital Health System - Fuld Campus	Trenton	99%	214
Carepoint Health - Hoboken UMC	Hoboken	99%	156
Centrastate Medical Center[2]	Freehold	99%	457
East Orange General Hospital[2]	East Orange	99%	179
Holy Name Medical Center[2]	Teaneck	99%	220
Hunterdon Medical Center[2]	Flemington	99%	176
Inspira Medical Center Elmer[2]	Elmer	99%	95
Inspira Medical Center Vineland[2]	Vineland	99%	144
Jersey Shore University Medical Center[2]	Neptune	99%	144
Kennedy Univ Hosp-Stratford Div	Stratford	99%	1175
Ocean Medical Center[2]	Brick	99%	210
Overlook Medical Center[2]	Summit	99%	164
Robert Wood Johnson University Hospital	New Brunswick	99%	523
Saint Clare's Hospital	Denville	99%	288
Saint Joseph's Regional Medical Center[2]	Paterson	99%	491
Saint Luke's Warren Hospital	Phillipsburg	99%	195
Trinitas Regional Medical Center[2]	Elizabeth	99%	75
VA New Jersey Health Care System	East Orange	99%	76
Valley Hospital[2]	Ridgewood	99%	194
Cooper University Hospital[2]	Camden	98%	130
Englewood Hospital & Medical Center	Englewood	98%	212
Hackensack University Medical Center	Hackensack	98%	451
Inspira Medical Center Woodbury	Woodbury	98%	361
Memorial Hospital of Salem County	Salem	98%	131
Our Lady of Lourdes Medical Center[2]	Camden	98%	122
Raritan Bay Medical Center[2]	Perth Amboy	98%	330
Shore Medical Center[2]	Somers Point	98%	186
University Hospital	Newark	98%	247
Carepoint Health - Christ Hospital	Jersey City	97%	240
Meadowlands Hospital Medical Center	Secaucus	97%	111
Morristown Medical Center[2]	Morristown	97%	156
Palisades Medical Center[2]	North Bergen	97%	157
Robert Wood Johnson Univ Hosp-Rahway	Rahway	97%	179
Newark Beth Israel Medical Center[2]	Newark	96%	157
Saint Michael's Medical Center[2]	Newark	96%	155
Somerset Medical Center[2]	Somerville	96%	103
Southern Ocean Medical Center	Manahawkin	96%	251
Newton Memorial Hospital[2]	Newton	95%	172
Community Medical Center[2]	Toms River	94%	198
Bergen Regional Medical Center	Paramus	84%	96

NOTE: Hospital profiles are in alphabetical order by state, then city, then hospital within the city; Rankings exclude hospitals with less than 25 cases except for patient surveys which excludes hospitals with less than 100 cases; (a) 100-299 cases; (1) The number of cases/patients is too few to report; (2) Data submitted were based on a sample of cases/patients; (3) Results are based on a shorter time period than required; (4) Data suppressed by CMS for one or more quarters; (5) Results are not available for this reporting period; (6) Fewer than 100 patients completed the HCAHPS survey; (7) No cases met the criteria for this measure; (8) The lower limit of the confidence interval cannot be calculated if the number of observed infections equals zero; (9) No data are available from the state/territory for this reporting period; (10) The scores shown reflect fewer than 50 completed surveys; (11) There were discrepancies in the data collection process; (12) This measure does not apply to this hospital for this reporting period; (13) Results cannot be calculated for this reporting period; (14) The results for this state are combined with nearby states to protect confidentiality; Please refer to the User's Guide for a full explanation of data.

Pregnancy and Delivery Care

Newborns whose Deliveries were Scheduled Early

Hospital Name	City	Rate	Cases
Carepoint Health - Christ Hospital[2]	Jersey City	0%	32
Chilton Medical Center	Pompton Plains	0%	133
Hackettstown Regional Medical Center	Hackettstown	0%	50
Hunterdon Medical Center[2]	Flemington	0%	28
Inspira Medical Center Elmer	Elmer	0%	25
Jersey Shore University Medical Center[2]	Neptune	0%	28
JFK Med Ctr-A M Yelencsics Comm Hosp	Edison	0%	412
Monmouth Medical Center[2]	Long Branch	0%	64
Morristown Medical Center	Morristown	0%	241
Newton Memorial Hospital	Newton	0%	58
Our Lady of Lourdes Medical Center[2]	Camden	0%	35
Overlook Medical Center[2]	Summit	0%	143
Robert W Johnson Univ Hosp-Hamilton	Hamilton	0%	153
Saint Clare's Hospital[2]	Denville	0%	27
Somerset Medical Center[2]	Somerville	0%	36
University Hospital[2]	Newark	0%	27
Newark Beth Israel Medical Center[2]	Newark	1%	581
Capital Health Medical Center - Hopewell[2]	Pennington	2%	40
Clara Maass Medical Center	Belleville	2%	190
Inspira Medical Center Vineland[2]	Vineland	2%	63
Cape Regional Medical Center[2]	Cape May CH	3%	34
Univ Med Ctr of Princeton-Plainsboro[2]	Plainsboro	3%	35
Community Medical Center[2]	Toms River	4%	27
Saint Mary's Hospital - Passaic[2]	Passaic	4%	47
Virtua West Jersey Hospitals Berlin[2]	Berlin	4%	109
Meadowlands Hospital Medical Center[2]	Secaucus	5%	38
Saint Peter's University Hospital[2]	New Brunswick	5%	95
Shore Medical Center[2]	Somers Point	5%	79
Trinitas Regional Medical Center[2]	Elizabeth	5%	202
Hackensack University Medical Center[2]	Hackensack	6%	156
Valley Hospital[2]	Ridgewood	6%	48
Kennedy Univ Hosp-Stratford Div[2]	Stratford	7%	29
Libertyhealth-Jersey City Med Ctr[2]	Jersey City	7%	44
Monmouth Medical Center - Southern Campus[2]	Lakewood	7%	30
Raritan Bay Medical Center[2]	Perth Amboy	8%	26
Saint Joseph's Regional Medical Center[2]	Paterson	9%	81
Holy Name Medical Center[2]	Teaneck	10%	51
Ocean Medical Center[2]	Brick	10%	50
Riverview Medical Center[2]	Red Bank	10%	39
Hackensack - Umc Mountainside[2]	Montclair	11%	35
Virtua Mem Hosp of Burlington County[2]	Mount Holly	11%	38
Englewood Hospital & Medical Center[2]	Englewood	12%	52
Atlanticare Regional Medical Center[2]	Atlantic City	17%	52
Saint Barnabas Medical Center[2]	Livingston	27%	75

Preventive Care

Immunization for Influenza

Hospital Name	City	Rate	Cases
Carepoint Health-Bayonne Hosp Ctr[2]	Bayonne	100%	564
Holy Name Medical Center[2]	Teaneck	100%	542
Riverview Medical Center[2]	Red Bank	100%	553
Chilton Medical Center[2]	Pompton Plains	99%	529
Libertyhealth-Jersey City Med Ctr[2]	Jersey City	99%	508
Memorial Hospital of Salem County[2]	Salem	99%	412
Monmouth Medical Center - Southern Campus[2]	Lakewood	99%	526
Ocean Medical Center[2]	Brick	99%	575
Saint Luke's Warren Hospital[2]	Phillipsburg	99%	604
Saint Peter's University Hospital[2]	New Brunswick	99%	461
Trinitas Regional Medical Center[2]	Elizabeth	99%	506
Bayshore Community Hospital[2]	Holmdel	98%	605
Cape Regional Medical Center[2]	Cape May CH	98%	553
Inspira Medical Center Woodbury[2]	Woodbury	98%	561
Newton Memorial Hospital[2]	Newton	98%	561
Our Lady of Lourdes Medical Center[2]	Camden	98%	558
Saint Michael's Medical Center[2]	Newark	98%	609
Virtua Mem Hosp of Burlington County[2]	Mount Holly	98%	522
Virtua West Jersey Hospitals Berlin[2]	Berlin	98%	532
Centrastate Medical Center[2]	Freehold	97%	509
Deborah Heart & Lung Center[2]	Browns Mills	97%	603
Hackettstown Regional Medical Center[2]	Hackettstown	97%	395
Kennedy Univ Hosp-Stratford Div[2]	Stratford	97%	595
Lourdes Med Ctr of Burlington County[2]	Willingboro	97%	583
Raritan Bay Medical Center[2]	Perth Amboy	97%	547
Robert W Johnson Univ Hosp-Hamilton[2]	Hamilton	97%	530
Univ Med Ctr of Princeton-Plainsboro[2]	Plainsboro	97%	515
Valley Hospital[2]	Ridgewood	97%	558
Carepoint Health - Christ Hospital[2]	Jersey City	96%	523
Clara Maass Medical Center[2]	Belleville	96%	549
Hunterdon Medical Center[2]	Flemington	96%	534
Saint Francis Medical Center[2]	Trenton	96%	470
Southern Ocean Medical Center[2]	Manahawkin	96%	569
Capital Health System - Fuld Campus[2]	Trenton	95%	583
Overlook Medical Center[2]	Summit	95%	587
Saint Clare's Hospital[2]	Denville	95%	535
Hackensack - Umc Mountainside[2]	Montclair	94%	508
Monmouth Medical Center[2]	Long Branch	94%	493
Inspira Medical Center Vineland[2]	Vineland	93%	495
Jersey Shore University Medical Center[2]	Neptune	93%	567
JFK Med Ctr-A M Yelencsics Comm Hosp[2]	Edison	93%	537
Robert Wood Johnson Univ Hosp-Rahway[2]	Rahway	93%	586
East Orange General Hospital[2]	East Orange	92%	607
Robert Wood Johnson University Hospital[2]	New Brunswick	92%	564
Saint Mary's Hospital - Passaic[2]	Passaic	91%	530
University Hospital[2]	Newark	91%	529
Inspira Medical Center Elmer[2]	Elmer	90%	341
Morristown Medical Center[2]	Morristown	90%	563
Saint Joseph's Regional Medical Center[2]	Paterson	90%	1053
Cooper University Hospital[2]	Camden	89%	565
Capital Health Medical Center - Hopewell[2]	Pennington	88%	500
Englewood Hospital & Medical Center[2]	Englewood	87%	552
Shore Medical Center[2]	Somers Point	86%	553
Newark Beth Israel Medical Center[2]	Newark	85%	516
Saint Barnabas Medical Center[2]	Livingston	85%	511
Bergen Regional Medical Center[2]	Paramus	84%	591
Somerset Medical Center[2]	Somerville	84%	578
Community Medical Center[2]	Toms River	83%	574
Carepoint Health - Hoboken UMC[2]	Hoboken	82%	465
Hackensack University Medical Center[2]	Hackensack	76%	493
Meadowlands Hospital Medical Center[2]	Secaucus	70%	378
Palisades Medical Center[2]	North Bergen	68%	501
Atlanticare Regional Medical Center[2]	Atlantic City	67%	551

Immunization for Pneumonia

Hospital Name	City	Rate	Cases
Carepoint Health-Bayonne Hosp Ctr[2]	Bayonne	100%	840
Holy Name Medical Center[2]	Teaneck	100%	642
Libertyhealth-Jersey City Med Ctr[2]	Jersey City	100%	536
Riverview Medical Center[2]	Red Bank	100%	689
Bayshore Community Hospital[2]	Holmdel	99%	916
Chilton Medical Center[2]	Pompton Plains	99%	741
Inspira Medical Center Woodbury[2]	Woodbury	99%	723
Memorial Hospital of Salem County[2]	Salem	99%	521
Ocean Medical Center[2]	Brick	99%	840
Univ Med Ctr of Princeton-Plainsboro[2]	Plainsboro	99%	558
Valley Hospital[2]	Ridgewood	99%	675
Raritan Bay Medical Center[2]	Perth Amboy	98%	692
Saint Luke's Warren Hospital[2]	Phillipsburg	98%	931
Southern Ocean Medical Center[2]	Manahawkin	98%	862
Cape Regional Medical Center[2]	Cape May CH	97%	751
Carepoint Health - Christ Hospital[2]	Jersey City	97%	672
Centrastate Medical Center[2]	Freehold	97%	569
Monmouth Medical Center - Southern Campus[2]	Lakewood	97%	687
Saint Francis Medical Center[2]	Trenton	97%	646
Saint Michael's Medical Center[2]	Newark	97%	932
Trinitas Regional Medical Center[2]	Elizabeth	97%	593
East Orange General Hospital[2]	East Orange	96%	905
Inspira Medical Center Vineland[2]	Vineland	96%	552
Jersey Shore University Medical Center[2]	Neptune	96%	652
Newton Memorial Hospital[2]	Newton	96%	732
Our Lady of Lourdes Medical Center[2]	Camden	96%	804
Saint Mary's Hospital - Passaic[2]	Passaic	96%	740
Saint Peter's University Hospital[2]	New Brunswick	96%	347
Virtua West Jersey Hospitals Berlin[2]	Berlin	96%	631
Carepoint Health - Hoboken UMC[2]	Hoboken	95%	421
Hunterdon Medical Center[2]	Flemington	95%	622
Kennedy Univ Hosp-Stratford Div[2]	Stratford	95%	815
Robert Wood Johnson Univ Hosp-Rahway[2]	Rahway	95%	946
Virtua Mem Hosp of Burlington County[2]	Mount Holly	95%	619
Inspira Medical Center Elmer[2]	Elmer	94%	402
Palisades Medical Center[2]	North Bergen	94%	588
Robert W Johnson Univ Hosp-Hamilton[2]	Hamilton	94%	719
Deborah Heart & Lung Center[2]	Browns Mills	93%	952
Hackensack - Umc Mountainside[2]	Montclair	93%	646
Hackettstown Regional Medical Center[2]	Hackettstown	93%	486
Robert Wood Johnson University Hospital[2]	New Brunswick	93%	612
Cooper University Hospital[2]	Camden	92%	606
Overlook Medical Center[2]	Summit	92%	513
Saint Joseph's Regional Medical Center[2]	Paterson	92%	1262
Capital Health System - Fuld Campus[2]	Trenton	91%	673
Clara Maass Medical Center[2]	Belleville	91%	697
Saint Clare's Hospital[2]	Denville	91%	693
Monmouth Medical Center[2]	Long Branch	90%	395
Shore Medical Center[2]	Somers Point	90%	683
Capital Health Medical Center - Hopewell[2]	Pennington	89%	457
Lourdes Med Ctr of Burlington County[2]	Willingboro	89%	797
Somerset Medical Center[2]	Somerville	89%	756
JFK Med Ctr-A M Yelencsics Comm Hosp[2]	Edison	88%	603
Hackensack University Medical Center[2]	Hackensack	86%	494
Morristown Medical Center[2]	Morristown	86%	508
Saint Barnabas Medical Center[2]	Livingston	85%	487
Community Medical Center[2]	Toms River	84%	825
Englewood Hospital & Medical Center[2]	Englewood	84%	634
Meadowlands Hospital Medical Center[2]	Secaucus	83%	363
Atlanticare Regional Medical Center[2]	Atlantic City	79%	627
Newark Beth Israel Medical Center[2]	Newark	78%	556
University Hospital[2]	Newark	78%	486
Bergen Regional Medical Center[2]	Paramus	74%	302

Stroke Care

Anticoagulation Therapy for Atrial Fibrillation

Hospital Name	City	Rate	Cases
Atlanticare Regional Medical Center	Atlantic City	100%	37
Englewood Hospital & Medical Center	Englewood	100%	40
Holy Name Medical Center	Teaneck	100%	35
JFK Med Ctr-A M Yelencsics Comm Hosp	Edison	100%	43
Kennedy Univ Hosp-Stratford Div[2]	Stratford	100%	33
Ocean Medical Center[2]	Brick	100%	47
Saint Barnabas Medical Center[2]	Livingston	100%	38
Valley Hospital	Ridgewood	100%	44
Virtua West Jersey Hospitals Berlin	Berlin	100%	26
Morristown Medical Center	Morristown	98%	41
Robert Wood Johnson University Hospital	New Brunswick	98%	53
Capital Health System - Fuld Campus	Trenton	97%	64
Jersey Shore University Medical Center	Neptune	97%	39
Saint Joseph's Regional Medical Center	Paterson	97%	36
Centrastate Medical Center[2]	Freehold	96%	26
Community Medical Center	Toms River	96%	51
Newton Memorial Hospital	Newton	96%	26
Overlook Medical Center	Summit	95%	62
Somerset Medical Center	Somerville	93%	30
Our Lady of Lourdes Medical Center	Camden	92%	25

Antithrombotic Therapy Timing

Hospital Name	City	Rate	Cases
Atlanticare Regional Medical Center	Atlantic City	100%	254
Capital Health Medical Center - Hopewell	Pennington	100%	117
Carepoint Health-Bayonne Hosp Ctr	Bayonne	100%	62
Clara Maass Medical Center	Belleville	100%	107
Hackensack - Umc Mountainside	Montclair	100%	87
Hackensack University Medical Center[2]	Hackensack	100%	92
Hackettstown Regional Medical Center	Hackettstown	100%	32
JFK Med Ctr-A M Yelencsics Comm Hosp	Edison	100%	236
Monmouth Medical Center - Southern Campus	Lakewood	100%	57
Morristown Medical Center	Morristown	100%	167
Overlook Medical Center	Summit	100%	267
Palisades Medical Center	North Bergen	100%	69
Raritan Bay Medical Center	Perth Amboy	100%	71
Saint Francis Medical Center	Trenton	100%	29
Southern Ocean Medical Center	Manahawkin	100%	70
Centrastate Medical Center[2]	Freehold	99%	134
Chilton Medical Center	Pompton Plains	99%	112
Holy Name Medical Center	Teaneck	99%	135
Hunterdon Medical Center	Flemington	99%	70
Inspira Medical Center Woodbury	Woodbury	99%	126
Jersey Shore University Medical Center	Neptune	99%	199
Kennedy Univ Hosp-Stratford Div[2]	Stratford	99%	308
Libertyhealth-Jersey City Med Ctr	Jersey City	99%	142
Monmouth Medical Center	Long Branch	99%	81
Ocean Medical Center[2]	Brick	99%	157
Riverview Medical Center	Red Bank	99%	96
Saint Peter's University Hospital	New Brunswick	99%	82
Shore Medical Center	Somers Point	99%	88
Valley Hospital	Ridgewood	99%	214
Bayshore Community Hospital	Holmdel	98%	91
Capital Health System - Fuld Campus	Trenton	98%	310
Carepoint Health - Hoboken UMC	Hoboken	98%	50
Cooper University Hospital[2]	Camden	98%	66
Englewood Hospital & Medical Center	Englewood	98%	155
Inspira Medical Center Vineland[2]	Vineland	98%	98
Memorial Hospital of Salem County	Salem	98%	41
Our Lady of Lourdes Medical Center	Camden	98%	144
Robert W Johnson Univ Hosp-Hamilton	Hamilton	98%	93
Saint Barnabas Medical Center[2]	Livingston	98%	216
Saint Clare's Hospital	Denville	98%	125
Saint Joseph's Regional Medical Center	Paterson	98%	256
University Hospital[2]	Newark	98%	59
Virtua Mem Hosp of Burlington County	Mount Holly	98%	140
Community Medical Center	Toms River	97%	275
East Orange General Hospital	East Orange	97%	74
Robert Wood Johnson University Hospital	New Brunswick	97%	203
Robert Wood Johnson Univ Hosp-Rahway	Rahway	97%	64
Saint Mary's Hospital - Passaic	Passaic	97%	70
Somerset Medical Center	Somerville	97%	176
Trinitas Regional Medical Center	Elizabeth	97%	125
Univ Med Ctr of Princeton-Plainsboro	Plainsboro	97%	104
Virtua West Jersey Hospitals Berlin	Berlin	97%	217
Cape Regional Medical Center	Cape May CH	96%	96
Newark Beth Israel Medical Center	Newark	96%	162
Newton Memorial Hospital	Newton	96%	98
Saint Michael's Medical Center	Newark	96%	70
Lourdes Med Ctr of Burlington County	Willingboro	95%	57
Inspira Medical Center Elmer	Elmer	93%	27
Carepoint Health - Christ Hospital	Jersey City	92%	65

NOTE: Hospital profiles are in alphabetical order by state, then city, then hospital within the city; Rankings exclude hospitals with less than 25 cases except for patient surveys which excludes hospitals with less than 100 cases; (a) 100-299 cases; (1) The number of cases/patients is too few to report; (2) Data submitted were based on a sample of cases/patients; (3) Results are based on a shorter time period than required; (4) Data suppressed by CMS for one or more quarters; (5) Results are not available for this reporting period; (6) Fewer than 100 patients completed the HCAHPS survey; (7) No cases met the criteria for this measure; (8) The lower limit of the confidence interval cannot be calculated if the number of observed infections equals zero; (9) No data are available from the state/territory for this reporting period; (10) The scores shown reflect fewer than 50 completed surveys; (11) There were discrepancies in the data collection process; (12) This measure does not apply to this hospital for this reporting period; (13) Results cannot be calculated for this reporting period; (14) The results for this state are combined with nearby states to protect confidentiality; Please refer to the User's Guide for a full explanation of data.

Assessed for Rehabilitation

Hospital Name	City	Rate	Cases
Atlanticare Regional Medical Center	Atlantic City	100%	325
Bayshore Community Hospital	Holmdel	100%	95
Capital Health System - Fuld Campus	Trenton	100%	529
Carepoint Health-Bayonne Hosp Ctr	Bayonne	100%	60
Carepoint Health - Hoboken UMC	Hoboken	100%	52
Chilton Medical Center	Pompton Plains	100%	131
Clara Maass Medical Center	Belleville	100%	138
Cooper University Hospital[2]	Camden	100%	86
Hackettstown Regional Medical Center	Hackettstown	100%	36
Inspira Medical Center Elmer	Elmer	100%	32
Libertyhealth-Jersey City Med Ctr	Jersey City	100%	173
Monmouth Medical Center - Southern Campus	Lakewood	100%	56
Morristown Medical Center	Morristown	100%	243
Ocean Medical Center[2]	Brick	100%	174
Overlook Medical Center	Summit	100%	428
Palisades Medical Center	North Bergen	100%	66
Raritan Bay Medical Center	Perth Amboy	100%	46
Riverview Medical Center	Red Bank	100%	128
Robert W Johnson Univ Hosp-Hamilton	Hamilton	100%	97
Saint Barnabas Medical Center[2]	Livingston	100%	286
Saint Joseph's Regional Medical Center	Paterson	100%	301
Shore Medical Center	Somers Point	100%	94
Valley Hospital	Ridgewood	100%	285
Virtua Mem Hosp of Burlington County	Mount Holly	100%	148
Capital Health Medical Center - Hopewell	Pennington	99%	150
Carepoint Health - Christ Hospital	Jersey City	99%	72
Community Medical Center	Toms River	99%	293
Monmouth Medical Center	Long Branch	99%	99
Robert Wood Johnson University Hospital	New Brunswick	99%	348
Saint Michael's Medical Center	Newark	99%	78
University Hospital[2]	Newark	99%	110
Holy Name Medical Center	Teaneck	98%	169
Inspira Medical Center Woodbury	Woodbury	98%	123
Jersey Shore University Medical Center	Neptune	98%	267
JFK Med Ctr-A M Yelencsics Comm Hosp	Edison	98%	338
Robert Wood Johnson Univ Hosp-Rahway	Rahway	98%	66
Saint Francis Medical Center	Trenton	98%	43
Saint Peter's University Hospital	New Brunswick	98%	104
Virtua West Jersey Hospitals Berlin	Berlin	98%	215
Centrastate Medical Center[2]	Freehold	97%	156
East Orange General Hospital	East Orange	97%	77
Hackensack - Umc Mountainside	Montclair	97%	106
Inspira Medical Center Vineland[2]	Vineland	97%	93
Southern Ocean Medical Center	Manahawkin	97%	73
Lourdes Med Ctr of Burlington County	Willingboro	96%	57
Saint Clare's Hospital	Denville	96%	139
Trinitas Regional Medical Center	Elizabeth	96%	139
Hunterdon Medical Center	Flemington	95%	78
Our Lady of Lourdes Medical Center	Camden	95%	154
Somerset Medical Center	Somerville	95%	212
Univ Med Ctr of Princeton-Plainsboro	Plainsboro	95%	119
Englewood Hospital & Medical Center	Englewood	94%	183
Hackensack University Medical Center[2]	Hackensack	94%	126
Kennedy Univ Hosp-Stratford Div[2]	Stratford	94%	362
Memorial Hospital of Salem County	Salem	93%	42
Newark Beth Israel Medical Center	Newark	92%	179
Newton Memorial Hospital	Newton	92%	99
Saint Mary's Hospital - Passaic	Passaic	88%	77
Cape Regional Medical Center	Cape May CH	86%	95

Discharged on Antithrombotic Therapy

Hospital Name	City	Rate	Cases
Atlanticare Regional Medical Center	Atlantic City	100%	271
Bayshore Community Hospital	Holmdel	100%	90
Capital Health Medical Center - Hopewell	Pennington	100%	126
Capital Health System - Fuld Campus	Trenton	100%	343
Carepoint Health-Bayonne Hosp Ctr	Bayonne	100%	56
Clara Maass Medical Center	Belleville	100%	110
Cooper University Hospital[2]	Camden	100%	70
Hackensack - Umc Mountainside	Montclair	100%	87
Hackensack University Medical Center[2]	Hackensack	100%	93
Hackettstown Regional Medical Center	Hackettstown	100%	34
Hunterdon Medical Center	Flemington	100%	71
Inspira Medical Center Elmer	Elmer	100%	30
Jersey Shore University Medical Center	Neptune	100%	205
JFK Med Ctr-A M Yelencsics Comm Hosp	Edison	100%	273
Kennedy Univ Hosp-Stratford Div[2]	Stratford	100%	325
Libertyhealth-Jersey City Med Ctr	Jersey City	100%	146
Lourdes Med Ctr of Burlington County	Willingboro	100%	56
Monmouth Medical Center	Long Branch	100%	85
Monmouth Medical Center - Southern Campus	Lakewood	100%	53
Morristown Medical Center	Morristown	100%	200
Ocean Medical Center[2]	Brick	100%	158
Palisades Medical Center	North Bergen	100%	57
Robert Wood Johnson University Hospital	New Brunswick	100%	279
Saint Barnabas Medical Center[2]	Livingston	100%	226
Saint Clare's Hospital	Denville	100%	120
Saint Francis Medical Center	Trenton	100%	38
Saint Peter's University Hospital	New Brunswick	100%	92
Shore Medical Center	Somers Point	100%	85
Southern Ocean Medical Center	Manahawkin	100%	72
University Hospital[2]	Newark	100%	72
Univ Med Ctr of Princeton-Plainsboro	Plainsboro	100%	98
Valley Hospital	Ridgewood	100%	248
Virtua Mem Hosp of Burlington County	Mount Holly	100%	145
Virtua West Jersey Hospitals Berlin	Berlin	100%	213
Englewood Hospital & Medical Center	Englewood	99%	163
Holy Name Medical Center	Teaneck	99%	150
Inspira Medical Center Vineland[2]	Vineland	99%	88
Our Lady of Lourdes Medical Center	Camden	99%	137
Overlook Medical Center	Summit	99%	311
Riverview Medical Center	Red Bank	99%	106
Chilton Medical Center	Pompton Plains	98%	117
Community Medical Center	Toms River	98%	248
Inspira Medical Center Woodbury	Woodbury	98%	119
Memorial Hospital of Salem County	Salem	98%	41
Newton Memorial Hospital	Newton	98%	93
Raritan Bay Medical Center	Perth Amboy	98%	45
Robert W Johnson Univ Hosp-Hamilton	Hamilton	98%	92
Trinitas Regional Medical Center	Elizabeth	98%	115
Cape Regional Medical Center	Cape May CH	97%	92
Centrastate Medical Center[2]	Freehold	97%	143
East Orange General Hospital	East Orange	97%	71
Newark Beth Israel Medical Center	Newark	97%	158
Saint Mary's Hospital - Passaic	Passaic	96%	67
Somerset Medical Center	Somerville	96%	180
Carepoint Health - Christ Hospital	Jersey City	95%	64
Saint Joseph's Regional Medical Center	Paterson	95%	259
Carepoint Health - Hoboken UMC	Hoboken	94%	49
Robert Wood Johnson Univ Hosp-Rahway	Rahway	94%	66
Saint Michael's Medical Center	Newark	88%	74

Discharged on Statin Medication

Hospital Name	City	Rate	Cases
Capital Health Medical Center - Hopewell	Pennington	100%	106
Carepoint Health-Bayonne Hosp Ctr	Bayonne	100%	49
Libertyhealth-Jersey City Med Ctr	Jersey City	100%	114
Monmouth Medical Center - Southern Campus	Lakewood	100%	38
Our Lady of Lourdes Medical Center	Camden	100%	108
Shore Medical Center	Somers Point	100%	76
University Hospital[2]	Newark	100%	45
Virtua Mem Hosp of Burlington County	Mount Holly	100%	107
Atlanticare Regional Medical Center	Atlantic City	99%	219
Capital Health System - Fuld Campus	Trenton	99%	253
Ocean Medical Center[2]	Brick	99%	119
Saint Barnabas Medical Center[2]	Livingston	99%	192
Saint Peter's University Hospital	New Brunswick	99%	71
Valley Hospital	Ridgewood	99%	196
Monmouth Medical Center	Long Branch	98%	64
Palisades Medical Center	North Bergen	98%	44
Bayshore Community Hospital	Holmdel	97%	63
Jersey Shore University Medical Center	Neptune	97%	163
Kennedy Univ Hosp-Stratford Div[2]	Stratford	97%	253
Morristown Medical Center	Morristown	97%	134
Raritan Bay Medical Center	Perth Amboy	97%	37
Robert Wood Johnson University Hospital	New Brunswick	97%	206
Saint Clare's Hospital	Denville	97%	93
Saint Francis Medical Center	Trenton	97%	33
Chilton Medical Center	Pompton Plains	96%	98
Cooper University Hospital[2]	Camden	96%	52
Englewood Hospital & Medical Center	Englewood	96%	125
Hackensack University Medical Center[2]	Hackensack	96%	79
Holy Name Medical Center	Teaneck	96%	125
Inspira Medical Center Vineland[2]	Vineland	96%	79
Inspira Medical Center Woodbury	Woodbury	96%	97
JFK Med Ctr-A M Yelencsics Comm Hosp	Edison	96%	213
Lourdes Med Ctr of Burlington County	Willingboro	96%	47
Robert W Johnson Univ Hosp-Hamilton	Hamilton	96%	69
Univ Med Ctr of Princeton-Plainsboro	Plainsboro	96%	77
Virtua West Jersey Hospitals Berlin	Berlin	96%	168
Centrastate Medical Center[2]	Freehold	95%	131
Clara Maass Medical Center	Belleville	95%	81
Riverview Medical Center	Red Bank	95%	77
Community Medical Center	Toms River	93%	177
Hunterdon Medical Center	Flemington	93%	61
Overlook Medical Center	Summit	93%	244
Saint Joseph's Regional Medical Center	Paterson	92%	202
Trinitas Regional Medical Center	Elizabeth	92%	99
Carepoint Health - Hoboken UMC	Hoboken	91%	34
Newton Memorial Hospital	Newton	90%	72
Hackensack - Umc Mountainside	Montclair	89%	64
Cape Regional Medical Center	Cape May CH	88%	69
Saint Michael's Medical Center	Newark	87%	63
Southern Ocean Medical Center	Manahawkin	87%	60
Robert Wood Johnson Univ Hosp-Rahway	Rahway	86%	44
Memorial Hospital of Salem County	Salem	85%	27
Carepoint Health - Christ Hospital	Jersey City	84%	56
Somerset Medical Center	Somerville	84%	122
East Orange General Hospital	East Orange	80%	44
Newark Beth Israel Medical Center	Newark	79%	133
Saint Mary's Hospital - Passaic	Passaic	75%	56

Thrombolytic Therapy Timing

Hospital Name	City	Rate	Cases
Morristown Medical Center	Morristown	100%	30
Kennedy Univ Hosp-Stratford Div[2]	Stratford	97%	31
Overlook Medical Center	Summit	95%	38
Valley Hospital	Ridgewood	93%	28
Robert Wood Johnson University Hospital	New Brunswick	91%	56
JFK Med Ctr-A M Yelencsics Comm Hosp	Edison	82%	45
Saint Joseph's Regional Medical Center	Paterson	30%	67

Venous Thromboembolism (VTE) Prophylaxis

Hospital Name	City	Rate	Cases
Capital Health System - Fuld Campus	Trenton	100%	579
Hunterdon Medical Center	Flemington	100%	80
Jersey Shore University Medical Center	Neptune	100%	315
Monmouth Medical Center - Southern Campus	Lakewood	100%	66
Raritan Bay Medical Center	Perth Amboy	100%	76
Capital Health Medical Center - Hopewell	Pennington	99%	153
Centrastate Medical Center[2]	Freehold	99%	167
Chilton Medical Center	Pompton Plains	99%	140
Kennedy Univ Hosp-Stratford Div[2]	Stratford	99%	386
Libertyhealth-Jersey City Med Ctr	Jersey City	99%	177
Saint Barnabas Medical Center[2]	Livingston	99%	301
Virtua West Jersey Hospitals Berlin	Berlin	99%	214
Monmouth Medical Center	Long Branch	98%	107
Ocean Medical Center[2]	Brick	98%	197
Overlook Medical Center	Summit	98%	477
Robert Wood Johnson University Hospital	New Brunswick	98%	371
Shore Medical Center	Somers Point	98%	95
Clara Maass Medical Center	Belleville	97%	148
JFK Med Ctr-A M Yelencsics Comm Hosp	Edison	97%	353
Morristown Medical Center	Morristown	97%	261
Our Lady of Lourdes Medical Center	Camden	97%	173
Saint Joseph's Regional Medical Center	Paterson	97%	330
University Hospital[2]	Newark	97%	119
Robert Wood Johnson Univ Hosp-Rahway	Rahway	96%	69
Saint Peter's University Hospital	New Brunswick	96%	102
Atlanticare Regional Medical Center	Atlantic City	95%	350
Bayshore Community Hospital	Holmdel	95%	102
Carepoint Health - Hoboken UMC	Hoboken	95%	57
Hackensack - Umc Mountainside	Montclair	95%	116
Hackettstown Regional Medical Center	Hackettstown	95%	38
Inspira Medical Center Woodbury	Woodbury	95%	130
Robert W Johnson Univ Hosp-Hamilton	Hamilton	95%	109
Saint Francis Medical Center	Trenton	95%	40
Valley Hospital	Ridgewood	95%	288
Carepoint Health-Bayonne Hosp Ctr	Bayonne	94%	67
Cooper University Hospital[2]	Camden	94%	88
Inspira Medical Center Vineland[2]	Vineland	94%	109
Riverview Medical Center	Red Bank	94%	134
Memorial Hospital of Salem County	Salem	93%	46
Saint Clare's Hospital	Denville	93%	149
Holy Name Medical Center	Teaneck	92%	178
Carepoint Health - Christ Hospital	Jersey City	91%	81
East Orange General Hospital	East Orange	91%	79
Virtua Mem Hosp of Burlington County	Mount Holly	91%	153
Newton Memorial Hospital	Newton	90%	105
Community Medical Center	Toms River	89%	320
Englewood Hospital & Medical Center	Englewood	88%	188
Inspira Medical Center Elmer	Elmer	88%	34
Palisades Medical Center	North Bergen	87%	76
Saint Michael's Medical Center	Newark	86%	77
Southern Ocean Medical Center	Manahawkin	86%	78
Trinitas Regional Medical Center	Elizabeth	86%	168
Cape Regional Medical Center	Cape May CH	85%	100
Univ Med Ctr of Princeton-Plainsboro	Plainsboro	83%	136
Hackensack University Medical Center[2]	Hackensack	79%	129
Somerset Medical Center	Somerville	79%	225
Lourdes Med Ctr of Burlington County	Willingboro	73%	56
Saint Mary's Hospital - Passaic	Passaic	72%	78
Newark Beth Israel Medical Center	Newark	68%	193

Written Stroke Educational Materials Given

Hospital Name	City	Rate	Cases
Atlanticare Regional Medical Center	Atlantic City	100%	162
Capital Health Medical Center - Hopewell	Pennington	100%	83
Capital Health System - Fuld Campus	Trenton	100%	200
Community Medical Center	Toms River	100%	117
Cooper University Hospital[2]	Camden	100%	50
Hackensack - Umc Mountainside	Montclair	100%	45
Libertyhealth-Jersey City Med Ctr	Jersey City	100%	94
Lourdes Med Ctr of Burlington County	Willingboro	100%	26
Monmouth Medical Center - Southern Campus	Lakewood	100%	26
Ocean Medical Center[2]	Brick	100%	42
Our Lady of Lourdes Medical Center	Camden	100%	77
Palisades Medical Center	North Bergen	100%	25
Robert Wood Johnson University Hospital	New Brunswick	100%	160

NOTE: Hospital profiles are in alphabetical order by state, then city, then hospital within the city; Rankings exclude hospitals with less than 25 cases except for patient surveys which excludes hospitals with less than 100 cases; (a) 100-299 cases; (1) The number of cases/patients is too few to report; (2) Data submitted were based on a sample of cases/patients; (3) Results are based on a shorter time period than required; (4) Data suppressed by CMS for one or more quarters; (5) Results are not available for this reporting period; (6) Fewer than 100 patients completed the HCAHPS survey; (7) No cases met the criteria for this measure; (8) The lower limit of the confidence interval cannot be calculated if the number of observed infections equals zero; (9) No data are available from the state/territory for this reporting period; (10) The scores shown reflect fewer than 50 completed surveys; (11) There were discrepancies in the data collection process; (12) This measure does not apply to this hospital for this reporting period; (13) Results cannot be calculated for this reporting period; (14) The results for this state are combined with nearby states to protect confidentiality; Please refer to the User's Guide for a full explanation of data.

Robert W Johnson Univ Hosp-Hamilton	Hamilton	100%	51
Robert Wood Johnson Univ Hosp-Rahway	Rahway	100%	33
Saint Francis Medical Center	Trenton	100%	25
Saint Michael's Medical Center	Newark	100%	47
Trinitas Regional Medical Center	Elizabeth	100%	71
University Hospital[2]	Newark	100%	46
Virtua Mem Hosp of Burlington County	Mount Holly	100%	65
JFK Med Ctr-A M Yelencsics Comm Hosp	Edison	99%	106
Saint Barnabas Medical Center[2]	Livingston	99%	143
Virtua West Jersey Hospitals Berlin	Berlin	99%	126
Saint Joseph's Regional Medical Center	Paterson	98%	153
Saint Peter's University Hospital	New Brunswick	98%	62
Clara Maass Medical Center	Belleville	97%	62
Jersey Shore University Medical Center	Neptune	97%	118
Monmouth Medical Center	Long Branch	97%	37
Newton Memorial Hospital	Newton	97%	59
Univ Med Ctr of Princeton-Plainsboro	Plainsboro	97%	68
Valley Hospital	Ridgewood	97%	139
Holy Name Medical Center	Teaneck	96%	77
Raritan Bay Medical Center	Perth Amboy	95%	38
Chilton Medical Center	Pompton Plains	94%	53
Riverview Medical Center	Red Bank	94%	50
Overlook Medical Center	Summit	93%	204
Saint Clare's Hospital	Denville	93%	67
Inspira Medical Center Woodbury	Woodbury	92%	78
Cape Regional Medical Center	Cape May CH	91%	57
East Orange General Hospital	East Orange	89%	46
Morristown Medical Center	Morristown	89%	106
Centrastate Medical Center[2]	Freehold	88%	75
Englewood Hospital & Medical Center	Englewood	87%	95
Kennedy Univ Hosp-Stratford Div[2]	Stratford	87%	196
Inspira Medical Center Vineland[2]	Vineland	86%	44
Shore Medical Center	Somers Point	86%	49
Bayshore Community Hospital	Holmdel	84%	44
Hackensack University Medical Center[2]	Hackensack	84%	62
Somerset Medical Center	Somerville	84%	95
Hunterdon Medical Center	Flemington	77%	31
Saint Mary's Hospital - Passaic	Passaic	77%	44
Carepoint Health - Christ Hospital	Jersey City	76%	25
Southern Ocean Medical Center	Manahawkin	72%	36
Newark Beth Israel Medical Center	Newark	65%	99

Surgical Care Improvement Project

Appropriate Beta Blocker Usage

Hospital Name	City	Rate	Cases
Carepoint Health-Bayonne Hosp Ctr	Bayonne	100%	41
Hackensack - Umc Mountainside	Montclair	100%	128
Hackettstown Regional Medical Center	Hackettstown	100%	72
Libertyhealth-Jersey City Med Ctr[2]	Jersey City	100%	174
Monmouth Medical Center - Southern Campus	Lakewood	100%	36
Newton Memorial Hospital	Newton	100%	84
Our Lady of Lourdes Medical Center[2]	Camden	100%	261
Robert Wood Johnson University Hospital[2]	New Brunswick	100%	645
Robert Wood Johnson Univ Hosp-Rahway	Rahway	100%	61
Saint Barnabas Medical Center[2]	Livingston	100%	262
Saint Francis Medical Center	Trenton	100%	97
Saint Luke's Warren Hospital[2]	Phillipsburg	100%	75
Saint Peter's University Hospital[2]	New Brunswick	100%	134
Valley Hospital[2]	Ridgewood	100%	292
Virtua West Jersey Hospitals Berlin[2]	Berlin	100%	966
Bayshore Community Hospital[2]	Holmdel	99%	73
Chilton Medical Center[2]	Pompton Plains	99%	125
Community Medical Center[2]	Toms River	99%	176
Inspira Medical Center Woodbury	Woodbury	99%	169
JFK Med Ctr-A M Yelencsics Comm Hosp[2]	Edison	99%	221
Lourdes Med Ctr of Burlington County[2]	Willingboro	99%	72
Ocean Medical Center[2]	Brick	99%	148
Overlook Medical Center[2]	Summit	99%	109
Saint Mary's Hospital - Passaic	Passaic	99%	127
Southern Ocean Medical Center	Manahawkin	99%	106
Univ Med Ctr of Princeton-Plainsboro[2]	Plainsboro	99%	109
Atlanticare Regional Medical Center[2]	Atlantic City	98%	327
Capital Health Medical Center - Hopewell	Pennington	98%	300
Clara Maass Medical Center[2]	Belleville	98%	84
Cooper University Hospital[2]	Camden	98%	171
Deborah Heart & Lung Center	Browns Mills	98%	183
Englewood Hospital & Medical Center[2]	Englewood	98%	407
Jersey Shore University Medical Center[2]	Neptune	98%	456
Kennedy Univ Hosp-Stratford Div[2]	Stratford	98%	350
Morristown Medical Center[2]	Morristown	98%	295
Saint Joseph's Regional Medical Center[2]	Paterson	98%	393
University Hospital[2]	Newark	98%	59
Cape Regional Medical Center	Cape May CH	97%	117
Carepoint Health - Christ Hospital	Jersey City	97%	37
Centrastate Medical Center[2]	Freehold	97%	208
Hackensack University Medical Center[2]	Hackensack	97%	217
Inspira Medical Center Vineland[2]	Vineland	97%	119
Robert W Johnson Univ Hosp-Hamilton[2]	Hamilton	97%	233
Shore Medical Center[2]	Somers Point	97%	181
Hunterdon Medical Center[2]	Flemington	96%	108
Inspira Medical Center Elmer[2]	Elmer	96%	54
Monmouth Medical Center[2]	Long Branch	96%	103
Newark Beth Israel Medical Center[2]	Newark	96%	192
Raritan Bay Medical Center	Perth Amboy	96%	118
Virtua Mem Hosp of Burlington County[2]	Mount Holly	96%	148
Holy Name Medical Center[2]	Teaneck	94%	123
Riverview Medical Center[2]	Red Bank	94%	142
Trinitas Regional Medical Center[2]	Elizabeth	93%	153
Capital Health System - Fuld Campus[2]	Trenton	92%	51
Saint Clare's Hospital	Denville	91%	182
Somerset Medical Center[2]	Somerville	90%	146
VA New Jersey Health Care System[2]	East Orange	89%	47
Saint Michael's Medical Center[2]	Newark	88%	174
Palisades Medical Center	North Bergen	87%	53

Appropriate VTP Within 24 Hours

Hospital Name	City	Rate	Cases
Capital Health System - Fuld Campus[2]	Trenton	100%	152
Carepoint Health - Hoboken UMC	Hoboken	100%	117
Chilton Medical Center[2]	Pompton Plains	100%	324
Clara Maass Medical Center[2]	Belleville	100%	376
Community Medical Center[2]	Toms River	100%	416
Hackettstown Regional Medical Center	Hackettstown	100%	239
Inspira Medical Center Vineland[2]	Vineland	100%	286
Libertyhealth-Jersey City Med Ctr[2]	Jersey City	100%	298
Our Lady of Lourdes Medical Center[2]	Camden	100%	227
Overlook Medical Center[2]	Summit	100%	415
Palisades Medical Center	North Bergen	100%	147
Robert Wood Johnson University Hospital[2]	New Brunswick	100%	948
Saint Luke's Warren Hospital[2]	Phillipsburg	100%	219
Saint Mary's Hospital - Passaic	Passaic	100%	222
Shore Medical Center[2]	Somers Point	100%	456
Valley Hospital[2]	Ridgewood	100%	416
Virtua West Jersey Hospitals Berlin[2]	Berlin	100%	2355
Atlanticare Regional Medical Center[2]	Atlantic City	99%	477
Bayshore Community Hospital[2]	Holmdel	99%	195
Cape Regional Medical Center	Cape May CH	99%	322
Capital Health Medical Center - Hopewell	Pennington	99%	799
Centrastate Medical Center[2]	Freehold	99%	544
Englewood Hospital & Medical Center[2]	Englewood	99%	736
Holy Name Medical Center[2]	Teaneck	99%	389
Hunterdon Medical Center[2]	Flemington	99%	301
Inspira Medical Center Elmer[2]	Elmer	99%	166
Inspira Medical Center Woodbury	Woodbury	99%	432
JFK Med Ctr-A M Yelencsics Comm Hosp[2]	Edison	99%	676
Kennedy Univ Hosp-Stratford Div[2]	Stratford	99%	879
Lourdes Med Ctr of Burlington County[2]	Willingboro	99%	200
Memorial Hospital of Salem County	Salem	99%	83
Monmouth Medical Center[2]	Long Branch	99%	404
Monmouth Medical Center - Southern Campus	Lakewood	99%	97
Morristown Medical Center[2]	Morristown	99%	481
Newark Beth Israel Medical Center[2]	Newark	99%	324
Newton Memorial Hospital	Newton	99%	261
Ocean Medical Center[2]	Brick	99%	393
Robert W Johnson Univ Hosp-Hamilton[2]	Hamilton	99%	571
Saint Francis Medical Center	Trenton	99%	128
Saint Joseph's Regional Medical Center[2]	Paterson	99%	760
Saint Peter's University Hospital[2]	New Brunswick	99%	388
University Hospital[2]	Newark	99%	258
Virtua Mem Hosp of Burlington County[2]	Mount Holly	99%	412
Carepoint Health-Bayonne Hosp Ctr	Bayonne	98%	130
Cooper University Hospital[2]	Camden	98%	326
Jersey Shore University Medical Center[2]	Neptune	98%	478
Robert Wood Johnson Univ Hosp-Rahway	Rahway	98%	152
Saint Clare's Hospital	Denville	98%	611
Trinitas Regional Medical Center[2]	Elizabeth	98%	430
Univ Med Ctr of Princeton-Plainsboro[2]	Plainsboro	98%	343
Hackensack University Medical Center[2]	Hackensack	97%	384
Raritan Bay Medical Center	Perth Amboy	97%	292
Riverview Medical Center[2]	Red Bank	97%	426
Saint Barnabas Medical Center[2]	Livingston	97%	500
Somerset Medical Center[2]	Somerville	97%	436
Southern Ocean Medical Center	Manahawkin	97%	253
Meadowlands Hospital Medical Center	Secaucus	96%	49
Saint Michael's Medical Center[2]	Newark	96%	351
VA New Jersey Health Care System[2]	East Orange	96%	112
Bergen Regional Medical Center	Paramus	95%	44
Carepoint Health - Christ Hospital	Jersey City	95%	132
Hackensack - Umc Mountainside	Montclair	95%	373
East Orange General Hospital	East Orange	94%	107

Controlled Postoperative Blood Glucose

Hospital Name	City	Rate	Cases
Cooper University Hospital[2]	Camden	100%	133
Libertyhealth-Jersey City Med Ctr[2]	Jersey City	100%	193
Saint Barnabas Medical Center[2]	Livingston	100%	170
Atlanticare Regional Medical Center[2]	Atlantic City	99%	135
Saint Mary's Hospital - Passaic	Passaic	99%	73
Newark Beth Israel Medical Center[2]	Newark	98%	153
Our Lady of Lourdes Medical Center[2]	Camden	98%	207
Valley Hospital[2]	Ridgewood	98%	171
Englewood Hospital & Medical Center[2]	Englewood	97%	231
Jersey Shore University Medical Center[2]	Neptune	97%	399
Robert Wood Johnson University Hospital[2]	New Brunswick	97%	618
Saint Joseph's Regional Medical Center[2]	Paterson	97%	237
Saint Francis Medical Center	Trenton	96%	85
Morristown Medical Center[2]	Morristown	95%	183
Deborah Heart & Lung Center	Browns Mills	94%	216
Saint Michael's Medical Center[2]	Newark	91%	112
Hackensack University Medical Center[2]	Hackensack	87%	134
University Hospital[2]	Newark	85%	48

Perioperative Temperature Management

Hospital Name	City	Rate	Cases
Atlanticare Regional Medical Center[2]	Atlantic City	100%	705
Bayshore Community Hospital[2]	Holmdel	100%	219
Bergen Regional Medical Center	Paramus	100%	46
Cape Regional Medical Center	Cape May CH	100%	358
Capital Health Medical Center - Hopewell	Pennington	100%	927
Carepoint Health - Christ Hospital	Jersey City	100%	163
Carepoint Health - Hoboken UMC	Hoboken	100%	141
Centrastate Medical Center[2]	Freehold	100%	662
Chilton Medical Center[2]	Pompton Plains	100%	365
Clara Maass Medical Center[2]	Belleville	100%	423
Community Medical Center[2]	Toms River	100%	481
Cooper University Hospital[2]	Camden	100%	474
Deborah Heart & Lung Center	Browns Mills	100%	107
East Orange General Hospital	East Orange	100%	113
Englewood Hospital & Medical Center[2]	Englewood	100%	830
Hackensack - Umc Mountainside	Montclair	100%	441
Hackettstown Regional Medical Center	Hackettstown	100%	266
Holy Name Medical Center[2]	Teaneck	100%	463
Inspira Medical Center Woodbury	Woodbury	100%	525
JFK Med Ctr-A M Yelencsics Comm Hosp[2]	Edison	100%	799
Kennedy Univ Hosp-Stratford Div[2]	Stratford	100%	1110
Libertyhealth-Jersey City Med Ctr[2]	Jersey City	100%	330
Lourdes Med Ctr of Burlington County[2]	Willingboro	100%	240
Meadowlands Hospital Medical Center	Secaucus	100%	64
Memorial Hospital of Salem County	Salem	100%	97
Monmouth Medical Center[2]	Long Branch	100%	453
Monmouth Medical Center - Southern Campus	Lakewood	100%	118
Morristown Medical Center[2]	Morristown	100%	649
Newark Beth Israel Medical Center[2]	Newark	100%	416
Newton Memorial Hospital	Newton	100%	299
Ocean Medical Center[2]	Brick	100%	409
Our Lady of Lourdes Medical Center[2]	Camden	100%	308
Overlook Medical Center[2]	Summit	100%	491
Palisades Medical Center	North Bergen	100%	171
Raritan Bay Medical Center	Perth Amboy	100%	355
Riverview Medical Center[2]	Red Bank	100%	474
Robert Wood Johnson University Hospital[2]	New Brunswick	100%	1141
Robert W Johnson Univ Hosp-Hamilton[2]	Hamilton	100%	624
Robert Wood Johnson Univ Hosp-Rahway	Rahway	100%	180
Saint Barnabas Medical Center[2]	Livingston	100%	612
Saint Clare's Hospital	Denville	100%	700
Saint Francis Medical Center	Trenton	100%	160
Saint Joseph's Regional Medical Center[2]	Paterson	100%	1052
Saint Luke's Warren Hospital[2]	Phillipsburg	100%	242
Saint Mary's Hospital - Passaic	Passaic	100%	331
Saint Michael's Medical Center[2]	Newark	100%	465
Saint Peter's University Hospital[2]	New Brunswick	100%	471
Shore Medical Center[2]	Somers Point	100%	592
Somerset Medical Center[2]	Somerville	100%	539
Southern Ocean Medical Center	Manahawkin	100%	286
Trinitas Regional Medical Center[2]	Elizabeth	100%	492
University Hospital[2]	Newark	100%	336
Univ Med Ctr of Princeton-Plainsboro[2]	Plainsboro	100%	408
Valley Hospital[2]	Ridgewood	100%	577
Virtua Mem Hosp of Burlington County[2]	Mount Holly	100%	504
Virtua West Jersey Hospitals Berlin[2]	Berlin	100%	3175
Capital Health System - Fuld Campus[2]	Trenton	99%	180
Carepoint Health-Bayonne Hosp Ctr	Bayonne	99%	145
Hackensack University Medical Center[2]	Hackensack	99%	489
Hunterdon Medical Center[2]	Flemington	99%	358
Inspira Medical Center Elmer[2]	Elmer	99%	175
Jersey Shore University Medical Center[2]	Neptune	99%	600
VA New Jersey Health Care System[2]	East Orange	99%	139
Inspira Medical Center Vineland[2]	Vineland	98%	345

Prophylactic Antibiotic Selection

Hospital Name	City	Rate	Cases
Atlanticare Regional Medical Center[2]	Atlantic City	100%	506
Cape Regional Medical Center	Cape May CH	100%	232
Capital Health Medical Center - Hopewell	Pennington	100%	473
Capital Health System - Fuld Campus[2]	Trenton	100%	58
Carepoint Health-Bayonne Hosp Ctr	Bayonne	100%	42
Centrastate Medical Center[2]	Freehold	100%	278
Clara Maass Medical Center[2]	Belleville	100%	252
Community Medical Center[2]	Toms River	100%	305

NOTE: Hospital profiles are in alphabetical order by state, then city, then hospital within the city; Rankings exclude hospitals with less than 25 cases except for patient surveys which excludes hospitals with less than 100 cases; (a) 100-299 cases; (1) The number of cases/patients is too few to report; (2) Data submitted were based on a sample of cases/patients; (3) Results are based on a shorter time period than required; (4) Data suppressed by CMS for one or more quarters; (5) Results are not available for this reporting period; (6) Fewer than 100 patients completed the HCAHPS survey; (7) No cases met the criteria for this measure; (8) The lower limit of the confidence interval cannot be calculated if the number of observed infections equals zero; (9) No data are available from the state/territory for this reporting period; (10) The scores shown reflect fewer than 50 completed surveys; (11) There were discrepancies in the data collection process; (12) This measure does not apply to this hospital for this reporting period; (13) Results cannot be calculated for this reporting period; (14) The results for this state are combined with nearby states to protect confidentiality; Please refer to the User's Guide for a full explanation of data.

Hospital Name	City	Rate	Cases
Cooper University Hospital[2]	Camden	100%	390
Deborah Heart & Lung Center	Browns Mills	100%	221
Hackensack - Umc Mountainside	Montclair	100%	214
Hackettstown Regional Medical Center	Hackettstown	100%	194
Hunterdon Medical Center[2]	Flemington	100%	219
Jersey Shore University Medical Center[2]	Neptune	100%	772
Libertyhealth-Jersey City Med Ctr[2]	Jersey City	100%	389
Lourdes Med Ctr of Burlington County[2]	Willingboro	100%	119
Ocean Medical Center[2]	Brick	100%	261
Saint Peter's University Hospital[2]	New Brunswick	100%	309
Shore Medical Center[2]	Somers Point	100%	404
Somerset Medical Center[2]	Somerville	100%	290
Univ Med Ctr of Princeton-Plainsboro[2]	Plainsboro	100%	260
Virtua West Jersey Hospitals Berlin[2]	Berlin	100%	2661
Carepoint Health - Hoboken UMC	Hoboken	99%	82
Chilton Medical Center[2]	Pompton Plains	99%	205
Englewood Hospital & Medical Center[2]	Englewood	99%	855
Hackensack University Medical Center[2]	Hackensack	99%	420
Inspira Medical Center Elmer[2]	Elmer	99%	114
Inspira Medical Center Vineland[2]	Vineland	99%	224
Inspira Medical Center Woodbury	Woodbury	99%	291
JFK Med Ctr-A M Yelencsics Comm Hosp[2]	Edison	99%	589
Kennedy Univ Hosp-Stratford Div[2]	Stratford	99%	700
Monmouth Medical Center[2]	Long Branch	99%	301
Morristown Medical Center[2]	Morristown	99%	603
Newark Beth Israel Medical Center[2]	Newark	99%	405
Newton Memorial Hospital	Newton	99%	186
Our Lady of Lourdes Medical Center[2]	Camden	99%	301
Overlook Medical Center[2]	Summit	99%	337
Robert Wood Johnson University Hospital[2]	New Brunswick	99%	1390
Robert Wood Johnson Univ Hosp-Rahway	Rahway	99%	80
Saint Barnabas Medical Center[2]	Livingston	99%	507
Saint Francis Medical Center	Trenton	99%	125
Saint Joseph's Regional Medical Center[2]	Paterson	99%	837
Saint Luke's Warren Hospital[2]	Phillipsburg	99%	128
Saint Michael's Medical Center[2]	Newark	99%	355
VA New Jersey Health Care System	East Orange	99%	88
Valley Hospital[2]	Ridgewood	99%	497
Virtua Mem Hosp of Burlington County[2]	Mount Holly	99%	279
Carepoint Health - Christ Hospital	Jersey City	98%	53
Holy Name Medical Center[2]	Teaneck	98%	311
Raritan Bay Medical Center	Perth Amboy	98%	164
Riverview Medical Center[2]	Red Bank	98%	308
Robert W Johnson Univ Hosp-Hamilton[2]	Hamilton	98%	466
Saint Clare's Hospital	Denville	98%	403
Bayshore Community Hospital[2]	Holmdel	97%	111
East Orange General Hospital	East Orange	97%	61
Saint Mary's Hospital - Passaic	Passaic	97%	210
Southern Ocean Medical Center	Manahawkin	97%	172
Trinitas Regional Medical Center[2]	Elizabeth	97%	230
Memorial Hospital of Salem County	Salem	96%	56
University Hospital[2]	Newark	95%	218
Meadowlands Hospital Medical Center	Secaucus	94%	34
Palisades Medical Center	North Bergen	93%	67

Prophylactic Antibiotic Selection (Outpatient)

Hospital Name	City	Rate	Cases
Community Medical Center	Toms River	100%	468
Deborah Heart & Lung Center	Browns Mills	100%	467
Monmouth Medical Center - Southern Campus	Lakewood	100%	40
Newton Memorial Hospital	Newton	100%	66
Ocean Medical Center	Brick	100%	208
Saint Luke's Warren Hospital	Phillipsburg	100%	67
Shore Medical Center	Somers Point	100%	149
Centrastate Medical Center	Freehold	99%	185
Chilton Medical Center	Pompton Plains	99%	83
Englewood Hospital & Medical Center	Englewood	99%	475
Jersey Shore University Medical Center	Neptune	99%	671
Morristown Medical Center	Morristown	99%	681
Newark Beth Israel Medical Center	Newark	99%	374
Our Lady of Lourdes Medical Center	Camden	99%	483
Overlook Medical Center	Summit	99%	493
Saint Barnabas Medical Center	Livingston	99%	897
Saint Francis Medical Center	Trenton	99%	261
Saint Michael's Medical Center	Newark	99%	183
Somerset Medical Center	Somerville	99%	181
Valley Hospital	Ridgewood	99%	596
Virtua Mem Hosp of Burlington County	Mount Holly	99%	181
Atlanticare Regional Medical Center	Atlantic City	98%	451
Cape Regional Medical Center	Cape May CH	98%	54
Cooper University Hospital	Camden	98%	356
Hackensack University Medical Center	Hackensack	98%	939
Holy Name Medical Center	Teaneck	98%	240
Hunterdon Medical Center	Flemington	98%	133
Monmouth Medical Center	Long Branch	98%	476
Riverview Medical Center	Red Bank	98%	328
Robert Wood Johnson University Hospital	New Brunswick	98%	931
Saint Peter's University Hospital	New Brunswick	98%	210
Trinitas Regional Medical Center	Elizabeth	98%	236
Univ Med Ctr of Princeton-Plainsboro	Plainsboro	98%	222
Virtua West Jersey Hospitals Berlin	Berlin	98%	352
Bayshore Community Hospital	Holmdel	97%	34
Carepoint Health-Bayonne Hosp Ctr	Bayonne	97%	29
Hackensack - Umc Mountainside	Montclair	97%	96
Hackettstown Regional Medical Center	Hackettstown	97%	68
Inspira Medical Center Elmer	Elmer	97%	91
Inspira Medical Center Vineland	Vineland	97%	324
Kennedy Univ Hosp-Stratford Div	Stratford	97%	252
Raritan Bay Medical Center	Perth Amboy	97%	74
Robert Wood Johnson Univ Hosp-Rahway	Rahway	97%	68
Saint Joseph's Regional Medical Center	Paterson	97%	266
Capital Health Medical Center - Hopewell	Pennington	95%	258
Carepoint Health - Christ Hospital	Jersey City	94%	72
Clara Maass Medical Center	Belleville	94%	162
JFK Med Ctr-A M Yelencsics Comm Hosp	Edison	94%	271
Libertyhealth-Jersey City Med Ctr	Jersey City	94%	78
Southern Ocean Medical Center	Manahawkin	92%	64
Inspira Medical Center Woodbury	Woodbury	90%	84
Lourdes Med Ctr of Burlington County	Willingboro	90%	42
Palisades Medical Center	North Bergen	90%	52
Carepoint Health - Hoboken UMC	Hoboken	88%	32
Meadowlands Hospital Medical Center	Secaucus	87%	119
Robert W Johnson Univ Hosp-Hamilton	Hamilton	86%	147
Saint Clare's Hospital	Denville	86%	207
Saint Mary's Hospital - Passaic	Passaic	86%	274
University Hospital	Newark	86%	157
Capital Health System - Fuld Campus	Trenton	84%	31

Prophylactic Antibiotic Stopped

Hospital Name	City	Rate	Cases
Carepoint Health - Christ Hospital	Jersey City	100%	52
Carepoint Health - Hoboken UMC	Hoboken	100%	82
Clara Maass Medical Center[2]	Belleville	100%	248
Hackensack - Umc Mountainside	Montclair	100%	199
Libertyhealth-Jersey City Med Ctr[2]	Jersey City	100%	368
Meadowlands Hospital Medical Center	Secaucus	100%	34
Overlook Medical Center[2]	Summit	100%	330
Saint Francis Medical Center	Trenton	100%	115
Virtua West Jersey Hospitals Berlin[2]	Berlin	100%	2645
Atlanticare Regional Medical Center[2]	Atlantic City	99%	500
Capital Health Medical Center - Hopewell	Pennington	99%	471
Chilton Medical Center[2]	Pompton Plains	99%	198
Englewood Hospital & Medical Center[2]	Englewood	99%	845
Hackettstown Regional Medical Center	Hackettstown	99%	190
Holy Name Medical Center[2]	Teaneck	99%	288
Inspira Medical Center Elmer[2]	Elmer	99%	109
Lourdes Med Ctr of Burlington County[2]	Willingboro	99%	119
Newton Memorial Hospital	Newton	99%	182
Riverview Medical Center[2]	Red Bank	99%	298
Robert Wood Johnson University Hospital[2]	New Brunswick	99%	1326
Saint Joseph's Regional Medical Center[2]	Paterson	99%	817
Shore Medical Center[2]	Somers Point	99%	393
Trinitas Regional Medical Center[2]	Elizabeth	99%	225
Valley Hospital[2]	Ridgewood	99%	492
Virtua Mem Hosp of Burlington County[2]	Mount Holly	99%	267
Bayshore Community Hospital[2]	Holmdel	98%	108
Cape Regional Medical Center	Cape May CH	98%	221
Capital Health System - Fuld Campus[2]	Trenton	98%	56
Community Medical Center[2]	Toms River	98%	293
Deborah Heart & Lung Center	Browns Mills	98%	215
Hackensack University Medical Center[2]	Hackensack	98%	392
Inspira Medical Center Woodbury	Woodbury	98%	284
JFK Med Ctr-A M Yelencsics Comm Hosp[2]	Edison	98%	567
Kennedy Univ Hosp-Stratford Div[2]	Stratford	98%	691
Morristown Medical Center[2]	Morristown	98%	569
Ocean Medical Center[2]	Brick	98%	253
Our Lady of Lourdes Medical Center[2]	Camden	98%	287
Saint Clare's Hospital	Denville	98%	397
Saint Luke's Warren Hospital[2]	Phillipsburg	98%	123
Saint Mary's Hospital - Passaic	Passaic	98%	180
Somerset Medical Center[2]	Somerville	98%	282
Southern Ocean Medical Center	Manahawkin	98%	160
Univ Med Ctr of Princeton-Plainsboro[2]	Plainsboro	98%	257
Centrastate Medical Center[2]	Freehold	97%	264
Hunterdon Medical Center[2]	Flemington	97%	212
Jersey Shore University Medical Center[2]	Neptune	97%	741
Newark Beth Israel Medical Center[2]	Newark	97%	380
Palisades Medical Center	North Bergen	97%	59
Robert W Johnson Univ Hosp-Hamilton[2]	Hamilton	97%	451
Robert Wood Johnson Univ Hosp-Rahway	Rahway	97%	75
Saint Barnabas Medical Center[2]	Livingston	97%	495
Saint Michael's Medical Center[2]	Newark	97%	348
Cooper University Hospital[2]	Camden	96%	372
Inspira Medical Center Vineland[2]	Vineland	96%	214
Monmouth Medical Center[2]	Long Branch	95%	294
Saint Peter's University Hospital[2]	New Brunswick	95%	305
University Hospital[2]	Newark	95%	211
VA New Jersey Health Care System	East Orange	95%	86
Memorial Hospital of Salem County	Salem	94%	54
Raritan Bay Medical Center	Perth Amboy	94%	154
East Orange General Hospital	East Orange	93%	55
Carepoint Health-Bayonne Hosp Ctr	Bayonne	90%	39

Prophylactic Antibiotic Timing

Hospital Name	City	Rate	Cases
Atlanticare Regional Medical Center[2]	Atlantic City	100%	508
Bayshore Community Hospital[2]	Holmdel	100%	111
Cape Regional Medical Center	Cape May CH	100%	232
Capital Health Medical Center - Hopewell	Pennington	100%	473
Capital Health System - Fuld Campus[2]	Trenton	100%	58
Carepoint Health-Bayonne Hosp Ctr	Bayonne	100%	42
Carepoint Health - Hoboken UMC	Hoboken	100%	82
Chilton Medical Center[2]	Pompton Plains	100%	205
Clara Maass Medical Center[2]	Belleville	100%	252
Community Medical Center[2]	Toms River	100%	305
Deborah Heart & Lung Center	Browns Mills	100%	221
Englewood Hospital & Medical Center[2]	Englewood	100%	857
Hackensack - Umc Mountainside	Montclair	100%	214
Hackettstown Regional Medical Center	Hackettstown	100%	194
Hunterdon Medical Center[2]	Flemington	100%	219
JFK Med Ctr-A M Yelencsics Comm Hosp[2]	Edison	100%	589
Kennedy Univ Hosp-Stratford Div[2]	Stratford	100%	700
Libertyhealth-Jersey City Med Ctr[2]	Jersey City	100%	388
Lourdes Med Ctr of Burlington County[2]	Willingboro	100%	119
Meadowlands Hospital Medical Center	Secaucus	100%	34
Monmouth Medical Center[2]	Long Branch	100%	301
Newark Beth Israel Medical Center[2]	Newark	100%	405
Ocean Medical Center[2]	Brick	100%	261
Our Lady of Lourdes Medical Center[2]	Camden	100%	301
Overlook Medical Center[2]	Summit	100%	336
Palisades Medical Center	North Bergen	100%	70
Robert Wood Johnson Univ Hosp-Rahway	Rahway	100%	80
Saint Barnabas Medical Center[2]	Livingston	100%	508
Saint Francis Medical Center	Trenton	100%	125
Saint Peter's University Hospital[2]	New Brunswick	100%	309
Shore Medical Center[2]	Somers Point	100%	404
Somerset Medical Center[2]	Somerville	100%	290
Trinitas Regional Medical Center[2]	Elizabeth	100%	230
University Hospital[2]	Newark	100%	221
Univ Med Ctr of Princeton-Plainsboro[2]	Plainsboro	100%	260
VA New Jersey Health Care System	East Orange	100%	88
Valley Hospital[2]	Ridgewood	100%	497
Virtua Mem Hosp of Burlington County[2]	Mount Holly	100%	279
Virtua West Jersey Hospitals Berlin[2]	Berlin	100%	2661
Centrastate Medical Center[2]	Freehold	99%	278
Hackensack University Medical Center[2]	Hackensack	99%	421
Holy Name Medical Center[2]	Teaneck	99%	311
Inspira Medical Center Elmer[2]	Elmer	99%	114
Inspira Medical Center Vineland[2]	Vineland	99%	224
Inspira Medical Center Woodbury	Woodbury	99%	291
Jersey Shore University Medical Center[2]	Neptune	99%	774
Morristown Medical Center[2]	Morristown	99%	604
Raritan Bay Medical Center	Perth Amboy	99%	164
Riverview Medical Center[2]	Red Bank	99%	308
Robert Wood Johnson University Hospital[2]	New Brunswick	99%	1390
Saint Clare's Hospital	Denville	99%	404
Saint Joseph's Regional Medical Center[2]	Paterson	99%	839
Saint Luke's Warren Hospital[2]	Phillipsburg	99%	129
Saint Mary's Hospital - Passaic	Passaic	99%	210
Saint Michael's Medical Center[2]	Newark	99%	355
Southern Ocean Medical Center	Manahawkin	99%	172
East Orange General Hospital	East Orange	98%	61
Memorial Hospital of Salem County	Salem	98%	57
Newton Memorial Hospital	Newton	98%	186
Robert W Johnson Univ Hosp-Hamilton[2]	Hamilton	98%	468
Cooper University Hospital[2]	Camden	97%	392
Carepoint Health - Christ Hospital	Jersey City	96%	53

Prophylactic Antibiotic Timing (Outpatient)

Hospital Name	City	Rate	Cases
Capital Health Medical Center - Hopewell	Pennington	100%	258
Carepoint Health - Hoboken UMC	Hoboken	100%	32
Deborah Heart & Lung Center	Browns Mills	100%	467
Hackensack - Umc Mountainside	Montclair	100%	96
Holy Name Medical Center	Teaneck	100%	241
Lourdes Med Ctr of Burlington County	Willingboro	100%	42
Monmouth Medical Center - Southern Campus	Lakewood	100%	40
Newton Memorial Hospital	Newton	100%	66
Univ Med Ctr of Princeton-Plainsboro	Plainsboro	100%	222
Centrastate Medical Center	Freehold	99%	129
Clara Maass Medical Center	Belleville	99%	164
Community Medical Center	Toms River	99%	459
Englewood Hospital & Medical Center	Englewood	99%	477
Inspira Medical Center Vineland	Vineland	99%	326
JFK Med Ctr-A M Yelencsics Comm Hosp	Edison	99%	273
Monmouth Medical Center	Long Branch	99%	470
Newark Beth Israel Medical Center	Newark	99%	375
Our Lady of Lourdes Medical Center	Camden	99%	483
Overlook Medical Center	Summit	99%	493
Riverview Medical Center	Red Bank	99%	328
Robert Wood Johnson University Hospital	New Brunswick	99%	932
Robert W Johnson Univ Hosp-Hamilton	Hamilton	99%	145
Robert Wood Johnson Univ Hosp-Rahway	Rahway	99%	68

NOTE: Hospital profiles are in alphabetical order by state, then city, then hospital within the city; Rankings exclude hospitals with less than 25 cases except for patient surveys which excludes hospitals with less than 100 cases; (a) 100-299 cases; (1) The number of cases/patients is too few to report; (2) Data submitted were based on a sample of cases/patients; (3) Results are based on a shorter time period than required; (4) Data suppressed by CMS for one or more quarters; (5) Results are not available for this reporting period; (6) Fewer than 100 patients completed the HCAHPS survey; (7) No cases met the criteria for this measure; (8) The lower limit of the confidence interval cannot be calculated if the number of observed infections equals zero; (9) No data are available from the state/territory for this reporting period; (10) The scores shown reflect fewer than 50 completed surveys; (11) There were discrepancies in the data collection process; (12) This measure does not apply to this hospital for this reporting period; (13) Results cannot be calculated for this reporting period; (14) The results for this state are combined with nearby states to protect confidentiality; Please refer to the User's Guide for a full explanation of data.

Saint Barnabas Medical Center	Livingston	99%	900
Saint Clare's Hospital	Denville	99%	209
Saint Francis Medical Center	Trenton	99%	260
Saint Mary's Hospital - Passaic	Passaic	99%	275
Saint Peter's University Hospital	New Brunswick	99%	210
Shore Medical Center	Somers Point	99%	149
Somerset Medical Center	Somerville	99%	182
Valley Hospital	Ridgewood	99%	598
Virtua West Jersey Hospitals Berlin	Berlin	99%	352
Atlanticare Regional Medical Center	Atlantic City	98%	450
Cape Regional Medical Center	Cape May CH	98%	54
Hackensack University Medical Center	Hackensack	98%	941
Hunterdon Medical Center	Flemington	98%	133
Jersey Shore University Medical Center	Neptune	98%	674
Meadowlands Hospital Medical Center	Secaucus	98%	119
Morristown Medical Center	Morristown	98%	683
Saint Joseph's Regional Medical Center	Paterson	98%	262
Saint Michael's Medical Center	Newark	98%	185
Southern Ocean Medical Center	Manahawkin	98%	64
Trinitas Regional Medical Center	Elizabeth	98%	238
University Hospital	Newark	98%	160
Virtua Mem Hosp of Burlington County	Mount Holly	98%	181
Bayshore Community Hospital	Holmdel	97%	34
Carepoint Health - Christ Hospital	Jersey City	97%	73
Hackettstown Regional Medical Center	Hackettstown	97%	69
Kennedy Univ Hosp-Stratford Div	Stratford	97%	253
Saint Luke's Warren Hospital	Phillipsburg	97%	65
Chilton Medical Center	Pompton Plains	96%	84
Cooper University Hospital	Camden	96%	358
Memorial Hospital of Salem County	Salem	96%	25
Palisades Medical Center	North Bergen	96%	53
Inspira Medical Center Elmer	Elmer	95%	95
Inspira Medical Center Woodbury	Woodbury	95%	84
Ocean Medical Center	Brick	95%	209
Libertyhealth-Jersey City Med Ctr	Jersey City	94%	82
Carepoint Health-Bayonne Hosp Ctr	Bayonne	93%	29
Raritan Bay Medical Center	Perth Amboy	92%	78
Capital Health System - Fuld Campus	Trenton	76%	38

Urinary Catheter Removal

Hospital Name	City	Rate	Cases
Bayshore Community Hospital[2]	Holmdel	100%	145
Capital Health Medical Center - Hopewell	Pennington	100%	603
Carepoint Health-Bayonne Hosp Ctr	Bayonne	100%	72
Carepoint Health - Hoboken UMC	Hoboken	100%	82
Centrastate Medical Center[2]	Freehold	100%	278
Chilton Medical Center[2]	Pompton Plains	100%	235
Clara Maass Medical Center[2]	Belleville	100%	244
Cooper University Hospital[2]	Camden	100%	324
Hackensack - Umc Mountainside	Montclair	100%	277
Hackettstown Regional Medical Center	Hackettstown	100%	178
Holy Name Medical Center[2]	Teaneck	100%	225
Inspira Medical Center Woodbury	Woodbury	100%	90
JFK Med Ctr-A M Yelencsics Comm Hosp[2]	Edison	100%	315
Libertyhealth-Jersey City Med Ctr[2]	Jersey City	100%	312
Monmouth Medical Center - Southern Campus	Lakewood	100%	39
Newark Beth Israel Medical Center[2]	Newark	100%	106
Overlook Medical Center[2]	Summit	100%	248
Palisades Medical Center	North Bergen	100%	79
Robert Wood Johnson University Hospital[2]	New Brunswick	100%	1096
Saint Francis Medical Center	Trenton	100%	110
Univ Med Ctr of Princeton-Plainsboro[2]	Plainsboro	100%	286
Valley Hospital[2]	Ridgewood	100%	420
Virtua West Jersey Hospitals Berlin[2]	Berlin	100%	1703
Deborah Heart & Lung Center	Browns Mills	99%	131
Englewood Hospital & Medical Center[2]	Englewood	99%	703
Hackensack University Medical Center[2]	Hackensack	99%	402
Inspira Medical Center Elmer[2]	Elmer	99%	139
Inspira Medical Center Vineland[2]	Vineland	99%	183
Monmouth Medical Center[2]	Long Branch	99%	239
Saint Mary's Hospital - Passaic	Passaic	99%	155
Trinitas Regional Medical Center[2]	Elizabeth	99%	252
Atlanticare Regional Medical Center[2]	Atlantic City	98%	322
Bergen Regional Medical Center	Paramus	98%	42
Cape Regional Medical Center	Cape May CH	98%	189
Jersey Shore University Medical Center[2]	Neptune	98%	532
Raritan Bay Medical Center	Perth Amboy	98%	200
Robert W Johnson Univ Hosp-Hamilton[2]	Hamilton	98%	461
Saint Joseph's Regional Medical Center[2]	Paterson	98%	662
Saint Luke's Warren Hospital[2]	Phillipsburg	98%	169
Shore Medical Center[2]	Somers Point	98%	199
Southern Ocean Medical Center	Manahawkin	98%	169
University Hospital[2]	Newark	98%	125
Carepoint Health - Christ Hospital	Jersey City	97%	88
Lourdes Med Ctr of Burlington County[2]	Willingboro	97%	131
Morristown Medical Center[2]	Morristown	97%	515
Ocean Medical Center[2]	Brick	97%	266
Saint Clare's Hospital	Denville	97%	435
Saint Peter's University Hospital[2]	New Brunswick	97%	136
Virtua Mem Hosp of Burlington County[2]	Mount Holly	97%	256
Kennedy Univ Hosp-Stratford Div[2]	Stratford	96%	390
Capital Health System - Fuld Campus[2]	Trenton	95%	111
Our Lady of Lourdes Medical Center[2]	Camden	95%	262
VA New Jersey Health Care System[2]	East Orange	95%	78
Memorial Hospital of Salem County	Salem	94%	34
Newton Memorial Hospital	Newton	94%	177
Riverview Medical Center[2]	Red Bank	94%	219
Community Medical Center[2]	Toms River	93%	120
Somerset Medical Center[2]	Somerville	93%	129
Robert Wood Johnson Univ Hosp-Rahway	Rahway	92%	62
Saint Barnabas Medical Center[2]	Livingston	91%	174
East Orange General Hospital	East Orange	90%	52
Saint Michael's Medical Center[2]	Newark	89%	131
Hunterdon Medical Center[2]	Flemington	88%	95

Survey of Patients' Hospital Experiences

Area Around Room 'Always' Quiet at Night

Hospital Name	City	Rate	Cases
Memorial Hospital of Salem County	Salem	63%	300+
Capital Health Medical Center - Hopewell	Pennington	61%	300+
Univ Med Ctr of Princeton-Plainsboro	Plainsboro	61%	300+
Saint Luke's Warren Hospital	Phillipsburg	60%	300+
Deborah Heart & Lung Center	Browns Mills	59%	300+
Morristown Medical Center	Morristown	59%	300+
East Orange General Hospital	East Orange	58%	300+
Meadowlands Hospital Medical Center	Secaucus	58%	300+
Saint Peter's University Hospital	New Brunswick	58%	300+
Virtua West Jersey Hospitals Berlin	Berlin	58%	300+
Capital Health System - Fuld Campus	Trenton	57%	300+
Hackensack - Umc Mountainside	Montclair	57%	300+
Centrastate Medical Center	Freehold	56%	300+
Chilton Medical Center	Pompton Plains	56%	300+
Shore Medical Center	Somers Point	56%	300+
University Hospital	Newark	56%	300+
Newark Beth Israel Medical Center	Newark	55%	300+
Our Lady of Lourdes Medical Center	Camden	55%	300+
Saint Clare's Hospital	Denville	55%	300+
Valley Hospital	Ridgewood	55%	300+
Bergen Regional Medical Center	Paramus	54%	(a)
Englewood Hospital & Medical Center	Englewood	54%	300+
Hackensack University Medical Center	Hackensack	54%	300+
Inspira Medical Center Vineland	Vineland	54%	300+
Jersey Shore University Medical Center	Neptune	54%	300+
Libertyhealth-Jersey City Med Ctr	Jersey City	54%	300+
Robert W Johnson Univ Hosp-Hamilton	Hamilton	54%	300+
Cape Regional Medical Center	Cape May CH	53%	300+
Carepoint Health - Christ Hospital	Jersey City	53%	300+
Palisades Medical Center	North Bergen	53%	300+
Raritan Bay Medical Center	Perth Amboy	53%	300+
Saint Barnabas Medical Center	Livingston	53%	300+
Saint Mary's Hospital - Passaic	Passaic	53%	300+
Somerset Medical Center	Somerville	53%	300+
Ocean Medical Center	Brick	52%	300+
Overlook Medical Center	Summit	52%	300+
Trinitas Regional Medical Center[11]	Elizabeth	52%	300+
Bayshore Community Hospital	Holmdel	51%	300+
Carepoint Health - Hoboken UMC	Hoboken	51%	300+
Holy Name Medical Center	Teaneck	51%	300+
Hunterdon Medical Center	Flemington	51%	300+
Riverview Medical Center	Red Bank	51%	300+
Saint Joseph's Regional Medical Center	Paterson	51%	300+
Saint Michael's Medical Center	Newark	51%	300+
Cooper University Hospital	Camden	50%	300+
Hackettstown Regional Medical Center	Hackettstown	50%	300+
JFK Med Ctr-A M Yelencsics Comm Hosp	Edison	50%	300+
Kennedy Univ Hosp-Stratford Div	Stratford	50%	300+
Robert Wood Johnson University Hospital	New Brunswick	50%	300+
Carepoint Health-Bayonne Hosp Ctr	Bayonne	49%	300+
Inspira Medical Center Woodbury	Woodbury	49%	300+
Monmouth Medical Center	Long Branch	49%	300+
Monmouth Medical Center - Southern Campus	Lakewood	49%	300+
Newton Memorial Hospital	Newton	49%	300+
Robert Wood Johnson Univ Hosp-Rahway	Rahway	49%	300+
Clara Maass Medical Center	Belleville	48%	300+
Community Medical Center	Toms River	48%	300+
Inspira Medical Center Elmer	Elmer	48%	300+
Saint Francis Medical Center	Trenton	48%	300+
Atlanticare Regional Medical Center	Atlantic City	47%	300+
Lourdes Med Ctr of Burlington County	Willingboro	47%	300+
Virtua Mem Hosp of Burlington County	Mount Holly	47%	300+
Southern Ocean Medical Center	Manahawkin	46%	300+

Doctors 'Always' Communicated Well

Hospital Name	City	Rate	Cases
Deborah Heart & Lung Center	Browns Mills	83%	300+
Valley Hospital	Ridgewood	83%	300+
Centrastate Medical Center	Freehold	82%	300+
Carepoint Health - Hoboken UMC	Hoboken	81%	300+
Hackensack - Umc Mountainside	Montclair	81%	300+
Hackensack University Medical Center	Hackensack	81%	300+
Hunterdon Medical Center	Flemington	81%	300+
Somerset Medical Center	Somerville	81%	300+
Memorial Hospital of Salem County	Salem	80%	300+
Riverview Medical Center	Red Bank	80%	300+
Saint Peter's University Hospital	New Brunswick	80%	300+
Shore Medical Center	Somers Point	80%	300+
Cape Regional Medical Center	Cape May CH	79%	300+
Saint Barnabas Medical Center	Livingston	79%	300+
Saint Luke's Warren Hospital	Phillipsburg	79%	300+
Univ Med Ctr of Princeton-Plainsboro	Plainsboro	79%	300+
Capital Health Medical Center - Hopewell	Pennington	78%	300+
Chilton Medical Center	Pompton Plains	78%	300+
East Orange General Hospital	East Orange	78%	300+
Englewood Hospital & Medical Center	Englewood	78%	300+
Holy Name Medical Center	Teaneck	78%	300+
Inspira Medical Center Elmer	Elmer	78%	300+
Inspira Medical Center Woodbury	Woodbury	78%	300+
JFK Med Ctr-A M Yelencsics Comm Hosp	Edison	78%	300+
Monmouth Medical Center	Long Branch	78%	300+
Overlook Medical Center	Summit	78%	300+
Robert Wood Johnson University Hospital	New Brunswick	78%	300+
Robert W Johnson Univ Hosp-Hamilton	Hamilton	78%	300+
Saint Joseph's Regional Medical Center	Paterson	78%	300+
Southern Ocean Medical Center	Manahawkin	78%	300+
Virtua West Jersey Hospitals Berlin	Berlin	78%	300+
Bayshore Community Hospital	Holmdel	77%	300+
Capital Health System - Fuld Campus	Trenton	77%	300+
Clara Maass Medical Center	Belleville	77%	300+
Cooper University Hospital	Camden	77%	300+
Jersey Shore University Medical Center	Neptune	77%	300+
Morristown Medical Center	Morristown	77%	300+
Newark Beth Israel Medical Center	Newark	77%	300+
Palisades Medical Center	North Bergen	77%	300+
Raritan Bay Medical Center	Perth Amboy	77%	300+
Saint Mary's Hospital - Passaic	Passaic	77%	300+
Carepoint Health-Bayonne Hosp Ctr	Bayonne	76%	300+
Community Medical Center	Toms River	76%	300+
Inspira Medical Center Vineland	Vineland	76%	300+
Kennedy Univ Hosp-Stratford Div	Stratford	76%	300+
Libertyhealth-Jersey City Med Ctr	Jersey City	76%	300+
Atlanticare Regional Medical Center	Atlantic City	75%	300+
Carepoint Health - Christ Hospital	Jersey City	75%	300+
Hackettstown Regional Medical Center	Hackettstown	75%	300+
Meadowlands Hospital Medical Center	Secaucus	75%	300+
Ocean Medical Center	Brick	75%	300+
Robert Wood Johnson Univ Hosp-Rahway	Rahway	75%	300+
Saint Clare's Hospital	Denville	75%	300+
Saint Francis Medical Center	Trenton	75%	300+
Trinitas Regional Medical Center[11]	Elizabeth	75%	300+
University Hospital	Newark	75%	300+
Virtua Mem Hosp of Burlington County	Mount Holly	75%	300+
Monmouth Medical Center - Southern Campus	Lakewood	74%	300+
Our Lady of Lourdes Medical Center	Camden	74%	300+
Saint Michael's Medical Center	Newark	73%	300+
Bergen Regional Medical Center	Paramus	68%	(a)
Lourdes Med Ctr of Burlington County	Willingboro	68%	300+
Newton Memorial Hospital	Newton	68%	300+

Home Recovery Information Given

Hospital Name	City	Rate	Cases
Deborah Heart & Lung Center	Browns Mills	89%	300+
Inspira Medical Center Elmer	Elmer	88%	300+
Atlanticare Regional Medical Center	Atlantic City	87%	300+
Centrastate Medical Center	Freehold	86%	300+
Cooper University Hospital	Camden	86%	300+
Riverview Medical Center	Red Bank	86%	300+
Saint Francis Medical Center	Trenton	86%	300+
Virtua West Jersey Hospitals Berlin	Berlin	86%	300+
Hackettstown Regional Medical Center	Hackettstown	85%	300+
Hunterdon Medical Center	Flemington	85%	300+
Inspira Medical Center Vineland	Vineland	85%	300+
Memorial Hospital of Salem County	Salem	85%	300+
Robert W Johnson Univ Hosp-Hamilton	Hamilton	85%	300+
Saint Clare's Hospital	Denville	85%	300+
Shore Medical Center	Somers Point	85%	300+
Carepoint Health - Hoboken UMC	Hoboken	84%	300+
Newton Memorial Hospital	Newton	84%	300+
Ocean Medical Center	Brick	84%	300+
Southern Ocean Medical Center	Manahawkin	84%	300+
Bayshore Community Hospital	Holmdel	83%	300+
Chilton Medical Center	Pompton Plains	83%	300+
Holy Name Medical Center	Teaneck	83%	300+
Robert Wood Johnson University Hospital	New Brunswick	83%	300+
Saint Peter's University Hospital	New Brunswick	83%	300+
Valley Hospital	Ridgewood	83%	300+
Capital Health Medical Center - Hopewell	Pennington	82%	300+
Carepoint Health-Bayonne Hosp Ctr	Bayonne	82%	300+
Community Medical Center	Toms River	82%	300+
Hackensack - Umc Mountainside	Montclair	82%	300+
Hackensack University Medical Center	Hackensack	82%	300+
Morristown Medical Center	Morristown	82%	300+

NOTE: Hospital profiles are in alphabetical order by state, then city, then hospital within the city; Rankings exclude hospitals with less than 25 cases except for patient surveys which excludes hospitals with less than 100 cases; (a) 100-299 cases; (1) The number of cases/patients is too few to report; (2) Data submitted were based on a sample of cases/patients; (3) Results are based on a shorter time period than required; (4) Data suppressed by CMS for one or more quarters; (5) Results are not available for this reporting period; (6) Fewer than 100 patients completed the HCAHPS survey; (7) No cases met the criteria for this measure; (8) The lower limit of the confidence interval cannot be calculated if the number of observed infections equals zero; (9) No data are available from the state/territory for this reporting period; (10) The scores shown reflect fewer than 50 completed surveys; (11) There were discrepancies in the data collection process; (12) This measure does not apply to this hospital for this reporting period; (13) Results cannot be calculated for this reporting period; (14) The results for this state are combined with nearby states to protect confidentiality; Please refer to the User's Guide for a full explanation of data.

Raritan Bay Medical Center	Perth Amboy	82%	300+
Saint Joseph's Regional Medical Center	Paterson	82%	300+
Saint Luke's Warren Hospital	Phillipsburg	82%	300+
Cape Regional Medical Center	Cape May CH	81%	300+
Capital Health System - Fuld Campus	Trenton	81%	300+
Jersey Shore University Medical Center	Neptune	81%	300+
Kennedy Univ Hosp-Stratford Div	Stratford	81%	300+
Monmouth Medical Center	Long Branch	81%	300+
Monmouth Medical Center - Southern Campus	Lakewood	81%	300+
Our Lady of Lourdes Medical Center	Camden	81%	300+
Somerset Medical Center	Somerville	81%	300+
Trinitas Regional Medical Center[11]	Elizabeth	81%	300+
Univ Med Ctr of Princeton-Plainsboro	Plainsboro	81%	300+
Carepoint Health - Christ Hospital	Jersey City	80%	300+
Clara Maass Medical Center	Belleville	80%	300+
East Orange General Hospital	East Orange	80%	300+
Inspira Medical Center Woodbury	Woodbury	80%	300+
Overlook Medical Center	Summit	80%	300+
Robert Wood Johnson Univ Hosp-Rahway	Rahway	80%	300+
Saint Barnabas Medical Center	Livingston	80%	300+
University Hospital	Newark	80%	300+
Lourdes Med Ctr of Burlington County	Willingboro	79%	300+
Libertyhealth-Jersey City Med Ctr	Jersey City	78%	300+
Meadowlands Hospital Medical Center	Secaucus	78%	300+
Newark Beth Israel Medical Center	Newark	78%	300+
Palisades Medical Center	North Bergen	78%	300+
Saint Mary's Hospital - Passaic	Passaic	78%	300+
Virtua Mem Hosp of Burlington County	Mount Holly	78%	300+
Englewood Hospital & Medical Center	Englewood	77%	300+
JFK Med Ctr-A M Yelencsics Comm Hosp	Edison	76%	300+
Bergen Regional Medical Center	Paramus	75%	(a)
Saint Michael's Medical Center	Newark	74%	300+

Hospital Given 9 or 10 on 10 Point Scale

Hospital Name	City	Rate	Cases
Deborah Heart & Lung Center	Browns Mills	82%	300+
Valley Hospital	Ridgewood	78%	300+
Morristown Medical Center	Morristown	77%	300+
Virtua West Jersey Hospitals Berlin	Berlin	76%	300+
Hackensack University Medical Center	Hackensack	75%	300+
Saint Peter's University Hospital	New Brunswick	75%	300+
Hunterdon Medical Center	Flemington	74%	300+
Univ Med Ctr of Princeton-Plainsboro	Plainsboro	74%	300+
Capital Health Medical Center - Hopewell	Pennington	72%	300+
Inspira Medical Center Elmer	Elmer	72%	300+
Jersey Shore University Medical Center	Neptune	72%	300+
Englewood Hospital & Medical Center	Englewood	70%	300+
Somerset Medical Center	Somerville	70%	300+
Centrastate Medical Center	Freehold	69%	300+
Capital Health System - Fuld Campus	Trenton	68%	300+
Holy Name Medical Center	Teaneck	68%	300+
Robert Wood Johnson University Hospital	New Brunswick	68%	300+
Saint Clare's Hospital	Denville	68%	300+
Shore Medical Center	Somers Point	68%	300+
Atlanticare Regional Medical Center	Atlantic City	67%	300+
Cooper University Hospital	Camden	67%	300+
Ocean Medical Center	Brick	67%	300+
Robert W Johnson Univ Hosp-Hamilton	Hamilton	67%	300+
Saint Barnabas Medical Center	Livingston	67%	300+
Carepoint Health - Hoboken UMC	Hoboken	66%	300+
Monmouth Medical Center	Long Branch	66%	300+
Overlook Medical Center	Summit	66%	300+
Hackensack - Umc Mountainside	Montclair	65%	300+
Saint Luke's Warren Hospital	Phillipsburg	65%	300+
Virtua Mem Hosp of Burlington County	Mount Holly	65%	300+
Chilton Medical Center	Pompton Plains	64%	300+
Our Lady of Lourdes Medical Center	Camden	64%	300+
Cape Regional Medical Center	Cape May CH	63%	300+
Hackettstown Regional Medical Center	Hackettstown	63%	300+
Kennedy Univ Hosp-Stratford Div	Stratford	63%	300+
Saint Joseph's Regional Medical Center	Paterson	63%	300+
Riverview Medical Center	Red Bank	62%	300+
Southern Ocean Medical Center	Manahawkin	62%	300+
Community Medical Center	Toms River	61%	300+
JFK Med Ctr-A M Yelencsics Comm Hosp	Edison	61%	300+
Bayshore Community Hospital	Holmdel	60%	300+
Inspira Medical Center Vineland	Vineland	60%	300+
Inspira Medical Center Woodbury	Woodbury	60%	300+
Libertyhealth-Jersey City Med Ctr	Jersey City	60%	300+
Newark Beth Israel Medical Center	Newark	60%	300+
Trinitas Regional Medical Center[11]	Elizabeth	60%	300+
Memorial Hospital of Salem County	Salem	59%	300+
Raritan Bay Medical Center	Perth Amboy	59%	300+
Robert Wood Johnson Univ Hosp-Rahway	Rahway	58%	300+
Saint Francis Medical Center	Trenton	58%	300+
University Hospital	Newark	58%	300+
Clara Maass Medical Center	Belleville	57%	300+
Monmouth Medical Center - Southern Campus	Lakewood	57%	300+
Palisades Medical Center	North Bergen	57%	300+
Saint Michael's Medical Center	Newark	57%	300+
Carepoint Health-Bayonne Hosp Ctr	Bayonne	56%	300+
Carepoint Health - Christ Hospital	Jersey City	56%	300+
Newton Memorial Hospital	Newton	56%	300+
Bergen Regional Medical Center	Paramus	55%	(a)
Meadowlands Hospital Medical Center	Secaucus	54%	300+
East Orange General Hospital	East Orange	52%	300+
Saint Mary's Hospital - Passaic	Passaic	52%	300+
Lourdes Med Ctr of Burlington County	Willingboro	46%	300+

Meds 'Always' Explained Before Given

Hospital Name	City	Rate	Cases
Deborah Heart & Lung Center	Browns Mills	70%	300+
Centrastate Medical Center	Freehold	68%	300+
Memorial Hospital of Salem County	Salem	66%	300+
Valley Hospital	Ridgewood	66%	300+
Virtua West Jersey Hospitals Berlin	Berlin	66%	300+
Hunterdon Medical Center	Flemington	65%	300+
Cape Regional Medical Center	Cape May CH	64%	300+
Chilton Medical Center	Pompton Plains	64%	300+
Jersey Shore University Medical Center	Neptune	64%	300+
Hackensack University Medical Center	Hackensack	63%	300+
Inspira Medical Center Elmer	Elmer	63%	300+
Monmouth Medical Center	Long Branch	63%	300+
Saint Peter's University Hospital	New Brunswick	63%	300+
Southern Ocean Medical Center	Manahawkin	63%	300+
Univ Med Ctr of Princeton-Plainsboro	Plainsboro	63%	300+
Bayshore Community Hospital	Holmdel	62%	300+
Capital Health System - Fuld Campus	Trenton	62%	300+
Community Medical Center	Toms River	62%	300+
Inspira Medical Center Woodbury	Woodbury	62%	300+
Ocean Medical Center	Brick	62%	300+
Our Lady of Lourdes Medical Center	Camden	62%	300+
Kennedy Univ Hosp-Stratford Div	Stratford	61%	300+
Saint Barnabas Medical Center	Livingston	61%	300+
Capital Health Medical Center - Hopewell	Pennington	60%	300+
Riverview Medical Center	Red Bank	60%	300+
Robert Wood Johnson University Hospital	New Brunswick	60%	300+
Robert W Johnson Univ Hosp-Hamilton	Hamilton	60%	300+
Saint Francis Medical Center	Trenton	60%	300+
Saint Luke's Warren Hospital	Phillipsburg	60%	300+
Shore Medical Center	Somers Point	60%	300+
Somerset Medical Center	Somerville	60%	300+
Inspira Medical Center Vineland	Vineland	59%	300+
Morristown Medical Center	Morristown	59%	300+
Holy Name Medical Center	Teaneck	58%	300+
JFK Med Ctr-A M Yelencsics Comm Hosp	Edison	58%	300+
Libertyhealth-Jersey City Med Ctr	Jersey City	58%	300+
Meadowlands Hospital Medical Center	Secaucus	58%	300+
Monmouth Medical Center - Southern Campus	Lakewood	58%	300+
Overlook Medical Center	Summit	58%	300+
Clara Maass Medical Center	Belleville	57%	300+
Newark Beth Israel Medical Center	Newark	57%	300+
Saint Joseph's Regional Medical Center	Paterson	57%	300+
Trinitas Regional Medical Center[11]	Elizabeth	57%	300+
Virtua Mem Hosp of Burlington County	Mount Holly	57%	300+
Cooper University Hospital	Camden	56%	300+
Englewood Hospital & Medical Center	Englewood	56%	300+
Hackensack - Umc Mountainside	Montclair	56%	300+
Lourdes Med Ctr of Burlington County	Willingboro	56%	300+
Raritan Bay Medical Center	Perth Amboy	56%	300+
Saint Clare's Hospital	Denville	56%	300+
East Orange General Hospital	East Orange	55%	300+
Newton Memorial Hospital	Newton	55%	300+
Palisades Medical Center	North Bergen	55%	300+
University Hospital	Newark	55%	300+
Atlanticare Regional Medical Center	Atlantic City	54%	300+
Carepoint Health-Bayonne Hosp Ctr	Bayonne	54%	300+
Carepoint Health - Christ Hospital	Jersey City	54%	300+
Robert Wood Johnson Univ Hosp-Rahway	Rahway	53%	300+
Saint Mary's Hospital - Passaic	Passaic	53%	300+
Carepoint Health - Hoboken UMC	Hoboken	51%	300+
Hackettstown Regional Medical Center	Hackettstown	51%	300+
Bergen Regional Medical Center	Paramus	50%	(a)
Saint Michael's Medical Center	Newark	50%	300+

Nurses 'Always' Communicated Well

Hospital Name	City	Rate	Cases
Saint Peter's University Hospital	New Brunswick	84%	300+
Valley Hospital	Ridgewood	84%	300+
Centrastate Medical Center	Freehold	83%	300+
Deborah Heart & Lung Center	Browns Mills	82%	300+
Virtua West Jersey Hospitals Berlin	Berlin	82%	300+
Hackensack University Medical Center	Hackensack	81%	300+
Hunterdon Medical Center	Flemington	81%	300+
Shore Medical Center	Somers Point	81%	300+
Cape Regional Medical Center	Cape May CH	80%	300+
Inspira Medical Center Elmer	Elmer	80%	300+
Inspira Medical Center Woodbury	Woodbury	80%	300+
Ocean Medical Center	Brick	80%	300+
Chilton Medical Center	Pompton Plains	79%	300+
Kennedy Univ Hosp-Stratford Div	Stratford	79%	300+
Memorial Hospital of Salem County	Salem	79%	300+
Robert W Johnson Univ Hosp-Hamilton	Hamilton	79%	300+
Somerset Medical Center	Somerville	79%	300+
Bayshore Community Hospital	Holmdel	78%	300+
Jersey Shore University Medical Center	Neptune	78%	300+
Morristown Medical Center	Morristown	78%	300+
Robert Wood Johnson University Hospital	New Brunswick	78%	300+
Southern Ocean Medical Center	Manahawkin	78%	300+
Virtua Mem Hosp of Burlington County	Mount Holly	78%	300+
Capital Health System - Fuld Campus	Trenton	77%	300+
Community Medical Center	Toms River	77%	300+
Monmouth Medical Center	Long Branch	77%	300+
Newton Memorial Hospital	Newton	77%	300+
Saint Luke's Warren Hospital	Phillipsburg	77%	300+
Univ Med Ctr of Princeton-Plainsboro	Plainsboro	77%	300+
Capital Health Medical Center - Hopewell	Pennington	76%	300+
Hackensack - Umc Mountainside	Montclair	76%	300+
JFK Med Ctr-A M Yelencsics Comm Hosp	Edison	76%	300+
Saint Barnabas Medical Center	Livingston	76%	300+
Saint Clare's Hospital	Denville	76%	300+
Saint Francis Medical Center	Trenton	76%	300+
Clara Maass Medical Center	Belleville	75%	300+
Cooper University Hospital	Camden	75%	300+
Englewood Hospital & Medical Center	Englewood	75%	300+
Our Lady of Lourdes Medical Center	Camden	75%	300+
Overlook Medical Center	Summit	75%	300+
Atlanticare Regional Medical Center	Atlantic City	74%	300+
Hackettstown Regional Medical Center	Hackettstown	74%	300+
Holy Name Medical Center	Teaneck	74%	300+
Inspira Medical Center Vineland	Vineland	74%	300+
Monmouth Medical Center - Southern Campus	Lakewood	74%	300+
Newark Beth Israel Medical Center	Newark	74%	300+
Raritan Bay Medical Center	Perth Amboy	74%	300+
Riverview Medical Center	Red Bank	74%	300+
Robert Wood Johnson Univ Hosp-Rahway	Rahway	74%	300+
Carepoint Health-Bayonne Hosp Ctr	Bayonne	73%	300+
Carepoint Health - Hoboken UMC	Hoboken	72%	300+
Libertyhealth-Jersey City Med Ctr	Jersey City	72%	300+
Saint Joseph's Regional Medical Center	Paterson	72%	300+
Palisades Medical Center	North Bergen	71%	300+
Saint Mary's Hospital - Passaic	Passaic	71%	300+
Carepoint Health - Christ Hospital	Jersey City	69%	300+
Meadowlands Hospital Medical Center	Secaucus	69%	300+
Trinitas Regional Medical Center[11]	Elizabeth	69%	300+
East Orange General Hospital	East Orange	68%	300+
Lourdes Med Ctr of Burlington County	Willingboro	68%	300+
University Hospital	Newark	68%	300+
Saint Michael's Medical Center	Newark	67%	300+
Bergen Regional Medical Center	Paramus	66%	(a)

Pain 'Always' Well Controlled

Hospital Name	City	Rate	Cases
Hackensack University Medical Center	Hackensack	76%	300+
Centrastate Medical Center	Freehold	75%	300+
Hunterdon Medical Center	Flemington	74%	300+
Memorial Hospital of Salem County	Salem	74%	300+
Saint Peter's University Hospital	New Brunswick	74%	300+
Valley Hospital	Ridgewood	74%	300+
Virtua West Jersey Hospitals Berlin	Berlin	74%	300+
Deborah Heart & Lung Center	Browns Mills	73%	300+
Inspira Medical Center Elmer	Elmer	73%	300+
Morristown Medical Center	Morristown	72%	300+
Ocean Medical Center	Brick	72%	300+
Southern Ocean Medical Center	Manahawkin	72%	300+
Community Medical Center	Toms River	71%	300+
Inspira Medical Center Woodbury	Woodbury	71%	300+
Robert W Johnson Univ Hosp-Hamilton	Hamilton	71%	300+
Cape Regional Medical Center	Cape May CH	70%	300+
Carepoint Health - Hoboken UMC	Hoboken	70%	300+
Chilton Medical Center	Pompton Plains	70%	300+
Hackettstown Regional Medical Center	Hackettstown	70%	300+
Monmouth Medical Center	Long Branch	70%	300+
Saint Francis Medical Center	Trenton	70%	300+
Saint Luke's Warren Hospital	Phillipsburg	70%	300+
Englewood Hospital & Medical Center	Englewood	69%	300+
Jersey Shore University Medical Center	Neptune	69%	300+
Kennedy Univ Hosp-Stratford Div	Stratford	69%	300+
Overlook Medical Center	Summit	69%	300+
Shore Medical Center	Somers Point	69%	300+
Somerset Medical Center	Somerville	69%	300+
Virtua Mem Hosp of Burlington County	Mount Holly	69%	300+
Bayshore Community Hospital	Holmdel	68%	300+
Capital Health Medical Center - Hopewell	Pennington	68%	300+
Cooper University Hospital	Camden	68%	300+
Hackensack - Umc Mountainside	Montclair	68%	300+
Holy Name Medical Center	Teaneck	68%	300+
Monmouth Medical Center - Southern Campus	Lakewood	68%	300+
Riverview Medical Center	Red Bank	68%	300+
Robert Wood Johnson University Hospital	New Brunswick	68%	300+
Saint Barnabas Medical Center	Livingston	68%	300+
Saint Clare's Hospital	Denville	68%	300+

NOTE: Hospital profiles are in alphabetical order by state, then city, then hospital within the city; Rankings exclude hospitals with less than 25 cases except for patient surveys which excludes hospitals with less than 100 cases; (a) 100-299 cases; (1) The number of cases/patients is too few to report; (2) Data submitted were based on a sample of cases/patients; (3) Results are based on a shorter time period than required; (4) Data suppressed by CMS for one or more quarters; (5) Results are not available for this reporting period; (6) Fewer than 100 patients completed the HCAHPS survey; (7) No cases met the criteria for this measure; (8) The lower limit of the confidence interval cannot be calculated if the number of observed infections equals zero; (9) No data are available from the state/territory for this reporting period; (10) The scores shown reflect fewer than 50 completed surveys; (11) There were discrepancies in the data collection process; (12) This measure does not apply to this hospital for this reporting period; (13) Results cannot be calculated for this reporting period; (14) The results for this state are combined with nearby states to protect confidentiality; Please refer to the User's Guide for a full explanation of data.

Hospital Name	City	Rate	Cases
Capital Health System - Fuld Campus	Trenton	67%	300+
JFK Med Ctr-A M Yelencsics Comm Hosp	Edison	67%	300+
Newark Beth Israel Medical Center	Newark	67%	300+
Newton Memorial Hospital	Newton	67%	300+
Clara Maass Medical Center	Belleville	66%	300+
Our Lady of Lourdes Medical Center	Camden	66%	300+
Raritan Bay Medical Center	Perth Amboy	66%	300+
Univ Med Ctr of Princeton-Plainsboro	Plainsboro	66%	300+
Inspira Medical Center Vineland	Vineland	65%	300+
Robert Wood Johnson Univ Hosp-Rahway	Rahway	65%	300+
Trinitas Regional Medical Center[11]	Elizabeth	65%	300+
Atlanticare Regional Medical Center	Atlantic City	63%	300+
Carepoint Health-Bayonne Hosp Ctr	Bayonne	63%	300+
East Orange General Hospital	East Orange	63%	300+
Libertyhealth-Jersey City Med Ctr	Jersey City	63%	300+
Lourdes Med Ctr of Burlington County	Willingboro	63%	300+
Meadowlands Hospital Medical Center	Secaucus	63%	300+
Saint Joseph's Regional Medical Center	Paterson	63%	300+
Palisades Medical Center	North Bergen	61%	300+
Saint Michael's Medical Center	Newark	61%	300+
University Hospital	Newark	61%	300+
Bergen Regional Medical Center	Paramus	60%	(a)
Carepoint Health - Christ Hospital	Jersey City	59%	300+
Saint Mary's Hospital - Passaic	Passaic	59%	300+

Room and Bathroom 'Always' Clean

Hospital Name	City	Rate	Cases
Virtua West Jersey Hospitals Berlin	Berlin	78%	300+
Centrastate Medical Center	Freehold	76%	300+
Deborah Heart & Lung Center	Browns Mills	76%	300+
JFK Med Ctr-A M Yelencsics Comm Hosp	Edison	76%	300+
Valley Hospital	Ridgewood	76%	300+
Capital Health Medical Center - Hopewell	Pennington	75%	300+
Inspira Medical Center Elmer	Elmer	75%	300+
Hackensack University Medical Center	Hackensack	74%	300+
Univ Med Ctr of Princeton-Plainsboro	Plainsboro	74%	300+
Morristown Medical Center	Morristown	73%	300+
Saint Peter's University Hospital	New Brunswick	73%	300+
Somerset Medical Center	Somerville	73%	300+
Libertyhealth-Jersey City Med Ctr	Jersey City	72%	300+
Monmouth Medical Center	Long Branch	72%	300+
Newton Memorial Hospital	Newton	72%	300+
Saint Barnabas Medical Center	Livingston	72%	300+
Shore Medical Center	Somers Point	72%	300+
Inspira Medical Center Vineland	Vineland	71%	300+
Memorial Hospital of Salem County	Salem	71%	300+
Saint Luke's Warren Hospital	Phillipsburg	71%	300+
Clara Maass Medical Center	Belleville	70%	300+
Hunterdon Medical Center	Flemington	70%	300+
Jersey Shore University Medical Center	Neptune	70%	300+
Meadowlands Hospital Medical Center	Secaucus	70%	300+
Monmouth Medical Center - Southern Campus	Lakewood	70%	300+
Ocean Medical Center	Brick	70%	300+
Saint Clare's Hospital	Denville	70%	300+
Saint Michael's Medical Center	Newark	70%	300+
Community Medical Center	Toms River	69%	300+
East Orange General Hospital	East Orange	69%	300+
Saint Joseph's Regional Medical Center	Paterson	69%	300+
Southern Ocean Medical Center	Manahawkin	69%	300+
Trinitas Regional Medical Center[11]	Elizabeth	69%	300+
Cape Regional Medical Center	Cape May CH	68%	300+
Chilton Medical Center	Pompton Plains	68%	300+
Englewood Hospital & Medical Center	Englewood	68%	300+
Holy Name Medical Center	Teaneck	68%	300+
Inspira Medical Center Woodbury	Woodbury	68%	300+
Kennedy Univ Hosp-Stratford Div	Stratford	68%	300+
Palisades Medical Center	North Bergen	68%	300+
Saint Francis Medical Center	Trenton	68%	300+
Capital Health System - Fuld Campus	Trenton	67%	300+
Carepoint Health - Hoboken UMC	Hoboken	67%	300+
Newark Beth Israel Medical Center	Newark	67%	300+
Robert W Johnson Univ Hosp-Hamilton	Hamilton	66%	300+
Atlanticare Regional Medical Center	Atlantic City	65%	300+
Our Lady of Lourdes Medical Center	Camden	65%	300+
Raritan Bay Medical Center	Perth Amboy	65%	300+
Carepoint Health-Bayonne Hosp Ctr	Bayonne	64%	300+
Hackensack - Umc Mountainside	Montclair	64%	300+
Overlook Medical Center	Summit	64%	300+
Robert Wood Johnson University Hospital	New Brunswick	64%	300+
Robert Wood Johnson Univ Hosp-Rahway	Rahway	64%	300+
Virtua Mem Hosp of Burlington County	Mount Holly	64%	300+
Bayshore Community Hospital	Holmdel	63%	300+
Cooper University Hospital	Camden	63%	300+
Riverview Medical Center	Red Bank	63%	300+
Lourdes Med Ctr of Burlington County	Willingboro	62%	300+
Saint Mary's Hospital - Passaic	Passaic	62%	300+
Carepoint Health - Christ Hospital	Jersey City	61%	300+
Hackettstown Regional Medical Center	Hackettstown	61%	300+
University Hospital	Newark	57%	300+
Bergen Regional Medical Center	Paramus	52%	(a)

Timely Help 'Always' Received

Hospital Name	City	Rate	Cases
Centrastate Medical Center	Freehold	70%	300+
Inspira Medical Center Elmer	Elmer	70%	300+
Virtua West Jersey Hospitals Berlin	Berlin	70%	300+
Deborah Heart & Lung Center	Browns Mills	69%	300+
Inspira Medical Center Woodbury	Woodbury	68%	300+
Saint Peter's University Hospital	New Brunswick	68%	300+
Cape Regional Medical Center	Cape May CH	67%	300+
Valley Hospital	Ridgewood	67%	300+
Carepoint Health - Hoboken UMC	Hoboken	66%	300+
Hackensack University Medical Center	Hackensack	66%	300+
Robert Wood Johnson University Hospital	New Brunswick	66%	300+
Chilton Medical Center	Pompton Plains	65%	300+
Jersey Shore University Medical Center	Neptune	65%	300+
Ocean Medical Center	Brick	65%	300+
Hunterdon Medical Center	Flemington	64%	300+
Robert W Johnson Univ Hosp-Hamilton	Hamilton	64%	300+
Shore Medical Center	Somers Point	64%	300+
Bayshore Community Hospital	Holmdel	63%	300+
Saint Luke's Warren Hospital	Phillipsburg	63%	300+
Somerset Medical Center	Somerville	63%	300+
Southern Ocean Medical Center	Manahawkin	63%	300+
Carepoint Health-Bayonne Hosp Ctr	Bayonne	62%	300+
Community Medical Center	Toms River	62%	300+
Kennedy Univ Hosp-Stratford Div	Stratford	62%	300+
Atlanticare Regional Medical Center	Atlantic City	61%	300+
Capital Health Medical Center - Hopewell	Pennington	61%	300+
Capital Health System - Fuld Campus	Trenton	61%	300+
Hackettstown Regional Medical Center	Hackettstown	61%	300+
Inspira Medical Center Vineland	Vineland	61%	300+
Memorial Hospital of Salem County	Salem	61%	300+
Robert Wood Johnson Univ Hosp-Rahway	Rahway	61%	300+
Cooper University Hospital	Camden	60%	300+
JFK Med Ctr-A M Yelencsics Comm Hosp	Edison	60%	300+
Meadowlands Hospital Medical Center	Secaucus	60%	300+
Newton Memorial Hospital	Newton	60%	300+
Saint Clare's Hospital	Denville	60%	300+
Univ Med Ctr of Princeton-Plainsboro	Plainsboro	60%	300+
Virtua Mem Hosp of Burlington County	Mount Holly	60%	300+
Hackensack - Umc Mountainside	Montclair	59%	300+
Monmouth Medical Center	Long Branch	59%	300+
Morristown Medical Center	Morristown	59%	300+
Our Lady of Lourdes Medical Center	Camden	59%	300+
Overlook Medical Center	Summit	59%	300+
Saint Barnabas Medical Center	Livingston	59%	300+
Clara Maass Medical Center	Belleville	58%	300+
Raritan Bay Medical Center	Perth Amboy	58%	300+
Lourdes Med Ctr of Burlington County	Willingboro	57%	300+
Saint Francis Medical Center	Trenton	57%	300+
Englewood Hospital & Medical Center	Englewood	56%	300+
Libertyhealth-Jersey City Med Ctr	Jersey City	56%	300+
Holy Name Medical Center	Teaneck	55%	300+
Riverview Medical Center	Red Bank	55%	300+
Carepoint Health - Christ Hospital	Jersey City	54%	300+
Palisades Medical Center	North Bergen	54%	300+
Trinitas Regional Medical Center[11]	Elizabeth	54%	300+
Saint Joseph's Regional Medical Center	Paterson	53%	300+
East Orange General Hospital	East Orange	52%	300+
Monmouth Medical Center - Southern Campus	Lakewood	52%	300+
Newark Beth Israel Medical Center	Newark	52%	300+
University Hospital	Newark	52%	300+
Saint Mary's Hospital - Passaic	Passaic	49%	300+
Saint Michael's Medical Center	Newark	49%	300+
Bergen Regional Medical Center	Paramus	44%	(a)

Would Definitely Recommend Hospital

Hospital Name	City	Rate	Cases
Deborah Heart & Lung Center	Browns Mills	87%	300+
Morristown Medical Center	Morristown	84%	300+
Valley Hospital	Ridgewood	81%	300+
Virtua West Jersey Hospitals Berlin	Berlin	81%	300+
Hackensack University Medical Center	Hackensack	80%	300+
Saint Peter's University Hospital	New Brunswick	79%	300+
Inspira Medical Center Elmer	Elmer	78%	300+
Hunterdon Medical Center	Flemington	77%	300+
Jersey Shore University Medical Center	Neptune	77%	300+
Univ Med Ctr of Princeton-Plainsboro	Plainsboro	76%	300+
Capital Health Medical Center - Hopewell	Pennington	75%	300+
Robert Wood Johnson University Hospital	New Brunswick	74%	300+
Centrastate Medical Center	Freehold	73%	300+
Shore Medical Center	Somers Point	73%	300+
Capital Health System - Fuld Campus	Trenton	72%	300+
Englewood Hospital & Medical Center	Englewood	72%	300+
Saint Barnabas Medical Center	Livingston	72%	300+
Holy Name Medical Center	Teaneck	71%	300+
Monmouth Medical Center	Long Branch	71%	300+
Somerset Medical Center	Somerville	71%	300+
Atlanticare Regional Medical Center	Atlantic City	70%	300+
Cooper University Hospital	Camden	70%	300+
Our Lady of Lourdes Medical Center	Camden	70%	300+
Overlook Medical Center	Summit	70%	300+
Saint Clare's Hospital	Denville	70%	300+
Hackensack - Umc Mountainside	Montclair	69%	300+
Ocean Medical Center	Brick	69%	300+
Robert W Johnson Univ Hosp-Hamilton	Hamilton	69%	300+
Riverview Medical Center	Red Bank	68%	300+
Cape Regional Medical Center	Cape May CH	66%	300+
Libertyhealth-Jersey City Med Ctr	Jersey City	66%	300+
Saint Joseph's Regional Medical Center	Paterson	66%	300+
Virtua Mem Hosp of Burlington County	Mount Holly	66%	300+
Carepoint Health - Hoboken UMC	Hoboken	65%	300+
Chilton Medical Center	Pompton Plains	64%	300+
Hackettstown Regional Medical Center	Hackettstown	64%	300+
Saint Luke's Warren Hospital	Phillipsburg	64%	300+
Southern Ocean Medical Center	Manahawkin	63%	300+
Kennedy Univ Hosp-Stratford Div	Stratford	62%	300+
Palisades Medical Center	North Bergen	62%	300+
University Hospital	Newark	62%	300+
Bergen Regional Medical Center	Paramus	61%	(a)
JFK Med Ctr-A M Yelencsics Comm Hosp	Edison	61%	300+
Robert Wood Johnson Univ Hosp-Rahway	Rahway	61%	300+
Saint Michael's Medical Center	Newark	61%	300+
Bayshore Community Hospital	Holmdel	60%	300+
Newark Beth Israel Medical Center	Newark	60%	300+
Clara Maass Medical Center	Belleville	59%	300+
Community Medical Center	Toms River	59%	300+
Inspira Medical Center Woodbury	Woodbury	59%	300+
Newton Memorial Hospital	Newton	58%	300+
Raritan Bay Medical Center	Perth Amboy	58%	300+
Saint Francis Medical Center	Trenton	58%	300+
Trinitas Regional Medical Center[11]	Elizabeth	58%	300+
Carepoint Health - Christ Hospital	Jersey City	57%	300+
Monmouth Medical Center - Southern Campus	Lakewood	57%	300+
Inspira Medical Center Vineland	Vineland	56%	300+
Meadowlands Hospital Medical Center	Secaucus	55%	300+
Carepoint Health-Bayonne Hosp Ctr	Bayonne	54%	300+
East Orange General Hospital	East Orange	54%	300+
Memorial Hospital of Salem County	Salem	53%	300+
Saint Mary's Hospital - Passaic	Passaic	52%	300+
Lourdes Med Ctr of Burlington County	Willingboro	45%	300+

Use of Medical Imaging

Cardiac Imaging Stress Test before OP Surgery

Hospital Name	City	Rate	Cases
Southern Ocean Medical Center	Manahawkin	0.7%	137
Saint Francis Medical Center	Trenton	1.3%	75
Capital Health System - Fuld Campus	Trenton	3.4%	175
Palisades Medical Center	North Bergen	3.8%	209
Carepoint Health - Christ Hospital	Jersey City	3.9%	181
University Hospital	Newark	3.9%	76
Hunterdon Medical Center	Flemington	4.1%	657
Kennedy Univ Hosp-Stratford Div	Stratford	4.1%	241
Deborah Heart & Lung Center	Browns Mills	4.2%	637
Centrastate Medical Center	Freehold	4.4%	249
Bayshore Community Hospital	Holmdel	4.5%	199
Englewood Hospital & Medical Center	Englewood	4.6%	1727
Atlanticare Regional Medical Center	Atlantic City	4.8%	913
Saint Peter's University Hospital	New Brunswick	4.8%	165
Inspira Medical Center Elmer	Elmer	4.9%	143
Saint Clare's Hospital	Denville	4.9%	648
Virtua Mem Hosp of Burlington County	Mount Holly	4.9%	285
Lourdes Med Ctr of Burlington County	Willingboro	5.0%	121
Capital Health Medical Center - Hopewell	Pennington	5.1%	396
JFK Med Ctr-A M Yelencsics Comm Hosp	Edison	5.1%	430
Raritan Bay Medical Center	Perth Amboy	5.1%	198
Trinitas Regional Medical Center	Elizabeth	5.1%	177
Univ Med Ctr of Princeton-Plainsboro	Plainsboro	5.1%	195
Newton Memorial Hospital	Newton	5.3%	114
Carepoint Health-Bayonne Hosp Ctr	Bayonne	5.4%	611
Overlook Medical Center	Summit	5.4%	1278
Inspira Medical Center Woodbury	Woodbury	5.6%	539
Our Lady of Lourdes Medical Center	Camden	5.6%	3039
Inspira Medical Center Vineland	Vineland	5.7%	192
Somerset Medical Center	Somerville	5.7%	507
Carepoint Health - Hoboken UMC	Hoboken	5.8%	121
Hackensack University Medical Center	Hackensack	5.8%	1609
Saint Joseph's Regional Medical Center	Paterson	6.0%	1951
Saint Michael's Medical Center	Newark	6.0%	302
Saint Barnabas Medical Center	Livingston	6.3%	1642
Riverview Medical Center	Red Bank	6.4%	249
Cooper University Hospital	Camden	6.5%	155
Holy Name Medical Center	Teaneck	6.5%	383
Morristown Medical Center	Morristown	6.5%	2195
Virtua West Jersey Hospitals Berlin	Berlin	6.7%	628
Chilton Medical Center	Pompton Plains	6.9%	145
Community Medical Center	Toms River	6.9%	203
Jersey Shore University Medical Center	Neptune	6.9%	403
Libertyhealth-Jersey City Med Ctr	Jersey City	7.0%	100

NOTE: Hospital profiles are in alphabetical order by state, then city, then hospital within the city; Rankings exclude hospitals with less than 25 cases except for patient surveys which excludes hospitals with less than 100 cases; (a) 100-299 cases; (1) The number of cases/patients is too few to report; (2) Data submitted were based on a sample of cases/patients; (3) Results are based on a shorter time period than required; (4) Data suppressed by CMS for one or more quarters; (5) Results are not available for this reporting period; (6) Fewer than 100 patients completed the HCAHPS survey; (7) No cases met the criteria for this measure; (8) The lower limit of the confidence interval cannot be calculated if the number of observed infections equals zero; (9) No data are available from the state/territory for this reporting period; (10) The scores shown reflect fewer than 50 completed surveys; (11) There were discrepancies in the data collection process; (12) This measure does not apply to this hospital for this reporting period; (13) Results cannot be calculated for this reporting period; (14) The results for this state are combined with nearby states to protect confidentiality; Please refer to the User's Guide for a full explanation of data.

Hospital Name	City	Rate	Cases
Newark Beth Israel Medical Center	Newark	7.0%	383
Valley Hospital	Ridgewood	7.0%	455
Monmouth Medical Center	Long Branch	7.2%	690
Robert W Johnson Univ Hosp-Hamilton	Hamilton	7.5%	80
Robert Wood Johnson Univ Hosp-Rahway	Rahway	7.5%	120
Robert Wood Johnson University Hospital	New Brunswick	7.6%	290
Ocean Medical Center	Brick	7.8%	154
Hackettstown Regional Medical Center	Hackettstown	8.8%	204
Cape Regional Medical Center	Cape May CH	9.6%	187
Saint Luke's Warren Hospital	Phillipsburg	10.4%	279
Clara Maass Medical Center	Belleville	11.4%	210
Shore Medical Center	Somers Point	11.4%	79

Combination Abdominal CT Scan

Hospital Name	City	Rate	Cases
Robert Wood Johnson University Hospital	New Brunswick	0.8%	723
Saint Luke's Warren Hospital	Phillipsburg	1.4%	814
Saint Peter's University Hospital	New Brunswick	1.6%	433
Virtua Mem Hosp of Burlington County	Mount Holly	1.7%	752
Virtua West Jersey Hospitals Berlin	Berlin	1.7%	1414
Newton Memorial Hospital	Newton	2.0%	637
Meadowlands Hospital Medical Center	Secaucus	2.3%	129
Atlanticare Regional Medical Center	Atlantic City	2.5%	1080
Robert W Johnson Univ Hosp-Hamilton	Hamilton	2.8%	1119
Trinitas Regional Medical Center	Elizabeth	2.8%	716
Hackensack University Medical Center	Hackensack	2.9%	2445
Deborah Heart & Lung Center	Browns Mills	3.2%	94
Lourdes Med Ctr of Burlington County	Willingboro	3.2%	747
Community Medical Center	Toms River	3.4%	1549
Centrastate Medical Center	Freehold	3.5%	944
Univ Med Ctr of Princeton-Plainsboro	Plainsboro	3.7%	644
Overlook Medical Center	Summit	3.8%	1486
Raritan Bay Medical Center	Perth Amboy	3.9%	824
Carepoint Health - Hoboken UMC	Hoboken	4.0%	272
Kennedy Univ Hosp-Stratford Div	Stratford	4.2%	2238
Southern Ocean Medical Center	Manahawkin	4.2%	914
Libertyhealth-Jersey City Med Ctr	Jersey City	4.3%	415
Capital Health System - Fuld Campus	Trenton	4.5%	550
Cooper University Hospital	Camden	4.6%	1285
Hunterdon Medical Center	Flemington	4.7%	849
Clara Maass Medical Center	Belleville	4.8%	598
Carepoint Health-Bayonne Hosp Ctr	Bayonne	4.9%	614
Morristown Medical Center	Morristown	4.9%	1860
Jersey Shore University Medical Center	Neptune	5.4%	1268
Riverview Medical Center	Red Bank	5.7%	1073
Robert Wood Johnson Univ Hosp-Rahway	Rahway	5.7%	546
Saint Clare's Hospital	Denville	5.7%	1599
Saint Mary's Hospital - Passaic	Passaic	5.9%	544
Saint Barnabas Medical Center	Livingston	6.1%	872
Bayshore Community Hospital	Holmdel	6.3%	856
Carepoint Health - Christ Hospital	Jersey City	6.8%	473
Saint Francis Medical Center	Trenton	6.9%	304
Inspira Medical Center Vineland	Vineland	7.2%	1113
Valley Hospital	Ridgewood	7.2%	2336
East Orange General Hospital	East Orange	7.4%	122
Ocean Medical Center	Brick	7.6%	1442
Holy Name Medical Center	Teaneck	7.8%	1314
Monmouth Medical Center	Long Branch	7.8%	617
Palisades Medical Center	North Bergen	7.8%	487
Shore Medical Center	Somers Point	8.1%	603
Monmouth Medical Center - Southern Campus	Lakewood	8.2%	478
Saint Michael's Medical Center	Newark	8.5%	471
Capital Health Medical Center - Hopewell	Pennington	8.8%	764
Inspira Medical Center Elmer	Elmer	9.0%	391
Memorial Hospital of Salem County	Salem	9.4%	413
Englewood Hospital & Medical Center	Englewood	10.2%	1615
Hackettstown Regional Medical Center	Hackettstown	11.4%	552
Our Lady of Lourdes Medical Center	Camden	11.7%	736
Saint Joseph's Regional Medical Center	Paterson	12.2%	1562
JFK Med Ctr-A M Yelencsics Comm Hosp	Edison	15.5%	1420
Newark Beth Israel Medical Center	Newark	16.1%	492
Hackensack - Umc Mountainside	Montclair	17.0%	788
Somerset Medical Center	Somerville	18.1%	936
Chilton Medical Center	Pompton Plains	26.0%	1176
Cape Regional Medical Center	Cape May CH	32.6%	858
University Hospital	Newark	40.5%	494

Combination Brain/Sinus CT Scan

Hospital Name	City	Rate	Cases
Cape Regional Medical Center	Cape May CH	0.4%	954
JFK Med Ctr-A M Yelencsics Comm Hosp	Edison	0.7%	1735
Riverview Medical Center	Red Bank	0.7%	831
Cooper University Hospital	Camden	0.9%	550
Univ Med Ctr of Princeton-Plainsboro	Plainsboro	0.9%	961
Virtua Mem Hosp of Burlington County	Mount Holly	1.2%	1163
Our Lady of Lourdes Medical Center	Camden	1.4%	937
Raritan Bay Medical Center	Perth Amboy	1.4%	984
Valley Hospital	Ridgewood	1.5%	1994
Centrastate Medical Center	Freehold	1.7%	1552
Overlook Medical Center	Summit	1.7%	1548
Robert W Johnson Univ Hosp-Hamilton	Hamilton	1.8%	1060
Somerset Medical Center	Somerville	1.9%	1046
Libertyhealth-Jersey City Med Ctr	Jersey City	2.0%	546
Clara Maass Medical Center	Belleville	2.1%	715
Holy Name Medical Center	Teaneck	2.1%	869
Morristown Medical Center	Morristown	2.1%	1187
University Hospital	Newark	2.1%	472
Bayshore Community Hospital	Holmdel	2.3%	554
Inspira Medical Center Woodbury	Woodbury	2.3%	1039
Lourdes Med Ctr of Burlington County	Willingboro	2.3%	1160
Newton Memorial Hospital	Newton	2.3%	619
Robert Wood Johnson University Hospital	New Brunswick	2.3%	1006
Robert Wood Johnson Univ Hosp-Rahway	Rahway	2.3%	565
Ocean Medical Center	Brick	2.4%	1780
Palisades Medical Center	North Bergen	2.4%	592
Hunterdon Medical Center	Flemington	2.5%	681
Inspira Medical Center Vineland	Vineland	2.5%	1285
Southern Ocean Medical Center	Manahawkin	2.5%	986
Monmouth Medical Center - Southern Campus	Lakewood	2.6%	880
Saint Joseph's Regional Medical Center	Paterson	2.6%	1606
Virtua West Jersey Hospitals Berlin	Berlin	2.6%	2274
Hackensack University Medical Center	Hackensack	2.7%	2005
Carepoint Health-Bayonne Hosp Ctr	Bayonne	2.9%	645
Englewood Hospital & Medical Center	Englewood	2.9%	1311
Community Medical Center	Toms River	3.0%	2215
Hackensack - Umc Mountainside	Montclair	3.1%	642
Saint Luke's Warren Hospital	Phillipsburg	3.2%	728
Jersey Shore University Medical Center	Neptune	3.9%	1556
Saint Clare's Hospital	Denville	4.0%	1219
Atlanticare Regional Medical Center	Atlantic City	4.1%	1415
Saint Michael's Medical Center	Newark	4.3%	416
Trinitas Regional Medical Center	Elizabeth	4.3%	635
Monmouth Medical Center	Long Branch	4.4%	566
Saint Barnabas Medical Center	Livingston	4.4%	1184
Shore Medical Center	Somers Point	4.4%	910
Kennedy Univ Hosp-Stratford Div	Stratford	4.7%	2341
Hackettstown Regional Medical Center	Hackettstown	5.0%	516
Carepoint Health - Christ Hospital	Jersey City	5.3%	490
Chilton Medical Center	Pompton Plains	5.3%	1064
Memorial Hospital of Salem County	Salem	5.3%	434
Capital Health System - Fuld Campus	Trenton	5.4%	654
Saint Peter's University Hospital	New Brunswick	5.7%	581
Saint Francis Medical Center	Trenton	5.8%	415
Bergen Regional Medical Center	Paramus	6.6%	151
Capital Health Medical Center - Hopewell	Pennington	6.6%	588

Combination Chest CT Scan

Hospital Name	City	Rate	Cases
East Orange General Hospital	East Orange	0.0%	51
Monmouth Medical Center - Southern Campus	Lakewood	0.0%	354
Saint Peter's University Hospital	New Brunswick	0.0%	162
Virtua Mem Hosp of Burlington County	Mount Holly	0.0%	285
Virtua West Jersey Hospitals Berlin	Berlin	0.0%	448
Centrastate Medical Center	Freehold	0.2%	457
Morristown Medical Center	Morristown	0.2%	1860
Robert W Johnson Univ Hosp-Hamilton	Hamilton	0.2%	489
Trinitas Regional Medical Center	Elizabeth	0.2%	414
Atlanticare Regional Medical Center	Atlantic City	0.3%	301
Bayshore Community Hospital	Holmdel	0.3%	600
Englewood Hospital & Medical Center	Englewood	0.3%	1298
JFK Med Ctr-A M Yelencsics Comm Hosp	Edison	0.3%	1086
Monmouth Medical Center	Long Branch	0.3%	625
Newton Memorial Hospital	Newton	0.3%	354
Saint Luke's Warren Hospital	Phillipsburg	0.3%	359
Deborah Heart & Lung Center	Browns Mills	0.4%	517
Robert Wood Johnson University Hospital	New Brunswick	0.4%	245
Cooper University Hospital	Camden	0.5%	1149
Memorial Hospital of Salem County	Salem	0.5%	217
Hackensack University Medical Center	Hackensack	0.6%	2957
Saint Mary's Hospital - Passaic	Passaic	0.6%	352
Jersey Shore University Medical Center	Neptune	0.7%	861
Lourdes Med Ctr of Burlington County	Willingboro	0.7%	277
Riverview Medical Center	Red Bank	0.7%	865
Inspira Medical Center Elmer	Elmer	0.8%	252
Saint Clare's Hospital	Denville	0.8%	915
Inspira Medical Center Vineland	Vineland	0.9%	641
Somerset Medical Center	Somerville	1.0%	763
University Hospital	Newark	1.2%	254
Raritan Bay Medical Center	Perth Amboy	1.3%	311
Univ Med Ctr of Princeton-Plainsboro	Plainsboro	1.3%	371
Cape Regional Medical Center	Cape May CH	1.4%	280
Hunterdon Medical Center	Flemington	1.4%	768
Palisades Medical Center	North Bergen	1.4%	213
Meadowlands Hospital Medical Center	Secaucus	1.6%	64
Kennedy Univ Hosp-Stratford Div	Stratford	2.0%	1399
Capital Health System - Fuld Campus	Trenton	2.5%	355
Ocean Medical Center	Brick	2.5%	1001
Community Medical Center	Toms River	2.6%	728
Overlook Medical Center	Summit	2.6%	1307
Robert Wood Johnson Univ Hosp-Rahway	Rahway	2.6%	340
Carepoint Health-Bayonne Hosp Ctr	Bayonne	3.0%	370
Carepoint Health - Christ Hospital	Jersey City	3.1%	223
Carepoint Health - Hoboken UMC	Hoboken	3.2%	124
Capital Health Medical Center - Hopewell	Pennington	3.9%	563
Hackettstown Regional Medical Center	Hackettstown	4.0%	351
Southern Ocean Medical Center	Manahawkin	4.3%	439
Newark Beth Israel Medical Center	Newark	4.5%	579
Shore Medical Center	Somers Point	4.5%	292
Libertyhealth-Jersey City Med Ctr	Jersey City	4.8%	147
Clara Maass Medical Center	Belleville	4.9%	142
Inspira Medical Center Woodbury	Woodbury	5.0%	260
Valley Hospital	Ridgewood	5.1%	2163
Holy Name Medical Center	Teaneck	5.8%	830
Saint Joseph's Regional Medical Center	Paterson	5.8%	807
Saint Barnabas Medical Center	Livingston	6.7%	329
Saint Michael's Medical Center	Newark	8.1%	197
Saint Francis Medical Center	Trenton	8.5%	153
Hackensack - Umc Mountainside	Montclair	10.4%	396
Our Lady of Lourdes Medical Center	Camden	13.5%	289
Chilton Medical Center	Pompton Plains	19.5%	691

Follow-up Mammogram/Ultrasound

A follow-up rate near zero may indicate missed cancer; a rate higher than 14% may mean there is unnecessary follow up.

Hospital Name	City	Rate	Cases
Trinitas Regional Medical Center	Elizabeth	3.9%	839
University Hospital	Newark	4.5%	467
Robert Wood Johnson Univ Hosp-Rahway	Rahway	5.1%	257
Monmouth Medical Center	Long Branch	5.7%	3045
East Orange General Hospital	East Orange	6.1%	229
Raritan Bay Medical Center	Perth Amboy	6.1%	933
Saint Joseph's Regional Medical Center	Paterson	6.2%	2192
Monmouth Medical Center - Southern Campus	Lakewood	6.3%	63
Robert W Johnson Univ Hosp-Hamilton	Hamilton	7.2%	1103
Saint Michael's Medical Center	Newark	7.4%	842
Capital Health Medical Center - Hopewell	Pennington	7.9%	1248
Capital Health System - Fuld Campus	Trenton	8.2%	281
Atlanticare Regional Medical Center	Atlantic City	8.4%	877
Univ Med Ctr of Princeton-Plainsboro	Plainsboro	8.4%	735
Valley Hospital	Ridgewood	8.8%	1714
Hackensack - Umc Mountainside	Montclair	9.1%	375
Saint Luke's Warren Hospital	Phillipsburg	9.3%	1164
Shore Medical Center	Somers Point	9.4%	672
Clara Maass Medical Center	Belleville	9.6%	407
JFK Med Ctr-A M Yelencsics Comm Hosp	Edison	9.6%	1992
Palisades Medical Center	North Bergen	10.0%	460
Lourdes Med Ctr of Burlington County	Willingboro	10.1%	477
Saint Francis Medical Center	Trenton	10.4%	367
Carepoint Health-Bayonne Hosp Ctr	Bayonne	10.5%	686
Hunterdon Medical Center	Flemington	10.5%	1637
Virtua Mem Hosp of Burlington County	Mount Holly	10.5%	306
Newark Beth Israel Medical Center	Newark	10.6%	642
Bayshore Community Hospital	Holmdel	10.9%	939
Hackettstown Regional Medical Center	Hackettstown	11.0%	710
Southern Ocean Medical Center	Manahawkin	11.0%	1348
Inspira Medical Center Vineland	Vineland	11.1%	1762
Newton Memorial Hospital	Newton	11.1%	315
Carepoint Health - Christ Hospital	Jersey City	11.4%	762
Memorial Hospital of Salem County	Salem	11.4%	361
Somerset Medical Center	Somerville	11.9%	1037
Centrastate Medical Center	Freehold	12.0%	1056
Our Lady of Lourdes Medical Center	Camden	12.3%	204
Saint Peter's University Hospital	New Brunswick	12.3%	324
Kennedy Univ Hosp-Stratford Div	Stratford	12.4%	953
Saint Clare's Hospital	Denville	12.7%	3032
Carepoint Health - Hoboken UMC	Hoboken	12.9%	287
Libertyhealth-Jersey City Med Ctr	Jersey City	13.0%	253
Hackensack University Medical Center	Hackensack	13.4%	3109
Saint Mary's Hospital - Passaic	Passaic	13.5%	592
Inspira Medical Center Elmer	Elmer	13.6%	619
Cooper University Hospital	Camden	14.0%	1622
Chilton Medical Center	Pompton Plains	14.1%	2408
Inspira Medical Center Woodbury	Woodbury	14.3%	244
Meadowlands Hospital Medical Center	Secaucus	14.3%	98
Community Medical Center	Toms River	15.3%	1132
Ocean Medical Center	Brick	16.4%	1198
Morristown Medical Center	Morristown	17.3%	1240
Riverview Medical Center	Red Bank	19.3%	848
Virtua West Jersey Hospitals Berlin	Berlin	19.3%	114
Englewood Hospital & Medical Center	Englewood	19.4%	3693
Overlook Medical Center	Summit	21.1%	920
Holy Name Medical Center	Teaneck	45.1%	1642

Lumbar Spine MRI for Low Back Pain

Hospital Name	City	Rate	Cases
Morristown Medical Center	Morristown	22.7%	110
Hackensack University Medical Center	Hackensack	27.9%	86
Somerset Medical Center	Somerville	28.2%	85
Valley Hospital	Ridgewood	28.5%	130
Inspira Medical Center Vineland	Vineland	30.5%	128
JFK Med Ctr-A M Yelencsics Comm Hosp	Edison	30.6%	216

NOTE: Hospital profiles are in alphabetical order by state, then city, then hospital within the city; Rankings exclude hospitals with less than 25 cases except for patient surveys which excludes hospitals with less than 100 cases; (a) 100-299 cases; (1) The number of cases/patients is too few to report; (2) Data submitted were based on a sample of cases/patients; (3) Results are based on a shorter time period than required; (4) Data suppressed by CMS for one or more quarters; (5) Results are not available for this reporting period; (6) Fewer than 100 patients completed the HCAHPS survey; (7) No cases met the criteria for this measure; (8) The lower limit of the confidence interval cannot be calculated if the number of observed infections equals zero; (9) No data are available from the state/territory for this reporting period; (10) The scores shown reflect fewer than 50 completed surveys; (11) There were discrepancies in the data collection process; (12) This measure does not apply to this hospital for this reporting period; (13) Results cannot be calculated for this reporting period; (14) The results for this state are combined with nearby states to protect confidentiality; Please refer to the User's Guide for a full explanation of data.

Chilton Medical Center	Pompton Plains	31.1%	151
Carepoint Health-Bayonne Hosp Ctr	Bayonne	31.3%	80
Englewood Hospital & Medical Center	Englewood	31.7%	189
Monmouth Medical Center	Long Branch	32.4%	68
Overlook Medical Center	Summit	32.4%	68
Holy Name Medical Center	Teaneck	33.0%	230
Kennedy Univ Hosp-Stratford Div	Stratford	33.3%	72
Saint Joseph's Regional Medical Center	Paterson	35.8%	187
Cooper University Hospital	Camden	35.9%	153
Bayshore Community Hospital	Holmdel	36.9%	84
Saint Luke's Warren Hospital	Phillipsburg	38.7%	75
Memorial Hospital of Salem County	Salem	38.8%	80
Ocean Medical Center	Brick	40.4%	52
Virtua West Jersey Hospitals Berlin	Berlin	41.0%	39
Saint Clare's Hospital	Denville	41.2%	51
Community Medical Center	Toms River	44.7%	38
Hackensack - Umc Mountainside	Montclair	47.1%	34
Newark Beth Israel Medical Center	Newark	47.1%	51
Capital Health Medical Center - Hopewell	Pennington	50.9%	53

NOTE: Hospital profiles are in alphabetical order by state, then city, then hospital within the city; Rankings exclude hospitals with less than 25 cases except for patient surveys which excludes hospitals with less than 100 cases; (a) 100-299 cases; (1) The number of cases/patients is too few to report; (2) Data submitted were based on a sample of cases/patients; (3) Results are based on a shorter time period than required; (4) Data suppressed by CMS for one or more quarters; (5) Results are not available for this reporting period; (6) Fewer than 100 patients completed the HCAHPS survey; (7) No cases met the criteria for this measure; (8) The lower limit of the confidence interval cannot be calculated if the number of observed infections equals zero; (9) No data are available from the state/territory for this reporting period; (10) The scores shown reflect fewer than 50 completed surveys; (11) There were discrepancies in the data collection process; (12) This measure does not apply to this hospital for this reporting period; (13) Results cannot be calculated for this reporting period; (14) The results for this state are combined with nearby states to protect confidentiality; Please refer to the User's Guide for a full explanation of data.

Atlanticare Regional Medical Center

1925 Pacific Ave
Atlantic City, NJ 08401
URL: www.atlanticare.org/acmc/index.html
Type: Acute Care Hospitals
Ownership: Voluntary non-profit - Other
Phone: 609-441-8020
Fax: 609-441-2108
Emergency Services: Yes
Beds: 442

Key Personnel:
CEO/President. . . . . Lori Herndon

Measure	Cases	This Hosp.	State Avg.	U.S. Avg.
Blood Clot Prevention and Treatment				
Anticoagulation Overlap Therapy[2]	250	100%	88%	93%
ICU Venous Thromboembolism Prophylaxis[2]	71	97%	93%	92%
Incidence of Potentially Preventable VTE[2]	64	6%	10%	10%
UFH with Dosages/Platelet Monitoring[2]	281	100%	99%	97%
Venous Thromboembolism Prophylaxis[2]	331	85%	83%	85%
Warfarin Therapy Discharge Instructions[2]	144	74%	77%	75%
Chest Pain/Possible Heart Attack Care				
Aspirin Given Within 24 Hours of Arrival[1,3]	-	-	98%	96%
Fibrinolytic Meds Within 30 Min. of Arrival[3,7]	-	-	63%	58%
Average Time to ECG (minutes)[1,3]	-	-	7	7
Average Time to Transfer (minutes)[3,7]	-	-	74	60
Children's Asthma Care				
Received Home Management Plan of Care	-	-	-	88%
Received Reliever Medication	-	-	-	100%
Received Systemic Corticosteroids	-	-	-	100%
Emergency Department				
Admittance Decision Time (minutes)[2]	810	167	148	98
Head CT Results Within 45 Min. of Arrival[7]	-	-	66%	57%
Patients Who Left ER Before Being Seen	>100k	2%	2%	2%
Time from ER Arrival to Admit. (minutes)[2]	810	340	355	274
Time from ER Arrival to Discharge (minutes)	395	142	152	134
Time in ER Before Being Evaluated (minutes)	429	23	32	26
Time to Pain Meds for Fractures (minutes)	180	56	58	57
Heart Attack Care				
Aspirin Given at Discharge[2]	341	100%	99%	99%
Fibrinolytic Meds Within 30 Min. of Arrival[2,7]	-	-	69%	54%
PCI Within 90 Minutes of Arrival[2]	81	95%	95%	96%
Statin Prescribed at Discharge[2]	322	100%	99%	98%
Heart Failure Care				
ACE Inhibitor or ARB for LVSD[2]	172	100%	98%	97%
Discharge Instructions Given[2]	446	99%	97%	94%
Evaluation of LVS Function[2]	563	100%	100%	99%
Medicare Spending				
Medicare Spending per Patient (ratio)	-	1.06	1.07	0.98
Pneumonia Care				
Appropriate Initial Antibiotic Given[2]	238	96%	98%	95%
Blood Culture Timing[2]	447	99%	99%	98%
Pregnancy and Delivery Care				
Newborn Deliveries Scheduled Early[2]	52	17%	3%	6%
Preventive Care				
Immunization for Influenza[2]	551	67%	93%	90%
Immunization for Pneumonia[2]	627	79%	94%	92%
Stroke Care				
Anticoagulation Therapy for Atrial Fibrillation	37	100%	97%	95%
Antithrombotic Therapy Timing	254	100%	98%	98%
Assessed for Rehabilitation	325	100%	98%	97%
Discharged on Antithrombotic Therapy	271	100%	99%	99%
Discharged on Statin Medication	219	99%	95%	94%
Thrombolytic Therapy Timing	21	95%	74%	66%
Venous Thromboembolism Prophylaxis	350	95%	94%	94%
Written Stroke Educational Materials Given	162	100%	94%	88%
Surgical Care Improvement Project				
Appropriate Beta Blocker Usage[2]	327	98%	98%	98%
Appropriate VTP Within 24 Hours[2]	477	99%	99%	98%
Controlled Postoperative Blood Glucose[2]	135	99%	97%	97%
Perioperative Temperature Management[2]	705	100%	100%	100%
Prophylactic Antibiotic Selection[2]	506	100%	99%	99%
Prophylactic Antibiotic Selection (Outpatient)	451	98%	97%	98%
Prophylactic Antibiotic Stopped[2]	500	99%	98%	98%
Prophylactic Antibiotic Timing[2]	508	100%	99%	99%
Prophylactic Antibiotic Timing (Outpatient)	450	98%	98%	98%
Urinary Catheter Removal[2]	322	98%	98%	97%
Survey of Patients' Hospital Experiences				
Area Around Room 'Always' Quiet at Night	300+	47%	53%	61%
Doctors 'Always' Communicated Well	300+	75%	77%	82%
Home Recovery Information Given	300+	87%	82%	85%
Hospital Given 9 or 10 on 10 Point Scale	300+	67%	64%	71%
Meds 'Always' Explained Before Given	300+	54%	59%	64%
Nurses 'Always' Communicated Well	300+	74%	76%	79%
Pain 'Always' Well Controlled	300+	63%	68%	71%
Room and Bathroom 'Always' Clean	300+	65%	68%	73%
Timely Help 'Always' Received	300+	61%	60%	68%
Would Definitely Recommend Hospital	300+	70%	66%	71%
Use of Medical Imaging				
Cardiac Imaging Stress Test before Surgery	913	4.8%	5.8%	5.3%
Combination Abdominal CT Scan	1,080	2.5%	7.4%	10.5%
Combination Brain/Sinus CT Scan	1,415	4.1%	2.8%	2.7%
Combination Chest CT Scan	301	0.3%	2.4%	2.7%
Follow-up Mammogram/Ultrasound	877	8.4%	12.5%	8.8%
Lumbar Spine MRI for Low Back Pain[1]	-	-	32.9%	37.2%

Carepoint Health - Bayonne Hospital Center

29 East 29th St
Bayonne, NJ 07002
URL: www.bayonnemedicalcenter.org
Type: Acute Care Hospitals
Ownership: Voluntary non-profit - Private
Phone: 201-858-5000
Fax: 201-858-7355
Emergency Services: Yes
Beds: 278

Key Personnel:
Pediatric In-Patient Care . . . . S Aly, MD
Radiology. . . . . Q Chew, MD
Chairman/CEO . . . . Daniel A. Kane
Quality Assurance . . . . Eileen Konecko
CEO/President. . . . . Mark Spektor

Measure	Cases	This Hosp.	State Avg.	U.S. Avg.
Blood Clot Prevention and Treatment				
Anticoagulation Overlap Therapy[2]	20	100%	88%	93%
ICU Venous Thromboembolism Prophylaxis[2]	90	100%	93%	92%
Incidence of Potentially Preventable VTE[1,2]	-	-	10%	10%
UFH with Dosages/Platelet Monitoring[2]	24	100%	99%	97%
Venous Thromboembolism Prophylaxis[2]	429	100%	83%	85%
Warfarin Therapy Discharge Instructions[2]	13	100%	77%	75%
Chest Pain/Possible Heart Attack Care				
Aspirin Given Within 24 Hours of Arrival[3,7]	-	-	98%	96%
Fibrinolytic Meds Within 30 Min. of Arrival[5]	-	-	63%	58%
Average Time to ECG (minutes)[3,7]	-	-	7	7
Average Time to Transfer (minutes)[5]	-	-	74	60
Children's Asthma Care				
Received Home Management Plan of Care	-	-	-	88%
Received Reliever Medication	-	-	-	100%
Received Systemic Corticosteroids	-	-	-	100%
Emergency Department				
Admittance Decision Time (minutes)[2]	745	149	148	98
Head CT Results Within 45 Min. of Arrival[1]	-	-	66%	57%
Patients Who Left ER Before Being Seen	28,516	2%	2%	2%
Time from ER Arrival to Admit. (minutes)[2]	749	332	355	274
Time from ER Arrival to Discharge (minutes)	401	164	152	134
Time in ER Before Being Evaluated (minutes)	444	31	32	26
Time to Pain Meds for Fractures (minutes)	66	58	58	57
Heart Attack Care				
Aspirin Given at Discharge	156	100%	99%	99%
Fibrinolytic Meds Within 30 Min. of Arrival[7]	-	-	69%	54%
PCI Within 90 Minutes of Arrival[1]	-	-	95%	96%
Statin Prescribed at Discharge	145	100%	99%	98%
Heart Failure Care				
ACE Inhibitor or ARB for LVSD[2]	61	100%	98%	97%
Discharge Instructions Given[2]	168	100%	97%	94%
Evaluation of LVS Function[2]	264	100%	100%	99%
Medicare Spending				
Medicare Spending per Patient (ratio)	-	1.13	1.07	0.98
Pneumonia Care				
Appropriate Initial Antibiotic Given[2]	71	100%	98%	95%
Blood Culture Timing[2]	133	100%	99%	98%
Pregnancy and Delivery Care				
Newborn Deliveries Scheduled Early[2,7]	-	-	3%	6%
Preventive Care				
Immunization for Influenza[2]	564	100%	93%	90%
Immunization for Pneumonia[2]	840	100%	94%	92%
Stroke Care				
Anticoagulation Therapy for Atrial Fibrillation[1]	-	-	97%	95%
Antithrombotic Therapy Timing	62	100%	98%	98%
Assessed for Rehabilitation	60	100%	98%	97%
Discharged on Antithrombotic Therapy	56	100%	99%	99%
Discharged on Statin Medication	49	100%	95%	94%
Thrombolytic Therapy Timing[1]	-	-	74%	66%
Venous Thromboembolism Prophylaxis	67	94%	94%	94%
Written Stroke Educational Materials Given	21	100%	94%	88%
Surgical Care Improvement Project				
Appropriate Beta Blocker Usage	41	100%	98%	98%
Appropriate VTP Within 24 Hours	130	98%	99%	98%
Controlled Postoperative Blood Glucose[7]	-	-	97%	97%
Perioperative Temperature Management	145	99%	100%	100%
Prophylactic Antibiotic Selection	42	100%	99%	99%
Prophylactic Antibiotic Selection (Outpatient)	29	97%	97%	98%
Prophylactic Antibiotic Stopped	39	90%	98%	98%
Prophylactic Antibiotic Timing	42	100%	99%	99%
Prophylactic Antibiotic Timing (Outpatient)	29	93%	98%	98%
Urinary Catheter Removal	72	100%	98%	97%
Survey of Patients' Hospital Experiences				
Area Around Room 'Always' Quiet at Night	300+	49%	53%	61%
Doctors 'Always' Communicated Well	300+	76%	77%	82%
Home Recovery Information Given	300+	82%	82%	85%
Hospital Given 9 or 10 on 10 Point Scale	300+	56%	64%	71%
Meds 'Always' Explained Before Given	300+	54%	59%	64%
Nurses 'Always' Communicated Well	300+	73%	76%	79%
Pain 'Always' Well Controlled	300+	63%	68%	71%
Room and Bathroom 'Always' Clean	300+	64%	68%	73%
Timely Help 'Always' Received	300+	62%	60%	68%
Would Definitely Recommend Hospital	300+	54%	66%	71%
Use of Medical Imaging				
Cardiac Imaging Stress Test before Surgery	611	5.4%	5.8%	5.3%
Combination Abdominal CT Scan	614	4.9%	7.4%	10.5%
Combination Brain/Sinus CT Scan	645	2.9%	2.8%	2.7%
Combination Chest CT Scan	370	3.0%	2.4%	2.7%
Follow-up Mammogram/Ultrasound	686	10.5%	12.5%	8.8%
Lumbar Spine MRI for Low Back Pain	80	31.3%	32.9%	37.2%

Clara Maass Medical Center

One Clara Maas Drive
Belleville, NJ 07109
E-mail: info@sbhcs.com
URL: www.sbhcs.com/hospitals
Type: Acute Care Hospitals
Ownership: Voluntary non-profit - Private
Phone: 973-450-2002
Fax: 973-450-0181
Emergency Services: Yes
Beds: 445

Key Personnel:
Intensive Care Unit. . . . . Ronnie Castro
Anesthesiology. . . . . Jose A Dtetres-Palacio, MD
Operating Room. . . . . Sue Gallina
Radiology. . . . . James A Heimann
Infection Control. . . . . Edward S Johnson
Quality Assurance . . . . Margaret Nielson
Emergency Room . . . . Karen Palletello, MD
Cardiac Laboratory. . . . . Michelle Witwick

Measure	Cases	This Hosp.	State Avg.	U.S. Avg.
Blood Clot Prevention and Treatment				
Anticoagulation Overlap Therapy[2]	77	64%	88%	93%
ICU Venous Thromboembolism Prophylaxis[2]	61	82%	93%	92%
Incidence of Potentially Preventable VTE[2]	27	33%	10%	10%
UFH with Dosages/Platelet Monitoring[1,2]	-	-	99%	97%
Venous Thromboembolism Prophylaxis[2]	408	71%	83%	85%
Warfarin Therapy Discharge Instructions[2]	40	62%	77%	75%
Chest Pain/Possible Heart Attack Care				
Aspirin Given Within 24 Hours of Arrival[5]	-	-	98%	96%
Fibrinolytic Meds Within 30 Min. of Arrival[5]	-	-	63%	58%
Average Time to ECG (minutes)[5]	-	-	7	7
Average Time to Transfer (minutes)[5]	-	-	74	60
Children's Asthma Care				
Received Home Management Plan of Care	-	-	-	88%
Received Reliever Medication	-	-	-	100%
Received Systemic Corticosteroids	-	-	-	100%
Emergency Department				
Admittance Decision Time (minutes)[2]	233	227	148	98

NOTE: Hospital profiles are in alphabetical order by state, then city, then hospital within the city; Rankings exclude hospitals with less than 25 cases except for patient surveys which excludes hospitals with less than 100 cases; (a) 100-299 cases; (1) The number of cases/patients is too few to report; (2) Data submitted were based on a sample of cases/patients; (3) Results are based on a shorter time period than required; (4) Data suppressed by CMS for one or more quarters; (5) Results are not available for this reporting period; (6) Fewer than 100 patients completed the HCAHPS survey; (7) No cases met the criteria for this measure; (8) The lower limit of the confidence interval cannot be calculated if the number of observed infections equals zero; (9) No data are available from the state/territory for this reporting period; (10) The scores shown reflect fewer than 50 completed surveys; (11) There were discrepancies in the data collection process; (12) This measure does not apply to this hospital for this reporting period; (13) Results cannot be calculated for this reporting period; (14) The results for this state are combined with nearby states to protect confidentiality; Please refer to the User's Guide for a full explanation of data.

Measure	Cases	This Hosp.	State Avg.	U.S. Avg.
Head CT Results Within 45 Min. of Arrival[1]	-	-	66%	57%
Patients Who Left ER Before Being Seen	39,658	3%	2%	2%
Time from ER Arrival to Admit. (minutes)[2]	233	522	355	274
Time from ER Arrival to Discharge (minutes)	344	152	152	134
Time in ER Before Being Evaluated (minutes)	432	48	32	26
Time to Pain Meds for Fractures (minutes)	250	72	58	57
Heart Attack Care				
Aspirin Given at Discharge[2]	203	100%	99%	99%
Fibrinolytic Meds Within 30 Min. of Arrival[2,7]	-	-	69%	54%
PCI Within 90 Minutes of Arrival[2]	35	97%	95%	96%
Statin Prescribed at Discharge[2]	207	100%	99%	98%
Heart Failure Care				
ACE Inhibitor or ARB for LVSD[2]	81	100%	98%	97%
Discharge Instructions Given[2]	229	100%	97%	94%
Evaluation of LVS Function[2]	309	100%	100%	99%
Medicare Spending				
Medicare Spending per Patient (ratio)	-	1.13	1.07	0.98
Pneumonia Care				
Appropriate Initial Antibiotic Given[2]	125	98%	98%	95%
Blood Culture Timing[2]	196	100%	99%	98%
Pregnancy and Delivery Care				
Newborn Deliveries Scheduled Early	190	2%	3%	6%
Preventive Care				
Immunization for Influenza[2]	549	96%	93%	90%
Immunization for Pneumonia[2]	697	91%	94%	92%
Stroke Care				
Anticoagulation Therapy for Atrial Fibrillation	16	100%	97%	95%
Antithrombotic Therapy Timing	107	100%	98%	98%
Assessed for Rehabilitation	138	100%	98%	97%
Discharged on Antithrombotic Therapy	110	100%	99%	99%
Discharged on Statin Medication	81	95%	95%	94%
Thrombolytic Therapy Timing[1]	-	-	74%	66%
Venous Thromboembolism Prophylaxis	148	97%	94%	94%
Written Stroke Educational Materials Given	62	97%	94%	88%
Surgical Care Improvement Project				
Appropriate Beta Blocker Usage[2]	84	98%	98%	98%
Appropriate VTP Within 24 Hours[2]	376	100%	99%	98%
Controlled Postoperative Blood Glucose[2,7]	-	-	97%	97%
Perioperative Temperature Management[2]	423	100%	100%	100%
Prophylactic Antibiotic Selection[2]	252	100%	99%	99%
Prophylactic Antibiotic Selection (Outpatient)	162	94%	97%	98%
Prophylactic Antibiotic Stopped[2]	248	100%	98%	98%
Prophylactic Antibiotic Timing[2]	252	100%	99%	99%
Prophylactic Antibiotic Timing (Outpatient)	164	99%	98%	98%
Urinary Catheter Removal[2]	244	100%	98%	97%
Survey of Patients' Hospital Experiences				
Area Around Room 'Always' Quiet at Night	300+	48%	53%	61%
Doctors 'Always' Communicated Well	300+	77%	77%	82%
Home Recovery Information Given	300+	80%	82%	85%
Hospital Given 9 or 10 on 10 Point Scale	300+	57%	64%	71%
Meds 'Always' Explained Before Given	300+	57%	59%	64%
Nurses 'Always' Communicated Well	300+	75%	76%	79%
Pain 'Always' Well Controlled	300+	66%	68%	71%
Room and Bathroom 'Always' Clean	300+	70%	68%	73%
Timely Help 'Always' Received	300+	58%	60%	68%
Would Definitely Recommend Hospital	300+	59%	66%	71%
Use of Medical Imaging				
Cardiac Imaging Stress Test before Surgery	210	11.4%	5.8%	5.3%
Combination Abdominal CT Scan	598	4.8%	7.4%	10.5%
Combination Brain/Sinus CT Scan	715	2.1%	2.8%	2.7%
Combination Chest CT Scan	142	4.9%	2.4%	2.7%
Follow-up Mammogram/Ultrasound	407	9.6%	12.5%	8.8%
Lumbar Spine MRI for Low Back Pain[1]	-	-	32.9%	37.2%

Virtua West Jersey Hospitals Berlin

Whitehorse Pike & Townsend Avenue Phone: 856-322-3200
Berlin, NJ 08009 Fax: 609-265-9514
URL: www.virtua.org
Type: Acute Care Hospitals Emergency Services: Yes
Ownership: Voluntary non-profit - Private Beds: 92

Key Personnel:
CEO/President................ Gary Long
Emergency Room .... Eileen Singer

Measure	Cases	This Hosp.	State Avg.	U.S. Avg.
Blood Clot Prevention and Treatment				
Anticoagulation Overlap Therapy[2]	268	95%	88%	93%
ICU Venous Thromboembolism Prophylaxis[2]	51	92%	93%	92%
Incidence of Potentially Preventable VTE[2]	54	11%	10%	10%
UFH with Dosages/Platelet Monitoring[2]	232	94%	99%	97%
Venous Thromboembolism Prophylaxis[2]	381	80%	83%	85%
Warfarin Therapy Discharge Instructions[2]	185	90%	77%	75%
Chest Pain/Possible Heart Attack Care				
Aspirin Given Within 24 Hours of Arrival	77	100%	98%	96%
Fibrinolytic Meds Within 30 Min. of Arrival[7]	-	-	63%	58%
Average Time to ECG (minutes)	78	4	7	7
Average Time to Transfer (minutes)[1]	-	-	74	60
Children's Asthma Care				
Received Home Management Plan of Care	-	-	-	88%
Received Reliever Medication	-	-	-	100%
Received Systemic Corticosteroids	-	-	-	100%
Emergency Department				
Admittance Decision Time (minutes)[2]	611	148	148	98
Head CT Results Within 45 Min. of Arrival	60	70%	66%	57%
Patients Who Left ER Before Being Seen	>100k	1%	2%	2%
Time from ER Arrival to Admit. (minutes)[2]	612	330	355	274
Time from ER Arrival to Discharge (minutes)	401	118	152	134
Time in ER Before Being Evaluated (minutes)	381	44	32	26
Time to Pain Meds for Fractures (minutes)	282	33	58	57
Heart Attack Care				
Aspirin Given at Discharge	340	100%	99%	99%
Fibrinolytic Meds Within 30 Min. of Arrival[7]	-	-	69%	54%
PCI Within 90 Minutes of Arrival	51	94%	95%	96%
Statin Prescribed at Discharge	333	99%	99%	98%
Heart Failure Care				
ACE Inhibitor or ARB for LVSD	153	100%	98%	97%
Discharge Instructions Given	531	96%	97%	94%
Evaluation of LVS Function	746	100%	100%	99%
Medicare Spending				
Medicare Spending per Patient (ratio)	-	1.04	1.07	0.98
Pneumonia Care				
Appropriate Initial Antibiotic Given	497	97%	98%	95%
Blood Culture Timing	956	100%	99%	98%
Pregnancy and Delivery Care				
Newborn Deliveries Scheduled Early[2]	109	4%	3%	6%
Preventive Care				
Immunization for Influenza[2]	532	98%	93%	90%
Immunization for Pneumonia[2]	631	96%	94%	92%
Stroke Care				
Anticoagulation Therapy for Atrial Fibrillation	26	100%	97%	95%
Antithrombotic Therapy Timing	217	97%	98%	98%
Assessed for Rehabilitation	215	98%	98%	97%
Discharged on Antithrombotic Therapy	213	100%	99%	99%
Discharged on Statin Medication	168	96%	95%	94%
Thrombolytic Therapy Timing[1]	-	-	74%	66%
Venous Thromboembolism Prophylaxis	214	99%	94%	94%
Written Stroke Educational Materials Given	126	99%	94%	88%
Surgical Care Improvement Project				
Appropriate Beta Blocker Usage[2]	966	100%	98%	98%
Appropriate VTP Within 24 Hours[2]	2,355	100%	99%	98%
Controlled Postoperative Blood Glucose[2,7]	-	-	97%	97%
Perioperative Temperature Management[2]	3,175	100%	100%	100%
Prophylactic Antibiotic Selection[2]	2,661	100%	99%	99%
Prophylactic Antibiotic Selection (Outpatient)	352	98%	97%	98%
Prophylactic Antibiotic Stopped[2]	2,645	100%	98%	98%
Prophylactic Antibiotic Timing[2]	2,661	100%	99%	99%
Prophylactic Antibiotic Timing (Outpatient)	352	99%	98%	98%
Urinary Catheter Removal[2]	1,703	100%	98%	97%
Survey of Patients' Hospital Experiences				
Area Around Room 'Always' Quiet at Night	300+	58%	53%	61%
Doctors 'Always' Communicated Well	300+	78%	77%	82%
Home Recovery Information Given	300+	86%	82%	85%
Hospital Given 9 or 10 on 10 Point Scale	300+	76%	64%	71%
Meds 'Always' Explained Before Given	300+	66%	59%	64%
Nurses 'Always' Communicated Well	300+	82%	76%	79%
Pain 'Always' Well Controlled	300+	74%	68%	71%
Room and Bathroom 'Always' Clean	300+	78%	68%	73%
Timely Help 'Always' Received	300+	70%	60%	68%
Would Definitely Recommend Hospital	300+	81%	66%	71%
Use of Medical Imaging				
Cardiac Imaging Stress Test before Surgery	628	6.7%	5.8%	5.3%
Combination Abdominal CT Scan	1,414	1.7%	7.4%	10.5%
Combination Brain/Sinus CT Scan	2,274	2.6%	2.8%	2.7%
Combination Chest CT Scan	448	0.0%	2.4%	2.7%
Follow-up Mammogram/Ultrasound	114	19.3%	12.5%	8.8%
Lumbar Spine MRI for Low Back Pain	39	41.0%	32.9%	37.2%

Ocean Medical Center

425 Jack Martin Blvd Phone: 732-840-2200
Brick, NJ 08724 Fax: 732-840-3284
URL: www.meridianhealth.com/mcoc.cfm/ind
Type: Acute Care Hospitals Emergency Services: Yes
Ownership: Voluntary non-profit - Other Beds: 281

Key Personnel:
Cardiac Laboratory........... P Insantolino
CEO/President............... Dean Q. Lin, MHA, MBA, FACHE
Radiology.................. Regina Mulholland
Chief of Medical Staff.......... David Neckritz, DO
Quality Assurance .... Carole Page
Pediatric In-Patient Care .... Jacquie Stanley, RN
Operating Room............. Patricia Tharp, RN
Infection Control............. Nancy Wagner, RN

Measure	Cases	This Hosp.	State Avg.	U.S. Avg.
Blood Clot Prevention and Treatment				
Anticoagulation Overlap Therapy[2]	82	94%	88%	93%
ICU Venous Thromboembolism Prophylaxis[2]	49	100%	93%	92%
Incidence of Potentially Preventable VTE[2]	24	8%	10%	10%
UFH with Dosages/Platelet Monitoring[2]	44	100%	99%	97%
Venous Thromboembolism Prophylaxis[2]	402	91%	83%	85%
Warfarin Therapy Discharge Instructions[2]	54	81%	77%	75%
Chest Pain/Possible Heart Attack Care				
Aspirin Given Within 24 Hours of Arrival	25	100%	98%	96%
Fibrinolytic Meds Within 30 Min. of Arrival[7]	-	-	63%	58%
Average Time to ECG (minutes)	27	6	7	7
Average Time to Transfer (minutes)[1]	-	-	74	60
Children's Asthma Care				
Received Home Management Plan of Care	-	-	-	88%
Received Reliever Medication	-	-	-	100%
Received Systemic Corticosteroids	-	-	-	100%
Emergency Department				
Admittance Decision Time (minutes)[2]	874	73	148	98
Head CT Results Within 45 Min. of Arrival	29	79%	66%	57%
Patients Who Left ER Before Being Seen	78,458	1%	2%	2%
Time from ER Arrival to Admit. (minutes)[2]	874	261	355	274
Time from ER Arrival to Discharge (minutes)	390	94	152	134
Time in ER Before Being Evaluated (minutes)	428	21	32	26
Time to Pain Meds for Fractures (minutes)	185	51	58	57
Heart Attack Care				
Aspirin Given at Discharge	135	99%	99%	99%
Fibrinolytic Meds Within 30 Min. of Arrival[1]	-	-	69%	54%
PCI Within 90 Minutes of Arrival	40	95%	95%	96%
Statin Prescribed at Discharge	129	98%	99%	98%
Heart Failure Care				
ACE Inhibitor or ARB for LVSD[2]	70	91%	98%	97%
Discharge Instructions Given[2]	181	91%	97%	94%
Evaluation of LVS Function[2]	292	98%	100%	99%
Medicare Spending				
Medicare Spending per Patient (ratio)	-	1.10	1.07	0.98
Pneumonia Care				
Appropriate Initial Antibiotic Given[2]	115	97%	98%	95%
Blood Culture Timing[2]	210	99%	99%	98%
Pregnancy and Delivery Care				
Newborn Deliveries Scheduled Early[2]	50	10%	3%	6%
Preventive Care				
Immunization for Influenza[2]	575	99%	93%	90%
Immunization for Pneumonia[2]	840	99%	94%	92%
Stroke Care				
Anticoagulation Therapy for Atrial Fibrillation[2]	47	100%	97%	95%
Antithrombotic Therapy Timing[2]	157	99%	98%	98%
Assessed for Rehabilitation[2]	174	100%	98%	97%

NOTE: Hospital profiles are in alphabetical order by state, then city, then hospital within the city; Rankings exclude hospitals with less than 25 cases except for patient surveys which excludes hospitals with less than 100 cases; (a) 100-299 cases; (1) The number of cases/patients is too few to report; (2) Data submitted were based on a sample of cases/patients; (3) Results are based on a shorter time period than required; (4) Data suppressed by CMS for one or more quarters; (5) Results are not available for this reporting period; (6) Fewer than 100 patients completed the HCAHPS survey; (7) No cases met the criteria for this measure; (8) The lower limit of the confidence interval cannot be calculated if the number of observed infections equals zero; (9) No data are available from the state/territory for this reporting period; (10) The scores shown reflect fewer than 50 completed surveys; (11) There were discrepancies in the data collection process; (12) This measure does not apply to this hospital for this reporting period; (13) Results cannot be calculated for this reporting period; (14) The results for this state are combined with nearby states to protect confidentiality; Please refer to the User's Guide for a full explanation of data.

Discharged on Antithrombotic Therapy[2]	158	100%	99%	99%
Discharged on Statin Medication[2]	119	99%	95%	94%
Thrombolytic Therapy Timing[2]	13	100%	74%	66%
Venous Thromboembolism Prophylaxis[2]	197	98%	94%	94%
Written Stroke Educational Materials Given[2]	42	100%	94%	88%
Surgical Care Improvement Project				
Appropriate Beta Blocker Usage[2]	148	99%	98%	98%
Appropriate VTP Within 24 Hours[2]	393	99%	99%	98%
Controlled Postoperative Blood Glucose[2,7]	-	-	97%	97%
Perioperative Temperature Management[2]	409	100%	100%	100%
Prophylactic Antibiotic Selection[2]	261	100%	99%	99%
Prophylactic Antibiotic Selection (Outpatient)	208	100%	97%	98%
Prophylactic Antibiotic Stopped[2]	253	98%	98%	98%
Prophylactic Antibiotic Timing[2]	261	100%	99%	99%
Prophylactic Antibiotic Timing (Outpatient)	209	95%	98%	98%
Urinary Catheter Removal[2]	266	97%	98%	97%
Survey of Patients' Hospital Experiences				
Area Around Room 'Always' Quiet at Night	300+	52%	53%	61%
Doctors 'Always' Communicated Well	300+	75%	77%	82%
Home Recovery Information Given	300+	84%	82%	85%
Hospital Given 9 or 10 on 10 Point Scale	300+	67%	64%	71%
Meds 'Always' Explained Before Given	300+	62%	59%	64%
Nurses 'Always' Communicated Well	300+	80%	76%	79%
Pain 'Always' Well Controlled	300+	72%	68%	71%
Room and Bathroom 'Always' Clean	300+	70%	68%	73%
Timely Help 'Always' Received	300+	65%	60%	68%
Would Definitely Recommend Hospital	300+	69%	66%	71%
Use of Medical Imaging				
Cardiac Imaging Stress Test before Surgery	154	7.8%	5.8%	5.3%
Combination Abdominal CT Scan	1,442	7.6%	7.4%	10.5%
Combination Brain/Sinus CT Scan	1,780	2.4%	2.8%	2.7%
Combination Chest CT Scan	1,001	2.5%	2.4%	2.7%
Follow-up Mammogram/Ultrasound	1,198	16.4%	12.5%	8.8%
Lumbar Spine MRI for Low Back Pain	52	40.4%	32.9%	37.2%

Deborah Heart & Lung Center

200 Trenton Road
Browns Mills, NJ 08015
Type: Acute Care Hospitals
Ownership: Voluntary non-profit - Private
Phone: 609-893-6611
Fax: 609-893-0626
Emergency Services: No
Beds: 161

Key Personnel:
CEO/President. . . . . Joseph P. Chirichella
Radiology. . . . . Thomas C Gallagher
Chairman/CEO . . . . Paul J. Stendardi

Measure	Cases	This Hosp.	State Avg.	U.S. Avg.
Blood Clot Prevention and Treatment				
Anticoagulation Overlap Therapy[2]	18	83%	88%	93%
ICU Venous Thromboembolism Prophylaxis[2]	183	97%	93%	92%
Incidence of Potentially Preventable VTE[1,2]	-	-	10%	10%
UFH with Dosages/Platelet Monitoring[2]	31	100%	99%	97%
Venous Thromboembolism Prophylaxis[2]	277	88%	83%	85%
Warfarin Therapy Discharge Instructions[1,2]	-	-	77%	75%
Chest Pain/Possible Heart Attack Care				
Aspirin Given Within 24 Hours of Arrival[5]	-	-	98%	96%
Fibrinolytic Meds Within 30 Min. of Arrival[5]	-	-	63%	58%
Average Time to ECG (minutes)[5]	-	-	7	7
Average Time to Transfer (minutes)[5]	-	-	74	60
Children's Asthma Care				
Received Home Management Plan of Care	-	-	-	88%
Received Reliever Medication	-	-	-	100%
Received Systemic Corticosteroids	-	-	-	100%
Emergency Department				
Admittance Decision Time (minutes)[2,7]	-	-	148	98
Head CT Results Within 45 Min. of Arrival[5]	-	-	66%	57%
Patients Who Left ER Before Being Seen[5]	-	-	2%	2%
Time from ER Arrival to Admit. (minutes)[2,7]	-	-	355	274
Time from ER Arrival to Discharge (minutes)[5]	-	-	152	134
Time in ER Before Being Evaluated (minutes)[5]	-	-	32	26
Time to Pain Meds for Fractures (minutes)[5]	-	-	58	57
Heart Attack Care				
Aspirin Given at Discharge	337	100%	99%	99%
Fibrinolytic Meds Within 30 Min. of Arrival[7]	-	-	69%	54%
PCI Within 90 Minutes of Arrival[1]	-	-	95%	96%
Statin Prescribed at Discharge	326	100%	99%	98%
Heart Failure Care				
ACE Inhibitor or ARB for LVSD	150	99%	98%	97%
Discharge Instructions Given	333	100%	97%	94%
Evaluation of LVS Function	403	100%	100%	99%
Medicare Spending				
Medicare Spending per Patient (ratio)	-	0.99	1.07	0.98
Pneumonia Care				
Appropriate Initial Antibiotic Given[7]	-	-	98%	95%
Blood Culture Timing[7]	-	-	99%	98%
Pregnancy and Delivery Care				
Newborn Deliveries Scheduled Early[7]	-	-	3%	6%
Preventive Care				
Immunization for Influenza[2]	603	97%	93%	90%
Immunization for Pneumonia[2]	952	93%	94%	92%
Stroke Care				
Anticoagulation Therapy for Atrial Fibrillation[7]	-	-	97%	95%
Antithrombotic Therapy Timing[7]	-	-	98%	98%
Assessed for Rehabilitation[7]	-	-	98%	97%
Discharged on Antithrombotic Therapy[7]	-	-	99%	99%
Discharged on Statin Medication[7]	-	-	95%	94%
Thrombolytic Therapy Timing[7]	-	-	74%	66%
Venous Thromboembolism Prophylaxis[7]	-	-	94%	94%
Written Stroke Educational Materials Given[7]	-	-	94%	88%
Surgical Care Improvement Project				
Appropriate Beta Blocker Usage	183	98%	98%	98%
Appropriate VTP Within 24 Hours	11	55%	99%	98%
Controlled Postoperative Blood Glucose	216	94%	97%	97%
Perioperative Temperature Management	107	100%	100%	100%
Prophylactic Antibiotic Selection	221	100%	99%	99%
Prophylactic Antibiotic Selection (Outpatient)	467	100%	97%	98%
Prophylactic Antibiotic Stopped	215	98%	98%	98%
Prophylactic Antibiotic Timing	221	100%	99%	99%
Prophylactic Antibiotic Timing (Outpatient)	467	100%	98%	98%
Urinary Catheter Removal	131	99%	98%	97%
Survey of Patients' Hospital Experiences				
Area Around Room 'Always' Quiet at Night	300+	59%	53%	61%
Doctors 'Always' Communicated Well	300+	83%	77%	82%
Home Recovery Information Given	300+	89%	82%	85%
Hospital Given 9 or 10 on 10 Point Scale	300+	82%	64%	71%
Meds 'Always' Explained Before Given	300+	70%	59%	64%
Nurses 'Always' Communicated Well	300+	82%	76%	79%
Pain 'Always' Well Controlled	300+	73%	68%	71%
Room and Bathroom 'Always' Clean	300+	76%	68%	73%
Timely Help 'Always' Received	300+	69%	60%	68%
Would Definitely Recommend Hospital	300+	87%	66%	71%
Use of Medical Imaging				
Cardiac Imaging Stress Test before Surgery	637	4.2%	5.8%	5.3%
Combination Abdominal CT Scan	94	3.2%	7.4%	10.5%
Combination Brain/Sinus CT Scan[1]	-	-	2.8%	2.7%
Combination Chest CT Scan	517	0.4%	2.4%	2.7%
Follow-up Mammogram/Ultrasound[7]	-	-	12.5%	8.8%
Lumbar Spine MRI for Low Back Pain[7]	-	-	32.9%	37.2%

Cooper University Hospital

1 Cooper Plaza
Camden, NJ 08103
URL: www.cooperhealth.org
Type: Acute Care Hospitals
Ownership: Voluntary non-profit - Private
Phone: 856-342-2000
Fax: 856-342-3299
Emergency Services: Yes

Key Personnel:
Chief of Medical Staff. . . . . Raymond L Baraldi
Radiology. . . . . Eriberto T David
CEO/President. . . . . John P. Sheridan, Jr.

Measure	Cases	This Hosp.	State Avg.	U.S. Avg.
Blood Clot Prevention and Treatment				
Anticoagulation Overlap Therapy[2]	137	87%	88%	93%
ICU Venous Thromboembolism Prophylaxis[2]	76	92%	93%	92%
Incidence of Potentially Preventable VTE[2]	88	5%	10%	10%
UFH with Dosages/Platelet Monitoring[2]	154	100%	99%	97%
Venous Thromboembolism Prophylaxis[2]	302	86%	83%	85%
Warfarin Therapy Discharge Instructions[2]	93	92%	77%	75%
Chest Pain/Possible Heart Attack Care				
Aspirin Given Within 24 Hours of Arrival[5]	-	-	98%	96%
Fibrinolytic Meds Within 30 Min. of Arrival[5]	-	-	63%	58%
Average Time to ECG (minutes)[5]	-	-	7	7
Average Time to Transfer (minutes)[5]	-	-	74	60
Children's Asthma Care				
Received Home Management Plan of Care	-	-	-	88%
Received Reliever Medication	-	-	-	100%
Received Systemic Corticosteroids	-	-	-	100%
Emergency Department				
Admittance Decision Time (minutes)[2]	620	242	148	98
Head CT Results Within 45 Min. of Arrival	11	27%	66%	57%
Patients Who Left ER Before Being Seen	58,126	5%	2%	2%
Time from ER Arrival to Admit. (minutes)[2]	621	396	355	274
Time from ER Arrival to Discharge (minutes)	331	175	152	134
Time in ER Before Being Evaluated (minutes)	400	39	32	26
Time to Pain Meds for Fractures (minutes)	174	83	58	57
Heart Attack Care				
Aspirin Given at Discharge[2]	277	100%	99%	99%
Fibrinolytic Meds Within 30 Min. of Arrival[2,7]	-	-	69%	54%
PCI Within 90 Minutes of Arrival[2]	22	100%	95%	96%
Statin Prescribed at Discharge[2]	274	100%	99%	98%
Heart Failure Care				
ACE Inhibitor or ARB for LVSD[2]	120	100%	98%	97%
Discharge Instructions Given[2]	253	99%	97%	94%
Evaluation of LVS Function[2]	288	100%	100%	99%
Medicare Spending				
Medicare Spending per Patient (ratio)	-	1.03	1.07	0.98
Pneumonia Care				
Appropriate Initial Antibiotic Given[2]	57	100%	98%	95%
Blood Culture Timing[2]	130	98%	99%	98%
Pregnancy and Delivery Care				
Newborn Deliveries Scheduled Early[2]	22	5%	3%	6%
Preventive Care				
Immunization for Influenza[2]	565	89%	93%	90%
Immunization for Pneumonia[2]	606	92%	94%	92%
Stroke Care				
Anticoagulation Therapy for Atrial Fibrillation[2]	15	100%	97%	95%
Antithrombotic Therapy Timing[2]	66	98%	98%	98%
Assessed for Rehabilitation[2]	86	100%	98%	97%
Discharged on Antithrombotic Therapy[2]	70	100%	99%	99%
Discharged on Statin Medication[2]	52	96%	95%	94%
Thrombolytic Therapy Timing[1,2]	-	-	74%	66%
Venous Thromboembolism Prophylaxis[2]	88	94%	94%	94%
Written Stroke Educational Materials Given[2]	50	100%	94%	88%
Surgical Care Improvement Project				
Appropriate Beta Blocker Usage[2]	171	98%	98%	98%
Appropriate VTP Within 24 Hours[2]	326	98%	99%	98%
Controlled Postoperative Blood Glucose[2]	133	100%	97%	97%
Perioperative Temperature Management[2]	474	100%	100%	100%
Prophylactic Antibiotic Selection[2]	390	100%	99%	99%
Prophylactic Antibiotic Selection (Outpatient)	356	98%	97%	98%
Prophylactic Antibiotic Stopped[2]	372	96%	98%	98%
Prophylactic Antibiotic Timing[2]	392	97%	99%	99%
Prophylactic Antibiotic Timing (Outpatient)	358	96%	98%	98%
Urinary Catheter Removal[2]	324	100%	98%	97%
Survey of Patients' Hospital Experiences				
Area Around Room 'Always' Quiet at Night	300+	50%	53%	61%
Doctors 'Always' Communicated Well	300+	77%	77%	82%
Home Recovery Information Given	300+	86%	82%	85%
Hospital Given 9 or 10 on 10 Point Scale	300+	67%	64%	71%
Meds 'Always' Explained Before Given	300+	56%	59%	64%
Nurses 'Always' Communicated Well	300+	75%	76%	79%
Pain 'Always' Well Controlled	300+	68%	68%	71%
Room and Bathroom 'Always' Clean	300+	63%	68%	73%
Timely Help 'Always' Received	300+	60%	60%	68%
Would Definitely Recommend Hospital	300+	70%	66%	71%
Use of Medical Imaging				
Cardiac Imaging Stress Test before Surgery	155	6.5%	5.8%	5.3%
Combination Abdominal CT Scan	1,285	4.6%	7.4%	10.5%
Combination Brain/Sinus CT Scan	550	0.9%	2.8%	2.7%
Combination Chest CT Scan	1,149	0.5%	2.4%	2.7%
Follow-up Mammogram/Ultrasound	1,622	14.0%	12.5%	8.8%

NOTE: Hospital profiles are in alphabetical order by state, then city, then hospital within the city; Rankings exclude hospitals with less than 25 cases except for patient surveys which excludes hospitals with less than 100 cases; (a) 100-299 cases; (1) The number of cases/patients is too few to report; (2) Data submitted were based on a sample of cases/patients; (3) Results are based on a shorter time period than required; (4) Data suppressed by CMS for one or more quarters; (5) Results are not available for this reporting period; (6) Fewer than 100 patients completed the HCAHPS survey; (7) No cases met the criteria for this measure; (8) The lower limit of the confidence interval cannot be calculated if the number of observed infections equals zero; (9) No data are available from the state/territory for this reporting period; (10) The scores shown reflect fewer than 50 completed surveys; (11) There were discrepancies in the data collection process; (12) This measure does not apply to this hospital for this reporting period; (13) Results cannot be calculated for this reporting period; (14) The results for this state are combined with nearby states to protect confidentiality; Please refer to the User's Guide for a full explanation of data.

Measure	Cases	This Hosp.	State Avg.	U.S. Avg.
Lumbar Spine MRI for Low Back Pain	153	35.9%	32.9%	37.2%

Our Lady of Lourdes Medical Center

1600 Haddon Avenue Phone: 856-757-3500
Camden, NJ 08103
E-mail: info@lourdesnet.org
URL: www.lourdesnet.org
Type: Acute Care Hospitals Emergency Services: Yes
Ownership: Voluntary non-profit - Private Beds: 410
Key Personnel:
Chief of Medical Staff.......... John P Capelli, MD
CEO/President............... Alexander J. Hatala

Measure	Cases	This Hosp.	State Avg.	U.S. Avg.
Blood Clot Prevention and Treatment				
Anticoagulation Overlap Therapy[2]	113	93%	88%	93%
ICU Venous Thromboembolism Prophylaxis[2]	114	85%	93%	92%
Incidence of Potentially Preventable VTE[1,2]	-	-	10%	10%
UFH with Dosages/Platelet Monitoring[2]	120	100%	99%	97%
Venous Thromboembolism Prophylaxis[2]	355	82%	83%	85%
Warfarin Therapy Discharge Instructions[2]	73	78%	77%	75%
Chest Pain/Possible Heart Attack Care				
Aspirin Given Within 24 Hours of Arrival[1,3]	-	-	98%	96%
Fibrinolytic Meds Within 30 Min. of Arrival[3,7]	-	-	63%	58%
Average Time to ECG (minutes)[1,3]	-	-	7	7
Average Time to Transfer (minutes)[1,3]	-	-	74	60
Children's Asthma Care				
Received Home Management Plan of Care	-	-	-	88%
Received Reliever Medication	-	-	-	100%
Received Systemic Corticosteroids	-	-	-	100%
Emergency Department				
Admittance Decision Time (minutes)[2]	678	254	148	98
Head CT Results Within 45 Min. of Arrival	16	94%	66%	57%
Patients Who Left ER Before Being Seen	59,096	1%	2%	2%
Time from ER Arrival to Admit. (minutes)[2]	678	407	355	274
Time from ER Arrival to Discharge (minutes)	379	144	152	134
Time in ER Before Being Evaluated (minutes)	435	17	32	26
Time to Pain Meds for Fractures (minutes)	69	53	58	57
Heart Attack Care				
Aspirin Given at Discharge[2]	341	100%	99%	99%
Fibrinolytic Meds Within 30 Min. of Arrival[1,2]	-	-	69%	54%
PCI Within 90 Minutes of Arrival[2]	21	100%	95%	96%
Statin Prescribed at Discharge[2]	342	100%	99%	98%
Heart Failure Care				
ACE Inhibitor or ARB for LVSD[2]	86	100%	98%	97%
Discharge Instructions Given[2]	262	98%	97%	94%
Evaluation of LVS Function[2]	326	100%	100%	99%
Medicare Spending				
Medicare Spending per Patient (ratio)	-	1.03	1.07	0.98
Pneumonia Care				
Appropriate Initial Antibiotic Given[2]	82	100%	98%	95%
Blood Culture Timing[2]	122	98%	99%	98%
Pregnancy and Delivery Care				
Newborn Deliveries Scheduled Early[2]	35	0%	3%	6%
Preventive Care				
Immunization for Influenza[2]	558	98%	93%	90%
Immunization for Pneumonia[2]	804	96%	94%	92%
Stroke Care				
Anticoagulation Therapy for Atrial Fibrillation	25	92%	97%	95%
Antithrombotic Therapy Timing	144	98%	98%	98%
Assessed for Rehabilitation	154	95%	98%	97%
Discharged on Antithrombotic Therapy	137	99%	99%	99%
Discharged on Statin Medication	108	100%	95%	94%
Thrombolytic Therapy Timing[1]	-	-	74%	66%
Venous Thromboembolism Prophylaxis	173	97%	94%	94%
Written Stroke Educational Materials Given	77	100%	94%	88%
Surgical Care Improvement Project				
Appropriate Beta Blocker Usage[2]	261	100%	98%	98%
Appropriate VTP Within 24 Hours[2]	227	100%	99%	98%
Controlled Postoperative Blood Glucose[2]	207	98%	97%	97%
Perioperative Temperature Management[2]	308	100%	100%	100%
Prophylactic Antibiotic Selection[2]	301	99%	99%	99%
Prophylactic Antibiotic Selection (Outpatient)	483	99%	97%	98%
Prophylactic Antibiotic Stopped[2]	287	98%	98%	98%
Prophylactic Antibiotic Timing[2]	301	100%	99%	99%
Prophylactic Antibiotic Timing (Outpatient)	483	99%	98%	98%
Urinary Catheter Removal[2]	262	95%	98%	97%
Survey of Patients' Hospital Experiences				
Area Around Room 'Always' Quiet at Night	300+	55%	53%	61%
Doctors 'Always' Communicated Well	300+	74%	77%	82%
Home Recovery Information Given	300+	81%	82%	85%
Hospital Given 9 or 10 on 10 Point Scale	300+	64%	64%	71%
Meds 'Always' Explained Before Given	300+	62%	59%	64%
Nurses 'Always' Communicated Well	300+	75%	76%	79%
Pain 'Always' Well Controlled	300+	66%	68%	71%
Room and Bathroom 'Always' Clean	300+	65%	68%	73%
Timely Help 'Always' Received	300+	59%	60%	68%
Would Definitely Recommend Hospital	300+	70%	66%	71%
Use of Medical Imaging				
Cardiac Imaging Stress Test before Surgery	3,039	5.6%	5.8%	5.3%
Combination Abdominal CT Scan	736	11.7%	7.4%	10.5%
Combination Brain/Sinus CT Scan	937	1.4%	2.8%	2.7%
Combination Chest CT Scan	289	13.5%	2.4%	2.7%
Follow-up Mammogram/Ultrasound	204	12.3%	12.5%	8.8%
Lumbar Spine MRI for Low Back Pain[1]	-	-	32.9%	37.2%

Cape Regional Medical Center

Two Stone Harbor Blvd Phone: 609-463-2000
Cape May Court House, NJ 08210 Fax: 609-463-2379
URL: www.caperegional.com
Type: Acute Care Hospitals Emergency Services: Yes
Ownership: Voluntary non-profit - Private Beds: 272
Key Personnel:
CEO/President.............. Joanne Carrocino, FACHE
Emergency Room .... Michael Dudnick, MD
Quality Assurance .... Mary Fay
Intensive Care Unit............ Betsy Holz
Operating Room............. Shirley Lathbury
Chief of Medical Staff.......... David Tarantino, MD

Measure	Cases	This Hosp.	State Avg.	U.S. Avg.
Blood Clot Prevention and Treatment				
Anticoagulation Overlap Therapy[2]	63	76%	88%	93%
ICU Venous Thromboembolism Prophylaxis[2]	92	93%	93%	92%
Incidence of Potentially Preventable VTE[1,2]	-	-	10%	10%
UFH with Dosages/Platelet Monitoring[2]	66	100%	99%	97%
Venous Thromboembolism Prophylaxis[2]	348	80%	83%	85%
Warfarin Therapy Discharge Instructions[2]	48	88%	77%	75%
Chest Pain/Possible Heart Attack Care				
Aspirin Given Within 24 Hours of Arrival	117	99%	98%	96%
Fibrinolytic Meds Within 30 Min. of Arrival[1]	-	-	63%	58%
Average Time to ECG (minutes)	117	6	7	7
Average Time to Transfer (minutes)[1]	-	-	74	60
Children's Asthma Care				
Received Home Management Plan of Care	-	-	-	88%
Received Reliever Medication	-	-	-	100%
Received Systemic Corticosteroids	-	-	-	100%
Emergency Department				
Admittance Decision Time (minutes)[2]	969	152	148	98
Head CT Results Within 45 Min. of Arrival	43	79%	66%	57%
Patients Who Left ER Before Being Seen	47,206	0%	2%	2%
Time from ER Arrival to Admit. (minutes)[2]	976	298	355	274
Time from ER Arrival to Discharge (minutes)	383	125	152	134
Time in ER Before Being Evaluated (minutes)	431	19	32	26
Time to Pain Meds for Fractures (minutes)	101	57	58	57
Heart Attack Care				
Aspirin Given at Discharge	29	90%	99%	99%
Fibrinolytic Meds Within 30 Min. of Arrival[7]	-	-	69%	54%
PCI Within 90 Minutes of Arrival[7]	-	-	95%	96%
Statin Prescribed at Discharge	28	96%	99%	98%
Heart Failure Care				
ACE Inhibitor or ARB for LVSD	69	90%	98%	97%
Discharge Instructions Given	184	92%	97%	94%
Evaluation of LVS Function	238	98%	100%	99%
Medicare Spending				
Medicare Spending per Patient (ratio)	-	0.98	1.07	0.98
Pneumonia Care				
Appropriate Initial Antibiotic Given	206	97%	98%	95%
Blood Culture Timing	394	100%	99%	98%
Pregnancy and Delivery Care				
Newborn Deliveries Scheduled Early[2]	34	3%	3%	6%
Preventive Care				
Immunization for Influenza[2]	553	98%	93%	90%
Immunization for Pneumonia[2]	751	97%	94%	92%
Stroke Care				
Anticoagulation Therapy for Atrial Fibrillation	13	62%	97%	95%
Antithrombotic Therapy Timing	96	96%	98%	98%
Assessed for Rehabilitation	95	86%	98%	97%
Discharged on Antithrombotic Therapy	92	97%	99%	99%
Discharged on Statin Medication	69	88%	95%	94%
Thrombolytic Therapy Timing[7]	-	-	74%	66%
Venous Thromboembolism Prophylaxis	100	85%	94%	94%
Written Stroke Educational Materials Given	57	91%	94%	88%
Surgical Care Improvement Project				
Appropriate Beta Blocker Usage	117	97%	98%	98%
Appropriate VTP Within 24 Hours	322	99%	99%	98%
Controlled Postoperative Blood Glucose[7]	-	-	97%	97%
Perioperative Temperature Management	358	100%	100%	100%
Prophylactic Antibiotic Selection	232	100%	99%	99%
Prophylactic Antibiotic Selection (Outpatient)	54	98%	97%	98%
Prophylactic Antibiotic Stopped	221	98%	98%	98%
Prophylactic Antibiotic Timing	232	100%	99%	99%
Prophylactic Antibiotic Timing (Outpatient)	54	98%	98%	98%
Urinary Catheter Removal	189	98%	98%	97%
Survey of Patients' Hospital Experiences				
Area Around Room 'Always' Quiet at Night	300+	53%	53%	61%
Doctors 'Always' Communicated Well	300+	79%	77%	82%
Home Recovery Information Given	300+	81%	82%	85%
Hospital Given 9 or 10 on 10 Point Scale	300+	63%	64%	71%
Meds 'Always' Explained Before Given	300+	64%	59%	64%
Nurses 'Always' Communicated Well	300+	80%	76%	79%
Pain 'Always' Well Controlled	300+	70%	68%	71%
Room and Bathroom 'Always' Clean	300+	68%	68%	73%
Timely Help 'Always' Received	300+	67%	60%	68%
Would Definitely Recommend Hospital	300+	66%	66%	71%
Use of Medical Imaging				
Cardiac Imaging Stress Test before Surgery	187	9.6%	5.8%	5.3%
Combination Abdominal CT Scan	858	32.6%	7.4%	10.5%
Combination Brain/Sinus CT Scan	954	0.4%	2.8%	2.7%
Combination Chest CT Scan	280	1.4%	2.4%	2.7%
Follow-up Mammogram/Ultrasound[7]	-	-	12.5%	8.8%
Lumbar Spine MRI for Low Back Pain[1]	-	-	32.9%	37.2%

Saint Clare's Hospital

25 Pocono Road Phone: 973-625-6000
Denville, NJ 07834 Fax: 973-537-3959
URL: www.saintclares.org
Type: Acute Care Hospitals Emergency Services: Yes
Ownership: Voluntary non-profit - Church Beds: 331
Key Personnel:
CEO/President.............. Leslie D. Hirsch
Chief of Medical Staff.......... Stephen Papish

Measure	Cases	This Hosp.	State Avg.	U.S. Avg.
Blood Clot Prevention and Treatment				
Anticoagulation Overlap Therapy[2]	71	93%	88%	93%
ICU Venous Thromboembolism Prophylaxis[2]	68	94%	93%	92%
Incidence of Potentially Preventable VTE[2]	14	7%	10%	10%
UFH with Dosages/Platelet Monitoring[2]	93	99%	99%	97%
Venous Thromboembolism Prophylaxis[2]	348	80%	83%	85%
Warfarin Therapy Discharge Instructions[2]	46	96%	77%	75%
Chest Pain/Possible Heart Attack Care				
Aspirin Given Within 24 Hours of Arrival	26	100%	98%	96%
Fibrinolytic Meds Within 30 Min. of Arrival[1]	-	-	63%	58%
Average Time to ECG (minutes)	28	4	7	7
Average Time to Transfer (minutes)[1]	-	-	74	60
Children's Asthma Care				
Received Home Management Plan of Care	-	-	-	88%
Received Reliever Medication	-	-	-	100%
Received Systemic Corticosteroids	-	-	-	100%
Emergency Department				
Admittance Decision Time (minutes)[2]	737	203	148	98
Head CT Results Within 45 Min. of Arrival[1]	-	-	66%	57%

NOTE: Hospital profiles are in alphabetical order by state, then city, then hospital within the city; Rankings exclude hospitals with less than 25 cases except for patient surveys which excludes hospitals with less than 100 cases; (a) 100-299 cases; (1) The number of cases/patients is too few to report; (2) Data submitted were based on a sample of cases/patients; (3) Results are based on a shorter time period than required; (4) Data suppressed by CMS for one or more quarters; (5) Results are not available for this reporting period; (6) Fewer than 100 patients completed the HCAHPS survey; (7) No cases met the criteria for this measure; (8) The lower limit of the confidence interval cannot be calculated if the number of observed infections equals zero; (9) No data are available from the state/territory for this reporting period; (10) The scores shown reflect fewer than 50 completed surveys; (11) There were discrepancies in the data collection process; (12) This measure does not apply to this hospital for this reporting period; (13) Results cannot be calculated for this reporting period; (14) The results for this state are combined with nearby states to protect confidentiality; Please refer to the User's Guide for a full explanation of data.

Patients Who Left ER Before Being Seen	72,338	1%	2%	2%
Time from ER Arrival to Admit. (minutes)[2]	780	404	355	274
Time from ER Arrival to Discharge (minutes)	434	120	152	134
Time in ER Before Being Evaluated (minutes)	466	29	32	26
Time to Pain Meds for Fractures (minutes)	198	52	58	57
Heart Attack Care				
Aspirin Given at Discharge	137	99%	99%	99%
Fibrinolytic Meds Within 30 Min. of Arrival[1]	-	-	69%	54%
PCI Within 90 Minutes of Arrival	40	100%	95%	96%
Statin Prescribed at Discharge	136	98%	99%	98%
Heart Failure Care				
ACE Inhibitor or ARB for LVSD	95	97%	98%	97%
Discharge Instructions Given	297	98%	97%	94%
Evaluation of LVS Function	464	100%	100%	99%
Medicare Spending				
Medicare Spending per Patient (ratio)	-	1.07	1.07	0.98
Pneumonia Care				
Appropriate Initial Antibiotic Given	169	96%	98%	95%
Blood Culture Timing	288	99%	99%	98%
Pregnancy and Delivery Care				
Newborn Deliveries Scheduled Early[2]	27	0%	3%	6%
Preventive Care				
Immunization for Influenza[2]	535	95%	93%	90%
Immunization for Pneumonia[2]	693	91%	94%	92%
Stroke Care				
Anticoagulation Therapy for Atrial Fibrillation	15	100%	97%	95%
Antithrombotic Therapy Timing	125	98%	98%	98%
Assessed for Rehabilitation	139	96%	98%	97%
Discharged on Antithrombotic Therapy	120	100%	99%	99%
Discharged on Statin Medication	93	97%	95%	94%
Thrombolytic Therapy Timing[1]	-	-	74%	66%
Venous Thromboembolism Prophylaxis	149	93%	94%	94%
Written Stroke Educational Materials Given	67	93%	94%	88%
Surgical Care Improvement Project				
Appropriate Beta Blocker Usage	182	91%	98%	98%
Appropriate VTP Within 24 Hours	611	98%	99%	98%
Controlled Postoperative Blood Glucose[7]	-	-	97%	97%
Perioperative Temperature Management	700	100%	100%	100%
Prophylactic Antibiotic Selection	403	98%	99%	99%
Prophylactic Antibiotic Selection (Outpatient)	207	86%	97%	98%
Prophylactic Antibiotic Stopped	397	98%	98%	98%
Prophylactic Antibiotic Timing	404	99%	99%	99%
Prophylactic Antibiotic Timing (Outpatient)	209	99%	98%	98%
Urinary Catheter Removal	435	97%	98%	97%
Survey of Patients' Hospital Experiences				
Area Around Room 'Always' Quiet at Night	300+	55%	53%	61%
Doctors 'Always' Communicated Well	300+	75%	77%	82%
Home Recovery Information Given	300+	85%	82%	85%
Hospital Given 9 or 10 on 10 Point Scale	300+	68%	64%	71%
Meds 'Always' Explained Before Given	300+	56%	59%	64%
Nurses 'Always' Communicated Well	300+	76%	76%	79%
Pain 'Always' Well Controlled	300+	68%	68%	71%
Room and Bathroom 'Always' Clean	300+	70%	68%	73%
Timely Help 'Always' Received	300+	60%	60%	68%
Would Definitely Recommend Hospital	300+	70%	66%	71%
Use of Medical Imaging				
Cardiac Imaging Stress Test before Surgery	648	4.9%	5.8%	5.3%
Combination Abdominal CT Scan	1,599	5.7%	7.4%	10.5%
Combination Brain/Sinus CT Scan	1,219	4.0%	2.8%	2.7%
Combination Chest CT Scan	915	0.8%	2.4%	2.7%
Follow-up Mammogram/Ultrasound	3,032	12.7%	12.5%	8.8%
Lumbar Spine MRI for Low Back Pain	51	41.2%	32.9%	37.2%

East Orange General Hospital

300 Central Ave
East Orange, NJ 07018
URL: www.evh.org
Type: Acute Care Hospitals
Ownership: Voluntary non-profit - Private

Phone: 973-266-4401
Fax: 973-266-8488
Emergency Services: Yes
Beds: 211

Key Personnel:
Radiology. . . . . Jose P Barba
Chief of Medical Staff. . . . . Valentine Burroughs, MD, MBA
Quality Assurance . . . . Blach Campbell
Intensive Care Unit. . . . . Nancy Naspo, RN
Anesthesiology. . . . . Dr Owen Rhhman
President/CEO. . . . . Kevin J Slavin, FACHE
Infection Control. . . . . Aldyth Stanford, RN C
Emergency Room . . . . Eduardo Tinio, MSN RN

Measure	Cases	This Hosp.	State Avg.	U.S. Avg.
Blood Clot Prevention and Treatment				
Anticoagulation Overlap Therapy[2]	59	64%	88%	93%
ICU Venous Thromboembolism Prophylaxis[2]	65	89%	93%	92%
Incidence of Potentially Preventable VTE[2]	21	14%	10%	10%
UFH with Dosages/Platelet Monitoring[2]	28	100%	99%	97%
Venous Thromboembolism Prophylaxis[2]	425	80%	83%	85%
Warfarin Therapy Discharge Instructions[2]	33	76%	77%	75%
Chest Pain/Possible Heart Attack Care				
Aspirin Given Within 24 Hours of Arrival[1,3]	-	-	98%	96%
Fibrinolytic Meds Within 30 Min. of Arrival[3,7]	-	-	63%	58%
Average Time to ECG (minutes)[1,3]	-	-	7	7
Average Time to Transfer (minutes)[1,3]	-	-	74	60
Children's Asthma Care				
Received Home Management Plan of Care	-	-	-	88%
Received Reliever Medication	-	-	-	100%
Received Systemic Corticosteroids	-	-	-	100%
Emergency Department				
Admittance Decision Time (minutes)[2]	734	240	148	98
Head CT Results Within 45 Min. of Arrival[3,7]	-	-	66%	57%
Patients Who Left ER Before Being Seen	6,794	8%	2%	2%
Time from ER Arrival to Admit. (minutes)[2]	735	520	355	274
Time from ER Arrival to Discharge (minutes)	309	155	152	134
Time in ER Before Being Evaluated (minutes)	333	55	32	26
Time to Pain Meds for Fractures (minutes)	39	95	58	57
Heart Attack Care				
Aspirin Given at Discharge	54	93%	99%	99%
Fibrinolytic Meds Within 30 Min. of Arrival[7]	-	-	69%	54%
PCI Within 90 Minutes of Arrival[7]	-	-	95%	96%
Statin Prescribed at Discharge	48	96%	99%	98%
Heart Failure Care				
ACE Inhibitor or ARB for LVSD[2]	73	99%	98%	97%
Discharge Instructions Given[2]	169	68%	97%	94%
Evaluation of LVS Function[2]	244	99%	100%	99%
Medicare Spending				
Medicare Spending per Patient (ratio)	-	1.17	1.07	0.98
Pneumonia Care				
Appropriate Initial Antibiotic Given[2]	52	100%	98%	95%
Blood Culture Timing[2]	179	99%	99%	98%
Pregnancy and Delivery Care				
Newborn Deliveries Scheduled Early[7]	-	-	3%	6%
Preventive Care				
Immunization for Influenza[2]	607	92%	93%	90%
Immunization for Pneumonia[2]	905	96%	94%	92%
Stroke Care				
Anticoagulation Therapy for Atrial Fibrillation[1]	-	-	97%	95%
Antithrombotic Therapy Timing	74	97%	98%	98%
Assessed for Rehabilitation	77	97%	98%	97%
Discharged on Antithrombotic Therapy	71	97%	99%	99%
Discharged on Statin Medication	44	80%	95%	94%
Thrombolytic Therapy Timing[7]	-	-	74%	66%
Venous Thromboembolism Prophylaxis	79	91%	94%	94%
Written Stroke Educational Materials Given	46	89%	94%	88%
Surgical Care Improvement Project				
Appropriate Beta Blocker Usage	19	89%	98%	98%
Appropriate VTP Within 24 Hours	107	94%	99%	98%
Controlled Postoperative Blood Glucose[7]	-	-	97%	97%
Perioperative Temperature Management	113	100%	100%	100%
Prophylactic Antibiotic Selection	61	97%	99%	99%
Prophylactic Antibiotic Selection (Outpatient)	22	95%	97%	98%
Prophylactic Antibiotic Stopped	55	93%	98%	98%
Prophylactic Antibiotic Timing	61	98%	99%	99%
Prophylactic Antibiotic Timing (Outpatient)	22	100%	98%	98%
Urinary Catheter Removal	52	90%	98%	97%
Survey of Patients' Hospital Experiences				
Area Around Room 'Always' Quiet at Night	300+	58%	53%	61%
Doctors 'Always' Communicated Well	300+	78%	77%	82%
Home Recovery Information Given	300+	80%	82%	85%
Hospital Given 9 or 10 on 10 Point Scale	300+	52%	64%	71%
Meds 'Always' Explained Before Given	300+	55%	59%	64%
Nurses 'Always' Communicated Well	300+	68%	76%	79%
Pain 'Always' Well Controlled	300+	63%	68%	71%
Room and Bathroom 'Always' Clean	300+	69%	68%	73%
Timely Help 'Always' Received	300+	52%	60%	68%
Would Definitely Recommend Hospital	300+	54%	66%	71%
Use of Medical Imaging				
Cardiac Imaging Stress Test before Surgery[1]	-	-	5.8%	5.3%
Combination Abdominal CT Scan	122	7.4%	7.4%	10.5%
Combination Brain/Sinus CT Scan[1]	-	-	2.8%	2.7%
Combination Chest CT Scan	51	0.0%	2.4%	2.7%
Follow-up Mammogram/Ultrasound	229	6.1%	12.5%	8.8%
Lumbar Spine MRI for Low Back Pain[1]	-	-	32.9%	37.2%

VA New Jersey Health Care System

385 Tremont Avenue
East Orange, NJ 07018
URL: www1.va.gov/visns/visn03/eorginfo.asp
Type: Acute Care - VA
Ownership: Government Federal

Phone: 973-676-1000
Fax: 973-395-7062
Emergency Services: No
Beds: 791

Key Personnel:
Cardiac Laboratory. . . . . Steve Binenbaum, MD
Infection Control. . . . . Robert Eng, MD
Chief of Medical Staff. . . . . Steven L Lieberman, MD
Operating Room. . . . . George Machiedo, RN
CEO/President. . . . . Kenneth H Mizrach
Quality Assurance . . . . Linda Mowad, RN, PhD
Radiology. . . . . Jyoti Shah, MD

Measure	Cases	This Hosp.	State Avg.	U.S. Avg.
Blood Clot Prevention and Treatment				
Anticoagulation Overlap Therapy	-	-	88%	93%
ICU Venous Thromboembolism Prophylaxis	-	-	93%	92%
Incidence of Potentially Preventable VTE	-	-	10%	10%
UFH with Dosages/Platelet Monitoring	-	-	99%	97%
Venous Thromboembolism Prophylaxis	-	-	83%	85%
Warfarin Therapy Discharge Instructions	-	-	77%	75%
Chest Pain/Possible Heart Attack Care				
Aspirin Given Within 24 Hours of Arrival	-	-	98%	96%
Fibrinolytic Meds Within 30 Min. of Arrival	-	-	63%	58%
Average Time to ECG (minutes)	-	-	7	7
Average Time to Transfer (minutes)	-	-	74	60
Children's Asthma Care				
Received Home Management Plan of Care	-	-	-	88%
Received Reliever Medication	-	-	-	100%
Received Systemic Corticosteroids	-	-	-	100%
Emergency Department				
Admittance Decision Time (minutes)	-	-	148	98
Head CT Results Within 45 Min. of Arrival	-	-	66%	57%
Patients Who Left ER Before Being Seen	-	-	2%	2%
Time from ER Arrival to Admit. (minutes)	-	-	355	274
Time from ER Arrival to Discharge (minutes)	-	-	152	134
Time in ER Before Being Evaluated (minutes)	-	-	32	26
Time to Pain Meds for Fractures (minutes)	-	-	58	57
Heart Attack Care				
Aspirin Given at Discharge[5]	-	-	99%	99%
Fibrinolytic Meds Within 30 Min. of Arrival[5]	-	-	69%	54%
PCI Within 90 Minutes of Arrival[5]	-	-	95%	96%
Statin Prescribed at Discharge[5]	-	-	99%	98%
Heart Failure Care				
ACE Inhibitor or ARB for LVSD	49	94%	98%	97%
Discharge Instructions Given	68	93%	97%	94%
Evaluation of LVS Function	73	100%	100%	99%
Medicare Spending				
Medicare Spending per Patient (ratio)	-	-	1.07	0.98
Pneumonia Care				
Appropriate Initial Antibiotic Given	31	81%	98%	95%
Blood Culture Timing	76	99%	99%	98%
Pregnancy and Delivery Care				
Newborn Deliveries Scheduled Early	-	-	3%	6%
Preventive Care				
Immunization for Influenza[5]	-	-	93%	90%
Immunization for Pneumonia[5]	-	-	94%	92%
Stroke Care				
Anticoagulation Therapy for Atrial Fibrillation	-	-	97%	95%

NOTE: Hospital profiles are in alphabetical order by state, then city, then hospital within the city; Rankings exclude hospitals with less than 25 cases except for patient surveys which excludes hospitals with less than 100 cases; (a) 100-299 cases; (1) The number of cases/patients is too few to report; (2) Data submitted were based on a sample of cases/patients; (3) Results are based on a shorter time period than required; (4) Data suppressed by CMS for one or more quarters; (5) Results are not available for this reporting period; (6) Fewer than 100 patients completed the HCAHPS survey; (7) No cases met the criteria for this measure; (8) The lower limit of the confidence interval cannot be calculated if the number of observed infections equals zero; (9) No data are available from the state/territory for this reporting period; (10) The scores shown reflect fewer than 50 completed surveys; (11) There were discrepancies in the data collection process; (12) This measure does not apply to this hospital for this reporting period; (13) Results cannot be calculated for this reporting period; (14) The results for this state are combined with nearby states to protect confidentiality; Please refer to the User's Guide for a full explanation of data.

Measure	Cases	This Hosp.	State Avg.	U.S. Avg.
Antithrombotic Therapy Timing	-	-	98%	98%
Assessed for Rehabilitation	-	-	98%	97%
Discharged on Antithrombotic Therapy	-	-	99%	99%
Discharged on Statin Medication	-	-	95%	94%
Thrombolytic Therapy Timing	-	-	74%	66%
Venous Thromboembolism Prophylaxis	-	-	94%	94%
Written Stroke Educational Materials Given	-	-	94%	88%
Surgical Care Improvement Project				
Appropriate Beta Blocker Usage[2]	47	89%	98%	98%
Appropriate VTP Within 24 Hours[2]	112	96%	99%	98%
Controlled Postoperative Blood Glucose[5]	-	-	97%	97%
Perioperative Temperature Management[2]	139	99%	100%	100%
Prophylactic Antibiotic Selection	88	99%	99%	99%
Prophylactic Antibiotic Selection (Outpatient)	-	-	97%	98%
Prophylactic Antibiotic Stopped	86	95%	98%	98%
Prophylactic Antibiotic Timing	88	100%	99%	99%
Prophylactic Antibiotic Timing (Outpatient)	-	-	98%	98%
Urinary Catheter Removal[2]	78	95%	98%	97%
Survey of Patients' Hospital Experiences				
Area Around Room 'Always' Quiet at Night	-	-	53%	61%
Doctors 'Always' Communicated Well	-	-	77%	82%
Home Recovery Information Given	-	-	82%	85%
Hospital Given 9 or 10 on 10 Point Scale	-	-	64%	71%
Meds 'Always' Explained Before Given	-	-	59%	64%
Nurses 'Always' Communicated Well	-	-	76%	79%
Pain 'Always' Well Controlled	-	-	68%	71%
Room and Bathroom 'Always' Clean	-	-	68%	73%
Timely Help 'Always' Received	-	-	60%	68%
Would Definitely Recommend Hospital	-	-	66%	71%
Use of Medical Imaging				
Cardiac Imaging Stress Test before Surgery	-	-	5.8%	5.3%
Combination Abdominal CT Scan	-	-	7.4%	10.5%
Combination Brain/Sinus CT Scan	-	-	2.8%	2.7%
Combination Chest CT Scan	-	-	2.4%	2.7%
Follow-up Mammogram/Ultrasound	-	-	12.5%	8.8%
Lumbar Spine MRI for Low Back Pain	-	-	32.9%	37.2%

JFK Medical Center - A M Yelencsics Comm Hospital

65 James Street
Edison, NJ 08818
URL: www.jfkmc.org
Type: Acute Care Hospitals
Ownership: Voluntary non-profit - Private

Phone: 732-321-7000
Fax: 732-549 8532
Emergency Services: Yes

Key Personnel:
Radiology. . . . . Robert A Friedman, MD
Quality Assurance . . . . Lucy Gall
CEO/President. . . . . John P McGee
Chief of Medical Staff. . . . . Williams Oser
Operating Room. . . . . Tushar R Patel, RN
Pediatric Ambulatory Care . . . . . . Anthony Santor, MD
Pediatric In-Patient Care . . . . Anthony Santor, MD
Infection Control. . . . . John Sensokovic, MD

Measure	Cases	This Hosp.	State Avg.	U.S. Avg.
Blood Clot Prevention and Treatment				
Anticoagulation Overlap Therapy[2]	164	58%	88%	93%
ICU Venous Thromboembolism Prophylaxis[2]	73	67%	93%	92%
Incidence of Potentially Preventable VTE[2]	51	33%	10%	10%
UFH with Dosages/Platelet Monitoring[2]	133	95%	99%	97%
Venous Thromboembolism Prophylaxis[2]	435	45%	83%	85%
Warfarin Therapy Discharge Instructions[2]	81	27%	77%	75%
Chest Pain/Possible Heart Attack Care				
Aspirin Given Within 24 Hours of Arrival	11	91%	98%	96%
Fibrinolytic Meds Within 30 Min. of Arrival[3,7]	-	-	63%	58%
Average Time to ECG (minutes)[1]	-	-	7	7
Average Time to Transfer (minutes)[1,3]	-	-	74	60
Children's Asthma Care				
Received Home Management Plan of Care	-	-	-	88%
Received Reliever Medication	-	-	-	100%
Received Systemic Corticosteroids	-	-	-	100%
Emergency Department				
Admittance Decision Time (minutes)[2]	585	187	148	98
Head CT Results Within 45 Min. of Arrival	12	33%	66%	57%
Patients Who Left ER Before Being Seen	32,384	1%	2%	2%
Time from ER Arrival to Admit. (minutes)[2]	588	434	355	274
Time from ER Arrival to Discharge (minutes)	358	154	152	134
Time in ER Before Being Evaluated (minutes)	422	34	32	26
Time to Pain Meds for Fractures (minutes)	237	44	58	57
Heart Attack Care				
Aspirin Given at Discharge	265	100%	99%	99%
Fibrinolytic Meds Within 30 Min. of Arrival[7]	-	-	69%	54%
PCI Within 90 Minutes of Arrival	68	94%	95%	96%
Statin Prescribed at Discharge	261	100%	99%	98%
Heart Failure Care				
ACE Inhibitor or ARB for LVSD	138	97%	98%	97%
Discharge Instructions Given	348	90%	97%	94%
Evaluation of LVS Function	546	100%	100%	99%
Medicare Spending				
Medicare Spending per Patient (ratio)	-	1.17	1.07	0.98
Pneumonia Care				
Appropriate Initial Antibiotic Given	238	99%	98%	95%
Blood Culture Timing	545	100%	99%	98%
Pregnancy and Delivery Care				
Newborn Deliveries Scheduled Early	412	0%	3%	6%
Preventive Care				
Immunization for Influenza[2]	537	93%	93%	90%
Immunization for Pneumonia[2]	603	88%	94%	92%
Stroke Care				
Anticoagulation Therapy for Atrial Fibrillation	43	100%	97%	95%
Antithrombotic Therapy Timing	236	100%	98%	98%
Assessed for Rehabilitation	338	98%	98%	97%
Discharged on Antithrombotic Therapy	273	100%	99%	99%
Discharged on Statin Medication	213	96%	95%	94%
Thrombolytic Therapy Timing	45	82%	74%	66%
Venous Thromboembolism Prophylaxis	353	97%	94%	94%
Written Stroke Educational Materials Given	106	99%	94%	88%
Surgical Care Improvement Project				
Appropriate Beta Blocker Usage[2]	221	99%	98%	98%
Appropriate VTP Within 24 Hours[2]	676	99%	99%	98%
Controlled Postoperative Blood Glucose[2,7]	-	-	97%	97%
Perioperative Temperature Management[2]	799	100%	100%	100%
Prophylactic Antibiotic Selection[2]	589	99%	99%	99%
Prophylactic Antibiotic Selection (Outpatient)	271	94%	97%	98%
Prophylactic Antibiotic Stopped[2]	567	98%	98%	98%
Prophylactic Antibiotic Timing[2]	589	100%	99%	99%
Prophylactic Antibiotic Timing (Outpatient)	273	99%	98%	98%
Urinary Catheter Removal[2]	315	100%	98%	97%
Survey of Patients' Hospital Experiences				
Area Around Room 'Always' Quiet at Night	300+	50%	53%	61%
Doctors 'Always' Communicated Well	300+	78%	77%	82%
Home Recovery Information Given	300+	76%	82%	85%
Hospital Given 9 or 10 on 10 Point Scale	300+	61%	64%	71%
Meds 'Always' Explained Before Given	300+	58%	59%	64%
Nurses 'Always' Communicated Well	300+	76%	76%	79%
Pain 'Always' Well Controlled	300+	67%	68%	71%
Room and Bathroom 'Always' Clean	300+	76%	68%	73%
Timely Help 'Always' Received	300+	60%	60%	68%
Would Definitely Recommend Hospital	300+	61%	66%	71%
Use of Medical Imaging				
Cardiac Imaging Stress Test before Surgery	430	5.1%	5.8%	5.3%
Combination Abdominal CT Scan	1,420	15.5%	7.4%	10.5%
Combination Brain/Sinus CT Scan	1,735	0.7%	2.8%	2.7%
Combination Chest CT Scan	1,086	0.3%	2.4%	2.7%
Follow-up Mammogram/Ultrasound	1,992	9.6%	12.5%	8.8%
Lumbar Spine MRI for Low Back Pain	216	30.6%	32.9%	37.2%

Trinitas Regional Medical Center

225 Williamson Street
Elizabeth, NJ 07207
URL: www.trinitashospital.org
Type: Acute Care Hospitals
Ownership: Voluntary non-profit - Private

Phone: 908-994-5000
Fax: 908-994-5727
Emergency Services: Yes
Beds: 531

Key Personnel:
Pediatric In-Patient Care . . . . Cheryl Dickson, MD
Cardiac Laboratory. . . . . Gary S. Horan, FACHE
Radiology. . . . . Eugene Kennedy, MD
Chief of Medical Staff. . . . . William McHugh, MD
Anesthesiology. . . . . Leon Pirak, MD
Hemotology Center . . . . Stanley Pomerantz, MD
Emergency Room . . . . Maribeth Santillo, RN MS
Infection Control. . . . . Uwe Schmidt, MD

Measure	Cases	This Hosp.	State Avg.	U.S. Avg.
Blood Clot Prevention and Treatment				
Anticoagulation Overlap Therapy[2]	84	94%	88%	93%
ICU Venous Thromboembolism Prophylaxis[2]	86	95%	93%	92%
Incidence of Potentially Preventable VTE[2]	26	4%	10%	10%
UFH with Dosages/Platelet Monitoring[2]	31	97%	99%	97%
Venous Thromboembolism Prophylaxis[2]	418	80%	83%	85%
Warfarin Therapy Discharge Instructions[2]	53	81%	77%	75%
Chest Pain/Possible Heart Attack Care				
Aspirin Given Within 24 Hours of Arrival[1,3]	-	-	98%	96%
Fibrinolytic Meds Within 30 Min. of Arrival[3,7]	-	-	63%	58%
Average Time to ECG (minutes)[1,3]	-	-	7	7
Average Time to Transfer (minutes)[3,7]	-	-	74	60
Children's Asthma Care				
Received Home Management Plan of Care	-	-	-	88%
Received Reliever Medication	-	-	-	100%
Received Systemic Corticosteroids	-	-	-	100%
Emergency Department				
Admittance Decision Time (minutes)[2]	652	153	148	98
Head CT Results Within 45 Min. of Arrival[1]	-	-	66%	57%
Patients Who Left ER Before Being Seen	70,449	3%	2%	2%
Time from ER Arrival to Admit. (minutes)[2]	655	410	355	274
Time from ER Arrival to Discharge (minutes)	351	175	152	134
Time in ER Before Being Evaluated (minutes)	408	41	32	26
Time to Pain Meds for Fractures (minutes)	232	63	58	57
Heart Attack Care				
Aspirin Given at Discharge	121	99%	99%	99%
Fibrinolytic Meds Within 30 Min. of Arrival[7]	-	-	69%	54%
PCI Within 90 Minutes of Arrival	27	89%	95%	96%
Statin Prescribed at Discharge	123	98%	99%	98%
Heart Failure Care				
ACE Inhibitor or ARB for LVSD	157	83%	98%	97%
Discharge Instructions Given	342	92%	97%	94%
Evaluation of LVS Function	437	100%	100%	99%
Medicare Spending				
Medicare Spending per Patient (ratio)	-	1.14	1.07	0.98
Pneumonia Care				
Appropriate Initial Antibiotic Given[2]	54	96%	98%	95%
Blood Culture Timing[2]	75	99%	99%	98%
Pregnancy and Delivery Care				
Newborn Deliveries Scheduled Early[2]	202	5%	3%	6%
Preventive Care				
Immunization for Influenza[2]	506	99%	93%	90%
Immunization for Pneumonia[2]	593	97%	94%	92%
Stroke Care				
Anticoagulation Therapy for Atrial Fibrillation[1]	-	-	97%	95%
Antithrombotic Therapy Timing	125	97%	98%	98%
Assessed for Rehabilitation	139	96%	98%	97%
Discharged on Antithrombotic Therapy	115	98%	99%	99%
Discharged on Statin Medication	99	92%	95%	94%
Thrombolytic Therapy Timing	11	100%	74%	66%
Venous Thromboembolism Prophylaxis	168	86%	94%	94%
Written Stroke Educational Materials Given	71	100%	94%	88%
Surgical Care Improvement Project				
Appropriate Beta Blocker Usage[2]	153	93%	98%	98%
Appropriate VTP Within 24 Hours[2]	430	98%	99%	98%
Controlled Postoperative Blood Glucose[2,7]	-	-	97%	97%
Perioperative Temperature Management[2]	492	100%	100%	100%
Prophylactic Antibiotic Selection[2]	230	97%	99%	99%
Prophylactic Antibiotic Selection (Outpatient)	236	98%	97%	98%
Prophylactic Antibiotic Stopped[2]	225	99%	98%	98%
Prophylactic Antibiotic Timing[2]	230	100%	99%	99%
Prophylactic Antibiotic Timing (Outpatient)	238	98%	98%	98%
Urinary Catheter Removal[2]	252	99%	98%	97%
Survey of Patients' Hospital Experiences				
Area Around Room 'Always' Quiet at Night[11]	300+	52%	53%	61%
Doctors 'Always' Communicated Well[11]	300+	75%	77%	82%
Home Recovery Information Given[11]	300+	81%	82%	85%
Hospital Given 9 or 10 on 10 Point Scale[11]	300+	60%	64%	71%
Meds 'Always' Explained Before Given[11]	300+	57%	59%	64%

NOTE: Hospital profiles are in alphabetical order by state, then city, then hospital within the city; Rankings exclude hospitals with less than 25 cases except for patient surveys which excludes hospitals with less than 100 cases; (a) 100-299 cases; (1) The number of cases/patients is too few to report; (2) Data submitted were based on a sample of cases/patients; (3) Results are based on a shorter time period than required; (4) Data suppressed by CMS for one or more quarters; (5) Results are not available for this reporting period; (6) Fewer than 100 patients completed the HCAHPS survey; (7) No cases met the criteria for this measure; (8) The lower limit of the confidence interval cannot be calculated if the number of observed infections equals zero; (9) No data are available from the state/territory for this reporting period; (10) The scores shown reflect fewer than 50 completed surveys; (11) There were discrepancies in the data collection process; (12) This measure does not apply to this hospital for this reporting period; (13) Results cannot be calculated for this reporting period; (14) The results for this state are combined with nearby states to protect confidentiality; Please refer to the User's Guide for a full explanation of data.

Nurses 'Always' Communicated Well[11]	300+	69%	76%	79%
Pain 'Always' Well Controlled[11]	300+	65%	68%	71%
Room and Bathroom 'Always' Clean[11]	300+	69%	68%	73%
Timely Help 'Always' Received[11]	300+	54%	60%	68%
Would Definitely Recommend Hospital[11]	300+	58%	66%	71%
Use of Medical Imaging				
Cardiac Imaging Stress Test before Surgery	177	5.1%	5.8%	5.3%
Combination Abdominal CT Scan	716	2.8%	7.4%	10.5%
Combination Brain/Sinus CT Scan	635	4.3%	2.8%	2.7%
Combination Chest CT Scan	414	0.2%	2.4%	2.7%
Follow-up Mammogram/Ultrasound	839	3.9%	12.5%	8.8%
Lumbar Spine MRI for Low Back Pain[1]	-	-	32.9%	37.2%

Inspira Medical Center Elmer

501 West Front Street
Elmer, NJ 08318
Phone: 856-363-1000
Fax: 856-358-3248
URL: www.sjhs.com/content/sjhelmerhospit
Type: Acute Care Hospitals
Emergency Services: Yes
Ownership: Voluntary non-profit - Private
Beds: 88

Key Personnel:
Quality Assurance . . . . Donna Cross
CEO/President . . . . Chet Kaletkowski
Chief of Medical Staff . . . . William Mills
Emergency Room . . . . Stanley Zoyac

Measure	Cases	This Hosp.	State Avg.	U.S. Avg.
Blood Clot Prevention and Treatment				
Anticoagulation Overlap Therapy[2]	51	94%	88%	93%
ICU Venous Thromboembolism Prophylaxis[2]	50	78%	93%	92%
Incidence of Potentially Preventable VTE[1,2]	-	-	10%	10%
UFH with Dosages/Platelet Monitoring[2]	50	100%	99%	97%
Venous Thromboembolism Prophylaxis[2]	319	75%	83%	85%
Warfarin Therapy Discharge Instructions[2]	40	100%	77%	75%
Chest Pain/Possible Heart Attack Care				
Aspirin Given Within 24 Hours of Arrival	46	98%	98%	96%
Fibrinolytic Meds Within 30 Min. of Arrival[1]	-	-	63%	58%
Average Time to ECG (minutes)	47	5	7	7
Average Time to Transfer (minutes)[1]	-	-	74	60
Children's Asthma Care				
Received Home Management Plan of Care	-	-	-	88%
Received Reliever Medication	-	-	-	100%
Received Systemic Corticosteroids	-	-	-	100%
Emergency Department				
Admittance Decision Time (minutes)[2]	528	94	148	98
Head CT Results Within 45 Min. of Arrival[1]	-	-	66%	57%
Patients Who Left ER Before Being Seen	22,341	3%	2%	2%
Time from ER Arrival to Admit. (minutes)[2]	530	306	355	274
Time from ER Arrival to Discharge (minutes)	2,848	181	152	134
Time in ER Before Being Evaluated (minutes)	2,981	30	32	26
Time to Pain Meds for Fractures (minutes)	74	68	58	57
Heart Attack Care				
Aspirin Given at Discharge[2]	13	92%	99%	99%
Fibrinolytic Meds Within 30 Min. of Arrival[2,7]	-	-	69%	54%
PCI Within 90 Minutes of Arrival[2,7]	-	-	95%	96%
Statin Prescribed at Discharge[2]	11	73%	99%	98%
Heart Failure Care				
ACE Inhibitor or ARB for LVSD[2]	37	86%	98%	97%
Discharge Instructions Given[2]	114	100%	97%	94%
Evaluation of LVS Function[2]	135	99%	100%	99%
Medicare Spending				
Medicare Spending per Patient (ratio)	-	0.98	1.07	0.98
Pneumonia Care				
Appropriate Initial Antibiotic Given[2]	60	97%	98%	95%
Blood Culture Timing[2]	95	99%	99%	98%
Pregnancy and Delivery Care				
Newborn Deliveries Scheduled Early	25	0%	3%	6%
Preventive Care				
Immunization for Influenza[2]	341	90%	93%	90%
Immunization for Pneumonia[2]	402	94%	94%	92%
Stroke Care				
Anticoagulation Therapy for Atrial Fibrillation[1]	-	-	97%	95%
Antithrombotic Therapy Timing	27	93%	98%	98%
Assessed for Rehabilitation	32	100%	98%	97%
Discharged on Antithrombotic Therapy	30	100%	99%	99%
Discharged on Statin Medication	16	94%	95%	94%
Thrombolytic Therapy Timing[1]	-	-	74%	66%
Venous Thromboembolism Prophylaxis	34	88%	94%	94%
Written Stroke Educational Materials Given	20	80%	94%	88%
Surgical Care Improvement Project				
Appropriate Beta Blocker Usage[2]	54	96%	98%	98%
Appropriate VTP Within 24 Hours[2]	166	99%	99%	98%
Controlled Postoperative Blood Glucose[2,7]	-	-	97%	97%
Perioperative Temperature Management[2]	175	99%	100%	100%
Prophylactic Antibiotic Selection[2]	114	99%	99%	99%
Prophylactic Antibiotic Selection (Outpatient)	91	97%	97%	98%
Prophylactic Antibiotic Stopped[2]	109	99%	98%	98%
Prophylactic Antibiotic Timing[2]	114	99%	99%	99%
Prophylactic Antibiotic Timing (Outpatient)	95	95%	98%	98%
Urinary Catheter Removal[2]	139	99%	98%	97%
Survey of Patients' Hospital Experiences				
Area Around Room 'Always' Quiet at Night	300+	48%	53%	61%
Doctors 'Always' Communicated Well	300+	78%	77%	82%
Home Recovery Information Given	300+	88%	82%	85%
Hospital Given 9 or 10 on 10 Point Scale	300+	72%	64%	71%
Meds 'Always' Explained Before Given	300+	63%	59%	64%
Nurses 'Always' Communicated Well	300+	80%	76%	79%
Pain 'Always' Well Controlled	300+	73%	68%	71%
Room and Bathroom 'Always' Clean	300+	75%	68%	73%
Timely Help 'Always' Received	300+	70%	60%	68%
Would Definitely Recommend Hospital	300+	78%	66%	71%
Use of Medical Imaging				
Cardiac Imaging Stress Test before Surgery	143	4.9%	5.8%	5.3%
Combination Abdominal CT Scan	391	9.0%	7.4%	10.5%
Combination Brain/Sinus CT Scan[1]	-	-	2.8%	2.7%
Combination Chest CT Scan	252	0.8%	2.4%	2.7%
Follow-up Mammogram/Ultrasound	619	13.6%	12.5%	8.8%
Lumbar Spine MRI for Low Back Pain[1]	-	-	32.9%	37.2%

Englewood Hospital & Medical Center

350 Engle St
Englewood, NJ 07631
Phone: 201-894-3000
Fax: 201-894-4791
URL: www.englewoodhospital.com
Type: Acute Care Hospitals
Emergency Services: Yes
Ownership: Voluntary non-profit - Private
Beds: 547

Key Personnel:
Chief of Medical Staff . . . . Robert Adair
CEO/President . . . . Douglas A Duchak
Radiology . . . . Marina Gutwein
Hemotology Center . . . . Michael Schleider, MD

Measure	Cases	This Hosp.	State Avg.	U.S. Avg.
Blood Clot Prevention and Treatment				
Anticoagulation Overlap Therapy[2]	41	95%	88%	93%
ICU Venous Thromboembolism Prophylaxis[2]	55	100%	93%	92%
Incidence of Potentially Preventable VTE[1,2]	-	-	10%	10%
UFH with Dosages/Platelet Monitoring[2]	11	100%	99%	97%
Venous Thromboembolism Prophylaxis[2]	363	98%	83%	85%
Warfarin Therapy Discharge Instructions[2]	24	88%	77%	75%
Chest Pain/Possible Heart Attack Care				
Aspirin Given Within 24 Hours of Arrival[5]	-	-	98%	96%
Fibrinolytic Meds Within 30 Min. of Arrival[5]	-	-	63%	58%
Average Time to ECG (minutes)[5]	-	-	7	7
Average Time to Transfer (minutes)[5]	-	-	74	60
Children's Asthma Care				
Received Home Management Plan of Care	-	-	-	88%
Received Reliever Medication	-	-	-	100%
Received Systemic Corticosteroids	-	-	-	100%
Emergency Department				
Admittance Decision Time (minutes)[2]	659	194	148	98
Head CT Results Within 45 Min. of Arrival[1]	-	-	66%	57%
Patients Who Left ER Before Being Seen	47,790	1%	2%	2%
Time from ER Arrival to Admit. (minutes)[2]	659	392	355	274
Time from ER Arrival to Discharge (minutes)	413	176	152	134
Time in ER Before Being Evaluated (minutes)	428	36	32	26
Time to Pain Meds for Fractures (minutes)	182	79	58	57
Heart Attack Care				
Aspirin Given at Discharge	342	100%	99%	99%
Fibrinolytic Meds Within 30 Min. of Arrival[7]	-	-	69%	54%
PCI Within 90 Minutes of Arrival	33	91%	95%	96%
Statin Prescribed at Discharge	339	99%	99%	98%
Heart Failure Care				
ACE Inhibitor or ARB for LVSD	147	99%	98%	97%
Discharge Instructions Given	338	96%	97%	94%
Evaluation of LVS Function	481	99%	100%	99%
Medicare Spending				
Medicare Spending per Patient (ratio)	-	1.07	1.07	0.98
Pneumonia Care				
Appropriate Initial Antibiotic Given	122	99%	98%	95%
Blood Culture Timing	212	98%	99%	98%
Pregnancy and Delivery Care				
Newborn Deliveries Scheduled Early[2]	52	12%	3%	6%
Preventive Care				
Immunization for Influenza[2]	552	87%	93%	90%
Immunization for Pneumonia[2]	634	84%	94%	92%
Stroke Care				
Anticoagulation Therapy for Atrial Fibrillation	40	100%	97%	95%
Antithrombotic Therapy Timing	155	98%	98%	98%
Assessed for Rehabilitation	183	94%	98%	97%
Discharged on Antithrombotic Therapy	163	99%	99%	99%
Discharged on Statin Medication	125	96%	95%	94%
Thrombolytic Therapy Timing	23	43%	74%	66%
Venous Thromboembolism Prophylaxis	188	88%	94%	94%
Written Stroke Educational Materials Given	95	87%	94%	88%
Surgical Care Improvement Project				
Appropriate Beta Blocker Usage[2]	407	98%	98%	98%
Appropriate VTP Within 24 Hours[2]	736	99%	99%	98%
Controlled Postoperative Blood Glucose[2]	231	97%	97%	97%
Perioperative Temperature Management[2]	830	100%	100%	100%
Prophylactic Antibiotic Selection[2]	855	99%	99%	99%
Prophylactic Antibiotic Selection (Outpatient)	475	99%	97%	98%
Prophylactic Antibiotic Stopped[2]	845	99%	98%	98%
Prophylactic Antibiotic Timing[2]	857	100%	99%	99%
Prophylactic Antibiotic Timing (Outpatient)	477	99%	98%	98%
Urinary Catheter Removal[2]	703	99%	98%	97%
Survey of Patients' Hospital Experiences				
Area Around Room 'Always' Quiet at Night	300+	54%	53%	61%
Doctors 'Always' Communicated Well	300+	78%	77%	82%
Home Recovery Information Given	300+	77%	82%	85%
Hospital Given 9 or 10 on 10 Point Scale	300+	70%	64%	71%
Meds 'Always' Explained Before Given	300+	56%	59%	64%
Nurses 'Always' Communicated Well	300+	75%	76%	79%
Pain 'Always' Well Controlled	300+	69%	68%	71%
Room and Bathroom 'Always' Clean	300+	68%	68%	73%
Timely Help 'Always' Received	300+	56%	60%	68%
Would Definitely Recommend Hospital	300+	72%	66%	71%
Use of Medical Imaging				
Cardiac Imaging Stress Test before Surgery	1,727	4.6%	5.8%	5.3%
Combination Abdominal CT Scan	1,615	10.2%	7.4%	10.5%
Combination Brain/Sinus CT Scan	1,311	2.9%	2.8%	2.7%
Combination Chest CT Scan	1,298	0.3%	2.4%	2.7%
Follow-up Mammogram/Ultrasound	3,693	19.4%	12.5%	8.8%
Lumbar Spine MRI for Low Back Pain	189	31.7%	32.9%	37.2%

Hunterdon Medical Center

2100 Wescott Drive
Flemington, NJ 08822
Phone: 908-788-6100
Fax: 908-788-6111
URL: www.hunterdonhealthcare.org
Type: Acute Care Hospitals
Emergency Services: Yes
Ownership: Voluntary non-profit - Private
Beds: 176

Key Personnel:
Operating Room. . . . . Donna Cole, RN
Radiology. . . . . Brian Donnelly, MD
Quality Assurance . . . . Stephanie Dougherty
Pediatric Ambulatory Care . . . . . . Wayne Fellmeth, MD
Pediatric In-Patient Care . . . . Wayne Fellmeth, MD
Chief of Medical Staff . . . . Robert Pickoff, MD
Infection Control. . . . . Kathy Roye, RN
CEO/President. . . . . Robert P Wise

Measure	Cases	This Hosp.	State Avg.	U.S. Avg.
Blood Clot Prevention and Treatment				
Anticoagulation Overlap Therapy[2]	49	88%	88%	93%
ICU Venous Thromboembolism Prophylaxis[2]	62	97%	93%	92%

NOTE: Hospital profiles are in alphabetical order by state, then city, then hospital within the city; Rankings exclude hospitals with less than 25 cases except for patient surveys which excludes hospitals with less than 100 cases; (a) 100-299 cases; (1) The number of cases/patients is too few to report; (2) Data submitted were based on a sample of cases/patients; (3) Results are based on a shorter time period than required; (4) Data suppressed by CMS for one or more quarters; (5) Results are not available for this reporting period; (6) Fewer than 100 patients completed the HCAHPS survey; (7) No cases met the criteria for this measure; (8) The lower limit of the confidence interval cannot be calculated if the number of observed infections equals zero; (9) No data are available from the state/territory for this reporting period; (10) The scores shown reflect fewer than 50 completed surveys; (11) There were discrepancies in the data collection process; (12) This measure does not apply to this hospital for this reporting period; (13) Results cannot be calculated for this reporting period; (14) The results for this state are combined with nearby states to protect confidentiality; Please refer to the User's Guide for a full explanation of data.

Incidence of Potentially Preventable VTE[1,2]	-	-	10%	10%
UFH with Dosages/Platelet Monitoring[2]	34	94%	99%	97%
Venous Thromboembolism Prophylaxis[2]	410	93%	83%	85%
Warfarin Therapy Discharge Instructions[2]	29	93%	77%	75%
Chest Pain/Possible Heart Attack Care				
Aspirin Given Within 24 Hours of Arrival[1]	-	-	98%	96%
Fibrinolytic Meds Within 30 Min. of Arrival[3,7]	-	-	63%	58%
Average Time to ECG (minutes)[1]	-	-	7	7
Average Time to Transfer (minutes)[3,7]	-	-	74	60
Children's Asthma Care				
Received Home Management Plan of Care	-	-	-	88%
Received Reliever Medication	-	-	-	100%
Received Systemic Corticosteroids	-	-	-	100%
Emergency Department				
Admittance Decision Time (minutes)[2]	773	148	148	98
Head CT Results Within 45 Min. of Arrival[1]	-	-	66%	57%
Patients Who Left ER Before Being Seen	34,172	1%	2%	2%
Time from ER Arrival to Admit. (minutes)[2]	774	317	355	274
Time from ER Arrival to Discharge (minutes)	399	177	152	134
Time in ER Before Being Evaluated (minutes)	411	43	32	26
Time to Pain Meds for Fractures (minutes)	111	53	58	57
Heart Attack Care				
Aspirin Given at Discharge	104	100%	99%	99%
Fibrinolytic Meds Within 30 Min. of Arrival[7]	-	-	69%	54%
PCI Within 90 Minutes of Arrival	35	97%	95%	96%
Statin Prescribed at Discharge	105	100%	99%	98%
Heart Failure Care				
ACE Inhibitor or ARB for LVSD	43	100%	98%	97%
Discharge Instructions Given	120	91%	97%	94%
Evaluation of LVS Function	166	99%	100%	99%
Medicare Spending				
Medicare Spending per Patient (ratio)	-	1.02	1.07	0.98
Pneumonia Care				
Appropriate Initial Antibiotic Given[2]	106	100%	98%	95%
Blood Culture Timing[2]	176	99%	99%	98%
Pregnancy and Delivery Care				
Newborn Deliveries Scheduled Early[2]	28	0%	3%	6%
Preventive Care				
Immunization for Influenza[2]	534	96%	93%	90%
Immunization for Pneumonia[2]	622	95%	94%	92%
Stroke Care				
Anticoagulation Therapy for Atrial Fibrillation	14	100%	97%	95%
Antithrombotic Therapy Timing	70	99%	98%	98%
Assessed for Rehabilitation	78	95%	98%	97%
Discharged on Antithrombotic Therapy	71	100%	99%	99%
Discharged on Statin Medication	61	93%	95%	94%
Thrombolytic Therapy Timing[1]	-	-	74%	66%
Venous Thromboembolism Prophylaxis	80	100%	94%	94%
Written Stroke Educational Materials Given	31	77%	94%	88%
Surgical Care Improvement Project				
Appropriate Beta Blocker Usage[2]	108	96%	98%	98%
Appropriate VTP Within 24 Hours[2]	301	99%	99%	98%
Controlled Postoperative Blood Glucose[2,7]	-	-	97%	97%
Perioperative Temperature Management[2]	358	99%	100%	100%
Prophylactic Antibiotic Selection[2]	219	100%	99%	99%
Prophylactic Antibiotic Selection (Outpatient)	133	98%	97%	98%
Prophylactic Antibiotic Stopped[2]	212	97%	98%	98%
Prophylactic Antibiotic Timing[2]	219	100%	99%	99%
Prophylactic Antibiotic Timing (Outpatient)	133	98%	98%	98%
Urinary Catheter Removal[2]	95	88%	98%	97%
Survey of Patients' Hospital Experiences				
Area Around Room 'Always' Quiet at Night	300+	51%	53%	61%
Doctors 'Always' Communicated Well	300+	81%	77%	82%
Home Recovery Information Given	300+	85%	82%	85%
Hospital Given 9 or 10 on 10 Point Scale	300+	74%	64%	71%
Meds 'Always' Explained Before Given	300+	65%	59%	64%
Nurses 'Always' Communicated Well	300+	81%	76%	79%
Pain 'Always' Well Controlled	300+	74%	68%	71%
Room and Bathroom 'Always' Clean	300+	70%	68%	73%
Timely Help 'Always' Received	300+	64%	60%	68%
Would Definitely Recommend Hospital	300+	77%	66%	71%
Use of Medical Imaging				
Cardiac Imaging Stress Test before Surgery	657	4.1%	5.8%	5.3%
Combination Abdominal CT Scan	849	4.7%	7.4%	10.5%
Combination Brain/Sinus CT Scan	681	2.5%	2.8%	2.7%
Combination Chest CT Scan	768	1.4%	2.4%	2.7%
Follow-up Mammogram/Ultrasound	1,637	10.5%	12.5%	8.8%
Lumbar Spine MRI for Low Back Pain[7]	-	-	32.9%	37.2%

Centrastate Medical Center

901 West Main Street
Freehold, NJ 07728
URL: www.centrastate.com
Type: Acute Care Hospitals
Ownership: Voluntary non-profit - Private
Phone: 732-431-2000
Fax: 732-462-5129
Emergency Services: Yes
Beds: 271

Key Personnel:

Quality Assurance . . . . Janice De Young Breen, RN, APRN
Chief of Medical Staff. . . . . Jack H. Dworkin, MD, MBA, FACC
Patient Relations . . . . Laura Geisler, RN
CEO/President. . . . . John T Gribbin, FACHE
Chairman/CEO . . . . Joseph R. Iantosca

Measure	Cases	This Hosp.	State Avg.	U.S. Avg.
Blood Clot Prevention and Treatment				
Anticoagulation Overlap Therapy[2]	64	81%	88%	93%
ICU Venous Thromboembolism Prophylaxis[2]	67	99%	93%	92%
Incidence of Potentially Preventable VTE[2]	13	23%	10%	10%
UFH with Dosages/Platelet Monitoring[2]	68	100%	99%	97%
Venous Thromboembolism Prophylaxis[2]	449	99%	83%	85%
Warfarin Therapy Discharge Instructions[2]	38	18%	77%	75%
Chest Pain/Possible Heart Attack Care				
Aspirin Given Within 24 Hours of Arrival	117	100%	98%	96%
Fibrinolytic Meds Within 30 Min. of Arrival	18	83%	63%	58%
Average Time to ECG (minutes)	116	4	7	7
Average Time to Transfer (minutes)	19	64	74	60
Children's Asthma Care				
Received Home Management Plan of Care	-	-	-	88%
Received Reliever Medication	-	-	-	100%
Received Systemic Corticosteroids	-	-	-	100%
Emergency Department				
Admittance Decision Time (minutes)[2]	724	156	148	98
Head CT Results Within 45 Min. of Arrival	13	85%	66%	57%
Patients Who Left ER Before Being Seen	65,888	1%	2%	2%
Time from ER Arrival to Admit. (minutes)[2]	729	376	355	274
Time from ER Arrival to Discharge (minutes)	373	170	152	134
Time in ER Before Being Evaluated (minutes)	384	40	32	26
Time to Pain Meds for Fractures (minutes)	211	52	58	57
Heart Attack Care				
Aspirin Given at Discharge[2]	30	100%	99%	99%
Fibrinolytic Meds Within 30 Min. of Arrival[1,2]	-	-	69%	54%
PCI Within 90 Minutes of Arrival[2,7]	-	-	95%	96%
Statin Prescribed at Discharge[2]	30	100%	99%	98%
Heart Failure Care				
ACE Inhibitor or ARB for LVSD[2]	72	100%	98%	97%
Discharge Instructions Given[2]	182	96%	97%	94%
Evaluation of LVS Function[2]	293	100%	100%	99%
Medicare Spending				
Medicare Spending per Patient (ratio)	-	1.07	1.07	0.98
Pneumonia Care				
Appropriate Initial Antibiotic Given[2]	222	99%	98%	95%
Blood Culture Timing[2]	457	99%	99%	98%
Pregnancy and Delivery Care				
Newborn Deliveries Scheduled Early[2]	23	0%	3%	6%
Preventive Care				
Immunization for Influenza[2]	509	97%	93%	90%
Immunization for Pneumonia[2]	569	97%	94%	92%
Stroke Care				
Anticoagulation Therapy for Atrial Fibrillation[2]	26	96%	97%	95%
Antithrombotic Therapy Timing[2]	134	99%	98%	98%
Assessed for Rehabilitation[2]	156	97%	98%	97%
Discharged on Antithrombotic Therapy[2]	143	97%	99%	99%
Discharged on Statin Medication[2]	131	95%	95%	94%
Thrombolytic Therapy Timing[1,2]	-	-	74%	66%
Venous Thromboembolism Prophylaxis[2]	167	99%	94%	94%
Written Stroke Educational Materials Given[2]	75	88%	94%	88%
Surgical Care Improvement Project				
Appropriate Beta Blocker Usage[2]	208	97%	98%	98%
Appropriate VTP Within 24 Hours[2]	544	99%	99%	98%
Controlled Postoperative Blood Glucose[2,7]	-	-	97%	97%
Perioperative Temperature Management[2]	662	100%	100%	100%
Prophylactic Antibiotic Selection[2]	278	100%	99%	99%
Prophylactic Antibiotic Selection (Outpatient)	185	99%	97%	98%
Prophylactic Antibiotic Stopped[2]	264	97%	98%	98%
Prophylactic Antibiotic Timing[2]	278	99%	99%	99%
Prophylactic Antibiotic Timing (Outpatient)	129	99%	98%	98%
Urinary Catheter Removal[2]	278	100%	98%	97%
Survey of Patients' Hospital Experiences				
Area Around Room 'Always' Quiet at Night	300+	56%	53%	61%
Doctors 'Always' Communicated Well	300+	82%	77%	82%
Home Recovery Information Given	300+	86%	82%	85%
Hospital Given 9 or 10 on 10 Point Scale	300+	69%	64%	71%
Meds 'Always' Explained Before Given	300+	68%	59%	64%
Nurses 'Always' Communicated Well	300+	83%	76%	79%
Pain 'Always' Well Controlled	300+	75%	68%	71%
Room and Bathroom 'Always' Clean	300+	76%	68%	73%
Timely Help 'Always' Received	300+	70%	60%	68%
Would Definitely Recommend Hospital	300+	73%	66%	71%
Use of Medical Imaging				
Cardiac Imaging Stress Test before Surgery	249	4.4%	5.8%	5.3%
Combination Abdominal CT Scan	944	3.5%	7.4%	10.5%
Combination Brain/Sinus CT Scan	1,552	1.7%	2.8%	2.7%
Combination Chest CT Scan	457	0.2%	2.4%	2.7%
Follow-up Mammogram/Ultrasound	1,056	12.0%	12.5%	8.8%
Lumbar Spine MRI for Low Back Pain[7]	-	-	32.9%	37.2%

Hackensack University Medical Center

30 Prospect Ave
Hackensack, NJ 07601
URL: www.humed.com
Type: Acute Care Hospitals
Ownership: Voluntary non-profit - Private
Phone: 201-996-2000
Fax: 201-996-3452
Emergency Services: Yes
Beds: 614

Key Personnel:

Chief of Medical Staff . . . . Jeanne Aversa
Radiology. . . . . Helen Chimel
CEO/President. . . . . Robert C Garrett
Quality Assurance . . . . Audrey Murphy
Infection Control. . . . . Nancy Nelsen, RN
Operating Room. . . . . Doreen Santora, RN
Pediatric In-Patient Care . . . . Donald Stark

Measure	Cases	This Hosp.	State Avg.	U.S. Avg.
Blood Clot Prevention and Treatment				
Anticoagulation Overlap Therapy[2]	241	92%	88%	93%
ICU Venous Thromboembolism Prophylaxis[2]	54	87%	93%	92%
Incidence of Potentially Preventable VTE[2]	101	10%	10%	10%
UFH with Dosages/Platelet Monitoring[2]	240	100%	99%	97%
Venous Thromboembolism Prophylaxis[2]	398	69%	83%	85%
Warfarin Therapy Discharge Instructions[2]	128	77%	77%	75%
Chest Pain/Possible Heart Attack Care				
Aspirin Given Within 24 Hours of Arrival[1,3]	-	-	98%	96%
Fibrinolytic Meds Within 30 Min. of Arrival[5]	-	-	63%	58%
Average Time to ECG (minutes)[1,3]	-	-	7	7
Average Time to Transfer (minutes)[5]	-	-	74	60
Children's Asthma Care				
Received Home Management Plan of Care	-	-	-	88%
Received Reliever Medication	-	-	-	100%
Received Systemic Corticosteroids	-	-	-	100%
Emergency Department				
Admittance Decision Time (minutes)[2]	451	315	148	98
Head CT Results Within 45 Min. of Arrival[1]	-	-	66%	57%
Patients Who Left ER Before Being Seen	>100k	1%	2%	2%
Time from ER Arrival to Admit. (minutes)[2]	472	477	355	274
Time from ER Arrival to Discharge (minutes)	341	174	152	134
Time in ER Before Being Evaluated (minutes)	376	44	32	26
Time to Pain Meds for Fractures (minutes)	384	61	58	57
Heart Attack Care				
Aspirin Given at Discharge	603	100%	99%	99%
Fibrinolytic Meds Within 30 Min. of Arrival[7]	-	-	69%	54%
PCI Within 90 Minutes of Arrival	86	95%	95%	96%
Statin Prescribed at Discharge	602	100%	99%	98%
Heart Failure Care				

NOTE: Hospital profiles are in alphabetical order by state, then city, then hospital within the city; Rankings exclude hospitals with less than 25 cases except for patient surveys which excludes hospitals with less than 100 cases; (a) 100-299 cases; (1) The number of cases/patients is too few to report; (2) Data submitted were based on a sample of cases/patients; (3) Results are based on a shorter time period than required; (4) Data suppressed by CMS for one or more quarters; (5) Results are not available for this reporting period; (6) Fewer than 100 patients completed the HCAHPS survey; (7) No cases met the criteria for this measure; (8) The lower limit of the confidence interval cannot be calculated if the number of observed infections equals zero; (9) No data are available from the state/territory for this reporting period; (10) The scores shown reflect fewer than 50 completed surveys; (11) There were discrepancies in the data collection process; (12) This measure does not apply to this hospital for this reporting period; (13) Results cannot be calculated for this reporting period; (14) The results for this state are combined with nearby states to protect confidentiality; Please refer to the User's Guide for a full explanation of data.

ACE Inhibitor or ARB for LVSD	261	97%	98%	97%
Discharge Instructions Given	570	97%	97%	94%
Evaluation of LVS Function	812	100%	100%	99%
Medicare Spending				
Medicare Spending per Patient (ratio)	-	1.11	1.07	0.98
Pneumonia Care				
Appropriate Initial Antibiotic Given	356	96%	98%	95%
Blood Culture Timing	451	98%	99%	98%
Pregnancy and Delivery Care				
Newborn Deliveries Scheduled Early[2]	156	6%	3%	6%
Preventive Care				
Immunization for Influenza[2]	493	76%	93%	90%
Immunization for Pneumonia[2]	494	86%	94%	92%
Stroke Care				
Anticoagulation Therapy for Atrial Fibrillation[2]	17	88%	97%	95%
Antithrombotic Therapy Timing[2]	92	100%	98%	98%
Assessed for Rehabilitation[2]	126	94%	98%	97%
Discharged on Antithrombotic Therapy[2]	93	100%	99%	99%
Discharged on Statin Medication[2]	79	96%	95%	94%
Thrombolytic Therapy Timing[1,2]	-	-	74%	66%
Venous Thromboembolism Prophylaxis[2]	129	79%	94%	94%
Written Stroke Educational Materials Given[2]	62	84%	94%	88%
Surgical Care Improvement Project				
Appropriate Beta Blocker Usage[2]	217	97%	98%	98%
Appropriate VTP Within 24 Hours[2]	384	97%	99%	98%
Controlled Postoperative Blood Glucose[2]	134	87%	97%	97%
Perioperative Temperature Management[2]	489	99%	100%	100%
Prophylactic Antibiotic Selection[2]	420	99%	99%	99%
Prophylactic Antibiotic Selection (Outpatient)	939	98%	97%	98%
Prophylactic Antibiotic Stopped[2]	392	98%	98%	98%
Prophylactic Antibiotic Timing[2]	421	99%	99%	99%
Prophylactic Antibiotic Timing (Outpatient)	941	98%	98%	98%
Urinary Catheter Removal[2]	402	99%	98%	97%
Survey of Patients' Hospital Experiences				
Area Around Room 'Always' Quiet at Night	300+	54%	53%	61%
Doctors 'Always' Communicated Well	300+	81%	77%	82%
Home Recovery Information Given	300+	82%	82%	85%
Hospital Given 9 or 10 on 10 Point Scale	300+	75%	64%	71%
Meds 'Always' Explained Before Given	300+	63%	59%	64%
Nurses 'Always' Communicated Well	300+	81%	76%	79%
Pain 'Always' Well Controlled	300+	76%	68%	71%
Room and Bathroom 'Always' Clean	300+	74%	68%	73%
Timely Help 'Always' Received	300+	66%	60%	68%
Would Definitely Recommend Hospital	300+	80%	66%	71%
Use of Medical Imaging				
Cardiac Imaging Stress Test before Surgery	1,609	5.8%	5.8%	5.3%
Combination Abdominal CT Scan	2,445	2.9%	7.4%	10.5%
Combination Brain/Sinus CT Scan	2,005	2.7%	2.8%	2.7%
Combination Chest CT Scan	2,957	0.6%	2.4%	2.7%
Follow-up Mammogram/Ultrasound	3,109	13.4%	12.5%	8.8%
Lumbar Spine MRI for Low Back Pain	86	27.9%	32.9%	37.2%

Hackettstown Regional Medical Center

651 Willow Grove St
Hackettstown, NJ 07840
Phone: 908-852-5100
Fax: 908-850-6822
URL: www.hrmcnj.org
Type: Acute Care Hospitals
Emergency Services: Yes
Ownership: Voluntary non-profit - Church
Beds: 99

Key Personnel:
Anesthesiology . . . . Arnold Bodner, MD
CEO/President . . . . Jason C Coe, MBA
Pediatric In-Patient Care . . . . Adam Dick, MD
Quality Assurance . . . . Kim Foreman
Intensive Care Unit. . . . . Cathy Richardson
Emergency Room . . . . Chester Skiba
Chief of Medical Staff . . . . Leong-Hean Tan

Measure	Cases	This Hosp.	State Avg.	U.S. Avg.
Blood Clot Prevention and Treatment				
Anticoagulation Overlap Therapy[2]	24	83%	88%	93%
ICU Venous Thromboembolism Prophylaxis[2]	52	81%	93%	92%
Incidence of Potentially Preventable VTE[1,2]	-	-	10%	10%
UFH with Dosages/Platelet Monitoring[2]	29	100%	99%	97%
Venous Thromboembolism Prophylaxis[2]	314	77%	83%	85%
Warfarin Therapy Discharge Instructions[2]	15	100%	77%	75%
Chest Pain/Possible Heart Attack Care				
Aspirin Given Within 24 Hours of Arrival	19	100%	98%	96%
Fibrinolytic Meds Within 30 Min. of Arrival[1]	-	-	63%	58%
Average Time to ECG (minutes)	20	14	7	7
Average Time to Transfer (minutes)[7]	-	-	74	60
Children's Asthma Care				
Received Home Management Plan of Care	-	-	-	88%
Received Reliever Medication	-	-	-	100%
Received Systemic Corticosteroids	-	-	-	100%
Emergency Department				
Admittance Decision Time (minutes)[2]	499	117	148	98
Head CT Results Within 45 Min. of Arrival[5]	-	-	66%	57%
Patients Who Left ER Before Being Seen	21,898	1%	2%	2%
Time from ER Arrival to Admit. (minutes)[2]	569	287	355	274
Time from ER Arrival to Discharge (minutes)	360	127	152	134
Time in ER Before Being Evaluated (minutes)	383	26	32	26
Time to Pain Meds for Fractures (minutes)	98	76	58	57
Heart Attack Care				
Aspirin Given at Discharge	36	100%	99%	99%
Fibrinolytic Meds Within 30 Min. of Arrival[7]	-	-	69%	54%
PCI Within 90 Minutes of Arrival[7]	-	-	95%	96%
Statin Prescribed at Discharge	37	100%	99%	98%
Heart Failure Care				
ACE Inhibitor or ARB for LVSD	27	100%	98%	97%
Discharge Instructions Given	117	100%	97%	94%
Evaluation of LVS Function	188	100%	100%	99%
Medicare Spending				
Medicare Spending per Patient (ratio)	-	1.07	1.07	0.98
Pneumonia Care				
Appropriate Initial Antibiotic Given	107	100%	98%	95%
Blood Culture Timing	204	100%	99%	98%
Pregnancy and Delivery Care				
Newborn Deliveries Scheduled Early	50	0%	3%	6%
Preventive Care				
Immunization for Influenza[2]	395	97%	93%	90%
Immunization for Pneumonia[2]	486	93%	94%	92%
Stroke Care				
Anticoagulation Therapy for Atrial Fibrillation[1]	-	-	97%	95%
Antithrombotic Therapy Timing	32	100%	98%	98%
Assessed for Rehabilitation	36	100%	98%	97%
Discharged on Antithrombotic Therapy	34	100%	99%	99%
Discharged on Statin Medication	22	100%	95%	94%
Thrombolytic Therapy Timing[1]	-	-	74%	66%
Venous Thromboembolism Prophylaxis	38	95%	94%	94%
Written Stroke Educational Materials Given	21	100%	94%	88%
Surgical Care Improvement Project				
Appropriate Beta Blocker Usage	72	100%	98%	98%
Appropriate VTP Within 24 Hours	239	100%	99%	98%
Controlled Postoperative Blood Glucose[7]	-	-	97%	97%
Perioperative Temperature Management	266	100%	100%	100%
Prophylactic Antibiotic Selection	194	100%	99%	99%
Prophylactic Antibiotic Selection (Outpatient)	68	97%	97%	98%
Prophylactic Antibiotic Stopped	190	99%	98%	98%
Prophylactic Antibiotic Timing	194	100%	99%	99%
Prophylactic Antibiotic Timing (Outpatient)	69	97%	98%	98%
Urinary Catheter Removal	178	100%	98%	97%
Survey of Patients' Hospital Experiences				
Area Around Room 'Always' Quiet at Night	300+	50%	53%	61%
Doctors 'Always' Communicated Well	300+	75%	77%	82%
Home Recovery Information Given	300+	85%	82%	85%
Hospital Given 9 or 10 on 10 Point Scale	300+	63%	64%	71%
Meds 'Always' Explained Before Given	300+	51%	59%	64%
Nurses 'Always' Communicated Well	300+	74%	76%	79%
Pain 'Always' Well Controlled	300+	70%	68%	71%
Room and Bathroom 'Always' Clean	300+	61%	68%	73%
Timely Help 'Always' Received	300+	61%	60%	68%
Would Definitely Recommend Hospital	300+	64%	66%	71%
Use of Medical Imaging				
Cardiac Imaging Stress Test before Surgery	204	8.8%	5.8%	5.3%
Combination Abdominal CT Scan	552	11.4%	7.4%	10.5%
Combination Brain/Sinus CT Scan	516	5.0%	2.8%	2.7%
Combination Chest CT Scan	351	4.0%	2.4%	2.7%
Follow-up Mammogram/Ultrasound	710	11.0%	12.5%	8.8%
Lumbar Spine MRI for Low Back Pain[1]	-	-	32.9%	37.2%

Robert Wood Johnson University Hospital - Hamilton

One Hamilton Health Place
Hamilton, NJ 08690
Phone: 609-586-7900
Fax: 609-584-6429
URL: www.rwjhamilton.org
Type: Acute Care Hospitals
Emergency Services: Yes
Ownership: Voluntary non-profit - Private
Beds: 200

Key Personnel:
Pediatric In-Patient Care . . . . Dennis M Baiser
Pediatric Ambulatory Care . . . . . . David H Carver, MD
CEO/President. . . . . Anthony Cimino
Infection Control. . . . . Anne Dikon
Operating Room. . . . . Louis G Fares II
Chief of Medical Staff . . . . Mahmoud Ghusson
Quality Assurance . . . . Jan Stout
Radiology. . . . . Hae W Won Shin

Measure	Cases	This Hosp.	State Avg.	U.S. Avg.
Blood Clot Prevention and Treatment				
Anticoagulation Overlap Therapy[2]	98	81%	88%	93%
ICU Venous Thromboembolism Prophylaxis[2]	91	98%	93%	92%
Incidence of Potentially Preventable VTE[2]	13	23%	10%	10%
UFH with Dosages/Platelet Monitoring[2]	104	100%	99%	97%
Venous Thromboembolism Prophylaxis[2]	312	87%	83%	85%
Warfarin Therapy Discharge Instructions[2]	62	23%	77%	75%
Chest Pain/Possible Heart Attack Care				
Aspirin Given Within 24 Hours of Arrival[5]	-	-	98%	96%
Fibrinolytic Meds Within 30 Min. of Arrival[5]	-	-	63%	58%
Average Time to ECG (minutes)[5]	-	-	7	7
Average Time to Transfer (minutes)[5]	-	-	74	60
Children's Asthma Care				
Received Home Management Plan of Care	-	-	-	88%
Received Reliever Medication	-	-	-	100%
Received Systemic Corticosteroids	-	-	-	100%
Emergency Department				
Admittance Decision Time (minutes)[2]	777	110	148	98
Head CT Results Within 45 Min. of Arrival	16	88%	66%	57%
Patients Who Left ER Before Being Seen	56,257	1%	2%	2%
Time from ER Arrival to Admit. (minutes)[2]	829	332	355	274
Time from ER Arrival to Discharge (minutes)	356	169	152	134
Time in ER Before Being Evaluated (minutes)	375	43	32	26
Time to Pain Meds for Fractures (minutes)	164	49	58	57
Heart Attack Care				
Aspirin Given at Discharge	81	100%	99%	99%
Fibrinolytic Meds Within 30 Min. of Arrival[7]	-	-	69%	54%
PCI Within 90 Minutes of Arrival	33	91%	95%	96%
Statin Prescribed at Discharge	76	100%	99%	98%
Heart Failure Care				
ACE Inhibitor or ARB for LVSD	67	99%	98%	97%
Discharge Instructions Given	243	89%	97%	94%
Evaluation of LVS Function	333	100%	100%	99%
Medicare Spending				
Medicare Spending per Patient (ratio)	-	1.07	1.07	0.98
Pneumonia Care				
Appropriate Initial Antibiotic Given	209	95%	98%	95%
Blood Culture Timing	425	100%	99%	98%
Pregnancy and Delivery Care				
Newborn Deliveries Scheduled Early	153	0%	3%	6%
Preventive Care				
Immunization for Influenza[2]	530	97%	93%	90%
Immunization for Pneumonia[2]	719	94%	94%	92%
Stroke Care				
Anticoagulation Therapy for Atrial Fibrillation	14	71%	97%	95%
Antithrombotic Therapy Timing	93	98%	98%	98%
Assessed for Rehabilitation	97	100%	98%	97%
Discharged on Antithrombotic Therapy	92	98%	99%	99%
Discharged on Statin Medication	69	96%	95%	94%
Thrombolytic Therapy Timing[1]	-	-	74%	66%
Venous Thromboembolism Prophylaxis	109	95%	94%	94%
Written Stroke Educational Materials Given	51	100%	94%	88%
Surgical Care Improvement Project				
Appropriate Beta Blocker Usage[2]	233	97%	98%	98%

NOTE: Hospital profiles are in alphabetical order by state, then city, then hospital within the city; Rankings exclude hospitals with less than 25 cases except for patient surveys which excludes hospitals with less than 100 cases; (a) 100-299 cases; (1) The number of cases/patients is too few to report; (2) Data submitted were based on a sample of cases/patients; (3) Results are based on a shorter time period than required; (4) Data suppressed by CMS for one or more quarters; (5) Results are not available for this reporting period; (6) Fewer than 100 patients completed the HCAHPS survey; (7) No cases met the criteria for this measure; (8) The lower limit of the confidence interval cannot be calculated if the number of observed infections equals zero; (9) No data are available from the state/territory for this reporting period; (10) The scores shown reflect fewer than 50 completed surveys; (11) There were discrepancies in the data collection process; (12) This measure does not apply to this hospital for this reporting period; (13) Results cannot be calculated for this reporting period; (14) The results for this state are combined with nearby states to protect confidentiality; Please refer to the User's Guide for a full explanation of data.

Measure	Cases	This Hosp.	State Avg.	U.S. Avg.
Appropriate VTP Within 24 Hours[2]	571	99%	99%	98%
Controlled Postoperative Blood Glucose[2,7]	-	-	97%	97%
Perioperative Temperature Management[2]	624	100%	100%	100%
Prophylactic Antibiotic Selection[2]	466	98%	99%	99%
Prophylactic Antibiotic Selection (Outpatient)	147	86%	97%	98%
Prophylactic Antibiotic Stopped[2]	451	97%	98%	98%
Prophylactic Antibiotic Timing[2]	468	98%	99%	99%
Prophylactic Antibiotic Timing (Outpatient)	145	99%	98%	98%
Urinary Catheter Removal[2]	461	98%	98%	97%
Survey of Patients' Hospital Experiences				
Area Around Room 'Always' Quiet at Night	300+	54%	53%	61%
Doctors 'Always' Communicated Well	300+	78%	77%	82%
Home Recovery Information Given	300+	85%	82%	85%
Hospital Given 9 or 10 on 10 Point Scale	300+	67%	64%	71%
Meds 'Always' Explained Before Given	300+	60%	59%	64%
Nurses 'Always' Communicated Well	300+	79%	76%	79%
Pain 'Always' Well Controlled	300+	71%	68%	71%
Room and Bathroom 'Always' Clean	300+	66%	68%	73%
Timely Help 'Always' Received	300+	64%	60%	68%
Would Definitely Recommend Hospital	300+	69%	66%	71%
Use of Medical Imaging				
Cardiac Imaging Stress Test before Surgery	80	7.5%	5.8%	5.3%
Combination Abdominal CT Scan	1,119	2.8%	7.4%	10.5%
Combination Brain/Sinus CT Scan	1,060	1.8%	2.8%	2.7%
Combination Chest CT Scan	489	0.2%	2.4%	2.7%
Follow-up Mammogram/Ultrasound	1,103	7.2%	12.5%	8.8%
Lumbar Spine MRI for Low Back Pain[1]	-	-	32.9%	37.2%

Carepoint Health - Hoboken UMC

308 Willow Ave
Hoboken, NJ 07030
Phone: 201-418-1004
Fax: 201-418-1011
URL: www.bonsecoursnj.com
Type: Acute Care Hospitals
Emergency Services: Yes
Ownership: Voluntary non-profit - Church
Beds: 266

Key Personnel:
Pediatric In-Patient Care . . . . Ruth Braddock
Operating Room. . . . . Ira Jacobs, MD
CEO/President. . . . . Richard J Statuto

Measure	Cases	This Hosp.	State Avg.	U.S. Avg.
Blood Clot Prevention and Treatment				
Anticoagulation Overlap Therapy[2]	17	94%	88%	93%
ICU Venous Thromboembolism Prophylaxis[2]	42	95%	93%	92%
Incidence of Potentially Preventable VTE[1,2]	-	-	10%	10%
UFH with Dosages/Platelet Monitoring[2]	22	100%	99%	97%
Venous Thromboembolism Prophylaxis[2]	293	85%	83%	85%
Warfarin Therapy Discharge Instructions[2]	13	92%	77%	75%
Chest Pain/Possible Heart Attack Care				
Aspirin Given Within 24 Hours of Arrival	13	92%	98%	96%
Fibrinolytic Meds Within 30 Min. of Arrival[1]	-	-	63%	58%
Average Time to ECG (minutes)[1]	-	-	7	7
Average Time to Transfer (minutes)[1]	-	-	74	60
Children's Asthma Care				
Received Home Management Plan of Care	-	-	-	88%
Received Reliever Medication	-	-	-	100%
Received Systemic Corticosteroids	-	-	-	100%
Emergency Department				
Admittance Decision Time (minutes)[2]	550	133	148	98
Head CT Results Within 45 Min. of Arrival[1]	-	-	66%	57%
Patients Who Left ER Before Being Seen	40,186	2%	2%	2%
Time from ER Arrival to Admit. (minutes)[2]	564	350	355	274
Time from ER Arrival to Discharge (minutes)	293	148	152	134
Time in ER Before Being Evaluated (minutes)	277	34	32	26
Time to Pain Meds for Fractures (minutes)	109	54	58	57
Heart Attack Care				
Aspirin Given at Discharge	18	100%	99%	99%
Fibrinolytic Meds Within 30 Min. of Arrival[7]	-	-	69%	54%
PCI Within 90 Minutes of Arrival[7]	-	-	95%	96%
Statin Prescribed at Discharge	20	100%	99%	98%
Heart Failure Care				
ACE Inhibitor or ARB for LVSD	59	100%	98%	97%
Discharge Instructions Given	98	100%	97%	94%
Evaluation of LVS Function	144	100%	100%	99%
Medicare Spending				
Medicare Spending per Patient (ratio)	-	1.11	1.07	0.98
Pneumonia Care				
Appropriate Initial Antibiotic Given	85	99%	98%	95%
Blood Culture Timing	156	99%	99%	98%
Pregnancy and Delivery Care				
Newborn Deliveries Scheduled Early[2]	16	31%	3%	6%
Preventive Care				
Immunization for Influenza[2]	465	82%	93%	90%
Immunization for Pneumonia[2]	421	95%	94%	92%
Stroke Care				
Anticoagulation Therapy for Atrial Fibrillation[1]	-	-	97%	95%
Antithrombotic Therapy Timing	50	98%	98%	98%
Assessed for Rehabilitation	52	100%	98%	97%
Discharged on Antithrombotic Therapy	49	94%	99%	99%
Discharged on Statin Medication	34	91%	95%	94%
Thrombolytic Therapy Timing[1]	-	-	74%	66%
Venous Thromboembolism Prophylaxis	57	95%	94%	94%
Written Stroke Educational Materials Given	21	100%	94%	88%
Surgical Care Improvement Project				
Appropriate Beta Blocker Usage	22	100%	98%	98%
Appropriate VTP Within 24 Hours	117	100%	99%	98%
Controlled Postoperative Blood Glucose[7]	-	-	97%	97%
Perioperative Temperature Management	141	100%	100%	100%
Prophylactic Antibiotic Selection	82	99%	99%	99%
Prophylactic Antibiotic Selection (Outpatient)	32	88%	97%	98%
Prophylactic Antibiotic Stopped	82	100%	98%	98%
Prophylactic Antibiotic Timing	82	100%	99%	99%
Prophylactic Antibiotic Timing (Outpatient)	32	100%	98%	98%
Urinary Catheter Removal	82	100%	98%	97%
Survey of Patients' Hospital Experiences				
Area Around Room 'Always' Quiet at Night	300+	51%	53%	61%
Doctors 'Always' Communicated Well	300+	81%	77%	82%
Home Recovery Information Given	300+	84%	82%	85%
Hospital Given 9 or 10 on 10 Point Scale	300+	66%	64%	71%
Meds 'Always' Explained Before Given	300+	51%	59%	64%
Nurses 'Always' Communicated Well	300+	72%	76%	79%
Pain 'Always' Well Controlled	300+	70%	68%	71%
Room and Bathroom 'Always' Clean	300+	67%	68%	73%
Timely Help 'Always' Received	300+	66%	60%	68%
Would Definitely Recommend Hospital	300+	65%	66%	71%
Use of Medical Imaging				
Cardiac Imaging Stress Test before Surgery	121	5.8%	5.8%	5.3%
Combination Abdominal CT Scan	272	4.0%	7.4%	10.5%
Combination Brain/Sinus CT Scan[1]	-	-	2.8%	2.7%
Combination Chest CT Scan	124	3.2%	2.4%	2.7%
Follow-up Mammogram/Ultrasound	287	12.9%	12.5%	8.8%
Lumbar Spine MRI for Low Back Pain[1]	-	-	32.9%	37.2%

Bayshore Community Hospital

727 N Beers St
Holmdel, NJ 07733
Phone: 732-739-5900
Fax: 732-739-5887
E-mail: pr@bchs.com
URL: www.bchs.com
Type: Acute Care Hospitals
Emergency Services: Yes
Ownership: Proprietary
Beds: 174

Key Personnel:
Infection Control. . . . . Genevieve Anderson
Radiology. . . . . David Chun
Chief of Medical Staff. . . . . Gerald V Costa, MD
Pediatric In-Patient Care . . . . Sharon Haskins, RN
President . . . . Timothy J. Hogan, FACHE
Quality Assurance . . . . Carolina Nowaczyk
Cardiac Laboratory. . . . . Greg Sabo, RN

Measure	Cases	This Hosp.	State Avg.	U.S. Avg.
Blood Clot Prevention and Treatment				
Anticoagulation Overlap Therapy[2]	57	93%	88%	93%
ICU Venous Thromboembolism Prophylaxis[2]	92	99%	93%	92%
Incidence of Potentially Preventable VTE[2]	14	0%	10%	10%
UFH with Dosages/Platelet Monitoring[2]	56	100%	99%	97%
Venous Thromboembolism Prophylaxis[2]	406	91%	83%	85%
Warfarin Therapy Discharge Instructions[2]	36	97%	77%	75%
Chest Pain/Possible Heart Attack Care				
Aspirin Given Within 24 Hours of Arrival	72	100%	98%	96%
Fibrinolytic Meds Within 30 Min. of Arrival[1]	-	-	63%	58%
Average Time to ECG (minutes)	70	6	7	7
Average Time to Transfer (minutes)[1]	-	-	74	60
Children's Asthma Care				
Received Home Management Plan of Care	-	-	-	88%
Received Reliever Medication	-	-	-	100%
Received Systemic Corticosteroids	-	-	-	100%
Emergency Department				
Admittance Decision Time (minutes)[2]	1,011	148	148	98
Head CT Results Within 45 Min. of Arrival[1]	-	-	66%	57%
Patients Who Left ER Before Being Seen	33,080	0%	2%	2%
Time from ER Arrival to Admit. (minutes)[2]	1,011	324	355	274
Time from ER Arrival to Discharge (minutes)	365	141	152	134
Time in ER Before Being Evaluated (minutes)	429	22	32	26
Time to Pain Meds for Fractures (minutes)	197	48	58	57
Heart Attack Care				
Aspirin Given at Discharge	47	100%	99%	99%
Fibrinolytic Meds Within 30 Min. of Arrival[7]	-	-	69%	54%
PCI Within 90 Minutes of Arrival[7]	-	-	95%	96%
Statin Prescribed at Discharge	42	100%	99%	98%
Heart Failure Care				
ACE Inhibitor or ARB for LVSD	48	100%	98%	97%
Discharge Instructions Given	178	97%	97%	94%
Evaluation of LVS Function	270	100%	100%	99%
Medicare Spending				
Medicare Spending per Patient (ratio)	-	1.07	1.07	0.98
Pneumonia Care				
Appropriate Initial Antibiotic Given[2]	102	99%	98%	95%
Blood Culture Timing[2]	157	99%	99%	98%
Pregnancy and Delivery Care				
Newborn Deliveries Scheduled Early[7]	-	-	3%	6%
Preventive Care				
Immunization for Influenza[2]	605	98%	93%	90%
Immunization for Pneumonia[2]	916	99%	94%	92%
Stroke Care				
Anticoagulation Therapy for Atrial Fibrillation	18	100%	97%	95%
Antithrombotic Therapy Timing	91	98%	98%	98%
Assessed for Rehabilitation	95	100%	98%	97%
Discharged on Antithrombotic Therapy	90	100%	99%	99%
Discharged on Statin Medication	63	97%	95%	94%
Thrombolytic Therapy Timing[1]	-	-	74%	66%
Venous Thromboembolism Prophylaxis	102	95%	94%	94%
Written Stroke Educational Materials Given	44	84%	94%	88%
Surgical Care Improvement Project				
Appropriate Beta Blocker Usage[2]	73	99%	98%	98%
Appropriate VTP Within 24 Hours[2]	195	99%	99%	98%
Controlled Postoperative Blood Glucose[2,7]	-	-	97%	97%
Perioperative Temperature Management[2]	219	100%	100%	100%
Prophylactic Antibiotic Selection[2]	111	97%	99%	99%
Prophylactic Antibiotic Selection (Outpatient)	34	97%	97%	98%
Prophylactic Antibiotic Stopped[2]	108	98%	98%	98%
Prophylactic Antibiotic Timing[2]	111	100%	99%	99%
Prophylactic Antibiotic Timing (Outpatient)	34	97%	98%	98%
Urinary Catheter Removal[2]	145	100%	98%	97%
Survey of Patients' Hospital Experiences				
Area Around Room 'Always' Quiet at Night	300+	51%	53%	61%
Doctors 'Always' Communicated Well	300+	77%	77%	82%
Home Recovery Information Given	300+	83%	82%	85%
Hospital Given 9 or 10 on 10 Point Scale	300+	60%	64%	71%
Meds 'Always' Explained Before Given	300+	62%	59%	64%
Nurses 'Always' Communicated Well	300+	78%	76%	79%
Pain 'Always' Well Controlled	300+	68%	68%	71%
Room and Bathroom 'Always' Clean	300+	63%	68%	73%
Timely Help 'Always' Received	300+	63%	60%	68%
Would Definitely Recommend Hospital	300+	60%	66%	71%
Use of Medical Imaging				
Cardiac Imaging Stress Test before Surgery	199	4.5%	5.8%	5.3%
Combination Abdominal CT Scan	856	6.3%	7.4%	10.5%
Combination Brain/Sinus CT Scan	554	2.3%	2.8%	2.7%
Combination Chest CT Scan	600	0.3%	2.4%	2.7%
Follow-up Mammogram/Ultrasound	939	10.9%	12.5%	8.8%
Lumbar Spine MRI for Low Back Pain	84	36.9%	32.9%	37.2%

NOTE: Hospital profiles are in alphabetical order by state, then city, then hospital within the city; Rankings exclude hospitals with less than 25 cases except for patient surveys which excludes hospitals with less than 100 cases; (a) 100-299 cases; (1) The number of cases/patients is too few to report; (2) Data submitted were based on a sample of cases/patients; (3) Results are based on a shorter time period than required; (4) Data suppressed by CMS for one or more quarters; (5) Results are not available for this reporting period; (6) Fewer than 100 patients completed the HCAHPS survey; (7) No cases met the criteria for this measure; (8) The lower limit of the confidence interval cannot be calculated if the number of observed infections equals zero; (9) No data are available from the state/territory for this reporting period; (10) The scores shown reflect fewer than 50 completed surveys; (11) There were discrepancies in the data collection process; (12) This measure does not apply to this hospital for this reporting period; (13) Results cannot be calculated for this reporting period; (14) The results for this state are combined with nearby states to protect confidentiality; Please refer to the User's Guide for a full explanation of data.

Carepoint Health - Christ Hospital

176 Palisade Ave
Jersey City, NJ 07306
URL: www.christhospital.org
Type: Acute Care Hospitals
Ownership: Voluntary non-profit - Church

Phone: 201-795-8200
Fax: 201-795-8796

Emergency Services: Yes
Beds: 381

Key Personnel:
Operating Room. . . . . Mohamed Al-Bashir, RN
Pediatric In-Patient Care . . . . Carolyn Amato
Chief of Medical Staff . . . . Anthony C Antonacci, MD
Radiology. . . . . Eileen Concannon
CEO/President. . . . . Nizar Kifaieh
Pediatric Ambulatory Care . . . . . . Miriam McKinney, MD
Infection Control. . . . . Marguerite Morgan
Quality Assurance . . . . Barbara Vicari

Measure	Cases	This Hosp.	State Avg.	U.S. Avg.
Blood Clot Prevention and Treatment				
Anticoagulation Overlap Therapy[2]	54	80%	88%	93%
ICU Venous Thromboembolism Prophylaxis[2]	60	97%	93%	92%
Incidence of Potentially Preventable VTE[2]	17	6%	10%	10%
UFH with Dosages/Platelet Monitoring[2]	40	100%	99%	97%
Venous Thromboembolism Prophylaxis[2]	426	81%	83%	85%
Warfarin Therapy Discharge Instructions[2]	38	74%	77%	75%
Chest Pain/Possible Heart Attack Care				
Aspirin Given Within 24 Hours of Arrival[1,3]	-	-	98%	96%
Fibrinolytic Meds Within 30 Min. of Arrival[3,7]	-	-	63%	58%
Average Time to ECG (minutes)[1,3]	-	-	7	7
Average Time to Transfer (minutes)[3,7]	-	-	74	60
Children's Asthma Care				
Received Home Management Plan of Care	-	-	-	88%
Received Reliever Medication	-	-	-	100%
Received Systemic Corticosteroids	-	-	-	100%
Emergency Department				
Admittance Decision Time (minutes)[2]	674	82	148	98
Head CT Results Within 45 Min. of Arrival[1,3]	-	-	66%	57%
Patients Who Left ER Before Being Seen	48,971	2%	2%	2%
Time from ER Arrival to Admit. (minutes)[2]	709	339	355	274
Time from ER Arrival to Discharge (minutes)	360	145	152	134
Time in ER Before Being Evaluated (minutes)	423	32	32	26
Time to Pain Meds for Fractures (minutes)	92	73	58	57
Heart Attack Care				
Aspirin Given at Discharge	96	98%	99%	99%
Fibrinolytic Meds Within 30 Min. of Arrival[7]	-	-	69%	54%
PCI Within 90 Minutes of Arrival	25	96%	95%	96%
Statin Prescribed at Discharge	96	92%	99%	98%
Heart Failure Care				
ACE Inhibitor or ARB for LVSD	79	99%	98%	97%
Discharge Instructions Given	232	97%	97%	94%
Evaluation of LVS Function	300	99%	100%	99%
Medicare Spending				
Medicare Spending per Patient (ratio)	-	1.11	1.07	0.98
Pneumonia Care				
Appropriate Initial Antibiotic Given	123	93%	98%	95%
Blood Culture Timing	240	97%	99%	98%
Pregnancy and Delivery Care				
Newborn Deliveries Scheduled Early[2]	32	0%	3%	6%
Preventive Care				
Immunization for Influenza[2]	523	96%	93%	90%
Immunization for Pneumonia[2]	672	97%	94%	92%
Stroke Care				
Anticoagulation Therapy for Atrial Fibrillation[1]	-	-	97%	95%
Antithrombotic Therapy Timing	65	92%	98%	98%
Assessed for Rehabilitation	72	99%	98%	97%
Discharged on Antithrombotic Therapy	64	95%	99%	99%
Discharged on Statin Medication	56	84%	95%	94%
Thrombolytic Therapy Timing[1]	-	-	74%	66%
Venous Thromboembolism Prophylaxis	81	91%	94%	94%
Written Stroke Educational Materials Given	25	76%	94%	88%
Surgical Care Improvement Project				
Appropriate Beta Blocker Usage	37	97%	98%	98%
Appropriate VTP Within 24 Hours	132	95%	99%	98%
Controlled Postoperative Blood Glucose[7]	-	-	97%	97%
Perioperative Temperature Management	163	100%	100%	100%
Prophylactic Antibiotic Selection	53	98%	99%	99%
Prophylactic Antibiotic Selection (Outpatient)	72	94%	97%	98%
Prophylactic Antibiotic Stopped	52	100%	98%	98%
Prophylactic Antibiotic Timing	53	96%	99%	99%
Prophylactic Antibiotic Timing (Outpatient)	73	97%	98%	98%
Urinary Catheter Removal	88	97%	98%	97%
Survey of Patients' Hospital Experiences				
Area Around Room 'Always' Quiet at Night	300+	53%	53%	61%
Doctors 'Always' Communicated Well	300+	75%	77%	82%
Home Recovery Information Given	300+	80%	82%	85%
Hospital Given 9 or 10 on 10 Point Scale	300+	56%	64%	71%
Meds 'Always' Explained Before Given	300+	54%	59%	64%
Nurses 'Always' Communicated Well	300+	69%	76%	79%
Pain 'Always' Well Controlled	300+	59%	68%	71%
Room and Bathroom 'Always' Clean	300+	61%	68%	73%
Timely Help 'Always' Received	300+	54%	60%	68%
Would Definitely Recommend Hospital	300+	57%	66%	71%
Use of Medical Imaging				
Cardiac Imaging Stress Test before Surgery	181	3.9%	5.8%	5.3%
Combination Abdominal CT Scan	473	6.8%	7.4%	10.5%
Combination Brain/Sinus CT Scan	490	5.3%	2.8%	2.7%
Combination Chest CT Scan	223	3.1%	2.4%	2.7%
Follow-up Mammogram/Ultrasound	762	11.4%	12.5%	8.8%
Lumbar Spine MRI for Low Back Pain[1]	-	-	32.9%	37.2%

Libertyhealth - Jersey City Medical Center Campus

355 Grand Street
Jersey City, NJ 07302
E-mail: news@libertyhcs.org
URL: www.libertyhcs.org
Type: Acute Care Hospitals
Ownership: Voluntary non-profit - Private

Phone: 201-915-2000
Fax: 201-915-2038

Emergency Services: Yes
Beds: 609

Key Personnel:
Pediatric Ambulatory Care . . . . . . Richard Bonforte
Radiology. . . . . John Cholankeril, MD
Chief of Medical Staff . . . . Kenneth Garay, MD
Quality Assurance . . . . Kathleen Locklear
Chairman/CEO . . . . Harry Melendez
Operating Room. . . . . Judy Neumeyer, RN
Anesthesiology. . . . . Ion Pancu, MD
CEO/President. . . . . Josephan F. Scott, FACHE

Measure	Cases	This Hosp.	State Avg.	U.S. Avg.
Blood Clot Prevention and Treatment				
Anticoagulation Overlap Therapy[2]	89	87%	88%	93%
ICU Venous Thromboembolism Prophylaxis[2]	109	91%	93%	92%
Incidence of Potentially Preventable VTE[2]	42	7%	10%	10%
UFH with Dosages/Platelet Monitoring[2]	59	100%	99%	97%
Venous Thromboembolism Prophylaxis[2]	317	72%	83%	85%
Warfarin Therapy Discharge Instructions[2]	63	56%	77%	75%
Chest Pain/Possible Heart Attack Care				
Aspirin Given Within 24 Hours of Arrival[1,3]	-	-	98%	96%
Fibrinolytic Meds Within 30 Min. of Arrival[5]	-	-	63%	58%
Average Time to ECG (minutes)[1,3]	-	-	7	7
Average Time to Transfer (minutes)[5]	-	-	74	60
Children's Asthma Care				
Received Home Management Plan of Care	-	-	-	88%
Received Reliever Medication	-	-	-	100%
Received Systemic Corticosteroids	-	-	-	100%
Emergency Department				
Admittance Decision Time (minutes)[2]	581	198	148	98
Head CT Results Within 45 Min. of Arrival[1]	-	-	66%	57%
Patients Who Left ER Before Being Seen	86,863	4%	2%	2%
Time from ER Arrival to Admit. (minutes)[2]	736	508	355	274
Time from ER Arrival to Discharge (minutes)	364	184	152	134
Time in ER Before Being Evaluated (minutes)	420	36	32	26
Time to Pain Meds for Fractures (minutes)	120	69	58	57
Heart Attack Care				
Aspirin Given at Discharge	362	100%	99%	99%
Fibrinolytic Meds Within 30 Min. of Arrival[7]	-	-	69%	54%
PCI Within 90 Minutes of Arrival	37	92%	95%	96%
Statin Prescribed at Discharge	364	100%	99%	98%
Heart Failure Care				
ACE Inhibitor or ARB for LVSD[2]	140	100%	98%	97%
Discharge Instructions Given[2]	270	100%	97%	94%
Evaluation of LVS Function[2]	335	100%	100%	99%
Medicare Spending				
Medicare Spending per Patient (ratio)	-	1.12	1.07	0.98
Pneumonia Care				
Appropriate Initial Antibiotic Given[2]	94	100%	98%	95%
Blood Culture Timing[2]	206	100%	99%	98%
Pregnancy and Delivery Care				
Newborn Deliveries Scheduled Early[2]	44	7%	3%	6%
Preventive Care				
Immunization for Influenza[2]	508	99%	93%	90%
Immunization for Pneumonia[2]	536	100%	94%	92%
Stroke Care				
Anticoagulation Therapy for Atrial Fibrillation	15	100%	97%	95%
Antithrombotic Therapy Timing	142	99%	98%	98%
Assessed for Rehabilitation	173	100%	98%	97%
Discharged on Antithrombotic Therapy	146	100%	99%	99%
Discharged on Statin Medication	114	100%	95%	94%
Thrombolytic Therapy Timing	12	92%	74%	66%
Venous Thromboembolism Prophylaxis	177	99%	94%	94%
Written Stroke Educational Materials Given	94	100%	94%	88%
Surgical Care Improvement Project				
Appropriate Beta Blocker Usage[2]	174	100%	98%	98%
Appropriate VTP Within 24 Hours[2]	298	100%	99%	98%
Controlled Postoperative Blood Glucose[2]	193	100%	97%	97%
Perioperative Temperature Management[2]	330	100%	100%	100%
Prophylactic Antibiotic Selection[2]	389	100%	99%	99%
Prophylactic Antibiotic Selection (Outpatient)	78	94%	97%	98%
Prophylactic Antibiotic Stopped[2]	368	100%	98%	98%
Prophylactic Antibiotic Timing[2]	388	100%	99%	99%
Prophylactic Antibiotic Timing (Outpatient)	82	94%	98%	98%
Urinary Catheter Removal[2]	312	100%	98%	97%
Survey of Patients' Hospital Experiences				
Area Around Room 'Always' Quiet at Night	300+	54%	53%	61%
Doctors 'Always' Communicated Well	300+	76%	77%	82%
Home Recovery Information Given	300+	78%	82%	85%
Hospital Given 9 or 10 on 10 Point Scale	300+	60%	64%	71%
Meds 'Always' Explained Before Given	300+	58%	59%	64%
Nurses 'Always' Communicated Well	300+	72%	76%	79%
Pain 'Always' Well Controlled	300+	63%	68%	71%
Room and Bathroom 'Always' Clean	300+	72%	68%	73%
Timely Help 'Always' Received	300+	56%	60%	68%
Would Definitely Recommend Hospital	300+	66%	66%	71%
Use of Medical Imaging				
Cardiac Imaging Stress Test before Surgery	100	7.0%	5.8%	5.3%
Combination Abdominal CT Scan	415	4.3%	7.4%	10.5%
Combination Brain/Sinus CT Scan	546	2.0%	2.8%	2.7%
Combination Chest CT Scan	147	4.8%	2.4%	2.7%
Follow-up Mammogram/Ultrasound	253	13.0%	12.5%	8.8%
Lumbar Spine MRI for Low Back Pain[1]	-	-	32.9%	37.2%

Monmouth Medical Center - Southern Campus

600 River Ave
Lakewood, NJ 08701
URL: www.sbhcs.com
Type: Acute Care Hospitals
Ownership: Voluntary non-profit - Private

Phone: 732-363-1900
Fax: 732-886-4406

Emergency Services: Yes
Beds: 350

Key Personnel:
Infection Control. . . . . Carolyn Cox
Radiology. . . . . Robert Cranley, MD
Emergency Room . . . . William Dalsey, MD
CEO/President. . . . . Joe Hick
Pediatric Ambulatory Care . . . . . . Norman Indich, MD
Anesthesiology. . . . . Jitendra Jadav, MD
Chief of Medical Staff . . . . Eric Lennes, MD
Quality Assurance . . . . Joan Ruane

Measure	Cases	This Hosp.	State Avg.	U.S. Avg.
Blood Clot Prevention and Treatment				
Anticoagulation Overlap Therapy[2]	43	84%	88%	93%
ICU Venous Thromboembolism Prophylaxis[2]	51	84%	93%	92%
Incidence of Potentially Preventable VTE[1,2]	-	-	10%	10%
UFH with Dosages/Platelet Monitoring[2]	16	100%	99%	97%
Venous Thromboembolism Prophylaxis[2]	383	68%	83%	85%
Warfarin Therapy Discharge Instructions[2]	24	83%	77%	75%
Chest Pain/Possible Heart Attack Care				
Aspirin Given Within 24 Hours of Arrival[1]	-	-	98%	96%

NOTE: Hospital profiles are in alphabetical order by state, then city, then hospital within the city; Rankings exclude hospitals with less than 25 cases except for patient surveys which excludes hospitals with less than 100 cases; (a) 100-299 cases; (1) The number of cases/patients is too few to report; (2) Data submitted were based on a sample of cases/patients; (3) Results are based on a shorter time period than required; (4) Data suppressed by CMS for one or more quarters; (5) Results are not available for this reporting period; (6) Fewer than 100 patients completed the HCAHPS survey; (7) No cases met the criteria for this measure; (8) The lower limit of the confidence interval cannot be calculated if the number of observed infections equals zero; (9) No data are available from the state/territory for this reporting period; (10) The scores shown reflect fewer than 50 completed surveys; (11) There were discrepancies in the data collection process; (12) This measure does not apply to this hospital for this reporting period; (13) Results cannot be calculated for this reporting period; (14) The results for this state are combined with nearby states to protect confidentiality; Please refer to the User's Guide for a full explanation of data.

Fibrinolytic Meds Within 30 Min. of Arrival[1]	-	-	63%	58%
Average Time to ECG (minutes)[1]	-	-	7	7
Average Time to Transfer (minutes)[7]	-	-	74	60
Children's Asthma Care				
Received Home Management Plan of Care	-	-	-	88%
Received Reliever Medication	-	-	-	100%
Received Systemic Corticosteroids	-	-	-	100%
Emergency Department				
Admittance Decision Time (minutes)[2]	796	88	148	98
Head CT Results Within 45 Min. of Arrival[1]	-	-	66%	57%
Patients Who Left ER Before Being Seen	24,736	0%	2%	2%
Time from ER Arrival to Admit. (minutes)[2]	802	322	355	274
Time from ER Arrival to Discharge (minutes)	382	96	152	134
Time in ER Before Being Evaluated (minutes)	397	19	32	26
Time to Pain Meds for Fractures (minutes)	105	52	58	57
Heart Attack Care				
Aspirin Given at Discharge	57	100%	99%	99%
Fibrinolytic Meds Within 30 Min. of Arrival[1]	-	-	69%	54%
PCI Within 90 Minutes of Arrival[7]	-	-	95%	96%
Statin Prescribed at Discharge	57	98%	99%	98%
Heart Failure Care				
ACE Inhibitor or ARB for LVSD	69	100%	98%	97%
Discharge Instructions Given	173	100%	97%	94%
Evaluation of LVS Function	322	100%	100%	99%
Medicare Spending				
Medicare Spending per Patient (ratio)	-	1.10	1.07	0.98
Pneumonia Care				
Appropriate Initial Antibiotic Given	132	100%	98%	95%
Blood Culture Timing	221	100%	99%	98%
Pregnancy and Delivery Care				
Newborn Deliveries Scheduled Early[2]	30	7%	3%	6%
Preventive Care				
Immunization for Influenza[2]	526	99%	93%	90%
Immunization for Pneumonia[2]	687	97%	94%	92%
Stroke Care				
Anticoagulation Therapy for Atrial Fibrillation	13	100%	97%	95%
Antithrombotic Therapy Timing	57	100%	98%	98%
Assessed for Rehabilitation	56	100%	98%	97%
Discharged on Antithrombotic Therapy	53	100%	99%	99%
Discharged on Statin Medication	38	100%	95%	94%
Thrombolytic Therapy Timing[1]	-	-	74%	66%
Venous Thromboembolism Prophylaxis	66	100%	94%	94%
Written Stroke Educational Materials Given	26	100%	94%	88%
Surgical Care Improvement Project				
Appropriate Beta Blocker Usage	36	100%	98%	98%
Appropriate VTP Within 24 Hours	97	99%	99%	98%
Controlled Postoperative Blood Glucose[7]	-	-	97%	97%
Perioperative Temperature Management	118	100%	100%	100%
Prophylactic Antibiotic Selection	23	100%	99%	99%
Prophylactic Antibiotic Selection (Outpatient)	40	100%	97%	98%
Prophylactic Antibiotic Stopped	23	96%	98%	98%
Prophylactic Antibiotic Timing	23	100%	99%	99%
Prophylactic Antibiotic Timing (Outpatient)	40	100%	98%	98%
Urinary Catheter Removal	39	100%	98%	97%
Survey of Patients' Hospital Experiences				
Area Around Room 'Always' Quiet at Night	300+	49%	53%	61%
Doctors 'Always' Communicated Well	300+	74%	77%	82%
Home Recovery Information Given	300+	81%	82%	85%
Hospital Given 9 or 10 on 10 Point Scale	300+	57%	64%	71%
Meds 'Always' Explained Before Given	300+	58%	59%	64%
Nurses 'Always' Communicated Well	300+	74%	76%	79%
Pain 'Always' Well Controlled	300+	68%	68%	71%
Room and Bathroom 'Always' Clean	300+	70%	68%	73%
Timely Help 'Always' Received	300+	52%	60%	68%
Would Definitely Recommend Hospital	300+	57%	66%	71%
Use of Medical Imaging				
Cardiac Imaging Stress Test before Surgery[1]	-	-	5.8%	5.3%
Combination Abdominal CT Scan	478	8.2%	7.4%	10.5%
Combination Brain/Sinus CT Scan	880	2.6%	2.8%	2.7%
Combination Chest CT Scan	354	0.0%	2.4%	2.7%
Follow-up Mammogram/Ultrasound	63	6.3%	12.5%	8.8%
Lumbar Spine MRI for Low Back Pain[1]	-	-	32.9%	37.2%

Saint Barnabas Medical Center

94 Old Short Hills Road
Livingston, NJ 07039
Phone: 973-322-5000
Fax: 973-322-4346
E-mail: info@sbhcs.com
URL: www.saintbarnabas.com
Type: Acute Care Hospitals
Emergency Services: Yes
Ownership: Voluntary non-profit - Other
Beds: 597

Key Personnel:
CEO/President . . . . John F. Bonamo, MD, MS
Radiology . . . . Robert L Goodman, MD
Pediatric Ambulatory Care . . . . . . Agnes Hilbert
Cardiac Laboratory . . . . Maggie Lundberg
Pediatric In-Patient Care . . . . Susan Margolin, MD
Chief of Medical Staff . . . . Gregory Rokoszt DO JD
Intensive Care Unit . . . . Chris Ruhren
Patient Relations . . . . Heather Veltra

Measure	Cases	This Hosp.	State Avg.	U.S. Avg.
Blood Clot Prevention and Treatment				
Anticoagulation Overlap Therapy[2]	162	83%	88%	93%
ICU Venous Thromboembolism Prophylaxis[2]	58	91%	93%	92%
Incidence of Potentially Preventable VTE[2]	74	8%	10%	10%
UFH with Dosages/Platelet Monitoring[2]	95	97%	99%	97%
Venous Thromboembolism Prophylaxis[2]	389	76%	83%	85%
Warfarin Therapy Discharge Instructions[2]	97	82%	77%	75%
Chest Pain/Possible Heart Attack Care				
Aspirin Given Within 24 Hours of Arrival[1,3]	-	-	98%	96%
Fibrinolytic Meds Within 30 Min. of Arrival[3,7]	-	-	63%	58%
Average Time to ECG (minutes)[1,3]	-	-	7	7
Average Time to Transfer (minutes)[3,7]	-	-	74	60
Children's Asthma Care				
Received Home Management Plan of Care	-	-	-	88%
Received Reliever Medication	-	-	-	100%
Received Systemic Corticosteroids	-	-	-	100%
Emergency Department				
Admittance Decision Time (minutes)[2]	489	161	148	98
Head CT Results Within 45 Min. of Arrival[1]	-	-	66%	57%
Patients Who Left ER Before Being Seen	87,741	1%	2%	2%
Time from ER Arrival to Admit. (minutes)[2]	489	378	355	274
Time from ER Arrival to Discharge (minutes)	375	145	152	134
Time in ER Before Being Evaluated (minutes)	421	14	32	26
Time to Pain Meds for Fractures (minutes)	223	39	58	57
Heart Attack Care				
Aspirin Given at Discharge	241	100%	99%	99%
Fibrinolytic Meds Within 30 Min. of Arrival[7]	-	-	69%	54%
PCI Within 90 Minutes of Arrival	29	97%	95%	96%
Statin Prescribed at Discharge	233	100%	99%	98%
Heart Failure Care				
ACE Inhibitor or ARB for LVSD[2]	77	100%	98%	97%
Discharge Instructions Given[2]	248	99%	97%	94%
Evaluation of LVS Function[2]	325	100%	100%	99%
Medicare Spending				
Medicare Spending per Patient (ratio)	-	1.08	1.07	0.98
Pneumonia Care				
Appropriate Initial Antibiotic Given[2]	118	100%	98%	95%
Blood Culture Timing[2]	96	100%	99%	98%
Pregnancy and Delivery Care				
Newborn Deliveries Scheduled Early[2]	75	27%	3%	6%
Preventive Care				
Immunization for Influenza[2]	511	85%	93%	90%
Immunization for Pneumonia[2]	487	85%	94%	92%
Stroke Care				
Anticoagulation Therapy for Atrial Fibrillation[2]	38	100%	97%	95%
Antithrombotic Therapy Timing[2]	216	98%	98%	98%
Assessed for Rehabilitation[2]	286	100%	98%	97%
Discharged on Antithrombotic Therapy[2]	226	100%	99%	99%
Discharged on Statin Medication[2]	192	99%	95%	94%
Thrombolytic Therapy Timing[1,2]	-	-	74%	66%
Venous Thromboembolism Prophylaxis[2]	301	99%	94%	94%
Written Stroke Educational Materials Given[2]	143	99%	94%	88%
Surgical Care Improvement Project				
Appropriate Beta Blocker Usage[2]	262	100%	98%	98%
Appropriate VTP Within 24 Hours[2]	500	97%	99%	98%
Controlled Postoperative Blood Glucose[2]	170	100%	97%	97%
Perioperative Temperature Management[2]	612	100%	100%	100%
Prophylactic Antibiotic Selection[2]	507	99%	99%	99%
Prophylactic Antibiotic Selection (Outpatient)	897	99%	97%	98%
Prophylactic Antibiotic Stopped[2]	495	97%	98%	98%
Prophylactic Antibiotic Timing[2]	508	100%	99%	99%
Prophylactic Antibiotic Timing (Outpatient)	900	99%	98%	98%
Urinary Catheter Removal[2]	174	91%	98%	97%
Survey of Patients' Hospital Experiences				
Area Around Room 'Always' Quiet at Night	300+	53%	53%	61%
Doctors 'Always' Communicated Well	300+	79%	77%	82%
Home Recovery Information Given	300+	80%	82%	85%
Hospital Given 9 or 10 on 10 Point Scale	300+	67%	64%	71%
Meds 'Always' Explained Before Given	300+	61%	59%	64%
Nurses 'Always' Communicated Well	300+	76%	76%	79%
Pain 'Always' Well Controlled	300+	68%	68%	71%
Room and Bathroom 'Always' Clean	300+	72%	68%	73%
Timely Help 'Always' Received	300+	59%	60%	68%
Would Definitely Recommend Hospital	300+	72%	66%	71%
Use of Medical Imaging				
Cardiac Imaging Stress Test before Surgery	1,642	6.3%	5.8%	5.3%
Combination Abdominal CT Scan	872	6.1%	7.4%	10.5%
Combination Brain/Sinus CT Scan	1,184	4.4%	2.8%	2.7%
Combination Chest CT Scan	329	6.7%	2.4%	2.7%
Follow-up Mammogram/Ultrasound[7]	-	-	12.5%	8.8%
Lumbar Spine MRI for Low Back Pain[1]	-	-	32.9%	37.2%

Monmouth Medical Center

300 Second Avenue
Long Branch, NJ 07740
Phone: 732-222-5200
Fax: 732-923-6633
E-mail: info@sbhcs.com
URL: www.sbhcs.com
Type: Acute Care Hospitals
Emergency Services: Yes
Ownership: Voluntary non-profit - Private
Beds: 526

Key Personnel:
Pediatric Ambulatory Care . . . . . . Howard Fox, MD
Pediatric In-Patient Care . . . . Howard Fox, MD
Quality Assurance . . . . Pat Keating
Operating Room . . . . Jadd W Koury
Infection Control . . . . Nancy Nelsen
Radiology . . . . Soliman Rabbani, MD
Chief of Medical Staff . . . . Daniel Shine, MD
CEO/President . . . . David Wallace, MD

Measure	Cases	This Hosp.	State Avg.	U.S. Avg.
Blood Clot Prevention and Treatment				
Anticoagulation Overlap Therapy[2]	67	78%	88%	93%
ICU Venous Thromboembolism Prophylaxis[2]	67	96%	93%	92%
Incidence of Potentially Preventable VTE[2]	26	27%	10%	10%
UFH with Dosages/Platelet Monitoring[2]	50	98%	99%	97%
Venous Thromboembolism Prophylaxis[2]	367	81%	83%	85%
Warfarin Therapy Discharge Instructions[2]	36	97%	77%	75%
Chest Pain/Possible Heart Attack Care				
Aspirin Given Within 24 Hours of Arrival	13	100%	98%	96%
Fibrinolytic Meds Within 30 Min. of Arrival[7]	-	-	63%	58%
Average Time to ECG (minutes)	13	8	7	7
Average Time to Transfer (minutes)[7]	-	-	74	60
Children's Asthma Care				
Received Home Management Plan of Care	-	-	-	88%
Received Reliever Medication	-	-	-	100%
Received Systemic Corticosteroids	-	-	-	100%
Emergency Department				
Admittance Decision Time (minutes)[2]	369	139	148	98
Head CT Results Within 45 Min. of Arrival[1]	-	-	66%	57%
Patients Who Left ER Before Being Seen	51,193	1%	2%	2%
Time from ER Arrival to Admit. (minutes)[2]	372	308	355	274
Time from ER Arrival to Discharge (minutes)	394	134	152	134
Time in ER Before Being Evaluated (minutes)	342	24	32	26
Time to Pain Meds for Fractures (minutes)	258	68	58	57
Heart Attack Care				
Aspirin Given at Discharge	53	98%	99%	99%
Fibrinolytic Meds Within 30 Min. of Arrival[1]	-	-	69%	54%
PCI Within 90 Minutes of Arrival	12	83%	95%	96%
Statin Prescribed at Discharge	47	100%	99%	98%
Heart Failure Care				
ACE Inhibitor or ARB for LVSD[2]	55	98%	98%	97%
Discharge Instructions Given[2]	176	100%	97%	94%

NOTE: Hospital profiles are in alphabetical order by state, then city, then hospital within the city; Rankings exclude hospitals with less than 25 cases except for patient surveys which excludes hospitals with less than 100 cases; (a) 100-299 cases; (1) The number of cases/patients is too few to report; (2) Data submitted were based on a sample of cases/patients; (3) Results are based on a shorter time period than required; (4) Data suppressed by CMS for one or more quarters; (5) Results are not available for this reporting period; (6) Fewer than 100 patients completed the HCAHPS survey; (7) No cases met the criteria for this measure; (8) The lower limit of the confidence interval cannot be calculated if the number of observed infections equals zero; (9) No data are available from the state/territory for this reporting period; (10) The scores shown reflect fewer than 50 completed surveys; (11) There were discrepancies in the data collection process; (12) This measure does not apply to this hospital for this reporting period; (13) Results cannot be calculated for this reporting period; (14) The results for this state are combined with nearby states to protect confidentiality; Please refer to the User's Guide for a full explanation of data.

Measure	Cases	This Hosp.	State Avg.	U.S. Avg.
Evaluation of LVS Function[2]	256	100%	100%	99%
Medicare Spending				
Medicare Spending per Patient (ratio)	-	1.11	1.07	0.98
Pneumonia Care				
Appropriate Initial Antibiotic Given[2]	88	97%	98%	95%
Blood Culture Timing[2]	159	100%	99%	98%
Pregnancy and Delivery Care				
Newborn Deliveries Scheduled Early[2]	64	0%	3%	6%
Preventive Care				
Immunization for Influenza[2]	493	94%	93%	90%
Immunization for Pneumonia[2]	395	90%	94%	92%
Stroke Care				
Anticoagulation Therapy for Atrial Fibrillation[1]	-	-	97%	95%
Antithrombotic Therapy Timing	81	99%	98%	98%
Assessed for Rehabilitation	99	99%	98%	97%
Discharged on Antithrombotic Therapy	85	100%	99%	99%
Discharged on Statin Medication	64	98%	95%	94%
Thrombolytic Therapy Timing[1]	-	-	74%	66%
Venous Thromboembolism Prophylaxis	107	98%	94%	94%
Written Stroke Educational Materials Given	37	97%	94%	88%
Surgical Care Improvement Project				
Appropriate Beta Blocker Usage[2]	103	96%	98%	98%
Appropriate VTP Within 24 Hours[2]	404	99%	99%	98%
Controlled Postoperative Blood Glucose[2,7]	-	-	97%	97%
Perioperative Temperature Management[2]	453	100%	100%	100%
Prophylactic Antibiotic Selection[2]	301	99%	99%	99%
Prophylactic Antibiotic Selection (Outpatient)	476	98%	97%	98%
Prophylactic Antibiotic Stopped[2]	294	95%	98%	98%
Prophylactic Antibiotic Timing[2]	301	100%	99%	99%
Prophylactic Antibiotic Timing (Outpatient)	470	99%	98%	98%
Urinary Catheter Removal[2]	239	99%	98%	97%
Survey of Patients' Hospital Experiences				
Area Around Room 'Always' Quiet at Night	300+	49%	53%	61%
Doctors 'Always' Communicated Well	300+	78%	77%	82%
Home Recovery Information Given	300+	81%	82%	85%
Hospital Given 9 or 10 on 10 Point Scale	300+	66%	64%	71%
Meds 'Always' Explained Before Given	300+	63%	59%	64%
Nurses 'Always' Communicated Well	300+	77%	76%	79%
Pain 'Always' Well Controlled	300+	70%	68%	71%
Room and Bathroom 'Always' Clean	300+	72%	68%	73%
Timely Help 'Always' Received	300+	59%	60%	68%
Would Definitely Recommend Hospital	300+	71%	66%	71%
Use of Medical Imaging				
Cardiac Imaging Stress Test before Surgery	690	7.2%	5.8%	5.3%
Combination Abdominal CT Scan	617	7.8%	7.4%	10.5%
Combination Brain/Sinus CT Scan	566	4.4%	2.8%	2.7%
Combination Chest CT Scan	625	0.3%	2.4%	2.7%
Follow-up Mammogram/Ultrasound	3,045	5.7%	12.5%	8.8%
Lumbar Spine MRI for Low Back Pain	68	32.4%	32.9%	37.2%

Southern Ocean Medical Center

1140 Rt 72 W
Manahawkin, NJ 08050
Phone: 609-597-6011
Fax: 609-978-8920
E-mail: info@soch.com
URL: www.soch.com
Type: Acute Care Hospitals
Emergency Services: Yes
Ownership: Voluntary non-profit - Private
Beds: 144

Key Personnel:

President . . . . Joseph P Coyle
Anesthesiology. . . . . James Loftus, MD
Chief of Medical Staff . . . . Walter Miller
Infection Control. . . . . Marsha Prato
Cardiac Laboratory. . . . . Jenny Stump
Radiology. . . . . John Swidryk, MD
Emergency Room . . . . William Wild

Measure	Cases	This Hosp.	State Avg.	U.S. Avg.
Blood Clot Prevention and Treatment				
Anticoagulation Overlap Therapy[2]	63	92%	88%	93%
ICU Venous Thromboembolism Prophylaxis[2]	86	94%	93%	92%
Incidence of Potentially Preventable VTE[1,2]	-	-	10%	10%
UFH with Dosages/Platelet Monitoring[2]	44	100%	99%	97%
Venous Thromboembolism Prophylaxis[2]	395	87%	83%	85%
Warfarin Therapy Discharge Instructions[2]	35	91%	77%	75%
Chest Pain/Possible Heart Attack Care				
Aspirin Given Within 24 Hours of Arrival	115	98%	98%	96%
Fibrinolytic Meds Within 30 Min. of Arrival[7]	-	-	63%	58%
Average Time to ECG (minutes)	116	8	7	7
Average Time to Transfer (minutes)	27	76	74	60
Children's Asthma Care				
Received Home Management Plan of Care	-	-	-	88%
Received Reliever Medication	-	-	-	100%
Received Systemic Corticosteroids	-	-	-	100%
Emergency Department				
Admittance Decision Time (minutes)[2]	978	136	148	98
Head CT Results Within 45 Min. of Arrival	15	60%	66%	57%
Patients Who Left ER Before Being Seen	40,455	3%	2%	2%
Time from ER Arrival to Admit. (minutes)[2]	991	340	355	274
Time from ER Arrival to Discharge (minutes)	372	162	152	134
Time in ER Before Being Evaluated (minutes)	421	35	32	26
Time to Pain Meds for Fractures (minutes)	129	68	58	57
Heart Attack Care				
Aspirin Given at Discharge	36	89%	99%	99%
Fibrinolytic Meds Within 30 Min. of Arrival[7]	-	-	69%	54%
PCI Within 90 Minutes of Arrival[7]	-	-	95%	96%
Statin Prescribed at Discharge	33	94%	99%	98%
Heart Failure Care				
ACE Inhibitor or ARB for LVSD	55	96%	98%	97%
Discharge Instructions Given	158	96%	97%	94%
Evaluation of LVS Function	233	100%	100%	99%
Medicare Spending				
Medicare Spending per Patient (ratio)	-	1.04	1.07	0.98
Pneumonia Care				
Appropriate Initial Antibiotic Given	158	97%	98%	95%
Blood Culture Timing	251	96%	99%	98%
Pregnancy and Delivery Care				
Newborn Deliveries Scheduled Early[2]	16	6%	3%	6%
Preventive Care				
Immunization for Influenza[2]	569	96%	93%	90%
Immunization for Pneumonia[2]	862	98%	94%	92%
Stroke Care				
Anticoagulation Therapy for Atrial Fibrillation	11	100%	97%	95%
Antithrombotic Therapy Timing	70	100%	98%	98%
Assessed for Rehabilitation	73	97%	98%	97%
Discharged on Antithrombotic Therapy	72	100%	99%	99%
Discharged on Statin Medication	60	87%	95%	94%
Thrombolytic Therapy Timing[1]	-	-	74%	66%
Venous Thromboembolism Prophylaxis	78	86%	94%	94%
Written Stroke Educational Materials Given	36	72%	94%	88%
Surgical Care Improvement Project				
Appropriate Beta Blocker Usage	106	99%	98%	98%
Appropriate VTP Within 24 Hours	253	97%	99%	98%
Controlled Postoperative Blood Glucose[7]	-	-	97%	97%
Perioperative Temperature Management	286	100%	100%	100%
Prophylactic Antibiotic Selection	172	97%	99%	99%
Prophylactic Antibiotic Selection (Outpatient)	64	92%	97%	98%
Prophylactic Antibiotic Stopped	160	98%	98%	98%
Prophylactic Antibiotic Timing	172	99%	99%	99%
Prophylactic Antibiotic Timing (Outpatient)	64	98%	98%	98%
Urinary Catheter Removal	169	98%	98%	97%
Survey of Patients' Hospital Experiences				
Area Around Room 'Always' Quiet at Night	300+	46%	53%	61%
Doctors 'Always' Communicated Well	300+	78%	77%	82%
Home Recovery Information Given	300+	84%	82%	85%
Hospital Given 9 or 10 on 10 Point Scale	300+	62%	64%	71%
Meds 'Always' Explained Before Given	300+	63%	59%	64%
Nurses 'Always' Communicated Well	300+	78%	76%	79%
Pain 'Always' Well Controlled	300+	72%	68%	71%
Room and Bathroom 'Always' Clean	300+	69%	68%	73%
Timely Help 'Always' Received	300+	63%	60%	68%
Would Definitely Recommend Hospital	300+	63%	66%	71%
Use of Medical Imaging				
Cardiac Imaging Stress Test before Surgery	137	0.7%	5.8%	5.3%
Combination Abdominal CT Scan	914	4.2%	7.4%	10.5%
Combination Brain/Sinus CT Scan	986	2.5%	2.8%	2.7%
Combination Chest CT Scan	439	4.3%	2.4%	2.7%
Follow-up Mammogram/Ultrasound	1,348	11.0%	12.5%	8.8%
Lumbar Spine MRI for Low Back Pain[1]	-	-	32.9%	37.2%

Hackensack - Umc Mountainside

Bay & Highland Ave
Montclair, NJ 07042
Phone: 973-429-6000
Fax: 973-429-6001
E-mail: info@mountainsidehosp.com
URL: www.mountainsidenow.org
Type: Acute Care Hospitals
Emergency Services: Yes
Ownership: Voluntary non-profit - Private
Beds: 365

Key Personnel:

CEO/President. . . . . John Fromhold
Chief of Medical Staff . . . . Marjory Langer, MD
Pediatric In-Patient Care . . . . Ragheda Saba
Surgery . . . . Konstantin Walmsley, MD

Measure	Cases	This Hosp.	State Avg.	U.S. Avg.
Blood Clot Prevention and Treatment				
Anticoagulation Overlap Therapy[2]	61	100%	88%	93%
ICU Venous Thromboembolism Prophylaxis[2]	64	97%	93%	92%
Incidence of Potentially Preventable VTE[2]	12	0%	10%	10%
UFH with Dosages/Platelet Monitoring[2]	34	100%	99%	97%
Venous Thromboembolism Prophylaxis[2]	366	80%	83%	85%
Warfarin Therapy Discharge Instructions[2]	38	97%	77%	75%
Chest Pain/Possible Heart Attack Care				
Aspirin Given Within 24 Hours of Arrival[5]	-	-	98%	96%
Fibrinolytic Meds Within 30 Min. of Arrival[5]	-	-	63%	58%
Average Time to ECG (minutes)[5]	-	-	7	7
Average Time to Transfer (minutes)[5]	-	-	74	60
Children's Asthma Care				
Received Home Management Plan of Care	-	-	-	88%
Received Reliever Medication	-	-	-	100%
Received Systemic Corticosteroids	-	-	-	100%
Emergency Department				
Admittance Decision Time (minutes)[2]	707	146	148	98
Head CT Results Within 45 Min. of Arrival[1]	-	-	66%	57%
Patients Who Left ER Before Being Seen	40,261	1%	2%	2%
Time from ER Arrival to Admit. (minutes)[2]	711	322	355	274
Time from ER Arrival to Discharge (minutes)	441	155	152	134
Time in ER Before Being Evaluated (minutes)	459	63	32	26
Time to Pain Meds for Fractures (minutes)	118	72	58	57
Heart Attack Care				
Aspirin Given at Discharge	84	99%	99%	99%
Fibrinolytic Meds Within 30 Min. of Arrival[7]	-	-	69%	54%
PCI Within 90 Minutes of Arrival	28	100%	95%	96%
Statin Prescribed at Discharge	77	100%	99%	98%
Heart Failure Care				
ACE Inhibitor or ARB for LVSD	94	99%	98%	97%
Discharge Instructions Given	218	100%	97%	94%
Evaluation of LVS Function	333	100%	100%	99%
Medicare Spending				
Medicare Spending per Patient (ratio)	-	1.08	1.07	0.98
Pneumonia Care				
Appropriate Initial Antibiotic Given	140	100%	98%	95%
Blood Culture Timing	252	100%	99%	98%
Pregnancy and Delivery Care				
Newborn Deliveries Scheduled Early[2]	35	11%	3%	6%
Preventive Care				
Immunization for Influenza[2]	508	94%	93%	90%
Immunization for Pneumonia[2]	646	93%	94%	92%
Stroke Care				
Anticoagulation Therapy for Atrial Fibrillation[1]	-	-	97%	95%
Antithrombotic Therapy Timing	87	100%	98%	98%
Assessed for Rehabilitation	106	97%	98%	97%
Discharged on Antithrombotic Therapy	87	100%	99%	99%
Discharged on Statin Medication	64	89%	95%	94%
Thrombolytic Therapy Timing[1]	-	-	74%	66%
Venous Thromboembolism Prophylaxis	116	95%	94%	94%
Written Stroke Educational Materials Given	45	100%	94%	88%
Surgical Care Improvement Project				
Appropriate Beta Blocker Usage	128	100%	98%	98%
Appropriate VTP Within 24 Hours	373	95%	99%	98%
Controlled Postoperative Blood Glucose[7]	-	-	97%	97%
Perioperative Temperature Management	441	100%	100%	100%
Prophylactic Antibiotic Selection	214	100%	99%	99%
Prophylactic Antibiotic Selection (Outpatient)	96	97%	97%	98%

NOTE: Hospital profiles are in alphabetical order by state, then city, then hospital within the city; Rankings exclude hospitals with less than 25 cases except for patient surveys which excludes hospitals with less than 100 cases; (a) 100-299 cases; (1) The number of cases/patients is too few to report; (2) Data submitted were based on a sample of cases/patients; (3) Results are based on a shorter time period than required; (4) Data suppressed by CMS for one or more quarters; (5) Results are not available for this reporting period; (6) Fewer than 100 patients completed the HCAHPS survey; (7) No cases met the criteria for this measure; (8) The lower limit of the confidence interval cannot be calculated if the number of observed infections equals zero; (9) No data are available from the state/territory for this reporting period; (10) The scores shown reflect fewer than 50 completed surveys; (11) There were discrepancies in the data collection process; (12) This measure does not apply to this hospital for this reporting period; (13) Results cannot be calculated for this reporting period; (14) The results for this state are combined with nearby states to protect confidentiality; Please refer to the User's Guide for a full explanation of data.

Prophylactic Antibiotic Stopped	199	100%	98%	98%
Prophylactic Antibiotic Timing	214	100%	99%	99%
Prophylactic Antibiotic Timing (Outpatient)	96	100%	98%	98%
Urinary Catheter Removal	277	100%	98%	97%
Survey of Patients' Hospital Experiences				
Area Around Room 'Always' Quiet at Night	300+	57%	53%	61%
Doctors 'Always' Communicated Well	300+	81%	77%	82%
Home Recovery Information Given	300+	82%	82%	85%
Hospital Given 9 or 10 on 10 Point Scale	300+	65%	64%	71%
Meds 'Always' Explained Before Given	300+	56%	59%	64%
Nurses 'Always' Communicated Well	300+	76%	76%	79%
Pain 'Always' Well Controlled	300+	68%	68%	71%
Room and Bathroom 'Always' Clean	300+	64%	68%	73%
Timely Help 'Always' Received	300+	59%	60%	68%
Would Definitely Recommend Hospital	300+	69%	66%	71%
Use of Medical Imaging				
Cardiac Imaging Stress Test before Surgery[1]	-	-	5.8%	5.3%
Combination Abdominal CT Scan	788	17.0%	7.4%	10.5%
Combination Brain/Sinus CT Scan	642	3.1%	2.8%	2.7%
Combination Chest CT Scan	396	10.4%	2.4%	2.7%
Follow-up Mammogram/Ultrasound	375	9.1%	12.5%	8.8%
Lumbar Spine MRI for Low Back Pain	34	47.1%	32.9%	37.2%

Morristown Medical Center

100 Madison Ave Phone: 973-971-5450
Morristown, NJ 07962 Fax: 973-290-7259
URL: www.morristownmemorialhospital.org
Type: Acute Care Hospitals Emergency Services: Yes
Ownership: Voluntary non-profit - Private Beds: 629

Key Personnel:
Pediatric In-Patient Care . . . . Leonard Feld, MD
Emergency Room . . . . John M Kealey, MD
Infection Control. . . . . Albert Klainer, MD
Anesthesiology. . . . . John T Lapchak, MD
Radiology. . . . . Harry Stein
CEO/President. . . . . Joseph A Trunfio, PhD
Operating Room. . . . . Liz Wein

Measure	Cases	This Hosp.	State Avg.	U.S. Avg.
Blood Clot Prevention and Treatment				
Anticoagulation Overlap Therapy[2]	235	94%	88%	93%
ICU Venous Thromboembolism Prophylaxis[2]	85	94%	93%	92%
Incidence of Potentially Preventable VTE[2]	82	4%	10%	10%
UFH with Dosages/Platelet Monitoring[2]	248	100%	99%	97%
Venous Thromboembolism Prophylaxis[2]	344	76%	83%	85%
Warfarin Therapy Discharge Instructions[2]	152	80%	77%	75%
Chest Pain/Possible Heart Attack Care				
Aspirin Given Within 24 Hours of Arrival[1,3]	-	-	98%	96%
Fibrinolytic Meds Within 30 Min. of Arrival[5]	-	-	63%	58%
Average Time to ECG (minutes)[1,3]	-	-	7	7
Average Time to Transfer (minutes)[5]	-	-	74	60
Children's Asthma Care				
Received Home Management Plan of Care	-	-	-	88%
Received Reliever Medication	-	-	-	100%
Received Systemic Corticosteroids	-	-	-	100%
Emergency Department				
Admittance Decision Time (minutes)[2]	491	198	148	98
Head CT Results Within 45 Min. of Arrival[1]	-	-	66%	57%
Patients Who Left ER Before Being Seen	82,239	0%	2%	2%
Time from ER Arrival to Admit. (minutes)[2]	520	404	355	274
Time from ER Arrival to Discharge (minutes)	382	165	152	134
Time in ER Before Being Evaluated (minutes)	401	31	32	26
Time to Pain Meds for Fractures (minutes)	247	52	58	57
Heart Attack Care				
Aspirin Given at Discharge[2]	328	99%	99%	99%
Fibrinolytic Meds Within 30 Min. of Arrival[2,7]	-	-	69%	54%
PCI Within 90 Minutes of Arrival[2]	29	90%	95%	96%
Statin Prescribed at Discharge[2]	325	97%	99%	98%
Heart Failure Care				
ACE Inhibitor or ARB for LVSD[2]	131	85%	98%	97%
Discharge Instructions Given[2]	217	97%	97%	94%
Evaluation of LVS Function[2]	323	100%	100%	99%
Medicare Spending				
Medicare Spending per Patient (ratio)	-	1.06	1.07	0.98
Pneumonia Care				
Appropriate Initial Antibiotic Given[2]	99	95%	98%	95%
Blood Culture Timing[2]	156	97%	99%	98%
Pregnancy and Delivery Care				
Newborn Deliveries Scheduled Early	241	0%	3%	6%
Preventive Care				
Immunization for Influenza[2]	563	90%	93%	90%
Immunization for Pneumonia[2]	508	86%	94%	92%
Stroke Care				
Anticoagulation Therapy for Atrial Fibrillation	41	98%	97%	95%
Antithrombotic Therapy Timing	167	100%	98%	98%
Assessed for Rehabilitation	243	100%	98%	97%
Discharged on Antithrombotic Therapy	200	100%	99%	99%
Discharged on Statin Medication	134	97%	95%	94%
Thrombolytic Therapy Timing	30	100%	74%	66%
Venous Thromboembolism Prophylaxis	261	97%	94%	94%
Written Stroke Educational Materials Given	106	89%	94%	88%
Surgical Care Improvement Project				
Appropriate Beta Blocker Usage[2]	295	98%	98%	98%
Appropriate VTP Within 24 Hours[2]	481	99%	99%	98%
Controlled Postoperative Blood Glucose[2]	183	95%	97%	97%
Perioperative Temperature Management[2]	649	100%	100%	100%
Prophylactic Antibiotic Selection[2]	603	99%	99%	99%
Prophylactic Antibiotic Selection (Outpatient)	681	99%	97%	98%
Prophylactic Antibiotic Stopped[2]	569	98%	98%	98%
Prophylactic Antibiotic Timing[2]	604	99%	99%	99%
Prophylactic Antibiotic Timing (Outpatient)	683	98%	98%	98%
Urinary Catheter Removal[2]	515	97%	98%	97%
Survey of Patients' Hospital Experiences				
Area Around Room 'Always' Quiet at Night	300+	59%	53%	61%
Doctors 'Always' Communicated Well	300+	77%	77%	82%
Home Recovery Information Given	300+	82%	82%	85%
Hospital Given 9 or 10 on 10 Point Scale	300+	77%	64%	71%
Meds 'Always' Explained Before Given	300+	59%	59%	64%
Nurses 'Always' Communicated Well	300+	78%	76%	79%
Pain 'Always' Well Controlled	300+	72%	68%	71%
Room and Bathroom 'Always' Clean	300+	73%	68%	73%
Timely Help 'Always' Received	300+	59%	60%	68%
Would Definitely Recommend Hospital	300+	84%	66%	71%
Use of Medical Imaging				
Cardiac Imaging Stress Test before Surgery	2,195	6.5%	5.8%	5.3%
Combination Abdominal CT Scan	1,860	4.9%	7.4%	10.5%
Combination Brain/Sinus CT Scan	1,187	2.1%	2.8%	2.7%
Combination Chest CT Scan	1,860	0.2%	2.4%	2.7%
Follow-up Mammogram/Ultrasound	1,240	17.3%	12.5%	8.8%
Lumbar Spine MRI for Low Back Pain	110	22.7%	32.9%	37.2%

Virtua Memorial Hospital of Burlington County

175 Madison Ave Phone: 609-914-6200
Mount Holly, NJ 08060
URL: www.virtua.org
Type: Acute Care Hospitals Emergency Services: Yes
Ownership: Voluntary non-profit - Private Beds: 433

Key Personnel:
Chair/CEO . . . . Dennis Flanagan
Chief of Medical Staff. . . . . Alka Kohli, MD, MBA
CEO/President. . . . . Richard P Miller, FACHE

Measure	Cases	This Hosp.	State Avg.	U.S. Avg.
Blood Clot Prevention and Treatment				
Anticoagulation Overlap Therapy[2]	146	93%	88%	93%
ICU Venous Thromboembolism Prophylaxis[2]	67	97%	93%	92%
Incidence of Potentially Preventable VTE[2]	32	3%	10%	10%
UFH with Dosages/Platelet Monitoring[2]	126	92%	99%	97%
Venous Thromboembolism Prophylaxis[2]	414	91%	83%	85%
Warfarin Therapy Discharge Instructions[2]	113	60%	77%	75%
Chest Pain/Possible Heart Attack Care				
Aspirin Given Within 24 Hours of Arrival	28	100%	98%	96%
Fibrinolytic Meds Within 30 Min. of Arrival[7]	-	-	63%	58%
Average Time to ECG (minutes)	29	7	7	7
Average Time to Transfer (minutes)[1]	-	-	74	60
Children's Asthma Care				
Received Home Management Plan of Care	-	-	-	88%
Received Reliever Medication	-	-	-	100%
Received Systemic Corticosteroids	-	-	-	100%
Emergency Department				
Admittance Decision Time (minutes)[2]	625	207	148	98
Head CT Results Within 45 Min. of Arrival	20	70%	66%	57%
Patients Who Left ER Before Being Seen	69,134	0%	2%	2%
Time from ER Arrival to Admit. (minutes)[2]	633	337	355	274
Time from ER Arrival to Discharge (minutes)	362	124	152	134
Time in ER Before Being Evaluated (minutes)	389	57	32	26
Time to Pain Meds for Fractures (minutes)	148	68	58	57
Heart Attack Care				
Aspirin Given at Discharge	160	100%	99%	99%
Fibrinolytic Meds Within 30 Min. of Arrival[7]	-	-	69%	54%
PCI Within 90 Minutes of Arrival	39	90%	95%	96%
Statin Prescribed at Discharge	152	100%	99%	98%
Heart Failure Care				
ACE Inhibitor or ARB for LVSD	97	100%	98%	97%
Discharge Instructions Given	342	98%	97%	94%
Evaluation of LVS Function	484	100%	100%	99%
Medicare Spending				
Medicare Spending per Patient (ratio)	-	1.02	1.07	0.98
Pneumonia Care				
Appropriate Initial Antibiotic Given	238	97%	98%	95%
Blood Culture Timing	403	100%	99%	98%
Pregnancy and Delivery Care				
Newborn Deliveries Scheduled Early[2]	38	11%	3%	6%
Preventive Care				
Immunization for Influenza[2]	522	98%	93%	90%
Immunization for Pneumonia[2]	619	95%	94%	92%
Stroke Care				
Anticoagulation Therapy for Atrial Fibrillation	19	100%	97%	95%
Antithrombotic Therapy Timing	140	98%	98%	98%
Assessed for Rehabilitation	148	100%	98%	97%
Discharged on Antithrombotic Therapy	145	100%	99%	99%
Discharged on Statin Medication	107	100%	95%	94%
Thrombolytic Therapy Timing	14	86%	74%	66%
Venous Thromboembolism Prophylaxis	153	91%	94%	94%
Written Stroke Educational Materials Given	65	100%	94%	88%
Surgical Care Improvement Project				
Appropriate Beta Blocker Usage[2]	148	96%	98%	98%
Appropriate VTP Within 24 Hours[2]	412	99%	99%	98%
Controlled Postoperative Blood Glucose[2,7]	-	-	97%	97%
Perioperative Temperature Management[2]	504	100%	100%	100%
Prophylactic Antibiotic Selection[2]	279	99%	99%	99%
Prophylactic Antibiotic Selection (Outpatient)	181	99%	97%	98%
Prophylactic Antibiotic Stopped[2]	267	99%	98%	98%
Prophylactic Antibiotic Timing[2]	279	100%	99%	99%
Prophylactic Antibiotic Timing (Outpatient)	181	98%	98%	98%
Urinary Catheter Removal[2]	256	97%	98%	97%
Survey of Patients' Hospital Experiences				
Area Around Room 'Always' Quiet at Night	300+	47%	53%	61%
Doctors 'Always' Communicated Well	300+	75%	77%	82%
Home Recovery Information Given	300+	78%	82%	85%
Hospital Given 9 or 10 on 10 Point Scale	300+	65%	64%	71%
Meds 'Always' Explained Before Given	300+	57%	59%	64%
Nurses 'Always' Communicated Well	300+	78%	76%	79%
Pain 'Always' Well Controlled	300+	69%	68%	71%
Room and Bathroom 'Always' Clean	300+	64%	68%	73%
Timely Help 'Always' Received	300+	60%	60%	68%
Would Definitely Recommend Hospital	300+	66%	66%	71%
Use of Medical Imaging				
Cardiac Imaging Stress Test before Surgery	285	4.9%	5.8%	5.3%
Combination Abdominal CT Scan	752	1.7%	7.4%	10.5%
Combination Brain/Sinus CT Scan	1,163	1.2%	2.8%	2.7%
Combination Chest CT Scan	285	0.0%	2.4%	2.7%
Follow-up Mammogram/Ultrasound	306	10.5%	12.5%	8.8%
Lumbar Spine MRI for Low Back Pain[1]	-	-	32.9%	37.2%

Jersey Shore University Medical Center

1945 Rte 33 Phone: 732-776-4900
Neptune, NJ 07754 Fax: 732-776-4583
URL: www.meridianhealth.com
Type: Acute Care Hospitals Emergency Services: Yes
Ownership: Voluntary non-profit - Private Beds: 529

Key Personnel:
Radiology. Rajiv Biswal, MD

NOTE: Hospital profiles are in alphabetical order by state, then city, then hospital within the city; Rankings exclude hospitals with less than 25 cases except for patient surveys which excludes hospitals with less than 100 cases; (a) 100-299 cases; (1) The number of cases/patients is too few to report; (2) Data submitted were based on a sample of cases/patients; (3) Results are based on a shorter time period than required; (4) Data suppressed by CMS for one or more quarters; (5) Results are not available for this reporting period; (6) Fewer than 100 patients completed the HCAHPS survey; (7) No cases met the criteria for this measure; (8) The lower limit of the confidence interval cannot be calculated if the number of observed infections equals zero; (9) No data are available from the state/territory for this reporting period; (10) The scores shown reflect fewer than 50 completed surveys; (11) There were discrepancies in the data collection process; (12) This measure does not apply to this hospital for this reporting period; (13) Results cannot be calculated for this reporting period; (14) The results for this state are combined with nearby states to protect confidentiality; Please refer to the User's Guide for a full explanation of data.

Pediatric Ambulatory Care . . . . . . Joseph Bogdan, MD
Pediatric In-Patient Care . . . . Joseph Bogdan, MD
Infection Control. . . . . Elliott Frank, MD
Intensive Care Unit. . . . . Richard Hayder, RN
CEO/President. . . . . Steven G Littleson, FACHE
Chief of Medical Staff . . . . Ray Masterson, MD
Emergency Room . . . . Robert Sweeney, DO

Measure	Cases	This Hosp.	State Avg.	U.S. Avg.
Blood Clot Prevention and Treatment				
Anticoagulation Overlap Therapy[2]	128	96%	88%	93%
ICU Venous Thromboembolism Prophylaxis[2]	69	100%	93%	92%
Incidence of Potentially Preventable VTE[2]	30	3%	10%	10%
UFH with Dosages/Platelet Monitoring[2]	131	100%	99%	97%
Venous Thromboembolism Prophylaxis[2]	384	89%	83%	85%
Warfarin Therapy Discharge Instructions[2]	75	77%	77%	75%
Chest Pain/Possible Heart Attack Care				
Aspirin Given Within 24 Hours of Arrival[1,3]	-	-	98%	96%
Fibrinolytic Meds Within 30 Min. of Arrival[5]	-	-	63%	58%
Average Time to ECG (minutes)[1,3]	-	-	7	7
Average Time to Transfer (minutes)[5]	-	-	74	60
Children's Asthma Care				
Received Home Management Plan of Care	-	-	-	88%
Received Reliever Medication	-	-	-	100%
Received Systemic Corticosteroids	-	-	-	100%
Emergency Department				
Admittance Decision Time (minutes)[2]	721	136	148	98
Head CT Results Within 45 Min. of Arrival[1]	-	-	66%	57%
Patients Who Left ER Before Being Seen	88,610	3%	2%	2%
Time from ER Arrival to Admit. (minutes)[2]	730	352	355	274
Time from ER Arrival to Discharge (minutes)	389	170	152	134
Time in ER Before Being Evaluated (minutes)	430	55	32	26
Time to Pain Meds for Fractures (minutes)	221	68	58	57
Heart Attack Care				
Aspirin Given at Discharge	778	100%	99%	99%
Fibrinolytic Meds Within 30 Min. of Arrival[7]	-	-	69%	54%
PCI Within 90 Minutes of Arrival	86	98%	95%	96%
Statin Prescribed at Discharge	758	100%	99%	98%
Heart Failure Care				
ACE Inhibitor or ARB for LVSD[2]	103	98%	98%	97%
Discharge Instructions Given[2]	213	99%	97%	94%
Evaluation of LVS Function[2]	315	100%	100%	99%
Medicare Spending				
Medicare Spending per Patient (ratio)	-	1.08	1.07	0.98
Pneumonia Care				
Appropriate Initial Antibiotic Given[2]	74	99%	98%	95%
Blood Culture Timing[2]	144	99%	99%	98%
Pregnancy and Delivery Care				
Newborn Deliveries Scheduled Early[2]	28	0%	3%	6%
Preventive Care				
Immunization for Influenza[2]	567	93%	93%	90%
Immunization for Pneumonia[2]	652	96%	94%	92%
Stroke Care				
Anticoagulation Therapy for Atrial Fibrillation	39	97%	97%	95%
Antithrombotic Therapy Timing	199	99%	98%	98%
Assessed for Rehabilitation	267	98%	98%	97%
Discharged on Antithrombotic Therapy	205	100%	99%	99%
Discharged on Statin Medication	163	97%	95%	94%
Thrombolytic Therapy Timing	22	82%	74%	66%
Venous Thromboembolism Prophylaxis	315	100%	94%	94%
Written Stroke Educational Materials Given	118	97%	94%	88%
Surgical Care Improvement Project				
Appropriate Beta Blocker Usage[2]	456	98%	98%	98%
Appropriate VTP Within 24 Hours[2]	478	98%	99%	98%
Controlled Postoperative Blood Glucose[2]	399	97%	97%	97%
Perioperative Temperature Management[2]	600	99%	100%	100%
Prophylactic Antibiotic Selection[2]	772	100%	99%	99%
Prophylactic Antibiotic Selection (Outpatient)	671	99%	97%	98%
Prophylactic Antibiotic Stopped[2]	741	97%	98%	98%
Prophylactic Antibiotic Timing[2]	774	99%	99%	99%
Prophylactic Antibiotic Timing (Outpatient)	674	98%	98%	98%
Urinary Catheter Removal[2]	532	98%	98%	97%
Survey of Patients' Hospital Experiences				
Area Around Room 'Always' Quiet at Night	300+	54%	53%	61%
Doctors 'Always' Communicated Well	300+	77%	77%	82%
Home Recovery Information Given	300+	81%	82%	85%
Hospital Given 9 or 10 on 10 Point Scale	300+	72%	64%	71%
Meds 'Always' Explained Before Given	300+	64%	59%	64%
Nurses 'Always' Communicated Well	300+	78%	76%	79%
Pain 'Always' Well Controlled	300+	69%	68%	71%
Room and Bathroom 'Always' Clean	300+	70%	68%	73%
Timely Help 'Always' Received	300+	65%	60%	68%
Would Definitely Recommend Hospital	300+	77%	66%	71%
Use of Medical Imaging				
Cardiac Imaging Stress Test before Surgery	403	6.9%	5.8%	5.3%
Combination Abdominal CT Scan	1,268	5.4%	7.4%	10.5%
Combination Brain/Sinus CT Scan	1,556	3.9%	2.8%	2.7%
Combination Chest CT Scan	861	0.7%	2.4%	2.7%
Follow-up Mammogram/Ultrasound[7]	-	-	12.5%	8.8%
Lumbar Spine MRI for Low Back Pain[1]	-	-	32.9%	37.2%

Robert Wood Johnson University Hospital

One Robert Wood Johnson Pl Phone: 732-937-8900
New Brunswick, NJ 08901 Fax: 732-937-8837
URL: www.rwjuh.edu
Type: Acute Care Hospitals Emergency Services: Yes
Ownership: Voluntary non-profit - Private Beds: 160
Key Personnel:
Chief of Medical Staff. . . . . Peter Amenta, MD
Radiology. . . . . Leonard Bodner
CEO/President. . . . . Stephen K. Jones, FACHE
Cardiac Laboratory. . . . . Peter Scholz, MD

Measure	Cases	This Hosp.	State Avg.	U.S. Avg.
Blood Clot Prevention and Treatment				
Anticoagulation Overlap Therapy[2]	155	99%	88%	93%
ICU Venous Thromboembolism Prophylaxis[2]	79	97%	93%	92%
Incidence of Potentially Preventable VTE[2]	57	4%	10%	10%
UFH with Dosages/Platelet Monitoring[2]	172	95%	99%	97%
Venous Thromboembolism Prophylaxis[2]	339	98%	83%	85%
Warfarin Therapy Discharge Instructions[2]	91	100%	77%	75%
Chest Pain/Possible Heart Attack Care				
Aspirin Given Within 24 Hours of Arrival[5]	-	-	98%	96%
Fibrinolytic Meds Within 30 Min. of Arrival[5]	-	-	63%	58%
Average Time to ECG (minutes)[5]	-	-	7	7
Average Time to Transfer (minutes)[5]	-	-	74	60
Children's Asthma Care				
Received Home Management Plan of Care	-	-	-	88%
Received Reliever Medication	-	-	-	100%
Received Systemic Corticosteroids	-	-	-	100%
Emergency Department				
Admittance Decision Time (minutes)[2]	622	260	148	98
Head CT Results Within 45 Min. of Arrival[1]	-	-	66%	57%
Patients Who Left ER Before Being Seen	96,445	0%	2%	2%
Time from ER Arrival to Admit. (minutes)[2]	630	458	355	274
Time from ER Arrival to Discharge (minutes)	379	135	152	134
Time in ER Before Being Evaluated (minutes)	431	25	32	26
Time to Pain Meds for Fractures (minutes)	302	44	58	57
Heart Attack Care				
Aspirin Given at Discharge	797	99%	99%	99%
Fibrinolytic Meds Within 30 Min. of Arrival[7]	-	-	69%	54%
PCI Within 90 Minutes of Arrival	107	98%	95%	96%
Statin Prescribed at Discharge	759	100%	99%	98%
Heart Failure Care				
ACE Inhibitor or ARB for LVSD	321	99%	98%	97%
Discharge Instructions Given	748	99%	97%	94%
Evaluation of LVS Function	1,040	100%	100%	99%
Medicare Spending				
Medicare Spending per Patient (ratio)	-	1.09	1.07	0.98
Pneumonia Care				
Appropriate Initial Antibiotic Given	164	99%	98%	95%
Blood Culture Timing	523	99%	99%	98%
Pregnancy and Delivery Care				
Newborn Deliveries Scheduled Early[2]	24	4%	3%	6%
Preventive Care				
Immunization for Influenza[2]	564	92%	93%	90%
Immunization for Pneumonia[2]	612	93%	94%	92%
Stroke Care				
Anticoagulation Therapy for Atrial Fibrillation	53	98%	97%	95%
Antithrombotic Therapy Timing	203	97%	98%	98%
Assessed for Rehabilitation	348	99%	98%	97%
Discharged on Antithrombotic Therapy	279	100%	99%	99%
Discharged on Statin Medication	206	97%	95%	94%
Thrombolytic Therapy Timing	56	91%	74%	66%
Venous Thromboembolism Prophylaxis	371	98%	94%	94%
Written Stroke Educational Materials Given	160	100%	94%	88%
Surgical Care Improvement Project				
Appropriate Beta Blocker Usage[2]	645	100%	98%	98%
Appropriate VTP Within 24 Hours[2]	948	100%	99%	98%
Controlled Postoperative Blood Glucose[2]	618	97%	97%	97%
Perioperative Temperature Management[2]	1,141	100%	100%	100%
Prophylactic Antibiotic Selection[2]	1,390	99%	99%	99%
Prophylactic Antibiotic Selection (Outpatient)	931	98%	97%	98%
Prophylactic Antibiotic Stopped[2]	1,326	99%	98%	98%
Prophylactic Antibiotic Timing[2]	1,390	99%	99%	99%
Prophylactic Antibiotic Timing (Outpatient)	932	99%	98%	98%
Urinary Catheter Removal[2]	1,096	100%	98%	97%
Survey of Patients' Hospital Experiences				
Area Around Room 'Always' Quiet at Night	300+	50%	53%	61%
Doctors 'Always' Communicated Well	300+	78%	77%	82%
Home Recovery Information Given	300+	83%	82%	85%
Hospital Given 9 or 10 on 10 Point Scale	300+	68%	64%	71%
Meds 'Always' Explained Before Given	300+	60%	59%	64%
Nurses 'Always' Communicated Well	300+	78%	76%	79%
Pain 'Always' Well Controlled	300+	68%	68%	71%
Room and Bathroom 'Always' Clean	300+	64%	68%	73%
Timely Help 'Always' Received	300+	66%	60%	68%
Would Definitely Recommend Hospital	300+	74%	66%	71%
Use of Medical Imaging				
Cardiac Imaging Stress Test before Surgery	290	7.6%	5.8%	5.3%
Combination Abdominal CT Scan	723	0.8%	7.4%	10.5%
Combination Brain/Sinus CT Scan	1,006	2.3%	2.8%	2.7%
Combination Chest CT Scan	245	0.4%	2.4%	2.7%
Follow-up Mammogram/Ultrasound[7]	-	-	12.5%	8.8%
Lumbar Spine MRI for Low Back Pain[1]	-	-	32.9%	37.2%

Saint Peter's University Hospital

254 Easton Ave Phone: 732-745-8600
New Brunswick, NJ 08901 Fax: 732-220-8046
E-mail: info@saintpetersuh.com
URL: www.saintpetersuh.com
Type: Acute Care Hospitals Emergency Services: Yes
Ownership: Voluntary non-profit - Church Beds: 478
Key Personnel:
Pediatric Ambulatory Care . . . . . . William Bernstein, MD
Operating Room. . . . . Jackie Carey, RN
Infection Control. . . . . Amy Gram
Coronary Care . . . . Lois Hobratschk, RN
Quality Assurance . . . . Jan Lichtenberger, RN
Pediatric In-Patient Care . . . . Bipin Patel, MD
Radiology. . . . . Steven Schonfeld, MD
CEO/President. . . . . Sheryl Slanim

Measure	Cases	This Hosp.	State Avg.	U.S. Avg.
Blood Clot Prevention and Treatment				
Anticoagulation Overlap Therapy[2]	80	95%	88%	93%
ICU Venous Thromboembolism Prophylaxis[2]	66	98%	93%	92%
Incidence of Potentially Preventable VTE[2]	32	0%	10%	10%
UFH with Dosages/Platelet Monitoring[2]	84	99%	99%	97%
Venous Thromboembolism Prophylaxis[2]	357	98%	83%	85%
Warfarin Therapy Discharge Instructions[2]	55	89%	77%	75%
Chest Pain/Possible Heart Attack Care				
Aspirin Given Within 24 Hours of Arrival[1]	-	-	98%	96%
Fibrinolytic Meds Within 30 Min. of Arrival[3,7]	-	-	63%	58%
Average Time to ECG (minutes)[1]	-	-	7	7
Average Time to Transfer (minutes)[3,7]	-	-	74	60
Children's Asthma Care				
Received Home Management Plan of Care	185	97%	-	88%
Received Reliever Medication	186	100%	-	100%
Received Systemic Corticosteroids	186	100%	-	100%
Emergency Department				
Admittance Decision Time (minutes)[2]	454	164	148	98
Head CT Results Within 45 Min. of Arrival[1]	-	-	66%	57%

NOTE: *Hospital profiles are in alphabetical order by state, then city, then hospital within the city; Rankings exclude hospitals with less than 25 cases except for patient surveys which excludes hospitals with less than 100 cases; (a) 100-299 cases; (1) The number of cases/patients is too few to report; (2) Data submitted were based on a sample of cases/patients; (3) Results are based on a shorter time period than required; (4) Data suppressed by CMS for one or more quarters; (5) Results are not available for this reporting period; (6) Fewer than 100 patients completed the HCAHPS survey; (7) No cases met the criteria for this measure; (8) The lower limit of the confidence interval cannot be calculated if the number of observed infections equals zero; (9) No data are available from the state/territory for this reporting period; (10) The scores shown reflect fewer than 50 completed surveys; (11) There were discrepancies in the data collection process; (12) This measure does not apply to this hospital for this reporting period; (13) Results cannot be calculated for this reporting period; (14) The results for this state are combined with nearby states to protect confidentiality; Please refer to the User's Guide for a full explanation of data.*

Measure	Cases	This Hosp.	State Avg.	U.S. Avg.
Patients Who Left ER Before Being Seen	66,771	0%	2%	2%
Time from ER Arrival to Admit. (minutes)[2]	455	357	355	274
Time from ER Arrival to Discharge (minutes)	409	132	152	134
Time in ER Before Being Evaluated (minutes)	432	32	32	26
Time to Pain Meds for Fractures (minutes)	168	56	58	57
Heart Attack Care				
Aspirin Given at Discharge	79	100%	99%	99%
Fibrinolytic Meds Within 30 Min. of Arrival[7]	-	-	69%	54%
PCI Within 90 Minutes of Arrival[1]	-	-	95%	96%
Statin Prescribed at Discharge	83	100%	99%	98%
Heart Failure Care				
ACE Inhibitor or ARB for LVSD	68	100%	98%	97%
Discharge Instructions Given	213	99%	97%	94%
Evaluation of LVS Function	296	100%	100%	99%
Medicare Spending				
Medicare Spending per Patient (ratio)	-	1.06	1.07	0.98
Pneumonia Care				
Appropriate Initial Antibiotic Given[2]	129	98%	98%	95%
Blood Culture Timing[2]	289	100%	99%	98%
Pregnancy and Delivery Care				
Newborn Deliveries Scheduled Early[2]	95	5%	3%	6%
Preventive Care				
Immunization for Influenza[2]	461	99%	93%	90%
Immunization for Pneumonia[2]	347	96%	94%	92%
Stroke Care				
Anticoagulation Therapy for Atrial Fibrillation	14	100%	97%	95%
Antithrombotic Therapy Timing	82	99%	98%	98%
Assessed for Rehabilitation	104	98%	98%	97%
Discharged on Antithrombotic Therapy	92	100%	99%	99%
Discharged on Statin Medication	71	99%	95%	94%
Thrombolytic Therapy Timing[1]	-	-	74%	66%
Venous Thromboembolism Prophylaxis	102	96%	94%	94%
Written Stroke Educational Materials Given	62	98%	94%	88%
Surgical Care Improvement Project				
Appropriate Beta Blocker Usage[2]	134	100%	98%	98%
Appropriate VTP Within 24 Hours[2]	388	99%	99%	98%
Controlled Postoperative Blood Glucose[2,7]	-	-	97%	97%
Perioperative Temperature Management[2]	471	100%	100%	100%
Prophylactic Antibiotic Selection[2]	309	100%	99%	99%
Prophylactic Antibiotic Selection (Outpatient)	210	98%	97%	98%
Prophylactic Antibiotic Stopped[2]	305	95%	98%	98%
Prophylactic Antibiotic Timing[2]	309	100%	99%	99%
Prophylactic Antibiotic Timing (Outpatient)	210	99%	98%	98%
Urinary Catheter Removal[2]	136	97%	98%	97%
Survey of Patients' Hospital Experiences				
Area Around Room 'Always' Quiet at Night	300+	58%	53%	61%
Doctors 'Always' Communicated Well	300+	80%	77%	82%
Home Recovery Information Given	300+	83%	82%	85%
Hospital Given 9 or 10 on 10 Point Scale	300+	75%	64%	71%
Meds 'Always' Explained Before Given	300+	63%	59%	64%
Nurses 'Always' Communicated Well	300+	84%	76%	79%
Pain 'Always' Well Controlled	300+	74%	68%	71%
Room and Bathroom 'Always' Clean	300+	73%	68%	73%
Timely Help 'Always' Received	300+	68%	60%	68%
Would Definitely Recommend Hospital	300+	79%	66%	71%
Use of Medical Imaging				
Cardiac Imaging Stress Test before Surgery	165	4.8%	5.8%	5.3%
Combination Abdominal CT Scan	433	1.6%	7.4%	10.5%
Combination Brain/Sinus CT Scan	581	5.7%	2.8%	2.7%
Combination Chest CT Scan	162	0.0%	2.4%	2.7%
Follow-up Mammogram/Ultrasound	324	12.3%	12.5%	8.8%
Lumbar Spine MRI for Low Back Pain[1]	-	-	32.9%	37.2%

Newark Beth Israel Medical Center

201 Lyons Ave
Newark, NJ 07112
Phone: 973-926-7850
Fax: 973-926-8371
E-mail: info@sbhcs.com
URL: www.sbhcs.com
Type: Acute Care Hospitals
Emergency Services: Yes
Ownership: Voluntary non-profit - Private
Beds: 673

Key Personnel:

Hemotology Center . . . . Alice Cohen, MD
Cardiac Laboratory. . . . . Marc Cohen
Chief of Medical Staff . . . . Donald Greenfield
CEO/President. . . . . Paul A Mertz
Infection Control. . . . . Jeremias Murillo, MD
Quality Assurance . . . . Howard Previllile
Radiology. . . . . Richard Shoenfeld, MD
Pediatric In-Patient Care . . . . Jules A Titelbaum, MD

Measure	Cases	This Hosp.	State Avg.	U.S. Avg.
Blood Clot Prevention and Treatment				
Anticoagulation Overlap Therapy[2]	130	85%	88%	93%
ICU Venous Thromboembolism Prophylaxis[2]	79	87%	93%	92%
Incidence of Potentially Preventable VTE[2]	68	7%	10%	10%
UFH with Dosages/Platelet Monitoring[2]	110	100%	99%	97%
Venous Thromboembolism Prophylaxis[2]	437	68%	83%	85%
Warfarin Therapy Discharge Instructions[2]	80	72%	77%	75%
Chest Pain/Possible Heart Attack Care				
Aspirin Given Within 24 Hours of Arrival[3,7]	-	-	98%	96%
Fibrinolytic Meds Within 30 Min. of Arrival[5]	-	-	63%	58%
Average Time to ECG (minutes)[3,7]	-	-	7	7
Average Time to Transfer (minutes)[5]	-	-	74	60
Children's Asthma Care				
Received Home Management Plan of Care	-	-	-	88%
Received Reliever Medication	-	-	-	100%
Received Systemic Corticosteroids	-	-	-	100%
Emergency Department				
Admittance Decision Time (minutes)[2]	489	520	148	98
Head CT Results Within 45 Min. of Arrival[1]	-	-	66%	57%
Patients Who Left ER Before Being Seen	44,282	5%	2%	2%
Time from ER Arrival to Admit. (minutes)[2]	498	897	355	274
Time from ER Arrival to Discharge (minutes)	398	189	152	134
Time in ER Before Being Evaluated (minutes)	430	75	32	26
Time to Pain Meds for Fractures (minutes)	139	88	58	57
Heart Attack Care				
Aspirin Given at Discharge[2]	284	100%	99%	99%
Fibrinolytic Meds Within 30 Min. of Arrival[2,7]	-	-	69%	54%
PCI Within 90 Minutes of Arrival[2]	46	100%	95%	96%
Statin Prescribed at Discharge[2]	274	100%	99%	98%
Heart Failure Care				
ACE Inhibitor or ARB for LVSD[2]	126	100%	98%	97%
Discharge Instructions Given[2]	282	100%	97%	94%
Evaluation of LVS Function[2]	339	100%	100%	99%
Medicare Spending				
Medicare Spending per Patient (ratio)	-	1.12	1.07	0.98
Pneumonia Care				
Appropriate Initial Antibiotic Given[2]	92	99%	98%	95%
Blood Culture Timing[2]	157	96%	99%	98%
Pregnancy and Delivery Care				
Newborn Deliveries Scheduled Early[2]	581	1%	3%	6%
Preventive Care				
Immunization for Influenza[2]	516	85%	93%	90%
Immunization for Pneumonia[2]	556	78%	94%	92%
Stroke Care				
Anticoagulation Therapy for Atrial Fibrillation	19	95%	97%	95%
Antithrombotic Therapy Timing	162	96%	98%	98%
Assessed for Rehabilitation	179	92%	98%	97%
Discharged on Antithrombotic Therapy	158	97%	99%	99%
Discharged on Statin Medication	133	79%	95%	94%
Thrombolytic Therapy Timing[1]	-	-	74%	66%
Venous Thromboembolism Prophylaxis	193	68%	94%	94%
Written Stroke Educational Materials Given	99	65%	94%	88%
Surgical Care Improvement Project				
Appropriate Beta Blocker Usage[2]	192	96%	98%	98%
Appropriate VTP Within 24 Hours[2]	324	99%	99%	98%
Controlled Postoperative Blood Glucose[2]	153	98%	97%	97%
Perioperative Temperature Management[2]	416	100%	100%	100%
Prophylactic Antibiotic Selection[2]	405	99%	99%	99%
Prophylactic Antibiotic Selection (Outpatient)	374	99%	97%	98%
Prophylactic Antibiotic Stopped[2]	380	97%	98%	98%
Prophylactic Antibiotic Timing[2]	405	100%	99%	99%
Prophylactic Antibiotic Timing (Outpatient)	375	99%	98%	98%
Urinary Catheter Removal[2]	106	100%	98%	97%
Survey of Patients' Hospital Experiences				
Area Around Room 'Always' Quiet at Night	300+	55%	53%	61%
Doctors 'Always' Communicated Well	300+	77%	77%	82%
Home Recovery Information Given	300+	78%	82%	85%
Hospital Given 9 or 10 on 10 Point Scale	300+	60%	64%	71%
Meds 'Always' Explained Before Given	300+	57%	59%	64%
Nurses 'Always' Communicated Well	300+	74%	76%	79%
Pain 'Always' Well Controlled	300+	67%	68%	71%
Room and Bathroom 'Always' Clean	300+	67%	68%	73%
Timely Help 'Always' Received	300+	52%	60%	68%
Would Definitely Recommend Hospital	300+	60%	66%	71%
Use of Medical Imaging				
Cardiac Imaging Stress Test before Surgery	383	7.0%	5.8%	5.3%
Combination Abdominal CT Scan	492	16.1%	7.4%	10.5%
Combination Brain/Sinus CT Scan[1]	-	-	2.8%	2.7%
Combination Chest CT Scan	579	4.5%	2.4%	2.7%
Follow-up Mammogram/Ultrasound	642	10.6%	12.5%	8.8%
Lumbar Spine MRI for Low Back Pain	51	47.1%	32.9%	37.2%

Saint Michael's Medical Center

111 Central Avenue
Newark, NJ 07102
Phone: 973-877-5350
Fax: 973-877-5635
URL: www.cathedralhealth.org
Type: Acute Care Hospitals
Emergency Services: Yes
Ownership: Voluntary non-profit - Private
Beds: 357

Key Personnel:

CEO/President. . . . . Henry Amoroso
Chief of Medical Staff . . . . Nicholas Baranetsky, MD
Emergency Room . . . . Dwight Lee, MD
Radiology. . . . . Suresh Mody, MD
Quality Assurance . . . . Adel Natividad, RN

Measure	Cases	This Hosp.	State Avg.	U.S. Avg.
Blood Clot Prevention and Treatment				
Anticoagulation Overlap Therapy[2]	44	52%	88%	93%
ICU Venous Thromboembolism Prophylaxis[2]	91	93%	93%	92%
Incidence of Potentially Preventable VTE[2]	14	7%	10%	10%
UFH with Dosages/Platelet Monitoring[2]	23	100%	99%	97%
Venous Thromboembolism Prophylaxis[2]	332	71%	83%	85%
Warfarin Therapy Discharge Instructions[2]	25	56%	77%	75%
Chest Pain/Possible Heart Attack Care				
Aspirin Given Within 24 Hours of Arrival[5]	-	-	98%	96%
Fibrinolytic Meds Within 30 Min. of Arrival[5]	-	-	63%	58%
Average Time to ECG (minutes)[5]	-	-	7	7
Average Time to Transfer (minutes)[5]	-	-	74	60
Children's Asthma Care				
Received Home Management Plan of Care	-	-	-	88%
Received Reliever Medication	-	-	-	100%
Received Systemic Corticosteroids	-	-	-	100%
Emergency Department				
Admittance Decision Time (minutes)[2]	853	205	148	98
Head CT Results Within 45 Min. of Arrival[1]	-	-	66%	57%
Patients Who Left ER Before Being Seen	35,619	1%	2%	2%
Time from ER Arrival to Admit. (minutes)[2]	860	448	355	274
Time from ER Arrival to Discharge (minutes)	365	197	152	134
Time in ER Before Being Evaluated (minutes)	432	72	32	26
Time to Pain Meds for Fractures (minutes)	34	79	58	57
Heart Attack Care				
Aspirin Given at Discharge	162	98%	99%	99%
Fibrinolytic Meds Within 30 Min. of Arrival[7]	-	-	69%	54%
PCI Within 90 Minutes of Arrival	18	83%	95%	96%
Statin Prescribed at Discharge	169	97%	99%	98%
Heart Failure Care				
ACE Inhibitor or ARB for LVSD[2]	151	93%	98%	97%
Discharge Instructions Given[2]	252	99%	97%	94%
Evaluation of LVS Function[2]	315	99%	100%	99%
Medicare Spending				
Medicare Spending per Patient (ratio)	-	1.11	1.07	0.98
Pneumonia Care				
Appropriate Initial Antibiotic Given[2]	76	95%	98%	95%
Blood Culture Timing[2]	155	96%	99%	98%
Pregnancy and Delivery Care				
Newborn Deliveries Scheduled Early[7]	-	-	3%	6%
Preventive Care				
Immunization for Influenza[2]	609	98%	93%	90%
Immunization for Pneumonia[2]	932	97%	94%	92%
Stroke Care				
Anticoagulation Therapy for Atrial Fibrillation[1]	-	-	97%	95%
Antithrombotic Therapy Timing	70	96%	98%	98%

NOTE: Hospital profiles are in alphabetical order by state, then city, then hospital within the city; Rankings exclude hospitals with less than 25 cases except for patient surveys which excludes hospitals with less than 100 cases; (a) 100-299 cases; (1) The number of cases/patients is too few to report; (2) Data submitted were based on a sample of cases/patients; (3) Results are based on a shorter time period than required; (4) Data suppressed by CMS for one or more quarters; (5) Results are not available for this reporting period; (6) Fewer than 100 patients completed the HCAHPS survey; (7) No cases met the criteria for this measure; (8) The lower limit of the confidence interval cannot be calculated if the number of observed infections equals zero; (9) No data are available from the state/territory for this reporting period; (10) The scores shown reflect fewer than 50 completed surveys; (11) There were discrepancies in the data collection process; (12) This measure does not apply to this hospital for this reporting period; (13) Results cannot be calculated for this reporting period; (14) The results for this state are combined with nearby states to protect confidentiality; Please refer to the User's Guide for a full explanation of data.

Measure	Cases	This Hosp.	State Avg.	U.S. Avg.
Assessed for Rehabilitation	78	99%	98%	97%
Discharged on Antithrombotic Therapy	74	88%	99%	99%
Discharged on Statin Medication	63	87%	95%	94%
Thrombolytic Therapy Timing[1]	-	-	74%	66%
Venous Thromboembolism Prophylaxis	77	86%	94%	94%
Written Stroke Educational Materials Given	47	100%	94%	88%
Surgical Care Improvement Project				
Appropriate Beta Blocker Usage[2]	174	88%	98%	98%
Appropriate VTP Within 24 Hours[2]	351	96%	99%	98%
Controlled Postoperative Blood Glucose[2]	112	91%	97%	97%
Perioperative Temperature Management[2]	465	100%	100%	100%
Prophylactic Antibiotic Selection[2]	355	99%	99%	99%
Prophylactic Antibiotic Selection (Outpatient)	183	99%	97%	98%
Prophylactic Antibiotic Stopped[2]	348	97%	98%	98%
Prophylactic Antibiotic Timing[2]	355	99%	99%	99%
Prophylactic Antibiotic Timing (Outpatient)	185	98%	98%	98%
Urinary Catheter Removal[2]	131	89%	98%	97%
Survey of Patients' Hospital Experiences				
Area Around Room 'Always' Quiet at Night	300+	51%	53%	61%
Doctors 'Always' Communicated Well	300+	73%	77%	82%
Home Recovery Information Given	300+	74%	82%	85%
Hospital Given 9 or 10 on 10 Point Scale	300+	57%	64%	71%
Meds 'Always' Explained Before Given	300+	50%	59%	64%
Nurses 'Always' Communicated Well	300+	67%	76%	79%
Pain 'Always' Well Controlled	300+	61%	68%	71%
Room and Bathroom 'Always' Clean	300+	70%	68%	73%
Timely Help 'Always' Received	300+	49%	60%	68%
Would Definitely Recommend Hospital	300+	61%	66%	71%
Use of Medical Imaging				
Cardiac Imaging Stress Test before Surgery	302	6.0%	5.8%	5.3%
Combination Abdominal CT Scan	471	8.5%	7.4%	10.5%
Combination Brain/Sinus CT Scan	416	4.3%	2.8%	2.7%
Combination Chest CT Scan	197	8.1%	2.4%	2.7%
Follow-up Mammogram/Ultrasound	842	7.4%	12.5%	8.8%
Lumbar Spine MRI for Low Back Pain[1]	-	-	32.9%	37.2%

University Hospital

150 Bergen St
Newark, NJ 07103
E-mail: uhcontact@umdnj.edu
URL: www.theuniversityhospital.com
Type: Acute Care Hospitals
Ownership: Government - State
Phone: 973-972-5658
Fax: 973-972-6943
Emergency Services: Yes
Beds: 519

Key Personnel:
Chief of Medical Staff.......... Suzanne H. Atkin, MD, FACEP, FACP
Radiology.................. Stephen Baker, MD
Quality Assurance .... Ronald DeVos
Pediatric Ambulatory Care ...... Frank Desposito, MD
Pediatric In-Patient Care .... Frank Desposito, MD
CEO/President............... James R. Gonzalez, MPH, FACHE
Infection Control.............. Steve Udem, MD

Measure	Cases	This Hosp.	State Avg.	U.S. Avg.
Blood Clot Prevention and Treatment				
Anticoagulation Overlap Therapy[2]	95	97%	88%	93%
ICU Venous Thromboembolism Prophylaxis[2]	83	94%	93%	92%
Incidence of Potentially Preventable VTE[2]	61	7%	10%	10%
UFH with Dosages/Platelet Monitoring[2]	89	97%	99%	97%
Venous Thromboembolism Prophylaxis[2]	292	92%	83%	85%
Warfarin Therapy Discharge Instructions[2]	58	38%	77%	75%
Chest Pain/Possible Heart Attack Care				
Aspirin Given Within 24 Hours of Arrival[3,7]	-	-	98%	96%
Fibrinolytic Meds Within 30 Min. of Arrival[5]	-	-	63%	58%
Average Time to ECG (minutes)[3,7]	-	-	7	7
Average Time to Transfer (minutes)[5]	-	-	74	60
Children's Asthma Care				
Received Home Management Plan of Care	-	-	-	88%
Received Reliever Medication	-	-	-	100%
Received Systemic Corticosteroids	-	-	-	100%
Emergency Department				
Admittance Decision Time (minutes)[2]	648	234	148	98
Head CT Results Within 45 Min. of Arrival	15	7%	66%	57%
Patients Who Left ER Before Being Seen	96,588	9%	2%	2%
Time from ER Arrival to Admit. (minutes)[2]	649	546	355	274
Time from ER Arrival to Discharge (minutes)	289	252	152	134
Time in ER Before Being Evaluated (minutes)	327	90	32	26
Time to Pain Meds for Fractures (minutes)	179	115	58	57
Heart Attack Care				
Aspirin Given at Discharge	106	100%	99%	99%
Fibrinolytic Meds Within 30 Min. of Arrival[7]	-	-	69%	54%
PCI Within 90 Minutes of Arrival	22	82%	95%	96%
Statin Prescribed at Discharge	104	100%	99%	98%
Heart Failure Care				
ACE Inhibitor or ARB for LVSD	181	100%	98%	97%
Discharge Instructions Given	249	100%	97%	94%
Evaluation of LVS Function	288	100%	100%	99%
Medicare Spending				
Medicare Spending per Patient (ratio)	-	1.06	1.07	0.98
Pneumonia Care				
Appropriate Initial Antibiotic Given	91	100%	98%	95%
Blood Culture Timing	247	98%	99%	98%
Pregnancy and Delivery Care				
Newborn Deliveries Scheduled Early[2]	27	0%	3%	6%
Preventive Care				
Immunization for Influenza[2]	529	91%	93%	90%
Immunization for Pneumonia[2]	486	78%	94%	92%
Stroke Care				
Anticoagulation Therapy for Atrial Fibrillation[1,2]	-	-	97%	95%
Antithrombotic Therapy Timing[2]	59	98%	98%	98%
Assessed for Rehabilitation[2]	110	99%	98%	97%
Discharged on Antithrombotic Therapy[2]	72	100%	99%	99%
Discharged on Statin Medication[2]	45	100%	95%	94%
Thrombolytic Therapy Timing[1,2]	-	-	74%	66%
Venous Thromboembolism Prophylaxis[2]	119	97%	94%	94%
Written Stroke Educational Materials Given[2]	46	100%	94%	88%
Surgical Care Improvement Project				
Appropriate Beta Blocker Usage[2]	59	98%	98%	98%
Appropriate VTP Within 24 Hours[2]	258	99%	99%	98%
Controlled Postoperative Blood Glucose[2]	48	85%	97%	97%
Perioperative Temperature Management[2]	336	100%	100%	100%
Prophylactic Antibiotic Selection[2]	218	95%	99%	99%
Prophylactic Antibiotic Selection (Outpatient)	157	86%	97%	98%
Prophylactic Antibiotic Stopped[2]	211	95%	98%	98%
Prophylactic Antibiotic Timing[2]	221	100%	99%	99%
Prophylactic Antibiotic Timing (Outpatient)	160	98%	98%	98%
Urinary Catheter Removal[2]	125	98%	98%	97%
Survey of Patients' Hospital Experiences				
Area Around Room 'Always' Quiet at Night	300+	56%	53%	61%
Doctors 'Always' Communicated Well	300+	75%	77%	82%
Home Recovery Information Given	300+	80%	82%	85%
Hospital Given 9 or 10 on 10 Point Scale	300+	58%	64%	71%
Meds 'Always' Explained Before Given	300+	55%	59%	64%
Nurses 'Always' Communicated Well	300+	68%	76%	79%
Pain 'Always' Well Controlled	300+	61%	68%	71%
Room and Bathroom 'Always' Clean	300+	57%	68%	73%
Timely Help 'Always' Received	300+	52%	60%	68%
Would Definitely Recommend Hospital	300+	62%	66%	71%
Use of Medical Imaging				
Cardiac Imaging Stress Test before Surgery	76	3.9%	5.8%	5.3%
Combination Abdominal CT Scan	494	40.5%	7.4%	10.5%
Combination Brain/Sinus CT Scan	472	2.1%	2.8%	2.7%
Combination Chest CT Scan	254	1.2%	2.4%	2.7%
Follow-up Mammogram/Ultrasound	467	4.5%	12.5%	8.8%
Lumbar Spine MRI for Low Back Pain[1]	-	-	32.9%	37.2%

Newton Memorial Hospital

175 High St
Newton, NJ 07860
E-mail: bgrace@itsyourlife.com
URL: www.itsyourlife.com
Type: Acute Care Hospitals
Ownership: Voluntary non-profit - Private
Phone: 973-383-2121
Fax: 973-383-8973
Emergency Services: Yes
Beds: 162

Key Personnel:
Radiology.................. Harmar D Brereton
Quality Assurance .... Jean Jones
Chair/CEO.................. Karen J. Kessler
Administrator .... Andrew L. Kovach
Operating Room.............. Donna Oregan
Chief of Medical Staff.......... Jan Schwarz-Miller, MD, MPH
CEO/President............... Joseph A. Trunfio, MD

Measure	Cases	This Hosp.	State Avg.	U.S. Avg.
Blood Clot Prevention and Treatment				
Anticoagulation Overlap Therapy[2]	54	94%	88%	93%
ICU Venous Thromboembolism Prophylaxis[2]	78	92%	93%	92%
Incidence of Potentially Preventable VTE[1,2]	-	-	10%	10%
UFH with Dosages/Platelet Monitoring[2]	25	92%	99%	97%
Venous Thromboembolism Prophylaxis[2]	391	90%	83%	85%
Warfarin Therapy Discharge Instructions[2]	36	100%	77%	75%
Chest Pain/Possible Heart Attack Care				
Aspirin Given Within 24 Hours of Arrival[3]	32	100%	98%	96%
Fibrinolytic Meds Within 30 Min. of Arrival[1,3]	-	-	63%	58%
Average Time to ECG (minutes)[3]	32	8	7	7
Average Time to Transfer (minutes)[1,3]	-	-	74	60
Children's Asthma Care				
Received Home Management Plan of Care	-	-	-	88%
Received Reliever Medication	-	-	-	100%
Received Systemic Corticosteroids	-	-	-	100%
Emergency Department				
Admittance Decision Time (minutes)[2]	908	228	148	98
Head CT Results Within 45 Min. of Arrival[1]	-	-	66%	57%
Patients Who Left ER Before Being Seen	29,174	2%	2%	2%
Time from ER Arrival to Admit. (minutes)[2]	909	436	355	274
Time from ER Arrival to Discharge (minutes)	374	187	152	134
Time in ER Before Being Evaluated (minutes)	375	31	32	26
Time to Pain Meds for Fractures (minutes)	117	58	58	57
Heart Attack Care				
Aspirin Given at Discharge	36	94%	99%	99%
Fibrinolytic Meds Within 30 Min. of Arrival[7]	-	-	69%	54%
PCI Within 90 Minutes of Arrival[7]	-	-	95%	96%
Statin Prescribed at Discharge	36	94%	99%	98%
Heart Failure Care				
ACE Inhibitor or ARB for LVSD	48	98%	98%	97%
Discharge Instructions Given	189	99%	97%	94%
Evaluation of LVS Function	270	99%	100%	99%
Medicare Spending				
Medicare Spending per Patient (ratio)	-	0.98	1.07	0.98
Pneumonia Care				
Appropriate Initial Antibiotic Given[2]	99	96%	98%	95%
Blood Culture Timing[2]	172	95%	99%	98%
Pregnancy and Delivery Care				
Newborn Deliveries Scheduled Early	58	0%	3%	6%
Preventive Care				
Immunization for Influenza[2]	561	98%	93%	90%
Immunization for Pneumonia[2]	732	96%	94%	92%
Stroke Care				
Anticoagulation Therapy for Atrial Fibrillation	26	96%	97%	95%
Antithrombotic Therapy Timing	98	96%	98%	98%
Assessed for Rehabilitation	99	92%	98%	97%
Discharged on Antithrombotic Therapy	93	98%	99%	99%
Discharged on Statin Medication	72	90%	95%	94%
Thrombolytic Therapy Timing[1]	-	-	74%	66%
Venous Thromboembolism Prophylaxis	105	90%	94%	94%
Written Stroke Educational Materials Given	59	97%	94%	88%
Surgical Care Improvement Project				
Appropriate Beta Blocker Usage	84	100%	98%	98%
Appropriate VTP Within 24 Hours	261	99%	99%	98%
Controlled Postoperative Blood Glucose[7]	-	-	97%	97%
Perioperative Temperature Management	299	100%	100%	100%
Prophylactic Antibiotic Selection	186	99%	99%	99%
Prophylactic Antibiotic Selection (Outpatient)	66	100%	97%	98%
Prophylactic Antibiotic Stopped	182	99%	98%	98%
Prophylactic Antibiotic Timing	186	98%	99%	99%
Prophylactic Antibiotic Timing (Outpatient)	66	100%	98%	98%
Urinary Catheter Removal	177	94%	98%	97%
Survey of Patients' Hospital Experiences				
Area Around Room 'Always' Quiet at Night	300+	49%	53%	61%
Doctors 'Always' Communicated Well	300+	68%	77%	82%
Home Recovery Information Given	300+	84%	82%	85%
Hospital Given 9 or 10 on 10 Point Scale	300+	56%	64%	71%
Meds 'Always' Explained Before Given	300+	55%	59%	64%

NOTE: Hospital profiles are in alphabetical order by state, then city, then hospital within the city; Rankings exclude hospitals with less than 25 cases except for patient surveys which excludes hospitals with less than 100 cases; (a) 100-299 cases; (1) The number of cases/patients is too few to report; (2) Data submitted were based on a sample of cases/patients; (3) Results are based on a shorter time period than required; (4) Data suppressed by CMS for one or more quarters; (5) Results are not available for this reporting period; (6) Fewer than 100 patients completed the HCAHPS survey; (7) No cases met the criteria for this measure; (8) The lower limit of the confidence interval cannot be calculated if the number of observed infections equals zero; (9) No data are available from the state/territory for this reporting period; (10) The scores shown reflect fewer than 50 completed surveys; (11) There were discrepancies in the data collection process; (12) This measure does not apply to this hospital for this reporting period; (13) Results cannot be calculated for this reporting period; (14) The results for this state are combined with nearby states to protect confidentiality; Please refer to the User's Guide for a full explanation of data.

Measure	Cases	This Hosp.	State Avg.	U.S. Avg.
Nurses 'Always' Communicated Well	300+	77%	76%	79%
Pain 'Always' Well Controlled	300+	67%	68%	71%
Room and Bathroom 'Always' Clean	300+	72%	68%	73%
Timely Help 'Always' Received	300+	60%	60%	68%
Would Definitely Recommend Hospital	300+	58%	66%	71%
Use of Medical Imaging				
Cardiac Imaging Stress Test before Surgery	114	5.3%	5.8%	5.3%
Combination Abdominal CT Scan	637	2.0%	7.4%	10.5%
Combination Brain/Sinus CT Scan	619	2.3%	2.8%	2.7%
Combination Chest CT Scan	354	0.3%	2.4%	2.7%
Follow-up Mammogram/Ultrasound	315	11.1%	12.5%	8.8%
Lumbar Spine MRI for Low Back Pain[1]	-	-	32.9%	37.2%

Palisades Medical Center

7600 River Rd
North Bergen, NJ 07047
Phone: 201-854-5000
Fax: 201-854-5036
URL: www.palisadesmedical.org
Type: Acute Care Hospitals
Emergency Services: Yes
Ownership: Voluntary non-profit - Private
Beds: 202

Key Personnel:

Chief of Medical Staff.......... Maria Bornia, MD
President/CEO............... Bruce J Markowitz
Infection Control.............. Doreen McSharry
Intensive Care Unit............ Adel Namour
Pediatric In-Patient Care .... Chitra Sethi, MD
Anesthesiology................ Veena Sharma, MD
Operating Room.............. Donna Vaglio, RN

Measure	Cases	This Hosp.	State Avg.	U.S. Avg.
Blood Clot Prevention and Treatment				
Anticoagulation Overlap Therapy[2]	36	100%	88%	93%
ICU Venous Thromboembolism Prophylaxis[2]	39	90%	93%	92%
Incidence of Potentially Preventable VTE[2]	13	15%	10%	10%
UFH with Dosages/Platelet Monitoring[2]	24	100%	99%	97%
Venous Thromboembolism Prophylaxis[2]	402	70%	83%	85%
Warfarin Therapy Discharge Instructions[2]	19	100%	77%	75%
Chest Pain/Possible Heart Attack Care				
Aspirin Given Within 24 Hours of Arrival[1,3]	-	-	98%	96%
Fibrinolytic Meds Within 30 Min. of Arrival[3,7]	-	-	63%	58%
Average Time to ECG (minutes)[1,3]	-	-	7	7
Average Time to Transfer (minutes)[3,7]	-	-	74	60
Children's Asthma Care				
Received Home Management Plan of Care	-	-	-	88%
Received Reliever Medication	-	-	-	100%
Received Systemic Corticosteroids	-	-	-	100%
Emergency Department				
Admittance Decision Time (minutes)[2]	766	104	148	98
Head CT Results Within 45 Min. of Arrival[1]	-	-	66%	57%
Patients Who Left ER Before Being Seen	39,423	1%	2%	2%
Time from ER Arrival to Admit. (minutes)[2]	766	340	355	274
Time from ER Arrival to Discharge (minutes)	316	170	152	134
Time in ER Before Being Evaluated (minutes)	381	30	32	26
Time to Pain Meds for Fractures (minutes)	84	84	58	57
Heart Attack Care				
Aspirin Given at Discharge	39	100%	99%	99%
Fibrinolytic Meds Within 30 Min. of Arrival[7]	-	-	69%	54%
PCI Within 90 Minutes of Arrival[7]	-	-	95%	96%
Statin Prescribed at Discharge	35	91%	99%	98%
Heart Failure Care				
ACE Inhibitor or ARB for LVSD[2]	51	100%	98%	97%
Discharge Instructions Given[2]	171	99%	97%	94%
Evaluation of LVS Function[2]	259	98%	100%	99%
Medicare Spending				
Medicare Spending per Patient (ratio)	-	1.07	1.07	0.98
Pneumonia Care				
Appropriate Initial Antibiotic Given[2]	92	97%	98%	95%
Blood Culture Timing[2]	157	97%	99%	98%
Pregnancy and Delivery Care				
Newborn Deliveries Scheduled Early[2]	23	0%	3%	6%
Preventive Care				
Immunization for Influenza[2]	501	68%	93%	90%
Immunization for Pneumonia[2]	588	94%	94%	92%
Stroke Care				
Anticoagulation Therapy for Atrial Fibrillation[1]	-	-	97%	95%
Antithrombotic Therapy Timing	69	100%	98%	98%
Assessed for Rehabilitation	66	100%	98%	97%
Discharged on Antithrombotic Therapy	57	100%	99%	99%
Discharged on Statin Medication	44	98%	95%	94%
Thrombolytic Therapy Timing[7]	-	-	74%	66%
Venous Thromboembolism Prophylaxis	76	87%	94%	94%
Written Stroke Educational Materials Given	25	100%	94%	88%
Surgical Care Improvement Project				
Appropriate Beta Blocker Usage	53	87%	98%	98%
Appropriate VTP Within 24 Hours	147	100%	99%	98%
Controlled Postoperative Blood Glucose[7]	-	-	97%	97%
Perioperative Temperature Management	171	100%	100%	100%
Prophylactic Antibiotic Selection	67	93%	99%	99%
Prophylactic Antibiotic Selection (Outpatient)	52	90%	97%	98%
Prophylactic Antibiotic Stopped	59	97%	98%	98%
Prophylactic Antibiotic Timing	70	100%	99%	99%
Prophylactic Antibiotic Timing (Outpatient)	53	96%	98%	98%
Urinary Catheter Removal	79	100%	98%	97%
Survey of Patients' Hospital Experiences				
Area Around Room 'Always' Quiet at Night	300+	53%	53%	61%
Doctors 'Always' Communicated Well	300+	77%	77%	82%
Home Recovery Information Given	300+	78%	82%	85%
Hospital Given 9 or 10 on 10 Point Scale	300+	57%	64%	71%
Meds 'Always' Explained Before Given	300+	55%	59%	64%
Nurses 'Always' Communicated Well	300+	71%	76%	79%
Pain 'Always' Well Controlled	300+	61%	68%	71%
Room and Bathroom 'Always' Clean	300+	68%	68%	73%
Timely Help 'Always' Received	300+	54%	60%	68%
Would Definitely Recommend Hospital	300+	62%	66%	71%
Use of Medical Imaging				
Cardiac Imaging Stress Test before Surgery	209	3.8%	5.8%	5.3%
Combination Abdominal CT Scan	487	7.8%	7.4%	10.5%
Combination Brain/Sinus CT Scan	592	2.4%	2.8%	2.7%
Combination Chest CT Scan	213	1.4%	2.4%	2.7%
Follow-up Mammogram/Ultrasound	460	10.0%	12.5%	8.8%
Lumbar Spine MRI for Low Back Pain[1]	-	-	32.9%	37.2%

Bergen Regional Medical Center

230 East Ridgewood Ave
Paramus, NJ 07652
Phone: 201-967-4000
Fax: 201-967-4109
E-mail: webmaster@bergenregional.com
URL: www.bergenregional.com
Type: Acute Care Hospitals
Emergency Services: Yes
Ownership: Government - Local
Beds: 1,185

Key Personnel:

President.................. Susan Mendelowitz, RN, MPA, FACHE
Cardiology.................. Joseph W. Montagnino, MD
Radiology.................. Susan Rubinoff, MD
Hemotology Center .... Indu Sharma, MD
Pediatrics.................. Scott Zucker, MD

Measure	Cases	This Hosp.	State Avg.	U.S. Avg.
Blood Clot Prevention and Treatment				
Anticoagulation Overlap Therapy[1,2]	-	-	88%	93%
ICU Venous Thromboembolism Prophylaxis[2]	23	91%	93%	92%
Incidence of Potentially Preventable VTE[1,2]	-	-	10%	10%
UFH with Dosages/Platelet Monitoring[1,2]	-	-	99%	97%
Venous Thromboembolism Prophylaxis[2]	54	72%	83%	85%
Warfarin Therapy Discharge Instructions[1,2]	-	-	77%	75%
Chest Pain/Possible Heart Attack Care				
Aspirin Given Within 24 Hours of Arrival[1,3]	-	-	98%	96%
Fibrinolytic Meds Within 30 Min. of Arrival[3,7]	-	-	63%	58%
Average Time to ECG (minutes)[1,3]	-	-	7	7
Average Time to Transfer (minutes)[1,3]	-	-	74	60
Children's Asthma Care				
Received Home Management Plan of Care	-	-	-	88%
Received Reliever Medication	-	-	-	100%
Received Systemic Corticosteroids	-	-	-	100%
Emergency Department				
Admittance Decision Time (minutes)[2]	132	129	148	98
Head CT Results Within 45 Min. of Arrival[3,7]	-	-	66%	57%
Patients Who Left ER Before Being Seen	16,292	2%	2%	2%
Time from ER Arrival to Admit. (minutes)[2]	132	368	355	274
Time from ER Arrival to Discharge (minutes)	235	147	152	134
Time in ER Before Being Evaluated (minutes)	401	30	32	26
Time to Pain Meds for Fractures (minutes)	19	72	58	57
Heart Attack Care				
Aspirin Given at Discharge[1]	-	-	99%	99%
Fibrinolytic Meds Within 30 Min. of Arrival[7]	-	-	69%	54%
PCI Within 90 Minutes of Arrival[7]	-	-	95%	96%
Statin Prescribed at Discharge[1]	-	-	99%	98%
Heart Failure Care				
ACE Inhibitor or ARB for LVSD[1]	-	-	98%	97%
Discharge Instructions Given[1]	-	-	97%	94%
Evaluation of LVS Function[1]	-	-	100%	99%
Medicare Spending				
Medicare Spending per Patient (ratio)	-	1.06	1.07	0.98
Pneumonia Care				
Appropriate Initial Antibiotic Given	32	84%	98%	95%
Blood Culture Timing	96	84%	99%	98%
Pregnancy and Delivery Care				
Newborn Deliveries Scheduled Early[7]	-	-	3%	6%
Preventive Care				
Immunization for Influenza[2]	591	84%	93%	90%
Immunization for Pneumonia[2]	302	74%	94%	92%
Stroke Care				
Anticoagulation Therapy for Atrial Fibrillation[1]	-	-	97%	95%
Antithrombotic Therapy Timing[1]	-	-	98%	98%
Assessed for Rehabilitation[1]	-	-	98%	97%
Discharged on Antithrombotic Therapy[1]	-	-	99%	99%
Discharged on Statin Medication[1]	-	-	95%	94%
Thrombolytic Therapy Timing[1]	-	-	74%	66%
Venous Thromboembolism Prophylaxis[1]	-	-	94%	94%
Written Stroke Educational Materials Given[1]	-	-	94%	88%
Surgical Care Improvement Project				
Appropriate Beta Blocker Usage	12	75%	98%	98%
Appropriate VTP Within 24 Hours	44	95%	99%	98%
Controlled Postoperative Blood Glucose[7]	-	-	97%	97%
Perioperative Temperature Management	46	100%	100%	100%
Prophylactic Antibiotic Selection	18	94%	99%	99%
Prophylactic Antibiotic Selection (Outpatient)	14	43%	97%	98%
Prophylactic Antibiotic Stopped	17	100%	98%	98%
Prophylactic Antibiotic Timing	18	61%	99%	99%
Prophylactic Antibiotic Timing (Outpatient)[1]	-	-	98%	98%
Urinary Catheter Removal	42	98%	98%	97%
Survey of Patients' Hospital Experiences				
Area Around Room 'Always' Quiet at Night	(a)	54%	53%	61%
Doctors 'Always' Communicated Well	(a)	68%	77%	82%
Home Recovery Information Given	(a)	75%	82%	85%
Hospital Given 9 or 10 on 10 Point Scale	(a)	55%	64%	71%
Meds 'Always' Explained Before Given	(a)	50%	59%	64%
Nurses 'Always' Communicated Well	(a)	66%	76%	79%
Pain 'Always' Well Controlled	(a)	60%	68%	71%
Room and Bathroom 'Always' Clean	(a)	52%	68%	73%
Timely Help 'Always' Received	(a)	44%	60%	68%
Would Definitely Recommend Hospital	(a)	61%	66%	71%
Use of Medical Imaging				
Cardiac Imaging Stress Test before Surgery[1]	-	-	5.8%	5.3%
Combination Abdominal CT Scan[1]	-	-	7.4%	10.5%
Combination Brain/Sinus CT Scan	151	6.6%	2.8%	2.7%
Combination Chest CT Scan[1]	-	-	2.4%	2.7%
Follow-up Mammogram/Ultrasound[1]	-	-	12.5%	8.8%
Lumbar Spine MRI for Low Back Pain[1]	-	-	32.9%	37.2%

Saint Mary's Hospital - Passaic

350 Boulevard
Passaic, NJ 07055
Phone: 973-365-4300
Fax: 973-471-5531
URL: www.smh-nj.com
Type: Acute Care Hospitals
Emergency Services: Yes
Ownership: Voluntary non-profit - Church
Beds: 264

Measure	Cases	This Hosp.	State Avg.	U.S. Avg.
Blood Clot Prevention and Treatment				
Anticoagulation Overlap Therapy[2]	47	81%	88%	93%
ICU Venous Thromboembolism Prophylaxis[2]	86	88%	93%	92%
Incidence of Potentially Preventable VTE[2]	14	14%	10%	10%
UFH with Dosages/Platelet Monitoring[2]	56	98%	99%	97%
Venous Thromboembolism Prophylaxis[2]	389	76%	83%	85%

NOTE: Hospital profiles are in alphabetical order by state, then city, then hospital within the city; Rankings exclude hospitals with less than 25 cases except for patient surveys which excludes hospitals with less than 100 cases; (a) 100-299 cases; (1) The number of cases/patients is too few to report; (2) Data submitted were based on a sample of cases/patients; (3) Results are based on a shorter time period than required; (4) Data suppressed by CMS for one or more quarters; (5) Results are not available for this reporting period; (6) Fewer than 100 patients completed the HCAHPS survey; (7) No cases met the criteria for this measure; (8) The lower limit of the confidence interval cannot be calculated if the number of observed infections equals zero; (9) No data are available from the state/territory for this reporting period; (10) The scores shown reflect fewer than 50 completed surveys; (11) There were discrepancies in the data collection process; (12) This measure does not apply to this hospital for this reporting period; (13) Results cannot be calculated for this reporting period; (14) The results for this state are combined with nearby states to protect confidentiality; Please refer to the User's Guide for a full explanation of data.

Measure	Cases	This Hosp.	State Avg.	U.S. Avg.
Warfarin Therapy Discharge Instructions[2]	32	100%	77%	75%
Chest Pain/Possible Heart Attack Care				
Aspirin Given Within 24 Hours of Arrival[5]	-	-	98%	96%
Fibrinolytic Meds Within 30 Min. of Arrival[5]	-	-	63%	58%
Average Time to ECG (minutes)[5]	-	-	7	7
Average Time to Transfer (minutes)[5]	-	-	74	60
Children's Asthma Care				
Received Home Management Plan of Care	-	-	-	88%
Received Reliever Medication	-	-	-	100%
Received Systemic Corticosteroids	-	-	-	100%
Emergency Department				
Admittance Decision Time (minutes)[2]	471	90	148	98
Head CT Results Within 45 Min. of Arrival[7]	-	-	66%	57%
Patients Who Left ER Before Being Seen	33,703	1%	2%	2%
Time from ER Arrival to Admit. (minutes)[2]	632	270	355	274
Time from ER Arrival to Discharge (minutes)	338	154	152	134
Time in ER Before Being Evaluated (minutes)	404	35	32	26
Time to Pain Meds for Fractures (minutes)	92	67	58	57
Heart Attack Care				
Aspirin Given at Discharge	90	100%	99%	99%
Fibrinolytic Meds Within 30 Min. of Arrival[7]	-	-	69%	54%
PCI Within 90 Minutes of Arrival	25	100%	95%	96%
Statin Prescribed at Discharge	85	100%	99%	98%
Heart Failure Care				
ACE Inhibitor or ARB for LVSD[2]	95	100%	98%	97%
Discharge Instructions Given[2]	223	100%	97%	94%
Evaluation of LVS Function[2]	315	100%	100%	99%
Medicare Spending				
Medicare Spending per Patient (ratio)	-	1.11	1.07	0.98
Pneumonia Care				
Appropriate Initial Antibiotic Given[2]	112	98%	98%	95%
Blood Culture Timing[2]	182	100%	99%	98%
Pregnancy and Delivery Care				
Newborn Deliveries Scheduled Early[2]	47	4%	3%	6%
Preventive Care				
Immunization for Influenza[2]	530	91%	93%	90%
Immunization for Pneumonia[2]	740	96%	94%	92%
Stroke Care				
Anticoagulation Therapy for Atrial Fibrillation	13	100%	97%	95%
Antithrombotic Therapy Timing	70	97%	98%	98%
Assessed for Rehabilitation	77	88%	98%	97%
Discharged on Antithrombotic Therapy	67	96%	99%	99%
Discharged on Statin Medication	56	75%	95%	94%
Thrombolytic Therapy Timing	21	0%	74%	66%
Venous Thromboembolism Prophylaxis	78	72%	94%	94%
Written Stroke Educational Materials Given	44	77%	94%	88%
Surgical Care Improvement Project				
Appropriate Beta Blocker Usage	127	99%	98%	98%
Appropriate VTP Within 24 Hours	222	100%	99%	98%
Controlled Postoperative Blood Glucose	73	99%	97%	97%
Perioperative Temperature Management	331	100%	100%	100%
Prophylactic Antibiotic Selection	210	97%	99%	99%
Prophylactic Antibiotic Selection (Outpatient)	274	86%	97%	98%
Prophylactic Antibiotic Stopped	180	98%	98%	98%
Prophylactic Antibiotic Timing	210	99%	99%	99%
Prophylactic Antibiotic Timing (Outpatient)	275	99%	98%	98%
Urinary Catheter Removal	155	99%	98%	97%
Survey of Patients' Hospital Experiences				
Area Around Room 'Always' Quiet at Night	300+	53%	53%	61%
Doctors 'Always' Communicated Well	300+	77%	77%	82%
Home Recovery Information Given	300+	78%	82%	85%
Hospital Given 9 or 10 on 10 Point Scale	300+	52%	64%	71%
Meds 'Always' Explained Before Given	300+	53%	59%	64%
Nurses 'Always' Communicated Well	300+	71%	76%	79%
Pain 'Always' Well Controlled	300+	59%	68%	71%
Room and Bathroom 'Always' Clean	300+	62%	68%	73%
Timely Help 'Always' Received	300+	49%	60%	68%
Would Definitely Recommend Hospital	300+	52%	66%	71%
Use of Medical Imaging				
Cardiac Imaging Stress Test before Surgery[1]	-	-	5.8%	5.3%
Combination Abdominal CT Scan	544	5.9%	7.4%	10.5%
Combination Brain/Sinus CT Scan[1]	-	-	2.8%	2.7%
Combination Chest CT Scan	352	0.6%	2.4%	2.7%
Follow-up Mammogram/Ultrasound	592	13.5%	12.5%	8.8%
Lumbar Spine MRI for Low Back Pain[1]	-	-	32.9%	37.2%

Saint Joseph's Regional Medical Center

703 Main St
Paterson, NJ 07503
URL: www.sjhmc.org
Type: Acute Care Hospitals
Ownership: Voluntary non-profit - Church
Phone: 973-754-2010
Fax: 973-754-3900
Emergency Services: Yes
Beds: 642

Key Personnel:

Pediatric In-Patient Care . . . . Thomas Daley, MD
Patient Relations . . . . Maureen Eisner
Radiology. Thomas M Herskovic, MD
CEO/President. . . . . William A McDonald
Infection Control. . . . . Marie Rella
Pediatric Ambulatory Care . . . . . . Albert Sanz, MD
Operating Room. . . . . Alan Sori, MD

Measure	Cases	This Hosp.	State Avg.	U.S. Avg.
Blood Clot Prevention and Treatment				
Anticoagulation Overlap Therapy[2]	120	88%	88%	93%
ICU Venous Thromboembolism Prophylaxis[2]	158	91%	93%	92%
Incidence of Potentially Preventable VTE[2]	13	0%	10%	10%
UFH with Dosages/Platelet Monitoring[2]	36	100%	99%	97%
Venous Thromboembolism Prophylaxis[2]	731	86%	83%	85%
Warfarin Therapy Discharge Instructions[2]	98	98%	77%	75%
Chest Pain/Possible Heart Attack Care				
Aspirin Given Within 24 Hours of Arrival[5]	-	-	98%	96%
Fibrinolytic Meds Within 30 Min. of Arrival[5]	-	-	63%	58%
Average Time to ECG (minutes)[5]	-	-	7	7
Average Time to Transfer (minutes)[5]	-	-	74	60
Children's Asthma Care				
Received Home Management Plan of Care	-	-	-	88%
Received Reliever Medication	-	-	-	100%
Received Systemic Corticosteroids	-	-	-	100%
Emergency Department				
Admittance Decision Time (minutes)[2]	1,719	100	148	98
Head CT Results Within 45 Min. of Arrival	12	75%	66%	57%
Patients Who Left ER Before Being Seen	>100k	2%	2%	2%
Time from ER Arrival to Admit. (minutes)[2]	1,755	314	355	274
Time from ER Arrival to Discharge (minutes)	780	150	152	134
Time in ER Before Being Evaluated (minutes)	884	30	32	26
Time to Pain Meds for Fractures (minutes)	372	60	58	57
Heart Attack Care				
Aspirin Given at Discharge	518	99%	99%	99%
Fibrinolytic Meds Within 30 Min. of Arrival[7]	-	-	69%	54%
PCI Within 90 Minutes of Arrival	81	96%	95%	96%
Statin Prescribed at Discharge	507	98%	99%	98%
Heart Failure Care				
ACE Inhibitor or ARB for LVSD[2]	194	99%	98%	97%
Discharge Instructions Given[2]	480	97%	97%	94%
Evaluation of LVS Function[2]	658	100%	100%	99%
Medicare Spending				
Medicare Spending per Patient (ratio)	-	1.11	1.07	0.98
Pneumonia Care				
Appropriate Initial Antibiotic Given[2]	216	96%	98%	95%
Blood Culture Timing[2]	491	99%	99%	98%
Pregnancy and Delivery Care				
Newborn Deliveries Scheduled Early[2]	81	9%	3%	6%
Preventive Care				
Immunization for Influenza[2]	1,053	90%	93%	90%
Immunization for Pneumonia[2]	1,262	92%	94%	92%
Stroke Care				
Anticoagulation Therapy for Atrial Fibrillation	36	97%	97%	95%
Antithrombotic Therapy Timing	256	98%	98%	98%
Assessed for Rehabilitation	301	100%	98%	97%
Discharged on Antithrombotic Therapy	259	95%	99%	99%
Discharged on Statin Medication	202	92%	95%	94%
Thrombolytic Therapy Timing	67	30%	74%	66%
Venous Thromboembolism Prophylaxis	330	97%	94%	94%
Written Stroke Educational Materials Given	153	98%	94%	88%
Surgical Care Improvement Project				
Appropriate Beta Blocker Usage[2]	393	98%	98%	98%
Appropriate VTP Within 24 Hours[2]	760	99%	99%	98%
Controlled Postoperative Blood Glucose[2]	237	97%	97%	97%
Perioperative Temperature Management[2]	1,052	100%	100%	100%
Prophylactic Antibiotic Selection[2]	837	99%	99%	99%
Prophylactic Antibiotic Selection (Outpatient)	266	97%	97%	98%
Prophylactic Antibiotic Stopped[2]	817	99%	98%	98%
Prophylactic Antibiotic Timing[2]	839	99%	99%	99%
Prophylactic Antibiotic Timing (Outpatient)	262	98%	98%	98%
Urinary Catheter Removal[2]	662	98%	98%	97%
Survey of Patients' Hospital Experiences				
Area Around Room 'Always' Quiet at Night	300+	51%	53%	61%
Doctors 'Always' Communicated Well	300+	78%	77%	82%
Home Recovery Information Given	300+	82%	82%	85%
Hospital Given 9 or 10 on 10 Point Scale	300+	63%	64%	71%
Meds 'Always' Explained Before Given	300+	57%	59%	64%
Nurses 'Always' Communicated Well	300+	72%	76%	79%
Pain 'Always' Well Controlled	300+	63%	68%	71%
Room and Bathroom 'Always' Clean	300+	69%	68%	73%
Timely Help 'Always' Received	300+	53%	60%	68%
Would Definitely Recommend Hospital	300+	66%	66%	71%
Use of Medical Imaging				
Cardiac Imaging Stress Test before Surgery	1,951	6.0%	5.8%	5.3%
Combination Abdominal CT Scan	1,562	12.2%	7.4%	10.5%
Combination Brain/Sinus CT Scan	1,606	2.6%	2.8%	2.7%
Combination Chest CT Scan	807	5.8%	2.4%	2.7%
Follow-up Mammogram/Ultrasound	2,192	6.2%	12.5%	8.8%
Lumbar Spine MRI for Low Back Pain	187	35.8%	32.9%	37.2%

Capital Health Medical Center - Hopewell

One Capital Way
Pennington, NJ 08534
URL: www.capitalhealth.org
Type: Acute Care Hospitals
Ownership: Voluntary non-profit - Private
Phone: 609-303-4000
Fax: 609-695-8865
Emergency Services: Yes
Beds: 589

Key Personnel:

Pediatric Ambulatory Care . . . . . . Randi Axelrod, MD
Pediatric In-Patient Care . . . . Randi Axelrod, MD
Radiology. . . . . Robert Collins, MD
Operating Room. . . . . Ann Lando
CEO/President. . . . . Al Maghazehe, PhD, FACHE
Chief of Medical Staff . . . . Robert Remstein, DO
Infection Control. . . . . Dawn Rumovitz
Quality Assurance . . . . Molly Sullivan

Measure	Cases	This Hosp.	State Avg.	U.S. Avg.
Blood Clot Prevention and Treatment				
Anticoagulation Overlap Therapy[2]	76	95%	88%	93%
ICU Venous Thromboembolism Prophylaxis[2]	99	98%	93%	92%
Incidence of Potentially Preventable VTE[2]	28	0%	10%	10%
UFH with Dosages/Platelet Monitoring[2]	89	100%	99%	97%
Venous Thromboembolism Prophylaxis[2]	333	94%	83%	85%
Warfarin Therapy Discharge Instructions[2]	54	85%	77%	75%
Chest Pain/Possible Heart Attack Care				
Aspirin Given Within 24 Hours of Arrival	13	92%	98%	96%
Fibrinolytic Meds Within 30 Min. of Arrival[3,7]	-	-	63%	58%
Average Time to ECG (minutes)	13	2	7	7
Average Time to Transfer (minutes)[3,7]	-	-	74	60
Children's Asthma Care				
Received Home Management Plan of Care	-	-	-	88%
Received Reliever Medication	-	-	-	100%
Received Systemic Corticosteroids	-	-	-	100%
Emergency Department				
Admittance Decision Time (minutes)[2]	576	144	148	98
Head CT Results Within 45 Min. of Arrival[1]	-	-	66%	57%
Patients Who Left ER Before Being Seen	35,117	1%	2%	2%
Time from ER Arrival to Admit. (minutes)[2]	588	421	355	274
Time from ER Arrival to Discharge (minutes)	423	147	152	134
Time in ER Before Being Evaluated (minutes)	432	28	32	26
Time to Pain Meds for Fractures (minutes)	136	39	58	57
Heart Attack Care				
Aspirin Given at Discharge	62	100%	99%	99%
Fibrinolytic Meds Within 30 Min. of Arrival[7]	-	-	69%	54%
PCI Within 90 Minutes of Arrival	18	100%	95%	96%
Statin Prescribed at Discharge	55	98%	99%	98%
Heart Failure Care				
ACE Inhibitor or ARB for LVSD	49	98%	98%	97%

NOTE: Hospital profiles are in alphabetical order by state, then city, then hospital within the city; Rankings exclude hospitals with less than 25 cases except for patient surveys which excludes hospitals with less than 100 cases; (a) 100-299 cases; (1) The number of cases/patients is too few to report; (2) Data submitted were based on a sample of cases/patients; (3) Results are based on a shorter time period than required; (4) Data suppressed by CMS for one or more quarters; (5) Results are not available for this reporting period; (6) Fewer than 100 patients completed the HCAHPS survey; (7) No cases met the criteria for this measure; (8) The lower limit of the confidence interval cannot be calculated if the number of observed infections equals zero; (9) No data are available from the state/territory for this reporting period; (10) The scores shown reflect fewer than 50 completed surveys; (11) There were discrepancies in the data collection process; (12) This measure does not apply to this hospital for this reporting period; (13) Results cannot be calculated for this reporting period; (14) The results for this state are combined with nearby states to protect confidentiality; Please refer to the User's Guide for a full explanation of data.

Measure	Cases	This Hosp.	State Avg.	U.S. Avg.
Discharge Instructions Given	144	94%	97%	94%
Evaluation of LVS Function	181	100%	100%	99%
Medicare Spending				
Medicare Spending per Patient (ratio)	-	1.03	1.07	0.98
Pneumonia Care				
Appropriate Initial Antibiotic Given	103	97%	98%	95%
Blood Culture Timing	216	100%	99%	98%
Pregnancy and Delivery Care				
Newborn Deliveries Scheduled Early[2]	40	2%	3%	6%
Preventive Care				
Immunization for Influenza[2]	500	88%	93%	90%
Immunization for Pneumonia[2]	457	89%	94%	92%
Stroke Care				
Anticoagulation Therapy for Atrial Fibrillation	24	96%	97%	95%
Antithrombotic Therapy Timing	117	100%	98%	98%
Assessed for Rehabilitation	150	99%	98%	97%
Discharged on Antithrombotic Therapy	126	100%	99%	99%
Discharged on Statin Medication	106	100%	95%	94%
Thrombolytic Therapy Timing[1]	-	-	74%	66%
Venous Thromboembolism Prophylaxis	153	99%	94%	94%
Written Stroke Educational Materials Given	83	100%	94%	88%
Surgical Care Improvement Project				
Appropriate Beta Blocker Usage	300	98%	98%	98%
Appropriate VTP Within 24 Hours	799	99%	99%	98%
Controlled Postoperative Blood Glucose[7]	-	-	97%	97%
Perioperative Temperature Management	927	100%	100%	100%
Prophylactic Antibiotic Selection	473	100%	99%	99%
Prophylactic Antibiotic Selection (Outpatient)	258	95%	97%	98%
Prophylactic Antibiotic Stopped	471	99%	98%	98%
Prophylactic Antibiotic Timing	473	100%	99%	99%
Prophylactic Antibiotic Timing (Outpatient)	258	100%	98%	98%
Urinary Catheter Removal	603	100%	98%	97%
Survey of Patients' Hospital Experiences				
Area Around Room 'Always' Quiet at Night	300+	61%	53%	61%
Doctors 'Always' Communicated Well	300+	78%	77%	82%
Home Recovery Information Given	300+	82%	82%	85%
Hospital Given 9 or 10 on 10 Point Scale	300+	72%	64%	71%
Meds 'Always' Explained Before Given	300+	60%	59%	64%
Nurses 'Always' Communicated Well	300+	76%	76%	79%
Pain 'Always' Well Controlled	300+	68%	68%	71%
Room and Bathroom 'Always' Clean	300+	75%	68%	73%
Timely Help 'Always' Received	300+	61%	60%	68%
Would Definitely Recommend Hospital	300+	75%	66%	71%
Use of Medical Imaging				
Cardiac Imaging Stress Test before Surgery	396	5.1%	5.8%	5.3%
Combination Abdominal CT Scan	764	8.8%	7.4%	10.5%
Combination Brain/Sinus CT Scan	588	6.6%	2.8%	2.7%
Combination Chest CT Scan	563	3.9%	2.4%	2.7%
Follow-up Mammogram/Ultrasound	1,248	7.9%	12.5%	8.8%
Lumbar Spine MRI for Low Back Pain	53	50.9%	32.9%	37.2%

Raritan Bay Medical Center

530 New Brunswick Ave
Perth Amboy, NJ 08861
Phone: 732-442-3700
Fax: 732-324-4994
URL: www.rbmc.org
Type: Acute Care Hospitals
Emergency Services: Yes
Ownership: Voluntary non-profit - Private
Beds: 522

Key Personnel:

Pediatric Ambulatory Care . . . . . . Norman Barofsky, MD
Pediatric In-Patient Care . . . . Norman Barofsky, MD
CEO/President. . . . . Michael R. D'Agnes
Operating Room. . . . . Geraldine DiGiovanni, RN
Radiology. . . . . Alvin Kravet, MD
Quality Assurance . . . . Erich Kreher
Chief of Medical Staff . . . . John Middleton, MD
Infection Control. . . . . John R Middleton, MD

Measure	Cases	This Hosp.	State Avg.	U.S. Avg.
Blood Clot Prevention and Treatment				
Anticoagulation Overlap Therapy[2]	103	81%	88%	93%
ICU Venous Thromboembolism Prophylaxis[2]	108	85%	93%	92%
Incidence of Potentially Preventable VTE[2]	32	22%	10%	10%
UFH with Dosages/Platelet Monitoring[2]	79	97%	99%	97%
Venous Thromboembolism Prophylaxis[2]	381	75%	83%	85%
Warfarin Therapy Discharge Instructions[2]	64	56%	77%	75%
Chest Pain/Possible Heart Attack Care				
Aspirin Given Within 24 Hours of Arrival[1,3]	-	-	98%	96%
Fibrinolytic Meds Within 30 Min. of Arrival[1,3]	-	-	63%	58%
Average Time to ECG (minutes)[1,3]	-	-	7	7
Average Time to Transfer (minutes)[1,3]	-	-	74	60
Children's Asthma Care				
Received Home Management Plan of Care	-	-	-	88%
Received Reliever Medication	-	-	-	100%
Received Systemic Corticosteroids	-	-	-	100%
Emergency Department				
Admittance Decision Time (minutes)[2]	802	130	148	98
Head CT Results Within 45 Min. of Arrival	21	14%	66%	57%
Patients Who Left ER Before Being Seen	48,708	2%	2%	2%
Time from ER Arrival to Admit. (minutes)[2]	802	376	355	274
Time from ER Arrival to Discharge (minutes)	366	130	152	134
Time in ER Before Being Evaluated (minutes)	405	69	32	26
Time to Pain Meds for Fractures (minutes)	151	72	58	57
Heart Attack Care				
Aspirin Given at Discharge	231	95%	99%	99%
Fibrinolytic Meds Within 30 Min. of Arrival[7]	-	-	69%	54%
PCI Within 90 Minutes of Arrival	43	79%	95%	96%
Statin Prescribed at Discharge	244	95%	99%	98%
Heart Failure Care				
ACE Inhibitor or ARB for LVSD[2]	125	94%	98%	97%
Discharge Instructions Given[2]	289	98%	97%	94%
Evaluation of LVS Function[2]	466	98%	100%	99%
Medicare Spending				
Medicare Spending per Patient (ratio)	-	1.07	1.07	0.98
Pneumonia Care				
Appropriate Initial Antibiotic Given[2]	173	95%	98%	95%
Blood Culture Timing[2]	330	98%	99%	98%
Pregnancy and Delivery Care				
Newborn Deliveries Scheduled Early[2]	26	8%	3%	6%
Preventive Care				
Immunization for Influenza[2]	547	97%	93%	90%
Immunization for Pneumonia[2]	692	98%	94%	92%
Stroke Care				
Anticoagulation Therapy for Atrial Fibrillation[1]	-	-	97%	95%
Antithrombotic Therapy Timing	71	100%	98%	98%
Assessed for Rehabilitation	46	100%	98%	97%
Discharged on Antithrombotic Therapy	45	98%	99%	99%
Discharged on Statin Medication	37	97%	95%	94%
Thrombolytic Therapy Timing[1]	-	-	74%	66%
Venous Thromboembolism Prophylaxis	76	100%	94%	94%
Written Stroke Educational Materials Given	38	95%	94%	88%
Surgical Care Improvement Project				
Appropriate Beta Blocker Usage	118	96%	98%	98%
Appropriate VTP Within 24 Hours	292	97%	99%	98%
Controlled Postoperative Blood Glucose[7]	-	-	97%	97%
Perioperative Temperature Management	355	100%	100%	100%
Prophylactic Antibiotic Selection	164	98%	99%	99%
Prophylactic Antibiotic Selection (Outpatient)	74	97%	97%	98%
Prophylactic Antibiotic Stopped	154	94%	98%	98%
Prophylactic Antibiotic Timing	164	99%	99%	99%
Prophylactic Antibiotic Timing (Outpatient)	78	92%	98%	98%
Urinary Catheter Removal	200	98%	98%	97%
Survey of Patients' Hospital Experiences				
Area Around Room 'Always' Quiet at Night	300+	53%	53%	61%
Doctors 'Always' Communicated Well	300+	77%	77%	82%
Home Recovery Information Given	300+	82%	82%	85%
Hospital Given 9 or 10 on 10 Point Scale	300+	59%	64%	71%
Meds 'Always' Explained Before Given	300+	56%	59%	64%
Nurses 'Always' Communicated Well	300+	74%	76%	79%
Pain 'Always' Well Controlled	300+	66%	68%	71%
Room and Bathroom 'Always' Clean	300+	65%	68%	73%
Timely Help 'Always' Received	300+	58%	60%	68%
Would Definitely Recommend Hospital	300+	58%	66%	71%
Use of Medical Imaging				
Cardiac Imaging Stress Test before Surgery	198	5.1%	5.8%	5.3%
Combination Abdominal CT Scan	824	3.9%	7.4%	10.5%
Combination Brain/Sinus CT Scan	984	1.4%	2.8%	2.7%
Combination Chest CT Scan	311	1.3%	2.4%	2.7%
Follow-up Mammogram/Ultrasound	933	6.1%	12.5%	8.8%
Lumbar Spine MRI for Low Back Pain[1]	-	-	32.9%	37.2%

Saint Luke's Warren Hospital

185 Roseberry St
Phillipsburg, NJ 08865
Phone: 908-859-6700
Fax: 908-859-4546
URL: www.warrenhospital.org
Type: Acute Care Hospitals
Emergency Services: Yes
Ownership: Voluntary non-profit - Other
Beds: 214

Key Personnel:

Quality Assurance . . . . Barbara Balas
Chief of Medical Staff . . . . Frank Gilley, MD
Emergency Room . . . . Howard Swidler, MD
Administrator . . . . Alice J. Wilson, FACHE
President. . . . . Scott R. Wolfe

Measure	Cases	This Hosp.	State Avg.	U.S. Avg.
Blood Clot Prevention and Treatment				
Anticoagulation Overlap Therapy[2]	61	74%	88%	93%
ICU Venous Thromboembolism Prophylaxis[2]	88	99%	93%	92%
Incidence of Potentially Preventable VTE[2]	12	0%	10%	10%
UFH with Dosages/Platelet Monitoring[2]	38	100%	99%	97%
Venous Thromboembolism Prophylaxis[2]	390	97%	83%	85%
Warfarin Therapy Discharge Instructions[2]	39	62%	77%	75%
Chest Pain/Possible Heart Attack Care				
Aspirin Given Within 24 Hours of Arrival	43	100%	98%	96%
Fibrinolytic Meds Within 30 Min. of Arrival[7]	-	-	63%	58%
Average Time to ECG (minutes)	43	6	7	7
Average Time to Transfer (minutes)	16	68	74	60
Children's Asthma Care				
Received Home Management Plan of Care	-	-	-	88%
Received Reliever Medication	-	-	-	100%
Received Systemic Corticosteroids	-	-	-	100%
Emergency Department				
Admittance Decision Time (minutes)[2]	870	124	148	98
Head CT Results Within 45 Min. of Arrival	13	38%	66%	57%
Patients Who Left ER Before Being Seen	30,267	1%	2%	2%
Time from ER Arrival to Admit. (minutes)[2]	937	271	355	274
Time from ER Arrival to Discharge (minutes)	376	123	152	134
Time in ER Before Being Evaluated (minutes)	414	34	32	26
Time to Pain Meds for Fractures (minutes)	70	46	58	57
Heart Attack Care				
Aspirin Given at Discharge	11	100%	99%	99%
Fibrinolytic Meds Within 30 Min. of Arrival[7]	-	-	69%	54%
PCI Within 90 Minutes of Arrival[7]	-	-	95%	96%
Statin Prescribed at Discharge	11	100%	99%	98%
Heart Failure Care				
ACE Inhibitor or ARB for LVSD	21	100%	98%	97%
Discharge Instructions Given	96	100%	97%	94%
Evaluation of LVS Function	142	100%	100%	99%
Medicare Spending				
Medicare Spending per Patient (ratio)	-	1.02	1.07	0.98
Pneumonia Care				
Appropriate Initial Antibiotic Given	118	97%	98%	95%
Blood Culture Timing	195	99%	99%	98%
Pregnancy and Delivery Care				
Newborn Deliveries Scheduled Early[7]	-	-	3%	6%
Preventive Care				
Immunization for Influenza[2]	604	99%	93%	90%
Immunization for Pneumonia[2]	931	98%	94%	92%
Stroke Care				
Anticoagulation Therapy for Atrial Fibrillation[1]	-	-	97%	95%
Antithrombotic Therapy Timing	18	100%	98%	98%
Assessed for Rehabilitation	21	100%	98%	97%
Discharged on Antithrombotic Therapy	20	100%	99%	99%
Discharged on Statin Medication	14	86%	95%	94%
Thrombolytic Therapy Timing[7]	-	-	74%	66%
Venous Thromboembolism Prophylaxis	19	100%	94%	94%
Written Stroke Educational Materials Given[1]	-	-	94%	88%
Surgical Care Improvement Project				
Appropriate Beta Blocker Usage[2]	75	100%	98%	98%
Appropriate VTP Within 24 Hours[2]	219	100%	99%	98%
Controlled Postoperative Blood Glucose[2,7]	-	-	97%	97%
Perioperative Temperature Management[2]	242	100%	100%	100%
Prophylactic Antibiotic Selection[2]	128	99%	99%	99%

NOTE: Hospital profiles are in alphabetical order by state, then city, then hospital within the city; Rankings exclude hospitals with less than 25 cases except for patient surveys which excludes hospitals with less than 100 cases; (a) 100-299 cases; (1) The number of cases/patients is too few to report; (2) Data submitted were based on a sample of cases/patients; (3) Results are based on a shorter time period than required; (4) Data suppressed by CMS for one or more quarters; (5) Results are not available for this reporting period; (6) Fewer than 100 patients completed the HCAHPS survey; (7) No cases met the criteria for this measure; (8) The lower limit of the confidence interval cannot be calculated if the number of observed infections equals zero; (9) No data are available from the state/territory for this reporting period; (10) The scores shown reflect fewer than 50 completed surveys; (11) There were discrepancies in the data collection process; (12) This measure does not apply to this hospital for this reporting period; (13) Results cannot be calculated for this reporting period; (14) The results for this state are combined with nearby states to protect confidentiality; Please refer to the User's Guide for a full explanation of data.

Measure	Cases	This Hosp.	State Avg.	U.S. Avg.
Prophylactic Antibiotic Selection (Outpatient)	67	100%	97%	98%
Prophylactic Antibiotic Stopped[2]	123	98%	98%	98%
Prophylactic Antibiotic Timing[2]	129	99%	99%	99%
Prophylactic Antibiotic Timing (Outpatient)	65	97%	98%	98%
Urinary Catheter Removal[2]	169	98%	98%	97%
Survey of Patients' Hospital Experiences				
Area Around Room 'Always' Quiet at Night	300+	60%	53%	61%
Doctors 'Always' Communicated Well	300+	79%	77%	82%
Home Recovery Information Given	300+	82%	82%	85%
Hospital Given 9 or 10 on 10 Point Scale	300+	65%	64%	71%
Meds 'Always' Explained Before Given	300+	60%	59%	64%
Nurses 'Always' Communicated Well	300+	77%	76%	79%
Pain 'Always' Well Controlled	300+	70%	68%	71%
Room and Bathroom 'Always' Clean	300+	71%	68%	73%
Timely Help 'Always' Received	300+	63%	60%	68%
Would Definitely Recommend Hospital	300+	64%	66%	71%
Use of Medical Imaging				
Cardiac Imaging Stress Test before Surgery	279	10.4%	5.8%	5.3%
Combination Abdominal CT Scan	814	1.4%	7.4%	10.5%
Combination Brain/Sinus CT Scan	728	3.2%	2.8%	2.7%
Combination Chest CT Scan	359	0.3%	2.4%	2.7%
Follow-up Mammogram/Ultrasound	1,164	9.3%	12.5%	8.8%
Lumbar Spine MRI for Low Back Pain	75	38.7%	32.9%	37.2%

University Medical Center of Princeton at Plainsboro

One - Five Plainsboro Road Phone: 866-460-4776
Plainsboro, NJ 08536 Fax: 609-497-4991
URL: www.princetonhcs.org
Type: Acute Care Hospitals Emergency Services: Yes
Ownership: Voluntary non-profit - Private Beds: 396

Key Personnel:
Infection Control. . . . . Dr Alexander Ackley
Chief of Medical Staff. . . . . Henry Davison, MD
Radiology. . . . . Donald Denny, MD
Pediatric In-Patient Care . . . . Stephen E Hefler, MD
CEO/President. . . . . Mark Jones
Quality Assurance . . . . Debbie Lloyd
Operating Room. . . . . Kathy Raney

Measure	Cases	This Hosp.	State Avg.	U.S. Avg.
Blood Clot Prevention and Treatment				
Anticoagulation Overlap Therapy[2]	79	100%	88%	93%
ICU Venous Thromboembolism Prophylaxis[2]	44	93%	93%	92%
Incidence of Potentially Preventable VTE[2]	24	8%	10%	10%
UFH with Dosages/Platelet Monitoring[2]	36	100%	99%	97%
Venous Thromboembolism Prophylaxis[2]	340	88%	83%	85%
Warfarin Therapy Discharge Instructions[2]	52	94%	77%	75%
Chest Pain/Possible Heart Attack Care				
Aspirin Given Within 24 Hours of Arrival	12	100%	98%	96%
Fibrinolytic Meds Within 30 Min. of Arrival[7]	-	-	63%	58%
Average Time to ECG (minutes)	12	13	7	7
Average Time to Transfer (minutes)[1]	-	-	74	60
Children's Asthma Care				
Received Home Management Plan of Care	-	-	-	88%
Received Reliever Medication	-	-	-	100%
Received Systemic Corticosteroids	-	-	-	100%
Emergency Department				
Admittance Decision Time (minutes)[2]	587	88	148	98
Head CT Results Within 45 Min. of Arrival	13	77%	66%	57%
Patients Who Left ER Before Being Seen	42,162	3%	2%	2%
Time from ER Arrival to Admit. (minutes)[2]	589	300	355	274
Time from ER Arrival to Discharge (minutes)	392	158	152	134
Time in ER Before Being Evaluated (minutes)	427	27	32	26
Time to Pain Meds for Fractures (minutes)	124	55	58	57
Heart Attack Care				
Aspirin Given at Discharge	57	98%	99%	99%
Fibrinolytic Meds Within 30 Min. of Arrival[7]	-	-	69%	54%
PCI Within 90 Minutes of Arrival[1]	-	-	95%	96%
Statin Prescribed at Discharge	53	98%	99%	98%
Heart Failure Care				
ACE Inhibitor or ARB for LVSD[2]	57	95%	98%	97%
Discharge Instructions Given[2]	178	96%	97%	94%
Evaluation of LVS Function[2]	281	100%	100%	99%
Medicare Spending				
Medicare Spending per Patient (ratio)	-	1.07	1.07	0.98
Pneumonia Care				
Appropriate Initial Antibiotic Given[2]	92	98%	98%	95%
Blood Culture Timing[2]	172	100%	99%	98%
Pregnancy and Delivery Care				
Newborn Deliveries Scheduled Early[2]	35	3%	3%	6%
Preventive Care				
Immunization for Influenza[2]	515	97%	93%	90%
Immunization for Pneumonia[2]	558	99%	94%	92%
Stroke Care				
Anticoagulation Therapy for Atrial Fibrillation[1]	-	-	97%	95%
Antithrombotic Therapy Timing	104	97%	98%	98%
Assessed for Rehabilitation	119	95%	98%	97%
Discharged on Antithrombotic Therapy	98	100%	99%	99%
Discharged on Statin Medication	77	96%	95%	94%
Thrombolytic Therapy Timing	11	36%	74%	66%
Venous Thromboembolism Prophylaxis	136	83%	94%	94%
Written Stroke Educational Materials Given	68	97%	94%	88%
Surgical Care Improvement Project				
Appropriate Beta Blocker Usage[2]	109	99%	98%	98%
Appropriate VTP Within 24 Hours[2]	343	98%	99%	98%
Controlled Postoperative Blood Glucose[2,7]	-	-	97%	97%
Perioperative Temperature Management[2]	408	100%	100%	100%
Prophylactic Antibiotic Selection[2]	260	100%	99%	99%
Prophylactic Antibiotic Selection (Outpatient)	222	98%	97%	98%
Prophylactic Antibiotic Stopped[2]	257	98%	98%	98%
Prophylactic Antibiotic Timing[2]	260	100%	99%	99%
Prophylactic Antibiotic Timing (Outpatient)	222	100%	98%	98%
Urinary Catheter Removal[2]	286	100%	98%	97%
Survey of Patients' Hospital Experiences				
Area Around Room 'Always' Quiet at Night	300+	61%	53%	61%
Doctors 'Always' Communicated Well	300+	79%	77%	82%
Home Recovery Information Given	300+	81%	82%	85%
Hospital Given 9 or 10 on 10 Point Scale	300+	74%	64%	71%
Meds 'Always' Explained Before Given	300+	63%	59%	64%
Nurses 'Always' Communicated Well	300+	77%	76%	79%
Pain 'Always' Well Controlled	300+	66%	68%	71%
Room and Bathroom 'Always' Clean	300+	74%	68%	73%
Timely Help 'Always' Received	300+	60%	60%	68%
Would Definitely Recommend Hospital	300+	76%	66%	71%
Use of Medical Imaging				
Cardiac Imaging Stress Test before Surgery	195	5.1%	5.8%	5.3%
Combination Abdominal CT Scan	644	3.7%	7.4%	10.5%
Combination Brain/Sinus CT Scan	961	0.9%	2.8%	2.7%
Combination Chest CT Scan	371	1.3%	2.4%	2.7%
Follow-up Mammogram/Ultrasound	735	8.4%	12.5%	8.8%
Lumbar Spine MRI for Low Back Pain[1]	-	-	32.9%	37.2%

Chilton Medical Center

97 West Parkway Phone: 973-831-5000
Pompton Plains, NJ 07444 Fax: 973-831-5516
URL: www.chiltonmemorial.org
Type: Acute Care Hospitals Emergency Services: Yes
Ownership: Voluntary non-profit - Private Beds: 256

Key Personnel:
Emergency Room . . . . Amelia Bortelloni
Quality Assurance . . . . John Browne
Ambulatory Care . . . . Donna Kirby
Operating Room. . . . . Donna Kirby
Chief of Medical Staff. . . . . Joel Nizon, MD
Intensive Care Unit. . . . . Cindy O'Banks
Cardiac Laboratory. . . . . Dina Tortorelli
President/CEO. . . . . Joseph A. Trunfio, PhD

Measure	Cases	This Hosp.	State Avg.	U.S. Avg.
Blood Clot Prevention and Treatment				
Anticoagulation Overlap Therapy[2]	80	100%	88%	93%
ICU Venous Thromboembolism Prophylaxis[2]	46	100%	93%	92%
Incidence of Potentially Preventable VTE[2]	14	0%	10%	10%
UFH with Dosages/Platelet Monitoring[2]	22	100%	99%	97%
Venous Thromboembolism Prophylaxis[2]	404	100%	83%	85%
Warfarin Therapy Discharge Instructions[2]	49	100%	77%	75%
Chest Pain/Possible Heart Attack Care				
Aspirin Given Within 24 Hours of Arrival[1]	-	-	98%	96%
Fibrinolytic Meds Within 30 Min. of Arrival[3,7]	-	-	63%	58%
Average Time to ECG (minutes)[1]	-	-	7	7
Average Time to Transfer (minutes)[1,3]	-	-	74	60
Children's Asthma Care				
Received Home Management Plan of Care	-	-	-	88%
Received Reliever Medication	-	-	-	100%
Received Systemic Corticosteroids	-	-	-	100%
Emergency Department				
Admittance Decision Time (minutes)[2]	736	134	148	98
Head CT Results Within 45 Min. of Arrival[1]	-	-	66%	57%
Patients Who Left ER Before Being Seen	49,132	0%	2%	2%
Time from ER Arrival to Admit. (minutes)[2]	739	327	355	274
Time from ER Arrival to Discharge (minutes)	385	92	152	134
Time in ER Before Being Evaluated (minutes)	384	22	32	26
Time to Pain Meds for Fractures (minutes)	32	56	58	57
Heart Attack Care				
Aspirin Given at Discharge	128	100%	99%	99%
Fibrinolytic Meds Within 30 Min. of Arrival[7]	-	-	69%	54%
PCI Within 90 Minutes of Arrival	57	95%	95%	96%
Statin Prescribed at Discharge	136	100%	99%	98%
Heart Failure Care				
ACE Inhibitor or ARB for LVSD	77	100%	98%	97%
Discharge Instructions Given	199	97%	97%	94%
Evaluation of LVS Function	299	100%	100%	99%
Medicare Spending				
Medicare Spending per Patient (ratio)	-	1.09	1.07	0.98
Pneumonia Care				
Appropriate Initial Antibiotic Given[2]	97	99%	98%	95%
Blood Culture Timing[2]	166	100%	99%	98%
Pregnancy and Delivery Care				
Newborn Deliveries Scheduled Early	133	0%	3%	6%
Preventive Care				
Immunization for Influenza[2]	529	99%	93%	90%
Immunization for Pneumonia[2]	741	99%	94%	92%
Stroke Care				
Anticoagulation Therapy for Atrial Fibrillation	19	95%	97%	95%
Antithrombotic Therapy Timing	112	99%	98%	98%
Assessed for Rehabilitation	131	100%	98%	97%
Discharged on Antithrombotic Therapy	117	98%	99%	99%
Discharged on Statin Medication	98	96%	95%	94%
Thrombolytic Therapy Timing[1]	-	-	74%	66%
Venous Thromboembolism Prophylaxis	140	99%	94%	94%
Written Stroke Educational Materials Given	53	94%	94%	88%
Surgical Care Improvement Project				
Appropriate Beta Blocker Usage[2]	125	99%	98%	98%
Appropriate VTP Within 24 Hours[2]	324	100%	99%	98%
Controlled Postoperative Blood Glucose[2,7]	-	-	97%	97%
Perioperative Temperature Management[2]	365	100%	100%	100%
Prophylactic Antibiotic Selection[2]	205	99%	99%	99%
Prophylactic Antibiotic Selection (Outpatient)	83	99%	97%	98%
Prophylactic Antibiotic Stopped[2]	198	99%	98%	98%
Prophylactic Antibiotic Timing[2]	205	100%	99%	99%
Prophylactic Antibiotic Timing (Outpatient)	84	96%	98%	98%
Urinary Catheter Removal[2]	235	100%	98%	97%
Survey of Patients' Hospital Experiences				
Area Around Room 'Always' Quiet at Night	300+	56%	53%	61%
Doctors 'Always' Communicated Well	300+	78%	77%	82%
Home Recovery Information Given	300+	83%	82%	85%
Hospital Given 9 or 10 on 10 Point Scale	300+	64%	64%	71%
Meds 'Always' Explained Before Given	300+	64%	59%	64%
Nurses 'Always' Communicated Well	300+	79%	76%	79%
Pain 'Always' Well Controlled	300+	70%	68%	71%
Room and Bathroom 'Always' Clean	300+	68%	68%	73%
Timely Help 'Always' Received	300+	65%	60%	68%
Would Definitely Recommend Hospital	300+	64%	66%	71%
Use of Medical Imaging				
Cardiac Imaging Stress Test before Surgery	145	6.9%	5.8%	5.3%
Combination Abdominal CT Scan	1,176	26.0%	7.4%	10.5%
Combination Brain/Sinus CT Scan	1,064	5.3%	2.8%	2.7%
Combination Chest CT Scan	691	19.5%	2.4%	2.7%
Follow-up Mammogram/Ultrasound	2,408	14.1%	12.5%	8.8%
Lumbar Spine MRI for Low Back Pain	151	31.1%	32.9%	37.2%

NOTE: Hospital profiles are in alphabetical order by state, then city, then hospital within the city; Rankings exclude hospitals with less than 25 cases except for patient surveys which excludes hospitals with less than 100 cases; (a) 100-299 cases; (1) The number of cases/patients is too few to report; (2) Data submitted were based on a sample of cases/patients; (3) Results are based on a shorter time period than required; (4) Data suppressed by CMS for one or more quarters; (5) Results are not available for this reporting period; (6) Fewer than 100 patients completed the HCAHPS survey; (7) No cases met the criteria for this measure; (8) The lower limit of the confidence interval cannot be calculated if the number of observed infections equals zero; (9) No data are available from the state/territory for this reporting period; (10) The scores shown reflect fewer than 50 completed surveys; (11) There were discrepancies in the data collection process; (12) This measure does not apply to this hospital for this reporting period; (13) Results cannot be calculated for this reporting period; (14) The results for this state are combined with nearby states to protect confidentiality; Please refer to the User's Guide for a full explanation of data.

Robert Wood Johnson University Hospital at Rahway

865 Stone St
Rahway, NJ 07065
Phone: 732-381-4200
Fax: 732-499-6337
URL: www.rwjuhr.com/about/history.html
Type: Acute Care Hospitals
Emergency Services: Yes
Ownership: Voluntary non-profit - Private
Beds: 311

Key Personnel:
Emergency Room . . . . Michael Bernstein, MD, MBA
Infection Control . . . . Bessie Boyant
Quality Assurance . . . . Lucinda Glynn
Radiology. . . . . Gary Kronfeld, MD
Operating Room. . . . . Connie Saquing
CEO/President. . . . . Kirk C Tice
Surgery . . . . Anthony Tonzola, MD
Chief of Medical Staff . . . . David Wexler, MD

Measure	Cases	This Hosp.	State Avg.	U.S. Avg.
Blood Clot Prevention and Treatment				
Anticoagulation Overlap Therapy[2]	48	83%	88%	93%
ICU Venous Thromboembolism Prophylaxis[2]	96	86%	93%	92%
Incidence of Potentially Preventable VTE[2]	15	40%	10%	10%
UFH with Dosages/Platelet Monitoring[2]	27	96%	99%	97%
Venous Thromboembolism Prophylaxis[2]	407	59%	83%	85%
Warfarin Therapy Discharge Instructions[2]	26	100%	77%	75%
Chest Pain/Possible Heart Attack Care				
Aspirin Given Within 24 Hours of Arrival[1,3]	-	-	98%	96%
Fibrinolytic Meds Within 30 Min. of Arrival[3,7]	-	-	63%	58%
Average Time to ECG (minutes)[1,3]	-	-	7	7
Average Time to Transfer (minutes)[1,3]	-	-	74	60
Children's Asthma Care				
Received Home Management Plan of Care	-	-	-	88%
Received Reliever Medication	-	-	-	100%
Received Systemic Corticosteroids	-	-	-	100%
Emergency Department				
Admittance Decision Time (minutes)[2]	1,102	163	148	98
Head CT Results Within 45 Min. of Arrival[1]	-	-	66%	57%
Patients Who Left ER Before Being Seen	31,661	1%	2%	2%
Time from ER Arrival to Admit. (minutes)[2]	1,194	363	355	274
Time from ER Arrival to Discharge (minutes)	385	129	152	134
Time in ER Before Being Evaluated (minutes)	408	32	32	26
Time to Pain Meds for Fractures (minutes)	67	51	58	57
Heart Attack Care				
Aspirin Given at Discharge	68	100%	99%	99%
Fibrinolytic Meds Within 30 Min. of Arrival[7]	-	-	69%	54%
PCI Within 90 Minutes of Arrival	25	96%	95%	96%
Statin Prescribed at Discharge	66	100%	99%	98%
Heart Failure Care				
ACE Inhibitor or ARB for LVSD	78	100%	98%	97%
Discharge Instructions Given	176	98%	97%	94%
Evaluation of LVS Function	308	100%	100%	99%
Medicare Spending				
Medicare Spending per Patient (ratio)	-	1.15	1.07	0.98
Pneumonia Care				
Appropriate Initial Antibiotic Given	95	96%	98%	95%
Blood Culture Timing	179	97%	99%	98%
Pregnancy and Delivery Care				
Newborn Deliveries Scheduled Early[7]	-	-	3%	6%
Preventive Care				
Immunization for Influenza[2]	586	93%	93%	90%
Immunization for Pneumonia[2]	946	95%	94%	92%
Stroke Care				
Anticoagulation Therapy for Atrial Fibrillation[1]	-	-	97%	95%
Antithrombotic Therapy Timing	64	97%	98%	98%
Assessed for Rehabilitation	66	98%	98%	97%
Discharged on Antithrombotic Therapy	66	94%	99%	99%
Discharged on Statin Medication	44	86%	95%	94%
Thrombolytic Therapy Timing	12	42%	74%	66%
Venous Thromboembolism Prophylaxis	69	96%	94%	94%
Written Stroke Educational Materials Given	33	100%	94%	88%
Surgical Care Improvement Project				
Appropriate Beta Blocker Usage	61	100%	98%	98%
Appropriate VTP Within 24 Hours	152	98%	99%	98%
Controlled Postoperative Blood Glucose[7]	-	-	97%	97%
Perioperative Temperature Management	180	100%	100%	100%
Prophylactic Antibiotic Selection	80	99%	99%	99%
Prophylactic Antibiotic Selection (Outpatient)	68	97%	97%	98%
Prophylactic Antibiotic Stopped	75	97%	98%	98%
Prophylactic Antibiotic Timing	80	100%	99%	99%
Prophylactic Antibiotic Timing (Outpatient)	68	99%	98%	98%
Urinary Catheter Removal	62	92%	98%	97%
Survey of Patients' Hospital Experiences				
Area Around Room 'Always' Quiet at Night	300+	49%	53%	61%
Doctors 'Always' Communicated Well	300+	75%	77%	82%
Home Recovery Information Given	300+	80%	82%	85%
Hospital Given 9 or 10 on 10 Point Scale	300+	58%	64%	71%
Meds 'Always' Explained Before Given	300+	53%	59%	64%
Nurses 'Always' Communicated Well	300+	74%	76%	79%
Pain 'Always' Well Controlled	300+	65%	68%	71%
Room and Bathroom 'Always' Clean	300+	64%	68%	73%
Timely Help 'Always' Received	300+	61%	60%	68%
Would Definitely Recommend Hospital	300+	61%	66%	71%
Use of Medical Imaging				
Cardiac Imaging Stress Test before Surgery	120	7.5%	5.8%	5.3%
Combination Abdominal CT Scan	546	5.7%	7.4%	10.5%
Combination Brain/Sinus CT Scan	565	2.3%	2.8%	2.7%
Combination Chest CT Scan	340	2.6%	2.4%	2.7%
Follow-up Mammogram/Ultrasound	257	5.1%	12.5%	8.8%
Lumbar Spine MRI for Low Back Pain[1]	-	-	32.9%	37.2%

Riverview Medical Center

One Riverview Plaza
Red Bank, NJ 07701
Phone: 732-741-2700
Fax: 732-224-8408
URL: www.meridianhealth.com
Type: Acute Care Hospitals
Emergency Services: Yes
Ownership: Proprietary
Beds: 476

Key Personnel:
Emergency Room . . . . James Cameron
CEO/President. . . . . Timothy J Hogan, FACHE
Pediatric Ambulatory Care . . . . . . Robert Morgan, MD
Pediatric In-Patient Care . . . . Robert Morgan, MD
Radiology. . . . . John Parrella
Chief of Medical Staff. . . . . Richard Scott, MD

Measure	Cases	This Hosp.	State Avg.	U.S. Avg.
Blood Clot Prevention and Treatment				
Anticoagulation Overlap Therapy[2]	52	83%	88%	93%
ICU Venous Thromboembolism Prophylaxis[2]	74	96%	93%	92%
Incidence of Potentially Preventable VTE[1,2]	-	-	10%	10%
UFH with Dosages/Platelet Monitoring[2]	39	95%	99%	97%
Venous Thromboembolism Prophylaxis[2]	375	61%	83%	85%
Warfarin Therapy Discharge Instructions[2]	26	100%	77%	75%
Chest Pain/Possible Heart Attack Care				
Aspirin Given Within 24 Hours of Arrival[1]	-	-	98%	96%
Fibrinolytic Meds Within 30 Min. of Arrival[3,7]	-	-	63%	58%
Average Time to ECG (minutes)[1]	-	-	7	7
Average Time to Transfer (minutes)[3,7]	-	-	74	60
Children's Asthma Care				
Received Home Management Plan of Care	-	-	-	88%
Received Reliever Medication	-	-	-	100%
Received Systemic Corticosteroids	-	-	-	100%
Emergency Department				
Admittance Decision Time (minutes)[2]	755	121	148	98
Head CT Results Within 45 Min. of Arrival[1]	-	-	66%	57%
Patients Who Left ER Before Being Seen	42,147	2%	2%	2%
Time from ER Arrival to Admit. (minutes)[2]	755	364	355	274
Time from ER Arrival to Discharge (minutes)	386	149	152	134
Time in ER Before Being Evaluated (minutes)	428	29	32	26
Time to Pain Meds for Fractures (minutes)	171	48	58	57
Heart Attack Care				
Aspirin Given at Discharge	155	100%	99%	99%
Fibrinolytic Meds Within 30 Min. of Arrival[7]	-	-	69%	54%
PCI Within 90 Minutes of Arrival	51	96%	95%	96%
Statin Prescribed at Discharge	150	100%	99%	98%
Heart Failure Care				
ACE Inhibitor or ARB for LVSD[2]	41	100%	98%	97%
Discharge Instructions Given[2]	167	100%	97%	94%
Evaluation of LVS Function[2]	262	100%	100%	99%
Medicare Spending				
Medicare Spending per Patient (ratio)	-	1.06	1.07	0.98
Pneumonia Care				
Appropriate Initial Antibiotic Given[2]	123	100%	98%	95%
Blood Culture Timing[2]	198	100%	99%	98%
Pregnancy and Delivery Care				
Newborn Deliveries Scheduled Early[2]	39	10%	3%	6%
Preventive Care				
Immunization for Influenza[2]	553	100%	93%	90%
Immunization for Pneumonia[2]	689	100%	94%	92%
Stroke Care				
Anticoagulation Therapy for Atrial Fibrillation	18	100%	97%	95%
Antithrombotic Therapy Timing	96	99%	98%	98%
Assessed for Rehabilitation	128	100%	98%	97%
Discharged on Antithrombotic Therapy	106	99%	99%	99%
Discharged on Statin Medication	77	95%	95%	94%
Thrombolytic Therapy Timing	13	92%	74%	66%
Venous Thromboembolism Prophylaxis	134	94%	94%	94%
Written Stroke Educational Materials Given	50	94%	94%	88%
Surgical Care Improvement Project				
Appropriate Beta Blocker Usage[2]	142	94%	98%	98%
Appropriate VTP Within 24 Hours[2]	426	97%	99%	98%
Controlled Postoperative Blood Glucose[2,7]	-	-	97%	97%
Perioperative Temperature Management[2]	474	100%	100%	100%
Prophylactic Antibiotic Selection[2]	308	98%	99%	99%
Prophylactic Antibiotic Selection (Outpatient)	328	98%	97%	98%
Prophylactic Antibiotic Stopped[2]	298	99%	98%	98%
Prophylactic Antibiotic Timing[2]	308	99%	99%	99%
Prophylactic Antibiotic Timing (Outpatient)	328	99%	98%	98%
Urinary Catheter Removal[2]	219	94%	98%	97%
Survey of Patients' Hospital Experiences				
Area Around Room 'Always' Quiet at Night	300+	51%	53%	61%
Doctors 'Always' Communicated Well	300+	80%	77%	82%
Home Recovery Information Given	300+	86%	82%	85%
Hospital Given 9 or 10 on 10 Point Scale	300+	62%	64%	71%
Meds 'Always' Explained Before Given	300+	60%	59%	64%
Nurses 'Always' Communicated Well	300+	74%	76%	79%
Pain 'Always' Well Controlled	300+	68%	68%	71%
Room and Bathroom 'Always' Clean	300+	63%	68%	73%
Timely Help 'Always' Received	300+	55%	60%	68%
Would Definitely Recommend Hospital	300+	68%	66%	71%
Use of Medical Imaging				
Cardiac Imaging Stress Test before Surgery	249	6.4%	5.8%	5.3%
Combination Abdominal CT Scan	1,073	5.7%	7.4%	10.5%
Combination Brain/Sinus CT Scan	831	0.7%	2.8%	2.7%
Combination Chest CT Scan	865	0.7%	2.4%	2.7%
Follow-up Mammogram/Ultrasound	848	19.3%	12.5%	8.8%
Lumbar Spine MRI for Low Back Pain[1]	-	-	32.9%	37.2%

Valley Hospital

223 N Van Dien Avenue
Ridgewood, NJ 07450
Phone: 201-447-8000
Fax: 201-447-8732
E-mail: tvanmar@valleyhealth.com
URL: www.valleyhealth.com
Type: Acute Care Hospitals
Emergency Services: Yes
Ownership: Voluntary non-profit - Private
Beds: 442

Key Personnel:
Operating Room. . . . . Lorraine Butler, RN
Pediatric Ambulatory Care . . . . . . Joseph A Cannaliato, MD
Pediatric In-Patient Care . . . . Joseph A Cannaliato, MD
Infection Control. . . . . Terry Dannels, RN
Chief of Medical Staff. . . . . Marc S Melamed, MD
CEO/President. . . . . Audrey Meyers
Quality Assurance . . . . Virginia O'Malley, RN
Radiology. . . . . Louis Rambler, MD

Measure	Cases	This Hosp.	State Avg.	U.S. Avg.
Blood Clot Prevention and Treatment				
Anticoagulation Overlap Therapy[2]	246	73%	88%	93%
ICU Venous Thromboembolism Prophylaxis[2]	64	94%	93%	92%
Incidence of Potentially Preventable VTE[2]	72	21%	10%	10%
UFH with Dosages/Platelet Monitoring[2]	130	98%	99%	97%
Venous Thromboembolism Prophylaxis[2]	393	77%	83%	85%
Warfarin Therapy Discharge Instructions[2]	150	17%	77%	75%
Chest Pain/Possible Heart Attack Care				
Aspirin Given Within 24 Hours of Arrival[1,3]	-	-	98%	96%
Fibrinolytic Meds Within 30 Min. of Arrival[5]	-	-	63%	58%

NOTE: Hospital profiles are in alphabetical order by state, then city, then hospital within the city; Rankings exclude hospitals with less than 25 cases except for patient surveys which excludes hospitals with less than 100 cases; (a) 100-299 cases; (1) The number of cases/patients is too few to report; (2) Data submitted were based on a sample of cases/patients; (3) Results are based on a shorter time period than required; (4) Data suppressed by CMS for one or more quarters; (5) Results are not available for this reporting period; (6) Fewer than 100 patients completed the HCAHPS survey; (7) No cases met the criteria for this measure; (8) The lower limit of the confidence interval cannot be calculated if the number of observed infections equals zero; (9) No data are available from the state/territory for this reporting period; (10) The scores shown reflect fewer than 50 completed surveys; (11) There were discrepancies in the data collection process; (12) This measure does not apply to this hospital for this reporting period; (13) Results cannot be calculated for this reporting period; (14) The results for this state are combined with nearby states to protect confidentiality; Please refer to the User's Guide for a full explanation of data.

Measure	Cases	This Hosp.	State Avg.	U.S. Avg.
Average Time to ECG (minutes)[1,3]	-	-	7	7
Average Time to Transfer (minutes)[5]	-	-	74	60
Children's Asthma Care				
Received Home Management Plan of Care	-	-	-	88%
Received Reliever Medication	-	-	-	100%
Received Systemic Corticosteroids	-	-	-	100%
Emergency Department				
Admittance Decision Time (minutes)[2]	747	71	148	98
Head CT Results Within 45 Min. of Arrival[1]	-	-	66%	57%
Patients Who Left ER Before Being Seen	76,812	0%	2%	2%
Time from ER Arrival to Admit. (minutes)[2]	747	283	355	274
Time from ER Arrival to Discharge (minutes)	399	160	152	134
Time in ER Before Being Evaluated (minutes)	433	25	32	26
Time to Pain Meds for Fractures (minutes)	249	45	58	57
Heart Attack Care				
Aspirin Given at Discharge[2]	307	100%	99%	99%
Fibrinolytic Meds Within 30 Min. of Arrival[2,7]	-	-	69%	54%
PCI Within 90 Minutes of Arrival[2]	44	98%	95%	96%
Statin Prescribed at Discharge[2]	311	100%	99%	98%
Heart Failure Care				
ACE Inhibitor or ARB for LVSD[2]	94	100%	98%	97%
Discharge Instructions Given[2]	208	97%	97%	94%
Evaluation of LVS Function[2]	330	100%	100%	99%
Medicare Spending				
Medicare Spending per Patient (ratio)	-	1.09	1.07	0.98
Pneumonia Care				
Appropriate Initial Antibiotic Given[2]	88	99%	98%	95%
Blood Culture Timing[2]	194	99%	99%	98%
Pregnancy and Delivery Care				
Newborn Deliveries Scheduled Early[2]	48	6%	3%	6%
Preventive Care				
Immunization for Influenza[2]	558	97%	93%	90%
Immunization for Pneumonia[2]	675	99%	94%	92%
Stroke Care				
Anticoagulation Therapy for Atrial Fibrillation	44	100%	97%	95%
Antithrombotic Therapy Timing	214	99%	98%	98%
Assessed for Rehabilitation	285	100%	98%	97%
Discharged on Antithrombotic Therapy	248	100%	99%	99%
Discharged on Statin Medication	196	99%	95%	94%
Thrombolytic Therapy Timing	28	93%	74%	66%
Venous Thromboembolism Prophylaxis	288	95%	94%	94%
Written Stroke Educational Materials Given	139	97%	94%	88%
Surgical Care Improvement Project				
Appropriate Beta Blocker Usage[2]	292	100%	98%	98%
Appropriate VTP Within 24 Hours[2]	416	100%	99%	98%
Controlled Postoperative Blood Glucose[2]	171	98%	97%	97%
Perioperative Temperature Management[2]	577	100%	100%	100%
Prophylactic Antibiotic Selection[2]	497	99%	99%	99%
Prophylactic Antibiotic Selection (Outpatient)	596	99%	97%	98%
Prophylactic Antibiotic Stopped[2]	492	99%	98%	98%
Prophylactic Antibiotic Timing[2]	497	100%	99%	99%
Prophylactic Antibiotic Timing (Outpatient)	598	99%	98%	98%
Urinary Catheter Removal[2]	420	100%	98%	97%
Survey of Patients' Hospital Experiences				
Area Around Room 'Always' Quiet at Night	300+	55%	53%	61%
Doctors 'Always' Communicated Well	300+	83%	77%	82%
Home Recovery Information Given	300+	83%	82%	85%
Hospital Given 9 or 10 on 10 Point Scale	300+	78%	64%	71%
Meds 'Always' Explained Before Given	300+	66%	59%	64%
Nurses 'Always' Communicated Well	300+	84%	76%	79%
Pain 'Always' Well Controlled	300+	74%	68%	71%
Room and Bathroom 'Always' Clean	300+	76%	68%	73%
Timely Help 'Always' Received	300+	67%	60%	68%
Would Definitely Recommend Hospital	300+	81%	66%	71%
Use of Medical Imaging				
Cardiac Imaging Stress Test before Surgery	455	7.0%	5.8%	5.3%
Combination Abdominal CT Scan	2,336	7.2%	7.4%	10.5%
Combination Brain/Sinus CT Scan	1,994	1.5%	2.8%	2.7%
Combination Chest CT Scan	2,163	5.1%	2.4%	2.7%
Follow-up Mammogram/Ultrasound	1,714	8.8%	12.5%	8.8%
Lumbar Spine MRI for Low Back Pain	130	28.5%	32.9%	37.2%

Memorial Hospital of Salem County

310 Woodstown Road
Salem, NJ 08079
Phone: 856-935-1000
Fax: 856-935-3175
URL: www.mhshealth.com
Type: Acute Care Hospitals
Emergency Services: Yes
Ownership: Voluntary non-profit - Private
Beds: 140

Key Personnel:
CEO/President . . . . Robert Allen
Chief of Medical Staff . . . . John Amrien, MD
Emergency Room . . . . Jane Fleurantin, MD

Measure	Cases	This Hosp.	State Avg.	U.S. Avg.
Blood Clot Prevention and Treatment				
Anticoagulation Overlap Therapy[2]	39	92%	88%	93%
ICU Venous Thromboembolism Prophylaxis[2]	105	91%	93%	92%
Incidence of Potentially Preventable VTE[1,2]	-	-	10%	10%
UFH with Dosages/Platelet Monitoring[2]	20	60%	99%	97%
Venous Thromboembolism Prophylaxis[2]	334	90%	83%	85%
Warfarin Therapy Discharge Instructions[2]	27	93%	77%	75%
Chest Pain/Possible Heart Attack Care				
Aspirin Given Within 24 Hours of Arrival	32	94%	98%	96%
Fibrinolytic Meds Within 30 Min. of Arrival[1]	-	-	63%	58%
Average Time to ECG (minutes)	31	7	7	7
Average Time to Transfer (minutes)[1]	-	-	74	60
Children's Asthma Care				
Received Home Management Plan of Care	-	-	-	88%
Received Reliever Medication	-	-	-	100%
Received Systemic Corticosteroids	-	-	-	100%
Emergency Department				
Admittance Decision Time (minutes)[2]	692	123	148	98
Head CT Results Within 45 Min. of Arrival[1]	-	-	66%	57%
Patients Who Left ER Before Being Seen	21,079	1%	2%	2%
Time from ER Arrival to Admit. (minutes)[2]	696	283	355	274
Time from ER Arrival to Discharge (minutes)	364	139	152	134
Time in ER Before Being Evaluated (minutes)	422	18	32	26
Time to Pain Meds for Fractures (minutes)	82	68	58	57
Heart Attack Care				
Aspirin Given at Discharge[1]	-	-	99%	99%
Fibrinolytic Meds Within 30 Min. of Arrival[7]	-	-	69%	54%
PCI Within 90 Minutes of Arrival[7]	-	-	95%	96%
Statin Prescribed at Discharge[1]	-	-	99%	98%
Heart Failure Care				
ACE Inhibitor or ARB for LVSD	44	100%	98%	97%
Discharge Instructions Given	121	98%	97%	94%
Evaluation of LVS Function	143	99%	100%	99%
Medicare Spending				
Medicare Spending per Patient (ratio)	-	1.02	1.07	0.98
Pneumonia Care				
Appropriate Initial Antibiotic Given	60	98%	98%	95%
Blood Culture Timing	131	98%	99%	98%
Pregnancy and Delivery Care				
Newborn Deliveries Scheduled Early[1,2]	-	-	3%	6%
Preventive Care				
Immunization for Influenza[2]	412	99%	93%	90%
Immunization for Pneumonia[2]	521	99%	94%	92%
Stroke Care				
Anticoagulation Therapy for Atrial Fibrillation[1]	-	-	97%	95%
Antithrombotic Therapy Timing	41	98%	98%	98%
Assessed for Rehabilitation	42	93%	98%	97%
Discharged on Antithrombotic Therapy	41	98%	99%	99%
Discharged on Statin Medication	27	85%	95%	94%
Thrombolytic Therapy Timing[1]	-	-	74%	66%
Venous Thromboembolism Prophylaxis	46	93%	94%	94%
Written Stroke Educational Materials Given	21	86%	94%	88%
Surgical Care Improvement Project				
Appropriate Beta Blocker Usage	22	91%	98%	98%
Appropriate VTP Within 24 Hours	83	99%	99%	98%
Controlled Postoperative Blood Glucose[7]	-	-	97%	97%
Perioperative Temperature Management	97	100%	100%	100%
Prophylactic Antibiotic Selection	56	96%	99%	99%
Prophylactic Antibiotic Selection (Outpatient)	24	100%	97%	98%
Prophylactic Antibiotic Stopped	54	94%	98%	98%
Prophylactic Antibiotic Timing	57	98%	99%	99%
Prophylactic Antibiotic Timing (Outpatient)	25	96%	98%	98%
Urinary Catheter Removal	34	94%	98%	97%
Survey of Patients' Hospital Experiences				
Area Around Room 'Always' Quiet at Night	300+	63%	53%	61%
Doctors 'Always' Communicated Well	300+	80%	77%	82%
Home Recovery Information Given	300+	85%	82%	85%
Hospital Given 9 or 10 on 10 Point Scale	300+	59%	64%	71%
Meds 'Always' Explained Before Given	300+	66%	59%	64%
Nurses 'Always' Communicated Well	300+	79%	76%	79%
Pain 'Always' Well Controlled	300+	74%	68%	71%
Room and Bathroom 'Always' Clean	300+	71%	68%	73%
Timely Help 'Always' Received	300+	61%	60%	68%
Would Definitely Recommend Hospital	300+	53%	66%	71%
Use of Medical Imaging				
Cardiac Imaging Stress Test before Surgery[1]	-	-	5.8%	5.3%
Combination Abdominal CT Scan	413	9.4%	7.4%	10.5%
Combination Brain/Sinus CT Scan	434	5.3%	2.8%	2.7%
Combination Chest CT Scan	217	0.5%	2.4%	2.7%
Follow-up Mammogram/Ultrasound	361	11.4%	12.5%	8.8%
Lumbar Spine MRI for Low Back Pain	80	38.8%	32.9%	37.2%

Meadowlands Hospital Medical Center

55 Meadowlands Pkwy
Secaucus, NJ 07094
Phone: 201-392-3200
Fax: 201-392-3527
E-mail: news@libertyhcs.org
URL: www.libertyhcs.org/meadowlands
Type: Acute Care Hospitals
Emergency Services: Yes
Ownership: Proprietary
Beds: 230

Key Personnel:
Pediatric Ambulatory Care . . . . . . Azzam Baker, MD
Pediatric In-Patient Care . . . . Azzam Baker, MD
Operating Room. . . . . Denise Desouza
Quality Assurance . . . . Kathleen Locklear
Emergency Room . . . . Liz Ramirez

Measure	Cases	This Hosp.	State Avg.	U.S. Avg.
Blood Clot Prevention and Treatment				
Anticoagulation Overlap Therapy[2]	16	100%	88%	93%
ICU Venous Thromboembolism Prophylaxis[2]	75	92%	93%	92%
Incidence of Potentially Preventable VTE[1,2]	-	-	10%	10%
UFH with Dosages/Platelet Monitoring[2]	11	100%	99%	97%
Venous Thromboembolism Prophylaxis[2]	212	82%	83%	85%
Warfarin Therapy Discharge Instructions[2]	14	100%	77%	75%
Chest Pain/Possible Heart Attack Care				
Aspirin Given Within 24 Hours of Arrival[5]	-	-	98%	96%
Fibrinolytic Meds Within 30 Min. of Arrival[5]	-	-	63%	58%
Average Time to ECG (minutes)[5]	-	-	7	7
Average Time to Transfer (minutes)[5]	-	-	74	60
Children's Asthma Care				
Received Home Management Plan of Care	-	-	-	88%
Received Reliever Medication	-	-	-	100%
Received Systemic Corticosteroids	-	-	-	100%
Emergency Department				
Admittance Decision Time (minutes)[2]	532	144	148	98
Head CT Results Within 45 Min. of Arrival[1]	-	-	66%	57%
Patients Who Left ER Before Being Seen	20,593	1%	2%	2%
Time from ER Arrival to Admit. (minutes)[2]	533	277	355	274
Time from ER Arrival to Discharge (minutes)	400	125	152	134
Time in ER Before Being Evaluated (minutes)	430	24	32	26
Time to Pain Meds for Fractures (minutes)	29	50	58	57
Heart Attack Care				
Aspirin Given at Discharge[1]	-	-	99%	99%
Fibrinolytic Meds Within 30 Min. of Arrival[1]	-	-	69%	54%
PCI Within 90 Minutes of Arrival[7]	-	-	95%	96%
Statin Prescribed at Discharge	11	91%	99%	98%
Heart Failure Care				
ACE Inhibitor or ARB for LVSD[1]	-	-	98%	97%
Discharge Instructions Given	41	100%	97%	94%
Evaluation of LVS Function	46	96%	100%	99%
Medicare Spending				
Medicare Spending per Patient (ratio)	-	1.13	1.07	0.98
Pneumonia Care				
Appropriate Initial Antibiotic Given	62	97%	98%	95%
Blood Culture Timing	111	97%	99%	98%
Pregnancy and Delivery Care				
Newborn Deliveries Scheduled Early[2]	38	5%	3%	6%

NOTE: Hospital profiles are in alphabetical order by state, then city, then hospital within the city; Rankings exclude hospitals with less than 25 cases except for patient surveys which excludes hospitals with less than 100 cases; (a) 100-299 cases; (1) The number of cases/patients is too few to report; (2) Data submitted were based on a sample of cases/patients; (3) Results are based on a shorter time period than required; (4) Data suppressed by CMS for one or more quarters; (5) Results are not available for this reporting period; (6) Fewer than 100 patients completed the HCAHPS survey; (7) No cases met the criteria for this measure; (8) The lower limit of the confidence interval cannot be calculated if the number of observed infections equals zero; (9) No data are available from the state/territory for this reporting period; (10) The scores shown reflect fewer than 50 completed surveys; (11) There were discrepancies in the data collection process; (12) This measure does not apply to this hospital for this reporting period; (13) Results cannot be calculated for this reporting period; (14) The results for this state are combined with nearby states to protect confidentiality; Please refer to the User's Guide for a full explanation of data.

Measure	Cases	This Hosp.	State Avg.	U.S. Avg.
Preventive Care				
Immunization for Influenza[2]	378	70%	93%	90%
Immunization for Pneumonia[2]	363	83%	94%	92%
Stroke Care				
Anticoagulation Therapy for Atrial Fibrillation[1]	-	-	97%	95%
Antithrombotic Therapy Timing	17	100%	98%	98%
Assessed for Rehabilitation	21	90%	98%	97%
Discharged on Antithrombotic Therapy	19	89%	99%	99%
Discharged on Statin Medication	18	94%	95%	94%
Thrombolytic Therapy Timing[1]	-	-	74%	66%
Venous Thromboembolism Prophylaxis	22	91%	94%	94%
Written Stroke Educational Materials Given	18	100%	94%	88%
Surgical Care Improvement Project				
Appropriate Beta Blocker Usage[1]	-	-	98%	98%
Appropriate VTP Within 24 Hours	49	96%	99%	98%
Controlled Postoperative Blood Glucose[7]	-	-	97%	97%
Perioperative Temperature Management	64	100%	100%	100%
Prophylactic Antibiotic Selection	34	94%	99%	99%
Prophylactic Antibiotic Selection (Outpatient)	119	87%	97%	98%
Prophylactic Antibiotic Stopped	34	100%	98%	98%
Prophylactic Antibiotic Timing	34	100%	99%	99%
Prophylactic Antibiotic Timing (Outpatient)	119	98%	98%	98%
Urinary Catheter Removal	19	95%	98%	97%
Survey of Patients' Hospital Experiences				
Area Around Room 'Always' Quiet at Night	300+	58%	53%	61%
Doctors 'Always' Communicated Well	300+	75%	77%	82%
Home Recovery Information Given	300+	78%	82%	85%
Hospital Given 9 or 10 on 10 Point Scale	300+	54%	64%	71%
Meds 'Always' Explained Before Given	300+	58%	59%	64%
Nurses 'Always' Communicated Well	300+	69%	76%	79%
Pain 'Always' Well Controlled	300+	63%	68%	71%
Room and Bathroom 'Always' Clean	300+	70%	68%	73%
Timely Help 'Always' Received	300+	60%	60%	68%
Would Definitely Recommend Hospital	300+	55%	66%	71%
Use of Medical Imaging				
Cardiac Imaging Stress Test before Surgery[1]	-	-	5.8%	5.3%
Combination Abdominal CT Scan	129	2.3%	7.4%	10.5%
Combination Brain/Sinus CT Scan[1]	-	-	2.8%	2.7%
Combination Chest CT Scan	64	1.6%	2.4%	2.7%
Follow-up Mammogram/Ultrasound	98	14.3%	12.5%	8.8%
Lumbar Spine MRI for Low Back Pain[1]	-	-	32.9%	37.2%

Shore Medical Center

100 Medical Center Way
Somers Point, NJ 08244
Phone: 609-653-3545
Fax: 609-926-1987
URL: www.shorememorial.org
Type: Acute Care Hospitals
Emergency Services: Yes
Ownership: Voluntary non-profit - Private
Beds: 296

Key Personnel:
Chair/CEO . . . . Gerald J. Corcoran, Esq.
CEO/President. . . . . Ronald W. Johnson, MBA, FACHE
Operating Room. . . . . Cynthia Leggett, RN
Emergency Room . . . . Mark Liwoch
Chief of Medical Staff . . . . Jeanne M. Rowe, MD
Quality Assurance . . . . Angelo Sparagna

Measure	Cases	This Hosp.	State Avg.	U.S. Avg.
Blood Clot Prevention and Treatment				
Anticoagulation Overlap Therapy[2]	71	65%	88%	93%
ICU Venous Thromboembolism Prophylaxis[2]	65	95%	93%	92%
Incidence of Potentially Preventable VTE[2]	19	5%	10%	10%
UFH with Dosages/Platelet Monitoring[2]	103	100%	99%	97%
Venous Thromboembolism Prophylaxis[2]	373	84%	83%	85%
Warfarin Therapy Discharge Instructions[2]	44	48%	77%	75%
Chest Pain/Possible Heart Attack Care				
Aspirin Given Within 24 Hours of Arrival	59	100%	98%	96%
Fibrinolytic Meds Within 30 Min. of Arrival[7]	-	-	63%	58%
Average Time to ECG (minutes)	59	11	7	7
Average Time to Transfer (minutes)	31	80	74	60
Children's Asthma Care				
Received Home Management Plan of Care	-	-	-	88%
Received Reliever Medication	-	-	-	100%
Received Systemic Corticosteroids	-	-	-	100%
Emergency Department				
Admittance Decision Time (minutes)[2]	798	170	148	98
Head CT Results Within 45 Min. of Arrival	11	100%	66%	57%
Patients Who Left ER Before Being Seen	46,714	0%	2%	2%
Time from ER Arrival to Admit. (minutes)[2]	798	320	355	274
Time from ER Arrival to Discharge (minutes)	402	134	152	134
Time in ER Before Being Evaluated (minutes)	414	20	32	26
Time to Pain Meds for Fractures (minutes)	85	42	58	57
Heart Attack Care				
Aspirin Given at Discharge	31	97%	99%	99%
Fibrinolytic Meds Within 30 Min. of Arrival[7]	-	-	69%	54%
PCI Within 90 Minutes of Arrival[7]	-	-	95%	96%
Statin Prescribed at Discharge	30	93%	99%	98%
Heart Failure Care				
ACE Inhibitor or ARB for LVSD[2]	73	97%	98%	97%
Discharge Instructions Given[2]	218	91%	97%	94%
Evaluation of LVS Function[2]	269	99%	100%	99%
Medicare Spending				
Medicare Spending per Patient (ratio)	-	0.98	1.07	0.98
Pneumonia Care				
Appropriate Initial Antibiotic Given[2]	95	98%	98%	95%
Blood Culture Timing[2]	186	98%	99%	98%
Pregnancy and Delivery Care				
Newborn Deliveries Scheduled Early[2]	79	5%	3%	6%
Preventive Care				
Immunization for Influenza[2]	553	86%	93%	90%
Immunization for Pneumonia[2]	683	90%	94%	92%
Stroke Care				
Anticoagulation Therapy for Atrial Fibrillation[1]	-	-	97%	95%
Antithrombotic Therapy Timing	88	99%	98%	98%
Assessed for Rehabilitation	94	100%	98%	97%
Discharged on Antithrombotic Therapy	85	100%	99%	99%
Discharged on Statin Medication	76	100%	95%	94%
Thrombolytic Therapy Timing[1]	-	-	74%	66%
Venous Thromboembolism Prophylaxis	95	98%	94%	94%
Written Stroke Educational Materials Given	49	86%	94%	88%
Surgical Care Improvement Project				
Appropriate Beta Blocker Usage[2]	181	97%	98%	98%
Appropriate VTP Within 24 Hours[2]	456	100%	99%	98%
Controlled Postoperative Blood Glucose[2,7]	-	-	97%	97%
Perioperative Temperature Management[2]	592	100%	100%	100%
Prophylactic Antibiotic Selection[2]	404	100%	99%	99%
Prophylactic Antibiotic Selection (Outpatient)	149	100%	97%	98%
Prophylactic Antibiotic Stopped[2]	393	99%	98%	98%
Prophylactic Antibiotic Timing[2]	404	100%	99%	99%
Prophylactic Antibiotic Timing (Outpatient)	149	99%	98%	98%
Urinary Catheter Removal[2]	199	98%	98%	97%
Survey of Patients' Hospital Experiences				
Area Around Room 'Always' Quiet at Night	300+	56%	53%	61%
Doctors 'Always' Communicated Well	300+	80%	77%	82%
Home Recovery Information Given	300+	85%	82%	85%
Hospital Given 9 or 10 on 10 Point Scale	300+	68%	64%	71%
Meds 'Always' Explained Before Given	300+	60%	59%	64%
Nurses 'Always' Communicated Well	300+	81%	76%	79%
Pain 'Always' Well Controlled	300+	69%	68%	71%
Room and Bathroom 'Always' Clean	300+	72%	68%	73%
Timely Help 'Always' Received	300+	64%	60%	68%
Would Definitely Recommend Hospital	300+	73%	66%	71%
Use of Medical Imaging				
Cardiac Imaging Stress Test before Surgery	79	11.4%	5.8%	5.3%
Combination Abdominal CT Scan	603	8.1%	7.4%	10.5%
Combination Brain/Sinus CT Scan	910	4.4%	2.8%	2.7%
Combination Chest CT Scan	292	4.5%	2.4%	2.7%
Follow-up Mammogram/Ultrasound	672	9.4%	12.5%	8.8%
Lumbar Spine MRI for Low Back Pain[1]	-	-	32.9%	37.2%

Somerset Medical Center

110 Rehill Ave
Somerville, NJ 08876
Phone: 908-685-2200
Fax: 908-685-2894
URL: www.somersetmedicalcenter.com
Type: Acute Care Hospitals
Emergency Services: Yes
Ownership: Voluntary non-profit - Private
Beds: 364

Key Personnel:
Patient Relations . . . . Steve Dean
Radiology. . . . . Lawrence Gross, MD
CEO/President. . . . . Paul Huegel
Infection Control. . . . . Patricia Lafaro, RN
Quality Assurance . . . . Mary Lund
Emergency Room . . . . Dennis McGill, MD
Operating Room. . . . . Kristin Peterson
Chief of Medical Staff . . . . Richard Todd Paris, MD

Measure	Cases	This Hosp.	State Avg.	U.S. Avg.
Blood Clot Prevention and Treatment				
Anticoagulation Overlap Therapy[2]	122	85%	88%	93%
ICU Venous Thromboembolism Prophylaxis[2]	60	75%	93%	92%
Incidence of Potentially Preventable VTE[2]	22	32%	10%	10%
UFH with Dosages/Platelet Monitoring[2]	130	100%	99%	97%
Venous Thromboembolism Prophylaxis[2]	376	56%	83%	85%
Warfarin Therapy Discharge Instructions[2]	87	82%	77%	75%
Chest Pain/Possible Heart Attack Care				
Aspirin Given Within 24 Hours of Arrival[1,3]	-	-	98%	96%
Fibrinolytic Meds Within 30 Min. of Arrival[5]	-	-	63%	58%
Average Time to ECG (minutes)[1,3]	-	-	7	7
Average Time to Transfer (minutes)[5]	-	-	74	60
Children's Asthma Care				
Received Home Management Plan of Care	-	-	-	88%
Received Reliever Medication	-	-	-	100%
Received Systemic Corticosteroids	-	-	-	100%
Emergency Department				
Admittance Decision Time (minutes)[2]	810	144	148	98
Head CT Results Within 45 Min. of Arrival[1]	-	-	66%	57%
Patients Who Left ER Before Being Seen	54,695	1%	2%	2%
Time from ER Arrival to Admit. (minutes)[2]	819	436	355	274
Time from ER Arrival to Discharge (minutes)	406	161	152	134
Time in ER Before Being Evaluated (minutes)	396	37	32	26
Time to Pain Meds for Fractures (minutes)	138	56	58	57
Heart Attack Care				
Aspirin Given at Discharge[2]	217	98%	99%	99%
Fibrinolytic Meds Within 30 Min. of Arrival[2,7]	-	-	69%	54%
PCI Within 90 Minutes of Arrival[2]	64	100%	95%	96%
Statin Prescribed at Discharge[2]	206	97%	99%	98%
Heart Failure Care				
ACE Inhibitor or ARB for LVSD[2]	60	98%	98%	97%
Discharge Instructions Given[2]	210	100%	97%	94%
Evaluation of LVS Function[2]	308	100%	100%	99%
Medicare Spending				
Medicare Spending per Patient (ratio)	-	1.12	1.07	0.98
Pneumonia Care				
Appropriate Initial Antibiotic Given[2]	80	100%	98%	95%
Blood Culture Timing[2]	103	96%	99%	98%
Pregnancy and Delivery Care				
Newborn Deliveries Scheduled Early[2]	36	0%	3%	6%
Preventive Care				
Immunization for Influenza[2]	578	84%	93%	90%
Immunization for Pneumonia[2]	756	89%	94%	92%
Stroke Care				
Anticoagulation Therapy for Atrial Fibrillation	30	93%	97%	95%
Antithrombotic Therapy Timing	176	97%	98%	98%
Assessed for Rehabilitation	212	95%	98%	97%
Discharged on Antithrombotic Therapy	180	96%	99%	99%
Discharged on Statin Medication	122	84%	95%	94%
Thrombolytic Therapy Timing	13	77%	74%	66%
Venous Thromboembolism Prophylaxis	225	79%	94%	94%
Written Stroke Educational Materials Given	95	84%	94%	88%
Surgical Care Improvement Project				
Appropriate Beta Blocker Usage[2]	146	90%	98%	98%
Appropriate VTP Within 24 Hours[2]	436	97%	99%	98%
Controlled Postoperative Blood Glucose[2,7]	-	-	97%	97%
Perioperative Temperature Management[2]	539	100%	100%	100%
Prophylactic Antibiotic Selection[2]	290	100%	99%	99%
Prophylactic Antibiotic Selection (Outpatient)	181	99%	97%	98%
Prophylactic Antibiotic Stopped[2]	282	98%	98%	98%
Prophylactic Antibiotic Timing[2]	290	100%	99%	99%
Prophylactic Antibiotic Timing (Outpatient)	182	99%	98%	98%
Urinary Catheter Removal[2]	129	93%	98%	97%
Survey of Patients' Hospital Experiences				
Area Around Room 'Always' Quiet at Night	300+	53%	53%	61%
Doctors 'Always' Communicated Well	300+	81%	77%	82%

NOTE: Hospital profiles are in alphabetical order by state, then city, then hospital within the city; Rankings exclude hospitals with less than 25 cases except for patient surveys which excludes hospitals with less than 100 cases; (a) 100-299 cases; (1) The number of cases/patients is too few to report; (2) Data submitted were based on a sample of cases/patients; (3) Results are based on a shorter time period than required; (4) Data suppressed by CMS for one or more quarters; (5) Results are not available for this reporting period; (6) Fewer than 100 patients completed the HCAHPS survey; (7) No cases met the criteria for this measure; (8) The lower limit of the confidence interval cannot be calculated if the number of observed infections equals zero; (9) No data are available from the state/territory for this reporting period; (10) The scores shown reflect fewer than 50 completed surveys; (11) There were discrepancies in the data collection process; (12) This measure does not apply to this hospital for this reporting period; (13) Results cannot be calculated for this reporting period; (14) The results for this state are combined with nearby states to protect confidentiality; Please refer to the User's Guide for a full explanation of data.

Home Recovery Information Given	300+	81%	82%	85%
Hospital Given 9 or 10 on 10 Point Scale	300+	70%	64%	71%
Meds 'Always' Explained Before Given	300+	60%	59%	64%
Nurses 'Always' Communicated Well	300+	79%	76%	79%
Pain 'Always' Well Controlled	300+	69%	68%	71%
Room and Bathroom 'Always' Clean	300+	73%	68%	73%
Timely Help 'Always' Received	300+	63%	60%	68%
Would Definitely Recommend Hospital	300+	71%	66%	71%
Use of Medical Imaging				
Cardiac Imaging Stress Test before Surgery	507	5.7%	5.8%	5.3%
Combination Abdominal CT Scan	936	18.1%	7.4%	10.5%
Combination Brain/Sinus CT Scan	1,046	1.9%	2.8%	2.7%
Combination Chest CT Scan	763	1.0%	2.4%	2.7%
Follow-up Mammogram/Ultrasound	1,037	11.9%	12.5%	8.8%
Lumbar Spine MRI for Low Back Pain	85	28.2%	32.9%	37.2%

Kennedy University Hospital - Stratford Div

18 East Laurel Road
Stratford, NJ 08084
Phone: 856-346-6000
Fax: 856-346-6005
URL: www.kennedyhealth.org
Type: Acute Care Hospitals
Emergency Services: Yes
Ownership: Voluntary non-profit - Private
Beds: 236

Key Personnel:
Quality Assurance . . . . Dennis L Bush
Chief of Medical Staff. . . . . Daniel Herriman, MD, JD
Ambulatory Care . . . . Richard Koss
CEO/President. . . . . Richard E Murray

Measure	Cases	This Hosp.	State Avg.	U.S. Avg.
Blood Clot Prevention and Treatment				
Anticoagulation Overlap Therapy[2]	257	86%	88%	93%
ICU Venous Thromboembolism Prophylaxis[2]	78	99%	93%	92%
Incidence of Potentially Preventable VTE[2]	57	5%	10%	10%
UFH with Dosages/Platelet Monitoring[2]	270	100%	99%	97%
Venous Thromboembolism Prophylaxis[2]	330	96%	83%	85%
Warfarin Therapy Discharge Instructions[2]	154	76%	77%	75%
Chest Pain/Possible Heart Attack Care				
Aspirin Given Within 24 Hours of Arrival	149	99%	98%	96%
Fibrinolytic Meds Within 30 Min. of Arrival	14	50%	63%	58%
Average Time to ECG (minutes)	149	8	7	7
Average Time to Transfer (minutes)	22	85	74	60
Children's Asthma Care				
Received Home Management Plan of Care	-	-	-	88%
Received Reliever Medication	-	-	-	100%
Received Systemic Corticosteroids	-	-	-	100%
Emergency Department				
Admittance Decision Time (minutes)[2]	1,005	208	148	98
Head CT Results Within 45 Min. of Arrival[1]	-	-	66%	57%
Patients Who Left ER Before Being Seen	>100k	2%	2%	2%
Time from ER Arrival to Admit. (minutes)[2]	1,021	377	355	274
Time from ER Arrival to Discharge (minutes)	379	153	152	134
Time in ER Before Being Evaluated (minutes)	428	19	32	26
Time to Pain Meds for Fractures (minutes)	310	65	58	57
Heart Attack Care				
Aspirin Given at Discharge	117	100%	99%	99%
Fibrinolytic Meds Within 30 Min. of Arrival[7]	-	-	69%	54%
PCI Within 90 Minutes of Arrival[7]	-	-	95%	96%
Statin Prescribed at Discharge	115	99%	99%	98%
Heart Failure Care				
ACE Inhibitor or ARB for LVSD	155	95%	98%	97%
Discharge Instructions Given	657	97%	97%	94%
Evaluation of LVS Function	899	100%	100%	99%
Medicare Spending				
Medicare Spending per Patient (ratio)	-	1.02	1.07	0.98
Pneumonia Care				
Appropriate Initial Antibiotic Given	524	98%	98%	95%
Blood Culture Timing	1,175	99%	99%	98%
Pregnancy and Delivery Care				
Newborn Deliveries Scheduled Early[2]	29	7%	3%	6%
Preventive Care				
Immunization for Influenza[2]	595	97%	93%	90%
Immunization for Pneumonia[2]	815	95%	94%	92%
Stroke Care				
Anticoagulation Therapy for Atrial Fibrillation[2]	33	100%	97%	95%
Antithrombotic Therapy Timing[2]	308	99%	98%	98%
Assessed for Rehabilitation[2]	362	94%	98%	97%
Discharged on Antithrombotic Therapy[2]	325	100%	99%	99%
Discharged on Statin Medication[2]	253	97%	95%	94%
Thrombolytic Therapy Timing[2]	31	97%	74%	66%
Venous Thromboembolism Prophylaxis[2]	386	99%	94%	94%
Written Stroke Educational Materials Given[2]	196	87%	94%	88%
Surgical Care Improvement Project				
Appropriate Beta Blocker Usage[2]	350	98%	98%	98%
Appropriate VTP Within 24 Hours[2]	879	99%	99%	98%
Controlled Postoperative Blood Glucose[2,7]	-	-	97%	97%
Perioperative Temperature Management[2]	1,110	100%	100%	100%
Prophylactic Antibiotic Selection[2]	700	99%	99%	99%
Prophylactic Antibiotic Selection (Outpatient)	252	97%	97%	98%
Prophylactic Antibiotic Stopped[2]	691	98%	98%	98%
Prophylactic Antibiotic Timing[2]	700	100%	99%	99%
Prophylactic Antibiotic Timing (Outpatient)	253	97%	98%	98%
Urinary Catheter Removal[2]	390	96%	98%	97%
Survey of Patients' Hospital Experiences				
Area Around Room 'Always' Quiet at Night	300+	50%	53%	61%
Doctors 'Always' Communicated Well	300+	76%	77%	82%
Home Recovery Information Given	300+	81%	82%	85%
Hospital Given 9 or 10 on 10 Point Scale	300+	63%	64%	71%
Meds 'Always' Explained Before Given	300+	61%	59%	64%
Nurses 'Always' Communicated Well	300+	79%	76%	79%
Pain 'Always' Well Controlled	300+	69%	68%	71%
Room and Bathroom 'Always' Clean	300+	68%	68%	73%
Timely Help 'Always' Received	300+	62%	60%	68%
Would Definitely Recommend Hospital	300+	62%	66%	71%
Use of Medical Imaging				
Cardiac Imaging Stress Test before Surgery	241	4.1%	5.8%	5.3%
Combination Abdominal CT Scan	2,238	4.2%	7.4%	10.5%
Combination Brain/Sinus CT Scan	2,341	4.7%	2.8%	2.7%
Combination Chest CT Scan	1,399	2.0%	2.4%	2.7%
Follow-up Mammogram/Ultrasound	953	12.4%	12.5%	8.8%
Lumbar Spine MRI for Low Back Pain	72	33.3%	32.9%	37.2%

Overlook Medical Center

99 Beauvoir Avenue
Summit, NJ 07902
Phone: 908-522-2000
Fax: 908-273-5134
URL: www.atlantichealth.org
Type: Acute Care Hospitals
Emergency Services: Yes
Ownership: Voluntary non-profit - Other
Beds: 504

Key Personnel:
Quality Assurance . . . . Jennifer Athens
Chief of Medical Staff. . . . . Susan Cantor, MD
Pediatric Ambulatory Care . . . . . . Leonard Feid, MD
Pediatric In-Patient Care . . . . Leonard Feid, MD
CEO/President. . . . . Alan Lieber
Radiology. . . . . William Matuozzi, MD
Infection Control. . . . . Sonia McGaugh, MD
Operating Room. . . . . Dawn Petronio

Measure	Cases	This Hosp.	State Avg.	U.S. Avg.
Blood Clot Prevention and Treatment				
Anticoagulation Overlap Therapy[2]	144	97%	88%	93%
ICU Venous Thromboembolism Prophylaxis[2]	89	98%	93%	92%
Incidence of Potentially Preventable VTE[2]	33	3%	10%	10%
UFH with Dosages/Platelet Monitoring[2]	80	100%	99%	97%
Venous Thromboembolism Prophylaxis[2]	340	89%	83%	85%
Warfarin Therapy Discharge Instructions[2]	95	84%	77%	75%
Chest Pain/Possible Heart Attack Care				
Aspirin Given Within 24 Hours of Arrival[1,3]	-	-	98%	96%
Fibrinolytic Meds Within 30 Min. of Arrival[3,7]	-	-	63%	58%
Average Time to ECG (minutes)[1,3]	-	-	7	7
Average Time to Transfer (minutes)[1,3]	-	-	74	60
Children's Asthma Care				
Received Home Management Plan of Care	-	-	-	88%
Received Reliever Medication	-	-	-	100%
Received Systemic Corticosteroids	-	-	-	100%
Emergency Department				
Admittance Decision Time (minutes)[2]	465	149	148	98
Head CT Results Within 45 Min. of Arrival[1]	-	-	66%	57%
Patients Who Left ER Before Being Seen	92,424	1%	2%	2%
Time from ER Arrival to Admit. (minutes)[2]	504	372	355	274
Time from ER Arrival to Discharge (minutes)	403	151	152	134
Time in ER Before Being Evaluated (minutes)	387	32	32	26
Time to Pain Meds for Fractures (minutes)	263	64	58	57
Heart Attack Care				
Aspirin Given at Discharge	251	99%	99%	99%
Fibrinolytic Meds Within 30 Min. of Arrival[7]	-	-	69%	54%
PCI Within 90 Minutes of Arrival	44	100%	95%	96%
Statin Prescribed at Discharge	250	98%	99%	98%
Heart Failure Care				
ACE Inhibitor or ARB for LVSD[2]	92	100%	98%	97%
Discharge Instructions Given[2]	229	100%	97%	94%
Evaluation of LVS Function[2]	302	100%	100%	99%
Medicare Spending				
Medicare Spending per Patient (ratio)	-	1.05	1.07	0.98
Pneumonia Care				
Appropriate Initial Antibiotic Given[2]	94	96%	98%	95%
Blood Culture Timing[2]	164	99%	99%	98%
Pregnancy and Delivery Care				
Newborn Deliveries Scheduled Early[2]	143	0%	3%	6%
Preventive Care				
Immunization for Influenza[2]	587	95%	93%	90%
Immunization for Pneumonia[2]	513	92%	94%	92%
Stroke Care				
Anticoagulation Therapy for Atrial Fibrillation	62	95%	97%	95%
Antithrombotic Therapy Timing	267	100%	98%	98%
Assessed for Rehabilitation	428	100%	98%	97%
Discharged on Antithrombotic Therapy	311	99%	99%	99%
Discharged on Statin Medication	244	93%	95%	94%
Thrombolytic Therapy Timing	38	95%	74%	66%
Venous Thromboembolism Prophylaxis	477	98%	94%	94%
Written Stroke Educational Materials Given	204	93%	94%	88%
Surgical Care Improvement Project				
Appropriate Beta Blocker Usage[2]	109	99%	98%	98%
Appropriate VTP Within 24 Hours[2]	415	100%	99%	98%
Controlled Postoperative Blood Glucose[2,7]	-	-	97%	97%
Perioperative Temperature Management[2]	491	100%	100%	100%
Prophylactic Antibiotic Selection[2]	337	99%	99%	99%
Prophylactic Antibiotic Selection (Outpatient)	493	99%	97%	98%
Prophylactic Antibiotic Stopped[2]	330	100%	98%	98%
Prophylactic Antibiotic Timing[2]	336	100%	99%	99%
Prophylactic Antibiotic Timing (Outpatient)	493	99%	98%	98%
Urinary Catheter Removal[2]	248	100%	98%	97%
Survey of Patients' Hospital Experiences				
Area Around Room 'Always' Quiet at Night	300+	52%	53%	61%
Doctors 'Always' Communicated Well	300+	78%	77%	82%
Home Recovery Information Given	300+	80%	82%	85%
Hospital Given 9 or 10 on 10 Point Scale	300+	66%	64%	71%
Meds 'Always' Explained Before Given	300+	58%	59%	64%
Nurses 'Always' Communicated Well	300+	75%	76%	79%
Pain 'Always' Well Controlled	300+	69%	68%	71%
Room and Bathroom 'Always' Clean	300+	64%	68%	73%
Timely Help 'Always' Received	300+	59%	60%	68%
Would Definitely Recommend Hospital	300+	70%	66%	71%
Use of Medical Imaging				
Cardiac Imaging Stress Test before Surgery	1,278	5.4%	5.8%	5.3%
Combination Abdominal CT Scan	1,486	3.8%	7.4%	10.5%
Combination Brain/Sinus CT Scan	1,548	1.7%	2.8%	2.7%
Combination Chest CT Scan	1,307	2.6%	2.4%	2.7%
Follow-up Mammogram/Ultrasound	920	21.1%	12.5%	8.8%
Lumbar Spine MRI for Low Back Pain	68	32.4%	32.9%	37.2%

Holy Name Medical Center

718 Teaneck Rd
Teaneck, NJ 07666
Phone: 201-833-3000
Fax: 201-833-3230
URL: www.holyname.org
Type: Acute Care Hospitals
Emergency Services: Yes
Ownership: Voluntary non-profit - Other
Beds: 361

Key Personnel:
Pediatric Ambulatory Care . . . . . Dr. Harry Banschick
Radiology. . . . . Dr. Jacqueline Brunetti
Operating Room. . . . . Frank Chase
Pediatric In-Patient Care . . . . . . Larysa Dyrszka, MD
Chief of Medical Staff. . . . . Adam Jarrett, MD, MS, FACHE
Quality Assurance . . . . Paul Mendelowitz, MD
Emergency Room . . . . Richard Schwab, MD

NOTE: Hospital profiles are in alphabetical order by state, then city, then hospital within the city; Rankings exclude hospitals with less than 25 cases except for patient surveys which excludes hospitals with less than 100 cases; (a) 100-299 cases; (1) The number of cases/patients is too few to report; (2) Data submitted were based on a sample of cases/patients; (3) Results are based on a shorter time period than required; (4) Data suppressed by CMS for one or more quarters; (5) Results are not available for this reporting period; (6) Fewer than 100 patients completed the HCAHPS survey; (7) No cases met the criteria for this measure; (8) The lower limit of the confidence interval can not be calculated if the number of observed infections equals zero; (9) No data are available from the state/territory for this reporting period; (10) The scores shown reflect fewer than 50 completed surveys; (11) There were discrepancies in the data collection process; (12) This measure does not apply to this hospital for this reporting period; (13) Results cannot be calculated for this reporting period; (14) The results for this state are combined with nearby states to protect confidentiality; Please refer to the User's Guide for a full explanation of data.

Infection Control. . . . . Dr. Mihran Seferian

Measure	Cases	This Hosp.	State Avg.	U.S. Avg.
Blood Clot Prevention and Treatment				
Anticoagulation Overlap Therapy[2]	97	87%	88%	93%
ICU Venous Thromboembolism Prophylaxis[2]	38	92%	93%	92%
Incidence of Potentially Preventable VTE[2]	61	8%	10%	10%
UFH with Dosages/Platelet Monitoring[2]	80	100%	99%	97%
Venous Thromboembolism Prophylaxis[2]	433	77%	83%	85%
Warfarin Therapy Discharge Instructions[2]	51	100%	77%	75%
Chest Pain/Possible Heart Attack Care				
Aspirin Given Within 24 Hours of Arrival[1,3]	-	-	98%	96%
Fibrinolytic Meds Within 30 Min. of Arrival[3,7]	-	-	63%	58%
Average Time to ECG (minutes)[1,3]	-	-	7	7
Average Time to Transfer (minutes)[3,7]	-	-	74	60
Children's Asthma Care				
Received Home Management Plan of Care	-	-	-	88%
Received Reliever Medication	-	-	-	100%
Received Systemic Corticosteroids	-	-	-	100%
Emergency Department				
Admittance Decision Time (minutes)[2]	782	142	148	98
Head CT Results Within 45 Min. of Arrival[1]	-	-	66%	57%
Patients Who Left ER Before Being Seen	55,879	1%	2%	2%
Time from ER Arrival to Admit. (minutes)[2]	790	333	355	274
Time from ER Arrival to Discharge (minutes)	382	153	152	134
Time in ER Before Being Evaluated (minutes)	427	34	32	26
Time to Pain Meds for Fractures (minutes)	131	59	58	57
Heart Attack Care				
Aspirin Given at Discharge	190	100%	99%	99%
Fibrinolytic Meds Within 30 Min. of Arrival[7]	-	-	69%	54%
PCI Within 90 Minutes of Arrival	35	100%	95%	96%
Statin Prescribed at Discharge	191	100%	99%	98%
Heart Failure Care				
ACE Inhibitor or ARB for LVSD[2]	61	100%	98%	97%
Discharge Instructions Given[2]	217	100%	97%	94%
Evaluation of LVS Function[2]	316	100%	100%	99%
Medicare Spending				
Medicare Spending per Patient (ratio)	-	1.08	1.07	0.98
Pneumonia Care				
Appropriate Initial Antibiotic Given[2]	134	93%	98%	95%
Blood Culture Timing[2]	220	99%	99%	98%
Pregnancy and Delivery Care				
Newborn Deliveries Scheduled Early[2]	51	10%	3%	6%
Preventive Care				
Immunization for Influenza[2]	542	100%	93%	90%
Immunization for Pneumonia[2]	642	100%	94%	92%
Stroke Care				
Anticoagulation Therapy for Atrial Fibrillation	35	100%	97%	95%
Antithrombotic Therapy Timing	135	99%	98%	98%
Assessed for Rehabilitation	169	98%	98%	97%
Discharged on Antithrombotic Therapy	150	99%	99%	99%
Discharged on Statin Medication	125	96%	95%	94%
Thrombolytic Therapy Timing	17	94%	74%	66%
Venous Thromboembolism Prophylaxis	178	92%	94%	94%
Written Stroke Educational Materials Given	77	96%	94%	88%
Surgical Care Improvement Project				
Appropriate Beta Blocker Usage[2]	123	94%	98%	98%
Appropriate VTP Within 24 Hours[2]	389	99%	99%	98%
Controlled Postoperative Blood Glucose[2,7]	-	-	97%	97%
Perioperative Temperature Management[2]	463	100%	100%	100%
Prophylactic Antibiotic Selection[2]	311	98%	99%	99%
Prophylactic Antibiotic Selection (Outpatient)	240	98%	97%	98%
Prophylactic Antibiotic Stopped[2]	288	99%	98%	98%
Prophylactic Antibiotic Timing[2]	311	99%	99%	99%
Prophylactic Antibiotic Timing (Outpatient)	241	100%	98%	98%
Urinary Catheter Removal[2]	225	100%	98%	97%
Survey of Patients' Hospital Experiences				
Area Around Room 'Always' Quiet at Night	300+	51%	53%	61%
Doctors 'Always' Communicated Well	300+	78%	77%	82%
Home Recovery Information Given	300+	83%	82%	85%
Hospital Given 9 or 10 on 10 Point Scale	300+	68%	64%	71%
Meds 'Always' Explained Before Given	300+	58%	59%	64%
Nurses 'Always' Communicated Well	300+	74%	76%	79%
Pain 'Always' Well Controlled	300+	68%	68%	71%
Room and Bathroom 'Always' Clean	300+	68%	68%	73%
Timely Help 'Always' Received	300+	55%	60%	68%
Would Definitely Recommend Hospital	300+	71%	66%	71%
Use of Medical Imaging				
Cardiac Imaging Stress Test before Surgery	383	6.5%	5.8%	5.3%
Combination Abdominal CT Scan	1,314	7.8%	7.4%	10.5%
Combination Brain/Sinus CT Scan	869	2.1%	2.8%	2.7%
Combination Chest CT Scan	830	5.8%	2.4%	2.7%
Follow-up Mammogram/Ultrasound	1,642	45.1%	12.5%	8.8%
Lumbar Spine MRI for Low Back Pain	230	33.0%	32.9%	37.2%

Community Medical Center

99 Rt 37 West
Toms River, NJ 08755
E-mail: info@sbhcs.com
URL: www.sbhcs.com
Type: Acute Care Hospitals
Ownership: Voluntary non-profit - Private
Phone: 732-557-8000
Fax: 732-286-7066
Emergency Services: Yes
Beds: 587

Key Personnel:
Coronary Care . . . . R Saunders Craig
Chief of Medical Staff . . . . Frank Kelly, MD
Anesthesiology. . . . . Sang Kim
Operating Room. . . . . Elyce Milgazo
Emergency Room . . . . William Valfey
CEO/President. . . . . Nancy Woolen

Measure	Cases	This Hosp.	State Avg.	U.S. Avg.
Blood Clot Prevention and Treatment				
Anticoagulation Overlap Therapy[2]	198	85%	88%	93%
ICU Venous Thromboembolism Prophylaxis[2]	66	98%	93%	92%
Incidence of Potentially Preventable VTE[2]	19	5%	10%	10%
UFH with Dosages/Platelet Monitoring[2]	101	99%	99%	97%
Venous Thromboembolism Prophylaxis[2]	422	90%	83%	85%
Warfarin Therapy Discharge Instructions[2]	107	88%	77%	75%
Chest Pain/Possible Heart Attack Care				
Aspirin Given Within 24 Hours of Arrival	33	100%	98%	96%
Fibrinolytic Meds Within 30 Min. of Arrival[7]	-	-	63%	58%
Average Time to ECG (minutes)	32	8	7	7
Average Time to Transfer (minutes)	12	152	74	60
Children's Asthma Care				
Received Home Management Plan of Care	-	-	-	88%
Received Reliever Medication	-	-	-	100%
Received Systemic Corticosteroids	-	-	-	100%
Emergency Department				
Admittance Decision Time (minutes)[2]	829	162	148	98
Head CT Results Within 45 Min. of Arrival	14	79%	66%	57%
Patients Who Left ER Before Being Seen	95,465	1%	2%	2%
Time from ER Arrival to Admit. (minutes)[2]	829	442	355	274
Time from ER Arrival to Discharge (minutes)	360	158	152	134
Time in ER Before Being Evaluated (minutes)	424	50	32	26
Time to Pain Meds for Fractures (minutes)	162	82	58	57
Heart Attack Care				
Aspirin Given at Discharge[2]	235	100%	99%	99%
Fibrinolytic Meds Within 30 Min. of Arrival[2,7]	-	-	69%	54%
PCI Within 90 Minutes of Arrival[2]	46	100%	95%	96%
Statin Prescribed at Discharge[2]	206	100%	99%	98%
Heart Failure Care				
ACE Inhibitor or ARB for LVSD[2]	78	100%	98%	97%
Discharge Instructions Given[2]	192	100%	97%	94%
Evaluation of LVS Function[2]	312	100%	100%	99%
Medicare Spending				
Medicare Spending per Patient (ratio)	-	1.08	1.07	0.98
Pneumonia Care				
Appropriate Initial Antibiotic Given[2]	119	98%	98%	95%
Blood Culture Timing[2]	198	94%	99%	98%
Pregnancy and Delivery Care				
Newborn Deliveries Scheduled Early[2]	27	4%	3%	6%
Preventive Care				
Immunization for Influenza[2]	574	83%	93%	90%
Immunization for Pneumonia[2]	825	84%	94%	92%
Stroke Care				
Anticoagulation Therapy for Atrial Fibrillation	51	96%	97%	95%
Antithrombotic Therapy Timing	275	97%	98%	98%
Assessed for Rehabilitation	293	99%	98%	97%
Discharged on Antithrombotic Therapy	248	98%	99%	99%
Discharged on Statin Medication	177	93%	95%	94%
Thrombolytic Therapy Timing	11	100%	74%	66%
Venous Thromboembolism Prophylaxis	320	89%	94%	94%
Written Stroke Educational Materials Given	117	100%	94%	88%
Surgical Care Improvement Project				
Appropriate Beta Blocker Usage[2]	176	99%	98%	98%
Appropriate VTP Within 24 Hours[2]	416	100%	99%	98%
Controlled Postoperative Blood Glucose[2,7]	-	-	97%	97%
Perioperative Temperature Management[2]	481	100%	100%	100%
Prophylactic Antibiotic Selection[2]	305	100%	99%	99%
Prophylactic Antibiotic Selection (Outpatient)	468	100%	97%	98%
Prophylactic Antibiotic Stopped[2]	293	98%	98%	98%
Prophylactic Antibiotic Timing[2]	305	100%	99%	99%
Prophylactic Antibiotic Timing (Outpatient)	459	99%	98%	98%
Urinary Catheter Removal[2]	120	93%	98%	97%
Survey of Patients' Hospital Experiences				
Area Around Room 'Always' Quiet at Night	300+	48%	53%	61%
Doctors 'Always' Communicated Well	300+	76%	77%	82%
Home Recovery Information Given	300+	82%	82%	85%
Hospital Given 9 or 10 on 10 Point Scale	300+	61%	64%	71%
Meds 'Always' Explained Before Given	300+	62%	59%	64%
Nurses 'Always' Communicated Well	300+	77%	76%	79%
Pain 'Always' Well Controlled	300+	71%	68%	71%
Room and Bathroom 'Always' Clean	300+	69%	68%	73%
Timely Help 'Always' Received	300+	62%	60%	68%
Would Definitely Recommend Hospital	300+	59%	66%	71%
Use of Medical Imaging				
Cardiac Imaging Stress Test before Surgery	203	6.9%	5.8%	5.3%
Combination Abdominal CT Scan	1,549	3.4%	7.4%	10.5%
Combination Brain/Sinus CT Scan	2,215	3.0%	2.8%	2.7%
Combination Chest CT Scan	728	2.6%	2.4%	2.7%
Follow-up Mammogram/Ultrasound	1,132	15.3%	12.5%	8.8%
Lumbar Spine MRI for Low Back Pain	38	44.7%	32.9%	37.2%

Capital Health System - Fuld Campus

750 Brunswick Ave
Trenton, NJ 08638
URL: www.capitalhealth.org
Type: Acute Care Hospitals
Ownership: Voluntary non-profit - Private
Phone: 609-394-6000
Emergency Services: Yes
Beds: 589

Key Personnel:
Ambulatory Care . . . . Nathan Bosk
Cardiac Laboratory. . . . . Rita Brooks
Emergency Room . . . . Robert Fine, MD
CEO/President. . . . . Al Maghazehe, PhD, FACHE
Chief of Medical Staff . . . . Robert Remstein DO
Quality Assurance . . . . Molly Sullivan
Intensive Care Unit. . . . . Mary Wilcox
Hemotology Center . . . . Shirnett Williamson, MD

Measure	Cases	This Hosp.	State Avg.	U.S. Avg.
Blood Clot Prevention and Treatment				
Anticoagulation Overlap Therapy[2]	72	94%	88%	93%
ICU Venous Thromboembolism Prophylaxis[2]	148	99%	93%	92%
Incidence of Potentially Preventable VTE[2]	46	0%	10%	10%
UFH with Dosages/Platelet Monitoring[2]	75	100%	99%	97%
Venous Thromboembolism Prophylaxis[2]	302	94%	83%	85%
Warfarin Therapy Discharge Instructions[2]	47	72%	77%	75%
Chest Pain/Possible Heart Attack Care				
Aspirin Given Within 24 Hours of Arrival[1,3]	-	-	98%	96%
Fibrinolytic Meds Within 30 Min. of Arrival[5]	-	-	63%	58%
Average Time to ECG (minutes)[1,3]	-	-	7	7
Average Time to Transfer (minutes)[5]	-	-	74	60
Children's Asthma Care				
Received Home Management Plan of Care	-	-	-	88%
Received Reliever Medication	-	-	-	100%
Received Systemic Corticosteroids	-	-	-	100%
Emergency Department				
Admittance Decision Time (minutes)[2]	877	233	148	98
Head CT Results Within 45 Min. of Arrival[7]	-	-	66%	57%
Patients Who Left ER Before Being Seen	61,333	7%	2%	2%
Time from ER Arrival to Admit. (minutes)[2]	952	496	355	274
Time from ER Arrival to Discharge (minutes)	383	162	152	134

NOTE: Hospital profiles are in alphabetical order by state, then city, then hospital within the city; Rankings exclude hospitals with less than 25 cases except for patient surveys which excludes hospitals with less than 100 cases; (a) 100-299 cases; (1) The number of cases/patients is too few to report; (2) Data submitted were based on a sample of cases/patients; (3) Results are based on a shorter time period than required; (4) Data suppressed by CMS for one or more quarters; (5) Results are not available for this reporting period; (6) Fewer than 100 patients completed the HCAHPS survey; (7) No cases met the criteria for this measure; (8) The lower limit of the confidence interval cannot be calculated if the number of observed infections equals zero; (9) No data are available from the state/territory for this reporting period; (10) The scores shown reflect fewer than 50 completed surveys; (11) There were discrepancies in the data collection process; (12) This measure does not apply to this hospital for this reporting period; (13) Results cannot be calculated for this reporting period; (14) The results for this state are combined with nearby states to protect confidentiality; Please refer to the User's Guide for a full explanation of data.

Measure	Cases	This Hosp.	State Avg.	U.S. Avg.
Time in ER Before Being Evaluated (minutes)	432	33	32	26
Time to Pain Meds for Fractures (minutes)	65	78	58	57
Heart Attack Care				
Aspirin Given at Discharge	13	100%	99%	99%
Fibrinolytic Meds Within 30 Min. of Arrival[7]	-	-	69%	54%
PCI Within 90 Minutes of Arrival[7]		-	95%	96%
Statin Prescribed at Discharge	12	100%	99%	98%
Heart Failure Care				
ACE Inhibitor or ARB for LVSD	73	100%	98%	97%
Discharge Instructions Given	141	96%	97%	94%
Evaluation of LVS Function	187	100%	100%	99%
Medicare Spending				
Medicare Spending per Patient (ratio)	-	1.07	1.07	0.98
Pneumonia Care				
Appropriate Initial Antibiotic Given	106	98%	98%	95%
Blood Culture Timing	214	99%	99%	98%
Pregnancy and Delivery Care				
Newborn Deliveries Scheduled Early	21	0%	3%	6%
Preventive Care				
Immunization for Influenza[2]	583	95%	93%	90%
Immunization for Pneumonia[2]	673	91%	94%	92%
Stroke Care				
Anticoagulation Therapy for Atrial Fibrillation	64	97%	97%	95%
Antithrombotic Therapy Timing	310	98%	98%	98%
Assessed for Rehabilitation	529	100%	98%	97%
Discharged on Antithrombotic Therapy	343	100%	99%	99%
Discharged on Statin Medication	253	99%	95%	94%
Thrombolytic Therapy Timing	18	100%	74%	66%
Venous Thromboembolism Prophylaxis	579	100%	94%	94%
Written Stroke Educational Materials Given	200	100%	94%	88%
Surgical Care Improvement Project				
Appropriate Beta Blocker Usage[2]	51	92%	98%	98%
Appropriate VTP Within 24 Hours[2]	152	100%	99%	98%
Controlled Postoperative Blood Glucose[2,7]	-	-	97%	97%
Perioperative Temperature Management[2]	180	99%	100%	100%
Prophylactic Antibiotic Selection[2]	58	100%	99%	99%
Prophylactic Antibiotic Selection (Outpatient)	31	84%	97%	98%
Prophylactic Antibiotic Stopped[2]	56	98%	98%	98%
Prophylactic Antibiotic Timing[2]	58	100%	99%	99%
Prophylactic Antibiotic Timing (Outpatient)	38	76%	98%	98%
Urinary Catheter Removal[2]	111	95%	98%	97%
Survey of Patients' Hospital Experiences				
Area Around Room 'Always' Quiet at Night	300+	57%	53%	61%
Doctors 'Always' Communicated Well	300+	77%	77%	82%
Home Recovery Information Given	300+	81%	82%	85%
Hospital Given 9 or 10 on 10 Point Scale	300+	68%	64%	71%
Meds 'Always' Explained Before Given	300+	62%	59%	64%
Nurses 'Always' Communicated Well	300+	77%	76%	79%
Pain 'Always' Well Controlled	300+	67%	68%	71%
Room and Bathroom 'Always' Clean	300+	67%	68%	73%
Timely Help 'Always' Received	300+	61%	60%	68%
Would Definitely Recommend Hospital	300+	72%	66%	71%
Use of Medical Imaging				
Cardiac Imaging Stress Test before Surgery	175	3.4%	5.8%	5.3%
Combination Abdominal CT Scan	550	4.5%	7.4%	10.5%
Combination Brain/Sinus CT Scan	654	5.4%	2.8%	2.7%
Combination Chest CT Scan	355	2.5%	2.4%	2.7%
Follow-up Mammogram/Ultrasound	281	8.2%	12.5%	8.8%
Lumbar Spine MRI for Low Back Pain[1]	-	-	32.9%	37.2%

Saint Francis Medical Center

601 Hamilton Ave — Phone: 609-599-5000
Trenton, NJ 08629 — Fax: 609-599-6257
E-mail: info@stfrancismedical.com
URL: www.stfrancismedical.com
Type: Acute Care Hospitals — Emergency Services: Yes
Ownership: Voluntary non-profit - Private — Beds: 274

Key Personnel:
Operating Room. . . . . Claude Abouchedid, RN
Radiology. . . . . Eric Bosworth
CEO/President. . . . . Gerard J Jablonowski
Emergency Room . . . . Steven Katz, MD
Anesthesiology. . . . . Perry Loesberg, MD
Chief of Medical Staff. . . . . C James Romano, MD
Infection Control. . . . . Eileen Taylor
Quality Assurance . . . . Kathleen Vaccaro

Measure	Cases	This Hosp.	State Avg.	U.S. Avg.
Blood Clot Prevention and Treatment				
Anticoagulation Overlap Therapy[2]	42	98%	88%	93%
ICU Venous Thromboembolism Prophylaxis[2]	118	97%	93%	92%
Incidence of Potentially Preventable VTE[1,2]	-	-	10%	10%
UFH with Dosages/Platelet Monitoring[2]	42	100%	99%	97%
Venous Thromboembolism Prophylaxis[2]	309	92%	83%	85%
Warfarin Therapy Discharge Instructions[2]	31	100%	77%	75%
Chest Pain/Possible Heart Attack Care				
Aspirin Given Within 24 Hours of Arrival[5]	-	-	98%	96%
Fibrinolytic Meds Within 30 Min. of Arrival[5]	-	-	63%	58%
Average Time to ECG (minutes)[5]	-	-	7	7
Average Time to Transfer (minutes)[5]	-	-	74	60
Children's Asthma Care				
Received Home Management Plan of Care	-	-	-	88%
Received Reliever Medication	-	-	-	100%
Received Systemic Corticosteroids	-	-	-	100%
Emergency Department				
Admittance Decision Time (minutes)[2]	660	80	148	98
Head CT Results Within 45 Min. of Arrival[5]	-	-	66%	57%
Patients Who Left ER Before Being Seen	35,589	4%	2%	2%
Time from ER Arrival to Admit. (minutes)[2]	662	288	355	274
Time from ER Arrival to Discharge (minutes)	360	147	152	134
Time in ER Before Being Evaluated (minutes)	389	26	32	26
Time to Pain Meds for Fractures (minutes)	88	58	58	57
Heart Attack Care				
Aspirin Given at Discharge	291	99%	99%	99%
Fibrinolytic Meds Within 30 Min. of Arrival[7]	-	-	69%	54%
PCI Within 90 Minutes of Arrival	28	93%	95%	96%
Statin Prescribed at Discharge	281	100%	99%	98%
Heart Failure Care				
ACE Inhibitor or ARB for LVSD	67	100%	98%	97%
Discharge Instructions Given	142	100%	97%	94%
Evaluation of LVS Function	186	100%	100%	99%
Medicare Spending				
Medicare Spending per Patient (ratio)	-	1.11	1.07	0.98
Pneumonia Care				
Appropriate Initial Antibiotic Given	71	100%	98%	95%
Blood Culture Timing	121	100%	99%	98%
Pregnancy and Delivery Care				
Newborn Deliveries Scheduled Early[7]	-	-	3%	6%
Preventive Care				
Immunization for Influenza[2]	470	96%	93%	90%
Immunization for Pneumonia[2]	646	97%	94%	92%
Stroke Care				
Anticoagulation Therapy for Atrial Fibrillation[7]	-	-	97%	95%
Antithrombotic Therapy Timing	29	100%	98%	98%
Assessed for Rehabilitation	43	98%	98%	97%
Discharged on Antithrombotic Therapy	38	100%	99%	99%
Discharged on Statin Medication	33	97%	95%	94%
Thrombolytic Therapy Timing[7]	-	-	74%	66%
Venous Thromboembolism Prophylaxis	40	95%	94%	94%
Written Stroke Educational Materials Given	25	100%	94%	88%
Surgical Care Improvement Project				
Appropriate Beta Blocker Usage	97	100%	98%	98%
Appropriate VTP Within 24 Hours	128	99%	99%	98%
Controlled Postoperative Blood Glucose	85	96%	97%	97%
Perioperative Temperature Management	160	100%	100%	100%
Prophylactic Antibiotic Selection	125	99%	99%	99%
Prophylactic Antibiotic Selection (Outpatient)	261	99%	97%	98%
Prophylactic Antibiotic Stopped	115	100%	98%	98%
Prophylactic Antibiotic Timing	125	100%	99%	99%
Prophylactic Antibiotic Timing (Outpatient)	260	99%	98%	98%
Urinary Catheter Removal	110	100%	98%	97%
Survey of Patients' Hospital Experiences				
Area Around Room 'Always' Quiet at Night	300+	48%	53%	61%
Doctors 'Always' Communicated Well	300+	75%	77%	82%
Home Recovery Information Given	300+	86%	82%	85%
Hospital Given 9 or 10 on 10 Point Scale	300+	58%	64%	71%
Meds 'Always' Explained Before Given	300+	60%	59%	64%
Nurses 'Always' Communicated Well	300+	76%	76%	79%
Pain 'Always' Well Controlled	300+	70%	68%	71%
Room and Bathroom 'Always' Clean	300+	68%	68%	73%
Timely Help 'Always' Received	300+	57%	60%	68%
Would Definitely Recommend Hospital	300+	58%	66%	71%
Use of Medical Imaging				
Cardiac Imaging Stress Test before Surgery	75	1.3%	5.8%	5.3%
Combination Abdominal CT Scan	304	6.9%	7.4%	10.5%
Combination Brain/Sinus CT Scan	415	5.8%	2.8%	2.7%
Combination Chest CT Scan	153	8.5%	2.4%	2.7%
Follow-up Mammogram/Ultrasound	367	10.4%	12.5%	8.8%
Lumbar Spine MRI for Low Back Pain[1]	-	-	32.9%	37.2%

Inspira Medical Center Vineland

1505 W Sherman Ave — Phone: 856-641-6610
Vineland, NJ 08360 — Fax: 856-451-6998
URL: www.sjhs.com
Type: Acute Care Hospitals — Emergency Services: Yes
Ownership: Voluntary non-profit - Private — Beds: 262

Key Personnel:
CEO/President. . . . . John A. DiAngelo
Chief of Medical Staff. . . . . Steven Linn

Measure	Cases	This Hosp.	State Avg.	U.S. Avg.
Blood Clot Prevention and Treatment				
Anticoagulation Overlap Therapy[2]	78	96%	88%	93%
ICU Venous Thromboembolism Prophylaxis[2]	113	97%	93%	92%
Incidence of Potentially Preventable VTE[1,2]	-	-	10%	10%
UFH with Dosages/Platelet Monitoring[2]	74	99%	99%	97%
Venous Thromboembolism Prophylaxis[2]	379	93%	83%	85%
Warfarin Therapy Discharge Instructions[2]	58	86%	77%	75%
Chest Pain/Possible Heart Attack Care				
Aspirin Given Within 24 Hours of Arrival	152	99%	98%	96%
Fibrinolytic Meds Within 30 Min. of Arrival	13	69%	63%	58%
Average Time to ECG (minutes)	154	6	7	7
Average Time to Transfer (minutes)	25	69	74	60
Children's Asthma Care				
Received Home Management Plan of Care	-	-	-	88%
Received Reliever Medication	-	-	-	100%
Received Systemic Corticosteroids	-	-	-	100%
Emergency Department				
Admittance Decision Time (minutes)[2]	655	120	148	98
Head CT Results Within 45 Min. of Arrival	40	80%	66%	57%
Patients Who Left ER Before Being Seen	92,479	4%	2%	2%
Time from ER Arrival to Admit. (minutes)[2]	657	357	355	274
Time from ER Arrival to Discharge (minutes)	948	138	152	134
Time in ER Before Being Evaluated (minutes)	1,037	26	32	26
Time to Pain Meds for Fractures (minutes)	203	56	58	57
Heart Attack Care				
Aspirin Given at Discharge	47	100%	99%	99%
Fibrinolytic Meds Within 30 Min. of Arrival[7]	-	-	69%	54%
PCI Within 90 Minutes of Arrival[7]	-	-	95%	96%
Statin Prescribed at Discharge	48	92%	99%	98%
Heart Failure Care				
ACE Inhibitor or ARB for LVSD[2]	88	98%	98%	97%
Discharge Instructions Given[2]	201	100%	97%	94%
Evaluation of LVS Function[2]	261	100%	100%	99%
Medicare Spending				
Medicare Spending per Patient (ratio)	-	1.05	1.07	0.98
Pneumonia Care				
Appropriate Initial Antibiotic Given[2]	48	100%	98%	95%
Blood Culture Timing[2]	144	99%	99%	98%
Pregnancy and Delivery Care				
Newborn Deliveries Scheduled Early[2]	63	2%	3%	6%
Preventive Care				
Immunization for Influenza[2]	495	93%	93%	90%
Immunization for Pneumonia[2]	552	96%	94%	92%
Stroke Care				
Anticoagulation Therapy for Atrial Fibrillation[1,2]	-	-	97%	95%
Antithrombotic Therapy Timing[2]	98	98%	98%	98%
Assessed for Rehabilitation[2]	93	97%	98%	97%
Discharged on Antithrombotic Therapy[2]	88	99%	99%	99%
Discharged on Statin Medication[2]	79	96%	95%	94%
Thrombolytic Therapy Timing[1,2]	-	-	74%	66%
Venous Thromboembolism Prophylaxis[2]	109	94%	94%	94%
Written Stroke Educational Materials Given[2]	44	86%	94%	88%

NOTE: Hospital profiles are in alphabetical order by state, then city, then hospital within the city; Rankings exclude hospitals with less than 25 cases except for patient surveys which excludes hospitals with less than 100 cases; (a) 100-299 cases; (1) The number of cases/patients is too few to report; (2) Data submitted were based on a sample of cases/patients; (3) Results are based on a shorter time period than required; (4) Data suppressed by CMS for one or more quarters; (5) Results are not available for this reporting period; (6) Fewer than 100 patients completed the HCAHPS survey; (7) No cases met the criteria for this measure; (8) The lower limit of the confidence interval cannot be calculated if the number of observed infections equals zero; (9) No data are available from the state/territory for this reporting period; (10) The scores shown reflect fewer than 50 completed surveys; (11) There were discrepancies in the data collection process; (12) This measure does not apply to this hospital for this reporting period; (13) Results cannot be calculated for this reporting period; (14) The results for this state are combined with nearby states to protect confidentiality; Please refer to the User's Guide for a full explanation of data.

Surgical Care Improvement Project				
Appropriate Beta Blocker Usage[2]	119	97%	98%	98%
Appropriate VTP Within 24 Hours[2]	286	100%	99%	98%
Controlled Postoperative Blood Glucose[2,7]	-	-	97%	97%
Perioperative Temperature Management[2]	345	98%	100%	100%
Prophylactic Antibiotic Selection[2]	224	99%	99%	99%
Prophylactic Antibiotic Selection (Outpatient)	324	97%	97%	98%
Prophylactic Antibiotic Stopped[2]	214	96%	98%	98%
Prophylactic Antibiotic Timing[2]	224	99%	99%	99%
Prophylactic Antibiotic Timing (Outpatient)	326	99%	98%	98%
Urinary Catheter Removal[2]	183	99%	98%	97%
Survey of Patients' Hospital Experiences				
Area Around Room 'Always' Quiet at Night	300+	54%	53%	61%
Doctors 'Always' Communicated Well	300+	76%	77%	82%
Home Recovery Information Given	300+	85%	82%	85%
Hospital Given 9 or 10 on 10 Point Scale	300+	60%	64%	71%
Meds 'Always' Explained Before Given	300+	59%	59%	64%
Nurses 'Always' Communicated Well	300+	74%	76%	79%
Pain 'Always' Well Controlled	300+	65%	68%	71%
Room and Bathroom 'Always' Clean	300+	71%	68%	73%
Timely Help 'Always' Received	300+	61%	60%	68%
Would Definitely Recommend Hospital	300+	56%	66%	71%
Use of Medical Imaging				
Cardiac Imaging Stress Test before Surgery	192	5.7%	5.8%	5.3%
Combination Abdominal CT Scan	1,113	7.2%	7.4%	10.5%
Combination Brain/Sinus CT Scan	1,285	2.5%	2.8%	2.7%
Combination Chest CT Scan	641	0.9%	2.4%	2.7%
Follow-up Mammogram/Ultrasound	1,762	11.1%	12.5%	8.8%
Lumbar Spine MRI for Low Back Pain	128	30.5%	32.9%	37.2%

Lourdes Medical Center of Burlington County

218a Sunset Road
Willingboro, NJ 08046
Phone: 609-835-2900
Fax: 865-635-2493
E-mail: info@lourdesnet.org
URL: www.lourdesnet.org/lourdes
Type: Acute Care Hospitals
Emergency Services: Yes
Ownership: Voluntary non-profit - Private
Beds: 410

Key Personnel:
Quality Assurance . . . . Ruthann Enriques
Pediatric Ambulatory Care . . . . . . Gerald Fendrick, MD
Pediatric In-Patient Care . . . . Gerald Fendrick, MD
CEO/President. . . . . Alexander J. Hatala
Coronary Care . . . . Marianne Kraemer
Infection Control. . . . . Peggy McDermott
Chief of Medical Staff . . . . Alan Pope, MD
Radiology. . . . . Daniel Scott, MD

Measure	Cases	This Hosp.	State Avg.	U.S. Avg.
Blood Clot Prevention and Treatment				
Anticoagulation Overlap Therapy[2]	66	89%	88%	93%
ICU Venous Thromboembolism Prophylaxis[2]	108	85%	93%	92%
Incidence of Potentially Preventable VTE[2]	19	11%	10%	10%
UFH with Dosages/Platelet Monitoring[2]	54	100%	99%	97%
Venous Thromboembolism Prophylaxis[2]	301	66%	83%	85%
Warfarin Therapy Discharge Instructions[2]	47	70%	77%	75%
Chest Pain/Possible Heart Attack Care				
Aspirin Given Within 24 Hours of Arrival	661	98%	98%	96%
Fibrinolytic Meds Within 30 Min. of Arrival[1]	-	-	63%	58%
Average Time to ECG (minutes)	682	7	7	7
Average Time to Transfer (minutes)	30	66	74	60
Children's Asthma Care				
Received Home Management Plan of Care	-	-	-	88%
Received Reliever Medication	-	-	-	100%
Received Systemic Corticosteroids	-	-	-	100%
Emergency Department				
Admittance Decision Time (minutes)[2]	1,026	181	148	98
Head CT Results Within 45 Min. of Arrival	43	65%	66%	57%
Patients Who Left ER Before Being Seen	68,134	1%	2%	2%
Time from ER Arrival to Admit. (minutes)[2]	1,028	364	355	274
Time from ER Arrival to Discharge (minutes)	372	108	152	134
Time in ER Before Being Evaluated (minutes)	426	18	32	26
Time to Pain Meds for Fractures (minutes)	143	52	58	57
Heart Attack Care				
Aspirin Given at Discharge	18	100%	99%	99%
Fibrinolytic Meds Within 30 Min. of Arrival[7]	-	-	69%	54%
PCI Within 90 Minutes of Arrival[7]	-	-	95%	96%
Statin Prescribed at Discharge	17	100%	99%	98%
Heart Failure Care				
ACE Inhibitor or ARB for LVSD[2]	44	98%	98%	97%
Discharge Instructions Given[2]	164	95%	97%	94%
Evaluation of LVS Function[2]	205	100%	100%	99%
Medicare Spending				
Medicare Spending per Patient (ratio)	-	1.03	1.07	0.98
Pneumonia Care				
Appropriate Initial Antibiotic Given[2]	89	98%	98%	95%
Blood Culture Timing[2]	164	100%	99%	98%
Pregnancy and Delivery Care				
Newborn Deliveries Scheduled Early[7]	-	-	3%	6%
Preventive Care				
Immunization for Influenza[2]	583	97%	93%	90%
Immunization for Pneumonia[2]	797	89%	94%	92%
Stroke Care				
Anticoagulation Therapy for Atrial Fibrillation[1]	-	-	97%	95%
Antithrombotic Therapy Timing	57	95%	98%	98%
Assessed for Rehabilitation	57	96%	98%	97%
Discharged on Antithrombotic Therapy	56	100%	99%	99%
Discharged on Statin Medication	47	96%	95%	94%
Thrombolytic Therapy Timing[1]	-	-	74%	66%
Venous Thromboembolism Prophylaxis	56	73%	94%	94%
Written Stroke Educational Materials Given	26	100%	94%	88%
Surgical Care Improvement Project				
Appropriate Beta Blocker Usage[2]	72	99%	98%	98%
Appropriate VTP Within 24 Hours[2]	200	99%	99%	98%
Controlled Postoperative Blood Glucose[2,7]	-	-	97%	97%
Perioperative Temperature Management[2]	240	100%	100%	100%
Prophylactic Antibiotic Selection[2]	119	100%	99%	99%
Prophylactic Antibiotic Selection (Outpatient)	42	90%	97%	98%
Prophylactic Antibiotic Stopped[2]	119	99%	98%	98%
Prophylactic Antibiotic Timing[2]	119	100%	99%	99%
Prophylactic Antibiotic Timing (Outpatient)	42	100%	98%	98%
Urinary Catheter Removal[2]	131	97%	98%	97%
Survey of Patients' Hospital Experiences				
Area Around Room 'Always' Quiet at Night	300+	47%	53%	61%
Doctors 'Always' Communicated Well	300+	68%	77%	82%
Home Recovery Information Given	300+	79%	82%	85%
Hospital Given 9 or 10 on 10 Point Scale	300+	46%	64%	71%
Meds 'Always' Explained Before Given	300+	56%	59%	64%
Nurses 'Always' Communicated Well	300+	68%	76%	79%
Pain 'Always' Well Controlled	300+	63%	68%	71%
Room and Bathroom 'Always' Clean	300+	62%	68%	73%
Timely Help 'Always' Received	300+	57%	60%	68%
Would Definitely Recommend Hospital	300+	45%	66%	71%
Use of Medical Imaging				
Cardiac Imaging Stress Test before Surgery	121	5.0%	5.8%	5.3%
Combination Abdominal CT Scan	747	3.2%	7.4%	10.5%
Combination Brain/Sinus CT Scan	1,160	2.3%	2.8%	2.7%
Combination Chest CT Scan	277	0.7%	2.4%	2.7%
Follow-up Mammogram/Ultrasound	477	10.1%	12.5%	8.8%
Lumbar Spine MRI for Low Back Pain[1]	-	-	32.9%	37.2%

Inspira Medical Center Woodbury

509 N Broad St
Woodbury, NJ 08096
Phone: 856-845-0100
Fax: 856-251-0383
E-mail: humanresources@umhospital.org.
URL: www.umhospital.org
Type: Acute Care Hospitals
Emergency Services: Yes
Ownership: Voluntary non-profit - Private
Beds: 305

Key Personnel:
Chief of Medical Staff . . . . Jeffrey Bittner, MD
CEO/President. . . . . Eileen K Cardile, RN, MS, CAN
Pediatric In-Patient Care . . . . Lawrence Epple, MD
Quality Assurance . . . . Marla Maybrook
Operating Room. . . . . Cindy Quint, RN
Intensive Care Unit. . . . . Dennis Sacter
Infection Control. . . . . Paula Simplot
Radiology. . . . . Mary Welch

Measure	Cases	This Hosp.	State Avg.	U.S. Avg.
Blood Clot Prevention and Treatment				
Anticoagulation Overlap Therapy[2]	66	76%	88%	93%
ICU Venous Thromboembolism Prophylaxis[2]	61	95%	93%	92%
Incidence of Potentially Preventable VTE[1,2]	-	-	10%	10%
UFH with Dosages/Platelet Monitoring[2]	33	100%	99%	97%
Venous Thromboembolism Prophylaxis[2]	391	94%	83%	85%
Warfarin Therapy Discharge Instructions[2]	45	100%	77%	75%
Chest Pain/Possible Heart Attack Care				
Aspirin Given Within 24 Hours of Arrival[1]	-	-	98%	96%
Fibrinolytic Meds Within 30 Min. of Arrival[5]	-	-	63%	58%
Average Time to ECG (minutes)[1]	-	-	7	7
Average Time to Transfer (minutes)[5]	-	-	74	60
Children's Asthma Care				
Received Home Management Plan of Care	-	-	-	88%
Received Reliever Medication	-	-	-	100%
Received Systemic Corticosteroids	-	-	-	100%
Emergency Department				
Admittance Decision Time (minutes)[2]	932	82	148	98
Head CT Results Within 45 Min. of Arrival	32	91%	66%	57%
Patients Who Left ER Before Being Seen	59,663	2%	2%	2%
Time from ER Arrival to Admit. (minutes)[2]	932	347	355	274
Time from ER Arrival to Discharge (minutes)	390	176	152	134
Time in ER Before Being Evaluated (minutes)	429	32	32	26
Time to Pain Meds for Fractures (minutes)	132	62	58	57
Heart Attack Care				
Aspirin Given at Discharge	143	100%	99%	99%
Fibrinolytic Meds Within 30 Min. of Arrival[1]	-	-	69%	54%
PCI Within 90 Minutes of Arrival	68	99%	95%	96%
Statin Prescribed at Discharge	141	100%	99%	98%
Heart Failure Care				
ACE Inhibitor or ARB for LVSD	94	100%	98%	97%
Discharge Instructions Given	311	100%	97%	94%
Evaluation of LVS Function	383	100%	100%	99%
Medicare Spending				
Medicare Spending per Patient (ratio)	-	1.02	1.07	0.98
Pneumonia Care				
Appropriate Initial Antibiotic Given	197	99%	98%	95%
Blood Culture Timing	361	98%	99%	98%
Pregnancy and Delivery Care				
Newborn Deliveries Scheduled Early[2]	21	5%	3%	6%
Preventive Care				
Immunization for Influenza[2]	561	98%	93%	90%
Immunization for Pneumonia[2]	723	99%	94%	92%
Stroke Care				
Anticoagulation Therapy for Atrial Fibrillation	13	92%	97%	95%
Antithrombotic Therapy Timing	126	99%	98%	98%
Assessed for Rehabilitation	123	98%	98%	97%
Discharged on Antithrombotic Therapy	119	98%	99%	99%
Discharged on Statin Medication	97	96%	95%	94%
Thrombolytic Therapy Timing[1]	-	-	74%	66%
Venous Thromboembolism Prophylaxis	130	95%	94%	94%
Written Stroke Educational Materials Given	78	92%	94%	88%
Surgical Care Improvement Project				
Appropriate Beta Blocker Usage	169	99%	98%	98%
Appropriate VTP Within 24 Hours	432	99%	99%	98%
Controlled Postoperative Blood Glucose[7]	-	-	97%	97%
Perioperative Temperature Management	525	100%	100%	100%
Prophylactic Antibiotic Selection	291	99%	99%	99%
Prophylactic Antibiotic Selection (Outpatient)	84	90%	97%	98%
Prophylactic Antibiotic Stopped	284	98%	98%	98%
Prophylactic Antibiotic Timing	291	99%	99%	99%
Prophylactic Antibiotic Timing (Outpatient)	84	95%	98%	98%
Urinary Catheter Removal	90	100%	98%	97%
Survey of Patients' Hospital Experiences				
Area Around Room 'Always' Quiet at Night	300+	49%	53%	61%
Doctors 'Always' Communicated Well	300+	78%	77%	82%
Home Recovery Information Given	300+	80%	82%	85%
Hospital Given 9 or 10 on 10 Point Scale	300+	60%	64%	71%
Meds 'Always' Explained Before Given	300+	62%	59%	64%
Nurses 'Always' Communicated Well	300+	80%	76%	79%
Pain 'Always' Well Controlled	300+	71%	68%	71%
Room and Bathroom 'Always' Clean	300+	68%	68%	73%
Timely Help 'Always' Received	300+	68%	60%	68%
Would Definitely Recommend Hospital	300+	59%	66%	71%

NOTE: Hospital profiles are in alphabetical order by state, then city, then hospital within the city; Rankings exclude hospitals with less than 25 cases except for patient surveys which excludes hospitals with less than 100 cases; (a) 100-299 cases; (1) The number of cases/patients is too few to report; (2) Data submitted were based on a sample of cases/patients; (3) Results are based on a shorter time period than required; (4) Data suppressed by CMS for one or more quarters; (5) Results are not available for this reporting period; (6) Fewer than 100 patients completed the HCAHPS survey; (7) No cases met the criteria for this measure; (8) The lower limit of the confidence interval cannot be calculated if the number of observed infections equals zero; (9) No data are available from the state/territory for this reporting period; (10) The scores shown reflect fewer than 50 completed surveys; (11) There were discrepancies in the data collection process; (12) This measure does not apply to this hospital for this reporting period; (13) Results cannot be calculated for this reporting period; (14) The results for this state are combined with nearby states to protect confidentiality; Please refer to the User's Guide for a full explanation of data.

Use of Medical Imaging				
Cardiac Imaging Stress Test before Surgery	539	5.6%	5.8%	5.3%
Combination Abdominal CT Scan[1]	-	-	7.4%	10.5%
Combination Brain/Sinus CT Scan	1,039	2.3%	2.8%	2.7%
Combination Chest CT Scan	260	5.0%	2.4%	2.7%
Follow-up Mammogram/Ultrasound	244	14.3%	12.5%	8.8%
Lumbar Spine MRI for Low Back Pain[1]	-	-	32.9%	37.2%

NOTE: Hospital profiles are in alphabetical order by state, then city, then hospital within the city; Rankings exclude hospitals with less than 25 cases except for patient surveys which excludes hospitals with less than 100 cases; (a) 100-299 cases; (1) The number of cases/patients is too few to report; (2) Data submitted were based on a sample of cases/patients; (3) Results are based on a shorter time period than required; (4) Data suppressed by CMS for one or more quarters; (5) Results are not available for this reporting period; (6) Fewer than 100 patients completed the HCAHPS survey; (7) No cases met the criteria for this measure; (8) The lower limit of the confidence interval cannot be calculated if the number of observed infections equals zero; (9) No data are available from the state/territory for this reporting period; (10) The scores shown reflect fewer than 50 completed surveys; (11) There were discrepancies in the data collection process; (12) This measure does not apply to this hospital for this reporting period; (13) Results cannot be calculated for this reporting period; (14) The results for this state are combined with nearby states to protect confidentiality; Please refer to the User's Guide for a full explanation of data.

Blood Clot Prevention and Treatment

Anticoagulation Overlap Therapy

Hospital Name	City	Rate	Cases
Brooklyn Hosp Ctr at Downtown Campus[2]	Brooklyn	100%	94
Elmhurst Hospital Center[2]	Elmhurst	100%	36
F F Thompson Hospital[2]	Canandaigua	100%	35
Flushing Hospital Medical Center[2]	Flushing	100%	36
Glens Falls Hospital[2]	Glens Falls	100%	76
Hospital For Special Surgery[2]	New York	100%	37
Kenmore Mercy Hospital[2]	Kenmore	100%	73
Mary Imogene Bassett Hospital[2]	Cooperstown	100%	61
Northern Dutchess Hospital[2]	Rhinebeck	100%	26
Northern Westchester Hospital[2]	Mount Kisco	100%	30
Nyack Hospital[2]	Nyack	100%	47
NYU Hospitals Center[2]	New York	100%	94
Our Lady of Lourdes Memorial Hospital[2]	Binghamton	100%	62
Putnam Hospital Center[2]	Carmel	100%	34
Saint Charles Hospital[2]	Port Jefferson	100%	41
Saint Francis Hospital[2]	Poughkeepsie	100%	51
St John's Episcopal Hosp-South Shore[2]	Far Rockaway	100%	73
Saint Joseph Hospital[2]	Bethpage	100%	45
Saint Mary's Hospital at Amsterdam[2]	Amsterdam	100%	48
Sisters of Charity Hospital[2]	Buffalo	100%	143
Mercy Hospital[2]	Buffalo	99%	173
Saint Peter's Hospital[2]	Albany	99%	165
Westchester Medical Center[2]	Valhalla	99%	94
Arnot Ogden Medical Center[2]	Elmira	98%	55
Columbia Memorial Hospital[2]	Hudson	98%	41
Coney Island Hospital[2]	Brooklyn	98%	41
Cortland Regional Medical Center[2]	Cortland	98%	54
Good Samaritan Hospital of Suffern[2]	Suffern	98%	64
Highland Hospital[2]	Rochester	98%	98
Lincoln Medical & Mental Health Center[2]	Bronx	98%	58
Rochester General Hospital[2]	Rochester	98%	232
Staten Island University Hospital[2]	Staten Island	98%	204
White Plains Hospital Center[2]	White Plains	98%	127
Good Samaritan Hospital Medical Center[2]	West Islip	97%	168
Harlem Hospital Center[2]	New York	97%	38
Montefiore New Rochelle Hospital[2]	New Rochelle	97%	33
New York Community Hospital of Brooklyn[2]	Brooklyn	97%	29
Richmond University Medical Center[2]	Staten Island	97%	36
Saint Luke's Cornwall Hospital[2]	Newburgh	97%	75
Woodhull Medical & Mental Health Center[2]	Brooklyn	97%	29
Bellevue Hospital Center[2]	New York	96%	73
Cayuga Medical Center at Ithaca[2]	Ithaca	96%	47
Nathan Littauer Hospital[2]	Gloversville	96%	26
Saint Barnabas Hospital[2]	Bronx	96%	54
Univ Hosp SUNY Health Science Ctr[2]	Syracuse	96%	186
Faxton - Saint Luke's Healthcare[2]	Utica	95%	44
John T Mather Mem Hosp-Port Jefferson[2]	Port Jefferson	95%	95
Kaleida Health[2]	Buffalo	95%	308
New York Methodist Hospital[2]	Brooklyn	95%	197
Saint Catherine of Siena Hospital[2]	Smithtown	95%	80
Winthrop - University Hospital[2]	Mineola	95%	143
Champlain Valley Phys Hosp Med Ctr[2]	Plattsburgh	94%	86
Ellis Hospital[2]	Schenectady	94%	102
Maimonides Medical Center[2]	Brooklyn	94%	101
New York - Presbyterian Hospital[2]	New York	94%	395
Samaritan Hospital[2]	Troy	94%	33
Saratoga Hospital[2]	Saratoga Spgs	94%	71
Unity Hospital of Rochester[2]	Rochester	94%	120
Brookhaven Mem Hosp Med Ctr[2]	Patchogue	93%	115
Geneva General Hospital[2]	Geneva	93%	27
Huntington Hospital[2]	Huntington	93%	99
Orange Regional Medical Center[2]	Middletown	93%	132
United Health Services Hospitals[2]	Johnson City	93%	108
University Hospital - Stony Brook[2]	Stony Brook	93%	187
Bronx - Lebanon Hospital Center[2]	Bronx	92%	78
Corning Hospital[2]	Corning	92%	40
Forest Hills Hospital[2]	Forest Hills	92%	76
Jacobi Medical Center[2]	Bronx	92%	80
Mount Sinai Hospital[2]	New York	92%	319
Rome Memorial Hospital[2]	Rome	92%	36
Saint Joseph's Medical Center[2]	Yonkers	92%	26
Health Alliance Hospital Broadway Campus[2]	Kingston	91%	58
Albany Memorial Hospital[2]	Albany	90%	29
Crouse Hospital[2]	Syracuse	90%	97
Lawrence Hospital Center[2]	Bronxville	90%	81
North Shore University Hospital[2]	Manhasset	90%	271
Queens Hospital Center[2]	Jamaica	90%	67
South Nassau Communities Hospital[2]	Oceanside	90%	138
Vassar Brothers Medical Center[2]	Poughkeepsie	90%	98
Mercy Medical Center[2]	Rockville Centre	89%	65
Mount St Mary's Hosp & Health Ctr[2]	Lewiston	89%	37
Newark - Wayne Community Hospital[2]	Newark	89%	28
Saint Elizabeth Medical Center[2]	Utica	89%	56
Samaritan Medical Center[2]	Watertown	89%	47
Kingsbrook Jewish Medical Center[2]	Brooklyn	88%	49
Nassau University Medical Center[2]	East Meadow	88%	52
Olean General Hospital[2]	Olean	88%	56
Univ Hosp of Brooklyn-Downstate[2]	Brooklyn	88%	96
Erie County Medical Center[2]	Buffalo	87%	53
Saint Luke's Roosevelt Hospital[2]	New York	87%	218
Beth Israel Medical Center[2]	New York	86%	253
Kings County Hospital Center[2]	Brooklyn	86%	125
Long Island Jewish Medical Center[2]	New Hyde Park	86%	239
Wyckoff Heights Medical Center[2]	Brooklyn	86%	73
Hudson Valley Hospital Center[2]	Cortlandt Manor	85%	46
Lutheran Medical Center[2]	Brooklyn	85%	94
Saint Joseph's Hospital Health Center[2]	Syracuse	85%	211
Southampton Hospital[2]	Southampton	85%	27
Albany Medical Center Hospital[2]	Albany	84%	86
Montefiore Medical Center[2]	Bronx	84%	411
Jamaica Hospital Medical Center[2]	Jamaica	82%	65
New York Hosp Med Ctr of Queens[2]	Flushing	82%	173
Oneida Healthcare Center[2]	Oneida	82%	28
Peconic Bay Medical Center[2]	Riverhead	82%	44
Plainview Hospital[2]	Plainview	80%	92
Strong Memorial Hospital[2]	Rochester	80%	122
Glen Cove Hospital[2]	Glen Cove	79%	47
Lenox Hill Hospital[2]	New York	79%	192
Southside Hospital[2]	Bay Shore	79%	125
Woman's Christian Association[2]	Jamestown	79%	33
Saint John's Riverside Hospital[2]	Yonkers	73%	78
Saint Francis Hospital - Roslyn[2]	Roslyn	70%	92
Brookdale Hospital Medical Center[2]	Brooklyn	69%	52
Franklin Hospital[2]	Valley Stream	63%	63
Eastern Niagara Hospital[2]	Lockport	51%	41

ICU Venous Thromboembolism Prophylaxis

Hospital Name	City	Rate	Cases
Bellevue Hospital Center[2]	New York	100%	33
Chenango Memorial Hospital[2]	Norwich	100%	87
Columbia Memorial Hospital[2]	Hudson	100%	72
Coney Island Hospital[2]	Brooklyn	100%	56
Cortland Regional Medical Center[2]	Cortland	100%	76
Crouse Hospital[2]	Syracuse	100%	31
Glens Falls Hospital[2]	Glens Falls	100%	56
Jacobi Medical Center[2]	Bronx	100%	69
Lincoln Medical & Mental Health Center[2]	Bronx	100%	64
Lutheran Medical Center[2]	Brooklyn	100%	54
New York - Presbyterian Hospital[2]	New York	100%	63
New York Methodist Hospital[2]	Brooklyn	100%	44
North Central Bronx Hospital[2]	Bronx	100%	50
NYU Hospitals Center[2]	New York	100%	53
Oneida Healthcare Center[2]	Oneida	100%	58
Rochester General Hospital[2]	Rochester	100%	48
Saint Joseph Hospital[2]	Bethpage	100%	82
Saint Luke's Roosevelt Hospital[2]	New York	100%	38
South Nassau Communities Hospital[2]	Oceanside	100%	25
Woodhull Medical & Mental Health Center[2]	Brooklyn	100%	39
Auburn Community Hospital[2]	Auburn	99%	101
Bronx - Lebanon Hospital Center[2]	Bronx	99%	99
Faxton - Saint Luke's Healthcare[2]	Utica	99%	70
Kenmore Mercy Hospital[2]	Kenmore	99%	69
Lewis County General Hospital[2]	Lowville	99%	76
Rome Memorial Hospital[2]	Rome	99%	76
Saint Catherine of Siena Hospital[2]	Smithtown	99%	68
Saint Elizabeth Medical Center[2]	Utica	99%	104
Saint Francis Hospital[2]	Poughkeepsie	99%	120
Saint Mary's Hospital at Amsterdam[2]	Amsterdam	99%	76
Univ Hosp SUNY Health Science Ctr[2]	Syracuse	99%	153
Winthrop - University Hospital[2]	Mineola	99%	83
Albany Memorial Hospital[2]	Albany	98%	65
Bon Secours Community Hospital[2]	Port Jervis	98%	45
Claxton - Hepburn Medical Center[2]	Ogdensburg	98%	42
Community Memorial Hospital[2]	Hamilton	98%	50
Flushing Hospital Medical Center[2]	Flushing	98%	54
Forest Hills Hospital[2]	Forest Hills	98%	47
John T Mather Mem Hosp-Port Jefferson[2]	Port Jefferson	98%	82
Kings County Hospital Center[2]	Brooklyn	98%	55
Lawrence Hospital Center[2]	Bronxville	98%	45
Mary Imogene Bassett Hospital[2]	Cooperstown	98%	46
Mercy Medical Center[2]	Rockville Centre	98%	65
Metropolitan Hospital Center[2]	New York	98%	82
Montefiore New Rochelle Hospital[2]	New Rochelle	98%	46
Nathan Littauer Hospital[2]	Gloversville	98%	63
Newark - Wayne Community Hospital[2]	Newark	98%	42
Our Lady of Lourdes Memorial Hospital[2]	Binghamton	98%	40
Putnam Hospital Center[2]	Carmel	98%	48
Richmond University Medical Center[2]	Staten Island	98%	57
Saint Anthony Community Hospital[2]	Warwick	98%	43
Saint Barnabas Hospital[2]	Bronx	98%	55
Saint Charles Hospital[2]	Port Jefferson	98%	91
Saint Luke's Cornwall Hospital[2]	Newburgh	98%	61
Sisters of Charity Hospital[2]	Buffalo	98%	53
Jones Memorial Hospital[2]	Wellsville	97%	36
St John's Episcopal Hosp-South Shore[2]	Far Rockaway	97%	67
Saint Joseph's Medical Center[2]	Yonkers	97%	29
Staten Island University Hospital[2]	Staten Island	97%	65
Huntington Hospital[2]	Huntington	96%	45
Jamaica Hospital Medical Center[2]	Jamaica	96%	55
Kaleida Health[2]	Buffalo	96%	93
Nassau University Medical Center[2]	East Meadow	96%	51
Nyack Hospital[2]	Nyack	96%	53
Southampton Hospital[2]	Southampton	96%	53
Westchester Medical Center[2]	Valhalla	96%	138
Brookhaven Mem Hosp Med Ctr[2]	Patchogue	95%	99
Brooks Memorial Hospital[2]	Dunkirk	95%	40
Elmhurst Hospital Center[2]	Elmhurst	95%	42
Good Samaritan Hospital Medical Center[2]	West Islip	95%	42
Kingsbrook Jewish Medical Center[2]	Brooklyn	95%	75
Niagara Falls Memorial Medical Center[2]	Niagara Falls	95%	156
Oswego Hospital[2]	Oswego	95%	59
Unity Hospital of Rochester[2]	Rochester	95%	39
Cayuga Medical Center at Ithaca[2]	Ithaca	94%	95
Champlain Valley Phys Hosp Med Ctr[2]	Plattsburgh	94%	70
Glen Cove Hospital[2]	Glen Cove	94%	62
Phelps Memorial Hospital Assn[2]	Sleepy Hollow	94%	85
Vassar Brothers Medical Center[2]	Poughkeepsie	94%	72
Wyoming County Community Hospital[2]	Warsaw	94%	54
Arnot Ogden Medical Center[2]	Elmira	93%	55
Brooklyn Hosp Ctr at Downtown Campus[2]	Brooklyn	93%	46
Ellis Hospital[2]	Schenectady	93%	100
Erie County Medical Center[2]	Buffalo	93%	57
Franklin Hospital[2]	Valley Stream	93%	46
Hudson Valley Hospital Center[2]	Cortland Manor	93%	27
Mercy Hospital[2]	Buffalo	93%	45
North Shore University Hospital[2]	Manhasset	93%	109
Olean General Hospital[2]	Olean	93%	71
Saint James Mercy Hospital[2]	Hornell	93%	46
Saint Joseph's Hospital Health Center[2]	Syracuse	93%	55
Saint Mary's Hospital - Troy[2]	Troy	93%	68
Samaritan Medical Center[2]	Watertown	93%	45
Beth Israel Medical Center[2]	New York	92%	26
Peconic Bay Medical Center[2]	Riverhead	92%	49
Queens Hospital Center[2]	Jamaica	92%	37
Saint Peter's Hospital[2]	Albany	92%	75
United Health Services Hospitals[2]	Johnson City	92%	90
White Plains Hospital Center[2]	White Plains	92%	40
Brookdale Hospital Medical Center[2]	Brooklyn	91%	88
Eastern Niagara Hospital[2]	Lockport	91%	78
Saint Francis Hospital - Roslyn[2]	Roslyn	91%	114
Samaritan Hospital[2]	Troy	91%	76
F F Thompson Hospital[2]	Canandaigua	90%	92
Geneva General Hospital[2]	Geneva	90%	63
Harlem Hospital Center[2]	New York	90%	52
Health Alliance Hospital Broadway Campus[2]	Kingston	90%	50
Soldiers & Sailors Mem Hosp of Yates[2]	Penn Yan	90%	29
University Hospital - Stony Brook[2]	Stony Brook	90%	60
Wyckoff Heights Medical Center[2]	Brooklyn	90%	58
Clifton Springs Hospital & Clinic[2]	Clifton Springs	89%	84
Long Island Jewish Medical Center[2]	New Hyde Park	89%	84
Plainview Hospital[2]	Plainview	88%	57
Medina Memorial Hospital[2]	Medina	87%	55
Northern Dutchess Hospital[2]	Rhinebeck	87%	38
Mount St Mary's Hosp & Health Ctr[2]	Lewiston	86%	69
United Memorial Medical Center[2]	Batavia	86%	69
Canton - Potsdam Hospital[2]	Potsdam	84%	31
Corning Hospital[2]	Corning	84%	128
Southside Hospital[2]	Bay Shore	84%	63
Maimonides Medical Center[2]	Brooklyn	83%	59
Orange Regional Medical Center[2]	Middletown	83%	71
Northern Westchester Hospital[2]	Mount Kisco	82%	34
Saint Joseph's Hospital[2]	Elmira	82%	51
Strong Memorial Hospital[2]	Rochester	81%	54
Highland Hospital[2]	Rochester	80%	25
Albany Medical Center Hospital[2]	Albany	79%	81
Adirondack Medical Center[2]	Saranac Lake	78%	46
Aurelia Osborn Fox Memorial Hospital[2]	Oneonta	77%	39
Mount Sinai Hospital[2]	New York	76%	71
Lenox Hill Hospital[2]	New York	74%	43
Woman's Christian Association[2]	Jamestown	74%	88
Saint John's Riverside Hospital[2]	Yonkers	73%	56
Saratoga Hospital[2]	Saratoga Spgs	72%	53
Nicholas H Noyes Memorial Hospital[2]	Dansville	69%	45
Good Samaritan Hospital of Suffern[2]	Suffern	62%	85
New York Hosp Med Ctr of Queens[2]	Flushing	51%	57
Carthage Area Hospital[2]	Carthage	35%	63

Incidence of Potentially Preventable VTE

Hospital Name	City	Rate	Cases
Bellevue Hospital Center[2]	New York	0%	47
Brookhaven Mem Hosp Med Ctr[2]	Patchogue	0%	33
Flushing Hospital Medical Center[2]	Flushing	0%	25
Hospital For Special Surgery[2]	New York	0%	41
Nyack Hospital[2]	Nyack	0%	35
Saint Peter's Hospital[2]	Albany	0%	43
South Nassau Communities Hospital[2]	Oceanside	0%	33
Winthrop - University Hospital[2]	Mineola	0%	48
Wyckoff Heights Medical Center[2]	Brooklyn	0%	28

NOTE: Hospital profiles are in alphabetical order by state, then city, then hospital within the city; Rankings exclude hospitals with less than 25 cases except for patient surveys which excludes hospitals with less than 100 cases; (a) 100-299 cases; (1) The number of cases/patients is too few to report; (2) Data submitted were based on a sample of cases/patients; (3) Results are based on a shorter time period than required; (4) Data suppressed by CMS for one or more quarters; (5) Results are not available for this reporting period; (6) Fewer than 100 patients completed the HCAHPS survey; (7) No cases met the criteria for this measure; (8) The lower limit of the confidence interval cannot be calculated if the number of observed infections equals zero; (9) No data are available from the state/territory for this reporting period; (10) The scores shown reflect fewer than 50 completed surveys; (11) There were discrepancies in the data collection process; (12) This measure does not apply to this hospital for this reporting period; (13) Results cannot be calculated for this reporting period; (14) The results for this state are combined with nearby states to protect confidentiality; Please refer to the User's Guide for a full explanation of data.

Hospital Name	City	Rate	Cases
New York - Presbyterian Hospital[2]	New York	1%	133
Kings County Hospital Center[2]	Brooklyn	2%	65
New York Methodist Hospital[2]	Brooklyn	2%	54
Saint Barnabas Hospital[2]	Bronx	3%	29
Saint Luke's Roosevelt Hospital[2]	New York	3%	62
Southside Hospital[2]	Bay Shore	3%	30
Brooklyn Hosp Ctr at Downtown Campus[2]	Brooklyn	4%	26
Good Samaritan Hospital Medical Center[2]	West Islip	4%	28
Jacobi Medical Center[2]	Bronx	4%	49
Staten Island University Hospital[2]	Staten Island	4%	69
North Shore University Hospital[2]	Manhasset	6%	127
NYU Hospitals Center[2]	New York	6%	47
Plainview Hospital[2]	Plainview	6%	31
Westchester Medical Center[2]	Valhalla	6%	67
Nassau University Medical Center[2]	East Meadow	7%	28
Long Island Jewish Medical Center[2]	New Hyde Park	8%	83
Mount Sinai Hospital[2]	New York	8%	142
Univ Hosp SUNY Health Science Ctr[2]	Syracuse	9%	55
Mercy Hospital[2]	Buffalo	10%	31
Univ Hosp of Brooklyn-Downstate[2]	Brooklyn	10%	31
Kaleida Health[2]	Buffalo	11%	95
Crouse Hospital[2]	Syracuse	12%	25
United Health Services Hospitals[2]	Johnson City	12%	25
Unity Hospital of Rochester[2]	Rochester	12%	34
University Hospital - Stony Brook[2]	Stony Brook	12%	77
Brookdale Hospital Medical Center[2]	Brooklyn	13%	39
Maimonides Medical Center[2]	Brooklyn	15%	26
Lenox Hill Hospital[2]	New York	16%	85
Beth Israel Medical Center[2]	New York	17%	83
Rochester General Hospital[2]	Rochester	18%	40
Montefiore Medical Center[2]	Bronx	22%	235
Albany Medical Center Hospital[2]	Albany	24%	38
New York Hosp Med Ctr of Queens[2]	Flushing	24%	46
Saint Joseph's Hospital Health Center[2]	Syracuse	36%	36
Strong Memorial Hospital[2]	Rochester	44%	25
Good Samaritan Hospital of Suffern[2]	Suffern	48%	29

UFH with Dosages/Platelet Count Monitoring

Hospital Name	City	Rate	Cases
Bellevue Hospital Center[2]	New York	100%	84
Brookhaven Mem Hosp Med Ctr[2]	Patchogue	100%	84
Brooklyn Hosp Ctr at Downtown Campus[2]	Brooklyn	100%	58
Cayuga Medical Center at Ithaca[2]	Ithaca	100%	26
Cortland Regional Medical Center[2]	Cortland	100%	26
Faxton - Saint Luke's Healthcare[2]	Utica	100%	62
Flushing Hospital Medical Center[2]	Flushing	100%	28
Franklin Hospital[2]	Valley Stream	100%	39
Good Samaritan Hospital Medical Center[2]	West Islip	100%	30
Health Alliance Hospital Broadway Campus[2]	Kingston	100%	26
Highland Hospital[2]	Rochester	100%	36
Huntington Hospital[2]	Huntington	100%	70
Jamaica Hospital Medical Center[2]	Jamaica	100%	28
John T Mather Mem Hosp-Port Jefferson[2]	Port Jefferson	100%	57
Kaleida Health[2]	Buffalo	100%	171
Kenmore Mercy Hospital[2]	Kenmore	100%	31
Lawrence Hospital Center[2]	Bronxville	100%	33
Lutheran Medical Center[2]	Brooklyn	100%	73
Maimonides Medical Center[2]	Brooklyn	100%	119
Mary Imogene Bassett Hospital[2]	Cooperstown	100%	36
Mercy Hospital[2]	Buffalo	100%	57
Mercy Medical Center[2]	Rockville Centre	100%	34
Nassau University Medical Center[2]	East Meadow	100%	34
North Shore University Hospital[2]	Manhasset	100%	158
NYU Hospitals Center[2]	New York	100%	83
Olean General Hospital[2]	Olean	100%	53
Orange Regional Medical Center[2]	Middletown	100%	90
Queens Hospital Center[2]	Jamaica	100%	35
Rochester General Hospital[2]	Rochester	100%	133
St John's Episcopal Hosp-South Shore[2]	Far Rockaway	100%	31
Saint John's Riverside Hospital[2]	Yonkers	100%	67
Saint Joseph's Medical Center[2]	Yonkers	100%	27
Saint Luke's Cornwall Hospital[2]	Newburgh	100%	40
Saint Luke's Roosevelt Hospital[2]	New York	100%	82
Sisters of Charity Hospital[2]	Buffalo	100%	125
South Nassau Communities Hospital[2]	Oceanside	100%	74
Southampton Hospital[2]	Southampton	100%	26
Unity Hospital of Rochester[2]	Rochester	100%	33
White Plains Hospital Center[2]	White Plains	100%	105
Winthrop - University Hospital[2]	Mineola	100%	108
Beth Israel Medical Center[2]	New York	99%	131
Montefiore Medical Center[2]	Bronx	99%	252
New York - Presbyterian Hospital[2]	New York	99%	365
Saint Francis Hospital - Roslyn[2]	Roslyn	99%	106
Saint Joseph's Hospital Health Center[2]	Syracuse	99%	179
Univ Hosp SUNY Health Science Ctr[2]	Syracuse	99%	154
Bronx - Lebanon Hospital Center[2]	Bronx	98%	44
Ellis Hospital[2]	Schenectady	98%	57
Our Lady of Lourdes Memorial Hospital[2]	Binghamton	98%	40
Saint Elizabeth Medical Center[2]	Utica	98%	59
Southside Hospital[2]	Bay Shore	98%	41
Champlain Valley Phys Hosp Med Ctr[2]	Plattsburgh	97%	75
Eastern Niagara Hospital[2]	Lockport	97%	31
Saint Peter's Hospital[2]	Albany	97%	92
University Hospital - Stony Brook[2]	Stony Brook	96%	149
Westchester Medical Center[2]	Valhalla	96%	85
Wyckoff Heights Medical Center[2]	Brooklyn	96%	26
Erie County Medical Center[2]	Buffalo	92%	26
Lenox Hill Hospital[2]	New York	92%	145
Long Island Jewish Medical Center[2]	New Hyde Park	92%	159
New York Methodist Hospital[2]	Brooklyn	92%	25
Good Samaritan Hospital of Suffern[2]	Suffern	90%	30
New York Hosp Med Ctr of Queens[2]	Flushing	90%	126
Strong Memorial Hospital[2]	Rochester	86%	56
United Health Services Hospitals[2]	Johnson City	86%	42
Crouse Hospital[2]	Syracuse	85%	81
Brookdale Hospital Medical Center[2]	Brooklyn	79%	29
Univ Hosp of Brooklyn-Downstate[2]	Brooklyn	76%	49
Mount Sinai Hospital[2]	New York	72%	200
Jacobi Medical Center[2]	Bronx	58%	45
Staten Island University Hospital[2]	Staten Island	34%	151
Kings County Hospital Center[2]	Brooklyn	30%	40
Albany Medical Center Hospital[2]	Albany	23%	86
Mount St Mary's Hosp & Health Ctr[2]	Lewiston	4%	25

Venous Thromboembolism Prophylaxis

Hospital Name	City	Rate	Cases
Chenango Memorial Hospital[2]	Norwich	100%	326
Helen Hayes Hospital	W Haverstraw	100%	419
Hospital For Special Surgery[2]	New York	100%	169
Winifred Masterson Burke Rehab Hosp[2]	White Plains	100%	528
Woodhull Medical & Mental Health Center[2]	Brooklyn	100%	273
Columbia Memorial Hospital[2]	Hudson	99%	345
Coney Island Hospital[2]	Brooklyn	98%	370
Flushing Hospital Medical Center[2]	Flushing	98%	343
Lincoln Medical & Mental Health Center[2]	Bronx	98%	222
Sisters of Charity Hospital[2]	Buffalo	98%	366
Auburn Community Hospital[2]	Auburn	97%	343
Bronx - Lebanon Hospital Center[2]	Bronx	97%	425
Clifton Springs Hospital & Clinic[2]	Clifton Springs	97%	253
Crouse Hospital[2]	Syracuse	97%	300
Elmhurst Hospital Center[2]	Elmhurst	97%	322
Faxton - Saint Luke's Healthcare[2]	Utica	97%	403
Jacobi Medical Center[2]	Bronx	97%	307
Nyack Hospital[2]	Nyack	97%	345
NYU Hospitals Center[2]	New York	97%	305
Saint James Mercy Hospital[2]	Hornell	97%	92
St John's Episcopal Hosp-South Shore[2]	Far Rockaway	97%	409
Winthrop - University Hospital[2]	Mineola	97%	329
Arnot Ogden Medical Center[2]	Elmira	96%	338
Claxton - Hepburn Medical Center[2]	Ogdensburg	96%	190
Cortland Regional Medical Center[2]	Cortland	96%	328
Jamaica Hospital Medical Center[2]	Jamaica	96%	325
Jones Memorial Hospital[2]	Wellsville	96%	122
Metropolitan Hospital Center[2]	New York	96%	205
North Central Bronx Hospital[2]	Bronx	96%	340
Oneida Healthcare Center[2]	Oneida	96%	221
Saint Charles Hospital[2]	Port Jefferson	96%	337
Saint Francis Hospital[2]	Poughkeepsie	96%	295
Saint Mary's Hospital at Amsterdam[2]	Amsterdam	96%	345
Bon Secours Community Hospital[2]	Port Jervis	95%	266
Glens Falls Hospital[2]	Glens Falls	95%	332
Good Samaritan Hospital Medical Center[2]	West Islip	95%	417
New York - Presbyterian Hospital[2]	New York	95%	357
Saint Luke's Cornwall Hospital[2]	Newburgh	95%	363
Bellevue Hospital Center[2]	New York	94%	287
Community Memorial Hospital[2]	Hamilton	94%	211
Kings County Hospital Center[2]	Brooklyn	94%	293
Lewis County General Hospital[2]	Lowville	94%	87
Lutheran Medical Center[2]	Brooklyn	94%	375
Massena Memorial Hospital[2]	Massena	94%	207
Nassau University Medical Center[2]	East Meadow	94%	229
Newark - Wayne Community Hospital[2]	Newark	94%	292
Phelps Memorial Hospital Assn[2]	Sleepy Hollow	94%	341
Richmond University Medical Center[2]	Staten Island	94%	397
South Nassau Communities Hospital[2]	Oceanside	94%	424
Brookhaven Mem Hosp Med Ctr[2]	Patchogue	93%	539
Corning Hospital[2]	Corning	93%	460
Ellis Hospital[2]	Schenectady	93%	355
Kenmore Mercy Hospital[2]	Kenmore	93%	318
Lawrence Hospital Center[2]	Bronxville	93%	387
Maimonides Medical Center[2]	Brooklyn	93%	343
New York Community Hospital of Brooklyn[2]	Brooklyn	93%	458
Oswego Hospital[2]	Oswego	93%	336
Putnam Hospital Center[2]	Carmel	93%	336
Queens Hospital Center[2]	Jamaica	93%	391
Rochester General Hospital[2]	Rochester	93%	346
White Plains Hospital Center[2]	White Plains	93%	381
Kingsbrook Jewish Medical Center[2]	Brooklyn	92%	364
Niagara Falls Memorial Medical Center[2]	Niagara Falls	92%	217
Our Lady of Lourdes Memorial Hospital[2]	Binghamton	92%	356
Staten Island University Hospital[2]	Staten Island	92%	304
Eastern Niagara Hospital[2]	Lockport	91%	413
Geneva General Hospital[2]	Geneva	91%	328
Northern Dutchess Hospital[2]	Rhinebeck	91%	277
Northern Westchester Hospital[2]	Mount Kisco	91%	331
Saint Catherine of Siena Hospital[2]	Smithtown	91%	386
Wyoming County Community Hospital[2]	Warsaw	91%	185
Albany Memorial Hospital[2]	Albany	90%	344
Brooklyn Hosp Ctr at Downtown Campus[2]	Brooklyn	90%	393
Cayuga Medical Center at Ithaca[2]	Ithaca	90%	238
Champlain Valley Phys Hosp Med Ctr[2]	Plattsburgh	90%	419
Erie County Medical Center[2]	Buffalo	90%	256
Huntington Hospital[2]	Huntington	90%	363
Mount Sinai Hospital[2]	New York	90%	744
Saint Joseph Hospital[2]	Bethpage	90%	428
Soldiers & Sailors Mem Hosp of Yates[2]	Penn Yan	90%	86
Univ Hosp of Brooklyn-Downstate[2]	Brooklyn	90%	390
Alice Hyde Medical Center[2]	Malone	89%	185
Catskill Regional Medical Center[2]	Harris	89%	318
Highland Hospital[2]	Rochester	89%	320
Hudson Valley Hospital Center[2]	Cortlandt Manor	89%	422
New York Methodist Hospital[2]	Brooklyn	89%	384
North Shore University Hospital[2]	Manhasset	89%	635
Vassar Brothers Medical Center[2]	Poughkeepsie	89%	375
F F Thompson Hospital[2]	Canandaigua	88%	325
Harlem Hospital Center[2]	New York	88%	234
Mary Imogene Bassett Hospital[2]	Cooperstown	88%	507
Mercy Hospital[2]	Buffalo	88%	386
Rome Memorial Hospital[2]	Rome	88%	291
Saint Elizabeth Medical Center[2]	Utica	88%	329
Saint Joseph's Medical Center[2]	Yonkers	88%	345
Wyckoff Heights Medical Center[2]	Brooklyn	88%	388
Kaleida Health[2]	Buffalo	87%	294
Mercy Medical Center[2]	Rockville Centre	87%	389
Saint Anthony Community Hospital[2]	Warwick	87%	167
Saint Mary's Hospital - Troy[2]	Troy	87%	349
Unity Hospital of Rochester[2]	Rochester	87%	304
Univ Hosp SUNY Health Science Ctr[2]	Syracuse	87%	632
Glen Cove Hospital[2]	Glen Cove	86%	265
Nathan Littauer Hospital[2]	Gloversville	86%	234
Samaritan Medical Center[2]	Watertown	86%	377
United Health Services Hospitals[2]	Johnson City	86%	330
Saint Peter's Hospital[2]	Albany	85%	343
Westchester Medical Center[2]	Valhalla	85%	317
Aurelia Osborn Fox Memorial Hospital[2]	Oneonta	84%	255
Brookdale Hospital Medical Center[2]	Brooklyn	84%	360
Forest Hills Hospital[2]	Forest Hills	84%	373
John T Mather Mem Hosp-Port Jefferson[2]	Port Jefferson	84%	401
Montefiore Mount Vernon Hospital[2]	Mount Vernon	84%	331
Montefiore New Rochelle Hospital[2]	New Rochelle	84%	377
Mount St Mary's Hosp & Health Ctr[2]	Lewiston	84%	317
Olean General Hospital[2]	Olean	84%	360
Southampton Hospital[2]	Southampton	84%	326
United Memorial Medical Center[2]	Batavia	84%	263
Ira Davenport Memorial Hospital	Bath	83%	277
Peconic Bay Medical Center[2]	Riverhead	83%	348
Saint Joseph's Hospital Health Center[2]	Syracuse	83%	335
Medina Memorial Hospital[2]	Medina	82%	178
Saint Joseph's Hospital[2]	Elmira	82%	203
Saint Luke's Roosevelt Hospital[2]	New York	82%	311
University Hospital - Stony Brook[2]	Stony Brook	82%	329
Brooks Memorial Hospital[2]	Dunkirk	81%	199
Franklin Hospital[2]	Valley Stream	81%	331
Saint Francis Hospital - Roslyn[2]	Roslyn	81%	357
Saint Barnabas Hospital[2]	Bronx	80%	260
Beth Israel Medical Center[2]	New York	79%	346
Interfaith Medical Center[2]	Brooklyn	78%	304
Cobleskill Regional Hospital[2]	Cobleskill	77%	292
Lenox Hill Hospital[2]	New York	77%	299
Southside Hospital[2]	Bay Shore	77%	305
Strong Memorial Hospital[2]	Rochester	77%	321
Adirondack Medical Center[2]	Saranac Lake	76%	199
Plainview Hospital[2]	Plainview	76%	359
Samaritan Hospital[2]	Troy	75%	268
TLC Health Network[2]	Gowanda	75%	123
Canton - Potsdam Hospital[2]	Potsdam	73%	240
Long Island Jewish Medical Center[2]	New Hyde Park	73%	472
New York Hosp Med Ctr of Queens[2]	Flushing	73%	426
Montefiore Medical Center[2]	Bronx	72%	453
Orange Regional Medical Center[2]	Middletown	72%	351
Nicholas H Noyes Memorial Hospital[2]	Dansville	71%	115
Woman's Christian Association[2]	Jamestown	71%	332
Bertrand Chaffee Hospital[2]	Springville	69%	420
Health Alliance Hospital Broadway Campus[2]	Kingston	68%	379
Health Alliance Hosp Mary's Ave Campus[2]	Kingston	64%	125
Saratoga Hospital[2]	Saratoga Spgs	60%	291
Albany Medical Center Hospital[2]	Albany	58%	330
Saint John's Riverside Hospital[2]	Yonkers	57%	404
Eastern Long Island Hospital[2]	Greenport	55%	177
Sunnyview Hosp & Rehab Ctr[2]	Schenectady	54%	456
Good Samaritan Hospital of Suffern[2]	Suffern	49%	333
Carthage Area Hospital[2]	Carthage	33%	106
New York Eye & Ear Infirmary	New York	19%	143

NOTE: Hospital profiles are in alphabetical order by state, then city, then hospital within the city; Rankings exclude hospitals with less than 25 cases except for patient surveys which excludes hospitals with less than 100 cases; (a) 100-299 cases; (1) The number of cases/patients is too few to report; (2) Data submitted were based on a sample of cases/patients; (3) Results are based on a shorter time period than required; (4) Data suppressed by CMS for one or more quarters; (5) Results are not available for this reporting period; (6) Fewer than 100 patients completed the HCAHPS survey; (7) No cases met the criteria for this measure; (8) The lower limit of the confidence interval cannot be calculated if the number of observed infections equals zero; (9) No data are available from the state/territory for this reporting period; (10) The scores shown reflect fewer than 50 completed surveys; (11) There were discrepancies in the data collection process; (12) This measure does not apply to this hospital for this reporting period; (13) Results cannot be calculated for this reporting period; (14) The results for this state are combined with nearby states to protect confidentiality; Please refer to the User's Guide for a full explanation of data.

Westfield Memorial Hospital[2]	Westfield	8%	73

Warfarin Therapy Discharge Instructions

Hospital Name	City	Rate	Cases
Bronx - Lebanon Hospital Center[2]	Bronx	100%	61
Brooklyn Hosp Ctr at Downtown Campus[2]	Brooklyn	100%	55
Coney Island Hospital[2]	Brooklyn	100%	33
Good Samaritan Hospital of Suffern[2]	Suffern	100%	36
Hudson Valley Hospital Center[2]	Cortlandt Manor	100%	27
Lawrence Hospital Center[2]	Bronxville	100%	53
Saint Catherine of Siena Hospital[2]	Smithtown	100%	47
Saint Charles Hospital[2]	Port Jefferson	100%	25
Saint Francis Hospital[2]	Poughkeepsie	100%	30
St John's Episcopal Hosp-South Shore[2]	Far Rockaway	100%	29
Sisters of Charity Hospital[2]	Buffalo	100%	110
NYU Hospitals Center[2]	New York	99%	67
Saint Francis Hospital - Roslyn[2]	Roslyn	98%	58
Saint Luke's Cornwall Hospital[2]	Newburgh	98%	52
Nyack Hospital[2]	Nyack	97%	29
Saint John's Riverside Hospital[2]	Yonkers	97%	58
Vassar Brothers Medical Center[2]	Poughkeepsie	97%	70
Lincoln Medical & Mental Health Center[2]	Bronx	96%	52
New York Community Hospital of Brooklyn[2]	Brooklyn	96%	28
Oneida Healthcare Center[2]	Oneida	96%	26
Mary Imogene Bassett Hospital[2]	Cooperstown	95%	44
Mercy Hospital[2]	Buffalo	95%	93
New York Hosp Med Ctr of Queens[2]	Flushing	94%	107
Kenmore Mercy Hospital[2]	Kenmore	93%	58
Saratoga Hospital[2]	Saratoga Spgs	93%	60
South Nassau Communities Hospital[2]	Oceanside	93%	103
White Plains Hospital Center[2]	White Plains	93%	94
John T Mather Mem Hosp-Port Jefferson[2]	Port Jefferson	91%	75
Columbia Memorial Hospital[2]	Hudson	90%	31
Olean General Hospital[2]	Olean	90%	41
Orange Regional Medical Center[2]	Middletown	90%	92
F F Thompson Hospital[2]	Canandaigua	88%	26
Good Samaritan Hospital Medical Center[2]	West Islip	88%	111
New York Methodist Hospital[2]	Brooklyn	87%	132
Saint Joseph Hospital[2]	Bethpage	87%	31
Saint Elizabeth Medical Center[2]	Utica	86%	37
Champlain Valley Phys Hosp Med Ctr[2]	Plattsburgh	85%	75
Our Lady of Lourdes Memorial Hospital[2]	Binghamton	85%	47
Brookhaven Mem Hosp Med Ctr[2]	Patchogue	83%	76
Glens Falls Hospital[2]	Glens Falls	82%	50
Jamaica Hospital Medical Center[2]	Jamaica	80%	35
Saint Barnabas Hospital[2]	Bronx	80%	40
Mount Sinai Hospital[2]	New York	79%	222
Rome Memorial Hospital[2]	Rome	79%	28
Wyckoff Heights Medical Center[2]	Brooklyn	76%	54
Forest Hills Hospital[2]	Forest Hills	74%	50
New York - Presbyterian Hospital[2]	New York	74%	274
Highland Hospital[2]	Rochester	73%	64
Nassau University Medical Center[2]	East Meadow	73%	30
Albany Medical Center Hospital[2]	Albany	72%	64
Queens Hospital Center[2]	Jamaica	71%	56
Westchester Medical Center[2]	Valhalla	71%	58
Kaleida Health[2]	Buffalo	68%	218
Univ Hosp of Brooklyn-Downstate[2]	Brooklyn	68%	73
Maimonides Medical Center[2]	Brooklyn	61%	57
Staten Island University Hospital[2]	Staten Island	61%	129
Faxton - Saint Luke's Healthcare[2]	Utica	58%	31
Arnot Ogden Medical Center[2]	Elmira	56%	45
Unity Hospital of Rochester[2]	Rochester	55%	86
Crouse Hospital[2]	Syracuse	54%	69
Cortland Regional Medical Center[2]	Cortland	53%	45
Health Alliance Hospital Broadway Campus[2]	Kingston	51%	39
Kingsbrook Jewish Medical Center[2]	Brooklyn	48%	25
Rochester General Hospital[2]	Rochester	48%	180
Saint Mary's Hospital at Amsterdam[2]	Amsterdam	47%	34
Univ Hosp SUNY Health Science Ctr[2]	Syracuse	46%	134
Ellis Hospital[2]	Schenectady	45%	82
Lutheran Medical Center[2]	Brooklyn	45%	55
Mercy Medical Center[2]	Rockville Centre	45%	40
Corning Hospital[2]	Corning	44%	32
Montefiore Medical Center[2]	Bronx	43%	222
Winthrop - University Hospital[2]	Mineola	42%	97
Saint Peter's Hospital[2]	Albany	41%	127
Bellevue Hospital Center[2]	New York	35%	49
Franklin Hospital[2]	Valley Stream	34%	38
Beth Israel Medical Center[2]	New York	30%	179
Kings County Hospital Center[2]	Brooklyn	29%	107
Saint Luke's Roosevelt Hospital[2]	New York	25%	151
Brookdale Hospital Medical Center[2]	Brooklyn	23%	31
Woman's Christian Association[2]	Jamestown	23%	26
North Shore University Hospital[2]	Manhasset	20%	192
Samaritan Hospital[2]	Troy	19%	27
Strong Memorial Hospital[2]	Rochester	18%	92
University Hospital - Stony Brook[2]	Stony Brook	15%	144
Erie County Medical Center[2]	Buffalo	13%	30
Plainview Hospital[2]	Plainview	13%	63
Samaritan Medical Center[2]	Watertown	12%	40
Long Island Jewish Medical Center[2]	New Hyde Park	10%	166
Saint Joseph's Hospital Health Center[2]	Syracuse	10%	160
Cayuga Medical Center at Ithaca[2]	Ithaca	7%	44
Eastern Niagara Hospital[2]	Lockport	7%	30
Harlem Hospital Center[2]	New York	6%	31
Lenox Hill Hospital[2]	New York	4%	137
Huntington Hospital[2]	Huntington	3%	70
Peconic Bay Medical Center[2]	Riverhead	3%	32
Glen Cove Hospital[2]	Glen Cove	0%	30
Jacobi Medical Center[2]	Bronx	0%	51
Southside Hospital[2]	Bay Shore	0%	94
United Health Services Hospitals[2]	Johnson City	0%	78

Chest Pain/Possible Heart Attack Care

Aspirin Given Within 24 Hours of Arrival

Hospital Name	City	Rate	Cases
Canton - Potsdam Hospital	Potsdam	100%	70
Chenango Memorial Hospital	Norwich	100%	67
Claxton - Hepburn Medical Center	Ogdensburg	100%	79
Clifton Springs Hospital & Clinic	Clifton Springs	100%	29
Community Memorial Hospital	Hamilton	100%	29
Delaware Valley Hospital	Walton	100%	40
F F Thompson Hospital	Canandaigua	100%	58
Forest Hills Hospital	Forest Hills	100%	65
Glen Cove Hospital	Glen Cove	100%	28
Jacobi Medical Center	Bronx	100%	47
Jamaica Hospital Medical Center	Jamaica	100%	26
John T Mather Mem Hosp-Port Jefferson	Port Jefferson	100%	99
Jones Memorial Hospital	Wellsville	100%	43
Kenmore Mercy Hospital	Kenmore	100%	49
Lawrence Hospital Center	Bronxville	100%	78
Massena Memorial Hospital	Massena	100%	53
Medina Memorial Hospital	Medina	100%	63
Mercy Medical Center	Rockville Centre	100%	48
Mount Sinai Hospital	New York	100%	58
Nassau University Medical Center	East Meadow	100%	74
Northern Dutchess Hospital	Rhinebeck	100%	30
Northern Westchester Hospital	Mount Kisco	100%	73
Our Lady of Lourdes Memorial Hospital	Binghamton	100%	34
Plainview Hospital	Plainview	100%	87
Putnam Hospital Center	Carmel	100%	69
Richmond University Medical Center	Staten Island	100%	35
Saint Joseph's Medical Center	Yonkers	100%	37
Sisters of Charity Hospital	Buffalo	100%	75
Southampton Hospital	Southampton	100%	62
TLC Health Network	Gowanda	100%	43
Woodhull Medical & Mental Health Center	Brooklyn	100%	37
Brookhaven Mem Hosp Med Ctr	Patchogue	99%	72
Cortland Regional Medical Center	Cortland	99%	82
Queens Hospital Center	Jamaica	99%	219
Adirondack Medical Center	Saranac Lake	98%	54
Geneva General Hospital	Geneva	98%	41
Nyack Hospital	Nyack	98%	51
Saint James Mercy Hospital	Hornell	98%	58
Saint Joseph Hospital	Bethpage	98%	194
Saint Mary's Hospital at Amsterdam	Amsterdam	98%	83
Alice Hyde Medical Center	Malone	97%	104
Lewis County General Hospital	Lowville	97%	35
Olean General Hospital	Olean	97%	144
United Memorial Medical Center	Batavia	97%	146
Univ Hosp SUNY Health Science Ctr	Syracuse	97%	60
Wyoming County Community Hospital	Warsaw	97%	108
Bertrand Chaffee Hospital	Springville	96%	51
Brooks Memorial Hospital	Dunkirk	96%	81
Corning Hospital	Corning	96%	93
Ellenville Regional Hospital	Ellenville	96%	51
Glens Falls Hospital	Glens Falls	96%	28
Health Alliance Hospital Broadway Campus	Kingston	96%	54
Newark - Wayne Community Hospital[3]	Newark	96%	46
Nicholas H Noyes Memorial Hospital	Dansville	96%	49
Oneida Healthcare Center	Oneida	96%	47
St John's Episcopal Hosp-South Shore	Far Rockaway	96%	27
Samaritan Medical Center	Watertown	96%	143
Saratoga Hospital	Saratoga Spgs	96%	57
Wyckoff Heights Medical Center	Brooklyn	96%	55
Bon Secours Community Hospital	Port Jervis	95%	60
Little Falls Hospital	Little Falls	95%	39
Niagara Falls Memorial Medical Center	Niagara Falls	95%	43
Woman's Christian Association	Jamestown	95%	126
Columbia Memorial Hospital	Hudson	94%	63
Highland Hospital	Rochester	94%	35
Peconic Bay Medical Center	Riverhead	94%	94
Rome Memorial Hospital	Rome	94%	33
Saint Anthony Community Hospital	Warwick	94%	36
Nathan Littauer Hospital	Gloversville	93%	70
Oswego Hospital	Oswego	93%	119
Saint Mary's Hospital - Troy	Troy	93%	30
Auburn Community Hospital	Auburn	92%	117
Eastern Niagara Hospital	Lockport	92%	145
Franklin Hospital	Valley Stream	92%	88
Aurelia Osborn Fox Memorial Hospital	Oneonta	91%	44
Mount St Mary's Hosp & Health Ctr	Lewiston	91%	55
Westfield Memorial Hospital	Westfield	82%	93
Carthage Area Hospital	Carthage	66%	35

Average Time to ECG (minutes)

Hospital Name	City	Min.	Cases
Jamaica Hospital Medical Center	Jamaica	0	25
Eastern Niagara Hospital	Lockport	2	148
Putnam Hospital Center	Carmel	2	72
Northern Westchester Hospital	Mount Kisco	3	74
Nyack Hospital	Nyack	3	52
Claxton - Hepburn Medical Center	Ogdensburg	4	82
Community Memorial Hospital	Hamilton	4	31
Forest Hills Hospital	Forest Hills	4	63
Medina Memorial Hospital	Medina	4	57
Mount St Mary's Hosp & Health Ctr	Lewiston	4	57
Nicholas H Noyes Memorial Hospital	Dansville	4	51
Saint James Mercy Hospital	Hornell	4	61
Saratoga Hospital	Saratoga Spgs	4	58
Southampton Hospital	Southampton	4	62
Woman's Christian Association	Jamestown	4	128
Wyoming County Community Hospital	Warsaw	4	113
Corning Hospital	Corning	5	94
John T Mather Mem Hosp-Port Jefferson	Port Jefferson	5	101
Peconic Bay Medical Center	Riverhead	5	95
Saint Anthony Community Hospital	Warwick	5	36
Adirondack Medical Center	Saranac Lake	6	56
Health Alliance Hospital Broadway Campus	Kingston	6	55
Jones Memorial Hospital	Wellsville	6	46
Mercy Medical Center	Rockville Centre	6	49
Northern Dutchess Hospital	Rhinebeck	6	29
Olean General Hospital	Olean	6	147
Westfield Memorial Hospital	Westfield	6	104
Brookhaven Mem Hosp Med Ctr	Patchogue	7	72
Rome Memorial Hospital	Rome	7	33
Samaritan Medical Center	Watertown	7	146
TLC Health Network	Gowanda	7	44
United Memorial Medical Center	Batavia	7	148
Chenango Memorial Hospital	Norwich	8	72
Little Falls Hospital	Little Falls	8	49
Oneida Healthcare Center	Oneida	8	48
Saint Joseph Hospital	Bethpage	8	201
Univ Hosp SUNY Health Science Ctr	Syracuse	8	69
Geneva General Hospital	Geneva	9	43
Jacobi Medical Center	Bronx	9	44
Nathan Littauer Hospital	Gloversville	9	71
Niagara Falls Memorial Medical Center	Niagara Falls	9	44
Oswego Hospital	Oswego	9	124
Our Lady of Lourdes Memorial Hospital	Binghamton	9	35
Saint Mary's Hospital - Troy	Troy	9	31
Wyckoff Heights Medical Center	Brooklyn	9	54
Bertrand Chaffee Hospital	Springville	10	55
Carthage Area Hospital	Carthage	10	37
Delaware Valley Hospital	Walton	10	40
Glens Falls Hospital	Glens Falls	10	28
Lewis County General Hospital	Lowville	10	36
Plainview Hospital	Plainview	10	92
F F Thompson Hospital	Canandaigua	11	57
Glen Cove Hospital	Glen Cove	11	29
Massena Memorial Hospital	Massena	11	57
Bon Secours Community Hospital	Port Jervis	12	62
Brooks Memorial Hospital	Dunkirk	12	78
Lawrence Hospital Center	Bronxville	12	72
Mount Sinai Hospital	New York	12	58
Sisters of Charity Hospital	Buffalo	12	77
Woodhull Medical & Mental Health Center	Brooklyn	12	38
Montefiore New Rochelle Hospital	New Rochelle	13	25
Aurelia Osborn Fox Memorial Hospital	Oneonta	14	49
Newark - Wayne Community Hospital[3]	Newark	14	52
Queens Hospital Center	Jamaica	14	204
Kenmore Mercy Hospital	Kenmore	15	52
Saint Mary's Hospital at Amsterdam	Amsterdam	15	87
Alice Hyde Medical Center	Malone	16	105
Columbia Memorial Hospital	Hudson	16	66
Nassau University Medical Center	East Meadow	17	80
Saint Joseph's Medical Center	Yonkers	17	37
Cortland Regional Medical Center	Cortland	18	85
Auburn Community Hospital	Auburn	19	123
Canton - Potsdam Hospital	Potsdam	19	71
Highland Hospital	Rochester	19	36
Clifton Springs Hospital & Clinic	Clifton Springs	20	29
Franklin Hospital	Valley Stream	20	96
Ellenville Regional Hospital	Ellenville	23	57
St John's Episcopal Hosp-South Shore	Far Rockaway	24	28
Richmond University Medical Center	Staten Island	31	36

NOTE: Hospital profiles are in alphabetical order by state, then city, then hospital within the city; Rankings exclude hospitals with less than 25 cases except for patient surveys which excludes hospitals with less than 100 cases; (a) 100-299 cases; (1) The number of cases/patients is too few to report; (2) Data submitted were based on a sample of cases/patients; (3) Results are based on a shorter time period than required; (4) Data suppressed by CMS for one or more quarters; (5) Results are not available for this reporting period; (6) Fewer than 100 patients completed the HCAHPS survey; (7) No cases met the criteria for this measure; (8) The lower limit of the confidence interval cannot be calculated if the number of observed infections equals zero; (9) No data are available from the state/territory for this reporting period; (10) The scores shown reflect fewer than 50 completed surveys; (11) There were discrepancies in the data collection process; (12) This measure does not apply to this hospital for this reporting period; (13) Results cannot be calculated for this reporting period; (14) The results for this state are combined with nearby states to protect confidentiality; Please refer to the User's Guide for a full explanation of data.

Average Time to Transfer (minutes)

Hospital Name	City	Min.	Cases
Plainview Hospital	Plainview	56	32
John T Mather Mem Hosp-Port Jefferson	Port Jefferson	60	36
Saint Joseph Hospital	Bethpage	62	42
Brookhaven Mem Hosp Med Ctr	Patchogue	63	31
Mount Sinai Hospital	New York	70	28
Forest Hills Hospital	Forest Hills	75	27
Franklin Hospital	Valley Stream	90	34
Queens Hospital Center	Jamaica	97	25

Children's Asthma Care

Received Home Management Plan of Care

Hospital Name	City	Rate	Cases
New York - Presbyterian Hospital	New York	96%	411
University Hospital - Stony Brook[2]	Stony Brook	59%	177

Received Reliever Medication

Hospital Name	City	Rate	Cases
New York - Presbyterian Hospital	New York	100%	414
University Hospital - Stony Brook	Stony Brook	100%	177

Received Systemic Corticosteroids

Hospital Name	City	Rate	Cases
New York - Presbyterian Hospital	New York	100%	413
University Hospital - Stony Brook	Stony Brook	95%	176

Emergency Department

Admittance Decision Time (minutes)

Hospital Name	City	Min.	Cases
Northern Westchester Hospital[2]	Mount Kisco	38	575
Brooks Memorial Hospital[2]	Dunkirk	50	297
Westfield Memorial Hospital[2]	Westfield	55	85
Chenango Memorial Hospital[2]	Norwich	60	438
Bertrand Chaffee Hospital[2]	Springville	61	405
Delaware Valley Hospital[2]	Walton	61	304
Alice Hyde Medical Center[2]	Malone	64	418
Ira Davenport Memorial Hospital	Bath	65	401
Jones Memorial Hospital[2]	Wellsville	66	330
Saint Mary's Hospital at Amsterdam[2]	Amsterdam	66	573
Highland Hospital[2]	Rochester	67	368
Newark - Wayne Community Hospital[2]	Newark	68	383
Our Lady of Lourdes Memorial Hospital[2]	Binghamton	70	782
TLC Health Network[2]	Gowanda	70	289
Little Falls Hospital[2,3]	Little Falls	74	125
Nyack Hospital[2]	Nyack	76	803
Coney Island Hospital[2]	Brooklyn	77	772
Adirondack Medical Center[2]	Saranac Lake	78	270
Massena Memorial Hospital[2]	Massena	79	344
Glens Falls Hospital[2]	Glens Falls	81	700
Saint James Mercy Hospital[2]	Hornell	82	304
Canton - Potsdam Hospital[2]	Potsdam	83	415
Clifton Springs Hospital & Clinic[2]	Clifton Springs	83	509
Eastern Long Island Hospital[2]	Greenport	83	203
Olean General Hospital[2]	Olean	83	591
Eastern Niagara Hospital[2]	Lockport	84	816
Medina Memorial Hospital[2]	Medina	85	324
Carthage Area Hospital[2]	Carthage	90	168
Soldiers & Sailors Mem Hosp of Yates[2]	Penn Yan	90	341
Corning Hospital	Corning	92	2004
Woman's Christian Association[2]	Jamestown	92	559
Samaritan Medical Center[2]	Watertown	93	546
Bon Secours Community Hospital[2]	Port Jervis	94	472
Nicholas H Noyes Memorial Hospital[2]	Dansville	94	331
United Health Services Hospitals[2]	Johnson City	94	516
Claxton - Hepburn Medical Center[2]	Ogdensburg	95	283
Nathan Littauer Hospital[2]	Gloversville	95	468
United Memorial Medical Center[2]	Batavia	95	469
Wyoming County Community Hospital[2]	Warsaw	95	363
Lewis County General Hospital[2]	Lowville	98	306
Faxton - Saint Luke's Healthcare[2]	Utica	100	653
Rome Memorial Hospital[2]	Rome	100	359
Niagara Falls Memorial Medical Center[2]	Niagara Falls	102	803
Crouse Hospital[2]	Syracuse	104	404
Kenmore Mercy Hospital[2]	Kenmore	107	928
Saint John's Riverside Hospital[2]	Yonkers	107	911
F F Thompson Hospital[2]	Canandaigua	111	567
Cobleskill Regional Hospital[2]	Cobleskill	112	288
Northern Dutchess Hospital[2]	Rhinebeck	112	384
Ellis Hospital[2]	Schenectady	116	366
Lawrence Hospital Center[2]	Bronxville	116	844
Putnam Hospital Center[2]	Carmel	117	752
North Central Bronx Hospital[2]	Bronx	118	581
Sisters of Charity Hospital[2]	Buffalo	120	530
Univ Hosp SUNY Health Science Ctr[2]	Syracuse	120	505
Catskill Regional Medical Center[2]	Harris	122	373
Kaleida Health[2]	Buffalo	123	602
Oneida Healthcare Center[2]	Oneida	123	389
Saratoga Hospital[2]	Saratoga Spgs	123	491
Champlain Valley Phys Hosp Med Ctr[2]	Plattsburgh	125	586
Geneva General Hospital[2]	Geneva	128	419
NYU Hospitals Center[2]	New York	128	228
Lincoln Medical & Mental Health Center[2]	Bronx	129	913
Mount St Mary's Hosp & Health Ctr[2]	Lewiston	134	648
Saint Anthony Community Hospital[2]	Warwick	135	339
Lenox Hill Hospital[2]	New York	136	532
Auburn Community Hospital[2]	Auburn	138	364
Community Memorial Hospital[2]	Hamilton	140	547
Long Island Jewish Medical Center[2]	New Hyde Park	140	91
Harlem Hospital Center[2]	New York	142	608
Nassau University Medical Center[2]	East Meadow	142	513
Aurelia Osborn Fox Memorial Hospital[2]	Oneonta	144	362
Saint Peter's Hospital[2]	Albany	145	583
Saint Luke's Cornwall Hospital[2]	Newburgh	149	694
Arnot Ogden Medical Center[2]	Elmira	150	479
Erie County Medical Center[2]	Buffalo	150	407
Saint Mary's Hospital - Troy[2]	Troy	150	640
South Nassau Communities Hospital[2]	Oceanside	150	958
Unity Hospital of Rochester[2]	Rochester	150	482
Cayuga Medical Center at Ithaca[2]	Ithaca	151	368
Saint Francis Hospital[2]	Poughkeepsie	151	809
Kingsbrook Jewish Medical Center[2]	Brooklyn	152	1139
Orange Regional Medical Center[2]	Middletown	152	661
Phelps Memorial Hospital Assn[2]	Sleepy Hollow	155	580
Mercy Hospital[2]	Buffalo	156	693
Health Alliance Hospital Broadway Campus[2]	Kingston	171	812
Rochester General Hospital[2]	Rochester	172	659
Woodhull Medical & Mental Health Center[2]	Brooklyn	172	511
Good Samaritan Hospital of Suffern[2]	Suffern	173	556
Mary Imogene Bassett Hospital[2]	Cooperstown	174	276
Vassar Brothers Medical Center[2]	Poughkeepsie	174	663
Bellevue Hospital Center[2]	New York	175	539
Saint Joseph's Hospital[2]	Elmira	175	257
Bronx - Lebanon Hospital Center[2]	Bronx	176	997
Glen Cove Hospital[2]	Glen Cove	176	787
Wyckoff Heights Medical Center[2]	Brooklyn	176	968
Albany Medical Center Hospital[2]	Albany	180	489
Winthrop - University Hospital[2]	Mineola	181	252
Southampton Hospital[2]	Southampton	184	785
North Shore University Hospital[2]	Manhasset	185	878
Cortland Regional Medical Center[2]	Cortland	186	616
Metropolitan Hospital Center[2]	New York	186	646
Oswego Hospital[2]	Oswego	189	563
Columbia Memorial Hospital[2]	Hudson	191	795
Saint Joseph's Medical Center[2]	Yonkers	193	771
Samaritan Hospital[2]	Troy	193	633
University Hospital - Stony Brook[2]	Stony Brook	194	607
Plainview Hospital[2]	Plainview	202	312
Saint Catherine of Siena Hospital[2]	Smithtown	203	687
White Plains Hospital Center[2]	White Plains	203	727
Queens Hospital Center[2]	Jamaica	207	853
Strong Memorial Hospital[2]	Rochester	209	610
New York Methodist Hospital[2]	Brooklyn	214	621
Saint Elizabeth Medical Center[2]	Utica	220	790
Saint Joseph's Hospital Health Center[2]	Syracuse	223	557
Albany Memorial Hospital[2]	Albany	225	562
Westchester Medical Center[2]	Valhalla	227	417
Jamaica Hospital Medical Center[2]	Jamaica	228	875
Montefiore New Rochelle Hospital[2]	New Rochelle	230	798
Montefiore Mount Vernon Hospital[2]	Mount Vernon	233	554
Maimonides Medical Center[2]	Brooklyn	234	604
New York Community Hospital of Brooklyn[2]	Brooklyn	239	1017
Saint Joseph Hospital[2]	Bethpage	245	939
Mercy Medical Center[2]	Rockville Centre	250	641
Saint Luke's Roosevelt Hospital[2]	New York	250	524
Flushing Hospital Medical Center[2]	Flushing	254	656
Huntington Hospital[2]	Huntington	254	53
Interfaith Medical Center[2]	Brooklyn	264	387
Elmhurst Hospital Center[2]	Elmhurst	266	631
Beth Israel Medical Center[2]	New York	272	722
Franklin Hospital[2]	Valley Stream	275	452
Good Samaritan Hospital Medical Center[2]	West Islip	278	830
Univ Hosp of Brooklyn-Downstate[2]	Brooklyn	279	627
Brooklyn Hosp Ctr at Downtown Campus[2]	Brooklyn	282	781
Saint Barnabas Hospital[2]	Bronx	283	133
John T Mather Mem Hosp-Port Jefferson[2]	Port Jefferson	284	1110
Forest Hills Hospital[2]	Forest Hills	285	412
Peconic Bay Medical Center[2]	Riverhead	295	359
Hudson Valley Hospital Center[2]	Cortlandt Manor	302	882
Richmond University Medical Center[2]	Staten Island	310	540
Staten Island University Hospital[2]	Staten Island	316	814
Montefiore Medical Center[2]	Bronx	317	331
Mount Sinai Hospital[2]	New York	325	1417
Brookdale Hospital Medical Center[2]	Brooklyn	328	567
Southside Hospital[2]	Bay Shore	333	687
New York Hosp Med Ctr of Queens[2]	Flushing	340	615
New York - Presbyterian Hospital[2]	New York	346	529
Saint Charles Hospital[2]	Port Jefferson	359	329
Jacobi Medical Center[2]	Bronx	369	709
St John's Episcopal Hosp-South Shore[2]	Far Rockaway	394	1068
Saint Francis Hospital - Roslyn[2]	Roslyn	428	601
Lutheran Medical Center[2]	Brooklyn	482	755
Brookhaven Mem Hosp Med Ctr[2]	Patchogue	610	1105
Kings County Hospital Center[2]	Brooklyn	716	862

Head CT Results Within 45 Minutes of Arrival

Hospital Name	City	Rate	Cases
Peconic Bay Medical Center	Riverhead	69%	39
Woman's Christian Association	Jamestown	38%	47
Nassau University Medical Center	East Meadow	36%	25
Olean General Hospital	Olean	32%	25

Patients Who Left ER Before Being Seen

Hospital Name	City	Rate	Cases
Adirondack Medical Center	Saranac Lake	0%	13150
Bon Secours Community Hospital	Port Jervis	0%	27558
Carthage Area Hospital	Carthage	0%	23490
Catskill Reg Med Ctr-G Hermann Site	Callicoon	0%	4127
Clifton Fine Hospital	Star Lake	0%	1712
Cuba Memorial Hospital	Cuba	0%	4734
Delaware Valley Hospital	Walton	0%	5141
Elizabethtown Community Hospital	Elizabethtown	0%	5203
Glen Cove Hospital	Glen Cove	0%	21833
Health Alliance Hospital Broadway Campus	Kingston	0%	45763
Hudson Valley Hospital Center	Cortlandt Manor	0%	38801
John T Mather Mem Hosp-Port Jefferson	Port Jefferson	0%	43467
Jones Memorial Hospital	Wellsville	0%	12448
Lenox Hill Hospital	New York	0%	58040
Margaretville Memorial Hospital	Margaretville	0%	4427
Moses - Ludington Hospital	Ticonderoga	0%	6810
Nassau University Medical Center	East Meadow	0%	70752
North Shore University Hospital	Manhasset	0%	106881
Northern Westchester Hospital	Mount Kisco	0%	31029
Nyack Hospital	Nyack	0%	60163
O'Connor Hospital	Delhi	0%	6402
Saint Mary's Hospital - Troy	Troy	0%	31159
Saint Mary's Hospital at Amsterdam	Amsterdam	0%	33627
Soldiers & Sailors Mem Hosp of Yates	Penn Yan	0%	8487
United Memorial Medical Center	Batavia	0%	22439
Albany Memorial Hospital	Albany	1%	47589
Arnot Ogden Medical Center	Elmira	1%	47380
Brookhaven Mem Hosp Med Ctr	Patchogue	1%	6403
Brooks Memorial Hospital	Dunkirk	1%	21011
Canton - Potsdam Hospital	Potsdam	1%	25872
Catskill Regional Medical Center	Harris	1%	28759
Champlain Valley Phys Hosp Med Ctr	Plattsburgh	1%	51029
Claxton - Hepburn Medical Center	Ogdensburg	1%	19074
Cobleskill Regional Hospital	Cobleskill	1%	11189
Columbia Memorial Hospital	Hudson	1%	32329
Cortland Regional Medical Center	Cortland	1%	22603
Crouse Hospital	Syracuse	1%	40866
Eastern Long Island Hospital	Greenport	1%	9264
Eastern Niagara Hospital	Lockport	1%	22457
Ellenville Regional Hospital	Ellenville	1%	13022
Flushing Hospital Medical Center	Flushing	1%	43984
Forest Hills Hospital	Forest Hills	1%	49465
Franklin Hospital	Valley Stream	1%	44191
Geneva General Hospital	Geneva	1%	20715
Good Samaritan Hospital Medical Center	West Islip	1%	98746
Good Samaritan Hospital of Suffern	Suffern	1%	37594
Highland Hospital	Rochester	1%	39758
Huntington Hospital	Huntington	1%	51754
Kenmore Mercy Hospital	Kenmore	1%	30336
Kingsbrook Jewish Medical Center	Brooklyn	1%	38863
Lawrence Hospital Center	Bronxville	1%	33576
Long Island Jewish Medical Center	New Hyde Park	1%	117901
Lutheran Medical Center	Brooklyn	1%	61383
Mary Imogene Bassett Hospital	Cooperstown	1%	18539
Mercy Medical Center	Rockville Centre	1%	39066
Montefiore New Rochelle Hospital	New Rochelle	1%	36812
Mount St Mary's Hosp & Health Ctr	Lewiston	1%	22955
Newark - Wayne Community Hospital	Newark	1%	23624
Nicholas H Noyes Memorial Hospital	Dansville	1%	14269
Northern Dutchess Hospital	Rhinebeck	1%	14779
NYU Hospitals Center	New York	1%	41546
Orange Regional Medical Center	Middletown	1%	52032
Phelps Memorial Hospital Assn	Sleepy Hollow	1%	27156
Plainview Hospital	Plainview	1%	35043
Putnam Hospital Center	Carmel	1%	26984
Richmond University Medical Center	Staten Island	1%	62830
Rochester General Hospital	Rochester	1%	119866
Saint Anthony Community Hospital	Warwick	1%	13961
Saint Catherine of Siena Hospital	Smithtown	1%	32308
Saint Charles Hospital	Port Jefferson	1%	22881
Saint Francis Hospital	Poughkeepsie	1%	32365
Saint Francis Hospital - Roslyn	Roslyn	1%	22832
Saint James Mercy Hospital	Hornell	1%	18031

NOTE: Hospital profiles are in alphabetical order by state, then city, then hospital within the city; Rankings exclude hospitals with less than 25 cases except for patient surveys which excludes hospitals with less than 100 cases; (a) 100-299 cases; (1) The number of cases/patients is too few to report; (2) Data submitted were based on a sample of cases/patients; (3) Results are based on a shorter time period than required; (4) Data suppressed by CMS for one or more quarters; (5) Results are not available for this reporting period; (6) Fewer than 100 patients completed the HCAHPS survey; (7) No cases met the criteria for this measure; (8) The lower limit of the confidence interval cannot be calculated if the number of observed infections equals zero; (9) No data are available from the state/territory for this reporting period; (10) The scores shown reflect fewer than 50 completed surveys; (11) There were discrepancies in the data collection process; (12) This measure does not apply to this hospital for this reporting period; (13) Results cannot be calculated for this reporting period; (14) The results for this state are combined with nearby states to protect confidentiality; Please refer to the User's Guide for a full explanation of data.

Saint Joseph Hospital	Bethpage	1%	36749
Saint Luke's Cornwall Hospital	Newburgh	1%	60730
Saint Luke's Roosevelt Hospital	New York	1%	191732
Saint Peter's Hospital	Albany	1%	53163
Saratoga Hospital	Saratoga Spgs	1%	40517
Sisters of Charity Hospital	Buffalo	1%	70388
South Nassau Communities Hospital	Oceanside	1%	59020
Southampton Hospital	Southampton	1%	25879
Southside Hospital	Bay Shore	1%	72040
Staten Island University Hospital	Staten Island	1%	127897
University Hospital - Stony Brook	Stony Brook	1%	96596
Univ Hosp of Brooklyn-Downstate	Brooklyn	1%	124792
Vassar Brothers Medical Center	Poughkeepsie	1%	67406
Westchester Medical Center	Valhalla	1%	37728
Westfield Memorial Hospital	Westfield	1%	8733
White Plains Hospital Center	White Plains	1%	54942
Wyoming County Community Hospital	Warsaw	1%	11496
Albany Medical Center Hospital	Albany	2%	72219
Bertrand Chaffee Hospital	Springville	2%	8872
Cayuga Medical Center at Ithaca	Ithaca	2%	31946
Chenango Memorial Hospital	Norwich	2%	16225
Clifton Springs Hospital & Clinic	Clifton Springs	2%	10839
Community Memorial Hospital	Hamilton	2%	10293
Corning Hospital	Corning	2%	21536
Ellis Hospital	Schenectady	2%	90682
Faxton - Saint Luke's Healthcare	Utica	2%	36084
Jamaica Hospital Medical Center	Jamaica	2%	121957
Lewis County General Hospital	Lowville	2%	12148
Maimonides Medical Center	Brooklyn	2%	118313
Medina Memorial Hospital	Medina	2%	10038
Mercy Hospital	Buffalo	2%	78756
Montefiore Mount Vernon Hospital	Mount Vernon	2%	18198
Nathan Littauer Hospital	Gloversville	2%	24235
New York Community Hospital of Brooklyn	Brooklyn	2%	21748
New York Hosp Med Ctr of Queens	Flushing	2%	126534
New York Methodist Hospital	Brooklyn	2%	94093
North Central Bronx Hospital	Bronx	2%	57051
Olean General Hospital	Olean	2%	33492
Oneida Healthcare Center	Oneida	2%	26659
Our Lady of Lourdes Memorial Hospital	Binghamton	2%	44234
Peconic Bay Medical Center	Riverhead	2%	35555
Queens Hospital Center	Jamaica	2%	104444
River Hospital	Alexandria Bay	2%	8048
Rome Memorial Hospital	Rome	2%	27539
Saint Elizabeth Medical Center	Utica	2%	41082
Saint John's Riverside Hospital	Yonkers	2%	47535
Samaritan Hospital	Troy	2%	48222
Schuyler Hospital	Montour Falls	2%	9183
TLC Health Network	Gowanda	2%	11190
United Health Services Hospitals	Johnson City	2%	61775
Univ Hosp SUNY Health Science Ctr	Syracuse	2%	88216
Winthrop - University Hospital	Mineola	2%	71945
Woman's Christian Association	Jamestown	2%	37856
Alice Hyde Medical Center	Malone	3%	16235
Auburn Community Hospital	Auburn	3%	26859
Aurelia Osborn Fox Memorial Hospital	Oneonta	3%	17270
Coney Island Hospital	Brooklyn	3%	66160
Erie County Medical Center	Buffalo	3%	65644
F F Thompson Hospital	Canandaigua	3%	25978
Glens Falls Hospital	Glens Falls	3%	53621
Ira Davenport Memorial Hospital	Bath	3%	8614
Kaleida Health	Buffalo	3%	168175
Little Falls Hospital	Little Falls	3%	16225
Massena Memorial Hospital	Massena	3%	1607
Montefiore Medical Center	Bronx	3%	294198
Saint Joseph's Medical Center	Yonkers	3%	39611
Samaritan Medical Center	Watertown	3%	52842
Strong Memorial Hospital	Rochester	3%	101096
Unity Hospital of Rochester	Rochester	3%	47777
Wyckoff Heights Medical Center	Brooklyn	3%	86002
Bronx - Lebanon Hospital Center	Bronx	4%	127989
Elmhurst Hospital Center	Elmhurst	4%	91202
Lincoln Medical & Mental Health Center	Bronx	4%	171138
Metropolitan Hospital Center	New York	4%	65524
Mount Sinai Hospital	New York	4%	151936
Niagara Falls Memorial Medical Center	Niagara Falls	4%	31220
Oswego Hospital	Oswego	4%	25742
St John's Episcopal Hosp-South Shore	Far Rockaway	4%	46468
Saint Joseph's Hospital	Elmira	4%	14736
Saint Joseph's Hospital Health Center	Syracuse	4%	69863
Woodhull Medical & Mental Health Center	Brooklyn	4%	128765
Brookdale Hospital Medical Center	Brooklyn	5%	103259
Brooklyn Hosp Ctr at Downtown Campus	Brooklyn	5%	64589
Kings County Hospital Center	Brooklyn	5%	149539
New York - Presbyterian Hospital	New York	5%	258419
Beth Israel Medical Center	New York	6%	122000
Bellevue Hospital Center	New York	7%	102725
Interfaith Medical Center	Brooklyn	7%	42288
Jacobi Medical Center	Bronx	8%	112868
Saint Barnabas Hospital	Bronx	10%	95700
Harlem Hospital Center	New York	11%	74091

Time from ER Arrival to Being Admitted (minutes)

Hospital Name	City	Min.	Cases
Chenango Memorial Hospital[2]	Norwich	196	495
Massena Memorial Hospital[2]	Massena	202	344
Canton - Potsdam Hospital[2]	Potsdam	208	415
Elizabethtown Community Hospital[2,3]	Elizabethtown	210	31
Jones Memorial Hospital[2]	Wellsville	218	341
Soldiers & Sailors Mem Hosp of Yates[2]	Penn Yan	225	383
Ira Davenport Memorial Hospital	Bath	232	416
Bertrand Chaffee Hospital[2]	Springville	235	449
Saint Mary's Hospital at Amsterdam[2]	Amsterdam	235	577
Eastern Long Island Hospital[2]	Greenport	237	225
Wyoming County Community Hospital[2]	Warsaw	238	367
Delaware Valley Hospital[2]	Walton	239	304
Saint James Mercy Hospital[2]	Hornell	242	318
Nyack Hospital[2]	Nyack	244	804
Alice Hyde Medical Center[2]	Malone	246	418
Clifton Springs Hospital & Clinic[2]	Clifton Springs	247	510
Newark - Wayne Community Hospital[2]	Newark	248	385
Westfield Memorial Hospital[2]	Westfield	250	91
Adirondack Medical Center[2]	Saranac Lake	253	295
Corning Hospital	Corning	254	2046
Brooks Memorial Hospital[2]	Dunkirk	261	301
Carthage Area Hospital[2]	Carthage	268	197
Eastern Niagara Hospital[2]	Lockport	270	882
Northern Westchester Hospital[2]	Mount Kisco	270	578
Lewis County General Hospital[2]	Lowville	271	339
Bon Secours Community Hospital[2]	Port Jervis	274	476
Nicholas H Noyes Memorial Hospital[2]	Dansville	275	331
Claxton - Hepburn Medical Center[2]	Ogdensburg	276	283
Highland Hospital[2]	Rochester	276	368
United Memorial Medical Center[2]	Batavia	276	469
Northern Dutchess Hospital[2]	Rhinebeck	277	384
Little Falls Hospital[2,3]	Little Falls	278	127
Glens Falls Hospital[2]	Glens Falls	281	700
Olean General Hospital[2]	Olean	283	592
TLC Health Network[2]	Gowanda	285	299
Community Memorial Hospital[2]	Hamilton	286	572
Geneva General Hospital[2]	Geneva	286	450
Our Lady of Lourdes Memorial Hospital[2]	Binghamton	287	795
Saint Anthony Community Hospital[2]	Warwick	288	354
Saint Mary's Hospital - Troy[2]	Troy	288	641
Cobleskill Regional Hospital[2]	Cobleskill	293	326
Rome Memorial Hospital[2]	Rome	294	394
United Health Services Hospitals[2]	Johnson City	298	592
Saratoga Hospital[2]	Saratoga Spgs	302	501
Mount St Mary's Hosp & Health Ctr[2]	Lewiston	304	684
Putnam Hospital Center[2]	Carmel	305	752
Kenmore Mercy Hospital[2]	Kenmore	310	928
Nathan Littauer Hospital[2]	Gloversville	310	495
Arnot Ogden Medical Center[2]	Elmira	315	507
Catskill Regional Medical Center[2]	Harris	317	374
Saint John's Riverside Hospital[2]	Yonkers	318	934
Niagara Falls Memorial Medical Center[2]	Niagara Falls	319	806
Champlain Valley Phys Hosp Med Ctr[2]	Plattsburgh	320	607
Sisters of Charity Hospital[2]	Buffalo	326	531
Woman's Christian Association[2]	Jamestown	327	570
Cayuga Medical Center at Ithaca[2]	Ithaca	328	395
North Central Bronx Hospital[2]	Bronx	329	587
Nassau University Medical Center[2]	East Meadow	334	513
Medina Memorial Hospital[2]	Medina	335	326
Orange Regional Medical Center[2]	Middletown	338	665
Southampton Hospital[2]	Southampton	338	785
Aurelia Osborn Fox Memorial Hospital[2]	Oneonta	344	368
Glen Cove Hospital[2]	Glen Cove	346	787
Crouse Hospital[2]	Syracuse	349	414
F F Thompson Hospital[2]	Canandaigua	350	575
Saint Luke's Cornwall Hospital[2]	Newburgh	352	729
Univ Hosp SUNY Health Science Ctr[2]	Syracuse	352	532
NYU Hospitals Center[2]	New York	355	237
Unity Hospital of Rochester[2]	Rochester	355	487
Lawrence Hospital Center[2]	Bronxville	357	844
Saint Joseph's Hospital[2]	Elmira	359	276
Faxton - Saint Luke's Healthcare[2]	Utica	364	668
Phelps Memorial Hospital Assn[2]	Sleepy Hollow	364	583
Samaritan Medical Center[2]	Watertown	364	556
Vassar Brothers Medical Center[2]	Poughkeepsie	365	663
Coney Island Hospital[2]	Brooklyn	367	779
Cortland Regional Medical Center[2]	Cortland	368	617
Metropolitan Hospital Center[2]	New York	368	646
Oneida Healthcare Center[2]	Oneida	368	389
Ellis Hospital[2]	Schenectady	369	567
Saint Peter's Hospital[2]	Albany	370	586
Mary Imogene Bassett Hospital[2]	Cooperstown	372	511
Saint Catherine of Siena Hospital[2]	Smithtown	372	688
North Shore University Hospital[2]	Manhasset	374	933
Rochester General Hospital[2]	Rochester	376	660
Auburn Community Hospital[2]	Auburn	378	387
Saint Francis Hospital[2]	Poughkeepsie	383	809
Health Alliance Hospital Broadway Campus[2]	Kingston	386	1023
Westchester Medical Center[2]	Valhalla	388	494
Albany Medical Center Hospital[2]	Albany	389	494
Long Island Jewish Medical Center[2]	New Hyde Park	390	94
Plainview Hospital[2]	Plainview	390	332
Oswego Hospital[2]	Oswego	392	573
South Nassau Communities Hospital[2]	Oceanside	395	967
Kaleida Health[2]	Buffalo	398	606
Lenox Hill Hospital[2]	New York	400	536
Saint Joseph Hospital[2]	Bethpage	401	974
Mercy Hospital[2]	Buffalo	402	696
Montefiore New Rochelle Hospital[2]	New Rochelle	405	799
Samaritan Hospital[2]	Troy	410	700
Lincoln Medical & Mental Health Center[2]	Bronx	415	919
Huntington Hospital[2]	Huntington	416	65
White Plains Hospital Center[2]	White Plains	416	784
Harlem Hospital Center[2]	New York	420	608
Erie County Medical Center[2]	Buffalo	428	417
Columbia Memorial Hospital[2]	Hudson	431	794
Saint Elizabeth Medical Center[2]	Utica	433	823
Good Samaritan Hospital of Suffern[2]	Suffern	434	574
Saint Joseph's Medical Center[2]	Yonkers	434	779
Albany Memorial Hospital[2]	Albany	439	569
Hudson Valley Hospital Center[2]	Cortlandt Manor	447	882
Flushing Hospital Medical Center[2]	Flushing	448	656
Wyckoff Heights Medical Center[2]	Brooklyn	449	977
Saint Joseph's Hospital Health Center[2]	Syracuse	464	575
Woodhull Medical & Mental Health Center[2]	Brooklyn	464	514
Bronx - Lebanon Hospital Center[2]	Bronx	474	988
Winthrop - University Hospital[2]	Mineola	482	252
Good Samaritan Hospital Medical Center[2]	West Islip	483	877
Kingsbrook Jewish Medical Center[2]	Brooklyn	484	1140
Jamaica Hospital Medical Center[2]	Jamaica	486	878
Mercy Medical Center[2]	Rockville Centre	490	738
Saint Luke's Roosevelt Hospital[2]	New York	490	524
New York Community Hospital of Brooklyn[2]	Brooklyn	495	1017
Richmond University Medical Center[2]	Staten Island	497	553
Forest Hills Hospital[2]	Forest Hills	500	430
Brooklyn Hosp Ctr at Downtown Campus[2]	Brooklyn	503	783
Bellevue Hospital Center[2]	New York	506	547
University Hospital - Stony Brook[2]	Stony Brook	516	613
New York Methodist Hospital[2]	Brooklyn	520	622
Strong Memorial Hospital[2]	Rochester	523	613
Peconic Bay Medical Center[2]	Riverhead	529	590
Beth Israel Medical Center[2]	New York	530	723
Montefiore Mount Vernon Hospital[2]	Mount Vernon	531	554
Univ Hosp of Brooklyn-Downstate[2]	Brooklyn	533	627
Queens Hospital Center[2]	Jamaica	534	852
John T Mather Mem Hosp-Port Jefferson[2]	Port Jefferson	540	1110
Maimonides Medical Center[2]	Brooklyn	547	605
Franklin Hospital[2]	Valley Stream	548	482
Staten Island University Hospital[2]	Staten Island	548	815
Southside Hospital[2]	Bay Shore	554	687
Mount Sinai Hospital[2]	New York	568	1418
Saint Charles Hospital[2]	Port Jefferson	580	464
Montefiore Medical Center[2]	Bronx	599	791
Elmhurst Hospital Center[2]	Elmhurst	615	633
New York Hosp Med Ctr of Queens[2]	Flushing	616	615
Interfaith Medical Center[2]	Brooklyn	643	387
Saint Francis Hospital - Roslyn[2]	Roslyn	656	613
Brookdale Hospital Medical Center[2]	Brooklyn	671	568
Jacobi Medical Center[2]	Bronx	674	710
St John's Episcopal Hosp-South Shore[2]	Far Rockaway	702	1071
New York - Presbyterian Hospital[2]	New York	717	531
Saint Barnabas Hospital[2]	Bronx	736	134
Lutheran Medical Center[2]	Brooklyn	808	757
Brookhaven Mem Hosp Med Ctr[2]	Patchogue	809	1105
Kings County Hospital Center[2]	Brooklyn	1155	867

Time from ER Arrival to Discharge (minutes)

Hospital Name	City	Min.	Cases
Elizabethtown Community Hospital[3]	Elizabethtown	75	160
Ellenville Regional Hospital	Ellenville	80	348
Chenango Memorial Hospital	Norwich	85	437
Adirondack Medical Center	Saranac Lake	90	370
Eastern Long Island Hospital	Greenport	91	317
Bon Secours Community Hospital	Port Jervis	95	399
Community Memorial Hospital	Hamilton	100	877
Jones Memorial Hospital	Wellsville	100	381
Saint Mary's Hospital - Troy	Troy	101	377
Saint James Mercy Hospital	Hornell	103	386
Carthage Area Hospital	Carthage	104	324
Massena Memorial Hospital	Massena	106	372
Soldiers & Sailors Mem Hosp of Yates	Penn Yan	106	324
United Memorial Medical Center	Batavia	109	433
Wyoming County Community Hospital	Warsaw	109	475
Nicholas H Noyes Memorial Hospital	Dansville	110	385
Canton - Potsdam Hospital	Potsdam	111	1480
Claxton - Hepburn Medical Center	Ogdensburg	115	411
Lewis County General Hospital	Lowville	116	436
North Shore University Hospital	Manhasset	117	727
Cobleskill Regional Hospital	Cobleskill	118	336

NOTE: Hospital profiles are in alphabetical order by state, then city, then hospital within the city; Rankings exclude hospitals with less than 25 cases except for patient surveys which excludes hospitals with less than 100 cases; (a) 100-299 cases; (1) The number of cases/patients is too few to report; (2) Data submitted were based on a sample of cases/patients; (3) Results are based on a shorter time period than required; (4) Data suppressed by CMS for one or more quarters; (5) Results are not available for this reporting period; (6) Fewer than 100 patients completed the HCAHPS survey; (7) No cases met the criteria for this measure; (8) The lower limit of the confidence interval cannot be calculated if the number of observed infections equals zero; (9) No data are available from the state/territory for this reporting period; (10) The scores shown reflect fewer than 50 completed surveys; (11) There were discrepancies in the data collection process; (12) This measure does not apply to this hospital for this reporting period; (13) Results cannot be calculated for this reporting period; (14) The results for this state are combined with nearby states to protect confidentiality; Please refer to the User's Guide for a full explanation of data.

Mercy Hospital	Buffalo	122	406
Northern Dutchess Hospital	Rhinebeck	122	418
Saint Joseph's Medical Center	Yonkers	124	297
Bertrand Chaffee Hospital	Springville	125	212
Catskill Regional Medical Center	Harris	125	368
Richmond University Medical Center	Staten Island	125	330
Saint Luke's Cornwall Hospital	Newburgh	126	361
Southampton Hospital	Southampton	128	379
Brooks Memorial Hospital	Dunkirk	130	373
Saint Anthony Community Hospital	Warwick	132	390
Saint John's Riverside Hospital	Yonkers	133	388
Champlain Valley Phys Hosp Med Ctr	Plattsburgh	134	531
Hudson Valley Hospital Center	Cortlandt Manor	134	403
Geneva General Hospital	Geneva	135	349
Montefiore New Rochelle Hospital	New Rochelle	135	431
Northern Westchester Hospital	Mount Kisco	135	394
Rome Memorial Hospital	Rome	136	340
Saint Joseph's Hospital	Elmira	136	302
Little Falls Hospital[3]	Little Falls	137	80
Alice Hyde Medical Center	Malone	138	363
Brookhaven Mem Hosp Med Ctr	Patchogue	138	1058
Nyack Hospital	Nyack	138	389
Ira Davenport Memorial Hospital	Bath	140	250
Oneida Healthcare Center	Oneida	140	403
Samaritan Medical Center	Watertown	140	352
Saint Luke's Roosevelt Hospital	New York	141	400
Samaritan Hospital	Troy	141	387
Clifton Springs Hospital & Clinic	Clifton Springs	142	270
Ellis Hospital	Schenectady	142	394
Huntington Hospital	Huntington	142	335
Eastern Niagara Hospital	Lockport	143	380
Glen Cove Hospital	Glen Cove	143	373
Nassau University Medical Center	East Meadow	143	314
Albany Memorial Hospital	Albany	144	391
Health Alliance Hospital Broadway Campus	Kingston	145	285
Saint Mary's Hospital at Amsterdam	Amsterdam	145	369
Southside Hospital	Bay Shore	145	367
Newark - Wayne Community Hospital	Newark	146	346
Putnam Hospital Center	Carmel	146	443
Woman's Christian Association	Jamestown	146	357
Forest Hills Hospital	Forest Hills	147	377
Phelps Memorial Hospital Assn	Sleepy Hollow	147	369
Corning Hospital	Corning	148	683
Sisters of Charity Hospital	Buffalo	148	392
Flushing Hospital Medical Center	Flushing	149	390
Brookdale Hospital Medical Center	Brooklyn	150	346
Medina Memorial Hospital	Medina	150	356
Mercy Medical Center	Rockville Centre	151	394
New York Hosp Med Ctr of Queens	Flushing	151	380
Saint Charles Hospital	Port Jefferson	152	386
TLC Health Network	Gowanda	153	366
Franklin Hospital	Valley Stream	154	364
Peconic Bay Medical Center	Riverhead	154	394
Coney Island Hospital	Brooklyn	156	375
Lenox Hill Hospital	New York	156	371
Staten Island University Hospital	Staten Island	156	370
Plainview Hospital	Plainview	159	375
Saint Francis Hospital	Poughkeepsie	160	302
Nathan Littauer Hospital	Gloversville	162	344
University Hospital - Stony Brook	Stony Brook	162	223
Lincoln Medical & Mental Health Center	Bronx	163	341
Saint Joseph Hospital	Bethpage	163	436
Kenmore Mercy Hospital	Kenmore	164	387
Olean General Hospital	Olean	164	410
Saratoga Hospital	Saratoga Spgs	164	513
Arnot Ogden Medical Center	Elmira	167	318
Brooklyn Hosp Ctr at Downtown Campus	Brooklyn	168	443
Metropolitan Hospital Center	New York	169	310
Westfield Memorial Hospital	Westfield	169	374
Kingsbrook Jewish Medical Center	Brooklyn	170	380
New York Community Hospital of Brooklyn	Brooklyn	170	310
Saint Catherine of Siena Hospital	Smithtown	170	373
Good Samaritan Hospital Medical Center	West Islip	171	446
Univ Hosp of Brooklyn-Downstate	Brooklyn	171	331
Mount St Mary's Hosp & Health Ctr	Lewiston	172	337
Saint Elizabeth Medical Center	Utica	172	369
Harlem Hospital Center	New York	173	315
Glens Falls Hospital	Glens Falls	174	373
NYU Hospitals Center[3]	New York	174	120
Orange Regional Medical Center	Middletown	174	351
Lawrence Hospital Center	Bronxville	176	406
Highland Hospital	Rochester	177	367
Oswego Hospital	Oswego	177	337
Our Lady of Lourdes Memorial Hospital	Binghamton	177	389
Univ Hosp SUNY Health Science Ctr	Syracuse	177	571
Cortland Regional Medical Center	Cortland	181	353
Rochester General Hospital	Rochester	181	349
Auburn Community Hospital	Auburn	183	328
Mary Imogene Bassett Hospital	Cooperstown	183	515
United Health Services Hospitals	Johnson City	183	418
Wyckoff Heights Medical Center	Brooklyn	184	409
Columbia Memorial Hospital	Hudson	185	371
Niagara Falls Memorial Medical Center	Niagara Falls	186	292
Kaleida Health	Buffalo	187	955
North Central Bronx Hospital	Bronx	188	350
Aurelia Osborn Fox Memorial Hospital	Oneonta	189	409
Queens Hospital Center	Jamaica	190	418
Vassar Brothers Medical Center	Poughkeepsie	192	406
White Plains Hospital Center	White Plains	192	367
Mount Sinai Hospital	New York	193	707
Cayuga Medical Center at Ithaca	Ithaca	194	376
Westchester Medical Center	Valhalla	194	296
Montefiore Mount Vernon Hospital	Mount Vernon	195	382
John T Mather Mem Hosp-Port Jefferson	Port Jefferson	196	369
Unity Hospital of Rochester	Rochester	196	334
Good Samaritan Hospital of Suffern	Suffern	197	400
New York Methodist Hospital	Brooklyn	197	395
St John's Episcopal Hosp-South Shore	Far Rockaway	198	364
Bronx - Lebanon Hospital Center	Bronx	199	350
South Nassau Communities Hospital	Oceanside	203	409
Bellevue Hospital Center	New York	204	353
F F Thompson Hospital	Canandaigua	205	371
Saint Peter's Hospital	Albany	206	365
Crouse Hospital	Syracuse	207	338
Beth Israel Medical Center	New York	208	354
Long Island Jewish Medical Center	New Hyde Park	208	493
Elmhurst Hospital Center	Elmhurst	211	360
Maimonides Medical Center	Brooklyn	216	384
Winthrop - University Hospital	Mineola	219	364
Albany Medical Center Hospital	Albany	224	325
Jamaica Hospital Medical Center	Jamaica	229	370
Saint Joseph's Hospital Health Center	Syracuse	234	343
Woodhull Medical & Mental Health Center	Brooklyn	236	325
Faxton - Saint Luke's Healthcare	Utica	246	366
Jacobi Medical Center	Bronx	246	331
Kings County Hospital Center	Brooklyn	247	364
Strong Memorial Hospital	Rochester	250	338
New York - Presbyterian Hospital	New York	256	394
Saint Francis Hospital - Roslyn	Roslyn	266	348
Montefiore Medical Center	Bronx	270	374
Lutheran Medical Center	Brooklyn	271	359
Interfaith Medical Center	Brooklyn	274	377
Erie County Medical Center	Buffalo	282	306
Saint Barnabas Hospital[3]	Bronx	353	41

Time in ER Before Being Evaluated (minutes)

Hospital Name	City	Min.	Cases
Saint Anthony Community Hospital	Warwick	6	405
John T Mather Mem Hosp-Port Jefferson	Port Jefferson	7	414
Elizabethtown Community Hospital[3]	Elizabethtown	10	166
Glen Cove Hospital	Glen Cove	11	397
Orange Regional Medical Center	Middletown	12	412
Bon Secours Community Hospital	Port Jervis	13	444
Ellenville Regional Hospital	Ellenville	14	376
Catskill Regional Medical Center	Harris	16	397
Highland Hospital	Rochester	16	382
Northern Westchester Hospital	Mount Kisco	16	411
Nyack Hospital	Nyack	16	414
Staten Island University Hospital	Staten Island	17	407
Carthage Area Hospital	Carthage	18	392
Newark - Wayne Community Hospital	Newark	18	405
Saint Mary's Hospital at Amsterdam	Amsterdam	18	431
Crouse Hospital	Syracuse	19	402
Hudson Valley Hospital Center	Cortlandt Manor	19	408
Eastern Long Island Hospital	Greenport	20	396
Jones Memorial Hospital	Wellsville	20	404
Adirondack Medical Center	Saranac Lake	21	354
Chenango Memorial Hospital	Norwich	21	540
Lenox Hill Hospital	New York	21	373
Lutheran Medical Center	Brooklyn	21	407
Rochester General Hospital	Rochester	21	404
Saint Luke's Cornwall Hospital	Newburgh	21	361
Soldiers & Sailors Mem Hosp of Yates	Penn Yan	21	319
Wyoming County Community Hospital	Warsaw	21	519
Claxton - Hepburn Medical Center	Ogdensburg	22	481
Health Alliance Hospital Broadway Campus	Kingston	22	409
Richmond University Medical Center	Staten Island	22	427
Saint James Mercy Hospital	Hornell	22	406
Westfield Memorial Hospital	Westfield	22	481
Corning Hospital	Corning	23	762
Geneva General Hospital	Geneva	23	266
Saint Peter's Hospital	Albany	23	410
Canton - Potsdam Hospital	Potsdam	24	1600
Eastern Niagara Hospital	Lockport	24	412
Massena Memorial Hospital	Massena	24	406
Mercy Hospital	Buffalo	24	420
North Shore University Hospital	Manhasset	25	646
Olean General Hospital	Olean	25	472
Phelps Memorial Hospital Assn	Sleepy Hollow	25	411
Plainview Hospital	Plainview	25	362
Southampton Hospital	Southampton	25	402
Saint Luke's Roosevelt Hospital	New York	26	436
Sisters of Charity Hospital	Buffalo	26	417
United Memorial Medical Center	Batavia	26	494
Columbia Memorial Hospital	Hudson	27	404
Oswego Hospital	Oswego	27	356
Saint Mary's Hospital - Troy	Troy	27	399
Kenmore Mercy Hospital	Kenmore	28	407
Brookhaven Mem Hosp Med Ctr	Patchogue	29	1156
Bertrand Chaffee Hospital	Springville	30	289
Saint Joseph's Hospital	Elmira	30	376
Alice Hyde Medical Center	Malone	31	388
Clifton Springs Hospital & Clinic	Clifton Springs	31	391
Community Memorial Hospital	Hamilton	31	972
Good Samaritan Hospital of Suffern	Suffern	31	439
TLC Health Network	Gowanda	31	403
Montefiore New Rochelle Hospital	New Rochelle	32	454
Maimonides Medical Center	Brooklyn	33	408
Saint Francis Hospital	Poughkeepsie	33	388
Samaritan Medical Center	Watertown	33	382
Albany Memorial Hospital	Albany	34	406
Good Samaritan Hospital Medical Center	West Islip	34	408
Ira Davenport Memorial Hospital	Bath	34	287
Nicholas H Noyes Memorial Hospital	Dansville	34	407
Cortland Regional Medical Center	Cortland	35	457
Ellis Hospital	Schenectady	35	418
Erie County Medical Center	Buffalo	35	320
Huntington Hospital	Huntington	35	250
Lewis County General Hospital	Lowville	35	439
Medina Memorial Hospital	Medina	35	259
Nathan Littauer Hospital	Gloversville	35	372
Northern Dutchess Hospital	Rhinebeck	35	400
Oneida Healthcare Center	Oneida	35	423
Saint Catherine of Siena Hospital	Smithtown	35	400
Samaritan Hospital	Troy	35	426
Strong Memorial Hospital	Rochester	35	377
Unity Hospital of Rochester	Rochester	35	419
Westchester Medical Center	Valhalla	36	407
Cobleskill Regional Hospital	Cobleskill	37	217
Franklin Hospital	Valley Stream	37	371
Mary Imogene Bassett Hospital	Cooperstown	37	265
Albany Medical Center Hospital	Albany	38	251
Arnot Ogden Medical Center	Elmira	38	360
Saint Elizabeth Medical Center	Utica	38	406
Peconic Bay Medical Center	Riverhead	39	325
White Plains Hospital Center	White Plains	39	417
Saint Charles Hospital	Port Jefferson	40	382
Saint John's Riverside Hospital	Yonkers	40	407
Our Lady of Lourdes Memorial Hospital	Binghamton	41	408
Champlain Valley Phys Hosp Med Ctr	Plattsburgh	42	549
Flushing Hospital Medical Center	Flushing	42	432
Kaleida Health	Buffalo	42	1010
Little Falls Hospital[3]	Little Falls	42	96
New York Community Hospital of Brooklyn	Brooklyn	42	374
Putnam Hospital Center	Carmel	42	423
Forest Hills Hospital	Forest Hills	43	383
Saratoga Hospital	Saratoga Spgs	43	583
Cayuga Medical Center at Ithaca	Ithaca	44	397
Univ Hosp SUNY Health Science Ctr	Syracuse	44	549
Mercy Medical Center	Rockville Centre	45	417
Rome Memorial Hospital	Rome	45	373
Saint Joseph Hospital	Bethpage	45	519
Glens Falls Hospital	Glens Falls	46	438
Queens Hospital Center	Jamaica	46	464
Bronx - Lebanon Hospital Center	Bronx	47	432
Brookdale Hospital Medical Center	Brooklyn	47	420
United Health Services Hospitals	Johnson City	48	499
Lawrence Hospital Center	Bronxville	49	416
Metropolitan Hospital Center	New York	49	373
Mount Sinai Hospital	New York	49	933
Nassau University Medical Center	East Meadow	49	400
Bellevue Hospital Center	New York	50	399
Coney Island Hospital	Brooklyn	50	422
F F Thompson Hospital	Canandaigua	50	402
Woman's Christian Association	Jamestown	50	382
NYU Hospitals Center[3]	New York	51	116
Brooks Memorial Hospital	Dunkirk	52	406
Long Island Jewish Medical Center	New Hyde Park	52	519
Saint Francis Hospital - Roslyn	Roslyn	52	239
Saint Joseph's Medical Center	Yonkers	52	362
Kingsbrook Jewish Medical Center	Brooklyn	53	351
Jamaica Hospital Medical Center	Jamaica	55	292
Faxton - Saint Luke's Healthcare	Utica	56	404
Southside Hospital	Bay Shore	56	342
Aurelia Osborn Fox Memorial Hospital	Oneonta	58	465
St John's Episcopal Hosp-South Shore	Far Rockaway	58	417
Winthrop - University Hospital	Mineola	58	410
Montefiore Mount Vernon Hospital	Mount Vernon	59	457
South Nassau Communities Hospital	Oceanside	59	390
Auburn Community Hospital	Auburn	60	380
Mount St Mary's Hosp & Health Ctr	Lewiston	61	376
New York Hosp Med Ctr of Queens	Flushing	61	392
Vassar Brothers Medical Center	Poughkeepsie	61	368

NOTE: Hospital profiles are in alphabetical order by state, then city, then hospital within the city; Rankings exclude hospitals with less than 25 cases except for patient surveys which excludes hospitals with less than 100 cases; (a) 100-299 cases; (1) The number of cases/patients is too few to report; (2) Data submitted were based on a sample of cases/patients; (3) Results are based on a shorter time period than required; (4) Data suppressed by CMS for one or more quarters; (5) Results are not available for this reporting period; (6) Fewer than 100 patients completed the HCAHPS survey; (7) No cases met the criteria for this measure; (8) The lower limit of the confidence interval cannot be calculated if the number of observed infections equals zero; (9) No data are available from the state/territory for this reporting period; (10) The scores shown reflect fewer than 50 completed surveys; (11) There were discrepancies in the data collection process; (12) This measure does not apply to this hospital for this reporting period; (13) Results cannot be calculated for this reporting period; (14) The results for this state are combined with nearby states to protect confidentiality; Please refer to the User's Guide for a full explanation of data.

Hospital Name	City		Cases
University Hospital - Stony Brook	Stony Brook	63	158
New York Methodist Hospital	Brooklyn	66	345
Univ Hosp of Brooklyn-Downstate	Brooklyn	67	373
Niagara Falls Memorial Medical Center	Niagara Falls	69	393
Beth Israel Medical Center	New York	70	380
North Central Bronx Hospital	Bronx	73	383
Jacobi Medical Center	Bronx	77	358
Lincoln Medical & Mental Health Center	Bronx	82	377
Harlem Hospital Center	New York	83	337
Saint Joseph's Hospital Health Center	Syracuse	84	391
New York - Presbyterian Hospital	New York	85	378
Saint Barnabas Hospital	Bronx	86	60
Elmhurst Hospital Center	Elmhurst	88	381
Wyckoff Heights Medical Center	Brooklyn	95	434
Woodhull Medical & Mental Health Center	Brooklyn	112	267
Brooklyn Hosp Ctr at Downtown Campus	Brooklyn	114	412
Kings County Hospital Center	Brooklyn	114	380
Montefiore Medical Center	Bronx	114	378
Interfaith Medical Center	Brooklyn	125	449

Time to Pain Meds for Bone Fractures (minutes)

Hospital Name	City	Min.	Cases
Saint James Mercy Hospital	Hornell	31	53
Soldiers & Sailors Mem Hosp of Yates	Penn Yan	31	32
New York Methodist Hospital	Brooklyn	33	101
Nyack Hospital	Nyack	33	236
Jones Memorial Hospital	Wellsville	35	39
Massena Memorial Hospital	Massena	35	38
Bronx - Lebanon Hospital Center	Bronx	37	123
United Memorial Medical Center	Batavia	37	58
Wyoming County Community Hospital	Warsaw	38	60
Rochester General Hospital	Rochester	41	236
Northern Westchester Hospital	Mount Kisco	42	161
Claxton - Hepburn Medical Center	Ogdensburg	43	68
Ellenville Regional Hospital	Ellenville	43	62
Northern Dutchess Hospital	Rhinebeck	43	48
University Hospital - Stony Brook	Stony Brook	43	189
Brookhaven Mem Hosp Med Ctr	Patchogue	44	118
Jamaica Hospital Medical Center	Jamaica	44	234
Lincoln Medical & Mental Health Center	Bronx	44	168
Maimonides Medical Center	Brooklyn	44	383
Putnam Hospital Center	Carmel	44	104
Corning Hospital	Corning	45	87
Crouse Hospital	Syracuse	45	46
Huntington Hospital	Huntington	45	164
North Shore University Hospital	Manhasset	45	189
Catskill Regional Medical Center	Harris	46	102
Glen Cove Hospital	Glen Cove	46	65
Saint Anthony Community Hospital	Warwick	46	105
Saint Luke's Cornwall Hospital	Newburgh	46	165
TLC Health Network	Gowanda	46	58
Geneva General Hospital	Geneva	47	68
Health Alliance Hospital Broadway Campus	Kingston	47	151
Mercy Hospital	Buffalo	47	299
Chenango Memorial Hospital	Norwich	48	51
Phelps Memorial Hospital Assn	Sleepy Hollow	48	56
Saint Luke's Roosevelt Hospital	New York	48	389
Saratoga Hospital	Saratoga Spgs	48	88
Univ Hosp of Brooklyn-Downstate	Brooklyn	48	169
Adirondack Medical Center	Saranac Lake	49	75
Brookdale Hospital Medical Center	Brooklyn	50	171
Ellis Hospital	Schenectady	50	331
Newark - Wayne Community Hospital	Newark	50	70
Oneida Healthcare Center	Oneida	50	101
Coney Island Hospital	Brooklyn	51	181
Hudson Valley Hospital Center	Cortlandt Manor	51	181
Southside Hospital	Bay Shore	51	132
Bellevue Hospital Center	New York	52	101
Community Memorial Hospital	Hamilton	52	74
North Central Bronx Hospital	Bronx	52	54
Olean General Hospital	Olean	52	110
Carthage Area Hospital	Carthage	53	55
Good Samaritan Hospital of Suffern	Suffern	53	89
Saint Francis Hospital	Poughkeepsie	54	98
Vassar Brothers Medical Center	Poughkeepsie	54	113
Bon Secours Community Hospital	Port Jervis	55	65
Plainview Hospital	Plainview	55	76
Saint Mary's Hospital at Amsterdam	Amsterdam	55	131
Samaritan Medical Center	Watertown	55	151
Cortland Regional Medical Center	Cortland	56	91
Saint John's Riverside Hospital	Yonkers	56	110
Southampton Hospital	Southampton	56	180
Glens Falls Hospital	Glens Falls	57	219
John T Mather Mem Hosp-Port Jefferson	Port Jefferson	58	94
Mercy Medical Center	Rockville Centre	58	80
Richmond University Medical Center	Staten Island	58	80
Woodhull Medical & Mental Health Center	Brooklyn	58	180
Cayuga Medical Center at Ithaca	Ithaca	59	92
Orange Regional Medical Center	Middletown	59	224
Franklin Hospital	Valley Stream	60	67
Nicholas H Noyes Memorial Hospital	Dansville	60	59
Saint Mary's Hospital - Troy	Troy	60	64
Sisters of Charity Hospital	Buffalo	60	192
Canton - Potsdam Hospital	Potsdam	61	97
Arnot Ogden Medical Center	Elmira	62	32
Columbia Memorial Hospital	Hudson	62	42
Elmhurst Hospital Center	Elmhurst	62	157
Champlain Valley Phys Hosp Med Ctr	Plattsburgh	63	111
F F Thompson Hospital	Canandaigua	63	110
Flushing Hospital Medical Center	Flushing	63	55
Kenmore Mercy Hospital	Kenmore	63	143
White Plains Hospital Center	White Plains	63	159
Woman's Christian Association	Jamestown	63	121
Alice Hyde Medical Center	Malone	64	36
Jacobi Medical Center	Bronx	64	180
Kings County Hospital Center	Brooklyn	64	279
Staten Island University Hospital	Staten Island	64	183
Strong Memorial Hospital	Rochester	64	289
Niagara Falls Memorial Medical Center	Niagara Falls	65	52
Peconic Bay Medical Center	Riverhead	65	119
Saint Elizabeth Medical Center	Utica	65	118
Saint Joseph Hospital	Bethpage	65	67
Lenox Hill Hospital	New York	66	66
Saint Joseph's Hospital Health Center	Syracuse	66	111
Univ Hosp SUNY Health Science Ctr	Syracuse	66	249
Mount Sinai Hospital	New York	67	153
Albany Memorial Hospital	Albany	68	81
Highland Hospital	Rochester	68	87
Lewis County General Hospital	Lowville	68	41
Samaritan Hospital	Troy	68	106
Saint Catherine of Siena Hospital	Smithtown	70	152
Saint Peter's Hospital	Albany	70	77
Beth Israel Medical Center	New York	71	137
South Nassau Communities Hospital	Oceanside	71	165
Winthrop - University Hospital	Mineola	71	231
Metropolitan Hospital Center	New York	72	34
Montefiore New Rochelle Hospital	New Rochelle	72	79
Nathan Littauer Hospital	Gloversville	72	67
Good Samaritan Hospital Medical Center	West Islip	73	181
Medina Memorial Hospital	Medina	73	29
Saint Charles Hospital	Port Jefferson	73	139
United Health Services Hospitals	Johnson City	73	132
Forest Hills Hospital	Forest Hills	74	69
Lawrence Hospital Center	Bronxville	74	110
Long Island Jewish Medical Center	New Hyde Park	74	266
Oswego Hospital	Oswego	74	57
New York Hosp Med Ctr of Queens	Flushing	75	195
Rome Memorial Hospital	Rome	75	55
Brooks Memorial Hospital	Dunkirk	77	74
Eastern Niagara Hospital	Lockport	78	57
Albany Medical Center Hospital	Albany	79	199
Kaleida Health	Buffalo	79	358
New York - Presbyterian Hospital	New York	80	400
Unity Hospital of Rochester	Rochester	80	140
Aurelia Osborn Fox Memorial Hospital	Oneonta	81	42
Mount St Mary's Hosp & Health Ctr	Lewiston	82	126
Nassau University Medical Center	East Meadow	82	123
Saint Barnabas Hospital	Bronx	83	121
Our Lady of Lourdes Memorial Hospital	Binghamton	84	185
Saint Joseph's Medical Center	Yonkers	84	26
Clifton Springs Hospital & Clinic	Clifton Springs	86	30
Harlem Hospital Center	New York	86	42
Erie County Medical Center	Buffalo	89	33
Westchester Medical Center	Valhalla	89	211
Queens Hospital Center	Jamaica	90	95
Lutheran Medical Center	Brooklyn	92	211
Brooklyn Hosp Ctr at Downtown Campus	Brooklyn	94	122
Saint Francis Hospital - Roslyn	Roslyn	96	30
St John's Episcopal Hosp-South Shore	Far Rockaway	96	110
Mary Imogene Bassett Hospital	Cooperstown	98	27
Faxton - Saint Luke's Healthcare	Utica	106	105
Montefiore Medical Center	Bronx	114	382
Auburn Community Hospital	Auburn	122	90
Interfaith Medical Center	Brooklyn	133	43
Wyckoff Heights Medical Center	Brooklyn	148	82

Heart Attack Care

Aspirin Given at Discharge

Hospital Name	City	Rate	Cases
Albany Medical Center Hospital	Albany	100%	458
Albany VA Medical Center	Albany	100%	36
Bellevue Hospital Center	New York	100%	339
Bronx - Lebanon Hospital Center	Bronx	100%	152
Brookhaven Mem Hosp Med Ctr	Patchogue	100%	83
Brooklyn Hosp Ctr at Downtown Campus	Brooklyn	100%	44
Cayuga Medical Center at Ithaca	Ithaca	100%	91
Columbia Memorial Hospital	Hudson	100%	25
Ellis Hospital	Schenectady	100%	534
Elmhurst Hospital Center	Elmhurst	100%	277
Faxton - Saint Luke's Healthcare	Utica	100%	152
Forest Hills Hospital[2]	Forest Hills	100%	31
Glens Falls Hospital[2]	Glens Falls	100%	196
Good Samaritan Hospital Medical Center	West Islip	100%	256
Good Samaritan Hospital of Suffern	Suffern	100%	380
Harlem Hospital Center	New York	100%	28
Hudson Valley Hospital Center	Cortlandt Manor	100%	51
Jacobi Medical Center	Bronx	100%	38
Jamaica Hospital Medical Center[2]	Jamaica	100%	228
John T Mather Mem Hosp-Port Jefferson	Port Jefferson	100%	60
Kenmore Mercy Hospital	Kenmore	100%	61
Kings County Hospital Center	Brooklyn	100%	49
Lincoln Medical & Mental Health Center	Bronx	100%	63
Long Island Jewish Medical Center[2]	New Hyde Park	100%	296
Lutheran Medical Center	Brooklyn	100%	199
Mary Imogene Bassett Hospital	Cooperstown	100%	211
Mercy Medical Center	Rockville Centre	100%	78
Metropolitan Hospital Center	New York	100%	30
Mount St Mary's Hosp & Health Ctr	Lewiston	100%	34
Nassau University Medical Center	East Meadow	100%	27
New York - Presbyterian Hospital[2]	New York	100%	648
Nyack Hospital	Nyack	100%	30
NYU Hospitals Center	New York	100%	179
Phelps Memorial Hospital Assn	Sleepy Hollow	100%	29
Richmond University Medical Center	Staten Island	100%	51
Rome Memorial Hospital	Rome	100%	25
Saint Barnabas Hospital	Bronx	100%	68
Saint Charles Hospital	Port Jefferson	100%	26
Saint John's Riverside Hospital	Yonkers	100%	41
Saint Joseph Hospital[2]	Bethpage	100%	29
Saint Luke's Cornwall Hospital	Newburgh	100%	212
Saint Luke's Roosevelt Hospital[2]	New York	100%	282
Saint Mary's Hospital - Troy	Troy	100%	26
Saint Mary's Hospital at Amsterdam	Amsterdam	100%	28
Saint Peter's Hospital	Albany	100%	473
Sisters of Charity Hospital	Buffalo	100%	55
South Nassau Communities Hospital	Oceanside	100%	273
Staten Island University Hospital[2]	Staten Island	100%	276
Strong Memorial Hospital	Rochester	100%	691
Syracuse VA Medical Center	Syracuse	100%	40
United Health Services Hospitals	Johnson City	100%	528
Upstate New York VA Healthcare Sys	Buffalo	100%	90
VA New York Harbor Healthcare System	New York	100%	77
Westchester Medical Center[2]	Valhalla	100%	346
White Plains Hospital Center	White Plains	100%	159
Winthrop - University Hospital	Mineola	100%	460
Arnot Ogden Medical Center	Elmira	99%	278
Beth Israel Medical Center[2]	New York	99%	249
Brookdale Hospital Medical Center	Brooklyn	99%	169
Champlain Valley Phys Hosp Med Ctr	Plattsburgh	99%	360
Crouse Hospital	Syracuse	99%	165
Kaleida Health[2]	Buffalo	99%	510
Lenox Hill Hospital[2]	New York	99%	286
Maimonides Medical Center[2]	Brooklyn	99%	288
Mercy Hospital[2]	Buffalo	99%	304
New York Hosp Med Ctr of Queens[2]	Flushing	99%	275
New York Methodist Hospital	Brooklyn	99%	367
North Shore University Hospital[2]	Manhasset	99%	320
Orange Regional Medical Center	Middletown	99%	328
Our Lady of Lourdes Memorial Hospital	Binghamton	99%	74
Saint Catherine of Siena Hospital	Smithtown	99%	160
Saint Elizabeth Medical Center	Utica	99%	295
Saint Francis Hospital - Roslyn[2]	Roslyn	99%	338
Saint Joseph's Hospital Health Center	Syracuse	99%	1043
Southside Hospital[2]	Bay Shore	99%	271
Unity Hospital of Rochester	Rochester	99%	173
University Hospital - Stony Brook[2]	Stony Brook	99%	541
Univ Hosp of Brooklyn-Downstate[2]	Brooklyn	99%	253
Univ Hosp SUNY Health Science Ctr	Syracuse	99%	266
Vassar Brothers Medical Center	Poughkeepsie	99%	503
Huntington Hospital[2]	Huntington	98%	184
Mount Sinai Hospital[2]	New York	98%	320
Plainview Hospital[2]	Plainview	98%	57
Rochester General Hospital[2]	Rochester	98%	441
Saratoga Hospital	Saratoga Spgs	98%	41
Auburn Community Hospital	Auburn	97%	37
Franklin Hospital[2]	Valley Stream	97%	32
Glen Cove Hospital[2]	Glen Cove	97%	30
Highland Hospital	Rochester	97%	38
Interfaith Medical Center	Brooklyn	97%	37
Kingsbrook Jewish Medical Center	Brooklyn	97%	38
Samaritan Hospital	Troy	97%	153
Woodhull Medical & Mental Health Center	Brooklyn	97%	29
Wyckoff Heights Medical Center	Brooklyn	97%	37
Erie County Medical Center	Buffalo	96%	94
Montefiore New Rochelle Hospital	New Rochelle	95%	37
Health Alliance Hospital Broadway Campus	Kingston	94%	65
Woman's Christian Association	Jamestown	94%	33
Montefiore Medical Center[2]	Bronx	93%	370
Peconic Bay Medical Center	Riverhead	91%	32
F F Thompson Hospital	Canandaigua	89%	27
United Memorial Medical Center	Batavia	85%	27

NOTE: Hospital profiles are in alphabetical order by state, then city, then hospital within the city; Rankings exclude hospitals with less than 25 cases except for patient surveys which excludes hospitals with less than 100 cases; (a) 100-299 cases; (1) The number of cases/patients is too few to report; (2) Data submitted were based on a sample of cases/patients; (3) Results are based on a shorter time period than required; (4) Data suppressed by CMS for one or more quarters; (5) Results are not available for this reporting period; (6) Fewer than 100 patients completed the HCAHPS survey; (7) No cases met the criteria for this measure; (8) The lower limit of the confidence interval cannot be calculated if the number of observed infections equals zero; (9) No data are available from the state/territory for this reporting period; (10) The scores shown reflect fewer than 50 completed surveys; (11) There were discrepancies in the data collection process; (12) This measure does not apply to this hospital for this reporting period; (13) Results cannot be calculated for this reporting period; (14) The results for this state are combined with nearby states to protect confidentiality; Please refer to the User's Guide for a full explanation of data.

Hospital Name	City	Rate	Cases
Oswego Hospital	Oswego	83%	36
Eastern Niagara Hospital[2]	Lockport	79%	43

PCI Within 90 Minutes of Arrival

Hospital Name	City	Rate	Cases
Beth Israel Medical Center[2]	New York	100%	33
Bronx - Lebanon Hospital Center	Bronx	100%	46
Good Samaritan Hospital Medical Center	West Islip	100%	35
Good Samaritan Hospital of Suffern	Suffern	100%	49
Jamaica Hospital Medical Center[2]	Jamaica	100%	59
New York - Presbyterian Hospital[2]	New York	100%	36
New York Hosp Med Ctr of Queens[2]	Flushing	100%	51
Saint Luke's Cornwall Hospital	Newburgh	100%	35
South Nassau Communities Hospital	Oceanside	100%	52
Staten Island University Hospital[2]	Staten Island	100%	53
Strong Memorial Hospital	Rochester	100%	121
Westchester Medical Center[2]	Valhalla	100%	34
White Plains Hospital Center	White Plains	100%	36
Albany Medical Center Hospital	Albany	98%	82
Arnot Ogden Medical Center	Elmira	98%	40
Crouse Hospital	Syracuse	98%	49
Orange Regional Medical Center	Middletown	98%	59
Bellevue Hospital Center	New York	97%	31
Saint Peter's Hospital	Albany	97%	36
Southside Hospital[2]	Bay Shore	97%	38
University Hospital - Stony Brook[2]	Stony Brook	97%	77
Vassar Brothers Medical Center	Poughkeepsie	97%	73
Saint Luke's Roosevelt Hospital[2]	New York	96%	28
United Health Services Hospitals	Johnson City	96%	82
Ellis Hospital	Schenectady	95%	78
Unity Hospital of Rochester	Rochester	95%	40
Lutheran Medical Center	Brooklyn	94%	33
Rochester General Hospital[2]	Rochester	94%	53
Saint Joseph's Hospital Health Center	Syracuse	94%	152
Samaritan Hospital	Troy	94%	31
Brookdale Hospital Medical Center	Brooklyn	93%	28
Glens Falls Hospital[2]	Glens Falls	93%	44
New York Methodist Hospital	Brooklyn	93%	42
Winthrop - University Hospital	Mineola	93%	84
Maimonides Medical Center[2]	Brooklyn	92%	48
Saint Elizabeth Medical Center	Utica	92%	63
Champlain Valley Phys Hosp Med Ctr	Plattsburgh	91%	33
Univ Hosp of Brooklyn-Downstate[2]	Brooklyn	91%	34
Elmhurst Hospital Center	Elmhurst	90%	51
Huntington Hospital[2]	Huntington	90%	40
Kaleida Health[2]	Buffalo	89%	28
Long Island Jewish Medical Center[2]	New Hyde Park	88%	26
Montefiore Medical Center[2]	Bronx	88%	34
Saint Catherine of Siena Hospital	Smithtown	85%	27
Mercy Hospital[2]	Buffalo	78%	40

Statin Prescribed at Discharge

Hospital Name	City	Rate	Cases
Albany Medical Center Hospital	Albany	100%	447
Bellevue Hospital Center	New York	100%	330
Beth Israel Medical Center[2]	New York	100%	247
Bronx - Lebanon Hospital Center	Bronx	100%	152
Brooklyn Hosp Ctr at Downtown Campus	Brooklyn	100%	41
Forest Hills Hospital[2]	Forest Hills	100%	33
Good Samaritan Hospital Medical Center	West Islip	100%	254
Good Samaritan Hospital of Suffern	Suffern	100%	369
Harlem Hospital Center	New York	100%	25
Hudson Valley Hospital Center	Cortlandt Manor	100%	46
Jamaica Hospital Medical Center[2]	Jamaica	100%	229
John T Mather Mem Hosp-Port Jefferson	Port Jefferson	100%	59
Mary Imogene Bassett Hospital	Cooperstown	100%	197
Mercy Hospital[2]	Buffalo	100%	288
Mercy Medical Center	Rockville Centre	100%	77
Metropolitan Hospital Center	New York	100%	29
Montefiore New Rochelle Hospital	New Rochelle	100%	39
Mount St Mary's Hosp & Health Ctr	Lewiston	100%	34
New York - Presbyterian Hospital[2]	New York	100%	636
Nyack Hospital	Nyack	100%	28
NYU Hospitals Center	New York	100%	180
Phelps Memorial Hospital Assn	Sleepy Hollow	100%	25
Saint Barnabas Hospital	Bronx	100%	64
Saint John's Riverside Hospital	Yonkers	100%	41
Saint Luke's Cornwall Hospital	Newburgh	100%	204
Saint Peter's Hospital	Albany	100%	474
Samaritan Hospital	Troy	100%	154
Sisters of Charity Hospital	Buffalo	100%	50
South Nassau Communities Hospital	Oceanside	100%	272
Staten Island University Hospital[2]	Staten Island	100%	265
Syracuse VA Medical Center	Syracuse	100%	36
Vassar Brothers Medical Center	Poughkeepsie	100%	512
Westchester Medical Center[2]	Valhalla	100%	346
Arnot Ogden Medical Center	Elmira	99%	270
Brookhaven Mem Hosp Med Ctr	Patchogue	99%	82
Ellis Hospital	Schenectady	99%	522
Erie County Medical Center	Buffalo	99%	95
Glens Falls Hospital[2]	Glens Falls	99%	194
Long Island Jewish Medical Center[2]	New Hyde Park	99%	290
Lutheran Medical Center	Brooklyn	99%	199
Mount Sinai Hospital[2]	New York	99%	325
Rochester General Hospital[2]	Rochester	99%	413
Saint Catherine of Siena Hospital	Smithtown	99%	154
Saint Luke's Roosevelt Hospital[2]	New York	99%	285
United Health Services Hospitals	Johnson City	99%	504
White Plains Hospital Center	White Plains	99%	154
Winthrop - University Hospital	Mineola	99%	465
Cayuga Medical Center at Ithaca	Ithaca	98%	83
Elmhurst Hospital Center	Elmhurst	98%	280
Huntington Hospital[2]	Huntington	98%	186
Kings County Hospital Center	Brooklyn	98%	48
Lincoln Medical & Mental Health Center	Bronx	98%	65
Maimonides Medical Center[2]	Brooklyn	98%	294
New York Methodist Hospital	Brooklyn	98%	362
Orange Regional Medical Center	Middletown	98%	332
Saint Francis Hospital - Roslyn[2]	Roslyn	98%	347
Southside Hospital[2]	Bay Shore	98%	268
Strong Memorial Hospital	Rochester	98%	670
Unity Hospital of Rochester	Rochester	98%	172
Upstate New York VA Healthcare Sys	Buffalo	98%	95
Albany VA Medical Center	Albany	97%	36
Jacobi Medical Center	Bronx	97%	35
Kaleida Health[2]	Buffalo	97%	513
Kenmore Mercy Hospital	Kenmore	97%	61
New York Hosp Med Ctr of Queens[2]	Flushing	97%	281
North Shore University Hospital[2]	Manhasset	97%	311
Oswego Hospital	Oswego	97%	33
Our Lady of Lourdes Memorial Hospital	Binghamton	97%	64
Saint Elizabeth Medical Center	Utica	97%	291
University Hospital - Stony Brook[2]	Stony Brook	97%	535
Woodhull Medical & Mental Health Center	Brooklyn	97%	30
Champlain Valley Phys Hosp Med Ctr	Plattsburgh	96%	341
Lenox Hill Hospital[2]	New York	96%	284
Saint Joseph's Hospital Health Center	Syracuse	96%	1022
Saint Mary's Hospital - Troy	Troy	96%	28
Saint Mary's Hospital at Amsterdam	Amsterdam	96%	28
Univ Hosp of Brooklyn-Downstate[2]	Brooklyn	96%	256
VA New York Harbor Healthcare System	New York	96%	79
Brookdale Hospital Medical Center	Brooklyn	95%	175
Crouse Hospital	Syracuse	95%	166
Wyckoff Heights Medical Center	Brooklyn	95%	38
Faxton - Saint Luke's Healthcare	Utica	94%	149
Interfaith Medical Center	Brooklyn	94%	32
Kingsbrook Jewish Medical Center	Brooklyn	94%	35
Richmond University Medical Center	Staten Island	94%	53
Univ Hosp SUNY Health Science Ctr	Syracuse	93%	264
Highland Hospital	Rochester	92%	37
Queens Hospital Center	Jamaica	92%	25
Glen Cove Hospital[2]	Glen Cove	90%	29
Health Alliance Hospital Broadway Campus	Kingston	90%	61
Peconic Bay Medical Center	Riverhead	90%	30
Montefiore Medical Center[2]	Bronx	89%	365
Woman's Christian Association	Jamestown	89%	37
Columbia Memorial Hospital	Hudson	88%	25
Plainview Hospital[2]	Plainview	88%	51
Saratoga Hospital	Saratoga Spgs	87%	39
Lawrence Hospital Center	Bronxville	85%	26
Franklin Hospital[2]	Valley Stream	80%	35
Auburn Community Hospital	Auburn	76%	42
Eastern Niagara Hospital[2]	Lockport	73%	44

Heart Failure Care

ACE Inhibitor or ARB for LVSD

Hospital Name	City	Rate	Cases
Albany Medical Center Hospital	Albany	100%	125
Albany VA Medical Center	Albany	100%	30
Auburn Community Hospital	Auburn	100%	36
Bellevue Hospital Center	New York	100%	165
Brooklyn Hosp Ctr at Downtown Campus	Brooklyn	100%	141
Brooks Memorial Hospital	Dunkirk	100%	32
Columbia Memorial Hospital	Hudson	100%	28
Ellis Hospital	Schenectady	100%	129
Flushing Hospital Medical Center	Flushing	100%	34
Good Samaritan Hospital Medical Center[2]	West Islip	100%	98
Good Samaritan Hospital of Suffern	Suffern	100%	99
Hudson Valley Hospital Center[2]	Cortlandt Manor	100%	47
Interfaith Medical Center	Brooklyn	100%	64
Jamaica Hospital Medical Center[2]	Jamaica	100%	123
John T Mather Mem Hosp-Port Jefferson	Port Jefferson	100%	47
Kenmore Mercy Hospital[2]	Kenmore	100%	54
Kings County Hospital Center	Brooklyn	100%	333
Mercy Medical Center	Rockville Centre	100%	50
Mount St Mary's Hosp & Health Ctr	Lewiston	100%	36
Nassau University Medical Center	East Meadow	100%	78
Nathan Littauer Hospital	Gloversville	100%	26
New York Community Hospital of Brooklyn[2]	Brooklyn	100%	31
Niagara Falls Memorial Medical Center[2]	Niagara Falls	100%	34
North Central Bronx Hospital	Bronx	100%	44
Northern Westchester Hospital	Mount Kisco	100%	28
NYU Hospitals Center[2]	New York	100%	70
Olean General Hospital	Olean	100%	38
Orange Regional Medical Center[2]	Middletown	100%	81
Phelps Memorial Hospital Assn	Sleepy Hollow	100%	27
Putnam Hospital Center	Carmel	100%	31
Rome Memorial Hospital	Rome	100%	36
Saint Catherine of Siena Hospital	Smithtown	100%	54
Saint John's Riverside Hospital[2]	Yonkers	100%	54
Saint Luke's Cornwall Hospital	Newburgh	100%	91
Saint Mary's Hospital - Troy	Troy	100%	27
Samaritan Hospital	Troy	100%	42
Saratoga Hospital	Saratoga Spgs	100%	26
Sisters of Charity Hospital[2]	Buffalo	100%	77
Staten Island University Hospital[2]	Staten Island	100%	95
Strong Memorial Hospital	Rochester	100%	237
Beth Israel Medical Center[2]	New York	99%	86
Bronx - Lebanon Hospital Center[2]	Bronx	99%	166
Harlem Hospital Center	New York	99%	100
Kingsbrook Jewish Medical Center	Brooklyn	99%	135
Lincoln Medical & Mental Health Center	Bronx	99%	177
Long Island Jewish Medical Center[2]	New Hyde Park	99%	102
Mercy Hospital[2]	Buffalo	99%	69
New York - Presbyterian Hospital[2]	New York	99%	323
Saint Barnabas Hospital	Bronx	99%	147
Saint Peter's Hospital	Albany	99%	142
South Nassau Communities Hospital[2]	Oceanside	99%	97
Vassar Brothers Medical Center	Poughkeepsie	99%	116
Westchester Medical Center	Valhalla	99%	73
White Plains Hospital Center[2]	White Plains	99%	78
Jacobi Medical Center	Bronx	98%	86
Lutheran Medical Center	Brooklyn	98%	145
North Shore University Hospital[2]	Manhasset	98%	120
Northport VA Medical Center	Northport	98%	58
University Hospital - Stony Brook[2]	Stony Brook	98%	83
Univ Hosp SUNY Health Science Ctr	Syracuse	98%	127
Winthrop - University Hospital[2]	Mineola	98%	96
Arnot Ogden Medical Center	Elmira	97%	65
Brookhaven Mem Hosp Med Ctr	Patchogue	97%	78
Canton - Potsdam Hospital	Potsdam	97%	39
Faxton - Saint Luke's Healthcare	Utica	97%	117
Geneva General Hospital	Geneva	97%	31
Kaleida Health	Buffalo	97%	358
Maimonides Medical Center[2]	Brooklyn	97%	88
Mary Imogene Bassett Hospital	Cooperstown	97%	77
Montefiore Mount Vernon Hospital	Mount Vernon	97%	32
Mount Sinai Hospital[2]	New York	97%	192
Nyack Hospital	Nyack	97%	64
Saint Francis Hospital - Roslyn[2]	Roslyn	97%	128
St John's Episcopal Hosp-South Shore	Far Rockaway	97%	64
United Health Services Hospitals	Johnson City	97%	171
Woodhull Medical & Mental Health Center	Brooklyn	97%	116
Crouse Hospital[2]	Syracuse	96%	76
Lawrence Hospital Center[2]	Bronxville	96%	70
Metropolitan Hospital Center	New York	96%	47
Wyckoff Heights Medical Center[2]	Brooklyn	96%	161
Bronx VA Medical Center	Bronx	95%	61
Glens Falls Hospital[2]	Glens Falls	95%	62
Queens Hospital Center	Jamaica	95%	92
Rochester General Hospital[2]	Rochester	95%	149
Saint Joseph's Medical Center	Yonkers	95%	62
Saint Luke's Roosevelt Hospital[2]	New York	95%	144
VA New York Harbor Healthcare System	New York	95%	105
Coney Island Hospital	Brooklyn	94%	81
Forest Hills Hospital[2]	Forest Hills	94%	50
Richmond University Medical Center	Staten Island	94%	79
Saint Joseph's Hospital Health Center	Syracuse	94%	231
Syracuse VA Medical Center	Syracuse	94%	31
Univ Hosp of Brooklyn-Downstate[2]	Brooklyn	94%	144
Champlain Valley Phys Hosp Med Ctr	Plattsburgh	93%	45
Glen Cove Hospital[2]	Glen Cove	93%	29
Huntington Hospital[2]	Huntington	93%	54
Montefiore New Rochelle Hospital	New Rochelle	93%	57
Saint Elizabeth Medical Center	Utica	93%	146
Corning Hospital	Corning	92%	40
Elmhurst Hospital Center	Elmhurst	92%	120
Franklin Hospital[2]	Valley Stream	92%	59
New York Methodist Hospital[2]	Brooklyn	92%	140
Our Lady of Lourdes Memorial Hospital	Binghamton	92%	66
Southside Hospital[2]	Bay Shore	92%	77
Plainview Hospital[2]	Plainview	91%	45
Health Alliance Hospital Broadway Campus	Kingston	90%	88
New York Hosp Med Ctr of Queens[2]	Flushing	89%	83
Unity Hospital of Rochester[2]	Rochester	89%	57
Brookdale Hospital Medical Center[2]	Brooklyn	88%	133
Erie County Medical Center	Buffalo	88%	78
Saint Joseph Hospital[2]	Bethpage	88%	43
Cortland Regional Medical Center	Cortland	87%	31
Eastern Niagara Hospital[2]	Lockport	87%	31

NOTE: Hospital profiles are in alphabetical order by state, then city, then hospital within the city; Rankings exclude hospitals with less than 25 cases except for patient surveys which excludes hospitals with less than 100 cases; (a) 100-299 cases; (1) The number of cases/patients is too few to report; (2) Data submitted were based on a sample of cases/patients; (3) Results are based on a shorter time period than required; (4) Data suppressed by CMS for one or more quarters; (5) Results are not available for this reporting period; (6) Fewer than 100 patients completed the HCAHPS survey; (7) No cases met the criteria for this measure; (8) The lower limit of the confidence interval cannot be calculated if the number of observed infections equals zero; (9) No data are available from the state/territory for this reporting period; (10) The scores shown reflect fewer than 50 completed surveys; (11) There were discrepancies in the data collection process; (12) This measure does not apply to this hospital for this reporting period; (13) Results cannot be calculated for this reporting period; (14) The results for this state are combined with nearby states to protect confidentiality; Please refer to the User's Guide for a full explanation of data.

Hospital Name	City	Rate	Cases
Oswego Hospital	Oswego	86%	28
United Memorial Medical Center	Batavia	86%	44
Montefiore Medical Center[2]	Bronx	85%	230
Lenox Hill Hospital[2]	New York	84%	124
Upstate New York VA Healthcare Sys	Buffalo	83%	69
Samaritan Medical Center	Watertown	82%	34
Highland Hospital	Rochester	81%	85
Aurelia Osborn Fox Memorial Hospital	Oneonta	76%	33
Woman's Christian Association	Jamestown	72%	57
Peconic Bay Medical Center	Riverhead	58%	31

Discharge Instructions Given

Hospital Name	City	Rate	Cases
Albany VA Medical Center	Albany	100%	74
Bath VA Medical Center	Bath	100%	33
Bellevue Hospital Center	New York	100%	275
Beth Israel Medical Center[2]	New York	100%	235
Bon Secours Community Hospital	Port Jervis	100%	85
Brooklyn Hosp Ctr at Downtown Campus	Brooklyn	100%	307
Catskill Regional Medical Center	Harris	100%	73
Claxton - Hepburn Medical Center	Ogdensburg	100%	31
Columbia Memorial Hospital	Hudson	100%	101
Crouse Hospital[2]	Syracuse	100%	238
Good Samaritan Hospital Medical Center[2]	West Islip	100%	265
Good Samaritan Hospital of Suffern	Suffern	100%	225
Hudson Valley Hospital Center[2]	Cortlandt Manor	100%	182
Jacobi Medical Center	Bronx	100%	196
Jamaica Hospital Medical Center[2]	Jamaica	100%	264
Lawrence Hospital Center[2]	Bronxville	100%	257
Mercy Medical Center	Rockville Centre	100%	112
Nathan Littauer Hospital	Gloversville	100%	69
New York - Presbyterian Hospital[2]	New York	100%	804
New York Community Hospital of Brooklyn[2]	Brooklyn	100%	212
Niagara Falls Memorial Medical Center[2]	Niagara Falls	100%	129
North Central Bronx Hospital	Bronx	100%	95
Northern Dutchess Hospital	Rhinebeck	100%	44
Northern Westchester Hospital	Mount Kisco	100%	147
NYU Hospitals Center[2]	New York	100%	220
Phelps Memorial Hospital Assn	Sleepy Hollow	100%	76
Richmond University Medical Center	Staten Island	100%	154
Saint Anthony Community Hospital	Warwick	100%	40
Saint Charles Hospital	Port Jefferson	100%	54
Saint Francis Hospital	Poughkeepsie	100%	37
St John's Episcopal Hosp-South Shore	Far Rockaway	100%	176
Saint John's Riverside Hospital[2]	Yonkers	100%	198
Saint Joseph's Hospital	Elmira	100%	38
Saint Luke's Roosevelt Hospital[2]	New York	100%	276
Saint Peter's Hospital	Albany	100%	490
Strong Memorial Hospital	Rochester	100%	663
Syracuse VA Medical Center	Syracuse	100%	128
TLC Health Network	Gowanda	100%	36
Vassar Brothers Medical Center	Poughkeepsie	100%	390
White Plains Hospital Center[2]	White Plains	100%	219
Cortland Regional Medical Center	Cortland	99%	105
Elmhurst Hospital Center	Elmhurst	99%	260
Forest Hills Hospital[2]	Forest Hills	99%	195
Geneva General Hospital	Geneva	99%	111
Interfaith Medical Center	Brooklyn	99%	150
John T Mather Mem Hosp-Port Jefferson	Port Jefferson	99%	239
Lutheran Medical Center	Brooklyn	99%	290
Mercy Hospital[2]	Buffalo	99%	200
Nassau University Medical Center	East Meadow	99%	149
Northport VA Medical Center	Northport	99%	140
Our Lady of Lourdes Memorial Hospital	Binghamton	99%	270
Saint Catherine of Siena Hospital	Smithtown	99%	256
Saint Joseph Hospital[2]	Bethpage	99%	191
South Nassau Communities Hospital[2]	Oceanside	99%	211
Albany Memorial Hospital	Albany	98%	100
Flushing Hospital Medical Center	Flushing	98%	105
Franklin Hospital[2]	Valley Stream	98%	173
Highland Hospital	Rochester	98%	295
Kenmore Mercy Hospital[2]	Kenmore	98%	172
Kingsbrook Jewish Medical Center	Brooklyn	98%	245
Lincoln Medical & Mental Health Center	Bronx	98%	341
Massena Memorial Hospital	Massena	98%	49
Medina Memorial Hospital	Medina	98%	45
Putnam Hospital Center	Carmel	98%	118
Rochester General Hospital[2]	Rochester	98%	483
Saint Barnabas Hospital	Bronx	98%	262
Saint Joseph's Hospital Health Center	Syracuse	98%	717
Saint Joseph's Medical Center	Yonkers	98%	118
Saint Mary's Hospital - Troy	Troy	98%	94
Sisters of Charity Hospital[2]	Buffalo	98%	219
Southampton Hospital	Southampton	98%	95
Staten Island University Hospital[2]	Staten Island	98%	226
Unity Hospital of Rochester[2]	Rochester	98%	243
Woodhull Medical & Mental Health Center	Brooklyn	98%	188
Albany Medical Center Hospital	Albany	97%	298
Arnot Ogden Medical Center	Elmira	97%	198
Bronx VA Medical Center	Bronx	97%	131
Champlain Valley Phys Hosp Med Ctr	Plattsburgh	97%	233
Chenango Memorial Hospital	Norwich	97%	60
Cobleskill Regional Hospital	Cobleskill	97%	30
Glens Falls Hospital[2]	Glens Falls	97%	270
Health Alliance Hospital Broadway Campus	Kingston	97%	220
Queens Hospital Center	Jamaica	97%	250
Upstate New York VA Healthcare Sys	Buffalo	97%	165
VA New York Harbor Healthcare System	New York	97%	227
Westchester Medical Center	Valhalla	97%	183
Wyoming County Community Hospital	Warsaw	97%	35
Auburn Community Hospital	Auburn	96%	152
Coney Island Hospital	Brooklyn	96%	199
Delaware Valley Hospital	Walton	96%	25
Ellis Hospital	Schenectady	96%	419
Soldiers & Sailors Mem Hosp of Yates	Penn Yan	96%	28
Winthrop - University Hospital[2]	Mineola	96%	260
Brookhaven Mem Hosp Med Ctr	Patchogue	95%	311
Canton - Potsdam Hospital	Potsdam	95%	122
Faxton - Saint Luke's Healthcare	Utica	95%	241
Orange Regional Medical Center[2]	Middletown	95%	259
Saint Francis Hospital - Roslyn[2]	Roslyn	95%	314
Samaritan Hospital	Troy	95%	147
Brooks Memorial Hospital	Dunkirk	94%	83
Clifton Springs Hospital & Clinic[2]	Clifton Springs	94%	52
Erie County Medical Center	Buffalo	94%	212
Kaleida Health	Buffalo	94%	1002
Long Island Jewish Medical Center[2]	New Hyde Park	94%	248
Mary Imogene Bassett Hospital	Cooperstown	94%	188
Montefiore New Rochelle Hospital	New Rochelle	94%	158
Newark - Wayne Community Hospital	Newark	94%	105
North Shore University Hospital[2]	Manhasset	94%	275
Saint Luke's Cornwall Hospital	Newburgh	94%	279
Corning Hospital	Corning	93%	126
Eastern Long Island Hospital	Greenport	93%	46
Huntington Hospital[2]	Huntington	93%	201
Jones Memorial Hospital	Wellsville	93%	58
Montefiore Medical Center[2]	Bronx	93%	545
New York Methodist Hospital[2]	Brooklyn	93%	289
Nyack Hospital	Nyack	93%	184
Oneida Healthcare Center	Oneida	93%	44
Alice Hyde Medical Center	Malone	92%	90
Bronx - Lebanon Hospital Center[2]	Bronx	92%	325
F F Thompson Hospital	Canandaigua	92%	95
Glen Cove Hospital[2]	Glen Cove	92%	120
Kings County Hospital Center	Brooklyn	92%	553
Mount St Mary's Hosp & Health Ctr	Lewiston	92%	156
Southside Hospital[2]	Bay Shore	92%	221
Univ Hosp SUNY Health Science Ctr	Syracuse	92%	356
New York Hosp Med Ctr of Queens[2]	Flushing	91%	205
Mount Sinai Hospital[2]	New York	90%	473
Plainview Hospital[2]	Plainview	90%	192
Saint Mary's Hospital at Amsterdam[2]	Amsterdam	90%	160
United Health Services Hospitals	Johnson City	90%	411
Wyckoff Heights Medical Center[2]	Brooklyn	90%	298
Saratoga Hospital	Saratoga Spgs	89%	163
Adirondack Medical Center	Saranac Lake	87%	55
Metropolitan Hospital Center	New York	87%	116
Rome Memorial Hospital	Rome	87%	127
United Memorial Medical Center	Batavia	87%	129
Lenox Hill Hospital[2]	New York	86%	266
Samaritan Medical Center	Watertown	86%	189
Saint Elizabeth Medical Center	Utica	85%	307
University Hospital - Stony Brook[2]	Stony Brook	84%	227
Brookdale Hospital Medical Center[2]	Brooklyn	83%	278
Harlem Hospital Center	New York	83%	166
Eastern Niagara Hospital[2]	Lockport	82%	157
Woman's Christian Association	Jamestown	82%	224
Cayuga Medical Center at Ithaca	Ithaca	80%	65
Aurelia Osborn Fox Memorial Hospital	Oneonta	79%	103
Nicholas H Noyes Memorial Hospital	Dansville	79%	62
Univ Hosp of Brooklyn-Downstate[2]	Brooklyn	79%	268
Olean General Hospital	Olean	78%	97
Montefiore Mount Vernon Hospital	Mount Vernon	72%	75
Oswego Hospital	Oswego	71%	96
Maimonides Medical Center[2]	Brooklyn	68%	235
Lewis County General Hospital	Lowville	65%	34
Peconic Bay Medical Center	Riverhead	62%	138
Carthage Area Hospital	Carthage	6%	32

Evaluation of LVS Function

Hospital Name	City	Rate	Cases
Albany Medical Center Hospital	Albany	100%	354
Alice Hyde Medical Center	Malone	100%	109
Arnot Ogden Medical Center	Elmira	100%	242
Bath VA Medical Center	Bath	100%	36
Bellevue Hospital Center	New York	100%	294
Beth Israel Medical Center[2]	New York	100%	275
Bronx - Lebanon Hospital Center[2]	Bronx	100%	349
Bronx VA Medical Center	Bronx	100%	146
Brookhaven Mem Hosp Med Ctr	Patchogue	100%	435
Brooklyn Hosp Ctr at Downtown Campus	Brooklyn	100%	396
Champlain Valley Phys Hosp Med Ctr	Plattsburgh	100%	283
Chenango Memorial Hospital	Norwich	100%	64
Claxton - Hepburn Medical Center	Ogdensburg	100%	41
Cobleskill Regional Hospital	Cobleskill	100%	36
Community Memorial Hospital	Hamilton	100%	27
Coney Island Hospital	Brooklyn	100%	236
Corning Hospital	Corning	100%	186
Cortland Regional Medical Center	Cortland	100%	147
Ellis Hospital	Schenectady	100%	531
Elmhurst Hospital Center	Elmhurst	100%	286
Forest Hills Hospital[2]	Forest Hills	100%	247
Franklin Hospital[2]	Valley Stream	100%	216
Glens Falls Hospital[2]	Glens Falls	100%	327
Good Samaritan Hospital Medical Center[2]	West Islip	100%	344
Good Samaritan Hospital of Suffern	Suffern	100%	322
Highland Hospital	Rochester	100%	407
Hudson Valley Hospital Center[2]	Cortlandt Manor	100%	275
Huntington Hospital[2]	Huntington	100%	272
Interfaith Medical Center	Brooklyn	100%	171
Ira Davenport Memorial Hospital	Bath	100%	29
Jacobi Medical Center	Bronx	100%	242
Jamaica Hospital Medical Center[2]	Jamaica	100%	306
Jones Memorial Hospital	Wellsville	100%	69
Kaleida Health	Buffalo	100%	1275
Kenmore Mercy Hospital[2]	Kenmore	100%	238
Kings County Hospital Center	Brooklyn	100%	594
Lawrence Hospital Center[2]	Bronxville	100%	322
Lincoln Medical & Mental Health Center	Bronx	100%	365
Long Island Jewish Medical Center[2]	New Hyde Park	100%	296
Mary Imogene Bassett Hospital	Cooperstown	100%	219
Massena Memorial Hospital	Massena	100%	64
Mercy Hospital[2]	Buffalo	100%	291
Mercy Medical Center	Rockville Centre	100%	159
Metropolitan Hospital Center	New York	100%	126
Mount St Mary's Hosp & Health Ctr	Lewiston	100%	201
Nassau University Medical Center	East Meadow	100%	198
New York - Presbyterian Hospital[2]	New York	100%	947
New York Community Hospital of Brooklyn[2]	Brooklyn	100%	260
New York Methodist Hospital[2]	Brooklyn	100%	337
Niagara Falls Memorial Medical Center[2]	Niagara Falls	100%	160
North Central Bronx Hospital	Bronx	100%	105
North Shore University Hospital[2]	Manhasset	100%	343
Northern Dutchess Hospital	Rhinebeck	100%	68
Northern Westchester Hospital	Mount Kisco	100%	186
Northport VA Medical Center	Northport	100%	154
Nyack Hospital	Nyack	100%	262
NYU Hospitals Center[2]	New York	100%	282
Oneida Healthcare Center	Oneida	100%	65
Orange Regional Medical Center[2]	Middletown	100%	354
Oswego Hospital	Oswego	100%	126
Phelps Memorial Hospital Assn	Sleepy Hollow	100%	116
Plainview Hospital[2]	Plainview	100%	261
Putnam Hospital Center	Carmel	100%	157
Queens Hospital Center	Jamaica	100%	267
Richmond University Medical Center	Staten Island	100%	196
Rochester General Hospital[2]	Rochester	100%	563
Saint Anthony Community Hospital	Warwick	100%	53
Saint Barnabas Hospital	Bronx	100%	286
Saint Catherine of Siena Hospital	Smithtown	100%	389
Saint Charles Hospital	Port Jefferson	100%	53
Saint Francis Hospital	Poughkeepsie	100%	54
Saint Francis Hospital - Roslyn[2]	Roslyn	100%	378
Saint James Mercy Hospital	Hornell	100%	25
Saint John's Riverside Hospital[2]	Yonkers	100%	265
Saint Joseph's Hospital Health Center	Syracuse	100%	880
Saint Joseph's Medical Center	Yonkers	100%	183
Saint Luke's Cornwall Hospital	Newburgh	100%	370
Saint Mary's Hospital - Troy	Troy	100%	124
Saint Mary's Hospital at Amsterdam[2]	Amsterdam	100%	211
Saint Peter's Hospital	Albany	100%	584
Samaritan Hospital	Troy	100%	183
Samaritan Medical Center	Watertown	100%	227
Saratoga Hospital	Saratoga Spgs	100%	193
Schuyler Hospital	Montour Falls	100%	26
Sisters of Charity Hospital[2]	Buffalo	100%	291
Soldiers & Sailors Mem Hosp of Yates	Penn Yan	100%	37
South Nassau Communities Hospital[2]	Oceanside	100%	287
Southampton Hospital	Southampton	100%	123
Southside Hospital[2]	Bay Shore	100%	284
Staten Island University Hospital[2]	Staten Island	100%	287
Strong Memorial Hospital	Rochester	100%	746
United Memorial Medical Center	Batavia	100%	153
University Hospital - Stony Brook[2]	Stony Brook	100%	273
Univ Hosp of Brooklyn-Downstate[2]	Brooklyn	100%	286
Univ Hosp SUNY Health Science Ctr	Syracuse	100%	429
Upstate New York VA Healthcare Sys	Buffalo	100%	214
VA New York Harbor Healthcare System	New York	100%	236
Vassar Brothers Medical Center	Poughkeepsie	100%	484
Westchester Medical Center	Valhalla	100%	219
White Plains Hospital Center[2]	White Plains	100%	287
Winthrop - University Hospital[2]	Mineola	100%	323
Woodhull Medical & Mental Health Center	Brooklyn	100%	200

NOTE: Hospital profiles are in alphabetical order by state, then city, then hospital within the city; Rankings exclude hospitals with less than 25 cases except for patient surveys which excludes hospitals with less than 100 cases; (a) 100-299 cases; (1) The number of cases/patients is too few to report; (2) Data submitted were based on a sample of cases/patients; (3) Results are based on a shorter time period than required; (4) Data suppressed by CMS for one or more quarters; (5) Results are not available for this reporting period; (6) Fewer than 100 patients completed the HCAHPS survey; (7) No cases met the criteria for this measure; (8) The lower limit of the confidence interval cannot be calculated if the number of observed infections equals zero; (9) No data are available from the state/territory for this reporting period; (10) The scores shown reflect fewer than 50 completed surveys; (11) There were discrepancies in the data collection process; (12) This measure does not apply to this hospital for this reporting period; (13) Results cannot be calculated for this reporting period; (14) The results for this state are combined with nearby states to protect confidentiality; Please refer to the User's Guide for a full explanation of data.

Hospital Name	City	Rate	Cases
Adirondack Medical Center	Saranac Lake	99%	68
Albany Memorial Hospital	Albany	99%	129
Brookdale Hospital Medical Center[2]	Brooklyn	99%	311
Cayuga Medical Center at Ithaca	Ithaca	99%	80
Columbia Memorial Hospital	Hudson	99%	152
Crouse Hospital[2]	Syracuse	99%	307
Faxton - Saint Luke's Healthcare	Utica	99%	344
Flushing Hospital Medical Center	Flushing	99%	189
Glen Cove Hospital[2]	Glen Cove	99%	178
Harlem Hospital Center	New York	99%	188
Health Alliance Hospital Broadway Campus	Kingston	99%	298
John T Mather Mem Hosp-Port Jefferson	Port Jefferson	99%	356
Kingsbrook Jewish Medical Center	Brooklyn	99%	336
Lenox Hill Hospital[2]	New York	99%	310
Lutheran Medical Center	Brooklyn	99%	372
Maimonides Medical Center[2]	Brooklyn	99%	307
Medina Memorial Hospital	Medina	99%	68
Montefiore Medical Center[2]	Bronx	99%	659
Montefiore New Rochelle Hospital	New Rochelle	99%	268
New York Hosp Med Ctr of Queens[2]	Flushing	99%	284
Newark - Wayne Community Hospital	Newark	99%	140
Olean General Hospital	Olean	99%	141
St John's Episcopal Hosp-South Shore	Far Rockaway	99%	237
Saint Joseph Hospital[2]	Bethpage	99%	258
Saint Luke's Roosevelt Hospital[2]	New York	99%	312
Syracuse VA Medical Center	Syracuse	99%	134
United Health Services Hospitals	Johnson City	99%	495
Woman's Christian Association	Jamestown	99%	276
Wyckoff Heights Medical Center[2]	Brooklyn	99%	327
Albany VA Medical Center	Albany	98%	90
Auburn Community Hospital	Auburn	98%	189
Canton - Potsdam Hospital	Potsdam	98%	145
Clifton Springs Hospital & Clinic[2]	Clifton Springs	98%	61
Eastern Long Island Hospital	Greenport	98%	59
Eastern Niagara Hospital[2]	Lockport	98%	208
F F Thompson Hospital	Canandaigua	98%	124
Geneva General Hospital	Geneva	98%	160
Montefiore Mount Vernon Hospital	Mount Vernon	98%	97
Mount Sinai Hospital[2]	New York	98%	552
Our Lady of Lourdes Memorial Hospital	Binghamton	98%	344
Saint Elizabeth Medical Center	Utica	98%	419
Unity Hospital of Rochester[2]	Rochester	98%	303
Wyoming County Community Hospital	Warsaw	98%	57
Bon Secours Community Hospital	Port Jervis	97%	107
Brooks Memorial Hospital	Dunkirk	97%	128
Catskill Regional Medical Center	Harris	97%	122
Delaware Valley Hospital	Walton	97%	36
Erie County Medical Center	Buffalo	97%	270
Carthage Area Hospital	Carthage	95%	43
Rome Memorial Hospital	Rome	95%	174
TLC Health Network	Gowanda	94%	47
Nathan Littauer Hospital	Gloversville	92%	86
Saint Joseph's Hospital	Elmira	92%	50
Bertrand Chaffee Hospital[2]	Springville	91%	35
Aurelia Osborn Fox Memorial Hospital	Oneonta	90%	132
Little Falls Hospital	Little Falls	90%	30
Lewis County General Hospital	Lowville	89%	47
Peconic Bay Medical Center	Riverhead	89%	181
Nicholas H Noyes Memorial Hospital	Dansville	88%	77

Medicare Spending

Medicare Spending per Patient (ratio)

Hospital Name	City	Ratio	Cases
Ira Davenport Memorial Hospital	Bath	0.75	-
Lewis County General Hospital	Lowville	0.75	-
Saint James Mercy Hospital	Hornell	0.79	-
Canton - Potsdam Hospital	Potsdam	0.81	-
Chenango Memorial Hospital	Norwich	0.82	-
Samaritan Medical Center	Watertown	0.83	-
Alice Hyde Medical Center	Malone	0.84	-
Community Memorial Hospital	Hamilton	0.84	-
Clifton Springs Hospital & Clinic	Clifton Springs	0.85	-
Cobleskill Regional Hospital	Cobleskill	0.85	-
Medina Memorial Hospital	Medina	0.85	-
Nicholas H Noyes Memorial Hospital	Dansville	0.85	-
Claxton - Hepburn Medical Center	Ogdensburg	0.86	-
Lincoln Medical & Mental Health Center	Bronx	0.86	-
Massena Memorial Hospital	Massena	0.86	-
Aurelia Osborn Fox Memorial Hospital	Oneonta	0.87	-
F F Thompson Hospital	Canandaigua	0.87	-
Nathan Littauer Hospital	Gloversville	0.87	-
United Memorial Medical Center	Batavia	0.87	-
Wyoming County Community Hospital	Warsaw	0.87	-
Carthage Area Hospital	Carthage	0.88	-
Cayuga Medical Center at Ithaca	Ithaca	0.88	-
Corning Hospital	Corning	0.88	-
Niagara Falls Memorial Medical Center	Niagara Falls	0.88	-
Arnot Ogden Medical Center	Elmira	0.89	-
Auburn Community Hospital	Auburn	0.89	-
Cortland Regional Medical Center	Cortland	0.89	-
Kings County Hospital Center	Brooklyn	0.89	-
Newark - Wayne Community Hospital	Newark	0.89	-
Saint Joseph's Hospital	Elmira	0.89	-
Eastern Long Island Hospital	Greenport	0.90	-
Eastern Niagara Hospital	Lockport	0.90	-
Geneva General Hospital	Geneva	0.90	-
Highland Hospital	Rochester	0.90	-
Jones Memorial Hospital	Wellsville	0.90	-
Our Lady of Lourdes Memorial Hospital	Binghamton	0.90	-
Rome Memorial Hospital	Rome	0.90	-
Champlain Valley Phys Hosp Med Ctr	Plattsburgh	0.91	-
Metropolitan Hospital Center	New York	0.91	-
North Central Bronx Hospital	Bronx	0.91	-
Rochester General Hospital	Rochester	0.91	-
Saint Barnabas Hospital	Bronx	0.91	-
Saratoga Hospital	Saratoga Spgs	0.91	-
Unity Hospital of Rochester	Rochester	0.91	-
Adirondack Medical Center	Saranac Lake	0.92	-
Bronx - Lebanon Hospital Center	Bronx	0.92	-
Oneida Healthcare Center	Oneida	0.92	-
Saint Mary's Hospital at Amsterdam	Amsterdam	0.92	-
Bellevue Hospital Center	New York	0.93	-
Bon Secours Community Hospital	Port Jervis	0.93	-
Health Alliance Hosp Mary's Ave Campus	Kingston	0.93	-
Mary Imogene Bassett Hospital	Cooperstown	0.93	-
Olean General Hospital	Olean	0.93	-
Queens Hospital Center	Jamaica	0.93	-
Saint Mary's Hospital - Troy	Troy	0.93	-
Saint Peter's Hospital	Albany	0.93	-
Samaritan Hospital	Troy	0.93	-
United Health Services Hospitals	Johnson City	0.93	-
Crouse Hospital	Syracuse	0.94	-
New York Eye & Ear Infirmary	New York	0.94	-
Northern Dutchess Hospital	Rhinebeck	0.94	-
Saint John's Riverside Hospital	Yonkers	0.94	-
Saint Joseph's Hospital Health Center	Syracuse	0.94	-
Strong Memorial Hospital	Rochester	0.94	-
Woman's Christian Association	Jamestown	0.94	-
Woodhull Medical & Mental Health Center	Brooklyn	0.94	-
Brooks Memorial Hospital	Dunkirk	0.95	-
Erie County Medical Center	Buffalo	0.95	-
Glens Falls Hospital	Glens Falls	0.95	-
Mount St Mary's Hosp & Health Ctr	Lewiston	0.95	-
New York - Presbyterian Hospital	New York	0.95	-
Southampton Hospital	Southampton	0.95	-
Albany Medical Center Hospital	Albany	0.96	-
Harlem Hospital Center	New York	0.96	-
Health Alliance Hospital Broadway Campus	Kingston	0.96	-
Jacobi Medical Center	Bronx	0.96	-
Kaleida Health	Buffalo	0.96	-
Univ Hosp of Brooklyn-Downstate	Brooklyn	0.96	-
Albany Memorial Hospital	Albany	0.97	-
Ellis Hospital	Schenectady	0.97	-
Elmhurst Hospital Center	Elmhurst	0.97	-
Interfaith Medical Center	Brooklyn	0.97	-
Montefiore Medical Center	Bronx	0.97	-
Mount Sinai Hospital	New York	0.97	-
Northern Westchester Hospital	Mount Kisco	0.97	-
Saint Luke's Cornwall Hospital	Newburgh	0.97	-
Sisters of Charity Hospital	Buffalo	0.97	-
Brookdale Hospital Medical Center	Brooklyn	0.98	-
Faxton - Saint Luke's Healthcare	Utica	0.98	-
Peconic Bay Medical Center	Riverhead	0.98	-
Saint Elizabeth Medical Center	Utica	0.98	-
Saint Luke's Roosevelt Hospital	New York	0.98	-
University Hospital - Stony Brook	Stony Brook	0.98	-
Univ Hosp SUNY Health Science Ctr	Syracuse	0.98	-
Coney Island Hospital	Brooklyn	0.99	-
John T Mather Mem Hosp-Port Jefferson	Port Jefferson	0.99	-
Kenmore Mercy Hospital	Kenmore	0.99	-
Lenox Hill Hospital	New York	0.99	-
Long Island Jewish Medical Center	New Hyde Park	0.99	-
Mercy Hospital	Buffalo	0.99	-
Maimonides Medical Center	Brooklyn	1.00	-
North Shore University Hospital	Manhasset	1.00	-
Oswego Hospital	Oswego	1.00	-
Saint Francis Hospital - Roslyn	Roslyn	1.00	-
St John's Episcopal Hosp-South Shore	Far Rockaway	1.00	-
Wyckoff Heights Medical Center	Brooklyn	1.00	-
Brooklyn Hosp Ctr at Downtown Campus	Brooklyn	1.01	-
Columbia Memorial Hospital	Hudson	1.01	-
Jamaica Hospital Medical Center	Jamaica	1.01	-
New York Community Hospital of Brooklyn	Brooklyn	1.01	-
Putnam Hospital Center	Carmel	1.01	-
Vassar Brothers Medical Center	Poughkeepsie	1.01	-
Winthrop - University Hospital	Mineola	1.01	-
Beth Israel Medical Center	New York	1.02	-
Hospital For Special Surgery	New York	1.02	-
Huntington Hospital	Huntington	1.02	-
Phelps Memorial Hospital Assn	Sleepy Hollow	1.02	-
Richmond University Medical Center	Staten Island	1.02	-
Saint Anthony Community Hospital	Warwick	1.02	-
Saint Francis Hospital	Poughkeepsie	1.02	-
Staten Island University Hospital	Staten Island	1.02	-
Lutheran Medical Center	Brooklyn	1.03	-
Nassau University Medical Center	East Meadow	1.03	-
New York Hosp Med Ctr of Queens	Flushing	1.03	-
New York Methodist Hospital	Brooklyn	1.03	-
NYU Hospitals Center	New York	1.03	-
Saint Charles Hospital	Port Jefferson	1.03	-
TLC Health Network	Gowanda	1.03	-
White Plains Hospital Center	White Plains	1.03	-
Catskill Regional Medical Center	Harris	1.04	-
Flushing Hospital Medical Center	Flushing	1.04	-
Lawrence Hospital Center	Bronxville	1.04	-
Montefiore New Rochelle Hospital	New Rochelle	1.04	-
Saint Joseph's Medical Center	Yonkers	1.04	-
South Nassau Communities Hospital	Oceanside	1.04	-
Forest Hills Hospital	Forest Hills	1.05	-
Good Samaritan Hospital Medical Center	West Islip	1.05	-
Good Samaritan Hospital of Suffern	Suffern	1.05	-
Orange Regional Medical Center	Middletown	1.05	-
Plainview Hospital	Plainview	1.05	-
Saint Catherine of Siena Hospital	Smithtown	1.05	-
Bertrand Chaffee Hospital	Springville	1.06	-
Brookhaven Mem Hosp Med Ctr	Patchogue	1.06	-
Hudson Valley Hospital Center	Cortlandt Manor	1.06	-
Westchester Medical Center	Valhalla	1.06	-
Kingsbrook Jewish Medical Center	Brooklyn	1.07	-
Nyack Hospital	Nyack	1.07	-
Franklin Hospital	Valley Stream	1.08	-
Mercy Medical Center	Rockville Centre	1.08	-
Southside Hospital	Bay Shore	1.09	-
Saint Joseph Hospital	Bethpage	1.10	-
Montefiore Mount Vernon Hospital	Mount Vernon	1.14	-
Glen Cove Hospital	Glen Cove	1.16	-

Pneumonia Care

Appropriate Initial Antibiotic Given

Hospital Name	City	Rate	Cases
Alice Hyde Medical Center	Malone	100%	46
Brooks Memorial Hospital	Dunkirk	100%	33
Catskill Regional Medical Center	Harris	100%	77
Chenango Memorial Hospital	Norwich	100%	84
Clifton Springs Hospital & Clinic[2]	Clifton Springs	100%	56
Forest Hills Hospital[2]	Forest Hills	100%	92
Good Samaritan Hospital Medical Center[2]	West Islip	100%	90
Harlem Hospital Center	New York	100%	68
Jamaica Hospital Medical Center[2]	Jamaica	100%	68
Kenmore Mercy Hospital[2]	Kenmore	100%	88
Lincoln Medical & Mental Health Center	Bronx	100%	227
Mercy Hospital[2]	Buffalo	100%	82
Nassau University Medical Center[2]	East Meadow	100%	56
New York Community Hospital of Brooklyn[2]	Brooklyn	100%	74
Northern Westchester Hospital[2]	Mount Kisco	100%	96
Northport VA Medical Center	Northport	100%	29
Nyack Hospital[2]	Nyack	100%	90
NYU Hospitals Center[2]	New York	100%	57
Saint Francis Hospital	Poughkeepsie	100%	56
St John's Episcopal Hosp-South Shore[2]	Far Rockaway	100%	33
Saint Joseph's Medical Center	Yonkers	100%	57
Samaritan Hospital[2]	Troy	100%	93
Sisters of Charity Hospital[2]	Buffalo	100%	100
Southside Hospital[2]	Bay Shore	100%	90
Staten Island University Hospital[2]	Staten Island	100%	82
Strong Memorial Hospital[2]	Rochester	100%	52
United Health Services Hospitals	Johnson City	100%	167
VA New York Harbor Healthcare System	New York	100%	61
Albany Memorial Hospital[2]	Albany	99%	94
Brooklyn Hosp Ctr at Downtown Campus	Brooklyn	99%	108
Champlain Valley Phys Hosp Med Ctr	Plattsburgh	99%	144
Ellis Hospital	Schenectady	99%	234
Elmhurst Hospital Center[2]	Elmhurst	99%	118
Faxton - Saint Luke's Healthcare	Utica	99%	155
Hudson Valley Hospital Center[2]	Cortlandt Manor	99%	102
Kingsbrook Jewish Medical Center	Brooklyn	99%	107
Massena Memorial Hospital	Massena	99%	79
Our Lady of Lourdes Memorial Hospital	Binghamton	99%	197
Saint Catherine of Siena Hospital[2]	Smithtown	99%	89
Saint Luke's Roosevelt Hospital[2]	New York	99%	90
Samaritan Medical Center	Watertown	99%	131
South Nassau Communities Hospital[2]	Oceanside	99%	68
Vassar Brothers Medical Center[2]	Poughkeepsie	99%	212
Columbia Memorial Hospital[2]	Hudson	98%	122
Corning Hospital	Corning	98%	82
Health Alliance Hospital Broadway Campus	Kingston	98%	182
Huntington Hospital[2]	Huntington	98%	63
John T Mather Mem Hosp-Port Jefferson	Port Jefferson	98%	208
Kaleida Health[2]	Buffalo	98%	190

NOTE: Hospital profiles are in alphabetical order by state, then city, then hospital within the city; Rankings exclude hospitals with less than 25 cases except for patient surveys which excludes hospitals with less than 100 cases; (a) 100-299 cases; (1) The number of cases/patients is too few to report; (2) Data submitted were based on a sample of cases/patients; (3) Results are based on a shorter time period than required; (4) Data suppressed by CMS for one or more quarters; (5) Results are not available for this reporting period; (6) Fewer than 100 patients completed the HCAHPS survey; (7) No cases met the criteria for this measure; (8) The lower limit of the confidence interval cannot be calculated if the number of observed infections equals zero; (9) No data are available from the state/territory for this reporting period; (10) The scores shown reflect fewer than 50 completed surveys; (11) There were discrepancies in the data collection process; (12) This measure does not apply to this hospital for this reporting period; (13) Results cannot be calculated for this reporting period; (14) The results for this state are combined with nearby states to protect confidentiality; Please refer to the User's Guide for a full explanation of data.

Kings County Hospital Center	Brooklyn	98%	171
Metropolitan Hospital Center	New York	98%	65
North Central Bronx Hospital	Bronx	98%	57
Orange Regional Medical Center[2]	Middletown	98%	106
Phelps Memorial Hospital Assn	Sleepy Hollow	98%	81
Putnam Hospital Center	Carmel	98%	96
Saint Barnabas Hospital[2]	Bronx	98%	60
Saint Charles Hospital	Port Jefferson	98%	60
Saint Mary's Hospital - Troy	Troy	98%	85
Saint Mary's Hospital at Amsterdam[2]	Amsterdam	98%	56
Wyckoff Heights Medical Center[2]	Brooklyn	98%	91
Albany Medical Center Hospital	Albany	97%	103
Bath VA Medical Center	Bath	97%	32
Bellevue Hospital Center	New York	97%	65
Bon Secours Community Hospital	Port Jervis	97%	104
Bronx - Lebanon Hospital Center[2]	Bronx	97%	79
Claxton - Hepburn Medical Center	Ogdensburg	97%	38
Cortland Regional Medical Center[2]	Cortland	97%	115
Delaware Valley Hospital	Walton	97%	31
Elizabethtown Community Hospital	Elizabethtown	97%	30
F F Thompson Hospital	Canandaigua	97%	138
Geneva General Hospital	Geneva	97%	63
Jacobi Medical Center	Bronx	97%	72
Lutheran Medical Center	Brooklyn	97%	258
New York - Presbyterian Hospital[2]	New York	97%	221
New York Hosp Med Ctr of Queens[2]	Flushing	97%	91
New York Methodist Hospital[2]	Brooklyn	97%	102
Niagara Falls Memorial Medical Center[2]	Niagara Falls	97%	65
Northern Dutchess Hospital	Rhinebeck	97%	67
Queens Hospital Center	Jamaica	97%	234
Rochester General Hospital	Rochester	97%	318
Saint James Mercy Hospital	Hornell	97%	29
Saint Luke's Cornwall Hospital	Newburgh	97%	183
Saint Peter's Hospital[2]	Albany	97%	98
Soldiers & Sailors Mem Hosp of Yates	Penn Yan	97%	33
Southampton Hospital	Southampton	97%	92
Woodhull Medical & Mental Health Center	Brooklyn	97%	86
Wyoming County Community Hospital	Warsaw	97%	31
Bertrand Chaffee Hospital[2]	Springville	96%	76
Cobleskill Regional Hospital	Cobleskill	96%	49
Flushing Hospital Medical Center[2]	Flushing	96%	55
Glen Cove Hospital[2]	Glen Cove	96%	67
Glens Falls Hospital[2]	Glens Falls	96%	100
Highland Hospital[2]	Rochester	96%	167
Lenox Hill Hospital[2]	New York	96%	81
Mercy Medical Center	Rockville Centre	96%	95
Montefiore New Rochelle Hospital	New Rochelle	96%	76
Oswego Hospital[2]	Oswego	96%	81
Saint Joseph Hospital[2]	Bethpage	96%	121
Unity Hospital of Rochester[2]	Rochester	96%	118
Albany VA Medical Center	Albany	95%	42
Erie County Medical Center	Buffalo	95%	57
Jones Memorial Hospital	Wellsville	95%	39
Lawrence Hospital Center[2]	Bronxville	95%	119
Medina Memorial Hospital	Medina	95%	60
Mount St Mary's Hosp & Health Ctr	Lewiston	95%	100
Olean General Hospital[2]	Olean	95%	120
Saratoga Hospital[2]	Saratoga Spgs	95%	148
Upstate New York VA Healthcare Sys	Buffalo	95%	56
Arnot Ogden Medical Center	Elmira	94%	162
Canton - Potsdam Hospital	Potsdam	94%	85
Crouse Hospital[2]	Syracuse	94%	99
Maimonides Medical Center[2]	Brooklyn	94%	62
Newark - Wayne Community Hospital	Newark	94%	71
Richmond University Medical Center[2]	Staten Island	94%	65
Saint Francis Hospital - Roslyn	Roslyn	94%	159
Saint Joseph's Hospital Health Center	Syracuse	94%	334
Univ Hosp SUNY Health Science Ctr	Syracuse	94%	154
White Plains Hospital Center[2]	White Plains	94%	88
Beth Israel Medical Center[2]	New York	93%	113
Mary Imogene Bassett Hospital[2]	Cooperstown	93%	55
Mount Sinai Hospital[2]	New York	93%	164
Plainview Hospital[2]	Plainview	93%	87
Rome Memorial Hospital	Rome	93%	98
Schuyler Hospital	Montour Falls	93%	27
University Hospital - Stony Brook[2]	Stony Brook	93%	68
Brookdale Hospital Medical Center[2]	Brooklyn	92%	84
Brookhaven Mem Hosp Med Ctr	Patchogue	92%	275
Community Memorial Hospital	Hamilton	92%	53
Ellenville Regional Hospital	Ellenville	92%	25
Franklin Hospital[2]	Valley Stream	92%	80
Nicholas H Noyes Memorial Hospital	Dansville	92%	63
North Shore University Hospital[2]	Manhasset	92%	145
Saint Anthony Community Hospital	Warwick	92%	52
Auburn Community Hospital	Auburn	91%	145
Bronx VA Medical Center	Bronx	91%	34
Nathan Littauer Hospital	Gloversville	91%	116
Oneida Healthcare Center	Oneida	91%	56
Saint Joseph's Hospital[2]	Elmira	91%	127
Winthrop - University Hospital[2]	Mineola	91%	95
Long Island Jewish Medical Center[2]	New Hyde Park	90%	68
Montefiore Mount Vernon Hospital	Mount Vernon	90%	40
Saint Elizabeth Medical Center	Utica	90%	132
Syracuse VA Medical Center	Syracuse	90%	77
Cayuga Medical Center at Ithaca	Ithaca	89%	98
Eastern Long Island Hospital	Greenport	89%	27
Eastern Niagara Hospital[2]	Lockport	89%	92
Good Samaritan Hospital of Suffern	Suffern	89%	149
United Memorial Medical Center	Batavia	89%	111
Coney Island Hospital	Brooklyn	88%	103
Ira Davenport Memorial Hospital	Bath	88%	41
Saint John's Riverside Hospital[2]	Yonkers	88%	73
Westchester Medical Center	Valhalla	88%	26
Woman's Christian Association[2]	Jamestown	87%	82
Lewis County General Hospital	Lowville	86%	56
Montefiore Medical Center[2]	Bronx	86%	143
Univ Hosp of Brooklyn-Downstate[2]	Brooklyn	86%	42
Interfaith Medical Center	Brooklyn	85%	74
Peconic Bay Medical Center[2]	Riverhead	83%	105
Aurelia Osborn Fox Memorial Hospital	Oneonta	81%	84
TLC Health Network	Gowanda	81%	42
Adirondack Medical Center	Saranac Lake	79%	38
Little Falls Hospital	Little Falls	79%	72
Moses - Ludington Hospital	Ticonderoga	73%	26

Blood Culture Timing

Hospital Name	City	Rate	Cases
Brooklyn Hosp Ctr at Downtown Campus	Brooklyn	100%	326
Delaware Valley Hospital	Walton	100%	37
Elizabethtown Community Hospital	Elizabethtown	100%	31
Ellis Hospital	Schenectady	100%	530
Forest Hills Hospital[2]	Forest Hills	100%	166
Good Samaritan Hospital Medical Center[2]	West Islip	100%	147
Highland Hospital[2]	Rochester	100%	322
Jamaica Hospital Medical Center[2]	Jamaica	100%	101
Kenmore Mercy Hospital[2]	Kenmore	100%	168
New York Community Hospital of Brooklyn[2]	Brooklyn	100%	100
Newark - Wayne Community Hospital	Newark	100%	144
Nicholas H Noyes Memorial Hospital	Dansville	100%	64
Northern Westchester Hospital[2]	Mount Kisco	100%	177
Orange Regional Medical Center[2]	Middletown	100%	234
Our Lady of Lourdes Memorial Hospital	Binghamton	100%	385
Saint Anthony Community Hospital	Warwick	100%	101
Saint Mary's Hospital - Troy	Troy	100%	125
Sisters of Charity Hospital[2]	Buffalo	100%	185
South Nassau Communities Hospital[2]	Oceanside	100%	153
Staten Island University Hospital[2]	Staten Island	100%	188
Vassar Brothers Medical Center[2]	Poughkeepsie	100%	332
White Plains Hospital Center[2]	White Plains	100%	179
Albany Medical Center Hospital	Albany	99%	163
Albany VA Medical Center	Albany	99%	81
Arnot Ogden Medical Center	Elmira	99%	275
Bellevue Hospital Center	New York	99%	123
Beth Israel Medical Center[2]	New York	99%	220
Catskill Regional Medical Center	Harris	99%	216
Chenango Memorial Hospital	Norwich	99%	150
Claxton - Hepburn Medical Center	Ogdensburg	99%	68
Clifton Springs Hospital & Clinic[2]	Clifton Springs	99%	90
F F Thompson Hospital	Canandaigua	99%	256
Harlem Hospital Center	New York	99%	135
Hudson Valley Hospital Center[2]	Cortlandt Manor	99%	181
Kingsbrook Jewish Medical Center	Brooklyn	99%	322
Massena Memorial Hospital	Massena	99%	137
Mercy Hospital[2]	Buffalo	99%	134
Mercy Medical Center	Rockville Centre	99%	273
Montefiore Mount Vernon Hospital	Mount Vernon	99%	82
Northern Dutchess Hospital	Rhinebeck	99%	109
Nyack Hospital[2]	Nyack	99%	159
Saint Barnabas Hospital[2]	Bronx	99%	134
Saint John's Riverside Hospital[2]	Yonkers	99%	159
Saint Joseph Hospital[2]	Bethpage	99%	182
Saint Joseph's Hospital Health Center	Syracuse	99%	603
Saint Luke's Cornwall Hospital	Newburgh	99%	313
Saint Peter's Hospital[2]	Albany	99%	179
Saratoga Hospital[2]	Saratoga Spgs	99%	215
Southside Hospital[2]	Bay Shore	99%	174
Strong Memorial Hospital[2]	Rochester	99%	111
Syracuse VA Medical Center	Syracuse	99%	150
United Memorial Medical Center	Batavia	99%	181
University Hospital - Stony Brook[2]	Stony Brook	99%	131
VA New York Harbor Healthcare System	New York	99%	138
Winthrop - University Hospital[2]	Mineola	99%	172
Wyoming County Community Hospital	Warsaw	99%	98
Aurelia Osborn Fox Memorial Hospital	Oneonta	98%	110
Bon Secours Community Hospital	Port Jervis	98%	164
Crouse Hospital[2]	Syracuse	98%	132
Faxton - Saint Luke's Healthcare	Utica	98%	343
Geneva General Hospital	Geneva	98%	121
Glens Falls Hospital[2]	Glens Falls	98%	190
Health Alliance Hospital Broadway Campus	Kingston	98%	348
Huntington Hospital[2]	Huntington	98%	164
Ira Davenport Memorial Hospital	Bath	98%	60
John T Mather Mem Hosp-Port Jefferson	Port Jefferson	98%	384
Jones Memorial Hospital	Wellsville	98%	58
Lawrence Hospital Center[2]	Bronxville	98%	180
Lutheran Medical Center	Brooklyn	98%	407
Mary Imogene Bassett Hospital[2]	Cooperstown	98%	85
Mount Sinai Hospital[2]	New York	98%	297
New York Hosp Med Ctr of Queens[2]	Flushing	98%	213
New York Methodist Hospital[2]	Brooklyn	98%	63
Niagara Falls Memorial Medical Center[2]	Niagara Falls	98%	114
North Shore University Hospital[2]	Manhasset	98%	251
NYU Hospitals Center[2]	New York	98%	145
Oswego Hospital[2]	Oswego	98%	121
Phelps Memorial Hospital Assn	Sleepy Hollow	98%	171
Plainview Hospital[2]	Plainview	98%	161
Saint Catherine of Siena Hospital[2]	Smithtown	98%	173
Saint Charles Hospital	Port Jefferson	98%	132
Saint Francis Hospital - Roslyn	Roslyn	98%	187
St John's Episcopal Hosp-South Shore[2]	Far Rockaway	98%	123
Saint Joseph's Medical Center	Yonkers	98%	86
Saint Luke's Roosevelt Hospital[2]	New York	98%	190
Samaritan Medical Center	Watertown	98%	228
Southampton Hospital	Southampton	98%	187
TLC Health Network	Gowanda	98%	66
Upstate New York VA Healthcare Sys	Buffalo	98%	123
Adirondack Medical Center	Saranac Lake	97%	75
Bronx VA Medical Center	Bronx	97%	72
Champlain Valley Phys Hosp Med Ctr	Plattsburgh	97%	322
Eastern Long Island Hospital	Greenport	97%	59
Eastern Niagara Hospital[2]	Lockport	97%	115
Margaretville Memorial Hospital[2]	Margaretville	97%	30
New York - Presbyterian Hospital[2]	New York	97%	535
North Central Bronx Hospital	Bronx	97%	104
Olean General Hospital[2]	Olean	97%	227
Rochester General Hospital	Rochester	97%	569
Rome Memorial Hospital	Rome	97%	147
Saint Elizabeth Medical Center	Utica	97%	221
Saint James Mercy Hospital	Hornell	97%	79
Saint Mary's Hospital at Amsterdam[2]	Amsterdam	97%	129
United Health Services Hospitals	Johnson City	97%	379
Univ Hosp SUNY Health Science Ctr	Syracuse	97%	275
Auburn Community Hospital	Auburn	96%	146
Brookdale Hospital Medical Center[2]	Brooklyn	96%	181
Brookhaven Mem Hosp Med Ctr	Patchogue	96%	575
Corning Hospital	Corning	96%	150
Cortland Regional Medical Center[2]	Cortland	96%	235
Ellenville Regional Hospital	Ellenville	96%	26
Franklin Hospital[2]	Valley Stream	96%	142
Glen Cove Hospital[2]	Glen Cove	96%	131
Good Samaritan Hospital of Suffern	Suffern	96%	304
Kaleida Health[2]	Buffalo	96%	329
Lenox Hill Hospital[2]	New York	96%	159
Lincoln Medical & Mental Health Center	Bronx	96%	495
Medina Memorial Hospital	Medina	96%	94
Metropolitan Hospital Center	New York	96%	112
Montefiore New Rochelle Hospital	New Rochelle	96%	113
Mount St Mary's Hosp & Health Ctr	Lewiston	96%	142
Nathan Littauer Hospital	Gloversville	96%	194
Northport VA Medical Center	Northport	96%	53
Oneida Healthcare Center	Oneida	96%	54
Putnam Hospital Center	Carmel	96%	110
Schuyler Hospital	Montour Falls	96%	50
Albany Memorial Hospital[2]	Albany	95%	180
Alice Hyde Medical Center	Malone	95%	64
Brooks Memorial Hospital	Dunkirk	95%	96
Cayuga Medical Center at Ithaca	Ithaca	95%	153
Columbia Memorial Hospital[2]	Hudson	95%	237
Flushing Hospital Medical Center[2]	Flushing	95%	169
Long Island Jewish Medical Center[2]	New Hyde Park	95%	149
Saint Francis Hospital	Poughkeepsie	95%	105
Samaritan Hospital[2]	Troy	95%	153
Soldiers & Sailors Mem Hosp of Yates	Penn Yan	95%	60
Unity Hospital of Rochester[2]	Rochester	95%	160
Bath VA Medical Center	Bath	94%	50
Bronx - Lebanon Hospital Center[2]	Bronx	94%	186
Canton - Potsdam Hospital	Potsdam	94%	139
Coney Island Hospital	Brooklyn	94%	144
Erie County Medical Center	Buffalo	94%	198
Kings County Hospital Center	Brooklyn	94%	354
Richmond University Medical Center[2]	Staten Island	94%	142
Saint Joseph's Hospital[2]	Elmira	94%	241
Woman's Christian Association[2]	Jamestown	94%	139
Woodhull Medical & Mental Health Center	Brooklyn	94%	132
Wyckoff Heights Medical Center[2]	Brooklyn	94%	124
Community Memorial Hospital	Hamilton	93%	60
Jacobi Medical Center	Bronx	92%	185
Bertrand Chaffee Hospital[2]	Springville	91%	101
Elmhurst Hospital Center[2]	Elmhurst	91%	136
Nassau University Medical Center[2]	East Meadow	91%	118
Queens Hospital Center	Jamaica	91%	375
Westchester Medical Center	Valhalla	91%	65
Cobleskill Regional Hospital	Cobleskill	90%	52

NOTE: Hospital profiles are in alphabetical order by state, then city, then hospital within the city; Rankings exclude hospitals with less than 25 cases except for patient surveys which excludes hospitals with less than 100 cases; (a) 100-299 cases; (1) The number of cases/patients is too few to report; (2) Data submitted were based on a sample of cases/patients; (3) Results are based on a shorter time period than required; (4) Data suppressed by CMS for one or more quarters; (5) Results are not available for this reporting period; (6) Fewer than 100 patients completed the HCAHPS survey; (7) No cases met the criteria for this measure; (8) The lower limit of the confidence interval cannot be calculated if the number of observed infections equals zero; (9) No data are available from the state/territory for this reporting period; (10) The scores shown reflect fewer than 50 completed surveys; (11) There were discrepancies in the data collection process; (12) This measure does not apply to this hospital for this reporting period; (13) Results cannot be calculated for this reporting period; (14) The results for this state are combined with nearby states to protect confidentiality; Please refer to the User's Guide for a full explanation of data.

Maimonides Medical Center[2]	Brooklyn	90%	159
Univ Hosp of Brooklyn-Downstate[2]	Brooklyn	90%	114
Lewis County General Hospital	Lowville	88%	74
Peconic Bay Medical Center[2]	Riverhead	85%	166
Montefiore Medical Center[2]	Bronx	84%	283
Moses - Ludington Hospital	Ticonderoga	79%	28
Interfaith Medical Center	Brooklyn	71%	94
Little Falls Hospital	Little Falls	71%	80

Pregnancy and Delivery Care

Newborns whose Deliveries were Scheduled Early

Hospital Name	City	Rate	Cases
Beth Israel Medical Center[2]	New York	0%	82
Bronx - Lebanon Hospital Center[2]	Bronx	0%	26
Claxton - Hepburn Medical Center	Ogdensburg	0%	26
Good Samaritan Hospital Medical Center[2]	West Islip	0%	38
Jacobi Medical Center[2]	Bronx	0%	39
Kaleida Health[2]	Buffalo	0%	49
Lewis County General Hospital	Lowville	0%	28
Long Island Jewish Medical Center[2]	New Hyde Park	0%	43
Mary Imogene Bassett Hospital[2]	Cooperstown	0%	27
Nathan Littauer Hospital	Gloversville	0%	28
New York - Presbyterian Hospital[2]	New York	0%	56
New York Hosp Med Ctr of Queens[2]	Flushing	0%	112
North Shore University Hospital[2]	Manhasset	0%	56
Nyack Hospital[2]	Nyack	0%	38
Oswego Hospital[2]	Oswego	0%	29
Our Lady of Lourdes Memorial Hospital[2]	Binghamton	0%	32
Queens Hospital Center[2]	Jamaica	0%	26
Rochester General Hospital[2]	Rochester	0%	37
Rome Memorial Hospital[2]	Rome	0%	31
Saint Mary's Hospital at Amsterdam[2]	Amsterdam	0%	26
Saint Peter's Hospital[2]	Albany	0%	44
Staten Island University Hospital[2]	Staten Island	0%	54
Univ Hosp SUNY Health Science Ctr	Syracuse	0%	91
Vassar Brothers Medical Center[2]	Poughkeepsie	0%	125
White Plains Hospital Center[2]	White Plains	0%	35
Mercy Hospital	Buffalo	1%	155
Unity Hospital of Rochester	Rochester	1%	266
Brooklyn Hosp Ctr at Downtown Campus[2]	Brooklyn	2%	58
Crouse Hospital[2]	Syracuse	2%	49
Good Samaritan Hospital of Suffern[2]	Suffern	2%	48
New York Methodist Hospital[2]	Brooklyn	2%	125
NYU Hospitals Center[2]	New York	2%	64
Sisters of Charity Hospital	Buffalo	2%	148
Auburn Community Hospital	Auburn	3%	29
Ellis Hospital	Schenectady	3%	215
Flushing Hospital Medical Center[2]	Flushing	3%	65
Lawrence Hospital Center[2]	Bronxville	3%	36
Lenox Hill Hospital[2]	New York	3%	33
Lincoln Medical & Mental Health Center[2]	Bronx	3%	39
Nassau University Medical Center[2]	East Meadow	3%	31
Newark - Wayne Community Hospital[2]	Newark	3%	34
Northern Westchester Hospital	Mount Kisco	3%	126
Orange Regional Medical Center	Middletown	3%	197
Phelps Memorial Hospital Assn[2]	Sleepy Hollow	3%	30
Putnam Hospital Center	Carmel	3%	31
Winthrop - University Hospital[2]	Mineola	3%	114
Columbia Memorial Hospital[2]	Hudson	4%	27
Kings County Hospital Center[2]	Brooklyn	4%	25
Maimonides Medical Center[2]	Brooklyn	4%	104
Woman's Christian Association[2]	Jamestown	4%	26
Aurelia Osborn Fox Memorial Hospital	Oneonta	5%	38
Corning Hospital	Corning	5%	38
Mount St Mary's Hosp & Health Ctr[2]	Lewiston	5%	56
Peconic Bay Medical Center	Riverhead	5%	44
Saint Luke's Roosevelt Hospital[2]	New York	5%	55
Niagara Falls Memorial Medical Center[2]	Niagara Falls	6%	86
Saint John's Riverside Hospital[2]	Yonkers	6%	35
United Health Services Hospitals[2]	Johnson City	6%	49
United Memorial Medical Center[2]	Batavia	6%	35
Catskill Regional Medical Center[2]	Harris	7%	28
Highland Hospital[2]	Rochester	7%	30
Jamaica Hospital Medical Center[2]	Jamaica	7%	44
Montefiore Medical Center[2]	Bronx	7%	70
Woodhull Medical & Mental Health Center[2]	Brooklyn	7%	30
Faxton - Saint Luke's Healthcare[2]	Utica	8%	26
Saint Joseph's Hospital Health Center[2]	Syracuse	8%	26
Southampton Hospital[2]	Southampton	8%	50
University Hospital - Stony Brook[2]	Stony Brook	8%	37
Brooks Memorial Hospital[2]	Dunkirk	9%	56
Mercy Medical Center[2]	Rockville Centre	9%	34
Montefiore New Rochelle Hospital[2]	New Rochelle	9%	34
Mount Sinai Hospital[2]	New York	9%	55
Oneida Healthcare Center[2]	Oneida	9%	34
Richmond University Medical Center[2]	Staten Island	9%	58
Saint Anthony Community Hospital[2]	Warwick	9%	34
Cortland Regional Medical Center[2]	Cortland	11%	44
Lutheran Medical Center[2]	Brooklyn	12%	65
Nicholas H Noyes Memorial Hospital	Dansville	12%	25
Saint Luke's Cornwall Hospital	Newburgh	12%	109
Geneva General Hospital	Geneva	13%	31
Saint Catherine of Siena Hospital[2]	Smithtown	15%	26
Eastern Niagara Hospital	Lockport	16%	38
Brookdale Hospital Medical Center[2]	Brooklyn	17%	36
Cayuga Medical Center at Ithaca[2]	Ithaca	27%	26
Olean General Hospital[2]	Olean	28%	36
Alice Hyde Medical Center[2]	Malone	34%	38
Univ Hosp of Brooklyn-Downstate[2]	Brooklyn	44%	27

Preventive Care

Immunization for Influenza

Hospital Name	City	Rate	Cases
Saint James Mercy Hospital[2]	Hornell	100%	257
Community Memorial Hospital[2]	Hamilton	99%	759
New York - Presbyterian Hospital[2]	New York	99%	564
Northern Westchester Hospital[2]	Mount Kisco	99%	516
Phelps Memorial Hospital Assn[2]	Sleepy Hollow	99%	532
Saint John's Riverside Hospital[2]	Yonkers	99%	573
White Plains Hospital Center[2]	White Plains	99%	558
Winifred Masterson Burke Rehab Hosp[2]	White Plains	99%	397
Arnot Ogden Medical Center[2]	Elmira	98%	519
Beth Israel Medical Center[2]	New York	98%	549
Chenango Memorial Hospital[2]	Norwich	98%	491
Cobleskill Regional Hospital[2]	Cobleskill	98%	248
Hospital For Special Surgery[2]	New York	98%	619
Jamaica Hospital Medical Center[2]	Jamaica	98%	525
Jones Memorial Hospital[2]	Wellsville	98%	256
Lawrence Hospital Center[2]	Bronxville	98%	539
Mount Sinai Hospital[2]	New York	98%	1086
Saint Francis Hospital[2]	Poughkeepsie	98%	529
Wyckoff Heights Medical Center[2]	Brooklyn	98%	564
Wyoming County Community Hospital[2]	Warsaw	98%	321
Bertrand Chaffee Hospital[2]	Springville	97%	321
Clifton Springs Hospital & Clinic[2]	Clifton Springs	97%	282
F F Thompson Hospital[2]	Canandaigua	97%	439
Hudson Valley Hospital Center[2]	Cortlandt Manor	97%	512
John T Mather Mem Hosp-Port Jefferson[2]	Port Jefferson	97%	602
Mercy Medical Center[2]	Rockville Centre	97%	508
Nassau University Medical Center[2]	East Meadow	97%	540
Saint Anthony Community Hospital[2]	Warwick	97%	249
Saratoga Hospital[2]	Saratoga Spgs	97%	551
United Health Services Hospitals[2]	Johnson City	97%	624
Glen Cove Hospital[2]	Glen Cove	96%	593
Good Samaritan Hospital Medical Center[2]	West Islip	96%	615
Mercy Hospital[2]	Buffalo	96%	558
Montefiore New Rochelle Hospital[2]	New Rochelle	96%	499
Samaritan Medical Center[2]	Watertown	96%	450
Vassar Brothers Medical Center[2]	Poughkeepsie	96%	534
Columbia Memorial Hospital[2]	Hudson	95%	510
Cortland Regional Medical Center[2]	Cortland	95%	409
Eastern Long Island Hospital[2]	Greenport	95%	313
Ellis Hospital[2]	Schenectady	95%	523
Flushing Hospital Medical Center[2]	Flushing	95%	495
Forest Hills Hospital[2]	Forest Hills	95%	498
Glens Falls Hospital[2]	Glens Falls	95%	549
Huntington Hospital[2]	Huntington	95%	564
Ira Davenport Memorial Hospital	Bath	95%	284
Kenmore Mercy Hospital[2]	Kenmore	95%	639
Lincoln Medical & Mental Health Center[2]	Bronx	95%	511
Massena Memorial Hospital[2]	Massena	95%	264
Medina Memorial Hospital[2]	Medina	95%	301
Niagara Falls Memorial Medical Center[2]	Niagara Falls	95%	565
Nyack Hospital[2]	Nyack	95%	530
Saint Joseph's Medical Center[2]	Yonkers	95%	521
University Hospital - Stony Brook[2]	Stony Brook	95%	521
Bon Secours Community Hospital[2]	Port Jervis	94%	362
Catskill Regional Medical Center[2]	Harris	94%	386
Faxton - Saint Luke's Healthcare[2]	Utica	94%	537
Health Alliance Hospital Broadway Campus[2]	Kingston	94%	567
Highland Hospital[2]	Rochester	94%	488
Kingsbrook Jewish Medical Center[2]	Brooklyn	94%	627
Oneida Healthcare Center[2]	Oneida	94%	320
Putnam Hospital Center[2]	Carmel	94%	594
Saint Mary's Hospital - Troy[2]	Troy	94%	443
Sisters of Charity Hospital[2]	Buffalo	94%	521
Sunnyview Hosp & Rehab Ctr[2]	Schenectady	94%	316
VA Hudson Valley Healthcare System[2,3]	Montrose	94%	141
Albany Memorial Hospital[2]	Albany	93%	347
Bellevue Hospital Center[2]	New York	93%	342
Claxton - Hepburn Medical Center[2]	Ogdensburg	93%	267
Delaware Valley Hospital[2]	Walton	93%	184
North Shore University Hospital[2]	Manhasset	93%	882
Richmond University Medical Center[2]	Staten Island	93%	488
Southampton Hospital[2]	Southampton	93%	473
United Memorial Medical Center[2]	Batavia	93%	359
Unity Hospital of Rochester[2]	Rochester	93%	539
Univ Hosp SUNY Health Science Ctr[2]	Syracuse	93%	1076
Westchester Medical Center[2]	Valhalla	93%	541
Winthrop - University Hospital[2]	Mineola	93%	527
Alice Hyde Medical Center[2]	Malone	92%	264
Bath VA Medical Center[2,3]	Bath	92%	133
Brooklyn Hosp Ctr at Downtown Campus[2]	Brooklyn	92%	527
Corning Hospital	Corning	92%	1830
Elmhurst Hospital Center[2]	Elmhurst	92%	478
Northern Dutchess Hospital[2]	Rhinebeck	92%	348
Saint Joseph Hospital[2]	Bethpage	92%	609
Soldiers & Sailors Mem Hosp of Yates[2]	Penn Yan	92%	264
South Nassau Communities Hospital[2]	Oceanside	92%	730
Albany Medical Center Hospital[2]	Albany	91%	526
Crouse Hospital[2]	Syracuse	91%	502
Helen Hayes Hospital	W Haverstraw	91%	264
Nathan Littauer Hospital[2]	Gloversville	91%	320
Nicholas H Noyes Memorial Hospital[2]	Dansville	91%	256
Our Lady of Lourdes Memorial Hospital[2]	Binghamton	91%	555
Plainview Hospital[2]	Plainview	91%	553
Rome Memorial Hospital[2]	Rome	91%	373
Saint Mary's Hospital at Amsterdam[2]	Amsterdam	91%	481
Auburn Community Hospital[2]	Auburn	90%	442
Cayuga Medical Center at Ithaca[2]	Ithaca	90%	506
Mary Imogene Bassett Hospital[2]	Cooperstown	90%	553
New York Hosp Med Ctr of Queens[2]	Flushing	90%	503
Saint Luke's Roosevelt Hospital[2]	New York	90%	521
Lutheran Medical Center[2]	Brooklyn	89%	505
Olean General Hospital[2]	Olean	89%	539
Saint Charles Hospital[2]	Port Jefferson	89%	505
Saint Luke's Cornwall Hospital[2]	Newburgh	89%	556
Staten Island University Hospital[2]	Staten Island	89%	542
Franklin Hospital[2]	Valley Stream	88%	595
Good Samaritan Hospital of Suffern[2]	Suffern	88%	497
Harlem Hospital Center[2]	New York	88%	524
Kaleida Health[2]	Buffalo	88%	614
New York Community Hospital of Brooklyn[2]	Brooklyn	88%	580
Saint Barnabas Hospital[2]	Bronx	88%	526
Newark - Wayne Community Hospital[2]	Newark	87%	386
Oswego Hospital[2]	Oswego	87%	399
Saint Catherine of Siena Hospital[2]	Smithtown	87%	566
Woodhull Medical & Mental Health Center[2]	Brooklyn	87%	447
Bronx - Lebanon Hospital Center[2]	Bronx	86%	739
Champlain Valley Phys Hosp Med Ctr[2]	Plattsburgh	86%	600
Coney Island Hospital[2]	Brooklyn	86%	287
Eastern Niagara Hospital[2]	Lockport	86%	623
Erie County Medical Center[2]	Buffalo	86%	578
New York Methodist Hospital[2]	Brooklyn	86%	516
Aurelia Osborn Fox Memorial Hospital[2]	Oneonta	85%	330
Brooks Memorial Hospital[2]	Dunkirk	85%	260
Geneva General Hospital[2]	Geneva	85%	401
Peconic Bay Medical Center[2]	Riverhead	85%	570
Health Alliance Hosp Mary's Ave Campus[2]	Kingston	84%	292
Orange Regional Medical Center[2]	Middletown	84%	553
Saint Elizabeth Medical Center[2]	Utica	84%	596
Saint Joseph's Hospital[2]	Elmira	84%	466
Southside Hospital[2]	Bay Shore	84%	543
Brookhaven Mem Hosp Med Ctr[2]	Patchogue	83%	575
Lewis County General Hospital[2]	Lowville	82%	245
Queens Hospital Center[2]	Jamaica	82%	581
Westfield Memorial Hospital[2]	Westfield	81%	54
Canton - Potsdam Hospital[2]	Potsdam	79%	443
Saint Francis Hospital - Roslyn[2]	Roslyn	79%	624
Long Island Jewish Medical Center[2]	New Hyde Park	78%	1491
Saint Joseph's Hospital Health Center[2]	Syracuse	76%	561
Saint Peter's Hospital[2]	Albany	76%	569
NYU Hospitals Center[2]	New York	75%	578
Woman's Christian Association[2]	Jamestown	75%	530
Adirondack Medical Center[2]	Saranac Lake	74%	304
Univ Hosp of Brooklyn-Downstate[2]	Brooklyn	73%	547
Lenox Hill Hospital[2]	New York	72%	549
Strong Memorial Hospital[2]	Rochester	72%	519
Rochester General Hospital[2]	Rochester	69%	566
Kings County Hospital Center[2]	Brooklyn	68%	521
Metropolitan Hospital Center[2]	New York	68%	511
TLC Health Network[2]	Gowanda	67%	306
Brookdale Hospital Medical Center[2]	Brooklyn	66%	556
Maimonides Medical Center[2]	Brooklyn	66%	468
Samaritan Hospital[2]	Troy	66%	574
Montefiore Mount Vernon Hospital[2]	Mount Vernon	65%	316
St John's Episcopal Hosp-South Shore[2]	Far Rockaway	65%	532
Mount St Mary's Hosp & Health Ctr[2]	Lewiston	63%	489
Carthage Area Hospital[2]	Carthage	55%	279
North Central Bronx Hospital[2]	Bronx	53%	464
Interfaith Medical Center[2]	Brooklyn	52%	591
Jacobi Medical Center[2]	Bronx	48%	507
Montefiore Medical Center[2]	Bronx	33%	584
New York Eye & Ear Infirmary[2]	New York	16%	271

Immunization for Pneumonia

Hospital Name	City	Rate	Cases
Saint James Mercy Hospital[2]	Hornell	100%	280
Jones Memorial Hospital[2]	Wellsville	99%	311

NOTE: Hospital profiles are in alphabetical order by state, then city, then hospital within the city; Rankings exclude hospitals with less than 25 cases except for patient surveys which excludes hospitals with less than 100 cases; (a) 100-299 cases; (1) The number of cases/patients is too few to report; (2) Data submitted were based on a sample of cases/patients; (3) Results are based on a shorter time period than required; (4) Data suppressed by CMS for one or more quarters; (5) Results are not available for this reporting period; (6) Fewer than 100 patients completed the HCAHPS survey; (7) No cases met the criteria for this measure; (8) The lower limit of the confidence interval cannot be calculated if the number of observed infections equals zero; (9) No data are available from the state/territory for this reporting period; (10) The scores shown reflect fewer than 50 completed surveys; (11) There were discrepancies in the data collection process; (12) This measure does not apply to this hospital for this reporting period; (13) Results cannot be calculated for this reporting period; (14) The results for this state are combined with nearby states to protect confidentiality; Please refer to the User's Guide for a full explanation of data.

Hospital Name	City	Rate	Cases
Chenango Memorial Hospital[2]	Norwich	98%	616
Hudson Valley Hospital Center[2]	Cortlandt Manor	98%	692
Saint Francis Hospital[2]	Poughkeepsie	98%	665
Saint John's Riverside Hospital[2]	Yonkers	98%	742
United Memorial Medical Center[2]	Batavia	98%	458
Cortland Regional Medical Center[2]	Cortland	97%	425
Eastern Long Island Hospital[2]	Greenport	97%	266
Massena Memorial Hospital[2]	Massena	97%	319
VA Hudson Valley Healthcare System[2,3]	Montrose	97%	248
Vassar Brothers Medical Center[2]	Poughkeepsie	97%	630
White Plains Hospital Center[2]	White Plains	97%	641
Wyoming County Community Hospital[2]	Warsaw	97%	392
Bath VA Medical Center[2,3]	Bath	96%	329
Beth Israel Medical Center[2]	New York	96%	680
Corning Hospital	Corning	96%	2484
Forest Hills Hospital[2]	Forest Hills	96%	644
Mercy Medical Center[2]	Rockville Centre	96%	659
Northern Westchester Hospital[2]	Mount Kisco	96%	542
Nyack Hospital[2]	Nyack	96%	596
Phelps Memorial Hospital Assn[2]	Sleepy Hollow	96%	590
Putnam Hospital Center[2]	Carmel	96%	727
Saint Anthony Community Hospital[2]	Warwick	96%	326
Wyckoff Heights Medical Center[2]	Brooklyn	96%	585
Arnot Ogden Medical Center[2]	Elmira	95%	644
Delaware Valley Hospital[2]	Walton	95%	293
Ellis Hospital[2]	Schenectady	95%	625
F F Thompson Hospital[2]	Canandaigua	95%	587
Ira Davenport Memorial Hospital	Bath	95%	397
Lawrence Hospital Center[2]	Bronxville	95%	613
Lincoln Medical & Mental Health Center[2]	Bronx	95%	507
Medina Memorial Hospital[2]	Medina	95%	425
Montefiore New Rochelle Hospital[2]	New Rochelle	95%	641
Saratoga Hospital[2]	Saratoga Spgs	95%	624
Clifton Springs Hospital & Clinic[2]	Clifton Springs	94%	467
Community Memorial Hospital[2]	Hamilton	94%	1032
Helen Hayes Hospital	W Haverstraw	94%	507
John T Mather Mem Hosp-Port Jefferson[2]	Port Jefferson	94%	885
Mount Sinai Hospital[2]	New York	94%	1381
New York - Presbyterian Hospital[2]	New York	94%	562
Niagara Falls Memorial Medical Center[2]	Niagara Falls	94%	732
Saint Joseph's Medical Center[2]	Yonkers	94%	671
Saint Mary's Hospital at Amsterdam[2]	Amsterdam	94%	640
Samaritan Medical Center[2]	Watertown	94%	485
South Nassau Communities Hospital[2]	Oceanside	94%	824
Unity Hospital of Rochester[2]	Rochester	94%	696
Auburn Community Hospital[2]	Auburn	93%	610
Bertrand Chaffee Hospital[2]	Springville	93%	524
Claxton - Hepburn Medical Center[2]	Ogdensburg	93%	317
Cobleskill Regional Hospital[2]	Cobleskill	93%	409
Geneva General Hospital[2]	Geneva	93%	542
Harlem Hospital Center[2]	New York	93%	480
Huntington Hospital[2]	Huntington	93%	705
Kingsbrook Jewish Medical Center[2]	Brooklyn	93%	978
Sunnyview Hosp & Rehab Ctr[2]	Schenectady	93%	577
Alice Hyde Medical Center[2]	Malone	92%	346
Crouse Hospital[2]	Syracuse	92%	484
Good Samaritan Hospital Medical Center[2]	West Islip	92%	632
New York Community Hospital of Brooklyn[2]	Brooklyn	92%	943
Richmond University Medical Center[2]	Staten Island	92%	475
Saint Mary's Hospital - Troy[2]	Troy	92%	635
Soldiers & Sailors Mem Hosp of Yates[2]	Penn Yan	92%	379
Albany Medical Center Hospital[2]	Albany	91%	546
Bon Secours Community Hospital[2]	Port Jervis	91%	430
Cayuga Medical Center at Ithaca[2]	Ithaca	91%	520
Columbia Memorial Hospital[2]	Hudson	91%	712
Eastern Niagara Hospital[2]	Lockport	91%	845
Elmhurst Hospital Center[2]	Elmhurst	91%	446
Health Alliance Hospital Broadway Campus[2]	Kingston	91%	818
Hospital For Special Surgery[2]	New York	91%	680
Jamaica Hospital Medical Center[2]	Jamaica	91%	547
Northern Dutchess Hospital[2]	Rhinebeck	91%	429
Oneida Healthcare Center[2]	Oneida	91%	358
Saint Barnabas Hospital[2]	Bronx	91%	550
Saint Luke's Cornwall Hospital[2]	Newburgh	91%	666
United Health Services Hospitals[2]	Johnson City	91%	740
Albany Memorial Hospital[2]	Albany	90%	473
Catskill Regional Medical Center[2]	Harris	90%	412
Champlain Valley Phys Hosp Med Ctr[2]	Plattsburgh	90%	740
Coney Island Hospital[2]	Brooklyn	90%	534
Faxton - Saint Luke's Healthcare[2]	Utica	90%	693
Flushing Hospital Medical Center[2]	Flushing	90%	432
Franklin Hospital[2]	Valley Stream	90%	834
Glen Cove Hospital[2]	Glen Cove	90%	821
Good Samaritan Hospital of Suffern[2]	Suffern	90%	530
Kenmore Mercy Hospital[2]	Kenmore	90%	939
Mercy Hospital[2]	Buffalo	90%	702
Nathan Littauer Hospital[2]	Gloversville	90%	437
Sisters of Charity Hospital[2]	Buffalo	90%	596
Southampton Hospital[2]	Southampton	90%	563
University Hospital - Stony Brook[2]	Stony Brook	90%	534
Winthrop - University Hospital[2]	Mineola	90%	556
Woodhull Medical & Mental Health Center[2]	Brooklyn	90%	333
Highland Hospital[2]	Rochester	89%	561
Kaleida Health[2]	Buffalo	89%	699
Mary Imogene Bassett Hospital[2]	Cooperstown	89%	706
Rome Memorial Hospital[2]	Rome	89%	455
Saint Catherine of Siena Hospital[2]	Smithtown	89%	751
Staten Island University Hospital[2]	Staten Island	89%	607
Bellevue Hospital Center[2]	New York	88%	449
Bronx - Lebanon Hospital Center[2]	Bronx	88%	790
Brooklyn Hosp Ctr at Downtown Campus[2]	Brooklyn	88%	557
Glens Falls Hospital[2]	Glens Falls	88%	738
Nassau University Medical Center[2]	East Meadow	88%	417
New York Hosp Med Ctr of Queens[2]	Flushing	88%	617
Nicholas H Noyes Memorial Hospital[2]	Dansville	88%	292
Saint Joseph Hospital[2]	Bethpage	88%	965
Univ Hosp SUNY Health Science Ctr[2]	Syracuse	88%	1066
Brooks Memorial Hospital[2]	Dunkirk	87%	301
Erie County Medical Center[2]	Buffalo	87%	576
Our Lady of Lourdes Memorial Hospital[2]	Binghamton	87%	775
Queens Hospital Center[2]	Jamaica	87%	580
Saint Luke's Roosevelt Hospital[2]	New York	87%	589
Newark - Wayne Community Hospital[2]	Newark	86%	538
North Shore University Hospital[2]	Manhasset	86%	1054
Olean General Hospital[2]	Olean	85%	693
Oswego Hospital[2]	Oswego	85%	504
Plainview Hospital[2]	Plainview	85%	730
Saint Peter's Hospital[2]	Albany	85%	696
Southside Hospital[2]	Bay Shore	85%	563
TLC Health Network[2]	Gowanda	85%	318
New York Methodist Hospital[2]	Brooklyn	84%	559
Westchester Medical Center[2]	Valhalla	84%	438
Brookhaven Mem Hosp Med Ctr[2]	Patchogue	83%	756
Canton - Potsdam Hospital[2]	Potsdam	83%	450
Health Alliance Hosp Mary's Ave Campus[2]	Kingston	83%	436
Lewis County General Hospital[2]	Lowville	83%	254
Long Island Jewish Medical Center[2]	New Hyde Park	83%	881
Lutheran Medical Center[2]	Brooklyn	83%	581
Peconic Bay Medical Center[2]	Riverhead	83%	775
Saint Elizabeth Medical Center[2]	Utica	83%	889
Aurelia Osborn Fox Memorial Hospital[2]	Oneonta	82%	414
Orange Regional Medical Center[2]	Middletown	82%	670
St John's Episcopal Hosp-South Shore[2]	Far Rockaway	82%	692
Saint Joseph's Hospital[2]	Elmira	82%	460
Woman's Christian Association[2]	Jamestown	82%	661
Maimonides Medical Center[2]	Brooklyn	81%	456
Saint Charles Hospital[2]	Port Jefferson	81%	453
Winifred Masterson Burke Rehab Hosp[2]	White Plains	81%	675
Kings County Hospital Center[2]	Brooklyn	79%	516
Lenox Hill Hospital[2]	New York	79%	621
Saint Francis Hospital - Roslyn[2]	Roslyn	79%	1023
Univ Hosp of Brooklyn-Downstate[2]	Brooklyn	78%	615
Metropolitan Hospital Center[2]	New York	77%	457
Samaritan Hospital[2]	Troy	77%	779
Adirondack Medical Center[2]	Saranac Lake	75%	335
Strong Memorial Hospital[2]	Rochester	75%	523
NYU Hospitals Center[2]	New York	74%	550
Mount St Mary's Hosp & Health Ctr[2]	Lewiston	72%	647
Westfield Memorial Hospital[2]	Westfield	69%	91
Carthage Area Hospital[2]	Carthage	68%	308
Brookdale Hospital Medical Center[2]	Brooklyn	67%	639
Little Falls Hospital[2,3]	Little Falls	67%	108
Montefiore Mount Vernon Hospital[2]	Mount Vernon	67%	410
Rochester General Hospital[2]	Rochester	65%	755
Saint Joseph's Hospital Health Center[2]	Syracuse	64%	775
North Central Bronx Hospital[2]	Bronx	60%	466
Interfaith Medical Center[2]	Brooklyn	58%	627
Montefiore Medical Center[2]	Bronx	54%	718
Jacobi Medical Center[2]	Bronx	47%	463
New York Eye & Ear Infirmary[2]	New York	22%	182

Stroke Care

Anticoagulation Therapy for Atrial Fibrillation

Hospital Name	City	Rate	Cases
Huntington Hospital[2]	Huntington	100%	27
Kaleida Health	Buffalo	100%	153
Mount Sinai Hospital	New York	100%	52
New York - Presbyterian Hospital	New York	100%	97
South Nassau Communities Hospital	Oceanside	100%	34
Strong Memorial Hospital[2]	Rochester	100%	32
Ellis Hospital	Schenectady	99%	67
Faxton - Saint Luke's Healthcare	Utica	97%	38
Maimonides Medical Center	Brooklyn	97%	97
Saint Peter's Hospital	Albany	97%	35
Vassar Brothers Medical Center	Poughkeepsie	97%	35
Albany Medical Center Hospital	Albany	95%	62
Lutheran Medical Center	Brooklyn	92%	36
Montefiore Medical Center	Bronx	90%	92
Jamaica Hospital Medical Center	Jamaica	87%	30
United Health Services Hospitals	Johnson City	87%	31
Rochester General Hospital	Rochester	86%	59

Antithrombotic Therapy Timing

Hospital Name	City	Rate	Cases
Alice Hyde Medical Center	Malone	100%	26
Arnot Ogden Medical Center	Elmira	100%	96
Auburn Community Hospital	Auburn	100%	25
Beth Israel Medical Center[2]	New York	100%	98
Bronx - Lebanon Hospital Center	Bronx	100%	110
Brookhaven Mem Hosp Med Ctr	Patchogue	100%	107
Champlain Valley Phys Hosp Med Ctr	Plattsburgh	100%	74
Columbia Memorial Hospital	Hudson	100%	33
Coney Island Hospital	Brooklyn	100%	117
Crouse Hospital[2]	Syracuse	100%	73
Elmhurst Hospital Center	Elmhurst	100%	106
F F Thompson Hospital	Canandaigua	100%	58
Faxton - Saint Luke's Healthcare	Utica	100%	166
Flushing Hospital Medical Center	Flushing	100%	116
Forest Hills Hospital[2]	Forest Hills	100%	89
Geneva General Hospital	Geneva	100%	36
Glens Falls Hospital[2]	Glens Falls	100%	88
Good Samaritan Hospital Medical Center	West Islip	100%	156
Harlem Hospital Center	New York	100%	73
Hudson Valley Hospital Center	Cortlandt Manor	100%	54
Huntington Hospital[2]	Huntington	100%	97
Jacobi Medical Center	Bronx	100%	94
Kaleida Health	Buffalo	100%	788
Kenmore Mercy Hospital	Kenmore	100%	76
Mary Imogene Bassett Hospital	Cooperstown	100%	63
Mercy Hospital[2]	Buffalo	100%	81
Mercy Medical Center[2]	Rockville Centre	100%	99
Montefiore New Rochelle Hospital	New Rochelle	100%	80
Nassau University Medical Center[2]	East Meadow	100%	81
Newark - Wayne Community Hospital	Newark	100%	33
Niagara Falls Memorial Medical Center	Niagara Falls	100%	26
North Central Bronx Hospital	Bronx	100%	26
Northern Dutchess Hospital	Rhinebeck	100%	25
Nyack Hospital	Nyack	100%	124
Our Lady of Lourdes Memorial Hospital[2]	Binghamton	100%	76
Plainview Hospital[2]	Plainview	100%	78
Richmond University Medical Center[2]	Staten Island	100%	65
Rochester General Hospital	Rochester	100%	307
Saint Catherine of Siena Hospital	Smithtown	100%	97
Saint Charles Hospital	Port Jefferson	100%	28
Saint Francis Hospital	Poughkeepsie	100%	25
Saint Joseph's Hospital Health Center[2]	Syracuse	100%	42
Saint Joseph's Medical Center[2]	Yonkers	100%	35
Saint Mary's Hospital at Amsterdam[2]	Amsterdam	100%	36
Samaritan Hospital	Troy	100%	62
Samaritan Medical Center	Watertown	100%	57
Saratoga Hospital	Saratoga Spgs	100%	28
Southampton Hospital	Southampton	100%	38
Southside Hospital[2]	Bay Shore	100%	96
Staten Island University Hospital[2]	Staten Island	100%	74
Univ Hosp SUNY Health Science Ctr[2]	Syracuse	100%	71
White Plains Hospital Center	White Plains	100%	106
Brookdale Hospital Medical Center	Brooklyn	99%	165
Brooklyn Hosp Ctr at Downtown Campus	Brooklyn	99%	85
Ellis Hospital	Schenectady	99%	158
Franklin Hospital[2]	Valley Stream	99%	110
Health Alliance Hospital Broadway Campus	Kingston	99%	106
Highland Hospital[2]	Rochester	99%	80
Maimonides Medical Center	Brooklyn	99%	344
North Shore University Hospital[2]	Manhasset	99%	88
NYU Hospitals Center	New York	99%	72
St John's Episcopal Hosp-South Shore	Far Rockaway	99%	83
Saint John's Riverside Hospital[2]	Yonkers	99%	99
Saint Joseph Hospital	Bethpage	99%	124
Saint Luke's Cornwall Hospital	Newburgh	99%	87
Saint Luke's Roosevelt Hospital[2]	New York	99%	92
Saint Peter's Hospital	Albany	99%	161
Strong Memorial Hospital[2]	Rochester	99%	144
Unity Hospital of Rochester[2]	Rochester	99%	82
Univ Hosp of Brooklyn-Downstate[2]	Brooklyn	99%	92
Vassar Brothers Medical Center	Poughkeepsie	99%	156
Albany Memorial Hospital	Albany	98%	40
Lincoln Medical & Mental Health Center	Bronx	98%	110
Northern Westchester Hospital	Mount Kisco	98%	51
Orange Regional Medical Center	Middletown	98%	191
Phelps Memorial Hospital Assn	Sleepy Hollow	98%	42
Putnam Hospital Center	Carmel	98%	55
Saint Elizabeth Medical Center	Utica	98%	46
Sisters of Charity Hospital[2]	Buffalo	98%	66
University Hospital - Stony Brook[2]	Stony Brook	98%	59
Westchester Medical Center[2]	Valhalla	98%	51
Winthrop - University Hospital	Mineola	98%	181
Woodhull Medical & Mental Health Center	Brooklyn	98%	89
Albany Medical Center Hospital	Albany	97%	275
Claxton - Hepburn Medical Center	Ogdensburg	97%	30
Mount St Mary's Hosp & Health Ctr[2]	Lewiston	97%	63
Mount Sinai Hospital	New York	97%	275

NOTE: Hospital profiles are in alphabetical order by state, then city, then hospital within the city; Rankings exclude hospitals with less than 25 cases except for patient surveys which excludes hospitals with less than 100 cases; (a) 100-299 cases; (1) The number of cases/patients is too few to report; (2) Data submitted were based on a sample of cases/patients; (3) Results are based on a shorter time period than required; (4) Data suppressed by CMS for one or more quarters; (5) Results are not available for this reporting period; (6) Fewer than 100 patients completed the HCAHPS survey; (7) No cases met the criteria for this measure; (8) The lower limit of the confidence interval cannot be calculated if the number of observed infections equals zero; (9) No data are available from the state/territory for this reporting period; (10) The scores shown reflect fewer than 50 completed surveys; (11) There were discrepancies in the data collection process; (12) This measure does not apply to this hospital for this reporting period; (13) Results cannot be calculated for this reporting period; (14) The results for this state are combined with nearby states to protect confidentiality; Please refer to the User's Guide for a full explanation of data.

Hospital Name	City	Rate	Cases
New York - Presbyterian Hospital	New York	97%	547
United Health Services Hospitals	Johnson City	97%	151
Catskill Regional Medical Center	Harris	96%	27
Cayuga Medical Center at Ithaca	Ithaca	96%	55
Corning Hospital	Corning	96%	49
Glen Cove Hospital[2]	Glen Cove	96%	55
Good Samaritan Hospital of Suffern	Suffern	96%	105
Jamaica Hospital Medical Center	Jamaica	96%	246
Lawrence Hospital Center[2]	Bronxville	96%	91
Montefiore Medical Center	Bronx	96%	570
New York Community Hospital of Brooklyn	Brooklyn	96%	48
New York Hosp Med Ctr of Queens[2]	Flushing	96%	135
Queens Hospital Center	Jamaica	96%	80
Bellevue Hospital Center[2]	New York	95%	58
John T Mather Mem Hosp-Port Jefferson	Port Jefferson	95%	96
Saint Barnabas Hospital	Bronx	95%	97
Saint Francis Hospital - Roslyn[2]	Roslyn	95%	55
South Nassau Communities Hospital	Oceanside	95%	173
Kingsbrook Jewish Medical Center	Brooklyn	94%	111
Peconic Bay Medical Center[2]	Riverhead	94%	47
Saint Mary's Hospital - Troy	Troy	94%	34
Wyckoff Heights Medical Center	Brooklyn	94%	142
Long Island Jewish Medical Center[2]	New Hyde Park	93%	90
Woman's Christian Association	Jamestown	92%	39
Erie County Medical Center	Buffalo	91%	45
Kings County Hospital Center	Brooklyn	91%	198
Lenox Hill Hospital[2]	New York	90%	63
Lutheran Medical Center	Brooklyn	90%	147
New York Methodist Hospital[2]	Brooklyn	90%	132

Assessed for Rehabilitation

Hospital Name	City	Rate	Cases
Adirondack Medical Center	Saranac Lake	100%	25
Auburn Community Hospital	Auburn	100%	28
Beth Israel Medical Center[2]	New York	100%	108
Bronx - Lebanon Hospital Center	Bronx	100%	140
Brookdale Hospital Medical Center	Brooklyn	100%	194
Columbia Memorial Hospital	Hudson	100%	36
Corning Hospital	Corning	100%	64
Erie County Medical Center	Buffalo	100%	48
Faxton - Saint Luke's Healthcare	Utica	100%	237
Flushing Hospital Medical Center	Flushing	100%	114
Forest Hills Hospital[2]	Forest Hills	100%	102
Geneva General Hospital	Geneva	100%	38
Good Samaritan Hospital Medical Center	West Islip	100%	182
Kenmore Mercy Hospital	Kenmore	100%	91
Lutheran Medical Center	Brooklyn	100%	202
Mercy Hospital[2]	Buffalo	100%	104
Montefiore New Rochelle Hospital	New Rochelle	100%	84
Mount St Mary's Hosp & Health Ctr[2]	Lewiston	100%	62
New York Community Hospital of Brooklyn	Brooklyn	100%	63
Niagara Falls Memorial Medical Center	Niagara Falls	100%	25
Northern Dutchess Hospital	Rhinebeck	100%	30
Phelps Memorial Hospital Assn	Sleepy Hollow	100%	48
Richmond University Medical Center[2]	Staten Island	100%	86
Saint Charles Hospital	Port Jefferson	100%	34
Saint Francis Hospital	Poughkeepsie	100%	48
Saint Francis Hospital - Roslyn[2]	Roslyn	100%	67
St John's Episcopal Hosp-South Shore	Far Rockaway	100%	84
Saint Joseph Hospital	Bethpage	100%	116
Saint Joseph's Medical Center[2]	Yonkers	100%	38
Saint Luke's Cornwall Hospital	Newburgh	100%	101
Saint Mary's Hospital - Troy	Troy	100%	41
Saint Mary's Hospital at Amsterdam[2]	Amsterdam	100%	26
Saratoga Hospital	Saratoga Spgs	100%	33
Sisters of Charity Hospital[2]	Buffalo	100%	80
South Nassau Communities Hospital	Oceanside	100%	203
Vassar Brothers Medical Center	Poughkeepsie	100%	168
White Plains Hospital Center	White Plains	100%	149
Brookhaven Mem Hosp Med Ctr	Patchogue	99%	104
Ellis Hospital	Schenectady	99%	218
Glens Falls Hospital[2]	Glens Falls	99%	99
Health Alliance Hospital Broadway Campus	Kingston	99%	121
Highland Hospital[2]	Rochester	99%	99
John T Mather Mem Hosp-Port Jefferson	Port Jefferson	99%	106
Maimonides Medical Center	Brooklyn	99%	428
Mercy Medical Center[2]	Rockville Centre	99%	126
New York Hosp Med Ctr of Queens[2]	Flushing	99%	163
Northern Westchester Hospital	Mount Kisco	99%	72
Nyack Hospital	Nyack	99%	145
NYU Hospitals Center	New York	99%	117
Rochester General Hospital	Rochester	99%	366
Saint Barnabas Hospital	Bronx	99%	105
Strong Memorial Hospital[2]	Rochester	99%	229
Woodhull Medical & Mental Health Center	Brooklyn	99%	92
Albany Medical Center Hospital	Albany	98%	480
Franklin Hospital[2]	Valley Stream	98%	120
Jamaica Hospital Medical Center	Jamaica	98%	316
Kaleida Health	Buffalo	98%	989
Kings County Hospital Center	Brooklyn	98%	223
Mary Imogene Bassett Hospital	Cooperstown	98%	82
Nassau University Medical Center[2]	East Meadow	98%	99
New York - Presbyterian Hospital	New York	98%	968
Putnam Hospital Center	Carmel	98%	53
Saint Catherine of Siena Hospital	Smithtown	98%	99
Westchester Medical Center[2]	Valhalla	98%	128
Arnot Ogden Medical Center	Elmira	97%	117
Canton - Potsdam Hospital	Potsdam	97%	31
Claxton - Hepburn Medical Center	Ogdensburg	97%	29
Elmhurst Hospital Center	Elmhurst	97%	145
Huntington Hospital[2]	Huntington	97%	113
Long Island Jewish Medical Center[2]	New Hyde Park	97%	117
North Shore University Hospital[2]	Manhasset	97%	145
Orange Regional Medical Center	Middletown	97%	204
Samaritan Medical Center	Watertown	97%	58
Staten Island University Hospital[2]	Staten Island	97%	95
United Health Services Hospitals	Johnson City	97%	202
Univ Hosp SUNY Health Science Ctr[2]	Syracuse	97%	110
Catskill Regional Medical Center	Harris	96%	28
Champlain Valley Phys Hosp Med Ctr	Plattsburgh	96%	73
Crouse Hospital[2]	Syracuse	96%	106
Hudson Valley Hospital Center	Cortlandt Manor	96%	67
Metropolitan Hospital Center	New York	96%	26
New York Methodist Hospital[2]	Brooklyn	96%	151
University Hospital - Stony Brook[2]	Stony Brook	96%	109
F F Thompson Hospital	Canandaigua	95%	59
Montefiore Medical Center	Bronx	95%	712
Mount Sinai Hospital	New York	95%	368
Our Lady of Lourdes Memorial Hospital[2]	Binghamton	95%	86
Southside Hospital[2]	Bay Shore	95%	103
Harlem Hospital Center	New York	94%	82
Jacobi Medical Center	Bronx	94%	112
Saint Luke's Roosevelt Hospital[2]	New York	94%	127
Samaritan Hospital	Troy	94%	68
Winthrop - University Hospital	Mineola	94%	246
Albany Memorial Hospital	Albany	93%	41
Coney Island Hospital	Brooklyn	93%	121
Glen Cove Hospital[2]	Glen Cove	93%	59
Kingsbrook Jewish Medical Center	Brooklyn	93%	126
Lawrence Hospital Center[2]	Bronxville	93%	98
Lincoln Medical & Mental Health Center	Bronx	93%	148
Peconic Bay Medical Center[2]	Riverhead	93%	46
Saint Peter's Hospital	Albany	93%	185
Good Samaritan Hospital of Suffern	Suffern	92%	133
Montefiore Mount Vernon Hospital	Mount Vernon	92%	26
Plainview Hospital[2]	Plainview	92%	88
Unity Hospital of Rochester[2]	Rochester	92%	99
Wyckoff Heights Medical Center	Brooklyn	92%	151
Cayuga Medical Center at Ithaca	Ithaca	91%	65
Newark - Wayne Community Hospital	Newark	91%	45
Saint Elizabeth Medical Center	Utica	91%	57
Bellevue Hospital Center[2]	New York	90%	109
Lenox Hill Hospital[2]	New York	90%	94
Brooklyn Hosp Ctr at Downtown Campus	Brooklyn	89%	95
Saint John's Riverside Hospital[2]	Yonkers	87%	94
Univ Hosp of Brooklyn-Downstate[2]	Brooklyn	86%	100
Saint Joseph's Hospital Health Center[2]	Syracuse	85%	54
Southampton Hospital	Southampton	81%	48
Woman's Christian Association	Jamestown	76%	34
Queens Hospital Center	Jamaica	74%	78

Discharged on Antithrombotic Therapy

Hospital Name	City	Rate	Cases
Albany Medical Center Hospital	Albany	100%	334
Albany Memorial Hospital	Albany	100%	39
Auburn Community Hospital	Auburn	100%	27
Bellevue Hospital Center[2]	New York	100%	70
Beth Israel Medical Center[2]	New York	100%	94
Bronx - Lebanon Hospital Center	Bronx	100%	116
Brookdale Hospital Medical Center	Brooklyn	100%	153
Canton - Potsdam Hospital	Potsdam	100%	26
Crouse Hospital[2]	Syracuse	100%	88
Ellis Hospital	Schenectady	100%	183
Elmhurst Hospital Center	Elmhurst	100%	116
Erie County Medical Center	Buffalo	100%	42
F F Thompson Hospital	Canandaigua	100%	56
Forest Hills Hospital[2]	Forest Hills	100%	94
Geneva General Hospital	Geneva	100%	36
Glens Falls Hospital[2]	Glens Falls	100%	93
Good Samaritan Hospital Medical Center	West Islip	100%	149
Highland Hospital[2]	Rochester	100%	93
Hudson Valley Hospital Center	Cortlandt Manor	100%	62
Huntington Hospital[2]	Huntington	100%	99
Jacobi Medical Center	Bronx	100%	100
John T Mather Mem Hosp-Port Jefferson	Port Jefferson	100%	101
Kaleida Health	Buffalo	100%	877
Maimonides Medical Center	Brooklyn	100%	379
Mary Imogene Bassett Hospital	Cooperstown	100%	66
Mercy Medical Center[2]	Rockville Centre	100%	100
Montefiore New Rochelle Hospital	New Rochelle	100%	77
Mount Sinai Hospital	New York	100%	301
New York - Presbyterian Hospital	New York	100%	706
New York Community Hospital of Brooklyn	Brooklyn	100%	54
New York Methodist Hospital[2]	Brooklyn	100%	129
Newark - Wayne Community Hospital	Newark	100%	41
North Shore University Hospital[2]	Manhasset	100%	98
Northern Dutchess Hospital	Rhinebeck	100%	29
Northern Westchester Hospital	Mount Kisco	100%	68
NYU Hospitals Center	New York	100%	90
Peconic Bay Medical Center[2]	Riverhead	100%	44
Phelps Memorial Hospital Assn	Sleepy Hollow	100%	44
Queens Hospital Center	Jamaica	100%	71
Richmond University Medical Center[2]	Staten Island	100%	63
Saint Catherine of Siena Hospital	Smithtown	100%	87
Saint Charles Hospital	Port Jefferson	100%	29
Saint Francis Hospital - Roslyn[2]	Roslyn	100%	62
Saint Joseph's Medical Center[2]	Yonkers	100%	34
Saint Luke's Cornwall Hospital	Newburgh	100%	91
Saint Mary's Hospital - Troy	Troy	100%	40
Samaritan Hospital	Troy	100%	65
Samaritan Medical Center	Watertown	100%	57
Sisters of Charity Hospital[2]	Buffalo	100%	62
Staten Island University Hospital[2]	Staten Island	100%	77
Strong Memorial Hospital[2]	Rochester	100%	197
United Health Services Hospitals	Johnson City	100%	160
Unity Hospital of Rochester[2]	Rochester	100%	91
University Hospital - Stony Brook[2]	Stony Brook	100%	75
Univ Hosp SUNY Health Science Ctr[2]	Syracuse	100%	81
Westchester Medical Center[2]	Valhalla	100%	61
White Plains Hospital Center	White Plains	100%	132
Winthrop - University Hospital	Mineola	100%	197
Arnot Ogden Medical Center	Elmira	99%	101
Brookhaven Mem Hosp Med Ctr	Patchogue	99%	89
Champlain Valley Phys Hosp Med Ctr	Plattsburgh	99%	72
Coney Island Hospital	Brooklyn	99%	103
Faxton - Saint Luke's Healthcare	Utica	99%	196
Good Samaritan Hospital of Suffern	Suffern	99%	116
Jamaica Hospital Medical Center	Jamaica	99%	271
Kenmore Mercy Hospital	Kenmore	99%	77
Kings County Hospital Center	Brooklyn	99%	198
Lawrence Hospital Center[2]	Bronxville	99%	90
Lincoln Medical & Mental Health Center	Bronx	99%	113
Long Island Jewish Medical Center[2]	New Hyde Park	99%	103
Nassau University Medical Center[2]	East Meadow	99%	79
New York Hosp Med Ctr of Queens[2]	Flushing	99%	145
Orange Regional Medical Center	Middletown	99%	167
Rochester General Hospital	Rochester	99%	320
Saint Barnabas Hospital	Bronx	99%	94
Saint John's Riverside Hospital[2]	Yonkers	99%	84
Saint Peter's Hospital	Albany	99%	162
South Nassau Communities Hospital	Oceanside	99%	184
Cayuga Medical Center at Ithaca	Ithaca	98%	57
Corning Hospital	Corning	98%	62
Flushing Hospital Medical Center	Flushing	98%	103
Lutheran Medical Center	Brooklyn	98%	165
Mercy Hospital[2]	Buffalo	98%	81
Montefiore Medical Center	Bronx	98%	599
Mount St Mary's Hosp & Health Ctr[2]	Lewiston	98%	59
Nyack Hospital	Nyack	98%	128
Plainview Hospital[2]	Plainview	98%	83
Putnam Hospital Center	Carmel	98%	49
Saint Joseph's Hospital Health Center[2]	Syracuse	98%	47
Saint Luke's Roosevelt Hospital[2]	New York	98%	101
Southampton Hospital	Southampton	98%	43
Southside Hospital[2]	Bay Shore	98%	95
Univ Hosp of Brooklyn-Downstate[2]	Brooklyn	98%	91
Vassar Brothers Medical Center	Poughkeepsie	98%	152
Woodhull Medical & Mental Health Center	Brooklyn	98%	81
Claxton - Hepburn Medical Center	Ogdensburg	97%	29
Columbia Memorial Hospital	Hudson	97%	35
Health Alliance Hospital Broadway Campus	Kingston	97%	116
St John's Episcopal Hosp-South Shore	Far Rockaway	97%	74
Brooklyn Hosp Ctr at Downtown Campus	Brooklyn	96%	81
Harlem Hospital Center	New York	96%	70
Montefiore Mount Vernon Hospital	Mount Vernon	96%	25
Saint Elizabeth Medical Center	Utica	96%	49
Saint Joseph Hospital	Bethpage	96%	113
Saint Mary's Hospital at Amsterdam[2]	Amsterdam	96%	25
Kingsbrook Jewish Medical Center	Brooklyn	95%	105
Our Lady of Lourdes Memorial Hospital[2]	Binghamton	95%	79
Wyckoff Heights Medical Center	Brooklyn	95%	133
Woman's Christian Association	Jamestown	94%	33
Catskill Regional Medical Center	Harris	93%	27
Lenox Hill Hospital[2]	New York	93%	74
Saratoga Hospital	Saratoga Spgs	93%	29
Franklin Hospital[2]	Valley Stream	92%	106
Glen Cove Hospital[2]	Glen Cove	86%	56

Discharged on Statin Medication

Hospital Name	City	Rate	Cases
Bellevue Hospital Center[2]	New York	100%	52
Canton - Potsdam Hospital	Potsdam	100%	27
Forest Hills Hospital[2]	Forest Hills	100%	80

NOTE: Hospital profiles are in alphabetical order by state, then city, then hospital within the city; Rankings exclude hospitals with less than 25 cases except for patient surveys which excludes hospitals with less than 100 cases; (a) 100-299 cases; (1) The number of cases/patients is too few to report; (2) Data submitted were based on a sample of cases/patients; (3) Results are based on a shorter time period than required; (4) Data suppressed by CMS for one or more quarters; (5) Results are not available for this reporting period; (6) Fewer than 100 patients completed the HCAHPS survey; (7) No cases met the criteria for this measure; (8) The lower limit of the confidence interval cannot be calculated if the number of observed infections equals zero; (9) No data are available from the state/territory for this reporting period; (10) The scores shown reflect fewer than 50 completed surveys; (11) There were discrepancies in the data collection process; (12) This measure does not apply to this hospital for this reporting period; (13) Results cannot be calculated for this reporting period; (14) The results for this state are combined with nearby states to protect confidentiality; Please refer to the User's Guide for a full explanation of data.

Hospital Name	City	Rate	Cases
Good Samaritan Hospital Medical Center	West Islip	100%	113
Mount St Mary's Hosp & Health Ctr[2]	Lewiston	100%	45
New York Community Hospital of Brooklyn	Brooklyn	100%	50
North Shore University Hospital[2]	Manhasset	100%	82
Nyack Hospital	Nyack	100%	107
Phelps Memorial Hospital Assn	Sleepy Hollow	100%	29
Richmond University Medical Center[2]	Staten Island	100%	70
Saint Barnabas Hospital	Bronx	100%	78
Saint Catherine of Siena Hospital	Smithtown	100%	68
Saint Francis Hospital	Poughkeepsie	100%	29
Saint Luke's Roosevelt Hospital[2]	New York	100%	78
Univ Hosp SUNY Health Science Ctr[2]	Syracuse	100%	58
Bronx - Lebanon Hospital Center	Bronx	99%	93
Brookdale Hospital Medical Center	Brooklyn	99%	149
Elmhurst Hospital Center	Elmhurst	99%	84
Huntington Hospital[2]	Huntington	99%	76
Lincoln Medical & Mental Health Center	Bronx	99%	98
Mercy Medical Center[2]	Rockville Centre	99%	79
NYU Hospitals Center	New York	99%	73
Staten Island University Hospital[2]	Staten Island	99%	67
Strong Memorial Hospital[2]	Rochester	99%	140
Unity Hospital of Rochester[2]	Rochester	99%	74
Vassar Brothers Medical Center	Poughkeepsie	99%	126
White Plains Hospital Center	White Plains	99%	116
Beth Israel Medical Center[2]	New York	98%	65
Corning Hospital	Corning	98%	52
Ellis Hospital	Schenectady	98%	166
Harlem Hospital Center	New York	98%	65
Highland Hospital[2]	Rochester	98%	65
Hudson Valley Hospital Center	Cortlandt Manor	98%	52
Jamaica Hospital Medical Center	Jamaica	98%	204
Kaleida Health	Buffalo	98%	704
Kings County Hospital Center	Brooklyn	98%	175
Maimonides Medical Center	Brooklyn	98%	276
Montefiore New Rochelle Hospital	New Rochelle	98%	46
Mount Sinai Hospital	New York	98%	223
Nassau University Medical Center[2]	East Meadow	98%	63
New York - Presbyterian Hospital	New York	98%	563
New York Methodist Hospital[2]	Brooklyn	98%	114
Saint Francis Hospital - Roslyn[2]	Roslyn	98%	51
Columbia Memorial Hospital	Hudson	97%	31
John T Mather Mem Hosp-Port Jefferson	Port Jefferson	97%	73
Mary Imogene Bassett Hospital	Cooperstown	97%	59
South Nassau Communities Hospital	Oceanside	97%	150
Albany Medical Center Hospital	Albany	96%	246
Arnot Ogden Medical Center	Elmira	96%	72
Brookhaven Mem Hosp Med Ctr	Patchogue	96%	67
F F Thompson Hospital	Canandaigua	96%	46
Faxton - Saint Luke's Healthcare	Utica	96%	151
Geneva General Hospital	Geneva	96%	25
Glens Falls Hospital[2]	Glens Falls	96%	76
Jacobi Medical Center	Bronx	96%	74
New York Hosp Med Ctr of Queens[2]	Flushing	96%	118
Plainview Hospital[2]	Plainview	96%	69
Saint Joseph Hospital	Bethpage	96%	74
Southside Hospital[2]	Bay Shore	96%	77
Crouse Hospital[2]	Syracuse	95%	76
Lutheran Medical Center	Brooklyn	95%	129
Mercy Hospital[2]	Buffalo	95%	66
Northern Westchester Hospital	Mount Kisco	95%	41
Orange Regional Medical Center	Middletown	95%	147
Putnam Hospital Center	Carmel	95%	43
Rochester General Hospital	Rochester	95%	264
Saint Luke's Cornwall Hospital	Newburgh	95%	76
Winthrop - University Hospital	Mineola	95%	168
Erie County Medical Center	Buffalo	94%	33
Long Island Jewish Medical Center[2]	New Hyde Park	94%	85
Montefiore Medical Center	Bronx	94%	494
Newark - Wayne Community Hospital	Newark	94%	32
Our Lady of Lourdes Memorial Hospital[2]	Binghamton	94%	67
Peconic Bay Medical Center[2]	Riverhead	94%	33
Univ Hosp of Brooklyn-Downstate[2]	Brooklyn	94%	71
Coney Island Hospital	Brooklyn	93%	82
Franklin Hospital[2]	Valley Stream	93%	85
Saint Joseph's Medical Center[2]	Yonkers	93%	27
Samaritan Hospital	Troy	92%	50
Westchester Medical Center[2]	Valhalla	92%	51
Woodhull Medical & Mental Health Center	Brooklyn	92%	66
Wyckoff Heights Medical Center	Brooklyn	92%	111
St John's Episcopal Hosp-South Shore	Far Rockaway	91%	66
United Health Services Hospitals	Johnson City	91%	129
Albany Memorial Hospital	Albany	90%	29
Champlain Valley Phys Hosp Med Ctr	Plattsburgh	90%	59
Flushing Hospital Medical Center	Flushing	90%	82
Kenmore Mercy Hospital	Kenmore	90%	69
Southampton Hospital	Southampton	90%	39
University Hospital - Stony Brook[2]	Stony Brook	90%	51
Lawrence Hospital Center[2]	Bronxville	89%	79
Sisters of Charity Hospital[2]	Buffalo	89%	55
Saint Mary's Hospital - Troy	Troy	88%	32
Saint Peter's Hospital	Albany	88%	119
Samaritan Medical Center	Watertown	88%	48
Good Samaritan Hospital of Suffern	Suffern	87%	90
Kingsbrook Jewish Medical Center	Brooklyn	87%	91
Saint Joseph's Hospital Health Center[2]	Syracuse	87%	46
Brooklyn Hosp Ctr at Downtown Campus	Brooklyn	86%	71
Cayuga Medical Center at Ithaca	Ithaca	86%	44
Saint John's Riverside Hospital[2]	Yonkers	86%	73
Health Alliance Hospital Broadway Campus	Kingston	85%	84
Queens Hospital Center	Jamaica	85%	62
Lenox Hill Hospital[2]	New York	83%	54
Saratoga Hospital	Saratoga Spgs	82%	28
Glen Cove Hospital[2]	Glen Cove	79%	42
Saint Elizabeth Medical Center	Utica	77%	43
Woman's Christian Association	Jamestown	57%	30

Thrombolytic Therapy Timing

Hospital Name	City	Rate	Cases
Maimonides Medical Center	Brooklyn	93%	42
New York - Presbyterian Hospital	New York	93%	69
Strong Memorial Hospital[2]	Rochester	87%	31
Kaleida Health	Buffalo	85%	91
Jamaica Hospital Medical Center	Jamaica	83%	35
Rochester General Hospital	Rochester	77%	39
Ellis Hospital	Schenectady	72%	32
Montefiore Medical Center	Bronx	68%	57
Albany Medical Center Hospital	Albany	66%	29
Faxton - Saint Luke's Healthcare	Utica	65%	48
Lincoln Medical & Mental Health Center	Bronx	23%	30
Saint John's Riverside Hospital[2]	Yonkers	17%	29
Saint Joseph Hospital	Bethpage	7%	44

Venous Thromboembolism (VTE) Prophylaxis

Hospital Name	City	Rate	Cases
Bronx - Lebanon Hospital Center	Bronx	100%	161
Brookdale Hospital Medical Center	Brooklyn	100%	226
Claxton - Hepburn Medical Center	Ogdensburg	100%	29
Columbia Memorial Hospital	Hudson	100%	36
Coney Island Hospital	Brooklyn	100%	156
Forest Hills Hospital[2]	Forest Hills	100%	111
Good Samaritan Hospital Medical Center	West Islip	100%	213
Kaleida Health	Buffalo	100%	1052
North Central Bronx Hospital	Bronx	100%	26
Northern Westchester Hospital	Mount Kisco	100%	70
NYU Hospitals Center	New York	100%	100
Saint Catherine of Siena Hospital	Smithtown	100%	119
Saint Francis Hospital	Poughkeepsie	100%	49
Saint Mary's Hospital at Amsterdam[2]	Amsterdam	100%	39
Univ Hosp SUNY Health Science Ctr[2]	Syracuse	100%	108
Winthrop - University Hospital	Mineola	100%	258
Woodhull Medical & Mental Health Center	Brooklyn	100%	107
Arnot Ogden Medical Center	Elmira	99%	118
Crouse Hospital[2]	Syracuse	99%	99
Elmhurst Hospital Center	Elmhurst	99%	166
Jamaica Hospital Medical Center	Jamaica	99%	339
New York Community Hospital of Brooklyn	Brooklyn	99%	69
Nyack Hospital	Nyack	99%	150
Richmond University Medical Center[2]	Staten Island	99%	99
Saint Luke's Cornwall Hospital	Newburgh	99%	103
Westchester Medical Center[2]	Valhalla	99%	146
Flushing Hospital Medical Center	Flushing	98%	138
Lincoln Medical & Mental Health Center	Bronx	98%	172
Lutheran Medical Center	Brooklyn	98%	227
Nassau University Medical Center[2]	East Meadow	98%	118
Phelps Memorial Hospital Assn	Sleepy Hollow	98%	49
Putnam Hospital Center	Carmel	98%	60
Strong Memorial Hospital[2]	Rochester	98%	233
Cayuga Medical Center at Ithaca	Ithaca	97%	64
Ellis Hospital	Schenectady	97%	215
Faxton - Saint Luke's Healthcare	Utica	97%	245
Geneva General Hospital	Geneva	97%	36
John T Mather Mem Hosp-Port Jefferson	Port Jefferson	97%	115
Kings County Hospital Center	Brooklyn	97%	235
Mercy Medical Center[2]	Rockville Centre	97%	130
New York - Presbyterian Hospital	New York	97%	937
Saint Charles Hospital	Port Jefferson	97%	36
Saint Mary's Hospital - Troy	Troy	97%	37
Univ Hosp of Brooklyn-Downstate[2]	Brooklyn	97%	113
White Plains Hospital Center	White Plains	97%	148
Auburn Community Hospital	Auburn	96%	28
Brookhaven Mem Hosp Med Ctr	Patchogue	96%	132
Glens Falls Hospital[2]	Glens Falls	96%	93
Maimonides Medical Center	Brooklyn	96%	457
Metropolitan Hospital Center	New York	96%	27
Niagara Falls Memorial Medical Center	Niagara Falls	96%	28
South Nassau Communities Hospital	Oceanside	96%	226
Staten Island University Hospital[2]	Staten Island	96%	109
Corning Hospital	Corning	95%	62
Mary Imogene Bassett Hospital	Cooperstown	95%	82
Mercy Hospital[2]	Buffalo	95%	110
Mount Sinai Hospital	New York	95%	404
New York Methodist Hospital[2]	Brooklyn	95%	173
Saint Joseph's Medical Center[2]	Yonkers	95%	40
Saint Luke's Roosevelt Hospital[2]	New York	95%	135
United Health Services Hospitals	Johnson City	95%	217
Vassar Brothers Medical Center	Poughkeepsie	95%	190
Brooklyn Hosp Ctr at Downtown Campus	Brooklyn	94%	108
Catskill Regional Medical Center	Harris	94%	31
Harlem Hospital Center	New York	94%	89
Interfaith Medical Center	Brooklyn	94%	33
Mount St Mary's Hosp & Health Ctr[2]	Lewiston	94%	69
Peconic Bay Medical Center[2]	Riverhead	94%	48
Albany Medical Center Hospital	Albany	93%	517
Champlain Valley Phys Hosp Med Ctr	Plattsburgh	93%	82
Huntington Hospital[2]	Huntington	93%	120
Jacobi Medical Center	Bronx	93%	123
Kingsbrook Jewish Medical Center	Brooklyn	93%	136
Plainview Hospital[2]	Plainview	93%	90
Rochester General Hospital	Rochester	93%	396
Saint Barnabas Hospital	Bronx	93%	124
Saint Joseph's Hospital Health Center[2]	Syracuse	93%	56
Wyckoff Heights Medical Center	Brooklyn	93%	177
Kenmore Mercy Hospital	Kenmore	92%	92
Montefiore New Rochelle Hospital	New Rochelle	92%	97
North Shore University Hospital[2]	Manhasset	92%	157
Sisters of Charity Hospital[2]	Buffalo	92%	80
St John's Episcopal Hosp-South Shore	Far Rockaway	91%	100
Southside Hospital[2]	Bay Shore	91%	113
F F Thompson Hospital	Canandaigua	90%	62
Lawrence Hospital Center[2]	Bronxville	90%	119
New York Hosp Med Ctr of Queens[2]	Flushing	90%	178
Northern Dutchess Hospital	Rhinebeck	90%	29
Queens Hospital Center	Jamaica	90%	86
Saint Joseph Hospital	Bethpage	90%	130
Saint Peter's Hospital	Albany	90%	202
Alice Hyde Medical Center	Malone	89%	27
Canton - Potsdam Hospital	Potsdam	89%	27
Highland Hospital[2]	Rochester	89%	97
Saint Francis Hospital - Roslyn[2]	Roslyn	89%	64
Franklin Hospital[2]	Valley Stream	88%	130
Hudson Valley Hospital Center	Cortlandt Manor	88%	73
Saint Elizabeth Medical Center	Utica	88%	58
Health Alliance Hospital Broadway Campus	Kingston	87%	119
Lenox Hill Hospital[2]	New York	87%	98
Montefiore Mount Vernon Hospital	Mount Vernon	87%	30
Bellevue Hospital Center[2]	New York	86%	129
Montefiore Medical Center	Bronx	86%	767
Unity Hospital of Rochester[2]	Rochester	86%	98
Beth Israel Medical Center[2]	New York	85%	119
Long Island Jewish Medical Center[2]	New Hyde Park	85%	115
Newark - Wayne Community Hospital	Newark	84%	43
Our Lady of Lourdes Memorial Hospital[2]	Binghamton	84%	81
Orange Regional Medical Center	Middletown	83%	224
Saratoga Hospital	Saratoga Spgs	83%	29
University Hospital - Stony Brook[2]	Stony Brook	82%	114
Albany Memorial Hospital	Albany	80%	41
Samaritan Hospital	Troy	80%	71
Samaritan Medical Center	Watertown	80%	69
Erie County Medical Center	Buffalo	79%	57
Glen Cove Hospital[2]	Glen Cove	78%	67
Southampton Hospital	Southampton	78%	45
Saint John's Riverside Hospital[2]	Yonkers	69%	121
Woman's Christian Association	Jamestown	64%	42
Good Samaritan Hospital of Suffern	Suffern	53%	140

Written Stroke Educational Materials Given

Hospital Name	City	Rate	Cases
Arnot Ogden Medical Center	Elmira	100%	64
Brookdale Hospital Medical Center	Brooklyn	100%	82
Brooklyn Hosp Ctr at Downtown Campus	Brooklyn	100%	32
Coney Island Hospital	Brooklyn	100%	64
Elmhurst Hospital Center	Elmhurst	100%	63
Forest Hills Hospital[2]	Forest Hills	100%	43
Geneva General Hospital	Geneva	100%	25
Good Samaritan Hospital Medical Center	West Islip	100%	92
Hudson Valley Hospital Center	Cortlandt Manor	100%	34
Kingsbrook Jewish Medical Center	Brooklyn	100%	51
Lawrence Hospital Center[2]	Bronxville	100%	39
Mercy Medical Center[2]	Rockville Centre	100%	48
New York Community Hospital of Brooklyn	Brooklyn	100%	29
Northern Westchester Hospital	Mount Kisco	100%	47
Nyack Hospital	Nyack	100%	65
Richmond University Medical Center[2]	Staten Island	100%	42
Saint Catherine of Siena Hospital	Smithtown	100%	45
Saint Joseph Hospital	Bethpage	100%	60
Vassar Brothers Medical Center	Poughkeepsie	100%	92
Bronx - Lebanon Hospital Center	Bronx	99%	84
New York Hosp Med Ctr of Queens[2]	Flushing	99%	88
Corning Hospital	Corning	98%	44
Jamaica Hospital Medical Center	Jamaica	98%	123
Saint Barnabas Hospital	Bronx	98%	65
Saint Francis Hospital - Roslyn[2]	Roslyn	98%	42

NOTE: Hospital profiles are in alphabetical order by state, then city, then hospital within the city; Rankings exclude hospitals with less than 25 cases except for patient surveys which excludes hospitals with less than 100 cases; (a) 100-299 cases; (1) The number of cases/patients is too few to report; (2) Data submitted were based on a sample of cases/patients; (3) Results are based on a shorter time period than required; (4) Data suppressed by CMS for one or more quarters; (5) Results are not available for this reporting period; (6) Fewer than 100 patients completed the HCAHPS survey; (7) No cases met the criteria for this measure; (8) The lower limit of the confidence interval cannot be calculated if the number of observed infections equals zero; (9) No data are available from the state/territory for this reporting period; (10) The scores shown reflect fewer than 50 completed surveys; (11) There were discrepancies in the data collection process; (12) This measure does not apply to this hospital for this reporting period; (13) Results cannot be calculated for this reporting period; (14) The results for this state are combined with nearby states to protect confidentiality; Please refer to the User's Guide for a full explanation of data.

Saint Luke's Cornwall Hospital	Newburgh	98%	49
Woodhull Medical & Mental Health Center	Brooklyn	98%	40
John T Mather Mem Hosp-Port Jefferson	Port Jefferson	97%	61
Mary Imogene Bassett Hospital	Cooperstown	97%	61
Mount Sinai Hospital	New York	97%	191
Plainview Hospital[2]	Plainview	97%	34
Putnam Hospital Center	Carmel	97%	31
White Plains Hospital Center	White Plains	97%	60
Brookhaven Mem Hosp Med Ctr	Patchogue	96%	52
Crouse Hospital[2]	Syracuse	96%	57
Kaleida Health	Buffalo	96%	560
Montefiore New Rochelle Hospital	New Rochelle	96%	28
Nassau University Medical Center[2]	East Meadow	96%	49
Orange Regional Medical Center	Middletown	96%	85
University Hospital - Stony Brook[2]	Stony Brook	96%	47
F F Thompson Hospital	Canandaigua	95%	37
Lincoln Medical & Mental Health Center	Bronx	95%	83
New York - Presbyterian Hospital	New York	95%	551
NYU Hospitals Center	New York	95%	76
Flushing Hospital Medical Center	Flushing	94%	52
Our Lady of Lourdes Memorial Hospital[2]	Binghamton	94%	48
South Nassau Communities Hospital	Oceanside	93%	113
Lenox Hill Hospital[2]	New York	92%	59
Maimonides Medical Center	Brooklyn	92%	259
Sisters of Charity Hospital[2]	Buffalo	92%	51
Southampton Hospital	Southampton	92%	25
Staten Island University Hospital[2]	Staten Island	92%	50
Unity Hospital of Rochester[2]	Rochester	92%	62
Mercy Hospital[2]	Buffalo	90%	52
Mount St Mary's Hosp & Health Ctr[2]	Lewiston	90%	42
Univ Hosp SUNY Health Science Ctr[2]	Syracuse	90%	69
Health Alliance Hospital Broadway Campus	Kingston	89%	56
Lutheran Medical Center	Brooklyn	89%	84
Strong Memorial Hospital[2]	Rochester	88%	149
Winthrop - University Hospital	Mineola	88%	145
Highland Hospital[2]	Rochester	87%	55
Huntington Hospital[2]	Huntington	87%	54
Beth Israel Medical Center[2]	New York	86%	51
Faxton - Saint Luke's Healthcare	Utica	86%	100
North Shore University Hospital[2]	Manhasset	86%	78
St John's Episcopal Hosp-South Shore	Far Rockaway	86%	37
Saint John's Riverside Hospital[2]	Yonkers	86%	44
Kenmore Mercy Hospital	Kenmore	85%	47
Kings County Hospital Center	Brooklyn	85%	131
New York Methodist Hospital[2]	Brooklyn	84%	73
Univ Hosp of Brooklyn-Downstate[2]	Brooklyn	83%	41
Albany Medical Center Hospital	Albany	81%	274
Saint Peter's Hospital	Albany	81%	93
Wyckoff Heights Medical Center	Brooklyn	81%	93
Good Samaritan Hospital of Suffern	Suffern	80%	66
United Health Services Hospitals	Johnson City	80%	87
Westchester Medical Center[2]	Valhalla	80%	59
Glens Falls Hospital[2]	Glens Falls	79%	48
Rochester General Hospital	Rochester	79%	243
Montefiore Medical Center	Bronx	78%	370
Saint Luke's Roosevelt Hospital[2]	New York	76%	68
Franklin Hospital[2]	Valley Stream	74%	46
Ellis Hospital	Schenectady	73%	85
Samaritan Hospital	Troy	73%	37
Newark - Wayne Community Hospital	Newark	69%	26
Long Island Jewish Medical Center[2]	New Hyde Park	67%	67
Southside Hospital[2]	Bay Shore	67%	57
Champlain Valley Phys Hosp Med Ctr	Plattsburgh	63%	38
Queens Hospital Center	Jamaica	54%	54
Harlem Hospital Center	New York	50%	34
Saint Elizabeth Medical Center	Utica	50%	32
Cayuga Medical Center at Ithaca	Ithaca	32%	38
Jacobi Medical Center	Bronx	24%	38
Glen Cove Hospital[2]	Glen Cove	18%	28
Saint Joseph's Hospital Health Center[2]	Syracuse	9%	33
Samaritan Medical Center	Watertown	6%	36
Bellevue Hospital Center[2]	New York	0%	40

Surgical Care Improvement Project

Appropriate Beta Blocker Usage

Hospital Name	City	Rate	Cases
Chenango Memorial Hospital	Norwich	100%	39
Clifton Springs Hospital & Clinic[2]	Clifton Springs	100%	38
Columbia Memorial Hospital	Hudson	100%	71
Community Memorial Hospital	Hamilton	100%	169
Ellis Hospital[2]	Schenectady	100%	253
Forest Hills Hospital[2]	Forest Hills	100%	103
Geneva General Hospital	Geneva	100%	122
Glen Cove Hospital[2]	Glen Cove	100%	72
Hudson Valley Hospital Center[2]	Cortlandt Manor	100%	158
Nathan Littauer Hospital	Gloversville	100%	48
New York Community Hospital of Brooklyn[2]	Brooklyn	100%	31
Niagara Falls Memorial Medical Center[2]	Niagara Falls	100%	45
Northern Westchester Hospital[2]	Mount Kisco	100%	99
Nyack Hospital	Nyack	100%	122
Our Lady of Lourdes Memorial Hospital[2]	Binghamton	100%	90
Saint Anthony Community Hospital	Warwick	100%	44
Saint Charles Hospital[2]	Port Jefferson	100%	187
Saint Francis Hospital[2]	Poughkeepsie	100%	107
St John's Episcopal Hosp-South Shore[2]	Far Rockaway	100%	35
Saint Joseph's Hospital[2]	Elmira	100%	43
Saint Joseph's Medical Center	Yonkers	100%	25
Saint Mary's Hospital at Amsterdam[2]	Amsterdam	100%	75
South Nassau Communities Hospital[2]	Oceanside	100%	361
Staten Island University Hospital[2]	Staten Island	100%	211
Strong Memorial Hospital[2]	Rochester	100%	435
Unity Hospital of Rochester[2]	Rochester	100%	187
Vassar Brothers Medical Center[2]	Poughkeepsie	100%	267
White Plains Hospital Center[2]	White Plains	100%	162
Adirondack Medical Center[2]	Saranac Lake	99%	92
Albany Medical Center Hospital[2]	Albany	99%	165
Albany Memorial Hospital[2]	Albany	99%	67
Bellevue Hospital Center[2]	New York	99%	108
Brooklyn Hosp Ctr at Downtown Campus	Brooklyn	99%	137
Canton - Potsdam Hospital	Potsdam	99%	70
F F Thompson Hospital	Canandaigua	99%	141
Good Samaritan Hospital of Suffern[2]	Suffern	99%	292
Health Alliance Hosp Mary's Ave Campus	Kingston	99%	151
Highland Hospital[2]	Rochester	99%	236
John T Mather Mem Hosp-Port Jefferson	Port Jefferson	99%	168
Maimonides Medical Center[2]	Brooklyn	99%	334
Mary Imogene Bassett Hospital[2]	Cooperstown	99%	267
Montefiore New Rochelle Hospital	New Rochelle	99%	145
New York Hosp Med Ctr of Queens[2]	Flushing	99%	195
NYU Hospitals Center[2]	New York	99%	191
Phelps Memorial Hospital Assn[2]	Sleepy Hollow	99%	144
Putnam Hospital Center	Carmel	99%	255
Richmond University Medical Center[2]	Staten Island	99%	96
Rochester General Hospital[2]	Rochester	99%	954
Saint Francis Hospital - Roslyn[2]	Roslyn	99%	398
Saint Joseph's Hospital Health Center[2]	Syracuse	99%	309
United Health Services Hospitals	Johnson City	99%	595
Westchester Medical Center[2]	Valhalla	99%	322
Albany VA Medical Center[2]	Albany	98%	47
Arnot Ogden Medical Center[2]	Elmira	98%	306
Auburn Community Hospital	Auburn	98%	48
Aurelia Osborn Fox Memorial Hospital	Oneonta	98%	40
Cayuga Medical Center at Ithaca	Ithaca	98%	100
Champlain Valley Phys Hosp Med Ctr[2]	Plattsburgh	98%	261
Crouse Hospital[2]	Syracuse	98%	148
Elmhurst Hospital Center	Elmhurst	98%	66
Hospital For Special Surgery[2]	New York	98%	134
Kaleida Health[2]	Buffalo	98%	464
Lincoln Medical & Mental Health Center[2]	Bronx	98%	62
Long Island Jewish Medical Center[2]	New Hyde Park	98%	221
Mercy Hospital[2]	Buffalo	98%	323
Mount St Mary's Hosp & Health Ctr[2]	Lewiston	98%	97
New York - Presbyterian Hospital[2]	New York	98%	516
Orange Regional Medical Center[2]	Middletown	98%	177
Rome Memorial Hospital	Rome	98%	42
Saint Elizabeth Medical Center[2]	Utica	98%	506
Saint Joseph Hospital[2]	Bethpage	98%	98
Saint Luke's Cornwall Hospital[2]	Newburgh	98%	169
Saint Luke's Roosevelt Hospital[2]	New York	98%	208
Southside Hospital[2]	Bay Shore	98%	228
University Hospital - Stony Brook[2]	Stony Brook	98%	224
Univ Hosp SUNY Health Science Ctr[2]	Syracuse	98%	210
Winthrop - University Hospital[2]	Mineola	98%	453
Faxton - Saint Luke's Healthcare[2]	Utica	97%	120
Glens Falls Hospital[2]	Glens Falls	97%	220
Huntington Hospital[2]	Huntington	97%	122
Jamaica Hospital Medical Center[2]	Jamaica	97%	39
Kenmore Mercy Hospital[2]	Kenmore	97%	143
Lawrence Hospital Center[2]	Bronxville	97%	100
Lenox Hill Hospital[2]	New York	97%	263
Mercy Medical Center[2]	Rockville Centre	97%	99
Mount Sinai Hospital[2]	New York	97%	344
New York Methodist Hospital[2]	Brooklyn	97%	257
North Shore University Hospital[2]	Manhasset	97%	307
Northern Dutchess Hospital[2]	Rhinebeck	97%	91
Saint John's Riverside Hospital[2]	Yonkers	97%	138
Samaritan Medical Center	Watertown	97%	181
Saratoga Hospital[2]	Saratoga Spgs	97%	215
TLC Health Network	Gowanda	97%	36
Univ Hosp of Brooklyn-Downstate[2]	Brooklyn	97%	125
Upstate New York VA Healthcare Sys[2]	Buffalo	97%	95
Beth Israel Medical Center[2]	New York	96%	237
Brooks Memorial Hospital[2]	Dunkirk	96%	85
Good Samaritan Hospital Medical Center[2]	West Islip	96%	171
Lutheran Medical Center[2]	Brooklyn	96%	249
Newark - Wayne Community Hospital	Newark	96%	94
Saint Catherine of Siena Hospital[2]	Smithtown	96%	123
Saint Mary's Hospital - Troy[2]	Troy	96%	52
Saint Peter's Hospital[2]	Albany	96%	330
Sisters of Charity Hospital[2]	Buffalo	96%	193
Syracuse VA Medical Center[2]	Syracuse	96%	55
Brookhaven Mem Hosp Med Ctr	Patchogue	95%	82
Corning Hospital	Corning	95%	83
Plainview Hospital[2]	Plainview	95%	129
Southampton Hospital	Southampton	95%	56
Erie County Medical Center	Buffalo	94%	215
Health Alliance Hospital Broadway Campus	Kingston	94%	62
Kingsbrook Jewish Medical Center	Brooklyn	94%	52
Nassau University Medical Center[2]	East Meadow	94%	50
Peconic Bay Medical Center[2]	Riverhead	94%	201
Saint Barnabas Hospital[2]	Bronx	94%	32
Bronx - Lebanon Hospital Center[2]	Bronx	93%	81
Oneida Healthcare Center	Oneida	93%	42
United Memorial Medical Center	Batavia	93%	96
Nicholas H Noyes Memorial Hospital	Dansville	92%	53
Oswego Hospital	Oswego	92%	37
Catskill Regional Medical Center	Harris	91%	32
Claxton - Hepburn Medical Center	Ogdensburg	91%	33
Eastern Niagara Hospital[2]	Lockport	91%	32
Flushing Hospital Medical Center[2]	Flushing	91%	66
Jacobi Medical Center	Bronx	91%	75
Northport VA Medical Center[2]	Northport	91%	35
Samaritan Hospital[2]	Troy	91%	139
Woman's Christian Association[2]	Jamestown	91%	116
Metropolitan Hospital Center[2]	New York	90%	29
Olean General Hospital[2]	Olean	89%	100
Queens Hospital Center	Jamaica	88%	50
Wyckoff Heights Medical Center[2]	Brooklyn	88%	75
Montefiore Medical Center[2]	Bronx	87%	384
Brookdale Hospital Medical Center	Brooklyn	86%	56
Woodhull Medical & Mental Health Center[2]	Brooklyn	86%	29
Kings County Hospital Center[2]	Brooklyn	84%	56
Franklin Hospital[2]	Valley Stream	82%	80
VA New York Harbor Healthcare System[2]	New York	81%	63
Bronx VA Medical Center[2]	Bronx	74%	31

Appropriate VTP Within 24 Hours

Hospital Name	City	Rate	Cases
Beth Israel Medical Center[2]	New York	100%	442
Brooks Memorial Hospital[2]	Dunkirk	100%	247
Chenango Memorial Hospital	Norwich	100%	141
Community Memorial Hospital	Hamilton	100%	300
Ellis Hospital[2]	Schenectady	100%	452
Elmhurst Hospital Center	Elmhurst	100%	410
Forest Hills Hospital[2]	Forest Hills	100%	324
Health Alliance Hosp Mary's Ave Campus	Kingston	100%	338
Highland Hospital[2]	Rochester	100%	716
John T Mather Mem Hosp-Port Jefferson	Port Jefferson	100%	325
Jones Memorial Hospital	Wellsville	100%	61
Lewis County General Hospital	Lowville	100%	34
Lincoln Medical & Mental Health Center[2]	Bronx	100%	256
Massena Memorial Hospital	Massena	100%	59
Mercy Medical Center[2]	Rockville Centre	100%	318
Metropolitan Hospital Center[2]	New York	100%	207
Nassau University Medical Center[2]	East Meadow	100%	219
New York - Presbyterian Hospital[2]	New York	100%	879
New York Community Hospital of Brooklyn[2]	Brooklyn	100%	79
New York Hosp Med Ctr of Queens[2]	Flushing	100%	424
Northern Westchester Hospital[2]	Mount Kisco	100%	425
Nyack Hospital	Nyack	100%	491
NYU Hospitals Center[2]	New York	100%	492
Orange Regional Medical Center[2]	Middletown	100%	548
Phelps Memorial Hospital Assn[2]	Sleepy Hollow	100%	400
Rochester General Hospital[2]	Rochester	100%	1259
Saint Charles Hospital[2]	Port Jefferson	100%	590
Saint Francis Hospital[2]	Poughkeepsie	100%	347
Saint Francis Hospital - Roslyn[2]	Roslyn	100%	416
Saint Joseph's Hospital Health Center[2]	Syracuse	100%	494
Saint Joseph's Medical Center	Yonkers	100%	121
Saint Mary's Hospital at Amsterdam[2]	Amsterdam	100%	224
South Nassau Communities Hospital[2]	Oceanside	100%	903
Staten Island University Hospital[2]	Staten Island	100%	299
Strong Memorial Hospital[2]	Rochester	100%	395
Unity Hospital of Rochester[2]	Rochester	100%	422
University Hospital - Stony Brook[2]	Stony Brook	100%	319
Westchester Medical Center[2]	Valhalla	100%	359
Alice Hyde Medical Center	Malone	99%	100
Claxton - Hepburn Medical Center	Ogdensburg	99%	132
F F Thompson Hospital	Canandaigua	99%	443
Flushing Hospital Medical Center[2]	Flushing	99%	267
Franklin Hospital[2]	Valley Stream	99%	260
Glen Cove Hospital[2]	Glen Cove	99%	244
Hospital For Special Surgery[2]	New York	99%	562
Hudson Valley Hospital Center[2]	Cortlandt Manor	99%	396
Huntington Hospital[2]	Huntington	99%	299
Jacobi Medical Center	Bronx	99%	352
Kenmore Mercy Hospital[2]	Kenmore	99%	428
Kings County Hospital Center[2]	Brooklyn	99%	300
Kingsbrook Jewish Medical Center	Brooklyn	99%	165
Lutheran Medical Center[2]	Brooklyn	99%	577
Maimonides Medical Center[2]	Brooklyn	99%	454

NOTE: Hospital profiles are in alphabetical order by state, then city, then hospital within the city; Rankings exclude hospitals with less than 25 cases except for patient surveys which excludes hospitals with less than 100 cases; (a) 100-299 cases; (1) The number of cases/patients is too few to report; (2) Data submitted were based on a sample of cases/patients; (3) Results are based on a shorter time period than required; (4) Data suppressed by CMS for one or more quarters; (5) Results are not available for this reporting period; (6) Fewer than 100 patients completed the HCAHPS survey; (7) No cases met the criteria for this measure; (8) The lower limit of the confidence interval cannot be calculated if the number of observed infections equals zero; (9) No data are available from the state/territory for this reporting period; (10) The scores shown reflect fewer than 50 completed surveys; (11) There were discrepancies in the data collection process; (12) This measure does not apply to this hospital for this reporting period; (13) Results cannot be calculated for this reporting period; (14) The results for this state are combined with nearby states to protect confidentiality; Please refer to the User's Guide for a full explanation of data.

Hospital Name	City	Rate	Cases
Mercy Hospital[2]	Buffalo	99%	406
Mount St Mary's Hosp & Health Ctr[2]	Lewiston	99%	281
Mount Sinai Hospital[2]	New York	99%	748
Nathan Littauer Hospital	Gloversville	99%	135
Newark - Wayne Community Hospital	Newark	99%	237
Niagara Falls Memorial Medical Center[2]	Niagara Falls	99%	126
Northern Dutchess Hospital[2]	Rhinebeck	99%	282
Oneida Healthcare Center	Oneida	99%	155
Our Lady of Lourdes Memorial Hospital[2]	Binghamton	99%	278
Plainview Hospital[2]	Plainview	99%	317
Putnam Hospital Center	Carmel	99%	811
Richmond University Medical Center[2]	Staten Island	99%	333
Saint Anthony Community Hospital	Warwick	99%	136
Saint Joseph Hospital[2]	Bethpage	99%	241
Sisters of Charity Hospital[2]	Buffalo	99%	473
Syracuse VA Medical Center[2]	Syracuse	99%	117
TLC Health Network	Gowanda	99%	117
United Health Services Hospitals	Johnson City	99%	1124
Univ Hosp SUNY Health Science Ctr[2]	Syracuse	99%	442
VA New York Harbor Healthcare System[2]	New York	99%	136
Vassar Brothers Medical Center[2]	Poughkeepsie	99%	380
White Plains Hospital Center[2]	White Plains	99%	426
Albany VA Medical Center[2]	Albany	98%	110
Arnot Ogden Medical Center[2]	Elmira	98%	593
Bellevue Hospital Center[2]	New York	98%	207
Brooklyn Hosp Ctr at Downtown Campus	Brooklyn	98%	496
Catskill Regional Medical Center	Harris	98%	86
Cayuga Medical Center at Ithaca	Ithaca	98%	334
Champlain Valley Phys Hosp Med Ctr[2]	Plattsburgh	98%	442
Clifton Springs Hospital & Clinic[2]	Clifton Springs	98%	52
Corning Hospital	Corning	98%	229
Crouse Hospital[2]	Syracuse	98%	393
Geneva General Hospital	Geneva	98%	376
Harlem Hospital Center[2]	New York	98%	115
Jamaica Hospital Medical Center[2]	Jamaica	98%	241
Kaleida Health[2]	Buffalo	98%	678
Lawrence Hospital Center[2]	Bronxville	98%	311
Lenox Hill Hospital[2]	New York	98%	377
Long Island Jewish Medical Center[2]	New Hyde Park	98%	369
Mary Imogene Bassett Hospital[2]	Cooperstown	98%	402
New York Methodist Hospital[2]	Brooklyn	98%	493
North Central Bronx Hospital	Bronx	98%	50
North Shore University Hospital[2]	Manhasset	98%	525
Saint Joseph's Hospital[2]	Elmira	98%	109
Saint Luke's Roosevelt Hospital[2]	New York	98%	493
Saint Peter's Hospital[2]	Albany	98%	567
Southside Hospital[2]	Bay Shore	98%	355
United Memorial Medical Center	Batavia	98%	236
Univ Hosp of Brooklyn-Downstate[2]	Brooklyn	98%	311
Woodhull Medical & Mental Health Center[2]	Brooklyn	98%	181
Wyckoff Heights Medical Center[2]	Brooklyn	98%	224
Albany Medical Center Hospital[2]	Albany	97%	298
Canton - Potsdam Hospital	Potsdam	97%	201
Coney Island Hospital[2]	Brooklyn	97%	114
Good Samaritan Hospital Medical Center[2]	West Islip	97%	463
Good Samaritan Hospital of Suffern[2]	Suffern	97%	374
Interfaith Medical Center	Brooklyn	97%	71
Medina Memorial Hospital	Medina	97%	38
Montefiore New Rochelle Hospital	New Rochelle	97%	481
Olean General Hospital[2]	Olean	97%	277
Peconic Bay Medical Center[2]	Riverhead	97%	565
Saint Barnabas Hospital[2]	Bronx	97%	153
Saint Elizabeth Medical Center[2]	Utica	97%	709
Saint James Mercy Hospital	Hornell	97%	101
Saint John's Riverside Hospital[2]	Yonkers	97%	372
Saint Luke's Cornwall Hospital[2]	Newburgh	97%	457
Samaritan Medical Center	Watertown	97%	421
Saratoga Hospital[2]	Saratoga Spgs	97%	570
Winthrop - University Hospital[2]	Mineola	97%	509
Woman's Christian Association[2]	Jamestown	97%	239
Bronx - Lebanon Hospital Center[2]	Bronx	96%	350
Columbia Memorial Hospital	Hudson	96%	226
Oswego Hospital	Oswego	96%	157
Queens Hospital Center	Jamaica	96%	222
Rome Memorial Hospital	Rome	96%	161
Saint Mary's Hospital - Troy[2]	Troy	96%	158
Upstate New York VA Healthcare Sys[2]	Buffalo	96%	124
Albany Memorial Hospital[2]	Albany	95%	208
Aurelia Osborn Fox Memorial Hospital	Oneonta	95%	100
Bronx VA Medical Center[2]	Bronx	95%	84
Brookdale Hospital Medical Center	Brooklyn	95%	281
Eastern Long Island Hospital	Greenport	95%	39
Erie County Medical Center	Buffalo	95%	675
Montefiore Medical Center[2]	Bronx	95%	645
Northport VA Medical Center[2]	Northport	95%	92
Samaritan Hospital[2]	Troy	95%	359
Faxton - Saint Luke's Healthcare[2]	Utica	94%	352
Glens Falls Hospital[2]	Glens Falls	94%	468
Montefiore Mount Vernon Hospital	Mount Vernon	94%	51
Nicholas H Noyes Memorial Hospital	Dansville	94%	144
Southampton Hospital	Southampton	94%	137
Wyoming County Community Hospital	Warsaw	94%	84
Adirondack Medical Center[2]	Saranac Lake	93%	359
Auburn Community Hospital	Auburn	93%	181
Eastern Niagara Hospital[2]	Lockport	93%	123
Saint Catherine of Siena Hospital[2]	Smithtown	93%	310
Bon Secours Community Hospital	Port Jervis	92%	87
Brookhaven Mem Hosp Med Ctr	Patchogue	92%	228
Health Alliance Hospital Broadway Campus	Kingston	92%	164
St John's Episcopal Hosp-South Shore[2]	Far Rockaway	92%	146
Cortland Regional Medical Center	Cortland	89%	54

Controlled Postoperative Blood Glucose

Hospital Name	City	Rate	Cases
New York Hosp Med Ctr of Queens[2]	Flushing	100%	100
Univ Hosp of Brooklyn-Downstate[2]	Brooklyn	100%	71
Albany Medical Center Hospital[2]	Albany	99%	121
Arnot Ogden Medical Center[2]	Elmira	99%	84
Ellis Hospital[2]	Schenectady	99%	189
NYU Hospitals Center[2]	New York	99%	129
Rochester General Hospital[2]	Rochester	99%	583
Saint Elizabeth Medical Center[2]	Utica	99%	283
Winthrop - University Hospital[2]	Mineola	99%	368
Beth Israel Medical Center[2]	New York	98%	142
Good Samaritan Hospital of Suffern[2]	Suffern	98%	119
Mary Imogene Bassett Hospital[2]	Cooperstown	98%	97
Mount Sinai Hospital[2]	New York	98%	180
Saint Luke's Roosevelt Hospital[2]	New York	98%	124
Staten Island University Hospital[2]	Staten Island	98%	101
Strong Memorial Hospital[2]	Rochester	98%	440
Vassar Brothers Medical Center[2]	Poughkeepsie	98%	157
Champlain Valley Phys Hosp Med Ctr[2]	Plattsburgh	97%	100
Long Island Jewish Medical Center[2]	New Hyde Park	97%	150
North Shore University Hospital[2]	Manhasset	97%	158
Saint Peter's Hospital[2]	Albany	97%	222
United Health Services Hospitals	Johnson City	97%	225
Univ Hosp SUNY Health Science Ctr[2]	Syracuse	97%	95
Bellevue Hospital Center[2]	New York	96%	138
Kaleida Health[2]	Buffalo	96%	248
Montefiore Medical Center[2]	Bronx	96%	212
New York - Presbyterian Hospital[2]	New York	96%	335
New York Methodist Hospital[2]	Brooklyn	96%	98
Southside Hospital[2]	Bay Shore	96%	141
Lenox Hill Hospital[2]	New York	95%	137
Maimonides Medical Center[2]	Brooklyn	95%	170
Mercy Hospital[2]	Buffalo	95%	201
Saint Francis Hospital - Roslyn[2]	Roslyn	94%	232
Erie County Medical Center	Buffalo	92%	37
Saint Joseph's Hospital Health Center[2]	Syracuse	92%	192
Westchester Medical Center[2]	Valhalla	92%	237
University Hospital - Stony Brook[2]	Stony Brook	90%	123
VA New York Harbor Healthcare System[2]	New York	86%	44
Upstate New York VA Healthcare Sys[2]	Buffalo	84%	56

Perioperative Temperature Management

Hospital Name	City	Rate	Cases
Albany Medical Center Hospital[2]	Albany	100%	450
Albany Memorial Hospital[2]	Albany	100%	253
Alice Hyde Medical Center	Malone	100%	110
Arnot Ogden Medical Center[2]	Elmira	100%	686
Auburn Community Hospital	Auburn	100%	193
Bellevue Hospital Center[2]	New York	100%	258
Beth Israel Medical Center[2]	New York	100%	556
Bon Secours Community Hospital	Port Jervis	100%	94
Bronx - Lebanon Hospital Center[2]	Bronx	100%	392
Brookhaven Mem Hosp Med Ctr	Patchogue	100%	260
Brooklyn Hosp Ctr at Downtown Campus	Brooklyn	100%	565
Canton - Potsdam Hospital	Potsdam	100%	217
Cayuga Medical Center at Ithaca	Ithaca	100%	368
Champlain Valley Phys Hosp Med Ctr[2]	Plattsburgh	100%	564
Chenango Memorial Hospital	Norwich	100%	158
Clifton Springs Hospital & Clinic[2]	Clifton Springs	100%	91
Columbia Memorial Hospital	Hudson	100%	257
Community Memorial Hospital	Hamilton	100%	545
Coney Island Hospital[2]	Brooklyn	100%	135
Corning Hospital	Corning	100%	248
Cortland Regional Medical Center	Cortland	100%	70
Crouse Hospital[2]	Syracuse	100%	563
Eastern Long Island Hospital	Greenport	100%	40
Elmhurst Hospital Center	Elmhurst	100%	453
Erie County Medical Center	Buffalo	100%	771
F F Thompson Hospital	Canandaigua	100%	509
Faxton - Saint Luke's Healthcare[2]	Utica	100%	440
Flushing Hospital Medical Center[2]	Flushing	100%	332
Forest Hills Hospital[2]	Forest Hills	100%	376
Franklin Hospital[2]	Valley Stream	100%	280
Glen Cove Hospital[2]	Glen Cove	100%	258
Glens Falls Hospital[2]	Glens Falls	100%	602
Good Samaritan Hospital Medical Center[2]	West Islip	100%	554
Good Samaritan Hospital of Suffern[2]	Suffern	100%	473
Harlem Hospital Center[2]	New York	100%	138
Health Alliance Hosp Mary's Ave Campus	Kingston	100%	395
Highland Hospital[2]	Rochester	100%	816
Hospital For Special Surgery[2]	New York	100%	593
Hudson Valley Hospital Center[2]	Cortlandt Manor	100%	449
Huntington Hospital[2]	Huntington	100%	351
John T Mather Mem Hosp-Port Jefferson	Port Jefferson	100%	417
Kaleida Health[2]	Buffalo	100%	905
Kenmore Mercy Hospital[2]	Kenmore	100%	449
Kings County Hospital Center[2]	Brooklyn	100%	346
Lawrence Hospital Center[2]	Bronxville	100%	342
Lenox Hill Hospital[2]	New York	100%	584
Lewis County General Hospital	Lowville	100%	39
Lincoln Medical & Mental Health Center[2]	Bronx	100%	304
Long Island Jewish Medical Center[2]	New Hyde Park	100%	602
Lutheran Medical Center[2]	Brooklyn	100%	714
Maimonides Medical Center[2]	Brooklyn	100%	635
Mary Imogene Bassett Hospital[2]	Cooperstown	100%	508
Massena Memorial Hospital	Massena	100%	64
Mercy Medical Center[2]	Rockville Centre	100%	360
Metropolitan Hospital Center[2]	New York	100%	229
Mount St Mary's Hosp & Health Ctr[2]	Lewiston	100%	326
Mount Sinai Hospital[2]	New York	100%	989
Nassau University Medical Center[2]	East Meadow	100%	260
Nathan Littauer Hospital	Gloversville	100%	145
New York - Presbyterian Hospital[2]	New York	100%	1137
New York Community Hospital of Brooklyn[2]	Brooklyn	100%	83
New York Hosp Med Ctr of Queens[2]	Flushing	100%	489
New York Methodist Hospital[2]	Brooklyn	100%	601
Niagara Falls Memorial Medical Center[2]	Niagara Falls	100%	161
Nicholas H Noyes Memorial Hospital	Dansville	100%	161
North Shore University Hospital[2]	Manhasset	100%	704
Northern Dutchess Hospital[2]	Rhinebeck	100%	315
Northern Westchester Hospital[2]	Mount Kisco	100%	470
Nyack Hospital	Nyack	100%	544
NYU Hospitals Center[2]	New York	100%	579
Olean General Hospital[2]	Olean	100%	321
Oneida Healthcare Center	Oneida	100%	177
Orange Regional Medical Center[2]	Middletown	100%	629
Oswego Hospital	Oswego	100%	171
Our Lady of Lourdes Memorial Hospital[2]	Binghamton	100%	316
Peconic Bay Medical Center[2]	Riverhead	100%	601
Phelps Memorial Hospital Assn[2]	Sleepy Hollow	100%	483
Plainview Hospital[2]	Plainview	100%	400
Putnam Hospital Center	Carmel	100%	868
Queens Hospital Center	Jamaica	100%	268
Richmond University Medical Center[2]	Staten Island	100%	408
Saint Anthony Community Hospital	Warwick	100%	159
Saint Catherine of Siena Hospital[2]	Smithtown	100%	367
Saint Charles Hospital[2]	Port Jefferson	100%	616
Saint Elizabeth Medical Center[2]	Utica	100%	865
Saint Francis Hospital[2]	Poughkeepsie	100%	385
Saint Francis Hospital - Roslyn[2]	Roslyn	100%	670
Saint James Mercy Hospital	Hornell	100%	108
Saint Joseph Hospital[2]	Bethpage	100%	265
Saint Joseph's Hospital[2]	Elmira	100%	135
Saint Joseph's Medical Center	Yonkers	100%	132
Saint Luke's Roosevelt Hospital[2]	New York	100%	623
Saint Mary's Hospital - Troy[2]	Troy	100%	176
Saint Mary's Hospital at Amsterdam[2]	Amsterdam	100%	247
Saint Peter's Hospital[2]	Albany	100%	659
Samaritan Hospital[2]	Troy	100%	434
Samaritan Medical Center	Watertown	100%	526
Saratoga Hospital[2]	Saratoga Spgs	100%	719
Sisters of Charity Hospital[2]	Buffalo	100%	608
South Nassau Communities Hospital[2]	Oceanside	100%	988
Southampton Hospital	Southampton	100%	160
Southside Hospital[2]	Bay Shore	100%	454
Staten Island University Hospital[2]	Staten Island	100%	469
Strong Memorial Hospital[2]	Rochester	100%	588
Syracuse VA Medical Center[2]	Syracuse	100%	137
United Health Services Hospitals	Johnson City	100%	1421
United Memorial Medical Center	Batavia	100%	250
Unity Hospital of Rochester[2]	Rochester	100%	517
Univ Hosp of Brooklyn-Downstate[2]	Brooklyn	100%	361
VA New York Harbor Healthcare System[2]	New York	100%	171
Vassar Brothers Medical Center[2]	Poughkeepsie	100%	488
White Plains Hospital Center[2]	White Plains	100%	487
Winthrop - University Hospital[2]	Mineola	100%	637
Woodhull Medical & Mental Health Center[2]	Brooklyn	100%	216
Wyckoff Heights Medical Center[2]	Brooklyn	100%	274
Wyoming County Community Hospital	Warsaw	100%	90
Adirondack Medical Center[2]	Saranac Lake	99%	386
Albany VA Medical Center[2]	Albany	99%	140
Brookdale Hospital Medical Center	Brooklyn	99%	353
Brooks Memorial Hospital[2]	Dunkirk	99%	306
Catskill Regional Medical Center	Harris	99%	104
Claxton - Hepburn Medical Center	Ogdensburg	99%	144
Ellis Hospital[2]	Schenectady	99%	543
Health Alliance Hospital Broadway Campus	Kingston	99%	188
Interfaith Medical Center	Brooklyn	99%	77
Jacobi Medical Center	Bronx	99%	417

NOTE: Hospital profiles are in alphabetical order by state, then city, then hospital within the city; Rankings exclude hospitals with less than 25 cases except for patient surveys which excludes hospitals with less than 100 cases; (a) 100-299 cases; (1) The number of cases/patients is too few to report; (2) Data submitted were based on a sample of cases/patients; (3) Results are based on a shorter time period than required; (4) Data suppressed by CMS for one or more quarters; (5) Results are not available for this reporting period; (6) Fewer than 100 patients completed the HCAHPS survey; (7) No cases met the criteria for this measure; (8) The lower limit of the confidence interval cannot be calculated if the number of observed infections equals zero; (9) No data are available from the state/territory for this reporting period; (10) The scores shown reflect fewer than 50 completed surveys; (11) There were discrepancies in the data collection process; (12) This measure does not apply to this hospital for this reporting period; (13) Results cannot be calculated for this reporting period; (14) The results for this state are combined with nearby states to protect confidentiality; Please refer to the User's Guide for a full explanation of data.

Jamaica Hospital Medical Center[2]	Jamaica	99%	295
Jones Memorial Hospital	Wellsville	99%	72
Kingsbrook Jewish Medical Center	Brooklyn	99%	184
Mercy Hospital[2]	Buffalo	99%	694
Montefiore New Rochelle Hospital	New Rochelle	99%	519
Newark - Wayne Community Hospital	Newark	99%	273
Northport VA Medical Center[2]	Northport	99%	108
Rochester General Hospital[2]	Rochester	99%	1636
Rome Memorial Hospital	Rome	99%	179
Saint Barnabas Hospital[2]	Bronx	99%	184
St John's Episcopal Hosp-South Shore[2]	Far Rockaway	99%	163
Univ Hosp SUNY Health Science Ctr[2]	Syracuse	99%	531
Westchester Medical Center[2]	Valhalla	99%	478
Woman's Christian Association[2]	Jamestown	99%	342
North Central Bronx Hospital	Bronx	98%	55
Saint Joseph's Hospital Health Center[2]	Syracuse	98%	663
Saint Luke's Cornwall Hospital[2]	Newburgh	98%	523
University Hospital - Stony Brook[2]	Stony Brook	98%	435
Geneva General Hospital	Geneva	97%	462
Saint John's Riverside Hospital[2]	Yonkers	97%	461
Bronx VA Medical Center[2]	Bronx	96%	96
TLC Health Network	Gowanda	96%	122
Medina Memorial Hospital	Medina	95%	43
Montefiore Medical Center[2]	Bronx	95%	906
Montefiore Mount Vernon Hospital	Mount Vernon	95%	66
Upstate New York VA Healthcare Sys[2]	Buffalo	95%	178
Eastern Niagara Hospital[2]	Lockport	93%	131
Aurelia Osborn Fox Memorial Hospital	Oneonta	92%	110

Prophylactic Antibiotic Selection

Hospital Name	City	Rate	Cases
Albany Medical Center Hospital[2]	Albany	100%	369
Albany VA Medical Center	Albany	100%	79
Arnot Ogden Medical Center[2]	Elmira	100%	638
Aurelia Osborn Fox Memorial Hospital	Oneonta	100%	54
Bellevue Hospital Center[2]	New York	100%	279
Bon Secours Community Hospital	Port Jervis	100%	37
Bronx VA Medical Center	Bronx	100%	50
Brooklyn Hosp Ctr at Downtown Campus	Brooklyn	100%	372
Brooks Memorial Hospital[2]	Dunkirk	100%	262
Claxton - Hepburn Medical Center	Ogdensburg	100%	114
Community Memorial Hospital	Hamilton	100%	460
Ellis Hospital[2]	Schenectady	100%	543
Elmhurst Hospital Center	Elmhurst	100%	183
F F Thompson Hospital	Canandaigua	100%	430
Forest Hills Hospital[2]	Forest Hills	100%	246
Highland Hospital[2]	Rochester	100%	632
Hospital For Special Surgery[2]	New York	100%	412
Huntington Hospital[2]	Huntington	100%	205
Jones Memorial Hospital	Wellsville	100%	37
Kaleida Health[2]	Buffalo	100%	815
Kings County Hospital Center[2]	Brooklyn	100%	225
Mercy Hospital[2]	Buffalo	100%	594
North Central Bronx Hospital	Bronx	100%	25
Northern Dutchess Hospital[2]	Rhinebeck	100%	248
Northern Westchester Hospital[2]	Mount Kisco	100%	314
Saint Barnabas Hospital[2]	Bronx	100%	91
Saint Charles Hospital[2]	Port Jefferson	100%	459
Saint Francis Hospital - Roslyn[2]	Roslyn	100%	559
Saint Luke's Roosevelt Hospital[2]	New York	100%	567
Saint Mary's Hospital at Amsterdam[2]	Amsterdam	100%	166
South Nassau Communities Hospital[2]	Oceanside	100%	747
Staten Island University Hospital[2]	Staten Island	100%	343
Strong Memorial Hospital[2]	Rochester	100%	658
Vassar Brothers Medical Center[2]	Poughkeepsie	100%	457
White Plains Hospital Center[2]	White Plains	100%	304
Beth Israel Medical Center[2]	New York	99%	503
Bronx - Lebanon Hospital Center[2]	Bronx	99%	263
Catskill Regional Medical Center	Harris	99%	70
Champlain Valley Phys Hosp Med Ctr[2]	Plattsburgh	99%	489
Chenango Memorial Hospital	Norwich	99%	110
Columbia Memorial Hospital	Hudson	99%	157
Franklin Hospital[2]	Valley Stream	99%	186
Geneva General Hospital	Geneva	99%	356
Glens Falls Hospital[2]	Glens Falls	99%	379
Good Samaritan Hospital Medical Center[2]	West Islip	99%	311
Good Samaritan Hospital of Suffern[2]	Suffern	99%	432
Health Alliance Hosp Mary's Ave Campus	Kingston	99%	309
Hudson Valley Hospital Center[2]	Cortlandt Manor	99%	281
Jacobi Medical Center	Bronx	99%	156
John T Mather Mem Hosp-Port Jefferson	Port Jefferson	99%	208
Kenmore Mercy Hospital[2]	Kenmore	99%	294
Lincoln Medical & Mental Health Center[2]	Bronx	99%	152
Lutheran Medical Center[2]	Brooklyn	99%	489
Mary Imogene Bassett Hospital[2]	Cooperstown	99%	454
Mercy Medical Center[2]	Rockville Centre	99%	169
Montefiore New Rochelle Hospital	New Rochelle	99%	364
Mount St Mary's Hosp & Health Ctr[2]	Lewiston	99%	252
Mount Sinai Hospital[2]	New York	99%	676
New York - Presbyterian Hospital[2]	New York	99%	975
New York Hosp Med Ctr of Queens[2]	Flushing	99%	427
Newark - Wayne Community Hospital	Newark	99%	171
Niagara Falls Memorial Medical Center[2]	Niagara Falls	99%	77
North Shore University Hospital[2]	Manhasset	99%	546
Nyack Hospital[2]	Nyack	99%	333
NYU Hospitals Center[2]	New York	99%	473
Orange Regional Medical Center[2]	Middletown	99%	404
Oswego Hospital	Oswego	99%	103
Our Lady of Lourdes Memorial Hospital[2]	Binghamton	99%	196
Peconic Bay Medical Center[2]	Riverhead	99%	437
Phelps Memorial Hospital Assn[2]	Sleepy Hollow	99%	375
Plainview Hospital[2]	Plainview	99%	228
Putnam Hospital Center	Carmel	99%	640
Queens Hospital Center	Jamaica	99%	95
Rochester General Hospital[2]	Rochester	99%	1726
Saint Anthony Community Hospital	Warwick	99%	124
Saint Elizabeth Medical Center[2]	Utica	99%	934
Saint Francis Hospital[2]	Poughkeepsie	99%	169
Saint James Mercy Hospital	Hornell	99%	71
Saint Joseph Hospital[2]	Bethpage	99%	168
Saint Joseph's Hospital[2]	Elmira	99%	126
Saint Joseph's Hospital Health Center[2]	Syracuse	99%	600
Saint Joseph's Medical Center	Yonkers	99%	76
Saint Luke's Cornwall Hospital[2]	Newburgh	99%	364
Saint Peter's Hospital[2]	Albany	99%	669
Samaritan Hospital[2]	Troy	99%	294
Samaritan Medical Center	Watertown	99%	353
Saratoga Hospital[2]	Saratoga Spgs	99%	460
Sisters of Charity Hospital[2]	Buffalo	99%	413
Southside Hospital[2]	Bay Shore	99%	410
United Health Services Hospitals	Johnson City	99%	1020
Unity Hospital of Rochester[2]	Rochester	99%	337
Univ Hosp SUNY Health Science Ctr[2]	Syracuse	99%	340
Westchester Medical Center[2]	Valhalla	99%	453
Winthrop - University Hospital[2]	Mineola	99%	738
Adirondack Medical Center[2]	Saranac Lake	98%	219
Canton - Potsdam Hospital	Potsdam	98%	149
Cayuga Medical Center at Ithaca	Ithaca	98%	247
Coney Island Hospital[2]	Brooklyn	98%	60
Corning Hospital	Corning	98%	184
Crouse Hospital[2]	Syracuse	98%	397
Flushing Hospital Medical Center[2]	Flushing	98%	215
Glen Cove Hospital[2]	Glen Cove	98%	172
Kingsbrook Jewish Medical Center	Brooklyn	98%	96
Lawrence Hospital Center[2]	Bronxville	98%	219
Lenox Hill Hospital[2]	New York	98%	457
Long Island Jewish Medical Center[2]	New Hyde Park	98%	453
Maimonides Medical Center[2]	Brooklyn	98%	555
Nassau University Medical Center[2]	East Meadow	98%	146
Northport VA Medical Center	Northport	98%	66
Oneida Healthcare Center	Oneida	98%	88
Richmond University Medical Center[2]	Staten Island	98%	252
Syracuse VA Medical Center	Syracuse	98%	53
United Memorial Medical Center	Batavia	98%	188
University Hospital - Stony Brook[2]	Stony Brook	98%	383
Woman's Christian Association[2]	Jamestown	98%	249
Woodhull Medical & Mental Health Center[2]	Brooklyn	98%	124
Albany Memorial Hospital[2]	Albany	97%	137
Alice Hyde Medical Center	Malone	97%	77
Auburn Community Hospital	Auburn	97%	125
Brookdale Hospital Medical Center	Brooklyn	97%	90
Health Alliance Hospital Broadway Campus	Kingston	97%	72
Jamaica Hospital Medical Center[2]	Jamaica	97%	149
Nathan Littauer Hospital	Gloversville	97%	108
New York Community Hospital of Brooklyn[2]	Brooklyn	97%	37
New York Methodist Hospital[2]	Brooklyn	97%	489
Rome Memorial Hospital	Rome	97%	101
Saint John's Riverside Hospital[2]	Yonkers	97%	318
TLC Health Network	Gowanda	97%	102
Univ Hosp of Brooklyn-Downstate[2]	Brooklyn	97%	293
VA New York Harbor Healthcare System	New York	97%	92
Brookhaven Mem Hosp Med Ctr	Patchogue	96%	95
Clifton Springs Hospital & Clinic[2]	Clifton Springs	96%	51
Olean General Hospital[2]	Olean	96%	191
Saint Mary's Hospital - Troy[2]	Troy	96%	97
Wyckoff Heights Medical Center[2]	Brooklyn	96%	112
Massena Memorial Hospital	Massena	95%	44
Metropolitan Hospital Center[2]	New York	95%	146
Upstate New York VA Healthcare Sys	Buffalo	95%	132
Wyoming County Community Hospital	Warsaw	95%	64
Eastern Niagara Hospital[2]	Lockport	94%	66
Erie County Medical Center	Buffalo	94%	481
Faxton - Saint Luke's Healthcare[2]	Utica	94%	274
Harlem Hospital Center[2]	New York	94%	47
Montefiore Medical Center[2]	Bronx	94%	710
Montefiore Mount Vernon Hospital	Mount Vernon	94%	32
Saint Catherine of Siena Hospital[2]	Smithtown	94%	208
St John's Episcopal Hosp-South Shore[2]	Far Rockaway	93%	68
Cortland Regional Medical Center	Cortland	92%	39
Nicholas H Noyes Memorial Hospital	Dansville	91%	91
Southampton Hospital	Southampton	90%	84
Interfaith Medical Center	Brooklyn	82%	39

Prophylactic Antibiotic Selection (Outpatient)

Hospital Name	City	Rate	Cases
Brookhaven Mem Hosp Med Ctr	Patchogue	100%	53
Claxton - Hepburn Medical Center	Ogdensburg	100%	25
F F Thompson Hospital	Canandaigua	100%	84
Health Alliance Hosp Mary's Ave Campus	Kingston	100%	54
Hospital For Special Surgery	New York	100%	415
Kenmore Mercy Hospital	Kenmore	100%	558
Medina Memorial Hospital	Medina	100%	30
Mercy Hospital	Buffalo	100%	635
Montefiore New Rochelle Hospital	New Rochelle	100%	29
New York Methodist Hospital	Brooklyn	100%	93
Nyack Hospital	Nyack	100%	45
NYU Hospitals Center	New York	100%	734
Saint Joseph's Hospital	Elmira	100%	25
South Nassau Communities Hospital	Oceanside	100%	338
Strong Memorial Hospital	Rochester	100%	641
Unity Hospital of Rochester	Rochester	100%	518
Albany Medical Center Hospital	Albany	99%	713
Ellis Hospital	Schenectady	99%	617
Glens Falls Hospital	Glens Falls	99%	352
Highland Hospital	Rochester	99%	174
Huntington Hospital	Huntington	99%	299
John T Mather Mem Hosp-Port Jefferson	Port Jefferson	99%	149
Jones Memorial Hospital	Wellsville	99%	73
Kaleida Health	Buffalo	99%	1477
Kings County Hospital Center	Brooklyn	99%	158
Lincoln Medical & Mental Health Center	Bronx	99%	191
Niagara Falls Memorial Medical Center	Niagara Falls	99%	160
Northern Westchester Hospital	Mount Kisco	99%	360
Oswego Hospital	Oswego	99%	104
Rochester General Hospital	Rochester	99%	725
Saint Charles Hospital	Port Jefferson	99%	157
Saint Elizabeth Medical Center	Utica	99%	352
Saint Joseph's Hospital Health Center	Syracuse	99%	807
Saint Mary's Hospital at Amsterdam	Amsterdam	99%	280
Samaritan Medical Center	Watertown	99%	344
Saratoga Hospital	Saratoga Spgs	99%	285
Sisters of Charity Hospital	Buffalo	99%	553
Vassar Brothers Medical Center	Poughkeepsie	99%	501
Winthrop - University Hospital	Mineola	99%	921
Albany Memorial Hospital	Albany	98%	179
Arnot Ogden Medical Center	Elmira	98%	390
Champlain Valley Phys Hosp Med Ctr	Plattsburgh	98%	432
Good Samaritan Hospital Medical Center	West Islip	98%	593
Hudson Valley Hospital Center	Cortlandt Manor	98%	87
Jacobi Medical Center	Bronx	98%	121
Mary Imogene Bassett Hospital	Cooperstown	98%	281
Mount St Mary's Hosp & Health Ctr	Lewiston	98%	157
Mount Sinai Hospital	New York	98%	782
Newark - Wayne Community Hospital	Newark	98%	102
North Shore University Hospital	Manhasset	98%	299
Orange Regional Medical Center	Middletown	98%	378
Putnam Hospital Center	Carmel	98%	144
Richmond University Medical Center	Staten Island	98%	333
Saint Anthony Community Hospital	Warwick	98%	57
Saint Francis Hospital	Poughkeepsie	98%	173
Samaritan Hospital	Troy	98%	203
United Health Services Hospitals	Johnson City	98%	891
United Memorial Medical Center	Batavia	98%	59
Westchester Medical Center	Valhalla	98%	283
White Plains Hospital Center	White Plains	98%	356
Woodhull Medical & Mental Health Center	Brooklyn	98%	84
Auburn Community Hospital	Auburn	97%	95
Bellevue Hospital Center	New York	97%	104
Cayuga Medical Center at Ithaca	Ithaca	97%	98
Community Memorial Hospital	Hamilton	97%	39
Flushing Hospital Medical Center	Flushing	97%	133
Jamaica Hospital Medical Center	Jamaica	97%	67
Lawrence Hospital Center	Bronxville	97%	66
Lutheran Medical Center	Brooklyn	97%	117
Maimonides Medical Center	Brooklyn	97%	392
Mercy Medical Center	Rockville Centre	97%	65
Nathan Littauer Hospital	Gloversville	97%	211
New York - Presbyterian Hospital	New York	97%	1200
Olean General Hospital	Olean	97%	126
Oneida Healthcare Center	Oneida	97%	175
Our Lady of Lourdes Memorial Hospital	Binghamton	97%	280
Queens Hospital Center	Jamaica	97%	65
Saint Barnabas Hospital	Bronx	97%	95
Saint Francis Hospital - Roslyn	Roslyn	97%	472
Saint Peter's Hospital	Albany	97%	785
Southampton Hospital	Southampton	97%	29
Southside Hospital	Bay Shore	97%	104
Univ Hosp SUNY Health Science Ctr	Syracuse	97%	561
Adirondack Medical Center	Saranac Lake	96%	94
Alice Hyde Medical Center	Malone	96%	28
Beth Israel Medical Center	New York	96%	466
Bronx - Lebanon Hospital Center	Bronx	96%	171
Brookdale Hospital Medical Center	Brooklyn	96%	136

NOTE: Hospital profiles are in alphabetical order by state, then city, then hospital within the city; Rankings exclude hospitals with less than 25 cases except for patient surveys which excludes hospitals with less than 100 cases; (a) 100-299 cases; (1) The number of cases/patients is too few to report; (2) Data submitted were based on a sample of cases/patients; (3) Results are based on a shorter time period than required; (4) Data suppressed by CMS for one or more quarters; (5) Results are not available for this reporting period; (6) Fewer than 100 patients completed the HCAHPS survey; (7) No cases met the criteria for this measure; (8) The lower limit of the confidence interval cannot be calculated if the number of observed infections equals zero; (9) No data are available from the state/territory for this reporting period; (10) The scores shown reflect fewer than 50 completed surveys; (11) There were discrepancies in the data collection process; (12) This measure does not apply to this hospital for this reporting period; (13) Results cannot be calculated for this reporting period; (14) The results for this state are combined with nearby states to protect confidentiality; Please refer to the User's Guide for a full explanation of data.

Corning Hospital	Corning	96%	56
Crouse Hospital	Syracuse	96%	766
Forest Hills Hospital	Forest Hills	96%	67
New York Hosp Med Ctr of Queens	Flushing	96%	475
Phelps Memorial Hospital Assn	Sleepy Hollow	96%	116
Plainview Hospital	Plainview	96%	89
Saint Luke's Roosevelt Hospital	New York	96%	345
Saint Mary's Hospital - Troy	Troy	96%	73
Univ Hosp of Brooklyn-Downstate	Brooklyn	96%	291
Columbia Memorial Hospital	Hudson	95%	107
Coney Island Hospital	Brooklyn	95%	80
Cortland Regional Medical Center	Cortland	95%	64
Erie County Medical Center	Buffalo	95%	331
Good Samaritan Hospital of Suffern	Suffern	95%	200
Nassau University Medical Center	East Meadow	95%	38
Saint Luke's Cornwall Hospital	Newburgh	95%	197
Woman's Christian Association	Jamestown	95%	105
Elmhurst Hospital Center	Elmhurst	94%	105
Glen Cove Hospital	Glen Cove	94%	50
Harlem Hospital Center	New York	94%	82
Nicholas H Noyes Memorial Hospital	Dansville	94%	77
Wyckoff Heights Medical Center	Brooklyn	94%	68
Brooks Memorial Hospital	Dunkirk	93%	29
Lenox Hill Hospital	New York	93%	451
Northern Dutchess Hospital	Rhinebeck	93%	153
Saint John's Riverside Hospital	Yonkers	93%	76
Staten Island University Hospital	Staten Island	93%	201
Saint Catherine of Siena Hospital	Smithtown	92%	365
Eastern Niagara Hospital	Lockport	91%	53
Interfaith Medical Center	Brooklyn	91%	33
University Hospital - Stony Brook	Stony Brook	91%	438
Aurelia Osborn Fox Memorial Hospital	Oneonta	90%	69
Catskill Regional Medical Center	Harris	90%	63
Kingsbrook Jewish Medical Center	Brooklyn	90%	31
Saint Joseph's Medical Center	Yonkers	90%	41
Little Falls Hospital	Little Falls	89%	28
Metropolitan Hospital Center	New York	89%	55
Health Alliance Hospital Broadway Campus	Kingston	88%	59
Brooklyn Hosp Ctr at Downtown Campus	Brooklyn	87%	234
Long Island Jewish Medical Center	New Hyde Park	86%	310
Peconic Bay Medical Center	Riverhead	85%	81
Faxton - Saint Luke's Healthcare	Utica	80%	215
St John's Episcopal Hosp-South Shore	Far Rockaway	80%	40
Montefiore Medical Center	Bronx	64%	500

Prophylactic Antibiotic Stopped

Hospital Name	City	Rate	Cases
Albany VA Medical Center	Albany	100%	78
Arnot Ogden Medical Center[2]	Elmira	100%	623
Canton - Potsdam Hospital	Potsdam	100%	149
Clifton Springs Hospital & Clinic[2]	Clifton Springs	100%	48
Columbia Memorial Hospital	Hudson	100%	156
Community Memorial Hospital	Hamilton	100%	456
Coney Island Hospital[2]	Brooklyn	100%	60
Ellis Hospital[2]	Schenectady	100%	526
Geneva General Hospital	Geneva	100%	354
Highland Hospital[2]	Rochester	100%	622
Hospital For Special Surgery[2]	New York	100%	409
Hudson Valley Hospital Center[2]	Cortlandt Manor	100%	280
Jones Memorial Hospital	Wellsville	100%	32
Kenmore Mercy Hospital[2]	Kenmore	100%	293
Lawrence Hospital Center[2]	Bronxville	100%	216
Massena Memorial Hospital	Massena	100%	44
Mercy Hospital[2]	Buffalo	100%	582
New York Community Hospital of Brooklyn[2]	Brooklyn	100%	36
Northern Dutchess Hospital[2]	Rhinebeck	100%	248
Northern Westchester Hospital[2]	Mount Kisco	100%	304
Orange Regional Medical Center[2]	Middletown	100%	403
Phelps Memorial Hospital Assn[2]	Sleepy Hollow	100%	372
Putnam Hospital Center	Carmel	100%	636
Rochester General Hospital[2]	Rochester	100%	1698
Saint Anthony Community Hospital	Warwick	100%	120
Saint Barnabas Hospital[2]	Bronx	100%	88
Saint Charles Hospital[2]	Port Jefferson	100%	449
Saint Francis Hospital[2]	Poughkeepsie	100%	169
St John's Episcopal Hosp-South Shore[2]	Far Rockaway	100%	66
Saint Joseph's Hospital[2]	Elmira	100%	126
Saint Joseph's Medical Center	Yonkers	100%	73
Sisters of Charity Hospital[2]	Buffalo	100%	404
South Nassau Communities Hospital[2]	Oceanside	100%	732
Staten Island University Hospital[2]	Staten Island	100%	322
Strong Memorial Hospital[2]	Rochester	100%	641
White Plains Hospital Center[2]	White Plains	100%	294
Albany Medical Center Hospital[2]	Albany	99%	369
Bellevue Hospital Center[2]	New York	99%	272
Catskill Regional Medical Center	Harris	99%	70
Champlain Valley Phys Hosp Med Ctr[2]	Plattsburgh	99%	477
Chenango Memorial Hospital	Norwich	99%	108
Corning Hospital	Corning	99%	180
Elmhurst Hospital Center	Elmhurst	99%	167
F F Thompson Hospital	Canandaigua	99%	409
Faxton - Saint Luke's Healthcare[2]	Utica	99%	271
Forest Hills Hospital[2]	Forest Hills	99%	240
Glen Cove Hospital[2]	Glen Cove	99%	171
Good Samaritan Hospital Medical Center[2]	West Islip	99%	300
Health Alliance Hosp Mary's Ave Campus	Kingston	99%	304
John T Mather Mem Hosp-Port Jefferson	Port Jefferson	99%	206
Kings County Hospital Center[2]	Brooklyn	99%	202
Kingsbrook Jewish Medical Center	Brooklyn	99%	88
Maimonides Medical Center[2]	Brooklyn	99%	533
Mercy Medical Center[2]	Rockville Centre	99%	158
Montefiore New Rochelle Hospital	New Rochelle	99%	362
Nassau University Medical Center[2]	East Meadow	99%	141
New York Hosp Med Ctr of Queens[2]	Flushing	99%	402
Nicholas H Noyes Memorial Hospital	Dansville	99%	89
NYU Hospitals Center[2]	New York	99%	459
Plainview Hospital[2]	Plainview	99%	225
Saint John's Riverside Hospital[2]	Yonkers	99%	307
Saint Joseph Hospital[2]	Bethpage	99%	167
Saint Luke's Cornwall Hospital[2]	Newburgh	99%	353
Saint Mary's Hospital - Troy[2]	Troy	99%	92
Saint Mary's Hospital at Amsterdam[2]	Amsterdam	99%	162
Saint Peter's Hospital[2]	Albany	99%	669
Samaritan Medical Center	Watertown	99%	352
Unity Hospital of Rochester[2]	Rochester	99%	337
VA New York Harbor Healthcare System	New York	99%	90
Adirondack Medical Center[2]	Saranac Lake	98%	213
Bronx VA Medical Center	Bronx	98%	49
Brooks Memorial Hospital[2]	Dunkirk	98%	260
Crouse Hospital[2]	Syracuse	98%	384
Franklin Hospital[2]	Valley Stream	98%	176
Good Samaritan Hospital of Suffern[2]	Suffern	98%	423
Huntington Hospital[2]	Huntington	98%	200
Mary Imogene Bassett Hospital[2]	Cooperstown	98%	450
Mount Sinai Hospital[2]	New York	98%	658
New York Methodist Hospital[2]	Brooklyn	98%	445
Northport VA Medical Center	Northport	98%	63
Nyack Hospital	Nyack	98%	323
Rome Memorial Hospital	Rome	98%	98
Saint Elizabeth Medical Center[2]	Utica	98%	923
Saint Luke's Roosevelt Hospital[2]	New York	98%	557
Saratoga Hospital[2]	Saratoga Spgs	98%	447
Southside Hospital[2]	Bay Shore	98%	400
Syracuse VA Medical Center	Syracuse	98%	53
University Hospital - Stony Brook[2]	Stony Brook	98%	376
Univ Hosp of Brooklyn-Downstate[2]	Brooklyn	98%	282
Vassar Brothers Medical Center[2]	Poughkeepsie	98%	433
Winthrop - University Hospital[2]	Mineola	98%	716
Woodhull Medical & Mental Health Center[2]	Brooklyn	98%	122
Albany Memorial Hospital[2]	Albany	97%	132
Bon Secours Community Hospital	Port Jervis	97%	35
Brooklyn Hosp Ctr at Downtown Campus	Brooklyn	97%	355
Cayuga Medical Center at Ithaca	Ithaca	97%	244
Erie County Medical Center	Buffalo	97%	473
Jamaica Hospital Medical Center[2]	Jamaica	97%	145
Long Island Jewish Medical Center[2]	New Hyde Park	97%	447
Lutheran Medical Center[2]	Brooklyn	97%	474
New York - Presbyterian Hospital[2]	New York	97%	952
Our Lady of Lourdes Memorial Hospital[2]	Binghamton	97%	192
Saint Catherine of Siena Hospital[2]	Smithtown	97%	201
Saint Francis Hospital - Roslyn[2]	Roslyn	97%	550
Samaritan Hospital[2]	Troy	97%	291
Univ Hosp SUNY Health Science Ctr[2]	Syracuse	97%	322
Upstate New York VA Healthcare Sys	Buffalo	97%	130
Beth Israel Medical Center[2]	New York	96%	498
Claxton - Hepburn Medical Center	Ogdensburg	96%	113
Mount St Mary's Hosp & Health Ctr[2]	Lewiston	96%	252
Newark - Wayne Community Hospital	Newark	96%	164
Niagara Falls Memorial Medical Center[2]	Niagara Falls	96%	74
North Central Bronx Hospital	Bronx	96%	25
North Shore University Hospital[2]	Manhasset	96%	540
Oswego Hospital	Oswego	96%	97
United Health Services Hospitals	Johnson City	96%	992
Westchester Medical Center[2]	Valhalla	96%	419
Alice Hyde Medical Center	Malone	95%	74
Bronx - Lebanon Hospital Center[2]	Bronx	95%	255
Cortland Regional Medical Center	Cortland	95%	37
Glens Falls Hospital[2]	Glens Falls	95%	376
Jacobi Medical Center	Bronx	95%	146
Kaleida Health[2]	Buffalo	95%	807
Lenox Hill Hospital[2]	New York	95%	442
Lincoln Medical & Mental Health Center[2]	Bronx	95%	150
Nathan Littauer Hospital	Gloversville	95%	108
Peconic Bay Medical Center[2]	Riverhead	95%	432
Queens Hospital Center	Jamaica	95%	88
Richmond University Medical Center[2]	Staten Island	95%	249
Saint Joseph's Hospital Health Center[2]	Syracuse	95%	586
TLC Health Network	Gowanda	95%	102
Wyckoff Heights Medical Center[2]	Brooklyn	95%	98
Metropolitan Hospital Center[2]	New York	94%	141
Montefiore Mount Vernon Hospital	Mount Vernon	94%	32
Aurelia Osborn Fox Memorial Hospital	Oneonta	93%	54
Harlem Hospital Center[2]	New York	93%	44
Health Alliance Hospital Broadway Campus	Kingston	93%	69
Montefiore Medical Center[2]	Bronx	93%	701
Saint James Mercy Hospital	Hornell	93%	71
Brookhaven Mem Hosp Med Ctr	Patchogue	92%	88
Eastern Niagara Hospital[2]	Lockport	92%	66
United Memorial Medical Center	Batavia	92%	184
Woman's Christian Association[2]	Jamestown	92%	245
Wyoming County Community Hospital	Warsaw	92%	62
Auburn Community Hospital	Auburn	91%	120
Interfaith Medical Center	Brooklyn	91%	34
Oneida Healthcare Center	Oneida	91%	85
Flushing Hospital Medical Center[2]	Flushing	90%	210
Olean General Hospital[2]	Olean	90%	174
Southampton Hospital	Southampton	90%	82
Brookdale Hospital Medical Center	Brooklyn	88%	88

Prophylactic Antibiotic Timing

Hospital Name	City	Rate	Cases
Albany Medical Center Hospital[2]	Albany	100%	373
Arnot Ogden Medical Center[2]	Elmira	100%	638
Beth Israel Medical Center[2]	New York	100%	503
Bronx VA Medical Center	Bronx	100%	50
Brookhaven Mem Hosp Med Ctr	Patchogue	100%	96
Catskill Regional Medical Center	Harris	100%	70
Claxton - Hepburn Medical Center	Ogdensburg	100%	114
Columbia Memorial Hospital	Hudson	100%	157
Corning Hospital	Corning	100%	184
Cortland Regional Medical Center	Cortland	100%	39
Eastern Niagara Hospital[2]	Lockport	100%	66
Ellis Hospital[2]	Schenectady	100%	543
Forest Hills Hospital[2]	Forest Hills	100%	246
Geneva General Hospital	Geneva	100%	356
Harlem Hospital Center[2]	New York	100%	47
Highland Hospital[2]	Rochester	100%	638
Hospital For Special Surgery[2]	New York	100%	412
Hudson Valley Hospital Center[2]	Cortlandt Manor	100%	281
Jones Memorial Hospital	Wellsville	100%	37
Lawrence Hospital Center[2]	Bronxville	100%	219
Lutheran Medical Center[2]	Brooklyn	100%	489
Massena Memorial Hospital	Massena	100%	44
Montefiore Mount Vernon Hospital	Mount Vernon	100%	32
Montefiore New Rochelle Hospital	New Rochelle	100%	364
Nassau University Medical Center[2]	East Meadow	100%	146
Northern Dutchess Hospital[2]	Rhinebeck	100%	248
Northern Westchester Hospital[2]	Mount Kisco	100%	314
Nyack Hospital	Nyack	100%	333
Oneida Healthcare Center	Oneida	100%	88
Our Lady of Lourdes Memorial Hospital[2]	Binghamton	100%	196
Phelps Memorial Hospital Assn[2]	Sleepy Hollow	100%	375
Putnam Hospital Center	Carmel	100%	640
Queens Hospital Center	Jamaica	100%	95
Saint Anthony Community Hospital	Warwick	100%	124
Saint Charles Hospital[2]	Port Jefferson	100%	459
Saint Francis Hospital[2]	Poughkeepsie	100%	169
Saint James Mercy Hospital	Hornell	100%	71
St John's Episcopal Hosp-South Shore[2]	Far Rockaway	100%	68
Saint John's Riverside Hospital[2]	Yonkers	100%	318
Saint Luke's Cornwall Hospital[2]	Newburgh	100%	364
Saint Luke's Roosevelt Hospital[2]	New York	100%	568
South Nassau Communities Hospital[2]	Oceanside	100%	747
Staten Island University Hospital[2]	Staten Island	100%	343
Strong Memorial Hospital[2]	Rochester	100%	659
Vassar Brothers Medical Center[2]	Poughkeepsie	100%	457
White Plains Hospital Center[2]	White Plains	100%	304
Wyoming County Community Hospital	Warsaw	100%	64
Auburn Community Hospital	Auburn	99%	125
Bellevue Hospital Center[2]	New York	99%	279
Bronx - Lebanon Hospital Center[2]	Bronx	99%	263
Brooklyn Hosp Ctr at Downtown Campus	Brooklyn	99%	372
Brooks Memorial Hospital[2]	Dunkirk	99%	262
Champlain Valley Phys Hosp Med Ctr[2]	Plattsburgh	99%	490
Community Memorial Hospital	Hamilton	99%	461
Elmhurst Hospital Center	Elmhurst	99%	181
F F Thompson Hospital	Canandaigua	99%	431
Flushing Hospital Medical Center[2]	Flushing	99%	215
Franklin Hospital[2]	Valley Stream	99%	186
Glen Cove Hospital[2]	Glen Cove	99%	172
Good Samaritan Hospital of Suffern[2]	Suffern	99%	432
Health Alliance Hospital Broadway Campus	Kingston	99%	72
Health Alliance Hosp Mary's Ave Campus	Kingston	99%	309
Huntington Hospital[2]	Huntington	99%	206
Jacobi Medical Center	Bronx	99%	156
John T Mather Mem Hosp-Port Jefferson	Port Jefferson	99%	210
Kaleida Health[2]	Buffalo	99%	815
Kings County Hospital Center[2]	Brooklyn	99%	227
Kingsbrook Jewish Medical Center	Brooklyn	99%	96
Lenox Hill Hospital[2]	New York	99%	457
Lincoln Medical & Mental Health Center[2]	Bronx	99%	152
Long Island Jewish Medical Center[2]	New Hyde Park	99%	453
Mercy Hospital[2]	Buffalo	99%	596

NOTE: Hospital profiles are in alphabetical order by state, then city, then hospital within the city; Rankings exclude hospitals with less than 25 cases except for patient surveys which excludes hospitals with less than 100 cases; (a) 100-299 cases; (1) The number of cases/patients is too few to report; (2) Data submitted were based on a sample of cases/patients; (3) Results are based on a shorter time period than required; (4) Data suppressed by CMS for one or more quarters; (5) Results are not available for this reporting period; (6) Fewer than 100 patients completed the HCAHPS survey; (7) No cases met the criteria for this measure; (8) The lower limit of the confidence interval cannot be calculated if the number of observed infections equals zero; (9) No data are available from the state/territory for this reporting period; (10) The scores shown reflect fewer than 50 completed surveys; (11) There were discrepancies in the data collection process; (12) This measure does not apply to this hospital for this reporting period; (13) Results cannot be calculated for this reporting period; (14) The results for this state are combined with nearby states to protect confidentiality; Please refer to the User's Guide for a full explanation of data.

Mount Sinai Hospital[2]	New York	99%	675
New York - Presbyterian Hospital[2]	New York	99%	973
New York Methodist Hospital[2]	Brooklyn	99%	489
Niagara Falls Memorial Medical Center[2]	Niagara Falls	99%	77
North Shore University Hospital[2]	Manhasset	99%	549
NYU Hospitals Center[2]	New York	99%	472
Orange Regional Medical Center[2]	Middletown	99%	406
Plainview Hospital[2]	Plainview	99%	228
Richmond University Medical Center[2]	Staten Island	99%	252
Saint Elizabeth Medical Center[2]	Utica	99%	936
Saint Francis Hospital - Roslyn[2]	Roslyn	99%	560
Saint Joseph's Hospital Health Center[2]	Syracuse	99%	600
Saint Mary's Hospital - Troy[2]	Troy	99%	97
Saint Mary's Hospital at Amsterdam[2]	Amsterdam	99%	166
Saint Peter's Hospital[2]	Albany	99%	669
Saratoga Hospital[2]	Saratoga Spgs	99%	460
Sisters of Charity Hospital[2]	Buffalo	99%	414
Southampton Hospital	Southampton	99%	84
Southside Hospital[2]	Bay Shore	99%	411
United Health Services Hospitals	Johnson City	99%	1020
Unity Hospital of Rochester[2]	Rochester	99%	339
Westchester Medical Center[2]	Valhalla	99%	453
Brookdale Hospital Medical Center	Brooklyn	98%	90
Cayuga Medical Center at Ithaca	Ithaca	98%	247
Chenango Memorial Hospital	Norwich	98%	111
Erie County Medical Center	Buffalo	98%	482
Good Samaritan Hospital Medical Center[2]	West Islip	98%	311
Kenmore Mercy Hospital[2]	Kenmore	98%	296
Maimonides Medical Center[2]	Brooklyn	98%	560
Mary Imogene Bassett Hospital[2]	Cooperstown	98%	454
Mount St Mary's Hosp & Health Ctr[2]	Lewiston	98%	252
New York Hosp Med Ctr of Queens[2]	Flushing	98%	427
Northport VA Medical Center	Northport	98%	66
Oswego Hospital	Oswego	98%	103
Rochester General Hospital[2]	Rochester	98%	1732
Saint Barnabas Hospital[2]	Bronx	98%	91
Saint Joseph Hospital[2]	Bethpage	98%	169
United Memorial Medical Center	Batavia	98%	188
University Hospital - Stony Brook[2]	Stony Brook	98%	385
Winthrop - University Hospital[2]	Mineola	98%	742
Woman's Christian Association[2]	Jamestown	98%	252
Wyckoff Heights Medical Center[2]	Brooklyn	98%	112
Bon Secours Community Hospital	Port Jervis	97%	37
Canton - Potsdam Hospital	Potsdam	97%	149
Coney Island Hospital[2]	Brooklyn	97%	60
Crouse Hospital[2]	Syracuse	97%	397
Glens Falls Hospital[2]	Glens Falls	97%	379
Interfaith Medical Center	Brooklyn	97%	39
Nathan Littauer Hospital	Gloversville	97%	108
New York Community Hospital of Brooklyn[2]	Brooklyn	97%	37
Nicholas H Noyes Memorial Hospital	Dansville	97%	91
Olean General Hospital[2]	Olean	97%	192
Peconic Bay Medical Center[2]	Riverhead	97%	437
Saint Joseph's Hospital[2]	Elmira	97%	126
Saint Joseph's Medical Center	Yonkers	97%	76
Samaritan Medical Center	Watertown	97%	356
Albany Memorial Hospital[2]	Albany	96%	137
Alice Hyde Medical Center	Malone	96%	77
Aurelia Osborn Fox Memorial Hospital	Oneonta	96%	54
Clifton Springs Hospital & Clinic[2]	Clifton Springs	96%	52
Faxton - Saint Luke's Healthcare[2]	Utica	96%	274
Mercy Medical Center[2]	Rockville Centre	96%	169
North Central Bronx Hospital	Bronx	96%	26
Saint Catherine of Siena Hospital[2]	Smithtown	96%	209
Syracuse VA Medical Center	Syracuse	96%	53
Adirondack Medical Center[2]	Saranac Lake	95%	220
Jamaica Hospital Medical Center[2]	Jamaica	95%	151
Newark - Wayne Community Hospital	Newark	95%	171
Rome Memorial Hospital	Rome	95%	101
Samaritan Hospital[2]	Troy	95%	294
Univ Hosp of Brooklyn-Downstate[2]	Brooklyn	95%	299
Albany VA Medical Center	Albany	94%	79
Woodhull Medical & Mental Health Center[2]	Brooklyn	94%	126
TLC Health Network	Gowanda	93%	102
Univ Hosp SUNY Health Science Ctr[2]	Syracuse	93%	342
VA New York Harbor Healthcare System	New York	92%	93
Upstate New York VA Healthcare Sys	Buffalo	91%	133
Montefiore Medical Center[2]	Bronx	89%	724
Metropolitan Hospital Center[2]	New York	83%	154

Prophylactic Antibiotic Timing (Outpatient)

Hospital Name	City	Rate	Cases
Brookhaven Mem Hosp Med Ctr	Patchogue	100%	53
Ellis Hospital	Schenectady	100%	617
Elmhurst Hospital Center	Elmhurst	100%	105
Hospital For Special Surgery	New York	100%	415
John T Mather Mem Hosp-Port Jefferson	Port Jefferson	100%	147
Jones Memorial Hospital	Wellsville	100%	73
Lawrence Hospital Center	Bronxville	100%	66
Mercy Medical Center	Rockville Centre	100%	65
North Shore University Hospital	Manhasset	100%	299
Northern Westchester Hospital	Mount Kisco	100%	361
Nyack Hospital	Nyack	100%	45
Phelps Memorial Hospital Assn	Sleepy Hollow	100%	76
Saint Anthony Community Hospital	Warwick	100%	57
Saint Francis Hospital - Roslyn	Roslyn	100%	472
St John's Episcopal Hosp-South Shore	Far Rockaway	100%	40
Saint Joseph's Hospital	Elmira	100%	25
Saint Joseph's Medical Center	Yonkers	100%	41
Saint Luke's Cornwall Hospital	Newburgh	100%	197
Saint Mary's Hospital at Amsterdam	Amsterdam	100%	255
Southside Hospital	Bay Shore	100%	104
Woman's Christian Association	Jamestown	100%	105
Albany Medical Center Hospital	Albany	99%	715
Columbia Memorial Hospital	Hudson	99%	108
Forest Hills Hospital	Forest Hills	99%	67
Good Samaritan Hospital Medical Center	West Islip	99%	593
Highland Hospital	Rochester	99%	175
Huntington Hospital	Huntington	99%	299
Lincoln Medical & Mental Health Center	Bronx	99%	190
Lutheran Medical Center	Brooklyn	99%	118
Mercy Hospital	Buffalo	99%	635
Mount St Mary's Hosp & Health Ctr	Lewiston	99%	158
Niagara Falls Memorial Medical Center	Niagara Falls	99%	157
NYU Hospitals Center	New York	99%	734
Oneida Healthcare Center	Oneida	99%	176
Peconic Bay Medical Center	Riverhead	99%	82
Saint Catherine of Siena Hospital	Smithtown	99%	367
Saint Charles Hospital	Port Jefferson	99%	157
Saint Francis Hospital	Poughkeepsie	99%	174
Saint Joseph's Hospital Health Center	Syracuse	99%	807
Saint Luke's Roosevelt Hospital	New York	99%	343
Saint Peter's Hospital	Albany	99%	785
Saratoga Hospital	Saratoga Spgs	99%	279
Sisters of Charity Hospital	Buffalo	99%	554
South Nassau Communities Hospital	Oceanside	99%	338
Strong Memorial Hospital	Rochester	99%	640
United Health Services Hospitals	Johnson City	99%	891
Vassar Brothers Medical Center	Poughkeepsie	99%	502
White Plains Hospital Center	White Plains	99%	356
Winthrop - University Hospital	Mineola	99%	924
Arnot Ogden Medical Center	Elmira	98%	390
Bronx - Lebanon Hospital Center	Bronx	98%	55
Brookdale Hospital Medical Center	Brooklyn	98%	136
Champlain Valley Phys Hosp Med Ctr	Plattsburgh	98%	435
Crouse Hospital	Syracuse	98%	768
Eastern Niagara Hospital	Lockport	98%	54
Glen Cove Hospital	Glen Cove	98%	51
Good Samaritan Hospital of Suffern	Suffern	98%	203
Health Alliance Hosp Mary's Ave Campus	Kingston	98%	54
Hudson Valley Hospital Center	Cortlandt Manor	98%	89
Kaleida Health	Buffalo	98%	1462
Kenmore Mercy Hospital	Kenmore	98%	562
Mary Imogene Bassett Hospital	Cooperstown	98%	231
Nathan Littauer Hospital	Gloversville	98%	215
Orange Regional Medical Center	Middletown	98%	383
Our Lady of Lourdes Memorial Hospital	Binghamton	98%	265
Staten Island University Hospital	Staten Island	98%	178
United Memorial Medical Center	Batavia	98%	59
Bellevue Hospital Center	New York	97%	29
Beth Israel Medical Center	New York	97%	445
Brooks Memorial Hospital	Dunkirk	97%	30
Catskill Regional Medical Center	Harris	97%	63
Corning Hospital	Corning	97%	58
Glens Falls Hospital	Glens Falls	97%	353
Interfaith Medical Center	Brooklyn	97%	33
Kingsbrook Jewish Medical Center	Brooklyn	97%	30
Little Falls Hospital	Little Falls	97%	29
Long Island Jewish Medical Center	New Hyde Park	97%	315
Montefiore New Rochelle Hospital	New Rochelle	97%	30
Mount Sinai Hospital	New York	97%	765
New York - Presbyterian Hospital	New York	97%	1200
Putnam Hospital Center	Carmel	97%	144
Rochester General Hospital	Rochester	97%	734
Saint Mary's Hospital - Troy	Troy	97%	73
Samaritan Medical Center	Watertown	97%	238
Univ Hosp of Brooklyn-Downstate	Brooklyn	97%	289
Westchester Medical Center	Valhalla	97%	280
Alice Hyde Medical Center	Malone	96%	28
Claxton - Hepburn Medical Center	Ogdensburg	96%	26
Maimonides Medical Center	Brooklyn	96%	402
Newark - Wayne Community Hospital	Newark	96%	104
Northern Dutchess Hospital	Rhinebeck	96%	157
Oswego Hospital	Oswego	96%	104
Plainview Hospital	Plainview	96%	92
Saint Elizabeth Medical Center	Utica	96%	352
Saint John's Riverside Hospital	Yonkers	96%	77
University Hospital - Stony Brook	Stony Brook	96%	414
Community Memorial Hospital	Hamilton	95%	40
New York Hosp Med Ctr of Queens	Flushing	95%	477
New York Methodist Hospital	Brooklyn	95%	95
Richmond University Medical Center	Staten Island	95%	338
Saint Barnabas Hospital	Bronx	95%	95
Albany Memorial Hospital	Albany	94%	189
Erie County Medical Center	Buffalo	94%	319
Lenox Hill Hospital	New York	94%	455
Unity Hospital of Rochester	Rochester	94%	521
Olean General Hospital	Olean	93%	134
Samaritan Hospital	Troy	93%	210
Southampton Hospital	Southampton	93%	29
Auburn Community Hospital	Auburn	92%	99
F F Thompson Hospital	Canandaigua	92%	90
Faxton - Saint Luke's Healthcare	Utica	92%	222
Nicholas H Noyes Memorial Hospital	Dansville	92%	80
Cortland Regional Medical Center	Cortland	91%	69
Flushing Hospital Medical Center	Flushing	91%	138
Univ Hosp SUNY Health Science Ctr	Syracuse	91%	480
Harlem Hospital Center	New York	90%	62
Health Alliance Hospital Broadway Campus	Kingston	90%	61
Jacobi Medical Center	Bronx	90%	51
Adirondack Medical Center	Saranac Lake	89%	93
Woodhull Medical & Mental Health Center	Brooklyn	88%	25
Brooklyn Hosp Ctr at Downtown Campus	Brooklyn	87%	135
Nassau University Medical Center	East Meadow	87%	30
Cayuga Medical Center at Ithaca	Ithaca	86%	105
Montefiore Medical Center	Bronx	86%	534
Wyckoff Heights Medical Center	Brooklyn	84%	56
Aurelia Osborn Fox Memorial Hospital	Oneonta	82%	74
Jamaica Hospital Medical Center	Jamaica	81%	73
Geneva General Hospital	Geneva	7%	41

Urinary Catheter Removal

Hospital Name	City	Rate	Cases
Albany Memorial Hospital[2]	Albany	100%	120
Bellevue Hospital Center[2]	New York	100%	252
Bronx VA Medical Center[2]	Bronx	100%	69
Brooklyn Hosp Ctr at Downtown Campus	Brooklyn	100%	347
Chenango Memorial Hospital	Norwich	100%	113
Clifton Springs Hospital & Clinic[2]	Clifton Springs	100%	61
Coney Island Hospital[2]	Brooklyn	100%	87
Elmhurst Hospital Center	Elmhurst	100%	162
F F Thompson Hospital	Canandaigua	100%	387
Health Alliance Hosp Mary's Ave Campus	Kingston	100%	336
Hospital For Special Surgery[2]	New York	100%	485
Hudson Valley Hospital Center[2]	Cortland Manor	100%	323
John T Mather Mem Hosp-Port Jefferson	Port Jefferson	100%	145
Lincoln Medical & Mental Health Center[2]	Bronx	100%	125
Massena Memorial Hospital	Massena	100%	37
Mercy Medical Center[2]	Rockville Centre	100%	208
Metropolitan Hospital Center[2]	New York	100%	128
Nassau University Medical Center[2]	East Meadow	100%	97
New York Community Hospital of Brooklyn[2]	Brooklyn	100%	54
Niagara Falls Memorial Medical Center[2]	Niagara Falls	100%	66
Northern Dutchess Hospital[2]	Rhinebeck	100%	266
Northern Westchester Hospital[2]	Mount Kisco	100%	313
NYU Hospitals Center[2]	New York	100%	253
Putnam Hospital Center	Carmel	100%	553
Saint Charles Hospital[2]	Port Jefferson	100%	479
Saint Francis Hospital[2]	Poughkeepsie	100%	266
St John's Episcopal Hosp-South Shore[2]	Far Rockaway	100%	50
Saint John's Riverside Hospital[2]	Yonkers	100%	99
South Nassau Communities Hospital[2]	Oceanside	100%	736
Staten Island University Hospital[2]	Staten Island	100%	264
Strong Memorial Hospital[2]	Rochester	100%	665
Syracuse VA Medical Center[2]	Syracuse	100%	85
Unity Hospital of Rochester[2]	Rochester	100%	372
White Plains Hospital Center[2]	White Plains	100%	120
Albany Medical Center Hospital[2]	Albany	99%	194
Albany VA Medical Center[2]	Albany	99%	78
Canton - Potsdam Hospital	Potsdam	99%	103
Columbia Memorial Hospital	Hudson	99%	162
Highland Hospital[2]	Rochester	99%	634
Lutheran Medical Center[2]	Brooklyn	99%	321
Maimonides Medical Center[2]	Brooklyn	99%	455
Mercy Hospital[2]	Buffalo	99%	494
Mount St Mary's Hosp & Health Ctr[2]	Lewiston	99%	217
New York - Presbyterian Hospital[2]	New York	99%	668
Nyack Hospital	Nyack	99%	373
Phelps Memorial Hospital Assn[2]	Sleepy Hollow	99%	390
Saint Anthony Community Hospital	Warwick	99%	120
Saint Joseph Hospital[2]	Bethpage	99%	79
Saint Mary's Hospital at Amsterdam[2]	Amsterdam	99%	170
Winthrop - University Hospital[2]	Mineola	99%	594
Claxton - Hepburn Medical Center	Ogdensburg	98%	62
Forest Hills Hospital[2]	Forest Hills	98%	230
Good Samaritan Hospital Medical Center[2]	West Islip	98%	269
Harlem Hospital Center[2]	New York	98%	49
Jamaica Hospital Medical Center[2]	Jamaica	98%	123
Kingsbrook Jewish Medical Center	Brooklyn	98%	93
Lawrence Hospital Center[2]	Bronxville	98%	159
Nathan Littauer Hospital	Gloversville	98%	100
New York Hosp Med Ctr of Queens[2]	Flushing	98%	358
Orange Regional Medical Center[2]	Middletown	98%	421

NOTE: Hospital profiles are in alphabetical order by state, then city, then hospital within the city; Rankings exclude hospitals with less than 25 cases except for patient surveys which excludes hospitals with less than 100 cases; (a) 100-299 cases; (1) The number of cases/patients is too few to report; (2) Data submitted were based on a sample of cases/patients; (3) Results are based on a shorter time period than required; (4) Data suppressed by CMS for one or more quarters; (5) Results are not available for this reporting period; (6) Fewer than 100 patients completed the HCAHPS survey; (7) No cases met the criteria for this measure; (8) The lower limit of the confidence interval cannot be calculated if the number of observed infections equals zero; (9) No data are available from the state/territory for this reporting period; (10) The scores shown reflect fewer than 50 completed surveys; (11) There were discrepancies in the data collection process; (12) This measure does not apply to this hospital for this reporting period; (13) Results cannot be calculated for this reporting period; (14) The results for this state are combined with nearby states to protect confidentiality; Please refer to the User's Guide for a full explanation of data.

Richmond University Medical Center[2]	Staten Island	98%	118
Saint Catherine of Siena Hospital[2]	Smithtown	98%	218
Saint James Mercy Hospital	Hornell	98%	41
Sisters of Charity Hospital[2]	Buffalo	98%	308
University Hospital - Stony Brook[2]	Stony Brook	98%	326
Vassar Brothers Medical Center[2]	Poughkeepsie	98%	331
Bon Secours Community Hospital	Port Jervis	97%	33
Champlain Valley Phys Hosp Med Ctr[2]	Plattsburgh	97%	515
Ellis Hospital[2]	Schenectady	97%	290
Geneva General Hospital	Geneva	97%	199
Glen Cove Hospital[2]	Glen Cove	97%	210
Kenmore Mercy Hospital[2]	Kenmore	97%	119
Mary Imogene Bassett Hospital[2]	Cooperstown	97%	439
Montefiore Mount Vernon Hospital	Mount Vernon	97%	34
Montefiore New Rochelle Hospital	New Rochelle	97%	399
Mount Sinai Hospital[2]	New York	97%	501
Plainview Hospital[2]	Plainview	97%	207
Saint Joseph's Hospital Health Center[2]	Syracuse	97%	529
Saint Luke's Cornwall Hospital[2]	Newburgh	97%	106
Saint Luke's Roosevelt Hospital[2]	New York	97%	419
Saint Peter's Hospital[2]	Albany	97%	402
Samaritan Medical Center	Watertown	97%	292
Southside Hospital[2]	Bay Shore	97%	326
United Health Services Hospitals	Johnson City	97%	672
Adirondack Medical Center[2]	Saranac Lake	96%	249
Alice Hyde Medical Center	Malone	96%	83
Beth Israel Medical Center[2]	New York	96%	464
Bronx - Lebanon Hospital Center[2]	Bronx	96%	92
Brooks Memorial Hospital[2]	Dunkirk	96%	214
Corning Hospital	Corning	96%	165
Good Samaritan Hospital of Suffern[2]	Suffern	96%	379
Oswego Hospital	Oswego	96%	68
Rochester General Hospital[2]	Rochester	96%	1117
Samaritan Hospital[2]	Troy	96%	300
Saratoga Hospital[2]	Saratoga Spgs	96%	348
Univ Hosp of Brooklyn-Downstate[2]	Brooklyn	96%	227
Huntington Hospital[2]	Huntington	95%	86
Jacobi Medical Center	Bronx	95%	188
Kaleida Health[2]	Buffalo	95%	628
Newark - Wayne Community Hospital	Newark	95%	207
Nicholas H Noyes Memorial Hospital	Dansville	95%	115
North Shore University Hospital[2]	Manhasset	95%	438
Peconic Bay Medical Center[2]	Riverhead	95%	407
Queens Hospital Center	Jamaica	95%	65
Saint Mary's Hospital - Troy[2]	Troy	95%	118
Westchester Medical Center[2]	Valhalla	95%	374
Wyckoff Heights Medical Center[2]	Brooklyn	95%	96
Cayuga Medical Center at Ithaca	Ithaca	94%	303
Crouse Hospital[2]	Syracuse	94%	323
Flushing Hospital Medical Center[2]	Flushing	94%	94
Franklin Hospital[2]	Valley Stream	94%	114
Lenox Hill Hospital[2]	New York	94%	285
Long Island Jewish Medical Center[2]	New Hyde Park	94%	381
New York Methodist Hospital[2]	Brooklyn	94%	418
Our Lady of Lourdes Memorial Hospital[2]	Binghamton	94%	96
Southampton Hospital	Southampton	94%	48
Upstate New York VA Healthcare Sys[2]	Buffalo	94%	125
Auburn Community Hospital	Auburn	93%	128
Rome Memorial Hospital	Rome	93%	41
Erie County Medical Center	Buffalo	92%	554
Faxton - Saint Luke's Healthcare[2]	Utica	92%	147
VA New York Harbor Healthcare System[2]	New York	92%	110
Woman's Christian Association[2]	Jamestown	92%	65
Eastern Niagara Hospital[2]	Lockport	90%	40
Health Alliance Hospital Broadway Campus	Kingston	90%	89
Northport VA Medical Center[2]	Northport	90%	72
Saint Barnabas Hospital[2]	Bronx	90%	68
Saint Francis Hospital - Roslyn[2]	Roslyn	90%	521
TLC Health Network	Gowanda	90%	51
Arnot Ogden Medical Center[2]	Elmira	89%	216
Cortland Regional Medical Center	Cortland	89%	36
Kings County Hospital Center[2]	Brooklyn	89%	138
Saint Elizabeth Medical Center[2]	Utica	89%	383
United Memorial Medical Center	Batavia	89%	156
Woodhull Medical & Mental Health Center[2]	Brooklyn	89%	55
Oneida Healthcare Center	Oneida	88%	81
Brookhaven Mem Hosp Med Ctr	Patchogue	87%	183
Catskill Regional Medical Center	Harris	87%	39
Glens Falls Hospital[2]	Glens Falls	86%	149
Eastern Long Island Hospital	Greenport	84%	32
Interfaith Medical Center	Brooklyn	82%	28
Montefiore Medical Center[2]	Bronx	82%	541
Aurelia Osborn Fox Memorial Hospital	Oneonta	81%	88
Brookdale Hospital Medical Center	Brooklyn	79%	86
Univ Hosp SUNY Health Science Ctr[2]	Syracuse	78%	336
Olean General Hospital[2]	Olean	74%	117

Survey of Patients' Hospital Experiences

Area Around Room 'Always' Quiet at Night

Hospital Name	City	Rate	Cases
Gouverneur Hospital	Gouverneur	68%	(a)
New York Eye & Ear Infirmary	New York	68%	(a)
Community Memorial Hospital	Hamilton	65%	300+
Soldiers & Sailors Mem Hosp of Yates	Penn Yan	65%	(a)
Oneida Healthcare Center	Oneida	62%	300+
Ira Davenport Memorial Hospital	Bath	61%	(a)
Northern Westchester Hospital	Mount Kisco	61%	300+
Our Lady of Lourdes Memorial Hospital	Binghamton	61%	300+
Orange Regional Medical Center	Middletown	60%	300+
Montefiore Mount Vernon Hospital	Mount Vernon	59%	300+
Putnam Hospital Center	Carmel	59%	300+
Saint James Mercy Hospital	Hornell	59%	300+
Saint John's Riverside Hospital	Yonkers	59%	300+
Ellenville Regional Hospital	Ellenville	58%	(a)
Hospital For Special Surgery	New York	58%	300+
Univ Hosp of Brooklyn-Downstate	Brooklyn	58%	300+
Adirondack Medical Center	Saranac Lake	57%	300+
Bon Secours Community Hospital	Port Jervis	57%	300+
Carthage Area Hospital	Carthage	57%	(a)
Health Alliance Hosp Mary's Ave Campus	Kingston	57%	300+
Kingsbrook Jewish Medical Center	Brooklyn	57%	300+
Long Island Jewish Medical Center	New Hyde Park	57%	300+
Nathan Littauer Hospital	Gloversville	57%	300+
Phelps Memorial Hospital Assn	Sleepy Hollow	57%	300+
Highland Hospital	Rochester	56%	300+
Montefiore New Rochelle Hospital	New Rochelle	56%	300+
Mount St Mary's Hosp & Health Ctr	Lewiston	56%	300+
North Central Bronx Hospital	Bronx	56%	300+
Saint Anthony Community Hospital	Warwick	56%	300+
Samaritan Medical Center	Watertown	56%	300+
Bronx - Lebanon Hospital Center	Bronx	55%	300+
Brooklyn Hosp Ctr at Downtown Campus	Brooklyn	55%	300+
Canton - Potsdam Hospital	Potsdam	55%	300+
Harlem Hospital Center	New York	55%	300+
Hudson Valley Hospital Center	Cortlandt Manor	55%	300+
Jones Memorial Hospital	Wellsville	55%	300+
New York Community Hospital of Brooklyn	Brooklyn	55%	300+
Chenango Memorial Hospital	Norwich	54%	300+
Corning Hospital	Corning	54%	300+
Geneva General Hospital	Geneva	54%	300+
Lewis County General Hospital	Lowville	54%	300+
Little Falls Hospital	Little Falls	54%	(a)
Mercy Medical Center	Rockville Centre	54%	300+
Montefiore Medical Center	Bronx	54%	300+
Nicholas H Noyes Memorial Hospital	Dansville	54%	300+
Oswego Hospital	Oswego	54%	300+
White Plains Hospital Center	White Plains	54%	300+
Alice Hyde Medical Center	Malone	53%	300+
Bertrand Chaffee Hospital	Springville	53%	300+
Eastern Long Island Hospital	Greenport	53%	300+
Franklin Hospital	Valley Stream	53%	300+
Interfaith Medical Center	Brooklyn	53%	300+
Lawrence Hospital Center	Bronxville	53%	300+
New York - Presbyterian Hospital	New York	53%	300+
Schuyler Hospital	Montour Falls	53%	(a)
Sisters of Charity Hospital	Buffalo	53%	300+
Southampton Hospital	Southampton	53%	300+
Cayuga Medical Center at Ithaca	Ithaca	52%	300+
Glen Cove Hospital	Glen Cove	52%	300+
Huntington Hospital	Huntington	52%	300+
Massena Memorial Hospital	Massena	52%	300+
Mount Sinai Hospital	New York	52%	300+
Niagara Falls Memorial Medical Center	Niagara Falls	52%	300+
Saint Barnabas Hospital	Bronx	52%	300+
Saint Francis Hospital - Roslyn	Roslyn	52%	300+
Saint Luke's Roosevelt Hospital	New York	52%	300+
Saint Mary's Hospital at Amsterdam	Amsterdam	52%	300+
South Nassau Communities Hospital	Oceanside	52%	300+
Southside Hospital	Bay Shore	52%	300+
Vassar Brothers Medical Center	Poughkeepsie	52%	300+
Woodhull Medical & Mental Health Center	Brooklyn	52%	300+
Brookdale Hospital Medical Center	Brooklyn	51%	300+
Medina Memorial Hospital	Medina	51%	300+
North Shore University Hospital	Manhasset	51%	300+
Unity Hospital of Rochester	Rochester	51%	300+
Brooks Memorial Hospital	Dunkirk	50%	300+
Clifton Springs Hospital & Clinic	Clifton Springs	50%	300+
Coney Island Hospital	Brooklyn	50%	300+
Queens Hospital Center	Jamaica	50%	300+
Saint Francis Hospital	Poughkeepsie	50%	300+
St John's Episcopal Hosp-South Shore	Far Rockaway	50%	300+
Saratoga Hospital	Saratoga Spgs	50%	300+
Faxton - Saint Luke's Healthcare	Utica	49%	300+
Glens Falls Hospital	Glens Falls	49%	300+
Jamaica Hospital Medical Center	Jamaica	49%	300+
John T Mather Mem Hosp-Port Jefferson	Port Jefferson	49%	300+
Kings County Hospital Center	Brooklyn	49%	300+
Olean General Hospital	Olean	49%	300+
Saint Elizabeth Medical Center	Utica	49%	300+
Saint Joseph Hospital	Bethpage	49%	300+
Saint Joseph's Hospital	Elmira	49%	300+
Claxton - Hepburn Medical Center	Ogdensburg	48%	300+
Kenmore Mercy Hospital	Kenmore	48%	300+
Lenox Hill Hospital	New York	48%	300+
New York Hosp Med Ctr of Queens	Flushing	48%	300+
New York Methodist Hospital	Brooklyn	48%	300+
Newark - Wayne Community Hospital	Newark	48%	300+
Rome Memorial Hospital	Rome	48%	300+
Saint Joseph's Hospital Health Center	Syracuse	48%	300+
Saint Luke's Cornwall Hospital	Newburgh	48%	300+
Univ Hosp SUNY Health Science Ctr[11]	Syracuse	48%	300+
Catskill Regional Medical Center	Harris	47%	300+
Jacobi Medical Center	Bronx	47%	300+
NYU Hospitals Center	New York	47%	300+
Rochester General Hospital	Rochester	47%	300+
Saint Mary's Hospital - Troy	Troy	47%	(a)
Wyckoff Heights Medical Center	Brooklyn	47%	300+
Wyoming County Community Hospital	Warsaw	47%	300+
Arnot Ogden Medical Center	Elmira	46%	300+
Aurelia Osborn Fox Memorial Hospital	Oneonta	46%	300+
Champlain Valley Phys Hosp Med Ctr	Plattsburgh	46%	300+
Cobleskill Regional Hospital	Cobleskill	46%	(a)
Cortland Regional Medical Center	Cortland	46%	300+
Lincoln Medical & Mental Health Center	Bronx	46%	300+
Mary Imogene Bassett Hospital	Cooperstown	46%	300+
Richmond University Medical Center	Staten Island	46%	300+
Saint Charles Hospital	Port Jefferson	46%	300+
Saint Joseph's Medical Center	Yonkers	46%	300+
Winthrop - University Hospital	Mineola	46%	300+
Woman's Christian Association	Jamestown	46%	300+
Beth Israel Medical Center	New York	45%	300+
F F Thompson Hospital	Canandaigua	45%	300+
Good Samaritan Hospital Medical Center	West Islip	45%	300+
Metropolitan Hospital Center	New York	45%	300+
Northern Dutchess Hospital	Rhinebeck	45%	300+
Nyack Hospital	Nyack	45%	300+
Albany Medical Center Hospital	Albany	44%	300+
Brookhaven Mem Hosp Med Ctr	Patchogue	44%	300+
Crouse Hospital	Syracuse	44%	300+
Eastern Niagara Hospital	Lockport	44%	300+
Ellis Hospital	Schenectady	44%	300+
Albany Memorial Hospital	Albany	43%	300+
Auburn Community Hospital[11]	Auburn	43%	300+
Bellevue Hospital Center	New York	43%	300+
Columbia Memorial Hospital	Hudson	43%	300+
Elmhurst Hospital Center	Elmhurst	43%	300+
Erie County Medical Center	Buffalo	43%	300+
Health Alliance Hospital Broadway Campus	Kingston	43%	300+
Kaleida Health	Buffalo	43%	300+
Mercy Hospital	Buffalo	43%	300+
Strong Memorial Hospital	Rochester	43%	300+
United Memorial Medical Center	Batavia	43%	300+
University Hospital - Stony Brook	Stony Brook	43%	300+
Forest Hills Hospital[11]	Forest Hills	42%	300+
Saint Catherine of Siena Hospital	Smithtown	42%	300+
TLC Health Network	Gowanda	42%	(a)
Flushing Hospital Medical Center	Flushing	41%	300+
Good Samaritan Hospital of Suffern	Suffern	41%	300+
Lutheran Medical Center	Brooklyn	41%	300+
Maimonides Medical Center	Brooklyn	41%	300+
Plainview Hospital[11]	Plainview	41%	300+
Staten Island University Hospital	Staten Island	41%	300+
Peconic Bay Medical Center	Riverhead	40%	300+
United Health Services Hospitals	Johnson City	40%	300+
Nassau University Medical Center	East Meadow	39%	300+
Saint Peter's Hospital	Albany	38%	300+
Samaritan Hospital	Troy	37%	300+
Westchester Medical Center	Valhalla	37%	300+

Doctors 'Always' Communicated Well

Hospital Name	City	Rate	Cases
Gouverneur Hospital	Gouverneur	87%	(a)
Little Falls Hospital	Little Falls	87%	(a)
Adirondack Medical Center	Saranac Lake	86%	300+
Community Memorial Hospital	Hamilton	85%	300+
Northern Westchester Hospital	Mount Kisco	85%	300+
Schuyler Hospital	Montour Falls	85%	(a)
Clifton Springs Hospital & Clinic	Clifton Springs	84%	300+
Lewis County General Hospital	Lowville	84%	300+
Saint Francis Hospital - Roslyn	Roslyn	84%	300+
Putnam Hospital Center	Carmel	83%	300+
Highland Hospital	Rochester	82%	300+
Hospital For Special Surgery	New York	82%	300+
Hudson Valley Hospital Center	Cortlandt Manor	82%	300+
Jones Memorial Hospital	Wellsville	82%	300+
New York Eye & Ear Infirmary	New York	82%	(a)
Plainview Hospital[11]	Plainview	82%	300+
Saint John's Riverside Hospital	Yonkers	82%	300+

NOTE: Hospital profiles are in alphabetical order by state, then city, then hospital within the city; Rankings exclude hospitals with less than 25 cases except for patient surveys which excludes hospitals with less than 100 cases; (a) 100-299 cases; (1) The number of cases/patients is too few to report; (2) Data submitted were based on a sample of cases/patients; (3) Results are based on a shorter time period than required; (4) Data suppressed by CMS for one or more quarters; (5) Results are not available for this reporting period; (6) Fewer than 100 patients completed the HCAHPS survey; (7) No cases met the criteria for this measure; (8) The lower limit of the confidence interval cannot be calculated if the number of observed infections equals zero; (9) No data are available from the state/territory for this reporting period; (10) The scores shown reflect fewer than 50 completed surveys; (11) There were discrepancies in the data collection process; (12) This measure does not apply to this hospital for this reporting period; (13) Results cannot be calculated for this reporting period; (14) The results for this state are combined with nearby states to protect confidentiality; Please refer to the User's Guide for a full explanation of data.

White Plains Hospital Center	White Plains	82%	300+
Ira Davenport Memorial Hospital	Bath	81%	(a)
Montefiore Mount Vernon Hospital	Mount Vernon	81%	300+
New York - Presbyterian Hospital	New York	81%	300+
Oneida Healthcare Center	Oneida	81%	300+
Saratoga Hospital	Saratoga Spgs	81%	300+
Soldiers & Sailors Mem Hosp of Yates	Penn Yan	81%	(a)
Brooks Memorial Hospital	Dunkirk	80%	300+
Champlain Valley Phys Hosp Med Ctr	Plattsburgh	80%	300+
Claxton - Hepburn Medical Center	Ogdensburg	80%	300+
Eastern Long Island Hospital	Greenport	80%	300+
Geneva General Hospital	Geneva	80%	300+
Glen Cove Hospital	Glen Cove	80%	300+
Kenmore Mercy Hospital	Kenmore	80%	300+
Newark - Wayne Community Hospital	Newark	80%	300+
Northern Dutchess Hospital	Rhinebeck	80%	300+
Phelps Memorial Hospital Assn	Sleepy Hollow	80%	300+
Rochester General Hospital	Rochester	80%	300+
Saint Barnabas Hospital	Bronx	80%	300+
Southside Hospital	Bay Shore	80%	300+
Unity Hospital of Rochester	Rochester	80%	300+
Canton - Potsdam Hospital	Potsdam	79%	300+
Eastern Niagara Hospital	Lockport	79%	300+
Ellenville Regional Hospital	Ellenville	79%	(a)
Glens Falls Hospital	Glens Falls	79%	300+
Huntington Hospital	Huntington	79%	300+
John T Mather Mem Hosp-Port Jefferson	Port Jefferson	79%	300+
Lenox Hill Hospital	New York	79%	300+
Mercy Medical Center	Rockville Centre	79%	300+
Nathan Littauer Hospital	Gloversville	79%	300+
Nicholas H Noyes Memorial Hospital	Dansville	79%	300+
North Shore University Hospital	Manhasset	79%	300+
NYU Hospitals Center	New York	79%	300+
Saint Charles Hospital	Port Jefferson	79%	300+
Southampton Hospital	Southampton	79%	300+
Strong Memorial Hospital	Rochester	79%	300+
Univ Hosp of Brooklyn-Downstate	Brooklyn	79%	300+
Vassar Brothers Medical Center	Poughkeepsie	79%	300+
Winthrop - University Hospital	Mineola	79%	300+
Alice Hyde Medical Center	Malone	78%	300+
Arnot Ogden Medical Center	Elmira	78%	300+
Bertrand Chaffee Hospital	Springville	78%	300+
Catskill Regional Medical Center	Harris	78%	300+
Cayuga Medical Center at Ithaca	Ithaca	78%	300+
Corning Hospital	Corning	78%	300+
Ellis Hospital	Schenectady	78%	300+
Faxton - Saint Luke's Healthcare	Utica	78%	300+
Lawrence Hospital Center	Bronxville	78%	300+
Massena Memorial Hospital	Massena	78%	300+
Medina Memorial Hospital	Medina	78%	300+
Montefiore Medical Center	Bronx	78%	300+
Montefiore New Rochelle Hospital	New Rochelle	78%	300+
Mount St Mary's Hosp & Health Ctr	Lewiston	78%	300+
Mount Sinai Hospital	New York	78%	300+
New York Community Hospital of Brooklyn	Brooklyn	78%	300+
Samaritan Medical Center	Watertown	78%	300+
Bronx - Lebanon Hospital Center	Bronx	77%	300+
Cobleskill Regional Hospital	Cobleskill	77%	(a)
Crouse Hospital	Syracuse	77%	300+
Health Alliance Hosp Mary's Ave Campus	Kingston	77%	300+
Niagara Falls Memorial Medical Center	Niagara Falls	77%	300+
North Central Bronx Hospital	Bronx	77%	300+
Olean General Hospital	Olean	77%	300+
Our Lady of Lourdes Memorial Hospital	Binghamton	77%	300+
Rome Memorial Hospital	Rome	77%	300+
Saint Anthony Community Hospital	Warwick	77%	300+
Saint Elizabeth Medical Center	Utica	77%	300+
Saint Joseph Hospital	Bethpage	77%	300+
Saint Joseph's Hospital Health Center	Syracuse	77%	300+
Saint Mary's Hospital at Amsterdam	Amsterdam	77%	300+
South Nassau Communities Hospital	Oceanside	77%	300+
University Hospital - Stony Brook	Stony Brook	77%	300+
Wyoming County Community Hospital	Warsaw	77%	300+
Bellevue Hospital Center	New York	76%	300+
Brooklyn Hosp Ctr at Downtown Campus	Brooklyn	76%	300+
Columbia Memorial Hospital	Hudson	76%	300+
F F Thompson Hospital	Canandaigua	76%	300+
Interfaith Medical Center	Brooklyn	76%	300+
Kingsbrook Jewish Medical Center	Brooklyn	76%	300+
Long Island Jewish Medical Center	New Hyde Park	76%	300+
Orange Regional Medical Center	Middletown	76%	300+
Oswego Hospital	Oswego	76%	300+
Saint Luke's Cornwall Hospital	Newburgh	76%	300+
Bon Secours Community Hospital	Port Jervis	75%	300+
Franklin Hospital	Valley Stream	75%	300+
Good Samaritan Hospital Medical Center	West Islip	75%	300+
Good Samaritan Hospital of Suffern	Suffern	75%	300+
Jacobi Medical Center	Bronx	75%	300+
Kings County Hospital Center	Brooklyn	75%	300+
Mary Imogene Bassett Hospital	Cooperstown	75%	300+
Mercy Hospital	Buffalo	75%	300+
New York Methodist Hospital	Brooklyn	75%	300+
Nyack Hospital	Nyack	75%	300+
Queens Hospital Center	Jamaica	75%	300+
Richmond University Medical Center	Staten Island	75%	300+
Saint James Mercy Hospital	Hornell	75%	300+
Saint Joseph's Hospital	Elmira	75%	300+
Saint Joseph's Medical Center	Yonkers	75%	300+
Sisters of Charity Hospital	Buffalo	75%	300+
United Health Services Hospitals	Johnson City	75%	300+
United Memorial Medical Center	Batavia	75%	300+
Woman's Christian Association	Jamestown	75%	300+
Auburn Community Hospital[11]	Auburn	74%	300+
Coney Island Hospital	Brooklyn	74%	300+
Kaleida Health	Buffalo	74%	300+
Lincoln Medical & Mental Health Center	Bronx	74%	300+
New York Hosp Med Ctr of Queens	Flushing	74%	300+
Saint Catherine of Siena Hospital	Smithtown	74%	300+
Saint Francis Hospital	Poughkeepsie	74%	300+
Saint Mary's Hospital - Troy	Troy	74%	(a)
Saint Peter's Hospital	Albany	74%	300+
TLC Health Network	Gowanda	74%	(a)
Univ Hosp SUNY Health Science Ctr[11]	Syracuse	74%	300+
Brookhaven Mem Hosp Med Ctr	Patchogue	73%	300+
Health Alliance Hospital Broadway Campus	Kingston	73%	300+
Lutheran Medical Center	Brooklyn	73%	300+
St John's Episcopal Hosp-South Shore	Far Rockaway	73%	300+
Carthage Area Hospital	Carthage	72%	(a)
Chenango Memorial Hospital	Norwich	72%	300+
Jamaica Hospital Medical Center	Jamaica	72%	300+
Maimonides Medical Center	Brooklyn	72%	300+
Peconic Bay Medical Center	Riverhead	72%	300+
Albany Memorial Hospital	Albany	71%	300+
Aurelia Osborn Fox Memorial Hospital	Oneonta	71%	300+
Beth Israel Medical Center	New York	71%	300+
Elmhurst Hospital Center	Elmhurst	71%	300+
Metropolitan Hospital Center	New York	71%	300+
Saint Luke's Roosevelt Hospital	New York	71%	300+
Albany Medical Center Hospital	Albany	70%	300+
Westchester Medical Center	Valhalla	70%	300+
Woodhull Medical & Mental Health Center	Brooklyn	70%	300+
Wyckoff Heights Medical Center	Brooklyn	70%	300+
Brookdale Hospital Medical Center	Brooklyn	69%	300+
Erie County Medical Center	Buffalo	69%	300+
Forest Hills Hospital[11]	Forest Hills	69%	300+
Harlem Hospital Center	New York	69%	300+
Samaritan Hospital	Troy	69%	300+
Staten Island University Hospital	Staten Island	69%	300+
Cortland Regional Medical Center	Cortland	68%	300+
Flushing Hospital Medical Center	Flushing	64%	300+
Nassau University Medical Center	East Meadow	62%	300+

Home Recovery Information Given

Hospital Name	City	Rate	Cases
Soldiers & Sailors Mem Hosp of Yates	Penn Yan	93%	(a)
Clifton Springs Hospital & Clinic	Clifton Springs	91%	300+
Geneva General Hospital	Geneva	91%	300+
Little Falls Hospital	Little Falls	91%	(a)
Adirondack Medical Center	Saranac Lake	90%	300+
Carthage Area Hospital	Carthage	90%	(a)
Community Memorial Hospital	Hamilton	90%	300+
Health Alliance Hosp Mary's Ave Campus	Kingston	90%	300+
Hospital For Special Surgery	New York	90%	300+
John T Mather Mem Hosp-Port Jefferson	Port Jefferson	90%	300+
Northern Dutchess Hospital	Rhinebeck	90%	300+
Saint James Mercy Hospital	Hornell	90%	300+
Saint Mary's Hospital at Amsterdam	Amsterdam	90%	300+
Saratoga Hospital	Saratoga Spgs	90%	300+
TLC Health Network	Gowanda	90%	(a)
Claxton - Hepburn Medical Center	Ogdensburg	89%	300+
Cobleskill Regional Hospital	Cobleskill	89%	(a)
Newark - Wayne Community Hospital	Newark	89%	300+
Putnam Hospital Center	Carmel	89%	300+
Saint Francis Hospital - Roslyn	Roslyn	89%	300+
Saint Peter's Hospital	Albany	89%	300+
Unity Hospital of Rochester	Rochester	89%	300+
Brooks Memorial Hospital	Dunkirk	88%	300+
Crouse Hospital	Syracuse	88%	300+
Ellis Hospital	Schenectady	88%	300+
F F Thompson Hospital	Canandaigua	88%	300+
Glens Falls Hospital	Glens Falls	88%	300+
Highland Hospital	Rochester	88%	300+
Mary Imogene Bassett Hospital	Cooperstown	88%	300+
Northern Westchester Hospital	Mount Kisco	88%	300+
Oswego Hospital	Oswego	88%	300+
Our Lady of Lourdes Memorial Hospital	Binghamton	88%	300+
Saint Joseph's Hospital	Elmira	88%	300+
Saint Joseph's Hospital Health Center	Syracuse	88%	300+
Strong Memorial Hospital	Rochester	88%	300+
Arnot Ogden Medical Center	Elmira	87%	300+
Bertrand Chaffee Hospital	Springville	87%	300+
Hudson Valley Hospital Center	Cortlandt Manor	87%	300+
Kenmore Mercy Hospital	Kenmore	87%	300+
Lewis County General Hospital	Lowville	87%	300+
Phelps Memorial Hospital Assn	Sleepy Hollow	87%	300+
Rochester General Hospital	Rochester	87%	300+
Rome Memorial Hospital	Rome	87%	300+
Samaritan Medical Center	Watertown	87%	300+
Schuyler Hospital	Montour Falls	87%	(a)
Vassar Brothers Medical Center	Poughkeepsie	87%	300+
Aurelia Osborn Fox Memorial Hospital	Oneonta	86%	300+
Canton - Potsdam Hospital	Potsdam	86%	300+
Catskill Regional Medical Center	Harris	86%	300+
Champlain Valley Phys Hosp Med Ctr	Plattsburgh	86%	300+
Jones Memorial Hospital	Wellsville	86%	300+
Medina Memorial Hospital	Medina	86%	300+
Nathan Littauer Hospital	Gloversville	86%	300+
Nicholas H Noyes Memorial Hospital	Dansville	86%	300+
Saint Luke's Cornwall Hospital	Newburgh	86%	300+
United Health Services Hospitals	Johnson City	86%	300+
University Hospital - Stony Brook	Stony Brook	86%	300+
Univ Hosp SUNY Health Science Ctr[11]	Syracuse	86%	300+
White Plains Hospital Center	White Plains	86%	300+
Winthrop - University Hospital	Mineola	86%	300+
Woman's Christian Association	Jamestown	86%	300+
Cayuga Medical Center at Ithaca	Ithaca	85%	300+
Chenango Memorial Hospital	Norwich	85%	300+
Corning Hospital	Corning	85%	300+
Eastern Long Island Hospital	Greenport	85%	300+
Good Samaritan Hospital Medical Center	West Islip	85%	300+
Gouverneur Hospital	Gouverneur	85%	(a)
Mercy Medical Center	Rockville Centre	85%	300+
Oneida Healthcare Center	Oneida	85%	300+
Orange Regional Medical Center	Middletown	85%	300+
Saint Catherine of Siena Hospital	Smithtown	85%	300+
Saint Charles Hospital	Port Jefferson	85%	300+
Saint Francis Hospital	Poughkeepsie	85%	300+
Saint Mary's Hospital - Troy	Troy	85%	(a)
Albany Memorial Hospital	Albany	84%	300+
Brookhaven Mem Hosp Med Ctr	Patchogue	84%	300+
Kaleida Health	Buffalo	84%	300+
Mercy Hospital	Buffalo	84%	300+
Mount St Mary's Hosp & Health Ctr	Lewiston	84%	300+
Mount Sinai Hospital	New York	84%	300+
Peconic Bay Medical Center	Riverhead	84%	300+
United Memorial Medical Center	Batavia	84%	300+
Bon Secours Community Hospital	Port Jervis	83%	300+
Cortland Regional Medical Center	Cortland	83%	300+
Eastern Niagara Hospital	Lockport	83%	300+
Montefiore New Rochelle Hospital	New Rochelle	83%	300+
NYU Hospitals Center	New York	83%	300+
Olean General Hospital	Olean	83%	300+
Saint Joseph Hospital	Bethpage	83%	300+
Samaritan Hospital	Troy	83%	300+
Sisters of Charity Hospital	Buffalo	83%	300+
South Nassau Communities Hospital	Oceanside	83%	300+
Southampton Hospital	Southampton	83%	300+
Wyoming County Community Hospital	Warsaw	83%	300+
Albany Medical Center Hospital	Albany	82%	300+
Columbia Memorial Hospital	Hudson	82%	300+
Erie County Medical Center	Buffalo	82%	300+
Faxton - Saint Luke's Healthcare	Utica	82%	300+
Long Island Jewish Medical Center	New Hyde Park	82%	300+
Montefiore Medical Center	Bronx	82%	300+
Montefiore Mount Vernon Hospital	Mount Vernon	82%	300+
New York - Presbyterian Hospital	New York	82%	300+
New York Eye & Ear Infirmary	New York	82%	(a)
New York Hosp Med Ctr of Queens	Flushing	82%	300+
Niagara Falls Memorial Medical Center	Niagara Falls	82%	300+
Saint Elizabeth Medical Center	Utica	82%	300+
Auburn Community Hospital[11]	Auburn	81%	300+
Bronx - Lebanon Hospital Center	Bronx	81%	300+
Ellenville Regional Hospital	Ellenville	81%	(a)
Elmhurst Hospital Center	Elmhurst	81%	300+
North Shore University Hospital	Manhasset	81%	300+
Saint Anthony Community Hospital	Warwick	81%	300+
Saint John's Riverside Hospital	Yonkers	81%	300+
Saint Joseph's Medical Center	Yonkers	81%	300+
Alice Hyde Medical Center	Malone	80%	300+
Beth Israel Medical Center	New York	80%	300+
Coney Island Hospital	Brooklyn	80%	300+
Huntington Hospital	Huntington	80%	300+
Jacobi Medical Center	Bronx	80%	300+
Lawrence Hospital Center	Bronxville	80%	300+
Lutheran Medical Center	Brooklyn	80%	300+
Maimonides Medical Center	Brooklyn	80%	300+
Massena Memorial Hospital	Massena	80%	300+
Southside Hospital	Bay Shore	80%	300+
Westchester Medical Center	Valhalla	80%	300+
Bellevue Hospital Center	New York	79%	300+
Ira Davenport Memorial Hospital	Bath	79%	(a)
Kingsbrook Jewish Medical Center	Brooklyn	79%	300+
Woodhull Medical & Mental Health Center	Brooklyn	79%	300+

NOTE: Hospital profiles are in alphabetical order by state, then city, then hospital within the city; Rankings exclude hospitals with less than 25 cases except for patient surveys which excludes hospitals with less than 100 cases; (a) 100-299 cases; (1) The number of cases/patients is too few to report; (2) Data submitted were based on a sample of cases/patients; (3) Results are based on a shorter time period than required; (4) Data suppressed by CMS for one or more quarters; (5) Results are not available for this reporting period; (6) Fewer than 100 patients completed the HCAHPS survey; (7) No cases met the criteria for this measure; (8) The lower limit of the confidence interval cannot be calculated if the number of observed infections equals zero; (9) No data are available from the state/territory for this reporting period; (10) The scores shown reflect fewer than 50 completed surveys; (11) There were discrepancies in the data collection process; (12) This measure does not apply to this hospital for this reporting period; (13) Results cannot be calculated for this reporting period; (14) The results for this state are combined with nearby states to protect confidentiality; Please refer to the User's Guide for a full explanation of data.

Hospital Name	City	Rate	Cases
Flushing Hospital Medical Center	Flushing	78%	300+
Good Samaritan Hospital of Suffern	Suffern	78%	300+
New York Community Hospital of Brooklyn	Brooklyn	78%	300+
Plainview Hospital[11]	Plainview	78%	300+
Queens Hospital Center	Jamaica	78%	300+
Saint Luke's Roosevelt Hospital	New York	78%	300+
Glen Cove Hospital	Glen Cove	77%	300+
Jamaica Hospital Medical Center	Jamaica	77%	300+
Lincoln Medical & Mental Health Center	Bronx	77%	300+
New York Methodist Hospital	Brooklyn	77%	300+
Nyack Hospital	Nyack	77%	300+
Lenox Hill Hospital	New York	76%	300+
Metropolitan Hospital Center	New York	76%	300+
Saint Barnabas Hospital	Bronx	76%	300+
Brooklyn Hosp Ctr at Downtown Campus	Brooklyn	75%	300+
Franklin Hospital	Valley Stream	75%	300+
Health Alliance Hospital Broadway Campus	Kingston	75%	300+
Interfaith Medical Center	Brooklyn	75%	300+
Staten Island University Hospital	Staten Island	75%	300+
Univ Hosp of Brooklyn-Downstate	Brooklyn	75%	300+
Forest Hills Hospital[11]	Forest Hills	74%	300+
North Central Bronx Hospital	Bronx	74%	300+
Richmond University Medical Center	Staten Island	74%	300+
Harlem Hospital Center	New York	73%	300+
Wyckoff Heights Medical Center	Brooklyn	73%	300+
St John's Episcopal Hosp-South Shore	Far Rockaway	72%	300+
Nassau University Medical Center	East Meadow	71%	300+
Brookdale Hospital Medical Center	Brooklyn	70%	300+
Kings County Hospital Center	Brooklyn	70%	300+

Hospital Given 9 or 10 on 10 Point Scale

Hospital Name	City	Rate	Cases
Hospital For Special Surgery	New York	88%	300+
Community Memorial Hospital	Hamilton	82%	300+
Saint Francis Hospital - Roslyn	Roslyn	82%	300+
Northern Westchester Hospital	Mount Kisco	80%	300+
Putnam Hospital Center	Carmel	78%	300+
White Plains Hospital Center	White Plains	78%	300+
Health Alliance Hosp Mary's Ave Campus	Kingston	77%	300+
Eastern Long Island Hospital	Greenport	76%	300+
Highland Hospital	Rochester	75%	300+
Northern Dutchess Hospital	Rhinebeck	75%	300+
Clifton Springs Hospital & Clinic	Clifton Springs	74%	300+
John T Mather Mem Hosp-Port Jefferson	Port Jefferson	74%	300+
New York - Presbyterian Hospital	New York	74%	300+
Saratoga Hospital	Saratoga Spgs	74%	300+
Hudson Valley Hospital Center	Cortlandt Manor	73%	300+
Long Island Jewish Medical Center	New Hyde Park	73%	300+
Phelps Memorial Hospital Assn	Sleepy Hollow	73%	300+
Saint Joseph's Hospital Health Center	Syracuse	73%	300+
Strong Memorial Hospital	Rochester	73%	300+
Adirondack Medical Center	Saranac Lake	72%	300+
Little Falls Hospital	Little Falls	72%	(a)
North Shore University Hospital	Manhasset	72%	300+
Rochester General Hospital	Rochester	72%	300+
Soldiers & Sailors Mem Hosp of Yates	Penn Yan	72%	(a)
New York Eye & Ear Infirmary	New York	71%	(a)
NYU Hospitals Center	New York	71%	300+
Orange Regional Medical Center	Middletown	71%	300+
Glen Cove Hospital	Glen Cove	70%	300+
Huntington Hospital	Huntington	70%	300+
Kenmore Mercy Hospital	Kenmore	70%	300+
Lewis County General Hospital	Lowville	70%	300+
Saint Elizabeth Medical Center	Utica	70%	300+
Sisters of Charity Hospital	Buffalo	70%	300+
Vassar Brothers Medical Center	Poughkeepsie	70%	300+
Oneida Healthcare Center	Oneida	69%	300+
Our Lady of Lourdes Memorial Hospital	Binghamton	69%	300+
University Hospital - Stony Brook	Stony Brook	69%	300+
Cayuga Medical Center at Ithaca	Ithaca	68%	300+
Medina Memorial Hospital	Medina	68%	300+
Saint John's Riverside Hospital	Yonkers	68%	300+
Saint Mary's Hospital at Amsterdam	Amsterdam	68%	300+
Ellenville Regional Hospital	Ellenville	67%	(a)
Nathan Littauer Hospital	Gloversville	67%	300+
Saint Anthony Community Hospital	Warwick	67%	300+
Saint Charles Hospital	Port Jefferson	67%	300+
Southampton Hospital	Southampton	67%	300+
Canton - Potsdam Hospital	Potsdam	66%	300+
Glens Falls Hospital	Glens Falls	66%	300+
Jones Memorial Hospital	Wellsville	66%	300+
Mercy Medical Center	Rockville Centre	66%	300+
Mount St Mary's Hosp & Health Ctr	Lewiston	66%	300+
Mount Sinai Hospital	New York	66%	300+
Saint Peter's Hospital	Albany	66%	300+
South Nassau Communities Hospital	Oceanside	66%	300+
Unity Hospital of Rochester	Rochester	66%	300+
Arnot Ogden Medical Center	Elmira	65%	300+
Bertrand Chaffee Hospital	Springville	65%	300+
F F Thompson Hospital	Canandaigua	65%	300+
Lawrence Hospital Center	Bronxville	65%	300+
Samaritan Medical Center	Watertown	65%	300+
Winthrop - University Hospital	Mineola	65%	300+
Geneva General Hospital	Geneva	64%	300+
Gouverneur Hospital	Gouverneur	64%	(a)
Newark - Wayne Community Hospital	Newark	64%	300+
Rome Memorial Hospital	Rome	64%	300+
Albany Medical Center Hospital	Albany	63%	300+
Bon Secours Community Hospital	Port Jervis	63%	300+
Crouse Hospital	Syracuse	63%	300+
Franklin Hospital	Valley Stream	63%	300+
Montefiore Medical Center	Bronx	63%	300+
Plainview Hospital[11]	Plainview	63%	300+
Southside Hospital	Bay Shore	63%	300+
United Health Services Hospitals	Johnson City	63%	300+
Univ Hosp SUNY Health Science Ctr[11]	Syracuse	63%	300+
Faxton - Saint Luke's Healthcare	Utica	62%	300+
Mary Imogene Bassett Hospital	Cooperstown	62%	300+
Albany Memorial Hospital	Albany	61%	300+
Eastern Niagara Hospital	Lockport	61%	300+
Ellis Hospital	Schenectady	61%	300+
Ira Davenport Memorial Hospital	Bath	61%	(a)
New York Hosp Med Ctr of Queens	Flushing	61%	300+
Nicholas H Noyes Memorial Hospital	Dansville	61%	300+
Saint Mary's Hospital - Troy	Troy	61%	(a)
Brooks Memorial Hospital	Dunkirk	60%	300+
Carthage Area Hospital	Carthage	60%	(a)
Claxton - Hepburn Medical Center	Ogdensburg	60%	300+
Kaleida Health	Buffalo	60%	300+
Lenox Hill Hospital	New York	60%	300+
Oswego Hospital	Oswego	60%	300+
Saint Joseph's Hospital	Elmira	60%	300+
Erie County Medical Center	Buffalo	59%	300+
Massena Memorial Hospital	Massena	59%	300+
Saint James Mercy Hospital	Hornell	59%	300+
Saint Joseph Hospital	Bethpage	59%	300+
Saint Luke's Cornwall Hospital	Newburgh	59%	300+
Schuyler Hospital	Montour Falls	59%	(a)
Wyoming County Community Hospital	Warsaw	59%	300+
Bellevue Hospital Center	New York	58%	300+
Chenango Memorial Hospital	Norwich	58%	300+
Montefiore New Rochelle Hospital	New Rochelle	58%	300+
New York Methodist Hospital	Brooklyn	58%	300+
Saint Catherine of Siena Hospital	Smithtown	58%	300+
Saint Francis Hospital	Poughkeepsie	58%	300+
Champlain Valley Phys Hosp Med Ctr	Plattsburgh	57%	300+
Cobleskill Regional Hospital	Cobleskill	57%	(a)
Corning Hospital	Corning	57%	300+
Cortland Regional Medical Center	Cortland	57%	300+
Forest Hills Hospital[11]	Forest Hills	57%	300+
Good Samaritan Hospital Medical Center	West Islip	57%	300+
Good Samaritan Hospital of Suffern	Suffern	57%	300+
North Central Bronx Hospital	Bronx	57%	300+
Olean General Hospital	Olean	57%	300+
Staten Island University Hospital	Staten Island	57%	300+
Aurelia Osborn Fox Memorial Hospital	Oneonta	56%	300+
Bronx - Lebanon Hospital Center	Bronx	56%	300+
Brooklyn Hosp Ctr at Downtown Campus	Brooklyn	56%	300+
Mercy Hospital	Buffalo	56%	300+
Queens Hospital Center	Jamaica	56%	300+
Univ Hosp of Brooklyn-Downstate	Brooklyn	56%	300+
Beth Israel Medical Center	New York	55%	300+
Interfaith Medical Center	Brooklyn	55%	300+
Jacobi Medical Center	Bronx	55%	300+
Lutheran Medical Center	Brooklyn	55%	300+
Nyack Hospital	Nyack	55%	300+
TLC Health Network	Gowanda	55%	(a)
Catskill Regional Medical Center	Harris	54%	300+
Columbia Memorial Hospital	Hudson	54%	300+
Coney Island Hospital	Brooklyn	54%	300+
Maimonides Medical Center	Brooklyn	54%	300+
Saint Barnabas Hospital	Bronx	54%	300+
Auburn Community Hospital[11]	Auburn	53%	300+
Health Alliance Hospital Broadway Campus	Kingston	53%	300+
Kingsbrook Jewish Medical Center	Brooklyn	53%	300+
Niagara Falls Memorial Medical Center	Niagara Falls	53%	300+
Peconic Bay Medical Center	Riverhead	53%	300+
Saint Luke's Roosevelt Hospital	New York	53%	300+
Samaritan Hospital	Troy	53%	300+
Montefiore Mount Vernon Hospital	Mount Vernon	52%	300+
Alice Hyde Medical Center	Malone	51%	300+
New York Community Hospital of Brooklyn	Brooklyn	51%	300+
Saint Joseph's Medical Center	Yonkers	51%	300+
Woodhull Medical & Mental Health Center	Brooklyn	51%	300+
Brookhaven Mem Hosp Med Ctr	Patchogue	50%	300+
Kings County Hospital Center	Brooklyn	50%	300+
Lincoln Medical & Mental Health Center	Bronx	50%	300+
Metropolitan Hospital Center	New York	50%	300+
Westchester Medical Center	Valhalla	50%	300+
Woman's Christian Association	Jamestown	50%	300+
United Memorial Medical Center	Batavia	49%	300+
Wyckoff Heights Medical Center	Brooklyn	49%	300+
Elmhurst Hospital Center	Elmhurst	48%	300+
Jamaica Hospital Medical Center	Jamaica	47%	300+
Richmond University Medical Center	Staten Island	44%	300+
Flushing Hospital Medical Center	Flushing	43%	300+
Harlem Hospital Center	New York	43%	300+
St John's Episcopal Hosp-South Shore	Far Rockaway	43%	300+
Brookdale Hospital Medical Center	Brooklyn	41%	300+
Nassau University Medical Center	East Meadow	38%	300+

Meds 'Always' Explained Before Given

Hospital Name	City	Rate	Cases
White Plains Hospital Center	White Plains	73%	300+
Ellenville Regional Hospital	Ellenville	70%	(a)
Putnam Hospital Center	Carmel	70%	300+
Lewis County General Hospital	Lowville	69%	300+
Community Memorial Hospital	Hamilton	68%	300+
Northern Westchester Hospital	Mount Kisco	68%	300+
Hudson Valley Hospital Center	Cortlandt Manor	67%	300+
Northern Dutchess Hospital	Rhinebeck	67%	300+
Saint Mary's Hospital at Amsterdam	Amsterdam	67%	300+
Saratoga Hospital	Saratoga Spgs	67%	300+
Schuyler Hospital	Montour Falls	67%	(a)
Carthage Area Hospital	Carthage	66%	(a)
Geneva General Hospital	Geneva	66%	300+
Highland Hospital	Rochester	66%	300+
Newark - Wayne Community Hospital	Newark	66%	300+
Phelps Memorial Hospital Assn	Sleepy Hollow	66%	300+
Saint Francis Hospital - Roslyn	Roslyn	66%	300+
Adirondack Medical Center	Saranac Lake	65%	300+
Cayuga Medical Center at Ithaca	Ithaca	65%	300+
Hospital For Special Surgery	New York	65%	300+
Little Falls Hospital	Little Falls	65%	(a)
Nathan Littauer Hospital	Gloversville	65%	300+
Nicholas H Noyes Memorial Hospital	Dansville	65%	300+
Oneida Healthcare Center	Oneida	65%	300+
Vassar Brothers Medical Center	Poughkeepsie	65%	300+
Eastern Long Island Hospital	Greenport	64%	300+
Glens Falls Hospital	Glens Falls	64%	300+
Long Island Jewish Medical Center	New Hyde Park	64%	300+
New York Community Hospital of Brooklyn	Brooklyn	64%	300+
Rochester General Hospital	Rochester	64%	300+
Samaritan Medical Center	Watertown	64%	300+
Strong Memorial Hospital	Rochester	64%	300+
Jones Memorial Hospital	Wellsville	63%	300+
Mount Sinai Hospital	New York	63%	300+
NYU Hospitals Center	New York	63%	300+
Saint John's Riverside Hospital	Yonkers	63%	300+
Soldiers & Sailors Mem Hosp of Yates	Penn Yan	63%	(a)
United Health Services Hospitals	Johnson City	63%	300+
Bon Secours Community Hospital	Port Jervis	62%	300+
Canton - Potsdam Hospital	Potsdam	62%	300+
Ellis Hospital	Schenectady	62%	300+
F F Thompson Hospital	Canandaigua	62%	300+
Huntington Hospital	Huntington	62%	300+
Montefiore Mount Vernon Hospital	Mount Vernon	62%	300+
Orange Regional Medical Center	Middletown	62%	300+
Saint Charles Hospital	Port Jefferson	62%	300+
Southside Hospital	Bay Shore	62%	300+
Claxton - Hepburn Medical Center	Ogdensburg	61%	300+
Clifton Springs Hospital & Clinic	Clifton Springs	61%	300+
John T Mather Mem Hosp-Port Jefferson	Port Jefferson	61%	300+
Massena Memorial Hospital	Massena	61%	300+
Montefiore New Rochelle Hospital	New Rochelle	61%	300+
Oswego Hospital	Oswego	61%	300+
Saint James Mercy Hospital	Hornell	61%	300+
Southampton Hospital	Southampton	61%	300+
TLC Health Network	Gowanda	61%	(a)
Univ Hosp SUNY Health Science Ctr[11]	Syracuse	61%	300+
Brooks Memorial Hospital	Dunkirk	60%	300+
Catskill Regional Medical Center	Harris	60%	300+
Champlain Valley Phys Hosp Med Ctr	Plattsburgh	60%	300+
Cobleskill Regional Hospital	Cobleskill	60%	(a)
Cortland Regional Medical Center	Cortland	60%	300+
Health Alliance Hosp Mary's Ave Campus	Kingston	60%	300+
Kenmore Mercy Hospital	Kenmore	60%	300+
Mary Imogene Bassett Hospital	Cooperstown	60%	300+
Mercy Medical Center	Rockville Centre	60%	300+
New York - Presbyterian Hospital	New York	60%	300+
Our Lady of Lourdes Memorial Hospital	Binghamton	60%	300+
Plainview Hospital[11]	Plainview	60%	300+
Saint Elizabeth Medical Center	Utica	60%	300+
Saint Joseph's Hospital Health Center	Syracuse	60%	300+
University Hospital - Stony Brook	Stony Brook	60%	300+
Wyoming County Community Hospital	Warsaw	60%	300+
Alice Hyde Medical Center	Malone	59%	300+
Aurelia Osborn Fox Memorial Hospital	Oneonta	59%	300+
Faxton - Saint Luke's Healthcare	Utica	59%	300+
Ira Davenport Memorial Hospital	Bath	59%	(a)
Montefiore Medical Center	Bronx	59%	300+
North Shore University Hospital	Manhasset	59%	300+
Olean General Hospital	Olean	59%	300+

NOTE: Hospital profiles are in alphabetical order by state, then city, then hospital within the city; Rankings exclude hospitals with less than 25 cases except for patient surveys which excludes hospitals with less than 100 cases; (a) 100-299 cases; (1) The number of cases/patients is too few to report; (2) Data submitted were based on a sample of cases/patients; (3) Results are based on a shorter time period than required; (4) Data suppressed by CMS for one or more quarters; (5) Results are not available for this reporting period; (6) Fewer than 100 patients completed the HCAHPS survey; (7) No cases met the criteria for this measure; (8) The lower limit of the confidence interval cannot be calculated if the number of observed infections equals zero; (9) No data are available from the state/territory for this reporting period; (10) The scores shown reflect fewer than 50 completed surveys; (11) There were discrepancies in the data collection process; (12) This measure does not apply to this hospital for this reporting period; (13) Results cannot be calculated for this reporting period; (14) The results for this state are combined with nearby states to protect confidentiality; Please refer to the User's Guide for a full explanation of data.

Rome Memorial Hospital	Rome	59%	300+
Saint Anthony Community Hospital	Warwick	59%	300+
Saint Catherine of Siena Hospital	Smithtown	59%	300+
Sisters of Charity Hospital	Buffalo	59%	300+
Unity Hospital of Rochester	Rochester	59%	300+
Winthrop - University Hospital	Mineola	59%	300+
Albany Memorial Hospital	Albany	58%	300+
Arnot Ogden Medical Center	Elmira	58%	300+
Brooklyn Hosp Ctr at Downtown Campus	Brooklyn	58%	300+
Chenango Memorial Hospital	Norwich	58%	300+
Corning Hospital	Corning	58%	300+
Crouse Hospital	Syracuse	58%	300+
Glen Cove Hospital	Glen Cove	58%	300+
Lenox Hill Hospital	New York	58%	300+
Mount St Mary's Hosp & Health Ctr	Lewiston	58%	300+
New York Hosp Med Ctr of Queens	Flushing	58%	300+
Saint Joseph's Hospital	Elmira	58%	300+
Saint Peter's Hospital	Albany	58%	300+
Bertrand Chaffee Hospital	Springville	57%	300+
Columbia Memorial Hospital	Hudson	57%	300+
Coney Island Hospital	Brooklyn	57%	300+
Medina Memorial Hospital	Medina	57%	300+
Nyack Hospital	Nyack	57%	300+
Saint Barnabas Hospital	Bronx	57%	300+
Saint Joseph Hospital	Bethpage	57%	300+
Saint Mary's Hospital - Troy	Troy	57%	(a)
Univ Hosp of Brooklyn-Downstate	Brooklyn	57%	300+
Albany Medical Center Hospital	Albany	56%	300+
Auburn Community Hospital[11]	Auburn	56%	300+
Brookhaven Mem Hosp Med Ctr	Patchogue	56%	300+
Eastern Niagara Hospital	Lockport	56%	300+
Franklin Hospital	Valley Stream	56%	300+
Good Samaritan Hospital Medical Center	West Islip	56%	300+
Health Alliance Hospital Broadway Campus	Kingston	56%	300+
Lutheran Medical Center	Brooklyn	56%	300+
Mercy Hospital	Buffalo	56%	300+
New York Eye & Ear Infirmary	New York	56%	(a)
New York Methodist Hospital	Brooklyn	56%	300+
Queens Hospital Center	Jamaica	56%	300+
Saint Francis Hospital	Poughkeepsie	56%	300+
Saint Luke's Cornwall Hospital	Newburgh	56%	300+
South Nassau Communities Hospital	Oceanside	56%	300+
Staten Island University Hospital	Staten Island	56%	300+
Interfaith Medical Center	Brooklyn	55%	300+
Niagara Falls Memorial Medical Center	Niagara Falls	55%	300+
United Memorial Medical Center	Batavia	55%	300+
Kingsbrook Jewish Medical Center	Brooklyn	54%	300+
Lawrence Hospital Center	Bronxville	54%	300+
Maimonides Medical Center	Brooklyn	54%	300+
Bronx - Lebanon Hospital Center	Bronx	53%	300+
Forest Hills Hospital[11]	Forest Hills	53%	300+
Peconic Bay Medical Center	Riverhead	53%	300+
Richmond University Medical Center	Staten Island	53%	300+
Saint Joseph's Medical Center	Yonkers	53%	300+
Samaritan Hospital	Troy	53%	300+
Woman's Christian Association	Jamestown	53%	300+
Beth Israel Medical Center	New York	52%	300+
Erie County Medical Center	Buffalo	52%	300+
Good Samaritan Hospital of Suffern	Suffern	52%	300+
Gouverneur Hospital	Gouverneur	52%	(a)
Kaleida Health	Buffalo	52%	300+
Lincoln Medical & Mental Health Center	Bronx	52%	300+
North Central Bronx Hospital	Bronx	52%	300+
Bellevue Hospital Center	New York	51%	300+
Brookdale Hospital Medical Center	Brooklyn	51%	300+
Flushing Hospital Medical Center	Flushing	51%	300+
Jacobi Medical Center	Bronx	51%	300+
Kings County Hospital Center	Brooklyn	51%	300+
Saint Luke's Roosevelt Hospital	New York	51%	300+
Elmhurst Hospital Center	Elmhurst	50%	300+
St John's Episcopal Hosp-South Shore	Far Rockaway	50%	300+
Westchester Medical Center	Valhalla	49%	300+
Wyckoff Heights Medical Center	Brooklyn	48%	300+
Harlem Hospital Center	New York	47%	300+
Jamaica Hospital Medical Center	Jamaica	47%	300+
Woodhull Medical & Mental Health Center	Brooklyn	47%	300+
Metropolitan Hospital Center	New York	46%	300+
Nassau University Medical Center	East Meadow	45%	300+

Nurses 'Always' Communicated Well

Hospital Name	City	Rate	Cases
Community Memorial Hospital	Hamilton	85%	300+
Northern Westchester Hospital	Mount Kisco	84%	300+
Putnam Hospital Center	Carmel	84%	300+
White Plains Hospital Center	White Plains	83%	300+
Adirondack Medical Center	Saranac Lake	82%	300+
Hospital For Special Surgery	New York	82%	300+
Northern Dutchess Hospital	Rhinebeck	82%	300+
Saint Francis Hospital - Roslyn	Roslyn	82%	300+
Saratoga Hospital	Saratoga Spgs	82%	300+
Eastern Long Island Hospital	Greenport	81%	300+
Highland Hospital	Rochester	81%	300+
Hudson Valley Hospital Center	Cortlandt Manor	81%	300+
Huntington Hospital	Huntington	81%	300+
John T Mather Mem Hosp-Port Jefferson	Port Jefferson	81%	300+
Little Falls Hospital	Little Falls	81%	(a)
Newark - Wayne Community Hospital	Newark	81%	300+
Phelps Memorial Hospital Assn	Sleepy Hollow	81%	300+
Saint Elizabeth Medical Center	Utica	81%	300+
Cayuga Medical Center at Ithaca	Ithaca	80%	300+
Champlain Valley Phys Hosp Med Ctr	Plattsburgh	80%	300+
Ellenville Regional Hospital	Ellenville	80%	(a)
Glens Falls Hospital	Glens Falls	80%	300+
Health Alliance Hosp Mary's Ave Campus	Kingston	80%	300+
New York Eye & Ear Infirmary	New York	80%	(a)
Rochester General Hospital	Rochester	80%	300+
Saint John's Riverside Hospital	Yonkers	80%	300+
Saint Joseph's Hospital Health Center	Syracuse	80%	300+
Vassar Brothers Medical Center	Poughkeepsie	80%	300+
Canton - Potsdam Hospital	Potsdam	79%	300+
Cortland Regional Medical Center	Cortland	79%	300+
Glen Cove Hospital	Glen Cove	79%	300+
Kenmore Mercy Hospital	Kenmore	79%	300+
Nathan Littauer Hospital	Gloversville	79%	300+
North Shore University Hospital	Manhasset	79%	300+
NYU Hospitals Center	New York	79%	300+
Orange Regional Medical Center	Middletown	79%	300+
Plainview Hospital[11]	Plainview	79%	300+
Saint Anthony Community Hospital	Warwick	79%	300+
Samaritan Medical Center	Watertown	79%	300+
Soldiers & Sailors Mem Hosp of Yates	Penn Yan	79%	(a)
Arnot Ogden Medical Center	Elmira	78%	300+
Bertrand Chaffee Hospital	Springville	78%	300+
Bon Secours Community Hospital	Port Jervis	78%	300+
Clifton Springs Hospital & Clinic	Clifton Springs	78%	300+
Geneva General Hospital	Geneva	78%	300+
Jones Memorial Hospital	Wellsville	78%	300+
Lewis County General Hospital	Lowville	78%	300+
Long Island Jewish Medical Center	New Hyde Park	78%	300+
Massena Memorial Hospital	Massena	78%	300+
Oswego Hospital	Oswego	78%	300+
Rome Memorial Hospital	Rome	78%	300+
Saint Mary's Hospital at Amsterdam	Amsterdam	78%	300+
Southampton Hospital	Southampton	78%	300+
Southside Hospital	Bay Shore	78%	300+
Strong Memorial Hospital	Rochester	78%	300+
University Hospital - Stony Brook	Stony Brook	78%	300+
Columbia Memorial Hospital	Hudson	77%	300+
Corning Hospital	Corning	77%	300+
Medina Memorial Hospital	Medina	77%	300+
Mount Sinai Hospital	New York	77%	300+
Nicholas H Noyes Memorial Hospital	Dansville	77%	300+
Oneida Healthcare Center	Oneida	77%	300+
Saint James Mercy Hospital	Hornell	77%	300+
Alice Hyde Medical Center	Malone	76%	300+
Faxton - Saint Luke's Healthcare	Utica	76%	300+
New York - Presbyterian Hospital	New York	76%	300+
Our Lady of Lourdes Memorial Hospital	Binghamton	76%	300+
Saint Charles Hospital	Port Jefferson	76%	300+
Schuyler Hospital	Montour Falls	76%	(a)
Sisters of Charity Hospital	Buffalo	76%	300+
South Nassau Communities Hospital	Oceanside	76%	300+
United Health Services Hospitals	Johnson City	76%	300+
Unity Hospital of Rochester	Rochester	76%	300+
Wyoming County Community Hospital	Warsaw	76%	300+
Carthage Area Hospital	Carthage	75%	(a)
Claxton - Hepburn Medical Center	Ogdensburg	75%	300+
Eastern Niagara Hospital	Lockport	75%	300+
Ellis Hospital	Schenectady	75%	300+
Lawrence Hospital Center	Bronxville	75%	300+
Mercy Medical Center	Rockville Centre	75%	300+
Mount St Mary's Hosp & Health Ctr	Lewiston	75%	300+
Saint Mary's Hospital - Troy	Troy	75%	(a)
United Memorial Medical Center	Batavia	75%	300+
Winthrop - University Hospital	Mineola	75%	300+
Brooks Memorial Hospital	Dunkirk	74%	300+
Chenango Memorial Hospital	Norwich	74%	300+
Franklin Hospital	Valley Stream	74%	300+
Univ Hosp SUNY Health Science Ctr[11]	Syracuse	74%	300+
Albany Medical Center Hospital	Albany	73%	300+
Catskill Regional Medical Center	Harris	73%	300+
Crouse Hospital	Syracuse	73%	300+
F F Thompson Hospital	Canandaigua	73%	300+
Mary Imogene Bassett Hospital	Cooperstown	73%	300+
Mercy Hospital	Buffalo	73%	300+
Montefiore New Rochelle Hospital	New Rochelle	73%	300+
New York Community Hospital of Brooklyn	Brooklyn	73%	300+
Saint Catherine of Siena Hospital	Smithtown	73%	300+
Saint Joseph Hospital	Bethpage	73%	300+
Saint Peter's Hospital	Albany	73%	300+
Staten Island University Hospital	Staten Island	73%	300+
Albany Memorial Hospital	Albany	72%	300+
Auburn Community Hospital[11]	Auburn	72%	300+
Aurelia Osborn Fox Memorial Hospital	Oneonta	72%	300+
Brookhaven Mem Hosp Med Ctr	Patchogue	72%	300+
Ira Davenport Memorial Hospital	Bath	72%	(a)
Kaleida Health	Buffalo	72%	300+
Lenox Hill Hospital	New York	72%	300+
Montefiore Medical Center	Bronx	72%	300+
Montefiore Mount Vernon Hospital	Mount Vernon	72%	300+
New York Hosp Med Ctr of Queens	Flushing	72%	300+
Nyack Hospital	Nyack	72%	300+
Saint Francis Hospital	Poughkeepsie	72%	300+
Saint Luke's Cornwall Hospital	Newburgh	72%	300+
Good Samaritan Hospital Medical Center	West Islip	71%	300+
Gouverneur Hospital	Gouverneur	71%	(a)
Health Alliance Hospital Broadway Campus	Kingston	71%	300+
Interfaith Medical Center	Brooklyn	71%	300+
Kingsbrook Jewish Medical Center	Brooklyn	71%	300+
New York Methodist Hospital	Brooklyn	71%	300+
Olean General Hospital	Olean	71%	300+
TLC Health Network	Gowanda	71%	(a)
Univ Hosp of Brooklyn-Downstate	Brooklyn	71%	300+
Brooklyn Hosp Ctr at Downtown Campus	Brooklyn	70%	300+
Cobleskill Regional Hospital	Cobleskill	70%	(a)
Coney Island Hospital	Brooklyn	70%	300+
Niagara Falls Memorial Medical Center	Niagara Falls	70%	300+
Saint Joseph's Hospital	Elmira	70%	300+
Saint Joseph's Medical Center	Yonkers	70%	300+
Samaritan Hospital	Troy	70%	300+
Forest Hills Hospital[11]	Forest Hills	69%	300+
Peconic Bay Medical Center	Riverhead	69%	300+
Woman's Christian Association	Jamestown	69%	300+
Erie County Medical Center	Buffalo	68%	300+
Lutheran Medical Center	Brooklyn	68%	300+
Richmond University Medical Center	Staten Island	68%	300+
Saint Barnabas Hospital	Bronx	68%	300+
Bronx - Lebanon Hospital Center	Bronx	67%	300+
Good Samaritan Hospital of Suffern	Suffern	67%	300+
North Central Bronx Hospital	Bronx	67%	300+
Beth Israel Medical Center	New York	66%	300+
Queens Hospital Center	Jamaica	66%	300+
St John's Episcopal Hosp-South Shore	Far Rockaway	65%	300+
Saint Luke's Roosevelt Hospital	New York	65%	300+
Bellevue Hospital Center	New York	64%	300+
Jamaica Hospital Medical Center	Jamaica	64%	300+
Wyckoff Heights Medical Center	Brooklyn	64%	300+
Jacobi Medical Center	Bronx	63%	300+
Kings County Hospital Center	Brooklyn	63%	300+
Maimonides Medical Center	Brooklyn	63%	300+
Brookdale Hospital Medical Center	Brooklyn	62%	300+
Lincoln Medical & Mental Health Center	Bronx	62%	300+
Westchester Medical Center	Valhalla	62%	300+
Woodhull Medical & Mental Health Center	Brooklyn	61%	300+
Elmhurst Hospital Center	Elmhurst	60%	300+
Flushing Hospital Medical Center	Flushing	60%	300+
Harlem Hospital Center	New York	58%	300+
Metropolitan Hospital Center	New York	57%	300+
Nassau University Medical Center	East Meadow	57%	300+

Pain 'Always' Well Controlled

Hospital Name	City	Rate	Cases
Putnam Hospital Center	Carmel	79%	300+
Phelps Memorial Hospital Assn	Sleepy Hollow	77%	300+
White Plains Hospital Center	White Plains	77%	300+
Community Memorial Hospital	Hamilton	76%	300+
Health Alliance Hosp Mary's Ave Campus	Kingston	76%	300+
Hospital For Special Surgery	New York	76%	300+
Northern Westchester Hospital	Mount Kisco	76%	300+
Adirondack Medical Center	Saranac Lake	74%	300+
Bon Secours Community Hospital	Port Jervis	74%	300+
Hudson Valley Hospital Center	Cortlandt Manor	74%	300+
Jones Memorial Hospital	Wellsville	74%	300+
Saint Francis Hospital - Roslyn	Roslyn	74%	300+
Huntington Hospital	Huntington	73%	300+
Kenmore Mercy Hospital	Kenmore	73%	300+
Lewis County General Hospital	Lowville	73%	300+
Little Falls Hospital	Little Falls	73%	(a)
Nathan Littauer Hospital	Gloversville	73%	300+
Orange Regional Medical Center	Middletown	73%	300+
Plainview Hospital[11]	Plainview	73%	300+
Saratoga Hospital	Saratoga Spgs	73%	300+
Southampton Hospital	Southampton	73%	300+
Vassar Brothers Medical Center	Poughkeepsie	73%	300+
Geneva General Hospital	Geneva	72%	300+
Saint Elizabeth Medical Center	Utica	72%	300+
Saint John's Riverside Hospital	Yonkers	72%	300+
Sisters of Charity Hospital	Buffalo	72%	300+
Soldiers & Sailors Mem Hosp of Yates	Penn Yan	72%	(a)
Wyoming County Community Hospital	Warsaw	72%	300+
Bertrand Chaffee Hospital	Springville	71%	300+
Canton - Potsdam Hospital	Potsdam	71%	300+
Champlain Valley Phys Hosp Med Ctr	Plattsburgh	71%	300+

NOTE: Hospital profiles are in alphabetical order by state, then city, then hospital within the city; Rankings exclude hospitals with less than 25 cases except for patient surveys which excludes hospitals with less than 100 cases; (a) 100-299 cases; (1) The number of cases/patients is too few to report; (2) Data submitted were based on a sample of cases/patients; (3) Results are based on a shorter time period than required; (4) Data suppressed by CMS for one or more quarters; (5) Results are not available for this reporting period; (6) Fewer than 100 patients completed the HCAHPS survey; (7) No cases met the criteria for this measure; (8) The lower limit of the confidence interval cannot be calculated if the number of observed infections equals zero; (9) No data are available from the state/territory for this reporting period; (10) The scores shown reflect fewer than 50 completed surveys; (11) There were discrepancies in the data collection process; (12) This measure does not apply to this hospital for this reporting period; (13) Results cannot be calculated for this reporting period; (14) The results for this state are combined with nearby states to protect confidentiality; Please refer to the User's Guide for a full explanation of data.

Clifton Springs Hospital & Clinic	Clifton Springs	71%	300+
Cortland Regional Medical Center	Cortland	71%	300+
Glens Falls Hospital	Glens Falls	71%	300+
Highland Hospital	Rochester	71%	300+
John T Mather Mem Hosp-Port Jefferson	Port Jefferson	71%	300+
Northern Dutchess Hospital	Rhinebeck	71%	300+
Arnot Ogden Medical Center	Elmira	70%	300+
Cayuga Medical Center at Ithaca	Ithaca	70%	300+
Mercy Medical Center	Rockville Centre	70%	300+
Mount Sinai Hospital	New York	70%	300+
Nicholas H Noyes Memorial Hospital	Dansville	70%	300+
Saint Anthony Community Hospital	Warwick	70%	300+
Saint Charles Hospital	Port Jefferson	70%	300+
Saint Peter's Hospital	Albany	70%	300+
Samaritan Medical Center	Watertown	70%	300+
Alice Hyde Medical Center	Malone	69%	300+
Brooks Memorial Hospital	Dunkirk	69%	300+
Ellenville Regional Hospital	Ellenville	69%	(a)
Ellis Hospital	Schenectady	69%	300+
Glen Cove Hospital	Glen Cove	69%	300+
Oneida Healthcare Center	Oneida	69%	300+
Our Lady of Lourdes Memorial Hospital	Binghamton	69%	300+
Rochester General Hospital	Rochester	69%	300+
Rome Memorial Hospital	Rome	69%	300+
Saint Joseph Hospital	Bethpage	69%	300+
Saint Joseph's Hospital Health Center	Syracuse	69%	300+
South Nassau Communities Hospital	Oceanside	69%	300+
Southside Hospital	Bay Shore	69%	300+
Eastern Long Island Hospital	Greenport	68%	300+
Faxton - Saint Luke's Healthcare	Utica	68%	300+
Mercy Hospital	Buffalo	68%	300+
New York Eye & Ear Infirmary	New York	68%	(a)
Newark - Wayne Community Hospital	Newark	68%	300+
NYU Hospitals Center	New York	68%	300+
Oswego Hospital	Oswego	68%	300+
Saint Mary's Hospital at Amsterdam	Amsterdam	68%	300+
United Memorial Medical Center	Batavia	68%	300+
University Hospital - Stony Brook	Stony Brook	68%	300+
Winthrop - University Hospital	Mineola	68%	300+
Auburn Community Hospital[11]	Auburn	67%	300+
Claxton - Hepburn Medical Center	Ogdensburg	67%	300+
Corning Hospital	Corning	67%	300+
Eastern Niagara Hospital	Lockport	67%	300+
Lawrence Hospital Center	Bronxville	67%	300+
Massena Memorial Hospital	Massena	67%	300+
Medina Memorial Hospital	Medina	67%	300+
New York - Presbyterian Hospital	New York	67%	300+
New York Community Hospital of Brooklyn	Brooklyn	67%	300+
North Shore University Hospital	Manhasset	67%	300+
Saint Francis Hospital	Poughkeepsie	67%	300+
Saint James Mercy Hospital	Hornell	67%	300+
Saint Mary's Hospital - Troy	Troy	67%	(a)
United Health Services Hospitals	Johnson City	67%	300+
Columbia Memorial Hospital	Hudson	66%	300+
Crouse Hospital	Syracuse	66%	300+
Franklin Hospital	Valley Stream	66%	300+
Gouverneur Hospital	Gouverneur	66%	(a)
Montefiore New Rochelle Hospital	New Rochelle	66%	300+
Mount St Mary's Hosp & Health Ctr	Lewiston	66%	300+
Saint Luke's Cornwall Hospital	Newburgh	66%	300+
Strong Memorial Hospital	Rochester	66%	300+
TLC Health Network	Gowanda	66%	(a)
Albany Medical Center Hospital	Albany	65%	300+
Brookhaven Mem Hosp Med Ctr	Patchogue	65%	300+
Catskill Regional Medical Center	Harris	65%	300+
Coney Island Hospital	Brooklyn	65%	300+
F F Thompson Hospital	Canandaigua	65%	300+
Good Samaritan Hospital Medical Center	West Islip	65%	300+
Ira Davenport Memorial Hospital	Bath	65%	(a)
Kaleida Health	Buffalo	65%	300+
Long Island Jewish Medical Center	New Hyde Park	65%	300+
Montefiore Medical Center	Bronx	65%	300+
Montefiore Mount Vernon Hospital	Mount Vernon	65%	300+
Unity Hospital of Rochester	Rochester	65%	300+
Albany Memorial Hospital	Albany	64%	300+
Aurelia Osborn Fox Memorial Hospital	Oneonta	64%	300+
Chenango Memorial Hospital	Norwich	64%	300+
Mary Imogene Bassett Hospital	Cooperstown	64%	300+
Niagara Falls Memorial Medical Center	Niagara Falls	64%	300+
Nyack Hospital	Nyack	64%	300+
Olean General Hospital	Olean	64%	300+
Saint Catherine of Siena Hospital	Smithtown	64%	300+
Saint Joseph's Hospital	Elmira	64%	300+
Schuyler Hospital	Montour Falls	64%	(a)
Bronx - Lebanon Hospital Center	Bronx	63%	300+
Carthage Area Hospital	Carthage	63%	(a)
Interfaith Medical Center	Brooklyn	63%	300+
Lenox Hill Hospital	New York	63%	300+
Lutheran Medical Center	Brooklyn	63%	300+
New York Hosp Med Ctr of Queens	Flushing	63%	300+
Univ Hosp of Brooklyn-Downstate	Brooklyn	63%	300+
Univ Hosp SUNY Health Science Ctr[11]	Syracuse	63%	300+
Health Alliance Hospital Broadway Campus	Kingston	62%	300+
New York Methodist Hospital	Brooklyn	62%	300+
Saint Barnabas Hospital	Bronx	62%	300+
St John's Episcopal Hosp-South Shore	Far Rockaway	62%	300+
Samaritan Hospital	Troy	62%	300+
Woman's Christian Association	Jamestown	62%	300+
Brooklyn Hosp Ctr at Downtown Campus	Brooklyn	61%	300+
Forest Hills Hospital[11]	Forest Hills	61%	300+
Jacobi Medical Center	Bronx	61%	300+
Beth Israel Medical Center	New York	60%	300+
Good Samaritan Hospital of Suffern	Suffern	60%	300+
Kingsbrook Jewish Medical Center	Brooklyn	60%	300+
Peconic Bay Medical Center	Riverhead	60%	300+
Saint Luke's Roosevelt Hospital	New York	60%	300+
Erie County Medical Center	Buffalo	59%	300+
Richmond University Medical Center	Staten Island	59%	300+
North Central Bronx Hospital	Bronx	58%	300+
Staten Island University Hospital	Staten Island	58%	300+
Wyckoff Heights Medical Center	Brooklyn	58%	300+
Bellevue Hospital Center	New York	57%	300+
Lincoln Medical & Mental Health Center	Bronx	57%	300+
Maimonides Medical Center	Brooklyn	57%	300+
Queens Hospital Center	Jamaica	57%	300+
Kings County Hospital Center	Brooklyn	56%	300+
Westchester Medical Center	Valhalla	56%	300+
Woodhull Medical & Mental Health Center	Brooklyn	55%	300+
Jamaica Hospital Medical Center	Jamaica	54%	300+
Brookdale Hospital Medical Center	Brooklyn	53%	300+
Cobleskill Regional Hospital	Cobleskill	53%	(a)
Elmhurst Hospital Center	Elmhurst	53%	300+
Flushing Hospital Medical Center	Flushing	53%	300+
Metropolitan Hospital Center	New York	53%	300+
Saint Joseph's Medical Center	Yonkers	52%	300+
Nassau University Medical Center	East Meadow	51%	300+
Harlem Hospital Center	New York	50%	300+

Room and Bathroom 'Always' Clean

Hospital Name	City	Rate	Cases
Gouverneur Hospital	Gouverneur	87%	(a)
Soldiers & Sailors Mem Hosp of Yates	Penn Yan	86%	(a)
Community Memorial Hospital	Hamilton	83%	300+
Samaritan Medical Center	Watertown	83%	300+
Saint John's Riverside Hospital	Yonkers	82%	300+
Lewis County General Hospital	Lowville	81%	300+
Adirondack Medical Center	Saranac Lake	80%	300+
Hospital For Special Surgery	New York	80%	300+
Little Falls Hospital	Little Falls	80%	(a)
Wyoming County Community Hospital	Warsaw	80%	300+
Alice Hyde Medical Center	Malone	79%	300+
Carthage Area Hospital	Carthage	79%	(a)
Northern Westchester Hospital	Mount Kisco	79%	300+
Canton - Potsdam Hospital	Potsdam	78%	300+
Southampton Hospital	Southampton	78%	300+
Eastern Long Island Hospital	Greenport	77%	300+
Glens Falls Hospital	Glens Falls	77%	300+
Hudson Valley Hospital Center	Cortlandt Manor	77%	300+
Medina Memorial Hospital	Medina	77%	300+
Nathan Littauer Hospital	Gloversville	77%	300+
North Shore University Hospital	Manhasset	77%	300+
Olean General Hospital	Olean	77%	300+
Phelps Memorial Hospital Assn	Sleepy Hollow	77%	300+
Cobleskill Regional Hospital	Cobleskill	76%	(a)
Geneva General Hospital	Geneva	76%	300+
Health Alliance Hosp Mary's Ave Campus	Kingston	76%	300+
Oneida Healthcare Center	Oneida	76%	300+
Putnam Hospital Center	Carmel	76%	300+
Bertrand Chaffee Hospital	Springville	75%	300+
Cortland Regional Medical Center	Cortland	75%	300+
New York Eye & Ear Infirmary	New York	75%	(a)
Newark - Wayne Community Hospital	Newark	75%	300+
Saint Francis Hospital - Roslyn	Roslyn	75%	300+
Ellenville Regional Hospital	Ellenville	74%	(a)
Long Island Jewish Medical Center	New Hyde Park	74%	300+
Massena Memorial Hospital	Massena	74%	300+
Mount Sinai Hospital	New York	74%	300+
Rome Memorial Hospital	Rome	74%	300+
Saint Mary's Hospital at Amsterdam	Amsterdam	74%	300+
Corning Hospital	Corning	73%	300+
Ira Davenport Memorial Hospital	Bath	73%	(a)
New York Community Hospital of Brooklyn	Brooklyn	73%	300+
Orange Regional Medical Center	Middletown	73%	300+
Bon Secours Community Hospital	Port Jervis	72%	300+
Brooks Memorial Hospital	Dunkirk	72%	300+
F F Thompson Hospital	Canandaigua	72%	300+
Huntington Hospital	Huntington	72%	300+
Northern Dutchess Hospital	Rhinebeck	72%	300+
Saratoga Hospital	Saratoga Spgs	72%	300+
Champlain Valley Phys Hosp Med Ctr	Plattsburgh	71%	300+
Ellis Hospital	Schenectady	71%	300+
Franklin Hospital	Valley Stream	71%	300+
Interfaith Medical Center	Brooklyn	71%	300+
Our Lady of Lourdes Memorial Hospital	Binghamton	71%	300+
Saint Elizabeth Medical Center	Utica	71%	300+
United Memorial Medical Center	Batavia	71%	300+
White Plains Hospital Center	White Plains	71%	300+
Auburn Community Hospital[11]	Auburn	70%	300+
Coney Island Hospital	Brooklyn	70%	300+
Eastern Niagara Hospital	Lockport	70%	300+
Forest Hills Hospital[11]	Forest Hills	70%	300+
Glen Cove Hospital	Glen Cove	70%	300+
Lawrence Hospital Center	Bronxville	70%	300+
Montefiore Medical Center	Bronx	70%	300+
Mount St Mary's Hosp & Health Ctr	Lewiston	70%	300+
New York Hosp Med Ctr of Queens	Flushing	70%	300+
Nyack Hospital	Nyack	70%	300+
NYU Hospitals Center	New York	70%	300+
Oswego Hospital	Oswego	70%	300+
Saint Charles Hospital	Port Jefferson	70%	300+
United Health Services Hospitals	Johnson City	70%	300+
Winthrop - University Hospital	Mineola	70%	300+
Aurelia Osborn Fox Memorial Hospital	Oneonta	69%	300+
Claxton - Hepburn Medical Center	Ogdensburg	69%	300+
Highland Hospital	Rochester	69%	300+
Kingsbrook Jewish Medical Center	Brooklyn	69%	300+
North Central Bronx Hospital	Bronx	69%	300+
Saint Joseph's Hospital	Elmira	69%	300+
Chenango Memorial Hospital	Norwich	68%	300+
Good Samaritan Hospital Medical Center	West Islip	68%	300+
John T Mather Mem Hosp-Port Jefferson	Port Jefferson	68%	300+
Jones Memorial Hospital	Wellsville	68%	300+
Queens Hospital Center	Jamaica	68%	300+
Saint Barnabas Hospital	Bronx	68%	300+
Saint Joseph's Hospital Health Center	Syracuse	68%	300+
Saint Joseph's Medical Center	Yonkers	68%	300+
Saint Peter's Hospital	Albany	68%	300+
Southside Hospital	Bay Shore	68%	300+
Woodhull Medical & Mental Health Center	Brooklyn	68%	300+
Beth Israel Medical Center	New York	67%	300+
Brooklyn Hosp Ctr at Downtown Campus	Brooklyn	67%	300+
Cayuga Medical Center at Ithaca	Ithaca	67%	300+
Mary Imogene Bassett Hospital	Cooperstown	67%	300+
Mercy Medical Center	Rockville Centre	67%	300+
Plainview Hospital[11]	Plainview	67%	300+
TLC Health Network	Gowanda	67%	(a)
Vassar Brothers Medical Center	Poughkeepsie	67%	300+
Albany Medical Center Hospital	Albany	66%	300+
Arnot Ogden Medical Center	Elmira	66%	300+
Columbia Memorial Hospital	Hudson	66%	300+
Jacobi Medical Center	Bronx	66%	300+
New York - Presbyterian Hospital	New York	66%	300+
Saint Catherine of Siena Hospital	Smithtown	66%	300+
Saint James Mercy Hospital	Hornell	66%	300+
Strong Memorial Hospital	Rochester	66%	300+
Clifton Springs Hospital & Clinic	Clifton Springs	65%	300+
Saint Mary's Hospital - Troy	Troy	65%	(a)
South Nassau Communities Hospital	Oceanside	65%	300+
University Hospital - Stony Brook	Stony Brook	65%	300+
Faxton - Saint Luke's Healthcare	Utica	64%	300+
Kenmore Mercy Hospital	Kenmore	64%	300+
Rochester General Hospital	Rochester	64%	300+
St John's Episcopal Hosp-South Shore	Far Rockaway	64%	300+
Sisters of Charity Hospital	Buffalo	64%	300+
Kings County Hospital Center	Brooklyn	63%	300+
Peconic Bay Medical Center	Riverhead	63%	300+
Saint Anthony Community Hospital	Warwick	63%	300+
Saint Francis Hospital	Poughkeepsie	63%	300+
Saint Luke's Roosevelt Hospital	New York	63%	300+
Samaritan Hospital	Troy	63%	300+
Staten Island University Hospital	Staten Island	63%	300+
Univ Hosp SUNY Health Science Ctr[11]	Syracuse	63%	300+
Wyckoff Heights Medical Center	Brooklyn	63%	300+
Albany Memorial Hospital	Albany	62%	300+
Crouse Hospital	Syracuse	62%	300+
Jamaica Hospital Medical Center	Jamaica	62%	300+
Montefiore New Rochelle Hospital	New Rochelle	62%	300+
Saint Joseph Hospital	Bethpage	62%	300+
Lenox Hill Hospital	New York	61%	300+
Metropolitan Hospital Center	New York	61%	300+
Univ Hosp of Brooklyn-Downstate	Brooklyn	61%	300+
Bellevue Hospital Center	New York	60%	300+
Bronx - Lebanon Hospital Center	Bronx	60%	300+
Health Alliance Hospital Broadway Campus	Kingston	60%	300+
Kaleida Health	Buffalo	60%	300+
Niagara Falls Memorial Medical Center	Niagara Falls	60%	300+
Nicholas H Noyes Memorial Hospital	Dansville	60%	300+
Unity Hospital of Rochester	Rochester	60%	300+
Brookhaven Mem Hosp Med Ctr	Patchogue	59%	300+
Harlem Hospital Center	New York	59%	300+
Montefiore Mount Vernon Hospital	Mount Vernon	59%	300+
Nassau University Medical Center	East Meadow	59%	300+
Woman's Christian Association	Jamestown	59%	300+

NOTE: Hospital profiles are in alphabetical order by state, then city, then hospital within the city; Rankings exclude hospitals with less than 25 cases except for patient surveys which excludes hospitals with less than 100 cases; (a) 100-299 cases; (1) The number of cases/patients is too few to report; (2) Data submitted were based on a sample of cases/patients; (3) Results are based on a shorter time period than required; (4) Data suppressed by CMS for one or more quarters; (5) Results are not available for this reporting period; (6) Fewer than 100 patients completed the HCAHPS survey; (7) No cases met the criteria for this measure; (8) The lower limit of the confidence interval cannot be calculated if the number of observed infections equals zero; (9) No data are available from the state/territory for this reporting period; (10) The scores shown reflect fewer than 50 completed surveys; (11) There were discrepancies in the data collection process; (12) This measure does not apply to this hospital for this reporting period; (13) Results cannot be calculated for this reporting period; (14) The results for this state are combined with nearby states to protect confidentiality; Please refer to the User's Guide for a full explanation of data.

Flushing Hospital Medical Center	Flushing	58%	300+
Lincoln Medical & Mental Health Center	Bronx	58%	300+
New York Methodist Hospital	Brooklyn	58%	300+
Saint Luke's Cornwall Hospital	Newburgh	58%	300+
Elmhurst Hospital Center	Elmhurst	57%	300+
Good Samaritan Hospital of Suffern	Suffern	57%	300+
Lutheran Medical Center	Brooklyn	57%	300+
Brookdale Hospital Medical Center	Brooklyn	56%	300+
Erie County Medical Center	Buffalo	56%	300+
Schuyler Hospital	Montour Falls	56%	(a)
Catskill Regional Medical Center	Harris	55%	300+
Maimonides Medical Center	Brooklyn	55%	300+
Mercy Hospital	Buffalo	55%	300+
Richmond University Medical Center	Staten Island	55%	300+
Westchester Medical Center	Valhalla	50%	300+

Timely Help 'Always' Received

Hospital Name	City	Rate	Cases
Soldiers & Sailors Mem Hosp of Yates	Penn Yan	80%	(a)
Adirondack Medical Center	Saranac Lake	76%	300+
New York Eye & Ear Infirmary	New York	74%	(a)
Saratoga Hospital	Saratoga Spgs	74%	300+
Community Memorial Hospital	Hamilton	73%	300+
Ellenville Regional Hospital	Ellenville	73%	(a)
Northern Westchester Hospital	Mount Kisco	73%	300+
Saint James Mercy Hospital	Hornell	73%	300+
Clifton Springs Hospital & Clinic	Clifton Springs	72%	300+
Health Alliance Hosp Mary's Ave Campus	Kingston	72%	300+
Lewis County General Hospital	Lowville	72%	300+
Cayuga Medical Center at Ithaca	Ithaca	71%	300+
Hospital For Special Surgery	New York	71%	300+
Hudson Valley Hospital Center	Cortlandt Manor	71%	300+
Phelps Memorial Hospital Assn	Sleepy Hollow	71%	300+
Samaritan Medical Center	Watertown	71%	300+
Canton - Potsdam Hospital	Potsdam	70%	300+
John T Mather Mem Hosp-Port Jefferson	Port Jefferson	70%	300+
Glens Falls Hospital	Glens Falls	69%	300+
Gouverneur Hospital	Gouverneur	69%	(a)
Ira Davenport Memorial Hospital	Bath	69%	(a)
Little Falls Hospital	Little Falls	69%	(a)
Nicholas H Noyes Memorial Hospital	Dansville	69%	300+
Northern Dutchess Hospital	Rhinebeck	69%	300+
Putnam Hospital Center	Carmel	69%	300+
Alice Hyde Medical Center	Malone	68%	300+
Champlain Valley Phys Hosp Med Ctr	Plattsburgh	68%	300+
Eastern Long Island Hospital	Greenport	68%	300+
Jones Memorial Hospital	Wellsville	68%	300+
Nathan Littauer Hospital	Gloversville	68%	300+
Oneida Healthcare Center	Oneida	68%	300+
Saint Anthony Community Hospital	Warwick	68%	300+
Bertrand Chaffee Hospital	Springville	67%	300+
Carthage Area Hospital	Carthage	67%	(a)
Plainview Hospital[11]	Plainview	67%	300+
Saint Francis Hospital - Roslyn	Roslyn	67%	300+
Bon Secours Community Hospital	Port Jervis	66%	300+
Claxton - Hepburn Medical Center	Ogdensburg	66%	300+
Massena Memorial Hospital	Massena	66%	300+
Saint Elizabeth Medical Center	Utica	66%	300+
Saint John's Riverside Hospital	Yonkers	66%	300+
Southampton Hospital	Southampton	66%	300+
TLC Health Network	Gowanda	66%	(a)
White Plains Hospital Center	White Plains	66%	300+
Huntington Hospital	Huntington	65%	300+
Kenmore Mercy Hospital	Kenmore	65%	300+
Schuyler Hospital	Montour Falls	65%	(a)
Sisters of Charity Hospital	Buffalo	65%	300+
United Health Services Hospitals	Johnson City	65%	300+
Columbia Memorial Hospital	Hudson	64%	300+
Highland Hospital	Rochester	64%	300+
Mount Sinai Hospital	New York	64%	300+
Newark - Wayne Community Hospital	Newark	64%	300+
NYU Hospitals Center	New York	64%	300+
Orange Regional Medical Center	Middletown	64%	300+
Rochester General Hospital	Rochester	64%	300+
Saint Joseph's Hospital Health Center	Syracuse	64%	300+
University Hospital - Stony Brook	Stony Brook	64%	300+
Chenango Memorial Hospital	Norwich	63%	300+
Corning Hospital	Corning	63%	300+
Franklin Hospital	Valley Stream	63%	300+
Geneva General Hospital	Geneva	63%	300+
Glen Cove Hospital	Glen Cove	63%	300+
Montefiore New Rochelle Hospital	New Rochelle	63%	300+
Niagara Falls Memorial Medical Center	Niagara Falls	63%	300+
Saint Mary's Hospital at Amsterdam	Amsterdam	63%	300+
Strong Memorial Hospital	Rochester	63%	300+
Lawrence Hospital Center	Bronxville	62%	300+
Our Lady of Lourdes Memorial Hospital	Binghamton	62%	300+
Saint Mary's Hospital - Troy	Troy	62%	(a)
United Memorial Medical Center	Batavia	62%	300+
Long Island Jewish Medical Center	New Hyde Park	61%	300+
New York Community Hospital of Brooklyn	Brooklyn	61%	300+
North Shore University Hospital	Manhasset	61%	300+
Rome Memorial Hospital	Rome	61%	300+
Staten Island University Hospital	Staten Island	61%	300+
Vassar Brothers Medical Center	Poughkeepsie	61%	300+
Albany Medical Center Hospital	Albany	60%	300+
Arnot Ogden Medical Center	Elmira	60%	300+
Mercy Medical Center	Rockville Centre	60%	300+
Montefiore Mount Vernon Hospital	Mount Vernon	60%	300+
Oswego Hospital	Oswego	60%	300+
Saint Charles Hospital	Port Jefferson	60%	300+
Univ Hosp SUNY Health Science Ctr[11]	Syracuse	60%	300+
Brooks Memorial Hospital	Dunkirk	59%	300+
Coney Island Hospital	Brooklyn	59%	300+
Eastern Niagara Hospital	Lockport	59%	300+
Faxton - Saint Luke's Healthcare	Utica	59%	300+
Nyack Hospital	Nyack	59%	300+
Saint Joseph Hospital	Bethpage	59%	300+
South Nassau Communities Hospital	Oceanside	59%	300+
Wyoming County Community Hospital	Warsaw	59%	300+
Cobleskill Regional Hospital	Cobleskill	58%	(a)
Ellis Hospital	Schenectady	58%	300+
F F Thompson Hospital	Canandaigua	58%	300+
Medina Memorial Hospital	Medina	58%	300+
Aurelia Osborn Fox Memorial Hospital	Oneonta	57%	300+
Catskill Regional Medical Center	Harris	57%	300+
Cortland Regional Medical Center	Cortland	57%	300+
Mary Imogene Bassett Hospital	Cooperstown	57%	300+
New York - Presbyterian Hospital	New York	57%	300+
Unity Hospital of Rochester	Rochester	57%	300+
Winthrop - University Hospital	Mineola	57%	300+
Albany Memorial Hospital	Albany	56%	300+
Auburn Community Hospital[11]	Auburn	56%	300+
Lutheran Medical Center	Brooklyn	56%	300+
New York Hosp Med Ctr of Queens	Flushing	56%	300+
Saint Barnabas Hospital	Bronx	56%	300+
Saint Francis Hospital	Poughkeepsie	56%	300+
Saint Joseph's Hospital	Elmira	56%	300+
Saint Luke's Cornwall Hospital	Newburgh	56%	300+
Southside Hospital	Bay Shore	56%	300+
Forest Hills Hospital[11]	Forest Hills	55%	300+
Lenox Hill Hospital	New York	55%	300+
Peconic Bay Medical Center	Riverhead	55%	300+
Saint Catherine of Siena Hospital	Smithtown	55%	300+
Saint Peter's Hospital	Albany	55%	300+
Brookhaven Mem Hosp Med Ctr	Patchogue	54%	300+
Crouse Hospital	Syracuse	54%	300+
Kaleida Health	Buffalo	54%	300+
Mercy Hospital	Buffalo	54%	300+
Montefiore Medical Center	Bronx	54%	300+
Beth Israel Medical Center	New York	53%	300+
Mount St Mary's Hosp & Health Ctr	Lewiston	53%	300+
Richmond University Medical Center	Staten Island	53%	300+
Univ Hosp of Brooklyn-Downstate	Brooklyn	53%	300+
Woman's Christian Association	Jamestown	53%	300+
Bronx - Lebanon Hospital Center	Bronx	52%	300+
Brooklyn Hosp Ctr at Downtown Campus	Brooklyn	52%	300+
Olean General Hospital	Olean	52%	300+
Good Samaritan Hospital Medical Center	West Islip	51%	300+
Health Alliance Hospital Broadway Campus	Kingston	51%	300+
Kingsbrook Jewish Medical Center	Brooklyn	51%	300+
Samaritan Hospital	Troy	51%	300+
Bellevue Hospital Center	New York	50%	300+
Flushing Hospital Medical Center	Flushing	50%	300+
Erie County Medical Center	Buffalo	49%	300+
Good Samaritan Hospital of Suffern	Suffern	49%	300+
New York Methodist Hospital	Brooklyn	49%	300+
Westchester Medical Center	Valhalla	49%	300+
Maimonides Medical Center	Brooklyn	48%	300+
Saint Joseph's Medical Center	Yonkers	48%	300+
Wyckoff Heights Medical Center	Brooklyn	48%	300+
Elmhurst Hospital Center	Elmhurst	47%	300+
Jacobi Medical Center	Bronx	47%	300+
Jamaica Hospital Medical Center	Jamaica	47%	300+
North Central Bronx Hospital	Bronx	47%	300+
Queens Hospital Center	Jamaica	47%	300+
St John's Episcopal Hosp-South Shore	Far Rockaway	47%	300+
Lincoln Medical & Mental Health Center	Bronx	46%	300+
Interfaith Medical Center	Brooklyn	45%	300+
Saint Luke's Roosevelt Hospital	New York	45%	300+
Woodhull Medical & Mental Health Center	Brooklyn	44%	300+
Brookdale Hospital Medical Center	Brooklyn	43%	300+
Metropolitan Hospital Center	New York	41%	300+
Harlem Hospital Center	New York	39%	300+
Kings County Hospital Center	Brooklyn	39%	300+
Nassau University Medical Center	East Meadow	39%	300+

Would Definitely Recommend Hospital

Hospital Name	City	Rate	Cases
Hospital For Special Surgery	New York	92%	300+
Saint Francis Hospital - Roslyn	Roslyn	86%	300+
Northern Westchester Hospital	Mount Kisco	85%	300+
Eastern Long Island Hospital	Greenport	83%	300+
Clifton Springs Hospital & Clinic	Clifton Springs	82%	300+
Northern Dutchess Hospital	Rhinebeck	82%	300+
Community Memorial Hospital	Hamilton	81%	300+
White Plains Hospital Center	White Plains	81%	300+
Highland Hospital	Rochester	80%	300+
Phelps Memorial Hospital Assn	Sleepy Hollow	80%	300+
New York - Presbyterian Hospital	New York	79%	300+
Putnam Hospital Center	Carmel	79%	300+
Saint Joseph's Hospital Health Center	Syracuse	79%	300+
Strong Memorial Hospital	Rochester	79%	300+
Health Alliance Hosp Mary's Ave Campus	Kingston	78%	300+
John T Mather Mem Hosp-Port Jefferson	Port Jefferson	78%	300+
NYU Hospitals Center	New York	78%	300+
Rochester General Hospital	Rochester	78%	300+
Long Island Jewish Medical Center	New Hyde Park	77%	300+
North Shore University Hospital	Manhasset	77%	300+
Saratoga Hospital	Saratoga Spgs	76%	300+
Vassar Brothers Medical Center	Poughkeepsie	76%	300+
Glen Cove Hospital	Glen Cove	75%	300+
Hudson Valley Hospital Center	Cortlandt Manor	75%	300+
Little Falls Hospital	Little Falls	75%	(a)
New York Eye & Ear Infirmary	New York	75%	(a)
Our Lady of Lourdes Memorial Hospital	Binghamton	75%	300+
Saint Charles Hospital	Port Jefferson	75%	300+
University Hospital - Stony Brook	Stony Brook	75%	300+
Kenmore Mercy Hospital	Kenmore	74%	300+
Mount Sinai Hospital	New York	74%	300+
Adirondack Medical Center	Saranac Lake	73%	300+
Lewis County General Hospital	Lowville	73%	300+
Saint John's Riverside Hospital	Yonkers	73%	300+
Saint Peter's Hospital	Albany	73%	300+
Orange Regional Medical Center	Middletown	72%	300+
Saint Elizabeth Medical Center	Utica	72%	300+
Saint Mary's Hospital at Amsterdam	Amsterdam	72%	300+
Sisters of Charity Hospital	Buffalo	72%	300+
Winthrop - University Hospital	Mineola	72%	300+
Canton - Potsdam Hospital	Potsdam	71%	300+
Cayuga Medical Center at Ithaca	Ithaca	71%	300+
Ellenville Regional Hospital	Ellenville	71%	(a)
F F Thompson Hospital	Canandaigua	71%	300+
Huntington Hospital	Huntington	71%	300+
Mount St Mary's Hosp & Health Ctr	Lewiston	71%	300+
South Nassau Communities Hospital	Oceanside	71%	300+
Unity Hospital of Rochester	Rochester	71%	300+
Albany Medical Center Hospital	Albany	70%	300+
Arnot Ogden Medical Center	Elmira	70%	300+
Lenox Hill Hospital	New York	70%	300+
Medina Memorial Hospital	Medina	70%	300+
Southampton Hospital	Southampton	70%	300+
Ellis Hospital	Schenectady	69%	300+
Oneida Healthcare Center	Oneida	69%	300+
Southside Hospital	Bay Shore	69%	300+
Crouse Hospital	Syracuse	68%	300+
Lawrence Hospital Center	Bronxville	68%	300+
Mercy Medical Center	Rockville Centre	68%	300+
New York Hosp Med Ctr of Queens	Flushing	68%	300+
United Health Services Hospitals	Johnson City	68%	300+
Faxton - Saint Luke's Healthcare	Utica	67%	300+
Montefiore Medical Center	Bronx	67%	300+
Saint Anthony Community Hospital	Warwick	67%	300+
Schuyler Hospital	Montour Falls	67%	(a)
Bertrand Chaffee Hospital	Springville	66%	300+
Franklin Hospital	Valley Stream	66%	300+
Glens Falls Hospital	Glens Falls	66%	300+
Gouverneur Hospital	Gouverneur	66%	(a)
Kaleida Health	Buffalo	66%	300+
Mary Imogene Bassett Hospital	Cooperstown	66%	300+
Newark - Wayne Community Hospital	Newark	66%	300+
Saint Mary's Hospital - Troy	Troy	66%	(a)
Albany Memorial Hospital	Albany	65%	300+
Champlain Valley Phys Hosp Med Ctr	Plattsburgh	65%	300+
Claxton - Hepburn Medical Center	Ogdensburg	65%	300+
Jones Memorial Hospital	Wellsville	65%	300+
New York Methodist Hospital	Brooklyn	65%	300+
Queens Hospital Center	Jamaica	65%	300+
Samaritan Medical Center	Watertown	65%	300+
Univ Hosp SUNY Health Science Ctr[11]	Syracuse	65%	300+
Bellevue Hospital Center	New York	64%	300+
Rome Memorial Hospital	Rome	64%	300+
Soldiers & Sailors Mem Hosp of Yates	Penn Yan	64%	(a)
Univ Hosp of Brooklyn-Downstate	Brooklyn	64%	300+
Bon Secours Community Hospital	Port Jervis	63%	300+
Plainview Hospital[11]	Plainview	63%	300+
Carthage Area Hospital	Carthage	62%	(a)
Erie County Medical Center	Buffalo	62%	300+
Forest Hills Hospital[11]	Forest Hills	62%	300+
Nathan Littauer Hospital	Gloversville	62%	300+
Saint Luke's Cornwall Hospital	Newburgh	62%	300+
Beth Israel Medical Center	New York	61%	300+
Eastern Niagara Hospital	Lockport	61%	300+

NOTE: Hospital profiles are in alphabetical order by state, then city, then hospital within the city; Rankings exclude hospitals with less than 25 cases except for patient surveys which excludes hospitals with less than 100 cases; (a) 100-299 cases; (1) The number of cases/patients is too few to report; (2) Data submitted were based on a sample of cases/patients; (3) Results are based on a shorter time period than required; (4) Data suppressed by CMS for one or more quarters; (5) Results are not available for this reporting period; (6) Fewer than 100 patients completed the HCAHPS survey; (7) No cases met the criteria for this measure; (8) The lower limit of the confidence interval cannot be calculated if the number of observed infections equals zero; (9) No data are available from the state/territory for this reporting period; (10) The scores shown reflect fewer than 50 completed surveys; (11) There were discrepancies in the data collection process; (12) This measure does not apply to this hospital for this reporting period; (13) Results cannot be calculated for this reporting period; (14) The results for this state are combined with nearby states to protect confidentiality; Please refer to the User's Guide for a full explanation of data.

Hospital Name	City	Rate	Cases
Geneva General Hospital	Geneva	61%	300+
Good Samaritan Hospital Medical Center	West Islip	61%	300+
Maimonides Medical Center	Brooklyn	61%	300+
Nicholas H Noyes Memorial Hospital	Dansville	61%	300+
North Central Bronx Hospital	Bronx	61%	300+
Saint Francis Hospital	Poughkeepsie	61%	300+
Good Samaritan Hospital of Suffern	Suffern	60%	300+
Kings County Hospital Center	Brooklyn	60%	300+
Massena Memorial Hospital	Massena	60%	300+
Nyack Hospital	Nyack	60%	300+
Saint Catherine of Siena Hospital	Smithtown	60%	300+
Saint Joseph's Hospital	Elmira	60%	300+
Corning Hospital	Corning	59%	300+
Kingsbrook Jewish Medical Center	Brooklyn	59%	300+
Saint Joseph Hospital	Bethpage	59%	300+
Saint Luke's Roosevelt Hospital	New York	59%	300+
Brooks Memorial Hospital	Dunkirk	58%	300+
Jacobi Medical Center	Bronx	58%	300+
Montefiore New Rochelle Hospital	New Rochelle	58%	300+
Staten Island University Hospital	Staten Island	58%	300+
Aurelia Osborn Fox Memorial Hospital	Oneonta	57%	300+
Brooklyn Hosp Ctr at Downtown Campus	Brooklyn	57%	300+
Interfaith Medical Center	Brooklyn	57%	300+
Lutheran Medical Center	Brooklyn	57%	300+
Mercy Hospital	Buffalo	57%	300+
Peconic Bay Medical Center	Riverhead	57%	300+
Saint Barnabas Hospital	Bronx	57%	300+
Cobleskill Regional Hospital	Cobleskill	56%	(a)
Coney Island Hospital	Brooklyn	56%	300+
Cortland Regional Medical Center	Cortland	56%	300+
Metropolitan Hospital Center	New York	56%	300+
Olean General Hospital	Olean	56%	300+
Oswego Hospital	Oswego	56%	300+
Samaritan Hospital	Troy	56%	300+
TLC Health Network	Gowanda	56%	(a)
Bronx - Lebanon Hospital Center	Bronx	55%	300+
Chenango Memorial Hospital	Norwich	55%	300+
New York Community Hospital of Brooklyn	Brooklyn	55%	300+
Niagara Falls Memorial Medical Center	Niagara Falls	55%	300+
Saint James Mercy Hospital	Hornell	55%	300+
Wyoming County Community Hospital	Warsaw	55%	300+
Montefiore Mount Vernon Hospital	Mount Vernon	54%	300+
Westchester Medical Center	Valhalla	54%	300+
Lincoln Medical & Mental Health Center	Bronx	53%	300+
Saint Joseph's Medical Center	Yonkers	53%	300+
Woodhull Medical & Mental Health Center	Brooklyn	53%	300+
Auburn Community Hospital[11]	Auburn	52%	300+
Elmhurst Hospital Center	Elmhurst	52%	300+
Ira Davenport Memorial Hospital	Bath	52%	(a)
Brookhaven Mem Hosp Med Ctr	Patchogue	51%	300+
Catskill Regional Medical Center	Harris	51%	300+
Columbia Memorial Hospital	Hudson	51%	300+
Health Alliance Hospital Broadway Campus	Kingston	50%	300+
Wyckoff Heights Medical Center	Brooklyn	50%	300+
Flushing Hospital Medical Center	Flushing	49%	300+
Richmond University Medical Center	Staten Island	49%	300+
St John's Episcopal Hosp-South Shore	Far Rockaway	49%	300+
Woman's Christian Association	Jamestown	49%	300+
Alice Hyde Medical Center	Malone	47%	300+
Jamaica Hospital Medical Center	Jamaica	47%	300+
Harlem Hospital Center	New York	46%	300+
United Memorial Medical Center	Batavia	46%	300+
Brookdale Hospital Medical Center	Brooklyn	41%	300+
Nassau University Medical Center	East Meadow	39%	300+

Use of Medical Imaging

Cardiac Imaging Stress Test before OP Surgery

Hospital Name	City	Rate	Cases
Community Memorial Hospital	Hamilton	0.0%	73
Little Falls Hospital	Little Falls	0.0%	48
TLC Health Network	Gowanda	0.8%	121
Faxton - Saint Luke's Healthcare	Utica	1.6%	126
Auburn Community Hospital	Auburn	2.0%	51
Jones Memorial Hospital	Wellsville	2.0%	49
Huntington Hospital	Huntington	2.1%	47
F F Thompson Hospital	Canandaigua	2.2%	93
Erie County Medical Center	Buffalo	2.7%	146
Saint Joseph's Hospital Health Center	Syracuse	2.7%	369
Saratoga Hospital	Saratoga Spgs	2.7%	111
United Health Services Hospitals	Johnson City	2.8%	603
Saint Mary's Hospital - Troy	Troy	2.9%	69
Saint James Mercy Hospital	Hornell	3.1%	64
Vassar Brothers Medical Center	Poughkeepsie	3.1%	97
Brooklyn Hosp Ctr at Downtown Campus	Brooklyn	3.2%	63
Glens Falls Hospital	Glens Falls	3.2%	531
Champlain Valley Phys Hosp Med Ctr	Plattsburgh	3.3%	601
Mary Imogene Bassett Hospital	Cooperstown	3.3%	548
Crouse Hospital	Syracuse	3.4%	59
Rome Memorial Hospital	Rome	3.4%	148
Saint Peter's Hospital	Albany	3.4%	59
Aurelia Osborn Fox Memorial Hospital	Oneonta	3.5%	282
Corning Hospital	Corning	3.5%	141
New York Methodist Hospital	Brooklyn	3.5%	487
University Hospital - Stony Brook	Stony Brook	3.5%	455
Cayuga Medical Center at Ithaca	Ithaca	3.7%	214
Chenango Memorial Hospital	Norwich	3.7%	108
Saint Luke's Roosevelt Hospital	New York	3.8%	160
Massena Memorial Hospital	Massena	3.9%	155
St John's Episcopal Hosp-South Shore	Far Rockaway	3.9%	129
Oswego Hospital	Oswego	4.0%	253
Arnot Ogden Medical Center	Elmira	4.1%	1268
Saint Francis Hospital	Poughkeepsie	4.1%	148
Woman's Christian Association	Jamestown	4.1%	222
Northern Dutchess Hospital	Rhinebeck	4.2%	120
Claxton - Hepburn Medical Center	Ogdensburg	4.3%	254
Highland Hospital	Rochester	4.3%	235
Unity Hospital of Rochester	Rochester	4.3%	138
Strong Memorial Hospital	Rochester	4.5%	559
Medina Memorial Hospital	Medina	4.6%	65
Mount St Mary's Hosp & Health Ctr	Lewiston	4.7%	404
Saint Joseph's Medical Center	Yonkers	4.7%	64
Clifton Springs Hospital & Clinic	Clifton Springs	4.8%	62
Kaleida Health	Buffalo	4.8%	600
John T Mather Mem Hosp-Port Jefferson	Port Jefferson	4.9%	327
Adirondack Medical Center	Saranac Lake	5.1%	157
Geneva General Hospital	Geneva	5.1%	117
Long Island Jewish Medical Center	New Hyde Park	5.1%	334
Univ Hosp SUNY Health Science Ctr	Syracuse	5.1%	370
Cortland Regional Medical Center	Cortland	5.3%	300
Eastern Niagara Hospital	Lockport	5.3%	171
Oneida Healthcare Center	Oneida	5.3%	75
Hudson Valley Hospital Center	Cortlandt Manor	5.4%	514
Lawrence Hospital Center	Bronxville	5.4%	147
Good Samaritan Hospital of Suffern	Suffern	5.5%	73
Montefiore New Rochelle Hospital	New Rochelle	5.5%	55
Catskill Regional Medical Center	Harris	5.7%	106
South Nassau Communities Hospital	Oceanside	5.7%	209
Lewis County General Hospital	Lowville	5.9%	118
Orange Regional Medical Center	Middletown	6.0%	448
Rochester General Hospital	Rochester	6.0%	348
Southside Hospital	Bay Shore	6.0%	134
Columbia Memorial Hospital	Hudson	6.1%	326
Health Alliance Hosp Mary's Ave Campus	Kingston	6.1%	147
Northern Westchester Hospital	Mount Kisco	6.2%	889
Saint Francis Hospital - Roslyn	Roslyn	6.2%	2342
Canton - Potsdam Hospital	Potsdam	6.3%	400
New York - Presbyterian Hospital	New York	6.3%	646
Woodhull Medical & Mental Health Center	Brooklyn	6.3%	80
Saint Charles Hospital	Port Jefferson	6.5%	77
Albany Medical Center Hospital	Albany	6.7%	193
Niagara Falls Memorial Medical Center	Niagara Falls	6.7%	149
Saint John's Riverside Hospital	Yonkers	6.7%	134
Samaritan Hospital	Troy	6.7%	164
Olean General Hospital	Olean	6.8%	294
Health Alliance Hospital Broadway Campus	Kingston	7.3%	109
Phelps Memorial Hospital Assn	Sleepy Hollow	7.3%	82
North Shore University Hospital	Manhasset	7.4%	472
Saint Luke's Cornwall Hospital	Newburgh	7.6%	119
Mercy Hospital	Buffalo	7.7%	155
Beth Israel Medical Center	New York	7.8%	447
Mercy Medical Center	Rockville Centre	7.8%	102
Saint Elizabeth Medical Center	Utica	8.0%	175
Staten Island University Hospital	Staten Island	8.0%	402
Montefiore Medical Center	Bronx	8.2%	388
NYU Hospitals Center	New York	8.3%	1343
Alice Hyde Medical Center	Malone	8.4%	143
Mount Sinai Hospital	New York	8.4%	1193
Lenox Hill Hospital	New York	8.5%	484
White Plains Hospital Center	White Plains	8.5%	330
Richmond University Medical Center	Staten Island	8.6%	70
Kenmore Mercy Hospital	Kenmore	8.7%	92
Bon Secours Community Hospital	Port Jervis	8.9%	79
Wyckoff Heights Medical Center	Brooklyn	9.1%	66
Brookdale Hospital Medical Center	Brooklyn	9.7%	72
New York Hosp Med Ctr of Queens	Flushing	10.4%	192
Westchester Medical Center	Valhalla	10.6%	292
Jamaica Hospital Medical Center	Jamaica	12.3%	106
Sisters of Charity Hospital	Buffalo	13.4%	97
Univ Hosp of Brooklyn-Downstate	Brooklyn	15.1%	192

Combination Abdominal CT Scan

Hospital Name	City	Rate	Cases
Forest Hills Hospital	Forest Hills	0.0%	293
Margaretville Memorial Hospital	Margaretville	0.0%	103
Health Alliance Hospital Broadway Campus	Kingston	0.2%	463
Franklin Hospital	Valley Stream	0.3%	289
Southside Hospital	Bay Shore	0.4%	528
Claxton - Hepburn Medical Center	Ogdensburg	0.6%	494
Lutheran Medical Center	Brooklyn	0.7%	271
Saint Joseph's Hospital Health Center	Syracuse	0.7%	858
Delaware Valley Hospital	Walton	0.8%	123
New York Community Hospital of Brooklyn	Brooklyn	0.8%	132
Kings County Hospital Center	Brooklyn	0.9%	111
Plainview Hospital	Plainview	1.0%	381
Long Island Jewish Medical Center	New Hyde Park	1.2%	511
Saint Barnabas Hospital	Bronx	1.2%	166
Ellis Hospital	Schenectady	1.3%	1007
Massena Memorial Hospital	Massena	1.4%	430
Montefiore New Rochelle Hospital	New Rochelle	1.4%	213
Richmond University Medical Center	Staten Island	1.4%	286
Saint Joseph Hospital	Bethpage	1.4%	419
Eastern Niagara Hospital	Lockport	1.6%	248
Saint Anthony Community Hospital	Warwick	1.6%	250
Unity Hospital of Rochester	Rochester	1.6%	246
Maimonides Medical Center	Brooklyn	1.7%	1257
Woodhull Medical & Mental Health Center	Brooklyn	1.7%	60
Saratoga Hospital	Saratoga Spgs	1.9%	943
Winthrop - University Hospital	Mineola	1.9%	838
Good Samaritan Hospital Medical Center	West Islip	2.1%	1020
River Hospital	Alexandria Bay	2.1%	143
Oswego Hospital	Oswego	2.2%	598
White Plains Hospital Center	White Plains	2.2%	1530
John T Mather Mem Hosp-Port Jefferson	Port Jefferson	2.4%	874
Mercy Medical Center	Rockville Centre	2.4%	547
Queens Hospital Center	Jamaica	2.4%	167
Crouse Hospital	Syracuse	2.5%	685
Peconic Bay Medical Center	Riverhead	2.8%	605
Huntington Hospital	Huntington	3.0%	675
Montefiore Mount Vernon Hospital	Mount Vernon	3.0%	133
Cayuga Medical Center at Ithaca	Ithaca	3.1%	995
Kenmore Mercy Hospital	Kenmore	3.1%	458
United Memorial Medical Center	Batavia	3.2%	282
Niagara Falls Memorial Medical Center	Niagara Falls	3.3%	301
Sisters of Charity Hospital	Buffalo	3.3%	601
Catskill Regional Medical Center	Harris	3.4%	471
Saint Luke's Cornwall Hospital	Newburgh	3.4%	505
Saint Catherine of Siena Hospital	Smithtown	3.5%	484
Soldiers & Sailors Mem Hosp of Yates	Penn Yan	3.5%	173
Vassar Brothers Medical Center	Poughkeepsie	3.7%	970
Albany Memorial Hospital	Albany	3.8%	550
Little Falls Hospital	Little Falls	3.8%	316
Saint Francis Hospital - Roslyn	Roslyn	3.9%	597
Champlain Valley Phys Hosp Med Ctr	Plattsburgh	4.0%	1163
Lincoln Medical & Mental Health Center	Bronx	4.0%	175
Wyckoff Heights Medical Center	Brooklyn	4.0%	329
Chenango Memorial Hospital	Norwich	4.2%	286
Glens Falls Hospital	Glens Falls	4.2%	1559
Saint Joseph's Hospital	Elmira	4.2%	309
Ellenville Regional Hospital	Ellenville	4.4%	181
Orange Regional Medical Center	Middletown	4.5%	1345
Saint Charles Hospital	Port Jefferson	4.5%	199
Good Samaritan Hospital of Suffern	Suffern	4.6%	479
Putnam Hospital Center	Carmel	4.6%	522
Samaritan Hospital	Troy	4.6%	524
United Health Services Hospitals	Johnson City	4.6%	1274
Alice Hyde Medical Center	Malone	4.8%	434
Saint Mary's Hospital - Troy	Troy	4.9%	507
Moses - Ludington Hospital	Ticonderoga	5.0%	120
Schuyler Hospital	Montour Falls	5.0%	219
Montefiore Medical Center	Bronx	5.2%	1941
Elizabethtown Community Hospital	Elizabethtown	5.4%	130
Staten Island University Hospital	Staten Island	5.4%	1055
Nassau University Medical Center	East Meadow	5.5%	128
O'Connor Hospital	Delhi	5.5%	127
Bellevue Hospital Center	New York	5.6%	72
Kingsbrook Jewish Medical Center	Brooklyn	5.6%	213
Mount St Mary's Hosp & Health Ctr	Lewiston	5.6%	359
Flushing Hospital Medical Center	Flushing	5.8%	137
New York Methodist Hospital	Brooklyn	5.9%	460
Elmhurst Hospital Center	Elmhurst	6.0%	84
Saint Mary's Hospital at Amsterdam	Amsterdam	6.0%	688
Adirondack Medical Center	Saranac Lake	6.3%	400
Bertrand Chaffee Hospital	Springville	6.3%	128
Brookhaven Mem Hosp Med Ctr	Patchogue	6.4%	698
Cobleskill Regional Hospital	Cobleskill	6.4%	236
Cortland Regional Medical Center	Cortland	6.4%	708
Hudson Valley Hospital Center	Cortlandt Manor	6.4%	683
Arnot Ogden Medical Center	Elmira	6.6%	1235
Bronx - Lebanon Hospital Center	Bronx	6.7%	238
Mercy Hospital	Buffalo	6.8%	680
F F Thompson Hospital	Canandaigua	7.0%	329
New York Hosp Med Ctr of Queens	Flushing	7.0%	1006
Health Alliance Hosp Mary's Ave Campus	Kingston	7.1%	336
Northern Westchester Hospital	Mount Kisco	7.2%	446
Aurelia Osborn Fox Memorial Hospital	Oneonta	7.7%	376
Saint Luke's Roosevelt Hospital	New York	7.7%	626
Geneva General Hospital	Geneva	7.8%	373
Olean General Hospital	Olean	7.8%	667
Nathan Littauer Hospital	Gloversville	7.9%	405
Saint Peter's Hospital	Albany	8.0%	1111
South Nassau Communities Hospital	Oceanside	8.0%	725

NOTE: Hospital profiles are in alphabetical order by state, then city, then hospital within the city; Rankings exclude hospitals with less than 25 cases except for patient surveys which excludes hospitals with less than 100 cases; (a) 100-299 cases; (1) The number of cases/patients is too few to report; (2) Data submitted were based on a sample of cases/patients; (3) Results are based on a shorter time period than required; (4) Data suppressed by CMS for one or more quarters; (5) Results are not available for this reporting period; (6) Fewer than 100 patients completed the HCAHPS survey; (7) No cases met the criteria for this measure; (8) The lower limit of the confidence interval cannot be calculated if the number of observed infections equals zero; (9) No data are available from the state/territory for this reporting period; (10) The scores shown reflect fewer than 50 completed surveys; (11) There were discrepancies in the data collection process; (12) This measure does not apply to this hospital for this reporting period; (13) Results cannot be calculated for this reporting period; (14) The results for this state are combined with nearby states to protect confidentiality; Please refer to the User's Guide for a full explanation of data.

Rochester General Hospital	Rochester	8.2%	863
TLC Health Network	Gowanda	8.2%	195
Kaleida Health	Buffalo	8.3%	1273
Saint Francis Hospital	Poughkeepsie	8.4%	394
Glen Cove Hospital	Glen Cove	8.5%	414
Mary Imogene Bassett Hospital	Cooperstown	8.5%	586
Westfield Memorial Hospital	Westfield	8.6%	187
Albany Medical Center Hospital	Albany	8.9%	760
University Hospital - Stony Brook	Stony Brook	8.9%	1371
Erie County Medical Center	Buffalo	9.1%	416
Saint Elizabeth Medical Center	Utica	9.1%	528
Rome Memorial Hospital	Rome	9.2%	476
Northern Dutchess Hospital	Rhinebeck	9.3%	334
Ira Davenport Memorial Hospital	Bath	9.5%	168
Coney Island Hospital	Brooklyn	9.6%	83
Southampton Hospital	Southampton	9.6%	585
Univ Hosp of Brooklyn-Downstate	Brooklyn	9.6%	490
NYU Hospitals Center	New York	9.7%	515
Saint John's Riverside Hospital	Yonkers	10.1%	725
Oneida Healthcare Center	Oneida	10.5%	466
Woman's Christian Association	Jamestown	10.6%	556
Auburn Community Hospital	Auburn	10.8%	600
Medina Memorial Hospital	Medina	10.9%	129
Beth Israel Medical Center	New York	11.2%	1021
North Shore University Hospital	Manhasset	11.3%	3802
Lenox Hill Hospital	New York	11.5%	616
Mount Sinai Hospital	New York	11.5%	633
Brookdale Hospital Medical Center	Brooklyn	12.0%	166
Highland Hospital	Rochester	12.1%	447
Bon Secours Community Hospital	Port Jervis	12.2%	434
Jamaica Hospital Medical Center	Jamaica	12.3%	171
Univ Hosp SUNY Health Science Ctr	Syracuse	12.4%	1265
Carthage Area Hospital	Carthage	12.9%	233
Saint Joseph's Medical Center	Yonkers	13.5%	259
Corning Hospital	Corning	13.8%	818
Jones Memorial Hospital	Wellsville	14.2%	226
Community Memorial Hospital	Hamilton	14.6%	130
Harlem Hospital Center	New York	14.7%	75
Nyack Hospital	Nyack	14.7%	617
Eastern Long Island Hospital	Greenport	15.5%	264
Our Lady of Lourdes Memorial Hospital	Binghamton	15.6%	1447
Phelps Memorial Hospital Assn	Sleepy Hollow	15.9%	723
Faxton - Saint Luke's Healthcare	Utica	16.7%	336
Canton - Potsdam Hospital	Potsdam	17.7%	674
Wyoming County Community Hospital	Warsaw	17.9%	117
Columbia Memorial Hospital	Hudson	18.0%	840
Brooks Memorial Hospital	Dunkirk	18.2%	292
New York - Presbyterian Hospital	New York	18.3%	2257
Brooklyn Hosp Ctr at Downtown Campus	Brooklyn	18.7%	241
Lewis County General Hospital	Lowville	19.0%	253
Strong Memorial Hospital	Rochester	19.2%	983
Lawrence Hospital Center	Bronxville	20.7%	589
Saint James Mercy Hospital	Hornell	21.5%	275
Clifton Springs Hospital & Clinic	Clifton Springs	22.4%	246
Nicholas H Noyes Memorial Hospital	Dansville	23.2%	211
Jacobi Medical Center	Bronx	27.3%	99
Westchester Medical Center	Valhalla	27.5%	542
Newark - Wayne Community Hospital	Newark	29.0%	293
Samaritan Medical Center	Watertown	33.3%	757
Long Beach Medical Center	Long Beach	59.3%	81
St John's Episcopal Hosp-South Shore	Far Rockaway	71.0%	383

Combination Brain/Sinus CT Scan

Hospital Name	City	Rate	Cases
Catskill Reg Med Ctr-G Hermann Site	Callicoon	0.0%	43
Cobleskill Regional Hospital	Cobleskill	0.0%	152
Community Memorial Hospital	Hamilton	0.0%	131
Moses - Ludington Hospital	Ticonderoga	0.0%	148
Westchester Medical Center	Valhalla	0.4%	258
Jacobi Medical Center	Bronx	0.6%	158
Elizabethtown Community Hospital	Elizabethtown	0.7%	138
Little Falls Hospital	Little Falls	0.8%	247
Saint Mary's Hospital - Troy	Troy	0.8%	359
Montefiore Medical Center	Bronx	1.0%	1532
Canton - Potsdam Hospital	Potsdam	1.3%	371
Saint Catherine of Siena Hospital	Smithtown	1.3%	615
Woman's Christian Association	Jamestown	1.5%	550
Phelps Memorial Hospital Assn	Sleepy Hollow	1.6%	611
Saint Francis Hospital - Roslyn	Roslyn	1.6%	682
Alice Hyde Medical Center	Malone	1.7%	355
Lenox Hill Hospital	New York	1.7%	401
Saint Joseph's Medical Center	Yonkers	1.7%	350
Saint Peter's Hospital	Albany	1.7%	761
Sisters of Charity Hospital	Buffalo	1.7%	465
Mercy Hospital	Buffalo	1.8%	566
Forest Hills Hospital	Forest Hills	1.9%	411
Hudson Valley Hospital Center	Cortlandt Manor	1.9%	686
Saint Joseph Hospital	Bethpage	1.9%	904
Southampton Hospital	Southampton	2.0%	405
Mercy Medical Center	Rockville Centre	2.2%	601
Champlain Valley Phys Hosp Med Ctr	Plattsburgh	2.3%	786
Staten Island University Hospital	Staten Island	2.3%	771
Saint Elizabeth Medical Center	Utica	2.4%	583
New York - Presbyterian Hospital	New York	2.5%	1722
Orange Regional Medical Center	Middletown	2.5%	1341
Vassar Brothers Medical Center	Poughkeepsie	2.5%	1468
Glens Falls Hospital	Glens Falls	2.6%	1101
Arnot Ogden Medical Center	Elmira	2.7%	921
Columbia Memorial Hospital	Hudson	2.7%	708
Saint Joseph's Hospital Health Center	Syracuse	2.7%	1394
Rochester General Hospital	Rochester	2.8%	798
Saratoga Hospital	Saratoga Spgs	3.0%	821
Peconic Bay Medical Center	Riverhead	3.1%	702
University Hospital - Stony Brook	Stony Brook	3.1%	982
Univ Hosp SUNY Health Science Ctr	Syracuse	3.1%	1075
Saint John's Riverside Hospital	Yonkers	3.2%	634
Crouse Hospital	Syracuse	3.4%	875
Long Island Jewish Medical Center	New Hyde Park	3.5%	718
United Health Services Hospitals	Johnson City	3.5%	1187
Kaleida Health	Buffalo	3.6%	1309
Good Samaritan Hospital Medical Center	West Islip	3.9%	1247
North Shore University Hospital	Manhasset	3.9%	2036
Olean General Hospital	Olean	3.9%	592
St John's Episcopal Hosp-South Shore	Far Rockaway	3.9%	485
South Nassau Communities Hospital	Oceanside	3.9%	1002
Winthrop - University Hospital	Mineola	3.9%	674
NYU Hospitals Center	New York	4.0%	503
Ellis Hospital	Schenectady	4.1%	1128
John T Mather Mem Hosp-Port Jefferson	Port Jefferson	4.2%	721
Wyckoff Heights Medical Center	Brooklyn	4.3%	351
Good Samaritan Hospital of Suffern	Suffern	4.4%	563
Mount Sinai Hospital	New York	4.4%	778
Saint Mary's Hospital at Amsterdam	Amsterdam	4.4%	635
New York Methodist Hospital	Brooklyn	4.5%	463
Our Lady of Lourdes Memorial Hospital	Binghamton	4.5%	1054
Richmond University Medical Center	Staten Island	4.5%	309
Univ Hosp of Brooklyn-Downstate	Brooklyn	4.5%	490
Highland Hospital	Rochester	4.6%	454
Putnam Hospital Center	Carmel	4.6%	584
Cayuga Medical Center at Ithaca	Ithaca	4.7%	791
Huntington Hospital	Huntington	4.8%	958
Kings County Hospital Center	Brooklyn	4.9%	203
Nyack Hospital	Nyack	4.9%	818
White Plains Hospital Center	White Plains	4.9%	1520
Cortland Regional Medical Center	Cortland	5.0%	496
Kenmore Mercy Hospital	Kenmore	5.0%	340
Saint Francis Hospital	Poughkeepsie	5.0%	440
Saint Luke's Cornwall Hospital	Newburgh	5.0%	675
Samaritan Medical Center	Watertown	5.0%	585
Beth Israel Medical Center	New York	5.1%	1180
Oswego Hospital	Oswego	5.1%	434
Aurelia Osborn Fox Memorial Hospital	Oneonta	5.2%	424
Health Alliance Hospital Broadway Campus	Kingston	5.2%	674
Strong Memorial Hospital	Rochester	5.2%	716
Brookhaven Mem Hosp Med Ctr	Patchogue	5.3%	789
New York Hosp Med Ctr of Queens	Flushing	5.3%	1212
Jamaica Hospital Medical Center	Jamaica	5.6%	449
Mount St Mary's Hosp & Health Ctr	Lewiston	5.7%	316
Maimonides Medical Center	Brooklyn	5.9%	1015
Glen Cove Hospital	Glen Cove	6.1%	492
Massena Memorial Hospital	Massena	6.2%	274
Southside Hospital	Bay Shore	6.4%	903
Flushing Hospital Medical Center	Flushing	7.1%	336
Erie County Medical Center	Buffalo	7.3%	440
New York Community Hospital of Brooklyn	Brooklyn	7.4%	285
Saint Joseph's Hospital	Elmira	7.5%	279
Lincoln Medical & Mental Health Center	Bronx	7.8%	218
Coney Island Hospital	Brooklyn	9.3%	129
Lutheran Medical Center	Brooklyn	10.6%	555
Nassau University Medical Center	East Meadow	17.0%	264

Combination Chest CT Scan

Hospital Name	City	Rate	Cases
Alice Hyde Medical Center	Malone	0.0%	270
Aurelia Osborn Fox Memorial Hospital	Oneonta	0.0%	150
Brookdale Hospital Medical Center	Brooklyn	0.0%	117
Cayuga Medical Center at Ithaca	Ithaca	0.0%	527
Chenango Memorial Hospital	Norwich	0.0%	146
Delaware Valley Hospital	Walton	0.0%	53
Elizabethtown Community Hospital	Elizabethtown	0.0%	122
Ellenville Regional Hospital	Ellenville	0.0%	81
Elmhurst Hospital Center	Elmhurst	0.0%	47
Erie County Medical Center	Buffalo	0.0%	181
F F Thompson Hospital	Canandaigua	0.0%	167
Forest Hills Hospital	Forest Hills	0.0%	61
Health Alliance Hospital Broadway Campus	Kingston	0.0%	89
Health Alliance Hosp Mary's Ave Campus	Kingston	0.0%	268
Hospital For Special Surgery	New York	0.0%	63
Lutheran Medical Center	Brooklyn	0.0%	144
Margaretville Memorial Hospital	Margaretville	0.0%	56
Massena Memorial Hospital	Massena	0.0%	255
Mercy Medical Center	Rockville Centre	0.0%	357
Montefiore Mount Vernon Hospital	Mount Vernon	0.0%	75
Montefiore New Rochelle Hospital	New Rochelle	0.0%	87
New York Hosp Med Ctr of Queens	Flushing	0.0%	415
O'Connor Hospital	Delhi	0.0%	95
Queens Hospital Center	Jamaica	0.0%	117
Richmond University Medical Center	Staten Island	0.0%	123
River Hospital	Alexandria Bay	0.0%	64
Saint Anthony Community Hospital	Warwick	0.0%	167
Saint Barnabas Hospital	Bronx	0.0%	49
St John's Episcopal Hosp-South Shore	Far Rockaway	0.0%	224
Saint Joseph Hospital	Bethpage	0.0%	118
Saint Joseph's Hospital Health Center	Syracuse	0.0%	256
Saint Luke's Cornwall Hospital	Newburgh	0.0%	205
Saint Mary's Hospital - Troy	Troy	0.0%	196
Samaritan Hospital	Troy	0.0%	276
Soldiers & Sailors Mem Hosp of Yates	Penn Yan	0.0%	66
South Nassau Communities Hospital	Oceanside	0.0%	509
Southside Hospital	Bay Shore	0.0%	142
Wyckoff Heights Medical Center	Brooklyn	0.0%	125
Arnot Ogden Medical Center	Elmira	0.1%	685
Glens Falls Hospital	Glens Falls	0.1%	1115
Strong Memorial Hospital	Rochester	0.1%	684
White Plains Hospital Center	White Plains	0.1%	1519
Champlain Valley Phys Hosp Med Ctr	Plattsburgh	0.2%	989
Samaritan Medical Center	Watertown	0.2%	535
Southampton Hospital	Southampton	0.2%	525
Claxton - Hepburn Medical Center	Ogdensburg	0.3%	312
Glen Cove Hospital	Glen Cove	0.3%	385
Huntington Hospital	Huntington	0.3%	322
Mount St Mary's Hosp & Health Ctr	Lewiston	0.3%	326
NYU Hospitals Center	New York	0.3%	704
Phelps Memorial Hospital Assn	Sleepy Hollow	0.3%	646
Saint Mary's Hospital at Amsterdam	Amsterdam	0.3%	382
North Shore University Hospital	Manhasset	0.4%	3716
Sisters of Charity Hospital	Buffalo	0.4%	230
Univ Hosp of Brooklyn-Downstate	Brooklyn	0.4%	263
Winthrop - University Hospital	Mineola	0.4%	762
Eastern Long Island Hospital	Greenport	0.5%	193
Good Samaritan Hospital Medical Center	West Islip	0.5%	820
Good Samaritan Hospital of Suffern	Suffern	0.5%	222
University Hospital - Stony Brook	Stony Brook	0.5%	1373
John T Mather Mem Hosp-Port Jefferson	Port Jefferson	0.6%	678
Little Falls Hospital	Little Falls	0.6%	177
Geneva General Hospital	Geneva	0.7%	138
Orange Regional Medical Center	Middletown	0.7%	902
Peconic Bay Medical Center	Riverhead	0.7%	289
Saint James Mercy Hospital	Hornell	0.7%	151
Saint John's Riverside Hospital	Yonkers	0.7%	705
Saint Luke's Roosevelt Hospital	New York	0.7%	298
Jamaica Hospital Medical Center	Jamaica	0.8%	120
Lincoln Medical & Mental Health Center	Bronx	0.8%	132
Long Island Jewish Medical Center	New Hyde Park	0.8%	133
Saint Joseph's Hospital	Elmira	0.8%	123
Saint Joseph's Medical Center	Yonkers	0.8%	128
Catskill Regional Medical Center	Harris	0.9%	231
Mercy Hospital	Buffalo	0.9%	215
Putnam Hospital Center	Carmel	0.9%	460
Saratoga Hospital	Saratoga Spgs	0.9%	441
United Memorial Medical Center	Batavia	0.9%	110
Westchester Medical Center	Valhalla	0.9%	462
Albany Medical Center Hospital	Albany	1.0%	604
Corning Hospital	Corning	1.0%	504
Univ Hosp SUNY Health Science Ctr	Syracuse	1.0%	1254
Woman's Christian Association	Jamestown	1.0%	298
Eastern Niagara Hospital	Lockport	1.1%	180
Highland Hospital	Rochester	1.2%	170
Hudson Valley Hospital Center	Cortlandt Manor	1.2%	574
Kenmore Mercy Hospital	Kenmore	1.2%	169
Maimonides Medical Center	Brooklyn	1.3%	751
Mary Imogene Bassett Hospital	Cooperstown	1.3%	540
Northern Dutchess Hospital	Rhinebeck	1.3%	160
Oneida Healthcare Center	Oneida	1.3%	152
Plainview Hospital	Plainview	1.3%	78
Saint Francis Hospital - Roslyn	Roslyn	1.3%	683
Northern Westchester Hospital	Mount Kisco	1.4%	218
Saint Charles Hospital	Port Jefferson	1.4%	148
Albany Memorial Hospital	Albany	1.5%	264
New York - Presbyterian Hospital	New York	1.5%	2375
Cobleskill Regional Hospital	Cobleskill	1.7%	175
Nassau University Medical Center	East Meadow	1.7%	58
Montefiore Medical Center	Bronx	1.8%	1566
Canton - Potsdam Hospital	Potsdam	1.9%	473
Crouse Hospital	Syracuse	2.0%	350
Oswego Hospital	Oswego	2.0%	456
Clifton Springs Hospital & Clinic	Clifton Springs	2.1%	191
Schuyler Hospital	Montour Falls	2.2%	90
Franklin Hospital	Valley Stream	2.3%	87
Saint Elizabeth Medical Center	Utica	2.3%	301
Kingsbrook Jewish Medical Center	Brooklyn	2.4%	125
United Health Services Hospitals	Johnson City	2.4%	742
Carthage Area Hospital	Carthage	2.5%	120

NOTE: Hospital profiles are in alphabetical order by state, then city, then hospital within the city; Rankings exclude hospitals with less than 25 cases except for patient surveys which excludes hospitals with less than 100 cases; (a) 100-299 cases; (1) The number of cases/patients is too few to report; (2) Data submitted were based on a sample of cases/patients; (3) Results are based on a shorter time period than required; (4) Data suppressed by CMS for one or more quarters; (5) Results are not available for this reporting period; (6) Fewer than 100 patients completed the HCAHPS survey; (7) No cases met the criteria for this measure; (8) The lower limit of the confidence interval cannot be calculated if the number of observed infections equals zero; (9) No data are available from the state/territory for this reporting period; (10) The scores shown reflect fewer than 50 completed surveys; (11) There were discrepancies in the data collection process; (12) This measure does not apply to this hospital for this reporting period; (13) Results cannot be calculated for this reporting period; (14) The results for this state are combined with nearby states to protect confidentiality; Please refer to the User's Guide for a full explanation of data.

Hospital Name	City	Rate	Cases
Kings County Hospital Center	Brooklyn	2.7%	74
New York Methodist Hospital	Brooklyn	2.7%	370
Vassar Brothers Medical Center	Poughkeepsie	2.7%	297
Ellis Hospital	Schenectady	2.8%	742
Staten Island University Hospital	Staten Island	2.8%	740
Olean General Hospital	Olean	2.9%	210
Rome Memorial Hospital	Rome	3.0%	366
Brooklyn Hosp Ctr at Downtown Campus	Brooklyn	3.1%	127
TLC Health Network	Gowanda	3.3%	92
Bellevue Hospital Center	New York	3.4%	59
Cortland Regional Medical Center	Cortland	3.5%	287
Flushing Hospital Medical Center	Flushing	3.7%	54
Ira Davenport Memorial Hospital	Bath	3.8%	52
Lenox Hill Hospital	New York	4.1%	459
Auburn Community Hospital	Auburn	4.3%	210
Beth Israel Medical Center	New York	4.4%	708
Saint Catherine of Siena Hospital	Smithtown	4.4%	205
Adirondack Medical Center	Saranac Lake	4.5%	314
Moses - Ludington Hospital	Ticonderoga	4.5%	66
Nathan Littauer Hospital	Gloversville	4.5%	202
Brookhaven Mem Hosp Med Ctr	Patchogue	4.6%	434
Bon Secours Community Hospital	Port Jervis	4.7%	233
Bronx - Lebanon Hospital Center	Bronx	4.7%	86
Newark - Wayne Community Hospital	Newark	5.0%	181
Saint Peter's Hospital	Albany	5.1%	749
Columbia Memorial Hospital	Hudson	5.2%	796
Kaleida Health	Buffalo	6.2%	451
Rochester General Hospital	Rochester	6.4%	642
Community Memorial Hospital	Hamilton	6.9%	87
Niagara Falls Memorial Medical Center	Niagara Falls	7.1%	140
Lawrence Hospital Center	Bronxville	7.2%	389
Mount Sinai Hospital	New York	7.8%	193
Lewis County General Hospital	Lowville	8.6%	116
Nyack Hospital	Nyack	8.8%	430
Faxton - Saint Luke's Healthcare	Utica	9.0%	433
Nicholas H Noyes Memorial Hospital	Dansville	9.0%	122
Our Lady of Lourdes Memorial Hospital	Binghamton	10.8%	1076
Jones Memorial Hospital	Wellsville	11.6%	69
Saint Francis Hospital	Poughkeepsie	11.6%	146
Brooks Memorial Hospital	Dunkirk	15.3%	72
Jacobi Medical Center	Bronx	17.5%	97

Follow-up Mammogram/Ultrasound

A follow-up rate near zero may indicate missed cancer; a rate higher than 14% may mean there is unnecessary follow up.

Hospital Name	City	Rate	Cases
Community Memorial Hospital	Hamilton	1.1%	276
Rome Memorial Hospital	Rome	1.9%	432
Newark - Wayne Community Hospital	Newark	2.3%	221
North Central Bronx Hospital	Bronx	2.6%	114
Aurelia Osborn Fox Memorial Hospital	Oneonta	3.0%	807
Bon Secours Community Hospital	Port Jervis	3.2%	593
Canton - Potsdam Hospital	Potsdam	3.3%	1038
Jacobi Medical Center	Bronx	3.4%	291
Oneida Healthcare Center	Oneida	3.5%	375
Eastern Niagara Hospital	Lockport	4.3%	601
Woman's Christian Association	Jamestown	4.4%	1131
Cortland Regional Medical Center	Cortland	4.5%	597
F F Thompson Hospital	Canandaigua	4.5%	666
Montefiore Medical Center	Bronx	4.9%	3017
Samaritan Medical Center	Watertown	5.0%	1313
United Memorial Medical Center	Batavia	5.0%	321
Saratoga Hospital	Saratoga Spgs	5.1%	1086
Arnot Ogden Medical Center	Elmira	5.2%	1870
Brookdale Hospital Medical Center	Brooklyn	5.2%	287
Cayuga Medical Center at Ithaca	Ithaca	5.2%	1377
Crouse Hospital	Syracuse	5.2%	1151
Brooks Memorial Hospital	Dunkirk	5.3%	513
Erie County Medical Center	Buffalo	5.3%	94
Oswego Hospital	Oswego	5.4%	1631
Rochester General Hospital	Rochester	5.4%	423
TLC Health Network	Gowanda	5.4%	315
New York Methodist Hospital	Brooklyn	6.0%	910
Bronx - Lebanon Hospital Center	Bronx	6.2%	177
Westfield Memorial Hospital	Westfield	6.2%	290
Saint Elizabeth Medical Center	Utica	6.3%	736
Health Alliance Hosp Mary's Ave Campus	Kingston	6.4%	1493
Niagara Falls Memorial Medical Center	Niagara Falls	6.4%	691
Ira Davenport Memorial Hospital	Bath	6.5%	168
Wyckoff Heights Medical Center	Brooklyn	6.5%	434
New York - Presbyterian Hospital	New York	6.8%	2308
Margaretville Memorial Hospital	Margaretville	6.9%	101
O'Connor Hospital	Delhi	6.9%	259
Bellevue Hospital Center	New York	7.2%	97
Little Falls Hospital	Little Falls	7.2%	291
Lutheran Medical Center	Brooklyn	7.2%	166
Massena Memorial Hospital	Massena	7.3%	551
Montefiore Mount Vernon Hospital	Mount Vernon	7.3%	384
Saint Peter's Hospital	Albany	7.3%	1936
Saint Joseph's Hospital	Elmira	7.5%	495
Kenmore Mercy Hospital	Kenmore	7.7%	365
Schuyler Hospital	Montour Falls	7.7%	297
Saint Mary's Hospital - Troy	Troy	7.8%	734
Mercy Hospital	Buffalo	7.9%	608
Auburn Community Hospital	Auburn	8.0%	609
Champlain Valley Phys Hosp Med Ctr	Plattsburgh	8.0%	2587
Medina Memorial Hospital	Medina	8.0%	251
Ellis Hospital	Schenectady	8.1%	2162
Moses - Ludington Hospital	Ticonderoga	8.1%	161
Albany Memorial Hospital	Albany	8.2%	982
Columbia Memorial Hospital	Hudson	8.2%	1588
Jones Memorial Hospital	Wellsville	8.2%	404
River Hospital	Alexandria Bay	8.4%	131
Staten Island University Hospital	Staten Island	8.4%	2820
Saint James Mercy Hospital	Hornell	8.5%	260
Clifton Springs Hospital & Clinic	Clifton Springs	8.6%	348
Lewis County General Hospital	Lowville	8.7%	576
Mary Imogene Bassett Hospital	Cooperstown	8.9%	2084
Jamaica Hospital Medical Center	Jamaica	9.1%	363
Catskill Regional Medical Center	Harris	9.2%	262
Bertrand Chaffee Hospital	Springville	9.4%	171
Olean General Hospital	Olean	9.4%	234
Ellenville Regional Hospital	Ellenville	9.5%	116
Saint Anthony Community Hospital	Warwick	9.5%	411
Univ Hosp of Brooklyn-Downstate	Brooklyn	9.5%	944
Nathan Littauer Hospital	Gloversville	9.6%	698
Beth Israel Medical Center	New York	9.7%	1802
Kingsbrook Jewish Medical Center	Brooklyn	9.7%	268
Soldiers & Sailors Mem Hosp of Yates	Penn Yan	9.8%	305
Carthage Area Hospital	Carthage	9.9%	172
Sisters of Charity Hospital	Buffalo	10.0%	529
Glens Falls Hospital	Glens Falls	10.1%	1769
Highland Hospital	Rochester	10.1%	975
Northern Dutchess Hospital	Rhinebeck	10.3%	614
Woodhull Medical & Mental Health Center	Brooklyn	10.3%	126
Our Lady of Lourdes Memorial Hospital	Binghamton	10.6%	2596
Saint Barnabas Hospital	Bronx	10.6%	161
Alice Hyde Medical Center	Malone	10.7%	831
Saint Mary's Hospital at Amsterdam	Amsterdam	10.8%	1138
Kaleida Health	Buffalo	10.9%	764
Cobleskill Regional Hospital	Cobleskill	11.1%	451
Mount St Mary's Hosp & Health Ctr	Lewiston	11.1%	612
Nassau University Medical Center	East Meadow	11.2%	295
Brooklyn Hosp Ctr at Downtown Campus	Brooklyn	11.3%	301
Elizabethtown Community Hospital	Elizabethtown	11.4%	272
Strong Memorial Hospital	Rochester	11.7%	333
Albany Medical Center Hospital	Albany	12.3%	861
Samaritan Hospital	Troy	12.6%	499
Corning Hospital	Corning	12.8%	1163
North Shore University Hospital	Manhasset	12.8%	1996
Glen Cove Hospital	Glen Cove	13.0%	740
Orange Regional Medical Center	Middletown	13.1%	1615
Claxton - Hepburn Medical Center	Ogdensburg	13.9%	1129
Flushing Hospital Medical Center	Flushing	13.9%	101
Elmhurst Hospital Center	Elmhurst	14.0%	107
Saint Joseph's Hospital Health Center	Syracuse	14.2%	204
New York Hosp Med Ctr of Queens	Flushing	14.3%	1236
Nyack Hospital	Nyack	14.4%	749
Queens Hospital Center	Jamaica	14.5%	152
United Health Services Hospitals	Johnson City	14.6%	2343
Delaware Valley Hospital	Walton	14.7%	143
Geneva General Hospital	Geneva	14.7%	600
University Hospital - Stony Brook	Stony Brook	14.8%	1552
Univ Hosp SUNY Health Science Ctr	Syracuse	15.0%	1723
Faxton - Saint Luke's Healthcare	Utica	15.1%	1644
Maimonides Medical Center	Brooklyn	15.1%	631
Brookhaven Mem Hosp Med Ctr	Patchogue	15.4%	1315
Saint Joseph's Medical Center	Yonkers	15.4%	435
Saint Luke's Cornwall Hospital	Newburgh	15.5%	116
Southampton Hospital	Southampton	15.7%	1264
Good Samaritan Hospital Medical Center	West Islip	15.9%	2079
Harlem Hospital Center	New York	15.9%	88
Interfaith Medical Center	Brooklyn	15.9%	69
NYU Hospitals Center	New York	16.1%	1860
Peconic Bay Medical Center	Riverhead	16.2%	68
Chenango Memorial Hospital	Norwich	16.6%	709
Saint Francis Hospital	Poughkeepsie	16.9%	320
Hudson Valley Hospital Center	Cortlandt Manor	17.2%	1155
Vassar Brothers Medical Center	Poughkeepsie	17.5%	832
Forest Hills Hospital	Forest Hills	17.8%	73
Saint Luke's Roosevelt Hospital	New York	17.9%	190
Mount Sinai Hospital	New York	18.0%	1557
Eastern Long Island Hospital	Greenport	18.8%	320
Saint John's Riverside Hospital	Yonkers	18.9%	1694
Putnam Hospital Center	Carmel	19.6%	866
Nicholas H Noyes Memorial Hospital	Dansville	20.4%	289
Montefiore New Rochelle Hospital	New Rochelle	21.5%	135
Westchester Medical Center	Valhalla	22.5%	445
Phelps Memorial Hospital Assn	Sleepy Hollow	22.6%	1521
Lawrence Hospital Center	Bronxville	22.8%	605
Wyoming County Community Hospital	Warsaw	24.0%	146
Adirondack Medical Center	Saranac Lake	26.2%	804
St John's Episcopal Hosp-South Shore	Far Rockaway	26.4%	299
Saint Charles Hospital	Port Jefferson	28.9%	346
Winthrop - University Hospital	Mineola	29.6%	609
Good Samaritan Hospital of Suffern	Suffern	30.0%	434
Richmond University Medical Center	Staten Island	30.2%	149
Northern Westchester Hospital	Mount Kisco	32.8%	491
Mercy Medical Center	Rockville Centre	38.3%	738
Huntington Hospital	Huntington	41.1%	912
White Plains Hospital Center	White Plains	41.3%	2143
Long Beach Medical Center	Long Beach	41.4%	58
Saint Francis Hospital - Roslyn	Roslyn	45.9%	713
Saint Catherine of Siena Hospital	Smithtown	49.8%	261
John T Mather Mem Hosp-Port Jefferson	Port Jefferson	50.0%	2020
Lenox Hill Hospital	New York	54.4%	272
South Nassau Communities Hospital	Oceanside	60.6%	1184

Lumbar Spine MRI for Low Back Pain

Hospital Name	City	Rate	Cases
Montefiore Medical Center	Bronx	21.4%	131
NYU Hospitals Center	New York	23.6%	297
Canton - Potsdam Hospital	Potsdam	28.9%	121
Orange Regional Medical Center	Middletown	28.9%	83
Bon Secours Community Hospital	Port Jervis	29.3%	99
Glen Cove Hospital	Glen Cove	29.7%	91
Ellis Hospital	Schenectady	29.9%	67
Woman's Christian Association	Jamestown	29.9%	107
Aurelia Osborn Fox Memorial Hospital	Oneonta	30.0%	60
Arnot Ogden Medical Center	Elmira	30.4%	112
North Shore University Hospital	Manhasset	30.9%	330
Rome Memorial Hospital	Rome	30.9%	55
University Hospital - Stony Brook	Stony Brook	30.9%	94
Samaritan Medical Center	Watertown	31.7%	63
Albany Memorial Hospital	Albany	32.1%	56
Southampton Hospital	Southampton	32.1%	109
Hospital For Special Surgery	New York	32.4%	624
Staten Island University Hospital	Staten Island	32.5%	80
Our Lady of Lourdes Memorial Hospital	Binghamton	32.8%	174
Oswego Hospital	Oswego	32.9%	70
Alice Hyde Medical Center	Malone	33.3%	60
Hudson Valley Hospital Center	Cortlandt Manor	33.3%	123
New York - Presbyterian Hospital	New York	33.3%	132
Champlain Valley Phys Hosp Med Ctr	Plattsburgh	33.8%	154
Saratoga Hospital	Saratoga Spgs	34.1%	91
Columbia Memorial Hospital	Hudson	34.8%	112
Putnam Hospital Center	Carmel	34.8%	46
Kaleida Health	Buffalo	35.0%	60
Albany Medical Center Hospital	Albany	36.2%	47
Peconic Bay Medical Center	Riverhead	36.2%	69
Eastern Long Island Hospital	Greenport	36.5%	52
Lawrence Hospital Center	Bronxville	36.8%	87
Saint John's Riverside Hospital	Yonkers	36.8%	106
Beth Israel Medical Center	New York	36.9%	65
Saint Mary's Hospital at Amsterdam	Amsterdam	37.5%	64
Niagara Falls Memorial Medical Center	Niagara Falls	38.5%	65
F F Thompson Hospital	Canandaigua	38.8%	49
Claxton - Hepburn Medical Center	Ogdensburg	39.0%	41
Cayuga Medical Center at Ithaca	Ithaca	39.8%	118
Mary Imogene Bassett Hospital	Cooperstown	40.2%	127
Phelps Memorial Hospital Assn	Sleepy Hollow	40.3%	62
Chenango Memorial Hospital	Norwich	40.4%	52
Nathan Littauer Hospital	Gloversville	40.5%	84
Saint Joseph's Hospital	Elmira	40.7%	86
Saint Peter's Hospital	Albany	40.7%	59
Strong Memorial Hospital	Rochester	42.1%	38
Corning Hospital	Corning	44.1%	102
Mount St Mary's Hosp & Health Ctr	Lewiston	45.8%	59
Rochester General Hospital	Rochester	47.0%	66
Health Alliance Hospital Broadway Campus	Kingston	50.0%	32
Brooks Memorial Hospital	Dunkirk	52.5%	40

NOTE: Hospital profiles are in alphabetical order by state, then city, then hospital within the city; Rankings exclude hospitals with less than 25 cases except for patient surveys which excludes hospitals with less than 100 cases; (a) 100-299 cases; (1) The number of cases/patients is too few to report; (2) Data submitted were based on a sample of cases/patients; (3) Results are based on a shorter time period than required; (4) Data suppressed by CMS for one or more quarters; (5) Results are not available for this reporting period; (6) Fewer than 100 patients completed the HCAHPS survey; (7) No cases met the criteria for this measure; (8) The lower limit of the confidence interval cannot be calculated if the number of observed infections equals zero; (9) No data are available from the state/territory for this reporting period; (10) The scores shown reflect fewer than 50 completed surveys; (11) There were discrepancies in the data collection process; (12) This measure does not apply to this hospital for this reporting period; (13) Results cannot be calculated for this reporting period; (14) The results for this state are combined with nearby states to protect confidentiality; Please refer to the User's Guide for a full explanation of data.

Albany Medical Center Hospital

43 New Scotland Avenue Phone: 518-262-3125
Albany, NY 12208 Fax: 518-262-3398
Type: Acute Care Hospitals Emergency Services: Yes
Ownership: Voluntary non-profit - Private Beds: 651

Key Personnel:
CEO/President. . . . . James J Barba
Chief of Medical Staff. . . . . James Hoehn, MD
Quality Assurance . . . . Vickey Masta
Emergency Room . . . . Vincent Verdial, MD

Measure	Cases	This Hosp.	State Avg.	U.S. Avg.
Blood Clot Prevention and Treatment				
Anticoagulation Overlap Therapy[2]	86	84%	91%	93%
ICU Venous Thromboembolism Prophylaxis[2]	81	79%	92%	92%
Incidence of Potentially Preventable VTE[2]	38	24%	10%	10%
UFH with Dosages/Platelet Monitoring[2]	86	23%	92%	97%
Venous Thromboembolism Prophylaxis[2]	330	58%	87%	85%
Warfarin Therapy Discharge Instructions[2]	64	72%	59%	75%
Chest Pain/Possible Heart Attack Care				
Aspirin Given Within 24 Hours of Arrival[5]	-	-	97%	96%
Fibrinolytic Meds Within 30 Min. of Arrival[5]	-	-	54%	58%
Average Time to ECG (minutes)[5]	-	-	9	7
Average Time to Transfer (minutes)[5]	-	-	78	60
Children's Asthma Care				
Received Home Management Plan of Care	-	-	-	88%
Received Reliever Medication	-	-	-	100%
Received Systemic Corticosteroids	-	-	-	100%
Emergency Department				
Admittance Decision Time (minutes)[2]	489	180	154	98
Head CT Results Within 45 Min. of Arrival[7]	-	-	55%	57%
Patients Who Left ER Before Being Seen	72,219	2%	2%	2%
Time from ER Arrival to Admit. (minutes)[2]	494	389	378	274
Time from ER Arrival to Discharge (minutes)	325	224	156	134
Time in ER Before Being Evaluated (minutes)	251	38	35	26
Time to Pain Meds for Fractures (minutes)	199	79	61	57
Heart Attack Care				
Aspirin Given at Discharge	458	100%	99%	99%
Fibrinolytic Meds Within 30 Min. of Arrival[1]	-	-	46%	54%
PCI Within 90 Minutes of Arrival	82	98%	95%	96%
Statin Prescribed at Discharge	447	100%	98%	98%
Heart Failure Care				
ACE Inhibitor or ARB for LVSD	125	100%	96%	97%
Discharge Instructions Given	298	97%	95%	94%
Evaluation of LVS Function	354	100%	99%	99%
Medicare Spending				
Medicare Spending per Patient (ratio)	-	0.96	0.96	0.98
Pneumonia Care				
Appropriate Initial Antibiotic Given	103	97%	95%	95%
Blood Culture Timing	163	99%	97%	98%
Pregnancy and Delivery Care				
Newborn Deliveries Scheduled Early[2]	21	0%	4%	6%
Preventive Care				
Immunization for Influenza[2]	526	91%	88%	90%
Immunization for Pneumonia[2]	546	91%	88%	92%
Stroke Care				
Anticoagulation Therapy for Atrial Fibrillation	62	95%	96%	95%
Antithrombotic Therapy Timing	275	97%	98%	98%
Assessed for Rehabilitation	480	98%	97%	97%
Discharged on Antithrombotic Therapy	334	100%	99%	99%
Discharged on Statin Medication	246	96%	95%	94%
Thrombolytic Therapy Timing	29	66%	69%	66%
Venous Thromboembolism Prophylaxis	517	93%	94%	94%
Written Stroke Educational Materials Given	274	81%	86%	88%
Surgical Care Improvement Project				
Appropriate Beta Blocker Usage[2]	165	99%	97%	98%
Appropriate VTP Within 24 Hours[2]	298	97%	98%	98%
Controlled Postoperative Blood Glucose[2]	121	99%	97%	97%
Perioperative Temperature Management[2]	450	100%	100%	100%
Prophylactic Antibiotic Selection[2]	369	100%	99%	99%
Prophylactic Antibiotic Selection (Outpatient)	713	99%	97%	98%
Prophylactic Antibiotic Stopped[2]	369	99%	98%	98%
Prophylactic Antibiotic Timing[2]	373	100%	99%	99%
Prophylactic Antibiotic Timing (Outpatient)	715	99%	97%	98%
Urinary Catheter Removal[2]	194	99%	96%	97%
Survey of Patients' Hospital Experiences				
Area Around Room 'Always' Quiet at Night	300+	44%	51%	61%
Doctors 'Always' Communicated Well	300+	70%	77%	82%
Home Recovery Information Given	300+	82%	83%	85%
Hospital Given 9 or 10 on 10 Point Scale	300+	63%	63%	71%
Meds 'Always' Explained Before Given	300+	56%	59%	64%
Nurses 'Always' Communicated Well	300+	73%	75%	79%
Pain 'Always' Well Controlled	300+	65%	67%	71%
Room and Bathroom 'Always' Clean	300+	66%	69%	73%
Timely Help 'Always' Received	300+	60%	61%	68%
Would Definitely Recommend Hospital	300+	70%	65%	71%
Use of Medical Imaging				
Cardiac Imaging Stress Test before Surgery	193	6.7%	5.8%	5.3%
Combination Abdominal CT Scan	760	8.9%	8.2%	10.5%
Combination Brain/Sinus CT Scan[1]	-	-	3.6%	2.7%
Combination Chest CT Scan	604	1.0%	1.3%	2.7%
Follow-up Mammogram/Ultrasound	861	12.3%	13%	8.8%
Lumbar Spine MRI for Low Back Pain	47	36.2%	33.4%	37.2%

Albany Memorial Hospital

600 Northern Boulevard Phone: 518-471-3221
Albany, NY 12204 Fax: 518-449-4410
URL: www.nehealth.com
Type: Acute Care Hospitals Emergency Services: Yes
Ownership: Voluntary non-profit - Private Beds: 165

Key Personnel:
Quality Assurance . . . . Robert Allen
Cardiac Laboratory. . . . . John Bennett
CEO/President. . . . . Norman Dascher
Radiology. . . . . Michael P Gaber
Ambulatory Care . . . . Nanci Lombard
Infection Control. . . . . Anna McClane
Hemotology Center . . . . Marianne Roberto

Measure	Cases	This Hosp.	State Avg.	U.S. Avg.
Blood Clot Prevention and Treatment				
Anticoagulation Overlap Therapy[2]	29	90%	91%	93%
ICU Venous Thromboembolism Prophylaxis[2]	65	98%	92%	92%
Incidence of Potentially Preventable VTE[1,2]	-	-	10%	10%
UFH with Dosages/Platelet Monitoring[2]	14	100%	92%	97%
Venous Thromboembolism Prophylaxis[2]	344	90%	87%	85%
Warfarin Therapy Discharge Instructions[2]	23	96%	59%	75%
Chest Pain/Possible Heart Attack Care				
Aspirin Given Within 24 Hours of Arrival	22	100%	97%	96%
Fibrinolytic Meds Within 30 Min. of Arrival[7]	-	-	54%	58%
Average Time to ECG (minutes)	24	8	9	7
Average Time to Transfer (minutes)[1]	-	-	78	60
Children's Asthma Care				
Received Home Management Plan of Care	-	-	-	88%
Received Reliever Medication	-	-	-	100%
Received Systemic Corticosteroids	-	-	-	100%
Emergency Department				
Admittance Decision Time (minutes)[2]	562	225	154	98
Head CT Results Within 45 Min. of Arrival[1]	-	-	55%	57%
Patients Who Left ER Before Being Seen	47,589	1%	2%	2%
Time from ER Arrival to Admit. (minutes)[2]	569	439	378	274
Time from ER Arrival to Discharge (minutes)	391	144	156	134
Time in ER Before Being Evaluated (minutes)	406	34	35	26
Time to Pain Meds for Fractures (minutes)	81	68	61	57
Heart Attack Care				
Aspirin Given at Discharge	22	100%	99%	99%
Fibrinolytic Meds Within 30 Min. of Arrival[7]	-	-	46%	54%
PCI Within 90 Minutes of Arrival[7]	-	-	95%	96%
Statin Prescribed at Discharge	20	80%	98%	98%
Heart Failure Care				
ACE Inhibitor or ARB for LVSD	11	100%	96%	97%
Discharge Instructions Given	100	98%	95%	94%
Evaluation of LVS Function	129	99%	99%	99%
Medicare Spending				
Medicare Spending per Patient (ratio)	-	0.97	0.96	0.98
Pneumonia Care				
Appropriate Initial Antibiotic Given[2]	94	99%	95%	95%
Blood Culture Timing[2]	180	95%	97%	98%
Pregnancy and Delivery Care				
Newborn Deliveries Scheduled Early[7]	-	-	4%	6%
Preventive Care				
Immunization for Influenza[2]	347	93%	88%	90%
Immunization for Pneumonia[2]	473	90%	88%	92%
Stroke Care				
Anticoagulation Therapy for Atrial Fibrillation[1]	-	-	96%	95%
Antithrombotic Therapy Timing	40	98%	98%	98%
Assessed for Rehabilitation	41	93%	97%	97%
Discharged on Antithrombotic Therapy	39	100%	99%	99%
Discharged on Statin Medication	29	90%	95%	94%
Thrombolytic Therapy Timing[1]	-	-	69%	66%
Venous Thromboembolism Prophylaxis	41	80%	94%	94%
Written Stroke Educational Materials Given	22	73%	86%	88%
Surgical Care Improvement Project				
Appropriate Beta Blocker Usage[2]	67	99%	97%	98%
Appropriate VTP Within 24 Hours[2]	208	95%	98%	98%
Controlled Postoperative Blood Glucose[2,7]	-	-	97%	97%
Perioperative Temperature Management[2]	253	100%	100%	100%
Prophylactic Antibiotic Selection[2]	137	97%	99%	99%
Prophylactic Antibiotic Selection (Outpatient)	179	98%	97%	98%
Prophylactic Antibiotic Stopped[2]	132	97%	98%	98%
Prophylactic Antibiotic Timing[2]	137	96%	99%	99%
Prophylactic Antibiotic Timing (Outpatient)	189	94%	97%	98%
Urinary Catheter Removal[2]	120	100%	96%	97%
Survey of Patients' Hospital Experiences				
Area Around Room 'Always' Quiet at Night	300+	43%	51%	61%
Doctors 'Always' Communicated Well	300+	71%	77%	82%
Home Recovery Information Given	300+	84%	83%	85%
Hospital Given 9 or 10 on 10 Point Scale	300+	61%	63%	71%
Meds 'Always' Explained Before Given	300+	58%	59%	64%
Nurses 'Always' Communicated Well	300+	72%	75%	79%
Pain 'Always' Well Controlled	300+	64%	67%	71%
Room and Bathroom 'Always' Clean	300+	62%	69%	73%
Timely Help 'Always' Received	300+	56%	61%	68%
Would Definitely Recommend Hospital	300+	65%	65%	71%
Use of Medical Imaging				
Cardiac Imaging Stress Test before Surgery[1]	-	-	5.8%	5.3%
Combination Abdominal CT Scan	550	3.8%	8.2%	10.5%
Combination Brain/Sinus CT Scan[1]	-	-	3.6%	2.7%
Combination Chest CT Scan	264	1.5%	1.3%	2.7%
Follow-up Mammogram/Ultrasound	982	8.2%	13%	8.8%
Lumbar Spine MRI for Low Back Pain	56	32.1%	33.4%	37.2%

Albany VA Medical Center

113 Holland Avenue Phone: 518-626-5000
Albany, NY 12208 Fax: 518-626-5500
URL: www1.va.gov/visns/visn02/albany.cfm
Type: Acute Care - VA Emergency Services: No
Ownership: Government Federal Beds: 156

Key Personnel:
Chief of Medical Staff. . . . . Lourdes Irizarry, MD
Radiology. . . . . Vernon King
Operating Room. . . . . Kathy Kovarik
Quality Assurance . . . . Barbara Parker
Patient Relations . . . . Deborah Spath

Measure	Cases	This Hosp.	State Avg.	U.S. Avg.
Blood Clot Prevention and Treatment				
Anticoagulation Overlap Therapy	-	-	91%	93%
ICU Venous Thromboembolism Prophylaxis	-	-	92%	92%
Incidence of Potentially Preventable VTE	-	-	10%	10%
UFH with Dosages/Platelet Monitoring	-	-	92%	97%
Venous Thromboembolism Prophylaxis	-	-	87%	85%
Warfarin Therapy Discharge Instructions	-	-	59%	75%
Chest Pain/Possible Heart Attack Care				
Aspirin Given Within 24 Hours of Arrival	-	-	97%	96%
Fibrinolytic Meds Within 30 Min. of Arrival	-	-	54%	58%
Average Time to ECG (minutes)	-	-	9	7
Average Time to Transfer (minutes)	-	-	78	60
Children's Asthma Care				
Received Home Management Plan of Care	-	-	-	88%
Received Reliever Medication	-	-	-	100%
Received Systemic Corticosteroids	-	-	-	100%
Emergency Department				

NOTE: Hospital profiles are in alphabetical order by state, then city, then hospital within the city; Rankings exclude hospitals with less than 25 cases except for patient surveys which excludes hospitals with less than 100 cases; (a) 100-299 cases; (1) The number of cases/patients is too few to report; (2) Data submitted were based on a sample of cases/patients; (3) Results are based on a shorter time period than required; (4) Data suppressed by CMS for one or more quarters; (5) Results are not available for this reporting period; (6) Fewer than 100 patients completed the HCAHPS survey; (7) No cases met the criteria for this measure; (8) The lower limit of the confidence interval cannot be calculated if the number of observed infections equals zero; (9) No data are available from the state/territory for this reporting period; (10) The scores shown reflect fewer than 50 completed surveys; (11) There were discrepancies in the data collection process; (12) This measure does not apply to this hospital for this reporting period; (13) Results cannot be calculated for this reporting period; (14) The results for this state are combined with nearby states to protect confidentiality; Please refer to the User's Guide for a full explanation of data.

Admittance Decision Time (minutes)	-	-	154	98
Head CT Results Within 45 Min. of Arrival	-	-	55%	57%
Patients Who Left ER Before Being Seen	-	-	2%	2%
Time from ER Arrival to Admit. (minutes)	-	-	378	274
Time from ER Arrival to Discharge (minutes)	-	-	156	134
Time in ER Before Being Evaluated (minutes)	-	-	35	26
Time to Pain Meds for Fractures (minutes)	-	-	61	57
Heart Attack Care				
Aspirin Given at Discharge	36	100%	99%	99%
Fibrinolytic Meds Within 30 Min. of Arrival[5]	-	-	46%	54%
PCI Within 90 Minutes of Arrival[5]	-	-	95%	96%
Statin Prescribed at Discharge	36	97%	98%	98%
Heart Failure Care				
ACE Inhibitor or ARB for LVSD	30	100%	96%	97%
Discharge Instructions Given	74	100%	95%	94%
Evaluation of LVS Function	90	98%	99%	99%
Medicare Spending				
Medicare Spending per Patient (ratio)	-	-	0.96	0.98
Pneumonia Care				
Appropriate Initial Antibiotic Given	42	95%	95%	95%
Blood Culture Timing	81	99%	97%	98%
Pregnancy and Delivery Care				
Newborn Deliveries Scheduled Early	-	-	4%	6%
Preventive Care				
Immunization for Influenza[5]	-	-	88%	90%
Immunization for Pneumonia[5]	-	-	88%	92%
Stroke Care				
Anticoagulation Therapy for Atrial Fibrillation	-	-	96%	95%
Antithrombotic Therapy Timing	-	-	98%	98%
Assessed for Rehabilitation	-	-	97%	97%
Discharged on Antithrombotic Therapy	-	-	99%	99%
Discharged on Statin Medication	-	-	95%	94%
Thrombolytic Therapy Timing	-	-	69%	66%
Venous Thromboembolism Prophylaxis	-	-	94%	94%
Written Stroke Educational Materials Given	-	-	86%	88%
Surgical Care Improvement Project				
Appropriate Beta Blocker Usage[2]	47	98%	97%	98%
Appropriate VTP Within 24 Hours[2]	110	98%	98%	98%
Controlled Postoperative Blood Glucose[5]	-	-	97%	97%
Perioperative Temperature Management[2]	140	99%	100%	100%
Prophylactic Antibiotic Selection	79	100%	99%	99%
Prophylactic Antibiotic Selection (Outpatient)	-	-	97%	98%
Prophylactic Antibiotic Stopped	78	100%	98%	98%
Prophylactic Antibiotic Timing	79	94%	99%	99%
Prophylactic Antibiotic Timing (Outpatient)	-	-	97%	98%
Urinary Catheter Removal[2]	78	99%	96%	97%
Survey of Patients' Hospital Experiences				
Area Around Room 'Always' Quiet at Night	-	-	51%	61%
Doctors 'Always' Communicated Well	-	-	77%	82%
Home Recovery Information Given	-	-	83%	85%
Hospital Given 9 or 10 on 10 Point Scale	-	-	63%	71%
Meds 'Always' Explained Before Given	-	-	59%	64%
Nurses 'Always' Communicated Well	-	-	75%	79%
Pain 'Always' Well Controlled	-	-	67%	71%
Room and Bathroom 'Always' Clean	-	-	69%	73%
Timely Help 'Always' Received	-	-	61%	68%
Would Definitely Recommend Hospital	-	-	65%	71%
Use of Medical Imaging				
Cardiac Imaging Stress Test before Surgery	-	-	5.8%	5.3%
Combination Abdominal CT Scan	-	-	8.2%	10.5%
Combination Brain/Sinus CT Scan	-	-	3.6%	2.7%
Combination Chest CT Scan	-	-	1.3%	2.7%
Follow-up Mammogram/Ultrasound	-	-	13%	8.8%
Lumbar Spine MRI for Low Back Pain	-	-	33.4%	37.2%

Saint Peter's Hospital

315 South Manning Boulevard
Albany, NY 12208
Phone: 518-525-1550
Fax: 518-525-1961
URL: www.stpetershealthcare.org
Type: Acute Care Hospitals
Emergency Services: Yes
Ownership: Voluntary non-profit - Church
Beds: 442

Key Personnel:

Chief of Medical Staff.......... Robert Cella, MD
CEO/President............... Ann Errichetti, MD, MBA
Infection Control.............. Amy R Gram
Cardiac Laboratory............ David Jacob
Chair/CEO.................... Robert Johnson
Quality Assurance .... Judy Phaff
Intensive Care Unit............ Steven Richards
Radiology.................... Edward Vining

Measure	Cases	This Hosp.	State Avg.	U.S. Avg.
Blood Clot Prevention and Treatment				
Anticoagulation Overlap Therapy[2]	165	99%	91%	93%
ICU Venous Thromboembolism Prophylaxis[2]	75	92%	92%	92%
Incidence of Potentially Preventable VTE[2]	43	0%	10%	10%
UFH with Dosages/Platelet Monitoring[2]	92	97%	92%	97%
Venous Thromboembolism Prophylaxis[2]	343	85%	87%	85%
Warfarin Therapy Discharge Instructions[2]	127	41%	59%	75%
Chest Pain/Possible Heart Attack Care				
Aspirin Given Within 24 Hours of Arrival[5]	-	-	97%	96%
Fibrinolytic Meds Within 30 Min. of Arrival[5]	-	-	54%	58%
Average Time to ECG (minutes)[5]	-	-	9	7
Average Time to Transfer (minutes)[5]	-	-	78	60
Children's Asthma Care				
Received Home Management Plan of Care	-	-	-	88%
Received Reliever Medication	-	-	-	100%
Received Systemic Corticosteroids	-	-	-	100%
Emergency Department				
Admittance Decision Time (minutes)[2]	583	145	154	98
Head CT Results Within 45 Min. of Arrival[1]	-	-	55%	57%
Patients Who Left ER Before Being Seen	53,163	1%	2%	2%
Time from ER Arrival to Admit. (minutes)[2]	586	370	378	274
Time from ER Arrival to Discharge (minutes)	365	206	156	134
Time in ER Before Being Evaluated (minutes)	410	23	35	26
Time to Pain Meds for Fractures (minutes)	77	70	61	57
Heart Attack Care				
Aspirin Given at Discharge	473	100%	99%	99%
Fibrinolytic Meds Within 30 Min. of Arrival[7]	-	-	46%	54%
PCI Within 90 Minutes of Arrival	36	97%	95%	96%
Statin Prescribed at Discharge	474	100%	98%	98%
Heart Failure Care				
ACE Inhibitor or ARB for LVSD	142	99%	96%	97%
Discharge Instructions Given	490	100%	95%	94%
Evaluation of LVS Function	584	100%	99%	99%
Medicare Spending				
Medicare Spending per Patient (ratio)	-	0.93	0.96	0.98
Pneumonia Care				
Appropriate Initial Antibiotic Given[2]	98	97%	95%	95%
Blood Culture Timing[2]	179	99%	97%	98%
Pregnancy and Delivery Care				
Newborn Deliveries Scheduled Early[2]	44	0%	4%	6%
Preventive Care				
Immunization for Influenza[2]	569	76%	88%	90%
Immunization for Pneumonia[2]	696	85%	88%	92%
Stroke Care				
Anticoagulation Therapy for Atrial Fibrillation	35	97%	96%	95%
Antithrombotic Therapy Timing	161	99%	98%	98%
Assessed for Rehabilitation	185	93%	97%	97%
Discharged on Antithrombotic Therapy	162	99%	99%	99%
Discharged on Statin Medication	119	88%	95%	94%
Thrombolytic Therapy Timing	14	79%	69%	66%
Venous Thromboembolism Prophylaxis	202	90%	94%	94%
Written Stroke Educational Materials Given	93	81%	86%	88%
Surgical Care Improvement Project				
Appropriate Beta Blocker Usage[2]	330	96%	97%	98%
Appropriate VTP Within 24 Hours[2]	567	98%	98%	98%
Controlled Postoperative Blood Glucose[2]	222	97%	97%	97%
Perioperative Temperature Management[2]	659	100%	100%	100%
Prophylactic Antibiotic Selection[2]	669	99%	99%	99%
Prophylactic Antibiotic Selection (Outpatient)	785	97%	97%	98%
Prophylactic Antibiotic Stopped[2]	669	99%	98%	98%
Prophylactic Antibiotic Timing[2]	669	99%	99%	99%
Prophylactic Antibiotic Timing (Outpatient)	785	99%	97%	98%
Urinary Catheter Removal[2]	402	97%	96%	97%
Survey of Patients' Hospital Experiences				
Area Around Room 'Always' Quiet at Night	300+	38%	51%	61%
Doctors 'Always' Communicated Well	300+	74%	77%	82%
Home Recovery Information Given	300+	89%	83%	85%
Hospital Given 9 or 10 on 10 Point Scale	300+	66%	63%	71%
Meds 'Always' Explained Before Given	300+	58%	59%	64%
Nurses 'Always' Communicated Well	300+	73%	75%	79%
Pain 'Always' Well Controlled	300+	70%	67%	71%
Room and Bathroom 'Always' Clean	300+	68%	69%	73%
Timely Help 'Always' Received	300+	55%	61%	68%
Would Definitely Recommend Hospital	300+	73%	65%	71%
Use of Medical Imaging				
Cardiac Imaging Stress Test before Surgery	59	3.4%	5.8%	5.3%
Combination Abdominal CT Scan	1,111	8.0%	8.2%	10.5%
Combination Brain/Sinus CT Scan	761	1.7%	3.6%	2.7%
Combination Chest CT Scan	749	5.1%	1.3%	2.7%
Follow-up Mammogram/Ultrasound	1,936	7.3%	13%	8.8%
Lumbar Spine MRI for Low Back Pain	59	40.7%	33.4%	37.2%

River Hospital

4 Fuller Street
Alexandria Bay, NY 13607
Phone: 315-482-2511
Fax: 315-482-6308
URL: www.samaritanhealth.com
Type: Critical Access Hospitals
Emergency Services: Yes
Ownership: Voluntary non-profit - Private
Beds: 52

Key Personnel:

Surgery .... Kiri Brandy, MD
Emergency Room .... Philip A Chafe
Radiology.................. Ali Gharaqozloo, MD
Cardiology .... Fritz Roc, MD, FACC
Chief of Medical Staff.......... Lauren Roman, MD
Chairman/CEO .... Joseph Russell
CEO/President............... David Tinker

Measure	Cases	This Hosp.	State Avg.	U.S. Avg.
Blood Clot Prevention and Treatment				
Anticoagulation Overlap Therapy[5]	-	-	91%	93%
ICU Venous Thromboembolism Prophylaxis[5]	-	-	92%	92%
Incidence of Potentially Preventable VTE[5]	-	-	10%	10%
UFH with Dosages/Platelet Monitoring[5]	-	-	92%	97%
Venous Thromboembolism Prophylaxis[5]	-	-	87%	85%
Warfarin Therapy Discharge Instructions[5]	-	-	59%	75%
Chest Pain/Possible Heart Attack Care				
Aspirin Given Within 24 Hours of Arrival[3]	22	100%	97%	96%
Fibrinolytic Meds Within 30 Min. of Arrival[1,3]	-	-	54%	58%
Average Time to ECG (minutes)[3]	22	16	9	7
Average Time to Transfer (minutes)[1,3]	-	-	78	60
Children's Asthma Care				
Received Home Management Plan of Care	-	-	-	88%
Received Reliever Medication	-	-	-	100%
Received Systemic Corticosteroids	-	-	-	100%
Emergency Department				
Admittance Decision Time (minutes)[5]	-	-	154	98
Head CT Results Within 45 Min. of Arrival[5]	-	-	55%	57%
Patients Who Left ER Before Being Seen	8,048	2%	2%	2%
Time from ER Arrival to Admit. (minutes)[5]	-	-	378	274
Time from ER Arrival to Discharge (minutes)[5]	-	-	156	134
Time in ER Before Being Evaluated (minutes)[5]	-	-	35	26
Time to Pain Meds for Fractures (minutes)[1,3]	-	-	61	57
Heart Attack Care				
Aspirin Given at Discharge[5]	-	-	99%	99%
Fibrinolytic Meds Within 30 Min. of Arrival[5]	-	-	46%	54%
PCI Within 90 Minutes of Arrival[5]	-	-	95%	96%
Statin Prescribed at Discharge[5]	-	-	98%	98%
Heart Failure Care				
ACE Inhibitor or ARB for LVSD[3,7]	-	-	96%	97%
Discharge Instructions Given[1,3]	-	-	95%	94%
Evaluation of LVS Function[1,3]	-	-	99%	99%
Medicare Spending				
Medicare Spending per Patient (ratio)	-	-	0.96	0.98
Pneumonia Care				
Appropriate Initial Antibiotic Given[1]	-	-	95%	95%
Blood Culture Timing[1]	-	-	97%	98%
Pregnancy and Delivery Care				
Newborn Deliveries Scheduled Early[5]	-	-	4%	6%
Preventive Care				
Immunization for Influenza[5]	-	-	88%	90%
Immunization for Pneumonia[5]	-	-	88%	92%

NOTE: Hospital profiles are in alphabetical order by state, then city, then hospital within the city; Rankings exclude hospitals with less than 25 cases except for patient surveys which excludes hospitals with less than 100 cases; (a) 100-299 cases; (1) The number of cases/patients is too few to report; (2) Data submitted were based on a sample of cases/patients; (3) Results are based on a shorter time period than required; (4) Data suppressed by CMS for one or more quarters; (5) Results are not available for this reporting period; (6) Fewer than 100 patients completed the HCAHPS survey; (7) No cases met the criteria for this measure; (8) The lower limit of the confidence interval cannot be calculated if the number of observed infections equals zero; (9) No data are available from the state/territory for this reporting period; (10) The scores shown reflect fewer than 50 completed surveys; (11) There were discrepancies in the data collection process; (12) This measure does not apply to this hospital for this reporting period; (13) Results cannot be calculated for this reporting period; (14) The results for this state are combined with nearby states to protect confidentiality; Please refer to the User's Guide for a full explanation of data.

Stroke Care				
Anticoagulation Therapy for Atrial Fibrillation[5]	-	-	96%	95%
Antithrombotic Therapy Timing[5]	-	-	98%	98%
Assessed for Rehabilitation[5]	-	-	97%	97%
Discharged on Antithrombotic Therapy[5]	-	-	99%	99%
Discharged on Statin Medication[5]	-	-	95%	94%
Thrombolytic Therapy Timing[5]	-	-	69%	66%
Venous Thromboembolism Prophylaxis[5]	-	-	94%	94%
Written Stroke Educational Materials Given[5]	-	-	86%	88%
Surgical Care Improvement Project				
Appropriate Beta Blocker Usage[5]	-	-	97%	98%
Appropriate VTP Within 24 Hours[5]	-	-	98%	98%
Controlled Postoperative Blood Glucose[5]	-	-	97%	97%
Perioperative Temperature Management[5]	-	-	100%	100%
Prophylactic Antibiotic Selection[5]	-	-	99%	99%
Prophylactic Antibiotic Selection (Outpatient)[5]	-	-	97%	98%
Prophylactic Antibiotic Stopped[5]	-	-	98%	98%
Prophylactic Antibiotic Timing[5]	-	-	99%	99%
Prophylactic Antibiotic Timing (Outpatient)[5]	-	-	97%	98%
Urinary Catheter Removal[5]	-	-	96%	97%
Survey of Patients' Hospital Experiences				
Area Around Room 'Always' Quiet at Night[10]	<100	85%	51%	61%
Doctors 'Always' Communicated Well[10]	<100	97%	77%	82%
Home Recovery Information Given[10]	<100	80%	83%	85%
Hospital Given 9 or 10 on 10 Point Scale[10]	<100	67%	63%	71%
Meds 'Always' Explained Before Given[10]	<100	68%	59%	64%
Nurses 'Always' Communicated Well[10]	<100	86%	75%	79%
Pain 'Always' Well Controlled[10]	<100	91%	67%	71%
Room and Bathroom 'Always' Clean[10]	<100	82%	69%	73%
Timely Help 'Always' Received[10]	<100	87%	61%	68%
Would Definitely Recommend Hospital[10]	<100	77%	65%	71%
Use of Medical Imaging				
Cardiac Imaging Stress Test before Surgery[7]	-	-	5.8%	5.3%
Combination Abdominal CT Scan	143	2.1%	8.2%	10.5%
Combination Brain/Sinus CT Scan[1]	-	-	3.6%	2.7%
Combination Chest CT Scan	64	0.0%	1.3%	2.7%
Follow-up Mammogram/Ultrasound	131	8.4%	13%	8.8%
Lumbar Spine MRI for Low Back Pain[7]	-	-	33.4%	37.2%

Saint Mary's Hospital at Amsterdam

427 Guy Park Avenue
Amsterdam, NY 12010
Phone: 518-842-1900
Fax: 518-842-0107
E-mail: info@smha.org
URL: www.smha.org
Type: Acute Care Hospitals
Emergency Services: Yes
Ownership: Voluntary non-profit - Private
Beds: 143

Key Personnel:
CEO/President. . . . . Victor Giulianelli
Infection Control. . . . . Phyllis MacMillon
Intensive Care Unit. . . . . Nancy Mead
Operating Room. . . . . Theresa Moore, RN
Emergency Room . . . . Steve Okhravi
Quality Assurance . . . . Kathleen Picciocca
Chief of Medical Staff. . . . . Tim Shoen, MD

Measure	Cases	This Hosp.	State Avg.	U.S. Avg.
Blood Clot Prevention and Treatment				
Anticoagulation Overlap Therapy[2]	48	100%	91%	93%
ICU Venous Thromboembolism Prophylaxis[2]	76	99%	92%	92%
Incidence of Potentially Preventable VTE[1,2]	-	-	10%	10%
UFH with Dosages/Platelet Monitoring[2]	22	100%	92%	97%
Venous Thromboembolism Prophylaxis[2]	345	96%	87%	85%
Warfarin Therapy Discharge Instructions[2]	34	47%	59%	75%
Chest Pain/Possible Heart Attack Care				
Aspirin Given Within 24 Hours of Arrival	83	98%	97%	96%
Fibrinolytic Meds Within 30 Min. of Arrival[7]	-	-	54%	58%
Average Time to ECG (minutes)	87	15	9	7
Average Time to Transfer (minutes)	12	46	78	60
Children's Asthma Care				
Received Home Management Plan of Care	-	-	-	88%
Received Reliever Medication	-	-	-	100%
Received Systemic Corticosteroids	-	-	-	100%
Emergency Department				
Admittance Decision Time (minutes)[2]	573	66	154	98
Head CT Results Within 45 Min. of Arrival[1]	-	-	55%	57%
Patients Who Left ER Before Being Seen	33,627	0%	2%	2%
Time from ER Arrival to Admit. (minutes)[2]	577	235	378	274
Time from ER Arrival to Discharge (minutes)	369	145	156	134
Time in ER Before Being Evaluated (minutes)	431	18	35	26
Time to Pain Meds for Fractures (minutes)	131	55	61	57
Heart Attack Care				
Aspirin Given at Discharge	28	100%	99%	99%
Fibrinolytic Meds Within 30 Min. of Arrival[7]	-	-	46%	54%
PCI Within 90 Minutes of Arrival[7]	-	-	95%	96%
Statin Prescribed at Discharge	28	96%	98%	98%
Heart Failure Care				
ACE Inhibitor or ARB for LVSD[2]	21	100%	96%	97%
Discharge Instructions Given[2]	160	90%	95%	94%
Evaluation of LVS Function[2]	211	100%	99%	99%
Medicare Spending				
Medicare Spending per Patient (ratio)	-	0.92	0.96	0.98
Pneumonia Care				
Appropriate Initial Antibiotic Given[2]	56	98%	95%	95%
Blood Culture Timing[2]	129	97%	97%	98%
Pregnancy and Delivery Care				
Newborn Deliveries Scheduled Early[2]	26	0%	4%	6%
Preventive Care				
Immunization for Influenza[2]	481	91%	88%	90%
Immunization for Pneumonia[2]	640	94%	88%	92%
Stroke Care				
Anticoagulation Therapy for Atrial Fibrillation[1,2]	-	-	96%	95%
Antithrombotic Therapy Timing[2]	36	100%	98%	98%
Assessed for Rehabilitation[2]	26	100%	97%	97%
Discharged on Antithrombotic Therapy[2]	25	96%	99%	99%
Discharged on Statin Medication[2]	18	78%	95%	94%
Thrombolytic Therapy Timing[1,2]	-	-	69%	66%
Venous Thromboembolism Prophylaxis[2]	39	100%	94%	94%
Written Stroke Educational Materials Given[1,2]	-	-	86%	88%
Surgical Care Improvement Project				
Appropriate Beta Blocker Usage[2]	75	100%	97%	98%
Appropriate VTP Within 24 Hours[2]	224	100%	98%	98%
Controlled Postoperative Blood Glucose[2,7]	-	-	97%	97%
Perioperative Temperature Management[2]	247	100%	100%	100%
Prophylactic Antibiotic Selection[2]	166	100%	99%	99%
Prophylactic Antibiotic Selection (Outpatient)	280	99%	97%	98%
Prophylactic Antibiotic Stopped[2]	162	99%	98%	98%
Prophylactic Antibiotic Timing[2]	166	99%	99%	99%
Prophylactic Antibiotic Timing (Outpatient)	255	100%	97%	98%
Urinary Catheter Removal[2]	170	99%	96%	97%
Survey of Patients' Hospital Experiences				
Area Around Room 'Always' Quiet at Night	300+	52%	51%	61%
Doctors 'Always' Communicated Well	300+	77%	77%	82%
Home Recovery Information Given	300+	90%	83%	85%
Hospital Given 9 or 10 on 10 Point Scale	300+	68%	63%	71%
Meds 'Always' Explained Before Given	300+	67%	59%	64%
Nurses 'Always' Communicated Well	300+	78%	75%	79%
Pain 'Always' Well Controlled	300+	68%	67%	71%
Room and Bathroom 'Always' Clean	300+	74%	69%	73%
Timely Help 'Always' Received	300+	63%	61%	68%
Would Definitely Recommend Hospital	300+	72%	65%	71%
Use of Medical Imaging				
Cardiac Imaging Stress Test before Surgery[1]	-	-	5.8%	5.3%
Combination Abdominal CT Scan	688	6.0%	8.2%	10.5%
Combination Brain/Sinus CT Scan	635	4.4%	3.6%	2.7%
Combination Chest CT Scan	382	0.3%	1.3%	2.7%
Follow-up Mammogram/Ultrasound	1,138	10.8%	13%	8.8%
Lumbar Spine MRI for Low Back Pain	64	37.5%	33.4%	37.2%

Auburn Community Hospital

17 Lansing Street
Auburn, NY 13021
Phone: 315-255-7011
Fax: 315-255-7018
E-mail: amhinput@auburnhospital.org
URL: www.auburnhospital.org
Type: Acute Care Hospitals
Emergency Services: Yes
Ownership: Voluntary non-profit - Private
Beds: 99

Key Personnel:
Anesthesiology. . . . . Anthony Ascioti
CEO/President. . . . . Scott Berlucchi
Chief of Medical Staff. . . . . James F Blute III, MD
Emergency Room . . . . Kathy Kendrick
Pediatric In-Patient Care . . . . Farokkh Nawer, MD
Radiology. . . . . G Palmer
Ambulatory Care . . . . Lorissa Plis
Infection Control. . . . . Donna Wrobel

Measure	Cases	This Hosp.	State Avg.	U.S. Avg.
Blood Clot Prevention and Treatment				
Anticoagulation Overlap Therapy[2]	13	69%	91%	93%
ICU Venous Thromboembolism Prophylaxis[2]	101	99%	92%	92%
Incidence of Potentially Preventable VTE[1,2]	-	-	10%	10%
UFH with Dosages/Platelet Monitoring[1,2]	-	-	92%	97%
Venous Thromboembolism Prophylaxis[2]	343	97%	87%	85%
Warfarin Therapy Discharge Instructions[1,2]	-	-	59%	75%
Chest Pain/Possible Heart Attack Care				
Aspirin Given Within 24 Hours of Arrival	117	92%	97%	96%
Fibrinolytic Meds Within 30 Min. of Arrival[1]	-	-	54%	58%
Average Time to ECG (minutes)	123	19	9	7
Average Time to Transfer (minutes)[1]	-	-	78	60
Children's Asthma Care				
Received Home Management Plan of Care	-	-	-	88%
Received Reliever Medication	-	-	-	100%
Received Systemic Corticosteroids	-	-	-	100%
Emergency Department				
Admittance Decision Time (minutes)[2]	364	138	154	98
Head CT Results Within 45 Min. of Arrival[1]	-	-	55%	57%
Patients Who Left ER Before Being Seen	26,859	3%	2%	2%
Time from ER Arrival to Admit. (minutes)[2]	387	378	378	274
Time from ER Arrival to Discharge (minutes)	328	183	156	134
Time in ER Before Being Evaluated (minutes)	380	60	35	26
Time to Pain Meds for Fractures (minutes)	90	122	61	57
Heart Attack Care				
Aspirin Given at Discharge	37	97%	99%	99%
Fibrinolytic Meds Within 30 Min. of Arrival[7]	-	-	46%	54%
PCI Within 90 Minutes of Arrival[7]	-	-	95%	96%
Statin Prescribed at Discharge	42	76%	98%	98%
Heart Failure Care				
ACE Inhibitor or ARB for LVSD	36	100%	96%	97%
Discharge Instructions Given	152	96%	95%	94%
Evaluation of LVS Function	189	98%	99%	99%
Medicare Spending				
Medicare Spending per Patient (ratio)	-	0.89	0.96	0.98
Pneumonia Care				
Appropriate Initial Antibiotic Given	145	91%	95%	95%
Blood Culture Timing	146	96%	97%	98%
Pregnancy and Delivery Care				
Newborn Deliveries Scheduled Early	29	3%	4%	6%
Preventive Care				
Immunization for Influenza[2]	442	90%	88%	90%
Immunization for Pneumonia[2]	610	93%	88%	92%
Stroke Care				
Anticoagulation Therapy for Atrial Fibrillation[1]	-	-	96%	95%
Antithrombotic Therapy Timing	25	100%	98%	98%
Assessed for Rehabilitation	28	100%	97%	97%
Discharged on Antithrombotic Therapy	27	100%	99%	99%
Discharged on Statin Medication	15	100%	95%	94%
Thrombolytic Therapy Timing[1]	-	-	69%	66%
Venous Thromboembolism Prophylaxis	28	96%	94%	94%
Written Stroke Educational Materials Given	22	91%	86%	88%
Surgical Care Improvement Project				
Appropriate Beta Blocker Usage	48	98%	97%	98%
Appropriate VTP Within 24 Hours	181	93%	98%	98%
Controlled Postoperative Blood Glucose[7]	-	-	97%	97%
Perioperative Temperature Management	193	100%	100%	100%
Prophylactic Antibiotic Selection	125	97%	99%	99%
Prophylactic Antibiotic Selection (Outpatient)	95	97%	97%	98%
Prophylactic Antibiotic Stopped	120	91%	98%	98%
Prophylactic Antibiotic Timing	125	99%	99%	99%
Prophylactic Antibiotic Timing (Outpatient)	99	92%	97%	98%
Urinary Catheter Removal	128	93%	96%	97%
Survey of Patients' Hospital Experiences				
Area Around Room 'Always' Quiet at Night[11]	300+	43%	51%	61%
Doctors 'Always' Communicated Well[11]	300+	74%	77%	82%
Home Recovery Information Given[11]	300+	81%	83%	85%

NOTE: Hospital profiles are in alphabetical order by state, then city, then hospital within the city; Rankings exclude hospitals with less than 25 cases except for patient surveys which excludes hospitals with less than 100 cases; (a) 100-299 cases; (1) The number of cases/patients is too few to report; (2) Data submitted were based on a sample of cases/patients; (3) Results are based on a shorter time period than required; (4) Data suppressed by CMS for one or more quarters; (5) Results are not available for this reporting period; (6) Fewer than 100 patients completed the HCAHPS survey; (7) No cases met the criteria for this measure; (8) The lower limit of the confidence interval cannot be calculated if the number of observed infections equals zero; (9) No data are available from the state/territory for this reporting period; (10) The scores shown reflect fewer than 50 completed surveys; (11) There were discrepancies in the data collection process; (12) This measure does not apply to this hospital for this reporting period; (13) Results cannot be calculated for this reporting period; (14) The results for this state are combined with nearby states to protect confidentiality; Please refer to the User's Guide for a full explanation of data.

Measure	Cases	This Hosp.	State Avg.	U.S. Avg.
Hospital Given 9 or 10 on 10 Point Scale[11]	300+	53%	63%	71%
Meds 'Always' Explained Before Given[11]	300+	56%	59%	64%
Nurses 'Always' Communicated Well[11]	300+	72%	75%	79%
Pain 'Always' Well Controlled[11]	300+	67%	67%	71%
Room and Bathroom 'Always' Clean[11]	300+	70%	69%	73%
Timely Help 'Always' Received[11]	300+	56%	61%	68%
Would Definitely Recommend Hospital[11]	300+	52%	65%	71%
Use of Medical Imaging				
Cardiac Imaging Stress Test before Surgery	51	2.0%	5.8%	5.3%
Combination Abdominal CT Scan	600	10.8%	8.2%	10.5%
Combination Brain/Sinus CT Scan[1]	-	-	3.6%	2.7%
Combination Chest CT Scan	210	4.3%	1.3%	2.7%
Follow-up Mammogram/Ultrasound	609	8.0%	13%	8.8%
Lumbar Spine MRI for Low Back Pain[1]	-	-	33.4%	37.2%

United Memorial Medical Center

127 North Street
Batavia, NY 14020
Phone: 585-343-6030
Fax: 585-344-7345
URL: www.ummc.org
Type: Acute Care Hospitals
Emergency Services: Yes
Ownership: Voluntary non-profit - Private
Beds: 126

Key Personnel:

Chief of Medical Staff.......... Jin Yoi Chang, MD
Infection Control.............. Lorraine Goergen
President..................... Daniel P. Ireland
Chair/CEO.................... Betty Lapp
Emergency Room............. Esther Natla, RN
CEO .... Mark C Schoell
Operating Room.............. Debbie Vick
Quality Assurance............ Carole Wujcik

Measure	Cases	This Hosp.	State Avg.	U.S. Avg.
Blood Clot Prevention and Treatment				
Anticoagulation Overlap Therapy[2]	20	90%	91%	93%
ICU Venous Thromboembolism Prophylaxis[2]	69	86%	92%	92%
Incidence of Potentially Preventable VTE[1,2]	-	-	10%	10%
UFH with Dosages/Platelet Monitoring[2]	11	100%	92%	97%
Venous Thromboembolism Prophylaxis[2]	263	84%	87%	85%
Warfarin Therapy Discharge Instructions[2]	13	92%	59%	75%
Chest Pain/Possible Heart Attack Care				
Aspirin Given Within 24 Hours of Arrival	146	97%	97%	96%
Fibrinolytic Meds Within 30 Min. of Arrival[1]	-	-	54%	58%
Average Time to ECG (minutes)	148	7	9	7
Average Time to Transfer (minutes)[1]	-	-	78	60
Children's Asthma Care				
Received Home Management Plan of Care	-	-	-	88%
Received Reliever Medication	-	-	-	100%
Received Systemic Corticosteroids	-	-	-	100%
Emergency Department				
Admittance Decision Time (minutes)[2]	469	95	154	98
Head CT Results Within 45 Min. of Arrival[1]	-	-	55%	57%
Patients Who Left ER Before Being Seen	22,439	0%	2%	2%
Time from ER Arrival to Admit. (minutes)[2]	469	276	378	274
Time from ER Arrival to Discharge (minutes)	433	109	156	134
Time in ER Before Being Evaluated (minutes)	494	26	35	26
Time to Pain Meds for Fractures (minutes)	58	37	61	57
Heart Attack Care				
Aspirin Given at Discharge	27	85%	99%	99%
Fibrinolytic Meds Within 30 Min. of Arrival[7]	-	-	46%	54%
PCI Within 90 Minutes of Arrival[7]	-	-	95%	96%
Statin Prescribed at Discharge	24	92%	98%	98%
Heart Failure Care				
ACE Inhibitor or ARB for LVSD	44	86%	96%	97%
Discharge Instructions Given	129	87%	95%	94%
Evaluation of LVS Function	153	100%	99%	99%
Medicare Spending				
Medicare Spending per Patient (ratio)	-	0.87	0.96	0.98
Pneumonia Care				
Appropriate Initial Antibiotic Given	111	89%	95%	95%
Blood Culture Timing	181	99%	97%	98%
Pregnancy and Delivery Care				
Newborn Deliveries Scheduled Early[2]	35	6%	4%	6%
Preventive Care				
Immunization for Influenza[2]	359	93%	88%	90%
Immunization for Pneumonia[2]	458	98%	88%	92%
Stroke Care				
Anticoagulation Therapy for Atrial Fibrillation[7]	-	-	96%	95%
Antithrombotic Therapy Timing	12	100%	98%	98%
Assessed for Rehabilitation	12	100%	97%	97%
Discharged on Antithrombotic Therapy	12	100%	99%	99%
Discharged on Statin Medication[1]	-	-	95%	94%
Thrombolytic Therapy Timing[7]	-	-	69%	66%
Venous Thromboembolism Prophylaxis	13	85%	94%	94%
Written Stroke Educational Materials Given[1]	-	-	86%	88%
Surgical Care Improvement Project				
Appropriate Beta Blocker Usage	96	93%	97%	98%
Appropriate VTP Within 24 Hours	236	98%	98%	98%
Controlled Postoperative Blood Glucose[7]	-	-	97%	97%
Perioperative Temperature Management	250	100%	100%	100%
Prophylactic Antibiotic Selection	188	98%	99%	99%
Prophylactic Antibiotic Selection (Outpatient)	59	98%	97%	98%
Prophylactic Antibiotic Stopped	184	92%	98%	98%
Prophylactic Antibiotic Timing	188	98%	99%	99%
Prophylactic Antibiotic Timing (Outpatient)	59	98%	97%	98%
Urinary Catheter Removal	156	89%	96%	97%
Survey of Patients' Hospital Experiences				
Area Around Room 'Always' Quiet at Night	300+	43%	51%	61%
Doctors 'Always' Communicated Well	300+	75%	77%	82%
Home Recovery Information Given	300+	84%	83%	85%
Hospital Given 9 or 10 on 10 Point Scale	300+	49%	63%	71%
Meds 'Always' Explained Before Given	300+	55%	59%	64%
Nurses 'Always' Communicated Well	300+	75%	75%	79%
Pain 'Always' Well Controlled	300+	68%	67%	71%
Room and Bathroom 'Always' Clean	300+	71%	69%	73%
Timely Help 'Always' Received	300+	62%	61%	68%
Would Definitely Recommend Hospital	300+	46%	65%	71%
Use of Medical Imaging				
Cardiac Imaging Stress Test before Surgery[1]	-	-	5.8%	5.3%
Combination Abdominal CT Scan	282	3.2%	8.2%	10.5%
Combination Brain/Sinus CT Scan[1]	-	-	3.6%	2.7%
Combination Chest CT Scan	110	0.9%	1.3%	2.7%
Follow-up Mammogram/Ultrasound	321	5.0%	13%	8.8%
Lumbar Spine MRI for Low Back Pain[1]	-	-	33.4%	37.2%

Bath VA Medical Center

76 Veterans Ave.
Bath, NY 14810
Phone: 607-664-4000
Fax: 607-664-4756
URL: www1.va.gov/visns/visn02/bath.cfm
Type: Acute Care - VA
Emergency Services: No
Ownership: Government Federal
Beds: 440

Key Personnel:

Intensive Care Unit............ Alfred A Bibawy, MD
Chief of Medical Staff.......... Felipe Diaz
Emergency Room .... Anthony Gerbasi, DO
Quality Assurance .... Judy Harris, RN
Patient Relations .... Shirley A Pikula, MSN
Radiology.................... Richard White

Measure	Cases	This Hosp.	State Avg.	U.S. Avg.
Blood Clot Prevention and Treatment				
Anticoagulation Overlap Therapy	-	-	91%	93%
ICU Venous Thromboembolism Prophylaxis	-	-	92%	92%
Incidence of Potentially Preventable VTE	-	-	10%	10%
UFH with Dosages/Platelet Monitoring	-	-	92%	97%
Venous Thromboembolism Prophylaxis	-	-	87%	85%
Warfarin Therapy Discharge Instructions	-	-	59%	75%
Chest Pain/Possible Heart Attack Care				
Aspirin Given Within 24 Hours of Arrival	-	-	97%	96%
Fibrinolytic Meds Within 30 Min. of Arrival	-	-	54%	58%
Average Time to ECG (minutes)	-	-	9	7
Average Time to Transfer (minutes)	-	-	78	60
Children's Asthma Care				
Received Home Management Plan of Care	-	-	-	88%
Received Reliever Medication	-	-	-	100%
Received Systemic Corticosteroids	-	-	-	100%
Emergency Department				
Admittance Decision Time (minutes)	-	-	154	98
Head CT Results Within 45 Min. of Arrival	-	-	55%	57%
Patients Who Left ER Before Being Seen	-	-	2%	2%
Time from ER Arrival to Admit. (minutes)	-	-	378	274
Time from ER Arrival to Discharge (minutes)	-	-	156	134
Time in ER Before Being Evaluated (minutes)	-	-	35	26
Time to Pain Meds for Fractures (minutes)	-	-	61	57
Heart Attack Care				
Aspirin Given at Discharge[5]	-	-	99%	99%
Fibrinolytic Meds Within 30 Min. of Arrival[5]	-	-	46%	54%
PCI Within 90 Minutes of Arrival[5]	-	-	95%	96%
Statin Prescribed at Discharge[5]	-	-	98%	98%
Heart Failure Care				
ACE Inhibitor or ARB for LVSD[1]	11	91%	96%	97%
Discharge Instructions Given	33	100%	95%	94%
Evaluation of LVS Function	36	100%	99%	99%
Medicare Spending				
Medicare Spending per Patient (ratio)	-	-	0.96	0.98
Pneumonia Care				
Appropriate Initial Antibiotic Given	32	97%	95%	95%
Blood Culture Timing	50	94%	97%	98%
Pregnancy and Delivery Care				
Newborn Deliveries Scheduled Early	-	-	4%	6%
Preventive Care				
Immunization for Influenza[2,3]	133	92%	88%	90%
Immunization for Pneumonia[2,3]	329	96%	88%	92%
Stroke Care				
Anticoagulation Therapy for Atrial Fibrillation	-	-	96%	95%
Antithrombotic Therapy Timing	-	-	98%	98%
Assessed for Rehabilitation	-	-	97%	97%
Discharged on Antithrombotic Therapy	-	-	99%	99%
Discharged on Statin Medication	-	-	95%	94%
Thrombolytic Therapy Timing	-	-	69%	66%
Venous Thromboembolism Prophylaxis	-	-	94%	94%
Written Stroke Educational Materials Given	-	-	86%	88%
Surgical Care Improvement Project				
Appropriate Beta Blocker Usage[5]	-	-	97%	98%
Appropriate VTP Within 24 Hours[5]	-	-	98%	98%
Controlled Postoperative Blood Glucose[5]	-	-	97%	97%
Perioperative Temperature Management[5]	-	-	100%	100%
Prophylactic Antibiotic Selection[5]	-	-	99%	99%
Prophylactic Antibiotic Selection (Outpatient)	-	-	97%	98%
Prophylactic Antibiotic Stopped[5]	-	-	98%	98%
Prophylactic Antibiotic Timing[5]	-	-	99%	99%
Prophylactic Antibiotic Timing (Outpatient)	-	-	97%	98%
Urinary Catheter Removal[5]	-	-	96%	97%
Survey of Patients' Hospital Experiences				
Area Around Room 'Always' Quiet at Night	-	-	51%	61%
Doctors 'Always' Communicated Well	-	-	77%	82%
Home Recovery Information Given	-	-	83%	85%
Hospital Given 9 or 10 on 10 Point Scale	-	-	63%	71%
Meds 'Always' Explained Before Given	-	-	59%	64%
Nurses 'Always' Communicated Well	-	-	75%	79%
Pain 'Always' Well Controlled	-	-	67%	71%
Room and Bathroom 'Always' Clean	-	-	69%	73%
Timely Help 'Always' Received	-	-	61%	68%
Would Definitely Recommend Hospital	-	-	65%	71%
Use of Medical Imaging				
Cardiac Imaging Stress Test before Surgery	-	-	5.8%	5.3%
Combination Abdominal CT Scan	-	-	8.2%	10.5%
Combination Brain/Sinus CT Scan	-	-	3.6%	2.7%
Combination Chest CT Scan	-	-	1.3%	2.7%
Follow-up Mammogram/Ultrasound	-	-	13%	8.8%
Lumbar Spine MRI for Low Back Pain	-	-	33.4%	37.2%

Ira Davenport Memorial Hospital

7571 State Route 54
Bath, NY 14810
Phone: 607-776-8500
Fax: 607-776-8817
E-mail: prflb@idmh.org
URL: www.davenportandtaylor.org
Type: Acute Care Hospitals
Emergency Services: Yes
Ownership: Voluntary non-profit - Other
Beds: 66

Key Personnel:

Radiology.................... Wendy Baker
CEO/President............... James Watson

Measure	Cases	This Hosp.	State Avg.	U.S. Avg.
Blood Clot Prevention and Treatment				

NOTE: Hospital profiles are in alphabetical order by state, then city, then hospital within the city; Rankings exclude hospitals with less than 25 cases except for patient surveys which excludes hospitals with less than 100 cases; (a) 100-299 cases; (1) The number of cases/patients is too few to report; (2) Data submitted were based on a sample of cases/patients; (3) Results are based on a shorter time period than required; (4) Data suppressed by CMS for one or more quarters; (5) Results are not available for this reporting period; (6) Fewer than 100 patients completed the HCAHPS survey; (7) No cases met the criteria for this measure; (8) The lower limit of the confidence interval cannot be calculated if the number of observed infections equals zero; (9) No data are available from the state/territory for this reporting period; (10) The scores shown reflect fewer than 50 completed surveys; (11) There were discrepancies in the data collection process; (12) This measure does not apply to this hospital for this reporting period; (13) Results cannot be calculated for this reporting period; (14) The results for this state are combined with nearby states to protect confidentiality; Please refer to the User's Guide for a full explanation of data.

Measure	Cases	This Hosp.	State Avg.	U.S. Avg.
Anticoagulation Overlap Therapy[1]	-	-	91%	93%
ICU Venous Thromboembolism Prophylaxis[7]	-	-	92%	92%
Incidence of Potentially Preventable VTE[7]	-	-	10%	10%
UFH with Dosages/Platelet Monitoring[1]	-	-	92%	97%
Venous Thromboembolism Prophylaxis	277	83%	87%	85%
Warfarin Therapy Discharge Instructions[1]	-	-	59%	75%
Chest Pain/Possible Heart Attack Care				
Aspirin Given Within 24 Hours of Arrival	14	100%	97%	96%
Fibrinolytic Meds Within 30 Min. of Arrival[1,3]	-	-	54%	58%
Average Time to ECG (minutes)	14	17	9	7
Average Time to Transfer (minutes)[3,7]	-	-	78	60
Children's Asthma Care				
Received Home Management Plan of Care	-	-	-	88%
Received Reliever Medication	-	-	-	100%
Received Systemic Corticosteroids	-	-	-	100%
Emergency Department				
Admittance Decision Time (minutes)	401	65	154	98
Head CT Results Within 45 Min. of Arrival[1]	-	-	55%	57%
Patients Who Left ER Before Being Seen	8,614	3%	2%	2%
Time from ER Arrival to Admit. (minutes)	416	232	378	274
Time from ER Arrival to Discharge (minutes)	250	140	156	134
Time in ER Before Being Evaluated (minutes)	287	34	35	26
Time to Pain Meds for Fractures (minutes)	13	76	61	57
Heart Attack Care				
Aspirin Given at Discharge[1,3]	-	-	99%	99%
Fibrinolytic Meds Within 30 Min. of Arrival[3,7]	-	-	46%	54%
PCI Within 90 Minutes of Arrival[3,7]	-	-	95%	96%
Statin Prescribed at Discharge[1,3]	-	-	98%	98%
Heart Failure Care				
ACE Inhibitor or ARB for LVSD[1]	-	-	96%	97%
Discharge Instructions Given	23	100%	95%	94%
Evaluation of LVS Function	29	100%	99%	99%
Medicare Spending				
Medicare Spending per Patient (ratio)	-	0.75	0.96	0.98
Pneumonia Care				
Appropriate Initial Antibiotic Given	41	88%	95%	95%
Blood Culture Timing	60	98%	97%	98%
Pregnancy and Delivery Care				
Newborn Deliveries Scheduled Early[2,7]	-	-	4%	6%
Preventive Care				
Immunization for Influenza	284	95%	88%	90%
Immunization for Pneumonia	397	95%	88%	92%
Stroke Care				
Anticoagulation Therapy for Atrial Fibrillation[3,7]	-	-	96%	95%
Antithrombotic Therapy Timing[1,3]	-	-	98%	98%
Assessed for Rehabilitation[1,3]	-	-	97%	97%
Discharged on Antithrombotic Therapy[1,3]	-	-	99%	99%
Discharged on Statin Medication[1,3]	-	-	95%	94%
Thrombolytic Therapy Timing[3,7]	-	-	69%	66%
Venous Thromboembolism Prophylaxis[1,3]	-	-	94%	94%
Written Stroke Educational Materials Given[1,3]	-	-	86%	88%
Surgical Care Improvement Project				
Appropriate Beta Blocker Usage[1,3]	-	-	97%	98%
Appropriate VTP Within 24 Hours[1,3]	-	-	98%	98%
Controlled Postoperative Blood Glucose[3,7]	-	-	97%	97%
Perioperative Temperature Management[3]	11	100%	100%	100%
Prophylactic Antibiotic Selection[1,3]	-	-	99%	99%
Prophylactic Antibiotic Selection (Outpatient)[1]	-	-	97%	98%
Prophylactic Antibiotic Stopped[1,3]	-	-	98%	98%
Prophylactic Antibiotic Timing[1,3]	-	-	99%	99%
Prophylactic Antibiotic Timing (Outpatient)[1]	-	-	97%	98%
Urinary Catheter Removal[1,3]	-	-	96%	97%
Survey of Patients' Hospital Experiences				
Area Around Room 'Always' Quiet at Night	(a)	61%	51%	61%
Doctors 'Always' Communicated Well	(a)	81%	77%	82%
Home Recovery Information Given	(a)	79%	83%	85%
Hospital Given 9 or 10 on 10 Point Scale	(a)	61%	63%	71%
Meds 'Always' Explained Before Given	(a)	59%	59%	64%
Nurses 'Always' Communicated Well	(a)	72%	75%	79%
Pain 'Always' Well Controlled	(a)	65%	67%	71%
Room and Bathroom 'Always' Clean	(a)	73%	69%	73%
Timely Help 'Always' Received	(a)	69%	61%	68%
Would Definitely Recommend Hospital	(a)	52%	65%	71%
Use of Medical Imaging				
Cardiac Imaging Stress Test before Surgery[7]	-	-	5.8%	5.3%
Combination Abdominal CT Scan	168	9.5%	8.2%	10.5%
Combination Brain/Sinus CT Scan[1]	-	-	3.6%	2.7%
Combination Chest CT Scan	52	3.8%	1.3%	2.7%
Follow-up Mammogram/Ultrasound	168	6.5%	13%	8.8%
Lumbar Spine MRI for Low Back Pain[1]	-	-	33.4%	37.2%

Southside Hospital

301 East Main Street
Bay Shore, NY 11706
Phone: 631-968-3000
Fax: 631-968-3315
URL: www.northshorelij.com
Type: Acute Care Hospitals
Emergency Services: Yes
Ownership: Voluntary non-profit - Private
Beds: 377

Key Personnel:
CEO/President. . . . . Michael J Dowling
Chief of Medical Staff . . . . Jay Enden, MD
Pediatric Ambulatory Care . . . . . . James Fagin, MD
Infection Control. . . . . Bruce Farber, MD
Radiology. . . . . Mitchell Goldman, MD
Quality Assurance . . . . Donn Haber
Coronary Care . . . . Kathy Mann, RN
Operating Room. . . . . Linda Olander, RN

Measure	Cases	This Hosp.	State Avg.	U.S. Avg.
Blood Clot Prevention and Treatment				
Anticoagulation Overlap Therapy[2]	125	79%	91%	93%
ICU Venous Thromboembolism Prophylaxis[2]	63	84%	92%	92%
Incidence of Potentially Preventable VTE[2]	30	3%	10%	10%
UFH with Dosages/Platelet Monitoring[2]	41	98%	92%	97%
Venous Thromboembolism Prophylaxis[2]	305	77%	87%	85%
Warfarin Therapy Discharge Instructions[2]	94	0%	59%	75%
Chest Pain/Possible Heart Attack Care				
Aspirin Given Within 24 Hours of Arrival[3,7]	-	-	97%	96%
Fibrinolytic Meds Within 30 Min. of Arrival[5]	-	-	54%	58%
Average Time to ECG (minutes)[3,7]	-	-	9	7
Average Time to Transfer (minutes)[5]	-	-	78	60
Children's Asthma Care				
Received Home Management Plan of Care	-	-	-	88%
Received Reliever Medication	-	-	-	100%
Received Systemic Corticosteroids	-	-	-	100%
Emergency Department				
Admittance Decision Time (minutes)[2]	687	333	154	98
Head CT Results Within 45 Min. of Arrival	14	64%	55%	57%
Patients Who Left ER Before Being Seen	72,040	1%	2%	2%
Time from ER Arrival to Admit. (minutes)[2]	687	554	378	274
Time from ER Arrival to Discharge (minutes)	367	145	156	134
Time in ER Before Being Evaluated (minutes)	342	56	35	26
Time to Pain Meds for Fractures (minutes)	132	51	61	57
Heart Attack Care				
Aspirin Given at Discharge[2]	271	99%	99%	99%
Fibrinolytic Meds Within 30 Min. of Arrival[2,7]	-	-	46%	54%
PCI Within 90 Minutes of Arrival[2]	38	97%	95%	96%
Statin Prescribed at Discharge[2]	268	98%	98%	98%
Heart Failure Care				
ACE Inhibitor or ARB for LVSD[2]	77	92%	96%	97%
Discharge Instructions Given[2]	221	92%	95%	94%
Evaluation of LVS Function[2]	284	100%	99%	99%
Medicare Spending				
Medicare Spending per Patient (ratio)	-	1.09	0.96	0.98
Pneumonia Care				
Appropriate Initial Antibiotic Given[2]	90	100%	95%	95%
Blood Culture Timing[2]	174	99%	97%	98%
Pregnancy and Delivery Care				
Newborn Deliveries Scheduled Early[2]	21	5%	4%	6%
Preventive Care				
Immunization for Influenza[2]	543	84%	88%	90%
Immunization for Pneumonia[2]	563	85%	88%	92%
Stroke Care				
Anticoagulation Therapy for Atrial Fibrillation[2]	20	100%	96%	95%
Antithrombotic Therapy Timing[2]	96	100%	98%	98%
Assessed for Rehabilitation[2]	103	95%	97%	97%
Discharged on Antithrombotic Therapy[2]	95	98%	99%	99%
Discharged on Statin Medication[2]	77	96%	95%	94%
Thrombolytic Therapy Timing[2]	11	64%	69%	66%
Venous Thromboembolism Prophylaxis[2]	113	91%	94%	94%
Written Stroke Educational Materials Given[2]	57	67%	86%	88%
Surgical Care Improvement Project				
Appropriate Beta Blocker Usage[2]	228	98%	97%	98%
Appropriate VTP Within 24 Hours[2]	355	98%	98%	98%
Controlled Postoperative Blood Glucose[2]	141	96%	97%	97%
Perioperative Temperature Management[2]	454	100%	100%	100%
Prophylactic Antibiotic Selection[2]	410	99%	99%	99%
Prophylactic Antibiotic Selection (Outpatient)	104	97%	97%	98%
Prophylactic Antibiotic Stopped[2]	400	98%	98%	98%
Prophylactic Antibiotic Timing[2]	411	99%	99%	99%
Prophylactic Antibiotic Timing (Outpatient)	104	100%	97%	98%
Urinary Catheter Removal[2]	326	97%	96%	97%
Survey of Patients' Hospital Experiences				
Area Around Room 'Always' Quiet at Night	300+	52%	51%	61%
Doctors 'Always' Communicated Well	300+	80%	77%	82%
Home Recovery Information Given	300+	80%	83%	85%
Hospital Given 9 or 10 on 10 Point Scale	300+	63%	63%	71%
Meds 'Always' Explained Before Given	300+	62%	59%	64%
Nurses 'Always' Communicated Well	300+	78%	75%	79%
Pain 'Always' Well Controlled	300+	69%	67%	71%
Room and Bathroom 'Always' Clean	300+	68%	69%	73%
Timely Help 'Always' Received	300+	56%	61%	68%
Would Definitely Recommend Hospital	300+	69%	65%	71%
Use of Medical Imaging				
Cardiac Imaging Stress Test before Surgery	134	6.0%	5.8%	5.3%
Combination Abdominal CT Scan	528	0.4%	8.2%	10.5%
Combination Brain/Sinus CT Scan	903	6.4%	3.6%	2.7%
Combination Chest CT Scan	142	0.0%	1.3%	2.7%
Follow-up Mammogram/Ultrasound[7]	-	-	13%	8.8%
Lumbar Spine MRI for Low Back Pain[7]	-	-	33.4%	37.2%

Saint Joseph Hospital

4295 Hempstead Turnpike
Bethpage, NY 11714
Phone: 516-579-6000
Fax: 516-579-0739
URL: www.newislandhospital.org
Type: Acute Care Hospitals
Emergency Services: Yes
Ownership: Voluntary non-profit - Private
Beds: 223

Key Personnel:
Quality Assurance . . . . Kathy Ambrose, RN
Chief of Medical Staff . . . . Vincent P Anzalone, MD
President. . . . . Brahmbhatt Bimalkumar, MD
Coronary Care . . . . Alan Scheinbach, DO
Infection Control. . . . . Vijay Shah, MD
Radiology. . . . . Scott J Sherman, MD
Operating Room. . . . . Robert Sunshine, MD
Pediatric Ambulatory Care . . . . . . Behved Talebian

Measure	Cases	This Hosp.	State Avg.	U.S. Avg.
Blood Clot Prevention and Treatment				
Anticoagulation Overlap Therapy[2]	45	100%	91%	93%
ICU Venous Thromboembolism Prophylaxis[2]	82	100%	92%	92%
Incidence of Potentially Preventable VTE[2]	11	0%	10%	10%
UFH with Dosages/Platelet Monitoring[1,2]	-	-	92%	97%
Venous Thromboembolism Prophylaxis[2]	428	90%	87%	85%
Warfarin Therapy Discharge Instructions[2]	31	87%	59%	75%
Chest Pain/Possible Heart Attack Care				
Aspirin Given Within 24 Hours of Arrival	194	98%	97%	96%
Fibrinolytic Meds Within 30 Min. of Arrival[7]	-	-	54%	58%
Average Time to ECG (minutes)	201	8	9	7
Average Time to Transfer (minutes)	42	62	78	60
Children's Asthma Care				
Received Home Management Plan of Care	-	-	-	88%
Received Reliever Medication	-	-	-	100%
Received Systemic Corticosteroids	-	-	-	100%
Emergency Department				
Admittance Decision Time (minutes)[2]	939	245	154	98
Head CT Results Within 45 Min. of Arrival[1]	-	-	55%	57%
Patients Who Left ER Before Being Seen	36,749	1%	2%	2%
Time from ER Arrival to Admit. (minutes)[2]	974	401	378	274
Time from ER Arrival to Discharge (minutes)	436	163	156	134
Time in ER Before Being Evaluated (minutes)	519	45	35	26
Time to Pain Meds for Fractures (minutes)	67	65	61	57
Heart Attack Care				

NOTE: Hospital profiles are in alphabetical order by state, then city, then hospital within the city; Rankings exclude hospitals with less than 25 cases except for patient surveys which excludes hospitals with less than 100 cases; (a) 100-299 cases; (1) The number of cases/patients is too few to report; (2) Data submitted were based on a sample of cases/patients; (3) Results are based on a shorter time period than required; (4) Data suppressed by CMS for one or more quarters; (5) Results are not available for this reporting period; (6) Fewer than 100 patients completed the HCAHPS survey; (7) No cases met the criteria for this measure; (8) The lower limit of the confidence interval cannot be calculated if the number of observed infections equals zero; (9) No data are available from the state/territory for this reporting period; (10) The scores shown reflect fewer than 50 completed surveys; (11) There were discrepancies in the data collection process; (12) This measure does not apply to this hospital for this reporting period; (13) Results cannot be calculated for this reporting period; (14) The results for this state are combined with nearby states to protect confidentiality; Please refer to the User's Guide for a full explanation of data.

Aspirin Given at Discharge[2]	29	100%	99%	99%
Fibrinolytic Meds Within 30 Min. of Arrival[2,7]	-	-	46%	54%
PCI Within 90 Minutes of Arrival[2,7]	-	-	95%	96%
Statin Prescribed at Discharge[2]	17	88%	98%	98%
Heart Failure Care				
ACE Inhibitor or ARB for LVSD[2]	43	88%	96%	97%
Discharge Instructions Given[2]	191	99%	95%	94%
Evaluation of LVS Function[2]	258	99%	99%	99%
Medicare Spending				
Medicare Spending per Patient (ratio)	-	1.10	0.96	0.98
Pneumonia Care				
Appropriate Initial Antibiotic Given[2]	121	96%	95%	95%
Blood Culture Timing[2]	182	99%	97%	98%
Pregnancy and Delivery Care				
Newborn Deliveries Scheduled Early[7]	-	-	4%	6%
Preventive Care				
Immunization for Influenza[2]	609	92%	88%	90%
Immunization for Pneumonia[2]	965	88%	88%	92%
Stroke Care				
Anticoagulation Therapy for Atrial Fibrillation	24	88%	96%	95%
Antithrombotic Therapy Timing	124	99%	98%	98%
Assessed for Rehabilitation	116	100%	97%	97%
Discharged on Antithrombotic Therapy	113	96%	99%	99%
Discharged on Statin Medication	74	96%	95%	94%
Thrombolytic Therapy Timing	44	7%	69%	66%
Venous Thromboembolism Prophylaxis	130	90%	94%	94%
Written Stroke Educational Materials Given	60	100%	86%	88%
Surgical Care Improvement Project				
Appropriate Beta Blocker Usage[2]	98	98%	97%	98%
Appropriate VTP Within 24 Hours[2]	241	99%	98%	98%
Controlled Postoperative Blood Glucose[2,7]	-	-	97%	97%
Perioperative Temperature Management[2]	265	100%	100%	100%
Prophylactic Antibiotic Selection[2]	168	99%	99%	99%
Prophylactic Antibiotic Selection (Outpatient)	13	77%	97%	98%
Prophylactic Antibiotic Stopped[2]	167	99%	98%	98%
Prophylactic Antibiotic Timing[2]	169	98%	99%	99%
Prophylactic Antibiotic Timing (Outpatient)	14	93%	97%	98%
Urinary Catheter Removal[2]	79	99%	96%	97%
Survey of Patients' Hospital Experiences				
Area Around Room 'Always' Quiet at Night	300+	49%	51%	61%
Doctors 'Always' Communicated Well	300+	77%	77%	82%
Home Recovery Information Given	300+	83%	83%	85%
Hospital Given 9 or 10 on 10 Point Scale	300+	59%	63%	71%
Meds 'Always' Explained Before Given	300+	57%	59%	64%
Nurses 'Always' Communicated Well	300+	73%	75%	79%
Pain 'Always' Well Controlled	300+	69%	67%	71%
Room and Bathroom 'Always' Clean	300+	62%	69%	73%
Timely Help 'Always' Received	300+	59%	61%	68%
Would Definitely Recommend Hospital	300+	59%	65%	71%
Use of Medical Imaging				
Cardiac Imaging Stress Test before Surgery[7]	-	-	5.8%	5.3%
Combination Abdominal CT Scan	419	1.4%	8.2%	10.5%
Combination Brain/Sinus CT Scan	904	1.9%	3.6%	2.7%
Combination Chest CT Scan	118	0.0%	1.3%	2.7%
Follow-up Mammogram/Ultrasound[1]	-	-	13%	8.8%
Lumbar Spine MRI for Low Back Pain[1]	-	-	33.4%	37.2%

Our Lady of Lourdes Memorial Hospital

169 Riverside Drive
Binghamton, NY 13905
Phone: 607-798-5111
Fax: 607-798-7681
E-mail: info@lourdes.com
URL: www.lourdes.com
Type: Acute Care Hospitals
Emergency Services: Yes
Ownership: Voluntary non-profit - Private
Beds: 161

Key Personnel:

Operating Room. . . . . Michael W Barrett
Quality Assurance . . . . Kathy Connerton
Emergency Room . . . . Debra Hackett
CEO/President. . . . . John O'Neil
Pediatric In-Patient Care . . . . Suzanne Parsons
Radiology. . . . . Mike Shevach
Chief of Medical Staff. . . . . Robert Taylor, III

Measure	Cases	This Hosp.	State Avg.	U.S. Avg.
Blood Clot Prevention and Treatment				
Anticoagulation Overlap Therapy[2]	62	100%	91%	93%
ICU Venous Thromboembolism Prophylaxis[2]	40	98%	92%	92%
Incidence of Potentially Preventable VTE[2,7]	-	-	10%	10%
UFH with Dosages/Platelet Monitoring[2]	40	98%	92%	97%
Venous Thromboembolism Prophylaxis[2]	356	92%	87%	85%
Warfarin Therapy Discharge Instructions[2]	47	85%	59%	75%
Chest Pain/Possible Heart Attack Care				
Aspirin Given Within 24 Hours of Arrival	34	100%	97%	96%
Fibrinolytic Meds Within 30 Min. of Arrival[7]	-	-	54%	58%
Average Time to ECG (minutes)	35	9	9	7
Average Time to Transfer (minutes)	16	78	78	60
Children's Asthma Care				
Received Home Management Plan of Care	-	-	-	88%
Received Reliever Medication	-	-	-	100%
Received Systemic Corticosteroids	-	-	-	100%
Emergency Department				
Admittance Decision Time (minutes)[2]	782	70	154	98
Head CT Results Within 45 Min. of Arrival[1]	-	-	55%	57%
Patients Who Left ER Before Being Seen	44,234	2%	2%	2%
Time from ER Arrival to Admit. (minutes)[2]	795	287	378	274
Time from ER Arrival to Discharge (minutes)	389	177	156	134
Time in ER Before Being Evaluated (minutes)	408	41	35	26
Time to Pain Meds for Fractures (minutes)	185	84	61	57
Heart Attack Care				
Aspirin Given at Discharge	74	99%	99%	99%
Fibrinolytic Meds Within 30 Min. of Arrival[7]	-	-	46%	54%
PCI Within 90 Minutes of Arrival[7]	-	-	95%	96%
Statin Prescribed at Discharge	64	97%	98%	98%
Heart Failure Care				
ACE Inhibitor or ARB for LVSD	66	92%	96%	97%
Discharge Instructions Given	270	99%	95%	94%
Evaluation of LVS Function	344	98%	99%	99%
Medicare Spending				
Medicare Spending per Patient (ratio)	-	0.90	0.96	0.98
Pneumonia Care				
Appropriate Initial Antibiotic Given	197	99%	95%	95%
Blood Culture Timing	385	100%	97%	98%
Pregnancy and Delivery Care				
Newborn Deliveries Scheduled Early[2]	32	0%	4%	6%
Preventive Care				
Immunization for Influenza[2]	555	91%	88%	90%
Immunization for Pneumonia[2]	775	87%	88%	92%
Stroke Care				
Anticoagulation Therapy for Atrial Fibrillation[2]	11	91%	96%	95%
Antithrombotic Therapy Timing[2]	76	100%	98%	98%
Assessed for Rehabilitation[2]	86	95%	97%	97%
Discharged on Antithrombotic Therapy[2]	79	95%	99%	99%
Discharged on Statin Medication[2]	67	94%	95%	94%
Thrombolytic Therapy Timing[1,2]	-	-	69%	66%
Venous Thromboembolism Prophylaxis[2]	81	84%	94%	94%
Written Stroke Educational Materials Given[2]	48	94%	86%	88%
Surgical Care Improvement Project				
Appropriate Beta Blocker Usage[2]	90	100%	97%	98%
Appropriate VTP Within 24 Hours[2]	278	99%	98%	98%
Controlled Postoperative Blood Glucose[2,7]	-	-	97%	97%
Perioperative Temperature Management[2]	316	100%	100%	100%
Prophylactic Antibiotic Selection[2]	196	99%	99%	99%
Prophylactic Antibiotic Selection (Outpatient)	280	97%	97%	98%
Prophylactic Antibiotic Stopped[2]	192	97%	98%	98%
Prophylactic Antibiotic Timing[2]	196	100%	99%	99%
Prophylactic Antibiotic Timing (Outpatient)	265	98%	97%	98%
Urinary Catheter Removal[2]	96	94%	96%	97%
Survey of Patients' Hospital Experiences				
Area Around Room 'Always' Quiet at Night	300+	61%	51%	61%
Doctors 'Always' Communicated Well	300+	77%	77%	82%
Home Recovery Information Given	300+	88%	83%	85%
Hospital Given 9 or 10 on 10 Point Scale	300+	69%	63%	71%
Meds 'Always' Explained Before Given	300+	60%	59%	64%
Nurses 'Always' Communicated Well	300+	76%	75%	79%
Pain 'Always' Well Controlled	300+	69%	67%	71%
Room and Bathroom 'Always' Clean	300+	71%	69%	73%
Timely Help 'Always' Received	300+	62%	61%	68%
Would Definitely Recommend Hospital	300+	75%	65%	71%
Use of Medical Imaging				
Cardiac Imaging Stress Test before Surgery[1]	-	-	5.8%	5.3%
Combination Abdominal CT Scan	1,447	15.6%	8.2%	10.5%
Combination Brain/Sinus CT Scan	1,054	4.5%	3.6%	2.7%
Combination Chest CT Scan	1,076	10.8%	1.3%	2.7%
Follow-up Mammogram/Ultrasound	2,596	10.6%	13%	8.8%
Lumbar Spine MRI for Low Back Pain	174	32.8%	33.4%	37.2%

Bronx - Lebanon Hospital Center

1276 Fulton Avenue
Bronx, NY 10456
Phone: 212-588-7000
Fax: 718-299-5447
URL: www.bronx-leb.org
Type: Acute Care Hospitals
Emergency Services: Yes
Ownership: Proprietary
Beds: 847

Key Personnel:

Cardiac Laboratory. . . . . Jonathan N Bella, MD
Operating Room. . . . . John M Cosgrove, MD
CEO/President. . . . . Miguel Fuentes
Pediatric Ambulatory Care . . . . . . Ram Kairam, MD
Pediatric In-Patient Care . . . . Ram Kairam, MD
Anesthesiology. . . . . Dave Livingstone, MD
Infection Control. . . . . Victor Lorian, MD
Radiology. . . . . Harvey Stern, MD

Measure	Cases	This Hosp.	State Avg.	U.S. Avg.
Blood Clot Prevention and Treatment				
Anticoagulation Overlap Therapy[2]	78	92%	91%	93%
ICU Venous Thromboembolism Prophylaxis[2]	99	99%	92%	92%
Incidence of Potentially Preventable VTE[2]	12	75%	10%	10%
UFH with Dosages/Platelet Monitoring[2]	44	98%	92%	97%
Venous Thromboembolism Prophylaxis[2]	425	97%	87%	85%
Warfarin Therapy Discharge Instructions[2]	61	100%	59%	75%
Chest Pain/Possible Heart Attack Care				
Aspirin Given Within 24 Hours of Arrival[1,3]	-	-	97%	96%
Fibrinolytic Meds Within 30 Min. of Arrival[5]	-	-	54%	58%
Average Time to ECG (minutes)[1,3]	-	-	9	7
Average Time to Transfer (minutes)[5]	-	-	78	60
Children's Asthma Care				
Received Home Management Plan of Care	-	-	-	88%
Received Reliever Medication	-	-	-	100%
Received Systemic Corticosteroids	-	-	-	100%
Emergency Department				
Admittance Decision Time (minutes)[2]	997	176	154	98
Head CT Results Within 45 Min. of Arrival[1]	-	-	55%	57%
Patients Who Left ER Before Being Seen	>100k	4%	2%	2%
Time from ER Arrival to Admit. (minutes)[2]	988	474	378	274
Time from ER Arrival to Discharge (minutes)	350	199	156	134
Time in ER Before Being Evaluated (minutes)	432	47	35	26
Time to Pain Meds for Fractures (minutes)	123	37	61	57
Heart Attack Care				
Aspirin Given at Discharge	152	100%	99%	99%
Fibrinolytic Meds Within 30 Min. of Arrival[1]	-	-	46%	54%
PCI Within 90 Minutes of Arrival	46	100%	95%	96%
Statin Prescribed at Discharge	152	100%	98%	98%
Heart Failure Care				
ACE Inhibitor or ARB for LVSD[2]	166	99%	96%	97%
Discharge Instructions Given[2]	325	92%	95%	94%
Evaluation of LVS Function[2]	349	100%	99%	99%
Medicare Spending				
Medicare Spending per Patient (ratio)	-	0.92	0.96	0.98
Pneumonia Care				
Appropriate Initial Antibiotic Given[2]	79	97%	95%	95%
Blood Culture Timing[2]	186	94%	97%	98%
Pregnancy and Delivery Care				
Newborn Deliveries Scheduled Early[2]	26	0%	4%	6%
Preventive Care				
Immunization for Influenza[2]	739	86%	88%	90%
Immunization for Pneumonia[2]	790	88%	88%	92%
Stroke Care				
Anticoagulation Therapy for Atrial Fibrillation[1]	-	-	96%	95%
Antithrombotic Therapy Timing	110	100%	98%	98%
Assessed for Rehabilitation	140	100%	97%	97%
Discharged on Antithrombotic Therapy	116	100%	99%	99%
Discharged on Statin Medication	93	99%	95%	94%

NOTE: Hospital profiles are in alphabetical order by state, then city, then hospital within the city; Rankings exclude hospitals with less than 25 cases except for patient surveys which excludes hospitals with less than 100 cases; (a) 100-299 cases; (1) The number of cases/patients is too few to report; (2) Data submitted were based on a sample of cases/patients; (3) Results are based on a shorter time period than required; (4) Data suppressed by CMS for one or more quarters; (5) Results are not available for this reporting period; (6) Fewer than 100 patients completed the HCAHPS survey; (7) No cases met the criteria for this measure; (8) The lower limit of the confidence interval cannot be calculated if the number of observed infections equals zero; (9) No data are available from the state/territory for this reporting period; (10) The scores shown reflect fewer than 50 completed surveys; (11) There were discrepancies in the data collection process; (12) This measure does not apply to this hospital for this reporting period; (13) Results cannot be calculated for this reporting period; (14) The results for this state are combined with nearby states to protect confidentiality; Please refer to the User's Guide for a full explanation of data.

Measure	Cases	This Hosp.	State Avg.	U.S. Avg.
Thrombolytic Therapy Timing	14	100%	69%	66%
Venous Thromboembolism Prophylaxis	161	100%	94%	94%
Written Stroke Educational Materials Given	84	99%	86%	88%
Surgical Care Improvement Project				
Appropriate Beta Blocker Usage[2]	81	93%	97%	98%
Appropriate VTP Within 24 Hours[2]	350	96%	98%	98%
Controlled Postoperative Blood Glucose[2,7]	-	-	97%	97%
Perioperative Temperature Management[2]	392	100%	100%	100%
Prophylactic Antibiotic Selection[2]	263	99%	99%	99%
Prophylactic Antibiotic Selection (Outpatient)	171	96%	97%	98%
Prophylactic Antibiotic Stopped[2]	255	95%	98%	98%
Prophylactic Antibiotic Timing[2]	263	99%	99%	99%
Prophylactic Antibiotic Timing (Outpatient)	55	98%	97%	98%
Urinary Catheter Removal[2]	92	96%	96%	97%
Survey of Patients' Hospital Experiences				
Area Around Room 'Always' Quiet at Night	300+	55%	51%	61%
Doctors 'Always' Communicated Well	300+	77%	77%	82%
Home Recovery Information Given	300+	81%	83%	85%
Hospital Given 9 or 10 on 10 Point Scale	300+	56%	63%	71%
Meds 'Always' Explained Before Given	300+	53%	59%	64%
Nurses 'Always' Communicated Well	300+	67%	75%	79%
Pain 'Always' Well Controlled	300+	63%	67%	71%
Room and Bathroom 'Always' Clean	300+	60%	69%	73%
Timely Help 'Always' Received	300+	52%	61%	68%
Would Definitely Recommend Hospital	300+	55%	65%	71%
Use of Medical Imaging				
Cardiac Imaging Stress Test before Surgery[1]	-	-	5.8%	5.3%
Combination Abdominal CT Scan	238	6.7%	8.2%	10.5%
Combination Brain/Sinus CT Scan[1]	-	-	3.6%	2.7%
Combination Chest CT Scan	86	4.7%	1.3%	2.7%
Follow-up Mammogram/Ultrasound	177	6.2%	13%	8.8%
Lumbar Spine MRI for Low Back Pain[1]	-	-	33.4%	37.2%

Bronx VA Medical Center

130 West Kingsbridge Road
Bronx, NY 10468
Phone: 718-584-9000
Fax: 718-741-4491
URL: www.med.va.gov
Type: Acute Care - VA
Ownership: Government Federal
Emergency Services: No
Beds: 459

Key Personnel:
Operating Room. . . . . Avrora Alconaba
Infection Control. . . . . Sheldon Brown
Coronary Care . . . . Yvonne Burrus
Chief of Medical Staff. . . . . Dr Erik Langnoff
Emergency Room . . . . Steve Pastores, MD
Intensive Care Unit. . . . . R Siegel, MD
Radiology. . . . . In Sook Song, MD
Anesthesiology. . . . . Thomas Tagliente

Measure	Cases	This Hosp.	State Avg.	U.S. Avg.
Blood Clot Prevention and Treatment				
Anticoagulation Overlap Therapy	-	-	91%	93%
ICU Venous Thromboembolism Prophylaxis	-	-	92%	92%
Incidence of Potentially Preventable VTE	-	-	10%	10%
UFH with Dosages/Platelet Monitoring	-	-	92%	97%
Venous Thromboembolism Prophylaxis	-	-	87%	85%
Warfarin Therapy Discharge Instructions	-	-	59%	75%
Chest Pain/Possible Heart Attack Care				
Aspirin Given Within 24 Hours of Arrival	-	-	97%	96%
Fibrinolytic Meds Within 30 Min. of Arrival	-	-	54%	58%
Average Time to ECG (minutes)	-	-	9	7
Average Time to Transfer (minutes)	-	-	78	60
Children's Asthma Care				
Received Home Management Plan of Care	-	-	-	88%
Received Reliever Medication	-	-	-	100%
Received Systemic Corticosteroids	-	-	-	100%
Emergency Department				
Admittance Decision Time (minutes)	-	-	154	98
Head CT Results Within 45 Min. of Arrival	-	-	55%	57%
Patients Who Left ER Before Being Seen	-	-	2%	2%
Time from ER Arrival to Admit. (minutes)	-	-	378	274
Time from ER Arrival to Discharge (minutes)	-	-	156	134
Time in ER Before Being Evaluated (minutes)	-	-	35	26
Time to Pain Meds for Fractures (minutes)	-	-	61	57
Heart Attack Care				
Aspirin Given at Discharge[1]	12	100%	99%	99%
Fibrinolytic Meds Within 30 Min. of Arrival[5]	-	-	46%	54%
PCI Within 90 Minutes of Arrival[5]	-	-	95%	96%
Statin Prescribed at Discharge[1]	12	100%	98%	98%
Heart Failure Care				
ACE Inhibitor or ARB for LVSD	61	95%	96%	97%
Discharge Instructions Given	131	97%	95%	94%
Evaluation of LVS Function	146	100%	99%	99%
Medicare Spending				
Medicare Spending per Patient (ratio)	-	-	0.96	0.98
Pneumonia Care				
Appropriate Initial Antibiotic Given	34	91%	95%	95%
Blood Culture Timing	72	97%	97%	98%
Pregnancy and Delivery Care				
Newborn Deliveries Scheduled Early	-	-	4%	6%
Preventive Care				
Immunization for Influenza[5]	-	-	88%	90%
Immunization for Pneumonia[5]	-	-	88%	92%
Stroke Care				
Anticoagulation Therapy for Atrial Fibrillation	-	-	96%	95%
Antithrombotic Therapy Timing	-	-	98%	98%
Assessed for Rehabilitation	-	-	97%	97%
Discharged on Antithrombotic Therapy	-	-	99%	99%
Discharged on Statin Medication	-	-	95%	94%
Thrombolytic Therapy Timing	-	-	69%	66%
Venous Thromboembolism Prophylaxis	-	-	94%	94%
Written Stroke Educational Materials Given	-	-	86%	88%
Surgical Care Improvement Project				
Appropriate Beta Blocker Usage[2]	31	74%	97%	98%
Appropriate VTP Within 24 Hours[2]	84	95%	98%	98%
Controlled Postoperative Blood Glucose[1,2]	-	-	97%	97%
Perioperative Temperature Management[2]	96	96%	100%	100%
Prophylactic Antibiotic Selection	50	100%	99%	99%
Prophylactic Antibiotic Selection (Outpatient)	-	-	97%	98%
Prophylactic Antibiotic Stopped	49	98%	98%	98%
Prophylactic Antibiotic Timing	50	100%	99%	99%
Prophylactic Antibiotic Timing (Outpatient)	-	-	97%	98%
Urinary Catheter Removal[2]	69	100%	96%	97%
Survey of Patients' Hospital Experiences				
Area Around Room 'Always' Quiet at Night	-	-	51%	61%
Doctors 'Always' Communicated Well	-	-	77%	82%
Home Recovery Information Given	-	-	83%	85%
Hospital Given 9 or 10 on 10 Point Scale	-	-	63%	71%
Meds 'Always' Explained Before Given	-	-	59%	64%
Nurses 'Always' Communicated Well	-	-	75%	79%
Pain 'Always' Well Controlled	-	-	67%	71%
Room and Bathroom 'Always' Clean	-	-	69%	73%
Timely Help 'Always' Received	-	-	61%	68%
Would Definitely Recommend Hospital	-	-	65%	71%
Use of Medical Imaging				
Cardiac Imaging Stress Test before Surgery	-	-	5.8%	5.3%
Combination Abdominal CT Scan	-	-	8.2%	10.5%
Combination Brain/Sinus CT Scan	-	-	3.6%	2.7%
Combination Chest CT Scan	-	-	1.3%	2.7%
Follow-up Mammogram/Ultrasound	-	-	13%	8.8%
Lumbar Spine MRI for Low Back Pain	-	-	33.4%	37.2%

Jacobi Medical Center

1400 Pelham Parkway South
Bronx, NY 10461
Phone: 718-918-5000
Fax: 718-918-4607
URL: www.ci.nyc.ny.us/html/hhc
Type: Acute Care Hospitals
Ownership: Government - Local
Emergency Services: Yes
Beds: 527

Key Personnel:
Emergency Room . . . . Paul Gennis, MD
CEO/President. . . . . Joseph Orlando

Measure	Cases	This Hosp.	State Avg.	U.S. Avg.
Blood Clot Prevention and Treatment				
Anticoagulation Overlap Therapy[2]	80	92%	91%	93%
ICU Venous Thromboembolism Prophylaxis[2]	69	100%	92%	92%
Incidence of Potentially Preventable VTE[2]	49	4%	10%	10%
UFH with Dosages/Platelet Monitoring[2]	45	58%	92%	97%
Venous Thromboembolism Prophylaxis[2]	307	97%	87%	85%
Warfarin Therapy Discharge Instructions[2]	51	0%	59%	75%
Chest Pain/Possible Heart Attack Care				
Aspirin Given Within 24 Hours of Arrival	47	100%	97%	96%
Fibrinolytic Meds Within 30 Min. of Arrival[7]	-	-	54%	58%
Average Time to ECG (minutes)	44	9	9	7
Average Time to Transfer (minutes)[1]	-	-	78	60
Children's Asthma Care				
Received Home Management Plan of Care	-	-	-	88%
Received Reliever Medication	-	-	-	100%
Received Systemic Corticosteroids	-	-	-	100%
Emergency Department				
Admittance Decision Time (minutes)[2]	709	369	154	98
Head CT Results Within 45 Min. of Arrival[1]	-	-	55%	57%
Patients Who Left ER Before Being Seen	>100k	8%	2%	2%
Time from ER Arrival to Admit. (minutes)[2]	710	674	378	274
Time from ER Arrival to Discharge (minutes)	331	246	156	134
Time in ER Before Being Evaluated (minutes)	358	77	35	26
Time to Pain Meds for Fractures (minutes)	180	64	61	57
Heart Attack Care				
Aspirin Given at Discharge	38	100%	99%	99%
Fibrinolytic Meds Within 30 Min. of Arrival[7]	-	-	46%	54%
PCI Within 90 Minutes of Arrival[7]	-	-	95%	96%
Statin Prescribed at Discharge	35	97%	98%	98%
Heart Failure Care				
ACE Inhibitor or ARB for LVSD	86	98%	96%	97%
Discharge Instructions Given	196	100%	95%	94%
Evaluation of LVS Function	242	100%	99%	99%
Medicare Spending				
Medicare Spending per Patient (ratio)	-	0.96	0.96	0.98
Pneumonia Care				
Appropriate Initial Antibiotic Given	72	97%	95%	95%
Blood Culture Timing	185	92%	97%	98%
Pregnancy and Delivery Care				
Newborn Deliveries Scheduled Early[2]	39	0%	4%	6%
Preventive Care				
Immunization for Influenza[2]	507	48%	88%	90%
Immunization for Pneumonia[2]	463	47%	88%	92%
Stroke Care				
Anticoagulation Therapy for Atrial Fibrillation[1]	-	-	96%	95%
Antithrombotic Therapy Timing	94	100%	98%	98%
Assessed for Rehabilitation	112	94%	97%	97%
Discharged on Antithrombotic Therapy	100	100%	99%	99%
Discharged on Statin Medication	74	96%	95%	94%
Thrombolytic Therapy Timing[1]	-	-	69%	66%
Venous Thromboembolism Prophylaxis	123	93%	94%	94%
Written Stroke Educational Materials Given	38	24%	86%	88%
Surgical Care Improvement Project				
Appropriate Beta Blocker Usage	75	91%	97%	98%
Appropriate VTP Within 24 Hours	352	99%	98%	98%
Controlled Postoperative Blood Glucose[1]	-	-	97%	97%
Perioperative Temperature Management	417	99%	100%	100%
Prophylactic Antibiotic Selection	156	99%	99%	99%
Prophylactic Antibiotic Selection (Outpatient)	121	98%	97%	98%
Prophylactic Antibiotic Stopped	146	95%	98%	98%
Prophylactic Antibiotic Timing	156	99%	99%	99%
Prophylactic Antibiotic Timing (Outpatient)	51	90%	97%	98%
Urinary Catheter Removal	188	95%	96%	97%
Survey of Patients' Hospital Experiences				
Area Around Room 'Always' Quiet at Night	300+	47%	51%	61%
Doctors 'Always' Communicated Well	300+	75%	77%	82%
Home Recovery Information Given	300+	80%	83%	85%
Hospital Given 9 or 10 on 10 Point Scale	300+	55%	63%	71%
Meds 'Always' Explained Before Given	300+	51%	59%	64%
Nurses 'Always' Communicated Well	300+	63%	75%	79%
Pain 'Always' Well Controlled	300+	61%	67%	71%
Room and Bathroom 'Always' Clean	300+	66%	69%	73%
Timely Help 'Always' Received	300+	47%	61%	68%
Would Definitely Recommend Hospital	300+	58%	65%	71%
Use of Medical Imaging				
Cardiac Imaging Stress Test before Surgery[1]	-	-	5.8%	5.3%
Combination Abdominal CT Scan	99	27.3%	8.2%	10.5%
Combination Brain/Sinus CT Scan	158	0.6%	3.6%	2.7%

NOTE: Hospital profiles are in alphabetical order by state, then city, then hospital within the city; Rankings exclude hospitals with less than 25 cases except for patient surveys which excludes hospitals with less than 100 cases; (a) 100-299 cases; (1) The number of cases/patients is too few to report; (2) Data submitted were based on a sample of cases/patients; (3) Results are based on a shorter time period than required; (4) Data suppressed by CMS for one or more quarters; (5) Results are not available for this reporting period; (6) Fewer than 100 patients completed the HCAHPS survey; (7) No cases met the criteria for this measure; (8) The lower limit of the confidence interval cannot be calculated if the number of observed infections equals zero; (9) No data are available from the state/territory for this reporting period; (10) The scores shown reflect fewer than 50 completed surveys; (11) There were discrepancies in the data collection process; (12) This measure does not apply to this hospital for this reporting period; (13) Results cannot be calculated for this reporting period; (14) The results for this state are combined with nearby states to protect confidentiality; Please refer to the User's Guide for a full explanation of data.

Combination Chest CT Scan	97	17.5%	1.3%	2.7%
Follow-up Mammogram/Ultrasound	291	3.4%	13%	8.8%
Lumbar Spine MRI for Low Back Pain[1]	-	-	33.4%	37.2%

Lincoln Medical & Mental Health Center

234 East 149th Street
Bronx, NY 10451
Phone: 718-579-5000
Fax: 718-579-5319
URL: www.nyc.gov/html/hhc/lincoln
Type: Acute Care Hospitals
Emergency Services: Yes
Ownership: Government - Local
Beds: 595

Key Personnel:

Operating Room. . . . . Barbara Booker, RN
Quality Assurance . . . . David DeJesus
Radiology. . . . . Y Fayemi, MD
Infection Control. . . . . D Hewlett, MD
Pediatric Ambulatory Care . . . . . . R Kairam, MD
Pediatric In-Patient Care . . . . R Kairam, MD
CEO/President. . . . . Roberto Rodriguez
Chief of Medical Staff . . . . D Shine, MD

Measure	Cases	This Hosp.	State Avg.	U.S. Avg.
Blood Clot Prevention and Treatment				
Anticoagulation Overlap Therapy[2]	58	98%	91%	93%
ICU Venous Thromboembolism Prophylaxis[2]	64	100%	92%	92%
Incidence of Potentially Preventable VTE[2]	14	0%	10%	10%
UFH with Dosages/Platelet Monitoring[2]	11	100%	92%	97%
Venous Thromboembolism Prophylaxis[2]	222	98%	87%	85%
Warfarin Therapy Discharge Instructions[2]	52	96%	59%	75%
Chest Pain/Possible Heart Attack Care				
Aspirin Given Within 24 Hours of Arrival	17	100%	97%	96%
Fibrinolytic Meds Within 30 Min. of Arrival[1]	-	-	54%	58%
Average Time to ECG (minutes)	17	10	9	7
Average Time to Transfer (minutes)[7]	-	-	78	60
Children's Asthma Care				
Received Home Management Plan of Care	-	-	-	88%
Received Reliever Medication	-	-	-	100%
Received Systemic Corticosteroids	-	-	-	100%
Emergency Department				
Admittance Decision Time (minutes)[2]	913	129	154	98
Head CT Results Within 45 Min. of Arrival[1]	-	-	55%	57%
Patients Who Left ER Before Being Seen	>100k	4%	2%	2%
Time from ER Arrival to Admit. (minutes)[2]	919	415	378	274
Time from ER Arrival to Discharge (minutes)	341	163	156	134
Time in ER Before Being Evaluated (minutes)	377	82	35	26
Time to Pain Meds for Fractures (minutes)	168	44	61	57
Heart Attack Care				
Aspirin Given at Discharge	63	100%	99%	99%
Fibrinolytic Meds Within 30 Min. of Arrival[7]	-	-	46%	54%
PCI Within 90 Minutes of Arrival[7]	-	-	95%	96%
Statin Prescribed at Discharge	65	98%	98%	98%
Heart Failure Care				
ACE Inhibitor or ARB for LVSD	177	99%	96%	97%
Discharge Instructions Given	341	98%	95%	94%
Evaluation of LVS Function	365	100%	99%	99%
Medicare Spending				
Medicare Spending per Patient (ratio)	-	0.86	0.96	0.98
Pneumonia Care				
Appropriate Initial Antibiotic Given	227	100%	95%	95%
Blood Culture Timing	495	96%	97%	98%
Pregnancy and Delivery Care				
Newborn Deliveries Scheduled Early[2]	39	3%	4%	6%
Preventive Care				
Immunization for Influenza[2]	511	95%	88%	90%
Immunization for Pneumonia[2]	507	95%	88%	92%
Stroke Care				
Anticoagulation Therapy for Atrial Fibrillation	18	100%	96%	95%
Antithrombotic Therapy Timing	110	98%	98%	98%
Assessed for Rehabilitation	148	93%	97%	97%
Discharged on Antithrombotic Therapy	113	99%	99%	99%
Discharged on Statin Medication	98	99%	95%	94%
Thrombolytic Therapy Timing	30	23%	69%	66%
Venous Thromboembolism Prophylaxis	172	98%	94%	94%
Written Stroke Educational Materials Given	83	95%	86%	88%
Surgical Care Improvement Project				
Appropriate Beta Blocker Usage[2]	62	98%	97%	98%
Appropriate VTP Within 24 Hours[2]	256	100%	98%	98%
Controlled Postoperative Blood Glucose[2,7]	-	-	97%	97%
Perioperative Temperature Management[2]	304	100%	100%	100%
Prophylactic Antibiotic Selection[2]	152	99%	99%	99%
Prophylactic Antibiotic Selection (Outpatient)	191	99%	97%	98%
Prophylactic Antibiotic Stopped[2]	150	95%	98%	98%
Prophylactic Antibiotic Timing[2]	152	99%	99%	99%
Prophylactic Antibiotic Timing (Outpatient)	190	99%	97%	98%
Urinary Catheter Removal[2]	125	100%	96%	97%
Survey of Patients' Hospital Experiences				
Area Around Room 'Always' Quiet at Night	300+	46%	51%	61%
Doctors 'Always' Communicated Well	300+	74%	77%	82%
Home Recovery Information Given	300+	77%	83%	85%
Hospital Given 9 or 10 on 10 Point Scale	300+	50%	63%	71%
Meds 'Always' Explained Before Given	300+	52%	59%	64%
Nurses 'Always' Communicated Well	300+	62%	75%	79%
Pain 'Always' Well Controlled	300+	57%	67%	71%
Room and Bathroom 'Always' Clean	300+	58%	69%	73%
Timely Help 'Always' Received	300+	46%	61%	68%
Would Definitely Recommend Hospital	300+	53%	65%	71%
Use of Medical Imaging				
Cardiac Imaging Stress Test before Surgery[1]	-	-	5.8%	5.3%
Combination Abdominal CT Scan	175	4.0%	8.2%	10.5%
Combination Brain/Sinus CT Scan	218	7.8%	3.6%	2.7%
Combination Chest CT Scan	132	0.8%	1.3%	2.7%
Follow-up Mammogram/Ultrasound[7]	-	-	13%	8.8%
Lumbar Spine MRI for Low Back Pain[7]	-	-	33.4%	37.2%

Montefiore Medical Center

111 East 210th Street
Bronx, NY 10467
Phone: 718-920-4321
Fax: 718-920-2242
URL: www.montefiore.org
Type: Acute Care Hospitals
Emergency Services: Yes
Ownership: Voluntary non-profit - Private
Beds: 1,062

Key Personnel:

Radiology. . . . . E Stephen Amis, MD
Pediatrics. . . . . Judy L. Aschner, MD
Operating Room. . . . . Arnold Berlin, MD
Anesthesiology. . . . . Ellise Delphin, MD, MPH
Chief of Medical Staff . . . . Gary Kalkut, MD, MPH
Surgery . . . . Robert E. Michler, MD
Hemotology Center . . . . Roman Perez-Soler, MD
CEO/President. . . . . Steven M Safyer, MD

Measure	Cases	This Hosp.	State Avg.	U.S. Avg.
Blood Clot Prevention and Treatment				
Anticoagulation Overlap Therapy[2]	411	84%	91%	93%
ICU Venous Thromboembolism Prophylaxis[2]	22	91%	92%	92%
Incidence of Potentially Preventable VTE[2]	235	22%	10%	10%
UFH with Dosages/Platelet Monitoring[2]	252	99%	92%	97%
Venous Thromboembolism Prophylaxis[2]	453	72%	87%	85%
Warfarin Therapy Discharge Instructions[2]	222	43%	59%	75%
Chest Pain/Possible Heart Attack Care				
Aspirin Given Within 24 Hours of Arrival[5]	-	-	97%	96%
Fibrinolytic Meds Within 30 Min. of Arrival[5]	-	-	54%	58%
Average Time to ECG (minutes)[5]	-	-	9	7
Average Time to Transfer (minutes)[5]	-	-	78	60
Children's Asthma Care				
Received Home Management Plan of Care	-	-	-	88%
Received Reliever Medication	-	-	-	100%
Received Systemic Corticosteroids	-	-	-	100%
Emergency Department				
Admittance Decision Time (minutes)[2]	331	317	154	98
Head CT Results Within 45 Min. of Arrival[1]	-	-	55%	57%
Patients Who Left ER Before Being Seen	>100k	3%	2%	2%
Time from ER Arrival to Admit. (minutes)[2]	791	599	378	274
Time from ER Arrival to Discharge (minutes)	374	270	156	134
Time in ER Before Being Evaluated (minutes)	378	114	35	26
Time to Pain Meds for Fractures (minutes)	382	114	61	57
Heart Attack Care				
Aspirin Given at Discharge[2]	370	93%	99%	99%
Fibrinolytic Meds Within 30 Min. of Arrival[2,7]	-	-	46%	54%
PCI Within 90 Minutes of Arrival[2]	34	88%	95%	96%
Statin Prescribed at Discharge[2]	365	89%	98%	98%
Heart Failure Care				
ACE Inhibitor or ARB for LVSD[2]	230	85%	96%	97%
Discharge Instructions Given[2]	545	93%	95%	94%
Evaluation of LVS Function[2]	659	99%	99%	99%
Medicare Spending				
Medicare Spending per Patient (ratio)	-	0.97	0.96	0.98
Pneumonia Care				
Appropriate Initial Antibiotic Given[2]	143	86%	95%	95%
Blood Culture Timing[2]	283	84%	97%	98%
Pregnancy and Delivery Care				
Newborn Deliveries Scheduled Early[2]	70	7%	4%	6%
Preventive Care				
Immunization for Influenza[2]	584	33%	88%	90%
Immunization for Pneumonia[2]	718	54%	88%	92%
Stroke Care				
Anticoagulation Therapy for Atrial Fibrillation	92	90%	96%	95%
Antithrombotic Therapy Timing	570	96%	98%	98%
Assessed for Rehabilitation	712	95%	97%	97%
Discharged on Antithrombotic Therapy	599	98%	99%	99%
Discharged on Statin Medication	494	94%	95%	94%
Thrombolytic Therapy Timing	57	68%	69%	66%
Venous Thromboembolism Prophylaxis	767	86%	94%	94%
Written Stroke Educational Materials Given	370	78%	86%	88%
Surgical Care Improvement Project				
Appropriate Beta Blocker Usage[2]	384	87%	97%	98%
Appropriate VTP Within 24 Hours[2]	645	95%	98%	98%
Controlled Postoperative Blood Glucose[2]	212	96%	97%	97%
Perioperative Temperature Management[2]	906	95%	100%	100%
Prophylactic Antibiotic Selection[2]	710	94%	99%	99%
Prophylactic Antibiotic Selection (Outpatient)	500	64%	97%	98%
Prophylactic Antibiotic Stopped[2]	701	93%	98%	98%
Prophylactic Antibiotic Timing[2]	724	89%	99%	99%
Prophylactic Antibiotic Timing (Outpatient)	534	86%	97%	98%
Urinary Catheter Removal[2]	541	82%	96%	97%
Survey of Patients' Hospital Experiences				
Area Around Room 'Always' Quiet at Night	300+	54%	51%	61%
Doctors 'Always' Communicated Well	300+	78%	77%	82%
Home Recovery Information Given	300+	82%	83%	85%
Hospital Given 9 or 10 on 10 Point Scale	300+	63%	63%	71%
Meds 'Always' Explained Before Given	300+	59%	59%	64%
Nurses 'Always' Communicated Well	300+	72%	75%	79%
Pain 'Always' Well Controlled	300+	65%	67%	71%
Room and Bathroom 'Always' Clean	300+	70%	69%	73%
Timely Help 'Always' Received	300+	54%	61%	68%
Would Definitely Recommend Hospital	300+	67%	65%	71%
Use of Medical Imaging				
Cardiac Imaging Stress Test before Surgery	388	8.2%	5.8%	5.3%
Combination Abdominal CT Scan	1,941	5.2%	8.2%	10.5%
Combination Brain/Sinus CT Scan	1,532	1.0%	3.6%	2.7%
Combination Chest CT Scan	1,566	1.8%	1.3%	2.7%
Follow-up Mammogram/Ultrasound	3,017	4.9%	13%	8.8%
Lumbar Spine MRI for Low Back Pain	131	21.4%	33.4%	37.2%

North Central Bronx Hospital

3424 Kossuth Avenue & 210th Street
Phone: 212-519-5000
Bronx, NY 10467
URL: www.nyc.gov/html/hhc/ncbh/home.html
Type: Acute Care Hospitals
Emergency Services: Yes
Ownership: Government - Local
Beds: 202

Measure	Cases	This Hosp.	State Avg.	U.S. Avg.
Blood Clot Prevention and Treatment				
Anticoagulation Overlap Therapy[2]	20	95%	91%	93%
ICU Venous Thromboembolism Prophylaxis[2]	50	100%	92%	92%
Incidence of Potentially Preventable VTE[1,2]	-	-	10%	10%
UFH with Dosages/Platelet Monitoring[1,2]	-	-	92%	97%
Venous Thromboembolism Prophylaxis[2]	340	96%	87%	85%
Warfarin Therapy Discharge Instructions[2]	18	0%	59%	75%
Chest Pain/Possible Heart Attack Care				
Aspirin Given Within 24 Hours of Arrival[1,3]	-	-	97%	96%
Fibrinolytic Meds Within 30 Min. of Arrival[3,7]	-	-	54%	58%
Average Time to ECG (minutes)[1,3]	-	-	9	7
Average Time to Transfer (minutes)[1,3]	-	-	78	60
Children's Asthma Care				

NOTE: Hospital profiles are in alphabetical order by state, then city, then hospital within the city; Rankings exclude hospitals with less than 25 cases except for patient surveys which excludes hospitals with less than 100 cases; (a) 100-299 cases; (1) The number of cases/patients is too few to report; (2) Data submitted were based on a sample of cases/patients; (3) Results are based on a shorter time period than required; (4) Data suppressed by CMS for one or more quarters; (5) Results are not available for this reporting period; (6) Fewer than 100 patients completed the HCAHPS survey; (7) No cases met the criteria for this measure; (8) The lower limit of the confidence interval cannot be calculated if the number of observed infections equals zero; (9) No data are available from the state/territory for this reporting period; (10) The scores shown reflect fewer than 50 completed surveys; (11) There were discrepancies in the data collection process; (12) This measure does not apply to this hospital for this reporting period; (13) Results cannot be calculated for this reporting period; (14) The results for this state are combined with nearby states to protect confidentiality; Please refer to the User's Guide for a full explanation of data.

Measure	Cases	This Hosp.	State Avg.	U.S. Avg.
Received Home Management Plan of Care	-	-	-	88%
Received Reliever Medication	-	-	-	100%
Received Systemic Corticosteroids	-	-	-	100%
Emergency Department				
Admittance Decision Time (minutes)[2]	581	118	154	98
Head CT Results Within 45 Min. of Arrival[5]	-	-	55%	57%
Patients Who Left ER Before Being Seen	57,051	2%	2%	2%
Time from ER Arrival to Admit. (minutes)[2]	587	329	378	274
Time from ER Arrival to Discharge (minutes)	350	188	156	134
Time in ER Before Being Evaluated (minutes)	383	73	35	26
Time to Pain Meds for Fractures (minutes)	54	52	61	57
Heart Attack Care				
Aspirin Given at Discharge	14	100%	99%	99%
Fibrinolytic Meds Within 30 Min. of Arrival[7]	-	-	46%	54%
PCI Within 90 Minutes of Arrival[7]	-	-	95%	96%
Statin Prescribed at Discharge	13	100%	98%	98%
Heart Failure Care				
ACE Inhibitor or ARB for LVSD	44	100%	96%	97%
Discharge Instructions Given	95	100%	95%	94%
Evaluation of LVS Function	105	100%	99%	99%
Medicare Spending				
Medicare Spending per Patient (ratio)	-	0.91	0.96	0.98
Pneumonia Care				
Appropriate Initial Antibiotic Given	57	98%	95%	95%
Blood Culture Timing	104	97%	97%	98%
Pregnancy and Delivery Care				
Newborn Deliveries Scheduled Early[2]	18	0%	4%	6%
Preventive Care				
Immunization for Influenza[2]	464	53%	88%	90%
Immunization for Pneumonia[2]	466	60%	88%	92%
Stroke Care				
Anticoagulation Therapy for Atrial Fibrillation[7]	-	-	96%	95%
Antithrombotic Therapy Timing	26	100%	98%	98%
Assessed for Rehabilitation	24	67%	97%	97%
Discharged on Antithrombotic Therapy	23	100%	99%	99%
Discharged on Statin Medication	19	95%	95%	94%
Thrombolytic Therapy Timing[1]	-	-	69%	66%
Venous Thromboembolism Prophylaxis	26	100%	94%	94%
Written Stroke Educational Materials Given	16	0%	86%	88%
Surgical Care Improvement Project				
Appropriate Beta Blocker Usage[1]	-	-	97%	98%
Appropriate VTP Within 24 Hours	50	98%	98%	98%
Controlled Postoperative Blood Glucose[7]	-	-	97%	97%
Perioperative Temperature Management	55	98%	100%	100%
Prophylactic Antibiotic Selection	25	100%	99%	99%
Prophylactic Antibiotic Selection (Outpatient)	22	95%	97%	98%
Prophylactic Antibiotic Stopped	25	96%	98%	98%
Prophylactic Antibiotic Timing	26	96%	99%	99%
Prophylactic Antibiotic Timing (Outpatient)[1]	-	-	97%	98%
Urinary Catheter Removal	13	100%	96%	97%
Survey of Patients' Hospital Experiences				
Area Around Room 'Always' Quiet at Night	300+	56%	51%	61%
Doctors 'Always' Communicated Well	300+	77%	77%	82%
Home Recovery Information Given	300+	74%	83%	85%
Hospital Given 9 or 10 on 10 Point Scale	300+	57%	63%	71%
Meds 'Always' Explained Before Given	300+	52%	59%	64%
Nurses 'Always' Communicated Well	300+	67%	75%	79%
Pain 'Always' Well Controlled	300+	58%	67%	71%
Room and Bathroom 'Always' Clean	300+	69%	69%	73%
Timely Help 'Always' Received	300+	47%	61%	68%
Would Definitely Recommend Hospital	300+	61%	65%	71%
Use of Medical Imaging				
Cardiac Imaging Stress Test before Surgery[1]	-	-	5.8%	5.3%
Combination Abdominal CT Scan[1]	-	-	8.2%	10.5%
Combination Brain/Sinus CT Scan[1]	-	-	3.6%	2.7%
Combination Chest CT Scan[1]	-	-	1.3%	2.7%
Follow-up Mammogram/Ultrasound	114	2.6%	13%	8.8%
Lumbar Spine MRI for Low Back Pain[1]	-	-	33.4%	37.2%

Saint Barnabas Hospital

4422 Third Avenue
Bronx, NY 10457
Phone: 212-960-9000
Fax: 718-960-6615
URL: www.stbarnabashospital.org
Type: Acute Care Hospitals
Emergency Services: Yes
Ownership: Voluntary non-profit - Private
Beds: 461

Key Personnel:

Quality Assurance . . . . Toni Armada
Chief of Medical Staff. . . . . Jerry Balentine
Infection Control. . . . . Judith Berger, MD
CEO/President. . . . . Scott Cooper, MD
Operating Room. . . . . Stephen Di Russo, MD
Radiology. . . . . Rocco Ducchille, MD
Pediatric In-Patient Care . . . . . . David Rubin, MD
Chairman/CEO . . . . Victor R. Wright

Measure	Cases	This Hosp.	State Avg.	U.S. Avg.
Blood Clot Prevention and Treatment				
Anticoagulation Overlap Therapy[2]	54	96%	91%	93%
ICU Venous Thromboembolism Prophylaxis[2]	55	98%	92%	92%
Incidence of Potentially Preventable VTE[2]	29	3%	10%	10%
UFH with Dosages/Platelet Monitoring[2]	15	100%	92%	97%
Venous Thromboembolism Prophylaxis[2]	260	80%	87%	85%
Warfarin Therapy Discharge Instructions[2]	40	80%	59%	75%
Chest Pain/Possible Heart Attack Care				
Aspirin Given Within 24 Hours of Arrival[1,3]	-	-	97%	96%
Fibrinolytic Meds Within 30 Min. of Arrival[3,7]	-	-	54%	58%
Average Time to ECG (minutes)[1,3]	-	-	9	7
Average Time to Transfer (minutes)[3,7]	-	-	78	60
Children's Asthma Care				
Received Home Management Plan of Care	-	-	-	88%
Received Reliever Medication	-	-	-	100%
Received Systemic Corticosteroids	-	-	-	100%
Emergency Department				
Admittance Decision Time (minutes)[2]	133	283	154	98
Head CT Results Within 45 Min. of Arrival[1]	-	-	55%	57%
Patients Who Left ER Before Being Seen	95,700	10%	2%	2%
Time from ER Arrival to Admit. (minutes)[2]	134	736	378	274
Time from ER Arrival to Discharge (minutes)[3]	41	353	156	134
Time in ER Before Being Evaluated (minutes)	60	86	35	26
Time to Pain Meds for Fractures (minutes)	121	83	61	57
Heart Attack Care				
Aspirin Given at Discharge	68	100%	99%	99%
Fibrinolytic Meds Within 30 Min. of Arrival[7]	-	-	46%	54%
PCI Within 90 Minutes of Arrival	16	100%	95%	96%
Statin Prescribed at Discharge	64	100%	98%	98%
Heart Failure Care				
ACE Inhibitor or ARB for LVSD	147	99%	96%	97%
Discharge Instructions Given	262	98%	95%	94%
Evaluation of LVS Function	286	100%	99%	99%
Medicare Spending				
Medicare Spending per Patient (ratio)	-	0.91	0.96	0.98
Pneumonia Care				
Appropriate Initial Antibiotic Given[2]	60	98%	95%	95%
Blood Culture Timing[2]	134	99%	97%	98%
Pregnancy and Delivery Care				
Newborn Deliveries Scheduled Early[2]	19	11%	4%	6%
Preventive Care				
Immunization for Influenza[2]	526	88%	88%	90%
Immunization for Pneumonia[2]	550	91%	88%	92%
Stroke Care				
Anticoagulation Therapy for Atrial Fibrillation[1]	-	-	96%	95%
Antithrombotic Therapy Timing	97	95%	98%	98%
Assessed for Rehabilitation	105	99%	97%	97%
Discharged on Antithrombotic Therapy	94	99%	99%	99%
Discharged on Statin Medication	78	100%	95%	94%
Thrombolytic Therapy Timing[1]	-	-	69%	66%
Venous Thromboembolism Prophylaxis	124	93%	94%	94%
Written Stroke Educational Materials Given	65	98%	86%	88%
Surgical Care Improvement Project				
Appropriate Beta Blocker Usage[2]	32	94%	97%	98%
Appropriate VTP Within 24 Hours[2]	153	97%	98%	98%
Controlled Postoperative Blood Glucose[1,2]	-	-	97%	97%
Perioperative Temperature Management[2]	184	99%	100%	100%
Prophylactic Antibiotic Selection[2]	91	100%	99%	99%
Prophylactic Antibiotic Selection (Outpatient)	95	97%	97%	98%
Prophylactic Antibiotic Stopped[2]	88	100%	98%	98%
Prophylactic Antibiotic Timing[2]	91	98%	99%	99%
Prophylactic Antibiotic Timing (Outpatient)	95	95%	97%	98%
Urinary Catheter Removal[2]	68	90%	96%	97%
Survey of Patients' Hospital Experiences				
Area Around Room 'Always' Quiet at Night	300+	52%	51%	61%
Doctors 'Always' Communicated Well	300+	80%	77%	82%
Home Recovery Information Given	300+	76%	83%	85%
Hospital Given 9 or 10 on 10 Point Scale	300+	54%	63%	71%
Meds 'Always' Explained Before Given	300+	57%	59%	64%
Nurses 'Always' Communicated Well	300+	68%	75%	79%
Pain 'Always' Well Controlled	300+	62%	67%	71%
Room and Bathroom 'Always' Clean	300+	68%	69%	73%
Timely Help 'Always' Received	300+	56%	61%	68%
Would Definitely Recommend Hospital	300+	57%	65%	71%
Use of Medical Imaging				
Cardiac Imaging Stress Test before Surgery[1]	-	-	5.8%	5.3%
Combination Abdominal CT Scan	166	1.2%	8.2%	10.5%
Combination Brain/Sinus CT Scan[1]	-	-	3.6%	2.7%
Combination Chest CT Scan	49	0.0%	1.3%	2.7%
Follow-up Mammogram/Ultrasound	161	10.6%	13%	8.8%
Lumbar Spine MRI for Low Back Pain[1]	-	-	33.4%	37.2%

Lawrence Hospital Center

55 Palmer Avenue
Bronxville, NY 10708
Phone: 914-787-1000
Fax: 914-787-5154
URL: www.lawrencehealth.org
Type: Acute Care Hospitals
Emergency Services: Yes
Ownership: Voluntary non-profit - Other
Beds: 281

Key Personnel:

Emergency Room . . . . Nicholas Crimarco, RN
CEO/President. . . . . Edward M. Dinan
Quality Assurance . . . . Diane Lango
Pediatric In-Patient Care . . . . M Levitt, MD
Radiology. . . . . Louis Perez, MD

Measure	Cases	This Hosp.	State Avg.	U.S. Avg.
Blood Clot Prevention and Treatment				
Anticoagulation Overlap Therapy[2]	81	90%	91%	93%
ICU Venous Thromboembolism Prophylaxis[2]	45	98%	92%	92%
Incidence of Potentially Preventable VTE[1,2]	-	-	10%	10%
UFH with Dosages/Platelet Monitoring[2]	33	100%	92%	97%
Venous Thromboembolism Prophylaxis[2]	387	93%	87%	85%
Warfarin Therapy Discharge Instructions[2]	53	100%	59%	75%
Chest Pain/Possible Heart Attack Care				
Aspirin Given Within 24 Hours of Arrival	78	100%	97%	96%
Fibrinolytic Meds Within 30 Min. of Arrival[1]	-	-	54%	58%
Average Time to ECG (minutes)	72	12	9	7
Average Time to Transfer (minutes)	24	128	78	60
Children's Asthma Care				
Received Home Management Plan of Care	-	-	-	88%
Received Reliever Medication	-	-	-	100%
Received Systemic Corticosteroids	-	-	-	100%
Emergency Department				
Admittance Decision Time (minutes)[2]	844	116	154	98
Head CT Results Within 45 Min. of Arrival	11	73%	55%	57%
Patients Who Left ER Before Being Seen	33,576	1%	2%	2%
Time from ER Arrival to Admit. (minutes)[2]	844	357	378	274
Time from ER Arrival to Discharge (minutes)	406	176	156	134
Time in ER Before Being Evaluated (minutes)	416	49	35	26
Time to Pain Meds for Fractures (minutes)	110	74	61	57
Heart Attack Care				
Aspirin Given at Discharge	22	95%	99%	99%
Fibrinolytic Meds Within 30 Min. of Arrival[1]	-	-	46%	54%
PCI Within 90 Minutes of Arrival[7]	-	-	95%	96%
Statin Prescribed at Discharge	26	85%	98%	98%
Heart Failure Care				
ACE Inhibitor or ARB for LVSD[2]	70	96%	96%	97%
Discharge Instructions Given[2]	257	100%	95%	94%
Evaluation of LVS Function[2]	322	100%	99%	99%
Medicare Spending				
Medicare Spending per Patient (ratio)	-	1.04	0.96	0.98
Pneumonia Care				

NOTE: Hospital profiles are in alphabetical order by state, then city, then hospital within the city; Rankings exclude hospitals with less than 25 cases except for patient surveys which excludes hospitals with less than 100 cases; (a) 100-299 cases; (1) The number of cases/patients is too few to report; (2) Data submitted were based on a sample of cases/patients; (3) Results are based on a shorter time period than required; (4) Data suppressed by CMS for one or more quarters; (5) Results are not available for this reporting period; (6) Fewer than 100 patients completed the HCAHPS survey; (7) No cases met the criteria for this measure; (8) The lower limit of the confidence interval cannot be calculated if the number of observed infections equals zero; (9) No data are available from the state/territory for this reporting period; (10) The scores shown reflect fewer than 50 completed surveys; (11) There were discrepancies in the data collection process; (12) This measure does not apply to this hospital for this reporting period; (13) Results cannot be calculated for this reporting period; (14) The results for this state are combined with nearby states to protect confidentiality; Please refer to the User's Guide for a full explanation of data.

Measure	Cases	This Hosp.	State Avg.	U.S. Avg.
Appropriate Initial Antibiotic Given[2]	119	95%	95%	95%
Blood Culture Timing[2]	180	98%	97%	98%
Pregnancy and Delivery Care				
Newborn Deliveries Scheduled Early[2]	36	3%	4%	6%
Preventive Care				
Immunization for Influenza[2]	539	98%	88%	90%
Immunization for Pneumonia[2]	613	95%	88%	92%
Stroke Care				
Anticoagulation Therapy for Atrial Fibrillation[2]	19	100%	96%	95%
Antithrombotic Therapy Timing[2]	91	96%	98%	98%
Assessed for Rehabilitation[2]	98	93%	97%	97%
Discharged on Antithrombotic Therapy[2]	90	99%	99%	99%
Discharged on Statin Medication[2]	79	89%	95%	94%
Thrombolytic Therapy Timing[1,2]	-	-	69%	66%
Venous Thromboembolism Prophylaxis[2]	119	90%	94%	94%
Written Stroke Educational Materials Given[2]	39	100%	86%	88%
Surgical Care Improvement Project				
Appropriate Beta Blocker Usage[2]	100	97%	97%	98%
Appropriate VTP Within 24 Hours[2]	311	98%	98%	98%
Controlled Postoperative Blood Glucose[2,7]	-	-	97%	97%
Perioperative Temperature Management[2]	342	100%	100%	100%
Prophylactic Antibiotic Selection[2]	219	98%	99%	99%
Prophylactic Antibiotic Selection (Outpatient)	66	97%	97%	98%
Prophylactic Antibiotic Stopped[2]	216	100%	98%	98%
Prophylactic Antibiotic Timing[2]	219	100%	99%	99%
Prophylactic Antibiotic Timing (Outpatient)	66	100%	97%	98%
Urinary Catheter Removal[2]	159	98%	96%	97%
Survey of Patients' Hospital Experiences				
Area Around Room 'Always' Quiet at Night	300+	53%	51%	61%
Doctors 'Always' Communicated Well	300+	78%	77%	82%
Home Recovery Information Given	300+	80%	83%	85%
Hospital Given 9 or 10 on 10 Point Scale	300+	65%	63%	71%
Meds 'Always' Explained Before Given	300+	54%	59%	64%
Nurses 'Always' Communicated Well	300+	75%	75%	79%
Pain 'Always' Well Controlled	300+	67%	67%	71%
Room and Bathroom 'Always' Clean	300+	70%	69%	73%
Timely Help 'Always' Received	300+	62%	61%	68%
Would Definitely Recommend Hospital	300+	68%	65%	71%
Use of Medical Imaging				
Cardiac Imaging Stress Test before Surgery	147	5.4%	5.8%	5.3%
Combination Abdominal CT Scan	589	20.7%	8.2%	10.5%
Combination Brain/Sinus CT Scan[1]	-	-	3.6%	2.7%
Combination Chest CT Scan	389	7.2%	1.3%	2.7%
Follow-up Mammogram/Ultrasound	605	22.8%	13%	8.8%
Lumbar Spine MRI for Low Back Pain	87	36.8%	33.4%	37.2%

Brookdale Hospital Medical Center

Linden Boulevard at Brookdale Plaza
Brooklyn, NY 11212
Phone: 718-240-5966
Fax: 718-240-6496
E-mail: info@brookdale.edu
URL: www.brookdalehospital.org
Type: Acute Care Hospitals
Emergency Services: Yes
Ownership: Voluntary non-profit - Private
Beds: 529

Key Personnel:
Quality Assurance . . . . Louise Falet, RN
Chief of Medical Staff . . . . Estevan Garcia, MD
Coronary Care . . . . Trevor Grazette, RN
Infection Control . . . . Linda Jendresky
Operating Room . . . . Socorro Lucas, RN
Pediatric Ambulatory Care . . . . . . Myron Sokal, MD
CEO/President . . . . Mark E. Toney
Radiology . . . . I Akiva Wulkan, MD

Measure	Cases	This Hosp.	State Avg.	U.S. Avg.
Blood Clot Prevention and Treatment				
Anticoagulation Overlap Therapy[2]	52	69%	91%	93%
ICU Venous Thromboembolism Prophylaxis[2]	88	91%	92%	92%
Incidence of Potentially Preventable VTE[2]	39	13%	10%	10%
UFH with Dosages/Platelet Monitoring[2]	29	79%	92%	97%
Venous Thromboembolism Prophylaxis[2]	360	84%	87%	85%
Warfarin Therapy Discharge Instructions[2]	31	23%	59%	75%
Chest Pain/Possible Heart Attack Care				
Aspirin Given Within 24 Hours of Arrival[5]	-	-	97%	96%
Fibrinolytic Meds Within 30 Min. of Arrival[5]	-	-	54%	58%
Average Time to ECG (minutes)[5]	-	-	9	7
Average Time to Transfer (minutes)[5]	-	-	78	60
Children's Asthma Care				
Received Home Management Plan of Care	-	-	-	88%
Received Reliever Medication	-	-	-	100%
Received Systemic Corticosteroids	-	-	-	100%
Emergency Department				
Admittance Decision Time (minutes)[2]	567	328	154	98
Head CT Results Within 45 Min. of Arrival[7]	-	-	55%	57%
Patients Who Left ER Before Being Seen	>100k	5%	2%	2%
Time from ER Arrival to Admit. (minutes)[2]	568	671	378	274
Time from ER Arrival to Discharge (minutes)	346	150	156	134
Time in ER Before Being Evaluated (minutes)	420	47	35	26
Time to Pain Meds for Fractures (minutes)	171	50	61	57
Heart Attack Care				
Aspirin Given at Discharge	169	99%	99%	99%
Fibrinolytic Meds Within 30 Min. of Arrival[7]	-	-	46%	54%
PCI Within 90 Minutes of Arrival	28	93%	95%	96%
Statin Prescribed at Discharge	175	95%	98%	98%
Heart Failure Care				
ACE Inhibitor or ARB for LVSD[2]	133	88%	96%	97%
Discharge Instructions Given[2]	278	83%	95%	94%
Evaluation of LVS Function[2]	311	99%	99%	99%
Medicare Spending				
Medicare Spending per Patient (ratio)	-	0.98	0.96	0.98
Pneumonia Care				
Appropriate Initial Antibiotic Given[2]	84	92%	95%	95%
Blood Culture Timing[2]	181	96%	97%	98%
Pregnancy and Delivery Care				
Newborn Deliveries Scheduled Early[2]	36	17%	4%	6%
Preventive Care				
Immunization for Influenza[2]	556	66%	88%	90%
Immunization for Pneumonia[2]	639	67%	88%	92%
Stroke Care				
Anticoagulation Therapy for Atrial Fibrillation	19	100%	96%	95%
Antithrombotic Therapy Timing	165	99%	98%	98%
Assessed for Rehabilitation	194	100%	97%	97%
Discharged on Antithrombotic Therapy	153	100%	99%	99%
Discharged on Statin Medication	149	99%	95%	94%
Thrombolytic Therapy Timing[1]	-	-	69%	66%
Venous Thromboembolism Prophylaxis	226	100%	94%	94%
Written Stroke Educational Materials Given	82	100%	86%	88%
Surgical Care Improvement Project				
Appropriate Beta Blocker Usage	56	86%	97%	98%
Appropriate VTP Within 24 Hours	281	95%	98%	98%
Controlled Postoperative Blood Glucose[1]	-	-	97%	97%
Perioperative Temperature Management	353	99%	100%	100%
Prophylactic Antibiotic Selection	90	97%	99%	99%
Prophylactic Antibiotic Selection (Outpatient)	136	96%	97%	98%
Prophylactic Antibiotic Stopped	88	88%	98%	98%
Prophylactic Antibiotic Timing	90	98%	99%	99%
Prophylactic Antibiotic Timing (Outpatient)	136	98%	97%	98%
Urinary Catheter Removal	86	79%	96%	97%
Survey of Patients' Hospital Experiences				
Area Around Room 'Always' Quiet at Night	300+	51%	51%	61%
Doctors 'Always' Communicated Well	300+	69%	77%	82%
Home Recovery Information Given	300+	70%	83%	85%
Hospital Given 9 or 10 on 10 Point Scale	300+	41%	63%	71%
Meds 'Always' Explained Before Given	300+	51%	59%	64%
Nurses 'Always' Communicated Well	300+	62%	75%	79%
Pain 'Always' Well Controlled	300+	53%	67%	71%
Room and Bathroom 'Always' Clean	300+	56%	69%	73%
Timely Help 'Always' Received	300+	43%	61%	68%
Would Definitely Recommend Hospital	300+	41%	65%	71%
Use of Medical Imaging				
Cardiac Imaging Stress Test before Surgery	72	9.7%	5.8%	5.3%
Combination Abdominal CT Scan	166	12.0%	8.2%	10.5%
Combination Brain/Sinus CT Scan[1]	-	-	3.6%	2.7%
Combination Chest CT Scan	117	0.0%	1.3%	2.7%
Follow-up Mammogram/Ultrasound	287	5.2%	13%	8.8%
Lumbar Spine MRI for Low Back Pain[1]	-	-	33.4%	37.2%

Brooklyn Hospital Center at Downtown Campus

121 Dekalb Avenue
Brooklyn, NY 11201
Phone: 718-250-8000
Fax: 718-260-2730
URL: www.tbh.org
Type: Acute Care Hospitals
Emergency Services: Yes
Ownership: Voluntary non-profit - Private
Beds: 416

Key Personnel:
Chief of Medical Staff . . . . Gary Almedo Stephens, MD
CEO/President . . . . Richard B. Becker, MD
Pediatric In-Patient Care . . . . Kenneth Bromberg, MD
Infection Control . . . . Anne Goonan
Patient Relations . . . . Suzanne Nicolettie-Kras
Intensive Care Unit . . . . Reynaldo Rivera
Quality Assurance . . . . Robert Rosati
Radiology . . . . Mohsen Samii, MD

Measure	Cases	This Hosp.	State Avg.	U.S. Avg.
Blood Clot Prevention and Treatment				
Anticoagulation Overlap Therapy[2]	94	100%	91%	93%
ICU Venous Thromboembolism Prophylaxis[2]	46	93%	92%	92%
Incidence of Potentially Preventable VTE[2]	26	4%	10%	10%
UFH with Dosages/Platelet Monitoring[2]	58	100%	92%	97%
Venous Thromboembolism Prophylaxis[2]	393	90%	87%	85%
Warfarin Therapy Discharge Instructions[2]	55	100%	59%	75%
Chest Pain/Possible Heart Attack Care				
Aspirin Given Within 24 Hours of Arrival	20	100%	97%	96%
Fibrinolytic Meds Within 30 Min. of Arrival[3,7]	-	-	54%	58%
Average Time to ECG (minutes)	19	32	9	7
Average Time to Transfer (minutes)[1,3]	-	-	78	60
Children's Asthma Care				
Received Home Management Plan of Care	-	-	-	88%
Received Reliever Medication	-	-	-	100%
Received Systemic Corticosteroids	-	-	-	100%
Emergency Department				
Admittance Decision Time (minutes)[2]	781	282	154	98
Head CT Results Within 45 Min. of Arrival[1]	-	-	55%	57%
Patients Who Left ER Before Being Seen	64,589	5%	2%	2%
Time from ER Arrival to Admit. (minutes)[2]	783	503	378	274
Time from ER Arrival to Discharge (minutes)	443	168	156	134
Time in ER Before Being Evaluated (minutes)	412	114	35	26
Time to Pain Meds for Fractures (minutes)	122	94	61	57
Heart Attack Care				
Aspirin Given at Discharge	44	100%	99%	99%
Fibrinolytic Meds Within 30 Min. of Arrival[7]	-	-	46%	54%
PCI Within 90 Minutes of Arrival[7]	-	-	95%	96%
Statin Prescribed at Discharge	41	100%	98%	98%
Heart Failure Care				
ACE Inhibitor or ARB for LVSD	141	100%	96%	97%
Discharge Instructions Given	307	100%	95%	94%
Evaluation of LVS Function	396	100%	99%	99%
Medicare Spending				
Medicare Spending per Patient (ratio)	-	1.01	0.96	0.98
Pneumonia Care				
Appropriate Initial Antibiotic Given	108	99%	95%	95%
Blood Culture Timing	326	100%	97%	98%
Pregnancy and Delivery Care				
Newborn Deliveries Scheduled Early[2]	58	2%	4%	6%
Preventive Care				
Immunization for Influenza[2]	527	92%	88%	90%
Immunization for Pneumonia[2]	557	88%	88%	92%
Stroke Care				
Anticoagulation Therapy for Atrial Fibrillation[1]	-	-	96%	95%
Antithrombotic Therapy Timing	85	99%	98%	98%
Assessed for Rehabilitation	95	89%	97%	97%
Discharged on Antithrombotic Therapy	81	96%	99%	99%
Discharged on Statin Medication	71	86%	95%	94%
Thrombolytic Therapy Timing	11	27%	69%	66%
Venous Thromboembolism Prophylaxis	108	94%	94%	94%
Written Stroke Educational Materials Given	32	100%	86%	88%
Surgical Care Improvement Project				
Appropriate Beta Blocker Usage	137	99%	97%	98%
Appropriate VTP Within 24 Hours	496	98%	98%	98%
Controlled Postoperative Blood Glucose[7]	-	-	97%	97%
Perioperative Temperature Management	565	100%	100%	100%
Prophylactic Antibiotic Selection	372	100%	99%	99%

NOTE: Hospital profiles are in alphabetical order by state, then city, then hospital within the city; Rankings exclude hospitals with less than 25 cases except for patient surveys which excludes hospitals with less than 100 cases; (a) 100-299 cases; (1) The number of cases/patients is too few to report; (2) Data submitted were based on a sample of cases/patients; (3) Results are based on a shorter time period than required; (4) Data suppressed by CMS for one or more quarters; (5) Results are not available for this reporting period; (6) Fewer than 100 patients completed the HCAHPS survey; (7) No cases met the criteria for this measure; (8) The lower limit of the confidence interval cannot be calculated if the number of observed infections equals zero; (9) No data are available from the state/territory for this reporting period; (10) The scores shown reflect fewer than 50 completed surveys; (11) There were discrepancies in the data collection process; (12) This measure does not apply to this hospital for this reporting period; (13) Results cannot be calculated for this reporting period; (14) The results for this state are combined with nearby states to protect confidentiality; Please refer to the User's Guide for a full explanation of data.

Measure	Cases	This Hosp.	State Avg.	U.S. Avg.
Prophylactic Antibiotic Selection (Outpatient)	234	87%	97%	98%
Prophylactic Antibiotic Stopped	355	97%	98%	98%
Prophylactic Antibiotic Timing	372	99%	99%	99%
Prophylactic Antibiotic Timing (Outpatient)	135	87%	97%	98%
Urinary Catheter Removal	347	100%	96%	97%
Survey of Patients' Hospital Experiences				
Area Around Room 'Always' Quiet at Night	300+	55%	51%	61%
Doctors 'Always' Communicated Well	300+	76%	77%	82%
Home Recovery Information Given	300+	75%	83%	85%
Hospital Given 9 or 10 on 10 Point Scale	300+	56%	63%	71%
Meds 'Always' Explained Before Given	300+	58%	59%	64%
Nurses 'Always' Communicated Well	300+	70%	75%	79%
Pain 'Always' Well Controlled	300+	61%	67%	71%
Room and Bathroom 'Always' Clean	300+	67%	69%	73%
Timely Help 'Always' Received	300+	52%	61%	68%
Would Definitely Recommend Hospital	300+	57%	65%	71%
Use of Medical Imaging				
Cardiac Imaging Stress Test before Surgery	63	3.2%	5.8%	5.3%
Combination Abdominal CT Scan	241	18.7%	8.2%	10.5%
Combination Brain/Sinus CT Scan[1]	-	-	3.6%	2.7%
Combination Chest CT Scan	127	3.1%	1.3%	2.7%
Follow-up Mammogram/Ultrasound	301	11.3%	13%	8.8%
Lumbar Spine MRI for Low Back Pain[1]	-	-	33.4%	37.2%

Coney Island Hospital

2601 Ocean Parkway
Brooklyn, NY 11235
Phone: 718-616-3000
Fax: 718-616-4448
URL: www.coneyislandhospital.com
Type: Acute Care Hospitals
Emergency Services: Yes
Ownership: Government - Local
Beds: 450

Key Personnel:

Chief of Medical Staff.......... Sandor Friedman, MD
Radiology.................... B Khurana, MD
Quality Assurance .... Betsy Lograno
Coronary Care................ Jennifer Mitchener, RN
Infection Control.............. Rose Recco, MD
Pediatric Ambulatory Care ...... Warren Seigel, MD
Pediatric In-Patient Care .... Warren Seigel, MD
CEO/President............... Arthur Wagner, CEO

Measure	Cases	This Hosp.	State Avg.	U.S. Avg.
Blood Clot Prevention and Treatment				
Anticoagulation Overlap Therapy[2]	41	98%	91%	93%
ICU Venous Thromboembolism Prophylaxis[2]	56	100%	92%	92%
Incidence of Potentially Preventable VTE[2]	15	0%	10%	10%
UFH with Dosages/Platelet Monitoring[2]	17	100%	92%	97%
Venous Thromboembolism Prophylaxis[2]	370	98%	87%	85%
Warfarin Therapy Discharge Instructions[2]	33	100%	59%	75%
Chest Pain/Possible Heart Attack Care				
Aspirin Given Within 24 Hours of Arrival[1,3]	-	-	97%	96%
Fibrinolytic Meds Within 30 Min. of Arrival[1,3]	-	-	54%	58%
Average Time to ECG (minutes)[1,3]	-	-	9	7
Average Time to Transfer (minutes)[3,7]	-	-	78	60
Children's Asthma Care				
Received Home Management Plan of Care	-	-	-	88%
Received Reliever Medication	-	-	-	100%
Received Systemic Corticosteroids	-	-	-	100%
Emergency Department				
Admittance Decision Time (minutes)[2]	772	77	154	98
Head CT Results Within 45 Min. of Arrival[1,3]	-	-	55%	57%
Patients Who Left ER Before Being Seen	66,160	3%	2%	2%
Time from ER Arrival to Admit. (minutes)[2]	779	367	378	274
Time from ER Arrival to Discharge (minutes)	375	156	156	134
Time in ER Before Being Evaluated (minutes)	422	50	35	26
Time to Pain Meds for Fractures (minutes)	181	51	61	57
Heart Attack Care				
Aspirin Given at Discharge	23	100%	99%	99%
Fibrinolytic Meds Within 30 Min. of Arrival[1]	-	-	46%	54%
PCI Within 90 Minutes of Arrival[7]	-	-	95%	96%
Statin Prescribed at Discharge	21	100%	98%	98%
Heart Failure Care				
ACE Inhibitor or ARB for LVSD	81	94%	96%	97%
Discharge Instructions Given	199	96%	95%	94%
Evaluation of LVS Function	236	100%	99%	99%
Medicare Spending				
Medicare Spending per Patient (ratio)	-	0.99	0.96	0.98
Pneumonia Care				
Appropriate Initial Antibiotic Given	103	88%	95%	95%
Blood Culture Timing	144	94%	97%	98%
Pregnancy and Delivery Care				
Newborn Deliveries Scheduled Early[2]	20	5%	4%	6%
Preventive Care				
Immunization for Influenza[2]	287	86%	88%	90%
Immunization for Pneumonia[2]	534	90%	88%	92%
Stroke Care				
Anticoagulation Therapy for Atrial Fibrillation[1]	-	-	96%	95%
Antithrombotic Therapy Timing	117	100%	98%	98%
Assessed for Rehabilitation	121	93%	97%	97%
Discharged on Antithrombotic Therapy	103	99%	99%	99%
Discharged on Statin Medication	82	93%	95%	94%
Thrombolytic Therapy Timing[1]	-	-	69%	66%
Venous Thromboembolism Prophylaxis	156	100%	94%	94%
Written Stroke Educational Materials Given	64	100%	86%	88%
Surgical Care Improvement Project				
Appropriate Beta Blocker Usage[2]	13	92%	97%	98%
Appropriate VTP Within 24 Hours[2]	114	97%	98%	98%
Controlled Postoperative Blood Glucose[1,2]	-	-	97%	97%
Perioperative Temperature Management[2]	135	100%	100%	100%
Prophylactic Antibiotic Selection[2]	60	98%	99%	99%
Prophylactic Antibiotic Selection (Outpatient)	80	95%	97%	98%
Prophylactic Antibiotic Stopped[2]	60	100%	98%	98%
Prophylactic Antibiotic Timing[2]	60	97%	99%	99%
Prophylactic Antibiotic Timing (Outpatient)	14	100%	97%	98%
Urinary Catheter Removal[2]	87	100%	96%	97%
Survey of Patients' Hospital Experiences				
Area Around Room 'Always' Quiet at Night	300+	50%	51%	61%
Doctors 'Always' Communicated Well	300+	74%	77%	82%
Home Recovery Information Given	300+	80%	83%	85%
Hospital Given 9 or 10 on 10 Point Scale	300+	54%	63%	71%
Meds 'Always' Explained Before Given	300+	57%	59%	64%
Nurses 'Always' Communicated Well	300+	70%	75%	79%
Pain 'Always' Well Controlled	300+	65%	67%	71%
Room and Bathroom 'Always' Clean	300+	70%	69%	73%
Timely Help 'Always' Received	300+	59%	61%	68%
Would Definitely Recommend Hospital	300+	56%	65%	71%
Use of Medical Imaging				
Cardiac Imaging Stress Test before Surgery[1]	-	-	5.8%	5.3%
Combination Abdominal CT Scan	83	9.6%	8.2%	10.5%
Combination Brain/Sinus CT Scan	129	9.3%	3.6%	2.7%
Combination Chest CT Scan[1]	-	-	1.3%	2.7%
Follow-up Mammogram/Ultrasound[1]	-	-	13%	8.8%
Lumbar Spine MRI for Low Back Pain[1]	-	-	33.4%	37.2%

Interfaith Medical Center

1545 Atlantic Avenue
Brooklyn, NY 11213
Phone: 718-613-4000
Fax: 718-613-4101
URL: www.interfaithmedical.com
Type: Acute Care Hospitals
Emergency Services: Yes
Ownership: Voluntary non-profit - Private
Beds: 287

Key Personnel:

Quality Assurance .... Virginia Baron
Pediatric In-Patient Care .... Mary Bastawros, MD
Emergency Room .... K Chandramohan, MD
Infection Control.............. Paul Dobre, PharmD
Radiology.................... Richard Heiden, MD
CEO/President............... Michael S Kaminski
Chief of Medical Staff.......... Franklin Marsh, MD
Intensive Care Unit............ Joseph Quist, MD

Measure	Cases	This Hosp.	State Avg.	U.S. Avg.
Blood Clot Prevention and Treatment				
Anticoagulation Overlap Therapy[2]	22	100%	91%	93%
ICU Venous Thromboembolism Prophylaxis[2]	24	83%	92%	92%
Incidence of Potentially Preventable VTE[1,2]	-	-	10%	10%
UFH with Dosages/Platelet Monitoring[1,2]	-	-	92%	97%
Venous Thromboembolism Prophylaxis[2]	304	78%	87%	85%
Warfarin Therapy Discharge Instructions[2]	13	8%	59%	75%
Chest Pain/Possible Heart Attack Care				
Aspirin Given Within 24 Hours of Arrival[1,3]	-	-	97%	96%
Fibrinolytic Meds Within 30 Min. of Arrival[3,7]	-	-	54%	58%
Average Time to ECG (minutes)[1,3]	-	-	9	7
Average Time to Transfer (minutes)[1,3]	-	-	78	60
Children's Asthma Care				
Received Home Management Plan of Care	-	-	-	88%
Received Reliever Medication	-	-	-	100%
Received Systemic Corticosteroids	-	-	-	100%
Emergency Department				
Admittance Decision Time (minutes)[2]	387	264	154	98
Head CT Results Within 45 Min. of Arrival[1]	-	-	55%	57%
Patients Who Left ER Before Being Seen	42,288	7%	2%	2%
Time from ER Arrival to Admit. (minutes)[2]	387	643	378	274
Time from ER Arrival to Discharge (minutes)	377	274	156	134
Time in ER Before Being Evaluated (minutes)	449	125	35	26
Time to Pain Meds for Fractures (minutes)	43	133	61	57
Heart Attack Care				
Aspirin Given at Discharge	37	97%	99%	99%
Fibrinolytic Meds Within 30 Min. of Arrival[7]	-	-	46%	54%
PCI Within 90 Minutes of Arrival[7]	-	-	95%	96%
Statin Prescribed at Discharge	32	94%	98%	98%
Heart Failure Care				
ACE Inhibitor or ARB for LVSD	64	100%	96%	97%
Discharge Instructions Given	150	99%	95%	94%
Evaluation of LVS Function	171	100%	99%	99%
Medicare Spending				
Medicare Spending per Patient (ratio)	-	0.97	0.96	0.98
Pneumonia Care				
Appropriate Initial Antibiotic Given	74	85%	95%	95%
Blood Culture Timing	94	71%	97%	98%
Pregnancy and Delivery Care				
Newborn Deliveries Scheduled Early[7]	-	-	4%	6%
Preventive Care				
Immunization for Influenza[2]	591	52%	88%	90%
Immunization for Pneumonia[2]	627	58%	88%	92%
Stroke Care				
Anticoagulation Therapy for Atrial Fibrillation[1]	-	-	96%	95%
Antithrombotic Therapy Timing	12	100%	98%	98%
Assessed for Rehabilitation	23	70%	97%	97%
Discharged on Antithrombotic Therapy[1]	-	-	99%	99%
Discharged on Statin Medication	19	74%	95%	94%
Thrombolytic Therapy Timing[1]	-	-	69%	66%
Venous Thromboembolism Prophylaxis	33	94%	94%	94%
Written Stroke Educational Materials Given	16	0%	86%	88%
Surgical Care Improvement Project				
Appropriate Beta Blocker Usage[1]	-	-	97%	98%
Appropriate VTP Within 24 Hours	71	97%	98%	98%
Controlled Postoperative Blood Glucose[7]	-	-	97%	97%
Perioperative Temperature Management	77	99%	100%	100%
Prophylactic Antibiotic Selection	39	82%	99%	99%
Prophylactic Antibiotic Selection (Outpatient)	33	91%	97%	98%
Prophylactic Antibiotic Stopped	34	91%	98%	98%
Prophylactic Antibiotic Timing	39	97%	99%	99%
Prophylactic Antibiotic Timing (Outpatient)	33	97%	97%	98%
Urinary Catheter Removal	28	82%	96%	97%
Survey of Patients' Hospital Experiences				
Area Around Room 'Always' Quiet at Night	300+	53%	51%	61%
Doctors 'Always' Communicated Well	300+	76%	77%	82%
Home Recovery Information Given	300+	75%	83%	85%
Hospital Given 9 or 10 on 10 Point Scale	300+	55%	63%	71%
Meds 'Always' Explained Before Given	300+	55%	59%	64%
Nurses 'Always' Communicated Well	300+	71%	75%	79%
Pain 'Always' Well Controlled	300+	63%	67%	71%
Room and Bathroom 'Always' Clean	300+	71%	69%	73%
Timely Help 'Always' Received	300+	45%	61%	68%
Would Definitely Recommend Hospital	300+	57%	65%	71%
Use of Medical Imaging				
Cardiac Imaging Stress Test before Surgery[1]	-	-	5.8%	5.3%
Combination Abdominal CT Scan[1]	-	-	8.2%	10.5%
Combination Brain/Sinus CT Scan[1]	-	-	3.6%	2.7%
Combination Chest CT Scan[1]	-	-	1.3%	2.7%
Follow-up Mammogram/Ultrasound	69	15.9%	13%	8.8%
Lumbar Spine MRI for Low Back Pain[1]	-	-	33.4%	37.2%

NOTE: Hospital profiles are in alphabetical order by state, then city, then hospital within the city; Rankings exclude hospitals with less than 25 cases except for patient surveys which excludes hospitals with less than 100 cases; (a) 100-299 cases; (1) The number of cases/patients is too few to report; (2) Data submitted were based on a sample of cases/patients; (3) Results are based on a shorter time period than required; (4) Data suppressed by CMS for one or more quarters; (5) Results are not available for this reporting period; (6) Fewer than 100 patients completed the HCAHPS survey; (7) No cases met the criteria for this measure; (8) The lower limit of the confidence interval cannot be calculated if the number of observed infections equals zero; (9) No data are available from the state/territory for this reporting period; (10) The scores shown reflect fewer than 50 completed surveys; (11) There were discrepancies in the data collection process; (12) This measure does not apply to this hospital for this reporting period; (13) Results cannot be calculated for this reporting period; (14) The results for this state are combined with nearby states to protect confidentiality; Please refer to the User's Guide for a full explanation of data.

Kings County Hospital Center

451 Clarkson Avenue Phone: 718-245-3901
Brooklyn, NY 11203 Fax: 718-245-3019
URL: www.nyc.gov/html/hhc/html/facilities/kings.shtml
Type: Acute Care Hospitals Emergency Services: Yes
Ownership: Government - Local Beds: 627

Key Personnel:
CEO/President. . . . . Alan D Aviles
Radiology. . . . . Joshua Becker, MD
Pediatric In-Patient Care . . . . Leonard Glass, MD
Chief of Medical Staff. . . . . Stephan Kamholz, MD
Quality Assurance . . . . Audrey Phillips-Caesar
Infection Control. . . . . Stephen Seligman, MD
Operating Room. . . . . Connie Thomas

Measure	Cases	This Hosp.	State Avg.	U.S. Avg.
Blood Clot Prevention and Treatment				
Anticoagulation Overlap Therapy[2]	125	86%	91%	93%
ICU Venous Thromboembolism Prophylaxis[2]	55	98%	92%	92%
Incidence of Potentially Preventable VTE[2]	65	2%	10%	10%
UFH with Dosages/Platelet Monitoring[2]	40	30%	92%	97%
Venous Thromboembolism Prophylaxis[2]	293	94%	87%	85%
Warfarin Therapy Discharge Instructions[2]	107	29%	59%	75%
Chest Pain/Possible Heart Attack Care				
Aspirin Given Within 24 Hours of Arrival[3]	19	89%	97%	96%
Fibrinolytic Meds Within 30 Min. of Arrival[3,7]	-	-	54%	58%
Average Time to ECG (minutes)[3]	19	30	9	7
Average Time to Transfer (minutes)[1,3]	-	-	78	60
Children's Asthma Care				
Received Home Management Plan of Care	-	-	-	88%
Received Reliever Medication	-	-	-	100%
Received Systemic Corticosteroids	-	-	-	100%
Emergency Department				
Admittance Decision Time (minutes)[2]	862	716	154	98
Head CT Results Within 45 Min. of Arrival[1]	-	-	55%	57%
Patients Who Left ER Before Being Seen	>100k	5%	2%	2%
Time from ER Arrival to Admit. (minutes)[2]	867	1155	378	274
Time from ER Arrival to Discharge (minutes)	364	247	156	134
Time in ER Before Being Evaluated (minutes)	380	114	35	26
Time to Pain Meds for Fractures (minutes)	279	64	61	57
Heart Attack Care				
Aspirin Given at Discharge	49	100%	99%	99%
Fibrinolytic Meds Within 30 Min. of Arrival[1]	-	-	46%	54%
PCI Within 90 Minutes of Arrival[7]	-	-	95%	96%
Statin Prescribed at Discharge	48	98%	98%	98%
Heart Failure Care				
ACE Inhibitor or ARB for LVSD	333	100%	96%	97%
Discharge Instructions Given	553	92%	95%	94%
Evaluation of LVS Function	594	100%	99%	99%
Medicare Spending				
Medicare Spending per Patient (ratio)	-	0.89	0.96	0.98
Pneumonia Care				
Appropriate Initial Antibiotic Given	171	98%	95%	95%
Blood Culture Timing	354	94%	97%	98%
Pregnancy and Delivery Care				
Newborn Deliveries Scheduled Early[2]	25	4%	4%	6%
Preventive Care				
Immunization for Influenza[2]	521	68%	88%	90%
Immunization for Pneumonia[2]	516	79%	88%	92%
Stroke Care				
Anticoagulation Therapy for Atrial Fibrillation	15	100%	96%	95%
Antithrombotic Therapy Timing	198	91%	98%	98%
Assessed for Rehabilitation	223	98%	97%	97%
Discharged on Antithrombotic Therapy	198	99%	99%	99%
Discharged on Statin Medication	175	98%	95%	94%
Thrombolytic Therapy Timing	12	92%	69%	66%
Venous Thromboembolism Prophylaxis	235	97%	94%	94%
Written Stroke Educational Materials Given	131	85%	86%	88%
Surgical Care Improvement Project				
Appropriate Beta Blocker Usage[2]	56	84%	97%	98%
Appropriate VTP Within 24 Hours[2]	300	99%	98%	98%
Controlled Postoperative Blood Glucose[2,7]	-	-	97%	97%
Perioperative Temperature Management[2]	346	100%	100%	100%
Prophylactic Antibiotic Selection[2]	225	100%	99%	99%
Prophylactic Antibiotic Selection (Outpatient)	158	99%	97%	98%
Prophylactic Antibiotic Stopped[2]	202	99%	98%	98%
Prophylactic Antibiotic Timing[2]	227	99%	99%	99%
Prophylactic Antibiotic Timing (Outpatient)	23	96%	97%	98%
Urinary Catheter Removal[2]	138	89%	96%	97%
Survey of Patients' Hospital Experiences				
Area Around Room 'Always' Quiet at Night	300+	49%	51%	61%
Doctors 'Always' Communicated Well	300+	75%	77%	82%
Home Recovery Information Given	300+	70%	83%	85%
Hospital Given 9 or 10 on 10 Point Scale	300+	50%	63%	71%
Meds 'Always' Explained Before Given	300+	51%	59%	64%
Nurses 'Always' Communicated Well	300+	63%	75%	79%
Pain 'Always' Well Controlled	300+	56%	67%	71%
Room and Bathroom 'Always' Clean	300+	63%	69%	73%
Timely Help 'Always' Received	300+	39%	61%	68%
Would Definitely Recommend Hospital	300+	60%	65%	71%
Use of Medical Imaging				
Cardiac Imaging Stress Test before Surgery[1]	-	-	5.8%	5.3%
Combination Abdominal CT Scan	111	0.9%	8.2%	10.5%
Combination Brain/Sinus CT Scan	203	4.9%	3.6%	2.7%
Combination Chest CT Scan	74	2.7%	1.3%	2.7%
Follow-up Mammogram/Ultrasound[1]	-	-	13%	8.8%
Lumbar Spine MRI for Low Back Pain[1]	-	-	33.4%	37.2%

Kingsbrook Jewish Medical Center

585 Schenectady Avenue Phone: 718-604-5789
Brooklyn, NY 11203 Fax: 718-604-5243
E-mail: info@kjmc.org
URL: www.kingsbrook.org
Type: Acute Care Hospitals Emergency Services: Yes
Ownership: Voluntary non-profit - Private Beds: 864

Key Personnel:
CEO/President. . . . . Linda Brady, MD
Pediatric In-Patient Care . . . . Hua-Chin Chen, MD
Anesthesiology. . . . . Jay Lee, MD
Surgery . . . . William A Lois, MD
Quality Assurance . . . . Mary Marshall
Radiology. . . . . Kenneth Schwartz, MD
Chief of Medical Staff. . . . . Akbarali Virani, MD
Chair/CEO . . . . Berhane Wubshet, MD

Measure	Cases	This Hosp.	State Avg.	U.S. Avg.
Blood Clot Prevention and Treatment				
Anticoagulation Overlap Therapy[2]	49	88%	91%	93%
ICU Venous Thromboembolism Prophylaxis[2]	75	95%	92%	92%
Incidence of Potentially Preventable VTE[2]	14	7%	10%	10%
UFH with Dosages/Platelet Monitoring[2]	14	100%	92%	97%
Venous Thromboembolism Prophylaxis[2]	364	92%	87%	85%
Warfarin Therapy Discharge Instructions[2]	25	48%	59%	75%
Chest Pain/Possible Heart Attack Care				
Aspirin Given Within 24 Hours of Arrival	17	100%	97%	96%
Fibrinolytic Meds Within 30 Min. of Arrival[7]	-	-	54%	58%
Average Time to ECG (minutes)	17	9	9	7
Average Time to Transfer (minutes)[1]	-	-	78	60
Children's Asthma Care				
Received Home Management Plan of Care	-	-	-	88%
Received Reliever Medication	-	-	-	100%
Received Systemic Corticosteroids	-	-	-	100%
Emergency Department				
Admittance Decision Time (minutes)[2]	1,139	152	154	98
Head CT Results Within 45 Min. of Arrival[1,3]	-	-	55%	57%
Patients Who Left ER Before Being Seen	38,863	1%	2%	2%
Time from ER Arrival to Admit. (minutes)[2]	1,140	484	378	274
Time from ER Arrival to Discharge (minutes)	380	170	156	134
Time in ER Before Being Evaluated (minutes)	351	53	35	26
Time to Pain Meds for Fractures (minutes)	22	119	61	57
Heart Attack Care				
Aspirin Given at Discharge	38	97%	99%	99%
Fibrinolytic Meds Within 30 Min. of Arrival[7]	-	-	46%	54%
PCI Within 90 Minutes of Arrival[7]	-	-	95%	96%
Statin Prescribed at Discharge	35	94%	98%	98%
Heart Failure Care				
ACE Inhibitor or ARB for LVSD	135	99%	96%	97%
Discharge Instructions Given	245	98%	95%	94%
Evaluation of LVS Function	336	99%	99%	99%
Medicare Spending				
Medicare Spending per Patient (ratio)	-	1.07	0.96	0.98
Pneumonia Care				
Appropriate Initial Antibiotic Given	107	99%	95%	95%
Blood Culture Timing	322	99%	97%	98%
Pregnancy and Delivery Care				
Newborn Deliveries Scheduled Early[7]	-	-	4%	6%
Preventive Care				
Immunization for Influenza[2]	627	94%	88%	90%
Immunization for Pneumonia[2]	978	93%	88%	92%
Stroke Care				
Anticoagulation Therapy for Atrial Fibrillation	11	100%	96%	95%
Antithrombotic Therapy Timing	111	94%	98%	98%
Assessed for Rehabilitation	126	93%	97%	97%
Discharged on Antithrombotic Therapy	105	95%	99%	99%
Discharged on Statin Medication	91	87%	95%	94%
Thrombolytic Therapy Timing[1]	-	-	69%	66%
Venous Thromboembolism Prophylaxis	136	93%	94%	94%
Written Stroke Educational Materials Given	51	100%	86%	88%
Surgical Care Improvement Project				
Appropriate Beta Blocker Usage	52	94%	97%	98%
Appropriate VTP Within 24 Hours	165	99%	98%	98%
Controlled Postoperative Blood Glucose[7]	-	-	97%	97%
Perioperative Temperature Management	184	99%	100%	100%
Prophylactic Antibiotic Selection	96	98%	99%	99%
Prophylactic Antibiotic Selection (Outpatient)	31	90%	97%	98%
Prophylactic Antibiotic Stopped	88	99%	98%	98%
Prophylactic Antibiotic Timing	96	99%	99%	99%
Prophylactic Antibiotic Timing (Outpatient)	30	97%	97%	98%
Urinary Catheter Removal	93	98%	96%	97%
Survey of Patients' Hospital Experiences				
Area Around Room 'Always' Quiet at Night	300+	57%	51%	61%
Doctors 'Always' Communicated Well	300+	76%	77%	82%
Home Recovery Information Given	300+	79%	83%	85%
Hospital Given 9 or 10 on 10 Point Scale	300+	53%	63%	71%
Meds 'Always' Explained Before Given	300+	54%	59%	64%
Nurses 'Always' Communicated Well	300+	71%	75%	79%
Pain 'Always' Well Controlled	300+	60%	67%	71%
Room and Bathroom 'Always' Clean	300+	69%	69%	73%
Timely Help 'Always' Received	300+	51%	61%	68%
Would Definitely Recommend Hospital	300+	59%	65%	71%
Use of Medical Imaging				
Cardiac Imaging Stress Test before Surgery[1]	-	-	5.8%	5.3%
Combination Abdominal CT Scan	213	5.6%	8.2%	10.5%
Combination Brain/Sinus CT Scan[1]	-	-	3.6%	2.7%
Combination Chest CT Scan	125	2.4%	1.3%	2.7%
Follow-up Mammogram/Ultrasound	268	9.7%	13%	8.8%
Lumbar Spine MRI for Low Back Pain[1]	-	-	33.4%	37.2%

Lutheran Medical Center

150 55th Street Phone: 718-630-8000
Brooklyn, NY 11220 Fax: 718-630-8653
URL: www.lmcmc.com
Type: Acute Care Hospitals Emergency Services: Yes
Ownership: Voluntary non-profit - Private Beds: 476

Key Personnel:
Surgery . . . . George Ferzli
CEO/President. . . . . Wendy Z Goldstein
Radiology. . . . . Jayanth V. Rao, MD
Chief of Medical Staff. . . . . Beth G. Raucher, MD
Patient Relations . . . . Sheldon Rock
Pediatric Ambulatory Care . . . . . . Steven Shelov, MD
Emergency Room . . . . Bonnie Simmons, DO
Infection Control. . . . . Ernest Visconti, MD

Measure	Cases	This Hosp.	State Avg.	U.S. Avg.
Blood Clot Prevention and Treatment				
Anticoagulation Overlap Therapy[2]	94	85%	91%	93%
ICU Venous Thromboembolism Prophylaxis[2]	54	100%	92%	92%
Incidence of Potentially Preventable VTE[2]	22	5%	10%	10%
UFH with Dosages/Platelet Monitoring[2]	73	100%	92%	97%
Venous Thromboembolism Prophylaxis[2]	375	94%	87%	85%
Warfarin Therapy Discharge Instructions[2]	55	45%	59%	75%
Chest Pain/Possible Heart Attack Care				
Aspirin Given Within 24 Hours of Arrival[1,3]	-	-	97%	96%
Fibrinolytic Meds Within 30 Min. of Arrival[5]	-	-	54%	58%

NOTE: Hospital profiles are in alphabetical order by state, then city, then hospital within the city; Rankings exclude hospitals with less than 25 cases except for patient surveys which excludes hospitals with less than 100 cases; (a) 100-299 cases; (1) The number of cases/patients is too few to report; (2) Data submitted were based on a sample of cases/patients; (3) Results are based on a shorter time period than required; (4) Data suppressed by CMS for one or more quarters; (5) Results are not available for this reporting period; (6) Fewer than 100 patients completed the HCAHPS survey; (7) No cases met the criteria for this measure; (8) The lower limit of the confidence interval cannot be calculated if the number of observed infections equals zero; (9) No data are available from the state/territory for this reporting period; (10) The scores shown reflect fewer than 50 completed surveys; (11) There were discrepancies in the data collection process; (12) This measure does not apply to this hospital for this reporting period; (13) Results cannot be calculated for this reporting period; (14) The results for this state are combined with nearby states to protect confidentiality; Please refer to the User's Guide for a full explanation of data.

Measure	Cases	This Hosp.	State Avg.	U.S. Avg.
Average Time to ECG (minutes)[1,3]	-	-	9	7
Average Time to Transfer (minutes)[5]	-	-	78	60
Children's Asthma Care				
Received Home Management Plan of Care	-	-	-	88%
Received Reliever Medication	-	-	-	100%
Received Systemic Corticosteroids	-	-	-	100%
Emergency Department				
Admittance Decision Time (minutes)[2]	755	482	154	98
Head CT Results Within 45 Min. of Arrival[1,3]	-	-	55%	57%
Patients Who Left ER Before Being Seen	61,383	1%	2%	2%
Time from ER Arrival to Admit. (minutes)[2]	757	808	378	274
Time from ER Arrival to Discharge (minutes)	359	271	156	134
Time in ER Before Being Evaluated (minutes)	407	21	35	26
Time to Pain Meds for Fractures (minutes)	211	92	61	57
Heart Attack Care				
Aspirin Given at Discharge	199	100%	99%	99%
Fibrinolytic Meds Within 30 Min. of Arrival[7]	-	-	46%	54%
PCI Within 90 Minutes of Arrival	33	94%	95%	96%
Statin Prescribed at Discharge	199	99%	98%	98%
Heart Failure Care				
ACE Inhibitor or ARB for LVSD	145	98%	96%	97%
Discharge Instructions Given	290	99%	95%	94%
Evaluation of LVS Function	372	99%	99%	99%
Medicare Spending				
Medicare Spending per Patient (ratio)	-	1.03	0.96	0.98
Pneumonia Care				
Appropriate Initial Antibiotic Given	258	97%	95%	95%
Blood Culture Timing	407	98%	97%	98%
Pregnancy and Delivery Care				
Newborn Deliveries Scheduled Early[2]	65	12%	4%	6%
Preventive Care				
Immunization for Influenza[2]	505	89%	88%	90%
Immunization for Pneumonia[2]	581	83%	88%	92%
Stroke Care				
Anticoagulation Therapy for Atrial Fibrillation	36	92%	96%	95%
Antithrombotic Therapy Timing	147	90%	98%	98%
Assessed for Rehabilitation	202	100%	97%	97%
Discharged on Antithrombotic Therapy	165	98%	99%	99%
Discharged on Statin Medication	129	95%	95%	94%
Thrombolytic Therapy Timing	19	89%	69%	66%
Venous Thromboembolism Prophylaxis	227	98%	94%	94%
Written Stroke Educational Materials Given	84	89%	86%	88%
Surgical Care Improvement Project				
Appropriate Beta Blocker Usage[2]	249	96%	97%	98%
Appropriate VTP Within 24 Hours[2]	577	99%	98%	98%
Controlled Postoperative Blood Glucose[1,2]	-	-	97%	97%
Perioperative Temperature Management[2]	714	100%	100%	100%
Prophylactic Antibiotic Selection[2]	489	99%	99%	99%
Prophylactic Antibiotic Selection (Outpatient)	117	97%	97%	98%
Prophylactic Antibiotic Stopped[2]	474	97%	98%	98%
Prophylactic Antibiotic Timing[2]	489	100%	99%	99%
Prophylactic Antibiotic Timing (Outpatient)	118	99%	97%	98%
Urinary Catheter Removal[2]	321	99%	96%	97%
Survey of Patients' Hospital Experiences				
Area Around Room 'Always' Quiet at Night	300+	41%	51%	61%
Doctors 'Always' Communicated Well	300+	73%	77%	82%
Home Recovery Information Given	300+	80%	83%	85%
Hospital Given 9 or 10 on 10 Point Scale	300+	55%	63%	71%
Meds 'Always' Explained Before Given	300+	56%	59%	64%
Nurses 'Always' Communicated Well	300+	68%	75%	79%
Pain 'Always' Well Controlled	300+	63%	67%	71%
Room and Bathroom 'Always' Clean	300+	57%	69%	73%
Timely Help 'Always' Received	300+	56%	61%	68%
Would Definitely Recommend Hospital	300+	57%	65%	71%
Use of Medical Imaging				
Cardiac Imaging Stress Test before Surgery[1]	-	-	5.8%	5.3%
Combination Abdominal CT Scan	271	0.7%	8.2%	10.5%
Combination Brain/Sinus CT Scan	555	10.6%	3.6%	2.7%
Combination Chest CT Scan	144	0.0%	1.3%	2.7%
Follow-up Mammogram/Ultrasound	166	7.2%	13%	8.8%
Lumbar Spine MRI for Low Back Pain[1]	-	-	33.4%	37.2%

Maimonides Medical Center

4802 Tenth Avenue
Brooklyn, NY 11219
Phone: 718-283-6000
Fax: 718-283-8553
E-mail: info@maimonidesmed.org
URL: www.maimonidesmed.org
Type: Acute Care Hospitals
Emergency Services: Yes
Ownership: Voluntary non-profit - Private
Beds: 705

Key Personnel:
Radiology. . . . . Javier Beltran, MD
Surgery . . . . Patrick I. Borgen, MD
CEO/President. . . . . Pamela S Brier, MPH
Anesthesiology. . . . . Steven Konstadt, MD
Chief of Medical Staff . . . . Samuel Kopel, MD
Pediatrics. . . . . Danielle Laraque, MD
Emergency Room . . . . John Marshall, MD
Cardiology . . . . Jacob Shani, MD

Measure	Cases	This Hosp.	State Avg.	U.S. Avg.
Blood Clot Prevention and Treatment				
Anticoagulation Overlap Therapy[2]	101	94%	91%	93%
ICU Venous Thromboembolism Prophylaxis[2]	59	83%	92%	92%
Incidence of Potentially Preventable VTE[2]	26	15%	10%	10%
UFH with Dosages/Platelet Monitoring[2]	119	100%	92%	97%
Venous Thromboembolism Prophylaxis[2]	343	93%	87%	85%
Warfarin Therapy Discharge Instructions[2]	57	61%	59%	75%
Chest Pain/Possible Heart Attack Care				
Aspirin Given Within 24 Hours of Arrival[3,7]	-	-	97%	96%
Fibrinolytic Meds Within 30 Min. of Arrival[5]	-	-	54%	58%
Average Time to ECG (minutes)[3,7]	-	-	9	7
Average Time to Transfer (minutes)[5]	-	-	78	60
Children's Asthma Care				
Received Home Management Plan of Care	-	-	-	88%
Received Reliever Medication	-	-	-	100%
Received Systemic Corticosteroids	-	-	-	100%
Emergency Department				
Admittance Decision Time (minutes)[2]	604	234	154	98
Head CT Results Within 45 Min. of Arrival[7]	-	-	55%	57%
Patients Who Left ER Before Being Seen	>100k	2%	2%	2%
Time from ER Arrival to Admit. (minutes)[2]	605	547	378	274
Time from ER Arrival to Discharge (minutes)	384	216	156	134
Time in ER Before Being Evaluated (minutes)	408	33	35	26
Time to Pain Meds for Fractures (minutes)	383	44	61	57
Heart Attack Care				
Aspirin Given at Discharge[2]	288	99%	99%	99%
Fibrinolytic Meds Within 30 Min. of Arrival[2,7]	-	-	46%	54%
PCI Within 90 Minutes of Arrival[2]	48	92%	95%	96%
Statin Prescribed at Discharge[2]	294	98%	98%	98%
Heart Failure Care				
ACE Inhibitor or ARB for LVSD[2]	88	97%	96%	97%
Discharge Instructions Given[2]	235	68%	95%	94%
Evaluation of LVS Function[2]	307	99%	99%	99%
Medicare Spending				
Medicare Spending per Patient (ratio)	-	1.00	0.96	0.98
Pneumonia Care				
Appropriate Initial Antibiotic Given[2]	62	94%	95%	95%
Blood Culture Timing[2]	159	90%	97%	98%
Pregnancy and Delivery Care				
Newborn Deliveries Scheduled Early[2]	104	4%	4%	6%
Preventive Care				
Immunization for Influenza[2]	468	66%	88%	90%
Immunization for Pneumonia[2]	456	81%	88%	92%
Stroke Care				
Anticoagulation Therapy for Atrial Fibrillation	97	97%	96%	95%
Antithrombotic Therapy Timing	344	99%	98%	98%
Assessed for Rehabilitation	428	99%	97%	97%
Discharged on Antithrombotic Therapy	379	100%	99%	99%
Discharged on Statin Medication	276	98%	95%	94%
Thrombolytic Therapy Timing	42	93%	69%	66%
Venous Thromboembolism Prophylaxis	457	96%	94%	94%
Written Stroke Educational Materials Given	259	92%	86%	88%
Surgical Care Improvement Project				
Appropriate Beta Blocker Usage[2]	334	99%	97%	98%
Appropriate VTP Within 24 Hours[2]	454	99%	98%	98%
Controlled Postoperative Blood Glucose[2]	170	95%	97%	97%
Perioperative Temperature Management[2]	635	100%	100%	100%
Prophylactic Antibiotic Selection[2]	555	98%	99%	99%
Prophylactic Antibiotic Selection (Outpatient)	392	97%	97%	98%
Prophylactic Antibiotic Stopped[2]	533	99%	98%	98%
Prophylactic Antibiotic Timing[2]	560	98%	99%	99%
Prophylactic Antibiotic Timing (Outpatient)	402	96%	97%	98%
Urinary Catheter Removal[2]	455	99%	96%	97%
Survey of Patients' Hospital Experiences				
Area Around Room 'Always' Quiet at Night	300+	41%	51%	61%
Doctors 'Always' Communicated Well	300+	72%	77%	82%
Home Recovery Information Given	300+	80%	83%	85%
Hospital Given 9 or 10 on 10 Point Scale	300+	54%	63%	71%
Meds 'Always' Explained Before Given	300+	54%	59%	64%
Nurses 'Always' Communicated Well	300+	63%	75%	79%
Pain 'Always' Well Controlled	300+	57%	67%	71%
Room and Bathroom 'Always' Clean	300+	55%	69%	73%
Timely Help 'Always' Received	300+	48%	61%	68%
Would Definitely Recommend Hospital	300+	61%	65%	71%
Use of Medical Imaging				
Cardiac Imaging Stress Test before Surgery[1]	-	-	5.8%	5.3%
Combination Abdominal CT Scan	1,257	1.7%	8.2%	10.5%
Combination Brain/Sinus CT Scan	1,015	5.9%	3.6%	2.7%
Combination Chest CT Scan	751	1.3%	1.3%	2.7%
Follow-up Mammogram/Ultrasound	631	15.1%	13%	8.8%
Lumbar Spine MRI for Low Back Pain[1]	-	-	33.4%	37.2%

New York Community Hospital of Brooklyn

2525 Kings Highway
Brooklyn, NY 11229
Phone: 718-692-5302
Fax: 718-692-5368
URL: www.nych.com
Type: Acute Care Hospitals
Emergency Services: Yes
Ownership: Voluntary non-profit - Private
Beds: 134

Key Personnel:
Chief of Medical Staff . . . . Steve Nozad
CEO/President. . . . . Barry Stern
Chairman/CEO . . . . George Weinberger
Emergency Room . . . . Nermard Yonk, MD

Measure	Cases	This Hosp.	State Avg.	U.S. Avg.
Blood Clot Prevention and Treatment				
Anticoagulation Overlap Therapy[2]	29	97%	91%	93%
ICU Venous Thromboembolism Prophylaxis[2]	23	96%	92%	92%
Incidence of Potentially Preventable VTE[1,2]	-	-	10%	10%
UFH with Dosages/Platelet Monitoring[1,2]	-	-	92%	97%
Venous Thromboembolism Prophylaxis[2]	458	93%	87%	85%
Warfarin Therapy Discharge Instructions[2]	28	96%	59%	75%
Chest Pain/Possible Heart Attack Care				
Aspirin Given Within 24 Hours of Arrival	13	100%	97%	96%
Fibrinolytic Meds Within 30 Min. of Arrival[1,3]	-	-	54%	58%
Average Time to ECG (minutes)	11	12	9	7
Average Time to Transfer (minutes)[3,7]	-	-	78	60
Children's Asthma Care				
Received Home Management Plan of Care	-	-	-	88%
Received Reliever Medication	-	-	-	100%
Received Systemic Corticosteroids	-	-	-	100%
Emergency Department				
Admittance Decision Time (minutes)[2]	1,017	239	154	98
Head CT Results Within 45 Min. of Arrival[1]	-	-	55%	57%
Patients Who Left ER Before Being Seen	21,748	2%	2%	2%
Time from ER Arrival to Admit. (minutes)[2]	1,017	495	378	274
Time from ER Arrival to Discharge (minutes)	310	170	156	134
Time in ER Before Being Evaluated (minutes)	374	42	35	26
Time to Pain Meds for Fractures (minutes)	24	76	61	57
Heart Attack Care				
Aspirin Given at Discharge	24	100%	99%	99%
Fibrinolytic Meds Within 30 Min. of Arrival[7]	-	-	46%	54%
PCI Within 90 Minutes of Arrival[7]	-	-	95%	96%
Statin Prescribed at Discharge	22	100%	98%	98%
Heart Failure Care				
ACE Inhibitor or ARB for LVSD[2]	31	100%	96%	97%
Discharge Instructions Given[2]	212	100%	95%	94%
Evaluation of LVS Function[2]	260	100%	99%	99%
Medicare Spending				
Medicare Spending per Patient (ratio)	-	1.01	0.96	0.98
Pneumonia Care				

NOTE: Hospital profiles are in alphabetical order by state, then city, then hospital within the city; Rankings exclude hospitals with less than 25 cases except for patient surveys which excludes hospitals with less than 100 cases; (a) 100-299 cases; (1) The number of cases/patients is too few to report; (2) Data submitted were based on a sample of cases/patients; (3) Results are based on a shorter time period than required; (4) Data suppressed by CMS for one or more quarters; (5) Results are not available for this reporting period; (6) Fewer than 100 patients completed the HCAHPS survey; (7) No cases met the criteria for this measure; (8) The lower limit of the confidence interval cannot be calculated if the number of observed infections equals zero; (9) No data are available from the state/territory for this reporting period; (10) The scores shown reflect fewer than 50 completed surveys; (11) There were discrepancies in the data collection process; (12) This measure does not apply to this hospital for this reporting period; (13) Results cannot be calculated for this reporting period; (14) The results for this state are combined with nearby states to protect confidentiality; Please refer to the User's Guide for a full explanation of data.

Appropriate Initial Antibiotic Given[2]	74	100%	95%	95%
Blood Culture Timing[2]	100	100%	97%	98%
Pregnancy and Delivery Care				
Newborn Deliveries Scheduled Early[2,7]	-	-	4%	6%
Preventive Care				
Immunization for Influenza[2]	580	88%	88%	90%
Immunization for Pneumonia[2]	943	92%	88%	92%
Stroke Care				
Anticoagulation Therapy for Atrial Fibrillation[1]	-	-	96%	95%
Antithrombotic Therapy Timing	48	96%	98%	98%
Assessed for Rehabilitation	63	100%	97%	97%
Discharged on Antithrombotic Therapy	54	100%	99%	99%
Discharged on Statin Medication	50	100%	95%	94%
Thrombolytic Therapy Timing	11	100%	69%	66%
Venous Thromboembolism Prophylaxis	69	99%	94%	94%
Written Stroke Educational Materials Given	29	100%	86%	88%
Surgical Care Improvement Project				
Appropriate Beta Blocker Usage[2]	31	100%	97%	98%
Appropriate VTP Within 24 Hours[2]	79	100%	98%	98%
Controlled Postoperative Blood Glucose[2,7]	-	-	97%	97%
Perioperative Temperature Management[2]	83	100%	100%	100%
Prophylactic Antibiotic Selection[2]	37	97%	99%	99%
Prophylactic Antibiotic Selection (Outpatient)[1]	-	-	97%	98%
Prophylactic Antibiotic Stopped[2]	36	100%	98%	98%
Prophylactic Antibiotic Timing[2]	37	97%	99%	99%
Prophylactic Antibiotic Timing (Outpatient)[1]	-	-	97%	98%
Urinary Catheter Removal[2]	54	100%	96%	97%
Survey of Patients' Hospital Experiences				
Area Around Room 'Always' Quiet at Night	300+	55%	51%	61%
Doctors 'Always' Communicated Well	300+	78%	77%	82%
Home Recovery Information Given	300+	78%	83%	85%
Hospital Given 9 or 10 on 10 Point Scale	300+	51%	63%	71%
Meds 'Always' Explained Before Given	300+	64%	59%	64%
Nurses 'Always' Communicated Well	300+	73%	75%	79%
Pain 'Always' Well Controlled	300+	67%	67%	71%
Room and Bathroom 'Always' Clean	300+	73%	69%	73%
Timely Help 'Always' Received	300+	61%	61%	68%
Would Definitely Recommend Hospital	300+	55%	65%	71%
Use of Medical Imaging				
Cardiac Imaging Stress Test before Surgery[7]	-	-	5.8%	5.3%
Combination Abdominal CT Scan	132	0.8%	8.2%	10.5%
Combination Brain/Sinus CT Scan	285	7.4%	3.6%	2.7%
Combination Chest CT Scan[1]	-	-	1.3%	2.7%
Follow-up Mammogram/Ultrasound[7]	-	-	13%	8.8%
Lumbar Spine MRI for Low Back Pain[7]	-	-	33.4%	37.2%

New York Methodist Hospital

506 Sixth Street
Brooklyn, NY 11215
Phone: 718-780-3000
Fax: 718-780-3770
E-mail: lyn9001@nyp.org
URL: www.nym.org
Type: Acute Care Hospitals
Emergency Services: Yes
Ownership: Voluntary non-profit - Private
Beds: 576

Key Personnel:
Radiology. . . . . Steven Garner, MD
Operating Room. . . . . Joanne Lagnes, RN
Infection Control. . . . . Kathleen McNamara, RN
Quality Assurance . . . . Pamela Monastero
CEO/President. . . . . Mark J Mundy
Pediatric In-Patient Care . . . . Pramod Narula, MD
Chief of Medical Staff. . . . . Anthony Saleh, MD
Anesthesiology. . . . . Joseph Schianodicola, MD

Measure	Cases	This Hosp.	State Avg.	U.S. Avg.
Blood Clot Prevention and Treatment				
Anticoagulation Overlap Therapy[2]	197	95%	91%	93%
ICU Venous Thromboembolism Prophylaxis[2]	44	100%	92%	92%
Incidence of Potentially Preventable VTE[2]	54	2%	10%	10%
UFH with Dosages/Platelet Monitoring[2]	25	92%	92%	97%
Venous Thromboembolism Prophylaxis[2]	384	89%	87%	85%
Warfarin Therapy Discharge Instructions[2]	132	87%	59%	75%
Chest Pain/Possible Heart Attack Care				
Aspirin Given Within 24 Hours of Arrival[1,3]	-	-	97%	96%
Fibrinolytic Meds Within 30 Min. of Arrival[3,7]	-	-	54%	58%
Average Time to ECG (minutes)[1,3]	-	-	9	7
Average Time to Transfer (minutes)[3,7]	-	-	78	60
Children's Asthma Care				
Received Home Management Plan of Care	-	-	-	88%
Received Reliever Medication	-	-	-	100%
Received Systemic Corticosteroids	-	-	-	100%
Emergency Department				
Admittance Decision Time (minutes)[2]	621	214	154	98
Head CT Results Within 45 Min. of Arrival[7]	-	-	55%	57%
Patients Who Left ER Before Being Seen	94,093	2%	2%	2%
Time from ER Arrival to Admit. (minutes)[2]	622	520	378	274
Time from ER Arrival to Discharge (minutes)	395	197	156	134
Time in ER Before Being Evaluated (minutes)	345	66	35	26
Time to Pain Meds for Fractures (minutes)	101	33	61	57
Heart Attack Care				
Aspirin Given at Discharge	367	99%	99%	99%
Fibrinolytic Meds Within 30 Min. of Arrival[7]	-	-	46%	54%
PCI Within 90 Minutes of Arrival	42	93%	95%	96%
Statin Prescribed at Discharge	362	98%	98%	98%
Heart Failure Care				
ACE Inhibitor or ARB for LVSD[2]	140	92%	96%	97%
Discharge Instructions Given[2]	289	93%	95%	94%
Evaluation of LVS Function[2]	337	100%	99%	99%
Medicare Spending				
Medicare Spending per Patient (ratio)	-	1.03	0.96	0.98
Pneumonia Care				
Appropriate Initial Antibiotic Given[2]	102	97%	95%	95%
Blood Culture Timing[2]	63	98%	97%	98%
Pregnancy and Delivery Care				
Newborn Deliveries Scheduled Early[2]	125	2%	4%	6%
Preventive Care				
Immunization for Influenza[2]	516	86%	88%	90%
Immunization for Pneumonia[2]	559	84%	88%	92%
Stroke Care				
Anticoagulation Therapy for Atrial Fibrillation[2]	14	100%	96%	95%
Antithrombotic Therapy Timing[2]	132	90%	98%	98%
Assessed for Rehabilitation[2]	151	96%	97%	97%
Discharged on Antithrombotic Therapy[2]	129	100%	99%	99%
Discharged on Statin Medication[2]	114	98%	95%	94%
Thrombolytic Therapy Timing[1,2]	-	-	69%	66%
Venous Thromboembolism Prophylaxis[2]	173	95%	94%	94%
Written Stroke Educational Materials Given[2]	73	84%	86%	88%
Surgical Care Improvement Project				
Appropriate Beta Blocker Usage[2]	257	97%	97%	98%
Appropriate VTP Within 24 Hours[2]	493	98%	98%	98%
Controlled Postoperative Blood Glucose[2]	98	96%	97%	97%
Perioperative Temperature Management[2]	601	100%	100%	100%
Prophylactic Antibiotic Selection[2]	489	97%	99%	99%
Prophylactic Antibiotic Selection (Outpatient)	93	100%	97%	98%
Prophylactic Antibiotic Stopped[2]	445	98%	98%	98%
Prophylactic Antibiotic Timing[2]	489	99%	99%	99%
Prophylactic Antibiotic Timing (Outpatient)	95	95%	97%	98%
Urinary Catheter Removal[2]	418	94%	96%	97%
Survey of Patients' Hospital Experiences				
Area Around Room 'Always' Quiet at Night	300+	48%	51%	61%
Doctors 'Always' Communicated Well	300+	75%	77%	82%
Home Recovery Information Given	300+	77%	83%	85%
Hospital Given 9 or 10 on 10 Point Scale	300+	58%	63%	71%
Meds 'Always' Explained Before Given	300+	56%	59%	64%
Nurses 'Always' Communicated Well	300+	71%	75%	79%
Pain 'Always' Well Controlled	300+	62%	67%	71%
Room and Bathroom 'Always' Clean	300+	58%	69%	73%
Timely Help 'Always' Received	300+	49%	61%	68%
Would Definitely Recommend Hospital	300+	65%	65%	71%
Use of Medical Imaging				
Cardiac Imaging Stress Test before Surgery	487	3.5%	5.8%	5.3%
Combination Abdominal CT Scan	460	5.9%	8.2%	10.5%
Combination Brain/Sinus CT Scan	463	4.5%	3.6%	2.7%
Combination Chest CT Scan	370	2.7%	1.3%	2.7%
Follow-up Mammogram/Ultrasound	910	6.0%	13%	8.8%
Lumbar Spine MRI for Low Back Pain[1]	-	-	33.4%	37.2%

University Hospital of Brooklyn - Downstate Medical Center

445 Lenox Road
Brooklyn, NY 11203
Phone: 718-270-1000
Fax: 718-270-1815
URL: www.downstate.edu
Type: Acute Care Hospitals
Emergency Services: Yes
Ownership: Government - State
Beds: 406

Key Personnel:
Infection Control. . . . . Michael Augenbraun, MD
CEO/President. . . . . Debra Carey, MS
Cardiac Laboratory. . . . . Luther Clark, MD
Pediatric In-Patient Care . . . . Stanley Fisher, MD
Chief of Medical Staff . . . . Michael Lucchesi, MD
Quality Assurance . . . . TRUE Samms
Operating Room. . . . . Edward Serio, MBA
Radiology. . . . . David Stark, MD

Measure	Cases	This Hosp.	State Avg.	U.S. Avg.
Blood Clot Prevention and Treatment				
Anticoagulation Overlap Therapy[2]	96	88%	91%	93%
ICU Venous Thromboembolism Prophylaxis[2]	22	86%	92%	92%
Incidence of Potentially Preventable VTE[2]	31	10%	10%	10%
UFH with Dosages/Platelet Monitoring[2]	49	76%	92%	97%
Venous Thromboembolism Prophylaxis[2]	390	90%	87%	85%
Warfarin Therapy Discharge Instructions[2]	73	68%	59%	75%
Chest Pain/Possible Heart Attack Care				
Aspirin Given Within 24 Hours of Arrival[5]	-	-	97%	96%
Fibrinolytic Meds Within 30 Min. of Arrival[5]	-	-	54%	58%
Average Time to ECG (minutes)[5]	-	-	9	7
Average Time to Transfer (minutes)[5]	-	-	78	60
Children's Asthma Care				
Received Home Management Plan of Care	-	-	-	88%
Received Reliever Medication	-	-	-	100%
Received Systemic Corticosteroids	-	-	-	100%
Emergency Department				
Admittance Decision Time (minutes)[2]	627	279	154	98
Head CT Results Within 45 Min. of Arrival[1]	-	-	55%	57%
Patients Who Left ER Before Being Seen	>100k	1%	2%	2%
Time from ER Arrival to Admit. (minutes)[2]	627	533	378	274
Time from ER Arrival to Discharge (minutes)	331	171	156	134
Time in ER Before Being Evaluated (minutes)	373	67	35	26
Time to Pain Meds for Fractures (minutes)	169	48	61	57
Heart Attack Care				
Aspirin Given at Discharge[2]	253	99%	99%	99%
Fibrinolytic Meds Within 30 Min. of Arrival[2,7]	-	-	46%	54%
PCI Within 90 Minutes of Arrival[2]	34	91%	95%	96%
Statin Prescribed at Discharge[2]	256	96%	98%	98%
Heart Failure Care				
ACE Inhibitor or ARB for LVSD[2]	144	94%	96%	97%
Discharge Instructions Given[2]	268	79%	95%	94%
Evaluation of LVS Function[2]	286	100%	99%	99%
Medicare Spending				
Medicare Spending per Patient (ratio)	-	0.96	0.96	0.98
Pneumonia Care				
Appropriate Initial Antibiotic Given[2]	42	86%	95%	95%
Blood Culture Timing[2]	114	90%	97%	98%
Pregnancy and Delivery Care				
Newborn Deliveries Scheduled Early[2]	27	44%	4%	6%
Preventive Care				
Immunization for Influenza[2]	547	73%	88%	90%
Immunization for Pneumonia[2]	615	78%	88%	92%
Stroke Care				
Anticoagulation Therapy for Atrial Fibrillation[1,2]	-	-	96%	95%
Antithrombotic Therapy Timing[2]	92	99%	98%	98%
Assessed for Rehabilitation[2]	100	86%	97%	97%
Discharged on Antithrombotic Therapy[2]	91	98%	99%	99%
Discharged on Statin Medication[2]	71	94%	95%	94%
Thrombolytic Therapy Timing[2]	14	71%	69%	66%
Venous Thromboembolism Prophylaxis[2]	113	97%	94%	94%
Written Stroke Educational Materials Given[2]	41	83%	86%	88%
Surgical Care Improvement Project				
Appropriate Beta Blocker Usage[2]	125	97%	97%	98%
Appropriate VTP Within 24 Hours[2]	311	98%	98%	98%
Controlled Postoperative Blood Glucose[2]	71	100%	97%	97%
Perioperative Temperature Management[2]	361	100%	100%	100%

NOTE: Hospital profiles are in alphabetical order by state, then city, then hospital within the city; Rankings exclude hospitals with less than 25 cases except for patient surveys which excludes hospitals with less than 100 cases; (a) 100-299 cases; (1) The number of cases/patients is too few to report; (2) Data submitted were based on a sample of cases/patients; (3) Results are based on a shorter time period than required; (4) Data suppressed by CMS for one or more quarters; (5) Results are not available for this reporting period; (6) Fewer than 100 patients completed the HCAHPS survey; (7) No cases met the criteria for this measure; (8) The lower limit of the confidence interval cannot be calculated if the number of observed infections equals zero; (9) No data are available from the state/territory for this reporting period; (10) The scores shown reflect fewer than 50 completed surveys; (11) There were discrepancies in the data collection process; (12) This measure does not apply to this hospital for this reporting period; (13) Results cannot be calculated for this reporting period; (14) The results for this state are combined with nearby states to protect confidentiality; Please refer to the User's Guide for a full explanation of data.

Prophylactic Antibiotic Selection[2]	293	97%	99%	99%
Prophylactic Antibiotic Selection (Outpatient)	291	96%	97%	98%
Prophylactic Antibiotic Stopped[2]	282	98%	98%	98%
Prophylactic Antibiotic Timing[2]	299	95%	99%	99%
Prophylactic Antibiotic Timing (Outpatient)	289	97%	97%	98%
Urinary Catheter Removal[2]	227	96%	96%	97%
Survey of Patients' Hospital Experiences				
Area Around Room 'Always' Quiet at Night	300+	58%	51%	61%
Doctors 'Always' Communicated Well	300+	79%	77%	82%
Home Recovery Information Given	300+	75%	83%	85%
Hospital Given 9 or 10 on 10 Point Scale	300+	56%	63%	71%
Meds 'Always' Explained Before Given	300+	57%	59%	64%
Nurses 'Always' Communicated Well	300+	71%	75%	79%
Pain 'Always' Well Controlled	300+	63%	67%	71%
Room and Bathroom 'Always' Clean	300+	61%	69%	73%
Timely Help 'Always' Received	300+	53%	61%	68%
Would Definitely Recommend Hospital	300+	64%	65%	71%
Use of Medical Imaging				
Cardiac Imaging Stress Test before Surgery	192	15.1%	5.8%	5.3%
Combination Abdominal CT Scan	490	9.6%	8.2%	10.5%
Combination Brain/Sinus CT Scan	490	4.5%	3.6%	2.7%
Combination Chest CT Scan	263	0.4%	1.3%	2.7%
Follow-up Mammogram/Ultrasound	944	9.5%	13%	8.8%
Lumbar Spine MRI for Low Back Pain[1]	-	-	33.4%	37.2%

Woodhull Medical & Mental Health Center

760 Broadway
Brooklyn, NY 11206
Phone: 718-963-8100
Fax: 718-963-8501
URL: www.ci.nyc.ny.us
Type: Acute Care Hospitals
Emergency Services: Yes
Ownership: Government - Local
Key Personnel:
Chief of Medical Staff.......... Edward Fishkin
Infection Control.............. Rosalie Giardina
Anesthesiology.............. Stephan Petranker
Intensive Care Unit............ Stacie Stewart

Measure	Cases	This Hosp.	State Avg.	U.S. Avg.
Blood Clot Prevention and Treatment				
Anticoagulation Overlap Therapy[2]	29	97%	91%	93%
ICU Venous Thromboembolism Prophylaxis[2]	39	100%	92%	92%
Incidence of Potentially Preventable VTE[2]	17	0%	10%	10%
UFH with Dosages/Platelet Monitoring[2]	17	18%	92%	97%
Venous Thromboembolism Prophylaxis[2]	273	100%	87%	85%
Warfarin Therapy Discharge Instructions[2]	20	100%	59%	75%
Chest Pain/Possible Heart Attack Care				
Aspirin Given Within 24 Hours of Arrival	37	100%	97%	96%
Fibrinolytic Meds Within 30 Min. of Arrival[1]	-	-	54%	58%
Average Time to ECG (minutes)	38	12	9	7
Average Time to Transfer (minutes)[1]	-	-	78	60
Children's Asthma Care				
Received Home Management Plan of Care	-	-	-	88%
Received Reliever Medication	-	-	-	100%
Received Systemic Corticosteroids	-	-	-	100%
Emergency Department				
Admittance Decision Time (minutes)[2]	511	172	154	98
Head CT Results Within 45 Min. of Arrival[1]	-	-	55%	57%
Patients Who Left ER Before Being Seen	>100k	4%	2%	2%
Time from ER Arrival to Admit. (minutes)[2]	514	464	378	274
Time from ER Arrival to Discharge (minutes)	325	236	156	134
Time in ER Before Being Evaluated (minutes)	267	112	35	26
Time to Pain Meds for Fractures (minutes)	180	58	61	57
Heart Attack Care				
Aspirin Given at Discharge	29	97%	99%	99%
Fibrinolytic Meds Within 30 Min. of Arrival[1]	-	-	46%	54%
PCI Within 90 Minutes of Arrival[7]	-	-	95%	96%
Statin Prescribed at Discharge	30	97%	98%	98%
Heart Failure Care				
ACE Inhibitor or ARB for LVSD	116	97%	96%	97%
Discharge Instructions Given	188	98%	95%	94%
Evaluation of LVS Function	200	100%	99%	99%
Medicare Spending				
Medicare Spending per Patient (ratio)	-	0.94	0.96	0.98
Pneumonia Care				
Appropriate Initial Antibiotic Given	86	97%	95%	95%
Blood Culture Timing	132	94%	97%	98%
Pregnancy and Delivery Care				
Newborn Deliveries Scheduled Early[2]	30	7%	4%	6%
Preventive Care				
Immunization for Influenza[2]	447	87%	88%	90%
Immunization for Pneumonia[2]	333	90%	88%	92%
Stroke Care				
Anticoagulation Therapy for Atrial Fibrillation[1]	-	-	96%	95%
Antithrombotic Therapy Timing	89	98%	98%	98%
Assessed for Rehabilitation	92	99%	97%	97%
Discharged on Antithrombotic Therapy	81	98%	99%	99%
Discharged on Statin Medication	66	92%	95%	94%
Thrombolytic Therapy Timing[1]	-	-	69%	66%
Venous Thromboembolism Prophylaxis	107	100%	94%	94%
Written Stroke Educational Materials Given	40	98%	86%	88%
Surgical Care Improvement Project				
Appropriate Beta Blocker Usage[2]	29	86%	97%	98%
Appropriate VTP Within 24 Hours[2]	181	98%	98%	98%
Controlled Postoperative Blood Glucose[2,7]	-	-	97%	97%
Perioperative Temperature Management[2]	216	100%	100%	100%
Prophylactic Antibiotic Selection[2]	124	98%	99%	99%
Prophylactic Antibiotic Selection (Outpatient)	84	98%	97%	98%
Prophylactic Antibiotic Stopped[2]	122	98%	98%	98%
Prophylactic Antibiotic Timing[2]	126	94%	99%	99%
Prophylactic Antibiotic Timing (Outpatient)	25	88%	97%	98%
Urinary Catheter Removal[2]	55	89%	96%	97%
Survey of Patients' Hospital Experiences				
Area Around Room 'Always' Quiet at Night	300+	52%	51%	61%
Doctors 'Always' Communicated Well	300+	70%	77%	82%
Home Recovery Information Given	300+	79%	83%	85%
Hospital Given 9 or 10 on 10 Point Scale	300+	51%	63%	71%
Meds 'Always' Explained Before Given	300+	47%	59%	64%
Nurses 'Always' Communicated Well	300+	61%	75%	79%
Pain 'Always' Well Controlled	300+	55%	67%	71%
Room and Bathroom 'Always' Clean	300+	68%	69%	73%
Timely Help 'Always' Received	300+	44%	61%	68%
Would Definitely Recommend Hospital	300+	53%	65%	71%
Use of Medical Imaging				
Cardiac Imaging Stress Test before Surgery	80	6.3%	5.8%	5.3%
Combination Abdominal CT Scan	60	1.7%	8.2%	10.5%
Combination Brain/Sinus CT Scan[1]	-	-	3.6%	2.7%
Combination Chest CT Scan[1]	-	-	1.3%	2.7%
Follow-up Mammogram/Ultrasound	126	10.3%	13%	8.8%
Lumbar Spine MRI for Low Back Pain[1]	-	-	33.4%	37.2%

Wyckoff Heights Medical Center

374 Stockholm Street
Brooklyn, NY 11237
Phone: 718-963-7272
Fax: 718-963-7752
URL: www.wyckoffhospital.org
Type: Acute Care Hospitals
Emergency Services: Yes
Ownership: Voluntary non-profit - Other
Beds: 305
Key Personnel:
Chief of Medical Staff.......... Gustavo Del Toro, MD
Pediatric In-Patient Care .... Alvin Eden, MD
Pediatric Ambulatory Care ...... Sol Gourji, MD
Operating Room.............. Vivian Jager, RN
Quality Assurance .... Ruth Krauthamer, RN
CEO/President............... Ramon J. Rodriguez
Radiology.................. Mohsen Sanui
Infection Control.............. John Vernaloo, MD

Measure	Cases	This Hosp.	State Avg.	U.S. Avg.
Blood Clot Prevention and Treatment				
Anticoagulation Overlap Therapy[2]	73	86%	91%	93%
ICU Venous Thromboembolism Prophylaxis[2]	58	90%	92%	92%
Incidence of Potentially Preventable VTE[2]	28	0%	10%	10%
UFH with Dosages/Platelet Monitoring[2]	26	96%	92%	97%
Venous Thromboembolism Prophylaxis[2]	388	88%	87%	85%
Warfarin Therapy Discharge Instructions[2]	54	76%	59%	75%
Chest Pain/Possible Heart Attack Care				
Aspirin Given Within 24 Hours of Arrival	55	96%	97%	96%
Fibrinolytic Meds Within 30 Min. of Arrival[1]	-	-	54%	58%
Average Time to ECG (minutes)	54	9	9	7
Average Time to Transfer (minutes)[1]	-	-	78	60
Children's Asthma Care				
Received Home Management Plan of Care	-	-	-	88%
Received Reliever Medication	-	-	-	100%
Received Systemic Corticosteroids	-	-	-	100%
Emergency Department				
Admittance Decision Time (minutes)[2]	968	176	154	98
Head CT Results Within 45 Min. of Arrival[1]	-	-	55%	57%
Patients Who Left ER Before Being Seen	86,002	3%	2%	2%
Time from ER Arrival to Admit. (minutes)[2]	977	449	378	274
Time from ER Arrival to Discharge (minutes)	409	184	156	134
Time in ER Before Being Evaluated (minutes)	434	95	35	26
Time to Pain Meds for Fractures (minutes)	82	148	61	57
Heart Attack Care				
Aspirin Given at Discharge	37	97%	99%	99%
Fibrinolytic Meds Within 30 Min. of Arrival[7]	-	-	46%	54%
PCI Within 90 Minutes of Arrival[7]	-	-	95%	96%
Statin Prescribed at Discharge	38	95%	98%	98%
Heart Failure Care				
ACE Inhibitor or ARB for LVSD[2]	161	96%	96%	97%
Discharge Instructions Given[2]	298	90%	95%	94%
Evaluation of LVS Function[2]	327	99%	99%	99%
Medicare Spending				
Medicare Spending per Patient (ratio)	-	1.00	0.96	0.98
Pneumonia Care				
Appropriate Initial Antibiotic Given[2]	91	98%	95%	95%
Blood Culture Timing[2]	124	94%	97%	98%
Pregnancy and Delivery Care				
Newborn Deliveries Scheduled Early[2]	23	9%	4%	6%
Preventive Care				
Immunization for Influenza[2]	564	98%	88%	90%
Immunization for Pneumonia[2]	585	96%	88%	92%
Stroke Care				
Anticoagulation Therapy for Atrial Fibrillation	16	75%	96%	95%
Antithrombotic Therapy Timing	142	94%	98%	98%
Assessed for Rehabilitation	151	92%	97%	97%
Discharged on Antithrombotic Therapy	133	95%	99%	99%
Discharged on Statin Medication	111	92%	95%	94%
Thrombolytic Therapy Timing[1]	-	-	69%	66%
Venous Thromboembolism Prophylaxis	177	93%	94%	94%
Written Stroke Educational Materials Given	93	81%	86%	88%
Surgical Care Improvement Project				
Appropriate Beta Blocker Usage[2]	75	88%	97%	98%
Appropriate VTP Within 24 Hours[2]	224	98%	98%	98%
Controlled Postoperative Blood Glucose[2,7]	-	-	97%	97%
Perioperative Temperature Management[2]	274	100%	100%	100%
Prophylactic Antibiotic Selection[2]	112	96%	99%	99%
Prophylactic Antibiotic Selection (Outpatient)	68	94%	97%	98%
Prophylactic Antibiotic Stopped[2]	98	95%	98%	98%
Prophylactic Antibiotic Timing[2]	112	98%	99%	99%
Prophylactic Antibiotic Timing (Outpatient)	56	84%	97%	98%
Urinary Catheter Removal[2]	96	95%	96%	97%
Survey of Patients' Hospital Experiences				
Area Around Room 'Always' Quiet at Night	300+	47%	51%	61%
Doctors 'Always' Communicated Well	300+	70%	77%	82%
Home Recovery Information Given	300+	73%	83%	85%
Hospital Given 9 or 10 on 10 Point Scale	300+	49%	63%	71%
Meds 'Always' Explained Before Given	300+	48%	59%	64%
Nurses 'Always' Communicated Well	300+	64%	75%	79%
Pain 'Always' Well Controlled	300+	58%	67%	71%
Room and Bathroom 'Always' Clean	300+	63%	69%	73%
Timely Help 'Always' Received	300+	48%	61%	68%
Would Definitely Recommend Hospital	300+	50%	65%	71%
Use of Medical Imaging				
Cardiac Imaging Stress Test before Surgery	66	9.1%	5.8%	5.3%
Combination Abdominal CT Scan	329	4.0%	8.2%	10.5%
Combination Brain/Sinus CT Scan	351	4.3%	3.6%	2.7%
Combination Chest CT Scan	125	0.0%	1.3%	2.7%
Follow-up Mammogram/Ultrasound	434	6.5%	13%	8.8%
Lumbar Spine MRI for Low Back Pain[1]	-	-	33.4%	37.2%

NOTE: Hospital profiles are in alphabetical order by state, then city, then hospital within the city; Rankings exclude hospitals with less than 25 cases except for patient surveys which excludes hospitals with less than 100 cases; (a) 100-299 cases; (1) The number of cases/patients is too few to report; (2) Data submitted were based on a sample of cases/patients; (3) Results are based on a shorter time period than required; (4) Data suppressed by CMS for one or more quarters; (5) Results are not available for this reporting period; (6) Fewer than 100 patients completed the HCAHPS survey; (7) No cases met the criteria for this measure; (8) The lower limit of the confidence interval cannot be calculated if the number of observed infections equals zero; (9) No data are available from the state/territory for this reporting period; (10) The scores shown reflect fewer than 50 completed surveys; (11) There were discrepancies in the data collection process; (12) This measure does not apply to this hospital for this reporting period; (13) Results cannot be calculated for this reporting period; (14) The results for this state are combined with nearby states to protect confidentiality; Please refer to the User's Guide for a full explanation of data.

Erie County Medical Center

462 Grider Street
Buffalo, NY 14215
Phone: 716-898-3936
Fax: 716-898-5178
URL: www.ecmc.edu
Type: Acute Care Hospitals
Emergency Services: Yes
Ownership: Voluntary non-profit - Private
Beds: 550

Key Personnel:
Pediatric Ambulatory Care . . . . . . Melinda Cameron, MD
CEO/President. . . . . Richard C. Cleland, MPA, FACHE, NHA
Radiology. . . . . Robert R Conti
Quality Assurance . . . . Kitty Gazda
Infection Control. . . . . Charlene Lulow
Chief of Medical Staff. . . . . Brian M. Murray, MD
Operating Room. . . . . Jim Turner

Measure	Cases	This Hosp.	State Avg.	U.S. Avg.
Blood Clot Prevention and Treatment				
Anticoagulation Overlap Therapy[2]	53	87%	91%	93%
ICU Venous Thromboembolism Prophylaxis[2]	57	93%	92%	92%
Incidence of Potentially Preventable VTE[2]	23	26%	10%	10%
UFH with Dosages/Platelet Monitoring[2]	26	92%	92%	97%
Venous Thromboembolism Prophylaxis[2]	256	90%	87%	85%
Warfarin Therapy Discharge Instructions[2]	30	13%	59%	75%
Chest Pain/Possible Heart Attack Care				
Aspirin Given Within 24 Hours of Arrival[1,3]	-	-	97%	96%
Fibrinolytic Meds Within 30 Min. of Arrival[3,7]	-	-	54%	58%
Average Time to ECG (minutes)[1,3]	-	-	9	7
Average Time to Transfer (minutes)[1,3]	-	-	78	60
Children's Asthma Care				
Received Home Management Plan of Care	-	-	-	88%
Received Reliever Medication	-	-	-	100%
Received Systemic Corticosteroids	-	-	-	100%
Emergency Department				
Admittance Decision Time (minutes)[2]	407	150	154	98
Head CT Results Within 45 Min. of Arrival[1,3]	-	-	55%	57%
Patients Who Left ER Before Being Seen	65,644	3%	2%	2%
Time from ER Arrival to Admit. (minutes)[2]	417	428	378	274
Time from ER Arrival to Discharge (minutes)	306	282	156	134
Time in ER Before Being Evaluated (minutes)	320	35	35	26
Time to Pain Meds for Fractures (minutes)	33	89	61	57
Heart Attack Care				
Aspirin Given at Discharge	94	96%	99%	99%
Fibrinolytic Meds Within 30 Min. of Arrival[7]	-	-	46%	54%
PCI Within 90 Minutes of Arrival	13	92%	95%	96%
Statin Prescribed at Discharge	95	99%	98%	98%
Heart Failure Care				
ACE Inhibitor or ARB for LVSD	78	88%	96%	97%
Discharge Instructions Given	212	94%	95%	94%
Evaluation of LVS Function	270	97%	99%	99%
Medicare Spending				
Medicare Spending per Patient (ratio)	-	0.95	0.96	0.98
Pneumonia Care				
Appropriate Initial Antibiotic Given	57	95%	95%	95%
Blood Culture Timing	198	94%	97%	98%
Pregnancy and Delivery Care				
Newborn Deliveries Scheduled Early[7]	-	-	4%	6%
Preventive Care				
Immunization for Influenza[2]	578	86%	88%	90%
Immunization for Pneumonia[2]	576	87%	88%	92%
Stroke Care				
Anticoagulation Therapy for Atrial Fibrillation[1]	-	-	96%	95%
Antithrombotic Therapy Timing	45	91%	98%	98%
Assessed for Rehabilitation	48	100%	97%	97%
Discharged on Antithrombotic Therapy	42	100%	99%	99%
Discharged on Statin Medication	33	94%	95%	94%
Thrombolytic Therapy Timing[7]	-	-	69%	66%
Venous Thromboembolism Prophylaxis	57	79%	94%	94%
Written Stroke Educational Materials Given	20	100%	86%	88%
Surgical Care Improvement Project				
Appropriate Beta Blocker Usage	215	94%	97%	98%
Appropriate VTP Within 24 Hours	675	95%	98%	98%
Controlled Postoperative Blood Glucose	37	92%	97%	97%
Perioperative Temperature Management	771	100%	100%	100%
Prophylactic Antibiotic Selection	481	94%	99%	99%
Prophylactic Antibiotic Selection (Outpatient)	331	95%	97%	98%
Prophylactic Antibiotic Stopped	473	97%	98%	98%
Prophylactic Antibiotic Timing	482	98%	99%	99%
Prophylactic Antibiotic Timing (Outpatient)	319	94%	97%	98%
Urinary Catheter Removal	554	92%	96%	97%
Survey of Patients' Hospital Experiences				
Area Around Room 'Always' Quiet at Night	300+	43%	51%	61%
Doctors 'Always' Communicated Well	300+	69%	77%	82%
Home Recovery Information Given	300+	82%	83%	85%
Hospital Given 9 or 10 on 10 Point Scale	300+	59%	63%	71%
Meds 'Always' Explained Before Given	300+	52%	59%	64%
Nurses 'Always' Communicated Well	300+	68%	75%	79%
Pain 'Always' Well Controlled	300+	59%	67%	71%
Room and Bathroom 'Always' Clean	300+	56%	69%	73%
Timely Help 'Always' Received	300+	49%	61%	68%
Would Definitely Recommend Hospital	300+	62%	65%	71%
Use of Medical Imaging				
Cardiac Imaging Stress Test before Surgery	146	2.7%	5.8%	5.3%
Combination Abdominal CT Scan	416	9.1%	8.2%	10.5%
Combination Brain/Sinus CT Scan	440	7.3%	3.6%	2.7%
Combination Chest CT Scan	181	0.0%	1.3%	2.7%
Follow-up Mammogram/Ultrasound	94	5.3%	13%	8.8%
Lumbar Spine MRI for Low Back Pain[1]	-	-	33.4%	37.2%

Kaleida Health

726 Exchange Street, Suite 522
Buffalo, NY 14210
Phone: 716-859-8620
URL: www.kaleidahealth.org
Type: Acute Care Hospitals
Emergency Services: Yes
Ownership: Voluntary non-profit - Private

Key Personnel:
President/CEO. . . . . Jody L. Lomeo

Measure	Cases	This Hosp.	State Avg.	U.S. Avg.
Blood Clot Prevention and Treatment				
Anticoagulation Overlap Therapy[2]	308	95%	91%	93%
ICU Venous Thromboembolism Prophylaxis[2]	93	96%	92%	92%
Incidence of Potentially Preventable VTE[2]	95	11%	10%	10%
UFH with Dosages/Platelet Monitoring[2]	171	100%	92%	97%
Venous Thromboembolism Prophylaxis[2]	294	87%	87%	85%
Warfarin Therapy Discharge Instructions[2]	218	68%	59%	75%
Chest Pain/Possible Heart Attack Care				
Aspirin Given Within 24 Hours of Arrival	17	88%	97%	96%
Fibrinolytic Meds Within 30 Min. of Arrival[3,7]	-	-	54%	58%
Average Time to ECG (minutes)	20	14	9	7
Average Time to Transfer (minutes)[1,3]	-	-	78	60
Children's Asthma Care				
Received Home Management Plan of Care	-	-	-	88%
Received Reliever Medication	-	-	-	100%
Received Systemic Corticosteroids	-	-	-	100%
Emergency Department				
Admittance Decision Time (minutes)[2]	602	123	154	98
Head CT Results Within 45 Min. of Arrival[1]	-	-	55%	57%
Patients Who Left ER Before Being Seen	>100k	3%	2%	2%
Time from ER Arrival to Admit. (minutes)[2]	606	398	378	274
Time from ER Arrival to Discharge (minutes)	955	187	156	134
Time in ER Before Being Evaluated (minutes)	1,010	42	35	26
Time to Pain Meds for Fractures (minutes)	358	79	61	57
Heart Attack Care				
Aspirin Given at Discharge[2]	510	99%	99%	99%
Fibrinolytic Meds Within 30 Min. of Arrival[2,7]	-	-	46%	54%
PCI Within 90 Minutes of Arrival[2]	28	89%	95%	96%
Statin Prescribed at Discharge[2]	513	97%	98%	98%
Heart Failure Care				
ACE Inhibitor or ARB for LVSD	358	97%	96%	97%
Discharge Instructions Given	1,002	94%	95%	94%
Evaluation of LVS Function	1,275	100%	99%	99%
Medicare Spending				
Medicare Spending per Patient (ratio)	-	0.96	0.96	0.98
Pneumonia Care				
Appropriate Initial Antibiotic Given[2]	190	98%	95%	95%
Blood Culture Timing[2]	329	96%	97%	98%
Pregnancy and Delivery Care				
Newborn Deliveries Scheduled Early[2]	49	0%	4%	6%
Preventive Care				
Immunization for Influenza[2]	614	88%	88%	90%
Immunization for Pneumonia[2]	699	89%	88%	92%
Stroke Care				
Anticoagulation Therapy for Atrial Fibrillation	153	100%	96%	95%
Antithrombotic Therapy Timing	788	100%	98%	98%
Assessed for Rehabilitation	989	98%	97%	97%
Discharged on Antithrombotic Therapy	877	100%	99%	99%
Discharged on Statin Medication	704	98%	95%	94%
Thrombolytic Therapy Timing	91	85%	69%	66%
Venous Thromboembolism Prophylaxis	1,052	100%	94%	94%
Written Stroke Educational Materials Given	560	96%	86%	88%
Surgical Care Improvement Project				
Appropriate Beta Blocker Usage[2]	464	98%	97%	98%
Appropriate VTP Within 24 Hours[2]	678	98%	98%	98%
Controlled Postoperative Blood Glucose[2]	248	96%	97%	97%
Perioperative Temperature Management[2]	905	100%	100%	100%
Prophylactic Antibiotic Selection[2]	815	100%	99%	99%
Prophylactic Antibiotic Selection (Outpatient)	1,477	99%	97%	98%
Prophylactic Antibiotic Stopped[2]	807	95%	98%	98%
Prophylactic Antibiotic Timing[2]	815	99%	99%	99%
Prophylactic Antibiotic Timing (Outpatient)	1,462	98%	97%	98%
Urinary Catheter Removal[2]	628	95%	96%	97%
Survey of Patients' Hospital Experiences				
Area Around Room 'Always' Quiet at Night	300+	43%	51%	61%
Doctors 'Always' Communicated Well	300+	74%	77%	82%
Home Recovery Information Given	300+	84%	83%	85%
Hospital Given 9 or 10 on 10 Point Scale	300+	60%	63%	71%
Meds 'Always' Explained Before Given	300+	52%	59%	64%
Nurses 'Always' Communicated Well	300+	72%	75%	79%
Pain 'Always' Well Controlled	300+	65%	67%	71%
Room and Bathroom 'Always' Clean	300+	60%	69%	73%
Timely Help 'Always' Received	300+	54%	61%	68%
Would Definitely Recommend Hospital	300+	66%	65%	71%
Use of Medical Imaging				
Cardiac Imaging Stress Test before Surgery	600	4.8%	5.8%	5.3%
Combination Abdominal CT Scan	1,273	8.3%	8.2%	10.5%
Combination Brain/Sinus CT Scan	1,309	3.6%	3.6%	2.7%
Combination Chest CT Scan	451	6.2%	1.3%	2.7%
Follow-up Mammogram/Ultrasound	764	10.9%	13%	8.8%
Lumbar Spine MRI for Low Back Pain	60	35.0%	33.4%	37.2%

Mercy Hospital

565 Abbott Road
Buffalo, NY 14220
Phone: 716-826-7000
Fax: 716-828-2700
URL: www.chsbuffalo.org
Type: Acute Care Hospitals
Emergency Services: Yes
Ownership: Voluntary non-profit - Private
Beds: 349

Key Personnel:
Chief of Medical Staff. . . . . Timothy Gabryel, MD
Radiology. . . . . Margaret Jetter
Operating Room. . . . . Sharon Kimaid
Infection Control. . . . . Carole McCann
Quality Assurance . . . . Nancy Sheehan
CEO/President. . . . . Charles J. Urlaub

Measure	Cases	This Hosp.	State Avg.	U.S. Avg.
Blood Clot Prevention and Treatment				
Anticoagulation Overlap Therapy[2]	173	99%	91%	93%
ICU Venous Thromboembolism Prophylaxis[2]	45	93%	92%	92%
Incidence of Potentially Preventable VTE[2]	31	10%	10%	10%
UFH with Dosages/Platelet Monitoring[2]	57	100%	92%	97%
Venous Thromboembolism Prophylaxis[2]	386	88%	87%	85%
Warfarin Therapy Discharge Instructions[2]	93	95%	59%	75%
Chest Pain/Possible Heart Attack Care				
Aspirin Given Within 24 Hours of Arrival[5]	-	-	97%	96%
Fibrinolytic Meds Within 30 Min. of Arrival[5]	-	-	54%	58%
Average Time to ECG (minutes)[5]	-	-	9	7
Average Time to Transfer (minutes)[5]	-	-	78	60
Children's Asthma Care				
Received Home Management Plan of Care	-	-	-	88%
Received Reliever Medication	-	-	-	100%
Received Systemic Corticosteroids	-	-	-	100%
Emergency Department				
Admittance Decision Time (minutes)[2]	693	156	154	98

NOTE: Hospital profiles are in alphabetical order by state, then city, then hospital within the city; Rankings exclude hospitals with less than 25 cases except for patient surveys which excludes hospitals with less than 100 cases; (a) 100-299 cases; (1) The number of cases/patients is too few to report; (2) Data submitted were based on a sample of cases/patients; (3) Results are based on a shorter time period than required; (4) Data suppressed by CMS for one or more quarters; (5) Results are not available for this reporting period; (6) Fewer than 100 patients completed the HCAHPS survey; (7) No cases met the criteria for this measure; (8) The lower limit of the confidence interval cannot be calculated if the number of observed infections equals zero; (9) No data are available from the state/territory for this reporting period; (10) The scores shown reflect fewer than 50 completed surveys; (11) There were discrepancies in the data collection process; (12) This measure does not apply to this hospital for this reporting period; (13) Results cannot be calculated for this reporting period; (14) The results for this state are combined with nearby states to protect confidentiality; Please refer to the User's Guide for a full explanation of data.

Measure	Cases	This Hosp.	State Avg.	U.S. Avg.
Head CT Results Within 45 Min. of Arrival[3,7]	-	-	55%	57%
Patients Who Left ER Before Being Seen	78,756	2%	2%	2%
Time from ER Arrival to Admit. (minutes)[2]	696	402	378	274
Time from ER Arrival to Discharge (minutes)	406	122	156	134
Time in ER Before Being Evaluated (minutes)	420	24	35	26
Time to Pain Meds for Fractures (minutes)	299	47	61	57
Heart Attack Care				
Aspirin Given at Discharge[2]	304	99%	99%	99%
Fibrinolytic Meds Within 30 Min. of Arrival[1,2]	-	-	46%	54%
PCI Within 90 Minutes of Arrival[2]	40	78%	95%	96%
Statin Prescribed at Discharge[2]	288	100%	98%	98%
Heart Failure Care				
ACE Inhibitor or ARB for LVSD[2]	69	99%	96%	97%
Discharge Instructions Given[2]	200	99%	95%	94%
Evaluation of LVS Function[2]	291	100%	99%	99%
Medicare Spending				
Medicare Spending per Patient (ratio)	-	0.99	0.96	0.98
Pneumonia Care				
Appropriate Initial Antibiotic Given[2]	82	100%	95%	95%
Blood Culture Timing[2]	134	99%	97%	98%
Pregnancy and Delivery Care				
Newborn Deliveries Scheduled Early	155	1%	4%	6%
Preventive Care				
Immunization for Influenza[2]	558	96%	88%	90%
Immunization for Pneumonia[2]	702	90%	88%	92%
Stroke Care				
Anticoagulation Therapy for Atrial Fibrillation[2]	22	91%	96%	95%
Antithrombotic Therapy Timing[2]	81	100%	98%	98%
Assessed for Rehabilitation[2]	104	100%	97%	97%
Discharged on Antithrombotic Therapy[2]	81	98%	99%	99%
Discharged on Statin Medication[2]	66	95%	95%	94%
Thrombolytic Therapy Timing[2]	18	78%	69%	66%
Venous Thromboembolism Prophylaxis[2]	110	95%	94%	94%
Written Stroke Educational Materials Given[2]	52	90%	86%	88%
Surgical Care Improvement Project				
Appropriate Beta Blocker Usage[2]	323	98%	97%	98%
Appropriate VTP Within 24 Hours[2]	406	99%	98%	98%
Controlled Postoperative Blood Glucose[2]	201	95%	97%	97%
Perioperative Temperature Management[2]	694	99%	100%	100%
Prophylactic Antibiotic Selection[2]	594	100%	99%	99%
Prophylactic Antibiotic Selection (Outpatient)	635	100%	97%	98%
Prophylactic Antibiotic Stopped[2]	582	100%	98%	98%
Prophylactic Antibiotic Timing[2]	596	99%	99%	99%
Prophylactic Antibiotic Timing (Outpatient)	635	99%	97%	98%
Urinary Catheter Removal[2]	494	99%	96%	97%
Survey of Patients' Hospital Experiences				
Area Around Room 'Always' Quiet at Night	300+	43%	51%	61%
Doctors 'Always' Communicated Well	300+	75%	77%	82%
Home Recovery Information Given	300+	84%	83%	85%
Hospital Given 9 or 10 on 10 Point Scale	300+	56%	63%	71%
Meds 'Always' Explained Before Given	300+	56%	59%	64%
Nurses 'Always' Communicated Well	300+	73%	75%	79%
Pain 'Always' Well Controlled	300+	68%	67%	71%
Room and Bathroom 'Always' Clean	300+	55%	69%	73%
Timely Help 'Always' Received	300+	54%	61%	68%
Would Definitely Recommend Hospital	300+	57%	65%	71%
Use of Medical Imaging				
Cardiac Imaging Stress Test before Surgery	155	7.7%	5.8%	5.3%
Combination Abdominal CT Scan	680	6.8%	8.2%	10.5%
Combination Brain/Sinus CT Scan	566	1.8%	3.6%	2.7%
Combination Chest CT Scan	215	0.9%	1.3%	2.7%
Follow-up Mammogram/Ultrasound	608	7.9%	13%	8.8%
Lumbar Spine MRI for Low Back Pain[1]	-	-	33.4%	37.2%

Sisters of Charity Hospital

2157 Main Street
Buffalo, NY 14214
URL: www.chsbuffalo.org
Type: Acute Care Hospitals
Ownership: Voluntary non-profit - Church

Phone: 716-862-1000
Fax: 716-862-1809
Emergency Services: Yes
Beds: 413

Key Personnel:
CEO/President. . . . . Peter U. Bergmann, FACHE
Coronary Care . . . . Susan Cirbus
Pediatric Ambulatory Care . . . . . . Frank Giacobbe, MD
Pediatric In-Patient Care . . . . Frank Giacobbe, MD
Infection Control. . . . . Patricia Jones
Radiology. . . . . Michael Reilly
Chief of Medical Staff. . . . . Nady Shehata, MD
Quality Assurance . . . . Carolyn Yeates

Measure	Cases	This Hosp.	State Avg.	U.S. Avg.
Blood Clot Prevention and Treatment				
Anticoagulation Overlap Therapy[2]	143	100%	91%	93%
ICU Venous Thromboembolism Prophylaxis[2]	53	98%	92%	92%
Incidence of Potentially Preventable VTE[2]	13	0%	10%	10%
UFH with Dosages/Platelet Monitoring[2]	125	100%	92%	97%
Venous Thromboembolism Prophylaxis[2]	366	98%	87%	85%
Warfarin Therapy Discharge Instructions[2]	110	100%	59%	75%
Chest Pain/Possible Heart Attack Care				
Aspirin Given Within 24 Hours of Arrival	75	100%	97%	96%
Fibrinolytic Meds Within 30 Min. of Arrival[7]	-	-	54%	58%
Average Time to ECG (minutes)	77	12	9	7
Average Time to Transfer (minutes)	24	73	78	60
Children's Asthma Care				
Received Home Management Plan of Care	-	-	-	88%
Received Reliever Medication	-	-	-	100%
Received Systemic Corticosteroids	-	-	-	100%
Emergency Department				
Admittance Decision Time (minutes)[2]	530	120	154	98
Head CT Results Within 45 Min. of Arrival[1]	-	-	55%	57%
Patients Who Left ER Before Being Seen	70,388	1%	2%	2%
Time from ER Arrival to Admit. (minutes)[2]	531	326	378	274
Time from ER Arrival to Discharge (minutes)	392	148	156	134
Time in ER Before Being Evaluated (minutes)	417	26	35	26
Time to Pain Meds for Fractures (minutes)	192	60	61	57
Heart Attack Care				
Aspirin Given at Discharge	55	100%	99%	99%
Fibrinolytic Meds Within 30 Min. of Arrival[7]	-	-	46%	54%
PCI Within 90 Minutes of Arrival[7]	-	-	95%	96%
Statin Prescribed at Discharge	50	100%	98%	98%
Heart Failure Care				
ACE Inhibitor or ARB for LVSD[2]	77	100%	96%	97%
Discharge Instructions Given[2]	219	98%	95%	94%
Evaluation of LVS Function[2]	291	100%	99%	99%
Medicare Spending				
Medicare Spending per Patient (ratio)	-	0.97	0.96	0.98
Pneumonia Care				
Appropriate Initial Antibiotic Given[2]	100	100%	95%	95%
Blood Culture Timing[2]	185	100%	97%	98%
Pregnancy and Delivery Care				
Newborn Deliveries Scheduled Early	148	2%	4%	6%
Preventive Care				
Immunization for Influenza[2]	521	94%	88%	90%
Immunization for Pneumonia[2]	596	90%	88%	92%
Stroke Care				
Anticoagulation Therapy for Atrial Fibrillation[1,2]	-	-	96%	95%
Antithrombotic Therapy Timing[2]	66	98%	98%	98%
Assessed for Rehabilitation[2]	80	100%	97%	97%
Discharged on Antithrombotic Therapy[2]	62	100%	99%	99%
Discharged on Statin Medication[2]	55	89%	95%	94%
Thrombolytic Therapy Timing[1,2]	-	-	69%	66%
Venous Thromboembolism Prophylaxis[2]	80	92%	94%	94%
Written Stroke Educational Materials Given[2]	51	92%	86%	88%
Surgical Care Improvement Project				
Appropriate Beta Blocker Usage[2]	193	96%	97%	98%
Appropriate VTP Within 24 Hours[2]	473	99%	98%	98%
Controlled Postoperative Blood Glucose[2,7]	-	-	97%	97%
Perioperative Temperature Management[2]	608	100%	100%	100%
Prophylactic Antibiotic Selection[2]	413	99%	99%	99%
Prophylactic Antibiotic Selection (Outpatient)	553	99%	97%	98%
Prophylactic Antibiotic Stopped[2]	404	100%	98%	98%
Prophylactic Antibiotic Timing[2]	414	99%	99%	99%
Prophylactic Antibiotic Timing (Outpatient)	554	99%	97%	98%
Urinary Catheter Removal[2]	308	98%	96%	97%
Survey of Patients' Hospital Experiences				
Area Around Room 'Always' Quiet at Night	300+	53%	51%	61%
Doctors 'Always' Communicated Well	300+	75%	77%	82%
Home Recovery Information Given	300+	83%	83%	85%
Hospital Given 9 or 10 on 10 Point Scale	300+	70%	63%	71%
Meds 'Always' Explained Before Given	300+	59%	59%	64%
Nurses 'Always' Communicated Well	300+	76%	75%	79%
Pain 'Always' Well Controlled	300+	72%	67%	71%
Room and Bathroom 'Always' Clean	300+	64%	69%	73%
Timely Help 'Always' Received	300+	65%	61%	68%
Would Definitely Recommend Hospital	300+	72%	65%	71%
Use of Medical Imaging				
Cardiac Imaging Stress Test before Surgery	97	13.4%	5.8%	5.3%
Combination Abdominal CT Scan	601	3.3%	8.2%	10.5%
Combination Brain/Sinus CT Scan	465	1.7%	3.6%	2.7%
Combination Chest CT Scan	230	0.4%	1.3%	2.7%
Follow-up Mammogram/Ultrasound	529	10.0%	13%	8.8%
Lumbar Spine MRI for Low Back Pain[1]	-	-	33.4%	37.2%

Upstate New York VA Healthcare System - Western NY

3495 Bailey Avenue
Buffalo, NY 14215
URL: www.buffalo.va.gov
Type: Acute Care - VA
Ownership: Government Federal

Phone: 716-862-3611
Fax: 716-862-8759
Emergency Services: No
Beds: 288

Key Personnel:
Chief of Medical Staff. . . . . Ali El Solh, MD
Emergency Room . . . . Mukesh Nangia, MD
Infection Control. . . . . John Sellick, MD
Quality Assurance . . . . Kathryn Varkonda
Patient Relations . . . . Lizabeth M Weiss, RN, CNA
Operating Room. . . . . Israel Ziv, MD

Measure	Cases	This Hosp.	State Avg.	U.S. Avg.
Blood Clot Prevention and Treatment				
Anticoagulation Overlap Therapy	-	-	91%	93%
ICU Venous Thromboembolism Prophylaxis	-	-	92%	92%
Incidence of Potentially Preventable VTE	-	-	10%	10%
UFH with Dosages/Platelet Monitoring	-	-	92%	97%
Venous Thromboembolism Prophylaxis	-	-	87%	85%
Warfarin Therapy Discharge Instructions	-	-	59%	75%
Chest Pain/Possible Heart Attack Care				
Aspirin Given Within 24 Hours of Arrival	-	-	97%	96%
Fibrinolytic Meds Within 30 Min. of Arrival	-	-	54%	58%
Average Time to ECG (minutes)	-	-	9	7
Average Time to Transfer (minutes)	-	-	78	60
Children's Asthma Care				
Received Home Management Plan of Care	-	-	-	88%
Received Reliever Medication	-	-	-	100%
Received Systemic Corticosteroids	-	-	-	100%
Emergency Department				
Admittance Decision Time (minutes)	-	-	154	98
Head CT Results Within 45 Min. of Arrival	-	-	55%	57%
Patients Who Left ER Before Being Seen	-	-	2%	2%
Time from ER Arrival to Admit. (minutes)	-	-	378	274
Time from ER Arrival to Discharge (minutes)	-	-	156	134
Time in ER Before Being Evaluated (minutes)	-	-	35	26
Time to Pain Meds for Fractures (minutes)	-	-	61	57
Heart Attack Care				
Aspirin Given at Discharge	90	100%	99%	99%
Fibrinolytic Meds Within 30 Min. of Arrival[5]	-	-	46%	54%
PCI Within 90 Minutes of Arrival[1]	-	-	95%	96%
Statin Prescribed at Discharge	95	98%	98%	98%
Heart Failure Care				
ACE Inhibitor or ARB for LVSD	69	83%	96%	97%
Discharge Instructions Given	165	97%	95%	94%
Evaluation of LVS Function	214	100%	99%	99%
Medicare Spending				
Medicare Spending per Patient (ratio)	-	-	0.96	0.98
Pneumonia Care				
Appropriate Initial Antibiotic Given	56	95%	95%	95%
Blood Culture Timing	123	98%	97%	98%
Pregnancy and Delivery Care				
Newborn Deliveries Scheduled Early	-	-	4%	6%
Preventive Care				
Immunization for Influenza[5]	-	-	88%	90%
Immunization for Pneumonia[5]	-	-	88%	92%

NOTE: Hospital profiles are in alphabetical order by state, then city, then hospital within the city; Rankings exclude hospitals with less than 25 cases except for patient surveys which excludes hospitals with less than 100 cases; (a) 100-299 cases; (1) The number of cases/patients is too few to report; (2) Data submitted were based on a sample of cases/patients; (3) Results are based on a shorter time period than required; (4) Data suppressed by CMS for one or more quarters; (5) Results are not available for this reporting period; (6) Fewer than 100 patients completed the HCAHPS survey; (7) No cases met the criteria for this measure; (8) The lower limit of the confidence interval cannot be calculated if the number of observed infections equals zero; (9) No data are available from the state/territory for this reporting period; (10) The scores shown reflect fewer than 50 completed surveys; (11) There were discrepancies in the data collection process; (12) This measure does not apply to this hospital for this reporting period; (13) Results cannot be calculated for this reporting period; (14) The results for this state are combined with nearby states to protect confidentiality; Please refer to the User's Guide for a full explanation of data.

Measure	Cases	This Hosp.	State Avg.	U.S. Avg.
Stroke Care				
Anticoagulation Therapy for Atrial Fibrillation	-	-	96%	95%
Antithrombotic Therapy Timing	-	-	98%	98%
Assessed for Rehabilitation	-	-	97%	97%
Discharged on Antithrombotic Therapy	-	-	99%	99%
Discharged on Statin Medication	-	-	95%	94%
Thrombolytic Therapy Timing	-	-	69%	66%
Venous Thromboembolism Prophylaxis	-	-	94%	94%
Written Stroke Educational Materials Given	-	-	86%	88%
Surgical Care Improvement Project				
Appropriate Beta Blocker Usage[2]	95	97%	97%	98%
Appropriate VTP Within 24 Hours[2]	124	96%	98%	98%
Controlled Postoperative Blood Glucose[2]	56	84%	97%	97%
Perioperative Temperature Management[2]	178	95%	100%	100%
Prophylactic Antibiotic Selection	132	95%	99%	99%
Prophylactic Antibiotic Selection (Outpatient)	-	-	97%	98%
Prophylactic Antibiotic Stopped	130	97%	98%	98%
Prophylactic Antibiotic Timing	133	91%	99%	99%
Prophylactic Antibiotic Timing (Outpatient)	-	-	97%	98%
Urinary Catheter Removal[2]	125	94%	96%	97%
Survey of Patients' Hospital Experiences				
Area Around Room 'Always' Quiet at Night	-	-	51%	61%
Doctors 'Always' Communicated Well	-	-	77%	82%
Home Recovery Information Given	-	-	83%	85%
Hospital Given 9 or 10 on 10 Point Scale	-	-	63%	71%
Meds 'Always' Explained Before Given	-	-	59%	64%
Nurses 'Always' Communicated Well	-	-	75%	79%
Pain 'Always' Well Controlled	-	-	67%	71%
Room and Bathroom 'Always' Clean	-	-	69%	73%
Timely Help 'Always' Received	-	-	61%	68%
Would Definitely Recommend Hospital	-	-	65%	71%
Use of Medical Imaging				
Cardiac Imaging Stress Test before Surgery	-	-	5.8%	5.3%
Combination Abdominal CT Scan	-	-	8.2%	10.5%
Combination Brain/Sinus CT Scan	-	-	3.6%	2.7%
Combination Chest CT Scan	-	-	1.3%	2.7%
Follow-up Mammogram/Ultrasound	-	-	13%	8.8%
Lumbar Spine MRI for Low Back Pain	-	-	33.4%	37.2%

Catskill Regional Medical Center - G Hermann Site

8081 Route 97 Phone: 845-887-5530
Callicoon, NY 12723
Type: Critical Access Hospitals Emergency Services: No
Ownership: Government - Federal

Measure	Cases	This Hosp.	State Avg.	U.S. Avg.
Blood Clot Prevention and Treatment				
Anticoagulation Overlap Therapy[5]	-	-	91%	93%
ICU Venous Thromboembolism Prophylaxis[5]	-	-	92%	92%
Incidence of Potentially Preventable VTE[5]	-	-	10%	10%
UFH with Dosages/Platelet Monitoring[5]	-	-	92%	97%
Venous Thromboembolism Prophylaxis[5]	-	-	87%	85%
Warfarin Therapy Discharge Instructions[5]	-	-	59%	75%
Chest Pain/Possible Heart Attack Care				
Aspirin Given Within 24 Hours of Arrival	14	100%	97%	96%
Fibrinolytic Meds Within 30 Min. of Arrival[1]	-	-	54%	58%
Average Time to ECG (minutes)	13	10	9	7
Average Time to Transfer (minutes)[1]	-	-	78	60
Children's Asthma Care				
Received Home Management Plan of Care	-	-	-	88%
Received Reliever Medication	-	-	-	100%
Received Systemic Corticosteroids	-	-	-	100%
Emergency Department				
Admittance Decision Time (minutes)[5]	-	-	154	98
Head CT Results Within 45 Min. of Arrival[5]	-	-	55%	57%
Patients Who Left ER Before Being Seen	4,127	0%	2%	2%
Time from ER Arrival to Admit. (minutes)[5]	-	-	378	274
Time from ER Arrival to Discharge (minutes)[5]	-	-	156	134
Time in ER Before Being Evaluated (minutes)[5]	-	-	35	26
Time to Pain Meds for Fractures (minutes)[5]	-	-	61	57
Heart Attack Care				
Aspirin Given at Discharge[1,3]	-	-	99%	99%
Fibrinolytic Meds Within 30 Min. of Arrival[3,7]	-	-	46%	54%
PCI Within 90 Minutes of Arrival[3,7]	-	-	95%	96%
Statin Prescribed at Discharge[1,3]	-	-	98%	98%
Heart Failure Care				
ACE Inhibitor or ARB for LVSD[1,3]	-	-	96%	97%
Discharge Instructions Given[1,3]	-	-	95%	94%
Evaluation of LVS Function[1,3]	-	-	99%	99%
Medicare Spending				
Medicare Spending per Patient (ratio)	-	-	0.96	0.98
Pneumonia Care				
Appropriate Initial Antibiotic Given[1]	-	-	95%	95%
Blood Culture Timing[1]	-	-	97%	98%
Pregnancy and Delivery Care				
Newborn Deliveries Scheduled Early[5]	-	-	4%	6%
Preventive Care				
Immunization for Influenza[5]	-	-	88%	90%
Immunization for Pneumonia[5]	-	-	88%	92%
Stroke Care				
Anticoagulation Therapy for Atrial Fibrillation[5]	-	-	96%	95%
Antithrombotic Therapy Timing[5]	-	-	98%	98%
Assessed for Rehabilitation[5]	-	-	97%	97%
Discharged on Antithrombotic Therapy[5]	-	-	99%	99%
Discharged on Statin Medication[5]	-	-	95%	94%
Thrombolytic Therapy Timing[5]	-	-	69%	66%
Venous Thromboembolism Prophylaxis[5]	-	-	94%	94%
Written Stroke Educational Materials Given[5]	-	-	86%	88%
Surgical Care Improvement Project				
Appropriate Beta Blocker Usage[5]	-	-	97%	98%
Appropriate VTP Within 24 Hours[5]	-	-	98%	98%
Controlled Postoperative Blood Glucose[5]	-	-	97%	97%
Perioperative Temperature Management[5]	-	-	100%	100%
Prophylactic Antibiotic Selection[5]	-	-	99%	99%
Prophylactic Antibiotic Selection (Outpatient)[5]	-	-	97%	98%
Prophylactic Antibiotic Stopped[5]	-	-	98%	98%
Prophylactic Antibiotic Timing[5]	-	-	99%	99%
Prophylactic Antibiotic Timing (Outpatient)[5]	-	-	97%	98%
Urinary Catheter Removal[5]	-	-	96%	97%
Survey of Patients' Hospital Experiences				
Area Around Room 'Always' Quiet at Night[5]	-	-	51%	61%
Doctors 'Always' Communicated Well[5]	-	-	77%	82%
Home Recovery Information Given[5]	-	-	83%	85%
Hospital Given 9 or 10 on 10 Point Scale[5]	-	-	63%	71%
Meds 'Always' Explained Before Given[5]	-	-	59%	64%
Nurses 'Always' Communicated Well[5]	-	-	75%	79%
Pain 'Always' Well Controlled[5]	-	-	67%	71%
Room and Bathroom 'Always' Clean[5]	-	-	69%	73%
Timely Help 'Always' Received[5]	-	-	61%	68%
Would Definitely Recommend Hospital[5]	-	-	65%	71%
Use of Medical Imaging				
Cardiac Imaging Stress Test before Surgery[7]	-	-	5.8%	5.3%
Combination Abdominal CT Scan[1]	-	-	8.2%	10.5%
Combination Brain/Sinus CT Scan	43	0.0%	3.6%	2.7%
Combination Chest CT Scan[1]	-	-	1.3%	2.7%
Follow-up Mammogram/Ultrasound[7]	-	-	13%	8.8%
Lumbar Spine MRI for Low Back Pain[7]	-	-	33.4%	37.2%

Canandaigua VA Medical Center

400 Foot Hill Ave. Phone: 585-394-2000
Canandaigua, NY 14424 Fax: 585-393-8328
URL: www.va.gov
Type: Acute Care - VA Emergency Services: No
Ownership: Government Federal Beds: 251

Key Personnel:
Chief of Medical Staff.......... Robert Babcock, MD
Ambulatory Care............... Richard Beninegna, MD
Patient Relations............. Laurie Guererri
Quality Assurance............ Doug Nather, RN
Infection Control............. Marguerite Sutton

Measure	Cases	This Hosp.	State Avg.	U.S. Avg.
Blood Clot Prevention and Treatment				
Anticoagulation Overlap Therapy	-	-	91%	93%
ICU Venous Thromboembolism Prophylaxis	-	-	92%	92%
Incidence of Potentially Preventable VTE	-	-	10%	10%
UFH with Dosages/Platelet Monitoring	-	-	92%	97%
Venous Thromboembolism Prophylaxis	-	-	87%	85%
Warfarin Therapy Discharge Instructions	-	-	59%	75%
Chest Pain/Possible Heart Attack Care				
Aspirin Given Within 24 Hours of Arrival	-	-	97%	96%
Fibrinolytic Meds Within 30 Min. of Arrival	-	-	54%	58%
Average Time to ECG (minutes)	-	-	9	7
Average Time to Transfer (minutes)	-	-	78	60
Children's Asthma Care				
Received Home Management Plan of Care	-	-	-	88%
Received Reliever Medication	-	-	-	100%
Received Systemic Corticosteroids	-	-	-	100%
Emergency Department				
Admittance Decision Time (minutes)	-	-	154	98
Head CT Results Within 45 Min. of Arrival	-	-	55%	57%
Patients Who Left ER Before Being Seen	-	-	2%	2%
Time from ER Arrival to Admit. (minutes)	-	-	378	274
Time from ER Arrival to Discharge (minutes)	-	-	156	134
Time in ER Before Being Evaluated (minutes)	-	-	35	26
Time to Pain Meds for Fractures (minutes)	-	-	61	57
Heart Attack Care				
Aspirin Given at Discharge[5]	-	-	99%	99%
Fibrinolytic Meds Within 30 Min. of Arrival[5]	-	-	46%	54%
PCI Within 90 Minutes of Arrival[5]	-	-	95%	96%
Statin Prescribed at Discharge[5]	-	-	98%	98%
Heart Failure Care				
ACE Inhibitor or ARB for LVSD[5]	-	-	96%	97%
Discharge Instructions Given[5]	-	-	95%	94%
Evaluation of LVS Function[5]	-	-	99%	99%
Medicare Spending				
Medicare Spending per Patient (ratio)	-	-	0.96	0.98
Pneumonia Care				
Appropriate Initial Antibiotic Given[5]	-	-	95%	95%
Blood Culture Timing[5]	-	-	97%	98%
Pregnancy and Delivery Care				
Newborn Deliveries Scheduled Early	-	-	4%	6%
Preventive Care				
Immunization for Influenza[5]	-	-	88%	90%
Immunization for Pneumonia[5]	-	-	88%	92%
Stroke Care				
Anticoagulation Therapy for Atrial Fibrillation	-	-	96%	95%
Antithrombotic Therapy Timing	-	-	98%	98%
Assessed for Rehabilitation	-	-	97%	97%
Discharged on Antithrombotic Therapy	-	-	99%	99%
Discharged on Statin Medication	-	-	95%	94%
Thrombolytic Therapy Timing	-	-	69%	66%
Venous Thromboembolism Prophylaxis	-	-	94%	94%
Written Stroke Educational Materials Given	-	-	86%	88%
Surgical Care Improvement Project				
Appropriate Beta Blocker Usage[5]	-	-	97%	98%
Appropriate VTP Within 24 Hours[5]	-	-	98%	98%
Controlled Postoperative Blood Glucose[5]	-	-	97%	97%
Perioperative Temperature Management[5]	-	-	100%	100%
Prophylactic Antibiotic Selection[5]	-	-	99%	99%
Prophylactic Antibiotic Selection (Outpatient)	-	-	97%	98%
Prophylactic Antibiotic Stopped[5]	-	-	98%	98%
Prophylactic Antibiotic Timing[5]	-	-	99%	99%
Prophylactic Antibiotic Timing (Outpatient)	-	-	97%	98%
Urinary Catheter Removal[5]	-	-	96%	97%
Survey of Patients' Hospital Experiences				
Area Around Room 'Always' Quiet at Night	-	-	51%	61%
Doctors 'Always' Communicated Well	-	-	77%	82%
Home Recovery Information Given	-	-	83%	85%
Hospital Given 9 or 10 on 10 Point Scale	-	-	63%	71%
Meds 'Always' Explained Before Given	-	-	59%	64%
Nurses 'Always' Communicated Well	-	-	75%	79%
Pain 'Always' Well Controlled	-	-	67%	71%
Room and Bathroom 'Always' Clean	-	-	69%	73%
Timely Help 'Always' Received	-	-	61%	68%
Would Definitely Recommend Hospital	-	-	65%	71%
Use of Medical Imaging				
Cardiac Imaging Stress Test before Surgery	-	-	5.8%	5.3%
Combination Abdominal CT Scan	-	-	8.2%	10.5%

NOTE: Hospital profiles are in alphabetical order by state, then city, then hospital within the city; Rankings exclude hospitals with less than 25 cases except for patient surveys which excludes hospitals with less than 100 cases; (a) 100-299 cases; (1) The number of cases/patients is too few to report; (2) Data submitted were based on a sample of cases/patients; (3) Results are based on a shorter time period than required; (4) Data suppressed by CMS for one or more quarters; (5) Results are not available for this reporting period; (6) Fewer than 100 patients completed the HCAHPS survey; (7) No cases met the criteria for this measure; (8) The lower limit of the confidence interval cannot be calculated if the number of observed infections equals zero; (9) No data are available from the state/territory for this reporting period; (10) The scores shown reflect fewer than 50 completed surveys; (11) There were discrepancies in the data collection process; (12) This measure does not apply to this hospital for this reporting period; (13) Results cannot be calculated for this reporting period; (14) The results for this state are combined with nearby states to protect confidentiality; Please refer to the User's Guide for a full explanation of data.

Measure	Cases	This Hosp.	State Avg.	U.S. Avg.
Combination Brain/Sinus CT Scan	-	-	3.6%	2.7%
Combination Chest CT Scan	-	-	1.3%	2.7%
Follow-up Mammogram/Ultrasound	-	-	13%	8.8%
Lumbar Spine MRI for Low Back Pain	-	-	33.4%	37.2%

F F Thompson Hospital

350 Parrish Street
Canandaigua, NY 14424
Phone: 585-396-6000
Fax: 585-396-6477
URL: www.thompsonhealth.com
Type: Acute Care Hospitals
Emergency Services: Yes
Ownership: Voluntary non-profit - Private
Beds: 113

Key Personnel:
Chief of Medical Staff.......... R Douglas Alling, MD
Hemotology Center........... Susan Bonanni
Pediatric In-Patient Care....... Diana Ellison
Intensive Care Unit............ Donna Fulmer
Operating Room.............. Donna Fulmer
Infection Control.............. Gloria Karr
Quality Assurance............ Linda Neva
President/CEO............... Michael F. Stapleton, Jr

Measure	Cases	This Hosp.	State Avg.	U.S. Avg.
Blood Clot Prevention and Treatment				
Anticoagulation Overlap Therapy[2]	35	100%	91%	93%
ICU Venous Thromboembolism Prophylaxis[2]	92	90%	92%	92%
Incidence of Potentially Preventable VTE[1,2]	-	-	10%	10%
UFH with Dosages/Platelet Monitoring[1,2]	-	-	92%	97%
Venous Thromboembolism Prophylaxis[2]	325	88%	87%	85%
Warfarin Therapy Discharge Instructions[2]	26	88%	59%	75%
Chest Pain/Possible Heart Attack Care				
Aspirin Given Within 24 Hours of Arrival	58	100%	97%	96%
Fibrinolytic Meds Within 30 Min. of Arrival[7]	-	-	54%	58%
Average Time to ECG (minutes)	57	11	9	7
Average Time to Transfer (minutes)	24	65	78	60
Children's Asthma Care				
Received Home Management Plan of Care	-	-	-	88%
Received Reliever Medication	-	-	-	100%
Received Systemic Corticosteroids	-	-	-	100%
Emergency Department				
Admittance Decision Time (minutes)[2]	567	111	154	98
Head CT Results Within 45 Min. of Arrival[1]	-	-	55%	57%
Patients Who Left ER Before Being Seen	25,978	3%	2%	2%
Time from ER Arrival to Admit. (minutes)[2]	575	350	378	274
Time from ER Arrival to Discharge (minutes)	371	205	156	134
Time in ER Before Being Evaluated (minutes)	402	50	35	26
Time to Pain Meds for Fractures (minutes)	110	63	61	57
Heart Attack Care				
Aspirin Given at Discharge	27	89%	99%	99%
Fibrinolytic Meds Within 30 Min. of Arrival[7]	-	-	46%	54%
PCI Within 90 Minutes of Arrival[7]	-	-	95%	96%
Statin Prescribed at Discharge	23	96%	98%	98%
Heart Failure Care				
ACE Inhibitor or ARB for LVSD	24	96%	96%	97%
Discharge Instructions Given	95	92%	95%	94%
Evaluation of LVS Function	124	98%	99%	99%
Medicare Spending				
Medicare Spending per Patient (ratio)	-	0.87	0.96	0.98
Pneumonia Care				
Appropriate Initial Antibiotic Given	138	97%	95%	95%
Blood Culture Timing	256	99%	97%	98%
Pregnancy and Delivery Care				
Newborn Deliveries Scheduled Early[2]	20	0%	4%	6%
Preventive Care				
Immunization for Influenza[2]	439	97%	88%	90%
Immunization for Pneumonia[2]	587	95%	88%	92%
Stroke Care				
Anticoagulation Therapy for Atrial Fibrillation[1]	-	-	96%	95%
Antithrombotic Therapy Timing	58	100%	98%	98%
Assessed for Rehabilitation	59	95%	97%	97%
Discharged on Antithrombotic Therapy	56	100%	99%	99%
Discharged on Statin Medication	46	96%	95%	94%
Thrombolytic Therapy Timing[1]	-	-	69%	66%
Venous Thromboembolism Prophylaxis	62	90%	94%	94%
Written Stroke Educational Materials Given	37	95%	86%	88%
Surgical Care Improvement Project				
Appropriate Beta Blocker Usage	141	99%	97%	98%
Appropriate VTP Within 24 Hours	443	99%	98%	98%
Controlled Postoperative Blood Glucose[7]	-	-	97%	97%
Perioperative Temperature Management	509	100%	100%	100%
Prophylactic Antibiotic Selection	430	100%	99%	99%
Prophylactic Antibiotic Selection (Outpatient)	84	100%	97%	98%
Prophylactic Antibiotic Stopped	409	99%	98%	98%
Prophylactic Antibiotic Timing	431	99%	99%	99%
Prophylactic Antibiotic Timing (Outpatient)	90	92%	97%	98%
Urinary Catheter Removal	387	100%	96%	97%
Survey of Patients' Hospital Experiences				
Area Around Room 'Always' Quiet at Night	300+	45%	51%	61%
Doctors 'Always' Communicated Well	300+	76%	77%	82%
Home Recovery Information Given	300+	88%	83%	85%
Hospital Given 9 or 10 on 10 Point Scale	300+	65%	63%	71%
Meds 'Always' Explained Before Given	300+	62%	59%	64%
Nurses 'Always' Communicated Well	300+	73%	75%	79%
Pain 'Always' Well Controlled	300+	65%	67%	71%
Room and Bathroom 'Always' Clean	300+	72%	69%	73%
Timely Help 'Always' Received	300+	58%	61%	68%
Would Definitely Recommend Hospital	300+	71%	65%	71%
Use of Medical Imaging				
Cardiac Imaging Stress Test before Surgery	93	2.2%	5.8%	5.3%
Combination Abdominal CT Scan	329	7.0%	8.2%	10.5%
Combination Brain/Sinus CT Scan[1]	-	-	3.6%	2.7%
Combination Chest CT Scan	167	0.0%	1.3%	2.7%
Follow-up Mammogram/Ultrasound	666	4.5%	13%	8.8%
Lumbar Spine MRI for Low Back Pain	49	38.8%	33.4%	37.2%

Putnam Hospital Center

670 Stoneleigh Avenue
Carmel, NY 10512
Phone: 914-279-5711
Fax: 845-279-7482
E-mail: info@putnamhospital.org
URL: www.putnamhospital.org
Type: Acute Care Hospitals
Emergency Services: Yes
Ownership: Voluntary non-profit - Private
Beds: 164

Key Personnel:
Radiology................... Philip Amatulle

Measure	Cases	This Hosp.	State Avg.	U.S. Avg.
Blood Clot Prevention and Treatment				
Anticoagulation Overlap Therapy[2]	34	100%	91%	93%
ICU Venous Thromboembolism Prophylaxis[2]	48	98%	92%	92%
Incidence of Potentially Preventable VTE[1,2]	-	-	10%	10%
UFH with Dosages/Platelet Monitoring[2]	11	91%	92%	97%
Venous Thromboembolism Prophylaxis[2]	336	93%	87%	85%
Warfarin Therapy Discharge Instructions[2]	23	91%	59%	75%
Chest Pain/Possible Heart Attack Care				
Aspirin Given Within 24 Hours of Arrival	69	100%	97%	96%
Fibrinolytic Meds Within 30 Min. of Arrival	19	63%	54%	58%
Average Time to ECG (minutes)	72	2	9	7
Average Time to Transfer (minutes)[1]	-	-	78	60
Children's Asthma Care				
Received Home Management Plan of Care	-	-	-	88%
Received Reliever Medication	-	-	-	100%
Received Systemic Corticosteroids	-	-	-	100%
Emergency Department				
Admittance Decision Time (minutes)[2]	752	117	154	98
Head CT Results Within 45 Min. of Arrival[1]	-	-	55%	57%
Patients Who Left ER Before Being Seen	26,984	1%	2%	2%
Time from ER Arrival to Admit. (minutes)[2]	752	305	378	274
Time from ER Arrival to Discharge (minutes)	443	146	156	134
Time in ER Before Being Evaluated (minutes)	423	42	35	26
Time to Pain Meds for Fractures (minutes)	104	44	61	57
Heart Attack Care				
Aspirin Given at Discharge	20	100%	99%	99%
Fibrinolytic Meds Within 30 Min. of Arrival[7]	-	-	46%	54%
PCI Within 90 Minutes of Arrival[7]	-	-	95%	96%
Statin Prescribed at Discharge	23	100%	98%	98%
Heart Failure Care				
ACE Inhibitor or ARB for LVSD	31	100%	96%	97%
Discharge Instructions Given	118	98%	95%	94%
Evaluation of LVS Function	157	100%	99%	99%
Medicare Spending				
Medicare Spending per Patient (ratio)	-	1.01	0.96	0.98
Pneumonia Care				
Appropriate Initial Antibiotic Given	96	98%	95%	95%
Blood Culture Timing	110	96%	97%	98%
Pregnancy and Delivery Care				
Newborn Deliveries Scheduled Early	31	3%	4%	6%
Preventive Care				
Immunization for Influenza[2]	594	94%	88%	90%
Immunization for Pneumonia[2]	727	96%	88%	92%
Stroke Care				
Anticoagulation Therapy for Atrial Fibrillation[1]	-	-	96%	95%
Antithrombotic Therapy Timing	55	98%	98%	98%
Assessed for Rehabilitation	53	98%	97%	97%
Discharged on Antithrombotic Therapy	49	98%	99%	99%
Discharged on Statin Medication	43	95%	95%	94%
Thrombolytic Therapy Timing[1]	-	-	69%	66%
Venous Thromboembolism Prophylaxis	60	98%	94%	94%
Written Stroke Educational Materials Given	31	97%	86%	88%
Surgical Care Improvement Project				
Appropriate Beta Blocker Usage	255	99%	97%	98%
Appropriate VTP Within 24 Hours	811	99%	98%	98%
Controlled Postoperative Blood Glucose[7]	-	-	97%	97%
Perioperative Temperature Management	868	100%	100%	100%
Prophylactic Antibiotic Selection	640	99%	99%	99%
Prophylactic Antibiotic Selection (Outpatient)	144	98%	97%	98%
Prophylactic Antibiotic Stopped	636	100%	98%	98%
Prophylactic Antibiotic Timing	640	100%	99%	99%
Prophylactic Antibiotic Timing (Outpatient)	144	97%	97%	98%
Urinary Catheter Removal	553	100%	96%	97%
Survey of Patients' Hospital Experiences				
Area Around Room 'Always' Quiet at Night	300+	59%	51%	61%
Doctors 'Always' Communicated Well	300+	83%	77%	82%
Home Recovery Information Given	300+	89%	83%	85%
Hospital Given 9 or 10 on 10 Point Scale	300+	78%	63%	71%
Meds 'Always' Explained Before Given	300+	70%	59%	64%
Nurses 'Always' Communicated Well	300+	84%	75%	79%
Pain 'Always' Well Controlled	300+	79%	67%	71%
Room and Bathroom 'Always' Clean	300+	76%	69%	73%
Timely Help 'Always' Received	300+	69%	61%	68%
Would Definitely Recommend Hospital	300+	79%	65%	71%
Use of Medical Imaging				
Cardiac Imaging Stress Test before Surgery[1]	-	-	5.8%	5.3%
Combination Abdominal CT Scan	522	4.6%	8.2%	10.5%
Combination Brain/Sinus CT Scan	584	4.6%	3.6%	2.7%
Combination Chest CT Scan	460	0.9%	1.3%	2.7%
Follow-up Mammogram/Ultrasound	866	19.6%	13%	8.8%
Lumbar Spine MRI for Low Back Pain	46	34.8%	33.4%	37.2%

Carthage Area Hospital

1001 West Street
Carthage, NY 13619
Phone: 315-493-1000
Fax: 315-493-4231
E-mail: cahadmin@carthageareahospital.com
URL: www.carthagehospital.com
Type: Acute Care Hospitals
Emergency Services: Yes
Ownership: Voluntary non-profit - Private
Beds: 78

Key Personnel:
Cardiac Laboratory............ Mirza Ashraf, MD
CEO/President............... Walter Becker
Intensive Care Unit............ Paula Bigelow, RN
Chief of Medical Staff.......... Kenneth Fish, DO
Radiology.................. Daniel Gray
Infection Control.............. Patti Jahnke
Operating Room.............. Belinda Pearson, RN
Quality Assurance............ Jan Widrick

Measure	Cases	This Hosp.	State Avg.	U.S. Avg.
Blood Clot Prevention and Treatment				
Anticoagulation Overlap Therapy[1,2]	-	-	91%	93%
ICU Venous Thromboembolism Prophylaxis[2]	63	35%	92%	92%
Incidence of Potentially Preventable VTE[2,7]	-	-	10%	10%
UFH with Dosages/Platelet Monitoring[1,2]	-	-	92%	97%
Venous Thromboembolism Prophylaxis[2]	106	33%	87%	85%
Warfarin Therapy Discharge Instructions[1,2]	-	-	59%	75%
Chest Pain/Possible Heart Attack Care				
Aspirin Given Within 24 Hours of Arrival	35	66%	97%	96%

NOTE: Hospital profiles are in alphabetical order by state, then city, then hospital within the city; Rankings exclude hospitals with less than 25 cases except for patient surveys which excludes hospitals with less than 100 cases; (a) 100-299 cases; (1) The number of cases/patients is too few to report; (2) Data submitted were based on a sample of cases/patients; (3) Results are based on a shorter time period than required; (4) Data suppressed by CMS for one or more quarters; (5) Results are not available for this reporting period; (6) Fewer than 100 patients completed the HCAHPS survey; (7) No cases met the criteria for this measure; (8) The lower limit of the confidence interval cannot be calculated if the number of observed infections equals zero; (9) No data are available from the state/territory for this reporting period; (10) The scores shown reflect fewer than 50 completed surveys; (11) There were discrepancies in the data collection process; (12) This measure does not apply to this hospital for this reporting period; (13) Results cannot be calculated for this reporting period; (14) The results for this state are combined with nearby states to protect confidentiality; Please refer to the User's Guide for a full explanation of data.

Measure	Cases	This Hosp.	State Avg.	U.S. Avg.
Fibrinolytic Meds Within 30 Min. of Arrival[1]	-	-	54%	58%
Average Time to ECG (minutes)	37	10	9	7
Average Time to Transfer (minutes)[7]	-	-	78	60
Children's Asthma Care				
Received Home Management Plan of Care	-	-	-	88%
Received Reliever Medication	-	-	-	100%
Received Systemic Corticosteroids	-	-	-	100%
Emergency Department				
Admittance Decision Time (minutes)[2]	168	90	154	98
Head CT Results Within 45 Min. of Arrival[1]	-	-	55%	57%
Patients Who Left ER Before Being Seen	23,490	0%	2%	2%
Time from ER Arrival to Admit. (minutes)[2]	197	268	378	274
Time from ER Arrival to Discharge (minutes)	324	104	156	134
Time in ER Before Being Evaluated (minutes)	392	18	35	26
Time to Pain Meds for Fractures (minutes)	55	53	61	57
Heart Attack Care				
Aspirin Given at Discharge[1,3]	-	-	99%	99%
Fibrinolytic Meds Within 30 Min. of Arrival[3,7]	-	-	46%	54%
PCI Within 90 Minutes of Arrival[3,7]	-	-	95%	96%
Statin Prescribed at Discharge[1,3]	-	-	98%	98%
Heart Failure Care				
ACE Inhibitor or ARB for LVSD[1]	-	-	96%	97%
Discharge Instructions Given	32	6%	95%	94%
Evaluation of LVS Function	43	95%	99%	99%
Medicare Spending				
Medicare Spending per Patient (ratio)	-	0.88	0.96	0.98
Pneumonia Care				
Appropriate Initial Antibiotic Given	22	82%	95%	95%
Blood Culture Timing	23	78%	97%	98%
Pregnancy and Delivery Care				
Newborn Deliveries Scheduled Early[2]	21	5%	4%	6%
Preventive Care				
Immunization for Influenza[2]	279	55%	88%	90%
Immunization for Pneumonia[2]	308	68%	88%	92%
Stroke Care				
Anticoagulation Therapy for Atrial Fibrillation[1,3]	-	-	96%	95%
Antithrombotic Therapy Timing[1,3]	-	-	98%	98%
Assessed for Rehabilitation[1,3]	-	-	97%	97%
Discharged on Antithrombotic Therapy[1,3]	-	-	99%	99%
Discharged on Statin Medication[1,3]	-	-	95%	94%
Thrombolytic Therapy Timing[1,3]	-	-	69%	66%
Venous Thromboembolism Prophylaxis[1,3]	-	-	94%	94%
Written Stroke Educational Materials Given[1,3]	-	-	86%	88%
Surgical Care Improvement Project				
Appropriate Beta Blocker Usage[1]	-	-	97%	98%
Appropriate VTP Within 24 Hours	22	36%	98%	98%
Controlled Postoperative Blood Glucose[7]	-	-	97%	97%
Perioperative Temperature Management	24	96%	100%	100%
Prophylactic Antibiotic Selection[1]	-	-	99%	99%
Prophylactic Antibiotic Selection (Outpatient)	21	33%	97%	98%
Prophylactic Antibiotic Stopped	11	64%	98%	98%
Prophylactic Antibiotic Timing	13	62%	99%	99%
Prophylactic Antibiotic Timing (Outpatient)	21	38%	97%	98%
Urinary Catheter Removal[1]	-	-	96%	97%
Survey of Patients' Hospital Experiences				
Area Around Room 'Always' Quiet at Night	(a)	57%	51%	61%
Doctors 'Always' Communicated Well	(a)	72%	77%	82%
Home Recovery Information Given	(a)	90%	83%	85%
Hospital Given 9 or 10 on 10 Point Scale	(a)	60%	63%	71%
Meds 'Always' Explained Before Given	(a)	66%	59%	64%
Nurses 'Always' Communicated Well	(a)	75%	75%	79%
Pain 'Always' Well Controlled	(a)	63%	67%	71%
Room and Bathroom 'Always' Clean	(a)	79%	69%	73%
Timely Help 'Always' Received	(a)	67%	61%	68%
Would Definitely Recommend Hospital	(a)	62%	65%	71%
Use of Medical Imaging				
Cardiac Imaging Stress Test before Surgery[7]	-	-	5.8%	5.3%
Combination Abdominal CT Scan	233	12.9%	8.2%	10.5%
Combination Brain/Sinus CT Scan[1]	-	-	3.6%	2.7%
Combination Chest CT Scan	120	2.5%	1.3%	2.7%
Follow-up Mammogram/Ultrasound	172	9.9%	13%	8.8%
Lumbar Spine MRI for Low Back Pain[1]	-	-	33.4%	37.2%

Clifton Springs Hospital & Clinic

2 Coulter Road
Clifton Springs, NY 14432
Phone: 315-462-9561
Fax: 315-462-3492
Type: Acute Care Hospitals
Emergency Services: Yes
Ownership: Voluntary non-profit - Private
Beds: 262

Key Personnel:

CEO/President. . . . . John Galati
Operating Room. . . . . Betsy Kearney
Quality Assurance . . . . Sue Pettis
Cardiac Laboratory. . . . . Karen Pyle
Radiology. . . . . John Severins
Chief of Medical Staff. . . . . Lewis Zwich, MD

Measure	Cases	This Hosp.	State Avg.	U.S. Avg.
Blood Clot Prevention and Treatment				
Anticoagulation Overlap Therapy[2]	14	100%	91%	93%
ICU Venous Thromboembolism Prophylaxis[2]	84	89%	92%	92%
Incidence of Potentially Preventable VTE[1,2]	-	-	10%	10%
UFH with Dosages/Platelet Monitoring[1,2]	-	-	92%	97%
Venous Thromboembolism Prophylaxis[2]	253	97%	87%	85%
Warfarin Therapy Discharge Instructions[2]	12	100%	59%	75%
Chest Pain/Possible Heart Attack Care				
Aspirin Given Within 24 Hours of Arrival	29	100%	97%	96%
Fibrinolytic Meds Within 30 Min. of Arrival[1]	-	-	54%	58%
Average Time to ECG (minutes)	29	20	9	7
Average Time to Transfer (minutes)[1]	-	-	78	60
Children's Asthma Care				
Received Home Management Plan of Care	-	-	-	88%
Received Reliever Medication	-	-	-	100%
Received Systemic Corticosteroids	-	-	-	100%
Emergency Department				
Admittance Decision Time (minutes)[2]	509	83	154	98
Head CT Results Within 45 Min. of Arrival[1]	-	-	55%	57%
Patients Who Left ER Before Being Seen	10,839	2%	2%	2%
Time from ER Arrival to Admit. (minutes)[2]	510	247	378	274
Time from ER Arrival to Discharge (minutes)	270	142	156	134
Time in ER Before Being Evaluated (minutes)	391	31	35	26
Time to Pain Meds for Fractures (minutes)	30	86	61	57
Heart Attack Care				
Aspirin Given at Discharge[1]	-	-	99%	99%
Fibrinolytic Meds Within 30 Min. of Arrival[7]	-	-	46%	54%
PCI Within 90 Minutes of Arrival[7]	-	-	95%	96%
Statin Prescribed at Discharge[1]	-	-	98%	98%
Heart Failure Care				
ACE Inhibitor or ARB for LVSD[2]	14	100%	96%	97%
Discharge Instructions Given[2]	52	94%	95%	94%
Evaluation of LVS Function[2]	61	98%	99%	99%
Medicare Spending				
Medicare Spending per Patient (ratio)	-	0.85	0.96	0.98
Pneumonia Care				
Appropriate Initial Antibiotic Given[2]	56	100%	95%	95%
Blood Culture Timing[2]	90	99%	97%	98%
Pregnancy and Delivery Care				
Newborn Deliveries Scheduled Early[7]	-	-	4%	6%
Preventive Care				
Immunization for Influenza[2]	282	97%	88%	90%
Immunization for Pneumonia[2]	467	94%	88%	92%
Stroke Care				
Anticoagulation Therapy for Atrial Fibrillation[1,2]	-	-	96%	95%
Antithrombotic Therapy Timing[2]	18	100%	98%	98%
Assessed for Rehabilitation[2]	17	94%	97%	97%
Discharged on Antithrombotic Therapy[2]	17	94%	99%	99%
Discharged on Statin Medication[2]	12	92%	95%	94%
Thrombolytic Therapy Timing[1,2]	-	-	69%	66%
Venous Thromboembolism Prophylaxis[2]	18	100%	94%	94%
Written Stroke Educational Materials Given[2]	12	75%	86%	88%
Surgical Care Improvement Project				
Appropriate Beta Blocker Usage[2]	38	100%	97%	98%
Appropriate VTP Within 24 Hours[2]	52	98%	98%	98%
Controlled Postoperative Blood Glucose[2,7]	-	-	97%	97%
Perioperative Temperature Management[2]	91	100%	100%	100%
Prophylactic Antibiotic Selection[2]	51	96%	99%	99%
Prophylactic Antibiotic Selection (Outpatient)	15	100%	97%	98%
Prophylactic Antibiotic Stopped[2]	48	100%	98%	98%
Prophylactic Antibiotic Timing[2]	52	96%	99%	99%
Prophylactic Antibiotic Timing (Outpatient)	15	93%	97%	98%
Urinary Catheter Removal[2]	61	100%	96%	97%
Survey of Patients' Hospital Experiences				
Area Around Room 'Always' Quiet at Night	300+	50%	51%	61%
Doctors 'Always' Communicated Well	300+	84%	77%	82%
Home Recovery Information Given	300+	91%	83%	85%
Hospital Given 9 or 10 on 10 Point Scale	300+	74%	63%	71%
Meds 'Always' Explained Before Given	300+	61%	59%	64%
Nurses 'Always' Communicated Well	300+	78%	75%	79%
Pain 'Always' Well Controlled	300+	71%	67%	71%
Room and Bathroom 'Always' Clean	300+	65%	69%	73%
Timely Help 'Always' Received	300+	72%	61%	68%
Would Definitely Recommend Hospital	300+	82%	65%	71%
Use of Medical Imaging				
Cardiac Imaging Stress Test before Surgery	62	4.8%	5.8%	5.3%
Combination Abdominal CT Scan	246	22.4%	8.2%	10.5%
Combination Brain/Sinus CT Scan[1]	-	-	3.6%	2.7%
Combination Chest CT Scan	191	2.1%	1.3%	2.7%
Follow-up Mammogram/Ultrasound	348	8.6%	13%	8.8%
Lumbar Spine MRI for Low Back Pain[1]	-	-	33.4%	37.2%

Cobleskill Regional Hospital

178 Grandview Drive
Cobleskill, NY 12043
Phone: 518-254-3270
Fax: 518-234-4839
E-mail: customer.service@bassett.org.
URL: www.bassett.org
Type: Acute Care Hospitals
Emergency Services: Yes
Ownership: Voluntary non-profit - Private
Beds: 40

Key Personnel:

Infection Control. . . . . Irene Abbott
Radiology. . . . . Lawrence Barnowsky
President/CEO. . . . . Vance Brown
Quality Assurance . . . . Janet Gorton
Chief of Medical Staff. . . . . Bertine C McKenna, MD
Pediatric In-Patient Care . . . . Linda Rodriguez
Operating Room. . . . . Nancy Simmons-Dawley

Measure	Cases	This Hosp.	State Avg.	U.S. Avg.
Blood Clot Prevention and Treatment				
Anticoagulation Overlap Therapy[1,2]	-	-	91%	93%
ICU Venous Thromboembolism Prophylaxis[2,7]	-	-	92%	92%
Incidence of Potentially Preventable VTE[1,2]	-	-	10%	10%
UFH with Dosages/Platelet Monitoring[1,2]	-	-	92%	97%
Venous Thromboembolism Prophylaxis[2]	292	77%	87%	85%
Warfarin Therapy Discharge Instructions[1,2]	-	-	59%	75%
Chest Pain/Possible Heart Attack Care				
Aspirin Given Within 24 Hours of Arrival	11	100%	97%	96%
Fibrinolytic Meds Within 30 Min. of Arrival[5]	-	-	54%	58%
Average Time to ECG (minutes)	12	6	9	7
Average Time to Transfer (minutes)[5]	-	-	78	60
Children's Asthma Care				
Received Home Management Plan of Care	-	-	-	88%
Received Reliever Medication	-	-	-	100%
Received Systemic Corticosteroids	-	-	-	100%
Emergency Department				
Admittance Decision Time (minutes)[2]	288	112	154	98
Head CT Results Within 45 Min. of Arrival[3,7]	-	-	55%	57%
Patients Who Left ER Before Being Seen	11,189	1%	2%	2%
Time from ER Arrival to Admit. (minutes)[2]	326	293	378	274
Time from ER Arrival to Discharge (minutes)	336	118	156	134
Time in ER Before Being Evaluated (minutes)	217	37	35	26
Time to Pain Meds for Fractures (minutes)	24	71	61	57
Heart Attack Care				
Aspirin Given at Discharge[1,3]	-	-	99%	99%
Fibrinolytic Meds Within 30 Min. of Arrival[3,7]	-	-	46%	54%
PCI Within 90 Minutes of Arrival[3,7]	-	-	95%	96%
Statin Prescribed at Discharge[1,3]	-	-	98%	98%
Heart Failure Care				
ACE Inhibitor or ARB for LVSD[1]	-	-	96%	97%
Discharge Instructions Given	30	97%	95%	94%
Evaluation of LVS Function	36	100%	99%	99%
Medicare Spending				
Medicare Spending per Patient (ratio)	-	0.85	0.96	0.98
Pneumonia Care				

NOTE: Hospital profiles are in alphabetical order by state, then city, then hospital within the city; Rankings exclude hospitals with less than 25 cases except for patient surveys which excludes hospitals with less than 100 cases; (a) 100-299 cases; (1) The number of cases/patients is too few to report; (2) Data submitted were based on a sample of cases/patients; (3) Results are based on a shorter time period than required; (4) Data suppressed by CMS for one or more quarters; (5) Results are not available for this reporting period; (6) Fewer than 100 patients completed the HCAHPS survey; (7) No cases met the criteria for this measure; (8) The lower limit of the confidence interval cannot be calculated if the number of observed infections equals zero; (9) No data are available from the state/territory for this reporting period; (10) The scores shown reflect fewer than 50 completed surveys; (11) There were discrepancies in the data collection process; (12) This measure does not apply to this hospital for this reporting period; (13) Results cannot be calculated for this reporting period; (14) The results for this state are combined with nearby states to protect confidentiality; Please refer to the User's Guide for a full explanation of data.

Appropriate Initial Antibiotic Given	49	96%	95%	95%
Blood Culture Timing	52	90%	97%	98%
Pregnancy and Delivery Care				
Newborn Deliveries Scheduled Early[7]	-	-	4%	6%
Preventive Care				
Immunization for Influenza[2]	248	98%	88%	90%
Immunization for Pneumonia[2]	409	93%	88%	92%
Stroke Care				
Anticoagulation Therapy for Atrial Fibrillation[1]	-	-	96%	95%
Antithrombotic Therapy Timing[1]	-	-	98%	98%
Assessed for Rehabilitation[1]	-	-	97%	97%
Discharged on Antithrombotic Therapy[1]	-	-	99%	99%
Discharged on Statin Medication[1]	-	-	95%	94%
Thrombolytic Therapy Timing[1]	-	-	69%	66%
Venous Thromboembolism Prophylaxis[1]	-	-	94%	94%
Written Stroke Educational Materials Given[1]	-	-	86%	88%
Surgical Care Improvement Project				
Appropriate Beta Blocker Usage[5]	-	-	97%	98%
Appropriate VTP Within 24 Hours[5]	-	-	98%	98%
Controlled Postoperative Blood Glucose[5]	-	-	97%	97%
Perioperative Temperature Management[5]	-	-	100%	100%
Prophylactic Antibiotic Selection[5]	-	-	99%	99%
Prophylactic Antibiotic Selection (Outpatient)	12	100%	97%	98%
Prophylactic Antibiotic Stopped[5]	-	-	98%	98%
Prophylactic Antibiotic Timing[5]	-	-	99%	99%
Prophylactic Antibiotic Timing (Outpatient)[7]	-	-	97%	98%
Urinary Catheter Removal[5]	-	-	96%	97%
Survey of Patients' Hospital Experiences				
Area Around Room 'Always' Quiet at Night	(a)	46%	51%	61%
Doctors 'Always' Communicated Well	(a)	77%	77%	82%
Home Recovery Information Given	(a)	89%	83%	85%
Hospital Given 9 or 10 on 10 Point Scale	(a)	57%	63%	71%
Meds 'Always' Explained Before Given	(a)	60%	59%	64%
Nurses 'Always' Communicated Well	(a)	70%	75%	79%
Pain 'Always' Well Controlled	(a)	53%	67%	71%
Room and Bathroom 'Always' Clean	(a)	76%	69%	73%
Timely Help 'Always' Received	(a)	58%	61%	68%
Would Definitely Recommend Hospital	(a)	56%	65%	71%
Use of Medical Imaging				
Cardiac Imaging Stress Test before Surgery[1]	-	-	5.8%	5.3%
Combination Abdominal CT Scan	236	6.4%	8.2%	10.5%
Combination Brain/Sinus CT Scan	152	0.0%	3.6%	2.7%
Combination Chest CT Scan	175	1.7%	1.3%	2.7%
Follow-up Mammogram/Ultrasound	451	11.1%	13%	8.8%
Lumbar Spine MRI for Low Back Pain[1]	-	-	33.4%	37.2%

Mary Imogene Bassett Hospital

One Atwell Road
Cooperstown, NY 13326
Phone: 607-547-3456
Fax: 607-547-3921
Type: Acute Care Hospitals
Emergency Services: Yes
Ownership: Voluntary non-profit - Private
Beds: 180

Key Personnel:
Emergency Room . . . . Timothy J Barrett
CEO/President. . . . . William F Streck, MD

Measure	Cases	This Hosp.	State Avg.	U.S. Avg.
Blood Clot Prevention and Treatment				
Anticoagulation Overlap Therapy[2]	61	100%	91%	93%
ICU Venous Thromboembolism Prophylaxis[2]	46	98%	92%	92%
Incidence of Potentially Preventable VTE[1,2]	-	-	10%	10%
UFH with Dosages/Platelet Monitoring[2]	36	100%	92%	97%
Venous Thromboembolism Prophylaxis[2]	507	88%	87%	85%
Warfarin Therapy Discharge Instructions[2]	44	95%	59%	75%
Chest Pain/Possible Heart Attack Care				
Aspirin Given Within 24 Hours of Arrival[1,3]	-	-	97%	96%
Fibrinolytic Meds Within 30 Min. of Arrival[3,7]	-	-	54%	58%
Average Time to ECG (minutes)[1,3]	-	-	9	7
Average Time to Transfer (minutes)[3,7]	-	-	78	60
Children's Asthma Care				
Received Home Management Plan of Care	-	-	-	88%
Received Reliever Medication	-	-	-	100%
Received Systemic Corticosteroids	-	-	-	100%
Emergency Department				
Admittance Decision Time (minutes)[2]	276	174	154	98
Head CT Results Within 45 Min. of Arrival[1]	-	-	55%	57%
Patients Who Left ER Before Being Seen	18,539	1%	2%	2%
Time from ER Arrival to Admit. (minutes)[2]	511	372	378	274
Time from ER Arrival to Discharge (minutes)	515	183	156	134
Time in ER Before Being Evaluated (minutes)	265	37	35	26
Time to Pain Meds for Fractures (minutes)	27	98	61	57
Heart Attack Care				
Aspirin Given at Discharge	211	100%	99%	99%
Fibrinolytic Meds Within 30 Min. of Arrival[7]	-	-	46%	54%
PCI Within 90 Minutes of Arrival	14	71%	95%	96%
Statin Prescribed at Discharge	197	100%	98%	98%
Heart Failure Care				
ACE Inhibitor or ARB for LVSD	77	97%	96%	97%
Discharge Instructions Given	188	94%	95%	94%
Evaluation of LVS Function	219	100%	99%	99%
Medicare Spending				
Medicare Spending per Patient (ratio)	-	0.93	0.96	0.98
Pneumonia Care				
Appropriate Initial Antibiotic Given[2]	55	93%	95%	95%
Blood Culture Timing[2]	85	98%	97%	98%
Pregnancy and Delivery Care				
Newborn Deliveries Scheduled Early[2]	27	0%	4%	6%
Preventive Care				
Immunization for Influenza[2]	553	90%	88%	90%
Immunization for Pneumonia[2]	706	89%	88%	92%
Stroke Care				
Anticoagulation Therapy for Atrial Fibrillation[1]	-	-	96%	95%
Antithrombotic Therapy Timing	63	100%	98%	98%
Assessed for Rehabilitation	82	98%	97%	97%
Discharged on Antithrombotic Therapy	66	100%	99%	99%
Discharged on Statin Medication	59	97%	95%	94%
Thrombolytic Therapy Timing[1]	-	-	69%	66%
Venous Thromboembolism Prophylaxis	82	95%	94%	94%
Written Stroke Educational Materials Given	61	97%	86%	88%
Surgical Care Improvement Project				
Appropriate Beta Blocker Usage[2]	267	99%	97%	98%
Appropriate VTP Within 24 Hours[2]	402	98%	98%	98%
Controlled Postoperative Blood Glucose[2]	97	98%	97%	97%
Perioperative Temperature Management[2]	508	100%	100%	100%
Prophylactic Antibiotic Selection[2]	454	99%	99%	99%
Prophylactic Antibiotic Selection (Outpatient)	281	98%	97%	98%
Prophylactic Antibiotic Stopped[2]	450	98%	98%	98%
Prophylactic Antibiotic Timing[2]	454	98%	99%	99%
Prophylactic Antibiotic Timing (Outpatient)	231	98%	97%	98%
Urinary Catheter Removal[2]	439	97%	96%	97%
Survey of Patients' Hospital Experiences				
Area Around Room 'Always' Quiet at Night	300+	46%	51%	61%
Doctors 'Always' Communicated Well	300+	75%	77%	82%
Home Recovery Information Given	300+	88%	83%	85%
Hospital Given 9 or 10 on 10 Point Scale	300+	62%	63%	71%
Meds 'Always' Explained Before Given	300+	60%	59%	64%
Nurses 'Always' Communicated Well	300+	73%	75%	79%
Pain 'Always' Well Controlled	300+	64%	67%	71%
Room and Bathroom 'Always' Clean	300+	67%	69%	73%
Timely Help 'Always' Received	300+	57%	61%	68%
Would Definitely Recommend Hospital	300+	66%	65%	71%
Use of Medical Imaging				
Cardiac Imaging Stress Test before Surgery	548	3.3%	5.8%	5.3%
Combination Abdominal CT Scan	586	8.5%	8.2%	10.5%
Combination Brain/Sinus CT Scan[1]	-	-	3.6%	2.7%
Combination Chest CT Scan	540	1.3%	1.3%	2.7%
Follow-up Mammogram/Ultrasound	2,084	8.9%	13%	8.8%
Lumbar Spine MRI for Low Back Pain	127	40.2%	33.4%	37.2%

Corning Hospital

176 Denison Parkway East
Corning, NY 14830
Phone: 607-937-7200
URL: www.corninghospital.org
Type: Acute Care Hospitals
Emergency Services: Yes
Ownership: Voluntary non-profit - Private
Beds: 99

Key Personnel:
Anesthesiology. . . . . Tanguile Adaniel, MD, PhD
Hemotology Center . . . . Aref Agheli, MD
Emergency Room . . . . Gary Enders, MD
Chief of Medical Staff. . . . . Richard I Bennett, CPA
CEO/President. . . . . Shirley Magana
Radiology. . . . . Staci Thompson, CMPE
Chief of Medical Staff. . . . . Paul G VerValin, FACMPE

Measure	Cases	This Hosp.	State Avg.	U.S. Avg.
Blood Clot Prevention and Treatment				
Anticoagulation Overlap Therapy[2]	40	92%	91%	93%
ICU Venous Thromboembolism Prophylaxis[2]	128	84%	92%	92%
Incidence of Potentially Preventable VTE[1,2]	-	-	10%	10%
UFH with Dosages/Platelet Monitoring[1,2]	-	-	92%	97%
Venous Thromboembolism Prophylaxis[2]	460	93%	87%	85%
Warfarin Therapy Discharge Instructions[2]	32	44%	59%	75%
Chest Pain/Possible Heart Attack Care				
Aspirin Given Within 24 Hours of Arrival	93	96%	97%	96%
Fibrinolytic Meds Within 30 Min. of Arrival[1]	-	-	54%	58%
Average Time to ECG (minutes)	94	5	9	7
Average Time to Transfer (minutes)[1]	-	-	78	60
Children's Asthma Care				
Received Home Management Plan of Care	-	-	-	88%
Received Reliever Medication	-	-	-	100%
Received Systemic Corticosteroids	-	-	-	100%
Emergency Department				
Admittance Decision Time (minutes)	2,004	92	154	98
Head CT Results Within 45 Min. of Arrival[1]	-	-	55%	57%
Patients Who Left ER Before Being Seen	21,536	2%	2%	2%
Time from ER Arrival to Admit. (minutes)	2,046	254	378	274
Time from ER Arrival to Discharge (minutes)	683	148	156	134
Time in ER Before Being Evaluated (minutes)	762	23	35	26
Time to Pain Meds for Fractures (minutes)	87	45	61	57
Heart Attack Care				
Aspirin Given at Discharge	16	100%	99%	99%
Fibrinolytic Meds Within 30 Min. of Arrival[7]	-	-	46%	54%
PCI Within 90 Minutes of Arrival[7]	-	-	95%	96%
Statin Prescribed at Discharge	15	93%	98%	98%
Heart Failure Care				
ACE Inhibitor or ARB for LVSD	40	92%	96%	97%
Discharge Instructions Given	126	93%	95%	94%
Evaluation of LVS Function	186	100%	99%	99%
Medicare Spending				
Medicare Spending per Patient (ratio)	-	0.88	0.96	0.98
Pneumonia Care				
Appropriate Initial Antibiotic Given	82	98%	95%	95%
Blood Culture Timing	150	96%	97%	98%
Pregnancy and Delivery Care				
Newborn Deliveries Scheduled Early	38	5%	4%	6%
Preventive Care				
Immunization for Influenza	1,830	92%	88%	90%
Immunization for Pneumonia	2,484	96%	88%	92%
Stroke Care				
Anticoagulation Therapy for Atrial Fibrillation[1]	-	-	96%	95%
Antithrombotic Therapy Timing	49	96%	98%	98%
Assessed for Rehabilitation	64	100%	97%	97%
Discharged on Antithrombotic Therapy	62	98%	99%	99%
Discharged on Statin Medication	52	98%	95%	94%
Thrombolytic Therapy Timing	12	75%	69%	66%
Venous Thromboembolism Prophylaxis	62	95%	94%	94%
Written Stroke Educational Materials Given	44	98%	86%	88%
Surgical Care Improvement Project				
Appropriate Beta Blocker Usage	83	95%	97%	98%
Appropriate VTP Within 24 Hours	229	98%	98%	98%
Controlled Postoperative Blood Glucose[7]	-	-	97%	97%
Perioperative Temperature Management	248	100%	100%	100%
Prophylactic Antibiotic Selection	184	98%	99%	99%
Prophylactic Antibiotic Selection (Outpatient)	56	96%	97%	98%
Prophylactic Antibiotic Stopped	180	99%	98%	98%
Prophylactic Antibiotic Timing	184	100%	99%	99%
Prophylactic Antibiotic Timing (Outpatient)	58	97%	97%	98%
Urinary Catheter Removal	165	96%	96%	97%
Survey of Patients' Hospital Experiences				
Area Around Room 'Always' Quiet at Night	300+	54%	51%	61%
Doctors 'Always' Communicated Well	300+	78%	77%	82%
Home Recovery Information Given	300+	85%	83%	85%

NOTE: Hospital profiles are in alphabetical order by state, then city, then hospital within the city; Rankings exclude hospitals with less than 25 cases except for patient surveys which excludes hospitals with less than 100 cases; (a) 100-299 cases; (1) The number of cases/patients is too few to report; (2) Data submitted were based on a sample of cases/patients; (3) Results are based on a shorter time period than required; (4) Data suppressed by CMS for one or more quarters; (5) Results are not available for this reporting period; (6) Fewer than 100 patients completed the HCAHPS survey; (7) No cases met the criteria for this measure; (8) The lower limit of the confidence interval cannot be calculated if the number of observed infections equals zero; (9) No data are available from the state/territory for this reporting period; (10) The scores shown reflect fewer than 50 completed surveys; (11) There were discrepancies in the data collection process; (12) This measure does not apply to this hospital for this reporting period; (13) Results cannot be calculated for this reporting period; (14) The results for this state are combined with nearby states to protect confidentiality; Please refer to the User's Guide for a full explanation of data.

Measure	Cases	This Hosp.	State Avg.	U.S. Avg.
Hospital Given 9 or 10 on 10 Point Scale	300+	57%	63%	71%
Meds 'Always' Explained Before Given	300+	58%	59%	64%
Nurses 'Always' Communicated Well	300+	77%	75%	79%
Pain 'Always' Well Controlled	300+	67%	67%	71%
Room and Bathroom 'Always' Clean	300+	73%	69%	73%
Timely Help 'Always' Received	300+	63%	61%	68%
Would Definitely Recommend Hospital	300+	59%	65%	71%
Use of Medical Imaging				
Cardiac Imaging Stress Test before Surgery	141	3.5%	5.8%	5.3%
Combination Abdominal CT Scan	818	13.8%	8.2%	10.5%
Combination Brain/Sinus CT Scan[1]	-	-	3.6%	2.7%
Combination Chest CT Scan	504	1.0%	1.3%	2.7%
Follow-up Mammogram/Ultrasound	1,163	12.8%	13%	8.8%
Lumbar Spine MRI for Low Back Pain	102	44.1%	33.4%	37.2%

Cortland Regional Medical Center

134 Homer Avenue
Cortland, NY 13045
Phone: 607-756-3500
Fax: 607-756-3590
URL: www.cortlandhospitals.org
Type: Acute Care Hospitals
Emergency Services: Yes
Ownership: Voluntary non-profit - Private
Beds: 181

Key Personnel:
Cardiology . . . . Marc Baker, M.D.
Emergency Room . . . . Ralph Battles, MD
Pediatrics. . . . . Mohammad Djafari, M.D.
Radiology. . . . . Kirwin Gibbs, M.D.
Anesthesiology. . . . . Yuri Khibkin, M.D.
Chief of Medical Staff. . . . . Peter Martin
CEO/President. . . . . Brian Mitteer

Measure	Cases	This Hosp.	State Avg.	U.S. Avg.
Blood Clot Prevention and Treatment				
Anticoagulation Overlap Therapy[2]	54	98%	91%	93%
ICU Venous Thromboembolism Prophylaxis[2]	76	100%	92%	92%
Incidence of Potentially Preventable VTE[1,2]	-	-	10%	10%
UFH with Dosages/Platelet Monitoring[2]	29	100%	92%	97%
Venous Thromboembolism Prophylaxis[2]	328	96%	87%	85%
Warfarin Therapy Discharge Instructions[2]	45	53%	59%	75%
Chest Pain/Possible Heart Attack Care				
Aspirin Given Within 24 Hours of Arrival	82	99%	97%	96%
Fibrinolytic Meds Within 30 Min. of Arrival[1]	-	-	54%	58%
Average Time to ECG (minutes)	85	18	9	7
Average Time to Transfer (minutes)[1]	-	-	78	60
Children's Asthma Care				
Received Home Management Plan of Care	-	-	-	88%
Received Reliever Medication	-	-	-	100%
Received Systemic Corticosteroids	-	-	-	100%
Emergency Department				
Admittance Decision Time (minutes)[2]	616	186	154	98
Head CT Results Within 45 Min. of Arrival[1]	-	-	55%	57%
Patients Who Left ER Before Being Seen	22,603	1%	2%	2%
Time from ER Arrival to Admit. (minutes)[2]	617	368	378	274
Time from ER Arrival to Discharge (minutes)	353	181	156	134
Time in ER Before Being Evaluated (minutes)	457	35	35	26
Time to Pain Meds for Fractures (minutes)	91	56	61	57
Heart Attack Care				
Aspirin Given at Discharge[1]	-	-	99%	99%
Fibrinolytic Meds Within 30 Min. of Arrival[7]	-	-	46%	54%
PCI Within 90 Minutes of Arrival[7]	-	-	95%	96%
Statin Prescribed at Discharge[1]	-	-	98%	98%
Heart Failure Care				
ACE Inhibitor or ARB for LVSD	31	87%	96%	97%
Discharge Instructions Given	105	99%	95%	94%
Evaluation of LVS Function	147	100%	99%	99%
Medicare Spending				
Medicare Spending per Patient (ratio)	-	0.89	0.96	0.98
Pneumonia Care				
Appropriate Initial Antibiotic Given[2]	115	97%	95%	95%
Blood Culture Timing[2]	235	96%	97%	98%
Pregnancy and Delivery Care				
Newborn Deliveries Scheduled Early[2]	44	11%	4%	6%
Preventive Care				
Immunization for Influenza[2]	409	95%	88%	90%
Immunization for Pneumonia[2]	425	97%	88%	92%
Stroke Care				
Anticoagulation Therapy for Atrial Fibrillation[1]	-	-	96%	95%
Antithrombotic Therapy Timing[1]	-	-	98%	98%
Assessed for Rehabilitation	11	100%	97%	97%
Discharged on Antithrombotic Therapy[1]	-	-	99%	99%
Discharged on Statin Medication[1]	-	-	95%	94%
Thrombolytic Therapy Timing[1]	-	-	69%	66%
Venous Thromboembolism Prophylaxis	11	100%	94%	94%
Written Stroke Educational Materials Given[1]	-	-	86%	88%
Surgical Care Improvement Project				
Appropriate Beta Blocker Usage	15	100%	97%	98%
Appropriate VTP Within 24 Hours	54	89%	98%	98%
Controlled Postoperative Blood Glucose[7]	-	-	97%	97%
Perioperative Temperature Management	70	100%	100%	100%
Prophylactic Antibiotic Selection	39	92%	99%	99%
Prophylactic Antibiotic Selection (Outpatient)	64	95%	97%	98%
Prophylactic Antibiotic Stopped	37	95%	98%	98%
Prophylactic Antibiotic Timing	39	100%	99%	99%
Prophylactic Antibiotic Timing (Outpatient)	69	91%	97%	98%
Urinary Catheter Removal	36	89%	96%	97%
Survey of Patients' Hospital Experiences				
Area Around Room 'Always' Quiet at Night	300+	46%	51%	61%
Doctors 'Always' Communicated Well	300+	68%	77%	82%
Home Recovery Information Given	300+	83%	83%	85%
Hospital Given 9 or 10 on 10 Point Scale	300+	57%	63%	71%
Meds 'Always' Explained Before Given	300+	60%	59%	64%
Nurses 'Always' Communicated Well	300+	79%	75%	79%
Pain 'Always' Well Controlled	300+	71%	67%	71%
Room and Bathroom 'Always' Clean	300+	75%	69%	73%
Timely Help 'Always' Received	300+	57%	61%	68%
Would Definitely Recommend Hospital	300+	56%	65%	71%
Use of Medical Imaging				
Cardiac Imaging Stress Test before Surgery	300	5.3%	5.8%	5.3%
Combination Abdominal CT Scan	708	6.4%	8.2%	10.5%
Combination Brain/Sinus CT Scan	496	5.0%	3.6%	2.7%
Combination Chest CT Scan	287	3.5%	1.3%	2.7%
Follow-up Mammogram/Ultrasound	597	4.5%	13%	8.8%
Lumbar Spine MRI for Low Back Pain[1]	-	-	33.4%	37.2%

Hudson Valley Hospital Center

1980 Crompond Road
Cortlandt Manor, NY 10567
Phone: 914-734-3611
Fax: 914-736-3459
E-mail: hvhc@hvhc.org
URL: www.hvhc.org
Type: Acute Care Hospitals
Emergency Services: Yes
Ownership: Voluntary non-profit - Private
Beds: 120

Key Personnel:
Emergency Room . . . . Lindsay Aarstad, MD
Intensive Care Unit. . . . . Maria Diesta-Acbo
CEO/President. . . . . John C Federspiel
Radiology. . . . . Maurice R Poplausky
Chief of Medical Staff. . . . . Valerie Zarcone, MD

Measure	Cases	This Hosp.	State Avg.	U.S. Avg.
Blood Clot Prevention and Treatment				
Anticoagulation Overlap Therapy[2]	46	85%	91%	93%
ICU Venous Thromboembolism Prophylaxis[2]	27	93%	92%	92%
Incidence of Potentially Preventable VTE[1,2]	-	-	10%	10%
UFH with Dosages/Platelet Monitoring[2]	17	100%	92%	97%
Venous Thromboembolism Prophylaxis[2]	422	89%	87%	85%
Warfarin Therapy Discharge Instructions[2]	27	100%	59%	75%
Chest Pain/Possible Heart Attack Care				
Aspirin Given Within 24 Hours of Arrival[3]	21	100%	97%	96%
Fibrinolytic Meds Within 30 Min. of Arrival[1,3]	-	-	54%	58%
Average Time to ECG (minutes)[3]	18	6	9	7
Average Time to Transfer (minutes)[1,3]	-	-	78	60
Children's Asthma Care				
Received Home Management Plan of Care	-	-	-	88%
Received Reliever Medication	-	-	-	100%
Received Systemic Corticosteroids	-	-	-	100%
Emergency Department				
Admittance Decision Time (minutes)[2]	882	302	154	98
Head CT Results Within 45 Min. of Arrival	11	82%	55%	57%
Patients Who Left ER Before Being Seen	38,801	0%	2%	2%
Time from ER Arrival to Admit. (minutes)[2]	882	447	378	274
Time from ER Arrival to Discharge (minutes)	403	134	156	134
Time in ER Before Being Evaluated (minutes)	408	19	35	26
Time to Pain Meds for Fractures (minutes)	181	51	61	57
Heart Attack Care				
Aspirin Given at Discharge	51	100%	99%	99%
Fibrinolytic Meds Within 30 Min. of Arrival[1]	-	-	46%	54%
PCI Within 90 Minutes of Arrival[7]	-	-	95%	96%
Statin Prescribed at Discharge	46	100%	98%	98%
Heart Failure Care				
ACE Inhibitor or ARB for LVSD[2]	47	100%	96%	97%
Discharge Instructions Given[2]	182	100%	95%	94%
Evaluation of LVS Function[2]	275	100%	99%	99%
Medicare Spending				
Medicare Spending per Patient (ratio)	-	1.06	0.96	0.98
Pneumonia Care				
Appropriate Initial Antibiotic Given[2]	102	99%	95%	95%
Blood Culture Timing[2]	181	99%	97%	98%
Pregnancy and Delivery Care				
Newborn Deliveries Scheduled Early[2]	23	4%	4%	6%
Preventive Care				
Immunization for Influenza[2]	512	97%	88%	90%
Immunization for Pneumonia[2]	692	98%	88%	92%
Stroke Care				
Anticoagulation Therapy for Atrial Fibrillation	12	100%	96%	95%
Antithrombotic Therapy Timing	54	100%	98%	98%
Assessed for Rehabilitation	67	96%	97%	97%
Discharged on Antithrombotic Therapy	62	100%	99%	99%
Discharged on Statin Medication	52	98%	95%	94%
Thrombolytic Therapy Timing[1]	-	-	69%	66%
Venous Thromboembolism Prophylaxis	73	88%	94%	94%
Written Stroke Educational Materials Given	34	100%	86%	88%
Surgical Care Improvement Project				
Appropriate Beta Blocker Usage[2]	158	100%	97%	98%
Appropriate VTP Within 24 Hours[2]	396	99%	98%	98%
Controlled Postoperative Blood Glucose[2,7]	-	-	97%	97%
Perioperative Temperature Management[2]	449	100%	100%	100%
Prophylactic Antibiotic Selection[2]	281	99%	99%	99%
Prophylactic Antibiotic Selection (Outpatient)	87	98%	97%	98%
Prophylactic Antibiotic Stopped[2]	280	100%	98%	98%
Prophylactic Antibiotic Timing[2]	281	100%	99%	99%
Prophylactic Antibiotic Timing (Outpatient)	89	98%	97%	98%
Urinary Catheter Removal[2]	323	100%	96%	97%
Survey of Patients' Hospital Experiences				
Area Around Room 'Always' Quiet at Night	300+	55%	51%	61%
Doctors 'Always' Communicated Well	300+	82%	77%	82%
Home Recovery Information Given	300+	87%	83%	85%
Hospital Given 9 or 10 on 10 Point Scale	300+	73%	63%	71%
Meds 'Always' Explained Before Given	300+	67%	59%	64%
Nurses 'Always' Communicated Well	300+	81%	75%	79%
Pain 'Always' Well Controlled	300+	74%	67%	71%
Room and Bathroom 'Always' Clean	300+	77%	69%	73%
Timely Help 'Always' Received	300+	71%	61%	68%
Would Definitely Recommend Hospital	300+	75%	65%	71%
Use of Medical Imaging				
Cardiac Imaging Stress Test before Surgery	514	5.4%	5.8%	5.3%
Combination Abdominal CT Scan	683	6.4%	8.2%	10.5%
Combination Brain/Sinus CT Scan	686	1.9%	3.6%	2.7%
Combination Chest CT Scan	574	1.2%	1.3%	2.7%
Follow-up Mammogram/Ultrasound	1,155	17.2%	13%	8.8%
Lumbar Spine MRI for Low Back Pain	123	33.3%	33.4%	37.2%

Cuba Memorial Hospital

140 West Main Street
Cuba, NY 14727
Phone: 585-961-2000
Type: Critical Access Hospitals
Emergency Services: Yes
Ownership: Voluntary non-profit - Private

Measure	Cases	This Hosp.	State Avg.	U.S. Avg.
Blood Clot Prevention and Treatment				
Anticoagulation Overlap Therapy[5]	-	-	91%	93%
ICU Venous Thromboembolism Prophylaxis[5]	-	-	92%	92%
Incidence of Potentially Preventable VTE[5]	-	-	10%	10%
UFH with Dosages/Platelet Monitoring[5]	-	-	92%	97%
Venous Thromboembolism Prophylaxis[5]	-	-	87%	85%

NOTE: Hospital profiles are in alphabetical order by state, then city, then hospital within the city; Rankings exclude hospitals with less than 25 cases except for patient surveys which excludes hospitals with less than 100 cases; (a) 100-299 cases; (1) The number of cases/patients is too few to report; (2) Data submitted were based on a sample of cases/patients; (3) Results are based on a shorter time period than required; (4) Data suppressed by CMS for one or more quarters; (5) Results are not available for this reporting period; (6) Fewer than 100 patients completed the HCAHPS survey; (7) No cases met the criteria for this measure; (8) The lower limit of the confidence interval cannot be calculated if the number of observed infections equals zero; (9) No data are available from the state/territory for this reporting period; (10) The scores shown reflect fewer than 50 completed surveys; (11) There were discrepancies in the data collection process; (12) This measure does not apply to this hospital for this reporting period; (13) Results cannot be calculated for this reporting period; (14) The results for this state are combined with nearby states to protect confidentiality; Please refer to the User's Guide for a full explanation of data.

Measure	Cases	This Hosp.	State Avg.	U.S. Avg.
Warfarin Therapy Discharge Instructions[5]	-	-	59%	75%
Chest Pain/Possible Heart Attack Care				
Aspirin Given Within 24 Hours of Arrival[1,3]	-	-	97%	96%
Fibrinolytic Meds Within 30 Min. of Arrival[3,7]	-	-	54%	58%
Average Time to ECG (minutes)[1,3]	-	-	9	7
Average Time to Transfer (minutes)[3,7]	-	-	78	60
Children's Asthma Care				
Received Home Management Plan of Care	-	-	-	88%
Received Reliever Medication	-	-	-	100%
Received Systemic Corticosteroids	-	-	-	100%
Emergency Department				
Admittance Decision Time (minutes)[5]	-	-	154	98
Head CT Results Within 45 Min. of Arrival[5]	-	-	55%	57%
Patients Who Left ER Before Being Seen	4,734	0%	2%	2%
Time from ER Arrival to Admit. (minutes)[5]	-	-	378	274
Time from ER Arrival to Discharge (minutes)[5]	-	-	156	134
Time in ER Before Being Evaluated (minutes)[5]	-	-	35	26
Time to Pain Meds for Fractures (minutes)[5]	-	-	61	57
Heart Attack Care				
Aspirin Given at Discharge[5]	-	-	99%	99%
Fibrinolytic Meds Within 30 Min. of Arrival[5]	-	-	46%	54%
PCI Within 90 Minutes of Arrival[5]	-	-	95%	96%
Statin Prescribed at Discharge[5]	-	-	98%	98%
Heart Failure Care				
ACE Inhibitor or ARB for LVSD[5]	-	-	96%	97%
Discharge Instructions Given[5]	-	-	95%	94%
Evaluation of LVS Function[5]	-	-	99%	99%
Medicare Spending				
Medicare Spending per Patient (ratio)	-	-	0.96	0.98
Pneumonia Care				
Appropriate Initial Antibiotic Given	17	71%	95%	95%
Blood Culture Timing	16	100%	97%	98%
Pregnancy and Delivery Care				
Newborn Deliveries Scheduled Early[5]	-	-	4%	6%
Preventive Care				
Immunization for Influenza[5]	-	-	88%	90%
Immunization for Pneumonia[5]	-	-	88%	92%
Stroke Care				
Anticoagulation Therapy for Atrial Fibrillation[5]	-	-	96%	95%
Antithrombotic Therapy Timing[5]	-	-	98%	98%
Assessed for Rehabilitation[5]	-	-	97%	97%
Discharged on Antithrombotic Therapy[5]	-	-	99%	99%
Discharged on Statin Medication[5]	-	-	95%	94%
Thrombolytic Therapy Timing[5]	-	-	69%	66%
Venous Thromboembolism Prophylaxis[5]	-	-	94%	94%
Written Stroke Educational Materials Given[5]	-	-	86%	88%
Surgical Care Improvement Project				
Appropriate Beta Blocker Usage[5]	-	-	97%	98%
Appropriate VTP Within 24 Hours[5]	-	-	98%	98%
Controlled Postoperative Blood Glucose[5]	-	-	97%	97%
Perioperative Temperature Management[5]	-	-	100%	100%
Prophylactic Antibiotic Selection[5]	-	-	99%	99%
Prophylactic Antibiotic Selection (Outpatient)[5]	-	-	97%	98%
Prophylactic Antibiotic Stopped[5]	-	-	98%	98%
Prophylactic Antibiotic Timing[5]	-	-	99%	99%
Prophylactic Antibiotic Timing (Outpatient)[5]	-	-	97%	98%
Urinary Catheter Removal[5]	-	-	96%	97%
Survey of Patients' Hospital Experiences				
Area Around Room 'Always' Quiet at Night[5]	-	-	51%	61%
Doctors 'Always' Communicated Well[5]	-	-	77%	82%
Home Recovery Information Given[5]	-	-	83%	85%
Hospital Given 9 or 10 on 10 Point Scale[5]	-	-	63%	71%
Meds 'Always' Explained Before Given[5]	-	-	59%	64%
Nurses 'Always' Communicated Well[5]	-	-	75%	79%
Pain 'Always' Well Controlled[5]	-	-	67%	71%
Room and Bathroom 'Always' Clean[5]	-	-	69%	73%
Timely Help 'Always' Received[5]	-	-	61%	68%
Would Definitely Recommend Hospital[5]	-	-	65%	71%
Use of Medical Imaging				
Cardiac Imaging Stress Test before Surgery[7]	-	-	5.8%	5.3%
Combination Abdominal CT Scan[1]	-	-	8.2%	10.5%
Combination Brain/Sinus CT Scan[1]	-	-	3.6%	2.7%
Combination Chest CT Scan[1]	-	-	1.3%	2.7%
Follow-up Mammogram/Ultrasound[1]	-	-	13%	8.8%
Lumbar Spine MRI for Low Back Pain[7]	-	-	33.4%	37.2%

Nicholas H Noyes Memorial Hospital

111 Clara Barton Street
Dansville, NY 14437
Phone: 585-335-6001
Fax: 585-335-2769
E-mail: tingram@noyes-hospital.org
URL: www.noyes-health.org
Type: Acute Care Hospitals
Emergency Services: Yes
Ownership: Voluntary non-profit - Private
Beds: 72

Key Personnel:

Operating Room. . . . . Andree Brasser
Cardiac Laboratory. . . . . Syed Igbal, MD
Emergency Room . . . . Douglas Mayhle, MD
Radiology. . . . . Omar Qureshi
Infection Control. . . . . Mary Stewart
CEO/President. . . . . James Wissler
Chief of Medical Staff. . . . . Tony Witte, MD

Measure	Cases	This Hosp.	State Avg.	U.S. Avg.
Blood Clot Prevention and Treatment				
Anticoagulation Overlap Therapy[2]	14	93%	91%	93%
ICU Venous Thromboembolism Prophylaxis[2]	45	69%	92%	92%
Incidence of Potentially Preventable VTE[1,2]	-	-	10%	10%
UFH with Dosages/Platelet Monitoring[1,2]	-	-	92%	97%
Venous Thromboembolism Prophylaxis[2]	115	71%	87%	85%
Warfarin Therapy Discharge Instructions[2]	13	85%	59%	75%
Chest Pain/Possible Heart Attack Care				
Aspirin Given Within 24 Hours of Arrival	49	96%	97%	96%
Fibrinolytic Meds Within 30 Min. of Arrival[1]	-	-	54%	58%
Average Time to ECG (minutes)	51	4	9	7
Average Time to Transfer (minutes)[1]	-	-	78	60
Children's Asthma Care				
Received Home Management Plan of Care	-	-	-	88%
Received Reliever Medication	-	-	-	100%
Received Systemic Corticosteroids	-	-	-	100%
Emergency Department				
Admittance Decision Time (minutes)[2]	331	94	154	98
Head CT Results Within 45 Min. of Arrival[1]	-	-	55%	57%
Patients Who Left ER Before Being Seen	14,269	1%	2%	2%
Time from ER Arrival to Admit. (minutes)[2]	331	275	378	274
Time from ER Arrival to Discharge (minutes)	385	110	156	134
Time in ER Before Being Evaluated (minutes)	407	34	35	26
Time to Pain Meds for Fractures (minutes)	59	60	61	57
Heart Attack Care				
Aspirin Given at Discharge[1,3]	-	-	99%	99%
Fibrinolytic Meds Within 30 Min. of Arrival[3,7]	-	-	46%	54%
PCI Within 90 Minutes of Arrival[3,7]	-	-	95%	96%
Statin Prescribed at Discharge[1,3]	-	-	98%	98%
Heart Failure Care				
ACE Inhibitor or ARB for LVSD	12	67%	96%	97%
Discharge Instructions Given	62	79%	95%	94%
Evaluation of LVS Function	77	88%	99%	99%
Medicare Spending				
Medicare Spending per Patient (ratio)	-	0.85	0.96	0.98
Pneumonia Care				
Appropriate Initial Antibiotic Given	63	92%	95%	95%
Blood Culture Timing	64	100%	97%	98%
Pregnancy and Delivery Care				
Newborn Deliveries Scheduled Early	25	12%	4%	6%
Preventive Care				
Immunization for Influenza[2]	256	91%	88%	90%
Immunization for Pneumonia[2]	292	88%	88%	92%
Stroke Care				
Anticoagulation Therapy for Atrial Fibrillation[1]	-	-	96%	95%
Antithrombotic Therapy Timing[1]	-	-	98%	98%
Assessed for Rehabilitation	13	85%	97%	97%
Discharged on Antithrombotic Therapy[1]	-	-	99%	99%
Discharged on Statin Medication	11	64%	95%	94%
Thrombolytic Therapy Timing[1]	-	-	69%	66%
Venous Thromboembolism Prophylaxis	17	88%	94%	94%
Written Stroke Educational Materials Given[1]	-	-	86%	88%
Surgical Care Improvement Project				
Appropriate Beta Blocker Usage	53	92%	97%	98%
Appropriate VTP Within 24 Hours	144	94%	98%	98%
Controlled Postoperative Blood Glucose[7]	-	-	97%	97%
Perioperative Temperature Management	161	100%	100%	100%
Prophylactic Antibiotic Selection	91	91%	99%	99%
Prophylactic Antibiotic Selection (Outpatient)	77	94%	97%	98%
Prophylactic Antibiotic Stopped	89	99%	98%	98%
Prophylactic Antibiotic Timing	91	97%	99%	99%
Prophylactic Antibiotic Timing (Outpatient)	80	92%	97%	98%
Urinary Catheter Removal	115	95%	96%	97%
Survey of Patients' Hospital Experiences				
Area Around Room 'Always' Quiet at Night	300+	54%	51%	61%
Doctors 'Always' Communicated Well	300+	79%	77%	82%
Home Recovery Information Given	300+	86%	83%	85%
Hospital Given 9 or 10 on 10 Point Scale	300+	61%	63%	71%
Meds 'Always' Explained Before Given	300+	65%	59%	64%
Nurses 'Always' Communicated Well	300+	77%	75%	79%
Pain 'Always' Well Controlled	300+	70%	67%	71%
Room and Bathroom 'Always' Clean	300+	60%	69%	73%
Timely Help 'Always' Received	300+	69%	61%	68%
Would Definitely Recommend Hospital	300+	61%	65%	71%
Use of Medical Imaging				
Cardiac Imaging Stress Test before Surgery[1]	-	-	5.8%	5.3%
Combination Abdominal CT Scan	211	23.2%	8.2%	10.5%
Combination Brain/Sinus CT Scan[1]	-	-	3.6%	2.7%
Combination Chest CT Scan	122	9.0%	1.3%	2.7%
Follow-up Mammogram/Ultrasound	289	20.4%	13%	8.8%
Lumbar Spine MRI for Low Back Pain[7]	-	-	33.4%	37.2%

O'Connor Hospital

460 Andes Road
Delhi, NY 13753
Phone: 607-746-0300
Fax: 607-746-0347
E-mail: pvogt@catskill.net
URL: www.oconnorhospital.org
Type: Critical Access Hospitals
Emergency Services: Yes
Ownership: Voluntary non-profit - Private
Beds: 28

Key Personnel:

Chief of Medical Staff. . . . . George Block
CEO . . . . James "Jim" F. Dover, FACHE
Radiology. . . . . Richard Kaplan
Quality Assurance . . . . Jean Krzyston
Operating Room. . . . . Betsy Morales

Measure	Cases	This Hosp.	State Avg.	U.S. Avg.
Blood Clot Prevention and Treatment				
Anticoagulation Overlap Therapy[5]	-	-	91%	93%
ICU Venous Thromboembolism Prophylaxis[5]	-	-	92%	92%
Incidence of Potentially Preventable VTE[5]	-	-	10%	10%
UFH with Dosages/Platelet Monitoring[5]	-	-	92%	97%
Venous Thromboembolism Prophylaxis[5]	-	-	87%	85%
Warfarin Therapy Discharge Instructions[5]	-	-	59%	75%
Chest Pain/Possible Heart Attack Care				
Aspirin Given Within 24 Hours of Arrival[1,3]	-	-	97%	96%
Fibrinolytic Meds Within 30 Min. of Arrival[5]	-	-	54%	58%
Average Time to ECG (minutes)[1,3]	-	-	9	7
Average Time to Transfer (minutes)[5]	-	-	78	60
Children's Asthma Care				
Received Home Management Plan of Care	-	-	-	88%
Received Reliever Medication	-	-	-	100%
Received Systemic Corticosteroids	-	-	-	100%
Emergency Department				
Admittance Decision Time (minutes)[5]	-	-	154	98
Head CT Results Within 45 Min. of Arrival[1,3]	-	-	55%	57%
Patients Who Left ER Before Being Seen	6,402	0%	2%	2%
Time from ER Arrival to Admit. (minutes)[5]	-	-	378	274
Time from ER Arrival to Discharge (minutes)[5]	-	-	156	134
Time in ER Before Being Evaluated (minutes)[5]	-	-	35	26
Time to Pain Meds for Fractures (minutes)[5]	-	-	61	57
Heart Attack Care				
Aspirin Given at Discharge[5]	-	-	99%	99%
Fibrinolytic Meds Within 30 Min. of Arrival[5]	-	-	46%	54%
PCI Within 90 Minutes of Arrival[5]	-	-	95%	96%
Statin Prescribed at Discharge[5]	-	-	98%	98%
Heart Failure Care				
ACE Inhibitor or ARB for LVSD[1]	-	-	96%	97%
Discharge Instructions Given[1]	-	-	95%	94%

NOTE: Hospital profiles are in alphabetical order by state, then city, then hospital within the city; Rankings exclude hospitals with less than 25 cases except for patient surveys which excludes hospitals with less than 100 cases; (a) 100-299 cases; (1) The number of cases/patients is too few to report; (2) Data submitted were based on a sample of cases/patients; (3) Results are based on a shorter time period than required; (4) Data suppressed by CMS for one or more quarters; (5) Results are not available for this reporting period; (6) Fewer than 100 patients completed the HCAHPS survey; (7) No cases met the criteria for this measure; (8) The lower limit of the confidence interval cannot be calculated if the number of observed infections equals zero; (9) No data are available from the state/territory for this reporting period; (10) The scores shown reflect fewer than 50 completed surveys; (11) There were discrepancies in the data collection process; (12) This measure does not apply to this hospital for this reporting period; (13) Results cannot be calculated for this reporting period; (14) The results for this state are combined with nearby states to protect confidentiality; Please refer to the User's Guide for a full explanation of data.

Evaluation of LVS Function[1]	-	-	99%	99%
Medicare Spending				
Medicare Spending per Patient (ratio)	-	-	0.96	0.98
Pneumonia Care				
Appropriate Initial Antibiotic Given[1,2]	-	-	95%	95%
Blood Culture Timing[1,2]	-	-	97%	98%
Pregnancy and Delivery Care				
Newborn Deliveries Scheduled Early[5]	-	-	4%	6%
Preventive Care				
Immunization for Influenza[5]	-	-	88%	90%
Immunization for Pneumonia[5]	-	-	88%	92%
Stroke Care				
Anticoagulation Therapy for Atrial Fibrillation[5]	-	-	96%	95%
Antithrombotic Therapy Timing[5]	-	-	98%	98%
Assessed for Rehabilitation[5]	-	-	97%	97%
Discharged on Antithrombotic Therapy[5]	-	-	99%	99%
Discharged on Statin Medication[5]	-	-	95%	94%
Thrombolytic Therapy Timing[5]	-	-	69%	66%
Venous Thromboembolism Prophylaxis[5]	-	-	94%	94%
Written Stroke Educational Materials Given[5]	-	-	86%	88%
Surgical Care Improvement Project				
Appropriate Beta Blocker Usage[5]	-	-	97%	98%
Appropriate VTP Within 24 Hours[5]	-	-	98%	98%
Controlled Postoperative Blood Glucose[5]	-	-	97%	97%
Perioperative Temperature Management[5]	-	-	100%	100%
Prophylactic Antibiotic Selection[5]	-	-	99%	99%
Prophylactic Antibiotic Selection (Outpatient)[1,3]	-	-	97%	98%
Prophylactic Antibiotic Stopped[5]	-	-	98%	98%
Prophylactic Antibiotic Timing[5]	-	-	99%	99%
Prophylactic Antibiotic Timing (Outpatient)[3,7]	-	-	97%	98%
Urinary Catheter Removal[5]	-	-	96%	97%
Survey of Patients' Hospital Experiences				
Area Around Room 'Always' Quiet at Night[6]	<100	61%	51%	61%
Doctors 'Always' Communicated Well[6]	<100	82%	77%	82%
Home Recovery Information Given[6]	<100	94%	83%	85%
Hospital Given 9 or 10 on 10 Point Scale[6]	<100	87%	63%	71%
Meds 'Always' Explained Before Given[6]	<100	72%	59%	64%
Nurses 'Always' Communicated Well[6]	<100	88%	75%	79%
Pain 'Always' Well Controlled[6]	<100	81%	67%	71%
Room and Bathroom 'Always' Clean[6]	<100	92%	69%	73%
Timely Help 'Always' Received[6]	<100	90%	61%	68%
Would Definitely Recommend Hospital[6]	<100	86%	65%	71%
Use of Medical Imaging				
Cardiac Imaging Stress Test before Surgery[7]	-	-	5.8%	5.3%
Combination Abdominal CT Scan	127	5.5%	8.2%	10.5%
Combination Brain/Sinus CT Scan[1]	-	-	3.6%	2.7%
Combination Chest CT Scan	95	0.0%	1.3%	2.7%
Follow-up Mammogram/Ultrasound	259	6.9%	13%	8.8%
Lumbar Spine MRI for Low Back Pain[1]	-	-	33.4%	37.2%

Brooks Memorial Hospital

529 Central Avenue
Dunkirk, NY 14048
Phone: 716-366-1111
Fax: 716-363-7288
URL: www.brookshospital.org
Type: Acute Care Hospitals
Emergency Services: Yes
Ownership: Voluntary non-profit - Private
Beds: 99

Key Personnel:

Chief of Medical Staff. . . . . G Jay Bishop, MD
Intensive Care Unit. . . . . Karen Hurlacher
CEO/President. . . . . Richard H Ketcham
Quality Assurance . . . . Teresa Larson
Infection Control. . . . . Susan Lis, RN
Radiology. . . . . Sharon Muntz
Operating Room. . . . . Sallie Piazza, RN
Emergency Room . . . . John Radford, MD

Measure	Cases	This Hosp.	State Avg.	U.S. Avg.
Blood Clot Prevention and Treatment				
Anticoagulation Overlap Therapy[2]	11	100%	91%	93%
ICU Venous Thromboembolism Prophylaxis[2]	40	95%	92%	92%
Incidence of Potentially Preventable VTE[1,2]	-	-	10%	10%
UFH with Dosages/Platelet Monitoring[1,2]	-	-	92%	97%
Venous Thromboembolism Prophylaxis[2]	199	81%	87%	85%
Warfarin Therapy Discharge Instructions[1,2]	-	-	59%	75%
Chest Pain/Possible Heart Attack Care				
Aspirin Given Within 24 Hours of Arrival	81	96%	97%	96%
Fibrinolytic Meds Within 30 Min. of Arrival[1]	-	-	54%	58%
Average Time to ECG (minutes)	78	12	9	7
Average Time to Transfer (minutes)[1]	-	-	78	60
Children's Asthma Care				
Received Home Management Plan of Care	-	-	-	88%
Received Reliever Medication	-	-	-	100%
Received Systemic Corticosteroids	-	-	-	100%
Emergency Department				
Admittance Decision Time (minutes)[2]	297	50	154	98
Head CT Results Within 45 Min. of Arrival	20	50%	55%	57%
Patients Who Left ER Before Being Seen	21,011	1%	2%	2%
Time from ER Arrival to Admit. (minutes)[2]	301	261	378	274
Time from ER Arrival to Discharge (minutes)	373	130	156	134
Time in ER Before Being Evaluated (minutes)	406	52	35	26
Time to Pain Meds for Fractures (minutes)	74	77	61	57
Heart Attack Care				
Aspirin Given at Discharge[1]	-	-	99%	99%
Fibrinolytic Meds Within 30 Min. of Arrival[7]	-	-	46%	54%
PCI Within 90 Minutes of Arrival[7]	-	-	95%	96%
Statin Prescribed at Discharge[1]	-	-	98%	98%
Heart Failure Care				
ACE Inhibitor or ARB for LVSD	32	100%	96%	97%
Discharge Instructions Given	83	94%	95%	94%
Evaluation of LVS Function	128	97%	99%	99%
Medicare Spending				
Medicare Spending per Patient (ratio)	-	0.95	0.96	0.98
Pneumonia Care				
Appropriate Initial Antibiotic Given	33	100%	95%	95%
Blood Culture Timing	96	95%	97%	98%
Pregnancy and Delivery Care				
Newborn Deliveries Scheduled Early[2]	56	9%	4%	6%
Preventive Care				
Immunization for Influenza[2]	260	85%	88%	90%
Immunization for Pneumonia[2]	301	87%	88%	92%
Stroke Care				
Anticoagulation Therapy for Atrial Fibrillation[1]	-	-	96%	95%
Antithrombotic Therapy Timing[1]	-	-	98%	98%
Assessed for Rehabilitation	11	100%	97%	97%
Discharged on Antithrombotic Therapy[1]	-	-	99%	99%
Discharged on Statin Medication[1]	-	-	95%	94%
Thrombolytic Therapy Timing[1]	-	-	69%	66%
Venous Thromboembolism Prophylaxis	11	100%	94%	94%
Written Stroke Educational Materials Given[1]	-	-	86%	88%
Surgical Care Improvement Project				
Appropriate Beta Blocker Usage[2]	85	96%	97%	98%
Appropriate VTP Within 24 Hours[2]	247	100%	98%	98%
Controlled Postoperative Blood Glucose[2,7]	-	-	97%	97%
Perioperative Temperature Management[2]	306	99%	100%	100%
Prophylactic Antibiotic Selection[2]	262	100%	99%	99%
Prophylactic Antibiotic Selection (Outpatient)	29	93%	97%	98%
Prophylactic Antibiotic Stopped[2]	260	98%	98%	98%
Prophylactic Antibiotic Timing[2]	262	99%	99%	99%
Prophylactic Antibiotic Timing (Outpatient)	30	97%	97%	98%
Urinary Catheter Removal[2]	214	96%	96%	97%
Survey of Patients' Hospital Experiences				
Area Around Room 'Always' Quiet at Night	300+	50%	51%	61%
Doctors 'Always' Communicated Well	300+	80%	77%	82%
Home Recovery Information Given	300+	88%	83%	85%
Hospital Given 9 or 10 on 10 Point Scale	300+	60%	63%	71%
Meds 'Always' Explained Before Given	300+	60%	59%	64%
Nurses 'Always' Communicated Well	300+	74%	75%	79%
Pain 'Always' Well Controlled	300+	69%	67%	71%
Room and Bathroom 'Always' Clean	300+	72%	69%	73%
Timely Help 'Always' Received	300+	59%	61%	68%
Would Definitely Recommend Hospital	300+	58%	65%	71%
Use of Medical Imaging				
Cardiac Imaging Stress Test before Surgery[1]	-	-	5.8%	5.3%
Combination Abdominal CT Scan	292	18.2%	8.2%	10.5%
Combination Brain/Sinus CT Scan[1]	-	-	3.6%	2.7%
Combination Chest CT Scan	72	15.3%	1.3%	2.7%
Follow-up Mammogram/Ultrasound	513	5.3%	13%	8.8%
Lumbar Spine MRI for Low Back Pain	40	52.5%	33.4%	37.2%

Nassau University Medical Center

2201 Hempstead Turnpike
East Meadow, NY 11554
Phone: 516-572-0123
Fax: 516-572-5792
URL: www.numc.edu
Type: Acute Care Hospitals
Emergency Services: Yes
Ownership: Government - State
Beds: 1,500

Key Personnel:

Operating Room. . . . . LD George Angus, MD
Radiology. . . . . Paul Moh, MD
CEO/President. . . . . Victor F. Politi, MD, FACP, FACEP
Infection Control. . . . . Joanne Selva, MD
Quality Assurance . . . . Maureen P Shannon, RN MHA
Pediatric In-Patient Care . . . . Bella Silecchia, MD
Chief of Medical Staff. . . . . Steven J Walerstein, MD

Measure	Cases	This Hosp.	State Avg.	U.S. Avg.
Blood Clot Prevention and Treatment				
Anticoagulation Overlap Therapy[2]	52	88%	91%	93%
ICU Venous Thromboembolism Prophylaxis[2]	51	96%	92%	92%
Incidence of Potentially Preventable VTE[2]	28	7%	10%	10%
UFH with Dosages/Platelet Monitoring[2]	34	100%	92%	97%
Venous Thromboembolism Prophylaxis[2]	229	94%	87%	85%
Warfarin Therapy Discharge Instructions[2]	30	73%	59%	75%
Chest Pain/Possible Heart Attack Care				
Aspirin Given Within 24 Hours of Arrival	74	100%	97%	96%
Fibrinolytic Meds Within 30 Min. of Arrival[7]	-	-	54%	58%
Average Time to ECG (minutes)	80	17	9	7
Average Time to Transfer (minutes)[7]	-	-	78	60
Children's Asthma Care				
Received Home Management Plan of Care	-	-	-	88%
Received Reliever Medication	-	-	-	100%
Received Systemic Corticosteroids	-	-	-	100%
Emergency Department				
Admittance Decision Time (minutes)[2]	513	142	154	98
Head CT Results Within 45 Min. of Arrival	25	36%	55%	57%
Patients Who Left ER Before Being Seen	70,752	0%	2%	2%
Time from ER Arrival to Admit. (minutes)[2]	513	334	378	274
Time from ER Arrival to Discharge (minutes)	314	143	156	134
Time in ER Before Being Evaluated (minutes)	400	49	35	26
Time to Pain Meds for Fractures (minutes)	123	82	61	57
Heart Attack Care				
Aspirin Given at Discharge	27	100%	99%	99%
Fibrinolytic Meds Within 30 Min. of Arrival[7]	-	-	46%	54%
PCI Within 90 Minutes of Arrival[7]	-	-	95%	96%
Statin Prescribed at Discharge	23	100%	98%	98%
Heart Failure Care				
ACE Inhibitor or ARB for LVSD	78	100%	96%	97%
Discharge Instructions Given	149	99%	95%	94%
Evaluation of LVS Function	198	100%	99%	99%
Medicare Spending				
Medicare Spending per Patient (ratio)	-	1.03	0.96	0.98
Pneumonia Care				
Appropriate Initial Antibiotic Given[2]	56	100%	95%	95%
Blood Culture Timing[2]	118	91%	97%	98%
Pregnancy and Delivery Care				
Newborn Deliveries Scheduled Early[2]	31	3%	4%	6%
Preventive Care				
Immunization for Influenza[2]	540	97%	88%	90%
Immunization for Pneumonia[2]	417	88%	88%	92%
Stroke Care				
Anticoagulation Therapy for Atrial Fibrillation[2]	13	100%	96%	95%
Antithrombotic Therapy Timing[2]	81	100%	98%	98%
Assessed for Rehabilitation[2]	99	98%	97%	97%
Discharged on Antithrombotic Therapy[2]	79	99%	99%	99%
Discharged on Statin Medication[2]	63	98%	95%	94%
Thrombolytic Therapy Timing[2]	15	47%	69%	66%
Venous Thromboembolism Prophylaxis[2]	118	98%	94%	94%
Written Stroke Educational Materials Given[2]	49	96%	86%	88%
Surgical Care Improvement Project				
Appropriate Beta Blocker Usage[2]	50	94%	97%	98%
Appropriate VTP Within 24 Hours[2]	219	100%	98%	98%
Controlled Postoperative Blood Glucose[2,7]	-	-	97%	97%
Perioperative Temperature Management[2]	260	100%	100%	100%

NOTE: Hospital profiles are in alphabetical order by state, then city, then hospital within the city; Rankings exclude hospitals with less than 25 cases except for patient surveys which excludes hospitals with less than 100 cases; (a) 100-299 cases; (1) The number of cases/patients is too few to report; (2) Data submitted were based on a sample of cases/patients; (3) Results are based on a shorter time period than required; (4) Data suppressed by CMS for one or more quarters; (5) Results are not available for this reporting period; (6) Fewer than 100 patients completed the HCAHPS survey; (7) No cases met the criteria for this measure; (8) The lower limit of the confidence interval cannot be calculated if the number of observed infections equals zero; (9) No data are available from the state/territory for this reporting period; (10) The scores shown reflect fewer than 50 completed surveys; (11) There were discrepancies in the data collection process; (12) This measure does not apply to this hospital for this reporting period; (13) Results cannot be calculated for this reporting period; (14) The results for this state are combined with nearby states to protect confidentiality; Please refer to the User's Guide for a full explanation of data.

Measure	Cases	This Hosp.	State Avg.	U.S. Avg.
Prophylactic Antibiotic Selection[2]	146	98%	99%	99%
Prophylactic Antibiotic Selection (Outpatient)	38	95%	97%	98%
Prophylactic Antibiotic Stopped[2]	141	99%	98%	98%
Prophylactic Antibiotic Timing[2]	146	100%	99%	99%
Prophylactic Antibiotic Timing (Outpatient)	30	87%	97%	98%
Urinary Catheter Removal[2]	97	100%	96%	97%
Survey of Patients' Hospital Experiences				
Area Around Room 'Always' Quiet at Night	300+	39%	51%	61%
Doctors 'Always' Communicated Well	300+	62%	77%	82%
Home Recovery Information Given	300+	71%	83%	85%
Hospital Given 9 or 10 on 10 Point Scale	300+	38%	63%	71%
Meds 'Always' Explained Before Given	300+	45%	59%	64%
Nurses 'Always' Communicated Well	300+	57%	75%	79%
Pain 'Always' Well Controlled	300+	51%	67%	71%
Room and Bathroom 'Always' Clean	300+	59%	69%	73%
Timely Help 'Always' Received	300+	39%	61%	68%
Would Definitely Recommend Hospital	300+	39%	65%	71%
Use of Medical Imaging				
Cardiac Imaging Stress Test before Surgery[1]	-	-	5.8%	5.3%
Combination Abdominal CT Scan	128	5.5%	8.2%	10.5%
Combination Brain/Sinus CT Scan	264	17.0%	3.6%	2.7%
Combination Chest CT Scan	58	1.7%	1.3%	2.7%
Follow-up Mammogram/Ultrasound	295	11.2%	13%	8.8%
Lumbar Spine MRI for Low Back Pain[1]	-	-	33.4%	37.2%

Elizabethtown Community Hospital

75 Park Street
Elizabethtown, NY 12932
Phone: 518-873-6377
Fax: 518-873-2005
URL: www.ech.org
Type: Critical Access Hospitals
Emergency Services: Yes
Ownership: Voluntary non-profit - Private
Beds: 25

Key Personnel:
CEO/President. . . . . Rod Boula
Emergency Room . . . . Rob DeMuro, MD

Measure	Cases	This Hosp.	State Avg.	U.S. Avg.
Blood Clot Prevention and Treatment				
Anticoagulation Overlap Therapy[5]	-	-	91%	93%
ICU Venous Thromboembolism Prophylaxis[5]	-	-	92%	92%
Incidence of Potentially Preventable VTE[5]	-	-	10%	10%
UFH with Dosages/Platelet Monitoring[5]	-	-	92%	97%
Venous Thromboembolism Prophylaxis[5]	-	-	87%	85%
Warfarin Therapy Discharge Instructions[5]	-	-	59%	75%
Chest Pain/Possible Heart Attack Care				
Aspirin Given Within 24 Hours of Arrival	18	100%	97%	96%
Fibrinolytic Meds Within 30 Min. of Arrival[1]	-	-	54%	58%
Average Time to ECG (minutes)	18	6	9	7
Average Time to Transfer (minutes)[7]	-	-	78	60
Children's Asthma Care				
Received Home Management Plan of Care	-	-	-	88%
Received Reliever Medication	-	-	-	100%
Received Systemic Corticosteroids	-	-	-	100%
Emergency Department				
Admittance Decision Time (minutes)[2,3]	22	10	154	98
Head CT Results Within 45 Min. of Arrival[1,3]	-	-	55%	57%
Patients Who Left ER Before Being Seen	5,203	0%	2%	2%
Time from ER Arrival to Admit. (minutes)[2,3]	31	210	378	274
Time from ER Arrival to Discharge (minutes)[3]	160	75	156	134
Time in ER Before Being Evaluated (minutes)[3]	166	10	35	26
Time to Pain Meds for Fractures (minutes)[5]	-	-	61	57
Heart Attack Care				
Aspirin Given at Discharge[5]	-	-	99%	99%
Fibrinolytic Meds Within 30 Min. of Arrival[5]	-	-	46%	54%
PCI Within 90 Minutes of Arrival[5]	-	-	95%	96%
Statin Prescribed at Discharge[5]	-	-	98%	98%
Heart Failure Care				
ACE Inhibitor or ARB for LVSD[1]	-	-	96%	97%
Discharge Instructions Given[1]	-	-	95%	94%
Evaluation of LVS Function	11	82%	99%	99%
Medicare Spending				
Medicare Spending per Patient (ratio)	-	-	0.96	0.98
Pneumonia Care				
Appropriate Initial Antibiotic Given	30	97%	95%	95%
Blood Culture Timing	31	100%	97%	98%
Pregnancy and Delivery Care				
Newborn Deliveries Scheduled Early[5]	-	-	4%	6%
Preventive Care				
Immunization for Influenza[5]	-	-	88%	90%
Immunization for Pneumonia[5]	-	-	88%	92%
Stroke Care				
Anticoagulation Therapy for Atrial Fibrillation[5]	-	-	96%	95%
Antithrombotic Therapy Timing[5]	-	-	98%	98%
Assessed for Rehabilitation[5]	-	-	97%	97%
Discharged on Antithrombotic Therapy[5]	-	-	99%	99%
Discharged on Statin Medication[5]	-	-	95%	94%
Thrombolytic Therapy Timing[5]	-	-	69%	66%
Venous Thromboembolism Prophylaxis[5]	-	-	94%	94%
Written Stroke Educational Materials Given[5]	-	-	86%	88%
Surgical Care Improvement Project				
Appropriate Beta Blocker Usage[5]	-	-	97%	98%
Appropriate VTP Within 24 Hours[5]	-	-	98%	98%
Controlled Postoperative Blood Glucose[5]	-	-	97%	97%
Perioperative Temperature Management[5]	-	-	100%	100%
Prophylactic Antibiotic Selection[5]	-	-	99%	99%
Prophylactic Antibiotic Selection (Outpatient)[5]	-	-	97%	98%
Prophylactic Antibiotic Stopped[5]	-	-	98%	98%
Prophylactic Antibiotic Timing[5]	-	-	99%	99%
Prophylactic Antibiotic Timing (Outpatient)[5]	-	-	97%	98%
Urinary Catheter Removal[5]	-	-	96%	97%
Survey of Patients' Hospital Experiences				
Area Around Room 'Always' Quiet at Night[6]	<100	67%	51%	61%
Doctors 'Always' Communicated Well[6]	<100	89%	77%	82%
Home Recovery Information Given[6]	<100	84%	83%	85%
Hospital Given 9 or 10 on 10 Point Scale[6]	<100	75%	63%	71%
Meds 'Always' Explained Before Given[6]	<100	71%	59%	64%
Nurses 'Always' Communicated Well[6]	<100	88%	75%	79%
Pain 'Always' Well Controlled[6]	<100	67%	67%	71%
Room and Bathroom 'Always' Clean[6]	<100	64%	69%	73%
Timely Help 'Always' Received[6]	<100	77%	61%	68%
Would Definitely Recommend Hospital[6]	<100	76%	65%	71%
Use of Medical Imaging				
Cardiac Imaging Stress Test before Surgery[7]	-	-	5.8%	5.3%
Combination Abdominal CT Scan	130	5.4%	8.2%	10.5%
Combination Brain/Sinus CT Scan	138	0.7%	3.6%	2.7%
Combination Chest CT Scan	122	0.0%	1.3%	2.7%
Follow-up Mammogram/Ultrasound	272	11.4%	13%	8.8%
Lumbar Spine MRI for Low Back Pain[1]	-	-	33.4%	37.2%

Ellenville Regional Hospital

10 Healthy Way
Ellenville, NY 12428
Phone: 845-647-6400
Fax: 845-647-6450
URL: www.ellenvilleregional.org
Type: Critical Access Hospitals
Emergency Services: Yes
Ownership: Voluntary non-profit - Private
Beds: 35

Key Personnel:
Hemotology Center . . . . Eva Edwards, RN
Infection Control. . . . . Kathy Guido
Pediatric Ambulatory Care . . . . . . Kathy Guido
Quality Assurance . . . . Kathy Guido
Chief of Medical Staff. . . . . Charles Johnson
President/CEO. . . . . Steven L. Kelly, FACHE
Patient Relations . . . . Cecelia Krom
Emergency Room . . . . Cathy Quinn, RN

Measure	Cases	This Hosp.	State Avg.	U.S. Avg.
Blood Clot Prevention and Treatment				
Anticoagulation Overlap Therapy[5]	-	-	91%	93%
ICU Venous Thromboembolism Prophylaxis[5]	-	-	92%	92%
Incidence of Potentially Preventable VTE[5]	-	-	10%	10%
UFH with Dosages/Platelet Monitoring[5]	-	-	92%	97%
Venous Thromboembolism Prophylaxis[5]	-	-	87%	85%
Warfarin Therapy Discharge Instructions[5]	-	-	59%	75%
Chest Pain/Possible Heart Attack Care				
Aspirin Given Within 24 Hours of Arrival	51	96%	97%	96%
Fibrinolytic Meds Within 30 Min. of Arrival[1]	-	-	54%	58%
Average Time to ECG (minutes)	57	23	9	7
Average Time to Transfer (minutes)[1]	-	-	78	60
Children's Asthma Care				
Received Home Management Plan of Care	-	-	-	88%
Received Reliever Medication	-	-	-	100%
Received Systemic Corticosteroids	-	-	-	100%
Emergency Department				
Admittance Decision Time (minutes)[5]	-	-	154	98
Head CT Results Within 45 Min. of Arrival[1]	-	-	55%	57%
Patients Who Left ER Before Being Seen	13,022	1%	2%	2%
Time from ER Arrival to Admit. (minutes)[5]	-	-	378	274
Time from ER Arrival to Discharge (minutes)	348	80	156	134
Time in ER Before Being Evaluated (minutes)	376	14	35	26
Time to Pain Meds for Fractures (minutes)	62	43	61	57
Heart Attack Care				
Aspirin Given at Discharge[5]	-	-	99%	99%
Fibrinolytic Meds Within 30 Min. of Arrival[5]	-	-	46%	54%
PCI Within 90 Minutes of Arrival[5]	-	-	95%	96%
Statin Prescribed at Discharge[5]	-	-	98%	98%
Heart Failure Care				
ACE Inhibitor or ARB for LVSD[1]	-	-	96%	97%
Discharge Instructions Given	16	100%	95%	94%
Evaluation of LVS Function	16	100%	99%	99%
Medicare Spending				
Medicare Spending per Patient (ratio)	-	-	0.96	0.98
Pneumonia Care				
Appropriate Initial Antibiotic Given	25	92%	95%	95%
Blood Culture Timing	26	96%	97%	98%
Pregnancy and Delivery Care				
Newborn Deliveries Scheduled Early[5]	-	-	4%	6%
Preventive Care				
Immunization for Influenza[5]	-	-	88%	90%
Immunization for Pneumonia[5]	-	-	88%	92%
Stroke Care				
Anticoagulation Therapy for Atrial Fibrillation[5]	-	-	96%	95%
Antithrombotic Therapy Timing[5]	-	-	98%	98%
Assessed for Rehabilitation[5]	-	-	97%	97%
Discharged on Antithrombotic Therapy[5]	-	-	99%	99%
Discharged on Statin Medication[5]	-	-	95%	94%
Thrombolytic Therapy Timing[5]	-	-	69%	66%
Venous Thromboembolism Prophylaxis[5]	-	-	94%	94%
Written Stroke Educational Materials Given[5]	-	-	86%	88%
Surgical Care Improvement Project				
Appropriate Beta Blocker Usage[5]	-	-	97%	98%
Appropriate VTP Within 24 Hours[5]	-	-	98%	98%
Controlled Postoperative Blood Glucose[5]	-	-	97%	97%
Perioperative Temperature Management[5]	-	-	100%	100%
Prophylactic Antibiotic Selection[5]	-	-	99%	99%
Prophylactic Antibiotic Selection (Outpatient)[1,3]	-	-	97%	98%
Prophylactic Antibiotic Stopped[5]	-	-	98%	98%
Prophylactic Antibiotic Timing[5]	-	-	99%	99%
Prophylactic Antibiotic Timing (Outpatient)[1,3]	-	-	97%	98%
Urinary Catheter Removal[5]	-	-	96%	97%
Survey of Patients' Hospital Experiences				
Area Around Room 'Always' Quiet at Night	(a)	58%	51%	61%
Doctors 'Always' Communicated Well	(a)	79%	77%	82%
Home Recovery Information Given	(a)	81%	83%	85%
Hospital Given 9 or 10 on 10 Point Scale	(a)	67%	63%	71%
Meds 'Always' Explained Before Given	(a)	70%	59%	64%
Nurses 'Always' Communicated Well	(a)	80%	75%	79%
Pain 'Always' Well Controlled	(a)	69%	67%	71%
Room and Bathroom 'Always' Clean	(a)	74%	69%	73%
Timely Help 'Always' Received	(a)	73%	61%	68%
Would Definitely Recommend Hospital	(a)	71%	65%	71%
Use of Medical Imaging				
Cardiac Imaging Stress Test before Surgery[1]	-	-	5.8%	5.3%
Combination Abdominal CT Scan	181	4.4%	8.2%	10.5%
Combination Brain/Sinus CT Scan[1]	-	-	3.6%	2.7%
Combination Chest CT Scan	81	0.0%	1.3%	2.7%
Follow-up Mammogram/Ultrasound	116	9.5%	13%	8.8%
Lumbar Spine MRI for Low Back Pain[1]	-	-	33.4%	37.2%

NOTE: Hospital profiles are in alphabetical order by state, then city, then hospital within the city; Rankings exclude hospitals with less than 25 cases except for patient surveys which excludes hospitals with less than 100 cases; (a) 100-299 cases; (1) The number of cases/patients is too few to report; (2) Data submitted were based on a sample of cases/patients; (3) Results are based on a shorter time period than required; (4) Data suppressed by CMS for one or more quarters; (5) Results are not available for this reporting period; (6) Fewer than 100 patients completed the HCAHPS survey; (7) No cases met the criteria for this measure; (8) The lower limit of the confidence interval cannot be calculated if the number of observed infections equals zero; (9) No data are available from the state/territory for this reporting period; (10) The scores shown reflect fewer than 50 completed surveys; (11) There were discrepancies in the data collection process; (12) This measure does not apply to this hospital for this reporting period; (13) Results cannot be calculated for this reporting period; (14) The results for this state are combined with nearby states to protect confidentiality; Please refer to the User's Guide for a full explanation of data.

Elmhurst Hospital Center

79-01 Broadway
Elmhurst, NY 11373
URL: www.nyc.gov
Type: Acute Care Hospitals
Ownership: Government - Local
Phone: 718-334-1141
Fax: 718-334-1810
Emergency Services: Yes
Beds: 525

Key Personnel:
Anesthesiology. . . . . Kenneth Abrams, MD
Quality Assurance . . . . Beverly Carroll
Pediatric Ambulatory Care . . . . . . Melvin Gertner, MD
Pediatric In-Patient Care . . . . Melvin Gertner, MD
Intensive Care Unit. . . . . JoAnn Gull, RN
Radiology. . . . . David Hayt, MD
Emergency Room . . . . Stuart Kessler, MD
Operating Room. . . . . Anne McGann, RN

Measure	Cases	This Hosp.	State Avg.	U.S. Avg.
Blood Clot Prevention and Treatment				
Anticoagulation Overlap Therapy[2]	36	100%	91%	93%
ICU Venous Thromboembolism Prophylaxis[2]	42	95%	92%	92%
Incidence of Potentially Preventable VTE[1,2]	-	-	10%	10%
UFH with Dosages/Platelet Monitoring[2]	12	100%	92%	97%
Venous Thromboembolism Prophylaxis[2]	322	97%	87%	85%
Warfarin Therapy Discharge Instructions[2]	22	73%	59%	75%
Chest Pain/Possible Heart Attack Care				
Aspirin Given Within 24 Hours of Arrival	22	100%	97%	96%
Fibrinolytic Meds Within 30 Min. of Arrival[5]	-	-	54%	58%
Average Time to ECG (minutes)	22	10	9	7
Average Time to Transfer (minutes)[5]	-	-	78	60
Children's Asthma Care				
Received Home Management Plan of Care	-	-	-	88%
Received Reliever Medication	-	-	-	100%
Received Systemic Corticosteroids	-	-	-	100%
Emergency Department				
Admittance Decision Time (minutes)[2]	631	266	154	98
Head CT Results Within 45 Min. of Arrival[1,3]	-	-	55%	57%
Patients Who Left ER Before Being Seen	91,202	4%	2%	2%
Time from ER Arrival to Admit. (minutes)[2]	633	615	378	274
Time from ER Arrival to Discharge (minutes)	360	211	156	134
Time in ER Before Being Evaluated (minutes)	381	88	35	26
Time to Pain Meds for Fractures (minutes)	157	62	61	57
Heart Attack Care				
Aspirin Given at Discharge	277	100%	99%	99%
Fibrinolytic Meds Within 30 Min. of Arrival[7]	-	-	46%	54%
PCI Within 90 Minutes of Arrival	51	90%	95%	96%
Statin Prescribed at Discharge	280	98%	98%	98%
Heart Failure Care				
ACE Inhibitor or ARB for LVSD	120	92%	96%	97%
Discharge Instructions Given	260	99%	95%	94%
Evaluation of LVS Function	286	100%	99%	99%
Medicare Spending				
Medicare Spending per Patient (ratio)	-	0.97	0.96	0.98
Pneumonia Care				
Appropriate Initial Antibiotic Given[2]	118	99%	95%	95%
Blood Culture Timing[2]	136	91%	97%	98%
Pregnancy and Delivery Care				
Newborn Deliveries Scheduled Early[2]	24	0%	4%	6%
Preventive Care				
Immunization for Influenza[2]	478	92%	88%	90%
Immunization for Pneumonia[2]	446	91%	88%	92%
Stroke Care				
Anticoagulation Therapy for Atrial Fibrillation	16	100%	96%	95%
Antithrombotic Therapy Timing	106	100%	98%	98%
Assessed for Rehabilitation	145	97%	97%	97%
Discharged on Antithrombotic Therapy	116	100%	99%	99%
Discharged on Statin Medication	84	99%	95%	94%
Thrombolytic Therapy Timing	17	88%	69%	66%
Venous Thromboembolism Prophylaxis	166	99%	94%	94%
Written Stroke Educational Materials Given	63	100%	86%	88%
Surgical Care Improvement Project				
Appropriate Beta Blocker Usage	66	98%	97%	98%
Appropriate VTP Within 24 Hours	410	100%	98%	98%
Controlled Postoperative Blood Glucose[7]	-	-	97%	97%
Perioperative Temperature Management	453	100%	100%	100%
Prophylactic Antibiotic Selection	183	100%	99%	99%
Prophylactic Antibiotic Selection (Outpatient)	105	94%	97%	98%
Prophylactic Antibiotic Stopped	167	99%	98%	98%
Prophylactic Antibiotic Timing	181	99%	99%	99%
Prophylactic Antibiotic Timing (Outpatient)	105	100%	97%	98%
Urinary Catheter Removal	162	100%	96%	97%
Survey of Patients' Hospital Experiences				
Area Around Room 'Always' Quiet at Night	300+	43%	51%	61%
Doctors 'Always' Communicated Well	300+	71%	77%	82%
Home Recovery Information Given	300+	81%	83%	85%
Hospital Given 9 or 10 on 10 Point Scale	300+	48%	63%	71%
Meds 'Always' Explained Before Given	300+	50%	59%	64%
Nurses 'Always' Communicated Well	300+	60%	75%	79%
Pain 'Always' Well Controlled	300+	53%	67%	71%
Room and Bathroom 'Always' Clean	300+	57%	69%	73%
Timely Help 'Always' Received	300+	47%	61%	68%
Would Definitely Recommend Hospital	300+	52%	65%	71%
Use of Medical Imaging				
Cardiac Imaging Stress Test before Surgery[1]	-	-	5.8%	5.3%
Combination Abdominal CT Scan	84	6.0%	8.2%	10.5%
Combination Brain/Sinus CT Scan[1]	-	-	3.6%	2.7%
Combination Chest CT Scan	47	0.0%	1.3%	2.7%
Follow-up Mammogram/Ultrasound	107	14.0%	13%	8.8%
Lumbar Spine MRI for Low Back Pain[1]	-	-	33.4%	37.2%

Arnot Ogden Medical Center

600 Roe Avenue
Elmira, NY 14905
E-mail: chandrick@aomc.org
URL: www.arnothealth.org
Type: Acute Care Hospitals
Ownership: Voluntary non-profit - Private
Phone: 607-737-4100
Fax: 607-737-4447
Emergency Services: Yes
Beds: 256

Key Personnel:
CEO/President. . . . . Anthony J Cooper
Operating Room. . . . . Beverly Hulslander
Radiology. . . . . Edwin Hutsal, MD
Pediatric Ambulatory Care . . . . . . Kurt Kraus, MD
Pediatric In-Patient Care . . . . Kurt Kraus, MD
Quality Assurance . . . . Rita McCabe, RN
Patient Relations . . . . Elaine Sherhood
Chief of Medical Staff. . . . . Luis Tapia, MD

Measure	Cases	This Hosp.	State Avg.	U.S. Avg.
Blood Clot Prevention and Treatment				
Anticoagulation Overlap Therapy[2]	55	98%	91%	93%
ICU Venous Thromboembolism Prophylaxis[2]	55	93%	92%	92%
Incidence of Potentially Preventable VTE[1,2]	-	-	10%	10%
UFH with Dosages/Platelet Monitoring[2]	22	77%	92%	97%
Venous Thromboembolism Prophylaxis[2]	338	96%	87%	85%
Warfarin Therapy Discharge Instructions[2]	45	56%	59%	75%
Chest Pain/Possible Heart Attack Care				
Aspirin Given Within 24 Hours of Arrival[1,3]	-	-	97%	96%
Fibrinolytic Meds Within 30 Min. of Arrival[5]	-	-	54%	58%
Average Time to ECG (minutes)[1,3]	-	-	9	7
Average Time to Transfer (minutes)[5]	-	-	78	60
Children's Asthma Care				
Received Home Management Plan of Care	-	-	-	88%
Received Reliever Medication	-	-	-	100%
Received Systemic Corticosteroids	-	-	-	100%
Emergency Department				
Admittance Decision Time (minutes)[2]	479	150	154	98
Head CT Results Within 45 Min. of Arrival[1]	-	-	55%	57%
Patients Who Left ER Before Being Seen	47,380	1%	2%	2%
Time from ER Arrival to Admit. (minutes)[2]	507	315	378	274
Time from ER Arrival to Discharge (minutes)	318	167	156	134
Time in ER Before Being Evaluated (minutes)	360	38	35	26
Time to Pain Meds for Fractures (minutes)	32	62	61	57
Heart Attack Care				
Aspirin Given at Discharge	278	99%	99%	99%
Fibrinolytic Meds Within 30 Min. of Arrival[1]	-	-	46%	54%
PCI Within 90 Minutes of Arrival	40	98%	95%	96%
Statin Prescribed at Discharge	270	99%	98%	98%
Heart Failure Care				
ACE Inhibitor or ARB for LVSD	65	97%	96%	97%
Discharge Instructions Given	198	97%	95%	94%
Evaluation of LVS Function	242	100%	99%	99%
Medicare Spending				
Medicare Spending per Patient (ratio)	-	0.89	0.96	0.98
Pneumonia Care				
Appropriate Initial Antibiotic Given	162	94%	95%	95%
Blood Culture Timing	275	99%	97%	98%
Pregnancy and Delivery Care				
Newborn Deliveries Scheduled Early[2]	15	0%	4%	6%
Preventive Care				
Immunization for Influenza[2]	519	98%	88%	90%
Immunization for Pneumonia[2]	644	95%	88%	92%
Stroke Care				
Anticoagulation Therapy for Atrial Fibrillation	17	100%	96%	95%
Antithrombotic Therapy Timing	96	100%	98%	98%
Assessed for Rehabilitation	117	97%	97%	97%
Discharged on Antithrombotic Therapy	101	99%	99%	99%
Discharged on Statin Medication	72	96%	95%	94%
Thrombolytic Therapy Timing[1]	-	-	69%	66%
Venous Thromboembolism Prophylaxis	118	99%	94%	94%
Written Stroke Educational Materials Given	64	100%	86%	88%
Surgical Care Improvement Project				
Appropriate Beta Blocker Usage[2]	306	98%	97%	98%
Appropriate VTP Within 24 Hours[2]	593	98%	98%	98%
Controlled Postoperative Blood Glucose[2]	84	99%	97%	97%
Perioperative Temperature Management[2]	686	100%	100%	100%
Prophylactic Antibiotic Selection[2]	638	100%	99%	99%
Prophylactic Antibiotic Selection (Outpatient)	390	98%	97%	98%
Prophylactic Antibiotic Stopped[2]	623	100%	98%	98%
Prophylactic Antibiotic Timing[2]	638	100%	99%	99%
Prophylactic Antibiotic Timing (Outpatient)	390	98%	97%	98%
Urinary Catheter Removal[2]	216	89%	96%	97%
Survey of Patients' Hospital Experiences				
Area Around Room 'Always' Quiet at Night	300+	46%	51%	61%
Doctors 'Always' Communicated Well	300+	78%	77%	82%
Home Recovery Information Given	300+	87%	83%	85%
Hospital Given 9 or 10 on 10 Point Scale	300+	65%	63%	71%
Meds 'Always' Explained Before Given	300+	58%	59%	64%
Nurses 'Always' Communicated Well	300+	78%	75%	79%
Pain 'Always' Well Controlled	300+	70%	67%	71%
Room and Bathroom 'Always' Clean	300+	66%	69%	73%
Timely Help 'Always' Received	300+	60%	61%	68%
Would Definitely Recommend Hospital	300+	70%	65%	71%
Use of Medical Imaging				
Cardiac Imaging Stress Test before Surgery	1,268	4.1%	5.8%	5.3%
Combination Abdominal CT Scan	1,235	6.6%	8.2%	10.5%
Combination Brain/Sinus CT Scan	921	2.7%	3.6%	2.7%
Combination Chest CT Scan	685	0.1%	1.3%	2.7%
Follow-up Mammogram/Ultrasound	1,870	5.2%	13%	8.8%
Lumbar Spine MRI for Low Back Pain	112	30.4%	33.4%	37.2%

Saint Joseph's Hospital

555 Saint Joseph's Blvd
Elmira, NY 14902
URL: www.stjosephs.org
Type: Acute Care Hospitals
Ownership: Voluntary non-profit - Private
Phone: 607-733-6541
Fax: 607-737-7837
Emergency Services: Yes
Beds: 295

Key Personnel:
CEO/President. . . . . Marie Castagnaro SSJ
Quality Assurance . . . . Diane Giantiso
Intensive Care Unit. . . . . Antoinette Shields
Infection Control. . . . . Deb Woodard
Operating Room. . . . . Lori Youmans, RN

Measure	Cases	This Hosp.	State Avg.	U.S. Avg.
Blood Clot Prevention and Treatment				
Anticoagulation Overlap Therapy[2]	18	100%	91%	93%
ICU Venous Thromboembolism Prophylaxis[2]	51	82%	92%	92%
Incidence of Potentially Preventable VTE[1,2]	-	-	10%	10%
UFH with Dosages/Platelet Monitoring[1,2]	-	-	92%	97%
Venous Thromboembolism Prophylaxis[2]	203	82%	87%	85%
Warfarin Therapy Discharge Instructions[2]	12	50%	59%	75%
Chest Pain/Possible Heart Attack Care				
Aspirin Given Within 24 Hours of Arrival[5]	-	-	97%	96%
Fibrinolytic Meds Within 30 Min. of Arrival[5]	-	-	54%	58%
Average Time to ECG (minutes)[5]	-	-	9	7

NOTE: Hospital profiles are in alphabetical order by state, then city, then hospital within the city; Rankings exclude hospitals with less than 25 cases except for patient surveys which excludes hospitals with less than 100 cases; (a) 100-299 cases; (1) The number of cases/patients is too few to report; (2) Data submitted were based on a sample of cases/patients; (3) Results are based on a shorter time period than required; (4) Data suppressed by CMS for one or more quarters; (5) Results are not available for this reporting period; (6) Fewer than 100 patients completed the HCAHPS survey; (7) No cases met the criteria for this measure; (8) The lower limit of the confidence interval cannot be calculated if the number of observed infections equals zero; (9) No data are available from the state/territory for this reporting period; (10) The scores shown reflect fewer than 50 completed surveys; (11) There were discrepancies in the data collection process; (12) This measure does not apply to this hospital for this reporting period; (13) Results cannot be calculated for this reporting period; (14) The results for this state are combined with nearby states to protect confidentiality; Please refer to the User's Guide for a full explanation of data.

Measure	Cases	This Hosp.	State Avg.	U.S. Avg.
Average Time to Transfer (minutes)[5]	-	-	78	60
Children's Asthma Care				
Received Home Management Plan of Care	-	-	-	88%
Received Reliever Medication	-	-	-	100%
Received Systemic Corticosteroids	-	-	-	100%
Emergency Department				
Admittance Decision Time (minutes)[2]	257	175	154	98
Head CT Results Within 45 Min. of Arrival[1]	-	-	55%	57%
Patients Who Left ER Before Being Seen	14,736	4%	2%	2%
Time from ER Arrival to Admit. (minutes)[2]	276	359	378	274
Time from ER Arrival to Discharge (minutes)	302	136	156	134
Time in ER Before Being Evaluated (minutes)	376	30	35	26
Time to Pain Meds for Fractures (minutes)	20	96	61	57
Heart Attack Care				
Aspirin Given at Discharge	17	94%	99%	99%
Fibrinolytic Meds Within 30 Min. of Arrival[7]	-	-	46%	54%
PCI Within 90 Minutes of Arrival[7]	-	-	95%	96%
Statin Prescribed at Discharge	18	100%	98%	98%
Heart Failure Care				
ACE Inhibitor or ARB for LVSD	14	86%	96%	97%
Discharge Instructions Given	38	100%	95%	94%
Evaluation of LVS Function	50	92%	99%	99%
Medicare Spending				
Medicare Spending per Patient (ratio)	-	0.89	0.96	0.98
Pneumonia Care				
Appropriate Initial Antibiotic Given[2]	127	91%	95%	95%
Blood Culture Timing[2]	241	94%	97%	98%
Pregnancy and Delivery Care				
Newborn Deliveries Scheduled Early[7]	-	-	4%	6%
Preventive Care				
Immunization for Influenza[2]	466	84%	88%	90%
Immunization for Pneumonia[2]	460	82%	88%	92%
Stroke Care				
Anticoagulation Therapy for Atrial Fibrillation[7]	-	-	96%	95%
Antithrombotic Therapy Timing	11	100%	98%	98%
Assessed for Rehabilitation[1]	-	-	97%	97%
Discharged on Antithrombotic Therapy[1]	-	-	99%	99%
Discharged on Statin Medication[1]	-	-	95%	94%
Thrombolytic Therapy Timing[1]	-	-	69%	66%
Venous Thromboembolism Prophylaxis[1]	-	-	94%	94%
Written Stroke Educational Materials Given[1]	-	-	86%	88%
Surgical Care Improvement Project				
Appropriate Beta Blocker Usage[2]	43	100%	97%	98%
Appropriate VTP Within 24 Hours[2]	109	98%	98%	98%
Controlled Postoperative Blood Glucose[2,7]	-	-	97%	97%
Perioperative Temperature Management[2]	135	100%	100%	100%
Prophylactic Antibiotic Selection[2]	126	99%	99%	99%
Prophylactic Antibiotic Selection (Outpatient)	25	100%	97%	98%
Prophylactic Antibiotic Stopped[2]	126	100%	98%	98%
Prophylactic Antibiotic Timing[2]	126	97%	99%	99%
Prophylactic Antibiotic Timing (Outpatient)	25	100%	97%	98%
Urinary Catheter Removal[1,2]	-	-	96%	97%
Survey of Patients' Hospital Experiences				
Area Around Room 'Always' Quiet at Night	300+	49%	51%	61%
Doctors 'Always' Communicated Well	300+	75%	77%	82%
Home Recovery Information Given	300+	88%	83%	85%
Hospital Given 9 or 10 on 10 Point Scale	300+	60%	63%	71%
Meds 'Always' Explained Before Given	300+	58%	59%	64%
Nurses 'Always' Communicated Well	300+	70%	75%	79%
Pain 'Always' Well Controlled	300+	64%	67%	71%
Room and Bathroom 'Always' Clean	300+	69%	69%	73%
Timely Help 'Always' Received	300+	56%	61%	68%
Would Definitely Recommend Hospital	300+	60%	65%	71%
Use of Medical Imaging				
Cardiac Imaging Stress Test before Surgery[1]	-	-	5.8%	5.3%
Combination Abdominal CT Scan	309	4.2%	8.2%	10.5%
Combination Brain/Sinus CT Scan	279	7.5%	3.6%	2.7%
Combination Chest CT Scan	123	0.8%	1.3%	2.7%
Follow-up Mammogram/Ultrasound	495	7.5%	13%	8.8%
Lumbar Spine MRI for Low Back Pain	86	40.7%	33.4%	37.2%

Saint John's Episcopal Hospital at South Shore

327 Beach 19th Street
Far Rockaway, NY 11691
URL: www.ehs.org
Phone: 718-869-7000
Fax: 718-869-8507
Type: Acute Care Hospitals
Emergency Services: Yes
Ownership: Voluntary non-profit - Private
Beds: 332

Key Personnel:
CEO/President. . . . . Richard Brown
Coronary Care. . . . . Lynore Dupiton
Infection Control. . . . . Mary Anne Hauff
Operating Room. . . . . Gilbert Makabali, MD
Chief of Medical Staff. . . . . Raymond Pastore, MD
Radiology. . . . . Dennis Rossi, MD
Quality Assurance . . . . Carol Seaman
Pediatric In-Patient Care . . . . Allan Steinberg, MD

Measure	Cases	This Hosp.	State Avg.	U.S. Avg.
Blood Clot Prevention and Treatment				
Anticoagulation Overlap Therapy[2]	73	100%	91%	93%
ICU Venous Thromboembolism Prophylaxis[2]	67	97%	92%	92%
Incidence of Potentially Preventable VTE[2]	21	0%	10%	10%
UFH with Dosages/Platelet Monitoring[2]	31	100%	92%	97%
Venous Thromboembolism Prophylaxis[2]	409	97%	87%	85%
Warfarin Therapy Discharge Instructions[2]	29	100%	59%	75%
Chest Pain/Possible Heart Attack Care				
Aspirin Given Within 24 Hours of Arrival	27	96%	97%	96%
Fibrinolytic Meds Within 30 Min. of Arrival[7]	-	-	54%	58%
Average Time to ECG (minutes)	28	24	9	7
Average Time to Transfer (minutes)[7]	-	-	78	60
Children's Asthma Care				
Received Home Management Plan of Care	-	-	-	88%
Received Reliever Medication	-	-	-	100%
Received Systemic Corticosteroids	-	-	-	100%
Emergency Department				
Admittance Decision Time (minutes)[2]	1,068	394	154	98
Head CT Results Within 45 Min. of Arrival[1]	-	-	55%	57%
Patients Who Left ER Before Being Seen	46,468	4%	2%	2%
Time from ER Arrival to Admit. (minutes)[2]	1,071	702	378	274
Time from ER Arrival to Discharge (minutes)	364	198	156	134
Time in ER Before Being Evaluated (minutes)	417	58	35	26
Time to Pain Meds for Fractures (minutes)	110	96	61	57
Heart Attack Care				
Aspirin Given at Discharge	22	100%	99%	99%
Fibrinolytic Meds Within 30 Min. of Arrival[7]	-	-	46%	54%
PCI Within 90 Minutes of Arrival[7]	-	-	95%	96%
Statin Prescribed at Discharge	23	100%	98%	98%
Heart Failure Care				
ACE Inhibitor or ARB for LVSD	64	97%	96%	97%
Discharge Instructions Given	176	100%	95%	94%
Evaluation of LVS Function	237	99%	99%	99%
Medicare Spending				
Medicare Spending per Patient (ratio)	-	1.00	0.96	0.98
Pneumonia Care				
Appropriate Initial Antibiotic Given[2]	33	100%	95%	95%
Blood Culture Timing[2]	123	98%	97%	98%
Pregnancy and Delivery Care				
Newborn Deliveries Scheduled Early[2]	24	4%	4%	6%
Preventive Care				
Immunization for Influenza[2]	532	65%	88%	90%
Immunization for Pneumonia[2]	692	82%	88%	92%
Stroke Care				
Anticoagulation Therapy for Atrial Fibrillation	11	45%	96%	95%
Antithrombotic Therapy Timing	83	99%	98%	98%
Assessed for Rehabilitation	84	100%	97%	97%
Discharged on Antithrombotic Therapy	74	97%	99%	99%
Discharged on Statin Medication	66	91%	95%	94%
Thrombolytic Therapy Timing[1]	-	-	69%	66%
Venous Thromboembolism Prophylaxis	100	91%	94%	94%
Written Stroke Educational Materials Given	37	86%	86%	88%
Surgical Care Improvement Project				
Appropriate Beta Blocker Usage[2]	35	100%	97%	98%
Appropriate VTP Within 24 Hours[2]	146	92%	98%	98%
Controlled Postoperative Blood Glucose[2,7]	-	-	97%	97%
Perioperative Temperature Management[2]	163	99%	100%	100%
Prophylactic Antibiotic Selection[2]	68	93%	99%	99%
Prophylactic Antibiotic Selection (Outpatient)	40	80%	97%	98%
Prophylactic Antibiotic Stopped[2]	66	100%	98%	98%
Prophylactic Antibiotic Timing[2]	68	100%	99%	99%
Prophylactic Antibiotic Timing (Outpatient)	40	100%	97%	98%
Urinary Catheter Removal[2]	50	100%	96%	97%
Survey of Patients' Hospital Experiences				
Area Around Room 'Always' Quiet at Night	300+	50%	51%	61%
Doctors 'Always' Communicated Well	300+	73%	77%	82%
Home Recovery Information Given	300+	72%	83%	85%
Hospital Given 9 or 10 on 10 Point Scale	300+	43%	63%	71%
Meds 'Always' Explained Before Given	300+	50%	59%	64%
Nurses 'Always' Communicated Well	300+	65%	75%	79%
Pain 'Always' Well Controlled	300+	62%	67%	71%
Room and Bathroom 'Always' Clean	300+	64%	69%	73%
Timely Help 'Always' Received	300+	47%	61%	68%
Would Definitely Recommend Hospital	300+	49%	65%	71%
Use of Medical Imaging				
Cardiac Imaging Stress Test before Surgery	129	3.9%	5.8%	5.3%
Combination Abdominal CT Scan	383	71.0%	8.2%	10.5%
Combination Brain/Sinus CT Scan	485	3.9%	3.6%	2.7%
Combination Chest CT Scan	224	0.0%	1.3%	2.7%
Follow-up Mammogram/Ultrasound	299	26.4%	13%	8.8%
Lumbar Spine MRI for Low Back Pain[1]	-	-	33.4%	37.2%

Flushing Hospital Medical Center

45th Avenue & Parsons Boulevard
Flushing, NY 11355
URL: www.flushinghospital.org
Phone: 718-670-5000
Fax: 718-670-3077
Type: Acute Care Hospitals
Emergency Services: Yes
Ownership: Voluntary non-profit - Private
Beds: 325

Key Personnel:
Quality Assurance . . . . Dawn Lewis
Pediatric In-Patient Care . . . . Susana Rapaport, MD
Radiology. . . . . Glenn Schwartz, MD
CEO/President. . . . . Frederick I Weinbaum

Measure	Cases	This Hosp.	State Avg.	U.S. Avg.
Blood Clot Prevention and Treatment				
Anticoagulation Overlap Therapy[2]	36	100%	91%	93%
ICU Venous Thromboembolism Prophylaxis[2]	54	98%	92%	92%
Incidence of Potentially Preventable VTE[2]	25	0%	10%	10%
UFH with Dosages/Platelet Monitoring[2]	28	100%	92%	97%
Venous Thromboembolism Prophylaxis[2]	343	98%	87%	85%
Warfarin Therapy Discharge Instructions[2]	18	94%	59%	75%
Chest Pain/Possible Heart Attack Care				
Aspirin Given Within 24 Hours of Arrival[1,3]	-	-	97%	96%
Fibrinolytic Meds Within 30 Min. of Arrival[1,3]	-	-	54%	58%
Average Time to ECG (minutes)[1,3]	-	-	9	7
Average Time to Transfer (minutes)[3,7]	-	-	78	60
Children's Asthma Care				
Received Home Management Plan of Care	-	-	-	88%
Received Reliever Medication	-	-	-	100%
Received Systemic Corticosteroids	-	-	-	100%
Emergency Department				
Admittance Decision Time (minutes)[2]	656	254	154	98
Head CT Results Within 45 Min. of Arrival[1]	-	-	55%	57%
Patients Who Left ER Before Being Seen	43,984	1%	2%	2%
Time from ER Arrival to Admit. (minutes)[2]	656	448	378	274
Time from ER Arrival to Discharge (minutes)	390	149	156	134
Time in ER Before Being Evaluated (minutes)	432	42	35	26
Time to Pain Meds for Fractures (minutes)	55	63	61	57
Heart Attack Care				
Aspirin Given at Discharge	19	100%	99%	99%
Fibrinolytic Meds Within 30 Min. of Arrival[7]	-	-	46%	54%
PCI Within 90 Minutes of Arrival[7]	-	-	95%	96%
Statin Prescribed at Discharge	24	88%	98%	98%
Heart Failure Care				
ACE Inhibitor or ARB for LVSD	34	100%	96%	97%
Discharge Instructions Given	105	98%	95%	94%
Evaluation of LVS Function	189	99%	99%	99%
Medicare Spending				
Medicare Spending per Patient (ratio)	-	1.04	0.96	0.98
Pneumonia Care				
Appropriate Initial Antibiotic Given[2]	55	96%	95%	95%

NOTE: Hospital profiles are in alphabetical order by state, then city, then hospital within the city; Rankings exclude hospitals with less than 25 cases except for patient surveys which excludes hospitals with less than 100 cases; (a) 100-299 cases; (1) The number of cases/patients is too few to report; (2) Data submitted were based on a sample of cases/patients; (3) Results are based on a shorter time period than required; (4) Data suppressed by CMS for one or more quarters; (5) Results are not available for this reporting period; (6) Fewer than 100 patients completed the HCAHPS survey; (7) No cases met the criteria for this measure; (8) The lower limit of the confidence interval cannot be calculated if the number of observed infections equals zero; (9) No data are available from the state/territory for this reporting period; (10) The scores shown reflect fewer than 50 completed surveys; (11) There were discrepancies in the data collection process; (12) This measure does not apply to this hospital for this reporting period; (13) Results cannot be calculated for this reporting period; (14) The results for this state are combined with nearby states to protect confidentiality; Please refer to the User's Guide for a full explanation of data.

Measure	Cases	This Hosp.	State Avg.	U.S. Avg.
Blood Culture Timing[2]	169	95%	97%	98%
Pregnancy and Delivery Care				
Newborn Deliveries Scheduled Early[2]	65	3%	4%	6%
Preventive Care				
Immunization for Influenza[2]	495	95%	88%	90%
Immunization for Pneumonia[2]	432	90%	88%	92%
Stroke Care				
Anticoagulation Therapy for Atrial Fibrillation	12	100%	96%	95%
Antithrombotic Therapy Timing	116	100%	98%	98%
Assessed for Rehabilitation	114	100%	97%	97%
Discharged on Antithrombotic Therapy	103	98%	99%	99%
Discharged on Statin Medication	82	90%	95%	94%
Thrombolytic Therapy Timing	11	100%	69%	66%
Venous Thromboembolism Prophylaxis	138	98%	94%	94%
Written Stroke Educational Materials Given	52	94%	86%	88%
Surgical Care Improvement Project				
Appropriate Beta Blocker Usage[2]	66	91%	97%	98%
Appropriate VTP Within 24 Hours[2]	267	99%	98%	98%
Controlled Postoperative Blood Glucose[2,7]	-	-	97%	97%
Perioperative Temperature Management[2]	332	100%	100%	100%
Prophylactic Antibiotic Selection[2]	215	98%	99%	99%
Prophylactic Antibiotic Selection (Outpatient)	133	97%	97%	98%
Prophylactic Antibiotic Stopped[2]	210	90%	98%	98%
Prophylactic Antibiotic Timing[2]	215	99%	99%	99%
Prophylactic Antibiotic Timing (Outpatient)	138	91%	97%	98%
Urinary Catheter Removal[2]	94	94%	96%	97%
Survey of Patients' Hospital Experiences				
Area Around Room 'Always' Quiet at Night	300+	41%	51%	61%
Doctors 'Always' Communicated Well	300+	64%	77%	82%
Home Recovery Information Given	300+	78%	83%	85%
Hospital Given 9 or 10 on 10 Point Scale	300+	43%	63%	71%
Meds 'Always' Explained Before Given	300+	51%	59%	64%
Nurses 'Always' Communicated Well	300+	60%	75%	79%
Pain 'Always' Well Controlled	300+	53%	67%	71%
Room and Bathroom 'Always' Clean	300+	58%	69%	73%
Timely Help 'Always' Received	300+	50%	61%	68%
Would Definitely Recommend Hospital	300+	49%	65%	71%
Use of Medical Imaging				
Cardiac Imaging Stress Test before Surgery[1]	-	-	5.8%	5.3%
Combination Abdominal CT Scan	137	5.8%	8.2%	10.5%
Combination Brain/Sinus CT Scan	336	7.1%	3.6%	2.7%
Combination Chest CT Scan	54	3.7%	1.3%	2.7%
Follow-up Mammogram/Ultrasound	101	13.9%	13%	8.8%
Lumbar Spine MRI for Low Back Pain[1]	-	-	33.4%	37.2%

New York Hospital Medical Center of Queens

56-45 Main Street
Flushing, NY 11355
Phone: 718-670-1231
Fax: 718-661-7976
URL: www.nyhq.org
Type: Acute Care Hospitals
Emergency Services: Yes
Ownership: Voluntary non-profit - Other
Beds: 439

Key Personnel:

Pediatric In-Patient Care . . . . Joe Abularrage
Patient Relations . . . . Michael Grady, MD
CEO/President. . . . . Stephen S. Mills, FACHE
Infection Control. . . . . James J Rahal, MD
Chief of Medical Staff . . . . Stephen Rimar, MD, MBA
Anesthesiology. . . . . Peter Silverberg
Emergency Room . . . . Diane Sixsmith, MD
Radiology. . . . . William Wolff

Measure	Cases	This Hosp.	State Avg.	U.S. Avg.
Blood Clot Prevention and Treatment				
Anticoagulation Overlap Therapy[2]	173	82%	91%	93%
ICU Venous Thromboembolism Prophylaxis[2]	57	51%	92%	92%
Incidence of Potentially Preventable VTE[2]	46	24%	10%	10%
UFH with Dosages/Platelet Monitoring[2]	126	90%	92%	97%
Venous Thromboembolism Prophylaxis[2]	426	73%	87%	85%
Warfarin Therapy Discharge Instructions[2]	107	94%	59%	75%
Chest Pain/Possible Heart Attack Care				
Aspirin Given Within 24 Hours of Arrival[1,3]	-	-	97%	96%
Fibrinolytic Meds Within 30 Min. of Arrival[5]	-	-	54%	58%
Average Time to ECG (minutes)[1,3]	-	-	9	7
Average Time to Transfer (minutes)[5]	-	-	78	60
Children's Asthma Care				
Received Home Management Plan of Care	-	-	-	88%
Received Reliever Medication	-	-	-	100%
Received Systemic Corticosteroids	-	-	-	100%
Emergency Department				
Admittance Decision Time (minutes)[2]	615	340	154	98
Head CT Results Within 45 Min. of Arrival	23	57%	55%	57%
Patients Who Left ER Before Being Seen	>100k	2%	2%	2%
Time from ER Arrival to Admit. (minutes)[2]	615	616	378	274
Time from ER Arrival to Discharge (minutes)	380	151	156	134
Time in ER Before Being Evaluated (minutes)	392	61	35	26
Time to Pain Meds for Fractures (minutes)	195	75	61	57
Heart Attack Care				
Aspirin Given at Discharge[2]	275	99%	99%	99%
Fibrinolytic Meds Within 30 Min. of Arrival[2,7]	-	-	46%	54%
PCI Within 90 Minutes of Arrival[2]	51	100%	95%	96%
Statin Prescribed at Discharge[2]	281	97%	98%	98%
Heart Failure Care				
ACE Inhibitor or ARB for LVSD[2]	83	89%	96%	97%
Discharge Instructions Given[2]	205	91%	95%	94%
Evaluation of LVS Function[2]	284	99%	99%	99%
Medicare Spending				
Medicare Spending per Patient (ratio)	-	1.03	0.96	0.98
Pneumonia Care				
Appropriate Initial Antibiotic Given[2]	91	97%	95%	95%
Blood Culture Timing[2]	213	98%	97%	98%
Pregnancy and Delivery Care				
Newborn Deliveries Scheduled Early[2]	112	0%	4%	6%
Preventive Care				
Immunization for Influenza[2]	503	90%	88%	90%
Immunization for Pneumonia[2]	617	88%	88%	92%
Stroke Care				
Anticoagulation Therapy for Atrial Fibrillation[2]	19	100%	96%	95%
Antithrombotic Therapy Timing[2]	135	96%	98%	98%
Assessed for Rehabilitation[2]	163	99%	97%	97%
Discharged on Antithrombotic Therapy[2]	145	99%	99%	99%
Discharged on Statin Medication[2]	118	96%	95%	94%
Thrombolytic Therapy Timing[2]	13	85%	69%	66%
Venous Thromboembolism Prophylaxis[2]	178	90%	94%	94%
Written Stroke Educational Materials Given[2]	88	99%	86%	88%
Surgical Care Improvement Project				
Appropriate Beta Blocker Usage[2]	195	99%	97%	98%
Appropriate VTP Within 24 Hours[2]	424	100%	98%	98%
Controlled Postoperative Blood Glucose[2]	100	100%	97%	97%
Perioperative Temperature Management[2]	489	100%	100%	100%
Prophylactic Antibiotic Selection[2]	427	99%	99%	99%
Prophylactic Antibiotic Selection (Outpatient)	475	96%	97%	98%
Prophylactic Antibiotic Stopped[2]	402	99%	98%	98%
Prophylactic Antibiotic Timing[2]	427	98%	99%	99%
Prophylactic Antibiotic Timing (Outpatient)	477	95%	97%	98%
Urinary Catheter Removal[2]	358	98%	96%	97%
Survey of Patients' Hospital Experiences				
Area Around Room 'Always' Quiet at Night	300+	48%	51%	61%
Doctors 'Always' Communicated Well	300+	74%	77%	82%
Home Recovery Information Given	300+	82%	83%	85%
Hospital Given 9 or 10 on 10 Point Scale	300+	61%	63%	71%
Meds 'Always' Explained Before Given	300+	58%	59%	64%
Nurses 'Always' Communicated Well	300+	72%	75%	79%
Pain 'Always' Well Controlled	300+	63%	67%	71%
Room and Bathroom 'Always' Clean	300+	70%	69%	73%
Timely Help 'Always' Received	300+	56%	61%	68%
Would Definitely Recommend Hospital	300+	68%	65%	71%
Use of Medical Imaging				
Cardiac Imaging Stress Test before Surgery	192	10.4%	5.8%	5.3%
Combination Abdominal CT Scan	1,006	7.0%	8.2%	10.5%
Combination Brain/Sinus CT Scan	1,212	5.3%	3.6%	2.7%
Combination Chest CT Scan	415	0.0%	1.3%	2.7%
Follow-up Mammogram/Ultrasound	1,236	14.3%	13%	8.8%
Lumbar Spine MRI for Low Back Pain[1]	-	-	33.4%	37.2%

Forest Hills Hospital

102 - 01 66th Road
Forest Hills, NY 11375
Phone: 718-830-4000
Fax: 718-275-0950
URL: www.northshorelij.com
Type: Acute Care Hospitals
Emergency Services: Yes
Ownership: Voluntary non-profit - Other
Beds: 309

Key Personnel:

Chief of Medical Staff . . . . Gerard Brogan, MD
Quality Assurance . . . . Linda Dascher
Pediatric Ambulatory Care . . . . . . Reginald McLaughlin, MD
Pediatric In-Patient Care . . . . Reginald McLaughlin, MD
CEO/President. . . . . Geralyn Randazzo
Radiology. . . . . Kenneth Schwartz, MD
Operating Room. . . . . Moises Tenembaum
Infection Control. . . . . Cecilia Wilfingon

Measure	Cases	This Hosp.	State Avg.	U.S. Avg.
Blood Clot Prevention and Treatment				
Anticoagulation Overlap Therapy[2]	76	92%	91%	93%
ICU Venous Thromboembolism Prophylaxis[2]	47	98%	92%	92%
Incidence of Potentially Preventable VTE[2]	17	0%	10%	10%
UFH with Dosages/Platelet Monitoring[2]	22	91%	92%	97%
Venous Thromboembolism Prophylaxis[2]	373	84%	87%	85%
Warfarin Therapy Discharge Instructions[2]	50	74%	59%	75%
Chest Pain/Possible Heart Attack Care				
Aspirin Given Within 24 Hours of Arrival	65	100%	97%	96%
Fibrinolytic Meds Within 30 Min. of Arrival[7]	-	-	54%	58%
Average Time to ECG (minutes)	63	4	9	7
Average Time to Transfer (minutes)	27	75	78	60
Children's Asthma Care				
Received Home Management Plan of Care	-	-	-	88%
Received Reliever Medication	-	-	-	100%
Received Systemic Corticosteroids	-	-	-	100%
Emergency Department				
Admittance Decision Time (minutes)[2]	412	285	154	98
Head CT Results Within 45 Min. of Arrival	20	80%	55%	57%
Patients Who Left ER Before Being Seen	49,465	1%	2%	2%
Time from ER Arrival to Admit. (minutes)[2]	430	500	378	274
Time from ER Arrival to Discharge (minutes)	377	147	156	134
Time in ER Before Being Evaluated (minutes)	383	43	35	26
Time to Pain Meds for Fractures (minutes)	69	74	61	57
Heart Attack Care				
Aspirin Given at Discharge[2]	31	100%	99%	99%
Fibrinolytic Meds Within 30 Min. of Arrival[2,7]	-	-	46%	54%
PCI Within 90 Minutes of Arrival[2,7]	-	-	95%	96%
Statin Prescribed at Discharge[2]	33	100%	98%	98%
Heart Failure Care				
ACE Inhibitor or ARB for LVSD[2]	50	94%	96%	97%
Discharge Instructions Given[2]	195	99%	95%	94%
Evaluation of LVS Function[2]	247	100%	99%	99%
Medicare Spending				
Medicare Spending per Patient (ratio)	-	1.05	0.96	0.98
Pneumonia Care				
Appropriate Initial Antibiotic Given[2]	92	100%	95%	95%
Blood Culture Timing[2]	166	100%	97%	98%
Pregnancy and Delivery Care				
Newborn Deliveries Scheduled Early[2]	20	0%	4%	6%
Preventive Care				
Immunization for Influenza[2]	498	95%	88%	90%
Immunization for Pneumonia[2]	644	96%	88%	92%
Stroke Care				
Anticoagulation Therapy for Atrial Fibrillation[2]	17	100%	96%	95%
Antithrombotic Therapy Timing[2]	89	100%	98%	98%
Assessed for Rehabilitation[2]	102	100%	97%	97%
Discharged on Antithrombotic Therapy[2]	94	100%	99%	99%
Discharged on Statin Medication[2]	80	100%	95%	94%
Thrombolytic Therapy Timing[2]	13	100%	69%	66%
Venous Thromboembolism Prophylaxis[2]	111	100%	94%	94%
Written Stroke Educational Materials Given[2]	43	100%	86%	88%
Surgical Care Improvement Project				
Appropriate Beta Blocker Usage[2]	103	100%	97%	98%
Appropriate VTP Within 24 Hours[2]	324	100%	98%	98%
Controlled Postoperative Blood Glucose[2,7]	-	-	97%	97%
Perioperative Temperature Management[2]	376	100%	100%	100%
Prophylactic Antibiotic Selection[2]	246	100%	99%	99%

NOTE: Hospital profiles are in alphabetical order by state, then city, then hospital within the city; Rankings exclude hospitals with less than 25 cases except for patient surveys which excludes hospitals with less than 100 cases; (a) 100-299 cases; (1) The number of cases/patients is too few to report; (2) Data submitted were based on a sample of cases/patients; (3) Results are based on a shorter time period than required; (4) Data suppressed by CMS for one or more quarters; (5) Results are not available for this reporting period; (6) Fewer than 100 patients completed the HCAHPS survey; (7) No cases met the criteria for this measure; (8) The lower limit of the confidence interval cannot be calculated if the number of observed infections equals zero; (9) No data are available from the state/territory for this reporting period; (10) The scores shown reflect fewer than 50 completed surveys; (11) There were discrepancies in the data collection process; (12) This measure does not apply to this hospital for this reporting period; (13) Results cannot be calculated for this reporting period; (14) The results for this state are combined with nearby states to protect confidentiality; Please refer to the User's Guide for a full explanation of data.

Measure	Cases	This Hosp.	State Avg.	U.S. Avg.
Prophylactic Antibiotic Selection (Outpatient)	67	96%	97%	98%
Prophylactic Antibiotic Stopped[2]	240	99%	98%	98%
Prophylactic Antibiotic Timing[2]	246	100%	99%	99%
Prophylactic Antibiotic Timing (Outpatient)	67	99%	97%	98%
Urinary Catheter Removal[2]	230	98%	96%	97%
Survey of Patients' Hospital Experiences				
Area Around Room 'Always' Quiet at Night[11]	300+	42%	51%	61%
Doctors 'Always' Communicated Well[11]	300+	69%	77%	82%
Home Recovery Information Given[11]	300+	74%	83%	85%
Hospital Given 9 or 10 on 10 Point Scale[11]	300+	57%	63%	71%
Meds 'Always' Explained Before Given[11]	300+	53%	59%	64%
Nurses 'Always' Communicated Well[11]	300+	69%	75%	79%
Pain 'Always' Well Controlled[11]	300+	61%	67%	71%
Room and Bathroom 'Always' Clean[11]	300+	70%	69%	73%
Timely Help 'Always' Received[11]	300+	55%	61%	68%
Would Definitely Recommend Hospital[11]	300+	62%	65%	71%
Use of Medical Imaging				
Cardiac Imaging Stress Test before Surgery[1]	-	-	5.8%	5.3%
Combination Abdominal CT Scan	293	0.0%	8.2%	10.5%
Combination Brain/Sinus CT Scan	411	1.9%	3.6%	2.7%
Combination Chest CT Scan	61	0.0%	1.3%	2.7%
Follow-up Mammogram/Ultrasound	73	17.8%	13%	8.8%
Lumbar Spine MRI for Low Back Pain[1]	-	-	33.4%	37.2%

Geneva General Hospital

196 -198 North Street
Geneva, NY 14456
Phone: 315-787-4175
Fax: 315-787-4009
URL: www.flhealth.org
Type: Acute Care Hospitals
Emergency Services: Yes
Ownership: Voluntary non-profit - Private
Beds: 136

Key Personnel:

CEO/President. . . . . Jose Acevedo, MD, MBA
Infection Control. . . . . Marge Brinn
Operating Room. . . . . Rose Leo
Chief of Medical Staff. . . . . Jane McCaffrey, MD
Pediatric In-Patient Care . . . . Mary Jo Olmstead
Radiology. . . . . Rodolfo Queiroz
Quality Assurance . . . . Betty Scarnati
Intensive Care Unit. . . . . Barb Weinberg

Measure	Cases	This Hosp.	State Avg.	U.S. Avg.
Blood Clot Prevention and Treatment				
Anticoagulation Overlap Therapy[2]	27	93%	91%	93%
ICU Venous Thromboembolism Prophylaxis[2]	63	90%	92%	92%
Incidence of Potentially Preventable VTE[2,7]	-	-	10%	10%
UFH with Dosages/Platelet Monitoring[2]	11	100%	92%	97%
Venous Thromboembolism Prophylaxis[2]	328	91%	87%	85%
Warfarin Therapy Discharge Instructions[2]	20	90%	59%	75%
Chest Pain/Possible Heart Attack Care				
Aspirin Given Within 24 Hours of Arrival	41	98%	97%	96%
Fibrinolytic Meds Within 30 Min. of Arrival[1]	-	-	54%	58%
Average Time to ECG (minutes)	43	9	9	7
Average Time to Transfer (minutes)[1]	-	-	78	60
Children's Asthma Care				
Received Home Management Plan of Care	-	-	-	88%
Received Reliever Medication	-	-	-	100%
Received Systemic Corticosteroids	-	-	-	100%
Emergency Department				
Admittance Decision Time (minutes)[2]	419	128	154	98
Head CT Results Within 45 Min. of Arrival[1]	-	-	55%	57%
Patients Who Left ER Before Being Seen	20,715	1%	2%	2%
Time from ER Arrival to Admit. (minutes)[2]	450	286	378	274
Time from ER Arrival to Discharge (minutes)	349	135	156	134
Time in ER Before Being Evaluated (minutes)	266	23	35	26
Time to Pain Meds for Fractures (minutes)	68	47	61	57
Heart Attack Care				
Aspirin Given at Discharge	15	100%	99%	99%
Fibrinolytic Meds Within 30 Min. of Arrival[7]	-	-	46%	54%
PCI Within 90 Minutes of Arrival[7]	-	-	95%	96%
Statin Prescribed at Discharge	14	93%	98%	98%
Heart Failure Care				
ACE Inhibitor or ARB for LVSD	31	97%	96%	97%
Discharge Instructions Given	111	99%	95%	94%
Evaluation of LVS Function	160	98%	99%	99%
Medicare Spending				
Medicare Spending per Patient (ratio)	-	0.90	0.96	0.98
Pneumonia Care				
Appropriate Initial Antibiotic Given	63	97%	95%	95%
Blood Culture Timing	121	98%	97%	98%
Pregnancy and Delivery Care				
Newborn Deliveries Scheduled Early	31	13%	4%	6%
Preventive Care				
Immunization for Influenza[2]	401	85%	88%	90%
Immunization for Pneumonia[2]	542	93%	88%	92%
Stroke Care				
Anticoagulation Therapy for Atrial Fibrillation[1]	-	-	96%	95%
Antithrombotic Therapy Timing	36	100%	98%	98%
Assessed for Rehabilitation	38	100%	97%	97%
Discharged on Antithrombotic Therapy	36	100%	99%	99%
Discharged on Statin Medication	25	96%	95%	94%
Thrombolytic Therapy Timing[7]	-	-	69%	66%
Venous Thromboembolism Prophylaxis	36	97%	94%	94%
Written Stroke Educational Materials Given	25	100%	86%	88%
Surgical Care Improvement Project				
Appropriate Beta Blocker Usage	122	100%	97%	98%
Appropriate VTP Within 24 Hours	376	98%	98%	98%
Controlled Postoperative Blood Glucose[7]	-	-	97%	97%
Perioperative Temperature Management	462	97%	100%	100%
Prophylactic Antibiotic Selection	356	99%	99%	99%
Prophylactic Antibiotic Selection (Outpatient)	15	20%	97%	98%
Prophylactic Antibiotic Stopped	354	100%	98%	98%
Prophylactic Antibiotic Timing	356	100%	99%	99%
Prophylactic Antibiotic Timing (Outpatient)	41	7%	97%	98%
Urinary Catheter Removal	199	97%	96%	97%
Survey of Patients' Hospital Experiences				
Area Around Room 'Always' Quiet at Night	300+	54%	51%	61%
Doctors 'Always' Communicated Well	300+	80%	77%	82%
Home Recovery Information Given	300+	91%	83%	85%
Hospital Given 9 or 10 on 10 Point Scale	300+	64%	63%	71%
Meds 'Always' Explained Before Given	300+	66%	59%	64%
Nurses 'Always' Communicated Well	300+	78%	75%	79%
Pain 'Always' Well Controlled	300+	72%	67%	71%
Room and Bathroom 'Always' Clean	300+	76%	69%	73%
Timely Help 'Always' Received	300+	63%	61%	68%
Would Definitely Recommend Hospital	300+	61%	65%	71%
Use of Medical Imaging				
Cardiac Imaging Stress Test before Surgery	117	5.1%	5.8%	5.3%
Combination Abdominal CT Scan	373	7.8%	8.2%	10.5%
Combination Brain/Sinus CT Scan[1]	-	-	3.6%	2.7%
Combination Chest CT Scan	138	0.7%	1.3%	2.7%
Follow-up Mammogram/Ultrasound	600	14.7%	13%	8.8%
Lumbar Spine MRI for Low Back Pain[7]	-	-	33.4%	37.2%

Glen Cove Hospital

101 Saint Andrews Lane
Glen Cove, NY 11542
Phone: 516-674-7300
Fax: 516-674-7670
URL: www.northshorelij.com
Type: Acute Care Hospitals
Emergency Services: Yes
Ownership: Voluntary non-profit - Private
Beds: 265

Key Personnel:

Chief of Medical Staff. . . . . David L. Battinelli, MD
CEO/President. . . . . Michael J. Dowling
Pediatric Ambulatory Care . . . . . . James Fagin, MD
Infection Control. . . . . Bruce Farber, MD
Radiology. . . . . Mitchell Goldman, MD
Quality Assurance . . . . Donn Haber
Coronary Care . . . . Kathy Mann, RN
Operating Room. . . . . Linda Olander, RN

Measure	Cases	This Hosp.	State Avg.	U.S. Avg.
Blood Clot Prevention and Treatment				
Anticoagulation Overlap Therapy[2]	47	79%	91%	93%
ICU Venous Thromboembolism Prophylaxis[2]	62	94%	92%	92%
Incidence of Potentially Preventable VTE[2]	20	5%	10%	10%
UFH with Dosages/Platelet Monitoring[1,2]	-	-	92%	97%
Venous Thromboembolism Prophylaxis[2]	265	86%	87%	85%
Warfarin Therapy Discharge Instructions[2]	30	0%	59%	75%
Chest Pain/Possible Heart Attack Care				
Aspirin Given Within 24 Hours of Arrival	28	100%	97%	96%
Fibrinolytic Meds Within 30 Min. of Arrival[7]	-	-	54%	58%
Average Time to ECG (minutes)	29	11	9	7
Average Time to Transfer (minutes)[1]	-	-	78	60
Children's Asthma Care				
Received Home Management Plan of Care	-	-	-	88%
Received Reliever Medication	-	-	-	100%
Received Systemic Corticosteroids	-	-	-	100%
Emergency Department				
Admittance Decision Time (minutes)[2]	787	176	154	98
Head CT Results Within 45 Min. of Arrival[1]	-	-	55%	57%
Patients Who Left ER Before Being Seen	21,833	0%	2%	2%
Time from ER Arrival to Admit. (minutes)[2]	787	346	378	274
Time from ER Arrival to Discharge (minutes)	373	143	156	134
Time in ER Before Being Evaluated (minutes)	397	11	35	26
Time to Pain Meds for Fractures (minutes)	65	46	61	57
Heart Attack Care				
Aspirin Given at Discharge[2]	30	97%	99%	99%
Fibrinolytic Meds Within 30 Min. of Arrival[2,7]	-	-	46%	54%
PCI Within 90 Minutes of Arrival[2,7]	-	-	95%	96%
Statin Prescribed at Discharge[2]	29	90%	98%	98%
Heart Failure Care				
ACE Inhibitor or ARB for LVSD[2]	29	93%	96%	97%
Discharge Instructions Given[2]	120	92%	95%	94%
Evaluation of LVS Function[2]	178	99%	99%	99%
Medicare Spending				
Medicare Spending per Patient (ratio)	-	1.16	0.96	0.98
Pneumonia Care				
Appropriate Initial Antibiotic Given[2]	67	96%	95%	95%
Blood Culture Timing[2]	131	96%	97%	98%
Pregnancy and Delivery Care				
Newborn Deliveries Scheduled Early[7]	-	-	4%	6%
Preventive Care				
Immunization for Influenza[2]	593	96%	88%	90%
Immunization for Pneumonia[2]	821	90%	88%	92%
Stroke Care				
Anticoagulation Therapy for Atrial Fibrillation[1,2]	-	-	96%	95%
Antithrombotic Therapy Timing[2]	55	96%	98%	98%
Assessed for Rehabilitation[2]	59	93%	97%	97%
Discharged on Antithrombotic Therapy[2]	56	86%	99%	99%
Discharged on Statin Medication[2]	42	79%	95%	94%
Thrombolytic Therapy Timing[1,2]	-	-	69%	66%
Venous Thromboembolism Prophylaxis[2]	67	78%	94%	94%
Written Stroke Educational Materials Given[2]	28	18%	86%	88%
Surgical Care Improvement Project				
Appropriate Beta Blocker Usage[2]	72	100%	97%	98%
Appropriate VTP Within 24 Hours[2]	244	99%	98%	98%
Controlled Postoperative Blood Glucose[2,7]	-	-	97%	97%
Perioperative Temperature Management[2]	258	100%	100%	100%
Prophylactic Antibiotic Selection[2]	172	98%	99%	99%
Prophylactic Antibiotic Selection (Outpatient)	50	94%	97%	98%
Prophylactic Antibiotic Stopped[2]	171	99%	98%	98%
Prophylactic Antibiotic Timing[2]	172	99%	99%	99%
Prophylactic Antibiotic Timing (Outpatient)	51	98%	97%	98%
Urinary Catheter Removal[2]	210	97%	96%	97%
Survey of Patients' Hospital Experiences				
Area Around Room 'Always' Quiet at Night	300+	52%	51%	61%
Doctors 'Always' Communicated Well	300+	80%	77%	82%
Home Recovery Information Given	300+	77%	83%	85%
Hospital Given 9 or 10 on 10 Point Scale	300+	70%	63%	71%
Meds 'Always' Explained Before Given	300+	58%	59%	64%
Nurses 'Always' Communicated Well	300+	79%	75%	79%
Pain 'Always' Well Controlled	300+	69%	67%	71%
Room and Bathroom 'Always' Clean	300+	70%	69%	73%
Timely Help 'Always' Received	300+	63%	61%	68%
Would Definitely Recommend Hospital	300+	75%	65%	71%
Use of Medical Imaging				
Cardiac Imaging Stress Test before Surgery[1]	-	-	5.8%	5.3%
Combination Abdominal CT Scan	414	8.5%	8.2%	10.5%
Combination Brain/Sinus CT Scan	492	6.1%	3.6%	2.7%
Combination Chest CT Scan	385	0.3%	1.3%	2.7%
Follow-up Mammogram/Ultrasound	740	13.0%	13%	8.8%
Lumbar Spine MRI for Low Back Pain	91	29.7%	33.4%	37.2%

NOTE: Hospital profiles are in alphabetical order by state, then city, then hospital within the city; Rankings exclude hospitals with less than 25 cases except for patient surveys which excludes hospitals with less than 100 cases; (a) 100-299 cases; (1) The number of cases/patients is too few to report; (2) Data submitted were based on a sample of cases/patients; (3) Results are based on a shorter time period than required; (4) Data suppressed by CMS for one or more quarters; (5) Results are not available for this reporting period; (6) Fewer than 100 patients completed the HCAHPS survey; (7) No cases met the criteria for this measure; (8) The lower limit of the confidence interval cannot be calculated if the number of observed infections equals zero; (9) No data are available from the state/territory for this reporting period; (10) The scores shown reflect fewer than 50 completed surveys; (11) There were discrepancies in the data collection process; (12) This measure does not apply to this hospital for this reporting period; (13) Results cannot be calculated for this reporting period; (14) The results for this state are combined with nearby states to protect confidentiality; Please refer to the User's Guide for a full explanation of data.

Glens Falls Hospital

100 Park Street
Glens Falls, NY 12801
Phone: 518-926-1000
Fax: 518-926-1919
E-mail: mail@glensfallshosp.org
URL: www.glensfallshospital.org
Type: Acute Care Hospitals
Emergency Services: Yes
Ownership: Voluntary non-profit - Private
Beds: 410

Key Personnel:
Coronary Care . . . . Carol Forman
Radiology. . . . . Ed Hanchett
Pediatric Ambulatory Care . . . . . . Guy Lehine, MD
Operating Room. . . . . Nancy Lombard
Chief of Medical Staff . . . . Robert Pringle, MD, FACS
CEO/President. . . . . Dianne Shugrue
Infection Control. . . . . Kathkeen Sposato
Quality Assurance . . . . Phyllis Western

Measure	Cases	This Hosp.	State Avg.	U.S. Avg.
Blood Clot Prevention and Treatment				
Anticoagulation Overlap Therapy[2]	76	100%	91%	93%
ICU Venous Thromboembolism Prophylaxis[2]	56	100%	92%	92%
Incidence of Potentially Preventable VTE[2]	11	0%	10%	10%
UFH with Dosages/Platelet Monitoring[1,2]	-	-	92%	97%
Venous Thromboembolism Prophylaxis[2]	332	95%	87%	85%
Warfarin Therapy Discharge Instructions[2]	50	82%	59%	75%
Chest Pain/Possible Heart Attack Care				
Aspirin Given Within 24 Hours of Arrival	28	96%	97%	96%
Fibrinolytic Meds Within 30 Min. of Arrival[3,7]	-	-	54%	58%
Average Time to ECG (minutes)	28	10	9	7
Average Time to Transfer (minutes)[3,7]	-	-	78	60
Children's Asthma Care				
Received Home Management Plan of Care	-	-	-	88%
Received Reliever Medication	-	-	-	100%
Received Systemic Corticosteroids	-	-	-	100%
Emergency Department				
Admittance Decision Time (minutes)[2]	700	81	154	98
Head CT Results Within 45 Min. of Arrival	20	85%	55%	57%
Patients Who Left ER Before Being Seen	53,621	3%	2%	2%
Time from ER Arrival to Admit. (minutes)[2]	700	281	378	274
Time from ER Arrival to Discharge (minutes)	373	174	156	134
Time in ER Before Being Evaluated (minutes)	438	46	35	26
Time to Pain Meds for Fractures (minutes)	219	57	61	57
Heart Attack Care				
Aspirin Given at Discharge[2]	196	100%	99%	99%
Fibrinolytic Meds Within 30 Min. of Arrival[2,7]	-	-	46%	54%
PCI Within 90 Minutes of Arrival[2]	44	93%	95%	96%
Statin Prescribed at Discharge[2]	194	99%	98%	98%
Heart Failure Care				
ACE Inhibitor or ARB for LVSD[2]	62	95%	96%	97%
Discharge Instructions Given[2]	270	97%	95%	94%
Evaluation of LVS Function[2]	327	100%	99%	99%
Medicare Spending				
Medicare Spending per Patient (ratio)	-	0.95	0.96	0.98
Pneumonia Care				
Appropriate Initial Antibiotic Given[2]	100	96%	95%	95%
Blood Culture Timing[2]	190	98%	97%	98%
Pregnancy and Delivery Care				
Newborn Deliveries Scheduled Early[2]	23	4%	4%	6%
Preventive Care				
Immunization for Influenza[2]	549	95%	88%	90%
Immunization for Pneumonia[2]	738	88%	88%	92%
Stroke Care				
Anticoagulation Therapy for Atrial Fibrillation[2]	15	100%	96%	95%
Antithrombotic Therapy Timing[2]	88	100%	98%	98%
Assessed for Rehabilitation[2]	99	99%	97%	97%
Discharged on Antithrombotic Therapy[2]	93	100%	99%	99%
Discharged on Statin Medication[2]	76	96%	95%	94%
Thrombolytic Therapy Timing[1,2]	-	-	69%	66%
Venous Thromboembolism Prophylaxis[2]	93	96%	94%	94%
Written Stroke Educational Materials Given[2]	48	79%	86%	88%
Surgical Care Improvement Project				
Appropriate Beta Blocker Usage[2]	220	97%	97%	98%
Appropriate VTP Within 24 Hours[2]	468	94%	98%	98%
Controlled Postoperative Blood Glucose[2,7]	-	-	97%	97%
Perioperative Temperature Management[2]	602	100%	100%	100%
Prophylactic Antibiotic Selection[2]	379	99%	99%	99%
Prophylactic Antibiotic Selection (Outpatient)	352	99%	97%	98%
Prophylactic Antibiotic Stopped[2]	376	95%	98%	98%
Prophylactic Antibiotic Timing[2]	379	97%	99%	99%
Prophylactic Antibiotic Timing (Outpatient)	353	97%	97%	98%
Urinary Catheter Removal[2]	149	86%	96%	97%
Survey of Patients' Hospital Experiences				
Area Around Room 'Always' Quiet at Night	300+	49%	51%	61%
Doctors 'Always' Communicated Well	300+	79%	77%	82%
Home Recovery Information Given	300+	88%	83%	85%
Hospital Given 9 or 10 on 10 Point Scale	300+	66%	63%	71%
Meds 'Always' Explained Before Given	300+	64%	59%	64%
Nurses 'Always' Communicated Well	300+	80%	75%	79%
Pain 'Always' Well Controlled	300+	71%	67%	71%
Room and Bathroom 'Always' Clean	300+	77%	69%	73%
Timely Help 'Always' Received	300+	69%	61%	68%
Would Definitely Recommend Hospital	300+	66%	65%	71%
Use of Medical Imaging				
Cardiac Imaging Stress Test before Surgery	531	3.2%	5.8%	5.3%
Combination Abdominal CT Scan	1,559	4.2%	8.2%	10.5%
Combination Brain/Sinus CT Scan	1,101	2.6%	3.6%	2.7%
Combination Chest CT Scan	1,115	0.1%	1.3%	2.7%
Follow-up Mammogram/Ultrasound	1,769	10.1%	13%	8.8%
Lumbar Spine MRI for Low Back Pain[7]	-	-	33.4%	37.2%

Nathan Littauer Hospital

99 East State Street
Gloversville, NY 12078
Phone: 518-725-8621
Fax: 518-773-5757
E-mail: info@nlh.org
URL: www.nlh.org
Type: Acute Care Hospitals
Emergency Services: Yes
Ownership: Voluntary non-profit - Private
Beds: 208

Key Personnel:
Emergency Room . . . . Marie Born, RN
Infection Control. . . . . Melissa Bown, RN
Radiology. . . . . Jerome Brustein, MD
Chief of Medical Staff . . . . George Disney, MD
Operating Room. . . . . John Fox, DDS
Intensive Care Unit. . . . . Nancy Hisert, RN
CEO/President. . . . . Laurence E Kelly
Quality Assurance . . . . Diane Swartz

Measure	Cases	This Hosp.	State Avg.	U.S. Avg.
Blood Clot Prevention and Treatment				
Anticoagulation Overlap Therapy[2]	26	96%	91%	93%
ICU Venous Thromboembolism Prophylaxis[2]	63	98%	92%	92%
Incidence of Potentially Preventable VTE[1,2]	-	-	10%	10%
UFH with Dosages/Platelet Monitoring[1,2]	-	-	92%	97%
Venous Thromboembolism Prophylaxis[2]	234	86%	87%	85%
Warfarin Therapy Discharge Instructions[2]	23	74%	59%	75%
Chest Pain/Possible Heart Attack Care				
Aspirin Given Within 24 Hours of Arrival	70	93%	97%	96%
Fibrinolytic Meds Within 30 Min. of Arrival[1]	-	-	54%	58%
Average Time to ECG (minutes)	71	9	9	7
Average Time to Transfer (minutes)	13	71	78	60
Children's Asthma Care				
Received Home Management Plan of Care	-	-	-	88%
Received Reliever Medication	-	-	-	100%
Received Systemic Corticosteroids	-	-	-	100%
Emergency Department				
Admittance Decision Time (minutes)[2]	468	95	154	98
Head CT Results Within 45 Min. of Arrival[1]	-	-	55%	57%
Patients Who Left ER Before Being Seen	24,235	2%	2%	2%
Time from ER Arrival to Admit. (minutes)[2]	495	310	378	274
Time from ER Arrival to Discharge (minutes)	344	162	156	134
Time in ER Before Being Evaluated (minutes)	372	35	35	26
Time to Pain Meds for Fractures (minutes)	67	72	61	57
Heart Attack Care				
Aspirin Given at Discharge	17	88%	99%	99%
Fibrinolytic Meds Within 30 Min. of Arrival[7]	-	-	46%	54%
PCI Within 90 Minutes of Arrival[7]	-	-	95%	96%
Statin Prescribed at Discharge	17	88%	98%	98%
Heart Failure Care				
ACE Inhibitor or ARB for LVSD	26	100%	96%	97%
Discharge Instructions Given	69	100%	95%	94%
Evaluation of LVS Function	86	92%	99%	99%
Medicare Spending				
Medicare Spending per Patient (ratio)	-	0.87	0.96	0.98
Pneumonia Care				
Appropriate Initial Antibiotic Given	116	91%	95%	95%
Blood Culture Timing	194	96%	97%	98%
Pregnancy and Delivery Care				
Newborn Deliveries Scheduled Early	28	0%	4%	6%
Preventive Care				
Immunization for Influenza[2]	320	91%	88%	90%
Immunization for Pneumonia[2]	437	90%	88%	92%
Stroke Care				
Anticoagulation Therapy for Atrial Fibrillation[1]	-	-	96%	95%
Antithrombotic Therapy Timing	18	94%	98%	98%
Assessed for Rehabilitation	19	89%	97%	97%
Discharged on Antithrombotic Therapy	17	94%	99%	99%
Discharged on Statin Medication	16	81%	95%	94%
Thrombolytic Therapy Timing[1]	-	-	69%	66%
Venous Thromboembolism Prophylaxis	21	90%	94%	94%
Written Stroke Educational Materials Given[1]	-	-	86%	88%
Surgical Care Improvement Project				
Appropriate Beta Blocker Usage	48	100%	97%	98%
Appropriate VTP Within 24 Hours	135	99%	98%	98%
Controlled Postoperative Blood Glucose[7]	-	-	97%	97%
Perioperative Temperature Management	145	100%	100%	100%
Prophylactic Antibiotic Selection	108	97%	99%	99%
Prophylactic Antibiotic Selection (Outpatient)	211	97%	97%	98%
Prophylactic Antibiotic Stopped	108	95%	98%	98%
Prophylactic Antibiotic Timing	108	97%	99%	99%
Prophylactic Antibiotic Timing (Outpatient)	215	98%	97%	98%
Urinary Catheter Removal	100	98%	96%	97%
Survey of Patients' Hospital Experiences				
Area Around Room 'Always' Quiet at Night	300+	57%	51%	61%
Doctors 'Always' Communicated Well	300+	79%	77%	82%
Home Recovery Information Given	300+	86%	83%	85%
Hospital Given 9 or 10 on 10 Point Scale	300+	67%	63%	71%
Meds 'Always' Explained Before Given	300+	65%	59%	64%
Nurses 'Always' Communicated Well	300+	79%	75%	79%
Pain 'Always' Well Controlled	300+	73%	67%	71%
Room and Bathroom 'Always' Clean	300+	77%	69%	73%
Timely Help 'Always' Received	300+	68%	61%	68%
Would Definitely Recommend Hospital	300+	62%	65%	71%
Use of Medical Imaging				
Cardiac Imaging Stress Test before Surgery[1]	-	-	5.8%	5.3%
Combination Abdominal CT Scan	405	7.9%	8.2%	10.5%
Combination Brain/Sinus CT Scan[1]	-	-	3.6%	2.7%
Combination Chest CT Scan	202	4.5%	1.3%	2.7%
Follow-up Mammogram/Ultrasound	698	9.6%	13%	8.8%
Lumbar Spine MRI for Low Back Pain	84	40.5%	33.4%	37.2%

Gouverneur Hospital

77 West Barney Street
Gouverneur, NY 13642
Phone: 315-287-1000
Type: Critical Access Hospitals
Emergency Services: Yes
Ownership: Voluntary non-profit - Private

Measure	Cases	This Hosp.	State Avg.	U.S. Avg.
Blood Clot Prevention and Treatment				
Anticoagulation Overlap Therapy[5]	-	-	91%	93%
ICU Venous Thromboembolism Prophylaxis[5]	-	-	92%	92%
Incidence of Potentially Preventable VTE[5]	-	-	10%	10%
UFH with Dosages/Platelet Monitoring[5]	-	-	92%	97%
Venous Thromboembolism Prophylaxis[5]	-	-	87%	85%
Warfarin Therapy Discharge Instructions[5]	-	-	59%	75%
Chest Pain/Possible Heart Attack Care				
Aspirin Given Within 24 Hours of Arrival	-	-	97%	96%
Fibrinolytic Meds Within 30 Min. of Arrival	-	-	54%	58%
Average Time to ECG (minutes)	-	-	9	7
Average Time to Transfer (minutes)	-	-	78	60
Children's Asthma Care				
Received Home Management Plan of Care	-	-	-	88%
Received Reliever Medication	-	-	-	100%
Received Systemic Corticosteroids	-	-	-	100%

NOTE: Hospital profiles are in alphabetical order by state, then city, then hospital within the city; Rankings exclude hospitals with less than 25 cases except for patient surveys which excludes hospitals with less than 100 cases; (a) 100-299 cases; (1) The number of cases/patients is too few to report; (2) Data submitted were based on a sample of cases/patients; (3) Results are based on a shorter time period than required; (4) Data suppressed by CMS for one or more quarters; (5) Results are not available for this reporting period; (6) Fewer than 100 patients completed the HCAHPS survey; (7) No cases met the criteria for this measure; (8) The lower limit of the confidence interval cannot be calculated if the number of observed infections equals zero; (9) No data are available from the state/territory for this reporting period; (10) The scores shown reflect fewer than 50 completed surveys; (11) There were discrepancies in the data collection process; (12) This measure does not apply to this hospital for this reporting period; (13) Results cannot be calculated for this reporting period; (14) The results for this state are combined with nearby states to protect confidentiality; Please refer to the User's Guide for a full explanation of data.

Measure	Cases	This Hosp.	State Avg.	U.S. Avg.
Emergency Department				
Admittance Decision Time (minutes)[5]	-	-	154	98
Head CT Results Within 45 Min. of Arrival	-	-	55%	57%
Patients Who Left ER Before Being Seen	-	-	2%	2%
Time from ER Arrival to Admit. (minutes)[5]	-	-	378	274
Time from ER Arrival to Discharge (minutes)	-	-	156	134
Time in ER Before Being Evaluated (minutes)	-	-	35	26
Time to Pain Meds for Fractures (minutes)	-	-	61	57
Heart Attack Care				
Aspirin Given at Discharge[5]	-	-	99%	99%
Fibrinolytic Meds Within 30 Min. of Arrival[5]	-	-	46%	54%
PCI Within 90 Minutes of Arrival[5]	-	-	95%	96%
Statin Prescribed at Discharge[5]	-	-	98%	98%
Heart Failure Care				
ACE Inhibitor or ARB for LVSD[5]	-	-	96%	97%
Discharge Instructions Given[5]	-	-	95%	94%
Evaluation of LVS Function[5]	-	-	99%	99%
Medicare Spending				
Medicare Spending per Patient (ratio)	-	-	0.96	0.98
Pneumonia Care				
Appropriate Initial Antibiotic Given[5]	-	-	95%	95%
Blood Culture Timing[5]	-	-	97%	98%
Pregnancy and Delivery Care				
Newborn Deliveries Scheduled Early[5]	-	-	4%	6%
Preventive Care				
Immunization for Influenza[5]	-	-	88%	90%
Immunization for Pneumonia[5]	-	-	88%	92%
Stroke Care				
Anticoagulation Therapy for Atrial Fibrillation[5]	-	-	96%	95%
Antithrombotic Therapy Timing[5]	-	-	98%	98%
Assessed for Rehabilitation[5]	-	-	97%	97%
Discharged on Antithrombotic Therapy[5]	-	-	99%	99%
Discharged on Statin Medication[5]	-	-	95%	94%
Thrombolytic Therapy Timing[5]	-	-	69%	66%
Venous Thromboembolism Prophylaxis[5]	-	-	94%	94%
Written Stroke Educational Materials Given[5]	-	-	86%	88%
Surgical Care Improvement Project				
Appropriate Beta Blocker Usage[5]	-	-	97%	98%
Appropriate VTP Within 24 Hours[5]	-	-	98%	98%
Controlled Postoperative Blood Glucose[5]	-	-	97%	97%
Perioperative Temperature Management[5]	-	-	100%	100%
Prophylactic Antibiotic Selection[5]	-	-	99%	99%
Prophylactic Antibiotic Selection (Outpatient)	-	-	97%	98%
Prophylactic Antibiotic Stopped[5]	-	-	98%	98%
Prophylactic Antibiotic Timing[5]	-	-	99%	99%
Prophylactic Antibiotic Timing (Outpatient)	-	-	97%	98%
Urinary Catheter Removal[5]	-	-	96%	97%
Survey of Patients' Hospital Experiences				
Area Around Room 'Always' Quiet at Night	(a)	68%	51%	61%
Doctors 'Always' Communicated Well	(a)	87%	77%	82%
Home Recovery Information Given	(a)	85%	83%	85%
Hospital Given 9 or 10 on 10 Point Scale	(a)	64%	63%	71%
Meds 'Always' Explained Before Given	(a)	52%	59%	64%
Nurses 'Always' Communicated Well	(a)	71%	75%	79%
Pain 'Always' Well Controlled	(a)	66%	67%	71%
Room and Bathroom 'Always' Clean	(a)	87%	69%	73%
Timely Help 'Always' Received	(a)	69%	61%	68%
Would Definitely Recommend Hospital	(a)	66%	65%	71%
Use of Medical Imaging				
Cardiac Imaging Stress Test before Surgery	-	-	5.8%	5.3%
Combination Abdominal CT Scan	-	-	8.2%	10.5%
Combination Brain/Sinus CT Scan	-	-	3.6%	2.7%
Combination Chest CT Scan	-	-	1.3%	2.7%
Follow-up Mammogram/Ultrasound	-	-	13%	8.8%
Lumbar Spine MRI for Low Back Pain	-	-	33.4%	37.2%

TLC Health Network

100 Memorial Drive
Gowanda, NY 14070
E-mail: wssmith@kaleidahealth.org
Phone: 716-532-3377
Fax: 716-532-3774
Type: Acute Care Hospitals
Ownership: Voluntary non-profit - Private
Emergency Services: Yes
Beds: 65

Key Personnel:
CEO/President. . . . . James H Campbell
Radiology. Noel Chiantella
Cardiac Laboratory. . . . . Ellen Franz, RN
Infection Control. . . . . Ellen Franz, RN
Operating Room. . . . . Cindy Lille
Chief of Medical Staff. . . . . Ramiah Sathananthan, MD
Quality Assurance . . . . Karen Volk, RN

Measure	Cases	This Hosp.	State Avg.	U.S. Avg.
Blood Clot Prevention and Treatment				
Anticoagulation Overlap Therapy[1,2]	-	-	91%	93%
ICU Venous Thromboembolism Prophylaxis[2]	21	95%	92%	92%
Incidence of Potentially Preventable VTE[1,2]	-	-	10%	10%
UFH with Dosages/Platelet Monitoring[1,2]	-	-	92%	97%
Venous Thromboembolism Prophylaxis[2]	123	75%	87%	85%
Warfarin Therapy Discharge Instructions[1,2]	-	-	59%	75%
Chest Pain/Possible Heart Attack Care				
Aspirin Given Within 24 Hours of Arrival	43	100%	97%	96%
Fibrinolytic Meds Within 30 Min. of Arrival[1]	-	-	54%	58%
Average Time to ECG (minutes)	44	7	9	7
Average Time to Transfer (minutes)[7]	-	-	78	60
Children's Asthma Care				
Received Home Management Plan of Care	-	-	-	88%
Received Reliever Medication	-	-	-	100%
Received Systemic Corticosteroids	-	-	-	100%
Emergency Department				
Admittance Decision Time (minutes)[2]	289	70	154	98
Head CT Results Within 45 Min. of Arrival[1]	-	-	55%	57%
Patients Who Left ER Before Being Seen	11,190	2%	2%	2%
Time from ER Arrival to Admit. (minutes)[2]	299	285	378	274
Time from ER Arrival to Discharge (minutes)	366	153	156	134
Time in ER Before Being Evaluated (minutes)	403	31	35	26
Time to Pain Meds for Fractures (minutes)	58	46	61	57
Heart Attack Care				
Aspirin Given at Discharge[1,3]	-	-	99%	99%
Fibrinolytic Meds Within 30 Min. of Arrival[3,7]	-	-	46%	54%
PCI Within 90 Minutes of Arrival[3,7]	-	-	95%	96%
Statin Prescribed at Discharge[1,3]	-	-	98%	98%
Heart Failure Care				
ACE Inhibitor or ARB for LVSD[1]	-	-	96%	97%
Discharge Instructions Given	36	100%	95%	94%
Evaluation of LVS Function	47	94%	99%	99%
Medicare Spending				
Medicare Spending per Patient (ratio)	-	1.03	0.96	0.98
Pneumonia Care				
Appropriate Initial Antibiotic Given	42	81%	95%	95%
Blood Culture Timing	66	98%	97%	98%
Pregnancy and Delivery Care				
Newborn Deliveries Scheduled Early[7]	-	-	4%	6%
Preventive Care				
Immunization for Influenza[2]	306	67%	88%	90%
Immunization for Pneumonia[2]	318	85%	88%	92%
Stroke Care				
Anticoagulation Therapy for Atrial Fibrillation[1]	-	-	96%	95%
Antithrombotic Therapy Timing[1]	-	-	98%	98%
Assessed for Rehabilitation[1]	-	-	97%	97%
Discharged on Antithrombotic Therapy[1]	-	-	99%	99%
Discharged on Statin Medication[1]	-	-	95%	94%
Thrombolytic Therapy Timing[7]	-	-	69%	66%
Venous Thromboembolism Prophylaxis[1]	-	-	94%	94%
Written Stroke Educational Materials Given[1]	-	-	86%	88%
Surgical Care Improvement Project				
Appropriate Beta Blocker Usage	36	97%	97%	98%
Appropriate VTP Within 24 Hours	117	99%	98%	98%
Controlled Postoperative Blood Glucose[7]	-	-	97%	97%
Perioperative Temperature Management	122	96%	100%	100%
Prophylactic Antibiotic Selection	102	97%	99%	99%
Prophylactic Antibiotic Selection (Outpatient)[1]	-	-	97%	98%
Prophylactic Antibiotic Stopped	102	95%	98%	98%
Prophylactic Antibiotic Timing	102	93%	99%	99%
Prophylactic Antibiotic Timing (Outpatient)[1]	-	-	97%	98%
Urinary Catheter Removal	51	90%	96%	97%
Survey of Patients' Hospital Experiences				
Area Around Room 'Always' Quiet at Night	(a)	42%	51%	61%
Doctors 'Always' Communicated Well	(a)	74%	77%	82%
Home Recovery Information Given	(a)	90%	83%	85%
Hospital Given 9 or 10 on 10 Point Scale	(a)	55%	63%	71%
Meds 'Always' Explained Before Given	(a)	61%	59%	64%
Nurses 'Always' Communicated Well	(a)	71%	75%	79%
Pain 'Always' Well Controlled	(a)	66%	67%	71%
Room and Bathroom 'Always' Clean	(a)	67%	69%	73%
Timely Help 'Always' Received	(a)	66%	61%	68%
Would Definitely Recommend Hospital	(a)	56%	65%	71%
Use of Medical Imaging				
Cardiac Imaging Stress Test before Surgery	121	0.8%	5.8%	5.3%
Combination Abdominal CT Scan	195	8.2%	8.2%	10.5%
Combination Brain/Sinus CT Scan[1]	-	-	3.6%	2.7%
Combination Chest CT Scan	92	3.3%	1.3%	2.7%
Follow-up Mammogram/Ultrasound	315	5.4%	13%	8.8%
Lumbar Spine MRI for Low Back Pain[7]	-	-	33.4%	37.2%

Eastern Long Island Hospital

201 Manor Place
Greenport, NY 11944
URL: www.elih.org
Phone: 631-477-1000
Fax: 631-477-1746
Type: Acute Care Hospitals
Ownership: Voluntary non-profit - Private
Emergency Services: Yes
Beds: 90

Key Personnel:
Anesthesiology. . . . . Frank J Adipietro, MD
Chief of Medical Staff. . . . . Frank J Adipietro, MD
CEO/President. . . . . Paul J Connor III, III
Quality Assurance . . . . Tara Kraemer
Radiology. . . . . Anthony Mitarotondo
Operating Room. . . . . Joanne Rutkowsi

Measure	Cases	This Hosp.	State Avg.	U.S. Avg.
Blood Clot Prevention and Treatment				
Anticoagulation Overlap Therapy[1,2]	-	-	91%	93%
ICU Venous Thromboembolism Prophylaxis[2]	12	75%	92%	92%
Incidence of Potentially Preventable VTE[1,2]	-	-	10%	10%
UFH with Dosages/Platelet Monitoring[1,2]	-	-	92%	97%
Venous Thromboembolism Prophylaxis[2]	177	55%	87%	85%
Warfarin Therapy Discharge Instructions[1,2]	-	-	59%	75%
Chest Pain/Possible Heart Attack Care				
Aspirin Given Within 24 Hours of Arrival	13	100%	97%	96%
Fibrinolytic Meds Within 30 Min. of Arrival[1,3]	-	-	54%	58%
Average Time to ECG (minutes)	14	6	9	7
Average Time to Transfer (minutes)[1,3]	-	-	78	60
Children's Asthma Care				
Received Home Management Plan of Care	-	-	-	88%
Received Reliever Medication	-	-	-	100%
Received Systemic Corticosteroids	-	-	-	100%
Emergency Department				
Admittance Decision Time (minutes)[2]	203	83	154	98
Head CT Results Within 45 Min. of Arrival[1]	-	-	55%	57%
Patients Who Left ER Before Being Seen	9,264	1%	2%	2%
Time from ER Arrival to Admit. (minutes)[2]	225	237	378	274
Time from ER Arrival to Discharge (minutes)	317	91	156	134
Time in ER Before Being Evaluated (minutes)	396	20	35	26
Time to Pain Meds for Fractures (minutes)	13	56	61	57
Heart Attack Care				
Aspirin Given at Discharge[1]	-	-	99%	99%
Fibrinolytic Meds Within 30 Min. of Arrival[1]	-	-	46%	54%
PCI Within 90 Minutes of Arrival[7]	-	-	95%	96%
Statin Prescribed at Discharge[1]	-	-	98%	98%
Heart Failure Care				
ACE Inhibitor or ARB for LVSD[1]	-	-	96%	97%
Discharge Instructions Given	46	93%	95%	94%
Evaluation of LVS Function	59	98%	99%	99%
Medicare Spending				
Medicare Spending per Patient (ratio)	-	0.90	0.96	0.98
Pneumonia Care				
Appropriate Initial Antibiotic Given	27	89%	95%	95%
Blood Culture Timing	59	97%	97%	98%
Pregnancy and Delivery Care				
Newborn Deliveries Scheduled Early[7]	-	-	4%	6%
Preventive Care				
Immunization for Influenza[2]	313	95%	88%	90%
Immunization for Pneumonia[2]	266	97%	88%	92%
Stroke Care				

NOTE: Hospital profiles are in alphabetical order by state, then city, then hospital within the city; Rankings exclude hospitals with less than 25 cases except for patient surveys which excludes hospitals with less than 100 cases; (a) 100-299 cases; (1) The number of cases/patients is too few to report; (2) Data submitted were based on a sample of cases/patients; (3) Results are based on a shorter time period than required; (4) Data suppressed by CMS for one or more quarters; (5) Results are not available for this reporting period; (6) Fewer than 100 patients completed the HCAHPS survey; (7) No cases met the criteria for this measure; (8) The lower limit of the confidence interval cannot be calculated if the number of observed infections equals zero; (9) No data are available from the state/territory for this reporting period; (10) The scores shown reflect fewer than 50 completed surveys; (11) There were discrepancies in the data collection process; (12) This measure does not apply to this hospital for this reporting period; (13) Results cannot be calculated for this reporting period; (14) The results for this state are combined with nearby states to protect confidentiality; Please refer to the User's Guide for a full explanation of data.

Measure	Cases	This Hosp.	State Avg.	U.S. Avg.
Anticoagulation Therapy for Atrial Fibrillation[7]	-	-	96%	95%
Antithrombotic Therapy Timing[1]	-	-	98%	98%
Assessed for Rehabilitation[1]	-	-	97%	97%
Discharged on Antithrombotic Therapy[1]	-	-	99%	99%
Discharged on Statin Medication[1]	-	-	95%	94%
Thrombolytic Therapy Timing[7]	-	-	69%	66%
Venous Thromboembolism Prophylaxis[1]	-	-	94%	94%
Written Stroke Educational Materials Given[1]	-	-	86%	88%
Surgical Care Improvement Project				
Appropriate Beta Blocker Usage	17	88%	97%	98%
Appropriate VTP Within 24 Hours	39	95%	98%	98%
Controlled Postoperative Blood Glucose[7]	-	-	97%	97%
Perioperative Temperature Management	40	100%	100%	100%
Prophylactic Antibiotic Selection	22	91%	99%	99%
Prophylactic Antibiotic Selection (Outpatient)	17	100%	97%	98%
Prophylactic Antibiotic Stopped	22	77%	98%	98%
Prophylactic Antibiotic Timing	22	100%	99%	99%
Prophylactic Antibiotic Timing (Outpatient)	17	100%	97%	98%
Urinary Catheter Removal	32	84%	96%	97%
Survey of Patients' Hospital Experiences				
Area Around Room 'Always' Quiet at Night	300+	53%	51%	61%
Doctors 'Always' Communicated Well	300+	80%	77%	82%
Home Recovery Information Given	300+	85%	83%	85%
Hospital Given 9 or 10 on 10 Point Scale	300+	76%	63%	71%
Meds 'Always' Explained Before Given	300+	64%	59%	64%
Nurses 'Always' Communicated Well	300+	81%	75%	79%
Pain 'Always' Well Controlled	300+	68%	67%	71%
Room and Bathroom 'Always' Clean	300+	77%	69%	73%
Timely Help 'Always' Received	300+	68%	61%	68%
Would Definitely Recommend Hospital	300+	83%	65%	71%
Use of Medical Imaging				
Cardiac Imaging Stress Test before Surgery[7]	-	-	5.8%	5.3%
Combination Abdominal CT Scan	264	15.5%	8.2%	10.5%
Combination Brain/Sinus CT Scan[1]	-	-	3.6%	2.7%
Combination Chest CT Scan	193	0.5%	1.3%	2.7%
Follow-up Mammogram/Ultrasound	320	18.8%	13%	8.8%
Lumbar Spine MRI for Low Back Pain	52	36.5%	33.4%	37.2%

Community Memorial Hospital

150 Broad Street
Hamilton, NY 13346
Phone: 315-824-1100
Fax: 315-824-3182
URL: www.communitymemorial.org
Type: Acute Care Hospitals
Emergency Services: Yes
Ownership: Voluntary non-profit - Private
Beds: 88

Key Personnel:

Cardiology . . . . Raymond Carlson
CEO/President . . . . Sean Fadale
Pediatrics . . . . Jennifer Meyers
Anesthesiology . . . . David Rebuck
Radiology . . . . David Wellenstein

Measure	Cases	This Hosp.	State Avg.	U.S. Avg.
Blood Clot Prevention and Treatment				
Anticoagulation Overlap Therapy[1,2]	-	-	91%	93%
ICU Venous Thromboembolism Prophylaxis[2]	50	98%	92%	92%
Incidence of Potentially Preventable VTE[1,2]	-	-	10%	10%
UFH with Dosages/Platelet Monitoring[1,2]	-	-	92%	97%
Venous Thromboembolism Prophylaxis[2]	211	94%	87%	85%
Warfarin Therapy Discharge Instructions[1,2]	-	-	59%	75%
Chest Pain/Possible Heart Attack Care				
Aspirin Given Within 24 Hours of Arrival	29	100%	97%	96%
Fibrinolytic Meds Within 30 Min. of Arrival[1]	-	-	54%	58%
Average Time to ECG (minutes)	31	4	9	7
Average Time to Transfer (minutes)[7]	-	-	78	60
Children's Asthma Care				
Received Home Management Plan of Care	-	-	-	88%
Received Reliever Medication	-	-	-	100%
Received Systemic Corticosteroids	-	-	-	100%
Emergency Department				
Admittance Decision Time (minutes)[2]	547	140	154	98
Head CT Results Within 45 Min. of Arrival[1,3]	-	-	55%	57%
Patients Who Left ER Before Being Seen	10,293	2%	2%	2%
Time from ER Arrival to Admit. (minutes)[2]	572	286	378	274
Time from ER Arrival to Discharge (minutes)	877	100	156	134
Time in ER Before Being Evaluated (minutes)	972	31	35	26
Time to Pain Meds for Fractures (minutes)	74	52	61	57
Heart Attack Care				
Aspirin Given at Discharge[1,3]	-	-	99%	99%
Fibrinolytic Meds Within 30 Min. of Arrival[3,7]	-	-	46%	54%
PCI Within 90 Minutes of Arrival[3,7]	-	-	95%	96%
Statin Prescribed at Discharge[1,3]	-	-	98%	98%
Heart Failure Care				
ACE Inhibitor or ARB for LVSD[1]	-	-	96%	97%
Discharge Instructions Given	21	95%	95%	94%
Evaluation of LVS Function	27	100%	99%	99%
Medicare Spending				
Medicare Spending per Patient (ratio)	-	0.84	0.96	0.98
Pneumonia Care				
Appropriate Initial Antibiotic Given	53	92%	95%	95%
Blood Culture Timing	60	93%	97%	98%
Pregnancy and Delivery Care				
Newborn Deliveries Scheduled Early[7]	-	-	4%	6%
Preventive Care				
Immunization for Influenza[2]	759	99%	88%	90%
Immunization for Pneumonia[2]	1,032	94%	88%	92%
Stroke Care				
Anticoagulation Therapy for Atrial Fibrillation[3,7]	-	-	96%	95%
Antithrombotic Therapy Timing[1,3]	-	-	98%	98%
Assessed for Rehabilitation[1,3]	-	-	97%	97%
Discharged on Antithrombotic Therapy[1,3]	-	-	99%	99%
Discharged on Statin Medication[1,3]	-	-	95%	94%
Thrombolytic Therapy Timing[1,3]	-	-	69%	66%
Venous Thromboembolism Prophylaxis[1,3]	-	-	94%	94%
Written Stroke Educational Materials Given[1,3]	-	-	86%	88%
Surgical Care Improvement Project				
Appropriate Beta Blocker Usage	169	100%	97%	98%
Appropriate VTP Within 24 Hours	300	100%	98%	98%
Controlled Postoperative Blood Glucose[7]	-	-	97%	97%
Perioperative Temperature Management	545	100%	100%	100%
Prophylactic Antibiotic Selection	460	100%	99%	99%
Prophylactic Antibiotic Selection (Outpatient)	39	97%	97%	98%
Prophylactic Antibiotic Stopped	456	100%	98%	98%
Prophylactic Antibiotic Timing	461	99%	99%	99%
Prophylactic Antibiotic Timing (Outpatient)	40	95%	97%	98%
Urinary Catheter Removal	13	100%	96%	97%
Survey of Patients' Hospital Experiences				
Area Around Room 'Always' Quiet at Night	300+	65%	51%	61%
Doctors 'Always' Communicated Well	300+	85%	77%	82%
Home Recovery Information Given	300+	90%	83%	85%
Hospital Given 9 or 10 on 10 Point Scale	300+	82%	63%	71%
Meds 'Always' Explained Before Given	300+	68%	59%	64%
Nurses 'Always' Communicated Well	300+	85%	75%	79%
Pain 'Always' Well Controlled	300+	76%	67%	71%
Room and Bathroom 'Always' Clean	300+	83%	69%	73%
Timely Help 'Always' Received	300+	73%	61%	68%
Would Definitely Recommend Hospital	300+	81%	65%	71%
Use of Medical Imaging				
Cardiac Imaging Stress Test before Surgery	73	0.0%	5.8%	5.3%
Combination Abdominal CT Scan	130	14.6%	8.2%	10.5%
Combination Brain/Sinus CT Scan	131	0.0%	3.6%	2.7%
Combination Chest CT Scan	87	6.9%	1.3%	2.7%
Follow-up Mammogram/Ultrasound	276	1.1%	13%	8.8%
Lumbar Spine MRI for Low Back Pain[1]	-	-	33.4%	37.2%

Catskill Regional Medical Center

68 Harris Bushville Road
Harris, NY 12742
Phone: 845-794-3300
Fax: 845-794-3240
URL: www.crmcny.org
Type: Acute Care Hospitals
Emergency Services: Yes
Ownership: Voluntary non-profit - Private
Beds: 263

Key Personnel:

Quality Assurance . . . . Debra DeJesus
CEO/President . . . . Gerard J. Galarneau, MD
Chief of Medical Staff . . . . Gerard J. Galarneau, MD
Pediatric In-Patient Care . . . . Amarjit Gill, MD
Radiology . . . . George Osmur
Operating Room . . . . Dotty Schultz, RN
Chairman/CEO . . . . Darrell Supak

Measure	Cases	This Hosp.	State Avg.	U.S. Avg.
Blood Clot Prevention and Treatment				
Anticoagulation Overlap Therapy[2]	22	100%	91%	93%
ICU Venous Thromboembolism Prophylaxis[2]	14	79%	92%	92%
Incidence of Potentially Preventable VTE[1,2]	-	-	10%	10%
UFH with Dosages/Platelet Monitoring[2]	11	100%	92%	97%
Venous Thromboembolism Prophylaxis[2]	318	89%	87%	85%
Warfarin Therapy Discharge Instructions[2]	15	67%	59%	75%
Chest Pain/Possible Heart Attack Care				
Aspirin Given Within 24 Hours of Arrival	20	100%	97%	96%
Fibrinolytic Meds Within 30 Min. of Arrival[7]	-	-	54%	58%
Average Time to ECG (minutes)	20	10	9	7
Average Time to Transfer (minutes)[1]	-	-	78	60
Children's Asthma Care				
Received Home Management Plan of Care	-	-	-	88%
Received Reliever Medication	-	-	-	100%
Received Systemic Corticosteroids	-	-	-	100%
Emergency Department				
Admittance Decision Time (minutes)[2]	373	122	154	98
Head CT Results Within 45 Min. of Arrival[1]	-	-	55%	57%
Patients Who Left ER Before Being Seen	28,759	1%	2%	2%
Time from ER Arrival to Admit. (minutes)[2]	374	317	378	274
Time from ER Arrival to Discharge (minutes)	368	125	156	134
Time in ER Before Being Evaluated (minutes)	397	16	35	26
Time to Pain Meds for Fractures (minutes)	102	46	61	57
Heart Attack Care				
Aspirin Given at Discharge	22	100%	99%	99%
Fibrinolytic Meds Within 30 Min. of Arrival[7]	-	-	46%	54%
PCI Within 90 Minutes of Arrival[7]	-	-	95%	96%
Statin Prescribed at Discharge	20	95%	98%	98%
Heart Failure Care				
ACE Inhibitor or ARB for LVSD	24	83%	96%	97%
Discharge Instructions Given	73	100%	95%	94%
Evaluation of LVS Function	122	97%	99%	99%
Medicare Spending				
Medicare Spending per Patient (ratio)	-	1.04	0.96	0.98
Pneumonia Care				
Appropriate Initial Antibiotic Given	77	100%	95%	95%
Blood Culture Timing	216	99%	97%	98%
Pregnancy and Delivery Care				
Newborn Deliveries Scheduled Early[2]	28	7%	4%	6%
Preventive Care				
Immunization for Influenza[2]	386	94%	88%	90%
Immunization for Pneumonia[2]	412	90%	88%	92%
Stroke Care				
Anticoagulation Therapy for Atrial Fibrillation[1]	-	-	96%	95%
Antithrombotic Therapy Timing	27	96%	98%	98%
Assessed for Rehabilitation	28	96%	97%	97%
Discharged on Antithrombotic Therapy	27	93%	99%	99%
Discharged on Statin Medication	21	86%	95%	94%
Thrombolytic Therapy Timing[1]	-	-	69%	66%
Venous Thromboembolism Prophylaxis	31	94%	94%	94%
Written Stroke Educational Materials Given	15	67%	86%	88%
Surgical Care Improvement Project				
Appropriate Beta Blocker Usage	32	91%	97%	98%
Appropriate VTP Within 24 Hours	86	98%	98%	98%
Controlled Postoperative Blood Glucose[7]	-	-	97%	97%
Perioperative Temperature Management	104	99%	100%	100%
Prophylactic Antibiotic Selection	70	99%	99%	99%
Prophylactic Antibiotic Selection (Outpatient)	63	90%	97%	98%
Prophylactic Antibiotic Stopped	70	99%	98%	98%
Prophylactic Antibiotic Timing	70	100%	99%	99%
Prophylactic Antibiotic Timing (Outpatient)	63	97%	97%	98%
Urinary Catheter Removal	39	87%	96%	97%
Survey of Patients' Hospital Experiences				
Area Around Room 'Always' Quiet at Night	300+	47%	51%	61%
Doctors 'Always' Communicated Well	300+	78%	77%	82%
Home Recovery Information Given	300+	86%	83%	85%
Hospital Given 9 or 10 on 10 Point Scale	300+	54%	63%	71%
Meds 'Always' Explained Before Given	300+	60%	59%	64%
Nurses 'Always' Communicated Well	300+	73%	75%	79%
Pain 'Always' Well Controlled	300+	65%	67%	71%

NOTE: Hospital profiles are in alphabetical order by state, then city, then hospital within the city; Rankings exclude hospitals with less than 25 cases except for patient surveys which excludes hospitals with less than 100 cases; (a) 100-299 cases; (1) The number of cases/patients is too few to report; (2) Data submitted were based on a sample of cases/patients; (3) Results are based on a shorter time period than required; (4) Data suppressed by CMS for one or more quarters; (5) Results are not available for this reporting period; (6) Fewer than 100 patients completed the HCAHPS survey; (7) No cases met the criteria for this measure; (8) The lower limit of the confidence interval cannot be calculated if the number of observed infections equals zero; (9) No data are available from the state/territory for this reporting period; (10) The scores shown reflect fewer than 50 completed surveys; (11) There were discrepancies in the data collection process; (12) This measure does not apply to this hospital for this reporting period; (13) Results cannot be calculated for this reporting period; (14) The results for this state are combined with nearby states to protect confidentiality; Please refer to the User's Guide for a full explanation of data.

Measure	Cases	This Hosp.	State Avg.	U.S. Avg.
Room and Bathroom 'Always' Clean	300+	55%	69%	73%
Timely Help 'Always' Received	300+	57%	61%	68%
Would Definitely Recommend Hospital	300+	51%	65%	71%
Use of Medical Imaging				
Cardiac Imaging Stress Test before Surgery	106	5.7%	5.8%	5.3%
Combination Abdominal CT Scan	471	3.4%	8.2%	10.5%
Combination Brain/Sinus CT Scan[1]	-	-	3.6%	2.7%
Combination Chest CT Scan	231	0.9%	1.3%	2.7%
Follow-up Mammogram/Ultrasound	262	9.2%	13%	8.8%
Lumbar Spine MRI for Low Back Pain[1]	-	-	33.4%	37.2%

Saint James Mercy Hospital

411 Canisteo Street
Hornell, NY 14843
Phone: 607-324-8000
Fax: 607-324-8115
E-mail: info@stjamesmercy.org
URL: www.stjamesmercy.org
Type: Acute Care Hospitals
Emergency Services: Yes
Ownership: Voluntary non-profit - Church
Beds: 297

Key Personnel:
Chief of Medical Staff.......... John Carroll, MD
Operating Room............. Mary Jo Foreman
Chair/CEO.............. Mary Fran Wegman, Sr, RSM
Quality Assurance........... Linda Henshaw
Surgery.................... Gary Jones
Radiology.................. Amanda Kula
Patient Relations............ Kim Meacham
CEO/President............... Jennifer L. Sullivan

Measure	Cases	This Hosp.	State Avg.	U.S. Avg.
Blood Clot Prevention and Treatment				
Anticoagulation Overlap Therapy[2]	13	100%	91%	93%
ICU Venous Thromboembolism Prophylaxis[2]	46	93%	92%	92%
Incidence of Potentially Preventable VTE[1,2]	-	-	10%	10%
UFH with Dosages/Platelet Monitoring[1,2]	-	-	92%	97%
Venous Thromboembolism Prophylaxis[2]	92	97%	87%	85%
Warfarin Therapy Discharge Instructions[1,2]	-	-	59%	75%
Chest Pain/Possible Heart Attack Care				
Aspirin Given Within 24 Hours of Arrival	58	98%	97%	96%
Fibrinolytic Meds Within 30 Min. of Arrival[1]	-	-	54%	58%
Average Time to ECG (minutes)	61	4	9	7
Average Time to Transfer (minutes)[7]	-	-	78	60
Children's Asthma Care				
Received Home Management Plan of Care	-	-	-	88%
Received Reliever Medication	-	-	-	100%
Received Systemic Corticosteroids	-	-	-	100%
Emergency Department				
Admittance Decision Time (minutes)[2]	304	82	154	98
Head CT Results Within 45 Min. of Arrival[1]	-	-	55%	57%
Patients Who Left ER Before Being Seen	18,031	1%	2%	2%
Time from ER Arrival to Admit. (minutes)[2]	318	242	378	274
Time from ER Arrival to Discharge (minutes)	386	103	156	134
Time in ER Before Being Evaluated (minutes)	406	22	35	26
Time to Pain Meds for Fractures (minutes)	53	31	61	57
Heart Attack Care				
Aspirin Given at Discharge[1]	-	-	99%	99%
Fibrinolytic Meds Within 30 Min. of Arrival[7]	-	-	46%	54%
PCI Within 90 Minutes of Arrival[7]	-	-	95%	96%
Statin Prescribed at Discharge	11	91%	98%	98%
Heart Failure Care				
ACE Inhibitor or ARB for LVSD[1]	-	-	96%	97%
Discharge Instructions Given	19	95%	95%	94%
Evaluation of LVS Function	25	100%	99%	99%
Medicare Spending				
Medicare Spending per Patient (ratio)	-	0.79	0.96	0.98
Pneumonia Care				
Appropriate Initial Antibiotic Given	29	97%	95%	95%
Blood Culture Timing	79	97%	97%	98%
Pregnancy and Delivery Care				
Newborn Deliveries Scheduled Early	15	0%	4%	6%
Preventive Care				
Immunization for Influenza[2]	257	100%	88%	90%
Immunization for Pneumonia[2]	280	100%	88%	92%
Stroke Care				
Anticoagulation Therapy for Atrial Fibrillation[1]	-	-	96%	95%
Antithrombotic Therapy Timing[1]	-	-	98%	98%
Assessed for Rehabilitation[1]	-	-	97%	97%
Discharged on Antithrombotic Therapy[1]	-	-	99%	99%
Discharged on Statin Medication[1]	-	-	95%	94%
Thrombolytic Therapy Timing[7]	-	-	69%	66%
Venous Thromboembolism Prophylaxis[1]	-	-	94%	94%
Written Stroke Educational Materials Given[1]	-	-	86%	88%
Surgical Care Improvement Project				
Appropriate Beta Blocker Usage	24	100%	97%	98%
Appropriate VTP Within 24 Hours	101	97%	98%	98%
Controlled Postoperative Blood Glucose[7]	-	-	97%	97%
Perioperative Temperature Management	108	100%	100%	100%
Prophylactic Antibiotic Selection	71	99%	99%	99%
Prophylactic Antibiotic Selection (Outpatient)[1]	-	-	97%	98%
Prophylactic Antibiotic Stopped	71	93%	98%	98%
Prophylactic Antibiotic Timing	71	100%	99%	99%
Prophylactic Antibiotic Timing (Outpatient)[1]	-	-	97%	98%
Urinary Catheter Removal	41	98%	96%	97%
Survey of Patients' Hospital Experiences				
Area Around Room 'Always' Quiet at Night	300+	59%	51%	61%
Doctors 'Always' Communicated Well	300+	75%	77%	82%
Home Recovery Information Given	300+	90%	83%	85%
Hospital Given 9 or 10 on 10 Point Scale	300+	59%	63%	71%
Meds 'Always' Explained Before Given	300+	61%	59%	64%
Nurses 'Always' Communicated Well	300+	77%	75%	79%
Pain 'Always' Well Controlled	300+	67%	67%	71%
Room and Bathroom 'Always' Clean	300+	66%	69%	73%
Timely Help 'Always' Received	300+	73%	61%	68%
Would Definitely Recommend Hospital	300+	55%	65%	71%
Use of Medical Imaging				
Cardiac Imaging Stress Test before Surgery	64	3.1%	5.8%	5.3%
Combination Abdominal CT Scan	275	21.5%	8.2%	10.5%
Combination Brain/Sinus CT Scan[1]	-	-	3.6%	2.7%
Combination Chest CT Scan	151	0.7%	1.3%	2.7%
Follow-up Mammogram/Ultrasound	260	8.5%	13%	8.8%
Lumbar Spine MRI for Low Back Pain[7]	-	-	33.4%	37.2%

Columbia Memorial Hospital

71 Prospect Avenue
Hudson, NY 12534
Phone: 518-828-7601
Fax: 518-828-8243
E-mail: info@columbiamemorial.com
URL: www.columbiamemorial.com
Type: Acute Care Hospitals
Emergency Services: Yes
Ownership: Voluntary non-profit - Private
Beds: 103

Key Personnel:
Emergency Room............ Barbara Brady, RN
Operating Room............ Barbara Brady, MD
Cardiac Laboratory.......... H L Clinton
Pediatric In-Patient Care....... Sara Friess
Radiology.................. Tariq Gill
Infection Control............. Sherri Meyer, MD
CEO/President.............. Brian Rogoz
Intensive Care Unit........... Donald Tessitore

Measure	Cases	This Hosp.	State Avg.	U.S. Avg.
Blood Clot Prevention and Treatment				
Anticoagulation Overlap Therapy[2]	41	98%	91%	93%
ICU Venous Thromboembolism Prophylaxis[2]	72	100%	92%	92%
Incidence of Potentially Preventable VTE[1,2]	-	-	10%	10%
UFH with Dosages/Platelet Monitoring[2]	15	100%	92%	97%
Venous Thromboembolism Prophylaxis[2]	345	99%	87%	85%
Warfarin Therapy Discharge Instructions[2]	31	90%	59%	75%
Chest Pain/Possible Heart Attack Care				
Aspirin Given Within 24 Hours of Arrival	63	94%	97%	96%
Fibrinolytic Meds Within 30 Min. of Arrival[1]	-	-	54%	58%
Average Time to ECG (minutes)	66	16	9	7
Average Time to Transfer (minutes)[1]	-	-	78	60
Children's Asthma Care				
Received Home Management Plan of Care	-	-	-	88%
Received Reliever Medication	-	-	-	100%
Received Systemic Corticosteroids	-	-	-	100%
Emergency Department				
Admittance Decision Time (minutes)[2]	795	191	154	98
Head CT Results Within 45 Min. of Arrival	12	75%	55%	57%
Patients Who Left ER Before Being Seen	32,329	1%	2%	2%
Time from ER Arrival to Admit. (minutes)[2]	794	431	378	274
Time from ER Arrival to Discharge (minutes)	371	185	156	134
Time in ER Before Being Evaluated (minutes)	404	27	35	26
Time to Pain Meds for Fractures (minutes)	42	62	61	57
Heart Attack Care				
Aspirin Given at Discharge	25	100%	99%	99%
Fibrinolytic Meds Within 30 Min. of Arrival[7]	-	-	46%	54%
PCI Within 90 Minutes of Arrival[7]	-	-	95%	96%
Statin Prescribed at Discharge	25	88%	98%	98%
Heart Failure Care				
ACE Inhibitor or ARB for LVSD	28	100%	96%	97%
Discharge Instructions Given	101	100%	95%	94%
Evaluation of LVS Function	152	99%	99%	99%
Medicare Spending				
Medicare Spending per Patient (ratio)	-	1.01	0.96	0.98
Pneumonia Care				
Appropriate Initial Antibiotic Given[2]	122	98%	95%	95%
Blood Culture Timing[2]	237	95%	97%	98%
Pregnancy and Delivery Care				
Newborn Deliveries Scheduled Early[2]	27	4%	4%	6%
Preventive Care				
Immunization for Influenza[2]	510	95%	88%	90%
Immunization for Pneumonia[2]	712	91%	88%	92%
Stroke Care				
Anticoagulation Therapy for Atrial Fibrillation[1]	-	-	96%	95%
Antithrombotic Therapy Timing	33	100%	98%	98%
Assessed for Rehabilitation	36	100%	97%	97%
Discharged on Antithrombotic Therapy	35	97%	99%	99%
Discharged on Statin Medication	31	97%	95%	94%
Thrombolytic Therapy Timing[1]	-	-	69%	66%
Venous Thromboembolism Prophylaxis	36	100%	94%	94%
Written Stroke Educational Materials Given	14	100%	86%	88%
Surgical Care Improvement Project				
Appropriate Beta Blocker Usage	71	100%	97%	98%
Appropriate VTP Within 24 Hours	226	96%	98%	98%
Controlled Postoperative Blood Glucose[7]	-	-	97%	97%
Perioperative Temperature Management	257	100%	100%	100%
Prophylactic Antibiotic Selection	157	99%	99%	99%
Prophylactic Antibiotic Selection (Outpatient)	107	95%	97%	98%
Prophylactic Antibiotic Stopped	156	100%	98%	98%
Prophylactic Antibiotic Timing	157	100%	99%	99%
Prophylactic Antibiotic Timing (Outpatient)	108	99%	97%	98%
Urinary Catheter Removal	162	99%	96%	97%
Survey of Patients' Hospital Experiences				
Area Around Room 'Always' Quiet at Night	300+	43%	51%	61%
Doctors 'Always' Communicated Well	300+	76%	77%	82%
Home Recovery Information Given	300+	82%	83%	85%
Hospital Given 9 or 10 on 10 Point Scale	300+	54%	63%	71%
Meds 'Always' Explained Before Given	300+	57%	59%	64%
Nurses 'Always' Communicated Well	300+	77%	75%	79%
Pain 'Always' Well Controlled	300+	66%	67%	71%
Room and Bathroom 'Always' Clean	300+	66%	69%	73%
Timely Help 'Always' Received	300+	64%	61%	68%
Would Definitely Recommend Hospital	300+	51%	65%	71%
Use of Medical Imaging				
Cardiac Imaging Stress Test before Surgery	326	6.1%	5.8%	5.3%
Combination Abdominal CT Scan	840	18.0%	8.2%	10.5%
Combination Brain/Sinus CT Scan	708	2.7%	3.6%	2.7%
Combination Chest CT Scan	796	5.2%	1.3%	2.7%
Follow-up Mammogram/Ultrasound	1,588	8.2%	13%	8.8%
Lumbar Spine MRI for Low Back Pain	112	34.8%	33.4%	37.2%

Huntington Hospital

270 Park Avenue
Huntington, NY 11743
Phone: 631-351-2000
Fax: 631-351-2586
E-mail: staff@hunthosp.org
URL: www.hunthosp.org
Type: Acute Care Hospitals
Emergency Services: Yes
Ownership: Voluntary non-profit - Private
Beds: 408

Key Personnel:
Pediatric Ambulatory Care...... James Fagin, MD
Infection Control............. Bruce Farber, MD
Chief of Medical Staff.......... Noah Finkel, MD
CEO/President.............. J Ronald Gaudreault
Radiology.................. Mitchell Goldman, MD
Quality Assurance........... Donn Haber

NOTE: Hospital profiles are in alphabetical order by state, then city, then hospital within the city; Rankings exclude hospitals with less than 25 cases except for patient surveys which excludes hospitals with less than 100 cases; (a) 100-299 cases; (1) The number of cases/patients is too few to report; (2) Data submitted were based on a sample of cases/patients; (3) Results are based on a shorter time period than required; (4) Data suppressed by CMS for one or more quarters; (5) Results are not available for this reporting period; (6) Fewer than 100 patients completed the HCAHPS survey; (7) No cases met the criteria for this measure; (8) The lower limit of the confidence interval cannot be calculated if the number of observed infections equals zero; (9) No data are available from the state/territory for this reporting period; (10) The scores shown reflect fewer than 50 completed surveys; (11) There were discrepancies in the data collection process; (12) This measure does not apply to this hospital for this reporting period; (13) Results cannot be calculated for this reporting period; (14) The results for this state are combined with nearby states to protect confidentiality; Please refer to the User's Guide for a full explanation of data.

Coronary Care . . . . Kathy Mann, RN
Operating Room. . . . . Linda Olander, RN

Measure	Cases	This Hosp.	State Avg.	U.S. Avg.
Blood Clot Prevention and Treatment				
Anticoagulation Overlap Therapy[2]	99	93%	91%	93%
ICU Venous Thromboembolism Prophylaxis[2]	45	96%	92%	92%
Incidence of Potentially Preventable VTE[2]	15	20%	10%	10%
UFH with Dosages/Platelet Monitoring[2]	70	100%	92%	97%
Venous Thromboembolism Prophylaxis[2]	363	90%	87%	85%
Warfarin Therapy Discharge Instructions[2]	70	3%	59%	75%
Chest Pain/Possible Heart Attack Care				
Aspirin Given Within 24 Hours of Arrival[1,3]	-	-	97%	96%
Fibrinolytic Meds Within 30 Min. of Arrival[3,7]	-	-	54%	58%
Average Time to ECG (minutes)[1,3]	-	-	9	7
Average Time to Transfer (minutes)[3,7]	-	-	78	60
Children's Asthma Care				
Received Home Management Plan of Care	-	-	-	88%
Received Reliever Medication	-	-	-	100%
Received Systemic Corticosteroids	-	-	-	100%
Emergency Department				
Admittance Decision Time (minutes)[2]	53	254	154	98
Head CT Results Within 45 Min. of Arrival[1]	-	-	55%	57%
Patients Who Left ER Before Being Seen	51,754	1%	2%	2%
Time from ER Arrival to Admit. (minutes)[2]	65	416	378	274
Time from ER Arrival to Discharge (minutes)	335	142	156	134
Time in ER Before Being Evaluated (minutes)	250	35	35	26
Time to Pain Meds for Fractures (minutes)	164	45	61	57
Heart Attack Care				
Aspirin Given at Discharge[2]	184	98%	99%	99%
Fibrinolytic Meds Within 30 Min. of Arrival[2,7]	-	-	46%	54%
PCI Within 90 Minutes of Arrival[2]	40	90%	95%	96%
Statin Prescribed at Discharge[2]	186	98%	98%	98%
Heart Failure Care				
ACE Inhibitor or ARB for LVSD[2]	54	93%	96%	97%
Discharge Instructions Given[2]	201	93%	95%	94%
Evaluation of LVS Function[2]	272	100%	99%	99%
Medicare Spending				
Medicare Spending per Patient (ratio)	-	1.02	0.96	0.98
Pneumonia Care				
Appropriate Initial Antibiotic Given[2]	63	98%	95%	95%
Blood Culture Timing[2]	164	98%	97%	98%
Pregnancy and Delivery Care				
Newborn Deliveries Scheduled Early[2]	24	0%	4%	6%
Preventive Care				
Immunization for Influenza[2]	564	95%	88%	90%
Immunization for Pneumonia[2]	705	93%	88%	92%
Stroke Care				
Anticoagulation Therapy for Atrial Fibrillation[2]	27	100%	96%	95%
Antithrombotic Therapy Timing[2]	97	100%	98%	98%
Assessed for Rehabilitation[2]	113	97%	97%	97%
Discharged on Antithrombotic Therapy[2]	99	100%	99%	99%
Discharged on Statin Medication[2]	76	99%	95%	94%
Thrombolytic Therapy Timing[1,2]	-	-	69%	66%
Venous Thromboembolism Prophylaxis[2]	120	93%	94%	94%
Written Stroke Educational Materials Given[2]	54	87%	86%	88%
Surgical Care Improvement Project				
Appropriate Beta Blocker Usage[2]	122	97%	97%	98%
Appropriate VTP Within 24 Hours[2]	299	99%	98%	98%
Controlled Postoperative Blood Glucose[2,7]	-	-	97%	97%
Perioperative Temperature Management[2]	351	100%	100%	100%
Prophylactic Antibiotic Selection[2]	205	100%	99%	99%
Prophylactic Antibiotic Selection (Outpatient)	299	99%	97%	98%
Prophylactic Antibiotic Stopped[2]	200	98%	98%	98%
Prophylactic Antibiotic Timing[2]	206	99%	99%	99%
Prophylactic Antibiotic Timing (Outpatient)	299	99%	97%	98%
Urinary Catheter Removal[2]	86	95%	96%	97%
Survey of Patients' Hospital Experiences				
Area Around Room 'Always' Quiet at Night	300+	52%	51%	61%
Doctors 'Always' Communicated Well	300+	79%	77%	82%
Home Recovery Information Given	300+	80%	83%	85%
Hospital Given 9 or 10 on 10 Point Scale	300+	70%	63%	71%
Meds 'Always' Explained Before Given	300+	62%	59%	64%
Nurses 'Always' Communicated Well	300+	81%	75%	79%
Pain 'Always' Well Controlled	300+	73%	67%	71%
Room and Bathroom 'Always' Clean	300+	72%	69%	73%
Timely Help 'Always' Received	300+	65%	61%	68%
Would Definitely Recommend Hospital	300+	71%	65%	71%
Use of Medical Imaging				
Cardiac Imaging Stress Test before Surgery	47	2.1%	5.8%	5.3%
Combination Abdominal CT Scan	675	3.0%	8.2%	10.5%
Combination Brain/Sinus CT Scan	958	4.8%	3.6%	2.7%
Combination Chest CT Scan	322	0.3%	1.3%	2.7%
Follow-up Mammogram/Ultrasound	912	41.1%	13%	8.8%
Lumbar Spine MRI for Low Back Pain[1]	-	-	33.4%	37.2%

Cayuga Medical Center at Ithaca

101 Dates Drive
Ithaca, NY 14850
Phone: 607-274-4401
Fax: 607-274-4527
E-mail: bconner@cayugamed.org
URL: www.cayugamed.org
Type: Acute Care Hospitals
Emergency Services: Yes
Ownership: Voluntary non-profit - Private
Beds: 204

Key Personnel:
Radiology. . . . . William Caroll
Infection Control. . . . . Sandra Coaley, RN
Pediatric Ambulatory Care . . . . . . Terri Koski
Pediatric In-Patient Care . . . . Terri Koski
Quality Assurance . . . . Carol LaBorie
Coronary Care . . . . Sue McKelvey
President/CEO. . . . . John Rudd, MD
Chief of Medical Staff. . . . . Jeffrey Snedecker, MD

Measure	Cases	This Hosp.	State Avg.	U.S. Avg.
Blood Clot Prevention and Treatment				
Anticoagulation Overlap Therapy[2]	47	96%	91%	93%
ICU Venous Thromboembolism Prophylaxis[2]	95	94%	92%	92%
Incidence of Potentially Preventable VTE[1,2]	-	-	10%	10%
UFH with Dosages/Platelet Monitoring[2]	26	100%	92%	97%
Venous Thromboembolism Prophylaxis[2]	238	90%	87%	85%
Warfarin Therapy Discharge Instructions[2]	44	7%	59%	75%
Chest Pain/Possible Heart Attack Care				
Aspirin Given Within 24 Hours of Arrival[1]	-	-	97%	96%
Fibrinolytic Meds Within 30 Min. of Arrival[3,7]	-	-	54%	58%
Average Time to ECG (minutes)	11	6	9	7
Average Time to Transfer (minutes)[1,3]	-	-	78	60
Children's Asthma Care				
Received Home Management Plan of Care	-	-	-	88%
Received Reliever Medication	-	-	-	100%
Received Systemic Corticosteroids	-	-	-	100%
Emergency Department				
Admittance Decision Time (minutes)[2]	368	151	154	98
Head CT Results Within 45 Min. of Arrival[1]	-	-	55%	57%
Patients Who Left ER Before Being Seen	31,946	2%	2%	2%
Time from ER Arrival to Admit. (minutes)[2]	395	328	378	274
Time from ER Arrival to Discharge (minutes)	376	194	156	134
Time in ER Before Being Evaluated (minutes)	397	44	35	26
Time to Pain Meds for Fractures (minutes)	92	59	61	57
Heart Attack Care				
Aspirin Given at Discharge	91	100%	99%	99%
Fibrinolytic Meds Within 30 Min. of Arrival[7]	-	-	46%	54%
PCI Within 90 Minutes of Arrival	21	90%	95%	96%
Statin Prescribed at Discharge	83	98%	98%	98%
Heart Failure Care				
ACE Inhibitor or ARB for LVSD	24	100%	96%	97%
Discharge Instructions Given	65	80%	95%	94%
Evaluation of LVS Function	80	99%	99%	99%
Medicare Spending				
Medicare Spending per Patient (ratio)	-	0.88	0.96	0.98
Pneumonia Care				
Appropriate Initial Antibiotic Given	98	89%	95%	95%
Blood Culture Timing	153	95%	97%	98%
Pregnancy and Delivery Care				
Newborn Deliveries Scheduled Early[2]	26	27%	4%	6%
Preventive Care				
Immunization for Influenza[2]	506	90%	88%	90%
Immunization for Pneumonia[2]	520	91%	88%	92%
Stroke Care				
Anticoagulation Therapy for Atrial Fibrillation	11	91%	96%	95%
Antithrombotic Therapy Timing	55	96%	98%	98%
Assessed for Rehabilitation	65	91%	97%	97%
Discharged on Antithrombotic Therapy	57	98%	99%	99%
Discharged on Statin Medication	44	86%	95%	94%
Thrombolytic Therapy Timing[1]	-	-	69%	66%
Venous Thromboembolism Prophylaxis	64	97%	94%	94%
Written Stroke Educational Materials Given	38	32%	86%	88%
Surgical Care Improvement Project				
Appropriate Beta Blocker Usage	100	98%	97%	98%
Appropriate VTP Within 24 Hours	334	98%	98%	98%
Controlled Postoperative Blood Glucose[7]	-	-	97%	97%
Perioperative Temperature Management	368	100%	100%	100%
Prophylactic Antibiotic Selection	247	98%	99%	99%
Prophylactic Antibiotic Selection (Outpatient)	98	97%	97%	98%
Prophylactic Antibiotic Stopped	244	97%	98%	98%
Prophylactic Antibiotic Timing	247	98%	99%	99%
Prophylactic Antibiotic Timing (Outpatient)	105	86%	97%	98%
Urinary Catheter Removal	303	94%	96%	97%
Survey of Patients' Hospital Experiences				
Area Around Room 'Always' Quiet at Night	300+	52%	51%	61%
Doctors 'Always' Communicated Well	300+	78%	77%	82%
Home Recovery Information Given	300+	85%	83%	85%
Hospital Given 9 or 10 on 10 Point Scale	300+	68%	63%	71%
Meds 'Always' Explained Before Given	300+	65%	59%	64%
Nurses 'Always' Communicated Well	300+	80%	75%	79%
Pain 'Always' Well Controlled	300+	70%	67%	71%
Room and Bathroom 'Always' Clean	300+	67%	69%	73%
Timely Help 'Always' Received	300+	71%	61%	68%
Would Definitely Recommend Hospital	300+	71%	65%	71%
Use of Medical Imaging				
Cardiac Imaging Stress Test before Surgery	214	3.7%	5.8%	5.3%
Combination Abdominal CT Scan	995	3.1%	8.2%	10.5%
Combination Brain/Sinus CT Scan	791	4.7%	3.6%	2.7%
Combination Chest CT Scan	527	0.0%	1.3%	2.7%
Follow-up Mammogram/Ultrasound	1,377	5.2%	13%	8.8%
Lumbar Spine MRI for Low Back Pain	118	39.8%	33.4%	37.2%

Jamaica Hospital Medical Center

89th Avenue & Van Wyck Expressway
Jamaica, NY 11418
Phone: 718-262-6000
Fax: 718-657-0545
URL: www.jamaicahospital.org
Type: Acute Care Hospitals
Emergency Services: Yes
Ownership: Voluntary non-profit - Private
Beds: 424

Key Personnel:
Ambulatory Care . . . . Fred Beekman
Infection Control. . . . . Judy Fine
CEO/President. . . . . Bruce J. Flanz
Cardiac Laboratory. . . . . Robert Mendelson
Chief of Medical Staff . . . . Antonietta Morisca, MD
Pediatric Ambulatory Care . . . . . . Susan Rapaport, MD
Operating Room. . . . . Doreen Voda
Pediatric In-Patient Care . . . . Phyllis Weiner, MD

Measure	Cases	This Hosp.	State Avg.	U.S. Avg.
Blood Clot Prevention and Treatment				
Anticoagulation Overlap Therapy[2]	65	82%	91%	93%
ICU Venous Thromboembolism Prophylaxis[2]	55	96%	92%	92%
Incidence of Potentially Preventable VTE[2]	20	0%	10%	10%
UFH with Dosages/Platelet Monitoring[2]	28	100%	92%	97%
Venous Thromboembolism Prophylaxis[2]	325	96%	87%	85%
Warfarin Therapy Discharge Instructions[2]	35	80%	59%	75%
Chest Pain/Possible Heart Attack Care				
Aspirin Given Within 24 Hours of Arrival	26	100%	97%	96%
Fibrinolytic Meds Within 30 Min. of Arrival[7]	-	-	54%	58%
Average Time to ECG (minutes)	25	0	9	7
Average Time to Transfer (minutes)[1]	-	-	78	60
Children's Asthma Care				
Received Home Management Plan of Care	-	-	-	88%
Received Reliever Medication	-	-	-	100%
Received Systemic Corticosteroids	-	-	-	100%
Emergency Department				
Admittance Decision Time (minutes)[2]	875	228	154	98
Head CT Results Within 45 Min. of Arrival[1]	-	-	55%	57%
Patients Who Left ER Before Being Seen	>100k	2%	2%	2%

NOTE: Hospital profiles are in alphabetical order by state, then city, then hospital within the city; Rankings exclude hospitals with less than 25 cases except for patient surveys which excludes hospitals with less than 100 cases; (a) 100-299 cases; (1) The number of cases/patients is too few to report; (2) Data submitted were based on a sample of cases/patients; (3) Results are based on a shorter time period than required; (4) Data suppressed by CMS for one or more quarters; (5) Results are not available for this reporting period; (6) Fewer than 100 patients completed the HCAHPS survey; (7) No cases met the criteria for this measure; (8) The lower limit of the confidence interval cannot be calculated if the number of observed infections equals zero; (9) No data are available from the state/territory for this reporting period; (10) The scores shown reflect fewer than 50 completed surveys; (11) There were discrepancies in the data collection process; (12) This measure does not apply to this hospital for this reporting period; (13) Results cannot be calculated for this reporting period; (14) The results for this state are combined with nearby states to protect confidentiality; Please refer to the User's Guide for a full explanation of data.

Measure	Cases	This Hosp.	State Avg.	U.S. Avg.
Time from ER Arrival to Admit. (minutes)[2]	878	486	378	274
Time from ER Arrival to Discharge (minutes)	370	229	156	134
Time in ER Before Being Evaluated (minutes)	292	55	35	26
Time to Pain Meds for Fractures (minutes)	234	44	61	57
Heart Attack Care				
Aspirin Given at Discharge[2]	228	100%	99%	99%
Fibrinolytic Meds Within 30 Min. of Arrival[2,7]	-	-	46%	54%
PCI Within 90 Minutes of Arrival[2]	59	100%	95%	96%
Statin Prescribed at Discharge[2]	229	100%	98%	98%
Heart Failure Care				
ACE Inhibitor or ARB for LVSD[2]	123	100%	96%	97%
Discharge Instructions Given[2]	264	100%	95%	94%
Evaluation of LVS Function[2]	306	100%	99%	99%
Medicare Spending				
Medicare Spending per Patient (ratio)	-	1.01	0.96	0.98
Pneumonia Care				
Appropriate Initial Antibiotic Given[2]	68	100%	95%	95%
Blood Culture Timing[2]	101	100%	97%	98%
Pregnancy and Delivery Care				
Newborn Deliveries Scheduled Early[2]	44	7%	4%	6%
Preventive Care				
Immunization for Influenza[2]	525	98%	88%	90%
Immunization for Pneumonia[2]	547	91%	88%	92%
Stroke Care				
Anticoagulation Therapy for Atrial Fibrillation	30	87%	96%	95%
Antithrombotic Therapy Timing	246	96%	98%	98%
Assessed for Rehabilitation	316	98%	97%	97%
Discharged on Antithrombotic Therapy	271	99%	99%	99%
Discharged on Statin Medication	204	98%	95%	94%
Thrombolytic Therapy Timing	35	83%	69%	66%
Venous Thromboembolism Prophylaxis	339	99%	94%	94%
Written Stroke Educational Materials Given	123	98%	86%	88%
Surgical Care Improvement Project				
Appropriate Beta Blocker Usage[2]	39	97%	97%	98%
Appropriate VTP Within 24 Hours[2]	241	98%	98%	98%
Controlled Postoperative Blood Glucose[2,7]	-	-	97%	97%
Perioperative Temperature Management[2]	295	99%	100%	100%
Prophylactic Antibiotic Selection[2]	149	97%	99%	99%
Prophylactic Antibiotic Selection (Outpatient)	67	97%	97%	98%
Prophylactic Antibiotic Stopped[2]	145	97%	98%	98%
Prophylactic Antibiotic Timing[2]	151	95%	99%	99%
Prophylactic Antibiotic Timing (Outpatient)	73	81%	97%	98%
Urinary Catheter Removal[2]	123	98%	96%	97%
Survey of Patients' Hospital Experiences				
Area Around Room 'Always' Quiet at Night	300+	49%	51%	61%
Doctors 'Always' Communicated Well	300+	72%	77%	82%
Home Recovery Information Given	300+	77%	83%	85%
Hospital Given 9 or 10 on 10 Point Scale	300+	47%	63%	71%
Meds 'Always' Explained Before Given	300+	47%	59%	64%
Nurses 'Always' Communicated Well	300+	64%	75%	79%
Pain 'Always' Well Controlled	300+	54%	67%	71%
Room and Bathroom 'Always' Clean	300+	62%	69%	73%
Timely Help 'Always' Received	300+	47%	61%	68%
Would Definitely Recommend Hospital	300+	47%	65%	71%
Use of Medical Imaging				
Cardiac Imaging Stress Test before Surgery	106	12.3%	5.8%	5.3%
Combination Abdominal CT Scan	171	12.3%	8.2%	10.5%
Combination Brain/Sinus CT Scan	449	5.6%	3.6%	2.7%
Combination Chest CT Scan	120	0.8%	1.3%	2.7%
Follow-up Mammogram/Ultrasound	363	9.1%	13%	8.8%
Lumbar Spine MRI for Low Back Pain[1]	-	-	33.4%	37.2%

Queens Hospital Center

82-68 164th Street　　Phone: 718-883-3000
Jamaica, NY 11432
URL: www.nyc.gov/html/hhc/qhn/home.html
Type: Acute Care Hospitals　　Emergency Services: Yes
Ownership: Government - Local　　Beds: 408

Key Personnel:
Pediatric Ambulatory Care . . . . . . Hedda Acs, MD
Pediatric In-Patient Care . . . . Hedda Acs, MD
Chief of Medical Staff. . . . . Jean Bernard-Poulard, MD
Patient Relations . . . . Joan Gabriele, RN
CEO/President. . . . . Antonio Martin

Measure	Cases	This Hosp.	State Avg.	U.S. Avg.
Blood Clot Prevention and Treatment				
Anticoagulation Overlap Therapy[2]	67	90%	91%	93%
ICU Venous Thromboembolism Prophylaxis[2]	37	92%	92%	92%
Incidence of Potentially Preventable VTE[1,2]	-	-	10%	10%
UFH with Dosages/Platelet Monitoring[2]	35	100%	92%	97%
Venous Thromboembolism Prophylaxis[2]	391	93%	87%	85%
Warfarin Therapy Discharge Instructions[2]	56	71%	59%	75%
Chest Pain/Possible Heart Attack Care				
Aspirin Given Within 24 Hours of Arrival	219	99%	97%	96%
Fibrinolytic Meds Within 30 Min. of Arrival[7]	-	-	54%	58%
Average Time to ECG (minutes)	204	14	9	7
Average Time to Transfer (minutes)	25	97	78	60
Children's Asthma Care				
Received Home Management Plan of Care	-	-	-	88%
Received Reliever Medication	-	-	-	100%
Received Systemic Corticosteroids	-	-	-	100%
Emergency Department				
Admittance Decision Time (minutes)[2]	853	207	154	98
Head CT Results Within 45 Min. of Arrival[1]	-	-	55%	57%
Patients Who Left ER Before Being Seen	>100k	2%	2%	2%
Time from ER Arrival to Admit. (minutes)[2]	852	534	378	274
Time from ER Arrival to Discharge (minutes)	418	190	156	134
Time in ER Before Being Evaluated (minutes)	464	46	35	26
Time to Pain Meds for Fractures (minutes)	95	90	61	57
Heart Attack Care				
Aspirin Given at Discharge	23	100%	99%	99%
Fibrinolytic Meds Within 30 Min. of Arrival[7]	-	-	46%	54%
PCI Within 90 Minutes of Arrival[7]	-	-	95%	96%
Statin Prescribed at Discharge	25	92%	98%	98%
Heart Failure Care				
ACE Inhibitor or ARB for LVSD	92	95%	96%	97%
Discharge Instructions Given	250	97%	95%	94%
Evaluation of LVS Function	267	100%	99%	99%
Medicare Spending				
Medicare Spending per Patient (ratio)	-	0.93	0.96	0.98
Pneumonia Care				
Appropriate Initial Antibiotic Given	234	97%	95%	95%
Blood Culture Timing	375	91%	97%	98%
Pregnancy and Delivery Care				
Newborn Deliveries Scheduled Early[2]	26	0%	4%	6%
Preventive Care				
Immunization for Influenza[2]	581	82%	88%	90%
Immunization for Pneumonia[2]	580	87%	88%	92%
Stroke Care				
Anticoagulation Therapy for Atrial Fibrillation[1]	-	-	96%	95%
Antithrombotic Therapy Timing	80	96%	98%	98%
Assessed for Rehabilitation	78	74%	97%	97%
Discharged on Antithrombotic Therapy	71	100%	99%	99%
Discharged on Statin Medication	62	85%	95%	94%
Thrombolytic Therapy Timing[1]	-	-	69%	66%
Venous Thromboembolism Prophylaxis	86	90%	94%	94%
Written Stroke Educational Materials Given	54	54%	86%	88%
Surgical Care Improvement Project				
Appropriate Beta Blocker Usage	50	88%	97%	98%
Appropriate VTP Within 24 Hours	222	96%	98%	98%
Controlled Postoperative Blood Glucose[7]	-	-	97%	97%
Perioperative Temperature Management	268	100%	100%	100%
Prophylactic Antibiotic Selection	95	99%	99%	99%
Prophylactic Antibiotic Selection (Outpatient)	65	97%	97%	98%
Prophylactic Antibiotic Stopped	88	95%	98%	98%
Prophylactic Antibiotic Timing	95	100%	99%	99%
Prophylactic Antibiotic Timing (Outpatient)	24	83%	97%	98%
Urinary Catheter Removal	65	95%	96%	97%
Survey of Patients' Hospital Experiences				
Area Around Room 'Always' Quiet at Night	300+	50%	51%	61%
Doctors 'Always' Communicated Well	300+	75%	77%	82%
Home Recovery Information Given	300+	78%	83%	85%
Hospital Given 9 or 10 on 10 Point Scale	300+	56%	63%	71%
Meds 'Always' Explained Before Given	300+	56%	59%	64%
Nurses 'Always' Communicated Well	300+	66%	75%	79%
Pain 'Always' Well Controlled	300+	57%	67%	71%
Room and Bathroom 'Always' Clean	300+	68%	69%	73%
Timely Help 'Always' Received	300+	47%	61%	68%
Would Definitely Recommend Hospital	300+	65%	65%	71%
Use of Medical Imaging				
Cardiac Imaging Stress Test before Surgery[1]	-	-	5.8%	5.3%
Combination Abdominal CT Scan	167	2.4%	8.2%	10.5%
Combination Brain/Sinus CT Scan[1]	-	-	3.6%	2.7%
Combination Chest CT Scan	117	0.0%	1.3%	2.7%
Follow-up Mammogram/Ultrasound	152	14.5%	13%	8.8%
Lumbar Spine MRI for Low Back Pain[1]	-	-	33.4%	37.2%

Woman's Christian Association

207 Foote Avenue　　Phone: 716-487-0141
Jamestown, NY 14701　　Fax: 716-664-8336
URL: www.wcahospital.org
Type: Acute Care Hospitals　　Emergency Services: Yes
Ownership: Voluntary non-profit - Private　　Beds: 342

Key Personnel:
Patient Relations . . . . Diana Buttafarro
Pediatric In-Patient Care . . . . Virginia Campion, MD
Radiology. . . . . Eugene Graham
CEO/President. . . . . RonaldT Klizek, MD
Emergency Room . . . . Bonnie Stockwell
Quality Assurance . . . . Betsy Wright

Measure	Cases	This Hosp.	State Avg.	U.S. Avg.
Blood Clot Prevention and Treatment				
Anticoagulation Overlap Therapy[2]	33	79%	91%	93%
ICU Venous Thromboembolism Prophylaxis[2]	88	74%	92%	92%
Incidence of Potentially Preventable VTE[1,2]	-	-	10%	10%
UFH with Dosages/Platelet Monitoring[2]	13	100%	92%	97%
Venous Thromboembolism Prophylaxis[2]	332	71%	87%	85%
Warfarin Therapy Discharge Instructions[2]	26	23%	59%	75%
Chest Pain/Possible Heart Attack Care				
Aspirin Given Within 24 Hours of Arrival	126	95%	97%	96%
Fibrinolytic Meds Within 30 Min. of Arrival[1]	-	-	54%	58%
Average Time to ECG (minutes)	128	4	9	7
Average Time to Transfer (minutes)	19	78	78	60
Children's Asthma Care				
Received Home Management Plan of Care	-	-	-	88%
Received Reliever Medication	-	-	-	100%
Received Systemic Corticosteroids	-	-	-	100%
Emergency Department				
Admittance Decision Time (minutes)[2]	559	92	154	98
Head CT Results Within 45 Min. of Arrival	47	38%	55%	57%
Patients Who Left ER Before Being Seen	37,856	2%	2%	2%
Time from ER Arrival to Admit. (minutes)[2]	570	327	378	274
Time from ER Arrival to Discharge (minutes)	357	146	156	134
Time in ER Before Being Evaluated (minutes)	382	50	35	26
Time to Pain Meds for Fractures (minutes)	121	63	61	57
Heart Attack Care				
Aspirin Given at Discharge	33	94%	99%	99%
Fibrinolytic Meds Within 30 Min. of Arrival[1]	-	-	46%	54%
PCI Within 90 Minutes of Arrival[7]	-	-	95%	96%
Statin Prescribed at Discharge	37	89%	98%	98%
Heart Failure Care				
ACE Inhibitor or ARB for LVSD	57	72%	96%	97%
Discharge Instructions Given	224	82%	95%	94%
Evaluation of LVS Function	276	99%	99%	99%
Medicare Spending				
Medicare Spending per Patient (ratio)	-	0.94	0.96	0.98
Pneumonia Care				
Appropriate Initial Antibiotic Given[2]	82	87%	95%	95%
Blood Culture Timing[2]	139	94%	97%	98%
Pregnancy and Delivery Care				
Newborn Deliveries Scheduled Early[2]	26	4%	4%	6%
Preventive Care				
Immunization for Influenza[2]	530	75%	88%	90%
Immunization for Pneumonia[2]	661	82%	88%	92%
Stroke Care				
Anticoagulation Therapy for Atrial Fibrillation[1]	-	-	96%	95%
Antithrombotic Therapy Timing	39	92%	98%	98%
Assessed for Rehabilitation	34	76%	97%	97%
Discharged on Antithrombotic Therapy	33	94%	99%	99%
Discharged on Statin Medication	30	57%	95%	94%

NOTE: Hospital profiles are in alphabetical order by state, then city, then hospital within the city; Rankings exclude hospitals with less than 25 cases except for patient surveys which excludes hospitals with less than 100 cases; (a) 100-299 cases; (1) The number of cases/patients is too few to report; (2) Data submitted were based on a sample of cases/patients; (3) Results are based on a shorter time period than required; (4) Data suppressed by CMS for one or more quarters; (5) Results are not available for this reporting period; (6) Fewer than 100 patients completed the HCAHPS survey; (7) No cases met the criteria for this measure; (8) The lower limit of the confidence interval cannot be calculated if the number of observed infections equals zero; (9) No data are available from the state/territory for this reporting period; (10) The scores shown reflect fewer than 50 completed surveys; (11) There were discrepancies in the data collection process; (12) This measure does not apply to this hospital for this reporting period; (13) Results cannot be calculated for this reporting period; (14) The results for this state are combined with nearby states to protect confidentiality; Please refer to the User's Guide for a full explanation of data.

Thrombolytic Therapy Timing	12	0%	69%	66%
Venous Thromboembolism Prophylaxis	42	64%	94%	94%
Written Stroke Educational Materials Given	24	4%	86%	88%
Surgical Care Improvement Project				
Appropriate Beta Blocker Usage[2]	116	91%	97%	98%
Appropriate VTP Within 24 Hours[2]	239	97%	98%	98%
Controlled Postoperative Blood Glucose[2,7]	-	-	97%	97%
Perioperative Temperature Management[2]	342	99%	100%	100%
Prophylactic Antibiotic Selection[2]	249	98%	99%	99%
Prophylactic Antibiotic Selection (Outpatient)	105	95%	97%	98%
Prophylactic Antibiotic Stopped[2]	245	92%	98%	98%
Prophylactic Antibiotic Timing[2]	252	98%	99%	99%
Prophylactic Antibiotic Timing (Outpatient)	105	100%	97%	98%
Urinary Catheter Removal[2]	65	92%	96%	97%
Survey of Patients' Hospital Experiences				
Area Around Room 'Always' Quiet at Night	300+	46%	51%	61%
Doctors 'Always' Communicated Well	300+	75%	77%	82%
Home Recovery Information Given	300+	86%	83%	85%
Hospital Given 9 or 10 on 10 Point Scale	300+	50%	63%	71%
Meds 'Always' Explained Before Given	300+	53%	59%	64%
Nurses 'Always' Communicated Well	300+	69%	75%	79%
Pain 'Always' Well Controlled	300+	62%	67%	71%
Room and Bathroom 'Always' Clean	300+	59%	69%	73%
Timely Help 'Always' Received	300+	53%	61%	68%
Would Definitely Recommend Hospital	300+	49%	65%	71%
Use of Medical Imaging				
Cardiac Imaging Stress Test before Surgery	222	4.1%	5.8%	5.3%
Combination Abdominal CT Scan	556	10.6%	8.2%	10.5%
Combination Brain/Sinus CT Scan	550	1.5%	3.6%	2.7%
Combination Chest CT Scan	298	1.0%	1.3%	2.7%
Follow-up Mammogram/Ultrasound	1,131	4.4%	13%	8.8%
Lumbar Spine MRI for Low Back Pain	107	29.9%	33.4%	37.2%

United Health Services Hospitals

33-57 Harrison Street
Johnson City, NY 13790
URL: www.vhs.ent
Type: Acute Care Hospitals
Ownership: Voluntary non-profit - Private
Phone: 607-763-6000
Fax: 607-763-6789
Emergency Services: Yes
Beds: 516

Key Personnel:
Operating Room. . . . . Michael Aronis
Chief of Medical Staff . . . . Rajesh Dave, MD
Anesthesiology. . . . . Hank H. Kang, MD
Infection Control. . . . . Debbie Mack
Quality Assurance . . . . Roberta Rivero
CEO/President. . . . . Matthew J Salanger

Measure	Cases	This Hosp.	State Avg.	U.S. Avg.
Blood Clot Prevention and Treatment				
Anticoagulation Overlap Therapy[2]	108	93%	91%	93%
ICU Venous Thromboembolism Prophylaxis[2]	90	92%	92%	92%
Incidence of Potentially Preventable VTE[2]	25	12%	10%	10%
UFH with Dosages/Platelet Monitoring[2]	42	86%	92%	97%
Venous Thromboembolism Prophylaxis[2]	330	86%	87%	85%
Warfarin Therapy Discharge Instructions[2]	78	0%	59%	75%
Chest Pain/Possible Heart Attack Care				
Aspirin Given Within 24 Hours of Arrival[5]	-	-	97%	96%
Fibrinolytic Meds Within 30 Min. of Arrival[5]	-	-	54%	58%
Average Time to ECG (minutes)[5]	-	-	9	7
Average Time to Transfer (minutes)[5]	-	-	78	60
Children's Asthma Care				
Received Home Management Plan of Care	-	-	-	88%
Received Reliever Medication	-	-	-	100%
Received Systemic Corticosteroids	-	-	-	100%
Emergency Department				
Admittance Decision Time (minutes)[2]	516	94	154	98
Head CT Results Within 45 Min. of Arrival[1]	-	-	55%	57%
Patients Who Left ER Before Being Seen	61,775	2%	2%	2%
Time from ER Arrival to Admit. (minutes)[2]	592	298	378	274
Time from ER Arrival to Discharge (minutes)	418	183	156	134
Time in ER Before Being Evaluated (minutes)	499	48	35	26
Time to Pain Meds for Fractures (minutes)	132	73	61	57
Heart Attack Care				
Aspirin Given at Discharge	528	100%	99%	99%
Fibrinolytic Meds Within 30 Min. of Arrival[7]	-	-	46%	54%
PCI Within 90 Minutes of Arrival	82	96%	95%	96%
Statin Prescribed at Discharge	504	99%	98%	98%
Heart Failure Care				
ACE Inhibitor or ARB for LVSD	171	97%	96%	97%
Discharge Instructions Given	411	90%	95%	94%
Evaluation of LVS Function	495	99%	99%	99%
Medicare Spending				
Medicare Spending per Patient (ratio)	-	0.93	0.96	0.98
Pneumonia Care				
Appropriate Initial Antibiotic Given	167	100%	95%	95%
Blood Culture Timing	379	97%	97%	98%
Pregnancy and Delivery Care				
Newborn Deliveries Scheduled Early[2]	49	6%	4%	6%
Preventive Care				
Immunization for Influenza[2]	624	97%	88%	90%
Immunization for Pneumonia[2]	740	91%	88%	92%
Stroke Care				
Anticoagulation Therapy for Atrial Fibrillation	31	87%	96%	95%
Antithrombotic Therapy Timing	151	97%	98%	98%
Assessed for Rehabilitation	202	97%	97%	97%
Discharged on Antithrombotic Therapy	160	100%	99%	99%
Discharged on Statin Medication	129	91%	95%	94%
Thrombolytic Therapy Timing	13	77%	69%	66%
Venous Thromboembolism Prophylaxis	217	95%	94%	94%
Written Stroke Educational Materials Given	87	80%	86%	88%
Surgical Care Improvement Project				
Appropriate Beta Blocker Usage	595	99%	97%	98%
Appropriate VTP Within 24 Hours	1,124	99%	98%	98%
Controlled Postoperative Blood Glucose	225	97%	97%	97%
Perioperative Temperature Management	1,421	100%	100%	100%
Prophylactic Antibiotic Selection	1,020	99%	99%	99%
Prophylactic Antibiotic Selection (Outpatient)	891	98%	97%	98%
Prophylactic Antibiotic Stopped	992	96%	98%	98%
Prophylactic Antibiotic Timing	1,020	99%	99%	99%
Prophylactic Antibiotic Timing (Outpatient)	891	99%	97%	98%
Urinary Catheter Removal	672	97%	96%	97%
Survey of Patients' Hospital Experiences				
Area Around Room 'Always' Quiet at Night	300+	40%	51%	61%
Doctors 'Always' Communicated Well	300+	75%	77%	82%
Home Recovery Information Given	300+	86%	83%	85%
Hospital Given 9 or 10 on 10 Point Scale	300+	63%	63%	71%
Meds 'Always' Explained Before Given	300+	63%	59%	64%
Nurses 'Always' Communicated Well	300+	76%	75%	79%
Pain 'Always' Well Controlled	300+	67%	67%	71%
Room and Bathroom 'Always' Clean	300+	70%	69%	73%
Timely Help 'Always' Received	300+	65%	61%	68%
Would Definitely Recommend Hospital	300+	68%	65%	71%
Use of Medical Imaging				
Cardiac Imaging Stress Test before Surgery	603	2.8%	5.8%	5.3%
Combination Abdominal CT Scan	1,274	4.6%	8.2%	10.5%
Combination Brain/Sinus CT Scan	1,187	3.5%	3.6%	2.7%
Combination Chest CT Scan	742	2.4%	1.3%	2.7%
Follow-up Mammogram/Ultrasound	2,343	14.6%	13%	8.8%
Lumbar Spine MRI for Low Back Pain[7]	-	-	33.4%	37.2%

Kenmore Mercy Hospital

2950 Elmwood Avenue
Kenmore, NY 14217
URL: www.chsbuffalo.org
Type: Acute Care Hospitals
Ownership: Voluntary non-profit - Church
Phone: 716-447-6100
Fax: 716-447-6090
Emergency Services: Yes
Beds: 184

Key Personnel:
Radiology. . . . . Amina Akhtar
Chief of Medical Staff. . . . . James Fitzpatrick
Patient Relations . . . . Cheryl Haynes, RN
President/CEO. . . . . Joseph D. McDonald

Measure	Cases	This Hosp.	State Avg.	U.S. Avg.
Blood Clot Prevention and Treatment				
Anticoagulation Overlap Therapy[2]	73	100%	91%	93%
ICU Venous Thromboembolism Prophylaxis[2]	69	99%	92%	92%
Incidence of Potentially Preventable VTE[1,2]	-	-	10%	10%
UFH with Dosages/Platelet Monitoring[2]	31	100%	92%	97%
Venous Thromboembolism Prophylaxis[2]	318	93%	87%	85%
Warfarin Therapy Discharge Instructions[2]	58	93%	59%	75%
Chest Pain/Possible Heart Attack Care				
Aspirin Given Within 24 Hours of Arrival	49	100%	97%	96%
Fibrinolytic Meds Within 30 Min. of Arrival[7]	-	-	54%	58%
Average Time to ECG (minutes)	52	15	9	7
Average Time to Transfer (minutes)	16	83	78	60
Children's Asthma Care				
Received Home Management Plan of Care	-	-	-	88%
Received Reliever Medication	-	-	-	100%
Received Systemic Corticosteroids	-	-	-	100%
Emergency Department				
Admittance Decision Time (minutes)[2]	928	107	154	98
Head CT Results Within 45 Min. of Arrival[5]	-	-	55%	57%
Patients Who Left ER Before Being Seen	30,336	1%	2%	2%
Time from ER Arrival to Admit. (minutes)[2]	928	310	378	274
Time from ER Arrival to Discharge (minutes)	387	164	156	134
Time in ER Before Being Evaluated (minutes)	407	28	35	26
Time to Pain Meds for Fractures (minutes)	143	63	61	57
Heart Attack Care				
Aspirin Given at Discharge	61	100%	99%	99%
Fibrinolytic Meds Within 30 Min. of Arrival[1]	-	-	46%	54%
PCI Within 90 Minutes of Arrival[7]	-	-	95%	96%
Statin Prescribed at Discharge	61	97%	98%	98%
Heart Failure Care				
ACE Inhibitor or ARB for LVSD[2]	54	100%	96%	97%
Discharge Instructions Given[2]	172	98%	95%	94%
Evaluation of LVS Function[2]	238	100%	99%	99%
Medicare Spending				
Medicare Spending per Patient (ratio)	-	0.99	0.96	0.98
Pneumonia Care				
Appropriate Initial Antibiotic Given[2]	88	100%	95%	95%
Blood Culture Timing[2]	168	100%	97%	98%
Pregnancy and Delivery Care				
Newborn Deliveries Scheduled Early[7]	-	-	4%	6%
Preventive Care				
Immunization for Influenza[2]	639	95%	88%	90%
Immunization for Pneumonia[2]	939	90%	88%	92%
Stroke Care				
Anticoagulation Therapy for Atrial Fibrillation	17	100%	96%	95%
Antithrombotic Therapy Timing	76	100%	98%	98%
Assessed for Rehabilitation	91	100%	97%	97%
Discharged on Antithrombotic Therapy	77	99%	99%	99%
Discharged on Statin Medication	69	90%	95%	94%
Thrombolytic Therapy Timing[1]	-	-	69%	66%
Venous Thromboembolism Prophylaxis	92	92%	94%	94%
Written Stroke Educational Materials Given	47	85%	86%	88%
Surgical Care Improvement Project				
Appropriate Beta Blocker Usage[2]	143	97%	97%	98%
Appropriate VTP Within 24 Hours[2]	428	99%	98%	98%
Controlled Postoperative Blood Glucose[2,7]	-	-	97%	97%
Perioperative Temperature Management[2]	449	100%	100%	100%
Prophylactic Antibiotic Selection[2]	294	99%	99%	99%
Prophylactic Antibiotic Selection (Outpatient)	558	100%	97%	98%
Prophylactic Antibiotic Stopped[2]	293	100%	98%	98%
Prophylactic Antibiotic Timing[2]	296	98%	99%	99%
Prophylactic Antibiotic Timing (Outpatient)	562	98%	97%	98%
Urinary Catheter Removal[2]	119	97%	96%	97%
Survey of Patients' Hospital Experiences				
Area Around Room 'Always' Quiet at Night	300+	48%	51%	61%
Doctors 'Always' Communicated Well	300+	80%	77%	82%
Home Recovery Information Given	300+	87%	83%	85%
Hospital Given 9 or 10 on 10 Point Scale	300+	70%	63%	71%
Meds 'Always' Explained Before Given	300+	60%	59%	64%
Nurses 'Always' Communicated Well	300+	79%	75%	79%
Pain 'Always' Well Controlled	300+	73%	67%	71%
Room and Bathroom 'Always' Clean	300+	64%	69%	73%
Timely Help 'Always' Received	300+	65%	61%	68%
Would Definitely Recommend Hospital	300+	74%	65%	71%
Use of Medical Imaging				
Cardiac Imaging Stress Test before Surgery	92	8.7%	5.8%	5.3%
Combination Abdominal CT Scan	458	3.1%	8.2%	10.5%
Combination Brain/Sinus CT Scan	340	5.0%	3.6%	2.7%

NOTE: Hospital profiles are in alphabetical order by state, then city, then hospital within the city; Rankings exclude hospitals with less than 25 cases except for patient surveys which excludes hospitals with less than 100 cases; (a) 100-299 cases; (1) The number of cases/patients is too few to report; (2) Data submitted were based on a sample of cases/patients; (3) Results are based on a shorter time period than required; (4) Data suppressed by CMS for one or more quarters; (5) Results are not available for this reporting period; (6) Fewer than 100 patients completed the HCAHPS survey; (7) No cases met the criteria for this measure; (8) The lower limit of the confidence interval cannot be calculated if the number of observed infections equals zero; (9) No data are available from the state/territory for this reporting period; (10) The scores shown reflect fewer than 50 completed surveys; (11) There were discrepancies in the data collection process; (12) This measure does not apply to this hospital for this reporting period; (13) Results cannot be calculated for this reporting period; (14) The results for this state are combined with nearby states to protect confidentiality; Please refer to the User's Guide for a full explanation of data.

Combination Chest CT Scan	169	1.2%	1.3%	2.7%
Follow-up Mammogram/Ultrasound	365	7.7%	13%	8.8%
Lumbar Spine MRI for Low Back Pain[1]	-	-	33.4%	37.2%

Health Alliance Hospital Broadway Campus

396 Broadway
Kingston, NY 12401
URL: www.kingstonregionalhealth.org
Type: Acute Care Hospitals
Ownership: Voluntary non-profit - Private
Phone: 914-331-3131
Fax: 845-331-3238
Emergency Services: No
Beds: 150

Key Personnel:
Quality Assurance . . . . Sherie Ashdawn
Emergency Room . . . . Marc A Borenstein, MD
Chief of Medical Staff . . . . Frank Ehrlich
Anesthesiology. . . . . James Kikuoka, MD
Operating Room. . . . . Jane Lucente
Chair/CEO . . . . Kevin Ryan
CEO/President. . . . . David Scarpino
Radiology. . . . . Steven Schwartz, MD

Measure	Cases	This Hosp.	State Avg.	U.S. Avg.
Blood Clot Prevention and Treatment				
Anticoagulation Overlap Therapy[2]	58	91%	91%	93%
ICU Venous Thromboembolism Prophylaxis[2]	50	90%	92%	92%
Incidence of Potentially Preventable VTE[1,2]	-	-	10%	10%
UFH with Dosages/Platelet Monitoring[2]	26	100%	92%	97%
Venous Thromboembolism Prophylaxis[2]	379	68%	87%	85%
Warfarin Therapy Discharge Instructions[2]	39	51%	59%	75%
Chest Pain/Possible Heart Attack Care				
Aspirin Given Within 24 Hours of Arrival	54	96%	97%	96%
Fibrinolytic Meds Within 30 Min. of Arrival[1]	-	-	54%	58%
Average Time to ECG (minutes)	55	6	9	7
Average Time to Transfer (minutes)[1]	-	-	78	60
Children's Asthma Care				
Received Home Management Plan of Care	-	-	-	88%
Received Reliever Medication	-	-	-	100%
Received Systemic Corticosteroids	-	-	-	100%
Emergency Department				
Admittance Decision Time (minutes)[2]	812	171	154	98
Head CT Results Within 45 Min. of Arrival	18	33%	55%	57%
Patients Who Left ER Before Being Seen	45,763	0%	2%	2%
Time from ER Arrival to Admit. (minutes)[2]	1,023	386	378	274
Time from ER Arrival to Discharge (minutes)	285	145	156	134
Time in ER Before Being Evaluated (minutes)	409	22	35	26
Time to Pain Meds for Fractures (minutes)	151	47	61	57
Heart Attack Care				
Aspirin Given at Discharge	65	94%	99%	99%
Fibrinolytic Meds Within 30 Min. of Arrival[7]	-	-	46%	54%
PCI Within 90 Minutes of Arrival[7]	-	-	95%	96%
Statin Prescribed at Discharge	61	90%	98%	98%
Heart Failure Care				
ACE Inhibitor or ARB for LVSD	88	90%	96%	97%
Discharge Instructions Given	220	97%	95%	94%
Evaluation of LVS Function	298	99%	99%	99%
Medicare Spending				
Medicare Spending per Patient (ratio)	-	0.96	0.96	0.98
Pneumonia Care				
Appropriate Initial Antibiotic Given	182	98%	95%	95%
Blood Culture Timing	348	98%	97%	98%
Pregnancy and Delivery Care				
Newborn Deliveries Scheduled Early	21	0%	4%	6%
Preventive Care				
Immunization for Influenza[2]	567	94%	88%	90%
Immunization for Pneumonia[2]	818	91%	88%	92%
Stroke Care				
Anticoagulation Therapy for Atrial Fibrillation	24	96%	96%	95%
Antithrombotic Therapy Timing	106	99%	98%	98%
Assessed for Rehabilitation	121	99%	97%	97%
Discharged on Antithrombotic Therapy	116	97%	99%	99%
Discharged on Statin Medication	84	85%	95%	94%
Thrombolytic Therapy Timing	13	92%	69%	66%
Venous Thromboembolism Prophylaxis	119	87%	94%	94%
Written Stroke Educational Materials Given	56	89%	86%	88%
Surgical Care Improvement Project				
Appropriate Beta Blocker Usage	62	94%	97%	98%
Appropriate VTP Within 24 Hours	164	92%	98%	98%
Controlled Postoperative Blood Glucose[7]	-	-	97%	97%
Perioperative Temperature Management	188	99%	100%	100%
Prophylactic Antibiotic Selection	72	97%	99%	99%
Prophylactic Antibiotic Selection (Outpatient)	59	88%	97%	98%
Prophylactic Antibiotic Stopped	69	93%	98%	98%
Prophylactic Antibiotic Timing	72	99%	99%	99%
Prophylactic Antibiotic Timing (Outpatient)	61	90%	97%	98%
Urinary Catheter Removal	89	90%	96%	97%
Survey of Patients' Hospital Experiences				
Area Around Room 'Always' Quiet at Night	300+	43%	51%	61%
Doctors 'Always' Communicated Well	300+	73%	77%	82%
Home Recovery Information Given	300+	75%	83%	85%
Hospital Given 9 or 10 on 10 Point Scale	300+	53%	63%	71%
Meds 'Always' Explained Before Given	300+	56%	59%	64%
Nurses 'Always' Communicated Well	300+	71%	75%	79%
Pain 'Always' Well Controlled	300+	62%	67%	71%
Room and Bathroom 'Always' Clean	300+	60%	69%	73%
Timely Help 'Always' Received	300+	51%	61%	68%
Would Definitely Recommend Hospital	300+	50%	65%	71%
Use of Medical Imaging				
Cardiac Imaging Stress Test before Surgery	109	7.3%	5.8%	5.3%
Combination Abdominal CT Scan	463	0.2%	8.2%	10.5%
Combination Brain/Sinus CT Scan	674	5.2%	3.6%	2.7%
Combination Chest CT Scan	89	0.0%	1.3%	2.7%
Follow-up Mammogram/Ultrasound[7]	-	-	13%	8.8%
Lumbar Spine MRI for Low Back Pain	32	50.0%	33.4%	37.2%

Health Alliance Hospital Mary's Avenue Campus

105 Mary's Avenue
Kingston, NY 12401
E-mail: webmaster@benedictine.org
URL: www.benedictine.org
Type: Acute Care Hospitals
Ownership: Voluntary non-profit - Church
Phone: 845-338-2500
Fax: 845-334-3149
Emergency Services: Yes
Beds: 222

Key Personnel:
Radiology. . . . . Laurie Abrams
Anesthesiology. . . . . Martin Cascio, MD
Emergency Room . . . . Mamie Caton
Infection Control. . . . . Lorna DeGrazia, RN
CEO/President. . . . . Thomas A Dee
Quality Assurance . . . . Jim Hansen, RN
Chief of Medical Staff . . . . Rafael Olazagasti, MD
Intensive Care Unit. . . . . Marcie Truesdale, RN

Measure	Cases	This Hosp.	State Avg.	U.S. Avg.
Blood Clot Prevention and Treatment				
Anticoagulation Overlap Therapy[1,2]	-	-	91%	93%
ICU Venous Thromboembolism Prophylaxis[1,2]	-	-	92%	92%
Incidence of Potentially Preventable VTE[1,2]	-	-	10%	10%
UFH with Dosages/Platelet Monitoring[1,2]	-	-	92%	97%
Venous Thromboembolism Prophylaxis[2]	125	64%	87%	85%
Warfarin Therapy Discharge Instructions[1,2]	-	-	59%	75%
Chest Pain/Possible Heart Attack Care				
Aspirin Given Within 24 Hours of Arrival[5]	-	-	97%	96%
Fibrinolytic Meds Within 30 Min. of Arrival[5]	-	-	54%	58%
Average Time to ECG (minutes)[5]	-	-	9	7
Average Time to Transfer (minutes)[5]	-	-	78	60
Children's Asthma Care				
Received Home Management Plan of Care	-	-	-	88%
Received Reliever Medication	-	-	-	100%
Received Systemic Corticosteroids	-	-	-	100%
Emergency Department				
Admittance Decision Time (minutes)[2,7]	-	-	154	98
Head CT Results Within 45 Min. of Arrival[5]	-	-	55%	57%
Patients Who Left ER Before Being Seen[5]	-	-	2%	2%
Time from ER Arrival to Admit. (minutes)[2,7]	-	-	378	274
Time from ER Arrival to Discharge (minutes)[5]	-	-	156	134
Time in ER Before Being Evaluated (minutes)[5]	-	-	35	26
Time to Pain Meds for Fractures (minutes)[5]	-	-	61	57
Heart Attack Care				
Aspirin Given at Discharge[5]	-	-	99%	99%
Fibrinolytic Meds Within 30 Min. of Arrival[5]	-	-	46%	54%
PCI Within 90 Minutes of Arrival[5]	-	-	95%	96%
Statin Prescribed at Discharge[5]	-	-	98%	98%
Heart Failure Care				
ACE Inhibitor or ARB for LVSD[1,3]	-	-	96%	97%
Discharge Instructions Given[1,3]	-	-	95%	94%
Evaluation of LVS Function[1,3]	-	-	99%	99%
Medicare Spending				
Medicare Spending per Patient (ratio)	-	0.93	0.96	0.98
Pneumonia Care				
Appropriate Initial Antibiotic Given[1]	-	-	95%	95%
Blood Culture Timing[7]	-	-	97%	98%
Pregnancy and Delivery Care				
Newborn Deliveries Scheduled Early[7]	-	-	4%	6%
Preventive Care				
Immunization for Influenza[2]	292	84%	88%	90%
Immunization for Pneumonia[2]	436	83%	88%	92%
Stroke Care				
Anticoagulation Therapy for Atrial Fibrillation[7]	-	-	96%	95%
Antithrombotic Therapy Timing[1]	-	-	98%	98%
Assessed for Rehabilitation[1]	-	-	97%	97%
Discharged on Antithrombotic Therapy[1]	-	-	99%	99%
Discharged on Statin Medication[1]	-	-	95%	94%
Thrombolytic Therapy Timing[7]	-	-	69%	66%
Venous Thromboembolism Prophylaxis[1]	-	-	94%	94%
Written Stroke Educational Materials Given[7]	-	-	86%	88%
Surgical Care Improvement Project				
Appropriate Beta Blocker Usage	151	99%	97%	98%
Appropriate VTP Within 24 Hours	338	100%	98%	98%
Controlled Postoperative Blood Glucose[7]	-	-	97%	97%
Perioperative Temperature Management	395	100%	100%	100%
Prophylactic Antibiotic Selection	309	99%	99%	99%
Prophylactic Antibiotic Selection (Outpatient)	54	100%	97%	98%
Prophylactic Antibiotic Stopped	304	99%	98%	98%
Prophylactic Antibiotic Timing	309	99%	99%	99%
Prophylactic Antibiotic Timing (Outpatient)	54	98%	97%	98%
Urinary Catheter Removal	336	100%	96%	97%
Survey of Patients' Hospital Experiences				
Area Around Room 'Always' Quiet at Night	300+	57%	51%	61%
Doctors 'Always' Communicated Well	300+	77%	77%	82%
Home Recovery Information Given	300+	90%	83%	85%
Hospital Given 9 or 10 on 10 Point Scale	300+	77%	63%	71%
Meds 'Always' Explained Before Given	300+	60%	59%	64%
Nurses 'Always' Communicated Well	300+	80%	75%	79%
Pain 'Always' Well Controlled	300+	76%	67%	71%
Room and Bathroom 'Always' Clean	300+	76%	69%	73%
Timely Help 'Always' Received	300+	72%	61%	68%
Would Definitely Recommend Hospital	300+	78%	65%	71%
Use of Medical Imaging				
Cardiac Imaging Stress Test before Surgery	147	6.1%	5.8%	5.3%
Combination Abdominal CT Scan	336	7.1%	8.2%	10.5%
Combination Brain/Sinus CT Scan[1]	-	-	3.6%	2.7%
Combination Chest CT Scan	268	0.0%	1.3%	2.7%
Follow-up Mammogram/Ultrasound	1,493	6.4%	13%	8.8%
Lumbar Spine MRI for Low Back Pain[7]	-	-	33.4%	37.2%

Mount Saint Mary's Hospital & Health Center

5300 Military Road
Lewiston, NY 14092
URL: www.msmh.org
Type: Acute Care Hospitals
Ownership: Voluntary non-profit - Church
Phone: 716-297-4800
Fax: 716-298-2091
Emergency Services: Yes
Beds: 179

Key Personnel:
Patient Relations . . . . Barbara Bucci
Emergency Room . . . . Linda Dattaglia, MD
Chief of Medical Staff . . . . Domonic F Falsetti, MD
Pediatric Ambulatory Care . . . . . . T Kaul, MD
Cardiac Laboratory. . . . . John Macklasuo, MD
CEO/President. . . . . Judith A Maness
Quality Assurance . . . . Laurie Merletti

Measure	Cases	This Hosp.	State Avg.	U.S. Avg.
Blood Clot Prevention and Treatment				
Anticoagulation Overlap Therapy[2]	37	89%	91%	93%
ICU Venous Thromboembolism Prophylaxis[2]	69	86%	92%	92%
Incidence of Potentially Preventable VTE[1,2]	-	-	10%	10%
UFH with Dosages/Platelet Monitoring[2]	25	4%	92%	97%
Venous Thromboembolism Prophylaxis[2]	317	84%	87%	85%

NOTE: Hospital profiles are in alphabetical order by state, then city, then hospital within the city; Rankings exclude hospitals with less than 25 cases except for patient surveys which excludes hospitals with less than 100 cases; (a) 100-299 cases; (1) The number of cases/patients is too few to report; (2) Data submitted were based on a sample of cases/patients; (3) Results are based on a shorter time period than required; (4) Data suppressed by CMS for one or more quarters; (5) Results are not available for this reporting period; (6) Fewer than 100 patients completed the HCAHPS survey; (7) No cases met the criteria for this measure; (8) The lower limit of the confidence interval cannot be calculated if the number of observed infections equals zero; (9) No data are available from the state/territory for this reporting period; (10) The scores shown reflect fewer than 50 completed surveys; (11) There were discrepancies in the data collection process; (12) This measure does not apply to this hospital for this reporting period; (13) Results cannot be calculated for this reporting period; (14) The results for this state are combined with nearby states to protect confidentiality; Please refer to the User's Guide for a full explanation of data.

Measure	Cases	This Hosp.	State Avg.	U.S. Avg.
Warfarin Therapy Discharge Instructions[2]	24	21%	59%	75%
Chest Pain/Possible Heart Attack Care				
Aspirin Given Within 24 Hours of Arrival	55	91%	97%	96%
Fibrinolytic Meds Within 30 Min. of Arrival[1]	-	-	54%	58%
Average Time to ECG (minutes)	57	4	9	7
Average Time to Transfer (minutes)[7]	-	-	78	60
Children's Asthma Care				
Received Home Management Plan of Care	-	-	-	88%
Received Reliever Medication	-	-	-	100%
Received Systemic Corticosteroids	-	-	-	100%
Emergency Department				
Admittance Decision Time (minutes)[2]	648	134	154	98
Head CT Results Within 45 Min. of Arrival[1]	-	-	55%	57%
Patients Who Left ER Before Being Seen	22,955	1%	2%	2%
Time from ER Arrival to Admit. (minutes)[2]	684	304	378	274
Time from ER Arrival to Discharge (minutes)	337	172	156	134
Time in ER Before Being Evaluated (minutes)	376	61	35	26
Time to Pain Meds for Fractures (minutes)	126	82	61	57
Heart Attack Care				
Aspirin Given at Discharge	34	100%	99%	99%
Fibrinolytic Meds Within 30 Min. of Arrival[1]	-	-	46%	54%
PCI Within 90 Minutes of Arrival[7]	-	-	95%	96%
Statin Prescribed at Discharge	34	100%	98%	98%
Heart Failure Care				
ACE Inhibitor or ARB for LVSD	36	100%	96%	97%
Discharge Instructions Given	156	92%	95%	94%
Evaluation of LVS Function	201	100%	99%	99%
Medicare Spending				
Medicare Spending per Patient (ratio)	-	0.95	0.96	0.98
Pneumonia Care				
Appropriate Initial Antibiotic Given	100	95%	95%	95%
Blood Culture Timing	142	96%	97%	98%
Pregnancy and Delivery Care				
Newborn Deliveries Scheduled Early[2]	56	5%	4%	6%
Preventive Care				
Immunization for Influenza[2]	489	63%	88%	90%
Immunization for Pneumonia[2]	647	72%	88%	92%
Stroke Care				
Anticoagulation Therapy for Atrial Fibrillation[2]	12	92%	96%	95%
Antithrombotic Therapy Timing[2]	63	97%	98%	98%
Assessed for Rehabilitation[2]	62	100%	97%	97%
Discharged on Antithrombotic Therapy[2]	59	98%	99%	99%
Discharged on Statin Medication[2]	45	100%	95%	94%
Thrombolytic Therapy Timing[1,2]	-	-	69%	66%
Venous Thromboembolism Prophylaxis[2]	69	94%	94%	94%
Written Stroke Educational Materials Given[2]	42	90%	86%	88%
Surgical Care Improvement Project				
Appropriate Beta Blocker Usage[2]	97	98%	97%	98%
Appropriate VTP Within 24 Hours[2]	281	99%	98%	98%
Controlled Postoperative Blood Glucose[2,7]	-	-	97%	97%
Perioperative Temperature Management[2]	326	100%	100%	100%
Prophylactic Antibiotic Selection[2]	252	99%	99%	99%
Prophylactic Antibiotic Selection (Outpatient)	157	98%	97%	98%
Prophylactic Antibiotic Stopped[2]	252	96%	98%	98%
Prophylactic Antibiotic Timing[2]	252	98%	99%	99%
Prophylactic Antibiotic Timing (Outpatient)	158	99%	97%	98%
Urinary Catheter Removal[2]	217	99%	96%	97%
Survey of Patients' Hospital Experiences				
Area Around Room 'Always' Quiet at Night	300+	56%	51%	61%
Doctors 'Always' Communicated Well	300+	78%	77%	82%
Home Recovery Information Given	300+	84%	83%	85%
Hospital Given 9 or 10 on 10 Point Scale	300+	66%	63%	71%
Meds 'Always' Explained Before Given	300+	58%	59%	64%
Nurses 'Always' Communicated Well	300+	75%	75%	79%
Pain 'Always' Well Controlled	300+	66%	67%	71%
Room and Bathroom 'Always' Clean	300+	70%	69%	73%
Timely Help 'Always' Received	300+	53%	61%	68%
Would Definitely Recommend Hospital	300+	71%	65%	71%
Use of Medical Imaging				
Cardiac Imaging Stress Test before Surgery	404	4.7%	5.8%	5.3%
Combination Abdominal CT Scan	359	5.6%	8.2%	10.5%
Combination Brain/Sinus CT Scan	316	5.7%	3.6%	2.7%
Combination Chest CT Scan	326	0.3%	1.3%	2.7%
Follow-up Mammogram/Ultrasound	612	11.1%	13%	8.8%
Lumbar Spine MRI for Low Back Pain	59	45.8%	33.4%	37.2%

Little Falls Hospital

140 Burwell Street
Little Falls, NY 13365
E-mail: c.mowers@lfny.org
URL: www.lfhny.org
Type: Critical Access Hospitals
Ownership: Voluntary non-profit - Private
Phone: 315-823-5261
Fax: 315-823-5383
Emergency Services: Yes
Beds: 25

Key Personnel:
Emergency Room . . . . Rebecca Akers, RN, BSN
Intensive Care Unit. . . . . Heidi Camardello, BSN, CNOR
Operating Room. . . . . Tammy Hedrick, RN
Patient Relations . . . . Catherine Kunz, MS, CPHQ
Quality Assurance . . . . Catherine Kunz, RN, CPHQ
CEO/President. . . . . Michael L Ogden
Chief of Medical Staff . . . . L Andrew Rauscher, MD
Infection Control. . . . . Patty Seifried, RUN

Measure	Cases	This Hosp.	State Avg.	U.S. Avg.
Blood Clot Prevention and Treatment				
Anticoagulation Overlap Therapy[5]	-	-	91%	93%
ICU Venous Thromboembolism Prophylaxis[5]	-	-	92%	92%
Incidence of Potentially Preventable VTE[5]	-	-	10%	10%
UFH with Dosages/Platelet Monitoring[5]	-	-	92%	97%
Venous Thromboembolism Prophylaxis[5]	-	-	87%	85%
Warfarin Therapy Discharge Instructions[5]	-	-	59%	75%
Chest Pain/Possible Heart Attack Care				
Aspirin Given Within 24 Hours of Arrival	39	95%	97%	96%
Fibrinolytic Meds Within 30 Min. of Arrival[1]	-	-	54%	58%
Average Time to ECG (minutes)	49	8	9	7
Average Time to Transfer (minutes)	14	96	78	60
Children's Asthma Care				
Received Home Management Plan of Care	-	-	-	88%
Received Reliever Medication	-	-	-	100%
Received Systemic Corticosteroids	-	-	-	100%
Emergency Department				
Admittance Decision Time (minutes)[2,3]	125	74	154	98
Head CT Results Within 45 Min. of Arrival[1,3]	-	-	55%	57%
Patients Who Left ER Before Being Seen	16,225	3%	2%	2%
Time from ER Arrival to Admit. (minutes)[2,3]	127	278	378	274
Time from ER Arrival to Discharge (minutes)[3]	80	137	156	134
Time in ER Before Being Evaluated (minutes)[3]	96	42	35	26
Time to Pain Meds for Fractures (minutes)[3]	18	110	61	57
Heart Attack Care				
Aspirin Given at Discharge[5]	-	-	99%	99%
Fibrinolytic Meds Within 30 Min. of Arrival[5]	-	-	46%	54%
PCI Within 90 Minutes of Arrival[5]	-	-	95%	96%
Statin Prescribed at Discharge[5]	-	-	98%	98%
Heart Failure Care				
ACE Inhibitor or ARB for LVSD	16	75%	96%	97%
Discharge Instructions Given	24	88%	95%	94%
Evaluation of LVS Function	30	90%	99%	99%
Medicare Spending				
Medicare Spending per Patient (ratio)	-	-	0.96	0.98
Pneumonia Care				
Appropriate Initial Antibiotic Given	72	79%	95%	95%
Blood Culture Timing	80	71%	97%	98%
Pregnancy and Delivery Care				
Newborn Deliveries Scheduled Early[5]	-	-	4%	6%
Preventive Care				
Immunization for Influenza[5]	-	-	88%	90%
Immunization for Pneumonia[2,3]	108	67%	88%	92%
Stroke Care				
Anticoagulation Therapy for Atrial Fibrillation[5]	-	-	96%	95%
Antithrombotic Therapy Timing[5]	-	-	98%	98%
Assessed for Rehabilitation[5]	-	-	97%	97%
Discharged on Antithrombotic Therapy[5]	-	-	99%	99%
Discharged on Statin Medication[5]	-	-	95%	94%
Thrombolytic Therapy Timing[5]	-	-	69%	66%
Venous Thromboembolism Prophylaxis[5]	-	-	94%	94%
Written Stroke Educational Materials Given[5]	-	-	86%	88%
Surgical Care Improvement Project				
Appropriate Beta Blocker Usage[5]	-	-	97%	98%
Appropriate VTP Within 24 Hours[5]	-	-	98%	98%
Controlled Postoperative Blood Glucose[5]	-	-	97%	97%
Perioperative Temperature Management[5]	-	-	100%	100%
Prophylactic Antibiotic Selection[5]	-	-	99%	99%
Prophylactic Antibiotic Selection (Outpatient)	28	89%	97%	98%
Prophylactic Antibiotic Stopped[5]	-	-	98%	98%
Prophylactic Antibiotic Timing[5]	-	-	99%	99%
Prophylactic Antibiotic Timing (Outpatient)	29	97%	97%	98%
Urinary Catheter Removal[5]	-	-	96%	97%
Survey of Patients' Hospital Experiences				
Area Around Room 'Always' Quiet at Night	(a)	54%	51%	61%
Doctors 'Always' Communicated Well	(a)	87%	77%	82%
Home Recovery Information Given	(a)	91%	83%	85%
Hospital Given 9 or 10 on 10 Point Scale	(a)	72%	63%	71%
Meds 'Always' Explained Before Given	(a)	65%	59%	64%
Nurses 'Always' Communicated Well	(a)	81%	75%	79%
Pain 'Always' Well Controlled	(a)	73%	67%	71%
Room and Bathroom 'Always' Clean	(a)	80%	69%	73%
Timely Help 'Always' Received	(a)	69%	61%	68%
Would Definitely Recommend Hospital	(a)	75%	65%	71%
Use of Medical Imaging				
Cardiac Imaging Stress Test before Surgery	48	0.0%	5.8%	5.3%
Combination Abdominal CT Scan	316	3.8%	8.2%	10.5%
Combination Brain/Sinus CT Scan	247	0.8%	3.6%	2.7%
Combination Chest CT Scan	177	0.6%	1.3%	2.7%
Follow-up Mammogram/Ultrasound	291	7.2%	13%	8.8%
Lumbar Spine MRI for Low Back Pain[1]	-	-	33.4%	37.2%

Eastern Niagara Hospital

521 East Avenue
Lockport, NY 14094
URL: www.enhs.org
Type: Acute Care Hospitals
Ownership: Voluntary non-profit - Private
Phone: 716-514-5700
Fax: 716-514-5587
Emergency Services: Yes
Beds: 134

Key Personnel:
CEO/President. . . . . Clare A Haar
Emergency Room . . . . Michael Torres, MD

Measure	Cases	This Hosp.	State Avg.	U.S. Avg.
Blood Clot Prevention and Treatment				
Anticoagulation Overlap Therapy[2]	41	51%	91%	93%
ICU Venous Thromboembolism Prophylaxis[2]	78	91%	92%	92%
Incidence of Potentially Preventable VTE[1,2]	-	-	10%	10%
UFH with Dosages/Platelet Monitoring[2]	31	97%	92%	97%
Venous Thromboembolism Prophylaxis[2]	413	91%	87%	85%
Warfarin Therapy Discharge Instructions[2]	30	7%	59%	75%
Chest Pain/Possible Heart Attack Care				
Aspirin Given Within 24 Hours of Arrival	145	92%	97%	96%
Fibrinolytic Meds Within 30 Min. of Arrival	18	33%	54%	58%
Average Time to ECG (minutes)	148	2	9	7
Average Time to Transfer (minutes)[1]	-	-	78	60
Children's Asthma Care				
Received Home Management Plan of Care	-	-	-	88%
Received Reliever Medication	-	-	-	100%
Received Systemic Corticosteroids	-	-	-	100%
Emergency Department				
Admittance Decision Time (minutes)[2]	816	84	154	98
Head CT Results Within 45 Min. of Arrival	13	23%	55%	57%
Patients Who Left ER Before Being Seen	22,457	1%	2%	2%
Time from ER Arrival to Admit. (minutes)[2]	882	270	378	274
Time from ER Arrival to Discharge (minutes)	380	143	156	134
Time in ER Before Being Evaluated (minutes)	412	24	35	26
Time to Pain Meds for Fractures (minutes)	57	78	61	57
Heart Attack Care				
Aspirin Given at Discharge[2]	43	79%	99%	99%
Fibrinolytic Meds Within 30 Min. of Arrival[2,7]	-	-	46%	54%
PCI Within 90 Minutes of Arrival[2,7]	-	-	95%	96%
Statin Prescribed at Discharge[2]	44	73%	98%	98%
Heart Failure Care				
ACE Inhibitor or ARB for LVSD[2]	31	87%	96%	97%
Discharge Instructions Given[2]	157	82%	95%	94%
Evaluation of LVS Function[2]	208	98%	99%	99%
Medicare Spending				

NOTE: Hospital profiles are in alphabetical order by state, then city, then hospital within the city; Rankings exclude hospitals with less than 25 cases except for patient surveys which excludes hospitals with less than 100 cases; (a) 100-299 cases; (1) The number of cases/patients is too few to report; (2) Data submitted were based on a sample of cases/patients; (3) Results are based on a shorter time period than required; (4) Data suppressed by CMS for one or more quarters; (5) Results are not available for this reporting period; (6) Fewer than 100 patients completed the HCAHPS survey; (7) No cases met the criteria for this measure; (8) The lower limit of the confidence interval cannot be calculated if the number of observed infections equals zero; (9) No data are available from the state/territory for this reporting period; (10) The scores shown reflect fewer than 50 completed surveys; (11) There were discrepancies in the data collection process; (12) This measure does not apply to this hospital for this reporting period; (13) Results cannot be calculated for this reporting period; (14) The results for this state are combined with nearby states to protect confidentiality; Please refer to the User's Guide for a full explanation of data.

Measure	Cases	This Hosp.	State Avg.	U.S. Avg.
Medicare Spending per Patient (ratio)	-	0.90	0.96	0.98
Pneumonia Care				
Appropriate Initial Antibiotic Given[2]	92	89%	95%	95%
Blood Culture Timing[2]	115	97%	97%	98%
Pregnancy and Delivery Care				
Newborn Deliveries Scheduled Early	38	16%	4%	6%
Preventive Care				
Immunization for Influenza[2]	623	86%	88%	90%
Immunization for Pneumonia[2]	845	91%	88%	92%
Stroke Care				
Anticoagulation Therapy for Atrial Fibrillation[1,2]	-	-	96%	95%
Antithrombotic Therapy Timing[2]	19	79%	98%	98%
Assessed for Rehabilitation[2]	18	72%	97%	97%
Discharged on Antithrombotic Therapy[2]	17	82%	99%	99%
Discharged on Statin Medication[2]	16	75%	95%	94%
Thrombolytic Therapy Timing[1,2]	-	-	69%	66%
Venous Thromboembolism Prophylaxis[2]	18	83%	94%	94%
Written Stroke Educational Materials Given[2]	13	0%	86%	88%
Surgical Care Improvement Project				
Appropriate Beta Blocker Usage[2]	32	91%	97%	98%
Appropriate VTP Within 24 Hours[2]	123	93%	98%	98%
Controlled Postoperative Blood Glucose[2,7]	-	-	97%	97%
Perioperative Temperature Management[2]	131	93%	100%	100%
Prophylactic Antibiotic Selection[2]	66	94%	99%	99%
Prophylactic Antibiotic Selection (Outpatient)	53	91%	97%	98%
Prophylactic Antibiotic Stopped[2]	66	92%	98%	98%
Prophylactic Antibiotic Timing[2]	66	100%	99%	99%
Prophylactic Antibiotic Timing (Outpatient)	54	98%	97%	98%
Urinary Catheter Removal[2]	40	90%	96%	97%
Survey of Patients' Hospital Experiences				
Area Around Room 'Always' Quiet at Night	300+	44%	51%	61%
Doctors 'Always' Communicated Well	300+	79%	77%	82%
Home Recovery Information Given	300+	83%	83%	85%
Hospital Given 9 or 10 on 10 Point Scale	300+	61%	63%	71%
Meds 'Always' Explained Before Given	300+	56%	59%	64%
Nurses 'Always' Communicated Well	300+	75%	75%	79%
Pain 'Always' Well Controlled	300+	67%	67%	71%
Room and Bathroom 'Always' Clean	300+	70%	69%	73%
Timely Help 'Always' Received	300+	59%	61%	68%
Would Definitely Recommend Hospital	300+	61%	65%	71%
Use of Medical Imaging				
Cardiac Imaging Stress Test before Surgery	171	5.3%	5.8%	5.3%
Combination Abdominal CT Scan	248	1.6%	8.2%	10.5%
Combination Brain/Sinus CT Scan[1]	-	-	3.6%	2.7%
Combination Chest CT Scan	180	1.1%	1.3%	2.7%
Follow-up Mammogram/Ultrasound	601	4.3%	13%	8.8%
Lumbar Spine MRI for Low Back Pain[1]	-	-	33.4%	37.2%

Long Beach Medical Center

455 East Bay Drive
Long Beach, NY 11561
URL: www.lbmc.org
Phone: 516-897-1000
Fax: 516-897-1214

Type: Acute Care Hospitals
Ownership: Voluntary non-profit - Private
Emergency Services: Yes
Beds: 203

Key Personnel:
Chief of Medical Staff.......... Iqbal Jangda
CEO/President............... Douglas L Melzer

Measure	Cases	This Hosp.	State Avg.	U.S. Avg.
Blood Clot Prevention and Treatment				
Anticoagulation Overlap Therapy[5]	-	-	91%	93%
ICU Venous Thromboembolism Prophylaxis[5]	-	-	92%	92%
Incidence of Potentially Preventable VTE[5]	-	-	10%	10%
UFH with Dosages/Platelet Monitoring[5]	-	-	92%	97%
Venous Thromboembolism Prophylaxis[5]	-	-	87%	85%
Warfarin Therapy Discharge Instructions[5]	-	-	59%	75%
Chest Pain/Possible Heart Attack Care				
Aspirin Given Within 24 Hours of Arrival[5]	-	-	97%	96%
Fibrinolytic Meds Within 30 Min. of Arrival[5]	-	-	54%	58%
Average Time to ECG (minutes)[5]	-	-	9	7
Average Time to Transfer (minutes)[5]	-	-	78	60
Children's Asthma Care				
Received Home Management Plan of Care	-	-	-	88%
Received Reliever Medication	-	-	-	100%
Received Systemic Corticosteroids	-	-	-	100%
Emergency Department				
Admittance Decision Time (minutes)[5]	-	-	154	98
Head CT Results Within 45 Min. of Arrival[5]	-	-	55%	57%
Patients Who Left ER Before Being Seen[5]	-	-	2%	2%
Time from ER Arrival to Admit. (minutes)[5]	-	-	378	274
Time from ER Arrival to Discharge (minutes)[5]	-	-	156	134
Time in ER Before Being Evaluated (minutes)[5]	-	-	35	26
Time to Pain Meds for Fractures (minutes)[5]	-	-	61	57
Heart Attack Care				
Aspirin Given at Discharge[5]	-	-	99%	99%
Fibrinolytic Meds Within 30 Min. of Arrival[5]	-	-	46%	54%
PCI Within 90 Minutes of Arrival[5]	-	-	95%	96%
Statin Prescribed at Discharge[5]	-	-	98%	98%
Heart Failure Care				
ACE Inhibitor or ARB for LVSD[5]	-	-	96%	97%
Discharge Instructions Given[5]	-	-	95%	94%
Evaluation of LVS Function[5]	-	-	99%	99%
Medicare Spending				
Medicare Spending per Patient (ratio)	-	-	0.96	0.98
Pneumonia Care				
Appropriate Initial Antibiotic Given[5]	-	-	95%	95%
Blood Culture Timing[5]	-	-	97%	98%
Pregnancy and Delivery Care				
Newborn Deliveries Scheduled Early[5]	-	-	4%	6%
Preventive Care				
Immunization for Influenza[5]	-	-	88%	90%
Immunization for Pneumonia[5]	-	-	88%	92%
Stroke Care				
Anticoagulation Therapy for Atrial Fibrillation[5]	-	-	96%	95%
Antithrombotic Therapy Timing[5]	-	-	98%	98%
Assessed for Rehabilitation[5]	-	-	97%	97%
Discharged on Antithrombotic Therapy[5]	-	-	99%	99%
Discharged on Statin Medication[5]	-	-	95%	94%
Thrombolytic Therapy Timing[5]	-	-	69%	66%
Venous Thromboembolism Prophylaxis[5]	-	-	94%	94%
Written Stroke Educational Materials Given[5]	-	-	86%	88%
Surgical Care Improvement Project				
Appropriate Beta Blocker Usage[5]	-	-	97%	98%
Appropriate VTP Within 24 Hours[5]	-	-	98%	98%
Controlled Postoperative Blood Glucose[5]	-	-	97%	97%
Perioperative Temperature Management[5]	-	-	100%	100%
Prophylactic Antibiotic Selection[5]	-	-	99%	99%
Prophylactic Antibiotic Selection (Outpatient)[5]	-	-	97%	98%
Prophylactic Antibiotic Stopped[5]	-	-	98%	98%
Prophylactic Antibiotic Timing[5]	-	-	99%	99%
Prophylactic Antibiotic Timing (Outpatient)[5]	-	-	97%	98%
Urinary Catheter Removal[5]	-	-	96%	97%
Survey of Patients' Hospital Experiences				
Area Around Room 'Always' Quiet at Night[5]	-	-	51%	61%
Doctors 'Always' Communicated Well[5]	-	-	77%	82%
Home Recovery Information Given[5]	-	-	83%	85%
Hospital Given 9 or 10 on 10 Point Scale[5]	-	-	63%	71%
Meds 'Always' Explained Before Given[5]	-	-	59%	64%
Nurses 'Always' Communicated Well[5]	-	-	75%	79%
Pain 'Always' Well Controlled[5]	-	-	67%	71%
Room and Bathroom 'Always' Clean[5]	-	-	69%	73%
Timely Help 'Always' Received[5]	-	-	61%	68%
Would Definitely Recommend Hospital[5]	-	-	65%	71%
Use of Medical Imaging				
Cardiac Imaging Stress Test before Surgery[1]	-	-	5.8%	5.3%
Combination Abdominal CT Scan	81	59.3%	8.2%	10.5%
Combination Brain/Sinus CT Scan[1]	-	-	3.6%	2.7%
Combination Chest CT Scan[1]	-	-	1.3%	2.7%
Follow-up Mammogram/Ultrasound	58	41.4%	13%	8.8%
Lumbar Spine MRI for Low Back Pain[1]	-	-	33.4%	37.2%

Lewis County General Hospital

7785 North State Street
Lowville, NY 13367
URL: www.lcgh.net
Phone: 315-376-5200
Fax: 315-376-9317

Type: Acute Care Hospitals
Ownership: Government - Local
Emergency Services: Yes
Beds: 160

Key Personnel:
Infection Control............... Christopher Cole
Operating Room............... Earl Der
Intensive Care Unit............ Fern Lynclecker, RN
Quality Assurance .... Pamela Mc Cain
Chief of Medical Staff.......... Dr Daniel Pisaniello
Radiology..................... Cindy Sirois
CEO/President............... Charles Truax
Cardiac Laboratory............ Dr Manoj Vera

Measure	Cases	This Hosp.	State Avg.	U.S. Avg.
Blood Clot Prevention and Treatment				
Anticoagulation Overlap Therapy[1,2]	-	-	91%	93%
ICU Venous Thromboembolism Prophylaxis[2]	76	99%	92%	92%
Incidence of Potentially Preventable VTE[1,2]	-	-	10%	10%
UFH with Dosages/Platelet Monitoring[1,2]	-	-	92%	97%
Venous Thromboembolism Prophylaxis[2]	87	94%	87%	85%
Warfarin Therapy Discharge Instructions[1,2]	-	-	59%	75%
Chest Pain/Possible Heart Attack Care				
Aspirin Given Within 24 Hours of Arrival	35	97%	97%	96%
Fibrinolytic Meds Within 30 Min. of Arrival	13	46%	54%	58%
Average Time to ECG (minutes)	36	10	9	7
Average Time to Transfer (minutes)[7]	-	-	78	60
Children's Asthma Care				
Received Home Management Plan of Care	-	-	-	88%
Received Reliever Medication	-	-	-	100%
Received Systemic Corticosteroids	-	-	-	100%
Emergency Department				
Admittance Decision Time (minutes)[2]	306	98	154	98
Head CT Results Within 45 Min. of Arrival[1,3]	-	-	55%	57%
Patients Who Left ER Before Being Seen	12,148	2%	2%	2%
Time from ER Arrival to Admit. (minutes)[2]	339	271	378	274
Time from ER Arrival to Discharge (minutes)	436	116	156	134
Time in ER Before Being Evaluated (minutes)	439	35	35	26
Time to Pain Meds for Fractures (minutes)	41	68	61	57
Heart Attack Care				
Aspirin Given at Discharge[1]	-	-	99%	99%
Fibrinolytic Meds Within 30 Min. of Arrival[7]	-	-	46%	54%
PCI Within 90 Minutes of Arrival[7]	-	-	95%	96%
Statin Prescribed at Discharge[1]	-	-	98%	98%
Heart Failure Care				
ACE Inhibitor or ARB for LVSD	22	64%	96%	97%
Discharge Instructions Given	34	65%	95%	94%
Evaluation of LVS Function	47	89%	99%	99%
Medicare Spending				
Medicare Spending per Patient (ratio)	-	0.75	0.96	0.98
Pneumonia Care				
Appropriate Initial Antibiotic Given	56	86%	95%	95%
Blood Culture Timing	74	88%	97%	98%
Pregnancy and Delivery Care				
Newborn Deliveries Scheduled Early	28	0%	4%	6%
Preventive Care				
Immunization for Influenza[2]	245	82%	88%	90%
Immunization for Pneumonia[2]	254	83%	88%	92%
Stroke Care				
Anticoagulation Therapy for Atrial Fibrillation[1]	-	-	96%	95%
Antithrombotic Therapy Timing[1]	-	-	98%	98%
Assessed for Rehabilitation[1]	-	-	97%	97%
Discharged on Antithrombotic Therapy[1]	-	-	99%	99%
Discharged on Statin Medication[1]	-	-	95%	94%
Thrombolytic Therapy Timing[1]	-	-	69%	66%
Venous Thromboembolism Prophylaxis[1]	-	-	94%	94%
Written Stroke Educational Materials Given[1]	-	-	86%	88%
Surgical Care Improvement Project				
Appropriate Beta Blocker Usage[1]	-	-	97%	98%
Appropriate VTP Within 24 Hours	34	100%	98%	98%
Controlled Postoperative Blood Glucose[7]	-	-	97%	97%
Perioperative Temperature Management	39	100%	100%	100%
Prophylactic Antibiotic Selection	15	93%	99%	99%

NOTE: Hospital profiles are in alphabetical order by state, then city, then hospital within the city; Rankings exclude hospitals with less than 25 cases except for patient surveys which excludes hospitals with less than 100 cases; (a) 100-299 cases; (1) The number of cases/patients is too few to report; (2) Data submitted were based on a sample of cases/patients; (3) Results are based on a shorter time period than required; (4) Data suppressed by CMS for one or more quarters; (5) Results are not available for this reporting period; (6) Fewer than 100 patients completed the HCAHPS survey; (7) No cases met the criteria for this measure; (8) The lower limit of the confidence interval cannot be calculated if the number of observed infections equals zero; (9) No data are available from the state/territory for this reporting period; (10) The scores shown reflect fewer than 50 completed surveys; (11) There were discrepancies in the data collection process; (12) This measure does not apply to this hospital for this reporting period; (13) Results cannot be calculated for this reporting period; (14) The results for this state are combined with nearby states to protect confidentiality; Please refer to the User's Guide for a full explanation of data.

Measure	Cases	This Hosp.	State Avg.	U.S. Avg.
Prophylactic Antibiotic Selection (Outpatient)[5]	-	-	97%	98%
Prophylactic Antibiotic Stopped	15	100%	98%	98%
Prophylactic Antibiotic Timing	15	80%	99%	99%
Prophylactic Antibiotic Timing (Outpatient)[5]	-	-	97%	98%
Urinary Catheter Removal	14	71%	96%	97%
Survey of Patients' Hospital Experiences				
Area Around Room 'Always' Quiet at Night	300+	54%	51%	61%
Doctors 'Always' Communicated Well	300+	84%	77%	82%
Home Recovery Information Given	300+	87%	83%	85%
Hospital Given 9 or 10 on 10 Point Scale	300+	70%	63%	71%
Meds 'Always' Explained Before Given	300+	69%	59%	64%
Nurses 'Always' Communicated Well	300+	78%	75%	79%
Pain 'Always' Well Controlled	300+	73%	67%	71%
Room and Bathroom 'Always' Clean	300+	81%	69%	73%
Timely Help 'Always' Received	300+	72%	61%	68%
Would Definitely Recommend Hospital	300+	73%	65%	71%
Use of Medical Imaging				
Cardiac Imaging Stress Test before Surgery	118	5.9%	5.8%	5.3%
Combination Abdominal CT Scan	253	19.0%	8.2%	10.5%
Combination Brain/Sinus CT Scan[1]	-	-	3.6%	2.7%
Combination Chest CT Scan	116	8.6%	1.3%	2.7%
Follow-up Mammogram/Ultrasound	576	8.7%	13%	8.8%
Lumbar Spine MRI for Low Back Pain[1]	-	-	33.4%	37.2%

Alice Hyde Medical Center

133 Park Street
Malone, NY 12953
Phone: 518-483-3000
Fax: 518-481-2598
E-mail: support@alicehyde.com
URL: www.alicehyde.com
Type: Acute Care Hospitals
Emergency Services: Yes
Ownership: Voluntary non-profit - Other
Beds: 151

Key Personnel:

Radiology.................. Morris Brownman, RTR
CEO/President............... Douglas F. DiVello, MPH, FACHE
Chief of Medical Staff.......... Leonardo Dishman, MD
Operating Room............. Barb LaBombard
Coronary Care.............. Sharon Martin, RN
Infection Control............ Sandi Pfaff
Quality Assurance .... Jeanette Snell, RN
Pediatric In-Patient Care .... Ira Weissman, MD

Measure	Cases	This Hosp.	State Avg.	U.S. Avg.
Blood Clot Prevention and Treatment				
Anticoagulation Overlap Therapy[2]	22	86%	91%	93%
ICU Venous Thromboembolism Prophylaxis[2]	19	84%	92%	92%
Incidence of Potentially Preventable VTE[1,2]	-	-	10%	10%
UFH with Dosages/Platelet Monitoring[1,2]	-	-	92%	97%
Venous Thromboembolism Prophylaxis[2]	185	89%	87%	85%
Warfarin Therapy Discharge Instructions[2]	18	72%	59%	75%
Chest Pain/Possible Heart Attack Care				
Aspirin Given Within 24 Hours of Arrival	104	97%	97%	96%
Fibrinolytic Meds Within 30 Min. of Arrival[1]	-	-	54%	58%
Average Time to ECG (minutes)	105	16	9	7
Average Time to Transfer (minutes)[1]	-	-	78	60
Children's Asthma Care				
Received Home Management Plan of Care	-	-	-	88%
Received Reliever Medication	-	-	-	100%
Received Systemic Corticosteroids	-	-	-	100%
Emergency Department				
Admittance Decision Time (minutes)[2]	418	64	154	98
Head CT Results Within 45 Min. of Arrival[1]	-	-	55%	57%
Patients Who Left ER Before Being Seen	16,235	3%	2%	2%
Time from ER Arrival to Admit. (minutes)[2]	418	246	378	274
Time from ER Arrival to Discharge (minutes)	363	138	156	134
Time in ER Before Being Evaluated (minutes)	388	31	35	26
Time to Pain Meds for Fractures (minutes)	36	64	61	57
Heart Attack Care				
Aspirin Given at Discharge	21	100%	99%	99%
Fibrinolytic Meds Within 30 Min. of Arrival[7]	-	-	46%	54%
PCI Within 90 Minutes of Arrival[7]	-	-	95%	96%
Statin Prescribed at Discharge	22	82%	98%	98%
Heart Failure Care				
ACE Inhibitor or ARB for LVSD	17	94%	96%	97%
Discharge Instructions Given	90	92%	95%	94%
Evaluation of LVS Function	109	100%	99%	99%
Medicare Spending				
Medicare Spending per Patient (ratio)	-	0.84	0.96	0.98
Pneumonia Care				
Appropriate Initial Antibiotic Given	46	100%	95%	95%
Blood Culture Timing	64	95%	97%	98%
Pregnancy and Delivery Care				
Newborn Deliveries Scheduled Early[2]	38	34%	4%	6%
Preventive Care				
Immunization for Influenza[2]	264	92%	88%	90%
Immunization for Pneumonia[2]	346	92%	88%	92%
Stroke Care				
Anticoagulation Therapy for Atrial Fibrillation[1]	-	-	96%	95%
Antithrombotic Therapy Timing	26	100%	98%	98%
Assessed for Rehabilitation	24	83%	97%	97%
Discharged on Antithrombotic Therapy	22	100%	99%	99%
Discharged on Statin Medication	15	100%	95%	94%
Thrombolytic Therapy Timing[1]	-	-	69%	66%
Venous Thromboembolism Prophylaxis	27	89%	94%	94%
Written Stroke Educational Materials Given	16	38%	86%	88%
Surgical Care Improvement Project				
Appropriate Beta Blocker Usage	23	96%	97%	98%
Appropriate VTP Within 24 Hours	100	99%	98%	98%
Controlled Postoperative Blood Glucose[7]	-	-	97%	97%
Perioperative Temperature Management	110	100%	100%	100%
Prophylactic Antibiotic Selection	77	97%	99%	99%
Prophylactic Antibiotic Selection (Outpatient)	28	96%	97%	98%
Prophylactic Antibiotic Stopped	74	95%	98%	98%
Prophylactic Antibiotic Timing	77	96%	99%	99%
Prophylactic Antibiotic Timing (Outpatient)	28	96%	97%	98%
Urinary Catheter Removal	83	96%	96%	97%
Survey of Patients' Hospital Experiences				
Area Around Room 'Always' Quiet at Night	300+	53%	51%	61%
Doctors 'Always' Communicated Well	300+	78%	77%	82%
Home Recovery Information Given	300+	80%	83%	85%
Hospital Given 9 or 10 on 10 Point Scale	300+	51%	63%	71%
Meds 'Always' Explained Before Given	300+	59%	59%	64%
Nurses 'Always' Communicated Well	300+	76%	75%	79%
Pain 'Always' Well Controlled	300+	69%	67%	71%
Room and Bathroom 'Always' Clean	300+	79%	69%	73%
Timely Help 'Always' Received	300+	68%	61%	68%
Would Definitely Recommend Hospital	300+	47%	65%	71%
Use of Medical Imaging				
Cardiac Imaging Stress Test before Surgery	143	8.4%	5.8%	5.3%
Combination Abdominal CT Scan	434	4.8%	8.2%	10.5%
Combination Brain/Sinus CT Scan	355	1.7%	3.6%	2.7%
Combination Chest CT Scan	270	0.0%	1.3%	2.7%
Follow-up Mammogram/Ultrasound	831	10.7%	13%	8.8%
Lumbar Spine MRI for Low Back Pain	60	33.3%	33.4%	37.2%

North Shore University Hospital

300 Community Drive
Manhasset, NY 11030
Phone: 516-562-0100
Fax: 516-562-1395
URL: www.northshorelij.com
Type: Acute Care Hospitals
Emergency Services: Yes
Ownership: Voluntary non-profit - Private
Beds: 900

Key Personnel:

Anesthesiology............... John Di Capua, MD
CEO/President............... Michael J. Dowling
Pediatric Ambulatory Care ...... James Fagin, MD
Quality Assurance .... Donn Haber
Cardiac Laboratory............ Stanley Katz, MD
Radiology.................. Jason J. Naidich, MD, MBA
Pediatrics.................. Charles Schleien, MD, MBA
Chief of Medical Staff.......... Lawrence G Smith, MD

Measure	Cases	This Hosp.	State Avg.	U.S. Avg.
Blood Clot Prevention and Treatment				
Anticoagulation Overlap Therapy[2]	271	90%	91%	93%
ICU Venous Thromboembolism Prophylaxis[2]	109	93%	92%	92%
Incidence of Potentially Preventable VTE[2]	127	6%	10%	10%
UFH with Dosages/Platelet Monitoring[2]	158	100%	92%	97%
Venous Thromboembolism Prophylaxis[2]	635	89%	87%	85%
Warfarin Therapy Discharge Instructions[2]	192	20%	59%	75%
Chest Pain/Possible Heart Attack Care				
Aspirin Given Within 24 Hours of Arrival[1]	-	-	97%	96%
Fibrinolytic Meds Within 30 Min. of Arrival[3,7]	-	-	54%	58%
Average Time to ECG (minutes)[1]	-	-	9	7
Average Time to Transfer (minutes)[1,3]	-	-	78	60
Children's Asthma Care				
Received Home Management Plan of Care	-	-	-	88%
Received Reliever Medication	-	-	-	100%
Received Systemic Corticosteroids	-	-	-	100%
Emergency Department				
Admittance Decision Time (minutes)[2]	878	185	154	98
Head CT Results Within 45 Min. of Arrival[1]	-	-	55%	57%
Patients Who Left ER Before Being Seen	>100k	0%	2%	2%
Time from ER Arrival to Admit. (minutes)[2]	933	374	378	274
Time from ER Arrival to Discharge (minutes)	727	117	156	134
Time in ER Before Being Evaluated (minutes)	646	25	35	26
Time to Pain Meds for Fractures (minutes)	189	45	61	57
Heart Attack Care				
Aspirin Given at Discharge[2]	320	99%	99%	99%
Fibrinolytic Meds Within 30 Min. of Arrival[2,7]	-	-	46%	54%
PCI Within 90 Minutes of Arrival[2]	16	75%	95%	96%
Statin Prescribed at Discharge[2]	311	97%	98%	98%
Heart Failure Care				
ACE Inhibitor or ARB for LVSD[2]	120	98%	96%	97%
Discharge Instructions Given[2]	275	94%	95%	94%
Evaluation of LVS Function[2]	343	100%	99%	99%
Medicare Spending				
Medicare Spending per Patient (ratio)	-	1.00	0.96	0.98
Pneumonia Care				
Appropriate Initial Antibiotic Given[2]	145	92%	95%	95%
Blood Culture Timing[2]	251	98%	97%	98%
Pregnancy and Delivery Care				
Newborn Deliveries Scheduled Early[2]	56	0%	4%	6%
Preventive Care				
Immunization for Influenza[2]	882	93%	88%	90%
Immunization for Pneumonia[2]	1,054	86%	88%	92%
Stroke Care				
Anticoagulation Therapy for Atrial Fibrillation[2]	15	93%	96%	95%
Antithrombotic Therapy Timing[2]	88	99%	98%	98%
Assessed for Rehabilitation[2]	145	97%	97%	97%
Discharged on Antithrombotic Therapy[2]	98	100%	99%	99%
Discharged on Statin Medication[2]	82	100%	95%	94%
Thrombolytic Therapy Timing[1,2]	-	-	69%	66%
Venous Thromboembolism Prophylaxis[2]	157	92%	94%	94%
Written Stroke Educational Materials Given[2]	78	86%	86%	88%
Surgical Care Improvement Project				
Appropriate Beta Blocker Usage[2]	307	97%	97%	98%
Appropriate VTP Within 24 Hours[2]	525	98%	98%	98%
Controlled Postoperative Blood Glucose[2]	158	97%	97%	97%
Perioperative Temperature Management[2]	704	100%	100%	100%
Prophylactic Antibiotic Selection[2]	546	99%	99%	99%
Prophylactic Antibiotic Selection (Outpatient)	299	98%	97%	98%
Prophylactic Antibiotic Stopped[2]	540	96%	98%	98%
Prophylactic Antibiotic Timing[2]	549	99%	99%	99%
Prophylactic Antibiotic Timing (Outpatient)	299	100%	97%	98%
Urinary Catheter Removal[2]	438	95%	96%	97%
Survey of Patients' Hospital Experiences				
Area Around Room 'Always' Quiet at Night	300+	51%	51%	61%
Doctors 'Always' Communicated Well	300+	79%	77%	82%
Home Recovery Information Given	300+	81%	83%	85%
Hospital Given 9 or 10 on 10 Point Scale	300+	72%	63%	71%
Meds 'Always' Explained Before Given	300+	59%	59%	64%
Nurses 'Always' Communicated Well	300+	79%	75%	79%
Pain 'Always' Well Controlled	300+	67%	67%	71%
Room and Bathroom 'Always' Clean	300+	77%	69%	73%
Timely Help 'Always' Received	300+	61%	61%	68%
Would Definitely Recommend Hospital	300+	77%	65%	71%
Use of Medical Imaging				
Cardiac Imaging Stress Test before Surgery	472	7.4%	5.8%	5.3%
Combination Abdominal CT Scan	3,802	11.3%	8.2%	10.5%
Combination Brain/Sinus CT Scan	2,036	3.9%	3.6%	2.7%
Combination Chest CT Scan	3,716	0.4%	1.3%	2.7%
Follow-up Mammogram/Ultrasound	1,996	12.8%	13%	8.8%
Lumbar Spine MRI for Low Back Pain	330	30.9%	33.4%	37.2%

NOTE: Hospital profiles are in alphabetical order by state, then city, then hospital within the city; Rankings exclude hospitals with less than 25 cases except for patient surveys which excludes hospitals with less than 100 cases; (a) 100-299 cases; (1) The number of cases/patients is too few to report; (2) Data submitted were based on a sample of cases/patients; (3) Results are based on a shorter time period than required; (4) Data suppressed by CMS for one or more quarters; (5) Results are not available for this reporting period; (6) Fewer than 100 patients completed the HCAHPS survey; (7) No cases met the criteria for this measure; (8) The lower limit of the confidence interval cannot be calculated if the number of observed infections equals zero; (9) No data are available from the state/territory for this reporting period; (10) The scores shown reflect fewer than 50 completed surveys; (11) There were discrepancies in the data collection process; (12) This measure does not apply to this hospital for this reporting period; (13) Results cannot be calculated for this reporting period; (14) The results for this state are combined with nearby states to protect confidentiality; Please refer to the User's Guide for a full explanation of data.

Margaretville Memorial Hospital

42084 State Highway 28
Margaretville, NY 12455
Phone: 845-586-5631
Fax: 845-586-1638
Type: Critical Access Hospitals
Emergency Services: Yes
Ownership: Voluntary non-profit - Private
Beds: 15

Key Personnel:
Radiology. . . . . Tony Allen
Operating Room. . . . . Marilyn Donnelly, RN
Chief of Medical Staff. . . . . Susan Fiore, MD
CEO/President. . . . . Edmond Morache
Infection Control. . . . . Nora Todd, RN

Measure	Cases	This Hosp.	State Avg.	U.S. Avg.
Blood Clot Prevention and Treatment				
Anticoagulation Overlap Therapy[5]	-	-	91%	93%
ICU Venous Thromboembolism Prophylaxis[5]	-	-	92%	92%
Incidence of Potentially Preventable VTE[5]	-	-	10%	10%
UFH with Dosages/Platelet Monitoring[5]	-	-	92%	97%
Venous Thromboembolism Prophylaxis[5]	-	-	87%	85%
Warfarin Therapy Discharge Instructions[5]	-	-	59%	75%
Chest Pain/Possible Heart Attack Care				
Aspirin Given Within 24 Hours of Arrival[1]	-	-	97%	96%
Fibrinolytic Meds Within 30 Min. of Arrival[3,7]	-	-	54%	58%
Average Time to ECG (minutes)[1]	-	-	9	7
Average Time to Transfer (minutes)[1,3]	-	-	78	60
Children's Asthma Care				
Received Home Management Plan of Care	-	-	-	88%
Received Reliever Medication	-	-	-	100%
Received Systemic Corticosteroids	-	-	-	100%
Emergency Department				
Admittance Decision Time (minutes)[5]	-	-	154	98
Head CT Results Within 45 Min. of Arrival[3,7]	-	-	55%	57%
Patients Who Left ER Before Being Seen	4,427	0%	2%	2%
Time from ER Arrival to Admit. (minutes)[5]	-	-	378	274
Time from ER Arrival to Discharge (minutes)[5]	-	-	156	134
Time in ER Before Being Evaluated (minutes)[5]	-	-	35	26
Time to Pain Meds for Fractures (minutes)[1]	-	-	61	57
Heart Attack Care				
Aspirin Given at Discharge[5]	-	-	99%	99%
Fibrinolytic Meds Within 30 Min. of Arrival[5]	-	-	46%	54%
PCI Within 90 Minutes of Arrival[5]	-	-	95%	96%
Statin Prescribed at Discharge[5]	-	-	98%	98%
Heart Failure Care				
ACE Inhibitor or ARB for LVSD[1,3]	-	-	96%	97%
Discharge Instructions Given[1,3]	-	-	95%	94%
Evaluation of LVS Function[1,3]	-	-	99%	99%
Medicare Spending				
Medicare Spending per Patient (ratio)	-	-	0.96	0.98
Pneumonia Care				
Appropriate Initial Antibiotic Given[2]	24	88%	95%	95%
Blood Culture Timing[2]	30	97%	97%	98%
Pregnancy and Delivery Care				
Newborn Deliveries Scheduled Early[5]	-	-	4%	6%
Preventive Care				
Immunization for Influenza[5]	-	-	88%	90%
Immunization for Pneumonia[5]	-	-	88%	92%
Stroke Care				
Anticoagulation Therapy for Atrial Fibrillation[5]	-	-	96%	95%
Antithrombotic Therapy Timing[5]	-	-	98%	98%
Assessed for Rehabilitation[5]	-	-	97%	97%
Discharged on Antithrombotic Therapy[5]	-	-	99%	99%
Discharged on Statin Medication[5]	-	-	95%	94%
Thrombolytic Therapy Timing[5]	-	-	69%	66%
Venous Thromboembolism Prophylaxis[5]	-	-	94%	94%
Written Stroke Educational Materials Given[5]	-	-	86%	88%
Surgical Care Improvement Project				
Appropriate Beta Blocker Usage[5]	-	-	97%	98%
Appropriate VTP Within 24 Hours[5]	-	-	98%	98%
Controlled Postoperative Blood Glucose[5]	-	-	97%	97%
Perioperative Temperature Management[5]	-	-	100%	100%
Prophylactic Antibiotic Selection[5]	-	-	99%	99%
Prophylactic Antibiotic Selection (Outpatient)[5]	-	-	97%	98%
Prophylactic Antibiotic Stopped[5]	-	-	98%	98%
Prophylactic Antibiotic Timing[5]	-	-	99%	99%
Prophylactic Antibiotic Timing (Outpatient)[5]	-	-	97%	98%
Urinary Catheter Removal[5]	-	-	96%	97%
Survey of Patients' Hospital Experiences				
Area Around Room 'Always' Quiet at Night[6]	<100	61%	51%	61%
Doctors 'Always' Communicated Well[6]	<100	88%	77%	82%
Home Recovery Information Given[6]	<100	83%	83%	85%
Hospital Given 9 or 10 on 10 Point Scale[6]	<100	79%	63%	71%
Meds 'Always' Explained Before Given[6]	<100	74%	59%	64%
Nurses 'Always' Communicated Well[6]	<100	86%	75%	79%
Pain 'Always' Well Controlled[6]	<100	74%	67%	71%
Room and Bathroom 'Always' Clean[6]	<100	84%	69%	73%
Timely Help 'Always' Received[6]	<100	82%	61%	68%
Would Definitely Recommend Hospital[6]	<100	76%	65%	71%
Use of Medical Imaging				
Cardiac Imaging Stress Test before Surgery[1]	-	-	5.8%	5.3%
Combination Abdominal CT Scan	103	0.0%	8.2%	10.5%
Combination Brain/Sinus CT Scan[1]	-	-	3.6%	2.7%
Combination Chest CT Scan	56	0.0%	1.3%	2.7%
Follow-up Mammogram/Ultrasound	101	6.9%	13%	8.8%
Lumbar Spine MRI for Low Back Pain[7]	-	-	33.4%	37.2%

Massena Memorial Hospital

1 Hospital Drive
Massena, NY 13662
Phone: 315-764-1711
Fax: 315-769-4344
E-mail: mmh@northnet.org
URL: www.massenahospital.org
Type: Acute Care Hospitals
Emergency Services: Yes
Ownership: Government - Local
Beds: 50

Key Personnel:
Hemotology Center . . . . Marcia Cox, RN
Chief of Medical Staff. . . . . Nimesh Desai, MD
Infection Control. . . . . Denille Dillabough, RN
CEO/President. . . . . Charles F Fahd, II
Quality Assurance . . . . Betty MacDonald
Emergency Room . . . . Judy Markell, RN, BSN
Intensive Care Unit. . . . . Judy Markell, RN, BSN
Operating Room. . . . . Karen Wilkins, RN

Measure	Cases	This Hosp.	State Avg.	U.S. Avg.
Blood Clot Prevention and Treatment				
Anticoagulation Overlap Therapy[1,2]	-	-	91%	93%
ICU Venous Thromboembolism Prophylaxis[2]	17	88%	92%	92%
Incidence of Potentially Preventable VTE[1,2]	-	-	10%	10%
UFH with Dosages/Platelet Monitoring[1,2]	-	-	92%	97%
Venous Thromboembolism Prophylaxis[2]	207	94%	87%	85%
Warfarin Therapy Discharge Instructions[1,2]	-	-	59%	75%
Chest Pain/Possible Heart Attack Care				
Aspirin Given Within 24 Hours of Arrival	53	100%	97%	96%
Fibrinolytic Meds Within 30 Min. of Arrival[1]	-	-	54%	58%
Average Time to ECG (minutes)	57	11	9	7
Average Time to Transfer (minutes)[7]	-	-	78	60
Children's Asthma Care				
Received Home Management Plan of Care	-	-	-	88%
Received Reliever Medication	-	-	-	100%
Received Systemic Corticosteroids	-	-	-	100%
Emergency Department				
Admittance Decision Time (minutes)[2]	344	79	154	98
Head CT Results Within 45 Min. of Arrival[1]	-	-	55%	57%
Patients Who Left ER Before Being Seen	1,607	3%	2%	2%
Time from ER Arrival to Admit. (minutes)[2]	344	202	378	274
Time from ER Arrival to Discharge (minutes)	372	106	156	134
Time in ER Before Being Evaluated (minutes)	406	24	35	26
Time to Pain Meds for Fractures (minutes)	38	35	61	57
Heart Attack Care				
Aspirin Given at Discharge[1]	-	-	99%	99%
Fibrinolytic Meds Within 30 Min. of Arrival[7]	-	-	46%	54%
PCI Within 90 Minutes of Arrival[7]	-	-	95%	96%
Statin Prescribed at Discharge[1]	-	-	98%	98%
Heart Failure Care				
ACE Inhibitor or ARB for LVSD[1]	-	-	96%	97%
Discharge Instructions Given	49	98%	95%	94%
Evaluation of LVS Function	64	100%	99%	99%
Medicare Spending				
Medicare Spending per Patient (ratio)	-	0.86	0.96	0.98
Pneumonia Care				
Appropriate Initial Antibiotic Given	79	99%	95%	95%
Blood Culture Timing	137	99%	97%	98%
Pregnancy and Delivery Care				
Newborn Deliveries Scheduled Early[1,2]	-	-	4%	6%
Preventive Care				
Immunization for Influenza[2]	264	95%	88%	90%
Immunization for Pneumonia[2]	319	97%	88%	92%
Stroke Care				
Anticoagulation Therapy for Atrial Fibrillation[1]	-	-	96%	95%
Antithrombotic Therapy Timing	16	100%	98%	98%
Assessed for Rehabilitation	16	94%	97%	97%
Discharged on Antithrombotic Therapy	16	100%	99%	99%
Discharged on Statin Medication[1]	-	-	95%	94%
Thrombolytic Therapy Timing[1]	-	-	69%	66%
Venous Thromboembolism Prophylaxis	16	94%	94%	94%
Written Stroke Educational Materials Given	11	82%	86%	88%
Surgical Care Improvement Project				
Appropriate Beta Blocker Usage	13	100%	97%	98%
Appropriate VTP Within 24 Hours	59	100%	98%	98%
Controlled Postoperative Blood Glucose[7]	-	-	97%	97%
Perioperative Temperature Management	64	100%	100%	100%
Prophylactic Antibiotic Selection	44	95%	99%	99%
Prophylactic Antibiotic Selection (Outpatient)[3]	13	100%	97%	98%
Prophylactic Antibiotic Stopped	44	100%	98%	98%
Prophylactic Antibiotic Timing	44	100%	99%	99%
Prophylactic Antibiotic Timing (Outpatient)[3]	13	100%	97%	98%
Urinary Catheter Removal	37	100%	96%	97%
Survey of Patients' Hospital Experiences				
Area Around Room 'Always' Quiet at Night	300+	52%	51%	61%
Doctors 'Always' Communicated Well	300+	78%	77%	82%
Home Recovery Information Given	300+	80%	83%	85%
Hospital Given 9 or 10 on 10 Point Scale	300+	59%	63%	71%
Meds 'Always' Explained Before Given	300+	61%	59%	64%
Nurses 'Always' Communicated Well	300+	78%	75%	79%
Pain 'Always' Well Controlled	300+	67%	67%	71%
Room and Bathroom 'Always' Clean	300+	74%	69%	73%
Timely Help 'Always' Received	300+	66%	61%	68%
Would Definitely Recommend Hospital	300+	60%	65%	71%
Use of Medical Imaging				
Cardiac Imaging Stress Test before Surgery	155	3.9%	5.8%	5.3%
Combination Abdominal CT Scan	430	1.4%	8.2%	10.5%
Combination Brain/Sinus CT Scan	274	6.2%	3.6%	2.7%
Combination Chest CT Scan	255	0.0%	1.3%	2.7%
Follow-up Mammogram/Ultrasound	551	7.3%	13%	8.8%
Lumbar Spine MRI for Low Back Pain[1]	-	-	33.4%	37.2%

Medina Memorial Hospital

200 Ohio Street
Medina, NY 14103
Phone: 585-798-8111
Fax: 585-798-8107
E-mail: info@medinamemorial.org
URL: www.medinahospital.com
Type: Acute Care Hospitals
Emergency Services: Yes
Ownership: Voluntary non-profit - Private
Beds: 101

Key Personnel:
CEO/President. . . . . Delos M. Cosgrove
Emergency Room . . . . C Jay Ellie Jr, MD

Measure	Cases	This Hosp.	State Avg.	U.S. Avg.
Blood Clot Prevention and Treatment				
Anticoagulation Overlap Therapy[2]	21	76%	91%	93%
ICU Venous Thromboembolism Prophylaxis[2]	55	87%	92%	92%
Incidence of Potentially Preventable VTE[1,2]	-	-	10%	10%
UFH with Dosages/Platelet Monitoring[2]	12	100%	92%	97%
Venous Thromboembolism Prophylaxis[2]	178	82%	87%	85%
Warfarin Therapy Discharge Instructions[2]	15	87%	59%	75%
Chest Pain/Possible Heart Attack Care				
Aspirin Given Within 24 Hours of Arrival	63	100%	97%	96%
Fibrinolytic Meds Within 30 Min. of Arrival[1]	-	-	54%	58%
Average Time to ECG (minutes)	57	4	9	7
Average Time to Transfer (minutes)[1]	-	-	78	60
Children's Asthma Care				
Received Home Management Plan of Care	-	-	-	88%
Received Reliever Medication	-	-	-	100%
Received Systemic Corticosteroids	-	-	-	100%

NOTE: Hospital profiles are in alphabetical order by state, then city, then hospital within the city; Rankings exclude hospitals with less than 25 cases except for patient surveys which excludes hospitals with less than 100 cases; (a) 100-299 cases; (1) The number of cases/patients is too few to report; (2) Data submitted were based on a sample of cases/patients; (3) Results are based on a shorter time period than required; (4) Data suppressed by CMS for one or more quarters; (5) Results are not available for this reporting period; (6) Fewer than 100 patients completed the HCAHPS survey; (7) No cases met the criteria for this measure; (8) The lower limit of the confidence interval cannot be calculated if the number of observed infections equals zero; (9) No data are available from the state/territory for this reporting period; (10) The scores shown reflect fewer than 50 completed surveys; (11) There were discrepancies in the data collection process; (12) This measure does not apply to this hospital for this reporting period; (13) Results cannot be calculated for this reporting period; (14) The results for this state are combined with nearby states to protect confidentiality; Please refer to the User's Guide for a full explanation of data.

Measure	Cases	This Hosp.	State Avg.	U.S. Avg.
Emergency Department				
Admittance Decision Time (minutes)[2]	324	85	154	98
Head CT Results Within 45 Min. of Arrival	15	60%	55%	57%
Patients Who Left ER Before Being Seen	10,038	2%	2%	2%
Time from ER Arrival to Admit. (minutes)[2]	326	335	378	274
Time from ER Arrival to Discharge (minutes)	356	150	156	134
Time in ER Before Being Evaluated (minutes)	259	35	35	26
Time to Pain Meds for Fractures (minutes)	29	73	61	57
Heart Attack Care				
Aspirin Given at Discharge	20	100%	99%	99%
Fibrinolytic Meds Within 30 Min. of Arrival[7]	-	-	46%	54%
PCI Within 90 Minutes of Arrival[7]	-	-	95%	96%
Statin Prescribed at Discharge	21	95%	98%	98%
Heart Failure Care				
ACE Inhibitor or ARB for LVSD	11	100%	96%	97%
Discharge Instructions Given	45	98%	95%	94%
Evaluation of LVS Function	68	99%	99%	99%
Medicare Spending				
Medicare Spending per Patient (ratio)	-	0.85	0.96	0.98
Pneumonia Care				
Appropriate Initial Antibiotic Given	60	95%	95%	95%
Blood Culture Timing	94	96%	97%	98%
Pregnancy and Delivery Care				
Newborn Deliveries Scheduled Early[2,7]	-	-	4%	6%
Preventive Care				
Immunization for Influenza[2]	301	95%	88%	90%
Immunization for Pneumonia[2]	425	95%	88%	92%
Stroke Care				
Anticoagulation Therapy for Atrial Fibrillation[1]	-	-	96%	95%
Antithrombotic Therapy Timing	22	100%	98%	98%
Assessed for Rehabilitation	20	100%	97%	97%
Discharged on Antithrombotic Therapy	18	94%	99%	99%
Discharged on Statin Medication	13	92%	95%	94%
Thrombolytic Therapy Timing[1]	-	-	69%	66%
Venous Thromboembolism Prophylaxis	24	79%	94%	94%
Written Stroke Educational Materials Given[1]	-	-	86%	88%
Surgical Care Improvement Project				
Appropriate Beta Blocker Usage	23	96%	97%	98%
Appropriate VTP Within 24 Hours	38	97%	98%	98%
Controlled Postoperative Blood Glucose[7]	-	-	97%	97%
Perioperative Temperature Management	43	95%	100%	100%
Prophylactic Antibiotic Selection	24	100%	99%	99%
Prophylactic Antibiotic Selection (Outpatient)	30	100%	97%	98%
Prophylactic Antibiotic Stopped	21	95%	98%	98%
Prophylactic Antibiotic Timing	24	100%	99%	99%
Prophylactic Antibiotic Timing (Outpatient)[1]	-	-	97%	98%
Urinary Catheter Removal	17	94%	96%	97%
Survey of Patients' Hospital Experiences				
Area Around Room 'Always' Quiet at Night	300+	51%	51%	61%
Doctors 'Always' Communicated Well	300+	78%	77%	82%
Home Recovery Information Given	300+	86%	83%	85%
Hospital Given 9 or 10 on 10 Point Scale	300+	68%	63%	71%
Meds 'Always' Explained Before Given	300+	57%	59%	64%
Nurses 'Always' Communicated Well	300+	77%	75%	79%
Pain 'Always' Well Controlled	300+	67%	67%	71%
Room and Bathroom 'Always' Clean	300+	77%	69%	73%
Timely Help 'Always' Received	300+	58%	61%	68%
Would Definitely Recommend Hospital	300+	70%	65%	71%
Use of Medical Imaging				
Cardiac Imaging Stress Test before Surgery	65	4.6%	5.8%	5.3%
Combination Abdominal CT Scan	129	10.9%	8.2%	10.5%
Combination Brain/Sinus CT Scan[1]	-	-	3.6%	2.7%
Combination Chest CT Scan[1]	-	-	1.3%	2.7%
Follow-up Mammogram/Ultrasound	251	8.0%	13%	8.8%
Lumbar Spine MRI for Low Back Pain[1]	-	-	33.4%	37.2%

Orange Regional Medical Center

707 East Main Street
Middletown, NY 10940
Phone: 845-343-2424
Fax: 845-294-2105
URL: www.ormc.org
Type: Acute Care Hospitals
Emergency Services: Yes
Ownership: Voluntary non-profit - Private
Beds: 174
Key Personnel:
CEO/President. . . . . Scott Batulis
Radiology. . . . . Susan M Beatty
Chairman/CEO . . . . Rolland B. Peacock, III
Chief of Medical Staff. . . . . Olanrewaju O Somorin, MD

Measure	Cases	This Hosp.	State Avg.	U.S. Avg.
Blood Clot Prevention and Treatment				
Anticoagulation Overlap Therapy[2]	132	93%	91%	93%
ICU Venous Thromboembolism Prophylaxis[2]	71	83%	92%	92%
Incidence of Potentially Preventable VTE[2]	16	19%	10%	10%
UFH with Dosages/Platelet Monitoring[2]	90	100%	92%	97%
Venous Thromboembolism Prophylaxis[2]	351	72%	87%	85%
Warfarin Therapy Discharge Instructions[2]	92	90%	59%	75%
Chest Pain/Possible Heart Attack Care				
Aspirin Given Within 24 Hours of Arrival	16	100%	97%	96%
Fibrinolytic Meds Within 30 Min. of Arrival[7]	-	-	54%	58%
Average Time to ECG (minutes)	16	15	9	7
Average Time to Transfer (minutes)[7]	-	-	78	60
Children's Asthma Care				
Received Home Management Plan of Care	-	-	-	88%
Received Reliever Medication	-	-	-	100%
Received Systemic Corticosteroids	-	-	-	100%
Emergency Department				
Admittance Decision Time (minutes)[2]	661	152	154	98
Head CT Results Within 45 Min. of Arrival[1]	-	-	55%	57%
Patients Who Left ER Before Being Seen	52,032	1%	2%	2%
Time from ER Arrival to Admit. (minutes)[2]	665	338	378	274
Time from ER Arrival to Discharge (minutes)	351	174	156	134
Time in ER Before Being Evaluated (minutes)	412	12	35	26
Time to Pain Meds for Fractures (minutes)	224	59	61	57
Heart Attack Care				
Aspirin Given at Discharge	328	99%	99%	99%
Fibrinolytic Meds Within 30 Min. of Arrival[7]	-	-	46%	54%
PCI Within 90 Minutes of Arrival	59	98%	95%	96%
Statin Prescribed at Discharge	332	98%	98%	98%
Heart Failure Care				
ACE Inhibitor or ARB for LVSD[2]	81	100%	96%	97%
Discharge Instructions Given[2]	259	95%	95%	94%
Evaluation of LVS Function[2]	354	100%	99%	99%
Medicare Spending				
Medicare Spending per Patient (ratio)	-	1.05	0.96	0.98
Pneumonia Care				
Appropriate Initial Antibiotic Given[2]	106	98%	95%	95%
Blood Culture Timing[2]	234	100%	97%	98%
Pregnancy and Delivery Care				
Newborn Deliveries Scheduled Early	197	3%	4%	6%
Preventive Care				
Immunization for Influenza[2]	553	84%	88%	90%
Immunization for Pneumonia[2]	670	82%	88%	92%
Stroke Care				
Anticoagulation Therapy for Atrial Fibrillation	23	100%	96%	95%
Antithrombotic Therapy Timing	191	98%	98%	98%
Assessed for Rehabilitation	204	97%	97%	97%
Discharged on Antithrombotic Therapy	167	99%	99%	99%
Discharged on Statin Medication	147	95%	95%	94%
Thrombolytic Therapy Timing	11	45%	69%	66%
Venous Thromboembolism Prophylaxis	224	83%	94%	94%
Written Stroke Educational Materials Given	85	96%	86%	88%
Surgical Care Improvement Project				
Appropriate Beta Blocker Usage[2]	177	98%	97%	98%
Appropriate VTP Within 24 Hours[2]	548	100%	98%	98%
Controlled Postoperative Blood Glucose[2,7]	-	-	97%	97%
Perioperative Temperature Management[2]	629	100%	100%	100%
Prophylactic Antibiotic Selection[2]	404	99%	99%	99%
Prophylactic Antibiotic Selection (Outpatient)	378	98%	97%	98%
Prophylactic Antibiotic Stopped[2]	403	100%	98%	98%
Prophylactic Antibiotic Timing[2]	406	99%	99%	99%
Prophylactic Antibiotic Timing (Outpatient)	383	98%	97%	98%
Urinary Catheter Removal[2]	421	98%	96%	97%
Survey of Patients' Hospital Experiences				
Area Around Room 'Always' Quiet at Night	300+	60%	51%	61%
Doctors 'Always' Communicated Well	300+	76%	77%	82%
Home Recovery Information Given	300+	85%	83%	85%
Hospital Given 9 or 10 on 10 Point Scale	300+	71%	63%	71%
Meds 'Always' Explained Before Given	300+	62%	59%	64%
Nurses 'Always' Communicated Well	300+	79%	75%	79%
Pain 'Always' Well Controlled	300+	73%	67%	71%
Room and Bathroom 'Always' Clean	300+	73%	69%	73%
Timely Help 'Always' Received	300+	64%	61%	68%
Would Definitely Recommend Hospital	300+	72%	65%	71%
Use of Medical Imaging				
Cardiac Imaging Stress Test before Surgery	448	6.0%	5.8%	5.3%
Combination Abdominal CT Scan	1,345	4.5%	8.2%	10.5%
Combination Brain/Sinus CT Scan	1,341	2.5%	3.6%	2.7%
Combination Chest CT Scan	902	0.7%	1.3%	2.7%
Follow-up Mammogram/Ultrasound	1,615	13.1%	13%	8.8%
Lumbar Spine MRI for Low Back Pain	83	28.9%	33.4%	37.2%

Winthrop - University Hospital

259 First Street
Mineola, NY 11501
Phone: 516-663-0333
Fax: 516-663-2953
URL: www.winthrop.org
Type: Acute Care Hospitals
Emergency Services: Yes
Ownership: Voluntary non-profit - Private
Beds: 591
Key Personnel:
Chief of Medical Staff. . . . . Michael Ammazzalorso, MD
Quality Assurance . . . . Bruce Cohn
CEO/President. . . . . John F Collins
Infection Control. . . . . Burke Cunha, MD
Radiology. . . . . Orlando Ortiz
Pediatric Ambulatory Care . . . . . . Warren Rosenfeld, MD
Pediatric In-Patient Care . . . . Warren Rosenfeld, MD
Emergency Room . . . . Barry Rosenthal, MD

Measure	Cases	This Hosp.	State Avg.	U.S. Avg.
Blood Clot Prevention and Treatment				
Anticoagulation Overlap Therapy[2]	143	95%	91%	93%
ICU Venous Thromboembolism Prophylaxis[2]	83	99%	92%	92%
Incidence of Potentially Preventable VTE[2]	48	0%	10%	10%
UFH with Dosages/Platelet Monitoring[2]	108	100%	92%	97%
Venous Thromboembolism Prophylaxis[2]	329	97%	87%	85%
Warfarin Therapy Discharge Instructions[2]	97	42%	59%	75%
Chest Pain/Possible Heart Attack Care				
Aspirin Given Within 24 Hours of Arrival[5]	-	-	97%	96%
Fibrinolytic Meds Within 30 Min. of Arrival[5]	-	-	54%	58%
Average Time to ECG (minutes)[5]	-	-	9	7
Average Time to Transfer (minutes)[5]	-	-	78	60
Children's Asthma Care				
Received Home Management Plan of Care	-	-	-	88%
Received Reliever Medication	-	-	-	100%
Received Systemic Corticosteroids	-	-	-	100%
Emergency Department				
Admittance Decision Time (minutes)[2]	252	181	154	98
Head CT Results Within 45 Min. of Arrival[1,3]	-	-	55%	57%
Patients Who Left ER Before Being Seen	71,945	2%	2%	2%
Time from ER Arrival to Admit. (minutes)[2]	252	482	378	274
Time from ER Arrival to Discharge (minutes)	364	219	156	134
Time in ER Before Being Evaluated (minutes)	410	58	35	26
Time to Pain Meds for Fractures (minutes)	231	71	61	57
Heart Attack Care				
Aspirin Given at Discharge	460	100%	99%	99%
Fibrinolytic Meds Within 30 Min. of Arrival[7]	-	-	46%	54%
PCI Within 90 Minutes of Arrival	84	93%	95%	96%
Statin Prescribed at Discharge	465	99%	98%	98%
Heart Failure Care				
ACE Inhibitor or ARB for LVSD[2]	96	98%	96%	97%
Discharge Instructions Given[2]	260	96%	95%	94%
Evaluation of LVS Function[2]	323	100%	99%	99%
Medicare Spending				
Medicare Spending per Patient (ratio)	-	1.01	0.96	0.98
Pneumonia Care				
Appropriate Initial Antibiotic Given[2]	95	91%	95%	95%
Blood Culture Timing[2]	172	99%	97%	98%
Pregnancy and Delivery Care				
Newborn Deliveries Scheduled Early[2]	114	3%	4%	6%
Preventive Care				
Immunization for Influenza[2]	527	93%	88%	90%
Immunization for Pneumonia[2]	556	90%	88%	92%
Stroke Care				

NOTE: Hospital profiles are in alphabetical order by state, then city, then hospital within the city; Rankings exclude hospitals with less than 25 cases except for patient surveys which excludes hospitals with less than 100 cases; (a) 100-299 cases; (1) The number of cases/patients is too few to report; (2) Data submitted were based on a sample of cases/patients; (3) Results are based on a shorter time period than required; (4) Data suppressed by CMS for one or more quarters; (5) Results are not available for this reporting period; (6) Fewer than 100 patients completed the HCAHPS survey; (7) No cases met the criteria for this measure; (8) The lower limit of the confidence interval cannot be calculated if the number of observed infections equals zero; (9) No data are available from the state/territory for this reporting period; (10) The scores shown reflect fewer than 50 completed surveys; (11) There were discrepancies in the data collection process; (12) This measure does not apply to this hospital for this reporting period; (13) Results cannot be calculated for this reporting period; (14) The results for this state are combined with nearby states to protect confidentiality; Please refer to the User's Guide for a full explanation of data.

Measure	Cases	This Hosp.	State Avg.	U.S. Avg.
Anticoagulation Therapy for Atrial Fibrillation	22	100%	96%	95%
Antithrombotic Therapy Timing	181	98%	98%	98%
Assessed for Rehabilitation	246	94%	97%	97%
Discharged on Antithrombotic Therapy	197	100%	99%	99%
Discharged on Statin Medication	168	95%	95%	94%
Thrombolytic Therapy Timing	16	100%	69%	66%
Venous Thromboembolism Prophylaxis	258	100%	94%	94%
Written Stroke Educational Materials Given	145	88%	86%	88%
Surgical Care Improvement Project				
Appropriate Beta Blocker Usage[2]	453	98%	97%	98%
Appropriate VTP Within 24 Hours[2]	509	97%	98%	98%
Controlled Postoperative Blood Glucose[2]	368	99%	97%	97%
Perioperative Temperature Management[2]	637	100%	100%	100%
Prophylactic Antibiotic Selection[2]	738	99%	99%	99%
Prophylactic Antibiotic Selection (Outpatient)	921	99%	97%	98%
Prophylactic Antibiotic Stopped[2]	716	98%	98%	98%
Prophylactic Antibiotic Timing[2]	742	98%	99%	99%
Prophylactic Antibiotic Timing (Outpatient)	924	99%	97%	98%
Urinary Catheter Removal[2]	594	99%	96%	97%
Survey of Patients' Hospital Experiences				
Area Around Room 'Always' Quiet at Night	300+	46%	51%	61%
Doctors 'Always' Communicated Well	300+	79%	77%	82%
Home Recovery Information Given	300+	86%	83%	85%
Hospital Given 9 or 10 on 10 Point Scale	300+	65%	63%	71%
Meds 'Always' Explained Before Given	300+	59%	59%	64%
Nurses 'Always' Communicated Well	300+	75%	75%	79%
Pain 'Always' Well Controlled	300+	68%	67%	71%
Room and Bathroom 'Always' Clean	300+	70%	69%	73%
Timely Help 'Always' Received	300+	57%	61%	68%
Would Definitely Recommend Hospital	300+	72%	65%	71%
Use of Medical Imaging				
Cardiac Imaging Stress Test before Surgery[1]	-	-	5.8%	5.3%
Combination Abdominal CT Scan	838	1.9%	8.2%	10.5%
Combination Brain/Sinus CT Scan	674	3.9%	3.6%	2.7%
Combination Chest CT Scan	762	0.4%	1.3%	2.7%
Follow-up Mammogram/Ultrasound	609	29.6%	13%	8.8%
Lumbar Spine MRI for Low Back Pain[1]	-	-	33.4%	37.2%

Schuyler Hospital

220 Steuben Street
Montour Falls, NY 14865
URL: www.schuylerhospital.org
Type: Critical Access Hospitals
Ownership: Voluntary non-profit - Private
Phone: 607-530-7121
Fax: 607-535-2433
Emergency Services: Yes
Beds: 169

Key Personnel:

Radiology. . . . . Edwin Acosta
Infection Control. . . . . Dr Irene Alexandraki
Pediatric Ambulatory Care . . . . . . Dr Manuel Castellanos
Pediatric In-Patient Care . . . . Dr Manuel Castellanos
Coronary Care . . . . Jonathon Laurence
Chief of Medical Staff. . . . . Dr Willaim Saks
CEO/President. . . . . Richard Stelzer
Quality Assurance . . . . Rita Tague

Measure	Cases	This Hosp.	State Avg.	U.S. Avg.
Blood Clot Prevention and Treatment				
Anticoagulation Overlap Therapy[5]	-	-	91%	93%
ICU Venous Thromboembolism Prophylaxis[5]	-	-	92%	92%
Incidence of Potentially Preventable VTE[5]	-	-	10%	10%
UFH with Dosages/Platelet Monitoring[5]	-	-	92%	97%
Venous Thromboembolism Prophylaxis[5]	-	-	87%	85%
Warfarin Therapy Discharge Instructions[5]	-	-	59%	75%
Chest Pain/Possible Heart Attack Care				
Aspirin Given Within 24 Hours of Arrival[1,3]	-	-	97%	96%
Fibrinolytic Meds Within 30 Min. of Arrival[1,3]	-	-	54%	58%
Average Time to ECG (minutes)[1,3]	-	-	9	7
Average Time to Transfer (minutes)[1,3]	-	-	78	60
Children's Asthma Care				
Received Home Management Plan of Care	-	-	-	88%
Received Reliever Medication	-	-	-	100%
Received Systemic Corticosteroids	-	-	-	100%
Emergency Department				
Admittance Decision Time (minutes)[5]	-	-	154	98
Head CT Results Within 45 Min. of Arrival[5]	-	-	55%	57%
Patients Who Left ER Before Being Seen	9,183	2%	2%	2%
Time from ER Arrival to Admit. (minutes)[5]	-	-	378	274
Time from ER Arrival to Discharge (minutes)[5]	-	-	156	134
Time in ER Before Being Evaluated (minutes)[5]	-	-	35	26
Time to Pain Meds for Fractures (minutes)[5]	-	-	61	57
Heart Attack Care				
Aspirin Given at Discharge[1]	-	-	99%	99%
Fibrinolytic Meds Within 30 Min. of Arrival[3,7]	-	-	46%	54%
PCI Within 90 Minutes of Arrival[3,7]	-	-	95%	96%
Statin Prescribed at Discharge[1]	-	-	98%	98%
Heart Failure Care				
ACE Inhibitor or ARB for LVSD[1]	-	-	96%	97%
Discharge Instructions Given	14	100%	95%	94%
Evaluation of LVS Function	26	100%	99%	99%
Medicare Spending				
Medicare Spending per Patient (ratio)	-	-	0.96	0.98
Pneumonia Care				
Appropriate Initial Antibiotic Given	27	93%	95%	95%
Blood Culture Timing	50	96%	97%	98%
Pregnancy and Delivery Care				
Newborn Deliveries Scheduled Early[5]	-	-	4%	6%
Preventive Care				
Immunization for Influenza[5]	-	-	88%	90%
Immunization for Pneumonia[5]	-	-	88%	92%
Stroke Care				
Anticoagulation Therapy for Atrial Fibrillation[5]	-	-	96%	95%
Antithrombotic Therapy Timing[5]	-	-	98%	98%
Assessed for Rehabilitation[5]	-	-	97%	97%
Discharged on Antithrombotic Therapy[5]	-	-	99%	99%
Discharged on Statin Medication[5]	-	-	95%	94%
Thrombolytic Therapy Timing[5]	-	-	69%	66%
Venous Thromboembolism Prophylaxis[5]	-	-	94%	94%
Written Stroke Educational Materials Given[5]	-	-	86%	88%
Surgical Care Improvement Project				
Appropriate Beta Blocker Usage[5]	-	-	97%	98%
Appropriate VTP Within 24 Hours[5]	-	-	98%	98%
Controlled Postoperative Blood Glucose[5]	-	-	97%	97%
Perioperative Temperature Management[5]	-	-	100%	100%
Prophylactic Antibiotic Selection[5]	-	-	99%	99%
Prophylactic Antibiotic Selection (Outpatient)[1,3]	-	-	97%	98%
Prophylactic Antibiotic Stopped[5]	-	-	98%	98%
Prophylactic Antibiotic Timing[5]	-	-	99%	99%
Prophylactic Antibiotic Timing (Outpatient)[1,3]	-	-	97%	98%
Urinary Catheter Removal[5]	-	-	96%	97%
Survey of Patients' Hospital Experiences				
Area Around Room 'Always' Quiet at Night	(a)	53%	51%	61%
Doctors 'Always' Communicated Well	(a)	85%	77%	82%
Home Recovery Information Given	(a)	87%	83%	85%
Hospital Given 9 or 10 on 10 Point Scale	(a)	59%	63%	71%
Meds 'Always' Explained Before Given	(a)	67%	59%	64%
Nurses 'Always' Communicated Well	(a)	76%	75%	79%
Pain 'Always' Well Controlled	(a)	64%	67%	71%
Room and Bathroom 'Always' Clean	(a)	56%	69%	73%
Timely Help 'Always' Received	(a)	65%	61%	68%
Would Definitely Recommend Hospital	(a)	67%	65%	71%
Use of Medical Imaging				
Cardiac Imaging Stress Test before Surgery[1]	-	-	5.8%	5.3%
Combination Abdominal CT Scan	219	5.0%	8.2%	10.5%
Combination Brain/Sinus CT Scan[1]	-	-	3.6%	2.7%
Combination Chest CT Scan	90	2.2%	1.3%	2.7%
Follow-up Mammogram/Ultrasound	297	7.7%	13%	8.8%
Lumbar Spine MRI for Low Back Pain[1]	-	-	33.4%	37.2%

VA Hudson Valley Healthcare System

2094 Albany Post Road
Montrose, NY 10548
URL: www.va.gov
Type: Acute Care - VA
Ownership: Government Federal
Phone: 914-737-4400
Fax: 914-788-4244
Emergency Services: No

Key Personnel:

Chief of Medical Staff. . . . . Malati Kollali, MD
CEO/President. . . . . Michael A Sabo
Quality Assurance . . . . Mary Ann Tyner

Measure	Cases	This Hosp.	State Avg.	U.S. Avg.
Blood Clot Prevention and Treatment				
Anticoagulation Overlap Therapy	-	-	91%	93%
ICU Venous Thromboembolism Prophylaxis	-	-	92%	92%
Incidence of Potentially Preventable VTE	-	-	10%	10%
UFH with Dosages/Platelet Monitoring	-	-	92%	97%
Venous Thromboembolism Prophylaxis	-	-	87%	85%
Warfarin Therapy Discharge Instructions	-	-	59%	75%
Chest Pain/Possible Heart Attack Care				
Aspirin Given Within 24 Hours of Arrival	-	-	97%	96%
Fibrinolytic Meds Within 30 Min. of Arrival	-	-	54%	58%
Average Time to ECG (minutes)	-	-	9	7
Average Time to Transfer (minutes)	-	-	78	60
Children's Asthma Care				
Received Home Management Plan of Care	-	-	-	88%
Received Reliever Medication	-	-	-	100%
Received Systemic Corticosteroids	-	-	-	100%
Emergency Department				
Admittance Decision Time (minutes)	-	-	154	98
Head CT Results Within 45 Min. of Arrival	-	-	55%	57%
Patients Who Left ER Before Being Seen	-	-	2%	2%
Time from ER Arrival to Admit. (minutes)	-	-	378	274
Time from ER Arrival to Discharge (minutes)	-	-	156	134
Time in ER Before Being Evaluated (minutes)	-	-	35	26
Time to Pain Meds for Fractures (minutes)	-	-	61	57
Heart Attack Care				
Aspirin Given at Discharge[5]	-	-	99%	99%
Fibrinolytic Meds Within 30 Min. of Arrival[5]	-	-	46%	54%
PCI Within 90 Minutes of Arrival[5]	-	-	95%	96%
Statin Prescribed at Discharge[5]	-	-	98%	98%
Heart Failure Care				
ACE Inhibitor or ARB for LVSD[1]	-	-	96%	97%
Discharge Instructions Given[1]	20	100%	95%	94%
Evaluation of LVS Function[1]	23	100%	99%	99%
Medicare Spending				
Medicare Spending per Patient (ratio)	-	-	0.96	0.98
Pneumonia Care				
Appropriate Initial Antibiotic Given[1]	14	100%	95%	95%
Blood Culture Timing[1]	12	100%	97%	98%
Pregnancy and Delivery Care				
Newborn Deliveries Scheduled Early	-	-	4%	6%
Preventive Care				
Immunization for Influenza[2,3]	141	94%	88%	90%
Immunization for Pneumonia[2,3]	248	97%	88%	92%
Stroke Care				
Anticoagulation Therapy for Atrial Fibrillation	-	-	96%	95%
Antithrombotic Therapy Timing	-	-	98%	98%
Assessed for Rehabilitation	-	-	97%	97%
Discharged on Antithrombotic Therapy	-	-	99%	99%
Discharged on Statin Medication	-	-	95%	94%
Thrombolytic Therapy Timing	-	-	69%	66%
Venous Thromboembolism Prophylaxis	-	-	94%	94%
Written Stroke Educational Materials Given	-	-	86%	88%
Surgical Care Improvement Project				
Appropriate Beta Blocker Usage[5]	-	-	97%	98%
Appropriate VTP Within 24 Hours[5]	-	-	98%	98%
Controlled Postoperative Blood Glucose[5]	-	-	97%	97%
Perioperative Temperature Management[5]	-	-	100%	100%
Prophylactic Antibiotic Selection[5]	-	-	99%	99%
Prophylactic Antibiotic Selection (Outpatient)	-	-	97%	98%
Prophylactic Antibiotic Stopped[5]	-	-	98%	98%
Prophylactic Antibiotic Timing[5]	-	-	99%	99%
Prophylactic Antibiotic Timing (Outpatient)	-	-	97%	98%
Urinary Catheter Removal[5]	-	-	96%	97%
Survey of Patients' Hospital Experiences				
Area Around Room 'Always' Quiet at Night	-	-	51%	61%
Doctors 'Always' Communicated Well	-	-	77%	82%
Home Recovery Information Given	-	-	83%	85%
Hospital Given 9 or 10 on 10 Point Scale	-	-	63%	71%
Meds 'Always' Explained Before Given	-	-	59%	64%
Nurses 'Always' Communicated Well	-	-	75%	79%
Pain 'Always' Well Controlled	-	-	67%	71%
Room and Bathroom 'Always' Clean	-	-	69%	73%

NOTE: Hospital profiles are in alphabetical order by state, then city, then hospital within the city; Rankings exclude hospitals with less than 25 cases except for patient surveys which excludes hospitals with less than 100 cases; (a) 100-299 cases; (1) The number of cases/patients is too few to report; (2) Data submitted were based on a sample of cases/patients; (3) Results are based on a shorter time period than required; (4) Data suppressed by CMS for one or more quarters; (5) Results are not available for this reporting period; (6) Fewer than 100 patients completed the HCAHPS survey; (7) No cases met the criteria for this measure; (8) The lower limit of the confidence interval cannot be calculated if the number of observed infections equals zero; (9) No data are available from the state/territory for this reporting period; (10) The scores shown reflect fewer than 50 completed surveys; (11) There were discrepancies in the data collection process; (12) This measure does not apply to this hospital for this reporting period; (13) Results cannot be calculated for this reporting period; (14) The results for this state are combined with nearby states to protect confidentiality; Please refer to the User's Guide for a full explanation of data.

Measure	Cases	This Hosp.	State Avg.	U.S. Avg.
Timely Help 'Always' Received	-	-	61%	68%
Would Definitely Recommend Hospital	-	-	65%	71%
Use of Medical Imaging				
Cardiac Imaging Stress Test before Surgery	-	-	5.8%	5.3%
Combination Abdominal CT Scan	-	-	8.2%	10.5%
Combination Brain/Sinus CT Scan	-	-	3.6%	2.7%
Combination Chest CT Scan	-	-	1.3%	2.7%
Follow-up Mammogram/Ultrasound	-	-	13%	8.8%
Lumbar Spine MRI for Low Back Pain	-	-	33.4%	37.2%

Northern Westchester Hospital

400 East Main Street
Mount Kisco, NY 10549
E-mail: nwhmarketing@nwhc.net
URL: www.nwhc.net
Phone: 914-666-1200
Fax: 914-666-1163
Type: Acute Care Hospitals
Ownership: Voluntary non-profit - Private
Emergency Services: Yes
Beds: 233

Key Personnel:
Infection Control. . . . . Sonia Appel
Quality Assurance . . . . Lisa Hanrahan
Radiology. . . . . Peter Khouri, MD
Coronary Care . . . . Judy Kinkel, RN
Chief of Medical Staff. . . . . Marla Koroly, MD
Pediatric In-Patient Care . . . . Jill Ratner, MD
Operating Room. . . . . Susan Roy
CEO/President. . . . . Joel Seligman

Measure	Cases	This Hosp.	State Avg.	U.S. Avg.
Blood Clot Prevention and Treatment				
Anticoagulation Overlap Therapy[2]	30	100%	91%	93%
ICU Venous Thromboembolism Prophylaxis[2]	34	82%	92%	92%
Incidence of Potentially Preventable VTE[1,2]	-	-	10%	10%
UFH with Dosages/Platelet Monitoring[1,2]	-	-	92%	97%
Venous Thromboembolism Prophylaxis[2]	331	91%	87%	85%
Warfarin Therapy Discharge Instructions[2]	24	100%	59%	75%
Chest Pain/Possible Heart Attack Care				
Aspirin Given Within 24 Hours of Arrival	73	100%	97%	96%
Fibrinolytic Meds Within 30 Min. of Arrival[1]	-	-	54%	58%
Average Time to ECG (minutes)	74	3	9	7
Average Time to Transfer (minutes)	16	86	78	60
Children's Asthma Care				
Received Home Management Plan of Care	-	-	-	88%
Received Reliever Medication	-	-	-	100%
Received Systemic Corticosteroids	-	-	-	100%
Emergency Department				
Admittance Decision Time (minutes)[2]	575	38	154	98
Head CT Results Within 45 Min. of Arrival	13	46%	55%	57%
Patients Who Left ER Before Being Seen	31,029	0%	2%	2%
Time from ER Arrival to Admit. (minutes)[2]	578	270	378	274
Time from ER Arrival to Discharge (minutes)	394	135	156	134
Time in ER Before Being Evaluated (minutes)	411	16	35	26
Time to Pain Meds for Fractures (minutes)	161	42	61	57
Heart Attack Care				
Aspirin Given at Discharge	21	100%	99%	99%
Fibrinolytic Meds Within 30 Min. of Arrival[7]	-	-	46%	54%
PCI Within 90 Minutes of Arrival[7]	-	-	95%	96%
Statin Prescribed at Discharge	24	100%	98%	98%
Heart Failure Care				
ACE Inhibitor or ARB for LVSD	28	100%	96%	97%
Discharge Instructions Given	147	100%	95%	94%
Evaluation of LVS Function	186	100%	99%	99%
Medicare Spending				
Medicare Spending per Patient (ratio)	-	0.97	0.96	0.98
Pneumonia Care				
Appropriate Initial Antibiotic Given[2]	96	100%	95%	95%
Blood Culture Timing[2]	177	100%	97%	98%
Pregnancy and Delivery Care				
Newborn Deliveries Scheduled Early	126	3%	4%	6%
Preventive Care				
Immunization for Influenza[2]	516	99%	88%	90%
Immunization for Pneumonia[2]	542	96%	88%	92%
Stroke Care				
Anticoagulation Therapy for Atrial Fibrillation[1]	-	-	96%	95%
Antithrombotic Therapy Timing	51	98%	98%	98%
Assessed for Rehabilitation	72	99%	97%	97%
Discharged on Antithrombotic Therapy	68	100%	99%	99%
Discharged on Statin Medication	41	95%	95%	94%
Thrombolytic Therapy Timing	11	100%	69%	66%
Venous Thromboembolism Prophylaxis	70	100%	94%	94%
Written Stroke Educational Materials Given	47	100%	86%	88%
Surgical Care Improvement Project				
Appropriate Beta Blocker Usage[2]	99	100%	97%	98%
Appropriate VTP Within 24 Hours[2]	425	100%	98%	98%
Controlled Postoperative Blood Glucose[2,7]	-	-	97%	97%
Perioperative Temperature Management[2]	470	100%	100%	100%
Prophylactic Antibiotic Selection[2]	314	100%	99%	99%
Prophylactic Antibiotic Selection (Outpatient)	360	99%	97%	98%
Prophylactic Antibiotic Stopped[2]	304	100%	98%	98%
Prophylactic Antibiotic Timing[2]	314	100%	99%	99%
Prophylactic Antibiotic Timing (Outpatient)	361	100%	97%	98%
Urinary Catheter Removal[2]	313	100%	96%	97%
Survey of Patients' Hospital Experiences				
Area Around Room 'Always' Quiet at Night	300+	61%	51%	61%
Doctors 'Always' Communicated Well	300+	85%	77%	82%
Home Recovery Information Given	300+	88%	83%	85%
Hospital Given 9 or 10 on 10 Point Scale	300+	80%	63%	71%
Meds 'Always' Explained Before Given	300+	68%	59%	64%
Nurses 'Always' Communicated Well	300+	84%	75%	79%
Pain 'Always' Well Controlled	300+	76%	67%	71%
Room and Bathroom 'Always' Clean	300+	79%	69%	73%
Timely Help 'Always' Received	300+	73%	61%	68%
Would Definitely Recommend Hospital	300+	85%	65%	71%
Use of Medical Imaging				
Cardiac Imaging Stress Test before Surgery	889	6.2%	5.8%	5.3%
Combination Abdominal CT Scan	446	7.2%	8.2%	10.5%
Combination Brain/Sinus CT Scan[1]	-	-	3.6%	2.7%
Combination Chest CT Scan	218	1.4%	1.3%	2.7%
Follow-up Mammogram/Ultrasound	491	32.8%	13%	8.8%
Lumbar Spine MRI for Low Back Pain[1]	-	-	33.4%	37.2%

Montefiore Mount Vernon Hospital

12 North 7th Avenue
Mount Vernon, NY 10550
URL: www.sshsw.org
Phone: 914-664-8000
Fax: 914-664-1569
Type: Acute Care Hospitals
Ownership: Voluntary non-profit - Private
Emergency Services: Yes
Beds: 228

Key Personnel:
Cardiac Laboratory. . . . . Gariush Alaie, MD
Radiology. . . . . Mark Armstrong, MD
CEO/President. . . . . George Haskins
Quality Assurance . . . . Janice Mule
Chief of Medical Staff. . . . . Richard Petrillo, MD
Operating Room. . . . . Vicky Reed
Pediatric Ambulatory Care . . . . . . Lori Semel, MD
Pediatric In-Patient Care . . . . Lori Semel, MD

Measure	Cases	This Hosp.	State Avg.	U.S. Avg.
Blood Clot Prevention and Treatment				
Anticoagulation Overlap Therapy[2]	18	89%	91%	93%
ICU Venous Thromboembolism Prophylaxis[2]	19	89%	92%	92%
Incidence of Potentially Preventable VTE[1,2]	-	-	10%	10%
UFH with Dosages/Platelet Monitoring[1,2]	-	-	92%	97%
Venous Thromboembolism Prophylaxis[2]	331	84%	87%	85%
Warfarin Therapy Discharge Instructions[2]	13	77%	59%	75%
Chest Pain/Possible Heart Attack Care				
Aspirin Given Within 24 Hours of Arrival[1]	-	-	97%	96%
Fibrinolytic Meds Within 30 Min. of Arrival[1,3]	-	-	54%	58%
Average Time to ECG (minutes)[1]	-	-	9	7
Average Time to Transfer (minutes)[3,7]	-	-	78	60
Children's Asthma Care				
Received Home Management Plan of Care	-	-	-	88%
Received Reliever Medication	-	-	-	100%
Received Systemic Corticosteroids	-	-	-	100%
Emergency Department				
Admittance Decision Time (minutes)[2]	554	233	154	98
Head CT Results Within 45 Min. of Arrival[1]	-	-	55%	57%
Patients Who Left ER Before Being Seen	18,198	2%	2%	2%
Time from ER Arrival to Admit. (minutes)[2]	554	531	378	274
Time from ER Arrival to Discharge (minutes)	382	195	156	134
Time in ER Before Being Evaluated (minutes)	457	59	35	26
Time to Pain Meds for Fractures (minutes)	11	105	61	57
Heart Attack Care				
Aspirin Given at Discharge[1]	-	-	99%	99%
Fibrinolytic Meds Within 30 Min. of Arrival[7]	-	-	46%	54%
PCI Within 90 Minutes of Arrival[7]	-	-	95%	96%
Statin Prescribed at Discharge[1]	-	-	98%	98%
Heart Failure Care				
ACE Inhibitor or ARB for LVSD	32	97%	96%	97%
Discharge Instructions Given	75	72%	95%	94%
Evaluation of LVS Function	97	98%	99%	99%
Medicare Spending				
Medicare Spending per Patient (ratio)	-	1.14	0.96	0.98
Pneumonia Care				
Appropriate Initial Antibiotic Given	40	90%	95%	95%
Blood Culture Timing	82	99%	97%	98%
Pregnancy and Delivery Care				
Newborn Deliveries Scheduled Early[7]	-	-	4%	6%
Preventive Care				
Immunization for Influenza[2]	316	65%	88%	90%
Immunization for Pneumonia[2]	410	67%	88%	92%
Stroke Care				
Anticoagulation Therapy for Atrial Fibrillation[1]	-	-	96%	95%
Antithrombotic Therapy Timing	24	100%	98%	98%
Assessed for Rehabilitation	26	92%	97%	97%
Discharged on Antithrombotic Therapy	25	96%	99%	99%
Discharged on Statin Medication	20	95%	95%	94%
Thrombolytic Therapy Timing[1]	-	-	69%	66%
Venous Thromboembolism Prophylaxis	30	87%	94%	94%
Written Stroke Educational Materials Given	14	64%	86%	88%
Surgical Care Improvement Project				
Appropriate Beta Blocker Usage	21	95%	97%	98%
Appropriate VTP Within 24 Hours	51	94%	98%	98%
Controlled Postoperative Blood Glucose[7]	-	-	97%	97%
Perioperative Temperature Management	66	95%	100%	100%
Prophylactic Antibiotic Selection	32	94%	99%	99%
Prophylactic Antibiotic Selection (Outpatient)[1]	-	-	97%	98%
Prophylactic Antibiotic Stopped	32	94%	98%	98%
Prophylactic Antibiotic Timing	32	100%	99%	99%
Prophylactic Antibiotic Timing (Outpatient)[1]	-	-	97%	98%
Urinary Catheter Removal	34	97%	96%	97%
Survey of Patients' Hospital Experiences				
Area Around Room 'Always' Quiet at Night	300+	59%	51%	61%
Doctors 'Always' Communicated Well	300+	81%	77%	82%
Home Recovery Information Given	300+	82%	83%	85%
Hospital Given 9 or 10 on 10 Point Scale	300+	52%	63%	71%
Meds 'Always' Explained Before Given	300+	62%	59%	64%
Nurses 'Always' Communicated Well	300+	72%	75%	79%
Pain 'Always' Well Controlled	300+	65%	67%	71%
Room and Bathroom 'Always' Clean	300+	59%	69%	73%
Timely Help 'Always' Received	300+	60%	61%	68%
Would Definitely Recommend Hospital	300+	54%	65%	71%
Use of Medical Imaging				
Cardiac Imaging Stress Test before Surgery[1]	-	-	5.8%	5.3%
Combination Abdominal CT Scan	133	3.0%	8.2%	10.5%
Combination Brain/Sinus CT Scan[1]	-	-	3.6%	2.7%
Combination Chest CT Scan	75	0.0%	1.3%	2.7%
Follow-up Mammogram/Ultrasound	384	7.3%	13%	8.8%
Lumbar Spine MRI for Low Back Pain[1]	-	-	33.4%	37.2%

Long Island Jewish Medical Center

270 - 05 76th Avenue
New Hyde Park, NY 11040
URL: www.northshorelij.com
Phone: 718-470-7000
Fax: 516-465-2650
Type: Acute Care Hospitals
Ownership: Voluntary non-profit - Private
Emergency Services: Yes
Beds: 452

Key Personnel:
Radiology. . . . . Lawrence Davis, MD
Quality Assurance . . . . Dorothy Feildman
Pediatric Ambulatory Care . . . . . . Arthor Klein, MD
Coronary Care . . . . Denise Maye, RN
Chief of Medical Staff. . . . . Jeremy Roal
Cardiac Laboratory. . . . . Stacy E Rosen, MD FACC
Operating Room. . . . . Diane Simmons, RN
Infection Control. . . . . Carol Singer, MD

NOTE: Hospital profiles are in alphabetical order by state, then city, then hospital within the city; Rankings exclude hospitals with less than 25 cases except for patient surveys which excludes hospitals with less than 100 cases; (a) 100-299 cases; (1) The number of cases/patients is too few to report; (2) Data submitted were based on a sample of cases/patients; (3) Results are based on a shorter time period than required; (4) Data suppressed by CMS for one or more quarters; (5) Results are not available for this reporting period; (6) Fewer than 100 patients completed the HCAHPS survey; (7) No cases met the criteria for this measure; (8) The lower limit of the confidence interval cannot be calculated if the number of observed infections equals zero; (9) No data are available from the state/territory for this reporting period; (10) The scores shown reflect fewer than 50 completed surveys; (11) There were discrepancies in the data collection process; (12) This measure does not apply to this hospital for this reporting period; (13) Results cannot be calculated for this reporting period; (14) The results for this state are combined with nearby states to protect confidentiality; Please refer to the User's Guide for a full explanation of data.

Measure	Cases	This Hosp.	State Avg.	U.S. Avg.
Blood Clot Prevention and Treatment				
Anticoagulation Overlap Therapy[2]	239	86%	91%	93%
ICU Venous Thromboembolism Prophylaxis[2]	84	89%	92%	92%
Incidence of Potentially Preventable VTE[2]	83	8%	10%	10%
UFH with Dosages/Platelet Monitoring[2]	159	92%	92%	97%
Venous Thromboembolism Prophylaxis[2]	472	73%	87%	85%
Warfarin Therapy Discharge Instructions[2]	166	10%	59%	75%
Chest Pain/Possible Heart Attack Care				
Aspirin Given Within 24 Hours of Arrival[1,3]	-	-	97%	96%
Fibrinolytic Meds Within 30 Min. of Arrival[5]	-	-	54%	58%
Average Time to ECG (minutes)[1,3]	-	-	9	7
Average Time to Transfer (minutes)[5]	-	-	78	60
Children's Asthma Care				
Received Home Management Plan of Care	-	-	-	88%
Received Reliever Medication	-	-	-	100%
Received Systemic Corticosteroids	-	-	-	100%
Emergency Department				
Admittance Decision Time (minutes)[2]	91	140	154	98
Head CT Results Within 45 Min. of Arrival[1]	-	-	55%	57%
Patients Who Left ER Before Being Seen	>100k	1%	2%	2%
Time from ER Arrival to Admit. (minutes)[2]	94	390	378	274
Time from ER Arrival to Discharge (minutes)	493	208	156	134
Time in ER Before Being Evaluated (minutes)	519	52	35	26
Time to Pain Meds for Fractures (minutes)	266	74	61	57
Heart Attack Care				
Aspirin Given at Discharge[2]	296	100%	99%	99%
Fibrinolytic Meds Within 30 Min. of Arrival[2,7]	-	-	46%	54%
PCI Within 90 Minutes of Arrival[2]	26	88%	95%	96%
Statin Prescribed at Discharge[2]	290	99%	98%	98%
Heart Failure Care				
ACE Inhibitor or ARB for LVSD[2]	102	99%	96%	97%
Discharge Instructions Given[2]	248	94%	95%	94%
Evaluation of LVS Function[2]	296	100%	99%	99%
Medicare Spending				
Medicare Spending per Patient (ratio)	-	0.99	0.96	0.98
Pneumonia Care				
Appropriate Initial Antibiotic Given[2]	68	90%	95%	95%
Blood Culture Timing[2]	149	95%	97%	98%
Pregnancy and Delivery Care				
Newborn Deliveries Scheduled Early[2]	43	0%	4%	6%
Preventive Care				
Immunization for Influenza[2]	1,491	78%	88%	90%
Immunization for Pneumonia[2]	881	83%	88%	92%
Stroke Care				
Anticoagulation Therapy for Atrial Fibrillation[2]	11	91%	96%	95%
Antithrombotic Therapy Timing[2]	90	93%	98%	98%
Assessed for Rehabilitation[2]	117	97%	97%	97%
Discharged on Antithrombotic Therapy[2]	103	99%	99%	99%
Discharged on Statin Medication[2]	85	94%	95%	94%
Thrombolytic Therapy Timing[1,2]	-	-	69%	66%
Venous Thromboembolism Prophylaxis[2]	115	85%	94%	94%
Written Stroke Educational Materials Given[2]	67	67%	86%	88%
Surgical Care Improvement Project				
Appropriate Beta Blocker Usage[2]	221	98%	97%	98%
Appropriate VTP Within 24 Hours[2]	369	98%	98%	98%
Controlled Postoperative Blood Glucose[2]	150	97%	97%	97%
Perioperative Temperature Management[2]	602	100%	100%	100%
Prophylactic Antibiotic Selection[2]	453	98%	99%	99%
Prophylactic Antibiotic Selection (Outpatient)	310	86%	97%	98%
Prophylactic Antibiotic Stopped[2]	447	97%	98%	98%
Prophylactic Antibiotic Timing[2]	453	99%	99%	99%
Prophylactic Antibiotic Timing (Outpatient)	315	97%	97%	98%
Urinary Catheter Removal[2]	381	94%	96%	97%
Survey of Patients' Hospital Experiences				
Area Around Room 'Always' Quiet at Night	300+	57%	51%	61%
Doctors 'Always' Communicated Well	300+	76%	77%	82%
Home Recovery Information Given	300+	82%	83%	85%
Hospital Given 9 or 10 on 10 Point Scale	300+	73%	63%	71%
Meds 'Always' Explained Before Given	300+	64%	59%	64%
Nurses 'Always' Communicated Well	300+	78%	75%	79%
Pain 'Always' Well Controlled	300+	65%	67%	71%
Room and Bathroom 'Always' Clean	300+	74%	69%	73%
Timely Help 'Always' Received	300+	61%	61%	68%
Would Definitely Recommend Hospital	300+	77%	65%	71%
Use of Medical Imaging				
Cardiac Imaging Stress Test before Surgery	334	5.1%	5.8%	5.3%
Combination Abdominal CT Scan	511	1.2%	8.2%	10.5%
Combination Brain/Sinus CT Scan	718	3.5%	3.6%	2.7%
Combination Chest CT Scan	133	0.8%	1.3%	2.7%
Follow-up Mammogram/Ultrasound[7]	-	-	13%	8.8%
Lumbar Spine MRI for Low Back Pain[1]	-	-	33.4%	37.2%

Montefiore New Rochelle Hospital

16 Guion Place
New Rochelle, NY 10802
URL: www.ssmc.org
Type: Acute Care Hospitals
Ownership: Voluntary non-profit - Private
Phone: 914-632-5000
Fax: 914-637-1203
Emergency Services: Yes
Beds: 476

Key Personnel:
Operating Room. . . . . Irene Giarolo
Pediatric In-Patient Care . . . . Mark Glassman, MD
Ambulatory Care . . . . Ann Reyna
CEO/President. . . . . John R Spicer

Measure	Cases	This Hosp.	State Avg.	U.S. Avg.
Blood Clot Prevention and Treatment				
Anticoagulation Overlap Therapy[2]	33	97%	91%	93%
ICU Venous Thromboembolism Prophylaxis[2]	46	98%	92%	92%
Incidence of Potentially Preventable VTE[1,2]	-	-	10%	10%
UFH with Dosages/Platelet Monitoring[2]	12	0%	92%	97%
Venous Thromboembolism Prophylaxis[2]	377	84%	87%	85%
Warfarin Therapy Discharge Instructions[2]	17	24%	59%	75%
Chest Pain/Possible Heart Attack Care				
Aspirin Given Within 24 Hours of Arrival	24	100%	97%	96%
Fibrinolytic Meds Within 30 Min. of Arrival[1,3]	-	-	54%	58%
Average Time to ECG (minutes)	25	13	9	7
Average Time to Transfer (minutes)[3,7]	-	-	78	60
Children's Asthma Care				
Received Home Management Plan of Care	-	-	-	88%
Received Reliever Medication	-	-	-	100%
Received Systemic Corticosteroids	-	-	-	100%
Emergency Department				
Admittance Decision Time (minutes)[2]	798	230	154	98
Head CT Results Within 45 Min. of Arrival[1]	-	-	55%	57%
Patients Who Left ER Before Being Seen	36,812	1%	2%	2%
Time from ER Arrival to Admit. (minutes)[2]	799	405	378	274
Time from ER Arrival to Discharge (minutes)	431	135	156	134
Time in ER Before Being Evaluated (minutes)	454	32	35	26
Time to Pain Meds for Fractures (minutes)	79	72	61	57
Heart Attack Care				
Aspirin Given at Discharge	37	95%	99%	99%
Fibrinolytic Meds Within 30 Min. of Arrival[1]	-	-	46%	54%
PCI Within 90 Minutes of Arrival[7]	-	-	95%	96%
Statin Prescribed at Discharge	39	100%	98%	98%
Heart Failure Care				
ACE Inhibitor or ARB for LVSD	57	93%	96%	97%
Discharge Instructions Given	158	94%	95%	94%
Evaluation of LVS Function	268	99%	99%	99%
Medicare Spending				
Medicare Spending per Patient (ratio)	-	1.04	0.96	0.98
Pneumonia Care				
Appropriate Initial Antibiotic Given	76	96%	95%	95%
Blood Culture Timing	113	96%	97%	98%
Pregnancy and Delivery Care				
Newborn Deliveries Scheduled Early[2]	34	9%	4%	6%
Preventive Care				
Immunization for Influenza[2]	499	96%	88%	90%
Immunization for Pneumonia[2]	641	95%	88%	92%
Stroke Care				
Anticoagulation Therapy for Atrial Fibrillation	13	100%	96%	95%
Antithrombotic Therapy Timing	80	100%	98%	98%
Assessed for Rehabilitation	84	100%	97%	97%
Discharged on Antithrombotic Therapy	77	100%	99%	99%
Discharged on Statin Medication	46	98%	95%	94%
Thrombolytic Therapy Timing[1]	-	-	69%	66%
Venous Thromboembolism Prophylaxis	97	92%	94%	94%
Written Stroke Educational Materials Given	28	96%	86%	88%
Surgical Care Improvement Project				
Appropriate Beta Blocker Usage	145	99%	97%	98%
Appropriate VTP Within 24 Hours	481	97%	98%	98%
Controlled Postoperative Blood Glucose[7]	-	-	97%	97%
Perioperative Temperature Management	519	99%	100%	100%
Prophylactic Antibiotic Selection	364	99%	99%	99%
Prophylactic Antibiotic Selection (Outpatient)	29	100%	97%	98%
Prophylactic Antibiotic Stopped	362	99%	98%	98%
Prophylactic Antibiotic Timing	364	100%	99%	99%
Prophylactic Antibiotic Timing (Outpatient)	30	97%	97%	98%
Urinary Catheter Removal	399	97%	96%	97%
Survey of Patients' Hospital Experiences				
Area Around Room 'Always' Quiet at Night	300+	56%	51%	61%
Doctors 'Always' Communicated Well	300+	78%	77%	82%
Home Recovery Information Given	300+	83%	83%	85%
Hospital Given 9 or 10 on 10 Point Scale	300+	58%	63%	71%
Meds 'Always' Explained Before Given	300+	61%	59%	64%
Nurses 'Always' Communicated Well	300+	73%	75%	79%
Pain 'Always' Well Controlled	300+	66%	67%	71%
Room and Bathroom 'Always' Clean	300+	62%	69%	73%
Timely Help 'Always' Received	300+	63%	61%	68%
Would Definitely Recommend Hospital	300+	58%	65%	71%
Use of Medical Imaging				
Cardiac Imaging Stress Test before Surgery	55	5.5%	5.8%	5.3%
Combination Abdominal CT Scan	213	1.4%	8.2%	10.5%
Combination Brain/Sinus CT Scan[1]	-	-	3.6%	2.7%
Combination Chest CT Scan	87	0.0%	1.3%	2.7%
Follow-up Mammogram/Ultrasound	135	21.5%	13%	8.8%
Lumbar Spine MRI for Low Back Pain[1]	-	-	33.4%	37.2%

Bellevue Hospital Center

462 First Avenue
New York, NY 10016
URL: www.nyc.gov/html/hhc/html/facilities/bellevue.shtml
Type: Acute Care Hospitals
Ownership: Government - Local
Phone: 212-561-4132
Fax: 212-562-4009
Emergency Services: Yes
Beds: 809

Key Personnel:
CEO/President. . . . . Alan D Aviles
Infection Control. . . . . Robert Holzman, MD
Radiology. . . . . Albert Keegan, MD
Pediatric Ambulatory Care . . . . . . Wade Parks, MD
Pediatric In-Patient Care . . . . Wade Parks, MD
Chief of Medical Staff . . . . Joe Schickmer
Quality Assurance . . . . Susan Schnall, RN, CPHQ
Operating Room. . . . . Alex Stone, MD

Measure	Cases	This Hosp.	State Avg.	U.S. Avg.
Blood Clot Prevention and Treatment				
Anticoagulation Overlap Therapy[2]	73	96%	91%	93%
ICU Venous Thromboembolism Prophylaxis[2]	33	100%	92%	92%
Incidence of Potentially Preventable VTE[2]	47	0%	10%	10%
UFH with Dosages/Platelet Monitoring[2]	70	100%	92%	97%
Venous Thromboembolism Prophylaxis[2]	287	94%	87%	85%
Warfarin Therapy Discharge Instructions[2]	49	35%	59%	75%
Chest Pain/Possible Heart Attack Care				
Aspirin Given Within 24 Hours of Arrival[1,3]	-	-	97%	96%
Fibrinolytic Meds Within 30 Min. of Arrival[5]	-	-	54%	58%
Average Time to ECG (minutes)[1,3]	-	-	9	7
Average Time to Transfer (minutes)[5]	-	-	78	60
Children's Asthma Care				
Received Home Management Plan of Care	-	-	-	88%
Received Reliever Medication	-	-	-	100%
Received Systemic Corticosteroids	-	-	-	100%
Emergency Department				
Admittance Decision Time (minutes)[2]	539	175	154	98
Head CT Results Within 45 Min. of Arrival[7]	-	-	55%	57%
Patients Who Left ER Before Being Seen	>100k	7%	2%	2%
Time from ER Arrival to Admit. (minutes)[2]	547	506	378	274
Time from ER Arrival to Discharge (minutes)	353	204	156	134
Time in ER Before Being Evaluated (minutes)	399	50	35	26
Time to Pain Meds for Fractures (minutes)	101	52	61	57
Heart Attack Care				
Aspirin Given at Discharge	339	100%	99%	99%

NOTE: Hospital profiles are in alphabetical order by state, then city, then hospital within the city; Rankings exclude hospitals with less than 25 cases except for patient surveys which excludes hospitals with less than 100 cases; (a) 100-299 cases; (1) The number of cases/patients is too few to report; (2) Data submitted were based on a sample of cases/patients; (3) Results are based on a shorter time period than required; (4) Data suppressed by CMS for one or more quarters; (5) Results are not available for this reporting period; (6) Fewer than 100 patients completed the HCAHPS survey; (7) No cases met the criteria for this measure; (8) The lower limit of the confidence interval cannot be calculated if the number of observed infections equals zero; (9) No data are available from the state/territory for this reporting period; (10) The scores shown reflect fewer than 50 completed surveys; (11) There were discrepancies in the data collection process; (12) This measure does not apply to this hospital for this reporting period; (13) Results cannot be calculated for this reporting period; (14) The results for this state are combined with nearby states to protect confidentiality; Please refer to the User's Guide for a full explanation of data.

Measure	Cases	This Hosp.	State Avg.	U.S. Avg.
Fibrinolytic Meds Within 30 Min. of Arrival[7]	-	-	46%	54%
PCI Within 90 Minutes of Arrival	31	97%	95%	96%
Statin Prescribed at Discharge	330	100%	98%	98%
Heart Failure Care				
ACE Inhibitor or ARB for LVSD	165	100%	96%	97%
Discharge Instructions Given	275	100%	95%	94%
Evaluation of LVS Function	294	100%	99%	99%
Medicare Spending				
Medicare Spending per Patient (ratio)	-	0.93	0.96	0.98
Pneumonia Care				
Appropriate Initial Antibiotic Given	65	97%	95%	95%
Blood Culture Timing	123	99%	97%	98%
Pregnancy and Delivery Care				
Newborn Deliveries Scheduled Early[2]	16	0%	4%	6%
Preventive Care				
Immunization for Influenza[2]	342	93%	88%	90%
Immunization for Pneumonia[2]	449	88%	88%	92%
Stroke Care				
Anticoagulation Therapy for Atrial Fibrillation[1,2]	-	-	96%	95%
Antithrombotic Therapy Timing[2]	58	95%	98%	98%
Assessed for Rehabilitation[2]	109	90%	97%	97%
Discharged on Antithrombotic Therapy[2]	70	100%	99%	99%
Discharged on Statin Medication[2]	52	100%	95%	94%
Thrombolytic Therapy Timing[1,2]	-	-	69%	66%
Venous Thromboembolism Prophylaxis[2]	129	86%	94%	94%
Written Stroke Educational Materials Given[2]	40	0%	86%	88%
Surgical Care Improvement Project				
Appropriate Beta Blocker Usage[2]	108	99%	97%	98%
Appropriate VTP Within 24 Hours[2]	207	98%	98%	98%
Controlled Postoperative Blood Glucose[2]	138	96%	97%	97%
Perioperative Temperature Management[2]	258	100%	100%	100%
Prophylactic Antibiotic Selection[2]	279	100%	99%	99%
Prophylactic Antibiotic Selection (Outpatient)	104	97%	97%	98%
Prophylactic Antibiotic Stopped[2]	272	99%	98%	98%
Prophylactic Antibiotic Timing[2]	279	99%	99%	99%
Prophylactic Antibiotic Timing (Outpatient)	29	97%	97%	98%
Urinary Catheter Removal[2]	252	100%	96%	97%
Survey of Patients' Hospital Experiences				
Area Around Room 'Always' Quiet at Night	300+	43%	51%	61%
Doctors 'Always' Communicated Well	300+	76%	77%	82%
Home Recovery Information Given	300+	79%	83%	85%
Hospital Given 9 or 10 on 10 Point Scale	300+	58%	63%	71%
Meds 'Always' Explained Before Given	300+	51%	59%	64%
Nurses 'Always' Communicated Well	300+	64%	75%	79%
Pain 'Always' Well Controlled	300+	57%	67%	71%
Room and Bathroom 'Always' Clean	300+	60%	69%	73%
Timely Help 'Always' Received	300+	50%	61%	68%
Would Definitely Recommend Hospital	300+	64%	65%	71%
Use of Medical Imaging				
Cardiac Imaging Stress Test before Surgery[1]	-	-	5.8%	5.3%
Combination Abdominal CT Scan	72	5.6%	8.2%	10.5%
Combination Brain/Sinus CT Scan[1]	-	-	3.6%	2.7%
Combination Chest CT Scan	59	3.4%	1.3%	2.7%
Follow-up Mammogram/Ultrasound	97	7.2%	13%	8.8%
Lumbar Spine MRI for Low Back Pain[1]	-	-	33.4%	37.2%

Beth Israel Medical Center

First Avenue at 16th Street
New York, NY 10003
Phone: 212-420-2000
URL: www.wehealny.org
Type: Acute Care Hospitals
Emergency Services: Yes
Ownership: Voluntary non-profit - Private
Beds: 1,368

Key Personnel:
Chief of Medical Staff.......... David B Bernard, MD
Pediatric Ambulatory Care...... Richard Bonforte, MD
Pediatric In-Patient Care....... Richard Bonforte, MD
Quality Assurance............ Barb Challan
Patient Relations............ Kathryn Davis
Anesthesiology.............. Sundar Koppolu, MD
CEO/President.............. Harris Nagler, MD, FACS
Operating Room............. George J Todd, MD FACS

Measure	Cases	This Hosp.	State Avg.	U.S. Avg.
Blood Clot Prevention and Treatment				
Anticoagulation Overlap Therapy[2]	253	86%	91%	93%
ICU Venous Thromboembolism Prophylaxis[2]	26	92%	92%	92%
Incidence of Potentially Preventable VTE[2]	83	17%	10%	10%
UFH with Dosages/Platelet Monitoring[2]	131	99%	92%	97%
Venous Thromboembolism Prophylaxis[2]	346	79%	87%	85%
Warfarin Therapy Discharge Instructions[2]	179	30%	59%	75%
Chest Pain/Possible Heart Attack Care				
Aspirin Given Within 24 Hours of Arrival[5]	-	-	97%	96%
Fibrinolytic Meds Within 30 Min. of Arrival[5]	-	-	54%	58%
Average Time to ECG (minutes)[5]	-	-	9	7
Average Time to Transfer (minutes)[5]	-	-	78	60
Children's Asthma Care				
Received Home Management Plan of Care	-	-	-	88%
Received Reliever Medication	-	-	-	100%
Received Systemic Corticosteroids	-	-	-	100%
Emergency Department				
Admittance Decision Time (minutes)[2]	722	272	154	98
Head CT Results Within 45 Min. of Arrival[1]	-	-	55%	57%
Patients Who Left ER Before Being Seen	>100k	6%	2%	2%
Time from ER Arrival to Admit. (minutes)[2]	723	530	378	274
Time from ER Arrival to Discharge (minutes)	354	208	156	134
Time in ER Before Being Evaluated (minutes)	380	70	35	26
Time to Pain Meds for Fractures (minutes)	137	71	61	57
Heart Attack Care				
Aspirin Given at Discharge[2]	249	99%	99%	99%
Fibrinolytic Meds Within 30 Min. of Arrival[2,7]	-	-	46%	54%
PCI Within 90 Minutes of Arrival[2]	33	100%	95%	96%
Statin Prescribed at Discharge[2]	247	100%	98%	98%
Heart Failure Care				
ACE Inhibitor or ARB for LVSD[2]	86	99%	96%	97%
Discharge Instructions Given[2]	235	100%	95%	94%
Evaluation of LVS Function[2]	275	100%	99%	99%
Medicare Spending				
Medicare Spending per Patient (ratio)	-	1.02	0.96	0.98
Pneumonia Care				
Appropriate Initial Antibiotic Given[2]	113	93%	95%	95%
Blood Culture Timing[2]	220	99%	97%	98%
Pregnancy and Delivery Care				
Newborn Deliveries Scheduled Early[2]	82	0%	4%	6%
Preventive Care				
Immunization for Influenza[2]	549	98%	88%	90%
Immunization for Pneumonia[2]	680	96%	88%	92%
Stroke Care				
Anticoagulation Therapy for Atrial Fibrillation[2]	14	100%	96%	95%
Antithrombotic Therapy Timing[2]	98	100%	98%	98%
Assessed for Rehabilitation[2]	108	100%	97%	97%
Discharged on Antithrombotic Therapy[2]	94	100%	99%	99%
Discharged on Statin Medication[2]	65	98%	95%	94%
Thrombolytic Therapy Timing[1,2]	-	-	69%	66%
Venous Thromboembolism Prophylaxis[2]	119	85%	94%	94%
Written Stroke Educational Materials Given[2]	51	86%	86%	88%
Surgical Care Improvement Project				
Appropriate Beta Blocker Usage[2]	237	96%	97%	98%
Appropriate VTP Within 24 Hours[2]	442	100%	98%	98%
Controlled Postoperative Blood Glucose[2]	142	98%	97%	97%
Perioperative Temperature Management[2]	556	100%	100%	100%
Prophylactic Antibiotic Selection[2]	503	99%	99%	99%
Prophylactic Antibiotic Selection (Outpatient)	466	96%	97%	98%
Prophylactic Antibiotic Stopped[2]	498	96%	98%	98%
Prophylactic Antibiotic Timing[2]	503	100%	99%	99%
Prophylactic Antibiotic Timing (Outpatient)	445	97%	97%	98%
Urinary Catheter Removal[2]	464	96%	96%	97%
Survey of Patients' Hospital Experiences				
Area Around Room 'Always' Quiet at Night	300+	45%	51%	61%
Doctors 'Always' Communicated Well	300+	71%	77%	82%
Home Recovery Information Given	300+	80%	83%	85%
Hospital Given 9 or 10 on 10 Point Scale	300+	55%	63%	71%
Meds 'Always' Explained Before Given	300+	52%	59%	64%
Nurses 'Always' Communicated Well	300+	66%	75%	79%
Pain 'Always' Well Controlled	300+	60%	67%	71%
Room and Bathroom 'Always' Clean	300+	67%	69%	73%
Timely Help 'Always' Received	300+	53%	61%	68%
Would Definitely Recommend Hospital	300+	61%	65%	71%
Use of Medical Imaging				
Cardiac Imaging Stress Test before Surgery	447	7.8%	5.8%	5.3%
Combination Abdominal CT Scan	1,021	11.2%	8.2%	10.5%
Combination Brain/Sinus CT Scan	1,180	5.1%	3.6%	2.7%
Combination Chest CT Scan	708	4.4%	1.3%	2.7%
Follow-up Mammogram/Ultrasound	1,802	9.7%	13%	8.8%
Lumbar Spine MRI for Low Back Pain	65	36.9%	33.4%	37.2%

Harlem Hospital Center

506 Lenox Avenue
New York, NY 10037
Phone: 212-491-8400
URL: www.nyc.gov/hhc
Type: Acute Care Hospitals
Emergency Services: Yes
Ownership: Government - Local
Beds: 7,560

Key Personnel:
CEO/President................ Alan Aviles

Measure	Cases	This Hosp.	State Avg.	U.S. Avg.
Blood Clot Prevention and Treatment				
Anticoagulation Overlap Therapy[2]	38	97%	91%	93%
ICU Venous Thromboembolism Prophylaxis[2]	52	90%	92%	92%
Incidence of Potentially Preventable VTE[2]	11	9%	10%	10%
UFH with Dosages/Platelet Monitoring[2]	17	12%	92%	97%
Venous Thromboembolism Prophylaxis[2]	234	88%	87%	85%
Warfarin Therapy Discharge Instructions[2]	31	6%	59%	75%
Chest Pain/Possible Heart Attack Care				
Aspirin Given Within 24 Hours of Arrival[1,3]	-	-	97%	96%
Fibrinolytic Meds Within 30 Min. of Arrival[3,7]	-	-	54%	58%
Average Time to ECG (minutes)[1,3]	-	-	9	7
Average Time to Transfer (minutes)[3,7]	-	-	78	60
Children's Asthma Care				
Received Home Management Plan of Care	-	-	-	88%
Received Reliever Medication	-	-	-	100%
Received Systemic Corticosteroids	-	-	-	100%
Emergency Department				
Admittance Decision Time (minutes)[2]	608	142	154	98
Head CT Results Within 45 Min. of Arrival[1]	-	-	55%	57%
Patients Who Left ER Before Being Seen	74,091	11%	2%	2%
Time from ER Arrival to Admit. (minutes)[2]	608	420	378	274
Time from ER Arrival to Discharge (minutes)	315	173	156	134
Time in ER Before Being Evaluated (minutes)	337	83	35	26
Time to Pain Meds for Fractures (minutes)	42	86	61	57
Heart Attack Care				
Aspirin Given at Discharge	28	100%	99%	99%
Fibrinolytic Meds Within 30 Min. of Arrival[7]	-	-	46%	54%
PCI Within 90 Minutes of Arrival[7]	-	-	95%	96%
Statin Prescribed at Discharge	25	100%	98%	98%
Heart Failure Care				
ACE Inhibitor or ARB for LVSD	100	99%	96%	97%
Discharge Instructions Given	166	83%	95%	94%
Evaluation of LVS Function	188	99%	99%	99%
Medicare Spending				
Medicare Spending per Patient (ratio)	-	0.96	0.96	0.98
Pneumonia Care				
Appropriate Initial Antibiotic Given	68	100%	95%	95%
Blood Culture Timing	135	99%	97%	98%
Pregnancy and Delivery Care				
Newborn Deliveries Scheduled Early[2]	22	5%	4%	6%
Preventive Care				
Immunization for Influenza[2]	524	88%	88%	90%
Immunization for Pneumonia[2]	480	93%	88%	92%
Stroke Care				
Anticoagulation Therapy for Atrial Fibrillation[1]	-	-	96%	95%
Antithrombotic Therapy Timing	73	100%	98%	98%
Assessed for Rehabilitation	82	94%	97%	97%
Discharged on Antithrombotic Therapy	70	96%	99%	99%
Discharged on Statin Medication	65	98%	95%	94%
Thrombolytic Therapy Timing[1]	-	-	69%	66%
Venous Thromboembolism Prophylaxis	89	94%	94%	94%
Written Stroke Educational Materials Given	34	50%	86%	88%
Surgical Care Improvement Project				
Appropriate Beta Blocker Usage[2]	14	86%	97%	98%
Appropriate VTP Within 24 Hours[2]	115	98%	98%	98%
Controlled Postoperative Blood Glucose[2,7]	-	-	97%	97%

NOTE: Hospital profiles are in alphabetical order by state, then city, then hospital within the city; Rankings exclude hospitals with less than 25 cases except for patient surveys which excludes hospitals with less than 100 cases; (a) 100-299 cases; (1) The number of cases/patients is too few to report; (2) Data submitted were based on a sample of cases/patients; (3) Results are based on a shorter time period than required; (4) Data suppressed by CMS for one or more quarters; (5) Results are not available for this reporting period; (6) Fewer than 100 patients completed the HCAHPS survey; (7) No cases met the criteria for this measure; (8) The lower limit of the confidence interval cannot be calculated if the number of observed infections equals zero; (9) No data are available from the state/territory for this reporting period; (10) The scores shown reflect fewer than 50 completed surveys; (11) There were discrepancies in the data collection process; (12) This measure does not apply to this hospital for this reporting period; (13) Results cannot be calculated for this reporting period; (14) The results for this state are combined with nearby states to protect confidentiality; Please refer to the User's Guide for a full explanation of data.

Measure	Cases	This Hosp.	State Avg.	U.S. Avg.
Perioperative Temperature Management[2]	138	100%	100%	100%
Prophylactic Antibiotic Selection[2]	47	94%	99%	99%
Prophylactic Antibiotic Selection (Outpatient)	82	94%	97%	98%
Prophylactic Antibiotic Stopped[2]	44	93%	98%	98%
Prophylactic Antibiotic Timing[2]	47	100%	99%	99%
Prophylactic Antibiotic Timing (Outpatient)	62	90%	97%	98%
Urinary Catheter Removal[2]	49	98%	96%	97%
Survey of Patients' Hospital Experiences				
Area Around Room 'Always' Quiet at Night	300+	55%	51%	61%
Doctors 'Always' Communicated Well	300+	69%	77%	82%
Home Recovery Information Given	300+	73%	83%	85%
Hospital Given 9 or 10 on 10 Point Scale	300+	43%	63%	71%
Meds 'Always' Explained Before Given	300+	47%	59%	64%
Nurses 'Always' Communicated Well	300+	58%	75%	79%
Pain 'Always' Well Controlled	300+	50%	67%	71%
Room and Bathroom 'Always' Clean	300+	59%	69%	73%
Timely Help 'Always' Received	300+	39%	61%	68%
Would Definitely Recommend Hospital	300+	46%	65%	71%
Use of Medical Imaging				
Cardiac Imaging Stress Test before Surgery[1]	-	-	5.8%	5.3%
Combination Abdominal CT Scan	75	14.7%	8.2%	10.5%
Combination Brain/Sinus CT Scan[1]	-	-	3.6%	2.7%
Combination Chest CT Scan[1]	-	-	1.3%	2.7%
Follow-up Mammogram/Ultrasound	88	15.9%	13%	8.8%
Lumbar Spine MRI for Low Back Pain[1]	-	-	33.4%	37.2%

Hospital For Special Surgery

535 East 70th Street
New York, NY 10021
URL: www.hss.edu
Type: Acute Care Hospitals
Ownership: Voluntary non-profit - Private
Phone: 212-606-1000
Fax: 212-606-1961
Emergency Services: Yes
Beds: 160

Key Personnel:
Radiology. Ronald S Adler
Quality Assurance . . . . Susan Flics
Chief of Medical Staff. . . . . Thomas P Sculco, MD
CEO/President. . . . . Louis A. Shapiro
Chair/CEO. . . . . Kendrick R. Wilson

Measure	Cases	This Hosp.	State Avg.	U.S. Avg.
Blood Clot Prevention and Treatment				
Anticoagulation Overlap Therapy[2]	37	100%	91%	93%
ICU Venous Thromboembolism Prophylaxis[2,7]	-	-	92%	92%
Incidence of Potentially Preventable VTE[2]	41	0%	10%	10%
UFH with Dosages/Platelet Monitoring[1,2]	-	-	92%	97%
Venous Thromboembolism Prophylaxis[2]	169	100%	87%	85%
Warfarin Therapy Discharge Instructions[2]	13	100%	59%	75%
Chest Pain/Possible Heart Attack Care				
Aspirin Given Within 24 Hours of Arrival[5]	-	-	97%	96%
Fibrinolytic Meds Within 30 Min. of Arrival[5]	-	-	54%	58%
Average Time to ECG (minutes)[5]	-	-	9	7
Average Time to Transfer (minutes)[5]	-	-	78	60
Children's Asthma Care				
Received Home Management Plan of Care	-	-	-	88%
Received Reliever Medication	-	-	-	100%
Received Systemic Corticosteroids	-	-	-	100%
Emergency Department				
Admittance Decision Time (minutes)[2,7]	-	-	154	98
Head CT Results Within 45 Min. of Arrival[5]	-	-	55%	57%
Patients Who Left ER Before Being Seen[5]	-	-	2%	2%
Time from ER Arrival to Admit. (minutes)[2,7]	-	-	378	274
Time from ER Arrival to Discharge (minutes)[5]	-	-	156	134
Time in ER Before Being Evaluated (minutes)[5]	-	-	35	26
Time to Pain Meds for Fractures (minutes)[5]	-	-	61	57
Heart Attack Care				
Aspirin Given at Discharge[5]	-	-	99%	99%
Fibrinolytic Meds Within 30 Min. of Arrival[5]	-	-	46%	54%
PCI Within 90 Minutes of Arrival[5]	-	-	95%	96%
Statin Prescribed at Discharge[5]	-	-	98%	98%
Heart Failure Care				
ACE Inhibitor or ARB for LVSD[5]	-	-	96%	97%
Discharge Instructions Given[5]	-	-	95%	94%
Evaluation of LVS Function[5]	-	-	99%	99%
Medicare Spending				
Medicare Spending per Patient (ratio)	-	1.02	0.96	0.98
Pneumonia Care				
Appropriate Initial Antibiotic Given[5]	-	-	95%	95%
Blood Culture Timing[5]	-	-	97%	98%
Pregnancy and Delivery Care				
Newborn Deliveries Scheduled Early[7]	-	-	4%	6%
Preventive Care				
Immunization for Influenza[2]	619	98%	88%	90%
Immunization for Pneumonia[2]	680	91%	88%	92%
Stroke Care				
Anticoagulation Therapy for Atrial Fibrillation[5]	-	-	96%	95%
Antithrombotic Therapy Timing[5]	-	-	98%	98%
Assessed for Rehabilitation[5]	-	-	97%	97%
Discharged on Antithrombotic Therapy[5]	-	-	99%	99%
Discharged on Statin Medication[5]	-	-	95%	94%
Thrombolytic Therapy Timing[5]	-	-	69%	66%
Venous Thromboembolism Prophylaxis[5]	-	-	94%	94%
Written Stroke Educational Materials Given[5]	-	-	86%	88%
Surgical Care Improvement Project				
Appropriate Beta Blocker Usage[2]	134	98%	97%	98%
Appropriate VTP Within 24 Hours[2]	562	99%	98%	98%
Controlled Postoperative Blood Glucose[2,7]	-	-	97%	97%
Perioperative Temperature Management[2]	593	100%	100%	100%
Prophylactic Antibiotic Selection[2]	412	100%	99%	99%
Prophylactic Antibiotic Selection (Outpatient)	415	100%	97%	98%
Prophylactic Antibiotic Stopped[2]	409	100%	98%	98%
Prophylactic Antibiotic Timing[2]	412	100%	99%	99%
Prophylactic Antibiotic Timing (Outpatient)	415	100%	97%	98%
Urinary Catheter Removal[2]	485	100%	96%	97%
Survey of Patients' Hospital Experiences				
Area Around Room 'Always' Quiet at Night	300+	58%	51%	61%
Doctors 'Always' Communicated Well	300+	82%	77%	82%
Home Recovery Information Given	300+	90%	83%	85%
Hospital Given 9 or 10 on 10 Point Scale	300+	88%	63%	71%
Meds 'Always' Explained Before Given	300+	65%	59%	64%
Nurses 'Always' Communicated Well	300+	82%	75%	79%
Pain 'Always' Well Controlled	300+	76%	67%	71%
Room and Bathroom 'Always' Clean	300+	80%	69%	73%
Timely Help 'Always' Received	300+	71%	61%	68%
Would Definitely Recommend Hospital	300+	92%	65%	71%
Use of Medical Imaging				
Cardiac Imaging Stress Test before Surgery[7]	-	-	5.8%	5.3%
Combination Abdominal CT Scan[1]	-	-	8.2%	10.5%
Combination Brain/Sinus CT Scan[1]	-	-	3.6%	2.7%
Combination Chest CT Scan	63	0.0%	1.3%	2.7%
Follow-up Mammogram/Ultrasound[7]	-	-	13%	8.8%
Lumbar Spine MRI for Low Back Pain	624	32.4%	33.4%	37.2%

Lenox Hill Hospital

100 East 77th Street
New York, NY 10021
URL: www.lenoxhillhospital.org
Type: Acute Care Hospitals
Ownership: Voluntary non-profit - Private
Phone: 212-439-2345
Emergency Services: Yes
Beds: 652

Key Personnel:
Radiology. . . . . Eric L Charles
Patient Relations . . . . Michael Conroy
Quality Assurance . . . . Janice Fajardo
Pediatric Ambulatory Care . . . . . . Armand Grassi, MD
Operating Room. . . . . Richard Green, RN
Chair/CEO. . . . . William O. Hiltz
Infection Control. . . . . Sarah Petrello
Anesthesiology. . . . . James Richter, MD

Measure	Cases	This Hosp.	State Avg.	U.S. Avg.
Blood Clot Prevention and Treatment				
Anticoagulation Overlap Therapy[2]	192	79%	91%	93%
ICU Venous Thromboembolism Prophylaxis[2]	43	74%	92%	92%
Incidence of Potentially Preventable VTE[2]	85	16%	10%	10%
UFH with Dosages/Platelet Monitoring[2]	145	92%	92%	97%
Venous Thromboembolism Prophylaxis[2]	299	77%	87%	85%
Warfarin Therapy Discharge Instructions[2]	137	4%	59%	75%
Chest Pain/Possible Heart Attack Care				
Aspirin Given Within 24 Hours of Arrival[5]	-	-	97%	96%
Fibrinolytic Meds Within 30 Min. of Arrival[5]	-	-	54%	58%
Average Time to ECG (minutes)[5]	-	-	9	7
Average Time to Transfer (minutes)[5]	-	-	78	60
Children's Asthma Care				
Received Home Management Plan of Care	-	-	-	88%
Received Reliever Medication	-	-	-	100%
Received Systemic Corticosteroids	-	-	-	100%
Emergency Department				
Admittance Decision Time (minutes)[2]	532	136	154	98
Head CT Results Within 45 Min. of Arrival[1]	-	-	55%	57%
Patients Who Left ER Before Being Seen	58,040	0%	2%	2%
Time from ER Arrival to Admit. (minutes)[2]	536	400	378	274
Time from ER Arrival to Discharge (minutes)	371	156	156	134
Time in ER Before Being Evaluated (minutes)	373	21	35	26
Time to Pain Meds for Fractures (minutes)	66	66	61	57
Heart Attack Care				
Aspirin Given at Discharge[2]	286	99%	99%	99%
Fibrinolytic Meds Within 30 Min. of Arrival[2,7]	-	-	46%	54%
PCI Within 90 Minutes of Arrival[2]	12	92%	95%	96%
Statin Prescribed at Discharge[2]	284	96%	98%	98%
Heart Failure Care				
ACE Inhibitor or ARB for LVSD[2]	124	84%	96%	97%
Discharge Instructions Given[2]	266	86%	95%	94%
Evaluation of LVS Function[2]	310	99%	99%	99%
Medicare Spending				
Medicare Spending per Patient (ratio)	-	0.99	0.96	0.98
Pneumonia Care				
Appropriate Initial Antibiotic Given[2]	81	96%	95%	95%
Blood Culture Timing[2]	159	96%	97%	98%
Pregnancy and Delivery Care				
Newborn Deliveries Scheduled Early[2]	33	3%	4%	6%
Preventive Care				
Immunization for Influenza[2]	549	72%	88%	90%
Immunization for Pneumonia[2]	621	79%	88%	92%
Stroke Care				
Anticoagulation Therapy for Atrial Fibrillation[2]	14	100%	96%	95%
Antithrombotic Therapy Timing[2]	63	90%	98%	98%
Assessed for Rehabilitation[2]	94	90%	97%	97%
Discharged on Antithrombotic Therapy[2]	74	93%	99%	99%
Discharged on Statin Medication[2]	54	83%	95%	94%
Thrombolytic Therapy Timing[1,2]	-	-	69%	66%
Venous Thromboembolism Prophylaxis[2]	98	87%	94%	94%
Written Stroke Educational Materials Given[2]	59	92%	86%	88%
Surgical Care Improvement Project				
Appropriate Beta Blocker Usage[2]	263	97%	97%	98%
Appropriate VTP Within 24 Hours[2]	377	98%	98%	98%
Controlled Postoperative Blood Glucose[2]	137	95%	97%	97%
Perioperative Temperature Management[2]	584	100%	100%	100%
Prophylactic Antibiotic Selection[2]	457	98%	99%	99%
Prophylactic Antibiotic Selection (Outpatient)	451	93%	97%	98%
Prophylactic Antibiotic Stopped[2]	442	95%	98%	98%
Prophylactic Antibiotic Timing[2]	457	99%	99%	99%
Prophylactic Antibiotic Timing (Outpatient)	455	94%	97%	98%
Urinary Catheter Removal[2]	285	94%	96%	97%
Survey of Patients' Hospital Experiences				
Area Around Room 'Always' Quiet at Night	300+	48%	51%	61%
Doctors 'Always' Communicated Well	300+	79%	77%	82%
Home Recovery Information Given	300+	76%	83%	85%
Hospital Given 9 or 10 on 10 Point Scale	300+	60%	63%	71%
Meds 'Always' Explained Before Given	300+	58%	59%	64%
Nurses 'Always' Communicated Well	300+	72%	75%	79%
Pain 'Always' Well Controlled	300+	63%	67%	71%
Room and Bathroom 'Always' Clean	300+	61%	69%	73%
Timely Help 'Always' Received	300+	55%	61%	68%
Would Definitely Recommend Hospital	300+	70%	65%	71%
Use of Medical Imaging				
Cardiac Imaging Stress Test before Surgery	484	8.5%	5.8%	5.3%
Combination Abdominal CT Scan	616	11.5%	8.2%	10.5%
Combination Brain/Sinus CT Scan	401	1.7%	3.6%	2.7%
Combination Chest CT Scan	459	4.1%	1.3%	2.7%
Follow-up Mammogram/Ultrasound	272	54.4%	13%	8.8%
Lumbar Spine MRI for Low Back Pain[1]	-	-	33.4%	37.2%

NOTE: Hospital profiles are in alphabetical order by state, then city, then hospital within the city; Rankings exclude hospitals with less than 25 cases except for patient surveys which excludes hospitals with less than 100 cases; (a) 100-299 cases; (1) The number of cases/patients is too few to report; (2) Data submitted were based on a sample of cases/patients; (3) Results are based on a shorter time period than required; (4) Data suppressed by CMS for one or more quarters; (5) Results are not available for this reporting period; (6) Fewer than 100 patients completed the HCAHPS survey; (7) No cases met the criteria for this measure; (8) The lower limit of the confidence interval cannot be calculated if the number of observed infections equals zero; (9) No data are available from the state/territory for this reporting period; (10) The scores shown reflect fewer than 50 completed surveys; (11) There were discrepancies in the data collection process; (12) This measure does not apply to this hospital for this reporting period; (13) Results cannot be calculated for this reporting period; (14) The results for this state are combined with nearby states to protect confidentiality; Please refer to the User's Guide for a full explanation of data.

Metropolitan Hospital Center

1901 First Avenue
New York, NY 10029
URL: www.nymc.edu/metres/mhc
Type: Acute Care Hospitals
Ownership: Government - Local
Phone: 212-423-7554
Fax: 212-423-6180
Emergency Services: Yes
Beds: 341

Key Personnel:
Emergency Room . . . . Greg Almond, MD
Quality Assurance . . . . Sandy Bezacqua
Radiology. . . . . Matari Hussein, MD
Pediatric Ambulatory Care . . . . . . Sarla Inamdar, MD
Pediatric In-Patient Care . . . . Sarla Inamdar, MD
Anesthesiology. . . . . Joseph Lopez, MD
Infection Control. . . . . Joyce Luther
Chief of Medical Staff. . . . . Marcie Rubin, MPH, MBA

Measure	Cases	This Hosp.	State Avg.	U.S. Avg.
Blood Clot Prevention and Treatment				
Anticoagulation Overlap Therapy[2]	15	93%	91%	93%
ICU Venous Thromboembolism Prophylaxis[2]	82	98%	92%	92%
Incidence of Potentially Preventable VTE[1,2]	-	-	10%	10%
UFH with Dosages/Platelet Monitoring[1,2]	-	-	92%	97%
Venous Thromboembolism Prophylaxis[2]	205	96%	87%	85%
Warfarin Therapy Discharge Instructions[1,2]	-	-	59%	75%
Chest Pain/Possible Heart Attack Care				
Aspirin Given Within 24 Hours of Arrival[3]	11	100%	97%	96%
Fibrinolytic Meds Within 30 Min. of Arrival[3,7]	-	-	54%	58%
Average Time to ECG (minutes)[3]	11	9	9	7
Average Time to Transfer (minutes)[1,3]	-	-	78	60
Children's Asthma Care				
Received Home Management Plan of Care	-	-	-	88%
Received Reliever Medication	-	-	-	100%
Received Systemic Corticosteroids	-	-	-	100%
Emergency Department				
Admittance Decision Time (minutes)[2]	646	186	154	98
Head CT Results Within 45 Min. of Arrival[1,3]	-	-	55%	57%
Patients Who Left ER Before Being Seen	65,524	4%	2%	2%
Time from ER Arrival to Admit. (minutes)[2]	646	368	378	274
Time from ER Arrival to Discharge (minutes)	310	169	156	134
Time in ER Before Being Evaluated (minutes)	373	49	35	26
Time to Pain Meds for Fractures (minutes)	34	72	61	57
Heart Attack Care				
Aspirin Given at Discharge	30	100%	99%	99%
Fibrinolytic Meds Within 30 Min. of Arrival[7]	-	-	46%	54%
PCI Within 90 Minutes of Arrival[7]	-	-	95%	96%
Statin Prescribed at Discharge	29	100%	98%	98%
Heart Failure Care				
ACE Inhibitor or ARB for LVSD	47	96%	96%	97%
Discharge Instructions Given	116	87%	95%	94%
Evaluation of LVS Function	126	100%	99%	99%
Medicare Spending				
Medicare Spending per Patient (ratio)	-	0.91	0.96	0.98
Pneumonia Care				
Appropriate Initial Antibiotic Given	65	98%	95%	95%
Blood Culture Timing	112	96%	97%	98%
Pregnancy and Delivery Care				
Newborn Deliveries Scheduled Early[2]	15	7%	4%	6%
Preventive Care				
Immunization for Influenza[2]	511	68%	88%	90%
Immunization for Pneumonia[2]	457	77%	88%	92%
Stroke Care				
Anticoagulation Therapy for Atrial Fibrillation[1]	-	-	96%	95%
Antithrombotic Therapy Timing	23	96%	98%	98%
Assessed for Rehabilitation	26	96%	97%	97%
Discharged on Antithrombotic Therapy	24	100%	99%	99%
Discharged on Statin Medication	21	95%	95%	94%
Thrombolytic Therapy Timing[1]	-	-	69%	66%
Venous Thromboembolism Prophylaxis	27	96%	94%	94%
Written Stroke Educational Materials Given[1]	-	-	86%	88%
Surgical Care Improvement Project				
Appropriate Beta Blocker Usage[2]	29	90%	97%	98%
Appropriate VTP Within 24 Hours[2]	207	100%	98%	98%
Controlled Postoperative Blood Glucose[2,7]	-	-	97%	97%
Perioperative Temperature Management[2]	229	100%	100%	100%
Prophylactic Antibiotic Selection[2]	146	95%	99%	99%
Prophylactic Antibiotic Selection (Outpatient)	55	89%	97%	98%
Prophylactic Antibiotic Stopped[2]	141	94%	98%	98%
Prophylactic Antibiotic Timing[2]	154	83%	99%	99%
Prophylactic Antibiotic Timing (Outpatient)	20	55%	97%	98%
Urinary Catheter Removal[2]	128	100%	96%	97%
Survey of Patients' Hospital Experiences				
Area Around Room 'Always' Quiet at Night	300+	45%	51%	61%
Doctors 'Always' Communicated Well	300+	71%	77%	82%
Home Recovery Information Given	300+	76%	83%	85%
Hospital Given 9 or 10 on 10 Point Scale	300+	50%	63%	71%
Meds 'Always' Explained Before Given	300+	46%	59%	64%
Nurses 'Always' Communicated Well	300+	57%	75%	79%
Pain 'Always' Well Controlled	300+	53%	67%	71%
Room and Bathroom 'Always' Clean	300+	61%	69%	73%
Timely Help 'Always' Received	300+	41%	61%	68%
Would Definitely Recommend Hospital	300+	56%	65%	71%
Use of Medical Imaging				
Cardiac Imaging Stress Test before Surgery[1]	-	-	5.8%	5.3%
Combination Abdominal CT Scan[1]	-	-	8.2%	10.5%
Combination Brain/Sinus CT Scan[1]	-	-	3.6%	2.7%
Combination Chest CT Scan[1]	-	-	1.3%	2.7%
Follow-up Mammogram/Ultrasound[7]	-	-	13%	8.8%
Lumbar Spine MRI for Low Back Pain[1]	-	-	33.4%	37.2%

Mount Sinai Hospital

One Gustave L Levy Place
New York, NY 10029
URL: www.mountsinai.org
Type: Acute Care Hospitals
Ownership: Voluntary non-profit - Private
Phone: 212-241-7981
Fax: 212-987-1763
Emergency Services: Yes
Beds: 1,171

Key Personnel:
CEO/President. . . . . Kenneth L. Davis, MD
Radiology. . . . . Burton P Drayer, MD
Cardiac Laboratory. . . . . Valentin Fuster, MD, PhD
Quality Assurance . . . . Vivian Hammer
Emergency Room . . . . Andy S Jagoda, MD
Operating Room. . . . . Michael McCarry, RN, BS
Chief of Medical Staff. . . . . Ira S Nash, MD

Measure	Cases	This Hosp.	State Avg.	U.S. Avg.
Blood Clot Prevention and Treatment				
Anticoagulation Overlap Therapy[2]	319	92%	91%	93%
ICU Venous Thromboembolism Prophylaxis[2]	71	76%	92%	92%
Incidence of Potentially Preventable VTE[2]	142	8%	10%	10%
UFH with Dosages/Platelet Monitoring[2]	200	72%	92%	97%
Venous Thromboembolism Prophylaxis[2]	744	90%	87%	85%
Warfarin Therapy Discharge Instructions[2]	222	79%	59%	75%
Chest Pain/Possible Heart Attack Care				
Aspirin Given Within 24 Hours of Arrival	58	100%	97%	96%
Fibrinolytic Meds Within 30 Min. of Arrival[7]	-	-	54%	58%
Average Time to ECG (minutes)	58	12	9	7
Average Time to Transfer (minutes)	28	70	78	60
Children's Asthma Care				
Received Home Management Plan of Care	-	-	-	88%
Received Reliever Medication	-	-	-	100%
Received Systemic Corticosteroids	-	-	-	100%
Emergency Department				
Admittance Decision Time (minutes)[2]	1,417	325	154	98
Head CT Results Within 45 Min. of Arrival[1]	-	-	55%	57%
Patients Who Left ER Before Being Seen	>100k	4%	2%	2%
Time from ER Arrival to Admit. (minutes)[2]	1,418	568	378	274
Time from ER Arrival to Discharge (minutes)	707	193	156	134
Time in ER Before Being Evaluated (minutes)	933	49	35	26
Time to Pain Meds for Fractures (minutes)	153	67	61	57
Heart Attack Care				
Aspirin Given at Discharge[2]	320	98%	99%	99%
Fibrinolytic Meds Within 30 Min. of Arrival[2,7]	-	-	46%	54%
PCI Within 90 Minutes of Arrival[2]	16	81%	95%	96%
Statin Prescribed at Discharge[2]	325	99%	98%	98%
Heart Failure Care				
ACE Inhibitor or ARB for LVSD[2]	192	97%	96%	97%
Discharge Instructions Given[2]	473	90%	95%	94%
Evaluation of LVS Function[2]	552	98%	99%	99%
Medicare Spending				
Medicare Spending per Patient (ratio)	-	0.97	0.96	0.98
Pneumonia Care				
Appropriate Initial Antibiotic Given[2]	164	93%	95%	95%
Blood Culture Timing[2]	297	98%	97%	98%
Pregnancy and Delivery Care				
Newborn Deliveries Scheduled Early[2]	55	9%	4%	6%
Preventive Care				
Immunization for Influenza[2]	1,086	98%	88%	90%
Immunization for Pneumonia[2]	1,381	94%	88%	92%
Stroke Care				
Anticoagulation Therapy for Atrial Fibrillation	52	100%	96%	95%
Antithrombotic Therapy Timing	275	97%	98%	98%
Assessed for Rehabilitation	368	95%	97%	97%
Discharged on Antithrombotic Therapy	301	100%	99%	99%
Discharged on Statin Medication	223	98%	95%	94%
Thrombolytic Therapy Timing	21	90%	69%	66%
Venous Thromboembolism Prophylaxis	404	95%	94%	94%
Written Stroke Educational Materials Given	191	97%	86%	88%
Surgical Care Improvement Project				
Appropriate Beta Blocker Usage[2]	344	97%	97%	98%
Appropriate VTP Within 24 Hours[2]	748	99%	98%	98%
Controlled Postoperative Blood Glucose[2]	180	98%	97%	97%
Perioperative Temperature Management[2]	989	100%	100%	100%
Prophylactic Antibiotic Selection[2]	676	99%	99%	99%
Prophylactic Antibiotic Selection (Outpatient)	782	98%	97%	98%
Prophylactic Antibiotic Stopped[2]	658	98%	98%	98%
Prophylactic Antibiotic Timing[2]	675	99%	99%	99%
Prophylactic Antibiotic Timing (Outpatient)	765	97%	97%	98%
Urinary Catheter Removal[2]	501	97%	96%	97%
Survey of Patients' Hospital Experiences				
Area Around Room 'Always' Quiet at Night	300+	52%	51%	61%
Doctors 'Always' Communicated Well	300+	78%	77%	82%
Home Recovery Information Given	300+	84%	83%	85%
Hospital Given 9 or 10 on 10 Point Scale	300+	66%	63%	71%
Meds 'Always' Explained Before Given	300+	63%	59%	64%
Nurses 'Always' Communicated Well	300+	77%	75%	79%
Pain 'Always' Well Controlled	300+	70%	67%	71%
Room and Bathroom 'Always' Clean	300+	74%	69%	73%
Timely Help 'Always' Received	300+	64%	61%	68%
Would Definitely Recommend Hospital	300+	74%	65%	71%
Use of Medical Imaging				
Cardiac Imaging Stress Test before Surgery	1,193	8.4%	5.8%	5.3%
Combination Abdominal CT Scan	633	11.5%	8.2%	10.5%
Combination Brain/Sinus CT Scan	778	4.4%	3.6%	2.7%
Combination Chest CT Scan	193	7.8%	1.3%	2.7%
Follow-up Mammogram/Ultrasound	1,557	18.0%	13%	8.8%
Lumbar Spine MRI for Low Back Pain[1]	-	-	33.4%	37.2%

New York - Presbyterian Hospital

525 East 68th Street
New York, NY 10021
E-mail: publicaffairs@med.cornell.edu
URL: www.nyp.org
Type: Acute Care Hospitals
Ownership: Voluntary non-profit - Private
Phone: 212-746-4189
Fax: 212-821-0576
Emergency Services: Yes
Beds: 2,344

Key Personnel:
Patient Relations . . . . Andrea Colon
CEO . . . . Steven J. Corwin, MD
Operating Room. . . . . Robert L Jones, MD
Chief of Medical Staff. . . . . Richard S. Liebowitz, MD, MHS
Radiology. . . . . Lawrence Schwartz, MD
Pediatric In-Patient Care . . . . Lawrence Stanberry, MD
Quality Assurance . . . . Henry H. Ting, MD
Anesthesiology. . . . . Magaret Wood, MD

Measure	Cases	This Hosp.	State Avg.	U.S. Avg.
Blood Clot Prevention and Treatment				
Anticoagulation Overlap Therapy[2]	395	94%	91%	93%
ICU Venous Thromboembolism Prophylaxis[2]	63	100%	92%	92%
Incidence of Potentially Preventable VTE[2]	133	1%	10%	10%
UFH with Dosages/Platelet Monitoring[2]	365	99%	92%	97%
Venous Thromboembolism Prophylaxis[2]	357	95%	87%	85%
Warfarin Therapy Discharge Instructions[2]	274	74%	59%	75%
Chest Pain/Possible Heart Attack Care				
Aspirin Given Within 24 Hours of Arrival[1,3]	-	-	97%	96%
Fibrinolytic Meds Within 30 Min. of Arrival[3,7]	-	-	54%	58%

NOTE: Hospital profiles are in alphabetical order by state, then city, then hospital within the city; Rankings exclude hospitals with less than 25 cases except for patient surveys which excludes hospitals with less than 100 cases; (a) 100-299 cases; (1) The number of cases/patients is too few to report; (2) Data submitted were based on a sample of cases/patients; (3) Results are based on a shorter time period than required; (4) Data suppressed by CMS for one or more quarters; (5) Results are not available for this reporting period; (6) Fewer than 100 patients completed the HCAHPS survey; (7) No cases met the criteria for this measure; (8) The lower limit of the confidence interval cannot be calculated if the number of observed infections equals zero; (9) No data are available from the state/territory for this reporting period; (10) The scores shown reflect fewer than 50 completed surveys; (11) There were discrepancies in the data collection process; (12) This measure does not apply to this hospital for this reporting period; (13) Results cannot be calculated for this reporting period; (14) The results for this state are combined with nearby states to protect confidentiality; Please refer to the User's Guide for a full explanation of data.

Measure	Cases	This Hosp.	State Avg.	U.S. Avg.
Average Time to ECG (minutes)[1,3]	-	-	9	7
Average Time to Transfer (minutes)[1,3]	-	-	78	60
Children's Asthma Care				
Received Home Management Plan of Care	411	96%	-	88%
Received Reliever Medication	414	100%	-	100%
Received Systemic Corticosteroids	413	100%	-	100%
Emergency Department				
Admittance Decision Time (minutes)[2]	529	346	154	98
Head CT Results Within 45 Min. of Arrival	11	91%	55%	57%
Patients Who Left ER Before Being Seen	>100k	5%	2%	2%
Time from ER Arrival to Admit. (minutes)[2]	531	717	378	274
Time from ER Arrival to Discharge (minutes)	394	256	156	134
Time in ER Before Being Evaluated (minutes)	378	85	35	26
Time to Pain Meds for Fractures (minutes)	400	80	61	57
Heart Attack Care				
Aspirin Given at Discharge[2]	648	100%	99%	99%
Fibrinolytic Meds Within 30 Min. of Arrival[2,7]	-	-	46%	54%
PCI Within 90 Minutes of Arrival[2]	36	100%	95%	96%
Statin Prescribed at Discharge[2]	636	100%	98%	98%
Heart Failure Care				
ACE Inhibitor or ARB for LVSD[2]	323	99%	96%	97%
Discharge Instructions Given[2]	804	100%	95%	94%
Evaluation of LVS Function[2]	947	100%	99%	99%
Medicare Spending				
Medicare Spending per Patient (ratio)	-	0.95	0.96	0.98
Pneumonia Care				
Appropriate Initial Antibiotic Given[2]	221	97%	95%	95%
Blood Culture Timing[2]	535	97%	97%	98%
Pregnancy and Delivery Care				
Newborn Deliveries Scheduled Early[2]	56	0%	4%	6%
Preventive Care				
Immunization for Influenza[2]	564	99%	88%	90%
Immunization for Pneumonia[2]	562	94%	88%	92%
Stroke Care				
Anticoagulation Therapy for Atrial Fibrillation	97	100%	96%	95%
Antithrombotic Therapy Timing	547	97%	98%	98%
Assessed for Rehabilitation	968	98%	97%	97%
Discharged on Antithrombotic Therapy	706	100%	99%	99%
Discharged on Statin Medication	563	98%	95%	94%
Thrombolytic Therapy Timing	69	93%	69%	66%
Venous Thromboembolism Prophylaxis	937	97%	94%	94%
Written Stroke Educational Materials Given	551	95%	86%	88%
Surgical Care Improvement Project				
Appropriate Beta Blocker Usage[2]	516	98%	97%	98%
Appropriate VTP Within 24 Hours[2]	879	100%	98%	98%
Controlled Postoperative Blood Glucose[2]	335	96%	97%	97%
Perioperative Temperature Management[2]	1,137	100%	100%	100%
Prophylactic Antibiotic Selection[2]	975	99%	99%	99%
Prophylactic Antibiotic Selection (Outpatient)	1,200	97%	97%	98%
Prophylactic Antibiotic Stopped[2]	952	97%	98%	98%
Prophylactic Antibiotic Timing[2]	973	99%	99%	99%
Prophylactic Antibiotic Timing (Outpatient)	1,200	97%	97%	98%
Urinary Catheter Removal[2]	668	99%	96%	97%
Survey of Patients' Hospital Experiences				
Area Around Room 'Always' Quiet at Night	300+	53%	51%	61%
Doctors 'Always' Communicated Well	300+	81%	77%	82%
Home Recovery Information Given	300+	82%	83%	85%
Hospital Given 9 or 10 on 10 Point Scale	300+	74%	63%	71%
Meds 'Always' Explained Before Given	300+	60%	59%	64%
Nurses 'Always' Communicated Well	300+	76%	75%	79%
Pain 'Always' Well Controlled	300+	67%	67%	71%
Room and Bathroom 'Always' Clean	300+	66%	69%	73%
Timely Help 'Always' Received	300+	57%	61%	68%
Would Definitely Recommend Hospital	300+	79%	65%	71%
Use of Medical Imaging				
Cardiac Imaging Stress Test before Surgery	646	6.3%	5.8%	5.3%
Combination Abdominal CT Scan	2,257	18.3%	8.2%	10.5%
Combination Brain/Sinus CT Scan	1,722	2.5%	3.6%	2.7%
Combination Chest CT Scan	2,375	1.5%	1.3%	2.7%
Follow-up Mammogram/Ultrasound	2,308	6.8%	13%	8.8%
Lumbar Spine MRI for Low Back Pain	132	33.3%	33.4%	37.2%

New York Eye & Ear Infirmary

310 East 14th Street
New York, NY 10003
URL: www.nyee.edu
Type: Acute Care Hospitals
Ownership: Voluntary non-profit - Private
Phone: 212-979-4000
Fax: 212-228-0664
Emergency Services: No
Beds: 103

Key Personnel:
Anesthesiology. . . . . Robert Durell, MD
President . . . . Allan Fine
Radiology. . . . . Roy Holliday, MD
Quality Assurance . . . . Linda Klingos, RN
Infection Control. . . . . Mercy Nelson, RN
Ambulatory Care . . . . Ann Marie Palladino
Operating Room. . . . . Nitin Sheth, RN

Measure	Cases	This Hosp.	State Avg.	U.S. Avg.
Blood Clot Prevention and Treatment				
Anticoagulation Overlap Therapy[7]	-	-	91%	93%
ICU Venous Thromboembolism Prophylaxis[7]	-	-	92%	92%
Incidence of Potentially Preventable VTE[7]	-	-	10%	10%
UFH with Dosages/Platelet Monitoring[7]	-	-	92%	97%
Venous Thromboembolism Prophylaxis	143	19%	87%	85%
Warfarin Therapy Discharge Instructions[7]	-	-	59%	75%
Chest Pain/Possible Heart Attack Care				
Aspirin Given Within 24 Hours of Arrival[5]	-	-	97%	96%
Fibrinolytic Meds Within 30 Min. of Arrival[5]	-	-	54%	58%
Average Time to ECG (minutes)[5]	-	-	9	7
Average Time to Transfer (minutes)[5]	-	-	78	60
Children's Asthma Care				
Received Home Management Plan of Care	-	-	-	88%
Received Reliever Medication	-	-	-	100%
Received Systemic Corticosteroids	-	-	-	100%
Emergency Department				
Admittance Decision Time (minutes)[7]	-	-	154	98
Head CT Results Within 45 Min. of Arrival[5]	-	-	55%	57%
Patients Who Left ER Before Being Seen[5]	-	-	2%	2%
Time from ER Arrival to Admit. (minutes)[7]	-	-	378	274
Time from ER Arrival to Discharge (minutes)[5]	-	-	156	134
Time in ER Before Being Evaluated (minutes)[5]	-	-	35	26
Time to Pain Meds for Fractures (minutes)[5]	-	-	61	57
Heart Attack Care				
Aspirin Given at Discharge[5]	-	-	99%	99%
Fibrinolytic Meds Within 30 Min. of Arrival[5]	-	-	46%	54%
PCI Within 90 Minutes of Arrival[5]	-	-	95%	96%
Statin Prescribed at Discharge[5]	-	-	98%	98%
Heart Failure Care				
ACE Inhibitor or ARB for LVSD[5]	-	-	96%	97%
Discharge Instructions Given[5]	-	-	95%	94%
Evaluation of LVS Function[5]	-	-	99%	99%
Medicare Spending				
Medicare Spending per Patient (ratio)	-	0.94	0.96	0.98
Pneumonia Care				
Appropriate Initial Antibiotic Given[5]	-	-	95%	95%
Blood Culture Timing[5]	-	-	97%	98%
Pregnancy and Delivery Care				
Newborn Deliveries Scheduled Early[7]	-	-	4%	6%
Preventive Care				
Immunization for Influenza[2]	271	16%	88%	90%
Immunization for Pneumonia[2]	182	22%	88%	92%
Stroke Care				
Anticoagulation Therapy for Atrial Fibrillation[5]	-	-	96%	95%
Antithrombotic Therapy Timing[5]	-	-	98%	98%
Assessed for Rehabilitation[5]	-	-	97%	97%
Discharged on Antithrombotic Therapy[5]	-	-	99%	99%
Discharged on Statin Medication[5]	-	-	95%	94%
Thrombolytic Therapy Timing[5]	-	-	69%	66%
Venous Thromboembolism Prophylaxis[5]	-	-	94%	94%
Written Stroke Educational Materials Given[5]	-	-	86%	88%
Surgical Care Improvement Project				
Appropriate Beta Blocker Usage[5]	-	-	97%	98%
Appropriate VTP Within 24 Hours[5]	-	-	98%	98%
Controlled Postoperative Blood Glucose[5]	-	-	97%	97%
Perioperative Temperature Management[5]	-	-	100%	100%
Prophylactic Antibiotic Selection[5]	-	-	99%	99%
Prophylactic Antibiotic Selection (Outpatient)[5]	-	-	97%	98%
Prophylactic Antibiotic Stopped[5]	-	-	98%	98%
Prophylactic Antibiotic Timing[5]	-	-	99%	99%
Prophylactic Antibiotic Timing (Outpatient)[5]	-	-	97%	98%
Urinary Catheter Removal[5]	-	-	96%	97%
Survey of Patients' Hospital Experiences				
Area Around Room 'Always' Quiet at Night	(a)	68%	51%	61%
Doctors 'Always' Communicated Well	(a)	82%	77%	82%
Home Recovery Information Given	(a)	82%	83%	85%
Hospital Given 9 or 10 on 10 Point Scale	(a)	71%	63%	71%
Meds 'Always' Explained Before Given	(a)	56%	59%	64%
Nurses 'Always' Communicated Well	(a)	80%	75%	79%
Pain 'Always' Well Controlled	(a)	68%	67%	71%
Room and Bathroom 'Always' Clean	(a)	75%	69%	73%
Timely Help 'Always' Received	(a)	74%	61%	68%
Would Definitely Recommend Hospital	(a)	75%	65%	71%
Use of Medical Imaging				
Cardiac Imaging Stress Test before Surgery[7]	-	-	5.8%	5.3%
Combination Abdominal CT Scan[1]	-	-	8.2%	10.5%
Combination Brain/Sinus CT Scan[1]	-	-	3.6%	2.7%
Combination Chest CT Scan[1]	-	-	1.3%	2.7%
Follow-up Mammogram/Ultrasound[7]	-	-	13%	8.8%
Lumbar Spine MRI for Low Back Pain[7]	-	-	33.4%	37.2%

NYU Hospitals Center

550 First Avenue
New York, NY 10016
URL: www.med.nyu.edu
Type: Acute Care Hospitals
Ownership: Voluntary non-profit - Private
Phone: 212-263-7300
Fax: 212-263-6690
Emergency Services: Yes
Beds: 1,069

Key Personnel:
Quality Assurance . . . . John Bittoni
CEO/President. . . . . Robert I Grossman, MD
Chief of Medical Staff . . . . Andrew W Litt, MD
Operating Room. . . . . H Leon Patcher, RN
Radiology. . . . . Michael Recht, MD
Anesthesiology. . . . . Andrew D. Rosenberg, MD
Pediatric In-Patient Care . . . . . . Catherin Scott Manno, MD
Infection Control. . . . . Roger Wetherbee, MD

Measure	Cases	This Hosp.	State Avg.	U.S. Avg.
Blood Clot Prevention and Treatment				
Anticoagulation Overlap Therapy[2]	94	100%	91%	93%
ICU Venous Thromboembolism Prophylaxis[2]	53	100%	92%	92%
Incidence of Potentially Preventable VTE[2]	47	6%	10%	10%
UFH with Dosages/Platelet Monitoring[2]	83	100%	92%	97%
Venous Thromboembolism Prophylaxis[2]	305	97%	87%	85%
Warfarin Therapy Discharge Instructions[2]	67	99%	59%	75%
Chest Pain/Possible Heart Attack Care				
Aspirin Given Within 24 Hours of Arrival[5]	-	-	97%	96%
Fibrinolytic Meds Within 30 Min. of Arrival[5]	-	-	54%	58%
Average Time to ECG (minutes)[5]	-	-	9	7
Average Time to Transfer (minutes)[5]	-	-	78	60
Children's Asthma Care				
Received Home Management Plan of Care	18	94%	-	88%
Received Reliever Medication	18	100%	-	100%
Received Systemic Corticosteroids	18	100%	-	100%
Emergency Department				
Admittance Decision Time (minutes)[2]	228	128	154	98
Head CT Results Within 45 Min. of Arrival[5]	-	-	55%	57%
Patients Who Left ER Before Being Seen	41,546	1%	2%	2%
Time from ER Arrival to Admit. (minutes)[2]	237	355	378	274
Time from ER Arrival to Discharge (minutes)[3]	120	174	156	134
Time in ER Before Being Evaluated (minutes)[3]	116	51	35	26
Time to Pain Meds for Fractures (minutes)[1,3]	-	-	61	57
Heart Attack Care				
Aspirin Given at Discharge	179	100%	99%	99%
Fibrinolytic Meds Within 30 Min. of Arrival[7]	-	-	46%	54%
PCI Within 90 Minutes of Arrival	16	94%	95%	96%
Statin Prescribed at Discharge	180	100%	98%	98%
Heart Failure Care				
ACE Inhibitor or ARB for LVSD[2]	70	100%	96%	97%
Discharge Instructions Given[2]	220	100%	95%	94%
Evaluation of LVS Function[2]	282	100%	99%	99%
Medicare Spending				
Medicare Spending per Patient (ratio)	-	1.03	0.96	0.98

NOTE: Hospital profiles are in alphabetical order by state, then city, then hospital within the city; Rankings exclude hospitals with less than 25 cases except for patient surveys which excludes hospitals with less than 100 cases; (a) 100-299 cases; (1) The number of cases/patients is too few to report; (2) Data submitted were based on a sample of cases/patients; (3) Results are based on a shorter time period than required; (4) Data suppressed by CMS for one or more quarters; (5) Results are not available for this reporting period; (6) Fewer than 100 patients completed the HCAHPS survey; (7) No cases met the criteria for this measure; (8) The lower limit of the confidence interval cannot be calculated if the number of observed infections equals zero; (9) No data are available from the state/territory for this reporting period; (10) The scores shown reflect fewer than 50 completed surveys; (11) There were discrepancies in the data collection process; (12) This measure does not apply to this hospital for this reporting period; (13) Results cannot be calculated for this reporting period; (14) The results for this state are combined with nearby states to protect confidentiality; Please refer to the User's Guide for a full explanation of data.

Measure	Cases	This Hosp.	State Avg.	U.S. Avg.
Pneumonia Care				
Appropriate Initial Antibiotic Given[2]	57	100%	95%	95%
Blood Culture Timing[2]	145	98%	97%	98%
Pregnancy and Delivery Care				
Newborn Deliveries Scheduled Early[2]	64	2%	4%	6%
Preventive Care				
Immunization for Influenza[2]	578	75%	88%	90%
Immunization for Pneumonia[2]	550	74%	88%	92%
Stroke Care				
Anticoagulation Therapy for Atrial Fibrillation	15	100%	96%	95%
Antithrombotic Therapy Timing	72	99%	98%	98%
Assessed for Rehabilitation	117	99%	97%	97%
Discharged on Antithrombotic Therapy	90	100%	99%	99%
Discharged on Statin Medication	73	99%	95%	94%
Thrombolytic Therapy Timing[1]	-	-	69%	66%
Venous Thromboembolism Prophylaxis	100	100%	94%	94%
Written Stroke Educational Materials Given	76	95%	86%	88%
Surgical Care Improvement Project				
Appropriate Beta Blocker Usage[2]	191	99%	97%	98%
Appropriate VTP Within 24 Hours[2]	492	100%	98%	98%
Controlled Postoperative Blood Glucose[2]	129	99%	97%	97%
Perioperative Temperature Management[2]	579	100%	100%	100%
Prophylactic Antibiotic Selection[2]	473	99%	99%	99%
Prophylactic Antibiotic Selection (Outpatient)	734	100%	97%	98%
Prophylactic Antibiotic Stopped[2]	459	99%	98%	98%
Prophylactic Antibiotic Timing[2]	472	99%	99%	99%
Prophylactic Antibiotic Timing (Outpatient)	734	99%	97%	98%
Urinary Catheter Removal[2]	253	100%	96%	97%
Survey of Patients' Hospital Experiences				
Area Around Room 'Always' Quiet at Night	300+	47%	51%	61%
Doctors 'Always' Communicated Well	300+	79%	77%	82%
Home Recovery Information Given	300+	83%	83%	85%
Hospital Given 9 or 10 on 10 Point Scale	300+	71%	63%	71%
Meds 'Always' Explained Before Given	300+	63%	59%	64%
Nurses 'Always' Communicated Well	300+	79%	75%	79%
Pain 'Always' Well Controlled	300+	68%	67%	71%
Room and Bathroom 'Always' Clean	300+	70%	69%	73%
Timely Help 'Always' Received	300+	64%	61%	68%
Would Definitely Recommend Hospital	300+	78%	65%	71%
Use of Medical Imaging				
Cardiac Imaging Stress Test before Surgery	1,343	8.3%	5.8%	5.3%
Combination Abdominal CT Scan	515	9.7%	8.2%	10.5%
Combination Brain/Sinus CT Scan	503	4.0%	3.6%	2.7%
Combination Chest CT Scan	704	0.3%	1.3%	2.7%
Follow-up Mammogram/Ultrasound	1,860	16.1%	13%	8.8%
Lumbar Spine MRI for Low Back Pain	297	23.6%	33.4%	37.2%

Saint Luke's Roosevelt Hospital

1111 Amsterdam Avenue — Phone: 212-523-4000
New York, NY 10025 — Fax: 212-523-2617
URL: www.wehealny.org
Type: Acute Care Hospitals — Emergency Services: Yes
Ownership: Voluntary non-profit - Private — Beds: 1,354

Key Personnel:
Chief of Medical Staff.......... Robert Catalano
Quality Assurance .... Timothy Day
President .... Arthur A. Gianelli, MBA, MPH
Emergency Room .... Richard G Lanoix, MD
Infection Control.............. Bruce Polsky, MD
Anesthesiology............... Alan C. Santos, MD, MPH
Operating Room.............. George J Todd, MD/FACS
Surgery .... George J. Todd, MD, FACS

Measure	Cases	This Hosp.	State Avg.	U.S. Avg.
Blood Clot Prevention and Treatment				
Anticoagulation Overlap Therapy[2]	218	87%	91%	93%
ICU Venous Thromboembolism Prophylaxis[2]	38	100%	92%	92%
Incidence of Potentially Preventable VTE[2]	62	3%	10%	10%
UFH with Dosages/Platelet Monitoring[2]	82	100%	92%	97%
Venous Thromboembolism Prophylaxis[2]	311	82%	87%	85%
Warfarin Therapy Discharge Instructions[2]	151	25%	59%	75%
Chest Pain/Possible Heart Attack Care				
Aspirin Given Within 24 Hours of Arrival[5]	-	-	97%	96%
Fibrinolytic Meds Within 30 Min. of Arrival[5]	-	-	54%	58%
Average Time to ECG (minutes)[5]	-	-	9	7
Average Time to Transfer (minutes)[5]	-	-	78	60
Children's Asthma Care				
Received Home Management Plan of Care	-	-	-	88%
Received Reliever Medication	-	-	-	100%
Received Systemic Corticosteroids	-	-	-	100%
Emergency Department				
Admittance Decision Time (minutes)[2]	524	250	154	98
Head CT Results Within 45 Min. of Arrival[3,7]	-	-	55%	57%
Patients Who Left ER Before Being Seen	>100k	1%	2%	2%
Time from ER Arrival to Admit. (minutes)[2]	524	490	378	274
Time from ER Arrival to Discharge (minutes)	400	141	156	134
Time in ER Before Being Evaluated (minutes)	436	26	35	26
Time to Pain Meds for Fractures (minutes)	389	48	61	57
Heart Attack Care				
Aspirin Given at Discharge[2]	282	100%	99%	99%
Fibrinolytic Meds Within 30 Min. of Arrival[2,7]	-	-	46%	54%
PCI Within 90 Minutes of Arrival[2]	28	96%	95%	96%
Statin Prescribed at Discharge[2]	285	99%	98%	98%
Heart Failure Care				
ACE Inhibitor or ARB for LVSD[2]	144	95%	96%	97%
Discharge Instructions Given[2]	276	100%	95%	94%
Evaluation of LVS Function[2]	312	99%	99%	99%
Medicare Spending				
Medicare Spending per Patient (ratio)	-	0.98	0.96	0.98
Pneumonia Care				
Appropriate Initial Antibiotic Given[2]	90	99%	95%	95%
Blood Culture Timing[2]	190	98%	97%	98%
Pregnancy and Delivery Care				
Newborn Deliveries Scheduled Early[2]	55	5%	4%	6%
Preventive Care				
Immunization for Influenza[2]	521	90%	88%	90%
Immunization for Pneumonia[2]	589	87%	88%	92%
Stroke Care				
Anticoagulation Therapy for Atrial Fibrillation[2]	13	92%	96%	95%
Antithrombotic Therapy Timing[2]	92	99%	98%	98%
Assessed for Rehabilitation[2]	127	94%	97%	97%
Discharged on Antithrombotic Therapy[2]	101	98%	99%	99%
Discharged on Statin Medication[2]	78	100%	95%	94%
Thrombolytic Therapy Timing[2]	16	56%	69%	66%
Venous Thromboembolism Prophylaxis[2]	135	95%	94%	94%
Written Stroke Educational Materials Given[2]	68	76%	86%	88%
Surgical Care Improvement Project				
Appropriate Beta Blocker Usage[2]	208	98%	97%	98%
Appropriate VTP Within 24 Hours[2]	493	98%	98%	98%
Controlled Postoperative Blood Glucose[2]	124	98%	97%	97%
Perioperative Temperature Management[2]	623	100%	100%	100%
Prophylactic Antibiotic Selection[2]	567	100%	99%	99%
Prophylactic Antibiotic Selection (Outpatient)	345	96%	97%	98%
Prophylactic Antibiotic Stopped[2]	557	98%	98%	98%
Prophylactic Antibiotic Timing[2]	568	100%	99%	99%
Prophylactic Antibiotic Timing (Outpatient)	343	99%	97%	98%
Urinary Catheter Removal[2]	419	97%	96%	97%
Survey of Patients' Hospital Experiences				
Area Around Room 'Always' Quiet at Night	300+	52%	51%	61%
Doctors 'Always' Communicated Well	300+	71%	77%	82%
Home Recovery Information Given	300+	78%	83%	85%
Hospital Given 9 or 10 on 10 Point Scale	300+	53%	63%	71%
Meds 'Always' Explained Before Given	300+	51%	59%	64%
Nurses 'Always' Communicated Well	300+	65%	75%	79%
Pain 'Always' Well Controlled	300+	60%	67%	71%
Room and Bathroom 'Always' Clean	300+	63%	69%	73%
Timely Help 'Always' Received	300+	45%	61%	68%
Would Definitely Recommend Hospital	300+	59%	65%	71%
Use of Medical Imaging				
Cardiac Imaging Stress Test before Surgery	160	3.8%	5.8%	5.3%
Combination Abdominal CT Scan	626	7.7%	8.2%	10.5%
Combination Brain/Sinus CT Scan[1]	-	-	3.6%	2.7%
Combination Chest CT Scan	298	0.7%	1.3%	2.7%
Follow-up Mammogram/Ultrasound	190	17.9%	13%	8.8%
Lumbar Spine MRI for Low Back Pain[1]	-	-	33.4%	37.2%

VA New York Harbor Healthcare System

423 East 23rd Street — Phone: 212-686-7500
New York, NY 10010 — Fax: 212-951-3375
URL: www.nyharbor.va.gov
Type: Acute Care - VA — Emergency Services: No
Ownership: Government Federal — Beds: 350

Key Personnel:
Anesthesiology.............. Patrick Annello, MD
Radiology.................. Norma Ettenger, MD
Quality Assurance .... May Mayor, RN
Intensive Care Unit........... Elvira Miller
Operating Room............. Doris Richardson, RN
Chief of Medical Staff.......... Michael Simberkoff
Infection Control............. Michael Simberkoff, MD

Measure	Cases	This Hosp.	State Avg.	U.S. Avg.
Blood Clot Prevention and Treatment				
Anticoagulation Overlap Therapy	-	-	91%	93%
ICU Venous Thromboembolism Prophylaxis	-	-	92%	92%
Incidence of Potentially Preventable VTE	-	-	10%	10%
UFH with Dosages/Platelet Monitoring	-	-	92%	97%
Venous Thromboembolism Prophylaxis	-	-	87%	85%
Warfarin Therapy Discharge Instructions	-	-	59%	75%
Chest Pain/Possible Heart Attack Care				
Aspirin Given Within 24 Hours of Arrival	-	-	97%	96%
Fibrinolytic Meds Within 30 Min. of Arrival	-	-	54%	58%
Average Time to ECG (minutes)	-	-	9	7
Average Time to Transfer (minutes)	-	-	78	60
Children's Asthma Care				
Received Home Management Plan of Care	-	-	-	88%
Received Reliever Medication	-	-	-	100%
Received Systemic Corticosteroids	-	-	-	100%
Emergency Department				
Admittance Decision Time (minutes)	-	-	154	98
Head CT Results Within 45 Min. of Arrival	-	-	55%	57%
Patients Who Left ER Before Being Seen	-	-	2%	2%
Time from ER Arrival to Admit. (minutes)	-	-	378	274
Time from ER Arrival to Discharge (minutes)	-	-	156	134
Time in ER Before Being Evaluated (minutes)	-	-	35	26
Time to Pain Meds for Fractures (minutes)	-	-	61	57
Heart Attack Care				
Aspirin Given at Discharge	77	100%	99%	99%
Fibrinolytic Meds Within 30 Min. of Arrival[1]	-	-	46%	54%
PCI Within 90 Minutes of Arrival[1]	-	-	95%	96%
Statin Prescribed at Discharge	79	96%	98%	98%
Heart Failure Care				
ACE Inhibitor or ARB for LVSD	105	95%	96%	97%
Discharge Instructions Given	227	97%	95%	94%
Evaluation of LVS Function	236	100%	99%	99%
Medicare Spending				
Medicare Spending per Patient (ratio)	-	-	0.96	0.98
Pneumonia Care				
Appropriate Initial Antibiotic Given	61	100%	95%	95%
Blood Culture Timing	138	99%	97%	98%
Pregnancy and Delivery Care				
Newborn Deliveries Scheduled Early	-	-	4%	6%
Preventive Care				
Immunization for Influenza[5]	-	-	88%	90%
Immunization for Pneumonia[5]	-	-	88%	92%
Stroke Care				
Anticoagulation Therapy for Atrial Fibrillation	-	-	96%	95%
Antithrombotic Therapy Timing	-	-	98%	98%
Assessed for Rehabilitation	-	-	97%	97%
Discharged on Antithrombotic Therapy	-	-	99%	99%
Discharged on Statin Medication	-	-	95%	94%
Thrombolytic Therapy Timing	-	-	69%	66%
Venous Thromboembolism Prophylaxis	-	-	94%	94%
Written Stroke Educational Materials Given	-	-	86%	88%
Surgical Care Improvement Project				
Appropriate Beta Blocker Usage[2]	63	81%	97%	98%
Appropriate VTP Within 24 Hours[2]	136	99%	98%	98%
Controlled Postoperative Blood Glucose[2]	44	86%	97%	97%
Perioperative Temperature Management[2]	171	100%	100%	100%
Prophylactic Antibiotic Selection	92	97%	99%	99%
Prophylactic Antibiotic Selection (Outpatient)	-	-	97%	98%

NOTE: Hospital profiles are in alphabetical order by state, then city, then hospital within the city; Rankings exclude hospitals with less than 25 cases except for patient surveys which excludes hospitals with less than 100 cases; (a) 100-299 cases; (1) The number of cases/patients is too few to report; (2) Data submitted were based on a sample of cases/patients; (3) Results are based on a shorter time period than required; (4) Data suppressed by CMS for one or more quarters; (5) Results are not available for this reporting period; (6) Fewer than 100 patients completed the HCAHPS survey; (7) No cases met the criteria for this measure; (8) The lower limit of the confidence interval cannot be calculated if the number of observed infections equals zero; (9) No data are available from the state/territory for this reporting period; (10) The scores shown reflect fewer than 50 completed surveys; (11) There were discrepancies in the data collection process; (12) This measure does not apply to this hospital for this reporting period; (13) Results cannot be calculated for this reporting period; (14) The results for this state are combined with nearby states to protect confidentiality; Please refer to the User's Guide for a full explanation of data.

Measure	Cases	This Hosp.	State Avg.	U.S. Avg.
Prophylactic Antibiotic Stopped	90	99%	98%	98%
Prophylactic Antibiotic Timing	93	92%	99%	99%
Prophylactic Antibiotic Timing (Outpatient)	-	-	97%	98%
Urinary Catheter Removal[2]	110	92%	96%	97%
Survey of Patients' Hospital Experiences				
Area Around Room 'Always' Quiet at Night	-	-	51%	61%
Doctors 'Always' Communicated Well	-	-	77%	82%
Home Recovery Information Given	-	-	83%	85%
Hospital Given 9 or 10 on 10 Point Scale	-	-	63%	71%
Meds 'Always' Explained Before Given	-	-	59%	64%
Nurses 'Always' Communicated Well	-	-	75%	79%
Pain 'Always' Well Controlled	-	-	67%	71%
Room and Bathroom 'Always' Clean	-	-	69%	73%
Timely Help 'Always' Received	-	-	61%	68%
Would Definitely Recommend Hospital	-	-	65%	71%
Use of Medical Imaging				
Cardiac Imaging Stress Test before Surgery	-	-	5.8%	5.3%
Combination Abdominal CT Scan	-	-	8.2%	10.5%
Combination Brain/Sinus CT Scan	-	-	3.6%	2.7%
Combination Chest CT Scan	-	-	1.3%	2.7%
Follow-up Mammogram/Ultrasound	-	-	13%	8.8%
Lumbar Spine MRI for Low Back Pain	-	-	33.4%	37.2%

Newark - Wayne Community Hospital

111 Driving Park Avenue Phone: 315-332-2022
Newark, NY 14513
URL: www.viahealth.org/home_newarkwayne.cfm
Type: Acute Care Hospitals Emergency Services: Yes
Ownership: Voluntary non-profit - Private

Key Personnel:
Emergency Room .... Frank Edwards
CEO/President............... Annette Leahy
Chief of Medical Staff.......... Arun Nagpaul, MD

Measure	Cases	This Hosp.	State Avg.	U.S. Avg.
Blood Clot Prevention and Treatment				
Anticoagulation Overlap Therapy[2]	28	89%	91%	93%
ICU Venous Thromboembolism Prophylaxis[2]	42	98%	92%	92%
Incidence of Potentially Preventable VTE[1,2]	-	-	10%	10%
UFH with Dosages/Platelet Monitoring[1,2]	-	-	92%	97%
Venous Thromboembolism Prophylaxis[2]	292	94%	87%	85%
Warfarin Therapy Discharge Instructions[2]	19	63%	59%	75%
Chest Pain/Possible Heart Attack Care				
Aspirin Given Within 24 Hours of Arrival[3]	46	96%	97%	96%
Fibrinolytic Meds Within 30 Min. of Arrival[1,3]	-	-	54%	58%
Average Time to ECG (minutes)[3]	52	14	9	7
Average Time to Transfer (minutes)[1,3]	-	-	78	60
Children's Asthma Care				
Received Home Management Plan of Care	-	-	-	88%
Received Reliever Medication	-	-	-	100%
Received Systemic Corticosteroids	-	-	-	100%
Emergency Department				
Admittance Decision Time (minutes)[2]	383	68	154	98
Head CT Results Within 45 Min. of Arrival[5]	-	-	55%	57%
Patients Who Left ER Before Being Seen	23,624	1%	2%	2%
Time from ER Arrival to Admit. (minutes)[2]	385	248	378	274
Time from ER Arrival to Discharge (minutes)	346	146	156	134
Time in ER Before Being Evaluated (minutes)	405	18	35	26
Time to Pain Meds for Fractures (minutes)	70	50	61	57
Heart Attack Care				
Aspirin Given at Discharge	18	100%	99%	99%
Fibrinolytic Meds Within 30 Min. of Arrival[7]	-	-	46%	54%
PCI Within 90 Minutes of Arrival[7]	-	-	95%	96%
Statin Prescribed at Discharge	15	93%	98%	98%
Heart Failure Care				
ACE Inhibitor or ARB for LVSD	22	86%	96%	97%
Discharge Instructions Given	105	94%	95%	94%
Evaluation of LVS Function	140	99%	99%	99%
Medicare Spending				
Medicare Spending per Patient (ratio)	-	0.89	0.96	0.98
Pneumonia Care				
Appropriate Initial Antibiotic Given	71	94%	95%	95%
Blood Culture Timing	144	100%	97%	98%
Pregnancy and Delivery Care				
Newborn Deliveries Scheduled Early[2]	34	3%	4%	6%
Preventive Care				
Immunization for Influenza[2]	386	87%	88%	90%
Immunization for Pneumonia[2]	538	86%	88%	92%
Stroke Care				
Anticoagulation Therapy for Atrial Fibrillation[1]	-	-	96%	95%
Antithrombotic Therapy Timing	33	100%	98%	98%
Assessed for Rehabilitation	45	91%	97%	97%
Discharged on Antithrombotic Therapy	41	100%	99%	99%
Discharged on Statin Medication	32	94%	95%	94%
Thrombolytic Therapy Timing[1]	-	-	69%	66%
Venous Thromboembolism Prophylaxis	43	84%	94%	94%
Written Stroke Educational Materials Given	26	69%	86%	88%
Surgical Care Improvement Project				
Appropriate Beta Blocker Usage	94	96%	97%	98%
Appropriate VTP Within 24 Hours	237	99%	98%	98%
Controlled Postoperative Blood Glucose[7]	-	-	97%	97%
Perioperative Temperature Management	273	99%	100%	100%
Prophylactic Antibiotic Selection	171	99%	99%	99%
Prophylactic Antibiotic Selection (Outpatient)	102	98%	97%	98%
Prophylactic Antibiotic Stopped	164	96%	98%	98%
Prophylactic Antibiotic Timing	171	95%	99%	99%
Prophylactic Antibiotic Timing (Outpatient)	104	96%	97%	98%
Urinary Catheter Removal	207	95%	96%	97%
Survey of Patients' Hospital Experiences				
Area Around Room 'Always' Quiet at Night	300+	48%	51%	61%
Doctors 'Always' Communicated Well	300+	80%	77%	82%
Home Recovery Information Given	300+	89%	83%	85%
Hospital Given 9 or 10 on 10 Point Scale	300+	64%	63%	71%
Meds 'Always' Explained Before Given	300+	66%	59%	64%
Nurses 'Always' Communicated Well	300+	81%	75%	79%
Pain 'Always' Well Controlled	300+	68%	67%	71%
Room and Bathroom 'Always' Clean	300+	75%	69%	73%
Timely Help 'Always' Received	300+	64%	61%	68%
Would Definitely Recommend Hospital	300+	66%	65%	71%
Use of Medical Imaging				
Cardiac Imaging Stress Test before Surgery[1]	-	-	5.8%	5.3%
Combination Abdominal CT Scan	293	29.0%	8.2%	10.5%
Combination Brain/Sinus CT Scan[1]	-	-	3.6%	2.7%
Combination Chest CT Scan	181	5.0%	1.3%	2.7%
Follow-up Mammogram/Ultrasound	221	2.3%	13%	8.8%
Lumbar Spine MRI for Low Back Pain[1]	-	-	33.4%	37.2%

Saint Luke's Cornwall Hospital

70 Dubois Street Phone: 845-561-4400
Newburgh, NY 12550 Fax: 845-568-2902
URL: www.stlukeshospital.org
Type: Acute Care Hospitals Emergency Services: Yes
Ownership: Voluntary non-profit - Other Beds: 259

Key Personnel:
Radiology.................. Clifford Barker, MD
Quality Assurance .... Mary Kelley
Patient Relations .... Renita McGuiness
CEO/President.............. Robert S. Ross
Hemotology Center .... Kathy Sellick
Pediatric In-Patient Care .... Kathy Sellick
Cardiac Laboratory........... Nirav D Shah, MD
Operating Room............. Jackie Veerboom

Measure	Cases	This Hosp.	State Avg.	U.S. Avg.
Blood Clot Prevention and Treatment				
Anticoagulation Overlap Therapy[2]	75	97%	91%	93%
ICU Venous Thromboembolism Prophylaxis[2]	61	98%	92%	92%
Incidence of Potentially Preventable VTE[2]	17	6%	10%	10%
UFH with Dosages/Platelet Monitoring[2]	40	100%	92%	97%
Venous Thromboembolism Prophylaxis[2]	363	95%	87%	85%
Warfarin Therapy Discharge Instructions[2]	52	98%	59%	75%
Chest Pain/Possible Heart Attack Care				
Aspirin Given Within 24 Hours of Arrival	19	100%	97%	96%
Fibrinolytic Meds Within 30 Min. of Arrival[3,7]	-	-	54%	58%
Average Time to ECG (minutes)	20	4	9	7
Average Time to Transfer (minutes)[3,7]	-	-	78	60
Children's Asthma Care				
Received Home Management Plan of Care	-	-	-	88%
Received Reliever Medication	-	-	-	100%
Received Systemic Corticosteroids	-	-	-	100%
Emergency Department				
Admittance Decision Time (minutes)[2]	694	149	154	98
Head CT Results Within 45 Min. of Arrival[1]	-	-	55%	57%
Patients Who Left ER Before Being Seen	60,730	1%	2%	2%
Time from ER Arrival to Admit. (minutes)[2]	729	352	378	274
Time from ER Arrival to Discharge (minutes)	361	126	156	134
Time in ER Before Being Evaluated (minutes)	361	21	35	26
Time to Pain Meds for Fractures (minutes)	165	46	61	57
Heart Attack Care				
Aspirin Given at Discharge	212	100%	99%	99%
Fibrinolytic Meds Within 30 Min. of Arrival[7]	-	-	46%	54%
PCI Within 90 Minutes of Arrival	35	100%	95%	96%
Statin Prescribed at Discharge	204	100%	98%	98%
Heart Failure Care				
ACE Inhibitor or ARB for LVSD	91	100%	96%	97%
Discharge Instructions Given	279	94%	95%	94%
Evaluation of LVS Function	370	100%	99%	99%
Medicare Spending				
Medicare Spending per Patient (ratio)	-	0.97	0.96	0.98
Pneumonia Care				
Appropriate Initial Antibiotic Given	183	97%	95%	95%
Blood Culture Timing	313	99%	97%	98%
Pregnancy and Delivery Care				
Newborn Deliveries Scheduled Early	109	12%	4%	6%
Preventive Care				
Immunization for Influenza[2]	556	89%	88%	90%
Immunization for Pneumonia[2]	666	91%	88%	92%
Stroke Care				
Anticoagulation Therapy for Atrial Fibrillation	17	100%	96%	95%
Antithrombotic Therapy Timing	87	99%	98%	98%
Assessed for Rehabilitation	101	100%	97%	97%
Discharged on Antithrombotic Therapy	91	100%	99%	99%
Discharged on Statin Medication	76	95%	95%	94%
Thrombolytic Therapy Timing[1]	-	-	69%	66%
Venous Thromboembolism Prophylaxis	103	99%	94%	94%
Written Stroke Educational Materials Given	49	98%	86%	88%
Surgical Care Improvement Project				
Appropriate Beta Blocker Usage[2]	169	98%	97%	98%
Appropriate VTP Within 24 Hours[2]	457	97%	98%	98%
Controlled Postoperative Blood Glucose[2,7]	-	-	97%	97%
Perioperative Temperature Management[2]	523	98%	100%	100%
Prophylactic Antibiotic Selection[2]	364	99%	99%	99%
Prophylactic Antibiotic Selection (Outpatient)	197	95%	97%	98%
Prophylactic Antibiotic Stopped[2]	353	99%	98%	98%
Prophylactic Antibiotic Timing[2]	364	100%	99%	99%
Prophylactic Antibiotic Timing (Outpatient)	197	100%	97%	98%
Urinary Catheter Removal[2]	106	97%	96%	97%
Survey of Patients' Hospital Experiences				
Area Around Room 'Always' Quiet at Night	300+	48%	51%	61%
Doctors 'Always' Communicated Well	300+	76%	77%	82%
Home Recovery Information Given	300+	86%	83%	85%
Hospital Given 9 or 10 on 10 Point Scale	300+	59%	63%	71%
Meds 'Always' Explained Before Given	300+	56%	59%	64%
Nurses 'Always' Communicated Well	300+	72%	75%	79%
Pain 'Always' Well Controlled	300+	66%	67%	71%
Room and Bathroom 'Always' Clean	300+	58%	69%	73%
Timely Help 'Always' Received	300+	56%	61%	68%
Would Definitely Recommend Hospital	300+	62%	65%	71%
Use of Medical Imaging				
Cardiac Imaging Stress Test before Surgery	119	7.6%	5.8%	5.3%
Combination Abdominal CT Scan	505	3.4%	8.2%	10.5%
Combination Brain/Sinus CT Scan	675	5.0%	3.6%	2.7%
Combination Chest CT Scan	205	0.0%	1.3%	2.7%
Follow-up Mammogram/Ultrasound	116	15.5%	13%	8.8%
Lumbar Spine MRI for Low Back Pain[7]	-	-	33.4%	37.2%

NOTE: Hospital profiles are in alphabetical order by state, then city, then hospital within the city; Rankings exclude hospitals with less than 25 cases except for patient surveys which excludes hospitals with less than 100 cases; (a) 100-299 cases; (1) The number of cases/patients is too few to report; (2) Data submitted were based on a sample of cases/patients; (3) Results are based on a shorter time period than required; (4) Data suppressed by CMS for one or more quarters; (5) Results are not available for this reporting period; (6) Fewer than 100 patients completed the HCAHPS survey; (7) No cases met the criteria for this measure; (8) The lower limit of the confidence interval cannot be calculated if the number of observed infections equals zero; (9) No data are available from the state/territory for this reporting period; (10) The scores shown reflect fewer than 50 completed surveys; (11) There were discrepancies in the data collection process; (12) This measure does not apply to this hospital for this reporting period; (13) Results cannot be calculated for this reporting period; (14) The results for this state are combined with nearby states to protect confidentiality; Please refer to the User's Guide for a full explanation of data.

Niagara Falls Memorial Medical Center

621 Tenth Street
Niagara Falls, NY 14302
Phone: 716-278-4000
Fax: 716-278-4054
E-mail: healthbeat@nfmmc.org
URL: www.nfmmc.org
Type: Acute Care Hospitals
Emergency Services: Yes
Ownership: Voluntary non-profit - Other

Key Personnel:
Chief of Medical Staff.......... Vijay Bojedla, MD
Infection Control.............. Lorrianne Duthe
Hemotology Center........... Joseph F Gioia, MD
Emergency Room............ Laura Hickey, RN
Radiology................... Mark Perry
CEO/President............... Joseph A Ruffolo
Quality Assurance............ Karen Tunis-Manny

Measure	Cases	This Hosp.	State Avg.	U.S. Avg.
Blood Clot Prevention and Treatment				
Anticoagulation Overlap Therapy[2]	16	94%	91%	93%
ICU Venous Thromboembolism Prophylaxis[2]	156	95%	92%	92%
Incidence of Potentially Preventable VTE[1,2]	-	-	10%	10%
UFH with Dosages/Platelet Monitoring[1,2]	-	-	92%	97%
Venous Thromboembolism Prophylaxis[2]	217	92%	87%	85%
Warfarin Therapy Discharge Instructions[1,2]	-	-	59%	75%
Chest Pain/Possible Heart Attack Care				
Aspirin Given Within 24 Hours of Arrival	43	95%	97%	96%
Fibrinolytic Meds Within 30 Min. of Arrival[1]	-	-	54%	58%
Average Time to ECG (minutes)	44	9	9	7
Average Time to Transfer (minutes)[1]	-	-	78	60
Children's Asthma Care				
Received Home Management Plan of Care	-	-	-	88%
Received Reliever Medication	-	-	-	100%
Received Systemic Corticosteroids	-	-	-	100%
Emergency Department				
Admittance Decision Time (minutes)[2]	803	102	154	98
Head CT Results Within 45 Min. of Arrival[1]	-	-	55%	57%
Patients Who Left ER Before Being Seen	31,220	4%	2%	2%
Time from ER Arrival to Admit. (minutes)[2]	806	319	378	274
Time from ER Arrival to Discharge (minutes)	292	186	156	134
Time in ER Before Being Evaluated (minutes)	393	69	35	26
Time to Pain Meds for Fractures (minutes)	52	65	61	57
Heart Attack Care				
Aspirin Given at Discharge	19	100%	99%	99%
Fibrinolytic Meds Within 30 Min. of Arrival[7]	-	-	46%	54%
PCI Within 90 Minutes of Arrival[7]	-	-	95%	96%
Statin Prescribed at Discharge	18	94%	98%	98%
Heart Failure Care				
ACE Inhibitor or ARB for LVSD[2]	34	100%	96%	97%
Discharge Instructions Given[2]	129	100%	95%	94%
Evaluation of LVS Function[2]	160	100%	99%	99%
Medicare Spending				
Medicare Spending per Patient (ratio)	-	0.88	0.96	0.98
Pneumonia Care				
Appropriate Initial Antibiotic Given[2]	63	97%	95%	95%
Blood Culture Timing[2]	114	98%	97%	98%
Pregnancy and Delivery Care				
Newborn Deliveries Scheduled Early[2]	86	6%	4%	6%
Preventive Care				
Immunization for Influenza[2]	565	95%	88%	90%
Immunization for Pneumonia[2]	732	94%	88%	92%
Stroke Care				
Anticoagulation Therapy for Atrial Fibrillation[7]	-	-	96%	95%
Antithrombotic Therapy Timing	26	100%	98%	98%
Assessed for Rehabilitation	25	100%	97%	97%
Discharged on Antithrombotic Therapy	23	100%	99%	99%
Discharged on Statin Medication	20	100%	95%	94%
Thrombolytic Therapy Timing[7]	-	-	69%	66%
Venous Thromboembolism Prophylaxis	28	96%	94%	94%
Written Stroke Educational Materials Given	16	100%	86%	88%
Surgical Care Improvement Project				
Appropriate Beta Blocker Usage[2]	45	100%	97%	98%
Appropriate VTP Within 24 Hours[2]	126	99%	98%	98%
Controlled Postoperative Blood Glucose[2,7]	-	-	97%	97%
Perioperative Temperature Management[2]	161	100%	100%	100%
Prophylactic Antibiotic Selection[2]	77	99%	99%	99%
Prophylactic Antibiotic Selection (Outpatient)	160	99%	97%	98%
Prophylactic Antibiotic Stopped[2]	74	96%	98%	98%
Prophylactic Antibiotic Timing[2]	77	99%	99%	99%
Prophylactic Antibiotic Timing (Outpatient)	157	99%	97%	98%
Urinary Catheter Removal[2]	66	100%	96%	97%
Survey of Patients' Hospital Experiences				
Area Around Room 'Always' Quiet at Night	300+	52%	51%	61%
Doctors 'Always' Communicated Well	300+	77%	77%	82%
Home Recovery Information Given	300+	82%	83%	85%
Hospital Given 9 or 10 on 10 Point Scale	300+	53%	63%	71%
Meds 'Always' Explained Before Given	300+	55%	59%	64%
Nurses 'Always' Communicated Well	300+	70%	75%	79%
Pain 'Always' Well Controlled	300+	64%	67%	71%
Room and Bathroom 'Always' Clean	300+	60%	69%	73%
Timely Help 'Always' Received	300+	63%	61%	68%
Would Definitely Recommend Hospital	300+	55%	65%	71%
Use of Medical Imaging				
Cardiac Imaging Stress Test before Surgery	149	6.7%	5.8%	5.3%
Combination Abdominal CT Scan	301	3.3%	8.2%	10.5%
Combination Brain/Sinus CT Scan[1]	-	-	3.6%	2.7%
Combination Chest CT Scan	140	7.1%	1.3%	2.7%
Follow-up Mammogram/Ultrasound	691	6.4%	13%	8.8%
Lumbar Spine MRI for Low Back Pain	65	38.5%	33.4%	37.2%

Northport VA Medical Center

79 Middleville Road
Northport, NY 11768
Phone: 516-261-4400
Fax: 631-754-7933
URL: www.va.gov
Type: Acute Care - VA
Emergency Services: No
Ownership: Government Federal
Beds: 524

Key Personnel:
CEO/President............... James A Clark
Chief of Medical Staff.......... Mark Graber, MD
Radiology................... Margaret Johnstone, MD
Operating Room............. Mary Ann Loh, RN
Emergency Room............ Shirley Tansiongco, MD

Measure	Cases	This Hosp.	State Avg.	U.S. Avg.
Blood Clot Prevention and Treatment				
Anticoagulation Overlap Therapy	-	-	91%	93%
ICU Venous Thromboembolism Prophylaxis	-	-	92%	92%
Incidence of Potentially Preventable VTE	-	-	10%	10%
UFH with Dosages/Platelet Monitoring	-	-	92%	97%
Venous Thromboembolism Prophylaxis	-	-	87%	85%
Warfarin Therapy Discharge Instructions	-	-	59%	75%
Chest Pain/Possible Heart Attack Care				
Aspirin Given Within 24 Hours of Arrival	-	-	97%	96%
Fibrinolytic Meds Within 30 Min. of Arrival	-	-	54%	58%
Average Time to ECG (minutes)	-	-	9	7
Average Time to Transfer (minutes)	-	-	78	60
Children's Asthma Care				
Received Home Management Plan of Care	-	-	-	88%
Received Reliever Medication	-	-	-	100%
Received Systemic Corticosteroids	-	-	-	100%
Emergency Department				
Admittance Decision Time (minutes)	-	-	154	98
Head CT Results Within 45 Min. of Arrival	-	-	55%	57%
Patients Who Left ER Before Being Seen	-	-	2%	2%
Time from ER Arrival to Admit. (minutes)	-	-	378	274
Time from ER Arrival to Discharge (minutes)	-	-	156	134
Time in ER Before Being Evaluated (minutes)	-	-	35	26
Time to Pain Meds for Fractures (minutes)	-	-	61	57
Heart Attack Care				
Aspirin Given at Discharge[5]	-	-	99%	99%
Fibrinolytic Meds Within 30 Min. of Arrival[5]	-	-	46%	54%
PCI Within 90 Minutes of Arrival[5]	-	-	95%	96%
Statin Prescribed at Discharge[5]	-	-	98%	98%
Heart Failure Care				
ACE Inhibitor or ARB for LVSD	58	98%	96%	97%
Discharge Instructions Given	140	99%	95%	94%
Evaluation of LVS Function	154	100%	99%	99%
Medicare Spending				
Medicare Spending per Patient (ratio)	-	-	0.96	0.98
Pneumonia Care				
Appropriate Initial Antibiotic Given	29	100%	95%	95%
Blood Culture Timing	53	96%	97%	98%
Pregnancy and Delivery Care				
Newborn Deliveries Scheduled Early	-	-	4%	6%
Preventive Care				
Immunization for Influenza[5]	-	-	88%	90%
Immunization for Pneumonia[5]	-	-	88%	92%
Stroke Care				
Anticoagulation Therapy for Atrial Fibrillation	-	-	96%	95%
Antithrombotic Therapy Timing	-	-	98%	98%
Assessed for Rehabilitation	-	-	97%	97%
Discharged on Antithrombotic Therapy	-	-	99%	99%
Discharged on Statin Medication	-	-	95%	94%
Thrombolytic Therapy Timing	-	-	69%	66%
Venous Thromboembolism Prophylaxis	-	-	94%	94%
Written Stroke Educational Materials Given	-	-	86%	88%
Surgical Care Improvement Project				
Appropriate Beta Blocker Usage[2]	35	91%	97%	98%
Appropriate VTP Within 24 Hours[2]	92	95%	98%	98%
Controlled Postoperative Blood Glucose[5]	-	-	97%	97%
Perioperative Temperature Management[2]	108	99%	100%	100%
Prophylactic Antibiotic Selection	66	98%	99%	99%
Prophylactic Antibiotic Selection (Outpatient)	-	-	97%	98%
Prophylactic Antibiotic Stopped	63	98%	98%	98%
Prophylactic Antibiotic Timing	66	98%	99%	99%
Prophylactic Antibiotic Timing (Outpatient)	-	-	97%	98%
Urinary Catheter Removal[2]	72	90%	96%	97%
Survey of Patients' Hospital Experiences				
Area Around Room 'Always' Quiet at Night	-	-	51%	61%
Doctors 'Always' Communicated Well	-	-	77%	82%
Home Recovery Information Given	-	-	83%	85%
Hospital Given 9 or 10 on 10 Point Scale	-	-	63%	71%
Meds 'Always' Explained Before Given	-	-	59%	64%
Nurses 'Always' Communicated Well	-	-	75%	79%
Pain 'Always' Well Controlled	-	-	67%	71%
Room and Bathroom 'Always' Clean	-	-	69%	73%
Timely Help 'Always' Received	-	-	61%	68%
Would Definitely Recommend Hospital	-	-	65%	71%
Use of Medical Imaging				
Cardiac Imaging Stress Test before Surgery	-	-	5.8%	5.3%
Combination Abdominal CT Scan	-	-	8.2%	10.5%
Combination Brain/Sinus CT Scan	-	-	3.6%	2.7%
Combination Chest CT Scan	-	-	1.3%	2.7%
Follow-up Mammogram/Ultrasound	-	-	13%	8.8%
Lumbar Spine MRI for Low Back Pain	-	-	33.4%	37.2%

Chenango Memorial Hospital

179 North Broad Street
Norwich, NY 13815
Phone: 607-335-4111
Fax: 607-337-4284
URL: www.uhs.net
Type: Acute Care Hospitals
Emergency Services: Yes
Ownership: Voluntary non-profit - Private
Beds: 139

Key Personnel:
Emergency Room............ William Boudreau, MD
Patient Relations............ Julie Briggs, RN
Quality Assurance............ Shirley Caezza, RN, BSN
CEO/President............... Drake Lamen, MD
Chair/CEO.................. Robert Nassar
Chief of Medical Staff.......... David Race, MD
Operating Room............. Patty Roma
Infection Control.............. Dottie VanVliet, RN

Measure	Cases	This Hosp.	State Avg.	U.S. Avg.
Blood Clot Prevention and Treatment				
Anticoagulation Overlap Therapy[2]	12	100%	91%	93%
ICU Venous Thromboembolism Prophylaxis[2]	87	100%	92%	92%
Incidence of Potentially Preventable VTE[2,7]	-	-	10%	10%
UFH with Dosages/Platelet Monitoring[1,2]	-	-	92%	97%
Venous Thromboembolism Prophylaxis[2]	326	100%	87%	85%
Warfarin Therapy Discharge Instructions[1,2]	-	-	59%	75%
Chest Pain/Possible Heart Attack Care				
Aspirin Given Within 24 Hours of Arrival	67	100%	97%	96%
Fibrinolytic Meds Within 30 Min. of Arrival[1]	-	-	54%	58%
Average Time to ECG (minutes)	72	8	9	7
Average Time to Transfer (minutes)[7]	-	-	78	60

NOTE: Hospital profiles are in alphabetical order by state, then city, then hospital within the city; Rankings exclude hospitals with less than 25 cases except for patient surveys which excludes hospitals with less than 100 cases; (a) 100-299 cases; (1) The number of cases/patients is too few to report; (2) Data submitted were based on a sample of cases/patients; (3) Results are based on a shorter time period than required; (4) Data suppressed by CMS for one or more quarters; (5) Results are not available for this reporting period; (6) Fewer than 100 patients completed the HCAHPS survey; (7) No cases met the criteria for this measure; (8) The lower limit of the confidence interval cannot be calculated if the number of observed infections equals zero; (9) No data are available from the state/territory for this reporting period; (10) The scores shown reflect fewer than 50 completed surveys; (11) There were discrepancies in the data collection process; (12) This measure does not apply to this hospital for this reporting period; (13) Results cannot be calculated for this reporting period; (14) The results for this state are combined with nearby states to protect confidentiality; Please refer to the User's Guide for a full explanation of data.

Measure	Cases	This Hosp.	State Avg.	U.S. Avg.
Children's Asthma Care				
Received Home Management Plan of Care	-	-	-	88%
Received Reliever Medication	-	-	-	100%
Received Systemic Corticosteroids	-	-	-	100%
Emergency Department				
Admittance Decision Time (minutes)[2]	438	60	154	98
Head CT Results Within 45 Min. of Arrival[1]	-	-	55%	57%
Patients Who Left ER Before Being Seen	16,225	2%	2%	2%
Time from ER Arrival to Admit. (minutes)[2]	495	196	378	274
Time from ER Arrival to Discharge (minutes)	437	85	156	134
Time in ER Before Being Evaluated (minutes)	540	21	35	26
Time to Pain Meds for Fractures (minutes)	51	48	61	57
Heart Attack Care				
Aspirin Given at Discharge	21	100%	99%	99%
Fibrinolytic Meds Within 30 Min. of Arrival[7]	-	-	46%	54%
PCI Within 90 Minutes of Arrival[7]	-	-	95%	96%
Statin Prescribed at Discharge	16	81%	98%	98%
Heart Failure Care				
ACE Inhibitor or ARB for LVSD	20	100%	96%	97%
Discharge Instructions Given	60	97%	95%	94%
Evaluation of LVS Function	64	100%	99%	99%
Medicare Spending				
Medicare Spending per Patient (ratio)	-	0.82	0.96	0.98
Pneumonia Care				
Appropriate Initial Antibiotic Given	84	100%	95%	95%
Blood Culture Timing	150	99%	97%	98%
Pregnancy and Delivery Care				
Newborn Deliveries Scheduled Early	11	0%	4%	6%
Preventive Care				
Immunization for Influenza[2]	491	98%	88%	90%
Immunization for Pneumonia[2]	616	98%	88%	92%
Stroke Care				
Anticoagulation Therapy for Atrial Fibrillation[7]	-	-	96%	95%
Antithrombotic Therapy Timing[1]	-	-	98%	98%
Assessed for Rehabilitation[1]	-	-	97%	97%
Discharged on Antithrombotic Therapy[1]	-	-	99%	99%
Discharged on Statin Medication[1]	-	-	95%	94%
Thrombolytic Therapy Timing[7]	-	-	69%	66%
Venous Thromboembolism Prophylaxis[1]	-	-	94%	94%
Written Stroke Educational Materials Given[1]	-	-	86%	88%
Surgical Care Improvement Project				
Appropriate Beta Blocker Usage	39	100%	97%	98%
Appropriate VTP Within 24 Hours	141	100%	98%	98%
Controlled Postoperative Blood Glucose[7]	-	-	97%	97%
Perioperative Temperature Management	158	100%	100%	100%
Prophylactic Antibiotic Selection	110	99%	99%	99%
Prophylactic Antibiotic Selection (Outpatient)[1,3]	-	-	97%	98%
Prophylactic Antibiotic Stopped	108	99%	98%	98%
Prophylactic Antibiotic Timing	111	98%	99%	99%
Prophylactic Antibiotic Timing (Outpatient)[1,3]	-	-	97%	98%
Urinary Catheter Removal	113	100%	96%	97%
Survey of Patients' Hospital Experiences				
Area Around Room 'Always' Quiet at Night	300+	54%	51%	61%
Doctors 'Always' Communicated Well	300+	72%	77%	82%
Home Recovery Information Given	300+	85%	83%	85%
Hospital Given 9 or 10 on 10 Point Scale	300+	58%	63%	71%
Meds 'Always' Explained Before Given	300+	58%	59%	64%
Nurses 'Always' Communicated Well	300+	74%	75%	79%
Pain 'Always' Well Controlled	300+	64%	67%	71%
Room and Bathroom 'Always' Clean	300+	68%	69%	73%
Timely Help 'Always' Received	300+	63%	61%	68%
Would Definitely Recommend Hospital	300+	55%	65%	71%
Use of Medical Imaging				
Cardiac Imaging Stress Test before Surgery	108	3.7%	5.8%	5.3%
Combination Abdominal CT Scan	286	4.2%	8.2%	10.5%
Combination Brain/Sinus CT Scan[1]	-	-	3.6%	2.7%
Combination Chest CT Scan	146	0.0%	1.3%	2.7%
Follow-up Mammogram/Ultrasound	709	16.6%	13%	8.8%
Lumbar Spine MRI for Low Back Pain	52	40.4%	33.4%	37.2%

Nyack Hospital

160 North Midland Avenue
Nyack, NY 10960
URL: www.nyackhospital.org
Type: Acute Care Hospitals
Ownership: Voluntary non-profit - Other
Phone: 845-348-2000
Fax: 845-348-2160
Emergency Services: Yes
Beds: 375

Key Personnel:
Pediatric Ambulatory Care . . . . . . Mary Ann Clay, RN
CEO/President. . . . . David H Freed, DHA
Radiology. . . . . Mark Geller, MD
Infection Control. . . . . Joan Graham-Rauscher, BSN RN
Operating Room. . . . . Nancy Madura, RN
Quality Assurance . . . . Kathleen O'Keefe, CFNP
Coronary Care. . . . . Mary Ortiz
Chief of Medical Staff. . . . . Michael Rader, MD

Measure	Cases	This Hosp.	State Avg.	U.S. Avg.
Blood Clot Prevention and Treatment				
Anticoagulation Overlap Therapy[2]	47	100%	91%	93%
ICU Venous Thromboembolism Prophylaxis[2]	53	96%	92%	92%
Incidence of Potentially Preventable VTE[2]	35	0%	10%	10%
UFH with Dosages/Platelet Monitoring[1,2]	-	-	92%	97%
Venous Thromboembolism Prophylaxis[2]	345	97%	87%	85%
Warfarin Therapy Discharge Instructions[2]	29	97%	59%	75%
Chest Pain/Possible Heart Attack Care				
Aspirin Given Within 24 Hours of Arrival	51	98%	97%	96%
Fibrinolytic Meds Within 30 Min. of Arrival[7]	-	-	54%	58%
Average Time to ECG (minutes)	52	3	9	7
Average Time to Transfer (minutes)	12	56	78	60
Children's Asthma Care				
Received Home Management Plan of Care	-	-	-	88%
Received Reliever Medication	-	-	-	100%
Received Systemic Corticosteroids	-	-	-	100%
Emergency Department				
Admittance Decision Time (minutes)[2]	803	76	154	98
Head CT Results Within 45 Min. of Arrival	15	60%	55%	57%
Patients Who Left ER Before Being Seen	60,163	0%	2%	2%
Time from ER Arrival to Admit. (minutes)[2]	804	244	378	274
Time from ER Arrival to Discharge (minutes)	389	138	156	134
Time in ER Before Being Evaluated (minutes)	414	16	35	26
Time to Pain Meds for Fractures (minutes)	236	33	61	57
Heart Attack Care				
Aspirin Given at Discharge	30	100%	99%	99%
Fibrinolytic Meds Within 30 Min. of Arrival[7]	-	-	46%	54%
PCI Within 90 Minutes of Arrival[7]	-	-	95%	96%
Statin Prescribed at Discharge	28	100%	98%	98%
Heart Failure Care				
ACE Inhibitor or ARB for LVSD	64	97%	96%	97%
Discharge Instructions Given	184	93%	95%	94%
Evaluation of LVS Function	262	100%	99%	99%
Medicare Spending				
Medicare Spending per Patient (ratio)	-	1.07	0.96	0.98
Pneumonia Care				
Appropriate Initial Antibiotic Given[2]	90	100%	95%	95%
Blood Culture Timing[2]	159	99%	97%	98%
Pregnancy and Delivery Care				
Newborn Deliveries Scheduled Early[2]	38	0%	4%	6%
Preventive Care				
Immunization for Influenza[2]	530	95%	88%	90%
Immunization for Pneumonia[2]	596	96%	88%	92%
Stroke Care				
Anticoagulation Therapy for Atrial Fibrillation	23	100%	96%	95%
Antithrombotic Therapy Timing	124	100%	98%	98%
Assessed for Rehabilitation	145	99%	97%	97%
Discharged on Antithrombotic Therapy	128	98%	99%	99%
Discharged on Statin Medication	107	100%	95%	94%
Thrombolytic Therapy Timing[1]	-	-	69%	66%
Venous Thromboembolism Prophylaxis	150	99%	94%	94%
Written Stroke Educational Materials Given	65	100%	86%	88%
Surgical Care Improvement Project				
Appropriate Beta Blocker Usage	122	100%	97%	98%
Appropriate VTP Within 24 Hours	491	100%	98%	98%
Controlled Postoperative Blood Glucose[7]	-	-	97%	97%
Perioperative Temperature Management	544	100%	100%	100%
Prophylactic Antibiotic Selection	333	99%	99%	99%
Prophylactic Antibiotic Selection (Outpatient)	45	100%	97%	98%
Prophylactic Antibiotic Stopped	323	98%	98%	98%
Prophylactic Antibiotic Timing	333	100%	99%	99%
Prophylactic Antibiotic Timing (Outpatient)	45	100%	97%	98%
Urinary Catheter Removal	373	99%	96%	97%
Survey of Patients' Hospital Experiences				
Area Around Room 'Always' Quiet at Night	300+	45%	51%	61%
Doctors 'Always' Communicated Well	300+	75%	77%	82%
Home Recovery Information Given	300+	77%	83%	85%
Hospital Given 9 or 10 on 10 Point Scale	300+	55%	63%	71%
Meds 'Always' Explained Before Given	300+	57%	59%	64%
Nurses 'Always' Communicated Well	300+	72%	75%	79%
Pain 'Always' Well Controlled	300+	64%	67%	71%
Room and Bathroom 'Always' Clean	300+	70%	69%	73%
Timely Help 'Always' Received	300+	59%	61%	68%
Would Definitely Recommend Hospital	300+	60%	65%	71%
Use of Medical Imaging				
Cardiac Imaging Stress Test before Surgery[1]	-	-	5.8%	5.3%
Combination Abdominal CT Scan	617	14.7%	8.2%	10.5%
Combination Brain/Sinus CT Scan	818	4.9%	3.6%	2.7%
Combination Chest CT Scan	430	8.8%	1.3%	2.7%
Follow-up Mammogram/Ultrasound	749	14.4%	13%	8.8%
Lumbar Spine MRI for Low Back Pain[1]	-	-	33.4%	37.2%

South Nassau Communities Hospital

One Healthy Way
Oceanside, NY 11572
URL: www.southnassau.org
Type: Acute Care Hospitals
Ownership: Voluntary non-profit - Private
Phone: 516-632-3000
Fax: 516-632-3981
Emergency Services: Yes
Beds: 435

Key Personnel:
Radiology. . . . . Michael Burghardt
Chief of Medical Staff . . . . Linda Efferen, M.D., FACP, FCC
Infection Control. . . . . Judith Goldstein, MD
Cardiac Laboratory. . . . . Robert Kramer, MD
Pediatrics. . . . . Clara Mayoral, MD
CEO/President. . . . . Richard J. Murphy
Quality Assurance . . . . Ruth Ragusa
Operating Room. . . . . Mary Weiner

Measure	Cases	This Hosp.	State Avg.	U.S. Avg.
Blood Clot Prevention and Treatment				
Anticoagulation Overlap Therapy[2]	138	90%	91%	93%
ICU Venous Thromboembolism Prophylaxis[2]	25	100%	92%	92%
Incidence of Potentially Preventable VTE[2]	33	0%	10%	10%
UFH with Dosages/Platelet Monitoring[2]	74	100%	92%	97%
Venous Thromboembolism Prophylaxis[2]	424	94%	87%	85%
Warfarin Therapy Discharge Instructions[2]	103	93%	59%	75%
Chest Pain/Possible Heart Attack Care				
Aspirin Given Within 24 Hours of Arrival[1,3]	-	-	97%	96%
Fibrinolytic Meds Within 30 Min. of Arrival[3,7]	-	-	54%	58%
Average Time to ECG (minutes)[1,3]	-	-	9	7
Average Time to Transfer (minutes)[3,7]	-	-	78	60
Children's Asthma Care				
Received Home Management Plan of Care	-	-	-	88%
Received Reliever Medication	-	-	-	100%
Received Systemic Corticosteroids	-	-	-	100%
Emergency Department				
Admittance Decision Time (minutes)[2]	958	150	154	98
Head CT Results Within 45 Min. of Arrival[1]	-	-	55%	57%
Patients Who Left ER Before Being Seen	59,020	1%	2%	2%
Time from ER Arrival to Admit. (minutes)[2]	967	395	378	274
Time from ER Arrival to Discharge (minutes)	409	203	156	134
Time in ER Before Being Evaluated (minutes)	390	59	35	26
Time to Pain Meds for Fractures (minutes)	165	71	61	57
Heart Attack Care				
Aspirin Given at Discharge	273	100%	99%	99%
Fibrinolytic Meds Within 30 Min. of Arrival[7]	-	-	46%	54%
PCI Within 90 Minutes of Arrival	52	100%	95%	96%
Statin Prescribed at Discharge	272	100%	98%	98%
Heart Failure Care				
ACE Inhibitor or ARB for LVSD[2]	97	99%	96%	97%
Discharge Instructions Given[2]	211	99%	95%	94%
Evaluation of LVS Function[2]	287	100%	99%	99%
Medicare Spending				

NOTE: Hospital profiles are in alphabetical order by state, then city, then hospital within the city; Rankings exclude hospitals with less than 25 cases except for patient surveys which excludes hospitals with less than 100 cases; (a) 100-299 cases; (1) The number of cases/patients is too few to report; (2) Data submitted were based on a sample of cases/patients; (3) Results are based on a shorter time period than required; (4) Data suppressed by CMS for one or more quarters; (5) Results are not available for this reporting period; (6) Fewer than 100 patients completed the HCAHPS survey; (7) No cases met the criteria for this measure; (8) The lower limit of the confidence interval cannot be calculated if the number of observed infections equals zero; (9) No data are available from the state/territory for this reporting period; (10) The scores shown reflect fewer than 50 completed surveys; (11) There were discrepancies in the data collection process; (12) This measure does not apply to this hospital for this reporting period; (13) Results cannot be calculated for this reporting period; (14) The results for this state are combined with nearby states to protect confidentiality; Please refer to the User's Guide for a full explanation of data.

Measure	Cases	This Hosp.	State Avg.	U.S. Avg.
Medicare Spending per Patient (ratio)	-	1.04	0.96	0.98
Pneumonia Care				
Appropriate Initial Antibiotic Given[2]	68	99%	95%	95%
Blood Culture Timing[2]	153	100%	97%	98%
Pregnancy and Delivery Care				
Newborn Deliveries Scheduled Early[2]	22	5%	4%	6%
Preventive Care				
Immunization for Influenza[2]	730	92%	88%	90%
Immunization for Pneumonia[2]	824	94%	88%	92%
Stroke Care				
Anticoagulation Therapy for Atrial Fibrillation	34	100%	96%	95%
Antithrombotic Therapy Timing	173	95%	98%	98%
Assessed for Rehabilitation	203	100%	97%	97%
Discharged on Antithrombotic Therapy	184	99%	99%	99%
Discharged on Statin Medication	150	97%	95%	94%
Thrombolytic Therapy Timing	18	100%	69%	66%
Venous Thromboembolism Prophylaxis	226	96%	94%	94%
Written Stroke Educational Materials Given	113	93%	86%	88%
Surgical Care Improvement Project				
Appropriate Beta Blocker Usage[2]	361	100%	97%	98%
Appropriate VTP Within 24 Hours[2]	903	100%	98%	98%
Controlled Postoperative Blood Glucose[2,7]	-	-	97%	97%
Perioperative Temperature Management[2]	988	100%	100%	100%
Prophylactic Antibiotic Selection[2]	747	100%	99%	99%
Prophylactic Antibiotic Selection (Outpatient)	338	100%	97%	98%
Prophylactic Antibiotic Stopped[2]	732	100%	98%	98%
Prophylactic Antibiotic Timing[2]	747	100%	99%	99%
Prophylactic Antibiotic Timing (Outpatient)	338	99%	97%	98%
Urinary Catheter Removal[2]	736	100%	96%	97%
Survey of Patients' Hospital Experiences				
Area Around Room 'Always' Quiet at Night	300+	52%	51%	61%
Doctors 'Always' Communicated Well	300+	77%	77%	82%
Home Recovery Information Given	300+	83%	83%	85%
Hospital Given 9 or 10 on 10 Point Scale	300+	66%	63%	71%
Meds 'Always' Explained Before Given	300+	56%	59%	64%
Nurses 'Always' Communicated Well	300+	76%	75%	79%
Pain 'Always' Well Controlled	300+	69%	67%	71%
Room and Bathroom 'Always' Clean	300+	65%	69%	73%
Timely Help 'Always' Received	300+	59%	61%	68%
Would Definitely Recommend Hospital	300+	71%	65%	71%
Use of Medical Imaging				
Cardiac Imaging Stress Test before Surgery	209	5.7%	5.8%	5.3%
Combination Abdominal CT Scan	725	8.0%	8.2%	10.5%
Combination Brain/Sinus CT Scan	1,002	3.9%	3.6%	2.7%
Combination Chest CT Scan	509	0.0%	1.3%	2.7%
Follow-up Mammogram/Ultrasound	1,184	60.6%	13%	8.8%
Lumbar Spine MRI for Low Back Pain[1]	-	-	33.4%	37.2%

Claxton - Hepburn Medical Center

214 King Street
Ogdensburg, NY 13669
E-mail: info@chmed.org
URL: www.chmed.org
Type: Acute Care Hospitals
Ownership: Voluntary non-profit - Private
Phone: 315-393-3600
Fax: 315-393-8506
Emergency Services: Yes
Beds: 159

Key Personnel:
Operating Room. . . . . Lenette Deloney
Infection Control. . . . . Vicki Hockenbery, RN
Radiology. . . . . Angela Klimaszewski
Chief of Medical Staff. . . . . Michael Roark, MD
Cardiac Laboratory. . . . . Keith Warren
CEO/President. . . . . Mark Webster
Quality Assurance . . . . Robin Wood

Measure	Cases	This Hosp.	State Avg.	U.S. Avg.
Blood Clot Prevention and Treatment				
Anticoagulation Overlap Therapy[2]	14	86%	91%	93%
ICU Venous Thromboembolism Prophylaxis[2]	42	98%	92%	92%
Incidence of Potentially Preventable VTE[1,2]	-	-	10%	10%
UFH with Dosages/Platelet Monitoring[1,2]	-	-	92%	97%
Venous Thromboembolism Prophylaxis[2]	190	96%	87%	85%
Warfarin Therapy Discharge Instructions[2]	13	69%	59%	75%
Chest Pain/Possible Heart Attack Care				
Aspirin Given Within 24 Hours of Arrival	79	100%	97%	96%
Fibrinolytic Meds Within 30 Min. of Arrival	12	83%	54%	58%
Average Time to ECG (minutes)	82	4	9	7
Average Time to Transfer (minutes)[1]	-	-	78	60
Children's Asthma Care				
Received Home Management Plan of Care	-	-	-	88%
Received Reliever Medication	-	-	-	100%
Received Systemic Corticosteroids	-	-	-	100%
Emergency Department				
Admittance Decision Time (minutes)[2]	283	95	154	98
Head CT Results Within 45 Min. of Arrival[1]	-	-	55%	57%
Patients Who Left ER Before Being Seen	19,074	1%	2%	2%
Time from ER Arrival to Admit. (minutes)[2]	283	276	378	274
Time from ER Arrival to Discharge (minutes)	411	115	156	134
Time in ER Before Being Evaluated (minutes)	481	22	35	26
Time to Pain Meds for Fractures (minutes)	68	43	61	57
Heart Attack Care				
Aspirin Given at Discharge	13	100%	99%	99%
Fibrinolytic Meds Within 30 Min. of Arrival[1]	-	-	46%	54%
PCI Within 90 Minutes of Arrival[7]	-	-	95%	96%
Statin Prescribed at Discharge	12	100%	98%	98%
Heart Failure Care				
ACE Inhibitor or ARB for LVSD	18	89%	96%	97%
Discharge Instructions Given	31	100%	95%	94%
Evaluation of LVS Function	41	100%	99%	99%
Medicare Spending				
Medicare Spending per Patient (ratio)	-	0.86	0.96	0.98
Pneumonia Care				
Appropriate Initial Antibiotic Given	38	97%	95%	95%
Blood Culture Timing	68	99%	97%	98%
Pregnancy and Delivery Care				
Newborn Deliveries Scheduled Early	26	0%	4%	6%
Preventive Care				
Immunization for Influenza[2]	267	93%	88%	90%
Immunization for Pneumonia[2]	317	93%	88%	92%
Stroke Care				
Anticoagulation Therapy for Atrial Fibrillation[1]	-	-	96%	95%
Antithrombotic Therapy Timing	30	97%	98%	98%
Assessed for Rehabilitation	29	97%	97%	97%
Discharged on Antithrombotic Therapy	29	97%	99%	99%
Discharged on Statin Medication	20	95%	95%	94%
Thrombolytic Therapy Timing[1]	-	-	69%	66%
Venous Thromboembolism Prophylaxis	29	100%	94%	94%
Written Stroke Educational Materials Given	13	62%	86%	88%
Surgical Care Improvement Project				
Appropriate Beta Blocker Usage	33	91%	97%	98%
Appropriate VTP Within 24 Hours	132	99%	98%	98%
Controlled Postoperative Blood Glucose[7]	-	-	97%	97%
Perioperative Temperature Management	144	99%	100%	100%
Prophylactic Antibiotic Selection	114	100%	99%	99%
Prophylactic Antibiotic Selection (Outpatient)	25	100%	97%	98%
Prophylactic Antibiotic Stopped	113	96%	98%	98%
Prophylactic Antibiotic Timing	114	100%	99%	99%
Prophylactic Antibiotic Timing (Outpatient)	26	96%	97%	98%
Urinary Catheter Removal	62	98%	96%	97%
Survey of Patients' Hospital Experiences				
Area Around Room 'Always' Quiet at Night	300+	48%	51%	61%
Doctors 'Always' Communicated Well	300+	80%	77%	82%
Home Recovery Information Given	300+	89%	83%	85%
Hospital Given 9 or 10 on 10 Point Scale	300+	60%	63%	71%
Meds 'Always' Explained Before Given	300+	61%	59%	64%
Nurses 'Always' Communicated Well	300+	75%	75%	79%
Pain 'Always' Well Controlled	300+	67%	67%	71%
Room and Bathroom 'Always' Clean	300+	69%	69%	73%
Timely Help 'Always' Received	300+	66%	61%	68%
Would Definitely Recommend Hospital	300+	65%	65%	71%
Use of Medical Imaging				
Cardiac Imaging Stress Test before Surgery	254	4.3%	5.8%	5.3%
Combination Abdominal CT Scan	494	0.6%	8.2%	10.5%
Combination Brain/Sinus CT Scan[1]	-	-	3.6%	2.7%
Combination Chest CT Scan	312	0.3%	1.3%	2.7%
Follow-up Mammogram/Ultrasound	1,129	13.9%	13%	8.8%
Lumbar Spine MRI for Low Back Pain	41	39.0%	33.4%	37.2%

Olean General Hospital

515 Main Street
Olean, NY 14760
URL: www.ogh.org
Type: Acute Care Hospitals
Ownership: Proprietary
Phone: 716-373-2600
Fax: 716-375-6380
Emergency Services: Yes
Beds: 217

Key Personnel:
Pediatric Ambulatory Care . . . . . . Pat Allen
Quality Assurance . . . . Donna Brenneman
Chief of Medical Staff. . . . . Richard Decker, MD
President/CEO. . . . . Timothy Finan
Coronary Care . . . . Denise Fish
Radiology. . . . . Helen Layman
Infection Control. . . . . Cynthia Paxhia

Measure	Cases	This Hosp.	State Avg.	U.S. Avg.
Blood Clot Prevention and Treatment				
Anticoagulation Overlap Therapy[2]	56	88%	91%	93%
ICU Venous Thromboembolism Prophylaxis[2]	71	93%	92%	92%
Incidence of Potentially Preventable VTE[1,2]	-	-	10%	10%
UFH with Dosages/Platelet Monitoring[2]	53	100%	92%	97%
Venous Thromboembolism Prophylaxis[2]	360	84%	87%	85%
Warfarin Therapy Discharge Instructions[2]	41	90%	59%	75%
Chest Pain/Possible Heart Attack Care				
Aspirin Given Within 24 Hours of Arrival	144	97%	97%	96%
Fibrinolytic Meds Within 30 Min. of Arrival	20	65%	54%	58%
Average Time to ECG (minutes)	147	6	9	7
Average Time to Transfer (minutes)[1]	-	-	78	60
Children's Asthma Care				
Received Home Management Plan of Care	-	-	-	88%
Received Reliever Medication	-	-	-	100%
Received Systemic Corticosteroids	-	-	-	100%
Emergency Department				
Admittance Decision Time (minutes)[2]	591	83	154	98
Head CT Results Within 45 Min. of Arrival	25	32%	55%	57%
Patients Who Left ER Before Being Seen	33,492	2%	2%	2%
Time from ER Arrival to Admit. (minutes)[2]	592	283	378	274
Time from ER Arrival to Discharge (minutes)	410	164	156	134
Time in ER Before Being Evaluated (minutes)	472	25	35	26
Time to Pain Meds for Fractures (minutes)	110	52	61	57
Heart Attack Care				
Aspirin Given at Discharge	23	100%	99%	99%
Fibrinolytic Meds Within 30 Min. of Arrival[1]	-	-	46%	54%
PCI Within 90 Minutes of Arrival[7]	-	-	95%	96%
Statin Prescribed at Discharge	21	100%	98%	98%
Heart Failure Care				
ACE Inhibitor or ARB for LVSD	38	100%	96%	97%
Discharge Instructions Given	97	78%	95%	94%
Evaluation of LVS Function	141	99%	99%	99%
Medicare Spending				
Medicare Spending per Patient (ratio)	-	0.93	0.96	0.98
Pneumonia Care				
Appropriate Initial Antibiotic Given[2]	120	95%	95%	95%
Blood Culture Timing[2]	227	97%	97%	98%
Pregnancy and Delivery Care				
Newborn Deliveries Scheduled Early[2]	36	28%	4%	6%
Preventive Care				
Immunization for Influenza[2]	539	89%	88%	90%
Immunization for Pneumonia[2]	693	85%	88%	92%
Stroke Care				
Anticoagulation Therapy for Atrial Fibrillation[1]	-	-	96%	95%
Antithrombotic Therapy Timing	16	81%	98%	98%
Assessed for Rehabilitation	14	100%	97%	97%
Discharged on Antithrombotic Therapy	13	92%	99%	99%
Discharged on Statin Medication[1]	-	-	95%	94%
Thrombolytic Therapy Timing[1]	-	-	69%	66%
Venous Thromboembolism Prophylaxis	17	82%	94%	94%
Written Stroke Educational Materials Given[1]	-	-	86%	88%
Surgical Care Improvement Project				
Appropriate Beta Blocker Usage[2]	100	89%	97%	98%
Appropriate VTP Within 24 Hours[2]	277	97%	98%	98%
Controlled Postoperative Blood Glucose[2,7]	-	-	97%	97%
Perioperative Temperature Management[2]	321	100%	100%	100%
Prophylactic Antibiotic Selection[2]	191	96%	99%	99%
Prophylactic Antibiotic Selection (Outpatient)	126	97%	97%	98%

NOTE: Hospital profiles are in alphabetical order by state, then city, then hospital within the city; Rankings exclude hospitals with less than 25 cases except for patient surveys which excludes hospitals with less than 100 cases; (a) 100-299 cases; (1) The number of cases/patients is too few to report; (2) Data submitted were based on a sample of cases/patients; (3) Results are based on a shorter time period than required; (4) Data suppressed by CMS for one or more quarters; (5) Results are not available for this reporting period; (6) Fewer than 100 patients completed the HCAHPS survey; (7) No cases met the criteria for this measure; (8) The lower limit of the confidence interval cannot be calculated if the number of observed infections equals zero; (9) No data are available from the state/territory for this reporting period; (10) The scores shown reflect fewer than 50 completed surveys; (11) There were discrepancies in the data collection process; (12) This measure does not apply to this hospital for this reporting period; (13) Results cannot be calculated for this reporting period; (14) The results for this state are combined with nearby states to protect confidentiality; Please refer to the User's Guide for a full explanation of data.

Measure	Cases	This Hosp.	State Avg.	U.S. Avg.
Prophylactic Antibiotic Stopped[2]	174	90%	98%	98%
Prophylactic Antibiotic Timing[2]	192	97%	99%	99%
Prophylactic Antibiotic Timing (Outpatient)	134	93%	97%	98%
Urinary Catheter Removal[2]	117	74%	96%	97%
Survey of Patients' Hospital Experiences				
Area Around Room 'Always' Quiet at Night	300+	49%	51%	61%
Doctors 'Always' Communicated Well	300+	77%	77%	82%
Home Recovery Information Given	300+	83%	83%	85%
Hospital Given 9 or 10 on 10 Point Scale	300+	57%	63%	71%
Meds 'Always' Explained Before Given	300+	59%	59%	64%
Nurses 'Always' Communicated Well	300+	71%	75%	79%
Pain 'Always' Well Controlled	300+	64%	67%	71%
Room and Bathroom 'Always' Clean	300+	77%	69%	73%
Timely Help 'Always' Received	300+	52%	61%	68%
Would Definitely Recommend Hospital	300+	56%	65%	71%
Use of Medical Imaging				
Cardiac Imaging Stress Test before Surgery	294	6.8%	5.8%	5.3%
Combination Abdominal CT Scan	667	7.8%	8.2%	10.5%
Combination Brain/Sinus CT Scan	592	3.9%	3.6%	2.7%
Combination Chest CT Scan	210	2.9%	1.3%	2.7%
Follow-up Mammogram/Ultrasound	234	9.4%	13%	8.8%
Lumbar Spine MRI for Low Back Pain[1]	-	-	33.4%	37.2%

Oneida Healthcare Center

321 Genesee Street
Oneida, NY 13421
Phone: 315-363-6000
Fax: 315-361-2043
E-mail: info@oneidahealthcare.org
URL: www.oneidahealthcare.org
Type: Acute Care Hospitals
Emergency Services: Yes
Ownership: Voluntary non-profit - Other
Beds: 101

Key Personnel:
Chief of Medical Staff.......... Leonard Argentine, MD
Quality Assurance .... Susan Daley
Radiology.................. Roberto Goldberg, MD
President/CEO.............. Gene F Morreale
Hemotology Center .... Amy Ross
Operating Room............. Jeanette Suchewski
Pediatric Ambulatory Care ...... I Vanderhoof, MD
Pediatric In-Patient Care .... I Vanderhoof, MD

Measure	Cases	This Hosp.	State Avg.	U.S. Avg.
Blood Clot Prevention and Treatment				
Anticoagulation Overlap Therapy[2]	28	82%	91%	93%
ICU Venous Thromboembolism Prophylaxis[2]	58	100%	92%	92%
Incidence of Potentially Preventable VTE[1,2]	-	-	10%	10%
UFH with Dosages/Platelet Monitoring[2]	23	100%	92%	97%
Venous Thromboembolism Prophylaxis[2]	221	96%	87%	85%
Warfarin Therapy Discharge Instructions[2]	26	96%	59%	75%
Chest Pain/Possible Heart Attack Care				
Aspirin Given Within 24 Hours of Arrival	47	96%	97%	96%
Fibrinolytic Meds Within 30 Min. of Arrival[1]	-	-	54%	58%
Average Time to ECG (minutes)	48	8	9	7
Average Time to Transfer (minutes)[1]	-	-	78	60
Children's Asthma Care				
Received Home Management Plan of Care	-	-	-	88%
Received Reliever Medication	-	-	-	100%
Received Systemic Corticosteroids	-	-	-	100%
Emergency Department				
Admittance Decision Time (minutes)[2]	389	123	154	98
Head CT Results Within 45 Min. of Arrival[1]	-	-	55%	57%
Patients Who Left ER Before Being Seen	26,659	2%	2%	2%
Time from ER Arrival to Admit. (minutes)[2]	389	368	378	274
Time from ER Arrival to Discharge (minutes)	403	140	156	134
Time in ER Before Being Evaluated (minutes)	423	35	35	26
Time to Pain Meds for Fractures (minutes)	101	50	61	57
Heart Attack Care				
Aspirin Given at Discharge[1,3]	-	-	99%	99%
Fibrinolytic Meds Within 30 Min. of Arrival[1,3]	-	-	46%	54%
PCI Within 90 Minutes of Arrival[3,7]	-	-	95%	96%
Statin Prescribed at Discharge[1,3]	-	-	98%	98%
Heart Failure Care				
ACE Inhibitor or ARB for LVSD	23	100%	96%	97%
Discharge Instructions Given	44	93%	95%	94%
Evaluation of LVS Function	65	100%	99%	99%
Medicare Spending				
Medicare Spending per Patient (ratio)	-	0.92	0.96	0.98
Pneumonia Care				
Appropriate Initial Antibiotic Given	56	91%	95%	95%
Blood Culture Timing	54	96%	97%	98%
Pregnancy and Delivery Care				
Newborn Deliveries Scheduled Early[2]	34	9%	4%	6%
Preventive Care				
Immunization for Influenza[2]	320	94%	88%	90%
Immunization for Pneumonia[2]	358	91%	88%	92%
Stroke Care				
Anticoagulation Therapy for Atrial Fibrillation[1]	-	-	96%	95%
Antithrombotic Therapy Timing[1]	-	-	98%	98%
Assessed for Rehabilitation[1]	-	-	97%	97%
Discharged on Antithrombotic Therapy[1]	-	-	99%	99%
Discharged on Statin Medication[1]	-	-	95%	94%
Thrombolytic Therapy Timing[7]	-	-	69%	66%
Venous Thromboembolism Prophylaxis[1]	-	-	94%	94%
Written Stroke Educational Materials Given[1]	-	-	86%	88%
Surgical Care Improvement Project				
Appropriate Beta Blocker Usage	42	93%	97%	98%
Appropriate VTP Within 24 Hours	155	99%	98%	98%
Controlled Postoperative Blood Glucose[7]	-	-	97%	97%
Perioperative Temperature Management	177	100%	100%	100%
Prophylactic Antibiotic Selection	88	98%	99%	99%
Prophylactic Antibiotic Selection (Outpatient)	175	97%	97%	98%
Prophylactic Antibiotic Stopped	85	91%	98%	98%
Prophylactic Antibiotic Timing	88	100%	99%	99%
Prophylactic Antibiotic Timing (Outpatient)	176	99%	97%	98%
Urinary Catheter Removal	81	88%	96%	97%
Survey of Patients' Hospital Experiences				
Area Around Room 'Always' Quiet at Night	300+	62%	51%	61%
Doctors 'Always' Communicated Well	300+	81%	77%	82%
Home Recovery Information Given	300+	85%	83%	85%
Hospital Given 9 or 10 on 10 Point Scale	300+	69%	63%	71%
Meds 'Always' Explained Before Given	300+	65%	59%	64%
Nurses 'Always' Communicated Well	300+	77%	75%	79%
Pain 'Always' Well Controlled	300+	69%	67%	71%
Room and Bathroom 'Always' Clean	300+	76%	69%	73%
Timely Help 'Always' Received	300+	68%	61%	68%
Would Definitely Recommend Hospital	300+	69%	65%	71%
Use of Medical Imaging				
Cardiac Imaging Stress Test before Surgery	75	5.3%	5.8%	5.3%
Combination Abdominal CT Scan	466	10.5%	8.2%	10.5%
Combination Brain/Sinus CT Scan[1]	-	-	3.6%	2.7%
Combination Chest CT Scan	152	1.3%	1.3%	2.7%
Follow-up Mammogram/Ultrasound	375	3.5%	13%	8.8%
Lumbar Spine MRI for Low Back Pain[1]	-	-	33.4%	37.2%

Aurelia Osborn Fox Memorial Hospital

One Norton Avenue
Oneonta, NY 13820
Phone: 607-423-2000
Fax: 607-431-5006
E-mail: aofox@catskill.net
URL: www.foxcarenetwork.com
Type: Acute Care Hospitals
Emergency Services: Yes
Ownership: Voluntary non-profit - Other
Beds: 128

Key Personnel:
Chief of Medical Staff.......... David G Evelyn, MD
Cardiac Laboratory............. Jeff Hewings
Radiology.................... James McChesney
Operating Room............... Nancy Mitchell, RN
Emergency Room .... Francis Nolan, MD
Quality Assurance .... Donna L Schultes
Infection Control.............. Ruth Sickler, RN
Intensive Care Unit............ James Wheeling, MD

Measure	Cases	This Hosp.	State Avg.	U.S. Avg.
Blood Clot Prevention and Treatment				
Anticoagulation Overlap Therapy[2]	24	88%	91%	93%
ICU Venous Thromboembolism Prophylaxis[2]	39	77%	92%	92%
Incidence of Potentially Preventable VTE[1,2]	-	-	10%	10%
UFH with Dosages/Platelet Monitoring[2]	18	94%	92%	97%
Venous Thromboembolism Prophylaxis[2]	255	84%	87%	85%
Warfarin Therapy Discharge Instructions[2]	19	47%	59%	75%
Chest Pain/Possible Heart Attack Care				
Aspirin Given Within 24 Hours of Arrival	44	91%	97%	96%
Fibrinolytic Meds Within 30 Min. of Arrival[1]	-	-	54%	58%
Average Time to ECG (minutes)	49	14	9	7
Average Time to Transfer (minutes)	13	131	78	60
Children's Asthma Care				
Received Home Management Plan of Care	-	-	-	88%
Received Reliever Medication	-	-	-	100%
Received Systemic Corticosteroids	-	-	-	100%
Emergency Department				
Admittance Decision Time (minutes)[2]	362	144	154	98
Head CT Results Within 45 Min. of Arrival[1]	-	-	55%	57%
Patients Who Left ER Before Being Seen	17,270	3%	2%	2%
Time from ER Arrival to Admit. (minutes)[2]	368	344	378	274
Time from ER Arrival to Discharge (minutes)	409	189	156	134
Time in ER Before Being Evaluated (minutes)	465	58	35	26
Time to Pain Meds for Fractures (minutes)	42	81	61	57
Heart Attack Care				
Aspirin Given at Discharge	15	93%	99%	99%
Fibrinolytic Meds Within 30 Min. of Arrival[7]	-	-	46%	54%
PCI Within 90 Minutes of Arrival[7]	-	-	95%	96%
Statin Prescribed at Discharge	21	86%	98%	98%
Heart Failure Care				
ACE Inhibitor or ARB for LVSD	33	76%	96%	97%
Discharge Instructions Given	103	79%	95%	94%
Evaluation of LVS Function	132	90%	99%	99%
Medicare Spending				
Medicare Spending per Patient (ratio)	-	0.87	0.96	0.98
Pneumonia Care				
Appropriate Initial Antibiotic Given	84	81%	95%	95%
Blood Culture Timing	110	98%	97%	98%
Pregnancy and Delivery Care				
Newborn Deliveries Scheduled Early	38	5%	4%	6%
Preventive Care				
Immunization for Influenza[2]	330	85%	88%	90%
Immunization for Pneumonia[2]	414	82%	88%	92%
Stroke Care				
Anticoagulation Therapy for Atrial Fibrillation[1]	-	-	96%	95%
Antithrombotic Therapy Timing	14	93%	98%	98%
Assessed for Rehabilitation	14	93%	97%	97%
Discharged on Antithrombotic Therapy	13	69%	99%	99%
Discharged on Statin Medication	13	69%	95%	94%
Thrombolytic Therapy Timing[1]	-	-	69%	66%
Venous Thromboembolism Prophylaxis	15	80%	94%	94%
Written Stroke Educational Materials Given[1]	-	-	86%	88%
Surgical Care Improvement Project				
Appropriate Beta Blocker Usage	40	98%	97%	98%
Appropriate VTP Within 24 Hours	100	95%	98%	98%
Controlled Postoperative Blood Glucose[7]	-	-	97%	97%
Perioperative Temperature Management	110	92%	100%	100%
Prophylactic Antibiotic Selection	54	100%	99%	99%
Prophylactic Antibiotic Selection (Outpatient)	69	90%	97%	98%
Prophylactic Antibiotic Stopped	54	93%	98%	98%
Prophylactic Antibiotic Timing	54	96%	99%	99%
Prophylactic Antibiotic Timing (Outpatient)	74	82%	97%	98%
Urinary Catheter Removal	88	81%	96%	97%
Survey of Patients' Hospital Experiences				
Area Around Room 'Always' Quiet at Night	300+	46%	51%	61%
Doctors 'Always' Communicated Well	300+	71%	77%	82%
Home Recovery Information Given	300+	86%	83%	85%
Hospital Given 9 or 10 on 10 Point Scale	300+	56%	63%	71%
Meds 'Always' Explained Before Given	300+	59%	59%	64%
Nurses 'Always' Communicated Well	300+	72%	75%	79%
Pain 'Always' Well Controlled	300+	64%	67%	71%
Room and Bathroom 'Always' Clean	300+	69%	69%	73%
Timely Help 'Always' Received	300+	57%	61%	68%
Would Definitely Recommend Hospital	300+	57%	65%	71%
Use of Medical Imaging				
Cardiac Imaging Stress Test before Surgery	282	3.5%	5.8%	5.3%
Combination Abdominal CT Scan	376	7.7%	8.2%	10.5%
Combination Brain/Sinus CT Scan	424	5.2%	3.6%	2.7%
Combination Chest CT Scan	150	0.0%	1.3%	2.7%
Follow-up Mammogram/Ultrasound	807	3.0%	13%	8.8%
Lumbar Spine MRI for Low Back Pain	60	30.0%	33.4%	37.2%

NOTE: Hospital profiles are in alphabetical order by state, then city, then hospital within the city; Rankings exclude hospitals with less than 25 cases except for patient surveys which excludes hospitals with less than 100 cases; (a) 100-299 cases; (1) The number of cases/patients is too few to report; (2) Data submitted were based on a sample of cases/patients; (3) Results are based on a shorter time period than required; (4) Data suppressed by CMS for one or more quarters; (5) Results are not available for this reporting period; (6) Fewer than 100 patients completed the HCAHPS survey; (7) No cases met the criteria for this measure; (8) The lower limit of the confidence interval cannot be calculated if the number of observed infections equals zero; (9) No data are available from the state/territory for this reporting period; (10) The scores shown reflect fewer than 50 completed surveys; (11) There were discrepancies in the data collection process; (12) This measure does not apply to this hospital for this reporting period; (13) Results cannot be calculated for this reporting period; (14) The results for this state are combined with nearby states to protect confidentiality; Please refer to the User's Guide for a full explanation of data.

Oswego Hospital

110 West Sixth Street
Oswego, NY 13126
Phone: 315-349-5511
Fax: 315-349-5732
URL: www.oswegohealth.org
Type: Acute Care Hospitals
Emergency Services: Yes
Ownership: Voluntary non-profit - Private
Beds: 74

Key Personnel:
CEO/President. . . . . Ann C Gilpin
Radiology. . . . . Sudhir Guthikonda
Chief of Medical Staff. . . . . Patsy Iannolo, MD
Anesthesiology. . . . . Stanley Lubinga, MD
Emergency Room . . . . Michael Russell

Measure	Cases	This Hosp.	State Avg.	U.S. Avg.
Blood Clot Prevention and Treatment				
Anticoagulation Overlap Therapy[2]	21	90%	91%	93%
ICU Venous Thromboembolism Prophylaxis[2]	59	95%	92%	92%
Incidence of Potentially Preventable VTE[1,2]	-	-	10%	10%
UFH with Dosages/Platelet Monitoring[2]	23	96%	92%	97%
Venous Thromboembolism Prophylaxis[2]	336	93%	87%	85%
Warfarin Therapy Discharge Instructions[2]	15	87%	59%	75%
Chest Pain/Possible Heart Attack Care				
Aspirin Given Within 24 Hours of Arrival	119	93%	97%	96%
Fibrinolytic Meds Within 30 Min. of Arrival[1]	-	-	54%	58%
Average Time to ECG (minutes)	124	9	9	7
Average Time to Transfer (minutes)[1]	-	-	78	60
Children's Asthma Care				
Received Home Management Plan of Care	-	-	-	88%
Received Reliever Medication	-	-	-	100%
Received Systemic Corticosteroids	-	-	-	100%
Emergency Department				
Admittance Decision Time (minutes)[2]	563	189	154	98
Head CT Results Within 45 Min. of Arrival	11	45%	55%	57%
Patients Who Left ER Before Being Seen	25,742	4%	2%	2%
Time from ER Arrival to Admit. (minutes)[2]	573	392	378	274
Time from ER Arrival to Discharge (minutes)	337	177	156	134
Time in ER Before Being Evaluated (minutes)	356	27	35	26
Time to Pain Meds for Fractures (minutes)	57	74	61	57
Heart Attack Care				
Aspirin Given at Discharge	36	83%	99%	99%
Fibrinolytic Meds Within 30 Min. of Arrival[7]	-	-	46%	54%
PCI Within 90 Minutes of Arrival[7]	-	-	95%	96%
Statin Prescribed at Discharge	33	97%	98%	98%
Heart Failure Care				
ACE Inhibitor or ARB for LVSD	28	86%	96%	97%
Discharge Instructions Given	96	71%	95%	94%
Evaluation of LVS Function	126	100%	99%	99%
Medicare Spending				
Medicare Spending per Patient (ratio)	-	1.00	0.96	0.98
Pneumonia Care				
Appropriate Initial Antibiotic Given[2]	81	96%	95%	95%
Blood Culture Timing[2]	121	98%	97%	98%
Pregnancy and Delivery Care				
Newborn Deliveries Scheduled Early[2]	29	0%	4%	6%
Preventive Care				
Immunization for Influenza[2]	399	87%	88%	90%
Immunization for Pneumonia[2]	504	85%	88%	92%
Stroke Care				
Anticoagulation Therapy for Atrial Fibrillation[1]	-	-	96%	95%
Antithrombotic Therapy Timing	20	95%	98%	98%
Assessed for Rehabilitation	20	100%	97%	97%
Discharged on Antithrombotic Therapy	16	100%	99%	99%
Discharged on Statin Medication	15	67%	95%	94%
Thrombolytic Therapy Timing[1]	-	-	69%	66%
Venous Thromboembolism Prophylaxis	23	96%	94%	94%
Written Stroke Educational Materials Given[1]	-	-	86%	88%
Surgical Care Improvement Project				
Appropriate Beta Blocker Usage	37	92%	97%	98%
Appropriate VTP Within 24 Hours	157	96%	98%	98%
Controlled Postoperative Blood Glucose[7]	-	-	97%	97%
Perioperative Temperature Management	171	100%	100%	100%
Prophylactic Antibiotic Selection	103	99%	99%	99%
Prophylactic Antibiotic Selection (Outpatient)	104	99%	97%	98%
Prophylactic Antibiotic Stopped	97	96%	98%	98%
Prophylactic Antibiotic Timing	103	98%	99%	99%
Prophylactic Antibiotic Timing (Outpatient)	104	96%	97%	98%
Urinary Catheter Removal	68	96%	96%	97%
Survey of Patients' Hospital Experiences				
Area Around Room 'Always' Quiet at Night	300+	54%	51%	61%
Doctors 'Always' Communicated Well	300+	76%	77%	82%
Home Recovery Information Given	300+	88%	83%	85%
Hospital Given 9 or 10 on 10 Point Scale	300+	60%	63%	71%
Meds 'Always' Explained Before Given	300+	61%	59%	64%
Nurses 'Always' Communicated Well	300+	78%	75%	79%
Pain 'Always' Well Controlled	300+	68%	67%	71%
Room and Bathroom 'Always' Clean	300+	70%	69%	73%
Timely Help 'Always' Received	300+	60%	61%	68%
Would Definitely Recommend Hospital	300+	56%	65%	71%
Use of Medical Imaging				
Cardiac Imaging Stress Test before Surgery	253	4.0%	5.8%	5.3%
Combination Abdominal CT Scan	598	2.2%	8.2%	10.5%
Combination Brain/Sinus CT Scan	434	5.1%	3.6%	2.7%
Combination Chest CT Scan	456	2.0%	1.3%	2.7%
Follow-up Mammogram/Ultrasound	1,631	5.4%	13%	8.8%
Lumbar Spine MRI for Low Back Pain	70	32.9%	33.4%	37.2%

Brookhaven Memorial Hospital Medical Center

101 Hospital Road
Patchogue, NY 11772
Phone: 631-654-7100
Fax: 631-447-3714
E-mail: communityrelations@bmhmc.org
URL: www.brookhavenhospitalorg
Type: Acute Care Hospitals
Emergency Services: Yes
Ownership: Voluntary non-profit - Private
Beds: 321

Key Personnel:
Radiology. . . . . Scott Coyner
Pediatric Ambulatory Care . . . . . . Kenneth Huml, MD
Pediatric In-Patient Care . . . . Kenneth Huml, MD
CEO/President. . . . . Richard T. Margulis
Operating Room. . . . . Philip Messina
Quality Assurance . . . . Walter Metz
Chief of Medical Staff. . . . . Anthony J Shallash, MD
Infection Control. . . . . Doreen Virgil, RN

Measure	Cases	This Hosp.	State Avg.	U.S. Avg.
Blood Clot Prevention and Treatment				
Anticoagulation Overlap Therapy[2]	115	93%	91%	93%
ICU Venous Thromboembolism Prophylaxis[2]	99	95%	92%	92%
Incidence of Potentially Preventable VTE[2]	33	0%	10%	10%
UFH with Dosages/Platelet Monitoring[2]	84	100%	92%	97%
Venous Thromboembolism Prophylaxis[2]	539	93%	87%	85%
Warfarin Therapy Discharge Instructions[2]	76	83%	59%	75%
Chest Pain/Possible Heart Attack Care				
Aspirin Given Within 24 Hours of Arrival	72	99%	97%	96%
Fibrinolytic Meds Within 30 Min. of Arrival[1]	-	-	54%	58%
Average Time to ECG (minutes)	72	7	9	7
Average Time to Transfer (minutes)	31	63	78	60
Children's Asthma Care				
Received Home Management Plan of Care	-	-	-	88%
Received Reliever Medication	-	-	-	100%
Received Systemic Corticosteroids	-	-	-	100%
Emergency Department				
Admittance Decision Time (minutes)[2]	1,105	610	154	98
Head CT Results Within 45 Min. of Arrival	12	33%	55%	57%
Patients Who Left ER Before Being Seen	6,403	1%	2%	2%
Time from ER Arrival to Admit. (minutes)[2]	1,105	809	378	274
Time from ER Arrival to Discharge (minutes)	1,058	138	156	134
Time in ER Before Being Evaluated (minutes)	1,156	29	35	26
Time to Pain Meds for Fractures (minutes)	118	44	61	57
Heart Attack Care				
Aspirin Given at Discharge	83	100%	99%	99%
Fibrinolytic Meds Within 30 Min. of Arrival[7]	-	-	46%	54%
PCI Within 90 Minutes of Arrival[7]	-	-	95%	96%
Statin Prescribed at Discharge	82	99%	98%	98%
Heart Failure Care				
ACE Inhibitor or ARB for LVSD	78	97%	96%	97%
Discharge Instructions Given	311	95%	95%	94%
Evaluation of LVS Function	435	100%	99%	99%
Medicare Spending				
Medicare Spending per Patient (ratio)	-	1.06	0.96	0.98
Pneumonia Care				
Appropriate Initial Antibiotic Given	275	92%	95%	95%
Blood Culture Timing	575	96%	97%	98%
Pregnancy and Delivery Care				
Newborn Deliveries Scheduled Early[2,7]	-	-	4%	6%
Preventive Care				
Immunization for Influenza[2]	575	83%	88%	90%
Immunization for Pneumonia[2]	756	83%	88%	92%
Stroke Care				
Anticoagulation Therapy for Atrial Fibrillation[1]	-	-	96%	95%
Antithrombotic Therapy Timing	107	100%	98%	98%
Assessed for Rehabilitation	104	99%	97%	97%
Discharged on Antithrombotic Therapy	89	99%	99%	99%
Discharged on Statin Medication	67	96%	95%	94%
Thrombolytic Therapy Timing[1]	-	-	69%	66%
Venous Thromboembolism Prophylaxis	132	96%	94%	94%
Written Stroke Educational Materials Given	52	96%	86%	88%
Surgical Care Improvement Project				
Appropriate Beta Blocker Usage	82	95%	97%	98%
Appropriate VTP Within 24 Hours	228	92%	98%	98%
Controlled Postoperative Blood Glucose[7]	-	-	97%	97%
Perioperative Temperature Management	260	100%	100%	100%
Prophylactic Antibiotic Selection	95	96%	99%	99%
Prophylactic Antibiotic Selection (Outpatient)	53	100%	97%	98%
Prophylactic Antibiotic Stopped	88	92%	98%	98%
Prophylactic Antibiotic Timing	96	100%	99%	99%
Prophylactic Antibiotic Timing (Outpatient)	53	100%	97%	98%
Urinary Catheter Removal	183	87%	96%	97%
Survey of Patients' Hospital Experiences				
Area Around Room 'Always' Quiet at Night	300+	44%	51%	61%
Doctors 'Always' Communicated Well	300+	73%	77%	82%
Home Recovery Information Given	300+	84%	83%	85%
Hospital Given 9 or 10 on 10 Point Scale	300+	50%	63%	71%
Meds 'Always' Explained Before Given	300+	56%	59%	64%
Nurses 'Always' Communicated Well	300+	72%	75%	79%
Pain 'Always' Well Controlled	300+	65%	67%	71%
Room and Bathroom 'Always' Clean	300+	59%	69%	73%
Timely Help 'Always' Received	300+	54%	61%	68%
Would Definitely Recommend Hospital	300+	51%	65%	71%
Use of Medical Imaging				
Cardiac Imaging Stress Test before Surgery[1]	-	-	5.8%	5.3%
Combination Abdominal CT Scan	698	6.4%	8.2%	10.5%
Combination Brain/Sinus CT Scan	789	5.3%	3.6%	2.7%
Combination Chest CT Scan	434	4.6%	1.3%	2.7%
Follow-up Mammogram/Ultrasound	1,315	15.4%	13%	8.8%
Lumbar Spine MRI for Low Back Pain[1]	-	-	33.4%	37.2%

Soldiers & Sailors Memorial Hospital of Yates

418 North Main Street
Penn Yan, NY 14527
Phone: 315-787-4175
Fax: 315-531-2014
URL: www.flhealth.org
Type: Critical Access Hospitals
Emergency Services: Yes
Ownership: Voluntary non-profit - Private
Beds: 186

Key Personnel:
Chief of Medical Staff. . . . . Jose Acevedo, MD
President/CEO. . . . . Jose Acevedo, MD, MBA
Quality Assurance . . . . Sally Bittner
Infection Control. . . . . Marge Brinn, RN
Emergency Room . . . . Deb McCaig, RN, BSN
Operating Room. . . . . Cindy Presher
Radiology. . . . . Rodolfo Queiroz
Intensive Care Unit. . . . . Kelley Stout

Measure	Cases	This Hosp.	State Avg.	U.S. Avg.
Blood Clot Prevention and Treatment				
Anticoagulation Overlap Therapy[1,2]	-	-	91%	93%
ICU Venous Thromboembolism Prophylaxis[2]	29	90%	92%	92%
Incidence of Potentially Preventable VTE[1,2]	-	-	10%	10%
UFH with Dosages/Platelet Monitoring[1,2]	-	-	92%	97%
Venous Thromboembolism Prophylaxis[2]	86	90%	87%	85%
Warfarin Therapy Discharge Instructions[2,7]	-	-	59%	75%
Chest Pain/Possible Heart Attack Care				
Aspirin Given Within 24 Hours of Arrival	23	100%	97%	96%
Fibrinolytic Meds Within 30 Min. of Arrival[1,3]	-	-	54%	58%
Average Time to ECG (minutes)	23	9	9	7

NOTE: Hospital profiles are in alphabetical order by state, then city, then hospital within the city; Rankings exclude hospitals with less than 25 cases except for patient surveys which excludes hospitals with less than 100 cases; (a) 100-299 cases; (1) The number of cases/patients is too few to report; (2) Data submitted were based on a sample of cases/patients; (3) Results are based on a shorter time period than required; (4) Data suppressed by CMS for one or more quarters; (5) Results are not available for this reporting period; (6) Fewer than 100 patients completed the HCAHPS survey; (7) No cases met the criteria for this measure; (8) The lower limit of the confidence interval cannot be calculated if the number of observed infections equals zero; (9) No data are available from the state/territory for this reporting period; (10) The scores shown reflect fewer than 50 completed surveys; (11) There were discrepancies in the data collection process; (12) This measure does not apply to this hospital for this reporting period; (13) Results cannot be calculated for this reporting period; (14) The results for this state are combined with nearby states to protect confidentiality; Please refer to the User's Guide for a full explanation of data.

Measure	Cases	This Hosp.	State Avg.	U.S. Avg.
Average Time to Transfer (minutes)[1,3]	-	-	78	60
Children's Asthma Care				
Received Home Management Plan of Care	-	-	-	88%
Received Reliever Medication	-	-	-	100%
Received Systemic Corticosteroids	-	-	-	100%
Emergency Department				
Admittance Decision Time (minutes)[2]	341	90	154	98
Head CT Results Within 45 Min. of Arrival[1,3]	-	-	55%	57%
Patients Who Left ER Before Being Seen	8,487	0%	2%	2%
Time from ER Arrival to Admit. (minutes)[2]	383	225	378	274
Time from ER Arrival to Discharge (minutes)	324	106	156	134
Time in ER Before Being Evaluated (minutes)	319	21	35	26
Time to Pain Meds for Fractures (minutes)	32	31	61	57
Heart Attack Care				
Aspirin Given at Discharge[1]	-	-	99%	99%
Fibrinolytic Meds Within 30 Min. of Arrival[7]	-	-	46%	54%
PCI Within 90 Minutes of Arrival[7]	-	-	95%	96%
Statin Prescribed at Discharge[1]	-	-	98%	98%
Heart Failure Care				
ACE Inhibitor or ARB for LVSD[1]	-	-	96%	97%
Discharge Instructions Given	28	96%	95%	94%
Evaluation of LVS Function	37	100%	99%	99%
Medicare Spending				
Medicare Spending per Patient (ratio)	-	-	0.96	0.98
Pneumonia Care				
Appropriate Initial Antibiotic Given	33	97%	95%	95%
Blood Culture Timing	60	95%	97%	98%
Pregnancy and Delivery Care				
Newborn Deliveries Scheduled Early[7]	-	-	4%	6%
Preventive Care				
Immunization for Influenza[2]	264	92%	88%	90%
Immunization for Pneumonia[2]	379	92%	88%	92%
Stroke Care				
Anticoagulation Therapy for Atrial Fibrillation[5]	-	-	96%	95%
Antithrombotic Therapy Timing[5]	-	-	98%	98%
Assessed for Rehabilitation[5]	-	-	97%	97%
Discharged on Antithrombotic Therapy[5]	-	-	99%	99%
Discharged on Statin Medication[5]	-	-	95%	94%
Thrombolytic Therapy Timing[5]	-	-	69%	66%
Venous Thromboembolism Prophylaxis[5]	-	-	94%	94%
Written Stroke Educational Materials Given[5]	-	-	86%	88%
Surgical Care Improvement Project				
Appropriate Beta Blocker Usage[5]	-	-	97%	98%
Appropriate VTP Within 24 Hours[5]	-	-	98%	98%
Controlled Postoperative Blood Glucose[5]	-	-	97%	97%
Perioperative Temperature Management[5]	-	-	100%	100%
Prophylactic Antibiotic Selection[5]	-	-	99%	99%
Prophylactic Antibiotic Selection (Outpatient)[5]	-	-	97%	98%
Prophylactic Antibiotic Stopped[5]	-	-	98%	98%
Prophylactic Antibiotic Timing[5]	-	-	99%	99%
Prophylactic Antibiotic Timing (Outpatient)[5]	-	-	97%	98%
Urinary Catheter Removal[5]	-	-	96%	97%
Survey of Patients' Hospital Experiences				
Area Around Room 'Always' Quiet at Night	(a)	65%	51%	61%
Doctors 'Always' Communicated Well	(a)	81%	77%	82%
Home Recovery Information Given	(a)	93%	83%	85%
Hospital Given 9 or 10 on 10 Point Scale	(a)	72%	63%	71%
Meds 'Always' Explained Before Given	(a)	63%	59%	64%
Nurses 'Always' Communicated Well	(a)	79%	75%	79%
Pain 'Always' Well Controlled	(a)	72%	67%	71%
Room and Bathroom 'Always' Clean	(a)	86%	69%	73%
Timely Help 'Always' Received	(a)	80%	61%	68%
Would Definitely Recommend Hospital	(a)	64%	65%	71%
Use of Medical Imaging				
Cardiac Imaging Stress Test before Surgery[1]	-	-	5.8%	5.3%
Combination Abdominal CT Scan	173	3.5%	8.2%	10.5%
Combination Brain/Sinus CT Scan[1]	-	-	3.6%	2.7%
Combination Chest CT Scan	66	0.0%	1.3%	2.7%
Follow-up Mammogram/Ultrasound	305	9.8%	13%	8.8%
Lumbar Spine MRI for Low Back Pain[7]	-	-	33.4%	37.2%

Plainview Hospital

888 Old Country Road
Plainview, NY 11803
Phone: 516-719-3000
Fax: 516-719-2729
URL: www.nslij.com
Type: Acute Care Hospitals
Emergency Services: Yes
Ownership: Voluntary non-profit - Private
Beds: 239

Key Personnel:
CEO/President . . . . Michael J Dowling
Pediatric Ambulatory Care . . . . . . James Fagin, MD
Coronary Care . . . . Kathleen Gallo, RN PhD
Radiology. . . . . Howard Heimowitz, MD
Quality Assurance . . . . Jeffrey A Kraut
Patient Relations . . . . Sylvia Lester
Operating Room. . . . . Linda Olander, RN

Measure	Cases	This Hosp.	State Avg.	U.S. Avg.
Blood Clot Prevention and Treatment				
Anticoagulation Overlap Therapy[2]	92	80%	91%	93%
ICU Venous Thromboembolism Prophylaxis[2]	57	88%	92%	92%
Incidence of Potentially Preventable VTE[2]	31	6%	10%	10%
UFH with Dosages/Platelet Monitoring[2]	12	100%	92%	97%
Venous Thromboembolism Prophylaxis[2]	359	76%	87%	85%
Warfarin Therapy Discharge Instructions[2]	63	13%	59%	75%
Chest Pain/Possible Heart Attack Care				
Aspirin Given Within 24 Hours of Arrival	87	100%	97%	96%
Fibrinolytic Meds Within 30 Min. of Arrival[7]	-	-	54%	58%
Average Time to ECG (minutes)	92	10	9	7
Average Time to Transfer (minutes)	32	56	78	60
Children's Asthma Care				
Received Home Management Plan of Care	-	-	-	88%
Received Reliever Medication	-	-	-	100%
Received Systemic Corticosteroids	-	-	-	100%
Emergency Department				
Admittance Decision Time (minutes)[2]	312	202	154	98
Head CT Results Within 45 Min. of Arrival	17	71%	55%	57%
Patients Who Left ER Before Being Seen	35,043	1%	2%	2%
Time from ER Arrival to Admit. (minutes)[2]	332	390	378	274
Time from ER Arrival to Discharge (minutes)	375	159	156	134
Time in ER Before Being Evaluated (minutes)	362	25	35	26
Time to Pain Meds for Fractures (minutes)	76	55	61	57
Heart Attack Care				
Aspirin Given at Discharge[2]	57	98%	99%	99%
Fibrinolytic Meds Within 30 Min. of Arrival[2,7]	-	-	46%	54%
PCI Within 90 Minutes of Arrival[2,7]	-	-	95%	96%
Statin Prescribed at Discharge[2]	51	88%	98%	98%
Heart Failure Care				
ACE Inhibitor or ARB for LVSD[2]	45	91%	96%	97%
Discharge Instructions Given[2]	192	90%	95%	94%
Evaluation of LVS Function[2]	261	100%	99%	99%
Medicare Spending				
Medicare Spending per Patient (ratio)	-	1.05	0.96	0.98
Pneumonia Care				
Appropriate Initial Antibiotic Given[2]	87	93%	95%	95%
Blood Culture Timing[2]	161	98%	97%	98%
Pregnancy and Delivery Care				
Newborn Deliveries Scheduled Early[2]	13	0%	4%	6%
Preventive Care				
Immunization for Influenza[2]	553	91%	88%	90%
Immunization for Pneumonia[2]	730	85%	88%	92%
Stroke Care				
Anticoagulation Therapy for Atrial Fibrillation[2]	20	90%	96%	95%
Antithrombotic Therapy Timing[2]	78	100%	98%	98%
Assessed for Rehabilitation[2]	88	92%	97%	97%
Discharged on Antithrombotic Therapy[2]	83	98%	99%	99%
Discharged on Statin Medication[2]	69	96%	95%	94%
Thrombolytic Therapy Timing[1,2]	-	-	69%	66%
Venous Thromboembolism Prophylaxis[2]	90	93%	94%	94%
Written Stroke Educational Materials Given[2]	34	97%	86%	88%
Surgical Care Improvement Project				
Appropriate Beta Blocker Usage[2]	129	95%	97%	98%
Appropriate VTP Within 24 Hours[2]	317	99%	98%	98%
Controlled Postoperative Blood Glucose[2,7]	-	-	97%	97%
Perioperative Temperature Management[2]	400	100%	100%	100%
Prophylactic Antibiotic Selection[2]	228	99%	99%	99%
Prophylactic Antibiotic Selection (Outpatient)	89	96%	97%	98%
Prophylactic Antibiotic Stopped[2]	225	99%	98%	98%
Prophylactic Antibiotic Timing[2]	228	99%	99%	99%
Prophylactic Antibiotic Timing (Outpatient)	92	96%	97%	98%
Urinary Catheter Removal[2]	207	97%	96%	97%
Survey of Patients' Hospital Experiences				
Area Around Room 'Always' Quiet at Night[11]	300+	41%	51%	61%
Doctors 'Always' Communicated Well[11]	300+	82%	77%	82%
Home Recovery Information Given[11]	300+	78%	83%	85%
Hospital Given 9 or 10 on 10 Point Scale[11]	300+	63%	63%	71%
Meds 'Always' Explained Before Given[11]	300+	60%	59%	64%
Nurses 'Always' Communicated Well[11]	300+	79%	75%	79%
Pain 'Always' Well Controlled[11]	300+	73%	67%	71%
Room and Bathroom 'Always' Clean[11]	300+	67%	69%	73%
Timely Help 'Always' Received[11]	300+	67%	61%	68%
Would Definitely Recommend Hospital[11]	300+	63%	65%	71%
Use of Medical Imaging				
Cardiac Imaging Stress Test before Surgery[7]	-	-	5.8%	5.3%
Combination Abdominal CT Scan	381	1.0%	8.2%	10.5%
Combination Brain/Sinus CT Scan[1]	-	-	3.6%	2.7%
Combination Chest CT Scan	78	1.3%	1.3%	2.7%
Follow-up Mammogram/Ultrasound[7]	-	-	13%	8.8%
Lumbar Spine MRI for Low Back Pain[1]	-	-	33.4%	37.2%

Champlain Valley Physicians Hospital Medical Center

75 Beekman Street
Plattsburgh, NY 12901
Phone: 518-561-2000
Fax: 518-562-7302
URL: www.cvph.org
Type: Acute Care Hospitals
Emergency Services: Yes
Ownership: Voluntary non-profit - Private
Beds: 405

Key Personnel:
Chief of Medical Staff . . . . Kent Hall, MD
Radiology. . . . . Gary King
CEO/President. . . . . Stephens M Mundy

Measure	Cases	This Hosp.	State Avg.	U.S. Avg.
Blood Clot Prevention and Treatment				
Anticoagulation Overlap Therapy[2]	86	94%	91%	93%
ICU Venous Thromboembolism Prophylaxis[2]	70	94%	92%	92%
Incidence of Potentially Preventable VTE[1,2]	-	-	10%	10%
UFH with Dosages/Platelet Monitoring[2]	75	97%	92%	97%
Venous Thromboembolism Prophylaxis[2]	419	90%	87%	85%
Warfarin Therapy Discharge Instructions[2]	75	85%	59%	75%
Chest Pain/Possible Heart Attack Care				
Aspirin Given Within 24 Hours of Arrival[1]	-	-	97%	96%
Fibrinolytic Meds Within 30 Min. of Arrival[3,7]	-	-	54%	58%
Average Time to ECG (minutes)[1]	-	-	9	7
Average Time to Transfer (minutes)[3,7]	-	-	78	60
Children's Asthma Care				
Received Home Management Plan of Care	-	-	-	88%
Received Reliever Medication	-	-	-	100%
Received Systemic Corticosteroids	-	-	-	100%
Emergency Department				
Admittance Decision Time (minutes)[2]	586	125	154	98
Head CT Results Within 45 Min. of Arrival	16	50%	55%	57%
Patients Who Left ER Before Being Seen	51,029	1%	2%	2%
Time from ER Arrival to Admit. (minutes)[2]	607	320	378	274
Time from ER Arrival to Discharge (minutes)	531	134	156	134
Time in ER Before Being Evaluated (minutes)	549	42	35	26
Time to Pain Meds for Fractures (minutes)	111	63	61	57
Heart Attack Care				
Aspirin Given at Discharge	360	99%	99%	99%
Fibrinolytic Meds Within 30 Min. of Arrival[7]	-	-	46%	54%
PCI Within 90 Minutes of Arrival	33	91%	95%	96%
Statin Prescribed at Discharge	341	96%	98%	98%
Heart Failure Care				
ACE Inhibitor or ARB for LVSD	45	93%	96%	97%
Discharge Instructions Given	233	97%	95%	94%
Evaluation of LVS Function	283	100%	99%	99%
Medicare Spending				
Medicare Spending per Patient (ratio)	-	0.91	0.96	0.98
Pneumonia Care				
Appropriate Initial Antibiotic Given	144	99%	95%	95%
Blood Culture Timing	322	97%	97%	98%

NOTE: Hospital profiles are in alphabetical order by state, then city, then hospital within the city; Rankings exclude hospitals with less than 25 cases except for patient surveys which excludes hospitals with less than 100 cases; (a) 100-299 cases; (1) The number of cases/patients is too few to report; (2) Data submitted were based on a sample of cases/patients; (3) Results are based on a shorter time period than required; (4) Data suppressed by CMS for one or more quarters; (5) Results are not available for this reporting period; (6) Fewer than 100 patients completed the HCAHPS survey; (7) No cases met the criteria for this measure; (8) The lower limit of the confidence interval cannot be calculated if the number of observed infections equals zero; (9) No data are available from the state/territory for this reporting period; (10) The scores shown reflect fewer than 50 completed surveys; (11) There were discrepancies in the data collection process; (12) This measure does not apply to this hospital for this reporting period; (13) Results cannot be calculated for this reporting period; (14) The results for this state are combined with nearby states to protect confidentiality; Please refer to the User's Guide for a full explanation of data.

Pregnancy and Delivery Care				
Newborn Deliveries Scheduled Early[2]	17	18%	4%	6%
Preventive Care				
Immunization for Influenza[2]	600	86%	88%	90%
Immunization for Pneumonia[2]	740	90%	88%	92%
Stroke Care				
Anticoagulation Therapy for Atrial Fibrillation	11	100%	96%	95%
Antithrombotic Therapy Timing	74	100%	98%	98%
Assessed for Rehabilitation	73	96%	97%	97%
Discharged on Antithrombotic Therapy	72	99%	99%	99%
Discharged on Statin Medication	59	90%	95%	94%
Thrombolytic Therapy Timing[1]	-	-	69%	66%
Venous Thromboembolism Prophylaxis	82	93%	94%	94%
Written Stroke Educational Materials Given	38	63%	86%	88%
Surgical Care Improvement Project				
Appropriate Beta Blocker Usage[2]	261	98%	97%	98%
Appropriate VTP Within 24 Hours[2]	442	98%	98%	98%
Controlled Postoperative Blood Glucose[2]	100	97%	97%	97%
Perioperative Temperature Management[2]	564	100%	100%	100%
Prophylactic Antibiotic Selection[2]	489	99%	99%	99%
Prophylactic Antibiotic Selection (Outpatient)	432	98%	97%	98%
Prophylactic Antibiotic Stopped[2]	477	99%	98%	98%
Prophylactic Antibiotic Timing[2]	490	99%	99%	99%
Prophylactic Antibiotic Timing (Outpatient)	435	98%	97%	98%
Urinary Catheter Removal[2]	515	97%	96%	97%
Survey of Patients' Hospital Experiences				
Area Around Room 'Always' Quiet at Night	300+	46%	51%	61%
Doctors 'Always' Communicated Well	300+	80%	77%	82%
Home Recovery Information Given	300+	86%	83%	85%
Hospital Given 9 or 10 on 10 Point Scale	300+	57%	63%	71%
Meds 'Always' Explained Before Given	300+	60%	59%	64%
Nurses 'Always' Communicated Well	300+	80%	75%	79%
Pain 'Always' Well Controlled	300+	71%	67%	71%
Room and Bathroom 'Always' Clean	300+	71%	69%	73%
Timely Help 'Always' Received	300+	68%	61%	68%
Would Definitely Recommend Hospital	300+	65%	65%	71%
Use of Medical Imaging				
Cardiac Imaging Stress Test before Surgery	601	3.3%	5.8%	5.3%
Combination Abdominal CT Scan	1,163	4.0%	8.2%	10.5%
Combination Brain/Sinus CT Scan	786	2.3%	3.6%	2.7%
Combination Chest CT Scan	989	0.2%	1.3%	2.7%
Follow-up Mammogram/Ultrasound	2,587	8.0%	13%	8.8%
Lumbar Spine MRI for Low Back Pain	154	33.8%	33.4%	37.2%

John T Mather Memorial Hospital of Port Jefferson

75 North Country Road Phone: 631-473-1320
Port Jefferson, NY 11777 Fax: 631-473-7367
E-mail: publicaffairs@matherhospital.org
URL: www.matherhospital.com
Type: Acute Care Hospitals Emergency Services: Yes
Ownership: Voluntary non-profit - Private Beds: 248

Key Personnel:
Radiology. . . . . Huntley Alper, MD
Pediatric Ambulatory Care . . . . . . Martin Kaplan, MD
Pediatric In-Patient Care . . . . Martin Kaplan, MD
Operating Room. . . . . Colleen McCloy
Quality Assurance . . . . Kevin Murray
Emergency Room . . . . Mitchell Pollack
President . . . . Kenneth D. Roberts
Chief of Medical Staff . . . . Richard Savino, MD

Measure	Cases	This Hosp.	State Avg.	U.S. Avg.
Blood Clot Prevention and Treatment				
Anticoagulation Overlap Therapy[2]	95	95%	91%	93%
ICU Venous Thromboembolism Prophylaxis[2]	82	98%	92%	92%
Incidence of Potentially Preventable VTE[2]	18	6%	10%	10%
UFH with Dosages/Platelet Monitoring[2]	57	100%	92%	97%
Venous Thromboembolism Prophylaxis[2]	401	84%	87%	85%
Warfarin Therapy Discharge Instructions[2]	75	91%	59%	75%
Chest Pain/Possible Heart Attack Care				
Aspirin Given Within 24 Hours of Arrival	99	100%	97%	96%
Fibrinolytic Meds Within 30 Min. of Arrival[7]	-	-	54%	58%
Average Time to ECG (minutes)	101	5	9	7
Average Time to Transfer (minutes)	36	60	78	60
Children's Asthma Care				
Received Home Management Plan of Care	-	-	-	88%
Received Reliever Medication	-	-	-	100%
Received Systemic Corticosteroids	-	-	-	100%
Emergency Department				
Admittance Decision Time (minutes)[2]	1,110	284	154	98
Head CT Results Within 45 Min. of Arrival	11	91%	55%	57%
Patients Who Left ER Before Being Seen	43,467	0%	2%	2%
Time from ER Arrival to Admit. (minutes)[2]	1,110	540	378	274
Time from ER Arrival to Discharge (minutes)	369	196	156	134
Time in ER Before Being Evaluated (minutes)	414	7	35	26
Time to Pain Meds for Fractures (minutes)	94	58	61	57
Heart Attack Care				
Aspirin Given at Discharge	60	100%	99%	99%
Fibrinolytic Meds Within 30 Min. of Arrival[7]	-	-	46%	54%
PCI Within 90 Minutes of Arrival[7]	-	-	95%	96%
Statin Prescribed at Discharge	59	100%	98%	98%
Heart Failure Care				
ACE Inhibitor or ARB for LVSD	47	100%	96%	97%
Discharge Instructions Given	239	99%	95%	94%
Evaluation of LVS Function	356	99%	99%	99%
Medicare Spending				
Medicare Spending per Patient (ratio)	-	0.99	0.96	0.98
Pneumonia Care				
Appropriate Initial Antibiotic Given	208	98%	95%	95%
Blood Culture Timing	384	98%	97%	98%
Pregnancy and Delivery Care				
Newborn Deliveries Scheduled Early[7]	-	-	4%	6%
Preventive Care				
Immunization for Influenza[2]	602	97%	88%	90%
Immunization for Pneumonia[2]	885	94%	88%	92%
Stroke Care				
Anticoagulation Therapy for Atrial Fibrillation	17	100%	96%	95%
Antithrombotic Therapy Timing	96	95%	98%	98%
Assessed for Rehabilitation	106	99%	97%	97%
Discharged on Antithrombotic Therapy	101	100%	99%	99%
Discharged on Statin Medication	73	97%	95%	94%
Thrombolytic Therapy Timing	18	61%	69%	66%
Venous Thromboembolism Prophylaxis	115	97%	94%	94%
Written Stroke Educational Materials Given	61	97%	86%	88%
Surgical Care Improvement Project				
Appropriate Beta Blocker Usage	168	99%	97%	98%
Appropriate VTP Within 24 Hours	325	100%	98%	98%
Controlled Postoperative Blood Glucose[7]	-	-	97%	97%
Perioperative Temperature Management	417	100%	100%	100%
Prophylactic Antibiotic Selection	208	99%	99%	99%
Prophylactic Antibiotic Selection (Outpatient)	149	99%	97%	98%
Prophylactic Antibiotic Stopped	206	99%	98%	98%
Prophylactic Antibiotic Timing	210	99%	99%	99%
Prophylactic Antibiotic Timing (Outpatient)	147	100%	97%	98%
Urinary Catheter Removal	145	100%	96%	97%
Survey of Patients' Hospital Experiences				
Area Around Room 'Always' Quiet at Night	300+	49%	51%	61%
Doctors 'Always' Communicated Well	300+	79%	77%	82%
Home Recovery Information Given	300+	90%	83%	85%
Hospital Given 9 or 10 on 10 Point Scale	300+	74%	63%	71%
Meds 'Always' Explained Before Given	300+	61%	59%	64%
Nurses 'Always' Communicated Well	300+	81%	75%	79%
Pain 'Always' Well Controlled	300+	71%	67%	71%
Room and Bathroom 'Always' Clean	300+	68%	69%	73%
Timely Help 'Always' Received	300+	70%	61%	68%
Would Definitely Recommend Hospital	300+	78%	65%	71%
Use of Medical Imaging				
Cardiac Imaging Stress Test before Surgery	327	4.9%	5.8%	5.3%
Combination Abdominal CT Scan	874	2.4%	8.2%	10.5%
Combination Brain/Sinus CT Scan	721	4.2%	3.6%	2.7%
Combination Chest CT Scan	678	0.6%	1.3%	2.7%
Follow-up Mammogram/Ultrasound	2,020	50.0%	13%	8.8%
Lumbar Spine MRI for Low Back Pain[1]	-	-	33.4%	37.2%

Saint Charles Hospital

200 Belle Terre Road Phone: 631-474-6000
Port Jefferson, NY 11777 Fax: 631-474-6824
URL: www.stcharles.org
Type: Acute Care Hospitals Emergency Services: Yes
Ownership: Voluntary non-profit - Church Beds: 231

Key Personnel:
Operating Room. . . . . Margaret Fischer
CEO/President. . . . . Alan Guerci, MD
Pediatric Ambulatory Care . . . . . . Harvey Kolker, MD
Pediatric In-Patient Care . . . . Harvey Kolker, MD
Quality Assurance . . . . Dante Latorre
Chief of Medical Staff . . . . Patrick M. O'Shaughnessy, DO
Radiology. . . . . Albert Trachtenberg, MD
Patient Relations . . . . Debra Vion

Measure	Cases	This Hosp.	State Avg.	U.S. Avg.
Blood Clot Prevention and Treatment				
Anticoagulation Overlap Therapy[2]	41	100%	91%	93%
ICU Venous Thromboembolism Prophylaxis[2]	91	98%	92%	92%
Incidence of Potentially Preventable VTE[2]	11	9%	10%	10%
UFH with Dosages/Platelet Monitoring[2]	17	100%	92%	97%
Venous Thromboembolism Prophylaxis[2]	337	96%	87%	85%
Warfarin Therapy Discharge Instructions[2]	25	100%	59%	75%
Chest Pain/Possible Heart Attack Care				
Aspirin Given Within 24 Hours of Arrival	11	100%	97%	96%
Fibrinolytic Meds Within 30 Min. of Arrival[3,7]	-	-	54%	58%
Average Time to ECG (minutes)	12	16	9	7
Average Time to Transfer (minutes)[1,3]	-	-	78	60
Children's Asthma Care				
Received Home Management Plan of Care	-	-	-	88%
Received Reliever Medication	-	-	-	100%
Received Systemic Corticosteroids	-	-	-	100%
Emergency Department				
Admittance Decision Time (minutes)[2]	329	359	154	98
Head CT Results Within 45 Min. of Arrival[3,7]	-	-	55%	57%
Patients Who Left ER Before Being Seen	22,881	1%	2%	2%
Time from ER Arrival to Admit. (minutes)[2]	464	580	378	274
Time from ER Arrival to Discharge (minutes)	386	152	156	134
Time in ER Before Being Evaluated (minutes)	382	40	35	26
Time to Pain Meds for Fractures (minutes)	139	73	61	57
Heart Attack Care				
Aspirin Given at Discharge	26	100%	99%	99%
Fibrinolytic Meds Within 30 Min. of Arrival[7]	-	-	46%	54%
PCI Within 90 Minutes of Arrival[7]	-	-	95%	96%
Statin Prescribed at Discharge	21	100%	98%	98%
Heart Failure Care				
ACE Inhibitor or ARB for LVSD[1]	-	-	96%	97%
Discharge Instructions Given	54	100%	95%	94%
Evaluation of LVS Function	53	100%	99%	99%
Medicare Spending				
Medicare Spending per Patient (ratio)	-	1.03	0.96	0.98
Pneumonia Care				
Appropriate Initial Antibiotic Given	60	98%	95%	95%
Blood Culture Timing	132	98%	97%	98%
Pregnancy and Delivery Care				
Newborn Deliveries Scheduled Early[2]	19	0%	4%	6%
Preventive Care				
Immunization for Influenza[2]	505	89%	88%	90%
Immunization for Pneumonia[2]	453	81%	88%	92%
Stroke Care				
Anticoagulation Therapy for Atrial Fibrillation[1]	-	-	96%	95%
Antithrombotic Therapy Timing	28	100%	98%	98%
Assessed for Rehabilitation	34	100%	97%	97%
Discharged on Antithrombotic Therapy	29	100%	99%	99%
Discharged on Statin Medication	21	100%	95%	94%
Thrombolytic Therapy Timing[1]	-	-	69%	66%
Venous Thromboembolism Prophylaxis	36	97%	94%	94%
Written Stroke Educational Materials Given	17	100%	86%	88%
Surgical Care Improvement Project				
Appropriate Beta Blocker Usage[2]	187	100%	97%	98%
Appropriate VTP Within 24 Hours[2]	590	100%	98%	98%
Controlled Postoperative Blood Glucose[2,7]	-	-	97%	97%
Perioperative Temperature Management[2]	616	100%	100%	100%
Prophylactic Antibiotic Selection[2]	459	100%	99%	99%

NOTE: Hospital profiles are in alphabetical order by state, then city, then hospital within the city; Rankings exclude hospitals with less than 25 cases except for patient surveys which excludes hospitals with less than 100 cases; (a) 100-299 cases; (1) The number of cases/patients is too few to report; (2) Data submitted were based on a sample of cases/patients; (3) Results are based on a shorter time period than required; (4) Data suppressed by CMS for one or more quarters; (5) Results are not available for this reporting period; (6) Fewer than 100 patients completed the HCAHPS survey; (7) No cases met the criteria for this measure; (8) The lower limit of the confidence interval cannot be calculated if the number of observed infections equals zero; (9) No data are available from the state/territory for this reporting period; (10) The scores shown reflect fewer than 50 completed surveys; (11) There were discrepancies in the data collection process; (12) This measure does not apply to this hospital for this reporting period; (13) Results cannot be calculated for this reporting period; (14) The results for this state are combined with nearby states to protect confidentiality; Please refer to the User's Guide for a full explanation of data.

Measure	Cases	This Hosp.	State Avg.	U.S. Avg.
Prophylactic Antibiotic Selection (Outpatient)	157	99%	97%	98%
Prophylactic Antibiotic Stopped[2]	449	100%	98%	98%
Prophylactic Antibiotic Timing[2]	459	100%	99%	99%
Prophylactic Antibiotic Timing (Outpatient)	157	99%	97%	98%
Urinary Catheter Removal[2]	479	100%	96%	97%
Survey of Patients' Hospital Experiences				
Area Around Room 'Always' Quiet at Night	300+	46%	51%	61%
Doctors 'Always' Communicated Well	300+	79%	77%	82%
Home Recovery Information Given	300+	85%	83%	85%
Hospital Given 9 or 10 on 10 Point Scale	300+	67%	63%	71%
Meds 'Always' Explained Before Given	300+	62%	59%	64%
Nurses 'Always' Communicated Well	300+	76%	75%	79%
Pain 'Always' Well Controlled	300+	70%	67%	71%
Room and Bathroom 'Always' Clean	300+	70%	69%	73%
Timely Help 'Always' Received	300+	60%	61%	68%
Would Definitely Recommend Hospital	300+	75%	65%	71%
Use of Medical Imaging				
Cardiac Imaging Stress Test before Surgery	77	6.5%	5.8%	5.3%
Combination Abdominal CT Scan	199	4.5%	8.2%	10.5%
Combination Brain/Sinus CT Scan[1]	-	-	3.6%	2.7%
Combination Chest CT Scan	148	1.4%	1.3%	2.7%
Follow-up Mammogram/Ultrasound	346	28.9%	13%	8.8%
Lumbar Spine MRI for Low Back Pain[1]	-	-	33.4%	37.2%

Bon Secours Community Hospital

160 East Main Street Phone: 845-856-5351
Port Jervis, NY 12771 Fax: 845-858-7415
URL: www.bonsecourscommunityhosp.com
Type: Acute Care Hospitals Emergency Services: Yes
Ownership: Voluntary non-profit - Church Beds: 183

Key Personnel:
Cardiac Laboratory............ Fradrick Ayers
Radiology.................... Rachael Braunstein
Chief of Medical Staff.......... Richard J Daboul
Emergency Room .... David Israel
CEO .... Mary Leahy, M.D.

Measure	Cases	This Hosp.	State Avg.	U.S. Avg.
Blood Clot Prevention and Treatment				
Anticoagulation Overlap Therapy[2]	21	95%	91%	93%
ICU Venous Thromboembolism Prophylaxis[2]	45	98%	92%	92%
Incidence of Potentially Preventable VTE[1,2]	-	-	10%	10%
UFH with Dosages/Platelet Monitoring[2]	17	100%	92%	97%
Venous Thromboembolism Prophylaxis[2]	266	95%	87%	85%
Warfarin Therapy Discharge Instructions[2]	14	93%	59%	75%
Chest Pain/Possible Heart Attack Care				
Aspirin Given Within 24 Hours of Arrival	60	95%	97%	96%
Fibrinolytic Meds Within 30 Min. of Arrival	12	67%	54%	58%
Average Time to ECG (minutes)	62	12	9	7
Average Time to Transfer (minutes)[1]	-	-	78	60
Children's Asthma Care				
Received Home Management Plan of Care	-	-	-	88%
Received Reliever Medication	-	-	-	100%
Received Systemic Corticosteroids	-	-	-	100%
Emergency Department				
Admittance Decision Time (minutes)[2]	472	94	154	98
Head CT Results Within 45 Min. of Arrival[1,3]	-	-	55%	57%
Patients Who Left ER Before Being Seen	27,558	0%	2%	2%
Time from ER Arrival to Admit. (minutes)[2]	476	274	378	274
Time from ER Arrival to Discharge (minutes)	399	95	156	134
Time in ER Before Being Evaluated (minutes)	444	13	35	26
Time to Pain Meds for Fractures (minutes)	65	55	61	57
Heart Attack Care				
Aspirin Given at Discharge[1]	-	-	99%	99%
Fibrinolytic Meds Within 30 Min. of Arrival[7]	-	-	46%	54%
PCI Within 90 Minutes of Arrival[7]	-	-	95%	96%
Statin Prescribed at Discharge[1]	-	-	98%	98%
Heart Failure Care				
ACE Inhibitor or ARB for LVSD	22	100%	96%	97%
Discharge Instructions Given	85	100%	95%	94%
Evaluation of LVS Function	107	97%	99%	99%
Medicare Spending				
Medicare Spending per Patient (ratio)	-	0.93	0.96	0.98
Pneumonia Care				
Appropriate Initial Antibiotic Given	104	97%	95%	95%
Blood Culture Timing	164	98%	97%	98%
Pregnancy and Delivery Care				
Newborn Deliveries Scheduled Early[7]	-	-	4%	6%
Preventive Care				
Immunization for Influenza[2]	362	94%	88%	90%
Immunization for Pneumonia[2]	430	91%	88%	92%
Stroke Care				
Anticoagulation Therapy for Atrial Fibrillation[1]	-	-	96%	95%
Antithrombotic Therapy Timing	19	100%	98%	98%
Assessed for Rehabilitation	13	100%	97%	97%
Discharged on Antithrombotic Therapy	13	100%	99%	99%
Discharged on Statin Medication[1]	-	-	95%	94%
Thrombolytic Therapy Timing[1]	-	-	69%	66%
Venous Thromboembolism Prophylaxis	17	100%	94%	94%
Written Stroke Educational Materials Given[1]	-	-	86%	88%
Surgical Care Improvement Project				
Appropriate Beta Blocker Usage	23	100%	97%	98%
Appropriate VTP Within 24 Hours	87	92%	98%	98%
Controlled Postoperative Blood Glucose[7]	-	-	97%	97%
Perioperative Temperature Management	94	100%	100%	100%
Prophylactic Antibiotic Selection	37	100%	99%	99%
Prophylactic Antibiotic Selection (Outpatient)[1,3]	-	-	97%	98%
Prophylactic Antibiotic Stopped	35	97%	98%	98%
Prophylactic Antibiotic Timing	37	97%	99%	99%
Prophylactic Antibiotic Timing (Outpatient)[1,3]	-	-	97%	98%
Urinary Catheter Removal	33	97%	96%	97%
Survey of Patients' Hospital Experiences				
Area Around Room 'Always' Quiet at Night	300+	57%	51%	61%
Doctors 'Always' Communicated Well	300+	75%	77%	82%
Home Recovery Information Given	300+	83%	83%	85%
Hospital Given 9 or 10 on 10 Point Scale	300+	63%	63%	71%
Meds 'Always' Explained Before Given	300+	62%	59%	64%
Nurses 'Always' Communicated Well	300+	78%	75%	79%
Pain 'Always' Well Controlled	300+	74%	67%	71%
Room and Bathroom 'Always' Clean	300+	72%	69%	73%
Timely Help 'Always' Received	300+	66%	61%	68%
Would Definitely Recommend Hospital	300+	63%	65%	71%
Use of Medical Imaging				
Cardiac Imaging Stress Test before Surgery	79	8.9%	5.8%	5.3%
Combination Abdominal CT Scan	434	12.2%	8.2%	10.5%
Combination Brain/Sinus CT Scan[1]	-	-	3.6%	2.7%
Combination Chest CT Scan	233	4.7%	1.3%	2.7%
Follow-up Mammogram/Ultrasound	593	3.2%	13%	8.8%
Lumbar Spine MRI for Low Back Pain	99	29.3%	33.4%	37.2%

Canton - Potsdam Hospital

50 Leroy Street Phone: 315-265-3300
Potsdam, NY 13676 Fax: 315-265-2056
URL: www.cphospital.org
Type: Acute Care Hospitals Emergency Services: Yes
Ownership: Voluntary non-profit - Private Beds: 94

Key Personnel:
CEO/President............... David B Acker, FACHE
Chief of Medical Staff.......... G Michael Maresca, MD
Radiology.................... Mark Morales
Cardiac Laboratory............ Alexandru Stoian, MD
Operating Room.............. Marion Vandenheuvel
Infection Control............. Nancy Wood

Measure	Cases	This Hosp.	State Avg.	U.S. Avg.
Blood Clot Prevention and Treatment				
Anticoagulation Overlap Therapy[2]	22	91%	91%	93%
ICU Venous Thromboembolism Prophylaxis[2]	31	84%	92%	92%
Incidence of Potentially Preventable VTE[1,2]	-	-	10%	10%
UFH with Dosages/Platelet Monitoring[1,2]	-	-	92%	97%
Venous Thromboembolism Prophylaxis[2]	240	73%	87%	85%
Warfarin Therapy Discharge Instructions[2]	18	11%	59%	75%
Chest Pain/Possible Heart Attack Care				
Aspirin Given Within 24 Hours of Arrival	70	100%	97%	96%
Fibrinolytic Meds Within 30 Min. of Arrival[1]	-	-	54%	58%
Average Time to ECG (minutes)	71	19	9	7
Average Time to Transfer (minutes)[7]	-	-	78	60
Children's Asthma Care				
Received Home Management Plan of Care	-	-	-	88%
Received Reliever Medication	-	-	-	100%
Received Systemic Corticosteroids	-	-	-	100%
Emergency Department				
Admittance Decision Time (minutes)[2]	415	83	154	98
Head CT Results Within 45 Min. of Arrival[1]	-	-	55%	57%
Patients Who Left ER Before Being Seen	25,872	1%	2%	2%
Time from ER Arrival to Admit. (minutes)[2]	415	208	378	274
Time from ER Arrival to Discharge (minutes)	1,480	111	156	134
Time in ER Before Being Evaluated (minutes)	1,600	24	35	26
Time to Pain Meds for Fractures (minutes)	97	61	61	57
Heart Attack Care				
Aspirin Given at Discharge[1]	-	-	99%	99%
Fibrinolytic Meds Within 30 Min. of Arrival[7]	-	-	46%	54%
PCI Within 90 Minutes of Arrival[7]	-	-	95%	96%
Statin Prescribed at Discharge[1]	-	-	98%	98%
Heart Failure Care				
ACE Inhibitor or ARB for LVSD	39	97%	96%	97%
Discharge Instructions Given	122	95%	95%	94%
Evaluation of LVS Function	145	98%	99%	99%
Medicare Spending				
Medicare Spending per Patient (ratio)	-	0.81	0.96	0.98
Pneumonia Care				
Appropriate Initial Antibiotic Given	85	94%	95%	95%
Blood Culture Timing	139	94%	97%	98%
Pregnancy and Delivery Care				
Newborn Deliveries Scheduled Early	15	0%	4%	6%
Preventive Care				
Immunization for Influenza[2]	443	79%	88%	90%
Immunization for Pneumonia[2]	450	83%	88%	92%
Stroke Care				
Anticoagulation Therapy for Atrial Fibrillation[1]	-	-	96%	95%
Antithrombotic Therapy Timing	24	100%	98%	98%
Assessed for Rehabilitation	31	97%	97%	97%
Discharged on Antithrombotic Therapy	26	100%	99%	99%
Discharged on Statin Medication	27	100%	95%	94%
Thrombolytic Therapy Timing[1]	-	-	69%	66%
Venous Thromboembolism Prophylaxis	27	89%	94%	94%
Written Stroke Educational Materials Given	18	6%	86%	88%
Surgical Care Improvement Project				
Appropriate Beta Blocker Usage	70	99%	97%	98%
Appropriate VTP Within 24 Hours	201	97%	98%	98%
Controlled Postoperative Blood Glucose[7]	-	-	97%	97%
Perioperative Temperature Management	217	100%	100%	100%
Prophylactic Antibiotic Selection	149	98%	99%	99%
Prophylactic Antibiotic Selection (Outpatient)	23	96%	97%	98%
Prophylactic Antibiotic Stopped	149	100%	98%	98%
Prophylactic Antibiotic Timing	149	97%	99%	99%
Prophylactic Antibiotic Timing (Outpatient)	24	88%	97%	98%
Urinary Catheter Removal	103	99%	96%	97%
Survey of Patients' Hospital Experiences				
Area Around Room 'Always' Quiet at Night	300+	55%	51%	61%
Doctors 'Always' Communicated Well	300+	79%	77%	82%
Home Recovery Information Given	300+	86%	83%	85%
Hospital Given 9 or 10 on 10 Point Scale	300+	66%	63%	71%
Meds 'Always' Explained Before Given	300+	62%	59%	64%
Nurses 'Always' Communicated Well	300+	79%	75%	79%
Pain 'Always' Well Controlled	300+	71%	67%	71%
Room and Bathroom 'Always' Clean	300+	78%	69%	73%
Timely Help 'Always' Received	300+	70%	61%	68%
Would Definitely Recommend Hospital	300+	71%	65%	71%
Use of Medical Imaging				
Cardiac Imaging Stress Test before Surgery	400	6.3%	5.8%	5.3%
Combination Abdominal CT Scan	674	17.7%	8.2%	10.5%
Combination Brain/Sinus CT Scan	371	1.3%	3.6%	2.7%
Combination Chest CT Scan	473	1.9%	1.3%	2.7%
Follow-up Mammogram/Ultrasound	1,038	3.3%	13%	8.8%
Lumbar Spine MRI for Low Back Pain	121	28.9%	33.4%	37.2%

NOTE: Hospital profiles are in alphabetical order by state, then city, then hospital within the city; Rankings exclude hospitals with less than 25 cases except for patient surveys which excludes hospitals with less than 100 cases; (a) 100-299 cases; (1) The number of cases/patients is too few to report; (2) Data submitted were based on a sample of cases/patients; (3) Results are based on a shorter time period than required; (4) Data suppressed by CMS for one or more quarters; (5) Results are not available for this reporting period; (6) Fewer than 100 patients completed the HCAHPS survey; (7) No cases met the criteria for this measure; (8) The lower limit of the confidence interval cannot be calculated if the number of observed infections equals zero; (9) No data are available from the state/territory for this reporting period; (10) The scores shown reflect fewer than 50 completed surveys; (11) There were discrepancies in the data collection process; (12) This measure does not apply to this hospital for this reporting period; (13) Results cannot be calculated for this reporting period; (14) The results for this state are combined with nearby states to protect confidentiality; Please refer to the User's Guide for a full explanation of data.

Saint Francis Hospital

241 North Road
Poughkeepsie, NY 12601
URL: www.sfhhc.org
Type: Acute Care Hospitals
Ownership: Voluntary non-profit - Private
Phone: 845-483-5000
Fax: 845-485-3762
Emergency Services: Yes
Beds: 400

Key Personnel:
Anesthesiology. . . . . Leon Basil, MD
Operating Room. . . . . Terri Egitto
Chief of Medical Staff . . . . J Keith Fasta, MD
Infection Control. . . . . Stuart Feinstein, MD
Cardiac Laboratory. . . . . Anthony Messina, MD
CEO/President. . . . . Arthur Nizza, DSW
Quality Assurance . . . . Patricia Smith
Radiology. . . . . J. Louis Solis, MD

Measure	Cases	This Hosp.	State Avg.	U.S. Avg.
Blood Clot Prevention and Treatment				
Anticoagulation Overlap Therapy[2]	51	100%	91%	93%
ICU Venous Thromboembolism Prophylaxis[2]	120	99%	92%	92%
Incidence of Potentially Preventable VTE[2]	19	0%	10%	10%
UFH with Dosages/Platelet Monitoring[2]	17	100%	92%	97%
Venous Thromboembolism Prophylaxis[2]	295	96%	87%	85%
Warfarin Therapy Discharge Instructions[2]	30	100%	59%	75%
Chest Pain/Possible Heart Attack Care				
Aspirin Given Within 24 Hours of Arrival[3]	18	100%	97%	96%
Fibrinolytic Meds Within 30 Min. of Arrival[3,7]	-	-	54%	58%
Average Time to ECG (minutes)[3]	18	3	9	7
Average Time to Transfer (minutes)[1,3]	-	-	78	60
Children's Asthma Care				
Received Home Management Plan of Care	-	-	-	88%
Received Reliever Medication	-	-	-	100%
Received Systemic Corticosteroids	-	-	-	100%
Emergency Department				
Admittance Decision Time (minutes)[2]	809	151	154	98
Head CT Results Within 45 Min. of Arrival[7]	-	-	55%	57%
Patients Who Left ER Before Being Seen	32,365	1%	2%	2%
Time from ER Arrival to Admit. (minutes)[2]	809	383	378	274
Time from ER Arrival to Discharge (minutes)	302	160	156	134
Time in ER Before Being Evaluated (minutes)	388	33	35	26
Time to Pain Meds for Fractures (minutes)	98	54	61	57
Heart Attack Care				
Aspirin Given at Discharge[1]	-	-	99%	99%
Fibrinolytic Meds Within 30 Min. of Arrival[7]	-	-	46%	54%
PCI Within 90 Minutes of Arrival[7]	-	-	95%	96%
Statin Prescribed at Discharge	12	100%	98%	98%
Heart Failure Care				
ACE Inhibitor or ARB for LVSD[1]	-	-	96%	97%
Discharge Instructions Given	37	100%	95%	94%
Evaluation of LVS Function	54	100%	99%	99%
Medicare Spending				
Medicare Spending per Patient (ratio)	-	1.02	0.96	0.98
Pneumonia Care				
Appropriate Initial Antibiotic Given	56	100%	95%	95%
Blood Culture Timing	105	95%	97%	98%
Pregnancy and Delivery Care				
Newborn Deliveries Scheduled Early[7]	-	-	4%	6%
Preventive Care				
Immunization for Influenza[2]	529	98%	88%	90%
Immunization for Pneumonia[2]	665	98%	88%	92%
Stroke Care				
Anticoagulation Therapy for Atrial Fibrillation[1]	-	-	96%	95%
Antithrombotic Therapy Timing	25	100%	98%	98%
Assessed for Rehabilitation	48	100%	97%	97%
Discharged on Antithrombotic Therapy	22	100%	99%	99%
Discharged on Statin Medication	29	100%	95%	94%
Thrombolytic Therapy Timing[1]	-	-	69%	66%
Venous Thromboembolism Prophylaxis	49	100%	94%	94%
Written Stroke Educational Materials Given	22	100%	86%	88%
Surgical Care Improvement Project				
Appropriate Beta Blocker Usage[2]	107	100%	97%	98%
Appropriate VTP Within 24 Hours[2]	347	100%	98%	98%
Controlled Postoperative Blood Glucose[2,7]	-	-	97%	97%
Perioperative Temperature Management[2]	385	100%	100%	100%
Prophylactic Antibiotic Selection[2]	169	99%	99%	99%
Prophylactic Antibiotic Selection (Outpatient)	173	98%	97%	98%
Prophylactic Antibiotic Stopped[2]	169	100%	98%	98%
Prophylactic Antibiotic Timing[2]	169	100%	99%	99%
Prophylactic Antibiotic Timing (Outpatient)	174	99%	97%	98%
Urinary Catheter Removal[2]	266	100%	96%	97%
Survey of Patients' Hospital Experiences				
Area Around Room 'Always' Quiet at Night	300+	50%	51%	61%
Doctors 'Always' Communicated Well	300+	74%	77%	82%
Home Recovery Information Given	300+	85%	83%	85%
Hospital Given 9 or 10 on 10 Point Scale	300+	58%	63%	71%
Meds 'Always' Explained Before Given	300+	56%	59%	64%
Nurses 'Always' Communicated Well	300+	72%	75%	79%
Pain 'Always' Well Controlled	300+	67%	67%	71%
Room and Bathroom 'Always' Clean	300+	63%	69%	73%
Timely Help 'Always' Received	300+	56%	61%	68%
Would Definitely Recommend Hospital	300+	61%	65%	71%
Use of Medical Imaging				
Cardiac Imaging Stress Test before Surgery	148	4.1%	5.8%	5.3%
Combination Abdominal CT Scan	394	8.4%	8.2%	10.5%
Combination Brain/Sinus CT Scan	440	5.0%	3.6%	2.7%
Combination Chest CT Scan	146	11.6%	1.3%	2.7%
Follow-up Mammogram/Ultrasound	320	16.9%	13%	8.8%
Lumbar Spine MRI for Low Back Pain[1]	-	-	33.4%	37.2%

Vassar Brothers Medical Center

45 Reade Place
Poughkeepsie, NY 12601
URL: www.vasserbrothers.org
Type: Acute Care Hospitals
Ownership: Voluntary non-profit - Other
Phone: 845-454-8500
Fax: 845-437-3120
Emergency Services: Yes
Beds: 365

Key Personnel:
Anesthesiology. . . . . Richard Goldmann, MD
Infection Control. . . . . Mary Ann Magerl
Pediatric In-Patient Care . . . . . . Lawrence Schaeffer, MD
Chief of Medical Staff . . . . Lawrence Scheck, MD
Emergency Room . . . . David Weinreich
Intensive Care Unit. . . . . Carol Wilson
Radiology. . . . . Bryan Yen

Measure	Cases	This Hosp.	State Avg.	U.S. Avg.
Blood Clot Prevention and Treatment				
Anticoagulation Overlap Therapy[2]	98	90%	91%	93%
ICU Venous Thromboembolism Prophylaxis[2]	72	94%	92%	92%
Incidence of Potentially Preventable VTE[2]	14	7%	10%	10%
UFH with Dosages/Platelet Monitoring[2]	21	100%	92%	97%
Venous Thromboembolism Prophylaxis[2]	375	89%	87%	85%
Warfarin Therapy Discharge Instructions[2]	70	97%	59%	75%
Chest Pain/Possible Heart Attack Care				
Aspirin Given Within 24 Hours of Arrival[1,3]	-	-	97%	96%
Fibrinolytic Meds Within 30 Min. of Arrival[5]	-	-	54%	58%
Average Time to ECG (minutes)[1,3]	-	-	9	7
Average Time to Transfer (minutes)[5]	-	-	78	60
Children's Asthma Care				
Received Home Management Plan of Care	-	-	-	88%
Received Reliever Medication	-	-	-	100%
Received Systemic Corticosteroids	-	-	-	100%
Emergency Department				
Admittance Decision Time (minutes)[2]	663	174	154	98
Head CT Results Within 45 Min. of Arrival[1]	-	-	55%	57%
Patients Who Left ER Before Being Seen	67,406	1%	2%	2%
Time from ER Arrival to Admit. (minutes)[2]	663	365	378	274
Time from ER Arrival to Discharge (minutes)	406	192	156	134
Time in ER Before Being Evaluated (minutes)	368	61	35	26
Time to Pain Meds for Fractures (minutes)	113	54	61	57
Heart Attack Care				
Aspirin Given at Discharge	503	99%	99%	99%
Fibrinolytic Meds Within 30 Min. of Arrival[1]	-	-	46%	54%
PCI Within 90 Minutes of Arrival	73	97%	95%	96%
Statin Prescribed at Discharge	512	100%	98%	98%
Heart Failure Care				
ACE Inhibitor or ARB for LVSD	116	99%	96%	97%
Discharge Instructions Given	390	100%	95%	94%
Evaluation of LVS Function	484	100%	99%	99%
Medicare Spending				
Medicare Spending per Patient (ratio)	-	1.01	0.96	0.98
Pneumonia Care				
Appropriate Initial Antibiotic Given[2]	212	99%	95%	95%
Blood Culture Timing[2]	332	100%	97%	98%
Pregnancy and Delivery Care				
Newborn Deliveries Scheduled Early[2]	125	0%	4%	6%
Preventive Care				
Immunization for Influenza[2]	534	96%	88%	90%
Immunization for Pneumonia[2]	630	97%	88%	92%
Stroke Care				
Anticoagulation Therapy for Atrial Fibrillation	35	97%	96%	95%
Antithrombotic Therapy Timing	156	99%	98%	98%
Assessed for Rehabilitation	168	100%	97%	97%
Discharged on Antithrombotic Therapy	152	98%	99%	99%
Discharged on Statin Medication	126	99%	95%	94%
Thrombolytic Therapy Timing	15	80%	69%	66%
Venous Thromboembolism Prophylaxis	190	95%	94%	94%
Written Stroke Educational Materials Given	92	100%	86%	88%
Surgical Care Improvement Project				
Appropriate Beta Blocker Usage[2]	267	100%	97%	98%
Appropriate VTP Within 24 Hours[2]	380	99%	98%	98%
Controlled Postoperative Blood Glucose[2]	157	98%	97%	97%
Perioperative Temperature Management[2]	488	100%	100%	100%
Prophylactic Antibiotic Selection[2]	457	100%	99%	99%
Prophylactic Antibiotic Selection (Outpatient)	501	99%	97%	98%
Prophylactic Antibiotic Stopped[2]	433	98%	98%	98%
Prophylactic Antibiotic Timing[2]	457	100%	99%	99%
Prophylactic Antibiotic Timing (Outpatient)	502	99%	97%	98%
Urinary Catheter Removal[2]	331	98%	96%	97%
Survey of Patients' Hospital Experiences				
Area Around Room 'Always' Quiet at Night	300+	52%	51%	61%
Doctors 'Always' Communicated Well	300+	79%	77%	82%
Home Recovery Information Given	300+	87%	83%	85%
Hospital Given 9 or 10 on 10 Point Scale	300+	70%	63%	71%
Meds 'Always' Explained Before Given	300+	65%	59%	64%
Nurses 'Always' Communicated Well	300+	80%	75%	79%
Pain 'Always' Well Controlled	300+	73%	67%	71%
Room and Bathroom 'Always' Clean	300+	67%	69%	73%
Timely Help 'Always' Received	300+	61%	61%	68%
Would Definitely Recommend Hospital	300+	76%	65%	71%
Use of Medical Imaging				
Cardiac Imaging Stress Test before Surgery	97	3.1%	5.8%	5.3%
Combination Abdominal CT Scan	970	3.7%	8.2%	10.5%
Combination Brain/Sinus CT Scan	1,468	2.5%	3.6%	2.7%
Combination Chest CT Scan	297	2.7%	1.3%	2.7%
Follow-up Mammogram/Ultrasound	832	17.5%	13%	8.8%
Lumbar Spine MRI for Low Back Pain[1]	-	-	33.4%	37.2%

Northern Dutchess Hospital

6511 Springbrook Avenue
Rhinebeck, NY 12572
E-mail: ndinfo@health-quest.org
URL: www.health-quest.org
Type: Acute Care Hospitals
Ownership: Voluntary non-profit - Other
Phone: 845-871-3391
Fax: 845-876-7195
Emergency Services: Yes
Beds: 68

Key Personnel:
Patient Relations . . . . Jean Clarke
Pediatric In-Patient Care . . . . Jane Ferguson
CEO/President. . . . . Denise George
Intensive Care Unit. . . . . Kathleen Liston-Scott, RN
Operating Room. . . . . Gailri Richardson
Chief of Medical Staff . . . . Robert Rosenzweig, MD
Infection Control. . . . . Maija Wheeler
Radiology. . . . . Judy Zaho

Measure	Cases	This Hosp.	State Avg.	U.S. Avg.
Blood Clot Prevention and Treatment				
Anticoagulation Overlap Therapy[2]	26	100%	91%	93%
ICU Venous Thromboembolism Prophylaxis[2]	38	87%	92%	92%
Incidence of Potentially Preventable VTE[1,2]	-	-	10%	10%
UFH with Dosages/Platelet Monitoring[1,2]	-	-	92%	97%
Venous Thromboembolism Prophylaxis[2]	277	91%	87%	85%
Warfarin Therapy Discharge Instructions[2]	19	100%	59%	75%
Chest Pain/Possible Heart Attack Care				
Aspirin Given Within 24 Hours of Arrival	30	100%	97%	96%
Fibrinolytic Meds Within 30 Min. of Arrival[1]	-	-	54%	58%

NOTE: Hospital profiles are in alphabetical order by state, then city, then hospital within the city; Rankings exclude hospitals with less than 25 cases except for patient surveys which excludes hospitals with less than 100 cases; (a) 100-299 cases; (1) The number of cases/patients is too few to report; (2) Data submitted were based on a sample of cases/patients; (3) Results are based on a shorter time period than required; (4) Data suppressed by CMS for one or more quarters; (5) Results are not available for this reporting period; (6) Fewer than 100 patients completed the HCAHPS survey; (7) No cases met the criteria for this measure; (8) The lower limit of the confidence interval cannot be calculated if the number of observed infections equals zero; (9) No data are available from the state/territory for this reporting period; (10) The scores shown reflect fewer than 50 completed surveys; (11) There were discrepancies in the data collection process; (12) This measure does not apply to this hospital for this reporting period; (13) Results cannot be calculated for this reporting period; (14) The results for this state are combined with nearby states to protect confidentiality; Please refer to the User's Guide for a full explanation of data.

Measure	Cases	This Hosp.	State Avg.	U.S. Avg.
Average Time to ECG (minutes)	29	6	9	7
Average Time to Transfer (minutes)[1]	-	-	78	60
Children's Asthma Care				
Received Home Management Plan of Care	-	-	-	88%
Received Reliever Medication	-	-	-	100%
Received Systemic Corticosteroids	-	-	-	100%
Emergency Department				
Admittance Decision Time (minutes)[2]	384	112	154	98
Head CT Results Within 45 Min. of Arrival[1]	-	-	55%	57%
Patients Who Left ER Before Being Seen	14,779	1%	2%	2%
Time from ER Arrival to Admit. (minutes)[2]	384	277	378	274
Time from ER Arrival to Discharge (minutes)	418	122	156	134
Time in ER Before Being Evaluated (minutes)	400	35	35	26
Time to Pain Meds for Fractures (minutes)	48	43	61	57
Heart Attack Care				
Aspirin Given at Discharge[1]	-	-	99%	99%
Fibrinolytic Meds Within 30 Min. of Arrival[7]	-	-	46%	54%
PCI Within 90 Minutes of Arrival[7]	-	-	95%	96%
Statin Prescribed at Discharge[1]	-	-	98%	98%
Heart Failure Care				
ACE Inhibitor or ARB for LVSD	19	95%	96%	97%
Discharge Instructions Given	44	100%	95%	94%
Evaluation of LVS Function	68	100%	99%	99%
Medicare Spending				
Medicare Spending per Patient (ratio)	-	0.94	0.96	0.98
Pneumonia Care				
Appropriate Initial Antibiotic Given	67	97%	95%	95%
Blood Culture Timing	109	99%	97%	98%
Pregnancy and Delivery Care				
Newborn Deliveries Scheduled Early[2]	22	27%	4%	6%
Preventive Care				
Immunization for Influenza[2]	348	92%	88%	90%
Immunization for Pneumonia[2]	429	91%	88%	92%
Stroke Care				
Anticoagulation Therapy for Atrial Fibrillation[1]	-	-	96%	95%
Antithrombotic Therapy Timing	25	100%	98%	98%
Assessed for Rehabilitation	30	100%	97%	97%
Discharged on Antithrombotic Therapy	29	100%	99%	99%
Discharged on Statin Medication	21	90%	95%	94%
Thrombolytic Therapy Timing[1]	-	-	69%	66%
Venous Thromboembolism Prophylaxis	29	90%	94%	94%
Written Stroke Educational Materials Given	13	100%	86%	88%
Surgical Care Improvement Project				
Appropriate Beta Blocker Usage[2]	91	97%	97%	98%
Appropriate VTP Within 24 Hours[2]	282	99%	98%	98%
Controlled Postoperative Blood Glucose[2,7]	-	-	97%	97%
Perioperative Temperature Management[2]	315	100%	100%	100%
Prophylactic Antibiotic Selection[2]	248	100%	99%	99%
Prophylactic Antibiotic Selection (Outpatient)	153	93%	97%	98%
Prophylactic Antibiotic Stopped[2]	248	100%	98%	98%
Prophylactic Antibiotic Timing[2]	248	100%	99%	99%
Prophylactic Antibiotic Timing (Outpatient)	157	96%	97%	98%
Urinary Catheter Removal[2]	266	100%	96%	97%
Survey of Patients' Hospital Experiences				
Area Around Room 'Always' Quiet at Night	300+	45%	51%	61%
Doctors 'Always' Communicated Well	300+	80%	77%	82%
Home Recovery Information Given	300+	90%	83%	85%
Hospital Given 9 or 10 on 10 Point Scale	300+	75%	63%	71%
Meds 'Always' Explained Before Given	300+	67%	59%	64%
Nurses 'Always' Communicated Well	300+	82%	75%	79%
Pain 'Always' Well Controlled	300+	71%	67%	71%
Room and Bathroom 'Always' Clean	300+	72%	69%	73%
Timely Help 'Always' Received	300+	69%	61%	68%
Would Definitely Recommend Hospital	300+	82%	65%	71%
Use of Medical Imaging				
Cardiac Imaging Stress Test before Surgery	120	4.2%	5.8%	5.3%
Combination Abdominal CT Scan	334	9.3%	8.2%	10.5%
Combination Brain/Sinus CT Scan[1]	-	-	3.6%	2.7%
Combination Chest CT Scan	160	1.3%	1.3%	2.7%
Follow-up Mammogram/Ultrasound	614	10.3%	13%	8.8%
Lumbar Spine MRI for Low Back Pain[1]	-	-	33.4%	37.2%

Peconic Bay Medical Center

1300 Roanoke Avenue
Riverhead, NY 11901
E-mail: info@pbmedicalcenter.org
URL: www.pbmedicalcenter.org
Type: Acute Care Hospitals
Ownership: Voluntary non-profit - Private
Phone: 631-548-6000
Fax: 631-548-6048
Emergency Services: Yes
Beds: 214

Key Personnel:
Radiology. . . . . James Badia
Chief of Medical Staff. . . . . Samir Bute
CEO/President. . . . . Andrew J Mitchell, FACHE

Measure	Cases	This Hosp.	State Avg.	U.S. Avg.
Blood Clot Prevention and Treatment				
Anticoagulation Overlap Therapy[2]	44	82%	91%	93%
ICU Venous Thromboembolism Prophylaxis[2]	49	92%	92%	92%
Incidence of Potentially Preventable VTE[1,2]	-	-	10%	10%
UFH with Dosages/Platelet Monitoring[2]	24	96%	92%	97%
Venous Thromboembolism Prophylaxis[2]	348	83%	87%	85%
Warfarin Therapy Discharge Instructions[2]	32	3%	59%	75%
Chest Pain/Possible Heart Attack Care				
Aspirin Given Within 24 Hours of Arrival	94	94%	97%	96%
Fibrinolytic Meds Within 30 Min. of Arrival[1]	-	-	54%	58%
Average Time to ECG (minutes)	95	5	9	7
Average Time to Transfer (minutes)	18	61	78	60
Children's Asthma Care				
Received Home Management Plan of Care	-	-	-	88%
Received Reliever Medication	-	-	-	100%
Received Systemic Corticosteroids	-	-	-	100%
Emergency Department				
Admittance Decision Time (minutes)[2]	359	295	154	98
Head CT Results Within 45 Min. of Arrival	39	69%	55%	57%
Patients Who Left ER Before Being Seen	35,555	2%	2%	2%
Time from ER Arrival to Admit. (minutes)[2]	590	529	378	274
Time from ER Arrival to Discharge (minutes)	394	154	156	134
Time in ER Before Being Evaluated (minutes)	325	39	35	26
Time to Pain Meds for Fractures (minutes)	119	65	61	57
Heart Attack Care				
Aspirin Given at Discharge	32	91%	99%	99%
Fibrinolytic Meds Within 30 Min. of Arrival[7]	-	-	46%	54%
PCI Within 90 Minutes of Arrival[7]	-	-	95%	96%
Statin Prescribed at Discharge	30	90%	98%	98%
Heart Failure Care				
ACE Inhibitor or ARB for LVSD	31	58%	96%	97%
Discharge Instructions Given	138	62%	95%	94%
Evaluation of LVS Function	181	89%	99%	99%
Medicare Spending				
Medicare Spending per Patient (ratio)	-	0.98	0.96	0.98
Pneumonia Care				
Appropriate Initial Antibiotic Given[2]	105	83%	95%	95%
Blood Culture Timing[2]	166	85%	97%	98%
Pregnancy and Delivery Care				
Newborn Deliveries Scheduled Early	44	5%	4%	6%
Preventive Care				
Immunization for Influenza[2]	570	85%	88%	90%
Immunization for Pneumonia[2]	775	83%	88%	92%
Stroke Care				
Anticoagulation Therapy for Atrial Fibrillation[2]	11	100%	96%	95%
Antithrombotic Therapy Timing[2]	47	94%	98%	98%
Assessed for Rehabilitation[2]	46	93%	97%	97%
Discharged on Antithrombotic Therapy[2]	44	100%	99%	99%
Discharged on Statin Medication[2]	33	94%	95%	94%
Thrombolytic Therapy Timing[1,2]	-	-	69%	66%
Venous Thromboembolism Prophylaxis[2]	48	94%	94%	94%
Written Stroke Educational Materials Given[2]	23	100%	86%	88%
Surgical Care Improvement Project				
Appropriate Beta Blocker Usage[2]	201	94%	97%	98%
Appropriate VTP Within 24 Hours[2]	565	97%	98%	98%
Controlled Postoperative Blood Glucose[2,7]	-	-	97%	97%
Perioperative Temperature Management[2]	601	100%	100%	100%
Prophylactic Antibiotic Selection[2]	437	99%	99%	99%
Prophylactic Antibiotic Selection (Outpatient)	81	85%	97%	98%
Prophylactic Antibiotic Stopped[2]	432	95%	98%	98%
Prophylactic Antibiotic Timing[2]	437	97%	99%	99%
Prophylactic Antibiotic Timing (Outpatient)	82	99%	97%	98%
Urinary Catheter Removal[2]	407	95%	96%	97%
Survey of Patients' Hospital Experiences				
Area Around Room 'Always' Quiet at Night	300+	40%	51%	61%
Doctors 'Always' Communicated Well	300+	72%	77%	82%
Home Recovery Information Given	300+	84%	83%	85%
Hospital Given 9 or 10 on 10 Point Scale	300+	53%	63%	71%
Meds 'Always' Explained Before Given	300+	53%	59%	64%
Nurses 'Always' Communicated Well	300+	69%	75%	79%
Pain 'Always' Well Controlled	300+	60%	67%	71%
Room and Bathroom 'Always' Clean	300+	63%	69%	73%
Timely Help 'Always' Received	300+	55%	61%	68%
Would Definitely Recommend Hospital	300+	57%	65%	71%
Use of Medical Imaging				
Cardiac Imaging Stress Test before Surgery[7]	-	-	5.8%	5.3%
Combination Abdominal CT Scan	605	2.8%	8.2%	10.5%
Combination Brain/Sinus CT Scan	702	3.1%	3.6%	2.7%
Combination Chest CT Scan	289	0.7%	1.3%	2.7%
Follow-up Mammogram/Ultrasound	68	16.2%	13%	8.8%
Lumbar Spine MRI for Low Back Pain	69	36.2%	33.4%	37.2%

Highland Hospital

1000 South Avenue
Rochester, NY 14620
URL: www.urmc.rochester.edu
Type: Acute Care Hospitals
Ownership: Voluntary non-profit - Private
Phone: 585-473-2200
Fax: 585-341-6703
Emergency Services: Yes
Beds: 272

Key Personnel:
Chief of Medical Staff. . . . . Howard Beckman, MD
Pediatric Ambulatory Care . . . . . Veronica Guillet, MD
Pediatric In-Patient Care . . . . . . Veronica Guillet, MD
Quality Assurance . . . . Donna Johnston
Radiology. . . . . Francis Kelley, MD
Operating Room. . . . . Amy Matroniano, RN
Infection Control. . . . . Ann Marie Pettis, RN
CEO/President. . . . . William Remizowski

Measure	Cases	This Hosp.	State Avg.	U.S. Avg.
Blood Clot Prevention and Treatment				
Anticoagulation Overlap Therapy[2]	98	98%	91%	93%
ICU Venous Thromboembolism Prophylaxis[2]	25	80%	92%	92%
Incidence of Potentially Preventable VTE[2]	14	7%	10%	10%
UFH with Dosages/Platelet Monitoring[2]	36	100%	92%	97%
Venous Thromboembolism Prophylaxis[2]	320	89%	87%	85%
Warfarin Therapy Discharge Instructions[2]	64	73%	59%	75%
Chest Pain/Possible Heart Attack Care				
Aspirin Given Within 24 Hours of Arrival	35	94%	97%	96%
Fibrinolytic Meds Within 30 Min. of Arrival[7]	-	-	54%	58%
Average Time to ECG (minutes)	36	19	9	7
Average Time to Transfer (minutes)[1]	-	-	78	60
Children's Asthma Care				
Received Home Management Plan of Care	-	-	-	88%
Received Reliever Medication	-	-	-	100%
Received Systemic Corticosteroids	-	-	-	100%
Emergency Department				
Admittance Decision Time (minutes)[2]	368	67	154	98
Head CT Results Within 45 Min. of Arrival[7]	-	-	55%	57%
Patients Who Left ER Before Being Seen	39,758	1%	2%	2%
Time from ER Arrival to Admit. (minutes)[2]	368	276	378	274
Time from ER Arrival to Discharge (minutes)	367	177	156	134
Time in ER Before Being Evaluated (minutes)	382	16	35	26
Time to Pain Meds for Fractures (minutes)	87	68	61	57
Heart Attack Care				
Aspirin Given at Discharge	38	97%	99%	99%
Fibrinolytic Meds Within 30 Min. of Arrival[7]	-	-	46%	54%
PCI Within 90 Minutes of Arrival[7]	-	-	95%	96%
Statin Prescribed at Discharge	37	92%	98%	98%
Heart Failure Care				
ACE Inhibitor or ARB for LVSD	85	81%	96%	97%
Discharge Instructions Given	295	98%	95%	94%
Evaluation of LVS Function	407	100%	99%	99%
Medicare Spending				
Medicare Spending per Patient (ratio)	-	0.90	0.96	0.98
Pneumonia Care				
Appropriate Initial Antibiotic Given[2]	167	96%	95%	95%

NOTE: Hospital profiles are in alphabetical order by state, then city, then hospital within the city; Rankings exclude hospitals with less than 25 cases except for patient surveys which excludes hospitals with less than 100 cases; (a) 100-299 cases; (1) The number of cases/patients is too few to report; (2) Data submitted were based on a sample of cases/patients; (3) Results are based on a shorter time period than required; (4) Data suppressed by CMS for one or more quarters; (5) Results are not available for this reporting period; (6) Fewer than 100 patients completed the HCAHPS survey; (7) No cases met the criteria for this measure; (8) The lower limit of the confidence interval cannot be calculated if the number of observed infections equals zero; (9) No data are available from the state/territory for this reporting period; (10) The scores shown reflect fewer than 50 completed surveys; (11) There were discrepancies in the data collection process; (12) This measure does not apply to this hospital for this reporting period; (13) Results cannot be calculated for this reporting period; (14) The results for this state are combined with nearby states to protect confidentiality; Please refer to the User's Guide for a full explanation of data.

Measure	Cases	This Hosp.	State Avg.	U.S. Avg.
Blood Culture Timing[2]	322	100%	97%	98%
Pregnancy and Delivery Care				
Newborn Deliveries Scheduled Early[2]	30	7%	4%	6%
Preventive Care				
Immunization for Influenza[2]	488	94%	88%	90%
Immunization for Pneumonia[2]	561	89%	88%	92%
Stroke Care				
Anticoagulation Therapy for Atrial Fibrillation[1,2]	-	-	96%	95%
Antithrombotic Therapy Timing[2]	80	99%	98%	98%
Assessed for Rehabilitation[2]	99	99%	97%	97%
Discharged on Antithrombotic Therapy[2]	93	100%	99%	99%
Discharged on Statin Medication[2]	65	98%	95%	94%
Thrombolytic Therapy Timing[1,2]	-	-	69%	66%
Venous Thromboembolism Prophylaxis[2]	97	89%	94%	94%
Written Stroke Educational Materials Given[2]	55	87%	86%	88%
Surgical Care Improvement Project				
Appropriate Beta Blocker Usage[2]	236	99%	97%	98%
Appropriate VTP Within 24 Hours[2]	716	100%	98%	98%
Controlled Postoperative Blood Glucose[2,7]	-	-	97%	97%
Perioperative Temperature Management[2]	816	100%	100%	100%
Prophylactic Antibiotic Selection[2]	632	100%	99%	99%
Prophylactic Antibiotic Selection (Outpatient)	174	99%	97%	98%
Prophylactic Antibiotic Stopped[2]	622	100%	98%	98%
Prophylactic Antibiotic Timing[2]	638	100%	99%	99%
Prophylactic Antibiotic Timing (Outpatient)	175	99%	97%	98%
Urinary Catheter Removal[2]	634	99%	96%	97%
Survey of Patients' Hospital Experiences				
Area Around Room 'Always' Quiet at Night	300+	56%	51%	61%
Doctors 'Always' Communicated Well	300+	82%	77%	82%
Home Recovery Information Given	300+	88%	83%	85%
Hospital Given 9 or 10 on 10 Point Scale	300+	75%	63%	71%
Meds 'Always' Explained Before Given	300+	66%	59%	64%
Nurses 'Always' Communicated Well	300+	81%	75%	79%
Pain 'Always' Well Controlled	300+	71%	67%	71%
Room and Bathroom 'Always' Clean	300+	69%	69%	73%
Timely Help 'Always' Received	300+	64%	61%	68%
Would Definitely Recommend Hospital	300+	80%	65%	71%
Use of Medical Imaging				
Cardiac Imaging Stress Test before Surgery	235	4.3%	5.8%	5.3%
Combination Abdominal CT Scan	447	12.1%	8.2%	10.5%
Combination Brain/Sinus CT Scan	454	4.6%	3.6%	2.7%
Combination Chest CT Scan	170	1.2%	1.3%	2.7%
Follow-up Mammogram/Ultrasound	975	10.1%	13%	8.8%
Lumbar Spine MRI for Low Back Pain[7]			33.4%	37.2%

Monroe Community Hospital

435 East Henrietta Road
Rochester, NY 14620
Phone: 585-760-6500
Fax: 585-760-6066
E-mail: info@monroehosp.org
URL: www.monroehosp.org
Type: Acute Care Hospitals
Emergency Services: No
Ownership: Government - State
Beds: 566

Key Personnel:
Radiology. Antoinette Cavalieri
Infection Control. . . . . Paul Graman
Chief of Medical Staff. . . . . Paul Katz
Quality Assurance . . . . Tom Yale

Measure	Cases	This Hosp.	State Avg.	U.S. Avg.
Blood Clot Prevention and Treatment				
Anticoagulation Overlap Therapy[7]	-	-	91%	93%
ICU Venous Thromboembolism Prophylaxis[7]	-	-	92%	92%
Incidence of Potentially Preventable VTE[7]	-	-	10%	10%
UFH with Dosages/Platelet Monitoring[7]	-	-	92%	97%
Venous Thromboembolism Prophylaxis	16	6%	87%	85%
Warfarin Therapy Discharge Instructions[7]	-	-	59%	75%
Chest Pain/Possible Heart Attack Care				
Aspirin Given Within 24 Hours of Arrival	-	-	97%	96%
Fibrinolytic Meds Within 30 Min. of Arrival	-	-	54%	58%
Average Time to ECG (minutes)	-	-	9	7
Average Time to Transfer (minutes)	-	-	78	60
Children's Asthma Care				
Received Home Management Plan of Care	-	-	-	88%
Received Reliever Medication	-	-	-	100%
Received Systemic Corticosteroids	-	-	-	100%
Emergency Department				
Admittance Decision Time (minutes)[2,7]	-	-	154	98
Head CT Results Within 45 Min. of Arrival	-	-	55%	57%
Patients Who Left ER Before Being Seen	-	-	2%	2%
Time from ER Arrival to Admit. (minutes)[2,7]	-	-	378	274
Time from ER Arrival to Discharge (minutes)	-	-	156	134
Time in ER Before Being Evaluated (minutes)	-	-	35	26
Time to Pain Meds for Fractures (minutes)	-	-	61	57
Heart Attack Care				
Aspirin Given at Discharge[5]	-	-	99%	99%
Fibrinolytic Meds Within 30 Min. of Arrival[5]	-	-	46%	54%
PCI Within 90 Minutes of Arrival[5]	-	-	95%	96%
Statin Prescribed at Discharge[5]	-	-	98%	98%
Heart Failure Care				
ACE Inhibitor or ARB for LVSD[5]	-	-	96%	97%
Discharge Instructions Given[5]	-	-	95%	94%
Evaluation of LVS Function[5]	-	-	99%	99%
Medicare Spending				
Medicare Spending per Patient (ratio)[1]	-	-	0.96	0.98
Pneumonia Care				
Appropriate Initial Antibiotic Given[2,3]	-	-	95%	95%
Blood Culture Timing[2,3]	-	-	97%	98%
Pregnancy and Delivery Care				
Newborn Deliveries Scheduled Early[7]	-	-	4%	6%
Preventive Care				
Immunization for Influenza[2]	12	100%	88%	90%
Immunization for Pneumonia[2]	20	90%	88%	92%
Stroke Care				
Anticoagulation Therapy for Atrial Fibrillation[5]	-	-	96%	95%
Antithrombotic Therapy Timing[5]	-	-	98%	98%
Assessed for Rehabilitation[5]	-	-	97%	97%
Discharged on Antithrombotic Therapy[5]	-	-	99%	99%
Discharged on Statin Medication[5]	-	-	95%	94%
Thrombolytic Therapy Timing[5]	-	-	69%	66%
Venous Thromboembolism Prophylaxis[5]	-	-	94%	94%
Written Stroke Educational Materials Given[5]	-	-	86%	88%
Surgical Care Improvement Project				
Appropriate Beta Blocker Usage[5]	-	-	97%	98%
Appropriate VTP Within 24 Hours[5]	-	-	98%	98%
Controlled Postoperative Blood Glucose[5]	-	-	97%	97%
Perioperative Temperature Management[5]	-	-	100%	100%
Prophylactic Antibiotic Selection[5]	-	-	99%	99%
Prophylactic Antibiotic Selection (Outpatient)	-	-	97%	98%
Prophylactic Antibiotic Stopped[5]	-	-	98%	98%
Prophylactic Antibiotic Timing[5]	-	-	99%	99%
Prophylactic Antibiotic Timing (Outpatient)	-	-	97%	98%
Urinary Catheter Removal[5]	-	-	96%	97%
Survey of Patients' Hospital Experiences				
Area Around Room 'Always' Quiet at Night[1]	-	-	51%	61%
Doctors 'Always' Communicated Well[1]	-	-	77%	82%
Home Recovery Information Given[1]	-	-	83%	85%
Hospital Given 9 or 10 on 10 Point Scale[1]	-	-	63%	71%
Meds 'Always' Explained Before Given[1]	-	-	59%	64%
Nurses 'Always' Communicated Well[1]	-	-	75%	79%
Pain 'Always' Well Controlled[1]	-	-	67%	71%
Room and Bathroom 'Always' Clean[1]	-	-	69%	73%
Timely Help 'Always' Received[1]	-	-	61%	68%
Would Definitely Recommend Hospital[1]	-	-	65%	71%
Use of Medical Imaging				
Cardiac Imaging Stress Test before Surgery	-	-	5.8%	5.3%
Combination Abdominal CT Scan	-	-	8.2%	10.5%
Combination Brain/Sinus CT Scan	-	-	3.6%	2.7%
Combination Chest CT Scan	-	-	1.3%	2.7%
Follow-up Mammogram/Ultrasound	-	-	13%	8.8%
Lumbar Spine MRI for Low Back Pain	-	-	33.4%	37.2%

Rochester General Hospital

1425 Portland Avenue
Rochester, NY 14621
Phone: 585-922-4000
Fax: 585-922-4290
URL: www.rochestergeneral.org
Type: Acute Care Hospitals
Emergency Services: Yes
Ownership: Voluntary non-profit - Private
Beds: 528

Key Personnel:
Radiology. . . . . Jonathan Broder, MD
CEO/President. . . . . Mark Clement
Coronary Care . . . . Ronald Kirshner, MD
Pediatric Ambulatory Care . . . . . . David Siegal, MD
Pediatric In-Patient Care . . . . David Siegal, MD
Quality Assurance . . . . Mary Tribuzzi
Infection Control. . . . . Edward Walsh, MD
Chief of Medical Staff . . . . Georgianne Zigarowicz, MD

Measure	Cases	This Hosp.	State Avg.	U.S. Avg.
Blood Clot Prevention and Treatment				
Anticoagulation Overlap Therapy[2]	232	98%	91%	93%
ICU Venous Thromboembolism Prophylaxis[2]	48	100%	92%	92%
Incidence of Potentially Preventable VTE[2]	40	18%	10%	10%
UFH with Dosages/Platelet Monitoring[2]	133	100%	92%	97%
Venous Thromboembolism Prophylaxis[2]	346	93%	87%	85%
Warfarin Therapy Discharge Instructions[2]	180	48%	59%	75%
Chest Pain/Possible Heart Attack Care				
Aspirin Given Within 24 Hours of Arrival[5]	-	-	97%	96%
Fibrinolytic Meds Within 30 Min. of Arrival[5]	-	-	54%	58%
Average Time to ECG (minutes)[5]	-	-	9	7
Average Time to Transfer (minutes)[5]	-	-	78	60
Children's Asthma Care				
Received Home Management Plan of Care	-	-	-	88%
Received Reliever Medication	-	-	-	100%
Received Systemic Corticosteroids	-	-	-	100%
Emergency Department				
Admittance Decision Time (minutes)[2]	659	172	154	98
Head CT Results Within 45 Min. of Arrival	24	71%	55%	57%
Patients Who Left ER Before Being Seen	>100k	1%	2%	2%
Time from ER Arrival to Admit. (minutes)[2]	660	376	378	274
Time from ER Arrival to Discharge (minutes)	349	181	156	134
Time in ER Before Being Evaluated (minutes)	404	21	35	26
Time to Pain Meds for Fractures (minutes)	236	41	61	57
Heart Attack Care				
Aspirin Given at Discharge[2]	441	98%	99%	99%
Fibrinolytic Meds Within 30 Min. of Arrival[2,7]	-	-	46%	54%
PCI Within 90 Minutes of Arrival[2]	53	94%	95%	96%
Statin Prescribed at Discharge[2]	413	99%	98%	98%
Heart Failure Care				
ACE Inhibitor or ARB for LVSD[2]	149	95%	96%	97%
Discharge Instructions Given[2]	483	98%	95%	94%
Evaluation of LVS Function[2]	563	100%	99%	99%
Medicare Spending				
Medicare Spending per Patient (ratio)	-	0.91	0.96	0.98
Pneumonia Care				
Appropriate Initial Antibiotic Given	318	97%	95%	95%
Blood Culture Timing	569	97%	97%	98%
Pregnancy and Delivery Care				
Newborn Deliveries Scheduled Early[2]	37	0%	4%	6%
Preventive Care				
Immunization for Influenza[2]	566	69%	88%	90%
Immunization for Pneumonia[2]	755	65%	88%	92%
Stroke Care				
Anticoagulation Therapy for Atrial Fibrillation	59	86%	96%	95%
Antithrombotic Therapy Timing	307	100%	98%	98%
Assessed for Rehabilitation	366	99%	97%	97%
Discharged on Antithrombotic Therapy	320	99%	99%	99%
Discharged on Statin Medication	264	95%	95%	94%
Thrombolytic Therapy Timing	39	77%	69%	66%
Venous Thromboembolism Prophylaxis	396	93%	94%	94%
Written Stroke Educational Materials Given	243	79%	86%	88%
Surgical Care Improvement Project				
Appropriate Beta Blocker Usage[2]	954	99%	97%	98%
Appropriate VTP Within 24 Hours[2]	1,259	100%	98%	98%
Controlled Postoperative Blood Glucose[2]	583	99%	97%	97%
Perioperative Temperature Management[2]	1,636	99%	100%	100%
Prophylactic Antibiotic Selection[2]	1,726	99%	99%	99%

NOTE: Hospital profiles are in alphabetical order by state, then city, then hospital within the city; Rankings exclude hospitals with less than 25 cases except for patient surveys which excludes hospitals with less than 100 cases; (a) 100-299 cases; (1) The number of cases/patients is too few to report; (2) Data submitted were based on a sample of cases/patients; (3) Results are based on a shorter time period than required; (4) Data suppressed by CMS for one or more quarters; (5) Results are not available for this reporting period; (6) Fewer than 100 patients completed the HCAHPS survey; (7) No cases met the criteria for this measure; (8) The lower limit of the confidence interval cannot be calculated if the number of observed infections equals zero; (9) No data are available from the state/territory for this reporting period; (10) The scores shown reflect fewer than 50 completed surveys; (11) There were discrepancies in the data collection process; (12) This measure does not apply to this hospital for this reporting period; (13) Results cannot be calculated for this reporting period; (14) The results for this state are combined with nearby states to protect confidentiality; Please refer to the User's Guide for a full explanation of data.

Prophylactic Antibiotic Selection (Outpatient)	725	99%	97%	98%
Prophylactic Antibiotic Stopped[2]	1,698	100%	98%	98%
Prophylactic Antibiotic Timing[2]	1,732	98%	99%	99%
Prophylactic Antibiotic Timing (Outpatient)	734	97%	97%	98%
Urinary Catheter Removal[2]	1,117	96%	96%	97%
Survey of Patients' Hospital Experiences				
Area Around Room 'Always' Quiet at Night	300+	47%	51%	61%
Doctors 'Always' Communicated Well	300+	80%	77%	82%
Home Recovery Information Given	300+	87%	83%	85%
Hospital Given 9 or 10 on 10 Point Scale	300+	72%	63%	71%
Meds 'Always' Explained Before Given	300+	64%	59%	64%
Nurses 'Always' Communicated Well	300+	80%	75%	79%
Pain 'Always' Well Controlled	300+	69%	67%	71%
Room and Bathroom 'Always' Clean	300+	64%	69%	73%
Timely Help 'Always' Received	300+	64%	61%	68%
Would Definitely Recommend Hospital	300+	78%	65%	71%
Use of Medical Imaging				
Cardiac Imaging Stress Test before Surgery	348	6.0%	5.8%	5.3%
Combination Abdominal CT Scan	863	8.2%	8.2%	10.5%
Combination Brain/Sinus CT Scan	798	2.8%	3.6%	2.7%
Combination Chest CT Scan	642	6.4%	1.3%	2.7%
Follow-up Mammogram/Ultrasound	423	5.4%	13%	8.8%
Lumbar Spine MRI for Low Back Pain	66	47.0%	33.4%	37.2%

Strong Memorial Hospital

601 Elmwood Ave
Rochester, NY 14642
URL: www.urmc.rochester.edu
Type: Acute Care Hospitals
Ownership: Voluntary non-profit - Private

Phone: 585-275-2121
Fax: 585-256-3805
Emergency Services: Yes
Beds: 750

Key Personnel:
Quality Assurance .... Ted Case
CEO/President............... Steven I Goldstein
Chief of Medical Staff.......... Raymond J. Mayewski, M.D., F.A.C.P
Operating Room.............. Sandra Monacelli
Pediatric Ambulatory Care ...... Nina F Schor, MD, PhD
Pediatric In-Patient Care .... Nina F Schor, MD, PhD
Infection Control.............. John J Treanorn, MD
Radiology................... David Waldman, MD

Measure	Cases	This Hosp.	State Avg.	U.S. Avg.
Blood Clot Prevention and Treatment				
Anticoagulation Overlap Therapy[2]	122	80%	91%	93%
ICU Venous Thromboembolism Prophylaxis[2]	54	81%	92%	92%
Incidence of Potentially Preventable VTE[2]	25	44%	10%	10%
UFH with Dosages/Platelet Monitoring[2]	56	86%	92%	97%
Venous Thromboembolism Prophylaxis[2]	321	77%	87%	85%
Warfarin Therapy Discharge Instructions[2]	92	18%	59%	75%
Chest Pain/Possible Heart Attack Care				
Aspirin Given Within 24 Hours of Arrival[1,3]	-	-	97%	96%
Fibrinolytic Meds Within 30 Min. of Arrival[5]	-	-	54%	58%
Average Time to ECG (minutes)[1,3]	-	-	9	7
Average Time to Transfer (minutes)[5]	-	-	78	60
Children's Asthma Care				
Received Home Management Plan of Care	-	-	-	88%
Received Reliever Medication	-	-	-	100%
Received Systemic Corticosteroids	-	-	-	100%
Emergency Department				
Admittance Decision Time (minutes)[2]	610	209	154	98
Head CT Results Within 45 Min. of Arrival[7]	-	-	55%	57%
Patients Who Left ER Before Being Seen	>100k	3%	2%	2%
Time from ER Arrival to Admit. (minutes)[2]	613	523	378	274
Time from ER Arrival to Discharge (minutes)	338	250	156	134
Time in ER Before Being Evaluated (minutes)	377	35	35	26
Time to Pain Meds for Fractures (minutes)	289	64	61	57
Heart Attack Care				
Aspirin Given at Discharge	691	100%	99%	99%
Fibrinolytic Meds Within 30 Min. of Arrival[1]	-	-	46%	54%
PCI Within 90 Minutes of Arrival	121	100%	95%	96%
Statin Prescribed at Discharge	670	98%	98%	98%
Heart Failure Care				
ACE Inhibitor or ARB for LVSD	237	100%	96%	97%
Discharge Instructions Given	663	100%	95%	94%
Evaluation of LVS Function	746	100%	99%	99%
Medicare Spending				
Medicare Spending per Patient (ratio)	-	0.94	0.96	0.98
Pneumonia Care				
Appropriate Initial Antibiotic Given[2]	52	100%	95%	95%
Blood Culture Timing[2]	111	99%	97%	98%
Pregnancy and Delivery Care				
Newborn Deliveries Scheduled Early[2]	22	5%	4%	6%
Preventive Care				
Immunization for Influenza[2]	519	72%	88%	90%
Immunization for Pneumonia[2]	523	75%	88%	92%
Stroke Care				
Anticoagulation Therapy for Atrial Fibrillation[2]	32	100%	96%	95%
Antithrombotic Therapy Timing[2]	144	99%	98%	98%
Assessed for Rehabilitation[2]	229	99%	97%	97%
Discharged on Antithrombotic Therapy[2]	197	100%	99%	99%
Discharged on Statin Medication[2]	140	99%	95%	94%
Thrombolytic Therapy Timing[2]	31	87%	69%	66%
Venous Thromboembolism Prophylaxis[2]	233	98%	94%	94%
Written Stroke Educational Materials Given[2]	149	88%	86%	88%
Surgical Care Improvement Project				
Appropriate Beta Blocker Usage[2]	435	100%	97%	98%
Appropriate VTP Within 24 Hours[2]	395	100%	98%	98%
Controlled Postoperative Blood Glucose[2]	440	98%	97%	97%
Perioperative Temperature Management[2]	588	100%	100%	100%
Prophylactic Antibiotic Selection[2]	658	100%	99%	99%
Prophylactic Antibiotic Selection (Outpatient)	641	100%	97%	98%
Prophylactic Antibiotic Stopped[2]	641	100%	98%	98%
Prophylactic Antibiotic Timing[2]	659	100%	99%	99%
Prophylactic Antibiotic Timing (Outpatient)	640	99%	97%	98%
Urinary Catheter Removal[2]	665	100%	96%	97%
Survey of Patients' Hospital Experiences				
Area Around Room 'Always' Quiet at Night	300+	43%	51%	61%
Doctors 'Always' Communicated Well	300+	79%	77%	82%
Home Recovery Information Given	300+	88%	83%	85%
Hospital Given 9 or 10 on 10 Point Scale	300+	73%	63%	71%
Meds 'Always' Explained Before Given	300+	64%	59%	64%
Nurses 'Always' Communicated Well	300+	78%	75%	79%
Pain 'Always' Well Controlled	300+	66%	67%	71%
Room and Bathroom 'Always' Clean	300+	66%	69%	73%
Timely Help 'Always' Received	300+	63%	61%	68%
Would Definitely Recommend Hospital	300+	79%	65%	71%
Use of Medical Imaging				
Cardiac Imaging Stress Test before Surgery	559	4.5%	5.8%	5.3%
Combination Abdominal CT Scan	983	19.2%	8.2%	10.5%
Combination Brain/Sinus CT Scan	716	5.2%	3.6%	2.7%
Combination Chest CT Scan	684	0.1%	1.3%	2.7%
Follow-up Mammogram/Ultrasound	333	11.7%	13%	8.8%
Lumbar Spine MRI for Low Back Pain	38	42.1%	33.4%	37.2%

Unity Hospital of Rochester

1555 Long Pond Road
Rochester, NY 14626
URL: www.unityhealth.org
Type: Acute Care Hospitals
Ownership: Voluntary non-profit - Private

Phone: 585-723-7000
Emergency Services: Yes
Beds: 681

Measure	Cases	This Hosp.	State Avg.	U.S. Avg.
Blood Clot Prevention and Treatment				
Anticoagulation Overlap Therapy[2]	120	94%	91%	93%
ICU Venous Thromboembolism Prophylaxis[2]	39	95%	92%	92%
Incidence of Potentially Preventable VTE[2]	34	12%	10%	10%
UFH with Dosages/Platelet Monitoring[2]	33	100%	92%	97%
Venous Thromboembolism Prophylaxis[2]	304	87%	87%	85%
Warfarin Therapy Discharge Instructions[2]	86	55%	59%	75%
Chest Pain/Possible Heart Attack Care				
Aspirin Given Within 24 Hours of Arrival	24	96%	97%	96%
Fibrinolytic Meds Within 30 Min. of Arrival[3,7]	-	-	54%	58%
Average Time to ECG (minutes)	24	12	9	7
Average Time to Transfer (minutes)[1,3]	-	-	78	60
Children's Asthma Care				
Received Home Management Plan of Care	-	-	-	88%
Received Reliever Medication	-	-	-	100%
Received Systemic Corticosteroids	-	-	-	100%
Emergency Department				
Admittance Decision Time (minutes)[2]	482	150	154	98
Head CT Results Within 45 Min. of Arrival[1]	-	-	55%	57%
Patients Who Left ER Before Being Seen	47,777	3%	2%	2%
Time from ER Arrival to Admit. (minutes)[2]	487	355	378	274
Time from ER Arrival to Discharge (minutes)	334	196	156	134
Time in ER Before Being Evaluated (minutes)	419	35	35	26
Time to Pain Meds for Fractures (minutes)	140	80	61	57
Heart Attack Care				
Aspirin Given at Discharge	173	99%	99%	99%
Fibrinolytic Meds Within 30 Min. of Arrival[7]	-	-	46%	54%
PCI Within 90 Minutes of Arrival	40	95%	95%	96%
Statin Prescribed at Discharge	172	98%	98%	98%
Heart Failure Care				
ACE Inhibitor or ARB for LVSD[2]	57	89%	96%	97%
Discharge Instructions Given[2]	243	98%	95%	94%
Evaluation of LVS Function[2]	303	98%	99%	99%
Medicare Spending				
Medicare Spending per Patient (ratio)	-	0.91	0.96	0.98
Pneumonia Care				
Appropriate Initial Antibiotic Given[2]	118	96%	95%	95%
Blood Culture Timing[2]	160	95%	97%	98%
Pregnancy and Delivery Care				
Newborn Deliveries Scheduled Early	266	1%	4%	6%
Preventive Care				
Immunization for Influenza[2]	539	93%	88%	90%
Immunization for Pneumonia[2]	696	94%	88%	92%
Stroke Care				
Anticoagulation Therapy for Atrial Fibrillation[2]	11	100%	96%	95%
Antithrombotic Therapy Timing[2]	82	99%	98%	98%
Assessed for Rehabilitation[2]	99	92%	97%	97%
Discharged on Antithrombotic Therapy[2]	91	100%	99%	99%
Discharged on Statin Medication[2]	74	99%	95%	94%
Thrombolytic Therapy Timing[1,2]	-	-	69%	66%
Venous Thromboembolism Prophylaxis[2]	98	86%	94%	94%
Written Stroke Educational Materials Given[2]	62	92%	86%	88%
Surgical Care Improvement Project				
Appropriate Beta Blocker Usage[2]	187	100%	97%	98%
Appropriate VTP Within 24 Hours[2]	422	100%	98%	98%
Controlled Postoperative Blood Glucose[2,7]	-	-	97%	97%
Perioperative Temperature Management[2]	517	100%	100%	100%
Prophylactic Antibiotic Selection[2]	337	99%	99%	99%
Prophylactic Antibiotic Selection (Outpatient)	518	100%	97%	98%
Prophylactic Antibiotic Stopped[2]	337	99%	98%	98%
Prophylactic Antibiotic Timing[2]	339	99%	99%	99%
Prophylactic Antibiotic Timing (Outpatient)	521	94%	97%	98%
Urinary Catheter Removal[2]	372	100%	96%	97%
Survey of Patients' Hospital Experiences				
Area Around Room 'Always' Quiet at Night	300+	51%	51%	61%
Doctors 'Always' Communicated Well	300+	80%	77%	82%
Home Recovery Information Given	300+	89%	83%	85%
Hospital Given 9 or 10 on 10 Point Scale	300+	66%	63%	71%
Meds 'Always' Explained Before Given	300+	59%	59%	64%
Nurses 'Always' Communicated Well	300+	76%	75%	79%
Pain 'Always' Well Controlled	300+	65%	67%	71%
Room and Bathroom 'Always' Clean	300+	60%	69%	73%
Timely Help 'Always' Received	300+	57%	61%	68%
Would Definitely Recommend Hospital	300+	71%	65%	71%
Use of Medical Imaging				
Cardiac Imaging Stress Test before Surgery	138	4.3%	5.8%	5.3%
Combination Abdominal CT Scan	246	1.6%	8.2%	10.5%
Combination Brain/Sinus CT Scan[1]	-	-	3.6%	2.7%
Combination Chest CT Scan[1]	-	-	1.3%	2.7%
Follow-up Mammogram/Ultrasound[7]	-	-	13%	8.8%
Lumbar Spine MRI for Low Back Pain[7]	-	-	33.4%	37.2%

Mercy Medical Center

1000 North Village Avenue
Rockville Centre, NY 11570
URL: www.mercymedicalcenter.info
Type: Acute Care Hospitals
Ownership: Voluntary non-profit - Church

Phone: 516-705-2525
Fax: 516-705-2584
Emergency Services: Yes
Beds: 375

Key Personnel:
CEO/President............... Alan D Guerci, MD

NOTE: Hospital profiles are in alphabetical order by state, then city, then hospital within the city; Rankings exclude hospitals with less than 25 cases except for patient surveys which excludes hospitals with less than 100 cases; (a) 100-299 cases; (1) The number of cases/patients is too few to report; (2) Data submitted were based on a sample of cases/patients; (3) Results are based on a shorter time period than required; (4) Data suppressed by CMS for one or more quarters; (5) Results are not available for this reporting period; (6) Fewer than 100 patients completed the HCAHPS survey; (7) No cases met the criteria for this measure; (8) The lower limit of the confidence interval cannot be calculated if the number of observed infections equals zero; (9) No data are available from the state/territory for this reporting period; (10) The scores shown reflect fewer than 50 completed surveys; (11) There were discrepancies in the data collection process; (12) This measure does not apply to this hospital for this reporting period; (13) Results cannot be calculated for this reporting period; (14) The results for this state are combined with nearby states to protect confidentiality; Please refer to the User's Guide for a full explanation of data.

Quality Assurance . . . . Catherine Magoone, RN
Chief of Medical Staff . . . . John P Reilly, MD

Measure	Cases	This Hosp.	State Avg.	U.S. Avg.
Blood Clot Prevention and Treatment				
Anticoagulation Overlap Therapy[2]	65	89%	91%	93%
ICU Venous Thromboembolism Prophylaxis[2]	65	98%	92%	92%
Incidence of Potentially Preventable VTE[2]	22	5%	10%	10%
UFH with Dosages/Platelet Monitoring[2]	34	100%	92%	97%
Venous Thromboembolism Prophylaxis[2]	389	87%	87%	85%
Warfarin Therapy Discharge Instructions[2]	40	45%	59%	75%
Chest Pain/Possible Heart Attack Care				
Aspirin Given Within 24 Hours of Arrival	48	100%	97%	96%
Fibrinolytic Meds Within 30 Min. of Arrival[7]	-	-	54%	58%
Average Time to ECG (minutes)	49	6	9	7
Average Time to Transfer (minutes)	14	44	78	60
Children's Asthma Care				
Received Home Management Plan of Care	-	-	-	88%
Received Reliever Medication	-	-	-	100%
Received Systemic Corticosteroids	-	-	-	100%
Emergency Department				
Admittance Decision Time (minutes)[2]	641	250	154	98
Head CT Results Within 45 Min. of Arrival[1]	-	-	55%	57%
Patients Who Left ER Before Being Seen	39,066	1%	2%	2%
Time from ER Arrival to Admit. (minutes)[2]	738	490	378	274
Time from ER Arrival to Discharge (minutes)	394	151	156	134
Time in ER Before Being Evaluated (minutes)	417	45	35	26
Time to Pain Meds for Fractures (minutes)	80	58	61	57
Heart Attack Care				
Aspirin Given at Discharge	78	100%	99%	99%
Fibrinolytic Meds Within 30 Min. of Arrival[7]	-	-	46%	54%
PCI Within 90 Minutes of Arrival[7]	-	-	95%	96%
Statin Prescribed at Discharge	77	100%	98%	98%
Heart Failure Care				
ACE Inhibitor or ARB for LVSD	50	100%	96%	97%
Discharge Instructions Given	112	100%	95%	94%
Evaluation of LVS Function	159	100%	99%	99%
Medicare Spending				
Medicare Spending per Patient (ratio)	-	1.08	0.96	0.98
Pneumonia Care				
Appropriate Initial Antibiotic Given	95	96%	95%	95%
Blood Culture Timing	273	99%	97%	98%
Pregnancy and Delivery Care				
Newborn Deliveries Scheduled Early[2]	34	9%	4%	6%
Preventive Care				
Immunization for Influenza[2]	508	97%	88%	90%
Immunization for Pneumonia[2]	659	96%	88%	92%
Stroke Care				
Anticoagulation Therapy for Atrial Fibrillation[2]	21	95%	96%	95%
Antithrombotic Therapy Timing[2]	99	100%	98%	98%
Assessed for Rehabilitation[2]	126	99%	97%	97%
Discharged on Antithrombotic Therapy[2]	100	100%	99%	99%
Discharged on Statin Medication[2]	79	99%	95%	94%
Thrombolytic Therapy Timing[1,2]	-	-	69%	66%
Venous Thromboembolism Prophylaxis[2]	130	97%	94%	94%
Written Stroke Educational Materials Given[2]	48	100%	86%	88%
Surgical Care Improvement Project				
Appropriate Beta Blocker Usage[2]	99	97%	97%	98%
Appropriate VTP Within 24 Hours[2]	318	100%	98%	98%
Controlled Postoperative Blood Glucose[2,7]	-	-	97%	97%
Perioperative Temperature Management[2]	360	100%	100%	100%
Prophylactic Antibiotic Selection[2]	169	99%	99%	99%
Prophylactic Antibiotic Selection (Outpatient)	65	97%	97%	98%
Prophylactic Antibiotic Stopped[2]	158	99%	98%	98%
Prophylactic Antibiotic Timing[2]	169	96%	99%	99%
Prophylactic Antibiotic Timing (Outpatient)	65	100%	97%	98%
Urinary Catheter Removal[2]	208	100%	96%	97%
Survey of Patients' Hospital Experiences				
Area Around Room 'Always' Quiet at Night	300+	54%	51%	61%
Doctors 'Always' Communicated Well	300+	79%	77%	82%
Home Recovery Information Given	300+	85%	83%	85%
Hospital Given 9 or 10 on 10 Point Scale	300+	66%	63%	71%
Meds 'Always' Explained Before Given	300+	60%	59%	64%
Nurses 'Always' Communicated Well	300+	75%	75%	79%
Pain 'Always' Well Controlled	300+	70%	67%	71%
Room and Bathroom 'Always' Clean	300+	67%	69%	73%
Timely Help 'Always' Received	300+	60%	61%	68%
Would Definitely Recommend Hospital	300+	68%	65%	71%
Use of Medical Imaging				
Cardiac Imaging Stress Test before Surgery	102	7.8%	5.8%	5.3%
Combination Abdominal CT Scan	547	2.4%	8.2%	10.5%
Combination Brain/Sinus CT Scan	601	2.2%	3.6%	2.7%
Combination Chest CT Scan	357	0.0%	1.3%	2.7%
Follow-up Mammogram/Ultrasound	738	38.3%	13%	8.8%
Lumbar Spine MRI for Low Back Pain[1]	-	-	33.4%	37.2%

Rome Memorial Hospital

1500 North James Street
Rome, NY 13440
Phone: 315-338-7000
Fax: 315-338-7072
URL: www.romehosp.org
Type: Acute Care Hospitals
Emergency Services: Yes
Ownership: Voluntary non-profit - Private
Beds: 129

Key Personnel:
CEO/President . . . . Basil J. Ariglio
Operating Room . . . . Teresa Bell
Pediatric Ambulatory Care . . . . . . Laurie Elwell, DO
Pediatric In-Patient Care . . . . Laurie Elwell, DO
Infection Control . . . . LeAnna Grace
Chief of Medical Staff . . . . Marybeth McCall, MD
Quality Assurance . . . . Kathleen Ulrich
Radiology . . . . Amy Weakley

Measure	Cases	This Hosp.	State Avg.	U.S. Avg.
Blood Clot Prevention and Treatment				
Anticoagulation Overlap Therapy[2]	36	92%	91%	93%
ICU Venous Thromboembolism Prophylaxis[2]	76	99%	92%	92%
Incidence of Potentially Preventable VTE[1,2]	-	-	10%	10%
UFH with Dosages/Platelet Monitoring[2]	20	100%	92%	97%
Venous Thromboembolism Prophylaxis[2]	291	88%	87%	85%
Warfarin Therapy Discharge Instructions[2]	28	79%	59%	75%
Chest Pain/Possible Heart Attack Care				
Aspirin Given Within 24 Hours of Arrival	33	94%	97%	96%
Fibrinolytic Meds Within 30 Min. of Arrival[7]	-	-	54%	58%
Average Time to ECG (minutes)	33	7	9	7
Average Time to Transfer (minutes)[1]	-	-	78	60
Children's Asthma Care				
Received Home Management Plan of Care	-	-	-	88%
Received Reliever Medication	-	-	-	100%
Received Systemic Corticosteroids	-	-	-	100%
Emergency Department				
Admittance Decision Time (minutes)[2]	359	100	154	98
Head CT Results Within 45 Min. of Arrival[1]	-	-	55%	57%
Patients Who Left ER Before Being Seen	27,539	2%	2%	2%
Time from ER Arrival to Admit. (minutes)[2]	394	294	378	274
Time from ER Arrival to Discharge (minutes)	340	136	156	134
Time in ER Before Being Evaluated (minutes)	373	45	35	26
Time to Pain Meds for Fractures (minutes)	55	75	61	57
Heart Attack Care				
Aspirin Given at Discharge	25	100%	99%	99%
Fibrinolytic Meds Within 30 Min. of Arrival[7]	-	-	46%	54%
PCI Within 90 Minutes of Arrival[7]	-	-	95%	96%
Statin Prescribed at Discharge	21	81%	98%	98%
Heart Failure Care				
ACE Inhibitor or ARB for LVSD	36	100%	96%	97%
Discharge Instructions Given	127	87%	95%	94%
Evaluation of LVS Function	174	95%	99%	99%
Medicare Spending				
Medicare Spending per Patient (ratio)	-	0.90	0.96	0.98
Pneumonia Care				
Appropriate Initial Antibiotic Given	98	93%	95%	95%
Blood Culture Timing	147	97%	97%	98%
Pregnancy and Delivery Care				
Newborn Deliveries Scheduled Early[2]	31	0%	4%	6%
Preventive Care				
Immunization for Influenza[2]	373	91%	88%	90%
Immunization for Pneumonia[2]	455	89%	88%	92%
Stroke Care				
Anticoagulation Therapy for Atrial Fibrillation[1]	-	-	96%	95%
Antithrombotic Therapy Timing	16	100%	98%	98%
Assessed for Rehabilitation	15	100%	97%	97%
Discharged on Antithrombotic Therapy	12	100%	99%	99%
Discharged on Statin Medication	11	91%	95%	94%
Thrombolytic Therapy Timing[1]	-	-	69%	66%
Venous Thromboembolism Prophylaxis	19	95%	94%	94%
Written Stroke Educational Materials Given[1]	-	-	86%	88%
Surgical Care Improvement Project				
Appropriate Beta Blocker Usage	42	98%	97%	98%
Appropriate VTP Within 24 Hours	161	96%	98%	98%
Controlled Postoperative Blood Glucose[7]	-	-	97%	97%
Perioperative Temperature Management	179	99%	100%	100%
Prophylactic Antibiotic Selection	101	97%	99%	99%
Prophylactic Antibiotic Selection (Outpatient)	20	100%	97%	98%
Prophylactic Antibiotic Stopped	98	98%	98%	98%
Prophylactic Antibiotic Timing	101	95%	99%	99%
Prophylactic Antibiotic Timing (Outpatient)	20	90%	97%	98%
Urinary Catheter Removal	41	93%	96%	97%
Survey of Patients' Hospital Experiences				
Area Around Room 'Always' Quiet at Night	300+	48%	51%	61%
Doctors 'Always' Communicated Well	300+	77%	77%	82%
Home Recovery Information Given	300+	87%	83%	85%
Hospital Given 9 or 10 on 10 Point Scale	300+	64%	63%	71%
Meds 'Always' Explained Before Given	300+	59%	59%	64%
Nurses 'Always' Communicated Well	300+	78%	75%	79%
Pain 'Always' Well Controlled	300+	69%	67%	71%
Room and Bathroom 'Always' Clean	300+	74%	69%	73%
Timely Help 'Always' Received	300+	61%	61%	68%
Would Definitely Recommend Hospital	300+	64%	65%	71%
Use of Medical Imaging				
Cardiac Imaging Stress Test before Surgery	148	3.4%	5.8%	5.3%
Combination Abdominal CT Scan	476	9.2%	8.2%	10.5%
Combination Brain/Sinus CT Scan[1]	-	-	3.6%	2.7%
Combination Chest CT Scan	366	3.0%	1.3%	2.7%
Follow-up Mammogram/Ultrasound	432	1.9%	13%	8.8%
Lumbar Spine MRI for Low Back Pain	55	30.9%	33.4%	37.2%

Saint Francis Hospital - Roslyn

100 Port Washington Boulevard
Roslyn, NY 11576
Phone: 516-562-6000
Fax: 516-705-6661
URL: www.stfrancisheartcenter.com
Type: Acute Care Hospitals
Emergency Services: Yes
Ownership: Voluntary non-profit - Church
Beds: 279

Key Personnel:
Radiology . . . . Ken Goodman, MD
CEO/President . . . . Alan D Guerci, MD
Coronary Care . . . . Susan Knoeffler, RN NCC
Pediatric Ambulatory Care . . . . . . Donna Rebelo, RN NCC
Pediatric In-Patient Care . . . . Donna Rebelo, RN NCC
Chief of Medical Staff . . . . Lawrence A Reduto, MD
Quality Assurance . . . . Nonette Schafer, RN
Infection Control . . . . Marylou Solliday, RN

Measure	Cases	This Hosp.	State Avg.	U.S. Avg.
Blood Clot Prevention and Treatment				
Anticoagulation Overlap Therapy[2]	92	70%	91%	93%
ICU Venous Thromboembolism Prophylaxis[2]	114	91%	92%	92%
Incidence of Potentially Preventable VTE[2]	23	4%	10%	10%
UFH with Dosages/Platelet Monitoring[2]	106	99%	92%	97%
Venous Thromboembolism Prophylaxis[2]	357	81%	87%	85%
Warfarin Therapy Discharge Instructions[2]	58	98%	59%	75%
Chest Pain/Possible Heart Attack Care				
Aspirin Given Within 24 Hours of Arrival[3,7]	-	-	97%	96%
Fibrinolytic Meds Within 30 Min. of Arrival[5]	-	-	54%	58%
Average Time to ECG (minutes)[3,7]	-	-	9	7
Average Time to Transfer (minutes)[5]	-	-	78	60
Children's Asthma Care				
Received Home Management Plan of Care	-	-	-	88%
Received Reliever Medication	-	-	-	100%
Received Systemic Corticosteroids	-	-	-	100%
Emergency Department				
Admittance Decision Time (minutes)[2]	601	428	154	98
Head CT Results Within 45 Min. of Arrival[1]	-	-	55%	57%
Patients Who Left ER Before Being Seen	22,832	1%	2%	2%
Time from ER Arrival to Admit. (minutes)[2]	613	656	378	274

NOTE: Hospital profiles are in alphabetical order by state, then city, then hospital within the city; Rankings exclude hospitals with less than 25 cases except for patient surveys which excludes hospitals with less than 100 cases; (a) 100-299 cases; (1) The number of cases/patients is too few to report; (2) Data submitted were based on a sample of cases/patients; (3) Results are based on a shorter time period than required; (4) Data suppressed by CMS for one or more quarters; (5) Results are not available for this reporting period; (6) Fewer than 100 patients completed the HCAHPS survey; (7) No cases met the criteria for this measure; (8) The lower limit of the confidence interval cannot be calculated if the number of observed infections equals zero; (9) No data are available from the state/territory for this reporting period; (10) The scores shown reflect fewer than 50 completed surveys; (11) There were discrepancies in the data collection process; (12) This measure does not apply to this hospital for this reporting period; (13) Results cannot be calculated for this reporting period; (14) The results for this state are combined with nearby states to protect confidentiality; Please refer to the User's Guide for a full explanation of data.

Measure	Cases	This Hosp.	State Avg.	U.S. Avg.
Time from ER Arrival to Discharge (minutes)	348	266	156	134
Time in ER Before Being Evaluated (minutes)	239	52	35	26
Time to Pain Meds for Fractures (minutes)	30	96	61	57
Heart Attack Care				
Aspirin Given at Discharge[2]	338	99%	99%	99%
Fibrinolytic Meds Within 30 Min. of Arrival[2,7]	-	-	46%	54%
PCI Within 90 Minutes of Arrival[2]	13	85%	95%	96%
Statin Prescribed at Discharge[2]	347	98%	98%	98%
Heart Failure Care				
ACE Inhibitor or ARB for LVSD[2]	128	97%	96%	97%
Discharge Instructions Given[2]	314	95%	95%	94%
Evaluation of LVS Function[2]	378	100%	99%	99%
Medicare Spending				
Medicare Spending per Patient (ratio)	-	1.00	0.96	0.98
Pneumonia Care				
Appropriate Initial Antibiotic Given	159	94%	95%	95%
Blood Culture Timing	187	98%	97%	98%
Pregnancy and Delivery Care				
Newborn Deliveries Scheduled Early[7]	-	-	4%	6%
Preventive Care				
Immunization for Influenza[2]	624	79%	88%	90%
Immunization for Pneumonia[2]	1,023	79%	88%	92%
Stroke Care				
Anticoagulation Therapy for Atrial Fibrillation[2]	18	89%	96%	95%
Antithrombotic Therapy Timing[2]	55	95%	98%	98%
Assessed for Rehabilitation[2]	67	100%	97%	97%
Discharged on Antithrombotic Therapy[2]	62	100%	99%	99%
Discharged on Statin Medication[2]	51	98%	95%	94%
Thrombolytic Therapy Timing[2,7]	-	-	69%	66%
Venous Thromboembolism Prophylaxis[2]	64	89%	94%	94%
Written Stroke Educational Materials Given[2]	42	98%	86%	88%
Surgical Care Improvement Project				
Appropriate Beta Blocker Usage[2]	398	99%	97%	98%
Appropriate VTP Within 24 Hours[2]	416	100%	98%	98%
Controlled Postoperative Blood Glucose[2]	232	94%	97%	97%
Perioperative Temperature Management[2]	670	100%	100%	100%
Prophylactic Antibiotic Selection[2]	559	100%	99%	99%
Prophylactic Antibiotic Selection (Outpatient)	472	97%	97%	98%
Prophylactic Antibiotic Stopped[2]	550	97%	98%	98%
Prophylactic Antibiotic Timing[2]	560	99%	99%	99%
Prophylactic Antibiotic Timing (Outpatient)	472	100%	97%	98%
Urinary Catheter Removal[2]	521	90%	96%	97%
Survey of Patients' Hospital Experiences				
Area Around Room 'Always' Quiet at Night	300+	52%	51%	61%
Doctors 'Always' Communicated Well	300+	84%	77%	82%
Home Recovery Information Given	300+	89%	83%	85%
Hospital Given 9 or 10 on 10 Point Scale	300+	82%	63%	71%
Meds 'Always' Explained Before Given	300+	66%	59%	64%
Nurses 'Always' Communicated Well	300+	82%	75%	79%
Pain 'Always' Well Controlled	300+	74%	67%	71%
Room and Bathroom 'Always' Clean	300+	75%	69%	73%
Timely Help 'Always' Received	300+	67%	61%	68%
Would Definitely Recommend Hospital	300+	86%	65%	71%
Use of Medical Imaging				
Cardiac Imaging Stress Test before Surgery	2,342	6.2%	5.8%	5.3%
Combination Abdominal CT Scan	597	3.9%	8.2%	10.5%
Combination Brain/Sinus CT Scan	682	1.6%	3.6%	2.7%
Combination Chest CT Scan	683	1.3%	1.3%	2.7%
Follow-up Mammogram/Ultrasound	713	45.9%	13%	8.8%
Lumbar Spine MRI for Low Back Pain[1]	-	-	33.4%	37.2%

Adirondack Medical Center

2233 State Route 86
Saranac Lake, NY 12983
URL: www.amccares.org
Type: Acute Care Hospitals
Ownership: Voluntary non-profit - Other

Phone: 518-891-4141
Fax: 518-891-1191
Emergency Services: Yes
Beds: 97

Key Personnel:
Ambulatory Care . . . . Barbara Dukett, RN
CEO/President. . . . . Adirondack Health
Emergency Room . . . . Mary O'Connor, RN
Hemotology Center . . . . Michael Randolph
Anesthesiology. . . . . Richard Rowell, MD
Quality Assurance . . . . Doug Sarr, RN
Chief of Medical Staff . . . . W Roy Slanowhite, MD
Infection Control. . . . . Mim Tracy, RN

Measure	Cases	This Hosp.	State Avg.	U.S. Avg.
Blood Clot Prevention and Treatment				
Anticoagulation Overlap Therapy[2]	17	76%	91%	93%
ICU Venous Thromboembolism Prophylaxis[2]	46	78%	92%	92%
Incidence of Potentially Preventable VTE[2,7]	-	-	10%	10%
UFH with Dosages/Platelet Monitoring[2]	14	100%	92%	97%
Venous Thromboembolism Prophylaxis[2]	199	76%	87%	85%
Warfarin Therapy Discharge Instructions[2]	16	94%	59%	75%
Chest Pain/Possible Heart Attack Care				
Aspirin Given Within 24 Hours of Arrival	54	98%	97%	96%
Fibrinolytic Meds Within 30 Min. of Arrival	11	73%	54%	58%
Average Time to ECG (minutes)	56	6	9	7
Average Time to Transfer (minutes)[1]	-	-	78	60
Children's Asthma Care				
Received Home Management Plan of Care	-	-	-	88%
Received Reliever Medication	-	-	-	100%
Received Systemic Corticosteroids	-	-	-	100%
Emergency Department				
Admittance Decision Time (minutes)[2]	270	78	154	98
Head CT Results Within 45 Min. of Arrival[1]	-	-	55%	57%
Patients Who Left ER Before Being Seen	13,150	0%	2%	2%
Time from ER Arrival to Admit. (minutes)[2]	295	253	378	274
Time from ER Arrival to Discharge (minutes)	370	90	156	134
Time in ER Before Being Evaluated (minutes)	354	21	35	26
Time to Pain Meds for Fractures (minutes)	75	49	61	57
Heart Attack Care				
Aspirin Given at Discharge[1]	-	-	99%	99%
Fibrinolytic Meds Within 30 Min. of Arrival[7]	-	-	46%	54%
PCI Within 90 Minutes of Arrival[7]	-	-	95%	96%
Statin Prescribed at Discharge[1]	-	-	98%	98%
Heart Failure Care				
ACE Inhibitor or ARB for LVSD	20	85%	96%	97%
Discharge Instructions Given	55	87%	95%	94%
Evaluation of LVS Function	68	99%	99%	99%
Medicare Spending				
Medicare Spending per Patient (ratio)	-	0.92	0.96	0.98
Pneumonia Care				
Appropriate Initial Antibiotic Given	38	79%	95%	95%
Blood Culture Timing	75	97%	97%	98%
Pregnancy and Delivery Care				
Newborn Deliveries Scheduled Early	22	0%	4%	6%
Preventive Care				
Immunization for Influenza[2]	304	74%	88%	90%
Immunization for Pneumonia[2]	335	75%	88%	92%
Stroke Care				
Anticoagulation Therapy for Atrial Fibrillation[1]	-	-	96%	95%
Antithrombotic Therapy Timing	16	94%	98%	98%
Assessed for Rehabilitation	25	100%	97%	97%
Discharged on Antithrombotic Therapy	20	95%	99%	99%
Discharged on Statin Medication	17	76%	95%	94%
Thrombolytic Therapy Timing[1]	-	-	69%	66%
Venous Thromboembolism Prophylaxis	24	83%	94%	94%
Written Stroke Educational Materials Given	19	95%	86%	88%
Surgical Care Improvement Project				
Appropriate Beta Blocker Usage[2]	92	99%	97%	98%
Appropriate VTP Within 24 Hours[2]	359	93%	98%	98%
Controlled Postoperative Blood Glucose[2,7]	-	-	97%	97%
Perioperative Temperature Management[2]	386	99%	100%	100%
Prophylactic Antibiotic Selection[2]	219	98%	99%	99%
Prophylactic Antibiotic Selection (Outpatient)	94	96%	97%	98%
Prophylactic Antibiotic Stopped[2]	213	98%	98%	98%
Prophylactic Antibiotic Timing[2]	220	95%	99%	99%
Prophylactic Antibiotic Timing (Outpatient)	93	89%	97%	98%
Urinary Catheter Removal[2]	249	96%	96%	97%
Survey of Patients' Hospital Experiences				
Area Around Room 'Always' Quiet at Night	300+	57%	51%	61%
Doctors 'Always' Communicated Well	300+	86%	77%	82%
Home Recovery Information Given	300+	90%	83%	85%
Hospital Given 9 or 10 on 10 Point Scale	300+	72%	63%	71%
Meds 'Always' Explained Before Given	300+	65%	59%	64%
Nurses 'Always' Communicated Well	300+	82%	75%	79%
Pain 'Always' Well Controlled	300+	74%	67%	71%
Room and Bathroom 'Always' Clean	300+	80%	69%	73%
Timely Help 'Always' Received	300+	76%	61%	68%
Would Definitely Recommend Hospital	300+	73%	65%	71%
Use of Medical Imaging				
Cardiac Imaging Stress Test before Surgery	157	5.1%	5.8%	5.3%
Combination Abdominal CT Scan	400	6.3%	8.2%	10.5%
Combination Brain/Sinus CT Scan[1]	-	-	3.6%	2.7%
Combination Chest CT Scan	314	4.5%	1.3%	2.7%
Follow-up Mammogram/Ultrasound	804	26.2%	13%	8.8%
Lumbar Spine MRI for Low Back Pain[1]	-	-	33.4%	37.2%

Saratoga Hospital

211 Church Street
Saratoga Springs, NY 12866
URL: www.saratogacare.org
Type: Acute Care Hospitals
Ownership: Voluntary non-profit - Private

Phone: 518-587-3222
Fax: 518-583-8428
Emergency Services: Yes
Beds: 243

Key Personnel:
Intensive Care Unit. . . . . Diane Bartos
Emergency Room . . . . Timothy Brooks
CEO/President. . . . . Angelo Calbone
Patient Relations . . . . Noel Cook
Operating Room. . . . . Cathleen Hamel
Quality Assurance . . . . Kim Hedley
Chief of Medical Staff. . . . . Joyce L Peabody, MD

Measure	Cases	This Hosp.	State Avg.	U.S. Avg.
Blood Clot Prevention and Treatment				
Anticoagulation Overlap Therapy[2]	71	94%	91%	93%
ICU Venous Thromboembolism Prophylaxis[2]	53	72%	92%	92%
Incidence of Potentially Preventable VTE[1,2]	-	-	10%	10%
UFH with Dosages/Platelet Monitoring[1,2]	-	-	92%	97%
Venous Thromboembolism Prophylaxis[2]	291	60%	87%	85%
Warfarin Therapy Discharge Instructions[2]	60	93%	59%	75%
Chest Pain/Possible Heart Attack Care				
Aspirin Given Within 24 Hours of Arrival	57	96%	97%	96%
Fibrinolytic Meds Within 30 Min. of Arrival	15	60%	54%	58%
Average Time to ECG (minutes)	58	4	9	7
Average Time to Transfer (minutes)[1]	-	-	78	60
Children's Asthma Care				
Received Home Management Plan of Care	-	-	-	88%
Received Reliever Medication	-	-	-	100%
Received Systemic Corticosteroids	-	-	-	100%
Emergency Department				
Admittance Decision Time (minutes)[2]	491	123	154	98
Head CT Results Within 45 Min. of Arrival	19	79%	55%	57%
Patients Who Left ER Before Being Seen	40,517	1%	2%	2%
Time from ER Arrival to Admit. (minutes)[2]	501	302	378	274
Time from ER Arrival to Discharge (minutes)	513	164	156	134
Time in ER Before Being Evaluated (minutes)	583	43	35	26
Time to Pain Meds for Fractures (minutes)	88	48	61	57
Heart Attack Care				
Aspirin Given at Discharge	41	98%	99%	99%
Fibrinolytic Meds Within 30 Min. of Arrival[1]	-	-	46%	54%
PCI Within 90 Minutes of Arrival[7]	-	-	95%	96%
Statin Prescribed at Discharge	39	87%	98%	98%
Heart Failure Care				
ACE Inhibitor or ARB for LVSD	26	100%	96%	97%
Discharge Instructions Given	163	89%	95%	94%
Evaluation of LVS Function	193	100%	99%	99%
Medicare Spending				
Medicare Spending per Patient (ratio)	-	0.91	0.96	0.98
Pneumonia Care				
Appropriate Initial Antibiotic Given[2]	148	95%	95%	95%
Blood Culture Timing[2]	215	99%	97%	98%
Pregnancy and Delivery Care				
Newborn Deliveries Scheduled Early[2]	11	18%	4%	6%
Preventive Care				
Immunization for Influenza[2]	551	97%	88%	90%
Immunization for Pneumonia[2]	624	95%	88%	92%
Stroke Care				
Anticoagulation Therapy for Atrial Fibrillation[1]	-	-	96%	95%
Antithrombotic Therapy Timing	28	100%	98%	98%

NOTE: Hospital profiles are in alphabetical order by state, then city, then hospital within the city; Rankings exclude hospitals with less than 25 cases except for patient surveys which excludes hospitals with less than 100 cases; (a) 100-299 cases; (1) The number of cases/patients is too few to report; (2) Data submitted were based on a sample of cases/patients; (3) Results are based on a shorter time period than required; (4) Data suppressed by CMS for one or more quarters; (5) Results are not available for this reporting period; (6) Fewer than 100 patients completed the HCAHPS survey; (7) No cases met the criteria for this measure; (8) The lower limit of the confidence interval cannot be calculated if the number of observed infections equals zero; (9) No data are available from the state/territory for this reporting period; (10) The scores shown reflect fewer than 50 completed surveys; (11) There were discrepancies in the data collection process; (12) This measure does not apply to this hospital for this reporting period; (13) Results cannot be calculated for this reporting period; (14) The results for this state are combined with nearby states to protect confidentiality; Please refer to the User's Guide for a full explanation of data.

Measure	Cases	This Hosp.	State Avg.	U.S. Avg.
Assessed for Rehabilitation	33	100%	97%	97%
Discharged on Antithrombotic Therapy	29	93%	99%	99%
Discharged on Statin Medication	28	82%	95%	94%
Thrombolytic Therapy Timing[1]	-	-	69%	66%
Venous Thromboembolism Prophylaxis	29	83%	94%	94%
Written Stroke Educational Materials Given	22	45%	86%	88%
Surgical Care Improvement Project				
Appropriate Beta Blocker Usage[2]	215	97%	97%	98%
Appropriate VTP Within 24 Hours[2]	570	97%	98%	98%
Controlled Postoperative Blood Glucose[2,7]	-	-	97%	97%
Perioperative Temperature Management[2]	719	100%	100%	100%
Prophylactic Antibiotic Selection[2]	460	99%	99%	99%
Prophylactic Antibiotic Selection (Outpatient)	285	99%	97%	98%
Prophylactic Antibiotic Stopped[2]	447	98%	98%	98%
Prophylactic Antibiotic Timing[2]	460	99%	99%	99%
Prophylactic Antibiotic Timing (Outpatient)	279	99%	97%	98%
Urinary Catheter Removal[2]	348	96%	96%	97%
Survey of Patients' Hospital Experiences				
Area Around Room 'Always' Quiet at Night	300+	50%	51%	61%
Doctors 'Always' Communicated Well	300+	81%	77%	82%
Home Recovery Information Given	300+	90%	83%	85%
Hospital Given 9 or 10 on 10 Point Scale	300+	74%	63%	71%
Meds 'Always' Explained Before Given	300+	67%	59%	64%
Nurses 'Always' Communicated Well	300+	82%	75%	79%
Pain 'Always' Well Controlled	300+	73%	67%	71%
Room and Bathroom 'Always' Clean	300+	72%	69%	73%
Timely Help 'Always' Received	300+	74%	61%	68%
Would Definitely Recommend Hospital	300+	76%	65%	71%
Use of Medical Imaging				
Cardiac Imaging Stress Test before Surgery	111	2.7%	5.8%	5.3%
Combination Abdominal CT Scan	943	1.9%	8.2%	10.5%
Combination Brain/Sinus CT Scan	821	3.0%	3.6%	2.7%
Combination Chest CT Scan	441	0.9%	1.3%	2.7%
Follow-up Mammogram/Ultrasound	1,086	5.1%	13%	8.8%
Lumbar Spine MRI for Low Back Pain	91	34.1%	33.4%	37.2%

Ellis Hospital

1101 Nott Street
Schenectady, NY 12308
Phone: 518-243-4196
Fax: 518-243-4668
E-mail: webmaster@ellishospital.org
URL: www.ellishospital.org
Type: Acute Care Hospitals
Emergency Services: Yes
Ownership: Proprietary
Beds: 368

Key Personnel:
Cardiac Laboratory. . . . . Lewis Bergman
CEO/President. . . . . James W Connolly
Operating Room. . . . . Carmen Hercules, RN
Pediatric Ambulatory Care . . . . . Pashu Pati Kumar, MD
Chief of Medical Staff . . . . David M. Liebers, MD
Chair/CEO . . . . Deborah Mullaney
Radiology. . . . . Gary Wood, MD
Infection Control . . . . Peg Wyant

Measure	Cases	This Hosp.	State Avg.	U.S. Avg.
Blood Clot Prevention and Treatment				
Anticoagulation Overlap Therapy[2]	102	94%	91%	93%
ICU Venous Thromboembolism Prophylaxis[2]	100	93%	92%	92%
Incidence of Potentially Preventable VTE[2]	16	19%	10%	10%
UFH with Dosages/Platelet Monitoring[2]	57	98%	92%	97%
Venous Thromboembolism Prophylaxis[2]	355	93%	87%	85%
Warfarin Therapy Discharge Instructions[2]	82	45%	59%	75%
Chest Pain/Possible Heart Attack Care				
Aspirin Given Within 24 Hours of Arrival[1,3]	-	-	97%	96%
Fibrinolytic Meds Within 30 Min. of Arrival[3,7]	-	-	54%	58%
Average Time to ECG (minutes)[1,3]	-	-	9	7
Average Time to Transfer (minutes)[1,3]	-	-	78	60
Children's Asthma Care				
Received Home Management Plan of Care	-	-	-	88%
Received Reliever Medication	-	-	-	100%
Received Systemic Corticosteroids	-	-	-	100%
Emergency Department				
Admittance Decision Time (minutes)[2]	366	116	154	98
Head CT Results Within 45 Min. of Arrival	15	47%	55%	57%
Patients Who Left ER Before Being Seen	90,682	2%	2%	2%
Time from ER Arrival to Admit. (minutes)[2]	567	369	378	274
Time from ER Arrival to Discharge (minutes)	394	142	156	134
Time in ER Before Being Evaluated (minutes)	418	35	35	26
Time to Pain Meds for Fractures (minutes)	331	50	61	57
Heart Attack Care				
Aspirin Given at Discharge	534	100%	99%	99%
Fibrinolytic Meds Within 30 Min. of Arrival[7]	-	-	46%	54%
PCI Within 90 Minutes of Arrival	78	95%	95%	96%
Statin Prescribed at Discharge	522	99%	98%	98%
Heart Failure Care				
ACE Inhibitor or ARB for LVSD	129	100%	96%	97%
Discharge Instructions Given	419	96%	95%	94%
Evaluation of LVS Function	531	100%	99%	99%
Medicare Spending				
Medicare Spending per Patient (ratio)	-	0.97	0.96	0.98
Pneumonia Care				
Appropriate Initial Antibiotic Given	234	99%	95%	95%
Blood Culture Timing	530	100%	97%	98%
Pregnancy and Delivery Care				
Newborn Deliveries Scheduled Early	215	3%	4%	6%
Preventive Care				
Immunization for Influenza[2]	523	95%	88%	90%
Immunization for Pneumonia[2]	625	95%	88%	92%
Stroke Care				
Anticoagulation Therapy for Atrial Fibrillation	67	99%	96%	95%
Antithrombotic Therapy Timing	158	99%	98%	98%
Assessed for Rehabilitation	218	99%	97%	97%
Discharged on Antithrombotic Therapy	183	100%	99%	99%
Discharged on Statin Medication	166	98%	95%	94%
Thrombolytic Therapy Timing	32	72%	69%	66%
Venous Thromboembolism Prophylaxis	215	97%	94%	94%
Written Stroke Educational Materials Given	85	73%	86%	88%
Surgical Care Improvement Project				
Appropriate Beta Blocker Usage[2]	253	100%	97%	98%
Appropriate VTP Within 24 Hours[2]	452	100%	98%	98%
Controlled Postoperative Blood Glucose[2]	189	99%	97%	97%
Perioperative Temperature Management[2]	543	99%	100%	100%
Prophylactic Antibiotic Selection[2]	543	100%	99%	99%
Prophylactic Antibiotic Selection (Outpatient)	617	99%	97%	98%
Prophylactic Antibiotic Stopped[2]	526	100%	98%	98%
Prophylactic Antibiotic Timing[2]	543	100%	99%	99%
Prophylactic Antibiotic Timing (Outpatient)	617	100%	97%	98%
Urinary Catheter Removal[2]	290	97%	96%	97%
Survey of Patients' Hospital Experiences				
Area Around Room 'Always' Quiet at Night	300+	44%	51%	61%
Doctors 'Always' Communicated Well	300+	78%	77%	82%
Home Recovery Information Given	300+	88%	83%	85%
Hospital Given 9 or 10 on 10 Point Scale	300+	61%	63%	71%
Meds 'Always' Explained Before Given	300+	62%	59%	64%
Nurses 'Always' Communicated Well	300+	75%	75%	79%
Pain 'Always' Well Controlled	300+	69%	67%	71%
Room and Bathroom 'Always' Clean	300+	71%	69%	73%
Timely Help 'Always' Received	300+	58%	61%	68%
Would Definitely Recommend Hospital	300+	69%	65%	71%
Use of Medical Imaging				
Cardiac Imaging Stress Test before Surgery[1]	-	-	5.8%	5.3%
Combination Abdominal CT Scan	1,007	1.3%	8.2%	10.5%
Combination Brain/Sinus CT Scan	1,128	4.1%	3.6%	2.7%
Combination Chest CT Scan	742	2.8%	1.3%	2.7%
Follow-up Mammogram/Ultrasound	2,162	8.1%	13%	8.8%
Lumbar Spine MRI for Low Back Pain	67	29.9%	33.4%	37.2%

Sunnyview Hospital & Rehabilitation Center

1270 Belmont Avenue
Schenectady, NY 12308
Phone: 518-386-3580
Fax: 518-382-4533
URL: www.sunnyview.org
Type: Acute Care Hospitals
Emergency Services: No
Ownership: Voluntary non-profit - Private
Beds: 104

Key Personnel:
CEO/President. . . . . Robert Bylancik
Pediatric In-Patient Care . . . . George W Crawl, MD
Quality Assurance . . . . John Mackey
Chief of Medical Staff . . . . Gary Williams, MD

Measure	Cases	This Hosp.	State Avg.	U.S. Avg.
Blood Clot Prevention and Treatment				
Anticoagulation Overlap Therapy[1,2]	-	-	91%	93%
ICU Venous Thromboembolism Prophylaxis[2,7]	-	-	92%	92%
Incidence of Potentially Preventable VTE[2,7]	-	-	10%	10%
UFH with Dosages/Platelet Monitoring[2,7]	-	-	92%	97%
Venous Thromboembolism Prophylaxis[2]	456	54%	87%	85%
Warfarin Therapy Discharge Instructions[1,2]	-	-	59%	75%
Chest Pain/Possible Heart Attack Care				
Aspirin Given Within 24 Hours of Arrival[5]	-	-	97%	96%
Fibrinolytic Meds Within 30 Min. of Arrival[5]	-	-	54%	58%
Average Time to ECG (minutes)[5]	-	-	9	7
Average Time to Transfer (minutes)[5]	-	-	78	60
Children's Asthma Care				
Received Home Management Plan of Care	-	-	-	88%
Received Reliever Medication	-	-	-	100%
Received Systemic Corticosteroids	-	-	-	100%
Emergency Department				
Admittance Decision Time (minutes)[2,7]	-	-	154	98
Head CT Results Within 45 Min. of Arrival[5]	-	-	55%	57%
Patients Who Left ER Before Being Seen[5]	-	-	2%	2%
Time from ER Arrival to Admit. (minutes)[2,7]	-	-	378	274
Time from ER Arrival to Discharge (minutes)[5]	-	-	156	134
Time in ER Before Being Evaluated (minutes)[5]	-	-	35	26
Time to Pain Meds for Fractures (minutes)[5]	-	-	61	57
Heart Attack Care				
Aspirin Given at Discharge[5]	-	-	99%	99%
Fibrinolytic Meds Within 30 Min. of Arrival[5]	-	-	46%	54%
PCI Within 90 Minutes of Arrival[5]	-	-	95%	96%
Statin Prescribed at Discharge[5]	-	-	98%	98%
Heart Failure Care				
ACE Inhibitor or ARB for LVSD[5]	-	-	96%	97%
Discharge Instructions Given[5]	-	-	95%	94%
Evaluation of LVS Function[5]	-	-	99%	99%
Medicare Spending				
Medicare Spending per Patient (ratio)[1]	-	-	0.96	0.98
Pneumonia Care				
Appropriate Initial Antibiotic Given[5]	-	-	95%	95%
Blood Culture Timing[5]	-	-	97%	98%
Pregnancy and Delivery Care				
Newborn Deliveries Scheduled Early[2,7]	-	-	4%	6%
Preventive Care				
Immunization for Influenza[2]	316	94%	88%	90%
Immunization for Pneumonia[2]	577	93%	88%	92%
Stroke Care				
Anticoagulation Therapy for Atrial Fibrillation[5]	-	-	96%	95%
Antithrombotic Therapy Timing[5]	-	-	98%	98%
Assessed for Rehabilitation[5]	-	-	97%	97%
Discharged on Antithrombotic Therapy[5]	-	-	99%	99%
Discharged on Statin Medication[5]	-	-	95%	94%
Thrombolytic Therapy Timing[5]	-	-	69%	66%
Venous Thromboembolism Prophylaxis[5]	-	-	94%	94%
Written Stroke Educational Materials Given[5]	-	-	86%	88%
Surgical Care Improvement Project				
Appropriate Beta Blocker Usage[5]	-	-	97%	98%
Appropriate VTP Within 24 Hours[5]	-	-	98%	98%
Controlled Postoperative Blood Glucose[5]	-	-	97%	97%
Perioperative Temperature Management[5]	-	-	100%	100%
Prophylactic Antibiotic Selection[5]	-	-	99%	99%
Prophylactic Antibiotic Selection (Outpatient)[5]	-	-	97%	98%
Prophylactic Antibiotic Stopped[5]	-	-	98%	98%
Prophylactic Antibiotic Timing[5]	-	-	99%	99%
Prophylactic Antibiotic Timing (Outpatient)[5]	-	-	97%	98%
Urinary Catheter Removal[5]	-	-	96%	97%
Survey of Patients' Hospital Experiences				
Area Around Room 'Always' Quiet at Night[1]	-	-	51%	61%
Doctors 'Always' Communicated Well[1]	-	-	77%	82%
Home Recovery Information Given[1]	-	-	83%	85%
Hospital Given 9 or 10 on 10 Point Scale[1]	-	-	63%	71%
Meds 'Always' Explained Before Given[1]	-	-	59%	64%
Nurses 'Always' Communicated Well[1]	-	-	75%	79%
Pain 'Always' Well Controlled[1]	-	-	67%	71%
Room and Bathroom 'Always' Clean[1]	-	-	69%	73%

NOTE: Hospital profiles are in alphabetical order by state, then city, then hospital within the city; Rankings exclude hospitals with less than 25 cases except for patient surveys which excludes hospitals with less than 100 cases; (a) 100-299 cases; (1) The number of cases/patients is too few to report; (2) Data submitted were based on a sample of cases/patients; (3) Results are based on a shorter time period than required; (4) Data suppressed by CMS for one or more quarters; (5) Results are not available for this reporting period; (6) Fewer than 100 patients completed the HCAHPS survey; (7) No cases met the criteria for this measure; (8) The lower limit of the confidence interval cannot be calculated if the number of observed infections equals zero; (9) No data are available from the state/territory for this reporting period; (10) The scores shown reflect fewer than 50 completed surveys; (11) There were discrepancies in the data collection process; (12) This measure does not apply to this hospital for this reporting period; (13) Results cannot be calculated for this reporting period; (14) The results for this state are combined with nearby states to protect confidentiality; Please refer to the User's Guide for a full explanation of data.

Measure	Cases	This Hosp.	State Avg.	U.S. Avg.
Timely Help 'Always' Received[1]	-	-	61%	68%
Would Definitely Recommend Hospital[1]	-	-	65%	71%
Use of Medical Imaging				
Cardiac Imaging Stress Test before Surgery[7]	-	-	5.8%	5.3%
Combination Abdominal CT Scan[7]	-	-	8.2%	10.5%
Combination Brain/Sinus CT Scan[7]	-	-	3.6%	2.7%
Combination Chest CT Scan[7]	-	-	1.3%	2.7%
Follow-up Mammogram/Ultrasound[7]	-	-	13%	8.8%
Lumbar Spine MRI for Low Back Pain[7]	-	-	33.4%	37.2%

Phelps Memorial Hospital Assn

701 North Broadway
Sleepy Hollow, NY 10591
Phone: 914-366-3000
Fax: 914-366-1308
E-mail: msernatinger@pmhc.us
URL: www.phelpshospital.org
Type: Acute Care Hospitals
Emergency Services: Yes
Ownership: Voluntary non-profit - Other
Beds: 235

Key Personnel:
Quality Assurance . . . . Eileen Egan
Chief of Medical Staff . . . . Elio Ippolito, MD
Cardiac Laboratory. . . . . Kenneth Kaplan, MD
Radiology. . . . . Robert Perelman, MD
Operating Room. . . . . Robert Raniolo
CEO/President. . . . . Keith F Safian
Pediatric In-Patient Care . . . . Margaret Stillman, MD
Infection Control. . . . . Anita Watson

Measure	Cases	This Hosp.	State Avg.	U.S. Avg.
Blood Clot Prevention and Treatment				
Anticoagulation Overlap Therapy[2]	24	96%	91%	93%
ICU Venous Thromboembolism Prophylaxis[2]	85	94%	92%	92%
Incidence of Potentially Preventable VTE[1,2]	-	-	10%	10%
UFH with Dosages/Platelet Monitoring[1,2]	-	-	92%	97%
Venous Thromboembolism Prophylaxis[2]	341	94%	87%	85%
Warfarin Therapy Discharge Instructions[2]	13	100%	59%	75%
Chest Pain/Possible Heart Attack Care				
Aspirin Given Within 24 Hours of Arrival	23	100%	97%	96%
Fibrinolytic Meds Within 30 Min. of Arrival[7]	-	-	54%	58%
Average Time to ECG (minutes)	24	15	9	7
Average Time to Transfer (minutes)[1]	-	-	78	60
Children's Asthma Care				
Received Home Management Plan of Care	-	-	-	88%
Received Reliever Medication	-	-	-	100%
Received Systemic Corticosteroids	-	-	-	100%
Emergency Department				
Admittance Decision Time (minutes)[2]	580	155	154	98
Head CT Results Within 45 Min. of Arrival	13	92%	55%	57%
Patients Who Left ER Before Being Seen	27,156	1%	2%	2%
Time from ER Arrival to Admit. (minutes)[2]	583	364	378	274
Time from ER Arrival to Discharge (minutes)	369	147	156	134
Time in ER Before Being Evaluated (minutes)	411	25	35	26
Time to Pain Meds for Fractures (minutes)	56	48	61	57
Heart Attack Care				
Aspirin Given at Discharge	29	100%	99%	99%
Fibrinolytic Meds Within 30 Min. of Arrival[7]	-	-	46%	54%
PCI Within 90 Minutes of Arrival[7]	-	-	95%	96%
Statin Prescribed at Discharge	25	100%	98%	98%
Heart Failure Care				
ACE Inhibitor or ARB for LVSD	27	100%	96%	97%
Discharge Instructions Given	76	100%	95%	94%
Evaluation of LVS Function	116	100%	99%	99%
Medicare Spending				
Medicare Spending per Patient (ratio)	-	1.02	0.96	0.98
Pneumonia Care				
Appropriate Initial Antibiotic Given	81	98%	95%	95%
Blood Culture Timing	171	98%	97%	98%
Pregnancy and Delivery Care				
Newborn Deliveries Scheduled Early[2]	30	3%	4%	6%
Preventive Care				
Immunization for Influenza[2]	532	99%	88%	90%
Immunization for Pneumonia[2]	590	96%	88%	92%
Stroke Care				
Anticoagulation Therapy for Atrial Fibrillation	11	100%	96%	95%
Antithrombotic Therapy Timing	42	98%	98%	98%
Assessed for Rehabilitation	48	100%	97%	97%
Discharged on Antithrombotic Therapy	44	100%	99%	99%
Discharged on Statin Medication	29	100%	95%	94%
Thrombolytic Therapy Timing[1]	-	-	69%	66%
Venous Thromboembolism Prophylaxis	49	98%	94%	94%
Written Stroke Educational Materials Given	21	100%	86%	88%
Surgical Care Improvement Project				
Appropriate Beta Blocker Usage[2]	144	99%	97%	98%
Appropriate VTP Within 24 Hours[2]	400	100%	98%	98%
Controlled Postoperative Blood Glucose[2,7]	-	-	97%	97%
Perioperative Temperature Management[2]	483	100%	100%	100%
Prophylactic Antibiotic Selection[2]	375	99%	99%	99%
Prophylactic Antibiotic Selection (Outpatient)	116	96%	97%	98%
Prophylactic Antibiotic Stopped[2]	372	100%	98%	98%
Prophylactic Antibiotic Timing[2]	375	100%	99%	99%
Prophylactic Antibiotic Timing (Outpatient)	76	100%	97%	98%
Urinary Catheter Removal[2]	390	99%	96%	97%
Survey of Patients' Hospital Experiences				
Area Around Room 'Always' Quiet at Night	300+	57%	51%	61%
Doctors 'Always' Communicated Well	300+	80%	77%	82%
Home Recovery Information Given	300+	87%	83%	85%
Hospital Given 9 or 10 on 10 Point Scale	300+	73%	63%	71%
Meds 'Always' Explained Before Given	300+	66%	59%	64%
Nurses 'Always' Communicated Well	300+	81%	75%	79%
Pain 'Always' Well Controlled	300+	77%	67%	71%
Room and Bathroom 'Always' Clean	300+	77%	69%	73%
Timely Help 'Always' Received	300+	71%	61%	68%
Would Definitely Recommend Hospital	300+	80%	65%	71%
Use of Medical Imaging				
Cardiac Imaging Stress Test before Surgery	82	7.3%	5.8%	5.3%
Combination Abdominal CT Scan	723	15.9%	8.2%	10.5%
Combination Brain/Sinus CT Scan	611	1.6%	3.6%	2.7%
Combination Chest CT Scan	646	0.3%	1.3%	2.7%
Follow-up Mammogram/Ultrasound	1,521	22.6%	13%	8.8%
Lumbar Spine MRI for Low Back Pain	62	40.3%	33.4%	37.2%

Saint Catherine of Siena Hospital

50 Route 25a
Smithtown, NY 11787
Phone: 631-862-3000
Fax: 631-862-3768
URL: www.stcatherines.chsli.org
Type: Acute Care Hospitals
Emergency Services: Yes
Ownership: Voluntary non-profit - Church
Beds: 311

Key Personnel:
Anesthesiology. . . . . Anthony Bonono, MD
Radiology. . . . . Scott Coyne, MD
CEO/President. . . . . Vincent DiRubbio
Patient Relations . . . . Gana Edelstein
Chief of Medical Staff . . . . Jason Golbin, DO
Operating Room. . . . . Patrice Kelly
Emergency Room . . . . Michael Kennedy, DO
Infection Control. . . . . Catherine Shannon

Measure	Cases	This Hosp.	State Avg.	U.S. Avg.
Blood Clot Prevention and Treatment				
Anticoagulation Overlap Therapy[2]	80	95%	91%	93%
ICU Venous Thromboembolism Prophylaxis[2]	68	99%	92%	92%
Incidence of Potentially Preventable VTE[2]	13	15%	10%	10%
UFH with Dosages/Platelet Monitoring[2]	23	100%	92%	97%
Venous Thromboembolism Prophylaxis[2]	386	91%	87%	85%
Warfarin Therapy Discharge Instructions[2]	47	100%	59%	75%
Chest Pain/Possible Heart Attack Care				
Aspirin Given Within 24 Hours of Arrival[1,3]	-	-	97%	96%
Fibrinolytic Meds Within 30 Min. of Arrival[3,7]	-	-	54%	58%
Average Time to ECG (minutes)[1,3]	-	-	9	7
Average Time to Transfer (minutes)[1,3]	-	-	78	60
Children's Asthma Care				
Received Home Management Plan of Care	-	-	-	88%
Received Reliever Medication	-	-	-	100%
Received Systemic Corticosteroids	-	-	-	100%
Emergency Department				
Admittance Decision Time (minutes)[2]	687	203	154	98
Head CT Results Within 45 Min. of Arrival[1]	-	-	55%	57%
Patients Who Left ER Before Being Seen	32,308	1%	2%	2%
Time from ER Arrival to Admit. (minutes)[2]	688	372	378	274
Time from ER Arrival to Discharge (minutes)	373	170	156	134
Time in ER Before Being Evaluated (minutes)	400	35	35	26
Time to Pain Meds for Fractures (minutes)	152	70	61	57
Heart Attack Care				
Aspirin Given at Discharge	160	99%	99%	99%
Fibrinolytic Meds Within 30 Min. of Arrival[7]	-	-	46%	54%
PCI Within 90 Minutes of Arrival	27	85%	95%	96%
Statin Prescribed at Discharge	154	99%	98%	98%
Heart Failure Care				
ACE Inhibitor or ARB for LVSD	54	100%	96%	97%
Discharge Instructions Given	256	99%	95%	94%
Evaluation of LVS Function	389	100%	99%	99%
Medicare Spending				
Medicare Spending per Patient (ratio)	-	1.05	0.96	0.98
Pneumonia Care				
Appropriate Initial Antibiotic Given[2]	89	99%	95%	95%
Blood Culture Timing[2]	173	98%	97%	98%
Pregnancy and Delivery Care				
Newborn Deliveries Scheduled Early[2]	26	15%	4%	6%
Preventive Care				
Immunization for Influenza[2]	566	87%	88%	90%
Immunization for Pneumonia[2]	751	89%	88%	92%
Stroke Care				
Anticoagulation Therapy for Atrial Fibrillation	23	100%	96%	95%
Antithrombotic Therapy Timing	97	100%	98%	98%
Assessed for Rehabilitation	99	98%	97%	97%
Discharged on Antithrombotic Therapy	87	100%	99%	99%
Discharged on Statin Medication	68	100%	95%	94%
Thrombolytic Therapy Timing	11	82%	69%	66%
Venous Thromboembolism Prophylaxis	119	100%	94%	94%
Written Stroke Educational Materials Given	45	100%	86%	88%
Surgical Care Improvement Project				
Appropriate Beta Blocker Usage[2]	123	96%	97%	98%
Appropriate VTP Within 24 Hours[2]	310	93%	98%	98%
Controlled Postoperative Blood Glucose[2,7]	-	-	97%	97%
Perioperative Temperature Management[2]	367	100%	100%	100%
Prophylactic Antibiotic Selection[2]	208	94%	99%	99%
Prophylactic Antibiotic Selection (Outpatient)	365	92%	97%	98%
Prophylactic Antibiotic Stopped[2]	201	97%	98%	98%
Prophylactic Antibiotic Timing[2]	209	96%	99%	99%
Prophylactic Antibiotic Timing (Outpatient)	367	99%	97%	98%
Urinary Catheter Removal[2]	218	98%	96%	97%
Survey of Patients' Hospital Experiences				
Area Around Room 'Always' Quiet at Night	300+	42%	51%	61%
Doctors 'Always' Communicated Well	300+	74%	77%	82%
Home Recovery Information Given	300+	85%	83%	85%
Hospital Given 9 or 10 on 10 Point Scale	300+	58%	63%	71%
Meds 'Always' Explained Before Given	300+	59%	59%	64%
Nurses 'Always' Communicated Well	300+	73%	75%	79%
Pain 'Always' Well Controlled	300+	64%	67%	71%
Room and Bathroom 'Always' Clean	300+	66%	69%	73%
Timely Help 'Always' Received	300+	55%	61%	68%
Would Definitely Recommend Hospital	300+	60%	65%	71%
Use of Medical Imaging				
Cardiac Imaging Stress Test before Surgery[1]	-	-	5.8%	5.3%
Combination Abdominal CT Scan	484	3.5%	8.2%	10.5%
Combination Brain/Sinus CT Scan	615	1.3%	3.6%	2.7%
Combination Chest CT Scan	205	4.4%	1.3%	2.7%
Follow-up Mammogram/Ultrasound	261	49.8%	13%	8.8%
Lumbar Spine MRI for Low Back Pain[1]	-	-	33.4%	37.2%

Southampton Hospital

240 Meeting House Lane
Southampton, NY 11968
Phone: 516-726-8200
Fax: 631-283-2842
URL: www.southamptonhospital.org
Type: Acute Care Hospitals
Emergency Services: Yes
Ownership: Voluntary non-profit - Private
Beds: 168

Key Personnel:
Radiology. . . . . William R Brancaccio, MD
CEO/President. . . . . Robert S. Chaloner
Infection Control. . . . . Karen D'John
Quality Assurance . . . . Sharon DiSunno, RN, MS
Pediatrics. . . . . Alexandra Halitsky, MD
Operating Room. . . . . John Hubbell, RN
Chief of Medical Staff . . . . Fredric Weinbaum, MD
Emergency Room . . . . Dr Darren Wiggins

NOTE: Hospital profiles are in alphabetical order by state, then city, then hospital within the city; Rankings exclude hospitals with less than 25 cases except for patient surveys which excludes hospitals with less than 100 cases; (a) 100-299 cases; (1) The number of cases/patients is too few to report; (2) Data submitted were based on a sample of cases/patients; (3) Results are based on a shorter time period than required; (4) Data suppressed by CMS for one or more quarters; (5) Results are not available for this reporting period; (6) Fewer than 100 patients completed the HCAHPS survey; (7) No cases met the criteria for this measure; (8) The lower limit of the confidence interval cannot be calculated if the number of observed infections equals zero; (9) No data are available from the state/territory for this reporting period; (10) The scores shown reflect fewer than 50 completed surveys; (11) There were discrepancies in the data collection process; (12) This measure does not apply to this hospital for this reporting period; (13) Results cannot be calculated for this reporting period; (14) The results for this state are combined with nearby states to protect confidentiality; Please refer to the User's Guide for a full explanation of data.

Measure	Cases	This Hosp.	State Avg.	U.S. Avg.
Blood Clot Prevention and Treatment				
Anticoagulation Overlap Therapy[2]	27	85%	91%	93%
ICU Venous Thromboembolism Prophylaxis[2]	53	96%	92%	92%
Incidence of Potentially Preventable VTE[1,2]	-	-	10%	10%
UFH with Dosages/Platelet Monitoring[2]	26	100%	92%	97%
Venous Thromboembolism Prophylaxis[2]	326	84%	87%	85%
Warfarin Therapy Discharge Instructions[2]	15	80%	59%	75%
Chest Pain/Possible Heart Attack Care				
Aspirin Given Within 24 Hours of Arrival	62	100%	97%	96%
Fibrinolytic Meds Within 30 Min. of Arrival	13	85%	54%	58%
Average Time to ECG (minutes)	62	4	9	7
Average Time to Transfer (minutes)[1]	-	-	78	60
Children's Asthma Care				
Received Home Management Plan of Care	-	-	-	88%
Received Reliever Medication	-	-	-	100%
Received Systemic Corticosteroids	-	-	-	100%
Emergency Department				
Admittance Decision Time (minutes)[2]	785	184	154	98
Head CT Results Within 45 Min. of Arrival[1]	-	-	55%	57%
Patients Who Left ER Before Being Seen	25,879	1%	2%	2%
Time from ER Arrival to Admit. (minutes)[2]	785	338	378	274
Time from ER Arrival to Discharge (minutes)	379	128	156	134
Time in ER Before Being Evaluated (minutes)	402	25	35	26
Time to Pain Meds for Fractures (minutes)	180	56	61	57
Heart Attack Care				
Aspirin Given at Discharge	12	100%	99%	99%
Fibrinolytic Meds Within 30 Min. of Arrival[7]	-	-	46%	54%
PCI Within 90 Minutes of Arrival[7]	-	-	95%	96%
Statin Prescribed at Discharge	13	100%	98%	98%
Heart Failure Care				
ACE Inhibitor or ARB for LVSD	23	91%	96%	97%
Discharge Instructions Given	95	98%	95%	94%
Evaluation of LVS Function	123	100%	99%	99%
Medicare Spending				
Medicare Spending per Patient (ratio)	-	0.95	0.96	0.98
Pneumonia Care				
Appropriate Initial Antibiotic Given	92	97%	95%	95%
Blood Culture Timing	187	98%	97%	98%
Pregnancy and Delivery Care				
Newborn Deliveries Scheduled Early[2]	50	8%	4%	6%
Preventive Care				
Immunization for Influenza[2]	473	93%	88%	90%
Immunization for Pneumonia[2]	563	90%	88%	92%
Stroke Care				
Anticoagulation Therapy for Atrial Fibrillation	11	100%	96%	95%
Antithrombotic Therapy Timing	38	100%	98%	98%
Assessed for Rehabilitation	48	81%	97%	97%
Discharged on Antithrombotic Therapy	43	98%	99%	99%
Discharged on Statin Medication	39	90%	95%	94%
Thrombolytic Therapy Timing[1]	-	-	69%	66%
Venous Thromboembolism Prophylaxis	45	78%	94%	94%
Written Stroke Educational Materials Given	25	92%	86%	88%
Surgical Care Improvement Project				
Appropriate Beta Blocker Usage	56	95%	97%	98%
Appropriate VTP Within 24 Hours	137	94%	98%	98%
Controlled Postoperative Blood Glucose[7]	-	-	97%	97%
Perioperative Temperature Management	160	100%	100%	100%
Prophylactic Antibiotic Selection	84	90%	99%	99%
Prophylactic Antibiotic Selection (Outpatient)	29	97%	97%	98%
Prophylactic Antibiotic Stopped	82	90%	98%	98%
Prophylactic Antibiotic Timing	84	99%	99%	99%
Prophylactic Antibiotic Timing (Outpatient)	29	93%	97%	98%
Urinary Catheter Removal	48	94%	96%	97%
Survey of Patients' Hospital Experiences				
Area Around Room 'Always' Quiet at Night	300+	53%	51%	61%
Doctors 'Always' Communicated Well	300+	79%	77%	82%
Home Recovery Information Given	300+	83%	83%	85%
Hospital Given 9 or 10 on 10 Point Scale	300+	67%	63%	71%
Meds 'Always' Explained Before Given	300+	61%	59%	64%
Nurses 'Always' Communicated Well	300+	78%	75%	79%
Pain 'Always' Well Controlled	300+	73%	67%	71%
Room and Bathroom 'Always' Clean	300+	78%	69%	73%
Timely Help 'Always' Received	300+	66%	61%	68%
Would Definitely Recommend Hospital	300+	70%	65%	71%
Use of Medical Imaging				
Cardiac Imaging Stress Test before Surgery[1]	-	-	5.8%	5.3%
Combination Abdominal CT Scan	585	9.6%	8.2%	10.5%
Combination Brain/Sinus CT Scan	405	2.0%	3.6%	2.7%
Combination Chest CT Scan	525	0.2%	1.3%	2.7%
Follow-up Mammogram/Ultrasound	1,264	15.7%	13%	8.8%
Lumbar Spine MRI for Low Back Pain	109	32.1%	33.4%	37.2%

Bertrand Chaffee Hospital

224 East Main Street
Springville, NY 14141
Type: Acute Care Hospitals
Ownership: Voluntary non-profit - Private
Phone: 716-592-2871
Fax: 716-592-8105
Emergency Services: Yes
Beds: 49

Key Personnel:
Operating Room. . . . . Barbara Appleby
Radiology. . . . . Steven Christen
Pediatric Ambulatory Care . . . . . . Robbin Hansen
Chief of Medical Staff. . . . . Edwin Heidelberger
CEO/President. . . . . Steven Krisiak
Quality Assurance . . . . Linda Reehling
Infection Control. . . . . Barbara Whittemore

Measure	Cases	This Hosp.	State Avg.	U.S. Avg.
Blood Clot Prevention and Treatment				
Anticoagulation Overlap Therapy[1,2]	-	-	91%	93%
ICU Venous Thromboembolism Prophylaxis[2,7]	-	-	92%	92%
Incidence of Potentially Preventable VTE[2,7]	-	-	10%	10%
UFH with Dosages/Platelet Monitoring[1,2]	-	-	92%	97%
Venous Thromboembolism Prophylaxis[2]	420	69%	87%	85%
Warfarin Therapy Discharge Instructions[1,2]	-	-	59%	75%
Chest Pain/Possible Heart Attack Care				
Aspirin Given Within 24 Hours of Arrival	51	96%	97%	96%
Fibrinolytic Meds Within 30 Min. of Arrival[1]	-	-	54%	58%
Average Time to ECG (minutes)	55	10	9	7
Average Time to Transfer (minutes)[1]	-	-	78	60
Children's Asthma Care				
Received Home Management Plan of Care	-	-	-	88%
Received Reliever Medication	-	-	-	100%
Received Systemic Corticosteroids	-	-	-	100%
Emergency Department				
Admittance Decision Time (minutes)[2]	405	61	154	98
Head CT Results Within 45 Min. of Arrival[5]	-	-	55%	57%
Patients Who Left ER Before Being Seen	8,872	2%	2%	2%
Time from ER Arrival to Admit. (minutes)[2]	449	235	378	274
Time from ER Arrival to Discharge (minutes)	212	125	156	134
Time in ER Before Being Evaluated (minutes)	289	30	35	26
Time to Pain Meds for Fractures (minutes)[5]	-	-	61	57
Heart Attack Care				
Aspirin Given at Discharge[1,2]	-	-	99%	99%
Fibrinolytic Meds Within 30 Min. of Arrival[2,7]	-	-	46%	54%
PCI Within 90 Minutes of Arrival[2,7]	-	-	95%	96%
Statin Prescribed at Discharge[1,2]	-	-	98%	98%
Heart Failure Care				
ACE Inhibitor or ARB for LVSD[1,2]	-	-	96%	97%
Discharge Instructions Given[2]	18	89%	95%	94%
Evaluation of LVS Function[2]	35	91%	99%	99%
Medicare Spending				
Medicare Spending per Patient (ratio)	-	1.06	0.96	0.98
Pneumonia Care				
Appropriate Initial Antibiotic Given[2]	76	96%	95%	95%
Blood Culture Timing[2]	101	91%	97%	98%
Pregnancy and Delivery Care				
Newborn Deliveries Scheduled Early[7]	-	-	4%	6%
Preventive Care				
Immunization for Influenza[2]	321	97%	88%	90%
Immunization for Pneumonia[2]	524	93%	88%	92%
Stroke Care				
Anticoagulation Therapy for Atrial Fibrillation[5]	-	-	96%	95%
Antithrombotic Therapy Timing[5]	-	-	98%	98%
Assessed for Rehabilitation[5]	-	-	97%	97%
Discharged on Antithrombotic Therapy[5]	-	-	99%	99%
Discharged on Statin Medication[5]	-	-	95%	94%
Thrombolytic Therapy Timing[5]	-	-	69%	66%
Venous Thromboembolism Prophylaxis[5]	-	-	94%	94%
Written Stroke Educational Materials Given[5]	-	-	86%	88%
Surgical Care Improvement Project				
Appropriate Beta Blocker Usage[3,7]	-	-	97%	98%
Appropriate VTP Within 24 Hours[1,3]	-	-	98%	98%
Controlled Postoperative Blood Glucose[3,7]	-	-	97%	97%
Perioperative Temperature Management[1,3]	-	-	100%	100%
Prophylactic Antibiotic Selection[1,3]	-	-	99%	99%
Prophylactic Antibiotic Selection (Outpatient)[1,3]	-	-	97%	98%
Prophylactic Antibiotic Stopped[1,3]	-	-	98%	98%
Prophylactic Antibiotic Timing[1,3]	-	-	99%	99%
Prophylactic Antibiotic Timing (Outpatient)[1,3]	-	-	97%	98%
Urinary Catheter Removal[1,3]	-	-	96%	97%
Survey of Patients' Hospital Experiences				
Area Around Room 'Always' Quiet at Night	300+	53%	51%	61%
Doctors 'Always' Communicated Well	300+	78%	77%	82%
Home Recovery Information Given	300+	87%	83%	85%
Hospital Given 9 or 10 on 10 Point Scale	300+	65%	63%	71%
Meds 'Always' Explained Before Given	300+	57%	59%	64%
Nurses 'Always' Communicated Well	300+	78%	75%	79%
Pain 'Always' Well Controlled	300+	71%	67%	71%
Room and Bathroom 'Always' Clean	300+	75%	69%	73%
Timely Help 'Always' Received	300+	67%	61%	68%
Would Definitely Recommend Hospital	300+	66%	65%	71%
Use of Medical Imaging				
Cardiac Imaging Stress Test before Surgery[1]	-	-	5.8%	5.3%
Combination Abdominal CT Scan	128	6.3%	8.2%	10.5%
Combination Brain/Sinus CT Scan[1]	-	-	3.6%	2.7%
Combination Chest CT Scan[1]	-	-	1.3%	2.7%
Follow-up Mammogram/Ultrasound	171	9.4%	13%	8.8%
Lumbar Spine MRI for Low Back Pain[1]	-	-	33.4%	37.2%

Clifton Fine Hospital

1014 Oswegatchie Trail
Star Lake, NY 13690
Type: Critical Access Hospitals
Ownership: Voluntary non-profit - Private
Phone: 315-848-3351
Emergency Services: Yes

Measure	Cases	This Hosp.	State Avg.	U.S. Avg.
Blood Clot Prevention and Treatment				
Anticoagulation Overlap Therapy[5]	-	-	91%	93%
ICU Venous Thromboembolism Prophylaxis[5]	-	-	92%	92%
Incidence of Potentially Preventable VTE[5]	-	-	10%	10%
UFH with Dosages/Platelet Monitoring[5]	-	-	92%	97%
Venous Thromboembolism Prophylaxis[5]	-	-	87%	85%
Warfarin Therapy Discharge Instructions[5]	-	-	59%	75%
Chest Pain/Possible Heart Attack Care				
Aspirin Given Within 24 Hours of Arrival[1,3]	-	-	97%	96%
Fibrinolytic Meds Within 30 Min. of Arrival[1,3]	-	-	54%	58%
Average Time to ECG (minutes)[1,3]	-	-	9	7
Average Time to Transfer (minutes)[3,7]	-	-	78	60
Children's Asthma Care				
Received Home Management Plan of Care	-	-	-	88%
Received Reliever Medication	-	-	-	100%
Received Systemic Corticosteroids	-	-	-	100%
Emergency Department				
Admittance Decision Time (minutes)[5]	-	-	154	98
Head CT Results Within 45 Min. of Arrival[5]	-	-	55%	57%
Patients Who Left ER Before Being Seen	1,712	0%	2%	2%
Time from ER Arrival to Admit. (minutes)[5]	-	-	378	274
Time from ER Arrival to Discharge (minutes)[5]	-	-	156	134
Time in ER Before Being Evaluated (minutes)[5]	-	-	35	26
Time to Pain Meds for Fractures (minutes)[5]	-	-	61	57
Heart Attack Care				
Aspirin Given at Discharge[5]	-	-	99%	99%
Fibrinolytic Meds Within 30 Min. of Arrival[5]	-	-	46%	54%
PCI Within 90 Minutes of Arrival[5]	-	-	95%	96%
Statin Prescribed at Discharge[5]	-	-	98%	98%
Heart Failure Care				
ACE Inhibitor or ARB for LVSD[3,7]	-	-	96%	97%
Discharge Instructions Given[1,3]	-	-	95%	94%
Evaluation of LVS Function[1,3]	-	-	99%	99%

NOTE: Hospital profiles are in alphabetical order by state, then city, then hospital within the city; Rankings exclude hospitals with less than 25 cases except for patient surveys which excludes hospitals with less than 100 cases; (a) 100-299 cases; (1) The number of cases/patients is too few to report; (2) Data submitted were based on a sample of cases/patients; (3) Results are based on a shorter time period than required; (4) Data suppressed by CMS for one or more quarters; (5) Results are not available for this reporting period; (6) Fewer than 100 patients completed the HCAHPS survey; (7) No cases met the criteria for this measure; (8) The lower limit of the confidence interval cannot be calculated if the number of observed infections equals zero; (9) No data are available from the state/territory for this reporting period; (10) The scores shown reflect fewer than 50 completed surveys; (11) There were discrepancies in the data collection process; (12) This measure does not apply to this hospital for this reporting period; (13) Results cannot be calculated for this reporting period; (14) The results for this state are combined with nearby states to protect confidentiality; Please refer to the User's Guide for a full explanation of data.

Measure	Cases	This Hosp.	State Avg.	U.S. Avg.
Medicare Spending				
Medicare Spending per Patient (ratio)	-	-	0.96	0.98
Pneumonia Care				
Appropriate Initial Antibiotic Given[1]	-	-	95%	95%
Blood Culture Timing[1]	-	-	97%	98%
Pregnancy and Delivery Care				
Newborn Deliveries Scheduled Early[5]	-	-	4%	6%
Preventive Care				
Immunization for Influenza[5]	-	-	88%	90%
Immunization for Pneumonia[5]	-	-	88%	92%
Stroke Care				
Anticoagulation Therapy for Atrial Fibrillation[5]	-	-	96%	95%
Antithrombotic Therapy Timing[5]	-	-	98%	98%
Assessed for Rehabilitation[5]	-	-	97%	97%
Discharged on Antithrombotic Therapy[5]	-	-	99%	99%
Discharged on Statin Medication[5]	-	-	95%	94%
Thrombolytic Therapy Timing[5]	-	-	69%	66%
Venous Thromboembolism Prophylaxis[5]	-	-	94%	94%
Written Stroke Educational Materials Given[5]	-	-	86%	88%
Surgical Care Improvement Project				
Appropriate Beta Blocker Usage[5]	-	-	97%	98%
Appropriate VTP Within 24 Hours[5]	-	-	98%	98%
Controlled Postoperative Blood Glucose[5]	-	-	97%	97%
Perioperative Temperature Management[5]	-	-	100%	100%
Prophylactic Antibiotic Selection[5]	-	-	99%	99%
Prophylactic Antibiotic Selection (Outpatient)[5]	-	-	97%	98%
Prophylactic Antibiotic Stopped[5]	-	-	98%	98%
Prophylactic Antibiotic Timing[5]	-	-	99%	99%
Prophylactic Antibiotic Timing (Outpatient)[5]	-	-	97%	98%
Urinary Catheter Removal[5]	-	-	96%	97%
Survey of Patients' Hospital Experiences				
Area Around Room 'Always' Quiet at Night[10]	<100	38%	51%	61%
Doctors 'Always' Communicated Well[10]	<100	82%	77%	82%
Home Recovery Information Given[10]	<100	83%	83%	85%
Hospital Given 9 or 10 on 10 Point Scale[10]	<100	82%	63%	71%
Meds 'Always' Explained Before Given[10]	<100	39%	59%	64%
Nurses 'Always' Communicated Well[10]	<100	73%	75%	79%
Pain 'Always' Well Controlled[10]	<100	86%	67%	71%
Room and Bathroom 'Always' Clean[10]	<100	94%	69%	73%
Timely Help 'Always' Received[10]	<100	75%	61%	68%
Would Definitely Recommend Hospital[10]	<100	83%	65%	71%
Use of Medical Imaging				
Cardiac Imaging Stress Test before Surgery[7]	-	-	5.8%	5.3%
Combination Abdominal CT Scan[1]	-	-	8.2%	10.5%
Combination Brain/Sinus CT Scan[1]	-	-	3.6%	2.7%
Combination Chest CT Scan[1]	-	-	1.3%	2.7%
Follow-up Mammogram/Ultrasound[7]	-	-	13%	8.8%
Lumbar Spine MRI for Low Back Pain[7]	-	-	33.4%	37.2%

Richmond University Medical Center

355 Bard Avenue
Staten Island, NY 10304
Phone: 718-818-1234
URL: www.rumcsi.org
Type: Acute Care Hospitals
Emergency Services: Yes
Ownership: Voluntary non-profit - Private

Key Personnel:
Chief of Medical Staff.......... Edward Arsura
Anesthesiology............... Pietro Carpenito, M.D.
Radiology................... Michael T. Mantello, M.D.
Pediatrics.................. Brian McMahon, M.D.
CEO/President............... Daniel J. Messina, Ph.D., FACHE, L
Pediatric In-Patient Care .... Simon Rabinowitz

Measure	Cases	This Hosp.	State Avg.	U.S. Avg.
Blood Clot Prevention and Treatment				
Anticoagulation Overlap Therapy[2]	36	97%	91%	93%
ICU Venous Thromboembolism Prophylaxis[2]	57	98%	92%	92%
Incidence of Potentially Preventable VTE[2]	16	0%	10%	10%
UFH with Dosages/Platelet Monitoring[2]	15	100%	92%	97%
Venous Thromboembolism Prophylaxis[2]	397	94%	87%	85%
Warfarin Therapy Discharge Instructions[2]	16	69%	59%	75%
Chest Pain/Possible Heart Attack Care				
Aspirin Given Within 24 Hours of Arrival	35	100%	97%	96%
Fibrinolytic Meds Within 30 Min. of Arrival[7]	-	-	54%	58%
Average Time to ECG (minutes)	36	31	9	7
Average Time to Transfer (minutes)	19	104	78	60
Children's Asthma Care				
Received Home Management Plan of Care	-	-	-	88%
Received Reliever Medication	-	-	-	100%
Received Systemic Corticosteroids	-	-	-	100%
Emergency Department				
Admittance Decision Time (minutes)[2]	540	310	154	98
Head CT Results Within 45 Min. of Arrival[1]	-	-	55%	57%
Patients Who Left ER Before Being Seen	62,830	1%	2%	2%
Time from ER Arrival to Admit. (minutes)[2]	553	497	378	274
Time from ER Arrival to Discharge (minutes)	330	125	156	134
Time in ER Before Being Evaluated (minutes)	427	22	35	26
Time to Pain Meds for Fractures (minutes)	80	58	61	57
Heart Attack Care				
Aspirin Given at Discharge	51	100%	99%	99%
Fibrinolytic Meds Within 30 Min. of Arrival[7]	-	-	46%	54%
PCI Within 90 Minutes of Arrival[7]	-	-	95%	96%
Statin Prescribed at Discharge	53	94%	98%	98%
Heart Failure Care				
ACE Inhibitor or ARB for LVSD	79	94%	96%	97%
Discharge Instructions Given	154	100%	95%	94%
Evaluation of LVS Function	196	100%	99%	99%
Medicare Spending				
Medicare Spending per Patient (ratio)	-	1.02	0.96	0.98
Pneumonia Care				
Appropriate Initial Antibiotic Given[2]	65	94%	95%	95%
Blood Culture Timing[2]	142	94%	97%	98%
Pregnancy and Delivery Care				
Newborn Deliveries Scheduled Early[2]	58	9%	4%	6%
Preventive Care				
Immunization for Influenza[2]	488	93%	88%	90%
Immunization for Pneumonia[2]	475	92%	88%	92%
Stroke Care				
Anticoagulation Therapy for Atrial Fibrillation[1,2]	-	-	96%	95%
Antithrombotic Therapy Timing[2]	65	100%	98%	98%
Assessed for Rehabilitation[2]	86	100%	97%	97%
Discharged on Antithrombotic Therapy[2]	63	100%	99%	99%
Discharged on Statin Medication[2]	60	100%	95%	94%
Thrombolytic Therapy Timing[1,2]	-	-	69%	66%
Venous Thromboembolism Prophylaxis[2]	99	99%	94%	94%
Written Stroke Educational Materials Given[2]	42	100%	86%	88%
Surgical Care Improvement Project				
Appropriate Beta Blocker Usage[2]	96	99%	97%	98%
Appropriate VTP Within 24 Hours[2]	333	99%	98%	98%
Controlled Postoperative Blood Glucose[2,7]	-	-	97%	97%
Perioperative Temperature Management[2]	408	100%	100%	100%
Prophylactic Antibiotic Selection[2]	252	98%	99%	99%
Prophylactic Antibiotic Selection (Outpatient)	333	98%	97%	98%
Prophylactic Antibiotic Stopped[2]	249	95%	98%	98%
Prophylactic Antibiotic Timing[2]	252	99%	99%	99%
Prophylactic Antibiotic Timing (Outpatient)	338	95%	97%	98%
Urinary Catheter Removal[2]	118	98%	96%	97%
Survey of Patients' Hospital Experiences				
Area Around Room 'Always' Quiet at Night	300+	46%	51%	61%
Doctors 'Always' Communicated Well	300+	75%	77%	82%
Home Recovery Information Given	300+	74%	83%	85%
Hospital Given 9 or 10 on 10 Point Scale	300+	44%	63%	71%
Meds 'Always' Explained Before Given	300+	53%	59%	64%
Nurses 'Always' Communicated Well	300+	68%	75%	79%
Pain 'Always' Well Controlled	300+	59%	67%	71%
Room and Bathroom 'Always' Clean	300+	55%	69%	73%
Timely Help 'Always' Received	300+	53%	61%	68%
Would Definitely Recommend Hospital	300+	49%	65%	71%
Use of Medical Imaging				
Cardiac Imaging Stress Test before Surgery	70	8.6%	5.8%	5.3%
Combination Abdominal CT Scan	286	1.4%	8.2%	10.5%
Combination Brain/Sinus CT Scan	309	4.5%	3.6%	2.7%
Combination Chest CT Scan	123	0.0%	1.3%	2.7%
Follow-up Mammogram/Ultrasound	149	30.2%	13%	8.8%
Lumbar Spine MRI for Low Back Pain[7]	-	-	33.4%	37.2%

Staten Island University Hospital

475 Seaview Avenue
Staten Island, NY 10305
Phone: 718-226-9000
Fax: 718-226-8966
E-mail: webmaster@siuh.edu
URL: www.siuh.edu
Type: Acute Care Hospitals
Emergency Services: Yes
Ownership: Voluntary non-profit - Private
Beds: 813

Key Personnel:
Pediatric Ambulatory Care ...... Lawrence Bodenstein, MD
CEO/President............... Anthony C. Ferreri
Infection Control............. Jordan b Glaser, MD
Quality Assurance .... Donn Haber
Coronary Care.............. Kathy Mann, RN
Operating Room............. Joseph T McGinn, RN
Chief of Medical Staff .... Mark Raden, MD
Radiology.................. Mark Raden, MD

Measure	Cases	This Hosp.	State Avg.	U.S. Avg.
Blood Clot Prevention and Treatment				
Anticoagulation Overlap Therapy[2]	204	98%	91%	93%
ICU Venous Thromboembolism Prophylaxis[2]	65	97%	92%	92%
Incidence of Potentially Preventable VTE[2]	69	4%	10%	10%
UFH with Dosages/Platelet Monitoring[2]	151	34%	92%	97%
Venous Thromboembolism Prophylaxis[2]	304	92%	87%	85%
Warfarin Therapy Discharge Instructions[2]	129	61%	59%	75%
Chest Pain/Possible Heart Attack Care				
Aspirin Given Within 24 Hours of Arrival[1,3]	-	-	97%	96%
Fibrinolytic Meds Within 30 Min. of Arrival[3,7]	-	-	54%	58%
Average Time to ECG (minutes)[1,3]	-	-	9	7
Average Time to Transfer (minutes)[3,7]	-	-	78	60
Children's Asthma Care				
Received Home Management Plan of Care	-	-	-	88%
Received Reliever Medication	-	-	-	100%
Received Systemic Corticosteroids	-	-	-	100%
Emergency Department				
Admittance Decision Time (minutes)[2]	814	316	154	98
Head CT Results Within 45 Min. of Arrival[1]	-	-	55%	57%
Patients Who Left ER Before Being Seen	>100k	1%	2%	2%
Time from ER Arrival to Admit. (minutes)[2]	815	548	378	274
Time from ER Arrival to Discharge (minutes)	370	156	156	134
Time in ER Before Being Evaluated (minutes)	407	17	35	26
Time to Pain Meds for Fractures (minutes)	183	64	61	57
Heart Attack Care				
Aspirin Given at Discharge[2]	276	100%	99%	99%
Fibrinolytic Meds Within 30 Min. of Arrival[2,7]	-	-	46%	54%
PCI Within 90 Minutes of Arrival[2]	53	100%	95%	96%
Statin Prescribed at Discharge[2]	265	100%	98%	98%
Heart Failure Care				
ACE Inhibitor or ARB for LVSD[2]	95	100%	96%	97%
Discharge Instructions Given[2]	226	98%	95%	94%
Evaluation of LVS Function[2]	287	100%	99%	99%
Medicare Spending				
Medicare Spending per Patient (ratio)	-	1.02	0.96	0.98
Pneumonia Care				
Appropriate Initial Antibiotic Given[2]	82	100%	95%	95%
Blood Culture Timing[2]	188	100%	97%	98%
Pregnancy and Delivery Care				
Newborn Deliveries Scheduled Early[2]	54	0%	4%	6%
Preventive Care				
Immunization for Influenza[2]	542	89%	88%	90%
Immunization for Pneumonia[2]	607	89%	88%	92%
Stroke Care				
Anticoagulation Therapy for Atrial Fibrillation[1,2]	-	-	96%	95%
Antithrombotic Therapy Timing[2]	74	100%	98%	98%
Assessed for Rehabilitation[2]	95	97%	97%	97%
Discharged on Antithrombotic Therapy[2]	77	100%	99%	99%
Discharged on Statin Medication[2]	67	99%	95%	94%
Thrombolytic Therapy Timing[1,2]	-	-	69%	66%
Venous Thromboembolism Prophylaxis[2]	109	96%	94%	94%
Written Stroke Educational Materials Given[2]	50	92%	86%	88%
Surgical Care Improvement Project				
Appropriate Beta Blocker Usage[2]	211	100%	97%	98%
Appropriate VTP Within 24 Hours[2]	299	100%	98%	98%
Controlled Postoperative Blood Glucose[2]	101	98%	97%	97%
Perioperative Temperature Management[2]	469	100%	100%	100%

NOTE: Hospital profiles are in alphabetical order by state, then city, then hospital within the city; Rankings exclude hospitals with less than 25 cases except for patient surveys which excludes hospitals with less than 100 cases; (a) 100-299 cases; (1) The number of cases/patients is too few to report; (2) Data submitted were based on a sample of cases/patients; (3) Results are based on a shorter time period than required; (4) Data suppressed by CMS for one or more quarters; (5) Results are not available for this reporting period; (6) Fewer than 100 patients completed the HCAHPS survey; (7) No cases met the criteria for this measure; (8) The lower limit of the confidence interval cannot be calculated if the number of observed infections equals zero; (9) No data are available from the state/territory for this reporting period; (10) The scores shown reflect fewer than 50 completed surveys; (11) There were discrepancies in the data collection process; (12) This measure does not apply to this hospital for this reporting period; (13) Results cannot be calculated for this reporting period; (14) The results for this state are combined with nearby states to protect confidentiality; Please refer to the User's Guide for a full explanation of data.

Prophylactic Antibiotic Selection[2]	343	100%	99%	99%
Prophylactic Antibiotic Selection (Outpatient)	201	93%	97%	98%
Prophylactic Antibiotic Stopped[2]	322	100%	98%	98%
Prophylactic Antibiotic Timing[2]	343	100%	99%	99%
Prophylactic Antibiotic Timing (Outpatient)	178	98%	97%	98%
Urinary Catheter Removal[2]	264	100%	96%	97%
Survey of Patients' Hospital Experiences				
Area Around Room 'Always' Quiet at Night	300+	41%	51%	61%
Doctors 'Always' Communicated Well	300+	69%	77%	82%
Home Recovery Information Given	300+	75%	83%	85%
Hospital Given 9 or 10 on 10 Point Scale	300+	57%	63%	71%
Meds 'Always' Explained Before Given	300+	56%	59%	64%
Nurses 'Always' Communicated Well	300+	73%	75%	79%
Pain 'Always' Well Controlled	300+	58%	67%	71%
Room and Bathroom 'Always' Clean	300+	63%	69%	73%
Timely Help 'Always' Received	300+	61%	61%	68%
Would Definitely Recommend Hospital	300+	58%	65%	71%
Use of Medical Imaging				
Cardiac Imaging Stress Test before Surgery	402	8.0%	5.8%	5.3%
Combination Abdominal CT Scan	1,055	5.4%	8.2%	10.5%
Combination Brain/Sinus CT Scan	771	2.3%	3.6%	2.7%
Combination Chest CT Scan	740	2.8%	1.3%	2.7%
Follow-up Mammogram/Ultrasound	2,820	8.4%	13%	8.8%
Lumbar Spine MRI for Low Back Pain	80	32.5%	33.4%	37.2%

University Hospital - Stony Brook

Health Sciences Center Suny
Stony Brook, NY 11794
Phone: 631-444-4000
Fax: 631-444-4724
URL: www.stonybrookmedicalcenter.org
Type: Acute Care Hospitals
Emergency Services: Yes
Ownership: Government - State
Beds: 540

Key Personnel:

Operating Room. . . . . Faith Buck
Pediatric Ambulatory Care . . . . . . Richard Fine, MD
Pediatric In-Patient Care . . . . Richard Fine, MD
Chief of Medical Staff . . . . Joseph Laver, MD
CEO . . . . L. Reuven Pasternak, MD, MPH, MBA
Radiology. . . . . Mark Schweitzer, MD, FRCPSC
Infection Control. . . . . Francina Sing
CEO/President. . . . . Steven Strongwater, MD

Measure	Cases	This Hosp.	State Avg.	U.S. Avg.
Blood Clot Prevention and Treatment				
Anticoagulation Overlap Therapy[2]	187	93%	91%	93%
ICU Venous Thromboembolism Prophylaxis[2]	60	90%	92%	92%
Incidence of Potentially Preventable VTE[2]	77	12%	10%	10%
UFH with Dosages/Platelet Monitoring[2]	149	96%	92%	97%
Venous Thromboembolism Prophylaxis[2]	329	82%	87%	85%
Warfarin Therapy Discharge Instructions[2]	144	15%	59%	75%
Chest Pain/Possible Heart Attack Care				
Aspirin Given Within 24 Hours of Arrival[5]	-	-	97%	96%
Fibrinolytic Meds Within 30 Min. of Arrival[5]	-	-	54%	58%
Average Time to ECG (minutes)[5]	-	-	9	7
Average Time to Transfer (minutes)[5]	-	-	78	60
Children's Asthma Care				
Received Home Management Plan of Care[2]	177	59%	-	88%
Received Reliever Medication	177	100%	-	100%
Received Systemic Corticosteroids	176	95%	-	100%
Emergency Department				
Admittance Decision Time (minutes)[2]	607	194	154	98
Head CT Results Within 45 Min. of Arrival[1]	-	-	55%	57%
Patients Who Left ER Before Being Seen	96,596	1%	2%	2%
Time from ER Arrival to Admit. (minutes)[2]	613	516	378	274
Time from ER Arrival to Discharge (minutes)	223	162	156	134
Time in ER Before Being Evaluated (minutes)	158	63	35	26
Time to Pain Meds for Fractures (minutes)	189	43	61	57
Heart Attack Care				
Aspirin Given at Discharge[2]	541	99%	99%	99%
Fibrinolytic Meds Within 30 Min. of Arrival[2,7]	-	-	46%	54%
PCI Within 90 Minutes of Arrival[2]	77	97%	95%	96%
Statin Prescribed at Discharge[2]	535	97%	98%	98%
Heart Failure Care				
ACE Inhibitor or ARB for LVSD[2]	83	98%	96%	97%
Discharge Instructions Given[2]	227	84%	95%	94%
Evaluation of LVS Function[2]	273	100%	99%	99%
Medicare Spending				
Medicare Spending per Patient (ratio)	-	0.98	0.96	0.98
Pneumonia Care				
Appropriate Initial Antibiotic Given[2]	68	93%	95%	95%
Blood Culture Timing[2]	131	99%	97%	98%
Pregnancy and Delivery Care				
Newborn Deliveries Scheduled Early[2]	37	8%	4%	6%
Preventive Care				
Immunization for Influenza[2]	521	95%	88%	90%
Immunization for Pneumonia[2]	534	90%	88%	92%
Stroke Care				
Anticoagulation Therapy for Atrial Fibrillation[1,2]	-	-	96%	95%
Antithrombotic Therapy Timing[2]	59	98%	98%	98%
Assessed for Rehabilitation[2]	109	96%	97%	97%
Discharged on Antithrombotic Therapy[2]	75	100%	99%	99%
Discharged on Statin Medication[2]	51	90%	95%	94%
Thrombolytic Therapy Timing[1,2]	-	-	69%	66%
Venous Thromboembolism Prophylaxis[2]	114	82%	94%	94%
Written Stroke Educational Materials Given[2]	47	96%	86%	88%
Surgical Care Improvement Project				
Appropriate Beta Blocker Usage[2]	224	98%	97%	98%
Appropriate VTP Within 24 Hours[2]	319	100%	98%	98%
Controlled Postoperative Blood Glucose[2]	123	90%	97%	97%
Perioperative Temperature Management[2]	435	98%	100%	100%
Prophylactic Antibiotic Selection[2]	383	98%	99%	99%
Prophylactic Antibiotic Selection (Outpatient)	438	91%	97%	98%
Prophylactic Antibiotic Stopped[2]	376	98%	98%	98%
Prophylactic Antibiotic Timing[2]	385	98%	99%	99%
Prophylactic Antibiotic Timing (Outpatient)	414	96%	97%	98%
Urinary Catheter Removal[2]	326	98%	96%	97%
Survey of Patients' Hospital Experiences				
Area Around Room 'Always' Quiet at Night	300+	43%	51%	61%
Doctors 'Always' Communicated Well	300+	77%	77%	82%
Home Recovery Information Given	300+	86%	83%	85%
Hospital Given 9 or 10 on 10 Point Scale	300+	69%	63%	71%
Meds 'Always' Explained Before Given	300+	60%	59%	64%
Nurses 'Always' Communicated Well	300+	78%	75%	79%
Pain 'Always' Well Controlled	300+	68%	67%	71%
Room and Bathroom 'Always' Clean	300+	65%	69%	73%
Timely Help 'Always' Received	300+	64%	61%	68%
Would Definitely Recommend Hospital	300+	75%	65%	71%
Use of Medical Imaging				
Cardiac Imaging Stress Test before Surgery	455	3.5%	5.8%	5.3%
Combination Abdominal CT Scan	1,371	8.9%	8.2%	10.5%
Combination Brain/Sinus CT Scan	982	3.1%	3.6%	2.7%
Combination Chest CT Scan	1,373	0.5%	1.3%	2.7%
Follow-up Mammogram/Ultrasound	1,552	14.8%	13%	8.8%
Lumbar Spine MRI for Low Back Pain	94	30.9%	33.4%	37.2%

Good Samaritan Hospital of Suffern

255 Lafayette Avenue
Suffern, NY 10901
Phone: 914-368-5000
Fax: 845-368-5430
URL: www.goodsamhosp.org
Type: Acute Care Hospitals
Emergency Services: Yes
Ownership: Voluntary non-profit - Church
Beds: 370

Key Personnel:

Operating Room. . . . . Nancy Berger
Chief of Medical Staff. . . . . William Cors, MD
Infection Control. . . . . Eileen Englebracht
Radiology. . . . . Scott G Luchs, MD
Quality Assurance . . . . Maureen Reynolds
Pediatric Ambulatory Care . . . . . . Richard Snop
Pediatric In-Patient Care . . . . Richard Snop

Measure	Cases	This Hosp.	State Avg.	U.S. Avg.
Blood Clot Prevention and Treatment				
Anticoagulation Overlap Therapy[2]	64	98%	91%	93%
ICU Venous Thromboembolism Prophylaxis[2]	85	62%	92%	92%
Incidence of Potentially Preventable VTE[2]	29	48%	10%	10%
UFH with Dosages/Platelet Monitoring[2]	30	90%	92%	97%
Venous Thromboembolism Prophylaxis[2]	333	49%	87%	85%
Warfarin Therapy Discharge Instructions[2]	36	100%	59%	75%
Chest Pain/Possible Heart Attack Care				
Aspirin Given Within 24 Hours of Arrival[1]	-	-	97%	96%
Fibrinolytic Meds Within 30 Min. of Arrival[5]	-	-	54%	58%
Average Time to ECG (minutes)[1]	-	-	9	7
Average Time to Transfer (minutes)[5]	-	-	78	60
Children's Asthma Care				
Received Home Management Plan of Care	-	-	-	88%
Received Reliever Medication	-	-	-	100%
Received Systemic Corticosteroids	-	-	-	100%
Emergency Department				
Admittance Decision Time (minutes)[2]	556	173	154	98
Head CT Results Within 45 Min. of Arrival[1]	-	-	55%	57%
Patients Who Left ER Before Being Seen	37,594	1%	2%	2%
Time from ER Arrival to Admit. (minutes)[2]	574	434	378	274
Time from ER Arrival to Discharge (minutes)	400	197	156	134
Time in ER Before Being Evaluated (minutes)	439	31	35	26
Time to Pain Meds for Fractures (minutes)	89	53	61	57
Heart Attack Care				
Aspirin Given at Discharge	380	100%	99%	99%
Fibrinolytic Meds Within 30 Min. of Arrival[7]	-	-	46%	54%
PCI Within 90 Minutes of Arrival	49	100%	95%	96%
Statin Prescribed at Discharge	369	100%	98%	98%
Heart Failure Care				
ACE Inhibitor or ARB for LVSD	99	100%	96%	97%
Discharge Instructions Given	225	100%	95%	94%
Evaluation of LVS Function	322	100%	99%	99%
Medicare Spending				
Medicare Spending per Patient (ratio)	-	1.05	0.96	0.98
Pneumonia Care				
Appropriate Initial Antibiotic Given	149	89%	95%	95%
Blood Culture Timing	304	96%	97%	98%
Pregnancy and Delivery Care				
Newborn Deliveries Scheduled Early[2]	48	2%	4%	6%
Preventive Care				
Immunization for Influenza[2]	497	88%	88%	90%
Immunization for Pneumonia[2]	530	90%	88%	92%
Stroke Care				
Anticoagulation Therapy for Atrial Fibrillation	20	85%	96%	95%
Antithrombotic Therapy Timing	105	96%	98%	98%
Assessed for Rehabilitation	133	92%	97%	97%
Discharged on Antithrombotic Therapy	116	99%	99%	99%
Discharged on Statin Medication	90	87%	95%	94%
Thrombolytic Therapy Timing[1]	-	-	69%	66%
Venous Thromboembolism Prophylaxis	140	53%	94%	94%
Written Stroke Educational Materials Given	66	80%	86%	88%
Surgical Care Improvement Project				
Appropriate Beta Blocker Usage[2]	292	99%	97%	98%
Appropriate VTP Within 24 Hours[2]	374	97%	98%	98%
Controlled Postoperative Blood Glucose[2]	119	98%	97%	97%
Perioperative Temperature Management[2]	473	100%	100%	100%
Prophylactic Antibiotic Selection[2]	432	99%	99%	99%
Prophylactic Antibiotic Selection (Outpatient)	200	95%	97%	98%
Prophylactic Antibiotic Stopped[2]	423	98%	98%	98%
Prophylactic Antibiotic Timing[2]	432	99%	99%	99%
Prophylactic Antibiotic Timing (Outpatient)	203	98%	97%	98%
Urinary Catheter Removal[2]	379	96%	96%	97%
Survey of Patients' Hospital Experiences				
Area Around Room 'Always' Quiet at Night	300+	41%	51%	61%
Doctors 'Always' Communicated Well	300+	75%	77%	82%
Home Recovery Information Given	300+	78%	83%	85%
Hospital Given 9 or 10 on 10 Point Scale	300+	57%	63%	71%
Meds 'Always' Explained Before Given	300+	52%	59%	64%
Nurses 'Always' Communicated Well	300+	67%	75%	79%
Pain 'Always' Well Controlled	300+	60%	67%	71%
Room and Bathroom 'Always' Clean	300+	57%	69%	73%
Timely Help 'Always' Received	300+	49%	61%	68%
Would Definitely Recommend Hospital	300+	60%	65%	71%
Use of Medical Imaging				
Cardiac Imaging Stress Test before Surgery	73	5.5%	5.8%	5.3%
Combination Abdominal CT Scan	479	4.6%	8.2%	10.5%
Combination Brain/Sinus CT Scan	563	4.4%	3.6%	2.7%
Combination Chest CT Scan	222	0.5%	1.3%	2.7%
Follow-up Mammogram/Ultrasound	434	30.0%	13%	8.8%
Lumbar Spine MRI for Low Back Pain[1]	-	-	33.4%	37.2%

NOTE: Hospital profiles are in alphabetical order by state, then city, then hospital within the city; Rankings exclude hospitals with less than 25 cases except for patient surveys which excludes hospitals with less than 100 cases; (a) 100-299 cases; (1) The number of cases/patients is too few to report; (2) Data submitted were based on a sample of cases/patients; (3) Results are based on a shorter time period than required; (4) Data suppressed by CMS for one or more quarters; (5) Results are not available for this reporting period; (6) Fewer than 100 patients completed the HCAHPS survey; (7) No cases met the criteria for this measure; (8) The lower limit of the confidence interval cannot be calculated if the number of observed infections equals zero; (9) No data are available from the state/territory for this reporting period; (10) The scores shown reflect fewer than 50 completed surveys; (11) There were discrepancies in the data collection process; (12) This measure does not apply to this hospital for this reporting period; (13) Results cannot be calculated for this reporting period; (14) The results for this state are combined with nearby states to protect confidentiality; Please refer to the User's Guide for a full explanation of data.

Crouse Hospital

736 Irving Avenue
Syracuse, NY 13210
Phone: 315-470-7449
Fax: 315-470-7232
URL: www.crouse.org
Type: Acute Care Hospitals
Emergency Services: Yes
Ownership: Voluntary non-profit - Private
Beds: 566

Key Personnel:

CEO/President. . . . . Kimberly Boynton
Pediatric Ambulatory Care . . . . . . Winston Gaum, MD
Pediatric In-Patient Care . . . . Winston Gaum, MD
Chief of Medical Staff . . . . Paul Kronenberg, MD
Quality Assurance . . . . Ron Press
Radiology. . . . . Stuart Singer
Operating Room. . . . . Tammy Tenerovicz
Infection Control. . . . . James Turchik, MD

Measure	Cases	This Hosp.	State Avg.	U.S. Avg.
Blood Clot Prevention and Treatment				
Anticoagulation Overlap Therapy[2]	97	90%	91%	93%
ICU Venous Thromboembolism Prophylaxis[2]	31	100%	92%	92%
Incidence of Potentially Preventable VTE[2]	25	12%	10%	10%
UFH with Dosages/Platelet Monitoring[2]	81	85%	92%	97%
Venous Thromboembolism Prophylaxis[2]	300	97%	87%	85%
Warfarin Therapy Discharge Instructions[2]	69	54%	59%	75%
Chest Pain/Possible Heart Attack Care				
Aspirin Given Within 24 Hours of Arrival[5]	-	-	97%	96%
Fibrinolytic Meds Within 30 Min. of Arrival[5]	-	-	54%	58%
Average Time to ECG (minutes)[5]	-	-	9	7
Average Time to Transfer (minutes)[5]	-	-	78	60
Children's Asthma Care				
Received Home Management Plan of Care	-	-	-	88%
Received Reliever Medication	-	-	-	100%
Received Systemic Corticosteroids	-	-	-	100%
Emergency Department				
Admittance Decision Time (minutes)[2]	404	104	154	98
Head CT Results Within 45 Min. of Arrival[1]	-	-	55%	57%
Patients Who Left ER Before Being Seen	40,866	1%	2%	2%
Time from ER Arrival to Admit. (minutes)[2]	414	349	378	274
Time from ER Arrival to Discharge (minutes)	338	207	156	134
Time in ER Before Being Evaluated (minutes)	402	19	35	26
Time to Pain Meds for Fractures (minutes)	46	45	61	57
Heart Attack Care				
Aspirin Given at Discharge	165	99%	99%	99%
Fibrinolytic Meds Within 30 Min. of Arrival[7]	-	-	46%	54%
PCI Within 90 Minutes of Arrival	49	98%	95%	96%
Statin Prescribed at Discharge	166	95%	98%	98%
Heart Failure Care				
ACE Inhibitor or ARB for LVSD[2]	76	96%	96%	97%
Discharge Instructions Given[2]	238	100%	95%	94%
Evaluation of LVS Function[2]	307	99%	99%	99%
Medicare Spending				
Medicare Spending per Patient (ratio)	-	0.94	0.96	0.98
Pneumonia Care				
Appropriate Initial Antibiotic Given[2]	99	94%	95%	95%
Blood Culture Timing[2]	132	98%	97%	98%
Pregnancy and Delivery Care				
Newborn Deliveries Scheduled Early[2]	49	2%	4%	6%
Preventive Care				
Immunization for Influenza[2]	502	91%	88%	90%
Immunization for Pneumonia[2]	484	92%	88%	92%
Stroke Care				
Anticoagulation Therapy for Atrial Fibrillation[2]	11	100%	96%	95%
Antithrombotic Therapy Timing[2]	73	100%	98%	98%
Assessed for Rehabilitation[2]	106	96%	97%	97%
Discharged on Antithrombotic Therapy[2]	88	100%	99%	99%
Discharged on Statin Medication[2]	76	95%	95%	94%
Thrombolytic Therapy Timing[2]	13	92%	69%	66%
Venous Thromboembolism Prophylaxis[2]	99	99%	94%	94%
Written Stroke Educational Materials Given[2]	57	96%	86%	88%
Surgical Care Improvement Project				
Appropriate Beta Blocker Usage[2]	148	98%	97%	98%
Appropriate VTP Within 24 Hours[2]	393	98%	98%	98%
Controlled Postoperative Blood Glucose[2,7]	-	-	97%	97%
Perioperative Temperature Management[2]	563	100%	100%	100%
Prophylactic Antibiotic Selection[2]	397	98%	99%	99%
Prophylactic Antibiotic Selection (Outpatient)	766	96%	97%	98%
Prophylactic Antibiotic Stopped[2]	384	98%	98%	98%
Prophylactic Antibiotic Timing[2]	397	97%	99%	99%
Prophylactic Antibiotic Timing (Outpatient)	768	98%	97%	98%
Urinary Catheter Removal[2]	323	94%	96%	97%
Survey of Patients' Hospital Experiences				
Area Around Room 'Always' Quiet at Night	300+	44%	51%	61%
Doctors 'Always' Communicated Well	300+	77%	77%	82%
Home Recovery Information Given	300+	88%	83%	85%
Hospital Given 9 or 10 on 10 Point Scale	300+	63%	63%	71%
Meds 'Always' Explained Before Given	300+	58%	59%	64%
Nurses 'Always' Communicated Well	300+	73%	75%	79%
Pain 'Always' Well Controlled	300+	66%	67%	71%
Room and Bathroom 'Always' Clean	300+	62%	69%	73%
Timely Help 'Always' Received	300+	54%	61%	68%
Would Definitely Recommend Hospital	300+	68%	65%	71%
Use of Medical Imaging				
Cardiac Imaging Stress Test before Surgery	59	3.4%	5.8%	5.3%
Combination Abdominal CT Scan	685	2.5%	8.2%	10.5%
Combination Brain/Sinus CT Scan	875	3.4%	3.6%	2.7%
Combination Chest CT Scan	350	2.0%	1.3%	2.7%
Follow-up Mammogram/Ultrasound	1,151	5.2%	13%	8.8%
Lumbar Spine MRI for Low Back Pain[7]	-	-	33.4%	37.2%

Saint Joseph's Hospital Health Center

301 Prospect Avenue
Syracuse, NY 13203
Phone: 315-448-5111
Fax: 315-703-2129
E-mail: community.relations@sjhsyr.org
URL: www.sjhsyr.org
Type: Acute Care Hospitals
Emergency Services: Yes
Ownership: Voluntary non-profit - Private
Beds: 431

Key Personnel:

Coronary Care . . . . AnneMarie Czyz, RN
Operating Room. . . . . Kim Murray, RN
CEO/President. . . . . Kathryn H. Ruscitto
Chief of Medical Staff . . . . Sandra Sulik, MD
Emergency Room . . . . Sarah Tubbert, RN
Radiology. . . . . Robert Whitmarsh

Measure	Cases	This Hosp.	State Avg.	U.S. Avg.
Blood Clot Prevention and Treatment				
Anticoagulation Overlap Therapy[2]	211	85%	91%	93%
ICU Venous Thromboembolism Prophylaxis[2]	55	93%	92%	92%
Incidence of Potentially Preventable VTE[2]	36	36%	10%	10%
UFH with Dosages/Platelet Monitoring[2]	179	99%	92%	97%
Venous Thromboembolism Prophylaxis[2]	335	83%	87%	85%
Warfarin Therapy Discharge Instructions[2]	160	10%	59%	75%
Chest Pain/Possible Heart Attack Care				
Aspirin Given Within 24 Hours of Arrival[5]	-	-	97%	96%
Fibrinolytic Meds Within 30 Min. of Arrival[5]	-	-	54%	58%
Average Time to ECG (minutes)[5]	-	-	9	7
Average Time to Transfer (minutes)[5]	-	-	78	60
Children's Asthma Care				
Received Home Management Plan of Care	-	-	-	88%
Received Reliever Medication	-	-	-	100%
Received Systemic Corticosteroids	-	-	-	100%
Emergency Department				
Admittance Decision Time (minutes)[2]	557	223	154	98
Head CT Results Within 45 Min. of Arrival[1]	-	-	55%	57%
Patients Who Left ER Before Being Seen	69,863	4%	2%	2%
Time from ER Arrival to Admit. (minutes)[2]	575	464	378	274
Time from ER Arrival to Discharge (minutes)	343	234	156	134
Time in ER Before Being Evaluated (minutes)	391	84	35	26
Time to Pain Meds for Fractures (minutes)	111	66	61	57
Heart Attack Care				
Aspirin Given at Discharge	1,043	99%	99%	99%
Fibrinolytic Meds Within 30 Min. of Arrival[1]	-	-	46%	54%
PCI Within 90 Minutes of Arrival	152	94%	95%	96%
Statin Prescribed at Discharge	1,022	96%	98%	98%
Heart Failure Care				
ACE Inhibitor or ARB for LVSD	231	94%	96%	97%
Discharge Instructions Given	717	98%	95%	94%
Evaluation of LVS Function	880	100%	99%	99%
Medicare Spending				
Medicare Spending per Patient (ratio)	-	0.94	0.96	0.98
Pneumonia Care				
Appropriate Initial Antibiotic Given	334	94%	95%	95%
Blood Culture Timing	603	99%	97%	98%
Pregnancy and Delivery Care				
Newborn Deliveries Scheduled Early[2]	26	8%	4%	6%
Preventive Care				
Immunization for Influenza[2]	561	76%	88%	90%
Immunization for Pneumonia[2]	775	64%	88%	92%
Stroke Care				
Anticoagulation Therapy for Atrial Fibrillation[1,2]	-	-	96%	95%
Antithrombotic Therapy Timing[2]	42	100%	98%	98%
Assessed for Rehabilitation[2]	54	85%	97%	97%
Discharged on Antithrombotic Therapy[2]	47	98%	99%	99%
Discharged on Statin Medication[2]	46	87%	95%	94%
Thrombolytic Therapy Timing[1,2]	-	-	69%	66%
Venous Thromboembolism Prophylaxis[2]	56	93%	94%	94%
Written Stroke Educational Materials Given[2]	33	9%	86%	88%
Surgical Care Improvement Project				
Appropriate Beta Blocker Usage[2]	309	99%	97%	98%
Appropriate VTP Within 24 Hours[2]	494	100%	98%	98%
Controlled Postoperative Blood Glucose[2]	192	92%	97%	97%
Perioperative Temperature Management[2]	663	98%	100%	100%
Prophylactic Antibiotic Selection[2]	600	99%	99%	99%
Prophylactic Antibiotic Selection (Outpatient)	807	99%	97%	98%
Prophylactic Antibiotic Stopped[2]	586	95%	98%	98%
Prophylactic Antibiotic Timing[2]	600	99%	99%	99%
Prophylactic Antibiotic Timing (Outpatient)	807	99%	97%	98%
Urinary Catheter Removal[2]	529	97%	96%	97%
Survey of Patients' Hospital Experiences				
Area Around Room 'Always' Quiet at Night	300+	48%	51%	61%
Doctors 'Always' Communicated Well	300+	77%	77%	82%
Home Recovery Information Given	300+	88%	83%	85%
Hospital Given 9 or 10 on 10 Point Scale	300+	73%	63%	71%
Meds 'Always' Explained Before Given	300+	60%	59%	64%
Nurses 'Always' Communicated Well	300+	80%	75%	79%
Pain 'Always' Well Controlled	300+	69%	67%	71%
Room and Bathroom 'Always' Clean	300+	68%	69%	73%
Timely Help 'Always' Received	300+	64%	61%	68%
Would Definitely Recommend Hospital	300+	79%	65%	71%
Use of Medical Imaging				
Cardiac Imaging Stress Test before Surgery	369	2.7%	5.8%	5.3%
Combination Abdominal CT Scan	858	0.7%	8.2%	10.5%
Combination Brain/Sinus CT Scan	1,394	2.7%	3.6%	2.7%
Combination Chest CT Scan	256	0.0%	1.3%	2.7%
Follow-up Mammogram/Ultrasound	204	14.2%	13%	8.8%
Lumbar Spine MRI for Low Back Pain[7]	-	-	33.4%	37.2%

Syracuse VA Medical Center

800 Irving Ave.
Syracuse, NY 13210
Phone: 315-425-4400
Fax: 315-425-4375
URL: www1.va.gov/visns/visn02
Type: Acute Care - VA
Emergency Services: No
Ownership: Government Federal
Beds: 164

Key Personnel:

Quality Assurance . . . . Marcia Dawley
Patient Relations . . . . Kerry Grant
Chief of Medical Staff . . . . William H Marx, DO, FACS
Operating Room. . . . . Brenda Rudy

Measure	Cases	This Hosp.	State Avg.	U.S. Avg.
Blood Clot Prevention and Treatment				
Anticoagulation Overlap Therapy	-	-	91%	93%
ICU Venous Thromboembolism Prophylaxis	-	-	92%	92%
Incidence of Potentially Preventable VTE	-	-	10%	10%
UFH with Dosages/Platelet Monitoring	-	-	92%	97%
Venous Thromboembolism Prophylaxis	-	-	87%	85%
Warfarin Therapy Discharge Instructions	-	-	59%	75%
Chest Pain/Possible Heart Attack Care				
Aspirin Given Within 24 Hours of Arrival	-	-	97%	96%
Fibrinolytic Meds Within 30 Min. of Arrival	-	-	54%	58%
Average Time to ECG (minutes)	-	-	9	7
Average Time to Transfer (minutes)	-	-	78	60
Children's Asthma Care				
Received Home Management Plan of Care	-	-	-	88%

NOTE: Hospital profiles are in alphabetical order by state, then city, then hospital within the city; Rankings exclude hospitals with less than 25 cases except for patient surveys which excludes hospitals with less than 100 cases; (a) 100-299 cases; (1) The number of cases/patients is too few to report; (2) Data submitted were based on a sample of cases/patients; (3) Results are based on a shorter time period than required; (4) Data suppressed by CMS for one or more quarters; (5) Results are not available for this reporting period; (6) Fewer than 100 patients completed the HCAHPS survey; (7) No cases met the criteria for this measure; (8) The lower limit of the confidence interval cannot be calculated if the number of observed infections equals zero; (9) No data are available from the state/territory for this reporting period; (10) The scores shown reflect fewer than 50 completed surveys; (11) There were discrepancies in the data collection process; (12) This measure does not apply to this hospital for this reporting period; (13) Results cannot be calculated for this reporting period; (14) The results for this state are combined with nearby states to protect confidentiality; Please refer to the User's Guide for a full explanation of data.

Measure	Cases	This Hosp.	State Avg.	U.S. Avg.
Received Reliever Medication	-	-	-	100%
Received Systemic Corticosteroids	-	-	-	100%
Emergency Department				
Admittance Decision Time (minutes)	-	-	154	98
Head CT Results Within 45 Min. of Arrival	-	-	55%	57%
Patients Who Left ER Before Being Seen	-	-	2%	2%
Time from ER Arrival to Admit. (minutes)	-	-	378	274
Time from ER Arrival to Discharge (minutes)	-	-	156	134
Time in ER Before Being Evaluated (minutes)	-	-	35	26
Time to Pain Meds for Fractures (minutes)	-	-	61	57
Heart Attack Care				
Aspirin Given at Discharge	40	100%	99%	99%
Fibrinolytic Meds Within 30 Min. of Arrival[5]	-	-	46%	54%
PCI Within 90 Minutes of Arrival[1]	-	-	95%	96%
Statin Prescribed at Discharge	36	100%	98%	98%
Heart Failure Care				
ACE Inhibitor or ARB for LVSD	31	94%	96%	97%
Discharge Instructions Given	128	100%	95%	94%
Evaluation of LVS Function	134	99%	99%	99%
Medicare Spending				
Medicare Spending per Patient (ratio)	-	-	0.96	0.98
Pneumonia Care				
Appropriate Initial Antibiotic Given	77	90%	95%	95%
Blood Culture Timing	150	99%	97%	98%
Pregnancy and Delivery Care				
Newborn Deliveries Scheduled Early	-	-	4%	6%
Preventive Care				
Immunization for Influenza[5]	-	-	88%	90%
Immunization for Pneumonia[5]	-	-	88%	92%
Stroke Care				
Anticoagulation Therapy for Atrial Fibrillation	-	-	96%	95%
Antithrombotic Therapy Timing	-	-	98%	98%
Assessed for Rehabilitation	-	-	97%	97%
Discharged on Antithrombotic Therapy	-	-	99%	99%
Discharged on Statin Medication	-	-	95%	94%
Thrombolytic Therapy Timing	-	-	69%	66%
Venous Thromboembolism Prophylaxis	-	-	94%	94%
Written Stroke Educational Materials Given	-	-	86%	88%
Surgical Care Improvement Project				
Appropriate Beta Blocker Usage[2]	55	96%	97%	98%
Appropriate VTP Within 24 Hours[2]	117	99%	98%	98%
Controlled Postoperative Blood Glucose[5]	-	-	97%	97%
Perioperative Temperature Management[2]	137	100%	100%	100%
Prophylactic Antibiotic Selection	53	98%	99%	99%
Prophylactic Antibiotic Selection (Outpatient)	-	-	97%	98%
Prophylactic Antibiotic Stopped	53	98%	98%	98%
Prophylactic Antibiotic Timing	53	96%	99%	99%
Prophylactic Antibiotic Timing (Outpatient)	-	-	97%	98%
Urinary Catheter Removal[2]	85	100%	96%	97%
Survey of Patients' Hospital Experiences				
Area Around Room 'Always' Quiet at Night	-	-	51%	61%
Doctors 'Always' Communicated Well	-	-	77%	82%
Home Recovery Information Given	-	-	83%	85%
Hospital Given 9 or 10 on 10 Point Scale	-	-	63%	71%
Meds 'Always' Explained Before Given	-	-	59%	64%
Nurses 'Always' Communicated Well	-	-	75%	79%
Pain 'Always' Well Controlled	-	-	67%	71%
Room and Bathroom 'Always' Clean	-	-	69%	73%
Timely Help 'Always' Received	-	-	61%	68%
Would Definitely Recommend Hospital	-	-	65%	71%
Use of Medical Imaging				
Cardiac Imaging Stress Test before Surgery	-	-	5.8%	5.3%
Combination Abdominal CT Scan	-	-	8.2%	10.5%
Combination Brain/Sinus CT Scan	-	-	3.6%	2.7%
Combination Chest CT Scan	-	-	1.3%	2.7%
Follow-up Mammogram/Ultrasound	-	-	13%	8.8%
Lumbar Spine MRI for Low Back Pain	-	-	33.4%	37.2%

University Hospital SUNY Health Science Center

750 East Adams Street
Syracuse, NY 13210
URL: www.upstate.edu
Phone: 315-473-4240
Fax: 315-464-4838
Type: Acute Care Hospitals
Ownership: Government - State
Emergency Services: Yes
Beds: 356

Key Personnel:
Operating Room. . . . . Paul Cunningham, MD
CEO/President. . . . . Gregory L. Eastwood, MD
Quality Assurance . . . . Theresa Gagnon
Emergency Room . . . . Richard Hunt, MD
Infection Control. . . . . Fred Rose, MD
Chief of Medical Staff. . . . . Anthony P. Weiss, MD, MBA

Measure	Cases	This Hosp.	State Avg.	U.S. Avg.
Blood Clot Prevention and Treatment				
Anticoagulation Overlap Therapy[2]	186	96%	91%	93%
ICU Venous Thromboembolism Prophylaxis[2]	153	99%	92%	92%
Incidence of Potentially Preventable VTE[2]	55	9%	10%	10%
UFH with Dosages/Platelet Monitoring[2]	154	99%	92%	97%
Venous Thromboembolism Prophylaxis[2]	632	87%	87%	85%
Warfarin Therapy Discharge Instructions[2]	134	46%	59%	75%
Chest Pain/Possible Heart Attack Care				
Aspirin Given Within 24 Hours of Arrival	60	97%	97%	96%
Fibrinolytic Meds Within 30 Min. of Arrival[3,7]	-	-	54%	58%
Average Time to ECG (minutes)	69	8	9	7
Average Time to Transfer (minutes)[3,7]	-	-	78	60
Children's Asthma Care				
Received Home Management Plan of Care	-	-	-	88%
Received Reliever Medication	-	-	-	100%
Received Systemic Corticosteroids	-	-	-	100%
Emergency Department				
Admittance Decision Time (minutes)[2]	505	120	154	98
Head CT Results Within 45 Min. of Arrival[1]	-	-	55%	57%
Patients Who Left ER Before Being Seen	88,216	2%	2%	2%
Time from ER Arrival to Admit. (minutes)[2]	532	352	378	274
Time from ER Arrival to Discharge (minutes)	571	177	156	134
Time in ER Before Being Evaluated (minutes)	549	44	35	26
Time to Pain Meds for Fractures (minutes)	249	66	61	57
Heart Attack Care				
Aspirin Given at Discharge	266	99%	99%	99%
Fibrinolytic Meds Within 30 Min. of Arrival[7]	-	-	46%	54%
PCI Within 90 Minutes of Arrival	22	91%	95%	96%
Statin Prescribed at Discharge	264	93%	98%	98%
Heart Failure Care				
ACE Inhibitor or ARB for LVSD	127	98%	96%	97%
Discharge Instructions Given	356	92%	95%	94%
Evaluation of LVS Function	429	100%	99%	99%
Medicare Spending				
Medicare Spending per Patient (ratio)	-	0.98	0.96	0.98
Pneumonia Care				
Appropriate Initial Antibiotic Given	154	94%	95%	95%
Blood Culture Timing	275	97%	97%	98%
Pregnancy and Delivery Care				
Newborn Deliveries Scheduled Early	91	0%	4%	6%
Preventive Care				
Immunization for Influenza[2]	1,076	93%	88%	90%
Immunization for Pneumonia[2]	1,066	88%	88%	92%
Stroke Care				
Anticoagulation Therapy for Atrial Fibrillation[2]	19	100%	96%	95%
Antithrombotic Therapy Timing[2]	71	100%	98%	98%
Assessed for Rehabilitation[2]	110	97%	97%	97%
Discharged on Antithrombotic Therapy[2]	81	100%	99%	99%
Discharged on Statin Medication[2]	58	100%	95%	94%
Thrombolytic Therapy Timing[1,2]	-	-	69%	66%
Venous Thromboembolism Prophylaxis[2]	108	100%	94%	94%
Written Stroke Educational Materials Given[2]	69	90%	86%	88%
Surgical Care Improvement Project				
Appropriate Beta Blocker Usage[2]	210	98%	97%	98%
Appropriate VTP Within 24 Hours[2]	442	99%	98%	98%
Controlled Postoperative Blood Glucose[2]	95	97%	97%	97%
Perioperative Temperature Management[2]	531	99%	100%	100%
Prophylactic Antibiotic Selection[2]	340	99%	99%	99%
Prophylactic Antibiotic Selection (Outpatient)	561	97%	97%	98%
Prophylactic Antibiotic Stopped[2]	322	97%	98%	98%
Prophylactic Antibiotic Timing[2]	342	93%	99%	99%
Prophylactic Antibiotic Timing (Outpatient)	480	91%	97%	98%
Urinary Catheter Removal[2]	336	78%	96%	97%
Survey of Patients' Hospital Experiences				
Area Around Room 'Always' Quiet at Night[11]	300+	48%	51%	61%
Doctors 'Always' Communicated Well[11]	300+	74%	77%	82%
Home Recovery Information Given[11]	300+	86%	83%	85%
Hospital Given 9 or 10 on 10 Point Scale[11]	300+	63%	63%	71%
Meds 'Always' Explained Before Given[11]	300+	61%	59%	64%
Nurses 'Always' Communicated Well[11]	300+	74%	75%	79%
Pain 'Always' Well Controlled[11]	300+	63%	67%	71%
Room and Bathroom 'Always' Clean[11]	300+	63%	69%	73%
Timely Help 'Always' Received[11]	300+	60%	61%	68%
Would Definitely Recommend Hospital[11]	300+	65%	65%	71%
Use of Medical Imaging				
Cardiac Imaging Stress Test before Surgery	370	5.1%	5.8%	5.3%
Combination Abdominal CT Scan	1,265	12.4%	8.2%	10.5%
Combination Brain/Sinus CT Scan	1,075	3.1%	3.6%	2.7%
Combination Chest CT Scan	1,254	1.0%	1.3%	2.7%
Follow-up Mammogram/Ultrasound	1,723	15.0%	13%	8.8%
Lumbar Spine MRI for Low Back Pain[1]	-	-	33.4%	37.2%

Moses - Ludington Hospital

1019 Wicker Street
Ticonderoga, NY 12883
Phone: 518-585-2831
Fax: 518-585-2576
E-mail: catherine.larsen@tenethealth.com
URL: www.tenethealth.com/dmcmodesto
Type: Critical Access Hospitals
Ownership: Voluntary non-profit - Private
Emergency Services: Yes
Beds: 99

Key Personnel:
Radiology. . . . . Valerie Brace
Infection Control. . . . . Pat Chamberlain, DON
CEO/President. . . . . Diane Hart
Chief of Medical Staff . . . . Robert Holterman, MD
Operating Room. . . . . Nancy LaTour
Quality Assurance . . . . Lynne Reale

Measure	Cases	This Hosp.	State Avg.	U.S. Avg.
Blood Clot Prevention and Treatment				
Anticoagulation Overlap Therapy[5]	-	-	91%	93%
ICU Venous Thromboembolism Prophylaxis[5]	-	-	92%	92%
Incidence of Potentially Preventable VTE[5]	-	-	10%	10%
UFH with Dosages/Platelet Monitoring[5]	-	-	92%	97%
Venous Thromboembolism Prophylaxis[5]	-	-	87%	85%
Warfarin Therapy Discharge Instructions[5]	-	-	59%	75%
Chest Pain/Possible Heart Attack Care				
Aspirin Given Within 24 Hours of Arrival	21	86%	97%	96%
Fibrinolytic Meds Within 30 Min. of Arrival[1]	-	-	54%	58%
Average Time to ECG (minutes)	23	16	9	7
Average Time to Transfer (minutes)[1]	-	-	78	60
Children's Asthma Care				
Received Home Management Plan of Care	-	-	-	88%
Received Reliever Medication	-	-	-	100%
Received Systemic Corticosteroids	-	-	-	100%
Emergency Department				
Admittance Decision Time (minutes)[5]	-	-	154	98
Head CT Results Within 45 Min. of Arrival[1,3]	-	-	55%	57%
Patients Who Left ER Before Being Seen	6,810	0%	2%	2%
Time from ER Arrival to Admit. (minutes)[5]	-	-	378	274
Time from ER Arrival to Discharge (minutes)[5]	-	-	156	134
Time in ER Before Being Evaluated (minutes)[5]	-	-	35	26
Time to Pain Meds for Fractures (minutes)[1]	-	-	61	57
Heart Attack Care				
Aspirin Given at Discharge[3,7]	-	-	99%	99%
Fibrinolytic Meds Within 30 Min. of Arrival[3,7]	-	-	46%	54%
PCI Within 90 Minutes of Arrival[3,7]	-	-	95%	96%
Statin Prescribed at Discharge[3,7]	-	-	98%	98%
Heart Failure Care				
ACE Inhibitor or ARB for LVSD[7]	-	-	96%	97%
Discharge Instructions Given	16	100%	95%	94%
Evaluation of LVS Function	23	74%	99%	99%
Medicare Spending				
Medicare Spending per Patient (ratio)	-	-	0.96	0.98
Pneumonia Care				
Appropriate Initial Antibiotic Given	26	73%	95%	95%

NOTE: Hospital profiles are in alphabetical order by state, then city, then hospital within the city; Rankings exclude hospitals with less than 25 cases except for patient surveys which excludes hospitals with less than 100 cases; (a) 100-299 cases; (1) The number of cases/patients is too few to report; (2) Data submitted were based on a sample of cases/patients; (3) Results are based on a shorter time period than required; (4) Data suppressed by CMS for one or more quarters; (5) Results are not available for this reporting period; (6) Fewer than 100 patients completed the HCAHPS survey; (7) No cases met the criteria for this measure; (8) The lower limit of the confidence interval cannot be calculated if the number of observed infections equals zero; (9) No data are available from the state/territory for this reporting period; (10) The scores shown reflect fewer than 50 completed surveys; (11) There were discrepancies in the data collection process; (12) This measure does not apply to this hospital for this reporting period; (13) Results cannot be calculated for this reporting period; (14) The results for this state are combined with nearby states to protect confidentiality; Please refer to the User's Guide for a full explanation of data.

Blood Culture Timing	28	79%	97%	98%
Pregnancy and Delivery Care				
Newborn Deliveries Scheduled Early[5]	-	-	4%	6%
Preventive Care				
Immunization for Influenza[5]	-	-	88%	90%
Immunization for Pneumonia[5]	-	-	88%	92%
Stroke Care				
Anticoagulation Therapy for Atrial Fibrillation[5]	-	-	96%	95%
Antithrombotic Therapy Timing[5]	-	-	98%	98%
Assessed for Rehabilitation[5]	-	-	97%	97%
Discharged on Antithrombotic Therapy[5]	-	-	99%	99%
Discharged on Statin Medication[5]	-	-	95%	94%
Thrombolytic Therapy Timing[5]	-	-	69%	66%
Venous Thromboembolism Prophylaxis[5]	-	-	94%	94%
Written Stroke Educational Materials Given[5]	-	-	86%	88%
Surgical Care Improvement Project				
Appropriate Beta Blocker Usage[5]	-	-	97%	98%
Appropriate VTP Within 24 Hours[5]	-	-	98%	98%
Controlled Postoperative Blood Glucose[5]	-	-	97%	97%
Perioperative Temperature Management[5]	-	-	100%	100%
Prophylactic Antibiotic Selection[5]	-	-	99%	99%
Prophylactic Antibiotic Selection (Outpatient)[5]	-	-	97%	98%
Prophylactic Antibiotic Stopped[5]	-	-	98%	98%
Prophylactic Antibiotic Timing[5]	-	-	99%	99%
Prophylactic Antibiotic Timing (Outpatient)[5]	-	-	97%	98%
Urinary Catheter Removal[5]	-	-	96%	97%
Survey of Patients' Hospital Experiences				
Area Around Room 'Always' Quiet at Night[6]	<100	55%	51%	61%
Doctors 'Always' Communicated Well[6]	<100	83%	77%	82%
Home Recovery Information Given[6]	<100	83%	83%	85%
Hospital Given 9 or 10 on 10 Point Scale[6]	<100	72%	63%	71%
Meds 'Always' Explained Before Given[6]	<100	76%	59%	64%
Nurses 'Always' Communicated Well[6]	<100	81%	75%	79%
Pain 'Always' Well Controlled[6]	<100	70%	67%	71%
Room and Bathroom 'Always' Clean[6]	<100	81%	69%	73%
Timely Help 'Always' Received[6]	<100	82%	61%	68%
Would Definitely Recommend Hospital[6]	<100	66%	65%	71%
Use of Medical Imaging				
Cardiac Imaging Stress Test before Surgery[7]	-	-	5.8%	5.3%
Combination Abdominal CT Scan	120	5.0%	8.2%	10.5%
Combination Brain/Sinus CT Scan	148	0.0%	3.6%	2.7%
Combination Chest CT Scan	66	4.5%	1.3%	2.7%
Follow-up Mammogram/Ultrasound	161	8.1%	13%	8.8%
Lumbar Spine MRI for Low Back Pain[7]	-	-	33.4%	37.2%

Saint Mary's Hospital - Troy

1300 Massachusetts Avenue
Troy, NY 12180
Phone: 518-272-5000
Fax: 518-268-5257
E-mail: info@setonhealth.org
URL: www.setonhealth.org
Type: Acute Care Hospitals
Emergency Services: Yes
Ownership: Voluntary non-profit - Private
Beds: 201

Key Personnel:
Quality Assurance . . . . Carol Crucetti
Infection Control . . . . Mary Beth Farley
Pediatric In-Patient Care . . . . Colleen Hatman, RN
Radiology . . . . Patti Nazarko
Chief of Medical Staff . . . . Richard Rubin, MD
Operating Room . . . . Debra Shumelda
CEO/President . . . . Scott St George

Measure	Cases	This Hosp.	State Avg.	U.S. Avg.
Blood Clot Prevention and Treatment				
Anticoagulation Overlap Therapy[2]	18	94%	91%	93%
ICU Venous Thromboembolism Prophylaxis[2]	68	93%	92%	92%
Incidence of Potentially Preventable VTE[1,2]	-	-	10%	10%
UFH with Dosages/Platelet Monitoring[1,2]	-	-	92%	97%
Venous Thromboembolism Prophylaxis[2]	349	87%	87%	85%
Warfarin Therapy Discharge Instructions[2]	15	47%	59%	75%
Chest Pain/Possible Heart Attack Care				
Aspirin Given Within 24 Hours of Arrival	30	93%	97%	96%
Fibrinolytic Meds Within 30 Min. of Arrival[7]	-	-	54%	58%
Average Time to ECG (minutes)	31	9	9	7
Average Time to Transfer (minutes)	16	55	78	60
Children's Asthma Care				
Received Home Management Plan of Care	-	-	-	88%
Received Reliever Medication	-	-	-	100%
Received Systemic Corticosteroids	-	-	-	100%
Emergency Department				
Admittance Decision Time (minutes)[2]	640	150	154	98
Head CT Results Within 45 Min. of Arrival[1]	-	-	55%	57%
Patients Who Left ER Before Being Seen	31,159	0%	2%	2%
Time from ER Arrival to Admit. (minutes)[2]	641	288	378	274
Time from ER Arrival to Discharge (minutes)	377	101	156	134
Time in ER Before Being Evaluated (minutes)	399	27	35	26
Time to Pain Meds for Fractures (minutes)	64	60	61	57
Heart Attack Care				
Aspirin Given at Discharge	26	100%	99%	99%
Fibrinolytic Meds Within 30 Min. of Arrival[7]	-	-	46%	54%
PCI Within 90 Minutes of Arrival[7]	-	-	95%	96%
Statin Prescribed at Discharge	28	96%	98%	98%
Heart Failure Care				
ACE Inhibitor or ARB for LVSD	27	100%	96%	97%
Discharge Instructions Given	94	98%	95%	94%
Evaluation of LVS Function	124	100%	99%	99%
Medicare Spending				
Medicare Spending per Patient (ratio)	-	0.93	0.96	0.98
Pneumonia Care				
Appropriate Initial Antibiotic Given	85	98%	95%	95%
Blood Culture Timing	125	100%	97%	98%
Pregnancy and Delivery Care				
Newborn Deliveries Scheduled Early[7]	-	-	4%	6%
Preventive Care				
Immunization for Influenza[2]	443	94%	88%	90%
Immunization for Pneumonia[2]	635	92%	88%	92%
Stroke Care				
Anticoagulation Therapy for Atrial Fibrillation[1]	-	-	96%	95%
Antithrombotic Therapy Timing	34	94%	98%	98%
Assessed for Rehabilitation	41	100%	97%	97%
Discharged on Antithrombotic Therapy	40	100%	99%	99%
Discharged on Statin Medication	32	88%	95%	94%
Thrombolytic Therapy Timing[1]	-	-	69%	66%
Venous Thromboembolism Prophylaxis	37	97%	94%	94%
Written Stroke Educational Materials Given	22	95%	86%	88%
Surgical Care Improvement Project				
Appropriate Beta Blocker Usage[2]	52	96%	97%	98%
Appropriate VTP Within 24 Hours[2]	158	96%	98%	98%
Controlled Postoperative Blood Glucose[2,7]	-	-	97%	97%
Perioperative Temperature Management[2]	176	100%	100%	100%
Prophylactic Antibiotic Selection[2]	97	96%	99%	99%
Prophylactic Antibiotic Selection (Outpatient)	73	96%	97%	98%
Prophylactic Antibiotic Stopped[2]	92	99%	98%	98%
Prophylactic Antibiotic Timing[2]	97	99%	99%	99%
Prophylactic Antibiotic Timing (Outpatient)	73	97%	97%	98%
Urinary Catheter Removal[2]	118	95%	96%	97%
Survey of Patients' Hospital Experiences				
Area Around Room 'Always' Quiet at Night	(a)	47%	51%	61%
Doctors 'Always' Communicated Well	(a)	74%	77%	82%
Home Recovery Information Given	(a)	85%	83%	85%
Hospital Given 9 or 10 on 10 Point Scale	(a)	61%	63%	71%
Meds 'Always' Explained Before Given	(a)	57%	59%	64%
Nurses 'Always' Communicated Well	(a)	75%	75%	79%
Pain 'Always' Well Controlled	(a)	67%	67%	71%
Room and Bathroom 'Always' Clean	(a)	65%	69%	73%
Timely Help 'Always' Received	(a)	62%	61%	68%
Would Definitely Recommend Hospital	(a)	66%	65%	71%
Use of Medical Imaging				
Cardiac Imaging Stress Test before Surgery	69	2.9%	5.8%	5.3%
Combination Abdominal CT Scan	507	4.9%	8.2%	10.5%
Combination Brain/Sinus CT Scan	359	0.8%	3.6%	2.7%
Combination Chest CT Scan	196	0.0%	1.3%	2.7%
Follow-up Mammogram/Ultrasound	734	7.8%	13%	8.8%
Lumbar Spine MRI for Low Back Pain[1]	-	-	33.4%	37.2%

Samaritan Hospital

2215 Burdett Avenue
Troy, NY 12180
Phone: 518-271-3225
Fax: 518-271-3781
URL: www.nehealth.com
Type: Acute Care Hospitals
Emergency Services: Yes
Ownership: Voluntary non-profit - Private
Beds: 238

Key Personnel:
Chief of Medical Staff . . . . John A Collins
Patient Relations . . . . Norman E Dascher, Jr, CHE
CEO/President . . . . James K Reed, MD

Measure	Cases	This Hosp.	State Avg.	U.S. Avg.
Blood Clot Prevention and Treatment				
Anticoagulation Overlap Therapy[2]	33	94%	91%	93%
ICU Venous Thromboembolism Prophylaxis[2]	76	91%	92%	92%
Incidence of Potentially Preventable VTE[1,2]	-	-	10%	10%
UFH with Dosages/Platelet Monitoring[2]	13	100%	92%	97%
Venous Thromboembolism Prophylaxis[2]	268	75%	87%	85%
Warfarin Therapy Discharge Instructions[2]	27	19%	59%	75%
Chest Pain/Possible Heart Attack Care				
Aspirin Given Within 24 Hours of Arrival[1,3]	-	-	97%	96%
Fibrinolytic Meds Within 30 Min. of Arrival[5]	-	-	54%	58%
Average Time to ECG (minutes)[1,3]	-	-	9	7
Average Time to Transfer (minutes)[5]	-	-	78	60
Children's Asthma Care				
Received Home Management Plan of Care	-	-	-	88%
Received Reliever Medication	-	-	-	100%
Received Systemic Corticosteroids	-	-	-	100%
Emergency Department				
Admittance Decision Time (minutes)[2]	633	193	154	98
Head CT Results Within 45 Min. of Arrival[1]	-	-	55%	57%
Patients Who Left ER Before Being Seen	48,222	2%	2%	2%
Time from ER Arrival to Admit. (minutes)[2]	700	410	378	274
Time from ER Arrival to Discharge (minutes)	387	141	156	134
Time in ER Before Being Evaluated (minutes)	426	35	35	26
Time to Pain Meds for Fractures (minutes)	106	68	61	57
Heart Attack Care				
Aspirin Given at Discharge	153	97%	99%	99%
Fibrinolytic Meds Within 30 Min. of Arrival[7]	-	-	46%	54%
PCI Within 90 Minutes of Arrival	31	94%	95%	96%
Statin Prescribed at Discharge	154	100%	98%	98%
Heart Failure Care				
ACE Inhibitor or ARB for LVSD	42	100%	96%	97%
Discharge Instructions Given	147	95%	95%	94%
Evaluation of LVS Function	183	100%	99%	99%
Medicare Spending				
Medicare Spending per Patient (ratio)	-	0.93	0.96	0.98
Pneumonia Care				
Appropriate Initial Antibiotic Given[2]	93	100%	95%	95%
Blood Culture Timing[2]	153	95%	97%	98%
Pregnancy and Delivery Care				
Newborn Deliveries Scheduled Early[7]	-	-	4%	6%
Preventive Care				
Immunization for Influenza[2]	574	66%	88%	90%
Immunization for Pneumonia[2]	779	77%	88%	92%
Stroke Care				
Anticoagulation Therapy for Atrial Fibrillation	15	100%	96%	95%
Antithrombotic Therapy Timing	62	100%	98%	98%
Assessed for Rehabilitation	68	94%	97%	97%
Discharged on Antithrombotic Therapy	65	100%	99%	99%
Discharged on Statin Medication	50	92%	95%	94%
Thrombolytic Therapy Timing[1]	-	-	69%	66%
Venous Thromboembolism Prophylaxis	71	80%	94%	94%
Written Stroke Educational Materials Given	37	73%	86%	88%
Surgical Care Improvement Project				
Appropriate Beta Blocker Usage[2]	139	91%	97%	98%
Appropriate VTP Within 24 Hours[2]	359	95%	98%	98%
Controlled Postoperative Blood Glucose[2,7]	-	-	97%	97%
Perioperative Temperature Management[2]	434	100%	100%	100%
Prophylactic Antibiotic Selection[2]	294	99%	99%	99%
Prophylactic Antibiotic Selection (Outpatient)	203	98%	97%	98%
Prophylactic Antibiotic Stopped[2]	291	97%	98%	98%
Prophylactic Antibiotic Timing[2]	294	95%	99%	99%
Prophylactic Antibiotic Timing (Outpatient)	210	93%	97%	98%

NOTE: Hospital profiles are in alphabetical order by state, then city, then hospital within the city; Rankings exclude hospitals with less than 25 cases except for patient surveys which excludes hospitals with less than 100 cases; (a) 100-299 cases; (1) The number of cases/patients is too few to report; (2) Data submitted were based on a sample of cases/patients; (3) Results are based on a shorter time period than required; (4) Data suppressed by CMS for one or more quarters; (5) Results are not available for this reporting period; (6) Fewer than 100 patients completed the HCAHPS survey; (7) No cases met the criteria for this measure; (8) The lower limit of the confidence interval cannot be calculated if the number of observed infections equals zero; (9) No data are available from the state/territory for this reporting period; (10) The scores shown reflect fewer than 50 completed surveys; (11) There were discrepancies in the data collection process; (12) This measure does not apply to this hospital for this reporting period; (13) Results cannot be calculated for this reporting period; (14) The results for this state are combined with nearby states to protect confidentiality; Please refer to the User's Guide for a full explanation of data.

Urinary Catheter Removal[2]	300	96%	96%	97%
Survey of Patients' Hospital Experiences				
Area Around Room 'Always' Quiet at Night	300+	37%	51%	61%
Doctors 'Always' Communicated Well	300+	69%	77%	82%
Home Recovery Information Given	300+	83%	83%	85%
Hospital Given 9 or 10 on 10 Point Scale	300+	53%	63%	71%
Meds 'Always' Explained Before Given	300+	53%	59%	64%
Nurses 'Always' Communicated Well	300+	70%	75%	79%
Pain 'Always' Well Controlled	300+	62%	67%	71%
Room and Bathroom 'Always' Clean	300+	63%	69%	73%
Timely Help 'Always' Received	300+	51%	61%	68%
Would Definitely Recommend Hospital	300+	56%	65%	71%
Use of Medical Imaging				
Cardiac Imaging Stress Test before Surgery	164	6.7%	5.8%	5.3%
Combination Abdominal CT Scan	524	4.6%	8.2%	10.5%
Combination Brain/Sinus CT Scan[1]	-	-	3.6%	2.7%
Combination Chest CT Scan	276	0.0%	1.3%	2.7%
Follow-up Mammogram/Ultrasound	499	12.6%	13%	8.8%
Lumbar Spine MRI for Low Back Pain[1]	-	-	33.4%	37.2%

Faxton - Saint Luke's Healthcare

1656 Champlin Avenue
Utica, NY 13503
Phone: 315-798-6000
Type: Acute Care Hospitals
Emergency Services: Yes
Ownership: Voluntary non-profit - Private

Measure	Cases	This Hosp.	State Avg.	U.S. Avg.
Blood Clot Prevention and Treatment				
Anticoagulation Overlap Therapy[2]	44	95%	91%	93%
ICU Venous Thromboembolism Prophylaxis[2]	70	99%	92%	92%
Incidence of Potentially Preventable VTE[1,2]	-	-	10%	10%
UFH with Dosages/Platelet Monitoring[2]	62	100%	92%	97%
Venous Thromboembolism Prophylaxis[2]	403	97%	87%	85%
Warfarin Therapy Discharge Instructions[2]	31	58%	59%	75%
Chest Pain/Possible Heart Attack Care				
Aspirin Given Within 24 Hours of Arrival[1,3]	-	-	97%	96%
Fibrinolytic Meds Within 30 Min. of Arrival[3,7]	-	-	54%	58%
Average Time to ECG (minutes)[1,3]	-	-	9	7
Average Time to Transfer (minutes)[3,7]	-	-	78	60
Children's Asthma Care				
Received Home Management Plan of Care	-	-	-	88%
Received Reliever Medication	-	-	-	100%
Received Systemic Corticosteroids	-	-	-	100%
Emergency Department				
Admittance Decision Time (minutes)[2]	653	100	154	98
Head CT Results Within 45 Min. of Arrival[1]	-	-	55%	57%
Patients Who Left ER Before Being Seen	36,084	2%	2%	2%
Time from ER Arrival to Admit. (minutes)[2]	668	364	378	274
Time from ER Arrival to Discharge (minutes)	366	246	156	134
Time in ER Before Being Evaluated (minutes)	404	56	35	26
Time to Pain Meds for Fractures (minutes)	105	106	61	57
Heart Attack Care				
Aspirin Given at Discharge	152	100%	99%	99%
Fibrinolytic Meds Within 30 Min. of Arrival[7]	-	-	46%	54%
PCI Within 90 Minutes of Arrival	20	85%	95%	96%
Statin Prescribed at Discharge	149	94%	98%	98%
Heart Failure Care				
ACE Inhibitor or ARB for LVSD	117	97%	96%	97%
Discharge Instructions Given	241	95%	95%	94%
Evaluation of LVS Function	344	99%	99%	99%
Medicare Spending				
Medicare Spending per Patient (ratio)	-	0.98	0.96	0.98
Pneumonia Care				
Appropriate Initial Antibiotic Given	155	99%	95%	95%
Blood Culture Timing	343	98%	97%	98%
Pregnancy and Delivery Care				
Newborn Deliveries Scheduled Early[2]	26	8%	4%	6%
Preventive Care				
Immunization for Influenza[2]	537	94%	88%	90%
Immunization for Pneumonia[2]	693	90%	88%	92%
Stroke Care				
Anticoagulation Therapy for Atrial Fibrillation	38	97%	96%	95%
Antithrombotic Therapy Timing	166	100%	98%	98%
Assessed for Rehabilitation	237	100%	97%	97%
Discharged on Antithrombotic Therapy	196	99%	99%	99%
Discharged on Statin Medication	151	96%	95%	94%
Thrombolytic Therapy Timing	48	65%	69%	66%
Venous Thromboembolism Prophylaxis	245	97%	94%	94%
Written Stroke Educational Materials Given	100	86%	86%	88%
Surgical Care Improvement Project				
Appropriate Beta Blocker Usage[2]	120	97%	97%	98%
Appropriate VTP Within 24 Hours[2]	352	94%	98%	98%
Controlled Postoperative Blood Glucose[2,7]	-	-	97%	97%
Perioperative Temperature Management[2]	440	100%	100%	100%
Prophylactic Antibiotic Selection[2]	274	94%	99%	99%
Prophylactic Antibiotic Selection (Outpatient)	215	80%	97%	98%
Prophylactic Antibiotic Stopped[2]	271	99%	98%	98%
Prophylactic Antibiotic Timing[2]	274	96%	99%	99%
Prophylactic Antibiotic Timing (Outpatient)	222	92%	97%	98%
Urinary Catheter Removal[2]	147	92%	96%	97%
Survey of Patients' Hospital Experiences				
Area Around Room 'Always' Quiet at Night	300+	49%	51%	61%
Doctors 'Always' Communicated Well	300+	78%	77%	82%
Home Recovery Information Given	300+	82%	83%	85%
Hospital Given 9 or 10 on 10 Point Scale	300+	62%	63%	71%
Meds 'Always' Explained Before Given	300+	59%	59%	64%
Nurses 'Always' Communicated Well	300+	76%	75%	79%
Pain 'Always' Well Controlled	300+	68%	67%	71%
Room and Bathroom 'Always' Clean	300+	64%	69%	73%
Timely Help 'Always' Received	300+	59%	61%	68%
Would Definitely Recommend Hospital	300+	67%	65%	71%
Use of Medical Imaging				
Cardiac Imaging Stress Test before Surgery	126	1.6%	5.8%	5.3%
Combination Abdominal CT Scan	336	16.7%	8.2%	10.5%
Combination Brain/Sinus CT Scan[1]	-	-	3.6%	2.7%
Combination Chest CT Scan	433	9.0%	1.3%	2.7%
Follow-up Mammogram/Ultrasound	1,644	15.1%	13%	8.8%
Lumbar Spine MRI for Low Back Pain[7]	-	-	33.4%	37.2%

Saint Elizabeth Medical Center

2209 Genesee Street
Utica, NY 13501
Phone: 315-798-8100
Fax: 315-734-3008
E-mail: marketing@stemc.org
URL: www.stemc.org
Type: Acute Care Hospitals
Emergency Services: Yes
Ownership: Voluntary non-profit - Private
Beds: 201

Key Personnel:

Chief of Medical Staff.......... Albert D'Accurzio, MD
Emergency Room .... Anna Giannico
Quality Assurance .... Christine Holehan, RN
Pediatric Ambulatory Care ...... Waleed Kaashmire
President/CEO.............. Scott H. Perra, FACHE
Operating Room.............. Robert Scholefield, RN,MS

Measure	Cases	This Hosp.	State Avg.	U.S. Avg.
Blood Clot Prevention and Treatment				
Anticoagulation Overlap Therapy[2]	56	89%	91%	93%
ICU Venous Thromboembolism Prophylaxis[2]	104	99%	92%	92%
Incidence of Potentially Preventable VTE[2]	12	0%	10%	10%
UFH with Dosages/Platelet Monitoring[2]	59	98%	92%	97%
Venous Thromboembolism Prophylaxis[2]	329	88%	87%	85%
Warfarin Therapy Discharge Instructions[2]	37	86%	59%	75%
Chest Pain/Possible Heart Attack Care				
Aspirin Given Within 24 Hours of Arrival[5]	-	-	97%	96%
Fibrinolytic Meds Within 30 Min. of Arrival[5]	-	-	54%	58%
Average Time to ECG (minutes)[5]	-	-	9	7
Average Time to Transfer (minutes)[5]	-	-	78	60
Children's Asthma Care				
Received Home Management Plan of Care	-	-	-	88%
Received Reliever Medication	-	-	-	100%
Received Systemic Corticosteroids	-	-	-	100%
Emergency Department				
Admittance Decision Time (minutes)[2]	790	220	154	98
Head CT Results Within 45 Min. of Arrival[5]	-	-	55%	57%
Patients Who Left ER Before Being Seen	41,082	2%	2%	2%
Time from ER Arrival to Admit. (minutes)[2]	823	433	378	274
Time from ER Arrival to Discharge (minutes)	369	172	156	134
Time in ER Before Being Evaluated (minutes)	406	38	35	26
Time to Pain Meds for Fractures (minutes)	118	65	61	57
Heart Attack Care				
Aspirin Given at Discharge	295	99%	99%	99%
Fibrinolytic Meds Within 30 Min. of Arrival[1]	-	-	46%	54%
PCI Within 90 Minutes of Arrival	63	92%	95%	96%
Statin Prescribed at Discharge	291	97%	98%	98%
Heart Failure Care				
ACE Inhibitor or ARB for LVSD	146	93%	96%	97%
Discharge Instructions Given	307	85%	95%	94%
Evaluation of LVS Function	419	98%	99%	99%
Medicare Spending				
Medicare Spending per Patient (ratio)	-	0.98	0.96	0.98
Pneumonia Care				
Appropriate Initial Antibiotic Given	132	90%	95%	95%
Blood Culture Timing	221	97%	97%	98%
Pregnancy and Delivery Care				
Newborn Deliveries Scheduled Early[7]	-	-	4%	6%
Preventive Care				
Immunization for Influenza[2]	596	84%	88%	90%
Immunization for Pneumonia[2]	889	83%	88%	92%
Stroke Care				
Anticoagulation Therapy for Atrial Fibrillation[1]	-	-	96%	95%
Antithrombotic Therapy Timing	46	98%	98%	98%
Assessed for Rehabilitation	57	91%	97%	97%
Discharged on Antithrombotic Therapy	49	96%	99%	99%
Discharged on Statin Medication	43	77%	95%	94%
Thrombolytic Therapy Timing[1]	-	-	69%	66%
Venous Thromboembolism Prophylaxis	58	88%	94%	94%
Written Stroke Educational Materials Given	32	50%	86%	88%
Surgical Care Improvement Project				
Appropriate Beta Blocker Usage[2]	506	98%	97%	98%
Appropriate VTP Within 24 Hours[2]	709	97%	98%	98%
Controlled Postoperative Blood Glucose[2]	283	99%	97%	97%
Perioperative Temperature Management[2]	865	100%	100%	100%
Prophylactic Antibiotic Selection[2]	934	99%	99%	99%
Prophylactic Antibiotic Selection (Outpatient)	352	99%	97%	98%
Prophylactic Antibiotic Stopped[2]	923	98%	98%	98%
Prophylactic Antibiotic Timing[2]	936	99%	99%	99%
Prophylactic Antibiotic Timing (Outpatient)	352	96%	97%	98%
Urinary Catheter Removal[2]	383	89%	96%	97%
Survey of Patients' Hospital Experiences				
Area Around Room 'Always' Quiet at Night	300+	49%	51%	61%
Doctors 'Always' Communicated Well	300+	77%	77%	82%
Home Recovery Information Given	300+	82%	83%	85%
Hospital Given 9 or 10 on 10 Point Scale	300+	70%	63%	71%
Meds 'Always' Explained Before Given	300+	60%	59%	64%
Nurses 'Always' Communicated Well	300+	81%	75%	79%
Pain 'Always' Well Controlled	300+	72%	67%	71%
Room and Bathroom 'Always' Clean	300+	71%	69%	73%
Timely Help 'Always' Received	300+	66%	61%	68%
Would Definitely Recommend Hospital	300+	72%	65%	71%
Use of Medical Imaging				
Cardiac Imaging Stress Test before Surgery	175	8.0%	5.8%	5.3%
Combination Abdominal CT Scan	528	9.1%	8.2%	10.5%
Combination Brain/Sinus CT Scan	583	2.4%	3.6%	2.7%
Combination Chest CT Scan	301	2.3%	1.3%	2.7%
Follow-up Mammogram/Ultrasound	736	6.3%	13%	8.8%
Lumbar Spine MRI for Low Back Pain[7]	-	-	33.4%	37.2%

Westchester Medical Center

100 Woods Rd
Valhalla, NY 10595
Phone: 914-285-7017
URL: www.wcmc.com
Type: Acute Care Hospitals
Emergency Services: Yes
Ownership: Govt - Hospital Dist/Auth
Beds: 635

Key Personnel:

Chief of Medical Staff.......... Renee Garrick, MD
Pediatric Ambulatory Care ...... Michael Gerwitz, MD
CEO/President.............. Michael D Israel
Quality Assurance .... Michael Lauria
Radiology................. Chitti R Moorthy, MD
Operating Room.............. John Savino, MD
Infection Control............. Gary Wormser, MD

Measure	Cases	This Hosp.	State Avg.	U.S. Avg.

NOTE: Hospital profiles are in alphabetical order by state, then city, then hospital within the city; Rankings exclude hospitals with less than 25 cases except for patient surveys which excludes hospitals with less than 100 cases; (a) 100-299 cases; (1) The number of cases/patients is too few to report; (2) Data submitted were based on a sample of cases/patients; (3) Results are based on a shorter time period than required; (4) Data suppressed by CMS for one or more quarters; (5) Results are not available for this reporting period; (6) Fewer than 100 patients completed the HCAHPS survey; (7) No cases met the criteria for this measure; (8) The lower limit of the confidence interval cannot be calculated if the number of observed infections equals zero; (9) No data are available from the state/territory for this reporting period; (10) The scores shown reflect fewer than 50 completed surveys; (11) There were discrepancies in the data collection process; (12) This measure does not apply to this hospital for this reporting period; (13) Results cannot be calculated for this reporting period; (14) The results for this state are combined with nearby states to protect confidentiality; Please refer to the User's Guide for a full explanation of data.

Blood Clot Prevention and Treatment				
Anticoagulation Overlap Therapy[2]	94	99%	91%	93%
ICU Venous Thromboembolism Prophylaxis[2]	138	96%	92%	92%
Incidence of Potentially Preventable VTE[2]	67	6%	10%	10%
UFH with Dosages/Platelet Monitoring[2]	85	96%	92%	97%
Venous Thromboembolism Prophylaxis[2]	317	85%	87%	85%
Warfarin Therapy Discharge Instructions[2]	58	71%	59%	75%
Chest Pain/Possible Heart Attack Care				
Aspirin Given Within 24 Hours of Arrival[1,3]	-	-	97%	96%
Fibrinolytic Meds Within 30 Min. of Arrival[5]	-	-	54%	58%
Average Time to ECG (minutes)[1,3]	-	-	9	7
Average Time to Transfer (minutes)[5]	-	-	78	60
Children's Asthma Care				
Received Home Management Plan of Care	-	-	-	88%
Received Reliever Medication	-	-	-	100%
Received Systemic Corticosteroids	-	-	-	100%
Emergency Department				
Admittance Decision Time (minutes)[2]	417	227	154	98
Head CT Results Within 45 Min. of Arrival[1,3]	-	-	55%	57%
Patients Who Left ER Before Being Seen	37,728	1%	2%	2%
Time from ER Arrival to Admit. (minutes)[2]	494	388	378	274
Time from ER Arrival to Discharge (minutes)	296	194	156	134
Time in ER Before Being Evaluated (minutes)	407	36	35	26
Time to Pain Meds for Fractures (minutes)	211	89	61	57
Heart Attack Care				
Aspirin Given at Discharge[2]	346	100%	99%	99%
Fibrinolytic Meds Within 30 Min. of Arrival[2,7]	-	-	46%	54%
PCI Within 90 Minutes of Arrival[2]	34	100%	95%	96%
Statin Prescribed at Discharge[2]	346	100%	98%	98%
Heart Failure Care				
ACE Inhibitor or ARB for LVSD	73	99%	96%	97%
Discharge Instructions Given	183	97%	95%	94%
Evaluation of LVS Function	219	100%	99%	99%
Medicare Spending				
Medicare Spending per Patient (ratio)	-	1.06	0.96	0.98
Pneumonia Care				
Appropriate Initial Antibiotic Given	26	88%	95%	95%
Blood Culture Timing	65	91%	97%	98%
Pregnancy and Delivery Care				
Newborn Deliveries Scheduled Early[2]	17	0%	4%	6%
Preventive Care				
Immunization for Influenza[2]	541	93%	88%	90%
Immunization for Pneumonia[2]	438	84%	88%	92%
Stroke Care				
Anticoagulation Therapy for Atrial Fibrillation[2]	13	100%	96%	95%
Antithrombotic Therapy Timing[2]	51	98%	98%	98%
Assessed for Rehabilitation[2]	128	98%	97%	97%
Discharged on Antithrombotic Therapy[2]	61	100%	99%	99%
Discharged on Statin Medication[2]	51	92%	95%	94%
Thrombolytic Therapy Timing[1,2]	-	-	69%	66%
Venous Thromboembolism Prophylaxis[2]	146	99%	94%	94%
Written Stroke Educational Materials Given[2]	59	80%	86%	88%
Surgical Care Improvement Project				
Appropriate Beta Blocker Usage[2]	322	99%	97%	98%
Appropriate VTP Within 24 Hours[2]	359	100%	98%	98%
Controlled Postoperative Blood Glucose[2]	237	92%	97%	97%
Perioperative Temperature Management[2]	478	99%	100%	100%
Prophylactic Antibiotic Selection[2]	453	99%	99%	99%
Prophylactic Antibiotic Selection (Outpatient)	283	98%	97%	98%
Prophylactic Antibiotic Stopped[2]	419	96%	98%	98%
Prophylactic Antibiotic Timing[2]	453	99%	99%	99%
Prophylactic Antibiotic Timing (Outpatient)	280	97%	97%	98%
Urinary Catheter Removal[2]	374	95%	96%	97%
Survey of Patients' Hospital Experiences				
Area Around Room 'Always' Quiet at Night	300+	37%	51%	61%
Doctors 'Always' Communicated Well	300+	70%	77%	82%
Home Recovery Information Given	300+	80%	83%	85%
Hospital Given 9 or 10 on 10 Point Scale	300+	50%	63%	71%
Meds 'Always' Explained Before Given	300+	49%	59%	64%
Nurses 'Always' Communicated Well	300+	62%	75%	79%
Pain 'Always' Well Controlled	300+	56%	67%	71%
Room and Bathroom 'Always' Clean	300+	50%	69%	73%
Timely Help 'Always' Received	300+	49%	61%	68%
Would Definitely Recommend Hospital	300+	54%	65%	71%
Use of Medical Imaging				
Cardiac Imaging Stress Test before Surgery	292	10.6%	5.8%	5.3%
Combination Abdominal CT Scan	542	27.5%	8.2%	10.5%
Combination Brain/Sinus CT Scan	258	0.4%	3.6%	2.7%
Combination Chest CT Scan	462	0.9%	1.3%	2.7%
Follow-up Mammogram/Ultrasound	445	22.5%	13%	8.8%
Lumbar Spine MRI for Low Back Pain[1]	-	-	33.4%	37.2%

Franklin Hospital

900 Franklin Avenue
Valley Stream, NY 11580
Phone: 516-256-6000
Fax: 516-256-6053
URL: www.northshorelij.com
Type: Acute Care Hospitals
Emergency Services: Yes
Ownership: Voluntary non-profit - Private
Beds: 305

Key Personnel:

Quality Assurance . . . . Roberta Dixon, RN
CEO/President. . . . . Michael J Dowling
Pediatric Ambulatory Care . . . . . . James Fagin, MD
Infection Control. . . . . Bruce Farber, MD
Radiology. . . . . Mitchell Goldman, MD
Coronary Care . . . . Kathy Mann, RN
Operating Room. . . . . Linda Olander, RN
Chief of Medical Staff . . . . Leonard Timpone, MD

Measure	Cases	This Hosp.	State Avg.	U.S. Avg.
Blood Clot Prevention and Treatment				
Anticoagulation Overlap Therapy[2]	63	63%	91%	93%
ICU Venous Thromboembolism Prophylaxis[2]	46	93%	92%	92%
Incidence of Potentially Preventable VTE[1,2]	-	-	10%	10%
UFH with Dosages/Platelet Monitoring[2]	39	100%	92%	97%
Venous Thromboembolism Prophylaxis[2]	331	81%	87%	85%
Warfarin Therapy Discharge Instructions[2]	38	34%	59%	75%
Chest Pain/Possible Heart Attack Care				
Aspirin Given Within 24 Hours of Arrival	88	92%	97%	96%
Fibrinolytic Meds Within 30 Min. of Arrival[7]	-	-	54%	58%
Average Time to ECG (minutes)	96	20	9	7
Average Time to Transfer (minutes)	34	90	78	60
Children's Asthma Care				
Received Home Management Plan of Care	-	-	-	88%
Received Reliever Medication	-	-	-	100%
Received Systemic Corticosteroids	-	-	-	100%
Emergency Department				
Admittance Decision Time (minutes)[2]	452	275	154	98
Head CT Results Within 45 Min. of Arrival	16	56%	55%	57%
Patients Who Left ER Before Being Seen	44,191	1%	2%	2%
Time from ER Arrival to Admit. (minutes)[2]	482	548	378	274
Time from ER Arrival to Discharge (minutes)	364	154	156	134
Time in ER Before Being Evaluated (minutes)	371	37	35	26
Time to Pain Meds for Fractures (minutes)	67	60	61	57
Heart Attack Care				
Aspirin Given at Discharge[2]	32	97%	99%	99%
Fibrinolytic Meds Within 30 Min. of Arrival[2,7]	-	-	46%	54%
PCI Within 90 Minutes of Arrival[2,7]	-	-	95%	96%
Statin Prescribed at Discharge[2]	35	80%	98%	98%
Heart Failure Care				
ACE Inhibitor or ARB for LVSD[2]	59	92%	96%	97%
Discharge Instructions Given[2]	173	98%	95%	94%
Evaluation of LVS Function[2]	216	100%	99%	99%
Medicare Spending				
Medicare Spending per Patient (ratio)	-	1.08	0.96	0.98
Pneumonia Care				
Appropriate Initial Antibiotic Given[2]	80	92%	95%	95%
Blood Culture Timing[2]	142	96%	97%	98%
Pregnancy and Delivery Care				
Newborn Deliveries Scheduled Early[7]	-	-	4%	6%
Preventive Care				
Immunization for Influenza[2]	595	88%	88%	90%
Immunization for Pneumonia[2]	834	90%	88%	92%
Stroke Care				
Anticoagulation Therapy for Atrial Fibrillation[2]	11	91%	96%	95%
Antithrombotic Therapy Timing[2]	110	99%	98%	98%
Assessed for Rehabilitation[2]	120	98%	97%	97%
Discharged on Antithrombotic Therapy[2]	106	92%	99%	99%
Discharged on Statin Medication[2]	85	93%	95%	94%
Thrombolytic Therapy Timing[1,2]	-	-	69%	66%
Venous Thromboembolism Prophylaxis[2]	130	88%	94%	94%
Written Stroke Educational Materials Given[2]	46	74%	86%	88%
Surgical Care Improvement Project				
Appropriate Beta Blocker Usage[2]	80	82%	97%	98%
Appropriate VTP Within 24 Hours[2]	260	99%	98%	98%
Controlled Postoperative Blood Glucose[2,7]	-	-	97%	97%
Perioperative Temperature Management[2]	280	100%	100%	100%
Prophylactic Antibiotic Selection[2]	186	99%	99%	99%
Prophylactic Antibiotic Selection (Outpatient)	12	100%	97%	98%
Prophylactic Antibiotic Stopped[2]	176	98%	98%	98%
Prophylactic Antibiotic Timing[2]	186	99%	99%	99%
Prophylactic Antibiotic Timing (Outpatient)	12	100%	97%	98%
Urinary Catheter Removal[2]	114	94%	96%	97%
Survey of Patients' Hospital Experiences				
Area Around Room 'Always' Quiet at Night	300+	53%	51%	61%
Doctors 'Always' Communicated Well	300+	75%	77%	82%
Home Recovery Information Given	300+	75%	83%	85%
Hospital Given 9 or 10 on 10 Point Scale	300+	63%	63%	71%
Meds 'Always' Explained Before Given	300+	56%	59%	64%
Nurses 'Always' Communicated Well	300+	74%	75%	79%
Pain 'Always' Well Controlled	300+	66%	67%	71%
Room and Bathroom 'Always' Clean	300+	71%	69%	73%
Timely Help 'Always' Received	300+	63%	61%	68%
Would Definitely Recommend Hospital	300+	66%	65%	71%
Use of Medical Imaging				
Cardiac Imaging Stress Test before Surgery[1]	-	-	5.8%	5.3%
Combination Abdominal CT Scan	289	0.3%	8.2%	10.5%
Combination Brain/Sinus CT Scan[1]	-	-	3.6%	2.7%
Combination Chest CT Scan	87	2.3%	1.3%	2.7%
Follow-up Mammogram/Ultrasound[7]	-	-	13%	8.8%
Lumbar Spine MRI for Low Back Pain[1]	-	-	33.4%	37.2%

Delaware Valley Hospital

1 Titus Place
Walton, NY 13856
Phone: 607-865-2100
Fax: 607-865-8482
URL: www.uhs.net
Type: Critical Access Hospitals
Emergency Services: Yes
Ownership: Voluntary non-profit - Private
Beds: 25

Key Personnel:

Anesthesiology. . . . . Michael Branigan, CRIIA
Pediatrics. . . . . Susan Converse, FNP
Chief of Medical Staff . . . . Rajesh Dave, MD
Emergency Room . . . . Mary Doig, RN
Quality Assurance . . . . Deborah Hitt
Infection Control. . . . . Christina Jones, RN
Operating Room. . . . . Cathy Phraner, RN
CEO/President. . . . . Paul Summers

Measure	Cases	This Hosp.	State Avg.	U.S. Avg.
Blood Clot Prevention and Treatment				
Anticoagulation Overlap Therapy[5]	-	-	91%	93%
ICU Venous Thromboembolism Prophylaxis[5]	-	-	92%	92%
Incidence of Potentially Preventable VTE[5]	-	-	10%	10%
UFH with Dosages/Platelet Monitoring[5]	-	-	92%	97%
Venous Thromboembolism Prophylaxis[5]	-	-	87%	85%
Warfarin Therapy Discharge Instructions[5]	-	-	59%	75%
Chest Pain/Possible Heart Attack Care				
Aspirin Given Within 24 Hours of Arrival	40	100%	97%	96%
Fibrinolytic Meds Within 30 Min. of Arrival[1]	-	-	54%	58%
Average Time to ECG (minutes)	40	10	9	7
Average Time to Transfer (minutes)[1]	-	-	78	60
Children's Asthma Care				
Received Home Management Plan of Care	-	-	-	88%
Received Reliever Medication	-	-	-	100%
Received Systemic Corticosteroids	-	-	-	100%
Emergency Department				
Admittance Decision Time (minutes)[2]	304	61	154	98
Head CT Results Within 45 Min. of Arrival[5]	-	-	55%	57%
Patients Who Left ER Before Being Seen	5,141	0%	2%	2%
Time from ER Arrival to Admit. (minutes)[2]	304	239	378	274
Time from ER Arrival to Discharge (minutes)[5]	-	-	156	134
Time in ER Before Being Evaluated (minutes)[5]	-	-	35	26
Time to Pain Meds for Fractures (minutes)[5]	-	-	61	57

NOTE: Hospital profiles are in alphabetical order by state, then city, then hospital within the city; Rankings exclude hospitals with less than 25 cases except for patient surveys which excludes hospitals with less than 100 cases; (a) 100-299 cases; (1) The number of cases/patients is too few to report; (2) Data submitted were based on a sample of cases/patients; (3) Results are based on a shorter time period than required; (4) Data suppressed by CMS for one or more quarters; (5) Results are not available for this reporting period; (6) Fewer than 100 patients completed the HCAHPS survey; (7) No cases met the criteria for this measure; (8) The lower limit of the confidence interval cannot be calculated if the number of observed infections equals zero; (9) No data are available from the state/territory for this reporting period; (10) The scores shown reflect fewer than 50 completed surveys; (11) There were discrepancies in the data collection process; (12) This measure does not apply to this hospital for this reporting period; (13) Results cannot be calculated for this reporting period; (14) The results for this state are combined with nearby states to protect confidentiality; Please refer to the User's Guide for a full explanation of data.

Measure	Cases	This Hosp.	State Avg.	U.S. Avg.
Heart Attack Care				
Aspirin Given at Discharge[5]	-	-	99%	99%
Fibrinolytic Meds Within 30 Min. of Arrival[5]	-	-	46%	54%
PCI Within 90 Minutes of Arrival[5]	-	-	95%	96%
Statin Prescribed at Discharge[5]	-	-	98%	98%
Heart Failure Care				
ACE Inhibitor or ARB for LVSD[1]	-	-	96%	97%
Discharge Instructions Given	25	96%	95%	94%
Evaluation of LVS Function	36	97%	99%	99%
Medicare Spending				
Medicare Spending per Patient (ratio)	-	-	0.96	0.98
Pneumonia Care				
Appropriate Initial Antibiotic Given	31	97%	95%	95%
Blood Culture Timing	37	100%	97%	98%
Pregnancy and Delivery Care				
Newborn Deliveries Scheduled Early[5]	-	-	4%	6%
Preventive Care				
Immunization for Influenza[2]	184	93%	88%	90%
Immunization for Pneumonia[2]	293	95%	88%	92%
Stroke Care				
Anticoagulation Therapy for Atrial Fibrillation[5]	-	-	96%	95%
Antithrombotic Therapy Timing[5]	-	-	98%	98%
Assessed for Rehabilitation[5]	-	-	97%	97%
Discharged on Antithrombotic Therapy[5]	-	-	99%	99%
Discharged on Statin Medication[5]	-	-	95%	94%
Thrombolytic Therapy Timing[5]	-	-	69%	66%
Venous Thromboembolism Prophylaxis[5]	-	-	94%	94%
Written Stroke Educational Materials Given[5]	-	-	86%	88%
Surgical Care Improvement Project				
Appropriate Beta Blocker Usage[5]	-	-	97%	98%
Appropriate VTP Within 24 Hours[5]	-	-	98%	98%
Controlled Postoperative Blood Glucose[5]	-	-	97%	97%
Perioperative Temperature Management[5]	-	-	100%	100%
Prophylactic Antibiotic Selection[5]	-	-	99%	99%
Prophylactic Antibiotic Selection (Outpatient)[5]	-	-	97%	98%
Prophylactic Antibiotic Stopped[5]	-	-	98%	98%
Prophylactic Antibiotic Timing[5]	-	-	99%	99%
Prophylactic Antibiotic Timing (Outpatient)[5]	-	-	97%	98%
Urinary Catheter Removal[5]	-	-	96%	97%
Survey of Patients' Hospital Experiences				
Area Around Room 'Always' Quiet at Night[6]	<100	67%	51%	61%
Doctors 'Always' Communicated Well[6]	<100	84%	77%	82%
Home Recovery Information Given[6]	<100	84%	83%	85%
Hospital Given 9 or 10 on 10 Point Scale[6]	<100	72%	63%	71%
Meds 'Always' Explained Before Given[6]	<100	71%	59%	64%
Nurses 'Always' Communicated Well[6]	<100	83%	75%	79%
Pain 'Always' Well Controlled[6]	<100	78%	67%	71%
Room and Bathroom 'Always' Clean[6]	<100	91%	69%	73%
Timely Help 'Always' Received[6]	<100	75%	61%	68%
Would Definitely Recommend Hospital[6]	<100	77%	65%	71%
Use of Medical Imaging				
Cardiac Imaging Stress Test before Surgery[7]	-	-	5.8%	5.3%
Combination Abdominal CT Scan	123	0.8%	8.2%	10.5%
Combination Brain/Sinus CT Scan[1]	-	-	3.6%	2.7%
Combination Chest CT Scan	53	0.0%	1.3%	2.7%
Follow-up Mammogram/Ultrasound	143	14.7%	13%	8.8%
Lumbar Spine MRI for Low Back Pain[1]	-	-	33.4%	37.2%

Wyoming County Community Hospital

400 North Main Street
Warsaw, NY 14569
Phone: 585-786-2233
Fax: 585-786-1222
URL: www.wccns.net
Type: Acute Care Hospitals
Emergency Services: Yes
Ownership: Government - Local
Beds: 264

Key Personnel:

Infection Control. . . . . Connie Almeter
Quality Assurance . . . . Peggy Cunningham
CEO/President. . . . . Donald T. Eichenauer
Operating Room. . . . . Cynthia Elbow
Cardiac Laboratory. . . . . Lori Merrill
Emergency Room . . . . Brian Meyers
Radiology. . . . . Margaret Morgan Hise
Chief of Medical Staff. . . . . Dr. Scott Treutlein

Measure	Cases	This Hosp.	State Avg.	U.S. Avg.
Blood Clot Prevention and Treatment				
Anticoagulation Overlap Therapy[2]	17	100%	91%	93%
ICU Venous Thromboembolism Prophylaxis[2]	54	94%	92%	92%
Incidence of Potentially Preventable VTE[1,2]	-	-	10%	10%
UFH with Dosages/Platelet Monitoring[2]	13	100%	92%	97%
Venous Thromboembolism Prophylaxis[2]	185	91%	87%	85%
Warfarin Therapy Discharge Instructions[1,2]	-	-	59%	75%
Chest Pain/Possible Heart Attack Care				
Aspirin Given Within 24 Hours of Arrival	108	97%	97%	96%
Fibrinolytic Meds Within 30 Min. of Arrival[1]	-	-	54%	58%
Average Time to ECG (minutes)	113	4	9	7
Average Time to Transfer (minutes)[7]	-	-	78	60
Children's Asthma Care				
Received Home Management Plan of Care	-	-	-	88%
Received Reliever Medication	-	-	-	100%
Received Systemic Corticosteroids	-	-	-	100%
Emergency Department				
Admittance Decision Time (minutes)[2]	363	95	154	98
Head CT Results Within 45 Min. of Arrival[1]	-	-	55%	57%
Patients Who Left ER Before Being Seen	11,496	1%	2%	2%
Time from ER Arrival to Admit. (minutes)[2]	367	238	378	274
Time from ER Arrival to Discharge (minutes)	475	109	156	134
Time in ER Before Being Evaluated (minutes)	519	21	35	26
Time to Pain Meds for Fractures (minutes)	60	38	61	57
Heart Attack Care				
Aspirin Given at Discharge[1]	-	-	99%	99%
Fibrinolytic Meds Within 30 Min. of Arrival[7]	-	-	46%	54%
PCI Within 90 Minutes of Arrival[7]	-	-	95%	96%
Statin Prescribed at Discharge[1]	-	-	98%	98%
Heart Failure Care				
ACE Inhibitor or ARB for LVSD	15	93%	96%	97%
Discharge Instructions Given	35	97%	95%	94%
Evaluation of LVS Function	57	98%	99%	99%
Medicare Spending				
Medicare Spending per Patient (ratio)	-	0.87	0.96	0.98
Pneumonia Care				
Appropriate Initial Antibiotic Given	31	97%	95%	95%
Blood Culture Timing	98	99%	97%	98%
Pregnancy and Delivery Care				
Newborn Deliveries Scheduled Early	15	0%	4%	6%
Preventive Care				
Immunization for Influenza[2]	321	98%	88%	90%
Immunization for Pneumonia[2]	392	97%	88%	92%
Stroke Care				
Anticoagulation Therapy for Atrial Fibrillation[1]	-	-	96%	95%
Antithrombotic Therapy Timing[1]	-	-	98%	98%
Assessed for Rehabilitation[1]	-	-	97%	97%
Discharged on Antithrombotic Therapy[1]	-	-	99%	99%
Discharged on Statin Medication[1]	-	-	95%	94%
Thrombolytic Therapy Timing[1]	-	-	69%	66%
Venous Thromboembolism Prophylaxis[1]	-	-	94%	94%
Written Stroke Educational Materials Given[1]	-	-	86%	88%
Surgical Care Improvement Project				
Appropriate Beta Blocker Usage	22	100%	97%	98%
Appropriate VTP Within 24 Hours	84	94%	98%	98%
Controlled Postoperative Blood Glucose[7]	-	-	97%	97%
Perioperative Temperature Management	90	100%	100%	100%
Prophylactic Antibiotic Selection	64	95%	99%	99%
Prophylactic Antibiotic Selection (Outpatient)	17	100%	97%	98%
Prophylactic Antibiotic Stopped	62	92%	98%	98%
Prophylactic Antibiotic Timing	64	100%	99%	99%
Prophylactic Antibiotic Timing (Outpatient)	17	100%	97%	98%
Urinary Catheter Removal	15	93%	96%	97%
Survey of Patients' Hospital Experiences				
Area Around Room 'Always' Quiet at Night	300+	47%	51%	61%
Doctors 'Always' Communicated Well	300+	77%	77%	82%
Home Recovery Information Given	300+	83%	83%	85%
Hospital Given 9 or 10 on 10 Point Scale	300+	59%	63%	71%
Meds 'Always' Explained Before Given	300+	60%	59%	64%
Nurses 'Always' Communicated Well	300+	76%	75%	79%
Pain 'Always' Well Controlled	300+	72%	67%	71%
Room and Bathroom 'Always' Clean	300+	80%	69%	73%
Timely Help 'Always' Received	300+	59%	61%	68%
Would Definitely Recommend Hospital	300+	55%	65%	71%
Use of Medical Imaging				
Cardiac Imaging Stress Test before Surgery[1]	-	-	5.8%	5.3%
Combination Abdominal CT Scan	117	17.9%	8.2%	10.5%
Combination Brain/Sinus CT Scan[1]	-	-	3.6%	2.7%
Combination Chest CT Scan[1]	-	-	1.3%	2.7%
Follow-up Mammogram/Ultrasound	146	24.0%	13%	8.8%
Lumbar Spine MRI for Low Back Pain[1]	-	-	33.4%	37.2%

Saint Anthony Community Hospital

15 - 19 Maple Avenue
Warwick, NY 10990
Phone: 845-986-2276
Fax: 845-986-2687
URL: www.stanthonycommunityhosp.org
Type: Acute Care Hospitals
Emergency Services: Yes
Ownership: Voluntary non-profit - Church
Beds: 73

Key Personnel:

Radiology. . . . . Patricia Barnes
CEO/President. . . . . Stephen Majetich, SC

Measure	Cases	This Hosp.	State Avg.	U.S. Avg.
Blood Clot Prevention and Treatment				
Anticoagulation Overlap Therapy[2]	13	85%	91%	93%
ICU Venous Thromboembolism Prophylaxis[2]	43	98%	92%	92%
Incidence of Potentially Preventable VTE[1,2]	-	-	10%	10%
UFH with Dosages/Platelet Monitoring[1,2]	-	-	92%	97%
Venous Thromboembolism Prophylaxis[2]	167	87%	87%	85%
Warfarin Therapy Discharge Instructions[1,2]	-	-	59%	75%
Chest Pain/Possible Heart Attack Care				
Aspirin Given Within 24 Hours of Arrival	36	94%	97%	96%
Fibrinolytic Meds Within 30 Min. of Arrival[7]	-	-	54%	58%
Average Time to ECG (minutes)	36	5	9	7
Average Time to Transfer (minutes)[1]	-	-	78	60
Children's Asthma Care				
Received Home Management Plan of Care	-	-	-	88%
Received Reliever Medication	-	-	-	100%
Received Systemic Corticosteroids	-	-	-	100%
Emergency Department				
Admittance Decision Time (minutes)[2]	339	135	154	98
Head CT Results Within 45 Min. of Arrival[1]	-	-	55%	57%
Patients Who Left ER Before Being Seen	13,961	1%	2%	2%
Time from ER Arrival to Admit. (minutes)[2]	354	288	378	274
Time from ER Arrival to Discharge (minutes)	390	132	156	134
Time in ER Before Being Evaluated (minutes)	405	6	35	26
Time to Pain Meds for Fractures (minutes)	105	46	61	57
Heart Attack Care				
Aspirin Given at Discharge[1]	-	-	99%	99%
Fibrinolytic Meds Within 30 Min. of Arrival[7]	-	-	46%	54%
PCI Within 90 Minutes of Arrival[7]	-	-	95%	96%
Statin Prescribed at Discharge[1]	-	-	98%	98%
Heart Failure Care				
ACE Inhibitor or ARB for LVSD[1]	-	-	96%	97%
Discharge Instructions Given	40	100%	95%	94%
Evaluation of LVS Function	53	100%	99%	99%
Medicare Spending				
Medicare Spending per Patient (ratio)	-	1.02	0.96	0.98
Pneumonia Care				
Appropriate Initial Antibiotic Given	52	92%	95%	95%
Blood Culture Timing	101	100%	97%	98%
Pregnancy and Delivery Care				
Newborn Deliveries Scheduled Early[2]	34	9%	4%	6%
Preventive Care				
Immunization for Influenza[2]	249	97%	88%	90%
Immunization for Pneumonia[2]	326	96%	88%	92%
Stroke Care				
Anticoagulation Therapy for Atrial Fibrillation[1,2]	-	-	96%	95%
Antithrombotic Therapy Timing[2]	13	92%	98%	98%
Assessed for Rehabilitation[2]	15	100%	97%	97%
Discharged on Antithrombotic Therapy[2]	14	100%	99%	99%
Discharged on Statin Medication[1,2]	-	-	95%	94%
Thrombolytic Therapy Timing[1,2]	-	-	69%	66%
Venous Thromboembolism Prophylaxis[2]	17	100%	94%	94%
Written Stroke Educational Materials Given[1,2]	-	-	86%	88%
Surgical Care Improvement Project				

NOTE: Hospital profiles are in alphabetical order by state, then city, then hospital within the city; Rankings exclude hospitals with less than 25 cases except for patient surveys which excludes hospitals with less than 100 cases; (a) 100-299 cases; (1) The number of cases/patients is too few to report; (2) Data submitted were based on a sample of cases/patients; (3) Results are based on a shorter time period than required; (4) Data suppressed by CMS for one or more quarters; (5) Results are not available for this reporting period; (6) Fewer than 100 patients completed the HCAHPS survey; (7) No cases met the criteria for this measure; (8) The lower limit of the confidence interval cannot be calculated if the number of observed infections equals zero; (9) No data are available from the state/territory for this reporting period; (10) The scores shown reflect fewer than 50 completed surveys; (11) There were discrepancies in the data collection process; (12) This measure does not apply to this hospital for this reporting period; (13) Results cannot be calculated for this reporting period; (14) The results for this state are combined with nearby states to protect confidentiality; Please refer to the User's Guide for a full explanation of data.

Measure	Cases	This Hosp.	State Avg.	U.S. Avg.
Appropriate Beta Blocker Usage	44	100%	97%	98%
Appropriate VTP Within 24 Hours	136	99%	98%	98%
Controlled Postoperative Blood Glucose[7]	-	-	97%	97%
Perioperative Temperature Management	159	100%	100%	100%
Prophylactic Antibiotic Selection	124	99%	99%	99%
Prophylactic Antibiotic Selection (Outpatient)	57	98%	97%	98%
Prophylactic Antibiotic Stopped	120	100%	98%	98%
Prophylactic Antibiotic Timing	124	100%	99%	99%
Prophylactic Antibiotic Timing (Outpatient)	57	100%	97%	98%
Urinary Catheter Removal	120	99%	96%	97%
Survey of Patients' Hospital Experiences				
Area Around Room 'Always' Quiet at Night	300+	56%	51%	61%
Doctors 'Always' Communicated Well	300+	77%	77%	82%
Home Recovery Information Given	300+	81%	83%	85%
Hospital Given 9 or 10 on 10 Point Scale	300+	67%	63%	71%
Meds 'Always' Explained Before Given	300+	59%	59%	64%
Nurses 'Always' Communicated Well	300+	79%	75%	79%
Pain 'Always' Well Controlled	300+	70%	67%	71%
Room and Bathroom 'Always' Clean	300+	63%	69%	73%
Timely Help 'Always' Received	300+	68%	61%	68%
Would Definitely Recommend Hospital	300+	67%	65%	71%
Use of Medical Imaging				
Cardiac Imaging Stress Test before Surgery[1]	-	-	5.8%	5.3%
Combination Abdominal CT Scan	250	1.6%	8.2%	10.5%
Combination Brain/Sinus CT Scan[1]	-	-	3.6%	2.7%
Combination Chest CT Scan	167	0.0%	1.3%	2.7%
Follow-up Mammogram/Ultrasound	411	9.5%	13%	8.8%
Lumbar Spine MRI for Low Back Pain[1]	-	-	33.4%	37.2%

Samaritan Medical Center

830 Washington Street
Watertown, NY 13601
URL: www.samaritanhealth.com
Type: Acute Care Hospitals
Ownership: Voluntary non-profit - Other
Phone: 315-785-4121
Fax: 315-785-4343
Emergency Services: Yes
Beds: 287

Key Personnel:
Pediatric In-Patient Care .... Robert Bacsik, MD
CEO/President............... Thomas H Carman
Radiology.................. Gary L Robbins, MD
Operating Room............. Bonnie Trudeau
Chief of Medical Staff.......... Leverne R Vandewall, MD

Measure	Cases	This Hosp.	State Avg.	U.S. Avg.
Blood Clot Prevention and Treatment				
Anticoagulation Overlap Therapy[2]	47	89%	91%	93%
ICU Venous Thromboembolism Prophylaxis[2]	45	93%	92%	92%
Incidence of Potentially Preventable VTE[1,2]	-	-	10%	10%
UFH with Dosages/Platelet Monitoring[2]	23	100%	92%	97%
Venous Thromboembolism Prophylaxis[2]	377	86%	87%	85%
Warfarin Therapy Discharge Instructions[2]	40	12%	59%	75%
Chest Pain/Possible Heart Attack Care				
Aspirin Given Within 24 Hours of Arrival	143	96%	97%	96%
Fibrinolytic Meds Within 30 Min. of Arrival	15	33%	54%	58%
Average Time to ECG (minutes)	146	7	9	7
Average Time to Transfer (minutes)[1]	-	-	78	60
Children's Asthma Care				
Received Home Management Plan of Care	-	-	-	88%
Received Reliever Medication	-	-	-	100%
Received Systemic Corticosteroids	-	-	-	100%
Emergency Department				
Admittance Decision Time (minutes)[2]	546	93	154	98
Head CT Results Within 45 Min. of Arrival[1]	-	-	55%	57%
Patients Who Left ER Before Being Seen	52,842	3%	2%	2%
Time from ER Arrival to Admit. (minutes)[2]	556	364	378	274
Time from ER Arrival to Discharge (minutes)	352	140	156	134
Time in ER Before Being Evaluated (minutes)	382	33	35	26
Time to Pain Meds for Fractures (minutes)	151	55	61	57
Heart Attack Care				
Aspirin Given at Discharge	17	100%	99%	99%
Fibrinolytic Meds Within 30 Min. of Arrival[1]	-	-	46%	54%
PCI Within 90 Minutes of Arrival[7]	-	-	95%	96%
Statin Prescribed at Discharge	17	82%	98%	98%
Heart Failure Care				
ACE Inhibitor or ARB for LVSD	34	82%	96%	97%
Discharge Instructions Given	189	86%	95%	94%
Evaluation of LVS Function	227	100%	99%	99%
Medicare Spending				
Medicare Spending per Patient (ratio)	-	0.83	0.96	0.98
Pneumonia Care				
Appropriate Initial Antibiotic Given	131	99%	95%	95%
Blood Culture Timing	228	98%	97%	98%
Pregnancy and Delivery Care				
Newborn Deliveries Scheduled Early[2]	21	0%	4%	6%
Preventive Care				
Immunization for Influenza[2]	450	96%	88%	90%
Immunization for Pneumonia[2]	485	94%	88%	92%
Stroke Care				
Anticoagulation Therapy for Atrial Fibrillation	16	88%	96%	95%
Antithrombotic Therapy Timing	57	100%	98%	98%
Assessed for Rehabilitation	58	97%	97%	97%
Discharged on Antithrombotic Therapy	57	100%	99%	99%
Discharged on Statin Medication	48	88%	95%	94%
Thrombolytic Therapy Timing[1]	-	-	69%	66%
Venous Thromboembolism Prophylaxis	69	80%	94%	94%
Written Stroke Educational Materials Given	36	6%	86%	88%
Surgical Care Improvement Project				
Appropriate Beta Blocker Usage	181	97%	97%	98%
Appropriate VTP Within 24 Hours	421	97%	98%	98%
Controlled Postoperative Blood Glucose[7]	-	-	97%	97%
Perioperative Temperature Management	526	100%	100%	100%
Prophylactic Antibiotic Selection	353	99%	99%	99%
Prophylactic Antibiotic Selection (Outpatient)	344	99%	97%	98%
Prophylactic Antibiotic Stopped	352	99%	98%	98%
Prophylactic Antibiotic Timing	356	97%	99%	99%
Prophylactic Antibiotic Timing (Outpatient)	238	97%	97%	98%
Urinary Catheter Removal	292	97%	96%	97%
Survey of Patients' Hospital Experiences				
Area Around Room 'Always' Quiet at Night	300+	56%	51%	61%
Doctors 'Always' Communicated Well	300+	78%	77%	82%
Home Recovery Information Given	300+	87%	83%	85%
Hospital Given 9 or 10 on 10 Point Scale	300+	65%	63%	71%
Meds 'Always' Explained Before Given	300+	64%	59%	64%
Nurses 'Always' Communicated Well	300+	79%	75%	79%
Pain 'Always' Well Controlled	300+	70%	67%	71%
Room and Bathroom 'Always' Clean	300+	83%	69%	73%
Timely Help 'Always' Received	300+	71%	61%	68%
Would Definitely Recommend Hospital	300+	65%	65%	71%
Use of Medical Imaging				
Cardiac Imaging Stress Test before Surgery[7]	-	-	5.8%	5.3%
Combination Abdominal CT Scan	757	33.3%	8.2%	10.5%
Combination Brain/Sinus CT Scan	585	5.0%	3.6%	2.7%
Combination Chest CT Scan	535	0.2%	1.3%	2.7%
Follow-up Mammogram/Ultrasound	1,313	5.0%	13%	8.8%
Lumbar Spine MRI for Low Back Pain	63	31.7%	33.4%	37.2%

Jones Memorial Hospital

191 North Main Street
Wellsville, NY 14895
URL: www.jmhny.org
Type: Acute Care Hospitals
Ownership: Voluntary non-profit - Private
Phone: 585-593-1100
Fax: 585-596-4005
Emergency Services: Yes
Beds: 70

Key Personnel:
Emergency Room .... Mona Carbon
Operating Room............. James H Edmonston, RN
Anesthesiology.............. Mark Elliot
Quality Assurance .... Cheryl Feeman
Quality Assurance .... Cheryl Macafee

Measure	Cases	This Hosp.	State Avg.	U.S. Avg.
Blood Clot Prevention and Treatment				
Anticoagulation Overlap Therapy[2]	11	100%	91%	93%
ICU Venous Thromboembolism Prophylaxis[2]	36	97%	92%	92%
Incidence of Potentially Preventable VTE[2,7]	-	-	10%	10%
UFH with Dosages/Platelet Monitoring[1,2]	-	-	92%	97%
Venous Thromboembolism Prophylaxis[2]	122	96%	87%	85%
Warfarin Therapy Discharge Instructions[1,2]	-	-	59%	75%
Chest Pain/Possible Heart Attack Care				
Aspirin Given Within 24 Hours of Arrival	43	100%	97%	96%
Fibrinolytic Meds Within 30 Min. of Arrival[1]	-	-	54%	58%
Average Time to ECG (minutes)	46	6	9	7
Average Time to Transfer (minutes)[7]	-	-	78	60
Children's Asthma Care				
Received Home Management Plan of Care	-	-	-	88%
Received Reliever Medication	-	-	-	100%
Received Systemic Corticosteroids	-	-	-	100%
Emergency Department				
Admittance Decision Time (minutes)[2]	330	66	154	98
Head CT Results Within 45 Min. of Arrival[1]	-	-	55%	57%
Patients Who Left ER Before Being Seen	12,448	0%	2%	2%
Time from ER Arrival to Admit. (minutes)[2]	341	218	378	274
Time from ER Arrival to Discharge (minutes)	381	100	156	134
Time in ER Before Being Evaluated (minutes)	404	20	35	26
Time to Pain Meds for Fractures (minutes)	39	35	61	57
Heart Attack Care				
Aspirin Given at Discharge[1]	-	-	99%	99%
Fibrinolytic Meds Within 30 Min. of Arrival[7]	-	-	46%	54%
PCI Within 90 Minutes of Arrival[7]	-	-	95%	96%
Statin Prescribed at Discharge[1]	-	-	98%	98%
Heart Failure Care				
ACE Inhibitor or ARB for LVSD	18	100%	96%	97%
Discharge Instructions Given	58	93%	95%	94%
Evaluation of LVS Function	69	100%	99%	99%
Medicare Spending				
Medicare Spending per Patient (ratio)	-	0.90	0.96	0.98
Pneumonia Care				
Appropriate Initial Antibiotic Given	39	95%	95%	95%
Blood Culture Timing	58	98%	97%	98%
Pregnancy and Delivery Care				
Newborn Deliveries Scheduled Early	22	0%	4%	6%
Preventive Care				
Immunization for Influenza[2]	256	98%	88%	90%
Immunization for Pneumonia[2]	311	99%	88%	92%
Stroke Care				
Anticoagulation Therapy for Atrial Fibrillation[1]	-	-	96%	95%
Antithrombotic Therapy Timing[1]	-	-	98%	98%
Assessed for Rehabilitation[1]	-	-	97%	97%
Discharged on Antithrombotic Therapy[1]	-	-	99%	99%
Discharged on Statin Medication[1]	-	-	95%	94%
Thrombolytic Therapy Timing[1]	-	-	69%	66%
Venous Thromboembolism Prophylaxis[1]	-	-	94%	94%
Written Stroke Educational Materials Given[1]	-	-	86%	88%
Surgical Care Improvement Project				
Appropriate Beta Blocker Usage	24	100%	97%	98%
Appropriate VTP Within 24 Hours	61	100%	98%	98%
Controlled Postoperative Blood Glucose[7]	-	-	97%	97%
Perioperative Temperature Management	72	99%	100%	100%
Prophylactic Antibiotic Selection	37	100%	99%	99%
Prophylactic Antibiotic Selection (Outpatient)	73	99%	97%	98%
Prophylactic Antibiotic Stopped	32	100%	98%	98%
Prophylactic Antibiotic Timing	37	100%	99%	99%
Prophylactic Antibiotic Timing (Outpatient)	73	100%	97%	98%
Urinary Catheter Removal	22	100%	96%	97%
Survey of Patients' Hospital Experiences				
Area Around Room 'Always' Quiet at Night	300+	55%	51%	61%
Doctors 'Always' Communicated Well	300+	82%	77%	82%
Home Recovery Information Given	300+	86%	83%	85%
Hospital Given 9 or 10 on 10 Point Scale	300+	66%	63%	71%
Meds 'Always' Explained Before Given	300+	63%	59%	64%
Nurses 'Always' Communicated Well	300+	78%	75%	79%
Pain 'Always' Well Controlled	300+	74%	67%	71%
Room and Bathroom 'Always' Clean	300+	68%	69%	73%
Timely Help 'Always' Received	300+	68%	61%	68%
Would Definitely Recommend Hospital	300+	65%	65%	71%
Use of Medical Imaging				
Cardiac Imaging Stress Test before Surgery	49	2.0%	5.8%	5.3%
Combination Abdominal CT Scan	226	14.2%	8.2%	10.5%
Combination Brain/Sinus CT Scan[1]	-	-	3.6%	2.7%
Combination Chest CT Scan	69	11.6%	1.3%	2.7%
Follow-up Mammogram/Ultrasound	404	8.2%	13%	8.8%
Lumbar Spine MRI for Low Back Pain[1]	-	-	33.4%	37.2%

NOTE: Hospital profiles are in alphabetical order by state, then city, then hospital within the city; Rankings exclude hospitals with less than 25 cases except for patient surveys which excludes hospitals with less than 100 cases; (a) 100-299 cases; (1) The number of cases/patients is too few to report; (2) Data submitted were based on a sample of cases/patients; (3) Results are based on a shorter time period than required; (4) Data suppressed by CMS for one or more quarters; (5) Results are not available for this reporting period; (6) Fewer than 100 patients completed the HCAHPS survey; (7) No cases met the criteria for this measure; (8) The lower limit of the confidence interval cannot be calculated if the number of observed infections equals zero; (9) No data are available from the state/territory for this reporting period; (10) The scores shown reflect fewer than 50 completed surveys; (11) There were discrepancies in the data collection process; (12) This measure does not apply to this hospital for this reporting period; (13) Results cannot be calculated for this reporting period; (14) The results for this state are combined with nearby states to protect confidentiality; Please refer to the User's Guide for a full explanation of data.

Helen Hayes Hospital

51 North Route 9w
West Haverstraw, NY 10993
E-mail: info@helenhayeshospital.org
URL: www.helenhayeshospital.org
Type: Acute Care Hospitals
Ownership: Government - Local
Phone: 845-786-4000
Fax: 845-947-3097
Emergency Services: No
Beds: 155

Key Personnel:
Patient Relations . . . . Mary Bianco
Infection Control. . . . . Liz Brown, RN
CEO/President. . . . . Val S Gray
Ambulatory Care . . . . Bruce Marshall
Chief of Medical Staff. . . . . John Pellicone, MD

Measure	Cases	This Hosp.	State Avg.	U.S. Avg.
Blood Clot Prevention and Treatment				
Anticoagulation Overlap Therapy[7]	-	-	91%	93%
ICU Venous Thromboembolism Prophylaxis[7]	-	-	92%	92%
Incidence of Potentially Preventable VTE[7]	-	-	10%	10%
UFH with Dosages/Platelet Monitoring[7]	-	-	92%	97%
Venous Thromboembolism Prophylaxis	419	100%	87%	85%
Warfarin Therapy Discharge Instructions[7]	-	-	59%	75%
Chest Pain/Possible Heart Attack Care				
Aspirin Given Within 24 Hours of Arrival[5]	-	-	97%	96%
Fibrinolytic Meds Within 30 Min. of Arrival[5]	-	-	54%	58%
Average Time to ECG (minutes)[5]	-	-	9	7
Average Time to Transfer (minutes)[5]	-	-	78	60
Children's Asthma Care				
Received Home Management Plan of Care	-	-	-	88%
Received Reliever Medication	-	-	-	100%
Received Systemic Corticosteroids	-	-	-	100%
Emergency Department				
Admittance Decision Time (minutes)[7]	-	-	154	98
Head CT Results Within 45 Min. of Arrival[5]	-	-	55%	57%
Patients Who Left ER Before Being Seen[5]	-	-	2%	2%
Time from ER Arrival to Admit. (minutes)[7]	-	-	378	274
Time from ER Arrival to Discharge (minutes)[5]	-	-	156	134
Time in ER Before Being Evaluated (minutes)[5]	-	-	35	26
Time to Pain Meds for Fractures (minutes)[5]	-	-	61	57
Heart Attack Care				
Aspirin Given at Discharge[5]	-	-	99%	99%
Fibrinolytic Meds Within 30 Min. of Arrival[5]	-	-	46%	54%
PCI Within 90 Minutes of Arrival[5]	-	-	95%	96%
Statin Prescribed at Discharge[5]	-	-	98%	98%
Heart Failure Care				
ACE Inhibitor or ARB for LVSD[5]	-	-	96%	97%
Discharge Instructions Given[5]	-	-	95%	94%
Evaluation of LVS Function[5]	-	-	99%	99%
Medicare Spending				
Medicare Spending per Patient (ratio)	-	-	0.96	0.98
Pneumonia Care				
Appropriate Initial Antibiotic Given[5]	-	-	95%	95%
Blood Culture Timing[5]	-	-	97%	98%
Pregnancy and Delivery Care				
Newborn Deliveries Scheduled Early[7]	-	-	4%	6%
Preventive Care				
Immunization for Influenza	264	91%	88%	90%
Immunization for Pneumonia	507	94%	88%	92%
Stroke Care				
Anticoagulation Therapy for Atrial Fibrillation[5]	-	-	96%	95%
Antithrombotic Therapy Timing[5]	-	-	98%	98%
Assessed for Rehabilitation[5]	-	-	97%	97%
Discharged on Antithrombotic Therapy[5]	-	-	99%	99%
Discharged on Statin Medication[5]	-	-	95%	94%
Thrombolytic Therapy Timing[5]	-	-	69%	66%
Venous Thromboembolism Prophylaxis[5]	-	-	94%	94%
Written Stroke Educational Materials Given[5]	-	-	86%	88%
Surgical Care Improvement Project				
Appropriate Beta Blocker Usage[5]	-	-	97%	98%
Appropriate VTP Within 24 Hours[5]	-	-	98%	98%
Controlled Postoperative Blood Glucose[5]	-	-	97%	97%
Perioperative Temperature Management[5]	-	-	100%	100%
Prophylactic Antibiotic Selection[5]	-	-	99%	99%
Prophylactic Antibiotic Selection (Outpatient)[5]	-	-	97%	98%
Prophylactic Antibiotic Stopped[5]	-	-	98%	98%
Prophylactic Antibiotic Timing[5]	-	-	99%	99%
Prophylactic Antibiotic Timing (Outpatient)[5]	-	-	97%	98%
Urinary Catheter Removal[5]	-	-	96%	97%
Survey of Patients' Hospital Experiences				
Area Around Room 'Always' Quiet at Night[1]	-	-	51%	61%
Doctors 'Always' Communicated Well[1]	-	-	77%	82%
Home Recovery Information Given[1]	-	-	83%	85%
Hospital Given 9 or 10 on 10 Point Scale[1]	-	-	63%	71%
Meds 'Always' Explained Before Given[1]	-	-	59%	64%
Nurses 'Always' Communicated Well[1]	-	-	75%	79%
Pain 'Always' Well Controlled[1]	-	-	67%	71%
Room and Bathroom 'Always' Clean[1]	-	-	69%	73%
Timely Help 'Always' Received[1]	-	-	61%	68%
Would Definitely Recommend Hospital[1]	-	-	65%	71%
Use of Medical Imaging				
Cardiac Imaging Stress Test before Surgery[7]	-	-	5.8%	5.3%
Combination Abdominal CT Scan[7]	-	-	8.2%	10.5%
Combination Brain/Sinus CT Scan[7]	-	-	3.6%	2.7%
Combination Chest CT Scan[7]	-	-	1.3%	2.7%
Follow-up Mammogram/Ultrasound[7]	-	-	13%	8.8%
Lumbar Spine MRI for Low Back Pain[7]	-	-	33.4%	37.2%

Good Samaritan Hospital Medical Center

1000 Montauk Highway
West Islip, NY 11795
URL: www.good-samaritan-hospital.org
Type: Acute Care Hospitals
Ownership: Voluntary non-profit - Church
Phone: 631-376-3000
Fax: 631-376-3893
Emergency Services: Yes
Beds: 437

Key Personnel:
CEO/President. . . . . William Allison
Infection Control. . . . . Franes Edwards, RN
Operating Room. . . . . John W Francfort, MD
Pediatric Ambulatory Care . . . . . . Barry Goldberg, MD
Quality Assurance . . . . Fred B Landon
Chief of Medical Staff. . . . . Kenneth Long
Radiology. . . . . Matthew Rifkin, MD

Measure	Cases	This Hosp.	State Avg.	U.S. Avg.
Blood Clot Prevention and Treatment				
Anticoagulation Overlap Therapy[2]	168	97%	91%	93%
ICU Venous Thromboembolism Prophylaxis[2]	42	95%	92%	92%
Incidence of Potentially Preventable VTE[2]	28	4%	10%	10%
UFH with Dosages/Platelet Monitoring[2]	30	100%	92%	97%
Venous Thromboembolism Prophylaxis[2]	417	95%	87%	85%
Warfarin Therapy Discharge Instructions[2]	111	88%	59%	75%
Chest Pain/Possible Heart Attack Care				
Aspirin Given Within 24 Hours of Arrival[1]	-	-	97%	96%
Fibrinolytic Meds Within 30 Min. of Arrival[3,7]	-	-	54%	58%
Average Time to ECG (minutes)[1]	-	-	9	7
Average Time to Transfer (minutes)[3,7]	-	-	78	60
Children's Asthma Care				
Received Home Management Plan of Care	-	-	-	88%
Received Reliever Medication	-	-	-	100%
Received Systemic Corticosteroids	-	-	-	100%
Emergency Department				
Admittance Decision Time (minutes)[2]	830	278	154	98
Head CT Results Within 45 Min. of Arrival[1]	-	-	55%	57%
Patients Who Left ER Before Being Seen	98,746	1%	2%	2%
Time from ER Arrival to Admit. (minutes)[2]	877	483	378	274
Time from ER Arrival to Discharge (minutes)	446	171	156	134
Time in ER Before Being Evaluated (minutes)	408	34	35	26
Time to Pain Meds for Fractures (minutes)	181	73	61	57
Heart Attack Care				
Aspirin Given at Discharge	256	100%	99%	99%
Fibrinolytic Meds Within 30 Min. of Arrival[7]	-	-	46%	54%
PCI Within 90 Minutes of Arrival	35	100%	95%	96%
Statin Prescribed at Discharge	254	100%	98%	98%
Heart Failure Care				
ACE Inhibitor or ARB for LVSD[2]	98	100%	96%	97%
Discharge Instructions Given[2]	265	100%	95%	94%
Evaluation of LVS Function[2]	344	100%	99%	99%
Medicare Spending				
Medicare Spending per Patient (ratio)	-	1.05	0.96	0.98
Pneumonia Care				
Appropriate Initial Antibiotic Given[2]	90	100%	95%	95%
Blood Culture Timing[2]	147	100%	97%	98%
Pregnancy and Delivery Care				
Newborn Deliveries Scheduled Early[2]	38	0%	4%	6%
Preventive Care				
Immunization for Influenza[2]	615	96%	88%	90%
Immunization for Pneumonia[2]	632	92%	88%	92%
Stroke Care				
Anticoagulation Therapy for Atrial Fibrillation	23	100%	96%	95%
Antithrombotic Therapy Timing	156	100%	98%	98%
Assessed for Rehabilitation	182	100%	97%	97%
Discharged on Antithrombotic Therapy	149	100%	99%	99%
Discharged on Statin Medication	113	100%	95%	94%
Thrombolytic Therapy Timing	16	100%	69%	66%
Venous Thromboembolism Prophylaxis	213	100%	94%	94%
Written Stroke Educational Materials Given	92	100%	86%	88%
Surgical Care Improvement Project				
Appropriate Beta Blocker Usage[2]	171	96%	97%	98%
Appropriate VTP Within 24 Hours[2]	463	97%	98%	98%
Controlled Postoperative Blood Glucose[2,7]	-	-	97%	97%
Perioperative Temperature Management[2]	554	100%	100%	100%
Prophylactic Antibiotic Selection[2]	311	99%	99%	99%
Prophylactic Antibiotic Selection (Outpatient)	593	98%	97%	98%
Prophylactic Antibiotic Stopped[2]	300	99%	98%	98%
Prophylactic Antibiotic Timing[2]	311	98%	99%	99%
Prophylactic Antibiotic Timing (Outpatient)	593	99%	97%	98%
Urinary Catheter Removal[2]	269	98%	96%	97%
Survey of Patients' Hospital Experiences				
Area Around Room 'Always' Quiet at Night	300+	45%	51%	61%
Doctors 'Always' Communicated Well	300+	75%	77%	82%
Home Recovery Information Given	300+	85%	83%	85%
Hospital Given 9 or 10 on 10 Point Scale	300+	57%	63%	71%
Meds 'Always' Explained Before Given	300+	56%	59%	64%
Nurses 'Always' Communicated Well	300+	71%	75%	79%
Pain 'Always' Well Controlled	300+	65%	67%	71%
Room and Bathroom 'Always' Clean	300+	68%	69%	73%
Timely Help 'Always' Received	300+	51%	61%	68%
Would Definitely Recommend Hospital	300+	61%	65%	71%
Use of Medical Imaging				
Cardiac Imaging Stress Test before Surgery[1]	-	-	5.8%	5.3%
Combination Abdominal CT Scan	1,020	2.1%	8.2%	10.5%
Combination Brain/Sinus CT Scan	1,247	3.9%	3.6%	2.7%
Combination Chest CT Scan	820	0.5%	1.3%	2.7%
Follow-up Mammogram/Ultrasound	2,079	15.9%	13%	8.8%
Lumbar Spine MRI for Low Back Pain[1]	-	-	33.4%	37.2%

Westfield Memorial Hospital

189 East Main Street
Westfield, NY 14787
URL: www.wmhinc.org
Type: Acute Care Hospitals
Ownership: Voluntary non-profit - Private
Phone: 716-326-4921
Fax: 716-326-3802
Emergency Services: Yes
Beds: 32

Key Personnel:
Chief of Medical Staff. . . . . Russell Ellwell, MD
Anesthesiology. . . . . Russell Elwell, MD
Radiology. . . . . Zhengming Gu
Infection Control. . . . . Gail Hiddell
CEO/President. . . . . Mary Larowe
Operating Room. . . . . Kathy Petroff
Emergency Room . . . . Grant Stephenson, MD
Quality Assurance . . . . Patricia Uldrich

Measure	Cases	This Hosp.	State Avg.	U.S. Avg.
Blood Clot Prevention and Treatment				
Anticoagulation Overlap Therapy[1,2]	-	-	91%	93%
ICU Venous Thromboembolism Prophylaxis[2,7]	-	-	92%	92%
Incidence of Potentially Preventable VTE[2,7]	-	-	10%	10%
UFH with Dosages/Platelet Monitoring[2,7]	-	-	92%	97%
Venous Thromboembolism Prophylaxis[2]	73	8%	87%	85%
Warfarin Therapy Discharge Instructions[1,2]	-	-	59%	75%
Chest Pain/Possible Heart Attack Care				
Aspirin Given Within 24 Hours of Arrival	93	82%	97%	96%
Fibrinolytic Meds Within 30 Min. of Arrival[1]	-	-	54%	58%
Average Time to ECG (minutes)	104	6	9	7
Average Time to Transfer (minutes)	12	124	78	60
Children's Asthma Care				

NOTE: Hospital profiles are in alphabetical order by state, then city, then hospital within the city; Rankings exclude hospitals with less than 25 cases except for patient surveys which excludes hospitals with less than 100 cases; (a) 100-299 cases; (1) The number of cases/patients is too few to report; (2) Data submitted were based on a sample of cases/patients; (3) Results are based on a shorter time period than required; (4) Data suppressed by CMS for one or more quarters; (5) Results are not available for this reporting period; (6) Fewer than 100 patients completed the HCAHPS survey; (7) No cases met the criteria for this measure; (8) The lower limit of the confidence interval cannot be calculated if the number of observed infections equals zero; (9) No data are available from the state/territory for this reporting period; (10) The scores shown reflect fewer than 50 completed surveys; (11) There were discrepancies in the data collection process; (12) This measure does not apply to this hospital for this reporting period; (13) Results cannot be calculated for this reporting period; (14) The results for this state are combined with nearby states to protect confidentiality; Please refer to the User's Guide for a full explanation of data.

Measure	Cases	This Hosp.	State Avg.	U.S. Avg.
Received Home Management Plan of Care	-	-	-	88%
Received Reliever Medication	-	-	-	100%
Received Systemic Corticosteroids	-	-	-	100%
Emergency Department				
Admittance Decision Time (minutes)[2]	85	55	154	98
Head CT Results Within 45 Min. of Arrival[1]	-	-	55%	57%
Patients Who Left ER Before Being Seen	8,733	1%	2%	2%
Time from ER Arrival to Admit. (minutes)[2]	91	250	378	274
Time from ER Arrival to Discharge (minutes)	374	169	156	134
Time in ER Before Being Evaluated (minutes)	481	22	35	26
Time to Pain Meds for Fractures (minutes)	16	64	61	57
Heart Attack Care				
Aspirin Given at Discharge[5]	-	-	99%	99%
Fibrinolytic Meds Within 30 Min. of Arrival[5]	-	-	46%	54%
PCI Within 90 Minutes of Arrival[5]	-	-	95%	96%
Statin Prescribed at Discharge[5]	-	-	98%	98%
Heart Failure Care				
ACE Inhibitor or ARB for LVSD[2,3]	-	-	96%	97%
Discharge Instructions Given[1,2]	-	-	95%	94%
Evaluation of LVS Function[1,2]	-	-	99%	99%
Medicare Spending				
Medicare Spending per Patient (ratio)[1]	-	-	0.96	0.98
Pneumonia Care				
Appropriate Initial Antibiotic Given[2,7]	-	-	95%	95%
Blood Culture Timing[2,7]	-	-	97%	98%
Pregnancy and Delivery Care				
Newborn Deliveries Scheduled Early[7]	-	-	4%	6%
Preventive Care				
Immunization for Influenza[2]	54	81%	88%	90%
Immunization for Pneumonia[2]	91	69%	88%	92%
Stroke Care				
Anticoagulation Therapy for Atrial Fibrillation[5]	-	-	96%	95%
Antithrombotic Therapy Timing[5]	-	-	98%	98%
Assessed for Rehabilitation[5]	-	-	97%	97%
Discharged on Antithrombotic Therapy[5]	-	-	99%	99%
Discharged on Statin Medication[5]	-	-	95%	94%
Thrombolytic Therapy Timing[5]	-	-	69%	66%
Venous Thromboembolism Prophylaxis[5]	-	-	94%	94%
Written Stroke Educational Materials Given[5]	-	-	86%	88%
Surgical Care Improvement Project				
Appropriate Beta Blocker Usage[2,3]	-	-	97%	98%
Appropriate VTP Within 24 Hours[1,2]	-	-	98%	98%
Controlled Postoperative Blood Glucose[2,3]	-	-	97%	97%
Perioperative Temperature Management[1,2]	-	-	100%	100%
Prophylactic Antibiotic Selection[1,2]	-	-	99%	99%
Prophylactic Antibiotic Selection (Outpatient)[5]	-	-	97%	98%
Prophylactic Antibiotic Stopped[1,2]	-	-	98%	98%
Prophylactic Antibiotic Timing[1,2]	-	-	99%	99%
Prophylactic Antibiotic Timing (Outpatient)[5]	-	-	97%	98%
Urinary Catheter Removal[2,3]	-	-	96%	97%
Survey of Patients' Hospital Experiences				
Area Around Room 'Always' Quiet at Night[10]	<100	78%	51%	61%
Doctors 'Always' Communicated Well[10]	<100	84%	77%	82%
Home Recovery Information Given[10]	<100	83%	83%	85%
Hospital Given 9 or 10 on 10 Point Scale[10]	<100	88%	63%	71%
Meds 'Always' Explained Before Given[10]	<100	72%	59%	64%
Nurses 'Always' Communicated Well[10]	<100	89%	75%	79%
Pain 'Always' Well Controlled[10]	<100	88%	67%	71%
Room and Bathroom 'Always' Clean[10]	<100	80%	69%	73%
Timely Help 'Always' Received[10]	<100	90%	61%	68%
Would Definitely Recommend Hospital[10]	<100	90%	65%	71%
Use of Medical Imaging				
Cardiac Imaging Stress Test before Surgery[1]	-	-	5.8%	5.3%
Combination Abdominal CT Scan	187	8.6%	8.2%	10.5%
Combination Brain/Sinus CT Scan[1]	-	-	3.6%	2.7%
Combination Chest CT Scan[1]	-	-	1.3%	2.7%
Follow-up Mammogram/Ultrasound	290	6.2%	13%	8.8%
Lumbar Spine MRI for Low Back Pain[7]	-	-	33.4%	37.2%

White Plains Hospital Center

41 East Post R0ad
White Plains, NY 10601
Phone: 914-681-0600
Fax: 914-681-2902
E-mail: wphcmail@wphospital.org
URL: www.wphospital.org
Type: Acute Care Hospitals
Emergency Services: Yes
Ownership: Voluntary non-profit - Private
Beds: 307

Key Personnel:
Pediatric Ambulatory Care . . . . . . Scott D Bookner, MD
Infection Control. . . . . Arthur L Forni, MD
President . . . . Susan Fox
Operating Room. . . . . Lynn G Josephson, MD
Radiology. . . . . Paul T Khoury, MD
Chief of Medical Staff. . . . . Michael Palumbo, MD
Quality Assurance . . . . Ellen Perlman
CEO . . . . Jon B Schandler

Measure	Cases	This Hosp.	State Avg.	U.S. Avg.
Blood Clot Prevention and Treatment				
Anticoagulation Overlap Therapy[2]	127	98%	91%	93%
ICU Venous Thromboembolism Prophylaxis[2]	40	92%	92%	92%
Incidence of Potentially Preventable VTE[2]	22	5%	10%	10%
UFH with Dosages/Platelet Monitoring[2]	105	100%	92%	97%
Venous Thromboembolism Prophylaxis[2]	381	93%	87%	85%
Warfarin Therapy Discharge Instructions[2]	94	93%	59%	75%
Chest Pain/Possible Heart Attack Care				
Aspirin Given Within 24 Hours of Arrival	16	100%	97%	96%
Fibrinolytic Meds Within 30 Min. of Arrival[3,7]	-	-	54%	58%
Average Time to ECG (minutes)	17	7	9	7
Average Time to Transfer (minutes)[1,3]	-	-	78	60
Children's Asthma Care				
Received Home Management Plan of Care	-	-	-	88%
Received Reliever Medication	-	-	-	100%
Received Systemic Corticosteroids	-	-	-	100%
Emergency Department				
Admittance Decision Time (minutes)[2]	727	203	154	98
Head CT Results Within 45 Min. of Arrival	11	82%	55%	57%
Patients Who Left ER Before Being Seen	54,942	1%	2%	2%
Time from ER Arrival to Admit. (minutes)[2]	784	416	378	274
Time from ER Arrival to Discharge (minutes)	367	192	156	134
Time in ER Before Being Evaluated (minutes)	417	39	35	26
Time to Pain Meds for Fractures (minutes)	159	63	61	57
Heart Attack Care				
Aspirin Given at Discharge	159	100%	99%	99%
Fibrinolytic Meds Within 30 Min. of Arrival[7]	-	-	46%	54%
PCI Within 90 Minutes of Arrival	36	100%	95%	96%
Statin Prescribed at Discharge	154	99%	98%	98%
Heart Failure Care				
ACE Inhibitor or ARB for LVSD[2]	78	99%	96%	97%
Discharge Instructions Given[2]	219	100%	95%	94%
Evaluation of LVS Function[2]	287	100%	99%	99%
Medicare Spending				
Medicare Spending per Patient (ratio)	-	1.03	0.96	0.98
Pneumonia Care				
Appropriate Initial Antibiotic Given[2]	88	94%	95%	95%
Blood Culture Timing[2]	179	100%	97%	98%
Pregnancy and Delivery Care				
Newborn Deliveries Scheduled Early[2]	35	0%	4%	6%
Preventive Care				
Immunization for Influenza[2]	558	99%	88%	90%
Immunization for Pneumonia[2]	641	97%	88%	92%
Stroke Care				
Anticoagulation Therapy for Atrial Fibrillation	24	100%	96%	95%
Antithrombotic Therapy Timing	106	100%	98%	98%
Assessed for Rehabilitation	149	100%	97%	97%
Discharged on Antithrombotic Therapy	132	100%	99%	99%
Discharged on Statin Medication	116	99%	95%	94%
Thrombolytic Therapy Timing	22	91%	69%	66%
Venous Thromboembolism Prophylaxis	148	97%	94%	94%
Written Stroke Educational Materials Given	60	97%	86%	88%
Surgical Care Improvement Project				
Appropriate Beta Blocker Usage[2]	162	100%	97%	98%
Appropriate VTP Within 24 Hours[2]	426	99%	98%	98%
Controlled Postoperative Blood Glucose[2,7]	-	-	97%	97%
Perioperative Temperature Management[2]	487	100%	100%	100%
Prophylactic Antibiotic Selection[2]	304	100%	99%	99%
Prophylactic Antibiotic Selection (Outpatient)	356	98%	97%	98%
Prophylactic Antibiotic Stopped[2]	294	100%	98%	98%
Prophylactic Antibiotic Timing[2]	304	100%	99%	99%
Prophylactic Antibiotic Timing (Outpatient)	356	99%	97%	98%
Urinary Catheter Removal[2]	120	100%	96%	97%
Survey of Patients' Hospital Experiences				
Area Around Room 'Always' Quiet at Night	300+	54%	51%	61%
Doctors 'Always' Communicated Well	300+	82%	77%	82%
Home Recovery Information Given	300+	86%	83%	85%
Hospital Given 9 or 10 on 10 Point Scale	300+	78%	63%	71%
Meds 'Always' Explained Before Given	300+	73%	59%	64%
Nurses 'Always' Communicated Well	300+	83%	75%	79%
Pain 'Always' Well Controlled	300+	77%	67%	71%
Room and Bathroom 'Always' Clean	300+	71%	69%	73%
Timely Help 'Always' Received	300+	66%	61%	68%
Would Definitely Recommend Hospital	300+	81%	65%	71%
Use of Medical Imaging				
Cardiac Imaging Stress Test before Surgery	330	8.5%	5.8%	5.3%
Combination Abdominal CT Scan	1,530	2.2%	8.2%	10.5%
Combination Brain/Sinus CT Scan	1,520	4.9%	3.6%	2.7%
Combination Chest CT Scan	1,519	0.1%	1.3%	2.7%
Follow-up Mammogram/Ultrasound	2,143	41.3%	13%	8.8%
Lumbar Spine MRI for Low Back Pain[7]	-	-	33.4%	37.2%

Winifred Masterson Burke Rehabilitation Hospital

785 Mamaroneck Avenue
White Plains, NY 10605
Phone: 914-597-2232
Fax: 914-597-2757
E-mail: web@burke.org
URL: www.burke.org
Type: Acute Care Hospitals
Emergency Services: No
Ownership: Voluntary non-profit - Private
Beds: 150

Key Personnel:
Quality Assurance . . . . Christine Reicke
Infection Control. . . . . Lois Van Fleet
CEO . . . . Mary Beth Walsh, MD
Chief of Medical Staff. . . . . Mary Beth Walsh, MD

Measure	Cases	This Hosp.	State Avg.	U.S. Avg.
Blood Clot Prevention and Treatment				
Anticoagulation Overlap Therapy[2,7]	-	-	91%	93%
ICU Venous Thromboembolism Prophylaxis[2,7]	-	-	92%	92%
Incidence of Potentially Preventable VTE[2,7]	-	-	10%	10%
UFH with Dosages/Platelet Monitoring[2,7]	-	-	92%	97%
Venous Thromboembolism Prophylaxis[2]	528	100%	87%	85%
Warfarin Therapy Discharge Instructions[2,7]	-	-	59%	75%
Chest Pain/Possible Heart Attack Care				
Aspirin Given Within 24 Hours of Arrival[5]	-	-	97%	96%
Fibrinolytic Meds Within 30 Min. of Arrival[5]	-	-	54%	58%
Average Time to ECG (minutes)[5]	-	-	9	7
Average Time to Transfer (minutes)[5]	-	-	78	60
Children's Asthma Care				
Received Home Management Plan of Care	-	-	-	88%
Received Reliever Medication	-	-	-	100%
Received Systemic Corticosteroids	-	-	-	100%
Emergency Department				
Admittance Decision Time (minutes)[2,7]	-	-	154	98
Head CT Results Within 45 Min. of Arrival[5]	-	-	55%	57%
Patients Who Left ER Before Being Seen[5]	-	-	2%	2%
Time from ER Arrival to Admit. (minutes)[2,7]	-	-	378	274
Time from ER Arrival to Discharge (minutes)[5]	-	-	156	134
Time in ER Before Being Evaluated (minutes)[5]	-	-	35	26
Time to Pain Meds for Fractures (minutes)[5]	-	-	61	57
Heart Attack Care				
Aspirin Given at Discharge[5]	-	-	99%	99%
Fibrinolytic Meds Within 30 Min. of Arrival[5]	-	-	46%	54%
PCI Within 90 Minutes of Arrival[5]	-	-	95%	96%
Statin Prescribed at Discharge[5]	-	-	98%	98%
Heart Failure Care				
ACE Inhibitor or ARB for LVSD[5]	-	-	96%	97%
Discharge Instructions Given[5]	-	-	95%	94%
Evaluation of LVS Function[5]	-	-	99%	99%
Medicare Spending				
Medicare Spending per Patient (ratio)	-	-	0.96	0.98

NOTE: Hospital profiles are in alphabetical order by state, then city, then hospital within the city; Rankings exclude hospitals with less than 25 cases except for patient surveys which excludes hospitals with less than 100 cases; (a) 100-299 cases; (1) The number of cases/patients is too few to report; (2) Data submitted were based on a sample of cases/patients; (3) Results are based on a shorter time period than required; (4) Data suppressed by CMS for one or more quarters; (5) Results are not available for this reporting period; (6) Fewer than 100 patients completed the HCAHPS survey; (7) No cases met the criteria for this measure; (8) The lower limit of the confidence interval cannot be calculated if the number of observed infections equals zero; (9) No data are available from the state/territory for this reporting period; (10) The scores shown reflect fewer than 50 completed surveys; (11) There were discrepancies in the data collection process; (12) This measure does not apply to this hospital for this reporting period; (13) Results cannot be calculated for this reporting period; (14) The results for this state are combined with nearby states to protect confidentiality; Please refer to the User's Guide for a full explanation of data.

Measure	Cases	This Hosp.	State Avg.	U.S. Avg.
Pneumonia Care				
Appropriate Initial Antibiotic Given[5]	-	-	95%	95%
Blood Culture Timing[5]	-	-	97%	98%
Pregnancy and Delivery Care				
Newborn Deliveries Scheduled Early[2,7]	-	-	4%	6%
Preventive Care				
Immunization for Influenza[2]	397	99%	88%	90%
Immunization for Pneumonia[2]	675	81%	88%	92%
Stroke Care				
Anticoagulation Therapy for Atrial Fibrillation[5]	-	-	96%	95%
Antithrombotic Therapy Timing[5]	-	-	98%	98%
Assessed for Rehabilitation[5]	-	-	97%	97%
Discharged on Antithrombotic Therapy[5]	-	-	99%	99%
Discharged on Statin Medication[5]	-	-	95%	94%
Thrombolytic Therapy Timing[5]	-	-	69%	66%
Venous Thromboembolism Prophylaxis[5]	-	-	94%	94%
Written Stroke Educational Materials Given[5]	-	-	86%	88%
Surgical Care Improvement Project				
Appropriate Beta Blocker Usage[5]	-	-	97%	98%
Appropriate VTP Within 24 Hours[5]	-	-	98%	98%
Controlled Postoperative Blood Glucose[5]	-	-	97%	97%
Perioperative Temperature Management[5]	-	-	100%	100%
Prophylactic Antibiotic Selection[5]	-	-	99%	99%
Prophylactic Antibiotic Selection (Outpatient)[5]	-	-	97%	98%
Prophylactic Antibiotic Stopped[5]	-	-	98%	98%
Prophylactic Antibiotic Timing[5]	-	-	99%	99%
Prophylactic Antibiotic Timing (Outpatient)[5]	-	-	97%	98%
Urinary Catheter Removal[5]	-	-	96%	97%
Survey of Patients' Hospital Experiences				
Area Around Room 'Always' Quiet at Night[1]	-	-	51%	61%
Doctors 'Always' Communicated Well[1]	-	-	77%	82%
Home Recovery Information Given[1]	-	-	83%	85%
Hospital Given 9 or 10 on 10 Point Scale[1]	-	-	63%	71%
Meds 'Always' Explained Before Given[1]	-	-	59%	64%
Nurses 'Always' Communicated Well[1]	-	-	75%	79%
Pain 'Always' Well Controlled[1]	-	-	67%	71%
Room and Bathroom 'Always' Clean[1]	-	-	69%	73%
Timely Help 'Always' Received[1]	-	-	61%	68%
Would Definitely Recommend Hospital[1]	-	-	65%	71%
Use of Medical Imaging				
Cardiac Imaging Stress Test before Surgery[7]	-	-	5.8%	5.3%
Combination Abdominal CT Scan[7]	-	-	8.2%	10.5%
Combination Brain/Sinus CT Scan[7]	-	-	3.6%	2.7%
Combination Chest CT Scan[7]	-	-	1.3%	2.7%
Follow-up Mammogram/Ultrasound[7]	-	-	13%	8.8%
Lumbar Spine MRI for Low Back Pain[7]	-	-	33.4%	37.2%

Saint John's Riverside Hospital

976 North Broadway
Yonkers, NY 10701
Phone: 914-964-4444
URL: www.riversidehealth.org
Type: Acute Care Hospitals
Emergency Services: Yes
Ownership: Voluntary non-profit - Private
Beds: 407

Measure	Cases	This Hosp.	State Avg.	U.S. Avg.
Blood Clot Prevention and Treatment				
Anticoagulation Overlap Therapy[2]	78	73%	91%	93%
ICU Venous Thromboembolism Prophylaxis[2]	56	73%	92%	92%
Incidence of Potentially Preventable VTE[2]	15	60%	10%	10%
UFH with Dosages/Platelet Monitoring[2]	67	100%	92%	97%
Venous Thromboembolism Prophylaxis[2]	404	57%	87%	85%
Warfarin Therapy Discharge Instructions[2]	58	97%	59%	75%
Chest Pain/Possible Heart Attack Care				
Aspirin Given Within 24 Hours of Arrival[3]	22	100%	97%	96%
Fibrinolytic Meds Within 30 Min. of Arrival[3,7]	-	-	54%	58%
Average Time to ECG (minutes)[3]	21	8	9	7
Average Time to Transfer (minutes)[3]	13	74	78	60
Children's Asthma Care				
Received Home Management Plan of Care	-	-	-	88%
Received Reliever Medication	-	-	-	100%
Received Systemic Corticosteroids	-	-	-	100%
Emergency Department				
Admittance Decision Time (minutes)[2]	911	107	154	98
Head CT Results Within 45 Min. of Arrival	16	6%	55%	57%
Patients Who Left ER Before Being Seen	47,535	2%	2%	2%
Time from ER Arrival to Admit. (minutes)[2]	934	318	378	274
Time from ER Arrival to Discharge (minutes)	388	133	156	134
Time in ER Before Being Evaluated (minutes)	407	40	35	26
Time to Pain Meds for Fractures (minutes)	110	56	61	57
Heart Attack Care				
Aspirin Given at Discharge	41	100%	99%	99%
Fibrinolytic Meds Within 30 Min. of Arrival[7]	-	-	46%	54%
PCI Within 90 Minutes of Arrival[7]	-	-	95%	96%
Statin Prescribed at Discharge	41	100%	98%	98%
Heart Failure Care				
ACE Inhibitor or ARB for LVSD[2]	54	100%	96%	97%
Discharge Instructions Given[2]	198	100%	95%	94%
Evaluation of LVS Function[2]	265	100%	99%	99%
Medicare Spending				
Medicare Spending per Patient (ratio)	-	0.94	0.96	0.98
Pneumonia Care				
Appropriate Initial Antibiotic Given[2]	73	88%	95%	95%
Blood Culture Timing[2]	159	99%	97%	98%
Pregnancy and Delivery Care				
Newborn Deliveries Scheduled Early[2]	35	6%	4%	6%
Preventive Care				
Immunization for Influenza[2]	573	99%	88%	90%
Immunization for Pneumonia[2]	742	98%	88%	92%
Stroke Care				
Anticoagulation Therapy for Atrial Fibrillation[2]	12	83%	96%	95%
Antithrombotic Therapy Timing[2]	99	99%	98%	98%
Assessed for Rehabilitation[2]	94	87%	97%	97%
Discharged on Antithrombotic Therapy[2]	84	99%	99%	99%
Discharged on Statin Medication[2]	73	86%	95%	94%
Thrombolytic Therapy Timing[2]	29	17%	69%	66%
Venous Thromboembolism Prophylaxis[2]	121	69%	94%	94%
Written Stroke Educational Materials Given[2]	44	86%	86%	88%
Surgical Care Improvement Project				
Appropriate Beta Blocker Usage[2]	138	97%	97%	98%
Appropriate VTP Within 24 Hours[2]	372	97%	98%	98%
Controlled Postoperative Blood Glucose[2,7]	-	-	97%	97%
Perioperative Temperature Management[2]	461	97%	100%	100%
Prophylactic Antibiotic Selection[2]	318	97%	99%	99%
Prophylactic Antibiotic Selection (Outpatient)	76	93%	97%	98%
Prophylactic Antibiotic Stopped[2]	307	99%	98%	98%
Prophylactic Antibiotic Timing[2]	318	100%	99%	99%
Prophylactic Antibiotic Timing (Outpatient)	77	96%	97%	98%
Urinary Catheter Removal[2]	99	100%	96%	97%
Survey of Patients' Hospital Experiences				
Area Around Room 'Always' Quiet at Night	300+	59%	51%	61%
Doctors 'Always' Communicated Well	300+	82%	77%	82%
Home Recovery Information Given	300+	81%	83%	85%
Hospital Given 9 or 10 on 10 Point Scale	300+	68%	63%	71%
Meds 'Always' Explained Before Given	300+	63%	59%	64%
Nurses 'Always' Communicated Well	300+	80%	75%	79%
Pain 'Always' Well Controlled	300+	72%	67%	71%
Room and Bathroom 'Always' Clean	300+	82%	69%	73%
Timely Help 'Always' Received	300+	66%	61%	68%
Would Definitely Recommend Hospital	300+	73%	65%	71%
Use of Medical Imaging				
Cardiac Imaging Stress Test before Surgery	134	6.7%	5.8%	5.3%
Combination Abdominal CT Scan	725	10.1%	8.2%	10.5%
Combination Brain/Sinus CT Scan	634	3.2%	3.6%	2.7%
Combination Chest CT Scan	705	0.7%	1.3%	2.7%
Follow-up Mammogram/Ultrasound	1,694	18.9%	13%	8.8%
Lumbar Spine MRI for Low Back Pain	106	36.8%	33.4%	37.2%

Saint Joseph's Medical Center

127 South Broadway
Yonkers, NY 10701
Phone: 914-378-7000
Fax: 914-965-4838
URL: www.saintjosephs.org
Type: Acute Care Hospitals
Emergency Services: Yes
Ownership: Voluntary non-profit - Private
Beds: 194

Key Personnel:
Quality Assurance . . . . Francis Casola
Chief of Medical Staff . . . . Nicholas E DeRobertis
Coronary Care . . . . Melvyn Pleiberg
Pediatric Ambulatory Care . . . . . . Sami E Sayegh, MD
Pediatric In-Patient Care . . . . Sami E Sayegh, MD
President/CEO. . . . . Michael J Spicer, FACHE

Measure	Cases	This Hosp.	State Avg.	U.S. Avg.
Blood Clot Prevention and Treatment				
Anticoagulation Overlap Therapy[2]	26	92%	91%	93%
ICU Venous Thromboembolism Prophylaxis[2]	29	97%	92%	92%
Incidence of Potentially Preventable VTE[1,2]	-	-	10%	10%
UFH with Dosages/Platelet Monitoring[2]	27	100%	92%	97%
Venous Thromboembolism Prophylaxis[2]	345	88%	87%	85%
Warfarin Therapy Discharge Instructions[2]	16	100%	59%	75%
Chest Pain/Possible Heart Attack Care				
Aspirin Given Within 24 Hours of Arrival	37	100%	97%	96%
Fibrinolytic Meds Within 30 Min. of Arrival[7]	-	-	54%	58%
Average Time to ECG (minutes)	37	17	9	7
Average Time to Transfer (minutes)	13	125	78	60
Children's Asthma Care				
Received Home Management Plan of Care	-	-	-	88%
Received Reliever Medication	-	-	-	100%
Received Systemic Corticosteroids	-	-	-	100%
Emergency Department				
Admittance Decision Time (minutes)[2]	771	193	154	98
Head CT Results Within 45 Min. of Arrival[1]	-	-	55%	57%
Patients Who Left ER Before Being Seen	39,611	3%	2%	2%
Time from ER Arrival to Admit. (minutes)[2]	779	434	378	274
Time from ER Arrival to Discharge (minutes)	297	124	156	134
Time in ER Before Being Evaluated (minutes)	362	52	35	26
Time to Pain Meds for Fractures (minutes)	26	84	61	57
Heart Attack Care				
Aspirin Given at Discharge	12	92%	99%	99%
Fibrinolytic Meds Within 30 Min. of Arrival[7]	-	-	46%	54%
PCI Within 90 Minutes of Arrival[7]	-	-	95%	96%
Statin Prescribed at Discharge	13	92%	98%	98%
Heart Failure Care				
ACE Inhibitor or ARB for LVSD	62	95%	96%	97%
Discharge Instructions Given	118	98%	95%	94%
Evaluation of LVS Function	183	100%	99%	99%
Medicare Spending				
Medicare Spending per Patient (ratio)	-	1.04	0.96	0.98
Pneumonia Care				
Appropriate Initial Antibiotic Given	57	100%	95%	95%
Blood Culture Timing	86	98%	97%	98%
Pregnancy and Delivery Care				
Newborn Deliveries Scheduled Early[7]	-	-	4%	6%
Preventive Care				
Immunization for Influenza[2]	521	95%	88%	90%
Immunization for Pneumonia[2]	671	94%	88%	92%
Stroke Care				
Anticoagulation Therapy for Atrial Fibrillation[1,2]	-	-	96%	95%
Antithrombotic Therapy Timing[2]	35	100%	98%	98%
Assessed for Rehabilitation[2]	38	100%	97%	97%
Discharged on Antithrombotic Therapy[2]	34	100%	99%	99%
Discharged on Statin Medication[2]	27	93%	95%	94%
Thrombolytic Therapy Timing[1,2]	-	-	69%	66%
Venous Thromboembolism Prophylaxis[2]	40	95%	94%	94%
Written Stroke Educational Materials Given[2]	17	94%	86%	88%
Surgical Care Improvement Project				
Appropriate Beta Blocker Usage	25	100%	97%	98%
Appropriate VTP Within 24 Hours	121	100%	98%	98%
Controlled Postoperative Blood Glucose[7]	-	-	97%	97%
Perioperative Temperature Management	132	100%	100%	100%
Prophylactic Antibiotic Selection	76	99%	99%	99%
Prophylactic Antibiotic Selection (Outpatient)	41	90%	97%	98%
Prophylactic Antibiotic Stopped	73	100%	98%	98%
Prophylactic Antibiotic Timing	76	97%	99%	99%
Prophylactic Antibiotic Timing (Outpatient)	41	100%	97%	98%
Urinary Catheter Removal[1]	-	-	96%	97%
Survey of Patients' Hospital Experiences				
Area Around Room 'Always' Quiet at Night	300+	46%	51%	61%
Doctors 'Always' Communicated Well	300+	75%	77%	82%
Home Recovery Information Given	300+	81%	83%	85%
Hospital Given 9 or 10 on 10 Point Scale	300+	51%	63%	71%

NOTE: Hospital profiles are in alphabetical order by state, then city, then hospital within the city; Rankings exclude hospitals with less than 25 cases except for patient surveys which excludes hospitals with less than 100 cases; (a) 100-299 cases; (1) The number of cases/patients is too few to report; (2) Data submitted were based on a sample of cases/patients; (3) Results are based on a shorter time period than required; (4) Data suppressed by CMS for one or more quarters; (5) Results are not available for this reporting period; (6) Fewer than 100 patients completed the HCAHPS survey; (7) No cases met the criteria for this measure; (8) The lower limit of the confidence interval cannot be calculated if the number of observed infections equals zero; (9) No data are available from the state/territory for this reporting period; (10) The scores shown reflect fewer than 50 completed surveys; (11) There were discrepancies in the data collection process; (12) This measure does not apply to this hospital for this reporting period; (13) Results cannot be calculated for this reporting period; (14) The results for this state are combined with nearby states to protect confidentiality; Please refer to the User's Guide for a full explanation of data.

Meds 'Always' Explained Before Given	300+	53%	59%	64%
Nurses 'Always' Communicated Well	300+	70%	75%	79%
Pain 'Always' Well Controlled	300+	52%	67%	71%
Room and Bathroom 'Always' Clean	300+	68%	69%	73%
Timely Help 'Always' Received	300+	48%	61%	68%
Would Definitely Recommend Hospital	300+	53%	65%	71%
Use of Medical Imaging				
Cardiac Imaging Stress Test before Surgery	64	4.7%	5.8%	5.3%
Combination Abdominal CT Scan	259	13.5%	8.2%	10.5%
Combination Brain/Sinus CT Scan	350	1.7%	3.6%	2.7%
Combination Chest CT Scan	128	0.8%	1.3%	2.7%
Follow-up Mammogram/Ultrasound	435	15.4%	13%	8.8%
Lumbar Spine MRI for Low Back Pain[1]	-	-	33.4%	37.2%

NOTE: Hospital profiles are in alphabetical order by state, then city, then hospital within the city; Rankings exclude hospitals with less than 25 cases except for patient surveys which excludes hospitals with less than 100 cases; (a) 100-299 cases; (1) The number of cases/patients is too few to report; (2) Data submitted were based on a sample of cases/patients; (3) Results are based on a shorter time period than required; (4) Data suppressed by CMS for one or more quarters; (5) Results are not available for this reporting period; (6) Fewer than 100 patients completed the HCAHPS survey; (7) No cases met the criteria for this measure; (8) The lower limit of the confidence interval cannot be calculated if the number of observed infections equals zero; (9) No data are available from the state/territory for this reporting period; (10) The scores shown reflect fewer than 50 completed surveys; (11) There were discrepancies in the data collection process; (12) This measure does not apply to this hospital for this reporting period; (13) Results cannot be calculated for this reporting period; (14) The results for this state are combined with nearby states to protect confidentiality; Please refer to the User's Guide for a full explanation of data.

Blood Clot Prevention and Treatment

Anticoagulation Overlap Therapy

Hospital Name	City	Rate	Cases
Carolinas Medical Center - University[2]	Charlotte	100%	53
Duke Regional Hospital[2]	Durham	100%	96
Duke University Hospital[2]	Durham	100%	153
Hugh Chatham Memorial Hospital[2]	Elkin	100%	31
Medwest Haywood[2]	Clyde	100%	46
Northern Hospital of Surry County[2]	Mount Airy	100%	34
Novant Health Brunswick Medical Center[2]	Supply	100%	27
Novant Health Forsyth Medical Center[2]	Winston-Salem	100%	235
Novant Health Huntersville Medical Center[2]	Huntersville	100%	41
Novant Health Rowan Medical Center[2]	Salisbury	100%	42
Onslow Memorial Hospital[2]	Jacksonville	100%	27
Stanly Regional Medical Center[2]	Albemarle	100%	25
Wakemed - Cary Hospital[2]	Cary	100%	87
Wakemed - Raleigh Campus[2]	Raleigh	100%	169
Wayne Memorial Hospital[2]	Goldsboro	100%	57
Wilkes Regional Medical Center[2]	N Wilkesboro	100%	27
Carolinas Medical Center - Northeast[2]	Concord	99%	180
Caromont Regional Medical Center[2]	Gastonia	99%	136
High Point Regional Hospital[2]	High Point	99%	86
Novant Health Presbyterian Medical Center[2]	Charlotte	99%	140
Rex Hospital[2]	Raleigh	99%	125
Cape Fear Valley Medical Center[2]	Fayetteville	98%	205
Carolinas Med Ctr/Behaviorial Health[2]	Charlotte	98%	220
Frye Regional Medical Center[2]	Hickory	98%	85
Lake Norman Regional Medical Center[2]	Mooresville	98%	53
Mem Mission Hosp & Asheville Surg Ctr[2]	Asheville	98%	250
University of North Carolina Hospital[2]	Chapel Hill	98%	116
The Moses H Cone Memorial Hospital[2]	Greensboro	97%	284
Presbyterian Hospital Matthews[2]	Matthews	97%	69
Medwest Harris[2]	Sylva	96%	27
North Carolina Baptist Hospital[2]	Winston-Salem	96%	251
Vidant Medical Center[2]	Greenville	96%	193
Watauga Medical Center[2]	Boone	96%	27
Caldwell Memorial Hospital[2]	Lenoir	95%	39
Carolina East Medical Center[2]	New Bern	95%	64
Carolinas Medical Center - Pineville[2]	Charlotte	95%	148
Duke Health Raleigh Hospital[2]	Raleigh	95%	65
Maria Parham Medical Center[2]	Henderson	95%	44
Nash General Hospital[2]	Rocky Mount	95%	78
New Hanover Regional Medical Center[2]	Wilmington	95%	170
Randolph Hospital[2]	Asheboro	95%	42
Wilson Medical Center[2]	Wilson	95%	41
Carolinas Medical Center - Lincoln[2]	Lincolnton	94%	36
Scotland Memorial Hospital[2]	Laurinburg	94%	36
Johnston Memorial Hospital[2]	Smithfield	91%	43
Catawba Valley Medical Center[2]	Hickory	90%	30
Lenoir Memorial Hospital[2]	Kinston	90%	68
Carolinas Medical Center - Union[2]	Monroe	89%	36
Margaret R Pardee Memorial Hospital[2]	Hendersonville	89%	65
Carteret General Hospital[2]	Morehead City	88%	49
Columbus Regional Healthcare System[2]	Whiteville	87%	30
Firsthealth Moore Regional Hospital[2]	Pinehurst	87%	170
Cleveland Regional Medical Center[2]	Shelby	85%	60
Iredell Memorial Hospital[2]	Statesville	81%	59
CMC - Blue Ridge[2]	Morganton	80%	75
Southeastern Regional Medical Center[2]	Lumberton	75%	122
Albemarle Hospital Authority[2]	Elizabeth City	73%	45
Betsy Johnson Regional Hospital[2]	Dunn	71%	35
Halifax Regional Medical Center[2]	Roanoke Rapids	65%	49
Alamance Regional Medical Center[2]	Burlington	62%	56

ICU Venous Thromboembolism Prophylaxis

Hospital Name	City	Rate	Cases
Davis Regional Medical Center[2]	Statesville	100%	69
Hugh Chatham Memorial Hospital[2]	Elkin	100%	110
Northern Hospital of Surry County[2]	Mount Airy	100%	62
Novant Health Brunswick Medical Center[2]	Supply	100%	50
Novant Health Forsyth Medical Center[2]	Winston-Salem	100%	199
Novant Health Franklin Medical Center[2]	Louisburg	100%	36
Novant Health Presbyterian Medical Center[2]	Charlotte	100%	44
Novant Health Thomasville Medical Center[2]	Thomasville	100%	105
Stanly Regional Medical Center[2]	Albemarle	100%	86
Vidant Medical Center[2]	Greenville	100%	79
Wakemed - Cary Hospital[2]	Cary	100%	34
Wakemed - Raleigh Campus[2]	Raleigh	100%	126
Catawba Valley Medical Center[2]	Hickory	99%	79
Wilkes Regional Medical Center[2]	N Wilkesboro	99%	126
Carolinas Medical Center - Lincoln[2]	Lincolnton	98%	114
Carolinas Medical Center - University[2]	Charlotte	98%	61
Frye Regional Medical Center[2]	Hickory	98%	125
The Mcdowell Hospital[2]	Marion	98%	48
Nash General Hospital[2]	Rocky Mount	98%	54
Scotland Memorial Hospital[2]	Laurinburg	98%	45
Carolinas Medical Center - Northeast[2]	Concord	97%	61
Carolinas Medical Center - Union[2]	Monroe	97%	58
Columbus Regional Healthcare System[2]	Whiteville	97%	75
Lake Norman Regional Medical Center[2]	Mooresville	97%	59
Margaret R Pardee Memorial Hospital[2]	Hendersonville	97%	37
Medwest Harris[2]	Sylva	97%	35
The Moses H Cone Memorial Hospital[2]	Greensboro	97%	116
Presbyterian Hospital Matthews[2]	Matthews	97%	35
Vidant Beaufort Hospital[2]	Washington	97%	31
Angel Medical Center[2]	Franklin	96%	55
Cape Fear Valley Medical Center[2]	Fayetteville	96%	56
Carolinas Med Ctr/Behaviorial Health[2]	Charlotte	96%	170
Novant Health Huntersville Medical Center[2]	Huntersville	96%	45
Novant Health Rowan Medical Center[2]	Salisbury	96%	81
Onslow Memorial Hospital[2]	Jacksonville	96%	46
Vidant Duplin Hospital[2]	Kenansville	96%	83
Carolinas Medical Center - Pineville[2]	Charlotte	95%	151
Duke Health Raleigh Hospital[2]	Raleigh	95%	80
Halifax Regional Medical Center[2]	Roanoke Rapids	95%	81
New Hanover Regional Medical Center[2]	Wilmington	95%	87
North Carolina Baptist Hospital[2]	Winston-Salem	95%	115
Spruce Pine Community Hospital[2]	Spruce Pine	95%	56
Vidant Roanoke Chowan Hospital[2]	Ahoskie	95%	85
Duke University Hospital[2]	Durham	94%	101
Johnston Memorial Hospital[2]	Smithfield	94%	52
Lexington Memorial Hospital[2]	Lexington	94%	54
Martin General Hospital[2]	Williamston	94%	71
Medwest Haywood[2]	Clyde	94%	54
Vidant Edgecombe Hospital[2]	Tarboro	94%	65
Caldwell Memorial Hospital[2]	Lenoir	93%	110
Duke Regional Hospital[2]	Durham	93%	44
Kings Mountain Hospital[2]	Kings Mountain	93%	61
Person Memorial Hospital[2]	Roxboro	93%	55
Carolina East Medical Center[2]	New Bern	91%	75
Caromont Regional Medical Center[2]	Gastonia	91%	64
Carteret General Hospital[2]	Morehead City	91%	55
Cleveland Regional Medical Center[2]	Shelby	91%	110
Rex Hospital[2]	Raleigh	91%	68
University of North Carolina Hospital[2]	Chapel Hill	91%	56
High Point Regional Hospital[2]	High Point	90%	51
Mem Mission Hosp & Asheville Surg Ctr[2]	Asheville	90%	84
Park Ridge Health[2]	Hendersonville	90%	39
Iredell Memorial Hospital[2]	Statesville	89%	104
Murphy Medical Center[2]	Murphy	89%	111
Watauga Medical Center[2]	Boone	89%	105
CMC - Blue Ridge[2]	Morganton	87%	99
Firsthealth Moore Regional Hospital[2]	Pinehurst	87%	85
Maria Parham Medical Center[2]	Henderson	87%	60
Albemarle Hospital Authority[2]	Elizabeth City	86%	90
Central Carolina Hospital[2]	Sanford	86%	65
Wayne Memorial Hospital[2]	Goldsboro	86%	35
Sandhills Regional Medical Center[2]	Hamlet	85%	46
Randolph Hospital[2]	Asheboro	84%	75
Sampson Regional Medical Center[2]	Clinton	82%	56
Alamance Regional Medical Center[2]	Burlington	81%	75
Rutherford Hospital[2]	Rutherfordton	81%	68
Lenoir Memorial Hospital[2]	Kinston	80%	79
Morehead Memorial Hospital[2]	Eden	79%	72
Wilson Medical Center[2]	Wilson	77%	57
Southeastern Regional Medical Center[2]	Lumberton	75%	32
Betsy Johnson Regional Hospital[2]	Dunn	73%	71
Granville Health Systems[2]	Oxford	68%	139

Incidence of Potentially Preventable VTE

Hospital Name	City	Rate	Cases
Novant Health Forsyth Medical Center[2]	Winston-Salem	0%	64
New Hanover Regional Medical Center[2]	Wilmington	2%	50
Vidant Medical Center[2]	Greenville	3%	64
Duke Health Raleigh Hospital[2]	Raleigh	4%	25
University of North Carolina Hospital[2]	Chapel Hill	4%	56
Novant Health Presbyterian Medical Center[2]	Charlotte	6%	32
Nash General Hospital[2]	Rocky Mount	7%	30
The Moses H Cone Memorial Hospital[2]	Greensboro	10%	52
North Carolina Baptist Hospital[2]	Winston-Salem	10%	69
Carolinas Med Ctr/Behaviorial Health[2]	Charlotte	12%	77
Duke University Hospital[2]	Durham	12%	82
Carolinas Medical Center - Pineville[2]	Charlotte	13%	30
Carolinas Medical Center - Northeast[2]	Concord	15%	46
Cape Fear Valley Medical Center[2]	Fayetteville	18%	38
Mem Mission Hosp & Asheville Surg Ctr[2]	Asheville	18%	50
Firsthealth Moore Regional Hospital[2]	Pinehurst	21%	34

UFH with Dosages/Platelet Count Monitoring

Hospital Name	City	Rate	Cases
Cape Fear Valley Medical Center[2]	Fayetteville	100%	38
Carolina East Medical Center[2]	New Bern	100%	25
Carolinas Medical Center - Northeast[2]	Concord	100%	154
Carolinas Medical Center - Pineville[2]	Charlotte	100%	88
Carolinas Med Ctr/Behaviorial Health[2]	Charlotte	100%	155
Caromont Regional Medical Center[2]	Gastonia	100%	80
Cleveland Regional Medical Center[2]	Shelby	100%	35
Duke Regional Hospital[2]	Durham	100%	51
Firsthealth Moore Regional Hospital[2]	Pinehurst	100%	66
Frye Regional Medical Center[2]	Hickory	100%	38
Halifax Regional Medical Center[2]	Roanoke Rapids	100%	25
High Point Regional Hospital[2]	High Point	100%	47
Lenoir Memorial Hospital[2]	Kinston	100%	37
Mem Mission Hosp & Asheville Surg Ctr[2]	Asheville	100%	126
The Moses H Cone Memorial Hospital[2]	Greensboro	100%	227
Novant Health Forsyth Medical Center[2]	Winston-Salem	100%	72
Novant Health Presbyterian Medical Center[2]	Charlotte	100%	97
Novant Health Rowan Medical Center[2]	Salisbury	100%	25
Presbyterian Hospital Matthews[2]	Matthews	100%	58
Rex Hospital[2]	Raleigh	100%	37
Southeastern Regional Medical Center[2]	Lumberton	100%	60
University of North Carolina Hospital[2]	Chapel Hill	100%	152
Vidant Medical Center[2]	Greenville	100%	163
Wakemed - Raleigh Campus[2]	Raleigh	100%	94
North Carolina Baptist Hospital[2]	Winston-Salem	99%	194
Albemarle Hospital Authority[2]	Elizabeth City	97%	38
Wilson Medical Center[2]	Wilson	96%	26
New Hanover Regional Medical Center[2]	Wilmington	95%	39
Alamance Regional Medical Center[2]	Burlington	80%	54
Duke University Hospital[2]	Durham	51%	174
Caldwell Memorial Hospital[2]	Lenoir	47%	43

Venous Thromboembolism Prophylaxis

Hospital Name	City	Rate	Cases
North Carolina Specialty Hospital[2]	Durham	100%	353
Novant Health Forsyth Medical Center[2]	Winston-Salem	100%	617
Novant Health Park Hospital[2]	Winston-Salem	100%	55
Davis Regional Medical Center[2]	Statesville	99%	207
The Mcdowell Hospital[2]	Marion	99%	174
Stanly Regional Medical Center[2]	Albemarle	99%	239
Wilkes Regional Medical Center[2]	N Wilkesboro	99%	274
Northern Hospital of Surry County[2]	Mount Airy	98%	336
Novant Health Franklin Medical Center[2]	Louisburg	98%	165
Presbyterian Hospital Matthews[2]	Matthews	98%	444
Vidant Medical Center[2]	Greenville	98%	360
Martin General Hospital[2]	Williamston	97%	204
Medwest Swain[2,3]	Bryson City	97%	34
Novant Health Brunswick Medical Center[2]	Supply	97%	342
Transylvania Regional Hospital[2]	Brevard	97%	189
Carolinas Medical Center - University[2]	Charlotte	96%	329
Medwest Haywood[2]	Clyde	96%	326
Novant Health Charlotte Ortho Hosp[2]	Charlotte	96%	206
Carolinas Medical Center - Union[2]	Monroe	95%	333
Lexington Memorial Hospital[2]	Lexington	95%	206
The Moses H Cone Memorial Hospital[2]	Greensboro	95%	1015
Carolinas Medical Center - Lincoln[2]	Lincolnton	94%	249
Carolinas Medical Center - Pineville[2]	Charlotte	94%	509
Caromont Regional Medical Center[2]	Gastonia	94%	351
Medwest Harris[2]	Sylva	94%	188
Novant Health Huntersville Medical Center[2]	Huntersville	94%	352
Park Ridge Health[2]	Hendersonville	94%	217
Person Memorial Hospital[2]	Roxboro	94%	164
Sampson Regional Medical Center[2]	Clinton	94%	255
Caldwell Memorial Hospital[2]	Lenoir	93%	246
Cape Fear Valley Medical Center[2]	Fayetteville	93%	383
Cherokee Indian Hospital Authority	Cherokee	93%	70
Duke Health Raleigh Hospital[2]	Raleigh	93%	306
Novant Health Rowan Medical Center[2]	Salisbury	93%	319
Novant Health Thomasville Medical Center[2]	Thomasville	93%	163
Onslow Memorial Hospital[2]	Jacksonville	93%	402
Hugh Chatham Memorial Hospital[2]	Elkin	92%	255
Novant Health Presbyterian Medical Center[2]	Charlotte	92%	366
Spruce Pine Community Hospital[2]	Spruce Pine	92%	135
Vidant Duplin Hospital[2]	Kenansville	92%	128
Vidant Edgecombe Hospital[2]	Tarboro	92%	307
Anson Community Hospital[2]	Wadesboro	91%	188
CMC - Blue Ridge[2]	Morganton	91%	456
Duke Regional Hospital[2]	Durham	91%	344
Frye Regional Medical Center[2]	Hickory	91%	322
Nash General Hospital[2]	Rocky Mount	91%	359
Rex Hospital[2]	Raleigh	91%	299
Angel Medical Center[2]	Franklin	90%	174
Catawba Valley Medical Center[2]	Hickory	90%	304
Halifax Regional Medical Center[2]	Roanoke Rapids	89%	489
High Point Regional Hospital[2]	High Point	89%	313
Murphy Medical Center[2]	Murphy	89%	254
Randolph Hospital[2]	Asheboro	89%	394
Scotland Memorial Hospital[2]	Laurinburg	89%	364
Carolinas Medical Center - Northeast[2]	Concord	88%	327
Carolinas Med Ctr/Behaviorial Health[2]	Charlotte	88%	272
J Arthur Dosher Memorial Hospital[2,3]	Southport	88%	69
Lake Norman Regional Medical Center[2]	Mooresville	88%	293
New Hanover Regional Medical Center[2]	Wilmington	88%	326
Vidant Roanoke Chowan Hospital[2]	Ahoskie	88%	233
Wakemed - Raleigh Campus[2]	Raleigh	88%	344
Central Carolina Hospital[2]	Sanford	87%	341
Cleveland Regional Medical Center[2]	Shelby	87%	296
North Carolina Baptist Hospital[2]	Winston-Salem	87%	312
Vidant Beaufort Hospital[2]	Washington	87%	211
Watauga Medical Center[2]	Boone	87%	245

NOTE: Hospital profiles are in alphabetical order by state, then city, then hospital within the city; Rankings exclude hospitals with less than 25 cases except for patient surveys which excludes hospitals with less than 100 cases; (a) 100-299 cases; (1) The number of cases/patients is too few to report; (2) Data submitted were based on a sample of cases/patients; (3) Results are based on a shorter time period than required; (4) Data suppressed by CMS for one or more quarters; (5) Results are not available for this reporting period; (6) Fewer than 100 patients completed the HCAHPS survey; (7) No cases met the criteria for this measure; (8) The lower limit of the confidence interval cannot be calculated if the number of observed infections equals zero; (9) No data are available from the state/territory for this reporting period; (10) The scores shown reflect fewer than 50 completed surveys; (11) There were discrepancies in the data collection process; (12) This measure does not apply to this hospital for this reporting period; (13) Results cannot be calculated for this reporting period; (14) The results for this state are combined with nearby states to protect confidentiality; Please refer to the User's Guide for a full explanation of data.

Carteret General Hospital[2]	Morehead City	86%	338
Columbus Regional Healthcare System[2]	Whiteville	86%	357
Margaret R Pardee Memorial Hospital[2]	Hendersonville	86%	362
Wakemed - Cary Hospital[2]	Cary	86%	370
Mem Mission Hosp & Asheville Surg Ctr[2]	Asheville	85%	352
Duke University Hospital[2]	Durham	84%	348
Iredell Memorial Hospital[2]	Statesville	84%	353
Southeastern Regional Medical Center[2]	Lumberton	83%	370
Carolina East Medical Center[2]	New Bern	82%	332
Johnston Memorial Hospital[2]	Smithfield	82%	300
Firsthealth Moore Regional Hospital[2]	Pinehurst	81%	316
Rutherford Hospital[2]	Rutherfordton	81%	325
Kings Mountain Hospital[2]	Kings Mountain	79%	129
Albemarle Hospital Authority[2]	Elizabeth City	78%	418
Wilson Medical Center[2]	Wilson	78%	391
Maria Parham Medical Center[2]	Henderson	76%	416
Morehead Memorial Hospital[2]	Eden	76%	391
Wayne Memorial Hospital[2]	Goldsboro	74%	363
Alamance Regional Medical Center[2]	Burlington	73%	324
University of North Carolina Hospital[2]	Chapel Hill	73%	310
Granville Health Systems[2]	Oxford	62%	502
Betsy Johnson Regional Hospital[2]	Dunn	61%	475
Lenoir Memorial Hospital[2]	Kinston	61%	384
Sandhills Regional Medical Center[2]	Hamlet	56%	162

Warfarin Therapy Discharge Instructions

Hospital Name	City	Rate	Cases
Carolina East Medical Center[2]	New Bern	100%	51
Hugh Chatham Memorial Hospital[2]	Elkin	100%	27
Novant Health Forsyth Medical Center[2]	Winston-Salem	100%	204
Wakemed - Cary Hospital[2]	Cary	100%	59
Wakemed - Raleigh Campus[2]	Raleigh	100%	126
Cape Fear Valley Medical Center[2]	Fayetteville	99%	160
Wayne Memorial Hospital[2]	Goldsboro	98%	41
Firsthealth Moore Regional Hospital[2]	Pinehurst	97%	126
Margaret R Pardee Memorial Hospital[2]	Hendersonville	97%	37
Scotland Memorial Hospital[2]	Laurinburg	97%	30
Caromont Regional Medical Center[2]	Gastonia	95%	105
Frye Regional Medical Center[2]	Hickory	95%	66
Mem Mission Hosp & Asheville Surg Ctr[2]	Asheville	95%	177
Nash General Hospital[2]	Rocky Mount	95%	42
North Carolina Baptist Hospital[2]	Winston-Salem	95%	212
Carolinas Medical Center - Pineville[2]	Charlotte	92%	110
High Point Regional Hospital[2]	High Point	92%	62
Halifax Regional Medical Center[2]	Roanoke Rapids	91%	35
Novant Health Huntersville Medical Center[2]	Huntersville	91%	35
Rex Hospital[2]	Raleigh	91%	96
Cleveland Regional Medical Center[2]	Shelby	90%	50
Duke University Hospital[2]	Durham	90%	101
Lake Norman Regional Medical Center[2]	Mooresville	90%	39
The Moses H Cone Memorial Hospital[2]	Greensboro	90%	214
Southeastern Regional Medical Center[2]	Lumberton	90%	86
Albemarle Hospital Authority[2]	Elizabeth City	88%	32
Medwest Haywood[2]	Clyde	88%	33
Duke Regional Hospital[2]	Durham	85%	73
Novant Health Rowan Medical Center[2]	Salisbury	84%	25
Carolinas Medical Center - Northeast[2]	Concord	83%	144
Carolinas Medical Center - University[2]	Charlotte	82%	51
Presbyterian Hospital Matthews[2]	Matthews	79%	53
CMC - Blue Ridge[2]	Morganton	78%	54
Carolinas Medical Center - Lincoln[2]	Lincolnton	76%	29
Iredell Memorial Hospital[2]	Statesville	74%	46
Wilson Medical Center[2]	Wilson	70%	30
Duke Health Raleigh Hospital[2]	Raleigh	68%	50
Novant Health Presbyterian Medical Center[2]	Charlotte	66%	94
University of North Carolina Hospital[2]	Chapel Hill	64%	91
Johnston Memorial Hospital[2]	Smithfield	63%	27
Lenoir Memorial Hospital[2]	Kinston	59%	46
Maria Parham Medical Center[2]	Henderson	55%	31
Carteret General Hospital[2]	Morehead City	44%	32
Carolinas Med Ctr/Behavioral Health[2]	Charlotte	43%	169
Vidant Medical Center[2]	Greenville	30%	122
New Hanover Regional Medical Center[2]	Wilmington	27%	117
Alamance Regional Medical Center[2]	Burlington	11%	37

Chest Pain/Possible Heart Attack Care

Aspirin Given Within 24 Hours of Arrival

Hospital Name	City	Rate	Cases
Caldwell Memorial Hospital	Lenoir	100%	75
Carolinas Medical Center - Pineville	Charlotte	100%	25
Carolinas Medical Center - University	Charlotte	100%	65
Central Carolina Hospital	Sanford	100%	66
Cleveland Regional Medical Center	Shelby	100%	132
Firsthealth Montgomery Memorial Hospital	Troy	100%	43
Granville Health Systems	Oxford	100%	44
Johnston Memorial Hospital	Smithfield	100%	178
Lake Norman Regional Medical Center	Mooresville	100%	40
Margaret R Pardee Memorial Hospital	Hendersonville	100%	60
Novant Health Franklin Medical Center	Louisburg	100%	60
Novant Health Thomasville Medical Center	Thomasville	100%	35
Person Memorial Hospital	Roxboro	100%	56
Presbyterian Hospital Matthews	Matthews	100%	42
Scotland Memorial Hospital	Laurinburg	100%	28
Vidant Beaufort Hospital	Washington	100%	45
Wakemed - Cary Hospital	Cary	100%	171
Watauga Medical Center	Boone	100%	47
Wilkes Regional Medical Center	N Wilkesboro	100%	90
Carolinas Medical Center - Lincoln	Lincolnton	99%	136
Hugh Chatham Memorial Hospital	Elkin	99%	159
Lexington Memorial Hospital	Lexington	99%	105
Nash General Hospital	Rocky Mount	99%	225
Northern Hospital of Surry County	Mount Airy	99%	132
Spruce Pine Community Hospital	Spruce Pine	99%	75
Vidant Duplin Hospital	Kenansville	99%	84
Alamance Regional Medical Center	Burlington	98%	53
Betsy Johnson Regional Hospital	Dunn	98%	173
CMC - Blue Ridge	Morganton	98%	88
Martin General Hospital	Williamston	98%	43
Morehead Memorial Hospital	Eden	98%	105
Murphy Medical Center	Murphy	98%	107
Novant Health Brunswick Medical Center	Supply	98%	48
Randolph Hospital	Asheboro	98%	94
Vidant Edgecombe Hospital	Tarboro	98%	86
Vidant Roanoke Chowan Hospital	Ahoskie	98%	46
Wakemed - Raleigh Campus	Raleigh	98%	84
Catawba Valley Medical Center	Hickory	97%	33
Columbus Regional Healthcare System	Whiteville	97%	86
Iredell Memorial Hospital	Statesville	97%	59
Maria Parham Medical Center	Henderson	97%	97
Medwest Haywood	Clyde	97%	60
Novant Health Huntersville Medical Center	Huntersville	97%	36
Park Ridge Health	Hendersonville	97%	30
Wayne Memorial Hospital	Goldsboro	97%	280
Carolinas Medical Center - Union	Monroe	96%	208
Kings Mountain Hospital	Kings Mountain	96%	53
The Mcdowell Hospital	Marion	96%	71
Rutherford Hospital	Rutherfordton	96%	101
Transylvania Regional Hospital	Brevard	96%	46
Albemarle Hospital Authority	Elizabeth City	95%	63
Anson Community Hospital	Wadesboro	95%	79
Onslow Memorial Hospital	Jacksonville	95%	151
Vidant Chowan Hospital	Edenton	95%	83
Angel Medical Center	Franklin	94%	48
Ashe Memorial Hospital	Jefferson	94%	77
Halifax Regional Medical Center	Roanoke Rapids	94%	229
Lenoir Memorial Hospital	Kinston	94%	64
Stanly Regional Medical Center	Albemarle	94%	72
Carteret General Hospital	Morehead City	93%	68
Sampson Regional Medical Center	Clinton	91%	202
Wilson Medical Center	Wilson	90%	78
J Arthur Dosher Memorial Hospital	Southport	86%	50

Fibrinolytic Meds Within 30 Minutes of Arrival

Hospital Name	City	Rate	Cases
Nash General Hospital	Rocky Mount	90%	29
Wayne Memorial Hospital	Goldsboro	83%	35

Average Time to ECG (minutes)

Hospital Name	City	Min.	Cases
Novant Health Brunswick Medical Center	Supply	0	50
Person Memorial Hospital	Roxboro	0	57
Novant Health Franklin Medical Center	Louisburg	1	64
Stanly Regional Medical Center	Albemarle	1	79
Johnston Memorial Hospital	Smithfield	2	183
Novant Health Huntersville Medical Center	Huntersville	2	36
Lenoir Memorial Hospital	Kinston	3	67
Novant Health Thomasville Medical Center	Thomasville	3	37
Presbyterian Hospital Matthews	Matthews	3	42
Carolinas Medical Center - Lincoln	Lincolnton	4	138
Carolinas Medical Center - Union	Monroe	4	213
Central Carolina Hospital	Sanford	4	70
Iredell Memorial Hospital	Statesville	4	64
J Arthur Dosher Memorial Hospital	Southport	4	50
Albemarle Hospital Authority	Elizabeth City	5	66
Carolinas Medical Center - Pineville	Charlotte	5	25
Carolinas Medical Center - University	Charlotte	5	67
Halifax Regional Medical Center	Roanoke Rapids	5	236
Margaret R Pardee Memorial Hospital	Hendersonville	5	61
Wakemed - Cary Hospital	Cary	5	175
Wilkes Regional Medical Center	N Wilkesboro	5	97
Cleveland Regional Medical Center	Shelby	6	135
Hugh Chatham Memorial Hospital	Elkin	6	170
Lake Norman Regional Medical Center	Mooresville	6	40
The Mcdowell Hospital	Marion	6	70
Murphy Medical Center	Murphy	6	110
Spruce Pine Community Hospital	Spruce Pine	6	78
Transylvania Regional Hospital	Brevard	6	47
Wakemed - Raleigh Campus	Raleigh	6	91
Watauga Medical Center	Boone	6	50
Anson Community Hospital	Wadesboro	7	83
Betsy Johnson Regional Hospital	Dunn	7	195
Columbus Regional Healthcare System	Whiteville	7	88
Kings Mountain Hospital	Kings Mountain	7	54
Morehead Memorial Hospital	Eden	7	105
Wayne Memorial Hospital	Goldsboro	7	292
Caldwell Memorial Hospital	Lenoir	8	78
Carteret General Hospital	Morehead City	8	69
CMC - Blue Ridge	Morganton	8	88
Martin General Hospital	Williamston	8	44
Nash General Hospital	Rocky Mount	8	231
Randolph Hospital	Asheboro	8	93
Rutherford Hospital	Rutherfordton	8	104
Scotland Memorial Hospital	Laurinburg	8	29
Alamance Regional Medical Center	Burlington	9	53
Catawba Valley Medical Center	Hickory	9	32
Firsthealth Montgomery Memorial Hospital	Troy	9	44
Vidant Duplin Hospital	Kenansville	9	87
Maria Parham Medical Center	Henderson	10	101
Northern Hospital of Surry County	Mount Airy	10	141
Onslow Memorial Hospital	Jacksonville	10	154
Sampson Regional Medical Center	Clinton	10	205
Vidant Chowan Hospital	Edenton	10	87
Ashe Memorial Hospital	Jefferson	11	78
Lexington Memorial Hospital	Lexington	11	104
Medwest Haywood	Clyde	11	60
Vidant Beaufort Hospital	Washington	11	47
Granville Health Systems	Oxford	12	47
Vidant Roanoke Chowan Hospital	Ahoskie	12	48
Wilson Medical Center	Wilson	12	81
Angel Medical Center	Franklin	13	51
Vidant Edgecombe Hospital	Tarboro	16	92

Average Time to Transfer (minutes)

Hospital Name	City	Min.	Cases
Caldwell Memorial Hospital	Lenoir	36	25
CMC - Blue Ridge	Morganton	36	31
Cleveland Regional Medical Center	Shelby	37	29
Wakemed - Cary Hospital	Cary	44	30
Carolinas Medical Center - Union	Monroe	46	48
Carolinas Medical Center - Lincoln	Lincolnton	48	26

Children's Asthma Care

Received Home Management Plan of Care

Hospital Name	City	Rate	Cases
Carolinas Med Ctr/Behavioral Health	Charlotte	97%	359
Novant Health Presbyterian Medical Center	Charlotte	97%	159
Carolinas Medical Center - Northeast	Concord	95%	87
Wilson Medical Center	Wilson	92%	26
Firsthealth Moore Regional Hospital	Pinehurst	89%	55
Mem Mission Hosp & Asheville Surg Ctr	Asheville	83%	58
North Carolina Baptist Hospital	Winston-Salem	66%	195

Received Reliever Medication

Hospital Name	City	Rate	Cases
Carolinas Medical Center - Northeast	Concord	100%	87
Carolinas Med Ctr/Behavioral Health	Charlotte	100%	360
Firsthealth Moore Regional Hospital	Pinehurst	100%	56
Mem Mission Hosp & Asheville Surg Ctr	Asheville	100%	58
North Carolina Baptist Hospital	Winston-Salem	100%	197
Novant Health Presbyterian Medical Center	Charlotte	100%	158
Wilson Medical Center	Wilson	100%	29

Received Systemic Corticosteroids

Hospital Name	City	Rate	Cases
Carolinas Medical Center - Northeast	Concord	100%	87
Carolinas Med Ctr/Behavioral Health	Charlotte	100%	354
Firsthealth Moore Regional Hospital	Pinehurst	100%	56
Mem Mission Hosp & Asheville Surg Ctr	Asheville	100%	58
Novant Health Presbyterian Medical Center	Charlotte	100%	156
Wilson Medical Center	Wilson	100%	29
North Carolina Baptist Hospital	Winston-Salem	99%	196

Emergency Department

Admittance Decision Time (minutes)

Hospital Name	City	Min.	Cases
Vidant Roanoke Chowan Hospital[2]	Ahoskie	34	379
Vidant Chowan Hospital[2]	Edenton	36	284
Vidant Duplin Hospital[2]	Kenansville	48	222
Wilkes Regional Medical Center[2]	N Wilkesboro	48	637
Cherokee Indian Hospital Authority[2]	Cherokee	50	289
Ashe Memorial Hospital[2]	Jefferson	51	455
Davis Regional Medical Center[2]	Statesville	51	433
The Mcdowell Hospital[2]	Marion	51	488
Vidant Beaufort Hospital[2]	Washington	52	243
Anson Community Hospital[2]	Wadesboro	55	256

NOTE: Hospital profiles are in alphabetical order by state, then city, then hospital within the city; Rankings exclude hospitals with less than 25 cases except for patient surveys which excludes hospitals with less than 100 cases; (a) 100-299 cases; (1) The number of cases/patients is too few to report; (2) Data submitted were based on a sample of cases/patients; (3) Results are based on a shorter time period than required; (4) Data suppressed by CMS for one or more quarters; (5) Results are not available for this reporting period; (6) Fewer than 100 patients completed the HCAHPS survey; (7) No cases met the criteria for this measure; (8) The lower limit of the confidence interval cannot be calculated if the number of observed infections equals zero; (9) No data are available from the state/territory for this reporting period; (10) The scores shown reflect fewer than 50 completed surveys; (11) There were discrepancies in the data collection process; (12) This measure does not apply to this hospital for this reporting period; (13) Results cannot be calculated for this reporting period; (14) The results for this state are combined with nearby states to protect confidentiality; Please refer to the User's Guide for a full explanation of data.

Sandhills Regional Medical Center[2]	Hamlet	56	387
Catawba Valley Medical Center[2]	Hickory	59	414
Person Memorial Hospital[2]	Roxboro	59	481
J Arthur Dosher Memorial Hospital[2,3]	Southport	61	297
Margaret R Pardee Memorial Hospital[2]	Hendersonville	62	822
Transylvania Regional Hospital[2,3]	Brevard	63	344
Hugh Chatham Memorial Hospital[2]	Elkin	65	679
Vidant Bertie Hospital	Windsor	65	354
Chatham Hospital	Siler City	68	436
Johnston Memorial Hospital[2]	Smithfield	68	470
Medwest Swain[2]	Bryson City	69	340
Iredell Memorial Hospital[2]	Statesville	70	631
Wayne Memorial Hospital[2]	Goldsboro	70	567
Lexington Memorial Hospital[2]	Lexington	71	69
Frye Regional Medical Center[2]	Hickory	73	637
Medwest Harris[2]	Sylva	74	296
Kings Mountain Hospital[2]	Kings Mountain	75	429
Lake Norman Regional Medical Center[2]	Mooresville	75	565
Spruce Pine Community Hospital[2]	Spruce Pine	75	450
Medwest Haywood[2]	Clyde	77	604
Carolinas Medical Center - Lincoln[2]	Lincolnton	78	441
Vidant Pungo Hospital	Belhaven	78	402
Novant Health Thomasville Medical Center[2]	Thomasville	79	455
Vidant Edgecombe Hospital[2]	Tarboro	79	277
High Point Regional Hospital[2]	High Point	80	659
North Carolina Baptist Hospital[2]	Winston-Salem	80	162
Carolinas Medical Center - University[2]	Charlotte	81	347
Granville Health Systems[2]	Oxford	83	741
Carolinas Medical Center - Pineville[2]	Charlotte	85	653
Albemarle Hospital Authority[2]	Elizabeth City	92	746
Northern Hospital of Surry County[2]	Mount Airy	97	632
Carolinas Medical Center - Northeast[2]	Concord	99	541
Morehead Memorial Hospital[2]	Eden	100	652
Caromont Regional Medical Center[2]	Gastonia	104	834
Maria Parham Medical Center[2]	Henderson	105	487
Carolinas Med Ctr/Behavioral Health[2]	Charlotte	108	256
Carolinas Medical Center - Union[2]	Monroe	110	424
Park Ridge Health[2]	Hendersonville	110	163
Southeastern Regional Medical Center[2]	Lumberton	111	776
Carteret General Hospital[2]	Morehead City	113	681
Sampson Regional Medical Center[2]	Clinton	113	375
Murphy Medical Center[2]	Murphy	115	616
Cleveland Regional Medical Center[2]	Shelby	116	718
Central Carolina Hospital[2]	Sanford	117	671
Novant Health Franklin Medical Center[2]	Louisburg	117	587
Angel Medical Center[2]	Franklin	119	690
Martin General Hospital[2]	Williamston	120	371
Randolph Hospital[2]	Asheboro	122	643
Firsthealth Moore Regional Hospital[2]	Pinehurst	125	658
Novant Health Brunswick Medical Center[2]	Supply	128	626
Halifax Regional Medical Center[2]	Roanoke Rapids	129	774
Novant Health Forsyth Medical Center[2]	Winston-Salem	131	1311
Scotland Memorial Hospital[2]	Laurinburg	132	688
Stanly Regional Medical Center[2]	Albemarle	133	560
Lenoir Memorial Hospital[2]	Kinston	134	813
Mem Mission Hosp & Asheville Surg Ctr[2]	Asheville	134	390
Onslow Memorial Hospital[2]	Jacksonville	134	550
Watauga Medical Center[2]	Boone	134	458
Novant Health Presbyterian Medical Center[2]	Charlotte	138	521
Alamance Regional Medical Center[2]	Burlington	140	749
Columbus Regional Healthcare System[2]	Whiteville	142	647
The Moses H Cone Memorial Hospital[2]	Greensboro	148	610
New Hanover Regional Medical Center[2]	Wilmington	148	577
CMC - Blue Ridge[2]	Morganton	151	643
Novant Health Huntersville Medical Center[2]	Huntersville	152	713
Novant Health Rowan Medical Center[2]	Salisbury	152	840
Betsy Johnson Regional Hospital[2]	Dunn	154	840
Wakemed - Cary Hospital[2]	Cary	154	510
Duke University Hospital[2]	Durham	157	433
Vidant Medical Center[2]	Greenville	158	318
Rutherford Hospital[2]	Rutherfordton	160	715
Wakemed - Raleigh Campus[2]	Raleigh	160	409
Carolina East Medical Center[2]	New Bern	163	496
Duke Health Raleigh Hospital[2]	Raleigh	165	531
Nash General Hospital[2]	Rocky Mount	172	619
The Outer Banks Hospital[2]	Nags Head	175	221
University of North Carolina Hospital[2]	Chapel Hill	180	344
Caldwell Memorial Hospital[2]	Lenoir	190	486
Presbyterian Hospital Matthews[2]	Matthews	201	806
Cape Fear Valley Medical Center[2]	Fayetteville	217	733
Rex Hospital[2]	Raleigh	230	447
Wilson Medical Center[2]	Wilson	240	640
Duke Regional Hospital[2]	Durham	274	631

Head CT Results Within 45 Minutes of Arrival

Hospital Name	City	Rate	Cases
Central Carolina Hospital	Sanford	96%	28
Halifax Regional Medical Center	Roanoke Rapids	86%	29
Carolinas Medical Center - Pineville	Charlotte	84%	25
Carteret General Hospital	Morehead City	84%	25
Novant Health Rowan Medical Center	Salisbury	84%	25
Novant Health Huntersville Medical Center	Huntersville	80%	25
Wakemed - Cary Hospital	Cary	77%	31
Iredell Memorial Hospital	Statesville	63%	27
Nash General Hospital	Rocky Mount	56%	25
Carolinas Medical Center - University	Charlotte	46%	26
Southeastern Regional Medical Center	Lumberton	19%	27
Sampson Regional Medical Center	Clinton	13%	30

Patients Who Left ER Before Being Seen

Hospital Name	City	Rate	Cases
Albemarle Hospital Authority	Elizabeth City	0%	45913
Caromont Regional Medical Center	Gastonia	0%	104892
Hugh Chatham Memorial Hospital	Elkin	0%	31611
Northern Hospital of Surry County	Mount Airy	0%	37312
Angel Medical Center	Franklin	1%	14614
Anson Community Hospital	Wadesboro	1%	13332
Cape Fear Valley Medical Center	Fayetteville	1%	135522
Carteret General Hospital	Morehead City	1%	42244
Cleveland Regional Medical Center	Shelby	1%	66046
Firsthealth Montgomery Memorial Hospital	Troy	1%	14706
Firsthealth Moore Regional Hospital	Pinehurst	1%	66453
Lake Norman Regional Medical Center	Mooresville	1%	25403
Novant Health Brunswick Medical Center	Supply	1%	27522
Novant Health Presbyterian Medical Center	Charlotte	1%	91499
Presbyterian Hospital Matthews	Matthews	1%	48064
Scotland Memorial Hospital	Laurinburg	1%	45809
Vidant Bertie Hospital	Windsor	1%	10057
Vidant Roanoke Chowan Hospital	Ahoskie	1%	21582
Wilkes Regional Medical Center	N Wilkesboro	1%	32584
Carolinas Medical Center - Lincoln	Lincolnton	2%	47931
Carolinas Medical Center - Northeast	Concord	2%	101954
Carolinas Medical Center - Pineville	Charlotte	2%	118245
Carolinas Medical Center - Union	Monroe	2%	69504
Carolinas Medical Center - University	Charlotte	2%	88110
Central Carolina Hospital	Sanford	2%	38456
CMC - Blue Ridge	Morganton	2%	62201
Davis Regional Medical Center	Statesville	2%	26197
Frye Regional Medical Center	Hickory	2%	40470
J Arthur Dosher Memorial Hospital	Southport	2%	13000
Johnston Memorial Hospital	Smithfield	2%	83804
Kings Mountain Hospital	Kings Mountain	2%	30439
Maria Parham Medical Center	Henderson	2%	40989
Medwest Haywood	Clyde	2%	25737
Novant Health Forsyth Medical Center	Winston-Salem	2%	119140
Novant Health Huntersville Medical Center	Huntersville	2%	34445
Park Ridge Health	Hendersonville	2%	23339
Rex Hospital	Raleigh	2%	61807
Saint Luke's Hospital	Columbus	2%	10185
Sampson Regional Medical Center	Clinton	2%	34137
Sandhills Regional Medical Center	Hamlet	2%	12093
Spruce Pine Community Hospital	Spruce Pine	2%	14040
University of North Carolina Hospital	Chapel Hill	2%	71342
Vidant Beaufort Hospital	Washington	2%	23050
Vidant Medical Center	Greenville	2%	71963
Watauga Medical Center	Boone	2%	21320
Betsy Johnson Regional Hospital	Dunn	3%	46652
Cape Fear Valley - Bladen County Hospital	Elizabethtown	3%	16312
Carolina East Medical Center	New Bern	3%	40541
Duke Health Raleigh Hospital	Raleigh	3%	41388
Granville Health Systems	Oxford	3%	16659
Halifax Regional Medical Center	Roanoke Rapids	3%	41623
High Point Regional Hospital	High Point	3%	64666
Lenoir Memorial Hospital	Kinston	3%	102938
The Mcdowell Hospital	Marion	3%	23111
Medwest Harris	Sylva	3%	16972
Mem Mission Hosp & Asheville Surg Ctr	Asheville	3%	105514
The Moses H Cone Memorial Hospital	Greensboro	3%	204780
Murphy Medical Center	Murphy	3%	16581
Nash General Hospital	Rocky Mount	3%	67049
New Hanover Regional Medical Center	Wilmington	3%	122587
North Carolina Baptist Hospital	Winston-Salem	3%	112357
Novant Health Franklin Medical Center	Louisburg	3%	20253
Novant Health Rowan Medical Center	Salisbury	3%	47921
Novant Health Thomasville Medical Center	Thomasville	3%	37409
Onslow Memorial Hospital	Jacksonville	3%	66634
Person Memorial Hospital	Roxboro	3%	20871
Stanly Regional Medical Center	Albemarle	3%	35578
Transylvania Regional Hospital	Brevard	3%	15901
Vidant Chowan Hospital	Edenton	3%	15065
Vidant Edgecombe Hospital	Tarboro	3%	27523
Wakemed - Cary Hospital	Cary	3%	63664
Ashe Memorial Hospital	Jefferson	4%	10655
Caldwell Memorial Hospital	Lenoir	4%	29806
Carolinas Med Ctr/Behavioral Health	Charlotte	4%	98110
Catawba Valley Medical Center	Hickory	4%	46937
Columbus Regional Healthcare System	Whiteville	4%	30722
Lexington Memorial Hospital	Lexington	4%	37800
Martin General Hospital	Williamston	4%	14226
Morehead Memorial Hospital	Eden	4%	34048
Southeastern Regional Medical Center	Lumberton	4%	68375
Wayne Memorial Hospital	Goldsboro	4%	61964
Wilson Medical Center	Wilson	4%	50781
Alamance Regional Medical Center	Burlington	5%	55193
Iredell Memorial Hospital	Statesville	5%	46067
Randolph Hospital	Asheboro	5%	41808
Rutherford Hospital	Rutherfordton	5%	25329
Vidant Duplin Hospital	Kenansville	5%	21992
Wakemed - Raleigh Campus	Raleigh	5%	171569
Duke Regional Hospital	Durham	6%	67524
Margaret R Pardee Memorial Hospital	Hendersonville	6%	30896
Duke University Hospital	Durham	8%	74344

Time from ER Arrival to Being Admitted (minutes)

Hospital Name	City	Min.	Cases
Vidant Pungo Hospital	Belhaven	196	434
Cherokee Indian Hospital Authority[2]	Cherokee	213	289
Davis Regional Medical Center[2]	Statesville	215	433
Kings Mountain Hospital[2]	Kings Mountain	215	435
Lake Norman Regional Medical Center[2]	Mooresville	220	566
Medwest Swain[2]	Bryson City	220	340
Person Memorial Hospital[2]	Roxboro	225	487
Wilkes Regional Medical Center[2]	N Wilkesboro	225	637
Ashe Memorial Hospital[2]	Jefferson	228	455
Vidant Bertie Hospital	Windsor	233	355
Albemarle Hospital Authority[2]	Elizabeth City	234	748
Vidant Roanoke Chowan Hospital[2]	Ahoskie	234	380
Medwest Harris[2]	Sylva	240	296
Carolinas Medical Center - Lincoln[2]	Lincolnton	243	446
Cleveland Regional Medical Center[2]	Shelby	245	724
The Mcdowell Hospital[2]	Marion	246	498
Frye Regional Medical Center[2]	Hickory	248	637
Hugh Chatham Memorial Hospital[2]	Elkin	248	680
Vidant Chowan Hospital[2]	Edenton	248	295
Wayne Memorial Hospital[2]	Goldsboro	252	604
Lexington Memorial Hospital[2]	Lexington	257	396
Murphy Medical Center[2]	Murphy	260	706
Central Carolina Hospital[2]	Sanford	261	671
Spruce Pine Community Hospital[2]	Spruce Pine	265	451
J Arthur Dosher Memorial Hospital[2,3]	Southport	266	341
Vidant Duplin Hospital[2]	Kenansville	266	238
Angel Medical Center[2]	Franklin	268	721
Carolinas Medical Center - Pineville[2]	Charlotte	269	713
Transylvania Regional Hospital[2,3]	Brevard	272	404
Johnston Memorial Hospital[2]	Smithfield	273	477
Carolinas Medical Center - University[2]	Charlotte	276	390
Granville Health Systems[2]	Oxford	276	746
Iredell Memorial Hospital[2]	Statesville	278	705
Park Ridge Health[2]	Hendersonville	278	178
Medwest Haywood[2]	Clyde	279	637
Carolinas Medical Center - Northeast[2]	Concord	280	564
Catawba Valley Medical Center[2]	Hickory	280	598
Margaret R Pardee Memorial Hospital[2]	Hendersonville	280	822
Sandhills Regional Medical Center[2]	Hamlet	280	396
Caromont Regional Medical Center[2]	Gastonia	281	841
Sampson Regional Medical Center[2]	Clinton	283	377
Watauga Medical Center[2]	Boone	283	478
Carolinas Med Ctr/Behavioral Health[2]	Charlotte	284	276
Anson Community Hospital[2]	Wadesboro	285	323
Novant Health Brunswick Medical Center[2]	Supply	286	626
Scotland Memorial Hospital[2]	Laurinburg	286	692
Firsthealth Moore Regional Hospital[2]	Pinehurst	293	660
Chatham Hospital	Siler City	295	466
Martin General Hospital[2]	Williamston	295	413
Novant Health Thomasville Medical Center[2]	Thomasville	296	482
Northern Hospital of Surry County[2]	Mount Airy	297	640
Novant Health Franklin Medical Center[2]	Louisburg	301	617
Vidant Beaufort Hospital[2]	Washington	301	249
Carolinas Medical Center - Union[2]	Monroe	306	481
Novant Health Forsyth Medical Center[2]	Winston-Salem	309	1325
Vidant Edgecombe Hospital[2]	Tarboro	310	283
Rutherford Hospital[2]	Rutherfordton	311	755
Carteret General Hospital[2]	Morehead City	314	682
Morehead Memorial Hospital[2]	Eden	316	652
Caldwell Memorial Hospital[2]	Lenoir	317	489
CMC - Blue Ridge[2]	Morganton	317	858
Novant Health Huntersville Medical Center[2]	Huntersville	317	720
Stanly Regional Medical Center[2]	Albemarle	317	560
New Hanover Regional Medical Center[2]	Wilmington	318	578
Novant Health Presbyterian Medical Center[2]	Charlotte	320	521
North Carolina Baptist Hospital[2]	Winston-Salem	322	193
Maria Parham Medical Center[2]	Henderson	326	498
Randolph Hospital[2]	Asheboro	329	644
Halifax Regional Medical Center[2]	Roanoke Rapids	330	785
High Point Regional Hospital[2]	High Point	330	659
Mem Mission Hosp & Asheville Surg Ctr[2]	Asheville	332	432
Carolina East Medical Center[2]	New Bern	336	666
Columbus Regional Healthcare System[2]	Whiteville	340	660
Alamance Regional Medical Center[2]	Burlington	343	1023
Novant Health Rowan Medical Center[2]	Salisbury	348	866
The Outer Banks Hospital[2]	Nags Head	350	226
Lenoir Memorial Hospital[2]	Kinston	354	816
Wakemed - Cary Hospital[2]	Cary	360	511

NOTE: Hospital profiles are in alphabetical order by state, then city, then hospital within the city; Rankings exclude hospitals with less than 25 cases except for patient surveys which excludes hospitals with less than 100 cases; (a) 100-299 cases; (1) The number of cases/patients is too few to report; (2) Data submitted were based on a sample of cases/patients; (3) Results are based on a shorter time period than required; (4) Data suppressed by CMS for one or more quarters; (5) Results are not available for this reporting period; (6) Fewer than 100 patients completed the HCAHPS survey; (7) No cases met the criteria for this measure; (8) The lower limit of the confidence interval cannot be calculated if the number of observed infections equals zero; (9) No data are available from the state/territory for this reporting period; (10) The scores shown reflect fewer than 50 completed surveys; (11) There were discrepancies in the data collection process; (12) This measure does not apply to this hospital for this reporting period; (13) Results cannot be calculated for this reporting period; (14) The results for this state are combined with nearby states to protect confidentiality; Please refer to the User's Guide for a full explanation of data.

Hospital Name	City	Min.	Cases
Nash General Hospital[2]	Rocky Mount	368	625
Vidant Medical Center[2]	Greenville	371	336
The Moses H Cone Memorial Hospital[2]	Greensboro	378	616
Betsy Johnson Regional Hospital[2]	Dunn	381	881
Presbyterian Hospital Matthews[2]	Matthews	397	833
Onslow Memorial Hospital[2]	Jacksonville	400	550
Rex Hospital[2]	Raleigh	405	459
Wakemed - Raleigh Campus[2]	Raleigh	405	416
Duke Health Raleigh Hospital[2]	Raleigh	432	629
Southeastern Regional Medical Center[2]	Lumberton	432	779
Duke University Hospital[2]	Durham	454	434
Wilson Medical Center[2]	Wilson	456	658
University of North Carolina Hospital[2]	Chapel Hill	465	353
Cape Fear Valley Medical Center[2]	Fayetteville	484	735
Duke Regional Hospital[2]	Durham	484	632

Time from ER Arrival to Discharge (minutes)

Hospital Name	City	Min.	Cases
Albemarle Hospital Authority	Elizabeth City	67	525
Alleghany County Memorial Hospital	Sparta	84	867
Davis Regional Medical Center	Statesville	108	649
Person Memorial Hospital	Roxboro	110	362
Cleveland Regional Medical Center	Shelby	113	363
Kings Mountain Hospital	Kings Mountain	114	358
J Arthur Dosher Memorial Hospital[3]	Southport	116	372
Vidant Bertie Hospital	Windsor	116	368
Lake Norman Regional Medical Center	Mooresville	117	594
Wilkes Regional Medical Center	N Wilkesboro	117	356
CMC - Blue Ridge	Morganton	121	662
Sandhills Regional Medical Center	Hamlet	122	338
Anson Community Hospital	Wadesboro	123	339
Sampson Regional Medical Center	Clinton	124	427
Caldwell Memorial Hospital	Lenoir	128	362
Central Carolina Hospital	Sanford	128	368
Rutherford Hospital	Rutherfordton	128	407
Firsthealth Moore Regional Hospital	Pinehurst	129	391
Scotland Memorial Hospital	Laurinburg	129	438
Park Ridge Health	Hendersonville	130	998
Angel Medical Center	Franklin	132	538
Hugh Chatham Memorial Hospital	Elkin	132	383
Vidant Roanoke Chowan Hospital	Ahoskie	132	386
Northern Hospital of Surry County	Mount Airy	133	432
Novant Health Brunswick Medical Center	Supply	133	452
Medwest Harris	Sylva	134	344
Frye Regional Medical Center	Hickory	136	432
Spruce Pine Community Hospital	Spruce Pine	136	408
Martin General Hospital	Williamston	137	363
The Mcdowell Hospital	Marion	137	413
Lexington Memorial Hospital	Lexington	138	328
Novant Health Thomasville Medical Center	Thomasville	138	453
Johnston Memorial Hospital	Smithfield	140	363
Wilson Medical Center	Wilson	144	372
Ashe Memorial Hospital	Jefferson	145	353
New Hanover Regional Medical Center	Wilmington	146	394
Novant Health Franklin Medical Center	Louisburg	146	441
Stanly Regional Medical Center	Albemarle	146	352
Betsy Johnson Regional Hospital	Dunn	150	565
Carteret General Hospital	Morehead City	150	374
Maria Parham Medical Center	Henderson	150	388
Morehead Memorial Hospital	Eden	150	399
Carolinas Medical Center - Union	Monroe	151	343
Novant Health Huntersville Medical Center	Huntersville	152	439
Medwest Haywood	Clyde	153	337
Granville Health Systems	Oxford	154	600
Watauga Medical Center	Boone	154	342
Transylvania Regional Hospital[3]	Brevard	156	386
Novant Health Forsyth Medical Center	Winston-Salem	157	1204
Duke Health Raleigh Hospital	Raleigh	158	389
Novant Health Presbyterian Medical Center	Charlotte	158	467
Carolinas Medical Center - University	Charlotte	159	352
Vidant Chowan Hospital	Edenton	159	360
Carolinas Medical Center - Pineville	Charlotte	160	669
Wayne Memorial Hospital	Goldsboro	161	345
Carolinas Medical Center - Lincoln	Lincolnton	162	344
Murphy Medical Center	Murphy	162	1120
Carolinas Medical Center - Northeast	Concord	163	342
Vidant Edgecombe Hospital	Tarboro	163	381
Margaret R Pardee Memorial Hospital	Hendersonville	165	359
North Carolina Baptist Hospital	Winston-Salem	165	347
Vidant Duplin Hospital	Kenansville	166	400
Wakemed - Cary Hospital	Cary	166	431
Novant Health Rowan Medical Center	Salisbury	168	447
Columbus Regional Healthcare System	Whiteville	169	365
Iredell Memorial Hospital	Statesville	169	379
Vidant Beaufort Hospital	Washington	174	411
Nash General Hospital	Rocky Mount	177	463
Catawba Valley Medical Center	Hickory	179	470
Vidant Medical Center	Greenville	179	371
Halifax Regional Medical Center	Roanoke Rapids	181	1047
Presbyterian Hospital Matthews	Matthews	181	466
Carolinas Med Ctr/Behavioral Health	Charlotte	183	291
Caromont Regional Medical Center	Gastonia	183	392
Lenoir Memorial Hospital	Kinston	185	567
Onslow Memorial Hospital	Jacksonville	185	1649
Rex Hospital	Raleigh	190	414
Randolph Hospital	Asheboro	191	362
Duke Regional Hospital	Durham	192	386
Mem Mission Hosp & Asheville Surg Ctr	Asheville	193	381
The Moses H Cone Memorial Hospital	Greensboro	193	1441
Wakemed - Raleigh Campus	Raleigh	194	428
Alamance Regional Medical Center	Burlington	203	395
Cape Fear Valley Medical Center	Fayetteville	203	322
High Point Regional Hospital	High Point	204	338
Carolina East Medical Center	New Bern	208	511
Southeastern Regional Medical Center	Lumberton	250	332
Duke University Hospital	Durham	263	609
University of North Carolina Hospital	Chapel Hill	282	370

Time in ER Before Being Evaluated (minutes)

Hospital Name	City	Min.	Cases
Albemarle Hospital Authority	Elizabeth City	2	562
Lake Norman Regional Medical Center	Mooresville	10	633
Maria Parham Medical Center	Henderson	14	431
Vidant Roanoke Chowan Hospital	Ahoskie	16	426
Alleghany County Memorial Hospital	Sparta	17	965
Carteret General Hospital	Morehead City	17	405
Cleveland Regional Medical Center	Shelby	18	298
Person Memorial Hospital	Roxboro	18	402
Granville Health Systems	Oxford	20	806
Hugh Chatham Memorial Hospital	Elkin	20	429
Presbyterian Hospital Matthews	Matthews	21	518
Stanly Regional Medical Center	Albemarle	21	376
Sampson Regional Medical Center	Clinton	22	475
Kings Mountain Hospital	Kings Mountain	23	323
Novant Health Forsyth Medical Center	Winston-Salem	23	1268
Novant Health Presbyterian Medical Center	Charlotte	23	480
Wilkes Regional Medical Center	N Wilkesboro	23	380
Cape Fear Valley Medical Center	Fayetteville	24	390
Firsthealth Moore Regional Hospital	Pinehurst	24	422
Northern Hospital of Surry County	Mount Airy	24	475
Central Carolina Hospital	Sanford	25	399
Novant Health Huntersville Medical Center	Huntersville	25	479
Vidant Bertie Hospital	Windsor	25	406
Betsy Johnson Regional Hospital	Dunn	26	515
Davis Regional Medical Center	Statesville	27	702
The Mcdowell Hospital	Marion	27	438
Medwest Haywood	Clyde	29	395
Novant Health Brunswick Medical Center	Supply	29	480
Angel Medical Center	Franklin	30	570
Anson Community Hospital	Wadesboro	30	348
Sandhills Regional Medical Center	Hamlet	30	380
Novant Health Franklin Medical Center	Louisburg	31	464
Medwest Harris	Sylva	32	383
Rutherford Hospital	Rutherfordton	32	414
Carolina East Medical Center	New Bern	33	320
Vidant Medical Center	Greenville	34	402
Caldwell Memorial Hospital	Lenoir	35	387
Carolinas Medical Center - Union	Monroe	35	371
Duke Health Raleigh Hospital	Raleigh	35	379
Martin General Hospital	Williamston	35	389
Novant Health Thomasville Medical Center	Thomasville	35	478
Onslow Memorial Hospital	Jacksonville	35	1808
Spruce Pine Community Hospital	Spruce Pine	35	440
Watauga Medical Center	Boone	35	381
Carolinas Medical Center - University	Charlotte	36	373
Carolinas Medical Center - Northeast	Concord	37	362
Novant Health Rowan Medical Center	Salisbury	37	479
Murphy Medical Center	Murphy	38	1235
North Carolina Baptist Hospital	Winston-Salem	38	180
Wakemed - Cary Hospital	Cary	38	432
CMC - Blue Ridge	Morganton	39	698
J Arthur Dosher Memorial Hospital[3]	Southport	39	383
Johnston Memorial Hospital	Smithfield	39	391
Vidant Chowan Hospital	Edenton	39	388
Vidant Edgecombe Hospital	Tarboro	39	349
Ashe Memorial Hospital	Jefferson	41	377
Frye Regional Medical Center	Hickory	41	469
The Moses H Cone Memorial Hospital	Greensboro	41	1526
Transylvania Regional Hospital[3]	Brevard	41	392
Carolinas Medical Center - Pineville	Charlotte	43	702
Caromont Regional Medical Center	Gastonia	43	431
Rex Hospital	Raleigh	43	429
Park Ridge Health	Hendersonville	45	1228
Carolinas Med Ctr/Behavioral Health	Charlotte	46	374
Mem Mission Hosp & Asheville Surg Ctr	Asheville	46	423
Morehead Memorial Hospital	Eden	46	422
Randolph Hospital	Asheboro	46	402
Columbus Regional Healthcare System	Whiteville	49	397
Iredell Memorial Hospital	Statesville	49	210
Vidant Beaufort Hospital	Washington	49	347
Vidant Duplin Hospital	Kenansville	51	239
Lexington Memorial Hospital	Lexington	53	294
High Point Regional Hospital	High Point	54	408
Scotland Memorial Hospital	Laurinburg	56	462
Wilson Medical Center	Wilson	57	397
Duke University Hospital	Durham	58	680
Wakemed - Raleigh Campus	Raleigh	58	406
Wayne Memorial Hospital	Goldsboro	58	275
Lenoir Memorial Hospital	Kinston	59	601
Margaret R Pardee Memorial Hospital	Hendersonville	59	399
University of North Carolina Hospital	Chapel Hill	59	383
Carolinas Medical Center - Lincoln	Lincolnton	60	377
Halifax Regional Medical Center	Roanoke Rapids	64	1152
New Hanover Regional Medical Center	Wilmington	69	405
Duke Regional Hospital	Durham	71	413
Catawba Valley Medical Center	Hickory	73	351
Nash General Hospital	Rocky Mount	74	360
Alamance Regional Medical Center	Burlington	98	329
Southeastern Regional Medical Center	Lumberton	98	278

Time to Pain Meds for Bone Fractures (minutes)

Hospital Name	City	Min.	Cases
Albemarle Hospital Authority	Elizabeth City	29	138
Vidant Medical Center	Greenville	40	167
Johnston Memorial Hospital	Smithfield	47	234
Lake Norman Regional Medical Center	Mooresville	47	133
Vidant Roanoke Chowan Hospital	Ahoskie	49	66
Wilkes Regional Medical Center	N Wilkesboro	49	135
Person Memorial Hospital	Roxboro	50	50
Cleveland Regional Medical Center	Shelby	52	146
Wakemed - Cary Hospital	Cary	52	250
The Mcdowell Hospital	Marion	54	61
Sampson Regional Medical Center	Clinton	54	50
Vidant Beaufort Hospital	Washington	54	88
Betsy Johnson Regional Hospital	Dunn	55	130
North Carolina Baptist Hospital	Winston-Salem	56	279
Novant Health Huntersville Medical Center	Huntersville	56	121
Carolinas Medical Center - University	Charlotte	58	206
Halifax Regional Medical Center	Roanoke Rapids	58	86
Hugh Chatham Memorial Hospital	Elkin	58	86
Novant Health Presbyterian Medical Center	Charlotte	58	178
CMC - Blue Ridge	Morganton	59	161
Frye Regional Medical Center	Hickory	59	99
Maria Parham Medical Center	Henderson	59	76
Northern Hospital of Surry County	Mount Airy	60	100
Novant Health Rowan Medical Center	Salisbury	60	126
Novant Health Thomasville Medical Center	Thomasville	60	86
Park Ridge Health	Hendersonville	60	70
Rex Hospital	Raleigh	60	120
Wakemed - Raleigh Campus	Raleigh	61	476
Firsthealth Moore Regional Hospital	Pinehurst	62	252
Novant Health Forsyth Medical Center	Winston-Salem	62	285
Novant Health Franklin Medical Center	Louisburg	62	62
Central Carolina Hospital	Sanford	63	165
Stanly Regional Medical Center	Albemarle	63	199
Murphy Medical Center	Murphy	64	100
Anson Community Hospital	Wadesboro	65	28
Medwest Haywood	Clyde	65	77
The Moses H Cone Memorial Hospital	Greensboro	65	513
High Point Regional Hospital	High Point	66	123
Angel Medical Center	Franklin	67	95
Carolinas Med Ctr/Behavioral Health	Charlotte	67	304
Davis Regional Medical Center	Statesville	67	61
Lexington Memorial Hospital	Lexington	67	117
Onslow Memorial Hospital	Jacksonville	67	201
Presbyterian Hospital Matthews	Matthews	68	189
Margaret R Pardee Memorial Hospital	Hendersonville	69	107
Martin General Hospital	Williamston	69	45
University of North Carolina Hospital	Chapel Hill	69	103
Carolinas Medical Center - Pineville	Charlotte	70	326
Carolinas Medical Center - Union	Monroe	70	205
Iredell Memorial Hospital	Statesville	70	95
Granville Health Systems	Oxford	71	62
Randolph Hospital	Asheboro	71	190
Scotland Memorial Hospital	Laurinburg	71	131
Carolinas Medical Center - Northeast	Concord	72	292
Caromont Regional Medical Center	Gastonia	72	244
Carteret General Hospital	Morehead City	72	118
J Arthur Dosher Memorial Hospital	Southport	72	40
Rutherford Hospital	Rutherfordton	72	105
Medwest Harris	Sylva	74	108
Watauga Medical Center	Boone	74	134
Wayne Memorial Hospital	Goldsboro	75	153
Caldwell Memorial Hospital	Lenoir	76	79
Cape Fear Valley Medical Center	Fayetteville	76	334
Kings Mountain Hospital	Kings Mountain	76	65
Nash General Hospital	Rocky Mount	76	222
Carolinas Medical Center - Lincoln	Lincolnton	77	165
Novant Health Brunswick Medical Center	Supply	77	96
Vidant Duplin Hospital	Kenansville	77	49
Wilson Medical Center	Wilson	77	113
Carolina East Medical Center	New Bern	78	102
Mem Mission Hosp & Asheville Surg Ctr	Asheville	78	264

NOTE: Hospital profiles are in alphabetical order by state, then city, then hospital within the city; Rankings exclude hospitals with less than 25 cases except for patient surveys which excludes hospitals with less than 100 cases; (a) 100-299 cases; (1) The number of cases/patients is too few to report; (2) Data submitted were based on a sample of cases/patients; (3) Results are based on a shorter time period than required; (4) Data suppressed by CMS for one or more quarters; (5) Results are not available for this reporting period; (6) Fewer than 100 patients completed the HCAHPS survey; (7) No cases met the criteria for this measure; (8) The lower limit of the confidence interval cannot be calculated if the number of observed infections equals zero; (9) No data are available from the state/territory for this reporting period; (10) The scores shown reflect fewer than 50 completed surveys; (11) There were discrepancies in the data collection process; (12) This measure does not apply to this hospital for this reporting period; (13) Results cannot be calculated for this reporting period; (14) The results for this state are combined with nearby states to protect confidentiality; Please refer to the User's Guide for a full explanation of data.

Duke University Hospital	Durham	80	220
New Hanover Regional Medical Center	Wilmington	81	396
Spruce Pine Community Hospital	Spruce Pine	81	84
Vidant Edgecombe Hospital	Tarboro	84	56
Vidant Chowan Hospital	Edenton	87	54
Duke Regional Hospital	Durham	93	87
Duke Health Raleigh Hospital	Raleigh	94	56
Southeastern Regional Medical Center	Lumberton	95	175
Lenoir Memorial Hospital	Kinston	96	174
Morehead Memorial Hospital	Eden	99	93
Alamance Regional Medical Center	Burlington	101	232
Catawba Valley Medical Center	Hickory	102	186
Columbus Regional Healthcare System	Whiteville	102	77
Transylvania Regional Hospital[3]	Brevard	113	57

Heart Attack Care

Aspirin Given at Discharge

Hospital Name	City	Rate	Cases
Asheville - Oteen VA Medical Center	Asheville	100%	59
Cape Fear Valley Medical Center	Fayetteville	100%	681
Carolinas Medical Center - Northeast	Concord	100%	454
Carolinas Medical Center - Pineville	Charlotte	100%	399
Caromont Regional Medical Center	Gastonia	100%	474
Cleveland Regional Medical Center	Shelby	100%	35
CMC - Blue Ridge	Morganton	100%	44
Duke Health Raleigh Hospital	Raleigh	100%	54
Duke Regional Hospital	Durham	100%	217
Duke University Hospital	Durham	100%	660
Durham VA Medical Center	Durham	100%	60
Firsthealth Moore Regional Hospital[2]	Pinehurst	100%	323
Frye Regional Medical Center[2]	Hickory	100%	360
High Point Regional Hospital	High Point	100%	475
Lake Norman Regional Medical Center	Mooresville	100%	40
Mem Mission Hosp & Asheville Surg Ctr[2]	Asheville	100%	312
The Moses H Cone Memorial Hospital	Greensboro	100%	901
Nash General Hospital	Rocky Mount	100%	113
North Carolina Baptist Hospital	Winston-Salem	100%	690
Novant Health Forsyth Medical Center	Winston-Salem	100%	685
Novant Health Presbyterian Medical Center	Charlotte	100%	448
Novant Health Rowan Medical Center	Salisbury	100%	234
Presbyterian Hospital Matthews	Matthews	100%	116
Randolph Hospital	Asheboro	100%	30
Rex Hospital[2]	Raleigh	100%	419
Scotland Memorial Hospital	Laurinburg	100%	39
Southeastern Regional Medical Center	Lumberton	100%	247
Stanly Regional Medical Center	Albemarle	100%	44
University of North Carolina Hospital[2]	Chapel Hill	100%	256
Vidant Medical Center	Greenville	100%	1231
Wakemed - Cary Hospital	Cary	100%	54
Wakemed - Raleigh Campus	Raleigh	100%	1397
Watauga Medical Center	Boone	100%	68
Alamance Regional Medical Center	Burlington	99%	189
Albemarle Hospital Authority	Elizabeth City	99%	79
Carolina East Medical Center	New Bern	99%	397
Carolinas Med Ctr/Behavioral Health	Charlotte	99%	856
New Hanover Regional Medical Center	Wilmington	99%	812
Catawba Valley Medical Center	Hickory	98%	63
Iredell Memorial Hospital	Statesville	98%	98
Wilson Medical Center	Wilson	98%	80
Lenoir Memorial Hospital	Kinston	97%	69
Margaret R Pardee Memorial Hospital	Hendersonville	97%	39
Wayne Memorial Hospital	Goldsboro	97%	38
Carteret General Hospital	Morehead City	96%	57
Johnston Memorial Hospital	Smithfield	96%	27
Maria Parham Medical Center	Henderson	96%	25
Morehead Memorial Hospital	Eden	91%	34

PCI Within 90 Minutes of Arrival

Hospital Name	City	Rate	Cases
Carolinas Medical Center - Pineville	Charlotte	100%	69
Caromont Regional Medical Center	Gastonia	100%	93
Duke Regional Hospital	Durham	100%	38
High Point Regional Hospital	High Point	100%	50
Mem Mission Hosp & Asheville Surg Ctr[2]	Asheville	100%	31
Novant Health Forsyth Medical Center	Winston-Salem	100%	124
Novant Health Presbyterian Medical Center	Charlotte	100%	55
Novant Health Rowan Medical Center	Salisbury	100%	49
University of North Carolina Hospital[2]	Chapel Hill	100%	31
Carolinas Medical Center - Northeast	Concord	99%	83
Duke University Hospital	Durham	99%	78
The Moses H Cone Memorial Hospital	Greensboro	99%	147
Vidant Medical Center	Greenville	99%	68
Carolinas Med Ctr/Behavioral Health	Charlotte	98%	116
Frye Regional Medical Center[2]	Hickory	98%	85
Rex Hospital[2]	Raleigh	98%	56
Wakemed - Raleigh Campus	Raleigh	98%	117
Firsthealth Moore Regional Hospital[2]	Pinehurst	97%	36
New Hanover Regional Medical Center	Wilmington	97%	175
North Carolina Baptist Hospital	Winston-Salem	97%	69
Cape Fear Valley Medical Center	Fayetteville	96%	127
Carolina East Medical Center	New Bern	94%	54
Southeastern Regional Medical Center	Lumberton	89%	45

Statin Prescribed at Discharge

Hospital Name	City	Rate	Cases
Cape Fear Valley Medical Center	Fayetteville	100%	651
Carolinas Medical Center - Northeast	Concord	100%	439
Carolinas Medical Center - Pineville	Charlotte	100%	386
Caromont Regional Medical Center	Gastonia	100%	444
Duke Regional Hospital	Durham	100%	208
Duke University Hospital	Durham	100%	634
Firsthealth Moore Regional Hospital[2]	Pinehurst	100%	316
High Point Regional Hospital	High Point	100%	459
Iredell Memorial Hospital	Statesville	100%	91
Lake Norman Regional Medical Center	Mooresville	100%	36
Margaret R Pardee Memorial Hospital	Hendersonville	100%	37
Mem Mission Hosp & Asheville Surg Ctr[2]	Asheville	100%	303
The Moses H Cone Memorial Hospital	Greensboro	100%	854
Nash General Hospital	Rocky Mount	100%	98
New Hanover Regional Medical Center	Wilmington	100%	780
Novant Health Forsyth Medical Center	Winston-Salem	100%	656
Novant Health Presbyterian Medical Center	Charlotte	100%	423
Novant Health Rowan Medical Center	Salisbury	100%	204
Presbyterian Hospital Matthews	Matthews	100%	115
Vidant Medical Center	Greenville	100%	1212
Wakemed - Cary Hospital	Cary	100%	47
Alamance Regional Medical Center	Burlington	99%	175
Carolinas Med Ctr/Behavioral Health	Charlotte	99%	849
Catawba Valley Medical Center	Hickory	99%	68
Frye Regional Medical Center[2]	Hickory	99%	356
North Carolina Baptist Hospital	Winston-Salem	99%	684
University of North Carolina Hospital[2]	Chapel Hill	99%	249
Wakemed - Raleigh Campus	Raleigh	99%	1360
CMC - Blue Ridge	Morganton	98%	50
Duke Health Raleigh Hospital	Raleigh	98%	48
Durham VA Medical Center	Durham	98%	56
Rex Hospital[2]	Raleigh	98%	400
Cleveland Regional Medical Center	Shelby	97%	36
Johnston Memorial Hospital	Smithfield	97%	31
Southeastern Regional Medical Center	Lumberton	97%	242
Watauga Medical Center	Boone	97%	65
Carolina East Medical Center	New Bern	96%	371
Maria Parham Medical Center	Henderson	96%	25
Albemarle Hospital Authority	Elizabeth City	95%	79
Scotland Memorial Hospital	Laurinburg	95%	40
Randolph Hospital	Asheboro	94%	33
Asheville - Oteen VA Medical Center	Asheville	93%	58
Wilson Medical Center	Wilson	93%	76
Wayne Memorial Hospital	Goldsboro	92%	39
Lenoir Memorial Hospital	Kinston	90%	68
Stanly Regional Medical Center	Albemarle	89%	38
Carteret General Hospital	Morehead City	81%	64
Morehead Memorial Hospital	Eden	79%	33

Heart Failure Care

ACE Inhibitor or ARB for LVSD

Hospital Name	City	Rate	Cases
Carolinas Medical Center - Lincoln	Lincolnton	100%	31
Carolinas Medical Center - University	Charlotte	100%	70
Caromont Regional Medical Center	Gastonia	100%	149
Catawba Valley Medical Center	Hickory	100%	27
Central Carolina Hospital	Sanford	100%	45
Davis Regional Medical Center	Statesville	100%	30
Duke Health Raleigh Hospital	Raleigh	100%	52
Duke University Hospital	Durham	100%	295
Granville Health Systems	Oxford	100%	29
High Point Regional Hospital	High Point	100%	144
Lake Norman Regional Medical Center	Mooresville	100%	46
Lexington Memorial Hospital	Lexington	100%	31
The Mcdowell Hospital	Marion	100%	45
Medwest Harris	Sylva	100%	30
The Moses H Cone Memorial Hospital	Greensboro	100%	357
Northern Hospital of Surry County	Mount Airy	100%	32
Novant Health Brunswick Medical Center	Supply	100%	42
Novant Health Forsyth Medical Center[2]	Winston-Salem	100%	256
Novant Health Huntersville Medical Center	Huntersville	100%	39
Novant Health Presbyterian Medical Center	Charlotte	100%	205
Novant Health Rowan Medical Center	Salisbury	100%	62
Novant Health Thomasville Medical Center	Thomasville	100%	26
Park Ridge Health	Hendersonville	100%	31
Presbyterian Hospital Matthews	Matthews	100%	64
Vidant Beaufort Hospital	Washington	100%	35
Wakemed - Cary Hospital	Cary	100%	62
Wakemed - Raleigh Campus	Raleigh	100%	390
Cape Fear Valley Medical Center	Fayetteville	99%	355
Carolina East Medical Center	New Bern	99%	125
Carolinas Medical Center - Pineville	Charlotte	99%	150
Cleveland Regional Medical Center	Shelby	99%	79
Halifax Regional Medical Center	Roanoke Rapids	99%	81
Johnston Memorial Hospital	Smithfield	99%	73
New Hanover Regional Medical Center	Wilmington	99%	320
North Carolina Baptist Hospital	Winston-Salem	99%	294
Rex Hospital[2]	Raleigh	99%	121
Scotland Memorial Hospital	Laurinburg	99%	82
Vidant Medical Center	Greenville	99%	501
Carolinas Medical Center - Northeast	Concord	98%	208
Carolinas Med Ctr/Behavioral Health	Charlotte	98%	285
Duke Regional Hospital	Durham	98%	125
Durham VA Medical Center	Durham	98%	83
Firsthealth Moore Regional Hospital[2]	Pinehurst	98%	100
Iredell Memorial Hospital	Statesville	98%	93
Margaret R Pardee Memorial Hospital	Hendersonville	98%	63
Maria Parham Medical Center	Henderson	98%	91
Mem Mission Hosp & Asheville Surg Ctr	Asheville	98%	352
Onslow Memorial Hospital	Jacksonville	98%	57
Stanly Regional Medical Center	Albemarle	98%	57
Vidant Edgecombe Hospital	Tarboro	98%	58
Vidant Roanoke Chowan Hospital	Ahoskie	98%	42
Alamance Regional Medical Center	Burlington	97%	109
Albemarle Hospital Authority	Elizabeth City	97%	109
Fayetteville NC VA Medical Center	Fayetteville	97%	33
Martin General Hospital	Williamston	97%	33
Person Memorial Hospital	Roxboro	97%	30
University of North Carolina Hospital[2]	Chapel Hill	97%	103
CMC - Blue Ridge	Morganton	96%	50
Frye Regional Medical Center	Hickory	96%	72
Rutherford Hospital	Rutherfordton	96%	52
Sampson Regional Medical Center	Clinton	96%	47
Wayne Memorial Hospital	Goldsboro	96%	171
Carolinas Medical Center - Union	Monroe	95%	102
Carteret General Hospital	Morehead City	95%	55
Nash General Hospital	Rocky Mount	95%	166
Randolph Hospital[2]	Asheboro	95%	61
Asheville - Oteen VA Medical Center	Asheville	94%	51
Betsy Johnson Regional Hospital	Dunn	94%	70
Lenoir Memorial Hospital	Kinston	94%	53
Morehead Memorial Hospital	Eden	94%	62
Vidant Duplin Hospital	Kenansville	94%	35
Wilson Medical Center	Wilson	94%	82
Southeastern Regional Medical Center	Lumberton	92%	204
Columbus Regional Healthcare System	Whiteville	86%	28

Discharge Instructions Given

Hospital Name	City	Rate	Cases
Carolinas Medical Center - Pineville	Charlotte	100%	435
Carolinas Medical Center - University	Charlotte	100%	152
Central Carolina Hospital	Sanford	100%	162
Charles A Cannon Jr Memorial Hospital	Linville	100%	27
Davis Regional Medical Center	Statesville	100%	101
Fayetteville NC VA Medical Center	Fayetteville	100%	74
High Point Regional Hospital	High Point	100%	432
Lake Norman Regional Medical Center	Mooresville	100%	121
The Mcdowell Hospital	Marion	100%	80
The Moses H Cone Memorial Hospital	Greensboro	100%	1197
Novant Health Brunswick Medical Center	Supply	100%	127
Novant Health Forsyth Medical Center[2]	Winston-Salem	100%	818
Novant Health Franklin Medical Center	Louisburg	100%	60
Onslow Memorial Hospital	Jacksonville	100%	149
Park Ridge Health	Hendersonville	100%	62
Presbyterian Hospital Matthews	Matthews	100%	179
Spruce Pine Community Hospital	Spruce Pine	100%	52
Vidant Bertie Hospital	Windsor	100%	28
Vidant Chowan Hospital	Edenton	100%	67
Vidant Duplin Hospital	Kenansville	100%	88
Vidant Roanoke Chowan Hospital	Ahoskie	100%	124
WG (Bill) Hefner Salisbury VA Med Ctr	Salisbury	100%	57
Carolinas Medical Center - Lincoln	Lincolnton	99%	124
Carolinas Medical Center - Union	Monroe	99%	279
Duke Health Raleigh Hospital	Raleigh	99%	152
Duke University Hospital	Durham	99%	736
Durham VA Medical Center	Durham	99%	232
Nash General Hospital	Rocky Mount	99%	436
New Hanover Regional Medical Center	Wilmington	99%	914
Novant Health Rowan Medical Center	Salisbury	99%	196
Novant Health Thomasville Medical Center	Thomasville	99%	84
Angel Medical Center	Franklin	98%	46
Caldwell Memorial Hospital	Lenoir	98%	48
Cape Fear Valley Medical Center	Fayetteville	98%	1018
Caromont Regional Medical Center	Gastonia	98%	516
Catawba Valley Medical Center	Hickory	98%	88
Duke Regional Hospital	Durham	98%	350
Margaret R Pardee Memorial Hospital	Hendersonville	98%	148
Mem Mission Hosp & Asheville Surg Ctr	Asheville	98%	845
Person Memorial Hospital	Roxboro	98%	90
University of North Carolina Hospital[2]	Chapel Hill	98%	237
Vidant Edgecombe Hospital	Tarboro	98%	195
Vidant Medical Center	Greenville	98%	1081
Wakemed - Cary Hospital	Cary	98%	238
Wilkes Regional Medical Center	N Wilkesboro	98%	83

NOTE: Hospital profiles are in alphabetical order by state, then city, then hospital within the city; Rankings exclude hospitals with less than 25 cases except for patient surveys which excludes hospitals with less than 100 cases; (a) 100-299 cases; (1) The number of cases/patients is too few to report; (2) Data submitted were based on a sample of cases/patients; (3) Results are based on a shorter time period than required; (4) Data suppressed by CMS for one or more quarters; (5) Results are not available for this reporting period; (6) Fewer than 100 patients completed the HCAHPS survey; (7) No cases met the criteria for this measure; (8) The lower limit of the confidence interval cannot be calculated if the number of observed infections equals zero; (9) No data are available from the state/territory for this reporting period; (10) The scores shown reflect fewer than 50 completed surveys; (11) There were discrepancies in the data collection process; (12) This measure does not apply to this hospital for this reporting period; (13) Results cannot be calculated for this reporting period; (14) The results for this state are combined with nearby states to protect confidentiality; Please refer to the User's Guide for a full explanation of data.

Carolinas Medical Center - Northeast	Concord	97%	552
Carolinas Med Ctr/Behavioral Health	Charlotte	97%	635
Chatham Hospital	Siler City	97%	37
Granville Health Systems	Oxford	97%	66
Novant Health Presbyterian Medical Center	Charlotte	97%	524
Sandhills Regional Medical Center	Hamlet	97%	88
Vidant Beaufort Hospital	Washington	97%	87
Wakemed - Raleigh Campus	Raleigh	97%	977
Wayne Memorial Hospital	Goldsboro	97%	368
Alamance Regional Medical Center	Burlington	96%	312
Cleveland Regional Medical Center	Shelby	96%	231
Firsthealth Moore Regional Hospital[2]	Pinehurst	96%	284
Kings Mountain Hospital	Kings Mountain	96%	54
Randolph Hospital[2]	Asheboro	96%	190
Scotland Memorial Hospital	Laurinburg	96%	272
Southeastern Regional Medical Center	Lumberton	96%	586
CMC - Blue Ridge	Morganton	95%	130
Frye Regional Medical Center	Hickory	95%	189
Stanly Regional Medical Center	Albemarle	95%	201
Johnston Memorial Hospital	Smithfield	94%	264
Lenoir Memorial Hospital	Kinston	94%	293
Northern Hospital of Surry County	Mount Airy	94%	94
Maria Parham Medical Center	Henderson	93%	181
Novant Health Huntersville Medical Center	Huntersville	93%	87
Rex Hospital[2]	Raleigh	93%	330
Sampson Regional Medical Center	Clinton	92%	144
Halifax Regional Medical Center	Roanoke Rapids	91%	211
Hugh Chatham Memorial Hospital	Elkin	91%	115
North Carolina Baptist Hospital	Winston-Salem	91%	641
Ashe Memorial Hospital	Jefferson	90%	31
Asheville - Oteen VA Medical Center	Asheville	90%	113
Lexington Memorial Hospital	Lexington	90%	94
Medwest Haywood	Clyde	90%	89
Betsy Johnson Regional Hospital	Dunn	89%	194
Wilson Medical Center	Wilson	89%	224
Carteret General Hospital	Morehead City	88%	126
Martin General Hospital	Williamston	88%	86
Columbus Regional Healthcare System	Whiteville	86%	107
Iredell Memorial Hospital	Statesville	86%	241
Medwest Harris	Sylva	86%	76
Watauga Medical Center	Boone	86%	59
Rutherford Hospital	Rutherfordton	85%	152
Albemarle Hospital Authority	Elizabeth City	83%	202
Carolina East Medical Center	New Bern	83%	350
Morehead Memorial Hospital	Eden	83%	172
Murphy Medical Center	Murphy	82%	49
J Arthur Dosher Memorial Hospital	Southport	81%	27
Anson Community Hospital	Wadesboro	79%	28

Evaluation of LVS Function

Hospital Name	City	Rate	Cases
Alamance Regional Medical Center	Burlington	100%	421
Albemarle Hospital Authority	Elizabeth City	100%	246
Asheville - Oteen VA Medical Center	Asheville	100%	117
Caldwell Memorial Hospital	Lenoir	100%	66
Cape Fear Valley Medical Center	Fayetteville	100%	1174
Carolina East Medical Center	New Bern	100%	410
Carolinas Medical Center - Northeast	Concord	100%	644
Carolinas Medical Center - Pineville	Charlotte	100%	502
Carolinas Medical Center - Union	Monroe	100%	337
Carolinas Medical Center - University	Charlotte	100%	169
Carolinas Med Ctr/Behavioral Health	Charlotte	100%	715
Caromont Regional Medical Center	Gastonia	100%	588
Carteret General Hospital	Morehead City	100%	188
Catawba Valley Medical Center	Hickory	100%	110
Central Carolina Hospital	Sanford	100%	207
Charles A Cannon Jr Memorial Hospital	Linville	100%	46
Cleveland Regional Medical Center	Shelby	100%	284
Davis Regional Medical Center	Statesville	100%	108
Duke Health Raleigh Hospital	Raleigh	100%	163
Duke Regional Hospital	Durham	100%	427
Duke University Hospital	Durham	100%	831
Durham VA Medical Center	Durham	100%	235
Firsthealth Moore Regional Hospital[2]	Pinehurst	100%	329
Frye Regional Medical Center	Hickory	100%	222
Halifax Regional Medical Center	Roanoke Rapids	100%	258
High Point Regional Hospital	High Point	100%	555
Iredell Memorial Hospital	Statesville	100%	292
Johnston Memorial Hospital	Smithfield	100%	335
Kings Mountain Hospital	Kings Mountain	100%	65
Lake Norman Regional Medical Center	Mooresville	100%	149
Lenoir Memorial Hospital	Kinston	100%	343
Margaret R Pardee Memorial Hospital	Hendersonville	100%	219
Maria Parham Medical Center	Henderson	100%	212
Martin General Hospital	Williamston	100%	102
The Mcdowell Hospital	Marion	100%	100
Medwest Harris	Sylva	100%	98
Medwest Haywood	Clyde	100%	125
Medwest Swain	Bryson City	100%	26
Mem Mission Hosp & Asheville Surg Ctr	Asheville	100%	1030
The Moses H Cone Memorial Hospital	Greensboro	100%	1423
New Hanover Regional Medical Center	Wilmington	100%	1138
North Carolina Baptist Hospital	Winston-Salem	100%	744
Northern Hospital of Surry County	Mount Airy	100%	121
Novant Health Brunswick Medical Center	Supply	100%	146
Novant Health Forsyth Medical Center[2]	Winston-Salem	100%	983
Novant Health Franklin Medical Center	Louisburg	100%	76
Novant Health Huntersville Medical Center	Huntersville	100%	103
Novant Health Presbyterian Medical Center	Charlotte	100%	612
Novant Health Rowan Medical Center	Salisbury	100%	245
Novant Health Thomasville Medical Center	Thomasville	100%	110
Park Ridge Health	Hendersonville	100%	92
Presbyterian Hospital Matthews	Matthews	100%	211
Rex Hospital[2]	Raleigh	100%	406
Saint Luke's Hospital	Columbus	100%	36
Sandhills Regional Medical Center	Hamlet	100%	104
Scotland Memorial Hospital	Laurinburg	100%	307
Southeastern Regional Medical Center	Lumberton	100%	672
Spruce Pine Community Hospital	Spruce Pine	100%	59
Stanly Regional Medical Center	Albemarle	100%	249
Transylvania Regional Hospital	Brevard	100%	40
University of North Carolina Hospital[2]	Chapel Hill	100%	270
Vidant Bertie Hospital	Windsor	100%	44
Vidant Duplin Hospital	Kenansville	100%	107
Vidant Edgecombe Hospital	Tarboro	100%	240
Vidant Medical Center	Greenville	100%	1211
Vidant Roanoke Chowan Hospital	Ahoskie	100%	146
Wakemed - Cary Hospital	Cary	100%	294
Wakemed - Raleigh Campus	Raleigh	100%	1143
Watauga Medical Center	Boone	100%	83
Wilkes Regional Medical Center	N Wilkesboro	100%	120
Wilson Medical Center	Wilson	100%	279
Betsy Johnson Regional Hospital	Dunn	99%	240
Carolinas Medical Center - Lincoln	Lincolnton	99%	155
CMC - Blue Ridge	Morganton	99%	158
Fayetteville NC VA Medical Center	Fayetteville	99%	76
Granville Health Systems	Oxford	99%	82
Hugh Chatham Memorial Hospital	Elkin	99%	146
Lexington Memorial Hospital	Lexington	99%	118
Nash General Hospital	Rocky Mount	99%	504
Onslow Memorial Hospital	Jacksonville	99%	171
Randolph Hospital[2]	Asheboro	99%	245
Rutherford Hospital	Rutherfordton	99%	185
Sampson Regional Medical Center	Clinton	99%	183
Vidant Beaufort Hospital	Washington	99%	101
Vidant Chowan Hospital	Edenton	99%	85
Wayne Memorial Hospital	Goldsboro	99%	416
Angel Medical Center	Franklin	98%	56
Murphy Medical Center	Murphy	98%	65
Person Memorial Hospital	Roxboro	98%	93
WG (Bill) Hefner Salisbury VA Med Ctr	Salisbury	98%	61
Morehead Memorial Hospital	Eden	97%	227
Columbus Regional Healthcare System	Whiteville	96%	135
Chatham Hospital	Siler City	95%	42
Anson Community Hospital	Wadesboro	94%	35
Ashe Memorial Hospital	Jefferson	94%	36
J Arthur Dosher Memorial Hospital	Southport	87%	39

Medicare Spending

Medicare Spending per Patient (ratio)

Hospital Name	City	Ratio	Cases
Cherokee Indian Hospital Authority	Cherokee	0.70	-
Sandhills Regional Medical Center	Hamlet	0.85	-
Sampson Regional Medical Center	Clinton	0.87	-
Scotland Memorial Hospital	Laurinburg	0.87	-
Kings Mountain Hospital	Kings Mountain	0.88	-
Morehead Memorial Hospital	Eden	0.88	-
Murphy Medical Center	Murphy	0.88	-
Granville Health Systems	Oxford	0.89	-
Martin General Hospital	Williamston	0.89	-
Person Memorial Hospital	Roxboro	0.89	-
Spruce Pine Community Hospital	Spruce Pine	0.89	-
Vidant Duplin Hospital	Kenansville	0.89	-
Carolina East Medical Center	New Bern	0.90	-
Stanly Regional Medical Center	Albemarle	0.90	-
Albemarle Hospital Authority	Elizabeth City	0.91	-
Carteret General Hospital	Morehead City	0.91	-
Davis Regional Medical Center	Statesville	0.91	-
Vidant Roanoke Chowan Hospital	Ahoskie	0.91	-
CMC - Blue Ridge	Morganton	0.92	-
Firsthealth Moore Regional Hospital	Pinehurst	0.92	-
Lexington Memorial Hospital	Lexington	0.92	-
Maria Parham Medical Center	Henderson	0.92	-
Southeastern Regional Medical Center	Lumberton	0.92	-
Vidant Edgecombe Hospital	Tarboro	0.92	-
Alamance Regional Medical Center	Burlington	0.93	-
Betsy Johnson Regional Hospital	Dunn	0.93	-
Caromont Regional Medical Center	Gastonia	0.93	-
Hugh Chatham Memorial Hospital	Elkin	0.93	-
Iredell Memorial Hospital	Statesville	0.93	-
Medwest Haywood	Clyde	0.93	-
North Carolina Specialty Hospital	Durham	0.93	-
Novant Health Park Hospital	Winston-Salem	0.93	-
Rutherford Hospital	Rutherfordton	0.93	-
University of North Carolina Hospital	Chapel Hill	0.93	-
Anson Community Hospital	Wadesboro	0.94	-
Cape Fear Valley Medical Center	Fayetteville	0.94	-
Central Carolina Hospital	Sanford	0.94	-
Cleveland Regional Medical Center	Shelby	0.94	-
Lake Norman Regional Medical Center	Mooresville	0.94	-
Novant Health Brunswick Medical Center	Supply	0.94	-
Presbyterian Hospital Matthews	Matthews	0.94	-
Rex Hospital	Raleigh	0.94	-
Vidant Beaufort Hospital	Washington	0.94	-
Vidant Medical Center	Greenville	0.94	-
Carolinas Medical Center - Northeast	Concord	0.95	-
Carolinas Medical Center - Pineville	Charlotte	0.95	-
Duke University Hospital	Durham	0.95	-
Lenoir Memorial Hospital	Kinston	0.95	-
North Carolina Baptist Hospital	Winston-Salem	0.95	-
Watauga Medical Center	Boone	0.95	-
Wilkes Regional Medical Center	N Wilkesboro	0.95	-
Medwest Harris	Sylva	0.96	-
The Moses H Cone Memorial Hospital	Greensboro	0.96	-
New Hanover Regional Medical Center	Wilmington	0.96	-
Northern Hospital of Surry County	Mount Airy	0.96	-
Novant Health Charlotte Ortho Hosp	Charlotte	0.96	-
Novant Health Thomasville Medical Center	Thomasville	0.96	-
Randolph Hospital	Asheboro	0.96	-
Wakemed - Cary Hospital	Cary	0.96	-
Carolinas Medical Center - Union	Monroe	0.97	-
Duke Regional Hospital	Durham	0.97	-
Frye Regional Medical Center	Hickory	0.97	-
Johnston Memorial Hospital	Smithfield	0.97	-
Margaret R Pardee Memorial Hospital	Hendersonville	0.97	-
The Mcdowell Hospital	Marion	0.97	-
Novant Health Forsyth Medical Center	Winston-Salem	0.97	-
Onslow Memorial Hospital	Jacksonville	0.97	-
Park Ridge Health	Hendersonville	0.97	-
Carolinas Medical Center - University	Charlotte	0.98	-
Columbus Regional Healthcare System	Whiteville	0.98	-
High Point Regional Hospital	High Point	0.98	-
Nash General Hospital	Rocky Mount	0.98	-
Novant Health Huntersville Medical Center	Huntersville	0.98	-
Wayne Memorial Hospital	Goldsboro	0.98	-
Wilson Medical Center	Wilson	0.98	-
Carolinas Med Ctr/Behavioral Health	Charlotte	0.99	-
Catawba Valley Medical Center	Hickory	0.99	-
Duke Health Raleigh Hospital	Raleigh	0.99	-
Halifax Regional Medical Center	Roanoke Rapids	0.99	-
Mem Mission Hosp & Asheville Surg Ctr	Asheville	0.99	-
Novant Health Presbyterian Medical Center	Charlotte	0.99	-
Novant Health Rowan Medical Center	Salisbury	0.99	-
Carolinas Medical Center - Lincoln	Lincolnton	1.00	-
Wakemed - Raleigh Campus	Raleigh	1.00	-
Caldwell Memorial Hospital	Lenoir	1.03	-
Novant Health Franklin Medical Center	Louisburg	1.05	-

Pneumonia Care

Appropriate Initial Antibiotic Given

Hospital Name	City	Rate	Cases
Duke Regional Hospital	Durham	100%	214
Medwest Swain	Bryson City	100%	33
Novant Health Forsyth Medical Center[2]	Winston-Salem	100%	712
Novant Health Franklin Medical Center	Louisburg	100%	43
Novant Health Huntersville Medical Center	Huntersville	100%	115
Novant Health Thomasville Medical Center	Thomasville	100%	65
The Outer Banks Hospital	Nags Head	100%	55
Transylvania Regional Hospital	Brevard	100%	55
Vidant Duplin Hospital	Kenansville	100%	60
Vidant Roanoke Chowan Hospital	Ahoskie	100%	69
Cape Fear Valley Medical Center	Fayetteville	99%	451
Carolinas Medical Center - Pineville	Charlotte	99%	250
Carolinas Medical Center - University	Charlotte	99%	115
Caromont Regional Medical Center	Gastonia	99%	478
Cleveland Regional Medical Center	Shelby	99%	174
Davis Regional Medical Center	Statesville	99%	89
Duke Health Raleigh Hospital	Raleigh	99%	102
Lake Norman Regional Medical Center	Mooresville	99%	89
Lexington Memorial Hospital	Lexington	99%	123
Margaret R Pardee Memorial Hospital	Hendersonville	99%	141
Medwest Harris	Sylva	99%	100
The Moses H Cone Memorial Hospital	Greensboro	99%	535
Novant Health Brunswick Medical Center	Supply	99%	112
Novant Health Presbyterian Medical Center	Charlotte	99%	184
Park Ridge Health	Hendersonville	99%	90
Presbyterian Hospital Matthews	Matthews	99%	206
Randolph Hospital[2]	Asheboro	99%	93
Spruce Pine Community Hospital	Spruce Pine	99%	79

NOTE: Hospital profiles are in alphabetical order by state, then city, then hospital within the city; Rankings exclude hospitals with less than 25 cases except for patient surveys which excludes hospitals with less than 100 cases; (a) 100-299 cases; (1) The number of cases/patients is too few to report; (2) Data submitted were based on a sample of cases/patients; (3) Results are based on a shorter time period than required; (4) Data suppressed by CMS for one or more quarters; (5) Results are not available for this reporting period; (6) Fewer than 100 patients completed the HCAHPS survey; (7) No cases met the criteria for this measure; (8) The lower limit of the confidence interval cannot be calculated if the number of observed infections equals zero; (9) No data are available from the state/territory for this reporting period; (10) The scores shown reflect fewer than 50 completed surveys; (11) There were discrepancies in the data collection process; (12) This measure does not apply to this hospital for this reporting period; (13) Results cannot be calculated for this reporting period; (14) The results for this state are combined with nearby states to protect confidentiality; Please refer to the User's Guide for a full explanation of data.

Vidant Medical Center	Greenville	99%	228
Wakemed - Cary Hospital	Cary	99%	132
Wayne Memorial Hospital	Goldsboro	99%	149
Betsy Johnson Regional Hospital	Dunn	98%	165
Caldwell Memorial Hospital	Lenoir	98%	100
Carteret General Hospital	Morehead City	98%	143
Central Carolina Hospital	Sanford	98%	130
Durham VA Medical Center	Durham	98%	42
Hugh Chatham Memorial Hospital	Elkin	98%	139
Nash General Hospital[2]	Rocky Mount	98%	131
Northern Hospital of Surry County	Mount Airy	98%	143
Novant Health Rowan Medical Center	Salisbury	98%	180
Rex Hospital[2]	Raleigh	98%	179
Saint Luke's Hospital	Columbus	98%	47
Scotland Memorial Hospital	Laurinburg	98%	138
Southeastern Regional Medical Center	Lumberton	98%	221
Wakemed - Raleigh Campus	Raleigh	98%	155
Alamance Regional Medical Center	Burlington	97%	215
Carolinas Med Ctr/Behaviorial Health	Charlotte	97%	171
CMC - Blue Ridge	Morganton	97%	218
Fayetteville NC VA Medical Center	Fayetteville	97%	30
Mem Mission Hosp & Asheville Surg Ctr[2]	Asheville	97%	35
New Hanover Regional Medical Center	Wilmington	97%	328
North Carolina Baptist Hospital	Winston-Salem	97%	247
Stanly Regional Medical Center	Albemarle	97%	126
Vidant Chowan Hospital	Edenton	97%	35
Vidant Edgecombe Hospital	Tarboro	97%	70
Carolinas Medical Center - Lincoln	Lincolnton	96%	186
Carolinas Medical Center - Northeast	Concord	96%	306
Carolinas Medical Center - Union	Monroe	96%	189
The Mcdowell Hospital	Marion	96%	73
Onslow Memorial Hospital	Jacksonville	96%	158
Sandhills Regional Medical Center	Hamlet	96%	52
University of North Carolina Hospital[2]	Chapel Hill	96%	46
Catawba Valley Medical Center	Hickory	95%	170
Duke University Hospital	Durham	95%	81
Firsthealth Moore Regional Hospital[2]	Pinehurst	95%	111
High Point Regional Hospital	High Point	95%	254
Kings Mountain Hospital	Kings Mountain	95%	44
Maria Parham Medical Center	Henderson	95%	91
Medwest Haywood	Clyde	95%	146
Murphy Medical Center	Murphy	95%	80
Watauga Medical Center	Boone	95%	110
Angel Medical Center	Franklin	94%	63
Frye Regional Medical Center[2]	Hickory	94%	134
Granville Health Systems	Oxford	94%	62
Iredell Memorial Hospital	Statesville	94%	197
Lenoir Memorial Hospital	Kinston	94%	126
Martin General Hospital	Williamston	94%	35
Person Memorial Hospital	Roxboro	94%	54
Sampson Regional Medical Center	Clinton	94%	83
Wilkes Regional Medical Center	N Wilkesboro	94%	159
Ashe Memorial Hospital	Jefferson	93%	99
Asheville - Oteen VA Medical Center	Asheville	93%	75
Halifax Regional Medical Center	Roanoke Rapids	93%	159
Morehead Memorial Hospital	Eden	93%	206
Wilson Medical Center	Wilson	93%	169
Albemarle Hospital Authority	Elizabeth City	92%	65
J Arthur Dosher Memorial Hospital	Southport	92%	36
Rutherford Hospital	Rutherfordton	92%	139
Alleghany County Memorial Hospital	Sparta	91%	67
Carolina East Medical Center	New Bern	91%	189
Columbus Regional Healthcare System	Whiteville	91%	101
Johnston Memorial Hospital	Smithfield	91%	181
Chatham Hospital	Siler City	90%	40
Vidant Beaufort Hospital	Washington	90%	62
WG (Bill) Hefner Salisbury VA Med Ctr	Salisbury	88%	52
Charles A Cannon Jr Memorial Hospital	Linville	87%	39

Blood Culture Timing

Hospital Name	City	Rate	Cases
Caldwell Memorial Hospital	Lenoir	100%	209
Caromont Regional Medical Center	Gastonia	100%	986
Davis Regional Medical Center	Statesville	100%	162
Fayetteville NC VA Medical Center	Fayetteville	100%	42
Firsthealth Montgomery Memorial Hospital	Troy	100%	41
Kings Mountain Hospital	Kings Mountain	100%	53
Medwest Harris	Sylva	100%	156
Medwest Swain	Bryson City	100%	54
Novant Health Brunswick Medical Center	Supply	100%	190
Novant Health Forsyth Medical Center[2]	Winston-Salem	100%	1344
Novant Health Franklin Medical Center	Louisburg	100%	83
Novant Health Huntersville Medical Center	Huntersville	100%	162
Novant Health Presbyterian Medical Center	Charlotte	100%	315
Novant Health Rowan Medical Center	Salisbury	100%	281
Novant Health Thomasville Medical Center	Thomasville	100%	145
Pender Memorial Hospital[3]	Burgaw	100%	25
Person Memorial Hospital	Roxboro	100%	103
Presbyterian Hospital Matthews	Matthews	100%	323
Saint Luke's Hospital	Columbus	100%	80
Stanly Regional Medical Center	Albemarle	100%	214
Transylvania Regional Hospital	Brevard	100%	89
Vidant Bertie Hospital	Windsor	100%	26
Alleghany County Memorial Hospital	Sparta	99%	78
Cape Fear Valley Medical Center	Fayetteville	99%	803
Carolinas Medical Center - Northeast	Concord	99%	642
Carolinas Medical Center - Pineville	Charlotte	99%	445
Carteret General Hospital	Morehead City	99%	245
Central Carolina Hospital	Sanford	99%	160
Cleveland Regional Medical Center	Shelby	99%	192
Columbus Regional Healthcare System	Whiteville	99%	156
Duke Regional Hospital	Durham	99%	422
Duke University Hospital	Durham	99%	265
Firsthealth Moore Regional Hospital[2]	Pinehurst	99%	197
Halifax Regional Medical Center	Roanoke Rapids	99%	233
Margaret R Pardee Memorial Hospital	Hendersonville	99%	225
Medwest Haywood	Clyde	99%	237
Morehead Memorial Hospital	Eden	99%	320
The Moses H Cone Memorial Hospital	Greensboro	99%	524
New Hanover Regional Medical Center	Wilmington	99%	695
Northern Hospital of Surry County	Mount Airy	99%	239
The Outer Banks Hospital	Nags Head	99%	71
Rex Hospital[2]	Raleigh	99%	306
Scotland Memorial Hospital	Laurinburg	99%	214
University of North Carolina Hospital[2]	Chapel Hill	99%	103
Vidant Roanoke Chowan Hospital	Ahoskie	99%	142
WG (Bill) Hefner Salisbury VA Med Ctr	Salisbury	99%	35
Wilkes Regional Medical Center	N Wilkesboro	99%	349
Angel Medical Center	Franklin	98%	93
Asheville - Oteen VA Medical Center	Asheville	98%	131
Betsy Johnson Regional Hospital	Dunn	98%	226
Carolina East Medical Center	New Bern	98%	345
Carolinas Medical Center - Lincoln	Lincolnton	98%	256
Carolinas Med Ctr/Behaviorial Health	Charlotte	98%	192
CMC - Blue Ridge	Morganton	98%	368
Duke Health Raleigh Hospital	Raleigh	98%	176
Durham VA Medical Center	Durham	98%	111
Frye Regional Medical Center[2]	Hickory	98%	195
High Point Regional Hospital	High Point	98%	395
Hugh Chatham Memorial Hospital	Elkin	98%	209
Johnston Memorial Hospital	Smithfield	98%	279
Lake Norman Regional Medical Center	Mooresville	98%	166
Lexington Memorial Hospital	Lexington	98%	221
The Mcdowell Hospital	Marion	98%	129
Nash General Hospital[2]	Rocky Mount	98%	253
North Carolina Baptist Hospital	Winston-Salem	98%	729
Onslow Memorial Hospital	Jacksonville	98%	266
Park Ridge Health	Hendersonville	98%	152
Sampson Regional Medical Center	Clinton	98%	139
Spruce Pine Community Hospital	Spruce Pine	98%	150
Vidant Edgecombe Hospital	Tarboro	98%	122
Carolinas Medical Center - Union	Monroe	97%	300
Catawba Valley Medical Center	Hickory	97%	238
Chatham Hospital	Siler City	97%	62
Mem Mission Hosp & Asheville Surg Ctr[2]	Asheville	97%	156
Randolph Hospital[2]	Asheboro	97%	131
Sandhills Regional Medical Center	Hamlet	97%	66
Wakemed - Raleigh Campus	Raleigh	97%	394
Watauga Medical Center	Boone	97%	177
Albemarle Hospital Authority	Elizabeth City	96%	141
Anson Community Hospital	Wadesboro	96%	27
Lenoir Memorial Hospital	Kinston	96%	184
Maria Parham Medical Center	Henderson	96%	173
Murphy Medical Center	Murphy	96%	117
Rutherford Hospital	Rutherfordton	96%	265
Vidant Chowan Hospital	Edenton	96%	52
Vidant Medical Center	Greenville	96%	540
Wakemed - Cary Hospital	Cary	96%	248
Iredell Memorial Hospital	Statesville	95%	253
Martin General Hospital	Williamston	95%	77
Vidant Duplin Hospital	Kenansville	95%	105
Wayne Memorial Hospital	Goldsboro	95%	169
Ashe Memorial Hospital	Jefferson	94%	63
Carolinas Medical Center - University	Charlotte	94%	195
Granville Health Systems	Oxford	94%	80
Charles A Cannon Jr Memorial Hospital	Linville	93%	44
Southeastern Regional Medical Center	Lumberton	92%	363
Wilson Medical Center	Wilson	91%	319
Alamance Regional Medical Center	Burlington	90%	309
Vidant Beaufort Hospital	Washington	90%	99
Pioneer Community Hospital of Stokes	Danbury	88%	25
J Arthur Dosher Memorial Hospital	Southport	87%	53

Pregnancy and Delivery Care

Newborns whose Deliveries were Scheduled Early

Hospital Name	City	Rate	Cases
Betsy Johnson Regional Hospital	Dunn	0%	47
Caldwell Memorial Hospital[2]	Lenoir	0%	47
Carolinas Medical Center - Lincoln	Lincolnton	0%	33
Carolinas Medical Center - Pineville	Charlotte	0%	252
Carolinas Medical Center - Union	Monroe	0%	82
Carolinas Medical Center - University	Charlotte	0%	105
CMC - Blue Ridge[2]	Morganton	0%	84
Columbus Regional Healthcare System[2]	Whiteville	0%	46
Firsthealth Moore Regional Hospital[2]	Pinehurst	0%	29
Johnston Memorial Hospital[2]	Smithfield	0%	26
Margaret R Pardee Memorial Hospital	Hendersonville	0%	32
Morehead Memorial Hospital	Eden	0%	47
Northern Hospital of Surry County	Mount Airy	0%	48
Novant Health Huntersville Medical Center[2]	Huntersville	0%	39
Randolph Hospital	Asheboro	0%	68
Rex Hospital[2]	Raleigh	0%	79
University of North Carolina Hospital[2]	Chapel Hill	0%	52
Vidant Roanoke Chowan Hospital	Ahoskie	0%	36
Wakemed - Raleigh Campus[2]	Raleigh	0%	64
Wayne Memorial Hospital[2]	Goldsboro	0%	26
Cape Fear Valley Medical Center[2]	Fayetteville	1%	85
Carolinas Med Ctr/Behaviorial Health	Charlotte	1%	248
Catawba Valley Medical Center	Hickory	1%	159
Cleveland Memorial Hospital	Shelby	1%	211
Lenoir Memorial Hospital	Kinston	1%	79
The Moses H Cone Memorial Hospital	Greensboro	1%	576
Novant Health Presbyterian Medical Center[2]	Charlotte	1%	110
Stanly Regional Medical Center[2]	Albemarle	1%	118
Albemarle Hospital Authority[2]	Elizabeth City	2%	63
Carolinas Medical Center - Northeast	Concord	2%	198
Caromont Regional Medical Center	Gastonia	2%	177
Duke University Hospital[2]	Durham	2%	112
Mem Mission Hosp & Asheville Surg Ctr[2]	Asheville	2%	40
Novant Health Rowan Medical Center[2]	Salisbury	2%	40
Southeastern Regional Medical Center[2]	Lumberton	2%	120
Vidant Duplin Hospital	Kenansville	2%	60
High Point Regional Hospital	High Point	3%	143
Nash General Hospital	Rocky Mount	3%	125
Onslow Memorial Hospital[2]	Jacksonville	3%	35
Wakemed - Cary Hospital[2]	Cary	3%	39
Carolina East Medical Center	New Bern	4%	119
Carteret General Hospital	Morehead City	4%	48
Novant Health Forsyth Medical Center[2]	Winston-Salem	4%	118
Vidant Medical Center[2]	Greenville	4%	159
Alamance Regional Medical Center	Burlington	5%	82
Duke Regional Hospital	Durham	5%	155
New Hanover Regional Medical Center[2]	Wilmington	5%	40
Scotland Memorial Hospital[2]	Laurinburg	5%	37
Vidant Edgecombe Hospital[2]	Tarboro	5%	43
Davis Regional Medical Center	Statesville	6%	31
Central Carolina Hospital[2]	Sanford	7%	29
Granville Health Systems	Oxford	7%	29
Novant Health Brunswick Medical Center[2]	Supply	8%	25
Sampson Regional Medical Center	Clinton	8%	25
Vidant Beaufort Hospital	Washington	8%	36
Hugh Chatham Memorial Hospital	Elkin	9%	45
Watauga Medical Center	Boone	9%	32
Halifax Regional Medical Center	Roanoke Rapids	12%	74
Wilson Medical Center[2]	Wilson	12%	33
Lexington Memorial Hospital[2]	Lexington	15%	72
Iredell Memorial Hospital[2]	Statesville	16%	44
Novant Health Thomasville Medical Center[2]	Thomasville	21%	52
Medwest Harris[2]	Sylva	34%	32

Preventive Care

Immunization for Influenza

Hospital Name	City	Rate	Cases
Davis Regional Medical Center[2]	Statesville	100%	334
North Carolina Specialty Hospital[2]	Durham	100%	304
Person Memorial Hospital[2]	Roxboro	100%	292
CMC - Blue Ridge[2]	Morganton	99%	738
Lake Norman Regional Medical Center[2]	Mooresville	99%	628
Martin General Hospital[2]	Williamston	99%	295
Northern Hospital of Surry County[2]	Mount Airy	99%	410
Novant Health Franklin Medical Center[2]	Louisburg	99%	346
Novant Health Park Hospital	Winston-Salem	99%	344
Spruce Pine Community Hospital[2]	Spruce Pine	99%	297
Angel Medical Center[2]	Franklin	98%	451
Duke Health Raleigh Hospital[2]	Raleigh	98%	615
Hugh Chatham Memorial Hospital[2]	Elkin	98%	478
Novant Health Brunswick Medical Center[2]	Supply	98%	469
Novant Health Huntersville Medical Center[2]	Huntersville	98%	584
Novant Health Thomasville Medical Center[2]	Thomasville	98%	476
University of North Carolina Hospital[2]	Chapel Hill	98%	534
Vidant Pungo Hospital	Belhaven	98%	254
Caldwell Memorial Hospital[2]	Lenoir	97%	341
Cape Fear Valley Medical Center[2]	Fayetteville	97%	504
High Point Regional Hospital[2]	High Point	97%	544
Margaret R Pardee Memorial Hospital[2]	Hendersonville	97%	619
Maria Parham Medical Center[2]	Henderson	97%	432
The Mcdowell Hospital[2]	Marion	97%	291
Novant Health Presbyterian Medical Center[2]	Charlotte	97%	642
Presbyterian Hospital Matthews[2]	Matthews	97%	576

NOTE: Hospital profiles are in alphabetical order by state, then city, then hospital within the city; Rankings exclude hospitals with less than 25 cases except for patient surveys which excludes hospitals with less than 100 cases; (a) 100-299 cases; (1) The number of cases/patients is too few to report; (2) Data submitted were based on a sample of cases/patients; (3) Results are based on a shorter time period than required; (4) Data suppressed by CMS for one or more quarters; (5) Results are not available for this reporting period; (6) Fewer than 100 patients completed the HCAHPS survey; (7) No cases met the criteria for this measure; (8) The lower limit of the confidence interval cannot be calculated if the number of observed infections equals zero; (9) No data are available from the state/territory for this reporting period; (10) The scores shown reflect fewer than 50 completed surveys; (11) There were discrepancies in the data collection process; (12) This measure does not apply to this hospital for this reporting period; (13) Results cannot be calculated for this reporting period; (14) The results for this state are combined with nearby states to protect confidentiality; Please refer to the User's Guide for a full explanation of data.

Hospital Name	City	Rate	Cases
Anson Community Hospital[2]	Wadesboro	96%	232
Betsy Johnson Regional Hospital[2]	Dunn	96%	623
Caromont Regional Medical Center[2]	Gastonia	96%	560
Frye Regional Medical Center[2]	Hickory	96%	612
Johnston Memorial Hospital[2]	Smithfield	96%	536
Medwest Swain[2]	Bryson City	96%	151
Mem Mission Hosp & Asheville Surg Ctr[2]	Asheville	96%	564
Novant Health Charlotte Ortho Hosp[2]	Charlotte	96%	412
Wayne Memorial Hospital[2]	Goldsboro	96%	498
Wilson Medical Center[2]	Wilson	96%	509
Carolinas Medical Center - Lincoln[2]	Lincolnton	95%	371
Carolinas Medical Center - Northeast[2]	Concord	95%	515
Carolinas Medical Center - Pineville[2]	Charlotte	95%	1050
Carolinas Medical Center - University[2]	Charlotte	95%	496
Cleveland Regional Medical Center[2]	Shelby	95%	523
Kings Mountain Hospital[2]	Kings Mountain	95%	298
Morehead Memorial Hospital[2]	Eden	95%	477
Novant Health Rowan Medical Center[2]	Salisbury	95%	678
Park Ridge Health[2]	Hendersonville	95%	322
Rutherford Hospital[2]	Rutherfordton	95%	575
Wilkes Regional Medical Center[2]	N Wilkesboro	95%	412
Albemarle Hospital Authority[2]	Elizabeth City	94%	517
Lexington Memorial Hospital[2]	Lexington	94%	343
Rex Hospital[2]	Raleigh	94%	545
Sampson Regional Medical Center[2]	Clinton	94%	376
Scotland Memorial Hospital[2]	Laurinburg	94%	559
Carolinas Medical Center - Union[2]	Monroe	93%	518
Carolinas Med Ctr/Behavioral Health[2]	Charlotte	93%	463
Firsthealth Moore Regional Hospital[2]	Pinehurst	93%	583
Halifax Regional Medical Center[2]	Roanoke Rapids	93%	536
Sandhills Regional Medical Center[2]	Hamlet	93%	286
Vidant Edgecombe Hospital[2]	Tarboro	93%	386
Vidant Roanoke Chowan Hospital[2]	Ahoskie	93%	429
Wakemed - Raleigh Campus[2]	Raleigh	93%	520
Alamance Regional Medical Center[2]	Burlington	92%	555
Iredell Memorial Hospital[2]	Statesville	92%	583
Murphy Medical Center[2]	Murphy	92%	493
Ashe Memorial Hospital[2]	Jefferson	91%	402
Vidant Medical Center[2]	Greenville	91%	541
Watauga Medical Center[2]	Boone	91%	363
Carolina East Medical Center[2]	New Bern	90%	569
Catawba Valley Medical Center[2]	Hickory	90%	525
Medwest Harris[2]	Sylva	90%	346
The Moses H Cone Memorial Hospital[2]	Greensboro	90%	538
Pioneer Community Hospital of Stokes	Danbury	90%	167
Wakemed - Cary Hospital[2]	Cary	90%	513
Columbus Regional Healthcare System[2]	Whiteville	89%	446
North Carolina Baptist Hospital[2]	Winston-Salem	89%	567
Novant Health Forsyth Medical Center[2]	Winston-Salem	89%	1027
Randolph Hospital[2]	Asheboro	89%	543
Carteret General Hospital[2]	Morehead City	88%	528
Granville Health Systems[2]	Oxford	88%	445
Medwest Haywood[2]	Clyde	88%	521
New Hanover Regional Medical Center[2]	Wilmington	87%	570
Vidant Beaufort Hospital[2]	Washington	87%	323
Onslow Memorial Hospital[2]	Jacksonville	86%	486
Lenoir Memorial Hospital[2]	Kinston	84%	545
Southeastern Regional Medical Center[2]	Lumberton	84%	526
Chatham Hospital	Siler City	83%	242
Nash General Hospital[2]	Rocky Mount	83%	581
Stanly Regional Medical Center[2]	Albemarle	83%	435
Central Carolina Hospital[2]	Sanford	82%	508
Vidant Duplin Hospital[2]	Kenansville	81%	354
Cherokee Indian Hospital Authority[2]	Cherokee	79%	187
Duke University Hospital[2]	Durham	78%	585
Duke Regional Hospital[2]	Durham	75%	582
J Arthur Dosher Memorial Hospital[2]	Southport	72%	298
Fayetteville NC VA Medical Center[2,3]	Fayetteville	38%	134

Immunization for Pneumonia

Hospital Name	City	Rate	Cases
Martin General Hospital[2]	Williamston	100%	414
North Carolina Specialty Hospital[2]	Durham	100%	610
Northern Hospital of Surry County[2]	Mount Airy	100%	553
Novant Health Brunswick Medical Center[2]	Supply	100%	614
Novant Health Park Hospital	Winston-Salem	100%	385
Person Memorial Hospital[2]	Roxboro	100%	458
Spruce Pine Community Hospital[2]	Spruce Pine	100%	415
Angel Medical Center[2]	Franklin	99%	697
Caldwell Memorial Hospital[2]	Lenoir	99%	468
CMC - Blue Ridge[2]	Morganton	99%	970
Davis Regional Medical Center[2]	Statesville	99%	358
High Point Regional Hospital[2]	High Point	99%	701
Maria Parham Medical Center[2]	Henderson	99%	612
Novant Health Huntersville Medical Center[2]	Huntersville	99%	688
Presbyterian Hospital Matthews[2]	Matthews	99%	734
Carolinas Medical Center - Pineville[2]	Charlotte	98%	1265
Caromont Regional Medical Center[2]	Gastonia	98%	712
Duke Health Raleigh Hospital[2]	Raleigh	98%	840
Hugh Chatham Memorial Hospital[2]	Elkin	98%	562
Kings Mountain Hospital[2]	Kings Mountain	98%	445
Lake Norman Regional Medical Center[2]	Mooresville	98%	623
Novant Health Franklin Medical Center[2]	Louisburg	98%	548
Novant Health Rowan Medical Center[2]	Salisbury	98%	861
Novant Health Thomasville Medical Center[2]	Thomasville	98%	637
Wilkes Regional Medical Center[2]	N Wilkesboro	98%	540
Cape Fear Valley Medical Center[2]	Fayetteville	97%	622
Carolinas Medical Center - University[2]	Charlotte	97%	447
Cleveland Regional Medical Center[2]	Shelby	97%	677
Novant Health Charlotte Ortho Hosp[2]	Charlotte	97%	550
Novant Health Presbyterian Medical Center[2]	Charlotte	97%	604
Scotland Memorial Hospital[2]	Laurinburg	97%	703
Ashe Memorial Hospital[2]	Jefferson	96%	483
Carolinas Medical Center - Northeast[2]	Concord	96%	673
Carolinas Medical Center - Union[2]	Monroe	96%	637
Carolinas Med Ctr/Behavioral Health[2]	Charlotte	96%	429
Johnston Memorial Hospital[2]	Smithfield	96%	630
Margaret R Pardee Memorial Hospital[2]	Hendersonville	96%	939
Medwest Swain[2]	Bryson City	96%	263
Park Ridge Health[2]	Hendersonville	96%	370
Rutherford Hospital[2]	Rutherfordton	96%	763
Vidant Pungo Hospital	Belhaven	96%	436
Wayne Memorial Hospital[2]	Goldsboro	96%	659
Anson Community Hospital[2]	Wadesboro	95%	318
Betsy Johnson Regional Hospital[2]	Dunn	95%	798
Carolinas Medical Center - Lincoln[2]	Lincolnton	95%	482
Cherokee Indian Hospital Authority[2]	Cherokee	95%	223
Columbus Regional Healthcare System[2]	Whiteville	95%	577
Frye Regional Medical Center[2]	Hickory	95%	870
Granville Health Systems[2]	Oxford	95%	775
Lenoir Memorial Hospital[2]	Kinston	95%	738
Medwest Harris[2]	Sylva	95%	414
Novant Health Forsyth Medical Center[2]	Winston-Salem	95%	1353
Sandhills Regional Medical Center[2]	Hamlet	95%	374
Stanly Regional Medical Center[2]	Albemarle	95%	522
Wilson Medical Center[2]	Wilson	95%	665
Firsthealth Moore Regional Hospital[2]	Pinehurst	94%	799
Lexington Memorial Hospital[2]	Lexington	94%	421
Sampson Regional Medical Center[2]	Clinton	93%	439
University of North Carolina Hospital[2]	Chapel Hill	93%	446
Vidant Roanoke Chowan Hospital[2]	Ahoskie	93%	453
Carteret General Hospital[2]	Morehead City	92%	671
Halifax Regional Medical Center[2]	Roanoke Rapids	92%	777
Mem Mission Hosp & Asheville Surg Ctr[2]	Asheville	92%	733
Morehead Memorial Hospital[2]	Eden	92%	629
The Moses H Cone Memorial Hospital[2]	Greensboro	92%	692
Transylvania Regional Hospital[2,3]	Brevard	92%	421
Albemarle Hospital Authority[2]	Elizabeth City	91%	743
Medwest Haywood[2]	Clyde	91%	667
Vidant Edgecombe Hospital[2]	Tarboro	91%	499
Wakemed - Cary Hospital[2]	Cary	91%	512
Wakemed - Raleigh Campus[2]	Raleigh	91%	562
Watauga Medical Center[2]	Boone	91%	465
The Mcdowell Hospital[2]	Marion	90%	416
Rex Hospital[2]	Raleigh	90%	633
Murphy Medical Center[2]	Murphy	89%	715
New Hanover Regional Medical Center[2]	Wilmington	89%	664
Iredell Memorial Hospital[2]	Statesville	88%	795
Onslow Memorial Hospital[2]	Jacksonville	88%	449
Southeastern Regional Medical Center[2]	Lumberton	88%	700
Vidant Beaufort Hospital[2]	Washington	88%	377
Vidant Medical Center[2]	Greenville	88%	650
Catawba Valley Medical Center[2]	Hickory	87%	541
Chatham Hospital	Siler City	86%	384
North Carolina Baptist Hospital[2]	Winston-Salem	86%	658
Randolph Hospital[2]	Asheboro	86%	716
Carolina East Medical Center[2]	New Bern	85%	750
Central Carolina Hospital[2]	Sanford	85%	611
Duke Regional Hospital[2]	Durham	85%	698
Pioneer Community Hospital of Stokes	Danbury	85%	241
Duke University Hospital[2]	Durham	84%	599
J Arthur Dosher Memorial Hospital[2,3]	Southport	84%	355
Alamance Regional Medical Center[2]	Burlington	83%	847
Vidant Duplin Hospital[2]	Kenansville	82%	338
Nash General Hospital[2]	Rocky Mount	80%	734
Fayetteville NC VA Medical Center[2,3]	Fayetteville	50%	236

Stroke Care

Anticoagulation Therapy for Atrial Fibrillation

Hospital Name	City	Rate	Cases
Carolinas Medical Center - Northeast	Concord	100%	49
Carolinas Medical Center - Pineville	Charlotte	100%	26
Carolinas Med Ctr/Behavioral Health	Charlotte	100%	43
Caromont Regional Medical Center	Gastonia	100%	35
Firsthealth Moore Regional Hospital	Pinehurst	100%	47
Frye Regional Medical Center	Hickory	100%	25
High Point Regional Hospital	High Point	100%	29
Novant Health Forsyth Medical Center	Winston-Salem	100%	65
Novant Health Rowan Medical Center	Salisbury	100%	29
Duke University Hospital	Durham	97%	31
Mem Mission Hosp & Asheville Surg Ctr	Asheville	97%	101
Cape Fear Valley Medical Center	Fayetteville	96%	25
Vidant Medical Center	Greenville	95%	59
The Moses H Cone Memorial Hospital	Greensboro	92%	111
New Hanover Regional Medical Center	Wilmington	92%	60
Wakemed - Raleigh Campus	Raleigh	91%	87

Antithrombotic Therapy Timing

Hospital Name	City	Rate	Cases
Albemarle Hospital Authority	Elizabeth City	100%	87
Betsy Johnson Regional Hospital	Dunn	100%	81
Cape Fear Valley Medical Center	Fayetteville	100%	312
Carolinas Medical Center - Lincoln	Lincolnton	100%	46
Carolinas Medical Center - Northeast	Concord	100%	251
Carolinas Medical Center - Pineville	Charlotte	100%	198
Carolinas Medical Center - Union	Monroe	100%	95
Carolinas Medical Center - University	Charlotte	100%	85
Carolinas Med Ctr/Behavioral Health	Charlotte	100%	279
Caromont Regional Medical Center	Gastonia	100%	252
Carteret General Hospital	Morehead City	100%	70
Central Carolina Hospital	Sanford	100%	71
Firsthealth Moore Regional Hospital	Pinehurst	100%	288
High Point Regional Hospital	High Point	100%	209
Hugh Chatham Memorial Hospital	Elkin	100%	37
Lake Norman Regional Medical Center	Mooresville	100%	40
Medwest Haywood	Clyde	100%	57
Northern Hospital of Surry County	Mount Airy	100%	29
Novant Health Brunswick Medical Center	Supply	100%	64
Novant Health Forsyth Medical Center	Winston-Salem	100%	443
Novant Health Huntersville Medical Center	Huntersville	100%	55
Novant Health Thomasville Medical Center	Thomasville	100%	48
Onslow Memorial Hospital	Jacksonville	100%	74
Park Ridge Health[2]	Hendersonville	100%	29
Randolph Hospital[2]	Asheboro	100%	78
Rex Hospital[2]	Raleigh	100%	96
Rutherford Hospital	Rutherfordton	100%	77
Stanly Regional Medical Center	Albemarle	100%	39
Vidant Beaufort Hospital	Washington	100%	56
Vidant Duplin Hospital	Kenansville	100%	36
Vidant Roanoke Chowan Hospital	Ahoskie	100%	57
Wakemed - Cary Hospital	Cary	100%	132
Wilkes Regional Medical Center	N Wilkesboro	100%	41
Carolina East Medical Center	New Bern	99%	149
Catawba Valley Medical Center	Hickory	99%	95
Cleveland Regional Medical Center	Shelby	99%	87
Duke Health Raleigh Hospital	Raleigh	99%	69
Duke University Hospital	Durham	99%	211
Halifax Regional Medical Center	Roanoke Rapids	99%	71
Iredell Memorial Hospital	Statesville	99%	78
North Carolina Baptist Hospital[2]	Winston-Salem	99%	74
Novant Health Presbyterian Medical Center	Charlotte	99%	207
Presbyterian Hospital Matthews	Matthews	99%	116
Southeastern Regional Medical Center	Lumberton	99%	141
Wakemed - Raleigh Campus	Raleigh	99%	438
Alamance Regional Medical Center	Burlington	98%	160
CMC - Blue Ridge	Morganton	98%	66
Lenoir Memorial Hospital	Kinston	98%	66
Maria Parham Medical Center	Henderson	98%	85
Martin General Hospital	Williamston	98%	43
Mem Mission Hosp & Asheville Surg Ctr	Asheville	98%	352
Morehead Memorial Hospital	Eden	98%	53
Nash General Hospital	Rocky Mount	98%	173
Novant Health Rowan Medical Center	Salisbury	98%	161
Sampson Regional Medical Center	Clinton	98%	48
Vidant Edgecombe Hospital	Tarboro	98%	49
Lexington Memorial Hospital	Lexington	97%	62
Margaret R Pardee Memorial Hospital	Hendersonville	97%	77
The Moses H Cone Memorial Hospital	Greensboro	97%	588
Scotland Memorial Hospital	Laurinburg	97%	66
Wayne Memorial Hospital	Goldsboro	97%	124
Frye Regional Medical Center	Hickory	96%	143
New Hanover Regional Medical Center	Wilmington	96%	327
Vidant Medical Center	Greenville	96%	390
Watauga Medical Center	Boone	96%	55
Wilson Medical Center	Wilson	96%	111
Duke Regional Hospital	Durham	95%	173
University of North Carolina Hospital[2]	Chapel Hill	93%	28
Caldwell Memorial Hospital	Lenoir	92%	50
Kings Mountain Hospital	Kings Mountain	92%	26
Columbus Regional Healthcare System	Whiteville	91%	46
Johnston Memorial Hospital	Smithfield	90%	42

Assessed for Rehabilitation

Hospital Name	City	Rate	Cases
Cape Fear Valley Medical Center	Fayetteville	100%	351
Carolinas Medical Center - Northeast	Concord	100%	337
Carolinas Medical Center - Pineville	Charlotte	100%	206
Carolinas Medical Center - Union	Monroe	100%	101
Caromont Regional Medical Center	Gastonia	100%	291
Catawba Valley Medical Center	Hickory	100%	104

NOTE: Hospital profiles are in alphabetical order by state, then city, then hospital within the city; Rankings exclude hospitals with less than 25 cases except for patient surveys which excludes hospitals with less than 100 cases; (a) 100-299 cases; (1) The number of cases/patients is too few to report; (2) Data submitted were based on a sample of cases/patients; (3) Results are based on a shorter time period than required; (4) Data suppressed by CMS for one or more quarters; (5) Results are not available for this reporting period; (6) Fewer than 100 patients completed the HCAHPS survey; (7) No cases met the criteria for this measure; (8) The lower limit of the confidence interval cannot be calculated if the number of observed infections equals zero; (9) No data are available from the state/territory for this reporting period; (10) The scores shown reflect fewer than 50 completed surveys; (11) There were discrepancies in the data collection process; (12) This measure does not apply to this hospital for this reporting period; (13) Results cannot be calculated for this reporting period; (14) The results for this state are combined with nearby states to protect confidentiality; Please refer to the User's Guide for a full explanation of data.

Hospital Name	City	Rate	Cases
Central Carolina Hospital	Sanford	100%	74
Duke Regional Hospital	Durham	100%	213
Duke University Hospital	Durham	100%	332
Firsthealth Moore Regional Hospital	Pinehurst	100%	324
Frye Regional Medical Center	Hickory	100%	149
High Point Regional Hospital	High Point	100%	244
Hugh Chatham Memorial Hospital	Elkin	100%	37
Johnston Memorial Hospital	Smithfield	100%	43
Kings Mountain Hospital	Kings Mountain	100%	29
The Mcdowell Hospital	Marion	100%	26
Mem Mission Hosp & Asheville Surg Ctr	Asheville	100%	576
Northern Hospital of Surry County	Mount Airy	100%	29
Novant Health Brunswick Medical Center	Supply	100%	68
Novant Health Forsyth Medical Center	Winston-Salem	100%	625
Novant Health Huntersville Medical Center	Huntersville	100%	79
Novant Health Presbyterian Medical Center	Charlotte	100%	316
Novant Health Rowan Medical Center	Salisbury	100%	200
Novant Health Thomasville Medical Center	Thomasville	100%	59
Park Ridge Health[2]	Hendersonville	100%	37
Randolph Hospital[2]	Asheboro	100%	85
Stanly Regional Medical Center	Albemarle	100%	55
University of North Carolina Hospital[2]	Chapel Hill	100%	102
Vidant Duplin Hospital	Kenansville	100%	38
Vidant Edgecombe Hospital	Tarboro	100%	54
Wilkes Regional Medical Center	N Wilkesboro	100%	40
Carolinas Medical Center - University	Charlotte	99%	94
Carolinas Med Ctr/Behaviorial Health	Charlotte	99%	589
Cleveland Regional Medical Center	Shelby	99%	104
Duke Health Raleigh Hospital	Raleigh	99%	85
Iredell Memorial Hospital	Statesville	99%	79
Maria Parham Medical Center	Henderson	99%	72
Presbyterian Hospital Matthews	Matthews	99%	117
Southeastern Regional Medical Center	Lumberton	99%	139
Vidant Medical Center	Greenville	99%	608
Wakemed - Cary Hospital	Cary	99%	141
Wilson Medical Center	Wilson	99%	94
Alamance Regional Medical Center	Burlington	98%	164
Caldwell Memorial Hospital	Lenoir	98%	44
Carolinas Medical Center - Lincoln	Lincolnton	98%	48
Lake Norman Regional Medical Center	Mooresville	98%	45
Martin General Hospital	Williamston	98%	42
Nash General Hospital	Rocky Mount	98%	189
Rex Hospital[2]	Raleigh	98%	125
Sampson Regional Medical Center	Clinton	98%	44
Wakemed - Raleigh Campus	Raleigh	98%	573
Carteret General Hospital	Morehead City	97%	67
CMC - Blue Ridge	Morganton	97%	74
Medwest Haywood	Clyde	97%	62
The Moses H Cone Memorial Hospital	Greensboro	97%	715
Onslow Memorial Hospital	Jacksonville	97%	71
Rutherford Hospital	Rutherfordton	97%	77
Watauga Medical Center	Boone	97%	61
Wayne Memorial Hospital	Goldsboro	97%	145
Lexington Memorial Hospital	Lexington	96%	70
Margaret R Pardee Memorial Hospital	Hendersonville	95%	85
New Hanover Regional Medical Center	Wilmington	95%	435
Scotland Memorial Hospital	Laurinburg	95%	63
Albemarle Hospital Authority	Elizabeth City	93%	95
Carolina East Medical Center	New Bern	93%	152
Betsy Johnson Regional Hospital	Dunn	92%	66
Halifax Regional Medical Center	Roanoke Rapids	92%	62
Lenoir Memorial Hospital	Kinston	92%	61
North Carolina Baptist Hospital[2]	Winston-Salem	92%	148
Morehead Memorial Hospital	Eden	89%	54
Vidant Roanoke Chowan Hospital	Ahoskie	89%	57
Columbus Regional Healthcare System	Whiteville	88%	43
Vidant Beaufort Hospital	Washington	87%	53

Discharged on Antithrombotic Therapy

Hospital Name	City	Rate	Cases
Albemarle Hospital Authority	Elizabeth City	100%	93
Betsy Johnson Regional Hospital	Dunn	100%	63
Cape Fear Valley Medical Center	Fayetteville	100%	307
Carolinas Medical Center - Northeast	Concord	100%	306
Carolinas Medical Center - Pineville	Charlotte	100%	200
Carolinas Medical Center - Union	Monroe	100%	98
Carolinas Medical Center - University	Charlotte	100%	92
Carolinas Med Ctr/Behaviorial Health	Charlotte	100%	344
Caromont Regional Medical Center	Gastonia	100%	259
Catawba Valley Medical Center	Hickory	100%	103
Central Carolina Hospital	Sanford	100%	73
Cleveland Regional Medical Center	Shelby	100%	101
Duke Health Raleigh Hospital	Raleigh	100%	76
Duke Regional Hospital	Durham	100%	190
Duke University Hospital	Durham	100%	246
Firsthealth Moore Regional Hospital	Pinehurst	100%	299
Frye Regional Medical Center	Hickory	100%	149
High Point Regional Hospital	High Point	100%	228
Hugh Chatham Memorial Hospital	Elkin	100%	37
Iredell Memorial Hospital	Statesville	100%	78
Lenoir Memorial Hospital	Kinston	100%	57
Lexington Memorial Hospital	Lexington	100%	68
Maria Parham Medical Center	Henderson	100%	72
Martin General Hospital	Williamston	100%	42
Medwest Haywood	Clyde	100%	62
Mem Mission Hosp & Asheville Surg Ctr	Asheville	100%	470
North Carolina Baptist Hospital[2]	Winston-Salem	100%	105
Northern Hospital of Surry County	Mount Airy	100%	29
Novant Health Brunswick Medical Center	Supply	100%	67
Novant Health Forsyth Medical Center	Winston-Salem	100%	511
Novant Health Huntersville Medical Center	Huntersville	100%	74
Novant Health Presbyterian Medical Center	Charlotte	100%	241
Novant Health Rowan Medical Center	Salisbury	100%	187
Novant Health Thomasville Medical Center	Thomasville	100%	59
Presbyterian Hospital Matthews	Matthews	100%	113
Rex Hospital[2]	Raleigh	100%	113
Rutherford Hospital	Rutherfordton	100%	75
Sampson Regional Medical Center	Clinton	100%	44
Scotland Memorial Hospital	Laurinburg	100%	62
Vidant Beaufort Hospital	Washington	100%	53
Vidant Medical Center	Greenville	100%	461
Wakemed - Cary Hospital	Cary	100%	134
Wakemed - Raleigh Campus	Raleigh	100%	485
Watauga Medical Center	Boone	100%	59
Wilkes Regional Medical Center	N Wilkesboro	100%	37
Carolina East Medical Center	New Bern	99%	150
CMC - Blue Ridge	Morganton	99%	72
Margaret R Pardee Memorial Hospital	Hendersonville	99%	83
The Moses H Cone Memorial Hospital	Greensboro	99%	638
Nash General Hospital	Rocky Mount	99%	178
Onslow Memorial Hospital	Jacksonville	99%	69
Randolph Hospital[2]	Asheboro	99%	79
Wayne Memorial Hospital	Goldsboro	99%	136
Wilson Medical Center	Wilson	99%	94
Alamance Regional Medical Center	Burlington	98%	164
Caldwell Memorial Hospital	Lenoir	98%	44
Carteret General Hospital	Morehead City	98%	66
Columbus Regional Healthcare System	Whiteville	98%	42
Johnston Memorial Hospital	Smithfield	98%	43
Lake Norman Regional Medical Center	Mooresville	98%	45
Southeastern Regional Medical Center	Lumberton	98%	131
Stanly Regional Medical Center	Albemarle	98%	54
Vidant Edgecombe Hospital	Tarboro	98%	53
Vidant Roanoke Chowan Hospital	Ahoskie	98%	53
Park Ridge Health[2]	Hendersonville	97%	35
Vidant Duplin Hospital	Kenansville	97%	36
Carolinas Medical Center - Lincoln	Lincolnton	96%	48
Morehead Memorial Hospital	Eden	96%	52
New Hanover Regional Medical Center	Wilmington	94%	371
Halifax Regional Medical Center	Roanoke Rapids	92%	62
Kings Mountain Hospital	Kings Mountain	82%	28
University of North Carolina Hospital[2]	Chapel Hill	80%	56

Discharged on Statin Medication

Hospital Name	City	Rate	Cases
Carolinas Medical Center - University	Charlotte	100%	71
Caromont Regional Medical Center	Gastonia	100%	196
Catawba Valley Medical Center	Hickory	100%	71
Central Carolina Hospital	Sanford	100%	56
Firsthealth Moore Regional Hospital	Pinehurst	100%	244
High Point Regional Hospital	High Point	100%	197
Hugh Chatham Memorial Hospital	Elkin	100%	26
Maria Parham Medical Center	Henderson	100%	49
Novant Health Forsyth Medical Center	Winston-Salem	100%	372
Novant Health Huntersville Medical Center	Huntersville	100%	52
Novant Health Presbyterian Medical Center	Charlotte	100%	175
Novant Health Rowan Medical Center	Salisbury	100%	135
Novant Health Thomasville Medical Center	Thomasville	100%	49
Presbyterian Hospital Matthews	Matthews	100%	87
Vidant Duplin Hospital	Kenansville	100%	30
Wakemed - Cary Hospital	Cary	100%	90
Cape Fear Valley Medical Center	Fayetteville	99%	234
Carolinas Medical Center - Pineville	Charlotte	99%	154
Carolinas Medical Center - Union	Monroe	99%	72
Duke University Hospital	Durham	98%	185
Scotland Memorial Hospital	Laurinburg	98%	52
Vidant Medical Center	Greenville	98%	368
Frye Regional Medical Center	Hickory	97%	118
Lake Norman Regional Medical Center	Mooresville	97%	34
Rex Hospital[2]	Raleigh	97%	79
University of North Carolina Hospital[2]	Chapel Hill	97%	37
Wakemed - Raleigh Campus	Raleigh	97%	390
Carolinas Medical Center - Northeast	Concord	96%	242
Carolinas Med Ctr/Behaviorial Health	Charlotte	96%	287
Duke Health Raleigh Hospital	Raleigh	96%	56
Duke Regional Hospital	Durham	96%	154
Nash General Hospital	Rocky Mount	96%	138
Novant Health Brunswick Medical Center	Supply	96%	54
Carolinas Medical Center - Lincoln	Lincolnton	95%	39
Lexington Memorial Hospital	Lexington	95%	55
North Carolina Baptist Hospital[2]	Winston-Salem	95%	79
Onslow Memorial Hospital	Jacksonville	95%	59
Vidant Edgecombe Hospital	Tarboro	95%	38
Martin General Hospital	Williamston	94%	33
Medwest Haywood	Clyde	94%	48
Watauga Medical Center	Boone	94%	47
Iredell Memorial Hospital	Statesville	93%	58
Mem Mission Hosp & Asheville Surg Ctr	Asheville	93%	328
Rutherford Hospital	Rutherfordton	93%	61
Vidant Beaufort Hospital	Washington	93%	43
Wilkes Regional Medical Center	N Wilkesboro	93%	30
Carolina East Medical Center	New Bern	92%	119
Carteret General Hospital	Morehead City	92%	53
Cleveland Regional Medical Center	Shelby	92%	86
Johnston Memorial Hospital	Smithfield	92%	37
New Hanover Regional Medical Center	Wilmington	92%	271
Randolph Hospital[2]	Asheboro	92%	64
Alamance Regional Medical Center	Burlington	91%	118
The Moses H Cone Memorial Hospital	Greensboro	91%	461
Southeastern Regional Medical Center	Lumberton	90%	105
Stanly Regional Medical Center	Albemarle	89%	38
Park Ridge Health[2]	Hendersonville	88%	25
Vidant Roanoke Chowan Hospital	Ahoskie	88%	43
Wayne Memorial Hospital	Goldsboro	88%	110
Wilson Medical Center	Wilson	88%	78
Sampson Regional Medical Center	Clinton	84%	32
Albemarle Hospital Authority	Elizabeth City	82%	72
CMC - Blue Ridge	Morganton	81%	63
Halifax Regional Medical Center	Roanoke Rapids	80%	50
Caldwell Memorial Hospital	Lenoir	77%	35
Lenoir Memorial Hospital	Kinston	72%	50
Margaret R Pardee Memorial Hospital	Hendersonville	72%	65
Betsy Johnson Regional Hospital	Dunn	68%	57
Columbus Regional Healthcare System	Whiteville	63%	38
Kings Mountain Hospital	Kings Mountain	62%	26
Morehead Memorial Hospital	Eden	53%	49

Thrombolytic Therapy Timing

Hospital Name	City	Rate	Cases
Novant Health Forsyth Medical Center	Winston-Salem	100%	44
Carolinas Medical Center - Northeast	Concord	97%	29
Mem Mission Hosp & Asheville Surg Ctr	Asheville	96%	83
The Moses H Cone Memorial Hospital	Greensboro	83%	41
New Hanover Regional Medical Center	Wilmington	45%	33
Alamance Regional Medical Center	Burlington	0%	69

Venous Thromboembolism (VTE) Prophylaxis

Hospital Name	City	Rate	Cases
Carolinas Medical Center - Lincoln	Lincolnton	100%	40
Carolinas Medical Center - Union	Monroe	100%	87
Carolinas Med Ctr/Behaviorial Health	Charlotte	100%	609
Caromont Regional Medical Center	Gastonia	100%	303
Central Carolina Hospital	Sanford	100%	70
Duke Health Raleigh Hospital	Raleigh	100%	79
Hugh Chatham Memorial Hospital	Elkin	100%	28
Lake Norman Regional Medical Center	Mooresville	100%	41
Martin General Hospital	Williamston	100%	40
The Mcdowell Hospital	Marion	100%	26
Northern Hospital of Surry County	Mount Airy	100%	28
Novant Health Brunswick Medical Center	Supply	100%	71
Novant Health Presbyterian Medical Center	Charlotte	100%	329
Stanly Regional Medical Center	Albemarle	100%	45
Wilkes Regional Medical Center	N Wilkesboro	100%	43
Cape Fear Valley Medical Center	Fayetteville	99%	366
Carolinas Medical Center - University	Charlotte	99%	81
Catawba Valley Medical Center	Hickory	99%	110
Novant Health Forsyth Medical Center	Winston-Salem	99%	644
Onslow Memorial Hospital	Jacksonville	99%	68
Presbyterian Hospital Matthews	Matthews	99%	120
Vidant Medical Center	Greenville	99%	647
Carolinas Medical Center - Pineville	Charlotte	98%	199
Firsthealth Moore Regional Hospital	Pinehurst	98%	319
The Moses H Cone Memorial Hospital	Greensboro	98%	743
Novant Health Huntersville Medical Center	Huntersville	98%	59
Novant Health Thomasville Medical Center	Thomasville	98%	47
Vidant Roanoke Chowan Hospital	Ahoskie	98%	59
Wakemed - Raleigh Campus	Raleigh	98%	564
Carolinas Medical Center - Northeast	Concord	97%	314
Carteret General Hospital	Morehead City	97%	67
Maria Parham Medical Center	Henderson	97%	79
Nash General Hospital	Rocky Mount	97%	191
Novant Health Rowan Medical Center	Salisbury	97%	185
Park Ridge Health[2]	Hendersonville	97%	30
Rex Hospital[2]	Raleigh	97%	118
Scotland Memorial Hospital	Laurinburg	97%	63
University of North Carolina Hospital[2]	Chapel Hill	97%	100
Wakemed - Cary Hospital	Cary	97%	119
CMC - Blue Ridge	Morganton	96%	71
High Point Regional Hospital	High Point	96%	242
Medwest Haywood	Clyde	96%	54
Rutherford Hospital	Rutherfordton	96%	76
Vidant Beaufort Hospital	Washington	96%	55

NOTE: Hospital profiles are in alphabetical order by state, then city, then hospital within the city; Rankings exclude hospitals with less than 25 cases except for patient surveys which excludes hospitals with less than 100 cases; (a) 100-299 cases; (1) The number of cases/patients is too few to report; (2) Data submitted were based on a sample of cases/patients; (3) Results are based on a shorter time period than required; (4) Data suppressed by CMS for one or more quarters; (5) Results are not available for this reporting period; (6) Fewer than 100 patients completed the HCAHPS survey; (7) No cases met the criteria for this measure; (8) The lower limit of the confidence interval cannot be calculated if the number of observed infections equals zero; (9) No data are available from the state/territory for this reporting period; (10) The scores shown reflect fewer than 50 completed surveys; (11) There were discrepancies in the data collection process; (12) This measure does not apply to this hospital for this reporting period; (13) Results cannot be calculated for this reporting period; (14) The results for this state are combined with nearby states to protect confidentiality; Please refer to the User's Guide for a full explanation of data.

Hospital Name	City	Rate	Cases
Duke Regional Hospital	Durham	95%	207
Duke University Hospital	Durham	95%	361
Frye Regional Medical Center	Hickory	95%	152
Iredell Memorial Hospital	Statesville	95%	75
Mem Mission Hosp & Asheville Surg Ctr	Asheville	95%	598
Caldwell Memorial Hospital	Lenoir	94%	50
Vidant Edgecombe Hospital	Tarboro	94%	48
Cleveland Regional Medical Center	Shelby	93%	88
Lexington Memorial Hospital	Lexington	93%	56
Margaret R Pardee Memorial Hospital	Hendersonville	93%	81
New Hanover Regional Medical Center	Wilmington	93%	444
North Carolina Baptist Hospital[2]	Winston-Salem	93%	138
Halifax Regional Medical Center	Roanoke Rapids	91%	70
Vidant Duplin Hospital	Kenansville	91%	35
Sampson Regional Medical Center	Clinton	90%	48
Southeastern Regional Medical Center	Lumberton	90%	148
Columbus Regional Healthcare System	Whiteville	89%	47
Alamance Regional Medical Center	Burlington	88%	151
Randolph Hospital[2]	Asheboro	88%	88
Albemarle Hospital Authority	Elizabeth City	87%	87
Wayne Memorial Hospital	Goldsboro	87%	144
Wilson Medical Center	Wilson	87%	108
Carolina East Medical Center	New Bern	85%	136
Johnston Memorial Hospital	Smithfield	85%	40
Watauga Medical Center	Boone	85%	60
Lenoir Memorial Hospital	Kinston	75%	67
Morehead Memorial Hospital	Eden	66%	50
Betsy Johnson Regional Hospital	Dunn	60%	80

Written Stroke Educational Materials Given

Hospital Name	City	Rate	Cases
Carolinas Medical Center - Northeast	Concord	100%	217
Caromont Regional Medical Center	Gastonia	100%	173
Catawba Valley Medical Center	Hickory	100%	56
Central Carolina Hospital	Sanford	100%	42
Medwest Haywood	Clyde	100%	35
Novant Health Brunswick Medical Center	Supply	100%	45
Novant Health Thomasville Medical Center	Thomasville	100%	33
Scotland Memorial Hospital	Laurinburg	100%	41
Southeastern Regional Medical Center	Lumberton	100%	75
Firsthealth Moore Regional Hospital	Pinehurst	99%	187
High Point Regional Hospital	High Point	99%	120
Novant Health Forsyth Medical Center	Winston-Salem	99%	350
Presbyterian Hospital Matthews	Matthews	99%	70
Wakemed - Cary Hospital	Cary	99%	83
Carolinas Medical Center - University	Charlotte	98%	57
Cleveland Regional Medical Center	Shelby	98%	63
Novant Health Rowan Medical Center	Salisbury	98%	112
Wayne Memorial Hospital	Goldsboro	98%	83
Hugh Chatham Memorial Hospital	Elkin	97%	31
Novant Health Huntersville Medical Center	Huntersville	97%	60
Novant Health Presbyterian Medical Center	Charlotte	97%	201
Stanly Regional Medical Center	Albemarle	97%	36
Carolinas Medical Center - Union	Monroe	96%	55
Lake Norman Regional Medical Center	Mooresville	96%	28
Maria Parham Medical Center	Henderson	96%	45
University of North Carolina Hospital[2]	Chapel Hill	96%	56
Cape Fear Valley Medical Center	Fayetteville	95%	184
Iredell Memorial Hospital	Statesville	95%	43
Carolinas Med Ctr/Behaviorial Health	Charlotte	94%	304
Frye Regional Medical Center	Hickory	94%	86
Margaret R Pardee Memorial Hospital	Hendersonville	94%	36
Wakemed - Raleigh Campus	Raleigh	94%	298
Watauga Medical Center	Boone	94%	33
Duke Health Raleigh Hospital	Raleigh	93%	45
Martin General Hospital	Williamston	93%	30
Morehead Memorial Hospital	Eden	93%	27
Carolinas Medical Center - Pineville	Charlotte	92%	122
Onslow Memorial Hospital	Jacksonville	92%	49
Duke Regional Hospital	Durham	91%	123
Rex Hospital[2]	Raleigh	91%	82
Duke University Hospital	Durham	90%	214
Lexington Memorial Hospital	Lexington	90%	40
Carolinas Medical Center - Lincoln	Lincolnton	89%	35
Nash General Hospital	Rocky Mount	89%	95
Rutherford Hospital	Rutherfordton	88%	43
Mem Mission Hosp & Asheville Surg Ctr	Asheville	87%	291
New Hanover Regional Medical Center	Wilmington	87%	242
Wilson Medical Center	Wilson	83%	47
Carolina East Medical Center	New Bern	81%	96
The Moses H Cone Memorial Hospital	Greensboro	80%	416
North Carolina Baptist Hospital[2]	Winston-Salem	79%	87
Vidant Duplin Hospital	Kenansville	78%	27
Johnston Memorial Hospital	Smithfield	77%	30
CMC - Blue Ridge	Morganton	74%	35
Vidant Medical Center	Greenville	73%	349
Vidant Beaufort Hospital	Washington	70%	27
Vidant Roanoke Chowan Hospital	Ahoskie	70%	37
Alamance Regional Medical Center	Burlington	69%	107
Albemarle Hospital Authority	Elizabeth City	69%	61
Randolph Hospital[2]	Asheboro	64%	45

Hospital Name	City	Rate	Cases
Vidant Edgecombe Hospital	Tarboro	45%	33
Betsy Johnson Regional Hospital	Dunn	44%	43
Carteret General Hospital	Morehead City	44%	34
Halifax Regional Medical Center	Roanoke Rapids	28%	29
Sampson Regional Medical Center	Clinton	23%	26
Lenoir Memorial Hospital	Kinston	14%	42

Surgical Care Improvement Project

Appropriate Beta Blocker Usage

Hospital Name	City	Rate	Cases
Albemarle Hospital Authority	Elizabeth City	100%	58
Caldwell Memorial Hospital	Lenoir	100%	66
Carolinas Medical Center - Pineville[2]	Charlotte	100%	689
CMC - Blue Ridge	Morganton	100%	85
Davis Regional Medical Center	Statesville	100%	37
Duke Health Raleigh Hospital	Raleigh	100%	323
Hugh Chatham Memorial Hospital	Elkin	100%	59
Margaret R Pardee Memorial Hospital	Hendersonville	100%	257
Maria Parham Medical Center	Henderson	100%	32
Martin General Hospital	Williamston	100%	27
New Hanover Regional Medical Center[2]	Wilmington	100%	741
North Carolina Specialty Hospital[2]	Durham	100%	51
Novant Health Brunswick Medical Center	Supply	100%	137
Novant Health Charlotte Ortho Hosp[2]	Charlotte	100%	416
Novant Health Forsyth Medical Center[2]	Winston-Salem	100%	1076
Novant Health Park Hospital[2]	Winston-Salem	100%	103
Novant Health Presbyterian Medical Center[2]	Charlotte	100%	435
Novant Health Rowan Medical Center[2]	Salisbury	100%	159
Onslow Memorial Hospital	Jacksonville	100%	65
Presbyterian Hospital Matthews[2]	Matthews	100%	132
Rutherford Hospital	Rutherfordton	100%	92
Saint Luke's Hospital	Columbus	100%	63
Southeastern Regional Medical Center	Lumberton	100%	104
Transylvania Regional Hospital	Brevard	100%	34
University of North Carolina Hospital[2]	Chapel Hill	100%	183
Vidant Medical Center[2]	Greenville	100%	963
WG (Bill) Hefner Salisbury VA Med Ctr[2]	Salisbury	100%	35
Wakemed - Cary Hospital	Cary	100%	189
Wakemed - Raleigh Campus[2]	Raleigh	100%	600
Wilkes Regional Medical Center	N Wilkesboro	100%	62
Cape Fear Valley Medical Center[2]	Fayetteville	99%	380
Carolina East Medical Center	New Bern	99%	442
Carolinas Medical Center - Lincoln	Lincolnton	99%	70
Caromont Regional Medical Center	Gastonia	99%	494
Catawba Valley Medical Center	Hickory	99%	169
Cleveland Regional Medical Center[2]	Shelby	99%	137
Duke Regional Hospital[2]	Durham	99%	280
Duke University Hospital[2]	Durham	99%	424
Firsthealth Moore Regional Hospital[2]	Pinehurst	99%	307
Iredell Memorial Hospital[2]	Statesville	99%	118
Lenoir Memorial Hospital	Kinston	99%	73
Mem Mission Hosp & Asheville Surg Ctr[2]	Asheville	99%	319
The Moses H Cone Memorial Hospital	Greensboro	99%	1348
North Carolina Baptist Hospital[2]	Winston-Salem	99%	340
Northern Hospital of Surry County	Mount Airy	99%	88
Novant Health Huntersville Medical Center[2]	Huntersville	99%	192
Rex Hospital[2]	Raleigh	99%	374
Watauga Medical Center	Boone	99%	75
Carolinas Medical Center - Northeast[2]	Concord	98%	496
Carolinas Medical Center - Union[2]	Monroe	98%	108
Carolinas Med Ctr/Behaviorial Health[2]	Charlotte	98%	544
Carteret General Hospital	Morehead City	98%	177
Columbus Regional Healthcare System	Whiteville	98%	64
Frye Regional Medical Center[2]	Hickory	98%	259
High Point Regional Hospital[2]	High Point	98%	159
Lexington Memorial Hospital	Lexington	98%	65
Randolph Hospital[2]	Asheboro	98%	97
Wayne Memorial Hospital[2]	Goldsboro	98%	159
Wilson Medical Center[2]	Wilson	98%	117
Asheville - Oteen VA Medical Center[2]	Asheville	97%	187
Durham VA Medical Center[2]	Durham	97%	123
Person Memorial Hospital	Roxboro	97%	35
Sampson Regional Medical Center	Clinton	97%	37
Vidant Beaufort Hospital	Washington	97%	58
Vidant Chowan Hospital	Edenton	97%	39
Alamance Regional Medical Center	Burlington	96%	211
Carolinas Medical Center - University[2]	Charlotte	96%	52
Halifax Regional Medical Center	Roanoke Rapids	96%	165
Johnston Memorial Hospital	Smithfield	96%	169
Lake Norman Regional Medical Center	Mooresville	96%	94
Novant Health Thomasville Medical Center	Thomasville	96%	54
The Outer Banks Hospital	Nags Head	96%	45
Stanly Regional Medical Center	Albemarle	96%	51
Central Carolina Hospital	Sanford	95%	43
Nash General Hospital[2]	Rocky Mount	95%	171
Vidant Edgecombe Hospital	Tarboro	95%	40
Vidant Roanoke Chowan Hospital	Ahoskie	95%	39
Granville Health Systems	Oxford	94%	62
Medwest Harris	Sylva	94%	49
Murphy Medical Center	Murphy	94%	53
Park Ridge Health	Hendersonville	94%	70
Scotland Memorial Hospital	Laurinburg	94%	90
Medwest Haywood	Clyde	93%	107
J Arthur Dosher Memorial Hospital[2]	Southport	92%	40
Betsy Johnson Regional Hospital	Dunn	86%	36

Appropriate VTP Within 24 Hours

Hospital Name	City	Rate	Cases
Caldwell Memorial Hospital	Lenoir	100%	230
Carolinas Medical Center - Pineville[2]	Charlotte	100%	1989
Caromont Regional Medical Center	Gastonia	100%	1006
Cleveland Regional Medical Center[2]	Shelby	100%	496
Duke Regional Hospital[2]	Durham	100%	888
Duke University Hospital[2]	Durham	100%	1141
Hugh Chatham Memorial Hospital	Elkin	100%	236
Margaret R Pardee Memorial Hospital	Hendersonville	100%	816
Martin General Hospital	Williamston	100%	74
The Mcdowell Hospital	Marion	100%	43
Mem Mission Hosp & Asheville Surg Ctr[2]	Asheville	100%	546
Murphy Medical Center	Murphy	100%	162
New Hanover Regional Medical Center[2]	Wilmington	100%	1292
North Carolina Baptist Hospital[2]	Winston-Salem	100%	482
North Carolina Specialty Hospital[2]	Durham	100%	229
Novant Health Brunswick Medical Center	Supply	100%	402
Novant Health Charlotte Ortho Hosp[2]	Charlotte	100%	1462
Novant Health Park Hospital[2]	Winston-Salem	100%	361
Novant Health Rowan Medical Center[2]	Salisbury	100%	617
The Outer Banks Hospital	Nags Head	100%	151
Spruce Pine Community Hospital	Spruce Pine	100%	54
University of North Carolina Hospital[2]	Chapel Hill	100%	389
Vidant Edgecombe Hospital	Tarboro	100%	128
Vidant Medical Center[2]	Greenville	100%	1279
Vidant Roanoke Chowan Hospital	Ahoskie	100%	165
Albemarle Hospital Authority	Elizabeth City	99%	150
Asheville - Oteen VA Medical Center[2]	Asheville	99%	398
Cape Fear Valley Medical Center[2]	Fayetteville	99%	691
Carolinas Medical Center - Lincoln	Lincolnton	99%	202
Carolinas Medical Center - Union[2]	Monroe	99%	425
CMC - Blue Ridge	Morganton	99%	294
Columbus Regional Healthcare System	Whiteville	99%	172
Duke Health Raleigh Hospital	Raleigh	99%	1135
Durham VA Medical Center[2]	Durham	99%	183
Firsthealth Moore Regional Hospital[2]	Pinehurst	99%	478
Frye Regional Medical Center[2]	Hickory	99%	333
Granville Health Systems	Oxford	99%	145
Iredell Memorial Hospital[2]	Statesville	99%	369
Lake Norman Regional Medical Center	Mooresville	99%	299
Maria Parham Medical Center	Henderson	99%	147
The Moses H Cone Memorial Hospital	Greensboro	99%	3173
Novant Health Forsyth Medical Center[2]	Winston-Salem	99%	2369
Novant Health Huntersville Medical Center[2]	Huntersville	99%	564
Novant Health Presbyterian Medical Center[2]	Charlotte	99%	738
Presbyterian Hospital Matthews[2]	Matthews	99%	448
Rex Hospital[2]	Raleigh	99%	685
Rutherford Hospital	Rutherfordton	99%	281
Scotland Memorial Hospital	Laurinburg	99%	360
Stanly Regional Medical Center	Albemarle	99%	163
Vidant Chowan Hospital	Edenton	99%	120
Wakemed - Cary Hospital	Cary	99%	625
Wakemed - Raleigh Campus[2]	Raleigh	99%	677
Wilkes Regional Medical Center	N Wilkesboro	99%	198
Angel Medical Center	Franklin	98%	66
Carolinas Medical Center - Northeast[2]	Concord	98%	1031
Carolinas Medical Center - University[2]	Charlotte	98%	241
Carolinas Med Ctr/Behaviorial Health[2]	Charlotte	98%	843
Carteret General Hospital	Morehead City	98%	524
Catawba Valley Medical Center	Hickory	98%	637
Davis Regional Medical Center	Statesville	98%	113
Medwest Haywood	Clyde	98%	316
Northern Hospital of Surry County	Mount Airy	98%	249
Onslow Memorial Hospital	Jacksonville	98%	230
Person Memorial Hospital	Roxboro	98%	120
Randolph Hospital[2]	Asheboro	98%	317
Saint Luke's Hospital	Columbus	98%	195
Southeastern Regional Medical Center	Lumberton	98%	210
Transylvania Regional Hospital	Brevard	98%	127
Watauga Medical Center	Boone	98%	273
Wayne Memorial Hospital[2]	Goldsboro	98%	532
Wilson Medical Center[2]	Wilson	98%	430
Betsy Johnson Regional Hospital	Dunn	97%	137
Carolina East Medical Center	New Bern	97%	972
Halifax Regional Medical Center	Roanoke Rapids	97%	404
Lenoir Memorial Hospital	Kinston	97%	220
Lexington Memorial Hospital	Lexington	97%	241
Medwest Harris	Sylva	97%	176
Nash General Hospital[2]	Rocky Mount	97%	508
Novant Health Thomasville Medical Center	Thomasville	97%	176
Park Ridge Health	Hendersonville	97%	295
Vidant Beaufort Hospital	Washington	97%	202
WG (Bill) Hefner Salisbury VA Med Ctr[2]	Salisbury	97%	145

NOTE: Hospital profiles are in alphabetical order by state, then city, then hospital within the city; Rankings exclude hospitals with less than 25 cases except for patient surveys which excludes hospitals with less than 100 cases; (a) 100-299 cases; (1) The number of cases/patients is too few to report; (2) Data submitted were based on a sample of cases/patients; (3) Results are based on a shorter time period than required; (4) Data suppressed by CMS for one or more quarters; (5) Results are not available for this reporting period; (6) Fewer than 100 patients completed the HCAHPS survey; (7) No cases met the criteria for this measure; (8) The lower limit of the confidence interval cannot be calculated if the number of observed infections equals zero; (9) No data are available from the state/territory for this reporting period; (10) The scores shown reflect fewer than 50 completed surveys; (11) There were discrepancies in the data collection process; (12) This measure does not apply to this hospital for this reporting period; (13) Results cannot be calculated for this reporting period; (14) The results for this state are combined with nearby states to protect confidentiality; Please refer to the User's Guide for a full explanation of data.

Hospital Name	City	Rate	Cases
Alamance Regional Medical Center	Burlington	96%	666
Central Carolina Hospital	Sanford	96%	150
Johnston Memorial Hospital	Smithfield	96%	363
High Point Regional Hospital[2]	High Point	94%	295
J Arthur Dosher Memorial Hospital[2]	Southport	94%	142
Kings Mountain Hospital	Kings Mountain	93%	30
Novant Health Franklin Medical Center	Louisburg	92%	38
Sampson Regional Medical Center	Clinton	92%	120
Morehead Memorial Hospital	Eden	91%	104
Ashe Memorial Hospital	Jefferson	84%	32

Controlled Postoperative Blood Glucose

Hospital Name	City	Rate	Cases
Asheville - Oteen VA Medical Center[2]	Asheville	100%	65
Carolinas Medical Center - Pineville[2]	Charlotte	100%	165
Caromont Regional Medical Center	Gastonia	100%	188
Mem Mission Hosp & Asheville Surg Ctr[2]	Asheville	100%	197
Carolinas Med Ctr/Behavioral Health[2]	Charlotte	99%	412
Duke Regional Hospital[2]	Durham	99%	75
Duke University Hospital[2]	Durham	99%	185
The Moses H Cone Memorial Hospital	Greensboro	99%	435
Novant Health Forsyth Medical Center[2]	Winston-Salem	99%	449
Novant Health Presbyterian Medical Center[2]	Charlotte	99%	333
University of North Carolina Hospital[2]	Chapel Hill	99%	85
Vidant Medical Center[2]	Greenville	99%	564
Carolinas Medical Center - Northeast[2]	Concord	98%	208
Durham VA Medical Center[2]	Durham	98%	126
Firsthealth Moore Regional Hospital[2]	Pinehurst	98%	182
New Hanover Regional Medical Center[2]	Wilmington	98%	435
Rex Hospital[2]	Raleigh	98%	246
Southeastern Regional Medical Center	Lumberton	98%	40
Wakemed - Raleigh Campus[2]	Raleigh	98%	448
Cape Fear Valley Medical Center[2]	Fayetteville	97%	160
Carolina East Medical Center	New Bern	97%	172
High Point Regional Hospital[2]	High Point	97%	96
Frye Regional Medical Center[2]	Hickory	95%	311
North Carolina Baptist Hospital[2]	Winston-Salem	95%	212

Perioperative Temperature Management

Hospital Name	City	Rate	Cases
Alamance Regional Medical Center	Burlington	100%	736
Albemarle Hospital Authority	Elizabeth City	100%	167
Angel Medical Center	Franklin	100%	78
Ashe Memorial Hospital	Jefferson	100%	31
Asheville - Oteen VA Medical Center[2]	Asheville	100%	435
Betsy Johnson Regional Hospital	Dunn	100%	152
Caldwell Memorial Hospital	Lenoir	100%	270
Cape Fear Valley Medical Center[2]	Fayetteville	100%	959
Carolina East Medical Center	New Bern	100%	1092
Carolinas Medical Center - Lincoln	Lincolnton	100%	218
Carolinas Medical Center - Northeast[2]	Concord	100%	1279
Carolinas Medical Center - Pineville[2]	Charlotte	100%	2492
Carolinas Medical Center - Union[2]	Monroe	100%	457
Carolinas Medical Center - University[2]	Charlotte	100%	284
Carolinas Med Ctr/Behavioral Health[2]	Charlotte	100%	1154
Caromont Regional Medical Center	Gastonia	100%	1153
Carteret General Hospital	Morehead City	100%	676
Catawba Valley Medical Center	Hickory	100%	748
Central Carolina Hospital	Sanford	100%	177
Cleveland Regional Medical Center[2]	Shelby	100%	543
CMC - Blue Ridge	Morganton	100%	321
Columbus Regional Healthcare System	Whiteville	100%	203
Davis Regional Medical Center	Statesville	100%	119
Duke Health Raleigh Hospital	Raleigh	100%	1225
Duke Regional Hospital[2]	Durham	100%	990
Durham VA Medical Center[2]	Durham	100%	211
Firsthealth Moore Regional Hospital[2]	Pinehurst	100%	623
Granville Health Systems	Oxford	100%	213
High Point Regional Hospital[2]	High Point	100%	358
Hugh Chatham Memorial Hospital	Elkin	100%	266
Iredell Memorial Hospital[2]	Statesville	100%	403
J Arthur Dosher Memorial Hospital[2]	Southport	100%	155
Johnston Memorial Hospital	Smithfield	100%	448
Kings Mountain Hospital	Kings Mountain	100%	33
Lake Norman Regional Medical Center	Mooresville	100%	367
Lenoir Memorial Hospital	Kinston	100%	250
Margaret R Pardee Memorial Hospital	Hendersonville	100%	890
Maria Parham Medical Center	Henderson	100%	151
Martin General Hospital	Williamston	100%	83
The Mcdowell Hospital	Marion	100%	48
Medwest Harris	Sylva	100%	184
Medwest Haywood	Clyde	100%	338
Mem Mission Hosp & Asheville Surg Ctr[2]	Asheville	100%	715
Morehead Memorial Hospital	Eden	100%	118
The Moses H Cone Memorial Hospital	Greensboro	100%	3847
Murphy Medical Center	Murphy	100%	171
Nash General Hospital[2]	Rocky Mount	100%	547
New Hanover Regional Medical Center[2]	Wilmington	100%	1616
North Carolina Specialty Hospital[2]	Durham	100%	240
Northern Hospital of Surry County	Mount Airy	100%	267
Novant Health Brunswick Medical Center	Supply	100%	470
Novant Health Charlotte Ortho Hosp[2]	Charlotte	100%	1574
Novant Health Forsyth Medical Center[2]	Winston-Salem	100%	2597
Novant Health Franklin Medical Center	Louisburg	100%	41
Novant Health Huntersville Medical Center[2]	Huntersville	100%	684
Novant Health Park Hospital[2]	Winston-Salem	100%	432
Novant Health Presbyterian Medical Center[2]	Charlotte	100%	926
Novant Health Rowan Medical Center[2]	Salisbury	100%	681
Novant Health Thomasville Medical Center	Thomasville	100%	188
Onslow Memorial Hospital	Jacksonville	100%	259
The Outer Banks Hospital	Nags Head	100%	151
Park Ridge Health	Hendersonville	100%	324
Person Memorial Hospital	Roxboro	100%	131
Presbyterian Hospital Matthews[2]	Matthews	100%	496
Randolph Hospital[2]	Asheboro	100%	344
Rex Hospital[2]	Raleigh	100%	813
Rutherford Hospital	Rutherfordton	100%	316
Saint Luke's Hospital	Columbus	100%	230
Sampson Regional Medical Center	Clinton	100%	133
Sandhills Regional Medical Center	Hamlet	100%	25
Scotland Memorial Hospital	Laurinburg	100%	376
Southeastern Regional Medical Center	Lumberton	100%	270
Spruce Pine Community Hospital	Spruce Pine	100%	60
Transylvania Regional Hospital	Brevard	100%	158
University of North Carolina Hospital[2]	Chapel Hill	100%	508
Vidant Beaufort Hospital	Washington	100%	218
Vidant Chowan Hospital	Edenton	100%	130
Vidant Duplin Hospital	Kenansville	100%	30
Vidant Edgecombe Hospital	Tarboro	100%	141
Vidant Medical Center[2]	Greenville	100%	1713
Vidant Roanoke Chowan Hospital	Ahoskie	100%	172
Wakemed - Cary Hospital	Cary	100%	679
Wakemed - Raleigh Campus[2]	Raleigh	100%	883
Watauga Medical Center	Boone	100%	293
Wayne Memorial Hospital[2]	Goldsboro	100%	573
Wilkes Regional Medical Center	N Wilkesboro	100%	210
Wilson Medical Center[2]	Wilson	100%	489
Duke University Hospital[2]	Durham	99%	1376
Frye Regional Medical Center[2]	Hickory	99%	484
North Carolina Baptist Hospital[2]	Winston-Salem	99%	656
Stanly Regional Medical Center	Albemarle	99%	185
WG (Bill) Hefner Salisbury VA Med Ctr[2]	Salisbury	99%	164
Halifax Regional Medical Center	Roanoke Rapids	98%	472
Lexington Memorial Hospital	Lexington	98%	251

Prophylactic Antibiotic Selection

Hospital Name	City	Rate	Cases
Asheville - Oteen VA Medical Center	Asheville	100%	396
Caldwell Memorial Hospital	Lenoir	100%	217
Carolinas Medical Center - Northeast[2]	Concord	100%	1178
Carolinas Medical Center - Pineville[2]	Charlotte	100%	2261
Carolinas Medical Center - Union[2]	Monroe	100%	305
Carolinas Medical Center - University[2]	Charlotte	100%	176
Caromont Regional Medical Center	Gastonia	100%	893
Cleveland Regional Medical Center[2]	Shelby	100%	405
Duke Regional Hospital[2]	Durham	100%	909
Duke University Hospital[2]	Durham	100%	1127
Granville Health Systems	Oxford	100%	136
Hugh Chatham Memorial Hospital	Elkin	100%	212
Johnston Memorial Hospital	Smithfield	100%	270
Margaret R Pardee Memorial Hospital	Hendersonville	100%	657
Mem Mission Hosp & Asheville Surg Ctr[2]	Asheville	100%	615
The Moses H Cone Memorial Hospital	Greensboro	100%	2831
Murphy Medical Center	Murphy	100%	144
North Carolina Specialty Hospital[2]	Durham	100%	155
Novant Health Brunswick Medical Center	Supply	100%	351
Novant Health Charlotte Ortho Hosp[2]	Charlotte	100%	1402
Novant Health Forsyth Medical Center[2]	Winston-Salem	100%	2215
Novant Health Franklin Medical Center	Louisburg	100%	25
Novant Health Huntersville Medical Center[2]	Huntersville	100%	509
Novant Health Park Hospital[2]	Winston-Salem	100%	226
Novant Health Presbyterian Medical Center[2]	Charlotte	100%	721
Novant Health Rowan Medical Center[2]	Salisbury	100%	539
The Outer Banks Hospital	Nags Head	100%	124
Person Memorial Hospital	Roxboro	100%	98
Presbyterian Hospital Matthews[2]	Matthews	100%	360
Rutherford Hospital	Rutherfordton	100%	217
Saint Luke's Hospital	Columbus	100%	203
Scotland Memorial Hospital	Laurinburg	100%	257
Spruce Pine Community Hospital	Spruce Pine	100%	39
University of North Carolina Hospital[2]	Chapel Hill	100%	307
Vidant Chowan Hospital	Edenton	100%	100
Vidant Edgecombe Hospital	Tarboro	100%	96
Vidant Medical Center[2]	Greenville	100%	1490
Vidant Roanoke Chowan Hospital	Ahoskie	100%	122
Wakemed - Cary Hospital	Cary	100%	362
Wakemed - Raleigh Campus[2]	Raleigh	100%	1002
Watauga Medical Center	Boone	100%	218
Wayne Memorial Hospital[2]	Goldsboro	100%	386
Wilson Medical Center[2]	Wilson	100%	373
Betsy Johnson Regional Hospital	Dunn	99%	79
Cape Fear Valley Medical Center[2]	Fayetteville	99%	807
Carolinas Medical Center - Lincoln	Lincolnton	99%	142
Carolinas Med Ctr/Behavioral Health[2]	Charlotte	99%	1053
Carteret General Hospital	Morehead City	99%	475
Catawba Valley Medical Center	Hickory	99%	543
CMC - Blue Ridge	Morganton	99%	195
Davis Regional Medical Center	Statesville	99%	76
Duke Health Raleigh Hospital	Raleigh	99%	854
Firsthealth Moore Regional Hospital[2]	Pinehurst	99%	589
Frye Regional Medical Center[2]	Hickory	99%	580
Halifax Regional Medical Center	Roanoke Rapids	99%	342
Iredell Memorial Hospital[2]	Statesville	99%	261
J Arthur Dosher Memorial Hospital[2]	Southport	99%	112
Lake Norman Regional Medical Center	Mooresville	99%	254
Medwest Harris	Sylva	99%	125
Medwest Haywood	Clyde	99%	233
New Hanover Regional Medical Center[2]	Wilmington	99%	1654
North Carolina Baptist Hospital[2]	Winston-Salem	99%	577
Northern Hospital of Surry County	Mount Airy	99%	182
Novant Health Thomasville Medical Center	Thomasville	99%	120
Onslow Memorial Hospital	Jacksonville	99%	172
Rex Hospital[2]	Raleigh	99%	739
Transylvania Regional Hospital	Brevard	99%	118
Wilkes Regional Medical Center	N Wilkesboro	99%	155
Albemarle Hospital Authority	Elizabeth City	98%	99
Angel Medical Center	Franklin	98%	48
Carolina East Medical Center	New Bern	98%	914
Durham VA Medical Center	Durham	98%	217
High Point Regional Hospital[2]	High Point	98%	319
Lexington Memorial Hospital	Lexington	98%	200
Maria Parham Medical Center	Henderson	98%	55
Nash General Hospital[2]	Rocky Mount	98%	430
Park Ridge Health	Hendersonville	98%	218
Randolph Hospital[2]	Asheboro	98%	217
Stanly Regional Medical Center	Albemarle	98%	125
Alamance Regional Medical Center	Burlington	97%	516
Central Carolina Hospital	Sanford	97%	93
Sampson Regional Medical Center	Clinton	97%	89
Southeastern Regional Medical Center	Lumberton	97%	159
Vidant Beaufort Hospital	Washington	97%	163
Columbus Regional Healthcare System	Whiteville	96%	69
Morehead Memorial Hospital	Eden	96%	74
Lenoir Memorial Hospital	Kinston	95%	158
Martin General Hospital	Williamston	95%	73
WG (Bill) Hefner Salisbury VA Med Ctr	Salisbury	87%	68

Prophylactic Antibiotic Selection (Outpatient)

Hospital Name	City	Rate	Cases
Davis Regional Medical Center	Statesville	100%	237
Lexington Memorial Hospital	Lexington	100%	83
Medwest Haywood	Clyde	100%	277
North Carolina Specialty Hospital	Durham	100%	187
Northern Hospital of Surry County	Mount Airy	100%	42
Novant Health Charlotte Ortho Hosp	Charlotte	100%	623
Novant Health Forsyth Medical Center	Winston-Salem	100%	1434
Novant Health Huntersville Medical Center	Huntersville	100%	219
Novant Health Park Hospital	Winston-Salem	100%	311
Novant Health Presbyterian Medical Center	Charlotte	100%	1320
Novant Health Rowan Medical Center	Salisbury	100%	360
Presbyterian Hospital Matthews	Matthews	100%	261
Sandhills Regional Medical Center	Hamlet	100%	93
Vidant Edgecombe Hospital	Tarboro	100%	122
Betsy Johnson Regional Hospital	Dunn	99%	71
Carolinas Medical Center - Northeast	Concord	99%	849
Carolinas Medical Center - University	Charlotte	99%	346
Carolinas Med Ctr/Behavioral Health	Charlotte	99%	1341
Caromont Regional Medical Center	Gastonia	99%	689
Catawba Valley Medical Center	Hickory	99%	548
Duke Regional Hospital	Durham	99%	524
Duke University Hospital	Durham	99%	947
Firsthealth Moore Regional Hospital	Pinehurst	99%	632
Frye Regional Medical Center	Hickory	99%	474
Johnston Memorial Hospital	Smithfield	99%	279
Lake Norman Regional Medical Center	Mooresville	99%	331
Margaret R Pardee Memorial Hospital	Hendersonville	99%	216
Mem Mission Hosp & Asheville Surg Ctr	Asheville	99%	988
North Carolina Baptist Hospital	Winston-Salem	99%	630
Novant Health Brunswick Medical Center	Supply	99%	103
Onslow Memorial Hospital	Jacksonville	99%	211
Park Ridge Health	Hendersonville	99%	157
Rex Hospital	Raleigh	99%	1069
University of North Carolina Hospital	Chapel Hill	99%	688
Wakemed - Raleigh Campus	Raleigh	99%	814
Caldwell Memorial Hospital	Lenoir	98%	92
Carolinas Medical Center - Pineville	Charlotte	98%	1259
Carteret General Hospital	Morehead City	98%	129
Duke Health Raleigh Hospital	Raleigh	98%	548
Halifax Regional Medical Center	Roanoke Rapids	98%	121
Medwest Harris	Sylva	98%	112
The Moses H Cone Memorial Hospital	Greensboro	98%	896
New Hanover Regional Medical Center	Wilmington	98%	700

NOTE: Hospital profiles are in alphabetical order by state, then city, then hospital within the city; Rankings exclude hospitals with less than 25 cases except for patient surveys which excludes hospitals with less than 100 cases; (a) 100-299 cases; (1) The number of cases/patients is too few to report; (2) Data submitted were based on a sample of cases/patients; (3) Results are based on a shorter time period than required; (4) Data suppressed by CMS for one or more quarters; (5) Results are not available for this reporting period; (6) Fewer than 100 patients completed the HCAHPS survey; (7) No cases met the criteria for this measure; (8) The lower limit of the confidence interval cannot be calculated if the number of observed infections equals zero; (9) No data are available from the state/territory for this reporting period; (10) The scores shown reflect fewer than 50 completed surveys; (11) There were discrepancies in the data collection process; (12) This measure does not apply to this hospital for this reporting period; (13) Results cannot be calculated for this reporting period; (14) The results for this state are combined with nearby states to protect confidentiality; Please refer to the User's Guide for a full explanation of data.

Hospital Name	City	Rate	Cases
Novant Health Thomasville Medical Center	Thomasville	98%	97
Randolph Hospital	Asheboro	98%	109
Transylvania Regional Hospital	Brevard	98%	50
Watauga Medical Center	Boone	98%	164
Wayne Memorial Hospital	Goldsboro	98%	310
Albemarle Hospital Authority	Elizabeth City	97%	235
Cape Fear Valley Medical Center	Fayetteville	97%	416
Carolinas Medical Center - Lincoln	Lincolnton	97%	31
Carolinas Medical Center - Union	Monroe	97%	64
Columbus Regional Healthcare System	Whiteville	97%	33
Hugh Chatham Memorial Hospital	Elkin	97%	73
The Mcdowell Hospital	Marion	97%	87
Wilkes Regional Medical Center	N Wilkesboro	97%	35
Wilson Medical Center	Wilson	97%	148
Central Carolina Hospital	Sanford	96%	127
Nash General Hospital	Rocky Mount	96%	434
Vidant Medical Center	Greenville	96%	1315
High Point Regional Hospital	High Point	95%	432
Southeastern Regional Medical Center	Lumberton	95%	147
Stanly Regional Medical Center	Albemarle	95%	81
Wakemed - Cary Hospital	Cary	95%	352
Cleveland Regional Medical Center	Shelby	94%	177
CMC - Blue Ridge	Morganton	94%	250
Scotland Memorial Hospital	Laurinburg	94%	35
Vidant Chowan Hospital	Edenton	94%	33
Granville Health Systems	Oxford	93%	90
Iredell Memorial Hospital	Statesville	93%	107
Lenoir Memorial Hospital	Kinston	93%	84
Vidant Beaufort Hospital	Washington	91%	105
Alamance Regional Medical Center	Burlington	90%	226
Maria Parham Medical Center	Henderson	88%	67
Carolina East Medical Center	New Bern	87%	693

Hospital Name	City	Rate	Cases
Novant Health Presbyterian Medical Center[2]	Charlotte	98%	692
The Outer Banks Hospital	Nags Head	98%	120
Rex Hospital[2]	Raleigh	98%	723
Wakemed - Raleigh Campus[2]	Raleigh	98%	898
Wayne Memorial Hospital[2]	Goldsboro	98%	355
Carolinas Medical Center - Union[2]	Monroe	97%	296
Carolinas Med Ctr/Behavioral Health[2]	Charlotte	97%	1014
Davis Regional Medical Center	Statesville	97%	67
Iredell Memorial Hospital[2]	Statesville	97%	251
Lexington Memorial Hospital	Lexington	97%	194
Medwest Haywood	Clyde	97%	221
Northern Hospital of Surry County	Mount Airy	97%	179
Sampson Regional Medical Center	Clinton	97%	89
Watauga Medical Center	Boone	97%	213
Asheville - Oteen VA Medical Center	Asheville	96%	389
Johnston Memorial Hospital	Smithfield	96%	262
Novant Health Franklin Medical Center	Louisburg	96%	25
Novant Health Thomasville Medical Center	Thomasville	96%	114
Stanly Regional Medical Center	Albemarle	96%	121
Vidant Beaufort Hospital	Washington	96%	162
Vidant Chowan Hospital	Edenton	96%	99
Alamance Regional Medical Center	Burlington	95%	504
Carolina East Medical Center	New Bern	95%	884
Durham VA Medical Center	Durham	95%	212
Granville Health Systems	Oxford	95%	129
Lenoir Memorial Hospital	Kinston	95%	151
Saint Luke's Hospital	Columbus	95%	203
Spruce Pine Community Hospital	Spruce Pine	95%	38
WG (Bill) Hefner Salisbury VA Med Ctr	Salisbury	95%	65
Betsy Johnson Regional Hospital	Dunn	94%	72
Central Carolina Hospital	Sanford	93%	91
Park Ridge Health	Hendersonville	92%	210
Morehead Memorial Hospital	Eden	89%	71

Hospital Name	City	Rate	Cases
Medwest Harris	Sylva	99%	126
Mem Mission Hosp & Asheville Surg Ctr[2]	Asheville	99%	618
Morehead Memorial Hospital	Eden	99%	76
Murphy Medical Center	Murphy	99%	144
Nash General Hospital[2]	Rocky Mount	99%	431
New Hanover Regional Medical Center[2]	Wilmington	99%	1654
Northern Hospital of Surry County	Mount Airy	99%	182
Novant Health Brunswick Medical Center	Supply	99%	351
Onslow Memorial Hospital	Jacksonville	99%	172
Park Ridge Health	Hendersonville	99%	218
Presbyterian Hospital Matthews[2]	Matthews	99%	360
Randolph Hospital[2]	Asheboro	99%	217
Saint Luke's Hospital	Columbus	99%	208
Scotland Memorial Hospital	Laurinburg	99%	257
Southeastern Regional Medical Center	Lumberton	99%	159
University of North Carolina Hospital[2]	Chapel Hill	99%	308
Wakemed - Cary Hospital	Cary	99%	362
Wakemed - Raleigh Campus[2]	Raleigh	99%	1004
Watauga Medical Center	Boone	99%	219
Wayne Memorial Hospital[2]	Goldsboro	99%	387
Angel Medical Center	Franklin	98%	49
Carolina East Medical Center	New Bern	98%	915
Carolinas Med Ctr/Behavioral Health[2]	Charlotte	98%	1056
Duke Health Raleigh Hospital	Raleigh	98%	854
Frye Regional Medical Center[2]	Hickory	98%	584
The Outer Banks Hospital	Nags Head	98%	124
Person Memorial Hospital	Roxboro	98%	98
Sampson Regional Medical Center	Clinton	98%	89
Stanly Regional Medical Center	Albemarle	98%	126
Vidant Roanoke Chowan Hospital	Ahoskie	98%	122
J Arthur Dosher Memorial Hospital[2]	Southport	97%	112
Lexington Memorial Hospital	Lexington	97%	200
North Carolina Baptist Hospital[2]	Winston-Salem	97%	579
WG (Bill) Hefner Salisbury VA Med Ctr	Salisbury	88%	69

Prophylactic Antibiotic Stopped

Hospital Name	City	Rate	Cases
Albemarle Hospital Authority	Elizabeth City	100%	95
Angel Medical Center	Franklin	100%	48
Caldwell Memorial Hospital	Lenoir	100%	199
Carolinas Medical Center - Pineville[2]	Charlotte	100%	2222
Caromont Regional Medical Center	Gastonia	100%	857
Carteret General Hospital	Morehead City	100%	471
Columbus Regional Healthcare System	Whiteville	100%	67
Hugh Chatham Memorial Hospital	Elkin	100%	212
Lake Norman Regional Medical Center	Mooresville	100%	254
Margaret R Pardee Memorial Hospital	Hendersonville	100%	642
Maria Parham Medical Center	Henderson	100%	54
Medwest Harris	Sylva	100%	123
New Hanover Regional Medical Center[2]	Wilmington	100%	1626
North Carolina Baptist Hospital[2]	Winston-Salem	100%	571
North Carolina Specialty Hospital[2]	Durham	100%	155
Novant Health Charlotte Ortho Hosp[2]	Charlotte	100%	1376
Novant Health Forsyth Medical Center[2]	Winston-Salem	100%	2139
Novant Health Huntersville Medical Center[2]	Huntersville	100%	498
Novant Health Rowan Medical Center[2]	Salisbury	100%	517
Person Memorial Hospital	Roxboro	100%	96
Rutherford Hospital	Rutherfordton	100%	212
Southeastern Regional Medical Center	Lumberton	100%	159
Transylvania Regional Hospital	Brevard	100%	112
Vidant Edgecombe Hospital	Tarboro	100%	94
Vidant Medical Center[2]	Greenville	100%	1456
Vidant Roanoke Chowan Hospital	Ahoskie	100%	120
Cape Fear Valley Medical Center[2]	Fayetteville	99%	796
Catawba Valley Medical Center	Hickory	99%	536
Cleveland Regional Medical Center[2]	Shelby	99%	403
CMC - Blue Ridge	Morganton	99%	176
Duke Health Raleigh Hospital	Raleigh	99%	844
Duke University Hospital[2]	Durham	99%	1100
Firsthealth Moore Regional Hospital[2]	Pinehurst	99%	573
High Point Regional Hospital[2]	High Point	99%	291
J Arthur Dosher Memorial Hospital[2]	Southport	99%	109
Martin General Hospital	Williamston	99%	71
Mem Mission Hosp & Asheville Surg Ctr[2]	Asheville	99%	596
The Moses H Cone Memorial Hospital	Greensboro	99%	2769
Murphy Medical Center	Murphy	99%	139
Novant Health Brunswick Medical Center	Supply	99%	340
Novant Health Park Hospital[2]	Winston-Salem	99%	222
Onslow Memorial Hospital	Jacksonville	99%	167
Presbyterian Hospital Matthews[2]	Matthews	99%	353
Randolph Hospital[2]	Asheboro	99%	213
Scotland Memorial Hospital	Laurinburg	99%	237
University of North Carolina Hospital[2]	Chapel Hill	99%	295
Wakemed - Cary Hospital	Cary	99%	340
Wilkes Regional Medical Center	N Wilkesboro	99%	153
Wilson Medical Center[2]	Wilson	99%	367
Carolinas Medical Center - Lincoln	Lincolnton	98%	126
Carolinas Medical Center - Northeast[2]	Concord	98%	1139
Carolinas Medical Center - University[2]	Charlotte	98%	167
Duke Regional Hospital[2]	Durham	98%	895
Frye Regional Medical Center[2]	Hickory	98%	565
Halifax Regional Medical Center	Roanoke Rapids	98%	332
Nash General Hospital[2]	Rocky Mount	98%	428

Prophylactic Antibiotic Timing

Hospital Name	City	Rate	Cases
Caldwell Memorial Hospital	Lenoir	100%	219
Cape Fear Valley Medical Center[2]	Fayetteville	100%	808
Carolinas Medical Center - Lincoln	Lincolnton	100%	142
Carolinas Medical Center - Northeast[2]	Concord	100%	1179
Carolinas Medical Center - Pineville[2]	Charlotte	100%	2261
Carolinas Medical Center - University[2]	Charlotte	100%	176
Caromont Regional Medical Center	Gastonia	100%	893
Carteret General Hospital	Morehead City	100%	475
Cleveland Regional Medical Center[2]	Shelby	100%	405
CMC - Blue Ridge	Morganton	100%	195
Duke University Hospital[2]	Durham	100%	1131
Firsthealth Moore Regional Hospital[2]	Pinehurst	100%	591
Hugh Chatham Memorial Hospital	Elkin	100%	212
Lake Norman Regional Medical Center	Mooresville	100%	254
Margaret R Pardee Memorial Hospital	Hendersonville	100%	657
Maria Parham Medical Center	Henderson	100%	55
Medwest Haywood	Clyde	100%	233
The Moses H Cone Memorial Hospital	Greensboro	100%	2836
North Carolina Specialty Hospital[2]	Durham	100%	155
Novant Health Charlotte Ortho Hosp[2]	Charlotte	100%	1403
Novant Health Forsyth Medical Center[2]	Winston-Salem	100%	2217
Novant Health Franklin Medical Center	Louisburg	100%	25
Novant Health Huntersville Medical Center[2]	Huntersville	100%	509
Novant Health Park Hospital[2]	Winston-Salem	100%	226
Novant Health Presbyterian Medical Center[2]	Charlotte	100%	722
Novant Health Rowan Medical Center[2]	Salisbury	100%	539
Novant Health Thomasville Medical Center	Thomasville	100%	120
Rex Hospital[2]	Raleigh	100%	739
Rutherford Hospital	Rutherfordton	100%	217
Spruce Pine Community Hospital	Spruce Pine	100%	39
Transylvania Regional Hospital	Brevard	100%	118
Vidant Beaufort Hospital	Washington	100%	163
Vidant Chowan Hospital	Edenton	100%	100
Vidant Edgecombe Hospital	Tarboro	100%	96
Vidant Medical Center[2]	Greenville	100%	1490
Wilkes Regional Medical Center	N Wilkesboro	100%	155
Wilson Medical Center[2]	Wilson	100%	375
Alamance Regional Medical Center	Burlington	99%	516
Albemarle Hospital Authority	Elizabeth City	99%	99
Asheville - Oteen VA Medical Center	Asheville	99%	396
Betsy Johnson Regional Hospital	Dunn	99%	79
Carolinas Medical Center - Union[2]	Monroe	99%	305
Catawba Valley Medical Center	Hickory	99%	543
Central Carolina Hospital	Sanford	99%	93
Columbus Regional Healthcare System	Whiteville	99%	70
Davis Regional Medical Center	Statesville	99%	76
Duke Regional Hospital[2]	Durham	99%	909
Durham VA Medical Center	Durham	99%	218
Granville Health Systems	Oxford	99%	136
Halifax Regional Medical Center	Roanoke Rapids	99%	342
High Point Regional Hospital[2]	High Point	99%	319
Iredell Memorial Hospital[2]	Statesville	99%	261
Johnston Memorial Hospital	Smithfield	99%	270
Lenoir Memorial Hospital	Kinston	99%	158
Martin General Hospital	Williamston	99%	73

Prophylactic Antibiotic Timing (Outpatient)

Hospital Name	City	Rate	Cases
Alamance Regional Medical Center	Burlington	100%	226
Caromont Regional Medical Center	Gastonia	100%	689
Davis Regional Medical Center	Statesville	100%	237
Frye Regional Medical Center	Hickory	100%	474
Hugh Chatham Memorial Hospital	Elkin	100%	73
Johnston Memorial Hospital	Smithfield	100%	280
Lake Norman Regional Medical Center	Mooresville	100%	330
Mem Mission Hosp & Asheville Surg Ctr	Asheville	100%	984
The Moses H Cone Memorial Hospital	Greensboro	100%	895
North Carolina Specialty Hospital	Durham	100%	187
Novant Health Brunswick Medical Center	Supply	100%	103
Novant Health Charlotte Ortho Hosp	Charlotte	100%	623
Novant Health Forsyth Medical Center	Winston-Salem	100%	1436
Novant Health Huntersville Medical Center	Huntersville	100%	219
Novant Health Presbyterian Medical Center	Charlotte	100%	1309
Novant Health Rowan Medical Center	Salisbury	100%	360
Presbyterian Hospital Matthews	Matthews	100%	262
Randolph Hospital	Asheboro	100%	109
Sandhills Regional Medical Center	Hamlet	100%	93
Scotland Memorial Hospital	Laurinburg	100%	35
Vidant Beaufort Hospital	Washington	100%	102
Watauga Medical Center	Boone	100%	164
Betsy Johnson Regional Hospital	Dunn	99%	71
Carolinas Medical Center - Northeast	Concord	99%	856
Carolinas Medical Center - Pineville	Charlotte	99%	1265
Carolinas Medical Center - University	Charlotte	99%	349
Carolinas Med Ctr/Behavioral Health	Charlotte	99%	1280
Catawba Valley Medical Center	Hickory	99%	551
Duke Health Raleigh Hospital	Raleigh	99%	548
Duke Regional Hospital	Durham	99%	525
Duke University Hospital	Durham	99%	748
Iredell Memorial Hospital	Statesville	99%	108
Lenoir Memorial Hospital	Kinston	99%	85
Lexington Memorial Hospital	Lexington	99%	84
Margaret R Pardee Memorial Hospital	Hendersonville	99%	217
Maria Parham Medical Center	Henderson	99%	67
Nash General Hospital	Rocky Mount	99%	434
Novant Health Park Hospital	Winston-Salem	99%	311
Novant Health Thomasville Medical Center	Thomasville	99%	98
Rex Hospital	Raleigh	99%	1069
Wakemed - Cary Hospital	Cary	99%	354
Albemarle Hospital Authority	Elizabeth City	98%	154
Caldwell Memorial Hospital	Lenoir	98%	93
Carteret General Hospital	Morehead City	98%	131
Central Carolina Hospital	Sanford	98%	127
Cleveland Regional Medical Center	Shelby	98%	177
Firsthealth Moore Regional Hospital	Pinehurst	98%	633
Granville Health Systems	Oxford	98%	90
Medwest Harris	Sylva	98%	113
Medwest Haywood	Clyde	98%	279
Northern Hospital of Surry County	Mount Airy	98%	43
Onslow Memorial Hospital	Jacksonville	98%	213
Stanly Regional Medical Center	Albemarle	98%	81
University of North Carolina Hospital	Chapel Hill	98%	681

NOTE: Hospital profiles are in alphabetical order by state, then city, then hospital within the city; Rankings exclude hospitals with less than 25 cases except for patient surveys which excludes hospitals with less than 100 cases; (a) 100-299 cases; (1) The number of cases/patients is too few to report; (2) Data submitted were based on a sample of cases/patients; (3) Results are based on a shorter time period than required; (4) Data suppressed by CMS for one or more quarters; (5) Results are not available for this reporting period; (6) Fewer than 100 patients completed the HCAHPS survey; (7) No cases met the criteria for this measure; (8) The lower limit of the confidence interval cannot be calculated if the number of observed infections equals zero; (9) No data are available from the state/territory for this reporting period; (10) The scores shown reflect fewer than 50 completed surveys; (11) There were discrepancies in the data collection process; (12) This measure does not apply to this hospital for this reporting period; (13) Results cannot be calculated for this reporting period; (14) The results for this state are combined with nearby states to protect confidentiality; Please refer to the User's Guide for a full explanation of data.

Vidant Edgecombe Hospital	Tarboro	98%	125
Wakemed - Raleigh Campus	Raleigh	98%	809
Wayne Memorial Hospital	Goldsboro	98%	310
Wilson Medical Center	Wilson	98%	149
Cape Fear Valley Medical Center	Fayetteville	97%	426
Carolina East Medical Center	New Bern	97%	695
High Point Regional Hospital	High Point	97%	434
The Mcdowell Hospital	Marion	97%	86
North Carolina Baptist Hospital	Winston-Salem	97%	631
Vidant Chowan Hospital	Edenton	97%	34
Vidant Medical Center	Greenville	97%	1322
Wilkes Regional Medical Center	N Wilkesboro	97%	36
CMC - Blue Ridge	Morganton	95%	259
New Hanover Regional Medical Center	Wilmington	95%	718
Park Ridge Health	Hendersonville	95%	154
Southeastern Regional Medical Center	Lumberton	95%	153
Halifax Regional Medical Center	Roanoke Rapids	94%	121
Carolinas Medical Center - Lincoln	Lincolnton	91%	32
Carolinas Medical Center - Union	Monroe	91%	65
Columbus Regional Healthcare System	Whiteville	91%	35

Urinary Catheter Removal

Hospital Name	City	Rate	Cases
Caldwell Memorial Hospital	Lenoir	100%	182
Carolinas Medical Center - Lincoln	Lincolnton	100%	92
Carolinas Medical Center - Pineville[2]	Charlotte	100%	1843
Caromont Regional Medical Center	Gastonia	100%	930
Cleveland Regional Medical Center[2]	Shelby	100%	230
CMC - Blue Ridge	Morganton	100%	251
Duke Health Raleigh Hospital	Raleigh	100%	940
Duke University Hospital[2]	Durham	100%	1085
Hugh Chatham Memorial Hospital	Elkin	100%	29
J Arthur Dosher Memorial Hospital[2]	Southport	100%	123
Lake Norman Regional Medical Center	Mooresville	100%	228
Margaret R Pardee Memorial Hospital	Hendersonville	100%	582
North Carolina Baptist Hospital[2]	Winston-Salem	100%	494
North Carolina Specialty Hospital[2]	Durham	100%	233
Northern Hospital of Surry County	Mount Airy	100%	90
Novant Health Charlotte Ortho Hosp[2]	Charlotte	100%	1363
Novant Health Forsyth Medical Center[2]	Winston-Salem	100%	2226
Novant Health Franklin Medical Center	Louisburg	100%	31
Novant Health Park Hospital[2]	Winston-Salem	100%	168
The Outer Banks Hospital	Nags Head	100%	137
Transylvania Regional Hospital	Brevard	100%	41
Vidant Chowan Hospital	Edenton	100%	100
Vidant Medical Center[2]	Greenville	100%	893
Vidant Roanoke Chowan Hospital	Ahoskie	100%	54
Wakemed - Raleigh Campus[2]	Raleigh	100%	912
Albemarle Hospital Authority	Elizabeth City	99%	99
Duke Regional Hospital[2]	Durham	99%	853
Firsthealth Moore Regional Hospital[2]	Pinehurst	99%	581
Frye Regional Medical Center[2]	Hickory	99%	563
High Point Regional Hospital[2]	High Point	99%	292
Iredell Memorial Hospital[2]	Statesville	99%	243
Johnston Memorial Hospital	Smithfield	99%	289
Mem Mission Hosp & Asheville Surg Ctr[2]	Asheville	99%	373
New Hanover Regional Medical Center[2]	Wilmington	99%	1199
Novant Health Brunswick Medical Center	Supply	99%	316
Novant Health Huntersville Medical Center[2]	Huntersville	99%	438
Park Ridge Health	Hendersonville	99%	159
Presbyterian Hospital Matthews[2]	Matthews	99%	374
Randolph Hospital[2]	Asheboro	99%	75
Rex Hospital[2]	Raleigh	99%	762
Rutherford Hospital	Rutherfordton	99%	70
Scotland Memorial Hospital	Laurinburg	99%	285
Southeastern Regional Medical Center	Lumberton	99%	177
Stanly Regional Medical Center	Albemarle	99%	130
University of North Carolina Hospital[2]	Chapel Hill	99%	286
Wakemed - Cary Hospital	Cary	99%	418
Wayne Memorial Hospital[2]	Goldsboro	99%	337
Wilkes Regional Medical Center	N Wilkesboro	99%	176
Angel Medical Center	Franklin	98%	63
Asheville - Oteen VA Medical Center[2]	Asheville	98%	396
Cape Fear Valley Medical Center[2]	Fayetteville	98%	639
Carolinas Medical Center - Northeast[2]	Concord	98%	1111
Carolinas Medical Center - Union[2]	Monroe	98%	227
Carolinas Medical Center - University[2]	Charlotte	98%	81
Durham VA Medical Center[2]	Durham	98%	146
Medwest Harris	Sylva	98%	138
The Moses H Cone Memorial Hospital	Greensboro	98%	3104
Murphy Medical Center	Murphy	98%	134
Nash General Hospital[2]	Rocky Mount	98%	313
Novant Health Presbyterian Medical Center[2]	Charlotte	98%	509
Novant Health Rowan Medical Center[2]	Salisbury	98%	236
Onslow Memorial Hospital	Jacksonville	98%	184
Person Memorial Hospital	Roxboro	98%	118
Wilson Medical Center[2]	Wilson	98%	321
Catawba Valley Medical Center	Hickory	97%	575
Central Carolina Hospital	Sanford	97%	103
Columbus Regional Healthcare System	Whiteville	97%	116
Lexington Memorial Hospital	Lexington	97%	204
Novant Health Thomasville Medical Center	Thomasville	97%	108
Saint Luke's Hospital	Columbus	97%	145
Vidant Edgecombe Hospital	Tarboro	97%	71
WG (Bill) Hefner Salisbury VA Med Ctr[2]	Salisbury	97%	60
Alamance Regional Medical Center	Burlington	96%	578
Betsy Johnson Regional Hospital	Dunn	96%	113
Carolina East Medical Center	New Bern	96%	941
Carolinas Med Ctr/Behaviorial Health[2]	Charlotte	96%	713
Davis Regional Medical Center	Statesville	96%	55
Maria Parham Medical Center	Henderson	96%	73
Sampson Regional Medical Center	Clinton	96%	104
Carteret General Hospital	Morehead City	95%	151
Granville Health Systems	Oxford	95%	165
Halifax Regional Medical Center	Roanoke Rapids	95%	80
Vidant Beaufort Hospital	Washington	94%	109
Morehead Memorial Hospital	Eden	92%	61
Medwest Haywood	Clyde	91%	81
Lenoir Memorial Hospital	Kinston	89%	84
Watauga Medical Center	Boone	89%	75

Survey of Patients' Hospital Experiences

Area Around Room 'Always' Quiet at Night

Hospital Name	City	Rate	Cases
Vidant Bertie Hospital	Windsor	85%	(a)
North Carolina Specialty Hospital	Durham	82%	300+
Anson Community Hospital	Wadesboro	76%	(a)
Carolinas Medical Center - Lincoln	Lincolnton	75%	300+
Sandhills Regional Medical Center	Hamlet	75%	(a)
Hugh Chatham Memorial Hospital	Elkin	74%	300+
New Hanover Regional Medical Center	Wilmington	73%	300+
Novant Health Park Hospital	Winston-Salem	73%	300+
Johnston Memorial Hospital	Smithfield	72%	300+
Southeastern Regional Medical Center	Lumberton	72%	300+
Spruce Pine Community Hospital	Spruce Pine	72%	300+
Martin General Hospital	Williamston	70%	300+
Scotland Memorial Hospital	Laurinburg	70%	300+
Cleveland Regional Medical Center	Shelby	69%	300+
Pender Memorial Hospital	Burgaw	69%	(a)
Person Memorial Hospital	Roxboro	69%	300+
Kings Mountain Hospital	Kings Mountain	68%	300+
Novant Health Brunswick Medical Center	Supply	68%	300+
Betsy Johnson Regional Hospital	Dunn	67%	300+
Carolinas Medical Center - Pineville	Charlotte	67%	300+
The Mcdowell Hospital	Marion	67%	300+
Transylvania Regional Hospital	Brevard	67%	300+
Vidant Duplin Hospital	Kenansville	67%	300+
Vidant Edgecombe Hospital	Tarboro	67%	300+
Carolinas Medical Center - Union	Monroe	66%	300+
Medwest Harris	Sylva	66%	300+
Randolph Hospital	Asheboro	66%	300+
Rutherford Hospital	Rutherfordton	66%	300+
Wakemed - Raleigh Campus	Raleigh	66%	300+
Ashe Memorial Hospital	Jefferson	65%	300+
Firsthealth Moore Regional Hospital	Pinehurst	65%	300+
Halifax Regional Medical Center	Roanoke Rapids	65%	300+
Northern Hospital of Surry County	Mount Airy	65%	300+
The Outer Banks Hospital	Nags Head	65%	300+
University of North Carolina Hospital	Chapel Hill	65%	300+
Vidant Roanoke Chowan Hospital	Ahoskie	65%	300+
Carolinas Medical Center - Northeast	Concord	64%	300+
Carolinas Medical Center - University	Charlotte	64%	300+
Carteret General Hospital	Morehead City	64%	300+
Chatham Hospital	Siler City	64%	(a)
CMC - Blue Ridge	Morganton	64%	300+
Duke Health Raleigh Hospital	Raleigh	64%	300+
Mem Mission Hosp & Asheville Surg Ctr	Asheville	64%	300+
North Carolina Baptist Hospital	Winston-Salem	64%	300+
Sampson Regional Medical Center	Clinton	64%	300+
Vidant Chowan Hospital	Edenton	64%	300+
Carolinas Med Ctr/Behaviorial Health	Charlotte	63%	300+
Park Ridge Health[11]	Hendersonville	63%	300+
Vidant Beaufort Hospital	Washington	63%	300+
Albemarle Hospital Authority	Elizabeth City	62%	300+
Columbus Regional Healthcare System	Whiteville	62%	300+
Davis Regional Medical Center	Statesville	62%	300+
Granville Health Systems	Oxford	62%	300+
Stanly Regional Medical Center	Albemarle	62%	300+
Wayne Memorial Hospital	Goldsboro	62%	300+
Wilkes Regional Medical Center	N Wilkesboro	62%	300+
Carolina East Medical Center	New Bern	61%	300+
Central Carolina Hospital	Sanford	61%	300+
Frye Regional Medical Center	Hickory	61%	300+
Margaret R Pardee Memorial Hospital	Hendersonville	61%	300+
Maria Parham Medical Center	Henderson	61%	300+
Medwest Haywood	Clyde	61%	300+
Novant Health Franklin Medical Center	Louisburg	61%	(a)
Rex Hospital	Raleigh	61%	300+
Caldwell Memorial Hospital	Lenoir	60%	300+
Novant Health Charlotte Ortho Hosp	Charlotte	60%	300+
Vidant Medical Center	Greenville	60%	300+
Wakemed - Cary Hospital	Cary	60%	300+
Wilson Medical Center	Wilson	60%	300+
High Point Regional Hospital	High Point	59%	300+
Iredell Memorial Hospital	Statesville	59%	300+
J Arthur Dosher Memorial Hospital	Southport	59%	300+
Novant Health Huntersville Medical Center	Huntersville	59%	300+
Alamance Regional Medical Center	Burlington	58%	300+
Catawba Valley Medical Center	Hickory	58%	300+
The Moses H Cone Memorial Hospital	Greensboro	58%	300+
Nash General Hospital	Rocky Mount	58%	300+
Saint Luke's Hospital	Columbus	58%	(a)
Cape Fear Valley Medical Center	Fayetteville	57%	300+
Caromont Regional Medical Center	Gastonia	57%	300+
Duke University Hospital	Durham	56%	300+
Lake Norman Regional Medical Center	Mooresville	56%	300+
Novant Health Presbyterian Medical Center	Charlotte	56%	300+
Novant Health Rowan Medical Center	Salisbury	56%	300+
Novant Health Thomasville Medical Center	Thomasville	56%	300+
Presbyterian Hospital Matthews	Matthews	56%	300+
Angel Medical Center	Franklin	55%	300+
Duke Regional Hospital	Durham	55%	300+
Lenoir Memorial Hospital	Kinston	55%	300+
Lexington Memorial Hospital	Lexington	55%	300+
Morehead Memorial Hospital	Eden	54%	300+
Murphy Medical Center	Murphy	53%	300+
Novant Health Forsyth Medical Center	Winston-Salem	53%	300+
Onslow Memorial Hospital	Jacksonville	51%	300+
Watauga Medical Center	Boone	51%	300+

Doctors 'Always' Communicated Well

Hospital Name	City	Rate	Cases
Vidant Bertie Hospital	Windsor	94%	(a)
Chatham Hospital	Siler City	92%	(a)
Anson Community Hospital	Wadesboro	90%	(a)
Ashe Memorial Hospital	Jefferson	89%	300+
The Mcdowell Hospital	Marion	88%	300+
North Carolina Specialty Hospital	Durham	88%	300+
The Outer Banks Hospital	Nags Head	88%	300+
Kings Mountain Hospital	Kings Mountain	87%	300+
Novant Health Park Hospital	Winston-Salem	87%	300+
Rex Hospital	Raleigh	87%	300+
Sandhills Regional Medical Center	Hamlet	87%	(a)
Spruce Pine Community Hospital	Spruce Pine	87%	300+
Vidant Beaufort Hospital	Washington	87%	300+
Angel Medical Center	Franklin	86%	300+
Carolinas Medical Center - Northeast	Concord	86%	300+
Carolinas Medical Center - University	Charlotte	86%	300+
Firsthealth Moore Regional Hospital	Pinehurst	86%	300+
Medwest Haywood	Clyde	86%	300+
Mem Mission Hosp & Asheville Surg Ctr	Asheville	86%	300+
New Hanover Regional Medical Center	Wilmington	86%	300+
Vidant Chowan Hospital	Edenton	86%	300+
Caldwell Memorial Hospital	Lenoir	85%	300+
Carolinas Medical Center - Pineville	Charlotte	85%	300+
Cleveland Regional Medical Center	Shelby	85%	300+
Columbus Regional Healthcare System	Whiteville	85%	300+
Duke Regional Hospital	Durham	85%	300+
Park Ridge Health[11]	Hendersonville	85%	300+
Pender Memorial Hospital	Burgaw	85%	(a)
Saint Luke's Hospital	Columbus	85%	(a)
Vidant Edgecombe Hospital	Tarboro	85%	300+
Vidant Roanoke Chowan Hospital	Ahoskie	85%	300+
Wilson Medical Center	Wilson	85%	300+
Carolinas Medical Center - Lincoln	Lincolnton	84%	300+
Caromont Regional Medical Center	Gastonia	84%	300+
Catawba Valley Medical Center	Hickory	84%	300+
Central Carolina Hospital	Sanford	84%	300+
Duke Health Raleigh Hospital	Raleigh	84%	300+
Hugh Chatham Memorial Hospital	Elkin	84%	300+
Martin General Hospital	Williamston	84%	300+
Murphy Medical Center	Murphy	84%	300+
Sampson Regional Medical Center	Clinton	84%	300+
Scotland Memorial Hospital	Laurinburg	84%	300+
University of North Carolina Hospital	Chapel Hill	84%	300+
Carolina East Medical Center	New Bern	83%	300+
Carolinas Medical Center - Union	Monroe	83%	300+
Carteret General Hospital	Morehead City	83%	300+
Frye Regional Medical Center	Hickory	83%	300+
J Arthur Dosher Memorial Hospital	Southport	83%	300+
Morehead Memorial Hospital	Eden	83%	300+
Novant Health Charlotte Ortho Hosp	Charlotte	83%	300+
Novant Health Huntersville Medical Center	Huntersville	83%	300+
Rutherford Hospital	Rutherfordton	83%	300+
Vidant Duplin Hospital	Kenansville	83%	300+
Vidant Medical Center	Greenville	83%	300+
Albemarle Hospital Authority	Elizabeth City	82%	300+
Duke University Hospital	Durham	82%	300+
Granville Health Systems	Oxford	82%	300+
Halifax Regional Medical Center	Roanoke Rapids	82%	300+
Iredell Memorial Hospital	Statesville	82%	300+

NOTE: Hospital profiles are in alphabetical order by state, then city, then hospital within the city; Rankings exclude hospitals with less than 25 cases except for patient surveys which excludes hospitals with less than 100 cases; (a) 100-299 cases; (1) The number of cases/patients is too few to report; (2) Data submitted were based on a sample of cases/patients; (3) Results are based on a shorter time period than required; (4) Data suppressed by CMS for one or more quarters; (5) Results are not available for this reporting period; (6) Fewer than 100 patients completed the HCAHPS survey; (7) No cases met the criteria for this measure; (8) The lower limit of the confidence interval cannot be calculated if the number of observed infections equals zero; (9) No data are available from the state/territory for this reporting period; (10) The scores shown reflect fewer than 50 completed surveys; (11) There were discrepancies in the data collection process; (12) This measure does not apply to this hospital for this reporting period; (13) Results cannot be calculated for this reporting period; (14) The results for this state are combined with nearby states to protect confidentiality; Please refer to the User's Guide for a full explanation of data.

Hospital Name	City	Rate	Cases
Margaret R Pardee Memorial Hospital	Hendersonville	82%	300+
Maria Parham Medical Center	Henderson	82%	300+
Medwest Harris	Sylva	82%	300+
The Moses H Cone Memorial Hospital	Greensboro	82%	300+
Person Memorial Hospital	Roxboro	82%	300+
Randolph Hospital	Asheboro	82%	300+
Southeastern Regional Medical Center	Lumberton	82%	300+
Stanly Regional Medical Center	Albemarle	82%	300+
Transylvania Regional Hospital	Brevard	82%	300+
Wilkes Regional Medical Center	N Wilkesboro	82%	300+
Alamance Regional Medical Center	Burlington	81%	300+
Carolinas Med Ctr/Behaviorial Health	Charlotte	81%	300+
High Point Regional Hospital	High Point	81%	300+
Johnston Memorial Hospital	Smithfield	81%	300+
Lake Norman Regional Medical Center	Mooresville	81%	300+
Novant Health Brunswick Medical Center	Supply	81%	300+
Wakemed - Raleigh Campus	Raleigh	81%	300+
CMC - Blue Ridge	Morganton	80%	300+
Lexington Memorial Hospital	Lexington	80%	300+
Nash General Hospital	Rocky Mount	80%	300+
Onslow Memorial Hospital	Jacksonville	80%	300+
Wayne Memorial Hospital	Goldsboro	80%	300+
Betsy Johnson Regional Hospital	Dunn	79%	300+
Davis Regional Medical Center	Statesville	79%	300+
North Carolina Baptist Hospital	Winston-Salem	79%	300+
Novant Health Forsyth Medical Center	Winston-Salem	79%	300+
Novant Health Presbyterian Medical Center	Charlotte	79%	300+
Novant Health Thomasville Medical Center	Thomasville	79%	300+
Presbyterian Hospital Matthews	Matthews	79%	300+
Wakemed - Cary Hospital	Cary	79%	300+
Watauga Medical Center	Boone	79%	300+
Lenoir Memorial Hospital	Kinston	78%	300+
Northern Hospital of Surry County	Mount Airy	78%	300+
Novant Health Rowan Medical Center	Salisbury	78%	300+
Cape Fear Valley Medical Center	Fayetteville	77%	300+
Novant Health Franklin Medical Center	Louisburg	70%	(a)

Home Recovery Information Given

Hospital Name	City	Rate	Cases
The Outer Banks Hospital	Nags Head	92%	300+
Carolinas Medical Center - Pineville	Charlotte	91%	300+
Mem Mission Hosp & Asheville Surg Ctr	Asheville	91%	300+
Vidant Bertie Hospital	Windsor	91%	(a)
Vidant Chowan Hospital	Edenton	91%	300+
Carolinas Medical Center - Lincoln	Lincolnton	90%	300+
Carolinas Medical Center - Northeast	Concord	90%	300+
Cleveland Regional Medical Center	Shelby	90%	300+
University of North Carolina Hospital	Chapel Hill	90%	300+
Vidant Beaufort Hospital	Washington	90%	300+
Vidant Medical Center	Greenville	90%	300+
Wilson Medical Center	Wilson	90%	300+
Ashe Memorial Hospital	Jefferson	89%	300+
Carolinas Medical Center - Union	Monroe	89%	300+
Caromont Regional Medical Center	Gastonia	89%	300+
CMC - Blue Ridge	Morganton	89%	300+
Firsthealth Moore Regional Hospital	Pinehurst	89%	300+
Frye Regional Medical Center	Hickory	89%	300+
J Arthur Dosher Memorial Hospital	Southport	89%	300+
Johnston Memorial Hospital	Smithfield	89%	300+
North Carolina Specialty Hospital	Durham	89%	300+
Novant Health Charlotte Ortho Hosp	Charlotte	89%	300+
Rex Hospital	Raleigh	89%	300+
Wakemed - Cary Hospital	Cary	89%	300+
Anson Community Hospital	Wadesboro	88%	(a)
Betsy Johnson Regional Hospital	Dunn	88%	300+
Carolinas Medical Center - University	Charlotte	88%	300+
Carolinas Med Ctr/Behaviorial Health	Charlotte	88%	300+
Duke Health Raleigh Hospital	Raleigh	88%	300+
Duke University Hospital	Durham	88%	300+
Kings Mountain Hospital	Kings Mountain	88%	300+
Margaret R Pardee Memorial Hospital	Hendersonville	88%	300+
The Mcdowell Hospital	Marion	88%	300+
New Hanover Regional Medical Center	Wilmington	88%	300+
Northern Hospital of Surry County	Mount Airy	88%	300+
Saint Luke's Hospital	Columbus	88%	(a)
Vidant Duplin Hospital	Kenansville	88%	300+
Vidant Edgecombe Hospital	Tarboro	88%	300+
Vidant Roanoke Chowan Hospital	Ahoskie	88%	300+
Wayne Memorial Hospital	Goldsboro	88%	300+
Alamance Regional Medical Center	Burlington	87%	300+
Carolina East Medical Center	New Bern	87%	300+
Catawba Valley Medical Center	Hickory	87%	300+
Columbus Regional Healthcare System	Whiteville	87%	300+
Maria Parham Medical Center	Henderson	87%	300+
Morehead Memorial Hospital	Eden	87%	300+
Park Ridge Health[11]	Hendersonville	87%	300+
Pender Memorial Hospital	Burgaw	87%	(a)
Sandhills Regional Medical Center	Hamlet	87%	(a)
Scotland Memorial Hospital	Laurinburg	87%	300+
Stanly Regional Medical Center	Albemarle	87%	300+
Wakemed - Raleigh Campus	Raleigh	87%	300+
Albemarle Hospital Authority	Elizabeth City	86%	300+
Caldwell Memorial Hospital	Lenoir	86%	300+
Halifax Regional Medical Center	Roanoke Rapids	86%	300+
Iredell Memorial Hospital	Statesville	86%	300+
Medwest Harris	Sylva	86%	300+
Medwest Haywood	Clyde	86%	300+
North Carolina Baptist Hospital	Winston-Salem	86%	300+
Novant Health Franklin Medical Center	Louisburg	86%	(a)
Novant Health Huntersville Medical Center	Huntersville	86%	300+
Novant Health Park Hospital	Winston-Salem	86%	300+
Onslow Memorial Hospital	Jacksonville	86%	300+
Randolph Hospital	Asheboro	86%	300+
Southeastern Regional Medical Center	Lumberton	86%	300+
Transylvania Regional Hospital	Brevard	86%	300+
Chatham Hospital	Siler City	85%	(a)
Duke Regional Hospital	Durham	85%	300+
Granville Health Systems	Oxford	85%	300+
Hugh Chatham Memorial Hospital	Elkin	85%	300+
Martin General Hospital	Williamston	85%	300+
The Moses H Cone Memorial Hospital	Greensboro	85%	300+
Nash General Hospital	Rocky Mount	85%	300+
Spruce Pine Community Hospital	Spruce Pine	85%	300+
Wilkes Regional Medical Center	N Wilkesboro	85%	300+
Carteret General Hospital	Morehead City	84%	300+
Lake Norman Regional Medical Center	Mooresville	84%	300+
Lenoir Memorial Hospital	Kinston	84%	300+
Novant Health Brunswick Medical Center	Supply	84%	300+
Sampson Regional Medical Center	Clinton	84%	300+
Watauga Medical Center	Boone	84%	300+
Angel Medical Center	Franklin	83%	300+
Central Carolina Hospital	Sanford	83%	300+
High Point Regional Hospital	High Point	83%	300+
Murphy Medical Center	Murphy	83%	300+
Novant Health Thomasville Medical Center	Thomasville	83%	300+
Person Memorial Hospital	Roxboro	83%	300+
Rutherford Hospital	Rutherfordton	83%	300+
Lexington Memorial Hospital	Lexington	82%	300+
Novant Health Forsyth Medical Center	Winston-Salem	82%	300+
Novant Health Presbyterian Medical Center	Charlotte	82%	300+
Presbyterian Hospital Matthews	Matthews	82%	300+
Cape Fear Valley Medical Center	Fayetteville	81%	300+
Davis Regional Medical Center	Statesville	81%	300+
Novant Health Rowan Medical Center	Salisbury	81%	300+

Hospital Given 9 or 10 on 10 Point Scale

Hospital Name	City	Rate	Cases
North Carolina Specialty Hospital	Durham	88%	300+
Novant Health Park Hospital	Winston-Salem	84%	300+
Carolinas Medical Center - Lincoln	Lincolnton	82%	300+
Firsthealth Moore Regional Hospital	Pinehurst	82%	300+
The Outer Banks Hospital	Nags Head	82%	300+
Park Ridge Health[11]	Hendersonville	81%	300+
University of North Carolina Hospital	Chapel Hill	81%	300+
Carolinas Medical Center - Northeast	Concord	79%	300+
Carolinas Medical Center - Pineville	Charlotte	79%	300+
Chatham Hospital	Siler City	79%	(a)
Hugh Chatham Memorial Hospital	Elkin	79%	300+
New Hanover Regional Medical Center	Wilmington	79%	300+
Vidant Chowan Hospital	Edenton	79%	300+
Mem Mission Hosp & Asheville Surg Ctr	Asheville	78%	300+
Saint Luke's Hospital	Columbus	78%	(a)
Spruce Pine Community Hospital	Spruce Pine	78%	300+
Carolinas Medical Center - University	Charlotte	77%	300+
Cleveland Regional Medical Center	Shelby	77%	300+
Duke University Hospital	Durham	77%	300+
Rex Hospital	Raleigh	77%	300+
Ashe Memorial Hospital	Jefferson	76%	300+
Carolinas Medical Center - Union	Monroe	76%	300+
Kings Mountain Hospital	Kings Mountain	76%	300+
North Carolina Baptist Hospital	Winston-Salem	76%	300+
Novant Health Huntersville Medical Center	Huntersville	76%	300+
Vidant Bertie Hospital	Windsor	76%	(a)
Transylvania Regional Hospital	Brevard	75%	300+
Vidant Medical Center	Greenville	75%	300+
Carolina East Medical Center	New Bern	74%	300+
Carolinas Med Ctr/Behaviorial Health	Charlotte	74%	300+
Caromont Regional Medical Center	Gastonia	74%	300+
Duke Health Raleigh Hospital	Raleigh	74%	300+
High Point Regional Hospital	High Point	74%	300+
Iredell Memorial Hospital	Statesville	74%	300+
The Mcdowell Hospital	Marion	74%	300+
Vidant Edgecombe Hospital	Tarboro	74%	300+
Angel Medical Center	Franklin	73%	300+
Sandhills Regional Medical Center	Hamlet	73%	(a)
Frye Regional Medical Center	Hickory	72%	300+
Johnston Memorial Hospital	Smithfield	72%	300+
The Moses H Cone Memorial Hospital	Greensboro	72%	300+
Scotland Memorial Hospital	Laurinburg	72%	300+
Vidant Beaufort Hospital	Washington	72%	300+
Catawba Valley Medical Center	Hickory	71%	300+
CMC - Blue Ridge	Morganton	71%	300+
Novant Health Brunswick Medical Center	Supply	71%	300+
Vidant Roanoke Chowan Hospital	Ahoskie	71%	300+
Wakemed - Cary Hospital	Cary	71%	300+
Wakemed - Raleigh Campus	Raleigh	71%	300+
Wilson Medical Center	Wilson	71%	300+
Anson Community Hospital	Wadesboro	70%	(a)
Duke Regional Hospital	Durham	70%	300+
J Arthur Dosher Memorial Hospital	Southport	70%	300+
Margaret R Pardee Memorial Hospital	Hendersonville	70%	300+
Presbyterian Hospital Matthews	Matthews	70%	300+
Randolph Hospital	Asheboro	70%	300+
Stanly Regional Medical Center	Albemarle	70%	300+
Betsy Johnson Regional Hospital	Dunn	69%	300+
Columbus Regional Healthcare System	Whiteville	69%	300+
Medwest Harris	Sylva	69%	300+
Medwest Haywood	Clyde	69%	300+
Northern Hospital of Surry County	Mount Airy	69%	300+
Vidant Duplin Hospital	Kenansville	69%	300+
Alamance Regional Medical Center	Burlington	68%	300+
Carteret General Hospital	Morehead City	68%	300+
Morehead Memorial Hospital	Eden	68%	300+
Novant Health Forsyth Medical Center	Winston-Salem	68%	300+
Novant Health Thomasville Medical Center	Thomasville	68%	300+
Wilkes Regional Medical Center	N Wilkesboro	68%	300+
Novant Health Charlotte Ortho Hosp	Charlotte	67%	300+
Novant Health Presbyterian Medical Center	Charlotte	67%	300+
Rutherford Hospital	Rutherfordton	67%	300+
Southeastern Regional Medical Center	Lumberton	67%	300+
Albemarle Hospital Authority	Elizabeth City	66%	300+
Davis Regional Medical Center	Statesville	66%	300+
Pender Memorial Hospital	Burgaw	66%	(a)
Nash General Hospital	Rocky Mount	65%	300+
Wayne Memorial Hospital	Goldsboro	65%	300+
Caldwell Memorial Hospital	Lenoir	64%	300+
Martin General Hospital	Williamston	64%	300+
Person Memorial Hospital	Roxboro	63%	300+
Lake Norman Regional Medical Center	Mooresville	62%	300+
Maria Parham Medical Center	Henderson	62%	300+
Murphy Medical Center	Murphy	62%	300+
Cape Fear Valley Medical Center	Fayetteville	61%	300+
Central Carolina Hospital	Sanford	61%	300+
Halifax Regional Medical Center	Roanoke Rapids	61%	300+
Sampson Regional Medical Center	Clinton	61%	300+
Granville Health Systems	Oxford	60%	300+
Lenoir Memorial Hospital	Kinston	60%	300+
Watauga Medical Center	Boone	60%	300+
Lexington Memorial Hospital	Lexington	59%	300+
Novant Health Rowan Medical Center	Salisbury	59%	300+
Onslow Memorial Hospital	Jacksonville	58%	300+
Novant Health Franklin Medical Center	Louisburg	52%	(a)

Meds 'Always' Explained Before Given

Hospital Name	City	Rate	Cases
Vidant Bertie Hospital	Windsor	82%	(a)
North Carolina Specialty Hospital	Durham	81%	300+
The Outer Banks Hospital	Nags Head	76%	300+
Carteret General Hospital	Morehead City	73%	300+
The Mcdowell Hospital	Marion	73%	300+
Mem Mission Hosp & Asheville Surg Ctr	Asheville	73%	300+
Chatham Hospital	Siler City	72%	(a)
Pender Memorial Hospital	Burgaw	72%	(a)
Sandhills Regional Medical Center	Hamlet	72%	(a)
Vidant Edgecombe Hospital	Tarboro	72%	300+
Cleveland Regional Medical Center	Shelby	71%	300+
Carolinas Medical Center - Lincoln	Lincolnton	70%	300+
Firsthealth Moore Regional Hospital	Pinehurst	70%	300+
New Hanover Regional Medical Center	Wilmington	70%	300+
Spruce Pine Community Hospital	Spruce Pine	70%	300+
Transylvania Regional Hospital	Brevard	70%	300+
Vidant Chowan Hospital	Edenton	70%	300+
Anson Community Hospital	Wadesboro	69%	(a)
Ashe Memorial Hospital	Jefferson	69%	300+
Carolina East Medical Center	New Bern	69%	300+
Kings Mountain Hospital	Kings Mountain	69%	300+
Southeastern Regional Medical Center	Lumberton	69%	300+
Vidant Duplin Hospital	Kenansville	69%	300+
Carolinas Medical Center - Northeast	Concord	68%	300+
Halifax Regional Medical Center	Roanoke Rapids	68%	300+
Morehead Memorial Hospital	Eden	68%	300+
Rex Hospital	Raleigh	68%	300+
Scotland Memorial Hospital	Laurinburg	68%	300+
University of North Carolina Hospital	Chapel Hill	68%	300+
Vidant Roanoke Chowan Hospital	Ahoskie	68%	300+
Carolinas Medical Center - Union	Monroe	67%	300+
Carolinas Medical Center - University	Charlotte	67%	300+
Duke Health Raleigh Hospital	Raleigh	67%	300+
Medwest Harris	Sylva	67%	300+
Saint Luke's Hospital	Columbus	67%	(a)
Wilson Medical Center	Wilson	67%	300+
Alamance Regional Medical Center	Burlington	66%	300+
Carolinas Medical Center - Pineville	Charlotte	66%	300+

NOTE: Hospital profiles are in alphabetical order by state, then city, then hospital within the city; Rankings exclude hospitals with less than 25 cases except for patient surveys which excludes hospitals with less than 100 cases; (a) 100-299 cases; (1) The number of cases/patients is too few to report; (2) Data submitted were based on a sample of cases/patients; (3) Results are based on a shorter time period than required; (4) Data suppressed by CMS for one or more quarters; (5) Results are not available for this reporting period; (6) Fewer than 100 patients completed the HCAHPS survey; (7) No cases met the criteria for this measure; (8) The lower limit of the confidence interval cannot be calculated if the number of observed infections equals zero; (9) No data are available from the state/territory for this reporting period; (10) The scores shown reflect fewer than 50 completed surveys; (11) There were discrepancies in the data collection process; (12) This measure does not apply to this hospital for this reporting period; (13) Results cannot be calculated for this reporting period; (14) The results for this state are combined with nearby states to protect confidentiality; Please refer to the User's Guide for a full explanation of data.

Hospital Name	City	Rate	Cases
Hugh Chatham Memorial Hospital	Elkin	66%	300+
J Arthur Dosher Memorial Hospital	Southport	66%	300+
Johnston Memorial Hospital	Smithfield	66%	300+
Martin General Hospital	Williamston	66%	300+
Medwest Haywood	Clyde	66%	300+
Murphy Medical Center	Murphy	66%	300+
Onslow Memorial Hospital	Jacksonville	66%	300+
Randolph Hospital	Asheboro	66%	300+
Vidant Beaufort Hospital	Washington	66%	300+
Caromont Regional Medical Center	Gastonia	65%	300+
Catawba Valley Medical Center	Hickory	65%	300+
Central Carolina Hospital	Sanford	65%	300+
Columbus Regional Healthcare System	Whiteville	65%	300+
Granville Health Systems	Oxford	65%	300+
Novant Health Park Hospital	Winston-Salem	65%	300+
Sampson Regional Medical Center	Clinton	65%	300+
Vidant Medical Center	Greenville	65%	300+
Wakemed - Raleigh Campus	Raleigh	65%	300+
Wilkes Regional Medical Center	N Wilkesboro	65%	300+
Angel Medical Center	Franklin	64%	300+
Duke Regional Hospital	Durham	64%	300+
Duke University Hospital	Durham	64%	300+
Frye Regional Medical Center	Hickory	64%	300+
Nash General Hospital	Rocky Mount	64%	300+
Albemarle Hospital Authority	Elizabeth City	63%	300+
CMC - Blue Ridge	Morganton	63%	300+
High Point Regional Hospital	High Point	63%	300+
Iredell Memorial Hospital	Statesville	63%	300+
Maria Parham Medical Center	Henderson	63%	300+
North Carolina Baptist Hospital	Winston-Salem	63%	300+
Betsy Johnson Regional Hospital	Dunn	62%	300+
Cape Fear Valley Medical Center	Fayetteville	62%	300+
Carolinas Med Ctr/Behavioral Health	Charlotte	62%	300+
Lenoir Memorial Hospital	Kinston	62%	300+
Margaret R Pardee Memorial Hospital	Hendersonville	62%	300+
Novant Health Franklin Medical Center	Louisburg	62%	(a)
Park Ridge Health[11]	Hendersonville	62%	300+
Rutherford Hospital	Rutherfordton	62%	300+
Stanly Regional Medical Center	Albemarle	62%	300+
Wakemed - Cary Hospital	Cary	62%	300+
Wayne Memorial Hospital	Goldsboro	62%	300+
Caldwell Memorial Hospital	Lenoir	61%	300+
Watauga Medical Center	Boone	61%	300+
Davis Regional Medical Center	Statesville	60%	300+
Lake Norman Regional Medical Center	Mooresville	59%	300+
Lexington Memorial Hospital	Lexington	59%	300+
The Moses H Cone Memorial Hospital	Greensboro	59%	300+
Novant Health Brunswick Medical Center	Supply	59%	300+
Novant Health Huntersville Medical Center	Huntersville	59%	300+
Person Memorial Hospital	Roxboro	59%	300+
Northern Hospital of Surry County	Mount Airy	58%	300+
Novant Health Thomasville Medical Center	Thomasville	58%	300+
Novant Health Charlotte Ortho Hosp	Charlotte	57%	300+
Novant Health Rowan Medical Center	Salisbury	57%	300+
Presbyterian Hospital Matthews	Matthews	57%	300+
Novant Health Forsyth Medical Center	Winston-Salem	56%	300+
Novant Health Presbyterian Medical Center	Charlotte	56%	300+

Nurses 'Always' Communicated Well

Hospital Name	City	Rate	Cases
Vidant Bertie Hospital	Windsor	92%	(a)
North Carolina Specialty Hospital	Durham	90%	300+
Chatham Hospital	Siler City	89%	(a)
Anson Community Hospital	Wadesboro	88%	(a)
Ashe Memorial Hospital	Jefferson	87%	300+
Carteret General Hospital	Morehead City	86%	300+
New Hanover Regional Medical Center	Wilmington	86%	300+
Carolinas Medical Center - Lincoln	Lincolnton	85%	300+
Carolinas Medical Center - University	Charlotte	85%	300+
Firsthealth Moore Regional Hospital	Pinehurst	85%	300+
Novant Health Park Hospital	Winston-Salem	85%	300+
Spruce Pine Community Hospital	Spruce Pine	85%	300+
Carolina East Medical Center	New Bern	84%	300+
Cleveland Regional Medical Center	Shelby	84%	300+
Hugh Chatham Memorial Hospital	Elkin	84%	300+
The Mcdowell Hospital	Marion	84%	300+
The Outer Banks Hospital	Nags Head	84%	300+
Randolph Hospital	Asheboro	84%	300+
Sandhills Regional Medical Center	Hamlet	84%	(a)
Vidant Chowan Hospital	Edenton	84%	300+
Vidant Edgecombe Hospital	Tarboro	84%	300+
Kings Mountain Hospital	Kings Mountain	83%	300+
Mem Mission Hosp & Asheville Surg Ctr	Asheville	83%	300+
Pender Memorial Hospital	Burgaw	83%	(a)
Saint Luke's Hospital	Columbus	83%	(a)
Scotland Memorial Hospital	Laurinburg	83%	300+
Vidant Roanoke Chowan Hospital	Ahoskie	83%	300+
Wilson Medical Center	Wilson	83%	300+
Angel Medical Center	Franklin	82%	300+
Carolinas Medical Center - Northeast	Concord	82%	300+
Carolinas Medical Center - Pineville	Charlotte	82%	300+
Carolinas Medical Center - Union	Monroe	82%	300+
Caromont Regional Medical Center	Gastonia	82%	300+
Columbus Regional Healthcare System	Whiteville	82%	300+
J Arthur Dosher Memorial Hospital	Southport	82%	300+
Onslow Memorial Hospital	Jacksonville	82%	300+
Park Ridge Health[11]	Hendersonville	82%	300+
Rutherford Hospital	Rutherfordton	82%	300+
Southeastern Regional Medical Center	Lumberton	82%	300+
Transylvania Regional Hospital	Brevard	82%	300+
University of North Carolina Hospital	Chapel Hill	82%	300+
Wakemed - Raleigh Campus	Raleigh	82%	300+
Duke Health Raleigh Hospital	Raleigh	81%	300+
Duke Regional Hospital	Durham	81%	300+
Johnston Memorial Hospital	Smithfield	81%	300+
Martin General Hospital	Williamston	81%	300+
Medwest Haywood	Clyde	81%	300+
Sampson Regional Medical Center	Clinton	81%	300+
Vidant Beaufort Hospital	Washington	81%	300+
Catawba Valley Medical Center	Hickory	80%	300+
CMC - Blue Ridge	Morganton	80%	300+
Frye Regional Medical Center	Hickory	80%	300+
Halifax Regional Medical Center	Roanoke Rapids	80%	300+
High Point Regional Hospital	High Point	80%	300+
Medwest Harris	Sylva	80%	300+
Murphy Medical Center	Murphy	80%	300+
Vidant Medical Center	Greenville	80%	300+
Alamance Regional Medical Center	Burlington	79%	300+
Albemarle Hospital Authority	Elizabeth City	79%	300+
Betsy Johnson Regional Hospital	Dunn	79%	300+
Duke University Hospital	Durham	79%	300+
Iredell Memorial Hospital	Statesville	79%	300+
Maria Parham Medical Center	Henderson	79%	300+
Morehead Memorial Hospital	Eden	79%	300+
The Moses H Cone Memorial Hospital	Greensboro	79%	300+
Nash General Hospital	Rocky Mount	79%	300+
North Carolina Baptist Hospital	Winston-Salem	79%	300+
Northern Hospital of Surry County	Mount Airy	79%	300+
Vidant Duplin Hospital	Kenansville	79%	300+
Wakemed - Cary Hospital	Cary	79%	300+
Central Carolina Hospital	Sanford	78%	300+
Granville Health Systems	Oxford	78%	300+
Novant Health Brunswick Medical Center	Supply	78%	300+
Rex Hospital	Raleigh	78%	300+
Stanly Regional Medical Center	Albemarle	78%	300+
Wilkes Regional Medical Center	N Wilkesboro	78%	300+
Carolinas Med Ctr/Behavioral Health	Charlotte	77%	300+
Davis Regional Medical Center	Statesville	77%	300+
Lenoir Memorial Hospital	Kinston	77%	300+
Margaret R Pardee Memorial Hospital	Hendersonville	77%	300+
Novant Health Huntersville Medical Center	Huntersville	77%	300+
Wayne Memorial Hospital	Goldsboro	77%	300+
Cape Fear Valley Medical Center	Fayetteville	76%	300+
Novant Health Thomasville Medical Center	Thomasville	76%	300+
Caldwell Memorial Hospital	Lenoir	75%	300+
Person Memorial Hospital	Roxboro	75%	300+
Lake Norman Regional Medical Center	Mooresville	74%	300+
Lexington Memorial Hospital	Lexington	74%	300+
Novant Health Rowan Medical Center	Salisbury	74%	300+
Presbyterian Hospital Matthews	Matthews	74%	300+
Watauga Medical Center	Boone	74%	300+
Novant Health Forsyth Medical Center	Winston-Salem	73%	300+
Novant Health Charlotte Ortho Hosp	Charlotte	72%	300+
Novant Health Franklin Medical Center	Louisburg	72%	(a)
Novant Health Presbyterian Medical Center	Charlotte	72%	300+

Pain 'Always' Well Controlled

Hospital Name	City	Rate	Cases
Vidant Bertie Hospital	Windsor	82%	(a)
North Carolina Specialty Hospital	Durham	80%	300+
Ashe Memorial Hospital	Jefferson	78%	300+
Carolinas Medical Center - University	Charlotte	78%	300+
Carteret General Hospital	Morehead City	78%	300+
Cleveland Regional Medical Center	Shelby	78%	300+
Firsthealth Moore Regional Hospital	Pinehurst	78%	300+
The Mcdowell Hospital	Marion	78%	300+
New Hanover Regional Medical Center	Wilmington	78%	300+
The Outer Banks Hospital	Nags Head	78%	300+
Sandhills Regional Medical Center	Hamlet	78%	(a)
Columbus Regional Healthcare System	Whiteville	77%	300+
Randolph Hospital	Asheboro	77%	300+
Vidant Chowan Hospital	Edenton	77%	300+
Mem Mission Hosp & Asheville Surg Ctr	Asheville	76%	300+
Scotland Memorial Hospital	Laurinburg	76%	300+
Transylvania Regional Hospital	Brevard	76%	300+
Anson Community Hospital	Wadesboro	75%	(a)
Carolinas Medical Center - Lincoln	Lincolnton	75%	300+
Caromont Regional Medical Center	Gastonia	75%	300+
Medwest Harris	Sylva	75%	300+
Vidant Edgecombe Hospital	Tarboro	75%	300+
Vidant Roanoke Chowan Hospital	Ahoskie	75%	300+
Wakemed - Raleigh Campus	Raleigh	75%	300+
Wilson Medical Center	Wilson	75%	300+
Angel Medical Center	Franklin	74%	300+
Carolina East Medical Center	New Bern	74%	300+
Catawba Valley Medical Center	Hickory	74%	300+
Chatham Hospital	Siler City	74%	(a)
Halifax Regional Medical Center	Roanoke Rapids	74%	300+
Medwest Haywood	Clyde	74%	300+
University of North Carolina Hospital	Chapel Hill	74%	300+
Carolinas Medical Center - Northeast	Concord	73%	300+
CMC - Blue Ridge	Morganton	73%	300+
Martin General Hospital	Williamston	73%	300+
Novant Health Park Hospital	Winston-Salem	73%	300+
Spruce Pine Community Hospital	Spruce Pine	73%	300+
Wakemed - Cary Hospital	Cary	73%	300+
Alamance Regional Medical Center	Burlington	72%	300+
Carolinas Medical Center - Union	Monroe	72%	300+
Duke Health Raleigh Hospital	Raleigh	72%	300+
Duke Regional Hospital	Durham	72%	300+
High Point Regional Hospital	High Point	72%	300+
Johnston Memorial Hospital	Smithfield	72%	300+
Park Ridge Health[11]	Hendersonville	72%	300+
Saint Luke's Hospital	Columbus	72%	(a)
Sampson Regional Medical Center	Clinton	72%	300+
Vidant Beaufort Hospital	Washington	72%	300+
Carolinas Medical Center - Pineville	Charlotte	71%	300+
Carolinas Med Ctr/Behavioral Health	Charlotte	71%	300+
Central Carolina Hospital	Sanford	71%	300+
Duke University Hospital	Durham	71%	300+
Frye Regional Medical Center	Hickory	71%	300+
Hugh Chatham Memorial Hospital	Elkin	71%	300+
J Arthur Dosher Memorial Hospital	Southport	71%	300+
Morehead Memorial Hospital	Eden	71%	300+
Murphy Medical Center	Murphy	71%	300+
Nash General Hospital	Rocky Mount	71%	300+
Pender Memorial Hospital	Burgaw	71%	(a)
Southeastern Regional Medical Center	Lumberton	71%	300+
Vidant Medical Center	Greenville	71%	300+
Albemarle Hospital Authority	Elizabeth City	70%	300+
Cape Fear Valley Medical Center	Fayetteville	70%	300+
Iredell Memorial Hospital	Statesville	70%	300+
Kings Mountain Hospital	Kings Mountain	70%	300+
Northern Hospital of Surry County	Mount Airy	70%	300+
Novant Health Huntersville Medical Center	Huntersville	70%	300+
Vidant Duplin Hospital	Kenansville	70%	300+
Caldwell Memorial Hospital	Lenoir	69%	300+
Lexington Memorial Hospital	Lexington	69%	300+
Margaret R Pardee Memorial Hospital	Hendersonville	69%	300+
The Moses H Cone Memorial Hospital	Greensboro	69%	300+
Novant Health Brunswick Medical Center	Supply	69%	300+
Rutherford Hospital	Rutherfordton	69%	300+
Betsy Johnson Regional Hospital	Dunn	68%	300+
Granville Health Systems	Oxford	68%	300+
Maria Parham Medical Center	Henderson	68%	300+
North Carolina Baptist Hospital	Winston-Salem	68%	300+
Rex Hospital	Raleigh	68%	300+
Stanly Regional Medical Center	Albemarle	68%	300+
Watauga Medical Center	Boone	68%	300+
Davis Regional Medical Center	Statesville	67%	300+
Lake Norman Regional Medical Center	Mooresville	67%	300+
Lenoir Memorial Hospital	Kinston	67%	300+
Person Memorial Hospital	Roxboro	67%	300+
Wilkes Regional Medical Center	N Wilkesboro	67%	300+
Onslow Memorial Hospital	Jacksonville	66%	300+
Wayne Memorial Hospital	Goldsboro	66%	300+
Novant Health Forsyth Medical Center	Winston-Salem	65%	300+
Novant Health Presbyterian Medical Center	Charlotte	65%	300+
Presbyterian Hospital Matthews	Matthews	65%	300+
Novant Health Charlotte Ortho Hosp	Charlotte	64%	300+
Novant Health Thomasville Medical Center	Thomasville	64%	300+
Novant Health Franklin Medical Center	Louisburg	63%	(a)
Novant Health Rowan Medical Center	Salisbury	63%	300+

Room and Bathroom 'Always' Clean

Hospital Name	City	Rate	Cases
North Carolina Specialty Hospital	Durham	86%	300+
Hugh Chatham Memorial Hospital	Elkin	83%	300+
Vidant Chowan Hospital	Edenton	83%	300+
Anson Community Hospital	Wadesboro	82%	(a)
Ashe Memorial Hospital	Jefferson	82%	300+
Park Ridge Health[11]	Hendersonville	82%	300+
Chatham Hospital	Siler City	81%	(a)
Transylvania Regional Hospital	Brevard	81%	300+
Novant Health Brunswick Medical Center	Supply	80%	300+
Novant Health Park Hospital	Winston-Salem	79%	300+
The Outer Banks Hospital	Nags Head	78%	300+
Scotland Memorial Hospital	Laurinburg	78%	300+
Carolinas Medical Center - Lincoln	Lincolnton	77%	300+
Sandhills Regional Medical Center	Hamlet	77%	(a)
Vidant Edgecombe Hospital	Tarboro	77%	300+
Vidant Bertie Hospital	Windsor	76%	(a)
Firsthealth Moore Regional Hospital	Pinehurst	75%	300+

NOTE: Hospital profiles are in alphabetical order by state, then city, then hospital within the city; Rankings exclude hospitals with less than 25 cases except for patient surveys which excludes hospitals with less than 100 cases; (a) 100-299 cases; (1) The number of cases/patients is too few to report; (2) Data submitted were based on a sample of cases/patients; (3) Results are based on a shorter time period than required; (4) Data suppressed by CMS for one or more quarters; (5) Results are not available for this reporting period; (6) Fewer than 100 patients completed the HCAHPS survey; (7) No cases met the criteria for this measure; (8) The lower limit of the confidence interval cannot be calculated if the number of observed infections equals zero; (9) No data are available from the state/territory for this reporting period; (10) The scores shown reflect fewer than 50 completed surveys; (11) There were discrepancies in the data collection process; (12) This measure does not apply to this hospital for this reporting period; (13) Results cannot be calculated for this reporting period; (14) The results for this state are combined with nearby states to protect confidentiality; Please refer to the User's Guide for a full explanation of data.

J Arthur Dosher Memorial Hospital	Southport	75%	300+
Margaret R Pardee Memorial Hospital	Hendersonville	75%	300+
The Mcdowell Hospital	Marion	75%	300+
Morehead Memorial Hospital	Eden	75%	300+
The Moses H Cone Memorial Hospital	Greensboro	75%	300+
New Hanover Regional Medical Center	Wilmington	75%	300+
Northern Hospital of Surry County	Mount Airy	75%	300+
Rutherford Hospital	Rutherfordton	75%	300+
Central Carolina Hospital	Sanford	74%	300+
CMC - Blue Ridge	Morganton	74%	300+
Medwest Harris	Sylva	74%	300+
Saint Luke's Hospital	Columbus	74%	(a)
Alamance Regional Medical Center	Burlington	73%	300+
Carolina East Medical Center	New Bern	73%	300+
Carteret General Hospital	Morehead City	73%	300+
Columbus Regional Healthcare System	Whiteville	73%	300+
Novant Health Thomasville Medical Center	Thomasville	73%	300+
Randolph Hospital	Asheboro	73%	300+
Spruce Pine Community Hospital	Spruce Pine	73%	300+
Stanly Regional Medical Center	Albemarle	73%	300+
Watauga Medical Center	Boone	73%	300+
Caldwell Memorial Hospital	Lenoir	72%	300+
Carolinas Medical Center - Northeast	Concord	72%	300+
Carolinas Medical Center - Pineville	Charlotte	72%	300+
Caromont Regional Medical Center	Gastonia	72%	300+
Catawba Valley Medical Center	Hickory	72%	300+
Cleveland Regional Medical Center	Shelby	72%	300+
Kings Mountain Hospital	Kings Mountain	72%	300+
North Carolina Baptist Hospital	Winston-Salem	72%	300+
University of North Carolina Hospital	Chapel Hill	72%	300+
Vidant Beaufort Hospital	Washington	72%	300+
Vidant Medical Center	Greenville	72%	300+
Wayne Memorial Hospital	Goldsboro	72%	300+
Albemarle Hospital Authority	Elizabeth City	71%	300+
Carolinas Medical Center - Union	Monroe	71%	300+
Halifax Regional Medical Center	Roanoke Rapids	71%	300+
Lexington Memorial Hospital	Lexington	71%	300+
Vidant Duplin Hospital	Kenansville	71%	300+
Vidant Roanoke Chowan Hospital	Ahoskie	71%	300+
Angel Medical Center	Franklin	70%	300+
Davis Regional Medical Center	Statesville	70%	300+
High Point Regional Hospital	High Point	70%	300+
Lake Norman Regional Medical Center	Mooresville	70%	300+
Nash General Hospital	Rocky Mount	70%	300+
Pender Memorial Hospital	Burgaw	70%	(a)
Wilkes Regional Medical Center	N Wilkesboro	70%	300+
Duke Regional Hospital	Durham	69%	300+
Novant Health Huntersville Medical Center	Huntersville	69%	300+
Rex Hospital	Raleigh	69%	300+
Iredell Memorial Hospital	Statesville	68%	300+
Johnston Memorial Hospital	Smithfield	68%	300+
Lenoir Memorial Hospital	Kinston	68%	300+
Medwest Haywood	Clyde	68%	300+
Murphy Medical Center	Murphy	68%	300+
Presbyterian Hospital Matthews	Matthews	68%	300+
Southeastern Regional Medical Center	Lumberton	68%	300+
Wilson Medical Center	Wilson	68%	300+
Betsy Johnson Regional Hospital	Dunn	67%	300+
Novant Health Charlotte Ortho Hosp	Charlotte	67%	300+
Novant Health Rowan Medical Center	Salisbury	67%	300+
Onslow Memorial Hospital	Jacksonville	67%	300+
Frye Regional Medical Center	Hickory	66%	300+
Novant Health Presbyterian Medical Center	Charlotte	66%	300+
Wakemed - Cary Hospital	Cary	66%	300+
Cape Fear Valley Medical Center	Fayetteville	65%	300+
Carolinas Medical Center - University	Charlotte	65%	300+
Duke Health Raleigh Hospital	Raleigh	65%	300+
Maria Parham Medical Center	Henderson	65%	300+
Mem Mission Hosp & Asheville Surg Ctr	Asheville	65%	300+
Novant Health Franklin Medical Center	Louisburg	65%	(a)
Sampson Regional Medical Center	Clinton	65%	300+
Martin General Hospital	Williamston	64%	300+
Novant Health Forsyth Medical Center	Winston-Salem	63%	300+
Carolinas Med Ctr/Behavioral Health	Charlotte	62%	300+
Person Memorial Hospital	Roxboro	61%	300+
Duke University Hospital	Durham	60%	300+
Granville Health Systems	Oxford	57%	300+
Wakemed - Raleigh Campus	Raleigh	57%	300+

Timely Help 'Always' Received

Hospital Name	City	Rate	Cases
North Carolina Specialty Hospital	Durham	84%	300+
Vidant Bertie Hospital	Windsor	84%	(a)
The Outer Banks Hospital	Nags Head	81%	300+
Chatham Hospital	Siler City	80%	(a)
Ashe Memorial Hospital	Jefferson	78%	300+
Vidant Chowan Hospital	Edenton	78%	300+
Pender Memorial Hospital	Burgaw	77%	(a)
Transylvania Regional Hospital	Brevard	77%	300+
Firsthealth Moore Regional Hospital	Pinehurst	76%	300+
Novant Health Park Hospital	Winston-Salem	76%	300+
Angel Medical Center	Franklin	75%	300+
Carteret General Hospital	Morehead City	75%	300+
The Mcdowell Hospital	Marion	75%	300+
Saint Luke's Hospital	Columbus	75%	(a)
Carolina East Medical Center	New Bern	74%	300+
Carolinas Medical Center - Lincoln	Lincolnton	74%	300+
Cleveland Regional Medical Center	Shelby	73%	300+
Frye Regional Medical Center	Hickory	73%	300+
J Arthur Dosher Memorial Hospital	Southport	73%	300+
Kings Mountain Hospital	Kings Mountain	73%	300+
Southeastern Regional Medical Center	Lumberton	73%	300+
Vidant Edgecombe Hospital	Tarboro	73%	300+
Vidant Roanoke Chowan Hospital	Ahoskie	73%	300+
Carolinas Medical Center - University	Charlotte	72%	300+
Caromont Regional Medical Center	Gastonia	72%	300+
Hugh Chatham Memorial Hospital	Elkin	72%	300+
Medwest Harris	Sylva	72%	300+
Murphy Medical Center	Murphy	72%	300+
New Hanover Regional Medical Center	Wilmington	72%	300+
Spruce Pine Community Hospital	Spruce Pine	72%	300+
Vidant Beaufort Hospital	Washington	72%	300+
Columbus Regional Healthcare System	Whiteville	71%	300+
Medwest Haywood	Clyde	71%	300+
Mem Mission Hosp & Asheville Surg Ctr	Asheville	71%	300+
Randolph Hospital	Asheboro	71%	300+
Sandhills Regional Medical Center	Hamlet	71%	(a)
CMC - Blue Ridge	Morganton	70%	300+
Onslow Memorial Hospital	Jacksonville	70%	300+
Scotland Memorial Hospital	Laurinburg	70%	300+
Carolinas Medical Center - Northeast	Concord	69%	300+
Halifax Regional Medical Center	Roanoke Rapids	69%	300+
Park Ridge Health[11]	Hendersonville	69%	300+
Rutherford Hospital	Rutherfordton	69%	300+
Stanly Regional Medical Center	Albemarle	69%	300+
Wilson Medical Center	Wilson	69%	300+
Anson Community Hospital	Wadesboro	68%	(a)
Carolinas Medical Center - Union	Monroe	68%	300+
Martin General Hospital	Williamston	68%	300+
Albemarle Hospital Authority	Elizabeth City	67%	300+
Johnston Memorial Hospital	Smithfield	67%	300+
Nash General Hospital	Rocky Mount	67%	300+
Northern Hospital of Surry County	Mount Airy	67%	300+
University of North Carolina Hospital	Chapel Hill	67%	300+
Vidant Duplin Hospital	Kenansville	67%	300+
Wakemed - Raleigh Campus	Raleigh	67%	300+
Betsy Johnson Regional Hospital	Dunn	66%	300+
Duke Health Raleigh Hospital	Raleigh	66%	300+
Morehead Memorial Hospital	Eden	66%	300+
Rex Hospital	Raleigh	66%	300+
Alamance Regional Medical Center	Burlington	65%	300+
Carolinas Medical Center - Pineville	Charlotte	65%	300+
Granville Health Systems	Oxford	65%	300+
High Point Regional Hospital	High Point	65%	300+
Margaret R Pardee Memorial Hospital	Hendersonville	65%	300+
North Carolina Baptist Hospital	Winston-Salem	65%	300+
Sampson Regional Medical Center	Clinton	65%	300+
Vidant Medical Center	Greenville	65%	300+
Caldwell Memorial Hospital	Lenoir	64%	300+
Catawba Valley Medical Center	Hickory	64%	300+
Duke Regional Hospital	Durham	64%	300+
The Moses H Cone Memorial Hospital	Greensboro	64%	300+
Novant Health Huntersville Medical Center	Huntersville	64%	300+
Wakemed - Cary Hospital	Cary	64%	300+
Wayne Memorial Hospital	Goldsboro	64%	300+
Central Carolina Hospital	Sanford	63%	300+
Duke University Hospital	Durham	63%	300+
Maria Parham Medical Center	Henderson	63%	300+
Novant Health Brunswick Medical Center	Supply	63%	300+
Novant Health Thomasville Medical Center	Thomasville	63%	300+
Wilkes Regional Medical Center	N Wilkesboro	63%	300+
Cape Fear Valley Medical Center	Fayetteville	61%	300+
Carolinas Med Ctr/Behavioral Health	Charlotte	61%	300+
Iredell Memorial Hospital	Statesville	60%	300+
Lenoir Memorial Hospital	Kinston	60%	300+
Lexington Memorial Hospital	Lexington	60%	300+
Watauga Medical Center	Boone	60%	300+
Lake Norman Regional Medical Center	Mooresville	59%	300+
Novant Health Forsyth Medical Center	Winston-Salem	59%	300+
Novant Health Rowan Medical Center	Salisbury	59%	300+
Person Memorial Hospital	Roxboro	59%	300+
Davis Regional Medical Center	Statesville	58%	300+
Novant Health Presbyterian Medical Center	Charlotte	56%	300+
Novant Health Charlotte Ortho Hosp	Charlotte	55%	300+
Presbyterian Hospital Matthews	Matthews	55%	300+
Novant Health Franklin Medical Center	Louisburg	52%	(a)

Would Definitely Recommend Hospital

Hospital Name	City	Rate	Cases
North Carolina Specialty Hospital	Durham	91%	300+
Novant Health Park Hospital	Winston-Salem	89%	300+
Park Ridge Health[11]	Hendersonville	85%	300+
Duke University Hospital	Durham	84%	300+
Firsthealth Moore Regional Hospital	Pinehurst	84%	300+
Mem Mission Hosp & Asheville Surg Ctr	Asheville	83%	300+
University of North Carolina Hospital	Chapel Hill	83%	300+
Vidant Bertie Hospital	Windsor	82%	(a)
Carolinas Medical Center - Northeast	Concord	81%	300+
Carolinas Medical Center - Pineville	Charlotte	81%	300+
New Hanover Regional Medical Center	Wilmington	81%	300+
Novant Health Huntersville Medical Center	Huntersville	81%	300+
Carolinas Medical Center - University	Charlotte	80%	300+
Duke Health Raleigh Hospital	Raleigh	80%	300+
North Carolina Baptist Hospital	Winston-Salem	80%	300+
Rex Hospital	Raleigh	80%	300+
Vidant Medical Center	Greenville	80%	300+
Hugh Chatham Memorial Hospital	Elkin	79%	300+
The Outer Banks Hospital	Nags Head	79%	300+
Carolinas Medical Center - Lincoln	Lincolnton	78%	300+
Chatham Hospital	Siler City	78%	(a)
Wakemed - Raleigh Campus	Raleigh	78%	300+
The Moses H Cone Memorial Hospital	Greensboro	77%	300+
Wakemed - Cary Hospital	Cary	77%	300+
Carolina East Medical Center	New Bern	76%	300+
Catawba Valley Medical Center	Hickory	76%	300+
Saint Luke's Hospital	Columbus	76%	(a)
Duke Regional Hospital	Durham	75%	300+
Kings Mountain Hospital	Kings Mountain	75%	300+
Vidant Chowan Hospital	Edenton	75%	300+
Angel Medical Center	Franklin	74%	300+
Carolinas Medical Center - Union	Monroe	74%	300+
Frye Regional Medical Center	Hickory	74%	300+
High Point Regional Hospital	High Point	74%	300+
Iredell Memorial Hospital	Statesville	74%	300+
Novant Health Brunswick Medical Center	Supply	74%	300+
Novant Health Forsyth Medical Center	Winston-Salem	74%	300+
Presbyterian Hospital Matthews	Matthews	74%	300+
Transylvania Regional Hospital	Brevard	74%	300+
Vidant Edgecombe Hospital	Tarboro	74%	300+
Vidant Beaufort Hospital	Washington	73%	300+
Ashe Memorial Hospital	Jefferson	72%	300+
Carolinas Med Ctr/Behavioral Health	Charlotte	72%	300+
Cleveland Regional Medical Center	Shelby	72%	300+
Margaret R Pardee Memorial Hospital	Hendersonville	72%	300+
Spruce Pine Community Hospital	Spruce Pine	72%	300+
J Arthur Dosher Memorial Hospital	Southport	71%	300+
The Mcdowell Hospital	Marion	71%	300+
Novant Health Presbyterian Medical Center	Charlotte	71%	300+
CMC - Blue Ridge	Morganton	70%	300+
Carteret General Hospital	Morehead City	69%	300+
Medwest Haywood	Clyde	69%	300+
Morehead Memorial Hospital	Eden	69%	300+
Novant Health Charlotte Ortho Hosp	Charlotte	69%	300+
Sandhills Regional Medical Center	Hamlet	69%	(a)
Scotland Memorial Hospital	Laurinburg	69%	300+
Caromont Regional Medical Center	Gastonia	68%	300+
Johnston Memorial Hospital	Smithfield	68%	300+
Vidant Roanoke Chowan Hospital	Ahoskie	68%	300+
Davis Regional Medical Center	Statesville	67%	300+
Wilkes Regional Medical Center	N Wilkesboro	67%	300+
Albemarle Hospital Authority	Elizabeth City	66%	300+
Columbus Regional Healthcare System	Whiteville	66%	300+
Northern Hospital of Surry County	Mount Airy	66%	300+
Novant Health Thomasville Medical Center	Thomasville	66%	300+
Randolph Hospital	Asheboro	66%	300+
Alamance Regional Medical Center	Burlington	65%	300+
Pender Memorial Hospital	Burgaw	65%	(a)
Stanly Regional Medical Center	Albemarle	65%	300+
Anson Community Hospital	Wadesboro	64%	(a)
Betsy Johnson Regional Hospital	Dunn	64%	300+
Vidant Duplin Hospital	Kenansville	64%	300+
Watauga Medical Center	Boone	64%	300+
Medwest Harris	Sylva	63%	300+
Rutherford Hospital	Rutherfordton	63%	300+
Martin General Hospital	Williamston	62%	300+
Murphy Medical Center	Murphy	62%	300+
Southeastern Regional Medical Center	Lumberton	62%	300+
Caldwell Memorial Hospital	Lenoir	61%	300+
Lake Norman Regional Medical Center	Mooresville	61%	300+
Nash General Hospital	Rocky Mount	61%	300+
Central Carolina Hospital	Sanford	60%	300+
Granville Health Systems	Oxford	60%	300+
Maria Parham Medical Center	Henderson	60%	300+
Wilson Medical Center	Wilson	60%	300+
Cape Fear Valley Medical Center	Fayetteville	59%	300+
Lexington Memorial Hospital	Lexington	59%	300+
Person Memorial Hospital	Roxboro	59%	300+
Halifax Regional Medical Center	Roanoke Rapids	58%	300+
Lenoir Memorial Hospital	Kinston	57%	300+
Novant Health Franklin Medical Center	Louisburg	57%	(a)
Sampson Regional Medical Center	Clinton	57%	300+
Wayne Memorial Hospital	Goldsboro	57%	300+
Onslow Memorial Hospital	Jacksonville	56%	300+

NOTE: Hospital profiles are in alphabetical order by state, then city, then hospital within the city; Rankings exclude hospitals with less than 25 cases except for patient surveys which excludes hospitals with less than 100 cases; (a) 100-299 cases; (1) The number of cases/patients is too few to report; (2) Data submitted were based on a sample of cases/patients; (3) Results are based on a shorter time period than required; (4) Data suppressed by CMS for one or more quarters; (5) Results are not available for this reporting period; (6) Fewer than 100 patients completed the HCAHPS survey; (7) No cases met the criteria for this measure; (8) The lower limit of the confidence interval cannot be calculated if the number of observed infections equals zero; (9) No data are available from the state/territory for this reporting period; (10) The scores shown reflect fewer than 50 completed surveys; (11) There were discrepancies in the data collection process; (12) This measure does not apply to this hospital for this reporting period; (13) Results cannot be calculated for this reporting period; (14) The results for this state are combined with nearby states to protect confidentiality; Please refer to the User's Guide for a full explanation of data.

Novant Health Rowan Medical Center	Salisbury	55%	300+

Use of Medical Imaging

Cardiac Imaging Stress Test before OP Surgery

Hospital Name	City	Rate	Cases
Scotland Memorial Hospital	Laurinburg	0.0%	50
Central Carolina Hospital	Sanford	1.7%	119
Randolph Hospital	Asheboro	2.3%	130
Watauga Medical Center	Boone	2.6%	578
Spruce Pine Community Hospital	Spruce Pine	2.7%	113
Northern Hospital of Surry County	Mount Airy	2.9%	105
Vidant Edgecombe Hospital	Tarboro	2.9%	68
Hugh Chatham Memorial Hospital	Elkin	3.2%	94
Southeastern Regional Medical Center	Lumberton	3.3%	667
Iredell Memorial Hospital	Statesville	3.7%	321
Novant Health Franklin Medical Center	Louisburg	3.7%	54
Novant Health Presbyterian Medical Center	Charlotte	3.7%	1070
Angel Medical Center	Franklin	3.8%	210
Catawba Valley Medical Center	Hickory	3.8%	341
Mem Mission Hosp & Asheville Surg Ctr	Asheville	3.9%	2937
Vidant Chowan Hospital	Edenton	3.9%	127
Vidant Duplin Hospital	Kenansville	3.9%	102
Davis Regional Medical Center	Statesville	4.0%	50
Duke Regional Hospital	Durham	4.1%	339
Firsthealth Moore Regional Hospital	Pinehurst	4.1%	904
Medwest Haywood	Clyde	4.1%	464
Park Ridge Health	Hendersonville	4.1%	266
Onslow Memorial Hospital	Jacksonville	4.2%	142
Frye Regional Medical Center	Hickory	4.3%	1228
Maria Parham Medical Center	Henderson	4.3%	209
Morehead Memorial Hospital	Eden	4.3%	235
Sampson Regional Medical Center	Clinton	4.5%	352
Carolinas Medical Center - University	Charlotte	4.6%	457
The Moses H Cone Memorial Hospital	Greensboro	4.6%	963
Halifax Regional Medical Center	Roanoke Rapids	4.7%	275
Carolinas Medical Center - Lincoln	Lincolnton	4.8%	435
University of North Carolina Hospital	Chapel Hill	4.8%	498
Carolinas Medical Center - Northeast	Concord	4.9%	1566
Carteret General Hospital	Morehead City	4.9%	370
Nash General Hospital	Rocky Mount	4.9%	368
Stanly Regional Medical Center	Albemarle	4.9%	411
Cape Fear Valley Medical Center	Fayetteville	5.0%	501
Carolinas Medical Center - Union	Monroe	5.0%	740
Murphy Medical Center	Murphy	5.0%	120
North Carolina Baptist Hospital	Winston-Salem	5.0%	798
High Point Regional Hospital	High Point	5.2%	660
Kings Mountain Hospital	Kings Mountain	5.2%	115
Lake Norman Regional Medical Center	Mooresville	5.2%	153
Johnston Memorial Hospital	Smithfield	5.3%	225
Cleveland Regional Medical Center	Shelby	5.5%	687
Novant Health Huntersville Medical Center	Huntersville	5.6%	196
Albemarle Hospital Authority	Elizabeth City	5.7%	228
Carolinas Medical Center - Pineville	Charlotte	5.7%	1140
New Hanover Regional Medical Center	Wilmington	5.7%	3321
Novant Health Rowan Medical Center	Salisbury	5.7%	333
Medwest Harris	Sylva	5.8%	400
Novant Health Forsyth Medical Center	Winston-Salem	5.9%	945
Sandhills Regional Medical Center	Hamlet	5.9%	85
Margaret R Pardee Memorial Hospital	Hendersonville	6.1%	163
The Mcdowell Hospital	Marion	6.1%	196
Betsy Johnson Regional Hospital	Dunn	6.3%	80
Presbyterian Hospital Matthews	Matthews	6.3%	223
Transylvania Regional Hospital	Brevard	6.3%	478
Caromont Regional Medical Center	Gastonia	6.4%	482
Novant Health Brunswick Medical Center	Supply	6.4%	439
Vidant Roanoke Chowan Hospital	Ahoskie	6.4%	125
Carolinas Med Ctr/Behaviorial Health	Charlotte	6.5%	1254
Columbus Regional Healthcare System	Whiteville	6.6%	137
Duke Health Raleigh Hospital	Raleigh	6.6%	76
Wilkes Regional Medical Center	N Wilkesboro	6.6%	167
Duke University Hospital	Durham	6.7%	1516
Lexington Memorial Hospital	Lexington	6.7%	149
Rutherford Hospital	Rutherfordton	6.8%	281
Wakemed - Raleigh Campus	Raleigh	7.0%	2135
Carolina East Medical Center	New Bern	7.1%	564
Vidant Medical Center	Greenville	7.1%	536
Caldwell Memorial Hospital	Lenoir	7.3%	124
Granville Health Systems	Oxford	7.4%	136
Wakemed - Cary Hospital	Cary	7.4%	163
J Arthur Dosher Memorial Hospital	Southport	7.6%	264
CMC - Blue Ridge	Morganton	7.8%	374
Ashe Memorial Hospital	Jefferson	8.2%	73
Wayne Memorial Hospital	Goldsboro	8.3%	915
Lenoir Memorial Hospital	Kinston	8.9%	112
Wilson Medical Center	Wilson	8.9%	326
Rex Hospital	Raleigh	9.1%	253
Alamance Regional Medical Center	Burlington	9.2%	174

Combination Abdominal CT Scan

Hospital Name	City	Rate	Cases
Martin General Hospital	Williamston	0.0%	181
Central Carolina Hospital	Sanford	0.3%	676
Maria Parham Medical Center	Henderson	0.4%	697
Caldwell Memorial Hospital	Lenoir	0.8%	509
Duke Regional Hospital	Durham	0.9%	890
Catawba Valley Medical Center	Hickory	1.1%	972
Wakemed - Cary Hospital	Cary	1.1%	880
High Point Regional Hospital	High Point	1.2%	736
The Mcdowell Hospital	Marion	1.2%	427
Wayne Memorial Hospital	Goldsboro	1.2%	642
Morehead Memorial Hospital	Eden	1.3%	544
Vidant Medical Center	Greenville	1.7%	1574
Washington County Hospital	Plymouth	1.7%	115
Anson Community Hospital	Wadesboro	1.8%	167
Watauga Medical Center	Boone	1.8%	783
Carolinas Medical Center - Northeast	Concord	1.9%	2309
The Moses H Cone Memorial Hospital	Greensboro	1.9%	2131
Frye Regional Medical Center	Hickory	2.0%	927
Novant Health Thomasville Medical Center	Thomasville	2.2%	451
Betsy Johnson Regional Hospital	Dunn	2.3%	894
Lenoir Memorial Hospital	Kinston	2.3%	646
Cape Fear Valley Medical Center	Fayetteville	2.4%	1390
Carolinas Medical Center - Lincoln	Lincolnton	2.4%	793
Lexington Memorial Hospital	Lexington	2.8%	493
Vidant Duplin Hospital	Kenansville	2.8%	358
Hugh Chatham Memorial Hospital	Elkin	2.9%	694
Iredell Memorial Hospital	Statesville	2.9%	816
Novant Health Huntersville Medical Center	Huntersville	3.0%	922
Mem Mission Hosp & Asheville Surg Ctr	Asheville	3.1%	1467
Spruce Pine Community Hospital	Spruce Pine	3.1%	354
Transylvania Regional Hospital	Brevard	3.1%	680
Novant Health Franklin Medical Center	Louisburg	3.3%	272
Rex Hospital	Raleigh	3.3%	1414
CMC - Blue Ridge	Morganton	3.4%	903
Davis Regional Medical Center	Statesville	3.4%	378
Northern Hospital of Surry County	Mount Airy	3.4%	999
Southeastern Regional Medical Center	Lumberton	3.5%	1526
Vidant Edgecombe Hospital	Tarboro	3.5%	424
Carteret General Hospital	Morehead City	3.6%	1120
University of North Carolina Hospital	Chapel Hill	3.6%	2274
Carolinas Medical Center - University	Charlotte	3.7%	1011
Vidant Bertie Hospital	Windsor	3.7%	189
Alleghany County Memorial Hospital	Sparta	3.9%	155
Rutherford Hospital	Rutherfordton	3.9%	750
Presbyterian Hospital Matthews	Matthews	4.0%	1322
Carolinas Medical Center - Union	Monroe	4.1%	1475
Lake Norman Regional Medical Center	Mooresville	4.1%	612
Duke Health Raleigh Hospital	Raleigh	4.3%	1183
Novant Health Charlotte Ortho Hosp	Charlotte	4.3%	47
Vidant Beaufort Hospital	Washington	4.4%	591
Novant Health Presbyterian Medical Center	Charlotte	4.5%	1581
Onslow Memorial Hospital	Jacksonville	4.6%	606
Alamance Regional Medical Center	Burlington	4.7%	918
Duke University Hospital	Durham	4.9%	4568
Johnston Memorial Hospital	Smithfield	4.9%	1375
Carolinas Medical Center - Pineville	Charlotte	5.1%	2503
Novant Health Forsyth Medical Center	Winston-Salem	5.1%	2968
Wilson Medical Center	Wilson	5.1%	1122
Wakemed - Raleigh Campus	Raleigh	5.4%	1528
Caromont Regional Medical Center	Gastonia	5.6%	1757
Nash General Hospital	Rocky Mount	5.6%	987
Novant Health Brunswick Medical Center	Supply	5.7%	736
Wilkes Regional Medical Center	N Wilkesboro	5.7%	889
Angel Medical Center	Franklin	5.9%	509
J Arthur Dosher Memorial Hospital	Southport	5.9%	441
Granville Health Systems	Oxford	6.0%	335
Randolph Hospital	Asheboro	6.1%	377
Vidant Chowan Hospital	Edenton	6.1%	396
New Hanover Regional Medical Center	Wilmington	6.2%	2807
Vidant Roanoke Chowan Hospital	Ahoskie	6.4%	566
North Carolina Baptist Hospital	Winston-Salem	6.7%	2480
Carolina East Medical Center	New Bern	6.8%	968
Park Ridge Health	Hendersonville	7.3%	523
Firsthealth Moore Regional Hospital	Pinehurst	7.4%	1577
Firsthealth Montgomery Memorial Hospital	Troy	7.5%	173
Scotland Memorial Hospital	Laurinburg	8.0%	1231
Sampson Regional Medical Center	Clinton	8.1%	779
Margaret R Pardee Memorial Hospital	Hendersonville	8.5%	1220
Halifax Regional Medical Center	Roanoke Rapids	8.9%	852
Novant Health Rowan Medical Center	Salisbury	8.9%	653
Cape Fear Valley - Bladen County Hospital	Elizabethtown	9.6%	228
Columbus Regional Healthcare System	Whiteville	9.7%	720
Saint Luke's Hospital	Columbus	10.2%	255
Medwest Haywood	Clyde	10.4%	838
Person Memorial Hospital	Roxboro	10.5%	294
Albemarle Hospital Authority	Elizabeth City	10.7%	929
Carolinas Med Ctr/Behaviorial Health	Charlotte	11.4%	2029
Murphy Medical Center	Murphy	12.8%	649
Stanly Regional Medical Center	Albemarle	13.7%	1134
Kings Mountain Hospital	Kings Mountain	21.5%	200
Sandhills Regional Medical Center	Hamlet	21.8%	170
Cleveland Regional Medical Center	Shelby	25.8%	1095
Medwest Harris	Sylva	38.5%	574
Ashe Memorial Hospital	Jefferson	45.9%	331

Combination Brain/Sinus CT Scan

Hospital Name	City	Rate	Cases
Kings Mountain Hospital	Kings Mountain	0.4%	243
Frye Regional Medical Center	Hickory	0.5%	960
Angel Medical Center	Franklin	0.9%	442
Wayne Memorial Hospital	Goldsboro	0.9%	1033
Cleveland Regional Medical Center	Shelby	1.0%	1052
Duke Health Raleigh Hospital	Raleigh	1.0%	885
Columbus Regional Healthcare System	Whiteville	1.1%	696
Scotland Memorial Hospital	Laurinburg	1.2%	954
Transylvania Regional Hospital	Brevard	1.2%	748
Nash General Hospital	Rocky Mount	1.3%	1111
Alamance Regional Medical Center	Burlington	1.4%	972
CMC - Blue Ridge	Morganton	1.4%	777
Murphy Medical Center	Murphy	1.4%	573
Rex Hospital	Raleigh	1.4%	1232
Vidant Beaufort Hospital	Washington	1.4%	556
Carolinas Medical Center - Union	Monroe	1.5%	1286
Carolinas Med Ctr/Behaviorial Health	Charlotte	1.5%	1087
Caromont Regional Medical Center	Gastonia	1.5%	1654
Vidant Edgecombe Hospital	Tarboro	1.5%	752
Martin General Hospital	Williamston	1.6%	440
Wilkes Regional Medical Center	N Wilkesboro	1.6%	749
Carolina East Medical Center	New Bern	1.7%	1404
Albemarle Hospital Authority	Elizabeth City	1.8%	855
Carolinas Medical Center - University	Charlotte	1.8%	927
Catawba Valley Medical Center	Hickory	1.8%	831
Halifax Regional Medical Center	Roanoke Rapids	1.8%	1048
Hugh Chatham Memorial Hospital	Elkin	1.8%	672
Sampson Regional Medical Center	Clinton	1.8%	870
Maria Parham Medical Center	Henderson	2.0%	696
Caldwell Memorial Hospital	Lenoir	2.1%	574
Carolinas Medical Center - Northeast	Concord	2.1%	2004
J Arthur Dosher Memorial Hospital	Southport	2.1%	430
Vidant Medical Center	Greenville	2.1%	1468
Duke Regional Hospital	Durham	2.2%	1103
Medwest Harris	Sylva	2.2%	407
Carteret General Hospital	Morehead City	2.3%	919
Central Carolina Hospital	Sanford	2.3%	600
Novant Health Huntersville Medical Center	Huntersville	2.3%	747
Novant Health Rowan Medical Center	Salisbury	2.3%	1033
Park Ridge Health	Hendersonville	2.3%	571
Carolinas Medical Center - Pineville	Charlotte	2.4%	2049
North Carolina Baptist Hospital	Winston-Salem	2.4%	1080
Rutherford Hospital	Rutherfordton	2.4%	807
Johnston Memorial Hospital	Smithfield	2.5%	1426
Novant Health Brunswick Medical Center	Supply	2.5%	713
Novant Health Forsyth Medical Center	Winston-Salem	2.5%	2502
Firsthealth Moore Regional Hospital	Pinehurst	2.6%	1923
Vidant Duplin Hospital	Kenansville	2.6%	585
Margaret R Pardee Memorial Hospital	Hendersonville	2.8%	833
Duke University Hospital	Durham	2.9%	1554
Betsy Johnson Regional Hospital	Dunn	3.0%	1216
Mem Mission Hosp & Asheville Surg Ctr	Asheville	3.0%	1588
Iredell Memorial Hospital	Statesville	3.1%	833
High Point Regional Hospital	High Point	3.2%	1059
Lenoir Memorial Hospital	Kinston	3.2%	977
Vidant Roanoke Chowan Hospital	Ahoskie	3.2%	625
Wakemed - Raleigh Campus	Raleigh	3.3%	1837
Novant Health Presbyterian Medical Center	Charlotte	3.4%	1370
Onslow Memorial Hospital	Jacksonville	3.4%	849
Cape Fear Valley Medical Center	Fayetteville	3.5%	1817
The Moses H Cone Memorial Hospital	Greensboro	3.5%	2330
University of North Carolina Hospital	Chapel Hill	3.5%	992
Randolph Hospital	Asheboro	3.6%	1004
Presbyterian Hospital Matthews	Matthews	3.8%	1034
Wilson Medical Center	Wilson	3.8%	1454
Watauga Medical Center	Boone	3.9%	537
Vidant Chowan Hospital	Edenton	4.0%	453
Wakemed - Cary Hospital	Cary	4.0%	1221
New Hanover Regional Medical Center	Wilmington	4.4%	1975
Southeastern Regional Medical Center	Lumberton	4.4%	1269
Northern Hospital of Surry County	Mount Airy	4.7%	1065
Stanly Regional Medical Center	Albemarle	4.7%	971
Carolinas Medical Center - Lincoln	Lincolnton	5.1%	830
Davis Regional Medical Center	Statesville	5.4%	317
Sandhills Regional Medical Center	Hamlet	5.7%	298

Combination Chest CT Scan

Hospital Name	City	Rate	Cases
Anson Community Hospital	Wadesboro	0.0%	74
Betsy Johnson Regional Hospital	Dunn	0.0%	320
Caldwell Memorial Hospital	Lenoir	0.0%	378

NOTE: Hospital profiles are in alphabetical order by state, then city, then hospital within the city; Rankings exclude hospitals with less than 25 cases except for patient surveys which excludes hospitals with less than 100 cases; (a) 100-299 cases; (1) The number of cases/patients is too few to report; (2) Data submitted were based on a sample of cases/patients; (3) Results are based on a shorter time period than required; (4) Data suppressed by CMS for one or more quarters; (5) Results are not available for this reporting period; (6) Fewer than 100 patients completed the HCAHPS survey; (7) No cases met the criteria for this measure; (8) The lower limit of the confidence interval cannot be calculated if the number of observed infections equals zero; (9) No data are available from the state/territory for this reporting period; (10) The scores shown reflect fewer than 50 completed surveys; (11) There were discrepancies in the data collection process; (12) This measure does not apply to this hospital for this reporting period; (13) Results cannot be calculated for this reporting period; (14) The results for this state are combined with nearby states to protect confidentiality; Please refer to the User's Guide for a full explanation of data.

Carolina East Medical Center	New Bern	0.0%	297
Carolinas Med Ctr/Behavioral Health	Charlotte	0.0%	1577
Caromont Regional Medical Center	Gastonia	0.0%	710
Central Carolina Hospital	Sanford	0.0%	224
Duke Regional Hospital	Durham	0.0%	369
Duke University Hospital	Durham	0.0%	6920
Firsthealth Montgomery Memorial Hospital	Troy	0.0%	45
High Point Regional Hospital	High Point	0.0%	189
J Arthur Dosher Memorial Hospital	Southport	0.0%	221
Kings Mountain Hospital	Kings Mountain	0.0%	72
Lenoir Memorial Hospital	Kinston	0.0%	322
Martin General Hospital	Williamston	0.0%	55
The Mcdowell Hospital	Marion	0.0%	188
Morehead Memorial Hospital	Eden	0.0%	293
The Moses H Cone Memorial Hospital	Greensboro	0.0%	1288
Novant Health Charlotte Ortho Hosp	Charlotte	0.0%	87
Novant Health Huntersville Medical Center	Huntersville	0.0%	579
Novant Health Presbyterian Medical Center	Charlotte	0.0%	1098
Novant Health Thomasville Medical Center	Thomasville	0.0%	172
Onslow Memorial Hospital	Jacksonville	0.0%	416
Presbyterian Hospital Matthews	Matthews	0.0%	914
Randolph Hospital	Asheboro	0.0%	444
Vidant Duplin Hospital	Kenansville	0.0%	176
Vidant Medical Center	Greenville	0.0%	887
Alamance Regional Medical Center	Burlington	0.1%	709
Carolinas Medical Center - Pineville	Charlotte	0.1%	1335
Carolinas Medical Center - Union	Monroe	0.1%	766
Duke Health Raleigh Hospital	Raleigh	0.1%	1370
Novant Health Forsyth Medical Center	Winston-Salem	0.1%	1752
University of North Carolina Hospital	Chapel Hill	0.1%	2544
Carteret General Hospital	Morehead City	0.2%	515
CMC - Blue Ridge	Morganton	0.2%	456
Mem Mission Hosp & Asheville Surg Ctr	Asheville	0.2%	568
Northern Hospital of Surry County	Mount Airy	0.2%	483
Lake Norman Regional Medical Center	Mooresville	0.3%	388
Transylvania Regional Hospital	Brevard	0.3%	364
Watauga Medical Center	Boone	0.3%	606
Wilson Medical Center	Wilson	0.3%	982
Cape Fear Valley Medical Center	Fayetteville	0.4%	785
Lexington Memorial Hospital	Lexington	0.4%	266
Wakemed - Cary Hospital	Cary	0.4%	568
Wayne Memorial Hospital	Goldsboro	0.4%	245
Carolinas Medical Center - University	Charlotte	0.5%	367
Rutherford Hospital	Rutherfordton	0.5%	366
Sampson Regional Medical Center	Clinton	0.5%	427
Vidant Roanoke Chowan Hospital	Ahoskie	0.5%	189
Columbus Regional Healthcare System	Whiteville	0.6%	318
Davis Regional Medical Center	Statesville	0.6%	156
Firsthealth Moore Regional Hospital	Pinehurst	0.6%	978
North Carolina Baptist Hospital	Winston-Salem	0.6%	2676
Iredell Memorial Hospital	Statesville	0.8%	369
Novant Health Rowan Medical Center	Salisbury	0.8%	237
Vidant Chowan Hospital	Edenton	0.8%	237
Carolinas Medical Center - Lincoln	Lincolnton	0.9%	344
Vidant Edgecombe Hospital	Tarboro	0.9%	222
New Hanover Regional Medical Center	Wilmington	1.0%	1880
Wakemed - Raleigh Campus	Raleigh	1.1%	1007
Catawba Valley Medical Center	Hickory	1.3%	754
Hugh Chatham Memorial Hospital	Elkin	1.3%	305
Ashe Memorial Hospital	Jefferson	1.5%	131
Vidant Beaufort Hospital	Washington	1.6%	364
Maria Parham Medical Center	Henderson	1.9%	482
Angel Medical Center	Franklin	2.0%	307
Frye Regional Medical Center	Hickory	2.0%	851
Vidant Bertie Hospital	Windsor	2.0%	50
Carolinas Medical Center - Northeast	Concord	2.1%	2240
Alleghany County Memorial Hospital	Sparta	2.2%	45
Rex Hospital	Raleigh	2.2%	1432
Nash General Hospital	Rocky Mount	2.5%	278
Novant Health Franklin Medical Center	Louisburg	2.9%	104
Murphy Medical Center	Murphy	3.0%	236
Halifax Regional Medical Center	Roanoke Rapids	3.2%	554
Spruce Pine Community Hospital	Spruce Pine	3.6%	221
Wilkes Regional Medical Center	N Wilkesboro	3.6%	305
Scotland Memorial Hospital	Laurinburg	4.1%	465
Albemarle Hospital Authority	Elizabeth City	4.4%	524
Granville Health Systems	Oxford	4.5%	155
Cleveland Regional Medical Center	Shelby	5.1%	723
Margaret R Pardee Memorial Hospital	Hendersonville	5.1%	649
Park Ridge Health	Hendersonville	5.6%	215
Southeastern Regional Medical Center	Lumberton	5.6%	720
Novant Health Brunswick Medical Center	Supply	6.7%	344
Medwest Harris	Sylva	7.0%	572
Saint Luke's Hospital	Columbus	7.1%	85
Stanly Regional Medical Center	Albemarle	8.0%	587
Medwest Haywood	Clyde	8.6%	590
Johnston Memorial Hospital	Smithfield	8.8%	821
Person Memorial Hospital	Roxboro	11.3%	115
Cape Fear Valley - Bladen County Hospital	Elizabethtown	11.7%	77

Follow-up Mammogram/Ultrasound

A follow-up rate near zero may indicate missed cancer; a rate higher than 14% may mean there is unnecessary follow up.

Hospital Name	City	Rate	Cases
Hugh Chatham Memorial Hospital	Elkin	3.9%	918
Sampson Regional Medical Center	Clinton	4.0%	1405
Ashe Memorial Hospital	Jefferson	4.1%	753
Iredell Memorial Hospital	Statesville	4.1%	2148
Alleghany County Memorial Hospital	Sparta	4.3%	255
Angel Medical Center	Franklin	4.4%	1176
Scotland Memorial Hospital	Laurinburg	4.4%	1595
Stanly Regional Medical Center	Albemarle	4.4%	1621
Southeastern Regional Medical Center	Lumberton	4.7%	1078
Vidant Bertie Hospital	Windsor	4.7%	342
Vidant Roanoke Chowan Hospital	Ahoskie	4.8%	1243
Onslow Memorial Hospital	Jacksonville	4.9%	962
Central Carolina Hospital	Sanford	5.7%	1654
Martin General Hospital	Williamston	5.7%	540
Person Memorial Hospital	Roxboro	5.7%	664
Carolina East Medical Center	New Bern	5.8%	1149
Wilson Medical Center	Wilson	5.8%	2276
Rex Hospital	Raleigh	5.9%	3011
Halifax Regional Medical Center	Roanoke Rapids	6.1%	1908
Medwest Haywood	Clyde	6.1%	1639
Columbus Regional Healthcare System	Whiteville	6.3%	1357
Firsthealth Moore Regional Hospital	Pinehurst	6.4%	1487
Cape Fear Valley - Bladen County Hospital	Elizabethtown	6.5%	448
Vidant Edgecombe Hospital	Tarboro	6.6%	1182
Wakemed - Raleigh Campus	Raleigh	6.6%	1242
Alamance Regional Medical Center	Burlington	6.8%	2402
Transylvania Regional Hospital	Brevard	6.8%	940
The Mcdowell Hospital	Marion	6.9%	757
Morehead Memorial Hospital	Eden	6.9%	771
North Carolina Baptist Hospital	Winston-Salem	6.9%	1067
Novant Health Huntersville Medical Center	Huntersville	7.0%	471
Novant Health Presbyterian Medical Center	Charlotte	7.0%	1737
Carolinas Medical Center - Northeast	Concord	7.1%	4766
Carteret General Hospital	Morehead City	7.1%	1960
Presbyterian Hospital Matthews	Matthews	7.1%	1277
Spruce Pine Community Hospital	Spruce Pine	7.1%	574
Lake Norman Regional Medical Center	Mooresville	7.2%	1567
Randolph Hospital	Asheboro	7.2%	1187
Duke Health Raleigh Hospital	Raleigh	7.6%	529
Margaret R Pardee Memorial Hospital	Hendersonville	7.6%	2383
Caromont Regional Medical Center	Gastonia	7.7%	4071
Murphy Medical Center	Murphy	7.7%	1022
Saint Luke's Hospital	Columbus	7.7%	549
Maria Parham Medical Center	Henderson	7.8%	1308
Novant Health Forsyth Medical Center	Winston-Salem	7.8%	6259
Rutherford Hospital	Rutherfordton	8.0%	1794
Vidant Chowan Hospital	Edenton	8.0%	849
Washington County Hospital	Plymouth	8.0%	261
Watauga Medical Center	Boone	8.0%	1509
New Hanover Regional Medical Center	Wilmington	8.1%	3749
Vidant Duplin Hospital	Kenansville	8.1%	595
Novant Health Franklin Medical Center	Louisburg	8.3%	605
Wilkes Regional Medical Center	N Wilkesboro	8.3%	1476
Johnston Memorial Hospital	Smithfield	8.5%	1539
The Moses H Cone Memorial Hospital	Greensboro	8.5%	1780
High Point Regional Hospital	High Point	8.6%	370
Novant Health Thomasville Medical Center	Thomasville	8.7%	607
Wakemed - Cary Hospital	Cary	8.7%	598
J Arthur Dosher Memorial Hospital	Southport	8.8%	1373
Wayne Memorial Hospital	Goldsboro	9.0%	500
Davis Regional Medical Center	Statesville	9.2%	184
University of North Carolina Hospital	Chapel Hill	9.2%	2223
Duke University Hospital	Durham	9.3%	3296
Medwest Harris	Sylva	9.3%	1300
Anson Community Hospital	Wadesboro	9.4%	373
Carolinas Medical Center - Lincoln	Lincolnton	9.4%	970
Novant Health Brunswick Medical Center	Supply	9.4%	1618
Park Ridge Health	Hendersonville	9.9%	950
Lexington Memorial Hospital	Lexington	10.1%	794
Catawba Valley Medical Center	Hickory	10.2%	2676
Cape Fear Valley Medical Center	Fayetteville	10.4%	1125
Firsthealth Montgomery Memorial Hospital	Troy	10.4%	308
Mem Mission Hosp & Asheville Surg Ctr	Asheville	10.7%	291
CMC - Blue Ridge	Morganton	10.8%	1368
Novant Health Rowan Medical Center	Salisbury	11.2%	2153
Sandhills Regional Medical Center	Hamlet	11.3%	311
Albemarle Hospital Authority	Elizabeth City	11.4%	2017
Northern Hospital of Surry County	Mount Airy	11.7%	1146
Duke Regional Hospital	Durham	11.9%	714
Betsy Johnson Regional Hospital	Dunn	12.1%	832
Frye Regional Medical Center	Hickory	12.4%	2542
Caldwell Memorial Hospital	Lenoir	13.0%	1150
Kings Mountain Hospital	Kings Mountain	13.1%	350
Nash General Hospital	Rocky Mount	13.6%	1880
Granville Health Systems	Oxford	13.9%	532
Cleveland Regional Medical Center	Shelby	15.8%	1028

Lumbar Spine MRI for Low Back Pain

Hospital Name	City	Rate	Cases
Novant Health Brunswick Medical Center	Supply	22.9%	157
Presbyterian Hospital Matthews	Matthews	23.2%	82
J Arthur Dosher Memorial Hospital	Southport	24.6%	57
Columbus Regional Healthcare System	Whiteville	24.8%	141
Nash General Hospital	Rocky Mount	25.9%	201
Randolph Hospital	Asheboro	26.4%	163
Wakemed - Cary Hospital	Cary	26.7%	60
Central Carolina Hospital	Sanford	27.2%	103
University of North Carolina Hospital	Chapel Hill	28.4%	204
Angel Medical Center	Franklin	28.8%	59
Vidant Edgecombe Hospital	Tarboro	28.9%	135
Betsy Johnson Regional Hospital	Dunn	29.1%	103
Medwest Haywood	Clyde	29.1%	203
Scotland Memorial Hospital	Laurinburg	29.8%	141
Saint Luke's Hospital	Columbus	30.0%	60
Transylvania Regional Hospital	Brevard	30.2%	86
Carolinas Med Ctr/Behavioral Health	Charlotte	31.3%	163
Frye Regional Medical Center	Hickory	31.4%	236
High Point Regional Hospital	High Point	31.4%	70
Duke University Hospital	Durham	31.5%	356
Novant Health Charlotte Ortho Hosp	Charlotte	31.6%	79
Novant Health Presbyterian Medical Center	Charlotte	31.6%	187
Wilkes Regional Medical Center	N Wilkesboro	31.6%	133
Margaret R Pardee Memorial Hospital	Hendersonville	31.7%	259
Carolinas Medical Center - Northeast	Concord	31.9%	458
Vidant Beaufort Hospital	Washington	32.2%	118
Carolinas Medical Center - Pineville	Charlotte	32.4%	176
Park Ridge Health	Hendersonville	32.4%	111
Wilson Medical Center	Wilson	32.9%	167
Johnston Memorial Hospital	Smithfield	33.1%	178
Caromont Regional Medical Center	Gastonia	33.6%	399
Duke Health Raleigh Hospital	Raleigh	33.7%	252
CMC - Blue Ridge	Morganton	33.9%	112
Duke Regional Hospital	Durham	34.0%	106
Firsthealth Moore Regional Hospital	Pinehurst	35.0%	755
Vidant Medical Center	Greenville	35.0%	117
Sampson Regional Medical Center	Clinton	35.2%	165
Granville Health Systems	Oxford	35.3%	102
Northern Hospital of Surry County	Mount Airy	35.4%	130
Wakemed - Raleigh Campus	Raleigh	35.5%	76
Alamance Regional Medical Center	Burlington	35.8%	193
Hugh Chatham Memorial Hospital	Elkin	35.8%	109
Novant Health Rowan Medical Center	Salisbury	35.9%	276
Cleveland Regional Medical Center	Shelby	36.1%	144
Watauga Medical Center	Boone	36.1%	61
Catawba Valley Medical Center	Hickory	36.2%	127
Ashe Memorial Hospital	Jefferson	36.4%	55
Medwest Harris	Sylva	36.6%	142
Lenoir Memorial Hospital	Kinston	36.7%	158
Murphy Medical Center	Murphy	36.7%	109
Rex Hospital	Raleigh	36.8%	155
Wayne Memorial Hospital	Goldsboro	36.8%	304
Rutherford Hospital	Rutherfordton	37.1%	159
Lake Norman Regional Medical Center	Mooresville	37.2%	94
Southeastern Regional Medical Center	Lumberton	37.4%	230
Davis Regional Medical Center	Statesville	37.5%	104
New Hanover Regional Medical Center	Wilmington	37.6%	482
Novant Health Thomasville Medical Center	Thomasville	37.8%	45
Carolinas Medical Center - Union	Monroe	37.9%	87
Lexington Memorial Hospital	Lexington	37.9%	87
Cape Fear Valley Medical Center	Fayetteville	38.1%	84
Novant Health Huntersville Medical Center	Huntersville	38.5%	182
Mem Mission Hosp & Asheville Surg Ctr	Asheville	38.6%	220
Carolina East Medical Center	New Bern	38.8%	129
North Carolina Baptist Hospital	Winston-Salem	39.2%	166
Carolinas Medical Center - University	Charlotte	39.4%	71
Stanly Regional Medical Center	Albemarle	39.6%	106
Vidant Chowan Hospital	Edenton	40.2%	127
Halifax Regional Medical Center	Roanoke Rapids	41.2%	97
Vidant Roanoke Chowan Hospital	Ahoskie	41.4%	70
Novant Health Forsyth Medical Center	Winston-Salem	41.6%	351
The Moses H Cone Memorial Hospital	Greensboro	41.8%	153
Carolinas Medical Center - Lincoln	Lincolnton	41.9%	93
Morehead Memorial Hospital	Eden	42.0%	138
Albemarle Hospital Authority	Elizabeth City	42.2%	102
Carteret General Hospital	Morehead City	43.0%	165
Iredell Memorial Hospital	Statesville	43.0%	93
Kings Mountain Hospital	Kings Mountain	47.2%	36
Spruce Pine Community Hospital	Spruce Pine	48.0%	50

NOTE: Hospital profiles are in alphabetical order by state, then city, then hospital within the city; Rankings exclude hospitals with less than 25 cases except for patient surveys which excludes hospitals with less than 100 cases; (a) 100-299 cases; (1) The number of cases/patients is too few to report; (2) Data submitted were based on a sample of cases/patients; (3) Results are based on a shorter time period than required; (4) Data suppressed by CMS for one or more quarters; (5) Results are not available for this reporting period; (6) Fewer than 100 patients completed the HCAHPS survey; (7) No cases met the criteria for this measure; (8) The lower limit of the confidence interval cannot be calculated if the number of observed infections equals zero; (9) No data are available from the state/territory for this reporting period; (10) The scores shown reflect fewer than 50 completed surveys; (11) There were discrepancies in the data collection process; (12) This measure does not apply to this hospital for this reporting period; (13) Results cannot be calculated for this reporting period; (14) The results for this state are combined with nearby states to protect confidentiality; Please refer to the User's Guide for a full explanation of data.

Vidant Roanoke Chowan Hospital

500 S Academy St
Ahoskie, NC 27910
Phone: 252-209-3000
Fax: 252-209-3049
E-mail: lnewsome@uhseast.com
URL: www.uhseast.com
Type: Acute Care Hospitals
Emergency Services: Yes
Ownership: Voluntary non-profit - Private
Beds: 105

Key Personnel:
Radiology. . . . . Mark Adkins
Chief of Medical Staff. . . . . Robert Kahn
CEO/President. . . . . Susan S Lassiter

Measure	Cases	This Hosp.	State Avg.	U.S. Avg.
Blood Clot Prevention and Treatment				
Anticoagulation Overlap Therapy[2]	21	86%	94%	93%
ICU Venous Thromboembolism Prophylaxis[2]	85	95%	93%	92%
Incidence of Potentially Preventable VTE[1,2]	-	-	10%	10%
UFH with Dosages/Platelet Monitoring[2]	16	31%	95%	97%
Venous Thromboembolism Prophylaxis[2]	233	88%	88%	85%
Warfarin Therapy Discharge Instructions[2]	17	71%	81%	75%
Chest Pain/Possible Heart Attack Care				
Aspirin Given Within 24 Hours of Arrival	46	98%	97%	96%
Fibrinolytic Meds Within 30 Min. of Arrival[1]	-	-	66%	58%
Average Time to ECG (minutes)	48	12	7	7
Average Time to Transfer (minutes)[7]	-	-	45	60
Children's Asthma Care				
Received Home Management Plan of Care	-	-	89%	88%
Received Reliever Medication	-	-	100%	100%
Received Systemic Corticosteroids	-	-	100%	100%
Emergency Department				
Admittance Decision Time (minutes)[2]	379	34	107	98
Head CT Results Within 45 Min. of Arrival[1]	-	-	60%	57%
Patients Who Left ER Before Being Seen	21,582	1%	3%	2%
Time from ER Arrival to Admit. (minutes)[2]	380	234	300	274
Time from ER Arrival to Discharge (minutes)	386	132	152	134
Time in ER Before Being Evaluated (minutes)	426	16	34	26
Time to Pain Meds for Fractures (minutes)	66	49	67	57
Heart Attack Care				
Aspirin Given at Discharge[1]	-	-	100%	99%
Fibrinolytic Meds Within 30 Min. of Arrival[7]	-	-	75%	54%
PCI Within 90 Minutes of Arrival[7]	-	-	98%	96%
Statin Prescribed at Discharge[1]	-	-	99%	98%
Heart Failure Care				
ACE Inhibitor or ARB for LVSD	42	98%	98%	97%
Discharge Instructions Given	124	100%	96%	94%
Evaluation of LVS Function	146	100%	100%	99%
Medicare Spending				
Medicare Spending per Patient (ratio)	-	0.91	0.94	0.98
Pneumonia Care				
Appropriate Initial Antibiotic Given	69	100%	97%	95%
Blood Culture Timing	142	99%	98%	98%
Pregnancy and Delivery Care				
Newborn Deliveries Scheduled Early	36	0%	3%	6%
Preventive Care				
Immunization for Influenza[2]	429	93%	93%	90%
Immunization for Pneumonia[2]	453	93%	94%	92%
Stroke Care				
Anticoagulation Therapy for Atrial Fibrillation[1]	-	-	95%	95%
Antithrombotic Therapy Timing	57	100%	98%	98%
Assessed for Rehabilitation	57	89%	98%	97%
Discharged on Antithrombotic Therapy	53	98%	99%	99%
Discharged on Statin Medication	43	88%	94%	94%
Thrombolytic Therapy Timing[1]	-	-	64%	66%
Venous Thromboembolism Prophylaxis	59	98%	96%	94%
Written Stroke Educational Materials Given	37	70%	88%	88%
Surgical Care Improvement Project				
Appropriate Beta Blocker Usage	39	95%	99%	98%
Appropriate VTP Within 24 Hours	165	100%	99%	98%
Controlled Postoperative Blood Glucose[7]	-	-	98%	97%
Perioperative Temperature Management	172	100%	100%	100%
Prophylactic Antibiotic Selection	122	100%	99%	99%
Prophylactic Antibiotic Selection (Outpatient)	21	95%	98%	98%
Prophylactic Antibiotic Stopped	120	100%	99%	98%
Prophylactic Antibiotic Timing	122	98%	99%	99%
Prophylactic Antibiotic Timing (Outpatient)	21	100%	99%	98%
Urinary Catheter Removal	54	100%	99%	97%
Survey of Patients' Hospital Experiences				
Area Around Room 'Always' Quiet at Night	300+	65%	64%	61%
Doctors 'Always' Communicated Well	300+	85%	83%	82%
Home Recovery Information Given	300+	88%	87%	85%
Hospital Given 9 or 10 on 10 Point Scale	300+	71%	71%	71%
Meds 'Always' Explained Before Given	300+	68%	65%	64%
Nurses 'Always' Communicated Well	300+	83%	81%	79%
Pain 'Always' Well Controlled	300+	75%	72%	71%
Room and Bathroom 'Always' Clean	300+	71%	72%	73%
Timely Help 'Always' Received	300+	73%	68%	68%
Would Definitely Recommend Hospital	300+	68%	70%	71%
Use of Medical Imaging				
Cardiac Imaging Stress Test before Surgery	125	6.4%	5.4%	5.3%
Combination Abdominal CT Scan	566	6.4%	5.6%	10.5%
Combination Brain/Sinus CT Scan	625	3.2%	2.6%	2.7%
Combination Chest CT Scan	189	0.5%	1.3%	2.7%
Follow-up Mammogram/Ultrasound	1,243	4.8%	8%	8.8%
Lumbar Spine MRI for Low Back Pain	70	41.4%	34.7%	37.2%

Stanly Regional Medical Center

301 Yadkin St
Albemarle, NC 28001
Phone: 704-984-4000
Fax: 704-983-3562
URL: www.stanly.org
Type: Acute Care Hospitals
Emergency Services: Yes
Ownership: Voluntary non-profit - Private
Beds: 119

Key Personnel:
Chairman/CEO . . . . Larry Baucom
Radiology. . . . . Peter Gusmer
CEO/President. . . . . Roy Hinson
Chief of Medical Staff. . . . . Eric Johnsen
Emergency Room . . . . Judy Moore

Measure	Cases	This Hosp.	State Avg.	U.S. Avg.
Blood Clot Prevention and Treatment				
Anticoagulation Overlap Therapy[2]	25	100%	94%	93%
ICU Venous Thromboembolism Prophylaxis[2]	86	100%	93%	92%
Incidence of Potentially Preventable VTE[1,2]	-	-	10%	10%
UFH with Dosages/Platelet Monitoring[1,2]	-	-	95%	97%
Venous Thromboembolism Prophylaxis[2]	239	99%	88%	85%
Warfarin Therapy Discharge Instructions[2]	19	84%	81%	75%
Chest Pain/Possible Heart Attack Care				
Aspirin Given Within 24 Hours of Arrival	72	94%	97%	96%
Fibrinolytic Meds Within 30 Min. of Arrival[7]	-	-	66%	58%
Average Time to ECG (minutes)	79	1	7	7
Average Time to Transfer (minutes)	11	48	45	60
Children's Asthma Care				
Received Home Management Plan of Care	-	-	89%	88%
Received Reliever Medication	-	-	100%	100%
Received Systemic Corticosteroids	-	-	100%	100%
Emergency Department				
Admittance Decision Time (minutes)[2]	560	133	107	98
Head CT Results Within 45 Min. of Arrival	16	75%	60%	57%
Patients Who Left ER Before Being Seen	35,578	3%	3%	2%
Time from ER Arrival to Admit. (minutes)[2]	560	317	300	274
Time from ER Arrival to Discharge (minutes)	352	146	152	134
Time in ER Before Being Evaluated (minutes)	376	21	34	26
Time to Pain Meds for Fractures (minutes)	199	63	67	57
Heart Attack Care				
Aspirin Given at Discharge	42	100%	100%	99%
Fibrinolytic Meds Within 30 Min. of Arrival[7]	-	-	75%	54%
PCI Within 90 Minutes of Arrival[7]	-	-	98%	96%
Statin Prescribed at Discharge	38	89%	99%	98%
Heart Failure Care				
ACE Inhibitor or ARB for LVSD	57	98%	98%	97%
Discharge Instructions Given	201	95%	96%	94%
Evaluation of LVS Function	249	100%	100%	99%
Medicare Spending				
Medicare Spending per Patient (ratio)	-	0.90	0.94	0.98
Pneumonia Care				
Appropriate Initial Antibiotic Given	126	97%	97%	95%
Blood Culture Timing	214	100%	98%	98%
Pregnancy and Delivery Care				
Newborn Deliveries Scheduled Early[2]	118	1%	3%	6%
Preventive Care				
Immunization for Influenza[2]	435	83%	93%	90%
Immunization for Pneumonia[2]	522	95%	94%	92%
Stroke Care				
Anticoagulation Therapy for Atrial Fibrillation[1]	-	-	95%	95%
Antithrombotic Therapy Timing	39	100%	98%	98%
Assessed for Rehabilitation	55	100%	98%	97%
Discharged on Antithrombotic Therapy	54	98%	99%	99%
Discharged on Statin Medication	38	89%	94%	94%
Thrombolytic Therapy Timing	12	50%	64%	66%
Venous Thromboembolism Prophylaxis	45	100%	96%	94%
Written Stroke Educational Materials Given	36	97%	88%	88%
Surgical Care Improvement Project				
Appropriate Beta Blocker Usage	51	96%	99%	98%
Appropriate VTP Within 24 Hours	163	99%	99%	98%
Controlled Postoperative Blood Glucose[7]	-	-	98%	97%
Perioperative Temperature Management	185	99%	100%	100%
Prophylactic Antibiotic Selection	125	98%	99%	99%
Prophylactic Antibiotic Selection (Outpatient)	81	95%	98%	98%
Prophylactic Antibiotic Stopped	121	96%	99%	98%
Prophylactic Antibiotic Timing	126	98%	99%	99%
Prophylactic Antibiotic Timing (Outpatient)	81	98%	99%	98%
Urinary Catheter Removal	130	99%	99%	97%
Survey of Patients' Hospital Experiences				
Area Around Room 'Always' Quiet at Night	300+	62%	64%	61%
Doctors 'Always' Communicated Well	300+	82%	83%	82%
Home Recovery Information Given	300+	87%	87%	85%
Hospital Given 9 or 10 on 10 Point Scale	300+	70%	71%	71%
Meds 'Always' Explained Before Given	300+	62%	65%	64%
Nurses 'Always' Communicated Well	300+	78%	81%	79%
Pain 'Always' Well Controlled	300+	68%	72%	71%
Room and Bathroom 'Always' Clean	300+	73%	72%	73%
Timely Help 'Always' Received	300+	69%	68%	68%
Would Definitely Recommend Hospital	300+	65%	70%	71%
Use of Medical Imaging				
Cardiac Imaging Stress Test before Surgery	411	4.9%	5.4%	5.3%
Combination Abdominal CT Scan	1,134	13.7%	5.6%	10.5%
Combination Brain/Sinus CT Scan	971	4.7%	2.6%	2.7%
Combination Chest CT Scan	587	8.0%	1.3%	2.7%
Follow-up Mammogram/Ultrasound	1,621	4.4%	8%	8.8%
Lumbar Spine MRI for Low Back Pain	106	39.6%	34.7%	37.2%

Randolph Hospital

364 White Oak Street
Asheboro, NC 27204
Phone: 336-625-5151
Fax: 336-626-7664
E-mail: amt@randolphhospital.org
URL: www.randolphhospital.org
Type: Acute Care Hospitals
Emergency Services: Yes
Ownership: Voluntary non-profit - Private
Beds: 145

Key Personnel:
Radiology. . . . . Paul D Barry
CEO/President. . . . . Robert E Morrison
Chief of Medical Staff. . . . . Charles B West, MD

Measure	Cases	This Hosp.	State Avg.	U.S. Avg.
Blood Clot Prevention and Treatment				
Anticoagulation Overlap Therapy[2]	42	95%	94%	93%
ICU Venous Thromboembolism Prophylaxis[2]	75	84%	93%	92%
Incidence of Potentially Preventable VTE[1,2]	-	-	10%	10%
UFH with Dosages/Platelet Monitoring[1,2]	-	-	95%	97%
Venous Thromboembolism Prophylaxis[2]	394	89%	88%	85%
Warfarin Therapy Discharge Instructions[2]	24	79%	81%	75%
Chest Pain/Possible Heart Attack Care				
Aspirin Given Within 24 Hours of Arrival	94	98%	97%	96%
Fibrinolytic Meds Within 30 Min. of Arrival[7]	-	-	66%	58%
Average Time to ECG (minutes)	93	8	7	7
Average Time to Transfer (minutes)	22	52	45	60
Children's Asthma Care				
Received Home Management Plan of Care	-	-	89%	88%
Received Reliever Medication	-	-	100%	100%
Received Systemic Corticosteroids	-	-	100%	100%
Emergency Department				
Admittance Decision Time (minutes)[2]	643	122	107	98
Head CT Results Within 45 Min. of Arrival[1]	-	-	60%	57%

NOTE: Hospital profiles are in alphabetical order by state, then city, then hospital within the city; Rankings exclude hospitals with less than 25 cases except for patient surveys which excludes hospitals with less than 100 cases; (a) 100-299 cases; (1) The number of cases/patients is too few to report; (2) Data submitted were based on a sample of cases/patients; (3) Results are based on a shorter time period than required; (4) Data suppressed by CMS for one or more quarters; (5) Results are not available for this reporting period; (6) Fewer than 100 patients completed the HCAHPS survey; (7) No cases met the criteria for this measure; (8) The lower limit of the confidence interval cannot be calculated if the number of observed infections equals zero; (9) No data are available from the state/territory for this reporting period; (10) The scores shown reflect fewer than 50 completed surveys; (11) There were discrepancies in the data collection process; (12) This measure does not apply to this hospital for this reporting period; (13) Results cannot be calculated for this reporting period; (14) The results for this state are combined with nearby states to protect confidentiality; Please refer to the User's Guide for a full explanation of data.

Measure	Cases	This Hosp.	State Avg.	U.S. Avg.
Patients Who Left ER Before Being Seen	41,808	5%	3%	2%
Time from ER Arrival to Admit. (minutes)[2]	644	329	300	274
Time from ER Arrival to Discharge (minutes)	362	191	152	134
Time in ER Before Being Evaluated (minutes)	402	46	34	26
Time to Pain Meds for Fractures (minutes)	190	71	67	57
Heart Attack Care				
Aspirin Given at Discharge	30	100%	100%	99%
Fibrinolytic Meds Within 30 Min. of Arrival[7]	-	-	75%	54%
PCI Within 90 Minutes of Arrival[7]	-	-	98%	96%
Statin Prescribed at Discharge	33	94%	99%	98%
Heart Failure Care				
ACE Inhibitor or ARB for LVSD[2]	61	95%	98%	97%
Discharge Instructions Given[2]	190	96%	96%	94%
Evaluation of LVS Function[2]	245	99%	100%	99%
Medicare Spending				
Medicare Spending per Patient (ratio)	-	0.96	0.94	0.98
Pneumonia Care				
Appropriate Initial Antibiotic Given[2]	93	99%	97%	95%
Blood Culture Timing[2]	131	97%	98%	98%
Pregnancy and Delivery Care				
Newborn Deliveries Scheduled Early	68	0%	3%	6%
Preventive Care				
Immunization for Influenza[2]	543	89%	93%	90%
Immunization for Pneumonia[2]	716	86%	94%	92%
Stroke Care				
Anticoagulation Therapy for Atrial Fibrillation[2]	17	71%	95%	95%
Antithrombotic Therapy Timing[2]	78	100%	98%	98%
Assessed for Rehabilitation[2]	85	100%	98%	97%
Discharged on Antithrombotic Therapy[2]	79	99%	99%	99%
Discharged on Statin Medication[2]	64	92%	94%	94%
Thrombolytic Therapy Timing[1,2]	-	-	64%	66%
Venous Thromboembolism Prophylaxis[2]	88	88%	96%	94%
Written Stroke Educational Materials Given[2]	45	64%	88%	88%
Surgical Care Improvement Project				
Appropriate Beta Blocker Usage[2]	97	98%	99%	98%
Appropriate VTP Within 24 Hours[2]	317	98%	99%	98%
Controlled Postoperative Blood Glucose[2,7]	-	-	98%	97%
Perioperative Temperature Management[2]	344	100%	100%	100%
Prophylactic Antibiotic Selection[2]	217	98%	99%	99%
Prophylactic Antibiotic Selection (Outpatient)	109	98%	98%	98%
Prophylactic Antibiotic Stopped[2]	213	99%	99%	98%
Prophylactic Antibiotic Timing[2]	217	99%	99%	99%
Prophylactic Antibiotic Timing (Outpatient)	109	100%	99%	98%
Urinary Catheter Removal[2]	75	99%	99%	97%
Survey of Patients' Hospital Experiences				
Area Around Room 'Always' Quiet at Night	300+	66%	64%	61%
Doctors 'Always' Communicated Well	300+	82%	83%	82%
Home Recovery Information Given	300+	86%	87%	85%
Hospital Given 9 or 10 on 10 Point Scale	300+	70%	71%	71%
Meds 'Always' Explained Before Given	300+	66%	65%	64%
Nurses 'Always' Communicated Well	300+	84%	81%	79%
Pain 'Always' Well Controlled	300+	77%	72%	71%
Room and Bathroom 'Always' Clean	300+	73%	72%	73%
Timely Help 'Always' Received	300+	71%	68%	68%
Would Definitely Recommend Hospital	300+	66%	70%	71%
Use of Medical Imaging				
Cardiac Imaging Stress Test before Surgery	130	2.3%	5.4%	5.3%
Combination Abdominal CT Scan	377	6.1%	5.6%	10.5%
Combination Brain/Sinus CT Scan	1,004	3.6%	2.6%	2.7%
Combination Chest CT Scan	444	0.0%	1.3%	2.7%
Follow-up Mammogram/Ultrasound	1,187	7.2%	8%	8.8%
Lumbar Spine MRI for Low Back Pain	163	26.4%	34.7%	37.2%

Asheville - Oteen VA Medical Center

1100 Tunnel Road
Asheville, NC 28805
Phone: 828-298-7911
Fax: 828-299-2501
URL: www.asheville.va.gov
Type: Acute Care - VA
Emergency Services: No
Ownership: Government Federal

Key Personnel:
Chief of Medical Staff.......... MaryAnn Curl, MD
Emergency Room........... James Johnson, MD
Radiology.................. Keith Kohatsu, MD
CEO/President.............. Susan Pendergrass

Measure	Cases	This Hosp.	State Avg.	U.S. Avg.
Blood Clot Prevention and Treatment				
Anticoagulation Overlap Therapy	-	-	94%	93%
ICU Venous Thromboembolism Prophylaxis	-	-	93%	92%
Incidence of Potentially Preventable VTE	-	-	10%	10%
UFH with Dosages/Platelet Monitoring	-	-	95%	97%
Venous Thromboembolism Prophylaxis	-	-	88%	85%
Warfarin Therapy Discharge Instructions	-	-	81%	75%
Chest Pain/Possible Heart Attack Care				
Aspirin Given Within 24 Hours of Arrival	-	-	97%	96%
Fibrinolytic Meds Within 30 Min. of Arrival	-	-	66%	58%
Average Time to ECG (minutes)	-	-	7	7
Average Time to Transfer (minutes)	-	-	45	60
Children's Asthma Care				
Received Home Management Plan of Care	-	-	89%	88%
Received Reliever Medication	-	-	100%	100%
Received Systemic Corticosteroids	-	-	100%	100%
Emergency Department				
Admittance Decision Time (minutes)	-	-	107	98
Head CT Results Within 45 Min. of Arrival	-	-	60%	57%
Patients Who Left ER Before Being Seen	-	-	3%	2%
Time from ER Arrival to Admit. (minutes)	-	-	300	274
Time from ER Arrival to Discharge (minutes)	-	-	152	134
Time in ER Before Being Evaluated (minutes)	-	-	34	26
Time to Pain Meds for Fractures (minutes)	-	-	67	57
Heart Attack Care				
Aspirin Given at Discharge	59	100%	100%	99%
Fibrinolytic Meds Within 30 Min. of Arrival[5]	-	-	75%	54%
PCI Within 90 Minutes of Arrival[1]	-	-	98%	96%
Statin Prescribed at Discharge	58	93%	99%	98%
Heart Failure Care				
ACE Inhibitor or ARB for LVSD	51	94%	98%	97%
Discharge Instructions Given	113	90%	96%	94%
Evaluation of LVS Function	117	100%	100%	99%
Medicare Spending				
Medicare Spending per Patient (ratio)	-	-	0.94	0.98
Pneumonia Care				
Appropriate Initial Antibiotic Given	75	93%	97%	95%
Blood Culture Timing	131	98%	98%	98%
Pregnancy and Delivery Care				
Newborn Deliveries Scheduled Early	-	-	3%	6%
Preventive Care				
Immunization for Influenza[5]	-	-	93%	90%
Immunization for Pneumonia[5]	-	-	94%	92%
Stroke Care				
Anticoagulation Therapy for Atrial Fibrillation	-	-	95%	95%
Antithrombotic Therapy Timing	-	-	98%	98%
Assessed for Rehabilitation	-	-	98%	97%
Discharged on Antithrombotic Therapy	-	-	99%	99%
Discharged on Statin Medication	-	-	94%	94%
Thrombolytic Therapy Timing	-	-	64%	66%
Venous Thromboembolism Prophylaxis	-	-	96%	94%
Written Stroke Educational Materials Given	-	-	88%	88%
Surgical Care Improvement Project				
Appropriate Beta Blocker Usage[2]	187	97%	99%	98%
Appropriate VTP Within 24 Hours[2]	398	99%	99%	98%
Controlled Postoperative Blood Glucose[2]	65	100%	98%	97%
Perioperative Temperature Management[2]	435	100%	100%	100%
Prophylactic Antibiotic Selection	396	100%	99%	99%
Prophylactic Antibiotic Selection (Outpatient)	-	-	98%	98%
Prophylactic Antibiotic Stopped	389	96%	99%	98%
Prophylactic Antibiotic Timing	396	99%	99%	99%
Prophylactic Antibiotic Timing (Outpatient)	-	-	99%	98%
Urinary Catheter Removal[2]	396	98%	99%	97%
Survey of Patients' Hospital Experiences				
Area Around Room 'Always' Quiet at Night	-	-	64%	61%
Doctors 'Always' Communicated Well	-	-	83%	82%
Home Recovery Information Given	-	-	87%	85%
Hospital Given 9 or 10 on 10 Point Scale	-	-	71%	71%
Meds 'Always' Explained Before Given	-	-	65%	64%
Nurses 'Always' Communicated Well	-	-	81%	79%
Pain 'Always' Well Controlled	-	-	72%	71%
Room and Bathroom 'Always' Clean	-	-	72%	73%
Timely Help 'Always' Received	-	-	68%	68%
Would Definitely Recommend Hospital	-	-	70%	71%
Use of Medical Imaging				
Cardiac Imaging Stress Test before Surgery	-	-	5.4%	5.3%
Combination Abdominal CT Scan	-	-	5.6%	10.5%
Combination Brain/Sinus CT Scan	-	-	2.6%	2.7%
Combination Chest CT Scan	-	-	1.3%	2.7%
Follow-up Mammogram/Ultrasound	-	-	8%	8.8%
Lumbar Spine MRI for Low Back Pain	-	-	34.7%	37.2%

Memorial Mission Hospital & Asheville Surgery Center

509 Biltmore Ave
Asheville, NC 28801
Phone: 828-213-1111
Fax: 828-213-4404
URL: www.missionhospitals.org
Type: Acute Care Hospitals
Emergency Services: Yes
Ownership: Voluntary non-profit - Private
Beds: 800

Key Personnel:
Chief of Medical Staff.......... Alan S Baumgarten, MD
Cardiac Laboratory............ Karen Lemieux
CEO/President.............. Ronald A. Paulus, MD
Ambulatory Care .... Kristi Sink
Anesthesiology............... Ann Young, JD

Measure	Cases	This Hosp.	State Avg.	U.S. Avg.
Blood Clot Prevention and Treatment				
Anticoagulation Overlap Therapy[2]	250	98%	94%	93%
ICU Venous Thromboembolism Prophylaxis[2]	84	90%	93%	92%
Incidence of Potentially Preventable VTE[2]	50	18%	10%	10%
UFH with Dosages/Platelet Monitoring[2]	126	100%	95%	97%
Venous Thromboembolism Prophylaxis[2]	352	85%	88%	85%
Warfarin Therapy Discharge Instructions[2]	177	95%	81%	75%
Chest Pain/Possible Heart Attack Care				
Aspirin Given Within 24 Hours of Arrival[1,3]	-	-	97%	96%
Fibrinolytic Meds Within 30 Min. of Arrival[5]	-	-	66%	58%
Average Time to ECG (minutes)[1,3]	-	-	7	7
Average Time to Transfer (minutes)[5]	-	-	45	60
Children's Asthma Care				
Received Home Management Plan of Care	58	83%	89%	88%
Received Reliever Medication	58	100%	100%	100%
Received Systemic Corticosteroids	58	100%	100%	100%
Emergency Department				
Admittance Decision Time (minutes)[2]	390	134	107	98
Head CT Results Within 45 Min. of Arrival[1]	-	-	60%	57%
Patients Who Left ER Before Being Seen	>100k	3%	3%	2%
Time from ER Arrival to Admit. (minutes)[2]	432	332	300	274
Time from ER Arrival to Discharge (minutes)	381	193	152	134
Time in ER Before Being Evaluated (minutes)	423	46	34	26
Time to Pain Meds for Fractures (minutes)	264	78	67	57
Heart Attack Care				
Aspirin Given at Discharge[2]	312	100%	100%	99%
Fibrinolytic Meds Within 30 Min. of Arrival[1,2]	-	-	75%	54%
PCI Within 90 Minutes of Arrival[2]	31	100%	98%	96%
Statin Prescribed at Discharge[2]	303	100%	99%	98%
Heart Failure Care				
ACE Inhibitor or ARB for LVSD	352	98%	98%	97%
Discharge Instructions Given	845	98%	96%	94%
Evaluation of LVS Function	1,030	100%	100%	99%
Medicare Spending				
Medicare Spending per Patient (ratio)	-	0.99	0.94	0.98
Pneumonia Care				
Appropriate Initial Antibiotic Given[2]	35	97%	97%	95%
Blood Culture Timing[2]	156	97%	98%	98%
Pregnancy and Delivery Care				
Newborn Deliveries Scheduled Early[2]	40	2%	3%	6%
Preventive Care				
Immunization for Influenza[2]	564	96%	93%	90%
Immunization for Pneumonia[2]	733	92%	94%	92%
Stroke Care				
Anticoagulation Therapy for Atrial Fibrillation	101	97%	95%	95%
Antithrombotic Therapy Timing	352	98%	98%	98%
Assessed for Rehabilitation	576	100%	98%	97%
Discharged on Antithrombotic Therapy	470	100%	99%	99%
Discharged on Statin Medication	328	93%	94%	94%

NOTE: Hospital profiles are in alphabetical order by state, then city, then hospital within the city; Rankings exclude hospitals with less than 25 cases except for patient surveys which excludes hospitals with less than 100 cases; (a) 100-299 cases; (1) The number of cases/patients is too few to report; (2) Data submitted were based on a sample of cases/patients; (3) Results are based on a shorter time period than required; (4) Data suppressed by CMS for one or more quarters; (5) Results are not available for this reporting period; (6) Fewer than 100 patients completed the HCAHPS survey; (7) No cases met the criteria for this measure; (8) The lower limit of the confidence interval cannot be calculated if the number of observed infections equals zero; (9) No data are available from the state/territory for this reporting period; (10) The scores shown reflect fewer than 50 completed surveys; (11) There were discrepancies in the data collection process; (12) This measure does not apply to this hospital for this reporting period; (13) Results cannot be calculated for this reporting period; (14) The results for this state are combined with nearby states to protect confidentiality; Please refer to the User's Guide for a full explanation of data.

Measure	Cases	This Hosp.	State Avg.	U.S. Avg.
Thrombolytic Therapy Timing	83	96%	64%	66%
Venous Thromboembolism Prophylaxis	598	95%	96%	94%
Written Stroke Educational Materials Given	291	87%	88%	88%
Surgical Care Improvement Project				
Appropriate Beta Blocker Usage[2]	319	99%	99%	98%
Appropriate VTP Within 24 Hours[2]	546	100%	99%	98%
Controlled Postoperative Blood Glucose[2]	197	100%	98%	97%
Perioperative Temperature Management[2]	715	100%	100%	100%
Prophylactic Antibiotic Selection[2]	615	100%	99%	99%
Prophylactic Antibiotic Selection (Outpatient)	988	99%	98%	98%
Prophylactic Antibiotic Stopped[2]	596	99%	99%	98%
Prophylactic Antibiotic Timing[2]	618	99%	99%	99%
Prophylactic Antibiotic Timing (Outpatient)	984	100%	99%	98%
Urinary Catheter Removal[2]	373	99%	99%	97%
Survey of Patients' Hospital Experiences				
Area Around Room 'Always' Quiet at Night	300+	64%	64%	61%
Doctors 'Always' Communicated Well	300+	86%	83%	82%
Home Recovery Information Given	300+	91%	87%	85%
Hospital Given 9 or 10 on 10 Point Scale	300+	78%	71%	71%
Meds 'Always' Explained Before Given	300+	73%	65%	64%
Nurses 'Always' Communicated Well	300+	83%	81%	79%
Pain 'Always' Well Controlled	300+	76%	72%	71%
Room and Bathroom 'Always' Clean	300+	65%	72%	73%
Timely Help 'Always' Received	300+	71%	68%	68%
Would Definitely Recommend Hospital	300+	83%	70%	71%
Use of Medical Imaging				
Cardiac Imaging Stress Test before Surgery	2,937	3.9%	5.4%	5.3%
Combination Abdominal CT Scan	1,467	3.1%	5.6%	10.5%
Combination Brain/Sinus CT Scan	1,588	3.0%	2.6%	2.7%
Combination Chest CT Scan	568	0.2%	1.3%	2.7%
Follow-up Mammogram/Ultrasound	291	10.7%	8%	8.8%
Lumbar Spine MRI for Low Back Pain	220	38.6%	34.7%	37.2%

Vidant Pungo Hospital

210 East Water St
Belhaven, NC 27810
Phone: 252-943-2111
Fax: 252-944-2236
Type: Critical Access Hospitals
Emergency Services: Yes
Ownership: Voluntary non-profit - Private
Beds: 49

Key Personnel:
Chief of Medical Staff.......... Mark Beamer, MD
CEO/President.............. Kenneth Ragland

Measure	Cases	This Hosp.	State Avg.	U.S. Avg.
Blood Clot Prevention and Treatment				
Anticoagulation Overlap Therapy[5]	-	-	94%	93%
ICU Venous Thromboembolism Prophylaxis[5]	-	-	93%	92%
Incidence of Potentially Preventable VTE[5]	-	-	10%	10%
UFH with Dosages/Platelet Monitoring[5]	-	-	95%	97%
Venous Thromboembolism Prophylaxis[5]	-	-	88%	85%
Warfarin Therapy Discharge Instructions[5]	-	-	81%	75%
Chest Pain/Possible Heart Attack Care				
Aspirin Given Within 24 Hours of Arrival	-	-	97%	96%
Fibrinolytic Meds Within 30 Min. of Arrival	-	-	66%	58%
Average Time to ECG (minutes)	-	-	7	7
Average Time to Transfer (minutes)	-	-	45	60
Children's Asthma Care				
Received Home Management Plan of Care	-	-	89%	88%
Received Reliever Medication	-	-	100%	100%
Received Systemic Corticosteroids	-	-	100%	100%
Emergency Department				
Admittance Decision Time (minutes)	402	78	107	98
Head CT Results Within 45 Min. of Arrival	-	-	60%	57%
Patients Who Left ER Before Being Seen	-	-	3%	2%
Time from ER Arrival to Admit. (minutes)	434	196	300	274
Time from ER Arrival to Discharge (minutes)	-	-	152	134
Time in ER Before Being Evaluated (minutes)	-	-	34	26
Time to Pain Meds for Fractures (minutes)	-	-	67	57
Heart Attack Care				
Aspirin Given at Discharge[5]	-	-	100%	99%
Fibrinolytic Meds Within 30 Min. of Arrival[5]	-	-	75%	54%
PCI Within 90 Minutes of Arrival[5]	-	-	98%	96%
Statin Prescribed at Discharge[5]	-	-	99%	98%
Heart Failure Care				
ACE Inhibitor or ARB for LVSD[1]	-	-	98%	97%
Discharge Instructions Given	12	100%	96%	94%
Evaluation of LVS Function	20	100%	100%	99%
Medicare Spending				
Medicare Spending per Patient (ratio)	-	-	0.94	0.98
Pneumonia Care				
Appropriate Initial Antibiotic Given[1]	-	-	97%	95%
Blood Culture Timing	16	100%	98%	98%
Pregnancy and Delivery Care				
Newborn Deliveries Scheduled Early[5]	-	-	3%	6%
Preventive Care				
Immunization for Influenza	254	98%	93%	90%
Immunization for Pneumonia	436	96%	94%	92%
Stroke Care				
Anticoagulation Therapy for Atrial Fibrillation[5]	-	-	95%	95%
Antithrombotic Therapy Timing[5]	-	-	98%	98%
Assessed for Rehabilitation[5]	-	-	98%	97%
Discharged on Antithrombotic Therapy[5]	-	-	99%	99%
Discharged on Statin Medication[5]	-	-	94%	94%
Thrombolytic Therapy Timing[5]	-	-	64%	66%
Venous Thromboembolism Prophylaxis[5]	-	-	96%	94%
Written Stroke Educational Materials Given[5]	-	-	88%	88%
Surgical Care Improvement Project				
Appropriate Beta Blocker Usage[5]	-	-	99%	98%
Appropriate VTP Within 24 Hours[5]	-	-	99%	98%
Controlled Postoperative Blood Glucose[5]	-	-	98%	97%
Perioperative Temperature Management[5]	-	-	100%	100%
Prophylactic Antibiotic Selection[5]	-	-	99%	99%
Prophylactic Antibiotic Selection (Outpatient)	-	-	98%	98%
Prophylactic Antibiotic Stopped[5]	-	-	99%	98%
Prophylactic Antibiotic Timing[5]	-	-	99%	99%
Prophylactic Antibiotic Timing (Outpatient)	-	-	99%	98%
Urinary Catheter Removal[5]	-	-	99%	97%
Survey of Patients' Hospital Experiences				
Area Around Room 'Always' Quiet at Night[6]	<100	79%	64%	61%
Doctors 'Always' Communicated Well[6]	<100	78%	83%	82%
Home Recovery Information Given[6]	<100	90%	87%	85%
Hospital Given 9 or 10 on 10 Point Scale[6]	<100	81%	71%	71%
Meds 'Always' Explained Before Given[6]	<100	73%	65%	64%
Nurses 'Always' Communicated Well[6]	<100	81%	81%	79%
Pain 'Always' Well Controlled[6]	<100	77%	72%	71%
Room and Bathroom 'Always' Clean[6]	<100	79%	72%	73%
Timely Help 'Always' Received[6]	<100	76%	68%	68%
Would Definitely Recommend Hospital[6]	<100	69%	70%	71%
Use of Medical Imaging				
Cardiac Imaging Stress Test before Surgery	-	-	5.4%	5.3%
Combination Abdominal CT Scan	-	-	5.6%	10.5%
Combination Brain/Sinus CT Scan	-	-	2.6%	2.7%
Combination Chest CT Scan	-	-	1.3%	2.7%
Follow-up Mammogram/Ultrasound	-	-	8%	8.8%
Lumbar Spine MRI for Low Back Pain	-	-	34.7%	37.2%

Blowing Rock Hospital

418 Chestnut Drive
Blowing Rock, NC 28605
Phone: 828-295-3136
Fax: 828-295-6698
URL: www.blowingrockhospital.org
Type: Critical Access Hospitals
Emergency Services: Yes
Ownership: Voluntary non-profit - Private
Beds: 100

Key Personnel:
Chief of Medical Staff.......... Charles Davant, III
CEO/President.............. Alice Salthouse

Measure	Cases	This Hosp.	State Avg.	U.S. Avg.
Blood Clot Prevention and Treatment				
Anticoagulation Overlap Therapy[5]	-	-	94%	93%
ICU Venous Thromboembolism Prophylaxis[5]	-	-	93%	92%
Incidence of Potentially Preventable VTE[5]	-	-	10%	10%
UFH with Dosages/Platelet Monitoring[5]	-	-	95%	97%
Venous Thromboembolism Prophylaxis[5]	-	-	88%	85%
Warfarin Therapy Discharge Instructions[5]	-	-	81%	75%
Chest Pain/Possible Heart Attack Care				
Aspirin Given Within 24 Hours of Arrival	-	-	97%	96%
Fibrinolytic Meds Within 30 Min. of Arrival	-	-	66%	58%
Average Time to ECG (minutes)	-	-	7	7
Average Time to Transfer (minutes)	-	-	45	60
Children's Asthma Care				
Received Home Management Plan of Care	-	-	89%	88%
Received Reliever Medication	-	-	100%	100%
Received Systemic Corticosteroids	-	-	100%	100%
Emergency Department				
Admittance Decision Time (minutes)[5]	-	-	107	98
Head CT Results Within 45 Min. of Arrival	-	-	60%	57%
Patients Who Left ER Before Being Seen	-	-	3%	2%
Time from ER Arrival to Admit. (minutes)[5]	-	-	300	274
Time from ER Arrival to Discharge (minutes)	-	-	152	134
Time in ER Before Being Evaluated (minutes)	-	-	34	26
Time to Pain Meds for Fractures (minutes)	-	-	67	57
Heart Attack Care				
Aspirin Given at Discharge[5]	-	-	100%	99%
Fibrinolytic Meds Within 30 Min. of Arrival[5]	-	-	75%	54%
PCI Within 90 Minutes of Arrival[5]	-	-	98%	96%
Statin Prescribed at Discharge[5]	-	-	99%	98%
Heart Failure Care				
ACE Inhibitor or ARB for LVSD[5]	-	-	98%	97%
Discharge Instructions Given[5]	-	-	96%	94%
Evaluation of LVS Function[5]	-	-	100%	99%
Medicare Spending				
Medicare Spending per Patient (ratio)	-	-	0.94	0.98
Pneumonia Care				
Appropriate Initial Antibiotic Given[5]	-	-	97%	95%
Blood Culture Timing[5]	-	-	98%	98%
Pregnancy and Delivery Care				
Newborn Deliveries Scheduled Early[5]	-	-	3%	6%
Preventive Care				
Immunization for Influenza[5]	-	-	93%	90%
Immunization for Pneumonia[5]	-	-	94%	92%
Stroke Care				
Anticoagulation Therapy for Atrial Fibrillation[5]	-	-	95%	95%
Antithrombotic Therapy Timing[5]	-	-	98%	98%
Assessed for Rehabilitation[5]	-	-	98%	97%
Discharged on Antithrombotic Therapy[5]	-	-	99%	99%
Discharged on Statin Medication[5]	-	-	94%	94%
Thrombolytic Therapy Timing[5]	-	-	64%	66%
Venous Thromboembolism Prophylaxis[5]	-	-	96%	94%
Written Stroke Educational Materials Given[5]	-	-	88%	88%
Surgical Care Improvement Project				
Appropriate Beta Blocker Usage[5]	-	-	99%	98%
Appropriate VTP Within 24 Hours[5]	-	-	99%	98%
Controlled Postoperative Blood Glucose[5]	-	-	98%	97%
Perioperative Temperature Management[5]	-	-	100%	100%
Prophylactic Antibiotic Selection[5]	-	-	99%	99%
Prophylactic Antibiotic Selection (Outpatient)	-	-	98%	98%
Prophylactic Antibiotic Stopped[5]	-	-	99%	98%
Prophylactic Antibiotic Timing[5]	-	-	99%	99%
Prophylactic Antibiotic Timing (Outpatient)	-	-	99%	98%
Urinary Catheter Removal[5]	-	-	99%	97%
Survey of Patients' Hospital Experiences				
Area Around Room 'Always' Quiet at Night[5]	-	-	64%	61%
Doctors 'Always' Communicated Well[5]	-	-	83%	82%
Home Recovery Information Given[5]	-	-	87%	85%
Hospital Given 9 or 10 on 10 Point Scale[5]	-	-	71%	71%
Meds 'Always' Explained Before Given[5]	-	-	65%	64%
Nurses 'Always' Communicated Well[5]	-	-	81%	79%
Pain 'Always' Well Controlled[5]	-	-	72%	71%
Room and Bathroom 'Always' Clean[5]	-	-	72%	73%
Timely Help 'Always' Received[5]	-	-	68%	68%
Would Definitely Recommend Hospital[5]	-	-	70%	71%
Use of Medical Imaging				
Cardiac Imaging Stress Test before Surgery	-	-	5.4%	5.3%
Combination Abdominal CT Scan	-	-	5.6%	10.5%
Combination Brain/Sinus CT Scan	-	-	2.6%	2.7%
Combination Chest CT Scan	-	-	1.3%	2.7%
Follow-up Mammogram/Ultrasound	-	-	8%	8.8%
Lumbar Spine MRI for Low Back Pain	-	-	34.7%	37.2%

NOTE: Hospital profiles are in alphabetical order by state, then city, then hospital within the city; Rankings exclude hospitals with less than 25 cases except for patient surveys which excludes hospitals with less than 100 cases; (a) 100-299 cases; (1) The number of cases/patients is too few to report; (2) Data submitted were based on a sample of cases/patients; (3) Results are based on a shorter time period than required; (4) Data suppressed by CMS for one or more quarters; (5) Results are not available for this reporting period; (6) Fewer than 100 patients completed the HCAHPS survey; (7) No cases met the criteria for this measure; (8) The lower limit of the confidence interval cannot be calculated if the number of observed infections equals zero; (9) No data are available from the state/territory for this reporting period; (10) The scores shown reflect fewer than 50 completed surveys; (11) There were discrepancies in the data collection process; (12) This measure does not apply to this hospital for this reporting period; (13) Results cannot be calculated for this reporting period; (14) The results for this state are combined with nearby states to protect confidentiality; Please refer to the User's Guide for a full explanation of data.

Watauga Medical Center

336 Deerfield Road
Boone, NC 28607
Phone: 828-262-4100
Fax: 828-262-4103
URL: www.wataugamc.org
Type: Acute Care Hospitals
Emergency Services: Yes
Ownership: Government - Local
Beds: 127

Key Personnel:

Emergency Room . . . . Allen Brandon, MD
Infection Control. . . . . Anne Brown
Operating Room. . . . . Peggy Burdiss
Intensive Care Unit. . . . . Terry McGuire
Quality Assurance . . . . Maran Sigmon
CEO/President. . . . . Richard G Sparks

Measure	Cases	This Hosp.	State Avg.	U.S. Avg.
Blood Clot Prevention and Treatment				
Anticoagulation Overlap Therapy[2]	27	96%	94%	93%
ICU Venous Thromboembolism Prophylaxis[2]	105	89%	93%	92%
Incidence of Potentially Preventable VTE[1,2]	-	-	10%	10%
UFH with Dosages/Platelet Monitoring[2]	18	100%	95%	97%
Venous Thromboembolism Prophylaxis[2]	245	87%	88%	85%
Warfarin Therapy Discharge Instructions[2]	22	91%	81%	75%
Chest Pain/Possible Heart Attack Care				
Aspirin Given Within 24 Hours of Arrival	47	100%	97%	96%
Fibrinolytic Meds Within 30 Min. of Arrival[1]	-	-	66%	58%
Average Time to ECG (minutes)	50	6	7	7
Average Time to Transfer (minutes)[7]	-	-	45	60
Children's Asthma Care				
Received Home Management Plan of Care	-	-	89%	88%
Received Reliever Medication	-	-	100%	100%
Received Systemic Corticosteroids	-	-	100%	100%
Emergency Department				
Admittance Decision Time (minutes)[2]	458	134	107	98
Head CT Results Within 45 Min. of Arrival[1]	-	-	60%	57%
Patients Who Left ER Before Being Seen	21,320	2%	3%	2%
Time from ER Arrival to Admit. (minutes)[2]	478	283	300	274
Time from ER Arrival to Discharge (minutes)	342	154	152	134
Time in ER Before Being Evaluated (minutes)	381	35	34	26
Time to Pain Meds for Fractures (minutes)	134	74	67	57
Heart Attack Care				
Aspirin Given at Discharge	68	100%	100%	99%
Fibrinolytic Meds Within 30 Min. of Arrival[7]	-	-	75%	54%
PCI Within 90 Minutes of Arrival[1]	-	-	98%	96%
Statin Prescribed at Discharge	65	97%	99%	98%
Heart Failure Care				
ACE Inhibitor or ARB for LVSD	16	94%	98%	97%
Discharge Instructions Given	59	86%	96%	94%
Evaluation of LVS Function	83	100%	100%	99%
Medicare Spending				
Medicare Spending per Patient (ratio)	-	0.95	0.94	0.98
Pneumonia Care				
Appropriate Initial Antibiotic Given	110	95%	97%	95%
Blood Culture Timing	177	97%	98%	98%
Pregnancy and Delivery Care				
Newborn Deliveries Scheduled Early	32	9%	3%	6%
Preventive Care				
Immunization for Influenza[2]	363	91%	93%	90%
Immunization for Pneumonia[2]	465	91%	94%	92%
Stroke Care				
Anticoagulation Therapy for Atrial Fibrillation[1]	-	-	95%	95%
Antithrombotic Therapy Timing	55	96%	98%	98%
Assessed for Rehabilitation	61	97%	98%	97%
Discharged on Antithrombotic Therapy	59	100%	99%	99%
Discharged on Statin Medication	47	94%	94%	94%
Thrombolytic Therapy Timing[1]	-	-	64%	66%
Venous Thromboembolism Prophylaxis	60	85%	96%	94%
Written Stroke Educational Materials Given	33	94%	88%	88%
Surgical Care Improvement Project				
Appropriate Beta Blocker Usage	75	99%	99%	98%
Appropriate VTP Within 24 Hours	273	98%	99%	98%
Controlled Postoperative Blood Glucose[7]	-	-	98%	97%
Perioperative Temperature Management	293	100%	100%	100%
Prophylactic Antibiotic Selection	218	100%	99%	99%
Prophylactic Antibiotic Selection (Outpatient)	164	98%	98%	98%
Prophylactic Antibiotic Stopped	213	97%	99%	98%
Prophylactic Antibiotic Timing	219	99%	99%	99%
Prophylactic Antibiotic Timing (Outpatient)	164	100%	99%	98%
Urinary Catheter Removal	75	89%	99%	97%
Survey of Patients' Hospital Experiences				
Area Around Room 'Always' Quiet at Night	300+	51%	64%	61%
Doctors 'Always' Communicated Well	300+	79%	83%	82%
Home Recovery Information Given	300+	84%	87%	85%
Hospital Given 9 or 10 on 10 Point Scale	300+	60%	71%	71%
Meds 'Always' Explained Before Given	300+	61%	65%	64%
Nurses 'Always' Communicated Well	300+	74%	81%	79%
Pain 'Always' Well Controlled	300+	68%	72%	71%
Room and Bathroom 'Always' Clean	300+	73%	72%	73%
Timely Help 'Always' Received	300+	60%	68%	68%
Would Definitely Recommend Hospital	300+	64%	70%	71%
Use of Medical Imaging				
Cardiac Imaging Stress Test before Surgery	578	2.6%	5.4%	5.3%
Combination Abdominal CT Scan	783	1.8%	5.6%	10.5%
Combination Brain/Sinus CT Scan	537	3.9%	2.6%	2.7%
Combination Chest CT Scan	606	0.3%	1.3%	2.7%
Follow-up Mammogram/Ultrasound	1,509	8.0%	8%	8.8%
Lumbar Spine MRI for Low Back Pain	61	36.1%	34.7%	37.2%

Transylvania Regional Hospital

90 Hospital Drive PO Box 1116
Brevard, NC 28712
Phone: 828-883-5302
Fax: 828-883-5370
URL: www.tchospital.org
Type: Critical Access Hospitals
Emergency Services: Yes
Ownership: Voluntary non-profit - Private
Beds: 88

Key Personnel:

Radiology. . . . . Timothy P Desmond
Chief of Medical Staff. . . . . Carmelo Hernandez

Measure	Cases	This Hosp.	State Avg.	U.S. Avg.
Blood Clot Prevention and Treatment				
Anticoagulation Overlap Therapy[1,2]	-	-	94%	93%
ICU Venous Thromboembolism Prophylaxis[2]	24	92%	93%	92%
Incidence of Potentially Preventable VTE[2,7]	-	-	10%	10%
UFH with Dosages/Platelet Monitoring[2,7]	-	-	95%	97%
Venous Thromboembolism Prophylaxis[2]	189	97%	88%	85%
Warfarin Therapy Discharge Instructions[1,2]	-	-	81%	75%
Chest Pain/Possible Heart Attack Care				
Aspirin Given Within 24 Hours of Arrival	46	96%	97%	96%
Fibrinolytic Meds Within 30 Min. of Arrival[7]	-	-	66%	58%
Average Time to ECG (minutes)	47	6	7	7
Average Time to Transfer (minutes)	11	48	45	60
Children's Asthma Care				
Received Home Management Plan of Care	-	-	89%	88%
Received Reliever Medication	-	-	100%	100%
Received Systemic Corticosteroids	-	-	100%	100%
Emergency Department				
Admittance Decision Time (minutes)[2,3]	344	63	107	98
Head CT Results Within 45 Min. of Arrival[1,3]	-	-	60%	57%
Patients Who Left ER Before Being Seen	15,901	3%	3%	2%
Time from ER Arrival to Admit. (minutes)[2,3]	404	272	300	274
Time from ER Arrival to Discharge (minutes)[3]	386	156	152	134
Time in ER Before Being Evaluated (minutes)[3]	392	41	34	26
Time to Pain Meds for Fractures (minutes)[3]	57	113	67	57
Heart Attack Care				
Aspirin Given at Discharge[1,3]	-	-	100%	99%
Fibrinolytic Meds Within 30 Min. of Arrival[3,7]	-	-	75%	54%
PCI Within 90 Minutes of Arrival[3,7]	-	-	98%	96%
Statin Prescribed at Discharge[3,7]	-	-	99%	98%
Heart Failure Care				
ACE Inhibitor or ARB for LVSD	12	100%	98%	97%
Discharge Instructions Given	20	100%	96%	94%
Evaluation of LVS Function	40	100%	100%	99%
Medicare Spending				
Medicare Spending per Patient (ratio)	-	-	0.94	0.98
Pneumonia Care				
Appropriate Initial Antibiotic Given	55	100%	97%	95%
Blood Culture Timing	89	100%	98%	98%
Pregnancy and Delivery Care				
Newborn Deliveries Scheduled Early[2]	18	6%	3%	6%
Preventive Care				
Immunization for Influenza[5]	-	-	93%	90%
Immunization for Pneumonia[2,3]	421	92%	94%	92%
Stroke Care				
Anticoagulation Therapy for Atrial Fibrillation[1]	-	-	95%	95%
Antithrombotic Therapy Timing	18	100%	98%	98%
Assessed for Rehabilitation	20	100%	98%	97%
Discharged on Antithrombotic Therapy	17	100%	99%	99%
Discharged on Statin Medication	14	93%	94%	94%
Thrombolytic Therapy Timing[7]	-	-	64%	66%
Venous Thromboembolism Prophylaxis	19	100%	96%	94%
Written Stroke Educational Materials Given[1]	-	-	88%	88%
Surgical Care Improvement Project				
Appropriate Beta Blocker Usage	34	100%	99%	98%
Appropriate VTP Within 24 Hours	127	98%	99%	98%
Controlled Postoperative Blood Glucose[7]	-	-	98%	97%
Perioperative Temperature Management	158	100%	100%	100%
Prophylactic Antibiotic Selection	118	99%	99%	99%
Prophylactic Antibiotic Selection (Outpatient)	50	98%	98%	98%
Prophylactic Antibiotic Stopped	112	100%	99%	98%
Prophylactic Antibiotic Timing	118	100%	99%	99%
Prophylactic Antibiotic Timing (Outpatient)	23	96%	99%	98%
Urinary Catheter Removal	41	100%	99%	97%
Survey of Patients' Hospital Experiences				
Area Around Room 'Always' Quiet at Night	300+	67%	64%	61%
Doctors 'Always' Communicated Well	300+	82%	83%	82%
Home Recovery Information Given	300+	86%	87%	85%
Hospital Given 9 or 10 on 10 Point Scale	300+	75%	71%	71%
Meds 'Always' Explained Before Given	300+	70%	65%	64%
Nurses 'Always' Communicated Well	300+	82%	81%	79%
Pain 'Always' Well Controlled	300+	76%	72%	71%
Room and Bathroom 'Always' Clean	300+	81%	72%	73%
Timely Help 'Always' Received	300+	77%	68%	68%
Would Definitely Recommend Hospital	300+	74%	70%	71%
Use of Medical Imaging				
Cardiac Imaging Stress Test before Surgery	478	6.3%	5.4%	5.3%
Combination Abdominal CT Scan	680	3.1%	5.6%	10.5%
Combination Brain/Sinus CT Scan	748	1.2%	2.6%	2.7%
Combination Chest CT Scan	364	0.3%	1.3%	2.7%
Follow-up Mammogram/Ultrasound	940	6.8%	8%	8.8%
Lumbar Spine MRI for Low Back Pain	86	30.2%	34.7%	37.2%

Medwest Swain

45 Plateau Street
Bryson City, NC 28713
Phone: 828-488-2155
URL: www.westcarehealth.org
Type: Critical Access Hospitals
Emergency Services: Yes
Ownership: Voluntary non-profit - Private

Measure	Cases	This Hosp.	State Avg.	U.S. Avg.
Blood Clot Prevention and Treatment				
Anticoagulation Overlap Therapy[1,2]	-	-	94%	93%
ICU Venous Thromboembolism Prophylaxis[2,3]	-	-	93%	92%
Incidence of Potentially Preventable VTE[2,3]	-	-	10%	10%
UFH with Dosages/Platelet Monitoring[2,3]	-	-	95%	97%
Venous Thromboembolism Prophylaxis[2,3]	34	97%	88%	85%
Warfarin Therapy Discharge Instructions[1,2]	-	-	81%	75%
Chest Pain/Possible Heart Attack Care				
Aspirin Given Within 24 Hours of Arrival	-	-	97%	96%
Fibrinolytic Meds Within 30 Min. of Arrival	-	-	66%	58%
Average Time to ECG (minutes)	-	-	7	7
Average Time to Transfer (minutes)	-	-	45	60
Children's Asthma Care				
Received Home Management Plan of Care	-	-	89%	88%
Received Reliever Medication	-	-	100%	100%
Received Systemic Corticosteroids	-	-	100%	100%
Emergency Department				
Admittance Decision Time (minutes)[2]	340	69	107	98
Head CT Results Within 45 Min. of Arrival	-	-	60%	57%
Patients Who Left ER Before Being Seen	-	-	3%	2%
Time from ER Arrival to Admit. (minutes)[2]	340	220	300	274
Time from ER Arrival to Discharge (minutes)	-	-	152	134
Time in ER Before Being Evaluated (minutes)	-	-	34	26
Time to Pain Meds for Fractures (minutes)	-	-	67	57

NOTE: Hospital profiles are in alphabetical order by state, then city, then hospital within the city; Rankings exclude hospitals with less than 25 cases except for patient surveys which excludes hospitals with less than 100 cases; (a) 100-299 cases; (1) The number of cases/patients is too few to report; (2) Data submitted were based on a sample of cases/patients; (3) Results are based on a shorter time period than required; (4) Data suppressed by CMS for one or more quarters; (5) Results are not available for this reporting period; (6) Fewer than 100 patients completed the HCAHPS survey; (7) No cases met the criteria for this measure; (8) The lower limit of the confidence interval cannot be calculated if the number of observed infections equals zero; (9) No data are available from the state/territory for this reporting period; (10) The scores shown reflect fewer than 50 completed surveys; (11) There were discrepancies in the data collection process; (12) This measure does not apply to this hospital for this reporting period; (13) Results cannot be calculated for this reporting period; (14) The results for this state are combined with nearby states to protect confidentiality; Please refer to the User's Guide for a full explanation of data.

Measure	Cases	This Hosp.	State Avg.	U.S. Avg.
Heart Attack Care				
Aspirin Given at Discharge[1,3]	-	-	100%	99%
Fibrinolytic Meds Within 30 Min. of Arrival[3,7]	-	-	75%	54%
PCI Within 90 Minutes of Arrival[3,7]	-	-	98%	96%
Statin Prescribed at Discharge[1,3]	-	-	99%	98%
Heart Failure Care				
ACE Inhibitor or ARB for LVSD[1]	-	-	98%	97%
Discharge Instructions Given	22	86%	96%	94%
Evaluation of LVS Function	26	100%	100%	99%
Medicare Spending				
Medicare Spending per Patient (ratio)	-	-	0.94	0.98
Pneumonia Care				
Appropriate Initial Antibiotic Given	33	100%	97%	95%
Blood Culture Timing	54	100%	98%	98%
Pregnancy and Delivery Care				
Newborn Deliveries Scheduled Early[3,7]	-	-	3%	6%
Preventive Care				
Immunization for Influenza[2]	151	96%	93%	90%
Immunization for Pneumonia[2]	263	96%	94%	92%
Stroke Care				
Anticoagulation Therapy for Atrial Fibrillation[3,7]	-	-	95%	95%
Antithrombotic Therapy Timing[1,3]	-	-	98%	98%
Assessed for Rehabilitation[1,3]	-	-	98%	97%
Discharged on Antithrombotic Therapy[1,3]	-	-	99%	99%
Discharged on Statin Medication[1,3]	-	-	94%	94%
Thrombolytic Therapy Timing[3,7]	-	-	64%	66%
Venous Thromboembolism Prophylaxis[1,3]	-	-	96%	94%
Written Stroke Educational Materials Given[1,3]	-	-	88%	88%
Surgical Care Improvement Project				
Appropriate Beta Blocker Usage[5]	-	-	99%	98%
Appropriate VTP Within 24 Hours[5]	-	-	99%	98%
Controlled Postoperative Blood Glucose[5]	-	-	98%	97%
Perioperative Temperature Management[5]	-	-	100%	100%
Prophylactic Antibiotic Selection[5]	-	-	99%	99%
Prophylactic Antibiotic Selection (Outpatient)	-	-	98%	98%
Prophylactic Antibiotic Stopped[5]	-	-	99%	98%
Prophylactic Antibiotic Timing[5]	-	-	99%	99%
Prophylactic Antibiotic Timing (Outpatient)	-	-	99%	98%
Urinary Catheter Removal[5]	-	-	99%	97%
Survey of Patients' Hospital Experiences				
Area Around Room 'Always' Quiet at Night[5]	-	-	64%	61%
Doctors 'Always' Communicated Well[5]	-	-	83%	82%
Home Recovery Information Given[5]	-	-	87%	85%
Hospital Given 9 or 10 on 10 Point Scale[5]	-	-	71%	71%
Meds 'Always' Explained Before Given[5]	-	-	65%	64%
Nurses 'Always' Communicated Well[5]	-	-	81%	79%
Pain 'Always' Well Controlled[5]	-	-	72%	71%
Room and Bathroom 'Always' Clean[5]	-	-	72%	73%
Timely Help 'Always' Received[5]	-	-	68%	68%
Would Definitely Recommend Hospital[5]	-	-	70%	71%
Use of Medical Imaging				
Cardiac Imaging Stress Test before Surgery	-	-	5.4%	5.3%
Combination Abdominal CT Scan	-	-	5.6%	10.5%
Combination Brain/Sinus CT Scan	-	-	2.6%	2.7%
Combination Chest CT Scan	-	-	1.3%	2.7%
Follow-up Mammogram/Ultrasound	-	-	8%	8.8%
Lumbar Spine MRI for Low Back Pain	-	-	34.7%	37.2%

Pender Memorial Hospital

507 E Fremont St
Burgaw, NC 28425
URL: www.nhhn.org
Phone: 910-259-5451
Fax: 910-259-7136
Type: Critical Access Hospitals
Emergency Services: Yes
Ownership: Government - Local
Beds: 68

Key Personnel:

Chief of Medical Staff.......... Naseem Nasrallah, MD
Operating Room.............. Karenie Schaller
Anesthesiology............... Don Shinoskie
Quality Assurance .... Verna Walkins
Radiology................... Walter C Whitehurst, Jr

Measure	Cases	This Hosp.	State Avg.	U.S. Avg.
Blood Clot Prevention and Treatment				
Anticoagulation Overlap Therapy[5]	-	-	94%	93%
ICU Venous Thromboembolism Prophylaxis[5]	-	-	93%	92%
Incidence of Potentially Preventable VTE[5]	-	-	10%	10%
UFH with Dosages/Platelet Monitoring[5]	-	-	95%	97%
Venous Thromboembolism Prophylaxis[5]	-	-	88%	85%
Warfarin Therapy Discharge Instructions[5]	-	-	81%	75%
Chest Pain/Possible Heart Attack Care				
Aspirin Given Within 24 Hours of Arrival	-	-	97%	96%
Fibrinolytic Meds Within 30 Min. of Arrival	-	-	66%	58%
Average Time to ECG (minutes)	-	-	7	7
Average Time to Transfer (minutes)	-	-	45	60
Children's Asthma Care				
Received Home Management Plan of Care	-	-	89%	88%
Received Reliever Medication	-	-	100%	100%
Received Systemic Corticosteroids	-	-	100%	100%
Emergency Department				
Admittance Decision Time (minutes)[5]	-	-	107	98
Head CT Results Within 45 Min. of Arrival	-	-	60%	57%
Patients Who Left ER Before Being Seen	-	-	3%	2%
Time from ER Arrival to Admit. (minutes)[5]	-	-	300	274
Time from ER Arrival to Discharge (minutes)	-	-	152	134
Time in ER Before Being Evaluated (minutes)	-	-	34	26
Time to Pain Meds for Fractures (minutes)	-	-	67	57
Heart Attack Care				
Aspirin Given at Discharge[5]	-	-	100%	99%
Fibrinolytic Meds Within 30 Min. of Arrival[5]	-	-	75%	54%
PCI Within 90 Minutes of Arrival[5]	-	-	98%	96%
Statin Prescribed at Discharge[5]	-	-	99%	98%
Heart Failure Care				
ACE Inhibitor or ARB for LVSD[1,3]	-	-	98%	97%
Discharge Instructions Given[1,3]	-	-	96%	94%
Evaluation of LVS Function[3]	13	100%	100%	99%
Medicare Spending				
Medicare Spending per Patient (ratio)	-	-	0.94	0.98
Pneumonia Care				
Appropriate Initial Antibiotic Given[3]	18	94%	97%	95%
Blood Culture Timing[3]	25	100%	98%	98%
Pregnancy and Delivery Care				
Newborn Deliveries Scheduled Early[5]	-	-	3%	6%
Preventive Care				
Immunization for Influenza[5]			93%	90%
Immunization for Pneumonia[5]			94%	92%
Stroke Care				
Anticoagulation Therapy for Atrial Fibrillation[5]	-	-	95%	95%
Antithrombotic Therapy Timing[5]	-	-	98%	98%
Assessed for Rehabilitation[5]	-	-	98%	97%
Discharged on Antithrombotic Therapy[5]	-	-	99%	99%
Discharged on Statin Medication[5]	-	-	94%	94%
Thrombolytic Therapy Timing[5]	-	-	64%	66%
Venous Thromboembolism Prophylaxis[5]	-	-	96%	94%
Written Stroke Educational Materials Given[5]	-	-	88%	88%
Surgical Care Improvement Project				
Appropriate Beta Blocker Usage[3,7]	-	-	99%	98%
Appropriate VTP Within 24 Hours[1,3]	-	-	99%	98%
Controlled Postoperative Blood Glucose[3,7]	-	-	98%	97%
Perioperative Temperature Management[1,3]	-	-	100%	100%
Prophylactic Antibiotic Selection[1,3]	-	-	99%	99%
Prophylactic Antibiotic Selection (Outpatient)	-	-	98%	98%
Prophylactic Antibiotic Stopped[1,3]	-	-	99%	98%
Prophylactic Antibiotic Timing[1,3]	-	-	99%	99%
Prophylactic Antibiotic Timing (Outpatient)	-	-	99%	98%
Urinary Catheter Removal[1,3]	-	-	99%	97%
Survey of Patients' Hospital Experiences				
Area Around Room 'Always' Quiet at Night	(a)	69%	64%	61%
Doctors 'Always' Communicated Well	(a)	85%	83%	82%
Home Recovery Information Given	(a)	87%	87%	85%
Hospital Given 9 or 10 on 10 Point Scale	(a)	66%	71%	71%
Meds 'Always' Explained Before Given	(a)	72%	65%	64%
Nurses 'Always' Communicated Well	(a)	83%	81%	79%
Pain 'Always' Well Controlled	(a)	71%	72%	71%
Room and Bathroom 'Always' Clean	(a)	70%	72%	73%
Timely Help 'Always' Received	(a)	77%	68%	68%
Would Definitely Recommend Hospital	(a)	65%	70%	71%
Use of Medical Imaging				
Cardiac Imaging Stress Test before Surgery	-	-	5.4%	5.3%
Combination Abdominal CT Scan	-	-	5.6%	10.5%
Combination Brain/Sinus CT Scan	-	-	2.6%	2.7%
Combination Chest CT Scan	-	-	1.3%	2.7%
Follow-up Mammogram/Ultrasound	-	-	8%	8.8%
Lumbar Spine MRI for Low Back Pain	-	-	34.7%	37.2%

Alamance Regional Medical Center

1240 Huffman Mill Rd
Burlington, NC 27216
E-mail: info@armc.com
URL: www.armc.com
Phone: 336-538-7000
Fax: 336-538-7425
Type: Acute Care Hospitals
Emergency Services: Yes
Ownership: Voluntary non-profit - Private
Beds: 298

Key Personnel:

Chief of Medical Staff.......... Barbara Aldridge
Radiology.................. Geoffrey H Browne
CEO/President............... Preston Hammock
Emergency Room .... Linda Lawter

Measure	Cases	This Hosp.	State Avg.	U.S. Avg.
Blood Clot Prevention and Treatment				
Anticoagulation Overlap Therapy[2]	56	62%	94%	93%
ICU Venous Thromboembolism Prophylaxis[2]	75	81%	93%	92%
Incidence of Potentially Preventable VTE[1,2]	-	-	10%	10%
UFH with Dosages/Platelet Monitoring[2]	54	80%	95%	97%
Venous Thromboembolism Prophylaxis[2]	324	73%	88%	85%
Warfarin Therapy Discharge Instructions[2]	37	11%	81%	75%
Chest Pain/Possible Heart Attack Care				
Aspirin Given Within 24 Hours of Arrival	53	98%	97%	96%
Fibrinolytic Meds Within 30 Min. of Arrival[7]	-	-	66%	58%
Average Time to ECG (minutes)	53	9	7	7
Average Time to Transfer (minutes)	23	82	45	60
Children's Asthma Care				
Received Home Management Plan of Care	-	-	89%	88%
Received Reliever Medication	-	-	100%	100%
Received Systemic Corticosteroids	-	-	100%	100%
Emergency Department				
Admittance Decision Time (minutes)[2]	749	140	107	98
Head CT Results Within 45 Min. of Arrival	21	33%	60%	57%
Patients Who Left ER Before Being Seen	55,193	5%	3%	2%
Time from ER Arrival to Admit. (minutes)[2]	1,023	343	300	274
Time from ER Arrival to Discharge (minutes)	395	203	152	134
Time in ER Before Being Evaluated (minutes)	329	98	34	26
Time to Pain Meds for Fractures (minutes)	232	101	67	57
Heart Attack Care				
Aspirin Given at Discharge	189	99%	100%	99%
Fibrinolytic Meds Within 30 Min. of Arrival[7]	-	-	75%	54%
PCI Within 90 Minutes of Arrival	14	93%	98%	96%
Statin Prescribed at Discharge	175	99%	99%	98%
Heart Failure Care				
ACE Inhibitor or ARB for LVSD	109	97%	98%	97%
Discharge Instructions Given	312	96%	96%	94%
Evaluation of LVS Function	421	100%	100%	99%
Medicare Spending				
Medicare Spending per Patient (ratio)	-	0.93	0.94	0.98
Pneumonia Care				
Appropriate Initial Antibiotic Given	215	97%	97%	95%
Blood Culture Timing	309	90%	98%	98%
Pregnancy and Delivery Care				
Newborn Deliveries Scheduled Early	82	5%	3%	6%
Preventive Care				
Immunization for Influenza[2]	555	92%	93%	90%
Immunization for Pneumonia[2]	847	83%	94%	92%
Stroke Care				
Anticoagulation Therapy for Atrial Fibrillation	22	91%	95%	95%
Antithrombotic Therapy Timing	160	98%	98%	98%
Assessed for Rehabilitation	164	98%	98%	97%
Discharged on Antithrombotic Therapy	164	98%	99%	99%
Discharged on Statin Medication	118	91%	94%	94%
Thrombolytic Therapy Timing	69	0%	64%	66%
Venous Thromboembolism Prophylaxis	151	88%	96%	94%
Written Stroke Educational Materials Given	107	69%	88%	88%
Surgical Care Improvement Project				
Appropriate Beta Blocker Usage	211	96%	99%	98%

NOTE: Hospital profiles are in alphabetical order by state, then city, then hospital within the city; Rankings exclude hospitals with less than 25 cases except for patient surveys which excludes hospitals with less than 100 cases; (a) 100-299 cases; (1) The number of cases/patients is too few to report; (2) Data submitted were based on a sample of cases/patients; (3) Results are based on a shorter time period than required; (4) Data suppressed by CMS for one or more quarters; (5) Results are not available for this reporting period; (6) Fewer than 100 patients completed the HCAHPS survey; (7) No cases met the criteria for this measure; (8) The lower limit of the confidence interval cannot be calculated if the number of observed infections equals zero; (9) No data are available from the state/territory for this reporting period; (10) The scores shown reflect fewer than 50 completed surveys; (11) There were discrepancies in the data collection process; (12) This measure does not apply to this hospital for this reporting period; (13) Results cannot be calculated for this reporting period; (14) The results for this state are combined with nearby states to protect confidentiality; Please refer to the User's Guide for a full explanation of data.

Measure	Cases	This Hosp.	State Avg.	U.S. Avg.
Appropriate VTP Within 24 Hours	666	96%	99%	98%
Controlled Postoperative Blood Glucose[7]	-	-	98%	97%
Perioperative Temperature Management	736	100%	100%	100%
Prophylactic Antibiotic Selection	516	97%	99%	99%
Prophylactic Antibiotic Selection (Outpatient)	226	90%	98%	98%
Prophylactic Antibiotic Stopped	504	95%	99%	98%
Prophylactic Antibiotic Timing	516	99%	99%	99%
Prophylactic Antibiotic Timing (Outpatient)	226	100%	99%	98%
Urinary Catheter Removal	578	96%	99%	97%
Survey of Patients' Hospital Experiences				
Area Around Room 'Always' Quiet at Night	300+	58%	64%	61%
Doctors 'Always' Communicated Well	300+	81%	83%	82%
Home Recovery Information Given	300+	87%	87%	85%
Hospital Given 9 or 10 on 10 Point Scale	300+	68%	71%	71%
Meds 'Always' Explained Before Given	300+	66%	65%	64%
Nurses 'Always' Communicated Well	300+	79%	81%	79%
Pain 'Always' Well Controlled	300+	72%	72%	71%
Room and Bathroom 'Always' Clean	300+	73%	72%	73%
Timely Help 'Always' Received	300+	65%	68%	68%
Would Definitely Recommend Hospital	300+	65%	70%	71%
Use of Medical Imaging				
Cardiac Imaging Stress Test before Surgery	174	9.2%	5.4%	5.3%
Combination Abdominal CT Scan	918	4.7%	5.6%	10.5%
Combination Brain/Sinus CT Scan	972	1.4%	2.6%	2.7%
Combination Chest CT Scan	709	0.1%	1.3%	2.7%
Follow-up Mammogram/Ultrasound	2,402	6.8%	8%	8.8%
Lumbar Spine MRI for Low Back Pain	193	35.8%	34.7%	37.2%

Wakemed - Cary Hospital

1900 Kildare Farm Road
Cary, NC 27518
Phone: 919-350-2550
Fax: 919-233-2555
URL: www.wakemed.org
Type: Acute Care Hospitals
Emergency Services: Yes
Ownership: Voluntary non-profit - Private
Beds: 156

Key Personnel:
Infection Control. . . . . Robin Carver
Radiology. . . . . Libby Dove
Quality Assurance . . . . Maggie Driscol
CEO/President. . . . . Donald R. Gintzig, MD
Ambulatory Care . . . . Carolyn Knaup, RN, MHA
Chief of Medical Staff. . . . . H West Lawson
Operating Room. . . . . Maria Maag

Measure	Cases	This Hosp.	State Avg.	U.S. Avg.
Blood Clot Prevention and Treatment				
Anticoagulation Overlap Therapy[2]	87	100%	94%	93%
ICU Venous Thromboembolism Prophylaxis[2]	34	100%	93%	92%
Incidence of Potentially Preventable VTE[2]	14	0%	10%	10%
UFH with Dosages/Platelet Monitoring[2]	15	100%	95%	97%
Venous Thromboembolism Prophylaxis[2]	370	86%	88%	85%
Warfarin Therapy Discharge Instructions[2]	59	100%	81%	75%
Chest Pain/Possible Heart Attack Care				
Aspirin Given Within 24 Hours of Arrival	171	100%	97%	96%
Fibrinolytic Meds Within 30 Min. of Arrival[7]	-	-	66%	58%
Average Time to ECG (minutes)	175	5	7	7
Average Time to Transfer (minutes)	30	44	45	60
Children's Asthma Care				
Received Home Management Plan of Care	-	-	89%	88%
Received Reliever Medication	-	-	100%	100%
Received Systemic Corticosteroids	-	-	100%	100%
Emergency Department				
Admittance Decision Time (minutes)[2]	510	154	107	98
Head CT Results Within 45 Min. of Arrival	31	77%	60%	57%
Patients Who Left ER Before Being Seen	63,664	3%	3%	2%
Time from ER Arrival to Admit. (minutes)[2]	511	360	300	274
Time from ER Arrival to Discharge (minutes)	431	166	152	134
Time in ER Before Being Evaluated (minutes)	432	38	34	26
Time to Pain Meds for Fractures (minutes)	250	52	67	57
Heart Attack Care				
Aspirin Given at Discharge	54	100%	100%	99%
Fibrinolytic Meds Within 30 Min. of Arrival[7]	-	-	75%	54%
PCI Within 90 Minutes of Arrival[7]	-	-	98%	96%
Statin Prescribed at Discharge	47	100%	99%	98%
Heart Failure Care				
ACE Inhibitor or ARB for LVSD	62	100%	98%	97%
Discharge Instructions Given	238	98%	96%	94%
Evaluation of LVS Function	294	100%	100%	99%
Medicare Spending				
Medicare Spending per Patient (ratio)	-	0.96	0.94	0.98
Pneumonia Care				
Appropriate Initial Antibiotic Given	132	99%	97%	95%
Blood Culture Timing	248	96%	98%	98%
Pregnancy and Delivery Care				
Newborn Deliveries Scheduled Early[2]	39	3%	3%	6%
Preventive Care				
Immunization for Influenza[2]	513	90%	93%	90%
Immunization for Pneumonia[2]	512	91%	94%	92%
Stroke Care				
Anticoagulation Therapy for Atrial Fibrillation	11	100%	95%	95%
Antithrombotic Therapy Timing	132	100%	98%	98%
Assessed for Rehabilitation	141	99%	98%	97%
Discharged on Antithrombotic Therapy	134	100%	99%	99%
Discharged on Statin Medication	90	100%	94%	94%
Thrombolytic Therapy Timing[7]	-	-	64%	66%
Venous Thromboembolism Prophylaxis	119	97%	96%	94%
Written Stroke Educational Materials Given	83	99%	88%	88%
Surgical Care Improvement Project				
Appropriate Beta Blocker Usage	189	100%	99%	98%
Appropriate VTP Within 24 Hours	625	99%	99%	98%
Controlled Postoperative Blood Glucose[7]	-	-	98%	97%
Perioperative Temperature Management	679	100%	100%	100%
Prophylactic Antibiotic Selection	362	100%	99%	99%
Prophylactic Antibiotic Selection (Outpatient)	352	95%	98%	98%
Prophylactic Antibiotic Stopped	340	99%	99%	98%
Prophylactic Antibiotic Timing	362	99%	99%	99%
Prophylactic Antibiotic Timing (Outpatient)	354	99%	99%	98%
Urinary Catheter Removal	418	99%	99%	97%
Survey of Patients' Hospital Experiences				
Area Around Room 'Always' Quiet at Night	300+	60%	64%	61%
Doctors 'Always' Communicated Well	300+	79%	83%	82%
Home Recovery Information Given	300+	89%	87%	85%
Hospital Given 9 or 10 on 10 Point Scale	300+	71%	71%	71%
Meds 'Always' Explained Before Given	300+	62%	65%	64%
Nurses 'Always' Communicated Well	300+	79%	81%	79%
Pain 'Always' Well Controlled	300+	73%	72%	71%
Room and Bathroom 'Always' Clean	300+	66%	72%	73%
Timely Help 'Always' Received	300+	64%	68%	68%
Would Definitely Recommend Hospital	300+	77%	70%	71%
Use of Medical Imaging				
Cardiac Imaging Stress Test before Surgery	163	7.4%	5.4%	5.3%
Combination Abdominal CT Scan	880	1.1%	5.6%	10.5%
Combination Brain/Sinus CT Scan	1,221	4.0%	2.6%	2.7%
Combination Chest CT Scan	568	0.4%	1.3%	2.7%
Follow-up Mammogram/Ultrasound	598	8.7%	8%	8.8%
Lumbar Spine MRI for Low Back Pain	60	26.7%	34.7%	37.2%

University of North Carolina Hospital

101 Manning Drive
Chapel Hill, NC 27514
Phone: 919-966-4131
Fax: 919-966-3709
URL: www.unchealthcare.org
Type: Acute Care Hospitals
Emergency Services: Yes
Ownership: Government - State
Beds: 803

Key Personnel:
Quality Assurance . . . . Bette Brotherton
Chief of Medical Staff. . . . . Brian Goldstein, MD
Radiology. . . . . Joseph KT Lee, MD
CEO/President. . . . . Gary L Park
Infection Control. . . . . William Rutala
Pediatric Ambulatory Care . . . . . . Roberta Williams, MD
Pediatric In-Patient Care . . . . Roberta Williams, MD

Measure	Cases	This Hosp.	State Avg.	U.S. Avg.
Blood Clot Prevention and Treatment				
Anticoagulation Overlap Therapy[2]	116	98%	94%	93%
ICU Venous Thromboembolism Prophylaxis[2]	56	91%	93%	92%
Incidence of Potentially Preventable VTE[2]	56	4%	10%	10%
UFH with Dosages/Platelet Monitoring[2]	152	100%	95%	97%
Venous Thromboembolism Prophylaxis[2]	310	73%	88%	85%
Warfarin Therapy Discharge Instructions[2]	91	64%	81%	75%
Chest Pain/Possible Heart Attack Care				
Aspirin Given Within 24 Hours of Arrival[5]	-	-	97%	96%
Fibrinolytic Meds Within 30 Min. of Arrival[5]	-	-	66%	58%
Average Time to ECG (minutes)[5]	-	-	7	7
Average Time to Transfer (minutes)[5]	-	-	45	60
Children's Asthma Care				
Received Home Management Plan of Care	-	-	89%	88%
Received Reliever Medication	-	-	100%	100%
Received Systemic Corticosteroids	-	-	100%	100%
Emergency Department				
Admittance Decision Time (minutes)[2]	344	180	107	98
Head CT Results Within 45 Min. of Arrival[1]	-	-	60%	57%
Patients Who Left ER Before Being Seen	71,342	2%	3%	2%
Time from ER Arrival to Admit. (minutes)[2]	353	465	300	274
Time from ER Arrival to Discharge (minutes)	370	282	152	134
Time in ER Before Being Evaluated (minutes)	383	59	34	26
Time to Pain Meds for Fractures (minutes)	103	69	67	57
Heart Attack Care				
Aspirin Given at Discharge[2]	256	100%	100%	99%
Fibrinolytic Meds Within 30 Min. of Arrival[2,7]	-	-	75%	54%
PCI Within 90 Minutes of Arrival[2]	31	100%	98%	96%
Statin Prescribed at Discharge[2]	249	99%	99%	98%
Heart Failure Care				
ACE Inhibitor or ARB for LVSD[2]	103	97%	98%	97%
Discharge Instructions Given[2]	237	98%	96%	94%
Evaluation of LVS Function[2]	270	100%	100%	99%
Medicare Spending				
Medicare Spending per Patient (ratio)	-	0.93	0.94	0.98
Pneumonia Care				
Appropriate Initial Antibiotic Given[2]	46	96%	97%	95%
Blood Culture Timing[2]	103	99%	98%	98%
Pregnancy and Delivery Care				
Newborn Deliveries Scheduled Early[2]	52	0%	3%	6%
Preventive Care				
Immunization for Influenza[2]	534	98%	93%	90%
Immunization for Pneumonia[2]	446	93%	94%	92%
Stroke Care				
Anticoagulation Therapy for Atrial Fibrillation[1,2]	-	-	95%	95%
Antithrombotic Therapy Timing[2]	28	93%	98%	98%
Assessed for Rehabilitation[2]	102	100%	98%	97%
Discharged on Antithrombotic Therapy[2]	56	80%	99%	99%
Discharged on Statin Medication[2]	37	97%	94%	94%
Thrombolytic Therapy Timing[1,2]	-	-	64%	66%
Venous Thromboembolism Prophylaxis[2]	100	97%	96%	94%
Written Stroke Educational Materials Given[2]	56	96%	88%	88%
Surgical Care Improvement Project				
Appropriate Beta Blocker Usage[2]	183	100%	99%	98%
Appropriate VTP Within 24 Hours[2]	389	100%	99%	98%
Controlled Postoperative Blood Glucose[2]	85	99%	98%	97%
Perioperative Temperature Management[2]	508	100%	100%	100%
Prophylactic Antibiotic Selection[2]	307	100%	99%	99%
Prophylactic Antibiotic Selection (Outpatient)	688	99%	98%	98%
Prophylactic Antibiotic Stopped[2]	295	99%	99%	98%
Prophylactic Antibiotic Timing[2]	308	99%	99%	99%
Prophylactic Antibiotic Timing (Outpatient)	681	98%	99%	98%
Urinary Catheter Removal[2]	286	99%	99%	97%
Survey of Patients' Hospital Experiences				
Area Around Room 'Always' Quiet at Night	300+	65%	64%	61%
Doctors 'Always' Communicated Well	300+	84%	83%	82%
Home Recovery Information Given	300+	90%	87%	85%
Hospital Given 9 or 10 on 10 Point Scale	300+	81%	71%	71%
Meds 'Always' Explained Before Given	300+	68%	65%	64%
Nurses 'Always' Communicated Well	300+	82%	81%	79%
Pain 'Always' Well Controlled	300+	74%	72%	71%
Room and Bathroom 'Always' Clean	300+	72%	72%	73%
Timely Help 'Always' Received	300+	67%	68%	68%
Would Definitely Recommend Hospital	300+	83%	70%	71%
Use of Medical Imaging				
Cardiac Imaging Stress Test before Surgery	498	4.8%	5.4%	5.3%
Combination Abdominal CT Scan	2,274	3.6%	5.6%	10.5%
Combination Brain/Sinus CT Scan	992	3.5%	2.6%	2.7%
Combination Chest CT Scan	2,544	0.1%	1.3%	2.7%
Follow-up Mammogram/Ultrasound	2,223	9.2%	8%	8.8%

NOTE: Hospital profiles are in alphabetical order by state, then city, then hospital within the city; Rankings exclude hospitals with less than 25 cases except for patient surveys which excludes hospitals with less than 100 cases; (a) 100-299 cases; (1) The number of cases/patients is too few to report; (2) Data submitted were based on a sample of cases/patients; (3) Results are based on a shorter time period than required; (4) Data suppressed by CMS for one or more quarters; (5) Results are not available for this reporting period; (6) Fewer than 100 patients completed the HCAHPS survey; (7) No cases met the criteria for this measure; (8) The lower limit of the confidence interval cannot be calculated if the number of observed infections equals zero; (9) No data are available from the state/territory for this reporting period; (10) The scores shown reflect fewer than 50 completed surveys; (11) There were discrepancies in the data collection process; (12) This measure does not apply to this hospital for this reporting period; (13) Results cannot be calculated for this reporting period; (14) The results for this state are combined with nearby states to protect confidentiality; Please refer to the User's Guide for a full explanation of data.

Lumbar Spine MRI for Low Back Pain	204	28.4%	34.7%	37.2%

Carolinas Medical Center - Pineville

10628 Park Rd
Charlotte, NC 28210
Phone: 704-379-5000
Fax: 704-379-5695
URL: www.carolinashealthcare.org
Type: Acute Care Hospitals
Emergency Services: Yes
Ownership: Govt - Hospital Dist/Auth
Beds: 224

Key Personnel:

Intensive Care Unit. . . . . Anne Focht, RN
Emergency Room . . . . Stacey Gouzenne
Infection Control. . . . . Dona Haney
Anesthesiology. . . . . Carter Keith, MD
Quality Assurance . . . . Pat Presley
Operating Room. . . . . Carol Puckett
CEO . . . . Michael C. Tarwater
Chief of Medical Staff . . . . Fred Vermeulen

Measure	Cases	This Hosp.	State Avg.	U.S. Avg.
Blood Clot Prevention and Treatment				
Anticoagulation Overlap Therapy[2]	148	95%	94%	93%
ICU Venous Thromboembolism Prophylaxis[2]	151	95%	93%	92%
Incidence of Potentially Preventable VTE[2]	30	13%	10%	10%
UFH with Dosages/Platelet Monitoring[2]	88	100%	95%	97%
Venous Thromboembolism Prophylaxis[2]	509	94%	88%	85%
Warfarin Therapy Discharge Instructions[2]	110	92%	81%	75%
Chest Pain/Possible Heart Attack Care				
Aspirin Given Within 24 Hours of Arrival	25	100%	97%	96%
Fibrinolytic Meds Within 30 Min. of Arrival[3,7]	-	-	66%	58%
Average Time to ECG (minutes)	25	5	7	7
Average Time to Transfer (minutes)[1,3]	-	-	45	60
Children's Asthma Care				
Received Home Management Plan of Care	-	-	89%	88%
Received Reliever Medication	-	-	100%	100%
Received Systemic Corticosteroids	-	-	100%	100%
Emergency Department				
Admittance Decision Time (minutes)[2]	653	85	107	98
Head CT Results Within 45 Min. of Arrival	25	84%	60%	57%
Patients Who Left ER Before Being Seen	>100k	2%	3%	2%
Time from ER Arrival to Admit. (minutes)[2]	713	269	300	274
Time from ER Arrival to Discharge (minutes)	669	160	152	134
Time in ER Before Being Evaluated (minutes)	702	43	34	26
Time to Pain Meds for Fractures (minutes)	326	70	67	57
Heart Attack Care				
Aspirin Given at Discharge	399	100%	100%	99%
Fibrinolytic Meds Within 30 Min. of Arrival[7]	-	-	75%	54%
PCI Within 90 Minutes of Arrival	69	100%	98%	96%
Statin Prescribed at Discharge	386	100%	99%	98%
Heart Failure Care				
ACE Inhibitor or ARB for LVSD	150	99%	98%	97%
Discharge Instructions Given	435	100%	96%	94%
Evaluation of LVS Function	502	100%	100%	99%
Medicare Spending				
Medicare Spending per Patient (ratio)	-	0.95	0.94	0.98
Pneumonia Care				
Appropriate Initial Antibiotic Given	250	99%	97%	95%
Blood Culture Timing	445	99%	98%	98%
Pregnancy and Delivery Care				
Newborn Deliveries Scheduled Early	252	0%	3%	6%
Preventive Care				
Immunization for Influenza[2]	1,050	95%	93%	90%
Immunization for Pneumonia[2]	1,265	98%	94%	92%
Stroke Care				
Anticoagulation Therapy for Atrial Fibrillation	26	100%	95%	95%
Antithrombotic Therapy Timing	198	100%	98%	98%
Assessed for Rehabilitation	206	100%	98%	97%
Discharged on Antithrombotic Therapy	200	100%	99%	99%
Discharged on Statin Medication	154	99%	94%	94%
Thrombolytic Therapy Timing[7]	-	-	64%	66%
Venous Thromboembolism Prophylaxis	199	98%	96%	94%
Written Stroke Educational Materials Given	122	92%	88%	88%
Surgical Care Improvement Project				
Appropriate Beta Blocker Usage[2]	689	100%	99%	98%
Appropriate VTP Within 24 Hours[2]	1,989	100%	99%	98%
Controlled Postoperative Blood Glucose[2]	165	100%	98%	97%
Perioperative Temperature Management[2]	2,492	100%	100%	100%
Prophylactic Antibiotic Selection[2]	2,261	100%	99%	99%
Prophylactic Antibiotic Selection (Outpatient)	1,259	98%	98%	98%
Prophylactic Antibiotic Stopped[2]	2,222	100%	99%	98%
Prophylactic Antibiotic Timing[2]	2,261	100%	99%	99%
Prophylactic Antibiotic Timing (Outpatient)	1,265	99%	99%	98%
Urinary Catheter Removal[2]	1,843	100%	99%	97%
Survey of Patients' Hospital Experiences				
Area Around Room 'Always' Quiet at Night	300+	67%	64%	61%
Doctors 'Always' Communicated Well	300+	85%	83%	82%
Home Recovery Information Given	300+	91%	87%	85%
Hospital Given 9 or 10 on 10 Point Scale	300+	79%	71%	71%
Meds 'Always' Explained Before Given	300+	66%	65%	64%
Nurses 'Always' Communicated Well	300+	82%	81%	79%
Pain 'Always' Well Controlled	300+	71%	72%	71%
Room and Bathroom 'Always' Clean	300+	72%	72%	73%
Timely Help 'Always' Received	300+	65%	68%	68%
Would Definitely Recommend Hospital	300+	81%	70%	71%
Use of Medical Imaging				
Cardiac Imaging Stress Test before Surgery	1,140	5.7%	5.4%	5.3%
Combination Abdominal CT Scan	2,503	5.1%	5.6%	10.5%
Combination Brain/Sinus CT Scan	2,049	2.4%	2.6%	2.7%
Combination Chest CT Scan	1,335	0.1%	1.3%	2.7%
Follow-up Mammogram/Ultrasound[7]	-	-	8%	8.8%
Lumbar Spine MRI for Low Back Pain	176	32.4%	34.7%	37.2%

Carolinas Medical Center - University

8800 North Tyron Street
Charlotte, NC 28262
Phone: 704-548-6000
Type: Acute Care Hospitals
Emergency Services: Yes
Ownership: Govt - Hospital Dist/Auth

Measure	Cases	This Hosp.	State Avg.	U.S. Avg.
Blood Clot Prevention and Treatment				
Anticoagulation Overlap Therapy[2]	53	100%	94%	93%
ICU Venous Thromboembolism Prophylaxis[2]	61	98%	93%	92%
Incidence of Potentially Preventable VTE[1,2]	-	-	10%	10%
UFH with Dosages/Platelet Monitoring[1,2]	-	-	95%	97%
Venous Thromboembolism Prophylaxis[2]	329	96%	88%	85%
Warfarin Therapy Discharge Instructions[2]	51	82%	81%	75%
Chest Pain/Possible Heart Attack Care				
Aspirin Given Within 24 Hours of Arrival	65	100%	97%	96%
Fibrinolytic Meds Within 30 Min. of Arrival[7]	-	-	66%	58%
Average Time to ECG (minutes)	67	5	7	7
Average Time to Transfer (minutes)	17	40	45	60
Children's Asthma Care				
Received Home Management Plan of Care	-	-	89%	88%
Received Reliever Medication	-	-	100%	100%
Received Systemic Corticosteroids	-	-	100%	100%
Emergency Department				
Admittance Decision Time (minutes)[2]	347	81	107	98
Head CT Results Within 45 Min. of Arrival	26	46%	60%	57%
Patients Who Left ER Before Being Seen	88,110	2%	3%	2%
Time from ER Arrival to Admit. (minutes)[2]	390	276	300	274
Time from ER Arrival to Discharge (minutes)	352	159	152	134
Time in ER Before Being Evaluated (minutes)	373	36	34	26
Time to Pain Meds for Fractures (minutes)	206	58	67	57
Heart Attack Care				
Aspirin Given at Discharge	20	100%	100%	99%
Fibrinolytic Meds Within 30 Min. of Arrival[7]	-	-	75%	54%
PCI Within 90 Minutes of Arrival[7]	-	-	98%	96%
Statin Prescribed at Discharge	20	100%	99%	98%
Heart Failure Care				
ACE Inhibitor or ARB for LVSD	70	100%	98%	97%
Discharge Instructions Given	152	100%	96%	94%
Evaluation of LVS Function	169	100%	100%	99%
Medicare Spending				
Medicare Spending per Patient (ratio)	-	0.98	0.94	0.98
Pneumonia Care				
Appropriate Initial Antibiotic Given	115	99%	97%	95%
Blood Culture Timing	195	94%	98%	98%
Pregnancy and Delivery Care				
Newborn Deliveries Scheduled Early	105	0%	3%	6%
Preventive Care				
Immunization for Influenza[2]	496	95%	93%	90%
Immunization for Pneumonia[2]	447	97%	94%	92%
Stroke Care				
Anticoagulation Therapy for Atrial Fibrillation[1]	-	-	95%	95%
Antithrombotic Therapy Timing	85	100%	98%	98%
Assessed for Rehabilitation	94	99%	98%	97%
Discharged on Antithrombotic Therapy	92	100%	99%	99%
Discharged on Statin Medication	71	100%	94%	94%
Thrombolytic Therapy Timing[7]	-	-	64%	66%
Venous Thromboembolism Prophylaxis	81	99%	96%	94%
Written Stroke Educational Materials Given	57	98%	88%	88%
Surgical Care Improvement Project				
Appropriate Beta Blocker Usage[2]	52	96%	99%	98%
Appropriate VTP Within 24 Hours[2]	241	98%	99%	98%
Controlled Postoperative Blood Glucose[2,7]	-	-	98%	97%
Perioperative Temperature Management[2]	284	100%	100%	100%
Prophylactic Antibiotic Selection[2]	176	100%	99%	99%
Prophylactic Antibiotic Selection (Outpatient)	346	99%	98%	98%
Prophylactic Antibiotic Stopped[2]	167	98%	99%	98%
Prophylactic Antibiotic Timing[2]	176	100%	99%	99%
Prophylactic Antibiotic Timing (Outpatient)	349	99%	99%	98%
Urinary Catheter Removal[2]	81	98%	99%	97%
Survey of Patients' Hospital Experiences				
Area Around Room 'Always' Quiet at Night	300+	64%	64%	61%
Doctors 'Always' Communicated Well	300+	86%	83%	82%
Home Recovery Information Given	300+	88%	87%	85%
Hospital Given 9 or 10 on 10 Point Scale	300+	77%	71%	71%
Meds 'Always' Explained Before Given	300+	67%	65%	64%
Nurses 'Always' Communicated Well	300+	85%	81%	79%
Pain 'Always' Well Controlled	300+	78%	72%	71%
Room and Bathroom 'Always' Clean	300+	65%	72%	73%
Timely Help 'Always' Received	300+	72%	68%	68%
Would Definitely Recommend Hospital	300+	80%	70%	71%
Use of Medical Imaging				
Cardiac Imaging Stress Test before Surgery	457	4.6%	5.4%	5.3%
Combination Abdominal CT Scan	1,011	3.7%	5.6%	10.5%
Combination Brain/Sinus CT Scan	927	1.8%	2.6%	2.7%
Combination Chest CT Scan	367	0.5%	1.3%	2.7%
Follow-up Mammogram/Ultrasound[7]	-	-	8%	8.8%
Lumbar Spine MRI for Low Back Pain	71	39.4%	34.7%	37.2%

Carolinas Medical Center/Behaviorial Health

1000 Blythe Blvd
Charlotte, NC 28203
Phone: 704-355-2000
Fax: 704-355-4084
URL: www.carolinasmedicalcenter.org
Type: Acute Care Hospitals
Emergency Services: Yes
Ownership: Govt - Hospital Dist/Auth
Beds: 874

Key Personnel:

Radiology. . . . . John Baumann
Pediatric Ambulatory Care . . . . . . Leonard G Feld, MD, PhD
Pediatric In-Patient Care . . . . Leonard G Feld, MD, PhD
Operating Room. . . . . Frederick L Greene, MD, FACS
Infection Control. . . . . James M Horton, MD
CEO/President. . . . . W. Spencer Lilly
Chief of Medical Staff . . . . Roger A. Ray, MD
CEO . . . . Michael C. Tarwater, MHA

Measure	Cases	This Hosp.	State Avg.	U.S. Avg.
Blood Clot Prevention and Treatment				
Anticoagulation Overlap Therapy[2]	220	98%	94%	93%
ICU Venous Thromboembolism Prophylaxis[2]	170	96%	93%	92%
Incidence of Potentially Preventable VTE[2]	77	12%	10%	10%
UFH with Dosages/Platelet Monitoring[2]	155	100%	95%	97%
Venous Thromboembolism Prophylaxis[2]	272	88%	88%	85%
Warfarin Therapy Discharge Instructions[2]	169	43%	81%	75%
Chest Pain/Possible Heart Attack Care				
Aspirin Given Within 24 Hours of Arrival[5]	-	-	97%	96%
Fibrinolytic Meds Within 30 Min. of Arrival[5]	-	-	66%	58%
Average Time to ECG (minutes)[5]	-	-	7	7
Average Time to Transfer (minutes)[5]	-	-	45	60
Children's Asthma Care				
Received Home Management Plan of Care	359	97%	89%	88%
Received Reliever Medication	360	100%	100%	100%
Received Systemic Corticosteroids	354	100%	100%	100%

NOTE: Hospital profiles are in alphabetical order by state, then city, then hospital within the city; Rankings exclude hospitals with less than 25 cases except for patient surveys which excludes hospitals with less than 100 cases; (a) 100-299 cases; (1) The number of cases/patients is too few to report; (2) Data submitted were based on a sample of cases/patients; (3) Results are based on a shorter time period than required; (4) Data suppressed by CMS for one or more quarters; (5) Results are not available for this reporting period; (6) Fewer than 100 patients completed the HCAHPS survey; (7) No cases met the criteria for this measure; (8) The lower limit of the confidence interval cannot be calculated if the number of observed infections equals zero; (9) No data are available from the state/territory for this reporting period; (10) The scores shown reflect fewer than 50 completed surveys; (11) There were discrepancies in the data collection process; (12) This measure does not apply to this hospital for this reporting period; (13) Results cannot be calculated for this reporting period; (14) The results for this state are combined with nearby states to protect confidentiality; Please refer to the User's Guide for a full explanation of data.

Measure	Cases	This Hosp.	State Avg.	U.S. Avg.
Emergency Department				
Admittance Decision Time (minutes)[2]	256	108	107	98
Head CT Results Within 45 Min. of Arrival[1]	-	-	60%	57%
Patients Who Left ER Before Being Seen	98,110	4%	3%	2%
Time from ER Arrival to Admit. (minutes)[2]	276	284	300	274
Time from ER Arrival to Discharge (minutes)	291	183	152	134
Time in ER Before Being Evaluated (minutes)	374	46	34	26
Time to Pain Meds for Fractures (minutes)	304	67	67	57
Heart Attack Care				
Aspirin Given at Discharge	856	99%	100%	99%
Fibrinolytic Meds Within 30 Min. of Arrival[7]	-	-	75%	54%
PCI Within 90 Minutes of Arrival	116	98%	98%	96%
Statin Prescribed at Discharge	849	99%	99%	98%
Heart Failure Care				
ACE Inhibitor or ARB for LVSD	285	98%	98%	97%
Discharge Instructions Given	635	97%	96%	94%
Evaluation of LVS Function	715	100%	100%	99%
Medicare Spending				
Medicare Spending per Patient (ratio)	-	0.99	0.94	0.98
Pneumonia Care				
Appropriate Initial Antibiotic Given	171	97%	97%	95%
Blood Culture Timing	192	98%	98%	98%
Pregnancy and Delivery Care				
Newborn Deliveries Scheduled Early	248	1%	3%	6%
Preventive Care				
Immunization for Influenza[2]	463	93%	93%	90%
Immunization for Pneumonia[2]	429	96%	94%	92%
Stroke Care				
Anticoagulation Therapy for Atrial Fibrillation	43	100%	95%	95%
Antithrombotic Therapy Timing	279	100%	98%	98%
Assessed for Rehabilitation	589	99%	98%	97%
Discharged on Antithrombotic Therapy	344	100%	99%	99%
Discharged on Statin Medication	287	96%	94%	94%
Thrombolytic Therapy Timing	13	100%	64%	66%
Venous Thromboembolism Prophylaxis	609	100%	96%	94%
Written Stroke Educational Materials Given	304	94%	88%	88%
Surgical Care Improvement Project				
Appropriate Beta Blocker Usage[2]	544	98%	99%	98%
Appropriate VTP Within 24 Hours[2]	843	98%	99%	98%
Controlled Postoperative Blood Glucose[2]	412	99%	98%	97%
Perioperative Temperature Management[2]	1,154	100%	100%	100%
Prophylactic Antibiotic Selection[2]	1,053	99%	99%	99%
Prophylactic Antibiotic Selection (Outpatient)	1,341	99%	98%	98%
Prophylactic Antibiotic Stopped[2]	1,014	97%	99%	98%
Prophylactic Antibiotic Timing[2]	1,056	98%	99%	99%
Prophylactic Antibiotic Timing (Outpatient)	1,280	99%	99%	98%
Urinary Catheter Removal[2]	713	96%	99%	97%
Survey of Patients' Hospital Experiences				
Area Around Room 'Always' Quiet at Night	300+	63%	64%	61%
Doctors 'Always' Communicated Well	300+	81%	83%	82%
Home Recovery Information Given	300+	88%	87%	85%
Hospital Given 9 or 10 on 10 Point Scale	300+	74%	71%	71%
Meds 'Always' Explained Before Given	300+	62%	65%	64%
Nurses 'Always' Communicated Well	300+	77%	81%	79%
Pain 'Always' Well Controlled	300+	71%	72%	71%
Room and Bathroom 'Always' Clean	300+	62%	72%	73%
Timely Help 'Always' Received	300+	61%	68%	68%
Would Definitely Recommend Hospital	300+	72%	70%	71%
Use of Medical Imaging				
Cardiac Imaging Stress Test before Surgery	1,254	6.5%	5.4%	5.3%
Combination Abdominal CT Scan	2,029	11.4%	5.6%	10.5%
Combination Brain/Sinus CT Scan	1,087	1.5%	2.6%	2.7%
Combination Chest CT Scan	1,577	0.0%	1.3%	2.7%
Follow-up Mammogram/Ultrasound[7]	-	-	8%	8.8%
Lumbar Spine MRI for Low Back Pain	163	31.3%	34.7%	37.2%

Novant Health Charlotte Orthopedic Hospital

1901 Randolph Rd — Phone: 704-316-2000
Charlotte, NC 28207
URL: www.presbyterian.org
Type: Acute Care Hospitals — Emergency Services: Yes
Ownership: Voluntary non-profit - Other
Key Personnel:
Ambulatory Care . . . . Dean Swindle
Chief of Medical Staff . . . . Stephen L Wallenhaupt
CEO/President. . . . . Paul M Wiles

Measure	Cases	This Hosp.	State Avg.	U.S. Avg.
Blood Clot Prevention and Treatment				
Anticoagulation Overlap Therapy[1,2]	-	-	94%	93%
ICU Venous Thromboembolism Prophylaxis[2,7]	-	-	93%	92%
Incidence of Potentially Preventable VTE[1,2]	-	-	10%	10%
UFH with Dosages/Platelet Monitoring[2,7]	-	-	95%	97%
Venous Thromboembolism Prophylaxis[2]	206	96%	88%	85%
Warfarin Therapy Discharge Instructions[1,2]	-	-	81%	75%
Chest Pain/Possible Heart Attack Care				
Aspirin Given Within 24 Hours of Arrival[5]	-	-	97%	96%
Fibrinolytic Meds Within 30 Min. of Arrival[5]	-	-	66%	58%
Average Time to ECG (minutes)[5]	-	-	7	7
Average Time to Transfer (minutes)[5]	-	-	45	60
Children's Asthma Care				
Received Home Management Plan of Care	-	-	89%	88%
Received Reliever Medication	-	-	100%	100%
Received Systemic Corticosteroids	-	-	100%	100%
Emergency Department				
Admittance Decision Time (minutes)[2,7]	-	-	107	98
Head CT Results Within 45 Min. of Arrival[5]	-	-	60%	57%
Patients Who Left ER Before Being Seen[5]	-	-	3%	2%
Time from ER Arrival to Admit. (minutes)[2,7]	-	-	300	274
Time from ER Arrival to Discharge (minutes)[5]	-	-	152	134
Time in ER Before Being Evaluated (minutes)[5]	-	-	34	26
Time to Pain Meds for Fractures (minutes)[5]	-	-	67	57
Heart Attack Care				
Aspirin Given at Discharge[5]	-	-	100%	99%
Fibrinolytic Meds Within 30 Min. of Arrival[5]	-	-	75%	54%
PCI Within 90 Minutes of Arrival[5]	-	-	98%	96%
Statin Prescribed at Discharge[5]	-	-	99%	98%
Heart Failure Care				
ACE Inhibitor or ARB for LVSD[5]	-	-	98%	97%
Discharge Instructions Given[5]	-	-	96%	94%
Evaluation of LVS Function[5]	-	-	100%	99%
Medicare Spending				
Medicare Spending per Patient (ratio)	-	0.96	0.94	0.98
Pneumonia Care				
Appropriate Initial Antibiotic Given[5]	-	-	97%	95%
Blood Culture Timing[5]	-	-	98%	98%
Pregnancy and Delivery Care				
Newborn Deliveries Scheduled Early[7]	-	-	3%	6%
Preventive Care				
Immunization for Influenza[2]	412	96%	93%	90%
Immunization for Pneumonia[2]	550	97%	94%	92%
Stroke Care				
Anticoagulation Therapy for Atrial Fibrillation[5]	-	-	95%	95%
Antithrombotic Therapy Timing[5]	-	-	98%	98%
Assessed for Rehabilitation[5]	-	-	98%	97%
Discharged on Antithrombotic Therapy[5]	-	-	99%	99%
Discharged on Statin Medication[5]	-	-	94%	94%
Thrombolytic Therapy Timing[5]	-	-	64%	66%
Venous Thromboembolism Prophylaxis[5]	-	-	96%	94%
Written Stroke Educational Materials Given[5]	-	-	88%	88%
Surgical Care Improvement Project				
Appropriate Beta Blocker Usage[2]	416	100%	99%	98%
Appropriate VTP Within 24 Hours[2]	1,462	100%	99%	98%
Controlled Postoperative Blood Glucose[2,7]	-	-	98%	97%
Perioperative Temperature Management[2]	1,574	100%	100%	100%
Prophylactic Antibiotic Selection[2]	1,402	100%	99%	99%
Prophylactic Antibiotic Selection (Outpatient)	623	100%	98%	98%
Prophylactic Antibiotic Stopped[2]	1,376	100%	99%	98%
Prophylactic Antibiotic Timing[2]	1,403	100%	99%	99%
Prophylactic Antibiotic Timing (Outpatient)	623	100%	99%	98%
Urinary Catheter Removal[2]	1,363	100%	99%	97%
Survey of Patients' Hospital Experiences				
Area Around Room 'Always' Quiet at Night	300+	60%	64%	61%
Doctors 'Always' Communicated Well	300+	83%	83%	82%
Home Recovery Information Given	300+	89%	87%	85%
Hospital Given 9 or 10 on 10 Point Scale	300+	67%	71%	71%
Meds 'Always' Explained Before Given	300+	57%	65%	64%
Nurses 'Always' Communicated Well	300+	72%	81%	79%
Pain 'Always' Well Controlled	300+	64%	72%	71%
Room and Bathroom 'Always' Clean	300+	67%	72%	73%
Timely Help 'Always' Received	300+	55%	68%	68%
Would Definitely Recommend Hospital	300+	69%	70%	71%
Use of Medical Imaging				
Cardiac Imaging Stress Test before Surgery[7]	-	-	5.4%	5.3%
Combination Abdominal CT Scan	47	4.3%	5.6%	10.5%
Combination Brain/Sinus CT Scan[1]	-	-	2.6%	2.7%
Combination Chest CT Scan	87	0.0%	1.3%	2.7%
Follow-up Mammogram/Ultrasound[7]	-	-	8%	8.8%
Lumbar Spine MRI for Low Back Pain	79	31.6%	34.7%	37.2%

Novant Health Presbyterian Medical Center

200 Hawthorne Lane Box 33549 — Phone: 704-384-4000
Charlotte, NC 28233 — Fax: 704-384-4296
URL: www.presbyterian.org
Type: Acute Care Hospitals — Emergency Services: Yes
Ownership: Voluntary non-profit - Private — Beds: 547
Key Personnel:
Chief of Medical Staff. . . . . Paul Blake, MD
Pediatric Ambulatory Care . . . . . . Pat Campbell
Pediatric In-Patient Care . . . . Pat Campbell
Infection Control. . . . . Sandy Cox
Radiology. . . . . Shelly Hall
Coronary Care . . . . Mary Hopin
Quality Assurance . . . . Carol Mault
CEO/President. . . . . Harry L. Smith, Jr.

Measure	Cases	This Hosp.	State Avg.	U.S. Avg.
Blood Clot Prevention and Treatment				
Anticoagulation Overlap Therapy[2]	140	99%	94%	93%
ICU Venous Thromboembolism Prophylaxis[2]	44	100%	93%	92%
Incidence of Potentially Preventable VTE[2]	32	6%	10%	10%
UFH with Dosages/Platelet Monitoring[2]	97	100%	95%	97%
Venous Thromboembolism Prophylaxis[2]	366	92%	88%	85%
Warfarin Therapy Discharge Instructions[2]	94	66%	81%	75%
Chest Pain/Possible Heart Attack Care				
Aspirin Given Within 24 Hours of Arrival[3,7]	-	-	97%	96%
Fibrinolytic Meds Within 30 Min. of Arrival[5]	-	-	66%	58%
Average Time to ECG (minutes)[3,7]	-	-	7	7
Average Time to Transfer (minutes)[5]	-	-	45	60
Children's Asthma Care				
Received Home Management Plan of Care	159	97%	89%	88%
Received Reliever Medication	158	100%	100%	100%
Received Systemic Corticosteroids	156	100%	100%	100%
Emergency Department				
Admittance Decision Time (minutes)[2]	521	138	107	98
Head CT Results Within 45 Min. of Arrival[7]	-	-	60%	57%
Patients Who Left ER Before Being Seen	91,499	1%	3%	2%
Time from ER Arrival to Admit. (minutes)[2]	521	320	300	274
Time from ER Arrival to Discharge (minutes)	467	158	152	134
Time in ER Before Being Evaluated (minutes)	480	23	34	26
Time to Pain Meds for Fractures (minutes)	178	58	67	57
Heart Attack Care				
Aspirin Given at Discharge	448	100%	100%	99%
Fibrinolytic Meds Within 30 Min. of Arrival[7]	-	-	75%	54%
PCI Within 90 Minutes of Arrival	55	100%	98%	96%
Statin Prescribed at Discharge	423	100%	99%	98%
Heart Failure Care				
ACE Inhibitor or ARB for LVSD	205	100%	98%	97%
Discharge Instructions Given	524	97%	96%	94%
Evaluation of LVS Function	612	100%	100%	99%
Medicare Spending				
Medicare Spending per Patient (ratio)	-	0.99	0.94	0.98
Pneumonia Care				
Appropriate Initial Antibiotic Given	184	99%	97%	95%
Blood Culture Timing	315	100%	98%	98%
Pregnancy and Delivery Care				
Newborn Deliveries Scheduled Early[2]	110	1%	3%	6%
Preventive Care				
Immunization for Influenza[2]	642	97%	93%	90%
Immunization for Pneumonia[2]	604	97%	94%	92%
Stroke Care				
Anticoagulation Therapy for Atrial Fibrillation	23	100%	95%	95%

NOTE: Hospital profiles are in alphabetical order by state, then city, then hospital within the city; Rankings exclude hospitals with less than 25 cases except for patient surveys which excludes hospitals with less than 100 cases; (a) 100-299 cases; (1) The number of cases/patients is too few to report; (2) Data submitted were based on a sample of cases/patients; (3) Results are based on a shorter time period than required; (4) Data suppressed by CMS for one or more quarters; (5) Results are not available for this reporting period; (6) Fewer than 100 patients completed the HCAHPS survey; (7) No cases met the criteria for this measure; (8) The lower limit of the confidence interval cannot be calculated if the number of observed infections equals zero; (9) No data are available from the state/territory for this reporting period; (10) The scores shown reflect fewer than 50 completed surveys; (11) There were discrepancies in the data collection process; (12) This measure does not apply to this hospital for this reporting period; (13) Results cannot be calculated for this reporting period; (14) The results for this state are combined with nearby states to protect confidentiality; Please refer to the User's Guide for a full explanation of data.

Measure	Cases	This Hosp.	State Avg.	U.S. Avg.
Antithrombotic Therapy Timing	207	99%	98%	98%
Assessed for Rehabilitation	316	100%	98%	97%
Discharged on Antithrombotic Therapy	241	100%	99%	99%
Discharged on Statin Medication	175	100%	94%	94%
Thrombolytic Therapy Timing	13	100%	64%	66%
Venous Thromboembolism Prophylaxis	329	100%	96%	94%
Written Stroke Educational Materials Given	201	97%	88%	88%
Surgical Care Improvement Project				
Appropriate Beta Blocker Usage[2]	435	100%	99%	98%
Appropriate VTP Within 24 Hours[2]	738	99%	99%	98%
Controlled Postoperative Blood Glucose[2]	333	99%	98%	97%
Perioperative Temperature Management[2]	926	100%	100%	100%
Prophylactic Antibiotic Selection[2]	721	100%	99%	99%
Prophylactic Antibiotic Selection (Outpatient)	1,320	100%	98%	98%
Prophylactic Antibiotic Stopped[2]	692	98%	99%	98%
Prophylactic Antibiotic Timing[2]	722	100%	99%	99%
Prophylactic Antibiotic Timing (Outpatient)	1,309	100%	99%	98%
Urinary Catheter Removal[2]	509	98%	99%	97%
Survey of Patients' Hospital Experiences				
Area Around Room 'Always' Quiet at Night	300+	56%	64%	61%
Doctors 'Always' Communicated Well	300+	79%	83%	82%
Home Recovery Information Given	300+	82%	87%	85%
Hospital Given 9 or 10 on 10 Point Scale	300+	67%	71%	71%
Meds 'Always' Explained Before Given	300+	56%	65%	64%
Nurses 'Always' Communicated Well	300+	72%	81%	79%
Pain 'Always' Well Controlled	300+	65%	72%	71%
Room and Bathroom 'Always' Clean	300+	66%	72%	73%
Timely Help 'Always' Received	300+	56%	68%	68%
Would Definitely Recommend Hospital	300+	71%	70%	71%
Use of Medical Imaging				
Cardiac Imaging Stress Test before Surgery	1,070	3.7%	5.4%	5.3%
Combination Abdominal CT Scan	1,581	4.5%	5.6%	10.5%
Combination Brain/Sinus CT Scan	1,370	3.4%	2.6%	2.7%
Combination Chest CT Scan	1,098	0.0%	1.3%	2.7%
Follow-up Mammogram/Ultrasound	1,737	7.0%	8%	8.8%
Lumbar Spine MRI for Low Back Pain	187	31.6%	34.7%	37.2%

Cherokee Indian Hospital Authority

Caller Box C268
Cherokee, NC 28719
Type: Acute Care Hospitals
Ownership: Government - Federal
Phone: 704-497-9163
Fax: 828-497-5343
Emergency Services: Yes
Beds: 32

Measure	Cases	This Hosp.	State Avg.	U.S. Avg.
Blood Clot Prevention and Treatment				
Anticoagulation Overlap Therapy[7]	-	-	94%	93%
ICU Venous Thromboembolism Prophylaxis[7]	-	-	93%	92%
Incidence of Potentially Preventable VTE[7]	-	-	10%	10%
UFH with Dosages/Platelet Monitoring[7]	-	-	95%	97%
Venous Thromboembolism Prophylaxis	70	93%	88%	85%
Warfarin Therapy Discharge Instructions[7]	-	-	81%	75%
Chest Pain/Possible Heart Attack Care				
Aspirin Given Within 24 Hours of Arrival	-	-	97%	96%
Fibrinolytic Meds Within 30 Min. of Arrival	-	-	66%	58%
Average Time to ECG (minutes)	-	-	7	7
Average Time to Transfer (minutes)	-	-	45	60
Children's Asthma Care				
Received Home Management Plan of Care	-	-	89%	88%
Received Reliever Medication	-	-	100%	100%
Received Systemic Corticosteroids	-	-	100%	100%
Emergency Department				
Admittance Decision Time (minutes)[2]	289	50	107	98
Head CT Results Within 45 Min. of Arrival	-	-	60%	57%
Patients Who Left ER Before Being Seen	-	-	3%	2%
Time from ER Arrival to Admit. (minutes)[2]	289	213	300	274
Time from ER Arrival to Discharge (minutes)	-	-	152	134
Time in ER Before Being Evaluated (minutes)	-	-	34	26
Time to Pain Meds for Fractures (minutes)	-	-	67	57
Heart Attack Care				
Aspirin Given at Discharge[3,7]	-	-	100%	99%
Fibrinolytic Meds Within 30 Min. of Arrival[3,7]	-	-	75%	54%
PCI Within 90 Minutes of Arrival[3,7]	-	-	98%	96%
Statin Prescribed at Discharge[3,7]	-	-	99%	98%
Heart Failure Care				
ACE Inhibitor or ARB for LVSD[1]	-	-	98%	97%
Discharge Instructions Given[1]	-	-	96%	94%
Evaluation of LVS Function[1]	-	-	100%	99%
Medicare Spending				
Medicare Spending per Patient (ratio)	-	0.70	0.94	0.98
Pneumonia Care				
Appropriate Initial Antibiotic Given	12	92%	97%	95%
Blood Culture Timing	15	100%	98%	98%
Pregnancy and Delivery Care				
Newborn Deliveries Scheduled Early[7]	-	-	3%	6%
Preventive Care				
Immunization for Influenza[2]	187	79%	93%	90%
Immunization for Pneumonia[2]	223	95%	94%	92%
Stroke Care				
Anticoagulation Therapy for Atrial Fibrillation[5]	-	-	95%	95%
Antithrombotic Therapy Timing[5]	-	-	98%	98%
Assessed for Rehabilitation[5]	-	-	98%	97%
Discharged on Antithrombotic Therapy[5]	-	-	99%	99%
Discharged on Statin Medication[5]	-	-	94%	94%
Thrombolytic Therapy Timing[5]	-	-	64%	66%
Venous Thromboembolism Prophylaxis[5]	-	-	96%	94%
Written Stroke Educational Materials Given[5]	-	-	88%	88%
Surgical Care Improvement Project				
Appropriate Beta Blocker Usage[5]	-	-	99%	98%
Appropriate VTP Within 24 Hours[5]	-	-	99%	98%
Controlled Postoperative Blood Glucose[5]	-	-	98%	97%
Perioperative Temperature Management[5]	-	-	100%	100%
Prophylactic Antibiotic Selection[5]	-	-	99%	99%
Prophylactic Antibiotic Selection (Outpatient)	-	-	98%	98%
Prophylactic Antibiotic Stopped[5]	-	-	99%	98%
Prophylactic Antibiotic Timing[5]	-	-	99%	99%
Prophylactic Antibiotic Timing (Outpatient)	-	-	99%	98%
Urinary Catheter Removal[5]	-	-	99%	97%
Survey of Patients' Hospital Experiences				
Area Around Room 'Always' Quiet at Night[6]	<100	82%	64%	61%
Doctors 'Always' Communicated Well[6]	<100	86%	83%	82%
Home Recovery Information Given[6]	<100	82%	87%	85%
Hospital Given 9 or 10 on 10 Point Scale[6]	<100	74%	71%	71%
Meds 'Always' Explained Before Given[6]	<100	69%	65%	64%
Nurses 'Always' Communicated Well[6]	<100	83%	81%	79%
Pain 'Always' Well Controlled[6]	<100	78%	72%	71%
Room and Bathroom 'Always' Clean[6]	<100	82%	72%	73%
Timely Help 'Always' Received[6]	<100	86%	68%	68%
Would Definitely Recommend Hospital[6]	<100	57%	70%	71%
Use of Medical Imaging				
Cardiac Imaging Stress Test before Surgery	-	-	5.4%	5.3%
Combination Abdominal CT Scan	-	-	5.6%	10.5%
Combination Brain/Sinus CT Scan	-	-	2.6%	2.7%
Combination Chest CT Scan	-	-	1.3%	2.7%
Follow-up Mammogram/Ultrasound	-	-	8%	8.8%
Lumbar Spine MRI for Low Back Pain	-	-	34.7%	37.2%

Sampson Regional Medical Center

607 Beaman St
Clinton, NC 28328
URL: www.sampsonrmc.org
Type: Acute Care Hospitals
Ownership: Government - Local
Phone: 910-592-8511
Fax: 910-590-2321
Emergency Services: Yes
Beds: 146

Key Personnel:
Patient Relations . . . . Ann Butler
CEO/President. . . . . Larry H Chewning
Pediatric Ambulatory Care . . . . . . Sara Hesketh
Intensive Care Unit. . . . . Heidi Jackson
Operating Room. . . . . Lisa King
Quality Assurance . . . . Rebecca Mahler
Radiology. . . . . Verlon Salley
Emergency Room . . . . Laurie Smith

Measure	Cases	This Hosp.	State Avg.	U.S. Avg.
Blood Clot Prevention and Treatment				
Anticoagulation Overlap Therapy[2]	18	100%	94%	93%
ICU Venous Thromboembolism Prophylaxis[2]	56	82%	93%	92%
Incidence of Potentially Preventable VTE[1,2]	-	-	10%	10%
UFH with Dosages/Platelet Monitoring[2,7]	-	-	95%	97%
Venous Thromboembolism Prophylaxis[2]	255	94%	88%	85%
Warfarin Therapy Discharge Instructions[2]	11	18%	81%	75%
Chest Pain/Possible Heart Attack Care				
Aspirin Given Within 24 Hours of Arrival	202	91%	97%	96%
Fibrinolytic Meds Within 30 Min. of Arrival	12	67%	66%	58%
Average Time to ECG (minutes)	205	10	7	7
Average Time to Transfer (minutes)[1]	-	-	45	60
Children's Asthma Care				
Received Home Management Plan of Care	-	-	89%	88%
Received Reliever Medication	-	-	100%	100%
Received Systemic Corticosteroids	-	-	100%	100%
Emergency Department				
Admittance Decision Time (minutes)[2]	375	113	107	98
Head CT Results Within 45 Min. of Arrival	30	13%	60%	57%
Patients Who Left ER Before Being Seen	34,137	2%	3%	2%
Time from ER Arrival to Admit. (minutes)[2]	377	283	300	274
Time from ER Arrival to Discharge (minutes)	427	124	152	134
Time in ER Before Being Evaluated (minutes)	475	22	34	26
Time to Pain Meds for Fractures (minutes)	50	54	67	57
Heart Attack Care				
Aspirin Given at Discharge[1]	-	-	100%	99%
Fibrinolytic Meds Within 30 Min. of Arrival[7]	-	-	75%	54%
PCI Within 90 Minutes of Arrival[7]	-	-	98%	96%
Statin Prescribed at Discharge[1]	-	-	99%	98%
Heart Failure Care				
ACE Inhibitor or ARB for LVSD	47	96%	98%	97%
Discharge Instructions Given	144	92%	96%	94%
Evaluation of LVS Function	183	99%	100%	99%
Medicare Spending				
Medicare Spending per Patient (ratio)	-	0.87	0.94	0.98
Pneumonia Care				
Appropriate Initial Antibiotic Given	83	94%	97%	95%
Blood Culture Timing	139	98%	98%	98%
Pregnancy and Delivery Care				
Newborn Deliveries Scheduled Early	25	8%	3%	6%
Preventive Care				
Immunization for Influenza[2]	376	94%	93%	90%
Immunization for Pneumonia[2]	439	93%	94%	92%
Stroke Care				
Anticoagulation Therapy for Atrial Fibrillation[1]	-	-	95%	95%
Antithrombotic Therapy Timing	48	98%	98%	98%
Assessed for Rehabilitation	44	98%	98%	97%
Discharged on Antithrombotic Therapy	44	100%	99%	99%
Discharged on Statin Medication	32	84%	94%	94%
Thrombolytic Therapy Timing[1]	-	-	64%	66%
Venous Thromboembolism Prophylaxis	48	90%	96%	94%
Written Stroke Educational Materials Given	26	23%	88%	88%
Surgical Care Improvement Project				
Appropriate Beta Blocker Usage	37	97%	99%	98%
Appropriate VTP Within 24 Hours	120	92%	99%	98%
Controlled Postoperative Blood Glucose[7]	-	-	98%	97%
Perioperative Temperature Management	133	100%	100%	100%
Prophylactic Antibiotic Selection	89	97%	99%	99%
Prophylactic Antibiotic Selection (Outpatient)[1]	-	-	98%	98%
Prophylactic Antibiotic Stopped	89	97%	99%	98%
Prophylactic Antibiotic Timing	89	98%	99%	99%
Prophylactic Antibiotic Timing (Outpatient)[1]	-	-	99%	98%
Urinary Catheter Removal	104	96%	99%	97%
Survey of Patients' Hospital Experiences				
Area Around Room 'Always' Quiet at Night	300+	64%	64%	61%
Doctors 'Always' Communicated Well	300+	84%	83%	82%
Home Recovery Information Given	300+	84%	87%	85%
Hospital Given 9 or 10 on 10 Point Scale	300+	61%	71%	71%
Meds 'Always' Explained Before Given	300+	65%	65%	64%
Nurses 'Always' Communicated Well	300+	81%	81%	79%
Pain 'Always' Well Controlled	300+	72%	72%	71%
Room and Bathroom 'Always' Clean	300+	65%	72%	73%
Timely Help 'Always' Received	300+	65%	68%	68%
Would Definitely Recommend Hospital	300+	57%	70%	71%
Use of Medical Imaging				
Cardiac Imaging Stress Test before Surgery	352	4.5%	5.4%	5.3%
Combination Abdominal CT Scan	779	8.1%	5.6%	10.5%

NOTE: Hospital profiles are in alphabetical order by state, then city, then hospital within the city; Rankings exclude hospitals with less than 25 cases except for patient surveys which excludes hospitals with less than 100 cases; (a) 100-299 cases; (1) The number of cases/patients is too few to report; (2) Data submitted were based on a sample of cases/patients; (3) Results are based on a shorter time period than required; (4) Data suppressed by CMS for one or more quarters; (5) Results are not available for this reporting period; (6) Fewer than 100 patients completed the HCAHPS survey; (7) No cases met the criteria for this measure; (8) The lower limit of the confidence interval cannot be calculated if the number of observed infections equals zero; (9) No data are available from the state/territory for this reporting period; (10) The scores shown reflect fewer than 50 completed surveys; (11) There were discrepancies in the data collection process; (12) This measure does not apply to this hospital for this reporting period; (13) Results cannot be calculated for this reporting period; (14) The results for this state are combined with nearby states to protect confidentiality; Please refer to the User's Guide for a full explanation of data.

Measure	Cases	This Hosp.	State Avg.	U.S. Avg.
Combination Brain/Sinus CT Scan	870	1.8%	2.6%	2.7%
Combination Chest CT Scan	427	0.5%	1.3%	2.7%
Follow-up Mammogram/Ultrasound	1,405	4.0%	8%	8.8%
Lumbar Spine MRI for Low Back Pain	165	35.2%	34.7%	37.2%

Medwest Haywood

262 Leroy George Drive
Clyde, NC 28721
URL: www.haymed.org
Type: Acute Care Hospitals
Ownership: Govt - Hospital Dist/Auth
Phone: 828-456-7311
Fax: 828-452-8294
Emergency Services: Yes
Beds: 200

Key Personnel:
Chief of Medical Staff.......... Keturah C Bell, MD
Patient Relations .... Nancy Burleson
Emergency Room .... Ryan Davis
Radiology.................... Debera L Huderly
Quality Assurance .... David Love, MD
Operating Room.............. Alfred Mina, RN
President/CEO............... Janie Sinacore-Jaberg, FACHE
Infection Control.............. Dianne Warren

Measure	Cases	This Hosp.	State Avg.	U.S. Avg.
Blood Clot Prevention and Treatment				
Anticoagulation Overlap Therapy[2]	46	100%	94%	93%
ICU Venous Thromboembolism Prophylaxis[2]	54	94%	93%	92%
Incidence of Potentially Preventable VTE[1,2]	-	-	10%	10%
UFH with Dosages/Platelet Monitoring[2]	15	100%	95%	97%
Venous Thromboembolism Prophylaxis[2]	326	96%	88%	85%
Warfarin Therapy Discharge Instructions[2]	33	88%	81%	75%
Chest Pain/Possible Heart Attack Care				
Aspirin Given Within 24 Hours of Arrival	60	97%	97%	96%
Fibrinolytic Meds Within 30 Min. of Arrival[7]	-	-	66%	58%
Average Time to ECG (minutes)	60	11	7	7
Average Time to Transfer (minutes)	12	44	45	60
Children's Asthma Care				
Received Home Management Plan of Care	-	-	89%	88%
Received Reliever Medication	-	-	100%	100%
Received Systemic Corticosteroids	-	-	100%	100%
Emergency Department				
Admittance Decision Time (minutes)[2]	604	77	107	98
Head CT Results Within 45 Min. of Arrival[1]	-	-	60%	57%
Patients Who Left ER Before Being Seen	25,737	2%	3%	2%
Time from ER Arrival to Admit. (minutes)[2]	637	279	300	274
Time from ER Arrival to Discharge (minutes)	337	153	152	134
Time in ER Before Being Evaluated (minutes)	395	29	34	26
Time to Pain Meds for Fractures (minutes)	77	65	67	57
Heart Attack Care				
Aspirin Given at Discharge	24	96%	100%	99%
Fibrinolytic Meds Within 30 Min. of Arrival[7]	-	-	75%	54%
PCI Within 90 Minutes of Arrival[7]	-	-	98%	96%
Statin Prescribed at Discharge	19	95%	99%	98%
Heart Failure Care				
ACE Inhibitor or ARB for LVSD	24	92%	98%	97%
Discharge Instructions Given	89	90%	96%	94%
Evaluation of LVS Function	125	100%	100%	99%
Medicare Spending				
Medicare Spending per Patient (ratio)	-	0.93	0.94	0.98
Pneumonia Care				
Appropriate Initial Antibiotic Given	146	95%	97%	95%
Blood Culture Timing	237	99%	98%	98%
Pregnancy and Delivery Care				
Newborn Deliveries Scheduled Early[2]	11	9%	3%	6%
Preventive Care				
Immunization for Influenza[2]	521	88%	93%	90%
Immunization for Pneumonia[2]	667	91%	94%	92%
Stroke Care				
Anticoagulation Therapy for Atrial Fibrillation	16	94%	95%	95%
Antithrombotic Therapy Timing	57	100%	98%	98%
Assessed for Rehabilitation	62	97%	98%	97%
Discharged on Antithrombotic Therapy	62	100%	99%	99%
Discharged on Statin Medication	48	94%	94%	94%
Thrombolytic Therapy Timing[1]	-	-	64%	66%
Venous Thromboembolism Prophylaxis	54	96%	96%	94%
Written Stroke Educational Materials Given	35	100%	88%	88%
Surgical Care Improvement Project				
Appropriate Beta Blocker Usage	107	93%	99%	98%
Appropriate VTP Within 24 Hours	316	98%	99%	98%
Controlled Postoperative Blood Glucose[7]	-	-	98%	97%
Perioperative Temperature Management	338	100%	100%	100%
Prophylactic Antibiotic Selection	233	99%	99%	99%
Prophylactic Antibiotic Selection (Outpatient)	277	100%	98%	98%
Prophylactic Antibiotic Stopped	221	97%	99%	98%
Prophylactic Antibiotic Timing	233	100%	99%	99%
Prophylactic Antibiotic Timing (Outpatient)	279	98%	99%	98%
Urinary Catheter Removal	81	91%	99%	97%
Survey of Patients' Hospital Experiences				
Area Around Room 'Always' Quiet at Night	300+	61%	64%	61%
Doctors 'Always' Communicated Well	300+	86%	83%	82%
Home Recovery Information Given	300+	86%	87%	85%
Hospital Given 9 or 10 on 10 Point Scale	300+	69%	71%	71%
Meds 'Always' Explained Before Given	300+	66%	65%	64%
Nurses 'Always' Communicated Well	300+	81%	81%	79%
Pain 'Always' Well Controlled	300+	74%	72%	71%
Room and Bathroom 'Always' Clean	300+	68%	72%	73%
Timely Help 'Always' Received	300+	71%	68%	68%
Would Definitely Recommend Hospital	300+	69%	70%	71%
Use of Medical Imaging				
Cardiac Imaging Stress Test before Surgery	464	4.1%	5.4%	5.3%
Combination Abdominal CT Scan	838	10.4%	5.6%	10.5%
Combination Brain/Sinus CT Scan[1]	-	-	2.6%	2.7%
Combination Chest CT Scan	590	8.6%	1.3%	2.7%
Follow-up Mammogram/Ultrasound	1,639	6.1%	8%	8.8%
Lumbar Spine MRI for Low Back Pain	203	29.1%	34.7%	37.2%

Saint Luke's Hospital

101 Hospital Drive
Columbus, NC 28722
URL: www.saintlukeshospital.com
Type: Critical Access Hospitals
Ownership: Voluntary non-profit - Private
Phone: 828-894-3311
Fax: 828-894-2155
Emergency Services: Yes
Beds: 73

Key Personnel:
Operating Room.............. Laurann Adams
Radiology.................... Martin Black
Chief of Medical Staff.......... Todd Colson, MD
Emergency Room .... Lori Oliver
Patient Relations .... Sandra Page
CEO .... Ken Shull

Measure	Cases	This Hosp.	State Avg.	U.S. Avg.
Blood Clot Prevention and Treatment				
Anticoagulation Overlap Therapy[5]	-	-	94%	93%
ICU Venous Thromboembolism Prophylaxis[5]	-	-	93%	92%
Incidence of Potentially Preventable VTE[5]	-	-	10%	10%
UFH with Dosages/Platelet Monitoring[5]	-	-	95%	97%
Venous Thromboembolism Prophylaxis[5]	-	-	88%	85%
Warfarin Therapy Discharge Instructions[5]	-	-	81%	75%
Chest Pain/Possible Heart Attack Care				
Aspirin Given Within 24 Hours of Arrival[5]	-	-	97%	96%
Fibrinolytic Meds Within 30 Min. of Arrival[5]	-	-	66%	58%
Average Time to ECG (minutes)[5]	-	-	7	7
Average Time to Transfer (minutes)[5]	-	-	45	60
Children's Asthma Care				
Received Home Management Plan of Care	-	-	89%	88%
Received Reliever Medication	-	-	100%	100%
Received Systemic Corticosteroids	-	-	100%	100%
Emergency Department				
Admittance Decision Time (minutes)[5]	-	-	107	98
Head CT Results Within 45 Min. of Arrival[5]	-	-	60%	57%
Patients Who Left ER Before Being Seen	10,185	2%	3%	2%
Time from ER Arrival to Admit. (minutes)[5]	-	-	300	274
Time from ER Arrival to Discharge (minutes)[5]	-	-	152	134
Time in ER Before Being Evaluated (minutes)[5]	-	-	34	26
Time to Pain Meds for Fractures (minutes)[5]	-	-	67	57
Heart Attack Care				
Aspirin Given at Discharge[5]	-	-	100%	99%
Fibrinolytic Meds Within 30 Min. of Arrival[5]	-	-	75%	54%
PCI Within 90 Minutes of Arrival[5]	-	-	98%	96%
Statin Prescribed at Discharge[5]	-	-	99%	98%
Heart Failure Care				
ACE Inhibitor or ARB for LVSD[1]	-	-	98%	97%
Discharge Instructions Given	11	100%	96%	94%
Evaluation of LVS Function	36	100%	100%	99%
Medicare Spending				
Medicare Spending per Patient (ratio)	-	-	0.94	0.98
Pneumonia Care				
Appropriate Initial Antibiotic Given	47	98%	97%	95%
Blood Culture Timing	80	100%	98%	98%
Pregnancy and Delivery Care				
Newborn Deliveries Scheduled Early[5]	-	-	3%	6%
Preventive Care				
Immunization for Influenza[5]	-	-	93%	90%
Immunization for Pneumonia[5]	-	-	94%	92%
Stroke Care				
Anticoagulation Therapy for Atrial Fibrillation[5]	-	-	95%	95%
Antithrombotic Therapy Timing[5]	-	-	98%	98%
Assessed for Rehabilitation[5]	-	-	98%	97%
Discharged on Antithrombotic Therapy[5]	-	-	99%	99%
Discharged on Statin Medication[5]	-	-	94%	94%
Thrombolytic Therapy Timing[5]	-	-	64%	66%
Venous Thromboembolism Prophylaxis[5]	-	-	96%	94%
Written Stroke Educational Materials Given[5]	-	-	88%	88%
Surgical Care Improvement Project				
Appropriate Beta Blocker Usage	63	100%	99%	98%
Appropriate VTP Within 24 Hours	195	98%	99%	98%
Controlled Postoperative Blood Glucose[3,7]	-	-	98%	97%
Perioperative Temperature Management	230	100%	100%	100%
Prophylactic Antibiotic Selection	203	100%	99%	99%
Prophylactic Antibiotic Selection (Outpatient)[5]	-	-	98%	98%
Prophylactic Antibiotic Stopped	203	95%	99%	98%
Prophylactic Antibiotic Timing	208	99%	99%	99%
Prophylactic Antibiotic Timing (Outpatient)[5]	-	-	99%	98%
Urinary Catheter Removal	145	97%	99%	97%
Survey of Patients' Hospital Experiences				
Area Around Room 'Always' Quiet at Night	(a)	58%	64%	61%
Doctors 'Always' Communicated Well	(a)	85%	83%	82%
Home Recovery Information Given	(a)	88%	87%	85%
Hospital Given 9 or 10 on 10 Point Scale	(a)	78%	71%	71%
Meds 'Always' Explained Before Given	(a)	67%	65%	64%
Nurses 'Always' Communicated Well	(a)	83%	81%	79%
Pain 'Always' Well Controlled	(a)	72%	72%	71%
Room and Bathroom 'Always' Clean	(a)	74%	72%	73%
Timely Help 'Always' Received	(a)	75%	68%	68%
Would Definitely Recommend Hospital	(a)	76%	70%	71%
Use of Medical Imaging				
Cardiac Imaging Stress Test before Surgery[7]	-	-	5.4%	5.3%
Combination Abdominal CT Scan	255	10.2%	5.6%	10.5%
Combination Brain/Sinus CT Scan[1]	-	-	2.6%	2.7%
Combination Chest CT Scan	85	7.1%	1.3%	2.7%
Follow-up Mammogram/Ultrasound	549	7.7%	8%	8.8%
Lumbar Spine MRI for Low Back Pain	60	30.0%	34.7%	37.2%

Carolinas Medical Center - Northeast

920 Church Saint N
Concord, NC 28025
URL: www.northeastmedical.org
Type: Acute Care Hospitals
Ownership: Govt - Hospital Dist/Auth
Phone: 704-783-3000
Fax: 704-783-3579
Emergency Services: Yes
Beds: 457

Key Personnel:
Quality Assurance .... Leesa Bain
Infection Control.............. Pat Hinson
Radiology.................... Timothy O Jenkins, MD
Chief of Medical Staff.......... Roger A. Ray, MD
CEO .... Michael C. Tarwater
President.................... Phyllis Wingate

Measure	Cases	This Hosp.	State Avg.	U.S. Avg.
Blood Clot Prevention and Treatment				
Anticoagulation Overlap Therapy[2]	180	99%	94%	93%
ICU Venous Thromboembolism Prophylaxis[2]	61	97%	93%	92%
Incidence of Potentially Preventable VTE[2]	46	15%	10%	10%
UFH with Dosages/Platelet Monitoring[2]	154	100%	95%	97%
Venous Thromboembolism Prophylaxis[2]	327	88%	88%	85%
Warfarin Therapy Discharge Instructions[2]	144	83%	81%	75%
Chest Pain/Possible Heart Attack Care				
Aspirin Given Within 24 Hours of Arrival[1,3]	-	-	97%	96%

NOTE: Hospital profiles are in alphabetical order by state, then city, then hospital within the city; Rankings exclude hospitals with less than 25 cases except for patient surveys which excludes hospitals with less than 100 cases; (a) 100-299 cases; (1) The number of cases/patients is too few to report; (2) Data submitted were based on a sample of cases/patients; (3) Results are based on a shorter time period than required; (4) Data suppressed by CMS for one or more quarters; (5) Results are not available for this reporting period; (6) Fewer than 100 patients completed the HCAHPS survey; (7) No cases met the criteria for this measure; (8) The lower limit of the confidence interval cannot be calculated if the number of observed infections equals zero; (9) No data are available from the state/territory for this reporting period; (10) The scores shown reflect fewer than 50 completed surveys; (11) There were discrepancies in the data collection process; (12) This measure does not apply to this hospital for this reporting period; (13) Results cannot be calculated for this reporting period; (14) The results for this state are combined with nearby states to protect confidentiality; Please refer to the User's Guide for a full explanation of data.

Measure	Cases	This Hosp.	State Avg.	U.S. Avg.
Fibrinolytic Meds Within 30 Min. of Arrival[3,7]	-	-	66%	58%
Average Time to ECG (minutes)[1,3]	-	-	7	7
Average Time to Transfer (minutes)[3,7]	-	-	45	60
Children's Asthma Care				
Received Home Management Plan of Care	87	95%	89%	88%
Received Reliever Medication	87	100%	100%	100%
Received Systemic Corticosteroids	87	100%	100%	100%
Emergency Department				
Admittance Decision Time (minutes)[2]	541	99	107	98
Head CT Results Within 45 Min. of Arrival[1]	-	-	60%	57%
Patients Who Left ER Before Being Seen	>100k	2%	3%	2%
Time from ER Arrival to Admit. (minutes)[2]	564	280	300	274
Time from ER Arrival to Discharge (minutes)	342	163	152	134
Time in ER Before Being Evaluated (minutes)	362	37	34	26
Time to Pain Meds for Fractures (minutes)	292	72	67	57
Heart Attack Care				
Aspirin Given at Discharge	454	100%	100%	99%
Fibrinolytic Meds Within 30 Min. of Arrival[7]	-	-	75%	54%
PCI Within 90 Minutes of Arrival	83	99%	98%	96%
Statin Prescribed at Discharge	439	100%	99%	98%
Heart Failure Care				
ACE Inhibitor or ARB for LVSD	208	98%	98%	97%
Discharge Instructions Given	552	97%	96%	94%
Evaluation of LVS Function	644	100%	100%	99%
Medicare Spending				
Medicare Spending per Patient (ratio)	-	0.95	0.94	0.98
Pneumonia Care				
Appropriate Initial Antibiotic Given	306	96%	97%	95%
Blood Culture Timing	642	99%	98%	98%
Pregnancy and Delivery Care				
Newborn Deliveries Scheduled Early	198	2%	3%	6%
Preventive Care				
Immunization for Influenza[2]	515	95%	93%	90%
Immunization for Pneumonia[2]	673	96%	94%	92%
Stroke Care				
Anticoagulation Therapy for Atrial Fibrillation	49	100%	95%	95%
Antithrombotic Therapy Timing	251	100%	98%	98%
Assessed for Rehabilitation	337	100%	98%	97%
Discharged on Antithrombotic Therapy	306	100%	99%	99%
Discharged on Statin Medication	242	96%	94%	94%
Thrombolytic Therapy Timing	29	97%	64%	66%
Venous Thromboembolism Prophylaxis	314	97%	96%	94%
Written Stroke Educational Materials Given	217	100%	88%	88%
Surgical Care Improvement Project				
Appropriate Beta Blocker Usage[2]	496	98%	99%	98%
Appropriate VTP Within 24 Hours[2]	1,031	98%	99%	98%
Controlled Postoperative Blood Glucose[2]	208	98%	98%	97%
Perioperative Temperature Management[2]	1,279	100%	100%	100%
Prophylactic Antibiotic Selection[2]	1,178	100%	99%	99%
Prophylactic Antibiotic Selection (Outpatient)	849	99%	98%	98%
Prophylactic Antibiotic Stopped[2]	1,139	98%	99%	98%
Prophylactic Antibiotic Timing[2]	1,179	100%	99%	99%
Prophylactic Antibiotic Timing (Outpatient)	856	99%	99%	98%
Urinary Catheter Removal[2]	1,111	98%	99%	97%
Survey of Patients' Hospital Experiences				
Area Around Room 'Always' Quiet at Night	300+	64%	64%	61%
Doctors 'Always' Communicated Well	300+	86%	83%	82%
Home Recovery Information Given	300+	90%	87%	85%
Hospital Given 9 or 10 on 10 Point Scale	300+	79%	71%	71%
Meds 'Always' Explained Before Given	300+	68%	65%	64%
Nurses 'Always' Communicated Well	300+	82%	81%	79%
Pain 'Always' Well Controlled	300+	73%	72%	71%
Room and Bathroom 'Always' Clean	300+	72%	72%	73%
Timely Help 'Always' Received	300+	69%	68%	68%
Would Definitely Recommend Hospital	300+	81%	70%	71%
Use of Medical Imaging				
Cardiac Imaging Stress Test before Surgery	1,566	4.9%	5.4%	5.3%
Combination Abdominal CT Scan	2,309	1.9%	5.6%	10.5%
Combination Brain/Sinus CT Scan	2,004	2.1%	2.6%	2.7%
Combination Chest CT Scan	2,240	2.1%	1.3%	2.7%
Follow-up Mammogram/Ultrasound	4,766	7.1%	8%	8.8%
Lumbar Spine MRI for Low Back Pain	458	31.9%	34.7%	37.2%

Pioneer Community Hospital of Stokes

1570 Nc 8 & 89 Hwy North
Danbury, NC 27016
E-mail: llabine@wfubmc.edu
URL: www.wfubmc.edu/stokes
Phone: 336-593-2831
Fax: 336-593-5350
Type: Critical Access Hospitals
Ownership: Proprietary
Emergency Services: Yes
Beds: 93

Key Personnel:
Infection Control. . . . . Pam Boyles
Operating Room. . . . . Dana Mabe
Chief of Medical Staff . . . . Samuel C Newsome
CEO/President. . . . . Sandra Priddy
Anesthesiology. . . . . Bill Sawyer, CRNA
Emergency Room . . . . Wendy Tachardson

Measure	Cases	This Hosp.	State Avg.	U.S. Avg.
Blood Clot Prevention and Treatment				
Anticoagulation Overlap Therapy[5]	-	-	94%	93%
ICU Venous Thromboembolism Prophylaxis[5]	-	-	93%	92%
Incidence of Potentially Preventable VTE[5]	-	-	10%	10%
UFH with Dosages/Platelet Monitoring[5]	-	-	95%	97%
Venous Thromboembolism Prophylaxis[5]	-	-	88%	85%
Warfarin Therapy Discharge Instructions[5]	-	-	81%	75%
Chest Pain/Possible Heart Attack Care				
Aspirin Given Within 24 Hours of Arrival	-	-	97%	96%
Fibrinolytic Meds Within 30 Min. of Arrival	-	-	66%	58%
Average Time to ECG (minutes)	-	-	7	7
Average Time to Transfer (minutes)	-	-	45	60
Children's Asthma Care				
Received Home Management Plan of Care	-	-	89%	88%
Received Reliever Medication	-	-	100%	100%
Received Systemic Corticosteroids	-	-	100%	100%
Emergency Department				
Admittance Decision Time (minutes)[5]	-	-	107	98
Head CT Results Within 45 Min. of Arrival	-	-	60%	57%
Patients Who Left ER Before Being Seen	-	-	3%	2%
Time from ER Arrival to Admit. (minutes)[5]	-	-	300	274
Time from ER Arrival to Discharge (minutes)	-	-	152	134
Time in ER Before Being Evaluated (minutes)	-	-	34	26
Time to Pain Meds for Fractures (minutes)	-	-	67	57
Heart Attack Care				
Aspirin Given at Discharge[5]	-	-	100%	99%
Fibrinolytic Meds Within 30 Min. of Arrival[5]	-	-	75%	54%
PCI Within 90 Minutes of Arrival[5]	-	-	98%	96%
Statin Prescribed at Discharge[5]	-	-	99%	98%
Heart Failure Care				
ACE Inhibitor or ARB for LVSD[1]	-	-	98%	97%
Discharge Instructions Given	15	100%	96%	94%
Evaluation of LVS Function	19	79%	100%	99%
Medicare Spending				
Medicare Spending per Patient (ratio)	-	-	0.94	0.98
Pneumonia Care				
Appropriate Initial Antibiotic Given	20	65%	97%	95%
Blood Culture Timing	25	88%	98%	98%
Pregnancy and Delivery Care				
Newborn Deliveries Scheduled Early[5]	-	-	3%	6%
Preventive Care				
Immunization for Influenza	167	90%	93%	90%
Immunization for Pneumonia	241	85%	94%	92%
Stroke Care				
Anticoagulation Therapy for Atrial Fibrillation[5]	-	-	95%	95%
Antithrombotic Therapy Timing[5]	-	-	98%	98%
Assessed for Rehabilitation[5]	-	-	98%	97%
Discharged on Antithrombotic Therapy[5]	-	-	99%	99%
Discharged on Statin Medication[5]	-	-	94%	94%
Thrombolytic Therapy Timing[5]	-	-	64%	66%
Venous Thromboembolism Prophylaxis[5]	-	-	96%	94%
Written Stroke Educational Materials Given[5]	-	-	88%	88%
Surgical Care Improvement Project				
Appropriate Beta Blocker Usage[5]	-	-	99%	98%
Appropriate VTP Within 24 Hours[5]	-	-	99%	98%
Controlled Postoperative Blood Glucose[5]	-	-	98%	97%
Perioperative Temperature Management[5]	-	-	100%	100%
Prophylactic Antibiotic Selection[5]	-	-	99%	99%
Prophylactic Antibiotic Selection (Outpatient)	-	-	98%	98%
Prophylactic Antibiotic Stopped[5]	-	-	99%	98%
Prophylactic Antibiotic Timing[5]	-	-	99%	99%
Prophylactic Antibiotic Timing (Outpatient)	-	-	99%	98%
Urinary Catheter Removal[5]	-	-	99%	97%
Survey of Patients' Hospital Experiences				
Area Around Room 'Always' Quiet at Night[5]	-	-	64%	61%
Doctors 'Always' Communicated Well[5]	-	-	83%	82%
Home Recovery Information Given[5]	-	-	87%	85%
Hospital Given 9 or 10 on 10 Point Scale[5]	-	-	71%	71%
Meds 'Always' Explained Before Given[5]	-	-	65%	64%
Nurses 'Always' Communicated Well[5]	-	-	81%	79%
Pain 'Always' Well Controlled[5]	-	-	72%	71%
Room and Bathroom 'Always' Clean[5]	-	-	72%	73%
Timely Help 'Always' Received[5]	-	-	68%	68%
Would Definitely Recommend Hospital[5]	-	-	70%	71%
Use of Medical Imaging				
Cardiac Imaging Stress Test before Surgery	-	-	5.4%	5.3%
Combination Abdominal CT Scan	-	-	5.6%	10.5%
Combination Brain/Sinus CT Scan	-	-	2.6%	2.7%
Combination Chest CT Scan	-	-	1.3%	2.7%
Follow-up Mammogram/Ultrasound	-	-	8%	8.8%
Lumbar Spine MRI for Low Back Pain	-	-	34.7%	37.2%

Betsy Johnson Regional Hospital

800 Tilghman Dr
Dunn, NC 28334
E-mail: bjrh@bjrh.org
URL: www.bjrh.org
Phone: 910-892-7161
Fax: 910-892-5032
Type: Acute Care Hospitals
Ownership: Voluntary non-profit - Private
Emergency Services: Yes
Beds: 101

Key Personnel:
Radiology. . . . . David J Allison
CEO/President. . . . . Kenneth E Bryan, FACHE
Chief of Medical Staff . . . . Patrick Gray
Cardiac Laboratory. . . . . Betsy Johnson

Measure	Cases	This Hosp.	State Avg.	U.S. Avg.
Blood Clot Prevention and Treatment				
Anticoagulation Overlap Therapy[2]	35	71%	94%	93%
ICU Venous Thromboembolism Prophylaxis[2]	71	73%	93%	92%
Incidence of Potentially Preventable VTE[1,2]	-	-	10%	10%
UFH with Dosages/Platelet Monitoring[1,2]	-	-	95%	97%
Venous Thromboembolism Prophylaxis[2]	475	61%	88%	85%
Warfarin Therapy Discharge Instructions[2]	24	67%	81%	75%
Chest Pain/Possible Heart Attack Care				
Aspirin Given Within 24 Hours of Arrival	173	98%	97%	96%
Fibrinolytic Meds Within 30 Min. of Arrival[1]	-	-	66%	58%
Average Time to ECG (minutes)	195	7	7	7
Average Time to Transfer (minutes)[7]	-	-	45	60
Children's Asthma Care				
Received Home Management Plan of Care	-	-	89%	88%
Received Reliever Medication	-	-	100%	100%
Received Systemic Corticosteroids	-	-	100%	100%
Emergency Department				
Admittance Decision Time (minutes)[2]	840	154	107	98
Head CT Results Within 45 Min. of Arrival	23	61%	60%	57%
Patients Who Left ER Before Being Seen	46,652	3%	3%	2%
Time from ER Arrival to Admit. (minutes)[2]	881	381	300	274
Time from ER Arrival to Discharge (minutes)	565	150	152	134
Time in ER Before Being Evaluated (minutes)	515	26	34	26
Time to Pain Meds for Fractures (minutes)	130	55	67	57
Heart Attack Care				
Aspirin Given at Discharge[1]	-	-	100%	99%
Fibrinolytic Meds Within 30 Min. of Arrival[7]	-	-	75%	54%
PCI Within 90 Minutes of Arrival[7]	-	-	98%	96%
Statin Prescribed at Discharge[1]	-	-	99%	98%
Heart Failure Care				
ACE Inhibitor or ARB for LVSD	70	94%	98%	97%
Discharge Instructions Given	194	89%	96%	94%
Evaluation of LVS Function	240	99%	100%	99%
Medicare Spending				
Medicare Spending per Patient (ratio)	-	0.93	0.94	0.98
Pneumonia Care				
Appropriate Initial Antibiotic Given	165	98%	97%	95%

NOTE: Hospital profiles are in alphabetical order by state, then city, then hospital within the city; Rankings exclude hospitals with less than 25 cases except for patient surveys which excludes hospitals with less than 100 cases; (a) 100-299 cases; (1) The number of cases/patients is too few to report; (2) Data submitted were based on a sample of cases/patients; (3) Results are based on a shorter time period than required; (4) Data suppressed by CMS for one or more quarters; (5) Results are not available for this reporting period; (6) Fewer than 100 patients completed the HCAHPS survey; (7) No cases met the criteria for this measure; (8) The lower limit of the confidence interval cannot be calculated if the number of observed infections equals zero; (9) No data are available from the state/territory for this reporting period; (10) The scores shown reflect fewer than 50 completed surveys; (11) There were discrepancies in the data collection process; (12) This measure does not apply to this hospital for this reporting period; (13) Results cannot be calculated for this reporting period; (14) The results for this state are combined with nearby states to protect confidentiality; Please refer to the User's Guide for a full explanation of data.

Measure	Cases	This Hosp.	State Avg.	U.S. Avg.
Blood Culture Timing	226	98%	98%	98%
Pregnancy and Delivery Care				
Newborn Deliveries Scheduled Early	47	0%	3%	6%
Preventive Care				
Immunization for Influenza[2]	623	96%	93%	90%
Immunization for Pneumonia[2]	798	95%	94%	92%
Stroke Care				
Anticoagulation Therapy for Atrial Fibrillation[1]	-	-	95%	95%
Antithrombotic Therapy Timing	81	100%	98%	98%
Assessed for Rehabilitation	66	92%	98%	97%
Discharged on Antithrombotic Therapy	63	100%	99%	99%
Discharged on Statin Medication	57	68%	94%	94%
Thrombolytic Therapy Timing	11	0%	64%	66%
Venous Thromboembolism Prophylaxis	80	60%	96%	94%
Written Stroke Educational Materials Given	43	44%	88%	88%
Surgical Care Improvement Project				
Appropriate Beta Blocker Usage	36	86%	99%	98%
Appropriate VTP Within 24 Hours	137	97%	99%	98%
Controlled Postoperative Blood Glucose[7]	-	-	98%	97%
Perioperative Temperature Management	152	100%	100%	100%
Prophylactic Antibiotic Selection	79	99%	99%	99%
Prophylactic Antibiotic Selection (Outpatient)	71	99%	98%	98%
Prophylactic Antibiotic Stopped	72	94%	99%	98%
Prophylactic Antibiotic Timing	79	99%	99%	99%
Prophylactic Antibiotic Timing (Outpatient)	71	99%	99%	98%
Urinary Catheter Removal	113	96%	99%	97%
Survey of Patients' Hospital Experiences				
Area Around Room 'Always' Quiet at Night	300+	67%	64%	61%
Doctors 'Always' Communicated Well	300+	79%	83%	82%
Home Recovery Information Given	300+	88%	87%	85%
Hospital Given 9 or 10 on 10 Point Scale	300+	69%	71%	71%
Meds 'Always' Explained Before Given	300+	62%	65%	64%
Nurses 'Always' Communicated Well	300+	79%	81%	79%
Pain 'Always' Well Controlled	300+	68%	72%	71%
Room and Bathroom 'Always' Clean	300+	67%	72%	73%
Timely Help 'Always' Received	300+	66%	68%	68%
Would Definitely Recommend Hospital	300+	64%	70%	71%
Use of Medical Imaging				
Cardiac Imaging Stress Test before Surgery	80	6.3%	5.4%	5.3%
Combination Abdominal CT Scan	894	2.3%	5.6%	10.5%
Combination Brain/Sinus CT Scan	1,216	3.0%	2.6%	2.7%
Combination Chest CT Scan	320	0.0%	1.3%	2.7%
Follow-up Mammogram/Ultrasound	832	12.1%	8%	8.8%
Lumbar Spine MRI for Low Back Pain	103	29.1%	34.7%	37.2%

Duke Regional Hospital

3643 N Roxboro Road
Durham, NC 27704
Phone: 919-620-1078
Fax: 919-681-7925
URL: www.durhamregional.org
Type: Acute Care Hospitals
Emergency Services: Yes
Ownership: Government - Local
Beds: 369

Key Personnel:
Radiology. . . . . Mitchell Steven Anscher
Operating Room. . . . . Ralph Randal Bollinger
CEO/President. . . . . Katie Galbraith
Chief of Medical Staff . . . . Barbara Griffith, MD
Intensive Care Unit. . . . . Betty Hinshaw
Emergency Room . . . . Sarah A Stahmer, MD

Measure	Cases	This Hosp.	State Avg.	U.S. Avg.
Blood Clot Prevention and Treatment				
Anticoagulation Overlap Therapy[2]	96	100%	94%	93%
ICU Venous Thromboembolism Prophylaxis[2]	44	93%	93%	92%
Incidence of Potentially Preventable VTE[2]	14	7%	10%	10%
UFH with Dosages/Platelet Monitoring[2]	51	100%	95%	97%
Venous Thromboembolism Prophylaxis[2]	344	91%	88%	85%
Warfarin Therapy Discharge Instructions[2]	73	85%	81%	75%
Chest Pain/Possible Heart Attack Care				
Aspirin Given Within 24 Hours of Arrival[1,3]	-	-	97%	96%
Fibrinolytic Meds Within 30 Min. of Arrival[5]	-	-	66%	58%
Average Time to ECG (minutes)[1,3]	-	-	7	7
Average Time to Transfer (minutes)[5]	-	-	45	60
Children's Asthma Care				
Received Home Management Plan of Care	-	-	89%	88%
Received Reliever Medication	-	-	100%	100%
Received Systemic Corticosteroids	-	-	100%	100%
Emergency Department				
Admittance Decision Time (minutes)[2]	631	274	107	98
Head CT Results Within 45 Min. of Arrival[1]	-	-	60%	57%
Patients Who Left ER Before Being Seen	67,524	6%	3%	2%
Time from ER Arrival to Admit. (minutes)[2]	632	484	300	274
Time from ER Arrival to Discharge (minutes)	386	192	152	134
Time in ER Before Being Evaluated (minutes)	413	71	34	26
Time to Pain Meds for Fractures (minutes)	87	93	67	57
Heart Attack Care				
Aspirin Given at Discharge	217	100%	100%	99%
Fibrinolytic Meds Within 30 Min. of Arrival[7]	-	-	75%	54%
PCI Within 90 Minutes of Arrival	38	100%	98%	96%
Statin Prescribed at Discharge	208	100%	99%	98%
Heart Failure Care				
ACE Inhibitor or ARB for LVSD	125	98%	98%	97%
Discharge Instructions Given	350	98%	96%	94%
Evaluation of LVS Function	427	100%	100%	99%
Medicare Spending				
Medicare Spending per Patient (ratio)	-	0.97	0.94	0.98
Pneumonia Care				
Appropriate Initial Antibiotic Given	214	100%	97%	95%
Blood Culture Timing	422	99%	98%	98%
Pregnancy and Delivery Care				
Newborn Deliveries Scheduled Early	155	5%	3%	6%
Preventive Care				
Immunization for Influenza[2]	582	75%	93%	90%
Immunization for Pneumonia[2]	698	85%	94%	92%
Stroke Care				
Anticoagulation Therapy for Atrial Fibrillation	24	96%	95%	95%
Antithrombotic Therapy Timing	173	95%	98%	98%
Assessed for Rehabilitation	213	100%	98%	97%
Discharged on Antithrombotic Therapy	190	100%	99%	99%
Discharged on Statin Medication	154	96%	94%	94%
Thrombolytic Therapy Timing	17	88%	64%	66%
Venous Thromboembolism Prophylaxis	207	95%	96%	94%
Written Stroke Educational Materials Given	123	91%	88%	88%
Surgical Care Improvement Project				
Appropriate Beta Blocker Usage[2]	280	99%	99%	98%
Appropriate VTP Within 24 Hours[2]	888	100%	99%	98%
Controlled Postoperative Blood Glucose[2]	75	99%	98%	97%
Perioperative Temperature Management[2]	990	100%	100%	100%
Prophylactic Antibiotic Selection[2]	909	100%	99%	99%
Prophylactic Antibiotic Selection (Outpatient)	524	99%	98%	98%
Prophylactic Antibiotic Stopped[2]	895	98%	99%	98%
Prophylactic Antibiotic Timing[2]	909	99%	99%	99%
Prophylactic Antibiotic Timing (Outpatient)	525	99%	99%	98%
Urinary Catheter Removal[2]	853	99%	99%	97%
Survey of Patients' Hospital Experiences				
Area Around Room 'Always' Quiet at Night	300+	55%	64%	61%
Doctors 'Always' Communicated Well	300+	85%	83%	82%
Home Recovery Information Given	300+	85%	87%	85%
Hospital Given 9 or 10 on 10 Point Scale	300+	70%	71%	71%
Meds 'Always' Explained Before Given	300+	64%	65%	64%
Nurses 'Always' Communicated Well	300+	81%	81%	79%
Pain 'Always' Well Controlled	300+	72%	72%	71%
Room and Bathroom 'Always' Clean	300+	69%	72%	73%
Timely Help 'Always' Received	300+	64%	68%	68%
Would Definitely Recommend Hospital	300+	75%	70%	71%
Use of Medical Imaging				
Cardiac Imaging Stress Test before Surgery	339	4.1%	5.4%	5.3%
Combination Abdominal CT Scan	890	0.9%	5.6%	10.5%
Combination Brain/Sinus CT Scan	1,103	2.2%	2.6%	2.7%
Combination Chest CT Scan	369	0.0%	1.3%	2.7%
Follow-up Mammogram/Ultrasound	714	11.9%	8%	8.8%
Lumbar Spine MRI for Low Back Pain	106	34.0%	34.7%	37.2%

Duke University Hospital

PO Box 3708 Dumc Erwin Rd
Durham, NC 27710
Phone: 919-684-8111
Fax: 919-470-7376
URL: www.dukehealth.org
Type: Acute Care Hospitals
Emergency Services: Yes
Ownership: Proprietary
Beds: 1,019

Key Personnel:
Pediatric Ambulatory Care . . . . . . Clay Bordley, MD
Coronary Care. . . . . Christopher B Granger, MD
Chief of Medical Staff. . . . . Ian Greenwald, MD
Emergency Room . . . . Michael B Hocker, MD
Ambulatory Care . . . . Paul Newman
Anesthesiology. . . . . Anthony M Roche, MD
CEO/President. . . . . Kevin Sowers, RN, MSN
Radiology. . . . . Diana Voorhees, MD

Measure	Cases	This Hosp.	State Avg.	U.S. Avg.
Blood Clot Prevention and Treatment				
Anticoagulation Overlap Therapy[2]	153	100%	94%	93%
ICU Venous Thromboembolism Prophylaxis[2]	101	94%	93%	92%
Incidence of Potentially Preventable VTE[2]	82	12%	10%	10%
UFH with Dosages/Platelet Monitoring[2]	174	51%	95%	97%
Venous Thromboembolism Prophylaxis[2]	348	84%	88%	85%
Warfarin Therapy Discharge Instructions[2]	101	90%	81%	75%
Chest Pain/Possible Heart Attack Care				
Aspirin Given Within 24 Hours of Arrival[1]	-	-	97%	96%
Fibrinolytic Meds Within 30 Min. of Arrival[3,7]	-	-	66%	58%
Average Time to ECG (minutes)[1]	-	-	7	7
Average Time to Transfer (minutes)[3,7]	-	-	45	60
Children's Asthma Care				
Received Home Management Plan of Care	-	-	89%	88%
Received Reliever Medication	-	-	100%	100%
Received Systemic Corticosteroids	-	-	100%	100%
Emergency Department				
Admittance Decision Time (minutes)[2]	433	157	107	98
Head CT Results Within 45 Min. of Arrival[1]	-	-	60%	57%
Patients Who Left ER Before Being Seen	74,344	8%	3%	2%
Time from ER Arrival to Admit. (minutes)[2]	434	454	300	274
Time from ER Arrival to Discharge (minutes)	609	263	152	134
Time in ER Before Being Evaluated (minutes)	680	58	34	26
Time to Pain Meds for Fractures (minutes)	220	80	67	57
Heart Attack Care				
Aspirin Given at Discharge	660	100%	100%	99%
Fibrinolytic Meds Within 30 Min. of Arrival[7]	-	-	75%	54%
PCI Within 90 Minutes of Arrival	78	99%	98%	96%
Statin Prescribed at Discharge	634	100%	99%	98%
Heart Failure Care				
ACE Inhibitor or ARB for LVSD	295	100%	98%	97%
Discharge Instructions Given	736	99%	96%	94%
Evaluation of LVS Function	831	100%	100%	99%
Medicare Spending				
Medicare Spending per Patient (ratio)	-	0.95	0.94	0.98
Pneumonia Care				
Appropriate Initial Antibiotic Given	81	95%	97%	95%
Blood Culture Timing	265	99%	98%	98%
Pregnancy and Delivery Care				
Newborn Deliveries Scheduled Early[2]	112	2%	3%	6%
Preventive Care				
Immunization for Influenza[2]	585	78%	93%	90%
Immunization for Pneumonia[2]	599	84%	94%	92%
Stroke Care				
Anticoagulation Therapy for Atrial Fibrillation	31	97%	95%	95%
Antithrombotic Therapy Timing	211	99%	98%	98%
Assessed for Rehabilitation	332	100%	98%	97%
Discharged on Antithrombotic Therapy	246	100%	99%	99%
Discharged on Statin Medication	185	98%	94%	94%
Thrombolytic Therapy Timing	21	90%	64%	66%
Venous Thromboembolism Prophylaxis	361	95%	96%	94%
Written Stroke Educational Materials Given	214	90%	88%	88%
Surgical Care Improvement Project				
Appropriate Beta Blocker Usage[2]	424	99%	99%	98%
Appropriate VTP Within 24 Hours[2]	1,141	100%	99%	98%
Controlled Postoperative Blood Glucose[2]	185	99%	98%	97%
Perioperative Temperature Management[2]	1,376	99%	100%	100%
Prophylactic Antibiotic Selection[2]	1,127	100%	99%	99%

NOTE: Hospital profiles are in alphabetical order by state, then city, then hospital within the city; Rankings exclude hospitals with less than 25 cases except for patient surveys which excludes hospitals with less than 100 cases; (a) 100-299 cases; (1) The number of cases/patients is too few to report; (2) Data submitted were based on a sample of cases/patients; (3) Results are based on a shorter time period than required; (4) Data suppressed by CMS for one or more quarters; (5) Results are not available for this reporting period; (6) Fewer than 100 patients completed the HCAHPS survey; (7) No cases met the criteria for this measure; (8) The lower limit of the confidence interval cannot be calculated if the number of observed infections equals zero; (9) No data are available from the state/territory for this reporting period; (10) The scores shown reflect fewer than 50 completed surveys; (11) There were discrepancies in the data collection process; (12) This measure does not apply to this hospital for this reporting period; (13) Results cannot be calculated for this reporting period; (14) The results for this state are combined with nearby states to protect confidentiality; Please refer to the User's Guide for a full explanation of data.

Prophylactic Antibiotic Selection (Outpatient)	947	99%	98%	98%
Prophylactic Antibiotic Stopped[2]	1,100	99%	99%	98%
Prophylactic Antibiotic Timing[2]	1,131	100%	99%	99%
Prophylactic Antibiotic Timing (Outpatient)	748	99%	99%	98%
Urinary Catheter Removal[2]	1,085	100%	99%	97%
Survey of Patients' Hospital Experiences				
Area Around Room 'Always' Quiet at Night	300+	56%	64%	61%
Doctors 'Always' Communicated Well	300+	82%	83%	82%
Home Recovery Information Given	300+	88%	87%	85%
Hospital Given 9 or 10 on 10 Point Scale	300+	77%	71%	71%
Meds 'Always' Explained Before Given	300+	64%	65%	64%
Nurses 'Always' Communicated Well	300+	79%	81%	79%
Pain 'Always' Well Controlled	300+	71%	72%	71%
Room and Bathroom 'Always' Clean	300+	60%	72%	73%
Timely Help 'Always' Received	300+	63%	68%	68%
Would Definitely Recommend Hospital	300+	84%	70%	71%
Use of Medical Imaging				
Cardiac Imaging Stress Test before Surgery	1,516	6.7%	5.4%	5.3%
Combination Abdominal CT Scan	4,568	4.9%	5.6%	10.5%
Combination Brain/Sinus CT Scan	1,554	2.9%	2.6%	2.7%
Combination Chest CT Scan	6,920	0.0%	1.3%	2.7%
Follow-up Mammogram/Ultrasound	3,296	9.3%	8%	8.8%
Lumbar Spine MRI for Low Back Pain	356	31.5%	34.7%	37.2%

Durham VA Medical Center

508 Fulton Street
Durham, NC 27705
Phone: 919-286-0411
Fax: 919-286-6825
URL: www.va.gov/sta/guide/facility.asp?id=43
Type: Acute Care - VA
Emergency Services: No
Ownership: Government Federal
Beds: 232

Key Personnel:
Intensive Care Unit. . . . . Charles S Brudney, MD, BCh
Quality Assurance . . . . Rose Burk
CEO/President. . . . . Ralph T Gigliotti
Coronary Care . . . . David Holzer, RN
Operating Room. . . . . Lael Jackson, RN
Emergency Room . . . . Paul Matson, MD
Chief of Medical Staff. . . . . John Shelburne, MD
Infection Control. . . . . Kenneth R Wilson, MD

Measure	Cases	This Hosp.	State Avg.	U.S. Avg.
Blood Clot Prevention and Treatment				
Anticoagulation Overlap Therapy	-	-	94%	93%
ICU Venous Thromboembolism Prophylaxis	-	-	93%	92%
Incidence of Potentially Preventable VTE	-	-	10%	10%
UFH with Dosages/Platelet Monitoring	-	-	95%	97%
Venous Thromboembolism Prophylaxis	-	-	88%	85%
Warfarin Therapy Discharge Instructions	-	-	81%	75%
Chest Pain/Possible Heart Attack Care				
Aspirin Given Within 24 Hours of Arrival	-	-	97%	96%
Fibrinolytic Meds Within 30 Min. of Arrival	-	-	66%	58%
Average Time to ECG (minutes)	-	-	7	7
Average Time to Transfer (minutes)	-	-	45	60
Children's Asthma Care				
Received Home Management Plan of Care	-	-	89%	88%
Received Reliever Medication	-	-	100%	100%
Received Systemic Corticosteroids	-	-	100%	100%
Emergency Department				
Admittance Decision Time (minutes)	-	-	107	98
Head CT Results Within 45 Min. of Arrival	-	-	60%	57%
Patients Who Left ER Before Being Seen	-	-	3%	2%
Time from ER Arrival to Admit. (minutes)	-	-	300	274
Time from ER Arrival to Discharge (minutes)	-	-	152	134
Time in ER Before Being Evaluated (minutes)	-	-	34	26
Time to Pain Meds for Fractures (minutes)	-	-	67	57
Heart Attack Care				
Aspirin Given at Discharge	60	100%	100%	99%
Fibrinolytic Meds Within 30 Min. of Arrival[5]	-	-	75%	54%
PCI Within 90 Minutes of Arrival[1]	-	-	98%	96%
Statin Prescribed at Discharge	56	98%	99%	98%
Heart Failure Care				
ACE Inhibitor or ARB for LVSD	83	98%	98%	97%
Discharge Instructions Given	232	99%	96%	94%
Evaluation of LVS Function	235	100%	100%	99%
Medicare Spending				
Medicare Spending per Patient (ratio)	-	-	0.94	0.98
Pneumonia Care				
Appropriate Initial Antibiotic Given	42	98%	97%	95%
Blood Culture Timing	111	98%	98%	98%
Pregnancy and Delivery Care				
Newborn Deliveries Scheduled Early	-	-	3%	6%
Preventive Care				
Immunization for Influenza[5]	-	-	93%	90%
Immunization for Pneumonia[5]	-	-	94%	92%
Stroke Care				
Anticoagulation Therapy for Atrial Fibrillation	-	-	95%	95%
Antithrombotic Therapy Timing	-	-	98%	98%
Assessed for Rehabilitation	-	-	98%	97%
Discharged on Antithrombotic Therapy	-	-	99%	99%
Discharged on Statin Medication	-	-	94%	94%
Thrombolytic Therapy Timing	-	-	64%	66%
Venous Thromboembolism Prophylaxis	-	-	96%	94%
Written Stroke Educational Materials Given	-	-	88%	88%
Surgical Care Improvement Project				
Appropriate Beta Blocker Usage[2]	123	97%	99%	98%
Appropriate VTP Within 24 Hours[2]	183	99%	99%	98%
Controlled Postoperative Blood Glucose[2]	126	98%	98%	97%
Perioperative Temperature Management[2]	211	100%	100%	100%
Prophylactic Antibiotic Selection	217	98%	99%	99%
Prophylactic Antibiotic Selection (Outpatient)	-	-	98%	98%
Prophylactic Antibiotic Stopped	212	95%	99%	98%
Prophylactic Antibiotic Timing	218	99%	99%	99%
Prophylactic Antibiotic Timing (Outpatient)	-	-	99%	98%
Urinary Catheter Removal[2]	146	98%	99%	97%
Survey of Patients' Hospital Experiences				
Area Around Room 'Always' Quiet at Night	-	-	64%	61%
Doctors 'Always' Communicated Well	-	-	83%	82%
Home Recovery Information Given	-	-	87%	85%
Hospital Given 9 or 10 on 10 Point Scale	-	-	71%	71%
Meds 'Always' Explained Before Given	-	-	65%	64%
Nurses 'Always' Communicated Well	-	-	81%	79%
Pain 'Always' Well Controlled	-	-	72%	71%
Room and Bathroom 'Always' Clean	-	-	72%	73%
Timely Help 'Always' Received	-	-	68%	68%
Would Definitely Recommend Hospital	-	-	70%	71%
Use of Medical Imaging				
Cardiac Imaging Stress Test before Surgery	-	-	5.4%	5.3%
Combination Abdominal CT Scan	-	-	5.6%	10.5%
Combination Brain/Sinus CT Scan	-	-	2.6%	2.7%
Combination Chest CT Scan	-	-	1.3%	2.7%
Follow-up Mammogram/Ultrasound	-	-	8%	8.8%
Lumbar Spine MRI for Low Back Pain	-	-	34.7%	37.2%

North Carolina Specialty Hospital

3916 Ben Franklin Boulevard
Durham, NC 27704
Phone: 919-956-9300
Fax: 919-287-3237
URL: www.ncspecialty.com
Type: Acute Care Hospitals
Emergency Services: No
Ownership: Proprietary
Beds: 14

Key Personnel:
Chief of Medical Staff. . . . . Dr David Dellaero
Infection Control. . . . . Donna Lockamy
CEO . . . . Randi Shults

Measure	Cases	This Hosp.	State Avg.	U.S. Avg.
Blood Clot Prevention and Treatment				
Anticoagulation Overlap Therapy[1,2]	-	-	94%	93%
ICU Venous Thromboembolism Prophylaxis[2,7]	-	-	93%	92%
Incidence of Potentially Preventable VTE[1,2]	-	-	10%	10%
UFH with Dosages/Platelet Monitoring[2,7]	-	-	95%	97%
Venous Thromboembolism Prophylaxis[2]	353	100%	88%	85%
Warfarin Therapy Discharge Instructions[1,2]	-	-	81%	75%
Chest Pain/Possible Heart Attack Care				
Aspirin Given Within 24 Hours of Arrival[5]	-	-	97%	96%
Fibrinolytic Meds Within 30 Min. of Arrival[5]	-	-	66%	58%
Average Time to ECG (minutes)[5]	-	-	7	7
Average Time to Transfer (minutes)[5]	-	-	45	60
Children's Asthma Care				
Received Home Management Plan of Care	-	-	89%	88%
Received Reliever Medication	-	-	100%	100%
Received Systemic Corticosteroids	-	-	100%	100%
Emergency Department				
Admittance Decision Time (minutes)[2,7]	-	-	107	98
Head CT Results Within 45 Min. of Arrival[5]	-	-	60%	57%
Patients Who Left ER Before Being Seen[5]	-	-	3%	2%
Time from ER Arrival to Admit. (minutes)[2,7]	-	-	300	274
Time from ER Arrival to Discharge (minutes)[5]	-	-	152	134
Time in ER Before Being Evaluated (minutes)[5]	-	-	34	26
Time to Pain Meds for Fractures (minutes)[5]	-	-	67	57
Heart Attack Care				
Aspirin Given at Discharge[5]	-	-	100%	99%
Fibrinolytic Meds Within 30 Min. of Arrival[5]	-	-	75%	54%
PCI Within 90 Minutes of Arrival[5]	-	-	98%	96%
Statin Prescribed at Discharge[5]	-	-	99%	98%
Heart Failure Care				
ACE Inhibitor or ARB for LVSD[5]	-	-	98%	97%
Discharge Instructions Given[5]	-	-	96%	94%
Evaluation of LVS Function[5]	-	-	100%	99%
Medicare Spending				
Medicare Spending per Patient (ratio)	-	0.93	0.94	0.98
Pneumonia Care				
Appropriate Initial Antibiotic Given[5]	-	-	97%	95%
Blood Culture Timing[5]	-	-	98%	98%
Pregnancy and Delivery Care				
Newborn Deliveries Scheduled Early[7]	-	-	3%	6%
Preventive Care				
Immunization for Influenza[2]	304	100%	93%	90%
Immunization for Pneumonia[2]	610	100%	94%	92%
Stroke Care				
Anticoagulation Therapy for Atrial Fibrillation[5]	-	-	95%	95%
Antithrombotic Therapy Timing[5]	-	-	98%	98%
Assessed for Rehabilitation[5]	-	-	98%	97%
Discharged on Antithrombotic Therapy[5]	-	-	99%	99%
Discharged on Statin Medication[5]	-	-	94%	94%
Thrombolytic Therapy Timing[5]	-	-	64%	66%
Venous Thromboembolism Prophylaxis[5]	-	-	96%	94%
Written Stroke Educational Materials Given[5]	-	-	88%	88%
Surgical Care Improvement Project				
Appropriate Beta Blocker Usage[2]	51	100%	99%	98%
Appropriate VTP Within 24 Hours[2]	229	100%	99%	98%
Controlled Postoperative Blood Glucose[2,7]	-	-	98%	97%
Perioperative Temperature Management[2]	240	100%	100%	100%
Prophylactic Antibiotic Selection[2]	155	100%	99%	99%
Prophylactic Antibiotic Selection (Outpatient)	187	100%	98%	98%
Prophylactic Antibiotic Stopped[2]	155	100%	99%	98%
Prophylactic Antibiotic Timing[2]	155	100%	99%	99%
Prophylactic Antibiotic Timing (Outpatient)	187	100%	99%	98%
Urinary Catheter Removal[2]	233	100%	99%	97%
Survey of Patients' Hospital Experiences				
Area Around Room 'Always' Quiet at Night	300+	82%	64%	61%
Doctors 'Always' Communicated Well	300+	88%	83%	82%
Home Recovery Information Given	300+	89%	87%	85%
Hospital Given 9 or 10 on 10 Point Scale	300+	88%	71%	71%
Meds 'Always' Explained Before Given	300+	81%	65%	64%
Nurses 'Always' Communicated Well	300+	90%	81%	79%
Pain 'Always' Well Controlled	300+	80%	72%	71%
Room and Bathroom 'Always' Clean	300+	86%	72%	73%
Timely Help 'Always' Received	300+	84%	68%	68%
Would Definitely Recommend Hospital	300+	91%	70%	71%
Use of Medical Imaging				
Cardiac Imaging Stress Test before Surgery[7]	-	-	5.4%	5.3%
Combination Abdominal CT Scan[7]	-	-	5.6%	10.5%
Combination Brain/Sinus CT Scan[7]	-	-	2.6%	2.7%
Combination Chest CT Scan[7]	-	-	1.3%	2.7%
Follow-up Mammogram/Ultrasound[7]	-	-	8%	8.8%
Lumbar Spine MRI for Low Back Pain[7]	-	-	34.7%	37.2%

NOTE: Hospital profiles are in alphabetical order by state, then city, then hospital within the city; Rankings exclude hospitals with less than 25 cases except for patient surveys which excludes hospitals with less than 100 cases; (a) 100-299 cases; (1) The number of cases/patients is too few to report; (2) Data submitted were based on a sample of cases/patients; (3) Results are based on a shorter time period than required; (4) Data suppressed by CMS for one or more quarters; (5) Results are not available for this reporting period; (6) Fewer than 100 patients completed the HCAHPS survey; (7) No cases met the criteria for this measure; (8) The lower limit of the confidence interval cannot be calculated if the number of observed infections equals zero; (9) No data are available from the state/territory for this reporting period; (10) The scores shown reflect fewer than 50 completed surveys; (11) There were discrepancies in the data collection process; (12) This measure does not apply to this hospital for this reporting period; (13) Results cannot be calculated for this reporting period; (14) The results for this state are combined with nearby states to protect confidentiality; Please refer to the User's Guide for a full explanation of data.

Morehead Memorial Hospital

117 E Kings Highway
Eden, NC 27288
Phone: 336-623-9711
Fax: 336-623-6182
URL: www.morehead.org
Type: Acute Care Hospitals
Emergency Services: Yes
Ownership: Voluntary non-profit - Private
Beds: 108

Key Personnel:
Chief of Medical Staff . . . . Daphyne Anderson
President/CEO . . . . Cindy Bradley
Radiology . . . . David L Call
Patient Relations . . . . Linda Chambers
Intensive Care Unit . . . . Rose Cullom
Emergency Room . . . . Anne Mills
Quality Assurance . . . . Susan Netherland
Surgery . . . . Lisa Tucker

Measure	Cases	This Hosp.	State Avg.	U.S. Avg.
Blood Clot Prevention and Treatment				
Anticoagulation Overlap Therapy[2]	23	91%	94%	93%
ICU Venous Thromboembolism Prophylaxis[2]	72	79%	93%	92%
Incidence of Potentially Preventable VTE[1,2]	-	-	10%	10%
UFH with Dosages/Platelet Monitoring[1,2]	-	-	95%	97%
Venous Thromboembolism Prophylaxis[2]	391	76%	88%	85%
Warfarin Therapy Discharge Instructions[2]	15	100%	81%	75%
Chest Pain/Possible Heart Attack Care				
Aspirin Given Within 24 Hours of Arrival	105	98%	97%	96%
Fibrinolytic Meds Within 30 Min. of Arrival[7]	-	-	66%	58%
Average Time to ECG (minutes)	105	7	7	7
Average Time to Transfer (minutes)	12	58	45	60
Children's Asthma Care				
Received Home Management Plan of Care	-	-	89%	88%
Received Reliever Medication	-	-	100%	100%
Received Systemic Corticosteroids	-	-	100%	100%
Emergency Department				
Admittance Decision Time (minutes)[2]	652	100	107	98
Head CT Results Within 45 Min. of Arrival[1]	-	-	60%	57%
Patients Who Left ER Before Being Seen	34,048	4%	3%	2%
Time from ER Arrival to Admit. (minutes)[2]	652	316	300	274
Time from ER Arrival to Discharge (minutes)	399	150	152	134
Time in ER Before Being Evaluated (minutes)	422	46	34	26
Time to Pain Meds for Fractures (minutes)	93	99	67	57
Heart Attack Care				
Aspirin Given at Discharge	34	91%	100%	99%
Fibrinolytic Meds Within 30 Min. of Arrival[7]	-	-	75%	54%
PCI Within 90 Minutes of Arrival[7]	-	-	98%	96%
Statin Prescribed at Discharge	33	79%	99%	98%
Heart Failure Care				
ACE Inhibitor or ARB for LVSD	62	94%	98%	97%
Discharge Instructions Given	172	83%	96%	94%
Evaluation of LVS Function	227	97%	100%	99%
Medicare Spending				
Medicare Spending per Patient (ratio)	-	0.88	0.94	0.98
Pneumonia Care				
Appropriate Initial Antibiotic Given	206	93%	97%	95%
Blood Culture Timing	320	99%	98%	98%
Pregnancy and Delivery Care				
Newborn Deliveries Scheduled Early	47	0%	3%	6%
Preventive Care				
Immunization for Influenza[2]	477	95%	93%	90%
Immunization for Pneumonia[2]	629	92%	94%	92%
Stroke Care				
Anticoagulation Therapy for Atrial Fibrillation[1]	-	-	95%	95%
Antithrombotic Therapy Timing	53	98%	98%	98%
Assessed for Rehabilitation	54	89%	98%	97%
Discharged on Antithrombotic Therapy	52	96%	99%	99%
Discharged on Statin Medication	49	53%	94%	94%
Thrombolytic Therapy Timing[1]	-	-	64%	66%
Venous Thromboembolism Prophylaxis	50	66%	96%	94%
Written Stroke Educational Materials Given	27	93%	88%	88%
Surgical Care Improvement Project				
Appropriate Beta Blocker Usage	24	96%	99%	98%
Appropriate VTP Within 24 Hours	104	91%	99%	98%
Controlled Postoperative Blood Glucose[7]	-	-	98%	97%
Perioperative Temperature Management	118	100%	100%	100%
Prophylactic Antibiotic Selection	74	96%	99%	99%
Prophylactic Antibiotic Selection (Outpatient)[1,3]	-	-	98%	98%
Prophylactic Antibiotic Stopped	71	89%	99%	98%
Prophylactic Antibiotic Timing	76	99%	99%	99%
Prophylactic Antibiotic Timing (Outpatient)[1,3]	-	-	99%	98%
Urinary Catheter Removal	61	92%	99%	97%
Survey of Patients' Hospital Experiences				
Area Around Room 'Always' Quiet at Night	300+	54%	64%	61%
Doctors 'Always' Communicated Well	300+	83%	83%	82%
Home Recovery Information Given	300+	87%	87%	85%
Hospital Given 9 or 10 on 10 Point Scale	300+	68%	71%	71%
Meds 'Always' Explained Before Given	300+	68%	65%	64%
Nurses 'Always' Communicated Well	300+	79%	81%	79%
Pain 'Always' Well Controlled	300+	71%	72%	71%
Room and Bathroom 'Always' Clean	300+	75%	72%	73%
Timely Help 'Always' Received	300+	66%	68%	68%
Would Definitely Recommend Hospital	300+	69%	70%	71%
Use of Medical Imaging				
Cardiac Imaging Stress Test before Surgery	235	4.3%	5.4%	5.3%
Combination Abdominal CT Scan	544	1.3%	5.6%	10.5%
Combination Brain/Sinus CT Scan[1]	-	-	2.6%	2.7%
Combination Chest CT Scan	293	0.0%	1.3%	2.7%
Follow-up Mammogram/Ultrasound	771	6.9%	8%	8.8%
Lumbar Spine MRI for Low Back Pain	138	42.0%	34.7%	37.2%

Vidant Chowan Hospital

211 Virginia Rd
Edenton, NC 27932
Phone: 252-482-8451
Fax: 252-482-6224
URL: www.uhseast.com
Type: Critical Access Hospitals
Emergency Services: Yes
Ownership: Government - Local
Beds: 111

Key Personnel:
Chief of Medical Staff . . . . Robin Adams
Radiology . . . . Mark Adkins
CEO/President . . . . Jeffrey N Sackrison

Measure	Cases	This Hosp.	State Avg.	U.S. Avg.
Blood Clot Prevention and Treatment				
Anticoagulation Overlap Therapy[5]	-	-	94%	93%
ICU Venous Thromboembolism Prophylaxis[5]	-	-	93%	92%
Incidence of Potentially Preventable VTE[5]	-	-	10%	10%
UFH with Dosages/Platelet Monitoring[5]	-	-	95%	97%
Venous Thromboembolism Prophylaxis[5]	-	-	88%	85%
Warfarin Therapy Discharge Instructions[5]	-	-	81%	75%
Chest Pain/Possible Heart Attack Care				
Aspirin Given Within 24 Hours of Arrival	83	95%	97%	96%
Fibrinolytic Meds Within 30 Min. of Arrival[1]	-	-	66%	58%
Average Time to ECG (minutes)	87	10	7	7
Average Time to Transfer (minutes)[7]	-	-	45	60
Children's Asthma Care				
Received Home Management Plan of Care	-	-	89%	88%
Received Reliever Medication	-	-	100%	100%
Received Systemic Corticosteroids	-	-	100%	100%
Emergency Department				
Admittance Decision Time (minutes)[2]	284	36	107	98
Head CT Results Within 45 Min. of Arrival[1]	-	-	60%	57%
Patients Who Left ER Before Being Seen	15,065	3%	3%	2%
Time from ER Arrival to Admit. (minutes)[2]	295	248	300	274
Time from ER Arrival to Discharge (minutes)	360	159	152	134
Time in ER Before Being Evaluated (minutes)	388	39	34	26
Time to Pain Meds for Fractures (minutes)	54	87	67	57
Heart Attack Care				
Aspirin Given at Discharge[5]	-	-	100%	99%
Fibrinolytic Meds Within 30 Min. of Arrival[5]	-	-	75%	54%
PCI Within 90 Minutes of Arrival[5]	-	-	98%	96%
Statin Prescribed at Discharge[5]	-	-	99%	98%
Heart Failure Care				
ACE Inhibitor or ARB for LVSD	16	100%	98%	97%
Discharge Instructions Given	67	100%	96%	94%
Evaluation of LVS Function	85	99%	100%	99%
Medicare Spending				
Medicare Spending per Patient (ratio)	-	-	0.94	0.98
Pneumonia Care				
Appropriate Initial Antibiotic Given	35	97%	97%	95%
Blood Culture Timing	52	96%	98%	98%
Pregnancy and Delivery Care				
Newborn Deliveries Scheduled Early[5]	-	-	3%	6%
Preventive Care				
Immunization for Influenza[5]	-	-	93%	90%
Immunization for Pneumonia[5]	-	-	94%	92%
Stroke Care				
Anticoagulation Therapy for Atrial Fibrillation[5]	-	-	95%	95%
Antithrombotic Therapy Timing[5]	-	-	98%	98%
Assessed for Rehabilitation[5]	-	-	98%	97%
Discharged on Antithrombotic Therapy[5]	-	-	99%	99%
Discharged on Statin Medication[5]	-	-	94%	94%
Thrombolytic Therapy Timing[5]	-	-	64%	66%
Venous Thromboembolism Prophylaxis[5]	-	-	96%	94%
Written Stroke Educational Materials Given[5]	-	-	88%	88%
Surgical Care Improvement Project				
Appropriate Beta Blocker Usage	39	97%	99%	98%
Appropriate VTP Within 24 Hours	120	99%	99%	98%
Controlled Postoperative Blood Glucose[7]	-	-	98%	97%
Perioperative Temperature Management	130	100%	100%	100%
Prophylactic Antibiotic Selection	100	100%	99%	99%
Prophylactic Antibiotic Selection (Outpatient)	33	94%	98%	98%
Prophylactic Antibiotic Stopped	99	96%	99%	98%
Prophylactic Antibiotic Timing	100	100%	99%	99%
Prophylactic Antibiotic Timing (Outpatient)	34	97%	99%	98%
Urinary Catheter Removal	100	100%	99%	97%
Survey of Patients' Hospital Experiences				
Area Around Room 'Always' Quiet at Night	300+	64%	64%	61%
Doctors 'Always' Communicated Well	300+	86%	83%	82%
Home Recovery Information Given	300+	91%	87%	85%
Hospital Given 9 or 10 on 10 Point Scale	300+	79%	71%	71%
Meds 'Always' Explained Before Given	300+	70%	65%	64%
Nurses 'Always' Communicated Well	300+	84%	81%	79%
Pain 'Always' Well Controlled	300+	77%	72%	71%
Room and Bathroom 'Always' Clean	300+	83%	72%	73%
Timely Help 'Always' Received	300+	78%	68%	68%
Would Definitely Recommend Hospital	300+	75%	70%	71%
Use of Medical Imaging				
Cardiac Imaging Stress Test before Surgery	127	3.9%	5.4%	5.3%
Combination Abdominal CT Scan	396	6.1%	5.6%	10.5%
Combination Brain/Sinus CT Scan	453	4.0%	2.6%	2.7%
Combination Chest CT Scan	237	0.8%	1.3%	2.7%
Follow-up Mammogram/Ultrasound	849	8.0%	8%	8.8%
Lumbar Spine MRI for Low Back Pain	127	40.2%	34.7%	37.2%

Albemarle Hospital Authority

1144 N Road St
Elizabeth City, NC 27909
Phone: 252-335-0531
Fax: 252-384-4637
URL: www.albemarlehealth.org
Type: Acute Care Hospitals
Emergency Services: Yes
Ownership: Govt - Hospital Dist/Auth
Beds: 182

Key Personnel:
Radiology . . . . Annapurna C Rao, MD
Chief of Medical Staff . . . . Victor Sonnino
Pediatric In-Patient Care . . . . Connie Swartz, MD
Quality Assurance . . . . Richard Thompson
President . . . . Kenneth Wood

Measure	Cases	This Hosp.	State Avg.	U.S. Avg.
Blood Clot Prevention and Treatment				
Anticoagulation Overlap Therapy[2]	45	73%	94%	93%
ICU Venous Thromboembolism Prophylaxis[2]	90	86%	93%	92%
Incidence of Potentially Preventable VTE[1,2]	-	-	10%	10%
UFH with Dosages/Platelet Monitoring[2]	38	97%	95%	97%
Venous Thromboembolism Prophylaxis[2]	418	78%	88%	85%
Warfarin Therapy Discharge Instructions[2]	32	88%	81%	75%
Chest Pain/Possible Heart Attack Care				
Aspirin Given Within 24 Hours of Arrival	63	95%	97%	96%
Fibrinolytic Meds Within 30 Min. of Arrival	23	70%	66%	58%
Average Time to ECG (minutes)	66	5	7	7
Average Time to Transfer (minutes)[7]	-	-	45	60
Children's Asthma Care				
Received Home Management Plan of Care	-	-	89%	88%
Received Reliever Medication	-	-	100%	100%
Received Systemic Corticosteroids	-	-	100%	100%

NOTE: Hospital profiles are in alphabetical order by state, then city, then hospital within the city; Rankings exclude hospitals with less than 25 cases except for patient surveys which excludes hospitals with less than 100 cases; (a) 100-299 cases; (1) The number of cases/patients is too few to report; (2) Data submitted were based on a sample of cases/patients; (3) Results are based on a shorter time period than required; (4) Data suppressed by CMS for one or more quarters; (5) Results are not available for this reporting period; (6) Fewer than 100 patients completed the HCAHPS survey; (7) No cases met the criteria for this measure; (8) The lower limit of the confidence interval cannot be calculated if the number of observed infections equals zero; (9) No data are available from the state/territory for this reporting period; (10) The scores shown reflect fewer than 50 completed surveys; (11) There were discrepancies in the data collection process; (12) This measure does not apply to this hospital for this reporting period; (13) Results cannot be calculated for this reporting period; (14) The results for this state are combined with nearby states to protect confidentiality; Please refer to the User's Guide for a full explanation of data.

Emergency Department				
Admittance Decision Time (minutes)[2]	746	92	107	98
Head CT Results Within 45 Min. of Arrival	18	39%	60%	57%
Patients Who Left ER Before Being Seen	45,913	0%	3%	2%
Time from ER Arrival to Admit. (minutes)[2]	748	234	300	274
Time from ER Arrival to Discharge (minutes)	525	67	152	134
Time in ER Before Being Evaluated (minutes)	562	2	34	26
Time to Pain Meds for Fractures (minutes)	138	29	67	57
Heart Attack Care				
Aspirin Given at Discharge	79	99%	100%	99%
Fibrinolytic Meds Within 30 Min. of Arrival[1]	-	-	75%	54%
PCI Within 90 Minutes of Arrival[7]	-	-	98%	96%
Statin Prescribed at Discharge	79	95%	99%	98%
Heart Failure Care				
ACE Inhibitor or ARB for LVSD	109	97%	98%	97%
Discharge Instructions Given	202	83%	96%	94%
Evaluation of LVS Function	246	100%	100%	99%
Medicare Spending				
Medicare Spending per Patient (ratio)	-	0.91	0.94	0.98
Pneumonia Care				
Appropriate Initial Antibiotic Given	65	92%	97%	95%
Blood Culture Timing	141	96%	98%	98%
Pregnancy and Delivery Care				
Newborn Deliveries Scheduled Early[2]	63	2%	3%	6%
Preventive Care				
Immunization for Influenza[2]	517	94%	93%	90%
Immunization for Pneumonia[2]	743	91%	94%	92%
Stroke Care				
Anticoagulation Therapy for Atrial Fibrillation	16	100%	95%	95%
Antithrombotic Therapy Timing	87	100%	98%	98%
Assessed for Rehabilitation	95	93%	98%	97%
Discharged on Antithrombotic Therapy	93	100%	99%	99%
Discharged on Statin Medication	72	82%	94%	94%
Thrombolytic Therapy Timing[1]	-	-	64%	66%
Venous Thromboembolism Prophylaxis	87	87%	96%	94%
Written Stroke Educational Materials Given	61	69%	88%	88%
Surgical Care Improvement Project				
Appropriate Beta Blocker Usage	58	100%	99%	98%
Appropriate VTP Within 24 Hours	150	99%	99%	98%
Controlled Postoperative Blood Glucose[7]	-	-	98%	97%
Perioperative Temperature Management	167	100%	100%	100%
Prophylactic Antibiotic Selection	99	98%	99%	99%
Prophylactic Antibiotic Selection (Outpatient)	235	97%	98%	98%
Prophylactic Antibiotic Stopped	95	100%	99%	98%
Prophylactic Antibiotic Timing	99	99%	99%	99%
Prophylactic Antibiotic Timing (Outpatient)	154	98%	99%	98%
Urinary Catheter Removal	99	99%	99%	97%
Survey of Patients' Hospital Experiences				
Area Around Room 'Always' Quiet at Night	300+	62%	64%	61%
Doctors 'Always' Communicated Well	300+	82%	83%	82%
Home Recovery Information Given	300+	86%	87%	85%
Hospital Given 9 or 10 on 10 Point Scale	300+	66%	71%	71%
Meds 'Always' Explained Before Given	300+	63%	65%	64%
Nurses 'Always' Communicated Well	300+	79%	81%	79%
Pain 'Always' Well Controlled	300+	70%	72%	71%
Room and Bathroom 'Always' Clean	300+	71%	72%	73%
Timely Help 'Always' Received	300+	67%	68%	68%
Would Definitely Recommend Hospital	300+	66%	70%	71%
Use of Medical Imaging				
Cardiac Imaging Stress Test before Surgery	228	5.7%	5.4%	5.3%
Combination Abdominal CT Scan	929	10.7%	5.6%	10.5%
Combination Brain/Sinus CT Scan	855	1.8%	2.6%	2.7%
Combination Chest CT Scan	524	4.4%	1.3%	2.7%
Follow-up Mammogram/Ultrasound	2,017	11.4%	8%	8.8%
Lumbar Spine MRI for Low Back Pain	102	42.2%	34.7%	37.2%

Cape Fear Valley - Bladen County Hospital

501 South Poplar Street
Elizabethtown, NC 28337
Phone: 910-862-5100
Fax: 910-862-1241
URL: www.bchn.org

Type: Critical Access Hospitals
Emergency Services: Yes
Ownership: Voluntary non-profit - Private
Beds: 35

Key Personnel:

Quality Assurance . . . . Jim Burney
Radiology. . . . . Betty Carroll
Operating Room. . . . . Jennifer Dove
Pediatric In-Patient Care . . . . Martha Gooden
Chief of Medical Staff. . . . . Vicki Lanier, MD
Cardiac Laboratory. . . . . Brenda McLamb
CEO . . . . Michael Nagowski
Infection Control. . . . . Sandra Taylor, RN

Measure	Cases	This Hosp.	State Avg.	U.S. Avg.
Blood Clot Prevention and Treatment				
Anticoagulation Overlap Therapy[5]	-	-	94%	93%
ICU Venous Thromboembolism Prophylaxis[5]	-	-	93%	92%
Incidence of Potentially Preventable VTE[5]	-	-	10%	10%
UFH with Dosages/Platelet Monitoring[5]	-	-	95%	97%
Venous Thromboembolism Prophylaxis[5]	-	-	88%	85%
Warfarin Therapy Discharge Instructions[5]	-	-	81%	75%
Chest Pain/Possible Heart Attack Care				
Aspirin Given Within 24 Hours of Arrival[5]	-	-	97%	96%
Fibrinolytic Meds Within 30 Min. of Arrival[5]	-	-	66%	58%
Average Time to ECG (minutes)[5]	-	-	7	7
Average Time to Transfer (minutes)[5]	-	-	45	60
Children's Asthma Care				
Received Home Management Plan of Care	-	-	89%	88%
Received Reliever Medication	-	-	100%	100%
Received Systemic Corticosteroids	-	-	100%	100%
Emergency Department				
Admittance Decision Time (minutes)[5]	-	-	107	98
Head CT Results Within 45 Min. of Arrival[5]	-	-	60%	57%
Patients Who Left ER Before Being Seen	16,312	3%	3%	2%
Time from ER Arrival to Admit. (minutes)[5]	-	-	300	274
Time from ER Arrival to Discharge (minutes)[5]	-	-	152	134
Time in ER Before Being Evaluated (minutes)[5]	-	-	34	26
Time to Pain Meds for Fractures (minutes)[5]	-	-	67	57
Heart Attack Care				
Aspirin Given at Discharge[5]	-	-	100%	99%
Fibrinolytic Meds Within 30 Min. of Arrival[5]	-	-	75%	54%
PCI Within 90 Minutes of Arrival[5]	-	-	98%	96%
Statin Prescribed at Discharge[5]	-	-	99%	98%
Heart Failure Care				
ACE Inhibitor or ARB for LVSD[1,3]	-	-	98%	97%
Discharge Instructions Given[1,3]	-	-	96%	94%
Evaluation of LVS Function[1,3]	-	-	100%	99%
Medicare Spending				
Medicare Spending per Patient (ratio)	-	-	0.94	0.98
Pneumonia Care				
Appropriate Initial Antibiotic Given[1,3]	-	-	97%	95%
Blood Culture Timing[1,3]	-	-	98%	98%
Pregnancy and Delivery Care				
Newborn Deliveries Scheduled Early[5]	-	-	3%	6%
Preventive Care				
Immunization for Influenza[1,3]	-	-	93%	90%
Immunization for Pneumonia[1,3]	-	-	94%	92%
Stroke Care				
Anticoagulation Therapy for Atrial Fibrillation[5]	-	-	95%	95%
Antithrombotic Therapy Timing[5]	-	-	98%	98%
Assessed for Rehabilitation[5]	-	-	98%	97%
Discharged on Antithrombotic Therapy[5]	-	-	99%	99%
Discharged on Statin Medication[5]	-	-	94%	94%
Thrombolytic Therapy Timing[5]	-	-	64%	66%
Venous Thromboembolism Prophylaxis[5]	-	-	96%	94%
Written Stroke Educational Materials Given[5]	-	-	88%	88%
Surgical Care Improvement Project				
Appropriate Beta Blocker Usage[1,3]	-	-	99%	98%
Appropriate VTP Within 24 Hours[1,3]	-	-	99%	98%
Controlled Postoperative Blood Glucose[3,7]	-	-	98%	97%
Perioperative Temperature Management[1,3]	-	-	100%	100%
Prophylactic Antibiotic Selection[1,3]	-	-	99%	99%
Prophylactic Antibiotic Selection (Outpatient)[5]	-	-	98%	98%
Prophylactic Antibiotic Stopped[1,3]	-	-	99%	98%
Prophylactic Antibiotic Timing[1,3]	-	-	99%	99%
Prophylactic Antibiotic Timing (Outpatient)[5]	-	-	99%	98%
Urinary Catheter Removal[3,7]	-	-	99%	97%
Survey of Patients' Hospital Experiences				
Area Around Room 'Always' Quiet at Night[5]	-	-	64%	61%
Doctors 'Always' Communicated Well[5]	-	-	83%	82%
Home Recovery Information Given[5]	-	-	87%	85%
Hospital Given 9 or 10 on 10 Point Scale[5]	-	-	71%	71%
Meds 'Always' Explained Before Given[5]	-	-	65%	64%
Nurses 'Always' Communicated Well[5]	-	-	81%	79%
Pain 'Always' Well Controlled[5]	-	-	72%	71%
Room and Bathroom 'Always' Clean[5]	-	-	72%	73%
Timely Help 'Always' Received[5]	-	-	68%	68%
Would Definitely Recommend Hospital[5]	-	-	70%	71%
Use of Medical Imaging				
Cardiac Imaging Stress Test before Surgery[7]	-	-	5.4%	5.3%
Combination Abdominal CT Scan	228	9.6%	5.6%	10.5%
Combination Brain/Sinus CT Scan[1]	-	-	2.6%	2.7%
Combination Chest CT Scan	77	11.7%	1.3%	2.7%
Follow-up Mammogram/Ultrasound	448	6.5%	8%	8.8%
Lumbar Spine MRI for Low Back Pain[1]	-	-	34.7%	37.2%

Hugh Chatham Memorial Hospital

180 Parkwood Dr
Elkin, NC 28621
Phone: 336-527-7000
Fax: 336-835-9262
E-mail: info@hughchatham.org
URL: www.hughchatham.org

Type: Acute Care Hospitals
Emergency Services: Yes
Ownership: Voluntary non-profit - Private
Beds: 222

Key Personnel:

Chief of Medical Staff . . . . Evan Ballard
Radiology. . . . . Paul Beerman
CEO/President. . . . . Richard Osmus

Measure	Cases	This Hosp.	State Avg.	U.S. Avg.
Blood Clot Prevention and Treatment				
Anticoagulation Overlap Therapy[2]	31	100%	94%	93%
ICU Venous Thromboembolism Prophylaxis[2]	110	100%	93%	92%
Incidence of Potentially Preventable VTE[2,7]	-	-	10%	10%
UFH with Dosages/Platelet Monitoring[1,2]	-	-	95%	97%
Venous Thromboembolism Prophylaxis[2]	255	92%	88%	85%
Warfarin Therapy Discharge Instructions[2]	27	100%	81%	75%
Chest Pain/Possible Heart Attack Care				
Aspirin Given Within 24 Hours of Arrival	159	99%	97%	96%
Fibrinolytic Meds Within 30 Min. of Arrival[7]	-	-	66%	58%
Average Time to ECG (minutes)	170	6	7	7
Average Time to Transfer (minutes)[1]	-	-	45	60
Children's Asthma Care				
Received Home Management Plan of Care	-	-	89%	88%
Received Reliever Medication	-	-	100%	100%
Received Systemic Corticosteroids	-	-	100%	100%
Emergency Department				
Admittance Decision Time (minutes)[2]	679	65	107	98
Head CT Results Within 45 Min. of Arrival[1]	-	-	60%	57%
Patients Who Left ER Before Being Seen	31,611	0%	3%	2%
Time from ER Arrival to Admit. (minutes)[2]	680	248	300	274
Time from ER Arrival to Discharge (minutes)	383	132	152	134
Time in ER Before Being Evaluated (minutes)	429	20	34	26
Time to Pain Meds for Fractures (minutes)	86	58	67	57
Heart Attack Care				
Aspirin Given at Discharge	18	94%	100%	99%
Fibrinolytic Meds Within 30 Min. of Arrival[7]	-	-	75%	54%
PCI Within 90 Minutes of Arrival[7]	-	-	98%	96%
Statin Prescribed at Discharge	16	94%	99%	98%
Heart Failure Care				
ACE Inhibitor or ARB for LVSD	20	100%	98%	97%
Discharge Instructions Given	115	91%	96%	94%
Evaluation of LVS Function	146	99%	100%	99%
Medicare Spending				
Medicare Spending per Patient (ratio)	-	0.93	0.94	0.98
Pneumonia Care				
Appropriate Initial Antibiotic Given	139	98%	97%	95%
Blood Culture Timing	209	98%	98%	98%
Pregnancy and Delivery Care				
Newborn Deliveries Scheduled Early	45	9%	3%	6%
Preventive Care				
Immunization for Influenza[2]	478	98%	93%	90%
Immunization for Pneumonia[2]	562	98%	94%	92%
Stroke Care				

NOTE: Hospital profiles are in alphabetical order by state, then city, then hospital within the city; Rankings exclude hospitals with less than 25 cases except for patient surveys which excludes hospitals with less than 100 cases; (a) 100-299 cases; (1) The number of cases/patients is too few to report; (2) Data submitted were based on a sample of cases/patients; (3) Results are based on a shorter time period than required; (4) Data suppressed by CMS for one or more quarters; (5) Results are not available for this reporting period; (6) Fewer than 100 patients completed the HCAHPS survey; (7) No cases met the criteria for this measure; (8) The lower limit of the confidence interval cannot be calculated if the number of observed infections equals zero; (9) No data are available from the state/territory for this reporting period; (10) The scores shown reflect fewer than 50 completed surveys; (11) There were discrepancies in the data collection process; (12) This measure does not apply to this hospital for this reporting period; (13) Results cannot be calculated for this reporting period; (14) The results for this state are combined with nearby states to protect confidentiality; Please refer to the User's Guide for a full explanation of data.

Measure	Cases	This Hosp.	State Avg.	U.S. Avg.
Anticoagulation Therapy for Atrial Fibrillation[1]	-	-	95%	95%
Antithrombotic Therapy Timing	37	100%	98%	98%
Assessed for Rehabilitation	37	100%	98%	97%
Discharged on Antithrombotic Therapy	37	100%	99%	99%
Discharged on Statin Medication	26	100%	94%	94%
Thrombolytic Therapy Timing[7]	-	-	64%	66%
Venous Thromboembolism Prophylaxis	28	100%	96%	94%
Written Stroke Educational Materials Given	31	97%	88%	88%
Surgical Care Improvement Project				
Appropriate Beta Blocker Usage	59	100%	99%	98%
Appropriate VTP Within 24 Hours	236	100%	99%	98%
Controlled Postoperative Blood Glucose[7]	-	-	98%	97%
Perioperative Temperature Management	266	100%	100%	100%
Prophylactic Antibiotic Selection	212	100%	99%	99%
Prophylactic Antibiotic Selection (Outpatient)	73	97%	98%	98%
Prophylactic Antibiotic Stopped	212	100%	99%	98%
Prophylactic Antibiotic Timing	212	100%	99%	99%
Prophylactic Antibiotic Timing (Outpatient)	73	100%	99%	98%
Urinary Catheter Removal	29	100%	99%	97%
Survey of Patients' Hospital Experiences				
Area Around Room 'Always' Quiet at Night	300+	74%	64%	61%
Doctors 'Always' Communicated Well	300+	84%	83%	82%
Home Recovery Information Given	300+	85%	87%	85%
Hospital Given 9 or 10 on 10 Point Scale	300+	79%	71%	71%
Meds 'Always' Explained Before Given	300+	66%	65%	64%
Nurses 'Always' Communicated Well	300+	84%	81%	79%
Pain 'Always' Well Controlled	300+	71%	72%	71%
Room and Bathroom 'Always' Clean	300+	83%	72%	73%
Timely Help 'Always' Received	300+	72%	68%	68%
Would Definitely Recommend Hospital	300+	79%	70%	71%
Use of Medical Imaging				
Cardiac Imaging Stress Test before Surgery	94	3.2%	5.4%	5.3%
Combination Abdominal CT Scan	694	2.9%	5.6%	10.5%
Combination Brain/Sinus CT Scan	672	1.8%	2.6%	2.7%
Combination Chest CT Scan	305	1.3%	1.3%	2.7%
Follow-up Mammogram/Ultrasound	918	3.9%	8%	8.8%
Lumbar Spine MRI for Low Back Pain	109	35.8%	34.7%	37.2%

Cape Fear Valley Medical Center

1638 Owen Drive PO Box 2000
Fayetteville, NC 28302
URL: www.capefearvalley.com
Phone: 910-609-4000
Fax: 910-609-6160
Type: Acute Care Hospitals
Emergency Services: Yes
Ownership: Voluntary non-profit - Private
Beds: 616

Key Personnel:
Radiology.................. David J Allison
Operating Room.............. Ravinder K Annamaneni, RN
Infection Control............. Kathy Butler
Quality Assurance .... Harold Mayner
CEO/President............... Michael Nagowski
Pediatric In-Patient Care .... Clarito Pang
Chief of Medical Staff.......... Eugene Wright

Measure	Cases	This Hosp.	State Avg.	U.S. Avg.
Blood Clot Prevention and Treatment				
Anticoagulation Overlap Therapy[2]	205	98%	94%	93%
ICU Venous Thromboembolism Prophylaxis[2]	56	96%	93%	92%
Incidence of Potentially Preventable VTE[2]	38	18%	10%	10%
UFH with Dosages/Platelet Monitoring[2]	38	100%	95%	97%
Venous Thromboembolism Prophylaxis[2]	383	93%	88%	85%
Warfarin Therapy Discharge Instructions[2]	160	99%	81%	75%
Chest Pain/Possible Heart Attack Care				
Aspirin Given Within 24 Hours of Arrival	17	94%	97%	96%
Fibrinolytic Meds Within 30 Min. of Arrival[3,7]	-	-	66%	58%
Average Time to ECG (minutes)	18	14	7	7
Average Time to Transfer (minutes)[3,7]	-	-	45	60
Children's Asthma Care				
Received Home Management Plan of Care	-	-	89%	88%
Received Reliever Medication	-	-	100%	100%
Received Systemic Corticosteroids	-	-	100%	100%
Emergency Department				
Admittance Decision Time (minutes)[2]	733	217	107	98
Head CT Results Within 45 Min. of Arrival[1]	-	-	60%	57%
Patients Who Left ER Before Being Seen	>100k	1%	3%	2%
Time from ER Arrival to Admit. (minutes)[2]	735	484	300	274
Time from ER Arrival to Discharge (minutes)	322	203	152	134
Time in ER Before Being Evaluated (minutes)	390	24	34	26
Time to Pain Meds for Fractures (minutes)	334	76	67	57
Heart Attack Care				
Aspirin Given at Discharge	681	100%	100%	99%
Fibrinolytic Meds Within 30 Min. of Arrival[1]	-	-	75%	54%
PCI Within 90 Minutes of Arrival	127	96%	98%	96%
Statin Prescribed at Discharge	651	100%	99%	98%
Heart Failure Care				
ACE Inhibitor or ARB for LVSD	355	99%	98%	97%
Discharge Instructions Given	1,018	98%	96%	94%
Evaluation of LVS Function	1,174	100%	100%	99%
Medicare Spending				
Medicare Spending per Patient (ratio)	-	0.94	0.94	0.98
Pneumonia Care				
Appropriate Initial Antibiotic Given	451	99%	97%	95%
Blood Culture Timing	803	99%	98%	98%
Pregnancy and Delivery Care				
Newborn Deliveries Scheduled Early[2]	85	1%	3%	6%
Preventive Care				
Immunization for Influenza[2]	504	97%	93%	90%
Immunization for Pneumonia[2]	622	97%	94%	92%
Stroke Care				
Anticoagulation Therapy for Atrial Fibrillation	25	96%	95%	95%
Antithrombotic Therapy Timing	312	100%	98%	98%
Assessed for Rehabilitation	351	100%	98%	97%
Discharged on Antithrombotic Therapy	307	100%	99%	99%
Discharged on Statin Medication	234	99%	94%	94%
Thrombolytic Therapy Timing	14	100%	64%	66%
Venous Thromboembolism Prophylaxis	366	99%	96%	94%
Written Stroke Educational Materials Given	184	95%	88%	88%
Surgical Care Improvement Project				
Appropriate Beta Blocker Usage[2]	380	99%	99%	98%
Appropriate VTP Within 24 Hours[2]	691	99%	99%	98%
Controlled Postoperative Blood Glucose[2]	160	97%	98%	97%
Perioperative Temperature Management[2]	959	100%	100%	100%
Prophylactic Antibiotic Selection[2]	807	99%	99%	99%
Prophylactic Antibiotic Selection (Outpatient)	416	97%	98%	98%
Prophylactic Antibiotic Stopped[2]	796	99%	99%	98%
Prophylactic Antibiotic Timing[2]	808	100%	99%	99%
Prophylactic Antibiotic Timing (Outpatient)	426	97%	99%	98%
Urinary Catheter Removal[2]	639	98%	99%	97%
Survey of Patients' Hospital Experiences				
Area Around Room 'Always' Quiet at Night	300+	57%	64%	61%
Doctors 'Always' Communicated Well	300+	77%	83%	82%
Home Recovery Information Given	300+	81%	87%	85%
Hospital Given 9 or 10 on 10 Point Scale	300+	61%	71%	71%
Meds 'Always' Explained Before Given	300+	62%	65%	64%
Nurses 'Always' Communicated Well	300+	76%	81%	79%
Pain 'Always' Well Controlled	300+	70%	72%	71%
Room and Bathroom 'Always' Clean	300+	65%	72%	73%
Timely Help 'Always' Received	300+	61%	68%	68%
Would Definitely Recommend Hospital	300+	59%	70%	71%
Use of Medical Imaging				
Cardiac Imaging Stress Test before Surgery	501	5.0%	5.4%	5.3%
Combination Abdominal CT Scan	1,390	2.4%	5.6%	10.5%
Combination Brain/Sinus CT Scan	1,817	3.5%	2.6%	2.7%
Combination Chest CT Scan	785	0.4%	1.3%	2.7%
Follow-up Mammogram/Ultrasound	1,125	10.4%	8%	8.8%
Lumbar Spine MRI for Low Back Pain	84	38.1%	34.7%	37.2%

Fayetteville NC VA Medical Center

2300 Ramsey Street
Fayetteville, NC 28301
URL: www.va.gov/sta/guide/home.asp
Phone: 910-488-2120
Fax: 910-822-7927
Type: Acute Care - VA
Emergency Services: No
Ownership: Government Federal
Beds: 159

Key Personnel:
Chief of Medical Staff.......... Kanan Chatterje, MD
Quality Assurance .... Beatrice Olack, RN
CEO/President............... Bruce C Triplett

Measure	Cases	This Hosp.	State Avg.	U.S. Avg.
Blood Clot Prevention and Treatment				
Anticoagulation Overlap Therapy	-	-	94%	93%
ICU Venous Thromboembolism Prophylaxis	-	-	93%	92%
Incidence of Potentially Preventable VTE	-	-	10%	10%
UFH with Dosages/Platelet Monitoring	-	-	95%	97%
Venous Thromboembolism Prophylaxis	-	-	88%	85%
Warfarin Therapy Discharge Instructions	-	-	81%	75%
Chest Pain/Possible Heart Attack Care				
Aspirin Given Within 24 Hours of Arrival	-	-	97%	96%
Fibrinolytic Meds Within 30 Min. of Arrival	-	-	66%	58%
Average Time to ECG (minutes)	-	-	7	7
Average Time to Transfer (minutes)	-	-	45	60
Children's Asthma Care				
Received Home Management Plan of Care	-	-	89%	88%
Received Reliever Medication	-	-	100%	100%
Received Systemic Corticosteroids	-	-	100%	100%
Emergency Department				
Admittance Decision Time (minutes)	-	-	107	98
Head CT Results Within 45 Min. of Arrival	-	-	60%	57%
Patients Who Left ER Before Being Seen	-	-	3%	2%
Time from ER Arrival to Admit. (minutes)	-	-	300	274
Time from ER Arrival to Discharge (minutes)	-	-	152	134
Time in ER Before Being Evaluated (minutes)	-	-	34	26
Time to Pain Meds for Fractures (minutes)	-	-	67	57
Heart Attack Care				
Aspirin Given at Discharge[5]	-	-	100%	99%
Fibrinolytic Meds Within 30 Min. of Arrival[5]	-	-	75%	54%
PCI Within 90 Minutes of Arrival[5]	-	-	98%	96%
Statin Prescribed at Discharge[5]	-	-	99%	98%
Heart Failure Care				
ACE Inhibitor or ARB for LVSD	33	97%	98%	97%
Discharge Instructions Given	74	100%	96%	94%
Evaluation of LVS Function	76	99%	100%	99%
Medicare Spending				
Medicare Spending per Patient (ratio)	-	-	0.94	0.98
Pneumonia Care				
Appropriate Initial Antibiotic Given	30	97%	97%	95%
Blood Culture Timing	42	100%	98%	98%
Pregnancy and Delivery Care				
Newborn Deliveries Scheduled Early	-	-	3%	6%
Preventive Care				
Immunization for Influenza[2,3]	134	38%	93%	90%
Immunization for Pneumonia[2,3]	236	50%	94%	92%
Stroke Care				
Anticoagulation Therapy for Atrial Fibrillation	-	-	95%	95%
Antithrombotic Therapy Timing	-	-	98%	98%
Assessed for Rehabilitation	-	-	98%	97%
Discharged on Antithrombotic Therapy	-	-	99%	99%
Discharged on Statin Medication	-	-	94%	94%
Thrombolytic Therapy Timing	-	-	64%	66%
Venous Thromboembolism Prophylaxis	-	-	96%	94%
Written Stroke Educational Materials Given	-	-	88%	88%
Surgical Care Improvement Project				
Appropriate Beta Blocker Usage[5]	-	-	99%	98%
Appropriate VTP Within 24 Hours[5]	-	-	99%	98%
Controlled Postoperative Blood Glucose[5]	-	-	98%	97%
Perioperative Temperature Management[5]	-	-	100%	100%
Prophylactic Antibiotic Selection[5]	-	-	99%	99%
Prophylactic Antibiotic Selection (Outpatient)	-	-	98%	98%
Prophylactic Antibiotic Stopped[5]	-	-	99%	98%
Prophylactic Antibiotic Timing[5]	-	-	99%	99%
Prophylactic Antibiotic Timing (Outpatient)	-	-	99%	98%
Urinary Catheter Removal[5]	-	-	99%	97%
Survey of Patients' Hospital Experiences				
Area Around Room 'Always' Quiet at Night	-	-	64%	61%
Doctors 'Always' Communicated Well	-	-	83%	82%
Home Recovery Information Given	-	-	87%	85%
Hospital Given 9 or 10 on 10 Point Scale	-	-	71%	71%
Meds 'Always' Explained Before Given	-	-	65%	64%
Nurses 'Always' Communicated Well	-	-	81%	79%
Pain 'Always' Well Controlled	-	-	72%	71%
Room and Bathroom 'Always' Clean	-	-	72%	73%
Timely Help 'Always' Received	-	-	68%	68%

NOTE: Hospital profiles are in alphabetical order by state, then city, then hospital within the city; Rankings exclude hospitals with less than 25 cases except for patient surveys which excludes hospitals with less than 100 cases; (a) 100-299 cases; (1) The number of cases/patients is too few to report; (2) Data submitted were based on a sample of cases/patients; (3) Results are based on a shorter time period than required; (4) Data suppressed by CMS for one or more quarters; (5) Results are not available for this reporting period; (6) Fewer than 100 patients completed the HCAHPS survey; (7) No cases met the criteria for this measure; (8) The lower limit of the confidence interval cannot be calculated if the number of observed infections equals zero; (9) No data are available from the state/territory for this reporting period; (10) The scores shown reflect fewer than 50 completed surveys; (11) There were discrepancies in the data collection process; (12) This measure does not apply to this hospital for this reporting period; (13) Results cannot be calculated for this reporting period; (14) The results for this state are combined with nearby states to protect confidentiality; Please refer to the User's Guide for a full explanation of data.

Measure	Cases	This Hosp.	State Avg.	U.S. Avg.
Would Definitely Recommend Hospital	-	-	70%	71%
Use of Medical Imaging				
Cardiac Imaging Stress Test before Surgery	-	-	5.4%	5.3%
Combination Abdominal CT Scan	-	-	5.6%	10.5%
Combination Brain/Sinus CT Scan	-	-	2.6%	2.7%
Combination Chest CT Scan	-	-	1.3%	2.7%
Follow-up Mammogram/Ultrasound	-	-	8%	8.8%
Lumbar Spine MRI for Low Back Pain	-	-	34.7%	37.2%

Angel Medical Center

120 Riverview Saint PO Box 1209
Franklin, NC 28734
Phone: 828-524-8411
Fax: 828-369-4162
E-mail: amc@angelmed.org
URL: www.angelmed.org
Type: Critical Access Hospitals
Emergency Services: Yes
Ownership: Voluntary non-profit - Private
Beds: 52
Key Personnel:
Radiology. . . . . Robert Berger, MD
CEO/President. . . . . James B. Bross
Cardiac Laboratory. . . . . Michael J Kegan, MD
Chief of Medical Staff. . . . . Travis Petrieck, MD
Chairman/CEO . . . . Jan Unger

Measure	Cases	This Hosp.	State Avg.	U.S. Avg.
Blood Clot Prevention and Treatment				
Anticoagulation Overlap Therapy[2]	11	91%	94%	93%
ICU Venous Thromboembolism Prophylaxis[2]	55	96%	93%	92%
Incidence of Potentially Preventable VTE[2,7]	-	-	10%	10%
UFH with Dosages/Platelet Monitoring[2,7]	-	-	95%	97%
Venous Thromboembolism Prophylaxis[2]	174	90%	88%	85%
Warfarin Therapy Discharge Instructions[2]	11	100%	81%	75%
Chest Pain/Possible Heart Attack Care				
Aspirin Given Within 24 Hours of Arrival	48	94%	97%	96%
Fibrinolytic Meds Within 30 Min. of Arrival[1]	-	-	66%	58%
Average Time to ECG (minutes)	51	13	7	7
Average Time to Transfer (minutes)[7]	-	-	45	60
Children's Asthma Care				
Received Home Management Plan of Care	-	-	89%	88%
Received Reliever Medication	-	-	100%	100%
Received Systemic Corticosteroids	-	-	100%	100%
Emergency Department				
Admittance Decision Time (minutes)[2]	690	119	107	98
Head CT Results Within 45 Min. of Arrival	15	93%	60%	57%
Patients Who Left ER Before Being Seen	14,614	1%	3%	2%
Time from ER Arrival to Admit. (minutes)[2]	721	268	300	274
Time from ER Arrival to Discharge (minutes)	538	132	152	134
Time in ER Before Being Evaluated (minutes)	570	30	34	26
Time to Pain Meds for Fractures (minutes)	95	67	67	57
Heart Attack Care				
Aspirin Given at Discharge	12	92%	100%	99%
Fibrinolytic Meds Within 30 Min. of Arrival[7]	-	-	75%	54%
PCI Within 90 Minutes of Arrival[7]	-	-	98%	96%
Statin Prescribed at Discharge	12	100%	99%	98%
Heart Failure Care				
ACE Inhibitor or ARB for LVSD	24	100%	98%	97%
Discharge Instructions Given	46	98%	96%	94%
Evaluation of LVS Function	56	98%	100%	99%
Medicare Spending				
Medicare Spending per Patient (ratio)	-	-	0.94	0.98
Pneumonia Care				
Appropriate Initial Antibiotic Given	63	94%	97%	95%
Blood Culture Timing	93	98%	98%	98%
Pregnancy and Delivery Care				
Newborn Deliveries Scheduled Early[1,3]	-	-	3%	6%
Preventive Care				
Immunization for Influenza[2]	451	98%	93%	90%
Immunization for Pneumonia[2]	697	99%	94%	92%
Stroke Care				
Anticoagulation Therapy for Atrial Fibrillation[1]	-	-	95%	95%
Antithrombotic Therapy Timing	17	88%	98%	98%
Assessed for Rehabilitation	20	100%	98%	97%
Discharged on Antithrombotic Therapy	18	100%	99%	99%
Discharged on Statin Medication	18	89%	94%	94%
Thrombolytic Therapy Timing[7]	-	-	64%	66%
Venous Thromboembolism Prophylaxis	20	70%	96%	94%
Written Stroke Educational Materials Given[1]	-	-	88%	88%
Surgical Care Improvement Project				
Appropriate Beta Blocker Usage	14	100%	99%	98%
Appropriate VTP Within 24 Hours	66	98%	99%	98%
Controlled Postoperative Blood Glucose[7]	-	-	98%	97%
Perioperative Temperature Management	78	100%	100%	100%
Prophylactic Antibiotic Selection	48	98%	99%	99%
Prophylactic Antibiotic Selection (Outpatient)	20	90%	98%	98%
Prophylactic Antibiotic Stopped	48	100%	99%	98%
Prophylactic Antibiotic Timing	49	98%	99%	99%
Prophylactic Antibiotic Timing (Outpatient)	20	95%	99%	98%
Urinary Catheter Removal	63	98%	99%	97%
Survey of Patients' Hospital Experiences				
Area Around Room 'Always' Quiet at Night	300+	55%	64%	61%
Doctors 'Always' Communicated Well	300+	86%	83%	82%
Home Recovery Information Given	300+	83%	87%	85%
Hospital Given 9 or 10 on 10 Point Scale	300+	73%	71%	71%
Meds 'Always' Explained Before Given	300+	64%	65%	64%
Nurses 'Always' Communicated Well	300+	82%	81%	79%
Pain 'Always' Well Controlled	300+	74%	72%	71%
Room and Bathroom 'Always' Clean	300+	70%	72%	73%
Timely Help 'Always' Received	300+	75%	68%	68%
Would Definitely Recommend Hospital	300+	74%	70%	71%
Use of Medical Imaging				
Cardiac Imaging Stress Test before Surgery	210	3.8%	5.4%	5.3%
Combination Abdominal CT Scan	509	5.9%	5.6%	10.5%
Combination Brain/Sinus CT Scan	442	0.9%	2.6%	2.7%
Combination Chest CT Scan	307	2.0%	1.3%	2.7%
Follow-up Mammogram/Ultrasound	1,176	4.4%	8%	8.8%
Lumbar Spine MRI for Low Back Pain	59	28.8%	34.7%	37.2%

Caromont Regional Medical Center

2525 Court Dr
Gastonia, NC 28052
Phone: 704-834-4891
Fax: 704-834-2068
URL: www.caromont.org
Type: Acute Care Hospitals
Emergency Services: Yes
Ownership: Government - Local
Beds: 435
Key Personnel:
Intensive Care Unit. . . . . Kathy Abrams
Radiology. . . . . Gerald W Arney, MD
Emergency Room . . . . Carol Dare
Infection Control. . . . . Connie Ford
Operating Room. . . . . Rose O'Neill
Quality Assurance . . . . Martha Rockett
Chief of Medical Staff. . . . . H Thomason, MD
Anesthesiology. . . . . Thomas W Wingfield, MD

Measure	Cases	This Hosp.	State Avg.	U.S. Avg.
Blood Clot Prevention and Treatment				
Anticoagulation Overlap Therapy[2]	136	99%	94%	93%
ICU Venous Thromboembolism Prophylaxis[2]	64	91%	93%	92%
Incidence of Potentially Preventable VTE[2]	13	8%	10%	10%
UFH with Dosages/Platelet Monitoring[2]	80	100%	95%	97%
Venous Thromboembolism Prophylaxis[2]	351	94%	88%	85%
Warfarin Therapy Discharge Instructions[2]	105	95%	81%	75%
Chest Pain/Possible Heart Attack Care				
Aspirin Given Within 24 Hours of Arrival[5]	-	-	97%	96%
Fibrinolytic Meds Within 30 Min. of Arrival[5]	-	-	66%	58%
Average Time to ECG (minutes)[5]	-	-	7	7
Average Time to Transfer (minutes)[5]	-	-	45	60
Children's Asthma Care				
Received Home Management Plan of Care	-	-	89%	88%
Received Reliever Medication	-	-	100%	100%
Received Systemic Corticosteroids	-	-	100%	100%
Emergency Department				
Admittance Decision Time (minutes)[2]	834	104	107	98
Head CT Results Within 45 Min. of Arrival	17	76%	60%	57%
Patients Who Left ER Before Being Seen	>100k	0%	3%	2%
Time from ER Arrival to Admit. (minutes)[2]	841	281	300	274
Time from ER Arrival to Discharge (minutes)	392	183	152	134
Time in ER Before Being Evaluated (minutes)	431	43	34	26
Time to Pain Meds for Fractures (minutes)	244	72	67	57
Heart Attack Care				
Aspirin Given at Discharge	474	100%	100%	99%
Fibrinolytic Meds Within 30 Min. of Arrival[7]	-	-	75%	54%
PCI Within 90 Minutes of Arrival	93	100%	98%	96%
Statin Prescribed at Discharge	444	100%	99%	98%
Heart Failure Care				
ACE Inhibitor or ARB for LVSD	149	100%	98%	97%
Discharge Instructions Given	516	98%	96%	94%
Evaluation of LVS Function	588	100%	100%	99%
Medicare Spending				
Medicare Spending per Patient (ratio)	-	0.93	0.94	0.98
Pneumonia Care				
Appropriate Initial Antibiotic Given	478	99%	97%	95%
Blood Culture Timing	986	100%	98%	98%
Pregnancy and Delivery Care				
Newborn Deliveries Scheduled Early	177	2%	3%	6%
Preventive Care				
Immunization for Influenza[2]	560	96%	93%	90%
Immunization for Pneumonia[2]	712	98%	94%	92%
Stroke Care				
Anticoagulation Therapy for Atrial Fibrillation	35	100%	95%	95%
Antithrombotic Therapy Timing	252	100%	98%	98%
Assessed for Rehabilitation	291	100%	98%	97%
Discharged on Antithrombotic Therapy	259	100%	99%	99%
Discharged on Statin Medication	196	100%	94%	94%
Thrombolytic Therapy Timing	20	100%	64%	66%
Venous Thromboembolism Prophylaxis	303	100%	96%	94%
Written Stroke Educational Materials Given	173	100%	88%	88%
Surgical Care Improvement Project				
Appropriate Beta Blocker Usage	494	99%	99%	98%
Appropriate VTP Within 24 Hours	1,006	100%	99%	98%
Controlled Postoperative Blood Glucose	188	100%	98%	97%
Perioperative Temperature Management	1,153	100%	100%	100%
Prophylactic Antibiotic Selection	893	100%	99%	99%
Prophylactic Antibiotic Selection (Outpatient)	689	99%	98%	98%
Prophylactic Antibiotic Stopped	857	100%	99%	98%
Prophylactic Antibiotic Timing	893	100%	99%	99%
Prophylactic Antibiotic Timing (Outpatient)	689	100%	99%	98%
Urinary Catheter Removal	930	100%	99%	97%
Survey of Patients' Hospital Experiences				
Area Around Room 'Always' Quiet at Night	300+	57%	64%	61%
Doctors 'Always' Communicated Well	300+	84%	83%	82%
Home Recovery Information Given	300+	89%	87%	85%
Hospital Given 9 or 10 on 10 Point Scale	300+	74%	71%	71%
Meds 'Always' Explained Before Given	300+	65%	65%	64%
Nurses 'Always' Communicated Well	300+	82%	81%	79%
Pain 'Always' Well Controlled	300+	75%	72%	71%
Room and Bathroom 'Always' Clean	300+	72%	72%	73%
Timely Help 'Always' Received	300+	72%	68%	68%
Would Definitely Recommend Hospital	300+	68%	70%	71%
Use of Medical Imaging				
Cardiac Imaging Stress Test before Surgery	482	6.4%	5.4%	5.3%
Combination Abdominal CT Scan	1,757	5.6%	5.6%	10.5%
Combination Brain/Sinus CT Scan	1,654	1.5%	2.6%	2.7%
Combination Chest CT Scan	710	0.0%	1.3%	2.7%
Follow-up Mammogram/Ultrasound	4,071	7.7%	8%	8.8%
Lumbar Spine MRI for Low Back Pain	399	33.6%	34.7%	37.2%

Wayne Memorial Hospital

2700 Wayne Memorial Dr
Goldsboro, NC 27534
Phone: 919-736-1110
Fax: 919-731-6966
URL: www.waynehealth.org
Type: Acute Care Hospitals
Emergency Services: Yes
Ownership: Voluntary non-profit - Private
Beds: 316
Key Personnel:
Radiology. . . . . Lance Arnder
Surgery . . . . Dr. Greg Bauer
Chief of Medical Staff. . . . . Michael Johnson
CEO/President. . . . . J William Paugh

Measure	Cases	This Hosp.	State Avg.	U.S. Avg.
Blood Clot Prevention and Treatment				
Anticoagulation Overlap Therapy[2]	57	100%	94%	93%
ICU Venous Thromboembolism Prophylaxis[2]	35	86%	93%	92%
Incidence of Potentially Preventable VTE[1,2]	-	-	10%	10%
UFH with Dosages/Platelet Monitoring[2]	15	100%	95%	97%
Venous Thromboembolism Prophylaxis[2]	363	74%	88%	85%

NOTE: Hospital profiles are in alphabetical order by state, then city, then hospital within the city; Rankings exclude hospitals with less than 25 cases except for patient surveys which excludes hospitals with less than 100 cases; (a) 100-299 cases; (1) The number of cases/patients is too few to report; (2) Data submitted were based on a sample of cases/patients; (3) Results are based on a shorter time period than required; (4) Data suppressed by CMS for one or more quarters; (5) Results are not available for this reporting period; (6) Fewer than 100 patients completed the HCAHPS survey; (7) No cases met the criteria for this measure; (8) The lower limit of the confidence interval cannot be calculated if the number of observed infections equals zero; (9) No data are available from the state/territory for this reporting period; (10) The scores shown reflect fewer than 50 completed surveys; (11) There were discrepancies in the data collection process; (12) This measure does not apply to this hospital for this reporting period; (13) Results cannot be calculated for this reporting period; (14) The results for this state are combined with nearby states to protect confidentiality; Please refer to the User's Guide for a full explanation of data.

Warfarin Therapy Discharge Instructions[2]	41	98%	81%	75%
Chest Pain/Possible Heart Attack Care				
Aspirin Given Within 24 Hours of Arrival	280	97%	97%	96%
Fibrinolytic Meds Within 30 Min. of Arrival	35	83%	66%	58%
Average Time to ECG (minutes)	292	7	7	7
Average Time to Transfer (minutes)[7]	-	-	45	60
Children's Asthma Care				
Received Home Management Plan of Care	-	-	89%	88%
Received Reliever Medication	-	-	100%	100%
Received Systemic Corticosteroids	-	-	100%	100%
Emergency Department				
Admittance Decision Time (minutes)[2]	567	70	107	98
Head CT Results Within 45 Min. of Arrival	11	82%	60%	57%
Patients Who Left ER Before Being Seen	61,964	4%	3%	2%
Time from ER Arrival to Admit. (minutes)[2]	604	252	300	274
Time from ER Arrival to Discharge (minutes)	345	161	152	134
Time in ER Before Being Evaluated (minutes)	275	58	34	26
Time to Pain Meds for Fractures (minutes)	153	75	67	57
Heart Attack Care				
Aspirin Given at Discharge	38	97%	100%	99%
Fibrinolytic Meds Within 30 Min. of Arrival[7]	-	-	75%	54%
PCI Within 90 Minutes of Arrival[7]	-	-	98%	96%
Statin Prescribed at Discharge	39	92%	99%	98%
Heart Failure Care				
ACE Inhibitor or ARB for LVSD	171	96%	98%	97%
Discharge Instructions Given	368	97%	96%	94%
Evaluation of LVS Function	416	99%	100%	99%
Medicare Spending				
Medicare Spending per Patient (ratio)	-	0.98	0.94	0.98
Pneumonia Care				
Appropriate Initial Antibiotic Given	149	99%	97%	95%
Blood Culture Timing	169	95%	98%	98%
Pregnancy and Delivery Care				
Newborn Deliveries Scheduled Early[2]	26	0%	3%	6%
Preventive Care				
Immunization for Influenza[2]	498	96%	93%	90%
Immunization for Pneumonia[2]	659	96%	94%	92%
Stroke Care				
Anticoagulation Therapy for Atrial Fibrillation	14	86%	95%	95%
Antithrombotic Therapy Timing	124	97%	98%	98%
Assessed for Rehabilitation	145	97%	98%	97%
Discharged on Antithrombotic Therapy	136	99%	99%	99%
Discharged on Statin Medication	110	88%	94%	94%
Thrombolytic Therapy Timing	11	100%	64%	66%
Venous Thromboembolism Prophylaxis	144	87%	96%	94%
Written Stroke Educational Materials Given	83	98%	88%	88%
Surgical Care Improvement Project				
Appropriate Beta Blocker Usage[2]	159	98%	99%	98%
Appropriate VTP Within 24 Hours[2]	532	98%	99%	98%
Controlled Postoperative Blood Glucose[2,7]	-	-	98%	97%
Perioperative Temperature Management[2]	573	100%	100%	100%
Prophylactic Antibiotic Selection[2]	386	100%	99%	99%
Prophylactic Antibiotic Selection (Outpatient)	310	98%	98%	98%
Prophylactic Antibiotic Stopped[2]	355	98%	99%	98%
Prophylactic Antibiotic Timing[2]	387	99%	99%	99%
Prophylactic Antibiotic Timing (Outpatient)	310	98%	99%	98%
Urinary Catheter Removal[2]	337	99%	99%	97%
Survey of Patients' Hospital Experiences				
Area Around Room 'Always' Quiet at Night	300+	62%	64%	61%
Doctors 'Always' Communicated Well	300+	80%	83%	82%
Home Recovery Information Given	300+	88%	87%	85%
Hospital Given 9 or 10 on 10 Point Scale	300+	65%	71%	71%
Meds 'Always' Explained Before Given	300+	62%	65%	64%
Nurses 'Always' Communicated Well	300+	77%	81%	79%
Pain 'Always' Well Controlled	300+	66%	72%	71%
Room and Bathroom 'Always' Clean	300+	72%	72%	73%
Timely Help 'Always' Received	300+	64%	68%	68%
Would Definitely Recommend Hospital	300+	57%	70%	71%
Use of Medical Imaging				
Cardiac Imaging Stress Test before Surgery	915	8.3%	5.4%	5.3%
Combination Abdominal CT Scan	642	1.2%	5.6%	10.5%
Combination Brain/Sinus CT Scan	1,033	0.9%	2.6%	2.7%
Combination Chest CT Scan	245	0.4%	1.3%	2.7%
Follow-up Mammogram/Ultrasound	500	9.0%	8%	8.8%
Lumbar Spine MRI for Low Back Pain	304	36.8%	34.7%	37.2%

The Moses H Cone Memorial Hospital

1200 N Elm St
Greensboro, NC 27401
Phone: 336-832-7000
Fax: 336-832-6630
E-mail: comments@mosescone.com
URL: www.mosescone.com
Type: Acute Care Hospitals
Emergency Services: Yes
Ownership: Voluntary non-profit - Private
Beds: 536

Key Personnel:
Emergency Room . . . . Robert Beaton
Quality Assurance . . . . Ken Boggs
Chief of Medical Staff. . . . . Mary Jo Cagle, MD
Radiology. . . . . Judy Grzyva
Anesthesiology. . . . . Franklin Hatchett Jr, MD
Infection Control. . . . . Debbie Houston
Cardiac Laboratory. . . . . Tony Petrillo
CEO/President. . . . . Tim Rice

Measure	Cases	This Hosp.	State Avg.	U.S. Avg.
Blood Clot Prevention and Treatment				
Anticoagulation Overlap Therapy[2]	284	97%	94%	93%
ICU Venous Thromboembolism Prophylaxis[2]	116	97%	93%	92%
Incidence of Potentially Preventable VTE[2]	52	10%	10%	10%
UFH with Dosages/Platelet Monitoring[2]	227	100%	95%	97%
Venous Thromboembolism Prophylaxis[2]	1,015	95%	88%	85%
Warfarin Therapy Discharge Instructions[2]	214	90%	81%	75%
Chest Pain/Possible Heart Attack Care				
Aspirin Given Within 24 Hours of Arrival	11	100%	97%	96%
Fibrinolytic Meds Within 30 Min. of Arrival[3,7]	-	-	66%	58%
Average Time to ECG (minutes)	12	17	7	7
Average Time to Transfer (minutes)[3,7]	-	-	45	60
Children's Asthma Care				
Received Home Management Plan of Care	-	-	89%	88%
Received Reliever Medication	-	-	100%	100%
Received Systemic Corticosteroids	-	-	100%	100%
Emergency Department				
Admittance Decision Time (minutes)[2]	610	148	107	98
Head CT Results Within 45 Min. of Arrival[1]	-	-	60%	57%
Patients Who Left ER Before Being Seen	>100k	3%	3%	2%
Time from ER Arrival to Admit. (minutes)[2]	616	378	300	274
Time from ER Arrival to Discharge (minutes)	1,441	193	152	134
Time in ER Before Being Evaluated (minutes)	1,526	41	34	26
Time to Pain Meds for Fractures (minutes)	513	65	67	57
Heart Attack Care				
Aspirin Given at Discharge	901	100%	100%	99%
Fibrinolytic Meds Within 30 Min. of Arrival[7]	-	-	75%	54%
PCI Within 90 Minutes of Arrival	147	99%	98%	96%
Statin Prescribed at Discharge	854	100%	99%	98%
Heart Failure Care				
ACE Inhibitor or ARB for LVSD	357	100%	98%	97%
Discharge Instructions Given	1,197	100%	96%	94%
Evaluation of LVS Function	1,423	100%	100%	99%
Medicare Spending				
Medicare Spending per Patient (ratio)	-	0.96	0.94	0.98
Pneumonia Care				
Appropriate Initial Antibiotic Given	535	99%	97%	95%
Blood Culture Timing	524	99%	98%	98%
Pregnancy and Delivery Care				
Newborn Deliveries Scheduled Early	576	1%	3%	6%
Preventive Care				
Immunization for Influenza[2]	538	90%	93%	90%
Immunization for Pneumonia[2]	692	92%	94%	92%
Stroke Care				
Anticoagulation Therapy for Atrial Fibrillation	111	92%	95%	95%
Antithrombotic Therapy Timing	588	97%	98%	98%
Assessed for Rehabilitation	715	97%	98%	97%
Discharged on Antithrombotic Therapy	638	99%	99%	99%
Discharged on Statin Medication	461	91%	94%	94%
Thrombolytic Therapy Timing	41	83%	64%	66%
Venous Thromboembolism Prophylaxis	743	98%	96%	94%
Written Stroke Educational Materials Given	416	80%	88%	88%
Surgical Care Improvement Project				
Appropriate Beta Blocker Usage	1,348	99%	99%	98%
Appropriate VTP Within 24 Hours	3,173	99%	99%	98%
Controlled Postoperative Blood Glucose	435	99%	98%	97%
Perioperative Temperature Management	3,847	100%	100%	100%
Prophylactic Antibiotic Selection	2,831	100%	99%	99%
Prophylactic Antibiotic Selection (Outpatient)	896	98%	98%	98%
Prophylactic Antibiotic Stopped	2,769	99%	99%	98%
Prophylactic Antibiotic Timing	2,836	100%	99%	99%
Prophylactic Antibiotic Timing (Outpatient)	895	100%	99%	98%
Urinary Catheter Removal	3,104	98%	99%	97%
Survey of Patients' Hospital Experiences				
Area Around Room 'Always' Quiet at Night	300+	58%	64%	61%
Doctors 'Always' Communicated Well	300+	82%	83%	82%
Home Recovery Information Given	300+	85%	87%	85%
Hospital Given 9 or 10 on 10 Point Scale	300+	72%	71%	71%
Meds 'Always' Explained Before Given	300+	59%	65%	64%
Nurses 'Always' Communicated Well	300+	79%	81%	79%
Pain 'Always' Well Controlled	300+	69%	72%	71%
Room and Bathroom 'Always' Clean	300+	75%	72%	73%
Timely Help 'Always' Received	300+	64%	68%	68%
Would Definitely Recommend Hospital	300+	77%	70%	71%
Use of Medical Imaging				
Cardiac Imaging Stress Test before Surgery	963	4.6%	5.4%	5.3%
Combination Abdominal CT Scan	2,131	1.9%	5.6%	10.5%
Combination Brain/Sinus CT Scan	2,330	3.5%	2.6%	2.7%
Combination Chest CT Scan	1,288	0.0%	1.3%	2.7%
Follow-up Mammogram/Ultrasound	1,780	8.5%	8%	8.8%
Lumbar Spine MRI for Low Back Pain	153	41.8%	34.7%	37.2%

Vidant Medical Center

2100 Stantonsburg Rd
Greenville, NC 27835
Phone: 252-847-4100
Fax: 252-847-8170
URL: www.uhseast.com
Type: Acute Care Hospitals
Emergency Services: Yes
Ownership: Voluntary non-profit - Private
Beds: 745

Key Personnel:
Quality Assurance . . . . Nancy Aycock
Emergency Room . . . . Nick Benson, MD
Chief of Medical Staff. . . . . Ernest Larkin, MD
CEO/President. . . . . Steve Lawler
Pediatric In-Patient Care . . . . Ron Perkin, MD
Operating Room. . . . . Sanjay Saha
Anesthesiology. . . . . Joshua Schwartz, MD
Radiology. . . . . Michael Weaver, MD

Measure	Cases	This Hosp.	State Avg.	U.S. Avg.
Blood Clot Prevention and Treatment				
Anticoagulation Overlap Therapy[2]	193	96%	94%	93%
ICU Venous Thromboembolism Prophylaxis[2]	79	100%	93%	92%
Incidence of Potentially Preventable VTE[2]	64	3%	10%	10%
UFH with Dosages/Platelet Monitoring[2]	163	100%	95%	97%
Venous Thromboembolism Prophylaxis[2]	360	98%	88%	85%
Warfarin Therapy Discharge Instructions[2]	122	30%	81%	75%
Chest Pain/Possible Heart Attack Care				
Aspirin Given Within 24 Hours of Arrival[5]	-	-	97%	96%
Fibrinolytic Meds Within 30 Min. of Arrival[5]	-	-	66%	58%
Average Time to ECG (minutes)[5]	-	-	7	7
Average Time to Transfer (minutes)[5]	-	-	45	60
Children's Asthma Care				
Received Home Management Plan of Care	-	-	89%	88%
Received Reliever Medication	-	-	100%	100%
Received Systemic Corticosteroids	-	-	100%	100%
Emergency Department				
Admittance Decision Time (minutes)[2]	318	158	107	98
Head CT Results Within 45 Min. of Arrival[1]	-	-	60%	57%
Patients Who Left ER Before Being Seen	71,963	2%	3%	2%
Time from ER Arrival to Admit. (minutes)[2]	336	371	300	274
Time from ER Arrival to Discharge (minutes)	371	179	152	134
Time in ER Before Being Evaluated (minutes)	402	34	34	26
Time to Pain Meds for Fractures (minutes)	167	40	67	57
Heart Attack Care				
Aspirin Given at Discharge	1,231	100%	100%	99%
Fibrinolytic Meds Within 30 Min. of Arrival[1]	-	-	75%	54%
PCI Within 90 Minutes of Arrival	68	99%	98%	96%
Statin Prescribed at Discharge	1,212	100%	99%	98%

NOTE: Hospital profiles are in alphabetical order by state, then city, then hospital within the city; Rankings exclude hospitals with less than 25 cases except for patient surveys which excludes hospitals with less than 100 cases; (a) 100-299 cases; (1) The number of cases/patients is too few to report; (2) Data submitted were based on a sample of cases/patients; (3) Results are based on a shorter time period than required; (4) Data suppressed by CMS for one or more quarters; (5) Results are not available for this reporting period; (6) Fewer than 100 patients completed the HCAHPS survey; (7) No cases met the criteria for this measure; (8) The lower limit of the confidence interval cannot be calculated if the number of observed infections equals zero; (9) No data are available from the state/territory for this reporting period; (10) The scores shown reflect fewer than 50 completed surveys; (11) There were discrepancies in the data collection process; (12) This measure does not apply to this hospital for this reporting period; (13) Results cannot be calculated for this reporting period; (14) The results for this state are combined with nearby states to protect confidentiality; Please refer to the User's Guide for a full explanation of data.

Measure	Cases	This Hosp.	State Avg.	U.S. Avg.
Heart Failure Care				
ACE Inhibitor or ARB for LVSD	501	99%	98%	97%
Discharge Instructions Given	1,081	98%	96%	94%
Evaluation of LVS Function	1,211	100%	100%	99%
Medicare Spending				
Medicare Spending per Patient (ratio)	-	0.94	0.94	0.98
Pneumonia Care				
Appropriate Initial Antibiotic Given	228	99%	97%	95%
Blood Culture Timing	540	96%	98%	98%
Pregnancy and Delivery Care				
Newborn Deliveries Scheduled Early[2]	159	4%	3%	6%
Preventive Care				
Immunization for Influenza[2]	541	91%	93%	90%
Immunization for Pneumonia[2]	650	88%	94%	92%
Stroke Care				
Anticoagulation Therapy for Atrial Fibrillation	59	95%	95%	95%
Antithrombotic Therapy Timing	390	96%	98%	98%
Assessed for Rehabilitation	608	99%	98%	97%
Discharged on Antithrombotic Therapy	461	100%	99%	99%
Discharged on Statin Medication	368	98%	94%	94%
Thrombolytic Therapy Timing	20	75%	64%	66%
Venous Thromboembolism Prophylaxis	647	99%	96%	94%
Written Stroke Educational Materials Given	349	73%	88%	88%
Surgical Care Improvement Project				
Appropriate Beta Blocker Usage[2]	963	100%	99%	98%
Appropriate VTP Within 24 Hours[2]	1,279	100%	99%	98%
Controlled Postoperative Blood Glucose[2]	564	99%	98%	97%
Perioperative Temperature Management[2]	1,713	100%	100%	100%
Prophylactic Antibiotic Selection[2]	1,490	100%	99%	99%
Prophylactic Antibiotic Selection (Outpatient)	1,315	96%	98%	98%
Prophylactic Antibiotic Stopped[2]	1,456	100%	99%	98%
Prophylactic Antibiotic Timing[2]	1,490	100%	99%	99%
Prophylactic Antibiotic Timing (Outpatient)	1,322	97%	99%	98%
Urinary Catheter Removal[2]	893	100%	99%	97%
Survey of Patients' Hospital Experiences				
Area Around Room 'Always' Quiet at Night	300+	60%	64%	61%
Doctors 'Always' Communicated Well	300+	83%	83%	82%
Home Recovery Information Given	300+	90%	87%	85%
Hospital Given 9 or 10 on 10 Point Scale	300+	75%	71%	71%
Meds 'Always' Explained Before Given	300+	65%	65%	64%
Nurses 'Always' Communicated Well	300+	80%	81%	79%
Pain 'Always' Well Controlled	300+	71%	72%	71%
Room and Bathroom 'Always' Clean	300+	72%	72%	73%
Timely Help 'Always' Received	300+	65%	68%	68%
Would Definitely Recommend Hospital	300+	80%	70%	71%
Use of Medical Imaging				
Cardiac Imaging Stress Test before Surgery	536	7.1%	5.4%	5.3%
Combination Abdominal CT Scan	1,574	1.7%	5.6%	10.5%
Combination Brain/Sinus CT Scan	1,468	2.1%	2.6%	2.7%
Combination Chest CT Scan	887	0.0%	1.3%	2.7%
Follow-up Mammogram/Ultrasound[7]	-	-	8%	8.8%
Lumbar Spine MRI for Low Back Pain	117	35.0%	34.7%	37.2%

Sandhills Regional Medical Center

1000 West Hamlet Avenue
Hamlet, NC 28345
Phone: 910-958-2361
Fax: 910-205-8117
URL: www.hma-corp.com
Type: Acute Care Hospitals
Emergency Services: Yes
Ownership: Proprietary
Beds: 64

Key Personnel:
Chief of Medical Staff . . . . Gilbert D Arenas
Radiology. . . . . Robert B Groves
CEO/President. . . . . Michael McNair

Measure	Cases	This Hosp.	State Avg.	U.S. Avg.
Blood Clot Prevention and Treatment				
Anticoagulation Overlap Therapy[1,2]	-	-	94%	93%
ICU Venous Thromboembolism Prophylaxis[2]	46	85%	93%	92%
Incidence of Potentially Preventable VTE[2,7]	-	-	10%	10%
UFH with Dosages/Platelet Monitoring[1,2]	-	-	95%	97%
Venous Thromboembolism Prophylaxis[2]	162	56%	88%	85%
Warfarin Therapy Discharge Instructions[1,2]	-	-	81%	75%
Chest Pain/Possible Heart Attack Care				
Aspirin Given Within 24 Hours of Arrival	12	83%	97%	96%
Fibrinolytic Meds Within 30 Min. of Arrival[3,7]	-	-	66%	58%
Average Time to ECG (minutes)	12	5	7	7
Average Time to Transfer (minutes)[1,3]	-	-	45	60
Children's Asthma Care				
Received Home Management Plan of Care	-	-	89%	88%
Received Reliever Medication	-	-	100%	100%
Received Systemic Corticosteroids	-	-	100%	100%
Emergency Department				
Admittance Decision Time (minutes)[2]	387	56	107	98
Head CT Results Within 45 Min. of Arrival[1,3]	-	-	60%	57%
Patients Who Left ER Before Being Seen	12,093	2%	3%	2%
Time from ER Arrival to Admit. (minutes)[2]	396	280	300	274
Time from ER Arrival to Discharge (minutes)	338	122	152	134
Time in ER Before Being Evaluated (minutes)	380	30	34	26
Time to Pain Meds for Fractures (minutes)	23	69	67	57
Heart Attack Care				
Aspirin Given at Discharge[1]	-	-	100%	99%
Fibrinolytic Meds Within 30 Min. of Arrival[7]	-	-	75%	54%
PCI Within 90 Minutes of Arrival[7]	-	-	98%	96%
Statin Prescribed at Discharge[1]	-	-	99%	98%
Heart Failure Care				
ACE Inhibitor or ARB for LVSD	23	100%	98%	97%
Discharge Instructions Given	88	97%	96%	94%
Evaluation of LVS Function	104	100%	100%	99%
Medicare Spending				
Medicare Spending per Patient (ratio)	-	0.85	0.94	0.98
Pneumonia Care				
Appropriate Initial Antibiotic Given	52	96%	97%	95%
Blood Culture Timing	66	97%	98%	98%
Pregnancy and Delivery Care				
Newborn Deliveries Scheduled Early[7]	-	-	3%	6%
Preventive Care				
Immunization for Influenza[2]	286	93%	93%	90%
Immunization for Pneumonia[2]	374	95%	94%	92%
Stroke Care				
Anticoagulation Therapy for Atrial Fibrillation[1]	-	-	95%	95%
Antithrombotic Therapy Timing	18	94%	98%	98%
Assessed for Rehabilitation	15	100%	98%	97%
Discharged on Antithrombotic Therapy	15	100%	99%	99%
Discharged on Statin Medication	13	85%	94%	94%
Thrombolytic Therapy Timing[1]	-	-	64%	66%
Venous Thromboembolism Prophylaxis	19	42%	96%	94%
Written Stroke Educational Materials Given[1]	-	-	88%	88%
Surgical Care Improvement Project				
Appropriate Beta Blocker Usage[1]	-	-	99%	98%
Appropriate VTP Within 24 Hours	22	91%	99%	98%
Controlled Postoperative Blood Glucose[7]	-	-	98%	97%
Perioperative Temperature Management	25	100%	100%	100%
Prophylactic Antibiotic Selection	19	100%	99%	99%
Prophylactic Antibiotic Selection (Outpatient)	93	100%	98%	98%
Prophylactic Antibiotic Stopped	19	89%	99%	98%
Prophylactic Antibiotic Timing	19	100%	99%	99%
Prophylactic Antibiotic Timing (Outpatient)	93	100%	99%	98%
Urinary Catheter Removal[1]	-	-	99%	97%
Survey of Patients' Hospital Experiences				
Area Around Room 'Always' Quiet at Night	(a)	75%	64%	61%
Doctors 'Always' Communicated Well	(a)	87%	83%	82%
Home Recovery Information Given	(a)	87%	87%	85%
Hospital Given 9 or 10 on 10 Point Scale	(a)	73%	71%	71%
Meds 'Always' Explained Before Given	(a)	72%	65%	64%
Nurses 'Always' Communicated Well	(a)	84%	81%	79%
Pain 'Always' Well Controlled	(a)	78%	72%	71%
Room and Bathroom 'Always' Clean	(a)	77%	72%	73%
Timely Help 'Always' Received	(a)	71%	68%	68%
Would Definitely Recommend Hospital	(a)	69%	70%	71%
Use of Medical Imaging				
Cardiac Imaging Stress Test before Surgery	85	5.9%	5.4%	5.3%
Combination Abdominal CT Scan	170	21.8%	5.6%	10.5%
Combination Brain/Sinus CT Scan	298	5.7%	2.6%	2.7%
Combination Chest CT Scan[1]	-	-	1.3%	2.7%
Follow-up Mammogram/Ultrasound	311	11.3%	8%	8.8%
Lumbar Spine MRI for Low Back Pain[1]	-	-	34.7%	37.2%

Maria Parham Medical Center

PO Box 59
Henderson, NC 27536
Phone: 252-438-4143
Fax: 252-436-1114
E-mail: information@mphosp.org
URL: www.mphosp.org
Type: Acute Care Hospitals
Emergency Services: Yes
Ownership: Voluntary non-profit - Other
Beds: 102

Key Personnel:
Quality Assurance . . . . Margie Hentze
Radiology. . . . . Bonnie Howell
Cardiology . . . . Erin McIntyre
Intensive Care Unit. . . . . Debby Pearce
Emergency Room . . . . Jane Ryan
CEO . . . . Bob Singletary
Infection Control. . . . . Patsy Stainback, RN
Chief of Medical Staff . . . . Christa Sudipo

Measure	Cases	This Hosp.	State Avg.	U.S. Avg.
Blood Clot Prevention and Treatment				
Anticoagulation Overlap Therapy[2]	44	95%	94%	93%
ICU Venous Thromboembolism Prophylaxis[2]	60	87%	93%	92%
Incidence of Potentially Preventable VTE[1,2]	-	-	10%	10%
UFH with Dosages/Platelet Monitoring[2]	19	100%	95%	97%
Venous Thromboembolism Prophylaxis[2]	416	76%	88%	85%
Warfarin Therapy Discharge Instructions[2]	31	55%	81%	75%
Chest Pain/Possible Heart Attack Care				
Aspirin Given Within 24 Hours of Arrival	97	97%	97%	96%
Fibrinolytic Meds Within 30 Min. of Arrival[7]	-	-	66%	58%
Average Time to ECG (minutes)	101	10	7	7
Average Time to Transfer (minutes)	20	38	45	60
Children's Asthma Care				
Received Home Management Plan of Care	-	-	89%	88%
Received Reliever Medication	-	-	100%	100%
Received Systemic Corticosteroids	-	-	100%	100%
Emergency Department				
Admittance Decision Time (minutes)[2]	487	105	107	98
Head CT Results Within 45 Min. of Arrival	15	100%	60%	57%
Patients Who Left ER Before Being Seen	40,989	2%	3%	2%
Time from ER Arrival to Admit. (minutes)[2]	498	326	300	274
Time from ER Arrival to Discharge (minutes)	388	150	152	134
Time in ER Before Being Evaluated (minutes)	431	14	34	26
Time to Pain Meds for Fractures (minutes)	76	59	67	57
Heart Attack Care				
Aspirin Given at Discharge	25	96%	100%	99%
Fibrinolytic Meds Within 30 Min. of Arrival[7]	-	-	75%	54%
PCI Within 90 Minutes of Arrival[7]	-	-	98%	96%
Statin Prescribed at Discharge	25	96%	99%	98%
Heart Failure Care				
ACE Inhibitor or ARB for LVSD	91	98%	98%	97%
Discharge Instructions Given	181	93%	96%	94%
Evaluation of LVS Function	212	100%	100%	99%
Medicare Spending				
Medicare Spending per Patient (ratio)	-	0.92	0.94	0.98
Pneumonia Care				
Appropriate Initial Antibiotic Given	91	95%	97%	95%
Blood Culture Timing	173	96%	98%	98%
Pregnancy and Delivery Care				
Newborn Deliveries Scheduled Early[1,2]	-	-	3%	6%
Preventive Care				
Immunization for Influenza[2]	432	97%	93%	90%
Immunization for Pneumonia[2]	612	99%	94%	92%
Stroke Care				
Anticoagulation Therapy for Atrial Fibrillation[1]	-	-	95%	95%
Antithrombotic Therapy Timing	85	98%	98%	98%
Assessed for Rehabilitation	72	99%	98%	97%
Discharged on Antithrombotic Therapy	72	100%	99%	99%
Discharged on Statin Medication	49	100%	94%	94%
Thrombolytic Therapy Timing[7]	-	-	64%	66%
Venous Thromboembolism Prophylaxis	79	97%	96%	94%
Written Stroke Educational Materials Given	45	96%	88%	88%
Surgical Care Improvement Project				
Appropriate Beta Blocker Usage	32	100%	99%	98%
Appropriate VTP Within 24 Hours	147	99%	99%	98%
Controlled Postoperative Blood Glucose[7]	-	-	98%	97%
Perioperative Temperature Management	151	100%	100%	100%

NOTE: Hospital profiles are in alphabetical order by state, then city, then hospital within the city; Rankings exclude hospitals with less than 25 cases except for patient surveys which excludes hospitals with less than 100 cases; (a) 100-299 cases; (1) The number of cases/patients is too few to report; (2) Data submitted were based on a sample of cases/patients; (3) Results are based on a shorter time period than required; (4) Data suppressed by CMS for one or more quarters; (5) Results are not available for this reporting period; (6) Fewer than 100 patients completed the HCAHPS survey; (7) No cases met the criteria for this measure; (8) The lower limit of the confidence interval cannot be calculated if the number of observed infections equals zero; (9) No data are available from the state/territory for this reporting period; (10) The scores shown reflect fewer than 50 completed surveys; (11) There were discrepancies in the data collection process; (12) This measure does not apply to this hospital for this reporting period; (13) Results cannot be calculated for this reporting period; (14) The results for this state are combined with nearby states to protect confidentiality; Please refer to the User's Guide for a full explanation of data.

Measure	Cases	This Hosp.	State Avg.	U.S. Avg.
Prophylactic Antibiotic Selection	55	98%	99%	99%
Prophylactic Antibiotic Selection (Outpatient)	67	88%	98%	98%
Prophylactic Antibiotic Stopped	54	100%	99%	98%
Prophylactic Antibiotic Timing	55	100%	99%	99%
Prophylactic Antibiotic Timing (Outpatient)	67	99%	99%	98%
Urinary Catheter Removal	73	96%	99%	97%
Survey of Patients' Hospital Experiences				
Area Around Room 'Always' Quiet at Night	300+	61%	64%	61%
Doctors 'Always' Communicated Well	300+	82%	83%	82%
Home Recovery Information Given	300+	87%	87%	85%
Hospital Given 9 or 10 on 10 Point Scale	300+	62%	71%	71%
Meds 'Always' Explained Before Given	300+	63%	65%	64%
Nurses 'Always' Communicated Well	300+	79%	81%	79%
Pain 'Always' Well Controlled	300+	68%	72%	71%
Room and Bathroom 'Always' Clean	300+	65%	72%	73%
Timely Help 'Always' Received	300+	63%	68%	68%
Would Definitely Recommend Hospital	300+	60%	70%	71%
Use of Medical Imaging				
Cardiac Imaging Stress Test before Surgery	209	4.3%	5.4%	5.3%
Combination Abdominal CT Scan	697	0.4%	5.6%	10.5%
Combination Brain/Sinus CT Scan	696	2.0%	2.6%	2.7%
Combination Chest CT Scan	482	1.9%	1.3%	2.7%
Follow-up Mammogram/Ultrasound	1,308	7.8%	8%	8.8%
Lumbar Spine MRI for Low Back Pain[1]	-	-	34.7%	37.2%

Margaret R Pardee Memorial Hospital

800 N Justice St
Hendersonville, NC 28791
Phone: 828-696-1000
Fax: 828-696-1128
E-mail: tiffany.ervin@pardeehospital.org
URL: www.pardeehospital.org
Type: Acute Care Hospitals
Emergency Services: Yes
Ownership: Government - Local
Beds: 282

Key Personnel:
CEO/President. . . . . James R. Kirby, II
Chief of Medical Staff. . . . . Robert Kiskaddon, MD
Chair/CEO. . . . . William L. Moyer

Measure	Cases	This Hosp.	State Avg.	U.S. Avg.
Blood Clot Prevention and Treatment				
Anticoagulation Overlap Therapy[2]	65	89%	94%	93%
ICU Venous Thromboembolism Prophylaxis[2]	37	97%	93%	92%
Incidence of Potentially Preventable VTE[1,2]	-	-	10%	10%
UFH with Dosages/Platelet Monitoring[1,2]	-	-	95%	97%
Venous Thromboembolism Prophylaxis[2]	362	86%	88%	85%
Warfarin Therapy Discharge Instructions[2]	37	97%	81%	75%
Chest Pain/Possible Heart Attack Care				
Aspirin Given Within 24 Hours of Arrival	60	100%	97%	96%
Fibrinolytic Meds Within 30 Min. of Arrival[7]	-	-	66%	58%
Average Time to ECG (minutes)	61	5	7	7
Average Time to Transfer (minutes)	15	50	45	60
Children's Asthma Care				
Received Home Management Plan of Care	-	-	89%	88%
Received Reliever Medication	-	-	100%	100%
Received Systemic Corticosteroids	-	-	100%	100%
Emergency Department				
Admittance Decision Time (minutes)[2]	822	62	107	98
Head CT Results Within 45 Min. of Arrival[1]	-	-	60%	57%
Patients Who Left ER Before Being Seen	30,896	6%	3%	2%
Time from ER Arrival to Admit. (minutes)[2]	822	280	300	274
Time from ER Arrival to Discharge (minutes)	359	165	152	134
Time in ER Before Being Evaluated (minutes)	399	59	34	26
Time to Pain Meds for Fractures (minutes)	107	69	67	57
Heart Attack Care				
Aspirin Given at Discharge	39	97%	100%	99%
Fibrinolytic Meds Within 30 Min. of Arrival[7]	-	-	75%	54%
PCI Within 90 Minutes of Arrival[7]	-	-	98%	96%
Statin Prescribed at Discharge	37	100%	99%	98%
Heart Failure Care				
ACE Inhibitor or ARB for LVSD	63	98%	98%	97%
Discharge Instructions Given	148	98%	96%	94%
Evaluation of LVS Function	219	100%	100%	99%
Medicare Spending				
Medicare Spending per Patient (ratio)	-	0.97	0.94	0.98
Pneumonia Care				
Appropriate Initial Antibiotic Given	141	99%	97%	95%
Blood Culture Timing	225	99%	98%	98%
Pregnancy and Delivery Care				
Newborn Deliveries Scheduled Early	32	0%	3%	6%
Preventive Care				
Immunization for Influenza[2]	619	97%	93%	90%
Immunization for Pneumonia[2]	939	96%	94%	92%
Stroke Care				
Anticoagulation Therapy for Atrial Fibrillation	14	93%	95%	95%
Antithrombotic Therapy Timing	77	97%	98%	98%
Assessed for Rehabilitation	85	95%	98%	97%
Discharged on Antithrombotic Therapy	83	99%	99%	99%
Discharged on Statin Medication	65	72%	94%	94%
Thrombolytic Therapy Timing[1]	-	-	64%	66%
Venous Thromboembolism Prophylaxis	81	93%	96%	94%
Written Stroke Educational Materials Given	36	94%	88%	88%
Surgical Care Improvement Project				
Appropriate Beta Blocker Usage	257	100%	99%	98%
Appropriate VTP Within 24 Hours	816	100%	99%	98%
Controlled Postoperative Blood Glucose[7]	-	-	98%	97%
Perioperative Temperature Management	890	100%	100%	100%
Prophylactic Antibiotic Selection	657	100%	99%	99%
Prophylactic Antibiotic Selection (Outpatient)	216	99%	98%	98%
Prophylactic Antibiotic Stopped	642	100%	99%	98%
Prophylactic Antibiotic Timing	657	100%	99%	99%
Prophylactic Antibiotic Timing (Outpatient)	217	99%	99%	98%
Urinary Catheter Removal	582	100%	99%	97%
Survey of Patients' Hospital Experiences				
Area Around Room 'Always' Quiet at Night	300+	61%	64%	61%
Doctors 'Always' Communicated Well	300+	82%	83%	82%
Home Recovery Information Given	300+	88%	87%	85%
Hospital Given 9 or 10 on 10 Point Scale	300+	70%	71%	71%
Meds 'Always' Explained Before Given	300+	62%	65%	64%
Nurses 'Always' Communicated Well	300+	77%	81%	79%
Pain 'Always' Well Controlled	300+	69%	72%	71%
Room and Bathroom 'Always' Clean	300+	75%	72%	73%
Timely Help 'Always' Received	300+	65%	68%	68%
Would Definitely Recommend Hospital	300+	72%	70%	71%
Use of Medical Imaging				
Cardiac Imaging Stress Test before Surgery	163	6.1%	5.4%	5.3%
Combination Abdominal CT Scan	1,220	8.5%	5.6%	10.5%
Combination Brain/Sinus CT Scan	833	2.8%	2.6%	2.7%
Combination Chest CT Scan	649	5.1%	1.3%	2.7%
Follow-up Mammogram/Ultrasound	2,383	7.6%	8%	8.8%
Lumbar Spine MRI for Low Back Pain	259	31.7%	34.7%	37.2%

Park Ridge Health

100 Hospital Drive
Hendersonville, NC 28792
Phone: 828-684-8501
Fax: 828-681-2770
E-mail: parkridge@ahss.org
URL: www.parkridgehospital.org
Type: Acute Care Hospitals
Emergency Services: Yes
Ownership: Voluntary non-profit - Private
Beds: 103

Key Personnel:
CEO/President. . . . . Jimm Bunch
Emergency Room . . . . DeWayne Butcher, MD
Cardiac Laboratory. . . . . Melissa Byrd
Anesthesiology. . . . . Jeff Coston, MD
Intensive Care Unit. . . . . Lora Harris
Chief of Medical Staff. . . . . Clive Possinger, Jr, MD
Quality Assurance . . . . Duane Price
Infection Control. . . . . Paula Thum

Measure	Cases	This Hosp.	State Avg.	U.S. Avg.
Blood Clot Prevention and Treatment				
Anticoagulation Overlap Therapy[2]	18	100%	94%	93%
ICU Venous Thromboembolism Prophylaxis[2]	39	90%	93%	92%
Incidence of Potentially Preventable VTE[1,2]	-	-	10%	10%
UFH with Dosages/Platelet Monitoring[1,2]	-	-	95%	97%
Venous Thromboembolism Prophylaxis[2]	217	94%	88%	85%
Warfarin Therapy Discharge Instructions[1,2]	-	-	81%	75%
Chest Pain/Possible Heart Attack Care				
Aspirin Given Within 24 Hours of Arrival	30	97%	97%	96%
Fibrinolytic Meds Within 30 Min. of Arrival[7]	-	-	66%	58%
Average Time to ECG (minutes)	24	21	7	7
Average Time to Transfer (minutes)[1]	-	-	45	60
Children's Asthma Care				
Received Home Management Plan of Care	-	-	89%	88%
Received Reliever Medication	-	-	100%	100%
Received Systemic Corticosteroids	-	-	100%	100%
Emergency Department				
Admittance Decision Time (minutes)[2]	163	110	107	98
Head CT Results Within 45 Min. of Arrival[1]	-	-	60%	57%
Patients Who Left ER Before Being Seen	23,339	2%	3%	2%
Time from ER Arrival to Admit. (minutes)[2]	178	278	300	274
Time from ER Arrival to Discharge (minutes)	998	130	152	134
Time in ER Before Being Evaluated (minutes)	1,228	45	34	26
Time to Pain Meds for Fractures (minutes)	70	60	67	57
Heart Attack Care				
Aspirin Given at Discharge	11	100%	100%	99%
Fibrinolytic Meds Within 30 Min. of Arrival[7]	-	-	75%	54%
PCI Within 90 Minutes of Arrival[7]	-	-	98%	96%
Statin Prescribed at Discharge[1]	-	-	99%	98%
Heart Failure Care				
ACE Inhibitor or ARB for LVSD	31	100%	98%	97%
Discharge Instructions Given	62	100%	96%	94%
Evaluation of LVS Function	92	100%	100%	99%
Medicare Spending				
Medicare Spending per Patient (ratio)	-	0.97	0.94	0.98
Pneumonia Care				
Appropriate Initial Antibiotic Given	90	99%	97%	95%
Blood Culture Timing	152	98%	98%	98%
Pregnancy and Delivery Care				
Newborn Deliveries Scheduled Early[2]	23	48%	3%	6%
Preventive Care				
Immunization for Influenza[2]	322	95%	93%	90%
Immunization for Pneumonia[2]	370	96%	94%	92%
Stroke Care				
Anticoagulation Therapy for Atrial Fibrillation[1,2]	-	-	95%	95%
Antithrombotic Therapy Timing[2]	29	100%	98%	98%
Assessed for Rehabilitation[2]	37	100%	98%	97%
Discharged on Antithrombotic Therapy[2]	35	97%	99%	99%
Discharged on Statin Medication[2]	25	88%	94%	94%
Thrombolytic Therapy Timing[1,2]	-	-	64%	66%
Venous Thromboembolism Prophylaxis[2]	30	97%	96%	94%
Written Stroke Educational Materials Given[2]	18	72%	88%	88%
Surgical Care Improvement Project				
Appropriate Beta Blocker Usage	70	94%	99%	98%
Appropriate VTP Within 24 Hours	295	97%	99%	98%
Controlled Postoperative Blood Glucose[7]	-	-	98%	97%
Perioperative Temperature Management	324	100%	100%	100%
Prophylactic Antibiotic Selection	218	98%	99%	99%
Prophylactic Antibiotic Selection (Outpatient)	157	99%	98%	98%
Prophylactic Antibiotic Stopped	210	92%	99%	98%
Prophylactic Antibiotic Timing	218	99%	99%	99%
Prophylactic Antibiotic Timing (Outpatient)	154	95%	99%	98%
Urinary Catheter Removal	159	99%	99%	97%
Survey of Patients' Hospital Experiences				
Area Around Room 'Always' Quiet at Night[11]	300+	63%	64%	61%
Doctors 'Always' Communicated Well[11]	300+	85%	83%	82%
Home Recovery Information Given[11]	300+	87%	87%	85%
Hospital Given 9 or 10 on 10 Point Scale[11]	300+	81%	71%	71%
Meds 'Always' Explained Before Given[11]	300+	62%	65%	64%
Nurses 'Always' Communicated Well[11]	300+	82%	81%	79%
Pain 'Always' Well Controlled[11]	300+	72%	72%	71%
Room and Bathroom 'Always' Clean[11]	300+	82%	72%	73%
Timely Help 'Always' Received[11]	300+	69%	68%	68%
Would Definitely Recommend Hospital[11]	300+	85%	70%	71%
Use of Medical Imaging				
Cardiac Imaging Stress Test before Surgery	266	4.1%	5.4%	5.3%
Combination Abdominal CT Scan	523	7.3%	5.6%	10.5%
Combination Brain/Sinus CT Scan	571	2.3%	2.6%	2.7%
Combination Chest CT Scan	215	5.6%	1.3%	2.7%
Follow-up Mammogram/Ultrasound	950	9.9%	8%	8.8%
Lumbar Spine MRI for Low Back Pain	111	32.4%	34.7%	37.2%

NOTE: Hospital profiles are in alphabetical order by state, then city, then hospital within the city; Rankings exclude hospitals with less than 25 cases except for patient surveys which excludes hospitals with less than 100 cases; (a) 100-299 cases; (1) The number of cases/patients is too few to report; (2) Data submitted were based on a sample of cases/patients; (3) Results are based on a shorter time period than required; (4) Data suppressed by CMS for one or more quarters; (5) Results are not available for this reporting period; (6) Fewer than 100 patients completed the HCAHPS survey; (7) No cases met the criteria for this measure; (8) The lower limit of the confidence interval cannot be calculated if the number of observed infections equals zero; (9) No data are available from the state/territory for this reporting period; (10) The scores shown reflect fewer than 50 completed surveys; (11) There were discrepancies in the data collection process; (12) This measure does not apply to this hospital for this reporting period; (13) Results cannot be calculated for this reporting period; (14) The results for this state are combined with nearby states to protect confidentiality; Please refer to the User's Guide for a full explanation of data.

Catawba Valley Medical Center

810 Fairgrove Church Rd
Hickory, NC 28602
Phone: 828-326-3809
Fax: 828-326-3371
URL: www.catawbavalleymc.org
Type: Acute Care Hospitals
Emergency Services: Yes
Ownership: Voluntary non-profit - Other
Beds: 213

Key Personnel:
Quality Assurance . . . . Sarah Bailey, RN
Pediatric Ambulatory Care . . . . . . David Berry, MD
Radiology. . . . . Parks J Booker, MD
Operating Room. . . . . Peter Bradshaw, RN
President/CEO. . . . . J Anthony Rose
Chief of Medical Staff . . . . I Shenoy, MD
Infection Control. . . . . Dorothea Wyant

Measure	Cases	This Hosp.	State Avg.	U.S. Avg.
Blood Clot Prevention and Treatment				
Anticoagulation Overlap Therapy[2]	30	90%	94%	93%
ICU Venous Thromboembolism Prophylaxis[2]	79	99%	93%	92%
Incidence of Potentially Preventable VTE[1,2]	-	-	10%	10%
UFH with Dosages/Platelet Monitoring[2]	20	95%	95%	97%
Venous Thromboembolism Prophylaxis[2]	304	90%	88%	85%
Warfarin Therapy Discharge Instructions[2]	24	92%	81%	75%
Chest Pain/Possible Heart Attack Care				
Aspirin Given Within 24 Hours of Arrival	33	97%	97%	96%
Fibrinolytic Meds Within 30 Min. of Arrival[7]	-	-	66%	58%
Average Time to ECG (minutes)	32	9	7	7
Average Time to Transfer (minutes)	15	42	45	60
Children's Asthma Care				
Received Home Management Plan of Care	-	-	89%	88%
Received Reliever Medication	-	-	100%	100%
Received Systemic Corticosteroids	-	-	100%	100%
Emergency Department				
Admittance Decision Time (minutes)[2]	414	59	107	98
Head CT Results Within 45 Min. of Arrival[1]	-	-	60%	57%
Patients Who Left ER Before Being Seen	46,937	4%	3%	2%
Time from ER Arrival to Admit. (minutes)[2]	598	280	300	274
Time from ER Arrival to Discharge (minutes)	470	179	152	134
Time in ER Before Being Evaluated (minutes)	351	73	34	26
Time to Pain Meds for Fractures (minutes)	186	102	67	57
Heart Attack Care				
Aspirin Given at Discharge	63	98%	100%	99%
Fibrinolytic Meds Within 30 Min. of Arrival[7]	-	-	75%	54%
PCI Within 90 Minutes of Arrival[1]	-	-	98%	96%
Statin Prescribed at Discharge	68	99%	99%	98%
Heart Failure Care				
ACE Inhibitor or ARB for LVSD	27	100%	98%	97%
Discharge Instructions Given	88	98%	96%	94%
Evaluation of LVS Function	110	100%	100%	99%
Medicare Spending				
Medicare Spending per Patient (ratio)	-	0.99	0.94	0.98
Pneumonia Care				
Appropriate Initial Antibiotic Given	170	95%	97%	95%
Blood Culture Timing	238	97%	98%	98%
Pregnancy and Delivery Care				
Newborn Deliveries Scheduled Early	159	1%	3%	6%
Preventive Care				
Immunization for Influenza[2]	525	90%	93%	90%
Immunization for Pneumonia[2]	541	87%	94%	92%
Stroke Care				
Anticoagulation Therapy for Atrial Fibrillation	15	100%	95%	95%
Antithrombotic Therapy Timing	95	99%	98%	98%
Assessed for Rehabilitation	104	100%	98%	97%
Discharged on Antithrombotic Therapy	103	100%	99%	99%
Discharged on Statin Medication	71	100%	94%	94%
Thrombolytic Therapy Timing[1]	-	-	64%	66%
Venous Thromboembolism Prophylaxis	110	99%	96%	94%
Written Stroke Educational Materials Given	56	100%	88%	88%
Surgical Care Improvement Project				
Appropriate Beta Blocker Usage	169	99%	99%	98%
Appropriate VTP Within 24 Hours	637	98%	99%	98%
Controlled Postoperative Blood Glucose[7]	-	-	98%	97%
Perioperative Temperature Management	748	100%	100%	100%
Prophylactic Antibiotic Selection	543	99%	99%	99%
Prophylactic Antibiotic Selection (Outpatient)	548	99%	98%	98%
Prophylactic Antibiotic Stopped	536	99%	99%	98%
Prophylactic Antibiotic Timing	543	99%	99%	99%
Prophylactic Antibiotic Timing (Outpatient)	551	99%	99%	98%
Urinary Catheter Removal	575	97%	99%	97%
Survey of Patients' Hospital Experiences				
Area Around Room 'Always' Quiet at Night	300+	58%	64%	61%
Doctors 'Always' Communicated Well	300+	84%	83%	82%
Home Recovery Information Given	300+	87%	87%	85%
Hospital Given 9 or 10 on 10 Point Scale	300+	71%	71%	71%
Meds 'Always' Explained Before Given	300+	65%	65%	64%
Nurses 'Always' Communicated Well	300+	80%	81%	79%
Pain 'Always' Well Controlled	300+	74%	72%	71%
Room and Bathroom 'Always' Clean	300+	72%	72%	73%
Timely Help 'Always' Received	300+	64%	68%	68%
Would Definitely Recommend Hospital	300+	76%	70%	71%
Use of Medical Imaging				
Cardiac Imaging Stress Test before Surgery	341	3.8%	5.4%	5.3%
Combination Abdominal CT Scan	972	1.1%	5.6%	10.5%
Combination Brain/Sinus CT Scan	831	1.8%	2.6%	2.7%
Combination Chest CT Scan	754	1.3%	1.3%	2.7%
Follow-up Mammogram/Ultrasound	2,676	10.2%	8%	8.8%
Lumbar Spine MRI for Low Back Pain	127	36.2%	34.7%	37.2%

Frye Regional Medical Center

420 N Center St
Hickory, NC 28601
Phone: 828-322-6070
Fax: 828-345-5755
URL: www.fryemedctr.com
Type: Acute Care Hospitals
Emergency Services: Yes
Ownership: Proprietary
Beds: 355

Key Personnel:
Chief of Medical Staff . . . . Mark Anderson
Quality Assurance . . . . Linda Drum
Operating Room. . . . . Jan Fisk
CEO/President. . . . . Dennis Phillips
Radiology. . . . . Charles Scheil

Measure	Cases	This Hosp.	State Avg.	U.S. Avg.
Blood Clot Prevention and Treatment				
Anticoagulation Overlap Therapy[2]	85	98%	94%	93%
ICU Venous Thromboembolism Prophylaxis[2]	125	98%	93%	92%
Incidence of Potentially Preventable VTE[2]	12	8%	10%	10%
UFH with Dosages/Platelet Monitoring[2]	38	100%	95%	97%
Venous Thromboembolism Prophylaxis[2]	322	91%	88%	85%
Warfarin Therapy Discharge Instructions[2]	66	95%	81%	75%
Chest Pain/Possible Heart Attack Care				
Aspirin Given Within 24 Hours of Arrival[1,3]	-	-	97%	96%
Fibrinolytic Meds Within 30 Min. of Arrival[5]	-	-	66%	58%
Average Time to ECG (minutes)[1,3]	-	-	7	7
Average Time to Transfer (minutes)[5]	-	-	45	60
Children's Asthma Care				
Received Home Management Plan of Care	-	-	89%	88%
Received Reliever Medication	-	-	100%	100%
Received Systemic Corticosteroids	-	-	100%	100%
Emergency Department				
Admittance Decision Time (minutes)[2]	637	73	107	98
Head CT Results Within 45 Min. of Arrival	18	39%	60%	57%
Patients Who Left ER Before Being Seen	40,470	2%	3%	2%
Time from ER Arrival to Admit. (minutes)[2]	637	248	300	274
Time from ER Arrival to Discharge (minutes)	432	136	152	134
Time in ER Before Being Evaluated (minutes)	469	41	34	26
Time to Pain Meds for Fractures (minutes)	99	59	67	57
Heart Attack Care				
Aspirin Given at Discharge[2]	360	100%	100%	99%
Fibrinolytic Meds Within 30 Min. of Arrival[2,7]	-	-	75%	54%
PCI Within 90 Minutes of Arrival[2]	85	98%	98%	96%
Statin Prescribed at Discharge[2]	356	99%	99%	98%
Heart Failure Care				
ACE Inhibitor or ARB for LVSD	72	96%	98%	97%
Discharge Instructions Given	189	95%	96%	94%
Evaluation of LVS Function	222	100%	100%	99%
Medicare Spending				
Medicare Spending per Patient (ratio)	-	0.97	0.94	0.98
Pneumonia Care				
Appropriate Initial Antibiotic Given[2]	134	94%	97%	95%
Blood Culture Timing[2]	195	98%	98%	98%
Pregnancy and Delivery Care				
Newborn Deliveries Scheduled Early[2]	23	0%	3%	6%
Preventive Care				
Immunization for Influenza[2]	612	96%	93%	90%
Immunization for Pneumonia[2]	870	95%	94%	92%
Stroke Care				
Anticoagulation Therapy for Atrial Fibrillation	25	100%	95%	95%
Antithrombotic Therapy Timing	143	96%	98%	98%
Assessed for Rehabilitation	149	100%	98%	97%
Discharged on Antithrombotic Therapy	149	100%	99%	99%
Discharged on Statin Medication	118	97%	94%	94%
Thrombolytic Therapy Timing	12	83%	64%	66%
Venous Thromboembolism Prophylaxis	152	95%	96%	94%
Written Stroke Educational Materials Given	86	94%	88%	88%
Surgical Care Improvement Project				
Appropriate Beta Blocker Usage[2]	259	98%	99%	98%
Appropriate VTP Within 24 Hours[2]	333	99%	99%	98%
Controlled Postoperative Blood Glucose[2]	311	95%	98%	97%
Perioperative Temperature Management[2]	484	99%	100%	100%
Prophylactic Antibiotic Selection[2]	580	99%	99%	99%
Prophylactic Antibiotic Selection (Outpatient)	474	99%	98%	98%
Prophylactic Antibiotic Stopped[2]	565	98%	99%	98%
Prophylactic Antibiotic Timing[2]	584	98%	99%	99%
Prophylactic Antibiotic Timing (Outpatient)	474	100%	99%	98%
Urinary Catheter Removal[2]	563	99%	99%	97%
Survey of Patients' Hospital Experiences				
Area Around Room 'Always' Quiet at Night	300+	61%	64%	61%
Doctors 'Always' Communicated Well	300+	83%	83%	82%
Home Recovery Information Given	300+	89%	87%	85%
Hospital Given 9 or 10 on 10 Point Scale	300+	72%	71%	71%
Meds 'Always' Explained Before Given	300+	64%	65%	64%
Nurses 'Always' Communicated Well	300+	80%	81%	79%
Pain 'Always' Well Controlled	300+	71%	72%	71%
Room and Bathroom 'Always' Clean	300+	66%	72%	73%
Timely Help 'Always' Received	300+	73%	68%	68%
Would Definitely Recommend Hospital	300+	74%	70%	71%
Use of Medical Imaging				
Cardiac Imaging Stress Test before Surgery	1,228	4.3%	5.4%	5.3%
Combination Abdominal CT Scan	927	2.0%	5.6%	10.5%
Combination Brain/Sinus CT Scan	960	0.5%	2.6%	2.7%
Combination Chest CT Scan	851	2.0%	1.3%	2.7%
Follow-up Mammogram/Ultrasound	2,542	12.4%	8%	8.8%
Lumbar Spine MRI for Low Back Pain	236	31.4%	34.7%	37.2%

High Point Regional Hospital

601 N Elm Saint PO Box Hp-5
High Point, NC 27261
Phone: 336-878-6000
Fax: 336-878-6709
URL: www.highpointregional.com
Type: Acute Care Hospitals
Emergency Services: Yes
Ownership: Voluntary non-profit - Private
Beds: 400

Key Personnel:
CEO/President. . . . . Ernie Bovio
Radiology. . . . . Diane O'Connell, MD
Emergency Room . . . . Karen Olsen
Pediatric Ambulatory Care . . . . . . Allison Poston, MD
Operating Room. . . . . Denise Rhew
Anesthesiology. . . . . Kevin Speight, MD
Infection Control. . . . . Vicki Tutor
Chief of Medical Staff . . . . Dale Williams, MD

Measure	Cases	This Hosp.	State Avg.	U.S. Avg.
Blood Clot Prevention and Treatment				
Anticoagulation Overlap Therapy[2]	86	99%	94%	93%
ICU Venous Thromboembolism Prophylaxis[2]	51	90%	93%	92%
Incidence of Potentially Preventable VTE[2]	11	36%	10%	10%
UFH with Dosages/Platelet Monitoring[2]	47	100%	95%	97%
Venous Thromboembolism Prophylaxis[2]	313	89%	88%	85%
Warfarin Therapy Discharge Instructions[2]	62	92%	81%	75%
Chest Pain/Possible Heart Attack Care				
Aspirin Given Within 24 Hours of Arrival	20	100%	97%	96%
Fibrinolytic Meds Within 30 Min. of Arrival[3,7]	-	-	66%	58%
Average Time to ECG (minutes)	21	7	7	7
Average Time to Transfer (minutes)[3,7]	-	-	45	60
Children's Asthma Care				

NOTE: Hospital profiles are in alphabetical order by state, then city, then hospital within the city; Rankings exclude hospitals with less than 25 cases except for patient surveys which excludes hospitals with less than 100 cases; (a) 100-299 cases; (1) The number of cases/patients is too few to report; (2) Data submitted were based on a sample of cases/patients; (3) Results are based on a shorter time period than required; (4) Data suppressed by CMS for one or more quarters; (5) Results are not available for this reporting period; (6) Fewer than 100 patients completed the HCAHPS survey; (7) No cases met the criteria for this measure; (8) The lower limit of the confidence interval cannot be calculated if the number of observed infections equals zero; (9) No data are available from the state/territory for this reporting period; (10) The scores shown reflect fewer than 50 completed surveys; (11) There were discrepancies in the data collection process; (12) This measure does not apply to this hospital for this reporting period; (13) Results cannot be calculated for this reporting period; (14) The results for this state are combined with nearby states to protect confidentiality; Please refer to the User's Guide for a full explanation of data.

Measure	Cases	This Hosp.	State Avg.	U.S. Avg.
Received Home Management Plan of Care	-	-	89%	88%
Received Reliever Medication	-	-	100%	100%
Received Systemic Corticosteroids	-	-	100%	100%
Emergency Department				
Admittance Decision Time (minutes)[2]	659	80	107	98
Head CT Results Within 45 Min. of Arrival[1]	-	-	60%	57%
Patients Who Left ER Before Being Seen	64,666	3%	3%	2%
Time from ER Arrival to Admit. (minutes)[2]	659	330	300	274
Time from ER Arrival to Discharge (minutes)	338	204	152	134
Time in ER Before Being Evaluated (minutes)	408	54	34	26
Time to Pain Meds for Fractures (minutes)	123	66	67	57
Heart Attack Care				
Aspirin Given at Discharge	475	100%	100%	99%
Fibrinolytic Meds Within 30 Min. of Arrival[7]	-	-	75%	54%
PCI Within 90 Minutes of Arrival	50	100%	98%	96%
Statin Prescribed at Discharge	459	100%	99%	98%
Heart Failure Care				
ACE Inhibitor or ARB for LVSD	144	100%	98%	97%
Discharge Instructions Given	432	100%	96%	94%
Evaluation of LVS Function	555	100%	100%	99%
Medicare Spending				
Medicare Spending per Patient (ratio)	-	0.98	0.94	0.98
Pneumonia Care				
Appropriate Initial Antibiotic Given	254	95%	97%	95%
Blood Culture Timing	395	98%	98%	98%
Pregnancy and Delivery Care				
Newborn Deliveries Scheduled Early	143	3%	3%	6%
Preventive Care				
Immunization for Influenza[2]	544	97%	93%	90%
Immunization for Pneumonia[2]	701	99%	94%	92%
Stroke Care				
Anticoagulation Therapy for Atrial Fibrillation	29	100%	95%	95%
Antithrombotic Therapy Timing	209	100%	98%	98%
Assessed for Rehabilitation	244	100%	98%	97%
Discharged on Antithrombotic Therapy	228	100%	99%	99%
Discharged on Statin Medication	197	100%	94%	94%
Thrombolytic Therapy Timing	18	83%	64%	66%
Venous Thromboembolism Prophylaxis	242	96%	96%	94%
Written Stroke Educational Materials Given	120	99%	88%	88%
Surgical Care Improvement Project				
Appropriate Beta Blocker Usage[2]	159	98%	99%	98%
Appropriate VTP Within 24 Hours[2]	295	94%	99%	98%
Controlled Postoperative Blood Glucose[2]	96	97%	98%	97%
Perioperative Temperature Management[2]	358	100%	100%	100%
Prophylactic Antibiotic Selection[2]	319	98%	99%	99%
Prophylactic Antibiotic Selection (Outpatient)	432	95%	98%	98%
Prophylactic Antibiotic Stopped[2]	291	99%	99%	98%
Prophylactic Antibiotic Timing[2]	319	99%	99%	99%
Prophylactic Antibiotic Timing (Outpatient)	434	97%	99%	98%
Urinary Catheter Removal[2]	292	99%	99%	97%
Survey of Patients' Hospital Experiences				
Area Around Room 'Always' Quiet at Night	300+	59%	64%	61%
Doctors 'Always' Communicated Well	300+	81%	83%	82%
Home Recovery Information Given	300+	83%	87%	85%
Hospital Given 9 or 10 on 10 Point Scale	300+	74%	71%	71%
Meds 'Always' Explained Before Given	300+	63%	65%	64%
Nurses 'Always' Communicated Well	300+	80%	81%	79%
Pain 'Always' Well Controlled	300+	72%	72%	71%
Room and Bathroom 'Always' Clean	300+	70%	72%	73%
Timely Help 'Always' Received	300+	65%	68%	68%
Would Definitely Recommend Hospital	300+	74%	70%	71%
Use of Medical Imaging				
Cardiac Imaging Stress Test before Surgery	660	5.2%	5.4%	5.3%
Combination Abdominal CT Scan	736	1.2%	5.6%	10.5%
Combination Brain/Sinus CT Scan	1,059	3.2%	2.6%	2.7%
Combination Chest CT Scan	189	0.0%	1.3%	2.7%
Follow-up Mammogram/Ultrasound	370	8.6%	8%	8.8%
Lumbar Spine MRI for Low Back Pain	70	31.4%	34.7%	37.2%

Highlands Cashiers Hospital

190 Hospital Drive
Highlands, NC 28741
E-mail: ftaylor@hchospital.org
URL: www.hchospital.org
Type: Critical Access Hospitals
Ownership: Voluntary non-profit - Private

Phone: 828-526-1200
Fax: 828-526-1230

Emergency Services: Yes
Beds: 104

Key Personnel:
President/CEO. . . . . Craig B. Jones
Radiology. . . . . Rodney Stinnett
Chief of Medical Staff. . . . . David M Wheeler

Measure	Cases	This Hosp.	State Avg.	U.S. Avg.
Blood Clot Prevention and Treatment				
Anticoagulation Overlap Therapy[5]	-	-	94%	93%
ICU Venous Thromboembolism Prophylaxis[5]	-	-	93%	92%
Incidence of Potentially Preventable VTE[5]	-	-	10%	10%
UFH with Dosages/Platelet Monitoring[5]	-	-	95%	97%
Venous Thromboembolism Prophylaxis[5]	-	-	88%	85%
Warfarin Therapy Discharge Instructions[5]	-	-	81%	75%
Chest Pain/Possible Heart Attack Care				
Aspirin Given Within 24 Hours of Arrival	-	-	97%	96%
Fibrinolytic Meds Within 30 Min. of Arrival	-	-	66%	58%
Average Time to ECG (minutes)	-	-	7	7
Average Time to Transfer (minutes)	-	-	45	60
Children's Asthma Care				
Received Home Management Plan of Care	-	-	89%	88%
Received Reliever Medication	-	-	100%	100%
Received Systemic Corticosteroids	-	-	100%	100%
Emergency Department				
Admittance Decision Time (minutes)[5]	-	-	107	98
Head CT Results Within 45 Min. of Arrival	-	-	60%	57%
Patients Who Left ER Before Being Seen	-	-	3%	2%
Time from ER Arrival to Admit. (minutes)[5]	-	-	300	274
Time from ER Arrival to Discharge (minutes)	-	-	152	134
Time in ER Before Being Evaluated (minutes)	-	-	34	26
Time to Pain Meds for Fractures (minutes)	-	-	67	57
Heart Attack Care				
Aspirin Given at Discharge[5]	-	-	100%	99%
Fibrinolytic Meds Within 30 Min. of Arrival[5]	-	-	75%	54%
PCI Within 90 Minutes of Arrival[5]	-	-	98%	96%
Statin Prescribed at Discharge[5]	-	-	99%	98%
Heart Failure Care				
ACE Inhibitor or ARB for LVSD[1,3]	-	-	98%	97%
Discharge Instructions Given[1,3]	-	-	96%	94%
Evaluation of LVS Function[1,3]	-	-	100%	99%
Medicare Spending				
Medicare Spending per Patient (ratio)	-	-	0.94	0.98
Pneumonia Care				
Appropriate Initial Antibiotic Given[1,3]	-	-	97%	95%
Blood Culture Timing[1,3]	-	-	98%	98%
Pregnancy and Delivery Care				
Newborn Deliveries Scheduled Early[5]	-	-	3%	6%
Preventive Care				
Immunization for Influenza[5]	-	-	93%	90%
Immunization for Pneumonia[5]	-	-	94%	92%
Stroke Care				
Anticoagulation Therapy for Atrial Fibrillation[5]	-	-	95%	95%
Antithrombotic Therapy Timing[5]	-	-	98%	98%
Assessed for Rehabilitation[5]	-	-	98%	97%
Discharged on Antithrombotic Therapy[5]	-	-	99%	99%
Discharged on Statin Medication[5]	-	-	94%	94%
Thrombolytic Therapy Timing[5]	-	-	64%	66%
Venous Thromboembolism Prophylaxis[5]	-	-	96%	94%
Written Stroke Educational Materials Given[5]	-	-	88%	88%
Surgical Care Improvement Project				
Appropriate Beta Blocker Usage[5]	-	-	99%	98%
Appropriate VTP Within 24 Hours[5]	-	-	99%	98%
Controlled Postoperative Blood Glucose[5]	-	-	98%	97%
Perioperative Temperature Management[5]	-	-	100%	100%
Prophylactic Antibiotic Selection[5]	-	-	99%	99%
Prophylactic Antibiotic Selection (Outpatient)	-	-	98%	98%
Prophylactic Antibiotic Stopped[5]	-	-	99%	98%
Prophylactic Antibiotic Timing[5]	-	-	99%	99%
Prophylactic Antibiotic Timing (Outpatient)	-	-	99%	98%
Urinary Catheter Removal[5]	-	-	99%	97%
Survey of Patients' Hospital Experiences				
Area Around Room 'Always' Quiet at Night[5]	-	-	64%	61%
Doctors 'Always' Communicated Well[5]	-	-	83%	82%
Home Recovery Information Given[5]	-	-	87%	85%
Hospital Given 9 or 10 on 10 Point Scale[5]	-	-	71%	71%
Meds 'Always' Explained Before Given[5]	-	-	65%	64%
Nurses 'Always' Communicated Well[5]	-	-	81%	79%
Pain 'Always' Well Controlled[5]	-	-	72%	71%
Room and Bathroom 'Always' Clean[5]	-	-	72%	73%
Timely Help 'Always' Received[5]	-	-	68%	68%
Would Definitely Recommend Hospital[5]	-	-	70%	71%
Use of Medical Imaging				
Cardiac Imaging Stress Test before Surgery	-	-	5.4%	5.3%
Combination Abdominal CT Scan	-	-	5.6%	10.5%
Combination Brain/Sinus CT Scan	-	-	2.6%	2.7%
Combination Chest CT Scan	-	-	1.3%	2.7%
Follow-up Mammogram/Ultrasound	-	-	8%	8.8%
Lumbar Spine MRI for Low Back Pain	-	-	34.7%	37.2%

Novant Health Huntersville Medical Center

10030 Gilead Road
Huntersville, NC 28078
E-mail: hic@novanthealth.org
URL: www.presbyterian.org
Type: Acute Care Hospitals
Ownership: Voluntary non-profit - Private

Phone: 704-316-4000

Emergency Services: Yes

Key Personnel:
Operating Room. . . . . Rohit Bhasin
Chief of Medical Staff. . . . . David Cook
Pediatric In-Patient Care . . . . William Flannery
Radiology. . . . . Denis R. Lincoln, M.D.
CEO/President. . . . . Melissa Robson
Emergency Room . . . . Joshua Sarett
Anesthesiology. . . . . Jeffrey Welna

Measure	Cases	This Hosp.	State Avg.	U.S. Avg.
Blood Clot Prevention and Treatment				
Anticoagulation Overlap Therapy[2]	41	100%	94%	93%
ICU Venous Thromboembolism Prophylaxis[2]	45	96%	93%	92%
Incidence of Potentially Preventable VTE[1,2]	-	-	10%	10%
UFH with Dosages/Platelet Monitoring[1,2]	-	-	95%	97%
Venous Thromboembolism Prophylaxis[2]	352	94%	88%	85%
Warfarin Therapy Discharge Instructions[2]	35	91%	81%	75%
Chest Pain/Possible Heart Attack Care				
Aspirin Given Within 24 Hours of Arrival	36	97%	97%	96%
Fibrinolytic Meds Within 30 Min. of Arrival[7]	-	-	66%	58%
Average Time to ECG (minutes)	36	2	7	7
Average Time to Transfer (minutes)[1]	-	-	45	60
Children's Asthma Care				
Received Home Management Plan of Care	-	-	89%	88%
Received Reliever Medication	-	-	100%	100%
Received Systemic Corticosteroids	-	-	100%	100%
Emergency Department				
Admittance Decision Time (minutes)[2]	713	152	107	98
Head CT Results Within 45 Min. of Arrival	25	80%	60%	57%
Patients Who Left ER Before Being Seen	34,445	2%	3%	2%
Time from ER Arrival to Admit. (minutes)[2]	720	317	300	274
Time from ER Arrival to Discharge (minutes)	439	152	152	134
Time in ER Before Being Evaluated (minutes)	479	25	34	26
Time to Pain Meds for Fractures (minutes)	121	56	67	57
Heart Attack Care				
Aspirin Given at Discharge[1]	-	-	100%	99%
Fibrinolytic Meds Within 30 Min. of Arrival[7]	-	-	75%	54%
PCI Within 90 Minutes of Arrival[7]	-	-	98%	96%
Statin Prescribed at Discharge[1]	-	-	99%	98%
Heart Failure Care				
ACE Inhibitor or ARB for LVSD	39	100%	98%	97%
Discharge Instructions Given	87	93%	96%	94%
Evaluation of LVS Function	103	100%	100%	99%
Medicare Spending				
Medicare Spending per Patient (ratio)	-	0.98	0.94	0.98
Pneumonia Care				
Appropriate Initial Antibiotic Given	115	100%	97%	95%

NOTE: Hospital profiles are in alphabetical order by state, then city, then hospital within the city; Rankings exclude hospitals with less than 25 cases except for patient surveys which excludes hospitals with less than 100 cases; (a) 100-299 cases; (1) The number of cases/patients is too few to report; (2) Data submitted were based on a sample of cases/patients; (3) Results are based on a shorter time period than required; (4) Data suppressed by CMS for one or more quarters; (5) Results are not available for this reporting period; (6) Fewer than 100 patients completed the HCAHPS survey; (7) No cases met the criteria for this measure; (8) The lower limit of the confidence interval cannot be calculated if the number of observed infections equals zero; (9) No data are available from the state/territory for this reporting period; (10) The scores shown reflect fewer than 50 completed surveys; (11) There were discrepancies in the data collection process; (12) This measure does not apply to this hospital for this reporting period; (13) Results cannot be calculated for this reporting period; (14) The results for this state are combined with nearby states to protect confidentiality; Please refer to the User's Guide for a full explanation of data.

Measure	Cases	This Hosp.	State Avg.	U.S. Avg.
Blood Culture Timing	162	100%	98%	98%
Pregnancy and Delivery Care				
Newborn Deliveries Scheduled Early[2]	39	0%	3%	6%
Preventive Care				
Immunization for Influenza[2]	584	98%	93%	90%
Immunization for Pneumonia[2]	688	99%	94%	92%
Stroke Care				
Anticoagulation Therapy for Atrial Fibrillation	11	100%	95%	95%
Antithrombotic Therapy Timing	55	100%	98%	98%
Assessed for Rehabilitation	79	100%	98%	97%
Discharged on Antithrombotic Therapy	74	100%	99%	99%
Discharged on Statin Medication	52	100%	94%	94%
Thrombolytic Therapy Timing[7]	-	-	64%	66%
Venous Thromboembolism Prophylaxis	59	98%	96%	94%
Written Stroke Educational Materials Given	60	97%	88%	88%
Surgical Care Improvement Project				
Appropriate Beta Blocker Usage[2]	192	99%	99%	98%
Appropriate VTP Within 24 Hours[2]	564	99%	99%	98%
Controlled Postoperative Blood Glucose[2,7]	-	-	98%	97%
Perioperative Temperature Management[2]	684	100%	100%	100%
Prophylactic Antibiotic Selection[2]	509	100%	99%	99%
Prophylactic Antibiotic Selection (Outpatient)	219	100%	98%	98%
Prophylactic Antibiotic Stopped[2]	498	100%	99%	98%
Prophylactic Antibiotic Timing[2]	509	100%	99%	99%
Prophylactic Antibiotic Timing (Outpatient)	219	100%	99%	98%
Urinary Catheter Removal[2]	438	99%	99%	97%
Survey of Patients' Hospital Experiences				
Area Around Room 'Always' Quiet at Night	300+	59%	64%	61%
Doctors 'Always' Communicated Well	300+	83%	83%	82%
Home Recovery Information Given	300+	86%	87%	85%
Hospital Given 9 or 10 on 10 Point Scale	300+	76%	71%	71%
Meds 'Always' Explained Before Given	300+	59%	65%	64%
Nurses 'Always' Communicated Well	300+	77%	81%	79%
Pain 'Always' Well Controlled	300+	70%	72%	71%
Room and Bathroom 'Always' Clean	300+	69%	72%	73%
Timely Help 'Always' Received	300+	64%	68%	68%
Would Definitely Recommend Hospital	300+	81%	70%	71%
Use of Medical Imaging				
Cardiac Imaging Stress Test before Surgery	196	5.6%	5.4%	5.3%
Combination Abdominal CT Scan	922	3.0%	5.6%	10.5%
Combination Brain/Sinus CT Scan	747	2.3%	2.6%	2.7%
Combination Chest CT Scan	579	0.0%	1.3%	2.7%
Follow-up Mammogram/Ultrasound	471	7.0%	8%	8.8%
Lumbar Spine MRI for Low Back Pain	182	38.5%	34.7%	37.2%

Onslow Memorial Hospital

317 Western Boulevard
Jacksonville, NC 28540
Phone: 910-577-2345
Fax: 910-577-2858
URL: www.onslowmemorial.org
Type: Acute Care Hospitals
Emergency Services: Yes
Ownership: Govt - Hospital Dist/Auth
Beds: 162

Key Personnel:
Chairman/CEO . . . . Pat Alford
Cardiac Laboratory. . . . . Jean Brazell, RN
Infection Control. . . . . Gloria Horne, RN
Chief of Medical Staff. . . . . Scott Johnson, MD
Radiology. . . . . Joanne Offult
Pediatric In-Patient Care . . . . . . Angela Pollack, RN
Operating Room. . . . . Kathy Schumacker, RN
Quality Assurance . . . . Richard Thompson

Measure	Cases	This Hosp.	State Avg.	U.S. Avg.
Blood Clot Prevention and Treatment				
Anticoagulation Overlap Therapy[2]	27	100%	94%	93%
ICU Venous Thromboembolism Prophylaxis[2]	46	96%	93%	92%
Incidence of Potentially Preventable VTE[1,2]	-	-	10%	10%
UFH with Dosages/Platelet Monitoring[2]	14	100%	95%	97%
Venous Thromboembolism Prophylaxis[2]	402	93%	88%	85%
Warfarin Therapy Discharge Instructions[2]	20	100%	81%	75%
Chest Pain/Possible Heart Attack Care				
Aspirin Given Within 24 Hours of Arrival	151	95%	97%	96%
Fibrinolytic Meds Within 30 Min. of Arrival[1]	-	-	66%	58%
Average Time to ECG (minutes)	154	10	7	7
Average Time to Transfer (minutes)[1]	-	-	45	60
Children's Asthma Care				
Received Home Management Plan of Care	-	-	89%	88%
Received Reliever Medication	-	-	100%	100%
Received Systemic Corticosteroids	-	-	100%	100%
Emergency Department				
Admittance Decision Time (minutes)[2]	550	134	107	98
Head CT Results Within 45 Min. of Arrival	11	91%	60%	57%
Patients Who Left ER Before Being Seen	66,634	3%	3%	2%
Time from ER Arrival to Admit. (minutes)[2]	550	400	300	274
Time from ER Arrival to Discharge (minutes)	1,649	185	152	134
Time in ER Before Being Evaluated (minutes)	1,808	35	34	26
Time to Pain Meds for Fractures (minutes)	201	67	67	57
Heart Attack Care				
Aspirin Given at Discharge	12	92%	100%	99%
Fibrinolytic Meds Within 30 Min. of Arrival[7]	-	-	75%	54%
PCI Within 90 Minutes of Arrival[7]	-	-	98%	96%
Statin Prescribed at Discharge[1]	-	-	99%	98%
Heart Failure Care				
ACE Inhibitor or ARB for LVSD	57	98%	98%	97%
Discharge Instructions Given	149	100%	96%	94%
Evaluation of LVS Function	171	99%	100%	99%
Medicare Spending				
Medicare Spending per Patient (ratio)	-	0.97	0.94	0.98
Pneumonia Care				
Appropriate Initial Antibiotic Given	158	96%	97%	95%
Blood Culture Timing	266	98%	98%	98%
Pregnancy and Delivery Care				
Newborn Deliveries Scheduled Early[2]	35	3%	3%	6%
Preventive Care				
Immunization for Influenza[2]	486	86%	93%	90%
Immunization for Pneumonia[2]	449	88%	94%	92%
Stroke Care				
Anticoagulation Therapy for Atrial Fibrillation[1]	-	-	95%	95%
Antithrombotic Therapy Timing	74	100%	98%	98%
Assessed for Rehabilitation	71	97%	98%	97%
Discharged on Antithrombotic Therapy	69	99%	99%	99%
Discharged on Statin Medication	59	95%	94%	94%
Thrombolytic Therapy Timing[1]	-	-	64%	66%
Venous Thromboembolism Prophylaxis	68	99%	96%	94%
Written Stroke Educational Materials Given	49	92%	88%	88%
Surgical Care Improvement Project				
Appropriate Beta Blocker Usage	65	100%	99%	98%
Appropriate VTP Within 24 Hours	230	98%	99%	98%
Controlled Postoperative Blood Glucose[7]	-	-	98%	97%
Perioperative Temperature Management	259	100%	100%	100%
Prophylactic Antibiotic Selection	172	99%	99%	99%
Prophylactic Antibiotic Selection (Outpatient)	211	99%	98%	98%
Prophylactic Antibiotic Stopped	167	99%	99%	98%
Prophylactic Antibiotic Timing	172	99%	99%	99%
Prophylactic Antibiotic Timing (Outpatient)	213	98%	99%	98%
Urinary Catheter Removal	184	98%	99%	97%
Survey of Patients' Hospital Experiences				
Area Around Room 'Always' Quiet at Night	300+	51%	64%	61%
Doctors 'Always' Communicated Well	300+	80%	83%	82%
Home Recovery Information Given	300+	86%	87%	85%
Hospital Given 9 or 10 on 10 Point Scale	300+	58%	71%	71%
Meds 'Always' Explained Before Given	300+	66%	65%	64%
Nurses 'Always' Communicated Well	300+	82%	81%	79%
Pain 'Always' Well Controlled	300+	66%	72%	71%
Room and Bathroom 'Always' Clean	300+	67%	72%	73%
Timely Help 'Always' Received	300+	70%	68%	68%
Would Definitely Recommend Hospital	300+	56%	70%	71%
Use of Medical Imaging				
Cardiac Imaging Stress Test before Surgery	142	4.2%	5.4%	5.3%
Combination Abdominal CT Scan	606	4.6%	5.6%	10.5%
Combination Brain/Sinus CT Scan	849	3.4%	2.6%	2.7%
Combination Chest CT Scan	416	0.0%	1.3%	2.7%
Follow-up Mammogram/Ultrasound	962	4.9%	8%	8.8%
Lumbar Spine MRI for Low Back Pain[1]	-	-	34.7%	37.2%

Ashe Memorial Hospital

200 Hospital Ave
Jefferson, NC 28640
Phone: 336-246-7101
Fax: 336-846-0746
E-mail: info@ashememorial.org
URL: www.ashememorial.org
Type: Critical Access Hospitals
Emergency Services: Yes
Ownership: Voluntary non-profit - Private

Key Personnel:
Chief of Medical Staff. . . . . Norma Gross
Operating Room. . . . . Charles W Jones
Emergency Room . . . . Kina Jones, RN
Radiology. . . . . David McCune
Intensive Care Unit. . . . . Polly Osowitt, RN
Quality Assurance . . . . Leisa Powell
Infection Control. . . . . Shirlene Widner, RN
CEO/President. . . . . RD Williams

Measure	Cases	This Hosp.	State Avg.	U.S. Avg.
Blood Clot Prevention and Treatment				
Anticoagulation Overlap Therapy[5]	-	-	94%	93%
ICU Venous Thromboembolism Prophylaxis[5]	-	-	93%	92%
Incidence of Potentially Preventable VTE[5]	-	-	10%	10%
UFH with Dosages/Platelet Monitoring[5]	-	-	95%	97%
Venous Thromboembolism Prophylaxis[5]	-	-	88%	85%
Warfarin Therapy Discharge Instructions[5]	-	-	81%	75%
Chest Pain/Possible Heart Attack Care				
Aspirin Given Within 24 Hours of Arrival	77	94%	97%	96%
Fibrinolytic Meds Within 30 Min. of Arrival	12	67%	66%	58%
Average Time to ECG (minutes)	78	11	7	7
Average Time to Transfer (minutes)[7]	-	-	45	60
Children's Asthma Care				
Received Home Management Plan of Care	-	-	89%	88%
Received Reliever Medication	-	-	100%	100%
Received Systemic Corticosteroids	-	-	100%	100%
Emergency Department				
Admittance Decision Time (minutes)[2]	455	51	107	98
Head CT Results Within 45 Min. of Arrival[5]	-	-	60%	57%
Patients Who Left ER Before Being Seen	10,655	4%	3%	2%
Time from ER Arrival to Admit. (minutes)[2]	455	228	300	274
Time from ER Arrival to Discharge (minutes)	353	145	152	134
Time in ER Before Being Evaluated (minutes)	377	41	34	26
Time to Pain Meds for Fractures (minutes)[5]	-	-	67	57
Heart Attack Care				
Aspirin Given at Discharge[1,3]	-	-	100%	99%
Fibrinolytic Meds Within 30 Min. of Arrival[3,7]	-	-	75%	54%
PCI Within 90 Minutes of Arrival[3,7]	-	-	98%	96%
Statin Prescribed at Discharge[1,3]	-	-	99%	98%
Heart Failure Care				
ACE Inhibitor or ARB for LVSD[1]	-	-	98%	97%
Discharge Instructions Given	31	90%	96%	94%
Evaluation of LVS Function	36	94%	100%	99%
Medicare Spending				
Medicare Spending per Patient (ratio)	-	-	0.94	0.98
Pneumonia Care				
Appropriate Initial Antibiotic Given	99	93%	97%	95%
Blood Culture Timing	63	94%	98%	98%
Pregnancy and Delivery Care				
Newborn Deliveries Scheduled Early[5]	-	-	3%	6%
Preventive Care				
Immunization for Influenza[2]	402	91%	93%	90%
Immunization for Pneumonia[2]	483	96%	94%	92%
Stroke Care				
Anticoagulation Therapy for Atrial Fibrillation[5]	-	-	95%	95%
Antithrombotic Therapy Timing[5]	-	-	98%	98%
Assessed for Rehabilitation[5]	-	-	98%	97%
Discharged on Antithrombotic Therapy[5]	-	-	99%	99%
Discharged on Statin Medication[5]	-	-	94%	94%
Thrombolytic Therapy Timing[5]	-	-	64%	66%
Venous Thromboembolism Prophylaxis[5]	-	-	96%	94%
Written Stroke Educational Materials Given[5]	-	-	88%	88%
Surgical Care Improvement Project				
Appropriate Beta Blocker Usage[1]	-	-	99%	98%
Appropriate VTP Within 24 Hours	32	84%	99%	98%
Controlled Postoperative Blood Glucose[7]	-	-	98%	97%
Perioperative Temperature Management	31	100%	100%	100%

NOTE: Hospital profiles are in alphabetical order by state, then city, then hospital within the city; Rankings exclude hospitals with less than 25 cases except for patient surveys which excludes hospitals with less than 100 cases; (a) 100-299 cases; (1) The number of cases/patients is too few to report; (2) Data submitted were based on a sample of cases/patients; (3) Results are based on a shorter time period than required; (4) Data suppressed by CMS for one or more quarters; (5) Results are not available for this reporting period; (6) Fewer than 100 patients completed the HCAHPS survey; (7) No cases met the criteria for this measure; (8) The lower limit of the confidence interval cannot be calculated if the number of observed infections equals zero; (9) No data are available from the state/territory for this reporting period; (10) The scores shown reflect fewer than 50 completed surveys; (11) There were discrepancies in the data collection process; (12) This measure does not apply to this hospital for this reporting period; (13) Results cannot be calculated for this reporting period; (14) The results for this state are combined with nearby states to protect confidentiality; Please refer to the User's Guide for a full explanation of data.

Measure	Cases	This Hosp.	State Avg.	U.S. Avg.
Prophylactic Antibiotic Selection	11	100%	99%	99%
Prophylactic Antibiotic Selection (Outpatient)[1]	-	-	98%	98%
Prophylactic Antibiotic Stopped	11	100%	99%	98%
Prophylactic Antibiotic Timing	11	91%	99%	99%
Prophylactic Antibiotic Timing (Outpatient)	11	91%	99%	98%
Urinary Catheter Removal	16	100%	99%	97%
Survey of Patients' Hospital Experiences				
Area Around Room 'Always' Quiet at Night	300+	65%	64%	61%
Doctors 'Always' Communicated Well	300+	89%	83%	82%
Home Recovery Information Given	300+	89%	87%	85%
Hospital Given 9 or 10 on 10 Point Scale	300+	76%	71%	71%
Meds 'Always' Explained Before Given	300+	69%	65%	64%
Nurses 'Always' Communicated Well	300+	87%	81%	79%
Pain 'Always' Well Controlled	300+	78%	72%	71%
Room and Bathroom 'Always' Clean	300+	82%	72%	73%
Timely Help 'Always' Received	300+	78%	68%	68%
Would Definitely Recommend Hospital	300+	72%	70%	71%
Use of Medical Imaging				
Cardiac Imaging Stress Test before Surgery	73	8.2%	5.4%	5.3%
Combination Abdominal CT Scan	331	45.9%	5.6%	10.5%
Combination Brain/Sinus CT Scan[1]	-	-	2.6%	2.7%
Combination Chest CT Scan	131	1.5%	1.3%	2.7%
Follow-up Mammogram/Ultrasound	753	4.1%	8%	8.8%
Lumbar Spine MRI for Low Back Pain	55	36.4%	34.7%	37.2%

Vidant Duplin Hospital

401 N Main St
Kenansville, NC 28349
URL: www.dgh.org
Type: Acute Care Hospitals
Ownership: Government - Local
Phone: 910-296-0941
Fax: 910-296-2951
Emergency Services: Yes
Beds: 89

Key Personnel:
Anesthesiology. . . . . Elizabeth Brayton, MD
Quality Assurance . . . . Margaret Broadhurst
CEO/President. . . . . Harvey Case
Intensive Care Unit. . . . . Deborah Coombs
Emergency Room . . . . Brenda Grubbs
Operating Room. . . . . Dyrek Miller
Chief of Medical Staff. . . . . C Daniel Pate, Jr
Radiology. . . . . Barry Powers

Measure	Cases	This Hosp.	State Avg.	U.S. Avg.
Blood Clot Prevention and Treatment				
Anticoagulation Overlap Therapy[2]	16	81%	94%	93%
ICU Venous Thromboembolism Prophylaxis[2]	83	96%	93%	92%
Incidence of Potentially Preventable VTE[2,7]	-	-	10%	10%
UFH with Dosages/Platelet Monitoring[1,2]	-	-	95%	97%
Venous Thromboembolism Prophylaxis[2]	128	92%	88%	85%
Warfarin Therapy Discharge Instructions[2]	13	54%	81%	75%
Chest Pain/Possible Heart Attack Care				
Aspirin Given Within 24 Hours of Arrival	84	99%	97%	96%
Fibrinolytic Meds Within 30 Min. of Arrival[1]	-	-	66%	58%
Average Time to ECG (minutes)	87	9	7	7
Average Time to Transfer (minutes)[7]	-	-	45	60
Children's Asthma Care				
Received Home Management Plan of Care	-	-	89%	88%
Received Reliever Medication	-	-	100%	100%
Received Systemic Corticosteroids	-	-	100%	100%
Emergency Department				
Admittance Decision Time (minutes)[2]	222	48	107	98
Head CT Results Within 45 Min. of Arrival	19	47%	60%	57%
Patients Who Left ER Before Being Seen	21,992	5%	3%	2%
Time from ER Arrival to Admit. (minutes)[2]	238	266	300	274
Time from ER Arrival to Discharge (minutes)	400	166	152	134
Time in ER Before Being Evaluated (minutes)	239	51	34	26
Time to Pain Meds for Fractures (minutes)	49	77	67	57
Heart Attack Care				
Aspirin Given at Discharge[1]	-	-	100%	99%
Fibrinolytic Meds Within 30 Min. of Arrival[7]	-	-	75%	54%
PCI Within 90 Minutes of Arrival[7]	-	-	98%	96%
Statin Prescribed at Discharge[1]	-	-	99%	98%
Heart Failure Care				
ACE Inhibitor or ARB for LVSD	35	94%	98%	97%
Discharge Instructions Given	88	100%	96%	94%
Evaluation of LVS Function	107	100%	100%	99%
Medicare Spending				
Medicare Spending per Patient (ratio)	-	0.89	0.94	0.98
Pneumonia Care				
Appropriate Initial Antibiotic Given	60	100%	97%	95%
Blood Culture Timing	105	95%	98%	98%
Pregnancy and Delivery Care				
Newborn Deliveries Scheduled Early	60	2%	3%	6%
Preventive Care				
Immunization for Influenza[2]	354	81%	93%	90%
Immunization for Pneumonia[2]	338	82%	94%	92%
Stroke Care				
Anticoagulation Therapy for Atrial Fibrillation[1]	-	-	95%	95%
Antithrombotic Therapy Timing	36	100%	98%	98%
Assessed for Rehabilitation	38	100%	98%	97%
Discharged on Antithrombotic Therapy	36	97%	99%	99%
Discharged on Statin Medication	30	100%	94%	94%
Thrombolytic Therapy Timing[1]	-	-	64%	66%
Venous Thromboembolism Prophylaxis	35	91%	96%	94%
Written Stroke Educational Materials Given	27	78%	88%	88%
Surgical Care Improvement Project				
Appropriate Beta Blocker Usage[1]	-	-	99%	98%
Appropriate VTP Within 24 Hours	23	100%	99%	98%
Controlled Postoperative Blood Glucose[7]	-	-	98%	97%
Perioperative Temperature Management	30	100%	100%	100%
Prophylactic Antibiotic Selection	19	100%	99%	99%
Prophylactic Antibiotic Selection (Outpatient)[1]	-	-	98%	98%
Prophylactic Antibiotic Stopped	19	95%	99%	98%
Prophylactic Antibiotic Timing	19	100%	99%	99%
Prophylactic Antibiotic Timing (Outpatient)[1]	-	-	99%	98%
Urinary Catheter Removal[1]	-	-	99%	97%
Survey of Patients' Hospital Experiences				
Area Around Room 'Always' Quiet at Night	300+	67%	64%	61%
Doctors 'Always' Communicated Well	300+	83%	83%	82%
Home Recovery Information Given	300+	88%	87%	85%
Hospital Given 9 or 10 on 10 Point Scale	300+	69%	71%	71%
Meds 'Always' Explained Before Given	300+	69%	65%	64%
Nurses 'Always' Communicated Well	300+	79%	81%	79%
Pain 'Always' Well Controlled	300+	70%	72%	71%
Room and Bathroom 'Always' Clean	300+	71%	72%	73%
Timely Help 'Always' Received	300+	67%	68%	68%
Would Definitely Recommend Hospital	300+	64%	70%	71%
Use of Medical Imaging				
Cardiac Imaging Stress Test before Surgery	102	3.9%	5.4%	5.3%
Combination Abdominal CT Scan	358	2.8%	5.6%	10.5%
Combination Brain/Sinus CT Scan	585	2.6%	2.6%	2.7%
Combination Chest CT Scan	176	0.0%	1.3%	2.7%
Follow-up Mammogram/Ultrasound	595	8.1%	8%	8.8%
Lumbar Spine MRI for Low Back Pain[1]	-	-	34.7%	37.2%

Kings Mountain Hospital

706 W King St
Kings Mountain, NC 28086
Type: Acute Care Hospitals
Ownership: Govt - Hospital Dist/Auth
Phone: 704-739-3601
Fax: 704-739-0800
Emergency Services: Yes
Beds: 102

Key Personnel:
Operating Room. . . . . Jama Hammond, RN
Quality Assurance . . . . Nadine Harris
Chief of Medical Staff . . . . Austin Osemeka, MD
Emergency Room . . . . Lisa Rice
Anesthesiology. . . . . Gene Tom, MD
CEO/President. . . . . John Young

Measure	Cases	This Hosp.	State Avg.	U.S. Avg.
Blood Clot Prevention and Treatment				
Anticoagulation Overlap Therapy[1,2]	-	-	94%	93%
ICU Venous Thromboembolism Prophylaxis[2]	61	93%	93%	92%
Incidence of Potentially Preventable VTE[1,2]	-	-	10%	10%
UFH with Dosages/Platelet Monitoring[1,2]	-	-	95%	97%
Venous Thromboembolism Prophylaxis[2]	129	79%	88%	85%
Warfarin Therapy Discharge Instructions[1,2]	-	-	81%	75%
Chest Pain/Possible Heart Attack Care				
Aspirin Given Within 24 Hours of Arrival	53	96%	97%	96%
Fibrinolytic Meds Within 30 Min. of Arrival[7]	-	-	66%	58%
Average Time to ECG (minutes)	54	7	7	7
Average Time to Transfer (minutes)[1]	-	-	45	60
Children's Asthma Care				
Received Home Management Plan of Care	-	-	89%	88%
Received Reliever Medication	-	-	100%	100%
Received Systemic Corticosteroids	-	-	100%	100%
Emergency Department				
Admittance Decision Time (minutes)[2]	429	75	107	98
Head CT Results Within 45 Min. of Arrival[1]	-	-	60%	57%
Patients Who Left ER Before Being Seen	30,439	2%	3%	2%
Time from ER Arrival to Admit. (minutes)[2]	435	215	300	274
Time from ER Arrival to Discharge (minutes)	358	114	152	134
Time in ER Before Being Evaluated (minutes)	323	23	34	26
Time to Pain Meds for Fractures (minutes)	65	76	67	57
Heart Attack Care				
Aspirin Given at Discharge[1]	-	-	100%	99%
Fibrinolytic Meds Within 30 Min. of Arrival[7]	-	-	75%	54%
PCI Within 90 Minutes of Arrival[7]	-	-	98%	96%
Statin Prescribed at Discharge[1]	-	-	99%	98%
Heart Failure Care				
ACE Inhibitor or ARB for LVSD	12	92%	98%	97%
Discharge Instructions Given	54	96%	96%	94%
Evaluation of LVS Function	65	100%	100%	99%
Medicare Spending				
Medicare Spending per Patient (ratio)	-	0.88	0.94	0.98
Pneumonia Care				
Appropriate Initial Antibiotic Given	44	95%	97%	95%
Blood Culture Timing	53	100%	98%	98%
Pregnancy and Delivery Care				
Newborn Deliveries Scheduled Early[7]	-	-	3%	6%
Preventive Care				
Immunization for Influenza[2]	298	95%	93%	90%
Immunization for Pneumonia[2]	445	98%	94%	92%
Stroke Care				
Anticoagulation Therapy for Atrial Fibrillation[1]	-	-	95%	95%
Antithrombotic Therapy Timing	26	92%	98%	98%
Assessed for Rehabilitation	29	100%	98%	97%
Discharged on Antithrombotic Therapy	28	82%	99%	99%
Discharged on Statin Medication	26	62%	94%	94%
Thrombolytic Therapy Timing[1]	-	-	64%	66%
Venous Thromboembolism Prophylaxis	24	79%	96%	94%
Written Stroke Educational Materials Given	18	61%	88%	88%
Surgical Care Improvement Project				
Appropriate Beta Blocker Usage[1]	-	-	99%	98%
Appropriate VTP Within 24 Hours	30	93%	99%	98%
Controlled Postoperative Blood Glucose[7]	-	-	98%	97%
Perioperative Temperature Management	33	100%	100%	100%
Prophylactic Antibiotic Selection[1]	-	-	99%	99%
Prophylactic Antibiotic Selection (Outpatient)[1,3]	-	-	98%	98%
Prophylactic Antibiotic Stopped[1]	-	-	99%	98%
Prophylactic Antibiotic Timing[1]	-	-	99%	99%
Prophylactic Antibiotic Timing (Outpatient)[1,3]	-	-	99%	98%
Urinary Catheter Removal	15	100%	99%	97%
Survey of Patients' Hospital Experiences				
Area Around Room 'Always' Quiet at Night	300+	68%	64%	61%
Doctors 'Always' Communicated Well	300+	87%	83%	82%
Home Recovery Information Given	300+	88%	87%	85%
Hospital Given 9 or 10 on 10 Point Scale	300+	76%	71%	71%
Meds 'Always' Explained Before Given	300+	69%	65%	64%
Nurses 'Always' Communicated Well	300+	83%	81%	79%
Pain 'Always' Well Controlled	300+	70%	72%	71%
Room and Bathroom 'Always' Clean	300+	72%	72%	73%
Timely Help 'Always' Received	300+	73%	68%	68%
Would Definitely Recommend Hospital	300+	75%	70%	71%
Use of Medical Imaging				
Cardiac Imaging Stress Test before Surgery	115	5.2%	5.4%	5.3%
Combination Abdominal CT Scan	200	21.5%	5.6%	10.5%
Combination Brain/Sinus CT Scan	243	0.4%	2.6%	2.7%
Combination Chest CT Scan	72	0.0%	1.3%	2.7%
Follow-up Mammogram/Ultrasound	350	13.1%	8%	8.8%
Lumbar Spine MRI for Low Back Pain	36	47.2%	34.7%	37.2%

NOTE: Hospital profiles are in alphabetical order by state, then city, then hospital within the city; Rankings exclude hospitals with less than 25 cases except for patient surveys which excludes hospitals with less than 100 cases; (a) 100-299 cases; (1) The number of cases/patients is too few to report; (2) Data submitted were based on a sample of cases/patients; (3) Results are based on a shorter time period than required; (4) Data suppressed by CMS for one or more quarters; (5) Results are not available for this reporting period; (6) Fewer than 100 patients completed the HCAHPS survey; (7) No cases met the criteria for this measure; (8) The lower limit of the confidence interval cannot be calculated if the number of observed infections equals zero; (9) No data are available from the state/territory for this reporting period; (10) The scores shown reflect fewer than 50 completed surveys; (11) There were discrepancies in the data collection process; (12) This measure does not apply to this hospital for this reporting period; (13) Results cannot be calculated for this reporting period; (14) The results for this state are combined with nearby states to protect confidentiality; Please refer to the User's Guide for a full explanation of data.

Lenoir Memorial Hospital

100 Airport Rd
Kinston, NC 28501
Phone: 252-522-7000
Fax: 252-522-7007
E-mail: hr@lenoir.org
URL: www.lenoirmemorial.org
Type: Acute Care Hospitals
Emergency Services: Yes
Ownership: Voluntary non-profit - Private
Beds: 261

Key Personnel:
Coronary Care . . . . Jessica Baker, RN
CEO/President. . . . . Gary E Black
Radiology. . . . . Jeff Cartwright
Quality Assurance . . . . Donna Floyd
Pediatric In-Patient Care . . . . Nanci Hood, RN
Chief of Medical Staff. . . . . Donald Riddle, MD
Infection Control. . . . . Jody Robbins, RN
Operating Room. . . . . Gisela Stroud

Measure	Cases	This Hosp.	State Avg.	U.S. Avg.
Blood Clot Prevention and Treatment				
Anticoagulation Overlap Therapy[2]	68	90%	94%	93%
ICU Venous Thromboembolism Prophylaxis[2]	79	80%	93%	92%
Incidence of Potentially Preventable VTE[1,2]	-	-	10%	10%
UFH with Dosages/Platelet Monitoring[2]	37	100%	95%	97%
Venous Thromboembolism Prophylaxis[2]	384	61%	88%	85%
Warfarin Therapy Discharge Instructions[2]	46	59%	81%	75%
Chest Pain/Possible Heart Attack Care				
Aspirin Given Within 24 Hours of Arrival	64	94%	97%	96%
Fibrinolytic Meds Within 30 Min. of Arrival[1]	-	-	66%	58%
Average Time to ECG (minutes)	67	3	7	7
Average Time to Transfer (minutes)[1]	-	-	45	60
Children's Asthma Care				
Received Home Management Plan of Care	-	-	89%	88%
Received Reliever Medication	-	-	100%	100%
Received Systemic Corticosteroids	-	-	100%	100%
Emergency Department				
Admittance Decision Time (minutes)[2]	813	134	107	98
Head CT Results Within 45 Min. of Arrival	11	36%	60%	57%
Patients Who Left ER Before Being Seen	>100k	3%	3%	2%
Time from ER Arrival to Admit. (minutes)[2]	816	354	300	274
Time from ER Arrival to Discharge (minutes)	567	185	152	134
Time in ER Before Being Evaluated (minutes)	601	59	34	26
Time to Pain Meds for Fractures (minutes)	174	96	67	57
Heart Attack Care				
Aspirin Given at Discharge	69	97%	100%	99%
Fibrinolytic Meds Within 30 Min. of Arrival[7]	-	-	75%	54%
PCI Within 90 Minutes of Arrival[7]	-	-	98%	96%
Statin Prescribed at Discharge	68	90%	99%	98%
Heart Failure Care				
ACE Inhibitor or ARB for LVSD	53	94%	98%	97%
Discharge Instructions Given	293	94%	96%	94%
Evaluation of LVS Function	343	100%	100%	99%
Medicare Spending				
Medicare Spending per Patient (ratio)	-	0.95	0.94	0.98
Pneumonia Care				
Appropriate Initial Antibiotic Given	126	94%	97%	95%
Blood Culture Timing	184	96%	98%	98%
Pregnancy and Delivery Care				
Newborn Deliveries Scheduled Early	79	1%	3%	6%
Preventive Care				
Immunization for Influenza[2]	545	84%	93%	90%
Immunization for Pneumonia[2]	738	95%	94%	92%
Stroke Care				
Anticoagulation Therapy for Atrial Fibrillation[1]	-	-	95%	95%
Antithrombotic Therapy Timing	66	98%	98%	98%
Assessed for Rehabilitation	61	92%	98%	97%
Discharged on Antithrombotic Therapy	57	100%	99%	99%
Discharged on Statin Medication	50	72%	94%	94%
Thrombolytic Therapy Timing[1]	-	-	64%	66%
Venous Thromboembolism Prophylaxis	67	75%	96%	94%
Written Stroke Educational Materials Given	42	14%	88%	88%
Surgical Care Improvement Project				
Appropriate Beta Blocker Usage	73	99%	99%	98%
Appropriate VTP Within 24 Hours	220	97%	99%	98%
Controlled Postoperative Blood Glucose[7]	-	-	98%	97%
Perioperative Temperature Management	250	100%	100%	100%
Prophylactic Antibiotic Selection	158	95%	99%	99%
Prophylactic Antibiotic Selection (Outpatient)	84	93%	98%	98%
Prophylactic Antibiotic Stopped	151	95%	99%	98%
Prophylactic Antibiotic Timing	158	99%	99%	99%
Prophylactic Antibiotic Timing (Outpatient)	85	99%	99%	98%
Urinary Catheter Removal	84	89%	99%	97%
Survey of Patients' Hospital Experiences				
Area Around Room 'Always' Quiet at Night	300+	55%	64%	61%
Doctors 'Always' Communicated Well	300+	78%	83%	82%
Home Recovery Information Given	300+	84%	87%	85%
Hospital Given 9 or 10 on 10 Point Scale	300+	60%	71%	71%
Meds 'Always' Explained Before Given	300+	62%	65%	64%
Nurses 'Always' Communicated Well	300+	77%	81%	79%
Pain 'Always' Well Controlled	300+	67%	72%	71%
Room and Bathroom 'Always' Clean	300+	68%	72%	73%
Timely Help 'Always' Received	300+	60%	68%	68%
Would Definitely Recommend Hospital	300+	57%	70%	71%
Use of Medical Imaging				
Cardiac Imaging Stress Test before Surgery	112	8.9%	5.4%	5.3%
Combination Abdominal CT Scan	646	2.3%	5.6%	10.5%
Combination Brain/Sinus CT Scan	977	3.2%	2.6%	2.7%
Combination Chest CT Scan	322	0.0%	1.3%	2.7%
Follow-up Mammogram/Ultrasound[7]	-	-	8%	8.8%
Lumbar Spine MRI for Low Back Pain	158	36.7%	34.7%	37.2%

Scotland Memorial Hospital

500 Lauchwood Dr
Laurinburg, NC 28352
Phone: 910-291-7000
Fax: 910-291-7499
URL: www.scotlandhealth.org
Type: Acute Care Hospitals
Emergency Services: Yes
Ownership: Voluntary non-profit - Private
Beds: 154

Key Personnel:
Operating Room. . . . . Patricia Decker
Quality Assurance . . . . Lori Dove, RN
Pediatric Ambulatory Care . . . . . . Laura Gailey
Patient Relations . . . . Ronnie Norton
Chief of Medical Staff. . . . . Donna Richardson, MD
Radiology. . . . . Zim Townsend
Hemotology Center . . . . Camille Utter, RN
CEO/President. . . . . Greg Wood

Measure	Cases	This Hosp.	State Avg.	U.S. Avg.
Blood Clot Prevention and Treatment				
Anticoagulation Overlap Therapy[2]	36	94%	94%	93%
ICU Venous Thromboembolism Prophylaxis[2]	45	98%	93%	92%
Incidence of Potentially Preventable VTE[1,2]	-	-	10%	10%
UFH with Dosages/Platelet Monitoring[1,2]	-	-	95%	97%
Venous Thromboembolism Prophylaxis[2]	364	89%	88%	85%
Warfarin Therapy Discharge Instructions[2]	30	97%	81%	75%
Chest Pain/Possible Heart Attack Care				
Aspirin Given Within 24 Hours of Arrival	28	100%	97%	96%
Fibrinolytic Meds Within 30 Min. of Arrival[7]	-	-	66%	58%
Average Time to ECG (minutes)	29	8	7	7
Average Time to Transfer (minutes)	18	35	45	60
Children's Asthma Care				
Received Home Management Plan of Care	-	-	89%	88%
Received Reliever Medication	-	-	100%	100%
Received Systemic Corticosteroids	-	-	100%	100%
Emergency Department				
Admittance Decision Time (minutes)[2]	688	132	107	98
Head CT Results Within 45 Min. of Arrival[1]	-	-	60%	57%
Patients Who Left ER Before Being Seen	45,809	1%	3%	2%
Time from ER Arrival to Admit. (minutes)[2]	692	286	300	274
Time from ER Arrival to Discharge (minutes)	438	129	152	134
Time in ER Before Being Evaluated (minutes)	462	56	34	26
Time to Pain Meds for Fractures (minutes)	131	71	67	57
Heart Attack Care				
Aspirin Given at Discharge	39	100%	100%	99%
Fibrinolytic Meds Within 30 Min. of Arrival[7]	-	-	75%	54%
PCI Within 90 Minutes of Arrival[7]	-	-	98%	96%
Statin Prescribed at Discharge	40	95%	99%	98%
Heart Failure Care				
ACE Inhibitor or ARB for LVSD	82	99%	98%	97%
Discharge Instructions Given	272	96%	96%	94%
Evaluation of LVS Function	307	100%	100%	99%
Medicare Spending				
Medicare Spending per Patient (ratio)	-	0.87	0.94	0.98
Pneumonia Care				
Appropriate Initial Antibiotic Given	138	98%	97%	95%
Blood Culture Timing	214	99%	98%	98%
Pregnancy and Delivery Care				
Newborn Deliveries Scheduled Early[2]	37	5%	3%	6%
Preventive Care				
Immunization for Influenza[2]	559	94%	93%	90%
Immunization for Pneumonia[2]	703	97%	94%	92%
Stroke Care				
Anticoagulation Therapy for Atrial Fibrillation[1]	-	-	95%	95%
Antithrombotic Therapy Timing	66	97%	98%	98%
Assessed for Rehabilitation	63	95%	98%	97%
Discharged on Antithrombotic Therapy	62	100%	99%	99%
Discharged on Statin Medication	52	98%	94%	94%
Thrombolytic Therapy Timing[1]	-	-	64%	66%
Venous Thromboembolism Prophylaxis	63	97%	96%	94%
Written Stroke Educational Materials Given	41	100%	88%	88%
Surgical Care Improvement Project				
Appropriate Beta Blocker Usage	90	94%	99%	98%
Appropriate VTP Within 24 Hours	360	99%	99%	98%
Controlled Postoperative Blood Glucose[7]	-	-	98%	97%
Perioperative Temperature Management	376	100%	100%	100%
Prophylactic Antibiotic Selection	257	100%	99%	99%
Prophylactic Antibiotic Selection (Outpatient)	35	94%	98%	98%
Prophylactic Antibiotic Stopped	237	99%	99%	98%
Prophylactic Antibiotic Timing	257	99%	99%	99%
Prophylactic Antibiotic Timing (Outpatient)	35	100%	99%	98%
Urinary Catheter Removal	285	99%	99%	97%
Survey of Patients' Hospital Experiences				
Area Around Room 'Always' Quiet at Night	300+	70%	64%	61%
Doctors 'Always' Communicated Well	300+	84%	83%	82%
Home Recovery Information Given	300+	87%	87%	85%
Hospital Given 9 or 10 on 10 Point Scale	300+	72%	71%	71%
Meds 'Always' Explained Before Given	300+	68%	65%	64%
Nurses 'Always' Communicated Well	300+	83%	81%	79%
Pain 'Always' Well Controlled	300+	76%	72%	71%
Room and Bathroom 'Always' Clean	300+	78%	72%	73%
Timely Help 'Always' Received	300+	70%	68%	68%
Would Definitely Recommend Hospital	300+	69%	70%	71%
Use of Medical Imaging				
Cardiac Imaging Stress Test before Surgery	50	0.0%	5.4%	5.3%
Combination Abdominal CT Scan	1,231	8.0%	5.6%	10.5%
Combination Brain/Sinus CT Scan	954	1.2%	2.6%	2.7%
Combination Chest CT Scan	465	4.1%	1.3%	2.7%
Follow-up Mammogram/Ultrasound	1,595	4.4%	8%	8.8%
Lumbar Spine MRI for Low Back Pain	141	29.8%	34.7%	37.2%

Caldwell Memorial Hospital

321 Mulberry Saint Sw
Lenoir, NC 28645
Phone: 828-757-5100
Fax: 828-757-5512
E-mail: lsmith@caldwell_mem.org
URL: www.caldwellmemorial.org
Type: Acute Care Hospitals
Emergency Services: Yes
Ownership: Voluntary non-profit - Other
Beds: 110

Key Personnel:
President/CEO. . . . . Laura Easton, RN, MSN
Infection Control. . . . . Patricia Hicks, RN
Radiology. . . . . Ed Pearce, RRT
Operating Room. . . . . Thomas A Pezzi, RN
Chief of Medical Staff. . . . . John D Powell
Quality Assurance . . . . Kathy Proffitt

Measure	Cases	This Hosp.	State Avg.	U.S. Avg.
Blood Clot Prevention and Treatment				
Anticoagulation Overlap Therapy[2]	39	95%	94%	93%
ICU Venous Thromboembolism Prophylaxis[2]	110	93%	93%	92%
Incidence of Potentially Preventable VTE[2]	12	33%	10%	10%
UFH with Dosages/Platelet Monitoring[2]	43	47%	95%	97%
Venous Thromboembolism Prophylaxis[2]	246	93%	88%	85%
Warfarin Therapy Discharge Instructions[2]	24	88%	81%	75%
Chest Pain/Possible Heart Attack Care				
Aspirin Given Within 24 Hours of Arrival	75	100%	97%	96%
Fibrinolytic Meds Within 30 Min. of Arrival[7]	-	-	66%	58%

NOTE: Hospital profiles are in alphabetical order by state, then city, then hospital within the city; Rankings exclude hospitals with less than 25 cases except for patient surveys which excludes hospitals with less than 100 cases; (a) 100-299 cases; (1) The number of cases/patients is too few to report; (2) Data submitted were based on a sample of cases/patients; (3) Results are based on a shorter time period than required; (4) Data suppressed by CMS for one or more quarters; (5) Results are not available for this reporting period; (6) Fewer than 100 patients completed the HCAHPS survey; (7) No cases met the criteria for this measure; (8) The lower limit of the confidence interval cannot be calculated if the number of observed infections equals zero; (9) No data are available from the state/territory for this reporting period; (10) The scores shown reflect fewer than 50 completed surveys; (11) There were discrepancies in the data collection process; (12) This measure does not apply to this hospital for this reporting period; (13) Results cannot be calculated for this reporting period; (14) The results for this state are combined with nearby states to protect confidentiality; Please refer to the User's Guide for a full explanation of data.

Measure	Cases	This Hosp.	State Avg.	U.S. Avg.
Average Time to ECG (minutes)	78	8	7	7
Average Time to Transfer (minutes)	25	36	45	60
Children's Asthma Care				
Received Home Management Plan of Care	-	-	89%	88%
Received Reliever Medication	-	-	100%	100%
Received Systemic Corticosteroids	-	-	100%	100%
Emergency Department				
Admittance Decision Time (minutes)[2]	486	190	107	98
Head CT Results Within 45 Min. of Arrival	18	67%	60%	57%
Patients Who Left ER Before Being Seen	29,806	4%	3%	2%
Time from ER Arrival to Admit. (minutes)[2]	489	317	300	274
Time from ER Arrival to Discharge (minutes)	362	128	152	134
Time in ER Before Being Evaluated (minutes)	387	35	34	26
Time to Pain Meds for Fractures (minutes)	79	76	67	57
Heart Attack Care				
Aspirin Given at Discharge	15	100%	100%	99%
Fibrinolytic Meds Within 30 Min. of Arrival[7]	-	-	75%	54%
PCI Within 90 Minutes of Arrival[7]	-	-	98%	96%
Statin Prescribed at Discharge	12	100%	99%	98%
Heart Failure Care				
ACE Inhibitor or ARB for LVSD	11	100%	98%	97%
Discharge Instructions Given	48	98%	96%	94%
Evaluation of LVS Function	66	100%	100%	99%
Medicare Spending				
Medicare Spending per Patient (ratio)	-	1.03	0.94	0.98
Pneumonia Care				
Appropriate Initial Antibiotic Given	100	98%	97%	95%
Blood Culture Timing	209	100%	98%	98%
Pregnancy and Delivery Care				
Newborn Deliveries Scheduled Early[2]	47	0%	3%	6%
Preventive Care				
Immunization for Influenza[2]	341	97%	93%	90%
Immunization for Pneumonia[2]	468	99%	94%	92%
Stroke Care				
Anticoagulation Therapy for Atrial Fibrillation	13	69%	95%	95%
Antithrombotic Therapy Timing	50	92%	98%	98%
Assessed for Rehabilitation	44	98%	98%	97%
Discharged on Antithrombotic Therapy	44	98%	99%	99%
Discharged on Statin Medication	35	77%	94%	94%
Thrombolytic Therapy Timing[7]	-	-	64%	66%
Venous Thromboembolism Prophylaxis	50	94%	96%	94%
Written Stroke Educational Materials Given	18	0%	88%	88%
Surgical Care Improvement Project				
Appropriate Beta Blocker Usage	66	100%	99%	98%
Appropriate VTP Within 24 Hours	230	100%	99%	98%
Controlled Postoperative Blood Glucose[7]	-	-	98%	97%
Perioperative Temperature Management	270	100%	100%	100%
Prophylactic Antibiotic Selection	217	100%	99%	99%
Prophylactic Antibiotic Selection (Outpatient)	92	98%	98%	98%
Prophylactic Antibiotic Stopped	199	100%	99%	98%
Prophylactic Antibiotic Timing	219	100%	99%	99%
Prophylactic Antibiotic Timing (Outpatient)	93	98%	99%	98%
Urinary Catheter Removal	182	100%	99%	97%
Survey of Patients' Hospital Experiences				
Area Around Room 'Always' Quiet at Night	300+	60%	64%	61%
Doctors 'Always' Communicated Well	300+	85%	83%	82%
Home Recovery Information Given	300+	86%	87%	85%
Hospital Given 9 or 10 on 10 Point Scale	300+	64%	71%	71%
Meds 'Always' Explained Before Given	300+	61%	65%	64%
Nurses 'Always' Communicated Well	300+	75%	81%	79%
Pain 'Always' Well Controlled	300+	69%	72%	71%
Room and Bathroom 'Always' Clean	300+	72%	72%	73%
Timely Help 'Always' Received	300+	64%	68%	68%
Would Definitely Recommend Hospital	300+	61%	70%	71%
Use of Medical Imaging				
Cardiac Imaging Stress Test before Surgery	124	7.3%	5.4%	5.3%
Combination Abdominal CT Scan	509	0.8%	5.6%	10.5%
Combination Brain/Sinus CT Scan	574	2.1%	2.6%	2.7%
Combination Chest CT Scan	378	0.0%	1.3%	2.7%
Follow-up Mammogram/Ultrasound	1,150	13.0%	8%	8.8%
Lumbar Spine MRI for Low Back Pain[1]	-	-	34.7%	37.2%

Lexington Memorial Hospital

250 Hospital Drive PO Box 1817
Lexington, NC 27293
Phone: 336-248-5161
Fax: 336-248-4711
E-mail: info@lmh.cc
URL: www.lexingtonmemorial.com
Type: Acute Care Hospitals
Emergency Services: Yes
Ownership: Voluntary non-profit - Private
Beds: 94

Key Personnel:
Emergency Room . . . . Mark Bardou
Radiology. . . . . Ira E Bell, III
CEO/President. . . . . John Cashion
Coronary Care . . . . Kathryn A McFarland
Chief of Medical Staff . . . . Malin Sadler

Measure	Cases	This Hosp.	State Avg.	U.S. Avg.
Blood Clot Prevention and Treatment				
Anticoagulation Overlap Therapy[2]	15	80%	94%	93%
ICU Venous Thromboembolism Prophylaxis[2]	54	94%	93%	92%
Incidence of Potentially Preventable VTE[1,2]	-	-	10%	10%
UFH with Dosages/Platelet Monitoring[1,2]	-	-	95%	97%
Venous Thromboembolism Prophylaxis[2]	206	95%	88%	85%
Warfarin Therapy Discharge Instructions[2]	13	92%	81%	75%
Chest Pain/Possible Heart Attack Care				
Aspirin Given Within 24 Hours of Arrival	105	99%	97%	96%
Fibrinolytic Meds Within 30 Min. of Arrival[7]	-	-	66%	58%
Average Time to ECG (minutes)	104	11	7	7
Average Time to Transfer (minutes)	21	47	45	60
Children's Asthma Care				
Received Home Management Plan of Care	-	-	89%	88%
Received Reliever Medication	-	-	100%	100%
Received Systemic Corticosteroids	-	-	100%	100%
Emergency Department				
Admittance Decision Time (minutes)[2]	69	71	107	98
Head CT Results Within 45 Min. of Arrival	14	86%	60%	57%
Patients Who Left ER Before Being Seen	37,800	4%	3%	2%
Time from ER Arrival to Admit. (minutes)[2]	396	257	300	274
Time from ER Arrival to Discharge (minutes)	328	138	152	134
Time in ER Before Being Evaluated (minutes)	294	53	34	26
Time to Pain Meds for Fractures (minutes)	117	67	67	57
Heart Attack Care				
Aspirin Given at Discharge	14	100%	100%	99%
Fibrinolytic Meds Within 30 Min. of Arrival[7]	-	-	75%	54%
PCI Within 90 Minutes of Arrival[7]	-	-	98%	96%
Statin Prescribed at Discharge	13	100%	99%	98%
Heart Failure Care				
ACE Inhibitor or ARB for LVSD	31	100%	98%	97%
Discharge Instructions Given	94	90%	96%	94%
Evaluation of LVS Function	118	99%	100%	99%
Medicare Spending				
Medicare Spending per Patient (ratio)	-	0.92	0.94	0.98
Pneumonia Care				
Appropriate Initial Antibiotic Given	123	99%	97%	95%
Blood Culture Timing	221	98%	98%	98%
Pregnancy and Delivery Care				
Newborn Deliveries Scheduled Early[2]	72	15%	3%	6%
Preventive Care				
Immunization for Influenza[2]	343	94%	93%	90%
Immunization for Pneumonia[2]	421	94%	94%	92%
Stroke Care				
Anticoagulation Therapy for Atrial Fibrillation[1]	-	-	95%	95%
Antithrombotic Therapy Timing	62	97%	98%	98%
Assessed for Rehabilitation	70	96%	98%	97%
Discharged on Antithrombotic Therapy	68	100%	99%	99%
Discharged on Statin Medication	55	95%	94%	94%
Thrombolytic Therapy Timing[7]	-	-	64%	66%
Venous Thromboembolism Prophylaxis	56	93%	96%	94%
Written Stroke Educational Materials Given	40	90%	88%	88%
Surgical Care Improvement Project				
Appropriate Beta Blocker Usage	65	98%	99%	98%
Appropriate VTP Within 24 Hours	241	97%	99%	98%
Controlled Postoperative Blood Glucose[7]	-	-	98%	97%
Perioperative Temperature Management	251	98%	100%	100%
Prophylactic Antibiotic Selection	200	98%	99%	99%
Prophylactic Antibiotic Selection (Outpatient)	83	100%	98%	98%
Prophylactic Antibiotic Stopped	194	97%	99%	98%
Prophylactic Antibiotic Timing	200	97%	99%	99%
Prophylactic Antibiotic Timing (Outpatient)	84	99%	99%	98%
Urinary Catheter Removal	204	97%	99%	97%
Survey of Patients' Hospital Experiences				
Area Around Room 'Always' Quiet at Night	300+	55%	64%	61%
Doctors 'Always' Communicated Well	300+	80%	83%	82%
Home Recovery Information Given	300+	82%	87%	85%
Hospital Given 9 or 10 on 10 Point Scale	300+	59%	71%	71%
Meds 'Always' Explained Before Given	300+	59%	65%	64%
Nurses 'Always' Communicated Well	300+	74%	81%	79%
Pain 'Always' Well Controlled	300+	69%	72%	71%
Room and Bathroom 'Always' Clean	300+	71%	72%	73%
Timely Help 'Always' Received	300+	60%	68%	68%
Would Definitely Recommend Hospital	300+	59%	70%	71%
Use of Medical Imaging				
Cardiac Imaging Stress Test before Surgery	149	6.7%	5.4%	5.3%
Combination Abdominal CT Scan	493	2.8%	5.6%	10.5%
Combination Brain/Sinus CT Scan[1]	-	-	2.6%	2.7%
Combination Chest CT Scan	266	0.4%	1.3%	2.7%
Follow-up Mammogram/Ultrasound	794	10.1%	8%	8.8%
Lumbar Spine MRI for Low Back Pain	87	37.9%	34.7%	37.2%

Carolinas Medical Center - Lincoln

433 Mcalister Rd
Lincolnton, NC 28092
Phone: 980-212-2000
Fax: 704-732-5494
URL: www.lincolnmedical.org
Type: Acute Care Hospitals
Emergency Services: Yes
Ownership: Govt - Hospital Dist/Auth
Beds: 87

Key Personnel:
CEO/President. . . . . Peter W Acker
Radiology. . . . . Deborah Agisim
Operating Room. . . . . William Beutel, RN
Infection Control. . . . . Suzanne Gazzaway, RN
Quality Assurance . . . . Beth King
Intensive Care Unit. . . . . Anne Parker, RN
Emergency Room . . . . V Washington, MD
Chief of Medical Staff . . . . Larry Weems, MD

Measure	Cases	This Hosp.	State Avg.	U.S. Avg.
Blood Clot Prevention and Treatment				
Anticoagulation Overlap Therapy[2]	36	94%	94%	93%
ICU Venous Thromboembolism Prophylaxis[2]	114	98%	93%	92%
Incidence of Potentially Preventable VTE[1,2]	-	-	10%	10%
UFH with Dosages/Platelet Monitoring[2]	22	95%	95%	97%
Venous Thromboembolism Prophylaxis[2]	249	94%	88%	85%
Warfarin Therapy Discharge Instructions[2]	29	76%	81%	75%
Chest Pain/Possible Heart Attack Care				
Aspirin Given Within 24 Hours of Arrival	136	99%	97%	96%
Fibrinolytic Meds Within 30 Min. of Arrival[7]	-	-	66%	58%
Average Time to ECG (minutes)	138	4	7	7
Average Time to Transfer (minutes)	26	48	45	60
Children's Asthma Care				
Received Home Management Plan of Care	-	-	89%	88%
Received Reliever Medication	-	-	100%	100%
Received Systemic Corticosteroids	-	-	100%	100%
Emergency Department				
Admittance Decision Time (minutes)[2]	441	78	107	98
Head CT Results Within 45 Min. of Arrival[1]	-	-	60%	57%
Patients Who Left ER Before Being Seen	47,931	2%	3%	2%
Time from ER Arrival to Admit. (minutes)[2]	446	243	300	274
Time from ER Arrival to Discharge (minutes)	344	162	152	134
Time in ER Before Being Evaluated (minutes)	377	60	34	26
Time to Pain Meds for Fractures (minutes)	165	77	67	57
Heart Attack Care				
Aspirin Given at Discharge[1]	-	-	100%	99%
Fibrinolytic Meds Within 30 Min. of Arrival[7]	-	-	75%	54%
PCI Within 90 Minutes of Arrival[7]	-	-	98%	96%
Statin Prescribed at Discharge[1]	-	-	99%	98%
Heart Failure Care				
ACE Inhibitor or ARB for LVSD	31	100%	98%	97%
Discharge Instructions Given	124	99%	96%	94%
Evaluation of LVS Function	155	99%	100%	99%
Medicare Spending				
Medicare Spending per Patient (ratio)	-	1.00	0.94	0.98
Pneumonia Care				

NOTE: Hospital profiles are in alphabetical order by state, then city, then hospital within the city; Rankings exclude hospitals with less than 25 cases except for patient surveys which excludes hospitals with less than 100 cases; (a) 100-299 cases; (1) The number of cases/patients is too few to report; (2) Data submitted were based on a sample of cases/patients; (3) Results are based on a shorter time period than required; (4) Data suppressed by CMS for one or more quarters; (5) Results are not available for this reporting period; (6) Fewer than 100 patients completed the HCAHPS survey; (7) No cases met the criteria for this measure; (8) The lower limit of the confidence interval cannot be calculated if the number of observed infections equals zero; (9) No data are available from the state/territory for this reporting period; (10) The scores shown reflect fewer than 50 completed surveys; (11) There were discrepancies in the data collection process; (12) This measure does not apply to this hospital for this reporting period; (13) Results cannot be calculated for this reporting period; (14) The results for this state are combined with nearby states to protect confidentiality; Please refer to the User's Guide for a full explanation of data.

Measure	Cases	This Hosp.	State Avg.	U.S. Avg.
Appropriate Initial Antibiotic Given	186	96%	97%	95%
Blood Culture Timing	256	98%	98%	98%
Pregnancy and Delivery Care				
Newborn Deliveries Scheduled Early	33	0%	3%	6%
Preventive Care				
Immunization for Influenza[2]	371	95%	93%	90%
Immunization for Pneumonia[2]	482	95%	94%	92%
Stroke Care				
Anticoagulation Therapy for Atrial Fibrillation[1]	-	-	95%	95%
Antithrombotic Therapy Timing	46	100%	98%	98%
Assessed for Rehabilitation	48	98%	98%	97%
Discharged on Antithrombotic Therapy	48	96%	99%	99%
Discharged on Statin Medication	39	95%	94%	94%
Thrombolytic Therapy Timing[7]	-	-	64%	66%
Venous Thromboembolism Prophylaxis	40	100%	96%	94%
Written Stroke Educational Materials Given	35	89%	88%	88%
Surgical Care Improvement Project				
Appropriate Beta Blocker Usage	70	99%	99%	98%
Appropriate VTP Within 24 Hours	202	99%	99%	98%
Controlled Postoperative Blood Glucose[7]	-	-	98%	97%
Perioperative Temperature Management	218	100%	100%	100%
Prophylactic Antibiotic Selection	142	99%	99%	99%
Prophylactic Antibiotic Selection (Outpatient)	31	97%	98%	98%
Prophylactic Antibiotic Stopped	126	98%	99%	98%
Prophylactic Antibiotic Timing	142	100%	99%	99%
Prophylactic Antibiotic Timing (Outpatient)	32	91%	99%	98%
Urinary Catheter Removal	92	100%	99%	97%
Survey of Patients' Hospital Experiences				
Area Around Room 'Always' Quiet at Night	300+	75%	64%	61%
Doctors 'Always' Communicated Well	300+	84%	83%	82%
Home Recovery Information Given	300+	90%	87%	85%
Hospital Given 9 or 10 on 10 Point Scale	300+	82%	71%	71%
Meds 'Always' Explained Before Given	300+	70%	65%	64%
Nurses 'Always' Communicated Well	300+	85%	81%	79%
Pain 'Always' Well Controlled	300+	75%	72%	71%
Room and Bathroom 'Always' Clean	300+	77%	72%	73%
Timely Help 'Always' Received	300+	74%	68%	68%
Would Definitely Recommend Hospital	300+	78%	70%	71%
Use of Medical Imaging				
Cardiac Imaging Stress Test before Surgery	435	4.8%	5.4%	5.3%
Combination Abdominal CT Scan	793	2.4%	5.6%	10.5%
Combination Brain/Sinus CT Scan	830	5.1%	2.6%	2.7%
Combination Chest CT Scan	344	0.9%	1.3%	2.7%
Follow-up Mammogram/Ultrasound	970	9.4%	8%	8.8%
Lumbar Spine MRI for Low Back Pain	93	41.9%	34.7%	37.2%

Charles A Cannon Jr Memorial Hospital

434 Hospital Drive
Linville, NC 28646
Phone: 828-737-7000
Fax: 828-737-7491
URL: www.cannonmh.org
Type: Critical Access Hospitals
Emergency Services: Yes
Ownership: Voluntary non-profit - Private
Beds: 70

Key Personnel:
Chief of Medical Staff.......... Thomas Haizlip Jr, MD
Infection Control.............. Elizabeth Kress
Operating Room.............. Elizabeth Kress, RN
Quality Assurance .... Carmen Lacey
CEO/President............... Chuck Montooth
Emergency Room .... Terri Yoder
Intensive Care Unit............ Terri Yoder

Measure	Cases	This Hosp.	State Avg.	U.S. Avg.
Blood Clot Prevention and Treatment				
Anticoagulation Overlap Therapy[5]	-	-	94%	93%
ICU Venous Thromboembolism Prophylaxis[5]	-	-	93%	92%
Incidence of Potentially Preventable VTE[5]	-	-	10%	10%
UFH with Dosages/Platelet Monitoring[5]	-	-	95%	97%
Venous Thromboembolism Prophylaxis[5]	-	-	88%	85%
Warfarin Therapy Discharge Instructions[5]	-	-	81%	75%
Chest Pain/Possible Heart Attack Care				
Aspirin Given Within 24 Hours of Arrival	-	-	97%	96%
Fibrinolytic Meds Within 30 Min. of Arrival	-	-	66%	58%
Average Time to ECG (minutes)	-	-	7	7
Average Time to Transfer (minutes)	-	-	45	60
Children's Asthma Care				
Received Home Management Plan of Care	-	-	89%	88%
Received Reliever Medication	-	-	100%	100%
Received Systemic Corticosteroids	-	-	100%	100%
Emergency Department				
Admittance Decision Time (minutes)[5]	-	-	107	98
Head CT Results Within 45 Min. of Arrival	-	-	60%	57%
Patients Who Left ER Before Being Seen	-	-	3%	2%
Time from ER Arrival to Admit. (minutes)[5]	-	-	300	274
Time from ER Arrival to Discharge (minutes)	-	-	152	134
Time in ER Before Being Evaluated (minutes)	-	-	34	26
Time to Pain Meds for Fractures (minutes)	-	-	67	57
Heart Attack Care				
Aspirin Given at Discharge[5]	-	-	100%	99%
Fibrinolytic Meds Within 30 Min. of Arrival[5]	-	-	75%	54%
PCI Within 90 Minutes of Arrival[5]	-	-	98%	96%
Statin Prescribed at Discharge[5]	-	-	99%	98%
Heart Failure Care				
ACE Inhibitor or ARB for LVSD[1]	-	-	98%	97%
Discharge Instructions Given	27	100%	96%	94%
Evaluation of LVS Function	46	100%	100%	99%
Medicare Spending				
Medicare Spending per Patient (ratio)	-	-	0.94	0.98
Pneumonia Care				
Appropriate Initial Antibiotic Given	39	87%	97%	95%
Blood Culture Timing	44	93%	98%	98%
Pregnancy and Delivery Care				
Newborn Deliveries Scheduled Early[5]	-	-	3%	6%
Preventive Care				
Immunization for Influenza[5]	-	-	93%	90%
Immunization for Pneumonia[5]	-	-	94%	92%
Stroke Care				
Anticoagulation Therapy for Atrial Fibrillation[5]	-	-	95%	95%
Antithrombotic Therapy Timing[5]	-	-	98%	98%
Assessed for Rehabilitation[5]	-	-	98%	97%
Discharged on Antithrombotic Therapy[5]	-	-	99%	99%
Discharged on Statin Medication[5]	-	-	94%	94%
Thrombolytic Therapy Timing[5]	-	-	64%	66%
Venous Thromboembolism Prophylaxis[5]	-	-	96%	94%
Written Stroke Educational Materials Given[5]	-	-	88%	88%
Surgical Care Improvement Project				
Appropriate Beta Blocker Usage[5]	-	-	99%	98%
Appropriate VTP Within 24 Hours[5]	-	-	99%	98%
Controlled Postoperative Blood Glucose[5]	-	-	98%	97%
Perioperative Temperature Management[5]	-	-	100%	100%
Prophylactic Antibiotic Selection[5]	-	-	99%	99%
Prophylactic Antibiotic Selection (Outpatient)	-	-	98%	98%
Prophylactic Antibiotic Stopped[5]	-	-	99%	98%
Prophylactic Antibiotic Timing[5]	-	-	99%	99%
Prophylactic Antibiotic Timing (Outpatient)	-	-	99%	98%
Urinary Catheter Removal[5]	-	-	99%	97%
Survey of Patients' Hospital Experiences				
Area Around Room 'Always' Quiet at Night[5]	-	-	64%	61%
Doctors 'Always' Communicated Well[5]	-	-	83%	82%
Home Recovery Information Given[5]	-	-	87%	85%
Hospital Given 9 or 10 on 10 Point Scale[5]	-	-	71%	71%
Meds 'Always' Explained Before Given[5]	-	-	65%	64%
Nurses 'Always' Communicated Well[5]	-	-	81%	79%
Pain 'Always' Well Controlled[5]	-	-	72%	71%
Room and Bathroom 'Always' Clean[5]	-	-	72%	73%
Timely Help 'Always' Received[5]	-	-	68%	68%
Would Definitely Recommend Hospital[5]	-	-	70%	71%
Use of Medical Imaging				
Cardiac Imaging Stress Test before Surgery	-	-	5.4%	5.3%
Combination Abdominal CT Scan	-	-	5.6%	10.5%
Combination Brain/Sinus CT Scan	-	-	2.6%	2.7%
Combination Chest CT Scan	-	-	1.3%	2.7%
Follow-up Mammogram/Ultrasound	-	-	8%	8.8%
Lumbar Spine MRI for Low Back Pain	-	-	34.7%	37.2%

Novant Health Franklin Medical Center

100 Hospital Dr Box 609
Louisburg, NC 27549
Phone: 919-496-5131
Fax: 919-497-8018
URL: www.franklinregionalmedicalctr.com
Type: Acute Care Hospitals
Emergency Services: Yes
Ownership: Voluntary non-profit - Private
Beds: 85

Key Personnel:
Infection Control.............. Betty Bernette
Quality Assurance .... Betty Bernette
Operating Room.............. Chad D Caldwell
Radiology................... Paul C D'Angelo
Chief of Medical Staff.......... Grant Jenkins
CEO/President............... Mike McNair
Emergency Room .... Andrew Pacos
Anesthesiology............... Steve Ziegler

Measure	Cases	This Hosp.	State Avg.	U.S. Avg.
Blood Clot Prevention and Treatment				
Anticoagulation Overlap Therapy[1,2]	-	-	94%	93%
ICU Venous Thromboembolism Prophylaxis[2]	36	100%	93%	92%
Incidence of Potentially Preventable VTE[2,7]	-	-	10%	10%
UFH with Dosages/Platelet Monitoring[1,2]	-	-	95%	97%
Venous Thromboembolism Prophylaxis[2]	165	98%	88%	85%
Warfarin Therapy Discharge Instructions[1,2]	-	-	81%	75%
Chest Pain/Possible Heart Attack Care				
Aspirin Given Within 24 Hours of Arrival	60	100%	97%	96%
Fibrinolytic Meds Within 30 Min. of Arrival[7]	-	-	66%	58%
Average Time to ECG (minutes)	64	1	7	7
Average Time to Transfer (minutes)[7]	-	-	45	60
Children's Asthma Care				
Received Home Management Plan of Care	-	-	89%	88%
Received Reliever Medication	-	-	100%	100%
Received Systemic Corticosteroids	-	-	100%	100%
Emergency Department				
Admittance Decision Time (minutes)[2]	587	117	107	98
Head CT Results Within 45 Min. of Arrival[1]	-	-	60%	57%
Patients Who Left ER Before Being Seen	20,253	3%	3%	2%
Time from ER Arrival to Admit. (minutes)[2]	617	301	300	274
Time from ER Arrival to Discharge (minutes)	441	146	152	134
Time in ER Before Being Evaluated (minutes)	464	31	34	26
Time to Pain Meds for Fractures (minutes)	62	62	67	57
Heart Attack Care				
Aspirin Given at Discharge[1]	-	-	100%	99%
Fibrinolytic Meds Within 30 Min. of Arrival[7]	-	-	75%	54%
PCI Within 90 Minutes of Arrival[7]	-	-	98%	96%
Statin Prescribed at Discharge[1]	-	-	99%	98%
Heart Failure Care				
ACE Inhibitor or ARB for LVSD	24	96%	98%	97%
Discharge Instructions Given	60	100%	96%	94%
Evaluation of LVS Function	76	100%	100%	99%
Medicare Spending				
Medicare Spending per Patient (ratio)	-	1.05	0.94	0.98
Pneumonia Care				
Appropriate Initial Antibiotic Given	43	100%	97%	95%
Blood Culture Timing	83	100%	98%	98%
Pregnancy and Delivery Care				
Newborn Deliveries Scheduled Early[7]	-	-	3%	6%
Preventive Care				
Immunization for Influenza[2]	346	99%	93%	90%
Immunization for Pneumonia[2]	548	98%	94%	92%
Stroke Care				
Anticoagulation Therapy for Atrial Fibrillation[1]	-	-	95%	95%
Antithrombotic Therapy Timing	17	100%	98%	98%
Assessed for Rehabilitation	22	100%	98%	97%
Discharged on Antithrombotic Therapy	20	100%	99%	99%
Discharged on Statin Medication	15	93%	94%	94%
Thrombolytic Therapy Timing[7]	-	-	64%	66%
Venous Thromboembolism Prophylaxis	23	100%	96%	94%
Written Stroke Educational Materials Given	12	67%	88%	88%
Surgical Care Improvement Project				
Appropriate Beta Blocker Usage	11	100%	99%	98%
Appropriate VTP Within 24 Hours	38	92%	99%	98%
Controlled Postoperative Blood Glucose[7]	-	-	98%	97%
Perioperative Temperature Management	41	100%	100%	100%
Prophylactic Antibiotic Selection	25	100%	99%	99%

NOTE: Hospital profiles are in alphabetical order by state, then city, then hospital within the city; Rankings exclude hospitals with less than 25 cases except for patient surveys which excludes hospitals with less than 100 cases; (a) 100-299 cases; (1) The number of cases/patients is too few to report; (2) Data submitted were based on a sample of cases/patients; (3) Results are based on a shorter time period than required; (4) Data suppressed by CMS for one or more quarters; (5) Results are not available for this reporting period; (6) Fewer than 100 patients completed the HCAHPS survey; (7) No cases met the criteria for this measure; (8) The lower limit of the confidence interval cannot be calculated if the number of observed infections equals zero; (9) No data are available from the state/territory for this reporting period; (10) The scores shown reflect fewer than 50 completed surveys; (11) There were discrepancies in the data collection process; (12) This measure does not apply to this hospital for this reporting period; (13) Results cannot be calculated for this reporting period; (14) The results for this state are combined with nearby states to protect confidentiality; Please refer to the User's Guide for a full explanation of data.

Measure	Cases	This Hosp.	State Avg.	U.S. Avg.
Prophylactic Antibiotic Selection (Outpatient)[1,3]	-	-	98%	98%
Prophylactic Antibiotic Stopped	25	96%	99%	98%
Prophylactic Antibiotic Timing	25	100%	99%	99%
Prophylactic Antibiotic Timing (Outpatient)[1,3]	-	-	99%	98%
Urinary Catheter Removal	31	100%	99%	97%
Survey of Patients' Hospital Experiences				
Area Around Room 'Always' Quiet at Night	(a)	61%	64%	61%
Doctors 'Always' Communicated Well	(a)	70%	83%	82%
Home Recovery Information Given	(a)	86%	87%	85%
Hospital Given 9 or 10 on 10 Point Scale	(a)	52%	71%	71%
Meds 'Always' Explained Before Given	(a)	62%	65%	64%
Nurses 'Always' Communicated Well	(a)	72%	81%	79%
Pain 'Always' Well Controlled	(a)	63%	72%	71%
Room and Bathroom 'Always' Clean	(a)	65%	72%	73%
Timely Help 'Always' Received	(a)	52%	68%	68%
Would Definitely Recommend Hospital	(a)	57%	70%	71%
Use of Medical Imaging				
Cardiac Imaging Stress Test before Surgery	54	3.7%	5.4%	5.3%
Combination Abdominal CT Scan	272	3.3%	5.6%	10.5%
Combination Brain/Sinus CT Scan[1]	-	-	2.6%	2.7%
Combination Chest CT Scan	104	2.9%	1.3%	2.7%
Follow-up Mammogram/Ultrasound	605	8.3%	8%	8.8%
Lumbar Spine MRI for Low Back Pain[1]	-	-	34.7%	37.2%

Southeastern Regional Medical Center

300 W 27 Saint PO Box 1408
Lumberton, NC 28359
Phone: 910-671-5000
Fax: 910-671-5200
URL: www.srmc.org
Type: Acute Care Hospitals
Emergency Services: Yes
Ownership: Voluntary non-profit - Private
Beds: 403

Key Personnel:
CEO/President. . . . . Joann Anderson
Operating Room. . . . . Anette Dial
Infection Control. . . . . Dale Gifford
Coronary Care. . . . . Renee Hester
Cardiac Laboratory. . . . . Amy Kessenich
Quality Assurance . . . . Elizabeth Kirschling
Radiology. . . . . Jon Thorsten

Measure	Cases	This Hosp.	State Avg.	U.S. Avg.
Blood Clot Prevention and Treatment				
Anticoagulation Overlap Therapy[2]	122	75%	94%	93%
ICU Venous Thromboembolism Prophylaxis[2]	32	75%	93%	92%
Incidence of Potentially Preventable VTE[2]	11	9%	10%	10%
UFH with Dosages/Platelet Monitoring[2]	60	100%	95%	97%
Venous Thromboembolism Prophylaxis[2]	370	83%	88%	85%
Warfarin Therapy Discharge Instructions[2]	86	90%	81%	75%
Chest Pain/Possible Heart Attack Care				
Aspirin Given Within 24 Hours of Arrival[1]	-	-	97%	96%
Fibrinolytic Meds Within 30 Min. of Arrival[3,7]	-	-	66%	58%
Average Time to ECG (minutes)[1]	-	-	7	7
Average Time to Transfer (minutes)[3,7]	-	-	45	60
Children's Asthma Care				
Received Home Management Plan of Care	-	-	89%	88%
Received Reliever Medication	-	-	100%	100%
Received Systemic Corticosteroids	-	-	100%	100%
Emergency Department				
Admittance Decision Time (minutes)[2]	776	111	107	98
Head CT Results Within 45 Min. of Arrival	27	19%	60%	57%
Patients Who Left ER Before Being Seen	68,375	4%	3%	2%
Time from ER Arrival to Admit. (minutes)[2]	779	432	300	274
Time from ER Arrival to Discharge (minutes)	332	250	152	134
Time in ER Before Being Evaluated (minutes)	278	98	34	26
Time to Pain Meds for Fractures (minutes)	175	95	67	57
Heart Attack Care				
Aspirin Given at Discharge	247	100%	100%	99%
Fibrinolytic Meds Within 30 Min. of Arrival[7]	-	-	75%	54%
PCI Within 90 Minutes of Arrival	45	89%	98%	96%
Statin Prescribed at Discharge	242	97%	99%	98%
Heart Failure Care				
ACE Inhibitor or ARB for LVSD	204	92%	98%	97%
Discharge Instructions Given	586	96%	96%	94%
Evaluation of LVS Function	672	100%	100%	99%
Medicare Spending				
Medicare Spending per Patient (ratio)	-	0.92	0.94	0.98
Pneumonia Care				
Appropriate Initial Antibiotic Given	221	98%	97%	95%
Blood Culture Timing	363	92%	98%	98%
Pregnancy and Delivery Care				
Newborn Deliveries Scheduled Early[2]	120	2%	3%	6%
Preventive Care				
Immunization for Influenza[2]	526	84%	93%	90%
Immunization for Pneumonia[2]	700	88%	94%	92%
Stroke Care				
Anticoagulation Therapy for Atrial Fibrillation	16	88%	95%	95%
Antithrombotic Therapy Timing	141	99%	98%	98%
Assessed for Rehabilitation	139	99%	98%	97%
Discharged on Antithrombotic Therapy	131	98%	99%	99%
Discharged on Statin Medication	105	90%	94%	94%
Thrombolytic Therapy Timing	15	33%	64%	66%
Venous Thromboembolism Prophylaxis	148	90%	96%	94%
Written Stroke Educational Materials Given	75	100%	88%	88%
Surgical Care Improvement Project				
Appropriate Beta Blocker Usage	104	100%	99%	98%
Appropriate VTP Within 24 Hours	210	98%	99%	98%
Controlled Postoperative Blood Glucose	40	98%	98%	97%
Perioperative Temperature Management	270	100%	100%	100%
Prophylactic Antibiotic Selection	159	97%	99%	99%
Prophylactic Antibiotic Selection (Outpatient)	147	95%	98%	98%
Prophylactic Antibiotic Stopped	159	100%	99%	98%
Prophylactic Antibiotic Timing	159	99%	99%	99%
Prophylactic Antibiotic Timing (Outpatient)	153	95%	99%	98%
Urinary Catheter Removal	177	99%	99%	97%
Survey of Patients' Hospital Experiences				
Area Around Room 'Always' Quiet at Night	300+	72%	64%	61%
Doctors 'Always' Communicated Well	300+	82%	83%	82%
Home Recovery Information Given	300+	86%	87%	85%
Hospital Given 9 or 10 on 10 Point Scale	300+	67%	71%	71%
Meds 'Always' Explained Before Given	300+	69%	65%	64%
Nurses 'Always' Communicated Well	300+	82%	81%	79%
Pain 'Always' Well Controlled	300+	71%	72%	71%
Room and Bathroom 'Always' Clean	300+	68%	72%	73%
Timely Help 'Always' Received	300+	73%	68%	68%
Would Definitely Recommend Hospital	300+	62%	70%	71%
Use of Medical Imaging				
Cardiac Imaging Stress Test before Surgery	667	3.3%	5.4%	5.3%
Combination Abdominal CT Scan	1,526	3.5%	5.6%	10.5%
Combination Brain/Sinus CT Scan	1,269	4.4%	2.6%	2.7%
Combination Chest CT Scan	720	5.6%	1.3%	2.7%
Follow-up Mammogram/Ultrasound	1,078	4.7%	8%	8.8%
Lumbar Spine MRI for Low Back Pain	230	37.4%	34.7%	37.2%

The Mcdowell Hospital

430 Rankin Drive PO Box 730
Marion, NC 28752
Phone: 828-659-5000
Fax: 828-652-1626
URL: www.mcdhospital.org
Type: Acute Care Hospitals
Emergency Services: Yes
Ownership: Voluntary non-profit - Private
Beds: 65

Key Personnel:
CEO/President. . . . . Lynn Boggs
Operating Room. . . . . Lori Elam
Emergency Room . . . . Karen English, RN
Intensive Care Unit. . . . . Keisha Hastings
Radiology. . . . . Kelly McFarland
Pediatric Ambulatory Care . . . . . . Teresa Wall
Pediatric In-Patient Care . . . . Teresa Wall

Measure	Cases	This Hosp.	State Avg.	U.S. Avg.
Blood Clot Prevention and Treatment				
Anticoagulation Overlap Therapy[2]	18	100%	94%	93%
ICU Venous Thromboembolism Prophylaxis[2]	48	98%	93%	92%
Incidence of Potentially Preventable VTE[1,2]	-	-	10%	10%
UFH with Dosages/Platelet Monitoring[1,2]	-	-	95%	97%
Venous Thromboembolism Prophylaxis[2]	174	99%	88%	85%
Warfarin Therapy Discharge Instructions[2]	14	36%	81%	75%
Chest Pain/Possible Heart Attack Care				
Aspirin Given Within 24 Hours of Arrival	71	96%	97%	96%
Fibrinolytic Meds Within 30 Min. of Arrival[7]	-	-	66%	58%
Average Time to ECG (minutes)	70	6	7	7
Average Time to Transfer (minutes)	15	58	45	60
Children's Asthma Care				
Received Home Management Plan of Care	-	-	89%	88%
Received Reliever Medication	-	-	100%	100%
Received Systemic Corticosteroids	-	-	100%	100%
Emergency Department				
Admittance Decision Time (minutes)[2]	488	51	107	98
Head CT Results Within 45 Min. of Arrival[1]	-	-	60%	57%
Patients Who Left ER Before Being Seen	23,111	3%	3%	2%
Time from ER Arrival to Admit. (minutes)[2]	498	246	300	274
Time from ER Arrival to Discharge (minutes)	413	137	152	134
Time in ER Before Being Evaluated (minutes)	438	27	34	26
Time to Pain Meds for Fractures (minutes)	61	54	67	57
Heart Attack Care				
Aspirin Given at Discharge[1]	-	-	100%	99%
Fibrinolytic Meds Within 30 Min. of Arrival[7]	-	-	75%	54%
PCI Within 90 Minutes of Arrival[7]	-	-	98%	96%
Statin Prescribed at Discharge[1]	-	-	99%	98%
Heart Failure Care				
ACE Inhibitor or ARB for LVSD	45	100%	98%	97%
Discharge Instructions Given	80	100%	96%	94%
Evaluation of LVS Function	100	100%	100%	99%
Medicare Spending				
Medicare Spending per Patient (ratio)	-	0.97	0.94	0.98
Pneumonia Care				
Appropriate Initial Antibiotic Given	73	96%	97%	95%
Blood Culture Timing	129	98%	98%	98%
Pregnancy and Delivery Care				
Newborn Deliveries Scheduled Early	13	8%	3%	6%
Preventive Care				
Immunization for Influenza[2]	291	97%	93%	90%
Immunization for Pneumonia[2]	416	90%	94%	92%
Stroke Care				
Anticoagulation Therapy for Atrial Fibrillation[1]	-	-	95%	95%
Antithrombotic Therapy Timing	24	100%	98%	98%
Assessed for Rehabilitation	26	100%	98%	97%
Discharged on Antithrombotic Therapy	23	100%	99%	99%
Discharged on Statin Medication	22	95%	94%	94%
Thrombolytic Therapy Timing[1]	-	-	64%	66%
Venous Thromboembolism Prophylaxis	26	100%	96%	94%
Written Stroke Educational Materials Given	13	100%	88%	88%
Surgical Care Improvement Project				
Appropriate Beta Blocker Usage	11	100%	99%	98%
Appropriate VTP Within 24 Hours	43	100%	99%	98%
Controlled Postoperative Blood Glucose[7]	-	-	98%	97%
Perioperative Temperature Management	48	100%	100%	100%
Prophylactic Antibiotic Selection	22	100%	99%	99%
Prophylactic Antibiotic Selection (Outpatient)	87	97%	98%	98%
Prophylactic Antibiotic Stopped	17	94%	99%	98%
Prophylactic Antibiotic Timing	22	100%	99%	99%
Prophylactic Antibiotic Timing (Outpatient)	86	97%	99%	98%
Urinary Catheter Removal	14	100%	99%	97%
Survey of Patients' Hospital Experiences				
Area Around Room 'Always' Quiet at Night	300+	67%	64%	61%
Doctors 'Always' Communicated Well	300+	88%	83%	82%
Home Recovery Information Given	300+	88%	87%	85%
Hospital Given 9 or 10 on 10 Point Scale	300+	74%	71%	71%
Meds 'Always' Explained Before Given	300+	73%	65%	64%
Nurses 'Always' Communicated Well	300+	84%	81%	79%
Pain 'Always' Well Controlled	300+	78%	72%	71%
Room and Bathroom 'Always' Clean	300+	75%	72%	73%
Timely Help 'Always' Received	300+	75%	68%	68%
Would Definitely Recommend Hospital	300+	71%	70%	71%
Use of Medical Imaging				
Cardiac Imaging Stress Test before Surgery	196	6.1%	5.4%	5.3%
Combination Abdominal CT Scan	427	1.2%	5.6%	10.5%
Combination Brain/Sinus CT Scan[1]	-	-	2.6%	2.7%
Combination Chest CT Scan	188	0.0%	1.3%	2.7%
Follow-up Mammogram/Ultrasound	757	6.9%	8%	8.8%
Lumbar Spine MRI for Low Back Pain[7]	-	-	34.7%	37.2%

NOTE: Hospital profiles are in alphabetical order by state, then city, then hospital within the city; Rankings exclude hospitals with less than 25 cases except for patient surveys which excludes hospitals with less than 100 cases; (a) 100-299 cases; (1) The number of cases/patients is too few to report; (2) Data submitted were based on a sample of cases/patients; (3) Results are based on a shorter time period than required; (4) Data suppressed by CMS for one or more quarters; (5) Results are not available for this reporting period; (6) Fewer than 100 patients completed the HCAHPS survey; (7) No cases met the criteria for this measure; (8) The lower limit of the confidence interval cannot be calculated if the number of observed infections equals zero; (9) No data are available from the state/territory for this reporting period; (10) The scores shown reflect fewer than 50 completed surveys; (11) There were discrepancies in the data collection process; (12) This measure does not apply to this hospital for this reporting period; (13) Results cannot be calculated for this reporting period; (14) The results for this state are combined with nearby states to protect confidentiality; Please refer to the User's Guide for a full explanation of data.

Presbyterian Hospital Matthews

1500 Matthews Twnshp Prkwy Box 3310
Matthews, NC 28106
E-mail: tcthompson@ph.novanthealth.org
URL: www.presbyterian.org
Type: Acute Care Hospitals
Ownership: Voluntary non-profit - Other
Phone: 704-384-6500
Fax: 704-384-6515
Emergency Services: Yes
Beds: 94

Key Personnel:
Radiology. . . . . Steven M Genkins
Chief of Medical Staff. . . . . Thomas H Phillips

Measure	Cases	This Hosp.	State Avg.	U.S. Avg.
Blood Clot Prevention and Treatment				
Anticoagulation Overlap Therapy[2]	69	97%	94%	93%
ICU Venous Thromboembolism Prophylaxis[2]	35	97%	93%	92%
Incidence of Potentially Preventable VTE[1,2]	-	-	10%	10%
UFH with Dosages/Platelet Monitoring[2]	58	100%	95%	97%
Venous Thromboembolism Prophylaxis[2]	444	98%	88%	85%
Warfarin Therapy Discharge Instructions[2]	53	79%	81%	75%
Chest Pain/Possible Heart Attack Care				
Aspirin Given Within 24 Hours of Arrival	42	100%	97%	96%
Fibrinolytic Meds Within 30 Min. of Arrival[7]	-	-	66%	58%
Average Time to ECG (minutes)	42	3	7	7
Average Time to Transfer (minutes)	19	29	45	60
Children's Asthma Care				
Received Home Management Plan of Care	-	-	89%	88%
Received Reliever Medication	-	-	100%	100%
Received Systemic Corticosteroids	-	-	100%	100%
Emergency Department				
Admittance Decision Time (minutes)[2]	806	201	107	98
Head CT Results Within 45 Min. of Arrival	16	69%	60%	57%
Patients Who Left ER Before Being Seen	48,064	1%	3%	2%
Time from ER Arrival to Admit. (minutes)[2]	833	397	300	274
Time from ER Arrival to Discharge (minutes)	466	181	152	134
Time in ER Before Being Evaluated (minutes)	518	21	34	26
Time to Pain Meds for Fractures (minutes)	189	68	67	57
Heart Attack Care				
Aspirin Given at Discharge	116	100%	100%	99%
Fibrinolytic Meds Within 30 Min. of Arrival[7]	-	-	75%	54%
PCI Within 90 Minutes of Arrival[1]	-	-	98%	96%
Statin Prescribed at Discharge	115	100%	99%	98%
Heart Failure Care				
ACE Inhibitor or ARB for LVSD	64	100%	98%	97%
Discharge Instructions Given	179	100%	96%	94%
Evaluation of LVS Function	211	100%	100%	99%
Medicare Spending				
Medicare Spending per Patient (ratio)	-	0.94	0.94	0.98
Pneumonia Care				
Appropriate Initial Antibiotic Given	206	99%	97%	95%
Blood Culture Timing	323	100%	98%	98%
Pregnancy and Delivery Care				
Newborn Deliveries Scheduled Early[2]	23	0%	3%	6%
Preventive Care				
Immunization for Influenza[2]	576	97%	93%	90%
Immunization for Pneumonia[2]	734	99%	94%	92%
Stroke Care				
Anticoagulation Therapy for Atrial Fibrillation[1]	-	-	95%	95%
Antithrombotic Therapy Timing	116	99%	98%	98%
Assessed for Rehabilitation	117	99%	98%	97%
Discharged on Antithrombotic Therapy	113	100%	99%	99%
Discharged on Statin Medication	87	100%	94%	94%
Thrombolytic Therapy Timing[1]	-	-	64%	66%
Venous Thromboembolism Prophylaxis	120	99%	96%	94%
Written Stroke Educational Materials Given	70	99%	88%	88%
Surgical Care Improvement Project				
Appropriate Beta Blocker Usage[2]	132	100%	99%	98%
Appropriate VTP Within 24 Hours[2]	448	99%	99%	98%
Controlled Postoperative Blood Glucose[2,7]	-	-	98%	97%
Perioperative Temperature Management[2]	496	100%	100%	100%
Prophylactic Antibiotic Selection[2]	360	100%	99%	99%
Prophylactic Antibiotic Selection (Outpatient)	261	100%	98%	98%
Prophylactic Antibiotic Stopped[2]	353	99%	99%	98%
Prophylactic Antibiotic Timing[2]	360	99%	99%	99%
Prophylactic Antibiotic Timing (Outpatient)	262	100%	99%	98%
Urinary Catheter Removal[2]	374	99%	99%	97%
Survey of Patients' Hospital Experiences				
Area Around Room 'Always' Quiet at Night	300+	56%	64%	61%
Doctors 'Always' Communicated Well	300+	79%	83%	82%
Home Recovery Information Given	300+	82%	87%	85%
Hospital Given 9 or 10 on 10 Point Scale	300+	70%	71%	71%
Meds 'Always' Explained Before Given	300+	57%	65%	64%
Nurses 'Always' Communicated Well	300+	74%	81%	79%
Pain 'Always' Well Controlled	300+	65%	72%	71%
Room and Bathroom 'Always' Clean	300+	68%	72%	73%
Timely Help 'Always' Received	300+	55%	68%	68%
Would Definitely Recommend Hospital	300+	74%	70%	71%
Use of Medical Imaging				
Cardiac Imaging Stress Test before Surgery	223	6.3%	5.4%	5.3%
Combination Abdominal CT Scan	1,322	4.0%	5.6%	10.5%
Combination Brain/Sinus CT Scan	1,034	3.8%	2.6%	2.7%
Combination Chest CT Scan	914	0.0%	1.3%	2.7%
Follow-up Mammogram/Ultrasound	1,277	7.1%	8%	8.8%
Lumbar Spine MRI for Low Back Pain	82	23.2%	34.7%	37.2%

Davie County Hospital

223 Hospital St
Mocksville, NC 27028
URL: www.daviehospital.org
Type: Critical Access Hospitals
Ownership: Voluntary non-profit - Other
Phone: 336-751-8100
Fax: 336-751-8402
Emergency Services: Yes
Beds: 81

Key Personnel:
CEO/President. . . . . Donny Lambath

Measure	Cases	This Hosp.	State Avg.	U.S. Avg.
Blood Clot Prevention and Treatment				
Anticoagulation Overlap Therapy[5]	-	-	94%	93%
ICU Venous Thromboembolism Prophylaxis[5]	-	-	93%	92%
Incidence of Potentially Preventable VTE[5]	-	-	10%	10%
UFH with Dosages/Platelet Monitoring[5]	-	-	95%	97%
Venous Thromboembolism Prophylaxis[5]	-	-	88%	85%
Warfarin Therapy Discharge Instructions[5]	-	-	81%	75%
Chest Pain/Possible Heart Attack Care				
Aspirin Given Within 24 Hours of Arrival	-	-	97%	96%
Fibrinolytic Meds Within 30 Min. of Arrival	-	-	66%	58%
Average Time to ECG (minutes)	-	-	7	7
Average Time to Transfer (minutes)	-	-	45	60
Children's Asthma Care				
Received Home Management Plan of Care	-	-	89%	88%
Received Reliever Medication	-	-	100%	100%
Received Systemic Corticosteroids	-	-	100%	100%
Emergency Department				
Admittance Decision Time (minutes)[5]	-	-	107	98
Head CT Results Within 45 Min. of Arrival	-	-	60%	57%
Patients Who Left ER Before Being Seen	-	-	3%	2%
Time from ER Arrival to Admit. (minutes)[5]	-	-	300	274
Time from ER Arrival to Discharge (minutes)	-	-	152	134
Time in ER Before Being Evaluated (minutes)	-	-	34	26
Time to Pain Meds for Fractures (minutes)	-	-	67	57
Heart Attack Care				
Aspirin Given at Discharge[5]	-	-	100%	99%
Fibrinolytic Meds Within 30 Min. of Arrival[5]	-	-	75%	54%
PCI Within 90 Minutes of Arrival[5]	-	-	98%	96%
Statin Prescribed at Discharge[5]	-	-	99%	98%
Heart Failure Care				
ACE Inhibitor or ARB for LVSD[1]	-	-	98%	97%
Discharge Instructions Given[1]	-	-	96%	94%
Evaluation of LVS Function[1]	-	-	100%	99%
Medicare Spending				
Medicare Spending per Patient (ratio)	-	-	0.94	0.98
Pneumonia Care				
Appropriate Initial Antibiotic Given[1]	-	-	97%	95%
Blood Culture Timing[1]	-	-	98%	98%
Pregnancy and Delivery Care				
Newborn Deliveries Scheduled Early[5]	-	-	3%	6%
Preventive Care				
Immunization for Influenza[5]	-	-	93%	90%
Immunization for Pneumonia[5]	-	-	94%	92%
Stroke Care				
Anticoagulation Therapy for Atrial Fibrillation[5]	-	-	95%	95%
Antithrombotic Therapy Timing[5]	-	-	98%	98%
Assessed for Rehabilitation[5]	-	-	98%	97%
Discharged on Antithrombotic Therapy[5]	-	-	99%	99%
Discharged on Statin Medication[5]	-	-	94%	94%
Thrombolytic Therapy Timing[5]	-	-	64%	66%
Venous Thromboembolism Prophylaxis[5]	-	-	96%	94%
Written Stroke Educational Materials Given[5]	-	-	88%	88%
Surgical Care Improvement Project				
Appropriate Beta Blocker Usage[5]	-	-	99%	98%
Appropriate VTP Within 24 Hours[5]	-	-	99%	98%
Controlled Postoperative Blood Glucose[5]	-	-	98%	97%
Perioperative Temperature Management[5]	-	-	100%	100%
Prophylactic Antibiotic Selection[5]	-	-	99%	99%
Prophylactic Antibiotic Selection (Outpatient)	-	-	98%	98%
Prophylactic Antibiotic Stopped[5]	-	-	99%	98%
Prophylactic Antibiotic Timing[5]	-	-	99%	99%
Prophylactic Antibiotic Timing (Outpatient)	-	-	99%	98%
Urinary Catheter Removal[5]	-	-	99%	97%
Survey of Patients' Hospital Experiences				
Area Around Room 'Always' Quiet at Night[10]	<100	83%	64%	61%
Doctors 'Always' Communicated Well[10]	<100	79%	83%	82%
Home Recovery Information Given[10]	<100	73%	87%	85%
Hospital Given 9 or 10 on 10 Point Scale[10]	<100	66%	71%	71%
Meds 'Always' Explained Before Given[10]	<100	46%	65%	64%
Nurses 'Always' Communicated Well[10]	<100	73%	81%	79%
Pain 'Always' Well Controlled[10]	<100	77%	72%	71%
Room and Bathroom 'Always' Clean[10]	<100	69%	72%	73%
Timely Help 'Always' Received[10]	<100	80%	68%	68%
Would Definitely Recommend Hospital[10]	<100	66%	70%	71%
Use of Medical Imaging				
Cardiac Imaging Stress Test before Surgery	-	-	5.4%	5.3%
Combination Abdominal CT Scan	-	-	5.6%	10.5%
Combination Brain/Sinus CT Scan	-	-	2.6%	2.7%
Combination Chest CT Scan	-	-	1.3%	2.7%
Follow-up Mammogram/Ultrasound	-	-	8%	8.8%
Lumbar Spine MRI for Low Back Pain	-	-	34.7%	37.2%

Carolinas Medical Center - Union

600 Hospital Dr
Monroe, NC 28110
URL: www.carolinashealthcare.org/cmc-union
Type: Acute Care Hospitals
Ownership: Govt - Hospital Dist/Auth
Phone: 704-283-3100
Fax: 704-296-4175
Emergency Services: Yes
Beds: 157

Key Personnel:
Radiology. . . . . John Adams
Operating Room. . . . . Edward Bower
Cardiac Laboratory. . . . . Steve Dence
Coronary Care . . . . Steve Dence
Chief of Medical Staff. . . . . Dan Hagler
Infection Control. . . . . Janet Little
CEO/President. . . . . John Miller, Jr.
CEO . . . . Michael C. Tarwater

Measure	Cases	This Hosp.	State Avg.	U.S. Avg.
Blood Clot Prevention and Treatment				
Anticoagulation Overlap Therapy[2]	36	89%	94%	93%
ICU Venous Thromboembolism Prophylaxis[2]	58	97%	93%	92%
Incidence of Potentially Preventable VTE[1,2]	-	-	10%	10%
UFH with Dosages/Platelet Monitoring[2]	11	100%	95%	97%
Venous Thromboembolism Prophylaxis[2]	333	95%	88%	85%
Warfarin Therapy Discharge Instructions[2]	23	91%	81%	75%
Chest Pain/Possible Heart Attack Care				
Aspirin Given Within 24 Hours of Arrival	208	96%	97%	96%
Fibrinolytic Meds Within 30 Min. of Arrival[7]	-	-	66%	58%
Average Time to ECG (minutes)	213	4	7	7
Average Time to Transfer (minutes)	48	46	45	60
Children's Asthma Care				
Received Home Management Plan of Care	-	-	89%	88%
Received Reliever Medication	-	-	100%	100%
Received Systemic Corticosteroids	-	-	100%	100%
Emergency Department				
Admittance Decision Time (minutes)[2]	424	110	107	98
Head CT Results Within 45 Min. of Arrival	24	42%	60%	57%
Patients Who Left ER Before Being Seen	69,504	2%	3%	2%

NOTE: Hospital profiles are in alphabetical order by state, then city, then hospital within the city; Rankings exclude hospitals with less than 25 cases except for patient surveys which excludes hospitals with less than 100 cases; (a) 100-299 cases; (1) The number of cases/patients is too few to report; (2) Data submitted were based on a sample of cases/patients; (3) Results are based on a shorter time period than required; (4) Data suppressed by CMS for one or more quarters; (5) Results are not available for this reporting period; (6) Fewer than 100 patients completed the HCAHPS survey; (7) No cases met the criteria for this measure; (8) The lower limit of the confidence interval cannot be calculated if the number of observed infections equals zero; (9) No data are available from the state/territory for this reporting period; (10) The scores shown reflect fewer than 50 completed surveys; (11) There were discrepancies in the data collection process; (12) This measure does not apply to this hospital for this reporting period; (13) Results cannot be calculated for this reporting period; (14) The results for this state are combined with nearby states to protect confidentiality; Please refer to the User's Guide for a full explanation of data.

Measure	Cases	This Hosp.	State Avg.	U.S. Avg.
Time from ER Arrival to Admit. (minutes)[2]	481	306	300	274
Time from ER Arrival to Discharge (minutes)	343	151	152	134
Time in ER Before Being Evaluated (minutes)	371	35	34	26
Time to Pain Meds for Fractures (minutes)	205	70	67	57
Heart Attack Care				
Aspirin Given at Discharge	24	100%	100%	99%
Fibrinolytic Meds Within 30 Min. of Arrival[7]	-	-	75%	54%
PCI Within 90 Minutes of Arrival[7]	-	-	98%	96%
Statin Prescribed at Discharge	23	100%	99%	98%
Heart Failure Care				
ACE Inhibitor or ARB for LVSD	102	95%	98%	97%
Discharge Instructions Given	279	99%	96%	94%
Evaluation of LVS Function	337	100%	100%	99%
Medicare Spending				
Medicare Spending per Patient (ratio)	-	0.97	0.94	0.98
Pneumonia Care				
Appropriate Initial Antibiotic Given	189	96%	97%	95%
Blood Culture Timing	300	97%	98%	98%
Pregnancy and Delivery Care				
Newborn Deliveries Scheduled Early	82	0%	3%	6%
Preventive Care				
Immunization for Influenza[2]	518	93%	93%	90%
Immunization for Pneumonia[2]	637	96%	94%	92%
Stroke Care				
Anticoagulation Therapy for Atrial Fibrillation	14	100%	95%	95%
Antithrombotic Therapy Timing	95	100%	98%	98%
Assessed for Rehabilitation	101	100%	98%	97%
Discharged on Antithrombotic Therapy	98	100%	99%	99%
Discharged on Statin Medication	72	99%	94%	94%
Thrombolytic Therapy Timing[7]	-	-	64%	66%
Venous Thromboembolism Prophylaxis	87	100%	96%	94%
Written Stroke Educational Materials Given	55	96%	88%	88%
Surgical Care Improvement Project				
Appropriate Beta Blocker Usage[2]	108	98%	99%	98%
Appropriate VTP Within 24 Hours[2]	425	99%	99%	98%
Controlled Postoperative Blood Glucose[2,7]	-	-	98%	97%
Perioperative Temperature Management[2]	457	100%	100%	100%
Prophylactic Antibiotic Selection[2]	305	100%	99%	99%
Prophylactic Antibiotic Selection (Outpatient)	64	97%	98%	98%
Prophylactic Antibiotic Stopped[2]	296	97%	99%	98%
Prophylactic Antibiotic Timing[2]	305	99%	99%	99%
Prophylactic Antibiotic Timing (Outpatient)	65	91%	99%	98%
Urinary Catheter Removal[2]	227	98%	99%	97%
Survey of Patients' Hospital Experiences				
Area Around Room 'Always' Quiet at Night	300+	66%	64%	61%
Doctors 'Always' Communicated Well	300+	83%	83%	82%
Home Recovery Information Given	300+	89%	87%	85%
Hospital Given 9 or 10 on 10 Point Scale	300+	76%	71%	71%
Meds 'Always' Explained Before Given	300+	67%	65%	64%
Nurses 'Always' Communicated Well	300+	82%	81%	79%
Pain 'Always' Well Controlled	300+	72%	72%	71%
Room and Bathroom 'Always' Clean	300+	71%	72%	73%
Timely Help 'Always' Received	300+	68%	68%	68%
Would Definitely Recommend Hospital	300+	74%	70%	71%
Use of Medical Imaging				
Cardiac Imaging Stress Test before Surgery	740	5.0%	5.4%	5.3%
Combination Abdominal CT Scan	1,475	4.1%	5.6%	10.5%
Combination Brain/Sinus CT Scan	1,286	1.5%	2.6%	2.7%
Combination Chest CT Scan	766	0.1%	1.3%	2.7%
Follow-up Mammogram/Ultrasound[7]	-	-	8%	8.8%
Lumbar Spine MRI for Low Back Pain	87	37.9%	34.7%	37.2%

Lake Norman Regional Medical Center

171 Fairview Road
Mooresville, NC 28117
Phone: 704-660-4000
Fax: 704-660-4005
E-mail: information@lnrmc.hma-corp.com
URL: www.lnrmc.com
Type: Acute Care Hospitals
Emergency Services: Yes
Ownership: Proprietary
Beds: 117

Key Personnel:
Quality Assurance . . . . Ann Allen
Infection Control. . . . . Brynne Beaver
Operating Room. . . . . Michelle Bertsch
Chief of Medical Staff . . . . Steven Bradley, MD
Coronary Care . . . . Deborah Dickens
Radiology. . . . . Teresa Lother
Pediatric In-Patient Care . . . . Kristy Miller

Measure	Cases	This Hosp.	State Avg.	U.S. Avg.
Blood Clot Prevention and Treatment				
Anticoagulation Overlap Therapy[2]	53	98%	94%	93%
ICU Venous Thromboembolism Prophylaxis[2]	59	97%	93%	92%
Incidence of Potentially Preventable VTE[1,2]	-	-	10%	10%
UFH with Dosages/Platelet Monitoring[2]	17	100%	95%	97%
Venous Thromboembolism Prophylaxis[2]	293	88%	88%	85%
Warfarin Therapy Discharge Instructions[2]	39	90%	81%	75%
Chest Pain/Possible Heart Attack Care				
Aspirin Given Within 24 Hours of Arrival	40	100%	97%	96%
Fibrinolytic Meds Within 30 Min. of Arrival[7]	-	-	66%	58%
Average Time to ECG (minutes)	40	6	7	7
Average Time to Transfer (minutes)[1]	-	-	45	60
Children's Asthma Care				
Received Home Management Plan of Care	-	-	89%	88%
Received Reliever Medication	-	-	100%	100%
Received Systemic Corticosteroids	-	-	100%	100%
Emergency Department				
Admittance Decision Time (minutes)[2]	565	75	107	98
Head CT Results Within 45 Min. of Arrival	21	95%	60%	57%
Patients Who Left ER Before Being Seen	25,403	1%	3%	2%
Time from ER Arrival to Admit. (minutes)[2]	566	220	300	274
Time from ER Arrival to Discharge (minutes)	594	117	152	134
Time in ER Before Being Evaluated (minutes)	633	10	34	26
Time to Pain Meds for Fractures (minutes)	133	47	67	57
Heart Attack Care				
Aspirin Given at Discharge	40	100%	100%	99%
Fibrinolytic Meds Within 30 Min. of Arrival[7]	-	-	75%	54%
PCI Within 90 Minutes of Arrival[7]	-	-	98%	96%
Statin Prescribed at Discharge	36	100%	99%	98%
Heart Failure Care				
ACE Inhibitor or ARB for LVSD	46	100%	98%	97%
Discharge Instructions Given	121	100%	96%	94%
Evaluation of LVS Function	149	100%	100%	99%
Medicare Spending				
Medicare Spending per Patient (ratio)	-	0.94	0.94	0.98
Pneumonia Care				
Appropriate Initial Antibiotic Given	89	99%	97%	95%
Blood Culture Timing	166	98%	98%	98%
Pregnancy and Delivery Care				
Newborn Deliveries Scheduled Early[2]	24	0%	3%	6%
Preventive Care				
Immunization for Influenza[2]	628	99%	93%	90%
Immunization for Pneumonia[2]	623	98%	94%	92%
Stroke Care				
Anticoagulation Therapy for Atrial Fibrillation[1]	-	-	95%	95%
Antithrombotic Therapy Timing	40	100%	98%	98%
Assessed for Rehabilitation	45	98%	98%	97%
Discharged on Antithrombotic Therapy	45	98%	99%	99%
Discharged on Statin Medication	34	97%	94%	94%
Thrombolytic Therapy Timing[1]	-	-	64%	66%
Venous Thromboembolism Prophylaxis	41	100%	96%	94%
Written Stroke Educational Materials Given	28	96%	88%	88%
Surgical Care Improvement Project				
Appropriate Beta Blocker Usage	94	96%	99%	98%
Appropriate VTP Within 24 Hours	299	99%	99%	98%
Controlled Postoperative Blood Glucose[7]	-	-	98%	97%
Perioperative Temperature Management	367	100%	100%	100%
Prophylactic Antibiotic Selection	254	99%	99%	99%
Prophylactic Antibiotic Selection (Outpatient)	331	99%	98%	98%
Prophylactic Antibiotic Stopped	254	100%	99%	98%
Prophylactic Antibiotic Timing	254	100%	99%	99%
Prophylactic Antibiotic Timing (Outpatient)	330	100%	99%	98%
Urinary Catheter Removal	228	100%	99%	97%
Survey of Patients' Hospital Experiences				
Area Around Room 'Always' Quiet at Night	300+	56%	64%	61%
Doctors 'Always' Communicated Well	300+	81%	83%	82%
Home Recovery Information Given	300+	84%	87%	85%
Hospital Given 9 or 10 on 10 Point Scale	300+	62%	71%	71%
Meds 'Always' Explained Before Given	300+	59%	65%	64%
Nurses 'Always' Communicated Well	300+	74%	81%	79%
Pain 'Always' Well Controlled	300+	67%	72%	71%
Room and Bathroom 'Always' Clean	300+	70%	72%	73%
Timely Help 'Always' Received	300+	59%	68%	68%
Would Definitely Recommend Hospital	300+	61%	70%	71%
Use of Medical Imaging				
Cardiac Imaging Stress Test before Surgery	153	5.2%	5.4%	5.3%
Combination Abdominal CT Scan	612	4.1%	5.6%	10.5%
Combination Brain/Sinus CT Scan[1]	-	-	2.6%	2.7%
Combination Chest CT Scan	388	0.3%	1.3%	2.7%
Follow-up Mammogram/Ultrasound	1,567	7.2%	8%	8.8%
Lumbar Spine MRI for Low Back Pain	94	37.2%	34.7%	37.2%

Carteret General Hospital

3500 Arendell St
Morehead City, NC 28557
Phone: 252-808-6000
Fax: 252-808-6916
E-mail: pr@ccgh.org
URL: www.ccgh.org
Type: Acute Care Hospitals
Emergency Services: Yes
Ownership: Proprietary
Beds: 117

Key Personnel:
Operating Room. . . . . Michael Bell
Radiology. . . . . S Joseph Buff
Infection Control. . . . . Elaine Crittonton
Cardiac Laboratory. . . . . John Gould, MD
Chief of Medical Staff . . . . Dr. Mary Katherine Lawre, MD
Quality Assurance . . . . Martha Kenworthy, RN
CEO/President. . . . . Fred A Odell, III
Pediatric In-Patient Care . . . . Callie Young

Measure	Cases	This Hosp.	State Avg.	U.S. Avg.
Blood Clot Prevention and Treatment				
Anticoagulation Overlap Therapy[2]	49	88%	94%	93%
ICU Venous Thromboembolism Prophylaxis[2]	55	91%	93%	92%
Incidence of Potentially Preventable VTE[1,2]	-	-	10%	10%
UFH with Dosages/Platelet Monitoring[1,2]	-	-	95%	97%
Venous Thromboembolism Prophylaxis[2]	338	86%	88%	85%
Warfarin Therapy Discharge Instructions[2]	32	44%	81%	75%
Chest Pain/Possible Heart Attack Care				
Aspirin Given Within 24 Hours of Arrival	68	93%	97%	96%
Fibrinolytic Meds Within 30 Min. of Arrival[1]	-	-	66%	58%
Average Time to ECG (minutes)	69	8	7	7
Average Time to Transfer (minutes)[1]	-	-	45	60
Children's Asthma Care				
Received Home Management Plan of Care	-	-	89%	88%
Received Reliever Medication	-	-	100%	100%
Received Systemic Corticosteroids	-	-	100%	100%
Emergency Department				
Admittance Decision Time (minutes)[2]	681	113	107	98
Head CT Results Within 45 Min. of Arrival	25	84%	60%	57%
Patients Who Left ER Before Being Seen	42,244	1%	3%	2%
Time from ER Arrival to Admit. (minutes)[2]	682	314	300	274
Time from ER Arrival to Discharge (minutes)	374	150	152	134
Time in ER Before Being Evaluated (minutes)	405	17	34	26
Time to Pain Meds for Fractures (minutes)	118	72	67	57
Heart Attack Care				
Aspirin Given at Discharge	57	96%	100%	99%
Fibrinolytic Meds Within 30 Min. of Arrival[7]	-	-	75%	54%
PCI Within 90 Minutes of Arrival[7]	-	-	98%	96%
Statin Prescribed at Discharge	64	81%	99%	98%
Heart Failure Care				
ACE Inhibitor or ARB for LVSD	55	95%	98%	97%
Discharge Instructions Given	126	88%	96%	94%
Evaluation of LVS Function	188	100%	100%	99%
Medicare Spending				
Medicare Spending per Patient (ratio)	-	0.91	0.94	0.98
Pneumonia Care				
Appropriate Initial Antibiotic Given	143	98%	97%	95%
Blood Culture Timing	245	99%	98%	98%
Pregnancy and Delivery Care				
Newborn Deliveries Scheduled Early	48	4%	3%	6%
Preventive Care				
Immunization for Influenza[2]	528	88%	93%	90%
Immunization for Pneumonia[2]	671	92%	94%	92%
Stroke Care				

NOTE: Hospital profiles are in alphabetical order by state, then city, then hospital within the city; Rankings exclude hospitals with less than 25 cases except for patient surveys which excludes hospitals with less than 100 cases; (a) 100-299 cases; (1) The number of cases/patients is too few to report; (2) Data submitted were based on a sample of cases/patients; (3) Results are based on a shorter time period than required; (4) Data suppressed by CMS for one or more quarters; (5) Results are not available for this reporting period; (6) Fewer than 100 patients completed the HCAHPS survey; (7) No cases met the criteria for this measure; (8) The lower limit of the confidence interval cannot be calculated if the number of observed infections equals zero; (9) No data are available from the state/territory for this reporting period; (10) The scores shown reflect fewer than 50 completed surveys; (11) There were discrepancies in the data collection process; (12) This measure does not apply to this hospital for this reporting period; (13) Results cannot be calculated for this reporting period; (14) The results for this state are combined with nearby states to protect confidentiality; Please refer to the User's Guide for a full explanation of data.

Measure	Cases	This Hosp.	State Avg.	U.S. Avg.
Anticoagulation Therapy for Atrial Fibrillation[1]	-	-	95%	95%
Antithrombotic Therapy Timing	70	100%	98%	98%
Assessed for Rehabilitation	67	97%	98%	97%
Discharged on Antithrombotic Therapy	66	98%	99%	99%
Discharged on Statin Medication	53	92%	94%	94%
Thrombolytic Therapy Timing[7]	-	-	64%	66%
Venous Thromboembolism Prophylaxis	67	97%	96%	94%
Written Stroke Educational Materials Given	34	44%	88%	88%
Surgical Care Improvement Project				
Appropriate Beta Blocker Usage	177	98%	99%	98%
Appropriate VTP Within 24 Hours	524	98%	99%	98%
Controlled Postoperative Blood Glucose[7]	-	-	98%	97%
Perioperative Temperature Management	676	100%	100%	100%
Prophylactic Antibiotic Selection	475	99%	99%	99%
Prophylactic Antibiotic Selection (Outpatient)	129	98%	98%	98%
Prophylactic Antibiotic Stopped	471	100%	99%	98%
Prophylactic Antibiotic Timing	475	100%	99%	99%
Prophylactic Antibiotic Timing (Outpatient)	131	98%	99%	98%
Urinary Catheter Removal	151	95%	99%	97%
Survey of Patients' Hospital Experiences				
Area Around Room 'Always' Quiet at Night	300+	64%	64%	61%
Doctors 'Always' Communicated Well	300+	83%	83%	82%
Home Recovery Information Given	300+	84%	87%	85%
Hospital Given 9 or 10 on 10 Point Scale	300+	68%	71%	71%
Meds 'Always' Explained Before Given	300+	73%	65%	64%
Nurses 'Always' Communicated Well	300+	86%	81%	79%
Pain 'Always' Well Controlled	300+	78%	72%	71%
Room and Bathroom 'Always' Clean	300+	73%	72%	73%
Timely Help 'Always' Received	300+	75%	68%	68%
Would Definitely Recommend Hospital	300+	69%	70%	71%
Use of Medical Imaging				
Cardiac Imaging Stress Test before Surgery	370	4.9%	5.4%	5.3%
Combination Abdominal CT Scan	1,120	3.6%	5.6%	10.5%
Combination Brain/Sinus CT Scan	919	2.3%	2.6%	2.7%
Combination Chest CT Scan	515	0.2%	1.3%	2.7%
Follow-up Mammogram/Ultrasound	1,960	7.1%	8%	8.8%
Lumbar Spine MRI for Low Back Pain	165	43.0%	34.7%	37.2%

CMC - Blue Ridge

2201 S Sterling St
Morganton, NC 28655
URL: www.gracehcs.org
Type: Acute Care Hospitals
Ownership: Proprietary
Phone: 828-580-5000
Fax: 828-580-5509
Emergency Services: Yes
Beds: 269

Key Personnel:
CEO/President. . . . . Kenneth W Wood

Measure	Cases	This Hosp.	State Avg.	U.S. Avg.
Blood Clot Prevention and Treatment				
Anticoagulation Overlap Therapy[2]	75	80%	94%	93%
ICU Venous Thromboembolism Prophylaxis[2]	99	87%	93%	92%
Incidence of Potentially Preventable VTE[1,2]	-	-	10%	10%
UFH with Dosages/Platelet Monitoring[2]	18	100%	95%	97%
Venous Thromboembolism Prophylaxis[2]	456	91%	88%	85%
Warfarin Therapy Discharge Instructions[2]	54	78%	81%	75%
Chest Pain/Possible Heart Attack Care				
Aspirin Given Within 24 Hours of Arrival	88	98%	97%	96%
Fibrinolytic Meds Within 30 Min. of Arrival[7]	-	-	66%	58%
Average Time to ECG (minutes)	88	8	7	7
Average Time to Transfer (minutes)	31	36	45	60
Children's Asthma Care				
Received Home Management Plan of Care	-	-	89%	88%
Received Reliever Medication	-	-	100%	100%
Received Systemic Corticosteroids	-	-	100%	100%
Emergency Department				
Admittance Decision Time (minutes)[2]	643	151	107	98
Head CT Results Within 45 Min. of Arrival	20	55%	60%	57%
Patients Who Left ER Before Being Seen	62,201	2%	3%	2%
Time from ER Arrival to Admit. (minutes)[2]	858	317	300	274
Time from ER Arrival to Discharge (minutes)	662	121	152	134
Time in ER Before Being Evaluated (minutes)	698	39	34	26
Time to Pain Meds for Fractures (minutes)	161	59	67	57
Heart Attack Care				
Aspirin Given at Discharge	44	100%	100%	99%
Fibrinolytic Meds Within 30 Min. of Arrival[7]	-	-	75%	54%
PCI Within 90 Minutes of Arrival[7]	-	-	98%	96%
Statin Prescribed at Discharge	50	98%	99%	98%
Heart Failure Care				
ACE Inhibitor or ARB for LVSD	50	96%	98%	97%
Discharge Instructions Given	130	95%	96%	94%
Evaluation of LVS Function	158	99%	100%	99%
Medicare Spending				
Medicare Spending per Patient (ratio)	-	0.92	0.94	0.98
Pneumonia Care				
Appropriate Initial Antibiotic Given	218	97%	97%	95%
Blood Culture Timing	368	98%	98%	98%
Pregnancy and Delivery Care				
Newborn Deliveries Scheduled Early[2]	84	0%	3%	6%
Preventive Care				
Immunization for Influenza[2]	738	99%	93%	90%
Immunization for Pneumonia[2]	970	99%	94%	92%
Stroke Care				
Anticoagulation Therapy for Atrial Fibrillation	13	85%	95%	95%
Antithrombotic Therapy Timing	66	98%	98%	98%
Assessed for Rehabilitation	74	97%	98%	97%
Discharged on Antithrombotic Therapy	72	99%	99%	99%
Discharged on Statin Medication	63	81%	94%	94%
Thrombolytic Therapy Timing	13	38%	64%	66%
Venous Thromboembolism Prophylaxis	71	96%	96%	94%
Written Stroke Educational Materials Given	35	74%	88%	88%
Surgical Care Improvement Project				
Appropriate Beta Blocker Usage	85	100%	99%	98%
Appropriate VTP Within 24 Hours	294	99%	99%	98%
Controlled Postoperative Blood Glucose[7]	-	-	98%	97%
Perioperative Temperature Management	321	100%	100%	100%
Prophylactic Antibiotic Selection	195	99%	99%	99%
Prophylactic Antibiotic Selection (Outpatient)	250	94%	98%	98%
Prophylactic Antibiotic Stopped	176	99%	99%	98%
Prophylactic Antibiotic Timing	195	100%	99%	99%
Prophylactic Antibiotic Timing (Outpatient)	259	95%	99%	98%
Urinary Catheter Removal	251	100%	99%	97%
Survey of Patients' Hospital Experiences				
Area Around Room 'Always' Quiet at Night	300+	64%	64%	61%
Doctors 'Always' Communicated Well	300+	80%	83%	82%
Home Recovery Information Given	300+	89%	87%	85%
Hospital Given 9 or 10 on 10 Point Scale	300+	71%	71%	71%
Meds 'Always' Explained Before Given	300+	63%	65%	64%
Nurses 'Always' Communicated Well	300+	80%	81%	79%
Pain 'Always' Well Controlled	300+	73%	72%	71%
Room and Bathroom 'Always' Clean	300+	74%	72%	73%
Timely Help 'Always' Received	300+	70%	68%	68%
Would Definitely Recommend Hospital	300+	70%	70%	71%
Use of Medical Imaging				
Cardiac Imaging Stress Test before Surgery	374	7.8%	5.4%	5.3%
Combination Abdominal CT Scan	903	3.4%	5.6%	10.5%
Combination Brain/Sinus CT Scan	777	1.4%	2.6%	2.7%
Combination Chest CT Scan	456	0.2%	1.3%	2.7%
Follow-up Mammogram/Ultrasound	1,368	10.8%	8%	8.8%
Lumbar Spine MRI for Low Back Pain	112	33.9%	34.7%	37.2%

Northern Hospital of Surry County

830 Rockford St
Mount Airy, NC 27030
URL: www.northernhospital.com
Type: Acute Care Hospitals
Ownership: Govt - Hospital Dist/Auth
Phone: 336-719-7000
Fax: 336-789-3470
Emergency Services: Yes
Beds: 113

Key Personnel:
Infection Control. . . . . Debbie Borawski, RN
Quality Assurance . . . . Deborah Borawski
Coronary Care . . . . Randy Collins, RN
Operating Room. . . . . Terri Grace, RN
CEO/President. . . . . William James
Chief of Medical Staff. . . . . Bill Refvem, MD
Radiology. . . . . Eric S Scharling

Measure	Cases	This Hosp.	State Avg.	U.S. Avg.
Blood Clot Prevention and Treatment				
Anticoagulation Overlap Therapy[2]	34	100%	94%	93%
ICU Venous Thromboembolism Prophylaxis[2]	62	100%	93%	92%
Incidence of Potentially Preventable VTE[1,2]	-	-	10%	10%
UFH with Dosages/Platelet Monitoring[1,2]	-	-	95%	97%
Venous Thromboembolism Prophylaxis[2]	336	98%	88%	85%
Warfarin Therapy Discharge Instructions[2]	23	83%	81%	75%
Chest Pain/Possible Heart Attack Care				
Aspirin Given Within 24 Hours of Arrival	132	99%	97%	96%
Fibrinolytic Meds Within 30 Min. of Arrival[7]	-	-	66%	58%
Average Time to ECG (minutes)	141	10	7	7
Average Time to Transfer (minutes)	12	42	45	60
Children's Asthma Care				
Received Home Management Plan of Care	-	-	89%	88%
Received Reliever Medication	-	-	100%	100%
Received Systemic Corticosteroids	-	-	100%	100%
Emergency Department				
Admittance Decision Time (minutes)[2]	632	97	107	98
Head CT Results Within 45 Min. of Arrival	15	60%	60%	57%
Patients Who Left ER Before Being Seen	37,312	0%	3%	2%
Time from ER Arrival to Admit. (minutes)[2]	640	297	300	274
Time from ER Arrival to Discharge (minutes)	432	133	152	134
Time in ER Before Being Evaluated (minutes)	475	24	34	26
Time to Pain Meds for Fractures (minutes)	100	60	67	57
Heart Attack Care				
Aspirin Given at Discharge[1]	-	-	100%	99%
Fibrinolytic Meds Within 30 Min. of Arrival[7]	-	-	75%	54%
PCI Within 90 Minutes of Arrival[7]	-	-	98%	96%
Statin Prescribed at Discharge[1]	-	-	99%	98%
Heart Failure Care				
ACE Inhibitor or ARB for LVSD	32	100%	98%	97%
Discharge Instructions Given	94	94%	96%	94%
Evaluation of LVS Function	121	100%	100%	99%
Medicare Spending				
Medicare Spending per Patient (ratio)	-	0.96	0.94	0.98
Pneumonia Care				
Appropriate Initial Antibiotic Given	143	98%	97%	95%
Blood Culture Timing	239	99%	98%	98%
Pregnancy and Delivery Care				
Newborn Deliveries Scheduled Early	48	0%	3%	6%
Preventive Care				
Immunization for Influenza[2]	410	99%	93%	90%
Immunization for Pneumonia[2]	553	100%	94%	92%
Stroke Care				
Anticoagulation Therapy for Atrial Fibrillation[1]	-	-	95%	95%
Antithrombotic Therapy Timing	29	100%	98%	98%
Assessed for Rehabilitation	29	100%	98%	97%
Discharged on Antithrombotic Therapy	29	100%	99%	99%
Discharged on Statin Medication	21	100%	94%	94%
Thrombolytic Therapy Timing[7]	-	-	64%	66%
Venous Thromboembolism Prophylaxis	28	100%	96%	94%
Written Stroke Educational Materials Given	16	81%	88%	88%
Surgical Care Improvement Project				
Appropriate Beta Blocker Usage	88	99%	99%	98%
Appropriate VTP Within 24 Hours	249	98%	99%	98%
Controlled Postoperative Blood Glucose[7]	-	-	98%	97%
Perioperative Temperature Management	267	100%	100%	100%
Prophylactic Antibiotic Selection	182	99%	99%	99%
Prophylactic Antibiotic Selection (Outpatient)	42	100%	98%	98%
Prophylactic Antibiotic Stopped	179	97%	99%	98%
Prophylactic Antibiotic Timing	182	99%	99%	99%
Prophylactic Antibiotic Timing (Outpatient)	43	98%	99%	98%
Urinary Catheter Removal	90	100%	99%	97%
Survey of Patients' Hospital Experiences				
Area Around Room 'Always' Quiet at Night	300+	65%	64%	61%
Doctors 'Always' Communicated Well	300+	78%	83%	82%
Home Recovery Information Given	300+	88%	87%	85%
Hospital Given 9 or 10 on 10 Point Scale	300+	69%	71%	71%
Meds 'Always' Explained Before Given	300+	58%	65%	64%
Nurses 'Always' Communicated Well	300+	79%	81%	79%
Pain 'Always' Well Controlled	300+	70%	72%	71%
Room and Bathroom 'Always' Clean	300+	75%	72%	73%
Timely Help 'Always' Received	300+	67%	68%	68%
Would Definitely Recommend Hospital	300+	66%	70%	71%
Use of Medical Imaging				

NOTE: Hospital profiles are in alphabetical order by state, then city, then hospital within the city; Rankings exclude hospitals with less than 25 cases except for patient surveys which excludes hospitals with less than 100 cases; (a) 100-299 cases; (1) The number of cases/patients is too few to report; (2) Data submitted were based on a sample of cases/patients; (3) Results are based on a shorter time period than required; (4) Data suppressed by CMS for one or more quarters; (5) Results are not available for this reporting period; (6) Fewer than 100 patients completed the HCAHPS survey; (7) No cases met the criteria for this measure; (8) The lower limit of the confidence interval cannot be calculated if the number of observed infections equals zero; (9) No data are available from the state/territory for this reporting period; (10) The scores shown reflect fewer than 50 completed surveys; (11) There were discrepancies in the data collection process; (12) This measure does not apply to this hospital for this reporting period; (13) Results cannot be calculated for this reporting period; (14) The results for this state are combined with nearby states to protect confidentiality; Please refer to the User's Guide for a full explanation of data.

Cardiac Imaging Stress Test before Surgery	105	2.9%	5.4%	5.3%
Combination Abdominal CT Scan	999	3.4%	5.6%	10.5%
Combination Brain/Sinus CT Scan	1,065	4.7%	2.6%	2.7%
Combination Chest CT Scan	483	0.2%	1.3%	2.7%
Follow-up Mammogram/Ultrasound	1,146	11.7%	8%	8.8%
Lumbar Spine MRI for Low Back Pain	130	35.4%	34.7%	37.2%

Murphy Medical Center

3990 East Us Highway 64 Alt
Murphy, NC 28906
Type: Acute Care Hospitals
Ownership: Voluntary non-profit - Private
Phone: 828-837-8161
Fax: 828-835-7507
Emergency Services: Yes
Beds: 184

Key Personnel:

Quality Assurance . . . . Sherrie Maze
CEO/President. . . . . Mark Stevenson
Emergency Room . . . . Mark Walters, MD
Chief of Medical Staff. . . . . Steven Zimmer, MD

Measure	Cases	This Hosp.	State Avg.	U.S. Avg.
Blood Clot Prevention and Treatment				
Anticoagulation Overlap Therapy[2]	17	94%	94%	93%
ICU Venous Thromboembolism Prophylaxis[2]	111	89%	93%	92%
Incidence of Potentially Preventable VTE[1,2]	-	-	10%	10%
UFH with Dosages/Platelet Monitoring[1,2]	-	-	95%	97%
Venous Thromboembolism Prophylaxis[2]	254	89%	88%	85%
Warfarin Therapy Discharge Instructions[2]	12	75%	81%	75%
Chest Pain/Possible Heart Attack Care				
Aspirin Given Within 24 Hours of Arrival	107	98%	97%	96%
Fibrinolytic Meds Within 30 Min. of Arrival[1]	-	-	66%	58%
Average Time to ECG (minutes)	110	6	7	7
Average Time to Transfer (minutes)[1]	-	-	45	60
Children's Asthma Care				
Received Home Management Plan of Care	-	-	89%	88%
Received Reliever Medication	-	-	100%	100%
Received Systemic Corticosteroids	-	-	100%	100%
Emergency Department				
Admittance Decision Time (minutes)[2]	616	115	107	98
Head CT Results Within 45 Min. of Arrival	12	67%	60%	57%
Patients Who Left ER Before Being Seen	16,581	3%	3%	2%
Time from ER Arrival to Admit. (minutes)[2]	706	260	300	274
Time from ER Arrival to Discharge (minutes)	1,120	162	152	134
Time in ER Before Being Evaluated (minutes)	1,235	38	34	26
Time to Pain Meds for Fractures (minutes)	100	64	67	57
Heart Attack Care				
Aspirin Given at Discharge[1]	-	-	100%	99%
Fibrinolytic Meds Within 30 Min. of Arrival[7]	-	-	75%	54%
PCI Within 90 Minutes of Arrival[7]	-	-	98%	96%
Statin Prescribed at Discharge[1]	-	-	99%	98%
Heart Failure Care				
ACE Inhibitor or ARB for LVSD	23	87%	98%	97%
Discharge Instructions Given	49	82%	96%	94%
Evaluation of LVS Function	65	98%	100%	99%
Medicare Spending				
Medicare Spending per Patient (ratio)	-	0.88	0.94	0.98
Pneumonia Care				
Appropriate Initial Antibiotic Given	80	95%	97%	95%
Blood Culture Timing	117	96%	98%	98%
Pregnancy and Delivery Care				
Newborn Deliveries Scheduled Early[1]	-	-	3%	6%
Preventive Care				
Immunization for Influenza[2]	493	92%	93%	90%
Immunization for Pneumonia[2]	715	89%	94%	92%
Stroke Care				
Anticoagulation Therapy for Atrial Fibrillation[1]	-	-	95%	95%
Antithrombotic Therapy Timing	16	94%	98%	98%
Assessed for Rehabilitation	17	100%	98%	97%
Discharged on Antithrombotic Therapy	16	100%	99%	99%
Discharged on Statin Medication	12	92%	94%	94%
Thrombolytic Therapy Timing[1]	-	-	64%	66%
Venous Thromboembolism Prophylaxis	17	100%	96%	94%
Written Stroke Educational Materials Given[1]	-	-	88%	88%
Surgical Care Improvement Project				
Appropriate Beta Blocker Usage	53	94%	99%	98%
Appropriate VTP Within 24 Hours	162	100%	99%	98%
Controlled Postoperative Blood Glucose[7]	-	-	98%	97%
Perioperative Temperature Management	171	100%	100%	100%
Prophylactic Antibiotic Selection	144	100%	99%	99%
Prophylactic Antibiotic Selection (Outpatient)	11	91%	98%	98%
Prophylactic Antibiotic Stopped	139	99%	99%	98%
Prophylactic Antibiotic Timing	144	99%	99%	99%
Prophylactic Antibiotic Timing (Outpatient)	12	75%	99%	98%
Urinary Catheter Removal	134	98%	99%	97%
Survey of Patients' Hospital Experiences				
Area Around Room 'Always' Quiet at Night	300+	53%	64%	61%
Doctors 'Always' Communicated Well	300+	84%	83%	82%
Home Recovery Information Given	300+	83%	87%	85%
Hospital Given 9 or 10 on 10 Point Scale	300+	62%	71%	71%
Meds 'Always' Explained Before Given	300+	66%	65%	64%
Nurses 'Always' Communicated Well	300+	80%	81%	79%
Pain 'Always' Well Controlled	300+	71%	72%	71%
Room and Bathroom 'Always' Clean	300+	68%	72%	73%
Timely Help 'Always' Received	300+	72%	68%	68%
Would Definitely Recommend Hospital	300+	62%	70%	71%
Use of Medical Imaging				
Cardiac Imaging Stress Test before Surgery	120	5.0%	5.4%	5.3%
Combination Abdominal CT Scan	649	12.8%	5.6%	10.5%
Combination Brain/Sinus CT Scan	573	1.4%	2.6%	2.7%
Combination Chest CT Scan	236	3.0%	1.3%	2.7%
Follow-up Mammogram/Ultrasound	1,022	7.7%	8%	8.8%
Lumbar Spine MRI for Low Back Pain	109	36.7%	34.7%	37.2%

The Outer Banks Hospital

4800 South Croatan Highway
Nags Head, NC 27959
URL: www.theouterbankshospital.com
Type: Critical Access Hospitals
Ownership: Voluntary non-profit - Private
Phone: 252-449-4500
Emergency Services: Yes
Beds: 19

Key Personnel:

President . . . . Ronnie Sloan, FACHE

Measure	Cases	This Hosp.	State Avg.	U.S. Avg.
Blood Clot Prevention and Treatment				
Anticoagulation Overlap Therapy[5]	-	-	94%	93%
ICU Venous Thromboembolism Prophylaxis[5]	-	-	93%	92%
Incidence of Potentially Preventable VTE[5]	-	-	10%	10%
UFH with Dosages/Platelet Monitoring[5]	-	-	95%	97%
Venous Thromboembolism Prophylaxis[5]	-	-	88%	85%
Warfarin Therapy Discharge Instructions[5]	-	-	81%	75%
Chest Pain/Possible Heart Attack Care				
Aspirin Given Within 24 Hours of Arrival	-	-	97%	96%
Fibrinolytic Meds Within 30 Min. of Arrival	-	-	66%	58%
Average Time to ECG (minutes)	-	-	7	7
Average Time to Transfer (minutes)	-	-	45	60
Children's Asthma Care				
Received Home Management Plan of Care	-	-	89%	88%
Received Reliever Medication	-	-	100%	100%
Received Systemic Corticosteroids	-	-	100%	100%
Emergency Department				
Admittance Decision Time (minutes)[2]	221	175	107	98
Head CT Results Within 45 Min. of Arrival	-	-	60%	57%
Patients Who Left ER Before Being Seen	-	-	3%	2%
Time from ER Arrival to Admit. (minutes)[2]	226	350	300	274
Time from ER Arrival to Discharge (minutes)	-	-	152	134
Time in ER Before Being Evaluated (minutes)	-	-	34	26
Time to Pain Meds for Fractures (minutes)	-	-	67	57
Heart Attack Care				
Aspirin Given at Discharge[5]	-	-	100%	99%
Fibrinolytic Meds Within 30 Min. of Arrival[5]	-	-	75%	54%
PCI Within 90 Minutes of Arrival[5]	-	-	98%	96%
Statin Prescribed at Discharge[5]	-	-	99%	98%
Heart Failure Care				
ACE Inhibitor or ARB for LVSD[1]	-	-	98%	97%
Discharge Instructions Given	16	100%	96%	94%
Evaluation of LVS Function	19	100%	100%	99%
Medicare Spending				
Medicare Spending per Patient (ratio)	-	-	0.94	0.98
Pneumonia Care				
Appropriate Initial Antibiotic Given	55	100%	97%	95%
Blood Culture Timing	71	99%	98%	98%
Pregnancy and Delivery Care				
Newborn Deliveries Scheduled Early[5]	-	-	3%	6%
Preventive Care				
Immunization for Influenza[5]	-	-	93%	90%
Immunization for Pneumonia[5]	-	-	94%	92%
Stroke Care				
Anticoagulation Therapy for Atrial Fibrillation[5]	-	-	95%	95%
Antithrombotic Therapy Timing[5]	-	-	98%	98%
Assessed for Rehabilitation[5]	-	-	98%	97%
Discharged on Antithrombotic Therapy[5]	-	-	99%	99%
Discharged on Statin Medication[5]	-	-	94%	94%
Thrombolytic Therapy Timing[5]	-	-	64%	66%
Venous Thromboembolism Prophylaxis[5]	-	-	96%	94%
Written Stroke Educational Materials Given[5]	-	-	88%	88%
Surgical Care Improvement Project				
Appropriate Beta Blocker Usage	45	96%	99%	98%
Appropriate VTP Within 24 Hours	151	100%	99%	98%
Controlled Postoperative Blood Glucose[7]	-	-	98%	97%
Perioperative Temperature Management	151	100%	100%	100%
Prophylactic Antibiotic Selection	124	100%	99%	99%
Prophylactic Antibiotic Selection (Outpatient)	-	-	98%	98%
Prophylactic Antibiotic Stopped	120	98%	99%	98%
Prophylactic Antibiotic Timing	124	98%	99%	99%
Prophylactic Antibiotic Timing (Outpatient)	-	-	99%	98%
Urinary Catheter Removal	137	100%	99%	97%
Survey of Patients' Hospital Experiences				
Area Around Room 'Always' Quiet at Night	300+	65%	64%	61%
Doctors 'Always' Communicated Well	300+	88%	83%	82%
Home Recovery Information Given	300+	92%	87%	85%
Hospital Given 9 or 10 on 10 Point Scale	300+	82%	71%	71%
Meds 'Always' Explained Before Given	300+	76%	65%	64%
Nurses 'Always' Communicated Well	300+	84%	81%	79%
Pain 'Always' Well Controlled	300+	78%	72%	71%
Room and Bathroom 'Always' Clean	300+	78%	72%	73%
Timely Help 'Always' Received	300+	81%	68%	68%
Would Definitely Recommend Hospital	300+	79%	70%	71%
Use of Medical Imaging				
Cardiac Imaging Stress Test before Surgery	-	-	5.4%	5.3%
Combination Abdominal CT Scan	-	-	5.6%	10.5%
Combination Brain/Sinus CT Scan	-	-	2.6%	2.7%
Combination Chest CT Scan	-	-	1.3%	2.7%
Follow-up Mammogram/Ultrasound	-	-	8%	8.8%
Lumbar Spine MRI for Low Back Pain	-	-	34.7%	37.2%

Carolina East Medical Center

2000 Neuse Blvd
New Bern, NC 28560
URL: www.cravenhealthcare.org
Type: Acute Care Hospitals
Ownership: Govt - Hospital Dist/Auth
Phone: 252-633-8640
Fax: 252-633-8144
Emergency Services: Yes
Beds: 350

Key Personnel:

Quality Assurance . . . . Pam Burkett
Infection Control. . . . . Cathy Fischer
CEO/President. . . . . G Raymond Leggett III
Chief of Medical Staff . . . . Ron May, MD
Pediatric In-Patient Care . . . . Cyndi Morton, RN
Patient Relations . . . . Leslie Pittman
Operating Room. . . . . Robin Schaefer
Radiology. . . . . David Williams

Measure	Cases	This Hosp.	State Avg.	U.S. Avg.
Blood Clot Prevention and Treatment				
Anticoagulation Overlap Therapy[2]	64	95%	94%	93%
ICU Venous Thromboembolism Prophylaxis[2]	75	91%	93%	92%
Incidence of Potentially Preventable VTE[2]	16	19%	10%	10%
UFH with Dosages/Platelet Monitoring[2]	25	100%	95%	97%
Venous Thromboembolism Prophylaxis[2]	332	82%	88%	85%
Warfarin Therapy Discharge Instructions[2]	51	100%	81%	75%
Chest Pain/Possible Heart Attack Care				
Aspirin Given Within 24 Hours of Arrival	12	92%	97%	96%
Fibrinolytic Meds Within 30 Min. of Arrival[3,7]	-	-	66%	58%
Average Time to ECG (minutes)	12	0	7	7
Average Time to Transfer (minutes)[3,7]	-	-	45	60
Children's Asthma Care				

NOTE: Hospital profiles are in alphabetical order by state, then city, then hospital within the city; Rankings exclude hospitals with less than 25 cases except for patient surveys which excludes hospitals with less than 100 cases; (a) 100-299 cases; (1) The number of cases/patients is too few to report; (2) Data submitted were based on a sample of cases/patients; (3) Results are based on a shorter time period than required; (4) Data suppressed by CMS for one or more quarters; (5) Results are not available for this reporting period; (6) Fewer than 100 patients completed the HCAHPS survey; (7) No cases met the criteria for this measure; (8) The lower limit of the confidence interval cannot be calculated if the number of observed infections equals zero; (9) No data are available from the state/territory for this reporting period; (10) The scores shown reflect fewer than 50 completed surveys; (11) There were discrepancies in the data collection process; (12) This measure does not apply to this hospital for this reporting period; (13) Results cannot be calculated for this reporting period; (14) The results for this state are combined with nearby states to protect confidentiality; Please refer to the User's Guide for a full explanation of data.

Measure	Cases	This Hosp.	State Avg.	U.S. Avg.
Received Home Management Plan of Care	-	-	89%	88%
Received Reliever Medication	-	-	100%	100%
Received Systemic Corticosteroids	-	-	100%	100%
Emergency Department				
Admittance Decision Time (minutes)[2]	496	163	107	98
Head CT Results Within 45 Min. of Arrival	23	52%	60%	57%
Patients Who Left ER Before Being Seen	40,541	3%	3%	2%
Time from ER Arrival to Admit. (minutes)[2]	666	336	300	274
Time from ER Arrival to Discharge (minutes)	511	208	152	134
Time in ER Before Being Evaluated (minutes)	320	33	34	26
Time to Pain Meds for Fractures (minutes)	102	78	67	57
Heart Attack Care				
Aspirin Given at Discharge	397	99%	100%	99%
Fibrinolytic Meds Within 30 Min. of Arrival[7]	-	-	75%	54%
PCI Within 90 Minutes of Arrival	54	94%	98%	96%
Statin Prescribed at Discharge	371	96%	99%	98%
Heart Failure Care				
ACE Inhibitor or ARB for LVSD	125	99%	98%	97%
Discharge Instructions Given	350	83%	96%	94%
Evaluation of LVS Function	410	100%	100%	99%
Medicare Spending				
Medicare Spending per Patient (ratio)	-	0.90	0.94	0.98
Pneumonia Care				
Appropriate Initial Antibiotic Given	189	91%	97%	95%
Blood Culture Timing	345	98%	98%	98%
Pregnancy and Delivery Care				
Newborn Deliveries Scheduled Early	119	4%	3%	6%
Preventive Care				
Immunization for Influenza[2]	569	90%	93%	90%
Immunization for Pneumonia[2]	750	85%	94%	92%
Stroke Care				
Anticoagulation Therapy for Atrial Fibrillation	17	94%	95%	95%
Antithrombotic Therapy Timing	149	99%	98%	98%
Assessed for Rehabilitation	152	93%	98%	97%
Discharged on Antithrombotic Therapy	150	99%	99%	99%
Discharged on Statin Medication	119	92%	94%	94%
Thrombolytic Therapy Timing[1]	-	-	64%	66%
Venous Thromboembolism Prophylaxis	136	85%	96%	94%
Written Stroke Educational Materials Given	96	81%	88%	88%
Surgical Care Improvement Project				
Appropriate Beta Blocker Usage	442	99%	99%	98%
Appropriate VTP Within 24 Hours	972	97%	99%	98%
Controlled Postoperative Blood Glucose	172	97%	98%	97%
Perioperative Temperature Management	1,092	100%	100%	100%
Prophylactic Antibiotic Selection	914	98%	99%	99%
Prophylactic Antibiotic Selection (Outpatient)	693	87%	98%	98%
Prophylactic Antibiotic Stopped	884	95%	99%	98%
Prophylactic Antibiotic Timing	915	98%	99%	99%
Prophylactic Antibiotic Timing (Outpatient)	695	97%	99%	98%
Urinary Catheter Removal	941	96%	99%	97%
Survey of Patients' Hospital Experiences				
Area Around Room 'Always' Quiet at Night	300+	61%	64%	61%
Doctors 'Always' Communicated Well	300+	83%	83%	82%
Home Recovery Information Given	300+	87%	87%	85%
Hospital Given 9 or 10 on 10 Point Scale	300+	74%	71%	71%
Meds 'Always' Explained Before Given	300+	69%	65%	64%
Nurses 'Always' Communicated Well	300+	84%	81%	79%
Pain 'Always' Well Controlled	300+	74%	72%	71%
Room and Bathroom 'Always' Clean	300+	73%	72%	73%
Timely Help 'Always' Received	300+	74%	68%	68%
Would Definitely Recommend Hospital	300+	76%	70%	71%
Use of Medical Imaging				
Cardiac Imaging Stress Test before Surgery	564	7.1%	5.4%	5.3%
Combination Abdominal CT Scan	968	6.8%	5.6%	10.5%
Combination Brain/Sinus CT Scan	1,404	1.7%	2.6%	2.7%
Combination Chest CT Scan	297	0.0%	1.3%	2.7%
Follow-up Mammogram/Ultrasound	1,149	5.8%	8%	8.8%
Lumbar Spine MRI for Low Back Pain	129	38.8%	34.7%	37.2%

Wilkes Regional Medical Center

1370 West D St
North Wilkesboro, NC 28659
URL: www.wilkesregional.com
Type: Acute Care Hospitals
Ownership: Government - Local

Phone: 336-651-8100
Fax: 336-651-8196
Emergency Services: Yes
Beds: 120

Key Personnel:
Chief of Medical Staff.......... Susan Albert
Radiology.................. Gregory Evans
CEO/President.............. David Henson

Measure	Cases	This Hosp.	State Avg.	U.S. Avg.
Blood Clot Prevention and Treatment				
Anticoagulation Overlap Therapy[2]	27	100%	94%	93%
ICU Venous Thromboembolism Prophylaxis[2]	126	99%	93%	92%
Incidence of Potentially Preventable VTE[1,2]	-	-	10%	10%
UFH with Dosages/Platelet Monitoring[1,2]	-	-	95%	97%
Venous Thromboembolism Prophylaxis[2]	274	99%	88%	85%
Warfarin Therapy Discharge Instructions[2]	19	100%	81%	75%
Chest Pain/Possible Heart Attack Care				
Aspirin Given Within 24 Hours of Arrival	90	100%	97%	96%
Fibrinolytic Meds Within 30 Min. of Arrival[7]	-	-	66%	58%
Average Time to ECG (minutes)	97	5	7	7
Average Time to Transfer (minutes)[1]	-	-	45	60
Children's Asthma Care				
Received Home Management Plan of Care	-	-	89%	88%
Received Reliever Medication	-	-	100%	100%
Received Systemic Corticosteroids	-	-	100%	100%
Emergency Department				
Admittance Decision Time (minutes)[2]	637	48	107	98
Head CT Results Within 45 Min. of Arrival	20	60%	60%	57%
Patients Who Left ER Before Being Seen	32,584	1%	3%	2%
Time from ER Arrival to Admit. (minutes)[2]	637	225	300	274
Time from ER Arrival to Discharge (minutes)	356	117	152	134
Time in ER Before Being Evaluated (minutes)	380	23	34	26
Time to Pain Meds for Fractures (minutes)	135	49	67	57
Heart Attack Care				
Aspirin Given at Discharge[1]	-	-	100%	99%
Fibrinolytic Meds Within 30 Min. of Arrival[7]	-	-	75%	54%
PCI Within 90 Minutes of Arrival[7]	-	-	98%	96%
Statin Prescribed at Discharge[1]	-	-	99%	98%
Heart Failure Care				
ACE Inhibitor or ARB for LVSD	20	100%	98%	97%
Discharge Instructions Given	83	98%	96%	94%
Evaluation of LVS Function	120	100%	100%	99%
Medicare Spending				
Medicare Spending per Patient (ratio)	-	0.95	0.94	0.98
Pneumonia Care				
Appropriate Initial Antibiotic Given	159	94%	97%	95%
Blood Culture Timing	349	99%	98%	98%
Pregnancy and Delivery Care				
Newborn Deliveries Scheduled Early[2]	21	10%	3%	6%
Preventive Care				
Immunization for Influenza[2]	412	95%	93%	90%
Immunization for Pneumonia[2]	540	98%	94%	92%
Stroke Care				
Anticoagulation Therapy for Atrial Fibrillation[1]	-	-	95%	95%
Antithrombotic Therapy Timing	41	100%	98%	98%
Assessed for Rehabilitation	40	100%	98%	97%
Discharged on Antithrombotic Therapy	37	100%	99%	99%
Discharged on Statin Medication	30	93%	94%	94%
Thrombolytic Therapy Timing[1]	-	-	64%	66%
Venous Thromboembolism Prophylaxis	43	100%	96%	94%
Written Stroke Educational Materials Given	23	91%	88%	88%
Surgical Care Improvement Project				
Appropriate Beta Blocker Usage	62	100%	99%	98%
Appropriate VTP Within 24 Hours	198	99%	99%	98%
Controlled Postoperative Blood Glucose[7]	-	-	98%	97%
Perioperative Temperature Management	210	100%	100%	100%
Prophylactic Antibiotic Selection	155	99%	99%	99%
Prophylactic Antibiotic Selection (Outpatient)	35	97%	98%	98%
Prophylactic Antibiotic Stopped	153	99%	99%	98%
Prophylactic Antibiotic Timing	155	100%	99%	99%
Prophylactic Antibiotic Timing (Outpatient)	36	97%	99%	98%
Urinary Catheter Removal	176	99%	99%	97%
Survey of Patients' Hospital Experiences				
Area Around Room 'Always' Quiet at Night	300+	62%	64%	61%
Doctors 'Always' Communicated Well	300+	82%	83%	82%
Home Recovery Information Given	300+	85%	87%	85%
Hospital Given 9 or 10 on 10 Point Scale	300+	68%	71%	71%
Meds 'Always' Explained Before Given	300+	65%	65%	64%
Nurses 'Always' Communicated Well	300+	78%	81%	79%
Pain 'Always' Well Controlled	300+	67%	72%	71%
Room and Bathroom 'Always' Clean	300+	70%	72%	73%
Timely Help 'Always' Received	300+	63%	68%	68%
Would Definitely Recommend Hospital	300+	67%	70%	71%
Use of Medical Imaging				
Cardiac Imaging Stress Test before Surgery	167	6.6%	5.4%	5.3%
Combination Abdominal CT Scan	889	5.7%	5.6%	10.5%
Combination Brain/Sinus CT Scan	749	1.6%	2.6%	2.7%
Combination Chest CT Scan	305	3.6%	1.3%	2.7%
Follow-up Mammogram/Ultrasound	1,476	8.3%	8%	8.8%
Lumbar Spine MRI for Low Back Pain	133	31.6%	34.7%	37.2%

Granville Health Systems

College Saint Box 947
Oxford, NC 27565
Type: Acute Care Hospitals
Ownership: Government - Local

Phone: 919-690-3000
Fax: 919-690-1430
Emergency Services: Yes
Beds: 142

Key Personnel:
Quality Assurance .... Ann Barnes
Infection Control.............. Jeanette Briggs, RN
Intensive Care Unit............ Stephen Ertischeck, MD
Chief of Medical Staff.......... D. Michael Mahan, MD
Anesthesiology............... Allen Ng, MD
CEO/President............... Joe Pollard
Radiology................... Michael P Stoll, MD
Emergency Room .... Robert Walston, MD

Measure	Cases	This Hosp.	State Avg.	U.S. Avg.
Blood Clot Prevention and Treatment				
Anticoagulation Overlap Therapy[1,2]	-	-	94%	93%
ICU Venous Thromboembolism Prophylaxis[2]	139	68%	93%	92%
Incidence of Potentially Preventable VTE[1,2]	-	-	10%	10%
UFH with Dosages/Platelet Monitoring[1,2]	-	-	95%	97%
Venous Thromboembolism Prophylaxis[2]	502	62%	88%	85%
Warfarin Therapy Discharge Instructions[1,2]	-	-	81%	75%
Chest Pain/Possible Heart Attack Care				
Aspirin Given Within 24 Hours of Arrival	44	100%	97%	96%
Fibrinolytic Meds Within 30 Min. of Arrival[7]	-	-	66%	58%
Average Time to ECG (minutes)	47	12	7	7
Average Time to Transfer (minutes)[1]	-	-	45	60
Children's Asthma Care				
Received Home Management Plan of Care	-	-	89%	88%
Received Reliever Medication	-	-	100%	100%
Received Systemic Corticosteroids	-	-	100%	100%
Emergency Department				
Admittance Decision Time (minutes)[2]	741	83	107	98
Head CT Results Within 45 Min. of Arrival[1]	-	-	60%	57%
Patients Who Left ER Before Being Seen	16,659	3%	3%	2%
Time from ER Arrival to Admit. (minutes)[2]	746	276	300	274
Time from ER Arrival to Discharge (minutes)	600	154	152	134
Time in ER Before Being Evaluated (minutes)	806	20	34	26
Time to Pain Meds for Fractures (minutes)	62	71	67	57
Heart Attack Care				
Aspirin Given at Discharge	13	92%	100%	99%
Fibrinolytic Meds Within 30 Min. of Arrival[7]	-	-	75%	54%
PCI Within 90 Minutes of Arrival[7]	-	-	98%	96%
Statin Prescribed at Discharge	13	92%	99%	98%
Heart Failure Care				
ACE Inhibitor or ARB for LVSD	29	100%	98%	97%
Discharge Instructions Given	66	97%	96%	94%
Evaluation of LVS Function	82	99%	100%	99%
Medicare Spending				
Medicare Spending per Patient (ratio)	-	0.89	0.94	0.98
Pneumonia Care				
Appropriate Initial Antibiotic Given	62	94%	97%	95%
Blood Culture Timing	80	94%	98%	98%
Pregnancy and Delivery Care				

NOTE: Hospital profiles are in alphabetical order by state, then city, then hospital within the city; Rankings exclude hospitals with less than 25 cases except for patient surveys which excludes hospitals with less than 100 cases; (a) 100-299 cases; (1) The number of cases/patients is too few to report; (2) Data submitted were based on a sample of cases/patients; (3) Results are based on a shorter time period than required; (4) Data suppressed by CMS for one or more quarters; (5) Results are not available for this reporting period; (6) Fewer than 100 patients completed the HCAHPS survey; (7) No cases met the criteria for this measure; (8) The lower limit of the confidence interval cannot be calculated if the number of observed infections equals zero; (9) No data are available from the state/territory for this reporting period; (10) The scores shown reflect fewer than 50 completed surveys; (11) There were discrepancies in the data collection process; (12) This measure does not apply to this hospital for this reporting period; (13) Results cannot be calculated for this reporting period; (14) The results for this state are combined with nearby states to protect confidentiality; Please refer to the User's Guide for a full explanation of data.

Measure	Cases	This Hosp.	State Avg.	U.S. Avg.
Newborn Deliveries Scheduled Early	29	7%	3%	6%
Preventive Care				
Immunization for Influenza[2]	445	88%	93%	90%
Immunization for Pneumonia[2]	775	95%	94%	92%
Stroke Care				
Anticoagulation Therapy for Atrial Fibrillation[1]	-	-	95%	95%
Antithrombotic Therapy Timing	21	90%	98%	98%
Assessed for Rehabilitation	21	95%	98%	97%
Discharged on Antithrombotic Therapy	20	85%	99%	99%
Discharged on Statin Medication	17	82%	94%	94%
Thrombolytic Therapy Timing[1]	-	-	64%	66%
Venous Thromboembolism Prophylaxis	24	79%	96%	94%
Written Stroke Educational Materials Given	15	40%	88%	88%
Surgical Care Improvement Project				
Appropriate Beta Blocker Usage	62	94%	99%	98%
Appropriate VTP Within 24 Hours	145	99%	99%	98%
Controlled Postoperative Blood Glucose[7]	-	-	98%	97%
Perioperative Temperature Management	213	100%	100%	100%
Prophylactic Antibiotic Selection	136	100%	99%	99%
Prophylactic Antibiotic Selection (Outpatient)	90	93%	98%	98%
Prophylactic Antibiotic Stopped	129	95%	99%	98%
Prophylactic Antibiotic Timing	136	99%	99%	99%
Prophylactic Antibiotic Timing (Outpatient)	90	98%	99%	98%
Urinary Catheter Removal	165	95%	99%	97%
Survey of Patients' Hospital Experiences				
Area Around Room 'Always' Quiet at Night	300+	62%	64%	61%
Doctors 'Always' Communicated Well	300+	82%	83%	82%
Home Recovery Information Given	300+	85%	87%	85%
Hospital Given 9 or 10 on 10 Point Scale	300+	60%	71%	71%
Meds 'Always' Explained Before Given	300+	65%	65%	64%
Nurses 'Always' Communicated Well	300+	78%	81%	79%
Pain 'Always' Well Controlled	300+	68%	72%	71%
Room and Bathroom 'Always' Clean	300+	57%	72%	73%
Timely Help 'Always' Received	300+	65%	68%	68%
Would Definitely Recommend Hospital	300+	60%	70%	71%
Use of Medical Imaging				
Cardiac Imaging Stress Test before Surgery	136	7.4%	5.4%	5.3%
Combination Abdominal CT Scan	335	6.0%	5.6%	10.5%
Combination Brain/Sinus CT Scan[1]	-	-	2.6%	2.7%
Combination Chest CT Scan	155	4.5%	1.3%	2.7%
Follow-up Mammogram/Ultrasound	532	13.9%	8%	8.8%
Lumbar Spine MRI for Low Back Pain	102	35.3%	34.7%	37.2%

Firsthealth Moore Regional Hospital

155 Memorial Drive
Pinehurst, NC 28374
Phone: 910-715-1000
Fax: 910-715-1444
URL: www.firsthealth.org
Type: Acute Care Hospitals
Emergency Services: Yes
Ownership: Voluntary non-profit - Private
Beds: 395

Key Personnel:
Radiology. . . . . Ole S Aassar
Coronary Care . . . . Beverly Alphin
Quality Assurance . . . . Barbara Bennett
CEO/President. . . . . Charles T Frock
Infection Control. . . . . Jayne Lee
Cardiac Laboratory. . . . . Roger Noble
Chief of Medical Staff . . . . Ward S Oakley
Operating Room. . . . . Ken Schwann

Measure	Cases	This Hosp.	State Avg.	U.S. Avg.
Blood Clot Prevention and Treatment				
Anticoagulation Overlap Therapy[2]	170	87%	94%	93%
ICU Venous Thromboembolism Prophylaxis[2]	85	87%	93%	92%
Incidence of Potentially Preventable VTE[2]	34	21%	10%	10%
UFH with Dosages/Platelet Monitoring[2]	66	100%	95%	97%
Venous Thromboembolism Prophylaxis[2]	316	81%	88%	85%
Warfarin Therapy Discharge Instructions[2]	126	97%	81%	75%
Chest Pain/Possible Heart Attack Care				
Aspirin Given Within 24 Hours of Arrival[1,3]	-	-	97%	96%
Fibrinolytic Meds Within 30 Min. of Arrival[3,7]	-	-	66%	58%
Average Time to ECG (minutes)[1,3]	-	-	7	7
Average Time to Transfer (minutes)[3,7]	-	-	45	60
Children's Asthma Care				
Received Home Management Plan of Care	55	89%	89%	88%
Received Reliever Medication	56	100%	100%	100%
Received Systemic Corticosteroids	56	100%	100%	100%
Emergency Department				
Admittance Decision Time (minutes)[2]	658	125	107	98
Head CT Results Within 45 Min. of Arrival[1]	-	-	60%	57%
Patients Who Left ER Before Being Seen	66,453	1%	3%	2%
Time from ER Arrival to Admit. (minutes)[2]	660	293	300	274
Time from ER Arrival to Discharge (minutes)	391	129	152	134
Time in ER Before Being Evaluated (minutes)	422	24	34	26
Time to Pain Meds for Fractures (minutes)	252	62	67	57
Heart Attack Care				
Aspirin Given at Discharge[2]	323	100%	100%	99%
Fibrinolytic Meds Within 30 Min. of Arrival[2,7]	-	-	75%	54%
PCI Within 90 Minutes of Arrival[2]	36	97%	98%	96%
Statin Prescribed at Discharge[2]	316	100%	99%	98%
Heart Failure Care				
ACE Inhibitor or ARB for LVSD[2]	100	98%	98%	97%
Discharge Instructions Given[2]	284	96%	96%	94%
Evaluation of LVS Function[2]	329	100%	100%	99%
Medicare Spending				
Medicare Spending per Patient (ratio)	-	0.92	0.94	0.98
Pneumonia Care				
Appropriate Initial Antibiotic Given[2]	111	95%	97%	95%
Blood Culture Timing[2]	197	99%	98%	98%
Pregnancy and Delivery Care				
Newborn Deliveries Scheduled Early[2]	29	0%	3%	6%
Preventive Care				
Immunization for Influenza[2]	583	93%	93%	90%
Immunization for Pneumonia[2]	799	94%	94%	92%
Stroke Care				
Anticoagulation Therapy for Atrial Fibrillation	47	100%	95%	95%
Antithrombotic Therapy Timing	288	100%	98%	98%
Assessed for Rehabilitation	324	100%	98%	97%
Discharged on Antithrombotic Therapy	299	100%	99%	99%
Discharged on Statin Medication	244	100%	94%	94%
Thrombolytic Therapy Timing	15	100%	64%	66%
Venous Thromboembolism Prophylaxis	319	98%	96%	94%
Written Stroke Educational Materials Given	187	99%	88%	88%
Surgical Care Improvement Project				
Appropriate Beta Blocker Usage[2]	307	99%	99%	98%
Appropriate VTP Within 24 Hours[2]	478	99%	99%	98%
Controlled Postoperative Blood Glucose[2]	182	98%	98%	97%
Perioperative Temperature Management[2]	623	100%	100%	100%
Prophylactic Antibiotic Selection[2]	589	99%	99%	99%
Prophylactic Antibiotic Selection (Outpatient)	632	99%	98%	98%
Prophylactic Antibiotic Stopped[2]	573	99%	99%	98%
Prophylactic Antibiotic Timing[2]	591	100%	99%	99%
Prophylactic Antibiotic Timing (Outpatient)	633	98%	99%	98%
Urinary Catheter Removal[2]	581	99%	99%	97%
Survey of Patients' Hospital Experiences				
Area Around Room 'Always' Quiet at Night	300+	65%	64%	61%
Doctors 'Always' Communicated Well	300+	86%	83%	82%
Home Recovery Information Given	300+	89%	87%	85%
Hospital Given 9 or 10 on 10 Point Scale	300+	82%	71%	71%
Meds 'Always' Explained Before Given	300+	70%	65%	64%
Nurses 'Always' Communicated Well	300+	85%	81%	79%
Pain 'Always' Well Controlled	300+	78%	72%	71%
Room and Bathroom 'Always' Clean	300+	75%	72%	73%
Timely Help 'Always' Received	300+	76%	68%	68%
Would Definitely Recommend Hospital	300+	84%	70%	71%
Use of Medical Imaging				
Cardiac Imaging Stress Test before Surgery	904	4.1%	5.4%	5.3%
Combination Abdominal CT Scan	1,577	7.4%	5.6%	10.5%
Combination Brain/Sinus CT Scan	1,923	2.6%	2.6%	2.7%
Combination Chest CT Scan	978	0.6%	1.3%	2.7%
Follow-up Mammogram/Ultrasound	1,487	6.4%	8%	8.8%
Lumbar Spine MRI for Low Back Pain	755	35.0%	34.7%	37.2%

Washington County Hospital

958 Us Hwy 64 East
Plymouth, NC 27962
Phone: 252-793-4135
Fax: 252-793-1530
URL: www.wchonline.com
Type: Critical Access Hospitals
Emergency Services: Yes
Ownership: Proprietary
Beds: 49

Key Personnel:
Chief of Medical Staff . . . . Robert Benadale
CEO/President. . . . . Betty Bowen
Emergency Room . . . . Ann Davenport
Coronary Care . . . . Sandy Downs
CEO . . . . Cameron Highsmith
Quality Assurance . . . . Deborah Raebuck

Measure	Cases	This Hosp.	State Avg.	U.S. Avg.
Blood Clot Prevention and Treatment				
Anticoagulation Overlap Therapy[5]	-	-	94%	93%
ICU Venous Thromboembolism Prophylaxis[5]	-	-	93%	92%
Incidence of Potentially Preventable VTE[5]	-	-	10%	10%
UFH with Dosages/Platelet Monitoring[5]	-	-	95%	97%
Venous Thromboembolism Prophylaxis[5]	-	-	88%	85%
Warfarin Therapy Discharge Instructions[5]	-	-	81%	75%
Chest Pain/Possible Heart Attack Care				
Aspirin Given Within 24 Hours of Arrival[5]	-	-	97%	96%
Fibrinolytic Meds Within 30 Min. of Arrival[5]	-	-	66%	58%
Average Time to ECG (minutes)[5]	-	-	7	7
Average Time to Transfer (minutes)[5]	-	-	45	60
Children's Asthma Care				
Received Home Management Plan of Care	-	-	89%	88%
Received Reliever Medication	-	-	100%	100%
Received Systemic Corticosteroids	-	-	100%	100%
Emergency Department				
Admittance Decision Time (minutes)[5]	-	-	107	98
Head CT Results Within 45 Min. of Arrival[5]	-	-	60%	57%
Patients Who Left ER Before Being Seen[5]	-	-	3%	2%
Time from ER Arrival to Admit. (minutes)[5]	-	-	300	274
Time from ER Arrival to Discharge (minutes)[5]	-	-	152	134
Time in ER Before Being Evaluated (minutes)[5]	-	-	34	26
Time to Pain Meds for Fractures (minutes)[5]	-	-	67	57
Heart Attack Care				
Aspirin Given at Discharge[5]	-	-	100%	99%
Fibrinolytic Meds Within 30 Min. of Arrival[5]	-	-	75%	54%
PCI Within 90 Minutes of Arrival[5]	-	-	98%	96%
Statin Prescribed at Discharge[5]	-	-	99%	98%
Heart Failure Care				
ACE Inhibitor or ARB for LVSD[5]	-	-	98%	97%
Discharge Instructions Given[5]	-	-	96%	94%
Evaluation of LVS Function[5]	-	-	100%	99%
Medicare Spending				
Medicare Spending per Patient (ratio)	-	-	0.94	0.98
Pneumonia Care				
Appropriate Initial Antibiotic Given[5]	-	-	97%	95%
Blood Culture Timing[5]	-	-	98%	98%
Pregnancy and Delivery Care				
Newborn Deliveries Scheduled Early[5]	-	-	3%	6%
Preventive Care				
Immunization for Influenza[5]	-	-	93%	90%
Immunization for Pneumonia[5]	-	-	94%	92%
Stroke Care				
Anticoagulation Therapy for Atrial Fibrillation[5]	-	-	95%	95%
Antithrombotic Therapy Timing[5]	-	-	98%	98%
Assessed for Rehabilitation[5]	-	-	98%	97%
Discharged on Antithrombotic Therapy[5]	-	-	99%	99%
Discharged on Statin Medication[5]	-	-	94%	94%
Thrombolytic Therapy Timing[5]	-	-	64%	66%
Venous Thromboembolism Prophylaxis[5]	-	-	96%	94%
Written Stroke Educational Materials Given[5]	-	-	88%	88%
Surgical Care Improvement Project				
Appropriate Beta Blocker Usage[5]	-	-	99%	98%
Appropriate VTP Within 24 Hours[5]	-	-	99%	98%
Controlled Postoperative Blood Glucose[5]	-	-	98%	97%
Perioperative Temperature Management[5]	-	-	100%	100%
Prophylactic Antibiotic Selection[5]	-	-	99%	99%
Prophylactic Antibiotic Selection (Outpatient)[5]	-	-	98%	98%
Prophylactic Antibiotic Stopped[5]	-	-	99%	98%

NOTE: Hospital profiles are in alphabetical order by state, then city, then hospital within the city; Rankings exclude hospitals with less than 25 cases except for patient surveys which excludes hospitals with less than 100 cases; (a) 100-299 cases; (1) The number of cases/patients is too few to report; (2) Data submitted were based on a sample of cases/patients; (3) Results are based on a shorter time period than required; (4) Data suppressed by CMS for one or more quarters; (5) Results are not available for this reporting period; (6) Fewer than 100 patients completed the HCAHPS survey; (7) No cases met the criteria for this measure; (8) The lower limit of the confidence interval cannot be calculated if the number of observed infections equals zero; (9) No data are available from the state/territory for this reporting period; (10) The scores shown reflect fewer than 50 completed surveys; (11) There were discrepancies in the data collection process; (12) This measure does not apply to this hospital for this reporting period; (13) Results cannot be calculated for this reporting period; (14) The results for this state are combined with nearby states to protect confidentiality; Please refer to the User's Guide for a full explanation of data.

Measure	Cases	This Hosp.	State Avg.	U.S. Avg.
Prophylactic Antibiotic Timing[5]	-	-	99%	99%
Prophylactic Antibiotic Timing (Outpatient)[5]	-	-	99%	98%
Urinary Catheter Removal[5]	-	-	99%	97%
Survey of Patients' Hospital Experiences				
Area Around Room 'Always' Quiet at Night[5]	-	-	64%	61%
Doctors 'Always' Communicated Well[5]	-	-	83%	82%
Home Recovery Information Given[5]	-	-	87%	85%
Hospital Given 9 or 10 on 10 Point Scale[5]	-	-	71%	71%
Meds 'Always' Explained Before Given[5]	-	-	65%	64%
Nurses 'Always' Communicated Well[5]	-	-	81%	79%
Pain 'Always' Well Controlled[5]	-	-	72%	71%
Room and Bathroom 'Always' Clean[5]	-	-	72%	73%
Timely Help 'Always' Received[5]	-	-	68%	68%
Would Definitely Recommend Hospital[5]	-	-	70%	71%
Use of Medical Imaging				
Cardiac Imaging Stress Test before Surgery[1]	-	-	5.4%	5.3%
Combination Abdominal CT Scan	115	1.7%	5.6%	10.5%
Combination Brain/Sinus CT Scan[1]	-	-	2.6%	2.7%
Combination Chest CT Scan[1]	-	-	1.3%	2.7%
Follow-up Mammogram/Ultrasound	261	8.0%	8%	8.8%
Lumbar Spine MRI for Low Back Pain[1]	-	-	34.7%	37.2%

Duke Health Raleigh Hospital

3400 Wake Forest Rd
Raleigh, NC 27609
Phone: 919-954-3000
Fax: 919-954-3900
URL: www.raleighcommunityhospital.com
Type: Acute Care Hospitals
Emergency Services: Yes
Ownership: Voluntary non-profit - Private
Beds: 222

Key Personnel:

Radiology. . . . . Tedric Dale Boyse
Emergency Room . . . . Marc Calabrese
Anesthesiology. . . . . Randy Efird, MD
Chief of Medical Staff. . . . . Ted Kunstling
Quality Assurance . . . . Cindy Nordlund
Infection Control. . . . . Polly Patget
President. . . . . David Zaas, MD,MBA

Measure	Cases	This Hosp.	State Avg.	U.S. Avg.
Blood Clot Prevention and Treatment				
Anticoagulation Overlap Therapy[2]	65	95%	94%	93%
ICU Venous Thromboembolism Prophylaxis[2]	80	95%	93%	92%
Incidence of Potentially Preventable VTE[2]	25	4%	10%	10%
UFH with Dosages/Platelet Monitoring[2]	11	100%	95%	97%
Venous Thromboembolism Prophylaxis[2]	306	93%	88%	85%
Warfarin Therapy Discharge Instructions[2]	50	68%	81%	75%
Chest Pain/Possible Heart Attack Care				
Aspirin Given Within 24 Hours of Arrival	14	86%	97%	96%
Fibrinolytic Meds Within 30 Min. of Arrival[7]	-	-	66%	58%
Average Time to ECG (minutes)	14	9	7	7
Average Time to Transfer (minutes)[1]	-	-	45	60
Children's Asthma Care				
Received Home Management Plan of Care	-	-	89%	88%
Received Reliever Medication	-	-	100%	100%
Received Systemic Corticosteroids	-	-	100%	100%
Emergency Department				
Admittance Decision Time (minutes)[2]	531	165	107	98
Head CT Results Within 45 Min. of Arrival[1,3]	-	-	60%	57%
Patients Who Left ER Before Being Seen	41,388	3%	3%	2%
Time from ER Arrival to Admit. (minutes)[2]	629	432	300	274
Time from ER Arrival to Discharge (minutes)	389	158	152	134
Time in ER Before Being Evaluated (minutes)	379	35	34	26
Time to Pain Meds for Fractures (minutes)	56	94	67	57
Heart Attack Care				
Aspirin Given at Discharge	54	100%	100%	99%
Fibrinolytic Meds Within 30 Min. of Arrival[7]	-	-	75%	54%
PCI Within 90 Minutes of Arrival[1]	-	-	98%	96%
Statin Prescribed at Discharge	48	98%	99%	98%
Heart Failure Care				
ACE Inhibitor or ARB for LVSD	52	100%	98%	97%
Discharge Instructions Given	152	99%	96%	94%
Evaluation of LVS Function	163	100%	100%	99%
Medicare Spending				
Medicare Spending per Patient (ratio)	-	0.99	0.94	0.98
Pneumonia Care				
Appropriate Initial Antibiotic Given	102	99%	97%	95%
Blood Culture Timing	176	98%	98%	98%
Pregnancy and Delivery Care				
Newborn Deliveries Scheduled Early[7]	-	-	3%	6%
Preventive Care				
Immunization for Influenza[2]	615	98%	93%	90%
Immunization for Pneumonia[2]	840	98%	94%	92%
Stroke Care				
Anticoagulation Therapy for Atrial Fibrillation[1]	-	-	95%	95%
Antithrombotic Therapy Timing	69	99%	98%	98%
Assessed for Rehabilitation	85	99%	98%	97%
Discharged on Antithrombotic Therapy	76	100%	99%	99%
Discharged on Statin Medication	56	96%	94%	94%
Thrombolytic Therapy Timing[1]	-	-	64%	66%
Venous Thromboembolism Prophylaxis	79	100%	96%	94%
Written Stroke Educational Materials Given	45	93%	88%	88%
Surgical Care Improvement Project				
Appropriate Beta Blocker Usage	323	100%	99%	98%
Appropriate VTP Within 24 Hours	1,135	99%	99%	98%
Controlled Postoperative Blood Glucose[7]	-	-	98%	97%
Perioperative Temperature Management	1,225	100%	100%	100%
Prophylactic Antibiotic Selection	854	99%	99%	99%
Prophylactic Antibiotic Selection (Outpatient)	548	98%	98%	98%
Prophylactic Antibiotic Stopped	844	99%	99%	98%
Prophylactic Antibiotic Timing	854	98%	99%	99%
Prophylactic Antibiotic Timing (Outpatient)	548	99%	99%	98%
Urinary Catheter Removal	940	100%	99%	97%
Survey of Patients' Hospital Experiences				
Area Around Room 'Always' Quiet at Night	300+	64%	64%	61%
Doctors 'Always' Communicated Well	300+	84%	83%	82%
Home Recovery Information Given	300+	88%	87%	85%
Hospital Given 9 or 10 on 10 Point Scale	300+	74%	71%	71%
Meds 'Always' Explained Before Given	300+	67%	65%	64%
Nurses 'Always' Communicated Well	300+	81%	81%	79%
Pain 'Always' Well Controlled	300+	72%	72%	71%
Room and Bathroom 'Always' Clean	300+	65%	72%	73%
Timely Help 'Always' Received	300+	66%	68%	68%
Would Definitely Recommend Hospital	300+	80%	70%	71%
Use of Medical Imaging				
Cardiac Imaging Stress Test before Surgery	76	6.6%	5.4%	5.3%
Combination Abdominal CT Scan	1,183	4.3%	5.6%	10.5%
Combination Brain/Sinus CT Scan	885	1.0%	2.6%	2.7%
Combination Chest CT Scan	1,370	0.1%	1.3%	2.7%
Follow-up Mammogram/Ultrasound	529	7.6%	8%	8.8%
Lumbar Spine MRI for Low Back Pain	252	33.7%	34.7%	37.2%

Rex Hospital

4420 Lake Boone Trail
Raleigh, NC 27607
Phone: 919-784-3100
Fax: 919-784-3336
E-mail: healthnet@rexhealth.com
URL: www.rexhealth.com
Type: Acute Care Hospitals
Emergency Services: Yes
Ownership: Voluntary non-profit - Private
Beds: 660

Key Personnel:

Chief of Medical Staff. . . . . Linda Butler, MD
Operating Room. . . . . Jayne Byrd
Infection Control. . . . . Linda Calderone
Radiology. . . . . John Contrael
Chairman/CEO . . . . A. Dale Jenkins
Emergency Room . . . . Pat Nelson, RN
Quality Assurance . . . . Sue Sherman
CEO/President. . . . . David Strong

Measure	Cases	This Hosp.	State Avg.	U.S. Avg.
Blood Clot Prevention and Treatment				
Anticoagulation Overlap Therapy[2]	125	99%	94%	93%
ICU Venous Thromboembolism Prophylaxis[2]	68	91%	93%	92%
Incidence of Potentially Preventable VTE[2]	22	9%	10%	10%
UFH with Dosages/Platelet Monitoring[2]	37	100%	95%	97%
Venous Thromboembolism Prophylaxis[2]	299	91%	88%	85%
Warfarin Therapy Discharge Instructions[2]	96	91%	81%	75%
Chest Pain/Possible Heart Attack Care				
Aspirin Given Within 24 Hours of Arrival[3,7]	-	-	97%	96%
Fibrinolytic Meds Within 30 Min. of Arrival[5]	-	-	66%	58%
Average Time to ECG (minutes)[3,7]	-	-	7	7
Average Time to Transfer (minutes)[5]	-	-	45	60
Children's Asthma Care				
Received Home Management Plan of Care	-	-	89%	88%
Received Reliever Medication	-	-	100%	100%
Received Systemic Corticosteroids	-	-	100%	100%
Emergency Department				
Admittance Decision Time (minutes)[2]	447	230	107	98
Head CT Results Within 45 Min. of Arrival[1]	-	-	60%	57%
Patients Who Left ER Before Being Seen	61,807	2%	3%	2%
Time from ER Arrival to Admit. (minutes)[2]	459	405	300	274
Time from ER Arrival to Discharge (minutes)	414	190	152	134
Time in ER Before Being Evaluated (minutes)	429	43	34	26
Time to Pain Meds for Fractures (minutes)	120	60	67	57
Heart Attack Care				
Aspirin Given at Discharge[2]	419	100%	100%	99%
Fibrinolytic Meds Within 30 Min. of Arrival[2,7]	-	-	75%	54%
PCI Within 90 Minutes of Arrival[2]	56	98%	98%	96%
Statin Prescribed at Discharge[2]	400	98%	99%	98%
Heart Failure Care				
ACE Inhibitor or ARB for LVSD[2]	121	99%	98%	97%
Discharge Instructions Given[2]	330	93%	96%	94%
Evaluation of LVS Function[2]	406	100%	100%	99%
Medicare Spending				
Medicare Spending per Patient (ratio)	-	0.94	0.94	0.98
Pneumonia Care				
Appropriate Initial Antibiotic Given[2]	179	98%	97%	95%
Blood Culture Timing[2]	306	99%	98%	98%
Pregnancy and Delivery Care				
Newborn Deliveries Scheduled Early[2]	79	0%	3%	6%
Preventive Care				
Immunization for Influenza[2]	545	94%	93%	90%
Immunization for Pneumonia[2]	633	90%	94%	92%
Stroke Care				
Anticoagulation Therapy for Atrial Fibrillation[2]	18	100%	95%	95%
Antithrombotic Therapy Timing[2]	96	100%	98%	98%
Assessed for Rehabilitation[2]	125	98%	98%	97%
Discharged on Antithrombotic Therapy[2]	113	100%	99%	99%
Discharged on Statin Medication[2]	79	97%	94%	94%
Thrombolytic Therapy Timing[1,2]	-	-	64%	66%
Venous Thromboembolism Prophylaxis[2]	118	97%	96%	94%
Written Stroke Educational Materials Given[2]	82	91%	88%	88%
Surgical Care Improvement Project				
Appropriate Beta Blocker Usage[2]	374	99%	99%	98%
Appropriate VTP Within 24 Hours[2]	685	99%	99%	98%
Controlled Postoperative Blood Glucose[2]	246	98%	98%	97%
Perioperative Temperature Management[2]	813	100%	100%	100%
Prophylactic Antibiotic Selection[2]	739	99%	99%	99%
Prophylactic Antibiotic Selection (Outpatient)	1,069	99%	98%	98%
Prophylactic Antibiotic Stopped[2]	723	98%	99%	98%
Prophylactic Antibiotic Timing[2]	739	100%	99%	99%
Prophylactic Antibiotic Timing (Outpatient)	1,069	99%	99%	98%
Urinary Catheter Removal[2]	762	99%	99%	97%
Survey of Patients' Hospital Experiences				
Area Around Room 'Always' Quiet at Night	300+	61%	64%	61%
Doctors 'Always' Communicated Well	300+	87%	83%	82%
Home Recovery Information Given	300+	89%	87%	85%
Hospital Given 9 or 10 on 10 Point Scale	300+	77%	71%	71%
Meds 'Always' Explained Before Given	300+	68%	65%	64%
Nurses 'Always' Communicated Well	300+	78%	81%	79%
Pain 'Always' Well Controlled	300+	68%	72%	71%
Room and Bathroom 'Always' Clean	300+	69%	72%	73%
Timely Help 'Always' Received	300+	66%	68%	68%
Would Definitely Recommend Hospital	300+	80%	70%	71%
Use of Medical Imaging				
Cardiac Imaging Stress Test before Surgery	253	9.1%	5.4%	5.3%
Combination Abdominal CT Scan	1,414	3.3%	5.6%	10.5%
Combination Brain/Sinus CT Scan	1,232	1.4%	2.6%	2.7%
Combination Chest CT Scan	1,432	2.2%	1.3%	2.7%
Follow-up Mammogram/Ultrasound	3,011	5.9%	8%	8.8%
Lumbar Spine MRI for Low Back Pain	155	36.8%	34.7%	37.2%

NOTE: Hospital profiles are in alphabetical order by state, then city, then hospital within the city; Rankings exclude hospitals with less than 25 cases except for patient surveys which excludes hospitals with less than 100 cases; (a) 100-299 cases; (1) The number of cases/patients is too few to report; (2) Data submitted were based on a sample of cases/patients; (3) Results are based on a shorter time period than required; (4) Data suppressed by CMS for one or more quarters; (5) Results are not available for this reporting period; (6) Fewer than 100 patients completed the HCAHPS survey; (7) No cases met the criteria for this measure; (8) The lower limit of the confidence interval cannot be calculated if the number of observed infections equals zero; (9) No data are available from the state/territory for this reporting period; (10) The scores shown reflect fewer than 50 completed surveys; (11) There were discrepancies in the data collection process; (12) This measure does not apply to this hospital for this reporting period; (13) Results cannot be calculated for this reporting period; (14) The results for this state are combined with nearby states to protect confidentiality; Please refer to the User's Guide for a full explanation of data.

Wakemed - Raleigh Campus

3000 New Bern Ave
Raleigh, NC 27610
E-mail: staylor@wakemed.org
URL: www.wakemed.org
Type: Acute Care Hospitals
Ownership: Voluntary non-profit - Private
Phone: 919-350-8000
Fax: 919-350-8868
Emergency Services: Yes
Beds: 515

Key Personnel:
CEO/President. . . . . Donald R. Gintzig
Chief of Medical Staff. . . . . H West Lawson, MD

Measure	Cases	This Hosp.	State Avg.	U.S. Avg.
Blood Clot Prevention and Treatment				
Anticoagulation Overlap Therapy[2]	169	100%	94%	93%
ICU Venous Thromboembolism Prophylaxis[2]	126	100%	93%	92%
Incidence of Potentially Preventable VTE[2]	21	0%	10%	10%
UFH with Dosages/Platelet Monitoring[2]	94	100%	95%	97%
Venous Thromboembolism Prophylaxis[2]	344	88%	88%	85%
Warfarin Therapy Discharge Instructions[2]	126	100%	81%	75%
Chest Pain/Possible Heart Attack Care				
Aspirin Given Within 24 Hours of Arrival	84	98%	97%	96%
Fibrinolytic Meds Within 30 Min. of Arrival[3,7]	-	-	66%	58%
Average Time to ECG (minutes)	91	6	7	7
Average Time to Transfer (minutes)[3,7]	-	-	45	60
Children's Asthma Care				
Received Home Management Plan of Care	-	-	89%	88%
Received Reliever Medication	-	-	100%	100%
Received Systemic Corticosteroids	-	-	100%	100%
Emergency Department				
Admittance Decision Time (minutes)[2]	409	160	107	98
Head CT Results Within 45 Min. of Arrival[1]	-	-	60%	57%
Patients Who Left ER Before Being Seen	>100k	5%	3%	2%
Time from ER Arrival to Admit. (minutes)[2]	416	405	300	274
Time from ER Arrival to Discharge (minutes)	428	194	152	134
Time in ER Before Being Evaluated (minutes)	406	58	34	26
Time to Pain Meds for Fractures (minutes)	476	61	67	57
Heart Attack Care				
Aspirin Given at Discharge	1,397	100%	100%	99%
Fibrinolytic Meds Within 30 Min. of Arrival[7]	-	-	75%	54%
PCI Within 90 Minutes of Arrival	117	98%	98%	96%
Statin Prescribed at Discharge	1,360	99%	99%	98%
Heart Failure Care				
ACE Inhibitor or ARB for LVSD	390	100%	98%	97%
Discharge Instructions Given	977	97%	96%	94%
Evaluation of LVS Function	1,143	100%	100%	99%
Medicare Spending				
Medicare Spending per Patient (ratio)	-	1.00	0.94	0.98
Pneumonia Care				
Appropriate Initial Antibiotic Given	155	98%	97%	95%
Blood Culture Timing	394	97%	98%	98%
Pregnancy and Delivery Care				
Newborn Deliveries Scheduled Early[2]	64	0%	3%	6%
Preventive Care				
Immunization for Influenza[2]	520	93%	93%	90%
Immunization for Pneumonia[2]	562	91%	94%	92%
Stroke Care				
Anticoagulation Therapy for Atrial Fibrillation	87	91%	95%	95%
Antithrombotic Therapy Timing	438	99%	98%	98%
Assessed for Rehabilitation	573	98%	98%	97%
Discharged on Antithrombotic Therapy	485	100%	99%	99%
Discharged on Statin Medication	390	97%	94%	94%
Thrombolytic Therapy Timing	24	88%	64%	66%
Venous Thromboembolism Prophylaxis	564	98%	96%	94%
Written Stroke Educational Materials Given	298	94%	88%	88%
Surgical Care Improvement Project				
Appropriate Beta Blocker Usage[2]	600	100%	99%	98%
Appropriate VTP Within 24 Hours[2]	677	99%	99%	98%
Controlled Postoperative Blood Glucose[2]	448	98%	98%	97%
Perioperative Temperature Management[2]	883	100%	100%	100%
Prophylactic Antibiotic Selection[2]	1,002	100%	99%	99%
Prophylactic Antibiotic Selection (Outpatient)	814	99%	98%	98%
Prophylactic Antibiotic Stopped[2]	898	98%	99%	98%
Prophylactic Antibiotic Timing[2]	1,004	99%	99%	99%
Prophylactic Antibiotic Timing (Outpatient)	809	98%	99%	98%
Urinary Catheter Removal[2]	912	100%	99%	97%
Survey of Patients' Hospital Experiences				
Area Around Room 'Always' Quiet at Night	300+	66%	64%	61%
Doctors 'Always' Communicated Well	300+	81%	83%	82%
Home Recovery Information Given	300+	87%	87%	85%
Hospital Given 9 or 10 on 10 Point Scale	300+	71%	71%	71%
Meds 'Always' Explained Before Given	300+	65%	65%	64%
Nurses 'Always' Communicated Well	300+	82%	81%	79%
Pain 'Always' Well Controlled	300+	75%	72%	71%
Room and Bathroom 'Always' Clean	300+	57%	72%	73%
Timely Help 'Always' Received	300+	67%	68%	68%
Would Definitely Recommend Hospital	300+	78%	70%	71%
Use of Medical Imaging				
Cardiac Imaging Stress Test before Surgery	2,135	7.0%	5.4%	5.3%
Combination Abdominal CT Scan	1,528	5.4%	5.6%	10.5%
Combination Brain/Sinus CT Scan	1,837	3.3%	2.6%	2.7%
Combination Chest CT Scan	1,007	1.1%	1.3%	2.7%
Follow-up Mammogram/Ultrasound	1,242	6.6%	8%	8.8%
Lumbar Spine MRI for Low Back Pain	76	35.5%	34.7%	37.2%

Halifax Regional Medical Center

250 Smith Church Rd
Roanoke Rapids, NC 27870
URL: www.halifaxmedicalcenter.org
Type: Acute Care Hospitals
Ownership: Voluntary non-profit - Private
Phone: 252-535-8005
Fax: 252-535-8466
Emergency Services: Yes
Beds: 206

Key Personnel:
Intensive Care Unit. . . . . Merrie Bischoff, RN
Pediatric Ambulatory Care . . . . Paulette Ingram, MD
Pediatric In-Patient Care . . . . Paulette Ingram, MD
President/CEO. . . . . Will Mahone, V
Chief of Medical Staff. . . . . N Manikham
Infection Control. . . . . Sarah Pulley
Quality Assurance . . . . Margaret Rose

Measure	Cases	This Hosp.	State Avg.	U.S. Avg.
Blood Clot Prevention and Treatment				
Anticoagulation Overlap Therapy[2]	49	65%	94%	93%
ICU Venous Thromboembolism Prophylaxis[2]	81	95%	93%	92%
Incidence of Potentially Preventable VTE[2]	15	7%	10%	10%
UFH with Dosages/Platelet Monitoring[2]	25	100%	95%	97%
Venous Thromboembolism Prophylaxis[2]	489	89%	88%	85%
Warfarin Therapy Discharge Instructions[2]	35	91%	81%	75%
Chest Pain/Possible Heart Attack Care				
Aspirin Given Within 24 Hours of Arrival	229	94%	97%	96%
Fibrinolytic Meds Within 30 Min. of Arrival	21	43%	66%	58%
Average Time to ECG (minutes)	236	5	7	7
Average Time to Transfer (minutes)[7]	-	-	45	60
Children's Asthma Care				
Received Home Management Plan of Care	-	-	89%	88%
Received Reliever Medication	-	-	100%	100%
Received Systemic Corticosteroids	-	-	100%	100%
Emergency Department				
Admittance Decision Time (minutes)[2]	774	129	107	98
Head CT Results Within 45 Min. of Arrival	29	86%	60%	57%
Patients Who Left ER Before Being Seen	41,623	3%	3%	2%
Time from ER Arrival to Admit. (minutes)[2]	785	330	300	274
Time from ER Arrival to Discharge (minutes)	1,047	181	152	134
Time in ER Before Being Evaluated (minutes)	1,152	64	34	26
Time to Pain Meds for Fractures (minutes)	86	58	67	57
Heart Attack Care				
Aspirin Given at Discharge[1]	-	-	100%	99%
Fibrinolytic Meds Within 30 Min. of Arrival[7]	-	-	75%	54%
PCI Within 90 Minutes of Arrival[7]	-	-	98%	96%
Statin Prescribed at Discharge[1]	-	-	99%	98%
Heart Failure Care				
ACE Inhibitor or ARB for LVSD	81	99%	98%	97%
Discharge Instructions Given	211	91%	96%	94%
Evaluation of LVS Function	258	100%	100%	99%
Medicare Spending				
Medicare Spending per Patient (ratio)	-	0.99	0.94	0.98
Pneumonia Care				
Appropriate Initial Antibiotic Given	159	93%	97%	95%
Blood Culture Timing	233	99%	98%	98%
Pregnancy and Delivery Care				
Newborn Deliveries Scheduled Early	74	12%	3%	6%
Preventive Care				
Immunization for Influenza[2]	536	93%	93%	90%
Immunization for Pneumonia[2]	777	92%	94%	92%
Stroke Care				
Anticoagulation Therapy for Atrial Fibrillation[1]	-	-	95%	95%
Antithrombotic Therapy Timing	71	99%	98%	98%
Assessed for Rehabilitation	62	92%	98%	97%
Discharged on Antithrombotic Therapy	62	92%	99%	99%
Discharged on Statin Medication	50	80%	94%	94%
Thrombolytic Therapy Timing[1]	-	-	64%	66%
Venous Thromboembolism Prophylaxis	70	91%	96%	94%
Written Stroke Educational Materials Given	29	28%	88%	88%
Surgical Care Improvement Project				
Appropriate Beta Blocker Usage	165	96%	99%	98%
Appropriate VTP Within 24 Hours	404	97%	99%	98%
Controlled Postoperative Blood Glucose[7]	-	-	98%	97%
Perioperative Temperature Management	472	98%	100%	100%
Prophylactic Antibiotic Selection	342	99%	99%	99%
Prophylactic Antibiotic Selection (Outpatient)	121	98%	98%	98%
Prophylactic Antibiotic Stopped	332	98%	99%	98%
Prophylactic Antibiotic Timing	342	99%	99%	99%
Prophylactic Antibiotic Timing (Outpatient)	121	94%	99%	98%
Urinary Catheter Removal	80	95%	99%	97%
Survey of Patients' Hospital Experiences				
Area Around Room 'Always' Quiet at Night	300+	65%	64%	61%
Doctors 'Always' Communicated Well	300+	82%	83%	82%
Home Recovery Information Given	300+	86%	87%	85%
Hospital Given 9 or 10 on 10 Point Scale	300+	61%	71%	71%
Meds 'Always' Explained Before Given	300+	68%	65%	64%
Nurses 'Always' Communicated Well	300+	80%	81%	79%
Pain 'Always' Well Controlled	300+	74%	72%	71%
Room and Bathroom 'Always' Clean	300+	71%	72%	73%
Timely Help 'Always' Received	300+	69%	68%	68%
Would Definitely Recommend Hospital	300+	58%	70%	71%
Use of Medical Imaging				
Cardiac Imaging Stress Test before Surgery	275	4.7%	5.4%	5.3%
Combination Abdominal CT Scan	852	8.9%	5.6%	10.5%
Combination Brain/Sinus CT Scan	1,048	1.8%	2.6%	2.7%
Combination Chest CT Scan	554	3.2%	1.3%	2.7%
Follow-up Mammogram/Ultrasound	1,908	6.1%	8%	8.8%
Lumbar Spine MRI for Low Back Pain	97	41.2%	34.7%	37.2%

Nash General Hospital

2460 Curtis Ellis Drive
Rocky Mount, NC 27804
URL: www.nhcs.org
Type: Acute Care Hospitals
Ownership: Govt - Hospital Dist/Auth
Phone: 252-443-8000
Fax: 252-443-8067
Emergency Services: Yes
Beds: 280

Key Personnel:
Radiology. . . . . Gerald Capps
CEO/President. . . . . Larry Chewning
Operating Room. . . . . Tom Jenkins
Chief of Medical Staff . . . . Meera Kelley, MD
Infection Control. . . . . Wanda Lamm
Quality Assurance . . . . Sandi Paige
Emergency Room . . . . Jamie Parsons
Patient Relations . . . . Lita Watson

Measure	Cases	This Hosp.	State Avg.	U.S. Avg.
Blood Clot Prevention and Treatment				
Anticoagulation Overlap Therapy[2]	78	95%	94%	93%
ICU Venous Thromboembolism Prophylaxis[2]	54	98%	93%	92%
Incidence of Potentially Preventable VTE[2]	30	7%	10%	10%
UFH with Dosages/Platelet Monitoring[1,2]	-	-	95%	97%
Venous Thromboembolism Prophylaxis[2]	359	91%	88%	85%
Warfarin Therapy Discharge Instructions[2]	42	95%	81%	75%
Chest Pain/Possible Heart Attack Care				
Aspirin Given Within 24 Hours of Arrival	225	99%	97%	96%
Fibrinolytic Meds Within 30 Min. of Arrival	29	90%	66%	58%
Average Time to ECG (minutes)	231	8	7	7
Average Time to Transfer (minutes)[7]	-	-	45	60
Children's Asthma Care				
Received Home Management Plan of Care	-	-	89%	88%
Received Reliever Medication	-	-	100%	100%

NOTE: Hospital profiles are in alphabetical order by state, then city, then hospital within the city; Rankings exclude hospitals with less than 25 cases except for patient surveys which excludes hospitals with less than 100 cases; (a) 100-299 cases; (1) The number of cases/patients is too few to report; (2) Data submitted were based on a sample of cases/patients; (3) Results are based on a shorter time period than required; (4) Data suppressed by CMS for one or more quarters; (5) Results are not available for this reporting period; (6) Fewer than 100 patients completed the HCAHPS survey; (7) No cases met the criteria for this measure; (8) The lower limit of the confidence interval cannot be calculated if the number of observed infections equals zero; (9) No data are available from the state/territory for this reporting period; (10) The scores shown reflect fewer than 50 completed surveys; (11) There were discrepancies in the data collection process; (12) This measure does not apply to this hospital for this reporting period; (13) Results cannot be calculated for this reporting period; (14) The results for this state are combined with nearby states to protect confidentiality; Please refer to the User's Guide for a full explanation of data.

Measure	Cases	This Hosp.	State Avg.	U.S. Avg.
Received Systemic Corticosteroids	-	-	100%	100%
Emergency Department				
Admittance Decision Time (minutes)[2]	619	172	107	98
Head CT Results Within 45 Min. of Arrival	25	56%	60%	57%
Patients Who Left ER Before Being Seen	67,049	3%	3%	2%
Time from ER Arrival to Admit. (minutes)[2]	625	368	300	274
Time from ER Arrival to Discharge (minutes)	463	177	152	134
Time in ER Before Being Evaluated (minutes)	360	74	34	26
Time to Pain Meds for Fractures (minutes)	222	76	67	57
Heart Attack Care				
Aspirin Given at Discharge	113	100%	100%	99%
Fibrinolytic Meds Within 30 Min. of Arrival[7]	-	-	75%	54%
PCI Within 90 Minutes of Arrival[7]	-	-	98%	96%
Statin Prescribed at Discharge	98	100%	99%	98%
Heart Failure Care				
ACE Inhibitor or ARB for LVSD	166	95%	98%	97%
Discharge Instructions Given	436	99%	96%	94%
Evaluation of LVS Function	504	99%	100%	99%
Medicare Spending				
Medicare Spending per Patient (ratio)	-	0.98	0.94	0.98
Pneumonia Care				
Appropriate Initial Antibiotic Given[2]	131	98%	97%	95%
Blood Culture Timing[2]	253	98%	98%	98%
Pregnancy and Delivery Care				
Newborn Deliveries Scheduled Early	125	3%	3%	6%
Preventive Care				
Immunization for Influenza[2]	581	83%	93%	90%
Immunization for Pneumonia[2]	734	80%	94%	92%
Stroke Care				
Anticoagulation Therapy for Atrial Fibrillation	13	92%	95%	95%
Antithrombotic Therapy Timing	173	98%	98%	98%
Assessed for Rehabilitation	189	98%	98%	97%
Discharged on Antithrombotic Therapy	178	99%	99%	99%
Discharged on Statin Medication	138	96%	94%	94%
Thrombolytic Therapy Timing	13	100%	64%	66%
Venous Thromboembolism Prophylaxis	191	97%	96%	94%
Written Stroke Educational Materials Given	95	89%	88%	88%
Surgical Care Improvement Project				
Appropriate Beta Blocker Usage[2]	171	95%	99%	98%
Appropriate VTP Within 24 Hours[2]	508	97%	99%	98%
Controlled Postoperative Blood Glucose[2,7]	-	-	98%	97%
Perioperative Temperature Management[2]	547	100%	100%	100%
Prophylactic Antibiotic Selection[2]	430	98%	99%	99%
Prophylactic Antibiotic Selection (Outpatient)	434	96%	98%	98%
Prophylactic Antibiotic Stopped[2]	428	98%	99%	98%
Prophylactic Antibiotic Timing[2]	431	99%	99%	99%
Prophylactic Antibiotic Timing (Outpatient)	434	99%	99%	98%
Urinary Catheter Removal[2]	313	98%	99%	97%
Survey of Patients' Hospital Experiences				
Area Around Room 'Always' Quiet at Night	300+	58%	64%	61%
Doctors 'Always' Communicated Well	300+	80%	83%	82%
Home Recovery Information Given	300+	85%	87%	85%
Hospital Given 9 or 10 on 10 Point Scale	300+	65%	71%	71%
Meds 'Always' Explained Before Given	300+	64%	65%	64%
Nurses 'Always' Communicated Well	300+	79%	81%	79%
Pain 'Always' Well Controlled	300+	71%	72%	71%
Room and Bathroom 'Always' Clean	300+	70%	72%	73%
Timely Help 'Always' Received	300+	67%	68%	68%
Would Definitely Recommend Hospital	300+	61%	70%	71%
Use of Medical Imaging				
Cardiac Imaging Stress Test before Surgery	368	4.9%	5.4%	5.3%
Combination Abdominal CT Scan	987	5.6%	5.6%	10.5%
Combination Brain/Sinus CT Scan	1,111	1.3%	2.6%	2.7%
Combination Chest CT Scan	278	2.5%	1.3%	2.7%
Follow-up Mammogram/Ultrasound	1,880	13.6%	8%	8.8%
Lumbar Spine MRI for Low Back Pain	201	25.9%	34.7%	37.2%

Person Memorial Hospital

615 Ridge Rd
Roxboro, NC 27573
E-mail: c_brigham98@yahoo.com
URL: www.personhospital.com
Phone: 336-599-2121
Fax: 336-503-5765
Type: Acute Care Hospitals
Ownership: Voluntary non-profit - Private
Emergency Services: Yes
Beds: 110

Key Personnel:
Emergency Room .... Margaret Bowen
Quality Assurance .... Linda Braunstein
Operating Room.............. Ginny Campbell
Radiology.................... William L Hall
Anesthesiology.............. Rick Jacobs, MD
CEO/President............... Craig James
Chief of Medical Staff.......... Jeffrey C Kafer, MD
Infection Control.............. Donna Lungford

Measure	Cases	This Hosp.	State Avg.	U.S. Avg.
Blood Clot Prevention and Treatment				
Anticoagulation Overlap Therapy[2]	11	100%	94%	93%
ICU Venous Thromboembolism Prophylaxis[2]	55	93%	93%	92%
Incidence of Potentially Preventable VTE[1,2]	-	-	10%	10%
UFH with Dosages/Platelet Monitoring[1,2]	-	-	95%	97%
Venous Thromboembolism Prophylaxis[2]	164	94%	88%	85%
Warfarin Therapy Discharge Instructions[1,2]	-	-	81%	75%
Chest Pain/Possible Heart Attack Care				
Aspirin Given Within 24 Hours of Arrival	56	100%	97%	96%
Fibrinolytic Meds Within 30 Min. of Arrival[7]	-	-	66%	58%
Average Time to ECG (minutes)	57	0	7	7
Average Time to Transfer (minutes)[1]	-	-	45	60
Children's Asthma Care				
Received Home Management Plan of Care	-	-	89%	88%
Received Reliever Medication	-	-	100%	100%
Received Systemic Corticosteroids	-	-	100%	100%
Emergency Department				
Admittance Decision Time (minutes)[2]	481	59	107	98
Head CT Results Within 45 Min. of Arrival[1]	-	-	60%	57%
Patients Who Left ER Before Being Seen	20,871	3%	3%	2%
Time from ER Arrival to Admit. (minutes)[2]	487	225	300	274
Time from ER Arrival to Discharge (minutes)	362	110	152	134
Time in ER Before Being Evaluated (minutes)	402	18	34	26
Time to Pain Meds for Fractures (minutes)	50	50	67	57
Heart Attack Care				
Aspirin Given at Discharge[1]	-	-	100%	99%
Fibrinolytic Meds Within 30 Min. of Arrival[7]	-	-	75%	54%
PCI Within 90 Minutes of Arrival[7]	-	-	98%	96%
Statin Prescribed at Discharge[1]	-	-	99%	98%
Heart Failure Care				
ACE Inhibitor or ARB for LVSD	30	97%	98%	97%
Discharge Instructions Given	90	98%	96%	94%
Evaluation of LVS Function	93	98%	100%	99%
Medicare Spending				
Medicare Spending per Patient (ratio)	-	0.89	0.94	0.98
Pneumonia Care				
Appropriate Initial Antibiotic Given	54	94%	97%	95%
Blood Culture Timing	103	100%	98%	98%
Pregnancy and Delivery Care				
Newborn Deliveries Scheduled Early[7]	-	-	3%	6%
Preventive Care				
Immunization for Influenza[2]	292	100%	93%	90%
Immunization for Pneumonia[2]	458	100%	94%	92%
Stroke Care				
Anticoagulation Therapy for Atrial Fibrillation[7]	-	-	95%	95%
Antithrombotic Therapy Timing	16	94%	98%	98%
Assessed for Rehabilitation	13	85%	98%	97%
Discharged on Antithrombotic Therapy	13	92%	99%	99%
Discharged on Statin Medication[1]	-	-	94%	94%
Thrombolytic Therapy Timing[1]	-	-	64%	66%
Venous Thromboembolism Prophylaxis	15	100%	96%	94%
Written Stroke Educational Materials Given[1]	-	-	88%	88%
Surgical Care Improvement Project				
Appropriate Beta Blocker Usage	35	97%	99%	98%
Appropriate VTP Within 24 Hours	120	98%	99%	98%
Controlled Postoperative Blood Glucose[7]	-	-	98%	97%
Perioperative Temperature Management	131	100%	100%	100%
Prophylactic Antibiotic Selection	98	100%	99%	99%
Prophylactic Antibiotic Selection (Outpatient)	22	95%	98%	98%
Prophylactic Antibiotic Stopped	96	100%	99%	98%
Prophylactic Antibiotic Timing	98	98%	99%	99%
Prophylactic Antibiotic Timing (Outpatient)	22	100%	99%	98%
Urinary Catheter Removal	118	98%	99%	97%
Survey of Patients' Hospital Experiences				
Area Around Room 'Always' Quiet at Night	300+	69%	64%	61%
Doctors 'Always' Communicated Well	300+	82%	83%	82%
Home Recovery Information Given	300+	83%	87%	85%
Hospital Given 9 or 10 on 10 Point Scale	300+	63%	71%	71%
Meds 'Always' Explained Before Given	300+	59%	65%	64%
Nurses 'Always' Communicated Well	300+	75%	81%	79%
Pain 'Always' Well Controlled	300+	67%	72%	71%
Room and Bathroom 'Always' Clean	300+	61%	72%	73%
Timely Help 'Always' Received	300+	59%	68%	68%
Would Definitely Recommend Hospital	300+	59%	70%	71%
Use of Medical Imaging				
Cardiac Imaging Stress Test before Surgery[1]	-	-	5.4%	5.3%
Combination Abdominal CT Scan	294	10.5%	5.6%	10.5%
Combination Brain/Sinus CT Scan[1]	-	-	2.6%	2.7%
Combination Chest CT Scan	115	11.3%	1.3%	2.7%
Follow-up Mammogram/Ultrasound	664	5.7%	8%	8.8%
Lumbar Spine MRI for Low Back Pain[1]	-	-	34.7%	37.2%

Rutherford Hospital

288 South Ridgecrest Ave
Rutherfordton, NC 28139
URL: www.rutherfordhosp.org
Phone: 828-286-5000
Fax: 828-286-5207
Type: Acute Care Hospitals
Ownership: Voluntary non-profit - Private
Emergency Services: Yes
Beds: 143

Key Personnel:
Chief of Medical Staff.......... Dean Beckstrom
CEO/President............... David Bixler
Patient Relations .... Nancy Boffemmyer
CEO .... Cindy Buck
Radiology.................. Edward K Grishaw

Measure	Cases	This Hosp.	State Avg.	U.S. Avg.
Blood Clot Prevention and Treatment				
Anticoagulation Overlap Therapy[2]	23	91%	94%	93%
ICU Venous Thromboembolism Prophylaxis[2]	68	81%	93%	92%
Incidence of Potentially Preventable VTE[1,2]	-	-	10%	10%
UFH with Dosages/Platelet Monitoring[1,2]	-	-	95%	97%
Venous Thromboembolism Prophylaxis[2]	325	81%	88%	85%
Warfarin Therapy Discharge Instructions[2]	18	50%	81%	75%
Chest Pain/Possible Heart Attack Care				
Aspirin Given Within 24 Hours of Arrival	101	96%	97%	96%
Fibrinolytic Meds Within 30 Min. of Arrival[1]	-	-	66%	58%
Average Time to ECG (minutes)	104	8	7	7
Average Time to Transfer (minutes)	15	55	45	60
Children's Asthma Care				
Received Home Management Plan of Care	-	-	89%	88%
Received Reliever Medication	-	-	100%	100%
Received Systemic Corticosteroids	-	-	100%	100%
Emergency Department				
Admittance Decision Time (minutes)[2]	715	160	107	98
Head CT Results Within 45 Min. of Arrival	13	62%	60%	57%
Patients Who Left ER Before Being Seen	25,329	5%	3%	2%
Time from ER Arrival to Admit. (minutes)[2]	755	311	300	274
Time from ER Arrival to Discharge (minutes)	407	128	152	134
Time in ER Before Being Evaluated (minutes)	414	32	34	26
Time to Pain Meds for Fractures (minutes)	105	72	67	57
Heart Attack Care				
Aspirin Given at Discharge	12	100%	100%	99%
Fibrinolytic Meds Within 30 Min. of Arrival[7]	-	-	75%	54%
PCI Within 90 Minutes of Arrival[7]	-	-	98%	96%
Statin Prescribed at Discharge	13	77%	99%	98%
Heart Failure Care				
ACE Inhibitor or ARB for LVSD	52	96%	98%	97%
Discharge Instructions Given	152	85%	96%	94%
Evaluation of LVS Function	185	99%	100%	99%
Medicare Spending				
Medicare Spending per Patient (ratio)	-	0.93	0.94	0.98

NOTE: Hospital profiles are in alphabetical order by state, then city, then hospital within the city; Rankings exclude hospitals with less than 25 cases except for patient surveys which excludes hospitals with less than 100 cases; (a) 100-299 cases; (1) The number of cases/patients is too few to report; (2) Data submitted were based on a sample of cases/patients; (3) Results are based on a shorter time period than required; (4) Data suppressed by CMS for one or more quarters; (5) Results are not available for this reporting period; (6) Fewer than 100 patients completed the HCAHPS survey; (7) No cases met the criteria for this measure; (8) The lower limit of the confidence interval cannot be calculated if the number of observed infections equals zero; (9) No data are available from the state/territory for this reporting period; (10) The scores shown reflect fewer than 50 completed surveys; (11) There were discrepancies in the data collection process; (12) This measure does not apply to this hospital for this reporting period; (13) Results cannot be calculated for this reporting period; (14) The results for this state are combined with nearby states to protect confidentiality; Please refer to the User's Guide for a full explanation of data.

Measure	Cases	This Hosp.	State Avg.	U.S. Avg.
Pneumonia Care				
Appropriate Initial Antibiotic Given	139	92%	97%	95%
Blood Culture Timing	265	96%	98%	98%
Pregnancy and Delivery Care				
Newborn Deliveries Scheduled Early[2]	22	5%	3%	6%
Preventive Care				
Immunization for Influenza[2]	575	95%	93%	90%
Immunization for Pneumonia[2]	763	96%	94%	92%
Stroke Care				
Anticoagulation Therapy for Atrial Fibrillation	16	94%	95%	95%
Antithrombotic Therapy Timing	77	100%	98%	98%
Assessed for Rehabilitation	77	97%	98%	97%
Discharged on Antithrombotic Therapy	75	100%	99%	99%
Discharged on Statin Medication	61	93%	94%	94%
Thrombolytic Therapy Timing	17	0%	64%	66%
Venous Thromboembolism Prophylaxis	76	96%	96%	94%
Written Stroke Educational Materials Given	43	88%	88%	88%
Surgical Care Improvement Project				
Appropriate Beta Blocker Usage	92	100%	99%	98%
Appropriate VTP Within 24 Hours	281	99%	99%	98%
Controlled Postoperative Blood Glucose[7]	-	-	98%	97%
Perioperative Temperature Management	316	100%	100%	100%
Prophylactic Antibiotic Selection	217	100%	99%	99%
Prophylactic Antibiotic Selection (Outpatient)	21	95%	98%	98%
Prophylactic Antibiotic Stopped	212	100%	99%	98%
Prophylactic Antibiotic Timing	217	100%	99%	99%
Prophylactic Antibiotic Timing (Outpatient)	23	87%	99%	98%
Urinary Catheter Removal	70	99%	99%	97%
Survey of Patients' Hospital Experiences				
Area Around Room 'Always' Quiet at Night	300+	66%	64%	61%
Doctors 'Always' Communicated Well	300+	83%	83%	82%
Home Recovery Information Given	300+	83%	87%	85%
Hospital Given 9 or 10 on 10 Point Scale	300+	67%	71%	71%
Meds 'Always' Explained Before Given	300+	62%	65%	64%
Nurses 'Always' Communicated Well	300+	82%	81%	79%
Pain 'Always' Well Controlled	300+	69%	72%	71%
Room and Bathroom 'Always' Clean	300+	75%	72%	73%
Timely Help 'Always' Received	300+	69%	68%	68%
Would Definitely Recommend Hospital	300+	63%	70%	71%
Use of Medical Imaging				
Cardiac Imaging Stress Test before Surgery	281	6.8%	5.4%	5.3%
Combination Abdominal CT Scan	750	3.9%	5.6%	10.5%
Combination Brain/Sinus CT Scan	807	2.4%	2.6%	2.7%
Combination Chest CT Scan	366	0.5%	1.3%	2.7%
Follow-up Mammogram/Ultrasound	1,794	8.0%	8%	8.8%
Lumbar Spine MRI for Low Back Pain	159	37.1%	34.7%	37.2%

Novant Health Rowan Medical Center

612 Mocksville Ave
Salisbury, NC 28144
Phone: 704-210-5000
Fax: 704-210-5631
E-mail: webdoctor@rowan.org
URL: www.rowan.org
Type: Acute Care Hospitals
Emergency Services: Yes
Ownership: Voluntary non-profit - Private
Beds: 188

Key Personnel:
Radiology. . . . . Marvin Abdalah
Coronary Care . . . . Sabrina Adkins
Operating Room. . . . . William Birmingham
Quality Assurance . . . . David Cook
Patient Relations . . . . Julie Gainer
CEO/President. . . . . Jeff Lindsay
Chief of Medical Staff . . . . David Smith

Measure	Cases	This Hosp.	State Avg.	U.S. Avg.
Blood Clot Prevention and Treatment				
Anticoagulation Overlap Therapy[2]	42	100%	94%	93%
ICU Venous Thromboembolism Prophylaxis[2]	81	96%	93%	92%
Incidence of Potentially Preventable VTE[2]	14	0%	10%	10%
UFH with Dosages/Platelet Monitoring[2]	25	100%	95%	97%
Venous Thromboembolism Prophylaxis[2]	319	93%	88%	85%
Warfarin Therapy Discharge Instructions[2]	25	84%	81%	75%
Chest Pain/Possible Heart Attack Care				
Aspirin Given Within 24 Hours of Arrival[1,3]	-	-	97%	96%
Fibrinolytic Meds Within 30 Min. of Arrival[3,7]	-	-	66%	58%
Average Time to ECG (minutes)[1,3]	-	-	7	7
Average Time to Transfer (minutes)[1,3]	-	-	45	60
Children's Asthma Care				
Received Home Management Plan of Care[1]	-	-	89%	88%
Received Reliever Medication	11	100%	100%	100%
Received Systemic Corticosteroids	11	100%	100%	100%
Emergency Department				
Admittance Decision Time (minutes)[2]	840	152	107	98
Head CT Results Within 45 Min. of Arrival	25	84%	60%	57%
Patients Who Left ER Before Being Seen	47,921	3%	3%	2%
Time from ER Arrival to Admit. (minutes)[2]	866	348	300	274
Time from ER Arrival to Discharge (minutes)	447	168	152	134
Time in ER Before Being Evaluated (minutes)	479	37	34	26
Time to Pain Meds for Fractures (minutes)	126	60	67	57
Heart Attack Care				
Aspirin Given at Discharge	234	100%	100%	99%
Fibrinolytic Meds Within 30 Min. of Arrival[7]	-	-	75%	54%
PCI Within 90 Minutes of Arrival	49	100%	98%	96%
Statin Prescribed at Discharge	204	100%	99%	98%
Heart Failure Care				
ACE Inhibitor or ARB for LVSD	62	100%	98%	97%
Discharge Instructions Given	196	99%	96%	94%
Evaluation of LVS Function	245	100%	100%	99%
Medicare Spending				
Medicare Spending per Patient (ratio)	-	0.99	0.94	0.98
Pneumonia Care				
Appropriate Initial Antibiotic Given	180	98%	97%	95%
Blood Culture Timing	281	100%	98%	98%
Pregnancy and Delivery Care				
Newborn Deliveries Scheduled Early[2]	40	2%	3%	6%
Preventive Care				
Immunization for Influenza[2]	678	95%	93%	90%
Immunization for Pneumonia[2]	861	98%	94%	92%
Stroke Care				
Anticoagulation Therapy for Atrial Fibrillation	29	100%	95%	95%
Antithrombotic Therapy Timing	161	98%	98%	98%
Assessed for Rehabilitation	200	100%	98%	97%
Discharged on Antithrombotic Therapy	187	100%	99%	99%
Discharged on Statin Medication	135	100%	94%	94%
Thrombolytic Therapy Timing[1]	-	-	64%	66%
Venous Thromboembolism Prophylaxis	185	97%	96%	94%
Written Stroke Educational Materials Given	112	98%	88%	88%
Surgical Care Improvement Project				
Appropriate Beta Blocker Usage[2]	159	100%	99%	98%
Appropriate VTP Within 24 Hours[2]	617	100%	99%	98%
Controlled Postoperative Blood Glucose[2,7]	-	-	98%	97%
Perioperative Temperature Management[2]	681	100%	100%	100%
Prophylactic Antibiotic Selection[2]	539	100%	99%	99%
Prophylactic Antibiotic Selection (Outpatient)	360	100%	98%	98%
Prophylactic Antibiotic Stopped[2]	517	100%	99%	98%
Prophylactic Antibiotic Timing[2]	539	100%	99%	99%
Prophylactic Antibiotic Timing (Outpatient)	360	100%	99%	98%
Urinary Catheter Removal[2]	236	98%	99%	97%
Survey of Patients' Hospital Experiences				
Area Around Room 'Always' Quiet at Night	300+	56%	64%	61%
Doctors 'Always' Communicated Well	300+	78%	83%	82%
Home Recovery Information Given	300+	81%	87%	85%
Hospital Given 9 or 10 on 10 Point Scale	300+	59%	71%	71%
Meds 'Always' Explained Before Given	300+	57%	65%	64%
Nurses 'Always' Communicated Well	300+	74%	81%	79%
Pain 'Always' Well Controlled	300+	63%	72%	71%
Room and Bathroom 'Always' Clean	300+	67%	72%	73%
Timely Help 'Always' Received	300+	59%	68%	68%
Would Definitely Recommend Hospital	300+	55%	70%	71%
Use of Medical Imaging				
Cardiac Imaging Stress Test before Surgery	333	5.7%	5.4%	5.3%
Combination Abdominal CT Scan	653	8.9%	5.6%	10.5%
Combination Brain/Sinus CT Scan	1,033	2.3%	2.6%	2.7%
Combination Chest CT Scan	237	0.8%	1.3%	2.7%
Follow-up Mammogram/Ultrasound	2,153	11.2%	8%	8.8%
Lumbar Spine MRI for Low Back Pain	276	35.9%	34.7%	37.2%

W G (Bill) Hefner Salisbury VA Medical Center

1601 Brenner Avenue
Salisbury, NC 28144
Phone: 704-638-9000
Fax: 704-638-3395
URL: www.va.gov/sta/guide/home.asp
Type: Acute Care - VA
Emergency Services: No
Ownership: Government Federal
Beds: 429

Key Personnel:
Infection Control. . . . . Charles A De Comarmond
Operating Room. . . . . Charles Graham
Quality Assurance . . . . Beverly Hartsell
Radiology. . . . . Paul Karmin, MD
Chief of Medical Staff . . . . Subbarao Pemmaraju, MD

Measure	Cases	This Hosp.	State Avg.	U.S. Avg.
Blood Clot Prevention and Treatment				
Anticoagulation Overlap Therapy	-	-	94%	93%
ICU Venous Thromboembolism Prophylaxis	-	-	93%	92%
Incidence of Potentially Preventable VTE	-	-	10%	10%
UFH with Dosages/Platelet Monitoring	-	-	95%	97%
Venous Thromboembolism Prophylaxis	-	-	88%	85%
Warfarin Therapy Discharge Instructions	-	-	81%	75%
Chest Pain/Possible Heart Attack Care				
Aspirin Given Within 24 Hours of Arrival	-	-	97%	96%
Fibrinolytic Meds Within 30 Min. of Arrival	-	-	66%	58%
Average Time to ECG (minutes)	-	-	7	7
Average Time to Transfer (minutes)	-	-	45	60
Children's Asthma Care				
Received Home Management Plan of Care	-	-	89%	88%
Received Reliever Medication	-	-	100%	100%
Received Systemic Corticosteroids	-	-	100%	100%
Emergency Department				
Admittance Decision Time (minutes)	-	-	107	98
Head CT Results Within 45 Min. of Arrival	-	-	60%	57%
Patients Who Left ER Before Being Seen	-	-	3%	2%
Time from ER Arrival to Admit. (minutes)	-	-	300	274
Time from ER Arrival to Discharge (minutes)	-	-	152	134
Time in ER Before Being Evaluated (minutes)	-	-	34	26
Time to Pain Meds for Fractures (minutes)	-	-	67	57
Heart Attack Care				
Aspirin Given at Discharge[5]	-	-	100%	99%
Fibrinolytic Meds Within 30 Min. of Arrival[5]	-	-	75%	54%
PCI Within 90 Minutes of Arrival[5]	-	-	98%	96%
Statin Prescribed at Discharge[5]	-	-	99%	98%
Heart Failure Care				
ACE Inhibitor or ARB for LVSD[1]	21	76%	98%	97%
Discharge Instructions Given	57	100%	96%	94%
Evaluation of LVS Function	61	98%	100%	99%
Medicare Spending				
Medicare Spending per Patient (ratio)	-	-	0.94	0.98
Pneumonia Care				
Appropriate Initial Antibiotic Given	52	88%	97%	95%
Blood Culture Timing	95	99%	98%	98%
Pregnancy and Delivery Care				
Newborn Deliveries Scheduled Early	-	-	3%	6%
Preventive Care				
Immunization for Influenza[5]	-	-	93%	90%
Immunization for Pneumonia[5]	-	-	94%	92%
Stroke Care				
Anticoagulation Therapy for Atrial Fibrillation	-	-	95%	95%
Antithrombotic Therapy Timing	-	-	98%	98%
Assessed for Rehabilitation	-	-	98%	97%
Discharged on Antithrombotic Therapy	-	-	99%	99%
Discharged on Statin Medication	-	-	94%	94%
Thrombolytic Therapy Timing	-	-	64%	66%
Venous Thromboembolism Prophylaxis	-	-	96%	94%
Written Stroke Educational Materials Given	-	-	88%	88%
Surgical Care Improvement Project				
Appropriate Beta Blocker Usage[2]	35	100%	99%	98%
Appropriate VTP Within 24 Hours[2]	145	97%	99%	98%
Controlled Postoperative Blood Glucose[5]	-	-	98%	97%
Perioperative Temperature Management[2]	164	99%	100%	100%
Prophylactic Antibiotic Selection	68	87%	99%	99%
Prophylactic Antibiotic Selection (Outpatient)	-	-	98%	98%
Prophylactic Antibiotic Stopped	65	95%	99%	98%

NOTE: Hospital profiles are in alphabetical order by state, then city, then hospital within the city; Rankings exclude hospitals with less than 25 cases except for patient surveys which excludes hospitals with less than 100 cases; (a) 100-299 cases; (1) The number of cases/patients is too few to report; (2) Data submitted were based on a sample of cases/patients; (3) Results are based on a shorter time period than required; (4) Data suppressed by CMS for one or more quarters; (5) Results are not available for this reporting period; (6) Fewer than 100 patients completed the HCAHPS survey; (7) No cases met the criteria for this measure; (8) The lower limit of the confidence interval cannot be calculated if the number of observed infections equals zero; (9) No data are available from the state/territory for this reporting period; (10) The scores shown reflect fewer than 50 completed surveys; (11) There were discrepancies in the data collection process; (12) This measure does not apply to this hospital for this reporting period; (13) Results cannot be calculated for this reporting period; (14) The results for this state are combined with nearby states to protect confidentiality; Please refer to the User's Guide for a full explanation of data.

Measure	Cases	This Hosp.	State Avg.	U.S. Avg.
Prophylactic Antibiotic Timing	69	88%	99%	99%
Prophylactic Antibiotic Timing (Outpatient)	-	-	99%	98%
Urinary Catheter Removal[2]	60	97%	99%	97%
Survey of Patients' Hospital Experiences				
Area Around Room 'Always' Quiet at Night	-	-	64%	61%
Doctors 'Always' Communicated Well	-	-	83%	82%
Home Recovery Information Given	-	-	87%	85%
Hospital Given 9 or 10 on 10 Point Scale	-	-	71%	71%
Meds 'Always' Explained Before Given	-	-	65%	64%
Nurses 'Always' Communicated Well	-	-	81%	79%
Pain 'Always' Well Controlled	-	-	72%	71%
Room and Bathroom 'Always' Clean	-	-	72%	73%
Timely Help 'Always' Received	-	-	68%	68%
Would Definitely Recommend Hospital	-	-	70%	71%
Use of Medical Imaging				
Cardiac Imaging Stress Test before Surgery	-	-	5.4%	5.3%
Combination Abdominal CT Scan	-	-	5.6%	10.5%
Combination Brain/Sinus CT Scan	-	-	2.6%	2.7%
Combination Chest CT Scan	-	-	1.3%	2.7%
Follow-up Mammogram/Ultrasound	-	-	8%	8.8%
Lumbar Spine MRI for Low Back Pain	-	-	34.7%	37.2%

Central Carolina Hospital

1135 Carthage St
Sanford, NC 27330
Phone: 919-774-2100
Fax: 919-774-2295
URL: www.centralcarolinahosp.com
Type: Acute Care Hospitals
Emergency Services: Yes
Ownership: Voluntary non-profit - Private
Beds: 137

Key Personnel:
Operating Room. . . . . James B Collins III
Radiology. . . . . Douglas Dacko
CEO/President. . . . . Doug Dorris
Emergency Room . . . . Dean Flynn
Anesthesiology. . . . . Jill Hilburger, MD
Intensive Care Unit. . . . . Phyllis Poe, RN
Infection Control. . . . . Tawny Ramsperburger
Chief of Medical Staff. . . . . Joseph Tozi, MD

Measure	Cases	This Hosp.	State Avg.	U.S. Avg.
Blood Clot Prevention and Treatment				
Anticoagulation Overlap Therapy[1,2]	-	-	94%	93%
ICU Venous Thromboembolism Prophylaxis[2]	65	86%	93%	92%
Incidence of Potentially Preventable VTE[1,2]	-	-	10%	10%
UFH with Dosages/Platelet Monitoring[1,2]	-	-	95%	97%
Venous Thromboembolism Prophylaxis[2]	341	87%	88%	85%
Warfarin Therapy Discharge Instructions[1,2]	-	-	81%	75%
Chest Pain/Possible Heart Attack Care				
Aspirin Given Within 24 Hours of Arrival	66	100%	97%	96%
Fibrinolytic Meds Within 30 Min. of Arrival[1]	-	-	66%	58%
Average Time to ECG (minutes)	70	4	7	7
Average Time to Transfer (minutes)[1]	-	-	45	60
Children's Asthma Care				
Received Home Management Plan of Care	-	-	89%	88%
Received Reliever Medication	-	-	100%	100%
Received Systemic Corticosteroids	-	-	100%	100%
Emergency Department				
Admittance Decision Time (minutes)[2]	671	117	107	98
Head CT Results Within 45 Min. of Arrival	28	96%	60%	57%
Patients Who Left ER Before Being Seen	38,456	2%	3%	2%
Time from ER Arrival to Admit. (minutes)[2]	671	261	300	274
Time from ER Arrival to Discharge (minutes)	368	128	152	134
Time in ER Before Being Evaluated (minutes)	399	25	34	26
Time to Pain Meds for Fractures (minutes)	165	63	67	57
Heart Attack Care				
Aspirin Given at Discharge[1]	-	-	100%	99%
Fibrinolytic Meds Within 30 Min. of Arrival[7]	-	-	75%	54%
PCI Within 90 Minutes of Arrival[7]	-	-	98%	96%
Statin Prescribed at Discharge[1]	-	-	99%	98%
Heart Failure Care				
ACE Inhibitor or ARB for LVSD	45	100%	98%	97%
Discharge Instructions Given	162	100%	96%	94%
Evaluation of LVS Function	207	100%	100%	99%
Medicare Spending				
Medicare Spending per Patient (ratio)	-	0.94	0.94	0.98
Pneumonia Care				
Appropriate Initial Antibiotic Given	130	98%	97%	95%
Blood Culture Timing	160	99%	98%	98%
Pregnancy and Delivery Care				
Newborn Deliveries Scheduled Early[2]	29	7%	3%	6%
Preventive Care				
Immunization for Influenza[2]	508	82%	93%	90%
Immunization for Pneumonia[2]	611	85%	94%	92%
Stroke Care				
Anticoagulation Therapy for Atrial Fibrillation	12	100%	95%	95%
Antithrombotic Therapy Timing	71	100%	98%	98%
Assessed for Rehabilitation	74	100%	98%	97%
Discharged on Antithrombotic Therapy	73	100%	99%	99%
Discharged on Statin Medication	56	100%	94%	94%
Thrombolytic Therapy Timing[1]	-	-	64%	66%
Venous Thromboembolism Prophylaxis	70	100%	96%	94%
Written Stroke Educational Materials Given	42	100%	88%	88%
Surgical Care Improvement Project				
Appropriate Beta Blocker Usage	43	95%	99%	98%
Appropriate VTP Within 24 Hours	150	96%	99%	98%
Controlled Postoperative Blood Glucose[7]	-	-	98%	97%
Perioperative Temperature Management	177	100%	100%	100%
Prophylactic Antibiotic Selection	93	97%	99%	99%
Prophylactic Antibiotic Selection (Outpatient)	127	96%	98%	98%
Prophylactic Antibiotic Stopped	91	93%	99%	98%
Prophylactic Antibiotic Timing	93	99%	99%	99%
Prophylactic Antibiotic Timing (Outpatient)	127	98%	99%	98%
Urinary Catheter Removal	103	97%	99%	97%
Survey of Patients' Hospital Experiences				
Area Around Room 'Always' Quiet at Night	300+	61%	64%	61%
Doctors 'Always' Communicated Well	300+	84%	83%	82%
Home Recovery Information Given	300+	83%	87%	85%
Hospital Given 9 or 10 on 10 Point Scale	300+	61%	71%	71%
Meds 'Always' Explained Before Given	300+	65%	65%	64%
Nurses 'Always' Communicated Well	300+	78%	81%	79%
Pain 'Always' Well Controlled	300+	71%	72%	71%
Room and Bathroom 'Always' Clean	300+	74%	72%	73%
Timely Help 'Always' Received	300+	63%	68%	68%
Would Definitely Recommend Hospital	300+	60%	70%	71%
Use of Medical Imaging				
Cardiac Imaging Stress Test before Surgery	119	1.7%	5.4%	5.3%
Combination Abdominal CT Scan	676	0.3%	5.6%	10.5%
Combination Brain/Sinus CT Scan	600	2.3%	2.6%	2.7%
Combination Chest CT Scan	224	0.0%	1.3%	2.7%
Follow-up Mammogram/Ultrasound	1,654	5.7%	8%	8.8%
Lumbar Spine MRI for Low Back Pain	103	27.2%	34.7%	37.2%

Our Community Hospital

921 Junior High Road
Scotland Neck, NC 27874
Phone: 252-826-4144
Type: Critical Access Hospitals
Emergency Services: Yes
Ownership: Govt - Hospital Dist/Auth

Measure	Cases	This Hosp.	State Avg.	U.S. Avg.
Blood Clot Prevention and Treatment				
Anticoagulation Overlap Therapy[5]	-	-	94%	93%
ICU Venous Thromboembolism Prophylaxis[5]	-	-	93%	92%
Incidence of Potentially Preventable VTE[5]	-	-	10%	10%
UFH with Dosages/Platelet Monitoring[5]	-	-	95%	97%
Venous Thromboembolism Prophylaxis[5]	-	-	88%	85%
Warfarin Therapy Discharge Instructions[5]	-	-	81%	75%
Chest Pain/Possible Heart Attack Care				
Aspirin Given Within 24 Hours of Arrival	-	-	97%	96%
Fibrinolytic Meds Within 30 Min. of Arrival	-	-	66%	58%
Average Time to ECG (minutes)	-	-	7	7
Average Time to Transfer (minutes)	-	-	45	60
Children's Asthma Care				
Received Home Management Plan of Care	-	-	89%	88%
Received Reliever Medication	-	-	100%	100%
Received Systemic Corticosteroids	-	-	100%	100%
Emergency Department				
Admittance Decision Time (minutes)[5]	-	-	107	98
Head CT Results Within 45 Min. of Arrival	-	-	60%	57%
Patients Who Left ER Before Being Seen	-	-	3%	2%
Time from ER Arrival to Admit. (minutes)[5]	-	-	300	274
Time from ER Arrival to Discharge (minutes)	-	-	152	134
Time in ER Before Being Evaluated (minutes)	-	-	34	26
Time to Pain Meds for Fractures (minutes)	-	-	67	57
Heart Attack Care				
Aspirin Given at Discharge[5]	-	-	100%	99%
Fibrinolytic Meds Within 30 Min. of Arrival[5]	-	-	75%	54%
PCI Within 90 Minutes of Arrival[5]	-	-	98%	96%
Statin Prescribed at Discharge[5]	-	-	99%	98%
Heart Failure Care				
ACE Inhibitor or ARB for LVSD[5]	-	-	98%	97%
Discharge Instructions Given[5]	-	-	96%	94%
Evaluation of LVS Function[5]	-	-	100%	99%
Medicare Spending				
Medicare Spending per Patient (ratio)	-	-	0.94	0.98
Pneumonia Care				
Appropriate Initial Antibiotic Given[5]	-	-	97%	95%
Blood Culture Timing[5]	-	-	98%	98%
Pregnancy and Delivery Care				
Newborn Deliveries Scheduled Early[5]	-	-	3%	6%
Preventive Care				
Immunization for Influenza[5]	-	-	93%	90%
Immunization for Pneumonia[5]	-	-	94%	92%
Stroke Care				
Anticoagulation Therapy for Atrial Fibrillation[5]	-	-	95%	95%
Antithrombotic Therapy Timing[5]	-	-	98%	98%
Assessed for Rehabilitation[5]	-	-	98%	97%
Discharged on Antithrombotic Therapy[5]	-	-	99%	99%
Discharged on Statin Medication[5]	-	-	94%	94%
Thrombolytic Therapy Timing[5]	-	-	64%	66%
Venous Thromboembolism Prophylaxis[5]	-	-	96%	94%
Written Stroke Educational Materials Given[5]	-	-	88%	88%
Surgical Care Improvement Project				
Appropriate Beta Blocker Usage[5]	-	-	99%	98%
Appropriate VTP Within 24 Hours[5]	-	-	99%	98%
Controlled Postoperative Blood Glucose[5]	-	-	98%	97%
Perioperative Temperature Management[5]	-	-	100%	100%
Prophylactic Antibiotic Selection[5]	-	-	99%	99%
Prophylactic Antibiotic Selection (Outpatient)	-	-	98%	98%
Prophylactic Antibiotic Stopped[5]	-	-	99%	98%
Prophylactic Antibiotic Timing[5]	-	-	99%	99%
Prophylactic Antibiotic Timing (Outpatient)	-	-	99%	98%
Urinary Catheter Removal[5]	-	-	99%	97%
Survey of Patients' Hospital Experiences				
Area Around Room 'Always' Quiet at Night[5]	-	-	64%	61%
Doctors 'Always' Communicated Well[5]	-	-	83%	82%
Home Recovery Information Given[5]	-	-	87%	85%
Hospital Given 9 or 10 on 10 Point Scale[5]	-	-	71%	71%
Meds 'Always' Explained Before Given[5]	-	-	65%	64%
Nurses 'Always' Communicated Well[5]	-	-	81%	79%
Pain 'Always' Well Controlled[5]	-	-	72%	71%
Room and Bathroom 'Always' Clean[5]	-	-	72%	73%
Timely Help 'Always' Received[5]	-	-	68%	68%
Would Definitely Recommend Hospital[5]	-	-	70%	71%
Use of Medical Imaging				
Cardiac Imaging Stress Test before Surgery	-	-	5.4%	5.3%
Combination Abdominal CT Scan	-	-	5.6%	10.5%
Combination Brain/Sinus CT Scan	-	-	2.6%	2.7%
Combination Chest CT Scan	-	-	1.3%	2.7%
Follow-up Mammogram/Ultrasound	-	-	8%	8.8%
Lumbar Spine MRI for Low Back Pain	-	-	34.7%	37.2%

Cleveland Regional Medical Center

201 E Grover St
Shelby, NC 28150
Phone: 704-487-3000
Fax: 704-487-3290
URL: www.clevelandregional.org
Type: Acute Care Hospitals
Emergency Services: Yes
Ownership: Govt - Hospital Dist/Auth
Beds: 241

Key Personnel:
Chief of Medical Staff. . . . . Thomas Davis, MD
CEO/President. . . . . Brian Gwyn
Quality Assurance . . . . Pat Hartsoe
Infection Control. . . . . Brian Hudson
Pediatric In-Patient Care . . . . Nancy Porter

NOTE: Hospital profiles are in alphabetical order by state, then city, then hospital within the city; Rankings exclude hospitals with less than 25 cases except for patient surveys which excludes hospitals with less than 100 cases; (a) 100-299 cases; (1) The number of cases/patients is too few to report; (2) Data submitted were based on a sample of cases/patients; (3) Results are based on a shorter time period than required; (4) Data suppressed by CMS for one or more quarters; (5) Results are not available for this reporting period; (6) Fewer than 100 patients completed the HCAHPS survey; (7) No cases met the criteria for this measure; (8) The lower limit of the confidence interval cannot be calculated if the number of observed infections equals zero; (9) No data are available from the state/territory for this reporting period; (10) The scores shown reflect fewer than 50 completed surveys; (11) There were discrepancies in the data collection process; (12) This measure does not apply to this hospital for this reporting period; (13) Results cannot be calculated for this reporting period; (14) The results for this state are combined with nearby states to protect confidentiality; Please refer to the User's Guide for a full explanation of data.

Measure	Cases	This Hosp.	State Avg.	U.S. Avg.
Blood Clot Prevention and Treatment				
Anticoagulation Overlap Therapy[2]	60	85%	94%	93%
ICU Venous Thromboembolism Prophylaxis[2]	110	91%	93%	92%
Incidence of Potentially Preventable VTE[1,2]	-	-	10%	10%
UFH with Dosages/Platelet Monitoring[2]	35	100%	95%	97%
Venous Thromboembolism Prophylaxis[2]	296	87%	88%	85%
Warfarin Therapy Discharge Instructions[2]	50	90%	81%	75%
Chest Pain/Possible Heart Attack Care				
Aspirin Given Within 24 Hours of Arrival	132	100%	97%	96%
Fibrinolytic Meds Within 30 Min. of Arrival[7]	-	-	66%	58%
Average Time to ECG (minutes)	135	6	7	7
Average Time to Transfer (minutes)	29	37	45	60
Children's Asthma Care				
Received Home Management Plan of Care	-	-	89%	88%
Received Reliever Medication	-	-	100%	100%
Received Systemic Corticosteroids	-	-	100%	100%
Emergency Department				
Admittance Decision Time (minutes)[2]	718	116	107	98
Head CT Results Within 45 Min. of Arrival	18	83%	60%	57%
Patients Who Left ER Before Being Seen	66,046	1%	3%	2%
Time from ER Arrival to Admit. (minutes)[2]	724	245	300	274
Time from ER Arrival to Discharge (minutes)	363	113	152	134
Time in ER Before Being Evaluated (minutes)	298	18	34	26
Time to Pain Meds for Fractures (minutes)	146	52	67	57
Heart Attack Care				
Aspirin Given at Discharge	35	100%	100%	99%
Fibrinolytic Meds Within 30 Min. of Arrival[7]	-	-	75%	54%
PCI Within 90 Minutes of Arrival[7]	-	-	98%	96%
Statin Prescribed at Discharge	36	97%	99%	98%
Heart Failure Care				
ACE Inhibitor or ARB for LVSD	79	99%	98%	97%
Discharge Instructions Given	231	96%	96%	94%
Evaluation of LVS Function	284	100%	100%	99%
Medicare Spending				
Medicare Spending per Patient (ratio)	-	0.94	0.94	0.98
Pneumonia Care				
Appropriate Initial Antibiotic Given	174	99%	97%	95%
Blood Culture Timing	192	99%	98%	98%
Pregnancy and Delivery Care				
Newborn Deliveries Scheduled Early	211	1%	3%	6%
Preventive Care				
Immunization for Influenza[2]	523	95%	93%	90%
Immunization for Pneumonia[2]	677	97%	94%	92%
Stroke Care				
Anticoagulation Therapy for Atrial Fibrillation	13	100%	95%	95%
Antithrombotic Therapy Timing	87	99%	98%	98%
Assessed for Rehabilitation	104	99%	98%	97%
Discharged on Antithrombotic Therapy	101	100%	99%	99%
Discharged on Statin Medication	86	92%	94%	94%
Thrombolytic Therapy Timing[7]	-	-	64%	66%
Venous Thromboembolism Prophylaxis	88	93%	96%	94%
Written Stroke Educational Materials Given	63	98%	88%	88%
Surgical Care Improvement Project				
Appropriate Beta Blocker Usage[2]	137	99%	99%	98%
Appropriate VTP Within 24 Hours[2]	496	100%	99%	98%
Controlled Postoperative Blood Glucose[2,7]	-	-	98%	97%
Perioperative Temperature Management[2]	543	100%	100%	100%
Prophylactic Antibiotic Selection[2]	405	100%	99%	99%
Prophylactic Antibiotic Selection (Outpatient)	177	94%	98%	98%
Prophylactic Antibiotic Stopped[2]	403	99%	99%	98%
Prophylactic Antibiotic Timing[2]	405	100%	99%	99%
Prophylactic Antibiotic Timing (Outpatient)	177	98%	99%	98%
Urinary Catheter Removal[2]	230	100%	99%	97%
Survey of Patients' Hospital Experiences				
Area Around Room 'Always' Quiet at Night	300+	69%	64%	61%
Doctors 'Always' Communicated Well	300+	85%	83%	82%
Home Recovery Information Given	300+	90%	87%	85%
Hospital Given 9 or 10 on 10 Point Scale	300+	77%	71%	71%
Meds 'Always' Explained Before Given	300+	71%	65%	64%
Nurses 'Always' Communicated Well	300+	84%	81%	79%
Pain 'Always' Well Controlled	300+	78%	72%	71%
Room and Bathroom 'Always' Clean	300+	72%	72%	73%
Timely Help 'Always' Received	300+	73%	68%	68%
Would Definitely Recommend Hospital	300+	72%	70%	71%
Use of Medical Imaging				
Cardiac Imaging Stress Test before Surgery	687	5.5%	5.4%	5.3%
Combination Abdominal CT Scan	1,095	25.8%	5.6%	10.5%
Combination Brain/Sinus CT Scan	1,052	1.0%	2.6%	2.7%
Combination Chest CT Scan	723	5.1%	1.3%	2.7%
Follow-up Mammogram/Ultrasound	1,028	15.8%	8%	8.8%
Lumbar Spine MRI for Low Back Pain	144	36.1%	34.7%	37.2%

Chatham Hospital

475 Progress Blvd
Siler City, NC 27344
URL: www.chathamhospital.org
Type: Critical Access Hospitals
Ownership: Voluntary non-profit - Private
Phone: 919-663-2113
Fax: 919-663-2343
Emergency Services: Yes
Beds: 68

Key Personnel:

Anesthesiology. . . . . Daniel Caraher, CRNA
Emergency Room . . . . Wilbur Carter
Chief of Medical Staff. . . . . David Gibson
Operating Room. . . . . Donna Sessoms
CEO/President. . . . . Carol Straight
Radiology. . . . . Kenneth Winter

Measure	Cases	This Hosp.	State Avg.	U.S. Avg.
Blood Clot Prevention and Treatment				
Anticoagulation Overlap Therapy[5]	-	-	94%	93%
ICU Venous Thromboembolism Prophylaxis[5]	-	-	93%	92%
Incidence of Potentially Preventable VTE[5]	-	-	10%	10%
UFH with Dosages/Platelet Monitoring[5]	-	-	95%	97%
Venous Thromboembolism Prophylaxis[5]	-	-	88%	85%
Warfarin Therapy Discharge Instructions[5]	-	-	81%	75%
Chest Pain/Possible Heart Attack Care				
Aspirin Given Within 24 Hours of Arrival	-	-	97%	96%
Fibrinolytic Meds Within 30 Min. of Arrival	-	-	66%	58%
Average Time to ECG (minutes)	-	-	7	7
Average Time to Transfer (minutes)	-	-	45	60
Children's Asthma Care				
Received Home Management Plan of Care	-	-	89%	88%
Received Reliever Medication	-	-	100%	100%
Received Systemic Corticosteroids	-	-	100%	100%
Emergency Department				
Admittance Decision Time (minutes)	436	68	107	98
Head CT Results Within 45 Min. of Arrival	-	-	60%	57%
Patients Who Left ER Before Being Seen	-	-	3%	2%
Time from ER Arrival to Admit. (minutes)	466	295	300	274
Time from ER Arrival to Discharge (minutes)	-	-	152	134
Time in ER Before Being Evaluated (minutes)	-	-	34	26
Time to Pain Meds for Fractures (minutes)	-	-	67	57
Heart Attack Care				
Aspirin Given at Discharge[1]	-	-	100%	99%
Fibrinolytic Meds Within 30 Min. of Arrival[7]	-	-	75%	54%
PCI Within 90 Minutes of Arrival[7]	-	-	98%	96%
Statin Prescribed at Discharge[1]	-	-	99%	98%
Heart Failure Care				
ACE Inhibitor or ARB for LVSD	19	89%	98%	97%
Discharge Instructions Given	37	97%	96%	94%
Evaluation of LVS Function	42	95%	100%	99%
Medicare Spending				
Medicare Spending per Patient (ratio)	-	-	0.94	0.98
Pneumonia Care				
Appropriate Initial Antibiotic Given	40	90%	97%	95%
Blood Culture Timing	62	97%	98%	98%
Pregnancy and Delivery Care				
Newborn Deliveries Scheduled Early[7]	-	-	3%	6%
Preventive Care				
Immunization for Influenza	242	83%	93%	90%
Immunization for Pneumonia	384	86%	94%	92%
Stroke Care				
Anticoagulation Therapy for Atrial Fibrillation[5]	-	-	95%	95%
Antithrombotic Therapy Timing[5]	-	-	98%	98%
Assessed for Rehabilitation[5]	-	-	98%	97%
Discharged on Antithrombotic Therapy[5]	-	-	99%	99%
Discharged on Statin Medication[5]	-	-	94%	94%
Thrombolytic Therapy Timing[5]	-	-	64%	66%
Venous Thromboembolism Prophylaxis[5]	-	-	96%	94%
Written Stroke Educational Materials Given[5]	-	-	88%	88%
Surgical Care Improvement Project				
Appropriate Beta Blocker Usage[3,7]	-	-	99%	98%
Appropriate VTP Within 24 Hours[1,3]	-	-	99%	98%
Controlled Postoperative Blood Glucose[3,7]	-	-	98%	97%
Perioperative Temperature Management[1,3]	-	-	100%	100%
Prophylactic Antibiotic Selection[1,3]	-	-	99%	99%
Prophylactic Antibiotic Selection (Outpatient)	-	-	98%	98%
Prophylactic Antibiotic Stopped[1,3]	-	-	99%	98%
Prophylactic Antibiotic Timing[1,3]	-	-	99%	99%
Prophylactic Antibiotic Timing (Outpatient)	-	-	99%	98%
Urinary Catheter Removal[1,3]	-	-	99%	97%
Survey of Patients' Hospital Experiences				
Area Around Room 'Always' Quiet at Night	(a)	64%	64%	61%
Doctors 'Always' Communicated Well	(a)	92%	83%	82%
Home Recovery Information Given	(a)	85%	87%	85%
Hospital Given 9 or 10 on 10 Point Scale	(a)	79%	71%	71%
Meds 'Always' Explained Before Given	(a)	72%	65%	64%
Nurses 'Always' Communicated Well	(a)	89%	81%	79%
Pain 'Always' Well Controlled	(a)	74%	72%	71%
Room and Bathroom 'Always' Clean	(a)	81%	72%	73%
Timely Help 'Always' Received	(a)	80%	68%	68%
Would Definitely Recommend Hospital	(a)	78%	70%	71%
Use of Medical Imaging				
Cardiac Imaging Stress Test before Surgery	-	-	5.4%	5.3%
Combination Abdominal CT Scan	-	-	5.6%	10.5%
Combination Brain/Sinus CT Scan	-	-	2.6%	2.7%
Combination Chest CT Scan	-	-	1.3%	2.7%
Follow-up Mammogram/Ultrasound	-	-	8%	8.8%
Lumbar Spine MRI for Low Back Pain	-	-	34.7%	37.2%

Johnston Memorial Hospital

509 Bright Leaf Blvd
Smithfield, NC 27577
URL: www.johnstanmemorial.org
Type: Acute Care Hospitals
Ownership: Govt - Hospital Dist/Auth
Phone: 919-934-8171
Fax: 919-989-7297
Emergency Services: Yes
Beds: 175

Key Personnel:

Chief of Medical Staff. . . . . Dr Eric Gloss
CEO/President. . . . . Kevin L Rogols

Measure	Cases	This Hosp.	State Avg.	U.S. Avg.
Blood Clot Prevention and Treatment				
Anticoagulation Overlap Therapy[2]	43	91%	94%	93%
ICU Venous Thromboembolism Prophylaxis[2]	52	94%	93%	92%
Incidence of Potentially Preventable VTE[1,2]	-	-	10%	10%
UFH with Dosages/Platelet Monitoring[2]	19	95%	95%	97%
Venous Thromboembolism Prophylaxis[2]	300	82%	88%	85%
Warfarin Therapy Discharge Instructions[2]	27	63%	81%	75%
Chest Pain/Possible Heart Attack Care				
Aspirin Given Within 24 Hours of Arrival	178	100%	97%	96%
Fibrinolytic Meds Within 30 Min. of Arrival[7]	-	-	66%	58%
Average Time to ECG (minutes)	183	2	7	7
Average Time to Transfer (minutes)	22	26	45	60
Children's Asthma Care				
Received Home Management Plan of Care	-	-	89%	88%
Received Reliever Medication	-	-	100%	100%
Received Systemic Corticosteroids	-	-	100%	100%
Emergency Department				
Admittance Decision Time (minutes)[2]	470	68	107	98
Head CT Results Within 45 Min. of Arrival[1]	-	-	60%	57%
Patients Who Left ER Before Being Seen	83,804	2%	3%	2%
Time from ER Arrival to Admit. (minutes)[2]	477	273	300	274
Time from ER Arrival to Discharge (minutes)	363	140	152	134
Time in ER Before Being Evaluated (minutes)	391	39	34	26
Time to Pain Meds for Fractures (minutes)	234	47	67	57
Heart Attack Care				
Aspirin Given at Discharge	27	96%	100%	99%
Fibrinolytic Meds Within 30 Min. of Arrival[7]	-	-	75%	54%
PCI Within 90 Minutes of Arrival[7]	-	-	98%	96%
Statin Prescribed at Discharge	31	97%	99%	98%
Heart Failure Care				

NOTE: Hospital profiles are in alphabetical order by state, then city, then hospital within the city; Rankings exclude hospitals with less than 25 cases except for patient surveys which excludes hospitals with less than 100 cases; (a) 100-299 cases; (1) The number of cases/patients is too few to report; (2) Data submitted were based on a sample of cases/patients; (3) Results are based on a shorter time period than required; (4) Data suppressed by CMS for one or more quarters; (5) Results are not available for this reporting period; (6) Fewer than 100 patients completed the HCAHPS survey; (7) No cases met the criteria for this measure; (8) The lower limit of the confidence interval cannot be calculated if the number of observed infections equals zero; (9) No data are available from the state/territory for this reporting period; (10) The scores shown reflect fewer than 50 completed surveys; (11) There were discrepancies in the data collection process; (12) This measure does not apply to this hospital for this reporting period; (13) Results cannot be calculated for this reporting period; (14) The results for this state are combined with nearby states to protect confidentiality; Please refer to the User's Guide for a full explanation of data.

Measure	Cases	This Hosp.	State Avg.	U.S. Avg.
ACE Inhibitor or ARB for LVSD	73	99%	98%	97%
Discharge Instructions Given	264	94%	96%	94%
Evaluation of LVS Function	335	100%	100%	99%
Medicare Spending				
Medicare Spending per Patient (ratio)	-	0.97	0.94	0.98
Pneumonia Care				
Appropriate Initial Antibiotic Given	181	91%	97%	95%
Blood Culture Timing	279	98%	98%	98%
Pregnancy and Delivery Care				
Newborn Deliveries Scheduled Early[2]	26	0%	3%	6%
Preventive Care				
Immunization for Influenza[2]	536	96%	93%	90%
Immunization for Pneumonia[2]	630	96%	94%	92%
Stroke Care				
Anticoagulation Therapy for Atrial Fibrillation[1]	-	-	95%	95%
Antithrombotic Therapy Timing	42	90%	98%	98%
Assessed for Rehabilitation	43	100%	98%	97%
Discharged on Antithrombotic Therapy	43	98%	99%	99%
Discharged on Statin Medication	37	92%	94%	94%
Thrombolytic Therapy Timing[1]	-	-	64%	66%
Venous Thromboembolism Prophylaxis	40	85%	96%	94%
Written Stroke Educational Materials Given	30	77%	88%	88%
Surgical Care Improvement Project				
Appropriate Beta Blocker Usage	169	96%	99%	98%
Appropriate VTP Within 24 Hours	363	96%	99%	98%
Controlled Postoperative Blood Glucose[7]	-	-	98%	97%
Perioperative Temperature Management	448	100%	100%	100%
Prophylactic Antibiotic Selection	270	100%	99%	99%
Prophylactic Antibiotic Selection (Outpatient)	279	99%	98%	98%
Prophylactic Antibiotic Stopped	262	96%	99%	98%
Prophylactic Antibiotic Timing	270	99%	99%	99%
Prophylactic Antibiotic Timing (Outpatient)	280	100%	99%	98%
Urinary Catheter Removal	289	99%	99%	97%
Survey of Patients' Hospital Experiences				
Area Around Room 'Always' Quiet at Night	300+	72%	64%	61%
Doctors 'Always' Communicated Well	300+	81%	83%	82%
Home Recovery Information Given	300+	89%	87%	85%
Hospital Given 9 or 10 on 10 Point Scale	300+	72%	71%	71%
Meds 'Always' Explained Before Given	300+	66%	65%	64%
Nurses 'Always' Communicated Well	300+	81%	81%	79%
Pain 'Always' Well Controlled	300+	72%	72%	71%
Room and Bathroom 'Always' Clean	300+	68%	72%	73%
Timely Help 'Always' Received	300+	67%	68%	68%
Would Definitely Recommend Hospital	300+	68%	70%	71%
Use of Medical Imaging				
Cardiac Imaging Stress Test before Surgery	225	5.3%	5.4%	5.3%
Combination Abdominal CT Scan	1,375	4.9%	5.6%	10.5%
Combination Brain/Sinus CT Scan	1,426	2.5%	2.6%	2.7%
Combination Chest CT Scan	821	8.8%	1.3%	2.7%
Follow-up Mammogram/Ultrasound	1,539	8.5%	8%	8.8%
Lumbar Spine MRI for Low Back Pain	178	33.1%	34.7%	37.2%

J Arthur Dosher Memorial Hospital

924 Howe St
Southport, NC 28461
Phone: 910-457-3800
Fax: 910-457-3908
URL: www.dosher.org
Type: Critical Access Hospitals
Emergency Services: Yes
Ownership: Voluntary non-profit - Other
Beds: 64

Key Personnel:

Cardiology . . . . J.L. Aldrich, MD, FACC
Anesthesiology. . . . . Kami Anderson, MD
Radiology. . . . . Gail M Capel, MD
Pediatrics. . . . . Jugta Kahai, MD, FAAP
Chairman/CEO . . . . Sherri Marshall
Surgery . . . . Richard Scallion, MD
Quality Assurance . . . . Connie Shea
CEO/President. . . . . Tom Siemers, FACHE

Measure	Cases	This Hosp.	State Avg.	U.S. Avg.
Blood Clot Prevention and Treatment				
Anticoagulation Overlap Therapy[1,2]	-	-	94%	93%
ICU Venous Thromboembolism Prophylaxis[1,2]	-	-	93%	92%
Incidence of Potentially Preventable VTE[2,3]	-	-	10%	10%
UFH with Dosages/Platelet Monitoring[1,2]	-	-	95%	97%
Venous Thromboembolism Prophylaxis[2,3]	69	88%	88%	85%
Warfarin Therapy Discharge Instructions[1,2]	-	-	81%	75%
Chest Pain/Possible Heart Attack Care				
Aspirin Given Within 24 Hours of Arrival	50	86%	97%	96%
Fibrinolytic Meds Within 30 Min. of Arrival[1]	-	-	66%	58%
Average Time to ECG (minutes)	50	4	7	7
Average Time to Transfer (minutes)[1]	-	-	45	60
Children's Asthma Care				
Received Home Management Plan of Care	-	-	89%	88%
Received Reliever Medication	-	-	100%	100%
Received Systemic Corticosteroids	-	-	100%	100%
Emergency Department				
Admittance Decision Time (minutes)[2,3]	297	61	107	98
Head CT Results Within 45 Min. of Arrival[1]	-	-	60%	57%
Patients Who Left ER Before Being Seen	13,000	2%	3%	2%
Time from ER Arrival to Admit. (minutes)[2,3]	341	266	300	274
Time from ER Arrival to Discharge (minutes)[3]	372	116	152	134
Time in ER Before Being Evaluated (minutes)[3]	383	39	34	26
Time to Pain Meds for Fractures (minutes)	40	72	67	57
Heart Attack Care				
Aspirin Given at Discharge[3,7]	-	-	100%	99%
Fibrinolytic Meds Within 30 Min. of Arrival[3,7]	-	-	75%	54%
PCI Within 90 Minutes of Arrival[3,7]	-	-	98%	96%
Statin Prescribed at Discharge[1,3]	-	-	99%	98%
Heart Failure Care				
ACE Inhibitor or ARB for LVSD	11	91%	98%	97%
Discharge Instructions Given	27	81%	96%	94%
Evaluation of LVS Function	39	87%	100%	99%
Medicare Spending				
Medicare Spending per Patient (ratio)	-	-	0.94	0.98
Pneumonia Care				
Appropriate Initial Antibiotic Given	36	92%	97%	95%
Blood Culture Timing	53	87%	98%	98%
Pregnancy and Delivery Care				
Newborn Deliveries Scheduled Early[5]	-	-	3%	6%
Preventive Care				
Immunization for Influenza[2]	298	72%	93%	90%
Immunization for Pneumonia[2,3]	355	84%	94%	92%
Stroke Care				
Anticoagulation Therapy for Atrial Fibrillation[1,3]	-	-	95%	95%
Antithrombotic Therapy Timing[1,3]	-	-	98%	98%
Assessed for Rehabilitation[1,3]	-	-	98%	97%
Discharged on Antithrombotic Therapy[1,3]	-	-	99%	99%
Discharged on Statin Medication[1,3]	-	-	94%	94%
Thrombolytic Therapy Timing[3,7]	-	-	64%	66%
Venous Thromboembolism Prophylaxis[1,3]	-	-	96%	94%
Written Stroke Educational Materials Given[1,3]	-	-	88%	88%
Surgical Care Improvement Project				
Appropriate Beta Blocker Usage[2]	40	92%	99%	98%
Appropriate VTP Within 24 Hours[2]	142	94%	99%	98%
Controlled Postoperative Blood Glucose[2,7]	-	-	98%	97%
Perioperative Temperature Management[2]	155	100%	100%	100%
Prophylactic Antibiotic Selection[2]	112	99%	99%	99%
Prophylactic Antibiotic Selection (Outpatient)[1,3]	-	-	98%	98%
Prophylactic Antibiotic Stopped[2]	109	99%	99%	98%
Prophylactic Antibiotic Timing[2]	112	97%	99%	99%
Prophylactic Antibiotic Timing (Outpatient)[1,3]	-	-	99%	98%
Urinary Catheter Removal[2]	123	100%	99%	97%
Survey of Patients' Hospital Experiences				
Area Around Room 'Always' Quiet at Night	300+	59%	64%	61%
Doctors 'Always' Communicated Well	300+	83%	83%	82%
Home Recovery Information Given	300+	89%	87%	85%
Hospital Given 9 or 10 on 10 Point Scale	300+	70%	71%	71%
Meds 'Always' Explained Before Given	300+	66%	65%	64%
Nurses 'Always' Communicated Well	300+	82%	81%	79%
Pain 'Always' Well Controlled	300+	71%	72%	71%
Room and Bathroom 'Always' Clean	300+	75%	72%	73%
Timely Help 'Always' Received	300+	73%	68%	68%
Would Definitely Recommend Hospital	300+	71%	70%	71%
Use of Medical Imaging				
Cardiac Imaging Stress Test before Surgery	264	7.6%	5.4%	5.3%
Combination Abdominal CT Scan	441	5.9%	5.6%	10.5%
Combination Brain/Sinus CT Scan	430	2.1%	2.6%	2.7%
Combination Chest CT Scan	221	0.0%	1.3%	2.7%
Follow-up Mammogram/Ultrasound	1,373	8.8%	8%	8.8%
Lumbar Spine MRI for Low Back Pain	57	24.6%	34.7%	37.2%

Alleghany County Memorial Hospital

617 Doctors Street
Sparta, NC 28675
Phone: 336-372-5511
Fax: 336-372-8451
URL: www.amhsparta.org
Type: Critical Access Hospitals
Emergency Services: Yes
Ownership: Voluntary non-profit - Private
Beds: 25

Key Personnel:

Radiology. . . . . Paul Beerman, RT
Infection Control. . . . . Mary Jones, RN
CEO . . . . Brent Lammers
Patient Relations . . . . Miranda Miller
Operating Room. . . . . Pam Moss
Quality Assurance . . . . Jayne Phipps-Boger
Emergency Room . . . . Jeff Ray, MD
Chief of Medical Staff. . . . . Jeffrey Ray, MD

Measure	Cases	This Hosp.	State Avg.	U.S. Avg.
Blood Clot Prevention and Treatment				
Anticoagulation Overlap Therapy[5]	-	-	94%	93%
ICU Venous Thromboembolism Prophylaxis[5]	-	-	93%	92%
Incidence of Potentially Preventable VTE[5]	-	-	10%	10%
UFH with Dosages/Platelet Monitoring[5]	-	-	95%	97%
Venous Thromboembolism Prophylaxis[5]	-	-	88%	85%
Warfarin Therapy Discharge Instructions[5]	-	-	81%	75%
Chest Pain/Possible Heart Attack Care				
Aspirin Given Within 24 Hours of Arrival[5]	-	-	97%	96%
Fibrinolytic Meds Within 30 Min. of Arrival[5]	-	-	66%	58%
Average Time to ECG (minutes)[5]	-	-	7	7
Average Time to Transfer (minutes)[5]	-	-	45	60
Children's Asthma Care				
Received Home Management Plan of Care	-	-	89%	88%
Received Reliever Medication	-	-	100%	100%
Received Systemic Corticosteroids	-	-	100%	100%
Emergency Department				
Admittance Decision Time (minutes)[5]	-	-	107	98
Head CT Results Within 45 Min. of Arrival[1,3]	-	-	60%	57%
Patients Who Left ER Before Being Seen[5]	-	-	3%	2%
Time from ER Arrival to Admit. (minutes)[5]	-	-	300	274
Time from ER Arrival to Discharge (minutes)	867	84	152	134
Time in ER Before Being Evaluated (minutes)	965	17	34	26
Time to Pain Meds for Fractures (minutes)	23	33	67	57
Heart Attack Care				
Aspirin Given at Discharge[1,3]	-	-	100%	99%
Fibrinolytic Meds Within 30 Min. of Arrival[3,7]	-	-	75%	54%
PCI Within 90 Minutes of Arrival[3,7]	-	-	98%	96%
Statin Prescribed at Discharge[1,3]	-	-	99%	98%
Heart Failure Care				
ACE Inhibitor or ARB for LVSD[1]	-	-	98%	97%
Discharge Instructions Given	13	100%	96%	94%
Evaluation of LVS Function	16	100%	100%	99%
Medicare Spending				
Medicare Spending per Patient (ratio)	-	-	0.94	0.98
Pneumonia Care				
Appropriate Initial Antibiotic Given	67	91%	97%	95%
Blood Culture Timing	78	99%	98%	98%
Pregnancy and Delivery Care				
Newborn Deliveries Scheduled Early[5]	-	-	3%	6%
Preventive Care				
Immunization for Influenza[5]	-	-	93%	90%
Immunization for Pneumonia[5]	-	-	94%	92%
Stroke Care				
Anticoagulation Therapy for Atrial Fibrillation[5]	-	-	95%	95%
Antithrombotic Therapy Timing[5]	-	-	98%	98%
Assessed for Rehabilitation[5]	-	-	98%	97%
Discharged on Antithrombotic Therapy[5]	-	-	99%	99%
Discharged on Statin Medication[5]	-	-	94%	94%
Thrombolytic Therapy Timing[5]	-	-	64%	66%
Venous Thromboembolism Prophylaxis[5]	-	-	96%	94%
Written Stroke Educational Materials Given[5]	-	-	88%	88%
Surgical Care Improvement Project				
Appropriate Beta Blocker Usage[5]	-	-	99%	98%

NOTE: Hospital profiles are in alphabetical order by state, then city, then hospital within the city; Rankings exclude hospitals with less than 25 cases except for patient surveys which excludes hospitals with less than 100 cases; (a) 100-299 cases; (1) The number of cases/patients is too few to report; (2) Data submitted were based on a sample of cases/patients; (3) Results are based on a shorter time period than required; (4) Data suppressed by CMS for one or more quarters; (5) Results are not available for this reporting period; (6) Fewer than 100 patients completed the HCAHPS survey; (7) No cases met the criteria for this measure; (8) The lower limit of the confidence interval cannot be calculated if the number of observed infections equals zero; (9) No data are available from the state/territory for this reporting period; (10) The scores shown reflect fewer than 50 completed surveys; (11) There were discrepancies in the data collection process; (12) This measure does not apply to this hospital for this reporting period; (13) Results cannot be calculated for this reporting period; (14) The results for this state are combined with nearby states to protect confidentiality; Please refer to the User's Guide for a full explanation of data.

Measure	Cases	This Hosp.	State Avg.	U.S. Avg.
Appropriate VTP Within 24 Hours[5]	-	-	99%	98%
Controlled Postoperative Blood Glucose[5]	-	-	98%	97%
Perioperative Temperature Management[5]	-	-	100%	100%
Prophylactic Antibiotic Selection[5]	-	-	99%	99%
Prophylactic Antibiotic Selection (Outpatient)[1,3]	-	-	98%	98%
Prophylactic Antibiotic Stopped[5]	-	-	99%	98%
Prophylactic Antibiotic Timing[5]	-	-	99%	99%
Prophylactic Antibiotic Timing (Outpatient)[1,3]	-	-	99%	98%
Urinary Catheter Removal[5]	-	-	99%	97%
Survey of Patients' Hospital Experiences				
Area Around Room 'Always' Quiet at Night[6]	<100	62%	64%	61%
Doctors 'Always' Communicated Well[6]	<100	84%	83%	82%
Home Recovery Information Given[6]	<100	88%	87%	85%
Hospital Given 9 or 10 on 10 Point Scale[6]	<100	71%	71%	71%
Meds 'Always' Explained Before Given[6]	<100	75%	65%	64%
Nurses 'Always' Communicated Well[6]	<100	82%	81%	79%
Pain 'Always' Well Controlled[6]	<100	68%	72%	71%
Room and Bathroom 'Always' Clean[6]	<100	73%	72%	73%
Timely Help 'Always' Received[6]	<100	75%	68%	68%
Would Definitely Recommend Hospital[6]	<100	76%	70%	71%
Use of Medical Imaging				
Cardiac Imaging Stress Test before Surgery[7]	-	-	5.4%	5.3%
Combination Abdominal CT Scan	155	3.9%	5.6%	10.5%
Combination Brain/Sinus CT Scan[1]	-	-	2.6%	2.7%
Combination Chest CT Scan	45	2.2%	1.3%	2.7%
Follow-up Mammogram/Ultrasound	255	4.3%	8%	8.8%
Lumbar Spine MRI for Low Back Pain[1]	-	-	34.7%	37.2%

Spruce Pine Community Hospital

125 Hospital Dr
Spruce Pine, NC 28777
Phone: 828-765-4201
Fax: 828-765-0824
URL: www.spchospital.org
Type: Acute Care Hospitals
Emergency Services: Yes
Ownership: Voluntary non-profit - Other
Beds: 40

Key Personnel:
Quality Assurance .... John Brazil
Chief of Medical Staff.......... Jerry Cade, MD
Emergency Room .... Jerry Cade, MD
Patient Relations .... Jane Edwards
Anesthesiology................ Andrea Hinson
CEO/President................ Keith Holtsclaw
Infection Control.............. Mary Ann Johnson, RN
Intensive Care Unit............ Vicky Tolley, RN

Measure	Cases	This Hosp.	State Avg.	U.S. Avg.
Blood Clot Prevention and Treatment				
Anticoagulation Overlap Therapy[1,2]	-	-	94%	93%
ICU Venous Thromboembolism Prophylaxis[2]	56	95%	93%	92%
Incidence of Potentially Preventable VTE[2,7]	-	-	10%	10%
UFH with Dosages/Platelet Monitoring[1,2]	-	-	95%	97%
Venous Thromboembolism Prophylaxis[2]	135	92%	88%	85%
Warfarin Therapy Discharge Instructions[1,2]	-	-	81%	75%
Chest Pain/Possible Heart Attack Care				
Aspirin Given Within 24 Hours of Arrival	75	99%	97%	96%
Fibrinolytic Meds Within 30 Min. of Arrival[1]	-	-	66%	58%
Average Time to ECG (minutes)	78	6	7	7
Average Time to Transfer (minutes)[1]	-	-	45	60
Children's Asthma Care				
Received Home Management Plan of Care	-	-	89%	88%
Received Reliever Medication	-	-	100%	100%
Received Systemic Corticosteroids	-	-	100%	100%
Emergency Department				
Admittance Decision Time (minutes)[2]	450	75	107	98
Head CT Results Within 45 Min. of Arrival[1]	-	-	60%	57%
Patients Who Left ER Before Being Seen	14,040	2%	3%	2%
Time from ER Arrival to Admit. (minutes)[2]	451	265	300	274
Time from ER Arrival to Discharge (minutes)	408	136	152	134
Time in ER Before Being Evaluated (minutes)	440	35	34	26
Time to Pain Meds for Fractures (minutes)	84	81	67	57
Heart Attack Care				
Aspirin Given at Discharge[1]	-	-	100%	99%
Fibrinolytic Meds Within 30 Min. of Arrival[7]	-	-	75%	54%
PCI Within 90 Minutes of Arrival[7]	-	-	98%	96%
Statin Prescribed at Discharge[7]	-	-	99%	98%
Heart Failure Care				
ACE Inhibitor or ARB for LVSD	17	100%	98%	97%
Discharge Instructions Given	52	100%	96%	94%
Evaluation of LVS Function	59	100%	100%	99%
Medicare Spending				
Medicare Spending per Patient (ratio)	-	0.89	0.94	0.98
Pneumonia Care				
Appropriate Initial Antibiotic Given	79	99%	97%	95%
Blood Culture Timing	150	98%	98%	98%
Pregnancy and Delivery Care				
Newborn Deliveries Scheduled Early	13	0%	3%	6%
Preventive Care				
Immunization for Influenza[2]	297	99%	93%	90%
Immunization for Pneumonia[2]	415	100%	94%	92%
Stroke Care				
Anticoagulation Therapy for Atrial Fibrillation[1]	-	-	95%	95%
Antithrombotic Therapy Timing	12	100%	98%	98%
Assessed for Rehabilitation	12	100%	98%	97%
Discharged on Antithrombotic Therapy	11	100%	99%	99%
Discharged on Statin Medication[1]	-	-	94%	94%
Thrombolytic Therapy Timing[7]	-	-	64%	66%
Venous Thromboembolism Prophylaxis	12	100%	96%	94%
Written Stroke Educational Materials Given[1]	-	-	88%	88%
Surgical Care Improvement Project				
Appropriate Beta Blocker Usage	22	100%	99%	98%
Appropriate VTP Within 24 Hours	54	100%	99%	98%
Controlled Postoperative Blood Glucose[7]	-	-	98%	97%
Perioperative Temperature Management	60	100%	100%	100%
Prophylactic Antibiotic Selection	39	100%	99%	99%
Prophylactic Antibiotic Selection (Outpatient)[1,3]	-	-	98%	98%
Prophylactic Antibiotic Stopped	38	95%	99%	98%
Prophylactic Antibiotic Timing	39	100%	99%	99%
Prophylactic Antibiotic Timing (Outpatient)[1,3]	-	-	99%	98%
Urinary Catheter Removal	23	100%	99%	97%
Survey of Patients' Hospital Experiences				
Area Around Room 'Always' Quiet at Night	300+	72%	64%	61%
Doctors 'Always' Communicated Well	300+	87%	83%	82%
Home Recovery Information Given	300+	85%	87%	85%
Hospital Given 9 or 10 on 10 Point Scale	300+	78%	71%	71%
Meds 'Always' Explained Before Given	300+	70%	65%	64%
Nurses 'Always' Communicated Well	300+	85%	81%	79%
Pain 'Always' Well Controlled	300+	73%	72%	71%
Room and Bathroom 'Always' Clean	300+	73%	72%	73%
Timely Help 'Always' Received	300+	72%	68%	68%
Would Definitely Recommend Hospital	300+	72%	70%	71%
Use of Medical Imaging				
Cardiac Imaging Stress Test before Surgery	113	2.7%	5.4%	5.3%
Combination Abdominal CT Scan	354	3.1%	5.6%	10.5%
Combination Brain/Sinus CT Scan[1]	-	-	2.6%	2.7%
Combination Chest CT Scan	221	3.6%	1.3%	2.7%
Follow-up Mammogram/Ultrasound	574	7.1%	8%	8.8%
Lumbar Spine MRI for Low Back Pain	50	48.0%	34.7%	37.2%

Davis Regional Medical Center

218 Old Mocksbville Rd PO Box 1823
Statesville, NC 28687
Phone: 704-873-0281
Fax: 704-838-7289
URL: www.davisregional.com
Type: Acute Care Hospitals
Emergency Services: Yes
Ownership: Proprietary
Beds: 131

Key Personnel:
Emergency Room .... Tammy Brooks, RN
CEO .... Chad French
Chief of Medical Staff.......... Seema Garcha, MD
Cardiac Laboratory............ Kimberly Harrell
Infection Control.............. Amy Painter
Operating Room............... Gary Robinson, MD
Radiology.................... Andrew M Schneider

Measure	Cases	This Hosp.	State Avg.	U.S. Avg.
Blood Clot Prevention and Treatment				
Anticoagulation Overlap Therapy[2]	17	100%	94%	93%
ICU Venous Thromboembolism Prophylaxis[2]	69	100%	93%	92%
Incidence of Potentially Preventable VTE[1,2]	-	-	10%	10%
UFH with Dosages/Platelet Monitoring[1,2]	-	-	95%	97%
Venous Thromboembolism Prophylaxis[2]	207	99%	88%	85%
Warfarin Therapy Discharge Instructions[2]	14	100%	81%	75%
Chest Pain/Possible Heart Attack Care				
Aspirin Given Within 24 Hours of Arrival[1]	-	-	97%	96%
Fibrinolytic Meds Within 30 Min. of Arrival[1]	-	-	66%	58%
Average Time to ECG (minutes)	11	7	7	7
Average Time to Transfer (minutes)[7]	-	-	45	60
Children's Asthma Care				
Received Home Management Plan of Care	-	-	89%	88%
Received Reliever Medication	-	-	100%	100%
Received Systemic Corticosteroids	-	-	100%	100%
Emergency Department				
Admittance Decision Time (minutes)[2]	433	51	107	98
Head CT Results Within 45 Min. of Arrival[1]	-	-	60%	57%
Patients Who Left ER Before Being Seen	26,197	2%	3%	2%
Time from ER Arrival to Admit. (minutes)[2]	433	215	300	274
Time from ER Arrival to Discharge (minutes)	649	108	152	134
Time in ER Before Being Evaluated (minutes)	702	27	34	26
Time to Pain Meds for Fractures (minutes)	61	67	67	57
Heart Attack Care				
Aspirin Given at Discharge	16	100%	100%	99%
Fibrinolytic Meds Within 30 Min. of Arrival[7]	-	-	75%	54%
PCI Within 90 Minutes of Arrival[7]	-	-	98%	96%
Statin Prescribed at Discharge	17	100%	99%	98%
Heart Failure Care				
ACE Inhibitor or ARB for LVSD	30	100%	98%	97%
Discharge Instructions Given	101	100%	96%	94%
Evaluation of LVS Function	108	100%	100%	99%
Medicare Spending				
Medicare Spending per Patient (ratio)	-	0.91	0.94	0.98
Pneumonia Care				
Appropriate Initial Antibiotic Given	89	99%	97%	95%
Blood Culture Timing	162	100%	98%	98%
Pregnancy and Delivery Care				
Newborn Deliveries Scheduled Early	31	6%	3%	6%
Preventive Care				
Immunization for Influenza[2]	334	100%	93%	90%
Immunization for Pneumonia[2]	358	99%	94%	92%
Stroke Care				
Anticoagulation Therapy for Atrial Fibrillation[1]	-	-	95%	95%
Antithrombotic Therapy Timing	15	100%	98%	98%
Assessed for Rehabilitation	17	100%	98%	97%
Discharged on Antithrombotic Therapy	17	100%	99%	99%
Discharged on Statin Medication	17	100%	94%	94%
Thrombolytic Therapy Timing[7]	-	-	64%	66%
Venous Thromboembolism Prophylaxis	15	100%	96%	94%
Written Stroke Educational Materials Given	15	100%	88%	88%
Surgical Care Improvement Project				
Appropriate Beta Blocker Usage	37	100%	99%	98%
Appropriate VTP Within 24 Hours	113	98%	99%	98%
Controlled Postoperative Blood Glucose[7]	-	-	98%	97%
Perioperative Temperature Management	119	100%	100%	100%
Prophylactic Antibiotic Selection	76	99%	99%	99%
Prophylactic Antibiotic Selection (Outpatient)	237	100%	98%	98%
Prophylactic Antibiotic Stopped	67	97%	99%	98%
Prophylactic Antibiotic Timing	76	99%	99%	99%
Prophylactic Antibiotic Timing (Outpatient)	237	100%	99%	98%
Urinary Catheter Removal	55	96%	99%	97%
Survey of Patients' Hospital Experiences				
Area Around Room 'Always' Quiet at Night	300+	62%	64%	61%
Doctors 'Always' Communicated Well	300+	79%	83%	82%
Home Recovery Information Given	300+	81%	87%	85%
Hospital Given 9 or 10 on 10 Point Scale	300+	66%	71%	71%
Meds 'Always' Explained Before Given	300+	60%	65%	64%
Nurses 'Always' Communicated Well	300+	77%	81%	79%
Pain 'Always' Well Controlled	300+	67%	72%	71%
Room and Bathroom 'Always' Clean	300+	70%	72%	73%
Timely Help 'Always' Received	300+	58%	68%	68%
Would Definitely Recommend Hospital	300+	67%	70%	71%
Use of Medical Imaging				
Cardiac Imaging Stress Test before Surgery	50	4.0%	5.4%	5.3%
Combination Abdominal CT Scan	378	3.4%	5.6%	10.5%
Combination Brain/Sinus CT Scan	317	5.4%	2.6%	2.7%
Combination Chest CT Scan	156	0.6%	1.3%	2.7%

NOTE: Hospital profiles are in alphabetical order by state, then city, then hospital within the city; Rankings exclude hospitals with less than 25 cases except for patient surveys which excludes hospitals with less than 100 cases; (a) 100-299 cases; (1) The number of cases/patients is too few to report; (2) Data submitted were based on a sample of cases/patients; (3) Results are based on a shorter time period than required; (4) Data suppressed by CMS for one or more quarters; (5) Results are not available for this reporting period; (6) Fewer than 100 patients completed the HCAHPS survey; (7) No cases met the criteria for this measure; (8) The lower limit of the confidence interval cannot be calculated if the number of observed infections equals zero; (9) No data are available from the state/territory for this reporting period; (10) The scores shown reflect fewer than 50 completed surveys; (11) There were discrepancies in the data collection process; (12) This measure does not apply to this hospital for this reporting period; (13) Results cannot be calculated for this reporting period; (14) The results for this state are combined with nearby states to protect confidentiality; Please refer to the User's Guide for a full explanation of data.

Follow-up Mammogram/Ultrasound	184	9.2%	8%	8.8%
Lumbar Spine MRI for Low Back Pain	104	37.5%	34.7%	37.2%

Iredell Memorial Hospital

557 Brookdale Dr PO Box 1828
Statesville, NC 28677
URL: www.iredellmemorial.org
Phone: 704-873-5661
Fax: 704-872-7924
Type: Acute Care Hospitals
Ownership: Voluntary non-profit - Private
Emergency Services: Yes
Beds: 247

Key Personnel:
Intensive Care Unit. . . . . Eddie Bass, RN
Radiology. . . . . Reid D Breckwoldt
Emergency Room . . . . James Bryant, MD
Infection Control. . . . . Sylvia Chapman
Chief of Medical Staff . . . . Anthony Mebech
Operating Room. . . . . Cindy Miller
CEO/President. . . . . Ed Rush
Quality Assurance . . . . Tracy Thomas

Measure	Cases	This Hosp.	State Avg.	U.S. Avg.
Blood Clot Prevention and Treatment				
Anticoagulation Overlap Therapy[2]	59	81%	94%	93%
ICU Venous Thromboembolism Prophylaxis[2]	104	89%	93%	92%
Incidence of Potentially Preventable VTE[2]	21	5%	10%	10%
UFH with Dosages/Platelet Monitoring[2]	22	100%	95%	97%
Venous Thromboembolism Prophylaxis[2]	353	84%	88%	85%
Warfarin Therapy Discharge Instructions[2]	46	74%	81%	75%
Chest Pain/Possible Heart Attack Care				
Aspirin Given Within 24 Hours of Arrival	59	97%	97%	96%
Fibrinolytic Meds Within 30 Min. of Arrival[1]	-	-	66%	58%
Average Time to ECG (minutes)	64	4	7	7
Average Time to Transfer (minutes)	20	50	45	60
Children's Asthma Care				
Received Home Management Plan of Care	-	-	89%	88%
Received Reliever Medication	-	-	100%	100%
Received Systemic Corticosteroids	-	-	100%	100%
Emergency Department				
Admittance Decision Time (minutes)[2]	631	70	107	98
Head CT Results Within 45 Min. of Arrival	27	63%	60%	57%
Patients Who Left ER Before Being Seen	46,067	5%	3%	2%
Time from ER Arrival to Admit. (minutes)[2]	705	278	300	274
Time from ER Arrival to Discharge (minutes)	379	169	152	134
Time in ER Before Being Evaluated (minutes)	210	49	34	26
Time to Pain Meds for Fractures (minutes)	95	70	67	57
Heart Attack Care				
Aspirin Given at Discharge	98	98%	100%	99%
Fibrinolytic Meds Within 30 Min. of Arrival[7]	-	-	75%	54%
PCI Within 90 Minutes of Arrival	20	100%	98%	96%
Statin Prescribed at Discharge	91	100%	99%	98%
Heart Failure Care				
ACE Inhibitor or ARB for LVSD	93	98%	98%	97%
Discharge Instructions Given	241	86%	96%	94%
Evaluation of LVS Function	292	100%	100%	99%
Medicare Spending				
Medicare Spending per Patient (ratio)	-	0.93	0.94	0.98
Pneumonia Care				
Appropriate Initial Antibiotic Given	197	94%	97%	95%
Blood Culture Timing	253	95%	98%	98%
Pregnancy and Delivery Care				
Newborn Deliveries Scheduled Early[2]	44	16%	3%	6%
Preventive Care				
Immunization for Influenza[2]	583	92%	93%	90%
Immunization for Pneumonia[2]	795	88%	94%	92%
Stroke Care				
Anticoagulation Therapy for Atrial Fibrillation[1]	-	-	95%	95%
Antithrombotic Therapy Timing	78	99%	98%	98%
Assessed for Rehabilitation	79	99%	98%	97%
Discharged on Antithrombotic Therapy	78	100%	99%	99%
Discharged on Statin Medication	58	93%	94%	94%
Thrombolytic Therapy Timing[1]	-	-	64%	66%
Venous Thromboembolism Prophylaxis	75	95%	96%	94%
Written Stroke Educational Materials Given	43	95%	88%	88%
Surgical Care Improvement Project				
Appropriate Beta Blocker Usage[2]	118	99%	99%	98%
Appropriate VTP Within 24 Hours[2]	369	99%	99%	98%
Controlled Postoperative Blood Glucose[2,7]	-	-	98%	97%
Perioperative Temperature Management[2]	403	100%	100%	100%
Prophylactic Antibiotic Selection[2]	261	99%	99%	99%
Prophylactic Antibiotic Selection (Outpatient)	107	93%	98%	98%
Prophylactic Antibiotic Stopped[2]	251	97%	99%	98%
Prophylactic Antibiotic Timing[2]	261	99%	99%	99%
Prophylactic Antibiotic Timing (Outpatient)	108	99%	99%	98%
Urinary Catheter Removal[2]	243	99%	99%	97%
Survey of Patients' Hospital Experiences				
Area Around Room 'Always' Quiet at Night	300+	59%	64%	61%
Doctors 'Always' Communicated Well	300+	82%	83%	82%
Home Recovery Information Given	300+	86%	87%	85%
Hospital Given 9 or 10 on 10 Point Scale	300+	74%	71%	71%
Meds 'Always' Explained Before Given	300+	63%	65%	64%
Nurses 'Always' Communicated Well	300+	79%	81%	79%
Pain 'Always' Well Controlled	300+	70%	72%	71%
Room and Bathroom 'Always' Clean	300+	68%	72%	73%
Timely Help 'Always' Received	300+	60%	68%	68%
Would Definitely Recommend Hospital	300+	74%	70%	71%
Use of Medical Imaging				
Cardiac Imaging Stress Test before Surgery	321	3.7%	5.4%	5.3%
Combination Abdominal CT Scan	816	2.9%	5.6%	10.5%
Combination Brain/Sinus CT Scan	833	3.1%	2.6%	2.7%
Combination Chest CT Scan	369	0.8%	1.3%	2.7%
Follow-up Mammogram/Ultrasound	2,148	4.1%	8%	8.8%
Lumbar Spine MRI for Low Back Pain	93	43.0%	34.7%	37.2%

Novant Health Brunswick Medical Center

1 Medical Center Dr PO Box 139
Supply, NC 28462
URL: www.brunswickcommunityhospital.com
Phone: 910-755-8121
Fax: 910-755-1200
Type: Acute Care Hospitals
Ownership: Voluntary non-profit - Other
Emergency Services: Yes
Beds: 60

Key Personnel:
Quality Assurance . . . . Sherry Cappellino
Emergency Room . . . . Warren Faulk
Chief of Medical Staff . . . . Robert Haffler
CEO/President. . . . . Shelbourn Stevens

Measure	Cases	This Hosp.	State Avg.	U.S. Avg.
Blood Clot Prevention and Treatment				
Anticoagulation Overlap Therapy[2]	27	100%	94%	93%
ICU Venous Thromboembolism Prophylaxis[2]	50	100%	93%	92%
Incidence of Potentially Preventable VTE[2,7]	-	-	10%	10%
UFH with Dosages/Platelet Monitoring[2,7]	-	-	95%	97%
Venous Thromboembolism Prophylaxis[2]	342	97%	88%	85%
Warfarin Therapy Discharge Instructions[2]	24	96%	81%	75%
Chest Pain/Possible Heart Attack Care				
Aspirin Given Within 24 Hours of Arrival	48	98%	97%	96%
Fibrinolytic Meds Within 30 Min. of Arrival[7]	-	-	66%	58%
Average Time to ECG (minutes)	50	0	7	7
Average Time to Transfer (minutes)[1]	-	-	45	60
Children's Asthma Care				
Received Home Management Plan of Care	-	-	89%	88%
Received Reliever Medication	-	-	100%	100%
Received Systemic Corticosteroids	-	-	100%	100%
Emergency Department				
Admittance Decision Time (minutes)[2]	626	128	107	98
Head CT Results Within 45 Min. of Arrival[1]	-	-	60%	57%
Patients Who Left ER Before Being Seen	27,522	1%	3%	2%
Time from ER Arrival to Admit. (minutes)[2]	626	286	300	274
Time from ER Arrival to Discharge (minutes)	452	133	152	134
Time in ER Before Being Evaluated (minutes)	480	29	34	26
Time to Pain Meds for Fractures (minutes)	96	77	67	57
Heart Attack Care				
Aspirin Given at Discharge	11	100%	100%	99%
Fibrinolytic Meds Within 30 Min. of Arrival[7]	-	-	75%	54%
PCI Within 90 Minutes of Arrival[7]	-	-	98%	96%
Statin Prescribed at Discharge[1]	-	-	99%	98%
Heart Failure Care				
ACE Inhibitor or ARB for LVSD	42	100%	98%	97%
Discharge Instructions Given	127	100%	96%	94%
Evaluation of LVS Function	146	100%	100%	99%
Medicare Spending				
Medicare Spending per Patient (ratio)	-	0.94	0.94	0.98
Pneumonia Care				
Appropriate Initial Antibiotic Given	112	99%	97%	95%
Blood Culture Timing	190	100%	98%	98%
Pregnancy and Delivery Care				
Newborn Deliveries Scheduled Early[2]	25	8%	3%	6%
Preventive Care				
Immunization for Influenza[2]	469	98%	93%	90%
Immunization for Pneumonia[2]	614	100%	94%	92%
Stroke Care				
Anticoagulation Therapy for Atrial Fibrillation	17	100%	95%	95%
Antithrombotic Therapy Timing	64	100%	98%	98%
Assessed for Rehabilitation	68	100%	98%	97%
Discharged on Antithrombotic Therapy	67	100%	99%	99%
Discharged on Statin Medication	54	96%	94%	94%
Thrombolytic Therapy Timing[1]	-	-	64%	66%
Venous Thromboembolism Prophylaxis	71	100%	96%	94%
Written Stroke Educational Materials Given	45	100%	88%	88%
Surgical Care Improvement Project				
Appropriate Beta Blocker Usage	137	100%	99%	98%
Appropriate VTP Within 24 Hours	402	100%	99%	98%
Controlled Postoperative Blood Glucose[7]	-	-	98%	97%
Perioperative Temperature Management	470	100%	100%	100%
Prophylactic Antibiotic Selection	351	100%	99%	99%
Prophylactic Antibiotic Selection (Outpatient)	103	99%	98%	98%
Prophylactic Antibiotic Stopped	340	99%	99%	98%
Prophylactic Antibiotic Timing	351	99%	99%	99%
Prophylactic Antibiotic Timing (Outpatient)	103	100%	99%	98%
Urinary Catheter Removal	316	99%	99%	97%
Survey of Patients' Hospital Experiences				
Area Around Room 'Always' Quiet at Night	300+	68%	64%	61%
Doctors 'Always' Communicated Well	300+	81%	83%	82%
Home Recovery Information Given	300+	84%	87%	85%
Hospital Given 9 or 10 on 10 Point Scale	300+	71%	71%	71%
Meds 'Always' Explained Before Given	300+	59%	65%	64%
Nurses 'Always' Communicated Well	300+	78%	81%	79%
Pain 'Always' Well Controlled	300+	69%	72%	71%
Room and Bathroom 'Always' Clean	300+	80%	72%	73%
Timely Help 'Always' Received	300+	63%	68%	68%
Would Definitely Recommend Hospital	300+	74%	70%	71%
Use of Medical Imaging				
Cardiac Imaging Stress Test before Surgery	439	6.4%	5.4%	5.3%
Combination Abdominal CT Scan	736	5.7%	5.6%	10.5%
Combination Brain/Sinus CT Scan	713	2.5%	2.6%	2.7%
Combination Chest CT Scan	344	6.7%	1.3%	2.7%
Follow-up Mammogram/Ultrasound	1,618	9.4%	8%	8.8%
Lumbar Spine MRI for Low Back Pain	157	22.9%	34.7%	37.2%

Medwest Harris

68 Hospital Rd
Sylva, NC 28779
URL: www.westcare.org
Phone: 828-586-7000
Fax: 828-586-7467
Type: Acute Care Hospitals
Ownership: Voluntary non-profit - Private
Emergency Services: Yes
Beds: 86

Key Personnel:
Quality Assurance . . . . Debra Bennett
Radiology. . . . . Jacky Bradley
Emergency Room . . . . Katrina Coggins
Infection Control. . . . . Alice Gibson
Cardiac Laboratory. . . . . Earl Haddock, MD
Operating Room. . . . . Nora Myers
CEO/President. . . . . Mike Poore
Chief of Medical Staff . . . . David Zimmerman

Measure	Cases	This Hosp.	State Avg.	U.S. Avg.
Blood Clot Prevention and Treatment				
Anticoagulation Overlap Therapy[2]	27	96%	94%	93%
ICU Venous Thromboembolism Prophylaxis[2]	35	97%	93%	92%
Incidence of Potentially Preventable VTE[1,2]	-	-	10%	10%
UFH with Dosages/Platelet Monitoring[1,2]	-	-	95%	97%
Venous Thromboembolism Prophylaxis[2]	188	94%	88%	85%
Warfarin Therapy Discharge Instructions[2]	16	69%	81%	75%
Chest Pain/Possible Heart Attack Care				
Aspirin Given Within 24 Hours of Arrival	17	100%	97%	96%
Fibrinolytic Meds Within 30 Min. of Arrival[1,3]	-	-	66%	58%

NOTE: Hospital profiles are in alphabetical order by state, then city, then hospital within the city; Rankings exclude hospitals with less than 25 cases except for patient surveys which excludes hospitals with less than 100 cases; (a) 100-299 cases; (1) The number of cases/patients is too few to report; (2) Data submitted were based on a sample of cases/patients; (3) Results are based on a shorter time period than required; (4) Data suppressed by CMS for one or more quarters; (5) Results are not available for this reporting period; (6) Fewer than 100 patients completed the HCAHPS survey; (7) No cases met the criteria for this measure; (8) The lower limit of the confidence interval cannot be calculated if the number of observed infections equals zero; (9) No data are available from the state/territory for this reporting period; (10) The scores shown reflect fewer than 50 completed surveys; (11) There were discrepancies in the data collection process; (12) This measure does not apply to this hospital for this reporting period; (13) Results cannot be calculated for this reporting period; (14) The results for this state are combined with nearby states to protect confidentiality; Please refer to the User's Guide for a full explanation of data.

Average Time to ECG (minutes)	16	16	7	7
Average Time to Transfer (minutes)[1,3]	-	-	45	60
Children's Asthma Care				
Received Home Management Plan of Care	-	-	89%	88%
Received Reliever Medication	-	-	100%	100%
Received Systemic Corticosteroids	-	-	100%	100%
Emergency Department				
Admittance Decision Time (minutes)[2]	296	74	107	98
Head CT Results Within 45 Min. of Arrival[1]	-	-	60%	57%
Patients Who Left ER Before Being Seen	16,972	3%	3%	2%
Time from ER Arrival to Admit. (minutes)[2]	296	240	300	274
Time from ER Arrival to Discharge (minutes)	344	134	152	134
Time in ER Before Being Evaluated (minutes)	383	32	34	26
Time to Pain Meds for Fractures (minutes)	108	74	67	57
Heart Attack Care				
Aspirin Given at Discharge[1]	-	-	100%	99%
Fibrinolytic Meds Within 30 Min. of Arrival[7]	-	-	75%	54%
PCI Within 90 Minutes of Arrival[7]	-	-	98%	96%
Statin Prescribed at Discharge[1]	-	-	99%	98%
Heart Failure Care				
ACE Inhibitor or ARB for LVSD	30	100%	98%	97%
Discharge Instructions Given	76	86%	96%	94%
Evaluation of LVS Function	98	100%	100%	99%
Medicare Spending				
Medicare Spending per Patient (ratio)	-	0.96	0.94	0.98
Pneumonia Care				
Appropriate Initial Antibiotic Given	100	99%	97%	95%
Blood Culture Timing	156	100%	98%	98%
Pregnancy and Delivery Care				
Newborn Deliveries Scheduled Early[2]	32	34%	3%	6%
Preventive Care				
Immunization for Influenza[2]	346	90%	93%	90%
Immunization for Pneumonia[2]	414	95%	94%	92%
Stroke Care				
Anticoagulation Therapy for Atrial Fibrillation[1]	-	-	95%	95%
Antithrombotic Therapy Timing	19	100%	98%	98%
Assessed for Rehabilitation	23	100%	98%	97%
Discharged on Antithrombotic Therapy	23	100%	99%	99%
Discharged on Statin Medication	17	94%	94%	94%
Thrombolytic Therapy Timing[1]	-	-	64%	66%
Venous Thromboembolism Prophylaxis	19	95%	96%	94%
Written Stroke Educational Materials Given	12	75%	88%	88%
Surgical Care Improvement Project				
Appropriate Beta Blocker Usage	49	94%	99%	98%
Appropriate VTP Within 24 Hours	176	97%	99%	98%
Controlled Postoperative Blood Glucose[7]	-	-	98%	97%
Perioperative Temperature Management	184	100%	100%	100%
Prophylactic Antibiotic Selection	125	99%	99%	99%
Prophylactic Antibiotic Selection (Outpatient)	112	98%	98%	98%
Prophylactic Antibiotic Stopped	123	100%	99%	98%
Prophylactic Antibiotic Timing	126	99%	99%	99%
Prophylactic Antibiotic Timing (Outpatient)	113	98%	99%	98%
Urinary Catheter Removal	138	98%	99%	97%
Survey of Patients' Hospital Experiences				
Area Around Room 'Always' Quiet at Night	300+	66%	64%	61%
Doctors 'Always' Communicated Well	300+	82%	83%	82%
Home Recovery Information Given	300+	86%	87%	85%
Hospital Given 9 or 10 on 10 Point Scale	300+	69%	71%	71%
Meds 'Always' Explained Before Given	300+	67%	65%	64%
Nurses 'Always' Communicated Well	300+	80%	81%	79%
Pain 'Always' Well Controlled	300+	75%	72%	71%
Room and Bathroom 'Always' Clean	300+	74%	72%	73%
Timely Help 'Always' Received	300+	72%	68%	68%
Would Definitely Recommend Hospital	300+	63%	70%	71%
Use of Medical Imaging				
Cardiac Imaging Stress Test before Surgery	400	5.8%	5.4%	5.3%
Combination Abdominal CT Scan	574	38.5%	5.6%	10.5%
Combination Brain/Sinus CT Scan	407	2.2%	2.6%	2.7%
Combination Chest CT Scan	572	7.0%	1.3%	2.7%
Follow-up Mammogram/Ultrasound	1,300	9.3%	8%	8.8%
Lumbar Spine MRI for Low Back Pain	142	36.6%	34.7%	37.2%

Vidant Edgecombe Hospital

111 Hospital Dr
Tarboro, NC 27886
Phone: 252-641-7700
URL: www.vidanthealth.com/edgecombe
Type: Acute Care Hospitals
Emergency Services: Yes
Ownership: Government - Local

Key Personnel:
CEO/President. . . . . Wick Baker
Radiology. . . . . Michael McLaughlin, MD
Chief of Medical Staff . . . . Jose D. Riojas

Measure	Cases	This Hosp.	State Avg.	U.S. Avg.
Blood Clot Prevention and Treatment				
Anticoagulation Overlap Therapy[2]	22	95%	94%	93%
ICU Venous Thromboembolism Prophylaxis[2]	65	94%	93%	92%
Incidence of Potentially Preventable VTE[1,2]	-	-	10%	10%
UFH with Dosages/Platelet Monitoring[1,2]	-	-	95%	97%
Venous Thromboembolism Prophylaxis[2]	307	92%	88%	85%
Warfarin Therapy Discharge Instructions[2]	13	38%	81%	75%
Chest Pain/Possible Heart Attack Care				
Aspirin Given Within 24 Hours of Arrival	86	98%	97%	96%
Fibrinolytic Meds Within 30 Min. of Arrival[1]	-	-	66%	58%
Average Time to ECG (minutes)	92	16	7	7
Average Time to Transfer (minutes)[7]	-	-	45	60
Children's Asthma Care				
Received Home Management Plan of Care	-	-	89%	88%
Received Reliever Medication	-	-	100%	100%
Received Systemic Corticosteroids	-	-	100%	100%
Emergency Department				
Admittance Decision Time (minutes)[2]	277	79	107	98
Head CT Results Within 45 Min. of Arrival[1]	-	-	60%	57%
Patients Who Left ER Before Being Seen	27,523	3%	3%	2%
Time from ER Arrival to Admit. (minutes)[2]	283	310	300	274
Time from ER Arrival to Discharge (minutes)	381	163	152	134
Time in ER Before Being Evaluated (minutes)	349	39	34	26
Time to Pain Meds for Fractures (minutes)	56	84	67	57
Heart Attack Care				
Aspirin Given at Discharge	14	100%	100%	99%
Fibrinolytic Meds Within 30 Min. of Arrival[7]	-	-	75%	54%
PCI Within 90 Minutes of Arrival[7]	-	-	98%	96%
Statin Prescribed at Discharge	15	93%	99%	98%
Heart Failure Care				
ACE Inhibitor or ARB for LVSD	58	98%	98%	97%
Discharge Instructions Given	195	98%	96%	94%
Evaluation of LVS Function	240	100%	100%	99%
Medicare Spending				
Medicare Spending per Patient (ratio)	-	0.92	0.94	0.98
Pneumonia Care				
Appropriate Initial Antibiotic Given	70	97%	97%	95%
Blood Culture Timing	122	98%	98%	98%
Pregnancy and Delivery Care				
Newborn Deliveries Scheduled Early[2]	43	5%	3%	6%
Preventive Care				
Immunization for Influenza[2]	386	93%	93%	90%
Immunization for Pneumonia[2]	499	91%	94%	92%
Stroke Care				
Anticoagulation Therapy for Atrial Fibrillation[1]	-	-	95%	95%
Antithrombotic Therapy Timing	49	98%	98%	98%
Assessed for Rehabilitation	54	100%	98%	97%
Discharged on Antithrombotic Therapy	53	98%	99%	99%
Discharged on Statin Medication	38	95%	94%	94%
Thrombolytic Therapy Timing[1]	-	-	64%	66%
Venous Thromboembolism Prophylaxis	48	94%	96%	94%
Written Stroke Educational Materials Given	33	45%	88%	88%
Surgical Care Improvement Project				
Appropriate Beta Blocker Usage	40	95%	99%	98%
Appropriate VTP Within 24 Hours	128	100%	99%	98%
Controlled Postoperative Blood Glucose[7]	-	-	98%	97%
Perioperative Temperature Management	141	100%	100%	100%
Prophylactic Antibiotic Selection	96	100%	99%	99%
Prophylactic Antibiotic Selection (Outpatient)	122	100%	98%	98%
Prophylactic Antibiotic Stopped	94	100%	99%	98%
Prophylactic Antibiotic Timing	96	100%	99%	99%
Prophylactic Antibiotic Timing (Outpatient)	125	98%	99%	98%
Urinary Catheter Removal	71	97%	99%	97%
Survey of Patients' Hospital Experiences				
Area Around Room 'Always' Quiet at Night	300+	67%	64%	61%
Doctors 'Always' Communicated Well	300+	85%	83%	82%
Home Recovery Information Given	300+	88%	87%	85%
Hospital Given 9 or 10 on 10 Point Scale	300+	74%	71%	71%
Meds 'Always' Explained Before Given	300+	72%	65%	64%
Nurses 'Always' Communicated Well	300+	84%	81%	79%
Pain 'Always' Well Controlled	300+	75%	72%	71%
Room and Bathroom 'Always' Clean	300+	77%	72%	73%
Timely Help 'Always' Received	300+	73%	68%	68%
Would Definitely Recommend Hospital	300+	74%	70%	71%
Use of Medical Imaging				
Cardiac Imaging Stress Test before Surgery	68	2.9%	5.4%	5.3%
Combination Abdominal CT Scan	424	3.5%	5.6%	10.5%
Combination Brain/Sinus CT Scan	752	1.5%	2.6%	2.7%
Combination Chest CT Scan	222	0.9%	1.3%	2.7%
Follow-up Mammogram/Ultrasound	1,182	6.6%	8%	8.8%
Lumbar Spine MRI for Low Back Pain	135	28.9%	34.7%	37.2%

Novant Health Thomasville Medical Center

207 Old Lexington Rd Box 789
Thomasville, NC 27360
Phone: 336-472-2000
Fax: 336-476-2534
URL: www.thomasvillemedicalcenter.org
Type: Acute Care Hospitals
Emergency Services: Yes
Ownership: Voluntary non-profit - Private
Beds: 81

Key Personnel:
Radiology. . . . . Sam Thomas Auringer, MD
CEO/President. . . . . Kathie Johnson
Chief of Medical Staff . . . . Richard Kirsch
Operating Room. . . . . Lynn Maxwell
Infection Control. . . . . Martha Musselman, RN
Quality Assurance . . . . Martha Musselman, RN

Measure	Cases	This Hosp.	State Avg.	U.S. Avg.
Blood Clot Prevention and Treatment				
Anticoagulation Overlap Therapy[2]	12	100%	94%	93%
ICU Venous Thromboembolism Prophylaxis[2]	105	100%	93%	92%
Incidence of Potentially Preventable VTE[1,2]	-	-	10%	10%
UFH with Dosages/Platelet Monitoring[1,2]	-	-	95%	97%
Venous Thromboembolism Prophylaxis[2]	163	93%	88%	85%
Warfarin Therapy Discharge Instructions[2]	12	92%	81%	75%
Chest Pain/Possible Heart Attack Care				
Aspirin Given Within 24 Hours of Arrival	35	100%	97%	96%
Fibrinolytic Meds Within 30 Min. of Arrival[7]	-	-	66%	58%
Average Time to ECG (minutes)	37	3	7	7
Average Time to Transfer (minutes)	12	38	45	60
Children's Asthma Care				
Received Home Management Plan of Care	16	100%	89%	88%
Received Reliever Medication	16	100%	100%	100%
Received Systemic Corticosteroids	16	100%	100%	100%
Emergency Department				
Admittance Decision Time (minutes)[2]	455	79	107	98
Head CT Results Within 45 Min. of Arrival	11	82%	60%	57%
Patients Who Left ER Before Being Seen	37,409	3%	3%	2%
Time from ER Arrival to Admit. (minutes)[2]	482	296	300	274
Time from ER Arrival to Discharge (minutes)	453	138	152	134
Time in ER Before Being Evaluated (minutes)	478	35	34	26
Time to Pain Meds for Fractures (minutes)	86	60	67	57
Heart Attack Care				
Aspirin Given at Discharge	11	100%	100%	99%
Fibrinolytic Meds Within 30 Min. of Arrival[7]	-	-	75%	54%
PCI Within 90 Minutes of Arrival[7]	-	-	98%	96%
Statin Prescribed at Discharge[1]	-	-	99%	98%
Heart Failure Care				
ACE Inhibitor or ARB for LVSD	26	100%	98%	97%
Discharge Instructions Given	84	99%	96%	94%
Evaluation of LVS Function	110	100%	100%	99%
Medicare Spending				
Medicare Spending per Patient (ratio)	-	0.96	0.94	0.98
Pneumonia Care				
Appropriate Initial Antibiotic Given	65	100%	97%	95%
Blood Culture Timing	145	100%	98%	98%
Pregnancy and Delivery Care				
Newborn Deliveries Scheduled Early[2]	52	21%	3%	6%

NOTE: Hospital profiles are in alphabetical order by state, then city, then hospital within the city; Rankings exclude hospitals with less than 25 cases except for patient surveys which excludes hospitals with less than 100 cases; (a) 100-299 cases; (1) The number of cases/patients is too few to report; (2) Data submitted were based on a sample of cases/patients; (3) Results are based on a shorter time period than required; (4) Data suppressed by CMS for one or more quarters; (5) Results are not available for this reporting period; (6) Fewer than 100 patients completed the HCAHPS survey; (7) No cases met the criteria for this measure; (8) The lower limit of the confidence interval cannot be calculated if the number of observed infections equals zero; (9) No data are available from the state/territory for this reporting period; (10) The scores shown reflect fewer than 50 completed surveys; (11) There were discrepancies in the data collection process; (12) This measure does not apply to this hospital for this reporting period; (13) Results cannot be calculated for this reporting period; (14) The results for this state are combined with nearby states to protect confidentiality; Please refer to the User's Guide for a full explanation of data.

Measure	Cases	This Hosp.	State Avg.	U.S. Avg.
Preventive Care				
Immunization for Influenza[2]	476	98%	93%	90%
Immunization for Pneumonia[2]	637	98%	94%	92%
Stroke Care				
Anticoagulation Therapy for Atrial Fibrillation[1]	-	-	95%	95%
Antithrombotic Therapy Timing	48	100%	98%	98%
Assessed for Rehabilitation	59	100%	98%	97%
Discharged on Antithrombotic Therapy	59	100%	99%	99%
Discharged on Statin Medication	49	100%	94%	94%
Thrombolytic Therapy Timing[1]	-	-	64%	66%
Venous Thromboembolism Prophylaxis	47	98%	96%	94%
Written Stroke Educational Materials Given	33	100%	88%	88%
Surgical Care Improvement Project				
Appropriate Beta Blocker Usage	54	96%	99%	98%
Appropriate VTP Within 24 Hours	176	97%	99%	98%
Controlled Postoperative Blood Glucose[7]	-	-	98%	97%
Perioperative Temperature Management	188	100%	100%	100%
Prophylactic Antibiotic Selection	120	99%	99%	99%
Prophylactic Antibiotic Selection (Outpatient)	97	98%	98%	98%
Prophylactic Antibiotic Stopped	114	96%	99%	98%
Prophylactic Antibiotic Timing	120	100%	99%	99%
Prophylactic Antibiotic Timing (Outpatient)	98	99%	99%	98%
Urinary Catheter Removal	108	97%	99%	97%
Survey of Patients' Hospital Experiences				
Area Around Room 'Always' Quiet at Night	300+	56%	64%	61%
Doctors 'Always' Communicated Well	300+	79%	83%	82%
Home Recovery Information Given	300+	83%	87%	85%
Hospital Given 9 or 10 on 10 Point Scale	300+	68%	71%	71%
Meds 'Always' Explained Before Given	300+	58%	65%	64%
Nurses 'Always' Communicated Well	300+	76%	81%	79%
Pain 'Always' Well Controlled	300+	64%	72%	71%
Room and Bathroom 'Always' Clean	300+	73%	72%	73%
Timely Help 'Always' Received	300+	63%	68%	68%
Would Definitely Recommend Hospital	300+	66%	70%	71%
Use of Medical Imaging				
Cardiac Imaging Stress Test before Surgery[1]	-	-	5.4%	5.3%
Combination Abdominal CT Scan	451	2.2%	5.6%	10.5%
Combination Brain/Sinus CT Scan[1]	-	-	2.6%	2.7%
Combination Chest CT Scan	172	0.0%	1.3%	2.7%
Follow-up Mammogram/Ultrasound	607	8.7%	8%	8.8%
Lumbar Spine MRI for Low Back Pain	45	37.8%	34.7%	37.2%

Firsthealth Montgomery Memorial Hospital

520 Allen Street
Troy, NC 27371
Phone: 910-572-1301
Fax: 910-572-4140
URL: www.firsthealth.org
Type: Critical Access Hospitals
Emergency Services: Yes
Ownership: Voluntary non-profit - Private
Beds: 55

Key Personnel:
Radiology.................... Jacob Abraham
Chief of Medical Staff.......... Gilbert D Arenas
CEO/President............... Kerry Hensley

Measure	Cases	This Hosp.	State Avg.	U.S. Avg.
Blood Clot Prevention and Treatment				
Anticoagulation Overlap Therapy[5]	-	-	94%	93%
ICU Venous Thromboembolism Prophylaxis[5]	-	-	93%	92%
Incidence of Potentially Preventable VTE[5]	-	-	10%	10%
UFH with Dosages/Platelet Monitoring[5]	-	-	95%	97%
Venous Thromboembolism Prophylaxis[5]	-	-	88%	85%
Warfarin Therapy Discharge Instructions[5]	-	-	81%	75%
Chest Pain/Possible Heart Attack Care				
Aspirin Given Within 24 Hours of Arrival	43	100%	97%	96%
Fibrinolytic Meds Within 30 Min. of Arrival[7]	-	-	66%	58%
Average Time to ECG (minutes)	44	9	7	7
Average Time to Transfer (minutes)[1]	-	-	45	60
Children's Asthma Care				
Received Home Management Plan of Care	-	-	89%	88%
Received Reliever Medication	-	-	100%	100%
Received Systemic Corticosteroids	-	-	100%	100%
Emergency Department				
Admittance Decision Time (minutes)[5]	-	-	107	98
Head CT Results Within 45 Min. of Arrival[5]	-	-	60%	57%
Patients Who Left ER Before Being Seen	14,706	1%	3%	2%
Time from ER Arrival to Admit. (minutes)[5]	-	-	300	274
Time from ER Arrival to Discharge (minutes)[5]	-	-	152	134
Time in ER Before Being Evaluated (minutes)[5]	-	-	34	26
Time to Pain Meds for Fractures (minutes)	16	54	67	57
Heart Attack Care				
Aspirin Given at Discharge[1,3]	-	-	100%	99%
Fibrinolytic Meds Within 30 Min. of Arrival[3,7]	-	-	75%	54%
PCI Within 90 Minutes of Arrival[3,7]	-	-	98%	96%
Statin Prescribed at Discharge[1,3]	-	-	99%	98%
Heart Failure Care				
ACE Inhibitor or ARB for LVSD[1,3]	-	-	98%	97%
Discharge Instructions Given[1,3]	-	-	96%	94%
Evaluation of LVS Function[1,3]	-	-	100%	99%
Medicare Spending				
Medicare Spending per Patient (ratio)	-	-	0.94	0.98
Pneumonia Care				
Appropriate Initial Antibiotic Given	15	100%	97%	95%
Blood Culture Timing	41	100%	98%	98%
Pregnancy and Delivery Care				
Newborn Deliveries Scheduled Early[5]	-	-	3%	6%
Preventive Care				
Immunization for Influenza[5]	-	-	93%	90%
Immunization for Pneumonia[5]	-	-	94%	92%
Stroke Care				
Anticoagulation Therapy for Atrial Fibrillation[5]	-	-	95%	95%
Antithrombotic Therapy Timing[5]	-	-	98%	98%
Assessed for Rehabilitation[5]	-	-	98%	97%
Discharged on Antithrombotic Therapy[5]	-	-	99%	99%
Discharged on Statin Medication[5]	-	-	94%	94%
Thrombolytic Therapy Timing[5]	-	-	64%	66%
Venous Thromboembolism Prophylaxis[5]	-	-	96%	94%
Written Stroke Educational Materials Given[5]	-	-	88%	88%
Surgical Care Improvement Project				
Appropriate Beta Blocker Usage[5]	-	-	99%	98%
Appropriate VTP Within 24 Hours[5]	-	-	99%	98%
Controlled Postoperative Blood Glucose[5]	-	-	98%	97%
Perioperative Temperature Management[5]	-	-	100%	100%
Prophylactic Antibiotic Selection[5]	-	-	99%	99%
Prophylactic Antibiotic Selection (Outpatient)[5]	-	-	98%	98%
Prophylactic Antibiotic Stopped[5]	-	-	99%	98%
Prophylactic Antibiotic Timing[5]	-	-	99%	99%
Prophylactic Antibiotic Timing (Outpatient)[5]	-	-	99%	98%
Urinary Catheter Removal[5]	-	-	99%	97%
Survey of Patients' Hospital Experiences				
Area Around Room 'Always' Quiet at Night[5]	-	-	64%	61%
Doctors 'Always' Communicated Well[5]	-	-	83%	82%
Home Recovery Information Given[5]	-	-	87%	85%
Hospital Given 9 or 10 on 10 Point Scale[5]	-	-	71%	71%
Meds 'Always' Explained Before Given[5]	-	-	65%	64%
Nurses 'Always' Communicated Well[5]	-	-	81%	79%
Pain 'Always' Well Controlled[5]	-	-	72%	71%
Room and Bathroom 'Always' Clean[5]	-	-	72%	73%
Timely Help 'Always' Received[5]	-	-	68%	68%
Would Definitely Recommend Hospital[5]	-	-	70%	71%
Use of Medical Imaging				
Cardiac Imaging Stress Test before Surgery[1]	-	-	5.4%	5.3%
Combination Abdominal CT Scan	173	7.5%	5.6%	10.5%
Combination Brain/Sinus CT Scan[1]	-	-	2.6%	2.7%
Combination Chest CT Scan	45	0.0%	1.3%	2.7%
Follow-up Mammogram/Ultrasound	308	10.4%	8%	8.8%
Lumbar Spine MRI for Low Back Pain[1]	-	-	34.7%	37.2%

Anson Community Hospital

500 Morven Road
Wadesboro, NC 28170
Phone: 704-694-5131
Fax: 704-694-3900
URL: www.carolinashealthcare.org/facilities/hospitals/anson
Type: Acute Care Hospitals
Emergency Services: Yes
Ownership: Govt - Hospital Dist/Auth
Beds: 125

Key Personnel:
Operating Room.............. Christie Grooms
Emergency Room .... Maureen Lear
Chief of Medical Staff.......... Roger A. Ray, MD
CEO/President............... Frederick G Thompson, PhD
Quality Assurance .... Carol Williams, RN

Measure	Cases	This Hosp.	State Avg.	U.S. Avg.
Blood Clot Prevention and Treatment				
Anticoagulation Overlap Therapy[2]	13	100%	94%	93%
ICU Venous Thromboembolism Prophylaxis[2,7]	-	-	93%	92%
Incidence of Potentially Preventable VTE[1,2]	-	-	10%	10%
UFH with Dosages/Platelet Monitoring[1,2]	-	-	95%	97%
Venous Thromboembolism Prophylaxis[2]	188	91%	88%	85%
Warfarin Therapy Discharge Instructions[1,2]	-	-	81%	75%
Chest Pain/Possible Heart Attack Care				
Aspirin Given Within 24 Hours of Arrival	79	95%	97%	96%
Fibrinolytic Meds Within 30 Min. of Arrival[1]	-	-	66%	58%
Average Time to ECG (minutes)	83	7	7	7
Average Time to Transfer (minutes)[7]	-	-	45	60
Children's Asthma Care				
Received Home Management Plan of Care	-	-	89%	88%
Received Reliever Medication	-	-	100%	100%
Received Systemic Corticosteroids	-	-	100%	100%
Emergency Department				
Admittance Decision Time (minutes)[2]	256	55	107	98
Head CT Results Within 45 Min. of Arrival	13	38%	60%	57%
Patients Who Left ER Before Being Seen	13,332	1%	3%	2%
Time from ER Arrival to Admit. (minutes)[2]	323	285	300	274
Time from ER Arrival to Discharge (minutes)	339	123	152	134
Time in ER Before Being Evaluated (minutes)	348	30	34	26
Time to Pain Meds for Fractures (minutes)	28	65	67	57
Heart Attack Care				
Aspirin Given at Discharge[1]	-	-	100%	99%
Fibrinolytic Meds Within 30 Min. of Arrival[7]	-	-	75%	54%
PCI Within 90 Minutes of Arrival[7]	-	-	98%	96%
Statin Prescribed at Discharge[1]	-	-	99%	98%
Heart Failure Care				
ACE Inhibitor or ARB for LVSD	14	100%	98%	97%
Discharge Instructions Given	28	79%	96%	94%
Evaluation of LVS Function	35	94%	100%	99%
Medicare Spending				
Medicare Spending per Patient (ratio)	-	0.94	0.94	0.98
Pneumonia Care				
Appropriate Initial Antibiotic Given	23	96%	97%	95%
Blood Culture Timing	27	96%	98%	98%
Pregnancy and Delivery Care				
Newborn Deliveries Scheduled Early[7]	-	-	3%	6%
Preventive Care				
Immunization for Influenza[2]	232	96%	93%	90%
Immunization for Pneumonia[2]	318	95%	94%	92%
Stroke Care				
Anticoagulation Therapy for Atrial Fibrillation[1,2]	-	-	95%	95%
Antithrombotic Therapy Timing[2]	12	92%	98%	98%
Assessed for Rehabilitation[2]	12	83%	98%	97%
Discharged on Antithrombotic Therapy[2]	12	92%	99%	99%
Discharged on Statin Medication[2]	12	92%	94%	94%
Thrombolytic Therapy Timing[2,7]	-	-	64%	66%
Venous Thromboembolism Prophylaxis[2]	11	91%	96%	94%
Written Stroke Educational Materials Given[1,2]	-	-	88%	88%
Surgical Care Improvement Project				
Appropriate Beta Blocker Usage[3,7]	-	-	99%	98%
Appropriate VTP Within 24 Hours[1,3]	-	-	99%	98%
Controlled Postoperative Blood Glucose[3,7]	-	-	98%	97%
Perioperative Temperature Management[1,3]	-	-	100%	100%
Prophylactic Antibiotic Selection[1,3]	-	-	99%	99%
Prophylactic Antibiotic Selection (Outpatient)[1,3]	-	-	98%	98%
Prophylactic Antibiotic Stopped[1,3]	-	-	99%	98%
Prophylactic Antibiotic Timing[1,3]	-	-	99%	99%
Prophylactic Antibiotic Timing (Outpatient)[1,3]	-	-	99%	98%
Urinary Catheter Removal[3,7]	-	-	99%	97%
Survey of Patients' Hospital Experiences				
Area Around Room 'Always' Quiet at Night	(a)	76%	64%	61%
Doctors 'Always' Communicated Well	(a)	90%	83%	82%
Home Recovery Information Given	(a)	88%	87%	85%
Hospital Given 9 or 10 on 10 Point Scale	(a)	70%	71%	71%
Meds 'Always' Explained Before Given	(a)	69%	65%	64%
Nurses 'Always' Communicated Well	(a)	88%	81%	79%
Pain 'Always' Well Controlled	(a)	75%	72%	71%

NOTE: Hospital profiles are in alphabetical order by state, then city, then hospital within the city; Rankings exclude hospitals with less than 25 cases except for patient surveys which excludes hospitals with less than 100 cases; (a) 100-299 cases; (1) The number of cases/patients is too few to report; (2) Data submitted were based on a sample of cases/patients; (3) Results are based on a shorter time period than required; (4) Data suppressed by CMS for one or more quarters; (5) Results are not available for this reporting period; (6) Fewer than 100 patients completed the HCAHPS survey; (7) No cases met the criteria for this measure; (8) The lower limit of the confidence interval cannot be calculated if the number of observed infections equals zero; (9) No data are available from the state/territory for this reporting period; (10) The scores shown reflect fewer than 50 completed surveys; (11) There were discrepancies in the data collection process; (12) This measure does not apply to this hospital for this reporting period; (13) Results cannot be calculated for this reporting period; (14) The results for this state are combined with nearby states to protect confidentiality; Please refer to the User's Guide for a full explanation of data.

Room and Bathroom 'Always' Clean	(a)	82%	72%	73%
Timely Help 'Always' Received	(a)	68%	68%	68%
Would Definitely Recommend Hospital	(a)	64%	70%	71%
Use of Medical Imaging				
Cardiac Imaging Stress Test before Surgery[1]	-	-	5.4%	5.3%
Combination Abdominal CT Scan	167	1.8%	5.6%	10.5%
Combination Brain/Sinus CT Scan[1]	-	-	2.6%	2.7%
Combination Chest CT Scan	74	0.0%	1.3%	2.7%
Follow-up Mammogram/Ultrasound	373	9.4%	8%	8.8%
Lumbar Spine MRI for Low Back Pain[1]	-	-	34.7%	37.2%

Vidant Beaufort Hospital

628 E 12th St Phone: 252-975-4100
Washington, NC 27889
Type: Acute Care Hospitals Emergency Services: Yes
Ownership: Voluntary non-profit - Private

Measure	Cases	This Hosp.	State Avg.	U.S. Avg.
Blood Clot Prevention and Treatment				
Anticoagulation Overlap Therapy[1,2]	-	-	94%	93%
ICU Venous Thromboembolism Prophylaxis[2]	31	97%	93%	92%
Incidence of Potentially Preventable VTE[1,2]	-	-	10%	10%
UFH with Dosages/Platelet Monitoring[1,2]	-	-	95%	97%
Venous Thromboembolism Prophylaxis[2]	211	87%	88%	85%
Warfarin Therapy Discharge Instructions[1,2]	-	-	81%	75%
Chest Pain/Possible Heart Attack Care				
Aspirin Given Within 24 Hours of Arrival	45	100%	97%	96%
Fibrinolytic Meds Within 30 Min. of Arrival[1]	-	-	66%	58%
Average Time to ECG (minutes)	47	11	7	7
Average Time to Transfer (minutes)[7]	-	-	45	60
Children's Asthma Care				
Received Home Management Plan of Care	-	-	89%	88%
Received Reliever Medication	-	-	100%	100%
Received Systemic Corticosteroids	-	-	100%	100%
Emergency Department				
Admittance Decision Time (minutes)[2]	243	52	107	98
Head CT Results Within 45 Min. of Arrival	15	53%	60%	57%
Patients Who Left ER Before Being Seen	23,050	2%	3%	2%
Time from ER Arrival to Admit. (minutes)[2]	249	301	300	274
Time from ER Arrival to Discharge (minutes)	411	174	152	134
Time in ER Before Being Evaluated (minutes)	347	49	34	26
Time to Pain Meds for Fractures (minutes)	88	54	67	57
Heart Attack Care				
Aspirin Given at Discharge[1]	-	-	100%	99%
Fibrinolytic Meds Within 30 Min. of Arrival[7]	-	-	75%	54%
PCI Within 90 Minutes of Arrival[7]	-	-	98%	96%
Statin Prescribed at Discharge[1]	-	-	99%	98%
Heart Failure Care				
ACE Inhibitor or ARB for LVSD	35	100%	98%	97%
Discharge Instructions Given	87	97%	96%	94%
Evaluation of LVS Function	101	99%	100%	99%
Medicare Spending				
Medicare Spending per Patient (ratio)	-	0.94	0.94	0.98
Pneumonia Care				
Appropriate Initial Antibiotic Given	62	90%	97%	95%
Blood Culture Timing	99	90%	98%	98%
Pregnancy and Delivery Care				
Newborn Deliveries Scheduled Early	36	8%	3%	6%
Preventive Care				
Immunization for Influenza[2]	323	87%	93%	90%
Immunization for Pneumonia[2]	377	88%	94%	92%
Stroke Care				
Anticoagulation Therapy for Atrial Fibrillation[1]	-	-	95%	95%
Antithrombotic Therapy Timing	56	100%	98%	98%
Assessed for Rehabilitation	53	87%	98%	97%
Discharged on Antithrombotic Therapy	53	100%	99%	99%
Discharged on Statin Medication	43	93%	94%	94%
Thrombolytic Therapy Timing[1]	-	-	64%	66%
Venous Thromboembolism Prophylaxis	55	96%	96%	94%
Written Stroke Educational Materials Given	27	70%	88%	88%
Surgical Care Improvement Project				
Appropriate Beta Blocker Usage	58	97%	99%	98%
Appropriate VTP Within 24 Hours	202	97%	99%	98%
Controlled Postoperative Blood Glucose[7]	-	-	98%	97%
Perioperative Temperature Management	218	100%	100%	100%
Prophylactic Antibiotic Selection	163	97%	99%	99%
Prophylactic Antibiotic Selection (Outpatient)	105	91%	98%	98%
Prophylactic Antibiotic Stopped	162	96%	99%	98%
Prophylactic Antibiotic Timing	163	100%	99%	99%
Prophylactic Antibiotic Timing (Outpatient)	102	100%	99%	98%
Urinary Catheter Removal	109	94%	99%	97%
Survey of Patients' Hospital Experiences				
Area Around Room 'Always' Quiet at Night	300+	63%	64%	61%
Doctors 'Always' Communicated Well	300+	87%	83%	82%
Home Recovery Information Given	300+	90%	87%	85%
Hospital Given 9 or 10 on 10 Point Scale	300+	72%	71%	71%
Meds 'Always' Explained Before Given	300+	66%	65%	64%
Nurses 'Always' Communicated Well	300+	81%	81%	79%
Pain 'Always' Well Controlled	300+	72%	72%	71%
Room and Bathroom 'Always' Clean	300+	72%	72%	73%
Timely Help 'Always' Received	300+	72%	68%	68%
Would Definitely Recommend Hospital	300+	73%	70%	71%
Use of Medical Imaging				
Cardiac Imaging Stress Test before Surgery[1]	-	-	5.4%	5.3%
Combination Abdominal CT Scan	591	4.4%	5.6%	10.5%
Combination Brain/Sinus CT Scan	556	1.4%	2.6%	2.7%
Combination Chest CT Scan	364	1.6%	1.3%	2.7%
Follow-up Mammogram/Ultrasound[7]	-	-	8%	8.8%
Lumbar Spine MRI for Low Back Pain	118	32.2%	34.7%	37.2%

Columbus Regional Healthcare System

500 Jefferson St Phone: 910-642-8011
Whiteville, NC 28472 Fax: 910-640-9305
E-mail: tpriest@crhealthcare.org
URL: www.crhealthcare.org
Type: Acute Care Hospitals Emergency Services: Yes
Ownership: Voluntary non-profit - Other Beds: 154

Key Personnel:
Radiology. . . . . Demir Bastug, MD
Emergency Room . . . . Paul DO, MD
Anesthesiology. . . . . Robin Dimitrious, MD
Operating Room. . . . . Luis E Donayre
Infection Control. . . . . Miranda Dufour, RN
Chief of Medical Staff . . . . V Wade Hash, MD
CEO/President. . . . . Henry Hawthorne, III
Quality Assurance . . . . W Hardy Ledbetter

Measure	Cases	This Hosp.	State Avg.	U.S. Avg.
Blood Clot Prevention and Treatment				
Anticoagulation Overlap Therapy[2]	30	87%	94%	93%
ICU Venous Thromboembolism Prophylaxis[2]	75	97%	93%	92%
Incidence of Potentially Preventable VTE[1,2]	-	-	10%	10%
UFH with Dosages/Platelet Monitoring[1,2]	-	-	95%	97%
Venous Thromboembolism Prophylaxis[2]	357	86%	88%	85%
Warfarin Therapy Discharge Instructions[2]	21	100%	81%	75%
Chest Pain/Possible Heart Attack Care				
Aspirin Given Within 24 Hours of Arrival	86	97%	97%	96%
Fibrinolytic Meds Within 30 Min. of Arrival	12	25%	66%	58%
Average Time to ECG (minutes)	88	7	7	7
Average Time to Transfer (minutes)[1]	-	-	45	60
Children's Asthma Care				
Received Home Management Plan of Care	-	-	89%	88%
Received Reliever Medication	-	-	100%	100%
Received Systemic Corticosteroids	-	-	100%	100%
Emergency Department				
Admittance Decision Time (minutes)[2]	647	142	107	98
Head CT Results Within 45 Min. of Arrival[1]	-	-	60%	57%
Patients Who Left ER Before Being Seen	30,722	4%	3%	2%
Time from ER Arrival to Admit. (minutes)[2]	660	340	300	274
Time from ER Arrival to Discharge (minutes)	365	169	152	134
Time in ER Before Being Evaluated (minutes)	397	49	34	26
Time to Pain Meds for Fractures (minutes)	77	102	67	57
Heart Attack Care				
Aspirin Given at Discharge[1]	-	-	100%	99%
Fibrinolytic Meds Within 30 Min. of Arrival[7]	-	-	75%	54%
PCI Within 90 Minutes of Arrival[7]	-	-	98%	96%
Statin Prescribed at Discharge[1]	-	-	99%	98%
Heart Failure Care				
ACE Inhibitor or ARB for LVSD	28	86%	98%	97%
Discharge Instructions Given	107	86%	96%	94%
Evaluation of LVS Function	135	96%	100%	99%
Medicare Spending				
Medicare Spending per Patient (ratio)	-	0.98	0.94	0.98
Pneumonia Care				
Appropriate Initial Antibiotic Given	101	91%	97%	95%
Blood Culture Timing	156	99%	98%	98%
Pregnancy and Delivery Care				
Newborn Deliveries Scheduled Early[2]	46	0%	3%	6%
Preventive Care				
Immunization for Influenza[2]	446	89%	93%	90%
Immunization for Pneumonia[2]	577	95%	94%	92%
Stroke Care				
Anticoagulation Therapy for Atrial Fibrillation[1]	-	-	95%	95%
Antithrombotic Therapy Timing	46	91%	98%	98%
Assessed for Rehabilitation	43	88%	98%	97%
Discharged on Antithrombotic Therapy	42	98%	99%	99%
Discharged on Statin Medication	38	63%	94%	94%
Thrombolytic Therapy Timing[1]	-	-	64%	66%
Venous Thromboembolism Prophylaxis	47	89%	96%	94%
Written Stroke Educational Materials Given	24	58%	88%	88%
Surgical Care Improvement Project				
Appropriate Beta Blocker Usage	64	98%	99%	98%
Appropriate VTP Within 24 Hours	172	99%	99%	98%
Controlled Postoperative Blood Glucose[7]	-	-	98%	97%
Perioperative Temperature Management	203	100%	100%	100%
Prophylactic Antibiotic Selection	69	96%	99%	99%
Prophylactic Antibiotic Selection (Outpatient)	33	97%	98%	98%
Prophylactic Antibiotic Stopped	67	100%	99%	98%
Prophylactic Antibiotic Timing	70	99%	99%	99%
Prophylactic Antibiotic Timing (Outpatient)	35	91%	99%	98%
Urinary Catheter Removal	116	97%	99%	97%
Survey of Patients' Hospital Experiences				
Area Around Room 'Always' Quiet at Night	300+	62%	64%	61%
Doctors 'Always' Communicated Well	300+	85%	83%	82%
Home Recovery Information Given	300+	87%	87%	85%
Hospital Given 9 or 10 on 10 Point Scale	300+	69%	71%	71%
Meds 'Always' Explained Before Given	300+	65%	65%	64%
Nurses 'Always' Communicated Well	300+	82%	81%	79%
Pain 'Always' Well Controlled	300+	77%	72%	71%
Room and Bathroom 'Always' Clean	300+	73%	72%	73%
Timely Help 'Always' Received	300+	71%	68%	68%
Would Definitely Recommend Hospital	300+	66%	70%	71%
Use of Medical Imaging				
Cardiac Imaging Stress Test before Surgery	137	6.6%	5.4%	5.3%
Combination Abdominal CT Scan	720	9.7%	5.6%	10.5%
Combination Brain/Sinus CT Scan	696	1.1%	2.6%	2.7%
Combination Chest CT Scan	318	0.6%	1.3%	2.7%
Follow-up Mammogram/Ultrasound	1,357	6.3%	8%	8.8%
Lumbar Spine MRI for Low Back Pain	141	24.8%	34.7%	37.2%

Martin General Hospital

310 S Mccaskey Rd PO Box 1128 Phone: 252-809-6179
Williamston, NC 27892 Fax: 252-809-6283
E-mail: billi_wynn@chs.net
URL: www.martingeneral.com
Type: Acute Care Hospitals Emergency Services: Yes
Ownership: Government - Local Beds: 49

Key Personnel:
Chief of Medical Staff . . . . Domingo Cue, MD
Cardiac Laboratory. . . . . Harold Finn
Radiology. . . . . Raymond Hassett
Emergency Room . . . . Thomas Hunter
Infection Control. . . . . Tonya Perry
CEO/President. . . . . David Sanders
Operating Room. . . . . Bonnie Speller, RN

Measure	Cases	This Hosp.	State Avg.	U.S. Avg.
Blood Clot Prevention and Treatment				
Anticoagulation Overlap Therapy[1,2]	-	-	94%	93%
ICU Venous Thromboembolism Prophylaxis[2]	71	94%	93%	92%
Incidence of Potentially Preventable VTE[1,2]	-	-	10%	10%
UFH with Dosages/Platelet Monitoring[2,7]	-	-	95%	97%
Venous Thromboembolism Prophylaxis[2]	204	97%	88%	85%

NOTE: Hospital profiles are in alphabetical order by state, then city, then hospital within the city; Rankings exclude hospitals with less than 25 cases except for patient surveys which excludes hospitals with less than 100 cases; (a) 100-299 cases; (1) The number of cases/patients is too few to report; (2) Data submitted were based on a sample of cases/patients; (3) Results are based on a shorter time period than required; (4) Data suppressed by CMS for one or more quarters; (5) Results are not available for this reporting period; (6) Fewer than 100 patients completed the HCAHPS survey; (7) No cases met the criteria for this measure; (8) The lower limit of the confidence interval cannot be calculated if the number of observed infections equals zero; (9) No data are available from the state/territory for this reporting period; (10) The scores shown reflect fewer than 50 completed surveys; (11) There were discrepancies in the data collection process; (12) This measure does not apply to this hospital for this reporting period; (13) Results cannot be calculated for this reporting period; (14) The results for this state are combined with nearby states to protect confidentiality; Please refer to the User's Guide for a full explanation of data.

Measure	Cases	This Hosp.	State Avg.	U.S. Avg.
Warfarin Therapy Discharge Instructions[1,2]	-	-	81%	75%
Chest Pain/Possible Heart Attack Care				
Aspirin Given Within 24 Hours of Arrival	43	98%	97%	96%
Fibrinolytic Meds Within 30 Min. of Arrival[1]	-	-	66%	58%
Average Time to ECG (minutes)	44	8	7	7
Average Time to Transfer (minutes)[1]	-	-	45	60
Children's Asthma Care				
Received Home Management Plan of Care	-	-	89%	88%
Received Reliever Medication	-	-	100%	100%
Received Systemic Corticosteroids	-	-	100%	100%
Emergency Department				
Admittance Decision Time (minutes)[2]	371	120	107	98
Head CT Results Within 45 Min. of Arrival[1]	-	-	60%	57%
Patients Who Left ER Before Being Seen	14,226	4%	3%	2%
Time from ER Arrival to Admit. (minutes)[2]	413	295	300	274
Time from ER Arrival to Discharge (minutes)	363	137	152	134
Time in ER Before Being Evaluated (minutes)	389	35	34	26
Time to Pain Meds for Fractures (minutes)	45	69	67	57
Heart Attack Care				
Aspirin Given at Discharge[1]	-	-	100%	99%
Fibrinolytic Meds Within 30 Min. of Arrival[7]	-	-	75%	54%
PCI Within 90 Minutes of Arrival[7]	-	-	98%	96%
Statin Prescribed at Discharge[1]	-	-	99%	98%
Heart Failure Care				
ACE Inhibitor or ARB for LVSD	33	97%	98%	97%
Discharge Instructions Given	86	88%	96%	94%
Evaluation of LVS Function	102	100%	100%	99%
Medicare Spending				
Medicare Spending per Patient (ratio)	-	0.89	0.94	0.98
Pneumonia Care				
Appropriate Initial Antibiotic Given	35	94%	97%	95%
Blood Culture Timing	77	95%	98%	98%
Pregnancy and Delivery Care				
Newborn Deliveries Scheduled Early[2]	20	0%	3%	6%
Preventive Care				
Immunization for Influenza[2]	295	99%	93%	90%
Immunization for Pneumonia[2]	414	100%	94%	92%
Stroke Care				
Anticoagulation Therapy for Atrial Fibrillation[1]	-	-	95%	95%
Antithrombotic Therapy Timing	43	98%	98%	98%
Assessed for Rehabilitation	42	98%	98%	97%
Discharged on Antithrombotic Therapy	42	100%	99%	99%
Discharged on Statin Medication	33	94%	94%	94%
Thrombolytic Therapy Timing[1]	-	-	64%	66%
Venous Thromboembolism Prophylaxis	40	100%	96%	94%
Written Stroke Educational Materials Given	30	93%	88%	88%
Surgical Care Improvement Project				
Appropriate Beta Blocker Usage	27	100%	99%	98%
Appropriate VTP Within 24 Hours	74	100%	99%	98%
Controlled Postoperative Blood Glucose[7]	-	-	98%	97%
Perioperative Temperature Management	83	100%	100%	100%
Prophylactic Antibiotic Selection	73	95%	99%	99%
Prophylactic Antibiotic Selection (Outpatient)	12	100%	98%	98%
Prophylactic Antibiotic Stopped	71	99%	99%	98%
Prophylactic Antibiotic Timing	73	99%	99%	99%
Prophylactic Antibiotic Timing (Outpatient)	12	100%	99%	98%
Urinary Catheter Removal[1]	-	-	99%	97%
Survey of Patients' Hospital Experiences				
Area Around Room 'Always' Quiet at Night	300+	70%	64%	61%
Doctors 'Always' Communicated Well	300+	84%	83%	82%
Home Recovery Information Given	300+	85%	87%	85%
Hospital Given 9 or 10 on 10 Point Scale	300+	64%	71%	71%
Meds 'Always' Explained Before Given	300+	66%	65%	64%
Nurses 'Always' Communicated Well	300+	81%	81%	79%
Pain 'Always' Well Controlled	300+	73%	72%	71%
Room and Bathroom 'Always' Clean	300+	64%	72%	73%
Timely Help 'Always' Received	300+	68%	68%	68%
Would Definitely Recommend Hospital	300+	62%	70%	71%
Use of Medical Imaging				
Cardiac Imaging Stress Test before Surgery[1]	-	-	5.4%	5.3%
Combination Abdominal CT Scan	181	0.0%	5.6%	10.5%
Combination Brain/Sinus CT Scan	440	1.6%	2.6%	2.7%
Combination Chest CT Scan	55	0.0%	1.3%	2.7%
Follow-up Mammogram/Ultrasound	540	5.7%	8%	8.8%
Lumbar Spine MRI for Low Back Pain[1]	-	-	34.7%	37.2%

New Hanover Regional Medical Center

2131 S 17th Saint Box 9000
Wilmington, NC 28402
URL: www.nhrmc.org
Phone: 910-343-7000
Fax: 910-343-7220
Type: Acute Care Hospitals
Emergency Services: Yes
Ownership: Government - Local
Beds: 628

Key Personnel:
CEO/President. . . . . Jack Barto
Radiology. . . . . Neal L Beard, MD
Chief of Medical Staff. . . . . Pat Canover
Pediatric Ambulatory Care . . . . . . Mary Forehand, MD
Pediatric In-Patient Care . . . . Mary Forehand, MD
Operating Room. . . . . Carolyn Knaup
Infection Control. . . . . Patricia Schlegel, RN
Quality Assurance . . . . Patricia Wheeler

Measure	Cases	This Hosp.	State Avg.	U.S. Avg.
Blood Clot Prevention and Treatment				
Anticoagulation Overlap Therapy[2]	170	95%	94%	93%
ICU Venous Thromboembolism Prophylaxis[2]	87	95%	93%	92%
Incidence of Potentially Preventable VTE[2]	50	2%	10%	10%
UFH with Dosages/Platelet Monitoring[2]	39	95%	95%	97%
Venous Thromboembolism Prophylaxis[2]	326	88%	88%	85%
Warfarin Therapy Discharge Instructions[2]	117	27%	81%	75%
Chest Pain/Possible Heart Attack Care				
Aspirin Given Within 24 Hours of Arrival[3,7]	-	-	97%	96%
Fibrinolytic Meds Within 30 Min. of Arrival[5]	-	-	66%	58%
Average Time to ECG (minutes)[1,3]	-	-	7	7
Average Time to Transfer (minutes)[5]	-	-	45	60
Children's Asthma Care				
Received Home Management Plan of Care	-	-	89%	88%
Received Reliever Medication	-	-	100%	100%
Received Systemic Corticosteroids	-	-	100%	100%
Emergency Department				
Admittance Decision Time (minutes)[2]	577	148	107	98
Head CT Results Within 45 Min. of Arrival	13	15%	60%	57%
Patients Who Left ER Before Being Seen	>100k	3%	3%	2%
Time from ER Arrival to Admit. (minutes)[2]	578	318	300	274
Time from ER Arrival to Discharge (minutes)	394	146	152	134
Time in ER Before Being Evaluated (minutes)	405	69	34	26
Time to Pain Meds for Fractures (minutes)	396	81	67	57
Heart Attack Care				
Aspirin Given at Discharge	812	99%	100%	99%
Fibrinolytic Meds Within 30 Min. of Arrival[7]	-	-	75%	54%
PCI Within 90 Minutes of Arrival	175	97%	98%	96%
Statin Prescribed at Discharge	780	100%	99%	98%
Heart Failure Care				
ACE Inhibitor or ARB for LVSD	320	99%	98%	97%
Discharge Instructions Given	914	99%	96%	94%
Evaluation of LVS Function	1,138	100%	100%	99%
Medicare Spending				
Medicare Spending per Patient (ratio)	-	0.96	0.94	0.98
Pneumonia Care				
Appropriate Initial Antibiotic Given	328	97%	97%	95%
Blood Culture Timing	695	99%	98%	98%
Pregnancy and Delivery Care				
Newborn Deliveries Scheduled Early[2]	40	5%	3%	6%
Preventive Care				
Immunization for Influenza[2]	570	87%	93%	90%
Immunization for Pneumonia[2]	664	89%	94%	92%
Stroke Care				
Anticoagulation Therapy for Atrial Fibrillation	60	92%	95%	95%
Antithrombotic Therapy Timing	327	96%	98%	98%
Assessed for Rehabilitation	435	95%	98%	97%
Discharged on Antithrombotic Therapy	371	94%	99%	99%
Discharged on Statin Medication	271	92%	94%	94%
Thrombolytic Therapy Timing	33	45%	64%	66%
Venous Thromboembolism Prophylaxis	444	93%	96%	94%
Written Stroke Educational Materials Given	242	87%	88%	88%
Surgical Care Improvement Project				
Appropriate Beta Blocker Usage[2]	741	100%	99%	98%
Appropriate VTP Within 24 Hours[2]	1,292	100%	99%	98%
Controlled Postoperative Blood Glucose[2]	435	98%	98%	97%
Perioperative Temperature Management[2]	1,616	100%	100%	100%
Prophylactic Antibiotic Selection[2]	1,654	99%	99%	99%
Prophylactic Antibiotic Selection (Outpatient)	700	98%	98%	98%
Prophylactic Antibiotic Stopped[2]	1,626	100%	99%	98%
Prophylactic Antibiotic Timing[2]	1,654	99%	99%	99%
Prophylactic Antibiotic Timing (Outpatient)	718	95%	99%	98%
Urinary Catheter Removal[2]	1,199	99%	99%	97%
Survey of Patients' Hospital Experiences				
Area Around Room 'Always' Quiet at Night	300+	73%	64%	61%
Doctors 'Always' Communicated Well	300+	86%	83%	82%
Home Recovery Information Given	300+	88%	87%	85%
Hospital Given 9 or 10 on 10 Point Scale	300+	79%	71%	71%
Meds 'Always' Explained Before Given	300+	70%	65%	64%
Nurses 'Always' Communicated Well	300+	86%	81%	79%
Pain 'Always' Well Controlled	300+	78%	72%	71%
Room and Bathroom 'Always' Clean	300+	75%	72%	73%
Timely Help 'Always' Received	300+	72%	68%	68%
Would Definitely Recommend Hospital	300+	81%	70%	71%
Use of Medical Imaging				
Cardiac Imaging Stress Test before Surgery	3,321	5.7%	5.4%	5.3%
Combination Abdominal CT Scan	2,807	6.2%	5.6%	10.5%
Combination Brain/Sinus CT Scan	1,975	4.4%	2.6%	2.7%
Combination Chest CT Scan	1,880	1.0%	1.3%	2.7%
Follow-up Mammogram/Ultrasound	3,749	8.1%	8%	8.8%
Lumbar Spine MRI for Low Back Pain	482	37.6%	34.7%	37.2%

Wilson Medical Center

1705 S Tarboro St
Wilson, NC 27893
URL: www.wilmed.org/contact.asp
Phone: 252-399-8040
Fax: 252-399-8778
Type: Acute Care Hospitals
Emergency Services: Yes
Ownership: Voluntary non-profit - Private
Beds: 317

Key Personnel:
Emergency Room . . . . Suzie Bass, RN
CEO/President. . . . . Bill Caldwell
Radiology. . . . . Paul Guay, MD
Operating Room. . . . . Glenda Mitchell, RN
Pediatric Ambulatory Care . . . . . . Robert Pope, MD
Pediatric In-Patient Care . . . . Robert Pope, MD
Quality Assurance . . . . Jane Rosenmarkel
Chief of Medical Staff. . . . . Roger Thurman, MD

Measure	Cases	This Hosp.	State Avg.	U.S. Avg.
Blood Clot Prevention and Treatment				
Anticoagulation Overlap Therapy[2]	41	95%	94%	93%
ICU Venous Thromboembolism Prophylaxis[2]	57	77%	93%	92%
Incidence of Potentially Preventable VTE[2]	13	15%	10%	10%
UFH with Dosages/Platelet Monitoring[2]	26	96%	95%	97%
Venous Thromboembolism Prophylaxis[2]	391	78%	88%	85%
Warfarin Therapy Discharge Instructions[2]	30	70%	81%	75%
Chest Pain/Possible Heart Attack Care				
Aspirin Given Within 24 Hours of Arrival	78	90%	97%	96%
Fibrinolytic Meds Within 30 Min. of Arrival	11	55%	66%	58%
Average Time to ECG (minutes)	81	12	7	7
Average Time to Transfer (minutes)[1]	-	-	45	60
Children's Asthma Care				
Received Home Management Plan of Care	26	92%	89%	88%
Received Reliever Medication	29	100%	100%	100%
Received Systemic Corticosteroids	29	100%	100%	100%
Emergency Department				
Admittance Decision Time (minutes)[2]	640	240	107	98
Head CT Results Within 45 Min. of Arrival	22	59%	60%	57%
Patients Who Left ER Before Being Seen	50,781	4%	3%	2%
Time from ER Arrival to Admit. (minutes)[2]	658	456	300	274
Time from ER Arrival to Discharge (minutes)	372	144	152	134
Time in ER Before Being Evaluated (minutes)	397	57	34	26
Time to Pain Meds for Fractures (minutes)	113	77	67	57
Heart Attack Care				
Aspirin Given at Discharge	80	98%	100%	99%
Fibrinolytic Meds Within 30 Min. of Arrival[7]	-	-	75%	54%
PCI Within 90 Minutes of Arrival[7]	-	-	98%	96%
Statin Prescribed at Discharge	76	93%	99%	98%
Heart Failure Care				

NOTE: Hospital profiles are in alphabetical order by state, then city, then hospital within the city; Rankings exclude hospitals with less than 25 cases except for patient surveys which excludes hospitals with less than 100 cases; (a) 100-299 cases; (1) The number of cases/patients is too few to report; (2) Data submitted were based on a sample of cases/patients; (3) Results are based on a shorter time period than required; (4) Data suppressed by CMS for one or more quarters; (5) Results are not available for this reporting period; (6) Fewer than 100 patients completed the HCAHPS survey; (7) No cases met the criteria for this measure; (8) The lower limit of the confidence interval cannot be calculated if the number of observed infections equals zero; (9) No data are available from the state/territory for this reporting period; (10) The scores shown reflect fewer than 50 completed surveys; (11) There were discrepancies in the data collection process; (12) This measure does not apply to this hospital for this reporting period; (13) Results cannot be calculated for this reporting period; (14) The results for this state are combined with nearby states to protect confidentiality; Please refer to the User's Guide for a full explanation of data.

Measure	Cases	This Hosp.	State Avg.	U.S. Avg.
ACE Inhibitor or ARB for LVSD	82	94%	98%	97%
Discharge Instructions Given	224	89%	96%	94%
Evaluation of LVS Function	279	100%	100%	99%
Medicare Spending				
Medicare Spending per Patient (ratio)	-	0.98	0.94	0.98
Pneumonia Care				
Appropriate Initial Antibiotic Given	169	93%	97%	95%
Blood Culture Timing	319	91%	98%	98%
Pregnancy and Delivery Care				
Newborn Deliveries Scheduled Early[2]	33	12%	3%	6%
Preventive Care				
Immunization for Influenza[2]	509	96%	93%	90%
Immunization for Pneumonia[2]	665	95%	94%	92%
Stroke Care				
Anticoagulation Therapy for Atrial Fibrillation[1]	-	-	95%	95%
Antithrombotic Therapy Timing	111	96%	98%	98%
Assessed for Rehabilitation	94	99%	98%	97%
Discharged on Antithrombotic Therapy	94	99%	99%	99%
Discharged on Statin Medication	78	88%	94%	94%
Thrombolytic Therapy Timing[1]	-	-	64%	66%
Venous Thromboembolism Prophylaxis	108	87%	96%	94%
Written Stroke Educational Materials Given	47	83%	88%	88%
Surgical Care Improvement Project				
Appropriate Beta Blocker Usage[2]	117	98%	99%	98%
Appropriate VTP Within 24 Hours[2]	430	98%	99%	98%
Controlled Postoperative Blood Glucose[2,7]	-	-	98%	97%
Perioperative Temperature Management[2]	489	100%	100%	100%
Prophylactic Antibiotic Selection[2]	373	100%	99%	99%
Prophylactic Antibiotic Selection (Outpatient)	148	97%	98%	98%
Prophylactic Antibiotic Stopped[2]	367	99%	99%	98%
Prophylactic Antibiotic Timing[2]	375	100%	99%	99%
Prophylactic Antibiotic Timing (Outpatient)	149	98%	99%	98%
Urinary Catheter Removal[2]	321	98%	99%	97%
Survey of Patients' Hospital Experiences				
Area Around Room 'Always' Quiet at Night	300+	60%	64%	61%
Doctors 'Always' Communicated Well	300+	85%	83%	82%
Home Recovery Information Given	300+	90%	87%	85%
Hospital Given 9 or 10 on 10 Point Scale	300+	71%	71%	71%
Meds 'Always' Explained Before Given	300+	67%	65%	64%
Nurses 'Always' Communicated Well	300+	83%	81%	79%
Pain 'Always' Well Controlled	300+	75%	72%	71%
Room and Bathroom 'Always' Clean	300+	68%	72%	73%
Timely Help 'Always' Received	300+	69%	68%	68%
Would Definitely Recommend Hospital	300+	60%	70%	71%
Use of Medical Imaging				
Cardiac Imaging Stress Test before Surgery	326	8.9%	5.4%	5.3%
Combination Abdominal CT Scan	1,122	5.1%	5.6%	10.5%
Combination Brain/Sinus CT Scan	1,454	3.8%	2.6%	2.7%
Combination Chest CT Scan	982	0.3%	1.3%	2.7%
Follow-up Mammogram/Ultrasound	2,276	5.8%	8%	8.8%
Lumbar Spine MRI for Low Back Pain	167	32.9%	34.7%	37.2%

Vidant Bertie Hospital

1403 South Kings Street
Windsor, NC 27983
Phone: 252-794-6600
Fax: 252-794-6641
E-mail: tmullen@coastalnet.com
URL: www.vidanthealth.com/bertie
Type: Critical Access Hospitals
Emergency Services: Yes
Ownership: Voluntary non-profit - Private
Beds: 15

Key Personnel:
Chief of Medical Staff . . . . V Ballance
CEO/President . . . . Jeffery Fackrison
Emergency Room . . . . Pat Taylor

Measure	Cases	This Hosp.	State Avg.	U.S. Avg.
Blood Clot Prevention and Treatment				
Anticoagulation Overlap Therapy[5]	-	-	94%	93%
ICU Venous Thromboembolism Prophylaxis[5]	-	-	93%	92%
Incidence of Potentially Preventable VTE[5]	-	-	10%	10%
UFH with Dosages/Platelet Monitoring[5]	-	-	95%	97%
Venous Thromboembolism Prophylaxis[5]	-	-	88%	85%
Warfarin Therapy Discharge Instructions[5]	-	-	81%	75%
Chest Pain/Possible Heart Attack Care				
Aspirin Given Within 24 Hours of Arrival	11	91%	97%	96%
Fibrinolytic Meds Within 30 Min. of Arrival[1]	-	-	66%	58%
Average Time to ECG (minutes)	11	16	7	7
Average Time to Transfer (minutes)[1]	-	-	45	60
Children's Asthma Care				
Received Home Management Plan of Care	-	-	89%	88%
Received Reliever Medication	-	-	100%	100%
Received Systemic Corticosteroids	-	-	100%	100%
Emergency Department				
Admittance Decision Time (minutes)	354	65	107	98
Head CT Results Within 45 Min. of Arrival[1]	-	-	60%	57%
Patients Who Left ER Before Being Seen	10,057	1%	3%	2%
Time from ER Arrival to Admit. (minutes)	355	233	300	274
Time from ER Arrival to Discharge (minutes)	368	116	152	134
Time in ER Before Being Evaluated (minutes)	406	25	34	26
Time to Pain Meds for Fractures (minutes)	24	46	67	57
Heart Attack Care				
Aspirin Given at Discharge[5]	-	-	100%	99%
Fibrinolytic Meds Within 30 Min. of Arrival[5]	-	-	75%	54%
PCI Within 90 Minutes of Arrival[5]	-	-	98%	96%
Statin Prescribed at Discharge[5]	-	-	99%	98%
Heart Failure Care				
ACE Inhibitor or ARB for LVSD	11	100%	98%	97%
Discharge Instructions Given	28	100%	96%	94%
Evaluation of LVS Function	44	100%	100%	99%
Medicare Spending				
Medicare Spending per Patient (ratio)	-	-	0.94	0.98
Pneumonia Care				
Appropriate Initial Antibiotic Given	11	100%	97%	95%
Blood Culture Timing	26	100%	98%	98%
Pregnancy and Delivery Care				
Newborn Deliveries Scheduled Early[5]	-	-	3%	6%
Preventive Care				
Immunization for Influenza[5]	-	-	93%	90%
Immunization for Pneumonia[5]	-	-	94%	92%
Stroke Care				
Anticoagulation Therapy for Atrial Fibrillation[5]	-	-	95%	95%
Antithrombotic Therapy Timing[5]	-	-	98%	98%
Assessed for Rehabilitation[5]	-	-	98%	97%
Discharged on Antithrombotic Therapy[5]	-	-	99%	99%
Discharged on Statin Medication[5]	-	-	94%	94%
Thrombolytic Therapy Timing[5]	-	-	64%	66%
Venous Thromboembolism Prophylaxis[5]	-	-	96%	94%
Written Stroke Educational Materials Given[5]	-	-	88%	88%
Surgical Care Improvement Project				
Appropriate Beta Blocker Usage[5]	-	-	99%	98%
Appropriate VTP Within 24 Hours[5]	-	-	99%	98%
Controlled Postoperative Blood Glucose[5]	-	-	98%	97%
Perioperative Temperature Management[5]	-	-	100%	100%
Prophylactic Antibiotic Selection[5]	-	-	99%	99%
Prophylactic Antibiotic Selection (Outpatient)	14	100%	98%	98%
Prophylactic Antibiotic Stopped[5]	-	-	99%	98%
Prophylactic Antibiotic Timing[5]	-	-	99%	99%
Prophylactic Antibiotic Timing (Outpatient)[7]	-	-	99%	98%
Urinary Catheter Removal[5]	-	-	99%	97%
Survey of Patients' Hospital Experiences				
Area Around Room 'Always' Quiet at Night	(a)	85%	64%	61%
Doctors 'Always' Communicated Well	(a)	94%	83%	82%
Home Recovery Information Given	(a)	91%	87%	85%
Hospital Given 9 or 10 on 10 Point Scale	(a)	76%	71%	71%
Meds 'Always' Explained Before Given	(a)	82%	65%	64%
Nurses 'Always' Communicated Well	(a)	92%	81%	79%
Pain 'Always' Well Controlled	(a)	82%	72%	71%
Room and Bathroom 'Always' Clean	(a)	76%	72%	73%
Timely Help 'Always' Received	(a)	84%	68%	68%
Would Definitely Recommend Hospital	(a)	82%	70%	71%
Use of Medical Imaging				
Cardiac Imaging Stress Test before Surgery[7]	-	-	5.4%	5.3%
Combination Abdominal CT Scan	189	3.7%	5.6%	10.5%
Combination Brain/Sinus CT Scan[1]	-	-	2.6%	2.7%
Combination Chest CT Scan	50	2.0%	1.3%	2.7%
Follow-up Mammogram/Ultrasound	342	4.7%	8%	8.8%
Lumbar Spine MRI for Low Back Pain[7]	-	-	34.7%	37.2%

North Carolina Baptist Hospital

Medical Center Boulevard
Winston-Salem, NC 27157
Phone: 336-716-2011
Fax: 336-716-6841
URL: www.wfubmc.edu
Type: Acute Care Hospitals
Emergency Services: Yes
Ownership: Voluntary non-profit - Private
Beds: 1,238

Key Personnel:
Operating Room. . . . . Willa M Abbott
Radiology. . . . . Allen D Elster, MD
Emergency Room . . . . Patricia Johnson
CEO/President. . . . . John D McConnell, MD
Anesthesiology. . . . . Raymond Roy, MD
Infection Control. . . . . Robert Sherertz, MD
Patient Relations . . . . Amanda F Smith
Quality Assurance . . . . Jerold Smith

Measure	Cases	This Hosp.	State Avg.	U.S. Avg.
Blood Clot Prevention and Treatment				
Anticoagulation Overlap Therapy[2]	251	96%	94%	93%
ICU Venous Thromboembolism Prophylaxis[2]	115	95%	93%	92%
Incidence of Potentially Preventable VTE[2]	69	10%	10%	10%
UFH with Dosages/Platelet Monitoring[2]	194	99%	95%	97%
Venous Thromboembolism Prophylaxis[2]	312	87%	88%	85%
Warfarin Therapy Discharge Instructions[2]	212	95%	81%	75%
Chest Pain/Possible Heart Attack Care				
Aspirin Given Within 24 Hours of Arrival[5]	-	-	97%	96%
Fibrinolytic Meds Within 30 Min. of Arrival[5]	-	-	66%	58%
Average Time to ECG (minutes)[5]	-	-	7	7
Average Time to Transfer (minutes)[5]	-	-	45	60
Children's Asthma Care				
Received Home Management Plan of Care	195	66%	89%	88%
Received Reliever Medication	197	100%	100%	100%
Received Systemic Corticosteroids	196	99%	100%	100%
Emergency Department				
Admittance Decision Time (minutes)[2]	162	80	107	98
Head CT Results Within 45 Min. of Arrival[7]	-	-	60%	57%
Patients Who Left ER Before Being Seen	>100k	3%	3%	2%
Time from ER Arrival to Admit. (minutes)[2]	193	322	300	274
Time from ER Arrival to Discharge (minutes)	347	165	152	134
Time in ER Before Being Evaluated (minutes)	180	38	34	26
Time to Pain Meds for Fractures (minutes)	279	56	67	57
Heart Attack Care				
Aspirin Given at Discharge	690	100%	100%	99%
Fibrinolytic Meds Within 30 Min. of Arrival[7]	-	-	75%	54%
PCI Within 90 Minutes of Arrival	69	97%	98%	96%
Statin Prescribed at Discharge	684	99%	99%	98%
Heart Failure Care				
ACE Inhibitor or ARB for LVSD	294	99%	98%	97%
Discharge Instructions Given	641	91%	96%	94%
Evaluation of LVS Function	744	100%	100%	99%
Medicare Spending				
Medicare Spending per Patient (ratio)	-	0.95	0.94	0.98
Pneumonia Care				
Appropriate Initial Antibiotic Given	247	97%	97%	95%
Blood Culture Timing	729	98%	98%	98%
Pregnancy and Delivery Care				
Newborn Deliveries Scheduled Early[7]	-	-	3%	6%
Preventive Care				
Immunization for Influenza[2]	567	89%	93%	90%
Immunization for Pneumonia[2]	658	86%	94%	92%
Stroke Care				
Anticoagulation Therapy for Atrial Fibrillation[2]	17	76%	95%	95%
Antithrombotic Therapy Timing[2]	74	99%	98%	98%
Assessed for Rehabilitation[2]	148	92%	98%	97%
Discharged on Antithrombotic Therapy[2]	105	100%	99%	99%
Discharged on Statin Medication[2]	79	95%	94%	94%
Thrombolytic Therapy Timing[1,2]	-	-	64%	66%
Venous Thromboembolism Prophylaxis[2]	138	93%	96%	94%
Written Stroke Educational Materials Given[2]	87	79%	88%	88%
Surgical Care Improvement Project				
Appropriate Beta Blocker Usage[2]	340	99%	99%	98%
Appropriate VTP Within 24 Hours[2]	482	100%	99%	98%
Controlled Postoperative Blood Glucose[2]	212	95%	98%	97%
Perioperative Temperature Management[2]	656	99%	100%	100%
Prophylactic Antibiotic Selection[2]	577	99%	99%	99%

NOTE: Hospital profiles are in alphabetical order by state, then city, then hospital within the city; Rankings exclude hospitals with less than 25 cases except for patient surveys which excludes hospitals with less than 100 cases; (a) 100-299 cases; (1) The number of cases/patients is too few to report; (2) Data submitted were based on a sample of cases/patients; (3) Results are based on a shorter time period than required; (4) Data suppressed by CMS for one or more quarters; (5) Results are not available for this reporting period; (6) Fewer than 100 patients completed the HCAHPS survey; (7) No cases met the criteria for this measure; (8) The lower limit of the confidence interval cannot be calculated if the number of observed infections equals zero; (9) No data are available from the state/territory for this reporting period; (10) The scores shown reflect fewer than 50 completed surveys; (11) There were discrepancies in the data collection process; (12) This measure does not apply to this hospital for this reporting period; (13) Results cannot be calculated for this reporting period; (14) The results for this state are combined with nearby states to protect confidentiality; Please refer to the User's Guide for a full explanation of data.

Prophylactic Antibiotic Selection (Outpatient)	630	99%	98%	98%
Prophylactic Antibiotic Stopped[2]	571	100%	99%	98%
Prophylactic Antibiotic Timing[2]	579	97%	99%	99%
Prophylactic Antibiotic Timing (Outpatient)	631	97%	99%	98%
Urinary Catheter Removal[2]	494	100%	99%	97%
Survey of Patients' Hospital Experiences				
Area Around Room 'Always' Quiet at Night	300+	64%	64%	61%
Doctors 'Always' Communicated Well	300+	79%	83%	82%
Home Recovery Information Given	300+	86%	87%	85%
Hospital Given 9 or 10 on 10 Point Scale	300+	76%	71%	71%
Meds 'Always' Explained Before Given	300+	63%	65%	64%
Nurses 'Always' Communicated Well	300+	79%	81%	79%
Pain 'Always' Well Controlled	300+	68%	72%	71%
Room and Bathroom 'Always' Clean	300+	72%	72%	73%
Timely Help 'Always' Received	300+	65%	68%	68%
Would Definitely Recommend Hospital	300+	80%	70%	71%
Use of Medical Imaging				
Cardiac Imaging Stress Test before Surgery	798	5.0%	5.4%	5.3%
Combination Abdominal CT Scan	2,480	6.7%	5.6%	10.5%
Combination Brain/Sinus CT Scan	1,080	2.4%	2.6%	2.7%
Combination Chest CT Scan	2,676	0.6%	1.3%	2.7%
Follow-up Mammogram/Ultrasound	1,067	6.9%	8%	8.8%
Lumbar Spine MRI for Low Back Pain	166	39.2%	34.7%	37.2%

Novant Health Forsyth Medical Center

3333 Silas Creek Parkway
Winston-Salem, NC 27103
Phone: 336-718-5000
Fax: 336-718-9863
URL: www.forsythmedicalcenter.org
Type: Acute Care Hospitals
Emergency Services: Yes
Ownership: Voluntary non-profit - Private
Beds: 921

Key Personnel:
Radiology. . . . . Sam Thomas Auringer
Emergency Room . . . . Paul Horton, MD
CEO/President. . . . . Jeffrey T. Lindsay
Anesthesiology. . . . . Suresh Penkar, MD
Chief of Medical Staff. . . . . Stephen L Wallenhaupt, MD
Quality Assurance . . . . Harold Whitt

Measure	Cases	This Hosp.	State Avg.	U.S. Avg.
Blood Clot Prevention and Treatment				
Anticoagulation Overlap Therapy[2]	235	100%	94%	93%
ICU Venous Thromboembolism Prophylaxis[2]	199	100%	93%	92%
Incidence of Potentially Preventable VTE[2]	64	0%	10%	10%
UFH with Dosages/Platelet Monitoring[2]	72	100%	95%	97%
Venous Thromboembolism Prophylaxis[2]	617	100%	88%	85%
Warfarin Therapy Discharge Instructions[2]	204	100%	81%	75%
Chest Pain/Possible Heart Attack Care				
Aspirin Given Within 24 Hours of Arrival	13	100%	97%	96%
Fibrinolytic Meds Within 30 Min. of Arrival[3,7]	-	-	66%	58%
Average Time to ECG (minutes)	13	5	7	7
Average Time to Transfer (minutes)[1,3]	-	-	45	60
Children's Asthma Care				
Received Home Management Plan of Care	-	-	89%	88%
Received Reliever Medication	-	-	100%	100%
Received Systemic Corticosteroids	-	-	100%	100%
Emergency Department				
Admittance Decision Time (minutes)[2]	1,311	131	107	98
Head CT Results Within 45 Min. of Arrival[1]	-	-	60%	57%
Patients Who Left ER Before Being Seen	>100k	2%	3%	2%
Time from ER Arrival to Admit. (minutes)[2]	1,325	309	300	274
Time from ER Arrival to Discharge (minutes)	1,204	157	152	134
Time in ER Before Being Evaluated (minutes)	1,268	23	34	26
Time to Pain Meds for Fractures (minutes)	285	62	67	57
Heart Attack Care				
Aspirin Given at Discharge	685	100%	100%	99%
Fibrinolytic Meds Within 30 Min. of Arrival[7]	-	-	75%	54%
PCI Within 90 Minutes of Arrival	124	100%	98%	96%
Statin Prescribed at Discharge	656	100%	99%	98%
Heart Failure Care				
ACE Inhibitor or ARB for LVSD[2]	256	100%	98%	97%
Discharge Instructions Given[2]	818	100%	96%	94%
Evaluation of LVS Function[2]	983	100%	100%	99%
Medicare Spending				
Medicare Spending per Patient (ratio)	-	0.97	0.94	0.98
Pneumonia Care				
Appropriate Initial Antibiotic Given[2]	712	100%	97%	95%
Blood Culture Timing[2]	1,344	100%	98%	98%
Pregnancy and Delivery Care				
Newborn Deliveries Scheduled Early[2]	118	4%	3%	6%
Preventive Care				
Immunization for Influenza[2]	1,027	89%	93%	90%
Immunization for Pneumonia[2]	1,353	95%	94%	92%
Stroke Care				
Anticoagulation Therapy for Atrial Fibrillation	65	100%	95%	95%
Antithrombotic Therapy Timing	443	100%	98%	98%
Assessed for Rehabilitation	625	100%	98%	97%
Discharged on Antithrombotic Therapy	511	100%	99%	99%
Discharged on Statin Medication	372	100%	94%	94%
Thrombolytic Therapy Timing	44	100%	64%	66%
Venous Thromboembolism Prophylaxis	644	99%	96%	94%
Written Stroke Educational Materials Given	350	99%	88%	88%
Surgical Care Improvement Project				
Appropriate Beta Blocker Usage[2]	1,076	100%	99%	98%
Appropriate VTP Within 24 Hours[2]	2,369	99%	99%	98%
Controlled Postoperative Blood Glucose[2]	449	99%	98%	97%
Perioperative Temperature Management[2]	2,597	100%	100%	100%
Prophylactic Antibiotic Selection[2]	2,215	100%	99%	99%
Prophylactic Antibiotic Selection (Outpatient)	1,434	100%	98%	98%
Prophylactic Antibiotic Stopped[2]	2,139	100%	99%	98%
Prophylactic Antibiotic Timing[2]	2,217	100%	99%	99%
Prophylactic Antibiotic Timing (Outpatient)	1,436	100%	99%	98%
Urinary Catheter Removal[2]	2,226	100%	99%	97%
Survey of Patients' Hospital Experiences				
Area Around Room 'Always' Quiet at Night	300+	53%	64%	61%
Doctors 'Always' Communicated Well	300+	79%	83%	82%
Home Recovery Information Given	300+	82%	87%	85%
Hospital Given 9 or 10 on 10 Point Scale	300+	68%	71%	71%
Meds 'Always' Explained Before Given	300+	56%	65%	64%
Nurses 'Always' Communicated Well	300+	73%	81%	79%
Pain 'Always' Well Controlled	300+	65%	72%	71%
Room and Bathroom 'Always' Clean	300+	63%	72%	73%
Timely Help 'Always' Received	300+	59%	68%	68%
Would Definitely Recommend Hospital	300+	74%	70%	71%
Use of Medical Imaging				
Cardiac Imaging Stress Test before Surgery	945	5.9%	5.4%	5.3%
Combination Abdominal CT Scan	2,968	5.1%	5.6%	10.5%
Combination Brain/Sinus CT Scan	2,502	2.5%	2.6%	2.7%
Combination Chest CT Scan	1,752	0.1%	1.3%	2.7%
Follow-up Mammogram/Ultrasound	6,259	7.8%	8%	8.8%
Lumbar Spine MRI for Low Back Pain	351	41.6%	34.7%	37.2%

Novant Health Park Hospital

1950 S Hawthorne Rd
Winston-Salem, NC 27103
Phone: 336-718-0600
Fax: 336-718-0384
URL: www.novanthealth.org
Type: Acute Care Hospitals
Emergency Services: No
Ownership: Voluntary non-profit - Other
Beds: 22

Key Personnel:
CEO/President. . . . . Timothy S Shelton, Jr

Measure	Cases	This Hosp.	State Avg.	U.S. Avg.
Blood Clot Prevention and Treatment				
Anticoagulation Overlap Therapy[2,7]	-	-	94%	93%
ICU Venous Thromboembolism Prophylaxis[2,7]	-	-	93%	92%
Incidence of Potentially Preventable VTE[1,2]	-	-	10%	10%
UFH with Dosages/Platelet Monitoring[1,2]	-	-	95%	97%
Venous Thromboembolism Prophylaxis[2]	55	100%	88%	85%
Warfarin Therapy Discharge Instructions[1,2]	-	-	81%	75%
Chest Pain/Possible Heart Attack Care				
Aspirin Given Within 24 Hours of Arrival[5]	-	-	97%	96%
Fibrinolytic Meds Within 30 Min. of Arrival[5]	-	-	66%	58%
Average Time to ECG (minutes)[5]	-	-	7	7
Average Time to Transfer (minutes)[5]	-	-	45	60
Children's Asthma Care				
Received Home Management Plan of Care	-	-	89%	88%
Received Reliever Medication	-	-	100%	100%
Received Systemic Corticosteroids	-	-	100%	100%
Emergency Department				
Admittance Decision Time (minutes)[7]	-	-	107	98
Head CT Results Within 45 Min. of Arrival[5]	-	-	60%	57%
Patients Who Left ER Before Being Seen[5]	-	-	3%	2%
Time from ER Arrival to Admit. (minutes)[7]	-	-	300	274
Time from ER Arrival to Discharge (minutes)[5]	-	-	152	134
Time in ER Before Being Evaluated (minutes)[5]	-	-	34	26
Time to Pain Meds for Fractures (minutes)[5]	-	-	67	57
Heart Attack Care				
Aspirin Given at Discharge[5]	-	-	100%	99%
Fibrinolytic Meds Within 30 Min. of Arrival[5]	-	-	75%	54%
PCI Within 90 Minutes of Arrival[5]	-	-	98%	96%
Statin Prescribed at Discharge[5]	-	-	99%	98%
Heart Failure Care				
ACE Inhibitor or ARB for LVSD[5]	-	-	98%	97%
Discharge Instructions Given[5]	-	-	96%	94%
Evaluation of LVS Function[5]	-	-	100%	99%
Medicare Spending				
Medicare Spending per Patient (ratio)	-	0.93	0.94	0.98
Pneumonia Care				
Appropriate Initial Antibiotic Given[5]	-	-	97%	95%
Blood Culture Timing[5]	-	-	98%	98%
Pregnancy and Delivery Care				
Newborn Deliveries Scheduled Early[7]	-	-	3%	6%
Preventive Care				
Immunization for Influenza	344	99%	93%	90%
Immunization for Pneumonia	385	100%	94%	92%
Stroke Care				
Anticoagulation Therapy for Atrial Fibrillation[5]	-	-	95%	95%
Antithrombotic Therapy Timing[5]	-	-	98%	98%
Assessed for Rehabilitation[5]	-	-	98%	97%
Discharged on Antithrombotic Therapy[5]	-	-	99%	99%
Discharged on Statin Medication[5]	-	-	94%	94%
Thrombolytic Therapy Timing[5]	-	-	64%	66%
Venous Thromboembolism Prophylaxis[5]	-	-	96%	94%
Written Stroke Educational Materials Given[5]	-	-	88%	88%
Surgical Care Improvement Project				
Appropriate Beta Blocker Usage[2]	103	100%	99%	98%
Appropriate VTP Within 24 Hours[2]	361	100%	99%	98%
Controlled Postoperative Blood Glucose[2,7]	-	-	98%	97%
Perioperative Temperature Management[2]	432	100%	100%	100%
Prophylactic Antibiotic Selection[2]	226	100%	99%	99%
Prophylactic Antibiotic Selection (Outpatient)	311	100%	98%	98%
Prophylactic Antibiotic Stopped[2]	222	99%	99%	98%
Prophylactic Antibiotic Timing[2]	226	100%	99%	99%
Prophylactic Antibiotic Timing (Outpatient)	311	99%	99%	98%
Urinary Catheter Removal[2]	168	100%	99%	97%
Survey of Patients' Hospital Experiences				
Area Around Room 'Always' Quiet at Night	300+	73%	64%	61%
Doctors 'Always' Communicated Well	300+	87%	83%	82%
Home Recovery Information Given	300+	86%	87%	85%
Hospital Given 9 or 10 on 10 Point Scale	300+	84%	71%	71%
Meds 'Always' Explained Before Given	300+	65%	65%	64%
Nurses 'Always' Communicated Well	300+	85%	81%	79%
Pain 'Always' Well Controlled	300+	73%	72%	71%
Room and Bathroom 'Always' Clean	300+	79%	72%	73%
Timely Help 'Always' Received	300+	76%	68%	68%
Would Definitely Recommend Hospital	300+	89%	70%	71%
Use of Medical Imaging				
Cardiac Imaging Stress Test before Surgery[7]	-	-	5.4%	5.3%
Combination Abdominal CT Scan[1]	-	-	5.6%	10.5%
Combination Brain/Sinus CT Scan[7]	-	-	2.6%	2.7%
Combination Chest CT Scan[7]	-	-	1.3%	2.7%
Follow-up Mammogram/Ultrasound[7]	-	-	8%	8.8%
Lumbar Spine MRI for Low Back Pain[7]	-	-	34.7%	37.2%

Yadkin Valley Community Hospital

624 West Main St
Yadkinville, NC 27055
Phone: 336-679-2041
Fax: 336-679-6717
E-mail: llabine@wfubmc.edu
Type: Critical Access Hospitals
Emergency Services: Yes
Ownership: Proprietary
Beds: 22

Key Personnel:
Radiology. . . . . Paul J Beerman
CEO . . . . Shawn Bright
Ambulatory Care . . . . Sharon Hill

NOTE: Hospital profiles are in alphabetical order by state, then city, then hospital within the city; Rankings exclude hospitals with less than 25 cases except for patient surveys which excludes hospitals with less than 100 cases; (a) 100-299 cases; (1) The number of cases/patients is too few to report; (2) Data submitted were based on a sample of cases/patients; (3) Results are based on a shorter time period than required; (4) Data suppressed by CMS for one or more quarters; (5) Results are not available for this reporting period; (6) Fewer than 100 patients completed the HCAHPS survey; (7) No cases met the criteria for this measure; (8) The lower limit of the confidence interval cannot be calculated if the number of observed infections equals zero; (9) No data are available from the state/territory for this reporting period; (10) The scores shown reflect fewer than 50 completed surveys; (11) There were discrepancies in the data collection process; (12) This measure does not apply to this hospital for this reporting period; (13) Results cannot be calculated for this reporting period; (14) The results for this state are combined with nearby states to protect confidentiality; Please refer to the User's Guide for a full explanation of data.

Quality Assurance . . . . Lance Labine
Chief of Medical Staff . . . . James S McGrath
Emergency Room . . . . Lisa Miller
Anesthesiology. . . . . Elizabeth Randleman
Infection Control . . . . Ellen Reece

Measure	Cases	This Hosp.	State Avg.	U.S. Avg.
Blood Clot Prevention and Treatment				
Anticoagulation Overlap Therapy[5]	-	-	94%	93%
ICU Venous Thromboembolism Prophylaxis[5]	-	-	93%	92%
Incidence of Potentially Preventable VTE[5]	-	-	10%	10%
UFH with Dosages/Platelet Monitoring[5]	-	-	95%	97%
Venous Thromboembolism Prophylaxis[5]	-	-	88%	85%
Warfarin Therapy Discharge Instructions[5]	-	-	81%	75%
Chest Pain/Possible Heart Attack Care				
Aspirin Given Within 24 Hours of Arrival	-	-	97%	96%
Fibrinolytic Meds Within 30 Min. of Arrival	-	-	66%	58%
Average Time to ECG (minutes)	-	-	7	7
Average Time to Transfer (minutes)	-	-	45	60
Children's Asthma Care				
Received Home Management Plan of Care	-	-	89%	88%
Received Reliever Medication	-	-	100%	100%
Received Systemic Corticosteroids	-	-	100%	100%
Emergency Department				
Admittance Decision Time (minutes)[5]	-	-	107	98
Head CT Results Within 45 Min. of Arrival	-	-	60%	57%
Patients Who Left ER Before Being Seen	-	-	3%	2%
Time from ER Arrival to Admit. (minutes)[5]	-	-	300	274
Time from ER Arrival to Discharge (minutes)	-	-	152	134
Time in ER Before Being Evaluated (minutes)	-	-	34	26
Time to Pain Meds for Fractures (minutes)	-	-	67	57
Heart Attack Care				
Aspirin Given at Discharge[5]	-	-	100%	99%
Fibrinolytic Meds Within 30 Min. of Arrival[5]	-	-	75%	54%
PCI Within 90 Minutes of Arrival[5]	-	-	98%	96%
Statin Prescribed at Discharge[5]	-	-	99%	98%
Heart Failure Care				
ACE Inhibitor or ARB for LVSD[5]	-	-	98%	97%
Discharge Instructions Given[5]	-	-	96%	94%
Evaluation of LVS Function[5]	-	-	100%	99%
Medicare Spending				
Medicare Spending per Patient (ratio)	-	-	0.94	0.98
Pneumonia Care				
Appropriate Initial Antibiotic Given[5]	-	-	97%	95%
Blood Culture Timing[5]	-	-	98%	98%
Pregnancy and Delivery Care				
Newborn Deliveries Scheduled Early[5]	-	-	3%	6%
Preventive Care				
Immunization for Influenza[5]	-	-	93%	90%
Immunization for Pneumonia[5]	-	-	94%	92%
Stroke Care				
Anticoagulation Therapy for Atrial Fibrillation[5]	-	-	95%	95%
Antithrombotic Therapy Timing[5]	-	-	98%	98%
Assessed for Rehabilitation[5]	-	-	98%	97%
Discharged on Antithrombotic Therapy[5]	-	-	99%	99%
Discharged on Statin Medication[5]	-	-	94%	94%
Thrombolytic Therapy Timing[5]	-	-	64%	66%
Venous Thromboembolism Prophylaxis[5]	-	-	96%	94%
Written Stroke Educational Materials Given[5]	-	-	88%	88%
Surgical Care Improvement Project				
Appropriate Beta Blocker Usage[5]	-	-	99%	98%
Appropriate VTP Within 24 Hours[5]	-	-	99%	98%
Controlled Postoperative Blood Glucose[5]	-	-	98%	97%
Perioperative Temperature Management[5]	-	-	100%	100%
Prophylactic Antibiotic Selection[5]	-	-	99%	99%
Prophylactic Antibiotic Selection (Outpatient)	-	-	98%	98%
Prophylactic Antibiotic Stopped[5]	-	-	99%	98%
Prophylactic Antibiotic Timing[5]	-	-	99%	99%
Prophylactic Antibiotic Timing (Outpatient)	-	-	99%	98%
Urinary Catheter Removal[5]	-	-	99%	97%
Survey of Patients' Hospital Experiences				
Area Around Room 'Always' Quiet at Night[5]	-	-	64%	61%
Doctors 'Always' Communicated Well[5]	-	-	83%	82%
Home Recovery Information Given[5]	-	-	87%	85%
Hospital Given 9 or 10 on 10 Point Scale[5]	-	-	71%	71%
Meds 'Always' Explained Before Given[5]	-	-	65%	64%
Nurses 'Always' Communicated Well[5]	-	-	81%	79%
Pain 'Always' Well Controlled[5]	-	-	72%	71%
Room and Bathroom 'Always' Clean[5]	-	-	72%	73%
Timely Help 'Always' Received[5]	-	-	68%	68%
Would Definitely Recommend Hospital[5]	-	-	70%	71%
Use of Medical Imaging				
Cardiac Imaging Stress Test before Surgery	-	-	5.4%	5.3%
Combination Abdominal CT Scan	-	-	5.6%	10.5%
Combination Brain/Sinus CT Scan	-	-	2.6%	2.7%
Combination Chest CT Scan	-	-	1.3%	2.7%
Follow-up Mammogram/Ultrasound	-	-	8%	8.8%
Lumbar Spine MRI for Low Back Pain	-	-	34.7%	37.2%

NOTE: Hospital profiles are in alphabetical order by state, then city, then hospital within the city; Rankings exclude hospitals with less than 25 cases except for patient surveys which excludes hospitals with less than 100 cases; (a) 100-299 cases; (1) The number of cases/patients is too few to report; (2) Data submitted were based on a sample of cases/patients; (3) Results are based on a shorter time period than required; (4) Data suppressed by CMS for one or more quarters; (5) Results are not available for this reporting period; (6) Fewer than 100 patients completed the HCAHPS survey; (7) No cases met the criteria for this measure; (8) The lower limit of the confidence interval cannot be calculated if the number of observed infections equals zero; (9) No data are available from the state/territory for this reporting period; (10) The scores shown reflect fewer than 50 completed surveys; (11) There were discrepancies in the data collection process; (12) This measure does not apply to this hospital for this reporting period; (13) Results cannot be calculated for this reporting period; (14) The results for this state are combined with nearby states to protect confidentiality; Please refer to the User's Guide for a full explanation of data.

Blood Clot Prevention and Treatment

Anticoagulation Overlap Therapy

Hospital Name	City	Rate	Cases
Adena Regional Medical Center[2]	Chillicothe	100%	69
Blanchard Valley Hospital[2]	Findlay	100%	61
Christ Hospital[2]	Cincinnati	100%	154
Clinton Memorial Hospital[2]	Wilmington	100%	26
Dublin Methodist Hospital[2]	Dublin	100%	33
Firelands Regional Medical Center[2]	Sandusky	100%	61
Grady Memorial Hospital[2]	Delaware	100%	25
Grant Medical Center[2]	Columbus	100%	134
Licking Memorial Hospital[2]	Newark	100%	53
Mercy Hospital Anderson[2]	Cincinnati	100%	69
Northside Medical Center[2]	Youngstown	100%	53
UH Geauga Medical Center[2]	Chardon	100%	64
University of Cincinnati Medical Center[2]	Cincinnati	100%	188
Doctors Hospital[2]	Columbus	99%	96
Good Samaritan Hospital[2]	Dayton	99%	145
Jewish Hospital[2]	Cincinnati	99%	85
University Hospitals Case Medical Center[2]	Cleveland	99%	202
Affinity Medical Center[2]	Massillon	98%	55
Akron General Medical Center[2]	Akron	98%	206
Ashtabula County Medical Center[2]	Ashtabula	98%	43
Atrium Medical Center[2]	Franklin	98%	118
Bethesda North[2]	Cincinnati	98%	139
Cleveland Clinic[2]	Cleveland	98%	400
Flower Hospital[2]	Sylvania	98%	48
Lake Health[2]	Concord	98%	140
Medcentral Health Sys Mansfield Hosp[2]	Mansfield	98%	58
Mercy Medical Center[2]	Canton	98%	162
Metrohealth System[2]	Cleveland	98%	116
Miami Valley Hospital[2]	Dayton	98%	242
Salem Regional Medical Center[2]	Salem	98%	41
Summa Western Reserve Hospital[2]	Cuyahoga Falls	98%	44
Trinity Med Ctr East & West[2]	Steubenville	98%	58
East Liverpool City Hospital[2]	East Liverpool	97%	33
Fort Hamilton Hughes Memorial Hospital[2]	Hamilton	97%	59
Kettering Medical Center[2]	Kettering	97%	144
Mercy Health - West Hospital[2]	Cincinnati	97%	33
Mercy Saint Vincent Medical Center[2]	Toledo	97%	134
Mount Carmel Saint Ann's[2]	Westerville	97%	103
Riverside Methodist Hospital[2]	Columbus	97%	278
Saint Luke's Hospital[2]	Maumee	97%	93
Southern Ohio Medical Center[2]	Portsmouth	97%	77
Wood County Hospital[2]	Bowling Green	97%	30
Grandview Hospital & Medical Center[2]	Dayton	96%	90
Indu & Raj Soin Medical Center[2]	Beaver Creek	96%	25
Mercy Hospital Fairfield[2]	Fairfield	96%	111
Mount Carmel West[2]	Columbus	96%	245
Springfield Regional Medical Center[2]	Springfield	96%	141
Sycamore Medical Center[2]	Miamisburg	96%	57
Wooster Community Hospital[2]	Wooster	96%	47
Fairfield Medical Center[2]	Lancaster	95%	76
Marion General Hospital[2]	Marion	95%	57
University of Toledo Medical Center[2]	Toledo	95%	81
East Ohio Regional Hospital[2]	Martins Ferry	94%	31
Good Samaritan Hospital[2]	Cincinnati	94%	167
Mercy Hospital Clermont[2]	Batavia	94%	33
Ohio State University Hospitals[2]	Columbus	94%	263
Saint Rita's Medical Center[2]	Lima	94%	99
University Hospitals Ahuja Medical Center[2]	Beachwood	94%	107
Fairview Hospital[2]	Cleveland	93%	130
Lutheran Hospital[2]	Cleveland	93%	30
Marymount Hospital[2]	Garfield Heights	93%	166
Fisher - Titus Hospital[2]	Norwalk	92%	25
Medina Hospital[2]	Medina	92%	64
Lima Memorial Health System[2]	Lima	91%	54
Saint Vincent Charity Medical Center[2]	Cleveland	91%	33
Upper Valley Medical Center[2]	Troy	91%	70
West Chester Hospital[2]	West Chester	91%	79
Euclid Hospital[2]	Euclid	90%	72
Southwest General Health Center[2]	Middleburg Hgts	90%	130
Aultman Hospital[2]	Canton	89%	205
Hillcrest Hospital[2]	Mayfield Heights	89%	205
Trumbull Memorial Hospital[2]	Warren	89%	72
Genesis Healthcare System[2]	Zanesville	88%	77
Parma Community General Hospital[2]	Parma	88%	88
Saint Elizabeth Boardman Health Center[2]	Boardman	88%	89
Mercy Saint Anne Hospital[2]	Toledo	87%	60
Saint John Medical Center[2]	Westlake	87%	71
South Pointe Hospital[2]	Warrensville Hgts	87%	102
UHHS Richmond Heights Hospital[2]	Richmond Hghts	84%	56
Lakewood Hospital[2]	Lakewood	83%	53
Summa Health Systems Hospitals[2]	Akron	83%	213
The Toledo Hospital[2]	Toledo	82%	143
Union Hospital[2]	Dover	82%	55
Alliance Community Hospital[2]	Alliance	81%	47
Knox Community Hospital[2]	Mount Vernon	81%	26
Saint Elizabeth Health Center[2]	Youngstown	80%	123
Univ Hosps-Elyria Med Ctr[2]	Elyria	76%	97
Marietta Memorial Hospital[2]	Marietta	69%	78
Summa Health System Barberton Hospital[2]	Barberton	69%	71
Mercy Saint Charles Hospital[2]	Oregon	66%	58
Saint Joseph Health Center[2]	Warren	66%	68
Mercy Regional Medical Center[2]	Lorain	57%	81
Robinson Memorial Hospital[2]	Ravenna	57%	58
Southeastern Ohio Regional Medical Center[2]	Cambridge	52%	31

ICU Venous Thromboembolism Prophylaxis

Hospital Name	City	Rate	Cases
Berger Hospital[2]	Circleville	100%	54
Doctors Hospital[2]	Columbus	100%	64
Euclid Hospital[2]	Euclid	100%	75
Flower Hospital[2]	Sylvania	100%	77
Greene Memorial Hospital[2]	Xenia	100%	55
Lutheran Hospital[2]	Cleveland	100%	46
Mercy Hospital Clermont[2]	Batavia	100%	81
O'Bleness Memorial Hospital[2]	Athens	100%	81
Southern Ohio Medical Center[2]	Portsmouth	100%	69
UHHS Memorial Hospital of Geneva[2]	Geneva	100%	40
Univ Hosps Conneaut Med Ctr[2]	Conneaut	100%	29
Upper Valley Medical Center[2]	Troy	100%	70
Akron General Medical Center[2]	Akron	99%	90
Atrium Medical Center[2]	Franklin	99%	107
Aultman Hospital[2]	Canton	99%	106
Blanchard Valley Hospital[2]	Findlay	99%	150
Lima Memorial Health System[2]	Lima	99%	162
Summa Western Reserve Hospital[2]	Cuyahoga Falls	99%	133
Sycamore Medical Center[2]	Miamisburg	99%	75
University of Toledo Medical Center[2]	Toledo	99%	82
Cleveland Clinic[2]	Cleveland	98%	84
Clinton Memorial Hospital[2]	Wilmington	98%	47
Fort Hamilton Hughes Memorial Hospital[2]	Hamilton	98%	90
Grant Medical Center[2]	Columbus	98%	51
Indu & Raj Soin Medical Center[2]	Beaver Creek	98%	86
Mercy Saint Anne Hospital[2]	Toledo	98%	111
Mount Carmel Saint Ann's[2]	Westerville	98%	40
Saint Vincent Charity Medical Center[2]	Cleveland	98%	119
Samaritan Regional Health System[2]	Ashland	98%	50
Summa Health Systems Hospitals[2]	Akron	98%	101
UHHS Richmond Heights Hospital[2]	Richmond Hghts	98%	154
Fairview Hospital[2]	Cleveland	97%	116
Good Samaritan Hospital[2]	Dayton	97%	100
Kettering Medical Center[2]	Kettering	97%	93
Medina Hospital[2]	Medina	97%	59
Memorial Hospital of Union County[2]	Marysville	97%	36
Mercy Saint Vincent Medical Center[2]	Toledo	97%	86
Northside Medical Center[2]	Youngstown	97%	91
Riverside Methodist Hospital[2]	Columbus	97%	121
South Pointe Hospital[2]	Warrensville Hgts	97%	120
University Hospitals Ahuja Medical Center[2]	Beachwood	97%	29
University of Cincinnati Medical Center[2]	Cincinnati	97%	110
Wood County Hospital[2]	Bowling Green	97%	35
Ashtabula County Medical Center[2]	Ashtabula	96%	56
Bay Park Community Hospital[2]	Oregon	96%	52
Bethesda North[2]	Cincinnati	96%	75
Fayette County Memorial Hospital	Washington Ch	96%	154
Grandview Hospital & Medical Center[2]	Dayton	96%	111
Hillcrest Hospital[2]	Mayfield Heights	96%	112
Mercer County Joint Twp Comm Hosp[2]	Coldwater	96%	25
Parma Community General Hospital[2]	Parma	96%	71
West Chester Hospital[2]	West Chester	96%	92
Wooster Community Hospital[2]	Wooster	96%	51
Affinity Medical Center[2]	Massillon	95%	181
Christ Hospital[2]	Cincinnati	95%	92
Community Hospitals & Wellness Centers	Bryan	95%	191
East Liverpool City Hospital[2]	East Liverpool	95%	61
Lake Health[2]	Concord	95%	56
Lakewood Hospital[2]	Lakewood	95%	78
Licking Memorial Hospital[2]	Newark	95%	63
Marymount Hospital[2]	Garfield Heights	95%	55
Mercy Health - West Hospital[2]	Cincinnati	95%	61
Mercy Hospital Fairfield[2]	Fairfield	95%	98
Union Hospital[2]	Dover	95%	60
University Hospitals Case Medical Center[2]	Cleveland	95%	95
Adena Regional Medical Center[2]	Chillicothe	94%	31
Mercy Hospital Anderson[2]	Cincinnati	94%	54
Miami Valley Hospital[2]	Dayton	94%	70
Ohio State University Hospitals[2]	Columbus	94%	66
Firelands Regional Medical Center[2]	Sandusky	93%	73
Good Samaritan Hospital[2]	Cincinnati	93%	91
Saint John Medical Center[2]	Westlake	93%	92
Wilson Memorial Hospital[2]	Sidney	93%	27
Dublin Methodist Hospital[2]	Dublin	92%	36
Trumbull Memorial Hospital[2]	Warren	92%	147
UH Geauga Medical Center[2]	Chardon	92%	103
Marietta Memorial Hospital[2]	Marietta	91%	77
Univ Hosps-Elyria Med Ctr[2]	Elyria	91%	98
Fisher - Titus Hospital[2]	Norwalk	90%	69
Mercy Medical Center[2]	Canton	90%	123
Alliance Community Hospital[2]	Alliance	89%	53
Fairfield Medical Center[2]	Lancaster	89%	89
Knox Community Hospital[2]	Mount Vernon	89%	71
Holzer Medical Center[2]	Gallipolis	88%	92
Marion General Hospital[2]	Marion	88%	72
Medcentral Health Sys Mansfield Hosp[2]	Mansfield	88%	99
Memorial Hospital[2]	Fremont	88%	43
Metrohealth System[2]	Cleveland	88%	92
Saint Luke's Hospital[2]	Maumee	88%	41
Salem Regional Medical Center[2]	Salem	88%	25
Southwest General Health Center[2]	Middleburg Hgts	88%	139
Mount Carmel West[2]	Columbus	87%	78
Saint Elizabeth Health Center[2]	Youngstown	87%	97
Springfield Regional Medical Center[2]	Springfield	87%	97
Jewish Hospital[2]	Cincinnati	86%	65
Saint Elizabeth Boardman Health Center[2]	Boardman	86%	64
Trinity Med Ctr East & West[2]	Steubenville	86%	74
Genesis Healthcare System[2]	Zanesville	85%	54
Saint Joseph Health Center[2]	Warren	84%	76
Summa Wadsworth - Rittman Hospital[2]	Wadsworth	84%	69
Madison County Hospital[2]	London	83%	42
Robinson Memorial Hospital[2]	Ravenna	83%	60
Saint Rita's Medical Center[2]	Lima	83%	114
Summa Health System Barberton Hospital[2]	Barberton	83%	161
Mercy Saint Charles Hospital[2]	Oregon	82%	68
The Toledo Hospital[2]	Toledo	81%	140
Wayne Hospital[2]	Greenville	81%	32
Bellevue Hospital[2]	Bellevue	80%	30
McCullough - Hyde Memorial Hospital[2]	Oxford	80%	30
Southeastern Ohio Regional Medical Center[2]	Cambridge	80%	60
East Ohio Regional Hospital[2]	Martins Ferry	71%	66
Mercy Regional Medical Center[2]	Lorain	60%	72
Coshocton County Memorial Hospital[2]	Coshocton	52%	27

Incidence of Potentially Preventable VTE

Hospital Name	City	Rate	Cases
Aultman Hospital[2]	Canton	0%	51
Grant Medical Center[2]	Columbus	0%	52
Metrohealth System[2]	Cleveland	0%	39
Ohio State University Hospitals[2]	Columbus	0%	77
University of Cincinnati Medical Center[2]	Cincinnati	1%	112
Cleveland Clinic[2]	Cleveland	2%	168
The Toledo Hospital[2]	Toledo	2%	46
Miami Valley Hospital[2]	Dayton	3%	73
Saint Elizabeth Health Center[2]	Youngstown	3%	34
Akron General Medical Center[2]	Akron	4%	50
Riverside Methodist Hospital[2]	Columbus	5%	75
University of Toledo Medical Center[2]	Toledo	5%	38
University Hospitals Case Medical Center[2]	Cleveland	6%	78
Mercy Saint Vincent Medical Center[2]	Toledo	7%	27
Christ Hospital[2]	Cincinnati	8%	25
Good Samaritan Hospital[2]	Cincinnati	8%	26
Saint Luke's Hospital[2]	Maumee	8%	26
Hillcrest Hospital[2]	Mayfield Heights	9%	46
Mount Carmel West[2]	Columbus	9%	78
Summa Health Systems Hospitals[2]	Akron	11%	47
Fairview Hospital[2]	Cleveland	16%	25

UFH with Dosages/Platelet Count Monitoring

Hospital Name	City	Rate	Cases
Adena Regional Medical Center[2]	Chillicothe	100%	48
Affinity Medical Center[2]	Massillon	100%	52
Akron General Medical Center[2]	Akron	100%	191
Atrium Medical Center[2]	Franklin	100%	95
Bethesda North[2]	Cincinnati	100%	142
Blanchard Valley Hospital[2]	Findlay	100%	49
Christ Hospital[2]	Cincinnati	100%	151
Cleveland Clinic[2]	Cleveland	100%	444
Doctors Hospital[2]	Columbus	100%	64
East Liverpool City Hospital[2]	East Liverpool	100%	29
East Ohio Regional Hospital[2]	Martins Ferry	100%	36
Euclid Hospital[2]	Euclid	100%	63
Fairfield Medical Center[2]	Lancaster	100%	72
Firelands Regional Medical Center[2]	Sandusky	100%	59
Flower Hospital[2]	Sylvania	100%	34
Fort Hamilton Hughes Memorial Hospital[2]	Hamilton	100%	35
Genesis Healthcare System[2]	Zanesville	100%	46
Good Samaritan Hospital[2]	Cincinnati	100%	152
Good Samaritan Hospital[2]	Dayton	100%	118
Grant Medical Center[2]	Columbus	100%	105
Hillcrest Hospital[2]	Mayfield Heights	100%	200
Jewish Hospital[2]	Cincinnati	100%	53
Kettering Medical Center[2]	Kettering	100%	67
Lake Health[2]	Concord	100%	109
Lakewood Hospital[2]	Lakewood	100%	31
Marietta Memorial Hospital[2]	Marietta	100%	39
Marymount Hospital[2]	Garfield Heights	100%	112
Medcentral Health Sys Mansfield Hosp[2]	Mansfield	100%	57
Mercy Health - West Hospital[2]	Cincinnati	100%	25
Mercy Hospital Anderson[2]	Cincinnati	100%	42

NOTE: Hospital profiles are in alphabetical order by state, then city, then hospital within the city; Rankings exclude hospitals with less than 25 cases except for patient surveys which excludes hospitals with less than 100 cases; (a) 100-299 cases; (1) The number of cases/patients is too few to report; (2) Data submitted were based on a sample of cases/patients; (3) Results are based on a shorter time period than required; (4) Data suppressed by CMS for one or more quarters; (5) Results are not available for this reporting period; (6) Fewer than 100 patients completed the HCAHPS survey; (7) No cases met the criteria for this measure; (8) The lower limit of the confidence interval cannot be calculated if the number of observed infections equals zero; (9) No data are available from the state/territory for this reporting period; (10) The scores shown reflect fewer than 50 completed surveys; (11) There were discrepancies in the data collection process; (12) This measure does not apply to this hospital for this reporting period; (13) Results cannot be calculated for this reporting period; (14) The results for this state are combined with nearby states to protect confidentiality; Please refer to the User's Guide for a full explanation of data.

Hospital Name	City	Rate	Cases
Mercy Hospital Fairfield[2]	Fairfield	100%	58
Mercy Medical Center[2]	Canton	100%	166
Mercy Saint Anne Hospital[2]	Toledo	100%	50
Mercy Saint Charles Hospital[2]	Oregon	100%	31
Mercy Saint Vincent Medical Center[2]	Toledo	100%	85
Metrohealth System[2]	Cleveland	100%	106
Miami Valley Hospital[2]	Dayton	100%	200
Mount Carmel Saint Ann's[2]	Westerville	100%	87
Mount Carmel West[2]	Columbus	100%	219
Northside Medical Center[2]	Youngstown	100%	43
Parma Community General Hospital[2]	Parma	100%	49
Riverside Methodist Hospital[2]	Columbus	100%	331
Saint Elizabeth Boardman Health Center[2]	Boardman	100%	50
Saint Elizabeth Health Center[2]	Youngstown	100%	65
Saint John Medical Center[2]	Westlake	100%	34
Saint Joseph Health Center[2]	Warren	100%	42
Saint Luke's Hospital[2]	Maumee	100%	71
Saint Rita's Medical Center[2]	Lima	100%	79
Salem Regional Medical Center[2]	Salem	100%	33
South Pointe Hospital[2]	Warrensville Hgts	100%	104
Southern Ohio Medical Center[2]	Portsmouth	100%	97
Southwest General Health Center[2]	Middleburg Hgts	100%	31
Springfield Regional Medical Center[2]	Springfield	100%	46
Summa Western Reserve Hospital[2]	Cuyahoga Falls	100%	28
Sycamore Medical Center[2]	Miamisburg	100%	29
Trinity Med Ctr East & West[2]	Steubenville	100%	57
UH Geauga Medical Center[2]	Chardon	100%	68
UHHS Richmond Heights Hospital[2]	Richmond Hghts	100%	42
Union Hospital[2]	Dover	100%	38
Univ Hosps-Elyria Med Ctr[2]	Elyria	100%	59
University Hospitals Ahuja Medical Center[2]	Beachwood	100%	99
University Hospitals Case Medical Center[2]	Cleveland	100%	217
University of Cincinnati Medical Center[2]	Cincinnati	100%	201
University of Toledo Medical Center[2]	Toledo	100%	94
Upper Valley Medical Center[2]	Troy	100%	27
West Chester Hospital[2]	West Chester	100%	66
Wooster Community Hospital[2]	Wooster	100%	38
Grandview Hospital & Medical Center[2]	Dayton	99%	77
Summa Health Systems Hospitals[2]	Akron	99%	189
The Toledo Hospital[2]	Toledo	99%	150
Alliance Community Hospital[2]	Alliance	98%	48
Fairview Hospital[2]	Cleveland	98%	82
Summa Health System Barberton Hospital[2]	Barberton	98%	59
Medina Hospital[2]	Medina	96%	47
Trumbull Memorial Hospital[2]	Warren	94%	54
Ohio State University Hospitals[2]	Columbus	93%	255
Fisher - Titus Hospital[2]	Norwalk	89%	35
Aultman Hospital[2]	Canton	79%	234
Lima Memorial Health System[2]	Lima	56%	48

Venous Thromboembolism Prophylaxis

Hospital Name	City	Rate	Cases
Belmont Community Hospital[2]	Bellaire	100%	74
Crystal Clinic Orthopaedic Center[2]	Akron	100%	188
Medical Center at Elizabeth Place[2]	Dayton	100%	26
Mercy Hospital of Defiance[2]	Defiance	100%	136
Mount Carmel New Albany Surgical Hospital[2]	New Albany	100%	121
Pomerene Hospital[2]	Millersburg	100%	84
Surgical Hospital at Southwoods	Youngstown	100%	156
Berger Hospital[2]	Circleville	99%	128
O'Bleness Memorial Hospital[2]	Athens	99%	165
Greene Memorial Hospital[2]	Xenia	98%	264
Indu & Raj Soin Medical Center[2]	Beaver Creek	98%	310
Summa Western Reserve Hospital[2]	Cuyahoga Falls	98%	299
Univ Hosps Conneaut Med Ctr[2]	Conneaut	98%	66
Blanchard Valley Hospital[2]	Findlay	97%	200
Grant Medical Center[2]	Columbus	97%	358
Mercy Hospital Clermont[2]	Batavia	97%	300
Mercy Memorial Hospital[2]	Urbana	97%	87
Ohio Valley Medical Center	Springfield	97%	129
Samaritan Regional Health System[2]	Ashland	97%	119
South Pointe Hospital[2]	Warrensville Hgts	97%	336
UHHS Memorial Hospital of Geneva[2]	Geneva	97%	98
Ashtabula County Medical Center[2]	Ashtabula	96%	270
Bluffton Hospital[2]	Bluffton	96%	46
Cleveland Clinic[2]	Cleveland	96%	347
Euclid Hospital[2]	Euclid	96%	259
Fort Hamilton Hughes Memorial Hospital[2]	Hamilton	96%	349
Sycamore Medical Center[2]	Miamisburg	96%	339
UH Geauga Medical Center[2]	Chardon	96%	339
UHHS Richmond Heights Hospital[2]	Richmond Hghts	96%	507
Dublin Methodist Hospital[2]	Dublin	95%	331
Firelands Regional Medical Center[2]	Sandusky	95%	331
Marymount Hospital[2]	Garfield Heights	95%	377
Mercy Health - West Hospital[2]	Cincinnati	95%	321
Mercy Hospital Anderson[2]	Cincinnati	95%	311
Mercy Tiffin Hospital[2]	Tiffin	95%	111
Saint Vincent Charity Medical Center[2]	Cleveland	95%	303
Southern Ohio Medical Center[2]	Portsmouth	95%	468
Southwest Regional Medical Center[2]	Georgetown	95%	75
Union Hospital[2]	Dover	95%	397
University Hospitals Ahuja Medical Center[2]	Beachwood	95%	357
Wood County Hospital[2]	Bowling Green	95%	218
Aultman Hospital[2]	Canton	94%	343
Good Samaritan Hospital[2]	Dayton	94%	331
Grandview Hospital & Medical Center[2]	Dayton	94%	332
Hardin Memorial Hospital[2,3]	Kenton	94%	49
Lima Memorial Health System[2]	Lima	94%	288
Memorial Hospital of Union County[2]	Marysville	94%	108
Mercy Willard Hospital[2]	Willard	94%	94
Upper Valley Medical Center[2]	Troy	94%	360
Licking Memorial Hospital[2]	Newark	93%	328
Memorial Hospital[2]	Fremont	93%	141
Mercer County Joint Twp Comm Hosp[2]	Coldwater	93%	82
University Hospitals Case Medical Center[2]	Cleveland	93%	334
West Chester Hospital[2]	West Chester	93%	284
Grady Memorial Hospital[2]	Delaware	92%	221
Kettering Medical Center[2]	Kettering	92%	326
Parma Community General Hospital[2]	Parma	92%	349
Adena Regional Medical Center[2]	Chillicothe	91%	361
Fairview Hospital[2]	Cleveland	91%	340
Fayette County Memorial Hospital	Washington Ch	91%	396
Flower Hospital[2]	Sylvania	91%	341
Good Samaritan Hospital[2]	Cincinnati	91%	302
Lake Health[2]	Concord	91%	331
Lutheran Hospital[2]	Cleveland	91%	240
Medina Hospital[2]	Medina	91%	299
Miami Valley Hospital[2]	Dayton	91%	350
Ohio State University Hospitals[2]	Columbus	91%	344
Summa Health Systems Hospitals[2]	Akron	91%	361
Van Wert County Hospital[2]	Van Wert	91%	85
Atrium Medical Center[2]	Franklin	90%	320
Institute For Orthopaedic Surgery[2]	Lima	90%	41
Lakewood Hospital[2]	Lakewood	90%	293
Mercy Hospital Fairfield[2]	Fairfield	90%	300
Northside Medical Center[2]	Youngstown	90%	415
Salem Regional Medical Center[2]	Salem	90%	335
University of Cincinnati Medical Center[2]	Cincinnati	90%	333
Akron General Medical Center[2]	Akron	89%	361
Bethesda North[2]	Cincinnati	89%	313
Community Hospitals & Wellness Centers	Bryan	89%	634
Fairfield Medical Center[2]	Lancaster	89%	284
Henry County Hospital[2]	Napoleon	89%	79
Riverside Methodist Hospital[2]	Columbus	89%	292
Trumbull Memorial Hospital[2]	Warren	89%	416
University of Toledo Medical Center[2]	Toledo	89%	322
Wooster Community Hospital[2]	Wooster	89%	297
Affinity Medical Center[2]	Massillon	88%	305
Springfield Regional Medical Center[2]	Springfield	88%	308
Summa Health System Barberton Hospital[2]	Barberton	88%	679
Clinton Memorial Hospital[2]	Wilmington	87%	243
Doctors Hospital[2]	Columbus	87%	369
Mercy Saint Vincent Medical Center[2]	Toledo	87%	314
Southwest General Health Center[2]	Middleburg Hgts	87%	315
East Liverpool City Hospital[2]	East Liverpool	86%	251
Fisher - Titus Hospital[2]	Norwalk	86%	262
Jewish Hospital[2]	Cincinnati	86%	355
Mercy Medical Center[2]	Canton	86%	309
Mercy Saint Anne Hospital[2]	Toledo	86%	340
Mercy Saint Charles Hospital[2]	Oregon	86%	345
Mount Carmel West[2]	Columbus	86%	310
Saint Rita's Medical Center[2]	Lima	86%	470
Hillcrest Hospital[2]	Mayfield Heights	85%	323
Saint John Medical Center[2]	Westlake	85%	288
Alliance Community Hospital[2]	Alliance	84%	240
Bay Park Community Hospital[2]	Oregon	84%	244
Holzer Medical Center[2]	Gallipolis	83%	347
Saint Elizabeth Boardman Health Center[2]	Boardman	83%	349
Christ Hospital[2]	Cincinnati	82%	300
Genesis Healthcare System[2]	Zanesville	81%	329
Grand Lake Health System[2]	Saint Marys	81%	188
Mercy Allen Hospital[2]	Oberlin	81%	85
Robinson Memorial Hospital[2]	Ravenna	81%	346
Knox Community Hospital[2]	Mount Vernon	80%	164
Medcentral Health Sys Mansfield Hosp[2]	Mansfield	80%	488
Saint Luke's Hospital[2]	Maumee	80%	346
Trinity Med Ctr East & West[2]	Steubenville	80%	415
Metrohealth System[2]	Cleveland	78%	294
Summa Wadsworth - Rittman Hospital[2]	Wadsworth	78%	227
Wilson Memorial Hospital[2]	Sidney	78%	127
Marion General Hospital[2]	Marion	77%	283
Morrow County Hospital[2]	Mount Gilead	77%	88
Mount Carmel Saint Ann's[2]	Westerville	75%	328
Saint Elizabeth Health Center[2]	Youngstown	75%	330
The Toledo Hospital[2]	Toledo	75%	270
Madison County Hospital[2]	London	74%	57
Marietta Memorial Hospital[2]	Marietta	74%	333
Southeastern Ohio Regional Medical Center[2]	Cambridge	74%	261
McCullough - Hyde Memorial Hospital[2]	Oxford	73%	246
Wayne Hospital[2]	Greenville	73%	138
Mary Rutan Hospital[2]	Bellefontaine	72%	92
Saint Joseph Health Center[2]	Warren	70%	354
Bellevue Hospital[2]	Bellevue	64%	76
East Ohio Regional Hospital[2]	Martins Ferry	64%	319
Univ Hosps-Elyria Med Ctr[2]	Elyria	60%	332
Coshocton County Memorial Hospital[2]	Coshocton	59%	153
Mercy Regional Medical Center[2]	Lorain	55%	321

Warfarin Therapy Discharge Instructions

Hospital Name	City	Rate	Cases
Adena Regional Medical Center[2]	Chillicothe	100%	63
Blanchard Valley Hospital[2]	Findlay	100%	49
Firelands Regional Medical Center[2]	Sandusky	100%	48
Licking Memorial Hospital[2]	Newark	100%	43
Marietta Memorial Hospital[2]	Marietta	100%	62
Mercy Health - West Hospital[2]	Cincinnati	100%	27
Saint Luke's Hospital[2]	Maumee	100%	66
Saint Vincent Charity Medical Center[2]	Cleveland	100%	26
Salem Regional Medical Center[2]	Salem	100%	35
Summa Western Reserve Hospital[2]	Cuyahoga Falls	100%	31
UH Geauga Medical Center[2]	Chardon	100%	45
Union Hospital[2]	Dover	100%	47
Upper Valley Medical Center[2]	Troy	100%	60
Wood County Hospital[2]	Bowling Green	100%	28
Kettering Medical Center[2]	Kettering	99%	101
Mercy Medical Center[2]	Canton	99%	122
Euclid Hospital[2]	Euclid	98%	40
Fort Hamilton Hughes Memorial Hospital[2]	Hamilton	98%	47
Good Samaritan Hospital[2]	Dayton	98%	107
Lima Memorial Health System[2]	Lima	98%	43
Mercy Hospital Anderson[2]	Cincinnati	98%	59
Grant Medical Center[2]	Columbus	97%	104
Northside Medical Center[2]	Youngstown	97%	37
Southwest General Health Center[2]	Middleburg Hgts	97%	98
Trinity Med Ctr East & West[2]	Steubenville	97%	32
Atrium Medical Center[2]	Franklin	96%	90
Mercy Saint Anne Hospital[2]	Toledo	96%	55
Southern Ohio Medical Center[2]	Portsmouth	96%	48
Miami Valley Hospital[2]	Dayton	95%	188
UHHS Richmond Heights Hospital[2]	Richmond Hghts	95%	44
Ashtabula County Medical Center[2]	Ashtabula	94%	34
Saint Joseph Health Center[2]	Warren	93%	42
University Hospitals Ahuja Medical Center[2]	Beachwood	93%	81
Doctors Hospital[2]	Columbus	92%	80
Saint Elizabeth Boardman Health Center[2]	Boardman	92%	65
Sycamore Medical Center[2]	Miamisburg	92%	39
Lake Health[2]	Concord	91%	118
Mercy Hospital Fairfield[2]	Fairfield	91%	87
Mercy Saint Vincent Medical Center[2]	Toledo	91%	102
University of Toledo Medical Center[2]	Toledo	91%	46
Riverside Methodist Hospital[2]	Columbus	90%	193
Cleveland Clinic[2]	Cleveland	89%	237
Mercy Hospital Clermont[2]	Batavia	88%	34
University of Cincinnati Medical Center[2]	Cincinnati	87%	125
Fairview Hospital[2]	Cleveland	86%	103
Saint Rita's Medical Center[2]	Lima	86%	80
University Hospitals Case Medical Center[2]	Cleveland	86%	138
Saint Elizabeth Health Center[2]	Youngstown	85%	91
Univ Hosps-Elyria Med Ctr[2]	Elyria	85%	71
Genesis Healthcare System[2]	Zanesville	82%	61
Medcentral Health Sys Mansfield Hosp[2]	Mansfield	81%	43
Parma Community General Hospital[2]	Parma	81%	43
Aultman Hospital[2]	Canton	80%	145
Marion General Hospital[2]	Marion	80%	41
Jewish Hospital[2]	Cincinnati	79%	66
Marymount Hospital[2]	Garfield Heights	77%	123
Saint John Medical Center[2]	Westlake	76%	42
Fairfield Medical Center[2]	Lancaster	75%	65
Affinity Medical Center[2]	Massillon	74%	35
Southeastern Ohio Regional Medical Center[2]	Cambridge	74%	27
East Liverpool City Hospital[2]	East Liverpool	72%	25
Hillcrest Hospital[2]	Mayfield Heights	72%	147
Akron General Medical Center[2]	Akron	70%	148
Grandview Hospital & Medical Center[2]	Dayton	69%	61
Flower Hospital[2]	Sylvania	66%	32
Mount Carmel Saint Ann's[2]	Westerville	66%	73
Good Samaritan Hospital[2]	Cincinnati	65%	140
South Pointe Hospital[2]	Warrensville Hgts	65%	65
West Chester Hospital[2]	West Chester	65%	60
Trumbull Memorial Hospital[2]	Warren	64%	55
Medina Hospital[2]	Medina	61%	44
Ohio State University Hospitals[2]	Columbus	60%	161
Robinson Memorial Hospital[2]	Ravenna	60%	50
Bethesda North[2]	Cincinnati	59%	92
Mount Carmel West[2]	Columbus	56%	165
Metrohealth System[2]	Cleveland	54%	87
Alliance Community Hospital[2]	Alliance	53%	36
Springfield Regional Medical Center[2]	Springfield	53%	101
Wooster Community Hospital[2]	Wooster	47%	36
Christ Hospital[2]	Cincinnati	46%	117
Mercy Saint Charles Hospital[2]	Oregon	42%	26
Mercy Regional Medical Center[2]	Lorain	32%	50
Lakewood Hospital[2]	Lakewood	23%	39

NOTE: Hospital profiles are in alphabetical order by state, then city, then hospital within the city; Rankings exclude hospitals with less than 25 cases except for patient surveys which excludes hospitals with less than 100 cases; (a) 100-299 cases; (1) The number of cases/patients is too few to report; (2) Data submitted were based on a sample of cases/patients; (3) Results are based on a shorter time period than required; (4) Data suppressed by CMS for one or more quarters; (5) Results are not available for this reporting period; (6) Fewer than 100 patients completed the HCAHPS survey; (7) No cases met the criteria for this measure; (8) The lower limit of the confidence interval cannot be calculated if the number of observed infections equals zero; (9) No data are available from the state/territory for this reporting period; (10) The scores shown reflect fewer than 50 completed surveys; (11) There were discrepancies in the data collection process; (12) This measure does not apply to this hospital for this reporting period; (13) Results cannot be calculated for this reporting period; (14) The results for this state are combined with nearby states to protect confidentiality; Please refer to the User's Guide for a full explanation of data.

Summa Health Systems Hospitals[2]	Akron	19%	143
The Toledo Hospital[2]	Toledo	19%	89
Summa Health System Barberton Hospital[2]	Barberton	0%	56

Chest Pain/Possible Heart Attack Care

Aspirin Given Within 24 Hours of Arrival

Hospital Name	City	Rate	Cases
Aultman Orrville Hospital	Orrville	100%	68
Berger Hospital	Circleville	100%	127
Clinton Memorial Hospital	Wilmington	100%	80
Community Hospitals & Wellness Centers	Montpelier	100%	26
Fostoria Community Hospital[3]	Fostoria	100%	47
Grady Memorial Hospital	Delaware	100%	42
Indu & Raj Soin Medical Center	Beaver Creek	100%	31
Marion General Hospital	Marion	100%	29
Mary Rutan Hospital	Bellefontaine	100%	131
Marymount Hospital	Garfield Heights	100%	74
Memorial Hospital of Union County	Marysville	100%	129
Mercer County Joint Twp Comm Hosp	Coldwater	100%	48
Mercy Hospital of Defiance	Defiance	100%	41
Mercy Saint Anne Hospital	Toledo	100%	42
Mercy Saint Charles Hospital	Oregon	100%	49
Summa Wadsworth - Rittman Hospital	Wadsworth	100%	68
Sycamore Medical Center	Miamisburg	100%	52
Union Hospital	Dover	100%	165
Univ Hosps Conneaut Med Ctr	Conneaut	100%	75
Upper Valley Medical Center	Troy	100%	74
Van Wert County Hospital	Van Wert	100%	77
Wood County Hospital	Bowling Green	100%	61
Wooster Community Hospital	Wooster	100%	222
East Liverpool City Hospital	East Liverpool	99%	95
Medina Hospital	Medina	99%	83
Mercy Hospital Clermont	Batavia	99%	77
Mercy Tiffin Hospital	Tiffin	99%	85
Salem Regional Medical Center	Salem	99%	79
Alliance Community Hospital	Alliance	98%	91
Bay Park Community Hospital	Oregon	98%	60
Diley Ridge Medical Center	Canal Wnchstr	98%	80
Flower Hospital	Sylvania	98%	50
H B Magruder Memorial Hospital	Port Clinton	98%	80
Saint Elizabeth Boardman Health Center	Boardman	98%	83
Southeastern Ohio Regional Medical Center	Cambridge	98%	122
UHHS Memorial Hospital of Geneva	Geneva	98%	80
Grant Medical Center	Columbus	97%	37
Robinson Memorial Hospital	Ravenna	97%	74
Summa Western Reserve Hospital	Cuyahoga Falls	97%	34
UHHS Richmond Heights Hospital	Richmond Hghts	97%	62
Wayne Hospital	Greenville	97%	115
Cleveland Clinic	Cleveland	96%	190
Lake Health	Concord	96%	28
O'Bleness Memorial Hospital	Athens	96%	120
Pomerene Hospital	Millersburg	96%	76
South Pointe Hospital	Warrensville Hgts	96%	98
Fulton County Health Center	Wauseon	95%	105
Grand Lake Health System	Saint Marys	95%	63
Samaritan Regional Health System	Ashland	95%	91
Bellevue Hospital	Bellevue	94%	84
Dublin Methodist Hospital	Dublin	94%	33
Euclid Hospital	Euclid	94%	54
Fisher - Titus Hospital	Norwalk	94%	50
Morrow County Hospital[3]	Mount Gilead	94%	31
Saint Joseph Health Center	Warren	94%	96
Southwest Regional Medical Center	Georgetown	94%	93
Adena Regional Medical Center	Chillicothe	93%	56
Ashtabula County Medical Center	Ashtabula	93%	60
Coshocton County Memorial Hospital	Coshocton	93%	81
Memorial Hospital	Fremont	93%	67
Fayette County Memorial Hospital	Washington Ch	90%	79
Univ Hosps-Elyria Med Ctr	Elyria	90%	29
Grandview Hospital & Medical Center	Dayton	88%	50
Wilson Memorial Hospital	Sidney	86%	58
Harrison Community Hospital[3]	Cadiz	82%	34
Madison County Hospital	London	80%	44
Medcentral Health Sys Mansfield Hosp	Mansfield	78%	36

Average Time to ECG (minutes)

Hospital Name	City	Min.	Cases
Adena Regional Medical Center	Chillicothe	1	55
Medina Hospital	Medina	1	83
Alliance Community Hospital	Alliance	2	88
Lake Health	Concord	2	31
Ashtabula County Medical Center	Ashtabula	3	59
Marion General Hospital	Marion	3	29
Mercer County Joint Twp Comm Hosp	Coldwater	3	49
Harrison Community Hospital[3]	Cadiz	4	33
Marymount Hospital	Garfield Heights	4	74
Mercy Hospital of Defiance	Defiance	4	42
Pomerene Hospital	Millersburg	4	77
Saint Elizabeth Boardman Health Center	Boardman	4	84
UHHS Memorial Hospital of Geneva	Geneva	4	85
Univ Hosps Conneaut Med Ctr	Conneaut	4	82
Upper Valley Medical Center	Troy	4	76
Bay Park Community Hospital	Oregon	5	62
Bellevue Hospital	Bellevue	5	88
Community Hospitals & Wellness Centers	Montpelier	5	27
Euclid Hospital	Euclid	5	53
Flower Hospital	Sylvania	5	53
Fostoria Community Hospital[3]	Fostoria	5	50
Grady Memorial Hospital	Delaware	5	44
Indu & Raj Soin Medical Center	Beaver Creek	5	31
Medcentral Health Sys Mansfield Hosp	Mansfield	5	36
Memorial Hospital	Fremont	5	74
Summa Wadsworth - Rittman Hospital	Wadsworth	5	71
Wooster Community Hospital	Wooster	5	229
Cleveland Clinic	Cleveland	6	197
Clinton Memorial Hospital	Wilmington	6	82
Fayette County Memorial Hospital	Washington Ch	6	82
Mary Rutan Hospital	Bellefontaine	6	134
Salem Regional Medical Center	Salem	6	81
Samaritan Regional Health System	Ashland	6	91
South Pointe Hospital	Warrensville Hgts	6	102
UHHS Richmond Heights Hospital	Richmond Hghts	6	68
Dublin Methodist Hospital	Dublin	7	33
Grand Lake Health System	Saint Marys	7	66
H B Magruder Memorial Hospital	Port Clinton	7	82
Memorial Hospital of Union County	Marysville	7	130
Mercy Tiffin Hospital	Tiffin	7	91
Sycamore Medical Center	Miamisburg	7	53
Wilson Memorial Hospital	Sidney	7	75
Aultman Orrville Hospital	Orrville	8	70
Diley Ridge Medical Center	Canal Wnchstr	8	82
Fisher - Titus Hospital	Norwalk	8	52
Fulton County Health Center	Wauseon	8	109
Grant Medical Center	Columbus	8	39
Mercy Saint Anne Hospital	Toledo	8	44
Mercy Saint Charles Hospital	Oregon	8	49
Southwest Regional Medical Center	Georgetown	8	96
Grandview Hospital & Medical Center	Dayton	9	52
Union Hospital	Dover	9	174
Van Wert County Hospital	Van Wert	9	80
Wayne Hospital	Greenville	9	122
Berger Hospital	Circleville	10	127
Coshocton County Memorial Hospital	Coshocton	10	83
Madison County Hospital	London	10	44
Robinson Memorial Hospital	Ravenna	10	77
Saint Joseph Health Center	Warren	10	98
Southeastern Ohio Regional Medical Center	Cambridge	10	125
Summa Western Reserve Hospital	Cuyahoga Falls	10	35
Univ Hosps-Elyria Med Ctr	Elyria	10	34
Wood County Hospital	Bowling Green	10	44
Mercy Hospital Clermont	Batavia	11	79
O'Bleness Memorial Hospital	Athens	14	126
East Liverpool City Hospital	East Liverpool	15	92
Morrow County Hospital[3]	Mount Gilead	15	31

Average Time to Transfer (minutes)

Hospital Name	City	Min.	Cases
Wooster Community Hospital	Wooster	30	30
Union Hospital	Dover	39	34
Mary Rutan Hospital	Bellefontaine	45	37
Salem Regional Medical Center	Salem	56	25
Adena Regional Medical Center	Chillicothe	57	25
Robinson Memorial Hospital	Ravenna	60	32
Saint Joseph Health Center	Warren	64	26
Upper Valley Medical Center	Troy	64	38
UHHS Richmond Heights Hospital	Richmond Hghts	66	28
East Liverpool City Hospital	East Liverpool	84	35

Children's Asthma Care

Received Home Management Plan of Care

Hospital Name	City	Rate	Cases
Cleveland Clinic	Cleveland	99%	74
The Toledo Hospital	Toledo	98%	115
Aultman Hospital	Canton	92%	25
Saint John Medical Center	Westlake	62%	34

Received Reliever Medication

Hospital Name	City	Rate	Cases
Aultman Hospital	Canton	100%	26
Cleveland Clinic	Cleveland	100%	75
Saint John Medical Center	Westlake	100%	35
The Toledo Hospital	Toledo	100%	116

Received Systemic Corticosteroids

Hospital Name	City	Rate	Cases
Cleveland Clinic	Cleveland	100%	74
Saint John Medical Center	Westlake	100%	35
The Toledo Hospital	Toledo	100%	116
Aultman Hospital	Canton	96%	26

Emergency Department

Admittance Decision Time (minutes)

Hospital Name	City	Min.	Cases
Mercy Willard Hospital[2]	Willard	35	402
Belmont Community Hospital[2]	Bellaire	39	61
Mercy Allen Hospital[2]	Oberlin	39	341
Mercy Hospital of Defiance[2]	Defiance	40	429
Mercy Tiffin Hospital[2]	Tiffin	41	262
Bluffton Hospital[2]	Bluffton	43	73
Alliance Community Hospital[2]	Alliance	46	311
Bellevue Hospital[2]	Bellevue	48	142
East Liverpool City Hospital[2]	East Liverpool	48	487
Community Hospitals & Wellness Centers	Bryan	50	776
Hardin Memorial Hospital[2,3]	Kenton	50	205
Univ Hosps Conneaut Med Ctr	Conneaut	50	279
Doctors Hospital[2]	Columbus	51	536
Madison County Hospital[2]	London	51	157
Memorial Hospital[2]	Fremont	55	315
Mercy Memorial Hospital[2]	Urbana	55	622
Fostoria Community Hospital[2,3]	Fostoria	56	82
Memorial Hospital of Union County[2]	Marysville	56	159
Firelands Regional Medical Center[2]	Sandusky	58	601
Union Hospital[2]	Dover	58	316
Wayne Hospital[2]	Greenville	58	257
Wood County Hospital[2]	Bowling Green	59	278
McCullough - Hyde Memorial Hospital[2]	Oxford	60	462
Southeastern Ohio Regional Medical Center[2]	Cambridge	60	558
Wilson Memorial Hospital[2]	Sidney	60	275
Ashtabula County Medical Center[2]	Ashtabula	61	545
Blanchard Valley Hospital[2]	Findlay	61	445
Fort Hamilton Hughes Memorial Hospital[2]	Hamilton	62	798
Fulton County Health Center[2]	Wauseon	62	136
Grand Lake Health System[2]	Saint Marys	63	241
Medcentral Health Sys Mansfield Hosp[2]	Mansfield	63	337
Mercer County Joint Twp Comm Hosp[2]	Coldwater	63	252
Mercy Health - West Hospital[2]	Cincinnati	63	767
Pomerene Hospital[2]	Millersburg	64	212
Samaritan Regional Health System[2]	Ashland	65	230
Licking Memorial Hospital[2]	Newark	67	736
Holzer Medical Center[2]	Gallipolis	68	442
Marion General Hospital[2]	Marion	68	517
O'Bleness Memorial Hospital[2]	Athens	68	286
Holzer Medical Center Jackson[2,3]	Jackson	69	107
Wooster Community Hospital[2]	Wooster	70	485
East Ohio Regional Hospital[2]	Martins Ferry	71	760
Mercy Saint Anne Hospital[2]	Toledo	71	642
Akron General Medical Center[2]	Akron	72	333
Salem Regional Medical Center[2]	Salem	72	471
Mary Rutan Hospital[2]	Bellefontaine	75	93
Univ Hosps-Elyria Med Ctr[2]	Elyria	75	467
West Chester Hospital[2]	West Chester	75	741
Aultman Hospital[2]	Canton	78	571
UHHS Memorial Hospital of Geneva[2]	Geneva	78	455
Van Wert County Hospital[2]	Van Wert	78	258
Trinity Med Ctr East & West[2]	Steubenville	79	907
Bay Park Community Hospital[2]	Oregon	80	327
Genesis Healthcare System[2]	Zanesville	80	618
Grady Memorial Hospital[2]	Delaware	80	441
Jewish Hospital[2]	Cincinnati	80	906
Saint Luke's Hospital[2]	Maumee	80	714
Affinity Medical Center[2]	Massillon	81	667
Flower Hospital[2]	Sylvania	81	721
Fairfield Medical Center[2]	Lancaster	82	496
Medina Hospital[2]	Medina	82	670
Lima Memorial Health System[2]	Lima	83	646
Mercy Medical Center[2]	Canton	83	866
Lutheran Hospital[2]	Cleveland	86	145
Mount Carmel Saint Ann's[2]	Westerville	87	314
The Toledo Hospital[2]	Toledo	88	441
Adena Regional Medical Center[2]	Chillicothe	89	441
Knox Community Hospital[2]	Mount Vernon	89	300
Clinton Memorial Hospital[2]	Wilmington	90	674
Euclid Hospital[2]	Euclid	93	597
University of Toledo Medical Center[2]	Toledo	93	614
Dublin Methodist Hospital[2]	Dublin	94	284
Robinson Memorial Hospital[2]	Ravenna	94	676
Coshocton County Memorial Hospital[2]	Coshocton	95	357
Marymount Hospital[2]	Garfield Heights	95	680
Summa Health Systems Hospitals[2]	Akron	95	654
UH Geauga Medical Center[2]	Chardon	95	569
UHHS Richmond Heights Hospital[2]	Richmond Hghts	96	844
South Pointe Hospital[2]	Warrensville Hgts	97	685
Fairview Hospital[2]	Cleveland	98	575
Mercy Regional Medical Center[2]	Lorain	98	665
Southwest Regional Medical Center[2]	Georgetown	98	333
Lake Health[2]	Concord	99	676

NOTE: Hospital profiles are in alphabetical order by state, then city, then hospital within the city; Rankings exclude hospitals with less than 25 cases except for patient surveys which excludes hospitals with less than 100 cases; (a) 100-299 cases; (1) The number of cases/patients is too few to report; (2) Data submitted were based on a sample of cases/patients; (3) Results are based on a shorter time period than required; (4) Data suppressed by CMS for one or more quarters; (5) Results are not available for this reporting period; (6) Fewer than 100 patients completed the HCAHPS survey; (7) No cases met the criteria for this measure; (8) The lower limit of the confidence interval cannot be calculated if the number of observed infections equals zero; (9) No data are available from the state/territory for this reporting period; (10) The scores shown reflect fewer than 50 completed surveys; (11) There were discrepancies in the data collection process; (12) This measure does not apply to this hospital for this reporting period; (13) Results cannot be calculated for this reporting period; (14) The results for this state are combined with nearby states to protect confidentiality; Please refer to the User's Guide for a full explanation of data.

Lakewood Hospital[2]	Lakewood	101	481
Saint John Medical Center[2]	Westlake	101	721
Bethesda North[2]	Cincinnati	102	716
Cleveland Clinic[2]	Cleveland	102	227
Indu & Raj Soin Medical Center[2]	Beaver Creek	102	598
Summa Health System Barberton Hospital[2]	Barberton	103	550
Saint Vincent Charity Medical Center[2]	Cleveland	104	490
Summa Wadsworth - Rittman Hospital[2]	Wadsworth	104	155
University of Cincinnati Medical Center[2]	Cincinnati	105	574
Mount Carmel West[2]	Columbus	106	413
Sycamore Medical Center[2]	Miamisburg	108	704
Saint Rita's Medical Center[2]	Lima	109	777
Southern Ohio Medical Center[2]	Portsmouth	110	691
Southwest General Health Center[2]	Middleburg Hgts	110	700
Summa Western Reserve Hospital[2]	Cuyahoga Falls	110	582
Fisher - Titus Hospital[2]	Norwalk	112	358
Hillcrest Hospital[2]	Mayfield Heights	112	523
Saint Joseph Health Center[2]	Warren	114	790
Mercy Hospital Anderson[2]	Cincinnati	116	760
Good Samaritan Hospital[2]	Cincinnati	118	528
Mercy Hospital Clermont[2]	Batavia	118	996
Miami Valley Hospital[2]	Dayton	118	595
Parma Community General Hospital[2]	Parma	121	768
Saint Elizabeth Boardman Health Center[2]	Boardman	122	988
Trumbull Memorial Hospital[2]	Warren	122	787
Marietta Memorial Hospital[2]	Marietta	125	597
Atrium Medical Center[2]	Franklin	126	700
Mercy Hospital Fairfield[2]	Fairfield	126	725
Mercy Saint Charles Hospital[2]	Oregon	127	786
Springfield Regional Medical Center[2]	Springfield	127	852
Greene Memorial Hospital[2]	Xenia	130	474
Northside Medical Center[2]	Youngstown	130	691
Upper Valley Medical Center[2]	Troy	133	781
Christ Hospital[2]	Cincinnati	135	437
Kettering Medical Center[2]	Kettering	137	506
Mercy Saint Vincent Medical Center[2]	Toledo	137	569
University Hospitals Ahuja Medical Center[2]	Beachwood	139	845
Good Samaritan Hospital[2]	Dayton	146	644
Ohio State University Hospitals[2]	Columbus	150	464
Saint Elizabeth Health Center[2]	Youngstown	158	630
Berger Hospital[2]	Circleville	170	186
Grandview Hospital & Medical Center[2]	Dayton	171	491
Metrohealth System[2]	Cleveland	179	682
Riverside Methodist Hospital[2]	Columbus	183	431
Grant Medical Center[2]	Columbus	192	476
University Hospitals Case Medical Center[2]	Cleveland	214	414

Head CT Results Within 45 Minutes of Arrival

Hospital Name	City	Rate	Cases
Marion General Hospital	Marion	93%	46
Univ Hosps-Elyria Med Ctr	Elyria	90%	30
Blanchard Valley Hospital	Findlay	88%	33
University Hospitals Ahuja Medical Center	Beachwood	88%	25
Adena Regional Medical Center	Chillicothe	85%	33
Fairfield Medical Center	Lancaster	78%	27
Trumbull Memorial Hospital	Warren	74%	31
UHHS Richmond Heights Hospital	Richmond Hghts	73%	41
O'Bleness Memorial Hospital	Athens	71%	38
Parma Community General Hospital	Parma	70%	27
Mercy Hospital Clermont	Batavia	67%	27
UH Geauga Medical Center	Chardon	64%	25
Lake Health	Concord	63%	43
Saint Joseph Health Center	Warren	55%	29
Springfield Regional Medical Center	Springfield	55%	47
Genesis Healthcare System	Zanesville	52%	65
Samaritan Regional Health System	Ashland	43%	28

Patients Who Left ER Before Being Seen

Hospital Name	City	Rate	Cases
Alliance Community Hospital	Alliance	0%	35590
Bellevue Hospital	Bellevue	0%	15798
Bethesda North	Cincinnati	0%	56381
Blanchard Valley Hospital	Findlay	0%	37072
Bluffton Hospital	Bluffton	0%	5993
Community Hospitals & Wellness Centers	Bryan	0%	12018
Community Hospitals & Wellness Centers	Montpelier	0%	4297
Diley Ridge Medical Center	Canal Wnchstr	0%	16657
Fisher - Titus Hospital	Norwalk	0%	27601
Fulton County Health Center	Wauseon	0%	16733
Henry County Hospital	Napoleon	0%	9597
Jewish Hospital	Cincinnati	0%	34009
McCullough - Hyde Memorial Hospital	Oxford	0%	16346
Mercer County Joint Twp Comm Hosp	Coldwater	0%	10953
Mercy Hospital of Defiance	Defiance	0%	9179
Mercy Tiffin Hospital	Tiffin	0%	17659
Pomerene Hospital	Millersburg	0%	12287
Summa Western Reserve Hospital	Cuyahoga Falls	0%	21960
UH Geauga Medical Center	Chardon	0%	19059
Van Wert County Hospital	Van Wert	0%	16847
West Chester Hospital	West Chester	0%	33830
Akron General Medical Center	Akron	1%	104024
Ashtabula County Medical Center	Ashtabula	1%	33970
Atrium Medical Center	Franklin	1%	63056
Bay Park Community Hospital	Oregon	1%	24918
Belmont Community Hospital	Bellaire	1%	6564
Berger Hospital	Circleville	1%	31657
Coshocton County Memorial Hospital	Coshocton	1%	26163
East Liverpool City Hospital	East Liverpool	1%	14120
Firelands Regional Medical Center	Sandusky	1%	47770
Flower Hospital	Sylvania	1%	33970
Fort Hamilton Hughes Memorial Hospital	Hamilton	1%	41683
Fostoria Community Hospital	Fostoria	1%	15481
Genesis Healthcare System	Zanesville	1%	71746
Good Samaritan Hospital	Cincinnati	1%	57935
Grady Memorial Hospital	Delaware	1%	26709
Grand Lake Health System	Saint Marys	1%	14624
Grandview Hospital & Medical Center	Dayton	1%	28606
Greene Memorial Hospital	Xenia	1%	26096
Hillcrest Hospital	Mayfield Heights	1%	58657
Hocking Valley Community Hospital	Logan	1%	10664
Indu & Raj Soin Medical Center	Beaver Creek	1%	21231
Kettering Medical Center	Kettering	1%	48897
Lake Health	Concord	1%	79051
Madison County Hospital	London	1%	13979
Marietta Memorial Hospital	Marietta	1%	42155
Marion General Hospital	Marion	1%	50286
Memorial Hospital	Fremont	1%	23151
Mercy Health - West Hospital	Cincinnati	1%	41240
Mercy Hospital Anderson	Cincinnati	1%	47437
Mercy Hospital Clermont	Batavia	1%	58862
Mercy Hospital Fairfield	Fairfield	1%	61969
Mercy Saint Anne Hospital	Toledo	1%	42599
Mercy Saint Charles Hospital	Oregon	1%	40704
Mount Carmel Saint Ann's	Westerville	1%	35332
Mount Carmel West	Columbus	1%	75444
Northside Medical Center	Youngstown	1%	30448
Parma Community General Hospital	Parma	1%	48933
Paulding County Hospital	Paulding	1%	4939
Saint Elizabeth Boardman Health Center	Boardman	1%	45446
Saint Elizabeth Health Center	Youngstown	1%	76635
Saint John Medical Center	Westlake	1%	37893
Saint Luke's Hospital	Maumee	1%	38428
Saint Vincent Charity Medical Center	Cleveland	1%	20021
Salem Regional Medical Center	Salem	1%	28115
Samaritan Regional Health System	Ashland	1%	27253
South Pointe Hospital	Warrensville Hgts	1%	40231
Southeastern Ohio Regional Medical Center	Cambridge	1%	30079
Southern Ohio Medical Center	Portsmouth	1%	50647
Southwest General Health Center	Middleburg Hgts	1%	61365
Southwest Regional Medical Center	Georgetown	1%	12130
Summa Health Systems Hospitals	Akron	1%	115988
Summa Wadsworth - Rittman Hospital	Wadsworth	1%	18661
Sycamore Medical Center	Miamisburg	1%	35599
Trinity Med Ctr East & West	Steubenville	1%	48285
UHHS Memorial Hospital of Geneva	Geneva	1%	14047
UHHS Richmond Heights Hospital	Richmond Hghts	1%	38376
Union Hospital	Dover	1%	45214
University Hospitals Ahuja Medical Center	Beachwood	1%	30917
Univ Hosps Conneaut Med Ctr	Conneaut	1%	13320
Wayne Hospital	Greenville	1%	22559
Wilson Memorial Hospital	Sidney	1%	28522
Wood County Hospital	Bowling Green	1%	25263
Wooster Community Hospital	Wooster	1%	33064
Adena Regional Medical Center	Chillicothe	2%	49699
Affinity Medical Center	Massillon	2%	27418
Aultman Hospital	Canton	2%	85812
Cleveland Clinic	Cleveland	2%	82229
Clinton Memorial Hospital	Wilmington	2%	33630
Doctors Hospital	Columbus	2%	83260
Dublin Methodist Hospital	Dublin	2%	36955
East Ohio Regional Hospital	Martins Ferry	2%	21328
Fairview Hospital	Cleveland	2%	78084
Knox Community Hospital	Mount Vernon	2%	27418
Lakewood Hospital	Lakewood	2%	36251
Lima Memorial Health System	Lima	2%	42306
Lutheran Hospital	Cleveland	2%	26918
Marymount Hospital	Garfield Heights	2%	50542
Medina Hospital	Medina	2%	22916
Mercy Memorial Hospital	Urbana	2%	17443
Mercy Regional Medical Center	Lorain	2%	49491
Metrohealth System	Cleveland	2%	104530
Miami Valley Hospital	Dayton	2%	125622
Riverside Methodist Hospital	Columbus	2%	89739
Saint Joseph Health Center	Warren	2%	72980
The Toledo Hospital	Toledo	2%	91991
Univ Hosps-Elyria Med Ctr	Elyria	2%	88075
University of Toledo Medical Center	Toledo	2%	27073
Christ Hospital	Cincinnati	3%	53595
Euclid Hospital	Euclid	3%	38473
Grant Medical Center	Columbus	3%	88369
Mary Rutan Hospital	Bellefontaine	3%	24325
Medcentral Health Sys Mansfield Hosp	Mansfield	3%	50461
Memorial Hospital of Union County	Marysville	3%	20531
Mercy Medical Center	Canton	3%	53464
Mercy Saint Vincent Medical Center	Toledo	3%	68188
O'Bleness Memorial Hospital	Athens	3%	28180
Upper Valley Medical Center	Troy	3%	44042
Good Samaritan Hospital	Dayton	4%	59399
Ohio State University Hospitals	Columbus	4%	121411
Robinson Memorial Hospital	Ravenna	4%	39345
Saint Rita's Medical Center	Lima	4%	58284
Springfield Regional Medical Center	Springfield	4%	65911
Trumbull Memorial Hospital	Warren	4%	40141
Fairfield Medical Center	Lancaster	5%	51343
Holzer Medical Center	Gallipolis	5%	22506
Licking Memorial Hospital	Newark	5%	58554
Summa Health System Barberton Hospital	Barberton	5%	38030
University of Cincinnati Medical Center	Cincinnati	5%	83638
University Hospitals Case Medical Center	Cleveland	10%	53978

Time from ER Arrival to Being Admitted (minutes)

Hospital Name	City	Min.	Cases
Mercy Hospital of Defiance[2]	Defiance	159	432
Fostoria Community Hospital[2,3]	Fostoria	173	93
Belmont Community Hospital[2]	Bellaire	178	122
Community Hospitals & Wellness Centers	Bryan	186	920
Bellevue Hospital[2]	Bellevue	191	159
Fulton County Health Center[2]	Wauseon	194	138
McCullough - Hyde Memorial Hospital[2]	Oxford	195	467
Alliance Community Hospital[2]	Alliance	196	312
Ashtabula County Medical Center[2]	Ashtabula	198	545
Mercer County Joint Twp Comm Hosp[2]	Coldwater	198	275
Mercy Allen Hospital[2]	Oberlin	198	346
Univ Hosps Conneaut Med Ctr	Conneaut	198	284
Pomerene Hospital[2]	Millersburg	199	231
Fort Hamilton Hughes Memorial Hospital[2]	Hamilton	202	801
Grand Lake Health System[2]	Saint Marys	203	259
Van Wert County Hospital[2]	Van Wert	203	386
Trinity Med Ctr East & West[2]	Steubenville	208	907
Mercy Willard Hospital[2]	Willard	211	433
Union Hospital[2]	Dover	215	663
Marion General Hospital[2]	Marion	219	517
Firelands Regional Medical Center[2]	Sandusky	220	627
Wood County Hospital[2]	Bowling Green	220	327
Memorial Hospital[2]	Fremont	221	322
Mercy Memorial Hospital[2]	Urbana	221	623
Southeastern Ohio Regional Medical Center[2]	Cambridge	221	573
Wooster Community Hospital[2]	Wooster	221	491
UHHS Richmond Heights Hospital[2]	Richmond Hghts	222	872
Bay Park Community Hospital[2]	Oregon	223	328
Hardin Memorial Hospital[2,3]	Kenton	225	205
Licking Memorial Hospital[2]	Newark	225	755
East Ohio Regional Hospital[2]	Martins Ferry	226	808
West Chester Hospital[2]	West Chester	226	745
Holzer Medical Center[2]	Gallipolis	229	464
Bluffton Hospital[2]	Bluffton	231	73
Clinton Memorial Hospital[2]	Wilmington	231	674
Univ Hosps-Elyria Med Ctr[2]	Elyria	231	468
Samaritan Regional Health System[2]	Ashland	232	234
East Liverpool City Hospital[2]	East Liverpool	233	503
Adena Regional Medical Center[2]	Chillicothe	234	516
Genesis Healthcare System[2]	Zanesville	238	624
Grady Memorial Hospital[2]	Delaware	238	441
Mercy Tiffin Hospital[2]	Tiffin	238	267
Wilson Memorial Hospital[2]	Sidney	240	275
Blanchard Valley Hospital[2]	Findlay	245	445
Flower Hospital[2]	Sylvania	247	721
Sycamore Medical Center[2]	Miamisburg	247	705
Madison County Hospital[2]	London	248	162
South Pointe Hospital[2]	Warrensville Hgts	250	695
Salem Regional Medical Center[2]	Salem	251	472
Fairfield Medical Center[2]	Lancaster	252	538
Holzer Medical Center Jackson[2,3]	Jackson	252	107
Lima Memorial Health System[2]	Lima	252	649
Mercy Saint Anne Hospital[2]	Toledo	252	650
Doctors Hospital[2]	Columbus	253	538
Miami Valley Hospital[2]	Dayton	253	601
Akron General Medical Center[2]	Akron	254	376
Mary Rutan Hospital[2]	Bellefontaine	254	177
Medcentral Health Sys Mansfield Hosp[2]	Mansfield	255	375
Bethesda North[2]	Cincinnati	256	729
Good Samaritan Hospital[2]	Cincinnati	256	531
Medina Hospital[2]	Medina	256	673
O'Bleness Memorial Hospital[2]	Athens	256	309
Saint John Medical Center[2]	Westlake	256	766
UHHS Memorial Hospital of Geneva[2]	Geneva	256	461
Indu & Raj Soin Medical Center[2]	Beaver Creek	257	599
Jewish Hospital[2]	Cincinnati	257	910
Mercy Health - West Hospital[2]	Cincinnati	258	770
UH Geauga Medical Center[2]	Chardon	260	577
Summa Wadsworth - Rittman Hospital[2]	Wadsworth	262	442
Upper Valley Medical Center[2]	Troy	263	787

NOTE: Hospital profiles are in alphabetical order by state, then city, then hospital within the city; Rankings exclude hospitals with less than 25 cases except for patient surveys which excludes hospitals with less than 100 cases; (a) 100-299 cases; (1) The number of cases/patients is too few to report; (2) Data submitted were based on a sample of cases/patients; (3) Results are based on a shorter time period than required; (4) Data suppressed by CMS for one or more quarters; (5) Results are not available for this reporting period; (6) Fewer than 100 patients completed the HCAHPS survey; (7) No cases met the criteria for this measure; (8) The lower limit of the confidence interval cannot be calculated if the number of observed infections equals zero; (9) No data are available from the state/territory for this reporting period; (10) The scores shown reflect fewer than 50 completed surveys; (11) There were discrepancies in the data collection process; (12) This measure does not apply to this hospital for this reporting period; (13) Results cannot be calculated for this reporting period; (14) The results for this state are combined with nearby states to protect confidentiality; Please refer to the User's Guide for a full explanation of data.

Hospital Name	City	Min.	Cases
Mount Carmel Saint Ann's[2]	Westerville	266	314
Wayne Hospital[2]	Greenville	266	302
Atrium Medical Center[2]	Franklin	267	716
Southwest Regional Medical Center[2]	Georgetown	268	342
Memorial Hospital of Union County[2]	Marysville	270	164
Fisher - Titus Hospital[2]	Norwalk	272	431
Knox Community Hospital[2]	Mount Vernon	273	328
The Toledo Hospital[2]	Toledo	273	456
Saint Vincent Charity Medical Center[2]	Cleveland	274	516
Aultman Hospital[2]	Canton	275	571
Greene Memorial Hospital[2]	Xenia	277	477
Dublin Methodist Hospital[2]	Dublin	279	285
Hillcrest Hospital[2]	Mayfield Heights	279	529
Robinson Memorial Hospital[2]	Ravenna	279	738
Kettering Medical Center[2]	Kettering	280	524
Summa Western Reserve Hospital[2]	Cuyahoga Falls	280	618
Southern Ohio Medical Center[2]	Portsmouth	281	692
Marymount Hospital[2]	Garfield Heights	284	703
Fairview Hospital[2]	Cleveland	289	576
Euclid Hospital[2]	Euclid	291	599
Mercy Regional Medical Center[2]	Lorain	292	667
Saint Rita's Medical Center[2]	Lima	292	790
Saint Luke's Hospital[2]	Maumee	293	714
Berger Hospital[2]	Circleville	294	301
Mercy Saint Charles Hospital[2]	Oregon	295	788
Lake Health[2]	Concord	297	677
Lutheran Hospital[2]	Cleveland	297	145
Mercy Hospital Fairfield[2]	Fairfield	297	725
Affinity Medical Center[2]	Massillon	299	709
Lakewood Hospital[2]	Lakewood	299	481
Coshocton County Memorial Hospital[2]	Coshocton	300	385
Mount Carmel West[2]	Columbus	300	413
Southwest General Health Center[2]	Middleburg Hgts	300	719
Saint Elizabeth Boardman Health Center[2]	Boardman	301	1005
Mercy Hospital Clermont[2]	Batavia	302	998
Mercy Medical Center[2]	Canton	302	872
Mercy Saint Vincent Medical Center[2]	Toledo	303	597
Cleveland Clinic[2]	Cleveland	304	228
Summa Health Systems Hospitals[2]	Akron	304	671
Summa Health System Barberton Hospital[2]	Barberton	305	804
Marietta Memorial Hospital[2]	Marietta	306	597
Good Samaritan Hospital[2]	Dayton	310	649
Mercy Hospital Anderson[2]	Cincinnati	312	762
Northside Medical Center[2]	Youngstown	315	693
Saint Joseph Health Center[2]	Warren	320	792
University of Toledo Medical Center[2]	Toledo	327	619
Springfield Regional Medical Center[2]	Springfield	329	853
Trumbull Memorial Hospital[2]	Warren	331	825
Riverside Methodist Hospital[2]	Columbus	332	431
University Hospitals Ahuja Medical Center[2]	Beachwood	332	848
Parma Community General Hospital[2]	Parma	333	795
Saint Elizabeth Health Center[2]	Youngstown	336	651
Grandview Hospital & Medical Center[2]	Dayton	340	521
Christ Hospital[2]	Cincinnati	353	437
Metrohealth System[2]	Cleveland	359	684
Grant Medical Center[2]	Columbus	360	476
Ohio State University Hospitals[2]	Columbus	363	467
University of Cincinnati Medical Center[2]	Cincinnati	370	583
University Hospitals Case Medical Center[2]	Cleveland	438	420

Time from ER Arrival to Discharge (minutes)

Hospital Name	City	Min.	Cases
Mercy Hospital of Defiance	Defiance	64	370
Aultman Orrville Hospital	Orrville	67	399
Belmont Community Hospital	Bellaire	68	352
Lodi Community Hospital	Lodi	70	293
Community Hospitals & Wellness Centers	Montpelier	72	390
Bay Park Community Hospital	Oregon	78	360
Ashtabula County Medical Center	Ashtabula	83	393
Alliance Community Hospital	Alliance	84	371
Univ Hosps Conneaut Med Ctr	Conneaut	84	398
Bluffton Hospital	Bluffton	85	361
McCullough - Hyde Memorial Hospital	Oxford	85	381
Van Wert County Hospital	Van Wert	91	365
Bellevue Hospital	Bellevue	92	340
Selby General Hospital	Marietta	93	1082
East Ohio Regional Hospital	Martins Ferry	98	368
UHHS Richmond Heights Hospital	Richmond Hghts	98	724
Fort Hamilton Hughes Memorial Hospital	Hamilton	100	387
Lima Memorial Health System	Lima	101	446
UHHS Memorial Hospital of Geneva	Geneva	102	355
Good Samaritan Hospital	Cincinnati	103	382
Mercer County Joint Twp Comm Hosp	Coldwater	104	342
Pomerene Hospital	Millersburg	104	370
Grand Lake Health System	Saint Marys	105	317
South Pointe Hospital	Warrensville Hgts	105	390
Coshocton County Memorial Hospital	Coshocton	106	363
The Toledo Hospital	Toledo	106	383
East Liverpool City Hospital	East Liverpool	107	330
Fulton County Health Center	Wauseon	107	341
Community Hospitals & Wellness Centers	Bryan	108	432
Mercy Health - West Hospital	Cincinnati	108	398
Memorial Hospital	Fremont	110	508
Trinity Med Ctr East & West	Steubenville	110	448
Clinton Memorial Hospital	Wilmington	111	351
Firelands Regional Medical Center	Sandusky	111	389
Mercy Saint Anne Hospital	Toledo	111	401
Akron General Medical Center	Akron	112	354
Berger Hospital	Circleville	112	366
Grady Memorial Hospital	Delaware	112	771
Madison County Hospital	London	112	338
Samaritan Regional Health System	Ashland	112	359
Univ Hosps-Elyria Med Ctr	Elyria	112	395
Marion General Hospital	Marion	113	361
Mercy Hospital Clermont	Batavia	114	378
Saint Joseph Health Center	Warren	114	390
Bethesda North	Cincinnati	115	377
Summa Wadsworth - Rittman Hospital	Wadsworth	116	354
Wooster Community Hospital	Wooster	116	371
Mary Rutan Hospital	Bellefontaine	117	341
Summa Health Systems Hospitals	Akron	118	387
Diley Ridge Medical Center	Canal Wnchstr	119	365
Union Hospital	Dover	119	383
Blanchard Valley Hospital	Findlay	121	361
Marymount Hospital	Garfield Heights	121	381
Wood County Hospital	Bowling Green	121	357
Knox Community Hospital	Mount Vernon	123	331
Saint Vincent Charity Medical Center	Cleveland	123	336
Salem Regional Medical Center	Salem	125	381
Southeastern Ohio Regional Medical Center	Cambridge	125	440
University of Toledo Medical Center	Toledo	126	433
Mercy Saint Charles Hospital	Oregon	127	381
Mercy Tiffin Hospital	Tiffin	127	409
Wilson Memorial Hospital	Sidney	127	376
Euclid Hospital	Euclid	128	375
Lutheran Hospital	Cleveland	128	373
Flower Hospital	Sylvania	129	403
Adena Regional Medical Center	Chillicothe	130	384
Cleveland Clinic	Cleveland	131	294
Northside Medical Center	Youngstown	131	381
Saint Elizabeth Health Center	Youngstown	132	356
Mercy Hospital Fairfield	Fairfield	134	397
West Chester Hospital	West Chester	135	392
Genesis Healthcare System	Zanesville	136	352
Saint John Medical Center	Westlake	136	356
Lakewood Hospital	Lakewood	137	377
UH Geauga Medical Center	Chardon	137	393
Sycamore Medical Center	Miamisburg	138	397
Marietta Memorial Hospital	Marietta	140	390
Doctors Hospital	Columbus	141	393
Fairview Hospital	Cleveland	141	407
Fisher - Titus Hospital	Norwalk	142	362
Greene Memorial Hospital	Xenia	142	419
Hillcrest Hospital	Mayfield Heights	144	384
Aultman Hospital	Canton	145	388
Jewish Hospital	Cincinnati	145	389
Atrium Medical Center	Franklin	146	395
Mercy Regional Medical Center	Lorain	146	374
Summa Western Reserve Hospital	Cuyahoga Falls	146	436
Indu & Raj Soin Medical Center	Beaver Creek	148	523
Southwest General Health Center	Middleburg Hgts	149	389
Lake Health	Concord	150	341
Licking Memorial Hospital	Newark	150	378
Parma Community General Hospital	Parma	152	346
Grant Medical Center	Columbus	153	427
Metrohealth System	Cleveland	153	368
Saint Elizabeth Boardman Health Center	Boardman	153	379
Grandview Hospital & Medical Center	Dayton	154	399
Wayne Hospital	Greenville	155	397
Southern Ohio Medical Center	Portsmouth	157	401
Miami Valley Hospital	Dayton	158	400
Medina Hospital	Medina	160	313
Trumbull Memorial Hospital	Warren	160	355
Dublin Methodist Hospital	Dublin	161	367
O'Bleness Memorial Hospital	Athens	161	413
Kettering Medical Center	Kettering	164	343
Memorial Hospital of Union County	Marysville	164	357
Mercy Hospital Anderson	Cincinnati	164	388
Robinson Memorial Hospital	Ravenna	164	357
Mount Carmel Saint Ann's	Westerville	165	355
Medcentral Health Sys Mansfield Hosp	Mansfield	168	575
Mount Carmel West	Columbus	168	687
Saint Luke's Hospital	Maumee	168	460
Saint Rita's Medical Center	Lima	168	438
University Hospitals Ahuja Medical Center	Beachwood	169	411
Springfield Regional Medical Center	Springfield	170	398
Christ Hospital	Cincinnati	172	392
Summa Health System Barberton Hospital	Barberton	172	774
Affinity Medical Center	Massillon	176	386
Upper Valley Medical Center	Troy	176	409
University of Cincinnati Medical Center	Cincinnati	177	361
Holzer Medical Center	Gallipolis	178	335
Mercy Saint Vincent Medical Center	Toledo	180	360
Ohio State University Hospitals	Columbus	184	321
Fairfield Medical Center	Lancaster	185	366
Mercy Medical Center	Canton	193	532
Southwest Regional Medical Center	Georgetown	200	142
Riverside Methodist Hospital	Columbus	203	319
Good Samaritan Hospital	Dayton	204	370
University Hospitals Case Medical Center	Cleveland	270	363

Time in ER Before Being Evaluated (minutes)

Hospital Name	City	Min.	Cases
Fort Hamilton Hughes Memorial Hospital	Hamilton	7	414
Harrison Community Hospital[3]	Cadiz	7	25
Lodi Community Hospital	Lodi	7	332
Mercy Hospital of Defiance	Defiance	9	419
Summa Health Systems Hospitals	Akron	9	425
Aultman Orrville Hospital	Orrville	10	432
Selby General Hospital	Marietta	10	1091
West Chester Hospital	West Chester	10	418
Cleveland Clinic	Cleveland	11	417
Marietta Memorial Hospital	Marietta	11	424
Mercy Hospital Clermont	Batavia	11	421
Blanchard Valley Hospital	Findlay	12	383
Bluffton Hospital	Bluffton	12	384
Wooster Community Hospital	Wooster	12	416
Community Hospitals & Wellness Centers	Montpelier	13	440
Lakewood Hospital	Lakewood	13	421
Mercy Hospital Anderson	Cincinnati	13	413
Mercy Hospital Fairfield	Fairfield	13	417
Ashtabula County Medical Center	Ashtabula	14	417
Atrium Medical Center	Franklin	14	420
McCullough - Hyde Memorial Hospital	Oxford	14	294
Southern Ohio Medical Center	Portsmouth	14	466
UH Geauga Medical Center	Chardon	14	405
UHHS Richmond Heights Hospital	Richmond Hghts	14	766
Greene Memorial Hospital	Xenia	15	451
Jewish Hospital	Cincinnati	15	413
Kettering Medical Center	Kettering	15	414
Miami Valley Hospital	Dayton	15	443
Sycamore Medical Center	Miamisburg	15	427
Flower Hospital	Sylvania	16	421
Fulton County Health Center	Wauseon	16	378
Indu & Raj Soin Medical Center	Beaver Creek	16	565
Lutheran Hospital	Cleveland	16	421
Northside Medical Center	Youngstown	16	421
Summa Wadsworth - Rittman Hospital	Wadsworth	16	336
Univ Hosps Conneaut Med Ctr	Conneaut	16	432
Community Hospitals & Wellness Centers	Bryan	17	493
Highland District Hospital[3]	Hillsboro	17	39
Medina Hospital	Medina	17	425
Memorial Hospital	Fremont	17	540
Mercer County Joint Twp Comm Hosp	Coldwater	17	382
Saint John Medical Center	Westlake	17	404
South Pointe Hospital	Warrensville Hgts	17	443
Southwest Regional Medical Center	Georgetown	17	249
UHHS Memorial Hospital of Geneva	Geneva	17	297
Bellevue Hospital	Bellevue	18	333
Grand Lake Health System	Saint Marys	18	387
Hillcrest Hospital	Mayfield Heights	18	438
Lima Memorial Health System	Lima	18	479
Marymount Hospital	Garfield Heights	18	428
Mount Carmel Saint Ann's	Westerville	18	388
Trumbull Memorial Hospital	Warren	18	418
Univ Hosps-Elyria Med Ctr	Elyria	18	426
Van Wert County Hospital	Van Wert	18	326
Akron General Medical Center	Akron	19	294
Clinton Memorial Hospital	Wilmington	19	397
Marion General Hospital	Marion	19	419
Saint Elizabeth Health Center	Youngstown	19	418
Summa Western Reserve Hospital	Cuyahoga Falls	19	464
Euclid Hospital	Euclid	20	415
Fairview Hospital	Cleveland	20	446
Grady Memorial Hospital	Delaware	20	840
Mercy Tiffin Hospital	Tiffin	20	432
Pomerene Hospital	Millersburg	20	363
Riverside Methodist Hospital	Columbus	20	419
Trinity Med Ctr East & West	Steubenville	20	402
Adena Regional Medical Center	Chillicothe	21	368
Christ Hospital	Cincinnati	21	421
Genesis Healthcare System	Zanesville	21	384
Alliance Community Hospital	Alliance	22	397
Kings Daughters Medical Center Ohio[3]	Portsmouth	22	40
Saint Elizabeth Boardman Health Center	Boardman	22	451
Southwest General Health Center	Middleburg Hgts	22	417
East Ohio Regional Hospital	Martins Ferry	24	400
Grandview Hospital & Medical Center	Dayton	24	433
Lake Health	Concord	25	303
Saint Joseph Health Center	Warren	25	423
Belmont Community Hospital	Bellaire	26	304
Mercy Health - West Hospital	Cincinnati	26	400
Mercy Saint Charles Hospital	Oregon	26	110

NOTE: Hospital profiles are in alphabetical order by state, then city, then hospital within the city; Rankings exclude hospitals with less than 25 cases except for patient surveys which excludes hospitals with less than 100 cases; (a) 100-299 cases; (1) The number of cases/patients is too few to report; (2) Data submitted were based on a sample of cases/patients; (3) Results are based on a shorter time period than required; (4) Data suppressed by CMS for one or more quarters; (5) Results are not available for this reporting period; (6) Fewer than 100 patients completed the HCAHPS survey; (7) No cases met the criteria for this measure; (8) The lower limit of the confidence interval cannot be calculated if the number of observed infections equals zero; (9) No data are available from the state/territory for this reporting period; (10) The scores shown reflect fewer than 50 completed surveys; (11) There were discrepancies in the data collection process; (12) This measure does not apply to this hospital for this reporting period; (13) Results cannot be calculated for this reporting period; (14) The results for this state are combined with nearby states to protect confidentiality; Please refer to the User's Guide for a full explanation of data.

Doctors Hospital	Columbus	27	434
Parma Community General Hospital	Parma	27	412
Samaritan Regional Health System	Ashland	27	402
The Toledo Hospital	Toledo	27	336
Wood County Hospital	Bowling Green	27	356
Madison County Hospital	London	28	343
Springfield Regional Medical Center	Springfield	28	423
Diley Ridge Medical Center	Canal Wnchstr	29	386
Mercy Regional Medical Center	Lorain	29	416
Mercy Saint Anne Hospital	Toledo	29	413
University of Cincinnati Medical Center	Cincinnati	29	400
Aultman Hospital	Canton	30	418
Berger Hospital	Circleville	30	401
East Liverpool City Hospital	East Liverpool	30	356
Good Samaritan Hospital	Dayton	30	412
Saint Rita's Medical Center	Lima	30	456
Saint Vincent Charity Medical Center	Cleveland	30	385
Wayne Hospital	Greenville	30	407
Fisher - Titus Hospital	Norwalk	31	391
Southeastern Ohio Regional Medical Center	Cambridge	31	426
University Hospitals Ahuja Medical Center	Beachwood	31	431
Bethesda North	Cincinnati	32	168
Salem Regional Medical Center	Salem	32	407
Firelands Regional Medical Center	Sandusky	34	401
Mary Rutan Hospital	Bellefontaine	34	383
Memorial Hospital of Union County	Marysville	34	337
Metrohealth System	Cleveland	34	420
Ohio State University Hospitals	Columbus	35	394
Union Hospital	Dover	35	428
Bay Park Community Hospital	Oregon	36	128
Coshocton County Memorial Hospital	Coshocton	36	374
Good Samaritan Hospital	Cincinnati	36	226
Knox Community Hospital	Mount Vernon	36	379
Robinson Memorial Hospital	Ravenna	36	158
Upper Valley Medical Center	Troy	36	442
Mercy Saint Vincent Medical Center	Toledo	37	407
Dublin Methodist Hospital	Dublin	38	413
Summa Health System Barberton Hospital	Barberton	40	268
Wilson Memorial Hospital	Sidney	40	383
Affinity Medical Center	Massillon	41	402
Mercy Medical Center	Canton	42	569
Saint Luke's Hospital	Maumee	42	499
O'Bleness Memorial Hospital	Athens	43	465
Mount Carmel West	Columbus	45	763
Fairfield Medical Center	Lancaster	47	406
University of Toledo Medical Center	Toledo	47	443
University Hospitals Case Medical Center	Cleveland	48	395
Holzer Medical Center	Gallipolis	49	374
Grant Medical Center	Columbus	56	454
Licking Memorial Hospital	Newark	56	383
Medcentral Health Sys Mansfield Hosp	Mansfield	71	616

Time to Pain Meds for Bone Fractures (minutes)

Hospital Name	City	Min.	Cases
Bluffton Hospital	Bluffton	30	26
Mercer County Joint Twp Comm Hosp	Coldwater	30	46
Alliance Community Hospital	Alliance	31	99
Hillcrest Hospital	Mayfield Heights	32	263
Miami Valley Hospital	Dayton	32	145
Madison County Hospital	London	36	39
McCullough - Hyde Memorial Hospital	Oxford	36	88
Bellevue Hospital	Bellevue	38	42
Trinity Med Ctr East & West	Steubenville	38	82
West Chester Hospital	West Chester	38	67
Univ Hosps-Elyria Med Ctr	Elyria	39	173
Ashtabula County Medical Center	Ashtabula	40	109
East Ohio Regional Hospital	Martins Ferry	40	65
Fort Hamilton Hughes Memorial Hospital	Hamilton	40	87
Marietta Memorial Hospital	Marietta	40	191
Medina Hospital	Medina	40	97
Wooster Community Hospital	Wooster	41	143
Fairview Hospital	Cleveland	42	264
Good Samaritan Hospital	Cincinnati	43	221
Wood County Hospital	Bowling Green	43	61
Bethesda North	Cincinnati	44	328
Samaritan Regional Health System	Ashland	44	111
Blanchard Valley Hospital	Findlay	45	149
Grady Memorial Hospital	Delaware	45	91
Grant Medical Center	Columbus	45	139
Marymount Hospital	Garfield Heights	45	119
Mercy Saint Anne Hospital	Toledo	45	69
Aultman Hospital	Canton	46	229
Cleveland Clinic	Cleveland	46	194
Saint Joseph Health Center	Warren	46	166
Summa Health Systems Hospitals	Akron	46	201
Summa Wadsworth - Rittman Hospital	Wadsworth	46	77
Lakewood Hospital	Lakewood	47	73
Mercy Hospital Anderson	Cincinnati	48	126
Northside Medical Center	Youngstown	48	67
South Pointe Hospital	Warrensville Hgts	48	88
Univ Hosps Conneaut Med Ctr	Conneaut	48	53
Jewish Hospital	Cincinnati	49	63
Marion General Hospital	Marion	49	157
Southwest General Health Center	Middleburg Hgts	49	156
UHHS Memorial Hospital of Geneva	Geneva	49	53
University of Cincinnati Medical Center	Cincinnati	49	55
Euclid Hospital	Euclid	50	54
Fulton County Health Center	Wauseon	50	70
Grand Lake Health System	Saint Marys	50	48
Indu & Raj Soin Medical Center	Beaver Creek	50	68
Lake Health	Concord	50	178
Mercy Health - West Hospital	Cincinnati	50	113
University Hospitals Ahuja Medical Center	Beachwood	50	114
Atrium Medical Center	Franklin	51	135
Bay Park Community Hospital	Oregon	51	69
Christ Hospital	Cincinnati	51	41
Lima Memorial Health System	Lima	51	58
Mercy Hospital Clermont	Batavia	51	126
Van Wert County Hospital	Van Wert	51	82
Adena Regional Medical Center	Chillicothe	52	146
UH Geauga Medical Center	Chardon	52	106
UHHS Richmond Heights Hospital	Richmond Hghts	52	73
Robinson Memorial Hospital	Ravenna	53	125
Saint John Medical Center	Westlake	54	133
Southern Ohio Medical Center	Portsmouth	54	119
Sycamore Medical Center	Miamisburg	54	102
The Toledo Hospital	Toledo	54	217
Community Hospitals & Wellness Centers	Bryan	55	41
Doctors Hospital	Columbus	55	337
Flower Hospital	Sylvania	55	147
Mary Rutan Hospital	Bellefontaine	55	107
Akron General Medical Center	Akron	56	181
Coshocton County Memorial Hospital	Coshocton	56	40
Fisher - Titus Hospital	Norwalk	56	110
Southeastern Ohio Regional Medical Center	Cambridge	56	101
Diley Ridge Medical Center	Canal Wnchstr	58	74
Knox Community Hospital	Mount Vernon	58	110
Mercy Saint Vincent Medical Center	Toledo	58	132
Pomerene Hospital	Millersburg	58	52
Saint Elizabeth Health Center	Youngstown	59	187
East Liverpool City Hospital	East Liverpool	60	156
Firelands Regional Medical Center	Sandusky	60	140
Licking Memorial Hospital	Newark	60	133
Mercy Medical Center	Canton	60	154
Mercy Tiffin Hospital	Tiffin	60	80
Salem Regional Medical Center	Salem	60	81
Wilson Memorial Hospital	Sidney	60	123
Berger Hospital	Circleville	61	75
Kettering Medical Center	Kettering	62	94
Memorial Hospital	Fremont	62	126
Memorial Hospital of Union County	Marysville	62	107
Mount Carmel Saint Ann's	Westerville	62	102
Dublin Methodist Hospital	Dublin	63	204
Genesis Healthcare System	Zanesville	64	214
Mercy Hospital Fairfield	Fairfield	64	135
Riverside Methodist Hospital	Columbus	64	134
Saint Vincent Charity Medical Center	Cleveland	64	54
Union Hospital	Dover	64	153
Clinton Memorial Hospital	Wilmington	65	116
Greene Memorial Hospital	Xenia	65	47
Parma Community General Hospital	Parma	65	145
Summa Health System Barberton Hospital	Barberton	65	35
Upper Valley Medical Center	Troy	65	118
Wayne Hospital	Greenville	66	96
Affinity Medical Center	Massillon	67	135
Lutheran Hospital	Cleveland	69	42
Fairfield Medical Center	Lancaster	70	94
Medcentral Health Sys Mansfield Hosp	Mansfield	71	143
O'Bleness Memorial Hospital	Athens	71	104
Good Samaritan Hospital	Dayton	72	75
Mercy Saint Charles Hospital	Oregon	72	74
Springfield Regional Medical Center	Springfield	72	292
Saint Elizabeth Boardman Health Center	Boardman	73	143
Trumbull Memorial Hospital	Warren	74	56
Ohio State University Hospitals	Columbus	76	80
Saint Luke's Hospital	Maumee	76	208
Mercy Regional Medical Center	Lorain	77	150
Mount Carmel West	Columbus	77	180
Grandview Hospital & Medical Center	Dayton	78	147
Summa Western Reserve Hospital	Cuyahoga Falls	78	73
Holzer Medical Center	Gallipolis	82	55
Saint Rita's Medical Center	Lima	86	187
University Hospitals Case Medical Center	Cleveland	100	39

Heart Attack Care

Aspirin Given at Discharge

Hospital Name	City	Rate	Cases
Adena Regional Medical Center[2]	Chillicothe	100%	249
Akron General Medical Center[2]	Akron	100%	290
Ashtabula County Medical Center	Ashtabula	100%	27
Atrium Medical Center	Franklin	100%	239
Aultman Hospital	Canton	100%	659
Bethesda North	Cincinnati	100%	371
Blanchard Valley Hospital	Findlay	100%	182
Christ Hospital[2]	Cincinnati	100%	314
Cincinnati VA Medical Center	Cincinnati	100%	49
Cleveland - Wade Park VA Medical Center	Cleveland	100%	27
Cleveland Clinic	Cleveland	100%	868
Community Hospitals & Wellness Centers	Bryan	100%	100
Dayton VA Medical Center	Dayton	100%	28
Doctors Hospital	Columbus	100%	166
Firelands Regional Medical Center	Sandusky	100%	138
Good Samaritan Hospital	Cincinnati	100%	244
Grandview Hospital & Medical Center	Dayton	100%	163
Grant Medical Center	Columbus	100%	335
Jewish Hospital	Cincinnati	100%	178
Kettering Medical Center	Kettering	100%	446
Lake Health	Concord	100%	290
Lima Memorial Health System	Lima	100%	281
Marion General Hospital	Marion	100%	204
Mercy Health - West Hospital	Cincinnati	100%	44
Mercy Hospital Anderson	Cincinnati	100%	348
Mercy Medical Center	Canton	100%	387
Mercy Saint Charles Hospital	Oregon	100%	29
Mercy Saint Vincent Medical Center	Toledo	100%	624
Miami Valley Hospital[2]	Dayton	100%	308
Northside Medical Center	Youngstown	100%	182
Ohio State University Hospitals[2]	Columbus	100%	279
Parma Community General Hospital	Parma	100%	288
Riverside Methodist Hospital[2]	Columbus	100%	299
Saint Elizabeth Boardman Health Center	Boardman	100%	36
Saint John Medical Center[2]	Westlake	100%	227
Saint Luke's Hospital	Maumee	100%	310
Southern Ohio Medical Center	Portsmouth	100%	295
Summa Health Systems Hospitals[2]	Akron	100%	307
The Toledo Hospital[2]	Toledo	100%	310
Trinity Med Ctr East & West	Steubenville	100%	269
Trumbull Memorial Hospital	Warren	100%	176
UH Geauga Medical Center	Chardon	100%	108
Union Hospital	Dover	100%	25
University Hospitals Ahuja Medical Center	Beachwood	100%	125
University Hospitals Case Medical Center	Cleveland	100%	396
Affinity Medical Center	Massillon	99%	106
Fairfield Medical Center	Lancaster	99%	285
Fairview Hospital	Cleveland	99%	285
Genesis Healthcare System	Zanesville	99%	429
Good Samaritan Hospital[2]	Dayton	99%	322
Hillcrest Hospital	Mayfield Heights	99%	307
Licking Memorial Hospital	Newark	99%	151
Marietta Memorial Hospital	Marietta	99%	151
Metrohealth System	Cleveland	99%	256
Mount Carmel West[2]	Columbus	99%	293
Saint Elizabeth Health Center	Youngstown	99%	537
Saint Rita's Medical Center	Lima	99%	472
Southwest General Health Center	Middleburg Hgts	99%	342
Univ Hosps-Elyria Med Ctr[2]	Elyria	99%	359
University of Cincinnati Medical Center	Cincinnati	99%	272
University of Toledo Medical Center[2]	Toledo	99%	209
East Ohio Regional Hospital	Martins Ferry	98%	42
Fort Hamilton Hughes Memorial Hospital	Hamilton	98%	140
Knox Community Hospital	Mount Vernon	98%	105
Lakewood Hospital	Lakewood	98%	62
Medcentral Health Sys Mansfield Hosp	Mansfield	98%	302
Mercy Hospital Fairfield	Fairfield	98%	389
Mount Carmel Saint Ann's	Westerville	98%	169
UHHS Richmond Heights Hospital	Richmond Hghts	98%	46
West Chester Hospital	West Chester	98%	216
Springfield Regional Medical Center	Springfield	97%	343
Summa Health System Barberton Hospital	Barberton	97%	119
Upper Valley Medical Center	Troy	97%	58
Holzer Medical Center	Gallipolis	96%	182
Marymount Hospital	Garfield Heights	96%	25
Mercy Regional Medical Center	Lorain	96%	323
Robinson Memorial Hospital	Ravenna	95%	38
Saint Vincent Charity Medical Center	Cleveland	94%	51
Saint Joseph Health Center	Warren	93%	29

PCI Within 90 Minutes of Arrival

Hospital Name	City	Rate	Cases
Akron General Medical Center[2]	Akron	100%	35
Blanchard Valley Hospital	Findlay	100%	46
Doctors Hospital	Columbus	100%	53
Fairfield Medical Center	Lancaster	100%	53
Fort Hamilton Hughes Memorial Hospital	Hamilton	100%	26
Good Samaritan Hospital	Cincinnati	100%	45
Licking Memorial Hospital	Newark	100%	60
Marion General Hospital	Marion	100%	38
Metrohealth System	Cleveland	100%	43
Miami Valley Hospital[2]	Dayton	100%	54
Mount Carmel West[2]	Columbus	100%	64
Parma Community General Hospital	Parma	100%	59

NOTE: Hospital profiles are in alphabetical order by state, then city, then hospital within the city; Rankings exclude hospitals with less than 25 cases except for patient surveys which excludes hospitals with less than 100 cases; (a) 100-299 cases; (1) The number of cases/patients is too few to report; (2) Data submitted were based on a sample of cases/patients; (3) Results are based on a shorter time period than required; (4) Data suppressed by CMS for one or more quarters; (5) Results are not available for this reporting period; (6) Fewer than 100 patients completed the HCAHPS survey; (7) No cases met the criteria for this measure; (8) The lower limit of the confidence interval cannot be calculated if the number of observed infections equals zero; (9) No data are available from the state/territory for this reporting period; (10) The scores shown reflect fewer than 50 completed surveys; (11) There were discrepancies in the data collection process; (12) This measure does not apply to this hospital for this reporting period; (13) Results cannot be calculated for this reporting period; (14) The results for this state are combined with nearby states to protect confidentiality; Please refer to the User's Guide for a full explanation of data.

Hospital Name	City	Rate	Cases
Riverside Methodist Hospital[2]	Columbus	100%	40
Saint Elizabeth Health Center	Youngstown	100%	73
Saint John Medical Center[2]	Westlake	100%	38
Saint Luke's Hospital	Maumee	100%	45
Southwest General Health Center	Middleburg Hgts	100%	51
University Hospitals Ahuja Medical Center	Beachwood	100%	36
University Hospitals Case Medical Center	Cleveland	100%	27
Aultman Hospital	Canton	99%	108
Grant Medical Center	Columbus	99%	71
Atrium Medical Center	Franklin	98%	55
Genesis Healthcare System	Zanesville	98%	60
Hillcrest Hospital	Mayfield Heights	98%	64
Kettering Medical Center	Kettering	98%	65
Lake Health	Concord	98%	64
Mercy Regional Medical Center	Lorain	98%	47
Mount Carmel Saint Ann's	Westerville	98%	42
Summa Health Systems Hospitals[2]	Akron	98%	52
Affinity Medical Center	Massillon	97%	36
Southern Ohio Medical Center	Portsmouth	97%	37
Bethesda North	Cincinnati	96%	75
Mercy Hospital Anderson	Cincinnati	96%	52
The Toledo Hospital[2]	Toledo	96%	28
West Chester Hospital	West Chester	96%	28
Grandview Hospital & Medical Center	Dayton	95%	37
Medcentral Health Sys Mansfield Hosp	Mansfield	95%	44
Saint Rita's Medical Center	Lima	94%	52
Springfield Regional Medical Center	Springfield	94%	52
Trumbull Memorial Hospital	Warren	94%	31
Univ Hosps-Elyria Med Ctr[2]	Elyria	94%	36
Mercy Hospital Fairfield	Fairfield	93%	57
Mercy Saint Vincent Medical Center	Toledo	93%	58
Trinity Med Ctr East & West	Steubenville	93%	30
Jewish Hospital	Cincinnati	92%	26
Mercy Medical Center	Canton	92%	75
University of Cincinnati Medical Center	Cincinnati	92%	40
Fairview Hospital	Cleveland	91%	56
Good Samaritan Hospital[2]	Dayton	90%	40
Knox Community Hospital	Mount Vernon	88%	26
Adena Regional Medical Center[2]	Chillicothe	87%	30
Holzer Medical Center	Gallipolis	84%	25

Statin Prescribed at Discharge

Hospital Name	City	Rate	Cases
Ashtabula County Medical Center	Ashtabula	100%	26
Atrium Medical Center	Franklin	100%	241
Aultman Hospital	Canton	100%	628
Blanchard Valley Hospital	Findlay	100%	179
Christ Hospital[2]	Cincinnati	100%	304
Cincinnati VA Medical Center	Cincinnati	100%	48
Cleveland - Wade Park VA Medical Center	Cleveland	100%	29
Cleveland Clinic	Cleveland	100%	834
Doctors Hospital	Columbus	100%	168
Fairview Hospital	Cleveland	100%	275
Fort Hamilton Hughes Memorial Hospital	Hamilton	100%	144
Good Samaritan Hospital[2]	Dayton	100%	304
Grant Medical Center	Columbus	100%	331
Hillcrest Hospital	Mayfield Heights	100%	303
Jewish Hospital	Cincinnati	100%	179
Lake Health	Concord	100%	286
Licking Memorial Hospital	Newark	100%	149
Marymount Hospital	Garfield Heights	100%	25
Mercy Health - West Hospital	Cincinnati	100%	43
Mercy Saint Vincent Medical Center	Toledo	100%	625
Miami Valley Hospital[2]	Dayton	100%	292
Parma Community General Hospital	Parma	100%	281
Riverside Methodist Hospital[2]	Columbus	100%	288
Saint Elizabeth Boardman Health Center	Boardman	100%	28
Saint John Medical Center[2]	Westlake	100%	219
Southern Ohio Medical Center	Portsmouth	100%	283
University Hospitals Case Medical Center	Cleveland	100%	380
University of Toledo Medical Center[2]	Toledo	100%	201
Affinity Medical Center	Massillon	99%	102
Fairfield Medical Center	Lancaster	99%	281
Firelands Regional Medical Center	Sandusky	99%	130
Good Samaritan Hospital	Cincinnati	99%	247
Kettering Medical Center	Kettering	99%	446
Lima Memorial Health System	Lima	99%	268
Marion General Hospital	Marion	99%	193
Mercy Hospital Anderson	Cincinnati	99%	333
Mercy Hospital Fairfield	Fairfield	99%	374
Metrohealth System	Cleveland	99%	255
Mount Carmel West[2]	Columbus	99%	288
Northside Medical Center	Youngstown	99%	178
Ohio State University Hospitals[2]	Columbus	99%	271
Saint Luke's Hospital	Maumee	99%	302
Southwest General Health Center	Middleburg Hgts	99%	333
The Toledo Hospital[2]	Toledo	99%	299
Trinity Med Ctr East & West	Steubenville	99%	268
Trumbull Memorial Hospital	Warren	99%	163
UH Geauga Medical Center	Chardon	99%	111
Univ Hosps-Elyria Med Ctr[2]	Elyria	99%	355
Adena Regional Medical Center[2]	Chillicothe	98%	247
Akron General Medical Center[2]	Akron	98%	283
Bethesda North	Cincinnati	98%	368
Community Hospitals & Wellness Centers	Bryan	98%	97
Genesis Healthcare System	Zanesville	98%	415
Grandview Hospital & Medical Center	Dayton	98%	165
Marietta Memorial Hospital	Marietta	98%	146
Mercy Medical Center	Canton	98%	360
Saint Rita's Medical Center	Lima	98%	451
Saint Vincent Charity Medical Center	Cleveland	98%	43
Springfield Regional Medical Center	Springfield	98%	347
Summa Health Systems Hospitals[2]	Akron	98%	303
University Hospitals Ahuja Medical Center	Beachwood	98%	122
Upper Valley Medical Center	Troy	98%	49
Dayton VA Medical Center	Dayton	97%	29
Holzer Medical Center	Gallipolis	97%	180
Knox Community Hospital	Mount Vernon	97%	99
Mercy Regional Medical Center	Lorain	97%	301
Robinson Memorial Hospital	Ravenna	97%	36
Saint Elizabeth Health Center	Youngstown	97%	534
University of Cincinnati Medical Center	Cincinnati	97%	259
Mercy Saint Charles Hospital	Oregon	96%	28
Mount Carmel Saint Ann's	Westerville	96%	161
West Chester Hospital	West Chester	96%	206
Lakewood Hospital	Lakewood	95%	57
Summa Health System Barberton Hospital	Barberton	93%	115
East Ohio Regional Hospital	Martins Ferry	92%	39
UHHS Richmond Heights Hospital	Richmond Hghts	91%	47
Medcentral Health Sys Mansfield Hosp	Mansfield	90%	302
Saint Joseph Health Center	Warren	83%	29

Heart Failure Care

ACE Inhibitor or ARB for LVSD

Hospital Name	City	Rate	Cases
Adena Regional Medical Center[2]	Chillicothe	100%	74
Affinity Medical Center	Massillon	100%	56
Akron General Medical Center[2]	Akron	100%	98
Ashtabula County Medical Center	Ashtabula	100%	27
Atrium Medical Center	Franklin	100%	54
Aultman Hospital	Canton	100%	203
Blanchard Valley Hospital	Findlay	100%	61
Christ Hospital	Cincinnati	100%	320
Doctors Hospital	Columbus	100%	99
East Liverpool City Hospital	East Liverpool	100%	36
Firelands Regional Medical Center	Sandusky	100%	86
Flower Hospital	Sylvania	100%	26
Fort Hamilton Hughes Memorial Hospital	Hamilton	100%	58
Grant Medical Center	Columbus	100%	152
Greene Memorial Hospital	Xenia	100%	33
Hillcrest Hospital	Mayfield Heights	100%	96
Indu & Raj Soin Medical Center	Beaver Creek	100%	30
Knox Community Hospital	Mount Vernon	100%	27
Lakewood Hospital	Lakewood	100%	35
Lima Memorial Health System	Lima	100%	59
Marietta Memorial Hospital	Marietta	100%	62
Marion General Hospital	Marion	100%	61
Mercy Health - West Hospital	Cincinnati	100%	49
Mercy Hospital Anderson	Cincinnati	100%	113
Mercy Hospital Clermont	Batavia	100%	34
Mercy Medical Center	Canton	100%	135
Mercy Saint Vincent Medical Center	Toledo	100%	244
Metrohealth System	Cleveland	100%	255
Mount Carmel Saint Ann's[2]	Westerville	100%	78
Mount Carmel West[2]	Columbus	100%	93
Northside Medical Center	Youngstown	100%	81
Parma Community General Hospital	Parma	100%	150
Riverside Methodist Hospital[2]	Columbus	100%	87
Saint Vincent Charity Medical Center[2]	Cleveland	100%	87
South Pointe Hospital	Warrensville Hgts	100%	99
Summa Western Reserve Hospital	Cuyahoga Falls	100%	25
Sycamore Medical Center	Miamisburg	100%	52
UH Geauga Medical Center	Chardon	100%	41
UHHS Richmond Heights Hospital	Richmond Hghts	100%	62
Union Hospital	Dover	100%	48
University Hospitals Ahuja Medical Center	Beachwood	100%	77
University Hospitals Case Medical Center[2]	Cleveland	100%	98
University of Cincinnati Medical Center	Cincinnati	100%	259
Upper Valley Medical Center	Troy	100%	78
Wood County Hospital	Bowling Green	100%	31
Cleveland - Wade Park VA Medical Center	Cleveland	99%	134
Cleveland Clinic[2]	Cleveland	99%	287
Fairview Hospital[2]	Cleveland	99%	161
Good Samaritan Hospital	Cincinnati	99%	134
Good Samaritan Hospital[2]	Dayton	99%	75
Jewish Hospital[2]	Cincinnati	99%	77
Licking Memorial Hospital	Newark	99%	82
Mercy Hospital Fairfield	Fairfield	99%	190
Miami Valley Hospital[2]	Dayton	99%	85
Southwest General Health Center	Middleburg Hgts	99%	105
Dayton VA Medical Center	Dayton	98%	45
Euclid Hospital	Euclid	98%	41
Kettering Medical Center	Kettering	98%	191
Marymount Hospital	Garfield Heights	98%	124
Saint Elizabeth Health Center[2]	Youngstown	98%	82
Saint Joseph Health Center[2]	Warren	98%	56
Saint Luke's Hospital	Maumee	98%	94
Southern Ohio Medical Center	Portsmouth	98%	94
Chillicothe VA Medical Center	Chillicothe	97%	31
Fairfield Medical Center	Lancaster	97%	87
Lake Health	Concord	97%	136
Mercy Regional Medical Center	Lorain	97%	90
Saint John Medical Center[2]	Westlake	97%	62
Trinity Med Ctr East & West	Steubenville	97%	136
Clinton Memorial Hospital	Wilmington	96%	28
Mercy Saint Charles Hospital	Oregon	96%	51
University of Toledo Medical Center[2]	Toledo	96%	81
Bethesda North	Cincinnati	95%	159
Ohio State University Hospitals[2]	Columbus	95%	122
Saint Elizabeth Boardman Health Center[2]	Boardman	95%	55
Southeastern Ohio Regional Medical Center	Cambridge	95%	37
The Toledo Hospital[2]	Toledo	95%	76
West Chester Hospital	West Chester	95%	59
Holzer Medical Center[2]	Gallipolis	94%	53
Univ Hosps-Elyria Med Ctr[2]	Elyria	94%	102
Cincinnati VA Medical Center	Cincinnati	93%	97
Grandview Hospital & Medical Center	Dayton	93%	87
Trumbull Memorial Hospital	Warren	93%	107
Wooster Community Hospital	Wooster	93%	43
Community Hospitals & Wellness Centers	Bryan	92%	36
Robinson Memorial Hospital	Ravenna	92%	60
Saint Rita's Medical Center	Lima	92%	140
Alliance Community Hospital	Alliance	91%	33
Genesis Healthcare System	Zanesville	91%	107
Medcentral Health Sys Mansfield Hosp	Mansfield	91%	90
Medina Hospital	Medina	91%	35
Summa Health Systems Hospitals[2]	Akron	91%	98
Fisher - Titus Hospital	Norwalk	90%	39
Mercy Saint Anne Hospital	Toledo	90%	51
Springfield Regional Medical Center	Springfield	89%	174
Summa Health System Barberton Hospital	Barberton	87%	91
East Ohio Regional Hospital	Martins Ferry	83%	29
Lutheran Hospital	Cleveland	78%	27

Discharge Instructions Given

Hospital Name	City	Rate	Cases
Barnesville Hospital Association	Barnesville	100%	38
Berger Hospital	Circleville	100%	57
Bethesda North	Cincinnati	100%	483
Blanchard Valley Hospital	Findlay	100%	101
Cincinnati VA Medical Center	Cincinnati	100%	165
Cleveland - Wade Park VA Medical Center	Cleveland	100%	350
Community Hospitals & Wellness Centers	Bryan	100%	73
Doctors Hospital	Columbus	100%	224
Dublin Methodist Hospital	Dublin	100%	57
Euclid Hospital	Euclid	100%	134
Fairview Hospital[2]	Cleveland	100%	425
Firelands Regional Medical Center	Sandusky	100%	201
Fort Hamilton Hughes Memorial Hospital	Hamilton	100%	162
Genesis Healthcare System	Zanesville	100%	328
Grady Memorial Hospital	Delaware	100%	64
Grant Medical Center	Columbus	100%	372
Hillcrest Hospital	Mayfield Heights	100%	375
Kettering Medical Center	Kettering	100%	412
Mary Rutan Hospital	Bellefontaine	100%	40
Marymount Hospital	Garfield Heights	100%	332
Mercy Hospital Clermont	Batavia	100%	148
Mercy Hospital Fairfield	Fairfield	100%	493
Mercy Memorial Hospital	Urbana	100%	35
Mercy Saint Vincent Medical Center	Toledo	100%	421
Mercy Tiffin Hospital	Tiffin	100%	43
Ohio State University Hospitals[2]	Columbus	100%	245
Parma Community General Hospital	Parma	100%	364
Pomerene Hospital	Millersburg	100%	30
Riverside Methodist Hospital[2]	Columbus	100%	239
Saint Elizabeth Boardman Health Center[2]	Boardman	100%	221
Saint Elizabeth Health Center[2]	Youngstown	100%	229
Saint Joseph Health Center[2]	Warren	100%	212
Salem Regional Medical Center	Salem	100%	89
Summa Wadsworth - Rittman Hospital	Wadsworth	100%	66
Summa Western Reserve Hospital	Cuyahoga Falls	100%	76
UH Geauga Medical Center	Chardon	100%	161
UHHS Memorial Hospital of Geneva	Geneva	100%	50
Union Hospital	Dover	100%	203
Wood County Hospital	Bowling Green	100%	70
Adena Regional Medical Center[2]	Chillicothe	99%	235
Atrium Medical Center	Franklin	99%	211
Chillicothe VA Medical Center	Chillicothe	99%	98
East Ohio Regional Hospital	Martins Ferry	99%	94
Good Samaritan Hospital	Cincinnati	99%	380
Greene Memorial Hospital	Xenia	99%	113

NOTE: Hospital profiles are in alphabetical order by state, then city, then hospital within the city; Rankings exclude hospitals with less than 25 cases except for patient surveys which excludes hospitals with less than 100 cases; (a) 100-299 cases; (1) The number of cases/patients is too few to report; (2) Data submitted were based on a sample of cases/patients; (3) Results are based on a shorter time period than required; (4) Data suppressed by CMS for one or more quarters; (5) Results are not available for this reporting period; (6) Fewer than 100 patients completed the HCAHPS survey; (7) No cases met the criteria for this measure; (8) The lower limit of the confidence interval cannot be calculated if the number of observed infections equals zero; (9) No data are available from the state/territory for this reporting period; (10) The scores shown reflect fewer than 50 completed surveys; (11) There were discrepancies in the data collection process; (12) This measure does not apply to this hospital for this reporting period; (13) Results cannot be calculated for this reporting period; (14) The results for this state are combined with nearby states to protect confidentiality; Please refer to the User's Guide for a full explanation of data.

Indu & Raj Soin Medical Center	Beaver Creek	99%	82
McCullough - Hyde Memorial Hospital	Oxford	99%	91
Mercy Saint Anne Hospital	Toledo	99%	137
Mercy Saint Charles Hospital	Oregon	99%	141
Robinson Memorial Hospital	Ravenna	99%	209
Saint Rita's Medical Center	Lima	99%	333
South Pointe Hospital	Warrensville Hgts	99%	259
Summa Health System Barberton Hospital	Barberton	99%	254
Sycamore Medical Center	Miamisburg	99%	143
Ashtabula County Medical Center	Ashtabula	98%	128
Christ Hospital	Cincinnati	98%	782
Flower Hospital	Sylvania	98%	125
Licking Memorial Hospital	Newark	98%	187
Memorial Hospital of Union County	Marysville	98%	51
Miami Valley Hospital[2]	Dayton	98%	231
Mount Carmel West[2]	Columbus	98%	247
Northside Medical Center	Youngstown	98%	213
Saint Luke's Hospital	Maumee	98%	223
UHHS Richmond Heights Hospital	Richmond Hghts	98%	216
Aultman Hospital	Canton	97%	508
Fayette County Memorial Hospital	Washington Ch	97%	29
Highland District Hospital	Hillsboro	97%	39
Lake Health	Concord	97%	449
Lima Memorial Health System	Lima	97%	174
Lutheran Hospital	Cleveland	97%	93
Marion General Hospital	Marion	97%	182
Medcentral Health Sys Mansfield Hosp	Mansfield	97%	220
Mercy Hospital of Defiance	Defiance	97%	31
Metrohealth System	Cleveland	97%	634
Mount Carmel Saint Ann's[2]	Westerville	97%	196
Saint Vincent Charity Medical Center[2]	Cleveland	97%	193
Samaritan Regional Health System	Ashland	97%	33
Southern Ohio Medical Center	Portsmouth	97%	278
Southwest General Health Center	Middleburg Hgts	97%	319
Trinity Med Ctr East & West	Steubenville	97%	327
University Hospitals Case Medical Center[2]	Cleveland	97%	244
Upper Valley Medical Center	Troy	97%	178
Good Samaritan Hospital[2]	Dayton	96%	238
Grand Lake Health System	Saint Marys	96%	53
Grandview Hospital & Medical Center	Dayton	96%	322
Marietta Memorial Hospital	Marietta	96%	189
Medina Hospital	Medina	96%	124
Mercy Health - West Hospital	Cincinnati	96%	138
Mercy Hospital Anderson	Cincinnati	96%	331
Wilson Memorial Hospital	Sidney	96%	54
Mercy Regional Medical Center	Lorain	95%	318
Summa Health Systems Hospitals[2]	Akron	95%	263
Cleveland Clinic[2]	Cleveland	94%	712
Fisher - Titus Hospital	Norwalk	94%	84
Knox Community Hospital	Mount Vernon	94%	87
Lakewood Hospital	Lakewood	94%	119
Southwest Regional Medical Center	Georgetown	94%	31
Univ Hosps-Elyria Med Ctr[2]	Elyria	94%	252
Wayne Hospital	Greenville	94%	65
Akron General Medical Center[2]	Akron	93%	259
Memorial Hospital	Fremont	93%	58
Mercer County Joint Twp Comm Hosp	Coldwater	93%	28
Mercy Medical Center	Canton	93%	344
University of Toledo Medical Center[2]	Toledo	93%	224
Wooster Community Hospital	Wooster	93%	120
University Hospitals Ahuja Medical Center	Beachwood	92%	235
Bellevue Hospital	Bellevue	91%	35
O'Bleness Memorial Hospital	Athens	91%	35
Clinton Memorial Hospital	Wilmington	90%	93
Dayton VA Medical Center	Dayton	90%	124
Fairfield Medical Center	Lancaster	89%	310
University of Cincinnati Medical Center	Cincinnati	89%	473
Jewish Hospital[2]	Cincinnati	88%	222
East Liverpool City Hospital	East Liverpool	87%	94
Saint John Medical Center[2]	Westlake	87%	190
Springfield Regional Medical Center	Springfield	87%	398
West Chester Hospital	West Chester	86%	186
Affinity Medical Center	Massillon	85%	134
Bay Park Community Hospital	Oregon	83%	77
H B Magruder Memorial Hospital	Port Clinton	83%	29
Trumbull Memorial Hospital	Warren	83%	358
The Toledo Hospital[2]	Toledo	81%	214
Southeastern Ohio Regional Medical Center	Cambridge	78%	100
Alliance Community Hospital	Alliance	75%	69
Coshocton County Memorial Hospital	Coshocton	75%	63
Holzer Medical Center[2]	Gallipolis	73%	160
Holzer Medical Center Jackson	Jackson	70%	33
Madison County Hospital	London	54%	35

Evaluation of LVS Function

Hospital Name	City	Rate	Cases
Adams County Regional Medical Center	Seaman	100%	26
Adena Regional Medical Center[2]	Chillicothe	100%	286
Affinity Medical Center	Massillon	100%	185
Akron General Medical Center[2]	Akron	100%	301
Ashtabula County Medical Center	Ashtabula	100%	187
Atrium Medical Center	Franklin	100%	261
Aultman Hospital	Canton	100%	679
Bay Park Community Hospital	Oregon	100%	111
Bellevue Hospital	Bellevue	100%	42
Berger Hospital	Circleville	100%	74
Bethesda North	Cincinnati	100%	608
Blanchard Valley Hospital	Findlay	100%	138
Chillicothe VA Medical Center	Chillicothe	100%	109
Christ Hospital	Cincinnati	100%	943
Cincinnati VA Medical Center	Cincinnati	100%	185
Cleveland - Wade Park VA Medical Center	Cleveland	100%	392
Cleveland Clinic[2]	Cleveland	100%	858
Community Hospitals & Wellness Centers	Bryan	100%	91
Dayton VA Medical Center	Dayton	100%	141
Doctors Hospital	Columbus	100%	267
Dublin Methodist Hospital	Dublin	100%	66
East Liverpool City Hospital	East Liverpool	100%	128
Euclid Hospital	Euclid	100%	220
Fairview Hospital[2]	Cleveland	100%	564
Firelands Regional Medical Center	Sandusky	100%	257
Fisher - Titus Hospital	Norwalk	100%	113
Flower Hospital	Sylvania	100%	184
Fort Hamilton Hughes Memorial Hospital	Hamilton	100%	233
Fostoria Community Hospital	Fostoria	100%	29
Genesis Healthcare System	Zanesville	100%	410
Good Samaritan Hospital	Cincinnati	100%	481
Good Samaritan Hospital[2]	Dayton	100%	305
Grady Memorial Hospital	Delaware	100%	81
Grand Lake Health System	Saint Marys	100%	89
Grandview Hospital & Medical Center	Dayton	100%	393
Grant Medical Center	Columbus	100%	460
Greene Memorial Hospital	Xenia	100%	137
H B Magruder Memorial Hospital	Port Clinton	100%	42
Hillcrest Hospital	Mayfield Heights	100%	513
Holzer Medical Center[2]	Gallipolis	100%	193
Holzer Medical Center Jackson	Jackson	100%	38
Indu & Raj Soin Medical Center	Beaver Creek	100%	113
Jewish Hospital[2]	Cincinnati	100%	304
Kettering Medical Center	Kettering	100%	533
Lake Health	Concord	100%	617
Lakewood Hospital	Lakewood	100%	199
Licking Memorial Hospital	Newark	100%	240
Lima Memorial Health System	Lima	100%	225
Marietta Memorial Hospital	Marietta	100%	252
Marion General Hospital	Marion	100%	231
Mary Rutan Hospital	Bellefontaine	100%	57
Marymount Hospital	Garfield Heights	100%	472
McCullough - Hyde Memorial Hospital	Oxford	100%	109
Medina Hospital	Medina	100%	187
Memorial Hospital of Union County	Marysville	100%	70
Mercer County Joint Twp Comm Hosp	Coldwater	100%	41
Mercy Health - West Hospital	Cincinnati	100%	171
Mercy Hospital Anderson	Cincinnati	100%	424
Mercy Hospital Clermont	Batavia	100%	183
Mercy Hospital Fairfield	Fairfield	100%	604
Mercy Hospital of Defiance	Defiance	100%	47
Mercy Medical Center	Canton	100%	452
Mercy Memorial Hospital	Urbana	100%	46
Mercy Saint Anne Hospital	Toledo	100%	181
Mercy Saint Charles Hospital	Oregon	100%	203
Mercy Saint Vincent Medical Center	Toledo	100%	522
Mercy Tiffin Hospital	Tiffin	100%	61
Metrohealth System	Cleveland	100%	701
Miami Valley Hospital[2]	Dayton	100%	287
Mount Carmel Saint Ann's[2]	Westerville	100%	265
Mount Carmel West[2]	Columbus	100%	312
Northside Medical Center	Youngstown	100%	291
O'Bleness Memorial Hospital	Athens	100%	46
Ohio State University Hospitals[2]	Columbus	100%	278
Parma Community General Hospital	Parma	100%	495
Pomerene Hospital	Millersburg	100%	36
Riverside Methodist Hospital[2]	Columbus	100%	306
Saint Elizabeth Boardman Health Center[2]	Boardman	100%	288
Saint Elizabeth Health Center[2]	Youngstown	100%	293
Saint Joseph Health Center[2]	Warren	100%	291
Saint Luke's Hospital	Maumee	100%	271
Saint Rita's Medical Center	Lima	100%	443
Saint Vincent Charity Medical Center[2]	Cleveland	100%	235
Samaritan Regional Health System	Ashland	100%	46
South Pointe Hospital	Warrensville Hgts	100%	327
Southeastern Ohio Regional Medical Center	Cambridge	100%	119
Southern Ohio Medical Center	Portsmouth	100%	349
Southwest General Health Center	Middleburg Hgts	100%	433
Summa Health System Barberton Hospital	Barberton	100%	331
Summa Wadsworth - Rittman Hospital	Wadsworth	100%	89
Sycamore Medical Center	Miamisburg	100%	189
The Toledo Hospital[2]	Toledo	100%	289
Trinity Med Ctr East & West	Steubenville	100%	491
Trumbull Memorial Hospital	Warren	100%	446
UH Geauga Medical Center	Chardon	100%	216
UHHS Memorial Hospital of Geneva	Geneva	100%	81
UHHS Richmond Heights Hospital	Richmond Hghts	100%	298
Union Hospital	Dover	100%	277
Univ Hosps-Elyria Med Ctr[2]	Elyria	100%	326
University Hospitals Ahuja Medical Center	Beachwood	100%	310
University Hospitals Case Medical Center[2]	Cleveland	100%	318
Univ Hosps Conneaut Med Ctr	Conneaut	100%	30
University of Cincinnati Medical Center	Cincinnati	100%	554
University of Toledo Medical Center[2]	Toledo	100%	281
Upper Valley Medical Center	Troy	100%	229
Wood County Hospital	Bowling Green	100%	86
East Ohio Regional Hospital	Martins Ferry	99%	144
Fairfield Medical Center	Lancaster	99%	377
Lutheran Hospital	Cleveland	99%	116
Memorial Hospital	Fremont	99%	77
Mercy Regional Medical Center	Lorain	99%	423
Robinson Memorial Hospital	Ravenna	99%	268
Saint John Medical Center[2]	Westlake	99%	268
Salem Regional Medical Center	Salem	99%	124
Summa Health Systems Hospitals[2]	Akron	99%	311
Summa Western Reserve Hospital	Cuyahoga Falls	99%	90
Wayne Hospital	Greenville	99%	86
West Chester Hospital	West Chester	99%	256
Wilson Memorial Hospital	Sidney	99%	72
Wooster Community Hospital	Wooster	99%	155
Clinton Memorial Hospital	Wilmington	98%	112
Fayette County Memorial Hospital	Washington Ch	98%	41
Medcentral Health Sys Mansfield Hosp	Mansfield	98%	289
Southwest Regional Medical Center	Georgetown	98%	65
Springfield Regional Medical Center	Springfield	98%	504
Alliance Community Hospital	Alliance	97%	101
Highland District Hospital	Hillsboro	97%	59
Knox Community Hospital	Mount Vernon	97%	111
Barnesville Hospital Association	Barnesville	96%	50
Morrow County Hospital	Mount Gilead	91%	33
Madison County Hospital	London	88%	43
Coshocton County Memorial Hospital	Coshocton	73%	84

Medicare Spending

Medicare Spending per Patient (ratio)

Hospital Name	City	Ratio	Cases
Glenbeigh	Rock Creek	0.85	-
Mercy Tiffin Hospital	Tiffin	0.87	-
Mount Carmel New Albany Surgical Hospital	New Albany	0.91	-
Grand Lake Health System	Saint Marys	0.93	-
Institute For Orthopaedic Surgery	Lima	0.93	-
Licking Memorial Hospital	Newark	0.93	-
Clinton Memorial Hospital	Wilmington	0.94	-
Crystal Clinic Orthopaedic Center	Akron	0.94	-
Genesis Healthcare System	Zanesville	0.94	-
Samaritan Regional Health System	Ashland	0.94	-
Mercy Hospital Clermont	Batavia	0.95	-
Wooster Community Hospital	Wooster	0.95	-
Jewish Hospital	Cincinnati	0.96	-
McCullough - Hyde Memorial Hospital	Oxford	0.96	-
Mercy Hospital Anderson	Cincinnati	0.96	-
Van Wert County Hospital	Van Wert	0.96	-
Blanchard Valley Hospital	Findlay	0.97	-
Greene Memorial Hospital	Xenia	0.97	-
Robinson Memorial Hospital	Ravenna	0.97	-
Saint Luke's Hospital	Maumee	0.97	-
East Liverpool City Hospital	East Liverpool	0.98	-
Good Samaritan Hospital	Cincinnati	0.98	-
Grandview Hospital & Medical Center	Dayton	0.98	-
Grant Medical Center	Columbus	0.98	-
Marion General Hospital	Marion	0.98	-
Metrohealth System	Cleveland	0.98	-
Summa Health System Barberton Hospital	Barberton	0.98	-
Sycamore Medical Center	Miamisburg	0.98	-
Ashtabula County Medical Center	Ashtabula	0.99	-
Cleveland Clinic	Cleveland	0.99	-
Grady Memorial Hospital	Delaware	0.99	-
Indu & Raj Soin Medical Center	Beaver Creek	0.99	-
Memorial Hospital of Union County	Marysville	0.99	-
Mercy Hospital Fairfield	Fairfield	0.99	-
Ohio Valley Medical Center	Springfield	0.99	-
Southeastern Ohio Regional Medical Center	Cambridge	0.99	-
Southwest Regional Medical Center	Georgetown	0.99	-
Fisher - Titus Hospital	Norwalk	1.00	-
Lima Memorial Health System	Lima	1.00	-
Memorial Hospital	Fremont	1.00	-
O'Bleness Memorial Hospital	Athens	1.00	-
Riverside Methodist Hospital	Columbus	1.00	-
Saint Rita's Medical Center	Lima	1.00	-
Surgical Hospital at Southwoods	Youngstown	1.00	-
The Toledo Hospital	Toledo	1.00	-
UH Geauga Medical Center	Chardon	1.00	-
University Hospitals Ahuja Medical Center	Beachwood	1.00	-
University Hospitals Case Medical Center	Cleveland	1.00	-
University of Cincinnati Medical Center	Cincinnati	1.00	-

NOTE: Hospital profiles are in alphabetical order by state, then city, then hospital within the city; Rankings exclude hospitals with less than 25 cases except for patient surveys which excludes hospitals with less than 100 cases; (a) 100-299 cases; (1) The number of cases/patients is too few to report; (2) Data submitted were based on a sample of cases/patients; (3) Results are based on a shorter time period than required; (4) Data suppressed by CMS for one or more quarters; (5) Results are not available for this reporting period; (6) Fewer than 100 patients completed the HCAHPS survey; (7) No cases met the criteria for this measure; (8) The lower limit of the confidence interval cannot be calculated if the number of observed infections equals zero; (9) No data are available from the state/territory for this reporting period; (10) The scores shown reflect fewer than 50 completed surveys; (11) There were discrepancies in the data collection process; (12) This measure does not apply to this hospital for this reporting period; (13) Results cannot be calculated for this reporting period; (14) The results for this state are combined with nearby states to protect confidentiality; Please refer to the User's Guide for a full explanation of data.

Wood County Hospital	Bowling Green	1.00	-
Adena Regional Medical Center	Chillicothe	1.01	-
Bellevue Hospital	Bellevue	1.01	-
Belmont Community Hospital	Bellaire	1.01	-
Christ Hospital	Cincinnati	1.01	-
Coshocton County Memorial Hospital	Coshocton	1.01	-
Doctors Hospital	Columbus	1.01	-
Dublin Methodist Hospital	Dublin	1.01	-
Fairfield Medical Center	Lancaster	1.01	-
Fort Hamilton Hughes Memorial Hospital	Hamilton	1.01	-
Lutheran Hospital	Cleveland	1.01	-
Madison County Hospital	London	1.01	-
Mercy Health - West Hospital	Cincinnati	1.01	-
Mount Carmel West	Columbus	1.01	-
Northside Medical Center	Youngstown	1.01	-
Ohio State University Hospitals	Columbus	1.01	-
Saint Vincent Charity Medical Center	Cleveland	1.01	-
Summa Western Reserve Hospital	Cuyahoga Falls	1.01	-
Wayne Hospital	Greenville	1.01	-
West Chester Hospital	West Chester	1.01	-
Atrium Medical Center	Franklin	1.02	-
Aultman Hospital	Canton	1.02	-
Bay Park Community Hospital	Oregon	1.02	-
Berger Hospital	Circleville	1.02	-
Bethesda North	Cincinnati	1.02	-
Hillcrest Hospital	Mayfield Heights	1.02	-
Kettering Medical Center	Kettering	1.02	-
Mary Rutan Hospital	Bellefontaine	1.02	-
Mount Carmel Saint Ann's	Westerville	1.02	-
Pomerene Hospital	Millersburg	1.02	-
Saint John Medical Center	Westlake	1.02	-
Summa Health Systems Hospitals	Akron	1.02	-
Trumbull Memorial Hospital	Warren	1.02	-
Union Hospital	Dover	1.02	-
Fairview Hospital	Cleveland	1.03	-
Knox Community Hospital	Mount Vernon	1.03	-
Lake Health	Concord	1.03	-
Marietta Memorial Hospital	Marietta	1.03	-
Mercy Saint Charles Hospital	Oregon	1.03	-
Mercy Saint Vincent Medical Center	Toledo	1.03	-
Miami Valley Hospital	Dayton	1.03	-
Salem Regional Medical Center	Salem	1.03	-
Univ Hosps-Elyria Med Ctr	Elyria	1.03	-
Upper Valley Medical Center	Troy	1.03	-
Affinity Medical Center	Massillon	1.04	-
Good Samaritan Hospital	Dayton	1.04	-
Medina Hospital	Medina	1.04	-
Mercy Hospital of Defiance	Defiance	1.04	-
Mercy Saint Anne Hospital	Toledo	1.04	-
Southwest General Health Center	Middleburg Hgts	1.04	-
University of Toledo Medical Center	Toledo	1.04	-
Akron General Medical Center	Akron	1.05	-
Firelands Regional Medical Center	Sandusky	1.05	-
Southern Ohio Medical Center	Portsmouth	1.05	-
East Ohio Regional Hospital	Martins Ferry	1.06	-
Flower Hospital	Sylvania	1.06	-
Medcentral Health Sys Mansfield Hosp	Mansfield	1.06	-
Saint Elizabeth Boardman Health Center	Boardman	1.06	-
Saint Elizabeth Health Center	Youngstown	1.06	-
Saint Joseph Health Center	Warren	1.06	-
Springfield Regional Medical Center	Springfield	1.06	-
Summa Wadsworth - Rittman Hospital	Wadsworth	1.06	-
Alliance Community Hospital	Alliance	1.07	-
Holzer Medical Center	Gallipolis	1.07	-
Marymount Hospital	Garfield Heights	1.07	-
South Pointe Hospital	Warrensville Hgts	1.07	-
UHHS Richmond Heights Hospital	Richmond Hghts	1.07	-
Lakewood Hospital	Lakewood	1.08	-
Mercy Medical Center	Canton	1.08	-
Mercy Regional Medical Center	Lorain	1.09	-
Euclid Hospital	Euclid	1.10	-
Mercer County Joint Twp Comm Hosp	Coldwater	1.10	-
Parma Community General Hospital	Parma	1.11	-
Community Hospitals & Wellness Centers	Bryan	1.12	-
Wilson Memorial Hospital	Sidney	1.13	-
Medical Center at Elizabeth Place	Dayton	1.16	-
Trinity Med Ctr East & West	Steubenville	1.17	-

Pneumonia Care

Appropriate Initial Antibiotic Given

Hospital Name	City	Rate	Cases
Adena Regional Medical Center[2]	Chillicothe	100%	113
Ashtabula County Medical Center	Ashtabula	100%	69
Atrium Medical Center[2]	Franklin	100%	75
Berger Hospital	Circleville	100%	65
Bucyrus Community Hospital	Bucyrus	100%	34
Christ Hospital[2]	Cincinnati	100%	53
Cincinnati VA Medical Center	Cincinnati	100%	61
Fayette County Memorial Hospital	Washington Ch	100%	44
Firelands Regional Medical Center	Sandusky	100%	107
Fostoria Community Hospital	Fostoria	100%	38
Greene Memorial Hospital	Xenia	100%	93
Hardin Memorial Hospital	Kenton	100%	38
Mary Rutan Hospital	Bellefontaine	100%	51
Mercy Hospital Fairfield	Fairfield	100%	211
Mercy Hospital of Defiance	Defiance	100%	45
Mercy Memorial Hospital	Urbana	100%	28
O'Bleness Memorial Hospital	Athens	100%	122
Ohio State University Hospitals[2]	Columbus	100%	37
Pomerene Hospital	Millersburg	100%	58
Saint Vincent Charity Medical Center[2]	Cleveland	100%	66
Samaritan Regional Health System	Ashland	100%	61
South Pointe Hospital	Warrensville Hgts	100%	108
Sycamore Medical Center	Miamisburg	100%	125
UH Geauga Medical Center	Chardon	100%	95
UHHS Memorial Hospital of Geneva	Geneva	100%	66
Union Hospital	Dover	100%	125
University Hospitals Ahuja Medical Center[2]	Beachwood	100%	77
Univ Hosps Conneaut Med Ctr	Conneaut	100%	26
Aultman Hospital	Canton	99%	410
Doctors Hospital	Columbus	99%	122
Good Samaritan Hospital[2]	Cincinnati	99%	99
Grant Medical Center[2]	Columbus	99%	88
Indu & Raj Soin Medical Center	Beaver Creek	99%	111
Lakewood Hospital	Lakewood	99%	82
Marietta Memorial Hospital[2]	Marietta	99%	82
Marymount Hospital	Garfield Heights	99%	180
Mercer County Joint Twp Comm Hosp	Coldwater	99%	77
Mercy Saint Vincent Medical Center	Toledo	99%	88
Mount Carmel West[2]	Columbus	99%	138
Saint John Medical Center[2]	Westlake	99%	77
Southeastern Ohio Regional Medical Center[2]	Cambridge	99%	86
Summa Health Systems Hospitals[2]	Akron	99%	89
University of Cincinnati Medical Center	Cincinnati	99%	136
Upper Valley Medical Center[2]	Troy	99%	106
Alliance Community Hospital[2]	Alliance	98%	89
Bethesda North[2]	Cincinnati	98%	127
Defiance Regional Medical Center	Defiance	98%	41
Euclid Hospital	Euclid	98%	82
Fisher - Titus Hospital	Norwalk	98%	106
Flower Hospital	Sylvania	98%	125
Genesis Healthcare System	Zanesville	98%	260
Grady Memorial Hospital	Delaware	98%	60
Grand Lake Health System	Saint Marys	98%	52
H B Magruder Memorial Hospital	Port Clinton	98%	40
Jewish Hospital[2]	Cincinnati	98%	96
Kettering Medical Center	Kettering	98%	193
Lake Health	Concord	98%	264
Licking Memorial Hospital[2]	Newark	98%	104
Marion General Hospital	Marion	98%	123
McCullough - Hyde Memorial Hospital	Oxford	98%	53
Mercy Hospital Clermont[2]	Batavia	98%	65
Mercy Saint Charles Hospital	Oregon	98%	96
Metrohealth System	Cleveland	98%	134
Northside Medical Center	Youngstown	98%	114
Riverside Methodist Hospital[2]	Columbus	98%	56
Saint Elizabeth Health Center[2]	Youngstown	98%	40
Summa Wadsworth - Rittman Hospital	Wadsworth	98%	120
Trumbull Memorial Hospital	Warren	98%	177
Van Wert County Hospital	Van Wert	98%	53
Wayne Hospital	Greenville	98%	54
Wood County Hospital	Bowling Green	98%	62
Wooster Community Hospital	Wooster	98%	122
Akron General Medical Center[2]	Akron	97%	68
Barnesville Hospital Association	Barnesville	97%	38
Clinton Memorial Hospital	Wilmington	97%	74
East Liverpool City Hospital	East Liverpool	97%	88
Fort Hamilton Hughes Memorial Hospital[2]	Hamilton	97%	71
Galion Community Hospital[2]	Galion	97%	67
Good Samaritan Hospital[2]	Dayton	97%	60
Grandview Hospital & Medical Center	Dayton	97%	155
Hillcrest Hospital	Mayfield Heights	97%	183
Lutheran Hospital	Cleveland	97%	37
Mercy Hospital Anderson	Cincinnati	97%	288
Mercy Regional Medical Center	Lorain	97%	208
Miami Valley Hospital[2]	Dayton	97%	74
Robinson Memorial Hospital[2]	Ravenna	97%	139
Southwest General Health Center	Middleburg Hgts	97%	227
Summa Health System Barberton Hospital	Barberton	97%	155
West Chester Hospital	West Chester	97%	146
Affinity Medical Center	Massillon	96%	114
Blanchard Valley Hospital	Findlay	96%	108
Fairview Hospital[2]	Cleveland	96%	167
Lima Memorial Health System	Lima	96%	107
Mercy Saint Anne Hospital	Toledo	96%	119
Mount Carmel Saint Ann's[2]	Westerville	96%	100
Saint Joseph Health Center[2]	Warren	96%	55
Saint Rita's Medical Center	Lima	96%	207
Salem Regional Medical Center	Salem	96%	140
Southern Ohio Medical Center	Portsmouth	96%	344
Springfield Regional Medical Center	Springfield	96%	310
Summa Western Reserve Hospital	Cuyahoga Falls	96%	96
UHHS Richmond Heights Hospital	Richmond Hghts	96%	113
Dublin Methodist Hospital	Dublin	95%	55
Holzer Medical Center Jackson	Jackson	95%	83
Memorial Hospital of Union County	Marysville	95%	44
Mercy Medical Center	Canton	95%	256
Cleveland Clinic	Cleveland	94%	84
Coshocton County Memorial Hospital	Coshocton	94%	62
Mercy Health - West Hospital	Cincinnati	94%	106
Mercy Tiffin Hospital	Tiffin	94%	70
Parma Community General Hospital	Parma	94%	268
Trinity Med Ctr East & West	Steubenville	94%	217
Univ Hosps-Elyria Med Ctr[2]	Elyria	94%	83
Bay Park Community Hospital	Oregon	93%	76
Cleveland - Wade Park VA Medical Center	Cleveland	93%	41
Community Hospitals & Wellness Centers	Bryan	93%	54
Fairfield Medical Center[2]	Lancaster	93%	87
Knox Community Hospital	Mount Vernon	93%	87
Medina Hospital	Medina	93%	121
Aultman Orrville Hospital	Orrville	92%	37
Chillicothe VA Medical Center	Chillicothe	92%	65
Southwest Regional Medical Center	Georgetown	92%	25
The Toledo Hospital[2]	Toledo	92%	63
University Hospitals Case Medical Center[2]	Cleveland	92%	51
Wilson Memorial Hospital	Sidney	92%	65
Adams County Regional Medical Center	Seaman	91%	56
Dayton VA Medical Center	Dayton	91%	47
Holzer Medical Center[2]	Gallipolis	91%	87
Saint Luke's Hospital[2]	Maumee	91%	89
Saint Elizabeth Boardman Health Center[2]	Boardman	90%	58
Medcentral Health Sys Mansfield Hosp	Mansfield	89%	189
East Ohio Regional Hospital	Martins Ferry	88%	126
Fulton County Health Center	Wauseon	88%	34
Hocking Valley Community Hospital	Logan	88%	43
Memorial Hospital	Fremont	88%	52
Mercy Willard Hospital	Willard	88%	32
Madison County Hospital	London	87%	55
Highland District Hospital[2]	Hillsboro	86%	72
Bellevue Hospital	Bellevue	85%	52
Belmont Community Hospital	Bellaire	85%	33
Mercy Allen Hospital	Oberlin	85%	33
Community Memorial Hospital	Hicksville	84%	25
Morrow County Hospital	Mount Gilead	84%	31
University of Toledo Medical Center[2]	Toledo	82%	38
Wyandot Memorial Hospital	Upper Sandusky	82%	28

Blood Culture Timing

Hospital Name	City	Rate	Cases
Ashtabula County Medical Center	Ashtabula	100%	145
Bay Park Community Hospital	Oregon	100%	123
Bucyrus Community Hospital	Bucyrus	100%	56
Coshocton County Memorial Hospital	Coshocton	100%	87
Defiance Regional Medical Center	Defiance	100%	57
Doctors Hospital	Columbus	100%	189
Fairfield Medical Center[2]	Lancaster	100%	184
Fostoria Community Hospital	Fostoria	100%	43
Genesis Healthcare System	Zanesville	100%	361
Grant Medical Center[2]	Columbus	100%	107
Greene Memorial Hospital	Xenia	100%	131
Hardin Memorial Hospital	Kenton	100%	45
Henry County Hospital	Napoleon	100%	28
Highland District Hospital[2]	Hillsboro	100%	92
Hillcrest Hospital	Mayfield Heights	100%	98
Indu & Raj Soin Medical Center	Beaver Creek	100%	169
Kettering Medical Center	Kettering	100%	433
Licking Memorial Hospital[2]	Newark	100%	122
Marion General Hospital	Marion	100%	214
Marymount Hospital	Garfield Heights	100%	255
Memorial Hospital	Fremont	100%	77
Mercy Health - West Hospital	Cincinnati	100%	177
Mercy Hospital of Defiance	Defiance	100%	71
Mercy Regional Medical Center	Lorain	100%	436
Miami Valley Hospital[2]	Dayton	100%	180
Pomerene Hospital	Millersburg	100%	100
Saint John Medical Center[2]	Westlake	100%	169
Southern Ohio Medical Center	Portsmouth	100%	553
Sycamore Medical Center	Miamisburg	100%	232
UH Geauga Medical Center	Chardon	100%	188
UHHS Memorial Hospital of Geneva	Geneva	100%	135
Adena Regional Medical Center[2]	Chillicothe	99%	167
Affinity Medical Center	Massillon	99%	219
Akron General Medical Center[2]	Akron	99%	150
Atrium Medical Center[2]	Franklin	99%	149
Berger Hospital	Circleville	99%	111
Bethesda North[2]	Cincinnati	99%	303
Chillicothe VA Medical Center	Chillicothe	99%	73
Dayton VA Medical Center	Dayton	99%	93
Fayette County Memorial Hospital	Washington Ch	99%	67
Firelands Regional Medical Center	Sandusky	99%	177
Flower Hospital	Sylvania	99%	192

NOTE: Hospital profiles are in alphabetical order by state, then city, then hospital within the city; Rankings exclude hospitals with less than 25 cases except for patient surveys which excludes hospitals with less than 100 cases; (a) 100-299 cases; (1) The number of cases/patients is too few to report; (2) Data submitted were based on a sample of cases/patients; (3) Results are based on a shorter time period than required; (4) Data suppressed by CMS for one or more quarters; (5) Results are not available for this reporting period; (6) Fewer than 100 patients completed the HCAHPS survey; (7) No cases met the criteria for this measure; (8) The lower limit of the confidence interval cannot be calculated if the number of observed infections equals zero; (9) No data are available from the state/territory for this reporting period; (10) The scores shown reflect fewer than 50 completed surveys; (11) There were discrepancies in the data collection process; (12) This measure does not apply to this hospital for this reporting period; (13) Results cannot be calculated for this reporting period; (14) The results for this state are combined with nearby states to protect confidentiality; Please refer to the User's Guide for a full explanation of data.

Fort Hamilton Hughes Memorial Hospital[2]	Hamilton	99%	118
Good Samaritan Hospital[2]	Cincinnati	99%	181
Grandview Hospital & Medical Center	Dayton	99%	240
Holzer Medical Center Jackson	Jackson	99%	97
Jewish Hospital[2]	Cincinnati	99%	149
Marietta Memorial Hospital[2]	Marietta	99%	142
Mary Rutan Hospital	Bellefontaine	99%	85
Memorial Hospital of Union County	Marysville	99%	72
Mercy Hospital Anderson	Cincinnati	99%	501
Mercy Hospital Clermont[2]	Batavia	99%	171
Mercy Hospital Fairfield	Fairfield	99%	433
Mercy Medical Center	Canton	99%	428
Mercy Saint Anne Hospital	Toledo	99%	205
Parma Community General Hospital	Parma	99%	401
Riverside Methodist Hospital[2]	Columbus	99%	79
Saint Elizabeth Boardman Health Center[2]	Boardman	99%	126
Southwest General Health Center	Middleburg Hgts	99%	517
Summa Health Systems Hospitals[2]	Akron	99%	140
Trinity Med Ctr East & West	Steubenville	99%	338
Trumbull Memorial Hospital	Warren	99%	265
UHHS Richmond Heights Hospital	Richmond Hghts	99%	222
Union Hospital	Dover	99%	199
Upper Valley Medical Center[2]	Troy	99%	180
Aultman Hospital	Canton	98%	807
Aultman Orrville Hospital	Orrville	98%	40
Blanchard Valley Hospital	Findlay	98%	163
Cincinnati VA Medical Center	Cincinnati	98%	122
Clinton Memorial Hospital	Wilmington	98%	124
Euclid Hospital	Euclid	98%	141
Fisher - Titus Hospital	Norwalk	98%	158
Good Samaritan Hospital[2]	Dayton	98%	140
Grand Lake Health System	Saint Marys	98%	64
H B Magruder Memorial Hospital	Port Clinton	98%	50
Holzer Medical Center[2]	Gallipolis	98%	102
Lakewood Hospital	Lakewood	98%	127
Medina Hospital	Medina	98%	201
Mercy Saint Charles Hospital	Oregon	98%	172
Mercy Saint Vincent Medical Center	Toledo	98%	186
Mount Carmel Saint Ann's[2]	Westerville	98%	128
Northside Medical Center	Youngstown	98%	217
Ohio State University Hospitals[2]	Columbus	98%	112
Saint Joseph Health Center[2]	Warren	98%	171
Saint Rita's Medical Center	Lima	98%	406
Saint Vincent Charity Medical Center[2]	Cleveland	98%	104
Salem Regional Medical Center	Salem	98%	166
Summa Health System Barberton Hospital	Barberton	98%	256
Summa Wadsworth - Rittman Hospital	Wadsworth	98%	171
Univ Hosps-Elyria Med Ctr[2]	Elyria	98%	94
University Hospitals Ahuja Medical Center[2]	Beachwood	98%	196
University Hospitals Case Medical Center[2]	Cleveland	98%	142
Univ Hosps Conneaut Med Ctr	Conneaut	98%	40
University of Cincinnati Medical Center	Cincinnati	98%	295
West Chester Hospital	West Chester	98%	260
Barnesville Hospital Association	Barnesville	97%	29
Belmont Community Hospital	Bellaire	97%	36
Christ Hospital[2]	Cincinnati	97%	114
Cleveland - Wade Park VA Medical Center	Cleveland	97%	94
Dublin Methodist Hospital	Dublin	97%	87
Fairview Hospital[2]	Cleveland	97%	307
Lake Health	Concord	97%	188
Lima Memorial Health System	Lima	97%	166
Medcentral Health Sys Mansfield Hosp	Mansfield	97%	360
Mercer County Joint Twp Comm Hosp	Coldwater	97%	78
Mercy Willard Hospital	Willard	97%	36
Samaritan Regional Health System	Ashland	97%	103
Southwest Regional Medical Center	Georgetown	97%	61
Springfield Regional Medical Center	Springfield	97%	455
Summa Western Reserve Hospital	Cuyahoga Falls	97%	143
The Toledo Hospital[2]	Toledo	97%	102
Wooster Community Hospital	Wooster	97%	189
Community Memorial Hospital	Hicksville	96%	25
Galion Community Hospital[2]	Galion	96%	85
Grady Memorial Hospital	Delaware	96%	83
Madison County Hospital	London	96%	51
Mercy Tiffin Hospital	Tiffin	96%	107
Mount Carmel West[2]	Columbus	96%	195
O'Bleness Memorial Hospital	Athens	96%	152
Saint Elizabeth Health Center[2]	Youngstown	96%	128
South Pointe Hospital	Warrensville Hgts	96%	122
Wilson Memorial Hospital	Sidney	96%	74
Alliance Community Hospital[2]	Alliance	95%	133
Cleveland Clinic	Cleveland	95%	176
East Liverpool City Hospital	East Liverpool	95%	155
Lutheran Hospital	Cleveland	95%	81
McCullough - Hyde Memorial Hospital	Oxford	95%	76
Metrohealth System	Cleveland	95%	165
Adams County Regional Medical Center	Seaman	94%	79
Community Hospitals & Wellness Centers	Bryan	94%	65
East Ohio Regional Hospital	Martins Ferry	94%	156
Knox Community Hospital	Mount Vernon	94%	145
Morrow County Hospital	Mount Gilead	94%	47
Trinity Hospital Twin City	Dennison	94%	31
University of Toledo Medical Center[2]	Toledo	94%	100
Hocking Valley Community Hospital	Logan	93%	57
Mercy Allen Hospital	Oberlin	93%	45
Mercy Memorial Hospital	Urbana	93%	55
Saint Luke's Hospital[2]	Maumee	93%	143
Southeastern Ohio Regional Medical Center[2]	Cambridge	93%	138
Van Wert County Hospital	Van Wert	93%	29
Bellevue Hospital	Bellevue	92%	59
Robinson Memorial Hospital[2]	Ravenna	92%	154
Selby General Hospital	Marietta	92%	25
Wayne Hospital	Greenville	92%	98
Wyandot Memorial Hospital	Upper Sandusky	92%	26
Wood County Hospital	Bowling Green	91%	94
Fulton County Health Center	Wauseon	88%	48
Pike Community Hospital[3]	Waverly	74%	38

Pregnancy and Delivery Care

Newborns whose Deliveries were Scheduled Early

Hospital Name	City	Rate	Cases
Adena Regional Medical Center[2]	Chillicothe	0%	27
Berger Hospital	Circleville	0%	38
Bethesda North[2]	Cincinnati	0%	50
Blanchard Valley Hospital[2]	Findlay	0%	29
Clinton Memorial Hospital	Wilmington	0%	52
Defiance Regional Medical Center[3]	Defiance	0%	44
Doctors Hospital	Columbus	0%	58
East Liverpool City Hospital	East Liverpool	0%	26
Fort Hamilton Hughes Memorial Hospital	Hamilton	0%	33
Grand Lake Health System[2]	Saint Marys	0%	26
Holzer Medical Center[2]	Gallipolis	0%	81
Licking Memorial Hospital[2]	Newark	0%	31
Mount Carmel West[2]	Columbus	0%	56
O'Bleness Memorial Hospital	Athens	0%	47
Southern Ohio Medical Center[2]	Portsmouth	0%	27
Atrium Medical Center	Franklin	1%	79
Good Samaritan Hospital	Dayton	1%	100
Grandview Hospital & Medical Center	Dayton	1%	83
Memorial Hospital of Union County	Marysville	1%	69
Mercy Hospital Anderson	Cincinnati	1%	153
Saint Elizabeth Health Center	Youngstown	1%	150
Southwest General Health Center	Middleburg Hgts	1%	110
Aultman Hospital	Canton	2%	125
Fairfield Medical Center[2]	Lancaster	2%	60
Good Samaritan Hospital[2]	Cincinnati	2%	59
Grant Medical Center	Columbus	2%	227
Marion General Hospital	Marion	2%	85
McCullough - Hyde Memorial Hospital	Oxford	2%	62
Miami Valley Hospital	Dayton	2%	400
Northside Medical Center[2]	Youngstown	2%	46
Riverside Methodist Hospital	Columbus	2%	532
Saint Luke's Hospital[2]	Maumee	2%	134
Trumbull Memorial Hospital[2]	Warren	2%	41
UH Geauga Medical Center	Chardon	2%	124
Upper Valley Medical Center	Troy	2%	52
Bellevue Hospital	Bellevue	3%	37
Dublin Methodist Hospital	Dublin	3%	181
Hillcrest Hospital[2]	Mayfield Heights	3%	63
Medina Hospital[2]	Medina	3%	69
Mercer County Joint Twp Comm Hosp	Coldwater	3%	36
Mercy Hospital Fairfield[2]	Fairfield	3%	38
University Hospitals Case Medical Center[2]	Cleveland	3%	60
Wooster Community Hospital[2]	Wooster	3%	35
Metrohealth System	Cleveland	4%	289
Mount Carmel Saint Ann's[2]	Westerville	4%	93
Saint John Medical Center[2]	Westlake	4%	28
Summa Health System Barberton Hospital	Barberton	4%	69
Trinity Med Ctr East & West	Steubenville	5%	38
Wilson Memorial Hospital	Sidney	5%	44
Fairview Hospital[2]	Cleveland	6%	50
Mercy Medical Center	Canton	6%	155
Mercy Saint Vincent Medical Center	Toledo	6%	68
Summa Health Systems Hospitals[2]	Akron	6%	34
Firelands Regional Medical Center	Sandusky	7%	72
Lima Memorial Health System[2]	Lima	7%	45
Mercy Tiffin Hospital[2]	Tiffin	7%	30
Ohio State University Hospitals[2]	Columbus	7%	41
Akron General Medical Center	Akron	8%	159
Grady Memorial Hospital	Delaware	8%	26
Mary Rutan Hospital	Bellefontaine	8%	25
Parma Community General Hospital	Parma	8%	59
Univ Hosps-Elyria Med Ctr[2]	Elyria	8%	25
University of Cincinnati Medical Center	Cincinnati	8%	121
Saint Joseph Health Center	Warren	9%	102
Samaritan Regional Health System[2]	Ashland	9%	44
Southeastern Ohio Regional Medical Center[2]	Cambridge	9%	56
Lake Health[2]	Concord	10%	52
Mercy Regional Medical Center[2]	Lorain	10%	29
Bay Park Community Hospital[2]	Oregon	11%	36
Genesis Healthcare System[2]	Zanesville	11%	37
Madison County Hospital	London	11%	28
Pomerene Hospital[2]	Millersburg	11%	28
The Toledo Hospital[2]	Toledo	11%	61
Indu & Raj Soin Medical Center	Beaver Creek	12%	25
Christ Hospital[2]	Cincinnati	13%	39
Community Hospitals & Wellness Centers	Bryan	13%	30
Robinson Memorial Hospital	Ravenna	13%	61
Mercy Saint Charles Hospital[2]	Oregon	15%	26
Saint Rita's Medical Center	Lima	15%	185
Kettering Medical Center	Kettering	17%	166
East Ohio Regional Hospital	Martins Ferry	19%	43
Knox Community Hospital	Mount Vernon	21%	34
Marietta Memorial Hospital	Marietta	22%	79
Ashtabula County Medical Center[2]	Ashtabula	26%	62
Fisher - Titus Hospital[2]	Norwalk	28%	36
Medcentral Health Sys Mansfield Hosp	Mansfield	32%	112

Preventive Care

Immunization for Influenza

Hospital Name	City	Rate	Cases
Adena Regional Medical Center[2]	Chillicothe	100%	563
Affinity Medical Center[2]	Massillon	100%	565
Atrium Medical Center[2]	Franklin	100%	619
Marymount Hospital[2]	Garfield Heights	100%	606
Summa Wadsworth - Rittman Hospital[2]	Wadsworth	100%	304
Upper Valley Medical Center[2]	Troy	100%	574
Berger Hospital[2]	Circleville	99%	289
Blanchard Valley Hospital[2]	Findlay	99%	501
Bluffton Hospital[2]	Bluffton	99%	154
Euclid Hospital[2]	Euclid	99%	556
Flower Hospital[2]	Sylvania	99%	548
Good Samaritan Hospital[2]	Dayton	99%	596
Grady Memorial Hospital[2]	Delaware	99%	369
Lake Health[2]	Concord	99%	525
Marietta Memorial Hospital[2]	Marietta	99%	567
Mercy Hospital Clermont[2]	Batavia	99%	591
Mercy Hospital of Defiance[2]	Defiance	99%	308
Surgical Hospital at Southwoods	Youngstown	99%	499
Trumbull Memorial Hospital[2]	Warren	99%	628
UHHS Memorial Hospital of Geneva[2]	Geneva	99%	295
Ashtabula County Medical Center[2]	Ashtabula	98%	481
Dublin Methodist Hospital[2]	Dublin	98%	480
Fairview Hospital[2]	Cleveland	98%	555
Greene Memorial Hospital[2]	Xenia	98%	329
Lima Memorial Health System[2]	Lima	98%	565
Marion General Hospital[2]	Marion	98%	539
Mary Rutan Hospital[2]	Bellefontaine	98%	240
Mercy Allen Hospital[2]	Oberlin	98%	243
Mercy Health - West Hospital[2]	Cincinnati	98%	509
Northside Medical Center[2]	Youngstown	98%	593
Ohio Valley Medical Center	Springfield	98%	393
Samaritan Regional Health System[2]	Ashland	98%	258
Southern Ohio Medical Center[2]	Portsmouth	98%	576
Summa Health Systems Hospitals[2]	Akron	98%	596
Summa Western Reserve Hospital[2]	Cuyahoga Falls	98%	466
Sycamore Medical Center[2]	Miamisburg	98%	572
UHHS Richmond Heights Hospital[2]	Richmond Hghts	98%	605
Union Hospital[2]	Dover	98%	510
Univ Hosps Conneaut Med Ctr	Conneaut	98%	197
Wooster Community Hospital[2]	Wooster	98%	480
Doctors Hospital[2]	Columbus	97%	547
Fort Hamilton Hughes Memorial Hospital[2]	Hamilton	97%	593
Indu & Raj Soin Medical Center[2]	Beaver Creek	97%	411
Jewish Hospital[2]	Cincinnati	97%	638
Lakewood Hospital[2]	Lakewood	97%	575
Licking Memorial Hospital[2]	Newark	97%	557
McCullough - Hyde Memorial Hospital[2]	Oxford	97%	315
Miami Valley Hospital[2]	Dayton	97%	573
Pomerene Hospital[2]	Millersburg	97%	231
Saint Elizabeth Boardman Health Center[2]	Boardman	97%	630
UH Geauga Medical Center[2]	Chardon	97%	550
University Hospitals Ahuja Medical Center[2]	Beachwood	97%	629
University Hospitals Case Medical Center[2]	Cleveland	97%	547
Wood County Hospital[2]	Bowling Green	97%	319
Aultman Hospital[2]	Canton	96%	553
Cleveland Clinic[2]	Cleveland	96%	577
East Liverpool City Hospital[2]	East Liverpool	96%	357
Hillcrest Hospital[2]	Mayfield Heights	96%	558
Institute For Orthopaedic Surgery[2]	Lima	96%	302
Kettering Medical Center[2]	Kettering	96%	556
Knox Community Hospital[2]	Mount Vernon	96%	283
Medina Hospital[2]	Medina	96%	528
Mercy Hospital Fairfield[2]	Fairfield	96%	581
Mercy Saint Charles Hospital[2]	Oregon	96%	579
Mercy Saint Vincent Medical Center[2]	Toledo	96%	581
Robinson Memorial Hospital[2]	Ravenna	96%	556
Salem Regional Medical Center[2]	Salem	96%	379
Summa Health System Barberton Hospital[2]	Barberton	96%	660

NOTE: Hospital profiles are in alphabetical order by state, then city, then hospital within the city; Rankings exclude hospitals with less than 25 cases except for patient surveys which excludes hospitals with less than 100 cases; (a) 100-299 cases; (1) The number of cases/patients is too few to report; (2) Data submitted were based on a sample of cases/patients; (3) Results are based on a shorter time period than required; (4) Data suppressed by CMS for one or more quarters; (5) Results are not available for this reporting period; (6) Fewer than 100 patients completed the HCAHPS survey; (7) No cases met the criteria for this measure; (8) The lower limit of the confidence interval cannot be calculated if the number of observed infections equals zero; (9) No data are available from the state/territory for this reporting period; (10) The scores shown reflect fewer than 50 completed surveys; (11) There were discrepancies in the data collection process; (12) This measure does not apply to this hospital for this reporting period; (13) Results cannot be calculated for this reporting period; (14) The results for this state are combined with nearby states to protect confidentiality; Please refer to the User's Guide for a full explanation of data.

Bay Park Community Hospital[2]	Oregon	95%	327
Community Hospitals & Wellness Centers	Bryan	95%	1032
Crystal Clinic Orthopaedic Center[2]	Akron	95%	431
Fisher - Titus Hospital[2]	Norwalk	95%	371
Grant Medical Center[2]	Columbus	95%	534
Lutheran Hospital[2]	Cleveland	95%	446
O'Bleness Memorial Hospital[2]	Athens	95%	321
Riverside Methodist Hospital[2]	Columbus	95%	547
Saint Joseph Health Center[2]	Warren	95%	570
Univ Hosps-Elyria Med Ctr[2]	Elyria	95%	598
Alliance Community Hospital[2]	Alliance	94%	308
Christ Hospital[2]	Cincinnati	94%	553
Firelands Regional Medical Center[2]	Sandusky	94%	564
Memorial Hospital[2]	Fremont	94%	268
Mercy Medical Center[2]	Canton	94%	761
Mercy Memorial Hospital[2]	Urbana	94%	324
Mercy Tiffin Hospital[2]	Tiffin	94%	258
Mount Carmel New Albany Surgical Hospital[2]	New Albany	94%	471
South Pointe Hospital[2]	Warrensville Hgts	94%	606
Southwest General Health Center[2]	Middleburg Hgts	94%	587
Southwest Regional Medical Center[2]	Georgetown	94%	299
Trinity Med Ctr East & West[2]	Steubenville	94%	606
Wayne Hospital[2]	Greenville	94%	272
West Chester Hospital[2]	West Chester	94%	638
Akron General Medical Center[2]	Akron	93%	540
Fairfield Medical Center[2]	Lancaster	93%	540
Grand Lake Health System[2]	Saint Marys	93%	261
Holzer Medical Center[2]	Gallipolis	93%	469
Mercy Regional Medical Center[2]	Lorain	93%	585
Mercy Saint Anne Hospital[2]	Toledo	93%	441
Southeastern Ohio Regional Medical Center[2]	Cambridge	93%	428
Mercer County Joint Twp Comm Hosp[2]	Coldwater	92%	232
Parma Community General Hospital[2]	Parma	92%	603
Saint Luke's Hospital[2]	Maumee	92%	586
Saint Rita's Medical Center[2]	Lima	92%	589
Grandview Hospital & Medical Center[2]	Dayton	91%	547
Medical Center at Elizabeth Place	Dayton	91%	201
Memorial Hospital of Union County[2]	Marysville	91%	251
Mercy Willard Hospital[2]	Willard	90%	273
Mount Carmel Saint Ann's[2]	Westerville	90%	462
Mount Carmel West[2]	Columbus	90%	518
Fulton County Health Center[2]	Wauseon	89%	246
Springfield Regional Medical Center[2]	Springfield	89%	566
Wilson Memorial Hospital[2]	Sidney	89%	255
Mercy Hospital Anderson[2]	Cincinnati	88%	578
East Ohio Regional Hospital[2]	Martins Ferry	87%	935
Morrow County Hospital[2,3]	Mount Gilead	87%	112
Clinton Memorial Hospital[2]	Wilmington	86%	599
Belmont Community Hospital[2]	Bellaire	85%	291
Coshocton County Memorial Hospital[2]	Coshocton	85%	258
Saint Elizabeth Health Center[2]	Youngstown	85%	577
Saint John Medical Center[2]	Westlake	85%	575
Three Gables Surgery Center	Proctorville	85%	34
Genesis Healthcare System[2]	Zanesville	84%	540
Good Samaritan Hospital[2]	Cincinnati	83%	517
Madison County Hospital[2]	London	83%	246
Metrohealth System[2]	Cleveland	83%	550
Saint Vincent Charity Medical Center[2]	Cleveland	83%	587
Bellevue Hospital[2]	Bellevue	82%	218
Fostoria Community Hospital[2]	Fostoria	82%	128
Chillicothe VA Medical Center[2,3]	Chillicothe	79%	140
Van Wert County Hospital[2]	Van Wert	79%	264
Ohio State University Hospitals[2]	Columbus	78%	530
The Toledo Hospital[2]	Toledo	78%	508
University of Toledo Medical Center[2]	Toledo	77%	597
Medcentral Health Sys Mansfield Hosp[2]	Mansfield	76%	568
Bethesda North[2]	Cincinnati	73%	546
University of Cincinnati Medical Center[2]	Cincinnati	67%	571
Fayette County Memorial Hospital	Washington Ch	62%	524
Glenbeigh	Rock Creek	55%	67

Immunization for Pneumonia

Hospital Name	City	Rate	Cases
Adena Regional Medical Center[2]	Chillicothe	100%	810
Atrium Medical Center[2]	Franklin	100%	783
Berger Hospital[2]	Circleville	100%	350
Blanchard Valley Hospital[2]	Findlay	100%	551
Hardin Memorial Hospital[2,3]	Kenton	100%	244
Kings Daughters Medical Center Ohio[3]	Portsmouth	100%	35
Bluffton Hospital[2]	Bluffton	99%	77
East Liverpool City Hospital[2]	East Liverpool	99%	490
Euclid Hospital[2]	Euclid	99%	822
Flower Hospital[2]	Sylvania	99%	716
Good Samaritan Hospital[2]	Dayton	99%	882
Grady Memorial Hospital[2]	Delaware	99%	545
Lake Health[2]	Concord	99%	725
Marietta Memorial Hospital[2]	Marietta	99%	729
Marymount Hospital[2]	Garfield Heights	99%	1018
Medina Hospital[2]	Medina	99%	687
Mercy Health - West Hospital[2]	Cincinnati	99%	759
Mercy Hospital Clermont[2]	Batavia	99%	846
Mercy Hospital of Defiance[2]	Defiance	99%	498
O'Bleness Memorial Hospital[2]	Athens	99%	364
Southern Ohio Medical Center[2]	Portsmouth	99%	783
Summa Wadsworth - Rittman Hospital[2]	Wadsworth	99%	478
Surgical Hospital at Southwoods	Youngstown	99%	502
Trumbull Memorial Hospital[2]	Warren	99%	863
UHHS Memorial Hospital of Geneva[2]	Geneva	99%	515
UHHS Richmond Heights Hospital[2]	Richmond Hghts	99%	1008
Upper Valley Medical Center[2]	Troy	99%	762
Ashtabula County Medical Center[2]	Ashtabula	98%	620
Barnesville Hospital Association[2,3]	Barnesville	98%	122
Bay Park Community Hospital[2]	Oregon	98%	413
Greene Memorial Hospital[2]	Xenia	98%	493
Holzer Medical Center[2]	Gallipolis	98%	643
Jewish Hospital[2]	Cincinnati	98%	939
Licking Memorial Hospital[2]	Newark	98%	698
Lima Memorial Health System[2]	Lima	98%	787
Marion General Hospital[2]	Marion	98%	713
Mary Rutan Hospital[2]	Bellefontaine	98%	292
McCullough - Hyde Memorial Hospital[2]	Oxford	98%	530
Northside Medical Center[2]	Youngstown	98%	809
Pomerene Hospital[2]	Millersburg	98%	212
Univ Hosps Conneaut Med Ctr	Conneaut	98%	350
Community Hospitals & Wellness Centers	Bryan	97%	1358
Doctors Hospital[2]	Columbus	97%	712
Fisher - Titus Hospital[2]	Norwalk	97%	490
Fort Hamilton Hughes Memorial Hospital[2]	Hamilton	97%	795
Indu & Raj Soin Medical Center[2]	Beaver Creek	97%	544
Memorial Hospital[2]	Fremont	97%	388
Samaritan Regional Health System[2]	Ashland	97%	336
Trihealth Evendale Hospital[2,3]	Cincinnati	97%	199
Union Hospital[2]	Dover	97%	707
Alliance Community Hospital[2]	Alliance	96%	447
Aultman Hospital[2]	Canton	96%	748
Dublin Methodist Hospital[2]	Dublin	96%	400
Firelands Regional Medical Center[2]	Sandusky	96%	831
Grant Medical Center[2]	Columbus	96%	625
Holzer Medical Center Jackson[2,3]	Jackson	96%	125
Lakewood Hospital[2]	Lakewood	96%	782
Mercy Medical Center[2]	Canton	96%	1009
Miami Valley Hospital[2]	Dayton	96%	627
Ohio Valley Medical Center	Springfield	96%	437
Parma Community General Hospital[2]	Parma	96%	929
Riverside Methodist Hospital[2]	Columbus	96%	681
Saint Elizabeth Boardman Health Center[2]	Boardman	96%	984
Saint Joseph Health Center[2]	Warren	96%	786
Salem Regional Medical Center[2]	Salem	96%	519
Southeastern Ohio Regional Medical Center[2]	Cambridge	96%	543
Sycamore Medical Center[2]	Miamisburg	96%	871
UH Geauga Medical Center[2]	Chardon	96%	683
University Hospitals Ahuja Medical Center[2]	Beachwood	96%	967
Wooster Community Hospital[2]	Wooster	96%	578
Cleveland Clinic[2]	Cleveland	95%	747
Fairfield Medical Center[2]	Lancaster	95%	730
Fairview Hospital[2]	Cleveland	95%	624
Mercy Allen Hospital[2]	Oberlin	95%	377
Mercy Saint Charles Hospital[2]	Oregon	95%	823
Univ Hosps-Elyria Med Ctr[2]	Elyria	95%	871
West Chester Hospital[2]	West Chester	95%	834
Christ Hospital[2]	Cincinnati	94%	707
East Ohio Regional Hospital[2]	Martins Ferry	94%	905
Hillcrest Hospital[2]	Mayfield Heights	94%	674
Institute For Orthopaedic Surgery[2]	Lima	94%	341
Lutheran Hospital[2]	Cleveland	94%	586
Mercy Hospital Fairfield[2]	Fairfield	94%	741
Mercy Memorial Hospital[2]	Urbana	94%	493
Mercy Tiffin Hospital[2]	Tiffin	94%	309
Saint Rita's Medical Center[2]	Lima	94%	736
South Pointe Hospital[2]	Warrensville Hgts	94%	1011
Southwest General Health Center[2]	Middleburg Hgts	94%	849
Summa Health Systems Hospitals[2]	Akron	94%	801
Summa Western Reserve Hospital[2]	Cuyahoga Falls	94%	747
University Hospitals Case Medical Center[2]	Cleveland	94%	663
Affinity Medical Center[2]	Massillon	93%	842
Grand Lake Health System[2]	Saint Marys	93%	347
Knox Community Hospital[2]	Mount Vernon	93%	339
Memorial Hospital of Union County[2]	Marysville	93%	254
Mercy Hospital Anderson[2]	Cincinnati	93%	735
Mercy Saint Vincent Medical Center[2]	Toledo	93%	672
Saint Luke's Hospital[2]	Maumee	93%	791
Southwest Regional Medical Center[2]	Georgetown	93%	483
Summa Health System Barberton Hospital[2]	Barberton	93%	931
Trinity Med Ctr East & West[2]	Steubenville	93%	845
Wayne Hospital[2]	Greenville	93%	361
Wood County Hospital[2]	Bowling Green	93%	393
Coshocton County Memorial Hospital[2]	Coshocton	92%	379
Genesis Healthcare System[2]	Zanesville	92%	702
Medcentral Health Sys Mansfield Hosp[2]	Mansfield	92%	704
Springfield Regional Medical Center[2]	Springfield	92%	844
Akron General Medical Center[2]	Akron	91%	680
Kettering Medical Center[2]	Kettering	91%	763
Mercer County Joint Twp Comm Hosp[2]	Coldwater	91%	241
Mercy Willard Hospital[2]	Willard	91%	434
Metrohealth System[2]	Cleveland	91%	519
Wilson Memorial Hospital[2]	Sidney	91%	290
Mercy Regional Medical Center[2]	Lorain	90%	770
Mercy Saint Anne Hospital[2]	Toledo	90%	650
Robinson Memorial Hospital[2]	Ravenna	90%	749
Clinton Memorial Hospital[2]	Wilmington	89%	691
Grandview Hospital & Medical Center[2]	Dayton	89%	638
Saint John Medical Center[2]	Westlake	89%	768
Van Wert County Hospital[2]	Van Wert	89%	373
Mount Carmel New Albany Surgical Hospital[2]	New Albany	88%	563
Chillicothe VA Medical Center[2,3]	Chillicothe	87%	280
Crystal Clinic Orthopaedic Center[2]	Akron	87%	562
Morrow County Hospital[2,3]	Mount Gilead	87%	255
Fulton County Health Center[2]	Wauseon	86%	280
Madison County Hospital[2]	London	86%	304
Saint Elizabeth Health Center[2]	Youngstown	85%	768
Saint Vincent Charity Medical Center[2]	Cleveland	85%	799
Belmont Community Hospital[2]	Bellaire	84%	370
Fostoria Community Hospital[2,3]	Fostoria	84%	155
Good Samaritan Hospital[2]	Cincinnati	84%	651
Mount Carmel West[2]	Columbus	83%	692
Bethesda North[2]	Cincinnati	80%	783
Mount Carmel Saint Ann's[2]	Westerville	80%	444
The Toledo Hospital[2]	Toledo	80%	563
University of Cincinnati Medical Center[2]	Cincinnati	80%	624
Glenbeigh	Rock Creek	78%	69
Medical Center at Elizabeth Place	Dayton	78%	209
Ohio State University Hospitals[2]	Columbus	77%	596
Fayette County Memorial Hospital	Washington Ch	75%	790
University of Toledo Medical Center[2]	Toledo	75%	723
Bellevue Hospital[2]	Bellevue	70%	226
Three Gables Surgery Center	Proctorville	59%	51

Stroke Care

Anticoagulation Therapy for Atrial Fibrillation

Hospital Name	City	Rate	Cases
Cleveland Clinic[2]	Cleveland	100%	34
Hillcrest Hospital	Mayfield Heights	100%	45
Mercy Medical Center	Canton	100%	28
Mercy Regional Medical Center	Lorain	100%	28
Southwest General Health Center	Middleburg Hgts	100%	28
Ohio State University Hospitals	Columbus	98%	54
Riverside Methodist Hospital	Columbus	98%	124
Bethesda North	Cincinnati	96%	25
Lake Health	Concord	93%	29
Akron General Medical Center	Akron	89%	36
Medcentral Health Sys Mansfield Hosp	Mansfield	62%	29

Antithrombotic Therapy Timing

Hospital Name	City	Rate	Cases
Affinity Medical Center	Massillon	100%	54
Ashtabula County Medical Center	Ashtabula	100%	41
Atrium Medical Center	Franklin	100%	96
Blanchard Valley Hospital	Findlay	100%	57
Christ Hospital[2]	Cincinnati	100%	77
Clinton Memorial Hospital	Wilmington	100%	31
Doctors Hospital	Columbus	100%	50
Dublin Methodist Hospital	Dublin	100%	26
Fairfield Medical Center	Lancaster	100%	72
Fisher - Titus Hospital	Norwalk	100%	51
Fort Hamilton Hughes Memorial Hospital	Hamilton	100%	62
Grant Medical Center[2]	Columbus	100%	80
Greene Memorial Hospital	Xenia	100%	32
Indu & Raj Soin Medical Center	Beaver Creek	100%	36
Lima Memorial Health System	Lima	100%	81
Marion General Hospital	Marion	100%	34
Medina Hospital	Medina	100%	47
Memorial Hospital	Fremont	100%	25
Mercy Health - West Hospital	Cincinnati	100%	42
Mercy Hospital Anderson[2]	Cincinnati	100%	116
Mercy Hospital Fairfield[2]	Fairfield	100%	100
Mercy Medical Center	Canton	100%	156
Mercy Saint Anne Hospital	Toledo	100%	42
Northside Medical Center	Youngstown	100%	75
Saint John Medical Center[2]	Westlake	100%	104
Saint Luke's Hospital	Maumee	100%	60
Saint Rita's Medical Center	Lima	100%	165
South Pointe Hospital	Warrensville Hgts	100%	62
Springfield Regional Medical Center[2]	Springfield	100%	108
Union Hospital	Dover	100%	47
Univ Hosps-Elyria Med Ctr	Elyria	100%	113
University Hospitals Case Medical Center[2]	Cleveland	100%	67
Upper Valley Medical Center	Troy	100%	73
Wooster Community Hospital	Wooster	100%	62
Aultman Hospital[2]	Canton	99%	87
Good Samaritan Hospital	Cincinnati	99%	170
Jewish Hospital[2]	Cincinnati	99%	88

NOTE: Hospital profiles are in alphabetical order by state, then city, then hospital within the city; Rankings exclude hospitals with less than 25 cases except for patient surveys which excludes hospitals with less than 100 cases; (a) 100-299 cases; (1) The number of cases/patients is too few to report; (2) Data submitted were based on a sample of cases/patients; (3) Results are based on a shorter time period than required; (4) Data suppressed by CMS for one or more quarters; (5) Results are not available for this reporting period; (6) Fewer than 100 patients completed the HCAHPS survey; (7) No cases met the criteria for this measure; (8) The lower limit of the confidence interval cannot be calculated if the number of observed infections equals zero; (9) No data are available from the state/territory for this reporting period; (10) The scores shown reflect fewer than 50 completed surveys; (11) There were discrepancies in the data collection process; (12) This measure does not apply to this hospital for this reporting period; (13) Results cannot be calculated for this reporting period; (14) The results for this state are combined with nearby states to protect confidentiality; Please refer to the User's Guide for a full explanation of data.

Hospital Name	City	Rate	Cases
Marietta Memorial Hospital	Marietta	99%	92
Marymount Hospital	Garfield Heights	99%	158
Mercy Regional Medical Center	Lorain	99%	148
Miami Valley Hospital[2]	Dayton	99%	85
Southern Ohio Medical Center	Portsmouth	99%	94
The Toledo Hospital[2]	Toledo	99%	80
Trinity Med Ctr East & West	Steubenville	99%	91
Trumbull Memorial Hospital	Warren	99%	81
West Chester Hospital	West Chester	99%	70
Bethesda North	Cincinnati	98%	190
Euclid Hospital	Euclid	98%	51
Fairview Hospital	Cleveland	98%	122
Genesis Healthcare System[2]	Zanesville	98%	51
Good Samaritan Hospital[2]	Dayton	98%	88
Lake Health	Concord	98%	194
Lakewood Hospital	Lakewood	98%	92
Licking Memorial Hospital	Newark	98%	45
Mercy Saint Charles Hospital	Oregon	98%	47
Mercy Saint Vincent Medical Center	Toledo	98%	156
Ohio State University Hospitals	Columbus	98%	251
Parma Community General Hospital	Parma	98%	121
Riverside Methodist Hospital	Columbus	98%	623
Saint Elizabeth Boardman Health Center	Boardman	98%	57
Saint Joseph Health Center[2]	Warren	98%	98
Summa Health System Barberton Hospital	Barberton	98%	59
Summa Health Systems Hospitals[2]	Akron	98%	94
UH Geauga Medical Center	Chardon	98%	47
UHHS Richmond Heights Hospital	Richmond Hghts	98%	48
Firelands Regional Medical Center	Sandusky	97%	72
Kettering Medical Center	Kettering	97%	184
Summa Western Reserve Hospital	Cuyahoga Falls	97%	32
Sycamore Medical Center	Miamisburg	97%	37
Cleveland Clinic[2]	Cleveland	96%	180
Flower Hospital	Sylvania	96%	69
Hillcrest Hospital	Mayfield Heights	96%	180
Medcentral Health Sys Mansfield Hosp	Mansfield	96%	113
Salem Regional Medical Center	Salem	96%	45
Southeastern Ohio Regional Medical Center	Cambridge	96%	28
Akron General Medical Center	Akron	95%	216
Mount Carmel Saint Ann's[2]	Westerville	95%	63
Robinson Memorial Hospital	Ravenna	95%	65
University Hospitals Ahuja Medical Center	Beachwood	95%	64
Holzer Medical Center	Gallipolis	94%	34
Metrohealth System	Cleveland	94%	189
Southwest General Health Center	Middleburg Hgts	94%	142
University of Cincinnati Medical Center[2]	Cincinnati	94%	80
University of Toledo Medical Center[2]	Toledo	94%	77
Adena Regional Medical Center[2]	Chillicothe	93%	96
Mount Carmel West[2]	Columbus	93%	108
Saint Elizabeth Health Center[2]	Youngstown	91%	101
Grandview Hospital & Medical Center	Dayton	90%	78

Assessed for Rehabilitation

Hospital Name	City	Rate	Cases
Atrium Medical Center	Franklin	100%	114
Blanchard Valley Hospital	Findlay	100%	66
Clinton Memorial Hospital	Wilmington	100%	30
Dublin Methodist Hospital	Dublin	100%	33
Euclid Hospital	Euclid	100%	53
Firelands Regional Medical Center	Sandusky	100%	76
Good Samaritan Hospital[2]	Dayton	100%	95
Grady Memorial Hospital	Delaware	100%	26
Grant Medical Center[2]	Columbus	100%	106
Greene Memorial Hospital	Xenia	100%	34
Indu & Raj Soin Medical Center	Beaver Creek	100%	34
Kettering Medical Center	Kettering	100%	237
Lakewood Hospital	Lakewood	100%	118
Licking Memorial Hospital	Newark	100%	63
Marion General Hospital	Marion	100%	39
Medina Hospital	Medina	100%	50
Memorial Hospital	Fremont	100%	25
Mercy Hospital Clermont	Batavia	100%	29
Mercy Hospital Fairfield[2]	Fairfield	100%	110
Mercy Regional Medical Center	Lorain	100%	160
Mercy Saint Vincent Medical Center	Toledo	100%	230
Northside Medical Center	Youngstown	100%	77
Ohio State University Hospitals	Columbus	100%	436
Parma Community General Hospital	Parma	100%	127
Saint John Medical Center[2]	Westlake	100%	110
South Pointe Hospital	Warrensville Hgts	100%	70
Summa Western Reserve Hospital	Cuyahoga Falls	100%	39
Sycamore Medical Center	Miamisburg	100%	50
Union Hospital	Dover	100%	47
University Hospitals Ahuja Medical Center	Beachwood	100%	68
Akron General Medical Center	Akron	99%	272
Christ Hospital[2]	Cincinnati	99%	106
Jewish Hospital[2]	Cincinnati	99%	118
Lake Health	Concord	99%	189
Mercy Hospital Anderson[2]	Cincinnati	99%	116
Miami Valley Hospital[2]	Dayton	99%	135
Riverside Methodist Hospital	Columbus	99%	992

Hospital Name	City	Rate	Cases
Saint Elizabeth Health Center[2]	Youngstown	99%	128
Southwest General Health Center	Middleburg Hgts	99%	170
University Hospitals Case Medical Center[2]	Cleveland	99%	127
Upper Valley Medical Center	Troy	99%	70
Aultman Hospital[2]	Canton	98%	114
Bethesda North	Cincinnati	98%	240
Cleveland Clinic[2]	Cleveland	98%	333
Doctors Hospital	Columbus	98%	50
Fairview Hospital	Cleveland	98%	145
Fisher - Titus Hospital	Norwalk	98%	58
Fort Hamilton Hughes Memorial Hospital	Hamilton	98%	60
Good Samaritan Hospital	Cincinnati	98%	201
Hillcrest Hospital	Mayfield Heights	98%	208
Lima Memorial Health System	Lima	98%	99
Mercy Medical Center	Canton	98%	170
Mercy Saint Anne Hospital	Toledo	98%	43
Metrohealth System	Cleveland	98%	289
Saint Joseph Health Center[2]	Warren	98%	98
Saint Luke's Hospital	Maumee	98%	63
Saint Rita's Medical Center	Lima	98%	190
Southern Ohio Medical Center	Portsmouth	98%	86
Trumbull Memorial Hospital	Warren	98%	87
UHHS Richmond Heights Hospital	Richmond Hghts	98%	52
University of Toledo Medical Center[2]	Toledo	98%	101
Wooster Community Hospital	Wooster	98%	63
Adena Regional Medical Center[2]	Chillicothe	97%	104
Grandview Hospital & Medical Center	Dayton	97%	97
The Toledo Hospital[2]	Toledo	97%	106
Univ Hosps-Elyria Med Ctr	Elyria	97%	108
Flower Hospital	Sylvania	96%	77
Genesis Healthcare System[2]	Zanesville	96%	70
Mount Carmel Saint Ann's[2]	Westerville	96%	78
Summa Health Systems Hospitals[2]	Akron	96%	112
University of Cincinnati Medical Center[2]	Cincinnati	96%	128
Fairfield Medical Center	Lancaster	95%	77
Marymount Hospital	Garfield Heights	95%	170
Mercy Health - West Hospital	Cincinnati	95%	41
West Chester Hospital	West Chester	95%	81
Medcentral Health Sys Mansfield Hosp	Mansfield	94%	123
Mount Carmel West[2]	Columbus	94%	151
Robinson Memorial Hospital	Ravenna	94%	67
Affinity Medical Center	Massillon	93%	56
Marietta Memorial Hospital	Marietta	93%	101
Mercy Saint Charles Hospital	Oregon	93%	42
Saint Elizabeth Boardman Health Center	Boardman	93%	58
Salem Regional Medical Center	Salem	93%	46
UH Geauga Medical Center	Chardon	92%	48
Holzer Medical Center	Gallipolis	90%	31
East Ohio Regional Hospital	Martins Ferry	89%	27
Springfield Regional Medical Center[2]	Springfield	89%	108
Ashtabula County Medical Center	Ashtabula	88%	50
Summa Health System Barberton Hospital	Barberton	88%	57
Trinity Med Ctr East & West	Steubenville	88%	81

Discharged on Antithrombotic Therapy

Hospital Name	City	Rate	Cases
Adena Regional Medical Center[2]	Chillicothe	100%	104
Affinity Medical Center	Massillon	100%	52
Atrium Medical Center	Franklin	100%	102
Aultman Hospital[2]	Canton	100%	92
Bethesda North	Cincinnati	100%	213
Blanchard Valley Hospital	Findlay	100%	58
Christ Hospital[2]	Cincinnati	100%	90
Cleveland Clinic[2]	Cleveland	100%	221
Clinton Memorial Hospital	Wilmington	100%	30
Doctors Hospital	Columbus	100%	47
Dublin Methodist Hospital	Dublin	100%	32
Euclid Hospital	Euclid	100%	48
Fairfield Medical Center	Lancaster	100%	72
Fisher - Titus Hospital	Norwalk	100%	58
Flower Hospital	Sylvania	100%	73
Genesis Healthcare System[2]	Zanesville	100%	56
Good Samaritan Hospital	Cincinnati	100%	179
Grady Memorial Hospital	Delaware	100%	25
Grant Medical Center[2]	Columbus	100%	79
Greene Memorial Hospital	Xenia	100%	32
Indu & Raj Soin Medical Center	Beaver Creek	100%	33
Jewish Hospital[2]	Cincinnati	100%	99
Kettering Medical Center	Kettering	100%	196
Lake Health	Concord	100%	184
Lakewood Hospital	Lakewood	100%	109
Licking Memorial Hospital	Newark	100%	63
Lima Memorial Health System	Lima	100%	88
Marietta Memorial Hospital	Marietta	100%	89
Marion General Hospital	Marion	100%	39
Medina Hospital	Medina	100%	48
Memorial Hospital	Fremont	100%	25
Mercy Health - West Hospital	Cincinnati	100%	37
Mercy Hospital Anderson[2]	Cincinnati	100%	114
Mercy Hospital Clermont	Batavia	100%	29
Mercy Hospital Fairfield[2]	Fairfield	100%	104

Hospital Name	City	Rate	Cases
Mercy Medical Center	Canton	100%	157
Mercy Saint Anne Hospital	Toledo	100%	37
Mercy Saint Vincent Medical Center	Toledo	100%	167
Miami Valley Hospital[2]	Dayton	100%	105
Northside Medical Center	Youngstown	100%	76
Riverside Methodist Hospital	Columbus	100%	779
Saint Elizabeth Boardman Health Center	Boardman	100%	58
Saint John Medical Center[2]	Westlake	100%	103
Saint Luke's Hospital	Maumee	100%	63
South Pointe Hospital	Warrensville Hgts	100%	66
Summa Health Systems Hospitals[2]	Akron	100%	98
Sycamore Medical Center	Miamisburg	100%	46
Trinity Med Ctr East & West	Steubenville	100%	80
UH Geauga Medical Center	Chardon	100%	48
Union Hospital	Dover	100%	42
University Hospitals Ahuja Medical Center	Beachwood	100%	66
University Hospitals Case Medical Center[2]	Cleveland	100%	93
Wooster Community Hospital	Wooster	100%	62
Akron General Medical Center	Akron	99%	237
Fairview Hospital	Cleveland	99%	126
Firelands Regional Medical Center	Sandusky	99%	70
Good Samaritan Hospital[2]	Dayton	99%	90
Marymount Hospital	Garfield Heights	99%	167
Mercy Regional Medical Center	Lorain	99%	150
Metrohealth System	Cleveland	99%	224
Mount Carmel Saint Ann's[2]	Westerville	99%	75
Saint Joseph Health Center[2]	Warren	99%	94
Southern Ohio Medical Center	Portsmouth	99%	84
The Toledo Hospital[2]	Toledo	99%	81
Trumbull Memorial Hospital	Warren	99%	83
Univ Hosps-Elyria Med Ctr	Elyria	99%	104
University of Cincinnati Medical Center[2]	Cincinnati	99%	88
University of Toledo Medical Center[2]	Toledo	99%	91
Upper Valley Medical Center	Troy	99%	68
West Chester Hospital	West Chester	99%	78
Fort Hamilton Hughes Memorial Hospital	Hamilton	98%	57
Grandview Hospital & Medical Center	Dayton	98%	84
Hillcrest Hospital	Mayfield Heights	98%	191
Mount Carmel West[2]	Columbus	98%	126
Ohio State University Hospitals	Columbus	98%	352
Parma Community General Hospital	Parma	98%	120
Saint Rita's Medical Center	Lima	98%	163
Salem Regional Medical Center	Salem	98%	44
UHHS Richmond Heights Hospital	Richmond Hghts	98%	46
Robinson Memorial Hospital	Ravenna	97%	66
Saint Elizabeth Health Center[2]	Youngstown	97%	105
Southwest General Health Center	Middleburg Hgts	97%	158
Summa Western Reserve Hospital	Cuyahoga Falls	97%	38
Summa Health System Barberton Hospital	Barberton	96%	56
Springfield Regional Medical Center[2]	Springfield	95%	101
Holzer Medical Center	Gallipolis	94%	31
Medcentral Health Sys Mansfield Hosp	Mansfield	94%	113
Mercy Saint Charles Hospital	Oregon	93%	41
Ashtabula County Medical Center	Ashtabula	92%	49

Discharged on Statin Medication

Hospital Name	City	Rate	Cases
Atrium Medical Center	Franklin	100%	83
Blanchard Valley Hospital	Findlay	100%	50
Doctors Hospital	Columbus	100%	41
Euclid Hospital	Euclid	100%	32
Good Samaritan Hospital[2]	Dayton	100%	63
Grant Medical Center[2]	Columbus	100%	68
Marion General Hospital	Marion	100%	30
Miami Valley Hospital[2]	Dayton	100%	82
Summa Western Reserve Hospital	Cuyahoga Falls	100%	30
Sycamore Medical Center	Miamisburg	100%	32
UHHS Richmond Heights Hospital	Richmond Hghts	100%	38
Union Hospital	Dover	100%	30
University Hospitals Ahuja Medical Center	Beachwood	100%	56
University Hospitals Case Medical Center[2]	Cleveland	100%	63
University of Cincinnati Medical Center[2]	Cincinnati	100%	66
Upper Valley Medical Center	Troy	100%	54
West Chester Hospital	West Chester	100%	66
Bethesda North	Cincinnati	99%	160
Cleveland Clinic[2]	Cleveland	99%	152
Good Samaritan Hospital	Cincinnati	99%	140
Kettering Medical Center	Kettering	99%	158
Lake Health	Concord	99%	123
Mercy Hospital Anderson[2]	Cincinnati	99%	99
Mercy Saint Vincent Medical Center	Toledo	99%	137
Ohio State University Hospitals	Columbus	99%	265
Parma Community General Hospital	Parma	99%	88
Riverside Methodist Hospital	Columbus	99%	578
Saint John Medical Center[2]	Westlake	99%	83
Akron General Medical Center	Akron	98%	177
Firelands Regional Medical Center	Sandusky	98%	55
Flower Hospital	Sylvania	98%	58
Fort Hamilton Hughes Memorial Hospital	Hamilton	98%	48
Hillcrest Hospital	Mayfield Heights	98%	165
Jewish Hospital[2]	Cincinnati	98%	84

NOTE: Hospital profiles are in alphabetical order by state, then city, then hospital within the city; Rankings exclude hospitals with less than 25 cases except for patient surveys which excludes hospitals with less than 100 cases; (a) 100-299 cases; (1) The number of cases/patients is too few to report; (2) Data submitted were based on a sample of cases/patients; (3) Results are based on a shorter time period than required; (4) Data suppressed by CMS for one or more quarters; (5) Results are not available for this reporting period; (6) Fewer than 100 patients completed the HCAHPS survey; (7) No cases met the criteria for this measure; (8) The lower limit of the confidence interval cannot be calculated if the number of observed infections equals zero; (9) No data are available from the state/territory for this reporting period; (10) The scores shown reflect fewer than 50 completed surveys; (11) There were discrepancies in the data collection process; (12) This measure does not apply to this hospital for this reporting period; (13) Results cannot be calculated for this reporting period; (14) The results for this state are combined with nearby states to protect confidentiality; Please refer to the User's Guide for a full explanation of data.

Hospital Name	City	Rate	Cases
Licking Memorial Hospital	Newark	98%	49
Metrohealth System	Cleveland	98%	189
Northside Medical Center	Youngstown	98%	66
Saint Rita's Medical Center	Lima	98%	132
South Pointe Hospital	Warrensville Hgts	98%	41
Southern Ohio Medical Center	Portsmouth	98%	65
Christ Hospital[2]	Cincinnati	97%	79
Fairview Hospital	Cleveland	97%	104
Mercy Health - West Hospital	Cincinnati	97%	30
Mount Carmel West[2]	Columbus	97%	97
Trumbull Memorial Hospital	Warren	97%	58
Adena Regional Medical Center[2]	Chillicothe	96%	85
Aultman Hospital[2]	Canton	96%	78
Grandview Hospital & Medical Center	Dayton	96%	68
Lakewood Hospital	Lakewood	96%	75
Saint Luke's Hospital	Maumee	96%	53
Wooster Community Hospital	Wooster	96%	52
Fairfield Medical Center	Lancaster	95%	55
Fisher - Titus Hospital	Norwalk	95%	42
Genesis Healthcare System[2]	Zanesville	95%	44
Mercy Medical Center	Canton	95%	122
Mount Carmel Saint Ann's[2]	Westerville	95%	57
Salem Regional Medical Center	Salem	95%	38
Univ Hosps-Elyria Med Ctr	Elyria	95%	81
Marymount Hospital	Garfield Heights	94%	124
Medina Hospital	Medina	94%	34
Mercy Hospital Fairfield[2]	Fairfield	94%	86
Mercy Saint Charles Hospital	Oregon	94%	34
Summa Health Systems Hospitals[2]	Akron	94%	66
The Toledo Hospital[2]	Toledo	94%	67
UH Geauga Medical Center	Chardon	94%	35
University of Toledo Medical Center[2]	Toledo	94%	70
Saint Elizabeth Health Center[2]	Youngstown	93%	88
Southwest General Health Center	Middleburg Hgts	93%	119
Mercy Regional Medical Center	Lorain	92%	127
Mercy Saint Anne Hospital	Toledo	92%	38
Lima Memorial Health System	Lima	90%	78
Saint Elizabeth Boardman Health Center	Boardman	89%	47
Saint Joseph Health Center[2]	Warren	87%	71
Ashtabula County Medical Center	Ashtabula	85%	39
Robinson Memorial Hospital	Ravenna	84%	58
Trinity Med Ctr East & West	Steubenville	84%	62
Affinity Medical Center	Massillon	82%	40
Marietta Memorial Hospital	Marietta	82%	82
Medcentral Health Sys Mansfield Hosp	Mansfield	82%	100
Springfield Regional Medical Center[2]	Springfield	77%	83
Summa Health System Barberton Hospital	Barberton	71%	45

Thrombolytic Therapy Timing

Hospital Name	City	Rate	Cases
Riverside Methodist Hospital	Columbus	94%	54
Mount Carmel West[2]	Columbus	88%	26

Venous Thromboembolism (VTE) Prophylaxis

Hospital Name	City	Rate	Cases
Blanchard Valley Hospital	Findlay	100%	63
Cleveland Clinic[2]	Cleveland	100%	349
Euclid Hospital	Euclid	100%	53
Fisher - Titus Hospital	Norwalk	100%	50
Grant Medical Center[2]	Columbus	100%	105
Greene Memorial Hospital	Xenia	100%	34
Riverside Methodist Hospital	Columbus	100%	1022
South Pointe Hospital	Warrensville Hgts	100%	70
University Hospitals Case Medical Center[2]	Cleveland	100%	122
Flower Hospital	Sylvania	99%	78
Kettering Medical Center	Kettering	99%	254
Lake Health	Concord	99%	199
Lakewood Hospital	Lakewood	99%	111
Mercy Medical Center	Canton	99%	171
Mercy Regional Medical Center	Lorain	99%	163
Miami Valley Hospital[2]	Dayton	99%	136
University of Cincinnati Medical Center[2]	Cincinnati	99%	137
Adena Regional Medical Center[2]	Chillicothe	98%	92
Doctors Hospital	Columbus	98%	50
Licking Memorial Hospital	Newark	98%	49
Lima Memorial Health System	Lima	98%	95
Mercy Health - West Hospital	Cincinnati	98%	42
Mercy Hospital Anderson[2]	Cincinnati	98%	122
Ohio State University Hospitals	Columbus	98%	430
Saint John Medical Center[2]	Westlake	98%	105
Southern Ohio Medical Center	Portsmouth	98%	92
Southwest General Health Center	Middleburg Hgts	98%	166
UH Geauga Medical Center	Chardon	98%	45
University Hospitals Ahuja Medical Center	Beachwood	98%	61
Wooster Community Hospital	Wooster	98%	63
Atrium Medical Center	Franklin	97%	114
Aultman Hospital[2]	Canton	97%	115
Bethesda North	Cincinnati	97%	231
Fairview Hospital	Cleveland	97%	151
Good Samaritan Hospital	Cincinnati	97%	199
Indu & Raj Soin Medical Center	Beaver Creek	97%	33
Marymount Hospital	Garfield Heights	97%	164
Mercy Saint Vincent Medical Center	Toledo	97%	273
Parma Community General Hospital	Parma	97%	125
Saint Rita's Medical Center	Lima	97%	186
Summa Western Reserve Hospital	Cuyahoga Falls	97%	36
Sycamore Medical Center	Miamisburg	97%	36
Upper Valley Medical Center	Troy	97%	70
Akron General Medical Center	Akron	96%	289
Christ Hospital[2]	Cincinnati	96%	103
Clinton Memorial Hospital	Wilmington	96%	28
Dublin Methodist Hospital	Dublin	96%	25
Fairfield Medical Center	Lancaster	96%	71
Hillcrest Hospital	Mayfield Heights	96%	215
Union Hospital	Dover	96%	53
Ashtabula County Medical Center	Ashtabula	95%	43
Fort Hamilton Hughes Memorial Hospital	Hamilton	95%	65
Medina Hospital	Medina	95%	38
Trumbull Memorial Hospital	Warren	95%	91
West Chester Hospital	West Chester	95%	80
Good Samaritan Hospital[2]	Dayton	94%	94
Marion General Hospital	Marion	94%	33
Summa Health Systems Hospitals[2]	Akron	94%	122
The Toledo Hospital[2]	Toledo	94%	115
Memorial Hospital	Fremont	93%	29
Mercy Hospital Fairfield[2]	Fairfield	93%	109
Springfield Regional Medical Center[2]	Springfield	93%	116
UHHS Richmond Heights Hospital	Richmond Hghts	93%	55
Jewish Hospital[2]	Cincinnati	92%	114
Mercy Saint Charles Hospital	Oregon	92%	50
Metrohealth System	Cleveland	92%	306
Northside Medical Center	Youngstown	92%	79
Affinity Medical Center	Massillon	91%	35
Holzer Medical Center	Gallipolis	91%	34
Saint Elizabeth Health Center[2]	Youngstown	91%	125
University of Toledo Medical Center[2]	Toledo	91%	113
Grandview Hospital & Medical Center	Dayton	90%	103
Genesis Healthcare System[2]	Zanesville	88%	72
Marietta Memorial Hospital	Marietta	88%	98
Mount Carmel West[2]	Columbus	88%	156
Saint Joseph Health Center[2]	Warren	88%	95
Saint Luke's Hospital	Maumee	86%	64
Firelands Regional Medical Center	Sandusky	85%	85
Mount Carmel Saint Ann's[2]	Westerville	85%	72
Salem Regional Medical Center	Salem	85%	48
Summa Health System Barberton Hospital	Barberton	84%	58
Trinity Med Ctr East & West	Steubenville	84%	95
Medcentral Health Sys Mansfield Hosp	Mansfield	82%	129
Mercy Saint Anne Hospital	Toledo	82%	44
Saint Elizabeth Boardman Health Center	Boardman	79%	58
Robinson Memorial Hospital	Ravenna	76%	59
Univ Hosps-Elyria Med Ctr	Elyria	67%	118
East Ohio Regional Hospital	Martins Ferry	58%	33

Written Stroke Educational Materials Given

Hospital Name	City	Rate	Cases
Adena Regional Medical Center[2]	Chillicothe	100%	70
Fairview Hospital	Cleveland	100%	62
Fisher - Titus Hospital	Norwalk	100%	29
Fort Hamilton Hughes Memorial Hospital	Hamilton	100%	35
Genesis Healthcare System[2]	Zanesville	100%	41
Good Samaritan Hospital	Cincinnati	100%	98
Kettering Medical Center	Kettering	100%	86
Lakewood Hospital	Lakewood	100%	50
Licking Memorial Hospital	Newark	100%	38
Marietta Memorial Hospital	Marietta	100%	60
Marymount Hospital	Garfield Heights	100%	107
Mercy Hospital Fairfield[2]	Fairfield	100%	65
Mercy Saint Vincent Medical Center	Toledo	100%	107
Saint Joseph Health Center[2]	Warren	100%	52
South Pointe Hospital	Warrensville Hgts	100%	37
Sycamore Medical Center	Miamisburg	100%	25
University Hospitals Case Medical Center[2]	Cleveland	100%	59
Wooster Community Hospital	Wooster	100%	28
Hillcrest Hospital	Mayfield Heights	99%	114
Lake Health	Concord	99%	120
Mercy Hospital Anderson[2]	Cincinnati	99%	76
Mercy Medical Center	Canton	99%	76
Riverside Methodist Hospital	Columbus	99%	474
Saint Rita's Medical Center	Lima	99%	108
Blanchard Valley Hospital	Findlay	98%	40
Christ Hospital[2]	Cincinnati	98%	46
Cleveland Clinic[2]	Cleveland	98%	125
Doctors Hospital	Columbus	98%	40
Grandview Hospital & Medical Center	Dayton	98%	55
Grant Medical Center[2]	Columbus	98%	65
Southern Ohio Medical Center	Portsmouth	98%	56
Atrium Medical Center	Franklin	97%	62
Flower Hospital	Sylvania	97%	37
Saint Elizabeth Boardman Health Center	Boardman	97%	39
UH Geauga Medical Center	Chardon	97%	32
Parma Community General Hospital	Parma	96%	54
Southwest General Health Center	Middleburg Hgts	96%	85
Firelands Regional Medical Center	Sandusky	95%	43
Saint John Medical Center[2]	Westlake	95%	61
Medina Hospital	Medina	94%	33
Springfield Regional Medical Center[2]	Springfield	94%	54
Univ Hosps-Elyria Med Ctr	Elyria	94%	65
Upper Valley Medical Center	Troy	94%	33
Ashtabula County Medical Center	Ashtabula	93%	28
Ohio State University Hospitals	Columbus	93%	183
Akron General Medical Center	Akron	92%	132
Bethesda North	Cincinnati	92%	151
University Hospitals Ahuja Medical Center	Beachwood	92%	38
Metrohealth System	Cleveland	91%	135
Miami Valley Hospital[2]	Dayton	90%	72
Trumbull Memorial Hospital	Warren	90%	51
Aultman Hospital[2]	Canton	89%	46
Jewish Hospital[2]	Cincinnati	89%	66
Mercy Regional Medical Center	Lorain	89%	64
University of Toledo Medical Center[2]	Toledo	86%	51
Medcentral Health Sys Mansfield Hosp	Mansfield	85%	52
Saint Luke's Hospital	Maumee	85%	48
Mount Carmel Saint Ann's[2]	Westerville	84%	44
Lima Memorial Health System	Lima	82%	55
Mount Carmel West[2]	Columbus	82%	62
University of Cincinnati Medical Center[2]	Cincinnati	81%	58
Good Samaritan Hospital[2]	Dayton	80%	45
Northside Medical Center	Youngstown	79%	42
Saint Elizabeth Health Center[2]	Youngstown	79%	53
Fairfield Medical Center	Lancaster	78%	55
Summa Health Systems Hospitals[2]	Akron	78%	50
The Toledo Hospital[2]	Toledo	78%	46
Salem Regional Medical Center	Salem	75%	32
Robinson Memorial Hospital	Ravenna	70%	40
West Chester Hospital	West Chester	62%	39
Mercy Saint Charles Hospital	Oregon	56%	25
Trinity Med Ctr East & West	Steubenville	44%	45
Summa Health System Barberton Hospital	Barberton	0%	35

Surgical Care Improvement Project

Appropriate Beta Blocker Usage

Hospital Name	City	Rate	Cases
Berger Hospital	Circleville	100%	104
Blanchard Valley Hospital[2]	Findlay	100%	227
Bucyrus Community Hospital[3]	Bucyrus	100%	28
Community Hospitals & Wellness Centers	Bryan	100%	111
Crystal Clinic Orthopaedic Center[2]	Akron	100%	156
Defiance Regional Medical Center[2]	Defiance	100%	52
Doctors Hospital[2]	Columbus	100%	154
East Ohio Regional Hospital	Martins Ferry	100%	107
Euclid Hospital[2]	Euclid	100%	81
Firelands Regional Medical Center[2]	Sandusky	100%	167
Fostoria Community Hospital	Fostoria	100%	26
Galion Community Hospital[3]	Galion	100%	37
Good Samaritan Hospital[2]	Dayton	100%	233
Greene Memorial Hospital	Xenia	100%	39
H B Magruder Memorial Hospital	Port Clinton	100%	25
Institute For Orthopaedic Surgery[2]	Lima	100%	56
Kettering Medical Center[2]	Kettering	100%	877
Lake Health[2]	Concord	100%	238
Marion General Hospital[2]	Marion	100%	137
Mary Rutan Hospital	Bellefontaine	100%	63
Marymount Hospital[2]	Garfield Heights	100%	124
Memorial Hospital	Fremont	100%	65
Mercy Allen Hospital	Oberlin	100%	27
Mercy Hospital Anderson[2]	Cincinnati	100%	208
Miami Valley Hospital[2]	Dayton	100%	276
Pomerene Hospital	Millersburg	100%	32
Saint Elizabeth Boardman Health Center[2]	Boardman	100%	128
Saint Luke's Hospital[2]	Maumee	100%	244
Samaritan Regional Health System	Ashland	100%	172
Selby General Hospital[2]	Marietta	100%	113
Southern Ohio Medical Center	Portsmouth	100%	247
Southwest General Health Center[2]	Middleburg Hgts	100%	371
Summa Wadsworth - Rittman Hospital	Wadsworth	100%	33
UH Geauga Medical Center[2]	Chardon	100%	170
UHHS Richmond Heights Hospital	Richmond Hghts	100%	61
Union Hospital[2]	Dover	100%	104
Upper Valley Medical Center	Troy	100%	63
Adena Regional Medical Center[2]	Chillicothe	99%	220
Akron General Medical Center[2]	Akron	99%	214
Atrium Medical Center[2]	Franklin	99%	205
Aultman Hospital[2]	Canton	99%	344
Bay Park Community Hospital	Oregon	99%	153
Christ Hospital[2]	Cincinnati	99%	358
Cleveland Clinic[2]	Cleveland	99%	356
Dublin Methodist Hospital	Dublin	99%	96
Fairview Hospital[2]	Cleveland	99%	209
Fisher - Titus Hospital	Norwalk	99%	90

NOTE: Hospital profiles are in alphabetical order by state, then city, then hospital within the city; Rankings exclude hospitals with less than 25 cases except for patient surveys which excludes hospitals with less than 100 cases; (a) 100-299 cases; (1) The number of cases/patients is too few to report; (2) Data submitted were based on a sample of cases/patients; (3) Results are based on a shorter time period than required; (4) Data suppressed by CMS for one or more quarters; (5) Results are not available for this reporting period; (6) Fewer than 100 patients completed the HCAHPS survey; (7) No cases met the criteria for this measure; (8) The lower limit of the confidence interval cannot be calculated if the number of observed infections equals zero; (9) No data are available from the state/territory for this reporting period; (10) The scores shown reflect fewer than 50 completed surveys; (11) There were discrepancies in the data collection process; (12) This measure does not apply to this hospital for this reporting period; (13) Results cannot be calculated for this reporting period; (14) The results for this state are combined with nearby states to protect confidentiality; Please refer to the User's Guide for a full explanation of data.

Flower Hospital[2]	Sylvania	99%	146
Fort Hamilton Hughes Memorial Hospital	Hamilton	99%	95
Grandview Hospital & Medical Center[2]	Dayton	99%	333
Grant Medical Center[2]	Columbus	99%	251
Lima Memorial Health System[2]	Lima	99%	202
Mercy Health - West Hospital[2]	Cincinnati	99%	131
Mount Carmel Saint Ann's[2]	Westerville	99%	179
Northside Medical Center	Youngstown	99%	279
Ohio Valley Medical Center	Springfield	99%	171
Parma Community General Hospital	Parma	99%	419
Riverside Methodist Hospital[2]	Columbus	99%	505
Saint John Medical Center[2]	Westlake	99%	162
Saint Vincent Charity Medical Center[2]	Cleveland	99%	152
South Pointe Hospital	Warrensville Hgts	99%	137
Southeastern Ohio Regional Medical Center	Cambridge	99%	85
Surgical Hospital at Southwoods	Youngstown	99%	140
Sycamore Medical Center[2]	Miamisburg	99%	154
Trinity Med Ctr East & West	Steubenville	99%	224
University Hospitals Case Medical Center[2]	Cleveland	99%	307
University of Cincinnati Medical Center[2]	Cincinnati	99%	261
University of Toledo Medical Center[2]	Toledo	99%	220
Affinity Medical Center	Massillon	98%	300
Alliance Community Hospital[2]	Alliance	98%	83
Ashtabula County Medical Center	Ashtabula	98%	49
Cincinnati VA Medical Center[2]	Cincinnati	98%	94
Fairfield Medical Center[2]	Lancaster	98%	317
Fulton County Health Center[2]	Wauseon	98%	99
Good Samaritan Hospital[2]	Cincinnati	98%	189
Hillcrest Hospital[2]	Mayfield Heights	98%	190
Knox Community Hospital	Mount Vernon	98%	101
Lakewood Hospital[2]	Lakewood	98%	269
Lutheran Hospital[2]	Cleveland	98%	82
Mercy Hospital Fairfield[2]	Fairfield	98%	200
Mercy Tiffin Hospital	Tiffin	98%	41
Metrohealth System[2]	Cleveland	98%	262
Mount Carmel New Albany Surgical Hospital[2]	New Albany	98%	175
Mount Carmel West[2]	Columbus	98%	373
O'Bleness Memorial Hospital	Athens	98%	43
Ohio State University Hospitals[2]	Columbus	98%	221
Saint Rita's Medical Center	Lima	98%	509
Springfield Regional Medical Center	Springfield	98%	245
Summa Health Systems Hospitals[2]	Akron	98%	195
Summa Western Reserve Hospital[2]	Cuyahoga Falls	98%	90
Trihealth Evendale Hospital[3]	Cincinnati	98%	62
Univ Hosps Conneaut Med Ctr	Conneaut	98%	48
West Chester Hospital	West Chester	98%	299
Bellevue Hospital	Bellevue	97%	34
Genesis Healthcare System[2]	Zanesville	97%	223
Grady Memorial Hospital	Delaware	97%	68
Holzer Medical Center	Gallipolis	97%	72
Holzer Medical Center Jackson	Jackson	97%	106
Licking Memorial Hospital	Newark	97%	117
Medcentral Health Sys Mansfield Hosp	Mansfield	97%	353
Medina Hospital[2]	Medina	97%	192
Memorial Hospital of Union County	Marysville	97%	39
Mercy Hospital Clermont[2]	Batavia	97%	77
Mercy Medical Center[2]	Canton	97%	257
Mercy Regional Medical Center[2]	Lorain	97%	270
Mercy Saint Anne Hospital[2]	Toledo	97%	64
Mercy Saint Charles Hospital[2]	Oregon	97%	119
Saint Elizabeth Health Center[2]	Youngstown	97%	148
The Toledo Hospital[2]	Toledo	97%	308
Univ Hosps-Elyria Med Ctr[2]	Elyria	97%	186
University Hospitals Ahuja Medical Center	Beachwood	97%	174
Wood County Hospital	Bowling Green	97%	110
Bethesda North[2]	Cincinnati	96%	182
Cleveland - Wade Park VA Medical Center[2]	Cleveland	96%	226
Clinton Memorial Hospital	Wilmington	96%	46
Indu & Raj Soin Medical Center	Beaver Creek	96%	26
McCullough - Hyde Memorial Hospital	Oxford	96%	26
Mercer County Joint Twp Comm Hosp	Coldwater	96%	25
Mercy Saint Vincent Medical Center[2]	Toledo	96%	293
Saint Joseph Health Center[2]	Warren	96%	119
Summa Health System Barberton Hospital	Barberton	96%	159
Wooster Community Hospital	Wooster	96%	139
Dayton VA Medical Center[2]	Dayton	95%	62
Trumbull Memorial Hospital	Warren	95%	247
Wilson Memorial Hospital	Sidney	95%	39
Jewish Hospital[2]	Cincinnati	94%	151
Marietta Memorial Hospital	Marietta	94%	119
Salem Regional Medical Center	Salem	94%	83
Wayne Hospital	Greenville	94%	51
Grand Lake Health System	Saint Marys	89%	45
Robinson Memorial Hospital[2]	Ravenna	89%	99
Van Wert County Hospital	Van Wert	87%	47
Coshocton County Memorial Hospital	Coshocton	86%	28
Madison County Hospital	London	85%	41
Medical Center at Elizabeth Place	Dayton	84%	32

Appropriate VTP Within 24 Hours

Hospital Name	City	Rate	Cases
Ashtabula County Medical Center	Ashtabula	100%	171
Aultman Hospital[2]	Canton	100%	541
Berger Hospital	Circleville	100%	289
Cincinnati VA Medical Center[2]	Cincinnati	100%	264
Community Memorial Hospital	Hicksville	100%	26
Defiance Regional Medical Center[2]	Defiance	100%	132
Euclid Hospital[2]	Euclid	100%	314
Firelands Regional Medical Center[2]	Sandusky	100%	321
Fisher - Titus Hospital	Norwalk	100%	254
Fostoria Community Hospital	Fostoria	100%	106
Fulton County Health Center[2]	Wauseon	100%	237
Good Samaritan Hospital[2]	Cincinnati	100%	304
Grandview Hospital & Medical Center[2]	Dayton	100%	768
Henry County Hospital	Napoleon	100%	54
Hocking Valley Community Hospital	Logan	100%	39
Institute For Orthopaedic Surgery[2]	Lima	100%	182
Kettering Medical Center[2]	Kettering	100%	1901
Kings Daughters Medical Center Ohio[3]	Portsmouth	100%	34
Lakewood Hospital[2]	Lakewood	100%	673
Marion General Hospital[2]	Marion	100%	323
Mary Rutan Hospital	Bellefontaine	100%	181
Marymount Hospital[2]	Garfield Heights	100%	301
Mercy Hospital Anderson[2]	Cincinnati	100%	754
Mercy Hospital Clermont[2]	Batavia	100%	285
Mercy Willard Hospital	Willard	100%	62
Miami Valley Hospital[2]	Dayton	100%	436
Riverside Methodist Hospital[2]	Columbus	100%	835
Saint Elizabeth Boardman Health Center[2]	Boardman	100%	365
Southwest Regional Medical Center	Georgetown	100%	29
Trihealth Evendale Hospital[3]	Cincinnati	100%	177
UH Geauga Medical Center[2]	Chardon	100%	423
UHHS Memorial Hospital of Geneva	Geneva	100%	49
Union Hospital[2]	Dover	100%	336
University Hospitals Ahuja Medical Center	Beachwood	100%	486
University Hospitals Case Medical Center[2]	Cleveland	100%	540
Univ Hosps Conneaut Med Ctr	Conneaut	100%	120
University of Cincinnati Medical Center[2]	Cincinnati	100%	577
Affinity Medical Center	Massillon	99%	445
Akron General Medical Center[2]	Akron	99%	471
Bay Park Community Hospital	Oregon	99%	304
Bethesda North[2]	Cincinnati	99%	315
Blanchard Valley Hospital[2]	Findlay	99%	543
Bucyrus Community Hospital	Bucyrus	99%	145
Christ Hospital[2]	Cincinnati	99%	529
Cleveland Clinic[2]	Cleveland	99%	447
Community Hospitals & Wellness Centers	Bryan	99%	227
Crystal Clinic Orthopaedic Center[2]	Akron	99%	474
Dayton VA Medical Center[2]	Dayton	99%	126
Doctors Hospital[2]	Columbus	99%	362
Fairfield Medical Center[2]	Lancaster	99%	491
Fort Hamilton Hughes Memorial Hospital	Hamilton	99%	279
Good Samaritan Hospital[2]	Dayton	99%	397
Grady Memorial Hospital	Delaware	99%	168
Grant Medical Center[2]	Columbus	99%	535
Greene Memorial Hospital	Xenia	99%	112
Hillcrest Hospital[2]	Mayfield Heights	99%	351
Licking Memorial Hospital	Newark	99%	313
Lutheran Hospital[2]	Cleveland	99%	319
Marietta Memorial Hospital	Marietta	99%	393
Medina Hospital[2]	Medina	99%	642
Mercy Health - West Hospital[2]	Cincinnati	99%	397
Mercy Hospital Fairfield[2]	Fairfield	99%	458
Mercy Regional Medical Center[2]	Lorain	99%	366
Ohio Valley Medical Center	Springfield	99%	475
Pomerene Hospital	Millersburg	99%	121
Saint John Medical Center[2]	Westlake	99%	411
Saint Vincent Charity Medical Center[2]	Cleveland	99%	378
Samaritan Regional Health System	Ashland	99%	480
Selby General Hospital[2]	Marietta	99%	369
Southeastern Ohio Regional Medical Center	Cambridge	99%	221
Southern Ohio Medical Center	Portsmouth	99%	395
Southwest General Health Center[2]	Middleburg Hgts	99%	839
Summa Wadsworth - Rittman Hospital	Wadsworth	99%	123
Summa Western Reserve Hospital[2]	Cuyahoga Falls	99%	301
Surgical Hospital at Southwoods	Youngstown	99%	559
Sycamore Medical Center[2]	Miamisburg	99%	497
UHHS Richmond Heights Hospital	Richmond Hghts	99%	197
Wayne Hospital	Greenville	99%	158
Wilson Memorial Hospital	Sidney	99%	156
Adena Regional Medical Center[2]	Chillicothe	98%	368
Atrium Medical Center[2]	Franklin	98%	364
Cleveland - Wade Park VA Medical Center[2]	Cleveland	98%	273
Dublin Methodist Hospital	Dublin	98%	272
East Liverpool City Hospital	East Liverpool	98%	53
Fairview Hospital[2]	Cleveland	98%	316
Flower Hospital[2]	Sylvania	98%	445
Galion Community Hospital	Galion	98%	127
Holzer Medical Center Jackson	Jackson	98%	257
Indu & Raj Soin Medical Center	Beaver Creek	98%	87
Jewish Hospital[2]	Cincinnati	98%	287
Lake Health[2]	Concord	98%	405
Lima Memorial Health System[2]	Lima	98%	172
McCullough - Hyde Memorial Hospital	Oxford	98%	152
Mercy Allen Hospital	Oberlin	98%	55
Mercy Hospital of Defiance	Defiance	98%	58
Mercy Memorial Hospital	Urbana	98%	50
Mercy Saint Anne Hospital[2]	Toledo	98%	242
Mount Carmel New Albany Surgical Hospital[2]	New Albany	98%	268
Northside Medical Center	Youngstown	98%	648
Ohio State University Hospitals[2]	Columbus	98%	345
Parma Community General Hospital	Parma	98%	904
Saint Joseph Health Center[2]	Warren	98%	369
Summa Health Systems Hospitals[2]	Akron	98%	254
The Toledo Hospital[2]	Toledo	98%	391
Upper Valley Medical Center	Troy	98%	263
West Chester Hospital	West Chester	98%	999
Wooster Community Hospital	Wooster	98%	376
Medcentral Health Sys Mansfield Hosp	Mansfield	97%	550
Mercy Tiffin Hospital	Tiffin	97%	148
Metrohealth System[2]	Cleveland	97%	540
Mount Carmel Saint Ann's[2]	Westerville	97%	321
Mount Carmel West[2]	Columbus	97%	642
O'Bleness Memorial Hospital	Athens	97%	173
Saint Elizabeth Health Center[2]	Youngstown	97%	382
Saint Luke's Hospital[2]	Maumee	97%	395
Saint Rita's Medical Center	Lima	97%	756
South Pointe Hospital	Warrensville Hgts	97%	280
Trinity Med Ctr East & West	Steubenville	97%	374
Trumbull Memorial Hospital	Warren	97%	523
Univ Hosps-Elyria Med Ctr[2]	Elyria	97%	455
University of Toledo Medical Center[2]	Toledo	97%	273
Wood County Hospital	Bowling Green	97%	280
Wyandot Memorial Hospital	Upper Sandusky	97%	33
Bellevue Hospital	Bellevue	96%	90
East Ohio Regional Hospital	Martins Ferry	96%	282
Genesis Healthcare System[2]	Zanesville	96%	315
Knox Community Hospital	Mount Vernon	96%	358
Mercy Medical Center[2]	Canton	96%	479
Mercy Saint Vincent Medical Center[2]	Toledo	96%	260
Robinson Memorial Hospital[2]	Ravenna	96%	306
Springfield Regional Medical Center	Springfield	96%	444
Summa Health System Barberton Hospital	Barberton	96%	481
Grand Lake Health System	Saint Marys	95%	131
Holzer Medical Center	Gallipolis	95%	129
Madison County Hospital	London	95%	99
Memorial Hospital of Union County	Marysville	95%	110
Mercer County Joint Twp Comm Hosp	Coldwater	95%	100
Mercy Saint Charles Hospital[2]	Oregon	95%	410
Salem Regional Medical Center	Salem	95%	207
Clinton Memorial Hospital	Wilmington	93%	124
Alliance Community Hospital[2]	Alliance	91%	204
Coshocton County Memorial Hospital	Coshocton	89%	75
Memorial Hospital	Fremont	89%	180
H B Magruder Memorial Hospital	Port Clinton	88%	69
Van Wert County Hospital	Van Wert	82%	80
Medical Center at Elizabeth Place	Dayton	72%	190

Controlled Postoperative Blood Glucose

Hospital Name	City	Rate	Cases
Affinity Medical Center	Massillon	100%	204
Akron General Medical Center[2]	Akron	100%	109
Doctors Hospital[2]	Columbus	100%	52
Fairview Hospital[2]	Cleveland	100%	108
Genesis Healthcare System[2]	Zanesville	100%	97
Hillcrest Hospital[2]	Mayfield Heights	100%	133
Marion General Hospital[2]	Marion	100%	29
Medcentral Health Sys Mansfield Hosp	Mansfield	100%	219
Ohio State University Hospitals[2]	Columbus	100%	135
Saint John Medical Center[2]	Westlake	100%	33
Trumbull Memorial Hospital	Warren	100%	74
Aultman Hospital[2]	Canton	99%	228
Good Samaritan Hospital[2]	Cincinnati	99%	136
Good Samaritan Hospital[2]	Dayton	99%	156
Grandview Hospital & Medical Center[2]	Dayton	99%	92
Mercy Hospital Anderson[2]	Cincinnati	99%	113
Mercy Hospital Fairfield[2]	Fairfield	99%	181
Metrohealth System[2]	Cleveland	99%	75
Mount Carmel West[2]	Columbus	99%	134
Springfield Regional Medical Center	Springfield	99%	173
Summa Health Systems Hospitals[2]	Akron	99%	138
Blanchard Valley Hospital[2]	Findlay	98%	43
Cleveland - Wade Park VA Medical Center[2]	Cleveland	98%	114
Kettering Medical Center[2]	Kettering	98%	325
Miami Valley Hospital[2]	Dayton	98%	139
Parma Community General Hospital	Parma	98%	82
Saint Luke's Hospital[2]	Maumee	98%	125
Saint Rita's Medical Center	Lima	98%	204
Southern Ohio Medical Center	Portsmouth	98%	87
University of Toledo Medical Center[2]	Toledo	98%	86

NOTE: Hospital profiles are in alphabetical order by state, then city, then hospital within the city; Rankings exclude hospitals with less than 25 cases except for patient surveys which excludes hospitals with less than 100 cases; (a) 100-299 cases; (1) The number of cases/patients is too few to report; (2) Data submitted were based on a sample of cases/patients; (3) Results are based on a shorter time period than required; (4) Data suppressed by CMS for one or more quarters; (5) Results are not available for this reporting period; (6) Fewer than 100 patients completed the HCAHPS survey; (7) No cases met the criteria for this measure; (8) The lower limit of the confidence interval cannot be calculated if the number of observed infections equals zero; (9) No data are available from the state/territory for this reporting period; (10) The scores shown reflect fewer than 50 completed surveys; (11) There were discrepancies in the data collection process; (12) This measure does not apply to this hospital for this reporting period; (13) Results cannot be calculated for this reporting period; (14) The results for this state are combined with nearby states to protect confidentiality; Please refer to the User's Guide for a full explanation of data.

Hospital Name	City	Rate	Cases
Atrium Medical Center[2]	Franklin	97%	76
Christ Hospital[2]	Cincinnati	97%	218
Lima Memorial Health System[2]	Lima	97%	187
Saint Vincent Charity Medical Center[2]	Cleveland	97%	33
The Toledo Hospital[2]	Toledo	97%	157
University Hospitals Ahuja Medical Center	Beachwood	97%	32
Adena Regional Medical Center[2]	Chillicothe	96%	57
Cleveland Clinic[2]	Cleveland	96%	253
Grant Medical Center[2]	Columbus	96%	137
Jewish Hospital[2]	Cincinnati	96%	49
Riverside Methodist Hospital[2]	Columbus	96%	285
Southwest General Health Center[2]	Middleburg Hgts	96%	55
University of Cincinnati Medical Center[2]	Cincinnati	96%	126
Mercy Medical Center[2]	Canton	95%	131
Northside Medical Center	Youngstown	95%	74
Trinity Med Ctr East & West	Steubenville	95%	101
University Hospitals Case Medical Center[2]	Cleveland	95%	164
Lake Health[2]	Concord	94%	88
Mercy Saint Vincent Medical Center[2]	Toledo	94%	234
Bethesda North[2]	Cincinnati	93%	119
Fairfield Medical Center[2]	Lancaster	93%	164
Mercy Regional Medical Center[2]	Lorain	93%	87
Firelands Regional Medical Center[2]	Sandusky	92%	26
Saint Elizabeth Health Center[2]	Youngstown	92%	141
Holzer Medical Center	Gallipolis	90%	30
Univ Hosps-Elyria Med Ctr[2]	Elyria	86%	28
Summa Health System Barberton Hospital	Barberton	84%	58

Perioperative Temperature Management

Hospital Name	City	Rate	Cases
Adena Regional Medical Center[2]	Chillicothe	100%	497
Affinity Medical Center	Massillon	100%	555
Akron General Medical Center[2]	Akron	100%	545
Alliance Community Hospital[2]	Alliance	100%	299
Ashtabula County Medical Center	Ashtabula	100%	200
Atrium Medical Center[2]	Franklin	100%	435
Aultman Hospital[2]	Canton	100%	729
Bay Park Community Hospital	Oregon	100%	356
Bellevue Hospital	Bellevue	100%	98
Berger Hospital	Circleville	100%	347
Blanchard Valley Hospital[2]	Findlay	100%	607
Christ Hospital[2]	Cincinnati	100%	800
Cincinnati VA Medical Center[2]	Cincinnati	100%	304
Cleveland Clinic[2]	Cleveland	100%	625
Clinton Memorial Hospital	Wilmington	100%	149
Community Hospitals & Wellness Centers	Bryan	100%	261
Community Memorial Hospital	Hicksville	100%	36
Crystal Clinic Orthopaedic Center[2]	Akron	100%	500
Dayton VA Medical Center[2]	Dayton	100%	161
Defiance Regional Medical Center[2]	Defiance	100%	135
Doctors Hospital[2]	Columbus	100%	445
Dublin Methodist Hospital	Dublin	100%	345
East Liverpool City Hospital	East Liverpool	100%	74
Euclid Hospital[2]	Euclid	100%	331
Fairfield Medical Center[2]	Lancaster	100%	584
Fairview Hospital[2]	Cleveland	100%	397
Firelands Regional Medical Center[2]	Sandusky	100%	469
Fisher - Titus Hospital	Norwalk	100%	280
Flower Hospital[2]	Sylvania	100%	473
Fort Hamilton Hughes Memorial Hospital	Hamilton	100%	335
Fostoria Community Hospital	Fostoria	100%	111
Fulton County Health Center[2]	Wauseon	100%	260
Galion Community Hospital	Galion	100%	145
Good Samaritan Hospital[2]	Cincinnati	100%	461
Good Samaritan Hospital[2]	Dayton	100%	498
Grady Memorial Hospital	Delaware	100%	188
Grand Lake Health System	Saint Marys	100%	145
Grandview Hospital & Medical Center[2]	Dayton	100%	885
Grant Medical Center[2]	Columbus	100%	639
Greene Memorial Hospital	Xenia	100%	117
Henry County Hospital	Napoleon	100%	68
Highland District Hospital	Hillsboro	100%	63
Hillcrest Hospital[2]	Mayfield Heights	100%	417
Hocking Valley Community Hospital	Logan	100%	44
Holzer Medical Center Jackson	Jackson	100%	276
Indu & Raj Soin Medical Center	Beaver Creek	100%	91
Institute For Orthopaedic Surgery[2]	Lima	100%	191
Jewish Hospital[2]	Cincinnati	100%	430
Kettering Medical Center[2]	Kettering	100%	2119
Kings Daughters Medical Center Ohio[3]	Portsmouth	100%	36
Knox Community Hospital	Mount Vernon	100%	374
Lake Health[2]	Concord	100%	523
Lakewood Hospital[2]	Lakewood	100%	743
Licking Memorial Hospital	Newark	100%	389
Lima Memorial Health System[2]	Lima	100%	260
Lutheran Hospital[2]	Cleveland	100%	337
Madison County Hospital	London	100%	110
Marietta Memorial Hospital	Marietta	100%	441
Marion General Hospital[2]	Marion	100%	372
Mary Rutan Hospital	Bellefontaine	100%	192
Marymount Hospital[2]	Garfield Heights	100%	348
McCullough - Hyde Memorial Hospital	Oxford	100%	179
Medcentral Health Sys Mansfield Hosp	Mansfield	100%	635
Medina Hospital[2]	Medina	100%	694
Memorial Hospital	Fremont	100%	192
Memorial Hospital of Union County	Marysville	100%	115
Mercer County Joint Twp Comm Hosp	Coldwater	100%	116
Mercy Allen Hospital	Oberlin	100%	61
Mercy Health - West Hospital[2]	Cincinnati	100%	447
Mercy Hospital Anderson[2]	Cincinnati	100%	831
Mercy Hospital Clermont[2]	Batavia	100%	295
Mercy Hospital Fairfield[2]	Fairfield	100%	624
Mercy Medical Center[2]	Canton	100%	582
Mercy Memorial Hospital	Urbana	100%	51
Mercy Regional Medical Center[2]	Lorain	100%	544
Mercy Saint Anne Hospital[2]	Toledo	100%	269
Mercy Saint Charles Hospital[2]	Oregon	100%	433
Mercy Saint Vincent Medical Center[2]	Toledo	100%	486
Mercy Willard Hospital	Willard	100%	62
Miami Valley Hospital[2]	Dayton	100%	637
Mount Carmel New Albany Surgical Hospital[2]	New Albany	100%	597
Mount Carmel Saint Ann's[2]	Westerville	100%	488
Mount Carmel West[2]	Columbus	100%	835
Northside Medical Center	Youngstown	100%	708
O'Bleness Memorial Hospital	Athens	100%	203
Ohio State University Hospitals[2]	Columbus	100%	415
Ohio Valley Medical Center	Springfield	100%	521
Parma Community General Hospital	Parma	100%	1019
Pomerene Hospital	Millersburg	100%	136
Riverside Methodist Hospital[2]	Columbus	100%	1052
Saint Elizabeth Boardman Health Center[2]	Boardman	100%	398
Saint Elizabeth Health Center[2]	Youngstown	100%	470
Saint John Medical Center[2]	Westlake	100%	440
Saint Joseph Health Center[2]	Warren	100%	399
Saint Luke's Hospital[2]	Maumee	100%	500
Saint Rita's Medical Center	Lima	100%	926
Saint Vincent Charity Medical Center[2]	Cleveland	100%	433
Salem Regional Medical Center	Salem	100%	239
Samaritan Regional Health System	Ashland	100%	525
Selby General Hospital[2]	Marietta	100%	398
South Pointe Hospital	Warrensville Hgts	100%	371
Southeastern Ohio Regional Medical Center	Cambridge	100%	248
Southern Ohio Medical Center	Portsmouth	100%	473
Southwest General Health Center[2]	Middleburg Hgts	100%	944
Springfield Regional Medical Center	Springfield	100%	572
Summa Health System Barberton Hospital	Barberton	100%	521
Summa Health Systems Hospitals[2]	Akron	100%	358
Summa Wadsworth - Rittman Hospital	Wadsworth	100%	134
Summa Western Reserve Hospital[2]	Cuyahoga Falls	100%	330
Surgical Hospital at Southwoods	Youngstown	100%	594
Sycamore Medical Center[2]	Miamisburg	100%	527
The Toledo Hospital[2]	Toledo	100%	554
Trihealth Evendale Hospital[3]	Cincinnati	100%	232
Trinity Med Ctr East & West	Steubenville	100%	468
Trumbull Memorial Hospital	Warren	100%	587
UH Geauga Medical Center[2]	Chardon	100%	493
UHHS Memorial Hospital of Geneva	Geneva	100%	50
UHHS Richmond Heights Hospital	Richmond Hghts	100%	214
Union Hospital[2]	Dover	100%	364
Univ Hosps-Elyria Med Ctr[2]	Elyria	100%	512
University Hospitals Ahuja Medical Center	Beachwood	100%	551
University Hospitals Case Medical Center[2]	Cleveland	100%	643
Univ Hosps Conneaut Med Ctr	Conneaut	100%	117
University of Cincinnati Medical Center[2]	Cincinnati	100%	653
University of Toledo Medical Center[2]	Toledo	100%	370
Upper Valley Medical Center	Troy	100%	291
Wayne Hospital	Greenville	100%	182
West Chester Hospital	West Chester	100%	1158
Wilson Memorial Hospital	Sidney	100%	167
Wood County Hospital	Bowling Green	100%	306
Wooster Community Hospital	Wooster	100%	434
Wyandot Memorial Hospital	Upper Sandusky	100%	46
Bethesda North[2]	Cincinnati	99%	434
Bucyrus Community Hospital	Bucyrus	99%	151
Cleveland - Wade Park VA Medical Center[2]	Cleveland	99%	470
Coshocton County Memorial Hospital	Coshocton	99%	93
East Ohio Regional Hospital	Martins Ferry	99%	313
Genesis Healthcare System[2]	Zanesville	99%	430
H B Magruder Memorial Hospital	Port Clinton	99%	74
Holzer Medical Center	Gallipolis	99%	154
Mercy Tiffin Hospital	Tiffin	99%	164
Metrohealth System[2]	Cleveland	99%	688
Robinson Memorial Hospital[2]	Ravenna	99%	359
Mercy Hospital of Defiance	Defiance	98%	64
Van Wert County Hospital	Van Wert	98%	130
Medical Center at Elizabeth Place	Dayton	97%	214
Southwest Regional Medical Center	Georgetown	97%	36

Prophylactic Antibiotic Selection

Hospital Name	City	Rate	Cases
Affinity Medical Center	Massillon	100%	570
Alliance Community Hospital[2]	Alliance	100%	211
Atrium Medical Center[2]	Franklin	100%	325
Aultman Hospital[2]	Canton	100%	682
Bellevue Hospital	Bellevue	100%	72
Berger Hospital	Circleville	100%	266
Bucyrus Community Hospital	Bucyrus	100%	126
Christ Hospital[2]	Cincinnati	100%	730
Crystal Clinic Orthopaedic Center[2]	Akron	100%	384
Doctors Hospital[2]	Columbus	100%	311
East Liverpool City Hospital	East Liverpool	100%	51
Euclid Hospital[2]	Euclid	100%	214
Firelands Regional Medical Center[2]	Sandusky	100%	306
Good Samaritan Hospital[2]	Dayton	100%	478
Grand Lake Health System	Saint Marys	100%	99
Grandview Hospital & Medical Center[2]	Dayton	100%	796
Grant Medical Center[2]	Columbus	100%	562
Greene Memorial Hospital	Xenia	100%	75
H B Magruder Memorial Hospital	Port Clinton	100%	51
Henry County Hospital	Napoleon	100%	63
Hocking Valley Community Hospital	Logan	100%	43
Holzer Medical Center	Gallipolis	100%	97
Holzer Medical Center Jackson	Jackson	100%	225
Indu & Raj Soin Medical Center	Beaver Creek	100%	32
Institute For Orthopaedic Surgery[2]	Lima	100%	178
Kettering Medical Center[2]	Kettering	100%	2151
Kings Daughters Medical Center Ohio[3]	Portsmouth	100%	33
Lakewood Hospital[2]	Lakewood	100%	483
Marion General Hospital[2]	Marion	100%	294
Marymount Hospital[2]	Garfield Heights	100%	232
McCullough - Hyde Memorial Hospital	Oxford	100%	137
Memorial Hospital	Fremont	100%	148
Mercy Health - West Hospital[2]	Cincinnati	100%	335
Mercy Hospital Anderson[2]	Cincinnati	100%	727
Mercy Hospital of Defiance	Defiance	100%	45
Mercy Medical Center[2]	Canton	100%	527
Mercy Memorial Hospital	Urbana	100%	47
Metrohealth System[2]	Cleveland	100%	541
Miami Valley Hospital[2]	Dayton	100%	510
Mount Carmel New Albany Surgical Hospital[2]	New Albany	100%	463
Mount Carmel West[2]	Columbus	100%	730
Ohio Valley Medical Center	Springfield	100%	440
Parma Community General Hospital	Parma	100%	845
Pomerene Hospital	Millersburg	100%	107
Saint Elizabeth Health Center[2]	Youngstown	100%	420
Saint Joseph Health Center[2]	Warren	100%	244
Saint Luke's Hospital[2]	Maumee	100%	444
Saint Rita's Medical Center	Lima	100%	616
Saint Vincent Charity Medical Center[2]	Cleveland	100%	333
Samaritan Regional Health System	Ashland	100%	481
Summa Health System Barberton Hospital	Barberton	100%	419
Summa Wadsworth - Rittman Hospital	Wadsworth	100%	103
Sycamore Medical Center[2]	Miamisburg	100%	368
Trihealth Evendale Hospital[3]	Cincinnati	100%	205
UH Geauga Medical Center[2]	Chardon	100%	361
UHHS Memorial Hospital of Geneva	Geneva	100%	37
Union Hospital[2]	Dover	100%	243
Univ Hosps Conneaut Med Ctr	Conneaut	100%	89
University of Cincinnati Medical Center[2]	Cincinnati	100%	515
Upper Valley Medical Center	Troy	100%	166
Adena Regional Medical Center[2]	Chillicothe	99%	373
Akron General Medical Center[2]	Akron	99%	470
Ashtabula County Medical Center	Ashtabula	99%	85
Bay Park Community Hospital	Oregon	99%	248
Bethesda North[2]	Cincinnati	99%	391
Blanchard Valley Hospital[2]	Findlay	99%	516
Cleveland Clinic[2]	Cleveland	99%	570
Clinton Memorial Hospital	Wilmington	99%	69
Dayton VA Medical Center	Dayton	99%	100
Defiance Regional Medical Center[2]	Defiance	99%	118
East Ohio Regional Hospital	Martins Ferry	99%	281
Fairfield Medical Center[2]	Lancaster	99%	552
Fairview Hospital[2]	Cleveland	99%	369
Fort Hamilton Hughes Memorial Hospital	Hamilton	99%	198
Fostoria Community Hospital	Fostoria	99%	110
Fulton County Health Center[2]	Wauseon	99%	216
Galion Community Hospital	Galion	99%	130
Genesis Healthcare System[2]	Zanesville	99%	379
Grady Memorial Hospital	Delaware	99%	104
Hillcrest Hospital[2]	Mayfield Heights	99%	402
Jewish Hospital[2]	Cincinnati	99%	327
Lake Health[2]	Concord	99%	398
Licking Memorial Hospital	Newark	99%	242
Lima Memorial Health System[2]	Lima	99%	289
Lutheran Hospital[2]	Cleveland	99%	224
Mary Rutan Hospital	Bellefontaine	99%	142
Medina Hospital[2]	Medina	99%	533
Mercy Hospital Clermont[2]	Batavia	99%	188
Mercy Hospital Fairfield[2]	Fairfield	99%	582
Mercy Regional Medical Center[2]	Lorain	99%	398
Mercy Saint Anne Hospital[2]	Toledo	99%	160
Mercy Saint Charles Hospital[2]	Oregon	99%	279
Mount Carmel Saint Ann's[2]	Westerville	99%	333

NOTE: Hospital profiles are in alphabetical order by state, then city, then hospital within the city; Rankings exclude hospitals with less than 25 cases except for patient surveys which excludes hospitals with less than 100 cases; (a) 100-299 cases; (1) The number of cases/patients is too few to report; (2) Data submitted were based on a sample of cases/patients; (3) Results are based on a shorter time period than required; (4) Data suppressed by CMS for one or more quarters; (5) Results are not available for this reporting period; (6) Fewer than 100 patients completed the HCAHPS survey; (7) No cases met the criteria for this measure; (8) The lower limit of the confidence interval cannot be calculated if the number of observed infections equals zero; (9) No data are available from the state/territory for this reporting period; (10) The scores shown reflect fewer than 50 completed surveys; (11) There were discrepancies in the data collection process; (12) This measure does not apply to this hospital for this reporting period; (13) Results cannot be calculated for this reporting period; (14) The results for this state are combined with nearby states to protect confidentiality; Please refer to the User's Guide for a full explanation of data.

Northside Medical Center	Youngstown	99%	621
O'Bleness Memorial Hospital	Athens	99%	120
Ohio State University Hospitals[2]	Columbus	99%	386
Riverside Methodist Hospital[2]	Columbus	99%	1012
Robinson Memorial Hospital[2]	Ravenna	99%	211
Saint Elizabeth Boardman Health Center[2]	Boardman	99%	240
Salem Regional Medical Center	Salem	99%	155
Selby General Hospital[2]	Marietta	99%	373
South Pointe Hospital	Warrensville Hgts	99%	227
Southern Ohio Medical Center	Portsmouth	99%	375
Southwest General Health Center[2]	Middleburg Hgts	99%	813
Springfield Regional Medical Center	Springfield	99%	359
Summa Health Systems Hospitals[2]	Akron	99%	340
Summa Western Reserve Hospital[2]	Cuyahoga Falls	99%	219
Surgical Hospital at Southwoods	Youngstown	99%	564
Trumbull Memorial Hospital	Warren	99%	450
UHHS Richmond Heights Hospital	Richmond Hghts	99%	150
Univ Hosps-Elyria Med Ctr[2]	Elyria	99%	355
University Hospitals Ahuja Medical Center	Beachwood	99%	395
University Hospitals Case Medical Center[2]	Cleveland	99%	540
West Chester Hospital	West Chester	99%	858
Wood County Hospital	Bowling Green	99%	210
Wooster Community Hospital	Wooster	99%	336
Cincinnati VA Medical Center	Cincinnati	98%	181
Cleveland - Wade Park VA Medical Center	Cleveland	98%	304
Community Hospitals & Wellness Centers	Bryan	98%	197
Dublin Methodist Hospital	Dublin	98%	121
Fisher - Titus Hospital	Norwalk	98%	223
Flower Hospital[2]	Sylvania	98%	321
Good Samaritan Hospital[2]	Cincinnati	98%	423
Mercy Allen Hospital	Oberlin	98%	56
Mercy Saint Vincent Medical Center[2]	Toledo	98%	441
The Toledo Hospital[2]	Toledo	98%	513
Trinity Med Ctr East & West	Steubenville	98%	383
Van Wert County Hospital	Van Wert	98%	42
Wayne Hospital	Greenville	98%	131
Wilson Memorial Hospital	Sidney	98%	114
Marietta Memorial Hospital	Marietta	97%	242
Medcentral Health Sys Mansfield Hosp	Mansfield	97%	629
Mercer County Joint Twp Comm Hosp	Coldwater	97%	86
Mercy Tiffin Hospital	Tiffin	97%	139
University of Toledo Medical Center[2]	Toledo	97%	310
Knox Community Hospital	Mount Vernon	96%	302
Memorial Hospital of Union County	Marysville	96%	92
Saint John Medical Center[2]	Westlake	96%	297
Madison County Hospital	London	95%	83
Medical Center at Elizabeth Place	Dayton	95%	149
Southeastern Ohio Regional Medical Center	Cambridge	95%	170
Wyandot Memorial Hospital	Upper Sandusky	95%	41
Community Memorial Hospital	Hicksville	91%	35
Mercy Willard Hospital	Willard	91%	46
Coshocton County Memorial Hospital	Coshocton	89%	62

Prophylactic Antibiotic Selection (Outpatient)

Hospital Name	City	Rate	Cases
Affinity Medical Center	Massillon	100%	135
Alliance Community Hospital	Alliance	100%	52
Ashtabula County Medical Center	Ashtabula	100%	72
Aultman Hospital	Canton	100%	772
Bluffton Hospital	Bluffton	100%	56
Cleveland Clinic	Cleveland	100%	1080
Crystal Clinic Orthopaedic Center	Akron	100%	504
Fort Hamilton Hughes Memorial Hospital	Hamilton	100%	107
Good Samaritan Hospital	Dayton	100%	488
Grady Memorial Hospital	Delaware	100%	39
Institute For Orthopaedic Surgery[3]	Lima	100%	47
Lima Memorial Health System	Lima	100%	434
Marion General Hospital	Marion	100%	159
Mary Rutan Hospital	Bellefontaine	100%	25
Mount Carmel New Albany Surgical Hospital	New Albany	100%	550
Northside Medical Center	Youngstown	100%	142
Saint Vincent Charity Medical Center	Cleveland	100%	238
South Pointe Hospital	Warrensville Hgts	100%	74
Surgical Hospital at Southwoods	Youngstown	100%	181
Three Gables Surgery Center	Proctorville	100%	26
Wayne Hospital	Greenville	100%	28
Akron General Medical Center	Akron	99%	586
Atrium Medical Center	Franklin	99%	312
Blanchard Valley Hospital	Findlay	99%	474
Christ Hospital	Cincinnati	99%	908
Doctors Hospital	Columbus	99%	139
Euclid Hospital	Euclid	99%	83
Fairview Hospital	Cleveland	99%	923
Good Samaritan Hospital	Cincinnati	99%	465
Grandview Hospital & Medical Center	Dayton	99%	409
Hillcrest Hospital	Mayfield Heights	99%	466
Lake Health	Concord	99%	295
Lutheran Hospital	Cleveland	99%	139
Marymount Hospital	Garfield Heights	99%	95
Memorial Hospital of Union County	Marysville	99%	87
Mercy Health - West Hospital	Cincinnati	99%	70
Mercy Medical Center	Canton	99%	716
Mercy Saint Anne Hospital	Toledo	99%	86
Mercy Saint Charles Hospital	Oregon	99%	80
Metrohealth System	Cleveland	99%	909
Miami Valley Hospital	Dayton	99%	769
Mount Carmel Saint Ann's	Westerville	99%	281
Ohio State University Hospitals	Columbus	99%	495
Robinson Memorial Hospital	Ravenna	99%	219
Salem Regional Medical Center	Salem	99%	76
UH Geauga Medical Center	Chardon	99%	187
UHHS Richmond Heights Hospital	Richmond Hghts	99%	81
Union Hospital	Dover	99%	118
University Hospitals Ahuja Medical Center	Beachwood	99%	251
University Hospitals Case Medical Center	Cleveland	99%	598
Dublin Methodist Hospital	Dublin	98%	329
Fairfield Medical Center	Lancaster	98%	283
Firelands Regional Medical Center	Sandusky	98%	327
Flower Hospital	Sylvania	98%	131
Fulton County Health Center	Wauseon	98%	97
Grant Medical Center	Columbus	98%	458
Kettering Medical Center	Kettering	98%	560
Marietta Memorial Hospital	Marietta	98%	260
Mercy Hospital Anderson	Cincinnati	98%	228
Mercy Saint Vincent Medical Center	Toledo	98%	635
O'Bleness Memorial Hospital	Athens	98%	176
Ohio Valley Medical Center	Springfield	98%	258
Riverside Methodist Hospital	Columbus	98%	617
Saint Elizabeth Health Center	Youngstown	98%	512
Saint John Medical Center	Westlake	98%	256
Saint Luke's Hospital	Maumee	98%	370
Saint Rita's Medical Center	Lima	98%	321
Southeastern Ohio Regional Medical Center	Cambridge	98%	84
Southwest General Health Center	Middleburg Hgts	98%	424
Summa Health Systems Hospitals	Akron	98%	694
Summa Wadsworth - Rittman Hospital	Wadsworth	98%	97
Summa Western Reserve Hospital	Cuyahoga Falls	98%	113
Trinity Med Ctr East & West	Steubenville	98%	264
University of Cincinnati Medical Center	Cincinnati	98%	525
Upper Valley Medical Center	Troy	98%	118
Wilson Memorial Hospital	Sidney	98%	90
Adena Regional Medical Center	Chillicothe	97%	385
Bay Park Community Hospital	Oregon	97%	37
Bethesda North	Cincinnati	97%	515
Jewish Hospital	Cincinnati	97%	150
Medcentral Health Sys Mansfield Hosp	Mansfield	97%	320
Medina Hospital	Medina	97%	103
Memorial Hospital	Fremont	97%	61
Mount Carmel West	Columbus	97%	610
Parma Community General Hospital	Parma	97%	177
Saint Joseph Health Center	Warren	97%	298
Summa Health System Barberton Hospital	Barberton	97%	98
Sycamore Medical Center	Miamisburg	97%	119
The Toledo Hospital	Toledo	97%	608
Trumbull Memorial Hospital	Warren	97%	310
Wood County Hospital	Bowling Green	97%	67
Wooster Community Hospital	Wooster	97%	211
Fisher - Titus Hospital	Norwalk	96%	89
Genesis Healthcare System	Zanesville	96%	346
H B Magruder Memorial Hospital	Port Clinton	96%	26
Holzer Medical Center	Gallipolis	96%	282
Indu & Raj Soin Medical Center	Beaver Creek	96%	144
Mercy Regional Medical Center	Lorain	96%	308
Southern Ohio Medical Center	Portsmouth	96%	184
Univ Hosps-Elyria Med Ctr	Elyria	96%	353
West Chester Hospital	West Chester	96%	260
Lakewood Hospital	Lakewood	95%	76
Mercy Hospital Clermont	Batavia	95%	104
Saint Elizabeth Boardman Health Center	Boardman	95%	63
University of Toledo Medical Center	Toledo	95%	253
McCullough - Hyde Memorial Hospital	Oxford	94%	33
Mercy Hospital Fairfield	Fairfield	94%	154
Licking Memorial Hospital	Newark	93%	59
Knox Community Hospital	Mount Vernon	91%	115
Samaritan Regional Health System	Ashland	91%	43
Clinton Memorial Hospital	Wilmington	89%	100
Community Hospitals & Wellness Centers	Bryan	89%	72
Medical Center at Elizabeth Place	Dayton	85%	98
Springfield Regional Medical Center	Springfield	84%	116
Bellevue Hospital	Bellevue	81%	53
Mercy Tiffin Hospital	Tiffin	74%	35
Highland District Hospital[3]	Hillsboro	71%	31

Prophylactic Antibiotic Stopped

Hospital Name	City	Rate	Cases
Aultman Hospital[2]	Canton	100%	666
Berger Hospital	Circleville	100%	260
Crystal Clinic Orthopaedic Center[2]	Akron	100%	381
Dayton VA Medical Center	Dayton	100%	100
Dublin Methodist Hospital	Dublin	100%	120
Euclid Hospital[2]	Euclid	100%	211
Firelands Regional Medical Center[2]	Sandusky	100%	305
Fostoria Community Hospital	Fostoria	100%	108
Good Samaritan Hospital[2]	Cincinnati	100%	413
Institute For Orthopaedic Surgery[2]	Lima	100%	178
Kettering Medical Center[2]	Kettering	100%	2122
Kings Daughters Medical Center Ohio[3]	Portsmouth	100%	33
Licking Memorial Hospital	Newark	100%	237
Lutheran Hospital[2]	Cleveland	100%	222
Marion General Hospital[2]	Marion	100%	289
Marymount Hospital[2]	Garfield Heights	100%	219
Mercy Allen Hospital	Oberlin	100%	55
Mercy Hospital Anderson[2]	Cincinnati	100%	717
Mercy Memorial Hospital	Urbana	100%	45
Mercy Saint Vincent Medical Center[2]	Toledo	100%	431
Mercy Willard Hospital	Willard	100%	46
Pomerene Hospital	Millersburg	100%	104
Saint Elizabeth Boardman Health Center[2]	Boardman	100%	237
Saint Joseph Health Center[2]	Warren	100%	237
Samaritan Regional Health System	Ashland	100%	479
Surgical Hospital at Southwoods	Youngstown	100%	561
Sycamore Medical Center[2]	Miamisburg	100%	366
Trihealth Evendale Hospital[3]	Cincinnati	100%	205
UH Geauga Medical Center[2]	Chardon	100%	348
UHHS Memorial Hospital of Geneva	Geneva	100%	35
Univ Hosps Conneaut Med Ctr	Conneaut	100%	89
Adena Regional Medical Center[2]	Chillicothe	99%	363
Akron General Medical Center[2]	Akron	99%	468
Atrium Medical Center[2]	Franklin	99%	302
Bay Park Community Hospital	Oregon	99%	241
Bethesda North[2]	Cincinnati	99%	379
Blanchard Valley Hospital[2]	Findlay	99%	505
Bucyrus Community Hospital	Bucyrus	99%	126
Cincinnati VA Medical Center	Cincinnati	99%	177
Community Hospitals & Wellness Centers	Bryan	99%	193
Defiance Regional Medical Center[2]	Defiance	99%	115
Doctors Hospital[2]	Columbus	99%	310
Fairview Hospital[2]	Cleveland	99%	362
Good Samaritan Hospital[2]	Dayton	99%	454
Grady Memorial Hospital	Delaware	99%	102
Grant Medical Center[2]	Columbus	99%	548
Greene Memorial Hospital	Xenia	99%	74
Hillcrest Hospital[2]	Mayfield Heights	99%	398
Lakewood Hospital[2]	Lakewood	99%	478
Mary Rutan Hospital	Bellefontaine	99%	139
Medical Center at Elizabeth Place	Dayton	99%	149
Medina Hospital[2]	Medina	99%	527
Mercy Health - West Hospital[2]	Cincinnati	99%	334
Mercy Hospital Clermont[2]	Batavia	99%	184
Mercy Saint Anne Hospital[2]	Toledo	99%	154
Mercy Tiffin Hospital	Tiffin	99%	135
Mount Carmel New Albany Surgical Hospital[2]	New Albany	99%	455
Ohio State University Hospitals[2]	Columbus	99%	375
Ohio Valley Medical Center	Springfield	99%	436
Saint Luke's Hospital[2]	Maumee	99%	443
Southern Ohio Medical Center	Portsmouth	99%	351
Southwest General Health Center[2]	Middleburg Hgts	99%	805
Summa Western Reserve Hospital[2]	Cuyahoga Falls	99%	216
Union Hospital[2]	Dover	99%	230
University Hospitals Ahuja Medical Center	Beachwood	99%	384
University Hospitals Case Medical Center[2]	Cleveland	99%	526
University of Toledo Medical Center[2]	Toledo	99%	287
Upper Valley Medical Center	Troy	99%	159
Wilson Memorial Hospital	Sidney	99%	109
Wood County Hospital	Bowling Green	99%	209
Wooster Community Hospital	Wooster	99%	333
Alliance Community Hospital[2]	Alliance	98%	209
Christ Hospital[2]	Cincinnati	98%	710
Fisher - Titus Hospital	Norwalk	98%	220
Fort Hamilton Hughes Memorial Hospital	Hamilton	98%	187
Grandview Hospital & Medical Center[2]	Dayton	98%	774
H B Magruder Memorial Hospital	Port Clinton	98%	47
Hocking Valley Community Hospital	Logan	98%	42
Jewish Hospital[2]	Cincinnati	98%	321
Lake Health[2]	Concord	98%	392
Lima Memorial Health System[2]	Lima	98%	282
Madison County Hospital	London	98%	82
Medcentral Health Sys Mansfield Hosp	Mansfield	98%	615
Mercer County Joint Twp Comm Hosp	Coldwater	98%	86
Mercy Hospital Fairfield[2]	Fairfield	98%	569
Mercy Hospital of Defiance	Defiance	98%	43
Mercy Medical Center[2]	Canton	98%	523
Mercy Saint Charles Hospital[2]	Oregon	98%	274
Miami Valley Hospital[2]	Dayton	98%	499
Mount Carmel West[2]	Columbus	98%	714
Northside Medical Center	Youngstown	98%	610
Parma Community General Hospital	Parma	98%	824
Riverside Methodist Hospital[2]	Columbus	98%	985
Saint Elizabeth Health Center[2]	Youngstown	98%	410
Saint John Medical Center[2]	Westlake	98%	288
Selby General Hospital[2]	Marietta	98%	367
Southeastern Ohio Regional Medical Center	Cambridge	98%	161
Trumbull Memorial Hospital	Warren	98%	431

NOTE: Hospital profiles are in alphabetical order by state, then city, then hospital within the city; Rankings exclude hospitals with less than 25 cases except for patient surveys which excludes hospitals with less than 100 cases; (a) 100-299 cases; (1) The number of cases/patients is too few to report; (2) Data submitted were based on a sample of cases/patients; (3) Results are based on a shorter time period than required; (4) Data suppressed by CMS for one or more quarters; (5) Results are not available for this reporting period; (6) Fewer than 100 patients completed the HCAHPS survey; (7) No cases met the criteria for this measure; (8) The lower limit of the confidence interval cannot be calculated if the number of observed infections equals zero; (9) No data are available from the state/territory for this reporting period; (10) The scores shown reflect fewer than 50 completed surveys; (11) There were discrepancies in the data collection process; (12) This measure does not apply to this hospital for this reporting period; (13) Results cannot be calculated for this reporting period; (14) The results for this state are combined with nearby states to protect confidentiality; Please refer to the User's Guide for a full explanation of data.

Hospital Name	City	Rate	Cases
Wayne Hospital	Greenville	98%	131
West Chester Hospital	West Chester	98%	852
Affinity Medical Center	Massillon	97%	554
Cleveland Clinic[2]	Cleveland	97%	554
East Ohio Regional Hospital	Martins Ferry	97%	276
Fairfield Medical Center[2]	Lancaster	97%	521
Flower Hospital[2]	Sylvania	97%	305
Grand Lake Health System	Saint Marys	97%	98
Holzer Medical Center Jackson	Jackson	97%	223
Indu & Raj Soin Medical Center	Beaver Creek	97%	32
Knox Community Hospital	Mount Vernon	97%	301
Marietta Memorial Hospital	Marietta	97%	224
Memorial Hospital	Fremont	97%	147
O'Bleness Memorial Hospital	Athens	97%	120
Robinson Memorial Hospital[2]	Ravenna	97%	209
Saint Rita's Medical Center	Lima	97%	599
Salem Regional Medical Center	Salem	97%	147
South Pointe Hospital	Warrensville Hgts	97%	226
Springfield Regional Medical Center	Springfield	97%	347
Summa Health System Barberton Hospital	Barberton	97%	395
The Toledo Hospital[2]	Toledo	97%	509
Trinity Med Ctr East & West	Steubenville	97%	372
UHHS Richmond Heights Hospital	Richmond Hghts	97%	146
University of Cincinnati Medical Center[2]	Cincinnati	97%	497
Ashtabula County Medical Center	Ashtabula	96%	76
Cleveland - Wade Park VA Medical Center	Cleveland	96%	297
Fulton County Health Center[2]	Wauseon	96%	215
McCullough - Hyde Memorial Hospital	Oxford	96%	135
Memorial Hospital of Union County	Marysville	96%	90
Metrohealth System[2]	Cleveland	96%	531
Mount Carmel Saint Ann's[2]	Westerville	96%	323
Saint Vincent Charity Medical Center[2]	Cleveland	96%	313
Genesis Healthcare System[2]	Zanesville	95%	368
Holzer Medical Center	Gallipolis	95%	95
Mercy Regional Medical Center[2]	Lorain	95%	395
Summa Health Systems Hospitals[2]	Akron	95%	320
Van Wert County Hospital	Van Wert	95%	39
East Liverpool City Hospital	East Liverpool	94%	49
Galion Community Hospital	Galion	94%	125
Bellevue Hospital	Bellevue	93%	68
Summa Wadsworth - Rittman Hospital	Wadsworth	93%	103
Clinton Memorial Hospital	Wilmington	92%	66
Univ Hosps-Elyria Med Ctr[2]	Elyria	92%	346
Henry County Hospital	Napoleon	89%	62
Community Memorial Hospital	Hicksville	88%	34
Wyandot Memorial Hospital	Upper Sandusky	78%	41
Coshocton County Memorial Hospital	Coshocton	70%	61

Prophylactic Antibiotic Timing

Hospital Name	City	Rate	Cases
Ashtabula County Medical Center	Ashtabula	100%	86
Bay Park Community Hospital	Oregon	100%	248
Berger Hospital	Circleville	100%	266
Bucyrus Community Hospital	Bucyrus	100%	126
Clinton Memorial Hospital	Wilmington	100%	72
Defiance Regional Medical Center[2]	Defiance	100%	118
Doctors Hospital[2]	Columbus	100%	312
East Liverpool City Hospital	East Liverpool	100%	53
Euclid Hospital[2]	Euclid	100%	214
Firelands Regional Medical Center[2]	Sandusky	100%	306
Fisher - Titus Hospital	Norwalk	100%	223
Fulton County Health Center[2]	Wauseon	100%	216
Good Samaritan Hospital[2]	Dayton	100%	478
Grant Medical Center[2]	Columbus	100%	562
Holzer Medical Center	Gallipolis	100%	97
Indu & Raj Soin Medical Center	Beaver Creek	100%	32
Institute For Orthopaedic Surgery[2]	Lima	100%	178
Kettering Medical Center[2]	Kettering	100%	2151
Lake Health[2]	Concord	100%	399
Lakewood Hospital[2]	Lakewood	100%	483
Licking Memorial Hospital	Newark	100%	242
Lutheran Hospital[2]	Cleveland	100%	224
Marion General Hospital[2]	Marion	100%	294
Mary Rutan Hospital	Bellefontaine	100%	142
Marymount Hospital[2]	Garfield Heights	100%	232
Medina Hospital[2]	Medina	100%	533
Mercy Allen Hospital	Oberlin	100%	56
Mercy Health - West Hospital[2]	Cincinnati	100%	335
Mercy Hospital of Defiance	Defiance	100%	45
Mercy Saint Anne Hospital[2]	Toledo	100%	160
Miami Valley Hospital[2]	Dayton	100%	511
Mount Carmel New Albany Surgical Hospital[2]	New Albany	100%	463
Mount Carmel Saint Ann's[2]	Westerville	100%	335
Mount Carmel West[2]	Columbus	100%	735
Northside Medical Center	Youngstown	100%	621
O'Bleness Memorial Hospital	Athens	100%	120
Pomerene Hospital	Millersburg	100%	107
Riverside Methodist Hospital[2]	Columbus	100%	1013
Saint Elizabeth Boardman Health Center[2]	Boardman	100%	240
Saint Joseph Health Center[2]	Warren	100%	244
Saint Vincent Charity Medical Center[2]	Cleveland	100%	333
Samaritan Regional Health System	Ashland	100%	481
South Pointe Hospital	Warrensville Hgts	100%	227
Southern Ohio Medical Center	Portsmouth	100%	375
Southwest General Health Center[2]	Middleburg Hgts	100%	813
Summa Health System Barberton Hospital	Barberton	100%	419
Summa Wadsworth - Rittman Hospital	Wadsworth	100%	103
Summa Western Reserve Hospital[2]	Cuyahoga Falls	100%	219
Surgical Hospital at Southwoods	Youngstown	100%	564
Sycamore Medical Center[2]	Miamisburg	100%	368
Trinity Med Ctr East & West	Steubenville	100%	384
Trumbull Memorial Hospital	Warren	100%	450
UHHS Memorial Hospital of Geneva	Geneva	100%	37
UHHS Richmond Heights Hospital	Richmond Hghts	100%	150
Union Hospital[2]	Dover	100%	243
University Hospitals Ahuja Medical Center	Beachwood	100%	396
University Hospitals Case Medical Center[2]	Cleveland	100%	541
Univ Hosps Conneaut Med Ctr	Conneaut	100%	89
Wood County Hospital	Bowling Green	100%	210
Adena Regional Medical Center[2]	Chillicothe	99%	372
Affinity Medical Center	Massillon	99%	570
Akron General Medical Center[2]	Akron	99%	471
Atrium Medical Center[2]	Franklin	99%	325
Aultman Hospital[2]	Canton	99%	683
Bellevue Hospital	Bellevue	99%	72
Blanchard Valley Hospital[2]	Findlay	99%	516
Christ Hospital[2]	Cincinnati	99%	732
Cleveland Clinic[2]	Cleveland	99%	570
Community Hospitals & Wellness Centers	Bryan	99%	197
Dayton VA Medical Center	Dayton	99%	102
Dublin Methodist Hospital	Dublin	99%	121
Fairfield Medical Center[2]	Lancaster	99%	552
Fairview Hospital[2]	Cleveland	99%	369
Flower Hospital[2]	Sylvania	99%	321
Fort Hamilton Hughes Memorial Hospital	Hamilton	99%	198
Fostoria Community Hospital	Fostoria	99%	110
Grady Memorial Hospital	Delaware	99%	104
Grandview Hospital & Medical Center[2]	Dayton	99%	796
Greene Memorial Hospital	Xenia	99%	75
Hillcrest Hospital[2]	Mayfield Heights	99%	403
Lima Memorial Health System[2]	Lima	99%	292
McCullough - Hyde Memorial Hospital	Oxford	99%	137
Medcentral Health Sys Mansfield Hosp	Mansfield	99%	629
Mercy Hospital Anderson[2]	Cincinnati	99%	727
Mercy Hospital Clermont[2]	Batavia	99%	188
Mercy Saint Charles Hospital[2]	Oregon	99%	279
Mercy Saint Vincent Medical Center[2]	Toledo	99%	442
Metrohealth System[2]	Cleveland	99%	541
Ohio State University Hospitals[2]	Columbus	99%	387
Ohio Valley Medical Center	Springfield	99%	440
Parma Community General Hospital	Parma	99%	845
Saint Elizabeth Health Center[2]	Youngstown	99%	421
Saint Luke's Hospital[2]	Maumee	99%	445
Saint Rita's Medical Center	Lima	99%	617
Springfield Regional Medical Center	Springfield	99%	359
Summa Health Systems Hospitals[2]	Akron	99%	341
The Toledo Hospital[2]	Toledo	99%	514
Trihealth Evendale Hospital[3]	Cincinnati	99%	205
UH Geauga Medical Center[2]	Chardon	99%	361
Univ Hosps-Elyria Med Ctr[2]	Elyria	99%	355
University of Toledo Medical Center[2]	Toledo	99%	312
Upper Valley Medical Center	Troy	99%	166
Alliance Community Hospital[2]	Alliance	98%	211
Crystal Clinic Orthopaedic Center[2]	Akron	98%	384
East Ohio Regional Hospital	Martins Ferry	98%	281
Genesis Healthcare System[2]	Zanesville	98%	381
Knox Community Hospital	Mount Vernon	98%	303
Memorial Hospital	Fremont	98%	148
Mercy Hospital Fairfield[2]	Fairfield	98%	583
Mercy Medical Center[2]	Canton	98%	527
Mercy Memorial Hospital	Urbana	98%	47
Mercy Regional Medical Center[2]	Lorain	98%	399
Saint John Medical Center[2]	Westlake	98%	298
University of Cincinnati Medical Center[2]	Cincinnati	98%	517
Wooster Community Hospital	Wooster	98%	337
Bethesda North[2]	Cincinnati	97%	391
Cincinnati VA Medical Center	Cincinnati	97%	181
Henry County Hospital	Napoleon	97%	63
Jewish Hospital[2]	Cincinnati	97%	328
Mercer County Joint Twp Comm Hosp	Coldwater	97%	86
Robinson Memorial Hospital[2]	Ravenna	97%	212
Salem Regional Medical Center	Salem	97%	155
West Chester Hospital	West Chester	97%	860
Galion Community Hospital	Galion	96%	130
H B Magruder Memorial Hospital	Port Clinton	96%	51
Marietta Memorial Hospital	Marietta	96%	242
Memorial Hospital of Union County	Marysville	96%	92
Mercy Tiffin Hospital	Tiffin	96%	139
Mercy Willard Hospital	Willard	96%	46
Wayne Hospital	Greenville	96%	131
Wilson Memorial Hospital	Sidney	96%	114
Cleveland - Wade Park VA Medical Center	Cleveland	95%	305
Hocking Valley Community Hospital	Logan	95%	43
Madison County Hospital	London	95%	83
Selby General Hospital[2]	Marietta	95%	373
Southeastern Ohio Regional Medical Center	Cambridge	95%	170
Grand Lake Health System	Saint Marys	94%	99
Kings Daughters Medical Center Ohio[3]	Portsmouth	94%	33
Good Samaritan Hospital[2]	Cincinnati	93%	425
Van Wert County Hospital	Van Wert	93%	42
Holzer Medical Center Jackson	Jackson	92%	228
Medical Center at Elizabeth Place	Dayton	92%	149
Coshocton County Memorial Hospital	Coshocton	90%	62
Community Memorial Hospital	Hicksville	89%	35
Wyandot Memorial Hospital	Upper Sandusky	78%	41

Prophylactic Antibiotic Timing (Outpatient)

Hospital Name	City	Rate	Cases
Akron General Medical Center	Akron	100%	586
Atrium Medical Center	Franklin	100%	312
Bay Park Community Hospital	Oregon	100%	37
Blanchard Valley Hospital	Findlay	100%	475
Bluffton Hospital	Bluffton	100%	56
Christ Hospital	Cincinnati	100%	838
Fairview Hospital	Cleveland	100%	832
Good Samaritan Hospital	Dayton	100%	488
Institute For Orthopaedic Surgery[3]	Lima	100%	47
Lutheran Hospital	Cleveland	100%	139
Mary Rutan Hospital	Bellefontaine	100%	25
McCullough - Hyde Memorial Hospital	Oxford	100%	33
Mount Carmel New Albany Surgical Hospital	New Albany	100%	550
Southeastern Ohio Regional Medical Center	Cambridge	100%	84
Southern Ohio Medical Center	Portsmouth	100%	184
Summa Health System Barberton Hospital	Barberton	100%	98
UH Geauga Medical Center	Chardon	100%	187
Union Hospital	Dover	100%	118
University Hospitals Ahuja Medical Center	Beachwood	100%	251
University Hospitals Case Medical Center	Cleveland	100%	518
Ashtabula County Medical Center	Ashtabula	99%	72
Crystal Clinic Orthopaedic Center	Akron	99%	505
Firelands Regional Medical Center	Sandusky	99%	329
Grant Medical Center	Columbus	99%	458
Lima Memorial Health System	Lima	99%	436
Mercy Hospital Anderson	Cincinnati	99%	229
Mercy Saint Anne Hospital	Toledo	99%	86
Mercy Saint Charles Hospital	Oregon	99%	81
Miami Valley Hospital	Dayton	99%	765
Mount Carmel Saint Ann's	Westerville	99%	283
Northside Medical Center	Youngstown	99%	143
O'Bleness Memorial Hospital	Athens	99%	178
Robinson Memorial Hospital	Ravenna	99%	192
Saint John Medical Center	Westlake	99%	258
Saint Vincent Charity Medical Center	Cleveland	99%	239
Southwest General Health Center	Middleburg Hgts	99%	425
Summa Wadsworth - Rittman Hospital	Wadsworth	99%	98
Summa Western Reserve Hospital	Cuyahoga Falls	99%	114
Surgical Hospital at Southwoods	Youngstown	99%	181
Trumbull Memorial Hospital	Warren	99%	310
UHHS Richmond Heights Hospital	Richmond Hghts	99%	72
Upper Valley Medical Center	Troy	99%	118
Adena Regional Medical Center	Chillicothe	98%	387
Aultman Hospital	Canton	98%	537
Bellevue Hospital	Bellevue	98%	54
Doctors Hospital	Columbus	98%	139
Euclid Hospital	Euclid	98%	83
Fulton County Health Center	Wauseon	98%	94
Hillcrest Hospital	Mayfield Heights	98%	469
Marion General Hospital	Marion	98%	162
Marymount Hospital	Garfield Heights	98%	90
Medina Hospital	Medina	98%	102
Mercy Hospital Clermont	Batavia	98%	87
Mercy Medical Center	Canton	98%	720
Metrohealth System	Cleveland	98%	761
Mount Carmel West	Columbus	98%	615
Ohio Valley Medical Center	Springfield	98%	260
Parma Community General Hospital	Parma	98%	177
Saint Rita's Medical Center	Lima	98%	321
Trinity Med Ctr East & West	Steubenville	98%	265
University of Toledo Medical Center	Toledo	98%	237
Wood County Hospital	Bowling Green	98%	65
Wooster Community Hospital	Wooster	98%	212
Affinity Medical Center	Massillon	97%	136
Cleveland Clinic	Cleveland	97%	563
Clinton Memorial Hospital	Wilmington	97%	103
Dublin Methodist Hospital	Dublin	97%	334
Fort Hamilton Hughes Memorial Hospital	Hamilton	97%	109
Grady Memorial Hospital	Delaware	97%	39
Grandview Hospital & Medical Center	Dayton	97%	409
Highland District Hospital[3]	Hillsboro	97%	32
Indu & Raj Soin Medical Center	Beaver Creek	97%	146
Jewish Hospital	Cincinnati	97%	152
Kettering Medical Center	Kettering	97%	561
Memorial Hospital of Union County	Marysville	97%	64

NOTE: Hospital profiles are in alphabetical order by state, then city, then hospital within the city; Rankings exclude hospitals with less than 25 cases except for patient surveys which excludes hospitals with less than 100 cases; (a) 100-299 cases; (1) The number of cases/patients is too few to report; (2) Data submitted were based on a sample of cases/patients; (3) Results are based on a shorter time period than required; (4) Data suppressed by CMS for one or more quarters; (5) Results are not available for this reporting period; (6) Fewer than 100 patients completed the HCAHPS survey; (7) No cases met the criteria for this measure; (8) The lower limit of the confidence interval cannot be calculated if the number of observed infections equals zero; (9) No data are available from the state/territory for this reporting period; (10) The scores shown reflect fewer than 50 completed surveys; (11) There were discrepancies in the data collection process; (12) This measure does not apply to this hospital for this reporting period; (13) Results cannot be calculated for this reporting period; (14) The results for this state are combined with nearby states to protect confidentiality; Please refer to the User's Guide for a full explanation of data.

Hospital Name	City	Rate	Cases
Ohio State University Hospitals	Columbus	97%	496
Riverside Methodist Hospital	Columbus	97%	624
Saint Elizabeth Health Center	Youngstown	97%	514
Summa Health Systems Hospitals	Akron	97%	698
Sycamore Medical Center	Miamisburg	97%	111
Univ Hosps-Elyria Med Ctr	Elyria	97%	330
University of Cincinnati Medical Center	Cincinnati	97%	502
Wilson Memorial Hospital	Sidney	97%	91
Bethesda North	Cincinnati	96%	525
Community Hospitals & Wellness Centers	Bryan	96%	74
Genesis Healthcare System	Zanesville	96%	354
Holzer Medical Center	Gallipolis	96%	288
Lake Health	Concord	96%	300
Mercy Health - West Hospital	Cincinnati	96%	71
Mercy Saint Vincent Medical Center	Toledo	96%	652
Salem Regional Medical Center	Salem	96%	79
South Pointe Hospital	Warrensville Hgts	96%	77
Three Gables Surgery Center	Proctorville	96%	27
West Chester Hospital	West Chester	96%	263
Fisher - Titus Hospital	Norwalk	95%	93
Good Samaritan Hospital	Cincinnati	95%	477
Marietta Memorial Hospital	Marietta	95%	255
Mercy Hospital Fairfield	Fairfield	95%	144
Saint Luke's Hospital	Maumee	95%	381
Fairfield Medical Center	Lancaster	94%	286
Medical Center at Elizabeth Place	Dayton	94%	98
Saint Joseph Health Center	Warren	94%	302
Springfield Regional Medical Center	Springfield	94%	119
Mercy Regional Medical Center	Lorain	93%	323
The Toledo Hospital	Toledo	93%	627
Flower Hospital	Sylvania	92%	131
Lakewood Hospital	Lakewood	91%	78
Alliance Community Hospital	Alliance	89%	57
Saint Elizabeth Boardman Health Center	Boardman	89%	65
Medcentral Health Sys Mansfield Hosp	Mansfield	88%	357
Memorial Hospital	Fremont	87%	70
Knox Community Hospital	Mount Vernon	86%	120
Licking Memorial Hospital	Newark	85%	40
Samaritan Regional Health System	Ashland	85%	48
Grand Lake Health System	Saint Marys	84%	25

Urinary Catheter Removal

Hospital Name	City	Rate	Cases
Ashtabula County Medical Center	Ashtabula	100%	65
Aultman Hospital[2]	Canton	100%	566
Berger Hospital	Circleville	100%	227
Community Hospitals & Wellness Centers	Bryan	100%	37
Dayton VA Medical Center[2]	Dayton	100%	33
Doctors Hospital[2]	Columbus	100%	323
East Liverpool City Hospital	East Liverpool	100%	38
Firelands Regional Medical Center[2]	Sandusky	100%	299
Fisher - Titus Hospital	Norwalk	100%	252
Flower Hospital[2]	Sylvania	100%	259
Fort Hamilton Hughes Memorial Hospital	Hamilton	100%	178
Grant Medical Center[2]	Columbus	100%	519
Henry County Hospital	Napoleon	100%	43
Hocking Valley Community Hospital	Logan	100%	42
Institute For Orthopaedic Surgery[2]	Lima	100%	39
Licking Memorial Hospital	Newark	100%	244
Lutheran Hospital[2]	Cleveland	100%	303
Marion General Hospital[2]	Marion	100%	234
Marymount Hospital[2]	Garfield Heights	100%	245
Mercer County Joint Twp Comm Hosp	Coldwater	100%	90
Mercy Allen Hospital	Oberlin	100%	54
Mercy Hospital Anderson[2]	Cincinnati	100%	521
Mercy Memorial Hospital	Urbana	100%	47
Mercy Saint Anne Hospital[2]	Toledo	100%	164
Pomerene Hospital	Millersburg	100%	88
Samaritan Regional Health System	Ashland	100%	389
Southern Ohio Medical Center	Portsmouth	100%	336
Surgical Hospital at Southwoods	Youngstown	100%	285
Trihealth Evendale Hospital[3]	Cincinnati	100%	128
UH Geauga Medical Center[2]	Chardon	100%	353
University Hospitals Ahuja Medical Center	Beachwood	100%	421
Univ Hosps Conneaut Med Ctr	Conneaut	100%	118
Affinity Medical Center	Massillon	99%	533
Atrium Medical Center[2]	Franklin	99%	265
Crystal Clinic Orthopaedic Center[2]	Akron	99%	92
Euclid Hospital[2]	Euclid	99%	185
Good Samaritan Hospital[2]	Dayton	99%	355
Kettering Medical Center[2]	Kettering	99%	1582
Lake Health[2]	Concord	99%	260
Lakewood Hospital[2]	Lakewood	99%	576
Medina Hospital[2]	Medina	99%	445
Memorial Hospital	Fremont	99%	156
Miami Valley Hospital[2]	Dayton	99%	416
Riverside Methodist Hospital[2]	Columbus	99%	812
Saint John Medical Center[2]	Westlake	99%	339
Saint Luke's Hospital[2]	Maumee	99%	202
Selby General Hospital[2]	Marietta	99%	244
South Pointe Hospital	Warrensville Hgts	99%	295
Summa Western Reserve Hospital[2]	Cuyahoga Falls	99%	174
Union Hospital[2]	Dover	99%	251
University Hospitals Case Medical Center[2]	Cleveland	99%	461
Adena Regional Medical Center[2]	Chillicothe	98%	253
Bay Park Community Hospital	Oregon	98%	262
Blanchard Valley Hospital[2]	Findlay	98%	323
Cleveland - Wade Park VA Medical Center[2]	Cleveland	98%	294
Cleveland Clinic[2]	Cleveland	98%	381
Fairfield Medical Center[2]	Lancaster	98%	464
Fairview Hospital[2]	Cleveland	98%	329
Grandview Hospital & Medical Center[2]	Dayton	98%	250
Greene Memorial Hospital	Xenia	98%	101
Hillcrest Hospital[2]	Mayfield Heights	98%	282
Lima Memorial Health System[2]	Lima	98%	184
Marietta Memorial Hospital	Marietta	98%	126
Mary Rutan Hospital	Bellefontaine	98%	106
Mercy Hospital Fairfield[2]	Fairfield	98%	451
Mercy Medical Center[2]	Canton	98%	442
Metrohealth System[2]	Cleveland	98%	524
Mount Carmel New Albany Surgical Hospital[2]	New Albany	98%	260
Parma Community General Hospital	Parma	98%	860
Saint Elizabeth Boardman Health Center[2]	Boardman	98%	309
Saint Vincent Charity Medical Center[2]	Cleveland	98%	318
Southwest General Health Center[2]	Middleburg Hgts	98%	669
The Toledo Hospital[2]	Toledo	98%	427
Trinity Med Ctr East & West	Steubenville	98%	312
UHHS Richmond Heights Hospital	Richmond Hghts	98%	164
Van Wert County Hospital	Van Wert	98%	55
Wayne Hospital	Greenville	98%	97
West Chester Hospital	West Chester	98%	815
Akron General Medical Center[2]	Akron	97%	311
Alliance Community Hospital[2]	Alliance	97%	61
Bucyrus Community Hospital	Bucyrus	97%	87
Christ Hospital[2]	Cincinnati	97%	491
Dublin Methodist Hospital	Dublin	97%	157
East Ohio Regional Hospital	Martins Ferry	97%	278
Good Samaritan Hospital[2]	Cincinnati	97%	267
Grady Memorial Hospital	Delaware	97%	120
H B Magruder Memorial Hospital	Port Clinton	97%	66
Holzer Medical Center Jackson	Jackson	97%	94
Mercy Hospital of Defiance	Defiance	97%	35
Mercy Saint Vincent Medical Center[2]	Toledo	97%	338
Northside Medical Center	Youngstown	97%	344
O'Bleness Memorial Hospital	Athens	97%	155
Ohio Valley Medical Center	Springfield	97%	250
Southwest Regional Medical Center	Georgetown	97%	32
Wilson Memorial Hospital	Sidney	97%	62
Wood County Hospital	Bowling Green	97%	223
Bellevue Hospital	Bellevue	96%	74
Bethesda North[2]	Cincinnati	96%	259
Clinton Memorial Hospital	Wilmington	96%	102
Mercy Hospital Clermont[2]	Batavia	96%	215
Mercy Regional Medical Center[2]	Lorain	96%	337
Robinson Memorial Hospital[2]	Ravenna	96%	240
Sycamore Medical Center[2]	Miamisburg	96%	212
University of Cincinnati Medical Center[2]	Cincinnati	96%	254
University of Toledo Medical Center[2]	Toledo	96%	281
Genesis Healthcare System[2]	Zanesville	95%	201
Madison County Hospital	London	95%	79
Mount Carmel Saint Ann's[2]	Westerville	95%	293
Mount Carmel West[2]	Columbus	95%	677
Ohio State University Hospitals[2]	Columbus	95%	338
Saint Joseph Health Center[2]	Warren	95%	265
Salem Regional Medical Center	Salem	95%	163
Univ Hosps-Elyria Med Ctr[2]	Elyria	95%	306
Upper Valley Medical Center	Troy	95%	86
Defiance Regional Medical Center[2]	Defiance	94%	36
Indu & Raj Soin Medical Center	Beaver Creek	94%	48
Mercy Health - West Hospital[2]	Cincinnati	94%	94
Medcentral Health Sys Mansfield Hosp	Mansfield	93%	384
Memorial Hospital of Union County	Marysville	93%	70
Mercy Willard Hospital	Willard	93%	44
Saint Elizabeth Health Center[2]	Youngstown	93%	347
Summa Health Systems Hospitals[2]	Akron	93%	231
Trumbull Memorial Hospital	Warren	93%	242
Wooster Community Hospital	Wooster	93%	56
Galion Community Hospital	Galion	92%	98
Knox Community Hospital	Mount Vernon	92%	236
Mercy Tiffin Hospital	Tiffin	92%	26
Grand Lake Health System	Saint Marys	91%	80
Holzer Medical Center	Gallipolis	91%	112
McCullough - Hyde Memorial Hospital	Oxford	91%	134
Saint Rita's Medical Center	Lima	89%	434
Southeastern Ohio Regional Medical Center	Cambridge	89%	102
Springfield Regional Medical Center	Springfield	89%	344
Mercy Saint Charles Hospital[2]	Oregon	88%	138
Jewish Hospital[2]	Cincinnati	86%	132
Summa Health System Barberton Hospital	Barberton	85%	138
Wyandot Memorial Hospital	Upper Sandusky	80%	30
Fulton County Health Center[2]	Wauseon	77%	31
Coshocton County Memorial Hospital	Coshocton	53%	34

Survey of Patients' Hospital Experiences

Area Around Room 'Always' Quiet at Night

Hospital Name	City	Rate	Cases
Surgical Hospital at Southwoods	Youngstown	84%	300+
Mount Carmel New Albany Surgical Hospital	New Albany	80%	300+
Bluffton Hospital	Bluffton	79%	(a)
Institute For Orthopaedic Surgery	Lima	79%	300+
Ohio Valley Medical Center	Springfield	79%	300+
Dublin Methodist Hospital	Dublin	76%	300+
Univ Hosps Conneaut Med Ctr	Conneaut	75%	(a)
Medical Center at Elizabeth Place	Dayton	74%	(a)
Mercy Willard Hospital	Willard	74%	(a)
Hardin Memorial Hospital	Kenton	71%	(a)
Fostoria Community Hospital	Fostoria	70%	(a)
Holzer Medical Center Jackson	Jackson	70%	(a)
West Chester Hospital	West Chester	70%	300+
Henry County Hospital	Napoleon	69%	(a)
Wood County Hospital	Bowling Green	69%	300+
Blanchard Valley Hospital	Findlay	68%	300+
Defiance Regional Medical Center	Defiance	68%	300+
Hocking Valley Community Hospital	Logan	68%	(a)
Indu & Raj Soin Medical Center	Beaver Creek	68%	300+
Southern Ohio Medical Center	Portsmouth	68%	300+
Community Memorial Hospital	Hicksville	67%	(a)
H B Magruder Memorial Hospital	Port Clinton	67%	300+
Saint Vincent Charity Medical Center	Cleveland	67%	300+
Doctors Hospital	Columbus	66%	300+
Memorial Hospital of Union County	Marysville	65%	300+
Morrow County Hospital	Mount Gilead	65%	(a)
Southeastern Ohio Regional Medical Center	Cambridge	65%	300+
Wooster Community Hospital	Wooster	65%	300+
Euclid Hospital	Euclid	64%	300+
Lutheran Hospital	Cleveland	64%	300+
Madison County Hospital	London	64%	(a)
Medcentral Health System Shelby Hospital	Shelby	64%	(a)
Mercy Hospital Fairfield	Fairfield	64%	300+
Atrium Medical Center[11]	Franklin	63%	300+
Aultman Orrville Hospital	Orrville	63%	(a)
Bellevue Hospital	Bellevue	63%	300+
Community Hospitals & Wellness Centers	Bryan	63%	300+
UHHS Memorial Hospital of Geneva	Geneva	63%	(a)
Mercy Hospital Clermont	Batavia	62%	300+
Mercy Hospital of Defiance	Defiance	62%	300+
Mercy Saint Anne Hospital	Toledo	62%	300+
Mercy Tiffin Hospital	Tiffin	62%	300+
Bay Park Community Hospital	Oregon	61%	300+
Grady Memorial Hospital	Delaware	61%	300+
Medcentral Health Sys Mansfield Hosp	Mansfield	61%	300+
Christ Hospital	Cincinnati	60%	300+
Fairview Hospital	Cleveland	60%	300+
Galion Community Hospital	Galion	60%	300+
Jewish Hospital	Cincinnati	60%	300+
Pomerene Hospital	Millersburg	60%	300+
Saint Elizabeth Boardman Health Center	Boardman	60%	300+
Samaritan Regional Health System	Ashland	60%	300+
Wilson Memorial Hospital[11]	Sidney	60%	300+
Good Samaritan Hospital	Cincinnati	59%	300+
Grand Lake Health System	Saint Marys	59%	300+
Miami Valley Hospital[11]	Dayton	59%	300+
Ohio State University Hospitals	Columbus	59%	300+
University of Cincinnati Medical Center	Cincinnati	59%	300+
Alliance Community Hospital	Alliance	58%	300+
Clinton Memorial Hospital	Wilmington	58%	300+
Grant Medical Center	Columbus	58%	300+
Licking Memorial Hospital	Newark	58%	300+
Marion General Hospital	Marion	58%	300+
Mary Rutan Hospital	Bellefontaine	58%	300+
McCullough - Hyde Memorial Hospital	Oxford	58%	300+
Medina Hospital	Medina	58%	300+
Memorial Hospital	Fremont	58%	300+
Univ Hosps-Elyria Med Ctr	Elyria	58%	300+
Van Wert County Hospital	Van Wert	58%	300+
Barnesville Hospital Association	Barnesville	57%	(a)
Cleveland Clinic	Cleveland	57%	300+
Crystal Clinic Orthopaedic Center	Akron	57%	300+
Fort Hamilton Hughes Memorial Hospital	Hamilton	57%	300+
Kettering Medical Center	Kettering	57%	300+
Mercy Saint Vincent Medical Center	Toledo	57%	300+
Saint Luke's Hospital	Maumee	57%	300+
Saint Rita's Medical Center	Lima	57%	300+
South Pointe Hospital	Warrensville Hgts	57%	300+
Summa Western Reserve Hospital	Cuyahoga Falls	57%	300+
The Toledo Hospital	Toledo	57%	300+
University Hospitals Case Medical Center	Cleveland	57%	300+
Wayne Hospital	Greenville	57%	300+
Adams County Regional Medical Center	Seaman	56%	(a)
Bucyrus Community Hospital	Bucyrus	56%	(a)
Fisher - Titus Hospital	Norwalk	56%	300+
Holzer Medical Center	Gallipolis	56%	300+
O'Bleness Memorial Hospital	Athens	56%	300+

NOTE: Hospital profiles are in alphabetical order by state, then city, then hospital within the city; Rankings exclude hospitals with less than 25 cases except for patient surveys which excludes hospitals with less than 100 cases; (a) 100-299 cases; (1) The number of cases/patients is too few to report; (2) Data submitted were based on a sample of cases/patients; (3) Results are based on a shorter time period than required; (4) Data suppressed by CMS for one or more quarters; (5) Results are not available for this reporting period; (6) Fewer than 100 patients completed the HCAHPS survey; (7) No cases met the criteria for this measure; (8) The lower limit of the confidence interval cannot be calculated if the number of observed infections equals zero; (9) No data are available from the state/territory for this reporting period; (10) The scores shown reflect fewer than 50 completed surveys; (11) There were discrepancies in the data collection process; (12) This measure does not apply to this hospital for this reporting period; (13) Results cannot be calculated for this reporting period; (14) The results for this state are combined with nearby states to protect confidentiality; Please refer to the User's Guide for a full explanation of data.

Selby General Hospital	Marietta	56%	300+
Mercer County Joint Twp Comm Hosp	Coldwater	55%	300+
Mercy Regional Medical Center[11]	Lorain	55%	300+
Mercy Saint Charles Hospital	Oregon	55%	300+
Sycamore Medical Center	Miamisburg	55%	300+
University Hospitals Ahuja Medical Center	Beachwood	55%	300+
Wyandot Memorial Hospital	Upper Sandusky	55%	(a)
Firelands Regional Medical Center	Sandusky	54%	300+
Fulton County Health Center	Wauseon	54%	300+
Lake Health	Concord	54%	300+
Lima Memorial Health System	Lima	54%	300+
Mercy Allen Hospital	Oberlin	54%	(a)
Metrohealth System	Cleveland	54%	300+
Mount Carmel Saint Ann's	Westerville	54%	300+
Saint John Medical Center	Westlake	54%	300+
Springfield Regional Medical Center	Springfield	54%	300+
Upper Valley Medical Center[11]	Troy	54%	300+
Affinity Medical Center	Massillon	53%	300+
Flower Hospital	Sylvania	53%	300+
Grandview Hospital & Medical Center	Dayton	53%	300+
Greene Memorial Hospital	Xenia	53%	300+
James Cancer Hosp & Solove Res Inst	Columbus	53%	300+
Lakewood Hospital	Lakewood	53%	300+
Mercy Hospital Anderson	Cincinnati	53%	300+
Riverside Methodist Hospital	Columbus	53%	300+
Southwest Regional Medical Center	Georgetown	53%	(a)
University of Toledo Medical Center	Toledo	53%	300+
Akron General Medical Center	Akron	52%	300+
Berger Hospital	Circleville	52%	300+
Bethesda North	Cincinnati	52%	300+
Coshocton County Memorial Hospital	Coshocton	52%	300+
East Liverpool City Hospital	East Liverpool	52%	300+
Fayette County Memorial Hospital	Washington Ch	52%	(a)
Good Samaritan Hospital[11]	Dayton	52%	300+
Highland District Hospital	Hillsboro	52%	(a)
Hillcrest Hospital	Mayfield Heights	52%	300+
Knox Community Hospital	Mount Vernon	52%	300+
Mercy Health - West Hospital	Cincinnati	52%	300+
Mount Carmel West	Columbus	52%	300+
Trinity Med Ctr East & West	Steubenville	52%	300+
UH Geauga Medical Center	Chardon	52%	300+
Aultman Hospital	Canton	51%	300+
Marymount Hospital	Garfield Heights	51%	300+
Robinson Memorial Hospital	Ravenna	51%	300+
Trumbull Memorial Hospital	Warren	51%	300+
UHHS Richmond Heights Hospital	Richmond Hghts	51%	300+
Union Hospital	Dover	51%	300+
Adena Regional Medical Center	Chillicothe	50%	300+
Ashtabula County Medical Center	Ashtabula	50%	300+
East Ohio Regional Hospital	Martins Ferry	50%	300+
Marietta Memorial Hospital	Marietta	50%	300+
Northside Medical Center	Youngstown	50%	300+
Saint Joseph Health Center	Warren	50%	300+
Fairfield Medical Center	Lancaster	48%	300+
Genesis Healthcare System	Zanesville	48%	300+
Parma Community General Hospital	Parma	47%	300+
Pike Community Hospital	Waverly	47%	(a)
Saint Elizabeth Health Center	Youngstown	47%	300+
Summa Health Systems Hospitals	Akron	47%	300+
Mercy Memorial Hospital	Urbana	46%	(a)
Salem Regional Medical Center	Salem	46%	300+
Mercy Medical Center	Canton	45%	300+
Summa Health System Barberton Hospital	Barberton	43%	300+
Southwest General Health Center	Middleburg Hgts	42%	300+
Summa Wadsworth - Rittman Hospital	Wadsworth	40%	300+

Doctors 'Always' Communicated Well

Hospital Name	City	Rate	Cases
H B Magruder Memorial Hospital	Port Clinton	91%	300+
Surgical Hospital at Southwoods	Youngstown	91%	300+
Mercy Willard Hospital	Willard	90%	(a)
Henry County Hospital	Napoleon	89%	(a)
Bluffton Hospital	Bluffton	88%	(a)
Community Memorial Hospital	Hicksville	88%	(a)
Institute For Orthopaedic Surgery	Lima	88%	300+
Bellevue Hospital	Bellevue	86%	300+
Defiance Regional Medical Center	Defiance	86%	300+
Fayette County Memorial Hospital	Washington Ch	86%	(a)
Hocking Valley Community Hospital	Logan	86%	(a)
Mercy Hospital of Defiance	Defiance	86%	300+
Aultman Orrville Hospital	Orrville	85%	(a)
Christ Hospital	Cincinnati	85%	300+
Fostoria Community Hospital	Fostoria	85%	(a)
Mount Carmel New Albany Surgical Hospital	New Albany	85%	300+
Univ Hosps Conneaut Med Ctr	Conneaut	85%	(a)
Barnesville Hospital Association	Barnesville	84%	(a)
Blanchard Valley Hospital	Findlay	84%	300+
Bucyrus Community Hospital	Bucyrus	84%	(a)
Community Hospitals & Wellness Centers	Bryan	84%	300+
Crystal Clinic Orthopaedic Center	Akron	84%	300+
Dublin Methodist Hospital	Dublin	84%	300+
Madison County Hospital	London	84%	(a)
Mary Rutan Hospital	Bellefontaine	84%	300+
Medcentral Health System Shelby Hospital	Shelby	84%	(a)
Memorial Hospital	Fremont	84%	300+
Samaritan Regional Health System	Ashland	84%	300+
Southern Ohio Medical Center	Portsmouth	84%	300+
UHHS Memorial Hospital of Geneva	Geneva	84%	(a)
James Cancer Hosp & Solove Res Inst	Columbus	83%	300+
McCullough - Hyde Memorial Hospital	Oxford	83%	300+
Morrow County Hospital	Mount Gilead	83%	(a)
Pomerene Hospital	Millersburg	83%	300+
Wood County Hospital	Bowling Green	83%	300+
Cleveland Clinic	Cleveland	82%	300+
Fairfield Medical Center	Lancaster	82%	300+
Fulton County Health Center	Wauseon	82%	300+
Galion Community Hospital	Galion	82%	300+
Grady Memorial Hospital	Delaware	82%	300+
Hardin Memorial Hospital	Kenton	82%	(a)
Lutheran Hospital	Cleveland	82%	300+
Medina Hospital	Medina	82%	300+
Mercer County Joint Twp Comm Hosp	Coldwater	82%	300+
Mercy Hospital Clermont	Batavia	82%	300+
Mercy Hospital Fairfield	Fairfield	82%	300+
O'Bleness Memorial Hospital	Athens	82%	300+
Ohio Valley Medical Center	Springfield	82%	300+
Pike Community Hospital	Waverly	82%	(a)
Saint Elizabeth Boardman Health Center	Boardman	82%	300+
Union Hospital	Dover	82%	300+
West Chester Hospital	West Chester	82%	300+
Wilson Memorial Hospital[11]	Sidney	82%	300+
Adams County Regional Medical Center	Seaman	81%	(a)
Alliance Community Hospital	Alliance	81%	300+
Good Samaritan Hospital	Cincinnati	81%	300+
Holzer Medical Center Jackson	Jackson	81%	(a)
Memorial Hospital of Union County	Marysville	81%	300+
Saint Vincent Charity Medical Center	Cleveland	81%	300+
Selby General Hospital	Marietta	81%	300+
Summa Western Reserve Hospital	Cuyahoga Falls	81%	300+
UH Geauga Medical Center	Chardon	81%	300+
Wooster Community Hospital	Wooster	81%	300+
Atrium Medical Center[11]	Franklin	80%	300+
Berger Hospital	Circleville	80%	300+
Firelands Regional Medical Center	Sandusky	80%	300+
Fisher - Titus Hospital	Norwalk	80%	300+
Grand Lake Health System	Saint Marys	80%	300+
Grandview Hospital & Medical Center	Dayton	80%	300+
Grant Medical Center	Columbus	80%	300+
Highland District Hospital	Hillsboro	80%	(a)
Holzer Medical Center	Gallipolis	80%	300+
Marion General Hospital	Marion	80%	300+
Mercy Tiffin Hospital	Tiffin	80%	300+
Northside Medical Center	Youngstown	80%	300+
South Pointe Hospital	Warrensville Hgts	80%	300+
Southeastern Ohio Regional Medical Center	Cambridge	80%	300+
UHHS Richmond Heights Hospital	Richmond Hghts	80%	300+
Upper Valley Medical Center[11]	Troy	80%	300+
Van Wert County Hospital	Van Wert	80%	300+
Wayne Hospital	Greenville	80%	300+
Affinity Medical Center	Massillon	79%	300+
Aultman Hospital	Canton	79%	300+
Bethesda North	Cincinnati	79%	300+
Doctors Hospital	Columbus	79%	300+
Euclid Hospital	Euclid	79%	300+
Fairview Hospital	Cleveland	79%	300+
Flower Hospital	Sylvania	79%	300+
Fort Hamilton Hughes Memorial Hospital	Hamilton	79%	300+
Hillcrest Hospital	Mayfield Heights	79%	300+
Kettering Medical Center	Kettering	79%	300+
Licking Memorial Hospital	Newark	79%	300+
Marymount Hospital	Garfield Heights	79%	300+
Medical Center at Elizabeth Place	Dayton	79%	(a)
Mercy Health - West Hospital	Cincinnati	79%	300+
Mercy Saint Anne Hospital	Toledo	79%	300+
Mount Carmel West	Columbus	79%	300+
Ohio State University Hospitals	Columbus	79%	300+
Parma Community General Hospital	Parma	79%	300+
Riverside Methodist Hospital	Columbus	79%	300+
Robinson Memorial Hospital	Ravenna	79%	300+
Saint Joseph Health Center	Warren	79%	300+
Southwest General Health Center	Middleburg Hgts	79%	300+
Springfield Regional Medical Center	Springfield	79%	300+
Sycamore Medical Center	Miamisburg	79%	300+
University Hospitals Ahuja Medical Center	Beachwood	79%	300+
University Hospitals Case Medical Center	Cleveland	79%	300+
Ashtabula County Medical Center	Ashtabula	78%	300+
Bay Park Community Hospital	Oregon	78%	300+
Clinton Memorial Hospital	Wilmington	78%	300+
Indu & Raj Soin Medical Center	Beaver Creek	78%	300+
Jewish Hospital	Cincinnati	78%	300+
Medcentral Health Sys Mansfield Hosp	Mansfield	78%	300+
Saint Elizabeth Health Center	Youngstown	78%	300+
Saint Luke's Hospital	Maumee	78%	300+
Salem Regional Medical Center	Salem	78%	300+
The Toledo Hospital	Toledo	78%	300+
Adena Regional Medical Center	Chillicothe	77%	300+
Akron General Medical Center	Akron	77%	300+
East Liverpool City Hospital	East Liverpool	77%	300+
East Ohio Regional Hospital	Martins Ferry	77%	300+
Good Samaritan Hospital[11]	Dayton	77%	300+
Marietta Memorial Hospital	Marietta	77%	300+
Mercy Hospital Anderson	Cincinnati	77%	300+
Miami Valley Hospital[11]	Dayton	77%	300+
Summa Health System Barberton Hospital	Barberton	77%	300+
Trinity Med Ctr East & West	Steubenville	77%	300+
Trumbull Memorial Hospital	Warren	77%	300+
Univ Hosps-Elyria Med Ctr	Elyria	77%	300+
Coshocton County Memorial Hospital	Coshocton	76%	300+
Lake Health	Concord	76%	300+
Mercy Medical Center	Canton	76%	300+
Mercy Memorial Hospital	Urbana	76%	(a)
Mercy Regional Medical Center[11]	Lorain	76%	300+
Metrohealth System	Cleveland	76%	300+
Mount Carmel Saint Ann's	Westerville	76%	300+
Saint Rita's Medical Center	Lima	76%	300+
Summa Health Systems Hospitals	Akron	76%	300+
Knox Community Hospital	Mount Vernon	75%	300+
Lakewood Hospital	Lakewood	75%	300+
Mercy Saint Vincent Medical Center	Toledo	75%	300+
Saint John Medical Center	Westlake	75%	300+
Summa Wadsworth - Rittman Hospital	Wadsworth	75%	300+
University of Cincinnati Medical Center	Cincinnati	75%	300+
Greene Memorial Hospital	Xenia	74%	300+
Lima Memorial Health System	Lima	74%	300+
Mercy Allen Hospital	Oberlin	74%	(a)
Mercy Saint Charles Hospital	Oregon	74%	300+
Southwest Regional Medical Center	Georgetown	74%	(a)
Genesis Healthcare System	Zanesville	73%	300+
University of Toledo Medical Center	Toledo	71%	300+
Wyandot Memorial Hospital	Upper Sandusky	71%	(a)

Home Recovery Information Given

Hospital Name	City	Rate	Cases
Bluffton Hospital	Bluffton	95%	(a)
Community Memorial Hospital	Hicksville	94%	(a)
Defiance Regional Medical Center	Defiance	93%	300+
Henry County Hospital	Napoleon	93%	(a)
Institute For Orthopaedic Surgery	Lima	93%	300+
UHHS Memorial Hospital of Geneva	Geneva	93%	(a)
Crystal Clinic Orthopaedic Center	Akron	92%	300+
Mount Carmel New Albany Surgical Hospital	New Albany	92%	300+
Surgical Hospital at Southwoods	Youngstown	92%	300+
Upper Valley Medical Center[11]	Troy	92%	300+
Euclid Hospital	Euclid	91%	300+
Galion Community Hospital	Galion	91%	300+
Good Samaritan Hospital[11]	Dayton	91%	300+
Hocking Valley Community Hospital	Logan	91%	(a)
Lutheran Hospital	Cleveland	91%	300+
Univ Hosps Conneaut Med Ctr	Conneaut	91%	(a)
Wilson Memorial Hospital[11]	Sidney	91%	300+
Wood County Hospital	Bowling Green	91%	300+
Bellevue Hospital	Bellevue	90%	300+
Cleveland Clinic	Cleveland	90%	300+
Fayette County Memorial Hospital	Washington Ch	90%	(a)
James Cancer Hosp & Solove Res Inst	Columbus	90%	300+
Medina Hospital	Medina	90%	300+
Mercy Hospital Fairfield	Fairfield	90%	300+
Miami Valley Hospital[11]	Dayton	90%	300+
Saint Vincent Charity Medical Center	Cleveland	90%	300+
Atrium Medical Center[11]	Franklin	89%	300+
Bethesda North	Cincinnati	89%	300+
Christ Hospital	Cincinnati	89%	300+
Doctors Hospital	Columbus	89%	300+
Dublin Methodist Hospital	Dublin	89%	300+
Flower Hospital	Sylvania	89%	300+
Grady Memorial Hospital	Delaware	89%	300+
Holzer Medical Center Jackson	Jackson	89%	(a)
Memorial Hospital of Union County	Marysville	89%	300+
Mercy Hospital Clermont	Batavia	89%	300+
Morrow County Hospital	Mount Gilead	89%	(a)
Samaritan Regional Health System	Ashland	89%	300+
Selby General Hospital	Marietta	89%	300+
Southeastern Ohio Regional Medical Center	Cambridge	89%	300+
Southern Ohio Medical Center	Portsmouth	89%	300+
The Toledo Hospital	Toledo	89%	300+
UH Geauga Medical Center	Chardon	89%	300+
Wooster Community Hospital	Wooster	89%	300+
Barnesville Hospital Association	Barnesville	88%	(a)
Bay Park Community Hospital	Oregon	88%	300+
Berger Hospital	Circleville	88%	300+
Community Hospitals & Wellness Centers	Bryan	88%	300+
Fairfield Medical Center	Lancaster	88%	300+
Fisher - Titus Hospital	Norwalk	88%	300+

NOTE: Hospital profiles are in alphabetical order by state, then city, then hospital within the city; Rankings exclude hospitals with less than 25 cases except for patient surveys which excludes hospitals with less than 100 cases; (a) 100-299 cases; (1) The number of cases/patients is too few to report; (2) Data submitted were based on a sample of cases/patients; (3) Results are based on a shorter time period than required; (4) Data suppressed by CMS for one or more quarters; (5) Results are not available for this reporting period; (6) Fewer than 100 patients completed the HCAHPS survey; (7) No cases met the criteria for this measure; (8) The lower limit of the confidence interval cannot be calculated if the number of observed infections equals zero; (9) No data are available from the state/territory for this reporting period; (10) The scores shown reflect fewer than 50 completed surveys; (11) There were discrepancies in the data collection process; (12) This measure does not apply to this hospital for this reporting period; (13) Results cannot be calculated for this reporting period; (14) The results for this state are combined with nearby states to protect confidentiality; Please refer to the User's Guide for a full explanation of data.

Hospital Name	City	Rate	Cases
Fostoria Community Hospital	Fostoria	88%	(a)
Good Samaritan Hospital	Cincinnati	88%	300+
Grant Medical Center	Columbus	88%	300+
Lima Memorial Health System	Lima	88%	300+
Marietta Memorial Hospital	Marietta	88%	300+
Memorial Hospital	Fremont	88%	300+
Mercer County Joint Twp Comm Hosp	Coldwater	88%	300+
Mercy Hospital of Defiance	Defiance	88%	300+
Mercy Saint Anne Hospital	Toledo	88%	300+
Mercy Willard Hospital	Willard	88%	(a)
Ohio Valley Medical Center	Springfield	88%	300+
Saint Joseph Health Center	Warren	88%	300+
Summa Western Reserve Hospital	Cuyahoga Falls	88%	300+
Trinity Med Ctr East & West	Steubenville	88%	300+
Affinity Medical Center	Massillon	87%	300+
Bucyrus Community Hospital	Bucyrus	87%	(a)
Hardin Memorial Hospital	Kenton	87%	(a)
Kettering Medical Center	Kettering	87%	300+
Lake Health	Concord	87%	300+
Lakewood Hospital	Lakewood	87%	300+
Marion General Hospital	Marion	87%	300+
Mercy Regional Medical Center[11]	Lorain	87%	300+
Mercy Saint Vincent Medical Center	Toledo	87%	300+
Mount Carmel Saint Ann's	Westerville	87%	300+
Mount Carmel West	Columbus	87%	300+
Ohio State University Hospitals	Columbus	87%	300+
Pomerene Hospital	Millersburg	87%	300+
Saint Rita's Medical Center	Lima	87%	300+
Southwest General Health Center	Middleburg Hgts	87%	300+
University Hospitals Case Medical Center	Cleveland	87%	300+
Akron General Medical Center	Akron	86%	300+
Alliance Community Hospital	Alliance	86%	300+
Genesis Healthcare System	Zanesville	86%	300+
Grandview Hospital & Medical Center	Dayton	86%	300+
H B Magruder Memorial Hospital	Port Clinton	86%	300+
Knox Community Hospital	Mount Vernon	86%	300+
Mary Rutan Hospital	Bellefontaine	86%	300+
McCullough - Hyde Memorial Hospital	Oxford	86%	300+
Medical Center at Elizabeth Place	Dayton	86%	(a)
Mercy Memorial Hospital	Urbana	86%	(a)
Mercy Saint Charles Hospital	Oregon	86%	300+
Northside Medical Center	Youngstown	86%	300+
Riverside Methodist Hospital	Columbus	86%	300+
Saint John Medical Center	Westlake	86%	300+
South Pointe Hospital	Warrensville Hgts	86%	300+
Summa Wadsworth - Rittman Hospital	Wadsworth	86%	300+
Sycamore Medical Center	Miamisburg	86%	300+
Trumbull Memorial Hospital	Warren	86%	300+
UHHS Richmond Heights Hospital	Richmond Hghts	86%	300+
Van Wert County Hospital	Van Wert	86%	300+
West Chester Hospital	West Chester	86%	300+
Blanchard Valley Hospital	Findlay	85%	300+
Clinton Memorial Hospital	Wilmington	85%	300+
Fairview Hospital	Cleveland	85%	300+
Grand Lake Health System	Saint Marys	85%	300+
Madison County Hospital	London	85%	(a)
Marymount Hospital	Garfield Heights	85%	300+
Medcentral Health Sys Mansfield Hosp	Mansfield	85%	300+
Medcentral Health System Shelby Hospital	Shelby	85%	(a)
Mercy Medical Center	Canton	85%	300+
O'Bleness Memorial Hospital	Athens	85%	300+
Saint Luke's Hospital	Maumee	85%	300+
Summa Health Systems Hospitals	Akron	85%	300+
Univ Hosps-Elyria Med Ctr	Elyria	85%	300+
Adena Regional Medical Center	Chillicothe	84%	300+
Ashtabula County Medical Center	Ashtabula	84%	300+
Aultman Hospital	Canton	84%	300+
Firelands Regional Medical Center	Sandusky	84%	300+
Fort Hamilton Hughes Memorial Hospital	Hamilton	84%	300+
Fulton County Health Center	Wauseon	84%	300+
Greene Memorial Hospital	Xenia	84%	300+
Holzer Medical Center	Gallipolis	84%	300+
Indu & Raj Soin Medical Center	Beaver Creek	84%	300+
Licking Memorial Hospital	Newark	84%	300+
Mercy Hospital Anderson	Cincinnati	84%	300+
Metrohealth System	Cleveland	84%	300+
Parma Community General Hospital	Parma	84%	300+
Springfield Regional Medical Center	Springfield	84%	300+
University Hospitals Ahuja Medical Center	Beachwood	84%	300+
Wyandot Memorial Hospital	Upper Sandusky	84%	(a)
Aultman Orrville Hospital	Orrville	83%	(a)
Highland District Hospital	Hillsboro	83%	(a)
Hillcrest Hospital	Mayfield Heights	83%	300+
Jewish Hospital	Cincinnati	83%	300+
Mercy Allen Hospital	Oberlin	83%	(a)
Mercy Health - West Hospital	Cincinnati	83%	300+
Mercy Tiffin Hospital	Tiffin	83%	300+
Union Hospital	Dover	83%	300+
University of Cincinnati Medical Center	Cincinnati	83%	300+
Wayne Hospital	Greenville	83%	300+
Adams County Regional Medical Center	Seaman	82%	(a)
East Ohio Regional Hospital	Martins Ferry	82%	300+
East Liverpool City Hospital	East Liverpool	81%	300+
Saint Elizabeth Boardman Health Center	Boardman	81%	300+
Saint Elizabeth Health Center	Youngstown	81%	300+
Salem Regional Medical Center	Salem	81%	300+
University of Toledo Medical Center	Toledo	81%	300+
Coshocton County Memorial Hospital	Coshocton	79%	300+
Pike Community Hospital	Waverly	79%	(a)
Robinson Memorial Hospital	Ravenna	79%	300+
Summa Health System Barberton Hospital	Barberton	79%	300+
Southwest Regional Medical Center	Georgetown	74%	(a)

Hospital Given 9 or 10 on 10 Point Scale

Hospital Name	City	Rate	Cases
Surgical Hospital at Southwoods	Youngstown	95%	300+
Institute For Orthopaedic Surgery	Lima	92%	300+
Bluffton Hospital	Bluffton	91%	(a)
Mount Carmel New Albany Surgical Hospital	New Albany	88%	300+
Community Memorial Hospital	Hicksville	87%	(a)
Mercy Willard Hospital	Willard	87%	(a)
Univ Hosps Conneaut Med Ctr	Conneaut	87%	(a)
Dublin Methodist Hospital	Dublin	86%	300+
Cleveland Clinic	Cleveland	84%	300+
H B Magruder Memorial Hospital	Port Clinton	84%	300+
Bellevue Hospital	Bellevue	83%	300+
Christ Hospital	Cincinnati	83%	300+
Defiance Regional Medical Center	Defiance	83%	300+
Henry County Hospital	Napoleon	83%	(a)
Mercy Hospital Fairfield	Fairfield	82%	300+
Ohio Valley Medical Center	Springfield	82%	300+
Indu & Raj Soin Medical Center	Beaver Creek	81%	300+
Community Hospitals & Wellness Centers	Bryan	80%	300+
Hocking Valley Community Hospital	Logan	80%	(a)
James Cancer Hosp & Solove Res Inst	Columbus	80%	300+
Medcentral Health System Shelby Hospital	Shelby	80%	(a)
Saint Elizabeth Boardman Health Center	Boardman	80%	300+
Fostoria Community Hospital	Fostoria	79%	(a)
West Chester Hospital	West Chester	79%	300+
Wooster Community Hospital	Wooster	79%	300+
Blanchard Valley Hospital	Findlay	78%	300+
Memorial Hospital of Union County	Marysville	78%	300+
Mercy Hospital of Defiance	Defiance	78%	300+
Morrow County Hospital	Mount Gilead	78%	(a)
Aultman Hospital	Canton	77%	300+
Barnesville Hospital Association	Barnesville	77%	(a)
Bay Park Community Hospital	Oregon	77%	300+
Fulton County Health Center	Wauseon	77%	300+
Kettering Medical Center	Kettering	77%	300+
Mercy Saint Anne Hospital	Toledo	77%	300+
UHHS Memorial Hospital of Geneva	Geneva	77%	(a)
Wood County Hospital	Bowling Green	77%	300+
Mercy Hospital Clermont	Batavia	76%	300+
Miami Valley Hospital[11]	Dayton	76%	300+
Riverside Methodist Hospital	Columbus	76%	300+
Sycamore Medical Center	Miamisburg	76%	300+
Crystal Clinic Orthopaedic Center	Akron	75%	300+
Flower Hospital	Sylvania	75%	300+
Grant Medical Center	Columbus	75%	300+
Holzer Medical Center Jackson	Jackson	75%	(a)
Summa Western Reserve Hospital	Cuyahoga Falls	75%	300+
Bucyrus Community Hospital	Bucyrus	74%	(a)
Fairview Hospital	Cleveland	74%	300+
Fisher - Titus Hospital	Norwalk	74%	300+
Grady Memorial Hospital	Delaware	74%	300+
Hardin Memorial Hospital	Kenton	74%	(a)
McCullough - Hyde Memorial Hospital	Oxford	74%	300+
Ohio State University Hospitals	Columbus	74%	300+
Southern Ohio Medical Center	Portsmouth	74%	300+
University Hospitals Case Medical Center	Cleveland	74%	300+
Aultman Orrville Hospital	Orrville	73%	(a)
Bethesda North	Cincinnati	73%	300+
Doctors Hospital	Columbus	73%	300+
Good Samaritan Hospital	Cincinnati	73%	300+
Madison County Hospital	London	73%	(a)
Mercer County Joint Twp Comm Hosp	Coldwater	73%	300+
Mercy Allen Hospital	Oberlin	73%	(a)
Mercy Tiffin Hospital	Tiffin	73%	300+
Pomerene Hospital	Millersburg	73%	300+
University Hospitals Ahuja Medical Center	Beachwood	73%	300+
Fairfield Medical Center	Lancaster	72%	300+
Galion Community Hospital	Galion	72%	300+
Grandview Hospital & Medical Center	Dayton	72%	300+
Lutheran Hospital	Cleveland	72%	300+
Mary Rutan Hospital	Bellefontaine	72%	300+
Mercy Saint Vincent Medical Center	Toledo	72%	300+
Saint John Medical Center	Westlake	72%	300+
Saint Rita's Medical Center	Lima	72%	300+
Saint Vincent Charity Medical Center	Cleveland	72%	300+
Selby General Hospital	Marietta	72%	300+
UH Geauga Medical Center	Chardon	72%	300+
Grand Lake Health System	Saint Marys	71%	300+
Mercy Hospital Anderson	Cincinnati	71%	300+
Mount Carmel West	Columbus	71%	300+
Saint Joseph Health Center	Warren	71%	300+
Saint Luke's Hospital	Maumee	71%	300+
Samaritan Regional Health System	Ashland	71%	300+
Akron General Medical Center	Akron	70%	300+
Alliance Community Hospital	Alliance	70%	300+
Atrium Medical Center[11]	Franklin	70%	300+
Firelands Regional Medical Center	Sandusky	70%	300+
Good Samaritan Hospital[11]	Dayton	70%	300+
Medcentral Health Sys Mansfield Hosp	Mansfield	70%	300+
South Pointe Hospital	Warrensville Hgts	70%	300+
The Toledo Hospital	Toledo	70%	300+
Union Hospital	Dover	70%	300+
Univ Hosps-Elyria Med Ctr	Elyria	70%	300+
Upper Valley Medical Center[11]	Troy	70%	300+
Van Wert County Hospital	Van Wert	70%	300+
Euclid Hospital	Euclid	69%	300+
Mercy Medical Center	Canton	69%	300+
Mount Carmel Saint Ann's	Westerville	69%	300+
Southwest General Health Center	Middleburg Hgts	69%	300+
Trinity Med Ctr East & West	Steubenville	69%	300+
Wyandot Memorial Hospital	Upper Sandusky	69%	(a)
Fayette County Memorial Hospital	Washington Ch	68%	(a)
Jewish Hospital	Cincinnati	68%	300+
Lake Health	Concord	68%	300+
Medina Hospital	Medina	68%	300+
Mercy Memorial Hospital	Urbana	68%	(a)
Southeastern Ohio Regional Medical Center	Cambridge	68%	300+
Wilson Memorial Hospital[11]	Sidney	68%	300+
Fort Hamilton Hughes Memorial Hospital	Hamilton	67%	300+
Hillcrest Hospital	Mayfield Heights	67%	300+
Marion General Hospital	Marion	67%	300+
Memorial Hospital	Fremont	67%	300+
Mercy Saint Charles Hospital	Oregon	67%	300+
Adams County Regional Medical Center	Seaman	66%	(a)
Adena Regional Medical Center	Chillicothe	66%	300+
Berger Hospital	Circleville	66%	300+
Lakewood Hospital	Lakewood	66%	300+
Lima Memorial Health System	Lima	66%	300+
Mercy Health - West Hospital	Cincinnati	66%	300+
Summa Health System Barberton Hospital	Barberton	66%	300+
Affinity Medical Center	Massillon	65%	300+
Holzer Medical Center	Gallipolis	65%	300+
Robinson Memorial Hospital	Ravenna	65%	300+
Saint Elizabeth Health Center	Youngstown	65%	300+
Summa Health Systems Hospitals	Akron	65%	300+
UHHS Richmond Heights Hospital	Richmond Hghts	65%	300+
Wayne Hospital	Greenville	65%	300+
East Liverpool City Hospital	East Liverpool	64%	300+
Knox Community Hospital	Mount Vernon	64%	300+
Licking Memorial Hospital	Newark	64%	300+
Marietta Memorial Hospital	Marietta	64%	300+
Marymount Hospital	Garfield Heights	64%	300+
Parma Community General Hospital	Parma	64%	300+
Springfield Regional Medical Center	Springfield	64%	300+
University of Cincinnati Medical Center	Cincinnati	64%	300+
Greene Memorial Hospital	Xenia	63%	300+
Northside Medical Center	Youngstown	63%	300+
East Ohio Regional Hospital	Martins Ferry	62%	300+
Genesis Healthcare System	Zanesville	62%	300+
Medical Center at Elizabeth Place	Dayton	62%	(a)
Mercy Regional Medical Center[11]	Lorain	62%	300+
Metrohealth System	Cleveland	62%	300+
O'Bleness Memorial Hospital	Athens	61%	300+
Salem Regional Medical Center	Salem	61%	300+
Ashtabula County Medical Center	Ashtabula	60%	300+
Clinton Memorial Hospital	Wilmington	60%	300+
Summa Wadsworth - Rittman Hospital	Wadsworth	59%	300+
Coshocton County Memorial Hospital	Coshocton	58%	300+
Trumbull Memorial Hospital	Warren	58%	300+
University of Toledo Medical Center	Toledo	58%	300+
Highland District Hospital	Hillsboro	56%	(a)
Pike Community Hospital	Waverly	53%	(a)
Southwest Regional Medical Center	Georgetown	51%	(a)

Meds 'Always' Explained Before Given

Hospital Name	City	Rate	Cases
Institute For Orthopaedic Surgery	Lima	80%	300+
Surgical Hospital at Southwoods	Youngstown	79%	300+
Morrow County Hospital	Mount Gilead	78%	(a)
Univ Hosps Conneaut Med Ctr	Conneaut	77%	(a)
Fostoria Community Hospital	Fostoria	73%	(a)
Henry County Hospital	Napoleon	72%	(a)
Fayette County Memorial Hospital	Washington Ch	71%	(a)
H B Magruder Memorial Hospital	Port Clinton	71%	300+
Hocking Valley Community Hospital	Logan	71%	(a)
Mount Carmel New Albany Surgical Hospital	New Albany	71%	300+
Hardin Memorial Hospital	Kenton	70%	(a)
Wood County Hospital	Bowling Green	70%	300+
Crystal Clinic Orthopaedic Center	Akron	69%	300+

NOTE: Hospital profiles are in alphabetical order by state, then city, then hospital within the city; Rankings exclude hospitals with less than 25 cases except for patient surveys which excludes hospitals with less than 100 cases; (a) 100-299 cases; (1) The number of cases/patients is too few to report; (2) Data submitted were based on a sample of cases/patients; (3) Results are based on a shorter time period than required; (4) Data suppressed by CMS for one or more quarters; (5) Results are not available for this reporting period; (6) Fewer than 100 patients completed the HCAHPS survey; (7) No cases met the criteria for this measure; (8) The lower limit of the confidence interval cannot be calculated if the number of observed infections equals zero; (9) No data are available from the state/territory for this reporting period; (10) The scores shown reflect fewer than 50 completed surveys; (11) There were discrepancies in the data collection process; (12) This measure does not apply to this hospital for this reporting period; (13) Results cannot be calculated for this reporting period; (14) The results for this state are combined with nearby states to protect confidentiality; Please refer to the User's Guide for a full explanation of data.

Barnesville Hospital Association	Barnesville	68%	(a)
Christ Hospital	Cincinnati	68%	300+
Euclid Hospital	Euclid	68%	300+
Galion Community Hospital	Galion	68%	300+
Grady Memorial Hospital	Delaware	68%	300+
James Cancer Hosp & Solove Res Inst	Columbus	68%	300+
Lutheran Hospital	Cleveland	68%	300+
Mercy Hospital Fairfield	Fairfield	68%	300+
Samaritan Regional Health System	Ashland	68%	300+
Adena Regional Medical Center	Chillicothe	67%	300+
Community Hospitals & Wellness Centers	Bryan	67%	300+
Holzer Medical Center Jackson	Jackson	67%	(a)
Madison County Hospital	London	67%	(a)
Medcentral Health System Shelby Hospital	Shelby	67%	(a)
Memorial Hospital of Union County	Marysville	67%	300+
Southern Ohio Medical Center	Portsmouth	67%	300+
Upper Valley Medical Center[11]	Troy	67%	300+
Bay Park Community Hospital	Oregon	66%	300+
Bellevue Hospital	Bellevue	66%	300+
Blanchard Valley Hospital	Findlay	66%	300+
Cleveland Clinic	Cleveland	66%	300+
Defiance Regional Medical Center	Defiance	66%	300+
Doctors Hospital	Columbus	66%	300+
Dublin Methodist Hospital	Dublin	66%	300+
Marion General Hospital	Marion	66%	300+
Mercy Hospital of Defiance	Defiance	66%	300+
O'Bleness Memorial Hospital	Athens	66%	300+
Ohio Valley Medical Center	Springfield	66%	300+
Southeastern Ohio Regional Medical Center	Cambridge	66%	300+
Alliance Community Hospital	Alliance	65%	300+
Bluffton Hospital	Bluffton	65%	(a)
Community Memorial Hospital	Hicksville	65%	(a)
East Ohio Regional Hospital	Martins Ferry	65%	300+
Fisher - Titus Hospital	Norwalk	65%	300+
Fort Hamilton Hughes Memorial Hospital	Hamilton	65%	300+
Grant Medical Center	Columbus	65%	300+
Mercy Hospital Anderson	Cincinnati	65%	300+
Mercy Hospital Clermont	Batavia	65%	300+
Mercy Tiffin Hospital	Tiffin	65%	300+
Ohio State University Hospitals	Columbus	65%	300+
Riverside Methodist Hospital	Columbus	65%	300+
Summa Western Reserve Hospital	Cuyahoga Falls	65%	300+
UHHS Memorial Hospital of Geneva	Geneva	65%	(a)
Univ Hosps-Elyria Med Ctr	Elyria	65%	300+
Wilson Memorial Hospital[11]	Sidney	65%	300+
Wooster Community Hospital	Wooster	65%	300+
Atrium Medical Center[11]	Franklin	64%	300+
Fairview Hospital	Cleveland	64%	300+
Firelands Regional Medical Center	Sandusky	64%	300+
Grand Lake Health System	Saint Marys	64%	300+
Lake Health	Concord	64%	300+
Medina Hospital	Medina	64%	300+
Memorial Hospital	Fremont	64%	300+
Mercer County Joint Twp Comm Hosp	Coldwater	64%	300+
Mercy Willard Hospital	Willard	64%	(a)
Pomerene Hospital	Millersburg	64%	300+
Saint Elizabeth Boardman Health Center	Boardman	64%	300+
Sycamore Medical Center	Miamisburg	64%	300+
University Hospitals Case Medical Center	Cleveland	64%	300+
West Chester Hospital	West Chester	64%	300+
Aultman Orrville Hospital	Orrville	63%	(a)
Fulton County Health Center	Wauseon	63%	300+
Hillcrest Hospital	Mayfield Heights	63%	300+
Mercy Saint Vincent Medical Center	Toledo	63%	300+
South Pointe Hospital	Warrensville Hgts	63%	300+
Trinity Med Ctr East & West	Steubenville	63%	300+
UH Geauga Medical Center	Chardon	63%	300+
UHHS Richmond Heights Hospital	Richmond Hghts	63%	300+
Akron General Medical Center	Akron	62%	300+
Ashtabula County Medical Center	Ashtabula	62%	300+
Flower Hospital	Sylvania	62%	300+
Indu & Raj Soin Medical Center	Beaver Creek	62%	300+
Jewish Hospital	Cincinnati	62%	300+
Lakewood Hospital	Lakewood	62%	300+
Licking Memorial Hospital	Newark	62%	300+
Mary Rutan Hospital	Bellefontaine	62%	300+
Marymount Hospital	Garfield Heights	62%	300+
Medcentral Health Sys Mansfield Hosp	Mansfield	62%	300+
Medical Center at Elizabeth Place	Dayton	62%	(a)
Mercy Health - West Hospital	Cincinnati	62%	300+
Mercy Memorial Hospital	Urbana	62%	(a)
Mercy Saint Anne Hospital	Toledo	62%	300+
Miami Valley Hospital[11]	Dayton	62%	300+
Saint Vincent Charity Medical Center	Cleveland	62%	300+
Selby General Hospital	Marietta	62%	300+
Summa Health System Barberton Hospital	Barberton	62%	300+
University Hospitals Ahuja Medical Center	Beachwood	62%	300+
Berger Hospital	Circleville	61%	300+
Fairfield Medical Center	Lancaster	61%	300+
Good Samaritan Hospital	Cincinnati	61%	300+
Good Samaritan Hospital[11]	Dayton	61%	300+
Kettering Medical Center	Kettering	61%	300+
McCullough - Hyde Memorial Hospital	Oxford	61%	300+
Metrohealth System	Cleveland	61%	300+
Saint John Medical Center	Westlake	61%	300+
Southwest General Health Center	Middleburg Hgts	61%	300+
Adams County Regional Medical Center	Seaman	60%	(a)
Coshocton County Memorial Hospital	Coshocton	60%	300+
Grandview Hospital & Medical Center	Dayton	60%	300+
Mercy Saint Charles Hospital	Oregon	60%	300+
Northside Medical Center	Youngstown	60%	300+
Robinson Memorial Hospital	Ravenna	60%	300+
Saint Elizabeth Health Center	Youngstown	60%	300+
Saint Luke's Hospital	Maumee	60%	300+
Saint Rita's Medical Center	Lima	60%	300+
Salem Regional Medical Center	Salem	60%	300+
The Toledo Hospital	Toledo	60%	300+
Wayne Hospital	Greenville	60%	300+
Wyandot Memorial Hospital	Upper Sandusky	60%	(a)
Aultman Hospital	Canton	59%	300+
East Liverpool City Hospital	East Liverpool	59%	300+
Greene Memorial Hospital	Xenia	59%	300+
Highland District Hospital	Hillsboro	59%	(a)
Holzer Medical Center	Gallipolis	59%	300+
Knox Community Hospital	Mount Vernon	59%	300+
Mercy Allen Hospital	Oberlin	59%	(a)
Saint Joseph Health Center	Warren	59%	300+
Summa Wadsworth - Rittman Hospital	Wadsworth	59%	300+
University of Cincinnati Medical Center	Cincinnati	59%	300+
Bethesda North	Cincinnati	58%	300+
Genesis Healthcare System	Zanesville	58%	300+
Lima Memorial Health System	Lima	58%	300+
Marietta Memorial Hospital	Marietta	58%	300+
Mercy Medical Center	Canton	58%	300+
Mercy Regional Medical Center[11]	Lorain	58%	300+
Mount Carmel West	Columbus	58%	300+
Pike Community Hospital	Waverly	58%	(a)
Springfield Regional Medical Center	Springfield	58%	300+
Trumbull Memorial Hospital	Warren	58%	300+
Union Hospital	Dover	58%	300+
University of Toledo Medical Center	Toledo	58%	300+
Van Wert County Hospital	Van Wert	58%	300+
Affinity Medical Center	Massillon	57%	300+
Bucyrus Community Hospital	Bucyrus	57%	(a)
Parma Community General Hospital	Parma	57%	300+
Clinton Memorial Hospital	Wilmington	56%	300+
Mount Carmel Saint Ann's	Westerville	56%	300+
Summa Health Systems Hospitals	Akron	55%	300+
Southwest Regional Medical Center	Georgetown	53%	(a)

Nurses 'Always' Communicated Well

Hospital Name	City	Rate	Cases
Surgical Hospital at Southwoods	Youngstown	95%	300+
Univ Hosps Conneaut Med Ctr	Conneaut	93%	(a)
Institute For Orthopaedic Surgery	Lima	92%	300+
Mercy Willard Hospital	Willard	89%	(a)
Bluffton Hospital	Bluffton	88%	(a)
Fostoria Community Hospital	Fostoria	88%	(a)
H B Magruder Memorial Hospital	Port Clinton	88%	300+
Barnesville Hospital Association	Barnesville	87%	(a)
Bellevue Hospital	Bellevue	87%	300+
Community Memorial Hospital	Hicksville	87%	(a)
Mount Carmel New Albany Surgical Hospital	New Albany	87%	300+
Hardin Memorial Hospital	Kenton	86%	(a)
Henry County Hospital	Napoleon	86%	(a)
Mercy Hospital of Defiance	Defiance	86%	300+
Morrow County Hospital	Mount Gilead	86%	(a)
UHHS Memorial Hospital of Geneva	Geneva	86%	(a)
Christ Hospital	Cincinnati	85%	300+
Defiance Regional Medical Center	Defiance	85%	300+
Dublin Methodist Hospital	Dublin	85%	300+
Hocking Valley Community Hospital	Logan	85%	(a)
Mercy Hospital Fairfield	Fairfield	85%	300+
Pomerene Hospital	Millersburg	85%	300+
Community Hospitals & Wellness Centers	Bryan	84%	300+
Crystal Clinic Orthopaedic Center	Akron	84%	300+
Fayette County Memorial Hospital	Washington Ch	84%	(a)
Mercy Hospital Clermont	Batavia	84%	300+
Ohio Valley Medical Center	Springfield	84%	300+
Blanchard Valley Hospital	Findlay	83%	300+
Cleveland Clinic	Cleveland	83%	300+
Holzer Medical Center Jackson	Jackson	83%	(a)
James Cancer Hosp & Solove Res Inst	Columbus	83%	300+
Medcentral Health System Shelby Hospital	Shelby	83%	(a)
Memorial Hospital of Union County	Marysville	83%	300+
Saint Elizabeth Boardman Health Center	Boardman	83%	300+
Samaritan Regional Health System	Ashland	83%	300+
Doctors Hospital	Columbus	82%	300+
Euclid Hospital	Euclid	82%	300+
Fort Hamilton Hughes Memorial Hospital	Hamilton	82%	300+
Grady Memorial Hospital	Delaware	82%	300+
Indu & Raj Soin Medical Center	Beaver Creek	82%	300+
Lutheran Hospital	Cleveland	82%	300+
Mary Rutan Hospital	Bellefontaine	82%	300+
Medcentral Health Sys Mansfield Hosp	Mansfield	82%	300+
Mercy Saint Anne Hospital	Toledo	82%	300+
Southeastern Ohio Regional Medical Center	Cambridge	82%	300+
Summa Western Reserve Hospital	Cuyahoga Falls	82%	300+
Sycamore Medical Center	Miamisburg	82%	300+
West Chester Hospital	West Chester	82%	300+
Wooster Community Hospital	Wooster	82%	300+
Aultman Orrville Hospital	Orrville	81%	(a)
Bay Park Community Hospital	Oregon	81%	300+
Fairfield Medical Center	Lancaster	81%	300+
Fisher - Titus Hospital	Norwalk	81%	300+
Grant Medical Center	Columbus	81%	300+
Lake Health	Concord	81%	300+
Madison County Hospital	London	81%	(a)
Mercer County Joint Twp Comm Hosp	Coldwater	81%	300+
Mercy Memorial Hospital	Urbana	81%	(a)
Ohio State University Hospitals	Columbus	81%	300+
Selby General Hospital	Marietta	81%	300+
Southern Ohio Medical Center	Portsmouth	81%	300+
UH Geauga Medical Center	Chardon	81%	300+
Union Hospital	Dover	81%	300+
Upper Valley Medical Center[11]	Troy	81%	300+
Wayne Hospital	Greenville	81%	300+
Wood County Hospital	Bowling Green	81%	300+
Ashtabula County Medical Center	Ashtabula	80%	300+
Atrium Medical Center[11]	Franklin	80%	300+
Fairview Hospital	Cleveland	80%	300+
Galion Community Hospital	Galion	80%	300+
Good Samaritan Hospital	Cincinnati	80%	300+
Good Samaritan Hospital[11]	Dayton	80%	300+
Grand Lake Health System	Saint Marys	80%	300+
Grandview Hospital & Medical Center	Dayton	80%	300+
Kettering Medical Center	Kettering	80%	300+
Marion General Hospital	Marion	80%	300+
Memorial Hospital	Fremont	80%	300+
Mercy Hospital Anderson	Cincinnati	80%	300+
Miami Valley Hospital[11]	Dayton	80%	300+
Riverside Methodist Hospital	Columbus	80%	300+
Saint Vincent Charity Medical Center	Cleveland	80%	300+
South Pointe Hospital	Warrensville Hgts	80%	300+
Southwest General Health Center	Middleburg Hgts	80%	300+
Univ Hosps-Elyria Med Ctr	Elyria	80%	300+
University Hospitals Case Medical Center	Cleveland	80%	300+
Van Wert County Hospital	Van Wert	80%	300+
Wilson Memorial Hospital[11]	Sidney	80%	300+
Akron General Medical Center	Akron	79%	300+
Coshocton County Memorial Hospital	Coshocton	79%	300+
Flower Hospital	Sylvania	79%	300+
Hillcrest Hospital	Mayfield Heights	79%	300+
Medical Center at Elizabeth Place	Dayton	79%	(a)
Medina Hospital	Medina	79%	300+
Mercy Saint Charles Hospital	Oregon	79%	300+
Mercy Tiffin Hospital	Tiffin	79%	300+
O'Bleness Memorial Hospital	Athens	79%	300+
Robinson Memorial Hospital	Ravenna	79%	300+
Saint Joseph Health Center	Warren	79%	300+
Saint Rita's Medical Center	Lima	79%	300+
Trinity Med Ctr East & West	Steubenville	79%	300+
Adena Regional Medical Center	Chillicothe	78%	300+
Alliance Community Hospital	Alliance	78%	300+
Aultman Hospital	Canton	78%	300+
Berger Hospital	Circleville	78%	300+
East Liverpool City Hospital	East Liverpool	78%	300+
Greene Memorial Hospital	Xenia	78%	300+
Jewish Hospital	Cincinnati	78%	300+
Knox Community Hospital	Mount Vernon	78%	300+
Lakewood Hospital	Lakewood	78%	300+
Licking Memorial Hospital	Newark	78%	300+
Marymount Hospital	Garfield Heights	78%	300+
McCullough - Hyde Memorial Hospital	Oxford	78%	300+
Mercy Health - West Hospital	Cincinnati	78%	300+
Mercy Saint Vincent Medical Center	Toledo	78%	300+
Mount Carmel West	Columbus	78%	300+
Parma Community General Hospital	Parma	78%	300+
UHHS Richmond Heights Hospital	Richmond Hghts	78%	300+
University Hospitals Ahuja Medical Center	Beachwood	78%	300+
Bethesda North	Cincinnati	77%	300+
Bucyrus Community Hospital	Bucyrus	77%	(a)
Firelands Regional Medical Center	Sandusky	77%	300+
Mercy Allen Hospital	Oberlin	77%	(a)
Northside Medical Center	Youngstown	77%	300+
Pike Community Hospital	Waverly	77%	(a)
Saint Elizabeth Health Center	Youngstown	77%	300+
Saint John Medical Center	Westlake	77%	300+
Springfield Regional Medical Center	Springfield	77%	300+
Summa Health System Barberton Hospital	Barberton	77%	300+
The Toledo Hospital	Toledo	77%	300+
Adams County Regional Medical Center	Seaman	76%	(a)
Affinity Medical Center	Massillon	76%	300+

NOTE: Hospital profiles are in alphabetical order by state, then city, then hospital within the city; Rankings exclude hospitals with less than 25 cases except for patient surveys which excludes hospitals with less than 100 cases; (a) 100-299 cases; (1) The number of cases/patients is too few to report; (2) Data submitted were based on a sample of cases/patients; (3) Results are based on a shorter time period than required; (4) Data suppressed by CMS for one or more quarters; (5) Results are not available for this reporting period; (6) Fewer than 100 patients completed the HCAHPS survey; (7) No cases met the criteria for this measure; (8) The lower limit of the confidence interval cannot be calculated if the number of observed infections equals zero; (9) No data are available from the state/territory for this reporting period; (10) The scores shown reflect fewer than 50 completed surveys; (11) There were discrepancies in the data collection process; (12) This measure does not apply to this hospital for this reporting period; (13) Results cannot be calculated for this reporting period; (14) The results for this state are combined with nearby states to protect confidentiality; Please refer to the User's Guide for a full explanation of data.

East Ohio Regional Hospital	Martins Ferry	76%	300+
Fulton County Health Center	Wauseon	76%	300+
Genesis Healthcare System	Zanesville	76%	300+
Lima Memorial Health System	Lima	76%	300+
Mercy Medical Center	Canton	76%	300+
Salem Regional Medical Center	Salem	76%	300+
University of Toledo Medical Center	Toledo	76%	300+
Clinton Memorial Hospital	Wilmington	75%	300+
Mercy Regional Medical Center[11]	Lorain	75%	300+
Metrohealth System	Cleveland	75%	300+
Mount Carmel Saint Ann's	Westerville	75%	300+
Saint Luke's Hospital	Maumee	75%	300+
Highland District Hospital	Hillsboro	74%	(a)
Marietta Memorial Hospital	Marietta	74%	300+
Summa Wadsworth - Rittman Hospital	Wadsworth	74%	300+
University of Cincinnati Medical Center	Cincinnati	74%	300+
Wyandot Memorial Hospital	Upper Sandusky	74%	(a)
Holzer Medical Center	Gallipolis	73%	300+
Summa Health Systems Hospitals	Akron	73%	300+
Trumbull Memorial Hospital	Warren	73%	300+
Southwest Regional Medical Center	Georgetown	72%	(a)

Pain 'Always' Well Controlled

Hospital Name	City	Rate	Cases
Surgical Hospital at Southwoods	Youngstown	87%	300+
Univ Hosps Conneaut Med Ctr	Conneaut	83%	(a)
Mercy Willard Hospital	Willard	82%	(a)
Bluffton Hospital	Bluffton	80%	(a)
Fostoria Community Hospital	Fostoria	79%	(a)
Mount Carmel New Albany Surgical Hospital	New Albany	79%	300+
Barnesville Hospital Association	Barnesville	78%	(a)
Institute For Orthopaedic Surgery	Lima	78%	300+
Defiance Regional Medical Center	Defiance	77%	300+
H B Magruder Memorial Hospital	Port Clinton	77%	300+
Hocking Valley Community Hospital	Logan	77%	(a)
Holzer Medical Center Jackson	Jackson	77%	(a)
Medcentral Health System Shelby Hospital	Shelby	77%	(a)
Morrow County Hospital	Mount Gilead	77%	(a)
Bellevue Hospital	Bellevue	76%	300+
Christ Hospital	Cincinnati	76%	300+
Southern Ohio Medical Center	Portsmouth	76%	300+
Bay Park Community Hospital	Oregon	75%	300+
Community Hospitals & Wellness Centers	Bryan	75%	300+
Mercy Hospital Fairfield	Fairfield	75%	300+
Bucyrus Community Hospital	Bucyrus	74%	(a)
Dublin Methodist Hospital	Dublin	74%	300+
Euclid Hospital	Euclid	74%	300+
Galion Community Hospital	Galion	74%	300+
Good Samaritan Hospital	Cincinnati	74%	300+
James Cancer Hosp & Solove Res Inst	Columbus	74%	300+
Medcentral Health Sys Mansfield Hosp	Mansfield	74%	300+
Memorial Hospital of Union County	Marysville	74%	300+
Wayne Hospital	Greenville	74%	300+
Fayette County Memorial Hospital	Washington Ch	73%	(a)
Fort Hamilton Hughes Memorial Hospital	Hamilton	73%	300+
Fulton County Health Center	Wauseon	73%	300+
Hardin Memorial Hospital	Kenton	73%	(a)
Henry County Hospital	Napoleon	73%	(a)
Medical Center at Elizabeth Place	Dayton	73%	(a)
Mercy Hospital of Defiance	Defiance	73%	300+
Ohio Valley Medical Center	Springfield	73%	300+
South Pointe Hospital	Warrensville Hgts	73%	300+
Southeastern Ohio Regional Medical Center	Cambridge	73%	300+
Summa Western Reserve Hospital	Cuyahoga Falls	73%	300+
Upper Valley Medical Center[11]	Troy	73%	300+
West Chester Hospital	West Chester	73%	300+
Wilson Memorial Hospital[11]	Sidney	73%	300+
Wood County Hospital	Bowling Green	73%	300+
Wooster Community Hospital	Wooster	73%	300+
Alliance Community Hospital	Alliance	72%	300+
Atrium Medical Center[11]	Franklin	72%	300+
Cleveland Clinic	Cleveland	72%	300+
Crystal Clinic Orthopaedic Center	Akron	72%	300+
Mercy Hospital Anderson	Cincinnati	72%	300+
Mercy Hospital Clermont	Batavia	72%	300+
Riverside Methodist Hospital	Columbus	72%	300+
Saint Elizabeth Boardman Health Center	Boardman	72%	300+
Saint Vincent Charity Medical Center	Cleveland	72%	300+
Samaritan Regional Health System	Ashland	72%	300+
Union Hospital	Dover	72%	300+
Aultman Hospital	Canton	71%	300+
Bethesda North	Cincinnati	71%	300+
Fairfield Medical Center	Lancaster	71%	300+
Fisher - Titus Hospital	Norwalk	71%	300+
Flower Hospital	Sylvania	71%	300+
Good Samaritan Hospital[11]	Dayton	71%	300+
Grady Memorial Hospital	Delaware	71%	300+
Grant Medical Center	Columbus	71%	300+
Indu & Raj Soin Medical Center	Beaver Creek	71%	300+
Lake Health	Concord	71%	300+
Madison County Hospital	London	71%	(a)
McCullough - Hyde Memorial Hospital	Oxford	71%	300+
Medina Hospital	Medina	71%	300+
Mercer County Joint Twp Comm Hosp	Coldwater	71%	300+
Miami Valley Hospital[11]	Dayton	71%	300+
Ohio State University Hospitals	Columbus	71%	300+
Springfield Regional Medical Center	Springfield	71%	300+
UH Geauga Medical Center	Chardon	71%	300+
Blanchard Valley Hospital	Findlay	70%	300+
Coshocton County Memorial Hospital	Coshocton	70%	300+
Doctors Hospital	Columbus	70%	300+
Fairview Hospital	Cleveland	70%	300+
Grand Lake Health System	Saint Marys	70%	300+
Hillcrest Hospital	Mayfield Heights	70%	300+
Jewish Hospital	Cincinnati	70%	300+
Kettering Medical Center	Kettering	70%	300+
Lutheran Hospital	Cleveland	70%	300+
Mercy Allen Hospital	Oberlin	70%	(a)
Mercy Medical Center	Canton	70%	300+
Mercy Saint Anne Hospital	Toledo	70%	300+
Mercy Tiffin Hospital	Tiffin	70%	300+
Mount Carmel West	Columbus	70%	300+
Robinson Memorial Hospital	Ravenna	70%	300+
Saint Joseph Health Center	Warren	70%	300+
Sycamore Medical Center	Miamisburg	70%	300+
Trinity Med Ctr East & West	Steubenville	70%	300+
University Hospitals Case Medical Center	Cleveland	70%	300+
Wyandot Memorial Hospital	Upper Sandusky	70%	(a)
Akron General Medical Center	Akron	69%	300+
Community Memorial Hospital	Hicksville	69%	(a)
Grandview Hospital & Medical Center	Dayton	69%	300+
Lakewood Hospital	Lakewood	69%	300+
Marion General Hospital	Marion	69%	300+
Marymount Hospital	Garfield Heights	69%	300+
Mercy Saint Vincent Medical Center	Toledo	69%	300+
Parma Community General Hospital	Parma	69%	300+
Saint Rita's Medical Center	Lima	69%	300+
Southwest General Health Center	Middleburg Hgts	69%	300+
The Toledo Hospital	Toledo	69%	300+
UHHS Richmond Heights Hospital	Richmond Hghts	69%	300+
Univ Hosps-Elyria Med Ctr	Elyria	69%	300+
Van Wert County Hospital	Van Wert	69%	300+
Ashtabula County Medical Center	Ashtabula	68%	300+
East Liverpool City Hospital	East Liverpool	68%	300+
East Ohio Regional Hospital	Martins Ferry	68%	300+
Licking Memorial Hospital	Newark	68%	300+
Memorial Hospital	Fremont	68%	300+
Mercy Memorial Hospital	Urbana	68%	(a)
Mercy Saint Charles Hospital	Oregon	68%	300+
Mount Carmel Saint Ann's	Westerville	68%	300+
Saint Elizabeth Health Center	Youngstown	68%	300+
Saint John Medical Center	Westlake	68%	300+
Selby General Hospital	Marietta	68%	300+
Summa Health System Barberton Hospital	Barberton	68%	300+
UHHS Memorial Hospital of Geneva	Geneva	68%	(a)
University Hospitals Ahuja Medical Center	Beachwood	68%	300+
Adena Regional Medical Center	Chillicothe	67%	300+
Affinity Medical Center	Massillon	67%	300+
Firelands Regional Medical Center	Sandusky	67%	300+
Knox Community Hospital	Mount Vernon	67%	300+
Lima Memorial Health System	Lima	67%	300+
Mary Rutan Hospital	Bellefontaine	67%	300+
Mercy Health - West Hospital	Cincinnati	67%	300+
Mercy Regional Medical Center[11]	Lorain	67%	300+
Northside Medical Center	Youngstown	67%	300+
O'Bleness Memorial Hospital	Athens	67%	300+
Pomerene Hospital	Millersburg	67%	300+
Summa Health Systems Hospitals	Akron	67%	300+
University of Cincinnati Medical Center	Cincinnati	67%	300+
Genesis Healthcare System	Zanesville	66%	300+
Marietta Memorial Hospital	Marietta	66%	300+
Metrohealth System	Cleveland	66%	300+
Summa Wadsworth - Rittman Hospital	Wadsworth	66%	300+
University of Toledo Medical Center	Toledo	66%	300+
Adams County Regional Medical Center	Seaman	65%	(a)
Berger Hospital	Circleville	65%	300+
Clinton Memorial Hospital	Wilmington	65%	300+
Greene Memorial Hospital	Xenia	65%	300+
Holzer Medical Center	Gallipolis	65%	300+
Saint Luke's Hospital	Maumee	65%	300+
Salem Regional Medical Center	Salem	65%	300+
Trumbull Memorial Hospital	Warren	65%	300+
Aultman Orrville Hospital	Orrville	63%	(a)
Pike Community Hospital	Waverly	63%	(a)
Highland District Hospital	Hillsboro	62%	(a)
Southwest Regional Medical Center	Georgetown	62%	(a)

Room and Bathroom 'Always' Clean

Hospital Name	City	Rate	Cases
Fostoria Community Hospital	Fostoria	94%	(a)
Community Memorial Hospital	Hicksville	91%	(a)
Surgical Hospital at Southwoods	Youngstown	90%	300+
H B Magruder Memorial Hospital	Port Clinton	89%	300+
Mercy Willard Hospital	Willard	88%	(a)
Univ Hosps Conneaut Med Ctr	Conneaut	87%	(a)
Wood County Hospital	Bowling Green	87%	300+
Grand Lake Health System	Saint Marys	86%	300+
Bluffton Hospital	Bluffton	85%	(a)
Holzer Medical Center Jackson	Jackson	85%	(a)
Institute For Orthopaedic Surgery	Lima	85%	300+
Morrow County Hospital	Mount Gilead	85%	(a)
Pomerene Hospital	Millersburg	85%	300+
Southeastern Ohio Regional Medical Center	Cambridge	85%	300+
Hardin Memorial Hospital	Kenton	84%	(a)
Madison County Hospital	London	84%	(a)
Mount Carmel New Albany Surgical Hospital	New Albany	84%	300+
Ashtabula County Medical Center	Ashtabula	83%	300+
Bellevue Hospital	Bellevue	83%	300+
Blanchard Valley Hospital	Findlay	83%	300+
Fairview Hospital	Cleveland	83%	300+
Fayette County Memorial Hospital	Washington Ch	83%	(a)
Hocking Valley Community Hospital	Logan	83%	(a)
Mercy Hospital of Defiance	Defiance	83%	300+
Barnesville Hospital Association	Barnesville	82%	(a)
Community Hospitals & Wellness Centers	Bryan	82%	300+
Alliance Community Hospital	Alliance	81%	300+
Aultman Orrville Hospital	Orrville	81%	(a)
Defiance Regional Medical Center	Defiance	81%	300+
Grady Memorial Hospital	Delaware	81%	300+
Henry County Hospital	Napoleon	81%	(a)
Medina Hospital	Medina	81%	300+
Mercy Hospital Fairfield	Fairfield	81%	300+
Mercy Tiffin Hospital	Tiffin	81%	300+
Southern Ohio Medical Center	Portsmouth	81%	300+
UHHS Memorial Hospital of Geneva	Geneva	81%	(a)
Firelands Regional Medical Center	Sandusky	80%	300+
Fulton County Health Center	Wauseon	80%	300+
Mercy Hospital Clermont	Batavia	80%	300+
Mercy Memorial Hospital	Urbana	80%	(a)
Ohio Valley Medical Center	Springfield	80%	300+
Selby General Hospital	Marietta	80%	300+
Wilson Memorial Hospital[11]	Sidney	80%	300+
Bucyrus Community Hospital	Bucyrus	79%	(a)
Fisher - Titus Hospital	Norwalk	79%	300+
Indu & Raj Soin Medical Center	Beaver Creek	79%	300+
Mary Rutan Hospital	Bellefontaine	79%	300+
Medcentral Health System Shelby Hospital	Shelby	79%	(a)
Wooster Community Hospital	Wooster	79%	300+
Cleveland Clinic	Cleveland	78%	300+
Coshocton County Memorial Hospital	Coshocton	78%	300+
Crystal Clinic Orthopaedic Center	Akron	78%	300+
Memorial Hospital	Fremont	78%	300+
Mercer County Joint Twp Comm Hosp	Coldwater	78%	300+
Union Hospital	Dover	78%	300+
Wyandot Memorial Hospital	Upper Sandusky	78%	(a)
Adams County Regional Medical Center	Seaman	77%	(a)
Dublin Methodist Hospital	Dublin	77%	300+
East Ohio Regional Hospital	Martins Ferry	77%	300+
Marymount Hospital	Garfield Heights	77%	300+
Mercy Saint Charles Hospital	Oregon	77%	300+
Clinton Memorial Hospital	Wilmington	76%	300+
Mercy Saint Anne Hospital	Toledo	76%	300+
Miami Valley Hospital[11]	Dayton	76%	300+
Samaritan Regional Health System	Ashland	76%	300+
South Pointe Hospital	Warrensville Hgts	76%	300+
Van Wert County Hospital	Van Wert	76%	300+
Lake Health	Concord	75%	300+
Marion General Hospital	Marion	75%	300+
Pike Community Hospital	Waverly	75%	(a)
Robinson Memorial Hospital	Ravenna	75%	300+
Saint Vincent Charity Medical Center	Cleveland	75%	300+
Wayne Hospital	Greenville	75%	300+
Atrium Medical Center[11]	Franklin	74%	300+
Bethesda North	Cincinnati	74%	300+
Lima Memorial Health System	Lima	74%	300+
Memorial Hospital of Union County	Marysville	74%	300+
Mercy Regional Medical Center[11]	Lorain	74%	300+
Mercy Saint Vincent Medical Center	Toledo	74%	300+
Springfield Regional Medical Center	Springfield	74%	300+
Upper Valley Medical Center[11]	Troy	74%	300+
West Chester Hospital	West Chester	74%	300+
Aultman Hospital	Canton	73%	300+
Christ Hospital	Cincinnati	73%	300+
East Liverpool City Hospital	East Liverpool	73%	300+
Grant Medical Center	Columbus	73%	300+
Medcentral Health Sys Mansfield Hosp	Mansfield	73%	300+
Mercy Allen Hospital	Oberlin	73%	(a)
O'Bleness Memorial Hospital	Athens	73%	300+
Salem Regional Medical Center	Salem	73%	300+
Summa Health System Barberton Hospital	Barberton	73%	300+
Sycamore Medical Center	Miamisburg	73%	300+
Univ Hosps-Elyria Med Ctr	Elyria	73%	300+
Bay Park Community Hospital	Oregon	72%	300+

NOTE: Hospital profiles are in alphabetical order by state, then city, then hospital within the city; Rankings exclude hospitals with less than 25 cases except for patient surveys which excludes hospitals with less than 100 cases; (a) 100-299 cases; (1) The number of cases/patients is too few to report; (2) Data submitted were based on a sample of cases/patients; (3) Results are based on a shorter time period than required; (4) Data suppressed by CMS for one or more quarters; (5) Results are not available for this reporting period; (6) Fewer than 100 patients completed the HCAHPS survey; (7) No cases met the criteria for this measure; (8) The lower limit of the confidence interval cannot be calculated if the number of observed infections equals zero; (9) No data are available from the state/territory for this reporting period; (10) The scores shown reflect fewer than 50 completed surveys; (11) There were discrepancies in the data collection process; (12) This measure does not apply to this hospital for this reporting period; (13) Results cannot be calculated for this reporting period; (14) The results for this state are combined with nearby states to protect confidentiality; Please refer to the User's Guide for a full explanation of data.

Doctors Hospital	Columbus	72%	300+
Fairfield Medical Center	Lancaster	72%	300+
Kettering Medical Center	Kettering	72%	300+
Lutheran Hospital	Cleveland	72%	300+
Trinity Med Ctr East & West	Steubenville	72%	300+
Flower Hospital	Sylvania	71%	300+
Galion Community Hospital	Galion	71%	300+
Good Samaritan Hospital	Cincinnati	71%	300+
Greene Memorial Hospital	Xenia	71%	300+
Hillcrest Hospital	Mayfield Heights	71%	300+
McCullough - Hyde Memorial Hospital	Oxford	71%	300+
Ohio State University Hospitals	Columbus	71%	300+
Riverside Methodist Hospital	Columbus	71%	300+
Saint Luke's Hospital	Maumee	71%	300+
Saint Rita's Medical Center	Lima	71%	300+
Summa Wadsworth - Rittman Hospital	Wadsworth	71%	300+
Berger Hospital	Circleville	70%	300+
Euclid Hospital	Euclid	70%	300+
Genesis Healthcare System	Zanesville	70%	300+
James Cancer Hosp & Solove Res Inst	Columbus	70%	300+
Lakewood Hospital	Lakewood	70%	300+
Marietta Memorial Hospital	Marietta	70%	300+
UH Geauga Medical Center	Chardon	70%	300+
Licking Memorial Hospital	Newark	69%	300+
Mercy Hospital Anderson	Cincinnati	69%	300+
Fort Hamilton Hughes Memorial Hospital	Hamilton	68%	300+
Grandview Hospital & Medical Center	Dayton	68%	300+
Holzer Medical Center	Gallipolis	68%	300+
Parma Community General Hospital	Parma	68%	300+
Saint Elizabeth Boardman Health Center	Boardman	68%	300+
Saint John Medical Center	Westlake	68%	300+
Summa Health Systems Hospitals	Akron	68%	300+
UHHS Richmond Heights Hospital	Richmond Hghts	68%	300+
Affinity Medical Center	Massillon	67%	300+
Jewish Hospital	Cincinnati	67%	300+
Mercy Health - West Hospital	Cincinnati	67%	300+
The Toledo Hospital	Toledo	67%	300+
University Hospitals Case Medical Center	Cleveland	67%	300+
Akron General Medical Center	Akron	66%	300+
Mercy Medical Center	Canton	66%	300+
Saint Joseph Health Center	Warren	66%	300+
Summa Western Reserve Hospital	Cuyahoga Falls	66%	300+
University Hospitals Ahuja Medical Center	Beachwood	66%	300+
Knox Community Hospital	Mount Vernon	65%	300+
Mount Carmel Saint Ann's	Westerville	65%	300+
Southwest General Health Center	Middleburg Hgts	65%	300+
University of Toledo Medical Center	Toledo	65%	300+
Southwest Regional Medical Center	Georgetown	64%	(a)
Adena Regional Medical Center	Chillicothe	63%	300+
Northside Medical Center	Youngstown	63%	300+
Highland District Hospital	Hillsboro	62%	(a)
Good Samaritan Hospital[11]	Dayton	61%	300+
Mount Carmel West	Columbus	61%	300+
Saint Elizabeth Health Center	Youngstown	61%	300+
University of Cincinnati Medical Center	Cincinnati	61%	300+
Medical Center at Elizabeth Place	Dayton	60%	(a)
Metrohealth System	Cleveland	59%	300+
Trumbull Memorial Hospital	Warren	58%	300+

Timely Help 'Always' Received

Hospital Name	City	Rate	Cases
Institute For Orthopaedic Surgery	Lima	91%	300+
Surgical Hospital at Southwoods	Youngstown	91%	300+
Univ Hosps Conneaut Med Ctr	Conneaut	91%	(a)
Bluffton Hospital	Bluffton	87%	(a)
H B Magruder Memorial Hospital	Port Clinton	87%	300+
Community Memorial Hospital	Hicksville	86%	(a)
Barnesville Hospital Association	Barnesville	84%	(a)
Fostoria Community Hospital	Fostoria	83%	(a)
Hocking Valley Community Hospital	Logan	83%	(a)
Holzer Medical Center Jackson	Jackson	81%	(a)
Medcentral Health System Shelby Hospital	Shelby	81%	(a)
Mercy Hospital of Defiance	Defiance	81%	300+
Mercy Willard Hospital	Willard	81%	(a)
Hardin Memorial Hospital	Kenton	80%	(a)
Mercer County Joint Twp Comm Hosp	Coldwater	79%	300+
Community Hospitals & Wellness Centers	Bryan	78%	300+
Defiance Regional Medical Center	Defiance	78%	300+
Morrow County Hospital	Mount Gilead	78%	(a)
UHHS Memorial Hospital of Geneva	Geneva	78%	(a)
Bellevue Hospital	Bellevue	77%	300+
Ohio Valley Medical Center	Springfield	77%	300+
Aultman Orrville Hospital	Orrville	76%	(a)
Henry County Hospital	Napoleon	76%	(a)
Memorial Hospital of Union County	Marysville	76%	300+
Samaritan Regional Health System	Ashland	76%	300+
Wood County Hospital	Bowling Green	76%	300+
Fayette County Memorial Hospital	Washington Ch	75%	(a)
Grand Lake Health System	Saint Marys	75%	300+
Mary Rutan Hospital	Bellefontaine	75%	300+
Mercy Hospital Fairfield	Fairfield	75%	300+
Mount Carmel New Albany Surgical Hospital	New Albany	75%	300+
Selby General Hospital	Marietta	75%	300+
Medical Center at Elizabeth Place	Dayton	74%	(a)
Mercy Memorial Hospital	Urbana	74%	(a)
Union Hospital	Dover	74%	300+
Van Wert County Hospital	Van Wert	74%	300+
Fulton County Health Center	Wauseon	73%	300+
Galion Community Hospital	Galion	73%	300+
Upper Valley Medical Center[11]	Troy	73%	300+
Wayne Hospital	Greenville	73%	300+
Ashtabula County Medical Center	Ashtabula	72%	300+
Bay Park Community Hospital	Oregon	72%	300+
Euclid Hospital	Euclid	72%	300+
Fairfield Medical Center	Lancaster	72%	300+
Madison County Hospital	London	72%	(a)
Medcentral Health Sys Mansfield Hosp	Mansfield	72%	300+
Southwest Regional Medical Center	Georgetown	72%	(a)
Wooster Community Hospital	Wooster	72%	300+
Christ Hospital	Cincinnati	71%	300+
Dublin Methodist Hospital	Dublin	71%	300+
Fort Hamilton Hughes Memorial Hospital	Hamilton	71%	300+
Good Samaritan Hospital	Cincinnati	71%	300+
Pomerene Hospital	Millersburg	71%	300+
Summa Western Reserve Hospital	Cuyahoga Falls	71%	300+
Bucyrus Community Hospital	Bucyrus	70%	(a)
Fisher - Titus Hospital	Norwalk	70%	300+
Knox Community Hospital	Mount Vernon	70%	300+
Memorial Hospital	Fremont	70%	300+
Mercy Allen Hospital	Oberlin	70%	(a)
Mercy Saint Anne Hospital	Toledo	70%	300+
Saint Rita's Medical Center	Lima	70%	300+
Southeastern Ohio Regional Medical Center	Cambridge	70%	300+
Univ Hosps-Elyria Med Ctr	Elyria	70%	300+
Wyandot Memorial Hospital	Upper Sandusky	70%	(a)
Aultman Hospital	Canton	69%	300+
Doctors Hospital	Columbus	69%	300+
Fairview Hospital	Cleveland	69%	300+
Indu & Raj Soin Medical Center	Beaver Creek	69%	300+
Mercy Tiffin Hospital	Tiffin	69%	300+
Wilson Memorial Hospital[11]	Sidney	69%	300+
Cleveland Clinic	Cleveland	68%	300+
Crystal Clinic Orthopaedic Center	Akron	68%	300+
Grady Memorial Hospital	Delaware	68%	300+
James Cancer Hosp & Solove Res Inst	Columbus	68%	300+
Lutheran Hospital	Cleveland	68%	300+
Marymount Hospital	Garfield Heights	68%	300+
Salem Regional Medical Center	Salem	68%	300+
Southern Ohio Medical Center	Portsmouth	68%	300+
Sycamore Medical Center	Miamisburg	68%	300+
Blanchard Valley Hospital	Findlay	67%	300+
Lake Health	Concord	67%	300+
Marion General Hospital	Marion	67%	300+
Mercy Hospital Anderson	Cincinnati	67%	300+
Mercy Hospital Clermont	Batavia	67%	300+
Mercy Saint Vincent Medical Center	Toledo	67%	300+
Parma Community General Hospital	Parma	67%	300+
Robinson Memorial Hospital	Ravenna	67%	300+
UH Geauga Medical Center	Chardon	67%	300+
Adena Regional Medical Center	Chillicothe	66%	300+
Berger Hospital	Circleville	66%	300+
Flower Hospital	Sylvania	66%	300+
Genesis Healthcare System	Zanesville	66%	300+
Grant Medical Center	Columbus	66%	300+
Licking Memorial Hospital	Newark	66%	300+
Mercy Saint Charles Hospital	Oregon	66%	300+
Ohio State University Hospitals	Columbus	66%	300+
Saint Elizabeth Boardman Health Center	Boardman	66%	300+
Saint Vincent Charity Medical Center	Cleveland	66%	300+
West Chester Hospital	West Chester	66%	300+
Bethesda North	Cincinnati	65%	300+
Firelands Regional Medical Center	Sandusky	65%	300+
Grandview Hospital & Medical Center	Dayton	65%	300+
Holzer Medical Center	Gallipolis	65%	300+
Kettering Medical Center	Kettering	65%	300+
Medina Hospital	Medina	65%	300+
Summa Health System Barberton Hospital	Barberton	65%	300+
Akron General Medical Center	Akron	64%	300+
Coshocton County Memorial Hospital	Coshocton	64%	300+
East Liverpool City Hospital	East Liverpool	64%	300+
Hillcrest Hospital	Mayfield Heights	64%	300+
Lakewood Hospital	Lakewood	64%	300+
Miami Valley Hospital[11]	Dayton	64%	300+
O'Bleness Memorial Hospital	Athens	64%	300+
Riverside Methodist Hospital	Columbus	64%	300+
Saint Joseph Health Center	Warren	64%	300+
Saint Luke's Hospital	Maumee	64%	300+
Southwest General Health Center	Middleburg Hgts	64%	300+
Trinity Med Ctr East & West	Steubenville	64%	300+
Adams County Regional Medical Center	Seaman	63%	(a)
Good Samaritan Hospital[11]	Dayton	63%	300+
Lima Memorial Health System	Lima	63%	300+
Marietta Memorial Hospital	Marietta	63%	300+
McCullough - Hyde Memorial Hospital	Oxford	63%	300+
Saint John Medical Center	Westlake	63%	300+
South Pointe Hospital	Warrensville Hgts	63%	300+
The Toledo Hospital	Toledo	63%	300+
UHHS Richmond Heights Hospital	Richmond Hghts	63%	300+
Alliance Community Hospital	Alliance	62%	300+
Mercy Regional Medical Center[11]	Lorain	62%	300+
Saint Elizabeth Health Center	Youngstown	62%	300+
East Ohio Regional Hospital	Martins Ferry	61%	300+
Greene Memorial Hospital	Xenia	61%	300+
Jewish Hospital	Cincinnati	61%	300+
Mount Carmel West	Columbus	61%	300+
Northside Medical Center	Youngstown	61%	300+
Summa Health Systems Hospitals	Akron	61%	300+
University Hospitals Case Medical Center	Cleveland	61%	300+
Affinity Medical Center	Massillon	60%	300+
Atrium Medical Center[11]	Franklin	60%	300+
Mercy Medical Center	Canton	60%	300+
Metrohealth System	Cleveland	60%	300+
Mount Carmel Saint Ann's	Westerville	60%	300+
Pike Community Hospital	Waverly	60%	(a)
Springfield Regional Medical Center	Springfield	60%	300+
Trumbull Memorial Hospital	Warren	59%	300+
Clinton Memorial Hospital	Wilmington	58%	300+
Highland District Hospital	Hillsboro	58%	(a)
Summa Wadsworth - Rittman Hospital	Wadsworth	58%	300+
University Hospitals Ahuja Medical Center	Beachwood	58%	300+
Mercy Health - West Hospital	Cincinnati	57%	300+
University of Cincinnati Medical Center	Cincinnati	56%	300+
University of Toledo Medical Center	Toledo	54%	300+

Would Definitely Recommend Hospital

Hospital Name	City	Rate	Cases
Surgical Hospital at Southwoods	Youngstown	96%	300+
Institute For Orthopaedic Surgery	Lima	92%	300+
Mount Carmel New Albany Surgical Hospital	New Albany	90%	300+
Bluffton Hospital	Bluffton	88%	(a)
Dublin Methodist Hospital	Dublin	88%	300+
Cleveland Clinic	Cleveland	87%	300+
Christ Hospital	Cincinnati	86%	300+
James Cancer Hosp & Solove Res Inst	Columbus	84%	300+
Univ Hosps Conneaut Med Ctr	Conneaut	84%	(a)
Mercy Hospital Fairfield	Fairfield	83%	300+
Mercy Willard Hospital	Willard	83%	(a)
Saint Elizabeth Boardman Health Center	Boardman	83%	300+
West Chester Hospital	West Chester	83%	300+
Defiance Regional Medical Center	Defiance	82%	300+
Indu & Raj Soin Medical Center	Beaver Creek	82%	300+
Bellevue Hospital	Bellevue	81%	300+
Kettering Medical Center	Kettering	81%	300+
Ohio Valley Medical Center	Springfield	81%	300+
Aultman Hospital	Canton	80%	300+
Community Memorial Hospital	Hicksville	80%	(a)
H B Magruder Memorial Hospital	Port Clinton	80%	300+
Henry County Hospital	Napoleon	80%	(a)
UHHS Memorial Hospital of Geneva	Geneva	80%	(a)
Mercy Saint Anne Hospital	Toledo	79%	300+
Miami Valley Hospital[11]	Dayton	79%	300+
Riverside Methodist Hospital	Columbus	79%	300+
University Hospitals Case Medical Center	Cleveland	79%	300+
Wooster Community Hospital	Wooster	79%	300+
Bay Park Community Hospital	Oregon	78%	300+
Crystal Clinic Orthopaedic Center	Akron	78%	300+
Medcentral Health System Shelby Hospital	Shelby	78%	(a)
Mercy Hospital Clermont	Batavia	78%	300+
Fairview Hospital	Cleveland	77%	300+
Good Samaritan Hospital	Cincinnati	77%	300+
Grant Medical Center	Columbus	77%	300+
Ohio State University Hospitals	Columbus	77%	300+
Saint Joseph Health Center	Warren	77%	300+
Community Hospitals & Wellness Centers	Bryan	76%	300+
Flower Hospital	Sylvania	76%	300+
Holzer Medical Center Jackson	Jackson	76%	(a)
Memorial Hospital of Union County	Marysville	76%	300+
Summa Western Reserve Hospital	Cuyahoga Falls	76%	300+
Bethesda North	Cincinnati	75%	300+
Fostoria Community Hospital	Fostoria	75%	(a)
Fulton County Health Center	Wauseon	75%	300+
Mercer County Joint Twp Comm Hosp	Coldwater	75%	300+
Mercy Hospital of Defiance	Defiance	75%	300+
Selby General Hospital	Marietta	75%	300+
Sycamore Medical Center	Miamisburg	75%	300+
University Hospitals Ahuja Medical Center	Beachwood	75%	300+
Akron General Medical Center	Akron	74%	300+
Barnesville Hospital Association	Barnesville	74%	(a)
Blanchard Valley Hospital	Findlay	74%	300+
Hocking Valley Community Hospital	Logan	74%	(a)
Mercy Medical Center	Canton	74%	300+
Morrow County Hospital	Mount Gilead	74%	(a)
Saint Rita's Medical Center	Lima	74%	300+

NOTE: Hospital profiles are in alphabetical order by state, then city, then hospital within the city; Rankings exclude hospitals with less than 25 cases except for patient surveys which excludes hospitals with less than 100 cases; (a) 100-299 cases; (1) The number of cases/patients is too few to report; (2) Data submitted were based on a sample of cases/patients; (3) Results are based on a shorter time period than required; (4) Data suppressed by CMS for one or more quarters; (5) Results are not available for this reporting period; (6) Fewer than 100 patients completed the HCAHPS survey; (7) No cases met the criteria for this measure; (8) The lower limit of the confidence interval cannot be calculated if the number of observed infections equals zero; (9) No data are available from the state/territory for this reporting period; (10) The scores shown reflect fewer than 50 completed surveys; (11) There were discrepancies in the data collection process; (12) This measure does not apply to this hospital for this reporting period; (13) Results cannot be calculated for this reporting period; (14) The results for this state are combined with nearby states to protect confidentiality; Please refer to the User's Guide for a full explanation of data.

Southwest General Health Center	Middleburg Hgts	74%	300+
UH Geauga Medical Center	Chardon	74%	300+
Wood County Hospital	Bowling Green	74%	300+
Grady Memorial Hospital	Delaware	73%	300+
Grandview Hospital & Medical Center	Dayton	73%	300+
Lutheran Hospital	Cleveland	73%	300+
McCullough - Hyde Memorial Hospital	Oxford	73%	300+
Mercy Saint Vincent Medical Center	Toledo	73%	300+
Saint John Medical Center	Westlake	73%	300+
The Toledo Hospital	Toledo	73%	300+
Doctors Hospital	Columbus	72%	300+
Fairfield Medical Center	Lancaster	72%	300+
Firelands Regional Medical Center	Sandusky	72%	300+
Good Samaritan Hospital[11]	Dayton	72%	300+
Jewish Hospital	Cincinnati	72%	300+
Mount Carmel West	Columbus	72%	300+
Saint Luke's Hospital	Maumee	72%	300+
Euclid Hospital	Euclid	71%	300+
Hillcrest Hospital	Mayfield Heights	71%	300+
Mercy Hospital Anderson	Cincinnati	71%	300+
Southern Ohio Medical Center	Portsmouth	71%	300+
Fisher - Titus Hospital	Norwalk	70%	300+
Galion Community Hospital	Galion	70%	300+
Hardin Memorial Hospital	Kenton	70%	(a)
Mercy Allen Hospital	Oberlin	70%	(a)
Mount Carmel Saint Ann's	Westerville	70%	300+
Saint Vincent Charity Medical Center	Cleveland	70%	300+
Summa Health Systems Hospitals	Akron	70%	300+
Trinity Med Ctr East & West	Steubenville	70%	300+
Atrium Medical Center[11]	Franklin	69%	300+
Grand Lake Health System	Saint Marys	69%	300+
Lake Health	Concord	69%	300+
Lima Memorial Health System	Lima	69%	300+
Saint Elizabeth Health Center	Youngstown	69%	300+
Samaritan Regional Health System	Ashland	69%	300+
Union Hospital	Dover	69%	300+
Univ Hosps-Elyria Med Ctr	Elyria	69%	300+
Aultman Orrville Hospital	Orrville	68%	(a)
Lakewood Hospital	Lakewood	68%	300+
Medina Hospital	Medina	68%	300+
Mercy Saint Charles Hospital	Oregon	68%	300+
South Pointe Hospital	Warrensville Hgts	68%	300+
Wilson Memorial Hospital[11]	Sidney	68%	300+
Wyandot Memorial Hospital	Upper Sandusky	68%	(a)
Alliance Community Hospital	Alliance	67%	300+
Fayette County Memorial Hospital	Washington Ch	67%	(a)
Madison County Hospital	London	67%	(a)
Mary Rutan Hospital	Bellefontaine	67%	300+
Mercy Tiffin Hospital	Tiffin	67%	300+
Southeastern Ohio Regional Medical Center	Cambridge	66%	300+
Summa Health System Barberton Hospital	Barberton	66%	300+
UHHS Richmond Heights Hospital	Richmond Hghts	66%	300+
Adena Regional Medical Center	Chillicothe	65%	300+
Affinity Medical Center	Massillon	65%	300+
Berger Hospital	Circleville	65%	300+
Fort Hamilton Hughes Memorial Hospital	Hamilton	65%	300+
Genesis Healthcare System	Zanesville	65%	300+
Marietta Memorial Hospital	Marietta	65%	300+
Marion General Hospital	Marion	65%	300+
Medcentral Health Sys Mansfield Hosp	Mansfield	65%	300+
Parma Community General Hospital	Parma	65%	300+
Holzer Medical Center	Gallipolis	64%	300+
Mercy Memorial Hospital	Urbana	64%	(a)
Metrohealth System	Cleveland	64%	300+
Pomerene Hospital	Millersburg	64%	300+
University of Cincinnati Medical Center	Cincinnati	64%	300+
Upper Valley Medical Center[11]	Troy	64%	300+
Licking Memorial Hospital	Newark	63%	300+
Marymount Hospital	Garfield Heights	63%	300+
Northside Medical Center	Youngstown	63%	300+
Van Wert County Hospital	Van Wert	63%	300+
East Ohio Regional Hospital	Martins Ferry	62%	300+
Greene Memorial Hospital	Xenia	62%	300+
Mercy Health - West Hospital	Cincinnati	62%	300+
Mercy Regional Medical Center[11]	Lorain	62%	300+
Adams County Regional Medical Center	Seaman	61%	(a)
Bucyrus Community Hospital	Bucyrus	61%	(a)
Memorial Hospital	Fremont	61%	300+
Robinson Memorial Hospital	Ravenna	61%	300+
Summa Wadsworth - Rittman Hospital	Wadsworth	61%	300+
Clinton Memorial Hospital	Wilmington	60%	300+
O'Bleness Memorial Hospital	Athens	60%	300+
Springfield Regional Medical Center	Springfield	60%	300+
Wayne Hospital	Greenville	60%	300+
Knox Community Hospital	Mount Vernon	59%	300+
Medical Center at Elizabeth Place	Dayton	59%	(a)
University of Toledo Medical Center	Toledo	59%	300+
Pike Community Hospital	Waverly	58%	(a)
Salem Regional Medical Center	Salem	58%	300+
Ashtabula County Medical Center	Ashtabula	56%	300+
Trumbull Memorial Hospital	Warren	56%	300+
East Liverpool City Hospital	East Liverpool	55%	300+
Southwest Regional Medical Center	Georgetown	52%	(a)
Highland District Hospital	Hillsboro	51%	(a)
Coshocton County Memorial Hospital	Coshocton	49%	300+

Use of Medical Imaging

Cardiac Imaging Stress Test before OP Surgery

Hospital Name	City	Rate	Cases
Coshocton County Memorial Hospital	Coshocton	0.9%	213
Univ Hosps Conneaut Med Ctr	Conneaut	1.7%	59
Holzer Medical Center	Gallipolis	2.0%	347
Mercy Tiffin Hospital	Tiffin	2.0%	198
UHHS Memorial Hospital of Geneva	Geneva	2.0%	101
Summa Health System Barberton Hospital	Barberton	2.1%	238
Saint Elizabeth Boardman Health Center	Boardman	2.3%	131
McCullough - Hyde Memorial Hospital	Oxford	2.5%	79
Wayne Hospital	Greenville	2.8%	463
Marion General Hospital	Marion	2.9%	70
Samaritan Regional Health System	Ashland	3.0%	237
Fairview Hospital	Cleveland	3.1%	96
Fostoria Community Hospital	Fostoria	3.1%	131
Metrohealth System	Cleveland	3.1%	449
East Liverpool City Hospital	East Liverpool	3.3%	215
Greene Memorial Hospital	Xenia	3.3%	122
Upper Valley Medical Center	Troy	3.3%	421
Adams County Regional Medical Center	Seaman	3.5%	57
Good Samaritan Hospital	Cincinnati	3.5%	865
Mercy Medical Center	Canton	3.5%	457
H B Magruder Memorial Hospital	Port Clinton	3.7%	164
Bellevue Hospital	Bellevue	3.9%	180
Marietta Memorial Hospital	Marietta	3.9%	593
Mercy Regional Medical Center	Lorain	4.0%	321
Southeastern Ohio Regional Medical Center	Cambridge	4.0%	250
Adena Regional Medical Center	Chillicothe	4.1%	756
Lutheran Hospital	Cleveland	4.1%	98
Mercy Health - West Hospital	Cincinnati	4.1%	97
Mercy Saint Vincent Medical Center	Toledo	4.1%	388
Christ Hospital	Cincinnati	4.2%	1580
Doctors Hospital	Columbus	4.2%	332
Galion Community Hospital	Galion	4.2%	165
Mercy Memorial Hospital	Urbana	4.2%	96
Mercy Willard Hospital	Willard	4.2%	144
Indu & Raj Soin Medical Center	Beaver Creek	4.3%	138
Licking Memorial Hospital	Newark	4.3%	277
Wood County Hospital	Bowling Green	4.4%	159
Ashtabula County Medical Center	Ashtabula	4.5%	289
The Toledo Hospital	Toledo	4.5%	1276
Trumbull Memorial Hospital	Warren	4.5%	201
Lima Memorial Health System	Lima	4.6%	787
Summa Health Systems Hospitals	Akron	4.6%	843
Euclid Hospital	Euclid	4.7%	86
Grant Medical Center	Columbus	4.7%	657
Saint Joseph Health Center	Warren	4.7%	192
Bethesda North	Cincinnati	4.8%	882
Good Samaritan Hospital	Dayton	4.8%	1242
Saint Elizabeth Health Center	Youngstown	4.8%	1187
West Chester Hospital	West Chester	4.8%	270
Henry County Hospital	Napoleon	4.9%	81
Kettering Medical Center	Kettering	4.9%	882
Southwest Regional Medical Center	Georgetown	4.9%	81
Fulton County Health Center	Wauseon	5.0%	280
Fairfield Medical Center	Lancaster	5.1%	156
Knox Community Hospital	Mount Vernon	5.1%	622
Univ Hosps-Elyria Med Ctr	Elyria	5.1%	1958
Wilson Memorial Hospital	Sidney	5.1%	295
Genesis Healthcare System	Zanesville	5.2%	482
Memorial Hospital	Fremont	5.2%	230
UH Geauga Medical Center	Chardon	5.2%	135
Van Wert County Hospital	Van Wert	5.2%	287
Fort Hamilton Hughes Memorial Hospital	Hamilton	5.3%	244
University of Cincinnati Medical Center	Cincinnati	5.3%	393
Saint Rita's Medical Center	Lima	5.4%	922
Sycamore Medical Center	Miamisburg	5.4%	480
Aultman Hospital	Canton	5.5%	817
Jewish Hospital	Cincinnati	5.5%	475
Affinity Medical Center	Massillon	5.6%	144
Berger Hospital	Circleville	5.6%	162
University Hospitals Case Medical Center	Cleveland	5.6%	676
University of Toledo Medical Center	Toledo	5.6%	233
Clinton Memorial Hospital	Wilmington	5.7%	229
Mercy Hospital Anderson	Cincinnati	5.7%	264
Mount Carmel Saint Ann's	Westerville	5.7%	421
Highland District Hospital	Hillsboro	5.8%	139
Akron General Medical Center	Akron	5.9%	883
Mercy Hospital Fairfield	Fairfield	5.9%	765
Mount Carmel West	Columbus	5.9%	870
Bay Park Community Hospital	Oregon	6.0%	333
Mercy Saint Charles Hospital	Oregon	6.0%	182
O'Bleness Memorial Hospital	Athens	6.0%	84
Parma Community General Hospital	Parma	6.0%	745
Riverside Methodist Hospital	Columbus	6.0%	1066
East Ohio Regional Hospital	Martins Ferry	6.1%	98
Saint Vincent Charity Medical Center	Cleveland	6.1%	214
Wooster Community Hospital	Wooster	6.2%	388
Mary Rutan Hospital	Bellefontaine	6.3%	96
Southwest General Health Center	Middleburg Hgts	6.3%	144
Fisher - Titus Hospital	Norwalk	6.4%	250
Grandview Hospital & Medical Center	Dayton	6.4%	718
Salem Regional Medical Center	Salem	6.4%	233
Springfield Regional Medical Center	Springfield	6.4%	574
Grady Memorial Hospital	Delaware	6.5%	168
Robinson Memorial Hospital	Ravenna	6.5%	418
Southern Ohio Medical Center	Portsmouth	6.5%	527
Trinity Hospital Twin City	Dennison	6.5%	77
Blanchard Valley Hospital	Findlay	6.6%	288
Cleveland Clinic	Cleveland	6.7%	4179
Fayette County Memorial Hospital	Washington Ch	6.7%	75
Mercy Hospital Clermont	Batavia	6.7%	165
Alliance Community Hospital	Alliance	6.8%	147
Dublin Methodist Hospital	Dublin	6.8%	74
Hillcrest Hospital	Mayfield Heights	6.8%	176
Miami Valley Hospital	Dayton	6.8%	1115
University Hospitals Ahuja Medical Center	Beachwood	6.8%	220
Lake Health	Concord	6.9%	173
Hocking Valley Community Hospital	Logan	7.0%	100
Firelands Regional Medical Center	Sandusky	7.3%	220
Northside Medical Center	Youngstown	7.3%	164
Saint Luke's Hospital	Maumee	7.3%	343
Medina Hospital	Medina	7.4%	242
Trinity Med Ctr East & West	Steubenville	7.5%	558
Marymount Hospital	Garfield Heights	7.6%	157
Atrium Medical Center	Franklin	7.9%	242
Saint John Medical Center	Westlake	8.0%	88
Union Hospital	Dover	8.3%	302
Mercy Saint Anne Hospital	Toledo	8.7%	104
Summa Wadsworth - Rittman Hospital	Wadsworth	8.7%	149
UHHS Richmond Heights Hospital	Richmond Hghts	8.7%	149
South Pointe Hospital	Warrensville Hgts	9.0%	67
Aultman Orrville Hospital	Orrville	9.2%	65
Summa Western Reserve Hospital	Cuyahoga Falls	9.2%	174
Flower Hospital	Sylvania	9.3%	129
Ohio State University Hospitals	Columbus	9.8%	610
Memorial Hospital of Union County	Marysville	10.3%	136
Pomerene Hospital	Millersburg	14.3%	133

Combination Abdominal CT Scan

Hospital Name	City	Rate	Cases
Henry County Hospital	Napoleon	0.6%	161
Medcentral Health Sys Mansfield Hosp	Mansfield	0.6%	1197
Mercy Hospital of Defiance	Defiance	0.7%	137
Doctors Hospital of Nelsonville	Nelsonville	1.0%	104
Mercy Saint Vincent Medical Center	Toledo	1.0%	414
Euclid Hospital	Euclid	1.2%	402
Diley Ridge Medical Center	Canal Wnchstr	1.3%	235
Lutheran Hospital	Cleveland	1.3%	230
Wooster Community Hospital	Wooster	1.4%	511
Holzer Medical Center Jackson	Jackson	1.5%	273
Ashtabula County Medical Center	Ashtabula	1.6%	608
Lakewood Hospital	Lakewood	1.6%	321
Mercy Allen Hospital	Oberlin	1.6%	191
Mercy Saint Anne Hospital	Toledo	1.9%	641
Ohio Valley Medical Center	Springfield	1.9%	53
Firelands Regional Medical Center	Sandusky	2.0%	982
UHHS Memorial Hospital of Geneva	Geneva	2.0%	445
Wayne Hospital	Greenville	2.0%	539
Grant Medical Center	Columbus	2.1%	1094
Mount Carmel West	Columbus	2.3%	1944
Southwest Regional Medical Center	Georgetown	2.3%	132
Flower Hospital	Sylvania	2.4%	576
Memorial Hospital of Union County	Marysville	2.4%	376
Northside Medical Center	Youngstown	2.4%	410
Trumbull Memorial Hospital	Warren	2.4%	740
Univ Hosps-Elyria Med Ctr	Elyria	2.4%	990
Lake Health	Concord	2.5%	1684
Doctors Hospital	Columbus	2.6%	494
Indu & Raj Soin Medical Center	Beaver Creek	2.6%	391
Mercy Regional Medical Center	Lorain	2.7%	1202
Coshocton County Memorial Hospital	Coshocton	2.9%	343
Dublin Methodist Hospital	Dublin	2.9%	446
Berger Hospital	Circleville	3.1%	557
Parma Community General Hospital	Parma	3.1%	1086
Springfield Regional Medical Center	Springfield	3.1%	1006
Madison County Hospital	London	3.2%	125
Mount Carmel Saint Ann's	Westerville	3.2%	743
Wood County Hospital	Bowling Green	3.2%	345
Fayette County Memorial Hospital	Washington Ch	3.3%	366
Licking Memorial Hospital	Newark	3.3%	1013
Summa Western Reserve Hospital	Cuyahoga Falls	3.3%	329
Adena Regional Medical Center	Chillicothe	3.5%	1269
Mercy Memorial Hospital	Urbana	3.5%	318

NOTE: Hospital profiles are in alphabetical order by state, then city, then hospital within the city; Rankings exclude hospitals with less than 25 cases except for patient surveys which excludes hospitals with less than 100 cases; (a) 100-299 cases; (1) The number of cases/patients is too few to report; (2) Data submitted were based on a sample of cases/patients; (3) Results are based on a shorter time period than required; (4) Data suppressed by CMS for one or more quarters; (5) Results are not available for this reporting period; (6) Fewer than 100 patients completed the HCAHPS survey; (7) No cases met the criteria for this measure; (8) The lower limit of the confidence interval cannot be calculated if the number of observed infections equals zero; (9) No data are available from the state/territory for this reporting period; (10) The scores shown reflect fewer than 50 completed surveys; (11) There were discrepancies in the data collection process; (12) This measure does not apply to this hospital for this reporting period; (13) Results cannot be calculated for this reporting period; (14) The results for this state are combined with nearby states to protect confidentiality; Please refer to the User's Guide for a full explanation of data.

Hospital Name	City	Rate	Cases
The Toledo Hospital	Toledo	3.5%	832
Fairfield Medical Center	Lancaster	3.6%	922
Summa Health System Barberton Hospital	Barberton	3.6%	471
Affinity Medical Center	Massillon	3.7%	433
Mercy Willard Hospital	Willard	3.7%	187
Barnesville Hospital Association	Barnesville	3.8%	132
Summa Wadsworth - Rittman Hospital	Wadsworth	3.8%	314
Akron General Medical Center	Akron	3.9%	1625
Greenfield Area Medical Center	Greenfield	4.0%	151
Robinson Memorial Hospital	Ravenna	4.0%	519
South Pointe Hospital	Warrensville Hgts	4.0%	572
Summa Health Systems Hospitals	Akron	4.2%	1259
Selby General Hospital	Marietta	4.3%	138
Community Hospitals & Wellness Centers	Montpelier	4.4%	45
Fairview Hospital	Cleveland	4.4%	1033
H B Magruder Memorial Hospital	Port Clinton	4.5%	397
Lodi Community Hospital	Lodi	4.5%	110
Mercy Hospital Anderson	Cincinnati	4.5%	1060
Mercy Hospital Clermont	Batavia	4.5%	785
Fort Hamilton Hughes Memorial Hospital	Hamilton	4.6%	658
University Hospitals Case Medical Center	Cleveland	4.6%	1959
Marymount Hospital	Garfield Heights	4.7%	654
Union Hospital	Dover	4.7%	705
Saint Luke's Hospital	Maumee	4.8%	871
UH Geauga Medical Center	Chardon	4.8%	565
Atrium Medical Center	Franklin	4.9%	991
Good Samaritan Hospital	Cincinnati	4.9%	1067
Riverside Methodist Hospital	Columbus	4.9%	1969
Good Samaritan Hospital	Dayton	5.0%	1148
Bay Park Community Hospital	Oregon	5.1%	294
University of Cincinnati Medical Center	Cincinnati	5.1%	925
Marion General Hospital	Marion	5.2%	618
Sycamore Medical Center	Miamisburg	5.2%	728
Community Hospitals & Wellness Centers	Bryan	5.3%	284
Kettering Medical Center	Kettering	5.3%	1305
Southeastern Ohio Regional Medical Center	Cambridge	5.3%	570
Jewish Hospital	Cincinnati	5.5%	814
Lima Memorial Health System	Lima	5.5%	690
Mercy Hospital Fairfield	Fairfield	5.5%	1034
Saint Elizabeth Health Center	Youngstown	5.5%	782
Mercy Medical Center	Canton	5.6%	1139
Hocking Valley Community Hospital	Logan	5.7%	230
Saint Vincent Charity Medical Center	Cleveland	5.7%	244
Morrow County Hospital	Mount Gilead	5.8%	260
Galion Community Hospital	Galion	5.9%	393
Blanchard Valley Hospital	Findlay	6.0%	922
Mercer County Joint Twp Comm Hosp	Coldwater	6.0%	250
Fulton County Health Center	Wauseon	6.1%	443
McCullough - Hyde Memorial Hospital	Oxford	6.1%	263
Univ Hosps Conneaut Med Ctr	Conneaut	6.1%	198
Aultman Hospital	Canton	6.2%	1502
Bluffton Hospital	Bluffton	6.2%	81
Genesis Healthcare System	Zanesville	6.3%	1552
Mercy Health - West Hospital	Cincinnati	6.3%	584
Trinity Hospital Twin City	Dennison	6.3%	159
Greene Memorial Hospital	Xenia	6.4%	342
O'Bleness Memorial Hospital	Athens	6.5%	339
Medina Hospital	Medina	6.8%	516
Grandview Hospital & Medical Center	Dayton	6.9%	1311
Christ Hospital	Cincinnati	7.2%	1712
Fisher - Titus Hospital	Norwalk	7.2%	414
Saint Elizabeth Boardman Health Center	Boardman	7.2%	769
Grady Memorial Hospital	Delaware	7.5%	334
Metrohealth System	Cleveland	7.5%	994
Mary Rutan Hospital	Bellefontaine	7.8%	477
University Hospitals Ahuja Medical Center	Beachwood	7.8%	438
Saint John Medical Center	Westlake	7.9%	624
Upper Valley Medical Center	Troy	7.9%	770
West Chester Hospital	West Chester	7.9%	391
Adams County Regional Medical Center	Seaman	8.0%	337
Fostoria Community Hospital	Fostoria	8.0%	261
Miami Valley Hospital	Dayton	8.1%	1776
Paulding County Hospital	Paulding	8.2%	146
Wilson Memorial Hospital	Sidney	8.5%	343
Ohio State University Hospitals	Columbus	8.7%	1536
Marietta Memorial Hospital	Marietta	8.8%	1563
Mercy Saint Charles Hospital	Oregon	8.9%	665
Pomerene Hospital	Millersburg	8.9%	168
Salem Regional Medical Center	Salem	9.1%	740
Bethesda North	Cincinnati	9.2%	1779
Hillcrest Hospital	Mayfield Heights	9.3%	1431
UHHS Richmond Heights Hospital	Richmond Hghts	9.6%	603
Southern Ohio Medical Center	Portsmouth	10.1%	1404
Community Memorial Hospital	Hicksville	10.3%	87
East Liverpool City Hospital	East Liverpool	10.7%	411
Highland District Hospital	Hillsboro	11.3%	389
University of Toledo Medical Center	Toledo	11.9%	538
Surgical Hospital at Southwoods	Youngstown	12.3%	106
Clinton Memorial Hospital	Wilmington	12.8%	545
Cleveland Clinic	Cleveland	13.0%	5813
Samaritan Regional Health System	Ashland	13.1%	473
Van Wert County Hospital	Van Wert	13.1%	314
Trinity Med Ctr East & West	Steubenville	14.9%	683
Saint Rita's Medical Center	Lima	15.2%	1324
Bellevue Hospital	Bellevue	15.5%	304
Southwest General Health Center	Middleburg Hgts	15.8%	1445
Memorial Hospital	Fremont	16.5%	375
Holzer Medical Center	Gallipolis	22.5%	993
Alliance Community Hospital	Alliance	23.8%	495
Grand Lake Health System	Saint Marys	24.0%	359
Aultman Orrville Hospital	Orrville	25.0%	116
Saint Joseph Health Center	Warren	26.4%	711
Knox Community Hospital	Mount Vernon	28.1%	754
Kings Daughters Medical Center Ohio	Portsmouth	28.6%	63
Harrison Community Hospital	Cadiz	29.6%	71
Mercy Tiffin Hospital	Tiffin	32.8%	357
East Ohio Regional Hospital	Martins Ferry	58.2%	306

Combination Brain/Sinus CT Scan

Hospital Name	City	Rate	Cases
Medical Center at Elizabeth Place	Dayton	0.0%	53
Marion General Hospital	Marion	0.2%	602
Good Samaritan Hospital	Cincinnati	0.3%	775
Fisher - Titus Hospital	Norwalk	0.4%	450
Mercy Willard Hospital	Willard	0.6%	176
Southwest Regional Medical Center	Georgetown	0.6%	169
Mercy Hospital Fairfield	Fairfield	0.9%	681
Bethesda North	Cincinnati	1.0%	1225
Mount Carmel West	Columbus	1.0%	1737
Licking Memorial Hospital	Newark	1.1%	724
Mercy Hospital Clermont	Batavia	1.1%	643
Mercy Hospital Anderson	Cincinnati	1.2%	581
Mercy Hospital of Defiance	Defiance	1.2%	173
Wood County Hospital	Bowling Green	1.2%	325
Galion Community Hospital	Galion	1.3%	388
Memorial Hospital of Union County	Marysville	1.3%	303
Mercy Health - West Hospital	Cincinnati	1.3%	382
Adams County Regional Medical Center	Seaman	1.4%	360
Alliance Community Hospital	Alliance	1.4%	566
Christ Hospital	Cincinnati	1.4%	898
Akron General Medical Center	Akron	1.5%	1293
Metrohealth System	Cleveland	1.5%	649
University of Toledo Medical Center	Toledo	1.5%	521
Salem Regional Medical Center	Salem	1.6%	577
The Toledo Hospital	Toledo	1.6%	690
Adena Regional Medical Center	Chillicothe	1.7%	871
Cleveland Clinic	Cleveland	1.7%	2131
Flower Hospital	Sylvania	1.7%	424
Good Samaritan Hospital	Dayton	1.7%	1169
Mercy Saint Anne Hospital	Toledo	1.7%	468
Saint Luke's Hospital	Maumee	1.7%	779
University of Cincinnati Medical Center	Cincinnati	1.7%	593
Wooster Community Hospital	Wooster	1.7%	523
Samaritan Regional Health System	Ashland	1.8%	494
Union Hospital	Dover	1.8%	562
Ashtabula County Medical Center	Ashtabula	1.9%	513
Mercy Saint Charles Hospital	Oregon	1.9%	537
Mercy Saint Vincent Medical Center	Toledo	1.9%	471
Euclid Hospital	Euclid	2.0%	649
Indu & Raj Soin Medical Center	Beaver Creek	2.0%	409
Mercy Regional Medical Center	Lorain	2.0%	955
Summa Health Systems Hospitals	Akron	2.0%	1085
Upper Valley Medical Center	Troy	2.0%	789
Wayne Hospital	Greenville	2.0%	547
Wilson Memorial Hospital	Sidney	2.0%	409
Aultman Hospital	Canton	2.1%	1365
Berger Hospital	Circleville	2.1%	528
Knox Community Hospital	Mount Vernon	2.2%	637
Medina Hospital	Medina	2.2%	582
Robinson Memorial Hospital	Ravenna	2.2%	538
Southeastern Ohio Regional Medical Center	Cambridge	2.2%	541
Atrium Medical Center	Franklin	2.3%	1020
Kettering Medical Center	Kettering	2.3%	1187
Lima Memorial Health System	Lima	2.3%	648
University Hospitals Ahuja Medical Center	Beachwood	2.5%	525
Sycamore Medical Center	Miamisburg	2.6%	696
Jewish Hospital	Cincinnati	2.7%	602
Univ Hosps-Elyria Med Ctr	Elyria	2.7%	916
Fairview Hospital	Cleveland	2.9%	693
Riverside Methodist Hospital	Columbus	2.9%	1290
Parma Community General Hospital	Parma	3.0%	760
Fairfield Medical Center	Lancaster	3.1%	891
Grant Medical Center	Columbus	3.1%	938
Medcentral Health Sys Mansfield Hosp	Mansfield	3.1%	1137
Trinity Med Ctr East & West	Steubenville	3.1%	718
UHHS Richmond Heights Hospital	Richmond Hghts	3.1%	720
Ohio State University Hospitals	Columbus	3.2%	816
Springfield Regional Medical Center	Springfield	3.2%	844
Marymount Hospital	Garfield Heights	3.3%	768
Mount Carmel Saint Ann's	Westerville	3.4%	715
Mercy Medical Center	Canton	3.6%	936
University Hospitals Case Medical Center	Cleveland	3.6%	726
Grandview Hospital & Medical Center	Dayton	3.7%	926
Genesis Healthcare System	Zanesville	3.9%	1065
Saint John Medical Center	Westlake	3.9%	670
Southern Ohio Medical Center	Portsmouth	3.9%	1222
Blanchard Valley Hospital	Findlay	4.0%	700
Lakewood Hospital	Lakewood	4.0%	424
South Pointe Hospital	Warrensville Hgts	4.0%	676
Firelands Regional Medical Center	Sandusky	4.3%	832
Lake Health	Concord	4.3%	1643
Saint Joseph Health Center	Warren	4.3%	828
Saint Rita's Medical Center	Lima	4.3%	1087
Miami Valley Hospital	Dayton	4.4%	2020
Trumbull Memorial Hospital	Warren	4.7%	620
East Liverpool City Hospital	East Liverpool	4.8%	501
Saint Elizabeth Boardman Health Center	Boardman	5.3%	702
Saint Elizabeth Health Center	Youngstown	5.3%	823
H B Magruder Memorial Hospital	Port Clinton	5.4%	389
Trinity Hospital Twin City	Dennison	5.4%	148
Hillcrest Hospital	Mayfield Heights	5.7%	1225
Southwest General Health Center	Middleburg Hgts	5.9%	1043
Affinity Medical Center	Massillon	6.1%	488
Marietta Memorial Hospital	Marietta	6.6%	1045
Saint Vincent Charity Medical Center	Cleveland	7.2%	223

Combination Chest CT Scan

Hospital Name	City	Rate	Cases
Affinity Medical Center	Massillon	0.0%	177
Ashtabula County Medical Center	Ashtabula	0.0%	414
Bay Park Community Hospital	Oregon	0.0%	207
Belmont Community Hospital	Bellaire	0.0%	53
Doctors Hospital of Nelsonville	Nelsonville	0.0%	51
East Ohio Regional Hospital	Martins Ferry	0.0%	212
Firelands Regional Medical Center	Sandusky	0.0%	627
Fort Hamilton Hughes Memorial Hospital	Hamilton	0.0%	358
H B Magruder Memorial Hospital	Port Clinton	0.0%	280
Henry County Hospital	Napoleon	0.0%	105
Hillcrest Hospital	Mayfield Heights	0.0%	1046
Hocking Valley Community Hospital	Logan	0.0%	93
Kettering Medical Center	Kettering	0.0%	826
Lodi Community Hospital	Lodi	0.0%	48
Lutheran Hospital	Cleveland	0.0%	56
Marion General Hospital	Marion	0.0%	182
McCullough - Hyde Memorial Hospital	Oxford	0.0%	179
Memorial Hospital of Union County	Marysville	0.0%	185
Mercy Hospital Anderson	Cincinnati	0.0%	699
Mercy Medical Center	Canton	0.0%	707
Northside Medical Center	Youngstown	0.0%	207
Robinson Memorial Hospital	Ravenna	0.0%	235
Saint Vincent Charity Medical Center	Cleveland	0.0%	142
Salem Regional Medical Center	Salem	0.0%	473
Summa Health Systems Hospitals	Akron	0.0%	870
Summa Wadsworth - Rittman Hospital	Wadsworth	0.0%	123
Summa Western Reserve Hospital	Cuyahoga Falls	0.0%	230
Surgical Hospital at Southwoods	Youngstown	0.0%	45
University of Toledo Medical Center	Toledo	0.0%	302
Wilson Memorial Hospital	Sidney	0.0%	238
Wooster Community Hospital	Wooster	0.0%	390
Cleveland Clinic	Cleveland	0.1%	6539
Southwest General Health Center	Middleburg Hgts	0.1%	854
University Hospitals Case Medical Center	Cleveland	0.1%	2664
Fairview Hospital	Cleveland	0.2%	603
Union Hospital	Dover	0.2%	470
Berger Hospital	Circleville	0.3%	295
Marymount Hospital	Garfield Heights	0.3%	320
Mercy Health - West Hospital	Cincinnati	0.3%	333
Mercy Hospital Clermont	Batavia	0.3%	701
Mercy Saint Vincent Medical Center	Toledo	0.3%	318
Ohio State University Hospitals	Columbus	0.3%	1417
Sycamore Medical Center	Miamisburg	0.3%	319
Univ Hosps-Elyria Med Ctr	Elyria	0.3%	327
University Hospitals Ahuja Medical Center	Beachwood	0.3%	330
Wayne Hospital	Greenville	0.3%	332
Bethesda North	Cincinnati	0.4%	1135
Genesis Healthcare System	Zanesville	0.4%	1532
Mount Carmel West	Columbus	0.4%	733
Summa Health System Barberton Hospital	Barberton	0.4%	225
Coshocton County Memorial Hospital	Coshocton	0.5%	220
Lake Health	Concord	0.5%	1082
UHHS Memorial Hospital of Geneva	Geneva	0.5%	422
Grant Medical Center	Columbus	0.6%	462
Medcentral Health Sys Mansfield Hosp	Mansfield	0.6%	693
Akron General Medical Center	Akron	0.7%	1151
Fayette County Memorial Hospital	Washington Ch	0.7%	152
Good Samaritan Hospital	Cincinnati	0.7%	751
Jewish Hospital	Cincinnati	0.7%	613
Lakewood Hospital	Lakewood	0.7%	134
Lima Memorial Health System	Lima	0.7%	289
Parma Community General Hospital	Parma	0.7%	757
Saint John Medical Center	Westlake	0.7%	451
Adena Regional Medical Center	Chillicothe	0.8%	745
Licking Memorial Hospital	Newark	0.8%	527

NOTE: Hospital profiles are in alphabetical order by state, then city, then hospital within the city; Rankings exclude hospitals with less than 25 cases except for patient surveys which excludes hospitals with less than 100 cases; (a) 100-299 cases; (1) The number of cases/patients is too few to report; (2) Data submitted were based on a sample of cases/patients; (3) Results are based on a shorter time period than required; (4) Data suppressed by CMS for one or more quarters; (5) Results are not available for this reporting period; (6) Fewer than 100 patients completed the HCAHPS survey; (7) No cases met the criteria for this measure; (8) The lower limit of the confidence interval cannot be calculated if the number of observed infections equals zero; (9) No data are available from the state/territory for this reporting period; (10) The scores shown reflect fewer than 50 completed surveys; (11) There were discrepancies in the data collection process; (12) This measure does not apply to this hospital for this reporting period; (13) Results cannot be calculated for this reporting period; (14) The results for this state are combined with nearby states to protect confidentiality; Please refer to the User's Guide for a full explanation of data.

Hospital Name	City	Rate	Cases
Mount Carmel Saint Ann's	Westerville	0.8%	265
O'Bleness Memorial Hospital	Athens	0.8%	125
Univ Hosps Conneaut Med Ctr	Conneaut	0.8%	124
University of Cincinnati Medical Center	Cincinnati	0.8%	1213
Fairfield Medical Center	Lancaster	0.9%	547
Medina Hospital	Medina	0.9%	317
Mercer County Joint Twp Comm Hosp	Coldwater	0.9%	117
Mercy Saint Anne Hospital	Toledo	0.9%	451
Doctors Hospital	Columbus	1.0%	314
Atrium Medical Center	Franklin	1.1%	824
Indu & Raj Soin Medical Center	Beaver Creek	1.1%	94
Christ Hospital	Cincinnati	1.2%	1522
Madison County Hospital	London	1.2%	82
Southwest Regional Medical Center	Georgetown	1.3%	75
West Chester Hospital	West Chester	1.3%	235
Riverside Methodist Hospital	Columbus	1.4%	1472
Saint Joseph Health Center	Warren	1.4%	491
Trumbull Memorial Hospital	Warren	1.4%	587
Barnesville Hospital Association	Barnesville	1.5%	134
Flower Hospital	Sylvania	1.5%	463
Grandview Hospital & Medical Center	Dayton	1.5%	537
Dublin Methodist Hospital	Dublin	1.6%	189
Fisher - Titus Hospital	Norwalk	1.6%	254
Good Samaritan Hospital	Dayton	1.6%	986
Greenfield Area Medical Center	Greenfield	1.6%	63
Highland District Hospital	Hillsboro	1.6%	192
Aultman Hospital	Canton	1.7%	1092
Blanchard Valley Hospital	Findlay	1.7%	473
The Toledo Hospital	Toledo	1.7%	459
Saint Luke's Hospital	Maumee	1.8%	487
Grady Memorial Hospital	Delaware	1.9%	211
Holzer Medical Center Jackson	Jackson	1.9%	53
Wood County Hospital	Bowling Green	2.0%	148
Mercy Hospital of Defiance	Defiance	2.1%	47
UHHS Richmond Heights Hospital	Richmond Hghts	2.1%	340
Mercy Willard Hospital	Willard	2.2%	138
Euclid Hospital	Euclid	2.4%	123
Metrohealth System	Cleveland	2.4%	931
Saint Rita's Medical Center	Lima	2.5%	731
Fostoria Community Hospital	Fostoria	2.8%	108
Trinity Hospital Twin City	Dennison	2.8%	71
Greene Memorial Hospital	Xenia	2.9%	139
UH Geauga Medical Center	Chardon	2.9%	448
Mercy Hospital Fairfield	Fairfield	3.0%	728
Southeastern Ohio Regional Medical Center	Cambridge	3.0%	427
South Pointe Hospital	Warrensville Hgts	3.1%	421
Springfield Regional Medical Center	Springfield	3.1%	485
Mercy Memorial Hospital	Urbana	3.6%	168
Miami Valley Hospital	Dayton	3.6%	1268
Upper Valley Medical Center	Troy	3.9%	611
Adams County Regional Medical Center	Seaman	4.2%	216
Fulton County Health Center	Wauseon	4.2%	166
Galion Community Hospital	Galion	4.2%	189
Mary Rutan Hospital	Bellefontaine	4.3%	258
Holzer Medical Center	Gallipolis	4.8%	705
Morrow County Hospital	Mount Gilead	5.0%	80
Trinity Med Ctr East & West	Steubenville	5.5%	436
Pomerene Hospital	Millersburg	6.2%	97
Community Hospitals & Wellness Centers	Bryan	6.7%	164
Van Wert County Hospital	Van Wert	7.1%	156
Grand Lake Health System	Saint Marys	7.2%	222
Saint Elizabeth Health Center	Youngstown	7.3%	412
Mercy Saint Charles Hospital	Oregon	7.4%	556
Mercy Tiffin Hospital	Tiffin	7.4%	204
Clinton Memorial Hospital	Wilmington	7.5%	320
Marietta Memorial Hospital	Marietta	7.6%	1104
Southern Ohio Medical Center	Portsmouth	7.8%	728
Knox Community Hospital	Mount Vernon	8.0%	424
Saint Elizabeth Boardman Health Center	Boardman	8.2%	441
Alliance Community Hospital	Alliance	8.5%	318
Memorial Hospital	Fremont	10.6%	236
Mercy Allen Hospital	Oberlin	10.7%	75
Mercy Regional Medical Center	Lorain	11.9%	496
Samaritan Regional Health System	Ashland	12.6%	206
East Liverpool City Hospital	East Liverpool	14.2%	233
Paulding County Hospital	Paulding	15.8%	76
Bellevue Hospital	Bellevue	19.1%	131

Follow-up Mammogram/Ultrasound

A follow-up rate near zero may indicate missed cancer; a rate higher than 14% may mean there is unnecessary follow up.

Hospital Name	City	Rate	Cases
Summa Wadsworth - Rittman Hospital	Wadsworth	1.4%	566
H B Magruder Memorial Hospital	Port Clinton	1.7%	463
Holzer Medical Center	Gallipolis	2.0%	1319
Licking Memorial Hospital	Newark	2.8%	1982
Grand Lake Health System	Saint Marys	3.0%	500
Henry County Hospital	Napoleon	3.5%	372
Atrium Medical Center	Franklin	3.9%	1362
Mercy Tiffin Hospital	Tiffin	3.9%	541
Surgical Hospital at Southwoods	Youngstown	4.3%	117
Euclid Hospital	Euclid	4.4%	361
Mercy Memorial Hospital	Urbana	4.5%	287
Fulton County Health Center	Wauseon	4.6%	655
Morrow County Hospital	Mount Gilead	4.6%	238
Univ Hosps-Elyria Med Ctr	Elyria	4.7%	635
Harrison Community Hospital	Cadiz	4.8%	84
Summa Health Systems Hospitals	Akron	5.0%	2600
Union Hospital	Dover	5.0%	866
Mercer County Joint Twp Comm Hosp	Coldwater	5.1%	391
Bluffton Hospital	Bluffton	5.2%	230
Kettering Medical Center	Kettering	5.2%	2972
Southwest General Health Center	Middleburg Hgts	5.2%	1610
Van Wert County Hospital	Van Wert	5.3%	340
Aultman Hospital	Canton	5.4%	1639
Mercy Hospital Fairfield	Fairfield	5.4%	1303
Robinson Memorial Hospital	Ravenna	5.4%	1000
Grant Medical Center	Columbus	5.5%	1608
Wooster Community Hospital	Wooster	5.5%	659
Clinton Memorial Hospital	Wilmington	5.6%	835
Mount Carmel Saint Ann's	Westerville	5.6%	1312
Samaritan Regional Health System	Ashland	5.6%	844
Marietta Memorial Hospital	Marietta	5.8%	1999
Salem Regional Medical Center	Salem	5.8%	1098
Wood County Hospital	Bowling Green	5.9%	444
Blanchard Valley Hospital	Findlay	6.0%	1562
Greene Memorial Hospital	Xenia	6.2%	485
Fairfield Medical Center	Lancaster	6.3%	1385
Grandview Hospital & Medical Center	Dayton	6.4%	1869
Mercy Hospital Anderson	Cincinnati	6.4%	1541
Lodi Community Hospital	Lodi	6.5%	138
Galion Community Hospital	Galion	6.6%	561
Lakewood Hospital	Lakewood	6.6%	558
Mount Carmel West	Columbus	6.6%	3189
Knox Community Hospital	Mount Vernon	6.7%	815
Mercy Health - West Hospital	Cincinnati	6.8%	879
Sycamore Medical Center	Miamisburg	6.8%	1373
Adena Regional Medical Center	Chillicothe	7.0%	1627
Community Memorial Hospital	Hicksville	7.0%	100
Memorial Hospital	Fremont	7.0%	717
Springfield Regional Medical Center	Springfield	7.0%	1130
Upper Valley Medical Center	Troy	7.0%	1605
Mercy Regional Medical Center	Lorain	7.1%	2141
Christ Hospital	Cincinnati	7.4%	3046
Grady Memorial Hospital	Delaware	7.4%	568
Greenfield Area Medical Center	Greenfield	7.4%	122
Parma Community General Hospital	Parma	7.5%	1802
Bay Park Community Hospital	Oregon	7.6%	593
Fostoria Community Hospital	Fostoria	7.6%	354
Saint Elizabeth Health Center	Youngstown	7.6%	460
Univ Hosps Conneaut Med Ctr	Conneaut	7.7%	233
Wayne Hospital	Greenville	7.7%	857
Coshocton County Memorial Hospital	Coshocton	7.9%	567
Fort Hamilton Hughes Memorial Hospital	Hamilton	7.9%	801
Saint Elizabeth Boardman Health Center	Boardman	7.9%	76
Dublin Methodist Hospital	Dublin	8.0%	561
O'Bleness Memorial Hospital	Athens	8.0%	389
Hocking Valley Community Hospital	Logan	8.1%	357
Firelands Regional Medical Center	Sandusky	8.5%	1759
Lake Health	Concord	8.5%	3409
Madison County Hospital	London	8.5%	235
Mercy Saint Anne Hospital	Toledo	8.5%	1334
Metrohealth System	Cleveland	8.5%	1960
The Toledo Hospital	Toledo	8.5%	2265
Marymount Hospital	Garfield Heights	8.6%	1029
Riverside Methodist Hospital	Columbus	8.6%	3935
Trinity Med Ctr East & West	Steubenville	8.6%	1101
University Hospitals Case Medical Center	Cleveland	8.7%	2080
Lutheran Hospital	Cleveland	8.8%	354
Fayette County Memorial Hospital	Washington Ch	8.9%	214
East Liverpool City Hospital	East Liverpool	9.0%	367
Pomerene Hospital	Millersburg	9.0%	233
Bellevue Hospital	Bellevue	9.1%	395
Good Samaritan Hospital	Cincinnati	9.1%	2338
Northside Medical Center	Youngstown	9.1%	660
Alliance Community Hospital	Alliance	9.2%	596
Lima Memorial Health System	Lima	9.2%	1176
Mercy Allen Hospital	Oberlin	9.2%	358
Saint Joseph Health Center	Warren	9.2%	641
Cleveland Clinic	Cleveland	9.3%	9962
Diley Ridge Medical Center	Canal Wnchstr	9.3%	226
Saint Luke's Hospital	Maumee	9.4%	1646
Akron General Medical Center	Akron	9.5%	3530
Genesis Healthcare System	Zanesville	9.5%	3053
Good Samaritan Hospital	Dayton	9.5%	2987
Doctors Hospital	Columbus	9.6%	572
Fisher - Titus Hospital	Norwalk	9.6%	758
Mercy Medical Center	Canton	9.7%	1795
Saint Rita's Medical Center	Lima	9.7%	2205
Flower Hospital	Sylvania	9.8%	754
Marion General Hospital	Marion	9.9%	841
Medcentral Health Sys Mansfield Hosp	Mansfield	9.9%	1702
Belmont Community Hospital	Bellaire	10.2%	137
Miami Valley Hospital	Dayton	10.2%	2292
Summa Health System Barberton Hospital	Barberton	10.3%	692
Affinity Medical Center	Massillon	10.4%	565
South Pointe Hospital	Warrensville Hgts	10.6%	836
Barnesville Hospital Association	Barnesville	10.7%	150
Southeastern Ohio Regional Medical Center	Cambridge	10.8%	850
Southwest Regional Medical Center	Georgetown	10.8%	231
Jewish Hospital	Cincinnati	10.9%	2879
Mercy Hospital Clermont	Batavia	10.9%	921
Highland District Hospital	Hillsboro	11.1%	325
Wilson Memorial Hospital	Sidney	11.1%	638
Ashtabula County Medical Center	Ashtabula	11.2%	819
Berger Hospital	Circleville	11.2%	552
Aultman Orrville Hospital	Orrville	11.3%	151
Hillcrest Hospital	Mayfield Heights	11.3%	1569
Mary Rutan Hospital	Bellefontaine	11.5%	738
Saint John Medical Center	Westlake	11.6%	602
Trumbull Memorial Hospital	Warren	11.6%	1729
UHHS Richmond Heights Hospital	Richmond Hghts	11.7%	873
University of Cincinnati Medical Center	Cincinnati	11.8%	1355
Fairview Hospital	Cleveland	11.9%	1433
Memorial Hospital of Union County	Marysville	12.0%	409
Doctors Hospital of Nelsonville	Nelsonville	12.4%	129
West Chester Hospital	West Chester	12.6%	214
Mercy Saint Charles Hospital	Oregon	13.0%	1075
Paulding County Hospital	Paulding	13.4%	194
Trinity Hospital Twin City	Dennison	13.4%	127
Adams County Regional Medical Center	Seaman	13.6%	184
Medina Hospital	Medina	14.3%	924
University of Toledo Medical Center	Toledo	14.3%	477
Southern Ohio Medical Center	Portsmouth	14.8%	1274
UH Geauga Medical Center	Chardon	15.0%	700
UHHS Memorial Hospital of Geneva	Geneva	15.6%	499
Mercy Saint Vincent Medical Center	Toledo	15.7%	414
McCullough - Hyde Memorial Hospital	Oxford	16.1%	299
Saint Vincent Charity Medical Center	Cleveland	17.3%	196
Ohio State University Hospitals	Columbus	17.9%	252
East Ohio Regional Hospital	Martins Ferry	19.0%	543
Mercy Willard Hospital	Willard	19.9%	281
Bethesda North	Cincinnati	20.9%	4143

Lumbar Spine MRI for Low Back Pain

Hospital Name	City	Rate	Cases
Upper Valley Medical Center	Troy	17.6%	68
Wood County Hospital	Bowling Green	19.7%	66
South Pointe Hospital	Warrensville Hgts	21.9%	64
Knox Community Hospital	Mount Vernon	24.4%	82
Memorial Hospital	Fremont	24.7%	93
Univ Hosps-Elyria Med Ctr	Elyria	24.7%	85
Grady Memorial Hospital	Delaware	25.0%	64
Saint Rita's Medical Center	Lima	25.3%	150
Marion General Hospital	Marion	25.4%	71
Crystal Clinic Orthopaedic Center	Akron	27.4%	84
Fisher - Titus Hospital	Norwalk	28.4%	116
Grant Medical Center	Columbus	28.5%	144
Summa Health Systems Hospitals	Akron	28.7%	209
Wayne Hospital	Greenville	29.0%	62
Akron General Medical Center	Akron	29.3%	239
Metrohealth System	Cleveland	29.6%	135
Medina Hospital	Medina	29.7%	91
O'Bleness Memorial Hospital	Athens	29.7%	74
West Chester Hospital	West Chester	29.7%	74
East Ohio Regional Hospital	Martins Ferry	30.2%	53
Mount Carmel New Albany Surgical Hospital	New Albany	30.5%	59
Trinity Med Ctr East & West	Steubenville	30.8%	156
Firelands Regional Medical Center	Sandusky	30.9%	204
Robinson Memorial Hospital	Ravenna	31.0%	100
Marymount Hospital	Garfield Heights	31.5%	89
Saint Joseph Health Center	Warren	31.5%	92
Cleveland Clinic	Cleveland	31.9%	661
Trumbull Memorial Hospital	Warren	32.0%	122
Adams County Regional Medical Center	Seaman	32.1%	56
Bethesda North	Cincinnati	32.1%	268
Highland District Hospital	Hillsboro	32.7%	49
Alliance Community Hospital	Alliance	32.8%	64
Holzer Medical Center	Gallipolis	32.8%	128
Doctors Hospital	Columbus	32.9%	73
Springfield Regional Medical Center	Springfield	32.9%	79
Miami Valley Hospital	Dayton	33.2%	214
Atrium Medical Center	Franklin	33.3%	165
Community Hospitals & Wellness Centers	Bryan	33.3%	120
The Toledo Hospital	Toledo	33.3%	123
Hillcrest Hospital	Mayfield Heights	33.7%	199
Mercy Saint Charles Hospital	Oregon	33.7%	101
Salem Regional Medical Center	Salem	33.7%	86
Blanchard Valley Hospital	Findlay	33.8%	222
Parma Community General Hospital	Parma	33.8%	145
University Hospitals Ahuja Medical Center	Beachwood	33.8%	65

NOTE: Hospital profiles are in alphabetical order by state, then city, then hospital within the city; Rankings exclude hospitals with less than 25 cases except for patient surveys which excludes hospitals with less than 100 cases; (a) 100-299 cases; (1) The number of cases/patients is too few to report; (2) Data submitted were based on a sample of cases/patients; (3) Results are based on a shorter time period than required; (4) Data suppressed by CMS for one or more quarters; (5) Results are not available for this reporting period; (6) Fewer than 100 patients completed the HCAHPS survey; (7) No cases met the criteria for this measure; (8) The lower limit of the confidence interval cannot be calculated if the number of observed infections equals zero; (9) No data are available from the state/territory for this reporting period; (10) The scores shown reflect fewer than 50 completed surveys; (11) There were discrepancies in the data collection process; (12) This measure does not apply to this hospital for this reporting period; (13) Results cannot be calculated for this reporting period; (14) The results for this state are combined with nearby states to protect confidentiality; Please refer to the User's Guide for a full explanation of data.

Ashtabula County Medical Center	Ashtabula	33.9%	56
Grandview Hospital & Medical Center	Dayton	33.9%	218
Marietta Memorial Hospital	Marietta	33.9%	410
Mercy Regional Medical Center	Lorain	33.9%	183
Medical Center at Elizabeth Place	Dayton	34.0%	103
Mercy Hospital Anderson	Cincinnati	34.5%	275
Riverside Methodist Hospital	Columbus	34.5%	342
Summa Health System Barberton Hospital	Barberton	34.5%	58
McCullough - Hyde Memorial Hospital	Oxford	34.6%	52
Saint Luke's Hospital	Maumee	34.9%	192
Sycamore Medical Center	Miamisburg	35.1%	57
Bay Park Community Hospital	Oregon	35.2%	54
Kettering Medical Center	Kettering	35.2%	219
Lima Memorial Health System	Lima	35.4%	99
Medcentral Health Sys Mansfield Hosp	Mansfield	35.4%	243
Mercy Saint Anne Hospital	Toledo	35.5%	93
Saint Elizabeth Boardman Health Center	Boardman	35.7%	56
Galion Community Hospital	Galion	35.8%	67
Coshocton County Memorial Hospital	Coshocton	35.9%	64
Lake Health	Concord	36.3%	237
Samaritan Regional Health System	Ashland	36.5%	63
Adena Regional Medical Center	Chillicothe	36.6%	287
Mercy Saint Vincent Medical Center	Toledo	36.6%	71
Union Hospital	Dover	36.9%	160
Genesis Healthcare System	Zanesville	37.0%	281
Wilson Memorial Hospital	Sidney	37.0%	54
Aultman Hospital	Canton	37.1%	205
Good Samaritan Hospital	Cincinnati	37.2%	172
Licking Memorial Hospital	Newark	37.2%	129
East Liverpool City Hospital	East Liverpool	37.3%	75
Fulton County Health Center	Wauseon	37.3%	51
University Hospitals Case Medical Center	Cleveland	37.3%	142
Grand Lake Health System	Saint Marys	37.7%	61
Ohio State University Hospitals	Columbus	37.7%	199
Mercy Hospital Clermont	Batavia	37.9%	116
Fairfield Medical Center	Lancaster	38.1%	197
University of Cincinnati Medical Center	Cincinnati	38.3%	107
Flower Hospital	Sylvania	38.4%	86
Summa Western Reserve Hospital	Cuyahoga Falls	38.4%	112
Southwest General Health Center	Middleburg Hgts	38.6%	145
Saint Elizabeth Health Center	Youngstown	38.9%	54
Mercy Medical Center	Canton	39.0%	172
Euclid Hospital	Euclid	39.6%	48
University of Toledo Medical Center	Toledo	39.6%	164
Clinton Memorial Hospital	Wilmington	39.8%	108
Mount Carmel West	Columbus	39.9%	173
Good Samaritan Hospital	Dayton	41.0%	244
Southern Ohio Medical Center	Portsmouth	41.1%	185
Jewish Hospital	Cincinnati	41.4%	133
UH Geauga Medical Center	Chardon	42.0%	88
Mercy Hospital Fairfield	Fairfield	42.3%	248
Christ Hospital	Cincinnati	43.4%	378
Mercy Health - West Hospital	Cincinnati	43.6%	117
Fort Hamilton Hughes Memorial Hospital	Hamilton	44.8%	87
Berger Hospital	Circleville	45.8%	59
Hocking Valley Community Hospital	Logan	46.5%	43
Bellevue Hospital	Bellevue	46.8%	47
Saint Vincent Charity Medical Center	Cleveland	48.1%	104
Indu & Raj Soin Medical Center	Beaver Creek	48.6%	35
Mount Carmel Saint Ann's	Westerville	49.1%	55

NOTE: Hospital profiles are in alphabetical order by state, then city, then hospital within the city; Rankings exclude hospitals with less than 25 cases except for patient surveys which excludes hospitals with less than 100 cases; (a) 100-299 cases; (1) The number of cases/patients is too few to report; (2) Data submitted were based on a sample of cases/patients; (3) Results are based on a shorter time period than required; (4) Data suppressed by CMS for one or more quarters; (5) Results are not available for this reporting period; (6) Fewer than 100 patients completed the HCAHPS survey; (7) No cases met the criteria for this measure; (8) The lower limit of the confidence interval cannot be calculated if the number of observed infections equals zero; (9) No data are available from the state/territory for this reporting period; (10) The scores shown reflect fewer than 50 completed surveys; (11) There were discrepancies in the data collection process; (12) This measure does not apply to this hospital for this reporting period; (13) Results cannot be calculated for this reporting period; (14) The results for this state are combined with nearby states to protect confidentiality; Please refer to the User's Guide for a full explanation of data.

Akron General Medical Center

400 Wabash Avenue
Akron, OH 44307
Phone: 330-344-6000
Fax: 330-376-4835
E-mail: jarmstrong@agmc.org
URL: www.akrongeneral.org
Type: Acute Care Hospitals
Emergency Services: Yes
Ownership: Voluntary non-profit - Private
Beds: 532

Key Personnel:

CEO/President. . . . . Alan Bleyer
Infection Control. . . . . Gary Bollin, MD
Quality Assurance . . . . Susan Carter
Chair/CEO . . . . William Frantz
Cardiac Laboratory. . . . . George I Litman, MD
Radiology. . . . . Marilyn Schultz, MD
Chief of Medical Staff. . . . . Richard J Streck, MD
Operating Room. . . . . Gary Tomcho, RN

Measure	Cases	This Hosp.	State Avg.	U.S. Avg.
Blood Clot Prevention and Treatment				
Anticoagulation Overlap Therapy[2]	206	98%	93%	93%
ICU Venous Thromboembolism Prophylaxis[2]	90	99%	93%	92%
Incidence of Potentially Preventable VTE[2]	50	4%	6%	10%
UFH with Dosages/Platelet Monitoring[2]	191	100%	98%	97%
Venous Thromboembolism Prophylaxis[2]	361	89%	88%	85%
Warfarin Therapy Discharge Instructions[2]	148	70%	79%	75%
Chest Pain/Possible Heart Attack Care				
Aspirin Given Within 24 Hours of Arrival[1,3]	-	-	97%	96%
Fibrinolytic Meds Within 30 Min. of Arrival[3,7]	-	-	44%	58%
Average Time to ECG (minutes)[1,3]	-	-	6	7
Average Time to Transfer (minutes)[1,3]	-	-	58	60
Children's Asthma Care				
Received Home Management Plan of Care	-	-	85%	88%
Received Reliever Medication	-	-	100%	100%
Received Systemic Corticosteroids	-	-	100%	100%
Emergency Department				
Admittance Decision Time (minutes)[2]	333	72	90	98
Head CT Results Within 45 Min. of Arrival[1]	-	-	63%	57%
Patients Who Left ER Before Being Seen	>100k	1%	2%	2%
Time from ER Arrival to Admit. (minutes)[2]	376	254	265	274
Time from ER Arrival to Discharge (minutes)	354	112	128	134
Time in ER Before Being Evaluated (minutes)	294	19	22	26
Time to Pain Meds for Fractures (minutes)	181	56	54	57
Heart Attack Care				
Aspirin Given at Discharge[2]	290	100%	99%	99%
Fibrinolytic Meds Within 30 Min. of Arrival[2,7]	-	-	80%	54%
PCI Within 90 Minutes of Arrival[2]	35	100%	97%	96%
Statin Prescribed at Discharge[2]	283	98%	98%	98%
Heart Failure Care				
ACE Inhibitor or ARB for LVSD[2]	98	100%	97%	97%
Discharge Instructions Given[2]	259	93%	96%	94%
Evaluation of LVS Function[2]	301	100%	100%	99%
Medicare Spending				
Medicare Spending per Patient (ratio)	-	1.05	1.01	0.98
Pneumonia Care				
Appropriate Initial Antibiotic Given[2]	68	97%	96%	95%
Blood Culture Timing[2]	150	99%	98%	98%
Pregnancy and Delivery Care				
Newborn Deliveries Scheduled Early	159	8%	5%	6%
Preventive Care				
Immunization for Influenza[2]	540	93%	93%	90%
Immunization for Pneumonia[2]	680	91%	94%	92%
Stroke Care				
Anticoagulation Therapy for Atrial Fibrillation	36	89%	95%	95%
Antithrombotic Therapy Timing	216	95%	98%	98%
Assessed for Rehabilitation	272	99%	98%	97%
Discharged on Antithrombotic Therapy	237	99%	99%	99%
Discharged on Statin Medication	177	98%	95%	94%
Thrombolytic Therapy Timing	19	89%	65%	66%
Venous Thromboembolism Prophylaxis	289	96%	95%	94%
Written Stroke Educational Materials Given	132	92%	92%	88%
Surgical Care Improvement Project				
Appropriate Beta Blocker Usage[2]	214	99%	98%	98%
Appropriate VTP Within 24 Hours[2]	471	99%	98%	98%
Controlled Postoperative Blood Glucose[2]	109	100%	97%	97%
Perioperative Temperature Management[2]	545	100%	100%	100%
Prophylactic Antibiotic Selection[2]	470	99%	99%	99%
Prophylactic Antibiotic Selection (Outpatient)	586	99%	98%	98%
Prophylactic Antibiotic Stopped[2]	468	99%	98%	98%
Prophylactic Antibiotic Timing[2]	471	99%	99%	99%
Prophylactic Antibiotic Timing (Outpatient)	586	100%	97%	98%
Urinary Catheter Removal[2]	311	97%	97%	97%
Survey of Patients' Hospital Experiences				
Area Around Room 'Always' Quiet at Night	300+	52%	58%	61%
Doctors 'Always' Communicated Well	300+	77%	80%	82%
Home Recovery Information Given	300+	86%	87%	85%
Hospital Given 9 or 10 on 10 Point Scale	300+	70%	72%	71%
Meds 'Always' Explained Before Given	300+	62%	64%	64%
Nurses 'Always' Communicated Well	300+	79%	81%	79%
Pain 'Always' Well Controlled	300+	69%	71%	71%
Room and Bathroom 'Always' Clean	300+	66%	75%	73%
Timely Help 'Always' Received	300+	64%	70%	68%
Would Definitely Recommend Hospital	300+	74%	71%	71%
Use of Medical Imaging				
Cardiac Imaging Stress Test before Surgery	883	5.9%	5.4%	5.3%
Combination Abdominal CT Scan	1,625	3.9%	7.1%	10.5%
Combination Brain/Sinus CT Scan	1,293	1.5%	2.8%	2.7%
Combination Chest CT Scan	1,151	0.7%	1.7%	2.7%
Follow-up Mammogram/Ultrasound	3,530	9.5%	8.7%	8.8%
Lumbar Spine MRI for Low Back Pain	239	29.3%	34.7%	37.2%

Crystal Clinic Orthopaedic Center

444 North Main Street
Akron, OH 44310
Phone: 330-668-4040
URL: www.crystalclinic.com
Type: Acute Care Hospitals
Emergency Services: No
Ownership: Proprietary

Key Personnel:

President/CEO. . . . . Ronald R Sutken, EdD

Measure	Cases	This Hosp.	State Avg.	U.S. Avg.
Blood Clot Prevention and Treatment				
Anticoagulation Overlap Therapy[1,2]	-	-	93%	93%
ICU Venous Thromboembolism Prophylaxis[2,7]	-	-	93%	92%
Incidence of Potentially Preventable VTE[1,2]	-	-	6%	10%
UFH with Dosages/Platelet Monitoring[1,2]	-	-	98%	97%
Venous Thromboembolism Prophylaxis[2]	188	100%	88%	85%
Warfarin Therapy Discharge Instructions[1,2]	-	-	79%	75%
Chest Pain/Possible Heart Attack Care				
Aspirin Given Within 24 Hours of Arrival[5]	-	-	97%	96%
Fibrinolytic Meds Within 30 Min. of Arrival[5]	-	-	44%	58%
Average Time to ECG (minutes)[5]	-	-	6	7
Average Time to Transfer (minutes)[5]	-	-	58	60
Children's Asthma Care				
Received Home Management Plan of Care	-	-	85%	88%
Received Reliever Medication	-	-	100%	100%
Received Systemic Corticosteroids	-	-	100%	100%
Emergency Department				
Admittance Decision Time (minutes)[2,7]	-	-	90	98
Head CT Results Within 45 Min. of Arrival[5]	-	-	63%	57%
Patients Who Left ER Before Being Seen[5]	-	-	2%	2%
Time from ER Arrival to Admit. (minutes)[2,7]	-	-	265	274
Time from ER Arrival to Discharge (minutes)[5]	-	-	128	134
Time in ER Before Being Evaluated (minutes)[5]	-	-	22	26
Time to Pain Meds for Fractures (minutes)[5]	-	-	54	57
Heart Attack Care				
Aspirin Given at Discharge[5]	-	-	99%	99%
Fibrinolytic Meds Within 30 Min. of Arrival[5]	-	-	80%	54%
PCI Within 90 Minutes of Arrival[5]	-	-	97%	96%
Statin Prescribed at Discharge[5]	-	-	98%	98%
Heart Failure Care				
ACE Inhibitor or ARB for LVSD[5]	-	-	97%	97%
Discharge Instructions Given[5]	-	-	96%	94%
Evaluation of LVS Function[5]	-	-	100%	99%
Medicare Spending				
Medicare Spending per Patient (ratio)	-	0.94	1.01	0.98
Pneumonia Care				
Appropriate Initial Antibiotic Given[5]	-	-	96%	95%
Blood Culture Timing[5]	-	-	98%	98%
Pregnancy and Delivery Care				
Newborn Deliveries Scheduled Early[7]	-	-	5%	6%
Preventive Care				
Immunization for Influenza[2]	431	95%	93%	90%
Immunization for Pneumonia[2]	562	87%	94%	92%
Stroke Care				
Anticoagulation Therapy for Atrial Fibrillation[5]	-	-	95%	95%
Antithrombotic Therapy Timing[5]	-	-	98%	98%
Assessed for Rehabilitation[5]	-	-	98%	97%
Discharged on Antithrombotic Therapy[5]	-	-	99%	99%
Discharged on Statin Medication[5]	-	-	95%	94%
Thrombolytic Therapy Timing[5]	-	-	65%	66%
Venous Thromboembolism Prophylaxis[5]	-	-	95%	94%
Written Stroke Educational Materials Given[5]	-	-	92%	88%
Surgical Care Improvement Project				
Appropriate Beta Blocker Usage[2]	156	100%	98%	98%
Appropriate VTP Within 24 Hours[2]	474	99%	98%	98%
Controlled Postoperative Blood Glucose[2,7]	-	-	97%	97%
Perioperative Temperature Management[2]	500	100%	100%	100%
Prophylactic Antibiotic Selection[2]	384	100%	99%	99%
Prophylactic Antibiotic Selection (Outpatient)	504	100%	98%	98%
Prophylactic Antibiotic Stopped[2]	381	100%	98%	98%
Prophylactic Antibiotic Timing[2]	384	98%	99%	99%
Prophylactic Antibiotic Timing (Outpatient)	505	99%	97%	98%
Urinary Catheter Removal[2]	92	99%	97%	97%
Survey of Patients' Hospital Experiences				
Area Around Room 'Always' Quiet at Night	300+	57%	58%	61%
Doctors 'Always' Communicated Well	300+	84%	80%	82%
Home Recovery Information Given	300+	92%	87%	85%
Hospital Given 9 or 10 on 10 Point Scale	300+	75%	72%	71%
Meds 'Always' Explained Before Given	300+	69%	64%	64%
Nurses 'Always' Communicated Well	300+	84%	81%	79%
Pain 'Always' Well Controlled	300+	72%	71%	71%
Room and Bathroom 'Always' Clean	300+	78%	75%	73%
Timely Help 'Always' Received	300+	68%	70%	68%
Would Definitely Recommend Hospital	300+	78%	71%	71%
Use of Medical Imaging				
Cardiac Imaging Stress Test before Surgery[7]	-	-	5.4%	5.3%
Combination Abdominal CT Scan[7]	-	-	7.1%	10.5%
Combination Brain/Sinus CT Scan[7]	-	-	2.8%	2.7%
Combination Chest CT Scan[7]	-	-	1.7%	2.7%
Follow-up Mammogram/Ultrasound[7]	-	-	8.7%	8.8%
Lumbar Spine MRI for Low Back Pain	84	27.4%	34.7%	37.2%

Summa Health Systems Hospitals

525 East Market Street
Akron, OH 44309
Phone: 330-375-3000
Fax: 330-375-7936
URL: www.summahealth.org
Type: Acute Care Hospitals
Emergency Services: Yes
Ownership: Voluntary non-profit - Private
Beds: 658

Key Personnel:

Infection Control. . . . . Ginnie Abell
Radiology. . . . . Daniel Finelli
CEO/President. . . . . Thomas Strauss
Chair/CEO . . . . Norman Wells, Jr.

Measure	Cases	This Hosp.	State Avg.	U.S. Avg.
Blood Clot Prevention and Treatment				
Anticoagulation Overlap Therapy[2]	213	83%	93%	93%
ICU Venous Thromboembolism Prophylaxis[2]	101	98%	93%	92%
Incidence of Potentially Preventable VTE[2]	47	11%	6%	10%
UFH with Dosages/Platelet Monitoring[2]	189	99%	98%	97%
Venous Thromboembolism Prophylaxis[2]	361	91%	88%	85%
Warfarin Therapy Discharge Instructions[2]	143	19%	79%	75%
Chest Pain/Possible Heart Attack Care				
Aspirin Given Within 24 Hours of Arrival[1,3]	-	-	97%	96%
Fibrinolytic Meds Within 30 Min. of Arrival[3,7]	-	-	44%	58%
Average Time to ECG (minutes)[1,3]	-	-	6	7
Average Time to Transfer (minutes)[3,7]	-	-	58	60
Children's Asthma Care				
Received Home Management Plan of Care	-	-	85%	88%
Received Reliever Medication	-	-	100%	100%
Received Systemic Corticosteroids	-	-	100%	100%
Emergency Department				
Admittance Decision Time (minutes)[2]	654	95	90	98

NOTE: Hospital profiles are in alphabetical order by state, then city, then hospital within the city; Rankings exclude hospitals with less than 25 cases except for patient surveys which excludes hospitals with less than 100 cases; (a) 100-299 cases; (1) The number of cases/patients is too few to report; (2) Data submitted were based on a sample of cases/patients; (3) Results are based on a shorter time period than required; (4) Data suppressed by CMS for one or more quarters; (5) Results are not available for this reporting period; (6) Fewer than 100 patients completed the HCAHPS survey; (7) No cases met the criteria for this measure; (8) The lower limit of the confidence interval cannot be calculated if the number of observed infections equals zero; (9) No data are available from the state/territory for this reporting period; (10) The scores shown reflect fewer than 50 completed surveys; (11) There were discrepancies in the data collection process; (12) This measure does not apply to this hospital for this reporting period; (13) Results cannot be calculated for this reporting period; (14) The results for this state are combined with nearby states to protect confidentiality; Please refer to the User's Guide for a full explanation of data.

Measure	Cases	This Hosp.	State Avg.	U.S. Avg.
Head CT Results Within 45 Min. of Arrival[1]	-	-	63%	57%
Patients Who Left ER Before Being Seen	>100k	1%	2%	2%
Time from ER Arrival to Admit. (minutes)[2]	671	304	265	274
Time from ER Arrival to Discharge (minutes)	387	118	128	134
Time in ER Before Being Evaluated (minutes)	425	9	22	26
Time to Pain Meds for Fractures (minutes)	201	46	54	57
Heart Attack Care				
Aspirin Given at Discharge[2]	307	100%	99%	99%
Fibrinolytic Meds Within 30 Min. of Arrival[2,7]	-	-	80%	54%
PCI Within 90 Minutes of Arrival[2]	52	98%	97%	96%
Statin Prescribed at Discharge[2]	303	98%	98%	98%
Heart Failure Care				
ACE Inhibitor or ARB for LVSD[2]	98	91%	97%	97%
Discharge Instructions Given[2]	263	95%	96%	94%
Evaluation of LVS Function[2]	311	99%	100%	99%
Medicare Spending				
Medicare Spending per Patient (ratio)	-	1.02	1.01	0.98
Pneumonia Care				
Appropriate Initial Antibiotic Given[2]	89	99%	96%	95%
Blood Culture Timing[2]	140	99%	98%	98%
Pregnancy and Delivery Care				
Newborn Deliveries Scheduled Early[2]	34	6%	5%	6%
Preventive Care				
Immunization for Influenza[2]	596	98%	93%	90%
Immunization for Pneumonia[2]	801	94%	94%	92%
Stroke Care				
Anticoagulation Therapy for Atrial Fibrillation[2]	20	100%	95%	95%
Antithrombotic Therapy Timing[2]	94	98%	98%	98%
Assessed for Rehabilitation[2]	112	96%	98%	97%
Discharged on Antithrombotic Therapy[2]	98	100%	99%	99%
Discharged on Statin Medication[2]	66	94%	95%	94%
Thrombolytic Therapy Timing[2]	15	87%	65%	66%
Venous Thromboembolism Prophylaxis[2]	122	94%	95%	94%
Written Stroke Educational Materials Given[2]	50	78%	92%	88%
Surgical Care Improvement Project				
Appropriate Beta Blocker Usage[2]	195	98%	98%	98%
Appropriate VTP Within 24 Hours[2]	254	98%	98%	98%
Controlled Postoperative Blood Glucose[2]	138	99%	97%	97%
Perioperative Temperature Management[2]	358	100%	100%	100%
Prophylactic Antibiotic Selection[2]	340	99%	99%	99%
Prophylactic Antibiotic Selection (Outpatient)	694	98%	98%	98%
Prophylactic Antibiotic Stopped[2]	320	95%	98%	98%
Prophylactic Antibiotic Timing[2]	341	99%	99%	99%
Prophylactic Antibiotic Timing (Outpatient)	698	97%	97%	98%
Urinary Catheter Removal[2]	231	93%	97%	97%
Survey of Patients' Hospital Experiences				
Area Around Room 'Always' Quiet at Night	300+	47%	58%	61%
Doctors 'Always' Communicated Well	300+	76%	80%	82%
Home Recovery Information Given	300+	85%	87%	85%
Hospital Given 9 or 10 on 10 Point Scale	300+	65%	72%	71%
Meds 'Always' Explained Before Given	300+	55%	64%	64%
Nurses 'Always' Communicated Well	300+	73%	81%	79%
Pain 'Always' Well Controlled	300+	67%	71%	71%
Room and Bathroom 'Always' Clean	300+	68%	75%	73%
Timely Help 'Always' Received	300+	61%	70%	68%
Would Definitely Recommend Hospital	300+	70%	71%	71%
Use of Medical Imaging				
Cardiac Imaging Stress Test before Surgery	843	4.6%	5.4%	5.3%
Combination Abdominal CT Scan	1,259	4.2%	7.1%	10.5%
Combination Brain/Sinus CT Scan	1,085	2.0%	2.8%	2.7%
Combination Chest CT Scan	870	0.0%	1.7%	2.7%
Follow-up Mammogram/Ultrasound	2,600	5.0%	8.7%	8.8%
Lumbar Spine MRI for Low Back Pain	209	28.7%	34.7%	37.2%

Alliance Community Hospital

200 East State Street
Alliance, OH 44601
E-mail: gayleb@achosp.org
URL: www.achosp.org
Type: Acute Care Hospitals
Ownership: Voluntary non-profit - Other
Phone: 330-596-7527
Fax: 330-596-7117
Emergency Services: Yes
Beds: 184

Key Personnel:
Emergency Room .... Timothy Billups, RN
Radiology.................. Gary L Dier
Quality Assurance .... Barb Dragomir
Chief of Medical Staff.......... Karen Gade-Pulido, MD
CEO/President.............. Stan W Jonas
Infection Control............... Tonia Martin
Operating Room.............. Debbie Percha
Intensive Care Unit............ Joe Sealak, RN

Measure	Cases	This Hosp.	State Avg.	U.S. Avg.
Blood Clot Prevention and Treatment				
Anticoagulation Overlap Therapy[2]	47	81%	93%	93%
ICU Venous Thromboembolism Prophylaxis[2]	53	89%	93%	92%
Incidence of Potentially Preventable VTE[1,2]	-	-	6%	10%
UFH with Dosages/Platelet Monitoring[2]	48	98%	98%	97%
Venous Thromboembolism Prophylaxis[2]	240	84%	88%	85%
Warfarin Therapy Discharge Instructions[2]	36	53%	79%	75%
Chest Pain/Possible Heart Attack Care				
Aspirin Given Within 24 Hours of Arrival	91	98%	97%	96%
Fibrinolytic Meds Within 30 Min. of Arrival[7]	-	-	44%	58%
Average Time to ECG (minutes)	88	2	6	7
Average Time to Transfer (minutes)	21	25	58	60
Children's Asthma Care				
Received Home Management Plan of Care	-	-	85%	88%
Received Reliever Medication	-	-	100%	100%
Received Systemic Corticosteroids	-	-	100%	100%
Emergency Department				
Admittance Decision Time (minutes)[2]	311	46	90	98
Head CT Results Within 45 Min. of Arrival	22	64%	63%	57%
Patients Who Left ER Before Being Seen	35,590	0%	2%	2%
Time from ER Arrival to Admit. (minutes)[2]	312	196	265	274
Time from ER Arrival to Discharge (minutes)	371	84	128	134
Time in ER Before Being Evaluated (minutes)	397	22	22	26
Time to Pain Meds for Fractures (minutes)	99	31	54	57
Heart Attack Care				
Aspirin Given at Discharge[1,3]	-	-	99%	99%
Fibrinolytic Meds Within 30 Min. of Arrival[3,7]	-	-	80%	54%
PCI Within 90 Minutes of Arrival[3,7]	-	-	97%	96%
Statin Prescribed at Discharge[1,3]	-	-	98%	98%
Heart Failure Care				
ACE Inhibitor or ARB for LVSD	33	91%	97%	97%
Discharge Instructions Given	69	75%	96%	94%
Evaluation of LVS Function	101	97%	100%	99%
Medicare Spending				
Medicare Spending per Patient (ratio)	-	1.07	1.01	0.98
Pneumonia Care				
Appropriate Initial Antibiotic Given[2]	89	98%	96%	95%
Blood Culture Timing[2]	133	95%	98%	98%
Pregnancy and Delivery Care				
Newborn Deliveries Scheduled Early[2]	21	5%	5%	6%
Preventive Care				
Immunization for Influenza[2]	308	94%	93%	90%
Immunization for Pneumonia[2]	447	96%	94%	92%
Stroke Care				
Anticoagulation Therapy for Atrial Fibrillation[1]	-	-	95%	95%
Antithrombotic Therapy Timing[1]	-	-	98%	98%
Assessed for Rehabilitation[1]	-	-	98%	97%
Discharged on Antithrombotic Therapy[1]	-	-	99%	99%
Discharged on Statin Medication[1]	-	-	95%	94%
Thrombolytic Therapy Timing[1]	-	-	65%	66%
Venous Thromboembolism Prophylaxis[1]	-	-	95%	94%
Written Stroke Educational Materials Given[1]	-	-	92%	88%
Surgical Care Improvement Project				
Appropriate Beta Blocker Usage[2]	83	98%	98%	98%
Appropriate VTP Within 24 Hours[2]	204	91%	98%	98%
Controlled Postoperative Blood Glucose[2,7]	-	-	97%	97%
Perioperative Temperature Management[2]	299	100%	100%	100%
Prophylactic Antibiotic Selection[2]	211	100%	99%	99%
Prophylactic Antibiotic Selection (Outpatient)	52	100%	98%	98%
Prophylactic Antibiotic Stopped[2]	209	98%	98%	98%
Prophylactic Antibiotic Timing[2]	211	98%	99%	99%
Prophylactic Antibiotic Timing (Outpatient)	57	89%	97%	98%
Urinary Catheter Removal[2]	61	97%	97%	97%
Survey of Patients' Hospital Experiences				
Area Around Room 'Always' Quiet at Night	300+	58%	58%	61%
Doctors 'Always' Communicated Well	300+	81%	80%	82%
Home Recovery Information Given	300+	86%	87%	85%
Hospital Given 9 or 10 on 10 Point Scale	300+	70%	72%	71%
Meds 'Always' Explained Before Given	300+	65%	64%	64%
Nurses 'Always' Communicated Well	300+	78%	81%	79%
Pain 'Always' Well Controlled	300+	72%	71%	71%
Room and Bathroom 'Always' Clean	300+	81%	75%	73%
Timely Help 'Always' Received	300+	62%	70%	68%
Would Definitely Recommend Hospital	300+	67%	71%	71%
Use of Medical Imaging				
Cardiac Imaging Stress Test before Surgery	147	6.8%	5.4%	5.3%
Combination Abdominal CT Scan	495	23.8%	7.1%	10.5%
Combination Brain/Sinus CT Scan	566	1.4%	2.8%	2.7%
Combination Chest CT Scan	318	8.5%	1.7%	2.7%
Follow-up Mammogram/Ultrasound	596	9.2%	8.7%	8.8%
Lumbar Spine MRI for Low Back Pain	64	32.8%	34.7%	37.2%

Samaritan Regional Health System

1025 Center St
Ashland, OH 44805
URL: www.samho.org
Type: Acute Care Hospitals
Ownership: Voluntary non-profit - Other
Phone: 419-289-0491
Fax: 419-207-2608
Emergency Services: Yes
Beds: 110

Key Personnel:
Radiology.................. Richard W Adams
CEO/President............... Danny Boggs
Chief of Medical Staff.......... Philip Myers

Measure	Cases	This Hosp.	State Avg.	U.S. Avg.
Blood Clot Prevention and Treatment				
Anticoagulation Overlap Therapy[1,2]	-	-	93%	93%
ICU Venous Thromboembolism Prophylaxis[2]	50	98%	93%	92%
Incidence of Potentially Preventable VTE[2,7]	-	-	6%	10%
UFH with Dosages/Platelet Monitoring[1,2]	-	-	98%	97%
Venous Thromboembolism Prophylaxis[2]	119	97%	88%	85%
Warfarin Therapy Discharge Instructions[1,2]	-	-	79%	75%
Chest Pain/Possible Heart Attack Care				
Aspirin Given Within 24 Hours of Arrival	91	95%	97%	96%
Fibrinolytic Meds Within 30 Min. of Arrival[1]	-	-	44%	58%
Average Time to ECG (minutes)	91	6	6	7
Average Time to Transfer (minutes)[1]	-	-	58	60
Children's Asthma Care				
Received Home Management Plan of Care	-	-	85%	88%
Received Reliever Medication	-	-	100%	100%
Received Systemic Corticosteroids	-	-	100%	100%
Emergency Department				
Admittance Decision Time (minutes)[2]	230	65	90	98
Head CT Results Within 45 Min. of Arrival	28	43%	63%	57%
Patients Who Left ER Before Being Seen	27,253	1%	2%	2%
Time from ER Arrival to Admit. (minutes)[2]	234	232	265	274
Time from ER Arrival to Discharge (minutes)	359	112	128	134
Time in ER Before Being Evaluated (minutes)	402	27	22	26
Time to Pain Meds for Fractures (minutes)	111	44	54	57
Heart Attack Care				
Aspirin Given at Discharge[1]	-	-	99%	99%
Fibrinolytic Meds Within 30 Min. of Arrival[7]	-	-	80%	54%
PCI Within 90 Minutes of Arrival[7]	-	-	97%	96%
Statin Prescribed at Discharge[1]	-	-	98%	98%
Heart Failure Care				
ACE Inhibitor or ARB for LVSD[1]	-	-	97%	97%
Discharge Instructions Given	33	97%	96%	94%
Evaluation of LVS Function	46	100%	100%	99%
Medicare Spending				
Medicare Spending per Patient (ratio)	-	0.94	1.01	0.98
Pneumonia Care				
Appropriate Initial Antibiotic Given	61	100%	96%	95%
Blood Culture Timing	103	97%	98%	98%
Pregnancy and Delivery Care				
Newborn Deliveries Scheduled Early[2]	44	9%	5%	6%
Preventive Care				
Immunization for Influenza[2]	258	98%	93%	90%
Immunization for Pneumonia[2]	336	97%	94%	92%
Stroke Care				
Anticoagulation Therapy for Atrial Fibrillation[7]	-	-	95%	95%
Antithrombotic Therapy Timing[1]	-	-	98%	98%

NOTE: Hospital profiles are in alphabetical order by state, then city, then hospital within the city; Rankings exclude hospitals with less than 25 cases except for patient surveys which excludes hospitals with less than 100 cases; (a) 100-299 cases; (1) The number of cases/patients is too few to report; (2) Data submitted were based on a sample of cases/patients; (3) Results are based on a shorter time period than required; (4) Data suppressed by CMS for one or more quarters; (5) Results are not available for this reporting period; (6) Fewer than 100 patients completed the HCAHPS survey; (7) No cases met the criteria for this measure; (8) The lower limit of the confidence interval cannot be calculated if the number of observed infections equals zero; (9) No data are available from the state/territory for this reporting period; (10) The scores shown reflect fewer than 50 completed surveys; (11) There were discrepancies in the data collection process; (12) This measure does not apply to this hospital for this reporting period; (13) Results cannot be calculated for this reporting period; (14) The results for this state are combined with nearby states to protect confidentiality; Please refer to the User's Guide for a full explanation of data.

Measure	Cases	This Hosp.	State Avg.	U.S. Avg.
Assessed for Rehabilitation[1]	-	-	98%	97%
Discharged on Antithrombotic Therapy[1]	-	-	99%	99%
Discharged on Statin Medication[1]	-	-	95%	94%
Thrombolytic Therapy Timing[1]	-	-	65%	66%
Venous Thromboembolism Prophylaxis[1]	-	-	95%	94%
Written Stroke Educational Materials Given[1]	-	-	92%	88%
Surgical Care Improvement Project				
Appropriate Beta Blocker Usage	172	100%	98%	98%
Appropriate VTP Within 24 Hours	480	99%	98%	98%
Controlled Postoperative Blood Glucose[7]	-	-	97%	97%
Perioperative Temperature Management	525	100%	100%	100%
Prophylactic Antibiotic Selection	481	100%	99%	99%
Prophylactic Antibiotic Selection (Outpatient)	43	91%	98%	98%
Prophylactic Antibiotic Stopped	479	100%	98%	98%
Prophylactic Antibiotic Timing	481	100%	99%	99%
Prophylactic Antibiotic Timing (Outpatient)	48	85%	97%	98%
Urinary Catheter Removal	389	100%	97%	97%
Survey of Patients' Hospital Experiences				
Area Around Room 'Always' Quiet at Night	300+	60%	58%	61%
Doctors 'Always' Communicated Well	300+	84%	80%	82%
Home Recovery Information Given	300+	89%	87%	85%
Hospital Given 9 or 10 on 10 Point Scale	300+	71%	72%	71%
Meds 'Always' Explained Before Given	300+	68%	64%	64%
Nurses 'Always' Communicated Well	300+	83%	81%	79%
Pain 'Always' Well Controlled	300+	72%	71%	71%
Room and Bathroom 'Always' Clean	300+	76%	75%	73%
Timely Help 'Always' Received	300+	76%	70%	68%
Would Definitely Recommend Hospital	300+	69%	71%	71%
Use of Medical Imaging				
Cardiac Imaging Stress Test before Surgery	237	3.0%	5.4%	5.3%
Combination Abdominal CT Scan	473	13.1%	7.1%	10.5%
Combination Brain/Sinus CT Scan	494	1.8%	2.8%	2.7%
Combination Chest CT Scan	206	12.6%	1.7%	2.7%
Follow-up Mammogram/Ultrasound	844	5.6%	8.7%	8.8%
Lumbar Spine MRI for Low Back Pain	63	36.5%	34.7%	37.2%

Ashtabula County Medical Center

2420 Lake Avenue
Ashtabula, OH 44004
Phone: 440-997-2262
Fax: 440-997-6644
URL: www.acmchealth.org
Type: Acute Care Hospitals
Emergency Services: Yes
Ownership: Voluntary non-profit - Private
Beds: 234

Key Personnel:
Operating Room. . . . . Lo Bruno
Infection Control. . . . . Cindy Callahan
Cardiac Laboratory. . . . . James Cho, MD
CEO/President. . . . . Kevin J Miller
Chief of Medical Staff. . . . . Timothy D O'Brien
Radiology. . . . . Jack Thome

Measure	Cases	This Hosp.	State Avg.	U.S. Avg.
Blood Clot Prevention and Treatment				
Anticoagulation Overlap Therapy[2]	43	98%	93%	93%
ICU Venous Thromboembolism Prophylaxis[2]	56	96%	93%	92%
Incidence of Potentially Preventable VTE[1,2]	-	-	6%	10%
UFH with Dosages/Platelet Monitoring[2]	18	89%	98%	97%
Venous Thromboembolism Prophylaxis[2]	270	96%	88%	85%
Warfarin Therapy Discharge Instructions[2]	34	94%	79%	75%
Chest Pain/Possible Heart Attack Care				
Aspirin Given Within 24 Hours of Arrival	60	93%	97%	96%
Fibrinolytic Meds Within 30 Min. of Arrival[7]	-	-	44%	58%
Average Time to ECG (minutes)	59	3	6	7
Average Time to Transfer (minutes)	21	112	58	60
Children's Asthma Care				
Received Home Management Plan of Care	-	-	85%	88%
Received Reliever Medication	-	-	100%	100%
Received Systemic Corticosteroids	-	-	100%	100%
Emergency Department				
Admittance Decision Time (minutes)[2]	545	61	90	98
Head CT Results Within 45 Min. of Arrival[1]	-	-	63%	57%
Patients Who Left ER Before Being Seen	33,970	1%	2%	2%
Time from ER Arrival to Admit. (minutes)[2]	545	198	265	274
Time from ER Arrival to Discharge (minutes)	393	83	128	134
Time in ER Before Being Evaluated (minutes)	417	14	22	26
Time to Pain Meds for Fractures (minutes)	109	40	54	57
Heart Attack Care				
Aspirin Given at Discharge	27	100%	99%	99%
Fibrinolytic Meds Within 30 Min. of Arrival[7]	-	-	80%	54%
PCI Within 90 Minutes of Arrival[7]	-	-	97%	96%
Statin Prescribed at Discharge	26	100%	98%	98%
Heart Failure Care				
ACE Inhibitor or ARB for LVSD	27	100%	97%	97%
Discharge Instructions Given	128	98%	96%	94%
Evaluation of LVS Function	187	100%	100%	99%
Medicare Spending				
Medicare Spending per Patient (ratio)	-	0.99	1.01	0.98
Pneumonia Care				
Appropriate Initial Antibiotic Given	69	100%	96%	95%
Blood Culture Timing	145	100%	98%	98%
Pregnancy and Delivery Care				
Newborn Deliveries Scheduled Early[2]	62	26%	5%	6%
Preventive Care				
Immunization for Influenza[2]	481	98%	93%	90%
Immunization for Pneumonia[2]	620	98%	94%	92%
Stroke Care				
Anticoagulation Therapy for Atrial Fibrillation	11	82%	95%	95%
Antithrombotic Therapy Timing	41	100%	98%	98%
Assessed for Rehabilitation	50	88%	98%	97%
Discharged on Antithrombotic Therapy	49	92%	99%	99%
Discharged on Statin Medication	39	85%	95%	94%
Thrombolytic Therapy Timing[1]	-	-	65%	66%
Venous Thromboembolism Prophylaxis	43	95%	95%	94%
Written Stroke Educational Materials Given	28	93%	92%	88%
Surgical Care Improvement Project				
Appropriate Beta Blocker Usage	49	98%	98%	98%
Appropriate VTP Within 24 Hours	171	100%	98%	98%
Controlled Postoperative Blood Glucose[7]	-	-	97%	97%
Perioperative Temperature Management	200	100%	100%	100%
Prophylactic Antibiotic Selection	85	99%	99%	99%
Prophylactic Antibiotic Selection (Outpatient)	72	100%	98%	98%
Prophylactic Antibiotic Stopped	76	96%	98%	98%
Prophylactic Antibiotic Timing	86	100%	99%	99%
Prophylactic Antibiotic Timing (Outpatient)	72	99%	97%	98%
Urinary Catheter Removal	65	100%	97%	97%
Survey of Patients' Hospital Experiences				
Area Around Room 'Always' Quiet at Night	300+	50%	58%	61%
Doctors 'Always' Communicated Well	300+	78%	80%	82%
Home Recovery Information Given	300+	84%	87%	85%
Hospital Given 9 or 10 on 10 Point Scale	300+	60%	72%	71%
Meds 'Always' Explained Before Given	300+	62%	64%	64%
Nurses 'Always' Communicated Well	300+	80%	81%	79%
Pain 'Always' Well Controlled	300+	68%	71%	71%
Room and Bathroom 'Always' Clean	300+	83%	75%	73%
Timely Help 'Always' Received	300+	72%	70%	68%
Would Definitely Recommend Hospital	300+	56%	71%	71%
Use of Medical Imaging				
Cardiac Imaging Stress Test before Surgery	289	4.5%	5.4%	5.3%
Combination Abdominal CT Scan	608	1.6%	7.1%	10.5%
Combination Brain/Sinus CT Scan	513	1.9%	2.8%	2.7%
Combination Chest CT Scan	414	0.0%	1.7%	2.7%
Follow-up Mammogram/Ultrasound	819	11.2%	8.7%	8.8%
Lumbar Spine MRI for Low Back Pain	56	33.9%	34.7%	37.2%

O'Bleness Memorial Hospital

55 Hospital Drive
Athens, OH 45701
Phone: 740-592-9233
Fax: 740-592-9200
URL: www.obleness.org
Type: Acute Care Hospitals
Emergency Services: Yes
Ownership: Voluntary non-profit - Other
Beds: 114

Key Personnel:
Radiology. . . . . Jeffrey S Benseler, DO
Operating Room. . . . . Shelly Cooper, RN
Chief of Medical Staff . . . . J Phillip Jones, DO
Infection Control. . . . . Donna Lofgren
CEO . . . . Greg Long
Quality Assurance . . . . Judy U Moffitt, RN, B
Pediatric Ambulatory Care . . . . . . Karen Montgomery-Reag, DO
Pediatric In-Patient Care . . . . Karen Montgomery-Reag, DO

Measure	Cases	This Hosp.	State Avg.	U.S. Avg.
Blood Clot Prevention and Treatment				
Anticoagulation Overlap Therapy[2]	18	100%	93%	93%
ICU Venous Thromboembolism Prophylaxis[2]	81	100%	93%	92%
Incidence of Potentially Preventable VTE[2,7]	-	-	6%	10%
UFH with Dosages/Platelet Monitoring[1,2]	-	-	98%	97%
Venous Thromboembolism Prophylaxis[2]	165	99%	88%	85%
Warfarin Therapy Discharge Instructions[2]	14	100%	79%	75%
Chest Pain/Possible Heart Attack Care				
Aspirin Given Within 24 Hours of Arrival	120	96%	97%	96%
Fibrinolytic Meds Within 30 Min. of Arrival[1]	-	-	44%	58%
Average Time to ECG (minutes)	126	14	6	7
Average Time to Transfer (minutes)[1]	-	-	58	60
Children's Asthma Care				
Received Home Management Plan of Care	-	-	85%	88%
Received Reliever Medication	-	-	100%	100%
Received Systemic Corticosteroids	-	-	100%	100%
Emergency Department				
Admittance Decision Time (minutes)[2]	286	68	90	98
Head CT Results Within 45 Min. of Arrival	38	71%	63%	57%
Patients Who Left ER Before Being Seen	28,180	3%	2%	2%
Time from ER Arrival to Admit. (minutes)[2]	309	256	265	274
Time from ER Arrival to Discharge (minutes)	413	161	128	134
Time in ER Before Being Evaluated (minutes)	465	43	22	26
Time to Pain Meds for Fractures (minutes)	104	71	54	57
Heart Attack Care				
Aspirin Given at Discharge[1]	-	-	99%	99%
Fibrinolytic Meds Within 30 Min. of Arrival[7]	-	-	80%	54%
PCI Within 90 Minutes of Arrival[7]	-	-	97%	96%
Statin Prescribed at Discharge[1]	-	-	98%	98%
Heart Failure Care				
ACE Inhibitor or ARB for LVSD	20	100%	97%	97%
Discharge Instructions Given	35	91%	96%	94%
Evaluation of LVS Function	46	100%	100%	99%
Medicare Spending				
Medicare Spending per Patient (ratio)	-	1.00	1.01	0.98
Pneumonia Care				
Appropriate Initial Antibiotic Given	122	100%	96%	95%
Blood Culture Timing	152	96%	98%	98%
Pregnancy and Delivery Care				
Newborn Deliveries Scheduled Early	47	0%	5%	6%
Preventive Care				
Immunization for Influenza[2]	321	95%	93%	90%
Immunization for Pneumonia[2]	364	99%	94%	92%
Stroke Care				
Anticoagulation Therapy for Atrial Fibrillation[1,3]	-	-	95%	95%
Antithrombotic Therapy Timing[1,3]	-	-	98%	98%
Assessed for Rehabilitation[1,3]	-	-	98%	97%
Discharged on Antithrombotic Therapy[1,3]	-	-	99%	99%
Discharged on Statin Medication[1,3]	-	-	95%	94%
Thrombolytic Therapy Timing[3,7]	-	-	65%	66%
Venous Thromboembolism Prophylaxis[1,3]	-	-	95%	94%
Written Stroke Educational Materials Given[1,3]	-	-	92%	88%
Surgical Care Improvement Project				
Appropriate Beta Blocker Usage	43	98%	98%	98%
Appropriate VTP Within 24 Hours	173	97%	98%	98%
Controlled Postoperative Blood Glucose[7]	-	-	97%	97%
Perioperative Temperature Management	203	100%	100%	100%
Prophylactic Antibiotic Selection	120	99%	99%	99%
Prophylactic Antibiotic Selection (Outpatient)	176	98%	98%	98%
Prophylactic Antibiotic Stopped	120	97%	98%	98%
Prophylactic Antibiotic Timing	120	100%	99%	99%
Prophylactic Antibiotic Timing (Outpatient)	178	99%	97%	98%
Urinary Catheter Removal	155	97%	97%	97%
Survey of Patients' Hospital Experiences				
Area Around Room 'Always' Quiet at Night	300+	56%	58%	61%
Doctors 'Always' Communicated Well	300+	82%	80%	82%
Home Recovery Information Given	300+	85%	87%	85%
Hospital Given 9 or 10 on 10 Point Scale	300+	61%	72%	71%
Meds 'Always' Explained Before Given	300+	66%	64%	64%
Nurses 'Always' Communicated Well	300+	79%	81%	79%
Pain 'Always' Well Controlled	300+	67%	71%	71%
Room and Bathroom 'Always' Clean	300+	73%	75%	73%

NOTE: Hospital profiles are in alphabetical order by state, then city, then hospital within the city; Rankings exclude hospitals with less than 25 cases except for patient surveys which excludes hospitals with less than 100 cases; (a) 100-299 cases; (1) The number of cases/patients is too few to report; (2) Data submitted were based on a sample of cases/patients; (3) Results are based on a shorter time period than required; (4) Data suppressed by CMS for one or more quarters; (5) Results are not available for this reporting period; (6) Fewer than 100 patients completed the HCAHPS survey; (7) No cases met the criteria for this measure; (8) The lower limit of the confidence interval cannot be calculated if the number of observed infections equals zero; (9) No data are available from the state/territory for this reporting period; (10) The scores shown reflect fewer than 50 completed surveys; (11) There were discrepancies in the data collection process; (12) This measure does not apply to this hospital for this reporting period; (13) Results cannot be calculated for this reporting period; (14) The results for this state are combined with nearby states to protect confidentiality; Please refer to the User's Guide for a full explanation of data.

Measure	Cases	This Hosp.	State Avg.	U.S. Avg.
Timely Help 'Always' Received	300+	64%	70%	68%
Would Definitely Recommend Hospital	300+	60%	71%	71%
Use of Medical Imaging				
Cardiac Imaging Stress Test before Surgery	84	6.0%	5.4%	5.3%
Combination Abdominal CT Scan	339	6.5%	7.1%	10.5%
Combination Brain/Sinus CT Scan[1]	-	-	2.8%	2.7%
Combination Chest CT Scan	125	0.8%	1.7%	2.7%
Follow-up Mammogram/Ultrasound	389	8.0%	8.7%	8.8%
Lumbar Spine MRI for Low Back Pain	74	29.7%	34.7%	37.2%

Summa Health System Barberton Hospital

155 5th Street N E
Barberton, OH 44203
Phone: 330-615-3000
Fax: 330-615-3033
URL: www.barbhosp.com
Type: Acute Care Hospitals
Emergency Services: Yes
Ownership: Proprietary
Beds: 311

Key Personnel:

Anesthesiology. . . . . James Cantoni, MD
Quality Assurance . . . . Mary Jo Goss
Radiology. . . . . Matthew Karlen, MD
Operating Room. . . . . Dean Majors, MD
Emergency Room . . . . Gregory Smith, MD
Chief of Medical Staff. . . . . Erik Steele, DO
CEO/President. . . . . Thomas Strauss
Chair/CEO . . . . Norman Wells, Jr.

Measure	Cases	This Hosp.	State Avg.	U.S. Avg.
Blood Clot Prevention and Treatment				
Anticoagulation Overlap Therapy[2]	71	69%	93%	93%
ICU Venous Thromboembolism Prophylaxis[2]	161	83%	93%	92%
Incidence of Potentially Preventable VTE[2]	15	33%	6%	10%
UFH with Dosages/Platelet Monitoring[2]	59	98%	98%	97%
Venous Thromboembolism Prophylaxis[2]	679	88%	88%	85%
Warfarin Therapy Discharge Instructions[2]	56	0%	79%	75%
Chest Pain/Possible Heart Attack Care				
Aspirin Given Within 24 Hours of Arrival	13	92%	97%	96%
Fibrinolytic Meds Within 30 Min. of Arrival[7]	-	-	44%	58%
Average Time to ECG (minutes)	13	5	6	7
Average Time to Transfer (minutes)[1]	-	-	58	60
Children's Asthma Care				
Received Home Management Plan of Care	-	-	85%	88%
Received Reliever Medication	-	-	100%	100%
Received Systemic Corticosteroids	-	-	100%	100%
Emergency Department				
Admittance Decision Time (minutes)[2]	550	103	90	98
Head CT Results Within 45 Min. of Arrival[1]	-	-	63%	57%
Patients Who Left ER Before Being Seen	38,030	5%	2%	2%
Time from ER Arrival to Admit. (minutes)[2]	804	305	265	274
Time from ER Arrival to Discharge (minutes)	774	172	128	134
Time in ER Before Being Evaluated (minutes)	268	40	22	26
Time to Pain Meds for Fractures (minutes)	35	65	54	57
Heart Attack Care				
Aspirin Given at Discharge	119	97%	99%	99%
Fibrinolytic Meds Within 30 Min. of Arrival[7]	-	-	80%	54%
PCI Within 90 Minutes of Arrival	16	94%	97%	96%
Statin Prescribed at Discharge	115	93%	98%	98%
Heart Failure Care				
ACE Inhibitor or ARB for LVSD	91	87%	97%	97%
Discharge Instructions Given	254	99%	96%	94%
Evaluation of LVS Function	331	100%	100%	99%
Medicare Spending				
Medicare Spending per Patient (ratio)	-	0.98	1.01	0.98
Pneumonia Care				
Appropriate Initial Antibiotic Given	155	97%	96%	95%
Blood Culture Timing	256	98%	98%	98%
Pregnancy and Delivery Care				
Newborn Deliveries Scheduled Early	69	4%	5%	6%
Preventive Care				
Immunization for Influenza[2]	660	96%	93%	90%
Immunization for Pneumonia[2]	931	93%	94%	92%
Stroke Care				
Anticoagulation Therapy for Atrial Fibrillation[1]	-	-	95%	95%
Antithrombotic Therapy Timing	59	98%	98%	98%
Assessed for Rehabilitation	57	88%	98%	97%
Discharged on Antithrombotic Therapy	56	96%	99%	99%
Discharged on Statin Medication	45	71%	95%	94%
Thrombolytic Therapy Timing	11	0%	65%	66%
Venous Thromboembolism Prophylaxis	58	84%	95%	94%
Written Stroke Educational Materials Given	35	0%	92%	88%
Surgical Care Improvement Project				
Appropriate Beta Blocker Usage	159	96%	98%	98%
Appropriate VTP Within 24 Hours	481	96%	98%	98%
Controlled Postoperative Blood Glucose	58	84%	97%	97%
Perioperative Temperature Management	521	100%	100%	100%
Prophylactic Antibiotic Selection	419	100%	99%	99%
Prophylactic Antibiotic Selection (Outpatient)	98	97%	98%	98%
Prophylactic Antibiotic Stopped	395	97%	98%	98%
Prophylactic Antibiotic Timing	419	100%	99%	99%
Prophylactic Antibiotic Timing (Outpatient)	98	100%	97%	98%
Urinary Catheter Removal	138	85%	97%	97%
Survey of Patients' Hospital Experiences				
Area Around Room 'Always' Quiet at Night	300+	43%	58%	61%
Doctors 'Always' Communicated Well	300+	77%	80%	82%
Home Recovery Information Given	300+	79%	87%	85%
Hospital Given 9 or 10 on 10 Point Scale	300+	66%	72%	71%
Meds 'Always' Explained Before Given	300+	62%	64%	64%
Nurses 'Always' Communicated Well	300+	77%	81%	79%
Pain 'Always' Well Controlled	300+	68%	71%	71%
Room and Bathroom 'Always' Clean	300+	73%	75%	73%
Timely Help 'Always' Received	300+	65%	70%	68%
Would Definitely Recommend Hospital	300+	66%	71%	71%
Use of Medical Imaging				
Cardiac Imaging Stress Test before Surgery	238	2.1%	5.4%	5.3%
Combination Abdominal CT Scan	471	3.6%	7.1%	10.5%
Combination Brain/Sinus CT Scan[1]	-	-	2.8%	2.7%
Combination Chest CT Scan	225	0.4%	1.7%	2.7%
Follow-up Mammogram/Ultrasound	692	10.3%	8.7%	8.8%
Lumbar Spine MRI for Low Back Pain	58	34.5%	34.7%	37.2%

Barnesville Hospital Association

639 West Main Street
Barnesville, OH 43713
Phone: 740-425-5101
Fax: 740-425-9213
E-mail: dcarroll@barnesvillehospital.com
URL: www.barnesvillehospital.com
Type: Critical Access Hospitals
Emergency Services: Yes
Ownership: Voluntary non-profit - Private
Beds: 25

Key Personnel:

Infection Control. . . . . JoAnn Barylak, RN
Emergency Room . . . . Michael Baum, MD
Quality Assurance . . . . Jane Hall, RN
Operating Room. . . . . Barb Mcmahon, RN
CEO/President. . . . . R Melvin Milburn
Radiology. . . . . Theresa Smith, DO
Chief of Medical Staff. . . . . PK Souri, MD
Intensive Care Unit. . . . . Joyce Weiss

Measure	Cases	This Hosp.	State Avg.	U.S. Avg.
Blood Clot Prevention and Treatment				
Anticoagulation Overlap Therapy[5]	-	-	93%	93%
ICU Venous Thromboembolism Prophylaxis[5]	-	-	93%	92%
Incidence of Potentially Preventable VTE[5]	-	-	6%	10%
UFH with Dosages/Platelet Monitoring[5]	-	-	98%	97%
Venous Thromboembolism Prophylaxis[5]	-	-	88%	85%
Warfarin Therapy Discharge Instructions[5]	-	-	79%	75%
Chest Pain/Possible Heart Attack Care				
Aspirin Given Within 24 Hours of Arrival[5]	-	-	97%	96%
Fibrinolytic Meds Within 30 Min. of Arrival[5]	-	-	44%	58%
Average Time to ECG (minutes)[5]	-	-	6	7
Average Time to Transfer (minutes)[5]	-	-	58	60
Children's Asthma Care				
Received Home Management Plan of Care	-	-	85%	88%
Received Reliever Medication	-	-	100%	100%
Received Systemic Corticosteroids	-	-	100%	100%
Emergency Department				
Admittance Decision Time (minutes)[5]	-	-	90	98
Head CT Results Within 45 Min. of Arrival[5]	-	-	63%	57%
Patients Who Left ER Before Being Seen[5]	-	-	2%	2%
Time from ER Arrival to Admit. (minutes)[5]	-	-	265	274
Time from ER Arrival to Discharge (minutes)[5]	-	-	128	134
Time in ER Before Being Evaluated (minutes)[5]	-	-	22	26
Time to Pain Meds for Fractures (minutes)[5]	-	-	54	57
Heart Attack Care				
Aspirin Given at Discharge	14	93%	99%	99%
Fibrinolytic Meds Within 30 Min. of Arrival[7]	-	-	80%	54%
PCI Within 90 Minutes of Arrival[7]	-	-	97%	96%
Statin Prescribed at Discharge[1]	-	-	98%	98%
Heart Failure Care				
ACE Inhibitor or ARB for LVSD	12	83%	97%	97%
Discharge Instructions Given	38	100%	96%	94%
Evaluation of LVS Function	50	96%	100%	99%
Medicare Spending				
Medicare Spending per Patient (ratio)	-	-	1.01	0.98
Pneumonia Care				
Appropriate Initial Antibiotic Given	38	97%	96%	95%
Blood Culture Timing	29	97%	98%	98%
Pregnancy and Delivery Care				
Newborn Deliveries Scheduled Early[5]	-	-	5%	6%
Preventive Care				
Immunization for Influenza[5]	-	-	93%	90%
Immunization for Pneumonia[2,3]	122	98%	94%	92%
Stroke Care				
Anticoagulation Therapy for Atrial Fibrillation[5]	-	-	95%	95%
Antithrombotic Therapy Timing[5]	-	-	98%	98%
Assessed for Rehabilitation[5]	-	-	98%	97%
Discharged on Antithrombotic Therapy[5]	-	-	99%	99%
Discharged on Statin Medication[5]	-	-	95%	94%
Thrombolytic Therapy Timing[5]	-	-	65%	66%
Venous Thromboembolism Prophylaxis[5]	-	-	95%	94%
Written Stroke Educational Materials Given[5]	-	-	92%	88%
Surgical Care Improvement Project				
Appropriate Beta Blocker Usage[5]	-	-	98%	98%
Appropriate VTP Within 24 Hours[5]	-	-	98%	98%
Controlled Postoperative Blood Glucose[5]	-	-	97%	97%
Perioperative Temperature Management[5]	-	-	100%	100%
Prophylactic Antibiotic Selection[5]	-	-	99%	99%
Prophylactic Antibiotic Selection (Outpatient)[5]	-	-	98%	98%
Prophylactic Antibiotic Stopped[5]	-	-	98%	98%
Prophylactic Antibiotic Timing[5]	-	-	99%	99%
Prophylactic Antibiotic Timing (Outpatient)[5]	-	-	97%	98%
Urinary Catheter Removal[5]	-	-	97%	97%
Survey of Patients' Hospital Experiences				
Area Around Room 'Always' Quiet at Night	(a)	57%	58%	61%
Doctors 'Always' Communicated Well	(a)	84%	80%	82%
Home Recovery Information Given	(a)	88%	87%	85%
Hospital Given 9 or 10 on 10 Point Scale	(a)	77%	72%	71%
Meds 'Always' Explained Before Given	(a)	68%	64%	64%
Nurses 'Always' Communicated Well	(a)	87%	81%	79%
Pain 'Always' Well Controlled	(a)	78%	71%	71%
Room and Bathroom 'Always' Clean	(a)	82%	75%	73%
Timely Help 'Always' Received	(a)	84%	70%	68%
Would Definitely Recommend Hospital	(a)	74%	71%	71%
Use of Medical Imaging				
Cardiac Imaging Stress Test before Surgery[1]	-	-	5.4%	5.3%
Combination Abdominal CT Scan	132	3.8%	7.1%	10.5%
Combination Brain/Sinus CT Scan[1]	-	-	2.8%	2.7%
Combination Chest CT Scan	134	1.5%	1.7%	2.7%
Follow-up Mammogram/Ultrasound	150	10.7%	8.7%	8.8%
Lumbar Spine MRI for Low Back Pain[1]	-	-	34.7%	37.2%

Mercy Hospital Clermont

3000 Hospital Drive
Batavia, OH 45103
Phone: 513-732-8278
Fax: 513-732-8361
URL: www.e-mercy.com
Type: Acute Care Hospitals
Emergency Services: Yes
Ownership: Voluntary non-profit - Church
Beds: 114

Key Personnel:

President/CEO. . . . . Yousuf J. Ahmad, DrPH, MHSA, MBA
Radiology. . . . . Richard G Cardella
Emergency Room . . . . Gayle Heintzelman
Anesthesiology. . . . . Ben Lee
Quality Assurance . . . . Patti Schroer
Chief of Medical Staff. . . . . Judy Stout

Measure	Cases	This Hosp.	State Avg.	U.S. Avg.

NOTE: Hospital profiles are in alphabetical order by state, then city, then hospital within the city; Rankings exclude hospitals with less than 25 cases except for patient surveys which excludes hospitals with less than 100 cases; (a) 100-299 cases; (1) The number of cases/patients is too few to report; (2) Data submitted were based on a sample of cases/patients; (3) Results are based on a shorter time period than required; (4) Data suppressed by CMS for one or more quarters; (5) Results are not available for this reporting period; (6) Fewer than 100 patients completed the HCAHPS survey; (7) No cases met the criteria for this measure; (8) The lower limit of the confidence interval cannot be calculated if the number of observed infections equals zero; (9) No data are available from the state/territory for this reporting period; (10) The scores shown reflect fewer than 50 completed surveys; (11) There were discrepancies in the data collection process; (12) This measure does not apply to this hospital for this reporting period; (13) Results cannot be calculated for this reporting period; (14) The results for this state are combined with nearby states to protect confidentiality; Please refer to the User's Guide for a full explanation of data.

Measure	Cases	This Hosp.	State Avg.	U.S. Avg.
Blood Clot Prevention and Treatment				
Anticoagulation Overlap Therapy[2]	33	94%	93%	93%
ICU Venous Thromboembolism Prophylaxis[2]	81	100%	93%	92%
Incidence of Potentially Preventable VTE[1,2]	-	-	6%	10%
UFH with Dosages/Platelet Monitoring[2]	16	100%	98%	97%
Venous Thromboembolism Prophylaxis[2]	300	97%	88%	85%
Warfarin Therapy Discharge Instructions[2]	34	88%	79%	75%
Chest Pain/Possible Heart Attack Care				
Aspirin Given Within 24 Hours of Arrival	77	99%	97%	96%
Fibrinolytic Meds Within 30 Min. of Arrival[7]	-	-	44%	58%
Average Time to ECG (minutes)	79	11	6	7
Average Time to Transfer (minutes)	17	65	58	60
Children's Asthma Care				
Received Home Management Plan of Care	-	-	85%	88%
Received Reliever Medication	-	-	100%	100%
Received Systemic Corticosteroids	-	-	100%	100%
Emergency Department				
Admittance Decision Time (minutes)[2]	996	118	90	98
Head CT Results Within 45 Min. of Arrival	27	67%	63%	57%
Patients Who Left ER Before Being Seen	58,862	1%	2%	2%
Time from ER Arrival to Admit. (minutes)[2]	998	302	265	274
Time from ER Arrival to Discharge (minutes)	378	114	128	134
Time in ER Before Being Evaluated (minutes)	421	11	22	26
Time to Pain Meds for Fractures (minutes)	126	51	54	57
Heart Attack Care				
Aspirin Given at Discharge	22	100%	99%	99%
Fibrinolytic Meds Within 30 Min. of Arrival[7]	-	-	80%	54%
PCI Within 90 Minutes of Arrival[7]	-	-	97%	96%
Statin Prescribed at Discharge	19	95%	98%	98%
Heart Failure Care				
ACE Inhibitor or ARB for LVSD	34	100%	97%	97%
Discharge Instructions Given	148	100%	96%	94%
Evaluation of LVS Function	183	100%	100%	99%
Medicare Spending				
Medicare Spending per Patient (ratio)	-	0.95	1.01	0.98
Pneumonia Care				
Appropriate Initial Antibiotic Given[2]	65	98%	96%	95%
Blood Culture Timing[2]	171	99%	98%	98%
Pregnancy and Delivery Care				
Newborn Deliveries Scheduled Early[7]	-	-	5%	6%
Preventive Care				
Immunization for Influenza[2]	591	99%	93%	90%
Immunization for Pneumonia[2]	846	99%	94%	92%
Stroke Care				
Anticoagulation Therapy for Atrial Fibrillation[1]	-	-	95%	95%
Antithrombotic Therapy Timing	24	100%	98%	98%
Assessed for Rehabilitation	29	100%	98%	97%
Discharged on Antithrombotic Therapy	29	100%	99%	99%
Discharged on Statin Medication	22	100%	95%	94%
Thrombolytic Therapy Timing[7]	-	-	65%	66%
Venous Thromboembolism Prophylaxis	21	100%	95%	94%
Written Stroke Educational Materials Given	19	100%	92%	88%
Surgical Care Improvement Project				
Appropriate Beta Blocker Usage[2]	77	97%	98%	98%
Appropriate VTP Within 24 Hours[2]	285	100%	98%	98%
Controlled Postoperative Blood Glucose[2,7]	-	-	97%	97%
Perioperative Temperature Management[2]	295	100%	100%	100%
Prophylactic Antibiotic Selection[2]	188	99%	99%	99%
Prophylactic Antibiotic Selection (Outpatient)	104	95%	98%	98%
Prophylactic Antibiotic Stopped[2]	184	99%	98%	98%
Prophylactic Antibiotic Timing[2]	188	99%	99%	99%
Prophylactic Antibiotic Timing (Outpatient)	87	98%	97%	98%
Urinary Catheter Removal[2]	215	96%	97%	97%
Survey of Patients' Hospital Experiences				
Area Around Room 'Always' Quiet at Night	300+	62%	58%	61%
Doctors 'Always' Communicated Well	300+	82%	80%	82%
Home Recovery Information Given	300+	89%	87%	85%
Hospital Given 9 or 10 on 10 Point Scale	300+	76%	72%	71%
Meds 'Always' Explained Before Given	300+	65%	64%	64%
Nurses 'Always' Communicated Well	300+	84%	81%	79%
Pain 'Always' Well Controlled	300+	72%	71%	71%
Room and Bathroom 'Always' Clean	300+	80%	75%	73%
Timely Help 'Always' Received	300+	67%	70%	68%
Would Definitely Recommend Hospital	300+	78%	71%	71%
Use of Medical Imaging				
Cardiac Imaging Stress Test before Surgery	165	6.7%	5.4%	5.3%
Combination Abdominal CT Scan	785	4.5%	7.1%	10.5%
Combination Brain/Sinus CT Scan	643	1.1%	2.8%	2.7%
Combination Chest CT Scan	701	0.3%	1.7%	2.7%
Follow-up Mammogram/Ultrasound	921	10.9%	8.7%	8.8%
Lumbar Spine MRI for Low Back Pain	116	37.9%	34.7%	37.2%

University Hospitals Ahuja Medical Center

3999 Richmond Road
Beachwood, OH 44122
Phone: 216-767-8793
URL: www.uhhospitals.org/ahuja
Type: Acute Care Hospitals
Emergency Services: Yes
Ownership: Voluntary non-profit - Private

Measure	Cases	This Hosp.	State Avg.	U.S. Avg.
Blood Clot Prevention and Treatment				
Anticoagulation Overlap Therapy[2]	107	94%	93%	93%
ICU Venous Thromboembolism Prophylaxis[2]	29	97%	93%	92%
Incidence of Potentially Preventable VTE[1,2]	-	-	6%	10%
UFH with Dosages/Platelet Monitoring[2]	99	100%	98%	97%
Venous Thromboembolism Prophylaxis[2]	357	95%	88%	85%
Warfarin Therapy Discharge Instructions[2]	81	93%	79%	75%
Chest Pain/Possible Heart Attack Care				
Aspirin Given Within 24 Hours of Arrival	18	100%	97%	96%
Fibrinolytic Meds Within 30 Min. of Arrival[3,7]	-	-	44%	58%
Average Time to ECG (minutes)	19	10	6	7
Average Time to Transfer (minutes)[3,7]	-	-	58	60
Children's Asthma Care				
Received Home Management Plan of Care	-	-	85%	88%
Received Reliever Medication	-	-	100%	100%
Received Systemic Corticosteroids	-	-	100%	100%
Emergency Department				
Admittance Decision Time (minutes)[2]	845	139	90	98
Head CT Results Within 45 Min. of Arrival	25	88%	63%	57%
Patients Who Left ER Before Being Seen	30,917	1%	2%	2%
Time from ER Arrival to Admit. (minutes)[2]	848	332	265	274
Time from ER Arrival to Discharge (minutes)	411	169	128	134
Time in ER Before Being Evaluated (minutes)	431	31	22	26
Time to Pain Meds for Fractures (minutes)	114	50	54	57
Heart Attack Care				
Aspirin Given at Discharge	125	100%	99%	99%
Fibrinolytic Meds Within 30 Min. of Arrival[7]	-	-	80%	54%
PCI Within 90 Minutes of Arrival	36	100%	97%	96%
Statin Prescribed at Discharge	122	98%	98%	98%
Heart Failure Care				
ACE Inhibitor or ARB for LVSD	77	100%	97%	97%
Discharge Instructions Given	235	92%	96%	94%
Evaluation of LVS Function	310	100%	100%	99%
Medicare Spending				
Medicare Spending per Patient (ratio)	-	1.00	1.01	0.98
Pneumonia Care				
Appropriate Initial Antibiotic Given[2]	77	100%	96%	95%
Blood Culture Timing[2]	196	98%	98%	98%
Pregnancy and Delivery Care				
Newborn Deliveries Scheduled Early[7]	-	-	5%	6%
Preventive Care				
Immunization for Influenza[2]	629	97%	93%	90%
Immunization for Pneumonia[2]	967	96%	94%	92%
Stroke Care				
Anticoagulation Therapy for Atrial Fibrillation	12	100%	95%	95%
Antithrombotic Therapy Timing	64	95%	98%	98%
Assessed for Rehabilitation	68	100%	98%	97%
Discharged on Antithrombotic Therapy	66	100%	99%	99%
Discharged on Statin Medication	56	100%	95%	94%
Thrombolytic Therapy Timing[7]	-	-	65%	66%
Venous Thromboembolism Prophylaxis	61	98%	95%	94%
Written Stroke Educational Materials Given	38	92%	92%	88%
Surgical Care Improvement Project				
Appropriate Beta Blocker Usage	174	97%	98%	98%
Appropriate VTP Within 24 Hours	486	100%	98%	98%
Controlled Postoperative Blood Glucose	32	97%	97%	97%
Perioperative Temperature Management	551	100%	100%	100%
Prophylactic Antibiotic Selection	395	99%	99%	99%
Prophylactic Antibiotic Selection (Outpatient)	251	99%	98%	98%
Prophylactic Antibiotic Stopped	384	99%	98%	98%
Prophylactic Antibiotic Timing	396	100%	99%	99%
Prophylactic Antibiotic Timing (Outpatient)	251	100%	97%	98%
Urinary Catheter Removal	421	100%	97%	97%
Survey of Patients' Hospital Experiences				
Area Around Room 'Always' Quiet at Night	300+	55%	58%	61%
Doctors 'Always' Communicated Well	300+	79%	80%	82%
Home Recovery Information Given	300+	84%	87%	85%
Hospital Given 9 or 10 on 10 Point Scale	300+	73%	72%	71%
Meds 'Always' Explained Before Given	300+	62%	64%	64%
Nurses 'Always' Communicated Well	300+	78%	81%	79%
Pain 'Always' Well Controlled	300+	68%	71%	71%
Room and Bathroom 'Always' Clean	300+	66%	75%	73%
Timely Help 'Always' Received	300+	58%	70%	68%
Would Definitely Recommend Hospital	300+	75%	71%	71%
Use of Medical Imaging				
Cardiac Imaging Stress Test before Surgery	220	6.8%	5.4%	5.3%
Combination Abdominal CT Scan	438	7.8%	7.1%	10.5%
Combination Brain/Sinus CT Scan	525	2.5%	2.8%	2.7%
Combination Chest CT Scan	330	0.3%	1.7%	2.7%
Follow-up Mammogram/Ultrasound[1]	-	-	8.7%	8.8%
Lumbar Spine MRI for Low Back Pain	65	33.8%	34.7%	37.2%

Indu & Raj Soin Medical Center

3535 Pentagon Park Blvd
Beaver Creek, OH 45431
Phone: 937-702-4000
Type: Acute Care Hospitals
Emergency Services: Yes
Ownership: Voluntary non-profit - Private

Measure	Cases	This Hosp.	State Avg.	U.S. Avg.
Blood Clot Prevention and Treatment				
Anticoagulation Overlap Therapy[2]	25	96%	93%	93%
ICU Venous Thromboembolism Prophylaxis[2]	86	98%	93%	92%
Incidence of Potentially Preventable VTE[1,2]	-	-	6%	10%
UFH with Dosages/Platelet Monitoring[1,2]	-	-	98%	97%
Venous Thromboembolism Prophylaxis[2]	310	98%	88%	85%
Warfarin Therapy Discharge Instructions[2]	17	76%	79%	75%
Chest Pain/Possible Heart Attack Care				
Aspirin Given Within 24 Hours of Arrival	31	100%	97%	96%
Fibrinolytic Meds Within 30 Min. of Arrival[7]	-	-	44%	58%
Average Time to ECG (minutes)	31	5	6	7
Average Time to Transfer (minutes)[1]	-	-	58	60
Children's Asthma Care				
Received Home Management Plan of Care	-	-	85%	88%
Received Reliever Medication	-	-	100%	100%
Received Systemic Corticosteroids	-	-	100%	100%
Emergency Department				
Admittance Decision Time (minutes)[2]	598	102	90	98
Head CT Results Within 45 Min. of Arrival	11	73%	63%	57%
Patients Who Left ER Before Being Seen	21,231	1%	2%	2%
Time from ER Arrival to Admit. (minutes)[2]	599	257	265	274
Time from ER Arrival to Discharge (minutes)	523	148	128	134
Time in ER Before Being Evaluated (minutes)	565	16	22	26
Time to Pain Meds for Fractures (minutes)	68	50	54	57
Heart Attack Care				
Aspirin Given at Discharge	17	100%	99%	99%
Fibrinolytic Meds Within 30 Min. of Arrival[7]	-	-	80%	54%
PCI Within 90 Minutes of Arrival[7]	-	-	97%	96%
Statin Prescribed at Discharge	16	100%	98%	98%
Heart Failure Care				
ACE Inhibitor or ARB for LVSD	30	100%	97%	97%
Discharge Instructions Given	82	99%	96%	94%
Evaluation of LVS Function	113	100%	100%	99%
Medicare Spending				
Medicare Spending per Patient (ratio)	-	0.99	1.01	0.98
Pneumonia Care				
Appropriate Initial Antibiotic Given	111	99%	96%	95%
Blood Culture Timing	169	100%	98%	98%
Pregnancy and Delivery Care				

NOTE: Hospital profiles are in alphabetical order by state, then city, then hospital within the city; Rankings exclude hospitals with less than 25 cases except for patient surveys which excludes hospitals with less than 100 cases; (a) 100-299 cases; (1) The number of cases/patients is too few to report; (2) Data submitted were based on a sample of cases/patients; (3) Results are based on a shorter time period than required; (4) Data suppressed by CMS for one or more quarters; (5) Results are not available for this reporting period; (6) Fewer than 100 patients completed the HCAHPS survey; (7) No cases met the criteria for this measure; (8) The lower limit of the confidence interval cannot be calculated if the number of observed infections equals zero; (9) No data are available from the state/territory for this reporting period; (10) The scores shown reflect fewer than 50 completed surveys; (11) There were discrepancies in the data collection process; (12) This measure does not apply to this hospital for this reporting period; (13) Results cannot be calculated for this reporting period; (14) The results for this state are combined with nearby states to protect confidentiality; Please refer to the User's Guide for a full explanation of data.

Measure	Cases	This Hosp.	State Avg.	U.S. Avg.
Newborn Deliveries Scheduled Early	25	12%	5%	6%
Preventive Care				
Immunization for Influenza[2]	411	97%	93%	90%
Immunization for Pneumonia[2]	544	97%	94%	92%
Stroke Care				
Anticoagulation Therapy for Atrial Fibrillation[1]	-	-	95%	95%
Antithrombotic Therapy Timing	36	100%	98%	98%
Assessed for Rehabilitation	34	100%	98%	97%
Discharged on Antithrombotic Therapy	33	100%	99%	99%
Discharged on Statin Medication	24	100%	95%	94%
Thrombolytic Therapy Timing[7]	-	-	65%	66%
Venous Thromboembolism Prophylaxis	33	97%	95%	94%
Written Stroke Educational Materials Given	24	100%	92%	88%
Surgical Care Improvement Project				
Appropriate Beta Blocker Usage	26	96%	98%	98%
Appropriate VTP Within 24 Hours	87	98%	98%	98%
Controlled Postoperative Blood Glucose[7]	-	-	97%	97%
Perioperative Temperature Management	91	100%	100%	100%
Prophylactic Antibiotic Selection	32	100%	99%	99%
Prophylactic Antibiotic Selection (Outpatient)	144	96%	98%	98%
Prophylactic Antibiotic Stopped	32	97%	98%	98%
Prophylactic Antibiotic Timing	32	100%	99%	99%
Prophylactic Antibiotic Timing (Outpatient)	146	97%	97%	98%
Urinary Catheter Removal	48	94%	97%	97%
Survey of Patients' Hospital Experiences				
Area Around Room 'Always' Quiet at Night	300+	68%	58%	61%
Doctors 'Always' Communicated Well	300+	78%	80%	82%
Home Recovery Information Given	300+	84%	87%	85%
Hospital Given 9 or 10 on 10 Point Scale	300+	81%	72%	71%
Meds 'Always' Explained Before Given	300+	62%	64%	64%
Nurses 'Always' Communicated Well	300+	82%	81%	79%
Pain 'Always' Well Controlled	300+	71%	71%	71%
Room and Bathroom 'Always' Clean	300+	79%	75%	73%
Timely Help 'Always' Received	300+	69%	70%	68%
Would Definitely Recommend Hospital	300+	82%	71%	71%
Use of Medical Imaging				
Cardiac Imaging Stress Test before Surgery	138	4.3%	5.4%	5.3%
Combination Abdominal CT Scan	391	2.6%	7.1%	10.5%
Combination Brain/Sinus CT Scan	409	2.0%	2.8%	2.7%
Combination Chest CT Scan	94	1.1%	1.7%	2.7%
Follow-up Mammogram/Ultrasound[7]	-	-	8.7%	8.8%
Lumbar Spine MRI for Low Back Pain	35	48.6%	34.7%	37.2%

Belmont Community Hospital

4697 Harrison Street
Bellaire, OH 43906
Phone: 740-671-1200
Fax: 740-671-1210
E-mail: webmaster@wheelinghospital.com
URL: www.wheelinghospital.com
Type: Acute Care Hospitals
Emergency Services: Yes
Ownership: Voluntary non-profit - Other
Beds: 99

Key Personnel:

Radiology. . . . . Eric R Balzano
Cardiology . . . . Devender K Batra, MD
Cardiology . . . . Edward K Chiu
Cardiology . . . . Adel E Fren
CEO/President. . . . . Gary Gold
Quality Assurance . . . . Diane Patt
Operating Room. . . . . Jean Thoburn

Measure	Cases	This Hosp.	State Avg.	U.S. Avg.
Blood Clot Prevention and Treatment				
Anticoagulation Overlap Therapy[1,2]	-	-	93%	93%
ICU Venous Thromboembolism Prophylaxis[2,7]	-	-	93%	92%
Incidence of Potentially Preventable VTE[1,2]	-	-	6%	10%
UFH with Dosages/Platelet Monitoring[1,2]	-	-	98%	97%
Venous Thromboembolism Prophylaxis[2]	74	100%	88%	85%
Warfarin Therapy Discharge Instructions[1,2]	-	-	79%	75%
Chest Pain/Possible Heart Attack Care				
Aspirin Given Within 24 Hours of Arrival	14	93%	97%	96%
Fibrinolytic Meds Within 30 Min. of Arrival[1]	-	-	44%	58%
Average Time to ECG (minutes)	13	4	6	7
Average Time to Transfer (minutes)[1]	-	-	58	60
Children's Asthma Care				
Received Home Management Plan of Care	-	-	85%	88%
Received Reliever Medication	-	-	100%	100%
Received Systemic Corticosteroids	-	-	100%	100%
Emergency Department				
Admittance Decision Time (minutes)[2]	61	39	90	98
Head CT Results Within 45 Min. of Arrival[1]	-	-	63%	57%
Patients Who Left ER Before Being Seen	6,564	1%	2%	2%
Time from ER Arrival to Admit. (minutes)[2]	122	178	265	274
Time from ER Arrival to Discharge (minutes)	352	68	128	134
Time in ER Before Being Evaluated (minutes)	304	26	22	26
Time to Pain Meds for Fractures (minutes)	22	58	54	57
Heart Attack Care				
Aspirin Given at Discharge[1]	-	-	99%	99%
Fibrinolytic Meds Within 30 Min. of Arrival[7]	-	-	80%	54%
PCI Within 90 Minutes of Arrival[7]	-	-	97%	96%
Statin Prescribed at Discharge[1]	-	-	98%	98%
Heart Failure Care				
ACE Inhibitor or ARB for LVSD[1]	-	-	97%	97%
Discharge Instructions Given	13	92%	96%	94%
Evaluation of LVS Function	19	95%	100%	99%
Medicare Spending				
Medicare Spending per Patient (ratio)	-	1.01	1.01	0.98
Pneumonia Care				
Appropriate Initial Antibiotic Given	33	85%	96%	95%
Blood Culture Timing	36	97%	98%	98%
Pregnancy and Delivery Care				
Newborn Deliveries Scheduled Early[7]	-	-	5%	6%
Preventive Care				
Immunization for Influenza[2]	291	85%	93%	90%
Immunization for Pneumonia[2]	370	84%	94%	92%
Stroke Care				
Anticoagulation Therapy for Atrial Fibrillation[3,7]	-	-	95%	95%
Antithrombotic Therapy Timing[1,3]	-	-	98%	98%
Assessed for Rehabilitation[1,3]	-	-	98%	97%
Discharged on Antithrombotic Therapy[1,3]	-	-	99%	99%
Discharged on Statin Medication[1,3]	-	-	95%	94%
Thrombolytic Therapy Timing[3,7]	-	-	65%	66%
Venous Thromboembolism Prophylaxis[1,3]	-	-	95%	94%
Written Stroke Educational Materials Given[1,3]	-	-	92%	88%
Surgical Care Improvement Project				
Appropriate Beta Blocker Usage[3,7]	-	-	98%	98%
Appropriate VTP Within 24 Hours[1,3]	-	-	98%	98%
Controlled Postoperative Blood Glucose[3,7]	-	-	97%	97%
Perioperative Temperature Management[1,3]	-	-	100%	100%
Prophylactic Antibiotic Selection[1,3]	-	-	99%	99%
Prophylactic Antibiotic Selection (Outpatient)[5]	-	-	98%	98%
Prophylactic Antibiotic Stopped[1,3]	-	-	98%	98%
Prophylactic Antibiotic Timing[1,3]	-	-	99%	99%
Prophylactic Antibiotic Timing (Outpatient)[5]	-	-	97%	98%
Urinary Catheter Removal[1,3]	-	-	97%	97%
Survey of Patients' Hospital Experiences				
Area Around Room 'Always' Quiet at Night[6]	<100	51%	58%	61%
Doctors 'Always' Communicated Well[6]	<100	76%	80%	82%
Home Recovery Information Given[6]	<100	78%	87%	85%
Hospital Given 9 or 10 on 10 Point Scale[6]	<100	69%	72%	71%
Meds 'Always' Explained Before Given[6]	<100	64%	64%	64%
Nurses 'Always' Communicated Well[6]	<100	81%	81%	79%
Pain 'Always' Well Controlled[6]	<100	78%	71%	71%
Room and Bathroom 'Always' Clean[6]	<100	86%	75%	73%
Timely Help 'Always' Received[6]	<100	80%	70%	68%
Would Definitely Recommend Hospital[6]	<100	72%	71%	71%
Use of Medical Imaging				
Cardiac Imaging Stress Test before Surgery[7]	-	-	5.4%	5.3%
Combination Abdominal CT Scan[1]	-	-	7.1%	10.5%
Combination Brain/Sinus CT Scan[1]	-	-	2.8%	2.7%
Combination Chest CT Scan	53	0.0%	1.7%	2.7%
Follow-up Mammogram/Ultrasound	137	10.2%	8.7%	8.8%
Lumbar Spine MRI for Low Back Pain[1]	-	-	34.7%	37.2%

Mary Rutan Hospital

205 Palmer Avenue
Bellefontaine, OH 43311
Phone: 937-592-4015
Fax: 937-592-7007
E-mail: pjmcbrien@maryrutan.org
Type: Acute Care Hospitals
Emergency Services: Yes
Ownership: Voluntary non-profit - Private
Beds: 105

Key Personnel:

President/CEO. . . . . Mandy Goble
Radiology. . . . . Therese Jones

Measure	Cases	This Hosp.	State Avg.	U.S. Avg.
Blood Clot Prevention and Treatment				
Anticoagulation Overlap Therapy[2]	12	83%	93%	93%
ICU Venous Thromboembolism Prophylaxis[2]	24	79%	93%	92%
Incidence of Potentially Preventable VTE[1,2]	-	-	6%	10%
UFH with Dosages/Platelet Monitoring[1,2]	-	-	98%	97%
Venous Thromboembolism Prophylaxis[2]	92	72%	88%	85%
Warfarin Therapy Discharge Instructions[2]	11	100%	79%	75%
Chest Pain/Possible Heart Attack Care				
Aspirin Given Within 24 Hours of Arrival	131	100%	97%	96%
Fibrinolytic Meds Within 30 Min. of Arrival[1]	-	-	44%	58%
Average Time to ECG (minutes)	134	6	6	7
Average Time to Transfer (minutes)	37	45	58	60
Children's Asthma Care				
Received Home Management Plan of Care	-	-	85%	88%
Received Reliever Medication	-	-	100%	100%
Received Systemic Corticosteroids	-	-	100%	100%
Emergency Department				
Admittance Decision Time (minutes)[2]	93	75	90	98
Head CT Results Within 45 Min. of Arrival	11	100%	63%	57%
Patients Who Left ER Before Being Seen	24,325	3%	2%	2%
Time from ER Arrival to Admit. (minutes)[2]	177	254	265	274
Time from ER Arrival to Discharge (minutes)	341	117	128	134
Time in ER Before Being Evaluated (minutes)	383	34	22	26
Time to Pain Meds for Fractures (minutes)	107	55	54	57
Heart Attack Care				
Aspirin Given at Discharge	20	100%	99%	99%
Fibrinolytic Meds Within 30 Min. of Arrival[7]	-	-	80%	54%
PCI Within 90 Minutes of Arrival[7]	-	-	97%	96%
Statin Prescribed at Discharge	20	100%	98%	98%
Heart Failure Care				
ACE Inhibitor or ARB for LVSD	23	96%	97%	97%
Discharge Instructions Given	40	100%	96%	94%
Evaluation of LVS Function	57	100%	100%	99%
Medicare Spending				
Medicare Spending per Patient (ratio)	-	1.02	1.01	0.98
Pneumonia Care				
Appropriate Initial Antibiotic Given	51	100%	96%	95%
Blood Culture Timing	85	99%	98%	98%
Pregnancy and Delivery Care				
Newborn Deliveries Scheduled Early	25	8%	5%	6%
Preventive Care				
Immunization for Influenza[2]	240	98%	93%	90%
Immunization for Pneumonia[2]	292	98%	94%	92%
Stroke Care				
Anticoagulation Therapy for Atrial Fibrillation[7]	-	-	95%	95%
Antithrombotic Therapy Timing	14	93%	98%	98%
Assessed for Rehabilitation	13	100%	98%	97%
Discharged on Antithrombotic Therapy	13	100%	99%	99%
Discharged on Statin Medication[1]	-	-	95%	94%
Thrombolytic Therapy Timing[7]	-	-	65%	66%
Venous Thromboembolism Prophylaxis	11	91%	95%	94%
Written Stroke Educational Materials Given[1]	-	-	92%	88%
Surgical Care Improvement Project				
Appropriate Beta Blocker Usage	63	100%	98%	98%
Appropriate VTP Within 24 Hours	181	100%	98%	98%
Controlled Postoperative Blood Glucose[7]	-	-	97%	97%
Perioperative Temperature Management	192	100%	100%	100%
Prophylactic Antibiotic Selection	142	99%	99%	99%
Prophylactic Antibiotic Selection (Outpatient)	25	100%	98%	98%
Prophylactic Antibiotic Stopped	139	99%	98%	98%
Prophylactic Antibiotic Timing	142	100%	99%	99%
Prophylactic Antibiotic Timing (Outpatient)	25	100%	97%	98%
Urinary Catheter Removal	106	98%	97%	97%

NOTE: Hospital profiles are in alphabetical order by state, then city, then hospital within the city; Rankings exclude hospitals with less than 25 cases except for patient surveys which excludes hospitals with less than 100 cases; (a) 100-299 cases; (1) The number of cases/patients is too few to report; (2) Data submitted were based on a sample of cases/patients; (3) Results are based on a shorter time period than required; (4) Data suppressed by CMS for one or more quarters; (5) Results are not available for this reporting period; (6) Fewer than 100 patients completed the HCAHPS survey; (7) No cases met the criteria for this measure; (8) The lower limit of the confidence interval cannot be calculated if the number of observed infections equals zero; (9) No data are available from the state/territory for this reporting period; (10) The scores shown reflect fewer than 50 completed surveys; (11) There were discrepancies in the data collection process; (12) This measure does not apply to this hospital for this reporting period; (13) Results cannot be calculated for this reporting period; (14) The results for this state are combined with nearby states to protect confidentiality; Please refer to the User's Guide for a full explanation of data.

Survey of Patients' Hospital Experiences				
Area Around Room 'Always' Quiet at Night	300+	58%	58%	61%
Doctors 'Always' Communicated Well	300+	84%	80%	82%
Home Recovery Information Given	300+	86%	87%	85%
Hospital Given 9 or 10 on 10 Point Scale	300+	72%	72%	71%
Meds 'Always' Explained Before Given	300+	62%	64%	64%
Nurses 'Always' Communicated Well	300+	82%	81%	79%
Pain 'Always' Well Controlled	300+	67%	71%	71%
Room and Bathroom 'Always' Clean	300+	79%	75%	73%
Timely Help 'Always' Received	300+	75%	70%	68%
Would Definitely Recommend Hospital	300+	67%	71%	71%
Use of Medical Imaging				
Cardiac Imaging Stress Test before Surgery	96	6.3%	5.4%	5.3%
Combination Abdominal CT Scan	477	7.8%	7.1%	10.5%
Combination Brain/Sinus CT Scan[1]	-	-	2.8%	2.7%
Combination Chest CT Scan	258	4.3%	1.7%	2.7%
Follow-up Mammogram/Ultrasound	738	11.5%	8.7%	8.8%
Lumbar Spine MRI for Low Back Pain[1]	-	-	34.7%	37.2%

Bellevue Hospital

1400 West Main Street
Bellevue, OH 44811
Phone: 419-483-4040
Fax: 419-483-9718
E-mail: webmaster@bellevuehospital.com
URL: www.bellevuehospital.com
Type: Acute Care Hospitals
Emergency Services: Yes
Ownership: Voluntary non-profit - Other
Beds: 64

Key Personnel:
Anesthesiology. . . . . Joseph E. Colizoli, MD
Quality Assurance . . . . Patricia Hetrick Semer
Chief of Medical Staff. . . . . Richard Kendall, MD
Infection Control. . . . . Susan Kistler
Operating Room. . . . . Tammi Lewis, RN
Chair/CEO . . . . Dean Miller
Radiology. . . . . David West, MD
Intensive Care Unit. . . . . Youngsook Yoon

Measure	Cases	This Hosp.	State Avg.	U.S. Avg.
Blood Clot Prevention and Treatment				
Anticoagulation Overlap Therapy[1,2]	-	-	93%	93%
ICU Venous Thromboembolism Prophylaxis[2]	30	80%	93%	92%
Incidence of Potentially Preventable VTE[1,2]	-	-	6%	10%
UFH with Dosages/Platelet Monitoring[1,2]	-	-	98%	97%
Venous Thromboembolism Prophylaxis[2]	76	64%	88%	85%
Warfarin Therapy Discharge Instructions[1,2]	-	-	79%	75%
Chest Pain/Possible Heart Attack Care				
Aspirin Given Within 24 Hours of Arrival	84	94%	97%	96%
Fibrinolytic Meds Within 30 Min. of Arrival[1]	-	-	44%	58%
Average Time to ECG (minutes)	88	5	6	7
Average Time to Transfer (minutes)	15	47	58	60
Children's Asthma Care				
Received Home Management Plan of Care	-	-	85%	88%
Received Reliever Medication	-	-	100%	100%
Received Systemic Corticosteroids	-	-	100%	100%
Emergency Department				
Admittance Decision Time (minutes)[2]	142	48	90	98
Head CT Results Within 45 Min. of Arrival[1]	-	-	63%	57%
Patients Who Left ER Before Being Seen	15,798	0%	2%	2%
Time from ER Arrival to Admit. (minutes)[2]	159	191	265	274
Time from ER Arrival to Discharge (minutes)	340	92	128	134
Time in ER Before Being Evaluated (minutes)	333	18	22	26
Time to Pain Meds for Fractures (minutes)	42	38	54	57
Heart Attack Care				
Aspirin Given at Discharge[1]	-	-	99%	99%
Fibrinolytic Meds Within 30 Min. of Arrival[7]	-	-	80%	54%
PCI Within 90 Minutes of Arrival[7]	-	-	97%	96%
Statin Prescribed at Discharge[1]	-	-	98%	98%
Heart Failure Care				
ACE Inhibitor or ARB for LVSD[1]	-	-	97%	97%
Discharge Instructions Given	35	91%	96%	94%
Evaluation of LVS Function	42	100%	100%	99%
Medicare Spending				
Medicare Spending per Patient (ratio)	-	1.01	1.01	0.98
Pneumonia Care				
Appropriate Initial Antibiotic Given	52	85%	96%	95%
Blood Culture Timing	59	92%	98%	98%
Pregnancy and Delivery Care				
Newborn Deliveries Scheduled Early	37	3%	5%	6%
Preventive Care				
Immunization for Influenza[2]	218	82%	93%	90%
Immunization for Pneumonia[2]	226	70%	94%	92%
Stroke Care				
Anticoagulation Therapy for Atrial Fibrillation[1]	-	-	95%	95%
Antithrombotic Therapy Timing	13	92%	98%	98%
Assessed for Rehabilitation	12	100%	98%	97%
Discharged on Antithrombotic Therapy	12	100%	99%	99%
Discharged on Statin Medication[1]	-	-	95%	94%
Thrombolytic Therapy Timing[1]	-	-	65%	66%
Venous Thromboembolism Prophylaxis	12	83%	95%	94%
Written Stroke Educational Materials Given[1]	-	-	92%	88%
Surgical Care Improvement Project				
Appropriate Beta Blocker Usage	34	97%	98%	98%
Appropriate VTP Within 24 Hours	90	96%	98%	98%
Controlled Postoperative Blood Glucose[7]	-	-	97%	97%
Perioperative Temperature Management	98	100%	100%	100%
Prophylactic Antibiotic Selection	72	100%	99%	99%
Prophylactic Antibiotic Selection (Outpatient)	53	81%	98%	98%
Prophylactic Antibiotic Stopped	68	93%	98%	98%
Prophylactic Antibiotic Timing	72	99%	99%	99%
Prophylactic Antibiotic Timing (Outpatient)	54	98%	97%	98%
Urinary Catheter Removal	74	96%	97%	97%
Survey of Patients' Hospital Experiences				
Area Around Room 'Always' Quiet at Night	300+	63%	58%	61%
Doctors 'Always' Communicated Well	300+	86%	80%	82%
Home Recovery Information Given	300+	90%	87%	85%
Hospital Given 9 or 10 on 10 Point Scale	300+	83%	72%	71%
Meds 'Always' Explained Before Given	300+	66%	64%	64%
Nurses 'Always' Communicated Well	300+	87%	81%	79%
Pain 'Always' Well Controlled	300+	76%	71%	71%
Room and Bathroom 'Always' Clean	300+	83%	75%	73%
Timely Help 'Always' Received	300+	77%	70%	68%
Would Definitely Recommend Hospital	300+	81%	71%	71%
Use of Medical Imaging				
Cardiac Imaging Stress Test before Surgery	180	3.9%	5.4%	5.3%
Combination Abdominal CT Scan	304	15.5%	7.1%	10.5%
Combination Brain/Sinus CT Scan[1]	-	-	2.8%	2.7%
Combination Chest CT Scan	131	19.1%	1.7%	2.7%
Follow-up Mammogram/Ultrasound	395	9.1%	8.7%	8.8%
Lumbar Spine MRI for Low Back Pain	47	46.8%	34.7%	37.2%

Bluffton Hospital

139 Garau Street
Bluffton, OH 45817
Phone: 419-358-9010
URL: www.bvhealthsystem.org
Type: Critical Access Hospitals
Emergency Services: Yes
Ownership: Voluntary non-profit - Private
Beds: 25

Key Personnel:
Administrator . . . . Bill Watkins

Measure	Cases	This Hosp.	State Avg.	U.S. Avg.
Blood Clot Prevention and Treatment				
Anticoagulation Overlap Therapy[1,2]	-	-	93%	93%
ICU Venous Thromboembolism Prophylaxis[1,2]	-	-	93%	92%
Incidence of Potentially Preventable VTE[2,7]	-	-	6%	10%
UFH with Dosages/Platelet Monitoring[2,7]	-	-	98%	97%
Venous Thromboembolism Prophylaxis[2]	46	96%	88%	85%
Warfarin Therapy Discharge Instructions[1,2]	-	-	79%	75%
Chest Pain/Possible Heart Attack Care				
Aspirin Given Within 24 Hours of Arrival[1]	-	-	97%	96%
Fibrinolytic Meds Within 30 Min. of Arrival[3,7]	-	-	44%	58%
Average Time to ECG (minutes)[1]	-	-	6	7
Average Time to Transfer (minutes)[1,3]	-	-	58	60
Children's Asthma Care				
Received Home Management Plan of Care	-	-	85%	88%
Received Reliever Medication	-	-	100%	100%
Received Systemic Corticosteroids	-	-	100%	100%
Emergency Department				
Admittance Decision Time (minutes)[2]	73	43	90	98
Head CT Results Within 45 Min. of Arrival[1]	-	-	63%	57%
Patients Who Left ER Before Being Seen	5,993	0%	2%	2%
Time from ER Arrival to Admit. (minutes)[2]	73	231	265	274
Time from ER Arrival to Discharge (minutes)	361	85	128	134
Time in ER Before Being Evaluated (minutes)	384	12	22	26
Time to Pain Meds for Fractures (minutes)	26	30	54	57
Heart Attack Care				
Aspirin Given at Discharge[5]	-	-	99%	99%
Fibrinolytic Meds Within 30 Min. of Arrival[5]	-	-	80%	54%
PCI Within 90 Minutes of Arrival[5]	-	-	97%	96%
Statin Prescribed at Discharge[5]	-	-	98%	98%
Heart Failure Care				
ACE Inhibitor or ARB for LVSD[1,3]	-	-	97%	97%
Discharge Instructions Given[1,3]	-	-	96%	94%
Evaluation of LVS Function[1,3]	-	-	100%	99%
Medicare Spending				
Medicare Spending per Patient (ratio)	-	-	1.01	0.98
Pneumonia Care				
Appropriate Initial Antibiotic Given[1]	-	-	96%	95%
Blood Culture Timing[1]	-	-	98%	98%
Pregnancy and Delivery Care				
Newborn Deliveries Scheduled Early[2]	16	0%	5%	6%
Preventive Care				
Immunization for Influenza[2]	154	99%	93%	90%
Immunization for Pneumonia[2]	77	99%	94%	92%
Stroke Care				
Anticoagulation Therapy for Atrial Fibrillation[3,7]	-	-	95%	95%
Antithrombotic Therapy Timing[1,3]	-	-	98%	98%
Assessed for Rehabilitation[1,3]	-	-	98%	97%
Discharged on Antithrombotic Therapy[1,3]	-	-	99%	99%
Discharged on Statin Medication[1,3]	-	-	95%	94%
Thrombolytic Therapy Timing[3,7]	-	-	65%	66%
Venous Thromboembolism Prophylaxis[1,3]	-	-	95%	94%
Written Stroke Educational Materials Given[3,7]	-	-	92%	88%
Surgical Care Improvement Project				
Appropriate Beta Blocker Usage[2,3]	-	-	98%	98%
Appropriate VTP Within 24 Hours[1,2]	-	-	98%	98%
Controlled Postoperative Blood Glucose[2,3]	-	-	97%	97%
Perioperative Temperature Management[1,2]	-	-	100%	100%
Prophylactic Antibiotic Selection[1,2]	-	-	99%	99%
Prophylactic Antibiotic Selection (Outpatient)	56	100%	98%	98%
Prophylactic Antibiotic Stopped[1,2]	-	-	98%	98%
Prophylactic Antibiotic Timing[1,2]	-	-	99%	99%
Prophylactic Antibiotic Timing (Outpatient)	56	100%	97%	98%
Urinary Catheter Removal[2,3]	-	-	97%	97%
Survey of Patients' Hospital Experiences				
Area Around Room 'Always' Quiet at Night	(a)	79%	58%	61%
Doctors 'Always' Communicated Well	(a)	88%	80%	82%
Home Recovery Information Given	(a)	95%	87%	85%
Hospital Given 9 or 10 on 10 Point Scale	(a)	91%	72%	71%
Meds 'Always' Explained Before Given	(a)	65%	64%	64%
Nurses 'Always' Communicated Well	(a)	88%	81%	79%
Pain 'Always' Well Controlled	(a)	80%	71%	71%
Room and Bathroom 'Always' Clean	(a)	85%	75%	73%
Timely Help 'Always' Received	(a)	87%	70%	68%
Would Definitely Recommend Hospital	(a)	88%	71%	71%
Use of Medical Imaging				
Cardiac Imaging Stress Test before Surgery[1]	-	-	5.4%	5.3%
Combination Abdominal CT Scan	81	6.2%	7.1%	10.5%
Combination Brain/Sinus CT Scan[1]	-	-	2.8%	2.7%
Combination Chest CT Scan[1]	-	-	1.7%	2.7%
Follow-up Mammogram/Ultrasound	230	5.2%	8.7%	8.8%
Lumbar Spine MRI for Low Back Pain[7]	-	-	34.7%	37.2%

Saint Elizabeth Boardman Health Center

8401 Market Street
Boardman, OH 44512
Phone: 330-729-2929
URL: www.ehealthconnection.com
Type: Acute Care Hospitals
Emergency Services: Yes
Ownership: Voluntary non-profit - Church

Key Personnel:
President/CEO. . . . . Bob Shroder

Measure	Cases	This Hosp.	State Avg.	U.S. Avg.
Blood Clot Prevention and Treatment				
Anticoagulation Overlap Therapy[2]	89	88%	93%	93%

NOTE: Hospital profiles are in alphabetical order by state, then city, then hospital within the city; Rankings exclude hospitals with less than 25 cases except for patient surveys which excludes hospitals with less than 100 cases; (a) 100-299 cases; (1) The number of cases/patients is too few to report; (2) Data submitted were based on a sample of cases/patients; (3) Results are based on a shorter time period than required; (4) Data suppressed by CMS for one or more quarters; (5) Results are not available for this reporting period; (6) Fewer than 100 patients completed the HCAHPS survey; (7) No cases met the criteria for this measure; (8) The lower limit of the confidence interval cannot be calculated if the number of observed infections equals zero; (9) No data are available from the state/territory for this reporting period; (10) The scores shown reflect fewer than 50 completed surveys; (11) There were discrepancies in the data collection process; (12) This measure does not apply to this hospital for this reporting period; (13) Results cannot be calculated for this reporting period; (14) The results for this state are combined with nearby states to protect confidentiality; Please refer to the User's Guide for a full explanation of data.

Measure	Cases	This Hosp.	State Avg.	U.S. Avg.
ICU Venous Thromboembolism Prophylaxis[2]	64	86%	93%	92%
Incidence of Potentially Preventable VTE[1,2]	-	-	6%	10%
UFH with Dosages/Platelet Monitoring[2]	50	100%	98%	97%
Venous Thromboembolism Prophylaxis[2]	349	83%	88%	85%
Warfarin Therapy Discharge Instructions[2]	65	92%	79%	75%
Chest Pain/Possible Heart Attack Care				
Aspirin Given Within 24 Hours of Arrival	83	98%	97%	96%
Fibrinolytic Meds Within 30 Min. of Arrival[1]	-	-	44%	58%
Average Time to ECG (minutes)	84	4	6	7
Average Time to Transfer (minutes)	24	40	58	60
Children's Asthma Care				
Received Home Management Plan of Care	-	-	85%	88%
Received Reliever Medication	-	-	100%	100%
Received Systemic Corticosteroids	-	-	100%	100%
Emergency Department				
Admittance Decision Time (minutes)[2]	988	122	90	98
Head CT Results Within 45 Min. of Arrival	16	12%	63%	57%
Patients Who Left ER Before Being Seen	45,446	1%	2%	2%
Time from ER Arrival to Admit. (minutes)[2]	1,005	301	265	274
Time from ER Arrival to Discharge (minutes)	379	153	128	134
Time in ER Before Being Evaluated (minutes)	451	22	22	26
Time to Pain Meds for Fractures (minutes)	143	73	54	57
Heart Attack Care				
Aspirin Given at Discharge	36	100%	99%	99%
Fibrinolytic Meds Within 30 Min. of Arrival[7]	-	-	80%	54%
PCI Within 90 Minutes of Arrival[7]	-	-	97%	96%
Statin Prescribed at Discharge	28	100%	98%	98%
Heart Failure Care				
ACE Inhibitor or ARB for LVSD[2]	55	95%	97%	97%
Discharge Instructions Given[2]	221	100%	96%	94%
Evaluation of LVS Function[2]	288	100%	100%	99%
Medicare Spending				
Medicare Spending per Patient (ratio)	-	1.06	1.01	0.98
Pneumonia Care				
Appropriate Initial Antibiotic Given[2]	58	90%	96%	95%
Blood Culture Timing[2]	126	99%	98%	98%
Pregnancy and Delivery Care				
Newborn Deliveries Scheduled Early[7]	-	-	5%	6%
Preventive Care				
Immunization for Influenza[2]	630	97%	93%	90%
Immunization for Pneumonia[2]	984	96%	94%	92%
Stroke Care				
Anticoagulation Therapy for Atrial Fibrillation[1]	-	-	95%	95%
Antithrombotic Therapy Timing	57	98%	98%	98%
Assessed for Rehabilitation	58	93%	98%	97%
Discharged on Antithrombotic Therapy	58	100%	99%	99%
Discharged on Statin Medication	47	89%	95%	94%
Thrombolytic Therapy Timing[7]	-	-	65%	66%
Venous Thromboembolism Prophylaxis	58	79%	95%	94%
Written Stroke Educational Materials Given	39	97%	92%	88%
Surgical Care Improvement Project				
Appropriate Beta Blocker Usage[2]	128	100%	98%	98%
Appropriate VTP Within 24 Hours[2]	365	100%	98%	98%
Controlled Postoperative Blood Glucose[2,7]	-	-	97%	97%
Perioperative Temperature Management[2]	398	100%	100%	100%
Prophylactic Antibiotic Selection[2]	240	99%	99%	99%
Prophylactic Antibiotic Selection (Outpatient)	63	95%	98%	98%
Prophylactic Antibiotic Stopped[2]	237	100%	98%	98%
Prophylactic Antibiotic Timing[2]	240	100%	99%	99%
Prophylactic Antibiotic Timing (Outpatient)	65	89%	97%	98%
Urinary Catheter Removal[2]	309	98%	97%	97%
Survey of Patients' Hospital Experiences				
Area Around Room 'Always' Quiet at Night	300+	60%	58%	61%
Doctors 'Always' Communicated Well	300+	82%	80%	82%
Home Recovery Information Given	300+	81%	87%	85%
Hospital Given 9 or 10 on 10 Point Scale	300+	80%	72%	71%
Meds 'Always' Explained Before Given	300+	64%	64%	64%
Nurses 'Always' Communicated Well	300+	83%	81%	79%
Pain 'Always' Well Controlled	300+	72%	71%	71%
Room and Bathroom 'Always' Clean	300+	68%	75%	73%
Timely Help 'Always' Received	300+	66%	70%	68%
Would Definitely Recommend Hospital	300+	83%	71%	71%
Use of Medical Imaging				
Cardiac Imaging Stress Test before Surgery	131	2.3%	5.4%	5.3%
Combination Abdominal CT Scan	769	7.2%	7.1%	10.5%
Combination Brain/Sinus CT Scan	702	5.3%	2.8%	2.7%
Combination Chest CT Scan	441	8.2%	1.7%	2.7%
Follow-up Mammogram/Ultrasound	76	7.9%	8.7%	8.8%
Lumbar Spine MRI for Low Back Pain	56	35.7%	34.7%	37.2%

Wood County Hospital

950 West Wooster Street
Bowling Green, OH 43402
E-mail: woodhosp@wcnet.org
URL: www.wch.net
Phone: 419-354-8900
Fax: 419-354-8957
Type: Acute Care Hospitals
Ownership: Voluntary non-profit - Private
Emergency Services: Yes
Beds: 162

Key Personnel:
Quality Assurance . . . . Steve Hunter
CEO/President. . . . . Stanley R Kordueki
Intensive Care Unit. . . . . Alan Mintz
Radiology. . . . . Sue Rayle
Pediatric In-Patient Care . . . . . . Lori Tuck
Infection Control. . . . . Louise White

Measure	Cases	This Hosp.	State Avg.	U.S. Avg.
Blood Clot Prevention and Treatment				
Anticoagulation Overlap Therapy[2]	30	97%	93%	93%
ICU Venous Thromboembolism Prophylaxis[2]	35	97%	93%	92%
Incidence of Potentially Preventable VTE[1,2]	-	-	6%	10%
UFH with Dosages/Platelet Monitoring[2]	21	100%	98%	97%
Venous Thromboembolism Prophylaxis[2]	218	95%	88%	85%
Warfarin Therapy Discharge Instructions[2]	28	100%	79%	75%
Chest Pain/Possible Heart Attack Care				
Aspirin Given Within 24 Hours of Arrival	61	100%	97%	96%
Fibrinolytic Meds Within 30 Min. of Arrival[1]	-	-	44%	58%
Average Time to ECG (minutes)	44	10	6	7
Average Time to Transfer (minutes)[1]	-	-	58	60
Children's Asthma Care				
Received Home Management Plan of Care	-	-	85%	88%
Received Reliever Medication	-	-	100%	100%
Received Systemic Corticosteroids	-	-	100%	100%
Emergency Department				
Admittance Decision Time (minutes)[2]	278	59	90	98
Head CT Results Within 45 Min. of Arrival[1]	-	-	63%	57%
Patients Who Left ER Before Being Seen	25,263	1%	2%	2%
Time from ER Arrival to Admit. (minutes)[2]	327	220	265	274
Time from ER Arrival to Discharge (minutes)	357	121	128	134
Time in ER Before Being Evaluated (minutes)	356	27	22	26
Time to Pain Meds for Fractures (minutes)	61	43	54	57
Heart Attack Care				
Aspirin Given at Discharge[1]	-	-	99%	99%
Fibrinolytic Meds Within 30 Min. of Arrival[7]	-	-	80%	54%
PCI Within 90 Minutes of Arrival[7]	-	-	97%	96%
Statin Prescribed at Discharge[1]	-	-	98%	98%
Heart Failure Care				
ACE Inhibitor or ARB for LVSD	31	100%	97%	97%
Discharge Instructions Given	70	100%	96%	94%
Evaluation of LVS Function	86	100%	100%	99%
Medicare Spending				
Medicare Spending per Patient (ratio)	-	1.00	1.01	0.98
Pneumonia Care				
Appropriate Initial Antibiotic Given	62	98%	96%	95%
Blood Culture Timing	94	91%	98%	98%
Pregnancy and Delivery Care				
Newborn Deliveries Scheduled Early	18	0%	5%	6%
Preventive Care				
Immunization for Influenza[2]	319	97%	93%	90%
Immunization for Pneumonia[2]	393	93%	94%	92%
Stroke Care				
Anticoagulation Therapy for Atrial Fibrillation[7]	-	-	95%	95%
Antithrombotic Therapy Timing	19	100%	98%	98%
Assessed for Rehabilitation	19	100%	98%	97%
Discharged on Antithrombotic Therapy	19	100%	99%	99%
Discharged on Statin Medication	12	92%	95%	94%
Thrombolytic Therapy Timing[7]	-	-	65%	66%
Venous Thromboembolism Prophylaxis	19	89%	95%	94%
Written Stroke Educational Materials Given	11	100%	92%	88%
Surgical Care Improvement Project				
Appropriate Beta Blocker Usage	110	97%	98%	98%
Appropriate VTP Within 24 Hours	280	97%	98%	98%
Controlled Postoperative Blood Glucose[7]	-	-	97%	97%
Perioperative Temperature Management	306	100%	100%	100%
Prophylactic Antibiotic Selection	210	99%	99%	99%
Prophylactic Antibiotic Selection (Outpatient)	67	97%	98%	98%
Prophylactic Antibiotic Stopped	209	99%	98%	98%
Prophylactic Antibiotic Timing	210	100%	99%	99%
Prophylactic Antibiotic Timing (Outpatient)	65	98%	97%	98%
Urinary Catheter Removal	223	97%	97%	97%
Survey of Patients' Hospital Experiences				
Area Around Room 'Always' Quiet at Night	300+	69%	58%	61%
Doctors 'Always' Communicated Well	300+	83%	80%	82%
Home Recovery Information Given	300+	91%	87%	85%
Hospital Given 9 or 10 on 10 Point Scale	300+	77%	72%	71%
Meds 'Always' Explained Before Given	300+	70%	64%	64%
Nurses 'Always' Communicated Well	300+	81%	81%	79%
Pain 'Always' Well Controlled	300+	73%	71%	71%
Room and Bathroom 'Always' Clean	300+	87%	75%	73%
Timely Help 'Always' Received	300+	76%	70%	68%
Would Definitely Recommend Hospital	300+	74%	71%	71%
Use of Medical Imaging				
Cardiac Imaging Stress Test before Surgery	159	4.4%	5.4%	5.3%
Combination Abdominal CT Scan	345	3.2%	7.1%	10.5%
Combination Brain/Sinus CT Scan	325	1.2%	2.8%	2.7%
Combination Chest CT Scan	148	2.0%	1.7%	2.7%
Follow-up Mammogram/Ultrasound	444	5.9%	8.7%	8.8%
Lumbar Spine MRI for Low Back Pain	66	19.7%	34.7%	37.2%

Community Hospitals & Wellness Centers

433 West High Street
Bryan, OH 43506
URL: www.chwchospital.com
Phone: 419-636-1131
Fax: 419-636-3100
Type: Acute Care Hospitals
Ownership: Voluntary non-profit - Other
Emergency Services: Yes
Beds: 131

Key Personnel:
Radiology. . . . . Darren Chao
Patient Relations . . . . Jan David, RN
CEO/President. . . . . Philip L Ennen
Coronary Care . . . . Marilyn Frank, RN
Operating Room. . . . . Kathy Lienberger, RN
Quality Assurance . . . . Sharon Mesnard, RN
Infection Control. . . . . Vickie Shaffer

Measure	Cases	This Hosp.	State Avg.	U.S. Avg.
Blood Clot Prevention and Treatment				
Anticoagulation Overlap Therapy[1]	-	-	93%	93%
ICU Venous Thromboembolism Prophylaxis	191	95%	93%	92%
Incidence of Potentially Preventable VTE[1]	-	-	6%	10%
UFH with Dosages/Platelet Monitoring[1]	-	-	98%	97%
Venous Thromboembolism Prophylaxis	634	89%	88%	85%
Warfarin Therapy Discharge Instructions[1]	-	-	79%	75%
Chest Pain/Possible Heart Attack Care				
Aspirin Given Within 24 Hours of Arrival[1,3]	-	-	97%	96%
Fibrinolytic Meds Within 30 Min. of Arrival[5]	-	-	44%	58%
Average Time to ECG (minutes)[1,3]	-	-	6	7
Average Time to Transfer (minutes)[5]	-	-	58	60
Children's Asthma Care				
Received Home Management Plan of Care	-	-	85%	88%
Received Reliever Medication	-	-	100%	100%
Received Systemic Corticosteroids	-	-	100%	100%
Emergency Department				
Admittance Decision Time (minutes)	776	50	90	98
Head CT Results Within 45 Min. of Arrival[1]	-	-	63%	57%
Patients Who Left ER Before Being Seen	12,018	0%	2%	2%
Time from ER Arrival to Admit. (minutes)	920	186	265	274
Time from ER Arrival to Discharge (minutes)	432	108	128	134
Time in ER Before Being Evaluated (minutes)	493	17	22	26
Time to Pain Meds for Fractures (minutes)	41	55	54	57
Heart Attack Care				
Aspirin Given at Discharge	100	100%	99%	99%
Fibrinolytic Meds Within 30 Min. of Arrival[7]	-	-	80%	54%
PCI Within 90 Minutes of Arrival	23	91%	97%	96%

NOTE: Hospital profiles are in alphabetical order by state, then city, then hospital within the city; Rankings exclude hospitals with less than 25 cases except for patient surveys which excludes hospitals with less than 100 cases; (a) 100-299 cases; (1) The number of cases/patients is too few to report; (2) Data submitted were based on a sample of cases/patients; (3) Results are based on a shorter time period than required; (4) Data suppressed by CMS for one or more quarters; (5) Results are not available for this reporting period; (6) Fewer than 100 patients completed the HCAHPS survey; (7) No cases met the criteria for this measure; (8) The lower limit of the confidence interval cannot be calculated if the number of observed infections equals zero; (9) No data are available from the state/territory for this reporting period; (10) The scores shown reflect fewer than 50 completed surveys; (11) There were discrepancies in the data collection process; (12) This measure does not apply to this hospital for this reporting period; (13) Results cannot be calculated for this reporting period; (14) The results for this state are combined with nearby states to protect confidentiality; Please refer to the User's Guide for a full explanation of data.

Measure	Cases	This Hosp.	State Avg.	U.S. Avg.
Statin Prescribed at Discharge	97	98%	98%	98%
Heart Failure Care				
ACE Inhibitor or ARB for LVSD	36	92%	97%	97%
Discharge Instructions Given	73	100%	96%	94%
Evaluation of LVS Function	91	100%	100%	99%
Medicare Spending				
Medicare Spending per Patient (ratio)	-	1.12	1.01	0.98
Pneumonia Care				
Appropriate Initial Antibiotic Given	54	93%	96%	95%
Blood Culture Timing	65	94%	98%	98%
Pregnancy and Delivery Care				
Newborn Deliveries Scheduled Early	30	13%	5%	6%
Preventive Care				
Immunization for Influenza	1,032	95%	93%	90%
Immunization for Pneumonia	1,358	97%	94%	92%
Stroke Care				
Anticoagulation Therapy for Atrial Fibrillation[1]	-	-	95%	95%
Antithrombotic Therapy Timing[1]	-	-	98%	98%
Assessed for Rehabilitation	11	100%	98%	97%
Discharged on Antithrombotic Therapy	11	100%	99%	99%
Discharged on Statin Medication[1]	-	-	95%	94%
Thrombolytic Therapy Timing[1]	-	-	65%	66%
Venous Thromboembolism Prophylaxis[1]	-	-	95%	94%
Written Stroke Educational Materials Given[1]	-	-	92%	88%
Surgical Care Improvement Project				
Appropriate Beta Blocker Usage	111	100%	98%	98%
Appropriate VTP Within 24 Hours	227	99%	98%	98%
Controlled Postoperative Blood Glucose[7]	-	-	97%	97%
Perioperative Temperature Management	261	100%	100%	100%
Prophylactic Antibiotic Selection	197	98%	99%	99%
Prophylactic Antibiotic Selection (Outpatient)	72	89%	98%	98%
Prophylactic Antibiotic Stopped	193	99%	98%	98%
Prophylactic Antibiotic Timing	197	99%	99%	99%
Prophylactic Antibiotic Timing (Outpatient)	74	96%	97%	98%
Urinary Catheter Removal	37	100%	97%	97%
Survey of Patients' Hospital Experiences				
Area Around Room 'Always' Quiet at Night	300+	63%	58%	61%
Doctors 'Always' Communicated Well	300+	84%	80%	82%
Home Recovery Information Given	300+	88%	87%	85%
Hospital Given 9 or 10 on 10 Point Scale	300+	80%	72%	71%
Meds 'Always' Explained Before Given	300+	67%	64%	64%
Nurses 'Always' Communicated Well	300+	84%	81%	79%
Pain 'Always' Well Controlled	300+	75%	71%	71%
Room and Bathroom 'Always' Clean	300+	82%	75%	73%
Timely Help 'Always' Received	300+	78%	70%	68%
Would Definitely Recommend Hospital	300+	76%	71%	71%
Use of Medical Imaging				
Cardiac Imaging Stress Test before Surgery[1]	-	-	5.4%	5.3%
Combination Abdominal CT Scan	284	5.3%	7.1%	10.5%
Combination Brain/Sinus CT Scan[1]	-	-	2.8%	2.7%
Combination Chest CT Scan	164	6.7%	1.7%	2.7%
Follow-up Mammogram/Ultrasound[7]	-	-	8.7%	8.8%
Lumbar Spine MRI for Low Back Pain	120	33.3%	34.7%	37.2%

Bucyrus Community Hospital

629 North Sandusky Avenue
Bucyrus, OH 44820
Phone: 419-562-4677
Fax: 419-562-6766
URL: www.bchonline.org
Type: Critical Access Hospitals
Emergency Services: Yes
Ownership: Voluntary non-profit - Other
Beds: 25

Key Personnel:
Chief of Medical Staff.......... Candy Christian
Operating Room............. Phyllis Crall
Quality Assurance............ Jeanne Perkins
Hemotology Center............ Joann Riedlinger
Emergency Room............ Larry Tincher
Infection Control............. Joyce Weaver
Cardiac Laboratory........... Tammi Wolfe, RN

Measure	Cases	This Hosp.	State Avg.	U.S. Avg.
Blood Clot Prevention and Treatment				
Anticoagulation Overlap Therapy[5]	-	-	93%	93%
ICU Venous Thromboembolism Prophylaxis[5]	-	-	93%	92%
Incidence of Potentially Preventable VTE[5]	-	-	6%	10%
UFH with Dosages/Platelet Monitoring[5]	-	-	98%	97%
Venous Thromboembolism Prophylaxis[5]	-	-	88%	85%
Warfarin Therapy Discharge Instructions[5]	-	-	79%	75%
Chest Pain/Possible Heart Attack Care				
Aspirin Given Within 24 Hours of Arrival	-	-	97%	96%
Fibrinolytic Meds Within 30 Min. of Arrival	-	-	44%	58%
Average Time to ECG (minutes)	-	-	6	7
Average Time to Transfer (minutes)	-	-	58	60
Children's Asthma Care				
Received Home Management Plan of Care	-	-	85%	88%
Received Reliever Medication	-	-	100%	100%
Received Systemic Corticosteroids	-	-	100%	100%
Emergency Department				
Admittance Decision Time (minutes)[5]	-	-	90	98
Head CT Results Within 45 Min. of Arrival	-	-	63%	57%
Patients Who Left ER Before Being Seen	-	-	2%	2%
Time from ER Arrival to Admit. (minutes)[5]	-	-	265	274
Time from ER Arrival to Discharge (minutes)	-	-	128	134
Time in ER Before Being Evaluated (minutes)	-	-	22	26
Time to Pain Meds for Fractures (minutes)	-	-	54	57
Heart Attack Care				
Aspirin Given at Discharge[1,3]	-	-	99%	99%
Fibrinolytic Meds Within 30 Min. of Arrival[3,7]	-	-	80%	54%
PCI Within 90 Minutes of Arrival[5]	-	-	97%	96%
Statin Prescribed at Discharge[3,7]	-	-	98%	98%
Heart Failure Care				
ACE Inhibitor or ARB for LVSD[7]	-	-	97%	97%
Discharge Instructions Given[1]	-	-	96%	94%
Evaluation of LVS Function	13	100%	100%	99%
Medicare Spending				
Medicare Spending per Patient (ratio)	-	-	1.01	0.98
Pneumonia Care				
Appropriate Initial Antibiotic Given	34	100%	96%	95%
Blood Culture Timing	56	100%	98%	98%
Pregnancy and Delivery Care				
Newborn Deliveries Scheduled Early[5]	-	-	5%	6%
Preventive Care				
Immunization for Influenza[5]	-	-	93%	90%
Immunization for Pneumonia[5]	-	-	94%	92%
Stroke Care				
Anticoagulation Therapy for Atrial Fibrillation[5]	-	-	95%	95%
Antithrombotic Therapy Timing[5]	-	-	98%	98%
Assessed for Rehabilitation[5]	-	-	98%	97%
Discharged on Antithrombotic Therapy[5]	-	-	99%	99%
Discharged on Statin Medication[5]	-	-	95%	94%
Thrombolytic Therapy Timing[5]	-	-	65%	66%
Venous Thromboembolism Prophylaxis[5]	-	-	95%	94%
Written Stroke Educational Materials Given[5]	-	-	92%	88%
Surgical Care Improvement Project				
Appropriate Beta Blocker Usage[3]	28	100%	98%	98%
Appropriate VTP Within 24 Hours	145	99%	98%	98%
Controlled Postoperative Blood Glucose[3,7]	-	-	97%	97%
Perioperative Temperature Management	151	99%	100%	100%
Prophylactic Antibiotic Selection	126	100%	99%	99%
Prophylactic Antibiotic Selection (Outpatient)	-	-	98%	98%
Prophylactic Antibiotic Stopped	126	99%	98%	98%
Prophylactic Antibiotic Timing	126	100%	99%	99%
Prophylactic Antibiotic Timing (Outpatient)	-	-	97%	98%
Urinary Catheter Removal	87	97%	97%	97%
Survey of Patients' Hospital Experiences				
Area Around Room 'Always' Quiet at Night	(a)	56%	58%	61%
Doctors 'Always' Communicated Well	(a)	84%	80%	82%
Home Recovery Information Given	(a)	87%	87%	85%
Hospital Given 9 or 10 on 10 Point Scale	(a)	74%	72%	71%
Meds 'Always' Explained Before Given	(a)	57%	64%	64%
Nurses 'Always' Communicated Well	(a)	77%	81%	79%
Pain 'Always' Well Controlled	(a)	74%	71%	71%
Room and Bathroom 'Always' Clean	(a)	79%	75%	73%
Timely Help 'Always' Received	(a)	70%	70%	68%
Would Definitely Recommend Hospital	(a)	61%	71%	71%
Use of Medical Imaging				
Cardiac Imaging Stress Test before Surgery	-	-	5.4%	5.3%
Combination Abdominal CT Scan	-	-	7.1%	10.5%
Combination Brain/Sinus CT Scan	-	-	2.8%	2.7%
Combination Chest CT Scan	-	-	1.7%	2.7%
Follow-up Mammogram/Ultrasound	-	-	8.7%	8.8%
Lumbar Spine MRI for Low Back Pain	-	-	34.7%	37.2%

Harrison Community Hospital

951 East Market Street
Cadiz, OH 43907
Phone: 740-942-4631
Fax: 740-942-2749
E-mail: hchosp@1st.net
URL: www.harrisoncommunity.com
Type: Critical Access Hospitals
Emergency Services: Yes
Ownership: Voluntary non-profit - Private
Beds: 48

Key Personnel:
Pediatrics................... Vaijanath Bhairappa, MD
CEO/President.............. Terry M Carson
Cardiology................... Joseph Gabis, MD
Anesthesiology.............. Shary Hillard
Emergency Room............ Ajit Modi, MD
Pulmonology................ Satyasagar Morisetty, MD
Operating Room.............. Anandhi Murthy
Chief of Medical Staff.......... Carole Patton

Measure	Cases	This Hosp.	State Avg.	U.S. Avg.
Blood Clot Prevention and Treatment				
Anticoagulation Overlap Therapy[5]	-	-	93%	93%
ICU Venous Thromboembolism Prophylaxis[5]	-	-	93%	92%
Incidence of Potentially Preventable VTE[5]	-	-	6%	10%
UFH with Dosages/Platelet Monitoring[5]	-	-	98%	97%
Venous Thromboembolism Prophylaxis[5]	-	-	88%	85%
Warfarin Therapy Discharge Instructions[5]	-	-	79%	75%
Chest Pain/Possible Heart Attack Care				
Aspirin Given Within 24 Hours of Arrival[3]	34	82%	97%	96%
Fibrinolytic Meds Within 30 Min. of Arrival[3,7]	-	-	44%	58%
Average Time to ECG (minutes)[3]	33	4	6	7
Average Time to Transfer (minutes)[1,3]	-	-	58	60
Children's Asthma Care				
Received Home Management Plan of Care	-	-	85%	88%
Received Reliever Medication	-	-	100%	100%
Received Systemic Corticosteroids	-	-	100%	100%
Emergency Department				
Admittance Decision Time (minutes)[5]	-	-	90	98
Head CT Results Within 45 Min. of Arrival[3,7]	-	-	63%	57%
Patients Who Left ER Before Being Seen[5]	-	-	2%	2%
Time from ER Arrival to Admit. (minutes)[5]	-	-	265	274
Time from ER Arrival to Discharge (minutes)[1,3]	-	-	128	134
Time in ER Before Being Evaluated (minutes)[3]	25	7	22	26
Time to Pain Meds for Fractures (minutes)[1,3]	-	-	54	57
Heart Attack Care				
Aspirin Given at Discharge[3,7]	-	-	99%	99%
Fibrinolytic Meds Within 30 Min. of Arrival[3,7]	-	-	80%	54%
PCI Within 90 Minutes of Arrival[5]	-	-	97%	96%
Statin Prescribed at Discharge[3,7]	-	-	98%	98%
Heart Failure Care				
ACE Inhibitor or ARB for LVSD[1]	-	-	97%	97%
Discharge Instructions Given	12	92%	96%	94%
Evaluation of LVS Function	13	54%	100%	99%
Medicare Spending				
Medicare Spending per Patient (ratio)	-	-	1.01	0.98
Pneumonia Care				
Appropriate Initial Antibiotic Given	19	68%	96%	95%
Blood Culture Timing	20	70%	98%	98%
Pregnancy and Delivery Care				
Newborn Deliveries Scheduled Early[5]	-	-	5%	6%
Preventive Care				
Immunization for Influenza[5]	-	-	93%	90%
Immunization for Pneumonia[5]	-	-	94%	92%
Stroke Care				
Anticoagulation Therapy for Atrial Fibrillation[3,7]	-	-	95%	95%
Antithrombotic Therapy Timing[1,3]	-	-	98%	98%
Assessed for Rehabilitation[1,3]	-	-	98%	97%
Discharged on Antithrombotic Therapy[1,3]	-	-	99%	99%
Discharged on Statin Medication[1,3]	-	-	95%	94%
Thrombolytic Therapy Timing[3,7]	-	-	65%	66%
Venous Thromboembolism Prophylaxis[1,3]	-	-	95%	94%
Written Stroke Educational Materials Given[3,7]	-	-	92%	88%

NOTE: Hospital profiles are in alphabetical order by state, then city, then hospital within the city; Rankings exclude hospitals with less than 25 cases except for patient surveys which excludes hospitals with less than 100 cases; (a) 100-299 cases; (1) The number of cases/patients is too few to report; (2) Data submitted were based on a sample of cases/patients; (3) Results are based on a shorter time period than required; (4) Data suppressed by CMS for one or more quarters; (5) Results are not available for this reporting period; (6) Fewer than 100 patients completed the HCAHPS survey; (7) No cases met the criteria for this measure; (8) The lower limit of the confidence interval cannot be calculated if the number of observed infections equals zero; (9) No data are available from the state/territory for this reporting period; (10) The scores shown reflect fewer than 50 completed surveys; (11) There were discrepancies in the data collection process; (12) This measure does not apply to this hospital for this reporting period; (13) Results cannot be calculated for this reporting period; (14) The results for this state are combined with nearby states to protect confidentiality; Please refer to the User's Guide for a full explanation of data.

Measure	Cases	This Hosp.	State Avg.	U.S. Avg.
Surgical Care Improvement Project				
Appropriate Beta Blocker Usage[1]	-	-	98%	98%
Appropriate VTP Within 24 Hours[1]	-	-	98%	98%
Controlled Postoperative Blood Glucose[7]	-	-	97%	97%
Perioperative Temperature Management[1]	-	-	100%	100%
Prophylactic Antibiotic Selection[1]	-	-	99%	99%
Prophylactic Antibiotic Selection (Outpatient)[5]	-	-	98%	98%
Prophylactic Antibiotic Stopped[1]	-	-	98%	98%
Prophylactic Antibiotic Timing[1]	-	-	99%	99%
Prophylactic Antibiotic Timing (Outpatient)[5]	-	-	97%	98%
Urinary Catheter Removal[1]	-	-	97%	97%
Survey of Patients' Hospital Experiences				
Area Around Room 'Always' Quiet at Night[5]	-	-	58%	61%
Doctors 'Always' Communicated Well[5]	-	-	80%	82%
Home Recovery Information Given[5]	-	-	87%	85%
Hospital Given 9 or 10 on 10 Point Scale[5]	-	-	72%	71%
Meds 'Always' Explained Before Given[5]	-	-	64%	64%
Nurses 'Always' Communicated Well[5]	-	-	81%	79%
Pain 'Always' Well Controlled[5]	-	-	71%	71%
Room and Bathroom 'Always' Clean[5]	-	-	75%	73%
Timely Help 'Always' Received[5]	-	-	70%	68%
Would Definitely Recommend Hospital[5]	-	-	71%	71%
Use of Medical Imaging				
Cardiac Imaging Stress Test before Surgery[1]	-	-	5.4%	5.3%
Combination Abdominal CT Scan	71	29.6%	7.1%	10.5%
Combination Brain/Sinus CT Scan[1]	-	-	2.8%	2.7%
Combination Chest CT Scan[1]	-	-	1.7%	2.7%
Follow-up Mammogram/Ultrasound	84	4.8%	8.7%	8.8%
Lumbar Spine MRI for Low Back Pain[1]	-	-	34.7%	37.2%

Southeastern Ohio Regional Medical Center

1341 North Clark Street
Cambridge, OH 43725
URL: www.seormc.org
Type: Acute Care Hospitals
Ownership: Voluntary non-profit - Private

Phone: 740-439-8111
Fax: 740-439-8175
Emergency Services: Yes
Beds: 209

Key Personnel:
Radiology. . . . . Shane Backus
President/CEO. . . . . Raymond M. Chorey, MD
Infection Control. . . . . Christine Daugherty, RN
Quality Assurance . . . . James Keller, MD
Cardiac Laboratory. . . . . Gilbert Kukielka, MD
Operating Room. . . . . Cathy McIntire, RN
Chief of Medical Staff. . . . . Brady Stonen, MD

Measure	Cases	This Hosp.	State Avg.	U.S. Avg.
Blood Clot Prevention and Treatment				
Anticoagulation Overlap Therapy[2]	31	52%	93%	93%
ICU Venous Thromboembolism Prophylaxis[2]	60	80%	93%	92%
Incidence of Potentially Preventable VTE[1,2]	-	-	6%	10%
UFH with Dosages/Platelet Monitoring[2]	23	100%	98%	97%
Venous Thromboembolism Prophylaxis[2]	261	74%	88%	85%
Warfarin Therapy Discharge Instructions[2]	27	74%	79%	75%
Chest Pain/Possible Heart Attack Care				
Aspirin Given Within 24 Hours of Arrival	122	98%	97%	96%
Fibrinolytic Meds Within 30 Min. of Arrival[7]	-	-	44%	58%
Average Time to ECG (minutes)	125	10	6	7
Average Time to Transfer (minutes)[1]	-	-	58	60
Children's Asthma Care				
Received Home Management Plan of Care	-	-	85%	88%
Received Reliever Medication	-	-	100%	100%
Received Systemic Corticosteroids	-	-	100%	100%
Emergency Department				
Admittance Decision Time (minutes)[2]	558	60	90	98
Head CT Results Within 45 Min. of Arrival[1]	-	-	63%	57%
Patients Who Left ER Before Being Seen	30,079	1%	2%	2%
Time from ER Arrival to Admit. (minutes)[2]	573	221	265	274
Time from ER Arrival to Discharge (minutes)	440	125	128	134
Time in ER Before Being Evaluated (minutes)	426	31	22	26
Time to Pain Meds for Fractures (minutes)	101	56	54	57
Heart Attack Care				
Aspirin Given at Discharge[1]	-	-	99%	99%
Fibrinolytic Meds Within 30 Min. of Arrival[7]	-	-	80%	54%
PCI Within 90 Minutes of Arrival[7]	-	-	97%	96%
Statin Prescribed at Discharge[1]	-	-	98%	98%
Heart Failure Care				
ACE Inhibitor or ARB for LVSD	37	95%	97%	97%
Discharge Instructions Given	100	78%	96%	94%
Evaluation of LVS Function	119	100%	100%	99%
Medicare Spending				
Medicare Spending per Patient (ratio)	-	0.99	1.01	0.98
Pneumonia Care				
Appropriate Initial Antibiotic Given[2]	86	99%	96%	95%
Blood Culture Timing[2]	138	93%	98%	98%
Pregnancy and Delivery Care				
Newborn Deliveries Scheduled Early[2]	56	9%	5%	6%
Preventive Care				
Immunization for Influenza[2]	428	93%	93%	90%
Immunization for Pneumonia[2]	543	96%	94%	92%
Stroke Care				
Anticoagulation Therapy for Atrial Fibrillation[1]	-	-	95%	95%
Antithrombotic Therapy Timing	28	96%	98%	98%
Assessed for Rehabilitation	24	83%	98%	97%
Discharged on Antithrombotic Therapy	24	100%	99%	99%
Discharged on Statin Medication	20	65%	95%	94%
Thrombolytic Therapy Timing[1]	-	-	65%	66%
Venous Thromboembolism Prophylaxis	24	54%	95%	94%
Written Stroke Educational Materials Given	13	62%	92%	88%
Surgical Care Improvement Project				
Appropriate Beta Blocker Usage	85	99%	98%	98%
Appropriate VTP Within 24 Hours	221	99%	98%	98%
Controlled Postoperative Blood Glucose[7]	-	-	97%	97%
Perioperative Temperature Management	248	100%	100%	100%
Prophylactic Antibiotic Selection	170	95%	99%	99%
Prophylactic Antibiotic Selection (Outpatient)	84	98%	98%	98%
Prophylactic Antibiotic Stopped	161	98%	98%	98%
Prophylactic Antibiotic Timing	170	95%	99%	99%
Prophylactic Antibiotic Timing (Outpatient)	84	100%	97%	98%
Urinary Catheter Removal	102	89%	97%	97%
Survey of Patients' Hospital Experiences				
Area Around Room 'Always' Quiet at Night	300+	65%	58%	61%
Doctors 'Always' Communicated Well	300+	80%	80%	82%
Home Recovery Information Given	300+	89%	87%	85%
Hospital Given 9 or 10 on 10 Point Scale	300+	68%	72%	71%
Meds 'Always' Explained Before Given	300+	66%	64%	64%
Nurses 'Always' Communicated Well	300+	82%	81%	79%
Pain 'Always' Well Controlled	300+	73%	71%	71%
Room and Bathroom 'Always' Clean	300+	85%	75%	73%
Timely Help 'Always' Received	300+	70%	70%	68%
Would Definitely Recommend Hospital	300+	66%	71%	71%
Use of Medical Imaging				
Cardiac Imaging Stress Test before Surgery	250	4.0%	5.4%	5.3%
Combination Abdominal CT Scan	570	5.3%	7.1%	10.5%
Combination Brain/Sinus CT Scan	541	2.2%	2.8%	2.7%
Combination Chest CT Scan	427	3.0%	1.7%	2.7%
Follow-up Mammogram/Ultrasound	850	10.8%	8.7%	8.8%
Lumbar Spine MRI for Low Back Pain[1]	-	-	34.7%	37.2%

Diley Ridge Medical Center

7911 Diley Road
Canal Winchester, OH 43110
URL: www.dileyridgemedicalcenter.com
Type: Acute Care Hospitals
Ownership: Voluntary non-profit - Private

Phone: 614-838-7910
Emergency Services: Yes

Measure	Cases	This Hosp.	State Avg.	U.S. Avg.
Blood Clot Prevention and Treatment				
Anticoagulation Overlap Therapy[1]	-	-	93%	93%
ICU Venous Thromboembolism Prophylaxis[7]	-	-	93%	92%
Incidence of Potentially Preventable VTE[7]	-	-	6%	10%
UFH with Dosages/Platelet Monitoring[1]	-	-	98%	97%
Venous Thromboembolism Prophylaxis[1]	-	-	88%	85%
Warfarin Therapy Discharge Instructions[1]	-	-	79%	75%
Chest Pain/Possible Heart Attack Care				
Aspirin Given Within 24 Hours of Arrival	80	98%	97%	96%
Fibrinolytic Meds Within 30 Min. of Arrival[7]	-	-	44%	58%
Average Time to ECG (minutes)	82	8	6	7
Average Time to Transfer (minutes)	11	39	58	60
Children's Asthma Care				
Received Home Management Plan of Care	-	-	85%	88%
Received Reliever Medication	-	-	100%	100%
Received Systemic Corticosteroids	-	-	100%	100%
Emergency Department				
Admittance Decision Time (minutes)[1,2]	-	-	90	98
Head CT Results Within 45 Min. of Arrival[1]	-	-	63%	57%
Patients Who Left ER Before Being Seen	16,657	0%	2%	2%
Time from ER Arrival to Admit. (minutes)[1,2]	-	-	265	274
Time from ER Arrival to Discharge (minutes)	365	119	128	134
Time in ER Before Being Evaluated (minutes)	386	29	22	26
Time to Pain Meds for Fractures (minutes)	74	58	54	57
Heart Attack Care				
Aspirin Given at Discharge[5]	-	-	99%	99%
Fibrinolytic Meds Within 30 Min. of Arrival[5]	-	-	80%	54%
PCI Within 90 Minutes of Arrival[5]	-	-	97%	96%
Statin Prescribed at Discharge[5]	-	-	98%	98%
Heart Failure Care				
ACE Inhibitor or ARB for LVSD[5]	-	-	97%	97%
Discharge Instructions Given[5]	-	-	96%	94%
Evaluation of LVS Function[5]	-	-	100%	99%
Medicare Spending				
Medicare Spending per Patient (ratio)[1]	-	-	1.01	0.98
Pneumonia Care				
Appropriate Initial Antibiotic Given[5]	-	-	96%	95%
Blood Culture Timing[5]	-	-	98%	98%
Pregnancy and Delivery Care				
Newborn Deliveries Scheduled Early[7]	-	-	5%	6%
Preventive Care				
Immunization for Influenza[1,2]	-	-	93%	90%
Immunization for Pneumonia[1,2]	-	-	94%	92%
Stroke Care				
Anticoagulation Therapy for Atrial Fibrillation[5]	-	-	95%	95%
Antithrombotic Therapy Timing[5]	-	-	98%	98%
Assessed for Rehabilitation[5]	-	-	98%	97%
Discharged on Antithrombotic Therapy[5]	-	-	99%	99%
Discharged on Statin Medication[5]	-	-	95%	94%
Thrombolytic Therapy Timing[5]	-	-	65%	66%
Venous Thromboembolism Prophylaxis[5]	-	-	95%	94%
Written Stroke Educational Materials Given[5]	-	-	92%	88%
Surgical Care Improvement Project				
Appropriate Beta Blocker Usage[5]	-	-	98%	98%
Appropriate VTP Within 24 Hours[5]	-	-	98%	98%
Controlled Postoperative Blood Glucose[5]	-	-	97%	97%
Perioperative Temperature Management[5]	-	-	100%	100%
Prophylactic Antibiotic Selection[5]	-	-	99%	99%
Prophylactic Antibiotic Selection (Outpatient)[5]	-	-	98%	98%
Prophylactic Antibiotic Stopped[5]	-	-	98%	98%
Prophylactic Antibiotic Timing[5]	-	-	99%	99%
Prophylactic Antibiotic Timing (Outpatient)[5]	-	-	97%	98%
Urinary Catheter Removal[5]	-	-	97%	97%
Survey of Patients' Hospital Experiences				
Area Around Room 'Always' Quiet at Night[1]	-	-	58%	61%
Doctors 'Always' Communicated Well[1]	-	-	80%	82%
Home Recovery Information Given[1]	-	-	87%	85%
Hospital Given 9 or 10 on 10 Point Scale[1]	-	-	72%	71%
Meds 'Always' Explained Before Given[1]	-	-	64%	64%
Nurses 'Always' Communicated Well[1]	-	-	81%	79%
Pain 'Always' Well Controlled[1]	-	-	71%	71%
Room and Bathroom 'Always' Clean[1]	-	-	75%	73%
Timely Help 'Always' Received[1]	-	-	70%	68%
Would Definitely Recommend Hospital[1]	-	-	71%	71%
Use of Medical Imaging				
Cardiac Imaging Stress Test before Surgery[7]	-	-	5.4%	5.3%
Combination Abdominal CT Scan	235	1.3%	7.1%	10.5%
Combination Brain/Sinus CT Scan[1]	-	-	2.8%	2.7%
Combination Chest CT Scan[1]	-	-	1.7%	2.7%
Follow-up Mammogram/Ultrasound	226	9.3%	8.7%	8.8%
Lumbar Spine MRI for Low Back Pain[1]	-	-	34.7%	37.2%

NOTE: Hospital profiles are in alphabetical order by state, then city, then hospital within the city; Rankings exclude hospitals with less than 25 cases except for patient surveys which excludes hospitals with less than 100 cases; (a) 100-299 cases; (1) The number of cases/patients is too few to report; (2) Data submitted were based on a sample of cases/patients; (3) Results are based on a shorter time period than required; (4) Data suppressed by CMS for one or more quarters; (5) Results are not available for this reporting period; (6) Fewer than 100 patients completed the HCAHPS survey; (7) No cases met the criteria for this measure; (8) The lower limit of the confidence interval cannot be calculated if the number of observed infections equals zero; (9) No data are available from the state/territory for this reporting period; (10) The scores shown reflect fewer than 50 completed surveys; (11) There were discrepancies in the data collection process; (12) This measure does not apply to this hospital for this reporting period; (13) Results cannot be calculated for this reporting period; (14) The results for this state are combined with nearby states to protect confidentiality; Please refer to the User's Guide for a full explanation of data.

Aultman Hospital

2600 Sixth Street Sw
Canton, OH 44710
Phone: 330-452-9911
Fax: 330-438-9811
URL: www.aultman.com
Type: Acute Care Hospitals
Emergency Services: Yes
Ownership: Voluntary non-profit - Other
Beds: 808

Key Personnel:
Operating Room. . . . . Elizabeth Edmunds, RN
Emergency Room . . . . Liz Edmunds, MD
Radiology. . . . . Liz Getz
Anesthesiology. . . . . Milton P Midis, MD
Infection Control . . . . Joan Pugnale
CEO/President. . . . . Edward Roth
Patient Relations . . . . Jennie Shisler
Chief of Medical Staff. . . . . Dr. Timothy O' Toole, MD

Measure	Cases	This Hosp.	State Avg.	U.S. Avg.
Blood Clot Prevention and Treatment				
Anticoagulation Overlap Therapy[2]	205	89%	93%	93%
ICU Venous Thromboembolism Prophylaxis[2]	106	99%	93%	92%
Incidence of Potentially Preventable VTE[2]	51	0%	6%	10%
UFH with Dosages/Platelet Monitoring[2]	234	79%	98%	97%
Venous Thromboembolism Prophylaxis[2]	343	94%	88%	85%
Warfarin Therapy Discharge Instructions[2]	145	80%	79%	75%
Chest Pain/Possible Heart Attack Care				
Aspirin Given Within 24 Hours of Arrival[1,3]	-	-	97%	96%
Fibrinolytic Meds Within 30 Min. of Arrival[3,7]	-	-	44%	58%
Average Time to ECG (minutes)[1,3]	-	-	6	7
Average Time to Transfer (minutes)[3,7]	-	-	58	60
Children's Asthma Care				
Received Home Management Plan of Care	25	92%	85%	88%
Received Reliever Medication	26	100%	100%	100%
Received Systemic Corticosteroids	26	96%	100%	100%
Emergency Department				
Admittance Decision Time (minutes)[2]	571	78	90	98
Head CT Results Within 45 Min. of Arrival	23	87%	63%	57%
Patients Who Left ER Before Being Seen	85,812	2%	2%	2%
Time from ER Arrival to Admit. (minutes)[2]	571	275	265	274
Time from ER Arrival to Discharge (minutes)	388	145	128	134
Time in ER Before Being Evaluated (minutes)	418	30	22	26
Time to Pain Meds for Fractures (minutes)	229	46	54	57
Heart Attack Care				
Aspirin Given at Discharge	659	100%	99%	99%
Fibrinolytic Meds Within 30 Min. of Arrival[7]	-	-	80%	54%
PCI Within 90 Minutes of Arrival	108	99%	97%	96%
Statin Prescribed at Discharge	628	100%	98%	98%
Heart Failure Care				
ACE Inhibitor or ARB for LVSD	203	100%	97%	97%
Discharge Instructions Given	508	97%	96%	94%
Evaluation of LVS Function	679	100%	100%	99%
Medicare Spending				
Medicare Spending per Patient (ratio)	-	1.02	1.01	0.98
Pneumonia Care				
Appropriate Initial Antibiotic Given	410	99%	96%	95%
Blood Culture Timing	807	98%	98%	98%
Pregnancy and Delivery Care				
Newborn Deliveries Scheduled Early	125	2%	5%	6%
Preventive Care				
Immunization for Influenza[2]	553	96%	93%	90%
Immunization for Pneumonia[2]	748	96%	94%	92%
Stroke Care				
Anticoagulation Therapy for Atrial Fibrillation[2]	11	100%	95%	95%
Antithrombotic Therapy Timing[2]	87	99%	98%	98%
Assessed for Rehabilitation[2]	114	98%	98%	97%
Discharged on Antithrombotic Therapy[2]	92	100%	99%	99%
Discharged on Statin Medication[2]	78	96%	95%	94%
Thrombolytic Therapy Timing[2,7]	-	-	65%	66%
Venous Thromboembolism Prophylaxis[2]	115	97%	95%	94%
Written Stroke Educational Materials Given[2]	46	89%	92%	88%
Surgical Care Improvement Project				
Appropriate Beta Blocker Usage[2]	344	99%	98%	98%
Appropriate VTP Within 24 Hours[2]	541	100%	98%	98%
Controlled Postoperative Blood Glucose[2]	228	99%	97%	97%
Perioperative Temperature Management[2]	729	100%	100%	100%
Prophylactic Antibiotic Selection[2]	682	100%	99%	99%
Prophylactic Antibiotic Selection (Outpatient)	772	100%	98%	98%
Prophylactic Antibiotic Stopped[2]	666	100%	98%	98%
Prophylactic Antibiotic Timing[2]	683	99%	99%	99%
Prophylactic Antibiotic Timing (Outpatient)	537	98%	97%	98%
Urinary Catheter Removal[2]	566	100%	97%	97%
Survey of Patients' Hospital Experiences				
Area Around Room 'Always' Quiet at Night	300+	51%	58%	61%
Doctors 'Always' Communicated Well	300+	79%	80%	82%
Home Recovery Information Given	300+	84%	87%	85%
Hospital Given 9 or 10 on 10 Point Scale	300+	77%	72%	71%
Meds 'Always' Explained Before Given	300+	59%	64%	64%
Nurses 'Always' Communicated Well	300+	78%	81%	79%
Pain 'Always' Well Controlled	300+	71%	71%	71%
Room and Bathroom 'Always' Clean	300+	73%	75%	73%
Timely Help 'Always' Received	300+	69%	70%	68%
Would Definitely Recommend Hospital	300+	80%	71%	71%
Use of Medical Imaging				
Cardiac Imaging Stress Test before Surgery	817	5.5%	5.4%	5.3%
Combination Abdominal CT Scan	1,502	6.2%	7.1%	10.5%
Combination Brain/Sinus CT Scan	1,365	2.1%	2.8%	2.7%
Combination Chest CT Scan	1,092	1.7%	1.7%	2.7%
Follow-up Mammogram/Ultrasound	1,639	5.4%	8.7%	8.8%
Lumbar Spine MRI for Low Back Pain	205	37.1%	34.7%	37.2%

Mercy Medical Center

1320 Mercy Drive Nw
Canton, OH 44708
Phone: 330-489-1001
Fax: 330-489-1127
URL: www.thequalityhospital.com
Type: Acute Care Hospitals
Emergency Services: Yes
Ownership: Voluntary non-profit - Church
Beds: 476

Key Personnel:
Pediatric In-Patient Care . . . . Mark Blaser, DO
CEO/President. . . . . Thomas E Cecconi, FACHE
Chief of Medical Staff. . . . . David L Gormsen, DO, F.A.C.E.P.
Operating Room. . . . . Laurie Hartline, RN
Coronary Care . . . . Allyson Kelly
Quality Assurance . . . . Tracey Majors, RN
Radiology. . . . . William Murphy, MD
Infection Control. . . . . Pat Nelson

Measure	Cases	This Hosp.	State Avg.	U.S. Avg.
Blood Clot Prevention and Treatment				
Anticoagulation Overlap Therapy[2]	162	98%	93%	93%
ICU Venous Thromboembolism Prophylaxis[2]	123	90%	93%	92%
Incidence of Potentially Preventable VTE[1,2]	-	-	6%	10%
UFH with Dosages/Platelet Monitoring[2]	166	100%	98%	97%
Venous Thromboembolism Prophylaxis[2]	309	86%	88%	85%
Warfarin Therapy Discharge Instructions[2]	122	99%	79%	75%
Chest Pain/Possible Heart Attack Care				
Aspirin Given Within 24 Hours of Arrival[5]	-	-	97%	96%
Fibrinolytic Meds Within 30 Min. of Arrival[5]	-	-	44%	58%
Average Time to ECG (minutes)[5]	-	-	6	7
Average Time to Transfer (minutes)[5]	-	-	58	60
Children's Asthma Care				
Received Home Management Plan of Care	-	-	85%	88%
Received Reliever Medication	-	-	100%	100%
Received Systemic Corticosteroids	-	-	100%	100%
Emergency Department				
Admittance Decision Time (minutes)[2]	866	83	90	98
Head CT Results Within 45 Min. of Arrival	12	75%	63%	57%
Patients Who Left ER Before Being Seen	53,464	3%	2%	2%
Time from ER Arrival to Admit. (minutes)[2]	872	302	265	274
Time from ER Arrival to Discharge (minutes)	532	193	128	134
Time in ER Before Being Evaluated (minutes)	569	42	22	26
Time to Pain Meds for Fractures (minutes)	154	60	54	57
Heart Attack Care				
Aspirin Given at Discharge	387	100%	99%	99%
Fibrinolytic Meds Within 30 Min. of Arrival[7]	-	-	80%	54%
PCI Within 90 Minutes of Arrival	75	92%	97%	96%
Statin Prescribed at Discharge	360	98%	98%	98%
Heart Failure Care				
ACE Inhibitor or ARB for LVSD	135	100%	97%	97%
Discharge Instructions Given	344	93%	96%	94%
Evaluation of LVS Function	452	100%	100%	99%
Medicare Spending				
Medicare Spending per Patient (ratio)	-	1.08	1.01	0.98
Pneumonia Care				
Appropriate Initial Antibiotic Given	256	95%	96%	95%
Blood Culture Timing	428	99%	98%	98%
Pregnancy and Delivery Care				
Newborn Deliveries Scheduled Early	155	6%	5%	6%
Preventive Care				
Immunization for Influenza[2]	761	94%	93%	90%
Immunization for Pneumonia[2]	1,009	96%	94%	92%
Stroke Care				
Anticoagulation Therapy for Atrial Fibrillation	28	100%	95%	95%
Antithrombotic Therapy Timing	156	100%	98%	98%
Assessed for Rehabilitation	170	98%	98%	97%
Discharged on Antithrombotic Therapy	157	100%	99%	99%
Discharged on Statin Medication	122	95%	95%	94%
Thrombolytic Therapy Timing[1]	-	-	65%	66%
Venous Thromboembolism Prophylaxis	171	99%	95%	94%
Written Stroke Educational Materials Given	76	99%	92%	88%
Surgical Care Improvement Project				
Appropriate Beta Blocker Usage[2]	257	97%	98%	98%
Appropriate VTP Within 24 Hours[2]	479	96%	98%	98%
Controlled Postoperative Blood Glucose[2]	131	95%	97%	97%
Perioperative Temperature Management[2]	582	100%	100%	100%
Prophylactic Antibiotic Selection[2]	527	100%	99%	99%
Prophylactic Antibiotic Selection (Outpatient)	716	99%	98%	98%
Prophylactic Antibiotic Stopped[2]	523	98%	98%	98%
Prophylactic Antibiotic Timing[2]	527	98%	99%	99%
Prophylactic Antibiotic Timing (Outpatient)	720	98%	97%	98%
Urinary Catheter Removal[2]	442	98%	97%	97%
Survey of Patients' Hospital Experiences				
Area Around Room 'Always' Quiet at Night	300+	45%	58%	61%
Doctors 'Always' Communicated Well	300+	76%	80%	82%
Home Recovery Information Given	300+	85%	87%	85%
Hospital Given 9 or 10 on 10 Point Scale	300+	69%	72%	71%
Meds 'Always' Explained Before Given	300+	58%	64%	64%
Nurses 'Always' Communicated Well	300+	76%	81%	79%
Pain 'Always' Well Controlled	300+	70%	71%	71%
Room and Bathroom 'Always' Clean	300+	66%	75%	73%
Timely Help 'Always' Received	300+	60%	70%	68%
Would Definitely Recommend Hospital	300+	74%	71%	71%
Use of Medical Imaging				
Cardiac Imaging Stress Test before Surgery	457	3.5%	5.4%	5.3%
Combination Abdominal CT Scan	1,139	5.6%	7.1%	10.5%
Combination Brain/Sinus CT Scan	936	3.6%	2.8%	2.7%
Combination Chest CT Scan	707	0.0%	1.7%	2.7%
Follow-up Mammogram/Ultrasound	1,795	9.7%	8.7%	8.8%
Lumbar Spine MRI for Low Back Pain	172	39.0%	34.7%	37.2%

UH Geauga Medical Center

13207 Ravenna Rd
Chardon, OH 44024
Phone: 440-269-6000
URL: www.uhgeauga.org
Type: Acute Care Hospitals
Emergency Services: Yes
Ownership: Voluntary non-profit - Private

Key Personnel:
CEO/President. . . . . Richard J Frenchie
Chief of Medical Staff. . . . . Donald Goddard

Measure	Cases	This Hosp.	State Avg.	U.S. Avg.
Blood Clot Prevention and Treatment				
Anticoagulation Overlap Therapy[2]	64	100%	93%	93%
ICU Venous Thromboembolism Prophylaxis[2]	103	92%	93%	92%
Incidence of Potentially Preventable VTE[1,2]	-	-	6%	10%
UFH with Dosages/Platelet Monitoring[2]	68	100%	98%	97%
Venous Thromboembolism Prophylaxis[2]	339	96%	88%	85%
Warfarin Therapy Discharge Instructions[2]	45	100%	79%	75%
Chest Pain/Possible Heart Attack Care				
Aspirin Given Within 24 Hours of Arrival[1,3]	-	-	97%	96%
Fibrinolytic Meds Within 30 Min. of Arrival[3,7]	-	-	44%	58%
Average Time to ECG (minutes)[1,3]	-	-	6	7
Average Time to Transfer (minutes)[3,7]	-	-	58	60
Children's Asthma Care				
Received Home Management Plan of Care	-	-	85%	88%
Received Reliever Medication	-	-	100%	100%

NOTE: Hospital profiles are in alphabetical order by state, then city, then hospital within the city; Rankings exclude hospitals with less than 25 cases except for patient surveys which excludes hospitals with less than 100 cases; (a) 100-299 cases; (1) The number of cases/patients is too few to report; (2) Data submitted were based on a sample of cases/patients; (3) Results are based on a shorter time period than required; (4) Data suppressed by CMS for one or more quarters; (5) Results are not available for this reporting period; (6) Fewer than 100 patients completed the HCAHPS survey; (7) No cases met the criteria for this measure; (8) The lower limit of the confidence interval cannot be calculated if the number of observed infections equals zero; (9) No data are available from the state/territory for this reporting period; (10) The scores shown reflect fewer than 50 completed surveys; (11) There were discrepancies in the data collection process; (12) This measure does not apply to this hospital for this reporting period; (13) Results cannot be calculated for this reporting period; (14) The results for this state are combined with nearby states to protect confidentiality; Please refer to the User's Guide for a full explanation of data.

Measure	Cases	This Hosp.	State Avg.	U.S. Avg.
Received Systemic Corticosteroids	-	-	100%	100%
Emergency Department				
Admittance Decision Time (minutes)[2]	569	95	90	98
Head CT Results Within 45 Min. of Arrival	25	64%	63%	57%
Patients Who Left ER Before Being Seen	19,059	0%	2%	2%
Time from ER Arrival to Admit. (minutes)[2]	577	260	265	274
Time from ER Arrival to Discharge (minutes)	393	137	128	134
Time in ER Before Being Evaluated (minutes)	405	14	22	26
Time to Pain Meds for Fractures (minutes)	106	52	54	57
Heart Attack Care				
Aspirin Given at Discharge	108	100%	99%	99%
Fibrinolytic Meds Within 30 Min. of Arrival[7]	-	-	80%	54%
PCI Within 90 Minutes of Arrival	22	91%	97%	96%
Statin Prescribed at Discharge	111	99%	98%	98%
Heart Failure Care				
ACE Inhibitor or ARB for LVSD	41	100%	97%	97%
Discharge Instructions Given	161	100%	96%	94%
Evaluation of LVS Function	216	100%	100%	99%
Medicare Spending				
Medicare Spending per Patient (ratio)	-	1.00	1.01	0.98
Pneumonia Care				
Appropriate Initial Antibiotic Given	95	100%	96%	95%
Blood Culture Timing	188	100%	98%	98%
Pregnancy and Delivery Care				
Newborn Deliveries Scheduled Early	124	2%	5%	6%
Preventive Care				
Immunization for Influenza[2]	550	97%	93%	90%
Immunization for Pneumonia[2]	683	96%	94%	92%
Stroke Care				
Anticoagulation Therapy for Atrial Fibrillation[1]	-	-	95%	95%
Antithrombotic Therapy Timing	47	98%	98%	98%
Assessed for Rehabilitation	48	92%	98%	97%
Discharged on Antithrombotic Therapy	48	100%	99%	99%
Discharged on Statin Medication	35	94%	95%	94%
Thrombolytic Therapy Timing	13	8%	65%	66%
Venous Thromboembolism Prophylaxis	45	98%	95%	94%
Written Stroke Educational Materials Given	32	97%	92%	88%
Surgical Care Improvement Project				
Appropriate Beta Blocker Usage[2]	170	100%	98%	98%
Appropriate VTP Within 24 Hours[2]	423	100%	98%	98%
Controlled Postoperative Blood Glucose[2,7]	-	-	97%	97%
Perioperative Temperature Management[2]	493	100%	100%	100%
Prophylactic Antibiotic Selection[2]	361	100%	99%	99%
Prophylactic Antibiotic Selection (Outpatient)	187	99%	98%	98%
Prophylactic Antibiotic Stopped[2]	348	100%	98%	98%
Prophylactic Antibiotic Timing[2]	361	99%	99%	99%
Prophylactic Antibiotic Timing (Outpatient)	187	100%	97%	98%
Urinary Catheter Removal[2]	353	100%	97%	97%
Survey of Patients' Hospital Experiences				
Area Around Room 'Always' Quiet at Night	300+	52%	58%	61%
Doctors 'Always' Communicated Well	300+	81%	80%	82%
Home Recovery Information Given	300+	89%	87%	85%
Hospital Given 9 or 10 on 10 Point Scale	300+	72%	72%	71%
Meds 'Always' Explained Before Given	300+	63%	64%	64%
Nurses 'Always' Communicated Well	300+	81%	81%	79%
Pain 'Always' Well Controlled	300+	71%	71%	71%
Room and Bathroom 'Always' Clean	300+	70%	75%	73%
Timely Help 'Always' Received	300+	67%	70%	68%
Would Definitely Recommend Hospital	300+	74%	71%	71%
Use of Medical Imaging				
Cardiac Imaging Stress Test before Surgery	135	5.2%	5.4%	5.3%
Combination Abdominal CT Scan	565	4.8%	7.1%	10.5%
Combination Brain/Sinus CT Scan[1]	-	-	2.8%	2.7%
Combination Chest CT Scan	448	2.9%	1.7%	2.7%
Follow-up Mammogram/Ultrasound	700	15.0%	8.7%	8.8%
Lumbar Spine MRI for Low Back Pain	88	42.0%	34.7%	37.2%

Adena Regional Medical Center

272 Hospital Road
Chillicothe, OH 45601
URL: www.adena.org
Type: Acute Care Hospitals
Ownership: Voluntary non-profit - Private
Phone: 740-779-7500
Fax: 740-779-7934
Emergency Services: Yes
Beds: 238

Key Personnel:
Operating Room. . . . . Damien Benjamin
Radiology. . . . . Bryan I Borland
Quality Assurance . . . . Patti Lamphear
Infection Control. . . . . Julie McCray
Chief of Medical Staff. . . . . Alan Shaw, MD
CEO/President. . . . . Mark Shuter FACHE
Cardiac Laboratory. . . . . Marla Weber

Measure	Cases	This Hosp.	State Avg.	U.S. Avg.
Blood Clot Prevention and Treatment				
Anticoagulation Overlap Therapy[2]	69	100%	93%	93%
ICU Venous Thromboembolism Prophylaxis[2]	31	94%	93%	92%
Incidence of Potentially Preventable VTE[2]	17	6%	6%	10%
UFH with Dosages/Platelet Monitoring[2]	48	100%	98%	97%
Venous Thromboembolism Prophylaxis[2]	361	91%	88%	85%
Warfarin Therapy Discharge Instructions[2]	63	100%	79%	75%
Chest Pain/Possible Heart Attack Care				
Aspirin Given Within 24 Hours of Arrival	56	93%	97%	96%
Fibrinolytic Meds Within 30 Min. of Arrival[1]	-	-	44%	58%
Average Time to ECG (minutes)	55	1	6	7
Average Time to Transfer (minutes)	25	57	58	60
Children's Asthma Care				
Received Home Management Plan of Care	-	-	85%	88%
Received Reliever Medication	-	-	100%	100%
Received Systemic Corticosteroids	-	-	100%	100%
Emergency Department				
Admittance Decision Time (minutes)[2]	441	89	90	98
Head CT Results Within 45 Min. of Arrival	33	85%	63%	57%
Patients Who Left ER Before Being Seen	49,699	2%	2%	2%
Time from ER Arrival to Admit. (minutes)[2]	516	234	265	274
Time from ER Arrival to Discharge (minutes)	384	130	128	134
Time in ER Before Being Evaluated (minutes)	368	21	22	26
Time to Pain Meds for Fractures (minutes)	146	52	54	57
Heart Attack Care				
Aspirin Given at Discharge[2]	249	100%	99%	99%
Fibrinolytic Meds Within 30 Min. of Arrival[2,7]	-	-	80%	54%
PCI Within 90 Minutes of Arrival[2]	30	87%	97%	96%
Statin Prescribed at Discharge[2]	247	98%	98%	98%
Heart Failure Care				
ACE Inhibitor or ARB for LVSD[2]	74	100%	97%	97%
Discharge Instructions Given[2]	235	99%	96%	94%
Evaluation of LVS Function[2]	286	100%	100%	99%
Medicare Spending				
Medicare Spending per Patient (ratio)	-	1.01	1.01	0.98
Pneumonia Care				
Appropriate Initial Antibiotic Given[2]	113	100%	96%	95%
Blood Culture Timing[2]	167	99%	98%	98%
Pregnancy and Delivery Care				
Newborn Deliveries Scheduled Early[2]	27	0%	5%	6%
Preventive Care				
Immunization for Influenza[2]	563	100%	93%	90%
Immunization for Pneumonia[2]	810	100%	94%	92%
Stroke Care				
Anticoagulation Therapy for Atrial Fibrillation[2]	12	83%	95%	95%
Antithrombotic Therapy Timing[2]	96	93%	98%	98%
Assessed for Rehabilitation[2]	104	97%	98%	97%
Discharged on Antithrombotic Therapy[2]	104	100%	99%	99%
Discharged on Statin Medication[2]	85	96%	95%	94%
Thrombolytic Therapy Timing[1,2]	-	-	65%	66%
Venous Thromboembolism Prophylaxis[2]	92	98%	95%	94%
Written Stroke Educational Materials Given[2]	70	100%	92%	88%
Surgical Care Improvement Project				
Appropriate Beta Blocker Usage[2]	220	99%	98%	98%
Appropriate VTP Within 24 Hours[2]	368	98%	98%	98%
Controlled Postoperative Blood Glucose[2]	57	96%	97%	97%
Perioperative Temperature Management[2]	497	100%	100%	100%
Prophylactic Antibiotic Selection[2]	373	99%	99%	99%
Prophylactic Antibiotic Selection (Outpatient)	385	97%	98%	98%
Prophylactic Antibiotic Stopped[2]	363	99%	98%	98%
Prophylactic Antibiotic Timing[2]	372	99%	99%	99%
Prophylactic Antibiotic Timing (Outpatient)	387	98%	97%	98%
Urinary Catheter Removal[2]	253	98%	97%	97%
Survey of Patients' Hospital Experiences				
Area Around Room 'Always' Quiet at Night	300+	50%	58%	61%
Doctors 'Always' Communicated Well	300+	77%	80%	82%
Home Recovery Information Given	300+	84%	87%	85%
Hospital Given 9 or 10 on 10 Point Scale	300+	66%	72%	71%
Meds 'Always' Explained Before Given	300+	67%	64%	64%
Nurses 'Always' Communicated Well	300+	78%	81%	79%
Pain 'Always' Well Controlled	300+	67%	71%	71%
Room and Bathroom 'Always' Clean	300+	63%	75%	73%
Timely Help 'Always' Received	300+	66%	70%	68%
Would Definitely Recommend Hospital	300+	65%	71%	71%
Use of Medical Imaging				
Cardiac Imaging Stress Test before Surgery	756	4.1%	5.4%	5.3%
Combination Abdominal CT Scan	1,269	3.5%	7.1%	10.5%
Combination Brain/Sinus CT Scan	871	1.7%	2.8%	2.7%
Combination Chest CT Scan	745	0.8%	1.7%	2.7%
Follow-up Mammogram/Ultrasound	1,627	7.0%	8.7%	8.8%
Lumbar Spine MRI for Low Back Pain	287	36.6%	34.7%	37.2%

Chillicothe VA Medical Center

17273 State Route 104
Chillicothe, OH 45601
URL: www.chillicothe.va.gov
Type: Acute Care - VA
Ownership: Government Federal
Phone: 740-773-1141
Emergency Services: No
Beds: 297

Key Personnel:
Infection Control. . . . . Teresa Davis, RN
Chief of Medical Staff. . . . . Deborah M Meesig, MD, JD
Emergency Room . . . . Thomas Oommen, MD

Measure	Cases	This Hosp.	State Avg.	U.S. Avg.
Blood Clot Prevention and Treatment				
Anticoagulation Overlap Therapy	-	-	93%	93%
ICU Venous Thromboembolism Prophylaxis	-	-	93%	92%
Incidence of Potentially Preventable VTE	-	-	6%	10%
UFH with Dosages/Platelet Monitoring	-	-	98%	97%
Venous Thromboembolism Prophylaxis	-	-	88%	85%
Warfarin Therapy Discharge Instructions	-	-	79%	75%
Chest Pain/Possible Heart Attack Care				
Aspirin Given Within 24 Hours of Arrival	-	-	97%	96%
Fibrinolytic Meds Within 30 Min. of Arrival	-	-	44%	58%
Average Time to ECG (minutes)	-	-	6	7
Average Time to Transfer (minutes)	-	-	58	60
Children's Asthma Care				
Received Home Management Plan of Care	-	-	85%	88%
Received Reliever Medication	-	-	100%	100%
Received Systemic Corticosteroids	-	-	100%	100%
Emergency Department				
Admittance Decision Time (minutes)	-	-	90	98
Head CT Results Within 45 Min. of Arrival	-	-	63%	57%
Patients Who Left ER Before Being Seen	-	-	2%	2%
Time from ER Arrival to Admit. (minutes)	-	-	265	274
Time from ER Arrival to Discharge (minutes)	-	-	128	134
Time in ER Before Being Evaluated (minutes)	-	-	22	26
Time to Pain Meds for Fractures (minutes)	-	-	54	57
Heart Attack Care				
Aspirin Given at Discharge[5]	-	-	99%	99%
Fibrinolytic Meds Within 30 Min. of Arrival[5]	-	-	80%	54%
PCI Within 90 Minutes of Arrival[5]	-	-	97%	96%
Statin Prescribed at Discharge[5]	-	-	98%	98%
Heart Failure Care				
ACE Inhibitor or ARB for LVSD	31	97%	97%	97%
Discharge Instructions Given	98	99%	96%	94%
Evaluation of LVS Function	109	100%	100%	99%
Medicare Spending				
Medicare Spending per Patient (ratio)	-	-	1.01	0.98
Pneumonia Care				
Appropriate Initial Antibiotic Given	65	92%	96%	95%
Blood Culture Timing	73	99%	98%	98%
Pregnancy and Delivery Care				

NOTE: Hospital profiles are in alphabetical order by state, then city, then hospital within the city; Rankings exclude hospitals with less than 25 cases except for patient surveys which excludes hospitals with less than 100 cases; (a) 100-299 cases; (1) The number of cases/patients is too few to report; (2) Data submitted were based on a sample of cases/patients; (3) Results are based on a shorter time period than required; (4) Data suppressed by CMS for one or more quarters; (5) Results are not available for this reporting period; (6) Fewer than 100 patients completed the HCAHPS survey; (7) No cases met the criteria for this measure; (8) The lower limit of the confidence interval cannot be calculated if the number of observed infections equals zero; (9) No data are available from the state/territory for this reporting period; (10) The scores shown reflect fewer than 50 completed surveys; (11) There were discrepancies in the data collection process; (12) This measure does not apply to this hospital for this reporting period; (13) Results cannot be calculated for this reporting period; (14) The results for this state are combined with nearby states to protect confidentiality; Please refer to the User's Guide for a full explanation of data.

Newborn Deliveries Scheduled Early	-	-	5%	6%
Preventive Care				
Immunization for Influenza[2,3]	140	79%	93%	90%
Immunization for Pneumonia[2,3]	280	87%	94%	92%
Stroke Care				
Anticoagulation Therapy for Atrial Fibrillation	-	-	95%	95%
Antithrombotic Therapy Timing	-	-	98%	98%
Assessed for Rehabilitation	-	-	98%	97%
Discharged on Antithrombotic Therapy	-	-	99%	99%
Discharged on Statin Medication	-	-	95%	94%
Thrombolytic Therapy Timing	-	-	65%	66%
Venous Thromboembolism Prophylaxis	-	-	95%	94%
Written Stroke Educational Materials Given	-	-	92%	88%
Surgical Care Improvement Project				
Appropriate Beta Blocker Usage[5]	-	-	98%	98%
Appropriate VTP Within 24 Hours[5]	-	-	98%	98%
Controlled Postoperative Blood Glucose[5]	-	-	97%	97%
Perioperative Temperature Management[5]	-	-	100%	100%
Prophylactic Antibiotic Selection[5]	-	-	99%	99%
Prophylactic Antibiotic Selection (Outpatient)	-	-	98%	98%
Prophylactic Antibiotic Stopped[5]	-	-	98%	98%
Prophylactic Antibiotic Timing[5]	-	-	99%	99%
Prophylactic Antibiotic Timing (Outpatient)	-	-	97%	98%
Urinary Catheter Removal[5]	-	-	97%	97%
Survey of Patients' Hospital Experiences				
Area Around Room 'Always' Quiet at Night	-	-	58%	61%
Doctors 'Always' Communicated Well	-	-	80%	82%
Home Recovery Information Given	-	-	87%	85%
Hospital Given 9 or 10 on 10 Point Scale	-	-	72%	71%
Meds 'Always' Explained Before Given	-	-	64%	64%
Nurses 'Always' Communicated Well	-	-	81%	79%
Pain 'Always' Well Controlled	-	-	71%	71%
Room and Bathroom 'Always' Clean	-	-	75%	73%
Timely Help 'Always' Received	-	-	70%	68%
Would Definitely Recommend Hospital	-	-	71%	71%
Use of Medical Imaging				
Cardiac Imaging Stress Test before Surgery	-	-	5.4%	5.3%
Combination Abdominal CT Scan	-	-	7.1%	10.5%
Combination Brain/Sinus CT Scan	-	-	2.8%	2.7%
Combination Chest CT Scan	-	-	1.7%	2.7%
Follow-up Mammogram/Ultrasound	-	-	8.7%	8.8%
Lumbar Spine MRI for Low Back Pain	-	-	34.7%	37.2%

Bethesda North

10500 Montgomery Road
Cincinnati, OH 45242
URL: www.trihealth.com
Type: Acute Care Hospitals
Ownership: Voluntary non-profit - Church
Phone: 513-865-1241
Fax: 513-745-1441
Emergency Services: Yes
Beds: 314

Key Personnel:
Cardiac Laboratory. . . . . Nancy Dallas
Chief of Medical Staff. . . . . Larry Johnsaw
CEO/President. . . . . John Prout
Emergency Room . . . . Bonnie Sheedy
Quality Assurance . . . . Tim Walters
Operating Room. . . . . Daniel Warmack

Measure	Cases	This Hosp.	State Avg.	U.S. Avg.
Blood Clot Prevention and Treatment				
Anticoagulation Overlap Therapy[2]	139	98%	93%	93%
ICU Venous Thromboembolism Prophylaxis[2]	75	96%	93%	92%
Incidence of Potentially Preventable VTE[2]	16	12%	6%	10%
UFH with Dosages/Platelet Monitoring[2]	142	100%	98%	97%
Venous Thromboembolism Prophylaxis[2]	313	89%	88%	85%
Warfarin Therapy Discharge Instructions[2]	92	59%	79%	75%
Chest Pain/Possible Heart Attack Care				
Aspirin Given Within 24 Hours of Arrival	14	86%	97%	96%
Fibrinolytic Meds Within 30 Min. of Arrival[3,7]	-	-	44%	58%
Average Time to ECG (minutes)	14	4	6	7
Average Time to Transfer (minutes)[3,7]	-	-	58	60
Children's Asthma Care				
Received Home Management Plan of Care	-	-	85%	88%
Received Reliever Medication	-	-	100%	100%
Received Systemic Corticosteroids	-	-	100%	100%
Emergency Department				
Admittance Decision Time (minutes)[2]	716	102	90	98
Head CT Results Within 45 Min. of Arrival	14	57%	63%	57%
Patients Who Left ER Before Being Seen	56,381	0%	2%	2%
Time from ER Arrival to Admit. (minutes)[2]	729	256	265	274
Time from ER Arrival to Discharge (minutes)	377	115	128	134
Time in ER Before Being Evaluated (minutes)	168	32	22	26
Time to Pain Meds for Fractures (minutes)	328	44	54	57
Heart Attack Care				
Aspirin Given at Discharge	371	100%	99%	99%
Fibrinolytic Meds Within 30 Min. of Arrival[7]	-	-	80%	54%
PCI Within 90 Minutes of Arrival	75	96%	97%	96%
Statin Prescribed at Discharge	368	98%	98%	98%
Heart Failure Care				
ACE Inhibitor or ARB for LVSD	159	95%	97%	97%
Discharge Instructions Given	483	100%	96%	94%
Evaluation of LVS Function	608	100%	100%	99%
Medicare Spending				
Medicare Spending per Patient (ratio)	-	1.02	1.01	0.98
Pneumonia Care				
Appropriate Initial Antibiotic Given[2]	127	98%	96%	95%
Blood Culture Timing[2]	303	99%	98%	98%
Pregnancy and Delivery Care				
Newborn Deliveries Scheduled Early[2]	50	0%	5%	6%
Preventive Care				
Immunization for Influenza[2]	546	73%	93%	90%
Immunization for Pneumonia[2]	783	80%	94%	92%
Stroke Care				
Anticoagulation Therapy for Atrial Fibrillation	25	96%	95%	95%
Antithrombotic Therapy Timing	190	98%	98%	98%
Assessed for Rehabilitation	240	98%	98%	97%
Discharged on Antithrombotic Therapy	213	100%	99%	99%
Discharged on Statin Medication	160	99%	95%	94%
Thrombolytic Therapy Timing	16	100%	65%	66%
Venous Thromboembolism Prophylaxis	231	97%	95%	94%
Written Stroke Educational Materials Given	151	92%	92%	88%
Surgical Care Improvement Project				
Appropriate Beta Blocker Usage[2]	182	96%	98%	98%
Appropriate VTP Within 24 Hours[2]	315	99%	98%	98%
Controlled Postoperative Blood Glucose[2]	119	93%	97%	97%
Perioperative Temperature Management[2]	434	99%	100%	100%
Prophylactic Antibiotic Selection[2]	391	99%	99%	99%
Prophylactic Antibiotic Selection (Outpatient)	515	97%	98%	98%
Prophylactic Antibiotic Stopped[2]	379	99%	98%	98%
Prophylactic Antibiotic Timing[2]	391	97%	99%	99%
Prophylactic Antibiotic Timing (Outpatient)	525	96%	97%	98%
Urinary Catheter Removal[2]	259	96%	97%	97%
Survey of Patients' Hospital Experiences				
Area Around Room 'Always' Quiet at Night	300+	52%	58%	61%
Doctors 'Always' Communicated Well	300+	79%	80%	82%
Home Recovery Information Given	300+	89%	87%	85%
Hospital Given 9 or 10 on 10 Point Scale	300+	73%	72%	71%
Meds 'Always' Explained Before Given	300+	58%	64%	64%
Nurses 'Always' Communicated Well	300+	77%	81%	79%
Pain 'Always' Well Controlled	300+	71%	71%	71%
Room and Bathroom 'Always' Clean	300+	74%	75%	73%
Timely Help 'Always' Received	300+	65%	70%	68%
Would Definitely Recommend Hospital	300+	75%	71%	71%
Use of Medical Imaging				
Cardiac Imaging Stress Test before Surgery	882	4.8%	5.4%	5.3%
Combination Abdominal CT Scan	1,779	9.2%	7.1%	10.5%
Combination Brain/Sinus CT Scan	1,225	1.0%	2.8%	2.7%
Combination Chest CT Scan	1,135	0.4%	1.7%	2.7%
Follow-up Mammogram/Ultrasound	4,143	20.9%	8.7%	8.8%
Lumbar Spine MRI for Low Back Pain	268	32.1%	34.7%	37.2%

Christ Hospital

2139 Auburn Avenue
Cincinnati, OH 45219
URL: www.thechristhospital.com
Type: Acute Care Hospitals
Ownership: Voluntary non-profit - Private
Phone: 513-585-2000
Fax: 513-585-4313
Emergency Services: Yes

Key Personnel:
Radiology. . . . . Richard Buddetein, MD
Infection Control. . . . . Corwin Dunn, MD
Chief of Medical Staff . . . . Berc Gawne, MD
CEO/President. . . . . Mike Keating
Operating Room. . . . . Jeff Morneanlt
Emergency Room . . . . Steven Yamaguschi, MD
Patient Relations . . . . Kathy Zimmerman

Measure	Cases	This Hosp.	State Avg.	U.S. Avg.
Blood Clot Prevention and Treatment				
Anticoagulation Overlap Therapy[2]	154	100%	93%	93%
ICU Venous Thromboembolism Prophylaxis[2]	92	95%	93%	92%
Incidence of Potentially Preventable VTE[2]	25	8%	6%	10%
UFH with Dosages/Platelet Monitoring[2]	151	100%	98%	97%
Venous Thromboembolism Prophylaxis[2]	300	82%	88%	85%
Warfarin Therapy Discharge Instructions[2]	117	46%	79%	75%
Chest Pain/Possible Heart Attack Care				
Aspirin Given Within 24 Hours of Arrival[5]	-	-	97%	96%
Fibrinolytic Meds Within 30 Min. of Arrival[5]	-	-	44%	58%
Average Time to ECG (minutes)[5]	-	-	6	7
Average Time to Transfer (minutes)[5]	-	-	58	60
Children's Asthma Care				
Received Home Management Plan of Care	-	-	85%	88%
Received Reliever Medication	-	-	100%	100%
Received Systemic Corticosteroids	-	-	100%	100%
Emergency Department				
Admittance Decision Time (minutes)[2]	437	135	90	98
Head CT Results Within 45 Min. of Arrival[1,3]	-	-	63%	57%
Patients Who Left ER Before Being Seen	53,595	3%	2%	2%
Time from ER Arrival to Admit. (minutes)[2]	437	353	265	274
Time from ER Arrival to Discharge (minutes)	392	172	128	134
Time in ER Before Being Evaluated (minutes)	421	21	22	26
Time to Pain Meds for Fractures (minutes)	41	51	54	57
Heart Attack Care				
Aspirin Given at Discharge[2]	314	100%	99%	99%
Fibrinolytic Meds Within 30 Min. of Arrival[2,7]	-	-	80%	54%
PCI Within 90 Minutes of Arrival[2]	23	100%	97%	96%
Statin Prescribed at Discharge[2]	304	100%	98%	98%
Heart Failure Care				
ACE Inhibitor or ARB for LVSD	320	100%	97%	97%
Discharge Instructions Given	782	98%	96%	94%
Evaluation of LVS Function	943	100%	100%	99%
Medicare Spending				
Medicare Spending per Patient (ratio)	-	1.01	1.01	0.98
Pneumonia Care				
Appropriate Initial Antibiotic Given[2]	53	100%	96%	95%
Blood Culture Timing[2]	114	97%	98%	98%
Pregnancy and Delivery Care				
Newborn Deliveries Scheduled Early[2]	39	13%	5%	6%
Preventive Care				
Immunization for Influenza[2]	553	94%	93%	90%
Immunization for Pneumonia[2]	707	94%	94%	92%
Stroke Care				
Anticoagulation Therapy for Atrial Fibrillation[2]	11	100%	95%	95%
Antithrombotic Therapy Timing[2]	77	100%	98%	98%
Assessed for Rehabilitation[2]	106	99%	98%	97%
Discharged on Antithrombotic Therapy[2]	90	100%	99%	99%
Discharged on Statin Medication[2]	79	97%	95%	94%
Thrombolytic Therapy Timing[1,2]	-	-	65%	66%
Venous Thromboembolism Prophylaxis[2]	103	96%	95%	94%
Written Stroke Educational Materials Given[2]	46	98%	92%	88%
Surgical Care Improvement Project				
Appropriate Beta Blocker Usage[2]	358	99%	98%	98%
Appropriate VTP Within 24 Hours[2]	529	99%	98%	98%
Controlled Postoperative Blood Glucose[2]	218	97%	97%	97%
Perioperative Temperature Management[2]	800	100%	100%	100%
Prophylactic Antibiotic Selection[2]	730	100%	99%	99%
Prophylactic Antibiotic Selection (Outpatient)	908	99%	98%	98%
Prophylactic Antibiotic Stopped[2]	710	98%	98%	98%
Prophylactic Antibiotic Timing[2]	732	99%	99%	99%
Prophylactic Antibiotic Timing (Outpatient)	838	100%	97%	98%
Urinary Catheter Removal[2]	491	97%	97%	97%
Survey of Patients' Hospital Experiences				
Area Around Room 'Always' Quiet at Night	300+	60%	58%	61%
Doctors 'Always' Communicated Well	300+	85%	80%	82%

NOTE: Hospital profiles are in alphabetical order by state, then city, then hospital within the city; Rankings exclude hospitals with less than 25 cases except for patient surveys which excludes hospitals with less than 100 cases; (a) 100-299 cases; (1) The number of cases/patients is too few to report; (2) Data submitted were based on a sample of cases/patients; (3) Results are based on a shorter time period than required; (4) Data suppressed by CMS for one or more quarters; (5) Results are not available for this reporting period; (6) Fewer than 100 patients completed the HCAHPS survey; (7) No cases met the criteria for this measure; (8) The lower limit of the confidence interval cannot be calculated if the number of observed infections equals zero; (9) No data are available from the state/territory for this reporting period; (10) The scores shown reflect fewer than 50 completed surveys; (11) There were discrepancies in the data collection process; (12) This measure does not apply to this hospital for this reporting period; (13) Results cannot be calculated for this reporting period; (14) The results for this state are combined with nearby states to protect confidentiality; Please refer to the User's Guide for a full explanation of data.

Home Recovery Information Given	300+	89%	87%	85%
Hospital Given 9 or 10 on 10 Point Scale	300+	83%	72%	71%
Meds 'Always' Explained Before Given	300+	68%	64%	64%
Nurses 'Always' Communicated Well	300+	85%	81%	79%
Pain 'Always' Well Controlled	300+	76%	71%	71%
Room and Bathroom 'Always' Clean	300+	73%	75%	73%
Timely Help 'Always' Received	300+	71%	70%	68%
Would Definitely Recommend Hospital	300+	86%	71%	71%
Use of Medical Imaging				
Cardiac Imaging Stress Test before Surgery	1,580	4.2%	5.4%	5.3%
Combination Abdominal CT Scan	1,712	7.2%	7.1%	10.5%
Combination Brain/Sinus CT Scan	898	1.4%	2.8%	2.7%
Combination Chest CT Scan	1,522	1.2%	1.7%	2.7%
Follow-up Mammogram/Ultrasound	3,046	7.4%	8.7%	8.8%
Lumbar Spine MRI for Low Back Pain	378	43.4%	34.7%	37.2%

Cincinnati VA Medical Center

3200 Vine Street
Cincinnati, OH 45220
URL: www.cincinnati.va.gov
Type: Acute Care - VA
Ownership: Government Federal

Phone: 513-861-3100
Fax: 513-475-6525
Emergency Services: No
Beds: 378

Key Personnel:

Operating Room. . . . . Robert Bower
Patient Relations . . . . Linda Dubois
Emergency Room . . . . James Huey, MD
CEO/President. . . . . Carlos B Lott, Jr
Hemotology Center . . . . Albert Muhleman, MD
Infection Control. . . . . Gary Roselle, MD
Chief of Medical Staff. . . . . Barbara K. Temeck
Quality Assurance . . . . Barbara Thomas, RN

Measure	Cases	This Hosp.	State Avg.	U.S. Avg.
Blood Clot Prevention and Treatment				
Anticoagulation Overlap Therapy	-	-	93%	93%
ICU Venous Thromboembolism Prophylaxis	-	-	93%	92%
Incidence of Potentially Preventable VTE	-	-	6%	10%
UFH with Dosages/Platelet Monitoring	-	-	98%	97%
Venous Thromboembolism Prophylaxis	-	-	88%	85%
Warfarin Therapy Discharge Instructions	-	-	79%	75%
Chest Pain/Possible Heart Attack Care				
Aspirin Given Within 24 Hours of Arrival	-	-	97%	96%
Fibrinolytic Meds Within 30 Min. of Arrival	-	-	44%	58%
Average Time to ECG (minutes)	-	-	6	7
Average Time to Transfer (minutes)	-	-	58	60
Children's Asthma Care				
Received Home Management Plan of Care	-	-	85%	88%
Received Reliever Medication	-	-	100%	100%
Received Systemic Corticosteroids	-	-	100%	100%
Emergency Department				
Admittance Decision Time (minutes)	-	-	90	98
Head CT Results Within 45 Min. of Arrival	-	-	63%	57%
Patients Who Left ER Before Being Seen	-	-	2%	2%
Time from ER Arrival to Admit. (minutes)	-	-	265	274
Time from ER Arrival to Discharge (minutes)	-	-	128	134
Time in ER Before Being Evaluated (minutes)	-	-	22	26
Time to Pain Meds for Fractures (minutes)	-	-	54	57
Heart Attack Care				
Aspirin Given at Discharge	49	100%	99%	99%
Fibrinolytic Meds Within 30 Min. of Arrival[5]	-	-	80%	54%
PCI Within 90 Minutes of Arrival[5]	-	-	97%	96%
Statin Prescribed at Discharge	48	100%	98%	98%
Heart Failure Care				
ACE Inhibitor or ARB for LVSD	97	93%	97%	97%
Discharge Instructions Given	165	100%	96%	94%
Evaluation of LVS Function	185	100%	100%	99%
Medicare Spending				
Medicare Spending per Patient (ratio)	-	-	1.01	0.98
Pneumonia Care				
Appropriate Initial Antibiotic Given	61	100%	96%	95%
Blood Culture Timing	122	98%	98%	98%
Pregnancy and Delivery Care				
Newborn Deliveries Scheduled Early	-	-	5%	6%
Preventive Care				
Immunization for Influenza[5]	-	-	93%	90%
Immunization for Pneumonia[5]	-	-	94%	92%
Stroke Care				
Anticoagulation Therapy for Atrial Fibrillation	-	-	95%	95%
Antithrombotic Therapy Timing	-	-	98%	98%
Assessed for Rehabilitation	-	-	98%	97%
Discharged on Antithrombotic Therapy	-	-	99%	99%
Discharged on Statin Medication	-	-	95%	94%
Thrombolytic Therapy Timing	-	-	65%	66%
Venous Thromboembolism Prophylaxis	-	-	95%	94%
Written Stroke Educational Materials Given	-	-	92%	88%
Surgical Care Improvement Project				
Appropriate Beta Blocker Usage[2]	94	98%	98%	98%
Appropriate VTP Within 24 Hours[2]	264	100%	98%	98%
Controlled Postoperative Blood Glucose[5]	-	-	97%	97%
Perioperative Temperature Management[2]	304	100%	100%	100%
Prophylactic Antibiotic Selection	181	98%	99%	99%
Prophylactic Antibiotic Selection (Outpatient)	-	-	98%	98%
Prophylactic Antibiotic Stopped	177	99%	98%	98%
Prophylactic Antibiotic Timing	181	97%	99%	99%
Prophylactic Antibiotic Timing (Outpatient)	-	-	97%	98%
Urinary Catheter Removal[1,2]	-	-	97%	97%
Survey of Patients' Hospital Experiences				
Area Around Room 'Always' Quiet at Night	-	-	58%	61%
Doctors 'Always' Communicated Well	-	-	80%	82%
Home Recovery Information Given	-	-	87%	85%
Hospital Given 9 or 10 on 10 Point Scale	-	-	72%	71%
Meds 'Always' Explained Before Given	-	-	64%	64%
Nurses 'Always' Communicated Well	-	-	81%	79%
Pain 'Always' Well Controlled	-	-	71%	71%
Room and Bathroom 'Always' Clean	-	-	75%	73%
Timely Help 'Always' Received	-	-	70%	68%
Would Definitely Recommend Hospital	-	-	71%	71%
Use of Medical Imaging				
Cardiac Imaging Stress Test before Surgery	-	-	5.4%	5.3%
Combination Abdominal CT Scan	-	-	7.1%	10.5%
Combination Brain/Sinus CT Scan	-	-	2.8%	2.7%
Combination Chest CT Scan	-	-	1.7%	2.7%
Follow-up Mammogram/Ultrasound	-	-	8.7%	8.8%
Lumbar Spine MRI for Low Back Pain	-	-	34.7%	37.2%

Good Samaritan Hospital

375 Dixmyth Avenue
Cincinnati, OH 45220
URL: www.trihealth.com
Type: Acute Care Hospitals
Ownership: Voluntary non-profit - Church

Phone: 513-862-2601
Fax: 513-872-3435
Emergency Services: Yes
Beds: 700

Key Personnel:

Chief of Medical Staff. . . . . Larry Johnstone
Emergency Room . . . . Jim Owen
CEO/President. . . . . John Prout

Measure	Cases	This Hosp.	State Avg.	U.S. Avg.
Blood Clot Prevention and Treatment				
Anticoagulation Overlap Therapy[2]	167	94%	93%	93%
ICU Venous Thromboembolism Prophylaxis[2]	91	93%	93%	92%
Incidence of Potentially Preventable VTE[2]	26	8%	6%	10%
UFH with Dosages/Platelet Monitoring[2]	152	100%	98%	97%
Venous Thromboembolism Prophylaxis[2]	302	91%	88%	85%
Warfarin Therapy Discharge Instructions[2]	140	65%	79%	75%
Chest Pain/Possible Heart Attack Care				
Aspirin Given Within 24 Hours of Arrival[1,3]	-	-	97%	96%
Fibrinolytic Meds Within 30 Min. of Arrival[3,7]	-	-	44%	58%
Average Time to ECG (minutes)[1,3]	-	-	6	7
Average Time to Transfer (minutes)[1,3]	-	-	58	60
Children's Asthma Care				
Received Home Management Plan of Care	-	-	85%	88%
Received Reliever Medication	-	-	100%	100%
Received Systemic Corticosteroids	-	-	100%	100%
Emergency Department				
Admittance Decision Time (minutes)[2]	528	118	90	98
Head CT Results Within 45 Min. of Arrival[1]	-	-	63%	57%
Patients Who Left ER Before Being Seen	57,935	1%	2%	2%
Time from ER Arrival to Admit. (minutes)[2]	531	256	265	274
Time from ER Arrival to Discharge (minutes)	382	103	128	134
Time in ER Before Being Evaluated (minutes)	226	36	22	26
Time to Pain Meds for Fractures (minutes)	221	43	54	57
Heart Attack Care				
Aspirin Given at Discharge	244	100%	99%	99%
Fibrinolytic Meds Within 30 Min. of Arrival[7]	-	-	80%	54%
PCI Within 90 Minutes of Arrival	45	100%	97%	96%
Statin Prescribed at Discharge	247	99%	98%	98%
Heart Failure Care				
ACE Inhibitor or ARB for LVSD	134	99%	97%	97%
Discharge Instructions Given	380	99%	96%	94%
Evaluation of LVS Function	481	100%	100%	99%
Medicare Spending				
Medicare Spending per Patient (ratio)	-	0.98	1.01	0.98
Pneumonia Care				
Appropriate Initial Antibiotic Given[2]	99	99%	96%	95%
Blood Culture Timing[2]	181	99%	98%	98%
Pregnancy and Delivery Care				
Newborn Deliveries Scheduled Early[2]	59	2%	5%	6%
Preventive Care				
Immunization for Influenza[2]	517	83%	93%	90%
Immunization for Pneumonia[2]	651	84%	94%	92%
Stroke Care				
Anticoagulation Therapy for Atrial Fibrillation	24	96%	95%	95%
Antithrombotic Therapy Timing	170	99%	98%	98%
Assessed for Rehabilitation	201	98%	98%	97%
Discharged on Antithrombotic Therapy	179	100%	99%	99%
Discharged on Statin Medication	140	99%	95%	94%
Thrombolytic Therapy Timing	16	88%	65%	66%
Venous Thromboembolism Prophylaxis	199	97%	95%	94%
Written Stroke Educational Materials Given	98	100%	92%	88%
Surgical Care Improvement Project				
Appropriate Beta Blocker Usage[2]	189	98%	98%	98%
Appropriate VTP Within 24 Hours[2]	304	100%	98%	98%
Controlled Postoperative Blood Glucose[2]	136	99%	97%	97%
Perioperative Temperature Management[2]	461	100%	100%	100%
Prophylactic Antibiotic Selection[2]	423	98%	99%	99%
Prophylactic Antibiotic Selection (Outpatient)	465	99%	98%	98%
Prophylactic Antibiotic Stopped[2]	413	100%	98%	98%
Prophylactic Antibiotic Timing[2]	425	93%	99%	99%
Prophylactic Antibiotic Timing (Outpatient)	477	95%	97%	98%
Urinary Catheter Removal[2]	267	97%	97%	97%
Survey of Patients' Hospital Experiences				
Area Around Room 'Always' Quiet at Night	300+	59%	58%	61%
Doctors 'Always' Communicated Well	300+	81%	80%	82%
Home Recovery Information Given	300+	88%	87%	85%
Hospital Given 9 or 10 on 10 Point Scale	300+	73%	72%	71%
Meds 'Always' Explained Before Given	300+	61%	64%	64%
Nurses 'Always' Communicated Well	300+	80%	81%	79%
Pain 'Always' Well Controlled	300+	74%	71%	71%
Room and Bathroom 'Always' Clean	300+	71%	75%	73%
Timely Help 'Always' Received	300+	71%	70%	68%
Would Definitely Recommend Hospital	300+	77%	71%	71%
Use of Medical Imaging				
Cardiac Imaging Stress Test before Surgery	865	3.5%	5.4%	5.3%
Combination Abdominal CT Scan	1,067	4.9%	7.1%	10.5%
Combination Brain/Sinus CT Scan	775	0.3%	2.8%	2.7%
Combination Chest CT Scan	751	0.7%	1.7%	2.7%
Follow-up Mammogram/Ultrasound	2,338	9.1%	8.7%	8.8%
Lumbar Spine MRI for Low Back Pain	172	37.2%	34.7%	37.2%

Jewish Hospital

4777 East Galbraith Road
Cincinnati, OH 45236
URL: www.jewishhospitalcincinnati.com
Type: Acute Care Hospitals
Ownership: Voluntary non-profit - Private

Phone: 513-686-3003
Fax: 513-585-6168
Emergency Services: Yes

Key Personnel:

CEO/President. . . . . Yousuf J. Ahmad, DrPH, MHSA, MBA
Hemotology Center . . . . E Randolph Broun, MD
Infection Control. . . . . Maria Clifton
Chief of Medical Staff . . . . David Dort
Radiology. . . . . Robert Lenobel, MD
Intensive Care Unit. . . . . Linda Miller
Operating Room. . . . . Pam Photiadis
Emergency Room . . . . Richard Regan

NOTE: Hospital profiles are in alphabetical order by state, then city, then hospital within the city; Rankings exclude hospitals with less than 25 cases except for patient surveys which excludes hospitals with less than 100 cases; (a) 100-299 cases; (1) The number of cases/patients is too few to report; (2) Data submitted were based on a sample of cases/patients; (3) Results are based on a shorter time period than required; (4) Data suppressed by CMS for one or more quarters; (5) Results are not available for this reporting period; (6) Fewer than 100 patients completed the HCAHPS survey; (7) No cases met the criteria for this measure; (8) The lower limit of the confidence interval cannot be calculated if the number of observed infections equals zero; (9) No data are available from the state/territory for this reporting period; (10) The scores shown reflect fewer than 50 completed surveys; (11) There were discrepancies in the data collection process; (12) This measure does not apply to this hospital for this reporting period; (13) Results cannot be calculated for this reporting period; (14) The results for this state are combined with nearby states to protect confidentiality; Please refer to the User's Guide for a full explanation of data.

Measure	Cases	This Hosp.	State Avg.	U.S. Avg.
Blood Clot Prevention and Treatment				
Anticoagulation Overlap Therapy[2]	85	99%	93%	93%
ICU Venous Thromboembolism Prophylaxis[2]	65	86%	93%	92%
Incidence of Potentially Preventable VTE[2]	15	0%	6%	10%
UFH with Dosages/Platelet Monitoring[2]	53	100%	98%	97%
Venous Thromboembolism Prophylaxis[2]	355	86%	88%	85%
Warfarin Therapy Discharge Instructions[2]	66	79%	79%	75%
Chest Pain/Possible Heart Attack Care				
Aspirin Given Within 24 Hours of Arrival[1,3]	-	-	97%	96%
Fibrinolytic Meds Within 30 Min. of Arrival[3,7]	-	-	44%	58%
Average Time to ECG (minutes)[1,3]	-	-	6	7
Average Time to Transfer (minutes)[3,7]	-	-	58	60
Children's Asthma Care				
Received Home Management Plan of Care	-	-	85%	88%
Received Reliever Medication	-	-	100%	100%
Received Systemic Corticosteroids	-	-	100%	100%
Emergency Department				
Admittance Decision Time (minutes)[2]	906	80	90	98
Head CT Results Within 45 Min. of Arrival[1]	-	-	63%	57%
Patients Who Left ER Before Being Seen	34,009	0%	2%	2%
Time from ER Arrival to Admit. (minutes)[2]	910	257	265	274
Time from ER Arrival to Discharge (minutes)	389	145	128	134
Time in ER Before Being Evaluated (minutes)	413	15	22	26
Time to Pain Meds for Fractures (minutes)	63	49	54	57
Heart Attack Care				
Aspirin Given at Discharge	178	100%	99%	99%
Fibrinolytic Meds Within 30 Min. of Arrival[7]	-	-	80%	54%
PCI Within 90 Minutes of Arrival	26	92%	97%	96%
Statin Prescribed at Discharge	179	100%	98%	98%
Heart Failure Care				
ACE Inhibitor or ARB for LVSD[2]	77	99%	97%	97%
Discharge Instructions Given[2]	222	88%	96%	94%
Evaluation of LVS Function[2]	304	100%	100%	99%
Medicare Spending				
Medicare Spending per Patient (ratio)	-	0.96	1.01	0.98
Pneumonia Care				
Appropriate Initial Antibiotic Given[2]	96	98%	96%	95%
Blood Culture Timing[2]	149	99%	98%	98%
Pregnancy and Delivery Care				
Newborn Deliveries Scheduled Early[7]	-	-	5%	6%
Preventive Care				
Immunization for Influenza[2]	638	97%	93%	90%
Immunization for Pneumonia[2]	939	98%	94%	92%
Stroke Care				
Anticoagulation Therapy for Atrial Fibrillation[2]	15	93%	95%	95%
Antithrombotic Therapy Timing[2]	88	99%	98%	98%
Assessed for Rehabilitation[2]	118	99%	98%	97%
Discharged on Antithrombotic Therapy[2]	99	100%	99%	99%
Discharged on Statin Medication[2]	84	98%	95%	94%
Thrombolytic Therapy Timing[1,2]	-	-	65%	66%
Venous Thromboembolism Prophylaxis[2]	114	92%	95%	94%
Written Stroke Educational Materials Given[2]	66	89%	92%	88%
Surgical Care Improvement Project				
Appropriate Beta Blocker Usage[2]	151	94%	98%	98%
Appropriate VTP Within 24 Hours[2]	287	98%	98%	98%
Controlled Postoperative Blood Glucose[2]	49	96%	97%	97%
Perioperative Temperature Management[2]	430	100%	100%	100%
Prophylactic Antibiotic Selection[2]	327	99%	99%	99%
Prophylactic Antibiotic Selection (Outpatient)	150	97%	98%	98%
Prophylactic Antibiotic Stopped[2]	321	98%	98%	98%
Prophylactic Antibiotic Timing[2]	328	97%	99%	99%
Prophylactic Antibiotic Timing (Outpatient)	152	97%	97%	98%
Urinary Catheter Removal[2]	132	86%	97%	97%
Survey of Patients' Hospital Experiences				
Area Around Room 'Always' Quiet at Night	300+	60%	58%	61%
Doctors 'Always' Communicated Well	300+	78%	80%	82%
Home Recovery Information Given	300+	83%	87%	85%
Hospital Given 9 or 10 on 10 Point Scale	300+	68%	72%	71%
Meds 'Always' Explained Before Given	300+	62%	64%	64%
Nurses 'Always' Communicated Well	300+	78%	81%	79%
Pain 'Always' Well Controlled	300+	70%	71%	71%
Room and Bathroom 'Always' Clean	300+	67%	75%	73%
Timely Help 'Always' Received	300+	61%	70%	68%
Would Definitely Recommend Hospital	300+	72%	71%	71%
Use of Medical Imaging				
Cardiac Imaging Stress Test before Surgery	475	5.5%	5.4%	5.3%
Combination Abdominal CT Scan	814	5.5%	7.1%	10.5%
Combination Brain/Sinus CT Scan	602	2.7%	2.8%	2.7%
Combination Chest CT Scan	613	0.7%	1.7%	2.7%
Follow-up Mammogram/Ultrasound	2,879	10.9%	8.7%	8.8%
Lumbar Spine MRI for Low Back Pain	133	41.4%	34.7%	37.2%

Mercy Health - West Hospital

3300 Mercy Health Blvd
Cincinnati, OH 45211
Phone: 513-215-5000
Fax: 513-853-5758
URL: www.e-mercy.com/west-hospital.aspx
Type: Acute Care Hospitals
Emergency Services: Yes
Ownership: Voluntary non-profit - Private
Beds: 269

Key Personnel:
Chief of Medical Staff. . . . . Dan Roth, MD
CEO/President. . . . . Michael Stephens, FACHE

Measure	Cases	This Hosp.	State Avg.	U.S. Avg.
Blood Clot Prevention and Treatment				
Anticoagulation Overlap Therapy[2]	33	97%	93%	93%
ICU Venous Thromboembolism Prophylaxis[2]	61	95%	93%	92%
Incidence of Potentially Preventable VTE[1,2]	-	-	6%	10%
UFH with Dosages/Platelet Monitoring[2]	25	100%	98%	97%
Venous Thromboembolism Prophylaxis[2]	321	95%	88%	85%
Warfarin Therapy Discharge Instructions[2]	27	100%	79%	75%
Chest Pain/Possible Heart Attack Care				
Aspirin Given Within 24 Hours of Arrival	17	94%	97%	96%
Fibrinolytic Meds Within 30 Min. of Arrival[3,7]	-	-	44%	58%
Average Time to ECG (minutes)	19	9	6	7
Average Time to Transfer (minutes)[1,3]	-	-	58	60
Children's Asthma Care				
Received Home Management Plan of Care	-	-	85%	88%
Received Reliever Medication	-	-	100%	100%
Received Systemic Corticosteroids	-	-	100%	100%
Emergency Department				
Admittance Decision Time (minutes)[2]	767	63	90	98
Head CT Results Within 45 Min. of Arrival[1]	-	-	63%	57%
Patients Who Left ER Before Being Seen	41,240	1%	2%	2%
Time from ER Arrival to Admit. (minutes)[2]	770	258	265	274
Time from ER Arrival to Discharge (minutes)	398	108	128	134
Time in ER Before Being Evaluated (minutes)	400	26	22	26
Time to Pain Meds for Fractures (minutes)	113	50	54	57
Heart Attack Care				
Aspirin Given at Discharge	44	100%	99%	99%
Fibrinolytic Meds Within 30 Min. of Arrival[7]	-	-	80%	54%
PCI Within 90 Minutes of Arrival[7]	-	-	97%	96%
Statin Prescribed at Discharge	43	100%	98%	98%
Heart Failure Care				
ACE Inhibitor or ARB for LVSD	49	100%	97%	97%
Discharge Instructions Given	138	96%	96%	94%
Evaluation of LVS Function	171	100%	100%	99%
Medicare Spending				
Medicare Spending per Patient (ratio)	-	1.01	1.01	0.98
Pneumonia Care				
Appropriate Initial Antibiotic Given	106	94%	96%	95%
Blood Culture Timing	177	100%	98%	98%
Pregnancy and Delivery Care				
Newborn Deliveries Scheduled Early[7]	-	-	5%	6%
Preventive Care				
Immunization for Influenza[2]	509	98%	93%	90%
Immunization for Pneumonia[2]	759	99%	94%	92%
Stroke Care				
Anticoagulation Therapy for Atrial Fibrillation[1]	-	-	95%	95%
Antithrombotic Therapy Timing	42	100%	98%	98%
Assessed for Rehabilitation	41	95%	98%	97%
Discharged on Antithrombotic Therapy	37	100%	99%	99%
Discharged on Statin Medication	30	97%	95%	94%
Thrombolytic Therapy Timing[1]	-	-	65%	66%
Venous Thromboembolism Prophylaxis	42	98%	95%	94%
Written Stroke Educational Materials Given	17	94%	92%	88%
Surgical Care Improvement Project				
Appropriate Beta Blocker Usage[2]	131	99%	98%	98%
Appropriate VTP Within 24 Hours[2]	397	99%	98%	98%
Controlled Postoperative Blood Glucose[1,2]	-	-	97%	97%
Perioperative Temperature Management[2]	447	100%	100%	100%
Prophylactic Antibiotic Selection[2]	335	100%	99%	99%
Prophylactic Antibiotic Selection (Outpatient)	70	99%	98%	98%
Prophylactic Antibiotic Stopped[2]	334	99%	98%	98%
Prophylactic Antibiotic Timing[2]	335	100%	99%	99%
Prophylactic Antibiotic Timing (Outpatient)	71	96%	97%	98%
Urinary Catheter Removal[2]	94	94%	97%	97%
Survey of Patients' Hospital Experiences				
Area Around Room 'Always' Quiet at Night	300+	52%	58%	61%
Doctors 'Always' Communicated Well	300+	79%	80%	82%
Home Recovery Information Given	300+	83%	87%	85%
Hospital Given 9 or 10 on 10 Point Scale	300+	66%	72%	71%
Meds 'Always' Explained Before Given	300+	62%	64%	64%
Nurses 'Always' Communicated Well	300+	78%	81%	79%
Pain 'Always' Well Controlled	300+	67%	71%	71%
Room and Bathroom 'Always' Clean	300+	67%	75%	73%
Timely Help 'Always' Received	300+	57%	70%	68%
Would Definitely Recommend Hospital	300+	62%	71%	71%
Use of Medical Imaging				
Cardiac Imaging Stress Test before Surgery	97	4.1%	5.4%	5.3%
Combination Abdominal CT Scan	584	6.3%	7.1%	10.5%
Combination Brain/Sinus CT Scan	382	1.3%	2.8%	2.7%
Combination Chest CT Scan	333	0.3%	1.7%	2.7%
Follow-up Mammogram/Ultrasound	879	6.8%	8.7%	8.8%
Lumbar Spine MRI for Low Back Pain	117	43.6%	34.7%	37.2%

Mercy Hospital Anderson

7500 State Road
Cincinnati, OH 45255
Phone: 513-624-4006
Fax: 513-624-3299
URL: www.e-mercy.com/mercy-hospital-anderson.aspx
Type: Acute Care Hospitals
Emergency Services: Yes
Ownership: Voluntary non-profit - Church
Beds: 186

Key Personnel:
Emergency Room . . . . Harry Boyce
Operating Room. . . . . Pam Brinks
Quality Assurance . . . . Dani Hext
Cardiac Laboratory. . . . . Terri Martin
Infection Control. . . . . Kathy Puthoff
CEO/President. . . . . Patricia Ann Schroer
Chief of Medical Staff . . . . Denberg Stanfield

Measure	Cases	This Hosp.	State Avg.	U.S. Avg.
Blood Clot Prevention and Treatment				
Anticoagulation Overlap Therapy[2]	69	100%	93%	93%
ICU Venous Thromboembolism Prophylaxis[2]	54	94%	93%	92%
Incidence of Potentially Preventable VTE[1,2]	-	-	6%	10%
UFH with Dosages/Platelet Monitoring[2]	42	100%	98%	97%
Venous Thromboembolism Prophylaxis[2]	311	95%	88%	85%
Warfarin Therapy Discharge Instructions[2]	59	98%	79%	75%
Chest Pain/Possible Heart Attack Care				
Aspirin Given Within 24 Hours of Arrival[5]	-	-	97%	96%
Fibrinolytic Meds Within 30 Min. of Arrival[5]	-	-	44%	58%
Average Time to ECG (minutes)[5]	-	-	6	7
Average Time to Transfer (minutes)[5]	-	-	58	60
Children's Asthma Care				
Received Home Management Plan of Care	-	-	85%	88%
Received Reliever Medication	-	-	100%	100%
Received Systemic Corticosteroids	-	-	100%	100%
Emergency Department				
Admittance Decision Time (minutes)[2]	760	116	90	98
Head CT Results Within 45 Min. of Arrival[1]	-	-	63%	57%
Patients Who Left ER Before Being Seen	47,437	1%	2%	2%
Time from ER Arrival to Admit. (minutes)[2]	762	312	265	274
Time from ER Arrival to Discharge (minutes)	388	164	128	134
Time in ER Before Being Evaluated (minutes)	413	13	22	26
Time to Pain Meds for Fractures (minutes)	126	48	54	57
Heart Attack Care				
Aspirin Given at Discharge	348	100%	99%	99%
Fibrinolytic Meds Within 30 Min. of Arrival[7]	-	-	80%	54%
PCI Within 90 Minutes of Arrival	52	96%	97%	96%
Statin Prescribed at Discharge	333	99%	98%	98%

NOTE: Hospital profiles are in alphabetical order by state, then city, then hospital within the city; Rankings exclude hospitals with less than 25 cases except for patient surveys which excludes hospitals with less than 100 cases; (a) 100-299 cases; (1) The number of cases/patients is too few to report; (2) Data submitted were based on a sample of cases/patients; (3) Results are based on a shorter time period than required; (4) Data suppressed by CMS for one or more quarters; (5) Results are not available for this reporting period; (6) Fewer than 100 patients completed the HCAHPS survey; (7) No cases met the criteria for this measure; (8) The lower limit of the confidence interval cannot be calculated if the number of observed infections equals zero; (9) No data are available from the state/territory for this reporting period; (10) The scores shown reflect fewer than 50 completed surveys; (11) There were discrepancies in the data collection process; (12) This measure does not apply to this hospital for this reporting period; (13) Results cannot be calculated for this reporting period; (14) The results for this state are combined with nearby states to protect confidentiality; Please refer to the User's Guide for a full explanation of data.

Measure	Cases	This Hosp.	State Avg.	U.S. Avg.
Heart Failure Care				
ACE Inhibitor or ARB for LVSD	113	100%	97%	97%
Discharge Instructions Given	331	96%	96%	94%
Evaluation of LVS Function	424	100%	100%	99%
Medicare Spending				
Medicare Spending per Patient (ratio)	-	0.96	1.01	0.98
Pneumonia Care				
Appropriate Initial Antibiotic Given	288	97%	96%	95%
Blood Culture Timing	501	99%	98%	98%
Pregnancy and Delivery Care				
Newborn Deliveries Scheduled Early	153	1%	5%	6%
Preventive Care				
Immunization for Influenza[2]	578	88%	93%	90%
Immunization for Pneumonia[2]	735	93%	94%	92%
Stroke Care				
Anticoagulation Therapy for Atrial Fibrillation[2]	13	100%	95%	95%
Antithrombotic Therapy Timing[2]	116	100%	98%	98%
Assessed for Rehabilitation[2]	116	99%	98%	97%
Discharged on Antithrombotic Therapy[2]	114	100%	99%	99%
Discharged on Statin Medication[2]	99	99%	95%	94%
Thrombolytic Therapy Timing[1,2]	-	-	65%	66%
Venous Thromboembolism Prophylaxis[2]	122	98%	95%	94%
Written Stroke Educational Materials Given[2]	76	99%	92%	88%
Surgical Care Improvement Project				
Appropriate Beta Blocker Usage[2]	208	100%	98%	98%
Appropriate VTP Within 24 Hours[2]	754	100%	98%	98%
Controlled Postoperative Blood Glucose[2]	113	99%	97%	97%
Perioperative Temperature Management[2]	831	100%	100%	100%
Prophylactic Antibiotic Selection[2]	727	100%	99%	99%
Prophylactic Antibiotic Selection (Outpatient)	228	98%	98%	98%
Prophylactic Antibiotic Stopped[2]	717	100%	98%	98%
Prophylactic Antibiotic Timing[2]	727	99%	99%	99%
Prophylactic Antibiotic Timing (Outpatient)	229	99%	97%	98%
Urinary Catheter Removal[2]	521	100%	97%	97%
Survey of Patients' Hospital Experiences				
Area Around Room 'Always' Quiet at Night	300+	53%	58%	61%
Doctors 'Always' Communicated Well	300+	77%	80%	82%
Home Recovery Information Given	300+	84%	87%	85%
Hospital Given 9 or 10 on 10 Point Scale	300+	71%	72%	71%
Meds 'Always' Explained Before Given	300+	65%	64%	64%
Nurses 'Always' Communicated Well	300+	80%	81%	79%
Pain 'Always' Well Controlled	300+	72%	71%	71%
Room and Bathroom 'Always' Clean	300+	69%	75%	73%
Timely Help 'Always' Received	300+	67%	70%	68%
Would Definitely Recommend Hospital	300+	71%	71%	71%
Use of Medical Imaging				
Cardiac Imaging Stress Test before Surgery	264	5.7%	5.4%	5.3%
Combination Abdominal CT Scan	1,060	4.5%	7.1%	10.5%
Combination Brain/Sinus CT Scan	581	1.2%	2.8%	2.7%
Combination Chest CT Scan	699	0.0%	1.7%	2.7%
Follow-up Mammogram/Ultrasound	1,541	6.4%	8.7%	8.8%
Lumbar Spine MRI for Low Back Pain	275	34.5%	34.7%	37.2%

Trihealth Evendale Hospital

3155 Glendale Milford Road Phone: 513-454-2222
Cincinnati, OH 45241
Type: Acute Care Hospitals Emergency Services: No
Ownership: Voluntary non-profit - Private

Measure	Cases	This Hosp.	State Avg.	U.S. Avg.
Blood Clot Prevention and Treatment				
Anticoagulation Overlap Therapy[3,7]	-	-	93%	93%
ICU Venous Thromboembolism Prophylaxis[3,7]	-	-	93%	92%
Incidence of Potentially Preventable VTE[3,7]	-	-	6%	10%
UFH with Dosages/Platelet Monitoring[3,7]	-	-	98%	97%
Venous Thromboembolism Prophylaxis[1,3]	-	-	88%	85%
Warfarin Therapy Discharge Instructions[3,7]	-	-	79%	75%
Chest Pain/Possible Heart Attack Care				
Aspirin Given Within 24 Hours of Arrival[5]	-	-	97%	96%
Fibrinolytic Meds Within 30 Min. of Arrival[5]	-	-	44%	58%
Average Time to ECG (minutes)[5]	-	-	6	7
Average Time to Transfer (minutes)[5]	-	-	58	60
Children's Asthma Care				
Received Home Management Plan of Care	-	-	85%	88%
Received Reliever Medication	-	-	100%	100%
Received Systemic Corticosteroids	-	-	100%	100%
Emergency Department				
Admittance Decision Time (minutes)[3,7]	-	-	90	98
Head CT Results Within 45 Min. of Arrival[5]	-	-	63%	57%
Patients Who Left ER Before Being Seen[5]	-	-	2%	2%
Time from ER Arrival to Admit. (minutes)[3,7]	-	-	265	274
Time from ER Arrival to Discharge (minutes)[5]	-	-	128	134
Time in ER Before Being Evaluated (minutes)[5]	-	-	22	26
Time to Pain Meds for Fractures (minutes)[5]	-	-	54	57
Heart Attack Care				
Aspirin Given at Discharge[5]	-	-	99%	99%
Fibrinolytic Meds Within 30 Min. of Arrival[5]	-	-	80%	54%
PCI Within 90 Minutes of Arrival[5]	-	-	97%	96%
Statin Prescribed at Discharge[5]	-	-	98%	98%
Heart Failure Care				
ACE Inhibitor or ARB for LVSD[5]	-	-	97%	97%
Discharge Instructions Given[5]	-	-	96%	94%
Evaluation of LVS Function[5]	-	-	100%	99%
Medicare Spending				
Medicare Spending per Patient (ratio)	-	-	1.01	0.98
Pneumonia Care				
Appropriate Initial Antibiotic Given[5]	-	-	96%	95%
Blood Culture Timing[5]	-	-	98%	98%
Pregnancy and Delivery Care				
Newborn Deliveries Scheduled Early[3,7]	-	-	5%	6%
Preventive Care				
Immunization for Influenza[5]	-	-	93%	90%
Immunization for Pneumonia[2,3]	199	97%	94%	92%
Stroke Care				
Anticoagulation Therapy for Atrial Fibrillation[5]	-	-	95%	95%
Antithrombotic Therapy Timing[5]	-	-	98%	98%
Assessed for Rehabilitation[5]	-	-	98%	97%
Discharged on Antithrombotic Therapy[5]	-	-	99%	99%
Discharged on Statin Medication[5]	-	-	95%	94%
Thrombolytic Therapy Timing[5]	-	-	65%	66%
Venous Thromboembolism Prophylaxis[5]	-	-	95%	94%
Written Stroke Educational Materials Given[5]	-	-	92%	88%
Surgical Care Improvement Project				
Appropriate Beta Blocker Usage[3]	62	98%	98%	98%
Appropriate VTP Within 24 Hours[3]	177	100%	98%	98%
Controlled Postoperative Blood Glucose[3,7]	-	-	97%	97%
Perioperative Temperature Management[3]	232	100%	100%	100%
Prophylactic Antibiotic Selection[3]	205	100%	99%	99%
Prophylactic Antibiotic Selection (Outpatient)[5]	-	-	98%	98%
Prophylactic Antibiotic Stopped[3]	205	100%	98%	98%
Prophylactic Antibiotic Timing[3]	205	99%	99%	99%
Prophylactic Antibiotic Timing (Outpatient)[5]	-	-	97%	98%
Urinary Catheter Removal[3]	128	100%	97%	97%
Survey of Patients' Hospital Experiences				
Area Around Room 'Always' Quiet at Night[5]	-	-	58%	61%
Doctors 'Always' Communicated Well[5]	-	-	80%	82%
Home Recovery Information Given[5]	-	-	87%	85%
Hospital Given 9 or 10 on 10 Point Scale[5]	-	-	72%	71%
Meds 'Always' Explained Before Given[5]	-	-	64%	64%
Nurses 'Always' Communicated Well[5]	-	-	81%	79%
Pain 'Always' Well Controlled[5]	-	-	71%	71%
Room and Bathroom 'Always' Clean[5]	-	-	75%	73%
Timely Help 'Always' Received[5]	-	-	70%	68%
Would Definitely Recommend Hospital[5]	-	-	71%	71%
Use of Medical Imaging				
Cardiac Imaging Stress Test before Surgery[7]	-	-	5.4%	5.3%
Combination Abdominal CT Scan[1]	-	-	7.1%	10.5%
Combination Brain/Sinus CT Scan[1]	-	-	2.8%	2.7%
Combination Chest CT Scan[1]	-	-	1.7%	2.7%
Follow-up Mammogram/Ultrasound[7]	-	-	8.7%	8.8%
Lumbar Spine MRI for Low Back Pain[1]	-	-	34.7%	37.2%

University of Cincinnati Medical Center

234 Goodman Street Phone: 513-584-1000
Cincinnati, OH 45219
URL: www.universityhospitalcincinnati.com
Type: Acute Care Hospitals Emergency Services: Yes
Ownership: Voluntary non-profit - Private
Key Personnel:
CEO/President. . . . . Lee Ann Liska
Chief of Medical Staff . . . . Keith Wilson, MD

Measure	Cases	This Hosp.	State Avg.	U.S. Avg.
Blood Clot Prevention and Treatment				
Anticoagulation Overlap Therapy[2]	188	100%	93%	93%
ICU Venous Thromboembolism Prophylaxis[2]	110	97%	93%	92%
Incidence of Potentially Preventable VTE[2]	112	1%	6%	10%
UFH with Dosages/Platelet Monitoring[2]	201	100%	98%	97%
Venous Thromboembolism Prophylaxis[2]	333	90%	88%	85%
Warfarin Therapy Discharge Instructions[2]	125	87%	79%	75%
Chest Pain/Possible Heart Attack Care				
Aspirin Given Within 24 Hours of Arrival[3,7]	-	-	97%	96%
Fibrinolytic Meds Within 30 Min. of Arrival[5]	-	-	44%	58%
Average Time to ECG (minutes)[3,7]	-	-	6	7
Average Time to Transfer (minutes)[5]	-	-	58	60
Children's Asthma Care				
Received Home Management Plan of Care	-	-	85%	88%
Received Reliever Medication	-	-	100%	100%
Received Systemic Corticosteroids	-	-	100%	100%
Emergency Department				
Admittance Decision Time (minutes)[2]	574	105	90	98
Head CT Results Within 45 Min. of Arrival[7]	-	-	63%	57%
Patients Who Left ER Before Being Seen	83,638	5%	2%	2%
Time from ER Arrival to Admit. (minutes)[2]	583	370	265	274
Time from ER Arrival to Discharge (minutes)	361	177	128	134
Time in ER Before Being Evaluated (minutes)	400	29	22	26
Time to Pain Meds for Fractures (minutes)	55	49	54	57
Heart Attack Care				
Aspirin Given at Discharge	272	99%	99%	99%
Fibrinolytic Meds Within 30 Min. of Arrival[7]	-	-	80%	54%
PCI Within 90 Minutes of Arrival	40	92%	97%	96%
Statin Prescribed at Discharge	259	97%	98%	98%
Heart Failure Care				
ACE Inhibitor or ARB for LVSD	259	100%	97%	97%
Discharge Instructions Given	473	89%	96%	94%
Evaluation of LVS Function	554	100%	100%	99%
Medicare Spending				
Medicare Spending per Patient (ratio)	-	1.00	1.01	0.98
Pneumonia Care				
Appropriate Initial Antibiotic Given	136	99%	96%	95%
Blood Culture Timing	295	98%	98%	98%
Pregnancy and Delivery Care				
Newborn Deliveries Scheduled Early	121	8%	5%	6%
Preventive Care				
Immunization for Influenza[2]	571	67%	93%	90%
Immunization for Pneumonia[2]	624	80%	94%	92%
Stroke Care				
Anticoagulation Therapy for Atrial Fibrillation[2]	13	92%	95%	95%
Antithrombotic Therapy Timing[2]	80	94%	98%	98%
Assessed for Rehabilitation[2]	128	96%	98%	97%
Discharged on Antithrombotic Therapy[2]	88	99%	99%	99%
Discharged on Statin Medication[2]	66	100%	95%	94%
Thrombolytic Therapy Timing[1,2]	-	-	65%	66%
Venous Thromboembolism Prophylaxis[2]	137	99%	95%	94%
Written Stroke Educational Materials Given[2]	58	81%	92%	88%
Surgical Care Improvement Project				
Appropriate Beta Blocker Usage[2]	261	99%	98%	98%
Appropriate VTP Within 24 Hours[2]	577	100%	98%	98%
Controlled Postoperative Blood Glucose[2]	126	96%	97%	97%
Perioperative Temperature Management[2]	653	100%	100%	100%
Prophylactic Antibiotic Selection[2]	515	100%	99%	99%
Prophylactic Antibiotic Selection (Outpatient)	525	98%	98%	98%
Prophylactic Antibiotic Stopped[2]	497	97%	98%	98%
Prophylactic Antibiotic Timing[2]	517	98%	99%	99%
Prophylactic Antibiotic Timing (Outpatient)	502	97%	97%	98%
Urinary Catheter Removal[2]	254	96%	97%	97%

NOTE: Hospital profiles are in alphabetical order by state, then city, then hospital within the city; Rankings exclude hospitals with less than 25 cases except for patient surveys which excludes hospitals with less than 100 cases; (a) 100-299 cases; (1) The number of cases/patients is too few to report; (2) Data submitted were based on a sample of cases/patients; (3) Results are based on a shorter time period than required; (4) Data suppressed by CMS for one or more quarters; (5) Results are not available for this reporting period; (6) Fewer than 100 patients completed the HCAHPS survey; (7) No cases met the criteria for this measure; (8) The lower limit of the confidence interval cannot be calculated if the number of observed infections equals zero; (9) No data are available from the state/territory for this reporting period; (10) The scores shown reflect fewer than 50 completed surveys; (11) There were discrepancies in the data collection process; (12) This measure does not apply to this hospital for this reporting period; (13) Results cannot be calculated for this reporting period; (14) The results for this state are combined with nearby states to protect confidentiality; Please refer to the User's Guide for a full explanation of data.

Measure	Cases	This Hosp.	State Avg.	U.S. Avg.
Survey of Patients' Hospital Experiences				
Area Around Room 'Always' Quiet at Night	300+	59%	58%	61%
Doctors 'Always' Communicated Well	300+	75%	80%	82%
Home Recovery Information Given	300+	83%	87%	85%
Hospital Given 9 or 10 on 10 Point Scale	300+	64%	72%	71%
Meds 'Always' Explained Before Given	300+	59%	64%	64%
Nurses 'Always' Communicated Well	300+	74%	81%	79%
Pain 'Always' Well Controlled	300+	67%	71%	71%
Room and Bathroom 'Always' Clean	300+	61%	75%	73%
Timely Help 'Always' Received	300+	56%	70%	68%
Would Definitely Recommend Hospital	300+	64%	71%	71%
Use of Medical Imaging				
Cardiac Imaging Stress Test before Surgery	393	5.3%	5.4%	5.3%
Combination Abdominal CT Scan	925	5.1%	7.1%	10.5%
Combination Brain/Sinus CT Scan	593	1.7%	2.8%	2.7%
Combination Chest CT Scan	1,213	0.8%	1.7%	2.7%
Follow-up Mammogram/Ultrasound	1,355	11.8%	8.7%	8.8%
Lumbar Spine MRI for Low Back Pain	107	38.3%	34.7%	37.2%

Berger Hospital

600 North Pickaway Street
Circleville, OH 43113
Phone: 740-420-8585
Fax: 740-474-1897
E-mail: pr@bergerhealth.com
URL: www.bergerhealth.com
Type: Acute Care Hospitals
Emergency Services: Yes
Ownership: Government - Local
Beds: 91

Key Personnel:

Emergency Room . . . . Bobby Dale, MD
Radiology. . . . . Laurian Dean, MD
Infection Control. . . . . Marilyn Frost, RN
Chief of Medical Staff . . . . Charles Hedges, MD
Intensive Care Unit. . . . . Joan King, RN
Operating Room. . . . . Bobbin Peters, RN
CEO/President. . . . . Larry W Thornhill
Quality Assurance . . . . Paul Westbrock

Measure	Cases	This Hosp.	State Avg.	U.S. Avg.
Blood Clot Prevention and Treatment				
Anticoagulation Overlap Therapy[2]	19	100%	93%	93%
ICU Venous Thromboembolism Prophylaxis[2]	54	100%	93%	92%
Incidence of Potentially Preventable VTE[1,2]	-	-	6%	10%
UFH with Dosages/Platelet Monitoring[1,2]	-	-	98%	97%
Venous Thromboembolism Prophylaxis[2]	128	99%	88%	85%
Warfarin Therapy Discharge Instructions[2]	13	100%	79%	75%
Chest Pain/Possible Heart Attack Care				
Aspirin Given Within 24 Hours of Arrival	127	100%	97%	96%
Fibrinolytic Meds Within 30 Min. of Arrival[7]	-	-	44%	58%
Average Time to ECG (minutes)	127	10	6	7
Average Time to Transfer (minutes)	11	52	58	60
Children's Asthma Care				
Received Home Management Plan of Care	-	-	85%	88%
Received Reliever Medication	-	-	100%	100%
Received Systemic Corticosteroids	-	-	100%	100%
Emergency Department				
Admittance Decision Time (minutes)[2]	186	170	90	98
Head CT Results Within 45 Min. of Arrival	17	76%	63%	57%
Patients Who Left ER Before Being Seen	31,657	1%	2%	2%
Time from ER Arrival to Admit. (minutes)[2]	301	294	265	274
Time from ER Arrival to Discharge (minutes)	366	112	128	134
Time in ER Before Being Evaluated (minutes)	401	30	22	26
Time to Pain Meds for Fractures (minutes)	75	61	54	57
Heart Attack Care				
Aspirin Given at Discharge[1]	-	-	99%	99%
Fibrinolytic Meds Within 30 Min. of Arrival[7]	-	-	80%	54%
PCI Within 90 Minutes of Arrival[7]	-	-	97%	96%
Statin Prescribed at Discharge[1]	-	-	98%	98%
Heart Failure Care				
ACE Inhibitor or ARB for LVSD[1]	-	-	97%	97%
Discharge Instructions Given	57	100%	96%	94%
Evaluation of LVS Function	74	100%	100%	99%
Medicare Spending				
Medicare Spending per Patient (ratio)	-	1.02	1.01	0.98
Pneumonia Care				
Appropriate Initial Antibiotic Given	65	100%	96%	95%
Blood Culture Timing	111	99%	98%	98%
Pregnancy and Delivery Care				
Newborn Deliveries Scheduled Early	38	0%	5%	6%
Preventive Care				
Immunization for Influenza[2]	289	99%	93%	90%
Immunization for Pneumonia[2]	350	100%	94%	92%
Stroke Care				
Anticoagulation Therapy for Atrial Fibrillation[1,3]	-	-	95%	95%
Antithrombotic Therapy Timing[1,3]	-	-	98%	98%
Assessed for Rehabilitation[1,3]	-	-	98%	97%
Discharged on Antithrombotic Therapy[1,3]	-	-	99%	99%
Discharged on Statin Medication[1,3]	-	-	95%	94%
Thrombolytic Therapy Timing[3,7]	-	-	65%	66%
Venous Thromboembolism Prophylaxis[1,3]	-	-	95%	94%
Written Stroke Educational Materials Given[1,3]	-	-	92%	88%
Surgical Care Improvement Project				
Appropriate Beta Blocker Usage	104	100%	98%	98%
Appropriate VTP Within 24 Hours	289	100%	98%	98%
Controlled Postoperative Blood Glucose[7]	-	-	97%	97%
Perioperative Temperature Management	347	100%	100%	100%
Prophylactic Antibiotic Selection	266	100%	99%	99%
Prophylactic Antibiotic Selection (Outpatient)	21	100%	98%	98%
Prophylactic Antibiotic Stopped	260	100%	98%	98%
Prophylactic Antibiotic Timing	266	100%	99%	99%
Prophylactic Antibiotic Timing (Outpatient)	21	100%	97%	98%
Urinary Catheter Removal	227	100%	97%	97%
Survey of Patients' Hospital Experiences				
Area Around Room 'Always' Quiet at Night	300+	52%	58%	61%
Doctors 'Always' Communicated Well	300+	80%	80%	82%
Home Recovery Information Given	300+	88%	87%	85%
Hospital Given 9 or 10 on 10 Point Scale	300+	66%	72%	71%
Meds 'Always' Explained Before Given	300+	61%	64%	64%
Nurses 'Always' Communicated Well	300+	78%	81%	79%
Pain 'Always' Well Controlled	300+	65%	71%	71%
Room and Bathroom 'Always' Clean	300+	70%	75%	73%
Timely Help 'Always' Received	300+	66%	70%	68%
Would Definitely Recommend Hospital	300+	65%	71%	71%
Use of Medical Imaging				
Cardiac Imaging Stress Test before Surgery	162	5.6%	5.4%	5.3%
Combination Abdominal CT Scan	557	3.1%	7.1%	10.5%
Combination Brain/Sinus CT Scan	528	2.1%	2.8%	2.7%
Combination Chest CT Scan	295	0.3%	1.7%	2.7%
Follow-up Mammogram/Ultrasound	552	11.2%	8.7%	8.8%
Lumbar Spine MRI for Low Back Pain	59	45.8%	34.7%	37.2%

Cleveland - Wade Park VA Medical Center

10701 East Blvd
Cleveland, OH 44106
Phone: 216-791-3800
Fax: 440-838-6017
URL: www.cleveland.va.gov
Type: Acute Care - VA
Emergency Services: No
Ownership: Government Federal
Beds: 688

Key Personnel:

Operating Room. . . . . Donald Benson, MD
Coronary Care . . . . Verena Briley-Hudson, RN
Chief of Medical Staff. . . . . Susan A. Fuehrer
CEO/President. . . . . William D Montatue
Radiology. . . . . MH Naheedy, MD
Quality Assurance . . . . Dora Rice, RN
Infection Control. . . . . Luis Rice

Measure	Cases	This Hosp.	State Avg.	U.S. Avg.
Blood Clot Prevention and Treatment				
Anticoagulation Overlap Therapy	-	-	93%	93%
ICU Venous Thromboembolism Prophylaxis	-	-	93%	92%
Incidence of Potentially Preventable VTE	-	-	6%	10%
UFH with Dosages/Platelet Monitoring	-	-	98%	97%
Venous Thromboembolism Prophylaxis	-	-	88%	85%
Warfarin Therapy Discharge Instructions	-	-	79%	75%
Chest Pain/Possible Heart Attack Care				
Aspirin Given Within 24 Hours of Arrival	-	-	97%	96%
Fibrinolytic Meds Within 30 Min. of Arrival	-	-	44%	58%
Average Time to ECG (minutes)	-	-	6	7
Average Time to Transfer (minutes)	-	-	58	60
Children's Asthma Care				
Received Home Management Plan of Care	-	-	85%	88%
Received Reliever Medication	-	-	100%	100%
Received Systemic Corticosteroids	-	-	100%	100%
Emergency Department				
Admittance Decision Time (minutes)	-	-	90	98
Head CT Results Within 45 Min. of Arrival	-	-	63%	57%
Patients Who Left ER Before Being Seen	-	-	2%	2%
Time from ER Arrival to Admit. (minutes)	-	-	265	274
Time from ER Arrival to Discharge (minutes)	-	-	128	134
Time in ER Before Being Evaluated (minutes)	-	-	22	26
Time to Pain Meds for Fractures (minutes)	-	-	54	57
Heart Attack Care				
Aspirin Given at Discharge	27	100%	99%	99%
Fibrinolytic Meds Within 30 Min. of Arrival[5]	-	-	80%	54%
PCI Within 90 Minutes of Arrival[1]	-	-	97%	96%
Statin Prescribed at Discharge	29	100%	98%	98%
Heart Failure Care				
ACE Inhibitor or ARB for LVSD	134	99%	97%	97%
Discharge Instructions Given	350	100%	96%	94%
Evaluation of LVS Function	392	100%	100%	99%
Medicare Spending				
Medicare Spending per Patient (ratio)	-	-	1.01	0.98
Pneumonia Care				
Appropriate Initial Antibiotic Given	41	93%	96%	95%
Blood Culture Timing	94	97%	98%	98%
Pregnancy and Delivery Care				
Newborn Deliveries Scheduled Early	-	-	5%	6%
Preventive Care				
Immunization for Influenza[5]	-	-	93%	90%
Immunization for Pneumonia[5]	-	-	94%	92%
Stroke Care				
Anticoagulation Therapy for Atrial Fibrillation	-	-	95%	95%
Antithrombotic Therapy Timing	-	-	98%	98%
Assessed for Rehabilitation	-	-	98%	97%
Discharged on Antithrombotic Therapy	-	-	99%	99%
Discharged on Statin Medication	-	-	95%	94%
Thrombolytic Therapy Timing	-	-	65%	66%
Venous Thromboembolism Prophylaxis	-	-	95%	94%
Written Stroke Educational Materials Given	-	-	92%	88%
Surgical Care Improvement Project				
Appropriate Beta Blocker Usage[2]	226	96%	98%	98%
Appropriate VTP Within 24 Hours[2]	273	98%	98%	98%
Controlled Postoperative Blood Glucose[2]	114	98%	97%	97%
Perioperative Temperature Management[2]	470	99%	100%	100%
Prophylactic Antibiotic Selection	304	98%	99%	99%
Prophylactic Antibiotic Selection (Outpatient)	-	-	98%	98%
Prophylactic Antibiotic Stopped	297	96%	98%	98%
Prophylactic Antibiotic Timing	305	95%	99%	99%
Prophylactic Antibiotic Timing (Outpatient)	-	-	97%	98%
Urinary Catheter Removal[2]	294	98%	97%	97%
Survey of Patients' Hospital Experiences				
Area Around Room 'Always' Quiet at Night	-	-	58%	61%
Doctors 'Always' Communicated Well	-	-	80%	82%
Home Recovery Information Given	-	-	87%	85%
Hospital Given 9 or 10 on 10 Point Scale	-	-	72%	71%
Meds 'Always' Explained Before Given	-	-	64%	64%
Nurses 'Always' Communicated Well	-	-	81%	79%
Pain 'Always' Well Controlled	-	-	71%	71%
Room and Bathroom 'Always' Clean	-	-	75%	73%
Timely Help 'Always' Received	-	-	70%	68%
Would Definitely Recommend Hospital	-	-	71%	71%
Use of Medical Imaging				
Cardiac Imaging Stress Test before Surgery	-	-	5.4%	5.3%
Combination Abdominal CT Scan	-	-	7.1%	10.5%
Combination Brain/Sinus CT Scan	-	-	2.8%	2.7%
Combination Chest CT Scan	-	-	1.7%	2.7%
Follow-up Mammogram/Ultrasound	-	-	8.7%	8.8%
Lumbar Spine MRI for Low Back Pain	-	-	34.7%	37.2%

NOTE: Hospital profiles are in alphabetical order by state, then city, then hospital within the city; Rankings exclude hospitals with less than 25 cases except for patient surveys which excludes hospitals with less than 100 cases; (a) 100-299 cases; (1) The number of cases/patients is too few to report; (2) Data submitted were based on a sample of cases/patients; (3) Results are based on a shorter time period than required; (4) Data suppressed by CMS for one or more quarters; (5) Results are not available for this reporting period; (6) Fewer than 100 patients completed the HCAHPS survey; (7) No cases met the criteria for this measure; (8) The lower limit of the confidence interval cannot be calculated if the number of observed infections equals zero; (9) No data are available from the state/territory for this reporting period; (10) The scores shown reflect fewer than 50 completed surveys; (11) There were discrepancies in the data collection process; (12) This measure does not apply to this hospital for this reporting period; (13) Results cannot be calculated for this reporting period; (14) The results for this state are combined with nearby states to protect confidentiality; Please refer to the User's Guide for a full explanation of data.

Cleveland Clinic

9500 Euclid Avenue
Cleveland, OH 44195
Phone: 216-444-2200
Fax: 216-445-7758
URL: www.clevelandclinic.org
Type: Acute Care Hospitals
Emergency Services: Yes
Ownership: Voluntary non-profit - Private
Beds: 1,113

Key Personnel:
Radiology. . . . . Gregory P Borkowski, MD
CEO/President. . . . . Delos M Cosgrove, MD
Chief of Medical Staff. . . . . Marc Harrison, MD
Quality Assurance . . . . J Michael Henderson, MD
Infection Control. . . . . David L Longworth, MD
Operating Room. . . . . Allan Siperstein, MD
Pediatric Ambulatory Care . . . . . . Robert Wyllie, MD
Pediatric In-Patient Care . . . . Robert Wyllie, MD

Measure	Cases	This Hosp.	State Avg.	U.S. Avg.
Blood Clot Prevention and Treatment				
Anticoagulation Overlap Therapy[2]	400	98%	93%	93%
ICU Venous Thromboembolism Prophylaxis[2]	84	98%	93%	92%
Incidence of Potentially Preventable VTE[2]	168	2%	6%	10%
UFH with Dosages/Platelet Monitoring[2]	444	100%	98%	97%
Venous Thromboembolism Prophylaxis[2]	347	96%	88%	85%
Warfarin Therapy Discharge Instructions[2]	237	89%	79%	75%
Chest Pain/Possible Heart Attack Care				
Aspirin Given Within 24 Hours of Arrival	190	96%	97%	96%
Fibrinolytic Meds Within 30 Min. of Arrival[7]	-	-	44%	58%
Average Time to ECG (minutes)	197	6	6	7
Average Time to Transfer (minutes)[1]	-	-	58	60
Children's Asthma Care				
Received Home Management Plan of Care	74	99%	85%	88%
Received Reliever Medication	75	100%	100%	100%
Received Systemic Corticosteroids	74	100%	100%	100%
Emergency Department				
Admittance Decision Time (minutes)[2]	227	102	90	98
Head CT Results Within 45 Min. of Arrival	11	91%	63%	57%
Patients Who Left ER Before Being Seen	82,229	2%	2%	2%
Time from ER Arrival to Admit. (minutes)[2]	228	304	265	274
Time from ER Arrival to Discharge (minutes)	294	131	128	134
Time in ER Before Being Evaluated (minutes)	417	11	22	26
Time to Pain Meds for Fractures (minutes)	194	46	54	57
Heart Attack Care				
Aspirin Given at Discharge	868	100%	99%	99%
Fibrinolytic Meds Within 30 Min. of Arrival[7]	-	-	80%	54%
PCI Within 90 Minutes of Arrival	13	92%	97%	96%
Statin Prescribed at Discharge	834	100%	98%	98%
Heart Failure Care				
ACE Inhibitor or ARB for LVSD[2]	287	99%	97%	97%
Discharge Instructions Given[2]	712	94%	96%	94%
Evaluation of LVS Function[2]	858	100%	100%	99%
Medicare Spending				
Medicare Spending per Patient (ratio)	-	0.99	1.01	0.98
Pneumonia Care				
Appropriate Initial Antibiotic Given	84	94%	96%	95%
Blood Culture Timing	176	95%	98%	98%
Pregnancy and Delivery Care				
Newborn Deliveries Scheduled Early[1]	-	-	5%	6%
Preventive Care				
Immunization for Influenza[2]	577	96%	93%	90%
Immunization for Pneumonia[2]	747	95%	94%	92%
Stroke Care				
Anticoagulation Therapy for Atrial Fibrillation[2]	34	100%	95%	95%
Antithrombotic Therapy Timing[2]	180	96%	98%	98%
Assessed for Rehabilitation[2]	333	98%	98%	97%
Discharged on Antithrombotic Therapy[2]	221	100%	99%	99%
Discharged on Statin Medication[2]	152	99%	95%	94%
Thrombolytic Therapy Timing[1,2]	-	-	65%	66%
Venous Thromboembolism Prophylaxis[2]	349	100%	95%	94%
Written Stroke Educational Materials Given[2]	125	98%	92%	88%
Surgical Care Improvement Project				
Appropriate Beta Blocker Usage[2]	356	99%	98%	98%
Appropriate VTP Within 24 Hours[2]	447	99%	98%	98%
Controlled Postoperative Blood Glucose[2]	253	96%	97%	97%
Perioperative Temperature Management[2]	625	100%	100%	100%
Prophylactic Antibiotic Selection[2]	570	99%	99%	99%
Prophylactic Antibiotic Selection (Outpatient)	1,080	100%	98%	98%
Prophylactic Antibiotic Stopped[2]	554	97%	98%	98%
Prophylactic Antibiotic Timing[2]	570	99%	99%	99%
Prophylactic Antibiotic Timing (Outpatient)	563	97%	97%	98%
Urinary Catheter Removal[2]	381	98%	97%	97%
Survey of Patients' Hospital Experiences				
Area Around Room 'Always' Quiet at Night	300+	57%	58%	61%
Doctors 'Always' Communicated Well	300+	82%	80%	82%
Home Recovery Information Given	300+	90%	87%	85%
Hospital Given 9 or 10 on 10 Point Scale	300+	84%	72%	71%
Meds 'Always' Explained Before Given	300+	66%	64%	64%
Nurses 'Always' Communicated Well	300+	83%	81%	79%
Pain 'Always' Well Controlled	300+	72%	71%	71%
Room and Bathroom 'Always' Clean	300+	78%	75%	73%
Timely Help 'Always' Received	300+	68%	70%	68%
Would Definitely Recommend Hospital	300+	87%	71%	71%
Use of Medical Imaging				
Cardiac Imaging Stress Test before Surgery	4,179	6.7%	5.4%	5.3%
Combination Abdominal CT Scan	5,813	13.0%	7.1%	10.5%
Combination Brain/Sinus CT Scan	2,131	1.7%	2.8%	2.7%
Combination Chest CT Scan	6,539	0.1%	1.7%	2.7%
Follow-up Mammogram/Ultrasound	9,962	9.3%	8.7%	8.8%
Lumbar Spine MRI for Low Back Pain	661	31.9%	34.7%	37.2%

Fairview Hospital

18101 Lorain Avenue
Cleveland, OH 44111
Phone: 216-476-7000
Fax: 216-476-7017
URL: www.fairviewhospital.org
Type: Acute Care Hospitals
Emergency Services: Yes
Ownership: Voluntary non-profit - Private
Beds: 511

Key Personnel:
Radiology. . . . . William Bishop, MD
Infection Control. . . . . KV Gopal, MD
Operating Room. . . . . Susan Keane, RN
Pediatric Ambulatory Care . . . . . . Sudhir Mehta, MD
Pediatric In-Patient Care . . . . Sudhir Mehta, MD
Quality Assurance . . . . Martha Mugford
CEO/President. . . . . Janice Murphy
Chief of Medical Staff. . . . . Michael Waggoner, MD

Measure	Cases	This Hosp.	State Avg.	U.S. Avg.
Blood Clot Prevention and Treatment				
Anticoagulation Overlap Therapy[2]	130	93%	93%	93%
ICU Venous Thromboembolism Prophylaxis[2]	116	97%	93%	92%
Incidence of Potentially Preventable VTE[2]	25	16%	6%	10%
UFH with Dosages/Platelet Monitoring[2]	82	98%	98%	97%
Venous Thromboembolism Prophylaxis[2]	340	91%	88%	85%
Warfarin Therapy Discharge Instructions[2]	103	86%	79%	75%
Chest Pain/Possible Heart Attack Care				
Aspirin Given Within 24 Hours of Arrival[1,3]	-	-	97%	96%
Fibrinolytic Meds Within 30 Min. of Arrival[3,7]	-	-	44%	58%
Average Time to ECG (minutes)[1,3]	-	-	6	7
Average Time to Transfer (minutes)[3,7]	-	-	58	60
Children's Asthma Care				
Received Home Management Plan of Care	-	-	85%	88%
Received Reliever Medication	-	-	100%	100%
Received Systemic Corticosteroids	-	-	100%	100%
Emergency Department				
Admittance Decision Time (minutes)[2]	575	98	90	98
Head CT Results Within 45 Min. of Arrival[1]	-	-	63%	57%
Patients Who Left ER Before Being Seen	78,084	2%	2%	2%
Time from ER Arrival to Admit. (minutes)[2]	576	289	265	274
Time from ER Arrival to Discharge (minutes)	407	141	128	134
Time in ER Before Being Evaluated (minutes)	446	20	22	26
Time to Pain Meds for Fractures (minutes)	264	42	54	57
Heart Attack Care				
Aspirin Given at Discharge	285	99%	99%	99%
Fibrinolytic Meds Within 30 Min. of Arrival[7]	-	-	80%	54%
PCI Within 90 Minutes of Arrival	56	91%	97%	96%
Statin Prescribed at Discharge	275	100%	98%	98%
Heart Failure Care				
ACE Inhibitor or ARB for LVSD[2]	161	99%	97%	97%
Discharge Instructions Given[2]	425	100%	96%	94%
Evaluation of LVS Function[2]	564	100%	100%	99%
Medicare Spending				
Medicare Spending per Patient (ratio)	-	1.03	1.01	0.98
Pneumonia Care				
Appropriate Initial Antibiotic Given[2]	167	96%	96%	95%
Blood Culture Timing[2]	307	97%	98%	98%
Pregnancy and Delivery Care				
Newborn Deliveries Scheduled Early[2]	50	6%	5%	6%
Preventive Care				
Immunization for Influenza[2]	555	98%	93%	90%
Immunization for Pneumonia[2]	624	95%	94%	92%
Stroke Care				
Anticoagulation Therapy for Atrial Fibrillation	14	100%	95%	95%
Antithrombotic Therapy Timing	122	98%	98%	98%
Assessed for Rehabilitation	145	98%	98%	97%
Discharged on Antithrombotic Therapy	126	99%	99%	99%
Discharged on Statin Medication	104	97%	95%	94%
Thrombolytic Therapy Timing[1]	-	-	65%	66%
Venous Thromboembolism Prophylaxis	151	97%	95%	94%
Written Stroke Educational Materials Given	62	100%	92%	88%
Surgical Care Improvement Project				
Appropriate Beta Blocker Usage[2]	209	99%	98%	98%
Appropriate VTP Within 24 Hours[2]	316	98%	98%	98%
Controlled Postoperative Blood Glucose[2]	108	100%	97%	97%
Perioperative Temperature Management[2]	397	100%	100%	100%
Prophylactic Antibiotic Selection[2]	369	99%	99%	99%
Prophylactic Antibiotic Selection (Outpatient)	923	99%	98%	98%
Prophylactic Antibiotic Stopped[2]	362	99%	98%	98%
Prophylactic Antibiotic Timing[2]	369	99%	99%	99%
Prophylactic Antibiotic Timing (Outpatient)	832	100%	97%	98%
Urinary Catheter Removal[2]	329	98%	97%	97%
Survey of Patients' Hospital Experiences				
Area Around Room 'Always' Quiet at Night	300+	60%	58%	61%
Doctors 'Always' Communicated Well	300+	79%	80%	82%
Home Recovery Information Given	300+	85%	87%	85%
Hospital Given 9 or 10 on 10 Point Scale	300+	74%	72%	71%
Meds 'Always' Explained Before Given	300+	64%	64%	64%
Nurses 'Always' Communicated Well	300+	80%	81%	79%
Pain 'Always' Well Controlled	300+	70%	71%	71%
Room and Bathroom 'Always' Clean	300+	83%	75%	73%
Timely Help 'Always' Received	300+	69%	70%	68%
Would Definitely Recommend Hospital	300+	77%	71%	71%
Use of Medical Imaging				
Cardiac Imaging Stress Test before Surgery	96	3.1%	5.4%	5.3%
Combination Abdominal CT Scan	1,033	4.4%	7.1%	10.5%
Combination Brain/Sinus CT Scan	693	2.9%	2.8%	2.7%
Combination Chest CT Scan	603	0.2%	1.7%	2.7%
Follow-up Mammogram/Ultrasound	1,433	11.9%	8.7%	8.8%
Lumbar Spine MRI for Low Back Pain[1]	-	-	34.7%	37.2%

Lutheran Hospital

1730 West 25th Street
Cleveland, OH 44113
Phone: 216-696-4300
Fax: 216-696-7397
URL: www.lutheranhospital.org
Type: Acute Care Hospitals
Emergency Services: Yes
Ownership: Voluntary non-profit - Private
Beds: 209

Key Personnel:
CEO/President. . . . . David F Perse
Operating Room. . . . . Bernard M Stulberg, MD

Measure	Cases	This Hosp.	State Avg.	U.S. Avg.
Blood Clot Prevention and Treatment				
Anticoagulation Overlap Therapy[2]	30	93%	93%	93%
ICU Venous Thromboembolism Prophylaxis[2]	46	100%	93%	92%
Incidence of Potentially Preventable VTE[1,2]	-	-	6%	10%
UFH with Dosages/Platelet Monitoring[2]	14	100%	98%	97%
Venous Thromboembolism Prophylaxis[2]	240	91%	88%	85%
Warfarin Therapy Discharge Instructions[2]	12	83%	79%	75%
Chest Pain/Possible Heart Attack Care				
Aspirin Given Within 24 Hours of Arrival[1]	-	-	97%	96%
Fibrinolytic Meds Within 30 Min. of Arrival[3,7]	-	-	44%	58%
Average Time to ECG (minutes)[1]	-	-	6	7
Average Time to Transfer (minutes)[1,3]	-	-	58	60
Children's Asthma Care				
Received Home Management Plan of Care	-	-	85%	88%
Received Reliever Medication	-	-	100%	100%

NOTE: Hospital profiles are in alphabetical order by state, then city, then hospital within the city; Rankings exclude hospitals with less than 25 cases except for patient surveys which excludes hospitals with less than 100 cases; (a) 100-299 cases; (1) The number of cases/patients is too few to report; (2) Data submitted were based on a sample of cases/patients; (3) Results are based on a shorter time period than required; (4) Data suppressed by CMS for one or more quarters; (5) Results are not available for this reporting period; (6) Fewer than 100 patients completed the HCAHPS survey; (7) No cases met the criteria for this measure; (8) The lower limit of the confidence interval cannot be calculated if the number of observed infections equals zero; (9) No data are available from the state/territory for this reporting period; (10) The scores shown reflect fewer than 50 completed surveys; (11) There were discrepancies in the data collection process; (12) This measure does not apply to this hospital for this reporting period; (13) Results cannot be calculated for this reporting period; (14) The results for this state are combined with nearby states to protect confidentiality; Please refer to the User's Guide for a full explanation of data.

Measure	Cases	This Hosp.	State Avg.	U.S. Avg.
Received Systemic Corticosteroids	-	-	100%	100%
Emergency Department				
Admittance Decision Time (minutes)[2]	145	86	90	98
Head CT Results Within 45 Min. of Arrival[1]	-	-	63%	57%
Patients Who Left ER Before Being Seen	26,918	2%	2%	2%
Time from ER Arrival to Admit. (minutes)[2]	145	297	265	274
Time from ER Arrival to Discharge (minutes)	373	128	128	134
Time in ER Before Being Evaluated (minutes)	421	16	22	26
Time to Pain Meds for Fractures (minutes)	42	69	54	57
Heart Attack Care				
Aspirin Given at Discharge[1]	-	-	99%	99%
Fibrinolytic Meds Within 30 Min. of Arrival[7]	-	-	80%	54%
PCI Within 90 Minutes of Arrival[7]	-	-	97%	96%
Statin Prescribed at Discharge[1]	-	-	98%	98%
Heart Failure Care				
ACE Inhibitor or ARB for LVSD	27	78%	97%	97%
Discharge Instructions Given	93	97%	96%	94%
Evaluation of LVS Function	116	99%	100%	99%
Medicare Spending				
Medicare Spending per Patient (ratio)	-	1.01	1.01	0.98
Pneumonia Care				
Appropriate Initial Antibiotic Given	37	97%	96%	95%
Blood Culture Timing	81	95%	98%	98%
Pregnancy and Delivery Care				
Newborn Deliveries Scheduled Early[7]	-	-	5%	6%
Preventive Care				
Immunization for Influenza[2]	446	95%	93%	90%
Immunization for Pneumonia[2]	586	94%	94%	92%
Stroke Care				
Anticoagulation Therapy for Atrial Fibrillation[1]	-	-	95%	95%
Antithrombotic Therapy Timing[1]	-	-	98%	98%
Assessed for Rehabilitation[1]	-	-	98%	97%
Discharged on Antithrombotic Therapy[1]	-	-	99%	99%
Discharged on Statin Medication[1]	-	-	95%	94%
Thrombolytic Therapy Timing[7]	-	-	65%	66%
Venous Thromboembolism Prophylaxis[1]	-	-	95%	94%
Written Stroke Educational Materials Given[1]	-	-	92%	88%
Surgical Care Improvement Project				
Appropriate Beta Blocker Usage[2]	82	98%	98%	98%
Appropriate VTP Within 24 Hours[2]	319	99%	98%	98%
Controlled Postoperative Blood Glucose[2,7]	-	-	97%	97%
Perioperative Temperature Management[2]	337	100%	100%	100%
Prophylactic Antibiotic Selection[2]	224	99%	99%	99%
Prophylactic Antibiotic Selection (Outpatient)	139	99%	98%	98%
Prophylactic Antibiotic Stopped[2]	222	100%	98%	98%
Prophylactic Antibiotic Timing[2]	224	100%	99%	99%
Prophylactic Antibiotic Timing (Outpatient)	139	100%	97%	98%
Urinary Catheter Removal[2]	303	100%	97%	97%
Survey of Patients' Hospital Experiences				
Area Around Room 'Always' Quiet at Night	300+	64%	58%	61%
Doctors 'Always' Communicated Well	300+	82%	80%	82%
Home Recovery Information Given	300+	91%	87%	85%
Hospital Given 9 or 10 on 10 Point Scale	300+	72%	72%	71%
Meds 'Always' Explained Before Given	300+	68%	64%	64%
Nurses 'Always' Communicated Well	300+	82%	81%	79%
Pain 'Always' Well Controlled	300+	70%	71%	71%
Room and Bathroom 'Always' Clean	300+	72%	75%	73%
Timely Help 'Always' Received	300+	68%	70%	68%
Would Definitely Recommend Hospital	300+	73%	71%	71%
Use of Medical Imaging				
Cardiac Imaging Stress Test before Surgery	98	4.1%	5.4%	5.3%
Combination Abdominal CT Scan	230	1.3%	7.1%	10.5%
Combination Brain/Sinus CT Scan[1]	-	-	2.8%	2.7%
Combination Chest CT Scan	56	0.0%	1.7%	2.7%
Follow-up Mammogram/Ultrasound	354	8.8%	8.7%	8.8%
Lumbar Spine MRI for Low Back Pain[1]	-	-	34.7%	37.2%

Metrohealth System

2500 Metrohealth Drive
Cleveland, OH 44109
Phone: 216-778-7089
Fax: 216-368-4678
URL: www.metrohealth.org
Type: Acute Care Hospitals
Emergency Services: Yes
Ownership: Voluntary non-profit - Other
Beds: 728

Key Personnel:
Quality Assurance . . . . Sandra Amin
Infection Control. . . . . Richard Blinkhorn, MD
CEO/President. . . . . Akram Boutros, MD
Chief of Medical Staff . . . . Alfred F. Connors, Jr., MD
Radiology. . . . . Robert Ferguson, MD
Operating Room. . . . . Mark A Malangoni, MD
Cardiac Laboratory. . . . . Norman Snow, MD
Pediatric In-Patient Care . . . . Margaret Stager, MD

Measure	Cases	This Hosp.	State Avg.	U.S. Avg.
Blood Clot Prevention and Treatment				
Anticoagulation Overlap Therapy[2]	116	98%	93%	93%
ICU Venous Thromboembolism Prophylaxis[2]	92	88%	93%	92%
Incidence of Potentially Preventable VTE[2]	39	0%	6%	10%
UFH with Dosages/Platelet Monitoring[2]	106	100%	98%	97%
Venous Thromboembolism Prophylaxis[2]	294	78%	88%	85%
Warfarin Therapy Discharge Instructions[2]	87	54%	79%	75%
Chest Pain/Possible Heart Attack Care				
Aspirin Given Within 24 Hours of Arrival[3,7]	-	-	97%	96%
Fibrinolytic Meds Within 30 Min. of Arrival[5]	-	-	44%	58%
Average Time to ECG (minutes)[3,7]	-	-	6	7
Average Time to Transfer (minutes)[5]	-	-	58	60
Children's Asthma Care				
Received Home Management Plan of Care	-	-	85%	88%
Received Reliever Medication	-	-	100%	100%
Received Systemic Corticosteroids	-	-	100%	100%
Emergency Department				
Admittance Decision Time (minutes)[2]	682	179	90	98
Head CT Results Within 45 Min. of Arrival[1]	-	-	63%	57%
Patients Who Left ER Before Being Seen	>100k	2%	2%	2%
Time from ER Arrival to Admit. (minutes)[2]	684	359	265	274
Time from ER Arrival to Discharge (minutes)	368	153	128	134
Time in ER Before Being Evaluated (minutes)	420	34	22	26
Time to Pain Meds for Fractures (minutes)	19	105	54	57
Heart Attack Care				
Aspirin Given at Discharge	256	99%	99%	99%
Fibrinolytic Meds Within 30 Min. of Arrival[7]	-	-	80%	54%
PCI Within 90 Minutes of Arrival	43	100%	97%	96%
Statin Prescribed at Discharge	255	99%	98%	98%
Heart Failure Care				
ACE Inhibitor or ARB for LVSD	255	100%	97%	97%
Discharge Instructions Given	634	97%	96%	94%
Evaluation of LVS Function	701	100%	100%	99%
Medicare Spending				
Medicare Spending per Patient (ratio)	-	0.98	1.01	0.98
Pneumonia Care				
Appropriate Initial Antibiotic Given	134	98%	96%	95%
Blood Culture Timing	165	95%	98%	98%
Pregnancy and Delivery Care				
Newborn Deliveries Scheduled Early	289	4%	5%	6%
Preventive Care				
Immunization for Influenza[2]	550	83%	93%	90%
Immunization for Pneumonia[2]	519	91%	94%	92%
Stroke Care				
Anticoagulation Therapy for Atrial Fibrillation	22	91%	95%	95%
Antithrombotic Therapy Timing	189	94%	98%	98%
Assessed for Rehabilitation	289	98%	98%	97%
Discharged on Antithrombotic Therapy	224	99%	99%	99%
Discharged on Statin Medication	189	98%	95%	94%
Thrombolytic Therapy Timing	23	96%	65%	66%
Venous Thromboembolism Prophylaxis	306	92%	95%	94%
Written Stroke Educational Materials Given	135	91%	92%	88%
Surgical Care Improvement Project				
Appropriate Beta Blocker Usage[2]	262	98%	98%	98%
Appropriate VTP Within 24 Hours[2]	540	97%	98%	98%
Controlled Postoperative Blood Glucose[2]	75	99%	97%	97%
Perioperative Temperature Management[2]	688	99%	100%	100%
Prophylactic Antibiotic Selection[2]	541	100%	99%	99%
Prophylactic Antibiotic Selection (Outpatient)	909	99%	98%	98%
Prophylactic Antibiotic Stopped[2]	531	96%	98%	98%
Prophylactic Antibiotic Timing[2]	541	99%	99%	99%
Prophylactic Antibiotic Timing (Outpatient)	761	98%	97%	98%
Urinary Catheter Removal[2]	524	98%	97%	97%
Survey of Patients' Hospital Experiences				
Area Around Room 'Always' Quiet at Night	300+	54%	58%	61%
Doctors 'Always' Communicated Well	300+	76%	80%	82%
Home Recovery Information Given	300+	84%	87%	85%
Hospital Given 9 or 10 on 10 Point Scale	300+	62%	72%	71%
Meds 'Always' Explained Before Given	300+	61%	64%	64%
Nurses 'Always' Communicated Well	300+	75%	81%	79%
Pain 'Always' Well Controlled	300+	66%	71%	71%
Room and Bathroom 'Always' Clean	300+	59%	75%	73%
Timely Help 'Always' Received	300+	60%	70%	68%
Would Definitely Recommend Hospital	300+	64%	71%	71%
Use of Medical Imaging				
Cardiac Imaging Stress Test before Surgery	449	3.1%	5.4%	5.3%
Combination Abdominal CT Scan	994	7.5%	7.1%	10.5%
Combination Brain/Sinus CT Scan	649	1.5%	2.8%	2.7%
Combination Chest CT Scan	931	2.4%	1.7%	2.7%
Follow-up Mammogram/Ultrasound	1,960	8.5%	8.7%	8.8%
Lumbar Spine MRI for Low Back Pain	135	29.6%	34.7%	37.2%

Saint Vincent Charity Medical Center

2351 East 22nd Street
Cleveland, OH 44115
Phone: 216-861-6200
Fax: 216-363-2796
Type: Acute Care Hospitals
Emergency Services: Yes
Ownership: Voluntary non-profit - Private
Beds: 492

Key Personnel:
Anesthesiology. . . . . John Bastulli, MD
Infection Control. . . . . Richard Chmielewski, MD
Emergency Room . . . . Gayle Galan, MD
Operating Room. . . . . Jo Ellen Horn
Quality Assurance . . . . Jane Jones
Chief of Medical Staff. . . . . Charity Kankan, MD
CEO/President. . . . . David F. Perse, MD
Radiology. . . . . Robert Porter, MD

Measure	Cases	This Hosp.	State Avg.	U.S. Avg.
Blood Clot Prevention and Treatment				
Anticoagulation Overlap Therapy[2]	33	91%	93%	93%
ICU Venous Thromboembolism Prophylaxis[2]	119	98%	93%	92%
Incidence of Potentially Preventable VTE[1,2]	-	-	6%	10%
UFH with Dosages/Platelet Monitoring[2]	23	100%	98%	97%
Venous Thromboembolism Prophylaxis[2]	303	95%	88%	85%
Warfarin Therapy Discharge Instructions[2]	26	100%	79%	75%
Chest Pain/Possible Heart Attack Care				
Aspirin Given Within 24 Hours of Arrival[1,3]	-	-	97%	96%
Fibrinolytic Meds Within 30 Min. of Arrival[5]	-	-	44%	58%
Average Time to ECG (minutes)[1,3]	-	-	6	7
Average Time to Transfer (minutes)[5]	-	-	58	60
Children's Asthma Care				
Received Home Management Plan of Care	-	-	85%	88%
Received Reliever Medication	-	-	100%	100%
Received Systemic Corticosteroids	-	-	100%	100%
Emergency Department				
Admittance Decision Time (minutes)[2]	490	104	90	98
Head CT Results Within 45 Min. of Arrival[1]	-	-	63%	57%
Patients Who Left ER Before Being Seen	20,021	1%	2%	2%
Time from ER Arrival to Admit. (minutes)[2]	516	274	265	274
Time from ER Arrival to Discharge (minutes)	336	123	128	134
Time in ER Before Being Evaluated (minutes)	385	30	22	26
Time to Pain Meds for Fractures (minutes)	54	64	54	57
Heart Attack Care				
Aspirin Given at Discharge	51	94%	99%	99%
Fibrinolytic Meds Within 30 Min. of Arrival[7]	-	-	80%	54%
PCI Within 90 Minutes of Arrival[1]	-	-	97%	96%
Statin Prescribed at Discharge	43	98%	98%	98%
Heart Failure Care				
ACE Inhibitor or ARB for LVSD[2]	87	100%	97%	97%
Discharge Instructions Given[2]	193	97%	96%	94%
Evaluation of LVS Function[2]	235	100%	100%	99%
Medicare Spending				
Medicare Spending per Patient (ratio)	-	1.01	1.01	0.98

NOTE: Hospital profiles are in alphabetical order by state, then city, then hospital within the city; Rankings exclude hospitals with less than 25 cases except for patient surveys which excludes hospitals with less than 100 cases; (a) 100-299 cases; (1) The number of cases/patients is too few to report; (2) Data submitted were based on a sample of cases/patients; (3) Results are based on a shorter time period than required; (4) Data suppressed by CMS for one or more quarters; (5) Results are not available for this reporting period; (6) Fewer than 100 patients completed the HCAHPS survey; (7) No cases met the criteria for this measure; (8) The lower limit of the confidence interval cannot be calculated if the number of observed infections equals zero; (9) No data are available from the state/territory for this reporting period; (10) The scores shown reflect fewer than 50 completed surveys; (11) There were discrepancies in the data collection process; (12) This measure does not apply to this hospital for this reporting period; (13) Results cannot be calculated for this reporting period; (14) The results for this state are combined with nearby states to protect confidentiality; Please refer to the User's Guide for a full explanation of data.

Measure	Cases	This Hosp.	State Avg.	U.S. Avg.
Pneumonia Care				
Appropriate Initial Antibiotic Given[2]	66	100%	96%	95%
Blood Culture Timing[2]	104	98%	98%	98%
Pregnancy and Delivery Care				
Newborn Deliveries Scheduled Early[7]	-	-	5%	6%
Preventive Care				
Immunization for Influenza[2]	587	83%	93%	90%
Immunization for Pneumonia[2]	799	85%	94%	92%
Stroke Care				
Anticoagulation Therapy for Atrial Fibrillation[7]	-	-	95%	95%
Antithrombotic Therapy Timing	20	95%	98%	98%
Assessed for Rehabilitation	21	100%	98%	97%
Discharged on Antithrombotic Therapy	21	100%	99%	99%
Discharged on Statin Medication	13	100%	95%	94%
Thrombolytic Therapy Timing[1]	-	-	65%	66%
Venous Thromboembolism Prophylaxis	23	96%	95%	94%
Written Stroke Educational Materials Given[1]	-	-	92%	88%
Surgical Care Improvement Project				
Appropriate Beta Blocker Usage[2]	152	99%	98%	98%
Appropriate VTP Within 24 Hours[2]	378	99%	98%	98%
Controlled Postoperative Blood Glucose[2]	33	97%	97%	97%
Perioperative Temperature Management[2]	433	100%	100%	100%
Prophylactic Antibiotic Selection[2]	333	100%	99%	99%
Prophylactic Antibiotic Selection (Outpatient)	238	100%	98%	98%
Prophylactic Antibiotic Stopped[2]	313	96%	98%	98%
Prophylactic Antibiotic Timing[2]	333	100%	99%	99%
Prophylactic Antibiotic Timing (Outpatient)	239	99%	97%	98%
Urinary Catheter Removal[2]	318	98%	97%	97%
Survey of Patients' Hospital Experiences				
Area Around Room 'Always' Quiet at Night	300+	67%	58%	61%
Doctors 'Always' Communicated Well	300+	81%	80%	82%
Home Recovery Information Given	300+	90%	87%	85%
Hospital Given 9 or 10 on 10 Point Scale	300+	72%	72%	71%
Meds 'Always' Explained Before Given	300+	62%	64%	64%
Nurses 'Always' Communicated Well	300+	80%	81%	79%
Pain 'Always' Well Controlled	300+	72%	71%	71%
Room and Bathroom 'Always' Clean	300+	75%	75%	73%
Timely Help 'Always' Received	300+	66%	70%	68%
Would Definitely Recommend Hospital	300+	70%	71%	71%
Use of Medical Imaging				
Cardiac Imaging Stress Test before Surgery	214	6.1%	5.4%	5.3%
Combination Abdominal CT Scan	244	5.7%	7.1%	10.5%
Combination Brain/Sinus CT Scan	223	7.2%	2.8%	2.7%
Combination Chest CT Scan	142	0.0%	1.7%	2.7%
Follow-up Mammogram/Ultrasound	196	17.3%	8.7%	8.8%
Lumbar Spine MRI for Low Back Pain	104	48.1%	34.7%	37.2%

University Hospitals Case Medical Center

11100 Euclid Avenue
Cleveland, OH 44106
Phone: 216-844-1000
Fax: 216-844-5805
URL: www.uhhs.com
Type: Acute Care Hospitals
Emergency Services: Yes
Ownership: Voluntary non-profit - Private
Beds: 1,032

Key Personnel:

Pediatric Ambulatory Care . . . . . . Ellis Avner, MD
Pediatric In-Patient Care . . . . Ellis Avner, MD
Operating Room. . . . . Cindy Danko
Radiology. . . . . Baz Debaz, MD
Infection Control. . . . . Michael Jacobs, MD
Chief of Medical Staff . . . . Pam Meyer
CEO . . . . Thomas F. Zenty, III

Measure	Cases	This Hosp.	State Avg.	U.S. Avg.
Blood Clot Prevention and Treatment				
Anticoagulation Overlap Therapy[2]	202	99%	93%	93%
ICU Venous Thromboembolism Prophylaxis[2]	95	95%	93%	92%
Incidence of Potentially Preventable VTE[2]	78	6%	6%	10%
UFH with Dosages/Platelet Monitoring[2]	217	100%	98%	97%
Venous Thromboembolism Prophylaxis[2]	334	93%	88%	85%
Warfarin Therapy Discharge Instructions[2]	138	86%	79%	75%
Chest Pain/Possible Heart Attack Care				
Aspirin Given Within 24 Hours of Arrival[1,3]	-	-	97%	96%
Fibrinolytic Meds Within 30 Min. of Arrival[5]	-	-	44%	58%
Average Time to ECG (minutes)[1,3]	-	-	6	7
Average Time to Transfer (minutes)[5]	-	-	58	60
Children's Asthma Care				
Received Home Management Plan of Care	-	-	85%	88%
Received Reliever Medication	-	-	100%	100%
Received Systemic Corticosteroids	-	-	100%	100%
Emergency Department				
Admittance Decision Time (minutes)[2]	414	214	90	98
Head CT Results Within 45 Min. of Arrival[1]	-	-	63%	57%
Patients Who Left ER Before Being Seen	53,978	10%	2%	2%
Time from ER Arrival to Admit. (minutes)[2]	420	438	265	274
Time from ER Arrival to Discharge (minutes)	363	270	128	134
Time in ER Before Being Evaluated (minutes)	395	48	22	26
Time to Pain Meds for Fractures (minutes)	39	100	54	57
Heart Attack Care				
Aspirin Given at Discharge	396	100%	99%	99%
Fibrinolytic Meds Within 30 Min. of Arrival[7]	-	-	80%	54%
PCI Within 90 Minutes of Arrival	27	100%	97%	96%
Statin Prescribed at Discharge	380	100%	98%	98%
Heart Failure Care				
ACE Inhibitor or ARB for LVSD[2]	98	100%	97%	97%
Discharge Instructions Given[2]	244	97%	96%	94%
Evaluation of LVS Function[2]	318	100%	100%	99%
Medicare Spending				
Medicare Spending per Patient (ratio)	-	1.00	1.01	0.98
Pneumonia Care				
Appropriate Initial Antibiotic Given[2]	51	92%	96%	95%
Blood Culture Timing[2]	142	98%	98%	98%
Pregnancy and Delivery Care				
Newborn Deliveries Scheduled Early[2]	60	3%	5%	6%
Preventive Care				
Immunization for Influenza[2]	547	97%	93%	90%
Immunization for Pneumonia[2]	663	94%	94%	92%
Stroke Care				
Anticoagulation Therapy for Atrial Fibrillation[1,2]	-	-	95%	95%
Antithrombotic Therapy Timing[2]	67	100%	98%	98%
Assessed for Rehabilitation[2]	127	99%	98%	97%
Discharged on Antithrombotic Therapy[2]	93	100%	99%	99%
Discharged on Statin Medication[2]	63	100%	95%	94%
Thrombolytic Therapy Timing[1,2]	-	-	65%	66%
Venous Thromboembolism Prophylaxis[2]	122	100%	95%	94%
Written Stroke Educational Materials Given[2]	59	100%	92%	88%
Surgical Care Improvement Project				
Appropriate Beta Blocker Usage[2]	307	99%	98%	98%
Appropriate VTP Within 24 Hours[2]	540	100%	98%	98%
Controlled Postoperative Blood Glucose[2]	164	95%	97%	97%
Perioperative Temperature Management[2]	643	100%	100%	100%
Prophylactic Antibiotic Selection[2]	540	99%	99%	99%
Prophylactic Antibiotic Selection (Outpatient)	598	99%	98%	98%
Prophylactic Antibiotic Stopped[2]	526	99%	98%	98%
Prophylactic Antibiotic Timing[2]	541	100%	99%	99%
Prophylactic Antibiotic Timing (Outpatient)	518	100%	97%	98%
Urinary Catheter Removal[2]	461	99%	97%	97%
Survey of Patients' Hospital Experiences				
Area Around Room 'Always' Quiet at Night	300+	57%	58%	61%
Doctors 'Always' Communicated Well	300+	79%	80%	82%
Home Recovery Information Given	300+	87%	87%	85%
Hospital Given 9 or 10 on 10 Point Scale	300+	74%	72%	71%
Meds 'Always' Explained Before Given	300+	64%	64%	64%
Nurses 'Always' Communicated Well	300+	80%	81%	79%
Pain 'Always' Well Controlled	300+	70%	71%	71%
Room and Bathroom 'Always' Clean	300+	67%	75%	73%
Timely Help 'Always' Received	300+	61%	70%	68%
Would Definitely Recommend Hospital	300+	79%	71%	71%
Use of Medical Imaging				
Cardiac Imaging Stress Test before Surgery	676	5.6%	5.4%	5.3%
Combination Abdominal CT Scan	1,959	4.6%	7.1%	10.5%
Combination Brain/Sinus CT Scan	726	3.6%	2.8%	2.7%
Combination Chest CT Scan	2,664	0.1%	1.7%	2.7%
Follow-up Mammogram/Ultrasound	2,080	8.7%	8.7%	8.8%
Lumbar Spine MRI for Low Back Pain	142	37.3%	34.7%	37.2%

Mercer County Joint Township Community Hospital

800 West Main Street
Coldwater, OH 45828
Phone: 419-678-4843
Fax: 419-678-3271
URL: www.mercer-health.com
Type: Acute Care Hospitals
Emergency Services: Yes
Ownership: Govt - Hospital Dist/Auth
Beds: 76

Key Personnel:

Chief of Medical Staff . . . . Franklin Holzer
CEO/President. . . . . Terrance Padden
Quality Assurance . . . . Karen Smalley
Emergency Room . . . . Ross Warren, DO

Measure	Cases	This Hosp.	State Avg.	U.S. Avg.
Blood Clot Prevention and Treatment				
Anticoagulation Overlap Therapy[2]	17	53%	93%	93%
ICU Venous Thromboembolism Prophylaxis[2]	25	96%	93%	92%
Incidence of Potentially Preventable VTE[2,7]	-	-	6%	10%
UFH with Dosages/Platelet Monitoring[1,2]	-	-	98%	97%
Venous Thromboembolism Prophylaxis[2]	82	93%	88%	85%
Warfarin Therapy Discharge Instructions[2]	15	100%	79%	75%
Chest Pain/Possible Heart Attack Care				
Aspirin Given Within 24 Hours of Arrival	48	100%	97%	96%
Fibrinolytic Meds Within 30 Min. of Arrival[1]	-	-	44%	58%
Average Time to ECG (minutes)	49	3	6	7
Average Time to Transfer (minutes)[1]	-	-	58	60
Children's Asthma Care				
Received Home Management Plan of Care	-	-	85%	88%
Received Reliever Medication	-	-	100%	100%
Received Systemic Corticosteroids	-	-	100%	100%
Emergency Department				
Admittance Decision Time (minutes)[2]	252	63	90	98
Head CT Results Within 45 Min. of Arrival[1]	-	-	63%	57%
Patients Who Left ER Before Being Seen	10,953	0%	2%	2%
Time from ER Arrival to Admit. (minutes)[2]	275	198	265	274
Time from ER Arrival to Discharge (minutes)	342	104	128	134
Time in ER Before Being Evaluated (minutes)	382	17	22	26
Time to Pain Meds for Fractures (minutes)	46	30	54	57
Heart Attack Care				
Aspirin Given at Discharge	12	92%	99%	99%
Fibrinolytic Meds Within 30 Min. of Arrival[7]	-	-	80%	54%
PCI Within 90 Minutes of Arrival[7]	-	-	97%	96%
Statin Prescribed at Discharge[1]	-	-	98%	98%
Heart Failure Care				
ACE Inhibitor or ARB for LVSD	21	100%	97%	97%
Discharge Instructions Given	28	93%	96%	94%
Evaluation of LVS Function	41	100%	100%	99%
Medicare Spending				
Medicare Spending per Patient (ratio)	-	1.10	1.01	0.98
Pneumonia Care				
Appropriate Initial Antibiotic Given	77	99%	96%	95%
Blood Culture Timing	78	97%	98%	98%
Pregnancy and Delivery Care				
Newborn Deliveries Scheduled Early	36	3%	5%	6%
Preventive Care				
Immunization for Influenza[2]	232	92%	93%	90%
Immunization for Pneumonia[2]	241	91%	94%	92%
Stroke Care				
Anticoagulation Therapy for Atrial Fibrillation[1]	-	-	95%	95%
Antithrombotic Therapy Timing	17	100%	98%	98%
Assessed for Rehabilitation	18	100%	98%	97%
Discharged on Antithrombotic Therapy	17	100%	99%	99%
Discharged on Statin Medication	13	77%	95%	94%
Thrombolytic Therapy Timing[1]	-	-	65%	66%
Venous Thromboembolism Prophylaxis	16	94%	95%	94%
Written Stroke Educational Materials Given	11	82%	92%	88%
Surgical Care Improvement Project				
Appropriate Beta Blocker Usage	25	96%	98%	98%
Appropriate VTP Within 24 Hours	100	95%	98%	98%
Controlled Postoperative Blood Glucose[7]	-	-	97%	97%
Perioperative Temperature Management	116	100%	100%	100%
Prophylactic Antibiotic Selection	86	97%	99%	99%
Prophylactic Antibiotic Selection (Outpatient)[1,3]	-	-	98%	98%
Prophylactic Antibiotic Stopped	86	98%	98%	98%
Prophylactic Antibiotic Timing	86	97%	99%	99%

NOTE: Hospital profiles are in alphabetical order by state, then city, then hospital within the city; Rankings exclude hospitals with less than 25 cases except for patient surveys which excludes hospitals with less than 100 cases; (a) 100-299 cases; (1) The number of cases/patients is too few to report; (2) Data submitted were based on a sample of cases/patients; (3) Results are based on a shorter time period than required; (4) Data suppressed by CMS for one or more quarters; (5) Results are not available for this reporting period; (6) Fewer than 100 patients completed the HCAHPS survey; (7) No cases met the criteria for this measure; (8) The lower limit of the confidence interval cannot be calculated if the number of observed infections equals zero; (9) No data are available from the state/territory for this reporting period; (10) The scores shown reflect fewer than 50 completed surveys; (11) There were discrepancies in the data collection process; (12) This measure does not apply to this hospital for this reporting period; (13) Results cannot be calculated for this reporting period; (14) The results for this state are combined with nearby states to protect confidentiality; Please refer to the User's Guide for a full explanation of data.

Measure	Cases	This Hosp.	State Avg.	U.S. Avg.
Prophylactic Antibiotic Timing (Outpatient)[3]	11	82%	97%	98%
Urinary Catheter Removal	90	100%	97%	97%
Survey of Patients' Hospital Experiences				
Area Around Room 'Always' Quiet at Night	300+	55%	58%	61%
Doctors 'Always' Communicated Well	300+	82%	80%	82%
Home Recovery Information Given	300+	88%	87%	85%
Hospital Given 9 or 10 on 10 Point Scale	300+	73%	72%	71%
Meds 'Always' Explained Before Given	300+	64%	64%	64%
Nurses 'Always' Communicated Well	300+	81%	81%	79%
Pain 'Always' Well Controlled	300+	71%	71%	71%
Room and Bathroom 'Always' Clean	300+	78%	75%	73%
Timely Help 'Always' Received	300+	79%	70%	68%
Would Definitely Recommend Hospital	300+	75%	71%	71%
Use of Medical Imaging				
Cardiac Imaging Stress Test before Surgery[1]	-	-	5.4%	5.3%
Combination Abdominal CT Scan	250	6.0%	7.1%	10.5%
Combination Brain/Sinus CT Scan[1]	-	-	2.8%	2.7%
Combination Chest CT Scan	117	0.9%	1.7%	2.7%
Follow-up Mammogram/Ultrasound	391	5.1%	8.7%	8.8%
Lumbar Spine MRI for Low Back Pain[1]	-	-	34.7%	37.2%

Doctors Hospital

5100 West Broad Street
Columbus, OH 43228
URL: www.columbusregional.com
Type: Acute Care Hospitals
Ownership: Voluntary non-profit - Church
Phone: 614-544-1000
Fax: 614-544-1710
Emergency Services: Yes
Beds: 478

Key Personnel:
Radiology. . . . . Thomas Anderson
Operating Room. . . . . Roberta Bannon, RN
Infection Control. . . . . Lee Chamberlin
Chief of Medical Staff. . . . . William Emlich, DO
CEO/President. . . . . Kreg Gruber
Pediatric Ambulatory Care . . . . . . Maureen Kollar, DO
Pediatric In-Patient Care . . . . Maureen Kollar, DO
Quality Assurance . . . . Kathy Kunkleman

Measure	Cases	This Hosp.	State Avg.	U.S. Avg.
Blood Clot Prevention and Treatment				
Anticoagulation Overlap Therapy[2]	96	99%	93%	93%
ICU Venous Thromboembolism Prophylaxis[2]	64	100%	93%	92%
Incidence of Potentially Preventable VTE[1,2]	-	-	6%	10%
UFH with Dosages/Platelet Monitoring[2]	64	100%	98%	97%
Venous Thromboembolism Prophylaxis[2]	369	87%	88%	85%
Warfarin Therapy Discharge Instructions[2]	80	92%	79%	75%
Chest Pain/Possible Heart Attack Care				
Aspirin Given Within 24 Hours of Arrival[1]	-	-	97%	96%
Fibrinolytic Meds Within 30 Min. of Arrival[3,7]	-	-	44%	58%
Average Time to ECG (minutes)[1]	-	-	6	7
Average Time to Transfer (minutes)[3,7]	-	-	58	60
Children's Asthma Care				
Received Home Management Plan of Care	-	-	85%	88%
Received Reliever Medication	-	-	100%	100%
Received Systemic Corticosteroids	-	-	100%	100%
Emergency Department				
Admittance Decision Time (minutes)[2]	536	51	90	98
Head CT Results Within 45 Min. of Arrival[1]	-	-	63%	57%
Patients Who Left ER Before Being Seen	83,260	2%	2%	2%
Time from ER Arrival to Admit. (minutes)[2]	538	253	265	274
Time from ER Arrival to Discharge (minutes)	393	141	128	134
Time in ER Before Being Evaluated (minutes)	434	27	22	26
Time to Pain Meds for Fractures (minutes)	337	55	54	57
Heart Attack Care				
Aspirin Given at Discharge	166	100%	99%	99%
Fibrinolytic Meds Within 30 Min. of Arrival[7]	-	-	80%	54%
PCI Within 90 Minutes of Arrival	53	100%	97%	96%
Statin Prescribed at Discharge	168	100%	98%	98%
Heart Failure Care				
ACE Inhibitor or ARB for LVSD	99	100%	97%	97%
Discharge Instructions Given	224	100%	96%	94%
Evaluation of LVS Function	267	100%	100%	99%
Medicare Spending				
Medicare Spending per Patient (ratio)	-	1.01	1.01	0.98
Pneumonia Care				
Appropriate Initial Antibiotic Given	122	99%	96%	95%
Blood Culture Timing	189	100%	98%	98%
Pregnancy and Delivery Care				
Newborn Deliveries Scheduled Early	58	0%	5%	6%
Preventive Care				
Immunization for Influenza[2]	547	97%	93%	90%
Immunization for Pneumonia[2]	712	97%	94%	92%
Stroke Care				
Anticoagulation Therapy for Atrial Fibrillation[1]	-	-	95%	95%
Antithrombotic Therapy Timing	50	100%	98%	98%
Assessed for Rehabilitation	50	98%	98%	97%
Discharged on Antithrombotic Therapy	47	100%	99%	99%
Discharged on Statin Medication	41	100%	95%	94%
Thrombolytic Therapy Timing[7]	-	-	65%	66%
Venous Thromboembolism Prophylaxis	50	98%	95%	94%
Written Stroke Educational Materials Given	40	98%	92%	88%
Surgical Care Improvement Project				
Appropriate Beta Blocker Usage[2]	154	100%	98%	98%
Appropriate VTP Within 24 Hours[2]	362	99%	98%	98%
Controlled Postoperative Blood Glucose[2]	52	100%	97%	97%
Perioperative Temperature Management[2]	445	100%	100%	100%
Prophylactic Antibiotic Selection[2]	311	100%	99%	99%
Prophylactic Antibiotic Selection (Outpatient)	139	99%	98%	98%
Prophylactic Antibiotic Stopped[2]	310	99%	98%	98%
Prophylactic Antibiotic Timing[2]	312	100%	99%	99%
Prophylactic Antibiotic Timing (Outpatient)	139	98%	97%	98%
Urinary Catheter Removal[2]	323	100%	97%	97%
Survey of Patients' Hospital Experiences				
Area Around Room 'Always' Quiet at Night	300+	66%	58%	61%
Doctors 'Always' Communicated Well	300+	79%	80%	82%
Home Recovery Information Given	300+	89%	87%	85%
Hospital Given 9 or 10 on 10 Point Scale	300+	73%	72%	71%
Meds 'Always' Explained Before Given	300+	66%	64%	64%
Nurses 'Always' Communicated Well	300+	82%	81%	79%
Pain 'Always' Well Controlled	300+	70%	71%	71%
Room and Bathroom 'Always' Clean	300+	72%	75%	73%
Timely Help 'Always' Received	300+	69%	70%	68%
Would Definitely Recommend Hospital	300+	72%	71%	71%
Use of Medical Imaging				
Cardiac Imaging Stress Test before Surgery	332	4.2%	5.4%	5.3%
Combination Abdominal CT Scan	494	2.6%	7.1%	10.5%
Combination Brain/Sinus CT Scan[1]	-	-	2.8%	2.7%
Combination Chest CT Scan	314	1.0%	1.7%	2.7%
Follow-up Mammogram/Ultrasound	572	9.6%	8.7%	8.8%
Lumbar Spine MRI for Low Back Pain	73	32.9%	34.7%	37.2%

Grant Medical Center

111 South Grant Avenue
Columbus, OH 43215
URL: www.ohiohealth.com
Type: Acute Care Hospitals
Ownership: Voluntary non-profit - Church
Phone: 614-566-9978
Fax: 614-566-8045
Emergency Services: Yes
Beds: 337

Key Personnel:
CEO/President. . . . . Michael Lawson

Measure	Cases	This Hosp.	State Avg.	U.S. Avg.
Blood Clot Prevention and Treatment				
Anticoagulation Overlap Therapy[2]	134	100%	93%	93%
ICU Venous Thromboembolism Prophylaxis[2]	51	98%	93%	92%
Incidence of Potentially Preventable VTE[2]	52	0%	6%	10%
UFH with Dosages/Platelet Monitoring[2]	105	100%	98%	97%
Venous Thromboembolism Prophylaxis[2]	358	97%	88%	85%
Warfarin Therapy Discharge Instructions[2]	104	97%	79%	75%
Chest Pain/Possible Heart Attack Care				
Aspirin Given Within 24 Hours of Arrival	37	97%	97%	96%
Fibrinolytic Meds Within 30 Min. of Arrival[3,7]	-	-	44%	58%
Average Time to ECG (minutes)	39	8	6	7
Average Time to Transfer (minutes)[1,3]	-	-	58	60
Children's Asthma Care				
Received Home Management Plan of Care	-	-	85%	88%
Received Reliever Medication	-	-	100%	100%
Received Systemic Corticosteroids	-	-	100%	100%
Emergency Department				
Admittance Decision Time (minutes)[2]	476	192	90	98
Head CT Results Within 45 Min. of Arrival[1]	-	-	63%	57%
Patients Who Left ER Before Being Seen	88,369	3%	2%	2%
Time from ER Arrival to Admit. (minutes)[2]	476	360	265	274
Time from ER Arrival to Discharge (minutes)	427	153	128	134
Time in ER Before Being Evaluated (minutes)	454	56	22	26
Time to Pain Meds for Fractures (minutes)	139	45	54	57
Heart Attack Care				
Aspirin Given at Discharge	335	100%	99%	99%
Fibrinolytic Meds Within 30 Min. of Arrival[1]	-	-	80%	54%
PCI Within 90 Minutes of Arrival	71	99%	97%	96%
Statin Prescribed at Discharge	331	100%	98%	98%
Heart Failure Care				
ACE Inhibitor or ARB for LVSD	152	100%	97%	97%
Discharge Instructions Given	372	100%	96%	94%
Evaluation of LVS Function	460	100%	100%	99%
Medicare Spending				
Medicare Spending per Patient (ratio)	-	0.98	1.01	0.98
Pneumonia Care				
Appropriate Initial Antibiotic Given[2]	88	99%	96%	95%
Blood Culture Timing[2]	107	100%	98%	98%
Pregnancy and Delivery Care				
Newborn Deliveries Scheduled Early	227	2%	5%	6%
Preventive Care				
Immunization for Influenza[2]	534	95%	93%	90%
Immunization for Pneumonia[2]	625	96%	94%	92%
Stroke Care				
Anticoagulation Therapy for Atrial Fibrillation[1,2]	-	-	95%	95%
Antithrombotic Therapy Timing[2]	80	100%	98%	98%
Assessed for Rehabilitation[2]	106	100%	98%	97%
Discharged on Antithrombotic Therapy[2]	79	100%	99%	99%
Discharged on Statin Medication[2]	68	100%	95%	94%
Thrombolytic Therapy Timing[1,2]	-	-	65%	66%
Venous Thromboembolism Prophylaxis[2]	105	100%	95%	94%
Written Stroke Educational Materials Given[2]	65	98%	92%	88%
Surgical Care Improvement Project				
Appropriate Beta Blocker Usage[2]	251	99%	98%	98%
Appropriate VTP Within 24 Hours[2]	535	99%	98%	98%
Controlled Postoperative Blood Glucose[2]	137	96%	97%	97%
Perioperative Temperature Management[2]	639	100%	100%	100%
Prophylactic Antibiotic Selection[2]	562	100%	99%	99%
Prophylactic Antibiotic Selection (Outpatient)	458	98%	98%	98%
Prophylactic Antibiotic Stopped[2]	548	99%	98%	98%
Prophylactic Antibiotic Timing[2]	562	100%	99%	99%
Prophylactic Antibiotic Timing (Outpatient)	458	99%	97%	98%
Urinary Catheter Removal[2]	519	100%	97%	97%
Survey of Patients' Hospital Experiences				
Area Around Room 'Always' Quiet at Night	300+	58%	58%	61%
Doctors 'Always' Communicated Well	300+	80%	80%	82%
Home Recovery Information Given	300+	88%	87%	85%
Hospital Given 9 or 10 on 10 Point Scale	300+	75%	72%	71%
Meds 'Always' Explained Before Given	300+	65%	64%	64%
Nurses 'Always' Communicated Well	300+	81%	81%	79%
Pain 'Always' Well Controlled	300+	71%	71%	71%
Room and Bathroom 'Always' Clean	300+	73%	75%	73%
Timely Help 'Always' Received	300+	66%	70%	68%
Would Definitely Recommend Hospital	300+	77%	71%	71%
Use of Medical Imaging				
Cardiac Imaging Stress Test before Surgery	657	4.7%	5.4%	5.3%
Combination Abdominal CT Scan	1,094	2.1%	7.1%	10.5%
Combination Brain/Sinus CT Scan	938	3.1%	2.8%	2.7%
Combination Chest CT Scan	462	0.6%	1.7%	2.7%
Follow-up Mammogram/Ultrasound	1,608	5.5%	8.7%	8.8%
Lumbar Spine MRI for Low Back Pain	144	28.5%	34.7%	37.2%

James Cancer Hospital & Solove Research Institute

300 West Tenth Avenue
Columbus, OH 43210
Type: Acute Care Hospitals
Ownership: Government - State
Phone: 614-293-3121
Emergency Services: Yes

Measure	Cases	This Hosp.	State Avg.	U.S. Avg.
Blood Clot Prevention and Treatment				
Anticoagulation Overlap Therapy[5]	-	-	93%	93%
ICU Venous Thromboembolism Prophylaxis[5]	-	-	93%	92%

NOTE: Hospital profiles are in alphabetical order by state, then city, then hospital within the city; Rankings exclude hospitals with less than 25 cases except for patient surveys which excludes hospitals with less than 100 cases; (a) 100-299 cases; (1) The number of cases/patients is too few to report; (2) Data submitted were based on a sample of cases/patients; (3) Results are based on a shorter time period than required; (4) Data suppressed by CMS for one or more quarters; (5) Results are not available for this reporting period; (6) Fewer than 100 patients completed the HCAHPS survey; (7) No cases met the criteria for this measure; (8) The lower limit of the confidence interval cannot be calculated if the number of observed infections equals zero; (9) No data are available from the state/territory for this reporting period; (10) The scores shown reflect fewer than 50 completed surveys; (11) There were discrepancies in the data collection process; (12) This measure does not apply to this hospital for this reporting period; (13) Results cannot be calculated for this reporting period; (14) The results for this state are combined with nearby states to protect confidentiality; Please refer to the User's Guide for a full explanation of data.

Measure	Cases	This Hosp.	State Avg.	U.S. Avg.
Incidence of Potentially Preventable VTE[5]	-	-	6%	10%
UFH with Dosages/Platelet Monitoring[5]	-	-	98%	97%
Venous Thromboembolism Prophylaxis[5]	-	-	88%	85%
Warfarin Therapy Discharge Instructions[5]	-	-	79%	75%
Chest Pain/Possible Heart Attack Care				
Aspirin Given Within 24 Hours of Arrival	-	-	97%	96%
Fibrinolytic Meds Within 30 Min. of Arrival	-	-	44%	58%
Average Time to ECG (minutes)	-	-	6	7
Average Time to Transfer (minutes)	-	-	58	60
Children's Asthma Care				
Received Home Management Plan of Care	-	-	85%	88%
Received Reliever Medication	-	-	100%	100%
Received Systemic Corticosteroids	-	-	100%	100%
Emergency Department				
Admittance Decision Time (minutes)[5]	-	-	90	98
Head CT Results Within 45 Min. of Arrival	-	-	63%	57%
Patients Who Left ER Before Being Seen	-	-	2%	2%
Time from ER Arrival to Admit. (minutes)[5]	-	-	265	274
Time from ER Arrival to Discharge (minutes)	-	-	128	134
Time in ER Before Being Evaluated (minutes)	-	-	22	26
Time to Pain Meds for Fractures (minutes)	-	-	54	57
Heart Attack Care				
Aspirin Given at Discharge[5]	-	-	99%	99%
Fibrinolytic Meds Within 30 Min. of Arrival[5]	-	-	80%	54%
PCI Within 90 Minutes of Arrival[5]	-	-	97%	96%
Statin Prescribed at Discharge[5]	-	-	98%	98%
Heart Failure Care				
ACE Inhibitor or ARB for LVSD[5]	-	-	97%	97%
Discharge Instructions Given[5]	-	-	96%	94%
Evaluation of LVS Function[5]	-	-	100%	99%
Medicare Spending				
Medicare Spending per Patient (ratio)	-	-	1.01	0.98
Pneumonia Care				
Appropriate Initial Antibiotic Given[5]	-	-	96%	95%
Blood Culture Timing[5]	-	-	98%	98%
Pregnancy and Delivery Care				
Newborn Deliveries Scheduled Early[5]	-	-	5%	6%
Preventive Care				
Immunization for Influenza[5]	-	-	93%	90%
Immunization for Pneumonia[5]	-	-	94%	92%
Stroke Care				
Anticoagulation Therapy for Atrial Fibrillation[5]	-	-	95%	95%
Antithrombotic Therapy Timing[5]	-	-	98%	98%
Assessed for Rehabilitation[5]	-	-	98%	97%
Discharged on Antithrombotic Therapy[5]	-	-	99%	99%
Discharged on Statin Medication[5]	-	-	95%	94%
Thrombolytic Therapy Timing[5]	-	-	65%	66%
Venous Thromboembolism Prophylaxis[5]	-	-	95%	94%
Written Stroke Educational Materials Given[5]	-	-	92%	88%
Surgical Care Improvement Project				
Appropriate Beta Blocker Usage[5]	-	-	98%	98%
Appropriate VTP Within 24 Hours[5]	-	-	98%	98%
Controlled Postoperative Blood Glucose[5]	-	-	97%	97%
Perioperative Temperature Management[5]	-	-	100%	100%
Prophylactic Antibiotic Selection[5]	-	-	99%	99%
Prophylactic Antibiotic Selection (Outpatient)	-	-	98%	98%
Prophylactic Antibiotic Stopped[5]	-	-	98%	98%
Prophylactic Antibiotic Timing[5]	-	-	99%	99%
Prophylactic Antibiotic Timing (Outpatient)	-	-	97%	98%
Urinary Catheter Removal[5]	-	-	97%	97%
Survey of Patients' Hospital Experiences				
Area Around Room 'Always' Quiet at Night	300+	53%	58%	61%
Doctors 'Always' Communicated Well	300+	83%	80%	82%
Home Recovery Information Given	300+	90%	87%	85%
Hospital Given 9 or 10 on 10 Point Scale	300+	80%	72%	71%
Meds 'Always' Explained Before Given	300+	68%	64%	64%
Nurses 'Always' Communicated Well	300+	83%	81%	79%
Pain 'Always' Well Controlled	300+	74%	71%	71%
Room and Bathroom 'Always' Clean	300+	70%	75%	73%
Timely Help 'Always' Received	300+	68%	70%	68%
Would Definitely Recommend Hospital	300+	84%	71%	71%
Use of Medical Imaging				
Cardiac Imaging Stress Test before Surgery	-	-	5.4%	5.3%
Combination Abdominal CT Scan	-	-	7.1%	10.5%
Combination Brain/Sinus CT Scan	-	-	2.8%	2.7%
Combination Chest CT Scan	-	-	1.7%	2.7%
Follow-up Mammogram/Ultrasound	-	-	8.7%	8.8%
Lumbar Spine MRI for Low Back Pain	-	-	34.7%	37.2%

Mount Carmel West

793 West State Street
Columbus, OH 43222
URL: www.mountcarmelhealth.com
Type: Acute Care Hospitals
Ownership: Voluntary non-profit - Other
Phone: 614-234-5000
Fax: 614-234-0456
Emergency Services: Yes
Beds: 523

Key Personnel:
Pediatric Ambulatory Care . . . . . . Craig Anderson, MD
Pediatric In-Patient Care . . . . . . Craig Anderson, MD
Chief of Medical Staff . . . . Edward Brand, MD
Operating Room. . . . . Vicki Carpenter
Infection Control . . . . Carol Elder
Radiology. . . . . Robert B. McGhee, MD
Quality Assurance . . . . Anita Morrison
President . . . . Richard Oberlander, D.O.

Measure	Cases	This Hosp.	State Avg.	U.S. Avg.
Blood Clot Prevention and Treatment				
Anticoagulation Overlap Therapy[2]	245	96%	93%	93%
ICU Venous Thromboembolism Prophylaxis[2]	78	87%	93%	92%
Incidence of Potentially Preventable VTE[2]	78	9%	6%	10%
UFH with Dosages/Platelet Monitoring[2]	219	100%	98%	97%
Venous Thromboembolism Prophylaxis[2]	310	86%	88%	85%
Warfarin Therapy Discharge Instructions[2]	165	56%	79%	75%
Chest Pain/Possible Heart Attack Care				
Aspirin Given Within 24 Hours of Arrival[1]	-	-	97%	96%
Fibrinolytic Meds Within 30 Min. of Arrival[3,7]	-	-	44%	58%
Average Time to ECG (minutes)[1]	-	-	6	7
Average Time to Transfer (minutes)[3,7]	-	-	58	60
Children's Asthma Care				
Received Home Management Plan of Care	-	-	85%	88%
Received Reliever Medication	-	-	100%	100%
Received Systemic Corticosteroids	-	-	100%	100%
Emergency Department				
Admittance Decision Time (minutes)[2]	413	106	90	98
Head CT Results Within 45 Min. of Arrival	14	50%	63%	57%
Patients Who Left ER Before Being Seen	75,444	1%	2%	2%
Time from ER Arrival to Admit. (minutes)[2]	413	300	265	274
Time from ER Arrival to Discharge (minutes)	687	168	128	134
Time in ER Before Being Evaluated (minutes)	763	45	22	26
Time to Pain Meds for Fractures (minutes)	180	77	54	57
Heart Attack Care				
Aspirin Given at Discharge[2]	293	99%	99%	99%
Fibrinolytic Meds Within 30 Min. of Arrival[2,7]	-	-	80%	54%
PCI Within 90 Minutes of Arrival[2]	64	100%	97%	96%
Statin Prescribed at Discharge[2]	288	99%	98%	98%
Heart Failure Care				
ACE Inhibitor or ARB for LVSD[2]	93	100%	97%	97%
Discharge Instructions Given[2]	247	98%	96%	94%
Evaluation of LVS Function[2]	312	100%	100%	99%
Medicare Spending				
Medicare Spending per Patient (ratio)	-	1.01	1.01	0.98
Pneumonia Care				
Appropriate Initial Antibiotic Given[2]	138	99%	96%	95%
Blood Culture Timing[2]	195	96%	98%	98%
Pregnancy and Delivery Care				
Newborn Deliveries Scheduled Early[2]	56	0%	5%	6%
Preventive Care				
Immunization for Influenza[2]	518	90%	93%	90%
Immunization for Pneumonia[2]	692	83%	94%	92%
Stroke Care				
Anticoagulation Therapy for Atrial Fibrillation[2]	20	100%	95%	95%
Antithrombotic Therapy Timing[2]	108	93%	98%	98%
Assessed for Rehabilitation[2]	151	94%	98%	97%
Discharged on Antithrombotic Therapy[2]	126	98%	99%	99%
Discharged on Statin Medication[2]	97	97%	95%	94%
Thrombolytic Therapy Timing[2]	26	88%	65%	66%
Venous Thromboembolism Prophylaxis[2]	156	88%	95%	94%
Written Stroke Educational Materials Given[2]	62	82%	92%	88%
Surgical Care Improvement Project				
Appropriate Beta Blocker Usage[2]	373	98%	98%	98%
Appropriate VTP Within 24 Hours[2]	642	97%	98%	98%
Controlled Postoperative Blood Glucose[2]	134	99%	97%	97%
Perioperative Temperature Management[2]	835	100%	100%	100%
Prophylactic Antibiotic Selection[2]	730	100%	99%	99%
Prophylactic Antibiotic Selection (Outpatient)	610	97%	98%	98%
Prophylactic Antibiotic Stopped[2]	714	98%	98%	98%
Prophylactic Antibiotic Timing[2]	735	100%	99%	99%
Prophylactic Antibiotic Timing (Outpatient)	615	98%	97%	98%
Urinary Catheter Removal[2]	677	95%	97%	97%
Survey of Patients' Hospital Experiences				
Area Around Room 'Always' Quiet at Night	300+	52%	58%	61%
Doctors 'Always' Communicated Well	300+	79%	80%	82%
Home Recovery Information Given	300+	87%	87%	85%
Hospital Given 9 or 10 on 10 Point Scale	300+	71%	72%	71%
Meds 'Always' Explained Before Given	300+	58%	64%	64%
Nurses 'Always' Communicated Well	300+	78%	81%	79%
Pain 'Always' Well Controlled	300+	70%	71%	71%
Room and Bathroom 'Always' Clean	300+	61%	75%	73%
Timely Help 'Always' Received	300+	61%	70%	68%
Would Definitely Recommend Hospital	300+	72%	71%	71%
Use of Medical Imaging				
Cardiac Imaging Stress Test before Surgery	870	5.9%	5.4%	5.3%
Combination Abdominal CT Scan	1,944	2.3%	7.1%	10.5%
Combination Brain/Sinus CT Scan	1,737	1.0%	2.8%	2.7%
Combination Chest CT Scan	733	0.4%	1.7%	2.7%
Follow-up Mammogram/Ultrasound	3,189	6.6%	8.7%	8.8%
Lumbar Spine MRI for Low Back Pain	173	39.9%	34.7%	37.2%

Ohio State University Hospitals

410 West 10th Avenue
Columbus, OH 43210
URL: www.jamesline.com
Type: Acute Care Hospitals
Ownership: Government - State
Phone: 614-293-9700
Fax: 614-293-3080
Emergency Services: Yes
Beds: 156

Key Personnel:
CEO . . . . Larry Anstine
Radiology. . . . . David Bates
Chief of Medical Staff . . . . William B Farrar
Quality Assurance . . . . Susan Moffatt-Bruce, MD,PhD

Measure	Cases	This Hosp.	State Avg.	U.S. Avg.
Blood Clot Prevention and Treatment				
Anticoagulation Overlap Therapy[2]	263	94%	93%	93%
ICU Venous Thromboembolism Prophylaxis[2]	66	94%	93%	92%
Incidence of Potentially Preventable VTE[2]	77	0%	6%	10%
UFH with Dosages/Platelet Monitoring[2]	255	93%	98%	97%
Venous Thromboembolism Prophylaxis[2]	344	91%	88%	85%
Warfarin Therapy Discharge Instructions[2]	161	60%	79%	75%
Chest Pain/Possible Heart Attack Care				
Aspirin Given Within 24 Hours of Arrival[1,3]	-	-	97%	96%
Fibrinolytic Meds Within 30 Min. of Arrival[3,7]	-	-	44%	58%
Average Time to ECG (minutes)[1,3]	-	-	6	7
Average Time to Transfer (minutes)[3,7]	-	-	58	60
Children's Asthma Care				
Received Home Management Plan of Care	-	-	85%	88%
Received Reliever Medication	-	-	100%	100%
Received Systemic Corticosteroids	-	-	100%	100%
Emergency Department				
Admittance Decision Time (minutes)[2]	464	150	90	98
Head CT Results Within 45 Min. of Arrival[1]	-	-	63%	57%
Patients Who Left ER Before Being Seen	>100k	4%	2%	2%
Time from ER Arrival to Admit. (minutes)[2]	467	363	265	274
Time from ER Arrival to Discharge (minutes)	321	184	128	134
Time in ER Before Being Evaluated (minutes)	394	35	22	26
Time to Pain Meds for Fractures (minutes)	80	76	54	57
Heart Attack Care				
Aspirin Given at Discharge[2]	279	100%	99%	99%
Fibrinolytic Meds Within 30 Min. of Arrival[1,2]	-	-	80%	54%
PCI Within 90 Minutes of Arrival[2]	12	92%	97%	96%
Statin Prescribed at Discharge[2]	271	99%	98%	98%
Heart Failure Care				

NOTE: Hospital profiles are in alphabetical order by state, then city, then hospital within the city; Rankings exclude hospitals with less than 25 cases except for patient surveys which excludes hospitals with less than 100 cases; (a) 100-299 cases; (1) The number of cases/patients is too few to report; (2) Data submitted were based on a sample of cases/patients; (3) Results are based on a shorter time period than required; (4) Data suppressed by CMS for one or more quarters; (5) Results are not available for this reporting period; (6) Fewer than 100 patients completed the HCAHPS survey; (7) No cases met the criteria for this measure; (8) The lower limit of the confidence interval cannot be calculated if the number of observed infections equals zero; (9) No data are available from the state/territory for this reporting period; (10) The scores shown reflect fewer than 50 completed surveys; (11) There were discrepancies in the data collection process; (12) This measure does not apply to this hospital for this reporting period; (13) Results cannot be calculated for this reporting period; (14) The results for this state are combined with nearby states to protect confidentiality; Please refer to the User's Guide for a full explanation of data.

Measure	Cases	This Hosp.	State Avg.	U.S. Avg.
ACE Inhibitor or ARB for LVSD[2]	122	95%	97%	97%
Discharge Instructions Given[2]	245	100%	96%	94%
Evaluation of LVS Function[2]	278	100%	100%	99%
Medicare Spending				
Medicare Spending per Patient (ratio)	-	1.01	1.01	0.98
Pneumonia Care				
Appropriate Initial Antibiotic Given[2]	37	100%	96%	95%
Blood Culture Timing[2]	112	98%	98%	98%
Pregnancy and Delivery Care				
Newborn Deliveries Scheduled Early[2]	41	7%	5%	6%
Preventive Care				
Immunization for Influenza[2]	530	78%	93%	90%
Immunization for Pneumonia[2]	596	77%	94%	92%
Stroke Care				
Anticoagulation Therapy for Atrial Fibrillation	54	98%	95%	95%
Antithrombotic Therapy Timing	251	98%	98%	98%
Assessed for Rehabilitation	436	100%	98%	97%
Discharged on Antithrombotic Therapy	352	98%	99%	99%
Discharged on Statin Medication	265	99%	95%	94%
Thrombolytic Therapy Timing	12	92%	65%	66%
Venous Thromboembolism Prophylaxis	430	98%	95%	94%
Written Stroke Educational Materials Given	183	93%	92%	88%
Surgical Care Improvement Project				
Appropriate Beta Blocker Usage[2]	221	98%	98%	98%
Appropriate VTP Within 24 Hours[2]	345	98%	98%	98%
Controlled Postoperative Blood Glucose[2]	135	100%	97%	97%
Perioperative Temperature Management[2]	415	100%	100%	100%
Prophylactic Antibiotic Selection[2]	386	99%	99%	99%
Prophylactic Antibiotic Selection (Outpatient)	495	99%	98%	98%
Prophylactic Antibiotic Stopped[2]	375	99%	98%	98%
Prophylactic Antibiotic Timing[2]	387	99%	99%	99%
Prophylactic Antibiotic Timing (Outpatient)	496	97%	97%	98%
Urinary Catheter Removal[2]	338	95%	97%	97%
Survey of Patients' Hospital Experiences				
Area Around Room 'Always' Quiet at Night	300+	59%	58%	61%
Doctors 'Always' Communicated Well	300+	79%	80%	82%
Home Recovery Information Given	300+	87%	87%	85%
Hospital Given 9 or 10 on 10 Point Scale	300+	74%	72%	71%
Meds 'Always' Explained Before Given	300+	65%	64%	64%
Nurses 'Always' Communicated Well	300+	81%	81%	79%
Pain 'Always' Well Controlled	300+	71%	71%	71%
Room and Bathroom 'Always' Clean	300+	71%	75%	73%
Timely Help 'Always' Received	300+	66%	70%	68%
Would Definitely Recommend Hospital	300+	77%	71%	71%
Use of Medical Imaging				
Cardiac Imaging Stress Test before Surgery	610	9.8%	5.4%	5.3%
Combination Abdominal CT Scan	1,536	8.7%	7.1%	10.5%
Combination Brain/Sinus CT Scan	816	3.2%	2.8%	2.7%
Combination Chest CT Scan	1,417	0.3%	1.7%	2.7%
Follow-up Mammogram/Ultrasound	252	17.9%	8.7%	8.8%
Lumbar Spine MRI for Low Back Pain	199	37.7%	34.7%	37.2%

Riverside Methodist Hospital

3535 Olentangy River Rd
Columbus, OH 43214
Phone: 614-566-5000
Fax: 614-566-6760
URL: www.ohiohealth.com
Type: Acute Care Hospitals
Emergency Services: Yes
Ownership: Voluntary non-profit - Private
Beds: 1,049

Key Personnel:

CEO/President. . . . . Bruce Hagen
Chief of Medical Staff. . . . . Mark Montoney, MD
Radiology. . . . . Kyle Sharp
Operating Room. . . . . Mary Spyros
Coronary Care . . . . Linda Wagner
Pediatric Ambulatory Care . . . . . . Patrick Wall, MD
Pediatric In-Patient Care . . . . Patrick Wall, MD
Cardiac Laboratory. . . . . Marty Yoder, RN

Measure	Cases	This Hosp.	State Avg.	U.S. Avg.
Blood Clot Prevention and Treatment				
Anticoagulation Overlap Therapy[2]	278	97%	93%	93%
ICU Venous Thromboembolism Prophylaxis[2]	121	97%	93%	92%
Incidence of Potentially Preventable VTE[2]	75	5%	6%	10%
UFH with Dosages/Platelet Monitoring[2]	331	100%	98%	97%
Venous Thromboembolism Prophylaxis[2]	292	89%	88%	85%
Warfarin Therapy Discharge Instructions[2]	193	90%	79%	75%
Chest Pain/Possible Heart Attack Care				
Aspirin Given Within 24 Hours of Arrival[1,3]	-	-	97%	96%
Fibrinolytic Meds Within 30 Min. of Arrival[5]	-	-	44%	58%
Average Time to ECG (minutes)[1,3]	-	-	6	7
Average Time to Transfer (minutes)[5]	-	-	58	60
Children's Asthma Care				
Received Home Management Plan of Care	-	-	85%	88%
Received Reliever Medication	-	-	100%	100%
Received Systemic Corticosteroids	-	-	100%	100%
Emergency Department				
Admittance Decision Time (minutes)[2]	431	183	90	98
Head CT Results Within 45 Min. of Arrival[1]	-	-	63%	57%
Patients Who Left ER Before Being Seen	89,739	2%	2%	2%
Time from ER Arrival to Admit. (minutes)[2]	431	332	265	274
Time from ER Arrival to Discharge (minutes)	319	203	128	134
Time in ER Before Being Evaluated (minutes)	419	20	22	26
Time to Pain Meds for Fractures (minutes)	134	64	54	57
Heart Attack Care				
Aspirin Given at Discharge[2]	299	100%	99%	99%
Fibrinolytic Meds Within 30 Min. of Arrival[2,7]	-	-	80%	54%
PCI Within 90 Minutes of Arrival[2]	40	100%	97%	96%
Statin Prescribed at Discharge[2]	288	100%	98%	98%
Heart Failure Care				
ACE Inhibitor or ARB for LVSD[2]	87	100%	97%	97%
Discharge Instructions Given[2]	239	100%	96%	94%
Evaluation of LVS Function[2]	306	100%	100%	99%
Medicare Spending				
Medicare Spending per Patient (ratio)	-	1.00	1.01	0.98
Pneumonia Care				
Appropriate Initial Antibiotic Given[2]	56	98%	96%	95%
Blood Culture Timing[2]	79	99%	98%	98%
Pregnancy and Delivery Care				
Newborn Deliveries Scheduled Early	532	2%	5%	6%
Preventive Care				
Immunization for Influenza[2]	547	95%	93%	90%
Immunization for Pneumonia[2]	681	96%	94%	92%
Stroke Care				
Anticoagulation Therapy for Atrial Fibrillation	124	98%	95%	95%
Antithrombotic Therapy Timing	623	98%	98%	98%
Assessed for Rehabilitation	992	99%	98%	97%
Discharged on Antithrombotic Therapy	779	100%	99%	99%
Discharged on Statin Medication	578	99%	95%	94%
Thrombolytic Therapy Timing	54	94%	65%	66%
Venous Thromboembolism Prophylaxis	1,022	100%	95%	94%
Written Stroke Educational Materials Given	474	99%	92%	88%
Surgical Care Improvement Project				
Appropriate Beta Blocker Usage[2]	505	99%	98%	98%
Appropriate VTP Within 24 Hours[2]	835	100%	98%	98%
Controlled Postoperative Blood Glucose[2]	285	96%	97%	97%
Perioperative Temperature Management[2]	1,052	100%	100%	100%
Prophylactic Antibiotic Selection[2]	1,012	99%	99%	99%
Prophylactic Antibiotic Selection (Outpatient)	617	98%	98%	98%
Prophylactic Antibiotic Stopped[2]	985	98%	98%	98%
Prophylactic Antibiotic Timing[2]	1,013	100%	99%	99%
Prophylactic Antibiotic Timing (Outpatient)	624	97%	97%	98%
Urinary Catheter Removal[2]	812	99%	97%	97%
Survey of Patients' Hospital Experiences				
Area Around Room 'Always' Quiet at Night	300+	53%	58%	61%
Doctors 'Always' Communicated Well	300+	79%	80%	82%
Home Recovery Information Given	300+	86%	87%	85%
Hospital Given 9 or 10 on 10 Point Scale	300+	76%	72%	71%
Meds 'Always' Explained Before Given	300+	65%	64%	64%
Nurses 'Always' Communicated Well	300+	80%	81%	79%
Pain 'Always' Well Controlled	300+	72%	71%	71%
Room and Bathroom 'Always' Clean	300+	71%	75%	73%
Timely Help 'Always' Received	300+	64%	70%	68%
Would Definitely Recommend Hospital	300+	79%	71%	71%
Use of Medical Imaging				
Cardiac Imaging Stress Test before Surgery	1,066	6.0%	5.4%	5.3%
Combination Abdominal CT Scan	1,969	4.9%	7.1%	10.5%
Combination Brain/Sinus CT Scan	1,290	2.9%	2.8%	2.7%
Combination Chest CT Scan	1,472	1.4%	1.7%	2.7%
Follow-up Mammogram/Ultrasound	3,935	8.6%	8.7%	8.8%
Lumbar Spine MRI for Low Back Pain	342	34.5%	34.7%	37.2%

Lake Health

7590 Auburn Road
Concord, OH 44077
Phone: 440-953-9600
URL: www.lakehealth.org
Type: Acute Care Hospitals
Emergency Services: Yes
Ownership: Voluntary non-profit - Private

Measure	Cases	This Hosp.	State Avg.	U.S. Avg.
Blood Clot Prevention and Treatment				
Anticoagulation Overlap Therapy[2]	140	98%	93%	93%
ICU Venous Thromboembolism Prophylaxis[2]	56	95%	93%	92%
Incidence of Potentially Preventable VTE[2]	12	0%	6%	10%
UFH with Dosages/Platelet Monitoring[2]	109	100%	98%	97%
Venous Thromboembolism Prophylaxis[2]	331	91%	88%	85%
Warfarin Therapy Discharge Instructions[2]	118	91%	79%	75%
Chest Pain/Possible Heart Attack Care				
Aspirin Given Within 24 Hours of Arrival	28	96%	97%	96%
Fibrinolytic Meds Within 30 Min. of Arrival[3,7]	-	-	44%	58%
Average Time to ECG (minutes)	31	2	6	7
Average Time to Transfer (minutes)[1,3]	-	-	58	60
Children's Asthma Care				
Received Home Management Plan of Care	-	-	85%	88%
Received Reliever Medication	-	-	100%	100%
Received Systemic Corticosteroids	-	-	100%	100%
Emergency Department				
Admittance Decision Time (minutes)[2]	676	99	90	98
Head CT Results Within 45 Min. of Arrival	43	63%	63%	57%
Patients Who Left ER Before Being Seen	79,051	1%	2%	2%
Time from ER Arrival to Admit. (minutes)[2]	677	297	265	274
Time from ER Arrival to Discharge (minutes)	341	150	128	134
Time in ER Before Being Evaluated (minutes)	303	25	22	26
Time to Pain Meds for Fractures (minutes)	178	50	54	57
Heart Attack Care				
Aspirin Given at Discharge	290	100%	99%	99%
Fibrinolytic Meds Within 30 Min. of Arrival[7]	-	-	80%	54%
PCI Within 90 Minutes of Arrival	64	98%	97%	96%
Statin Prescribed at Discharge	286	100%	98%	98%
Heart Failure Care				
ACE Inhibitor or ARB for LVSD	136	97%	97%	97%
Discharge Instructions Given	449	97%	96%	94%
Evaluation of LVS Function	617	100%	100%	99%
Medicare Spending				
Medicare Spending per Patient (ratio)	-	1.03	1.01	0.98
Pneumonia Care				
Appropriate Initial Antibiotic Given	264	98%	96%	95%
Blood Culture Timing	188	97%	98%	98%
Pregnancy and Delivery Care				
Newborn Deliveries Scheduled Early[2]	52	10%	5%	6%
Preventive Care				
Immunization for Influenza[2]	525	99%	93%	90%
Immunization for Pneumonia[2]	725	99%	94%	92%
Stroke Care				
Anticoagulation Therapy for Atrial Fibrillation	29	93%	95%	95%
Antithrombotic Therapy Timing	194	98%	98%	98%
Assessed for Rehabilitation	189	99%	98%	97%
Discharged on Antithrombotic Therapy	184	100%	99%	99%
Discharged on Statin Medication	123	99%	95%	94%
Thrombolytic Therapy Timing[1]	-	-	65%	66%
Venous Thromboembolism Prophylaxis	199	99%	95%	94%
Written Stroke Educational Materials Given	120	99%	92%	88%
Surgical Care Improvement Project				
Appropriate Beta Blocker Usage[2]	238	100%	98%	98%
Appropriate VTP Within 24 Hours[2]	405	98%	98%	98%
Controlled Postoperative Blood Glucose[2]	88	94%	97%	97%
Perioperative Temperature Management[2]	523	100%	100%	100%
Prophylactic Antibiotic Selection[2]	398	99%	99%	99%
Prophylactic Antibiotic Selection (Outpatient)	295	99%	98%	98%
Prophylactic Antibiotic Stopped[2]	392	98%	98%	98%
Prophylactic Antibiotic Timing[2]	399	100%	99%	99%

NOTE: Hospital profiles are in alphabetical order by state, then city, then hospital within the city; Rankings exclude hospitals with less than 25 cases except for patient surveys which excludes hospitals with less than 100 cases; (a) 100-299 cases; (1) The number of cases/patients is too few to report; (2) Data submitted were based on a sample of cases/patients; (3) Results are based on a shorter time period than required; (4) Data suppressed by CMS for one or more quarters; (5) Results are not available for this reporting period; (6) Fewer than 100 patients completed the HCAHPS survey; (7) No cases met the criteria for this measure; (8) The lower limit of the confidence interval cannot be calculated if the number of observed infections equals zero; (9) No data are available from the state/territory for this reporting period; (10) The scores shown reflect fewer than 50 completed surveys; (11) There were discrepancies in the data collection process; (12) This measure does not apply to this hospital for this reporting period; (13) Results cannot be calculated for this reporting period; (14) The results for this state are combined with nearby states to protect confidentiality; Please refer to the User's Guide for a full explanation of data.

Measure	Cases	This Hosp.	State Avg.	U.S. Avg.
Prophylactic Antibiotic Timing (Outpatient)	300	96%	97%	98%
Urinary Catheter Removal[2]	260	99%	97%	97%
Survey of Patients' Hospital Experiences				
Area Around Room 'Always' Quiet at Night	300+	54%	58%	61%
Doctors 'Always' Communicated Well	300+	76%	80%	82%
Home Recovery Information Given	300+	87%	87%	85%
Hospital Given 9 or 10 on 10 Point Scale	300+	68%	72%	71%
Meds 'Always' Explained Before Given	300+	64%	64%	64%
Nurses 'Always' Communicated Well	300+	81%	81%	79%
Pain 'Always' Well Controlled	300+	71%	71%	71%
Room and Bathroom 'Always' Clean	300+	75%	75%	73%
Timely Help 'Always' Received	300+	67%	70%	68%
Would Definitely Recommend Hospital	300+	69%	71%	71%
Use of Medical Imaging				
Cardiac Imaging Stress Test before Surgery	173	6.9%	5.4%	5.3%
Combination Abdominal CT Scan	1,684	2.5%	7.1%	10.5%
Combination Brain/Sinus CT Scan	1,643	4.3%	2.8%	2.7%
Combination Chest CT Scan	1,082	0.5%	1.7%	2.7%
Follow-up Mammogram/Ultrasound	3,409	8.5%	8.7%	8.8%
Lumbar Spine MRI for Low Back Pain	237	36.3%	34.7%	37.2%

University Hospitals Conneaut Medical Center

158 West Main Road
Conneaut, OH 44030
Phone: 440-593-1131
Fax: 440-593-5050
URL: www.uhhospitals.org/conneaut
Type: Critical Access Hospitals
Emergency Services: Yes
Ownership: Voluntary non-profit - Other
Beds: 86

Key Personnel:
CEO/President. . . . . William Lawrence

Measure	Cases	This Hosp.	State Avg.	U.S. Avg.
Blood Clot Prevention and Treatment				
Anticoagulation Overlap Therapy[1,2]	-	-	93%	93%
ICU Venous Thromboembolism Prophylaxis[2]	29	100%	93%	92%
Incidence of Potentially Preventable VTE[1,2]	-	-	6%	10%
UFH with Dosages/Platelet Monitoring[1,2]	-	-	98%	97%
Venous Thromboembolism Prophylaxis[2]	66	98%	88%	85%
Warfarin Therapy Discharge Instructions[1,2]	-	-	79%	75%
Chest Pain/Possible Heart Attack Care				
Aspirin Given Within 24 Hours of Arrival	75	100%	97%	96%
Fibrinolytic Meds Within 30 Min. of Arrival[7]	-	-	44%	58%
Average Time to ECG (minutes)	82	4	6	7
Average Time to Transfer (minutes)[1]	-	-	58	60
Children's Asthma Care				
Received Home Management Plan of Care	-	-	85%	88%
Received Reliever Medication	-	-	100%	100%
Received Systemic Corticosteroids	-	-	100%	100%
Emergency Department				
Admittance Decision Time (minutes)	279	50	90	98
Head CT Results Within 45 Min. of Arrival[3,7]	-	-	63%	57%
Patients Who Left ER Before Being Seen	13,320	1%	2%	2%
Time from ER Arrival to Admit. (minutes)	284	198	265	274
Time from ER Arrival to Discharge (minutes)	398	84	128	134
Time in ER Before Being Evaluated (minutes)	432	16	22	26
Time to Pain Meds for Fractures (minutes)	53	48	54	57
Heart Attack Care				
Aspirin Given at Discharge[1,3]	-	-	99%	99%
Fibrinolytic Meds Within 30 Min. of Arrival[3,7]	-	-	80%	54%
PCI Within 90 Minutes of Arrival[3,7]	-	-	97%	96%
Statin Prescribed at Discharge[1,3]	-	-	98%	98%
Heart Failure Care				
ACE Inhibitor or ARB for LVSD[1]	-	-	97%	97%
Discharge Instructions Given	20	100%	96%	94%
Evaluation of LVS Function	30	100%	100%	99%
Medicare Spending				
Medicare Spending per Patient (ratio)	-	-	1.01	0.98
Pneumonia Care				
Appropriate Initial Antibiotic Given	26	100%	96%	95%
Blood Culture Timing	40	98%	98%	98%
Pregnancy and Delivery Care				
Newborn Deliveries Scheduled Early[7]	-	-	5%	6%
Preventive Care				
Immunization for Influenza	197	98%	93%	90%
Immunization for Pneumonia	350	98%	94%	92%
Stroke Care				
Anticoagulation Therapy for Atrial Fibrillation[3,7]	-	-	95%	95%
Antithrombotic Therapy Timing[1,3]	-	-	98%	98%
Assessed for Rehabilitation[1,3]	-	-	98%	97%
Discharged on Antithrombotic Therapy[1,3]	-	-	99%	99%
Discharged on Statin Medication[1,3]	-	-	95%	94%
Thrombolytic Therapy Timing[3,7]	-	-	65%	66%
Venous Thromboembolism Prophylaxis[1,3]	-	-	95%	94%
Written Stroke Educational Materials Given[3,7]	-	-	92%	88%
Surgical Care Improvement Project				
Appropriate Beta Blocker Usage	48	98%	98%	98%
Appropriate VTP Within 24 Hours	120	100%	98%	98%
Controlled Postoperative Blood Glucose[7]	-	-	97%	97%
Perioperative Temperature Management	117	100%	100%	100%
Prophylactic Antibiotic Selection	89	100%	99%	99%
Prophylactic Antibiotic Selection (Outpatient)[5]	-	-	98%	98%
Prophylactic Antibiotic Stopped	89	100%	98%	98%
Prophylactic Antibiotic Timing	89	100%	99%	99%
Prophylactic Antibiotic Timing (Outpatient)[5]	-	-	97%	98%
Urinary Catheter Removal	118	100%	97%	97%
Survey of Patients' Hospital Experiences				
Area Around Room 'Always' Quiet at Night	(a)	75%	58%	61%
Doctors 'Always' Communicated Well	(a)	85%	80%	82%
Home Recovery Information Given	(a)	91%	87%	85%
Hospital Given 9 or 10 on 10 Point Scale	(a)	87%	72%	71%
Meds 'Always' Explained Before Given	(a)	77%	64%	64%
Nurses 'Always' Communicated Well	(a)	93%	81%	79%
Pain 'Always' Well Controlled	(a)	83%	71%	71%
Room and Bathroom 'Always' Clean	(a)	87%	75%	73%
Timely Help 'Always' Received	(a)	91%	70%	68%
Would Definitely Recommend Hospital	(a)	84%	71%	71%
Use of Medical Imaging				
Cardiac Imaging Stress Test before Surgery	59	1.7%	5.4%	5.3%
Combination Abdominal CT Scan	198	6.1%	7.1%	10.5%
Combination Brain/Sinus CT Scan[1]	-	-	2.8%	2.7%
Combination Chest CT Scan	124	0.8%	1.7%	2.7%
Follow-up Mammogram/Ultrasound	233	7.7%	8.7%	8.8%
Lumbar Spine MRI for Low Back Pain[1]	-	-	34.7%	37.2%

Coshocton County Memorial Hospital

1460 Orange Street
Coshocton, OH 43812
Phone: 740-622-6411
Fax: 740-623-4095
URL: www.ccmh.com
Type: Acute Care Hospitals
Emergency Services: Yes
Ownership: Voluntary non-profit - Private
Beds: 61

Key Personnel:
Quality Assurance . . . . Kathy Bauman, RN
Infection Control. . . . . Marjorie Erman
Chief of Medical Staff. . . . . Robert B. Gwinn, DO
Radiology. . . . . Linda J Magness, MD
Intensive Care Unit. . . . . Gwen Miller, RN
Emergency Room . . . . R Patel, MD
Operating Room. . . . . Judi Shaffer, RN
CEO . . . . Lorri S. Wildi

Measure	Cases	This Hosp.	State Avg.	U.S. Avg.
Blood Clot Prevention and Treatment				
Anticoagulation Overlap Therapy[1,2]	-	-	93%	93%
ICU Venous Thromboembolism Prophylaxis[2]	27	52%	93%	92%
Incidence of Potentially Preventable VTE[1,2]	-	-	6%	10%
UFH with Dosages/Platelet Monitoring[1,2]	-	-	98%	97%
Venous Thromboembolism Prophylaxis[2]	153	59%	88%	85%
Warfarin Therapy Discharge Instructions[1,2]	-	-	79%	75%
Chest Pain/Possible Heart Attack Care				
Aspirin Given Within 24 Hours of Arrival	81	93%	97%	96%
Fibrinolytic Meds Within 30 Min. of Arrival[1]	-	-	44%	58%
Average Time to ECG (minutes)	83	10	6	7
Average Time to Transfer (minutes)[1]	-	-	58	60
Children's Asthma Care				
Received Home Management Plan of Care	-	-	85%	88%
Received Reliever Medication	-	-	100%	100%
Received Systemic Corticosteroids	-	-	100%	100%
Emergency Department				
Admittance Decision Time (minutes)[2]	357	95	90	98
Head CT Results Within 45 Min. of Arrival[1]	-	-	63%	57%
Patients Who Left ER Before Being Seen	26,163	1%	2%	2%
Time from ER Arrival to Admit. (minutes)[2]	385	300	265	274
Time from ER Arrival to Discharge (minutes)	363	106	128	134
Time in ER Before Being Evaluated (minutes)	374	36	22	26
Time to Pain Meds for Fractures (minutes)	40	56	54	57
Heart Attack Care				
Aspirin Given at Discharge[1]	-	-	99%	99%
Fibrinolytic Meds Within 30 Min. of Arrival[7]	-	-	80%	54%
PCI Within 90 Minutes of Arrival[7]	-	-	97%	96%
Statin Prescribed at Discharge[1]	-	-	98%	98%
Heart Failure Care				
ACE Inhibitor or ARB for LVSD	11	64%	97%	97%
Discharge Instructions Given	63	75%	96%	94%
Evaluation of LVS Function	84	73%	100%	99%
Medicare Spending				
Medicare Spending per Patient (ratio)	-	1.01	1.01	0.98
Pneumonia Care				
Appropriate Initial Antibiotic Given	62	94%	96%	95%
Blood Culture Timing	87	100%	98%	98%
Pregnancy and Delivery Care				
Newborn Deliveries Scheduled Early[2]	11	0%	5%	6%
Preventive Care				
Immunization for Influenza[2]	258	85%	93%	90%
Immunization for Pneumonia[2]	379	92%	94%	92%
Stroke Care				
Anticoagulation Therapy for Atrial Fibrillation[1]	-	-	95%	95%
Antithrombotic Therapy Timing	19	84%	98%	98%
Assessed for Rehabilitation	18	100%	98%	97%
Discharged on Antithrombotic Therapy	18	83%	99%	99%
Discharged on Statin Medication	15	67%	95%	94%
Thrombolytic Therapy Timing[7]	-	-	65%	66%
Venous Thromboembolism Prophylaxis	16	50%	95%	94%
Written Stroke Educational Materials Given	11	55%	92%	88%
Surgical Care Improvement Project				
Appropriate Beta Blocker Usage	28	86%	98%	98%
Appropriate VTP Within 24 Hours	75	89%	98%	98%
Controlled Postoperative Blood Glucose[7]	-	-	97%	97%
Perioperative Temperature Management	93	99%	100%	100%
Prophylactic Antibiotic Selection	62	89%	99%	99%
Prophylactic Antibiotic Selection (Outpatient)	21	90%	98%	98%
Prophylactic Antibiotic Stopped	61	70%	98%	98%
Prophylactic Antibiotic Timing	62	90%	99%	99%
Prophylactic Antibiotic Timing (Outpatient)	21	100%	97%	98%
Urinary Catheter Removal	34	53%	97%	97%
Survey of Patients' Hospital Experiences				
Area Around Room 'Always' Quiet at Night	300+	52%	58%	61%
Doctors 'Always' Communicated Well	300+	76%	80%	82%
Home Recovery Information Given	300+	79%	87%	85%
Hospital Given 9 or 10 on 10 Point Scale	300+	58%	72%	71%
Meds 'Always' Explained Before Given	300+	60%	64%	64%
Nurses 'Always' Communicated Well	300+	79%	81%	79%
Pain 'Always' Well Controlled	300+	70%	71%	71%
Room and Bathroom 'Always' Clean	300+	78%	75%	73%
Timely Help 'Always' Received	300+	64%	70%	68%
Would Definitely Recommend Hospital	300+	49%	71%	71%
Use of Medical Imaging				
Cardiac Imaging Stress Test before Surgery	213	0.9%	5.4%	5.3%
Combination Abdominal CT Scan	343	2.9%	7.1%	10.5%
Combination Brain/Sinus CT Scan[1]	-	-	2.8%	2.7%
Combination Chest CT Scan	220	0.5%	1.7%	2.7%
Follow-up Mammogram/Ultrasound	567	7.9%	8.7%	8.8%
Lumbar Spine MRI for Low Back Pain	64	35.9%	34.7%	37.2%

Edwin Shaw Rehab Institute

330 Broadway East
Cuyahoga Falls, OH 44221
Phone: 330-436-0910
URL: www.akrongeneral.org
Type: Acute Care Hospitals
Emergency Services: No
Ownership: Government - Local

Measure	Cases	This Hosp.	State Avg.	U.S. Avg.
Blood Clot Prevention and Treatment				
Anticoagulation Overlap Therapy[5]	-	-	93%	93%

NOTE: Hospital profiles are in alphabetical order by state, then city, then hospital within the city; Rankings exclude hospitals with less than 25 cases except for patient surveys which excludes hospitals with less than 100 cases; (a) 100-299 cases; (1) The number of cases/patients is too few to report; (2) Data submitted were based on a sample of cases/patients; (3) Results are based on a shorter time period than required; (4) Data suppressed by CMS for one or more quarters; (5) Results are not available for this reporting period; (6) Fewer than 100 patients completed the HCAHPS survey; (7) No cases met the criteria for this measure; (8) The lower limit of the confidence interval cannot be calculated if the number of observed infections equals zero; (9) No data are available from the state/territory for this reporting period; (10) The scores shown reflect fewer than 50 completed surveys; (11) There were discrepancies in the data collection process; (12) This measure does not apply to this hospital for this reporting period; (13) Results cannot be calculated for this reporting period; (14) The results for this state are combined with nearby states to protect confidentiality; Please refer to the User's Guide for a full explanation of data.

Measure	Cases	This Hosp.	State Avg.	U.S. Avg.
ICU Venous Thromboembolism Prophylaxis[5]	-	-	93%	92%
Incidence of Potentially Preventable VTE[5]	-	-	6%	10%
UFH with Dosages/Platelet Monitoring[5]	-	-	98%	97%
Venous Thromboembolism Prophylaxis[5]	-	-	88%	85%
Warfarin Therapy Discharge Instructions[5]	-	-	79%	75%
Chest Pain/Possible Heart Attack Care				
Aspirin Given Within 24 Hours of Arrival	-	-	97%	96%
Fibrinolytic Meds Within 30 Min. of Arrival	-	-	44%	58%
Average Time to ECG (minutes)	-	-	6	7
Average Time to Transfer (minutes)	-	-	58	60
Children's Asthma Care				
Received Home Management Plan of Care	-	-	85%	88%
Received Reliever Medication	-	-	100%	100%
Received Systemic Corticosteroids	-	-	100%	100%
Emergency Department				
Admittance Decision Time (minutes)[5]	-	-	90	98
Head CT Results Within 45 Min. of Arrival	-	-	63%	57%
Patients Who Left ER Before Being Seen	-	-	2%	2%
Time from ER Arrival to Admit. (minutes)[5]	-	-	265	274
Time from ER Arrival to Discharge (minutes)	-	-	128	134
Time in ER Before Being Evaluated (minutes)	-	-	22	26
Time to Pain Meds for Fractures (minutes)	-	-	54	57
Heart Attack Care				
Aspirin Given at Discharge[5]	-	-	99%	99%
Fibrinolytic Meds Within 30 Min. of Arrival[5]	-	-	80%	54%
PCI Within 90 Minutes of Arrival[5]	-	-	97%	96%
Statin Prescribed at Discharge[5]	-	-	98%	98%
Heart Failure Care				
ACE Inhibitor or ARB for LVSD[5]	-	-	97%	97%
Discharge Instructions Given[5]	-	-	96%	94%
Evaluation of LVS Function[5]	-	-	100%	99%
Medicare Spending				
Medicare Spending per Patient (ratio)	-	-	1.01	0.98
Pneumonia Care				
Appropriate Initial Antibiotic Given[5]	-	-	96%	95%
Blood Culture Timing[5]	-	-	98%	98%
Pregnancy and Delivery Care				
Newborn Deliveries Scheduled Early[7]	-	-	5%	6%
Preventive Care				
Immunization for Influenza[5]	-	-	93%	90%
Immunization for Pneumonia[5]	-	-	94%	92%
Stroke Care				
Anticoagulation Therapy for Atrial Fibrillation[5]	-	-	95%	95%
Antithrombotic Therapy Timing[5]	-	-	98%	98%
Assessed for Rehabilitation[5]	-	-	98%	97%
Discharged on Antithrombotic Therapy[5]	-	-	99%	99%
Discharged on Statin Medication[5]	-	-	95%	94%
Thrombolytic Therapy Timing[5]	-	-	65%	66%
Venous Thromboembolism Prophylaxis[5]	-	-	95%	94%
Written Stroke Educational Materials Given[5]	-	-	92%	88%
Surgical Care Improvement Project				
Appropriate Beta Blocker Usage[5]	-	-	98%	98%
Appropriate VTP Within 24 Hours[5]	-	-	98%	98%
Controlled Postoperative Blood Glucose[5]	-	-	97%	97%
Perioperative Temperature Management[5]	-	-	100%	100%
Prophylactic Antibiotic Selection[5]	-	-	99%	99%
Prophylactic Antibiotic Selection (Outpatient)	-	-	98%	98%
Prophylactic Antibiotic Stopped[5]	-	-	98%	98%
Prophylactic Antibiotic Timing[5]	-	-	99%	99%
Prophylactic Antibiotic Timing (Outpatient)	-	-	97%	98%
Urinary Catheter Removal[5]	-	-	97%	97%
Survey of Patients' Hospital Experiences				
Area Around Room 'Always' Quiet at Night[1]	-	-	58%	61%
Doctors 'Always' Communicated Well[1]	-	-	80%	82%
Home Recovery Information Given[1]	-	-	87%	85%
Hospital Given 9 or 10 on 10 Point Scale[1]	-	-	72%	71%
Meds 'Always' Explained Before Given[1]	-	-	64%	64%
Nurses 'Always' Communicated Well[1]	-	-	81%	79%
Pain 'Always' Well Controlled[1]	-	-	71%	71%
Room and Bathroom 'Always' Clean[1]	-	-	75%	73%
Timely Help 'Always' Received[1]	-	-	70%	68%
Would Definitely Recommend Hospital[1]	-	-	71%	71%
Use of Medical Imaging				
Cardiac Imaging Stress Test before Surgery	-	-	5.4%	5.3%
Combination Abdominal CT Scan	-	-	7.1%	10.5%
Combination Brain/Sinus CT Scan	-	-	2.8%	2.7%
Combination Chest CT Scan	-	-	1.7%	2.7%
Follow-up Mammogram/Ultrasound	-	-	8.7%	8.8%
Lumbar Spine MRI for Low Back Pain	-	-	34.7%	37.2%

Summa Western Reserve Hospital

1900 23rd Street Phone: 330-971-7000
Cuyahoga Falls, OH 44223 Fax: 330-971-7155
URL: www.westernreservehospital.org
Type: Acute Care Hospitals Emergency Services: Yes
Ownership: Voluntary non-profit - Other Beds: 257
Key Personnel:
Radiology. . . . . GL Classen, DO
Quality Assurance . . . . Denise Haynes
Chief of Medical Staff. . . . . Leroy Refer
CEO/President. . . . . Kathleen Rice

Measure	Cases	This Hosp.	State Avg.	U.S. Avg.
Blood Clot Prevention and Treatment				
Anticoagulation Overlap Therapy[2]	44	98%	93%	93%
ICU Venous Thromboembolism Prophylaxis[2]	133	99%	93%	92%
Incidence of Potentially Preventable VTE[1,2]	-	-	6%	10%
UFH with Dosages/Platelet Monitoring[2]	28	100%	98%	97%
Venous Thromboembolism Prophylaxis[2]	299	98%	88%	85%
Warfarin Therapy Discharge Instructions[2]	31	100%	79%	75%
Chest Pain/Possible Heart Attack Care				
Aspirin Given Within 24 Hours of Arrival	34	97%	97%	96%
Fibrinolytic Meds Within 30 Min. of Arrival[7]	-	-	44%	58%
Average Time to ECG (minutes)	35	10	6	7
Average Time to Transfer (minutes)	19	56	58	60
Children's Asthma Care				
Received Home Management Plan of Care	-	-	85%	88%
Received Reliever Medication	-	-	100%	100%
Received Systemic Corticosteroids	-	-	100%	100%
Emergency Department				
Admittance Decision Time (minutes)[2]	582	110	90	98
Head CT Results Within 45 Min. of Arrival[1]	-	-	63%	57%
Patients Who Left ER Before Being Seen	21,960	0%	2%	2%
Time from ER Arrival to Admit. (minutes)[2]	618	280	265	274
Time from ER Arrival to Discharge (minutes)	436	146	128	134
Time in ER Before Being Evaluated (minutes)	464	19	22	26
Time to Pain Meds for Fractures (minutes)	73	78	54	57
Heart Attack Care				
Aspirin Given at Discharge[1]	-	-	99%	99%
Fibrinolytic Meds Within 30 Min. of Arrival[7]	-	-	80%	54%
PCI Within 90 Minutes of Arrival[7]	-	-	97%	96%
Statin Prescribed at Discharge[1]	-	-	98%	98%
Heart Failure Care				
ACE Inhibitor or ARB for LVSD	25	100%	97%	97%
Discharge Instructions Given	76	100%	96%	94%
Evaluation of LVS Function	90	99%	100%	99%
Medicare Spending				
Medicare Spending per Patient (ratio)	-	1.01	1.01	0.98
Pneumonia Care				
Appropriate Initial Antibiotic Given	96	96%	96%	95%
Blood Culture Timing	143	97%	98%	98%
Pregnancy and Delivery Care				
Newborn Deliveries Scheduled Early[7]	-	-	5%	6%
Preventive Care				
Immunization for Influenza[2]	466	98%	93%	90%
Immunization for Pneumonia[2]	747	94%	94%	92%
Stroke Care				
Anticoagulation Therapy for Atrial Fibrillation[1]	-	-	95%	95%
Antithrombotic Therapy Timing	32	97%	98%	98%
Assessed for Rehabilitation	39	100%	98%	97%
Discharged on Antithrombotic Therapy	38	97%	99%	99%
Discharged on Statin Medication	30	100%	95%	94%
Thrombolytic Therapy Timing[1]	-	-	65%	66%
Venous Thromboembolism Prophylaxis	36	97%	95%	94%
Written Stroke Educational Materials Given	20	95%	92%	88%
Surgical Care Improvement Project				
Appropriate Beta Blocker Usage[2]	90	98%	98%	98%
Appropriate VTP Within 24 Hours[2]	301	99%	98%	98%
Controlled Postoperative Blood Glucose[2,7]	-	-	97%	97%
Perioperative Temperature Management[2]	330	100%	100%	100%
Prophylactic Antibiotic Selection[2]	219	99%	99%	99%
Prophylactic Antibiotic Selection (Outpatient)	113	98%	98%	98%
Prophylactic Antibiotic Stopped[2]	216	99%	98%	98%
Prophylactic Antibiotic Timing[2]	219	100%	99%	99%
Prophylactic Antibiotic Timing (Outpatient)	114	99%	97%	98%
Urinary Catheter Removal[2]	174	99%	97%	97%
Survey of Patients' Hospital Experiences				
Area Around Room 'Always' Quiet at Night	300+	57%	58%	61%
Doctors 'Always' Communicated Well	300+	81%	80%	82%
Home Recovery Information Given	300+	88%	87%	85%
Hospital Given 9 or 10 on 10 Point Scale	300+	75%	72%	71%
Meds 'Always' Explained Before Given	300+	65%	64%	64%
Nurses 'Always' Communicated Well	300+	82%	81%	79%
Pain 'Always' Well Controlled	300+	73%	71%	71%
Room and Bathroom 'Always' Clean	300+	66%	75%	73%
Timely Help 'Always' Received	300+	71%	70%	68%
Would Definitely Recommend Hospital	300+	76%	71%	71%
Use of Medical Imaging				
Cardiac Imaging Stress Test before Surgery	174	9.2%	5.4%	5.3%
Combination Abdominal CT Scan	329	3.3%	7.1%	10.5%
Combination Brain/Sinus CT Scan[1]	-	-	2.8%	2.7%
Combination Chest CT Scan	230	0.0%	1.7%	2.7%
Follow-up Mammogram/Ultrasound[7]	-	-	8.7%	8.8%
Lumbar Spine MRI for Low Back Pain	112	38.4%	34.7%	37.2%

Dayton VA Medical Center

4100 West Third Street Phone: 937-268-6511
Dayton, OH 45428 Fax: 937-262-2170
URL: www.dayton.va.gov
Type: Acute Care - VA Emergency Services: No
Ownership: Government Federal Beds: 539
Key Personnel:
Ambulatory Care . . . . Ronald Beaulied, ACOS
CEO/President. . . . . Steven Cohen, MD
Chief of Medical Staff. . . . . Mark Murdock, MD

Measure	Cases	This Hosp.	State Avg.	U.S. Avg.
Blood Clot Prevention and Treatment				
Anticoagulation Overlap Therapy	-	-	93%	93%
ICU Venous Thromboembolism Prophylaxis	-	-	93%	92%
Incidence of Potentially Preventable VTE	-	-	6%	10%
UFH with Dosages/Platelet Monitoring	-	-	98%	97%
Venous Thromboembolism Prophylaxis	-	-	88%	85%
Warfarin Therapy Discharge Instructions	-	-	79%	75%
Chest Pain/Possible Heart Attack Care				
Aspirin Given Within 24 Hours of Arrival	-	-	97%	96%
Fibrinolytic Meds Within 30 Min. of Arrival	-	-	44%	58%
Average Time to ECG (minutes)	-	-	6	7
Average Time to Transfer (minutes)	-	-	58	60
Children's Asthma Care				
Received Home Management Plan of Care	-	-	85%	88%
Received Reliever Medication	-	-	100%	100%
Received Systemic Corticosteroids	-	-	100%	100%
Emergency Department				
Admittance Decision Time (minutes)	-	-	90	98
Head CT Results Within 45 Min. of Arrival	-	-	63%	57%
Patients Who Left ER Before Being Seen	-	-	2%	2%
Time from ER Arrival to Admit. (minutes)	-	-	265	274
Time from ER Arrival to Discharge (minutes)	-	-	128	134
Time in ER Before Being Evaluated (minutes)	-	-	22	26
Time to Pain Meds for Fractures (minutes)	-	-	54	57
Heart Attack Care				
Aspirin Given at Discharge	28	100%	99%	99%
Fibrinolytic Meds Within 30 Min. of Arrival[5]	-	-	80%	54%
PCI Within 90 Minutes of Arrival[5]	-	-	97%	96%
Statin Prescribed at Discharge	29	97%	98%	98%
Heart Failure Care				
ACE Inhibitor or ARB for LVSD	45	98%	97%	97%
Discharge Instructions Given	124	90%	96%	94%
Evaluation of LVS Function	141	100%	100%	99%

NOTE: Hospital profiles are in alphabetical order by state, then city, then hospital within the city; Rankings exclude hospitals with less than 25 cases except for patient surveys which excludes hospitals with less than 100 cases; (a) 100-299 cases; (1) The number of cases/patients is too few to report; (2) Data submitted were based on a sample of cases/patients; (3) Results are based on a shorter time period than required; (4) Data suppressed by CMS for one or more quarters; (5) Results are not available for this reporting period; (6) Fewer than 100 patients completed the HCAHPS survey; (7) No cases met the criteria for this measure; (8) The lower limit of the confidence interval cannot be calculated if the number of observed infections equals zero; (9) No data are available from the state/territory for this reporting period; (10) The scores shown reflect fewer than 50 completed surveys; (11) There were discrepancies in the data collection process; (12) This measure does not apply to this hospital for this reporting period; (13) Results cannot be calculated for this reporting period; (14) The results for this state are combined with nearby states to protect confidentiality; Please refer to the User's Guide for a full explanation of data.

Measure	Cases	This Hosp.	State Avg.	U.S. Avg.
Medicare Spending				
Medicare Spending per Patient (ratio)	-	-	1.01	0.98
Pneumonia Care				
Appropriate Initial Antibiotic Given	47	91%	96%	95%
Blood Culture Timing	93	99%	98%	98%
Pregnancy and Delivery Care				
Newborn Deliveries Scheduled Early	-	-	5%	6%
Preventive Care				
Immunization for Influenza[5]	-	-	93%	90%
Immunization for Pneumonia[5]	-	-	94%	92%
Stroke Care				
Anticoagulation Therapy for Atrial Fibrillation	-	-	95%	95%
Antithrombotic Therapy Timing	-	-	98%	98%
Assessed for Rehabilitation	-	-	98%	97%
Discharged on Antithrombotic Therapy	-	-	99%	99%
Discharged on Statin Medication	-	-	95%	94%
Thrombolytic Therapy Timing	-	-	65%	66%
Venous Thromboembolism Prophylaxis	-	-	95%	94%
Written Stroke Educational Materials Given	-	-	92%	88%
Surgical Care Improvement Project				
Appropriate Beta Blocker Usage[2]	62	95%	98%	98%
Appropriate VTP Within 24 Hours[2]	126	99%	98%	98%
Controlled Postoperative Blood Glucose[5]	-	-	97%	97%
Perioperative Temperature Management[2]	161	100%	100%	100%
Prophylactic Antibiotic Selection	100	99%	99%	99%
Prophylactic Antibiotic Selection (Outpatient)	-	-	98%	98%
Prophylactic Antibiotic Stopped	100	100%	98%	98%
Prophylactic Antibiotic Timing	102	99%	99%	99%
Prophylactic Antibiotic Timing (Outpatient)	-	-	97%	98%
Urinary Catheter Removal[2]	33	100%	97%	97%
Survey of Patients' Hospital Experiences				
Area Around Room 'Always' Quiet at Night	-	-	58%	61%
Doctors 'Always' Communicated Well	-	-	80%	82%
Home Recovery Information Given	-	-	87%	85%
Hospital Given 9 or 10 on 10 Point Scale	-	-	72%	71%
Meds 'Always' Explained Before Given	-	-	64%	64%
Nurses 'Always' Communicated Well	-	-	81%	79%
Pain 'Always' Well Controlled	-	-	71%	71%
Room and Bathroom 'Always' Clean	-	-	75%	73%
Timely Help 'Always' Received	-	-	70%	68%
Would Definitely Recommend Hospital	-	-	71%	71%
Use of Medical Imaging				
Cardiac Imaging Stress Test before Surgery	-	-	5.4%	5.3%
Combination Abdominal CT Scan	-	-	7.1%	10.5%
Combination Brain/Sinus CT Scan	-	-	2.8%	2.7%
Combination Chest CT Scan	-	-	1.7%	2.7%
Follow-up Mammogram/Ultrasound	-	-	8.7%	8.8%
Lumbar Spine MRI for Low Back Pain	-	-	34.7%	37.2%

Good Samaritan Hospital

2222 Philadelphia Drive
Dayton, OH 45406
Phone: 937-278-2612
Fax: 937-276-8244
URL: www.goodsamdayton.org
Type: Acute Care Hospitals
Emergency Services: Yes
Ownership: Voluntary non-profit - Church
Beds: 560

Key Personnel:

Emergency Room . . . . Richard Garrison, MD
Quality Assurance . . . . Mary Gutman
Infection Control. . . . . Sandy Iams
Radiology. . . . . Randall J Reilman, MD
CEO/President. . . . . Mark S Shaker
Chief of Medical Staff. . . . . Timothy B Sorg, MD
Pediatric Ambulatory Care . . . . . . G Youra, MD
Pediatric In-Patient Care . . . . G Youra, MD

Measure	Cases	This Hosp.	State Avg.	U.S. Avg.
Blood Clot Prevention and Treatment				
Anticoagulation Overlap Therapy[2]	145	99%	93%	93%
ICU Venous Thromboembolism Prophylaxis[2]	100	97%	93%	92%
Incidence of Potentially Preventable VTE[2]	20	10%	6%	10%
UFH with Dosages/Platelet Monitoring[2]	118	100%	98%	97%
Venous Thromboembolism Prophylaxis[2]	331	94%	88%	85%
Warfarin Therapy Discharge Instructions[2]	107	98%	79%	75%
Chest Pain/Possible Heart Attack Care				
Aspirin Given Within 24 Hours of Arrival[1,3]	-	-	97%	96%
Fibrinolytic Meds Within 30 Min. of Arrival[3,7]	-	-	44%	58%
Average Time to ECG (minutes)[1,3]	-	-	6	7
Average Time to Transfer (minutes)[3,7]	-	-	58	60
Children's Asthma Care				
Received Home Management Plan of Care	-	-	85%	88%
Received Reliever Medication	-	-	100%	100%
Received Systemic Corticosteroids	-	-	100%	100%
Emergency Department				
Admittance Decision Time (minutes)[2]	644	146	90	98
Head CT Results Within 45 Min. of Arrival	18	72%	63%	57%
Patients Who Left ER Before Being Seen	59,399	4%	2%	2%
Time from ER Arrival to Admit. (minutes)[2]	649	310	265	274
Time from ER Arrival to Discharge (minutes)	370	204	128	134
Time in ER Before Being Evaluated (minutes)	412	30	22	26
Time to Pain Meds for Fractures (minutes)	75	72	54	57
Heart Attack Care				
Aspirin Given at Discharge[2]	322	99%	99%	99%
Fibrinolytic Meds Within 30 Min. of Arrival[2,7]	-	-	80%	54%
PCI Within 90 Minutes of Arrival[2]	40	90%	97%	96%
Statin Prescribed at Discharge[2]	304	100%	98%	98%
Heart Failure Care				
ACE Inhibitor or ARB for LVSD[2]	75	99%	97%	97%
Discharge Instructions Given[2]	238	96%	96%	94%
Evaluation of LVS Function[2]	305	100%	100%	99%
Medicare Spending				
Medicare Spending per Patient (ratio)	-	1.04	1.01	0.98
Pneumonia Care				
Appropriate Initial Antibiotic Given[2]	60	97%	96%	95%
Blood Culture Timing[2]	140	98%	98%	98%
Pregnancy and Delivery Care				
Newborn Deliveries Scheduled Early	100	1%	5%	6%
Preventive Care				
Immunization for Influenza[2]	596	99%	93%	90%
Immunization for Pneumonia[2]	882	99%	94%	92%
Stroke Care				
Anticoagulation Therapy for Atrial Fibrillation[1,2]	-	-	95%	95%
Antithrombotic Therapy Timing[2]	88	98%	98%	98%
Assessed for Rehabilitation[2]	95	100%	98%	97%
Discharged on Antithrombotic Therapy[2]	90	99%	99%	99%
Discharged on Statin Medication[2]	63	100%	95%	94%
Thrombolytic Therapy Timing[1,2]	-	-	65%	66%
Venous Thromboembolism Prophylaxis[2]	94	94%	95%	94%
Written Stroke Educational Materials Given[2]	45	80%	92%	88%
Surgical Care Improvement Project				
Appropriate Beta Blocker Usage[2]	233	100%	98%	98%
Appropriate VTP Within 24 Hours[2]	397	99%	98%	98%
Controlled Postoperative Blood Glucose[2]	156	99%	97%	97%
Perioperative Temperature Management[2]	498	100%	100%	100%
Prophylactic Antibiotic Selection[2]	478	100%	99%	99%
Prophylactic Antibiotic Selection (Outpatient)	488	100%	98%	98%
Prophylactic Antibiotic Stopped[2]	454	99%	98%	98%
Prophylactic Antibiotic Timing[2]	478	100%	99%	99%
Prophylactic Antibiotic Timing (Outpatient)	488	100%	97%	98%
Urinary Catheter Removal[2]	355	99%	97%	97%
Survey of Patients' Hospital Experiences				
Area Around Room 'Always' Quiet at Night[11]	300+	52%	58%	61%
Doctors 'Always' Communicated Well[11]	300+	77%	80%	82%
Home Recovery Information Given[11]	300+	91%	87%	85%
Hospital Given 9 or 10 on 10 Point Scale[11]	300+	70%	72%	71%
Meds 'Always' Explained Before Given[11]	300+	61%	64%	64%
Nurses 'Always' Communicated Well[11]	300+	80%	81%	79%
Pain 'Always' Well Controlled[11]	300+	71%	71%	71%
Room and Bathroom 'Always' Clean[11]	300+	61%	75%	73%
Timely Help 'Always' Received[11]	300+	63%	70%	68%
Would Definitely Recommend Hospital[11]	300+	72%	71%	71%
Use of Medical Imaging				
Cardiac Imaging Stress Test before Surgery	1,242	4.8%	5.4%	5.3%
Combination Abdominal CT Scan	1,148	5.0%	7.1%	10.5%
Combination Brain/Sinus CT Scan	1,169	1.7%	2.8%	2.7%
Combination Chest CT Scan	986	1.6%	1.7%	2.7%
Follow-up Mammogram/Ultrasound	2,987	9.5%	8.7%	8.8%
Lumbar Spine MRI for Low Back Pain	244	41.0%	34.7%	37.2%

Grandview Hospital & Medical Center

405 Grand Avenue
Dayton, OH 45405
Phone: 937-723-3312
Fax: 937-461-0020
URL: www.kmcnetwork.org
Type: Acute Care Hospitals
Emergency Services: Yes
Ownership: Voluntary non-profit - Other
Beds: 452

Key Personnel:

Anesthesiology. . . . . Wayne Anderson, DO
Emergency Room . . . . Charles K MacIntosh, DO
Pediatric In-Patient Care . . . . Robert Myers, DO
CEO/President. . . . . Francisco J Perez
Chief of Medical Staff. . . . . Kevin Reid, DO
Quality Assurance . . . . Diane Setty
Radiology. . . . . David Volarich, DO

Measure	Cases	This Hosp.	State Avg.	U.S. Avg.
Blood Clot Prevention and Treatment				
Anticoagulation Overlap Therapy[2]	90	96%	93%	93%
ICU Venous Thromboembolism Prophylaxis[2]	111	96%	93%	92%
Incidence of Potentially Preventable VTE[2]	16	0%	6%	10%
UFH with Dosages/Platelet Monitoring[2]	77	99%	98%	97%
Venous Thromboembolism Prophylaxis[2]	332	94%	88%	85%
Warfarin Therapy Discharge Instructions[2]	61	69%	79%	75%
Chest Pain/Possible Heart Attack Care				
Aspirin Given Within 24 Hours of Arrival	50	88%	97%	96%
Fibrinolytic Meds Within 30 Min. of Arrival[7]	-	-	44%	58%
Average Time to ECG (minutes)	52	9	6	7
Average Time to Transfer (minutes)[7]	-	-	58	60
Children's Asthma Care				
Received Home Management Plan of Care	-	-	85%	88%
Received Reliever Medication	-	-	100%	100%
Received Systemic Corticosteroids	-	-	100%	100%
Emergency Department				
Admittance Decision Time (minutes)[2]	491	171	90	98
Head CT Results Within 45 Min. of Arrival[1]	-	-	63%	57%
Patients Who Left ER Before Being Seen	28,606	1%	2%	2%
Time from ER Arrival to Admit. (minutes)[2]	521	340	265	274
Time from ER Arrival to Discharge (minutes)	399	154	128	134
Time in ER Before Being Evaluated (minutes)	433	24	22	26
Time to Pain Meds for Fractures (minutes)	147	78	54	57
Heart Attack Care				
Aspirin Given at Discharge	163	100%	99%	99%
Fibrinolytic Meds Within 30 Min. of Arrival[7]	-	-	80%	54%
PCI Within 90 Minutes of Arrival	37	95%	97%	96%
Statin Prescribed at Discharge	165	98%	98%	98%
Heart Failure Care				
ACE Inhibitor or ARB for LVSD	87	93%	97%	97%
Discharge Instructions Given	322	96%	96%	94%
Evaluation of LVS Function	393	100%	100%	99%
Medicare Spending				
Medicare Spending per Patient (ratio)	-	0.98	1.01	0.98
Pneumonia Care				
Appropriate Initial Antibiotic Given	155	97%	96%	95%
Blood Culture Timing	240	99%	98%	98%
Pregnancy and Delivery Care				
Newborn Deliveries Scheduled Early	83	1%	5%	6%
Preventive Care				
Immunization for Influenza[2]	547	91%	93%	90%
Immunization for Pneumonia[2]	638	89%	94%	92%
Stroke Care				
Anticoagulation Therapy for Atrial Fibrillation	12	92%	95%	95%
Antithrombotic Therapy Timing	78	90%	98%	98%
Assessed for Rehabilitation	97	97%	98%	97%
Discharged on Antithrombotic Therapy	84	98%	99%	99%
Discharged on Statin Medication	68	96%	95%	94%
Thrombolytic Therapy Timing[1]	-	-	65%	66%
Venous Thromboembolism Prophylaxis	103	90%	95%	94%
Written Stroke Educational Materials Given	55	98%	92%	88%
Surgical Care Improvement Project				
Appropriate Beta Blocker Usage[2]	333	99%	98%	98%
Appropriate VTP Within 24 Hours[2]	768	100%	98%	98%
Controlled Postoperative Blood Glucose[2]	92	99%	97%	97%
Perioperative Temperature Management[2]	885	100%	100%	100%
Prophylactic Antibiotic Selection[2]	796	100%	99%	99%
Prophylactic Antibiotic Selection (Outpatient)	409	99%	98%	98%

NOTE: Hospital profiles are in alphabetical order by state, then city, then hospital within the city; Rankings exclude hospitals with less than 25 cases except for patient surveys which excludes hospitals with less than 100 cases; (a) 100-299 cases; (1) The number of cases/patients is too few to report; (2) Data submitted were based on a sample of cases/patients; (3) Results are based on a shorter time period than required; (4) Data suppressed by CMS for one or more quarters; (5) Results are not available for this reporting period; (6) Fewer than 100 patients completed the HCAHPS survey; (7) No cases met the criteria for this measure; (8) The lower limit of the confidence interval cannot be calculated if the number of observed infections equals zero; (9) No data are available from the state/territory for this reporting period; (10) The scores shown reflect fewer than 50 completed surveys; (11) There were discrepancies in the data collection process; (12) This measure does not apply to this hospital for this reporting period; (13) Results cannot be calculated for this reporting period; (14) The results for this state are combined with nearby states to protect confidentiality; Please refer to the User's Guide for a full explanation of data.

Measure	Cases	This Hosp.	State Avg.	U.S. Avg.
Prophylactic Antibiotic Stopped[2]	774	98%	98%	98%
Prophylactic Antibiotic Timing[2]	796	99%	99%	99%
Prophylactic Antibiotic Timing (Outpatient)	409	97%	97%	98%
Urinary Catheter Removal[2]	250	98%	97%	97%
Survey of Patients' Hospital Experiences				
Area Around Room 'Always' Quiet at Night	300+	53%	58%	61%
Doctors 'Always' Communicated Well	300+	80%	80%	82%
Home Recovery Information Given	300+	86%	87%	85%
Hospital Given 9 or 10 on 10 Point Scale	300+	72%	72%	71%
Meds 'Always' Explained Before Given	300+	60%	64%	64%
Nurses 'Always' Communicated Well	300+	80%	81%	79%
Pain 'Always' Well Controlled	300+	69%	71%	71%
Room and Bathroom 'Always' Clean	300+	68%	75%	73%
Timely Help 'Always' Received	300+	65%	70%	68%
Would Definitely Recommend Hospital	300+	73%	71%	71%
Use of Medical Imaging				
Cardiac Imaging Stress Test before Surgery	718	6.4%	5.4%	5.3%
Combination Abdominal CT Scan	1,311	6.9%	7.1%	10.5%
Combination Brain/Sinus CT Scan	926	3.7%	2.8%	2.7%
Combination Chest CT Scan	537	1.5%	1.7%	2.7%
Follow-up Mammogram/Ultrasound	1,869	6.4%	8.7%	8.8%
Lumbar Spine MRI for Low Back Pain	218	33.9%	34.7%	37.2%

Medical Center at Elizabeth Place

One Elizabeth Place Phone: 937-853-1053
Dayton, OH 45408
URL: www.mcep.us
Type: Acute Care Hospitals Emergency Services: Yes
Ownership: Government - Federal Beds: 26
Key Personnel:
CEO .... Alex Rintoul

Measure	Cases	This Hosp.	State Avg.	U.S. Avg.
Blood Clot Prevention and Treatment				
Anticoagulation Overlap Therapy[2,7]	-	-	93%	93%
ICU Venous Thromboembolism Prophylaxis[2,7]	-	-	93%	92%
Incidence of Potentially Preventable VTE[2,7]	-	-	6%	10%
UFH with Dosages/Platelet Monitoring[2,7]	-	-	98%	97%
Venous Thromboembolism Prophylaxis[2]	26	100%	88%	85%
Warfarin Therapy Discharge Instructions[2,7]	-	-	79%	75%
Chest Pain/Possible Heart Attack Care				
Aspirin Given Within 24 Hours of Arrival[5]	-	-	97%	96%
Fibrinolytic Meds Within 30 Min. of Arrival[5]	-	-	44%	58%
Average Time to ECG (minutes)[5]	-	-	6	7
Average Time to Transfer (minutes)[5]	-	-	58	60
Children's Asthma Care				
Received Home Management Plan of Care	-	-	85%	88%
Received Reliever Medication	-	-	100%	100%
Received Systemic Corticosteroids	-	-	100%	100%
Emergency Department				
Admittance Decision Time (minutes)[7]	-	-	90	98
Head CT Results Within 45 Min. of Arrival[5]	-	-	63%	57%
Patients Who Left ER Before Being Seen[5]	-	-	2%	2%
Time from ER Arrival to Admit. (minutes)[7]	-	-	265	274
Time from ER Arrival to Discharge (minutes)[5]	-	-	128	134
Time in ER Before Being Evaluated (minutes)[5]	-	-	22	26
Time to Pain Meds for Fractures (minutes)[5]	-	-	54	57
Heart Attack Care				
Aspirin Given at Discharge[5]	-	-	99%	99%
Fibrinolytic Meds Within 30 Min. of Arrival[5]	-	-	80%	54%
PCI Within 90 Minutes of Arrival[5]	-	-	97%	96%
Statin Prescribed at Discharge[5]	-	-	98%	98%
Heart Failure Care				
ACE Inhibitor or ARB for LVSD[5]	-	-	97%	97%
Discharge Instructions Given[5]	-	-	96%	94%
Evaluation of LVS Function[5]	-	-	100%	99%
Medicare Spending				
Medicare Spending per Patient (ratio)	-	1.16	1.01	0.98
Pneumonia Care				
Appropriate Initial Antibiotic Given[5]	-	-	96%	95%
Blood Culture Timing[5]	-	-	98%	98%
Pregnancy and Delivery Care				
Newborn Deliveries Scheduled Early[7]	-	-	5%	6%
Preventive Care				
Immunization for Influenza	201	91%	93%	90%
Immunization for Pneumonia	209	78%	94%	92%
Stroke Care				
Anticoagulation Therapy for Atrial Fibrillation[5]	-	-	95%	95%
Antithrombotic Therapy Timing[5]	-	-	98%	98%
Assessed for Rehabilitation[5]	-	-	98%	97%
Discharged on Antithrombotic Therapy[5]	-	-	99%	99%
Discharged on Statin Medication[5]	-	-	95%	94%
Thrombolytic Therapy Timing[5]	-	-	65%	66%
Venous Thromboembolism Prophylaxis[5]	-	-	95%	94%
Written Stroke Educational Materials Given[5]	-	-	92%	88%
Surgical Care Improvement Project				
Appropriate Beta Blocker Usage	32	84%	98%	98%
Appropriate VTP Within 24 Hours	190	72%	98%	98%
Controlled Postoperative Blood Glucose[7]	-	-	97%	97%
Perioperative Temperature Management	214	97%	100%	100%
Prophylactic Antibiotic Selection	149	95%	99%	99%
Prophylactic Antibiotic Selection (Outpatient)	98	85%	98%	98%
Prophylactic Antibiotic Stopped	149	99%	98%	98%
Prophylactic Antibiotic Timing	149	92%	99%	99%
Prophylactic Antibiotic Timing (Outpatient)	98	94%	97%	98%
Urinary Catheter Removal[1]	-	-	97%	97%
Survey of Patients' Hospital Experiences				
Area Around Room 'Always' Quiet at Night	(a)	74%	58%	61%
Doctors 'Always' Communicated Well	(a)	79%	80%	82%
Home Recovery Information Given	(a)	86%	87%	85%
Hospital Given 9 or 10 on 10 Point Scale	(a)	62%	72%	71%
Meds 'Always' Explained Before Given	(a)	62%	64%	64%
Nurses 'Always' Communicated Well	(a)	79%	81%	79%
Pain 'Always' Well Controlled	(a)	73%	71%	71%
Room and Bathroom 'Always' Clean	(a)	60%	75%	73%
Timely Help 'Always' Received	(a)	74%	70%	68%
Would Definitely Recommend Hospital	(a)	59%	71%	71%
Use of Medical Imaging				
Cardiac Imaging Stress Test before Surgery[7]	-	-	5.4%	5.3%
Combination Abdominal CT Scan[1]	-	-	7.1%	10.5%
Combination Brain/Sinus CT Scan	53	0.0%	2.8%	2.7%
Combination Chest CT Scan[1]	-	-	1.7%	2.7%
Follow-up Mammogram/Ultrasound[7]	-	-	8.7%	8.8%
Lumbar Spine MRI for Low Back Pain	103	34.0%	34.7%	37.2%

Miami Valley Hospital

One Wyoming Street Phone: 937-208-8000
Dayton, OH 45409 Fax: 937-341-8611
URL: www.miamivalleyhospital.com
Type: Acute Care Hospitals Emergency Services: Yes
Ownership: Voluntary non-profit - Private Beds: 848
Key Personnel:
Radiology.................... Larry D Buchanan, MD
Infection Control.............. Tim Collins
Quality Assurance .... Tim Collins
CEO/President................ James R Pancoast
Pediatric Ambulatory Care ...... William Spohn, MD
Pediatric In-Patient Care .... William Spohn, MD
Operating Room............... Randy Woods
Chief of Medical Staff.......... Howard Wunderlich, MD

Measure	Cases	This Hosp.	State Avg.	U.S. Avg.
Blood Clot Prevention and Treatment				
Anticoagulation Overlap Therapy[2]	242	98%	93%	93%
ICU Venous Thromboembolism Prophylaxis[2]	70	94%	93%	92%
Incidence of Potentially Preventable VTE[2]	73	3%	6%	10%
UFH with Dosages/Platelet Monitoring[2]	200	100%	98%	97%
Venous Thromboembolism Prophylaxis[2]	350	91%	88%	85%
Warfarin Therapy Discharge Instructions[2]	188	95%	79%	75%
Chest Pain/Possible Heart Attack Care				
Aspirin Given Within 24 Hours of Arrival[1,3]	-	-	97%	96%
Fibrinolytic Meds Within 30 Min. of Arrival[3,7]	-	-	44%	58%
Average Time to ECG (minutes)[1,3]	-	-	6	7
Average Time to Transfer (minutes)[3,7]	-	-	58	60
Children's Asthma Care				
Received Home Management Plan of Care	-	-	85%	88%
Received Reliever Medication	-	-	100%	100%
Received Systemic Corticosteroids	-	-	100%	100%
Emergency Department				
Admittance Decision Time (minutes)[2]	595	118	90	98
Head CT Results Within 45 Min. of Arrival[1]	-	-	63%	57%
Patients Who Left ER Before Being Seen	>100k	2%	2%	2%
Time from ER Arrival to Admit. (minutes)[2]	601	253	265	274
Time from ER Arrival to Discharge (minutes)	400	158	128	134
Time in ER Before Being Evaluated (minutes)	443	15	22	26
Time to Pain Meds for Fractures (minutes)	145	32	54	57
Heart Attack Care				
Aspirin Given at Discharge[2]	308	100%	99%	99%
Fibrinolytic Meds Within 30 Min. of Arrival[2,7]	-	-	80%	54%
PCI Within 90 Minutes of Arrival[2]	54	100%	97%	96%
Statin Prescribed at Discharge[2]	292	100%	98%	98%
Heart Failure Care				
ACE Inhibitor or ARB for LVSD[2]	85	99%	97%	97%
Discharge Instructions Given[2]	231	98%	96%	94%
Evaluation of LVS Function[2]	287	100%	100%	99%
Medicare Spending				
Medicare Spending per Patient (ratio)	-	1.03	1.01	0.98
Pneumonia Care				
Appropriate Initial Antibiotic Given[2]	74	97%	96%	95%
Blood Culture Timing[2]	180	100%	98%	98%
Pregnancy and Delivery Care				
Newborn Deliveries Scheduled Early	400	2%	5%	6%
Preventive Care				
Immunization for Influenza[2]	573	97%	93%	90%
Immunization for Pneumonia[2]	627	96%	94%	92%
Stroke Care				
Anticoagulation Therapy for Atrial Fibrillation[2]	11	100%	95%	95%
Antithrombotic Therapy Timing[2]	85	99%	98%	98%
Assessed for Rehabilitation[2]	135	99%	98%	97%
Discharged on Antithrombotic Therapy[2]	105	100%	99%	99%
Discharged on Statin Medication[2]	82	100%	95%	94%
Thrombolytic Therapy Timing[1,2]	-	-	65%	66%
Venous Thromboembolism Prophylaxis[2]	136	99%	95%	94%
Written Stroke Educational Materials Given[2]	72	90%	92%	88%
Surgical Care Improvement Project				
Appropriate Beta Blocker Usage[2]	276	100%	98%	98%
Appropriate VTP Within 24 Hours[2]	436	100%	98%	98%
Controlled Postoperative Blood Glucose[2]	139	98%	97%	97%
Perioperative Temperature Management[2]	637	100%	100%	100%
Prophylactic Antibiotic Selection[2]	510	100%	99%	99%
Prophylactic Antibiotic Selection (Outpatient)	769	99%	98%	98%
Prophylactic Antibiotic Stopped[2]	499	98%	98%	98%
Prophylactic Antibiotic Timing[2]	511	100%	99%	99%
Prophylactic Antibiotic Timing (Outpatient)	765	99%	97%	98%
Urinary Catheter Removal[2]	416	99%	97%	97%
Survey of Patients' Hospital Experiences				
Area Around Room 'Always' Quiet at Night[11]	300+	59%	58%	61%
Doctors 'Always' Communicated Well[11]	300+	77%	80%	82%
Home Recovery Information Given[11]	300+	90%	87%	85%
Hospital Given 9 or 10 on 10 Point Scale[11]	300+	76%	72%	71%
Meds 'Always' Explained Before Given[11]	300+	62%	64%	64%
Nurses 'Always' Communicated Well[11]	300+	80%	81%	79%
Pain 'Always' Well Controlled[11]	300+	71%	71%	71%
Room and Bathroom 'Always' Clean[11]	300+	76%	75%	73%
Timely Help 'Always' Received[11]	300+	64%	70%	68%
Would Definitely Recommend Hospital[11]	300+	79%	71%	71%
Use of Medical Imaging				
Cardiac Imaging Stress Test before Surgery	1,115	6.8%	5.4%	5.3%
Combination Abdominal CT Scan	1,776	8.1%	7.1%	10.5%
Combination Brain/Sinus CT Scan	2,020	4.4%	2.8%	2.7%
Combination Chest CT Scan	1,268	3.6%	1.7%	2.7%
Follow-up Mammogram/Ultrasound	2,292	10.2%	8.7%	8.8%
Lumbar Spine MRI for Low Back Pain	214	33.2%	34.7%	37.2%

Defiance Regional Medical Center

1200 Ralston Avenue Phone: 419-783-6955
Defiance, OH 43512 Fax: 419-783-6904
URL: www.promedica.org/defiance
Type: Critical Access Hospitals Emergency Services: Yes
Ownership: Voluntary non-profit - Private Beds: 61
Key Personnel:
Chief of Medical Staff.......... Robert Barnett, MD
Cardiac Laboratory............ Raza Hashmi, MD

NOTE: Hospital profiles are in alphabetical order by state, then city, then hospital within the city; Rankings exclude hospitals with less than 25 cases except for patient surveys which excludes hospitals with less than 100 cases; (a) 100-299 cases; (1) The number of cases/patients is too few to report; (2) Data submitted were based on a sample of cases/patients; (3) Results are based on a shorter time period than required; (4) Data suppressed by CMS for one or more quarters; (5) Results are not available for this reporting period; (6) Fewer than 100 patients completed the HCAHPS survey; (7) No cases met the criteria for this measure; (8) The lower limit of the confidence interval cannot be calculated if the number of observed infections equals zero; (9) No data are available from the state/territory for this reporting period; (10) The scores shown reflect fewer than 50 completed surveys; (11) There were discrepancies in the data collection process; (12) This measure does not apply to this hospital for this reporting period; (13) Results cannot be calculated for this reporting period; (14) The results for this state are combined with nearby states to protect confidentiality; Please refer to the User's Guide for a full explanation of data.

Coronary Care. . . . . Anne Minic, RN
Infection Control. . . . . Elizabeth Rettig
Quality Assurance . . . . Elizabeth Rettig, RN
Operating Room. . . . . LouAnn Walton, RN

Measure	Cases	This Hosp.	State Avg.	U.S. Avg.
Blood Clot Prevention and Treatment				
Anticoagulation Overlap Therapy[5]	-	-	93%	93%
ICU Venous Thromboembolism Prophylaxis[5]	-	-	93%	92%
Incidence of Potentially Preventable VTE[5]	-	-	6%	10%
UFH with Dosages/Platelet Monitoring[5]	-	-	98%	97%
Venous Thromboembolism Prophylaxis[5]	-	-	88%	85%
Warfarin Therapy Discharge Instructions[5]	-	-	79%	75%
Chest Pain/Possible Heart Attack Care				
Aspirin Given Within 24 Hours of Arrival	-	-	97%	96%
Fibrinolytic Meds Within 30 Min. of Arrival	-	-	44%	58%
Average Time to ECG (minutes)	-	-	6	7
Average Time to Transfer (minutes)	-	-	58	60
Children's Asthma Care				
Received Home Management Plan of Care	-	-	85%	88%
Received Reliever Medication	-	-	100%	100%
Received Systemic Corticosteroids	-	-	100%	100%
Emergency Department				
Admittance Decision Time (minutes)[5]	-	-	90	98
Head CT Results Within 45 Min. of Arrival	-	-	63%	57%
Patients Who Left ER Before Being Seen	-	-	2%	2%
Time from ER Arrival to Admit. (minutes)[5]	-	-	265	274
Time from ER Arrival to Discharge (minutes)	-	-	128	134
Time in ER Before Being Evaluated (minutes)	-	-	22	26
Time to Pain Meds for Fractures (minutes)	-	-	54	57
Heart Attack Care				
Aspirin Given at Discharge[1]	-	-	99%	99%
Fibrinolytic Meds Within 30 Min. of Arrival[7]	-	-	80%	54%
PCI Within 90 Minutes of Arrival[7]	-	-	97%	96%
Statin Prescribed at Discharge[1]	-	-	98%	98%
Heart Failure Care				
ACE Inhibitor or ARB for LVSD[1]	-	-	97%	97%
Discharge Instructions Given	16	88%	96%	94%
Evaluation of LVS Function	19	100%	100%	99%
Medicare Spending				
Medicare Spending per Patient (ratio)	-	-	1.01	0.98
Pneumonia Care				
Appropriate Initial Antibiotic Given	41	98%	96%	95%
Blood Culture Timing	57	100%	98%	98%
Pregnancy and Delivery Care				
Newborn Deliveries Scheduled Early[3]	44	0%	5%	6%
Preventive Care				
Immunization for Influenza[5]	-	-	93%	90%
Immunization for Pneumonia[5]	-	-	94%	92%
Stroke Care				
Anticoagulation Therapy for Atrial Fibrillation[5]	-	-	95%	95%
Antithrombotic Therapy Timing[5]	-	-	98%	98%
Assessed for Rehabilitation[5]	-	-	98%	97%
Discharged on Antithrombotic Therapy[5]	-	-	99%	99%
Discharged on Statin Medication[5]	-	-	95%	94%
Thrombolytic Therapy Timing[5]	-	-	65%	66%
Venous Thromboembolism Prophylaxis[5]	-	-	95%	94%
Written Stroke Educational Materials Given[5]	-	-	92%	88%
Surgical Care Improvement Project				
Appropriate Beta Blocker Usage[2]	52	100%	98%	98%
Appropriate VTP Within 24 Hours[2]	132	100%	98%	98%
Controlled Postoperative Blood Glucose[2,7]	-	-	97%	97%
Perioperative Temperature Management[2]	135	100%	100%	100%
Prophylactic Antibiotic Selection[2]	118	99%	99%	99%
Prophylactic Antibiotic Selection (Outpatient)	-	-	98%	98%
Prophylactic Antibiotic Stopped[2]	115	99%	98%	98%
Prophylactic Antibiotic Timing[2]	118	100%	99%	99%
Prophylactic Antibiotic Timing (Outpatient)	-	-	97%	98%
Urinary Catheter Removal[2]	36	94%	97%	97%
Survey of Patients' Hospital Experiences				
Area Around Room 'Always' Quiet at Night	300+	68%	58%	61%
Doctors 'Always' Communicated Well	300+	86%	80%	82%
Home Recovery Information Given	300+	93%	87%	85%
Hospital Given 9 or 10 on 10 Point Scale	300+	83%	72%	71%
Meds 'Always' Explained Before Given	300+	66%	64%	64%
Nurses 'Always' Communicated Well	300+	85%	81%	79%
Pain 'Always' Well Controlled	300+	77%	71%	71%
Room and Bathroom 'Always' Clean	300+	81%	75%	73%
Timely Help 'Always' Received	300+	78%	70%	68%
Would Definitely Recommend Hospital	300+	82%	71%	71%
Use of Medical Imaging				
Cardiac Imaging Stress Test before Surgery	-	-	5.4%	5.3%
Combination Abdominal CT Scan	-	-	7.1%	10.5%
Combination Brain/Sinus CT Scan	-	-	2.8%	2.7%
Combination Chest CT Scan	-	-	1.7%	2.7%
Follow-up Mammogram/Ultrasound	-	-	8.7%	8.8%
Lumbar Spine MRI for Low Back Pain	-	-	34.7%	37.2%

Mercy Hospital of Defiance

1404 East Second Street
Defiance, OH 43512
Phone: 419-782-8444
URL: www.mercyweb.org/mercy_defiance.aspx
Type: Acute Care Hospitals
Emergency Services: Yes
Ownership: Proprietary

Measure	Cases	This Hosp.	State Avg.	U.S. Avg.
Blood Clot Prevention and Treatment				
Anticoagulation Overlap Therapy[1,2]	-	-	93%	93%
ICU Venous Thromboembolism Prophylaxis[1,2]	-	-	93%	92%
Incidence of Potentially Preventable VTE[2,7]	-	-	6%	10%
UFH with Dosages/Platelet Monitoring[1,2]	-	-	98%	97%
Venous Thromboembolism Prophylaxis[2]	136	100%	88%	85%
Warfarin Therapy Discharge Instructions[1,2]	-	-	79%	75%
Chest Pain/Possible Heart Attack Care				
Aspirin Given Within 24 Hours of Arrival	41	100%	97%	96%
Fibrinolytic Meds Within 30 Min. of Arrival[1]	-	-	44%	58%
Average Time to ECG (minutes)	42	4	6	7
Average Time to Transfer (minutes)	11	65	58	60
Children's Asthma Care				
Received Home Management Plan of Care	-	-	85%	88%
Received Reliever Medication	-	-	100%	100%
Received Systemic Corticosteroids	-	-	100%	100%
Emergency Department				
Admittance Decision Time (minutes)[2]	429	40	90	98
Head CT Results Within 45 Min. of Arrival[1]	-	-	63%	57%
Patients Who Left ER Before Being Seen	9,179	0%	2%	2%
Time from ER Arrival to Admit. (minutes)[2]	432	159	265	274
Time from ER Arrival to Discharge (minutes)	370	64	128	134
Time in ER Before Being Evaluated (minutes)	419	9	22	26
Time to Pain Meds for Fractures (minutes)	23	31	54	57
Heart Attack Care				
Aspirin Given at Discharge[1]	-	-	99%	99%
Fibrinolytic Meds Within 30 Min. of Arrival[7]	-	-	80%	54%
PCI Within 90 Minutes of Arrival[7]	-	-	97%	96%
Statin Prescribed at Discharge[1]	-	-	98%	98%
Heart Failure Care				
ACE Inhibitor or ARB for LVSD	13	77%	97%	97%
Discharge Instructions Given	31	97%	96%	94%
Evaluation of LVS Function	47	100%	100%	99%
Medicare Spending				
Medicare Spending per Patient (ratio)	-	1.04	1.01	0.98
Pneumonia Care				
Appropriate Initial Antibiotic Given	45	100%	96%	95%
Blood Culture Timing	71	100%	98%	98%
Pregnancy and Delivery Care				
Newborn Deliveries Scheduled Early[7]	-	-	5%	6%
Preventive Care				
Immunization for Influenza[2]	308	99%	93%	90%
Immunization for Pneumonia[2]	498	99%	94%	92%
Stroke Care				
Anticoagulation Therapy for Atrial Fibrillation[1]	-	-	95%	95%
Antithrombotic Therapy Timing	16	100%	98%	98%
Assessed for Rehabilitation	18	100%	98%	97%
Discharged on Antithrombotic Therapy	17	94%	99%	99%
Discharged on Statin Medication[1]	-	-	95%	94%
Thrombolytic Therapy Timing[1]	-	-	65%	66%
Venous Thromboembolism Prophylaxis	16	100%	95%	94%
Written Stroke Educational Materials Given	13	100%	92%	88%
Surgical Care Improvement Project				
Appropriate Beta Blocker Usage	22	100%	98%	98%
Appropriate VTP Within 24 Hours	58	98%	98%	98%
Controlled Postoperative Blood Glucose[7]	-	-	97%	97%
Perioperative Temperature Management	64	98%	100%	100%
Prophylactic Antibiotic Selection	45	100%	99%	99%
Prophylactic Antibiotic Selection (Outpatient)[1]	-	-	98%	98%
Prophylactic Antibiotic Stopped	43	98%	98%	98%
Prophylactic Antibiotic Timing	45	100%	99%	99%
Prophylactic Antibiotic Timing (Outpatient)	11	91%	97%	98%
Urinary Catheter Removal	35	97%	97%	97%
Survey of Patients' Hospital Experiences				
Area Around Room 'Always' Quiet at Night	300+	62%	58%	61%
Doctors 'Always' Communicated Well	300+	86%	80%	82%
Home Recovery Information Given	300+	88%	87%	85%
Hospital Given 9 or 10 on 10 Point Scale	300+	78%	72%	71%
Meds 'Always' Explained Before Given	300+	66%	64%	64%
Nurses 'Always' Communicated Well	300+	86%	81%	79%
Pain 'Always' Well Controlled	300+	73%	71%	71%
Room and Bathroom 'Always' Clean	300+	83%	75%	73%
Timely Help 'Always' Received	300+	81%	70%	68%
Would Definitely Recommend Hospital	300+	75%	71%	71%
Use of Medical Imaging				
Cardiac Imaging Stress Test before Surgery[7]	-	-	5.4%	5.3%
Combination Abdominal CT Scan	137	0.7%	7.1%	10.5%
Combination Brain/Sinus CT Scan	173	1.2%	2.8%	2.7%
Combination Chest CT Scan	47	2.1%	1.7%	2.7%
Follow-up Mammogram/Ultrasound[7]	-	-	8.7%	8.8%
Lumbar Spine MRI for Low Back Pain[7]	-	-	34.7%	37.2%

Grady Memorial Hospital

561 West Central Avenue
Delaware, OH 43015
Phone: 740-368-5145
Fax: 740-368-5213
URL: www.gradyhospital.com
Type: Acute Care Hospitals
Emergency Services: Yes
Ownership: Voluntary non-profit - Private
Beds: 135

Key Personnel:

CEO . . . . Warren Kean
Chairman/CEO . . . . Denver Talley
CEO/President. . . . . Everett P Weber Jr

Measure	Cases	This Hosp.	State Avg.	U.S. Avg.
Blood Clot Prevention and Treatment				
Anticoagulation Overlap Therapy[2]	25	100%	93%	93%
ICU Venous Thromboembolism Prophylaxis[2]	21	86%	93%	92%
Incidence of Potentially Preventable VTE[1,2]	-	-	6%	10%
UFH with Dosages/Platelet Monitoring[2]	18	100%	98%	97%
Venous Thromboembolism Prophylaxis[2]	221	92%	88%	85%
Warfarin Therapy Discharge Instructions[2]	15	100%	79%	75%
Chest Pain/Possible Heart Attack Care				
Aspirin Given Within 24 Hours of Arrival	42	100%	97%	96%
Fibrinolytic Meds Within 30 Min. of Arrival[1]	-	-	44%	58%
Average Time to ECG (minutes)	44	5	6	7
Average Time to Transfer (minutes)[1]	-	-	58	60
Children's Asthma Care				
Received Home Management Plan of Care	-	-	85%	88%
Received Reliever Medication	-	-	100%	100%
Received Systemic Corticosteroids	-	-	100%	100%
Emergency Department				
Admittance Decision Time (minutes)[2]	441	80	90	98
Head CT Results Within 45 Min. of Arrival[1]	-	-	63%	57%
Patients Who Left ER Before Being Seen	26,709	1%	2%	2%
Time from ER Arrival to Admit. (minutes)[2]	441	238	265	274
Time from ER Arrival to Discharge (minutes)	771	112	128	134
Time in ER Before Being Evaluated (minutes)	840	20	22	26
Time to Pain Meds for Fractures (minutes)	91	45	54	57
Heart Attack Care				
Aspirin Given at Discharge[1]	-	-	99%	99%
Fibrinolytic Meds Within 30 Min. of Arrival[7]	-	-	80%	54%
PCI Within 90 Minutes of Arrival[7]	-	-	97%	96%
Statin Prescribed at Discharge[1]	-	-	98%	98%
Heart Failure Care				

NOTE: Hospital profiles are in alphabetical order by state, then city, then hospital within the city; Rankings exclude hospitals with less than 25 cases except for patient surveys which excludes hospitals with less than 100 cases; (a) 100-299 cases; (1) The number of cases/patients is too few to report; (2) Data submitted were based on a sample of cases/patients; (3) Results are based on a shorter time period than required; (4) Data suppressed by CMS for one or more quarters; (5) Results are not available for this reporting period; (6) Fewer than 100 patients completed the HCAHPS survey; (7) No cases met the criteria for this measure; (8) The lower limit of the confidence interval cannot be calculated if the number of observed infections equals zero; (9) No data are available from the state/territory for this reporting period; (10) The scores shown reflect fewer than 50 completed surveys; (11) There were discrepancies in the data collection process; (12) This measure does not apply to this hospital for this reporting period; (13) Results cannot be calculated for this reporting period; (14) The results for this state are combined with nearby states to protect confidentiality; Please refer to the User's Guide for a full explanation of data.

Measure	Cases	This Hosp.	State Avg.	U.S. Avg.
ACE Inhibitor or ARB for LVSD	19	100%	97%	97%
Discharge Instructions Given	64	100%	96%	94%
Evaluation of LVS Function	81	100%	100%	99%
Medicare Spending				
Medicare Spending per Patient (ratio)	-	0.99	1.01	0.98
Pneumonia Care				
Appropriate Initial Antibiotic Given	60	98%	96%	95%
Blood Culture Timing	83	96%	98%	98%
Pregnancy and Delivery Care				
Newborn Deliveries Scheduled Early	26	8%	5%	6%
Preventive Care				
Immunization for Influenza[2]	369	99%	93%	90%
Immunization for Pneumonia[2]	545	99%	94%	92%
Stroke Care				
Anticoagulation Therapy for Atrial Fibrillation[7]	-	-	95%	95%
Antithrombotic Therapy Timing	23	100%	98%	98%
Assessed for Rehabilitation	26	100%	98%	97%
Discharged on Antithrombotic Therapy	25	100%	99%	99%
Discharged on Statin Medication	22	100%	95%	94%
Thrombolytic Therapy Timing[7]	-	-	65%	66%
Venous Thromboembolism Prophylaxis	22	100%	95%	94%
Written Stroke Educational Materials Given	14	93%	92%	88%
Surgical Care Improvement Project				
Appropriate Beta Blocker Usage	68	97%	98%	98%
Appropriate VTP Within 24 Hours	168	99%	98%	98%
Controlled Postoperative Blood Glucose[7]	-	-	97%	97%
Perioperative Temperature Management	188	100%	100%	100%
Prophylactic Antibiotic Selection	104	99%	99%	99%
Prophylactic Antibiotic Selection (Outpatient)	39	100%	98%	98%
Prophylactic Antibiotic Stopped	102	99%	98%	98%
Prophylactic Antibiotic Timing	104	99%	99%	99%
Prophylactic Antibiotic Timing (Outpatient)	39	97%	97%	98%
Urinary Catheter Removal	120	97%	97%	97%
Survey of Patients' Hospital Experiences				
Area Around Room 'Always' Quiet at Night	300+	61%	58%	61%
Doctors 'Always' Communicated Well	300+	82%	80%	82%
Home Recovery Information Given	300+	89%	87%	85%
Hospital Given 9 or 10 on 10 Point Scale	300+	74%	72%	71%
Meds 'Always' Explained Before Given	300+	68%	64%	64%
Nurses 'Always' Communicated Well	300+	82%	81%	79%
Pain 'Always' Well Controlled	300+	71%	71%	71%
Room and Bathroom 'Always' Clean	300+	81%	75%	73%
Timely Help 'Always' Received	300+	68%	70%	68%
Would Definitely Recommend Hospital	300+	73%	71%	71%
Use of Medical Imaging				
Cardiac Imaging Stress Test before Surgery	168	6.5%	5.4%	5.3%
Combination Abdominal CT Scan	334	7.5%	7.1%	10.5%
Combination Brain/Sinus CT Scan[1]	-	-	2.8%	2.7%
Combination Chest CT Scan	211	1.9%	1.7%	2.7%
Follow-up Mammogram/Ultrasound	568	7.4%	8.7%	8.8%
Lumbar Spine MRI for Low Back Pain	64	25.0%	34.7%	37.2%

Trinity Hospital Twin City

819 North First Street
Dennison, OH 44621
Phone: 740-922-2800
Fax: 740-922-6945
URL: www.twincityhospital.org
Type: Critical Access Hospitals
Emergency Services: Yes
Ownership: Voluntary non-profit - Church
Beds: 25

Key Personnel:

Infection Control. . . . . Ruthann Belknap, RN
Operating Room. . . . . Ruthann Belknap, RN
Chief of Medical Staff. . . . . Tim McKnight, MD
Anesthesiology. . . . . Laura Rollandini
CEO/President. . . . . Frank Swinehart, CEO
Patient Relations . . . . Cindy Unrue
Emergency Room . . . . Sue Walters, RN
Intensive Care Unit. . . . . Tui Wanosik, RN

Measure	Cases	This Hosp.	State Avg.	U.S. Avg.
Blood Clot Prevention and Treatment				
Anticoagulation Overlap Therapy[5]	-	-	93%	93%
ICU Venous Thromboembolism Prophylaxis[5]	-	-	93%	92%
Incidence of Potentially Preventable VTE[5]	-	-	6%	10%
UFH with Dosages/Platelet Monitoring[5]	-	-	98%	97%
Venous Thromboembolism Prophylaxis[5]	-	-	88%	85%
Warfarin Therapy Discharge Instructions[5]	-	-	79%	75%
Chest Pain/Possible Heart Attack Care				
Aspirin Given Within 24 Hours of Arrival[5]	-	-	97%	96%
Fibrinolytic Meds Within 30 Min. of Arrival[5]	-	-	44%	58%
Average Time to ECG (minutes)[5]	-	-	6	7
Average Time to Transfer (minutes)[5]	-	-	58	60
Children's Asthma Care				
Received Home Management Plan of Care	-	-	85%	88%
Received Reliever Medication	-	-	100%	100%
Received Systemic Corticosteroids	-	-	100%	100%
Emergency Department				
Admittance Decision Time (minutes)[5]	-	-	90	98
Head CT Results Within 45 Min. of Arrival[5]	-	-	63%	57%
Patients Who Left ER Before Being Seen[5]	-	-	2%	2%
Time from ER Arrival to Admit. (minutes)[5]	-	-	265	274
Time from ER Arrival to Discharge (minutes)[5]	-	-	128	134
Time in ER Before Being Evaluated (minutes)[5]	-	-	22	26
Time to Pain Meds for Fractures (minutes)[5]	-	-	54	57
Heart Attack Care				
Aspirin Given at Discharge[1,3]	-	-	99%	99%
Fibrinolytic Meds Within 30 Min. of Arrival[3,7]	-	-	80%	54%
PCI Within 90 Minutes of Arrival[5]	-	-	97%	96%
Statin Prescribed at Discharge[1,3]	-	-	98%	98%
Heart Failure Care				
ACE Inhibitor or ARB for LVSD[1]	-	-	97%	97%
Discharge Instructions Given	14	100%	96%	94%
Evaluation of LVS Function	24	96%	100%	99%
Medicare Spending				
Medicare Spending per Patient (ratio)	-	-	1.01	0.98
Pneumonia Care				
Appropriate Initial Antibiotic Given	20	90%	96%	95%
Blood Culture Timing	31	94%	98%	98%
Pregnancy and Delivery Care				
Newborn Deliveries Scheduled Early[5]	-	-	5%	6%
Preventive Care				
Immunization for Influenza[5]	-	-	93%	90%
Immunization for Pneumonia[5]	-	-	94%	92%
Stroke Care				
Anticoagulation Therapy for Atrial Fibrillation[5]	-	-	95%	95%
Antithrombotic Therapy Timing[5]	-	-	98%	98%
Assessed for Rehabilitation[5]	-	-	98%	97%
Discharged on Antithrombotic Therapy[5]	-	-	99%	99%
Discharged on Statin Medication[5]	-	-	95%	94%
Thrombolytic Therapy Timing[5]	-	-	65%	66%
Venous Thromboembolism Prophylaxis[5]	-	-	95%	94%
Written Stroke Educational Materials Given[5]	-	-	92%	88%
Surgical Care Improvement Project				
Appropriate Beta Blocker Usage[5]	-	-	98%	98%
Appropriate VTP Within 24 Hours[5]	-	-	98%	98%
Controlled Postoperative Blood Glucose[5]	-	-	97%	97%
Perioperative Temperature Management[5]	-	-	100%	100%
Prophylactic Antibiotic Selection[5]	-	-	99%	99%
Prophylactic Antibiotic Selection (Outpatient)[5]	-	-	98%	98%
Prophylactic Antibiotic Stopped[5]	-	-	98%	98%
Prophylactic Antibiotic Timing[5]	-	-	99%	99%
Prophylactic Antibiotic Timing (Outpatient)[5]	-	-	97%	98%
Urinary Catheter Removal[5]	-	-	97%	97%
Survey of Patients' Hospital Experiences				
Area Around Room 'Always' Quiet at Night[6]	<100	69%	58%	61%
Doctors 'Always' Communicated Well[6]	<100	80%	80%	82%
Home Recovery Information Given[6]	<100	92%	87%	85%
Hospital Given 9 or 10 on 10 Point Scale[6]	<100	77%	72%	71%
Meds 'Always' Explained Before Given[6]	<100	64%	64%	64%
Nurses 'Always' Communicated Well[6]	<100	81%	81%	79%
Pain 'Always' Well Controlled[6]	<100	81%	71%	71%
Room and Bathroom 'Always' Clean[6]	<100	73%	75%	73%
Timely Help 'Always' Received[6]	<100	76%	70%	68%
Would Definitely Recommend Hospital[6]	<100	76%	71%	71%
Use of Medical Imaging				
Cardiac Imaging Stress Test before Surgery	77	6.5%	5.4%	5.3%
Combination Abdominal CT Scan	159	6.3%	7.1%	10.5%
Combination Brain/Sinus CT Scan	148	5.4%	2.8%	2.7%
Combination Chest CT Scan	71	2.8%	1.7%	2.7%
Follow-up Mammogram/Ultrasound	127	13.4%	8.7%	8.8%
Lumbar Spine MRI for Low Back Pain[1]	-	-	34.7%	37.2%

Union Hospital

659 Boulevard
Dover, OH 44622
Phone: 330-343-3311
Fax: 330-364-0951
URL: www.unionhospital.org
Type: Acute Care Hospitals
Emergency Services: Yes
Ownership: Voluntary non-profit - Other
Beds: 105

Key Personnel:

Radiology. . . . . Robert L Basista, DO
Chief of Medical Staff. . . . . Donald R Braden
Operating Room. . . . . Miguel Bravo, RN
Emergency Room . . . . Carma J Clarke, RN
Quality Assurance . . . . Cathy Corbett
CEO/President. . . . . William Harding
Pediatric Ambulatory Care . . . . . . Anita S Olmos, MD
Pediatric In-Patient Care . . . . Anita S Olmos, MD

Measure	Cases	This Hosp.	State Avg.	U.S. Avg.
Blood Clot Prevention and Treatment				
Anticoagulation Overlap Therapy[2]	55	82%	93%	93%
ICU Venous Thromboembolism Prophylaxis[2]	60	95%	93%	92%
Incidence of Potentially Preventable VTE[1,2]	-	-	6%	10%
UFH with Dosages/Platelet Monitoring[2]	38	100%	98%	97%
Venous Thromboembolism Prophylaxis[2]	397	95%	88%	85%
Warfarin Therapy Discharge Instructions[2]	47	100%	79%	75%
Chest Pain/Possible Heart Attack Care				
Aspirin Given Within 24 Hours of Arrival	165	100%	97%	96%
Fibrinolytic Meds Within 30 Min. of Arrival[7]	-	-	44%	58%
Average Time to ECG (minutes)	174	9	6	7
Average Time to Transfer (minutes)	34	39	58	60
Children's Asthma Care				
Received Home Management Plan of Care	-	-	85%	88%
Received Reliever Medication	-	-	100%	100%
Received Systemic Corticosteroids	-	-	100%	100%
Emergency Department				
Admittance Decision Time (minutes)[2]	316	58	90	98
Head CT Results Within 45 Min. of Arrival[1]	-	-	63%	57%
Patients Who Left ER Before Being Seen	45,214	1%	2%	2%
Time from ER Arrival to Admit. (minutes)[2]	663	215	265	274
Time from ER Arrival to Discharge (minutes)	383	119	128	134
Time in ER Before Being Evaluated (minutes)	428	35	22	26
Time to Pain Meds for Fractures (minutes)	153	64	54	57
Heart Attack Care				
Aspirin Given at Discharge	25	100%	99%	99%
Fibrinolytic Meds Within 30 Min. of Arrival[7]	-	-	80%	54%
PCI Within 90 Minutes of Arrival[7]	-	-	97%	96%
Statin Prescribed at Discharge	23	96%	98%	98%
Heart Failure Care				
ACE Inhibitor or ARB for LVSD	48	100%	97%	97%
Discharge Instructions Given	203	100%	96%	94%
Evaluation of LVS Function	277	100%	100%	99%
Medicare Spending				
Medicare Spending per Patient (ratio)	-	1.02	1.01	0.98
Pneumonia Care				
Appropriate Initial Antibiotic Given	125	100%	96%	95%
Blood Culture Timing	199	99%	98%	98%
Pregnancy and Delivery Care				
Newborn Deliveries Scheduled Early[2]	19	0%	5%	6%
Preventive Care				
Immunization for Influenza[2]	510	98%	93%	90%
Immunization for Pneumonia[2]	707	97%	94%	92%
Stroke Care				
Anticoagulation Therapy for Atrial Fibrillation[1]	-	-	95%	95%
Antithrombotic Therapy Timing	47	100%	98%	98%
Assessed for Rehabilitation	47	100%	98%	97%
Discharged on Antithrombotic Therapy	42	100%	99%	99%
Discharged on Statin Medication	30	100%	95%	94%
Thrombolytic Therapy Timing[7]	-	-	65%	66%
Venous Thromboembolism Prophylaxis	53	96%	95%	94%
Written Stroke Educational Materials Given	15	93%	92%	88%
Surgical Care Improvement Project				
Appropriate Beta Blocker Usage[2]	104	100%	98%	98%

NOTE: Hospital profiles are in alphabetical order by state, then city, then hospital within the city; Rankings exclude hospitals with less than 25 cases except for patient surveys which excludes hospitals with less than 100 cases; (a) 100-299 cases; (1) The number of cases/patients is too few to report; (2) Data submitted were based on a sample of cases/patients; (3) Results are based on a shorter time period than required; (4) Data suppressed by CMS for one or more quarters; (5) Results are not available for this reporting period; (6) Fewer than 100 patients completed the HCAHPS survey; (7) No cases met the criteria for this measure; (8) The lower limit of the confidence interval cannot be calculated if the number of observed infections equals zero; (9) No data are available from the state/territory for this reporting period; (10) The scores shown reflect fewer than 50 completed surveys; (11) There were discrepancies in the data collection process; (12) This measure does not apply to this hospital for this reporting period; (13) Results cannot be calculated for this reporting period; (14) The results for this state are combined with nearby states to protect confidentiality; Please refer to the User's Guide for a full explanation of data.

Measure	Cases	This Hosp.	State Avg.	U.S. Avg.
Appropriate VTP Within 24 Hours[2]	336	100%	98%	98%
Controlled Postoperative Blood Glucose[2,7]	-	-	97%	97%
Perioperative Temperature Management[2]	364	100%	100%	100%
Prophylactic Antibiotic Selection[2]	243	100%	99%	99%
Prophylactic Antibiotic Selection (Outpatient)	118	99%	98%	98%
Prophylactic Antibiotic Stopped[2]	230	99%	98%	98%
Prophylactic Antibiotic Timing[2]	243	100%	99%	99%
Prophylactic Antibiotic Timing (Outpatient)	118	100%	97%	98%
Urinary Catheter Removal[2]	251	99%	97%	97%
Survey of Patients' Hospital Experiences				
Area Around Room 'Always' Quiet at Night	300+	51%	58%	61%
Doctors 'Always' Communicated Well	300+	82%	80%	82%
Home Recovery Information Given	300+	83%	87%	85%
Hospital Given 9 or 10 on 10 Point Scale	300+	70%	72%	71%
Meds 'Always' Explained Before Given	300+	58%	64%	64%
Nurses 'Always' Communicated Well	300+	81%	81%	79%
Pain 'Always' Well Controlled	300+	72%	71%	71%
Room and Bathroom 'Always' Clean	300+	78%	75%	73%
Timely Help 'Always' Received	300+	74%	70%	68%
Would Definitely Recommend Hospital	300+	69%	71%	71%
Use of Medical Imaging				
Cardiac Imaging Stress Test before Surgery	302	8.3%	5.4%	5.3%
Combination Abdominal CT Scan	705	4.7%	7.1%	10.5%
Combination Brain/Sinus CT Scan	562	1.8%	2.8%	2.7%
Combination Chest CT Scan	470	0.2%	1.7%	2.7%
Follow-up Mammogram/Ultrasound	866	5.0%	8.7%	8.8%
Lumbar Spine MRI for Low Back Pain	160	36.9%	34.7%	37.2%

Dublin Methodist Hospital

7500 Hospital Avenue Phone: 614-544-8000
Dublin, OH 43016
URL: www.ohiohealth.com
Type: Acute Care Hospitals Emergency Services: Yes
Ownership: Voluntary non-profit - Private
Key Personnel:
President. . . . . Bruce P Hagan

Measure	Cases	This Hosp.	State Avg.	U.S. Avg.
Blood Clot Prevention and Treatment				
Anticoagulation Overlap Therapy[2]	33	100%	93%	93%
ICU Venous Thromboembolism Prophylaxis[2]	36	92%	93%	92%
Incidence of Potentially Preventable VTE[1,2]	-	-	6%	10%
UFH with Dosages/Platelet Monitoring[2]	19	100%	98%	97%
Venous Thromboembolism Prophylaxis[2]	331	95%	88%	85%
Warfarin Therapy Discharge Instructions[2]	24	100%	79%	75%
Chest Pain/Possible Heart Attack Care				
Aspirin Given Within 24 Hours of Arrival	33	94%	97%	96%
Fibrinolytic Meds Within 30 Min. of Arrival[7]	-	-	44%	58%
Average Time to ECG (minutes)	33	7	6	7
Average Time to Transfer (minutes)[1]	-	-	58	60
Children's Asthma Care				
Received Home Management Plan of Care	-	-	85%	88%
Received Reliever Medication	-	-	100%	100%
Received Systemic Corticosteroids	-	-	100%	100%
Emergency Department				
Admittance Decision Time (minutes)[2]	284	94	90	98
Head CT Results Within 45 Min. of Arrival[1]	-	-	63%	57%
Patients Who Left ER Before Being Seen	36,955	2%	2%	2%
Time from ER Arrival to Admit. (minutes)[2]	285	279	265	274
Time from ER Arrival to Discharge (minutes)	367	161	128	134
Time in ER Before Being Evaluated (minutes)	413	38	22	26
Time to Pain Meds for Fractures (minutes)	204	63	54	57
Heart Attack Care				
Aspirin Given at Discharge[1,3]	-	-	99%	99%
Fibrinolytic Meds Within 30 Min. of Arrival[3,7]	-	-	80%	54%
PCI Within 90 Minutes of Arrival[3,7]	-	-	97%	96%
Statin Prescribed at Discharge[1,3]	-	-	98%	98%
Heart Failure Care				
ACE Inhibitor or ARB for LVSD	21	100%	97%	97%
Discharge Instructions Given	57	100%	96%	94%
Evaluation of LVS Function	66	100%	100%	99%
Medicare Spending				
Medicare Spending per Patient (ratio)	-	1.01	1.01	0.98
Pneumonia Care				
Appropriate Initial Antibiotic Given	55	95%	96%	95%
Blood Culture Timing	87	97%	98%	98%
Pregnancy and Delivery Care				
Newborn Deliveries Scheduled Early	181	3%	5%	6%
Preventive Care				
Immunization for Influenza[2]	480	98%	93%	90%
Immunization for Pneumonia[2]	400	96%	94%	92%
Stroke Care				
Anticoagulation Therapy for Atrial Fibrillation[1]	-	-	95%	95%
Antithrombotic Therapy Timing	26	100%	98%	98%
Assessed for Rehabilitation	33	100%	98%	97%
Discharged on Antithrombotic Therapy	32	100%	99%	99%
Discharged on Statin Medication	22	100%	95%	94%
Thrombolytic Therapy Timing[7]	-	-	65%	66%
Venous Thromboembolism Prophylaxis	25	96%	95%	94%
Written Stroke Educational Materials Given	21	95%	92%	88%
Surgical Care Improvement Project				
Appropriate Beta Blocker Usage	96	99%	98%	98%
Appropriate VTP Within 24 Hours	272	98%	98%	98%
Controlled Postoperative Blood Glucose[7]	-	-	97%	97%
Perioperative Temperature Management	345	100%	100%	100%
Prophylactic Antibiotic Selection	121	98%	99%	99%
Prophylactic Antibiotic Selection (Outpatient)	329	98%	98%	98%
Prophylactic Antibiotic Stopped	120	100%	98%	98%
Prophylactic Antibiotic Timing	121	99%	99%	99%
Prophylactic Antibiotic Timing (Outpatient)	334	97%	97%	98%
Urinary Catheter Removal	157	97%	97%	97%
Survey of Patients' Hospital Experiences				
Area Around Room 'Always' Quiet at Night	300+	76%	58%	61%
Doctors 'Always' Communicated Well	300+	84%	80%	82%
Home Recovery Information Given	300+	89%	87%	85%
Hospital Given 9 or 10 on 10 Point Scale	300+	86%	72%	71%
Meds 'Always' Explained Before Given	300+	66%	64%	64%
Nurses 'Always' Communicated Well	300+	85%	81%	79%
Pain 'Always' Well Controlled	300+	74%	71%	71%
Room and Bathroom 'Always' Clean	300+	77%	75%	73%
Timely Help 'Always' Received	300+	71%	70%	68%
Would Definitely Recommend Hospital	300+	88%	71%	71%
Use of Medical Imaging				
Cardiac Imaging Stress Test before Surgery	74	6.8%	5.4%	5.3%
Combination Abdominal CT Scan	446	2.9%	7.1%	10.5%
Combination Brain/Sinus CT Scan[1]	-	-	2.8%	2.7%
Combination Chest CT Scan	189	1.6%	1.7%	2.7%
Follow-up Mammogram/Ultrasound	561	8.0%	8.7%	8.8%
Lumbar Spine MRI for Low Back Pain[1]	-	-	34.7%	37.2%

East Liverpool City Hospital

425 West 5th Street Phone: 330-385-7200
East Liverpool, OH 43920
URL: www.elch.org
Type: Acute Care Hospitals Emergency Services: Yes
Ownership: Voluntary non-profit - Private Beds: 199
Key Personnel:
President/CEO. . . . . Kenneth J. Cochran, RN, FACHE
Infection Control. . . . . Pamela Fox
Radiology. . . . . Boris A Karaman
Operating Room. . . . . Joseph Lach
Pediatric Ambulatory Care . . . . . . Helouise Mapa, MD
Pediatric In-Patient Care . . . . Helouise Mapa, MD
Quality Assurance . . . . Michelle Miller
Chief of Medical Staff. . . . . Mark W Swift

Measure	Cases	This Hosp.	State Avg.	U.S. Avg.
Blood Clot Prevention and Treatment				
Anticoagulation Overlap Therapy[2]	33	97%	93%	93%
ICU Venous Thromboembolism Prophylaxis[2]	61	95%	93%	92%
Incidence of Potentially Preventable VTE[1,2]	-	-	6%	10%
UFH with Dosages/Platelet Monitoring[2]	29	100%	98%	97%
Venous Thromboembolism Prophylaxis[2]	251	86%	88%	85%
Warfarin Therapy Discharge Instructions[2]	25	72%	79%	75%
Chest Pain/Possible Heart Attack Care				
Aspirin Given Within 24 Hours of Arrival	95	99%	97%	96%
Fibrinolytic Meds Within 30 Min. of Arrival[7]	-	-	44%	58%
Average Time to ECG (minutes)	92	15	6	7
Average Time to Transfer (minutes)	35	84	58	60
Children's Asthma Care				
Received Home Management Plan of Care	-	-	85%	88%
Received Reliever Medication	-	-	100%	100%
Received Systemic Corticosteroids	-	-	100%	100%
Emergency Department				
Admittance Decision Time (minutes)[2]	487	48	90	98
Head CT Results Within 45 Min. of Arrival	12	42%	63%	57%
Patients Who Left ER Before Being Seen	14,120	1%	2%	2%
Time from ER Arrival to Admit. (minutes)[2]	503	233	265	274
Time from ER Arrival to Discharge (minutes)	330	107	128	134
Time in ER Before Being Evaluated (minutes)	356	30	22	26
Time to Pain Meds for Fractures (minutes)	156	60	54	57
Heart Attack Care				
Aspirin Given at Discharge[1]	-	-	99%	99%
Fibrinolytic Meds Within 30 Min. of Arrival[7]	-	-	80%	54%
PCI Within 90 Minutes of Arrival[7]	-	-	97%	96%
Statin Prescribed at Discharge[1]	-	-	98%	98%
Heart Failure Care				
ACE Inhibitor or ARB for LVSD	36	100%	97%	97%
Discharge Instructions Given	94	87%	96%	94%
Evaluation of LVS Function	128	100%	100%	99%
Medicare Spending				
Medicare Spending per Patient (ratio)	-	0.98	1.01	0.98
Pneumonia Care				
Appropriate Initial Antibiotic Given	88	97%	96%	95%
Blood Culture Timing	155	95%	98%	98%
Pregnancy and Delivery Care				
Newborn Deliveries Scheduled Early	26	0%	5%	6%
Preventive Care				
Immunization for Influenza[2]	357	96%	93%	90%
Immunization for Pneumonia[2]	490	99%	94%	92%
Stroke Care				
Anticoagulation Therapy for Atrial Fibrillation[1]	-	-	95%	95%
Antithrombotic Therapy Timing	13	100%	98%	98%
Assessed for Rehabilitation	11	100%	98%	97%
Discharged on Antithrombotic Therapy	11	100%	99%	99%
Discharged on Statin Medication[1]	-	-	95%	94%
Thrombolytic Therapy Timing[1]	-	-	65%	66%
Venous Thromboembolism Prophylaxis[1]	-	-	95%	94%
Written Stroke Educational Materials Given[1]	-	-	92%	88%
Surgical Care Improvement Project				
Appropriate Beta Blocker Usage	14	93%	98%	98%
Appropriate VTP Within 24 Hours	53	98%	98%	98%
Controlled Postoperative Blood Glucose[7]	-	-	97%	97%
Perioperative Temperature Management	74	100%	100%	100%
Prophylactic Antibiotic Selection	51	100%	99%	99%
Prophylactic Antibiotic Selection (Outpatient)	21	100%	98%	98%
Prophylactic Antibiotic Stopped	49	94%	98%	98%
Prophylactic Antibiotic Timing	53	100%	99%	99%
Prophylactic Antibiotic Timing (Outpatient)	22	95%	97%	98%
Urinary Catheter Removal	38	100%	97%	97%
Survey of Patients' Hospital Experiences				
Area Around Room 'Always' Quiet at Night	300+	52%	58%	61%
Doctors 'Always' Communicated Well	300+	77%	80%	82%
Home Recovery Information Given	300+	81%	87%	85%
Hospital Given 9 or 10 on 10 Point Scale	300+	64%	72%	71%
Meds 'Always' Explained Before Given	300+	59%	64%	64%
Nurses 'Always' Communicated Well	300+	78%	81%	79%
Pain 'Always' Well Controlled	300+	68%	71%	71%
Room and Bathroom 'Always' Clean	300+	73%	75%	73%
Timely Help 'Always' Received	300+	64%	70%	68%
Would Definitely Recommend Hospital	300+	55%	71%	71%
Use of Medical Imaging				
Cardiac Imaging Stress Test before Surgery	215	3.3%	5.4%	5.3%
Combination Abdominal CT Scan	411	10.7%	7.1%	10.5%
Combination Brain/Sinus CT Scan	501	4.8%	2.8%	2.7%
Combination Chest CT Scan	233	14.2%	1.7%	2.7%
Follow-up Mammogram/Ultrasound	367	9.0%	8.7%	8.8%
Lumbar Spine MRI for Low Back Pain	75	37.3%	34.7%	37.2%

NOTE: Hospital profiles are in alphabetical order by state, then city, then hospital within the city; Rankings exclude hospitals with less than 25 cases except for patient surveys which excludes hospitals with less than 100 cases; (a) 100-299 cases; (1) The number of cases/patients is too few to report; (2) Data submitted were based on a sample of cases/patients; (3) Results are based on a shorter time period than required; (4) Data suppressed by CMS for one or more quarters; (5) Results are not available for this reporting period; (6) Fewer than 100 patients completed the HCAHPS survey; (7) No cases met the criteria for this measure; (8) The lower limit of the confidence interval cannot be calculated if the number of observed infections equals zero; (9) No data are available from the state/territory for this reporting period; (10) The scores shown reflect fewer than 50 completed surveys; (11) There were discrepancies in the data collection process; (12) This measure does not apply to this hospital for this reporting period; (13) Results cannot be calculated for this reporting period; (14) The results for this state are combined with nearby states to protect confidentiality; Please refer to the User's Guide for a full explanation of data.

University Hospitals - Elyria Medical Center

630 East River Street
Elyria, OH 44035
URL: www.emh-healthcare.org
Type: Acute Care Hospitals
Ownership: Voluntary non-profit - Private

Phone: 440-329-7500
Fax: 440-329-7505

Emergency Services: Yes
Beds: 348

Key Personnel:
Quality Assurance . . . . Sue Ballard
Chief of Medical Staff. . . . . Kenneth Bescak, MD
Infection Control. . . . . Peggy Gnizak
Emergency Room . . . . JoAnn Hozalski
Patient Relations . . . . Deb Jones
CEO/President. . . . . Kevin C Martin
Radiology. . . . . Eduardo Martinez

Measure	Cases	This Hosp.	State Avg.	U.S. Avg.
Blood Clot Prevention and Treatment				
Anticoagulation Overlap Therapy[2]	97	76%	93%	93%
ICU Venous Thromboembolism Prophylaxis[2]	98	91%	93%	92%
Incidence of Potentially Preventable VTE[2]	13	8%	6%	10%
UFH with Dosages/Platelet Monitoring[2]	59	100%	98%	97%
Venous Thromboembolism Prophylaxis[2]	332	60%	88%	85%
Warfarin Therapy Discharge Instructions[2]	71	85%	79%	75%
Chest Pain/Possible Heart Attack Care				
Aspirin Given Within 24 Hours of Arrival	29	90%	97%	96%
Fibrinolytic Meds Within 30 Min. of Arrival[7]	-	-	44%	58%
Average Time to ECG (minutes)	34	10	6	7
Average Time to Transfer (minutes)[7]	-	-	58	60
Children's Asthma Care				
Received Home Management Plan of Care	-	-	85%	88%
Received Reliever Medication	-	-	100%	100%
Received Systemic Corticosteroids	-	-	100%	100%
Emergency Department				
Admittance Decision Time (minutes)[2]	467	75	90	98
Head CT Results Within 45 Min. of Arrival	30	90%	63%	57%
Patients Who Left ER Before Being Seen	88,075	2%	2%	2%
Time from ER Arrival to Admit. (minutes)[2]	468	231	265	274
Time from ER Arrival to Discharge (minutes)	395	112	128	134
Time in ER Before Being Evaluated (minutes)	426	18	22	26
Time to Pain Meds for Fractures (minutes)	173	39	54	57
Heart Attack Care				
Aspirin Given at Discharge[2]	359	99%	99%	99%
Fibrinolytic Meds Within 30 Min. of Arrival[2,7]	-	-	80%	54%
PCI Within 90 Minutes of Arrival[2]	36	94%	97%	96%
Statin Prescribed at Discharge[2]	355	99%	98%	98%
Heart Failure Care				
ACE Inhibitor or ARB for LVSD[2]	102	94%	97%	97%
Discharge Instructions Given[2]	252	94%	96%	94%
Evaluation of LVS Function[2]	326	100%	100%	99%
Medicare Spending				
Medicare Spending per Patient (ratio)	-	1.03	1.01	0.98
Pneumonia Care				
Appropriate Initial Antibiotic Given[2]	83	94%	96%	95%
Blood Culture Timing[2]	94	98%	98%	98%
Pregnancy and Delivery Care				
Newborn Deliveries Scheduled Early[2]	25	8%	5%	6%
Preventive Care				
Immunization for Influenza[2]	598	95%	93%	90%
Immunization for Pneumonia[2]	871	95%	94%	92%
Stroke Care				
Anticoagulation Therapy for Atrial Fibrillation	18	89%	95%	95%
Antithrombotic Therapy Timing	113	100%	98%	98%
Assessed for Rehabilitation	108	97%	98%	97%
Discharged on Antithrombotic Therapy	104	99%	99%	99%
Discharged on Statin Medication	81	95%	95%	94%
Thrombolytic Therapy Timing	11	9%	65%	66%
Venous Thromboembolism Prophylaxis	118	67%	95%	94%
Written Stroke Educational Materials Given	65	94%	92%	88%
Surgical Care Improvement Project				
Appropriate Beta Blocker Usage[2]	186	97%	98%	98%
Appropriate VTP Within 24 Hours[2]	455	97%	98%	98%
Controlled Postoperative Blood Glucose[2]	28	86%	97%	97%
Perioperative Temperature Management[2]	512	100%	100%	100%
Prophylactic Antibiotic Selection[2]	355	99%	99%	99%
Prophylactic Antibiotic Selection (Outpatient)	353	96%	98%	98%
Prophylactic Antibiotic Stopped[2]	346	92%	98%	98%
Prophylactic Antibiotic Timing[2]	355	99%	99%	99%
Prophylactic Antibiotic Timing (Outpatient)	330	97%	97%	98%
Urinary Catheter Removal[2]	306	95%	97%	97%
Survey of Patients' Hospital Experiences				
Area Around Room 'Always' Quiet at Night	300+	58%	58%	61%
Doctors 'Always' Communicated Well	300+	77%	80%	82%
Home Recovery Information Given	300+	85%	87%	85%
Hospital Given 9 or 10 on 10 Point Scale	300+	70%	72%	71%
Meds 'Always' Explained Before Given	300+	65%	64%	64%
Nurses 'Always' Communicated Well	300+	80%	81%	79%
Pain 'Always' Well Controlled	300+	69%	71%	71%
Room and Bathroom 'Always' Clean	300+	73%	75%	73%
Timely Help 'Always' Received	300+	70%	70%	68%
Would Definitely Recommend Hospital	300+	69%	71%	71%
Use of Medical Imaging				
Cardiac Imaging Stress Test before Surgery	1,958	5.1%	5.4%	5.3%
Combination Abdominal CT Scan	990	2.4%	7.1%	10.5%
Combination Brain/Sinus CT Scan	916	2.7%	2.8%	2.7%
Combination Chest CT Scan	327	0.3%	1.7%	2.7%
Follow-up Mammogram/Ultrasound	635	4.7%	8.7%	8.8%
Lumbar Spine MRI for Low Back Pain	85	24.7%	34.7%	37.2%

Euclid Hospital

18901 Lake Shore Boulevard
Euclid, OH 44119
URL: www.euclidhospital.org
Type: Acute Care Hospitals
Ownership: Voluntary non-profit - Other

Phone: 216-531-9000
Fax: 216-692-7473

Emergency Services: Yes
Beds: 371

Key Personnel:
Chief of Medical Staff. . . . . Tommas Anton
Operating Room. . . . . Mark Janzen, MD
Radiology. . . . . Ellen Park
CEO/President. . . . . Lauren Rock

Measure	Cases	This Hosp.	State Avg.	U.S. Avg.
Blood Clot Prevention and Treatment				
Anticoagulation Overlap Therapy[2]	72	90%	93%	93%
ICU Venous Thromboembolism Prophylaxis[2]	75	100%	93%	92%
Incidence of Potentially Preventable VTE[2]	12	0%	6%	10%
UFH with Dosages/Platelet Monitoring[2]	63	100%	98%	97%
Venous Thromboembolism Prophylaxis[2]	259	96%	88%	85%
Warfarin Therapy Discharge Instructions[2]	40	98%	79%	75%
Chest Pain/Possible Heart Attack Care				
Aspirin Given Within 24 Hours of Arrival	54	94%	97%	96%
Fibrinolytic Meds Within 30 Min. of Arrival[7]	-	-	44%	58%
Average Time to ECG (minutes)	53	5	6	7
Average Time to Transfer (minutes)	11	55	58	60
Children's Asthma Care				
Received Home Management Plan of Care	-	-	85%	88%
Received Reliever Medication	-	-	100%	100%
Received Systemic Corticosteroids	-	-	100%	100%
Emergency Department				
Admittance Decision Time (minutes)[2]	597	93	90	98
Head CT Results Within 45 Min. of Arrival	22	82%	63%	57%
Patients Who Left ER Before Being Seen	38,473	3%	2%	2%
Time from ER Arrival to Admit. (minutes)[2]	599	291	265	274
Time from ER Arrival to Discharge (minutes)	375	128	128	134
Time in ER Before Being Evaluated (minutes)	415	20	22	26
Time to Pain Meds for Fractures (minutes)	54	50	54	57
Heart Attack Care				
Aspirin Given at Discharge[1]	-	-	99%	99%
Fibrinolytic Meds Within 30 Min. of Arrival[7]	-	-	80%	54%
PCI Within 90 Minutes of Arrival[7]	-	-	97%	96%
Statin Prescribed at Discharge[1]	-	-	98%	98%
Heart Failure Care				
ACE Inhibitor or ARB for LVSD	41	98%	97%	97%
Discharge Instructions Given	134	100%	96%	94%
Evaluation of LVS Function	220	100%	100%	99%
Medicare Spending				
Medicare Spending per Patient (ratio)	-	1.10	1.01	0.98
Pneumonia Care				
Appropriate Initial Antibiotic Given	82	98%	96%	95%
Blood Culture Timing	141	98%	98%	98%
Pregnancy and Delivery Care				
Newborn Deliveries Scheduled Early[7]	-	-	5%	6%
Preventive Care				
Immunization for Influenza[2]	556	99%	93%	90%
Immunization for Pneumonia[2]	822	99%	94%	92%
Stroke Care				
Anticoagulation Therapy for Atrial Fibrillation[1]	-	-	95%	95%
Antithrombotic Therapy Timing	51	98%	98%	98%
Assessed for Rehabilitation	53	100%	98%	97%
Discharged on Antithrombotic Therapy	48	100%	99%	99%
Discharged on Statin Medication	32	100%	95%	94%
Thrombolytic Therapy Timing[1]	-	-	65%	66%
Venous Thromboembolism Prophylaxis	53	100%	95%	94%
Written Stroke Educational Materials Given	16	100%	92%	88%
Surgical Care Improvement Project				
Appropriate Beta Blocker Usage[2]	81	100%	98%	98%
Appropriate VTP Within 24 Hours[2]	314	100%	98%	98%
Controlled Postoperative Blood Glucose[2,7]	-	-	97%	97%
Perioperative Temperature Management[2]	331	100%	100%	100%
Prophylactic Antibiotic Selection[2]	214	100%	99%	99%
Prophylactic Antibiotic Selection (Outpatient)	83	99%	98%	98%
Prophylactic Antibiotic Stopped[2]	211	100%	98%	98%
Prophylactic Antibiotic Timing[2]	214	100%	99%	99%
Prophylactic Antibiotic Timing (Outpatient)	83	98%	97%	98%
Urinary Catheter Removal[2]	185	99%	97%	97%
Survey of Patients' Hospital Experiences				
Area Around Room 'Always' Quiet at Night	300+	64%	58%	61%
Doctors 'Always' Communicated Well	300+	79%	80%	82%
Home Recovery Information Given	300+	91%	87%	85%
Hospital Given 9 or 10 on 10 Point Scale	300+	69%	72%	71%
Meds 'Always' Explained Before Given	300+	68%	64%	64%
Nurses 'Always' Communicated Well	300+	82%	81%	79%
Pain 'Always' Well Controlled	300+	74%	71%	71%
Room and Bathroom 'Always' Clean	300+	70%	75%	73%
Timely Help 'Always' Received	300+	72%	70%	68%
Would Definitely Recommend Hospital	300+	71%	71%	71%
Use of Medical Imaging				
Cardiac Imaging Stress Test before Surgery	86	4.7%	5.4%	5.3%
Combination Abdominal CT Scan	402	1.2%	7.1%	10.5%
Combination Brain/Sinus CT Scan	649	2.0%	2.8%	2.7%
Combination Chest CT Scan	123	2.4%	1.7%	2.7%
Follow-up Mammogram/Ultrasound	361	4.4%	8.7%	8.8%
Lumbar Spine MRI for Low Back Pain	48	39.6%	34.7%	37.2%

Mercy Hospital Fairfield

3000 Mack Road
Fairfield, OH 45014
URL: www.e-mercy.com/mercy-hospital-fairfield.aspx
Type: Acute Care Hospitals
Ownership: Voluntary non-profit - Church

Phone: 513-870-7197
Fax: 513-870-7065

Emergency Services: Yes
Beds: 167

Key Personnel:
CEO/President. . . . . Yousuf J. Ahmad
Chief of Medical Staff. . . . . Dan Roth, MD
Emergency Room . . . . Marla Yost

Measure	Cases	This Hosp.	State Avg.	U.S. Avg.
Blood Clot Prevention and Treatment				
Anticoagulation Overlap Therapy[2]	111	96%	93%	93%
ICU Venous Thromboembolism Prophylaxis[2]	98	95%	93%	92%
Incidence of Potentially Preventable VTE[2]	12	17%	6%	10%
UFH with Dosages/Platelet Monitoring[2]	58	100%	98%	97%
Venous Thromboembolism Prophylaxis[2]	300	90%	88%	85%
Warfarin Therapy Discharge Instructions[2]	87	91%	79%	75%
Chest Pain/Possible Heart Attack Care				
Aspirin Given Within 24 Hours of Arrival[1,3]	-	-	97%	96%
Fibrinolytic Meds Within 30 Min. of Arrival[3,7]	-	-	44%	58%
Average Time to ECG (minutes)[1,3]	-	-	6	7
Average Time to Transfer (minutes)[1,3]	-	-	58	60
Children's Asthma Care				
Received Home Management Plan of Care	-	-	85%	88%
Received Reliever Medication	-	-	100%	100%
Received Systemic Corticosteroids	-	-	100%	100%
Emergency Department				
Admittance Decision Time (minutes)[2]	725	126	90	98

NOTE: Hospital profiles are in alphabetical order by state, then city, then hospital within the city; Rankings exclude hospitals with less than 25 cases except for patient surveys which excludes hospitals with less than 100 cases; (a) 100-299 cases; (1) The number of cases/patients is too few to report; (2) Data submitted were based on a sample of cases/patients; (3) Results are based on a shorter time period than required; (4) Data suppressed by CMS for one or more quarters; (5) Results are not available for this reporting period; (6) Fewer than 100 patients completed the HCAHPS survey; (7) No cases met the criteria for this measure; (8) The lower limit of the confidence interval cannot be calculated if the number of observed infections equals zero; (9) No data are available from the state/territory for this reporting period; (10) The scores shown reflect fewer than 50 completed surveys; (11) There were discrepancies in the data collection process; (12) This measure does not apply to this hospital for this reporting period; (13) Results cannot be calculated for this reporting period; (14) The results for this state are combined with nearby states to protect confidentiality; Please refer to the User's Guide for a full explanation of data.

Measure	Cases	This Hosp.	State Avg.	U.S. Avg.
Head CT Results Within 45 Min. of Arrival[1]	-	-	63%	57%
Patients Who Left ER Before Being Seen	61,969	1%	2%	2%
Time from ER Arrival to Admit. (minutes)[2]	725	297	265	274
Time from ER Arrival to Discharge (minutes)	397	134	128	134
Time in ER Before Being Evaluated (minutes)	417	13	22	26
Time to Pain Meds for Fractures (minutes)	135	64	54	57
Heart Attack Care				
Aspirin Given at Discharge	389	98%	99%	99%
Fibrinolytic Meds Within 30 Min. of Arrival[7]	-	-	80%	54%
PCI Within 90 Minutes of Arrival	57	93%	97%	96%
Statin Prescribed at Discharge	374	99%	98%	98%
Heart Failure Care				
ACE Inhibitor or ARB for LVSD	190	99%	97%	97%
Discharge Instructions Given	493	100%	96%	94%
Evaluation of LVS Function	604	100%	100%	99%
Medicare Spending				
Medicare Spending per Patient (ratio)	-	0.99	1.01	0.98
Pneumonia Care				
Appropriate Initial Antibiotic Given	211	100%	96%	95%
Blood Culture Timing	433	99%	98%	98%
Pregnancy and Delivery Care				
Newborn Deliveries Scheduled Early[2]	38	3%	5%	6%
Preventive Care				
Immunization for Influenza[2]	581	96%	93%	90%
Immunization for Pneumonia[2]	741	94%	94%	92%
Stroke Care				
Anticoagulation Therapy for Atrial Fibrillation[2]	22	95%	95%	95%
Antithrombotic Therapy Timing[2]	100	100%	98%	98%
Assessed for Rehabilitation[2]	110	100%	98%	97%
Discharged on Antithrombotic Therapy[2]	104	100%	99%	99%
Discharged on Statin Medication[2]	86	94%	95%	94%
Thrombolytic Therapy Timing[1,2]	-	-	65%	66%
Venous Thromboembolism Prophylaxis[2]	109	93%	95%	94%
Written Stroke Educational Materials Given[2]	65	100%	92%	88%
Surgical Care Improvement Project				
Appropriate Beta Blocker Usage[2]	200	98%	98%	98%
Appropriate VTP Within 24 Hours[2]	458	99%	98%	98%
Controlled Postoperative Blood Glucose[2]	181	99%	97%	97%
Perioperative Temperature Management[2]	624	100%	100%	100%
Prophylactic Antibiotic Selection[2]	582	99%	99%	99%
Prophylactic Antibiotic Selection (Outpatient)	154	94%	98%	98%
Prophylactic Antibiotic Stopped[2]	569	98%	98%	98%
Prophylactic Antibiotic Timing[2]	583	98%	99%	99%
Prophylactic Antibiotic Timing (Outpatient)	144	95%	97%	98%
Urinary Catheter Removal[2]	451	98%	97%	97%
Survey of Patients' Hospital Experiences				
Area Around Room 'Always' Quiet at Night	300+	64%	58%	61%
Doctors 'Always' Communicated Well	300+	82%	80%	82%
Home Recovery Information Given	300+	90%	87%	85%
Hospital Given 9 or 10 on 10 Point Scale	300+	82%	72%	71%
Meds 'Always' Explained Before Given	300+	68%	64%	64%
Nurses 'Always' Communicated Well	300+	85%	81%	79%
Pain 'Always' Well Controlled	300+	75%	71%	71%
Room and Bathroom 'Always' Clean	300+	81%	75%	73%
Timely Help 'Always' Received	300+	75%	70%	68%
Would Definitely Recommend Hospital	300+	83%	71%	71%
Use of Medical Imaging				
Cardiac Imaging Stress Test before Surgery	765	5.9%	5.4%	5.3%
Combination Abdominal CT Scan	1,034	5.5%	7.1%	10.5%
Combination Brain/Sinus CT Scan	681	0.9%	2.8%	2.7%
Combination Chest CT Scan	728	3.0%	1.7%	2.7%
Follow-up Mammogram/Ultrasound	1,303	5.4%	8.7%	8.8%
Lumbar Spine MRI for Low Back Pain	248	42.3%	34.7%	37.2%

Blanchard Valley Hospital

1900 South Main Street
Findlay, OH 45840
Phone: 419-423-4500
Fax: 419-423-5358
URL: www.bvha.org
Type: Acute Care Hospitals
Emergency Services: Yes
Ownership: Voluntary non-profit - Other
Beds: 150

Key Personnel:

Radiology. . . . . Edward Bok
Operating Room. . . . . Eric Browning
Chairman/CEO . . . . Duane Jebbett
CEO/President. . . . . Scott Malaney
Chief of Medical Staff . . . . Richard Polder
Pediatric Ambulatory Care . . . . . . A Ritz, MD
Quality Assurance . . . . Sandy Shutt
Coronary Care . . . . Sherri Winegardner

Measure	Cases	This Hosp.	State Avg.	U.S. Avg.
Blood Clot Prevention and Treatment				
Anticoagulation Overlap Therapy[2]	61	100%	93%	93%
ICU Venous Thromboembolism Prophylaxis[2]	150	99%	93%	92%
Incidence of Potentially Preventable VTE[1,2]	-	-	6%	10%
UFH with Dosages/Platelet Monitoring[2]	49	100%	98%	97%
Venous Thromboembolism Prophylaxis[2]	200	97%	88%	85%
Warfarin Therapy Discharge Instructions[2]	49	100%	79%	75%
Chest Pain/Possible Heart Attack Care				
Aspirin Given Within 24 Hours of Arrival[1,3]	-	-	97%	96%
Fibrinolytic Meds Within 30 Min. of Arrival[3,7]	-	-	44%	58%
Average Time to ECG (minutes)[1,3]	-	-	6	7
Average Time to Transfer (minutes)[3,7]	-	-	58	60
Children's Asthma Care				
Received Home Management Plan of Care	-	-	85%	88%
Received Reliever Medication	-	-	100%	100%
Received Systemic Corticosteroids	-	-	100%	100%
Emergency Department				
Admittance Decision Time (minutes)[2]	445	61	90	98
Head CT Results Within 45 Min. of Arrival	33	88%	63%	57%
Patients Who Left ER Before Being Seen	37,072	0%	2%	2%
Time from ER Arrival to Admit. (minutes)[2]	445	245	265	274
Time from ER Arrival to Discharge (minutes)	361	121	128	134
Time in ER Before Being Evaluated (minutes)	383	12	22	26
Time to Pain Meds for Fractures (minutes)	149	45	54	57
Heart Attack Care				
Aspirin Given at Discharge	182	100%	99%	99%
Fibrinolytic Meds Within 30 Min. of Arrival[7]	-	-	80%	54%
PCI Within 90 Minutes of Arrival	46	100%	97%	96%
Statin Prescribed at Discharge	179	100%	98%	98%
Heart Failure Care				
ACE Inhibitor or ARB for LVSD	61	100%	97%	97%
Discharge Instructions Given	101	100%	96%	94%
Evaluation of LVS Function	138	100%	100%	99%
Medicare Spending				
Medicare Spending per Patient (ratio)	-	0.97	1.01	0.98
Pneumonia Care				
Appropriate Initial Antibiotic Given	108	96%	96%	95%
Blood Culture Timing	163	98%	98%	98%
Pregnancy and Delivery Care				
Newborn Deliveries Scheduled Early[2]	29	0%	5%	6%
Preventive Care				
Immunization for Influenza[2]	501	99%	93%	90%
Immunization for Pneumonia[2]	551	100%	94%	92%
Stroke Care				
Anticoagulation Therapy for Atrial Fibrillation[1]	-	-	95%	95%
Antithrombotic Therapy Timing	57	100%	98%	98%
Assessed for Rehabilitation	66	100%	98%	97%
Discharged on Antithrombotic Therapy	58	100%	99%	99%
Discharged on Statin Medication	50	100%	95%	94%
Thrombolytic Therapy Timing[7]	-	-	65%	66%
Venous Thromboembolism Prophylaxis	63	100%	95%	94%
Written Stroke Educational Materials Given	40	98%	92%	88%
Surgical Care Improvement Project				
Appropriate Beta Blocker Usage[2]	227	100%	98%	98%
Appropriate VTP Within 24 Hours[2]	543	99%	98%	98%
Controlled Postoperative Blood Glucose[2]	43	98%	97%	97%
Perioperative Temperature Management[2]	607	100%	100%	100%
Prophylactic Antibiotic Selection[2]	516	99%	99%	99%
Prophylactic Antibiotic Selection (Outpatient)	474	99%	98%	98%
Prophylactic Antibiotic Stopped[2]	505	99%	98%	98%
Prophylactic Antibiotic Timing[2]	516	99%	99%	99%
Prophylactic Antibiotic Timing (Outpatient)	475	100%	97%	98%
Urinary Catheter Removal[2]	323	98%	97%	97%
Survey of Patients' Hospital Experiences				
Area Around Room 'Always' Quiet at Night	300+	68%	58%	61%
Doctors 'Always' Communicated Well	300+	84%	80%	82%
Home Recovery Information Given	300+	85%	87%	85%
Hospital Given 9 or 10 on 10 Point Scale	300+	78%	72%	71%
Meds 'Always' Explained Before Given	300+	66%	64%	64%
Nurses 'Always' Communicated Well	300+	83%	81%	79%
Pain 'Always' Well Controlled	300+	70%	71%	71%
Room and Bathroom 'Always' Clean	300+	83%	75%	73%
Timely Help 'Always' Received	300+	67%	70%	68%
Would Definitely Recommend Hospital	300+	74%	71%	71%
Use of Medical Imaging				
Cardiac Imaging Stress Test before Surgery	288	6.6%	5.4%	5.3%
Combination Abdominal CT Scan	922	6.0%	7.1%	10.5%
Combination Brain/Sinus CT Scan	700	4.0%	2.8%	2.7%
Combination Chest CT Scan	473	1.7%	1.7%	2.7%
Follow-up Mammogram/Ultrasound	1,562	6.0%	8.7%	8.8%
Lumbar Spine MRI for Low Back Pain	222	33.8%	34.7%	37.2%

Fostoria Community Hospital

501 Van Buren Street
Fostoria, OH 44830
Phone: 419-435-7734
Fax: 419-436-6602
URL: www.promedica.org
Type: Critical Access Hospitals
Emergency Services: Yes
Ownership: Voluntary non-profit - Private
Beds: 66

Key Personnel:

CEO/President. . . . . Randy Oostra
Emergency Room . . . . Amy Preble
Chief of Medical Staff . . . . D Ross, MD

Measure	Cases	This Hosp.	State Avg.	U.S. Avg.
Blood Clot Prevention and Treatment				
Anticoagulation Overlap Therapy[5]	-	-	93%	93%
ICU Venous Thromboembolism Prophylaxis[5]	-	-	93%	92%
Incidence of Potentially Preventable VTE[5]	-	-	6%	10%
UFH with Dosages/Platelet Monitoring[5]	-	-	98%	97%
Venous Thromboembolism Prophylaxis[5]	-	-	88%	85%
Warfarin Therapy Discharge Instructions[5]	-	-	79%	75%
Chest Pain/Possible Heart Attack Care				
Aspirin Given Within 24 Hours of Arrival[3]	47	100%	97%	96%
Fibrinolytic Meds Within 30 Min. of Arrival[1,3]	-	-	44%	58%
Average Time to ECG (minutes)[3]	50	5	6	7
Average Time to Transfer (minutes)[1,3]	-	-	58	60
Children's Asthma Care				
Received Home Management Plan of Care	-	-	85%	88%
Received Reliever Medication	-	-	100%	100%
Received Systemic Corticosteroids	-	-	100%	100%
Emergency Department				
Admittance Decision Time (minutes)[2,3]	82	56	90	98
Head CT Results Within 45 Min. of Arrival[1,3]	-	-	63%	57%
Patients Who Left ER Before Being Seen	15,481	1%	2%	2%
Time from ER Arrival to Admit. (minutes)[2,3]	93	173	265	274
Time from ER Arrival to Discharge (minutes)[5]	-	-	128	134
Time in ER Before Being Evaluated (minutes)[5]	-	-	22	26
Time to Pain Meds for Fractures (minutes)[1,3]	-	-	54	57
Heart Attack Care				
Aspirin Given at Discharge[1]	-	-	99%	99%
Fibrinolytic Meds Within 30 Min. of Arrival[7]	-	-	80%	54%
PCI Within 90 Minutes of Arrival[7]	-	-	97%	96%
Statin Prescribed at Discharge[1]	-	-	98%	98%
Heart Failure Care				
ACE Inhibitor or ARB for LVSD[1]	-	-	97%	97%
Discharge Instructions Given	21	100%	96%	94%
Evaluation of LVS Function	29	100%	100%	99%
Medicare Spending				
Medicare Spending per Patient (ratio)	-	-	1.01	0.98
Pneumonia Care				
Appropriate Initial Antibiotic Given	38	100%	96%	95%
Blood Culture Timing	43	100%	98%	98%
Pregnancy and Delivery Care				
Newborn Deliveries Scheduled Early[7]	-	-	5%	6%
Preventive Care				
Immunization for Influenza[2]	128	82%	93%	90%
Immunization for Pneumonia[2,3]	155	84%	94%	92%
Stroke Care				
Anticoagulation Therapy for Atrial Fibrillation[1,3]	-	-	95%	95%
Antithrombotic Therapy Timing[1,3]	-	-	98%	98%

NOTE: Hospital profiles are in alphabetical order by state, then city, then hospital within the city; Rankings exclude hospitals with less than 25 cases except for patient surveys which excludes hospitals with less than 100 cases; (a) 100-299 cases; (1) The number of cases/patients is too few to report; (2) Data submitted were based on a sample of cases/patients; (3) Results are based on a shorter time period than required; (4) Data suppressed by CMS for one or more quarters; (5) Results are not available for this reporting period; (6) Fewer than 100 patients completed the HCAHPS survey; (7) No cases met the criteria for this measure; (8) The lower limit of the confidence interval cannot be calculated if the number of observed infections equals zero; (9) No data are available from the state/territory for this reporting period; (10) The scores shown reflect fewer than 50 completed surveys; (11) There were discrepancies in the data collection process; (12) This measure does not apply to this hospital for this reporting period; (13) Results cannot be calculated for this reporting period; (14) The results for this state are combined with nearby states to protect confidentiality; Please refer to the User's Guide for a full explanation of data.

Measure	Cases	This Hosp.	State Avg.	U.S. Avg.
Assessed for Rehabilitation[1,3]	-	-	98%	97%
Discharged on Antithrombotic Therapy[1,3]	-	-	99%	99%
Discharged on Statin Medication[1,3]	-	-	95%	94%
Thrombolytic Therapy Timing[3,7]	-	-	65%	66%
Venous Thromboembolism Prophylaxis[1,3]	-	-	95%	94%
Written Stroke Educational Materials Given[1,3]	-	-	92%	88%
Surgical Care Improvement Project				
Appropriate Beta Blocker Usage	26	100%	98%	98%
Appropriate VTP Within 24 Hours	106	100%	98%	98%
Controlled Postoperative Blood Glucose[7]	-	-	97%	97%
Perioperative Temperature Management	111	100%	100%	100%
Prophylactic Antibiotic Selection	110	99%	99%	99%
Prophylactic Antibiotic Selection (Outpatient)[1,3]	-	-	98%	98%
Prophylactic Antibiotic Stopped	108	100%	98%	98%
Prophylactic Antibiotic Timing	110	99%	99%	99%
Prophylactic Antibiotic Timing (Outpatient)[1,3]	-	-	97%	98%
Urinary Catheter Removal[1]	-	-	97%	97%
Survey of Patients' Hospital Experiences				
Area Around Room 'Always' Quiet at Night	(a)	70%	58%	61%
Doctors 'Always' Communicated Well	(a)	85%	80%	82%
Home Recovery Information Given	(a)	88%	87%	85%
Hospital Given 9 or 10 on 10 Point Scale	(a)	79%	72%	71%
Meds 'Always' Explained Before Given	(a)	73%	64%	64%
Nurses 'Always' Communicated Well	(a)	88%	81%	79%
Pain 'Always' Well Controlled	(a)	79%	71%	71%
Room and Bathroom 'Always' Clean	(a)	94%	75%	73%
Timely Help 'Always' Received	(a)	83%	70%	68%
Would Definitely Recommend Hospital	(a)	75%	71%	71%
Use of Medical Imaging				
Cardiac Imaging Stress Test before Surgery	131	3.1%	5.4%	5.3%
Combination Abdominal CT Scan	261	8.0%	7.1%	10.5%
Combination Brain/Sinus CT Scan[1]	-	-	2.8%	2.7%
Combination Chest CT Scan	108	2.8%	1.7%	2.7%
Follow-up Mammogram/Ultrasound	354	7.6%	8.7%	8.8%
Lumbar Spine MRI for Low Back Pain[1]	-	-	34.7%	37.2%

Atrium Medical Center

One Medical Center Drive
Franklin, OH 45005
URL: www.atriummedcenter.org
Type: Acute Care Hospitals
Ownership: Voluntary non-profit - Private
Phone: 513-420-5102
Emergency Services: Yes
Beds: 250

Key Personnel:
Radiology . . . . Chris Chung, MD
CEO/President . . . . McNeill Doug
Pediatric Ambulatory Care . . . . . . Diana E Small, MD

Measure	Cases	This Hosp.	State Avg.	U.S. Avg.
Blood Clot Prevention and Treatment				
Anticoagulation Overlap Therapy[2]	118	98%	93%	93%
ICU Venous Thromboembolism Prophylaxis[2]	107	99%	93%	92%
Incidence of Potentially Preventable VTE[2]	16	0%	6%	10%
UFH with Dosages/Platelet Monitoring[2]	95	100%	98%	97%
Venous Thromboembolism Prophylaxis[2]	320	90%	88%	85%
Warfarin Therapy Discharge Instructions[2]	90	96%	79%	75%
Chest Pain/Possible Heart Attack Care				
Aspirin Given Within 24 Hours of Arrival[1]	-	-	97%	96%
Fibrinolytic Meds Within 30 Min. of Arrival[3,7]	-	-	44%	58%
Average Time to ECG (minutes)[1]	-	-	6	7
Average Time to Transfer (minutes)[1,3]	-	-	58	60
Children's Asthma Care				
Received Home Management Plan of Care	-	-	85%	88%
Received Reliever Medication	-	-	100%	100%
Received Systemic Corticosteroids	-	-	100%	100%
Emergency Department				
Admittance Decision Time (minutes)[2]	700	126	90	98
Head CT Results Within 45 Min. of Arrival	15	100%	63%	57%
Patients Who Left ER Before Being Seen	63,056	1%	2%	2%
Time from ER Arrival to Admit. (minutes)[2]	716	267	265	274
Time from ER Arrival to Discharge (minutes)	395	146	128	134
Time in ER Before Being Evaluated (minutes)	420	14	22	26
Time to Pain Meds for Fractures (minutes)	135	51	54	57
Heart Attack Care				
Aspirin Given at Discharge	239	100%	99%	99%
Fibrinolytic Meds Within 30 Min. of Arrival[7]	-	-	80%	54%
PCI Within 90 Minutes of Arrival	55	98%	97%	96%
Statin Prescribed at Discharge	241	100%	98%	98%
Heart Failure Care				
ACE Inhibitor or ARB for LVSD	54	100%	97%	97%
Discharge Instructions Given	211	99%	96%	94%
Evaluation of LVS Function	261	100%	100%	99%
Medicare Spending				
Medicare Spending per Patient (ratio)	-	1.02	1.01	0.98
Pneumonia Care				
Appropriate Initial Antibiotic Given[2]	75	100%	96%	95%
Blood Culture Timing[2]	149	99%	98%	98%
Pregnancy and Delivery Care				
Newborn Deliveries Scheduled Early	79	1%	5%	6%
Preventive Care				
Immunization for Influenza[2]	619	100%	93%	90%
Immunization for Pneumonia[2]	783	100%	94%	92%
Stroke Care				
Anticoagulation Therapy for Atrial Fibrillation	14	100%	95%	95%
Antithrombotic Therapy Timing	96	100%	98%	98%
Assessed for Rehabilitation	114	100%	98%	97%
Discharged on Antithrombotic Therapy	102	100%	99%	99%
Discharged on Statin Medication	83	100%	95%	94%
Thrombolytic Therapy Timing[1]	-	-	65%	66%
Venous Thromboembolism Prophylaxis	114	97%	95%	94%
Written Stroke Educational Materials Given	62	97%	92%	88%
Surgical Care Improvement Project				
Appropriate Beta Blocker Usage[2]	205	99%	98%	98%
Appropriate VTP Within 24 Hours[2]	364	98%	98%	98%
Controlled Postoperative Blood Glucose[2]	76	97%	97%	97%
Perioperative Temperature Management[2]	435	100%	100%	100%
Prophylactic Antibiotic Selection[2]	325	100%	99%	99%
Prophylactic Antibiotic Selection (Outpatient)	312	99%	98%	98%
Prophylactic Antibiotic Stopped[2]	302	99%	98%	98%
Prophylactic Antibiotic Timing[2]	325	99%	99%	99%
Prophylactic Antibiotic Timing (Outpatient)	312	100%	97%	98%
Urinary Catheter Removal[2]	265	99%	97%	97%
Survey of Patients' Hospital Experiences				
Area Around Room 'Always' Quiet at Night[11]	300+	63%	58%	61%
Doctors 'Always' Communicated Well[11]	300+	80%	80%	82%
Home Recovery Information Given[11]	300+	89%	87%	85%
Hospital Given 9 or 10 on 10 Point Scale[11]	300+	70%	72%	71%
Meds 'Always' Explained Before Given[11]	300+	64%	64%	64%
Nurses 'Always' Communicated Well[11]	300+	80%	81%	79%
Pain 'Always' Well Controlled[11]	300+	72%	71%	71%
Room and Bathroom 'Always' Clean[11]	300+	74%	75%	73%
Timely Help 'Always' Received[11]	300+	60%	70%	68%
Would Definitely Recommend Hospital[11]	300+	69%	71%	71%
Use of Medical Imaging				
Cardiac Imaging Stress Test before Surgery	242	7.9%	5.4%	5.3%
Combination Abdominal CT Scan	991	4.9%	7.1%	10.5%
Combination Brain/Sinus CT Scan	1,020	2.3%	2.8%	2.7%
Combination Chest CT Scan	824	1.1%	1.7%	2.7%
Follow-up Mammogram/Ultrasound	1,362	3.9%	8.7%	8.8%
Lumbar Spine MRI for Low Back Pain	165	33.3%	34.7%	37.2%

Memorial Hospital

715 South Taft Avenue
Fremont, OH 43420
URL: www.freemontmemorial.org
Type: Acute Care Hospitals
Ownership: Voluntary non-profit - Other
Phone: 419-334-6617
Fax: 419-332-5875
Emergency Services: Yes
Beds: 186

Key Personnel:
Infection Control . . . . Tami Binger
Operating Room . . . . Michael E Grillis
Radiology . . . . Bruce L Hammond
Emergency Room . . . . Dana Levy
Anesthesiology . . . . Joseph Loskove, MD
Chief of Medical Staff . . . . Robert Marshall, MD
Surgery . . . . Emil Matei
Quality Assurance . . . . Brenda McClain

Measure	Cases	This Hosp.	State Avg.	U.S. Avg.
Blood Clot Prevention and Treatment				
Anticoagulation Overlap Therapy[2]	13	100%	93%	93%
ICU Venous Thromboembolism Prophylaxis[2]	43	88%	93%	92%
Incidence of Potentially Preventable VTE[1,2]	-	-	6%	10%
UFH with Dosages/Platelet Monitoring[1,2]	-	-	98%	97%
Venous Thromboembolism Prophylaxis[2]	141	93%	88%	85%
Warfarin Therapy Discharge Instructions[1,2]	-	-	79%	75%
Chest Pain/Possible Heart Attack Care				
Aspirin Given Within 24 Hours of Arrival	67	93%	97%	96%
Fibrinolytic Meds Within 30 Min. of Arrival[1]	-	-	44%	58%
Average Time to ECG (minutes)	74	5	6	7
Average Time to Transfer (minutes)[1]	-	-	58	60
Children's Asthma Care				
Received Home Management Plan of Care	-	-	85%	88%
Received Reliever Medication	-	-	100%	100%
Received Systemic Corticosteroids	-	-	100%	100%
Emergency Department				
Admittance Decision Time (minutes)[2]	315	55	90	98
Head CT Results Within 45 Min. of Arrival	14	64%	63%	57%
Patients Who Left ER Before Being Seen	23,151	1%	2%	2%
Time from ER Arrival to Admit. (minutes)[2]	322	221	265	274
Time from ER Arrival to Discharge (minutes)	508	110	128	134
Time in ER Before Being Evaluated (minutes)	540	17	22	26
Time to Pain Meds for Fractures (minutes)	126	62	54	57
Heart Attack Care				
Aspirin Given at Discharge[1]	-	-	99%	99%
Fibrinolytic Meds Within 30 Min. of Arrival[7]	-	-	80%	54%
PCI Within 90 Minutes of Arrival[7]	-	-	97%	96%
Statin Prescribed at Discharge[1]	-	-	98%	98%
Heart Failure Care				
ACE Inhibitor or ARB for LVSD	20	100%	97%	97%
Discharge Instructions Given	58	93%	96%	94%
Evaluation of LVS Function	77	99%	100%	99%
Medicare Spending				
Medicare Spending per Patient (ratio)	-	1.00	1.01	0.98
Pneumonia Care				
Appropriate Initial Antibiotic Given	52	88%	96%	95%
Blood Culture Timing	77	100%	98%	98%
Pregnancy and Delivery Care				
Newborn Deliveries Scheduled Early	21	0%	5%	6%
Preventive Care				
Immunization for Influenza[2]	268	94%	93%	90%
Immunization for Pneumonia[2]	388	97%	94%	92%
Stroke Care				
Anticoagulation Therapy for Atrial Fibrillation[1]	-	-	95%	95%
Antithrombotic Therapy Timing	25	100%	98%	98%
Assessed for Rehabilitation	25	100%	98%	97%
Discharged on Antithrombotic Therapy	25	100%	99%	99%
Discharged on Statin Medication	19	100%	95%	94%
Thrombolytic Therapy Timing[1]	-	-	65%	66%
Venous Thromboembolism Prophylaxis	29	93%	95%	94%
Written Stroke Educational Materials Given	12	100%	92%	88%
Surgical Care Improvement Project				
Appropriate Beta Blocker Usage	65	100%	98%	98%
Appropriate VTP Within 24 Hours	180	89%	98%	98%
Controlled Postoperative Blood Glucose[7]	-	-	97%	97%
Perioperative Temperature Management	192	100%	100%	100%
Prophylactic Antibiotic Selection	148	100%	99%	99%
Prophylactic Antibiotic Selection (Outpatient)	61	97%	98%	98%
Prophylactic Antibiotic Stopped	147	97%	98%	98%
Prophylactic Antibiotic Timing	148	98%	99%	99%
Prophylactic Antibiotic Timing (Outpatient)	70	87%	97%	98%
Urinary Catheter Removal	156	99%	97%	97%
Survey of Patients' Hospital Experiences				
Area Around Room 'Always' Quiet at Night	300+	58%	58%	61%
Doctors 'Always' Communicated Well	300+	84%	80%	82%
Home Recovery Information Given	300+	88%	87%	85%
Hospital Given 9 or 10 on 10 Point Scale	300+	67%	72%	71%
Meds 'Always' Explained Before Given	300+	64%	64%	64%
Nurses 'Always' Communicated Well	300+	80%	81%	79%
Pain 'Always' Well Controlled	300+	68%	71%	71%
Room and Bathroom 'Always' Clean	300+	78%	75%	73%
Timely Help 'Always' Received	300+	70%	70%	68%
Would Definitely Recommend Hospital	300+	61%	71%	71%

NOTE: Hospital profiles are in alphabetical order by state, then city, then hospital within the city; Rankings exclude hospitals with less than 25 cases except for patient surveys which excludes hospitals with less than 100 cases; (a) 100-299 cases; (1) The number of cases/patients is too few to report; (2) Data submitted were based on a sample of cases/patients; (3) Results are based on a shorter time period than required; (4) Data suppressed by CMS for one or more quarters; (5) Results are not available for this reporting period; (6) Fewer than 100 patients completed the HCAHPS survey; (7) No cases met the criteria for this measure; (8) The lower limit of the confidence interval cannot be calculated if the number of observed infections equals zero; (9) No data are available from the state/territory for this reporting period; (10) The scores shown reflect fewer than 50 completed surveys; (11) There were discrepancies in the data collection process; (12) This measure does not apply to this hospital for this reporting period; (13) Results cannot be calculated for this reporting period; (14) The results for this state are combined with nearby states to protect confidentiality; Please refer to the User's Guide for a full explanation of data.

Use of Medical Imaging				
Cardiac Imaging Stress Test before Surgery	230	5.2%	5.4%	5.3%
Combination Abdominal CT Scan	375	16.5%	7.1%	10.5%
Combination Brain/Sinus CT Scan[1]	-	-	2.8%	2.7%
Combination Chest CT Scan	236	10.6%	1.7%	2.7%
Follow-up Mammogram/Ultrasound	717	7.0%	8.7%	8.8%
Lumbar Spine MRI for Low Back Pain	93	24.7%	34.7%	37.2%

Galion Community Hospital

269 Portland Way South
Galion, OH 44833
Phone: 419-468-4841
Fax: 419-468-2381
URL: www.galionhospital.org
Type: Critical Access Hospitals
Emergency Services: Yes
Ownership: Voluntary non-profit - Church
Beds: 25

Key Personnel:
Chief of Medical Staff . . . . Julie C Beard
Quality Assurance . . . . Helen Burdine
Intensive Care Unit. . . . . Shirley Fitz
Radiology. . . . . James J Jerele
Patient Relations . . . . Rebecca Miller
Emergency Room . . . . John Schoettmer
CEO/President. . . . . LaMar Wyse

Measure	Cases	This Hosp.	State Avg.	U.S. Avg.
Blood Clot Prevention and Treatment				
Anticoagulation Overlap Therapy[5]	-	-	93%	93%
ICU Venous Thromboembolism Prophylaxis[5]	-	-	93%	92%
Incidence of Potentially Preventable VTE[5]	-	-	6%	10%
UFH with Dosages/Platelet Monitoring[5]	-	-	98%	97%
Venous Thromboembolism Prophylaxis[5]	-	-	88%	85%
Warfarin Therapy Discharge Instructions[5]	-	-	79%	75%
Chest Pain/Possible Heart Attack Care				
Aspirin Given Within 24 Hours of Arrival[5]	-	-	97%	96%
Fibrinolytic Meds Within 30 Min. of Arrival[5]	-	-	44%	58%
Average Time to ECG (minutes)[5]	-	-	6	7
Average Time to Transfer (minutes)[5]	-	-	58	60
Children's Asthma Care				
Received Home Management Plan of Care	-	-	85%	88%
Received Reliever Medication	-	-	100%	100%
Received Systemic Corticosteroids	-	-	100%	100%
Emergency Department				
Admittance Decision Time (minutes)[5]	-	-	90	98
Head CT Results Within 45 Min. of Arrival[5]	-	-	63%	57%
Patients Who Left ER Before Being Seen[5]	-	-	2%	2%
Time from ER Arrival to Admit. (minutes)[5]	-	-	265	274
Time from ER Arrival to Discharge (minutes)[5]	-	-	128	134
Time in ER Before Being Evaluated (minutes)[5]	-	-	22	26
Time to Pain Meds for Fractures (minutes)[5]	-	-	54	57
Heart Attack Care				
Aspirin Given at Discharge[1]	-	-	99%	99%
Fibrinolytic Meds Within 30 Min. of Arrival[3,7]	-	-	80%	54%
PCI Within 90 Minutes of Arrival[3,7]	-	-	97%	96%
Statin Prescribed at Discharge[1]	-	-	98%	98%
Heart Failure Care				
ACE Inhibitor or ARB for LVSD[1,2]	-	-	97%	97%
Discharge Instructions Given[2]	11	55%	96%	94%
Evaluation of LVS Function[2]	14	93%	100%	99%
Medicare Spending				
Medicare Spending per Patient (ratio)		-	1.01	0.98
Pneumonia Care				
Appropriate Initial Antibiotic Given[2]	67	97%	96%	95%
Blood Culture Timing[2]	85	96%	98%	98%
Pregnancy and Delivery Care				
Newborn Deliveries Scheduled Early[5]	-	-	5%	6%
Preventive Care				
Immunization for Influenza[5]	-	-	93%	90%
Immunization for Pneumonia[5]	-	-	94%	92%
Stroke Care				
Anticoagulation Therapy for Atrial Fibrillation[5]	-	-	95%	95%
Antithrombotic Therapy Timing[5]	-	-	98%	98%
Assessed for Rehabilitation[5]	-	-	98%	97%
Discharged on Antithrombotic Therapy[5]	-	-	99%	99%
Discharged on Statin Medication[5]	-	-	95%	94%
Thrombolytic Therapy Timing[5]	-	-	65%	66%
Venous Thromboembolism Prophylaxis[5]	-	-	95%	94%
Written Stroke Educational Materials Given[5]	-	-	92%	88%
Surgical Care Improvement Project				
Appropriate Beta Blocker Usage[3]	37	100%	98%	98%
Appropriate VTP Within 24 Hours	127	98%	98%	98%
Controlled Postoperative Blood Glucose[3,7]	-	-	97%	97%
Perioperative Temperature Management	145	100%	100%	100%
Prophylactic Antibiotic Selection	130	99%	99%	99%
Prophylactic Antibiotic Selection (Outpatient)[5]	-	-	98%	98%
Prophylactic Antibiotic Stopped	125	94%	98%	98%
Prophylactic Antibiotic Timing	130	96%	99%	99%
Prophylactic Antibiotic Timing (Outpatient)[5]	-	-	97%	98%
Urinary Catheter Removal	98	92%	97%	97%
Survey of Patients' Hospital Experiences				
Area Around Room 'Always' Quiet at Night	300+	60%	58%	61%
Doctors 'Always' Communicated Well	300+	82%	80%	82%
Home Recovery Information Given	300+	91%	87%	85%
Hospital Given 9 or 10 on 10 Point Scale	300+	72%	72%	71%
Meds 'Always' Explained Before Given	300+	68%	64%	64%
Nurses 'Always' Communicated Well	300+	80%	81%	79%
Pain 'Always' Well Controlled	300+	74%	71%	71%
Room and Bathroom 'Always' Clean	300+	71%	75%	73%
Timely Help 'Always' Received	300+	73%	70%	68%
Would Definitely Recommend Hospital	300+	70%	71%	71%
Use of Medical Imaging				
Cardiac Imaging Stress Test before Surgery	165	4.2%	5.4%	5.3%
Combination Abdominal CT Scan	393	5.9%	7.1%	10.5%
Combination Brain/Sinus CT Scan	388	1.3%	2.8%	2.7%
Combination Chest CT Scan	189	4.2%	1.7%	2.7%
Follow-up Mammogram/Ultrasound	561	6.6%	8.7%	8.8%
Lumbar Spine MRI for Low Back Pain	67	35.8%	34.7%	37.2%

Holzer Medical Center

100 Jackson Pike
Gallipolis, OH 45631
Phone: 740-446-5000
Fax: 740-446-5522
URL: www.holzer.org
Type: Acute Care Hospitals
Emergency Services: Yes
Ownership: Voluntary non-profit - Private
Beds: 269

Key Personnel:
Infection Control . . . . Nancy Childs, RN
Pediatric Ambulatory Care . . . . . . Cindy Harrison
Pediatric In-Patient Care . . . . Cindy Harrison
Quality Assurance . . . . Thomas Judy
Chief of Medical Staff. . . . . Dr. Christopher Meyer
CEO/President. . . . . Dr. T. Wanye Munro
Radiology. . . . . Mike Roe
Coronary Care . . . . Glenda Skinner

Measure	Cases	This Hosp.	State Avg.	U.S. Avg.
Blood Clot Prevention and Treatment				
Anticoagulation Overlap Therapy[2]	19	89%	93%	93%
ICU Venous Thromboembolism Prophylaxis[2]	92	88%	93%	92%
Incidence of Potentially Preventable VTE[1,2]	-	-	6%	10%
UFH with Dosages/Platelet Monitoring[1,2]	-	-	98%	97%
Venous Thromboembolism Prophylaxis[2]	347	83%	88%	85%
Warfarin Therapy Discharge Instructions[2]	16	31%	79%	75%
Chest Pain/Possible Heart Attack Care				
Aspirin Given Within 24 Hours of Arrival	17	88%	97%	96%
Fibrinolytic Meds Within 30 Min. of Arrival[3,7]	-	-	44%	58%
Average Time to ECG (minutes)	18	0	6	7
Average Time to Transfer (minutes)[3,7]	-	-	58	60
Children's Asthma Care				
Received Home Management Plan of Care	-	-	85%	88%
Received Reliever Medication	-	-	100%	100%
Received Systemic Corticosteroids	-	-	100%	100%
Emergency Department				
Admittance Decision Time (minutes)[2]	442	68	90	98
Head CT Results Within 45 Min. of Arrival[1]	-	-	63%	57%
Patients Who Left ER Before Being Seen	22,506	5%	2%	2%
Time from ER Arrival to Admit. (minutes)[2]	464	229	265	274
Time from ER Arrival to Discharge (minutes)	335	178	128	134
Time in ER Before Being Evaluated (minutes)	374	49	22	26
Time to Pain Meds for Fractures (minutes)	55	82	54	57
Heart Attack Care				
Aspirin Given at Discharge	182	96%	99%	99%
Fibrinolytic Meds Within 30 Min. of Arrival[7]	-	-	80%	54%
PCI Within 90 Minutes of Arrival	25	84%	97%	96%
Statin Prescribed at Discharge	180	97%	98%	98%
Heart Failure Care				
ACE Inhibitor or ARB for LVSD[2]	53	94%	97%	97%
Discharge Instructions Given[2]	160	73%	96%	94%
Evaluation of LVS Function[2]	193	100%	100%	99%
Medicare Spending				
Medicare Spending per Patient (ratio)	-	1.07	1.01	0.98
Pneumonia Care				
Appropriate Initial Antibiotic Given[2]	87	91%	96%	95%
Blood Culture Timing[2]	102	98%	98%	98%
Pregnancy and Delivery Care				
Newborn Deliveries Scheduled Early[2]	81	0%	5%	6%
Preventive Care				
Immunization for Influenza[2]	469	93%	93%	90%
Immunization for Pneumonia[2]	643	98%	94%	92%
Stroke Care				
Anticoagulation Therapy for Atrial Fibrillation[1]	-	-	95%	95%
Antithrombotic Therapy Timing	34	94%	98%	98%
Assessed for Rehabilitation	31	90%	98%	97%
Discharged on Antithrombotic Therapy	31	94%	99%	99%
Discharged on Statin Medication	24	96%	95%	94%
Thrombolytic Therapy Timing[1]	-	-	65%	66%
Venous Thromboembolism Prophylaxis	34	91%	95%	94%
Written Stroke Educational Materials Given	16	50%	92%	88%
Surgical Care Improvement Project				
Appropriate Beta Blocker Usage	72	97%	98%	98%
Appropriate VTP Within 24 Hours	129	95%	98%	98%
Controlled Postoperative Blood Glucose	30	90%	97%	97%
Perioperative Temperature Management	154	99%	100%	100%
Prophylactic Antibiotic Selection	97	100%	99%	99%
Prophylactic Antibiotic Selection (Outpatient)	282	96%	98%	98%
Prophylactic Antibiotic Stopped	95	95%	98%	98%
Prophylactic Antibiotic Timing	97	100%	99%	99%
Prophylactic Antibiotic Timing (Outpatient)	288	96%	97%	98%
Urinary Catheter Removal	112	91%	97%	97%
Survey of Patients' Hospital Experiences				
Area Around Room 'Always' Quiet at Night	300+	56%	58%	61%
Doctors 'Always' Communicated Well	300+	80%	80%	82%
Home Recovery Information Given	300+	84%	87%	85%
Hospital Given 9 or 10 on 10 Point Scale	300+	65%	72%	71%
Meds 'Always' Explained Before Given	300+	59%	64%	64%
Nurses 'Always' Communicated Well	300+	73%	81%	79%
Pain 'Always' Well Controlled	300+	65%	71%	71%
Room and Bathroom 'Always' Clean	300+	68%	75%	73%
Timely Help 'Always' Received	300+	65%	70%	68%
Would Definitely Recommend Hospital	300+	64%	71%	71%
Use of Medical Imaging				
Cardiac Imaging Stress Test before Surgery	347	2.0%	5.4%	5.3%
Combination Abdominal CT Scan	993	22.5%	7.1%	10.5%
Combination Brain/Sinus CT Scan[1]	-	-	2.8%	2.7%
Combination Chest CT Scan	705	4.8%	1.7%	2.7%
Follow-up Mammogram/Ultrasound	1,319	2.0%	8.7%	8.8%
Lumbar Spine MRI for Low Back Pain	128	32.8%	34.7%	37.2%

Marymount Hospital

12300 Mccracken Road
Garfield Heights, OH 44125
Phone: 216-581-0500
Fax: 216-587-8967
E-mail: marketing@marymount.org
URL: www.marymount.org
Type: Acute Care Hospitals
Emergency Services: Yes
Ownership: Voluntary non-profit - Private
Beds: 322

Key Personnel:
Radiology. . . . . Indu Agarwal
CEO/President. . . . . David J Kilarski
Chief of Medical Staff. . . . . Richard Ungvarsky, MD

Measure	Cases	This Hosp.	State Avg.	U.S. Avg.
Blood Clot Prevention and Treatment				
Anticoagulation Overlap Therapy[2]	166	93%	93%	93%
ICU Venous Thromboembolism Prophylaxis[2]	55	95%	93%	92%
Incidence of Potentially Preventable VTE[2]	18	6%	6%	10%
UFH with Dosages/Platelet Monitoring[2]	112	100%	98%	97%
Venous Thromboembolism Prophylaxis[2]	377	95%	88%	85%

NOTE: Hospital profiles are in alphabetical order by state, then city, then hospital within the city; Rankings exclude hospitals with less than 25 cases except for patient surveys which excludes hospitals with less than 100 cases; (a) 100-299 cases; (1) The number of cases/patients is too few to report; (2) Data submitted were based on a sample of cases/patients; (3) Results are based on a shorter time period than required; (4) Data suppressed by CMS for one or more quarters; (5) Results are not available for this reporting period; (6) Fewer than 100 patients completed the HCAHPS survey; (7) No cases met the criteria for this measure; (8) The lower limit of the confidence interval cannot be calculated if the number of observed infections equals zero; (9) No data are available from the state/territory for this reporting period; (10) The scores shown reflect fewer than 50 completed surveys; (11) There were discrepancies in the data collection process; (12) This measure does not apply to this hospital for this reporting period; (13) Results cannot be calculated for this reporting period; (14) The results for this state are combined with nearby states to protect confidentiality; Please refer to the User's Guide for a full explanation of data.

Warfarin Therapy Discharge Instructions[2]	123	77%	79%	75%
Chest Pain/Possible Heart Attack Care				
Aspirin Given Within 24 Hours of Arrival	74	100%	97%	96%
Fibrinolytic Meds Within 30 Min. of Arrival[7]	-	-	44%	58%
Average Time to ECG (minutes)	74	4	6	7
Average Time to Transfer (minutes)	15	58	58	60
Children's Asthma Care				
Received Home Management Plan of Care	-	-	85%	88%
Received Reliever Medication	-	-	100%	100%
Received Systemic Corticosteroids	-	-	100%	100%
Emergency Department				
Admittance Decision Time (minutes)[2]	680	95	90	98
Head CT Results Within 45 Min. of Arrival	16	56%	63%	57%
Patients Who Left ER Before Being Seen	50,542	2%	2%	2%
Time from ER Arrival to Admit. (minutes)[2]	703	284	265	274
Time from ER Arrival to Discharge (minutes)	381	121	128	134
Time in ER Before Being Evaluated (minutes)	428	18	22	26
Time to Pain Meds for Fractures (minutes)	119	45	54	57
Heart Attack Care				
Aspirin Given at Discharge	25	96%	99%	99%
Fibrinolytic Meds Within 30 Min. of Arrival[7]	-	-	80%	54%
PCI Within 90 Minutes of Arrival[7]	-	-	97%	96%
Statin Prescribed at Discharge	25	100%	98%	98%
Heart Failure Care				
ACE Inhibitor or ARB for LVSD	124	98%	97%	97%
Discharge Instructions Given	332	100%	96%	94%
Evaluation of LVS Function	472	100%	100%	99%
Medicare Spending				
Medicare Spending per Patient (ratio)	-	1.07	1.01	0.98
Pneumonia Care				
Appropriate Initial Antibiotic Given	180	99%	96%	95%
Blood Culture Timing	255	100%	98%	98%
Pregnancy and Delivery Care				
Newborn Deliveries Scheduled Early[7]	-	-	5%	6%
Preventive Care				
Immunization for Influenza[2]	606	100%	93%	90%
Immunization for Pneumonia[2]	1,018	99%	94%	92%
Stroke Care				
Anticoagulation Therapy for Atrial Fibrillation	24	100%	95%	95%
Antithrombotic Therapy Timing	158	99%	98%	98%
Assessed for Rehabilitation	170	95%	98%	97%
Discharged on Antithrombotic Therapy	167	99%	99%	99%
Discharged on Statin Medication	124	94%	95%	94%
Thrombolytic Therapy Timing[1]	-	-	65%	66%
Venous Thromboembolism Prophylaxis	164	97%	95%	94%
Written Stroke Educational Materials Given	107	100%	92%	88%
Surgical Care Improvement Project				
Appropriate Beta Blocker Usage[2]	124	100%	98%	98%
Appropriate VTP Within 24 Hours[2]	301	100%	98%	98%
Controlled Postoperative Blood Glucose[2,7]	-	-	97%	97%
Perioperative Temperature Management[2]	348	100%	100%	100%
Prophylactic Antibiotic Selection[2]	232	100%	99%	99%
Prophylactic Antibiotic Selection (Outpatient)	95	99%	98%	98%
Prophylactic Antibiotic Stopped[2]	219	100%	98%	98%
Prophylactic Antibiotic Timing[2]	232	100%	99%	99%
Prophylactic Antibiotic Timing (Outpatient)	90	98%	97%	98%
Urinary Catheter Removal[2]	245	100%	97%	97%
Survey of Patients' Hospital Experiences				
Area Around Room 'Always' Quiet at Night	300+	51%	58%	61%
Doctors 'Always' Communicated Well	300+	79%	80%	82%
Home Recovery Information Given	300+	85%	87%	85%
Hospital Given 9 or 10 on 10 Point Scale	300+	64%	72%	71%
Meds 'Always' Explained Before Given	300+	62%	64%	64%
Nurses 'Always' Communicated Well	300+	78%	81%	79%
Pain 'Always' Well Controlled	300+	69%	71%	71%
Room and Bathroom 'Always' Clean	300+	77%	75%	73%
Timely Help 'Always' Received	300+	68%	70%	68%
Would Definitely Recommend Hospital	300+	63%	71%	71%
Use of Medical Imaging				
Cardiac Imaging Stress Test before Surgery	157	7.6%	5.4%	5.3%
Combination Abdominal CT Scan	654	4.7%	7.1%	10.5%
Combination Brain/Sinus CT Scan	768	3.3%	2.8%	2.7%
Combination Chest CT Scan	320	0.3%	1.7%	2.7%
Follow-up Mammogram/Ultrasound	1,029	8.6%	8.7%	8.8%
Lumbar Spine MRI for Low Back Pain	89	31.5%	34.7%	37.2%

UHHS Memorial Hospital of Geneva

870 West Main Street
Geneva, OH 44041
Phone: 440-466-1141
Fax: 440-466-0903
URL: www.uhhospitals.org/geneva
Type: Critical Access Hospitals
Emergency Services: Yes
Ownership: Voluntary non-profit - Private
Beds: 46

Key Personnel:
Chief of Medical Staff.......... Emolyn Defensor, MD
Intensive Care Unit.......... Debra Greiner, RN
Emergency Room............ Sue Hopkins, RN
Operating Room............. Sue Hopkins, RN
Quality Assurance........... Laurie Lewis, ART
Infection Control............. Robert Malinowski, DO
CEO/President............... Thomas Zenty, III

Measure	Cases	This Hosp.	State Avg.	U.S. Avg.
Blood Clot Prevention and Treatment				
Anticoagulation Overlap Therapy[1,2]	-	-	93%	93%
ICU Venous Thromboembolism Prophylaxis[2]	40	100%	93%	92%
Incidence of Potentially Preventable VTE[2,7]	-	-	6%	10%
UFH with Dosages/Platelet Monitoring[1,2]	-	-	98%	97%
Venous Thromboembolism Prophylaxis[2]	98	97%	88%	85%
Warfarin Therapy Discharge Instructions[1,2]	-	-	79%	75%
Chest Pain/Possible Heart Attack Care				
Aspirin Given Within 24 Hours of Arrival	80	98%	97%	96%
Fibrinolytic Meds Within 30 Min. of Arrival[7]	-	-	44%	58%
Average Time to ECG (minutes)	85	4	6	7
Average Time to Transfer (minutes)	12	56	58	60
Children's Asthma Care				
Received Home Management Plan of Care	-	-	85%	88%
Received Reliever Medication	-	-	100%	100%
Received Systemic Corticosteroids	-	-	100%	100%
Emergency Department				
Admittance Decision Time (minutes)[2]	455	78	90	98
Head CT Results Within 45 Min. of Arrival[1]	-	-	63%	57%
Patients Who Left ER Before Being Seen	14,047	1%	2%	2%
Time from ER Arrival to Admit. (minutes)[2]	461	256	265	274
Time from ER Arrival to Discharge (minutes)	355	102	128	134
Time in ER Before Being Evaluated (minutes)	297	17	22	26
Time to Pain Meds for Fractures (minutes)	53	49	54	57
Heart Attack Care				
Aspirin Given at Discharge[1]	-	-	99%	99%
Fibrinolytic Meds Within 30 Min. of Arrival[7]	-	-	80%	54%
PCI Within 90 Minutes of Arrival[7]	-	-	97%	96%
Statin Prescribed at Discharge[1]	-	-	98%	98%
Heart Failure Care				
ACE Inhibitor or ARB for LVSD	12	92%	97%	97%
Discharge Instructions Given	50	100%	96%	94%
Evaluation of LVS Function	81	100%	100%	99%
Medicare Spending				
Medicare Spending per Patient (ratio)	-	-	1.01	0.98
Pneumonia Care				
Appropriate Initial Antibiotic Given	66	100%	96%	95%
Blood Culture Timing	135	100%	98%	98%
Pregnancy and Delivery Care				
Newborn Deliveries Scheduled Early[3,7]	-	-	5%	6%
Preventive Care				
Immunization for Influenza[2]	295	99%	93%	90%
Immunization for Pneumonia[2]	515	99%	94%	92%
Stroke Care				
Anticoagulation Therapy for Atrial Fibrillation[1]	-	-	95%	95%
Antithrombotic Therapy Timing[1]	-	-	98%	98%
Assessed for Rehabilitation[1]	-	-	98%	97%
Discharged on Antithrombotic Therapy[1]	-	-	99%	99%
Discharged on Statin Medication[1]	-	-	95%	94%
Thrombolytic Therapy Timing[7]	-	-	65%	66%
Venous Thromboembolism Prophylaxis[1]	-	-	95%	94%
Written Stroke Educational Materials Given[1]	-	-	92%	88%
Surgical Care Improvement Project				
Appropriate Beta Blocker Usage	17	100%	98%	98%
Appropriate VTP Within 24 Hours	49	100%	98%	98%
Controlled Postoperative Blood Glucose[7]	-	-	97%	97%
Perioperative Temperature Management	50	100%	100%	100%
Prophylactic Antibiotic Selection	37	100%	99%	99%
Prophylactic Antibiotic Selection (Outpatient)[1,3]	-	-	98%	98%
Prophylactic Antibiotic Stopped	35	100%	98%	98%
Prophylactic Antibiotic Timing	37	100%	99%	99%
Prophylactic Antibiotic Timing (Outpatient)[1,3]	-	-	97%	98%
Urinary Catheter Removal	12	100%	97%	97%
Survey of Patients' Hospital Experiences				
Area Around Room 'Always' Quiet at Night	(a)	63%	58%	61%
Doctors 'Always' Communicated Well	(a)	84%	80%	82%
Home Recovery Information Given	(a)	93%	87%	85%
Hospital Given 9 or 10 on 10 Point Scale	(a)	77%	72%	71%
Meds 'Always' Explained Before Given	(a)	65%	64%	64%
Nurses 'Always' Communicated Well	(a)	86%	81%	79%
Pain 'Always' Well Controlled	(a)	68%	71%	71%
Room and Bathroom 'Always' Clean	(a)	81%	75%	73%
Timely Help 'Always' Received	(a)	78%	70%	68%
Would Definitely Recommend Hospital	(a)	80%	71%	71%
Use of Medical Imaging				
Cardiac Imaging Stress Test before Surgery	101	2.0%	5.4%	5.3%
Combination Abdominal CT Scan	445	2.0%	7.1%	10.5%
Combination Brain/Sinus CT Scan[1]	-	-	2.8%	2.7%
Combination Chest CT Scan	422	0.5%	1.7%	2.7%
Follow-up Mammogram/Ultrasound	499	15.6%	8.7%	8.8%
Lumbar Spine MRI for Low Back Pain[1]	-	-	34.7%	37.2%

Southwest Regional Medical Center

425 Home Street
Georgetown, OH 45121
Phone: 513-378-7800
Fax: 937-378-7744
E-mail: c_beck@bcrhc.org
URL: www.browncountygeneralhospital.com
Type: Acute Care Hospitals
Emergency Services: Yes
Ownership: Proprietary
Beds: 127

Key Personnel:
Radiology................. Kevin A Aukerman, MD
CEO/President............. Bruce A Bennett
Intensive Care Unit........... Cindy Edmister
Operating Room............. Lisa Michael
Emergency Room........... Scott Walden, MD
Chief of Medical Staff.......... Todd Williams, MD
Infection Control............. Mino Wright, RN

Measure	Cases	This Hosp.	State Avg.	U.S. Avg.
Blood Clot Prevention and Treatment				
Anticoagulation Overlap Therapy[1,2]	-	-	93%	93%
ICU Venous Thromboembolism Prophylaxis[2]	14	100%	93%	92%
Incidence of Potentially Preventable VTE[2,7]	-	-	6%	10%
UFH with Dosages/Platelet Monitoring[1,2]	-	-	98%	97%
Venous Thromboembolism Prophylaxis[2]	75	95%	88%	85%
Warfarin Therapy Discharge Instructions[1,2]	-	-	79%	75%
Chest Pain/Possible Heart Attack Care				
Aspirin Given Within 24 Hours of Arrival	93	94%	97%	96%
Fibrinolytic Meds Within 30 Min. of Arrival[1]	-	-	44%	58%
Average Time to ECG (minutes)	96	8	6	7
Average Time to Transfer (minutes)[1]	-	-	58	60
Children's Asthma Care				
Received Home Management Plan of Care	-	-	85%	88%
Received Reliever Medication	-	-	100%	100%
Received Systemic Corticosteroids	-	-	100%	100%
Emergency Department				
Admittance Decision Time (minutes)[2]	333	98	90	98
Head CT Results Within 45 Min. of Arrival	13	62%	63%	57%
Patients Who Left ER Before Being Seen	12,130	1%	2%	2%
Time from ER Arrival to Admit. (minutes)[2]	342	268	265	274
Time from ER Arrival to Discharge (minutes)	142	200	128	134
Time in ER Before Being Evaluated (minutes)	249	17	22	26
Time to Pain Meds for Fractures (minutes)[3]	19	50	54	57
Heart Attack Care				
Aspirin Given at Discharge[1]	-	-	99%	99%
Fibrinolytic Meds Within 30 Min. of Arrival[7]	-	-	80%	54%
PCI Within 90 Minutes of Arrival[7]	-	-	97%	96%
Statin Prescribed at Discharge[1]	-	-	98%	98%
Heart Failure Care				
ACE Inhibitor or ARB for LVSD	13	100%	97%	97%

NOTE: Hospital profiles are in alphabetical order by state, then city, then hospital within the city; Rankings exclude hospitals with less than 25 cases except for patient surveys which excludes hospitals with less than 100 cases; (a) 100-299 cases; (1) The number of cases/patients is too few to report; (2) Data submitted were based on a sample of cases/patients; (3) Results are based on a shorter time period than required; (4) Data suppressed by CMS for one or more quarters; (5) Results are not available for this reporting period; (6) Fewer than 100 patients completed the HCAHPS survey; (7) No cases met the criteria for this measure; (8) The lower limit of the confidence interval cannot be calculated if the number of observed infections equals zero; (9) No data are available from the state/territory for this reporting period; (10) The scores shown reflect fewer than 50 completed surveys; (11) There were discrepancies in the data collection process; (12) This measure does not apply to this hospital for this reporting period; (13) Results cannot be calculated for this reporting period; (14) The results for this state are combined with nearby states to protect confidentiality; Please refer to the User's Guide for a full explanation of data.

Measure	Cases	This Hosp.	State Avg.	U.S. Avg.
Discharge Instructions Given	31	94%	96%	94%
Evaluation of LVS Function	65	98%	100%	99%
Medicare Spending				
Medicare Spending per Patient (ratio)	-	0.99	1.01	0.98
Pneumonia Care				
Appropriate Initial Antibiotic Given	25	92%	96%	95%
Blood Culture Timing	61	97%	98%	98%
Pregnancy and Delivery Care				
Newborn Deliveries Scheduled Early[7]	-	-	5%	6%
Preventive Care				
Immunization for Influenza[2]	299	94%	93%	90%
Immunization for Pneumonia[2]	483	93%	94%	92%
Stroke Care				
Anticoagulation Therapy for Atrial Fibrillation[7]	-	-	95%	95%
Antithrombotic Therapy Timing[1]	-	-	98%	98%
Assessed for Rehabilitation[1]	-	-	98%	97%
Discharged on Antithrombotic Therapy[1]	-	-	99%	99%
Discharged on Statin Medication[1]	-	-	95%	94%
Thrombolytic Therapy Timing[1]	-	-	65%	66%
Venous Thromboembolism Prophylaxis[1]	-	-	95%	94%
Written Stroke Educational Materials Given[1]	-	-	92%	88%
Surgical Care Improvement Project				
Appropriate Beta Blocker Usage	17	94%	98%	98%
Appropriate VTP Within 24 Hours	29	100%	98%	98%
Controlled Postoperative Blood Glucose[7]	-	-	97%	97%
Perioperative Temperature Management	36	97%	100%	100%
Prophylactic Antibiotic Selection	12	100%	99%	99%
Prophylactic Antibiotic Selection (Outpatient)	23	78%	98%	98%
Prophylactic Antibiotic Stopped	11	100%	98%	98%
Prophylactic Antibiotic Timing	12	100%	99%	99%
Prophylactic Antibiotic Timing (Outpatient)	20	90%	97%	98%
Urinary Catheter Removal	32	97%	97%	97%
Survey of Patients' Hospital Experiences				
Area Around Room 'Always' Quiet at Night	(a)	53%	58%	61%
Doctors 'Always' Communicated Well	(a)	74%	80%	82%
Home Recovery Information Given	(a)	74%	87%	85%
Hospital Given 9 or 10 on 10 Point Scale	(a)	51%	72%	71%
Meds 'Always' Explained Before Given	(a)	53%	64%	64%
Nurses 'Always' Communicated Well	(a)	72%	81%	79%
Pain 'Always' Well Controlled	(a)	62%	71%	71%
Room and Bathroom 'Always' Clean	(a)	64%	75%	73%
Timely Help 'Always' Received	(a)	72%	70%	68%
Would Definitely Recommend Hospital	(a)	52%	71%	71%
Use of Medical Imaging				
Cardiac Imaging Stress Test before Surgery	81	4.9%	5.4%	5.3%
Combination Abdominal CT Scan	132	2.3%	7.1%	10.5%
Combination Brain/Sinus CT Scan	169	0.6%	2.8%	2.7%
Combination Chest CT Scan	75	1.3%	1.7%	2.7%
Follow-up Mammogram/Ultrasound	231	10.8%	8.7%	8.8%
Lumbar Spine MRI for Low Back Pain[1]	-	-	34.7%	37.2%

Greenfield Area Medical Center

550 Mirabeau Street
Greenfield, OH 45123
Phone: 937-981-9400
Fax: 937-981-9499
URL: www.adena.org
Type: Critical Access Hospitals
Emergency Services: No
Ownership: Voluntary non-profit - Private
Beds: 46

Key Personnel:
Chief of Medical Staff .... Wayne W Beam Jr
Radiology .... Bryan I Borland
Emergency Room .... Kevin Dorothy
CEO/President .... Mark Shuter

Measure	Cases	This Hosp.	State Avg.	U.S. Avg.
Blood Clot Prevention and Treatment				
Anticoagulation Overlap Therapy	-	-	93%	93%
ICU Venous Thromboembolism Prophylaxis	-	-	93%	92%
Incidence of Potentially Preventable VTE	-	-	6%	10%
UFH with Dosages/Platelet Monitoring	-	-	98%	97%
Venous Thromboembolism Prophylaxis	-	-	88%	85%
Warfarin Therapy Discharge Instructions	-	-	79%	75%
Chest Pain/Possible Heart Attack Care				
Aspirin Given Within 24 Hours of Arrival[5]	-	-	97%	96%
Fibrinolytic Meds Within 30 Min. of Arrival[5]	-	-	44%	58%
Average Time to ECG (minutes)[5]	-	-	6	7
Average Time to Transfer (minutes)[5]	-	-	58	60
Children's Asthma Care				
Received Home Management Plan of Care	-	-	85%	88%
Received Reliever Medication	-	-	100%	100%
Received Systemic Corticosteroids	-	-	100%	100%
Emergency Department				
Admittance Decision Time (minutes)	-	-	90	98
Head CT Results Within 45 Min. of Arrival[5]	-	-	63%	57%
Patients Who Left ER Before Being Seen[5]	-	-	2%	2%
Time from ER Arrival to Admit. (minutes)	-	-	265	274
Time from ER Arrival to Discharge (minutes)[5]	-	-	128	134
Time in ER Before Being Evaluated (minutes)[5]	-	-	22	26
Time to Pain Meds for Fractures (minutes)[5]	-	-	54	57
Heart Attack Care				
Aspirin Given at Discharge	-	-	99%	99%
Fibrinolytic Meds Within 30 Min. of Arrival	-	-	80%	54%
PCI Within 90 Minutes of Arrival	-	-	97%	96%
Statin Prescribed at Discharge	-	-	98%	98%
Heart Failure Care				
ACE Inhibitor or ARB for LVSD	-	-	97%	97%
Discharge Instructions Given	-	-	96%	94%
Evaluation of LVS Function	-	-	100%	99%
Medicare Spending				
Medicare Spending per Patient (ratio)	-	-	1.01	0.98
Pneumonia Care				
Appropriate Initial Antibiotic Given	-	-	96%	95%
Blood Culture Timing	-	-	98%	98%
Pregnancy and Delivery Care				
Newborn Deliveries Scheduled Early	-	-	5%	6%
Preventive Care				
Immunization for Influenza	-	-	93%	90%
Immunization for Pneumonia	-	-	94%	92%
Stroke Care				
Anticoagulation Therapy for Atrial Fibrillation	-	-	95%	95%
Antithrombotic Therapy Timing	-	-	98%	98%
Assessed for Rehabilitation	-	-	98%	97%
Discharged on Antithrombotic Therapy	-	-	99%	99%
Discharged on Statin Medication	-	-	95%	94%
Thrombolytic Therapy Timing	-	-	65%	66%
Venous Thromboembolism Prophylaxis	-	-	95%	94%
Written Stroke Educational Materials Given	-	-	92%	88%
Surgical Care Improvement Project				
Appropriate Beta Blocker Usage	-	-	98%	98%
Appropriate VTP Within 24 Hours	-	-	98%	98%
Controlled Postoperative Blood Glucose	-	-	97%	97%
Perioperative Temperature Management	-	-	100%	100%
Prophylactic Antibiotic Selection	-	-	99%	99%
Prophylactic Antibiotic Selection (Outpatient)[5]	-	-	98%	98%
Prophylactic Antibiotic Stopped	-	-	98%	98%
Prophylactic Antibiotic Timing	-	-	99%	99%
Prophylactic Antibiotic Timing (Outpatient)[5]	-	-	97%	98%
Urinary Catheter Removal	-	-	97%	97%
Survey of Patients' Hospital Experiences				
Area Around Room 'Always' Quiet at Night	-	-	58%	61%
Doctors 'Always' Communicated Well	-	-	80%	82%
Home Recovery Information Given	-	-	87%	85%
Hospital Given 9 or 10 on 10 Point Scale	-	-	72%	71%
Meds 'Always' Explained Before Given	-	-	64%	64%
Nurses 'Always' Communicated Well	-	-	81%	79%
Pain 'Always' Well Controlled	-	-	71%	71%
Room and Bathroom 'Always' Clean	-	-	75%	73%
Timely Help 'Always' Received	-	-	70%	68%
Would Definitely Recommend Hospital	-	-	71%	71%
Use of Medical Imaging				
Cardiac Imaging Stress Test before Surgery[1]	-	-	5.4%	5.3%
Combination Abdominal CT Scan	151	4.0%	7.1%	10.5%
Combination Brain/Sinus CT Scan[1]	-	-	2.8%	2.7%
Combination Chest CT Scan	63	1.6%	1.7%	2.7%
Follow-up Mammogram/Ultrasound	122	7.4%	8.7%	8.8%
Lumbar Spine MRI for Low Back Pain[1]	-	-	34.7%	37.2%

Wayne Hospital

835 Sweitzer Street
Greenville, OH 45331
Phone: 937-547-5722
Fax: 937-547-5712
URL: www.waynehospital.com
Type: Acute Care Hospitals
Emergency Services: Yes
Ownership: Voluntary non-profit - Private
Beds: 92

Key Personnel:
Chief of Medical Staff .... James Appleman
Emergency Room .... Robert Girmann, DO
Operating Room .... Holly Lemar, RN
Infection Control .... Nancy Raffel
Quality Assurance .... Susan Weisenberger
Intensive Care Unit .... Shirley Winger, RN

Measure	Cases	This Hosp.	State Avg.	U.S. Avg.
Blood Clot Prevention and Treatment				
Anticoagulation Overlap Therapy[1,2]	-	-	93%	93%
ICU Venous Thromboembolism Prophylaxis[2]	32	81%	93%	92%
Incidence of Potentially Preventable VTE[1,2]	-	-	6%	10%
UFH with Dosages/Platelet Monitoring[1,2]	-	-	98%	97%
Venous Thromboembolism Prophylaxis[2]	138	73%	88%	85%
Warfarin Therapy Discharge Instructions[1,2]	-	-	79%	75%
Chest Pain/Possible Heart Attack Care				
Aspirin Given Within 24 Hours of Arrival	115	97%	97%	96%
Fibrinolytic Meds Within 30 Min. of Arrival[1]	-	-	44%	58%
Average Time to ECG (minutes)	122	9	6	7
Average Time to Transfer (minutes)[1]	-	-	58	60
Children's Asthma Care				
Received Home Management Plan of Care	-	-	85%	88%
Received Reliever Medication	-	-	100%	100%
Received Systemic Corticosteroids	-	-	100%	100%
Emergency Department				
Admittance Decision Time (minutes)[2]	257	58	90	98
Head CT Results Within 45 Min. of Arrival	19	53%	63%	57%
Patients Who Left ER Before Being Seen	22,559	1%	2%	2%
Time from ER Arrival to Admit. (minutes)[2]	302	266	265	274
Time from ER Arrival to Discharge (minutes)	397	155	128	134
Time in ER Before Being Evaluated (minutes)	407	30	22	26
Time to Pain Meds for Fractures (minutes)	96	66	54	57
Heart Attack Care				
Aspirin Given at Discharge[1]	-	-	99%	99%
Fibrinolytic Meds Within 30 Min. of Arrival[7]	-	-	80%	54%
PCI Within 90 Minutes of Arrival[7]	-	-	97%	96%
Statin Prescribed at Discharge[1]	-	-	98%	98%
Heart Failure Care				
ACE Inhibitor or ARB for LVSD	12	92%	97%	97%
Discharge Instructions Given	65	94%	96%	94%
Evaluation of LVS Function	86	99%	100%	99%
Medicare Spending				
Medicare Spending per Patient (ratio)	-	1.01	1.01	0.98
Pneumonia Care				
Appropriate Initial Antibiotic Given	54	98%	96%	95%
Blood Culture Timing	98	92%	98%	98%
Pregnancy and Delivery Care				
Newborn Deliveries Scheduled Early[2]	12	8%	5%	6%
Preventive Care				
Immunization for Influenza[2]	272	94%	93%	90%
Immunization for Pneumonia[2]	361	93%	94%	92%
Stroke Care				
Anticoagulation Therapy for Atrial Fibrillation[7]	-	-	95%	95%
Antithrombotic Therapy Timing[1]	-	-	98%	98%
Assessed for Rehabilitation[1]	-	-	98%	97%
Discharged on Antithrombotic Therapy[1]	-	-	99%	99%
Discharged on Statin Medication[1]	-	-	95%	94%
Thrombolytic Therapy Timing[1]	-	-	65%	66%
Venous Thromboembolism Prophylaxis[1]	-	-	95%	94%
Written Stroke Educational Materials Given[1]	-	-	92%	88%
Surgical Care Improvement Project				
Appropriate Beta Blocker Usage	51	94%	98%	98%
Appropriate VTP Within 24 Hours	158	99%	98%	98%
Controlled Postoperative Blood Glucose[7]	-	-	97%	97%
Perioperative Temperature Management	182	100%	100%	100%
Prophylactic Antibiotic Selection	131	98%	99%	99%
Prophylactic Antibiotic Selection (Outpatient)	28	100%	98%	98%
Prophylactic Antibiotic Stopped	131	98%	98%	98%

NOTE: Hospital profiles are in alphabetical order by state, then city, then hospital within the city; Rankings exclude hospitals with less than 25 cases except for patient surveys which excludes hospitals with less than 100 cases; (a) 100-299 cases; (1) The number of cases/patients is too few to report; (2) Data submitted were based on a sample of cases/patients; (3) Results are based on a shorter time period than required; (4) Data suppressed by CMS for one or more quarters; (5) Results are not available for this reporting period; (6) Fewer than 100 patients completed the HCAHPS survey; (7) No cases met the criteria for this measure; (8) The lower limit of the confidence interval cannot be calculated if the number of observed infections equals zero; (9) No data are available from the state/territory for this reporting period; (10) The scores shown reflect fewer than 50 completed surveys; (11) There were discrepancies in the data collection process; (12) This measure does not apply to this hospital for this reporting period; (13) Results cannot be calculated for this reporting period; (14) The results for this state are combined with nearby states to protect confidentiality; Please refer to the User's Guide for a full explanation of data.

Measure	Cases	This Hosp.	State Avg.	U.S. Avg.
Prophylactic Antibiotic Timing	131	96%	99%	99%
Prophylactic Antibiotic Timing (Outpatient)[1]	-	-	97%	98%
Urinary Catheter Removal	97	98%	97%	97%
Survey of Patients' Hospital Experiences				
Area Around Room 'Always' Quiet at Night	300+	57%	58%	61%
Doctors 'Always' Communicated Well	300+	80%	80%	82%
Home Recovery Information Given	300+	83%	87%	85%
Hospital Given 9 or 10 on 10 Point Scale	300+	65%	72%	71%
Meds 'Always' Explained Before Given	300+	60%	64%	64%
Nurses 'Always' Communicated Well	300+	81%	81%	79%
Pain 'Always' Well Controlled	300+	74%	71%	71%
Room and Bathroom 'Always' Clean	300+	75%	75%	73%
Timely Help 'Always' Received	300+	73%	70%	68%
Would Definitely Recommend Hospital	300+	60%	71%	71%
Use of Medical Imaging				
Cardiac Imaging Stress Test before Surgery	463	2.8%	5.4%	5.3%
Combination Abdominal CT Scan	539	2.0%	7.1%	10.5%
Combination Brain/Sinus CT Scan	547	2.0%	2.8%	2.7%
Combination Chest CT Scan	332	0.3%	1.7%	2.7%
Follow-up Mammogram/Ultrasound	857	7.7%	8.7%	8.8%
Lumbar Spine MRI for Low Back Pain	62	29.0%	34.7%	37.2%

Fort Hamilton Hughes Memorial Hospital

630 Eaton Avenue
Hamilton, OH 45013
Phone: 513-867-2000
Fax: 513-867-2620
URL: www.forthamiltonhospital.com
Type: Acute Care Hospitals
Emergency Services: Yes
Ownership: Voluntary non-profit - Private
Beds: 310

Key Personnel:
Quality Assurance . . . . Nancy Cohen
Operating Room. . . . . Cheryl Creach
Emergency Room . . . . Pam Klaber
Chief of Medical Staff . . . . H S Ramadas, MD
Pediatric In-Patient Care . . . . Marc Richardson, MD
CEO/President. . . . . Mark Smith
Radiology. . . . . Karen Wilson

Measure	Cases	This Hosp.	State Avg.	U.S. Avg.
Blood Clot Prevention and Treatment				
Anticoagulation Overlap Therapy[2]	59	97%	93%	93%
ICU Venous Thromboembolism Prophylaxis[2]	90	98%	93%	92%
Incidence of Potentially Preventable VTE[1,2]	-	-	6%	10%
UFH with Dosages/Platelet Monitoring[2]	35	100%	98%	97%
Venous Thromboembolism Prophylaxis[2]	349	96%	88%	85%
Warfarin Therapy Discharge Instructions[2]	47	98%	79%	75%
Chest Pain/Possible Heart Attack Care				
Aspirin Given Within 24 Hours of Arrival[1]	-	-	97%	96%
Fibrinolytic Meds Within 30 Min. of Arrival[3,7]	-	-	44%	58%
Average Time to ECG (minutes)[1]	-	-	6	7
Average Time to Transfer (minutes)[3,7]	-	-	58	60
Children's Asthma Care				
Received Home Management Plan of Care	-	-	85%	88%
Received Reliever Medication	-	-	100%	100%
Received Systemic Corticosteroids	-	-	100%	100%
Emergency Department				
Admittance Decision Time (minutes)[2]	798	62	90	98
Head CT Results Within 45 Min. of Arrival[1]	-	-	63%	57%
Patients Who Left ER Before Being Seen	41,683	1%	2%	2%
Time from ER Arrival to Admit. (minutes)[2]	801	202	265	274
Time from ER Arrival to Discharge (minutes)	387	100	128	134
Time in ER Before Being Evaluated (minutes)	414	7	22	26
Time to Pain Meds for Fractures (minutes)	87	40	54	57
Heart Attack Care				
Aspirin Given at Discharge	140	98%	99%	99%
Fibrinolytic Meds Within 30 Min. of Arrival[7]	-	-	80%	54%
PCI Within 90 Minutes of Arrival	26	100%	97%	96%
Statin Prescribed at Discharge	144	100%	98%	98%
Heart Failure Care				
ACE Inhibitor or ARB for LVSD	58	100%	97%	97%
Discharge Instructions Given	162	100%	96%	94%
Evaluation of LVS Function	233	100%	100%	99%
Medicare Spending				
Medicare Spending per Patient (ratio)	-	1.01	1.01	0.98
Pneumonia Care				
Appropriate Initial Antibiotic Given[2]	71	97%	96%	95%
Blood Culture Timing[2]	118	99%	98%	98%
Pregnancy and Delivery Care				
Newborn Deliveries Scheduled Early	33	0%	5%	6%
Preventive Care				
Immunization for Influenza[2]	593	97%	93%	90%
Immunization for Pneumonia[2]	795	97%	94%	92%
Stroke Care				
Anticoagulation Therapy for Atrial Fibrillation[1]	-	-	95%	95%
Antithrombotic Therapy Timing	62	100%	98%	98%
Assessed for Rehabilitation	60	98%	98%	97%
Discharged on Antithrombotic Therapy	57	98%	99%	99%
Discharged on Statin Medication	48	98%	95%	94%
Thrombolytic Therapy Timing[1]	-	-	65%	66%
Venous Thromboembolism Prophylaxis	65	95%	95%	94%
Written Stroke Educational Materials Given	35	100%	92%	88%
Surgical Care Improvement Project				
Appropriate Beta Blocker Usage	95	99%	98%	98%
Appropriate VTP Within 24 Hours	279	99%	98%	98%
Controlled Postoperative Blood Glucose[7]	-	-	97%	97%
Perioperative Temperature Management	335	100%	100%	100%
Prophylactic Antibiotic Selection	198	99%	99%	99%
Prophylactic Antibiotic Selection (Outpatient)	107	100%	98%	98%
Prophylactic Antibiotic Stopped	187	98%	98%	98%
Prophylactic Antibiotic Timing	198	99%	99%	99%
Prophylactic Antibiotic Timing (Outpatient)	109	97%	97%	98%
Urinary Catheter Removal	178	100%	97%	97%
Survey of Patients' Hospital Experiences				
Area Around Room 'Always' Quiet at Night	300+	57%	58%	61%
Doctors 'Always' Communicated Well	300+	79%	80%	82%
Home Recovery Information Given	300+	84%	87%	85%
Hospital Given 9 or 10 on 10 Point Scale	300+	67%	72%	71%
Meds 'Always' Explained Before Given	300+	65%	64%	64%
Nurses 'Always' Communicated Well	300+	82%	81%	79%
Pain 'Always' Well Controlled	300+	73%	71%	71%
Room and Bathroom 'Always' Clean	300+	68%	75%	73%
Timely Help 'Always' Received	300+	71%	70%	68%
Would Definitely Recommend Hospital	300+	65%	71%	71%
Use of Medical Imaging				
Cardiac Imaging Stress Test before Surgery	244	5.3%	5.4%	5.3%
Combination Abdominal CT Scan	658	4.6%	7.1%	10.5%
Combination Brain/Sinus CT Scan[1]	-	-	2.8%	2.7%
Combination Chest CT Scan	358	0.0%	1.7%	2.7%
Follow-up Mammogram/Ultrasound	801	7.9%	8.7%	8.8%
Lumbar Spine MRI for Low Back Pain	87	44.8%	34.7%	37.2%

Community Memorial Hospital

208 N Columbus St
Hicksville, OH 43526
Phone: 419-542-6692
URL: www.cmhosp.com
Type: Critical Access Hospitals
Emergency Services: Yes
Ownership: Govt - Hospital Dist/Auth

Measure	Cases	This Hosp.	State Avg.	U.S. Avg.
Blood Clot Prevention and Treatment				
Anticoagulation Overlap Therapy[1,3]	-	-	93%	93%
ICU Venous Thromboembolism Prophylaxis[3,7]	-	-	93%	92%
Incidence of Potentially Preventable VTE[3,7]	-	-	6%	10%
UFH with Dosages/Platelet Monitoring[3,7]	-	-	98%	97%
Venous Thromboembolism Prophylaxis[3,7]	-	-	88%	85%
Warfarin Therapy Discharge Instructions[1,3]	-	-	79%	75%
Chest Pain/Possible Heart Attack Care				
Aspirin Given Within 24 Hours of Arrival	17	100%	97%	96%
Fibrinolytic Meds Within 30 Min. of Arrival[7]	-	-	44%	58%
Average Time to ECG (minutes)	17	5	6	7
Average Time to Transfer (minutes)[1]	-	-	58	60
Children's Asthma Care				
Received Home Management Plan of Care	-	-	85%	88%
Received Reliever Medication	-	-	100%	100%
Received Systemic Corticosteroids	-	-	100%	100%
Emergency Department				
Admittance Decision Time (minutes)[5]	-	-	90	98
Head CT Results Within 45 Min. of Arrival[1,3]	-	-	63%	57%
Patients Who Left ER Before Being Seen[5]	-	-	2%	2%
Time from ER Arrival to Admit. (minutes)[5]	-	-	265	274
Time from ER Arrival to Discharge (minutes)[5]	-	-	128	134
Time in ER Before Being Evaluated (minutes)[5]	-	-	22	26
Time to Pain Meds for Fractures (minutes)[3]	22	36	54	57
Heart Attack Care				
Aspirin Given at Discharge[3,7]	-	-	99%	99%
Fibrinolytic Meds Within 30 Min. of Arrival[3,7]	-	-	80%	54%
PCI Within 90 Minutes of Arrival[3,7]	-	-	97%	96%
Statin Prescribed at Discharge[3,7]	-	-	98%	98%
Heart Failure Care				
ACE Inhibitor or ARB for LVSD[1]	-	-	97%	97%
Discharge Instructions Given	17	94%	96%	94%
Evaluation of LVS Function	24	83%	100%	99%
Medicare Spending				
Medicare Spending per Patient (ratio)	-	-	1.01	0.98
Pneumonia Care				
Appropriate Initial Antibiotic Given	25	84%	96%	95%
Blood Culture Timing	25	96%	98%	98%
Pregnancy and Delivery Care				
Newborn Deliveries Scheduled Early[5]	-	-	5%	6%
Preventive Care				
Immunization for Influenza[5]	-	-	93%	90%
Immunization for Pneumonia[5]	-	-	94%	92%
Stroke Care				
Anticoagulation Therapy for Atrial Fibrillation[3,7]	-	-	95%	95%
Antithrombotic Therapy Timing[1,3]	-	-	98%	98%
Assessed for Rehabilitation[1,3]	-	-	98%	97%
Discharged on Antithrombotic Therapy[1,3]	-	-	99%	99%
Discharged on Statin Medication[1,3]	-	-	95%	94%
Thrombolytic Therapy Timing[3,7]	-	-	65%	66%
Venous Thromboembolism Prophylaxis[1,3]	-	-	95%	94%
Written Stroke Educational Materials Given[1,3]	-	-	92%	88%
Surgical Care Improvement Project				
Appropriate Beta Blocker Usage	12	75%	98%	98%
Appropriate VTP Within 24 Hours	26	100%	98%	98%
Controlled Postoperative Blood Glucose[7]	-	-	97%	97%
Perioperative Temperature Management	36	100%	100%	100%
Prophylactic Antibiotic Selection	35	91%	99%	99%
Prophylactic Antibiotic Selection (Outpatient)[5]	-	-	98%	98%
Prophylactic Antibiotic Stopped	34	88%	98%	98%
Prophylactic Antibiotic Timing	35	89%	99%	99%
Prophylactic Antibiotic Timing (Outpatient)[5]	-	-	97%	98%
Urinary Catheter Removal[1]	-	-	97%	97%
Survey of Patients' Hospital Experiences				
Area Around Room 'Always' Quiet at Night	(a)	67%	58%	61%
Doctors 'Always' Communicated Well	(a)	88%	80%	82%
Home Recovery Information Given	(a)	94%	87%	85%
Hospital Given 9 or 10 on 10 Point Scale	(a)	87%	72%	71%
Meds 'Always' Explained Before Given	(a)	65%	64%	64%
Nurses 'Always' Communicated Well	(a)	87%	81%	79%
Pain 'Always' Well Controlled	(a)	69%	71%	71%
Room and Bathroom 'Always' Clean	(a)	91%	75%	73%
Timely Help 'Always' Received	(a)	86%	70%	68%
Would Definitely Recommend Hospital	(a)	80%	71%	71%
Use of Medical Imaging				
Cardiac Imaging Stress Test before Surgery[7]	-	-	5.4%	5.3%
Combination Abdominal CT Scan	87	10.3%	7.1%	10.5%
Combination Brain/Sinus CT Scan[1]	-	-	2.8%	2.7%
Combination Chest CT Scan[1]	-	-	1.7%	2.7%
Follow-up Mammogram/Ultrasound	100	7.0%	8.7%	8.8%
Lumbar Spine MRI for Low Back Pain[1]	-	-	34.7%	37.2%

Highland District Hospital

1275 North High Street
Hillsboro, OH 45133
Phone: 937-393-6100
Fax: 937-393-6278
E-mail: hdhadm@bright.net
URL: www.hdh.org
Type: Critical Access Hospitals
Emergency Services: Yes
Ownership: Govt - Hospital Dist/Auth
Beds: 65

Key Personnel:
Emergency Room . . . . Terri Balser
Quality Assurance . . . . Bob Barger
Surgery . . . . Steven Battaglia, MD
Radiology. . . . . Jeffrey Cushman
CEO/President. . . . . Paula Detterman

NOTE: Hospital profiles are in alphabetical order by state, then city, then hospital within the city; Rankings exclude hospitals with less than 25 cases except for patient surveys which excludes hospitals with less than 100 cases; (a) 100-299 cases; (1) The number of cases/patients is too few to report; (2) Data submitted were based on a sample of cases/patients; (3) Results are based on a shorter time period than required; (4) Data suppressed by CMS for one or more quarters; (5) Results are not available for this reporting period; (6) Fewer than 100 patients completed the HCAHPS survey; (7) No cases met the criteria for this measure; (8) The lower limit of the confidence interval cannot be calculated if the number of observed infections equals zero; (9) No data are available from the state/territory for this reporting period; (10) The scores shown reflect fewer than 50 completed surveys; (11) There were discrepancies in the data collection process; (12) This measure does not apply to this hospital for this reporting period; (13) Results cannot be calculated for this reporting period; (14) The results for this state are combined with nearby states to protect confidentiality; Please refer to the User's Guide for a full explanation of data.

Chief of Medical Staff . . . . David Gunderman

Measure	Cases	This Hosp.	State Avg.	U.S. Avg.
Blood Clot Prevention and Treatment				
Anticoagulation Overlap Therapy[5]	-	-	93%	93%
ICU Venous Thromboembolism Prophylaxis[5]	-	-	93%	92%
Incidence of Potentially Preventable VTE[5]	-	-	6%	10%
UFH with Dosages/Platelet Monitoring[5]	-	-	98%	97%
Venous Thromboembolism Prophylaxis[5]	-	-	88%	85%
Warfarin Therapy Discharge Instructions[5]	-	-	79%	75%
Chest Pain/Possible Heart Attack Care				
Aspirin Given Within 24 Hours of Arrival[5]	-	-	97%	96%
Fibrinolytic Meds Within 30 Min. of Arrival[5]	-	-	44%	58%
Average Time to ECG (minutes)[5]	-	-	6	7
Average Time to Transfer (minutes)[5]	-	-	58	60
Children's Asthma Care				
Received Home Management Plan of Care	-	-	85%	88%
Received Reliever Medication	-	-	100%	100%
Received Systemic Corticosteroids	-	-	100%	100%
Emergency Department				
Admittance Decision Time (minutes)[5]	-	-	90	98
Head CT Results Within 45 Min. of Arrival[5]	-	-	63%	57%
Patients Who Left ER Before Being Seen[5]	-	-	2%	2%
Time from ER Arrival to Admit. (minutes)[5]	-	-	265	274
Time from ER Arrival to Discharge (minutes)[3,7]	-	-	128	134
Time in ER Before Being Evaluated (minutes)[3]	39	17	22	26
Time to Pain Meds for Fractures (minutes)[1,3]	-	-	54	57
Heart Attack Care				
Aspirin Given at Discharge[1,3]	-	-	99%	99%
Fibrinolytic Meds Within 30 Min. of Arrival[3,7]	-	-	80%	54%
PCI Within 90 Minutes of Arrival[3,7]	-	-	97%	96%
Statin Prescribed at Discharge[1,3]	-	-	98%	98%
Heart Failure Care				
ACE Inhibitor or ARB for LVSD	12	100%	97%	97%
Discharge Instructions Given	39	97%	96%	94%
Evaluation of LVS Function	59	97%	100%	99%
Medicare Spending				
Medicare Spending per Patient (ratio)	-	-	1.01	0.98
Pneumonia Care				
Appropriate Initial Antibiotic Given[2]	72	86%	96%	95%
Blood Culture Timing[2]	92	100%	98%	98%
Pregnancy and Delivery Care				
Newborn Deliveries Scheduled Early[5]	-	-	5%	6%
Preventive Care				
Immunization for Influenza[5]	-	-	93%	90%
Immunization for Pneumonia[1,3]	-	-	94%	92%
Stroke Care				
Anticoagulation Therapy for Atrial Fibrillation[5]	-	-	95%	95%
Antithrombotic Therapy Timing[5]	-	-	98%	98%
Assessed for Rehabilitation[5]	-	-	98%	97%
Discharged on Antithrombotic Therapy[5]	-	-	99%	99%
Discharged on Statin Medication[5]	-	-	95%	94%
Thrombolytic Therapy Timing[5]	-	-	65%	66%
Venous Thromboembolism Prophylaxis[5]	-	-	95%	94%
Written Stroke Educational Materials Given[5]	-	-	92%	88%
Surgical Care Improvement Project				
Appropriate Beta Blocker Usage[1]	-	-	98%	98%
Appropriate VTP Within 24 Hours[1,3]	-	-	98%	98%
Controlled Postoperative Blood Glucose[3,7]	-	-	97%	97%
Perioperative Temperature Management	63	100%	100%	100%
Prophylactic Antibiotic Selection[1]	-	-	99%	99%
Prophylactic Antibiotic Selection (Outpatient)[3]	31	71%	98%	98%
Prophylactic Antibiotic Stopped[1]	-	-	98%	98%
Prophylactic Antibiotic Timing[1]	-	-	99%	99%
Prophylactic Antibiotic Timing (Outpatient)[3]	32	97%	97%	98%
Urinary Catheter Removal	14	100%	97%	97%
Survey of Patients' Hospital Experiences				
Area Around Room 'Always' Quiet at Night	(a)	52%	58%	61%
Doctors 'Always' Communicated Well	(a)	80%	80%	82%
Home Recovery Information Given	(a)	83%	87%	85%
Hospital Given 9 or 10 on 10 Point Scale	(a)	56%	72%	71%
Meds 'Always' Explained Before Given	(a)	59%	64%	64%
Nurses 'Always' Communicated Well	(a)	74%	81%	79%
Pain 'Always' Well Controlled	(a)	62%	71%	71%
Room and Bathroom 'Always' Clean	(a)	62%	75%	73%
Timely Help 'Always' Received	(a)	58%	70%	68%
Would Definitely Recommend Hospital	(a)	51%	71%	71%
Use of Medical Imaging				
Cardiac Imaging Stress Test before Surgery	139	5.8%	5.4%	5.3%
Combination Abdominal CT Scan	389	11.3%	7.1%	10.5%
Combination Brain/Sinus CT Scan[1]	-	-	2.8%	2.7%
Combination Chest CT Scan	192	1.6%	1.7%	2.7%
Follow-up Mammogram/Ultrasound	325	11.1%	8.7%	8.8%
Lumbar Spine MRI for Low Back Pain	49	32.7%	34.7%	37.2%

Holzer Medical Center Jackson

500 Burlington Road
Jackson, OH 45640
Phone: 740-395-8500
Type: Critical Access Hospitals
Emergency Services: Yes
Ownership: Voluntary non-profit - Private

Measure	Cases	This Hosp.	State Avg.	U.S. Avg.
Blood Clot Prevention and Treatment				
Anticoagulation Overlap Therapy[5]	-	-	93%	93%
ICU Venous Thromboembolism Prophylaxis[5]	-	-	93%	92%
Incidence of Potentially Preventable VTE[5]	-	-	6%	10%
UFH with Dosages/Platelet Monitoring[5]	-	-	98%	97%
Venous Thromboembolism Prophylaxis[5]	-	-	88%	85%
Warfarin Therapy Discharge Instructions[5]	-	-	79%	75%
Chest Pain/Possible Heart Attack Care				
Aspirin Given Within 24 Hours of Arrival[5]	-	-	97%	96%
Fibrinolytic Meds Within 30 Min. of Arrival[5]	-	-	44%	58%
Average Time to ECG (minutes)[5]	-	-	6	7
Average Time to Transfer (minutes)[5]	-	-	58	60
Children's Asthma Care				
Received Home Management Plan of Care	-	-	85%	88%
Received Reliever Medication	-	-	100%	100%
Received Systemic Corticosteroids	-	-	100%	100%
Emergency Department				
Admittance Decision Time (minutes)[2,3]	107	69	90	98
Head CT Results Within 45 Min. of Arrival[5]	-	-	63%	57%
Patients Who Left ER Before Being Seen[5]	-	-	2%	2%
Time from ER Arrival to Admit. (minutes)[2,3]	107	252	265	274
Time from ER Arrival to Discharge (minutes)[5]	-	-	128	134
Time in ER Before Being Evaluated (minutes)[5]	-	-	22	26
Time to Pain Meds for Fractures (minutes)[5]	-	-	54	57
Heart Attack Care				
Aspirin Given at Discharge[7]	-	-	99%	99%
Fibrinolytic Meds Within 30 Min. of Arrival[3,7]	-	-	80%	54%
PCI Within 90 Minutes of Arrival[3,7]	-	-	97%	96%
Statin Prescribed at Discharge[7]	-	-	98%	98%
Heart Failure Care				
ACE Inhibitor or ARB for LVSD[1]	-	-	97%	97%
Discharge Instructions Given	33	70%	96%	94%
Evaluation of LVS Function	38	100%	100%	99%
Medicare Spending				
Medicare Spending per Patient (ratio)	-	-	1.01	0.98
Pneumonia Care				
Appropriate Initial Antibiotic Given	83	95%	96%	95%
Blood Culture Timing	97	99%	98%	98%
Pregnancy and Delivery Care				
Newborn Deliveries Scheduled Early[3,7]	-	-	5%	6%
Preventive Care				
Immunization for Influenza[5]	-	-	93%	90%
Immunization for Pneumonia[2,3]	125	96%	94%	92%
Stroke Care				
Anticoagulation Therapy for Atrial Fibrillation[5]	-	-	95%	95%
Antithrombotic Therapy Timing[5]	-	-	98%	98%
Assessed for Rehabilitation[5]	-	-	98%	97%
Discharged on Antithrombotic Therapy[5]	-	-	99%	99%
Discharged on Statin Medication[5]	-	-	95%	94%
Thrombolytic Therapy Timing[5]	-	-	65%	66%
Venous Thromboembolism Prophylaxis[5]	-	-	95%	94%
Written Stroke Educational Materials Given[5]	-	-	92%	88%
Surgical Care Improvement Project				
Appropriate Beta Blocker Usage	106	97%	98%	98%
Appropriate VTP Within 24 Hours	257	98%	98%	98%
Controlled Postoperative Blood Glucose[3,7]	-	-	97%	97%
Perioperative Temperature Management	276	100%	100%	100%
Prophylactic Antibiotic Selection	225	100%	99%	99%
Prophylactic Antibiotic Selection (Outpatient)[5]	-	-	98%	98%
Prophylactic Antibiotic Stopped	223	97%	98%	98%
Prophylactic Antibiotic Timing	228	92%	99%	99%
Prophylactic Antibiotic Timing (Outpatient)[5]	-	-	97%	98%
Urinary Catheter Removal	94	97%	97%	97%
Survey of Patients' Hospital Experiences				
Area Around Room 'Always' Quiet at Night	(a)	70%	58%	61%
Doctors 'Always' Communicated Well	(a)	81%	80%	82%
Home Recovery Information Given	(a)	89%	87%	85%
Hospital Given 9 or 10 on 10 Point Scale	(a)	75%	72%	71%
Meds 'Always' Explained Before Given	(a)	67%	64%	64%
Nurses 'Always' Communicated Well	(a)	83%	81%	79%
Pain 'Always' Well Controlled	(a)	77%	71%	71%
Room and Bathroom 'Always' Clean	(a)	85%	75%	73%
Timely Help 'Always' Received	(a)	81%	70%	68%
Would Definitely Recommend Hospital	(a)	76%	71%	71%
Use of Medical Imaging				
Cardiac Imaging Stress Test before Surgery[1]	-	-	5.4%	5.3%
Combination Abdominal CT Scan	273	1.5%	7.1%	10.5%
Combination Brain/Sinus CT Scan[1]	-	-	2.8%	2.7%
Combination Chest CT Scan	53	1.9%	1.7%	2.7%
Follow-up Mammogram/Ultrasound[7]	-	-	8.7%	8.8%
Lumbar Spine MRI for Low Back Pain[7]	-	-	34.7%	37.2%

Hardin Memorial Hospital

921 East Franklin Street
Kenton, OH 43326
Phone: 419-673-0761
Fax: 419-673-1097
E-mail: publicrelations@hardinmemorial.org
URL: www.hardinmemorial.org
Type: Critical Access Hospitals
Emergency Services: Yes
Ownership: Voluntary non-profit - Private
Beds: 103

Key Personnel:

Operating Room. . . . . M Saadallah Abdulkarim, RN
Infection Control. . . . . Cindy Althouse, RN
Chief of Medical Staff. . . . . Katherine Johnson, MD
Emergency Room . . . . Roxanne Tackett

Measure	Cases	This Hosp.	State Avg.	U.S. Avg.
Blood Clot Prevention and Treatment				
Anticoagulation Overlap Therapy[1,2]	-	-	93%	93%
ICU Venous Thromboembolism Prophylaxis[2,3]	22	100%	93%	92%
Incidence of Potentially Preventable VTE[2,3]	-	-	6%	10%
UFH with Dosages/Platelet Monitoring[2,3]	-	-	98%	97%
Venous Thromboembolism Prophylaxis[2,3]	49	94%	88%	85%
Warfarin Therapy Discharge Instructions[1,2]	-	-	79%	75%
Chest Pain/Possible Heart Attack Care				
Aspirin Given Within 24 Hours of Arrival	-	-	97%	96%
Fibrinolytic Meds Within 30 Min. of Arrival	-	-	44%	58%
Average Time to ECG (minutes)	-	-	6	7
Average Time to Transfer (minutes)	-	-	58	60
Children's Asthma Care				
Received Home Management Plan of Care	-	-	85%	88%
Received Reliever Medication	-	-	100%	100%
Received Systemic Corticosteroids	-	-	100%	100%
Emergency Department				
Admittance Decision Time (minutes)[2,3]	205	50	90	98
Head CT Results Within 45 Min. of Arrival	-	-	63%	57%
Patients Who Left ER Before Being Seen	-	-	2%	2%
Time from ER Arrival to Admit. (minutes)[2,3]	205	225	265	274
Time from ER Arrival to Discharge (minutes)	-	-	128	134
Time in ER Before Being Evaluated (minutes)	-	-	22	26
Time to Pain Meds for Fractures (minutes)	-	-	54	57
Heart Attack Care				
Aspirin Given at Discharge[3,7]	-	-	99%	99%
Fibrinolytic Meds Within 30 Min. of Arrival[3,7]	-	-	80%	54%
PCI Within 90 Minutes of Arrival[3,7]	-	-	97%	96%
Statin Prescribed at Discharge[1,3]	-	-	98%	98%
Heart Failure Care				
ACE Inhibitor or ARB for LVSD[1]	-	-	97%	97%

NOTE: Hospital profiles are in alphabetical order by state, then city, then hospital within the city; Rankings exclude hospitals with less than 25 cases except for patient surveys which excludes hospitals with less than 100 cases; (a) 100-299 cases; (1) The number of cases/patients is too few to report; (2) Data submitted were based on a sample of cases/patients; (3) Results are based on a shorter time period than required; (4) Data suppressed by CMS for one or more quarters; (5) Results are not available for this reporting period; (6) Fewer than 100 patients completed the HCAHPS survey; (7) No cases met the criteria for this measure; (8) The lower limit of the confidence interval cannot be calculated if the number of observed infections equals zero; (9) No data are available from the state/territory for this reporting period; (10) The scores shown reflect fewer than 50 completed surveys; (11) There were discrepancies in the data collection process; (12) This measure does not apply to this hospital for this reporting period; (13) Results cannot be calculated for this reporting period; (14) The results for this state are combined with nearby states to protect confidentiality; Please refer to the User's Guide for a full explanation of data.

Discharge Instructions Given	20	100%	96%	94%
Evaluation of LVS Function	22	95%	100%	99%
Medicare Spending				
Medicare Spending per Patient (ratio)	-	-	1.01	0.98
Pneumonia Care				
Appropriate Initial Antibiotic Given	38	100%	96%	95%
Blood Culture Timing	45	100%	98%	98%
Pregnancy and Delivery Care				
Newborn Deliveries Scheduled Early[3,7]	-	-	5%	6%
Preventive Care				
Immunization for Influenza[5]	-	-	93%	90%
Immunization for Pneumonia[2,3]	244	100%	94%	92%
Stroke Care				
Anticoagulation Therapy for Atrial Fibrillation[3,7]	-	-	95%	95%
Antithrombotic Therapy Timing[3,7]	-	-	98%	98%
Assessed for Rehabilitation[3,7]	-	-	98%	97%
Discharged on Antithrombotic Therapy[3,7]	-	-	99%	99%
Discharged on Statin Medication[3,7]	-	-	95%	94%
Thrombolytic Therapy Timing[3,7]	-	-	65%	66%
Venous Thromboembolism Prophylaxis[3,7]	-	-	95%	94%
Written Stroke Educational Materials Given[3,7]	-	-	92%	88%
Surgical Care Improvement Project				
Appropriate Beta Blocker Usage[1]	-	-	98%	98%
Appropriate VTP Within 24 Hours	24	100%	98%	98%
Controlled Postoperative Blood Glucose[7]	-	-	97%	97%
Perioperative Temperature Management	24	100%	100%	100%
Prophylactic Antibiotic Selection	23	100%	99%	99%
Prophylactic Antibiotic Selection (Outpatient)	-	-	98%	98%
Prophylactic Antibiotic Stopped	23	100%	98%	98%
Prophylactic Antibiotic Timing	23	100%	99%	99%
Prophylactic Antibiotic Timing (Outpatient)	-	-	97%	98%
Urinary Catheter Removal[1]	-	-	97%	97%
Survey of Patients' Hospital Experiences				
Area Around Room 'Always' Quiet at Night	(a)	71%	58%	61%
Doctors 'Always' Communicated Well	(a)	82%	80%	82%
Home Recovery Information Given	(a)	87%	87%	85%
Hospital Given 9 or 10 on 10 Point Scale	(a)	74%	72%	71%
Meds 'Always' Explained Before Given	(a)	70%	64%	64%
Nurses 'Always' Communicated Well	(a)	86%	81%	79%
Pain 'Always' Well Controlled	(a)	73%	71%	71%
Room and Bathroom 'Always' Clean	(a)	84%	75%	73%
Timely Help 'Always' Received	(a)	80%	70%	68%
Would Definitely Recommend Hospital	(a)	70%	71%	71%
Use of Medical Imaging				
Cardiac Imaging Stress Test before Surgery	-	-	5.4%	5.3%
Combination Abdominal CT Scan	-	-	7.1%	10.5%
Combination Brain/Sinus CT Scan	-	-	2.8%	2.7%
Combination Chest CT Scan	-	-	1.7%	2.7%
Follow-up Mammogram/Ultrasound	-	-	8.7%	8.8%
Lumbar Spine MRI for Low Back Pain	-	-	34.7%	37.2%

Kettering Medical Center

3535 Southern Boulevard
Kettering, OH 45429
URL: www.khnetwork.org
Type: Acute Care Hospitals
Ownership: Voluntary non-profit - Church

Phone: 937-298-4331
Fax: 937-395-8355
Emergency Services: Yes
Beds: 522

Key Personnel:
CEO/President. . . . . Roy Chew, PhD
Chief of Medical Staff. . . . . R Gupta, MD
Radiology. . . . . Theodore Miller, MD
Quality Assurance . . . . Carolyn Peterson
Operating Room. . . . . Kae Quinlan
Infection Control. . . . . Sandy Shrader, MD
Pediatric Ambulatory Care . . . . . . Thomas Sorauf, MD
Pediatric In-Patient Care . . . . Thomas Sorauf, MD

Measure	Cases	This Hosp.	State Avg.	U.S. Avg.
Blood Clot Prevention and Treatment				
Anticoagulation Overlap Therapy[2]	144	97%	93%	93%
ICU Venous Thromboembolism Prophylaxis[2]	93	97%	93%	92%
Incidence of Potentially Preventable VTE[2]	23	0%	6%	10%
UFH with Dosages/Platelet Monitoring[2]	67	100%	98%	97%
Venous Thromboembolism Prophylaxis[2]	326	92%	88%	85%
Warfarin Therapy Discharge Instructions[2]	101	99%	79%	75%
Chest Pain/Possible Heart Attack Care				
Aspirin Given Within 24 Hours of Arrival[1,3]	-	-	97%	96%
Fibrinolytic Meds Within 30 Min. of Arrival[5]	-	-	44%	58%
Average Time to ECG (minutes)[1,3]	-	-	6	7
Average Time to Transfer (minutes)[5]	-	-	58	60
Children's Asthma Care				
Received Home Management Plan of Care	-	-	85%	88%
Received Reliever Medication	-	-	100%	100%
Received Systemic Corticosteroids	-	-	100%	100%
Emergency Department				
Admittance Decision Time (minutes)[2]	506	137	90	98
Head CT Results Within 45 Min. of Arrival[1]	-	-	63%	57%
Patients Who Left ER Before Being Seen	48,897	1%	2%	2%
Time from ER Arrival to Admit. (minutes)[2]	524	280	265	274
Time from ER Arrival to Discharge (minutes)	343	164	128	134
Time in ER Before Being Evaluated (minutes)	414	15	22	26
Time to Pain Meds for Fractures (minutes)	94	62	54	57
Heart Attack Care				
Aspirin Given at Discharge	446	100%	99%	99%
Fibrinolytic Meds Within 30 Min. of Arrival[7]	-	-	80%	54%
PCI Within 90 Minutes of Arrival	65	98%	97%	96%
Statin Prescribed at Discharge	446	99%	98%	98%
Heart Failure Care				
ACE Inhibitor or ARB for LVSD	191	98%	97%	97%
Discharge Instructions Given	412	100%	96%	94%
Evaluation of LVS Function	533	100%	100%	99%
Medicare Spending				
Medicare Spending per Patient (ratio)	-	1.02	1.01	0.98
Pneumonia Care				
Appropriate Initial Antibiotic Given	193	98%	96%	95%
Blood Culture Timing	433	100%	98%	98%
Pregnancy and Delivery Care				
Newborn Deliveries Scheduled Early	166	17%	5%	6%
Preventive Care				
Immunization for Influenza[2]	556	96%	93%	90%
Immunization for Pneumonia[2]	763	91%	94%	92%
Stroke Care				
Anticoagulation Therapy for Atrial Fibrillation	19	100%	95%	95%
Antithrombotic Therapy Timing	184	97%	98%	98%
Assessed for Rehabilitation	237	100%	98%	97%
Discharged on Antithrombotic Therapy	196	100%	99%	99%
Discharged on Statin Medication	158	99%	95%	94%
Thrombolytic Therapy Timing	20	100%	65%	66%
Venous Thromboembolism Prophylaxis	254	99%	95%	94%
Written Stroke Educational Materials Given	86	100%	92%	88%
Surgical Care Improvement Project				
Appropriate Beta Blocker Usage[2]	877	100%	98%	98%
Appropriate VTP Within 24 Hours[2]	1,901	100%	98%	98%
Controlled Postoperative Blood Glucose[2]	325	98%	97%	97%
Perioperative Temperature Management[2]	2,119	100%	100%	100%
Prophylactic Antibiotic Selection[2]	2,151	100%	99%	99%
Prophylactic Antibiotic Selection (Outpatient)	560	98%	98%	98%
Prophylactic Antibiotic Stopped[2]	2,122	100%	98%	98%
Prophylactic Antibiotic Timing[2]	2,151	100%	99%	99%
Prophylactic Antibiotic Timing (Outpatient)	561	97%	97%	98%
Urinary Catheter Removal[2]	1,582	99%	97%	97%
Survey of Patients' Hospital Experiences				
Area Around Room 'Always' Quiet at Night	300+	57%	58%	61%
Doctors 'Always' Communicated Well	300+	79%	80%	82%
Home Recovery Information Given	300+	87%	87%	85%
Hospital Given 9 or 10 on 10 Point Scale	300+	77%	72%	71%
Meds 'Always' Explained Before Given	300+	61%	64%	64%
Nurses 'Always' Communicated Well	300+	80%	81%	79%
Pain 'Always' Well Controlled	300+	70%	71%	71%
Room and Bathroom 'Always' Clean	300+	72%	75%	73%
Timely Help 'Always' Received	300+	65%	70%	68%
Would Definitely Recommend Hospital	300+	81%	71%	71%
Use of Medical Imaging				
Cardiac Imaging Stress Test before Surgery	882	4.9%	5.4%	5.3%
Combination Abdominal CT Scan	1,305	5.3%	7.1%	10.5%
Combination Brain/Sinus CT Scan	1,187	2.3%	2.8%	2.7%
Combination Chest CT Scan	826	0.0%	1.7%	2.7%
Follow-up Mammogram/Ultrasound	2,972	5.2%	8.7%	8.8%
Lumbar Spine MRI for Low Back Pain	219	35.2%	34.7%	37.2%

Lakewood Hospital

14519 Detroit Avenue
Lakewood, OH 44107
URL: www.lakewoodhospital.org
Type: Acute Care Hospitals
Ownership: Voluntary non-profit - Other

Phone: 216-521-4200
Fax: 216-227-2621
Emergency Services: Yes
Beds: 400

Key Personnel:
CEO/President. . . . . Jack Gustin, MBA
Chief of Medical Staff . . . . Marvin Shie III, MD

Measure	Cases	This Hosp.	State Avg.	U.S. Avg.
Blood Clot Prevention and Treatment				
Anticoagulation Overlap Therapy[2]	53	83%	93%	93%
ICU Venous Thromboembolism Prophylaxis[2]	78	95%	93%	92%
Incidence of Potentially Preventable VTE[1,2]	-	-	6%	10%
UFH with Dosages/Platelet Monitoring[2]	31	100%	98%	97%
Venous Thromboembolism Prophylaxis[2]	293	90%	88%	85%
Warfarin Therapy Discharge Instructions[2]	39	23%	79%	75%
Chest Pain/Possible Heart Attack Care				
Aspirin Given Within 24 Hours of Arrival[1,3]	-	-	97%	96%
Fibrinolytic Meds Within 30 Min. of Arrival[3,7]	-	-	44%	58%
Average Time to ECG (minutes)[1,3]	-	-	6	7
Average Time to Transfer (minutes)[1,3]	-	-	58	60
Children's Asthma Care				
Received Home Management Plan of Care	-	-	85%	88%
Received Reliever Medication	-	-	100%	100%
Received Systemic Corticosteroids	-	-	100%	100%
Emergency Department				
Admittance Decision Time (minutes)[2]	481	101	90	98
Head CT Results Within 45 Min. of Arrival[1]	-	-	63%	57%
Patients Who Left ER Before Being Seen	36,251	2%	2%	2%
Time from ER Arrival to Admit. (minutes)[2]	481	299	265	274
Time from ER Arrival to Discharge (minutes)	377	137	128	134
Time in ER Before Being Evaluated (minutes)	421	13	22	26
Time to Pain Meds for Fractures (minutes)	73	47	54	57
Heart Attack Care				
Aspirin Given at Discharge	62	98%	99%	99%
Fibrinolytic Meds Within 30 Min. of Arrival[7]	-	-	80%	54%
PCI Within 90 Minutes of Arrival	11	64%	97%	96%
Statin Prescribed at Discharge	57	95%	98%	98%
Heart Failure Care				
ACE Inhibitor or ARB for LVSD	35	100%	97%	97%
Discharge Instructions Given	119	94%	96%	94%
Evaluation of LVS Function	199	100%	100%	99%
Medicare Spending				
Medicare Spending per Patient (ratio)	-	1.08	1.01	0.98
Pneumonia Care				
Appropriate Initial Antibiotic Given	82	99%	96%	95%
Blood Culture Timing	127	98%	98%	98%
Pregnancy and Delivery Care				
Newborn Deliveries Scheduled Early[2]	23	0%	5%	6%
Preventive Care				
Immunization for Influenza[2]	575	97%	93%	90%
Immunization for Pneumonia[2]	782	96%	94%	92%
Stroke Care				
Anticoagulation Therapy for Atrial Fibrillation[1]	-	-	95%	95%
Antithrombotic Therapy Timing	92	98%	98%	98%
Assessed for Rehabilitation	118	100%	98%	97%
Discharged on Antithrombotic Therapy	109	100%	99%	99%
Discharged on Statin Medication	75	96%	95%	94%
Thrombolytic Therapy Timing[1]	-	-	65%	66%
Venous Thromboembolism Prophylaxis	111	99%	95%	94%
Written Stroke Educational Materials Given	50	100%	92%	88%
Surgical Care Improvement Project				
Appropriate Beta Blocker Usage[2]	269	98%	98%	98%
Appropriate VTP Within 24 Hours[2]	673	100%	98%	98%
Controlled Postoperative Blood Glucose[2,7]	-	-	97%	97%
Perioperative Temperature Management[2]	743	100%	100%	100%
Prophylactic Antibiotic Selection[2]	483	100%	99%	99%
Prophylactic Antibiotic Selection (Outpatient)	76	95%	98%	98%
Prophylactic Antibiotic Stopped[2]	478	99%	98%	98%

NOTE: Hospital profiles are in alphabetical order by state, then city, then hospital within the city; Rankings exclude hospitals with less than 25 cases except for patient surveys which excludes hospitals with less than 100 cases; (a) 100-299 cases; (1) The number of cases/patients is too few to report; (2) Data submitted were based on a sample of cases/patients; (3) Results are based on a shorter time period than required; (4) Data suppressed by CMS for one or more quarters; (5) Results are not available for this reporting period; (6) Fewer than 100 patients completed the HCAHPS survey; (7) No cases met the criteria for this measure; (8) The lower limit of the confidence interval cannot be calculated if the number of observed infections equals zero; (9) No data are available from the state/territory for this reporting period; (10) The scores shown reflect fewer than 50 completed surveys; (11) There were discrepancies in the data collection process; (12) This measure does not apply to this hospital for this reporting period; (13) Results cannot be calculated for this reporting period; (14) The results for this state are combined with nearby states to protect confidentiality; Please refer to the User's Guide for a full explanation of data.

Prophylactic Antibiotic Timing[2]	483	100%	99%	99%
Prophylactic Antibiotic Timing (Outpatient)	78	91%	97%	98%
Urinary Catheter Removal[2]	576	99%	97%	97%
Survey of Patients' Hospital Experiences				
Area Around Room 'Always' Quiet at Night	300+	53%	58%	61%
Doctors 'Always' Communicated Well	300+	75%	80%	82%
Home Recovery Information Given	300+	87%	87%	85%
Hospital Given 9 or 10 on 10 Point Scale	300+	66%	72%	71%
Meds 'Always' Explained Before Given	300+	62%	64%	64%
Nurses 'Always' Communicated Well	300+	78%	81%	79%
Pain 'Always' Well Controlled	300+	69%	71%	71%
Room and Bathroom 'Always' Clean	300+	70%	75%	73%
Timely Help 'Always' Received	300+	64%	70%	68%
Would Definitely Recommend Hospital	300+	68%	71%	71%
Use of Medical Imaging				
Cardiac Imaging Stress Test before Surgery[1]	-	-	5.4%	5.3%
Combination Abdominal CT Scan	321	1.6%	7.1%	10.5%
Combination Brain/Sinus CT Scan	424	4.0%	2.8%	2.7%
Combination Chest CT Scan	134	0.7%	1.7%	2.7%
Follow-up Mammogram/Ultrasound	558	6.6%	8.7%	8.8%
Lumbar Spine MRI for Low Back Pain[1]	-	-	34.7%	37.2%

Fairfield Medical Center

401 North Ewing Street
Lancaster, OH 43130
Phone: 740-687-8009
Fax: 740-687-8115
URL: www.fmchealth.org
Type: Acute Care Hospitals
Emergency Services: Yes
Ownership: Voluntary non-profit - Other
Beds: 229

Key Personnel:
Chief of Medical Staff.......... Sarah Alley, MD
Radiology.................. Ricardo B Barboza
Coronary Care.............. Anne Brown
Operating Room............. Steven D Cox
CEO .... Sky Gettys
Quality Assurance .... Roxanne Mathias
Pediatric In-Patient Care .... Dora Metzger
Cardiac Laboratory............ Misty Newsome

Measure	Cases	This Hosp.	State Avg.	U.S. Avg.
Blood Clot Prevention and Treatment				
Anticoagulation Overlap Therapy[2]	76	95%	93%	93%
ICU Venous Thromboembolism Prophylaxis[2]	89	89%	93%	92%
Incidence of Potentially Preventable VTE[1,2]	-	-	6%	10%
UFH with Dosages/Platelet Monitoring[2]	72	100%	98%	97%
Venous Thromboembolism Prophylaxis[2]	284	89%	88%	85%
Warfarin Therapy Discharge Instructions[2]	65	75%	79%	75%
Chest Pain/Possible Heart Attack Care				
Aspirin Given Within 24 Hours of Arrival[1]	-	-	97%	96%
Fibrinolytic Meds Within 30 Min. of Arrival[3,7]	-	-	44%	58%
Average Time to ECG (minutes)[1]	-	-	6	7
Average Time to Transfer (minutes)[3,7]	-	-	58	60
Children's Asthma Care				
Received Home Management Plan of Care	-	-	85%	88%
Received Reliever Medication	-	-	100%	100%
Received Systemic Corticosteroids	-	-	100%	100%
Emergency Department				
Admittance Decision Time (minutes)[2]	496	82	90	98
Head CT Results Within 45 Min. of Arrival	27	78%	63%	57%
Patients Who Left ER Before Being Seen	51,343	5%	2%	2%
Time from ER Arrival to Admit. (minutes)[2]	538	252	265	274
Time from ER Arrival to Discharge (minutes)	366	185	128	134
Time in ER Before Being Evaluated (minutes)	406	47	22	26
Time to Pain Meds for Fractures (minutes)	94	70	54	57
Heart Attack Care				
Aspirin Given at Discharge	285	99%	99%	99%
Fibrinolytic Meds Within 30 Min. of Arrival[7]	-	-	80%	54%
PCI Within 90 Minutes of Arrival	53	100%	97%	96%
Statin Prescribed at Discharge	281	99%	98%	98%
Heart Failure Care				
ACE Inhibitor or ARB for LVSD	87	97%	97%	97%
Discharge Instructions Given	310	89%	96%	94%
Evaluation of LVS Function	377	99%	100%	99%
Medicare Spending				
Medicare Spending per Patient (ratio)	-	1.01	1.01	0.98
Pneumonia Care				
Appropriate Initial Antibiotic Given[2]	87	93%	96%	95%
Blood Culture Timing[2]	184	100%	98%	98%
Pregnancy and Delivery Care				
Newborn Deliveries Scheduled Early[2]	60	2%	5%	6%
Preventive Care				
Immunization for Influenza[2]	540	93%	93%	90%
Immunization for Pneumonia[2]	730	95%	94%	92%
Stroke Care				
Anticoagulation Therapy for Atrial Fibrillation[1]	-	-	95%	95%
Antithrombotic Therapy Timing	72	100%	98%	98%
Assessed for Rehabilitation	77	95%	98%	97%
Discharged on Antithrombotic Therapy	72	100%	99%	99%
Discharged on Statin Medication	55	95%	95%	94%
Thrombolytic Therapy Timing[1]	-	-	65%	66%
Venous Thromboembolism Prophylaxis	71	96%	95%	94%
Written Stroke Educational Materials Given	55	78%	92%	88%
Surgical Care Improvement Project				
Appropriate Beta Blocker Usage[2]	317	98%	98%	98%
Appropriate VTP Within 24 Hours[2]	491	99%	98%	98%
Controlled Postoperative Blood Glucose[2]	164	93%	97%	97%
Perioperative Temperature Management[2]	584	100%	100%	100%
Prophylactic Antibiotic Selection[2]	552	99%	99%	99%
Prophylactic Antibiotic Selection (Outpatient)	283	98%	98%	98%
Prophylactic Antibiotic Stopped[2]	521	97%	98%	98%
Prophylactic Antibiotic Timing[2]	552	99%	99%	99%
Prophylactic Antibiotic Timing (Outpatient)	286	94%	97%	98%
Urinary Catheter Removal[2]	464	98%	97%	97%
Survey of Patients' Hospital Experiences				
Area Around Room 'Always' Quiet at Night	300+	48%	58%	61%
Doctors 'Always' Communicated Well	300+	82%	80%	82%
Home Recovery Information Given	300+	88%	87%	85%
Hospital Given 9 or 10 on 10 Point Scale	300+	72%	72%	71%
Meds 'Always' Explained Before Given	300+	61%	64%	64%
Nurses 'Always' Communicated Well	300+	81%	81%	79%
Pain 'Always' Well Controlled	300+	71%	71%	71%
Room and Bathroom 'Always' Clean	300+	72%	75%	73%
Timely Help 'Always' Received	300+	72%	70%	68%
Would Definitely Recommend Hospital	300+	72%	71%	71%
Use of Medical Imaging				
Cardiac Imaging Stress Test before Surgery	156	5.1%	5.4%	5.3%
Combination Abdominal CT Scan	922	3.6%	7.1%	10.5%
Combination Brain/Sinus CT Scan	891	3.1%	2.8%	2.7%
Combination Chest CT Scan	547	0.9%	1.7%	2.7%
Follow-up Mammogram/Ultrasound	1,385	6.3%	8.7%	8.8%
Lumbar Spine MRI for Low Back Pain	197	38.1%	34.7%	37.2%

Institute For Orthopaedic Surgery

801 Medical Drive, Suite B
Lima, OH 45804
Phone: 419-224-7586
URL: www.ioshospital.com
Type: Acute Care Hospitals
Emergency Services: No
Ownership: Proprietary

Key Personnel:
Cardiology.................. Paula Anike, DO
CEO/President............... Mark McDonald, MD

Measure	Cases	This Hosp.	State Avg.	U.S. Avg.
Blood Clot Prevention and Treatment				
Anticoagulation Overlap Therapy[2,7]	-	-	93%	93%
ICU Venous Thromboembolism Prophylaxis[2,7]	-	-	93%	92%
Incidence of Potentially Preventable VTE[2,7]	-	-	6%	10%
UFH with Dosages/Platelet Monitoring[2,7]	-	-	98%	97%
Venous Thromboembolism Prophylaxis[2]	41	90%	88%	85%
Warfarin Therapy Discharge Instructions[2,7]	-	-	79%	75%
Chest Pain/Possible Heart Attack Care				
Aspirin Given Within 24 Hours of Arrival[5]	-	-	97%	96%
Fibrinolytic Meds Within 30 Min. of Arrival[5]	-	-	44%	58%
Average Time to ECG (minutes)[5]	-	-	6	7
Average Time to Transfer (minutes)[5]	-	-	58	60
Children's Asthma Care				
Received Home Management Plan of Care	-	-	85%	88%
Received Reliever Medication	-	-	100%	100%
Received Systemic Corticosteroids	-	-	100%	100%
Emergency Department				
Admittance Decision Time (minutes)[2,7]	-	-	90	98
Head CT Results Within 45 Min. of Arrival[5]	-	-	63%	57%
Patients Who Left ER Before Being Seen[5]	-	-	2%	2%
Time from ER Arrival to Admit. (minutes)[2,7]	-	-	265	274
Time from ER Arrival to Discharge (minutes)[5]	-	-	128	134
Time in ER Before Being Evaluated (minutes)[5]	-	-	22	26
Time to Pain Meds for Fractures (minutes)[5]	-	-	54	57
Heart Attack Care				
Aspirin Given at Discharge[5]	-	-	99%	99%
Fibrinolytic Meds Within 30 Min. of Arrival[5]	-	-	80%	54%
PCI Within 90 Minutes of Arrival[5]	-	-	97%	96%
Statin Prescribed at Discharge[5]	-	-	98%	98%
Heart Failure Care				
ACE Inhibitor or ARB for LVSD[5]	-	-	97%	97%
Discharge Instructions Given[5]	-	-	96%	94%
Evaluation of LVS Function[5]	-	-	100%	99%
Medicare Spending				
Medicare Spending per Patient (ratio)	-	0.93	1.01	0.98
Pneumonia Care				
Appropriate Initial Antibiotic Given[5]	-	-	96%	95%
Blood Culture Timing[5]	-	-	98%	98%
Pregnancy and Delivery Care				
Newborn Deliveries Scheduled Early[7]	-	-	5%	6%
Preventive Care				
Immunization for Influenza[2]	302	96%	93%	90%
Immunization for Pneumonia[2]	341	94%	94%	92%
Stroke Care				
Anticoagulation Therapy for Atrial Fibrillation[5]	-	-	95%	95%
Antithrombotic Therapy Timing[5]	-	-	98%	98%
Assessed for Rehabilitation[5]	-	-	98%	97%
Discharged on Antithrombotic Therapy[5]	-	-	99%	99%
Discharged on Statin Medication[5]	-	-	95%	94%
Thrombolytic Therapy Timing[5]	-	-	65%	66%
Venous Thromboembolism Prophylaxis[5]	-	-	95%	94%
Written Stroke Educational Materials Given[5]	-	-	92%	88%
Surgical Care Improvement Project				
Appropriate Beta Blocker Usage[2]	56	100%	98%	98%
Appropriate VTP Within 24 Hours[2]	182	100%	98%	98%
Controlled Postoperative Blood Glucose[2,7]	-	-	97%	97%
Perioperative Temperature Management[2]	191	100%	100%	100%
Prophylactic Antibiotic Selection[2]	178	100%	99%	99%
Prophylactic Antibiotic Selection (Outpatient)[3]	47	100%	98%	98%
Prophylactic Antibiotic Stopped[2]	178	100%	98%	98%
Prophylactic Antibiotic Timing[2]	178	100%	99%	99%
Prophylactic Antibiotic Timing (Outpatient)[3]	47	100%	97%	98%
Urinary Catheter Removal[2]	39	100%	97%	97%
Survey of Patients' Hospital Experiences				
Area Around Room 'Always' Quiet at Night	300+	79%	58%	61%
Doctors 'Always' Communicated Well	300+	88%	80%	82%
Home Recovery Information Given	300+	93%	87%	85%
Hospital Given 9 or 10 on 10 Point Scale	300+	92%	72%	71%
Meds 'Always' Explained Before Given	300+	80%	64%	64%
Nurses 'Always' Communicated Well	300+	92%	81%	79%
Pain 'Always' Well Controlled	300+	78%	71%	71%
Room and Bathroom 'Always' Clean	300+	85%	75%	73%
Timely Help 'Always' Received	300+	91%	70%	68%
Would Definitely Recommend Hospital	300+	92%	71%	71%
Use of Medical Imaging				
Cardiac Imaging Stress Test before Surgery[7]	-	-	5.4%	5.3%
Combination Abdominal CT Scan[7]	-	-	7.1%	10.5%
Combination Brain/Sinus CT Scan[7]	-	-	2.8%	2.7%
Combination Chest CT Scan[7]	-	-	1.7%	2.7%
Follow-up Mammogram/Ultrasound[7]	-	-	8.7%	8.8%
Lumbar Spine MRI for Low Back Pain[7]	-	-	34.7%	37.2%

Lima Memorial Health System

1001 Bellefontaine Avenue
Lima, OH 45804
Phone: 419-998-4731
Fax: 419-998-4509
URL: www.limamemorial.org
Type: Acute Care Hospitals
Emergency Services: Yes
Ownership: Voluntary non-profit - Other
Beds: 308

Key Personnel:
Operating Room.............. Jeff Collins
Emergency Room .... Sue Fickel, RN, MS

NOTE: Hospital profiles are in alphabetical order by state, then city, then hospital within the city; Rankings exclude hospitals with less than 25 cases except for patient surveys which excludes hospitals with less than 100 cases; (a) 100-299 cases; (1) The number of cases/patients is too few to report; (2) Data submitted were based on a sample of cases/patients; (3) Results are based on a shorter time period than required; (4) Data suppressed by CMS for one or more quarters; (5) Results are not available for this reporting period; (6) Fewer than 100 patients completed the HCAHPS survey; (7) No cases met the criteria for this measure; (8) The lower limit of the confidence interval cannot be calculated if the number of observed infections equals zero; (9) No data are available from the state/territory for this reporting period; (10) The scores shown reflect fewer than 50 completed surveys; (11) There were discrepancies in the data collection process; (12) This measure does not apply to this hospital for this reporting period; (13) Results cannot be calculated for this reporting period; (14) The results for this state are combined with nearby states to protect confidentiality; Please refer to the User's Guide for a full explanation of data.

Quality Assurance . . . . Anita Good
Chief of Medical Staff. . . . . Jean Johns
Pediatric Ambulatory Care . . . . . . J Liggett, MD
Radiology. . . . . PK Malhotra, MD
CEO/President. . . . . Michael D. Swick

Measure	Cases	This Hosp.	State Avg.	U.S. Avg.
Blood Clot Prevention and Treatment				
Anticoagulation Overlap Therapy[2]	54	91%	93%	93%
ICU Venous Thromboembolism Prophylaxis[2]	162	99%	93%	92%
Incidence of Potentially Preventable VTE[1,2]	-	-	6%	10%
UFH with Dosages/Platelet Monitoring[2]	48	56%	98%	97%
Venous Thromboembolism Prophylaxis[2]	288	94%	88%	85%
Warfarin Therapy Discharge Instructions[2]	43	98%	79%	75%
Chest Pain/Possible Heart Attack Care				
Aspirin Given Within 24 Hours of Arrival[1,3]	-	-	97%	96%
Fibrinolytic Meds Within 30 Min. of Arrival[5]	-	-	44%	58%
Average Time to ECG (minutes)[1,3]	-	-	6	7
Average Time to Transfer (minutes)[5]	-	-	58	60
Children's Asthma Care				
Received Home Management Plan of Care	-	-	85%	88%
Received Reliever Medication	-	-	100%	100%
Received Systemic Corticosteroids	-	-	100%	100%
Emergency Department				
Admittance Decision Time (minutes)[2]	646	83	90	98
Head CT Results Within 45 Min. of Arrival	12	50%	63%	57%
Patients Who Left ER Before Being Seen	42,306	2%	2%	2%
Time from ER Arrival to Admit. (minutes)[2]	649	252	265	274
Time from ER Arrival to Discharge (minutes)	446	101	128	134
Time in ER Before Being Evaluated (minutes)	479	18	22	26
Time to Pain Meds for Fractures (minutes)	58	51	54	57
Heart Attack Care				
Aspirin Given at Discharge	281	100%	99%	99%
Fibrinolytic Meds Within 30 Min. of Arrival[7]	-	-	80%	54%
PCI Within 90 Minutes of Arrival	23	100%	97%	96%
Statin Prescribed at Discharge	268	99%	98%	98%
Heart Failure Care				
ACE Inhibitor or ARB for LVSD	59	100%	97%	97%
Discharge Instructions Given	174	97%	96%	94%
Evaluation of LVS Function	225	100%	100%	99%
Medicare Spending				
Medicare Spending per Patient (ratio)	-	1.00	1.01	0.98
Pneumonia Care				
Appropriate Initial Antibiotic Given	107	96%	96%	95%
Blood Culture Timing	166	97%	98%	98%
Pregnancy and Delivery Care				
Newborn Deliveries Scheduled Early[2]	45	7%	5%	6%
Preventive Care				
Immunization for Influenza[2]	565	98%	93%	90%
Immunization for Pneumonia[2]	787	98%	94%	92%
Stroke Care				
Anticoagulation Therapy for Atrial Fibrillation[1]	-	-	95%	95%
Antithrombotic Therapy Timing	81	100%	98%	98%
Assessed for Rehabilitation	99	98%	98%	97%
Discharged on Antithrombotic Therapy	88	100%	99%	99%
Discharged on Statin Medication	78	90%	95%	94%
Thrombolytic Therapy Timing[7]	-	-	65%	66%
Venous Thromboembolism Prophylaxis	95	98%	95%	94%
Written Stroke Educational Materials Given	55	82%	92%	88%
Surgical Care Improvement Project				
Appropriate Beta Blocker Usage[2]	202	99%	98%	98%
Appropriate VTP Within 24 Hours[2]	172	98%	98%	98%
Controlled Postoperative Blood Glucose[2]	187	97%	97%	97%
Perioperative Temperature Management[2]	260	100%	100%	100%
Prophylactic Antibiotic Selection[2]	289	99%	99%	99%
Prophylactic Antibiotic Selection (Outpatient)	434	100%	98%	98%
Prophylactic Antibiotic Stopped[2]	282	98%	98%	98%
Prophylactic Antibiotic Timing[2]	292	99%	99%	99%
Prophylactic Antibiotic Timing (Outpatient)	436	99%	97%	98%
Urinary Catheter Removal[2]	184	98%	97%	97%
Survey of Patients' Hospital Experiences				
Area Around Room 'Always' Quiet at Night	300+	54%	58%	61%
Doctors 'Always' Communicated Well	300+	74%	80%	82%
Home Recovery Information Given	300+	88%	87%	85%
Hospital Given 9 or 10 on 10 Point Scale	300+	66%	72%	71%
Meds 'Always' Explained Before Given	300+	58%	64%	64%
Nurses 'Always' Communicated Well	300+	76%	81%	79%
Pain 'Always' Well Controlled	300+	67%	71%	71%
Room and Bathroom 'Always' Clean	300+	74%	75%	73%
Timely Help 'Always' Received	300+	63%	70%	68%
Would Definitely Recommend Hospital	300+	69%	71%	71%
Use of Medical Imaging				
Cardiac Imaging Stress Test before Surgery	787	4.6%	5.4%	5.3%
Combination Abdominal CT Scan	690	5.5%	7.1%	10.5%
Combination Brain/Sinus CT Scan	648	2.3%	2.8%	2.7%
Combination Chest CT Scan	289	0.7%	1.7%	2.7%
Follow-up Mammogram/Ultrasound	1,176	9.2%	8.7%	8.8%
Lumbar Spine MRI for Low Back Pain	99	35.4%	34.7%	37.2%

Saint Rita's Medical Center

730 West Market Street
Lima, OH 45801
Phone: 419-227-3361
Fax: 419-226-9718
URL: www.stritas.org
Type: Acute Care Hospitals
Emergency Services: Yes
Ownership: Voluntary non-profit - Church
Beds: 424

Key Personnel:
Radiology. . . . . EV Bostick, MD
Infection Control. . . . . KM Griffith, MD
Chief of Medical Staff. . . . . DL Imler, DO
Pediatric Ambulatory Care . . . . . . JS Liggett, MD
Pediatric In-Patient Care . . . . JS Liggett, MD
Quality Assurance . . . . Cindy Mefferd
CEO/President. . . . . James P Reber
Operating Room. . . . . Jo Shough

Measure	Cases	This Hosp.	State Avg.	U.S. Avg.
Blood Clot Prevention and Treatment				
Anticoagulation Overlap Therapy[2]	99	94%	93%	93%
ICU Venous Thromboembolism Prophylaxis[2]	114	83%	93%	92%
Incidence of Potentially Preventable VTE[2]	12	8%	6%	10%
UFH with Dosages/Platelet Monitoring[2]	79	100%	98%	97%
Venous Thromboembolism Prophylaxis[2]	470	86%	88%	85%
Warfarin Therapy Discharge Instructions[2]	80	86%	79%	75%
Chest Pain/Possible Heart Attack Care				
Aspirin Given Within 24 Hours of Arrival[1]	-	-	97%	96%
Fibrinolytic Meds Within 30 Min. of Arrival[5]	-	-	44%	58%
Average Time to ECG (minutes)[1]	-	-	6	7
Average Time to Transfer (minutes)[5]	-	-	58	60
Children's Asthma Care				
Received Home Management Plan of Care	-	-	85%	88%
Received Reliever Medication	-	-	100%	100%
Received Systemic Corticosteroids	-	-	100%	100%
Emergency Department				
Admittance Decision Time (minutes)[2]	777	109	90	98
Head CT Results Within 45 Min. of Arrival	19	74%	63%	57%
Patients Who Left ER Before Being Seen	58,284	4%	2%	2%
Time from ER Arrival to Admit. (minutes)[2]	790	292	265	274
Time from ER Arrival to Discharge (minutes)	438	168	128	134
Time in ER Before Being Evaluated (minutes)	456	30	22	26
Time to Pain Meds for Fractures (minutes)	187	86	54	57
Heart Attack Care				
Aspirin Given at Discharge	472	99%	99%	99%
Fibrinolytic Meds Within 30 Min. of Arrival[7]	-	-	80%	54%
PCI Within 90 Minutes of Arrival	52	94%	97%	96%
Statin Prescribed at Discharge	451	98%	98%	98%
Heart Failure Care				
ACE Inhibitor or ARB for LVSD	140	92%	97%	97%
Discharge Instructions Given	333	99%	96%	94%
Evaluation of LVS Function	443	100%	100%	99%
Medicare Spending				
Medicare Spending per Patient (ratio)	-	1.00	1.01	0.98
Pneumonia Care				
Appropriate Initial Antibiotic Given	207	96%	96%	95%
Blood Culture Timing	406	98%	98%	98%
Pregnancy and Delivery Care				
Newborn Deliveries Scheduled Early	185	15%	5%	6%
Preventive Care				
Immunization for Influenza[2]	589	92%	93%	90%
Immunization for Pneumonia[2]	736	94%	94%	92%
Stroke Care				
Anticoagulation Therapy for Atrial Fibrillation[1]	-	-	95%	95%
Antithrombotic Therapy Timing	165	100%	98%	98%
Assessed for Rehabilitation	190	98%	98%	97%
Discharged on Antithrombotic Therapy	163	98%	99%	99%
Discharged on Statin Medication	132	98%	95%	94%
Thrombolytic Therapy Timing[1]	-	-	65%	66%
Venous Thromboembolism Prophylaxis	186	97%	95%	94%
Written Stroke Educational Materials Given	108	99%	92%	88%
Surgical Care Improvement Project				
Appropriate Beta Blocker Usage	509	98%	98%	98%
Appropriate VTP Within 24 Hours	756	97%	98%	98%
Controlled Postoperative Blood Glucose	204	98%	97%	97%
Perioperative Temperature Management	926	100%	100%	100%
Prophylactic Antibiotic Selection	616	100%	99%	99%
Prophylactic Antibiotic Selection (Outpatient)	321	98%	98%	98%
Prophylactic Antibiotic Stopped	599	97%	98%	98%
Prophylactic Antibiotic Timing	617	99%	99%	99%
Prophylactic Antibiotic Timing (Outpatient)	321	98%	97%	98%
Urinary Catheter Removal	434	89%	97%	97%
Survey of Patients' Hospital Experiences				
Area Around Room 'Always' Quiet at Night	300+	57%	58%	61%
Doctors 'Always' Communicated Well	300+	76%	80%	82%
Home Recovery Information Given	300+	87%	87%	85%
Hospital Given 9 or 10 on 10 Point Scale	300+	72%	72%	71%
Meds 'Always' Explained Before Given	300+	60%	64%	64%
Nurses 'Always' Communicated Well	300+	79%	81%	79%
Pain 'Always' Well Controlled	300+	69%	71%	71%
Room and Bathroom 'Always' Clean	300+	71%	75%	73%
Timely Help 'Always' Received	300+	70%	70%	68%
Would Definitely Recommend Hospital	300+	74%	71%	71%
Use of Medical Imaging				
Cardiac Imaging Stress Test before Surgery	922	5.4%	5.4%	5.3%
Combination Abdominal CT Scan	1,324	15.2%	7.1%	10.5%
Combination Brain/Sinus CT Scan	1,087	4.3%	2.8%	2.7%
Combination Chest CT Scan	731	2.5%	1.7%	2.7%
Follow-up Mammogram/Ultrasound	2,205	9.7%	8.7%	8.8%
Lumbar Spine MRI for Low Back Pain	150	25.3%	34.7%	37.2%

Lodi Community Hospital

225 Elyria Street
Lodi, OH 44254
Phone: 330-948-1222
Fax: 330-948-2614
URL: www.lodihospital.com
Type: Critical Access Hospitals
Emergency Services: Yes
Ownership: Voluntary non-profit - Private
Beds: 25

Key Personnel:
Chief of Medical Staff. . . . . Mary Hancock, MD
Patient Relations . . . . Dana Kocsis, RN
Operating Room. . . . . Molly Saal, RN
Emergency Room . . . . Christine Snow, RN
CEO/President. . . . . Thomas Whelan

Measure	Cases	This Hosp.	State Avg.	U.S. Avg.
Blood Clot Prevention and Treatment				
Anticoagulation Overlap Therapy[5]	-	-	93%	93%
ICU Venous Thromboembolism Prophylaxis[5]	-	-	93%	92%
Incidence of Potentially Preventable VTE[5]	-	-	6%	10%
UFH with Dosages/Platelet Monitoring[5]	-	-	98%	97%
Venous Thromboembolism Prophylaxis[5]	-	-	88%	85%
Warfarin Therapy Discharge Instructions[5]	-	-	79%	75%
Chest Pain/Possible Heart Attack Care				
Aspirin Given Within 24 Hours of Arrival[3]	16	100%	97%	96%
Fibrinolytic Meds Within 30 Min. of Arrival[3,7]	-	-	44%	58%
Average Time to ECG (minutes)[3]	16	6	6	7
Average Time to Transfer (minutes)[1,3]	-	-	58	60
Children's Asthma Care				
Received Home Management Plan of Care	-	-	85%	88%
Received Reliever Medication	-	-	100%	100%
Received Systemic Corticosteroids	-	-	100%	100%
Emergency Department				
Admittance Decision Time (minutes)[5]	-	-	90	98
Head CT Results Within 45 Min. of Arrival[5]	-	-	63%	57%
Patients Who Left ER Before Being Seen[5]	-	-	2%	2%

NOTE: Hospital profiles are in alphabetical order by state, then city, then hospital within the city; Rankings exclude hospitals with less than 25 cases except for patient surveys which excludes hospitals with less than 100 cases; (a) 100-299 cases; (1) The number of cases/patients is too few to report; (2) Data submitted were based on a sample of cases/patients; (3) Results are based on a shorter time period than required; (4) Data suppressed by CMS for one or more quarters; (5) Results are not available for this reporting period; (6) Fewer than 100 patients completed the HCAHPS survey; (7) No cases met the criteria for this measure; (8) The lower limit of the confidence interval cannot be calculated if the number of observed infections equals zero; (9) No data are available from the state/territory for this reporting period; (10) The scores shown reflect fewer than 50 completed surveys; (11) There were discrepancies in the data collection process; (12) This measure does not apply to this hospital for this reporting period; (13) Results cannot be calculated for this reporting period; (14) The results for this state are combined with nearby states to protect confidentiality; Please refer to the User's Guide for a full explanation of data.

Measure	Cases	This Hosp.	State Avg.	U.S. Avg.
Time from ER Arrival to Admit. (minutes)[5]	-	-	265	274
Time from ER Arrival to Discharge (minutes)	293	70	128	134
Time in ER Before Being Evaluated (minutes)	332	7	22	26
Time to Pain Meds for Fractures (minutes)[5]	-	-	54	57
Heart Attack Care				
Aspirin Given at Discharge[5]	-	-	99%	99%
Fibrinolytic Meds Within 30 Min. of Arrival[5]	-	-	80%	54%
PCI Within 90 Minutes of Arrival[5]	-	-	97%	96%
Statin Prescribed at Discharge[5]	-	-	98%	98%
Heart Failure Care				
ACE Inhibitor or ARB for LVSD[5]	-	-	97%	97%
Discharge Instructions Given[5]	-	-	96%	94%
Evaluation of LVS Function[5]	-	-	100%	99%
Medicare Spending				
Medicare Spending per Patient (ratio)	-	-	1.01	0.98
Pneumonia Care				
Appropriate Initial Antibiotic Given[1,3]	-	-	96%	95%
Blood Culture Timing[3]	12	100%	98%	98%
Pregnancy and Delivery Care				
Newborn Deliveries Scheduled Early[5]	-	-	5%	6%
Preventive Care				
Immunization for Influenza[5]	-	-	93%	90%
Immunization for Pneumonia[5]	-	-	94%	92%
Stroke Care				
Anticoagulation Therapy for Atrial Fibrillation[5]	-	-	95%	95%
Antithrombotic Therapy Timing[5]	-	-	98%	98%
Assessed for Rehabilitation[5]	-	-	98%	97%
Discharged on Antithrombotic Therapy[5]	-	-	99%	99%
Discharged on Statin Medication[5]	-	-	95%	94%
Thrombolytic Therapy Timing[5]	-	-	65%	66%
Venous Thromboembolism Prophylaxis[5]	-	-	95%	94%
Written Stroke Educational Materials Given[5]	-	-	92%	88%
Surgical Care Improvement Project				
Appropriate Beta Blocker Usage[5]	-	-	98%	98%
Appropriate VTP Within 24 Hours[5]	-	-	98%	98%
Controlled Postoperative Blood Glucose[5]	-	-	97%	97%
Perioperative Temperature Management[5]	-	-	100%	100%
Prophylactic Antibiotic Selection[5]	-	-	99%	99%
Prophylactic Antibiotic Selection (Outpatient)[5]	-	-	98%	98%
Prophylactic Antibiotic Stopped[5]	-	-	98%	98%
Prophylactic Antibiotic Timing[5]	-	-	99%	99%
Prophylactic Antibiotic Timing (Outpatient)[5]	-	-	97%	98%
Urinary Catheter Removal[5]	-	-	97%	97%
Survey of Patients' Hospital Experiences				
Area Around Room 'Always' Quiet at Night[10]	<100	64%	58%	61%
Doctors 'Always' Communicated Well[10]	<100	89%	80%	82%
Home Recovery Information Given[10]	<100	84%	87%	85%
Hospital Given 9 or 10 on 10 Point Scale[10]	<100	84%	72%	71%
Meds 'Always' Explained Before Given[10]	<100	68%	64%	64%
Nurses 'Always' Communicated Well[10]	<100	85%	81%	79%
Pain 'Always' Well Controlled[10]	<100	75%	71%	71%
Room and Bathroom 'Always' Clean[10]	<100	79%	75%	73%
Timely Help 'Always' Received[10]	<100	80%	70%	68%
Would Definitely Recommend Hospital[10]	<100	89%	71%	71%
Use of Medical Imaging				
Cardiac Imaging Stress Test before Surgery[1]	-	-	5.4%	5.3%
Combination Abdominal CT Scan	110	4.5%	7.1%	10.5%
Combination Brain/Sinus CT Scan[1]	-	-	2.8%	2.7%
Combination Chest CT Scan	48	0.0%	1.7%	2.7%
Follow-up Mammogram/Ultrasound	138	6.5%	8.7%	8.8%
Lumbar Spine MRI for Low Back Pain[1]	-	-	34.7%	37.2%

Hocking Valley Community Hospital

601 State Route 664n
Logan, OH 43138
Type: Critical Access Hospitals
Ownership: Voluntary non-profit - Other
Phone: 740-380-8000
Fax: 740-385-9771
Emergency Services: Yes
Beds: 93

Key Personnel:
Radiology. . . . . Robert Cox
Intensive Care Unit. . . . . Katy Daubenmeir
Infection Control. . . . . Connie Gaib
Quality Assurance . . . . Connie Gaib
Chief of Medical Staff. . . . . Prakash Kudlapur
Pediatric Ambulatory Care . . . . Rosario Labrador
Pediatric In-Patient Care . . . . Rosario Labrador
Operating Room. . . . . Mary Rosier

Measure	Cases	This Hosp.	State Avg.	U.S. Avg.
Blood Clot Prevention and Treatment				
Anticoagulation Overlap Therapy[5]	-	-	93%	93%
ICU Venous Thromboembolism Prophylaxis[5]	-	-	93%	92%
Incidence of Potentially Preventable VTE[5]	-	-	6%	10%
UFH with Dosages/Platelet Monitoring[5]	-	-	98%	97%
Venous Thromboembolism Prophylaxis[5]	-	-	88%	85%
Warfarin Therapy Discharge Instructions[5]	-	-	79%	75%
Chest Pain/Possible Heart Attack Care				
Aspirin Given Within 24 Hours of Arrival[5]	-	-	97%	96%
Fibrinolytic Meds Within 30 Min. of Arrival[5]	-	-	44%	58%
Average Time to ECG (minutes)[5]	-	-	6	7
Average Time to Transfer (minutes)[5]	-	-	58	60
Children's Asthma Care				
Received Home Management Plan of Care	-	-	85%	88%
Received Reliever Medication	-	-	100%	100%
Received Systemic Corticosteroids	-	-	100%	100%
Emergency Department				
Admittance Decision Time (minutes)[5]	-	-	90	98
Head CT Results Within 45 Min. of Arrival[5]	-	-	63%	57%
Patients Who Left ER Before Being Seen	10,664	1%	2%	2%
Time from ER Arrival to Admit. (minutes)[5]	-	-	265	274
Time from ER Arrival to Discharge (minutes)[5]	-	-	128	134
Time in ER Before Being Evaluated (minutes)[5]	-	-	22	26
Time to Pain Meds for Fractures (minutes)[5]	-	-	54	57
Heart Attack Care				
Aspirin Given at Discharge[7]	-	-	99%	99%
Fibrinolytic Meds Within 30 Min. of Arrival[7]	-	-	80%	54%
PCI Within 90 Minutes of Arrival[7]	-	-	97%	96%
Statin Prescribed at Discharge[7]	-	-	98%	98%
Heart Failure Care				
ACE Inhibitor or ARB for LVSD[1]	-	-	97%	97%
Discharge Instructions Given[1]	-	-	96%	94%
Evaluation of LVS Function	14	93%	100%	99%
Medicare Spending				
Medicare Spending per Patient (ratio)	-	-	1.01	0.98
Pneumonia Care				
Appropriate Initial Antibiotic Given	43	88%	96%	95%
Blood Culture Timing	57	93%	98%	98%
Pregnancy and Delivery Care				
Newborn Deliveries Scheduled Early[5]	-	-	5%	6%
Preventive Care				
Immunization for Influenza[5]	-	-	93%	90%
Immunization for Pneumonia[5]	-	-	94%	92%
Stroke Care				
Anticoagulation Therapy for Atrial Fibrillation[5]	-	-	95%	95%
Antithrombotic Therapy Timing[5]	-	-	98%	98%
Assessed for Rehabilitation[5]	-	-	98%	97%
Discharged on Antithrombotic Therapy[5]	-	-	99%	99%
Discharged on Statin Medication[5]	-	-	95%	94%
Thrombolytic Therapy Timing[5]	-	-	65%	66%
Venous Thromboembolism Prophylaxis[5]	-	-	95%	94%
Written Stroke Educational Materials Given[5]	-	-	92%	88%
Surgical Care Improvement Project				
Appropriate Beta Blocker Usage	23	100%	98%	98%
Appropriate VTP Within 24 Hours	39	100%	98%	98%
Controlled Postoperative Blood Glucose[7]	-	-	97%	97%
Perioperative Temperature Management	44	100%	100%	100%
Prophylactic Antibiotic Selection	43	100%	99%	99%
Prophylactic Antibiotic Selection (Outpatient)[5]	-	-	98%	98%
Prophylactic Antibiotic Stopped	42	98%	98%	98%
Prophylactic Antibiotic Timing	43	95%	99%	99%
Prophylactic Antibiotic Timing (Outpatient)[5]	-	-	97%	98%
Urinary Catheter Removal	42	100%	97%	97%
Survey of Patients' Hospital Experiences				
Area Around Room 'Always' Quiet at Night	(a)	68%	58%	61%
Doctors 'Always' Communicated Well	(a)	86%	80%	82%
Home Recovery Information Given	(a)	91%	87%	85%
Hospital Given 9 or 10 on 10 Point Scale	(a)	80%	72%	71%
Meds 'Always' Explained Before Given	(a)	71%	64%	64%
Nurses 'Always' Communicated Well	(a)	85%	81%	79%
Pain 'Always' Well Controlled	(a)	77%	71%	71%
Room and Bathroom 'Always' Clean	(a)	83%	75%	73%
Timely Help 'Always' Received	(a)	83%	70%	68%
Would Definitely Recommend Hospital	(a)	74%	71%	71%
Use of Medical Imaging				
Cardiac Imaging Stress Test before Surgery	100	7.0%	5.4%	5.3%
Combination Abdominal CT Scan	230	5.7%	7.1%	10.5%
Combination Brain/Sinus CT Scan[1]	-	-	2.8%	2.7%
Combination Chest CT Scan	93	0.0%	1.7%	2.7%
Follow-up Mammogram/Ultrasound	357	8.1%	8.7%	8.8%
Lumbar Spine MRI for Low Back Pain	43	46.5%	34.7%	37.2%

Madison County Hospital

210 North Main Street
London, OH 43140
Type: Acute Care Hospitals
Ownership: Voluntary non-profit - Private
Phone: 740-845-7000
Fax: 740-852-3315
Emergency Services: Yes
Beds: 102

Key Personnel:
Operating Room. . . . . AJ Beisler, RN
CEO . . . . Dana Engle
Quality Assurance . . . . Darla Howland
Pediatric Ambulatory Care . . . . . . Sooja Kim
Pediatric In-Patient Care . . . . Sooja Kim
Infection Control. . . . . Millie Newman
President . . . . Mike Quilter
Chief of Medical Staff. . . . . Michael Turner, MD

Measure	Cases	This Hosp.	State Avg.	U.S. Avg.
Blood Clot Prevention and Treatment				
Anticoagulation Overlap Therapy[1,2]	-	-	93%	93%
ICU Venous Thromboembolism Prophylaxis[2]	42	83%	93%	92%
Incidence of Potentially Preventable VTE[2,7]	-	-	6%	10%
UFH with Dosages/Platelet Monitoring[1,2]	-	-	98%	97%
Venous Thromboembolism Prophylaxis[2]	57	74%	88%	85%
Warfarin Therapy Discharge Instructions[1,2]	-	-	79%	75%
Chest Pain/Possible Heart Attack Care				
Aspirin Given Within 24 Hours of Arrival	44	80%	97%	96%
Fibrinolytic Meds Within 30 Min. of Arrival[7]	-	-	44%	58%
Average Time to ECG (minutes)	44	10	6	7
Average Time to Transfer (minutes)[1]	-	-	58	60
Children's Asthma Care				
Received Home Management Plan of Care	-	-	85%	88%
Received Reliever Medication	-	-	100%	100%
Received Systemic Corticosteroids	-	-	100%	100%
Emergency Department				
Admittance Decision Time (minutes)[2]	157	51	90	98
Head CT Results Within 45 Min. of Arrival[1]	-	-	63%	57%
Patients Who Left ER Before Being Seen	13,979	1%	2%	2%
Time from ER Arrival to Admit. (minutes)[2]	162	248	265	274
Time from ER Arrival to Discharge (minutes)	338	112	128	134
Time in ER Before Being Evaluated (minutes)	343	28	22	26
Time to Pain Meds for Fractures (minutes)	39	36	54	57
Heart Attack Care				
Aspirin Given at Discharge[3,7]	-	-	99%	99%
Fibrinolytic Meds Within 30 Min. of Arrival[3,7]	-	-	80%	54%
PCI Within 90 Minutes of Arrival[3,7]	-	-	97%	96%
Statin Prescribed at Discharge[3,7]	-	-	98%	98%
Heart Failure Care				
ACE Inhibitor or ARB for LVSD[1]	-	-	97%	97%
Discharge Instructions Given	35	54%	96%	94%
Evaluation of LVS Function	43	88%	100%	99%
Medicare Spending				
Medicare Spending per Patient (ratio)	-	1.01	1.01	0.98
Pneumonia Care				
Appropriate Initial Antibiotic Given	55	87%	96%	95%
Blood Culture Timing	51	96%	98%	98%
Pregnancy and Delivery Care				
Newborn Deliveries Scheduled Early	28	11%	5%	6%
Preventive Care				
Immunization for Influenza[2]	246	83%	93%	90%
Immunization for Pneumonia[2]	304	86%	94%	92%
Stroke Care				
Anticoagulation Therapy for Atrial Fibrillation[3,7]	-	-	95%	95%
Antithrombotic Therapy Timing[3,7]	-	-	98%	98%

NOTE: Hospital profiles are in alphabetical order by state, then city, then hospital within the city; Rankings exclude hospitals with less than 25 cases except for patient surveys which excludes hospitals with less than 100 cases; (a) 100-299 cases; (1) The number of cases/patients is too few to report; (2) Data submitted were based on a sample of cases/patients; (3) Results are based on a shorter time period than required; (4) Data suppressed by CMS for one or more quarters; (5) Results are not available for this reporting period; (6) Fewer than 100 patients completed the HCAHPS survey; (7) No cases met the criteria for this measure; (8) The lower limit of the confidence interval cannot be calculated if the number of observed infections equals zero; (9) No data are available from the state/territory for this reporting period; (10) The scores shown reflect fewer than 50 completed surveys; (11) There were discrepancies in the data collection process; (12) This measure does not apply to this hospital for this reporting period; (13) Results cannot be calculated for this reporting period; (14) The results for this state are combined with nearby states to protect confidentiality; Please refer to the User's Guide for a full explanation of data.

Measure	Cases	This Hosp.	State Avg.	U.S. Avg.
Assessed for Rehabilitation[1,3]	-	-	98%	97%
Discharged on Antithrombotic Therapy[1,3]	-	-	99%	99%
Discharged on Statin Medication[1,3]	-	-	95%	94%
Thrombolytic Therapy Timing[3,7]	-	-	65%	66%
Venous Thromboembolism Prophylaxis[1,3]	-	-	95%	94%
Written Stroke Educational Materials Given[1,3]	-	-	92%	88%
Surgical Care Improvement Project				
Appropriate Beta Blocker Usage	41	85%	98%	98%
Appropriate VTP Within 24 Hours	99	95%	98%	98%
Controlled Postoperative Blood Glucose[7]	-	-	97%	97%
Perioperative Temperature Management	110	100%	100%	100%
Prophylactic Antibiotic Selection	83	95%	99%	99%
Prophylactic Antibiotic Selection (Outpatient)[1,3]	-	-	98%	98%
Prophylactic Antibiotic Stopped	82	98%	98%	98%
Prophylactic Antibiotic Timing	83	95%	99%	99%
Prophylactic Antibiotic Timing (Outpatient)[1,3]	-	-	97%	98%
Urinary Catheter Removal	79	95%	97%	97%
Survey of Patients' Hospital Experiences				
Area Around Room 'Always' Quiet at Night	(a)	64%	58%	61%
Doctors 'Always' Communicated Well	(a)	84%	80%	82%
Home Recovery Information Given	(a)	85%	87%	85%
Hospital Given 9 or 10 on 10 Point Scale	(a)	73%	72%	71%
Meds 'Always' Explained Before Given	(a)	67%	64%	64%
Nurses 'Always' Communicated Well	(a)	81%	81%	79%
Pain 'Always' Well Controlled	(a)	71%	71%	71%
Room and Bathroom 'Always' Clean	(a)	84%	75%	73%
Timely Help 'Always' Received	(a)	72%	70%	68%
Would Definitely Recommend Hospital	(a)	67%	71%	71%
Use of Medical Imaging				
Cardiac Imaging Stress Test before Surgery[1]	-	-	5.4%	5.3%
Combination Abdominal CT Scan	125	3.2%	7.1%	10.5%
Combination Brain/Sinus CT Scan[1]	-	-	2.8%	2.7%
Combination Chest CT Scan	82	1.2%	1.7%	2.7%
Follow-up Mammogram/Ultrasound	235	8.5%	8.7%	8.8%
Lumbar Spine MRI for Low Back Pain[1]	-	-	34.7%	37.2%

Mercy Regional Medical Center

3700 Kolbe Road
Lorain, OH 44053
Phone: 440-960-4000
Type: Acute Care Hospitals
Emergency Services: Yes
Ownership: Voluntary non-profit - Private

Measure	Cases	This Hosp.	State Avg.	U.S. Avg.
Blood Clot Prevention and Treatment				
Anticoagulation Overlap Therapy[2]	81	57%	93%	93%
ICU Venous Thromboembolism Prophylaxis[2]	72	60%	93%	92%
Incidence of Potentially Preventable VTE[2]	16	0%	6%	10%
UFH with Dosages/Platelet Monitoring[1,2]	-	-	98%	97%
Venous Thromboembolism Prophylaxis[2]	321	55%	88%	85%
Warfarin Therapy Discharge Instructions[2]	50	32%	79%	75%
Chest Pain/Possible Heart Attack Care				
Aspirin Given Within 24 Hours of Arrival[1,3]	-	-	97%	96%
Fibrinolytic Meds Within 30 Min. of Arrival[3,7]	-	-	44%	58%
Average Time to ECG (minutes)[1,3]	-	-	6	7
Average Time to Transfer (minutes)[3,7]	-	-	58	60
Children's Asthma Care				
Received Home Management Plan of Care	-	-	85%	88%
Received Reliever Medication	-	-	100%	100%
Received Systemic Corticosteroids	-	-	100%	100%
Emergency Department				
Admittance Decision Time (minutes)[2]	665	98	90	98
Head CT Results Within 45 Min. of Arrival	14	71%	63%	57%
Patients Who Left ER Before Being Seen	49,491	2%	2%	2%
Time from ER Arrival to Admit. (minutes)[2]	667	292	265	274
Time from ER Arrival to Discharge (minutes)	374	146	128	134
Time in ER Before Being Evaluated (minutes)	416	29	22	26
Time to Pain Meds for Fractures (minutes)	150	77	54	57
Heart Attack Care				
Aspirin Given at Discharge	323	96%	99%	99%
Fibrinolytic Meds Within 30 Min. of Arrival[7]	-	-	80%	54%
PCI Within 90 Minutes of Arrival	47	98%	97%	96%
Statin Prescribed at Discharge	301	97%	98%	98%
Heart Failure Care				
ACE Inhibitor or ARB for LVSD	90	97%	97%	97%
Discharge Instructions Given	318	95%	96%	94%
Evaluation of LVS Function	423	99%	100%	99%
Medicare Spending				
Medicare Spending per Patient (ratio)	-	1.09	1.01	0.98
Pneumonia Care				
Appropriate Initial Antibiotic Given	208	97%	96%	95%
Blood Culture Timing	436	100%	98%	98%
Pregnancy and Delivery Care				
Newborn Deliveries Scheduled Early[2]	29	10%	5%	6%
Preventive Care				
Immunization for Influenza[2]	585	93%	93%	90%
Immunization for Pneumonia[2]	770	90%	94%	92%
Stroke Care				
Anticoagulation Therapy for Atrial Fibrillation	28	100%	95%	95%
Antithrombotic Therapy Timing	148	99%	98%	98%
Assessed for Rehabilitation	160	100%	98%	97%
Discharged on Antithrombotic Therapy	150	99%	99%	99%
Discharged on Statin Medication	127	92%	95%	94%
Thrombolytic Therapy Timing[1]	-	-	65%	66%
Venous Thromboembolism Prophylaxis	163	99%	95%	94%
Written Stroke Educational Materials Given	64	89%	92%	88%
Surgical Care Improvement Project				
Appropriate Beta Blocker Usage[2]	270	97%	98%	98%
Appropriate VTP Within 24 Hours[2]	366	99%	98%	98%
Controlled Postoperative Blood Glucose[2]	87	93%	97%	97%
Perioperative Temperature Management[2]	544	100%	100%	100%
Prophylactic Antibiotic Selection[2]	398	99%	99%	99%
Prophylactic Antibiotic Selection (Outpatient)	308	96%	98%	98%
Prophylactic Antibiotic Stopped[2]	395	95%	98%	98%
Prophylactic Antibiotic Timing[2]	399	98%	99%	99%
Prophylactic Antibiotic Timing (Outpatient)	323	93%	97%	98%
Urinary Catheter Removal[2]	337	96%	97%	97%
Survey of Patients' Hospital Experiences				
Area Around Room 'Always' Quiet at Night[11]	300+	55%	58%	61%
Doctors 'Always' Communicated Well[11]	300+	76%	80%	82%
Home Recovery Information Given[11]	300+	87%	87%	85%
Hospital Given 9 or 10 on 10 Point Scale[11]	300+	62%	72%	71%
Meds 'Always' Explained Before Given[11]	300+	58%	64%	64%
Nurses 'Always' Communicated Well[11]	300+	75%	81%	79%
Pain 'Always' Well Controlled[11]	300+	67%	71%	71%
Room and Bathroom 'Always' Clean[11]	300+	74%	75%	73%
Timely Help 'Always' Received[11]	300+	62%	70%	68%
Would Definitely Recommend Hospital[11]	300+	62%	71%	71%
Use of Medical Imaging				
Cardiac Imaging Stress Test before Surgery	321	4.0%	5.4%	5.3%
Combination Abdominal CT Scan	1,202	2.7%	7.1%	10.5%
Combination Brain/Sinus CT Scan	955	2.0%	2.8%	2.7%
Combination Chest CT Scan	496	11.9%	1.7%	2.7%
Follow-up Mammogram/Ultrasound	2,141	7.1%	8.7%	8.8%
Lumbar Spine MRI for Low Back Pain	183	33.9%	34.7%	37.2%

Medcentral Health System Mansfield Hospital

335 Glessner Avenue
Mansfield, OH 44903
Phone: 419-526-8000
Fax: 419-521-7960
E-mail: medcentral@medcentral.org
URL: www.medcentral.org
Type: Acute Care Hospitals
Emergency Services: Yes
Ownership: Voluntary non-profit - Private
Beds: 398

Key Personnel:

Radiology. . . . . Terry Baker
Pediatric In-Patient Care . . . . Susan Brown
Infection Control. . . . . Liz DeHaan
Coronary Care . . . . Patti Kastelic
CEO/President. . . . . James E Meyer
Operating Room. . . . . Linda Nelson
Chief of Medical Staff. . . . . Terry Weston, MD
Quality Assurance . . . . Janene Yeater

Measure	Cases	This Hosp.	State Avg.	U.S. Avg.
Blood Clot Prevention and Treatment				
Anticoagulation Overlap Therapy[2]	58	98%	93%	93%
ICU Venous Thromboembolism Prophylaxis[2]	99	88%	93%	92%
Incidence of Potentially Preventable VTE[1,2]	-	-	6%	10%
UFH with Dosages/Platelet Monitoring[2]	57	100%	98%	97%
Venous Thromboembolism Prophylaxis[2]	488	80%	88%	85%
Warfarin Therapy Discharge Instructions[2]	43	81%	79%	75%
Chest Pain/Possible Heart Attack Care				
Aspirin Given Within 24 Hours of Arrival	36	78%	97%	96%
Fibrinolytic Meds Within 30 Min. of Arrival[3,7]	-	-	44%	58%
Average Time to ECG (minutes)	36	5	6	7
Average Time to Transfer (minutes)[1,3]	-	-	58	60
Children's Asthma Care				
Received Home Management Plan of Care	-	-	85%	88%
Received Reliever Medication	-	-	100%	100%
Received Systemic Corticosteroids	-	-	100%	100%
Emergency Department				
Admittance Decision Time (minutes)[2]	337	63	90	98
Head CT Results Within 45 Min. of Arrival	14	29%	63%	57%
Patients Who Left ER Before Being Seen	50,461	3%	2%	2%
Time from ER Arrival to Admit. (minutes)[2]	375	255	265	274
Time from ER Arrival to Discharge (minutes)	575	168	128	134
Time in ER Before Being Evaluated (minutes)	616	71	22	26
Time to Pain Meds for Fractures (minutes)	143	71	54	57
Heart Attack Care				
Aspirin Given at Discharge	302	98%	99%	99%
Fibrinolytic Meds Within 30 Min. of Arrival[7]	-	-	80%	54%
PCI Within 90 Minutes of Arrival	44	95%	97%	96%
Statin Prescribed at Discharge	302	90%	98%	98%
Heart Failure Care				
ACE Inhibitor or ARB for LVSD	90	91%	97%	97%
Discharge Instructions Given	220	97%	96%	94%
Evaluation of LVS Function	289	98%	100%	99%
Medicare Spending				
Medicare Spending per Patient (ratio)	-	1.06	1.01	0.98
Pneumonia Care				
Appropriate Initial Antibiotic Given	189	89%	96%	95%
Blood Culture Timing	360	97%	98%	98%
Pregnancy and Delivery Care				
Newborn Deliveries Scheduled Early	112	32%	5%	6%
Preventive Care				
Immunization for Influenza[2]	568	76%	93%	90%
Immunization for Pneumonia[2]	704	92%	94%	92%
Stroke Care				
Anticoagulation Therapy for Atrial Fibrillation	29	62%	95%	95%
Antithrombotic Therapy Timing	113	96%	98%	98%
Assessed for Rehabilitation	123	94%	98%	97%
Discharged on Antithrombotic Therapy	113	94%	99%	99%
Discharged on Statin Medication	100	82%	95%	94%
Thrombolytic Therapy Timing[1]	-	-	65%	66%
Venous Thromboembolism Prophylaxis	129	82%	95%	94%
Written Stroke Educational Materials Given	52	85%	92%	88%
Surgical Care Improvement Project				
Appropriate Beta Blocker Usage	353	97%	98%	98%
Appropriate VTP Within 24 Hours	550	97%	98%	98%
Controlled Postoperative Blood Glucose	219	100%	97%	97%
Perioperative Temperature Management	635	100%	100%	100%
Prophylactic Antibiotic Selection	629	97%	99%	99%
Prophylactic Antibiotic Selection (Outpatient)	320	97%	98%	98%
Prophylactic Antibiotic Stopped	615	98%	98%	98%
Prophylactic Antibiotic Timing	629	99%	99%	99%
Prophylactic Antibiotic Timing (Outpatient)	357	88%	97%	98%
Urinary Catheter Removal	384	93%	97%	97%
Survey of Patients' Hospital Experiences				
Area Around Room 'Always' Quiet at Night	300+	61%	58%	61%
Doctors 'Always' Communicated Well	300+	78%	80%	82%
Home Recovery Information Given	300+	85%	87%	85%
Hospital Given 9 or 10 on 10 Point Scale	300+	70%	72%	71%
Meds 'Always' Explained Before Given	300+	62%	64%	64%
Nurses 'Always' Communicated Well	300+	82%	81%	79%
Pain 'Always' Well Controlled	300+	74%	71%	71%
Room and Bathroom 'Always' Clean	300+	73%	75%	73%
Timely Help 'Always' Received	300+	72%	70%	68%
Would Definitely Recommend Hospital	300+	65%	71%	71%
Use of Medical Imaging				
Cardiac Imaging Stress Test before Surgery[1]	-	-	5.4%	5.3%
Combination Abdominal CT Scan	1,197	0.6%	7.1%	10.5%

NOTE: Hospital profiles are in alphabetical order by state, then city, then hospital within the city; Rankings exclude hospitals with less than 25 cases except for patient surveys which excludes hospitals with less than 100 cases; (a) 100-299 cases; (1) The number of cases/patients is too few to report; (2) Data submitted were based on a sample of cases/patients; (3) Results are based on a shorter time period than required; (4) Data suppressed by CMS for one or more quarters; (5) Results are not available for this reporting period; (6) Fewer than 100 patients completed the HCAHPS survey; (7) No cases met the criteria for this measure; (8) The lower limit of the confidence interval cannot be calculated if the number of observed infections equals zero; (9) No data are available from the state/territory for this reporting period; (10) The scores shown reflect fewer than 50 completed surveys; (11) There were discrepancies in the data collection process; (12) This measure does not apply to this hospital for this reporting period; (13) Results cannot be calculated for this reporting period; (14) The results for this state are combined with nearby states to protect confidentiality; Please refer to the User's Guide for a full explanation of data.

Combination Brain/Sinus CT Scan	1,137	3.1%	2.8%	2.7%
Combination Chest CT Scan	693	0.6%	1.7%	2.7%
Follow-up Mammogram/Ultrasound	1,702	9.9%	8.7%	8.8%
Lumbar Spine MRI for Low Back Pain	243	35.4%	34.7%	37.2%

Marietta Memorial Hospital

401 Matthew Street
Marietta, OH 45750
Phone: 740-374-1400
Fax: 740-376-5045
URL: www.mmhospital.org
Type: Acute Care Hospitals
Emergency Services: Yes
Ownership: Voluntary non-profit - Other
Beds: 204

Key Personnel:
Infection Control. . . . . Suzanne Baker
Radiology. . . . . Steve Boker, MD
Operating Room. . . . . Bradley Carman
Chief of Medical Staff. . . . . Joseph Cooper, MD
Quality Assurance . . . . Bonnie Flannery
Pediatric Ambulatory Care . . . . . . William Jacoby, MD
Pediatric In-Patient Care . . . . William Jacoby, MD
CEO/President. . . . . Larry Unroe

Measure	Cases	This Hosp.	State Avg.	U.S. Avg.
Blood Clot Prevention and Treatment				
Anticoagulation Overlap Therapy[2]	78	69%	93%	93%
ICU Venous Thromboembolism Prophylaxis[2]	77	91%	93%	92%
Incidence of Potentially Preventable VTE[2]	15	13%	6%	10%
UFH with Dosages/Platelet Monitoring[2]	39	100%	98%	97%
Venous Thromboembolism Prophylaxis[2]	333	74%	88%	85%
Warfarin Therapy Discharge Instructions[2]	62	100%	79%	75%
Chest Pain/Possible Heart Attack Care				
Aspirin Given Within 24 Hours of Arrival[3]	14	100%	97%	96%
Fibrinolytic Meds Within 30 Min. of Arrival[3,7]	-	-	44%	58%
Average Time to ECG (minutes)[3]	14	1	6	7
Average Time to Transfer (minutes)[1,3]	-	-	58	60
Children's Asthma Care				
Received Home Management Plan of Care	-	-	85%	88%
Received Reliever Medication	-	-	100%	100%
Received Systemic Corticosteroids	-	-	100%	100%
Emergency Department				
Admittance Decision Time (minutes)[2]	597	125	90	98
Head CT Results Within 45 Min. of Arrival	21	43%	63%	57%
Patients Who Left ER Before Being Seen	42,155	1%	2%	2%
Time from ER Arrival to Admit. (minutes)[2]	597	306	265	274
Time from ER Arrival to Discharge (minutes)	390	140	128	134
Time in ER Before Being Evaluated (minutes)	424	11	22	26
Time to Pain Meds for Fractures (minutes)	191	40	54	57
Heart Attack Care				
Aspirin Given at Discharge	151	99%	99%	99%
Fibrinolytic Meds Within 30 Min. of Arrival[7]	-	-	80%	54%
PCI Within 90 Minutes of Arrival	24	100%	97%	96%
Statin Prescribed at Discharge	146	98%	98%	98%
Heart Failure Care				
ACE Inhibitor or ARB for LVSD	62	100%	97%	97%
Discharge Instructions Given	189	96%	96%	94%
Evaluation of LVS Function	252	100%	100%	99%
Medicare Spending				
Medicare Spending per Patient (ratio)	-	1.03	1.01	0.98
Pneumonia Care				
Appropriate Initial Antibiotic Given[2]	82	99%	96%	95%
Blood Culture Timing[2]	142	99%	98%	98%
Pregnancy and Delivery Care				
Newborn Deliveries Scheduled Early	79	22%	5%	6%
Preventive Care				
Immunization for Influenza[2]	567	99%	93%	90%
Immunization for Pneumonia[2]	729	99%	94%	92%
Stroke Care				
Anticoagulation Therapy for Atrial Fibrillation	15	87%	95%	95%
Antithrombotic Therapy Timing	92	99%	98%	98%
Assessed for Rehabilitation	101	93%	98%	97%
Discharged on Antithrombotic Therapy	89	100%	99%	99%
Discharged on Statin Medication	82	82%	95%	94%
Thrombolytic Therapy Timing[1]	-	-	65%	66%
Venous Thromboembolism Prophylaxis	98	88%	95%	94%
Written Stroke Educational Materials Given	60	100%	92%	88%
Surgical Care Improvement Project				
Appropriate Beta Blocker Usage	119	94%	98%	98%
Appropriate VTP Within 24 Hours	393	99%	98%	98%
Controlled Postoperative Blood Glucose[7]	-	-	97%	97%
Perioperative Temperature Management	441	100%	100%	100%
Prophylactic Antibiotic Selection	242	97%	99%	99%
Prophylactic Antibiotic Selection (Outpatient)	260	98%	98%	98%
Prophylactic Antibiotic Stopped	224	97%	98%	98%
Prophylactic Antibiotic Timing	242	96%	99%	99%
Prophylactic Antibiotic Timing (Outpatient)	255	95%	97%	98%
Urinary Catheter Removal	126	98%	97%	97%
Survey of Patients' Hospital Experiences				
Area Around Room 'Always' Quiet at Night	300+	50%	58%	61%
Doctors 'Always' Communicated Well	300+	77%	80%	82%
Home Recovery Information Given	300+	88%	87%	85%
Hospital Given 9 or 10 on 10 Point Scale	300+	64%	72%	71%
Meds 'Always' Explained Before Given	300+	58%	64%	64%
Nurses 'Always' Communicated Well	300+	74%	81%	79%
Pain 'Always' Well Controlled	300+	66%	71%	71%
Room and Bathroom 'Always' Clean	300+	70%	75%	73%
Timely Help 'Always' Received	300+	63%	70%	68%
Would Definitely Recommend Hospital	300+	65%	71%	71%
Use of Medical Imaging				
Cardiac Imaging Stress Test before Surgery	593	3.9%	5.4%	5.3%
Combination Abdominal CT Scan	1,563	8.8%	7.1%	10.5%
Combination Brain/Sinus CT Scan	1,045	6.6%	2.8%	2.7%
Combination Chest CT Scan	1,104	7.6%	1.7%	2.7%
Follow-up Mammogram/Ultrasound	1,999	5.8%	8.7%	8.8%
Lumbar Spine MRI for Low Back Pain	410	33.9%	34.7%	37.2%

Selby General Hospital

1106 Colegate Drive
Marietta, OH 45750
Phone: 740-568-2000
Fax: 740-568-2089
E-mail: ceo@selbygeneralhospital.com
URL: www.selbygeneralhospital.con
Type: Critical Access Hospitals
Emergency Services: Yes
Ownership: Voluntary non-profit - Private
Beds: 80

Key Personnel:
CEO/President. . . . . Kevin P Calhoun
Anesthesiology. . . . . Joseph Castle DO
Operating Room. . . . . Nancy Chandler
Emergency Room . . . . James Conde
Chief of Medical Staff. . . . . Charles Merrill
Intensive Care Unit. . . . . Angela Saffell, RN

Measure	Cases	This Hosp.	State Avg.	U.S. Avg.
Blood Clot Prevention and Treatment				
Anticoagulation Overlap Therapy[1,3]	-	-	93%	93%
ICU Venous Thromboembolism Prophylaxis[3,7]	-	-	93%	92%
Incidence of Potentially Preventable VTE[3,7]	-	-	6%	10%
UFH with Dosages/Platelet Monitoring[3,7]	-	-	98%	97%
Venous Thromboembolism Prophylaxis[3,7]	-	-	88%	85%
Warfarin Therapy Discharge Instructions[1,3]	-	-	79%	75%
Chest Pain/Possible Heart Attack Care				
Aspirin Given Within 24 Hours of Arrival[5]	-	-	97%	96%
Fibrinolytic Meds Within 30 Min. of Arrival[5]	-	-	44%	58%
Average Time to ECG (minutes)[5]	-	-	6	7
Average Time to Transfer (minutes)[5]	-	-	58	60
Children's Asthma Care				
Received Home Management Plan of Care	-	-	85%	88%
Received Reliever Medication	-	-	100%	100%
Received Systemic Corticosteroids	-	-	100%	100%
Emergency Department				
Admittance Decision Time (minutes)[5]	-	-	90	98
Head CT Results Within 45 Min. of Arrival[5]	-	-	63%	57%
Patients Who Left ER Before Being Seen[5]	-	-	2%	2%
Time from ER Arrival to Admit. (minutes)[5]	-	-	265	274
Time from ER Arrival to Discharge (minutes)	1,082	93	128	134
Time in ER Before Being Evaluated (minutes)	1,091	10	22	26
Time to Pain Meds for Fractures (minutes)[5]	-	-	54	57
Heart Attack Care				
Aspirin Given at Discharge[1,3]	-	-	99%	99%
Fibrinolytic Meds Within 30 Min. of Arrival[1,3]	-	-	80%	54%
PCI Within 90 Minutes of Arrival[3,7]	-	-	97%	96%
Statin Prescribed at Discharge[1,3]	-	-	98%	98%
Heart Failure Care				
ACE Inhibitor or ARB for LVSD[1]	-	-	97%	97%
Discharge Instructions Given	16	100%	96%	94%
Evaluation of LVS Function	16	100%	100%	99%
Medicare Spending				
Medicare Spending per Patient (ratio)	-	-	1.01	0.98
Pneumonia Care				
Appropriate Initial Antibiotic Given	21	71%	96%	95%
Blood Culture Timing	25	92%	98%	98%
Pregnancy and Delivery Care				
Newborn Deliveries Scheduled Early[3,7]	-	-	5%	6%
Preventive Care				
Immunization for Influenza[5]	-	-	93%	90%
Immunization for Pneumonia[5]	-	-	94%	92%
Stroke Care				
Anticoagulation Therapy for Atrial Fibrillation[3,7]	-	-	95%	95%
Antithrombotic Therapy Timing[3,7]	-	-	98%	98%
Assessed for Rehabilitation[1,3]	-	-	98%	97%
Discharged on Antithrombotic Therapy[3,7]	-	-	99%	99%
Discharged on Statin Medication[1,3]	-	-	95%	94%
Thrombolytic Therapy Timing[3,7]	-	-	65%	66%
Venous Thromboembolism Prophylaxis[1,3]	-	-	95%	94%
Written Stroke Educational Materials Given[1,3]	-	-	92%	88%
Surgical Care Improvement Project				
Appropriate Beta Blocker Usage[2]	113	100%	98%	98%
Appropriate VTP Within 24 Hours[2]	369	99%	98%	98%
Controlled Postoperative Blood Glucose[2,7]	-	-	97%	97%
Perioperative Temperature Management[2]	398	100%	100%	100%
Prophylactic Antibiotic Selection[2]	373	99%	99%	99%
Prophylactic Antibiotic Selection (Outpatient)[5]	-	-	98%	98%
Prophylactic Antibiotic Stopped[2]	367	98%	98%	98%
Prophylactic Antibiotic Timing[2]	373	95%	99%	99%
Prophylactic Antibiotic Timing (Outpatient)[5]	-	-	97%	98%
Urinary Catheter Removal[2]	244	99%	97%	97%
Survey of Patients' Hospital Experiences				
Area Around Room 'Always' Quiet at Night	300+	56%	58%	61%
Doctors 'Always' Communicated Well	300+	81%	80%	82%
Home Recovery Information Given	300+	89%	87%	85%
Hospital Given 9 or 10 on 10 Point Scale	300+	72%	72%	71%
Meds 'Always' Explained Before Given	300+	62%	64%	64%
Nurses 'Always' Communicated Well	300+	81%	81%	79%
Pain 'Always' Well Controlled	300+	68%	71%	71%
Room and Bathroom 'Always' Clean	300+	80%	75%	73%
Timely Help 'Always' Received	300+	75%	70%	68%
Would Definitely Recommend Hospital	300+	75%	71%	71%
Use of Medical Imaging				
Cardiac Imaging Stress Test before Surgery[1]	-	-	5.4%	5.3%
Combination Abdominal CT Scan	138	4.3%	7.1%	10.5%
Combination Brain/Sinus CT Scan[1]	-	-	2.8%	2.7%
Combination Chest CT Scan[1]	-	-	1.7%	2.7%
Follow-up Mammogram/Ultrasound[7]	-	-	8.7%	8.8%
Lumbar Spine MRI for Low Back Pain[1]	-	-	34.7%	37.2%

Marion General Hospital

1000 Mckinley Park Drive
Marion, OH 43302
Phone: 740-383-8400
URL: www.mariongeneral.com
Type: Acute Care Hospitals
Emergency Services: Yes
Ownership: Voluntary non-profit - Private

Key Personnel:
Chief of Medical Staff. . . . . Aaron M Fritz DO

Measure	Cases	This Hosp.	State Avg.	U.S. Avg.
Blood Clot Prevention and Treatment				
Anticoagulation Overlap Therapy[2]	57	95%	93%	93%
ICU Venous Thromboembolism Prophylaxis[2]	72	88%	93%	92%
Incidence of Potentially Preventable VTE[1,2]	-	-	6%	10%
UFH with Dosages/Platelet Monitoring[2]	23	100%	98%	97%
Venous Thromboembolism Prophylaxis[2]	283	77%	88%	85%
Warfarin Therapy Discharge Instructions[2]	41	80%	79%	75%
Chest Pain/Possible Heart Attack Care				
Aspirin Given Within 24 Hours of Arrival	29	100%	97%	96%
Fibrinolytic Meds Within 30 Min. of Arrival[7]	-	-	44%	58%
Average Time to ECG (minutes)	29	3	6	7
Average Time to Transfer (minutes)[1]	-	-	58	60

NOTE: Hospital profiles are in alphabetical order by state, then city, then hospital within the city; Rankings exclude hospitals with less than 25 cases except for patient surveys which excludes hospitals with less than 100 cases; (a) 100-299 cases; (1) The number of cases/patients is too few to report; (2) Data submitted were based on a sample of cases/patients; (3) Results are based on a shorter time period than required; (4) Data suppressed by CMS for one or more quarters; (5) Results are not available for this reporting period; (6) Fewer than 100 patients completed the HCAHPS survey; (7) No cases met the criteria for this measure; (8) The lower limit of the confidence interval cannot be calculated if the number of observed infections equals zero; (9) No data are available from the state/territory for this reporting period; (10) The scores shown reflect fewer than 50 completed surveys; (11) There were discrepancies in the data collection process; (12) This measure does not apply to this hospital for this reporting period; (13) Results cannot be calculated for this reporting period; (14) The results for this state are combined with nearby states to protect confidentiality; Please refer to the User's Guide for a full explanation of data.

Measure	Cases	This Hosp.	State Avg.	U.S. Avg.
Children's Asthma Care				
Received Home Management Plan of Care	-	-	85%	88%
Received Reliever Medication	-	-	100%	100%
Received Systemic Corticosteroids	-	-	100%	100%
Emergency Department				
Admittance Decision Time (minutes)[2]	517	68	90	98
Head CT Results Within 45 Min. of Arrival	46	93%	63%	57%
Patients Who Left ER Before Being Seen	50,286	1%	2%	2%
Time from ER Arrival to Admit. (minutes)[2]	517	219	265	274
Time from ER Arrival to Discharge (minutes)	361	113	128	134
Time in ER Before Being Evaluated (minutes)	419	19	22	26
Time to Pain Meds for Fractures (minutes)	157	49	54	57
Heart Attack Care				
Aspirin Given at Discharge	204	100%	99%	99%
Fibrinolytic Meds Within 30 Min. of Arrival[7]	-	-	80%	54%
PCI Within 90 Minutes of Arrival	38	100%	97%	96%
Statin Prescribed at Discharge	193	99%	98%	98%
Heart Failure Care				
ACE Inhibitor or ARB for LVSD	61	100%	97%	97%
Discharge Instructions Given	182	97%	96%	94%
Evaluation of LVS Function	231	100%	100%	99%
Medicare Spending				
Medicare Spending per Patient (ratio)	-	0.98	1.01	0.98
Pneumonia Care				
Appropriate Initial Antibiotic Given	123	98%	96%	95%
Blood Culture Timing	214	100%	98%	98%
Pregnancy and Delivery Care				
Newborn Deliveries Scheduled Early	85	2%	5%	6%
Preventive Care				
Immunization for Influenza[2]	539	98%	93%	90%
Immunization for Pneumonia[2]	713	98%	94%	92%
Stroke Care				
Anticoagulation Therapy for Atrial Fibrillation[1]	-	-	95%	95%
Antithrombotic Therapy Timing	34	100%	98%	98%
Assessed for Rehabilitation	39	100%	98%	97%
Discharged on Antithrombotic Therapy	39	100%	99%	99%
Discharged on Statin Medication	30	100%	95%	94%
Thrombolytic Therapy Timing[7]	-	-	65%	66%
Venous Thromboembolism Prophylaxis	33	94%	95%	94%
Written Stroke Educational Materials Given	22	100%	92%	88%
Surgical Care Improvement Project				
Appropriate Beta Blocker Usage[2]	137	100%	98%	98%
Appropriate VTP Within 24 Hours[2]	323	100%	98%	98%
Controlled Postoperative Blood Glucose[2]	29	100%	97%	97%
Perioperative Temperature Management[2]	372	100%	100%	100%
Prophylactic Antibiotic Selection[2]	294	100%	99%	99%
Prophylactic Antibiotic Selection (Outpatient)	159	100%	98%	98%
Prophylactic Antibiotic Stopped[2]	289	100%	98%	98%
Prophylactic Antibiotic Timing[2]	294	100%	99%	99%
Prophylactic Antibiotic Timing (Outpatient)	162	98%	97%	98%
Urinary Catheter Removal[2]	234	100%	97%	97%
Survey of Patients' Hospital Experiences				
Area Around Room 'Always' Quiet at Night	300+	58%	58%	61%
Doctors 'Always' Communicated Well	300+	80%	80%	82%
Home Recovery Information Given	300+	87%	87%	85%
Hospital Given 9 or 10 on 10 Point Scale	300+	67%	72%	71%
Meds 'Always' Explained Before Given	300+	66%	64%	64%
Nurses 'Always' Communicated Well	300+	80%	81%	79%
Pain 'Always' Well Controlled	300+	69%	71%	71%
Room and Bathroom 'Always' Clean	300+	75%	75%	73%
Timely Help 'Always' Received	300+	67%	70%	68%
Would Definitely Recommend Hospital	300+	65%	71%	71%
Use of Medical Imaging				
Cardiac Imaging Stress Test before Surgery	70	2.9%	5.4%	5.3%
Combination Abdominal CT Scan	618	5.2%	7.1%	10.5%
Combination Brain/Sinus CT Scan	602	0.2%	2.8%	2.7%
Combination Chest CT Scan	182	0.0%	1.7%	2.7%
Follow-up Mammogram/Ultrasound	841	9.9%	8.7%	8.8%
Lumbar Spine MRI for Low Back Pain	71	25.4%	34.7%	37.2%

East Ohio Regional Hospital

90 North Fourth Street
Martins Ferry, OH 43935
URL: www.eastohioregionalhospital.com
Type: Acute Care Hospitals
Ownership: Voluntary non-profit - Other

Phone: 740-633-4151
Fax: 740-633-4512
Emergency Services: Yes
Beds: 250

Measure	Cases	This Hosp.	State Avg.	U.S. Avg.
Blood Clot Prevention and Treatment				
Anticoagulation Overlap Therapy[2]	31	94%	93%	93%
ICU Venous Thromboembolism Prophylaxis[2]	66	71%	93%	92%
Incidence of Potentially Preventable VTE[1,2]	-	-	6%	10%
UFH with Dosages/Platelet Monitoring[2]	36	100%	98%	97%
Venous Thromboembolism Prophylaxis[2]	319	64%	88%	85%
Warfarin Therapy Discharge Instructions[2]	19	58%	79%	75%
Chest Pain/Possible Heart Attack Care				
Aspirin Given Within 24 Hours of Arrival	21	100%	97%	96%
Fibrinolytic Meds Within 30 Min. of Arrival[7]	-	-	44%	58%
Average Time to ECG (minutes)	21	5	6	7
Average Time to Transfer (minutes)	11	71	58	60
Children's Asthma Care				
Received Home Management Plan of Care	-	-	85%	88%
Received Reliever Medication	-	-	100%	100%
Received Systemic Corticosteroids	-	-	100%	100%
Emergency Department				
Admittance Decision Time (minutes)[2]	760	71	90	98
Head CT Results Within 45 Min. of Arrival	14	50%	63%	57%
Patients Who Left ER Before Being Seen	21,328	2%	2%	2%
Time from ER Arrival to Admit. (minutes)[2]	808	226	265	274
Time from ER Arrival to Discharge (minutes)	368	98	128	134
Time in ER Before Being Evaluated (minutes)	400	24	22	26
Time to Pain Meds for Fractures (minutes)	65	40	54	57
Heart Attack Care				
Aspirin Given at Discharge	42	98%	99%	99%
Fibrinolytic Meds Within 30 Min. of Arrival[7]	-	-	80%	54%
PCI Within 90 Minutes of Arrival[7]	-	-	97%	96%
Statin Prescribed at Discharge	39	92%	98%	98%
Heart Failure Care				
ACE Inhibitor or ARB for LVSD	29	83%	97%	97%
Discharge Instructions Given	94	99%	96%	94%
Evaluation of LVS Function	144	99%	100%	99%
Medicare Spending				
Medicare Spending per Patient (ratio)	-	1.06	1.01	0.98
Pneumonia Care				
Appropriate Initial Antibiotic Given	126	88%	96%	95%
Blood Culture Timing	156	94%	98%	98%
Pregnancy and Delivery Care				
Newborn Deliveries Scheduled Early	43	19%	5%	6%
Preventive Care				
Immunization for Influenza[2]	935	87%	93%	90%
Immunization for Pneumonia[2]	905	94%	94%	92%
Stroke Care				
Anticoagulation Therapy for Atrial Fibrillation[1]	-	-	95%	95%
Antithrombotic Therapy Timing	24	50%	98%	98%
Assessed for Rehabilitation	27	89%	98%	97%
Discharged on Antithrombotic Therapy	23	43%	99%	99%
Discharged on Statin Medication	23	61%	95%	94%
Thrombolytic Therapy Timing[1]	-	-	65%	66%
Venous Thromboembolism Prophylaxis	33	58%	95%	94%
Written Stroke Educational Materials Given	11	36%	92%	88%
Surgical Care Improvement Project				
Appropriate Beta Blocker Usage	107	100%	98%	98%
Appropriate VTP Within 24 Hours	282	96%	98%	98%
Controlled Postoperative Blood Glucose[7]	-	-	97%	97%
Perioperative Temperature Management	313	99%	100%	100%
Prophylactic Antibiotic Selection	281	99%	99%	99%
Prophylactic Antibiotic Selection (Outpatient)	18	100%	98%	98%
Prophylactic Antibiotic Stopped	276	97%	98%	98%
Prophylactic Antibiotic Timing	281	98%	99%	99%
Prophylactic Antibiotic Timing (Outpatient)	19	89%	97%	98%
Urinary Catheter Removal	278	97%	97%	97%
Survey of Patients' Hospital Experiences				
Area Around Room 'Always' Quiet at Night	300+	50%	58%	61%
Doctors 'Always' Communicated Well	300+	77%	80%	82%
Home Recovery Information Given	300+	82%	87%	85%
Hospital Given 9 or 10 on 10 Point Scale	300+	62%	72%	71%
Meds 'Always' Explained Before Given	300+	65%	64%	64%
Nurses 'Always' Communicated Well	300+	76%	81%	79%
Pain 'Always' Well Controlled	300+	68%	71%	71%
Room and Bathroom 'Always' Clean	300+	77%	75%	73%
Timely Help 'Always' Received	300+	61%	70%	68%
Would Definitely Recommend Hospital	300+	62%	71%	71%
Use of Medical Imaging				
Cardiac Imaging Stress Test before Surgery	98	6.1%	5.4%	5.3%
Combination Abdominal CT Scan	306	58.2%	7.1%	10.5%
Combination Brain/Sinus CT Scan[1]	-	-	2.8%	2.7%
Combination Chest CT Scan	212	0.0%	1.7%	2.7%
Follow-up Mammogram/Ultrasound	543	19.0%	8.7%	8.8%
Lumbar Spine MRI for Low Back Pain	53	30.2%	34.7%	37.2%

Memorial Hospital of Union County

500 London Avenue
Marysville, OH 43040
Type: Acute Care Hospitals
Ownership: Government - Local

Phone: 937-578-2289
Fax: 937-578-2806
Emergency Services: Yes
Beds: 82

Key Personnel:
Chief of Medical Staff. . . . . David T Applegate, MD
Infection Control. . . . . Filiberto Cavazos, MD
Operating Room. . . . . Karen Hall, RN
CEO/President. . . . . Olas A Hubbs, III
Emergency Room . . . . Sharon Walls, RN
Intensive Care Unit. . . . . Sharon Walls, RN
Quality Assurance . . . . Laurie Whittington

Measure	Cases	This Hosp.	State Avg.	U.S. Avg.
Blood Clot Prevention and Treatment				
Anticoagulation Overlap Therapy[2]	13	100%	93%	93%
ICU Venous Thromboembolism Prophylaxis[2]	36	97%	93%	92%
Incidence of Potentially Preventable VTE[1,2]	-	-	6%	10%
UFH with Dosages/Platelet Monitoring[1,2]	-	-	98%	97%
Venous Thromboembolism Prophylaxis[2]	108	94%	88%	85%
Warfarin Therapy Discharge Instructions[1,2]	-	-	79%	75%
Chest Pain/Possible Heart Attack Care				
Aspirin Given Within 24 Hours of Arrival	129	100%	97%	96%
Fibrinolytic Meds Within 30 Min. of Arrival[1]	-	-	44%	58%
Average Time to ECG (minutes)	130	7	6	7
Average Time to Transfer (minutes)	23	49	58	60
Children's Asthma Care				
Received Home Management Plan of Care	-	-	85%	88%
Received Reliever Medication	-	-	100%	100%
Received Systemic Corticosteroids	-	-	100%	100%
Emergency Department				
Admittance Decision Time (minutes)[2]	159	56	90	98
Head CT Results Within 45 Min. of Arrival	15	53%	63%	57%
Patients Who Left ER Before Being Seen	20,531	3%	2%	2%
Time from ER Arrival to Admit. (minutes)[2]	164	270	265	274
Time from ER Arrival to Discharge (minutes)	357	164	128	134
Time in ER Before Being Evaluated (minutes)	337	34	22	26
Time to Pain Meds for Fractures (minutes)	107	62	54	57
Heart Attack Care				
Aspirin Given at Discharge[1]	-	-	99%	99%
Fibrinolytic Meds Within 30 Min. of Arrival[7]	-	-	80%	54%
PCI Within 90 Minutes of Arrival[7]	-	-	97%	96%
Statin Prescribed at Discharge[1]	-	-	98%	98%
Heart Failure Care				
ACE Inhibitor or ARB for LVSD	20	95%	97%	97%
Discharge Instructions Given	51	98%	96%	94%
Evaluation of LVS Function	70	100%	100%	99%
Medicare Spending				
Medicare Spending per Patient (ratio)	-	0.99	1.01	0.98
Pneumonia Care				
Appropriate Initial Antibiotic Given	44	95%	96%	95%
Blood Culture Timing	72	99%	98%	98%
Pregnancy and Delivery Care				
Newborn Deliveries Scheduled Early	69	1%	5%	6%
Preventive Care				
Immunization for Influenza[2]	251	91%	93%	90%
Immunization for Pneumonia[2]	254	93%	94%	92%

NOTE: Hospital profiles are in alphabetical order by state, then city, then hospital within the city; Rankings exclude hospitals with less than 25 cases except for patient surveys which excludes hospitals with less than 100 cases; (a) 100-299 cases; (1) The number of cases/patients is too few to report; (2) Data submitted were based on a sample of cases/patients; (3) Results are based on a shorter time period than required; (4) Data suppressed by CMS for one or more quarters; (5) Results are not available for this reporting period; (6) Fewer than 100 patients completed the HCAHPS survey; (7) No cases met the criteria for this measure; (8) The lower limit of the confidence interval cannot be calculated if the number of observed infections equals zero; (9) No data are available from the state/territory for this reporting period; (10) The scores shown reflect fewer than 50 completed surveys; (11) There were discrepancies in the data collection process; (12) This measure does not apply to this hospital for this reporting period; (13) Results cannot be calculated for this reporting period; (14) The results for this state are combined with nearby states to protect confidentiality; Please refer to the User's Guide for a full explanation of data.

Measure	Cases	This Hosp.	State Avg.	U.S. Avg.
Stroke Care				
Anticoagulation Therapy for Atrial Fibrillation[7]	-	-	95%	95%
Antithrombotic Therapy Timing[1]	-	-	98%	98%
Assessed for Rehabilitation[1]	-	-	98%	97%
Discharged on Antithrombotic Therapy[1]	-	-	99%	99%
Discharged on Statin Medication[1]	-	-	95%	94%
Thrombolytic Therapy Timing[7]	-	-	65%	66%
Venous Thromboembolism Prophylaxis[1]	-	-	95%	94%
Written Stroke Educational Materials Given[1]	-	-	92%	88%
Surgical Care Improvement Project				
Appropriate Beta Blocker Usage	39	97%	98%	98%
Appropriate VTP Within 24 Hours	110	95%	98%	98%
Controlled Postoperative Blood Glucose[7]	-	-	97%	97%
Perioperative Temperature Management	115	100%	100%	100%
Prophylactic Antibiotic Selection	92	96%	99%	99%
Prophylactic Antibiotic Selection (Outpatient)	87	99%	98%	98%
Prophylactic Antibiotic Stopped	90	96%	98%	98%
Prophylactic Antibiotic Timing	92	96%	99%	99%
Prophylactic Antibiotic Timing (Outpatient)	64	97%	97%	98%
Urinary Catheter Removal	70	93%	97%	97%
Survey of Patients' Hospital Experiences				
Area Around Room 'Always' Quiet at Night	300+	65%	58%	61%
Doctors 'Always' Communicated Well	300+	81%	80%	82%
Home Recovery Information Given	300+	89%	87%	85%
Hospital Given 9 or 10 on 10 Point Scale	300+	78%	72%	71%
Meds 'Always' Explained Before Given	300+	67%	64%	64%
Nurses 'Always' Communicated Well	300+	83%	81%	79%
Pain 'Always' Well Controlled	300+	74%	71%	71%
Room and Bathroom 'Always' Clean	300+	74%	75%	73%
Timely Help 'Always' Received	300+	76%	70%	68%
Would Definitely Recommend Hospital	300+	76%	71%	71%
Use of Medical Imaging				
Cardiac Imaging Stress Test before Surgery	136	10.3%	5.4%	5.3%
Combination Abdominal CT Scan	376	2.4%	7.1%	10.5%
Combination Brain/Sinus CT Scan	303	1.3%	2.8%	2.7%
Combination Chest CT Scan	185	0.0%	1.7%	2.7%
Follow-up Mammogram/Ultrasound	409	12.0%	8.7%	8.8%
Lumbar Spine MRI for Low Back Pain[1]	-	-	34.7%	37.2%

Affinity Medical Center

875 Eighth Street Ne
Massillon, OH 44646
Phone: 330-837-6863
URL: www.affinitymedicalcenter.com
Type: Acute Care Hospitals
Emergency Services: Yes
Ownership: Proprietary
Beds: 451
Key Personnel:
CEO/President. . . . . Wendy Meighen

Measure	Cases	This Hosp.	State Avg.	U.S. Avg.
Blood Clot Prevention and Treatment				
Anticoagulation Overlap Therapy[2]	55	98%	93%	93%
ICU Venous Thromboembolism Prophylaxis[2]	181	95%	93%	92%
Incidence of Potentially Preventable VTE[1,2]	-	-	6%	10%
UFH with Dosages/Platelet Monitoring[2]	52	100%	98%	97%
Venous Thromboembolism Prophylaxis[2]	305	88%	88%	85%
Warfarin Therapy Discharge Instructions[2]	35	74%	79%	75%
Chest Pain/Possible Heart Attack Care				
Aspirin Given Within 24 Hours of Arrival[1,3]	-	-	97%	96%
Fibrinolytic Meds Within 30 Min. of Arrival[3,7]	-	-	44%	58%
Average Time to ECG (minutes)[1,3]	-	-	6	7
Average Time to Transfer (minutes)[3,7]	-	-	58	60
Children's Asthma Care				
Received Home Management Plan of Care	-	-	85%	88%
Received Reliever Medication	-	-	100%	100%
Received Systemic Corticosteroids	-	-	100%	100%
Emergency Department				
Admittance Decision Time (minutes)[2]	667	81	90	98
Head CT Results Within 45 Min. of Arrival[1]	-	-	63%	57%
Patients Who Left ER Before Being Seen	27,418	2%	2%	2%
Time from ER Arrival to Admit. (minutes)[2]	709	299	265	274
Time from ER Arrival to Discharge (minutes)	386	176	128	134
Time in ER Before Being Evaluated (minutes)	402	41	22	26
Time to Pain Meds for Fractures (minutes)	135	67	54	57
Heart Attack Care				
Aspirin Given at Discharge	106	99%	99%	99%
Fibrinolytic Meds Within 30 Min. of Arrival[7]	-	-	80%	54%
PCI Within 90 Minutes of Arrival	36	97%	97%	96%
Statin Prescribed at Discharge	102	99%	98%	98%
Heart Failure Care				
ACE Inhibitor or ARB for LVSD	56	100%	97%	97%
Discharge Instructions Given	134	85%	96%	94%
Evaluation of LVS Function	185	100%	100%	99%
Medicare Spending				
Medicare Spending per Patient (ratio)	-	1.04	1.01	0.98
Pneumonia Care				
Appropriate Initial Antibiotic Given	114	96%	96%	95%
Blood Culture Timing	219	99%	98%	98%
Pregnancy and Delivery Care				
Newborn Deliveries Scheduled Early[7]	-	-	5%	6%
Preventive Care				
Immunization for Influenza[2]	565	100%	93%	90%
Immunization for Pneumonia[2]	842	93%	94%	92%
Stroke Care				
Anticoagulation Therapy for Atrial Fibrillation[1]	-	-	95%	95%
Antithrombotic Therapy Timing	54	100%	98%	98%
Assessed for Rehabilitation	56	93%	98%	97%
Discharged on Antithrombotic Therapy	52	100%	99%	99%
Discharged on Statin Medication	40	82%	95%	94%
Thrombolytic Therapy Timing[1]	-	-	65%	66%
Venous Thromboembolism Prophylaxis	54	91%	95%	94%
Written Stroke Educational Materials Given	23	35%	92%	88%
Surgical Care Improvement Project				
Appropriate Beta Blocker Usage	300	98%	98%	98%
Appropriate VTP Within 24 Hours	445	99%	98%	98%
Controlled Postoperative Blood Glucose	204	100%	97%	97%
Perioperative Temperature Management	555	100%	100%	100%
Prophylactic Antibiotic Selection	570	100%	99%	99%
Prophylactic Antibiotic Selection (Outpatient)	135	100%	98%	98%
Prophylactic Antibiotic Stopped	554	97%	98%	98%
Prophylactic Antibiotic Timing	570	99%	99%	99%
Prophylactic Antibiotic Timing (Outpatient)	136	97%	97%	98%
Urinary Catheter Removal	533	99%	97%	97%
Survey of Patients' Hospital Experiences				
Area Around Room 'Always' Quiet at Night	300+	53%	58%	61%
Doctors 'Always' Communicated Well	300+	79%	80%	82%
Home Recovery Information Given	300+	87%	87%	85%
Hospital Given 9 or 10 on 10 Point Scale	300+	65%	72%	71%
Meds 'Always' Explained Before Given	300+	57%	64%	64%
Nurses 'Always' Communicated Well	300+	76%	81%	79%
Pain 'Always' Well Controlled	300+	67%	71%	71%
Room and Bathroom 'Always' Clean	300+	67%	75%	73%
Timely Help 'Always' Received	300+	60%	70%	68%
Would Definitely Recommend Hospital	300+	65%	71%	71%
Use of Medical Imaging				
Cardiac Imaging Stress Test before Surgery	144	5.6%	5.4%	5.3%
Combination Abdominal CT Scan	433	3.7%	7.1%	10.5%
Combination Brain/Sinus CT Scan	488	6.1%	2.8%	2.7%
Combination Chest CT Scan	177	0.0%	1.7%	2.7%
Follow-up Mammogram/Ultrasound	565	10.4%	8.7%	8.8%
Lumbar Spine MRI for Low Back Pain[1]	-	-	34.7%	37.2%

Saint Luke's Hospital

5901 Monclova Road
Maumee, OH 43537
Phone: 419-893-5900
Fax: 419-891-8079
URL: www.stlukeshospital.com
Type: Acute Care Hospitals
Emergency Services: Yes
Ownership: Voluntary non-profit - Other
Beds: 314
Key Personnel:
CEO/President. . . . . Frank J Bartell, III
Chief of Medical Staff. . . . . Stephen Bazelay, MD
Operating Room. . . . . Nadine Forton
Coronary Care . . . . Caroyln Gbur
Emergency Room . . . . Cheryl Herr
Quality Assurance . . . . Betsy Woodring
Pediatric Ambulatory Care . . . . . . Ursula Xanthakos, MD
Pediatric In-Patient Care . . . . Ursula Xanthakos, MD

Measure	Cases	This Hosp.	State Avg.	U.S. Avg.
Blood Clot Prevention and Treatment				
Anticoagulation Overlap Therapy[2]	93	97%	93%	93%
ICU Venous Thromboembolism Prophylaxis[2]	41	88%	93%	92%
Incidence of Potentially Preventable VTE[2]	26	8%	6%	10%
UFH with Dosages/Platelet Monitoring[2]	71	100%	98%	97%
Venous Thromboembolism Prophylaxis[2]	346	80%	88%	85%
Warfarin Therapy Discharge Instructions[2]	66	100%	79%	75%
Chest Pain/Possible Heart Attack Care				
Aspirin Given Within 24 Hours of Arrival[1,3]	-	-	97%	96%
Fibrinolytic Meds Within 30 Min. of Arrival[5]	-	-	44%	58%
Average Time to ECG (minutes)[1,3]	-	-	6	7
Average Time to Transfer (minutes)[5]	-	-	58	60
Children's Asthma Care				
Received Home Management Plan of Care	-	-	85%	88%
Received Reliever Medication	-	-	100%	100%
Received Systemic Corticosteroids	-	-	100%	100%
Emergency Department				
Admittance Decision Time (minutes)[2]	714	80	90	98
Head CT Results Within 45 Min. of Arrival[1]	-	-	63%	57%
Patients Who Left ER Before Being Seen	38,428	1%	2%	2%
Time from ER Arrival to Admit. (minutes)[2]	714	293	265	274
Time from ER Arrival to Discharge (minutes)	460	168	128	134
Time in ER Before Being Evaluated (minutes)	499	42	22	26
Time to Pain Meds for Fractures (minutes)	208	76	54	57
Heart Attack Care				
Aspirin Given at Discharge	310	100%	99%	99%
Fibrinolytic Meds Within 30 Min. of Arrival[7]	-	-	80%	54%
PCI Within 90 Minutes of Arrival	45	100%	97%	96%
Statin Prescribed at Discharge	302	99%	98%	98%
Heart Failure Care				
ACE Inhibitor or ARB for LVSD	94	98%	97%	97%
Discharge Instructions Given	223	98%	96%	94%
Evaluation of LVS Function	271	100%	100%	99%
Medicare Spending				
Medicare Spending per Patient (ratio)	-	0.97	1.01	0.98
Pneumonia Care				
Appropriate Initial Antibiotic Given[2]	89	91%	96%	95%
Blood Culture Timing[2]	143	93%	98%	98%
Pregnancy and Delivery Care				
Newborn Deliveries Scheduled Early[2]	134	2%	5%	6%
Preventive Care				
Immunization for Influenza[2]	586	92%	93%	90%
Immunization for Pneumonia[2]	791	93%	94%	92%
Stroke Care				
Anticoagulation Therapy for Atrial Fibrillation[1]	-	-	95%	95%
Antithrombotic Therapy Timing	60	100%	98%	98%
Assessed for Rehabilitation	63	98%	98%	97%
Discharged on Antithrombotic Therapy	63	100%	99%	99%
Discharged on Statin Medication	53	96%	95%	94%
Thrombolytic Therapy Timing[7]	-	-	65%	66%
Venous Thromboembolism Prophylaxis	64	86%	95%	94%
Written Stroke Educational Materials Given	48	85%	92%	88%
Surgical Care Improvement Project				
Appropriate Beta Blocker Usage[2]	244	100%	98%	98%
Appropriate VTP Within 24 Hours[2]	395	97%	98%	98%
Controlled Postoperative Blood Glucose[2]	125	98%	97%	97%
Perioperative Temperature Management[2]	500	100%	100%	100%
Prophylactic Antibiotic Selection[2]	444	100%	99%	99%
Prophylactic Antibiotic Selection (Outpatient)	370	98%	98%	98%
Prophylactic Antibiotic Stopped[2]	443	99%	98%	98%
Prophylactic Antibiotic Timing[2]	445	99%	99%	99%
Prophylactic Antibiotic Timing (Outpatient)	381	95%	97%	98%
Urinary Catheter Removal[2]	202	99%	97%	97%
Survey of Patients' Hospital Experiences				
Area Around Room 'Always' Quiet at Night	300+	57%	58%	61%
Doctors 'Always' Communicated Well	300+	78%	80%	82%
Home Recovery Information Given	300+	85%	87%	85%
Hospital Given 9 or 10 on 10 Point Scale	300+	71%	72%	71%
Meds 'Always' Explained Before Given	300+	60%	64%	64%
Nurses 'Always' Communicated Well	300+	75%	81%	79%
Pain 'Always' Well Controlled	300+	65%	71%	71%
Room and Bathroom 'Always' Clean	300+	71%	75%	73%
Timely Help 'Always' Received	300+	64%	70%	68%

NOTE: Hospital profiles are in alphabetical order by state, then city, then hospital within the city; Rankings exclude hospitals with less than 25 cases except for patient surveys which excludes hospitals with less than 100 cases; (a) 100-299 cases; (1) The number of cases/patients is too few to report; (2) Data submitted were based on a sample of cases/patients; (3) Results are based on a shorter time period than required; (4) Data suppressed by CMS for one or more quarters; (5) Results are not available for this reporting period; (6) Fewer than 100 patients completed the HCAHPS survey; (7) No cases met the criteria for this measure; (8) The lower limit of the confidence interval cannot be calculated if the number of observed infections equals zero; (9) No data are available from the state/territory for this reporting period; (10) The scores shown reflect fewer than 50 completed surveys; (11) There were discrepancies in the data collection process; (12) This measure does not apply to this hospital for this reporting period; (13) Results cannot be calculated for this reporting period; (14) The results for this state are combined with nearby states to protect confidentiality; Please refer to the User's Guide for a full explanation of data.

Would Definitely Recommend Hospital	300+	72%	71%	71%
Use of Medical Imaging				
Cardiac Imaging Stress Test before Surgery	343	7.3%	5.4%	5.3%
Combination Abdominal CT Scan	871	4.8%	7.1%	10.5%
Combination Brain/Sinus CT Scan	779	1.7%	2.8%	2.7%
Combination Chest CT Scan	487	1.8%	1.7%	2.7%
Follow-up Mammogram/Ultrasound	1,646	9.4%	8.7%	8.8%
Lumbar Spine MRI for Low Back Pain	192	34.9%	34.7%	37.2%

Hillcrest Hospital

6780 Mayfield Road
Mayfield Heights, OH 44124
Phone: 440-312-4500
Fax: 440-312-6407
URL: www.hillcresthospital.org
Type: Acute Care Hospitals
Emergency Services: Yes
Ownership: Voluntary non-profit - Private
Beds: 424

Key Personnel:
Emergency Room . . . . Peg McDonald
CEO/President. . . . . Delos Toby Cosgrove, MD

Measure	Cases	This Hosp.	State Avg.	U.S. Avg.
Blood Clot Prevention and Treatment				
Anticoagulation Overlap Therapy[2]	205	89%	93%	93%
ICU Venous Thromboembolism Prophylaxis[2]	112	96%	93%	92%
Incidence of Potentially Preventable VTE[2]	46	9%	6%	10%
UFH with Dosages/Platelet Monitoring[2]	200	100%	98%	97%
Venous Thromboembolism Prophylaxis[2]	323	85%	88%	85%
Warfarin Therapy Discharge Instructions[2]	147	72%	79%	75%
Chest Pain/Possible Heart Attack Care				
Aspirin Given Within 24 Hours of Arrival	13	85%	97%	96%
Fibrinolytic Meds Within 30 Min. of Arrival[3,7]	-	-	44%	58%
Average Time to ECG (minutes)	14	11	6	7
Average Time to Transfer (minutes)[3,7]	-	-	58	60
Children's Asthma Care				
Received Home Management Plan of Care	-	-	85%	88%
Received Reliever Medication	-	-	100%	100%
Received Systemic Corticosteroids	-	-	100%	100%
Emergency Department				
Admittance Decision Time (minutes)[2]	523	112	90	98
Head CT Results Within 45 Min. of Arrival[1]	-	-	63%	57%
Patients Who Left ER Before Being Seen	58,657	1%	2%	2%
Time from ER Arrival to Admit. (minutes)[2]	529	279	265	274
Time from ER Arrival to Discharge (minutes)	384	144	128	134
Time in ER Before Being Evaluated (minutes)	438	18	22	26
Time to Pain Meds for Fractures (minutes)	263	32	54	57
Heart Attack Care				
Aspirin Given at Discharge	307	99%	99%	99%
Fibrinolytic Meds Within 30 Min. of Arrival[7]	-	-	80%	54%
PCI Within 90 Minutes of Arrival	64	98%	97%	96%
Statin Prescribed at Discharge	303	100%	98%	98%
Heart Failure Care				
ACE Inhibitor or ARB for LVSD	96	100%	97%	97%
Discharge Instructions Given	375	100%	96%	94%
Evaluation of LVS Function	513	100%	100%	99%
Medicare Spending				
Medicare Spending per Patient (ratio)	-	1.02	1.01	0.98
Pneumonia Care				
Appropriate Initial Antibiotic Given	183	97%	96%	95%
Blood Culture Timing	98	100%	98%	98%
Pregnancy and Delivery Care				
Newborn Deliveries Scheduled Early[2]	63	3%	5%	6%
Preventive Care				
Immunization for Influenza[2]	558	96%	93%	90%
Immunization for Pneumonia[2]	674	94%	94%	92%
Stroke Care				
Anticoagulation Therapy for Atrial Fibrillation	45	100%	95%	95%
Antithrombotic Therapy Timing	180	96%	98%	98%
Assessed for Rehabilitation	208	98%	98%	97%
Discharged on Antithrombotic Therapy	191	98%	99%	99%
Discharged on Statin Medication	165	98%	95%	94%
Thrombolytic Therapy Timing	14	100%	65%	66%
Venous Thromboembolism Prophylaxis	215	96%	95%	94%
Written Stroke Educational Materials Given	114	99%	92%	88%
Surgical Care Improvement Project				
Appropriate Beta Blocker Usage[2]	190	98%	98%	98%
Appropriate VTP Within 24 Hours[2]	351	99%	98%	98%
Controlled Postoperative Blood Glucose[2]	133	100%	97%	97%
Perioperative Temperature Management[2]	417	100%	100%	100%
Prophylactic Antibiotic Selection[2]	402	99%	99%	99%
Prophylactic Antibiotic Selection (Outpatient)	466	99%	98%	98%
Prophylactic Antibiotic Stopped[2]	398	99%	98%	98%
Prophylactic Antibiotic Timing[2]	403	99%	99%	99%
Prophylactic Antibiotic Timing (Outpatient)	469	98%	97%	98%
Urinary Catheter Removal[2]	282	98%	97%	97%
Survey of Patients' Hospital Experiences				
Area Around Room 'Always' Quiet at Night	300+	52%	58%	61%
Doctors 'Always' Communicated Well	300+	79%	80%	82%
Home Recovery Information Given	300+	83%	87%	85%
Hospital Given 9 or 10 on 10 Point Scale	300+	67%	72%	71%
Meds 'Always' Explained Before Given	300+	63%	64%	64%
Nurses 'Always' Communicated Well	300+	79%	81%	79%
Pain 'Always' Well Controlled	300+	70%	71%	71%
Room and Bathroom 'Always' Clean	300+	71%	75%	73%
Timely Help 'Always' Received	300+	64%	70%	68%
Would Definitely Recommend Hospital	300+	71%	71%	71%
Use of Medical Imaging				
Cardiac Imaging Stress Test before Surgery	176	6.8%	5.4%	5.3%
Combination Abdominal CT Scan	1,431	9.3%	7.1%	10.5%
Combination Brain/Sinus CT Scan	1,225	5.7%	2.8%	2.7%
Combination Chest CT Scan	1,046	0.0%	1.7%	2.7%
Follow-up Mammogram/Ultrasound	1,569	11.3%	8.7%	8.8%
Lumbar Spine MRI for Low Back Pain	199	33.7%	34.7%	37.2%

Medina Hospital

1000 East Washington Street
Medina, OH 44256
Phone: 330-725-1000
Fax: 330-722-5812
Type: Acute Care Hospitals
Emergency Services: Yes
Ownership: Voluntary non-profit - Private
Beds: 118

Key Personnel:
Radiology. . . . . Gregory L Arko
Emergency Room . . . . Kim Bowen
CEO/President. . . . . Gary Hallman
Cardiac Laboratory. . . . . Sampath Ramanazartu
Chief of Medical Staff. . . . . Patrick Sziraky

Measure	Cases	This Hosp.	State Avg.	U.S. Avg.
Blood Clot Prevention and Treatment				
Anticoagulation Overlap Therapy[2]	64	92%	93%	93%
ICU Venous Thromboembolism Prophylaxis[2]	59	97%	93%	92%
Incidence of Potentially Preventable VTE[1,2]	-	-	6%	10%
UFH with Dosages/Platelet Monitoring[2]	47	96%	98%	97%
Venous Thromboembolism Prophylaxis[2]	299	91%	88%	85%
Warfarin Therapy Discharge Instructions[2]	44	61%	79%	75%
Chest Pain/Possible Heart Attack Care				
Aspirin Given Within 24 Hours of Arrival	83	99%	97%	96%
Fibrinolytic Meds Within 30 Min. of Arrival[7]	-	-	44%	58%
Average Time to ECG (minutes)	83	1	6	7
Average Time to Transfer (minutes)	20	75	58	60
Children's Asthma Care				
Received Home Management Plan of Care	-	-	85%	88%
Received Reliever Medication	-	-	100%	100%
Received Systemic Corticosteroids	-	-	100%	100%
Emergency Department				
Admittance Decision Time (minutes)[2]	670	82	90	98
Head CT Results Within 45 Min. of Arrival	15	87%	63%	57%
Patients Who Left ER Before Being Seen	22,916	2%	2%	2%
Time from ER Arrival to Admit. (minutes)[2]	673	256	265	274
Time from ER Arrival to Discharge (minutes)	313	160	128	134
Time in ER Before Being Evaluated (minutes)	425	17	22	26
Time to Pain Meds for Fractures (minutes)	97	40	54	57
Heart Attack Care				
Aspirin Given at Discharge[1]	-	-	99%	99%
Fibrinolytic Meds Within 30 Min. of Arrival[7]	-	-	80%	54%
PCI Within 90 Minutes of Arrival[7]	-	-	97%	96%
Statin Prescribed at Discharge[1]	-	-	98%	98%
Heart Failure Care				
ACE Inhibitor or ARB for LVSD	35	91%	97%	97%
Discharge Instructions Given	124	96%	96%	94%
Evaluation of LVS Function	187	100%	100%	99%
Medicare Spending				
Medicare Spending per Patient (ratio)	-	1.04	1.01	0.98
Pneumonia Care				
Appropriate Initial Antibiotic Given	121	93%	96%	95%
Blood Culture Timing	201	98%	98%	98%
Pregnancy and Delivery Care				
Newborn Deliveries Scheduled Early[2]	69	3%	5%	6%
Preventive Care				
Immunization for Influenza[2]	528	96%	93%	90%
Immunization for Pneumonia[2]	687	99%	94%	92%
Stroke Care				
Anticoagulation Therapy for Atrial Fibrillation[1]	-	-	95%	95%
Antithrombotic Therapy Timing	47	100%	98%	98%
Assessed for Rehabilitation	50	100%	98%	97%
Discharged on Antithrombotic Therapy	48	100%	99%	99%
Discharged on Statin Medication	34	94%	95%	94%
Thrombolytic Therapy Timing[1]	-	-	65%	66%
Venous Thromboembolism Prophylaxis	38	95%	95%	94%
Written Stroke Educational Materials Given	33	94%	92%	88%
Surgical Care Improvement Project				
Appropriate Beta Blocker Usage[2]	192	97%	98%	98%
Appropriate VTP Within 24 Hours[2]	642	99%	98%	98%
Controlled Postoperative Blood Glucose[2,7]	-	-	97%	97%
Perioperative Temperature Management[2]	694	100%	100%	100%
Prophylactic Antibiotic Selection[2]	533	99%	99%	99%
Prophylactic Antibiotic Selection (Outpatient)	103	97%	98%	98%
Prophylactic Antibiotic Stopped[2]	527	99%	98%	98%
Prophylactic Antibiotic Timing[2]	533	100%	99%	99%
Prophylactic Antibiotic Timing (Outpatient)	102	98%	97%	98%
Urinary Catheter Removal[2]	445	99%	97%	97%
Survey of Patients' Hospital Experiences				
Area Around Room 'Always' Quiet at Night	300+	58%	58%	61%
Doctors 'Always' Communicated Well	300+	82%	80%	82%
Home Recovery Information Given	300+	90%	87%	85%
Hospital Given 9 or 10 on 10 Point Scale	300+	68%	72%	71%
Meds 'Always' Explained Before Given	300+	64%	64%	64%
Nurses 'Always' Communicated Well	300+	79%	81%	79%
Pain 'Always' Well Controlled	300+	71%	71%	71%
Room and Bathroom 'Always' Clean	300+	81%	75%	73%
Timely Help 'Always' Received	300+	65%	70%	68%
Would Definitely Recommend Hospital	300+	68%	71%	71%
Use of Medical Imaging				
Cardiac Imaging Stress Test before Surgery	242	7.4%	5.4%	5.3%
Combination Abdominal CT Scan	516	6.8%	7.1%	10.5%
Combination Brain/Sinus CT Scan	582	2.2%	2.8%	2.7%
Combination Chest CT Scan	317	0.9%	1.7%	2.7%
Follow-up Mammogram/Ultrasound	924	14.3%	8.7%	8.8%
Lumbar Spine MRI for Low Back Pain	91	29.7%	34.7%	37.2%

Sycamore Medical Center

4000 Miamisburg - Centerville Road
Miamisburg, OH 45342
Phone: 937-384-8776
URL: www.khnetwork.org/sycamore
Type: Acute Care Hospitals
Emergency Services: Yes
Ownership: Voluntary non-profit - Church
Beds: 181

Key Personnel:
President . . . . Terri Day
CEO . . . . Fred Manchur

Measure	Cases	This Hosp.	State Avg.	U.S. Avg.
Blood Clot Prevention and Treatment				
Anticoagulation Overlap Therapy[2]	57	96%	93%	93%
ICU Venous Thromboembolism Prophylaxis[2]	75	99%	93%	92%
Incidence of Potentially Preventable VTE[1,2]	-	-	6%	10%
UFH with Dosages/Platelet Monitoring[2]	29	100%	98%	97%
Venous Thromboembolism Prophylaxis[2]	339	96%	88%	85%
Warfarin Therapy Discharge Instructions[2]	39	92%	79%	75%
Chest Pain/Possible Heart Attack Care				
Aspirin Given Within 24 Hours of Arrival	52	100%	97%	96%
Fibrinolytic Meds Within 30 Min. of Arrival[7]	-	-	44%	58%
Average Time to ECG (minutes)	53	7	6	7
Average Time to Transfer (minutes)	12	59	58	60
Children's Asthma Care				
Received Home Management Plan of Care	-	-	85%	88%

NOTE: Hospital profiles are in alphabetical order by state, then city, then hospital within the city; Rankings exclude hospitals with less than 25 cases except for patient surveys which excludes hospitals with less than 100 cases; (a) 100-299 cases; (1) The number of cases/patients is too few to report; (2) Data submitted were based on a sample of cases/patients; (3) Results are based on a shorter time period than required; (4) Data suppressed by CMS for one or more quarters; (5) Results are not available for this reporting period; (6) Fewer than 100 patients completed the HCAHPS survey; (7) No cases met the criteria for this measure; (8) The lower limit of the confidence interval cannot be calculated if the number of observed infections equals zero; (9) No data are available from the state/territory for this reporting period; (10) The scores shown reflect fewer than 50 completed surveys; (11) There were discrepancies in the data collection process; (12) This measure does not apply to this hospital for this reporting period; (13) Results cannot be calculated for this reporting period; (14) The results for this state are combined with nearby states to protect confidentiality; Please refer to the User's Guide for a full explanation of data.

Measure	Cases	This Hosp.	State Avg.	U.S. Avg.
Received Reliever Medication	-	-	100%	100%
Received Systemic Corticosteroids	-	-	100%	100%
Emergency Department				
Admittance Decision Time (minutes)[2]	704	108	90	98
Head CT Results Within 45 Min. of Arrival	11	27%	63%	57%
Patients Who Left ER Before Being Seen	35,599	1%	2%	2%
Time from ER Arrival to Admit. (minutes)[2]	705	247	265	274
Time from ER Arrival to Discharge (minutes)	397	138	128	134
Time in ER Before Being Evaluated (minutes)	427	15	22	26
Time to Pain Meds for Fractures (minutes)	102	54	54	57
Heart Attack Care				
Aspirin Given at Discharge	18	100%	99%	99%
Fibrinolytic Meds Within 30 Min. of Arrival[7]	-	-	80%	54%
PCI Within 90 Minutes of Arrival[7]	-	-	97%	96%
Statin Prescribed at Discharge	19	100%	98%	98%
Heart Failure Care				
ACE Inhibitor or ARB for LVSD	52	100%	97%	97%
Discharge Instructions Given	143	99%	96%	94%
Evaluation of LVS Function	189	100%	100%	99%
Medicare Spending				
Medicare Spending per Patient (ratio)	-	0.98	1.01	0.98
Pneumonia Care				
Appropriate Initial Antibiotic Given	125	100%	96%	95%
Blood Culture Timing	232	100%	98%	98%
Pregnancy and Delivery Care				
Newborn Deliveries Scheduled Early[7]	-	-	5%	6%
Preventive Care				
Immunization for Influenza[2]	572	98%	93%	90%
Immunization for Pneumonia[2]	871	96%	94%	92%
Stroke Care				
Anticoagulation Therapy for Atrial Fibrillation[1]	-	-	95%	95%
Antithrombotic Therapy Timing	37	97%	98%	98%
Assessed for Rehabilitation	50	100%	98%	97%
Discharged on Antithrombotic Therapy	46	100%	99%	99%
Discharged on Statin Medication	32	100%	95%	94%
Thrombolytic Therapy Timing[1]	-	-	65%	66%
Venous Thromboembolism Prophylaxis	36	97%	95%	94%
Written Stroke Educational Materials Given	25	100%	92%	88%
Surgical Care Improvement Project				
Appropriate Beta Blocker Usage[2]	154	99%	98%	98%
Appropriate VTP Within 24 Hours[2]	497	99%	98%	98%
Controlled Postoperative Blood Glucose[2,7]	-	-	97%	97%
Perioperative Temperature Management[2]	527	100%	100%	100%
Prophylactic Antibiotic Selection[2]	368	100%	99%	99%
Prophylactic Antibiotic Selection (Outpatient)	119	97%	98%	98%
Prophylactic Antibiotic Stopped[2]	366	100%	98%	98%
Prophylactic Antibiotic Timing[2]	368	100%	99%	99%
Prophylactic Antibiotic Timing (Outpatient)	111	97%	97%	98%
Urinary Catheter Removal[2]	212	96%	97%	97%
Survey of Patients' Hospital Experiences				
Area Around Room 'Always' Quiet at Night	300+	55%	58%	61%
Doctors 'Always' Communicated Well	300+	79%	80%	82%
Home Recovery Information Given	300+	86%	87%	85%
Hospital Given 9 or 10 on 10 Point Scale	300+	76%	72%	71%
Meds 'Always' Explained Before Given	300+	64%	64%	64%
Nurses 'Always' Communicated Well	300+	82%	81%	79%
Pain 'Always' Well Controlled	300+	70%	71%	71%
Room and Bathroom 'Always' Clean	300+	73%	75%	73%
Timely Help 'Always' Received	300+	68%	70%	68%
Would Definitely Recommend Hospital	300+	75%	71%	71%
Use of Medical Imaging				
Cardiac Imaging Stress Test before Surgery	480	5.4%	5.4%	5.3%
Combination Abdominal CT Scan	728	5.2%	7.1%	10.5%
Combination Brain/Sinus CT Scan	696	2.6%	2.8%	2.7%
Combination Chest CT Scan	319	0.3%	1.7%	2.7%
Follow-up Mammogram/Ultrasound	1,373	6.8%	8.7%	8.8%
Lumbar Spine MRI for Low Back Pain	57	35.1%	34.7%	37.2%

Southwest General Health Center

18697 Bagley Road
Middleburg Heights, OH 44130
URL: www.swgeneral.com
Type: Acute Care Hospitals
Ownership: Voluntary non-profit - Private
Phone: 440-816-8000
Fax: 440-816-5299
Emergency Services: Yes
Beds: 336

Key Personnel:
Radiology.................... Chris Blagojevic
Pediatric Ambulatory Care ...... Nancy Crow
Pediatric In-Patient Care .... Nancy Crow
Quality Assurance .... Sue Ferrante
Chief of Medical Staff.......... Dr Kulbir Pannu
CEO/President............... Thomas A. Selden
Coronary Care............... Robyn Szeles
Infection Control.............. Debbie Winar

Measure	Cases	This Hosp.	State Avg.	U.S. Avg.
Blood Clot Prevention and Treatment				
Anticoagulation Overlap Therapy[2]	130	90%	93%	93%
ICU Venous Thromboembolism Prophylaxis[2]	139	88%	93%	92%
Incidence of Potentially Preventable VTE[2]	23	9%	6%	10%
UFH with Dosages/Platelet Monitoring[2]	31	100%	98%	97%
Venous Thromboembolism Prophylaxis[2]	315	87%	88%	85%
Warfarin Therapy Discharge Instructions[2]	98	97%	79%	75%
Chest Pain/Possible Heart Attack Care				
Aspirin Given Within 24 Hours of Arrival	17	94%	97%	96%
Fibrinolytic Meds Within 30 Min. of Arrival[3,7]	-	-	44%	58%
Average Time to ECG (minutes)	21	6	6	7
Average Time to Transfer (minutes)[3,7]	-	-	58	60
Children's Asthma Care				
Received Home Management Plan of Care	-	-	85%	88%
Received Reliever Medication	-	-	100%	100%
Received Systemic Corticosteroids	-	-	100%	100%
Emergency Department				
Admittance Decision Time (minutes)[2]	700	110	90	98
Head CT Results Within 45 Min. of Arrival	15	100%	63%	57%
Patients Who Left ER Before Being Seen	61,365	1%	2%	2%
Time from ER Arrival to Admit. (minutes)[2]	719	300	265	274
Time from ER Arrival to Discharge (minutes)	389	149	128	134
Time in ER Before Being Evaluated (minutes)	417	22	22	26
Time to Pain Meds for Fractures (minutes)	156	49	54	57
Heart Attack Care				
Aspirin Given at Discharge	342	99%	99%	99%
Fibrinolytic Meds Within 30 Min. of Arrival[7]	-	-	80%	54%
PCI Within 90 Minutes of Arrival	51	100%	97%	96%
Statin Prescribed at Discharge	333	99%	98%	98%
Heart Failure Care				
ACE Inhibitor or ARB for LVSD	105	99%	97%	97%
Discharge Instructions Given	319	97%	96%	94%
Evaluation of LVS Function	433	100%	100%	99%
Medicare Spending				
Medicare Spending per Patient (ratio)	-	1.04	1.01	0.98
Pneumonia Care				
Appropriate Initial Antibiotic Given	227	97%	96%	95%
Blood Culture Timing	517	99%	98%	98%
Pregnancy and Delivery Care				
Newborn Deliveries Scheduled Early	110	1%	5%	6%
Preventive Care				
Immunization for Influenza[2]	587	94%	93%	90%
Immunization for Pneumonia[2]	849	94%	94%	92%
Stroke Care				
Anticoagulation Therapy for Atrial Fibrillation	28	100%	95%	95%
Antithrombotic Therapy Timing	142	94%	98%	98%
Assessed for Rehabilitation	170	99%	98%	97%
Discharged on Antithrombotic Therapy	158	97%	99%	99%
Discharged on Statin Medication	119	93%	95%	94%
Thrombolytic Therapy Timing	15	93%	65%	66%
Venous Thromboembolism Prophylaxis	166	98%	95%	94%
Written Stroke Educational Materials Given	85	96%	92%	88%
Surgical Care Improvement Project				
Appropriate Beta Blocker Usage[2]	371	100%	98%	98%
Appropriate VTP Within 24 Hours[2]	839	99%	98%	98%
Controlled Postoperative Blood Glucose[2]	55	96%	97%	97%
Perioperative Temperature Management[2]	944	100%	100%	100%
Prophylactic Antibiotic Selection[2]	813	99%	99%	99%
Prophylactic Antibiotic Selection (Outpatient)	424	98%	98%	98%
Prophylactic Antibiotic Stopped[2]	805	99%	98%	98%
Prophylactic Antibiotic Timing[2]	813	100%	99%	99%
Prophylactic Antibiotic Timing (Outpatient)	425	99%	97%	98%
Urinary Catheter Removal[2]	669	98%	97%	97%
Survey of Patients' Hospital Experiences				
Area Around Room 'Always' Quiet at Night	300+	42%	58%	61%
Doctors 'Always' Communicated Well	300+	79%	80%	82%
Home Recovery Information Given	300+	87%	87%	85%
Hospital Given 9 or 10 on 10 Point Scale	300+	69%	72%	71%
Meds 'Always' Explained Before Given	300+	61%	64%	64%
Nurses 'Always' Communicated Well	300+	80%	81%	79%
Pain 'Always' Well Controlled	300+	69%	71%	71%
Room and Bathroom 'Always' Clean	300+	65%	75%	73%
Timely Help 'Always' Received	300+	64%	70%	68%
Would Definitely Recommend Hospital	300+	74%	71%	71%
Use of Medical Imaging				
Cardiac Imaging Stress Test before Surgery	144	6.3%	5.4%	5.3%
Combination Abdominal CT Scan	1,445	15.8%	7.1%	10.5%
Combination Brain/Sinus CT Scan	1,043	5.9%	2.8%	2.7%
Combination Chest CT Scan	854	0.1%	1.7%	2.7%
Follow-up Mammogram/Ultrasound	1,610	5.2%	8.7%	8.8%
Lumbar Spine MRI for Low Back Pain	145	38.6%	34.7%	37.2%

Pomerene Hospital

981 Wooster Road
Millersburg, OH 44654
URL: www.pomerenehospital.org
Type: Acute Care Hospitals
Ownership: Government - Local
Phone: 330-674-1015
Fax: 330-674-9707
Emergency Services: Yes
Beds: 55

Key Personnel:
Anesthesiology............... Robert Anthony, MD
Operating Room............. Brian Black
Emergency Room .... Stan Boyd, MD
Quality Assurance .... Sandy Cunningham
Chairman/CEO .... Dan Mathie
Surgery..................... Leon Miller, MD
Chief of Medical Staff.......... Dr. Yasser Omran
Radiology................... Claudia M Rozuk, MD

Measure	Cases	This Hosp.	State Avg.	U.S. Avg.
Blood Clot Prevention and Treatment				
Anticoagulation Overlap Therapy[1,2]	-	-	93%	93%
ICU Venous Thromboembolism Prophylaxis[2]	23	100%	93%	92%
Incidence of Potentially Preventable VTE[1,2]	-	-	6%	10%
UFH with Dosages/Platelet Monitoring[1,2]	-	-	98%	97%
Venous Thromboembolism Prophylaxis[2]	84	100%	88%	85%
Warfarin Therapy Discharge Instructions[1,2]	-	-	79%	75%
Chest Pain/Possible Heart Attack Care				
Aspirin Given Within 24 Hours of Arrival	76	96%	97%	96%
Fibrinolytic Meds Within 30 Min. of Arrival[7]	-	-	44%	58%
Average Time to ECG (minutes)	77	4	6	7
Average Time to Transfer (minutes)[1]	-	-	58	60
Children's Asthma Care				
Received Home Management Plan of Care	-	-	85%	88%
Received Reliever Medication	-	-	100%	100%
Received Systemic Corticosteroids	-	-	100%	100%
Emergency Department				
Admittance Decision Time (minutes)[2]	212	64	90	98
Head CT Results Within 45 Min. of Arrival	11	64%	63%	57%
Patients Who Left ER Before Being Seen	12,287	0%	2%	2%
Time from ER Arrival to Admit. (minutes)[2]	231	199	265	274
Time from ER Arrival to Discharge (minutes)	370	104	128	134
Time in ER Before Being Evaluated (minutes)	363	20	22	26
Time to Pain Meds for Fractures (minutes)	52	58	54	57
Heart Attack Care				
Aspirin Given at Discharge[3,7]	-	-	99%	99%
Fibrinolytic Meds Within 30 Min. of Arrival[3,7]	-	-	80%	54%
PCI Within 90 Minutes of Arrival[3,7]	-	-	97%	96%
Statin Prescribed at Discharge[3,7]	-	-	98%	98%
Heart Failure Care				
ACE Inhibitor or ARB for LVSD	18	100%	97%	97%
Discharge Instructions Given	30	100%	96%	94%
Evaluation of LVS Function	36	100%	100%	99%
Medicare Spending				

NOTE: Hospital profiles are in alphabetical order by state, then city, then hospital within the city; Rankings exclude hospitals with less than 25 cases except for patient surveys which excludes hospitals with less than 100 cases; (a) 100-299 cases; (1) The number of cases/patients is too few to report; (2) Data submitted were based on a sample of cases/patients; (3) Results are based on a shorter time period than required; (4) Data suppressed by CMS for one or more quarters; (5) Results are not available for this reporting period; (6) Fewer than 100 patients completed the HCAHPS survey; (7) No cases met the criteria for this measure; (8) The lower limit of the confidence interval cannot be calculated if the number of observed infections equals zero; (9) No data are available from the state/territory for this reporting period; (10) The scores shown reflect fewer than 50 completed surveys; (11) There were discrepancies in the data collection process; (12) This measure does not apply to this hospital for this reporting period; (13) Results cannot be calculated for this reporting period; (14) The results for this state are combined with nearby states to protect confidentiality; Please refer to the User's Guide for a full explanation of data.

Measure	Cases	This Hosp.	State Avg.	U.S. Avg.
Medicare Spending per Patient (ratio)	-	1.02	1.01	0.98
Pneumonia Care				
Appropriate Initial Antibiotic Given	58	100%	96%	95%
Blood Culture Timing	100	100%	98%	98%
Pregnancy and Delivery Care				
Newborn Deliveries Scheduled Early[2]	28	11%	5%	6%
Preventive Care				
Immunization for Influenza[2]	231	97%	93%	90%
Immunization for Pneumonia[2]	212	98%	94%	92%
Stroke Care				
Anticoagulation Therapy for Atrial Fibrillation[7]	-	-	95%	95%
Antithrombotic Therapy Timing[1]	-	-	98%	98%
Assessed for Rehabilitation[1]	-	-	98%	97%
Discharged on Antithrombotic Therapy[1]	-	-	99%	99%
Discharged on Statin Medication[1]	-	-	95%	94%
Thrombolytic Therapy Timing[1]	-	-	65%	66%
Venous Thromboembolism Prophylaxis[1]	-	-	95%	94%
Written Stroke Educational Materials Given[1]	-	-	92%	88%
Surgical Care Improvement Project				
Appropriate Beta Blocker Usage	32	100%	98%	98%
Appropriate VTP Within 24 Hours	121	99%	98%	98%
Controlled Postoperative Blood Glucose[7]	-	-	97%	97%
Perioperative Temperature Management	136	100%	100%	100%
Prophylactic Antibiotic Selection	107	100%	99%	99%
Prophylactic Antibiotic Selection (Outpatient)	21	100%	98%	98%
Prophylactic Antibiotic Stopped	104	100%	98%	98%
Prophylactic Antibiotic Timing	107	100%	99%	99%
Prophylactic Antibiotic Timing (Outpatient)	21	100%	97%	98%
Urinary Catheter Removal	88	100%	97%	97%
Survey of Patients' Hospital Experiences				
Area Around Room 'Always' Quiet at Night	300+	60%	58%	61%
Doctors 'Always' Communicated Well	300+	83%	80%	82%
Home Recovery Information Given	300+	87%	87%	85%
Hospital Given 9 or 10 on 10 Point Scale	300+	73%	72%	71%
Meds 'Always' Explained Before Given	300+	64%	64%	64%
Nurses 'Always' Communicated Well	300+	85%	81%	79%
Pain 'Always' Well Controlled	300+	67%	71%	71%
Room and Bathroom 'Always' Clean	300+	85%	75%	73%
Timely Help 'Always' Received	300+	71%	70%	68%
Would Definitely Recommend Hospital	300+	64%	71%	71%
Use of Medical Imaging				
Cardiac Imaging Stress Test before Surgery	133	14.3%	5.4%	5.3%
Combination Abdominal CT Scan	168	8.9%	7.1%	10.5%
Combination Brain/Sinus CT Scan[1]	-	-	2.8%	2.7%
Combination Chest CT Scan	97	6.2%	1.7%	2.7%
Follow-up Mammogram/Ultrasound	233	9.0%	8.7%	8.8%
Lumbar Spine MRI for Low Back Pain[1]	-	-	34.7%	37.2%

Community Hospitals & Wellness Centers

909 East Snyder Avenue Phone: 419-485-3154
Montpelier, OH 43543
Type: Critical Access Hospitals Emergency Services: Yes
Ownership: Voluntary non-profit - Private

Measure	Cases	This Hosp.	State Avg.	U.S. Avg.
Blood Clot Prevention and Treatment				
Anticoagulation Overlap Therapy	-	-	93%	93%
ICU Venous Thromboembolism Prophylaxis	-	-	93%	92%
Incidence of Potentially Preventable VTE	-	-	6%	10%
UFH with Dosages/Platelet Monitoring	-	-	98%	97%
Venous Thromboembolism Prophylaxis	-	-	88%	85%
Warfarin Therapy Discharge Instructions	-	-	79%	75%
Chest Pain/Possible Heart Attack Care				
Aspirin Given Within 24 Hours of Arrival	26	100%	97%	96%
Fibrinolytic Meds Within 30 Min. of Arrival[7]	-	-	44%	58%
Average Time to ECG (minutes)	27	5	6	7
Average Time to Transfer (minutes)[1]	-	-	58	60
Children's Asthma Care				
Received Home Management Plan of Care	-	-	85%	88%
Received Reliever Medication	-	-	100%	100%
Received Systemic Corticosteroids	-	-	100%	100%
Emergency Department				
Admittance Decision Time (minutes)	-	-	90	98
Head CT Results Within 45 Min. of Arrival[1,3]	-	-	63%	57%
Patients Who Left ER Before Being Seen	4,297	0%	2%	2%
Time from ER Arrival to Admit. (minutes)	-	-	265	274
Time from ER Arrival to Discharge (minutes)	390	72	128	134
Time in ER Before Being Evaluated (minutes)	440	13	22	26
Time to Pain Meds for Fractures (minutes)[3]	15	46	54	57
Heart Attack Care				
Aspirin Given at Discharge	-	-	99%	99%
Fibrinolytic Meds Within 30 Min. of Arrival	-	-	80%	54%
PCI Within 90 Minutes of Arrival	-	-	97%	96%
Statin Prescribed at Discharge	-	-	98%	98%
Heart Failure Care				
ACE Inhibitor or ARB for LVSD	-	-	97%	97%
Discharge Instructions Given	-	-	96%	94%
Evaluation of LVS Function	-	-	100%	99%
Medicare Spending				
Medicare Spending per Patient (ratio)	-	-	1.01	0.98
Pneumonia Care				
Appropriate Initial Antibiotic Given	-	-	96%	95%
Blood Culture Timing	-	-	98%	98%
Pregnancy and Delivery Care				
Newborn Deliveries Scheduled Early	-	-	5%	6%
Preventive Care				
Immunization for Influenza	-	-	93%	90%
Immunization for Pneumonia	-	-	94%	92%
Stroke Care				
Anticoagulation Therapy for Atrial Fibrillation	-	-	95%	95%
Antithrombotic Therapy Timing	-	-	98%	98%
Assessed for Rehabilitation	-	-	98%	97%
Discharged on Antithrombotic Therapy	-	-	99%	99%
Discharged on Statin Medication	-	-	95%	94%
Thrombolytic Therapy Timing	-	-	65%	66%
Venous Thromboembolism Prophylaxis	-	-	95%	94%
Written Stroke Educational Materials Given	-	-	92%	88%
Surgical Care Improvement Project				
Appropriate Beta Blocker Usage	-	-	98%	98%
Appropriate VTP Within 24 Hours	-	-	98%	98%
Controlled Postoperative Blood Glucose	-	-	97%	97%
Perioperative Temperature Management	-	-	100%	100%
Prophylactic Antibiotic Selection	-	-	99%	99%
Prophylactic Antibiotic Selection (Outpatient)[5]	-	-	98%	98%
Prophylactic Antibiotic Stopped	-	-	98%	98%
Prophylactic Antibiotic Timing	-	-	99%	99%
Prophylactic Antibiotic Timing (Outpatient)[5]	-	-	97%	98%
Urinary Catheter Removal	-	-	97%	97%
Survey of Patients' Hospital Experiences				
Area Around Room 'Always' Quiet at Night	-	-	58%	61%
Doctors 'Always' Communicated Well	-	-	80%	82%
Home Recovery Information Given	-	-	87%	85%
Hospital Given 9 or 10 on 10 Point Scale	-	-	72%	71%
Meds 'Always' Explained Before Given	-	-	64%	64%
Nurses 'Always' Communicated Well	-	-	81%	79%
Pain 'Always' Well Controlled	-	-	71%	71%
Room and Bathroom 'Always' Clean	-	-	75%	73%
Timely Help 'Always' Received	-	-	70%	68%
Would Definitely Recommend Hospital	-	-	71%	71%
Use of Medical Imaging				
Cardiac Imaging Stress Test before Surgery[7]	-	-	5.4%	5.3%
Combination Abdominal CT Scan	45	4.4%	7.1%	10.5%
Combination Brain/Sinus CT Scan[1]	-	-	2.8%	2.7%
Combination Chest CT Scan[1]	-	-	1.7%	2.7%
Follow-up Mammogram/Ultrasound[7]	-	-	8.7%	8.8%
Lumbar Spine MRI for Low Back Pain[7]	-	-	34.7%	37.2%

Morrow County Hospital

651 West Marion Road Phone: 419-946-5015
Mount Gilead, OH 43338 Fax: 419-949-3144
URL: www.morrowcountyhospital.com
Type: Critical Access Hospitals Emergency Services: Yes
Ownership: Government - Local Beds: 79

Key Personnel:
Cardiology . . . . Imtiaz Ahmed
Emergency Room . . . . Mark Davis
CEO/President . . . . Diana D Fisher
Radiology . . . . Earnest Hetrick
Anesthesiology . . . . Vinod K Koduri, MD
Hemotology Center . . . . Tejas B Lodhawala
Intensive Care Unit . . . . Laura Mahle
Pulmonology . . . . Hiten G Shah

Measure	Cases	This Hosp.	State Avg.	U.S. Avg.
Blood Clot Prevention and Treatment				
Anticoagulation Overlap Therapy[1,2]	-	-	93%	93%
ICU Venous Thromboembolism Prophylaxis[2]	12	92%	93%	92%
Incidence of Potentially Preventable VTE[2,7]	-	-	6%	10%
UFH with Dosages/Platelet Monitoring[1,2]	-	-	98%	97%
Venous Thromboembolism Prophylaxis[2]	88	77%	88%	85%
Warfarin Therapy Discharge Instructions[1,2]	-	-	79%	75%
Chest Pain/Possible Heart Attack Care				
Aspirin Given Within 24 Hours of Arrival[3]	31	94%	97%	96%
Fibrinolytic Meds Within 30 Min. of Arrival[3,7]	-	-	44%	58%
Average Time to ECG (minutes)[3]	31	15	6	7
Average Time to Transfer (minutes)[1,3]	-	-	58	60
Children's Asthma Care				
Received Home Management Plan of Care	-	-	85%	88%
Received Reliever Medication	-	-	100%	100%
Received Systemic Corticosteroids	-	-	100%	100%
Emergency Department				
Admittance Decision Time (minutes)[5]	-	-	90	98
Head CT Results Within 45 Min. of Arrival[5]	-	-	63%	57%
Patients Who Left ER Before Being Seen[5]	-	-	2%	2%
Time from ER Arrival to Admit. (minutes)[5]	-	-	265	274
Time from ER Arrival to Discharge (minutes)[5]	-	-	128	134
Time in ER Before Being Evaluated (minutes)[5]	-	-	22	26
Time to Pain Meds for Fractures (minutes)[5]	-	-	54	57
Heart Attack Care				
Aspirin Given at Discharge[1]	-	-	99%	99%
Fibrinolytic Meds Within 30 Min. of Arrival[7]	-	-	80%	54%
PCI Within 90 Minutes of Arrival[7]	-	-	97%	96%
Statin Prescribed at Discharge[1]	-	-	98%	98%
Heart Failure Care				
ACE Inhibitor or ARB for LVSD[1]	-	-	97%	97%
Discharge Instructions Given	21	100%	96%	94%
Evaluation of LVS Function	33	91%	100%	99%
Medicare Spending				
Medicare Spending per Patient (ratio)	-	-	1.01	0.98
Pneumonia Care				
Appropriate Initial Antibiotic Given	31	84%	96%	95%
Blood Culture Timing	47	94%	98%	98%
Pregnancy and Delivery Care				
Newborn Deliveries Scheduled Early[5]	-	-	5%	6%
Preventive Care				
Immunization for Influenza[2,3]	112	87%	93%	90%
Immunization for Pneumonia[2,3]	255	87%	94%	92%
Stroke Care				
Anticoagulation Therapy for Atrial Fibrillation[3,7]	-	-	95%	95%
Antithrombotic Therapy Timing[1,3]	-	-	98%	98%
Assessed for Rehabilitation[1,3]	-	-	98%	97%
Discharged on Antithrombotic Therapy[1,3]	-	-	99%	99%
Discharged on Statin Medication[1,3]	-	-	95%	94%
Thrombolytic Therapy Timing[1,3]	-	-	65%	66%
Venous Thromboembolism Prophylaxis[3,7]	-	-	95%	94%
Written Stroke Educational Materials Given[1,3]	-	-	92%	88%
Surgical Care Improvement Project				
Appropriate Beta Blocker Usage[1]	-	-	98%	98%
Appropriate VTP Within 24 Hours	11	100%	98%	98%
Controlled Postoperative Blood Glucose[7]	-	-	97%	97%
Perioperative Temperature Management	16	100%	100%	100%
Prophylactic Antibiotic Selection	11	91%	99%	99%
Prophylactic Antibiotic Selection (Outpatient)[3,7]	-	-	98%	98%
Prophylactic Antibiotic Stopped	11	100%	98%	98%
Prophylactic Antibiotic Timing	11	91%	99%	99%
Prophylactic Antibiotic Timing (Outpatient)[3,7]	-	-	97%	98%
Urinary Catheter Removal	13	100%	97%	97%
Survey of Patients' Hospital Experiences				
Area Around Room 'Always' Quiet at Night	(a)	65%	58%	61%
Doctors 'Always' Communicated Well	(a)	83%	80%	82%

NOTE: Hospital profiles are in alphabetical order by state, then city, then hospital within the city; Rankings exclude hospitals with less than 25 cases except for patient surveys which excludes hospitals with less than 100 cases; (a) 100-299 cases; (1) The number of cases/patients is too few to report; (2) Data submitted were based on a sample of cases/patients; (3) Results are based on a shorter time period than required; (4) Data suppressed by CMS for one or more quarters; (5) Results are not available for this reporting period; (6) Fewer than 100 patients completed the HCAHPS survey; (7) No cases met the criteria for this measure; (8) The lower limit of the confidence interval cannot be calculated if the number of observed infections equals zero; (9) No data are available from the state/territory for this reporting period; (10) The scores shown reflect fewer than 50 completed surveys; (11) There were discrepancies in the data collection process; (12) This measure does not apply to this hospital for this reporting period; (13) Results cannot be calculated for this reporting period; (14) The results for this state are combined with nearby states to protect confidentiality; Please refer to the User's Guide for a full explanation of data.

Home Recovery Information Given	(a)	89%	87%	85%
Hospital Given 9 or 10 on 10 Point Scale	(a)	78%	72%	71%
Meds 'Always' Explained Before Given	(a)	78%	64%	64%
Nurses 'Always' Communicated Well	(a)	86%	81%	79%
Pain 'Always' Well Controlled	(a)	77%	71%	71%
Room and Bathroom 'Always' Clean	(a)	85%	75%	73%
Timely Help 'Always' Received	(a)	78%	70%	68%
Would Definitely Recommend Hospital	(a)	74%	71%	71%
Use of Medical Imaging				
Cardiac Imaging Stress Test before Surgery[1]	-	-	5.4%	5.3%
Combination Abdominal CT Scan	260	5.8%	7.1%	10.5%
Combination Brain/Sinus CT Scan[1]	-	-	2.8%	2.7%
Combination Chest CT Scan	80	5.0%	1.7%	2.7%
Follow-up Mammogram/Ultrasound	238	4.6%	8.7%	8.8%
Lumbar Spine MRI for Low Back Pain[1]	-	-	34.7%	37.2%

Knox Community Hospital

1330 Coshocton Road
Mount Vernon, OH 43050
Phone: 740-393-9000
Fax: 740-399-3130
Type: Acute Care Hospitals
Emergency Services: Yes
Ownership: Voluntary non-profit - Other
Beds: 115

Key Personnel:

Coronary Care . . . . Jaya Pala
Quality Assurance . . . . Peggy Penkhus
Chief of Medical Staff. . . . . Judy Schwartz
Emergency Room . . . . Lee Weiss
CEO/President. . . . . Bruce White
Radiology. . . . . Henry Windler

Measure	Cases	This Hosp.	State Avg.	U.S. Avg.
Blood Clot Prevention and Treatment				
Anticoagulation Overlap Therapy[2]	26	81%	93%	93%
ICU Venous Thromboembolism Prophylaxis[2]	71	89%	93%	92%
Incidence of Potentially Preventable VTE[2,7]	-	-	6%	10%
UFH with Dosages/Platelet Monitoring[1,2]	-	-	98%	97%
Venous Thromboembolism Prophylaxis[2]	164	80%	88%	85%
Warfarin Therapy Discharge Instructions[2]	16	56%	79%	75%
Chest Pain/Possible Heart Attack Care				
Aspirin Given Within 24 Hours of Arrival	16	100%	97%	96%
Fibrinolytic Meds Within 30 Min. of Arrival[3,7]	-	-	44%	58%
Average Time to ECG (minutes)	16	8	6	7
Average Time to Transfer (minutes)[3,7]	-	-	58	60
Children's Asthma Care				
Received Home Management Plan of Care	-	-	85%	88%
Received Reliever Medication	-	-	100%	100%
Received Systemic Corticosteroids	-	-	100%	100%
Emergency Department				
Admittance Decision Time (minutes)[2]	300	89	90	98
Head CT Results Within 45 Min. of Arrival	17	6%	63%	57%
Patients Who Left ER Before Being Seen	27,418	2%	2%	2%
Time from ER Arrival to Admit. (minutes)[2]	328	273	265	274
Time from ER Arrival to Discharge (minutes)	331	123	128	134
Time in ER Before Being Evaluated (minutes)	379	36	22	26
Time to Pain Meds for Fractures (minutes)	110	58	54	57
Heart Attack Care				
Aspirin Given at Discharge	105	98%	99%	99%
Fibrinolytic Meds Within 30 Min. of Arrival[7]	-	-	80%	54%
PCI Within 90 Minutes of Arrival	26	88%	97%	96%
Statin Prescribed at Discharge	99	97%	98%	98%
Heart Failure Care				
ACE Inhibitor or ARB for LVSD	27	100%	97%	97%
Discharge Instructions Given	87	94%	96%	94%
Evaluation of LVS Function	111	97%	100%	99%
Medicare Spending				
Medicare Spending per Patient (ratio)	-	1.03	1.01	0.98
Pneumonia Care				
Appropriate Initial Antibiotic Given	87	93%	96%	95%
Blood Culture Timing	145	94%	98%	98%
Pregnancy and Delivery Care				
Newborn Deliveries Scheduled Early	34	21%	5%	6%
Preventive Care				
Immunization for Influenza[2]	283	96%	93%	90%
Immunization for Pneumonia[2]	339	93%	94%	92%
Stroke Care				
Anticoagulation Therapy for Atrial Fibrillation[1]	-	-	95%	95%
Antithrombotic Therapy Timing[1]	-	-	98%	98%
Assessed for Rehabilitation[1]	-	-	98%	97%
Discharged on Antithrombotic Therapy[1]	-	-	99%	99%
Discharged on Statin Medication[1]	-	-	95%	94%
Thrombolytic Therapy Timing[1]	-	-	65%	66%
Venous Thromboembolism Prophylaxis[1]	-	-	95%	94%
Written Stroke Educational Materials Given[1]	-	-	92%	88%
Surgical Care Improvement Project				
Appropriate Beta Blocker Usage	101	98%	98%	98%
Appropriate VTP Within 24 Hours	358	96%	98%	98%
Controlled Postoperative Blood Glucose[7]	-	-	97%	97%
Perioperative Temperature Management	374	100%	100%	100%
Prophylactic Antibiotic Selection	302	96%	99%	99%
Prophylactic Antibiotic Selection (Outpatient)	115	91%	98%	98%
Prophylactic Antibiotic Stopped	301	97%	98%	98%
Prophylactic Antibiotic Timing	303	98%	99%	99%
Prophylactic Antibiotic Timing (Outpatient)	120	86%	97%	98%
Urinary Catheter Removal	236	92%	97%	97%
Survey of Patients' Hospital Experiences				
Area Around Room 'Always' Quiet at Night	300+	52%	58%	61%
Doctors 'Always' Communicated Well	300+	75%	80%	82%
Home Recovery Information Given	300+	86%	87%	85%
Hospital Given 9 or 10 on 10 Point Scale	300+	64%	72%	71%
Meds 'Always' Explained Before Given	300+	59%	64%	64%
Nurses 'Always' Communicated Well	300+	78%	81%	79%
Pain 'Always' Well Controlled	300+	67%	71%	71%
Room and Bathroom 'Always' Clean	300+	65%	75%	73%
Timely Help 'Always' Received	300+	70%	70%	68%
Would Definitely Recommend Hospital	300+	59%	71%	71%
Use of Medical Imaging				
Cardiac Imaging Stress Test before Surgery	622	5.1%	5.4%	5.3%
Combination Abdominal CT Scan	754	28.1%	7.1%	10.5%
Combination Brain/Sinus CT Scan	637	2.2%	2.8%	2.7%
Combination Chest CT Scan	424	8.0%	1.7%	2.7%
Follow-up Mammogram/Ultrasound	815	6.7%	8.7%	8.8%
Lumbar Spine MRI for Low Back Pain	82	24.4%	34.7%	37.2%

Henry County Hospital

1600 East Riverview Avenue
Napoleon, OH 43545
Phone: 419-592-4015
Fax: 419-592-4017
Type: Critical Access Hospitals
Emergency Services: Yes
Ownership: Voluntary non-profit - Private
Beds: 52

Key Personnel:

CEO . . . . Kim Bordenkircher
CEO/President. . . . . Kim Bordenkircher
Infection Control. . . . . Carol Borstelman
Emergency Room . . . . R Chesler, MD
Quality Assurance . . . . Tara Frease
Chief of Medical Staff. . . . . Stephen Knipe
Radiology. . . . . Edmundo A Somoza

Measure	Cases	This Hosp.	State Avg.	U.S. Avg.
Blood Clot Prevention and Treatment				
Anticoagulation Overlap Therapy[1,2]	-	-	93%	93%
ICU Venous Thromboembolism Prophylaxis[1,2]	-	-	93%	92%
Incidence of Potentially Preventable VTE[1,2]	-	-	6%	10%
UFH with Dosages/Platelet Monitoring[2,7]	-	-	98%	97%
Venous Thromboembolism Prophylaxis[2]	79	89%	88%	85%
Warfarin Therapy Discharge Instructions[1,2]	-	-	79%	75%
Chest Pain/Possible Heart Attack Care				
Aspirin Given Within 24 Hours of Arrival[5]	-	-	97%	96%
Fibrinolytic Meds Within 30 Min. of Arrival[5]	-	-	44%	58%
Average Time to ECG (minutes)[5]	-	-	6	7
Average Time to Transfer (minutes)[5]	-	-	58	60
Children's Asthma Care				
Received Home Management Plan of Care	-	-	85%	88%
Received Reliever Medication	-	-	100%	100%
Received Systemic Corticosteroids	-	-	100%	100%
Emergency Department				
Admittance Decision Time (minutes)[5]	-	-	90	98
Head CT Results Within 45 Min. of Arrival[5]	-	-	63%	57%
Patients Who Left ER Before Being Seen	9,597	0%	2%	2%
Time from ER Arrival to Admit. (minutes)[5]	-	-	265	274
Time from ER Arrival to Discharge (minutes)[5]	-	-	128	134
Time in ER Before Being Evaluated (minutes)[5]	-	-	22	26
Time to Pain Meds for Fractures (minutes)[5]	-	-	54	57
Heart Attack Care				
Aspirin Given at Discharge[5]	-	-	99%	99%
Fibrinolytic Meds Within 30 Min. of Arrival[5]	-	-	80%	54%
PCI Within 90 Minutes of Arrival[5]	-	-	97%	96%
Statin Prescribed at Discharge[5]	-	-	98%	98%
Heart Failure Care				
ACE Inhibitor or ARB for LVSD[1]	-	-	97%	97%
Discharge Instructions Given	13	77%	96%	94%
Evaluation of LVS Function	17	100%	100%	99%
Medicare Spending				
Medicare Spending per Patient (ratio)	-	-	1.01	0.98
Pneumonia Care				
Appropriate Initial Antibiotic Given	20	100%	96%	95%
Blood Culture Timing	28	100%	98%	98%
Pregnancy and Delivery Care				
Newborn Deliveries Scheduled Early[1,3]	-	-	5%	6%
Preventive Care				
Immunization for Influenza[5]	-	-	93%	90%
Immunization for Pneumonia[5]	-	-	94%	92%
Stroke Care				
Anticoagulation Therapy for Atrial Fibrillation[5]	-	-	95%	95%
Antithrombotic Therapy Timing[5]	-	-	98%	98%
Assessed for Rehabilitation[5]	-	-	98%	97%
Discharged on Antithrombotic Therapy[5]	-	-	99%	99%
Discharged on Statin Medication[5]	-	-	95%	94%
Thrombolytic Therapy Timing[5]	-	-	65%	66%
Venous Thromboembolism Prophylaxis[5]	-	-	95%	94%
Written Stroke Educational Materials Given[5]	-	-	92%	88%
Surgical Care Improvement Project				
Appropriate Beta Blocker Usage	24	100%	98%	98%
Appropriate VTP Within 24 Hours	54	100%	98%	98%
Controlled Postoperative Blood Glucose[7]	-	-	97%	97%
Perioperative Temperature Management	68	100%	100%	100%
Prophylactic Antibiotic Selection	63	100%	99%	99%
Prophylactic Antibiotic Selection (Outpatient)[5]	-	-	98%	98%
Prophylactic Antibiotic Stopped	62	89%	98%	98%
Prophylactic Antibiotic Timing	63	97%	99%	99%
Prophylactic Antibiotic Timing (Outpatient)[5]	-	-	97%	98%
Urinary Catheter Removal	43	100%	97%	97%
Survey of Patients' Hospital Experiences				
Area Around Room 'Always' Quiet at Night	(a)	69%	58%	61%
Doctors 'Always' Communicated Well	(a)	89%	80%	82%
Home Recovery Information Given	(a)	93%	87%	85%
Hospital Given 9 or 10 on 10 Point Scale	(a)	83%	72%	71%
Meds 'Always' Explained Before Given	(a)	72%	64%	64%
Nurses 'Always' Communicated Well	(a)	86%	81%	79%
Pain 'Always' Well Controlled	(a)	73%	71%	71%
Room and Bathroom 'Always' Clean	(a)	81%	75%	73%
Timely Help 'Always' Received	(a)	76%	70%	68%
Would Definitely Recommend Hospital	(a)	80%	71%	71%
Use of Medical Imaging				
Cardiac Imaging Stress Test before Surgery	81	4.9%	5.4%	5.3%
Combination Abdominal CT Scan	161	0.6%	7.1%	10.5%
Combination Brain/Sinus CT Scan[1]	-	-	2.8%	2.7%
Combination Chest CT Scan	105	0.0%	1.7%	2.7%
Follow-up Mammogram/Ultrasound	372	3.5%	8.7%	8.8%
Lumbar Spine MRI for Low Back Pain[1]	-	-	34.7%	37.2%

Doctors Hospital of Nelsonville

1950 Mount Saint Marys Drive
Nelsonville, OH 45764
Phone: 740-753-7300
Fax: 740-753-2197
Type: Critical Access Hospitals
Emergency Services: Yes
Ownership: Voluntary non-profit - Private
Beds: 50

Key Personnel:

Radiology. . . . . Richard W Adams
Chief of Medical Staff. . . . . Patricia A Bacon
Coronary Care . . . . Susan Bencley
Quality Assurance . . . . Robert Seamon
CEO/President. . . . . Steven Swart
Emergency Room . . . . Diane Viere

Measure	Cases	This Hosp.	State Avg.	U.S. Avg.
Blood Clot Prevention and Treatment				
Anticoagulation Overlap Therapy[5]	-	-	93%	93%

NOTE: Hospital profiles are in alphabetical order by state, then city, then hospital within the city; Rankings exclude hospitals with less than 25 cases except for patient surveys which excludes hospitals with less than 100 cases; (a) 100-299 cases; (1) The number of cases/patients is too few to report; (2) Data submitted were based on a sample of cases/patients; (3) Results are based on a shorter time period than required; (4) Data suppressed by CMS for one or more quarters; (5) Results are not available for this reporting period; (6) Fewer than 100 patients completed the HCAHPS survey; (7) No cases met the criteria for this measure; (8) The lower limit of the confidence interval cannot be calculated if the number of observed infections equals zero; (9) No data are available from the state/territory for this reporting period; (10) The scores shown reflect fewer than 50 completed surveys; (11) There were discrepancies in the data collection process; (12) This measure does not apply to this hospital for this reporting period; (13) Results cannot be calculated for this reporting period; (14) The results for this state are combined with nearby states to protect confidentiality; Please refer to the User's Guide for a full explanation of data.

Measure	Cases	This Hosp.	State Avg.	U.S. Avg.
ICU Venous Thromboembolism Prophylaxis[5]	-	-	93%	92%
Incidence of Potentially Preventable VTE[5]	-	-	6%	10%
UFH with Dosages/Platelet Monitoring[5]	-	-	98%	97%
Venous Thromboembolism Prophylaxis[5]	-	-	88%	85%
Warfarin Therapy Discharge Instructions[5]	-	-	79%	75%
Chest Pain/Possible Heart Attack Care				
Aspirin Given Within 24 Hours of Arrival[5]	-	-	97%	96%
Fibrinolytic Meds Within 30 Min. of Arrival[5]	-	-	44%	58%
Average Time to ECG (minutes)[5]	-	-	6	7
Average Time to Transfer (minutes)[5]	-	-	58	60
Children's Asthma Care				
Received Home Management Plan of Care	-	-	85%	88%
Received Reliever Medication	-	-	100%	100%
Received Systemic Corticosteroids	-	-	100%	100%
Emergency Department				
Admittance Decision Time (minutes)[5]	-	-	90	98
Head CT Results Within 45 Min. of Arrival[5]	-	-	63%	57%
Patients Who Left ER Before Being Seen[5]	-	-	2%	2%
Time from ER Arrival to Admit. (minutes)[5]	-	-	265	274
Time from ER Arrival to Discharge (minutes)[5]	-	-	128	134
Time in ER Before Being Evaluated (minutes)[5]	-	-	22	26
Time to Pain Meds for Fractures (minutes)[5]	-	-	54	57
Heart Attack Care				
Aspirin Given at Discharge[5]	-	-	99%	99%
Fibrinolytic Meds Within 30 Min. of Arrival[5]	-	-	80%	54%
PCI Within 90 Minutes of Arrival[5]	-	-	97%	96%
Statin Prescribed at Discharge[5]	-	-	98%	98%
Heart Failure Care				
ACE Inhibitor or ARB for LVSD[5]	-	-	97%	97%
Discharge Instructions Given[5]	-	-	96%	94%
Evaluation of LVS Function[5]	-	-	100%	99%
Medicare Spending				
Medicare Spending per Patient (ratio)	-	-	1.01	0.98
Pneumonia Care				
Appropriate Initial Antibiotic Given[5]	-	-	96%	95%
Blood Culture Timing[5]	-	-	98%	98%
Pregnancy and Delivery Care				
Newborn Deliveries Scheduled Early[5]	-	-	5%	6%
Preventive Care				
Immunization for Influenza[5]	-	-	93%	90%
Immunization for Pneumonia[5]	-	-	94%	92%
Stroke Care				
Anticoagulation Therapy for Atrial Fibrillation[5]	-	-	95%	95%
Antithrombotic Therapy Timing[5]	-	-	98%	98%
Assessed for Rehabilitation[5]	-	-	98%	97%
Discharged on Antithrombotic Therapy[5]	-	-	99%	99%
Discharged on Statin Medication[5]	-	-	95%	94%
Thrombolytic Therapy Timing[5]	-	-	65%	66%
Venous Thromboembolism Prophylaxis[5]	-	-	95%	94%
Written Stroke Educational Materials Given[5]	-	-	92%	88%
Surgical Care Improvement Project				
Appropriate Beta Blocker Usage[5]	-	-	98%	98%
Appropriate VTP Within 24 Hours[5]	-	-	98%	98%
Controlled Postoperative Blood Glucose[5]	-	-	97%	97%
Perioperative Temperature Management[5]	-	-	100%	100%
Prophylactic Antibiotic Selection[5]	-	-	99%	99%
Prophylactic Antibiotic Selection (Outpatient)[5]	-	-	98%	98%
Prophylactic Antibiotic Stopped[5]	-	-	98%	98%
Prophylactic Antibiotic Timing[5]	-	-	99%	99%
Prophylactic Antibiotic Timing (Outpatient)[5]	-	-	97%	98%
Urinary Catheter Removal[5]	-	-	97%	97%
Survey of Patients' Hospital Experiences				
Area Around Room 'Always' Quiet at Night[6]	<100	65%	58%	61%
Doctors 'Always' Communicated Well[6]	<100	78%	80%	82%
Home Recovery Information Given[6]	<100	88%	87%	85%
Hospital Given 9 or 10 on 10 Point Scale[6]	<100	76%	72%	71%
Meds 'Always' Explained Before Given[6]	<100	73%	64%	64%
Nurses 'Always' Communicated Well[6]	<100	85%	81%	79%
Pain 'Always' Well Controlled[6]	<100	69%	71%	71%
Room and Bathroom 'Always' Clean[6]	<100	85%	75%	73%
Timely Help 'Always' Received[6]	<100	75%	70%	68%
Would Definitely Recommend Hospital[6]	<100	78%	71%	71%
Use of Medical Imaging				
Cardiac Imaging Stress Test before Surgery[1]	-	-	5.4%	5.3%
Combination Abdominal CT Scan	104	1.0%	7.1%	10.5%
Combination Brain/Sinus CT Scan[1]	-	-	2.8%	2.7%
Combination Chest CT Scan	51	0.0%	1.7%	2.7%
Follow-up Mammogram/Ultrasound	129	12.4%	8.7%	8.8%
Lumbar Spine MRI for Low Back Pain[1]	-	-	34.7%	37.2%

Mount Carmel New Albany Surgical Hospital

7333 Smith's Mill Road
New Albany, OH 43054
Phone: 614-775-6600
URL: www.mountcarmelhealth.com
Type: Acute Care Hospitals
Emergency Services: No
Ownership: Proprietary

Measure	Cases	This Hosp.	State Avg.	U.S. Avg.
Blood Clot Prevention and Treatment				
Anticoagulation Overlap Therapy[1,2]	-	-	93%	93%
ICU Venous Thromboembolism Prophylaxis[2,7]	-	-	93%	92%
Incidence of Potentially Preventable VTE[1,2]	-	-	6%	10%
UFH with Dosages/Platelet Monitoring[2,7]	-	-	98%	97%
Venous Thromboembolism Prophylaxis[2]	121	100%	88%	85%
Warfarin Therapy Discharge Instructions[1,2]	-	-	79%	75%
Chest Pain/Possible Heart Attack Care				
Aspirin Given Within 24 Hours of Arrival[5]	-	-	97%	96%
Fibrinolytic Meds Within 30 Min. of Arrival[5]	-	-	44%	58%
Average Time to ECG (minutes)[5]	-	-	6	7
Average Time to Transfer (minutes)[5]	-	-	58	60
Children's Asthma Care				
Received Home Management Plan of Care	-	-	85%	88%
Received Reliever Medication	-	-	100%	100%
Received Systemic Corticosteroids	-	-	100%	100%
Emergency Department				
Admittance Decision Time (minutes)[2,7]	-	-	90	98
Head CT Results Within 45 Min. of Arrival[5]	-	-	63%	57%
Patients Who Left ER Before Being Seen[5]	-	-	2%	2%
Time from ER Arrival to Admit. (minutes)[2,7]	-	-	265	274
Time from ER Arrival to Discharge (minutes)[5]	-	-	128	134
Time in ER Before Being Evaluated (minutes)[5]	-	-	22	26
Time to Pain Meds for Fractures (minutes)[5]	-	-	54	57
Heart Attack Care				
Aspirin Given at Discharge[5]	-	-	99%	99%
Fibrinolytic Meds Within 30 Min. of Arrival[5]	-	-	80%	54%
PCI Within 90 Minutes of Arrival[5]	-	-	97%	96%
Statin Prescribed at Discharge[5]	-	-	98%	98%
Heart Failure Care				
ACE Inhibitor or ARB for LVSD[5]	-	-	97%	97%
Discharge Instructions Given[5]	-	-	96%	94%
Evaluation of LVS Function[5]	-	-	100%	99%
Medicare Spending				
Medicare Spending per Patient (ratio)	-	0.91	1.01	0.98
Pneumonia Care				
Appropriate Initial Antibiotic Given[5]	-	-	96%	95%
Blood Culture Timing[5]	-	-	98%	98%
Pregnancy and Delivery Care				
Newborn Deliveries Scheduled Early[7]	-	-	5%	6%
Preventive Care				
Immunization for Influenza[2]	471	94%	93%	90%
Immunization for Pneumonia[2]	563	88%	94%	92%
Stroke Care				
Anticoagulation Therapy for Atrial Fibrillation[5]	-	-	95%	95%
Antithrombotic Therapy Timing[5]	-	-	98%	98%
Assessed for Rehabilitation[5]	-	-	98%	97%
Discharged on Antithrombotic Therapy[5]	-	-	99%	99%
Discharged on Statin Medication[5]	-	-	95%	94%
Thrombolytic Therapy Timing[5]	-	-	65%	66%
Venous Thromboembolism Prophylaxis[5]	-	-	95%	94%
Written Stroke Educational Materials Given[5]	-	-	92%	88%
Surgical Care Improvement Project				
Appropriate Beta Blocker Usage[2]	175	98%	98%	98%
Appropriate VTP Within 24 Hours[2]	268	98%	98%	98%
Controlled Postoperative Blood Glucose[2,7]	-	-	97%	97%
Perioperative Temperature Management[2]	597	100%	100%	100%
Prophylactic Antibiotic Selection[2]	463	100%	99%	99%
Prophylactic Antibiotic Selection (Outpatient)	550	100%	98%	98%
Prophylactic Antibiotic Stopped[2]	455	99%	98%	98%
Prophylactic Antibiotic Timing[2]	463	100%	99%	99%
Prophylactic Antibiotic Timing (Outpatient)	550	100%	97%	98%
Urinary Catheter Removal[2]	260	98%	97%	97%
Survey of Patients' Hospital Experiences				
Area Around Room 'Always' Quiet at Night	300+	80%	58%	61%
Doctors 'Always' Communicated Well	300+	85%	80%	82%
Home Recovery Information Given	300+	92%	87%	85%
Hospital Given 9 or 10 on 10 Point Scale	300+	88%	72%	71%
Meds 'Always' Explained Before Given	300+	71%	64%	64%
Nurses 'Always' Communicated Well	300+	87%	81%	79%
Pain 'Always' Well Controlled	300+	79%	71%	71%
Room and Bathroom 'Always' Clean	300+	84%	75%	73%
Timely Help 'Always' Received	300+	75%	70%	68%
Would Definitely Recommend Hospital	300+	90%	71%	71%
Use of Medical Imaging				
Cardiac Imaging Stress Test before Surgery[7]	-	-	5.4%	5.3%
Combination Abdominal CT Scan[1]	-	-	7.1%	10.5%
Combination Brain/Sinus CT Scan[1]	-	-	2.8%	2.7%
Combination Chest CT Scan[1]	-	-	1.7%	2.7%
Follow-up Mammogram/Ultrasound[7]	-	-	8.7%	8.8%
Lumbar Spine MRI for Low Back Pain	59	30.5%	34.7%	37.2%

Licking Memorial Hospital

1320 West Main Street
Newark, OH 43055
Phone: 740-348-4000
Fax: 740-348-4055
URL: www.lmhealth.org
Type: Acute Care Hospitals
Emergency Services: Yes
Ownership: Voluntary non-profit - Private
Beds: 195

Key Personnel:

Quality Assurance .... Paula Alexander
Chief of Medical Staff .... Craig Cairns
Radiology.................... Subbarao Cherukuri, MD
Emergency Room .... Penny McCort
President/CEO............... Robert A Montagnese, C.P.A., M.H.A.,
Operating Room.............. Deborah Young, RN

Measure	Cases	This Hosp.	State Avg.	U.S. Avg.
Blood Clot Prevention and Treatment				
Anticoagulation Overlap Therapy[2]	53	100%	93%	93%
ICU Venous Thromboembolism Prophylaxis[2]	63	95%	93%	92%
Incidence of Potentially Preventable VTE[1,2]	-	-	6%	10%
UFH with Dosages/Platelet Monitoring[2]	16	100%	98%	97%
Venous Thromboembolism Prophylaxis[2]	328	93%	88%	85%
Warfarin Therapy Discharge Instructions[2]	43	100%	79%	75%
Chest Pain/Possible Heart Attack Care				
Aspirin Given Within 24 Hours of Arrival	16	100%	97%	96%
Fibrinolytic Meds Within 30 Min. of Arrival[7]	-	-	44%	58%
Average Time to ECG (minutes)	17	2	6	7
Average Time to Transfer (minutes)[7]	-	-	58	60
Children's Asthma Care				
Received Home Management Plan of Care	-	-	85%	88%
Received Reliever Medication	-	-	100%	100%
Received Systemic Corticosteroids	-	-	100%	100%
Emergency Department				
Admittance Decision Time (minutes)[2]	736	67	90	98
Head CT Results Within 45 Min. of Arrival	13	69%	63%	57%
Patients Who Left ER Before Being Seen	58,554	5%	2%	2%
Time from ER Arrival to Admit. (minutes)[2]	755	225	265	274
Time from ER Arrival to Discharge (minutes)	378	150	128	134
Time in ER Before Being Evaluated (minutes)	383	56	22	26
Time to Pain Meds for Fractures (minutes)	133	60	54	57
Heart Attack Care				
Aspirin Given at Discharge	151	99%	99%	99%
Fibrinolytic Meds Within 30 Min. of Arrival[1]	-	-	80%	54%
PCI Within 90 Minutes of Arrival	60	100%	97%	96%
Statin Prescribed at Discharge	149	100%	98%	98%
Heart Failure Care				
ACE Inhibitor or ARB for LVSD	82	99%	97%	97%
Discharge Instructions Given	187	98%	96%	94%
Evaluation of LVS Function	240	100%	100%	99%
Medicare Spending				

NOTE: Hospital profiles are in alphabetical order by state, then city, then hospital within the city; Rankings exclude hospitals with less than 25 cases except for patient surveys which excludes hospitals with less than 100 cases; (a) 100-299 cases; (1) The number of cases/patients is too few to report; (2) Data submitted were based on a sample of cases/patients; (3) Results are based on a shorter time period than required; (4) Data suppressed by CMS for one or more quarters; (5) Results are not available for this reporting period; (6) Fewer than 100 patients completed the HCAHPS survey; (7) No cases met the criteria for this measure; (8) The lower limit of the confidence interval cannot be calculated if the number of observed infections equals zero; (9) No data are available from the state/territory for this reporting period; (10) The scores shown reflect fewer than 50 completed surveys; (11) There were discrepancies in the data collection process; (12) This measure does not apply to this hospital for this reporting period; (13) Results cannot be calculated for this reporting period; (14) The results for this state are combined with nearby states to protect confidentiality; Please refer to the User's Guide for a full explanation of data.

Medicare Spending per Patient (ratio)	-	0.93	1.01	0.98
Pneumonia Care				
Appropriate Initial Antibiotic Given[2]	104	98%	96%	95%
Blood Culture Timing[2]	122	100%	98%	98%
Pregnancy and Delivery Care				
Newborn Deliveries Scheduled Early[2]	31	0%	5%	6%
Preventive Care				
Immunization for Influenza[2]	557	97%	93%	90%
Immunization for Pneumonia[2]	698	98%	94%	92%
Stroke Care				
Anticoagulation Therapy for Atrial Fibrillation	12	100%	95%	95%
Antithrombotic Therapy Timing	45	98%	98%	98%
Assessed for Rehabilitation	63	100%	98%	97%
Discharged on Antithrombotic Therapy	63	100%	99%	99%
Discharged on Statin Medication	49	98%	95%	94%
Thrombolytic Therapy Timing	12	75%	65%	66%
Venous Thromboembolism Prophylaxis	49	98%	95%	94%
Written Stroke Educational Materials Given	38	100%	92%	88%
Surgical Care Improvement Project				
Appropriate Beta Blocker Usage	117	97%	98%	98%
Appropriate VTP Within 24 Hours	313	99%	98%	98%
Controlled Postoperative Blood Glucose[7]	-	-	97%	97%
Perioperative Temperature Management	389	100%	100%	100%
Prophylactic Antibiotic Selection	242	99%	99%	99%
Prophylactic Antibiotic Selection (Outpatient)	59	93%	98%	98%
Prophylactic Antibiotic Stopped	237	100%	98%	98%
Prophylactic Antibiotic Timing	242	100%	99%	99%
Prophylactic Antibiotic Timing (Outpatient)	40	85%	97%	98%
Urinary Catheter Removal	244	100%	97%	97%
Survey of Patients' Hospital Experiences				
Area Around Room 'Always' Quiet at Night	300+	58%	58%	61%
Doctors 'Always' Communicated Well	300+	79%	80%	82%
Home Recovery Information Given	300+	84%	87%	85%
Hospital Given 9 or 10 on 10 Point Scale	300+	64%	72%	71%
Meds 'Always' Explained Before Given	300+	62%	64%	64%
Nurses 'Always' Communicated Well	300+	78%	81%	79%
Pain 'Always' Well Controlled	300+	68%	71%	71%
Room and Bathroom 'Always' Clean	300+	69%	75%	73%
Timely Help 'Always' Received	300+	66%	70%	68%
Would Definitely Recommend Hospital	300+	63%	71%	71%
Use of Medical Imaging				
Cardiac Imaging Stress Test before Surgery	277	4.3%	5.4%	5.3%
Combination Abdominal CT Scan	1,013	3.3%	7.1%	10.5%
Combination Brain/Sinus CT Scan	724	1.1%	2.8%	2.7%
Combination Chest CT Scan	527	0.8%	1.7%	2.7%
Follow-up Mammogram/Ultrasound	1,982	2.8%	8.7%	8.8%
Lumbar Spine MRI for Low Back Pain	129	37.2%	34.7%	37.2%

Fisher - Titus Hospital

272 Benedict Avenue
Norwalk, OH 44857
Phone: 419-668-8101
Fax: 419-663-6036
E-mail: jraboin@fimc.com
URL: www.fisher-titus.com
Type: Acute Care Hospitals
Emergency Services: Yes
Ownership: Voluntary non-profit - Private
Beds: 112

Key Personnel:

Operating Room. . . . . Souheil M Al-Jadda, RN
Infection Control. . . . . Rae Colahan, RN
Chief of Medical Staff. . . . . William B Cornell, MD
Radiology. . . . . William L Ferber, DO
CEO/President. . . . . Patrick J Martin
Quality Assurance . . . . Cherlie Spragg, RN
Pediatric Ambulatory Care . . . . . . Glenn Trippe
Pediatric In-Patient Care . . . . Glenn Trippe

Measure	Cases	This Hosp.	State Avg.	U.S. Avg.
Blood Clot Prevention and Treatment				
Anticoagulation Overlap Therapy[2]	25	92%	93%	93%
ICU Venous Thromboembolism Prophylaxis[2]	69	90%	93%	92%
Incidence of Potentially Preventable VTE[1,2]	-	-	6%	10%
UFH with Dosages/Platelet Monitoring[2]	35	89%	98%	97%
Venous Thromboembolism Prophylaxis[2]	262	86%	88%	85%
Warfarin Therapy Discharge Instructions[2]	18	94%	79%	75%
Chest Pain/Possible Heart Attack Care				
Aspirin Given Within 24 Hours of Arrival	50	94%	97%	96%
Fibrinolytic Meds Within 30 Min. of Arrival[7]	-	-	44%	58%
Average Time to ECG (minutes)	52	8	6	7
Average Time to Transfer (minutes)	22	74	58	60
Children's Asthma Care				
Received Home Management Plan of Care	-	-	85%	88%
Received Reliever Medication	-	-	100%	100%
Received Systemic Corticosteroids	-	-	100%	100%
Emergency Department				
Admittance Decision Time (minutes)[2]	358	112	90	98
Head CT Results Within 45 Min. of Arrival	13	77%	63%	57%
Patients Who Left ER Before Being Seen	27,601	0%	2%	2%
Time from ER Arrival to Admit. (minutes)[2]	431	272	265	274
Time from ER Arrival to Discharge (minutes)	362	142	128	134
Time in ER Before Being Evaluated (minutes)	391	31	22	26
Time to Pain Meds for Fractures (minutes)	110	56	54	57
Heart Attack Care				
Aspirin Given at Discharge[1]	-	-	99%	99%
Fibrinolytic Meds Within 30 Min. of Arrival[7]	-	-	80%	54%
PCI Within 90 Minutes of Arrival[7]	-	-	97%	96%
Statin Prescribed at Discharge[1]	-	-	98%	98%
Heart Failure Care				
ACE Inhibitor or ARB for LVSD	39	90%	97%	97%
Discharge Instructions Given	84	94%	96%	94%
Evaluation of LVS Function	113	100%	100%	99%
Medicare Spending				
Medicare Spending per Patient (ratio)	-	1.00	1.01	0.98
Pneumonia Care				
Appropriate Initial Antibiotic Given	106	98%	96%	95%
Blood Culture Timing	158	98%	98%	98%
Pregnancy and Delivery Care				
Newborn Deliveries Scheduled Early[2]	36	28%	5%	6%
Preventive Care				
Immunization for Influenza[2]	371	95%	93%	90%
Immunization for Pneumonia[2]	490	97%	94%	92%
Stroke Care				
Anticoagulation Therapy for Atrial Fibrillation[1]	-	-	95%	95%
Antithrombotic Therapy Timing	51	100%	98%	98%
Assessed for Rehabilitation	58	98%	98%	97%
Discharged on Antithrombotic Therapy	58	100%	99%	99%
Discharged on Statin Medication	42	95%	95%	94%
Thrombolytic Therapy Timing[1]	-	-	65%	66%
Venous Thromboembolism Prophylaxis	50	100%	95%	94%
Written Stroke Educational Materials Given	29	100%	92%	88%
Surgical Care Improvement Project				
Appropriate Beta Blocker Usage	90	99%	98%	98%
Appropriate VTP Within 24 Hours	254	100%	98%	98%
Controlled Postoperative Blood Glucose[7]	-	-	97%	97%
Perioperative Temperature Management	280	100%	100%	100%
Prophylactic Antibiotic Selection	223	98%	99%	99%
Prophylactic Antibiotic Selection (Outpatient)	89	96%	98%	98%
Prophylactic Antibiotic Stopped	220	98%	98%	98%
Prophylactic Antibiotic Timing	223	100%	99%	99%
Prophylactic Antibiotic Timing (Outpatient)	93	95%	97%	98%
Urinary Catheter Removal	252	100%	97%	97%
Survey of Patients' Hospital Experiences				
Area Around Room 'Always' Quiet at Night	300+	56%	58%	61%
Doctors 'Always' Communicated Well	300+	80%	80%	82%
Home Recovery Information Given	300+	88%	87%	85%
Hospital Given 9 or 10 on 10 Point Scale	300+	74%	72%	71%
Meds 'Always' Explained Before Given	300+	65%	64%	64%
Nurses 'Always' Communicated Well	300+	81%	81%	79%
Pain 'Always' Well Controlled	300+	71%	71%	71%
Room and Bathroom 'Always' Clean	300+	79%	75%	73%
Timely Help 'Always' Received	300+	70%	70%	68%
Would Definitely Recommend Hospital	300+	70%	71%	71%
Use of Medical Imaging				
Cardiac Imaging Stress Test before Surgery	250	6.4%	5.4%	5.3%
Combination Abdominal CT Scan	414	7.2%	7.1%	10.5%
Combination Brain/Sinus CT Scan	450	0.4%	2.8%	2.7%
Combination Chest CT Scan	254	1.6%	1.7%	2.7%
Follow-up Mammogram/Ultrasound	758	9.6%	8.7%	8.8%
Lumbar Spine MRI for Low Back Pain	116	28.4%	34.7%	37.2%

Mercy Allen Hospital

200 West Lorain Street
Oberlin, OH 44074
Phone: 440-775-1211
Fax: 440-775-9153
URL: www.ehealthconnection.com/lorain
Type: Critical Access Hospitals
Emergency Services: Yes
Ownership: Voluntary non-profit - Private
Beds: 25

Key Personnel:

Operating Room. . . . . Nancy Eastaugh
Patient Relations . . . . Dale Greathouse
Cardiac Laboratory. . . . . Geeth Mohan, MD
CEO/President. . . . . Jerome Morasko
Quality Assurance . . . . Kathy Neptune
Chief of Medical Staff. . . . . Georgia Newman, MD
Infection Control. . . . . Denise Perry
Radiology. . . . . Thomas Wu

Measure	Cases	This Hosp.	State Avg.	U.S. Avg.
Blood Clot Prevention and Treatment				
Anticoagulation Overlap Therapy[1,2]	-	-	93%	93%
ICU Venous Thromboembolism Prophylaxis[1,2]	-	-	93%	92%
Incidence of Potentially Preventable VTE[2,7]	-	-	6%	10%
UFH with Dosages/Platelet Monitoring[1,2]	-	-	98%	97%
Venous Thromboembolism Prophylaxis[2]	85	81%	88%	85%
Warfarin Therapy Discharge Instructions[1,2]	-	-	79%	75%
Chest Pain/Possible Heart Attack Care				
Aspirin Given Within 24 Hours of Arrival[5]	-	-	97%	96%
Fibrinolytic Meds Within 30 Min. of Arrival[5]	-	-	44%	58%
Average Time to ECG (minutes)[5]	-	-	6	7
Average Time to Transfer (minutes)[5]	-	-	58	60
Children's Asthma Care				
Received Home Management Plan of Care	-	-	85%	88%
Received Reliever Medication	-	-	100%	100%
Received Systemic Corticosteroids	-	-	100%	100%
Emergency Department				
Admittance Decision Time (minutes)[2]	341	39	90	98
Head CT Results Within 45 Min. of Arrival[5]	-	-	63%	57%
Patients Who Left ER Before Being Seen[5]	-	-	2%	2%
Time from ER Arrival to Admit. (minutes)[2]	346	198	265	274
Time from ER Arrival to Discharge (minutes)[5]	-	-	128	134
Time in ER Before Being Evaluated (minutes)[5]	-	-	22	26
Time to Pain Meds for Fractures (minutes)[5]	-	-	54	57
Heart Attack Care				
Aspirin Given at Discharge[3,7]	-	-	99%	99%
Fibrinolytic Meds Within 30 Min. of Arrival[1,3]	-	-	80%	54%
PCI Within 90 Minutes of Arrival[3,7]	-	-	97%	96%
Statin Prescribed at Discharge[3,7]	-	-	98%	98%
Heart Failure Care				
ACE Inhibitor or ARB for LVSD[1,3]	-	-	97%	97%
Discharge Instructions Given[1,3]	-	-	96%	94%
Evaluation of LVS Function[1,3]	-	-	100%	99%
Medicare Spending				
Medicare Spending per Patient (ratio)	-	-	1.01	0.98
Pneumonia Care				
Appropriate Initial Antibiotic Given	33	85%	96%	95%
Blood Culture Timing	45	93%	98%	98%
Pregnancy and Delivery Care				
Newborn Deliveries Scheduled Early[3,7]	-	-	5%	6%
Preventive Care				
Immunization for Influenza[2]	243	98%	93%	90%
Immunization for Pneumonia[2]	377	95%	94%	92%
Stroke Care				
Anticoagulation Therapy for Atrial Fibrillation[7]	-	-	95%	95%
Antithrombotic Therapy Timing[1]	-	-	98%	98%
Assessed for Rehabilitation[1]	-	-	98%	97%
Discharged on Antithrombotic Therapy[1]	-	-	99%	99%
Discharged on Statin Medication[1]	-	-	95%	94%
Thrombolytic Therapy Timing[7]	-	-	65%	66%
Venous Thromboembolism Prophylaxis[1]	-	-	95%	94%
Written Stroke Educational Materials Given[1]	-	-	92%	88%
Surgical Care Improvement Project				
Appropriate Beta Blocker Usage	27	100%	98%	98%
Appropriate VTP Within 24 Hours	55	98%	98%	98%
Controlled Postoperative Blood Glucose[7]	-	-	97%	97%
Perioperative Temperature Management	61	100%	100%	100%
Prophylactic Antibiotic Selection	56	98%	99%	99%

NOTE: Hospital profiles are in alphabetical order by state, then city, then hospital within the city; Rankings exclude hospitals with less than 25 cases except for patient surveys which excludes hospitals with less than 100 cases; (a) 100-299 cases; (1) The number of cases/patients is too few to report; (2) Data submitted were based on a sample of cases/patients; (3) Results are based on a shorter time period than required; (4) Data suppressed by CMS for one or more quarters; (5) Results are not available for this reporting period; (6) Fewer than 100 patients completed the HCAHPS survey; (7) No cases met the criteria for this measure; (8) The lower limit of the confidence interval cannot be calculated if the number of observed infections equals zero; (9) No data are available from the state/territory for this reporting period; (10) The scores shown reflect fewer than 50 completed surveys; (11) There were discrepancies in the data collection process; (12) This measure does not apply to this hospital for this reporting period; (13) Results cannot be calculated for this reporting period; (14) The results for this state are combined with nearby states to protect confidentiality; Please refer to the User's Guide for a full explanation of data.

Prophylactic Antibiotic Selection (Outpatient)[5]	-	-	98%	98%
Prophylactic Antibiotic Stopped	55	100%	98%	98%
Prophylactic Antibiotic Timing	56	100%	99%	99%
Prophylactic Antibiotic Timing (Outpatient)[5]	-	-	97%	98%
Urinary Catheter Removal	54	100%	97%	97%
Survey of Patients' Hospital Experiences				
Area Around Room 'Always' Quiet at Night	(a)	54%	58%	61%
Doctors 'Always' Communicated Well	(a)	74%	80%	82%
Home Recovery Information Given	(a)	83%	87%	85%
Hospital Given 9 or 10 on 10 Point Scale	(a)	73%	72%	71%
Meds 'Always' Explained Before Given	(a)	59%	64%	64%
Nurses 'Always' Communicated Well	(a)	77%	81%	79%
Pain 'Always' Well Controlled	(a)	70%	71%	71%
Room and Bathroom 'Always' Clean	(a)	73%	75%	73%
Timely Help 'Always' Received	(a)	70%	70%	68%
Would Definitely Recommend Hospital	(a)	70%	71%	71%
Use of Medical Imaging				
Cardiac Imaging Stress Test before Surgery[1]	-	-	5.4%	5.3%
Combination Abdominal CT Scan	191	1.6%	7.1%	10.5%
Combination Brain/Sinus CT Scan[1]	-	-	2.8%	2.7%
Combination Chest CT Scan	75	10.7%	1.7%	2.7%
Follow-up Mammogram/Ultrasound	358	9.2%	8.7%	8.8%
Lumbar Spine MRI for Low Back Pain[7]	-	-	34.7%	37.2%

Bay Park Community Hospital

2801 Bay Park Drive
Oregon, OH 43616
Phone: 419-690-7700
Fax: 419-690-7746
URL: www.promedica.org
Type: Acute Care Hospitals
Emergency Services: Yes
Ownership: Voluntary non-profit - Other
Beds: 70

Key Personnel:
Chief of Medical Staff. . . . . Bryan Badik
CEO/President. . . . . William M Mueller, FACHE

Measure	Cases	This Hosp.	State Avg.	U.S. Avg.
Blood Clot Prevention and Treatment				
Anticoagulation Overlap Therapy[2]	19	89%	93%	93%
ICU Venous Thromboembolism Prophylaxis[2]	52	96%	93%	92%
Incidence of Potentially Preventable VTE[1,2]	-	-	6%	10%
UFH with Dosages/Platelet Monitoring[1,2]	-	-	98%	97%
Venous Thromboembolism Prophylaxis[2]	244	84%	88%	85%
Warfarin Therapy Discharge Instructions[2]	12	33%	79%	75%
Chest Pain/Possible Heart Attack Care				
Aspirin Given Within 24 Hours of Arrival	60	98%	97%	96%
Fibrinolytic Meds Within 30 Min. of Arrival[7]	-	-	44%	58%
Average Time to ECG (minutes)	62	5	6	7
Average Time to Transfer (minutes)[1]	-	-	58	60
Children's Asthma Care				
Received Home Management Plan of Care	-	-	85%	88%
Received Reliever Medication	-	-	100%	100%
Received Systemic Corticosteroids	-	-	100%	100%
Emergency Department				
Admittance Decision Time (minutes)[2]	327	80	90	98
Head CT Results Within 45 Min. of Arrival[1]	-	-	63%	57%
Patients Who Left ER Before Being Seen	24,918	1%	2%	2%
Time from ER Arrival to Admit. (minutes)[2]	328	223	265	274
Time from ER Arrival to Discharge (minutes)	360	78	128	134
Time in ER Before Being Evaluated (minutes)	128	36	22	26
Time to Pain Meds for Fractures (minutes)	69	51	54	57
Heart Attack Care				
Aspirin Given at Discharge[1]	-	-	99%	99%
Fibrinolytic Meds Within 30 Min. of Arrival[7]	-	-	80%	54%
PCI Within 90 Minutes of Arrival[7]	-	-	97%	96%
Statin Prescribed at Discharge[1]	-	-	98%	98%
Heart Failure Care				
ACE Inhibitor or ARB for LVSD	21	95%	97%	97%
Discharge Instructions Given	77	83%	96%	94%
Evaluation of LVS Function	111	100%	100%	99%
Medicare Spending				
Medicare Spending per Patient (ratio)	-	1.02	1.01	0.98
Pneumonia Care				
Appropriate Initial Antibiotic Given	76	93%	96%	95%
Blood Culture Timing	123	100%	98%	98%
Pregnancy and Delivery Care				
Newborn Deliveries Scheduled Early[2]	36	11%	5%	6%
Preventive Care				
Immunization for Influenza[2]	327	95%	93%	90%
Immunization for Pneumonia[2]	413	98%	94%	92%
Stroke Care				
Anticoagulation Therapy for Atrial Fibrillation[1]	-	-	95%	95%
Antithrombotic Therapy Timing	22	100%	98%	98%
Assessed for Rehabilitation	21	100%	98%	97%
Discharged on Antithrombotic Therapy	20	95%	99%	99%
Discharged on Statin Medication	20	90%	95%	94%
Thrombolytic Therapy Timing[1]	-	-	65%	66%
Venous Thromboembolism Prophylaxis	22	73%	95%	94%
Written Stroke Educational Materials Given	15	60%	92%	88%
Surgical Care Improvement Project				
Appropriate Beta Blocker Usage	153	99%	98%	98%
Appropriate VTP Within 24 Hours	304	99%	98%	98%
Controlled Postoperative Blood Glucose[7]	-	-	97%	97%
Perioperative Temperature Management	356	100%	100%	100%
Prophylactic Antibiotic Selection	248	99%	99%	99%
Prophylactic Antibiotic Selection (Outpatient)	37	97%	98%	98%
Prophylactic Antibiotic Stopped	241	99%	98%	98%
Prophylactic Antibiotic Timing	248	100%	99%	99%
Prophylactic Antibiotic Timing (Outpatient)	37	100%	97%	98%
Urinary Catheter Removal	262	98%	97%	97%
Survey of Patients' Hospital Experiences				
Area Around Room 'Always' Quiet at Night	300+	61%	58%	61%
Doctors 'Always' Communicated Well	300+	78%	80%	82%
Home Recovery Information Given	300+	88%	87%	85%
Hospital Given 9 or 10 on 10 Point Scale	300+	77%	72%	71%
Meds 'Always' Explained Before Given	300+	66%	64%	64%
Nurses 'Always' Communicated Well	300+	81%	81%	79%
Pain 'Always' Well Controlled	300+	75%	71%	71%
Room and Bathroom 'Always' Clean	300+	72%	75%	73%
Timely Help 'Always' Received	300+	72%	70%	68%
Would Definitely Recommend Hospital	300+	78%	71%	71%
Use of Medical Imaging				
Cardiac Imaging Stress Test before Surgery	333	6.0%	5.4%	5.3%
Combination Abdominal CT Scan	294	5.1%	7.1%	10.5%
Combination Brain/Sinus CT Scan[1]	-	-	2.8%	2.7%
Combination Chest CT Scan	207	0.0%	1.7%	2.7%
Follow-up Mammogram/Ultrasound	593	7.6%	8.7%	8.8%
Lumbar Spine MRI for Low Back Pain	54	35.2%	34.7%	37.2%

Mercy Saint Charles Hospital

2600 Navarre Avenue
Oregon, OH 43616
Phone: 419-696-7200
URL: www.mercyweb.org/st_charles
Type: Acute Care Hospitals
Emergency Services: Yes
Ownership: Voluntary non-profit - Church
Beds: 390

Key Personnel:
President/CEO. . . . . Steven L Mickus

Measure	Cases	This Hosp.	State Avg.	U.S. Avg.
Blood Clot Prevention and Treatment				
Anticoagulation Overlap Therapy[2]	58	66%	93%	93%
ICU Venous Thromboembolism Prophylaxis[2]	68	82%	93%	92%
Incidence of Potentially Preventable VTE[1,2]	-	-	6%	10%
UFH with Dosages/Platelet Monitoring[2]	31	100%	98%	97%
Venous Thromboembolism Prophylaxis[2]	345	86%	88%	85%
Warfarin Therapy Discharge Instructions[2]	26	42%	79%	75%
Chest Pain/Possible Heart Attack Care				
Aspirin Given Within 24 Hours of Arrival	49	100%	97%	96%
Fibrinolytic Meds Within 30 Min. of Arrival[7]	-	-	44%	58%
Average Time to ECG (minutes)	49	8	6	7
Average Time to Transfer (minutes)	20	78	58	60
Children's Asthma Care				
Received Home Management Plan of Care	-	-	85%	88%
Received Reliever Medication	-	-	100%	100%
Received Systemic Corticosteroids	-	-	100%	100%
Emergency Department				
Admittance Decision Time (minutes)[2]	786	127	90	98
Head CT Results Within 45 Min. of Arrival	12	8%	63%	57%
Patients Who Left ER Before Being Seen	40,704	1%	2%	2%
Time from ER Arrival to Admit. (minutes)[2]	788	295	265	274
Time from ER Arrival to Discharge (minutes)	381	127	128	134
Time in ER Before Being Evaluated (minutes)	110	26	22	26
Time to Pain Meds for Fractures (minutes)	74	72	54	57
Heart Attack Care				
Aspirin Given at Discharge	29	100%	99%	99%
Fibrinolytic Meds Within 30 Min. of Arrival[7]	-	-	80%	54%
PCI Within 90 Minutes of Arrival[7]	-	-	97%	96%
Statin Prescribed at Discharge	28	96%	98%	98%
Heart Failure Care				
ACE Inhibitor or ARB for LVSD	51	96%	97%	97%
Discharge Instructions Given	141	99%	96%	94%
Evaluation of LVS Function	203	100%	100%	99%
Medicare Spending				
Medicare Spending per Patient (ratio)	-	1.03	1.01	0.98
Pneumonia Care				
Appropriate Initial Antibiotic Given	96	98%	96%	95%
Blood Culture Timing	172	98%	98%	98%
Pregnancy and Delivery Care				
Newborn Deliveries Scheduled Early[2]	26	15%	5%	6%
Preventive Care				
Immunization for Influenza[2]	579	96%	93%	90%
Immunization for Pneumonia[2]	823	95%	94%	92%
Stroke Care				
Anticoagulation Therapy for Atrial Fibrillation[1]	-	-	95%	95%
Antithrombotic Therapy Timing	47	98%	98%	98%
Assessed for Rehabilitation	42	93%	98%	97%
Discharged on Antithrombotic Therapy	41	93%	99%	99%
Discharged on Statin Medication	34	94%	95%	94%
Thrombolytic Therapy Timing[1]	-	-	65%	66%
Venous Thromboembolism Prophylaxis	50	92%	95%	94%
Written Stroke Educational Materials Given	25	56%	92%	88%
Surgical Care Improvement Project				
Appropriate Beta Blocker Usage[2]	119	97%	98%	98%
Appropriate VTP Within 24 Hours[2]	410	95%	98%	98%
Controlled Postoperative Blood Glucose[2,7]	-	-	97%	97%
Perioperative Temperature Management[2]	433	100%	100%	100%
Prophylactic Antibiotic Selection[2]	279	99%	99%	99%
Prophylactic Antibiotic Selection (Outpatient)	80	99%	98%	98%
Prophylactic Antibiotic Stopped[2]	274	98%	98%	98%
Prophylactic Antibiotic Timing[2]	279	99%	99%	99%
Prophylactic Antibiotic Timing (Outpatient)	81	99%	97%	98%
Urinary Catheter Removal[2]	138	88%	97%	97%
Survey of Patients' Hospital Experiences				
Area Around Room 'Always' Quiet at Night	300+	55%	58%	61%
Doctors 'Always' Communicated Well	300+	74%	80%	82%
Home Recovery Information Given	300+	86%	87%	85%
Hospital Given 9 or 10 on 10 Point Scale	300+	67%	72%	71%
Meds 'Always' Explained Before Given	300+	60%	64%	64%
Nurses 'Always' Communicated Well	300+	79%	81%	79%
Pain 'Always' Well Controlled	300+	68%	71%	71%
Room and Bathroom 'Always' Clean	300+	77%	75%	73%
Timely Help 'Always' Received	300+	66%	70%	68%
Would Definitely Recommend Hospital	300+	68%	71%	71%
Use of Medical Imaging				
Cardiac Imaging Stress Test before Surgery	182	6.0%	5.4%	5.3%
Combination Abdominal CT Scan	665	8.9%	7.1%	10.5%
Combination Brain/Sinus CT Scan	537	1.9%	2.8%	2.7%
Combination Chest CT Scan	556	7.4%	1.7%	2.7%
Follow-up Mammogram/Ultrasound	1,075	13.0%	8.7%	8.8%
Lumbar Spine MRI for Low Back Pain	101	33.7%	34.7%	37.2%

Aultman Orrville Hospital

832 South Main Street
Orrville, OH 44667
Phone: 330-682-3010
Fax: 330-683-2130
Type: Critical Access Hospitals
Emergency Services: Yes
Ownership: Voluntary non-profit - Private
Beds: 51

Key Personnel:
Operating Room. . . . . Laura Brelin
Emergency Room . . . . Michael Corko
Chief of Medical Staff . . . . Robert H Hutson
Infection Control. . . . . Jan Oberly, RN
Radiology. . . . . Karla Volke

Measure	Cases	This Hosp.	State Avg.	U.S. Avg.

NOTE: Hospital profiles are in alphabetical order by state, then city, then hospital within the city; Rankings exclude hospitals with less than 25 cases except for patient surveys which excludes hospitals with less than 100 cases; (a) 100-299 cases; (1) The number of cases/patients is too few to report; (2) Data submitted were based on a sample of cases/patients; (3) Results are based on a shorter time period than required; (4) Data suppressed by CMS for one or more quarters; (5) Results are not available for this reporting period; (6) Fewer than 100 patients completed the HCAHPS survey; (7) No cases met the criteria for this measure; (8) The lower limit of the confidence interval cannot be calculated if the number of observed infections equals zero; (9) No data are available from the state/territory for this reporting period; (10) The scores shown reflect fewer than 50 completed surveys; (11) There were discrepancies in the data collection process; (12) This measure does not apply to this hospital for this reporting period; (13) Results cannot be calculated for this reporting period; (14) The results for this state are combined with nearby states to protect confidentiality; Please refer to the User's Guide for a full explanation of data.

Blood Clot Prevention and Treatment				
Anticoagulation Overlap Therapy[5]	-	-	93%	93%
ICU Venous Thromboembolism Prophylaxis[5]	-	-	93%	92%
Incidence of Potentially Preventable VTE[5]	-	-	6%	10%
UFH with Dosages/Platelet Monitoring[5]	-	-	98%	97%
Venous Thromboembolism Prophylaxis[5]	-	-	88%	85%
Warfarin Therapy Discharge Instructions[5]	-	-	79%	75%
Chest Pain/Possible Heart Attack Care				
Aspirin Given Within 24 Hours of Arrival	68	100%	97%	96%
Fibrinolytic Meds Within 30 Min. of Arrival[7]	-	-	44%	58%
Average Time to ECG (minutes)	70	8	6	7
Average Time to Transfer (minutes)[7]	-	-	58	60
Children's Asthma Care				
Received Home Management Plan of Care	-	-	85%	88%
Received Reliever Medication	-	-	100%	100%
Received Systemic Corticosteroids	-	-	100%	100%
Emergency Department				
Admittance Decision Time (minutes)[5]	-	-	90	98
Head CT Results Within 45 Min. of Arrival[5]	-	-	63%	57%
Patients Who Left ER Before Being Seen[5]	-	-	2%	2%
Time from ER Arrival to Admit. (minutes)[5]	-	-	265	274
Time from ER Arrival to Discharge (minutes)	399	67	128	134
Time in ER Before Being Evaluated (minutes)	432	10	22	26
Time to Pain Meds for Fractures (minutes)[5]	-	-	54	57
Heart Attack Care				
Aspirin Given at Discharge[3,7]	-	-	99%	99%
Fibrinolytic Meds Within 30 Min. of Arrival[3,7]	-	-	80%	54%
PCI Within 90 Minutes of Arrival[3,7]	-	-	97%	96%
Statin Prescribed at Discharge[3,7]	-	-	98%	98%
Heart Failure Care				
ACE Inhibitor or ARB for LVSD	12	92%	97%	97%
Discharge Instructions Given	18	78%	96%	94%
Evaluation of LVS Function	18	83%	100%	99%
Medicare Spending				
Medicare Spending per Patient (ratio)	-	-	1.01	0.98
Pneumonia Care				
Appropriate Initial Antibiotic Given	37	92%	96%	95%
Blood Culture Timing	40	98%	98%	98%
Pregnancy and Delivery Care				
Newborn Deliveries Scheduled Early[1,3]	-	-	5%	6%
Preventive Care				
Immunization for Influenza[5]	-	-	93%	90%
Immunization for Pneumonia[5]	-	-	94%	92%
Stroke Care				
Anticoagulation Therapy for Atrial Fibrillation[5]	-	-	95%	95%
Antithrombotic Therapy Timing[5]	-	-	98%	98%
Assessed for Rehabilitation[5]	-	-	98%	97%
Discharged on Antithrombotic Therapy[5]	-	-	99%	99%
Discharged on Statin Medication[5]	-	-	95%	94%
Thrombolytic Therapy Timing[5]	-	-	65%	66%
Venous Thromboembolism Prophylaxis[5]	-	-	95%	94%
Written Stroke Educational Materials Given[5]	-	-	92%	88%
Surgical Care Improvement Project				
Appropriate Beta Blocker Usage[1]	-	-	98%	98%
Appropriate VTP Within 24 Hours	16	100%	98%	98%
Controlled Postoperative Blood Glucose[7]	-	-	97%	97%
Perioperative Temperature Management	19	100%	100%	100%
Prophylactic Antibiotic Selection	18	100%	99%	99%
Prophylactic Antibiotic Selection (Outpatient)[3]	17	100%	98%	98%
Prophylactic Antibiotic Stopped	18	100%	98%	98%
Prophylactic Antibiotic Timing	18	100%	99%	99%
Prophylactic Antibiotic Timing (Outpatient)[3]	17	100%	97%	98%
Urinary Catheter Removal[1]	-	-	97%	97%
Survey of Patients' Hospital Experiences				
Area Around Room 'Always' Quiet at Night	(a)	63%	58%	61%
Doctors 'Always' Communicated Well	(a)	85%	80%	82%
Home Recovery Information Given	(a)	83%	87%	85%
Hospital Given 9 or 10 on 10 Point Scale	(a)	73%	72%	71%
Meds 'Always' Explained Before Given	(a)	63%	64%	64%
Nurses 'Always' Communicated Well	(a)	81%	81%	79%
Pain 'Always' Well Controlled	(a)	63%	71%	71%
Room and Bathroom 'Always' Clean	(a)	81%	75%	73%
Timely Help 'Always' Received	(a)	76%	70%	68%
Would Definitely Recommend Hospital	(a)	68%	71%	71%
Use of Medical Imaging				
Cardiac Imaging Stress Test before Surgery	65	9.2%	5.4%	5.3%
Combination Abdominal CT Scan	116	25.0%	7.1%	10.5%
Combination Brain/Sinus CT Scan[1]	-	-	2.8%	2.7%
Combination Chest CT Scan[1]	-	-	1.7%	2.7%
Follow-up Mammogram/Ultrasound	151	11.3%	8.7%	8.8%
Lumbar Spine MRI for Low Back Pain[1]	-	-	34.7%	37.2%

McCullough - Hyde Memorial Hospital

110 North Poplar Street
Oxford, OH 45056
Phone: 513-523-2111
URL: www.mhmh.org
Type: Acute Care Hospitals
Emergency Services: Yes
Ownership: Voluntary non-profit - Private
Beds: 60

Key Personnel:
Radiology. Lynn Brown
Chief of Medical Staff. . . . . Bruce Gray, MD
CEO/President. . . . . Bryan D Henemann, FACHE
Chair/CEO . . . . Richard Norman

Measure	Cases	This Hosp.	State Avg.	U.S. Avg.
Blood Clot Prevention and Treatment				
Anticoagulation Overlap Therapy[2]	23	91%	93%	93%
ICU Venous Thromboembolism Prophylaxis[2]	30	80%	93%	92%
Incidence of Potentially Preventable VTE[1,2]	-	-	6%	10%
UFH with Dosages/Platelet Monitoring[1,2]	-	-	98%	97%
Venous Thromboembolism Prophylaxis[2]	246	73%	88%	85%
Warfarin Therapy Discharge Instructions[2]	18	83%	79%	75%
Chest Pain/Possible Heart Attack Care				
Aspirin Given Within 24 Hours of Arrival	19	100%	97%	96%
Fibrinolytic Meds Within 30 Min. of Arrival[7]	-	-	44%	58%
Average Time to ECG (minutes)	20	4	6	7
Average Time to Transfer (minutes)[1]	-	-	58	60
Children's Asthma Care				
Received Home Management Plan of Care	-	-	85%	88%
Received Reliever Medication	-	-	100%	100%
Received Systemic Corticosteroids	-	-	100%	100%
Emergency Department				
Admittance Decision Time (minutes)[2]	462	60	90	98
Head CT Results Within 45 Min. of Arrival[1]	-	-	63%	57%
Patients Who Left ER Before Being Seen	16,346	0%	2%	2%
Time from ER Arrival to Admit. (minutes)[2]	467	195	265	274
Time from ER Arrival to Discharge (minutes)	381	85	128	134
Time in ER Before Being Evaluated (minutes)	294	14	22	26
Time to Pain Meds for Fractures (minutes)	88	36	54	57
Heart Attack Care				
Aspirin Given at Discharge[1,3]	-	-	99%	99%
Fibrinolytic Meds Within 30 Min. of Arrival[3,7]	-	-	80%	54%
PCI Within 90 Minutes of Arrival[3,7]	-	-	97%	96%
Statin Prescribed at Discharge[1,3]	-	-	98%	98%
Heart Failure Care				
ACE Inhibitor or ARB for LVSD	19	95%	97%	97%
Discharge Instructions Given	91	99%	96%	94%
Evaluation of LVS Function	109	100%	100%	99%
Medicare Spending				
Medicare Spending per Patient (ratio)	-	0.96	1.01	0.98
Pneumonia Care				
Appropriate Initial Antibiotic Given	53	98%	96%	95%
Blood Culture Timing	76	95%	98%	98%
Pregnancy and Delivery Care				
Newborn Deliveries Scheduled Early	62	2%	5%	6%
Preventive Care				
Immunization for Influenza[2]	315	97%	93%	90%
Immunization for Pneumonia[2]	530	98%	94%	92%
Stroke Care				
Anticoagulation Therapy for Atrial Fibrillation[1]	-	-	95%	95%
Antithrombotic Therapy Timing	16	38%	98%	98%
Assessed for Rehabilitation	19	84%	98%	97%
Discharged on Antithrombotic Therapy	18	89%	99%	99%
Discharged on Statin Medication	19	58%	95%	94%
Thrombolytic Therapy Timing[1]	-	-	65%	66%
Venous Thromboembolism Prophylaxis	19	63%	95%	94%
Written Stroke Educational Materials Given[1]	-	-	92%	88%
Surgical Care Improvement Project				
Appropriate Beta Blocker Usage	26	96%	98%	98%
Appropriate VTP Within 24 Hours	152	98%	98%	98%
Controlled Postoperative Blood Glucose[7]	-	-	97%	97%
Perioperative Temperature Management	179	100%	100%	100%
Prophylactic Antibiotic Selection	137	100%	99%	99%
Prophylactic Antibiotic Selection (Outpatient)	33	94%	98%	98%
Prophylactic Antibiotic Stopped	135	96%	98%	98%
Prophylactic Antibiotic Timing	137	99%	99%	99%
Prophylactic Antibiotic Timing (Outpatient)	33	100%	97%	98%
Urinary Catheter Removal	134	91%	97%	97%
Survey of Patients' Hospital Experiences				
Area Around Room 'Always' Quiet at Night	300+	58%	58%	61%
Doctors 'Always' Communicated Well	300+	83%	80%	82%
Home Recovery Information Given	300+	86%	87%	85%
Hospital Given 9 or 10 on 10 Point Scale	300+	74%	72%	71%
Meds 'Always' Explained Before Given	300+	61%	64%	64%
Nurses 'Always' Communicated Well	300+	78%	81%	79%
Pain 'Always' Well Controlled	300+	71%	71%	71%
Room and Bathroom 'Always' Clean	300+	71%	75%	73%
Timely Help 'Always' Received	300+	63%	70%	68%
Would Definitely Recommend Hospital	300+	73%	71%	71%
Use of Medical Imaging				
Cardiac Imaging Stress Test before Surgery	79	2.5%	5.4%	5.3%
Combination Abdominal CT Scan	263	6.1%	7.1%	10.5%
Combination Brain/Sinus CT Scan[1]	-	-	2.8%	2.7%
Combination Chest CT Scan	179	0.0%	1.7%	2.7%
Follow-up Mammogram/Ultrasound	299	16.1%	8.7%	8.8%
Lumbar Spine MRI for Low Back Pain	52	34.6%	34.7%	37.2%

Parma Community General Hospital

7007 Powers Boulevard
Parma, OH 44129
Phone: 440-743-3000
Fax: 440-743-4092
E-mail: amatyas@parmahospital.org
URL: www.parmahopsital.org
Type: Acute Care Hospitals
Emergency Services: Yes
Ownership: Voluntary non-profit - Private
Beds: 348

Key Personnel:
Infection Control. . . . . Sara Barwacz
CEO/President. . . . . Terrence G. Deis
Coronary Care . . . . Carolyn Holy, RN
Radiology. . . . . Linda Nicklas
Chief of Medical Staff . . . . Tom Sidor, MD
Operating Room. . . . . Dale Winsberg
Quality Assurance . . . . Barbara Wojtala, RN

Measure	Cases	This Hosp.	State Avg.	U.S. Avg.
Blood Clot Prevention and Treatment				
Anticoagulation Overlap Therapy[2]	88	88%	93%	93%
ICU Venous Thromboembolism Prophylaxis[2]	71	96%	93%	92%
Incidence of Potentially Preventable VTE[2]	17	6%	6%	10%
UFH with Dosages/Platelet Monitoring[2]	49	100%	98%	97%
Venous Thromboembolism Prophylaxis[2]	349	92%	88%	85%
Warfarin Therapy Discharge Instructions[2]	43	81%	79%	75%
Chest Pain/Possible Heart Attack Care				
Aspirin Given Within 24 Hours of Arrival[1]	-	-	97%	96%
Fibrinolytic Meds Within 30 Min. of Arrival[3,7]	-	-	44%	58%
Average Time to ECG (minutes)[1]	-	-	6	7
Average Time to Transfer (minutes)[3,7]	-	-	58	60
Children's Asthma Care				
Received Home Management Plan of Care	-	-	85%	88%
Received Reliever Medication	-	-	100%	100%
Received Systemic Corticosteroids	-	-	100%	100%
Emergency Department				
Admittance Decision Time (minutes)[2]	768	121	90	98
Head CT Results Within 45 Min. of Arrival	27	70%	63%	57%
Patients Who Left ER Before Being Seen	48,933	1%	2%	2%
Time from ER Arrival to Admit. (minutes)[2]	795	333	265	274
Time from ER Arrival to Discharge (minutes)	346	152	128	134
Time in ER Before Being Evaluated (minutes)	412	27	22	26
Time to Pain Meds for Fractures (minutes)	145	65	54	57
Heart Attack Care				
Aspirin Given at Discharge	288	100%	99%	99%
Fibrinolytic Meds Within 30 Min. of Arrival[7]	-	-	80%	54%

NOTE: Hospital profiles are in alphabetical order by state, then city, then hospital within the city; Rankings exclude hospitals with less than 25 cases except for patient surveys which excludes hospitals with less than 100 cases; (a) 100-299 cases; (1) The number of cases/patients is too few to report; (2) Data submitted were based on a sample of cases/patients; (3) Results are based on a shorter time period than required; (4) Data suppressed by CMS for one or more quarters; (5) Results are not available for this reporting period; (6) Fewer than 100 patients completed the HCAHPS survey; (7) No cases met the criteria for this measure; (8) The lower limit of the confidence interval cannot be calculated if the number of observed infections equals zero; (9) No data are available from the state/territory for this reporting period; (10) The scores shown reflect fewer than 50 completed surveys; (11) There were discrepancies in the data collection process; (12) This measure does not apply to this hospital for this reporting period; (13) Results cannot be calculated for this reporting period; (14) The results for this state are combined with nearby states to protect confidentiality; Please refer to the User's Guide for a full explanation of data.

Measure	Cases	This Hosp.	State Avg.	U.S. Avg.
PCI Within 90 Minutes of Arrival	59	100%	97%	96%
Statin Prescribed at Discharge	281	100%	98%	98%
Heart Failure Care				
ACE Inhibitor or ARB for LVSD	150	100%	97%	97%
Discharge Instructions Given	364	100%	96%	94%
Evaluation of LVS Function	495	100%	100%	99%
Medicare Spending				
Medicare Spending per Patient (ratio)	-	1.11	1.01	0.98
Pneumonia Care				
Appropriate Initial Antibiotic Given	268	94%	96%	95%
Blood Culture Timing	401	99%	98%	98%
Pregnancy and Delivery Care				
Newborn Deliveries Scheduled Early	59	8%	5%	6%
Preventive Care				
Immunization for Influenza[2]	603	92%	93%	90%
Immunization for Pneumonia[2]	929	96%	94%	92%
Stroke Care				
Anticoagulation Therapy for Atrial Fibrillation	17	100%	95%	95%
Antithrombotic Therapy Timing	121	98%	98%	98%
Assessed for Rehabilitation	127	100%	98%	97%
Discharged on Antithrombotic Therapy	120	98%	99%	99%
Discharged on Statin Medication	88	99%	95%	94%
Thrombolytic Therapy Timing	23	0%	65%	66%
Venous Thromboembolism Prophylaxis	125	97%	95%	94%
Written Stroke Educational Materials Given	54	96%	92%	88%
Surgical Care Improvement Project				
Appropriate Beta Blocker Usage	419	99%	98%	98%
Appropriate VTP Within 24 Hours	904	98%	98%	98%
Controlled Postoperative Blood Glucose	82	98%	97%	97%
Perioperative Temperature Management	1,019	100%	100%	100%
Prophylactic Antibiotic Selection	845	100%	99%	99%
Prophylactic Antibiotic Selection (Outpatient)	177	97%	98%	98%
Prophylactic Antibiotic Stopped	824	98%	98%	98%
Prophylactic Antibiotic Timing	845	99%	99%	99%
Prophylactic Antibiotic Timing (Outpatient)	177	98%	97%	98%
Urinary Catheter Removal	860	98%	97%	97%
Survey of Patients' Hospital Experiences				
Area Around Room 'Always' Quiet at Night	300+	47%	58%	61%
Doctors 'Always' Communicated Well	300+	79%	80%	82%
Home Recovery Information Given	300+	84%	87%	85%
Hospital Given 9 or 10 on 10 Point Scale	300+	64%	72%	71%
Meds 'Always' Explained Before Given	300+	57%	64%	64%
Nurses 'Always' Communicated Well	300+	78%	81%	79%
Pain 'Always' Well Controlled	300+	69%	71%	71%
Room and Bathroom 'Always' Clean	300+	68%	75%	73%
Timely Help 'Always' Received	300+	67%	70%	68%
Would Definitely Recommend Hospital	300+	65%	71%	71%
Use of Medical Imaging				
Cardiac Imaging Stress Test before Surgery	745	6.0%	5.4%	5.3%
Combination Abdominal CT Scan	1,086	3.1%	7.1%	10.5%
Combination Brain/Sinus CT Scan	760	3.0%	2.8%	2.7%
Combination Chest CT Scan	757	0.7%	1.7%	2.7%
Follow-up Mammogram/Ultrasound	1,802	7.5%	8.7%	8.8%
Lumbar Spine MRI for Low Back Pain	145	33.8%	34.7%	37.2%

Paulding County Hospital

1035 West Wayne St.
Paulding, OH 45879
Phone: 419-399-4080
Fax: 419-399-5560
E-mail: pch@bright.net
URL: www.pauldingcountyhospital.com
Type: Critical Access Hospitals
Emergency Services: Yes
Ownership: Government - Local
Beds: 25

Key Personnel:
Quality Assurance . . . . Mary Hohenberger, RN
CEO . . . . Randy Ruge
Operating Room. . . . . Brent Savage, MD
Chief of Medical Staff . . . . Wendell Spangler, MD
Ambulatory Care . . . . Sherry Wilhelm, RN
Emergency Room . . . . Sherry Wilhelm, RN
Infection Control. . . . . Sherry Wilhelm, RN

Measure	Cases	This Hosp.	State Avg.	U.S. Avg.
Blood Clot Prevention and Treatment				
Anticoagulation Overlap Therapy[5]	-	-	93%	93%
ICU Venous Thromboembolism Prophylaxis[5]	-	-	93%	92%
Incidence of Potentially Preventable VTE[5]	-	-	6%	10%
UFH with Dosages/Platelet Monitoring[5]	-	-	98%	97%
Venous Thromboembolism Prophylaxis[5]	-	-	88%	85%
Warfarin Therapy Discharge Instructions[5]	-	-	79%	75%
Chest Pain/Possible Heart Attack Care				
Aspirin Given Within 24 Hours of Arrival[5]	-	-	97%	96%
Fibrinolytic Meds Within 30 Min. of Arrival[5]	-	-	44%	58%
Average Time to ECG (minutes)[5]	-	-	6	7
Average Time to Transfer (minutes)[5]	-	-	58	60
Children's Asthma Care				
Received Home Management Plan of Care	-	-	85%	88%
Received Reliever Medication	-	-	100%	100%
Received Systemic Corticosteroids	-	-	100%	100%
Emergency Department				
Admittance Decision Time (minutes)[5]	-	-	90	98
Head CT Results Within 45 Min. of Arrival[5]	-	-	63%	57%
Patients Who Left ER Before Being Seen	4,939	1%	2%	2%
Time from ER Arrival to Admit. (minutes)[5]	-	-	265	274
Time from ER Arrival to Discharge (minutes)[5]	-	-	128	134
Time in ER Before Being Evaluated (minutes)[5]	-	-	22	26
Time to Pain Meds for Fractures (minutes)[5]	-	-	54	57
Heart Attack Care				
Aspirin Given at Discharge[5]	-	-	99%	99%
Fibrinolytic Meds Within 30 Min. of Arrival[5]	-	-	80%	54%
PCI Within 90 Minutes of Arrival[5]	-	-	97%	96%
Statin Prescribed at Discharge[5]	-	-	98%	98%
Heart Failure Care				
ACE Inhibitor or ARB for LVSD[5]	-	-	97%	97%
Discharge Instructions Given[5]	-	-	96%	94%
Evaluation of LVS Function[5]	-	-	100%	99%
Medicare Spending				
Medicare Spending per Patient (ratio)	-	-	1.01	0.98
Pneumonia Care				
Appropriate Initial Antibiotic Given[5]	-	-	96%	95%
Blood Culture Timing[5]	-	-	98%	98%
Pregnancy and Delivery Care				
Newborn Deliveries Scheduled Early[3,7]	-	-	5%	6%
Preventive Care				
Immunization for Influenza[5]	-	-	93%	90%
Immunization for Pneumonia[5]	-	-	94%	92%
Stroke Care				
Anticoagulation Therapy for Atrial Fibrillation[5]	-	-	95%	95%
Antithrombotic Therapy Timing[5]	-	-	98%	98%
Assessed for Rehabilitation[5]	-	-	98%	97%
Discharged on Antithrombotic Therapy[5]	-	-	99%	99%
Discharged on Statin Medication[5]	-	-	95%	94%
Thrombolytic Therapy Timing[5]	-	-	65%	66%
Venous Thromboembolism Prophylaxis[5]	-	-	95%	94%
Written Stroke Educational Materials Given[5]	-	-	92%	88%
Surgical Care Improvement Project				
Appropriate Beta Blocker Usage[5]	-	-	98%	98%
Appropriate VTP Within 24 Hours[5]	-	-	98%	98%
Controlled Postoperative Blood Glucose[5]	-	-	97%	97%
Perioperative Temperature Management[5]	-	-	100%	100%
Prophylactic Antibiotic Selection[5]	-	-	99%	99%
Prophylactic Antibiotic Selection (Outpatient)[5]	-	-	98%	98%
Prophylactic Antibiotic Stopped[5]	-	-	98%	98%
Prophylactic Antibiotic Timing[5]	-	-	99%	99%
Prophylactic Antibiotic Timing (Outpatient)[5]	-	-	97%	98%
Urinary Catheter Removal[5]	-	-	97%	97%
Survey of Patients' Hospital Experiences				
Area Around Room 'Always' Quiet at Night[6]	<100	59%	58%	61%
Doctors 'Always' Communicated Well[6]	<100	89%	80%	82%
Home Recovery Information Given[6]	<100	88%	87%	85%
Hospital Given 9 or 10 on 10 Point Scale[6]	<100	82%	72%	71%
Meds 'Always' Explained Before Given[6]	<100	61%	64%	64%
Nurses 'Always' Communicated Well[6]	<100	86%	81%	79%
Pain 'Always' Well Controlled[6]	<100	86%	71%	71%
Room and Bathroom 'Always' Clean[6]	<100	83%	75%	73%
Timely Help 'Always' Received[6]	<100	78%	70%	68%
Would Definitely Recommend Hospital[6]	<100	77%	71%	71%
Use of Medical Imaging				
Cardiac Imaging Stress Test before Surgery[1]	-	-	5.4%	5.3%
Combination Abdominal CT Scan	146	8.2%	7.1%	10.5%
Combination Brain/Sinus CT Scan[1]	-	-	2.8%	2.7%
Combination Chest CT Scan	76	15.8%	1.7%	2.7%
Follow-up Mammogram/Ultrasound	194	13.4%	8.7%	8.8%
Lumbar Spine MRI for Low Back Pain[1]	-	-	34.7%	37.2%

H B Magruder Memorial Hospital

615 Fulton St
Port Clinton, OH 43452
Phone: 419-734-3131
Fax: 419-734-8217
URL: www.magruderhospital.com
Type: Critical Access Hospitals
Emergency Services: No
Ownership: Voluntary non-profit - Private
Beds: 98

Key Personnel:
Chief of Medical Staff . . . . Barry Cover, MD
Radiology. . . . . Sina Hazneci
Quality Assurance . . . . Michael Long
Emergency Room . . . . Julie Norway, RN
CEO/President. . . . . David Norwine, FACHE

Measure	Cases	This Hosp.	State Avg.	U.S. Avg.
Blood Clot Prevention and Treatment				
Anticoagulation Overlap Therapy[5]	-	-	93%	93%
ICU Venous Thromboembolism Prophylaxis[5]	-	-	93%	92%
Incidence of Potentially Preventable VTE[5]	-	-	6%	10%
UFH with Dosages/Platelet Monitoring[5]	-	-	98%	97%
Venous Thromboembolism Prophylaxis[5]	-	-	88%	85%
Warfarin Therapy Discharge Instructions[5]	-	-	79%	75%
Chest Pain/Possible Heart Attack Care				
Aspirin Given Within 24 Hours of Arrival	80	98%	97%	96%
Fibrinolytic Meds Within 30 Min. of Arrival[1]	-	-	44%	58%
Average Time to ECG (minutes)	82	7	6	7
Average Time to Transfer (minutes)[1]	-	-	58	60
Children's Asthma Care				
Received Home Management Plan of Care	-	-	85%	88%
Received Reliever Medication	-	-	100%	100%
Received Systemic Corticosteroids	-	-	100%	100%
Emergency Department				
Admittance Decision Time (minutes)[5]	-	-	90	98
Head CT Results Within 45 Min. of Arrival[5]	-	-	63%	57%
Patients Who Left ER Before Being Seen[5]	-	-	2%	2%
Time from ER Arrival to Admit. (minutes)[5]	-	-	265	274
Time from ER Arrival to Discharge (minutes)[5]	-	-	128	134
Time in ER Before Being Evaluated (minutes)[5]	-	-	22	26
Time to Pain Meds for Fractures (minutes)[5]	-	-	54	57
Heart Attack Care				
Aspirin Given at Discharge[5]	-	-	99%	99%
Fibrinolytic Meds Within 30 Min. of Arrival[5]	-	-	80%	54%
PCI Within 90 Minutes of Arrival[5]	-	-	97%	96%
Statin Prescribed at Discharge[5]	-	-	98%	98%
Heart Failure Care				
ACE Inhibitor or ARB for LVSD	13	85%	97%	97%
Discharge Instructions Given	29	83%	96%	94%
Evaluation of LVS Function	42	100%	100%	99%
Medicare Spending				
Medicare Spending per Patient (ratio)	-	-	1.01	0.98
Pneumonia Care				
Appropriate Initial Antibiotic Given	40	98%	96%	95%
Blood Culture Timing	50	98%	98%	98%
Pregnancy and Delivery Care				
Newborn Deliveries Scheduled Early[5]	-	-	5%	6%
Preventive Care				
Immunization for Influenza[5]	-	-	93%	90%
Immunization for Pneumonia[5]	-	-	94%	92%
Stroke Care				
Anticoagulation Therapy for Atrial Fibrillation[5]	-	-	95%	95%
Antithrombotic Therapy Timing[5]	-	-	98%	98%
Assessed for Rehabilitation[5]	-	-	98%	97%
Discharged on Antithrombotic Therapy[5]	-	-	99%	99%
Discharged on Statin Medication[5]	-	-	95%	94%
Thrombolytic Therapy Timing[5]	-	-	65%	66%
Venous Thromboembolism Prophylaxis[5]	-	-	95%	94%
Written Stroke Educational Materials Given[5]	-	-	92%	88%
Surgical Care Improvement Project				
Appropriate Beta Blocker Usage	25	100%	98%	98%

NOTE: Hospital profiles are in alphabetical order by state, then city, then hospital within the city; Rankings exclude hospitals with less than 25 cases except for patient surveys which excludes hospitals with less than 100 cases; (a) 100-299 cases; (1) The number of cases/patients is too few to report; (2) Data submitted were based on a sample of cases/patients; (3) Results are based on a shorter time period than required; (4) Data suppressed by CMS for one or more quarters; (5) Results are not available for this reporting period; (6) Fewer than 100 patients completed the HCAHPS survey; (7) No cases met the criteria for this measure; (8) The lower limit of the confidence interval cannot be calculated if the number of observed infections equals zero; (9) No data are available from the state/territory for this reporting period; (10) The scores shown reflect fewer than 50 completed surveys; (11) There were discrepancies in the data collection process; (12) This measure does not apply to this hospital for this reporting period; (13) Results cannot be calculated for this reporting period; (14) The results for this state are combined with nearby states to protect confidentiality; Please refer to the User's Guide for a full explanation of data.

Measure	Cases	This Hosp.	State Avg.	U.S. Avg.
Appropriate VTP Within 24 Hours	69	88%	98%	98%
Controlled Postoperative Blood Glucose[7]	-	-	97%	97%
Perioperative Temperature Management	74	99%	100%	100%
Prophylactic Antibiotic Selection	51	100%	99%	99%
Prophylactic Antibiotic Selection (Outpatient)	26	96%	98%	98%
Prophylactic Antibiotic Stopped	47	98%	98%	98%
Prophylactic Antibiotic Timing	51	96%	99%	99%
Prophylactic Antibiotic Timing (Outpatient)[1]	-	-	97%	98%
Urinary Catheter Removal	66	97%	97%	97%
Survey of Patients' Hospital Experiences				
Area Around Room 'Always' Quiet at Night	300+	67%	58%	61%
Doctors 'Always' Communicated Well	300+	91%	80%	82%
Home Recovery Information Given	300+	86%	87%	85%
Hospital Given 9 or 10 on 10 Point Scale	300+	84%	72%	71%
Meds 'Always' Explained Before Given	300+	71%	64%	64%
Nurses 'Always' Communicated Well	300+	88%	81%	79%
Pain 'Always' Well Controlled	300+	77%	71%	71%
Room and Bathroom 'Always' Clean	300+	89%	75%	73%
Timely Help 'Always' Received	300+	87%	70%	68%
Would Definitely Recommend Hospital	300+	80%	71%	71%
Use of Medical Imaging				
Cardiac Imaging Stress Test before Surgery	164	3.7%	5.4%	5.3%
Combination Abdominal CT Scan	397	4.5%	7.1%	10.5%
Combination Brain/Sinus CT Scan	389	5.4%	2.8%	2.7%
Combination Chest CT Scan	280	0.0%	1.7%	2.7%
Follow-up Mammogram/Ultrasound	463	1.7%	8.7%	8.8%
Lumbar Spine MRI for Low Back Pain[1]	-	-	34.7%	37.2%

Kings Daughters Medical Center Ohio

1901 Argonne Road
Portsmouth, OH 45662
Phone: 740-991-4000
Type: Acute Care Hospitals
Emergency Services: Yes
Ownership: Voluntary non-profit - Private

Measure	Cases	This Hosp.	State Avg.	U.S. Avg.
Blood Clot Prevention and Treatment				
Anticoagulation Overlap Therapy[3,7]	-	-	93%	93%
ICU Venous Thromboembolism Prophylaxis[3,7]	-	-	93%	92%
Incidence of Potentially Preventable VTE[3,7]	-	-	6%	10%
UFH with Dosages/Platelet Monitoring[3,7]	-	-	98%	97%
Venous Thromboembolism Prophylaxis[1,3]	-	-	88%	85%
Warfarin Therapy Discharge Instructions[3,7]	-	-	79%	75%
Chest Pain/Possible Heart Attack Care				
Aspirin Given Within 24 Hours of Arrival[1,3]	-	-	97%	96%
Fibrinolytic Meds Within 30 Min. of Arrival[5]	-	-	44%	58%
Average Time to ECG (minutes)[1,3]	-	-	6	7
Average Time to Transfer (minutes)[5]	-	-	58	60
Children's Asthma Care				
Received Home Management Plan of Care	-	-	85%	88%
Received Reliever Medication	-	-	100%	100%
Received Systemic Corticosteroids	-	-	100%	100%
Emergency Department				
Admittance Decision Time (minutes)[1,3]	-	-	90	98
Head CT Results Within 45 Min. of Arrival[5]	-	-	63%	57%
Patients Who Left ER Before Being Seen[5]	-	-	2%	2%
Time from ER Arrival to Admit. (minutes)[1,3]	-	-	265	274
Time from ER Arrival to Discharge (minutes)[3]	22	165	128	134
Time in ER Before Being Evaluated (minutes)[3]	40	22	22	26
Time to Pain Meds for Fractures (minutes)[5]	-	-	54	57
Heart Attack Care				
Aspirin Given at Discharge[5]	-	-	99%	99%
Fibrinolytic Meds Within 30 Min. of Arrival[5]	-	-	80%	54%
PCI Within 90 Minutes of Arrival[5]	-	-	97%	96%
Statin Prescribed at Discharge[5]	-	-	98%	98%
Heart Failure Care				
ACE Inhibitor or ARB for LVSD[5]	-	-	97%	97%
Discharge Instructions Given[5]	-	-	96%	94%
Evaluation of LVS Function[5]	-	-	100%	99%
Medicare Spending				
Medicare Spending per Patient (ratio)	-	-	1.01	0.98
Pneumonia Care				
Appropriate Initial Antibiotic Given[3,7]	-	-	96%	95%
Blood Culture Timing[3,7]	-	-	98%	98%
Pregnancy and Delivery Care				
Newborn Deliveries Scheduled Early[5]	-	-	5%	6%
Preventive Care				
Immunization for Influenza[5]	-	-	93%	90%
Immunization for Pneumonia[3]	35	100%	94%	92%
Stroke Care				
Anticoagulation Therapy for Atrial Fibrillation[5]	-	-	95%	95%
Antithrombotic Therapy Timing[5]	-	-	98%	98%
Assessed for Rehabilitation[5]	-	-	98%	97%
Discharged on Antithrombotic Therapy[5]	-	-	99%	99%
Discharged on Statin Medication[5]	-	-	95%	94%
Thrombolytic Therapy Timing[5]	-	-	65%	66%
Venous Thromboembolism Prophylaxis[5]	-	-	95%	94%
Written Stroke Educational Materials Given[5]	-	-	92%	88%
Surgical Care Improvement Project				
Appropriate Beta Blocker Usage[3]	15	100%	98%	98%
Appropriate VTP Within 24 Hours[3]	34	100%	98%	98%
Controlled Postoperative Blood Glucose[3,7]	-	-	97%	97%
Perioperative Temperature Management[3]	36	100%	100%	100%
Prophylactic Antibiotic Selection[3]	33	100%	99%	99%
Prophylactic Antibiotic Selection (Outpatient)[1,3]	-	-	98%	98%
Prophylactic Antibiotic Stopped[3]	33	100%	98%	98%
Prophylactic Antibiotic Timing[3]	33	94%	99%	99%
Prophylactic Antibiotic Timing (Outpatient)[1,3]	-	-	97%	98%
Urinary Catheter Removal[3]	24	100%	97%	97%
Survey of Patients' Hospital Experiences				
Area Around Room 'Always' Quiet at Night[5]	-	-	58%	61%
Doctors 'Always' Communicated Well[5]	-	-	80%	82%
Home Recovery Information Given[5]	-	-	87%	85%
Hospital Given 9 or 10 on 10 Point Scale[5]	-	-	72%	71%
Meds 'Always' Explained Before Given[5]	-	-	64%	64%
Nurses 'Always' Communicated Well[5]	-	-	81%	79%
Pain 'Always' Well Controlled[5]	-	-	71%	71%
Room and Bathroom 'Always' Clean[5]	-	-	75%	73%
Timely Help 'Always' Received[5]	-	-	70%	68%
Would Definitely Recommend Hospital[5]	-	-	71%	71%
Use of Medical Imaging				
Cardiac Imaging Stress Test before Surgery[1]	-	-	5.4%	5.3%
Combination Abdominal CT Scan	63	28.6%	7.1%	10.5%
Combination Brain/Sinus CT Scan[1]	-	-	2.8%	2.7%
Combination Chest CT Scan[1]	-	-	1.7%	2.7%
Follow-up Mammogram/Ultrasound[7]	-	-	8.7%	8.8%
Lumbar Spine MRI for Low Back Pain[1]	-	-	34.7%	37.2%

Southern Ohio Medical Center

1805 27th Street
Portsmouth, OH 45662
Phone: 740-356-5000
Fax: 740-353-5644
URL: www.somc.org
Type: Acute Care Hospitals
Emergency Services: Yes
Ownership: Voluntary non-profit - Other
Beds: 488

Key Personnel:

CEO/President. . . . . Randal M Arnett
Quality Assurance . . . . Rebecca Hall
Radiology. . . . . George Johnson, MD
Operating Room. . . . . Teresa Lute, RN
Infection Control. . . . . Randy Sosolik, MD
Pediatric Ambulatory Care . . . . . . Randy Sosolik, MD
Pediatric In-Patient Care . . . . Randy Sosolik, MD
Chief of Medical Staff. . . . . Kendall Stewart

Measure	Cases	This Hosp.	State Avg.	U.S. Avg.
Blood Clot Prevention and Treatment				
Anticoagulation Overlap Therapy[2]	77	97%	93%	93%
ICU Venous Thromboembolism Prophylaxis[2]	69	100%	93%	92%
Incidence of Potentially Preventable VTE[1,2]	-	-	6%	10%
UFH with Dosages/Platelet Monitoring[2]	97	100%	98%	97%
Venous Thromboembolism Prophylaxis[2]	468	95%	88%	85%
Warfarin Therapy Discharge Instructions[2]	48	96%	79%	75%
Chest Pain/Possible Heart Attack Care				
Aspirin Given Within 24 Hours of Arrival	19	100%	97%	96%
Fibrinolytic Meds Within 30 Min. of Arrival[7]	-	-	44%	58%
Average Time to ECG (minutes)	22	2	6	7
Average Time to Transfer (minutes)[7]	-	-	58	60
Children's Asthma Care				
Received Home Management Plan of Care	-	-	85%	88%
Received Reliever Medication	-	-	100%	100%
Received Systemic Corticosteroids	-	-	100%	100%
Emergency Department				
Admittance Decision Time (minutes)[2]	691	110	90	98
Head CT Results Within 45 Min. of Arrival	17	82%	63%	57%
Patients Who Left ER Before Being Seen	50,647	1%	2%	2%
Time from ER Arrival to Admit. (minutes)[2]	692	281	265	274
Time from ER Arrival to Discharge (minutes)	401	157	128	134
Time in ER Before Being Evaluated (minutes)	466	14	22	26
Time to Pain Meds for Fractures (minutes)	119	54	54	57
Heart Attack Care				
Aspirin Given at Discharge	295	100%	99%	99%
Fibrinolytic Meds Within 30 Min. of Arrival[7]	-	-	80%	54%
PCI Within 90 Minutes of Arrival	37	97%	97%	96%
Statin Prescribed at Discharge	283	100%	98%	98%
Heart Failure Care				
ACE Inhibitor or ARB for LVSD	94	98%	97%	97%
Discharge Instructions Given	278	97%	96%	94%
Evaluation of LVS Function	349	100%	100%	99%
Medicare Spending				
Medicare Spending per Patient (ratio)	-	1.05	1.01	0.98
Pneumonia Care				
Appropriate Initial Antibiotic Given	344	96%	96%	95%
Blood Culture Timing	553	100%	98%	98%
Pregnancy and Delivery Care				
Newborn Deliveries Scheduled Early[2]	27	0%	5%	6%
Preventive Care				
Immunization for Influenza[2]	576	98%	93%	90%
Immunization for Pneumonia[2]	783	99%	94%	92%
Stroke Care				
Anticoagulation Therapy for Atrial Fibrillation	14	100%	95%	95%
Antithrombotic Therapy Timing	94	99%	98%	98%
Assessed for Rehabilitation	86	98%	98%	97%
Discharged on Antithrombotic Therapy	84	99%	99%	99%
Discharged on Statin Medication	65	98%	95%	94%
Thrombolytic Therapy Timing[7]	-	-	65%	66%
Venous Thromboembolism Prophylaxis	92	98%	95%	94%
Written Stroke Educational Materials Given	56	98%	92%	88%
Surgical Care Improvement Project				
Appropriate Beta Blocker Usage	247	100%	98%	98%
Appropriate VTP Within 24 Hours	395	99%	98%	98%
Controlled Postoperative Blood Glucose	87	98%	97%	97%
Perioperative Temperature Management	473	100%	100%	100%
Prophylactic Antibiotic Selection	375	99%	99%	99%
Prophylactic Antibiotic Selection (Outpatient)	184	96%	98%	98%
Prophylactic Antibiotic Stopped	351	99%	98%	98%
Prophylactic Antibiotic Timing	375	100%	99%	99%
Prophylactic Antibiotic Timing (Outpatient)	184	100%	97%	98%
Urinary Catheter Removal	336	100%	97%	97%
Survey of Patients' Hospital Experiences				
Area Around Room 'Always' Quiet at Night	300+	68%	58%	61%
Doctors 'Always' Communicated Well	300+	84%	80%	82%
Home Recovery Information Given	300+	89%	87%	85%
Hospital Given 9 or 10 on 10 Point Scale	300+	74%	72%	71%
Meds 'Always' Explained Before Given	300+	67%	64%	64%
Nurses 'Always' Communicated Well	300+	81%	81%	79%
Pain 'Always' Well Controlled	300+	76%	71%	71%
Room and Bathroom 'Always' Clean	300+	81%	75%	73%
Timely Help 'Always' Received	300+	68%	70%	68%
Would Definitely Recommend Hospital	300+	71%	71%	71%
Use of Medical Imaging				
Cardiac Imaging Stress Test before Surgery	527	6.5%	5.4%	5.3%
Combination Abdominal CT Scan	1,404	10.1%	7.1%	10.5%
Combination Brain/Sinus CT Scan	1,222	3.9%	2.8%	2.7%
Combination Chest CT Scan	728	7.8%	1.7%	2.7%
Follow-up Mammogram/Ultrasound	1,274	14.8%	8.7%	8.8%
Lumbar Spine MRI for Low Back Pain	185	41.1%	34.7%	37.2%

NOTE: Hospital profiles are in alphabetical order by state, then city, then hospital within the city; Rankings exclude hospitals with less than 25 cases except for patient surveys which excludes hospitals with less than 100 cases; (a) 100-299 cases; (1) The number of cases/patients is too few to report; (2) Data submitted were based on a sample of cases/patients; (3) Results are based on a shorter time period than required; (4) Data suppressed by CMS for one or more quarters; (5) Results are not available for this reporting period; (6) Fewer than 100 patients completed the HCAHPS survey; (7) No cases met the criteria for this measure; (8) The lower limit of the confidence interval cannot be calculated if the number of observed infections equals zero; (9) No data are available from the state/territory for this reporting period; (10) The scores shown reflect fewer than 50 completed surveys; (11) There were discrepancies in the data collection process; (12) This measure does not apply to this hospital for this reporting period; (13) Results cannot be calculated for this reporting period; (14) The results for this state are combined with nearby states to protect confidentiality; Please refer to the User's Guide for a full explanation of data.

Three Gables Surgery Center

5897 County Road 107
Proctorville, OH 45669
Phone: 740-886-9911
Fax: 740-886-9922
URL: www.threegablessurgery.com
Type: Acute Care Hospitals
Emergency Services: No
Ownership: Proprietary
Key Personnel:
CEO/President. . . . . John Stone

Measure	Cases	This Hosp.	State Avg.	U.S. Avg.
Blood Clot Prevention and Treatment				
Anticoagulation Overlap Therapy[7]	-	-	93%	93%
ICU Venous Thromboembolism Prophylaxis[7]	-	-	93%	92%
Incidence of Potentially Preventable VTE[7]	-	-	6%	10%
UFH with Dosages/Platelet Monitoring[7]	-	-	98%	97%
Venous Thromboembolism Prophylaxis[1]	-	-	88%	85%
Warfarin Therapy Discharge Instructions[7]	-	-	79%	75%
Chest Pain/Possible Heart Attack Care				
Aspirin Given Within 24 Hours of Arrival[5]	-	-	97%	96%
Fibrinolytic Meds Within 30 Min. of Arrival[5]	-	-	44%	58%
Average Time to ECG (minutes)[5]	-	-	6	7
Average Time to Transfer (minutes)[5]	-	-	58	60
Children's Asthma Care				
Received Home Management Plan of Care	-	-	85%	88%
Received Reliever Medication	-	-	100%	100%
Received Systemic Corticosteroids	-	-	100%	100%
Emergency Department				
Admittance Decision Time (minutes)[7]	-	-	90	98
Head CT Results Within 45 Min. of Arrival[5]	-	-	63%	57%
Patients Who Left ER Before Being Seen[5]	-	-	2%	2%
Time from ER Arrival to Admit. (minutes)[7]	-	-	265	274
Time from ER Arrival to Discharge (minutes)[5]	-	-	128	134
Time in ER Before Being Evaluated (minutes)[5]	-	-	22	26
Time to Pain Meds for Fractures (minutes)[5]	-	-	54	57
Heart Attack Care				
Aspirin Given at Discharge[5]	-	-	99%	99%
Fibrinolytic Meds Within 30 Min. of Arrival[5]	-	-	80%	54%
PCI Within 90 Minutes of Arrival[5]	-	-	97%	96%
Statin Prescribed at Discharge[5]	-	-	98%	98%
Heart Failure Care				
ACE Inhibitor or ARB for LVSD[5]	-	-	97%	97%
Discharge Instructions Given[5]	-	-	96%	94%
Evaluation of LVS Function[5]	-	-	100%	99%
Medicare Spending				
Medicare Spending per Patient (ratio)[1]	-	-	1.01	0.98
Pneumonia Care				
Appropriate Initial Antibiotic Given[5]	-	-	96%	95%
Blood Culture Timing[5]	-	-	98%	98%
Pregnancy and Delivery Care				
Newborn Deliveries Scheduled Early[2,7]	-	-	5%	6%
Preventive Care				
Immunization for Influenza	34	85%	93%	90%
Immunization for Pneumonia	51	59%	94%	92%
Stroke Care				
Anticoagulation Therapy for Atrial Fibrillation[5]	-	-	95%	95%
Antithrombotic Therapy Timing[5]	-	-	98%	98%
Assessed for Rehabilitation[5]	-	-	98%	97%
Discharged on Antithrombotic Therapy[5]	-	-	99%	99%
Discharged on Statin Medication[5]	-	-	95%	94%
Thrombolytic Therapy Timing[5]	-	-	65%	66%
Venous Thromboembolism Prophylaxis[5]	-	-	95%	94%
Written Stroke Educational Materials Given[5]	-	-	92%	88%
Surgical Care Improvement Project				
Appropriate Beta Blocker Usage[5]	-	-	98%	98%
Appropriate VTP Within 24 Hours[5]	-	-	98%	98%
Controlled Postoperative Blood Glucose[5]	-	-	97%	97%
Perioperative Temperature Management[5]	-	-	100%	100%
Prophylactic Antibiotic Selection[5]	-	-	99%	99%
Prophylactic Antibiotic Selection (Outpatient)	26	100%	98%	98%
Prophylactic Antibiotic Stopped[5]	-	-	98%	98%
Prophylactic Antibiotic Timing[5]	-	-	99%	99%
Prophylactic Antibiotic Timing (Outpatient)	27	96%	97%	98%
Urinary Catheter Removal[5]	-	-	97%	97%
Survey of Patients' Hospital Experiences				
Area Around Room 'Always' Quiet at Night[10]	<100	87%	58%	61%
Doctors 'Always' Communicated Well[10]	<100	92%	80%	82%
Home Recovery Information Given[10]	<100	94%	87%	85%
Hospital Given 9 or 10 on 10 Point Scale[10]	<100	92%	72%	71%
Meds 'Always' Explained Before Given[10]	<100	89%	64%	64%
Nurses 'Always' Communicated Well[10]	<100	99%	81%	79%
Pain 'Always' Well Controlled[10]	<100	91%	71%	71%
Room and Bathroom 'Always' Clean[10]	<100	94%	75%	73%
Timely Help 'Always' Received[10]	<100	92%	70%	68%
Would Definitely Recommend Hospital[10]	<100	87%	71%	71%
Use of Medical Imaging				
Cardiac Imaging Stress Test before Surgery[7]	-	-	5.4%	5.3%
Combination Abdominal CT Scan[1]	-	-	7.1%	10.5%
Combination Brain/Sinus CT Scan[1]	-	-	2.8%	2.7%
Combination Chest CT Scan[1]	-	-	1.7%	2.7%
Follow-up Mammogram/Ultrasound[7]	-	-	8.7%	8.8%
Lumbar Spine MRI for Low Back Pain[1]	-	-	34.7%	37.2%

Robinson Memorial Hospital

6847 N Chestnut
Ravenna, OH 44266
Phone: 330-297-2300
Fax: 330-297-2949
URL: www.robinsonmemorial.org
Type: Acute Care Hospitals
Emergency Services: Yes
Ownership: Voluntary non-profit - Private
Beds: 285
Key Personnel:
Radiology. Edward Bury, Jr., MD
CEO/President. . . . . Stephen Colecchi
Anesthesiology. . . . . Paul Jones, DO
Chairman/CEO . . . . Gordon L. Ober
Surgery . . . . Edward Panzeter, MD
Emergency Room . . . . Julie Vesco, DO

Measure	Cases	This Hosp.	State Avg.	U.S. Avg.
Blood Clot Prevention and Treatment				
Anticoagulation Overlap Therapy[2]	58	57%	93%	93%
ICU Venous Thromboembolism Prophylaxis[2]	60	83%	93%	92%
Incidence of Potentially Preventable VTE[1,2]	-	-	6%	10%
UFH with Dosages/Platelet Monitoring[1,2]	-	-	98%	97%
Venous Thromboembolism Prophylaxis[2]	346	81%	88%	85%
Warfarin Therapy Discharge Instructions[2]	50	60%	79%	75%
Chest Pain/Possible Heart Attack Care				
Aspirin Given Within 24 Hours of Arrival	74	97%	97%	96%
Fibrinolytic Meds Within 30 Min. of Arrival[7]	-	-	44%	58%
Average Time to ECG (minutes)	77	10	6	7
Average Time to Transfer (minutes)	32	60	58	60
Children's Asthma Care				
Received Home Management Plan of Care	-	-	85%	88%
Received Reliever Medication	-	-	100%	100%
Received Systemic Corticosteroids	-	-	100%	100%
Emergency Department				
Admittance Decision Time (minutes)[2]	676	94	90	98
Head CT Results Within 45 Min. of Arrival[1]	-	-	63%	57%
Patients Who Left ER Before Being Seen	39,345	4%	2%	2%
Time from ER Arrival to Admit. (minutes)[2]	738	279	265	274
Time from ER Arrival to Discharge (minutes)	357	164	128	134
Time in ER Before Being Evaluated (minutes)	158	36	22	26
Time to Pain Meds for Fractures (minutes)	125	53	54	57
Heart Attack Care				
Aspirin Given at Discharge	38	95%	99%	99%
Fibrinolytic Meds Within 30 Min. of Arrival[7]	-	-	80%	54%
PCI Within 90 Minutes of Arrival[7]	-	-	97%	96%
Statin Prescribed at Discharge	36	97%	98%	98%
Heart Failure Care				
ACE Inhibitor or ARB for LVSD	60	92%	97%	97%
Discharge Instructions Given	209	99%	96%	94%
Evaluation of LVS Function	268	99%	100%	99%
Medicare Spending				
Medicare Spending per Patient (ratio)	-	0.97	1.01	0.98
Pneumonia Care				
Appropriate Initial Antibiotic Given[2]	139	97%	96%	95%
Blood Culture Timing[2]	154	92%	98%	98%
Pregnancy and Delivery Care				
Newborn Deliveries Scheduled Early	61	13%	5%	6%
Preventive Care				
Immunization for Influenza[2]	556	96%	93%	90%
Immunization for Pneumonia[2]	749	90%	94%	92%
Stroke Care				
Anticoagulation Therapy for Atrial Fibrillation	13	92%	95%	95%
Antithrombotic Therapy Timing	65	95%	98%	98%
Assessed for Rehabilitation	67	94%	98%	97%
Discharged on Antithrombotic Therapy	66	97%	99%	99%
Discharged on Statin Medication	58	84%	95%	94%
Thrombolytic Therapy Timing[1]	-	-	65%	66%
Venous Thromboembolism Prophylaxis	59	76%	95%	94%
Written Stroke Educational Materials Given	40	70%	92%	88%
Surgical Care Improvement Project				
Appropriate Beta Blocker Usage[2]	99	89%	98%	98%
Appropriate VTP Within 24 Hours[2]	306	96%	98%	98%
Controlled Postoperative Blood Glucose[2,7]	-	-	97%	97%
Perioperative Temperature Management[2]	359	99%	100%	100%
Prophylactic Antibiotic Selection[2]	211	99%	99%	99%
Prophylactic Antibiotic Selection (Outpatient)	219	99%	98%	98%
Prophylactic Antibiotic Stopped[2]	209	97%	98%	98%
Prophylactic Antibiotic Timing[2]	212	97%	99%	99%
Prophylactic Antibiotic Timing (Outpatient)	192	99%	97%	98%
Urinary Catheter Removal[2]	240	96%	97%	97%
Survey of Patients' Hospital Experiences				
Area Around Room 'Always' Quiet at Night	300+	51%	58%	61%
Doctors 'Always' Communicated Well	300+	79%	80%	82%
Home Recovery Information Given	300+	79%	87%	85%
Hospital Given 9 or 10 on 10 Point Scale	300+	65%	72%	71%
Meds 'Always' Explained Before Given	300+	60%	64%	64%
Nurses 'Always' Communicated Well	300+	79%	81%	79%
Pain 'Always' Well Controlled	300+	70%	71%	71%
Room and Bathroom 'Always' Clean	300+	75%	75%	73%
Timely Help 'Always' Received	300+	67%	70%	68%
Would Definitely Recommend Hospital	300+	61%	71%	71%
Use of Medical Imaging				
Cardiac Imaging Stress Test before Surgery	418	6.5%	5.4%	5.3%
Combination Abdominal CT Scan	519	4.0%	7.1%	10.5%
Combination Brain/Sinus CT Scan	538	2.2%	2.8%	2.7%
Combination Chest CT Scan	235	0.0%	1.7%	2.7%
Follow-up Mammogram/Ultrasound	1,000	5.4%	8.7%	8.8%
Lumbar Spine MRI for Low Back Pain	100	31.0%	34.7%	37.2%

UHHS Richmond Heights Hospital

27100 Chardon Road
Richmond Heights, OH 44143
Phone: 440-585-6170
Fax: 440-585-6341
URL: www.uhhospitals.org
Type: Acute Care Hospitals
Emergency Services: Yes
Ownership: Proprietary
Beds: 250
Key Personnel:
Patient Relations . . . . Paul A Bailey
Cardiac Laboratory. . . . . Larry Martin
Emergency Room . . . . Robin McCrone
Chief of Medical Staff . . . . David Rapkin, MD
CEO . . . . Thomas F. Zenty III

Measure	Cases	This Hosp.	State Avg.	U.S. Avg.
Blood Clot Prevention and Treatment				
Anticoagulation Overlap Therapy[2]	56	84%	93%	93%
ICU Venous Thromboembolism Prophylaxis[2]	154	98%	93%	92%
Incidence of Potentially Preventable VTE[1,2]	-	-	6%	10%
UFH with Dosages/Platelet Monitoring[2]	42	100%	98%	97%
Venous Thromboembolism Prophylaxis[2]	507	96%	88%	85%
Warfarin Therapy Discharge Instructions[2]	44	95%	79%	75%
Chest Pain/Possible Heart Attack Care				
Aspirin Given Within 24 Hours of Arrival	62	97%	97%	96%
Fibrinolytic Meds Within 30 Min. of Arrival[7]	-	-	44%	58%
Average Time to ECG (minutes)	68	6	6	7
Average Time to Transfer (minutes)	28	66	58	60
Children's Asthma Care				
Received Home Management Plan of Care	-	-	85%	88%
Received Reliever Medication	-	-	100%	100%
Received Systemic Corticosteroids	-	-	100%	100%
Emergency Department				
Admittance Decision Time (minutes)[2]	844	96	90	98
Head CT Results Within 45 Min. of Arrival	41	73%	63%	57%
Patients Who Left ER Before Being Seen	38,376	1%	2%	2%

NOTE: Hospital profiles are in alphabetical order by state, then city, then hospital within the city; Rankings exclude hospitals with less than 25 cases except for patient surveys which excludes hospitals with less than 100 cases; (a) 100-299 cases; (1) The number of cases/patients is too few to report; (2) Data submitted were based on a sample of cases/patients; (3) Results are based on a shorter time period than required; (4) Data suppressed by CMS for one or more quarters; (5) Results are not available for this reporting period; (6) Fewer than 100 patients completed the HCAHPS survey; (7) No cases met the criteria for this measure; (8) The lower limit of the confidence interval cannot be calculated if the number of observed infections equals zero; (9) No data are available from the state/territory for this reporting period; (10) The scores shown reflect fewer than 50 completed surveys; (11) There were discrepancies in the data collection process; (12) This measure does not apply to this hospital for this reporting period; (13) Results cannot be calculated for this reporting period; (14) The results for this state are combined with nearby states to protect confidentiality; Please refer to the User's Guide for a full explanation of data.

Measure	Cases	This Hosp.	State Avg.	U.S. Avg.
Time from ER Arrival to Admit. (minutes)[2]	872	222	265	274
Time from ER Arrival to Discharge (minutes)	724	98	128	134
Time in ER Before Being Evaluated (minutes)	766	14	22	26
Time to Pain Meds for Fractures (minutes)	73	52	54	57
Heart Attack Care				
Aspirin Given at Discharge	46	98%	99%	99%
Fibrinolytic Meds Within 30 Min. of Arrival[7]	-	-	80%	54%
PCI Within 90 Minutes of Arrival[7]	-	-	97%	96%
Statin Prescribed at Discharge	47	91%	98%	98%
Heart Failure Care				
ACE Inhibitor or ARB for LVSD	62	100%	97%	97%
Discharge Instructions Given	216	98%	96%	94%
Evaluation of LVS Function	298	100%	100%	99%
Medicare Spending				
Medicare Spending per Patient (ratio)	-	1.07	1.01	0.98
Pneumonia Care				
Appropriate Initial Antibiotic Given	113	96%	96%	95%
Blood Culture Timing	222	99%	98%	98%
Pregnancy and Delivery Care				
Newborn Deliveries Scheduled Early[7]	-	-	5%	6%
Preventive Care				
Immunization for Influenza[2]	605	98%	93%	90%
Immunization for Pneumonia[2]	1,008	99%	94%	92%
Stroke Care				
Anticoagulation Therapy for Atrial Fibrillation[1]	-	-	95%	95%
Antithrombotic Therapy Timing	48	98%	98%	98%
Assessed for Rehabilitation	52	98%	98%	97%
Discharged on Antithrombotic Therapy	46	98%	99%	99%
Discharged on Statin Medication	38	100%	95%	94%
Thrombolytic Therapy Timing[1]	-	-	65%	66%
Venous Thromboembolism Prophylaxis	55	93%	95%	94%
Written Stroke Educational Materials Given	23	96%	92%	88%
Surgical Care Improvement Project				
Appropriate Beta Blocker Usage	61	100%	98%	98%
Appropriate VTP Within 24 Hours	197	99%	98%	98%
Controlled Postoperative Blood Glucose[7]	-	-	97%	97%
Perioperative Temperature Management	214	100%	100%	100%
Prophylactic Antibiotic Selection	150	99%	99%	99%
Prophylactic Antibiotic Selection (Outpatient)	81	99%	98%	98%
Prophylactic Antibiotic Stopped	146	97%	98%	98%
Prophylactic Antibiotic Timing	150	100%	99%	99%
Prophylactic Antibiotic Timing (Outpatient)	72	99%	97%	98%
Urinary Catheter Removal	164	98%	97%	97%
Survey of Patients' Hospital Experiences				
Area Around Room 'Always' Quiet at Night	300+	51%	58%	61%
Doctors 'Always' Communicated Well	300+	80%	80%	82%
Home Recovery Information Given	300+	86%	87%	85%
Hospital Given 9 or 10 on 10 Point Scale	300+	65%	72%	71%
Meds 'Always' Explained Before Given	300+	63%	64%	64%
Nurses 'Always' Communicated Well	300+	78%	81%	79%
Pain 'Always' Well Controlled	300+	69%	71%	71%
Room and Bathroom 'Always' Clean	300+	68%	75%	73%
Timely Help 'Always' Received	300+	63%	70%	68%
Would Definitely Recommend Hospital	300+	66%	71%	71%
Use of Medical Imaging				
Cardiac Imaging Stress Test before Surgery	149	8.7%	5.4%	5.3%
Combination Abdominal CT Scan	603	9.6%	7.1%	10.5%
Combination Brain/Sinus CT Scan	720	3.1%	2.8%	2.7%
Combination Chest CT Scan	340	2.1%	1.7%	2.7%
Follow-up Mammogram/Ultrasound	873	11.7%	8.7%	8.8%
Lumbar Spine MRI for Low Back Pain[1]	-	-	34.7%	37.2%

Glenbeigh

2863 State Route 45
Rock Creek, OH 44084
Phone: 440-563-3400
Fax: 440-563-9619
E-mail: helen@glenbeigh.com
URL: www.glenbeigh.com
Type: Acute Care Hospitals
Emergency Services: No
Ownership: Voluntary non-profit - Private
Beds: 80

Key Personnel:
Infection Control. . . . . Renee Enstrom, RN
Quality Assurance . . . . Ruth Leslie, RN
Chief of Medical Staff . . . . Chester J Prusinski, DO
CEO/President. . . . . Pat Weston-Hall, LISW

Measure	Cases	This Hosp.	State Avg.	U.S. Avg.
Blood Clot Prevention and Treatment				
Anticoagulation Overlap Therapy[7]	-	-	93%	93%
ICU Venous Thromboembolism Prophylaxis[7]	-	-	93%	92%
Incidence of Potentially Preventable VTE[7]	-	-	6%	10%
UFH with Dosages/Platelet Monitoring[7]	-	-	98%	97%
Venous Thromboembolism Prophylaxis[7]	-	-	88%	85%
Warfarin Therapy Discharge Instructions[7]	-	-	79%	75%
Chest Pain/Possible Heart Attack Care				
Aspirin Given Within 24 Hours of Arrival[5]	-	-	97%	96%
Fibrinolytic Meds Within 30 Min. of Arrival[5]	-	-	44%	58%
Average Time to ECG (minutes)[5]	-	-	6	7
Average Time to Transfer (minutes)[5]	-	-	58	60
Children's Asthma Care				
Received Home Management Plan of Care	-	-	85%	88%
Received Reliever Medication	-	-	100%	100%
Received Systemic Corticosteroids	-	-	100%	100%
Emergency Department				
Admittance Decision Time (minutes)[7]	-	-	90	98
Head CT Results Within 45 Min. of Arrival[5]	-	-	63%	57%
Patients Who Left ER Before Being Seen[5]	-	-	2%	2%
Time from ER Arrival to Admit. (minutes)[7]	-	-	265	274
Time from ER Arrival to Discharge (minutes)[5]	-	-	128	134
Time in ER Before Being Evaluated (minutes)[5]	-	-	22	26
Time to Pain Meds for Fractures (minutes)[5]	-	-	54	57
Heart Attack Care				
Aspirin Given at Discharge[5]	-	-	99%	99%
Fibrinolytic Meds Within 30 Min. of Arrival[5]	-	-	80%	54%
PCI Within 90 Minutes of Arrival[5]	-	-	97%	96%
Statin Prescribed at Discharge[5]	-	-	98%	98%
Heart Failure Care				
ACE Inhibitor or ARB for LVSD[5]	-	-	97%	97%
Discharge Instructions Given[5]	-	-	96%	94%
Evaluation of LVS Function[5]	-	-	100%	99%
Medicare Spending				
Medicare Spending per Patient (ratio)		0.85	1.01	0.98
Pneumonia Care				
Appropriate Initial Antibiotic Given[5]	-	-	96%	95%
Blood Culture Timing[5]	-	-	98%	98%
Pregnancy and Delivery Care				
Newborn Deliveries Scheduled Early[7]	-	-	5%	6%
Preventive Care				
Immunization for Influenza	67	55%	93%	90%
Immunization for Pneumonia	69	78%	94%	92%
Stroke Care				
Anticoagulation Therapy for Atrial Fibrillation[5]	-	-	95%	95%
Antithrombotic Therapy Timing[5]	-	-	98%	98%
Assessed for Rehabilitation[5]	-	-	98%	97%
Discharged on Antithrombotic Therapy[5]	-	-	99%	99%
Discharged on Statin Medication[5]	-	-	95%	94%
Thrombolytic Therapy Timing[5]	-	-	65%	66%
Venous Thromboembolism Prophylaxis[5]	-	-	95%	94%
Written Stroke Educational Materials Given[5]	-	-	92%	88%
Surgical Care Improvement Project				
Appropriate Beta Blocker Usage[5]	-	-	98%	98%
Appropriate VTP Within 24 Hours[5]	-	-	98%	98%
Controlled Postoperative Blood Glucose[5]	-	-	97%	97%
Perioperative Temperature Management[5]	-	-	100%	100%
Prophylactic Antibiotic Selection[5]	-	-	99%	99%
Prophylactic Antibiotic Selection (Outpatient)[5]	-	-	98%	98%
Prophylactic Antibiotic Stopped[5]	-	-	98%	98%
Prophylactic Antibiotic Timing[5]	-	-	99%	99%
Prophylactic Antibiotic Timing (Outpatient)[5]	-	-	97%	98%
Urinary Catheter Removal[5]	-	-	97%	97%
Survey of Patients' Hospital Experiences				
Area Around Room 'Always' Quiet at Night[1]	-	-	58%	61%
Doctors 'Always' Communicated Well[1]	-	-	80%	82%
Home Recovery Information Given[1]	-	-	87%	85%
Hospital Given 9 or 10 on 10 Point Scale[1]	-	-	72%	71%
Meds 'Always' Explained Before Given[1]	-	-	64%	64%
Nurses 'Always' Communicated Well[1]	-	-	81%	79%
Pain 'Always' Well Controlled[1]	-	-	71%	71%
Room and Bathroom 'Always' Clean[1]	-	-	75%	73%
Timely Help 'Always' Received[1]	-	-	70%	68%
Would Definitely Recommend Hospital[1]	-	-	71%	71%
Use of Medical Imaging				
Cardiac Imaging Stress Test before Surgery[7]	-	-	5.4%	5.3%
Combination Abdominal CT Scan[7]	-	-	7.1%	10.5%
Combination Brain/Sinus CT Scan[7]	-	-	2.8%	2.7%
Combination Chest CT Scan[7]	-	-	1.7%	2.7%
Follow-up Mammogram/Ultrasound[7]	-	-	8.7%	8.8%
Lumbar Spine MRI for Low Back Pain[7]	-	-	34.7%	37.2%

Grand Lake Health System

200 Saint Clair Street
Saint Marys, OH 45885
Phone: 419-394-3335
Fax: 419-394-8485
Type: Acute Care Hospitals
Emergency Services: Yes
Ownership: Voluntary non-profit - Private
Beds: 130

Key Personnel:
Radiology. . . . . Ashni K Behal
Chief of Medical Staff . . . . Gregory Bergman
CEO/President. . . . . Kevin W. Harlan

Measure	Cases	This Hosp.	State Avg.	U.S. Avg.
Blood Clot Prevention and Treatment				
Anticoagulation Overlap Therapy[2]	20	95%	93%	93%
ICU Venous Thromboembolism Prophylaxis[2]	18	94%	93%	92%
Incidence of Potentially Preventable VTE[1,2]	-	-	6%	10%
UFH with Dosages/Platelet Monitoring[1,2]	-	-	98%	97%
Venous Thromboembolism Prophylaxis[2]	188	81%	88%	85%
Warfarin Therapy Discharge Instructions[2]	15	7%	79%	75%
Chest Pain/Possible Heart Attack Care				
Aspirin Given Within 24 Hours of Arrival	63	95%	97%	96%
Fibrinolytic Meds Within 30 Min. of Arrival[1]	-	-	44%	58%
Average Time to ECG (minutes)	66	7	6	7
Average Time to Transfer (minutes)[1]	-	-	58	60
Children's Asthma Care				
Received Home Management Plan of Care	-	-	85%	88%
Received Reliever Medication	-	-	100%	100%
Received Systemic Corticosteroids	-	-	100%	100%
Emergency Department				
Admittance Decision Time (minutes)[2]	241	63	90	98
Head CT Results Within 45 Min. of Arrival	12	58%	63%	57%
Patients Who Left ER Before Being Seen	14,624	1%	2%	2%
Time from ER Arrival to Admit. (minutes)[2]	259	203	265	274
Time from ER Arrival to Discharge (minutes)	317	105	128	134
Time in ER Before Being Evaluated (minutes)	387	18	22	26
Time to Pain Meds for Fractures (minutes)	48	50	54	57
Heart Attack Care				
Aspirin Given at Discharge	11	91%	99%	99%
Fibrinolytic Meds Within 30 Min. of Arrival[7]	-	-	80%	54%
PCI Within 90 Minutes of Arrival[7]	-	-	97%	96%
Statin Prescribed at Discharge	12	83%	98%	98%
Heart Failure Care				
ACE Inhibitor or ARB for LVSD	18	89%	97%	97%
Discharge Instructions Given	53	96%	96%	94%
Evaluation of LVS Function	89	100%	100%	99%
Medicare Spending				
Medicare Spending per Patient (ratio)	-	0.93	1.01	0.98
Pneumonia Care				
Appropriate Initial Antibiotic Given	52	98%	96%	95%
Blood Culture Timing	64	98%	98%	98%
Pregnancy and Delivery Care				
Newborn Deliveries Scheduled Early[2]	26	0%	5%	6%
Preventive Care				
Immunization for Influenza[2]	261	93%	93%	90%
Immunization for Pneumonia[2]	347	93%	94%	92%
Stroke Care				
Anticoagulation Therapy for Atrial Fibrillation[7]	-	-	95%	95%
Antithrombotic Therapy Timing[1]	-	-	98%	98%
Assessed for Rehabilitation	11	91%	98%	97%
Discharged on Antithrombotic Therapy	11	100%	99%	99%
Discharged on Statin Medication[1]	-	-	95%	94%
Thrombolytic Therapy Timing[1]	-	-	65%	66%
Venous Thromboembolism Prophylaxis[1]	-	-	95%	94%
Written Stroke Educational Materials Given[1]	-	-	92%	88%

NOTE: Hospital profiles are in alphabetical order by state, then city, then hospital within the city; Rankings exclude hospitals with less than 25 cases except for patient surveys which excludes hospitals with less than 100 cases; (a) 100-299 cases; (1) The number of cases/patients is too few to report; (2) Data submitted were based on a sample of cases/patients; (3) Results are based on a shorter time period than required; (4) Data suppressed by CMS for one or more quarters; (5) Results are not available for this reporting period; (6) Fewer than 100 patients completed the HCAHPS survey; (7) No cases met the criteria for this measure; (8) The lower limit of the confidence interval cannot be calculated if the number of observed infections equals zero; (9) No data are available from the state/territory for this reporting period; (10) The scores shown reflect fewer than 50 completed surveys; (11) There were discrepancies in the data collection process; (12) This measure does not apply to this hospital for this reporting period; (13) Results cannot be calculated for this reporting period; (14) The results for this state are combined with nearby states to protect confidentiality; Please refer to the User's Guide for a full explanation of data.

Measure	Cases	This Hosp.	State Avg.	U.S. Avg.
Surgical Care Improvement Project				
Appropriate Beta Blocker Usage	45	89%	98%	98%
Appropriate VTP Within 24 Hours	131	95%	98%	98%
Controlled Postoperative Blood Glucose[7]	-	-	97%	97%
Perioperative Temperature Management	145	100%	100%	100%
Prophylactic Antibiotic Selection	99	100%	99%	99%
Prophylactic Antibiotic Selection (Outpatient)	24	96%	98%	98%
Prophylactic Antibiotic Stopped	98	97%	98%	98%
Prophylactic Antibiotic Timing	99	94%	99%	99%
Prophylactic Antibiotic Timing (Outpatient)	25	84%	97%	98%
Urinary Catheter Removal	80	91%	97%	97%
Survey of Patients' Hospital Experiences				
Area Around Room 'Always' Quiet at Night	300+	59%	58%	61%
Doctors 'Always' Communicated Well	300+	80%	80%	82%
Home Recovery Information Given	300+	85%	87%	85%
Hospital Given 9 or 10 on 10 Point Scale	300+	71%	72%	71%
Meds 'Always' Explained Before Given	300+	64%	64%	64%
Nurses 'Always' Communicated Well	300+	80%	81%	79%
Pain 'Always' Well Controlled	300+	70%	71%	71%
Room and Bathroom 'Always' Clean	300+	86%	75%	73%
Timely Help 'Always' Received	300+	75%	70%	68%
Would Definitely Recommend Hospital	300+	69%	71%	71%
Use of Medical Imaging				
Cardiac Imaging Stress Test before Surgery[1]	-	-	5.4%	5.3%
Combination Abdominal CT Scan	359	24.0%	7.1%	10.5%
Combination Brain/Sinus CT Scan[1]	-	-	2.8%	2.7%
Combination Chest CT Scan	222	7.2%	1.7%	2.7%
Follow-up Mammogram/Ultrasound	500	3.0%	8.7%	8.8%
Lumbar Spine MRI for Low Back Pain	61	37.7%	34.7%	37.2%

Salem Regional Medical Center

1995 East State Street
Salem, OH 44460
Phone: 330-332-1551
Fax: 330-332-7691
E-mail: info@salemhosp.com
URL: www.salemhosp.com
Type: Acute Care Hospitals
Emergency Services: Yes
Ownership: Voluntary non-profit - Private
Beds: 183

Key Personnel:
Radiology. . . . . Peter L Apicella
Anesthesiology. . . . . James A Bachmeier, M.D.
Emergency Room . . . . Lisa A Bennett
Pediatrics. . . . . Richelle L Keleman, M.D.
CEO/President. . . . . Howard E Rohleder
Chief of Medical Staff. . . . . Marc Ucchino

Measure	Cases	This Hosp.	State Avg.	U.S. Avg.
Blood Clot Prevention and Treatment				
Anticoagulation Overlap Therapy[2]	41	98%	93%	93%
ICU Venous Thromboembolism Prophylaxis[2]	25	88%	93%	92%
Incidence of Potentially Preventable VTE[2,7]	-	-	6%	10%
UFH with Dosages/Platelet Monitoring[2]	33	100%	98%	97%
Venous Thromboembolism Prophylaxis[2]	335	90%	88%	85%
Warfarin Therapy Discharge Instructions[2]	35	100%	79%	75%
Chest Pain/Possible Heart Attack Care				
Aspirin Given Within 24 Hours of Arrival	79	99%	97%	96%
Fibrinolytic Meds Within 30 Min. of Arrival[7]	-	-	44%	58%
Average Time to ECG (minutes)	81	6	6	7
Average Time to Transfer (minutes)	25	56	58	60
Children's Asthma Care				
Received Home Management Plan of Care	-	-	85%	88%
Received Reliever Medication	-	-	100%	100%
Received Systemic Corticosteroids	-	-	100%	100%
Emergency Department				
Admittance Decision Time (minutes)[2]	471	72	90	98
Head CT Results Within 45 Min. of Arrival	19	63%	63%	57%
Patients Who Left ER Before Being Seen	28,115	1%	2%	2%
Time from ER Arrival to Admit. (minutes)[2]	472	251	265	274
Time from ER Arrival to Discharge (minutes)	381	125	128	134
Time in ER Before Being Evaluated (minutes)	407	32	22	26
Time to Pain Meds for Fractures (minutes)	81	60	54	57
Heart Attack Care				
Aspirin Given at Discharge	23	100%	99%	99%
Fibrinolytic Meds Within 30 Min. of Arrival[7]	-	-	80%	54%
PCI Within 90 Minutes of Arrival[7]	-	-	97%	96%
Statin Prescribed at Discharge	16	88%	98%	98%
Heart Failure Care				
ACE Inhibitor or ARB for LVSD	23	96%	97%	97%
Discharge Instructions Given	89	100%	96%	94%
Evaluation of LVS Function	124	99%	100%	99%
Medicare Spending				
Medicare Spending per Patient (ratio)	-	1.03	1.01	0.98
Pneumonia Care				
Appropriate Initial Antibiotic Given	140	96%	96%	95%
Blood Culture Timing	166	98%	98%	98%
Pregnancy and Delivery Care				
Newborn Deliveries Scheduled Early[1]	-	-	5%	6%
Preventive Care				
Immunization for Influenza[2]	379	96%	93%	90%
Immunization for Pneumonia[2]	519	96%	94%	92%
Stroke Care				
Anticoagulation Therapy for Atrial Fibrillation[1]	-	-	95%	95%
Antithrombotic Therapy Timing	45	96%	98%	98%
Assessed for Rehabilitation	46	93%	98%	97%
Discharged on Antithrombotic Therapy	44	98%	99%	99%
Discharged on Statin Medication	38	95%	95%	94%
Thrombolytic Therapy Timing[7]	-	-	65%	66%
Venous Thromboembolism Prophylaxis	48	85%	95%	94%
Written Stroke Educational Materials Given	32	75%	92%	88%
Surgical Care Improvement Project				
Appropriate Beta Blocker Usage	83	94%	98%	98%
Appropriate VTP Within 24 Hours	207	95%	98%	98%
Controlled Postoperative Blood Glucose[7]	-	-	97%	97%
Perioperative Temperature Management	239	100%	100%	100%
Prophylactic Antibiotic Selection	155	99%	99%	99%
Prophylactic Antibiotic Selection (Outpatient)	76	99%	98%	98%
Prophylactic Antibiotic Stopped	147	97%	98%	98%
Prophylactic Antibiotic Timing	155	97%	99%	99%
Prophylactic Antibiotic Timing (Outpatient)	79	96%	97%	98%
Urinary Catheter Removal	163	95%	97%	97%
Survey of Patients' Hospital Experiences				
Area Around Room 'Always' Quiet at Night	300+	46%	58%	61%
Doctors 'Always' Communicated Well	300+	78%	80%	82%
Home Recovery Information Given	300+	81%	87%	85%
Hospital Given 9 or 10 on 10 Point Scale	300+	61%	72%	71%
Meds 'Always' Explained Before Given	300+	60%	64%	64%
Nurses 'Always' Communicated Well	300+	76%	81%	79%
Pain 'Always' Well Controlled	300+	65%	71%	71%
Room and Bathroom 'Always' Clean	300+	73%	75%	73%
Timely Help 'Always' Received	300+	68%	70%	68%
Would Definitely Recommend Hospital	300+	58%	71%	71%
Use of Medical Imaging				
Cardiac Imaging Stress Test before Surgery	233	6.4%	5.4%	5.3%
Combination Abdominal CT Scan	740	9.1%	7.1%	10.5%
Combination Brain/Sinus CT Scan	577	1.6%	2.8%	2.7%
Combination Chest CT Scan	473	0.0%	1.7%	2.7%
Follow-up Mammogram/Ultrasound	1,098	5.8%	8.7%	8.8%
Lumbar Spine MRI for Low Back Pain	86	33.7%	34.7%	37.2%

Firelands Regional Medical Center

1111 Hayes Avenue
Sandusky, OH 44870
Phone: 419-557-7400
Fax: 419-557-6835
URL: www.firelands.com
Type: Acute Care Hospitals
Emergency Services: Yes
Ownership: Voluntary non-profit - Private
Beds: 325

Key Personnel:
Operating Room. . . . . Ann Arnold, RN
Pediatric Ambulatory Care . . . . . . Ann Arnold, RN
Quality Assurance . . . . Amy Bohn-Green, RN
Infection Control. . . . . Beth Frank
Pediatric In-Patient Care . . . . Linda Ricci, RN
CEO/President. . . . . Martin E. Tursky
Radiology. . . . . Mike Vickery
Chief of Medical Staff. . . . . Brenda Violette

Measure	Cases	This Hosp.	State Avg.	U.S. Avg.
Blood Clot Prevention and Treatment				
Anticoagulation Overlap Therapy[2]	61	100%	93%	93%
ICU Venous Thromboembolism Prophylaxis[2]	73	93%	93%	92%
Incidence of Potentially Preventable VTE[2]	13	0%	6%	10%
UFH with Dosages/Platelet Monitoring[2]	59	100%	98%	97%
Venous Thromboembolism Prophylaxis[2]	331	95%	88%	85%
Warfarin Therapy Discharge Instructions[2]	48	100%	79%	75%
Chest Pain/Possible Heart Attack Care				
Aspirin Given Within 24 Hours of Arrival	22	100%	97%	96%
Fibrinolytic Meds Within 30 Min. of Arrival[7]	-	-	44%	58%
Average Time to ECG (minutes)	24	5	6	7
Average Time to Transfer (minutes)	18	54	58	60
Children's Asthma Care				
Received Home Management Plan of Care	-	-	85%	88%
Received Reliever Medication	-	-	100%	100%
Received Systemic Corticosteroids	-	-	100%	100%
Emergency Department				
Admittance Decision Time (minutes)[2]	601	58	90	98
Head CT Results Within 45 Min. of Arrival[1]	-	-	63%	57%
Patients Who Left ER Before Being Seen	47,770	1%	2%	2%
Time from ER Arrival to Admit. (minutes)[2]	627	220	265	274
Time from ER Arrival to Discharge (minutes)	389	111	128	134
Time in ER Before Being Evaluated (minutes)	401	34	22	26
Time to Pain Meds for Fractures (minutes)	140	60	54	57
Heart Attack Care				
Aspirin Given at Discharge	138	100%	99%	99%
Fibrinolytic Meds Within 30 Min. of Arrival[7]	-	-	80%	54%
PCI Within 90 Minutes of Arrival	18	100%	97%	96%
Statin Prescribed at Discharge	130	99%	98%	98%
Heart Failure Care				
ACE Inhibitor or ARB for LVSD	86	100%	97%	97%
Discharge Instructions Given	201	100%	96%	94%
Evaluation of LVS Function	257	100%	100%	99%
Medicare Spending				
Medicare Spending per Patient (ratio)	-	1.05	1.01	0.98
Pneumonia Care				
Appropriate Initial Antibiotic Given	107	100%	96%	95%
Blood Culture Timing	177	99%	98%	98%
Pregnancy and Delivery Care				
Newborn Deliveries Scheduled Early	72	7%	5%	6%
Preventive Care				
Immunization for Influenza[2]	564	94%	93%	90%
Immunization for Pneumonia[2]	831	96%	94%	92%
Stroke Care				
Anticoagulation Therapy for Atrial Fibrillation[1]	-	-	95%	95%
Antithrombotic Therapy Timing	72	97%	98%	98%
Assessed for Rehabilitation	76	100%	98%	97%
Discharged on Antithrombotic Therapy	70	99%	99%	99%
Discharged on Statin Medication	55	98%	95%	94%
Thrombolytic Therapy Timing[1]	-	-	65%	66%
Venous Thromboembolism Prophylaxis	85	85%	95%	94%
Written Stroke Educational Materials Given	43	95%	92%	88%
Surgical Care Improvement Project				
Appropriate Beta Blocker Usage[2]	167	100%	98%	98%
Appropriate VTP Within 24 Hours[2]	321	100%	98%	98%
Controlled Postoperative Blood Glucose[2]	26	92%	97%	97%
Perioperative Temperature Management[2]	469	100%	100%	100%
Prophylactic Antibiotic Selection[2]	306	100%	99%	99%
Prophylactic Antibiotic Selection (Outpatient)	327	98%	98%	98%
Prophylactic Antibiotic Stopped[2]	305	100%	98%	98%
Prophylactic Antibiotic Timing[2]	306	100%	99%	99%
Prophylactic Antibiotic Timing (Outpatient)	329	99%	97%	98%
Urinary Catheter Removal[2]	299	100%	97%	97%
Survey of Patients' Hospital Experiences				
Area Around Room 'Always' Quiet at Night	300+	54%	58%	61%
Doctors 'Always' Communicated Well	300+	80%	80%	82%
Home Recovery Information Given	300+	84%	87%	85%
Hospital Given 9 or 10 on 10 Point Scale	300+	70%	72%	71%
Meds 'Always' Explained Before Given	300+	64%	64%	64%
Nurses 'Always' Communicated Well	300+	77%	81%	79%
Pain 'Always' Well Controlled	300+	67%	71%	71%
Room and Bathroom 'Always' Clean	300+	80%	75%	73%
Timely Help 'Always' Received	300+	65%	70%	68%
Would Definitely Recommend Hospital	300+	72%	71%	71%
Use of Medical Imaging				
Cardiac Imaging Stress Test before Surgery	220	7.3%	5.4%	5.3%
Combination Abdominal CT Scan	982	2.0%	7.1%	10.5%

NOTE: Hospital profiles are in alphabetical order by state, then city, then hospital within the city; Rankings exclude hospitals with less than 25 cases except for patient surveys which excludes hospitals with less than 100 cases; (a) 100-299 cases; (1) The number of cases/patients is too few to report; (2) Data submitted were based on a sample of cases/patients; (3) Results are based on a shorter time period than required; (4) Data suppressed by CMS for one or more quarters; (5) Results are not available for this reporting period; (6) Fewer than 100 patients completed the HCAHPS survey; (7) No cases met the criteria for this measure; (8) The lower limit of the confidence interval cannot be calculated if the number of observed infections equals zero; (9) No data are available from the state/territory for this reporting period; (10) The scores shown reflect fewer than 50 completed surveys; (11) There were discrepancies in the data collection process; (12) This measure does not apply to this hospital for this reporting period; (13) Results cannot be calculated for this reporting period; (14) The results for this state are combined with nearby states to protect confidentiality; Please refer to the User's Guide for a full explanation of data.

Combination Brain/Sinus CT Scan	832	4.3%	2.8%	2.7%
Combination Chest CT Scan	627	0.0%	1.7%	2.7%
Follow-up Mammogram/Ultrasound	1,759	8.5%	8.7%	8.8%
Lumbar Spine MRI for Low Back Pain	204	30.9%	34.7%	37.2%

Adams County Regional Medical Center

230 Medical Center Drive Phone: 937-386-3400
Seaman, OH 45679
URL: www.acrmc.com
Type: Critical Access Hospitals Emergency Services: Yes
Ownership: Government - Local
Key Personnel:
Emergency . . . . Olayinka Aina, MD
Surgery . . . . Tyler Campbell, MD
Imaging . . . . Thomas Heffernan, MD

Measure	Cases	This Hosp.	State Avg.	U.S. Avg.
Blood Clot Prevention and Treatment				
Anticoagulation Overlap Therapy[5]	-	-	93%	93%
ICU Venous Thromboembolism Prophylaxis[5]	-	-	93%	92%
Incidence of Potentially Preventable VTE[5]	-	-	6%	10%
UFH with Dosages/Platelet Monitoring[5]	-	-	98%	97%
Venous Thromboembolism Prophylaxis[5]	-	-	88%	85%
Warfarin Therapy Discharge Instructions[5]	-	-	79%	75%
Chest Pain/Possible Heart Attack Care				
Aspirin Given Within 24 Hours of Arrival[5]	-	-	97%	96%
Fibrinolytic Meds Within 30 Min. of Arrival[5]	-	-	44%	58%
Average Time to ECG (minutes)[5]	-	-	6	7
Average Time to Transfer (minutes)[5]	-	-	58	60
Children's Asthma Care				
Received Home Management Plan of Care	-	-	85%	88%
Received Reliever Medication	-	-	100%	100%
Received Systemic Corticosteroids	-	-	100%	100%
Emergency Department				
Admittance Decision Time (minutes)[5]	-	-	90	98
Head CT Results Within 45 Min. of Arrival[5]	-	-	63%	57%
Patients Who Left ER Before Being Seen[5]	-	-	2%	2%
Time from ER Arrival to Admit. (minutes)[5]	-	-	265	274
Time from ER Arrival to Discharge (minutes)[5]	-	-	128	134
Time in ER Before Being Evaluated (minutes)[5]	-	-	22	26
Time to Pain Meds for Fractures (minutes)[5]	-	-	54	57
Heart Attack Care				
Aspirin Given at Discharge[3,7]	-	-	99%	99%
Fibrinolytic Meds Within 30 Min. of Arrival[3,7]	-	-	80%	54%
PCI Within 90 Minutes of Arrival[3,7]	-	-	97%	96%
Statin Prescribed at Discharge[3,7]	-	-	98%	98%
Heart Failure Care				
ACE Inhibitor or ARB for LVSD[1]	-	-	97%	97%
Discharge Instructions Given	18	83%	96%	94%
Evaluation of LVS Function	26	100%	100%	99%
Medicare Spending				
Medicare Spending per Patient (ratio)	-	-	1.01	0.98
Pneumonia Care				
Appropriate Initial Antibiotic Given	56	91%	96%	95%
Blood Culture Timing	79	94%	98%	98%
Pregnancy and Delivery Care				
Newborn Deliveries Scheduled Early[5]	-	-	5%	6%
Preventive Care				
Immunization for Influenza[5]	-	-	93%	90%
Immunization for Pneumonia[5]	-	-	94%	92%
Stroke Care				
Anticoagulation Therapy for Atrial Fibrillation[5]	-	-	95%	95%
Antithrombotic Therapy Timing[5]	-	-	98%	98%
Assessed for Rehabilitation[5]	-	-	98%	97%
Discharged on Antithrombotic Therapy[5]	-	-	99%	99%
Discharged on Statin Medication[5]	-	-	95%	94%
Thrombolytic Therapy Timing[5]	-	-	65%	66%
Venous Thromboembolism Prophylaxis[5]	-	-	95%	94%
Written Stroke Educational Materials Given[5]	-	-	92%	88%
Surgical Care Improvement Project				
Appropriate Beta Blocker Usage[5]	-	-	98%	98%
Appropriate VTP Within 24 Hours[5]	-	-	98%	98%
Controlled Postoperative Blood Glucose[5]	-	-	97%	97%
Perioperative Temperature Management[5]	-	-	100%	100%
Prophylactic Antibiotic Selection[5]	-	-	99%	99%
Prophylactic Antibiotic Selection (Outpatient)[5]	-	-	98%	98%
Prophylactic Antibiotic Stopped[5]	-	-	98%	98%
Prophylactic Antibiotic Timing[5]	-	-	99%	99%
Prophylactic Antibiotic Timing (Outpatient)[5]	-	-	97%	98%
Urinary Catheter Removal[5]	-	-	97%	97%
Survey of Patients' Hospital Experiences				
Area Around Room 'Always' Quiet at Night	(a)	56%	58%	61%
Doctors 'Always' Communicated Well	(a)	81%	80%	82%
Home Recovery Information Given	(a)	82%	87%	85%
Hospital Given 9 or 10 on 10 Point Scale	(a)	66%	72%	71%
Meds 'Always' Explained Before Given	(a)	60%	64%	64%
Nurses 'Always' Communicated Well	(a)	76%	81%	79%
Pain 'Always' Well Controlled	(a)	65%	71%	71%
Room and Bathroom 'Always' Clean	(a)	77%	75%	73%
Timely Help 'Always' Received	(a)	63%	70%	68%
Would Definitely Recommend Hospital	(a)	61%	71%	71%
Use of Medical Imaging				
Cardiac Imaging Stress Test before Surgery	57	3.5%	5.4%	5.3%
Combination Abdominal CT Scan	337	8.0%	7.1%	10.5%
Combination Brain/Sinus CT Scan	360	1.4%	2.8%	2.7%
Combination Chest CT Scan	216	4.2%	1.7%	2.7%
Follow-up Mammogram/Ultrasound	184	13.6%	8.7%	8.8%
Lumbar Spine MRI for Low Back Pain	56	32.1%	34.7%	37.2%

Medcentral Health System Shelby Hospital

199 West Main Street Phone: 419-342-5015
Shelby, OH 44875 Fax: 419-521-7960
Type: Critical Access Hospitals Emergency Services: Yes
Ownership: Voluntary non-profit - Private Beds: 68
Key Personnel:
Radiology. Paul Buehrer
CEO/President. . . . . Jim Meyer

Measure	Cases	This Hosp.	State Avg.	U.S. Avg.
Blood Clot Prevention and Treatment				
Anticoagulation Overlap Therapy[5]	-	-	93%	93%
ICU Venous Thromboembolism Prophylaxis[5]	-	-	93%	92%
Incidence of Potentially Preventable VTE[5]	-	-	6%	10%
UFH with Dosages/Platelet Monitoring[5]	-	-	98%	97%
Venous Thromboembolism Prophylaxis[5]	-	-	88%	85%
Warfarin Therapy Discharge Instructions[5]	-	-	79%	75%
Chest Pain/Possible Heart Attack Care				
Aspirin Given Within 24 Hours of Arrival	-	-	97%	96%
Fibrinolytic Meds Within 30 Min. of Arrival	-	-	44%	58%
Average Time to ECG (minutes)	-	-	6	7
Average Time to Transfer (minutes)	-	-	58	60
Children's Asthma Care				
Received Home Management Plan of Care	-	-	85%	88%
Received Reliever Medication	-	-	100%	100%
Received Systemic Corticosteroids	-	-	100%	100%
Emergency Department				
Admittance Decision Time (minutes)[5]	-	-	90	98
Head CT Results Within 45 Min. of Arrival	-	-	63%	57%
Patients Who Left ER Before Being Seen	-	-	2%	2%
Time from ER Arrival to Admit. (minutes)[5]	-	-	265	274
Time from ER Arrival to Discharge (minutes)	-	-	128	134
Time in ER Before Being Evaluated (minutes)	-	-	22	26
Time to Pain Meds for Fractures (minutes)	-	-	54	57
Heart Attack Care				
Aspirin Given at Discharge[5]	-	-	99%	99%
Fibrinolytic Meds Within 30 Min. of Arrival[5]	-	-	80%	54%
PCI Within 90 Minutes of Arrival[5]	-	-	97%	96%
Statin Prescribed at Discharge[5]	-	-	98%	98%
Heart Failure Care				
ACE Inhibitor or ARB for LVSD[5]	-	-	97%	97%
Discharge Instructions Given[5]	-	-	96%	94%
Evaluation of LVS Function[5]	-	-	100%	99%
Medicare Spending				
Medicare Spending per Patient (ratio)	-	-	1.01	0.98
Pneumonia Care				
Appropriate Initial Antibiotic Given[5]	-	-	96%	95%
Blood Culture Timing[5]	-	-	98%	98%
Pregnancy and Delivery Care				
Newborn Deliveries Scheduled Early[1,3]	-	-	5%	6%
Preventive Care				
Immunization for Influenza[5]	-	-	93%	90%
Immunization for Pneumonia[5]	-	-	94%	92%
Stroke Care				
Anticoagulation Therapy for Atrial Fibrillation[5]	-	-	95%	95%
Antithrombotic Therapy Timing[5]	-	-	98%	98%
Assessed for Rehabilitation[5]	-	-	98%	97%
Discharged on Antithrombotic Therapy[5]	-	-	99%	99%
Discharged on Statin Medication[5]	-	-	95%	94%
Thrombolytic Therapy Timing[5]	-	-	65%	66%
Venous Thromboembolism Prophylaxis[5]	-	-	95%	94%
Written Stroke Educational Materials Given[5]	-	-	92%	88%
Surgical Care Improvement Project				
Appropriate Beta Blocker Usage[5]	-	-	98%	98%
Appropriate VTP Within 24 Hours[5]	-	-	98%	98%
Controlled Postoperative Blood Glucose[5]	-	-	97%	97%
Perioperative Temperature Management[5]	-	-	100%	100%
Prophylactic Antibiotic Selection[5]	-	-	99%	99%
Prophylactic Antibiotic Selection (Outpatient)	-	-	98%	98%
Prophylactic Antibiotic Stopped[5]	-	-	98%	98%
Prophylactic Antibiotic Timing[5]	-	-	99%	99%
Prophylactic Antibiotic Timing (Outpatient)	-	-	97%	98%
Urinary Catheter Removal[5]	-	-	97%	97%
Survey of Patients' Hospital Experiences				
Area Around Room 'Always' Quiet at Night	(a)	64%	58%	61%
Doctors 'Always' Communicated Well	(a)	84%	80%	82%
Home Recovery Information Given	(a)	85%	87%	85%
Hospital Given 9 or 10 on 10 Point Scale	(a)	80%	72%	71%
Meds 'Always' Explained Before Given	(a)	67%	64%	64%
Nurses 'Always' Communicated Well	(a)	83%	81%	79%
Pain 'Always' Well Controlled	(a)	77%	71%	71%
Room and Bathroom 'Always' Clean	(a)	79%	75%	73%
Timely Help 'Always' Received	(a)	81%	70%	68%
Would Definitely Recommend Hospital	(a)	78%	71%	71%
Use of Medical Imaging				
Cardiac Imaging Stress Test before Surgery	-	-	5.4%	5.3%
Combination Abdominal CT Scan	-	-	7.1%	10.5%
Combination Brain/Sinus CT Scan	-	-	2.8%	2.7%
Combination Chest CT Scan	-	-	1.7%	2.7%
Follow-up Mammogram/Ultrasound	-	-	8.7%	8.8%
Lumbar Spine MRI for Low Back Pain	-	-	34.7%	37.2%

Wilson Memorial Hospital

915 West Michigan Street Phone: 937-498-5418
Sidney, OH 45365 Fax: 937-497-8251
URL: www.wilsonhospital.com
Type: Acute Care Hospitals Emergency Services: Yes
Ownership: Voluntary non-profit - Other Beds: 112
Key Personnel:
Radiology. . . . . C H Bahng
Patient Relations . . . . Connie Burgess
Quality Assurance . . . . Elizabeth Custis
President/CEO. . . . . Mark Dooley
Emergency Room . . . . Fred Haussman
Intensive Care Unit. . . . . Linda Maurer
Chief of Medical Staff . . . . Robert McDevitt
Infection Control. . . . . Linda Smith, RN

Measure	Cases	This Hosp.	State Avg.	U.S. Avg.
Blood Clot Prevention and Treatment				
Anticoagulation Overlap Therapy[2]	14	93%	93%	93%
ICU Venous Thromboembolism Prophylaxis[2]	27	93%	93%	92%
Incidence of Potentially Preventable VTE[2,7]	-	-	6%	10%
UFH with Dosages/Platelet Monitoring[1,2]	-	-	98%	97%
Venous Thromboembolism Prophylaxis[2]	127	78%	88%	85%
Warfarin Therapy Discharge Instructions[2]	14	93%	79%	75%
Chest Pain/Possible Heart Attack Care				
Aspirin Given Within 24 Hours of Arrival	58	86%	97%	96%
Fibrinolytic Meds Within 30 Min. of Arrival[1]	-	-	44%	58%
Average Time to ECG (minutes)	75	7	6	7
Average Time to Transfer (minutes)[1]	-	-	58	60
Children's Asthma Care				
Received Home Management Plan of Care	-	-	85%	88%
Received Reliever Medication	-	-	100%	100%

NOTE: Hospital profiles are in alphabetical order by state, then city, then hospital within the city; Rankings exclude hospitals with less than 25 cases except for patient surveys which excludes hospitals with less than 100 cases; (a) 100-299 cases; (1) The number of cases/patients is too few to report; (2) Data submitted were based on a sample of cases/patients; (3) Results are based on a shorter time period than required; (4) Data suppressed by CMS for one or more quarters; (5) Results are not available for this reporting period; (6) Fewer than 100 patients completed the HCAHPS survey; (7) No cases met the criteria for this measure; (8) The lower limit of the confidence interval cannot be calculated if the number of observed infections equals zero; (9) No data are available from the state/territory for this reporting period; (10) The scores shown reflect fewer than 50 completed surveys; (11) There were discrepancies in the data collection process; (12) This measure does not apply to this hospital for this reporting period; (13) Results cannot be calculated for this reporting period; (14) The results for this state are combined with nearby states to protect confidentiality; Please refer to the User's Guide for a full explanation of data.

Measure	Cases	This Hosp.	State Avg.	U.S. Avg.
Received Systemic Corticosteroids	-	-	100%	100%
Emergency Department				
Admittance Decision Time (minutes)[2]	275	60	90	98
Head CT Results Within 45 Min. of Arrival	16	56%	63%	57%
Patients Who Left ER Before Being Seen	28,522	1%	2%	2%
Time from ER Arrival to Admit. (minutes)[2]	275	240	265	274
Time from ER Arrival to Discharge (minutes)	376	127	128	134
Time in ER Before Being Evaluated (minutes)	383	40	22	26
Time to Pain Meds for Fractures (minutes)	123	60	54	57
Heart Attack Care				
Aspirin Given at Discharge[1]	-	-	99%	99%
Fibrinolytic Meds Within 30 Min. of Arrival[7]	-	-	80%	54%
PCI Within 90 Minutes of Arrival[7]	-	-	97%	96%
Statin Prescribed at Discharge[1]	-	-	98%	98%
Heart Failure Care				
ACE Inhibitor or ARB for LVSD	13	85%	97%	97%
Discharge Instructions Given	54	96%	96%	94%
Evaluation of LVS Function	72	99%	100%	99%
Medicare Spending				
Medicare Spending per Patient (ratio)	-	1.13	1.01	0.98
Pneumonia Care				
Appropriate Initial Antibiotic Given	65	92%	96%	95%
Blood Culture Timing	74	96%	98%	98%
Pregnancy and Delivery Care				
Newborn Deliveries Scheduled Early	44	5%	5%	6%
Preventive Care				
Immunization for Influenza[2]	255	89%	93%	90%
Immunization for Pneumonia[2]	290	91%	94%	92%
Stroke Care				
Anticoagulation Therapy for Atrial Fibrillation[7]	-	-	95%	95%
Antithrombotic Therapy Timing	12	100%	98%	98%
Assessed for Rehabilitation	13	92%	98%	97%
Discharged on Antithrombotic Therapy	11	100%	99%	99%
Discharged on Statin Medication[1]	-	-	95%	94%
Thrombolytic Therapy Timing[7]	-	-	65%	66%
Venous Thromboembolism Prophylaxis	11	55%	95%	94%
Written Stroke Educational Materials Given[1]	-	-	92%	88%
Surgical Care Improvement Project				
Appropriate Beta Blocker Usage	39	95%	98%	98%
Appropriate VTP Within 24 Hours	156	99%	98%	98%
Controlled Postoperative Blood Glucose[7]	-	-	97%	97%
Perioperative Temperature Management	167	100%	100%	100%
Prophylactic Antibiotic Selection	114	98%	99%	99%
Prophylactic Antibiotic Selection (Outpatient)	90	98%	98%	98%
Prophylactic Antibiotic Stopped	109	99%	98%	98%
Prophylactic Antibiotic Timing	114	96%	99%	99%
Prophylactic Antibiotic Timing (Outpatient)	91	97%	97%	98%
Urinary Catheter Removal	62	97%	97%	97%
Survey of Patients' Hospital Experiences				
Area Around Room 'Always' Quiet at Night[11]	300+	60%	58%	61%
Doctors 'Always' Communicated Well[11]	300+	82%	80%	82%
Home Recovery Information Given[11]	300+	91%	87%	85%
Hospital Given 9 or 10 on 10 Point Scale[11]	300+	68%	72%	71%
Meds 'Always' Explained Before Given[11]	300+	65%	64%	64%
Nurses 'Always' Communicated Well[11]	300+	80%	81%	79%
Pain 'Always' Well Controlled[11]	300+	73%	71%	71%
Room and Bathroom 'Always' Clean[11]	300+	80%	75%	73%
Timely Help 'Always' Received[11]	300+	69%	70%	68%
Would Definitely Recommend Hospital[11]	300+	68%	71%	71%
Use of Medical Imaging				
Cardiac Imaging Stress Test before Surgery	295	5.1%	5.4%	5.3%
Combination Abdominal CT Scan	343	8.5%	7.1%	10.5%
Combination Brain/Sinus CT Scan	409	2.0%	2.8%	2.7%
Combination Chest CT Scan	238	0.0%	1.7%	2.7%
Follow-up Mammogram/Ultrasound	638	11.1%	8.7%	8.8%
Lumbar Spine MRI for Low Back Pain	54	37.0%	34.7%	37.2%

Ohio Valley Medical Center

100 West Main Street
Springfield, OH 45502
Phone: 937-521-3900
URL: www.ovmc-online.com
Type: Acute Care Hospitals
Emergency Services: No
Ownership: Voluntary non-profit - Private

Measure	Cases	This Hosp.	State Avg.	U.S. Avg.
Blood Clot Prevention and Treatment				
Anticoagulation Overlap Therapy[7]	-	-	93%	93%
ICU Venous Thromboembolism Prophylaxis[7]	-	-	93%	92%
Incidence of Potentially Preventable VTE[7]	-	-	6%	10%
UFH with Dosages/Platelet Monitoring[7]	-	-	98%	97%
Venous Thromboembolism Prophylaxis	129	97%	88%	85%
Warfarin Therapy Discharge Instructions[7]	-	-	79%	75%
Chest Pain/Possible Heart Attack Care				
Aspirin Given Within 24 Hours of Arrival[5]	-	-	97%	96%
Fibrinolytic Meds Within 30 Min. of Arrival[5]	-	-	44%	58%
Average Time to ECG (minutes)[5]	-	-	6	7
Average Time to Transfer (minutes)[5]	-	-	58	60
Children's Asthma Care				
Received Home Management Plan of Care	-	-	85%	88%
Received Reliever Medication	-	-	100%	100%
Received Systemic Corticosteroids	-	-	100%	100%
Emergency Department				
Admittance Decision Time (minutes)[7]	-	-	90	98
Head CT Results Within 45 Min. of Arrival[5]	-	-	63%	57%
Patients Who Left ER Before Being Seen[5]	-	-	2%	2%
Time from ER Arrival to Admit. (minutes)[7]	-	-	265	274
Time from ER Arrival to Discharge (minutes)[5]	-	-	128	134
Time in ER Before Being Evaluated (minutes)[5]	-	-	22	26
Time to Pain Meds for Fractures (minutes)[5]	-	-	54	57
Heart Attack Care				
Aspirin Given at Discharge[5]	-	-	99%	99%
Fibrinolytic Meds Within 30 Min. of Arrival[5]	-	-	80%	54%
PCI Within 90 Minutes of Arrival[5]	-	-	97%	96%
Statin Prescribed at Discharge[5]	-	-	98%	98%
Heart Failure Care				
ACE Inhibitor or ARB for LVSD[5]	-	-	97%	97%
Discharge Instructions Given[5]	-	-	96%	94%
Evaluation of LVS Function[5]	-	-	100%	99%
Medicare Spending				
Medicare Spending per Patient (ratio)	-	0.99	1.01	0.98
Pneumonia Care				
Appropriate Initial Antibiotic Given[5]	-	-	96%	95%
Blood Culture Timing[5]	-	-	98%	98%
Pregnancy and Delivery Care				
Newborn Deliveries Scheduled Early[7]	-	-	5%	6%
Preventive Care				
Immunization for Influenza	393	98%	93%	90%
Immunization for Pneumonia	437	96%	94%	92%
Stroke Care				
Anticoagulation Therapy for Atrial Fibrillation[5]	-	-	95%	95%
Antithrombotic Therapy Timing[5]	-	-	98%	98%
Assessed for Rehabilitation[5]	-	-	98%	97%
Discharged on Antithrombotic Therapy[5]	-	-	99%	99%
Discharged on Statin Medication[5]	-	-	95%	94%
Thrombolytic Therapy Timing[5]	-	-	65%	66%
Venous Thromboembolism Prophylaxis[5]	-	-	95%	94%
Written Stroke Educational Materials Given[5]	-	-	92%	88%
Surgical Care Improvement Project				
Appropriate Beta Blocker Usage	171	99%	98%	98%
Appropriate VTP Within 24 Hours	475	99%	98%	98%
Controlled Postoperative Blood Glucose[7]	-	-	97%	97%
Perioperative Temperature Management	521	100%	100%	100%
Prophylactic Antibiotic Selection	440	100%	99%	99%
Prophylactic Antibiotic Selection (Outpatient)	258	98%	98%	98%
Prophylactic Antibiotic Stopped	436	99%	98%	98%
Prophylactic Antibiotic Timing	440	99%	99%	99%
Prophylactic Antibiotic Timing (Outpatient)	260	98%	97%	98%
Urinary Catheter Removal	250	97%	97%	97%
Survey of Patients' Hospital Experiences				
Area Around Room 'Always' Quiet at Night	300+	79%	58%	61%
Doctors 'Always' Communicated Well	300+	82%	80%	82%
Home Recovery Information Given	300+	88%	87%	85%
Hospital Given 9 or 10 on 10 Point Scale	300+	82%	72%	71%
Meds 'Always' Explained Before Given	300+	66%	64%	64%
Nurses 'Always' Communicated Well	300+	84%	81%	79%
Pain 'Always' Well Controlled	300+	73%	71%	71%
Room and Bathroom 'Always' Clean	300+	80%	75%	73%
Timely Help 'Always' Received	300+	77%	70%	68%
Would Definitely Recommend Hospital	300+	81%	71%	71%
Use of Medical Imaging				
Cardiac Imaging Stress Test before Surgery[7]	-	-	5.4%	5.3%
Combination Abdominal CT Scan	53	1.9%	7.1%	10.5%
Combination Brain/Sinus CT Scan[1]	-	-	2.8%	2.7%
Combination Chest CT Scan[1]	-	-	1.7%	2.7%
Follow-up Mammogram/Ultrasound[7]	-	-	8.7%	8.8%
Lumbar Spine MRI for Low Back Pain[1]	-	-	34.7%	37.2%

Springfield Regional Medical Center

100 Medical Center Drive
Springfield, OH 45504
Phone: 937-523-1000
Fax: 937-328-8770
E-mail: comrel@communityhospital.com
URL: www.communityhospital.com
Type: Acute Care Hospitals
Emergency Services: Yes
Ownership: Voluntary non-profit - Private
Beds: 324

Key Personnel:
Operating Room. . . . . Tedros Andom
Intensive Care Unit. . . . . Penny Brubaker
Chief of Medical Staff . . . . Stephen Feagins, MD
Cardiac Laboratory. . . . . Chris Fritts
CEO/President. . . . . Paul Hiltz
Coronary Care . . . . Mary Ann Roberts
Quality Assurance . . . . Nancy Shively
Radiology. . . . . Jerry Tobler

Measure	Cases	This Hosp.	State Avg.	U.S. Avg.
Blood Clot Prevention and Treatment				
Anticoagulation Overlap Therapy[2]	141	96%	93%	93%
ICU Venous Thromboembolism Prophylaxis[2]	97	87%	93%	92%
Incidence of Potentially Preventable VTE[1,2]	-	-	6%	10%
UFH with Dosages/Platelet Monitoring[2]	46	100%	98%	97%
Venous Thromboembolism Prophylaxis[2]	308	88%	88%	85%
Warfarin Therapy Discharge Instructions[2]	101	53%	79%	75%
Chest Pain/Possible Heart Attack Care				
Aspirin Given Within 24 Hours of Arrival[1,3]	-	-	97%	96%
Fibrinolytic Meds Within 30 Min. of Arrival[5]	-	-	44%	58%
Average Time to ECG (minutes)[1,3]	-	-	6	7
Average Time to Transfer (minutes)[5]	-	-	58	60
Children's Asthma Care				
Received Home Management Plan of Care	-	-	85%	88%
Received Reliever Medication	-	-	100%	100%
Received Systemic Corticosteroids	-	-	100%	100%
Emergency Department				
Admittance Decision Time (minutes)[2]	852	127	90	98
Head CT Results Within 45 Min. of Arrival	47	55%	63%	57%
Patients Who Left ER Before Being Seen	65,911	4%	2%	2%
Time from ER Arrival to Admit. (minutes)[2]	853	329	265	274
Time from ER Arrival to Discharge (minutes)	398	170	128	134
Time in ER Before Being Evaluated (minutes)	423	28	22	26
Time to Pain Meds for Fractures (minutes)	292	72	54	57
Heart Attack Care				
Aspirin Given at Discharge	343	97%	99%	99%
Fibrinolytic Meds Within 30 Min. of Arrival[7]	-	-	80%	54%
PCI Within 90 Minutes of Arrival	52	94%	97%	96%
Statin Prescribed at Discharge	347	98%	98%	98%
Heart Failure Care				
ACE Inhibitor or ARB for LVSD	174	89%	97%	97%
Discharge Instructions Given	398	87%	96%	94%
Evaluation of LVS Function	504	98%	100%	99%
Medicare Spending				
Medicare Spending per Patient (ratio)	-	1.06	1.01	0.98
Pneumonia Care				
Appropriate Initial Antibiotic Given	310	96%	96%	95%
Blood Culture Timing	455	97%	98%	98%
Pregnancy and Delivery Care				
Newborn Deliveries Scheduled Early[2]	19	5%	5%	6%

NOTE: Hospital profiles are in alphabetical order by state, then city, then hospital within the city; Rankings exclude hospitals with less than 25 cases except for patient surveys which excludes hospitals with less than 100 cases; (a) 100-299 cases; (1) The number of cases/patients is too few to report; (2) Data submitted were based on a sample of cases/patients; (3) Results are based on a shorter time period than required; (4) Data suppressed by CMS for one or more quarters; (5) Results are not available for this reporting period; (6) Fewer than 100 patients completed the HCAHPS survey; (7) No cases met the criteria for this measure; (8) The lower limit of the confidence interval cannot be calculated if the number of observed infections equals zero; (9) No data are available from the state/territory for this reporting period; (10) The scores shown reflect fewer than 50 completed surveys; (11) There were discrepancies in the data collection process; (12) This measure does not apply to this hospital for this reporting period; (13) Results cannot be calculated for this reporting period; (14) The results for this state are combined with nearby states to protect confidentiality; Please refer to the User's Guide for a full explanation of data.

Preventive Care				
Immunization for Influenza[2]	566	89%	93%	90%
Immunization for Pneumonia[2]	844	92%	94%	92%
Stroke Care				
Anticoagulation Therapy for Atrial Fibrillation[2]	19	79%	95%	95%
Antithrombotic Therapy Timing[2]	108	100%	98%	98%
Assessed for Rehabilitation[2]	108	89%	98%	97%
Discharged on Antithrombotic Therapy[2]	101	95%	99%	99%
Discharged on Statin Medication[2]	83	77%	95%	94%
Thrombolytic Therapy Timing[1,2]	-	-	65%	66%
Venous Thromboembolism Prophylaxis[2]	116	93%	95%	94%
Written Stroke Educational Materials Given[2]	54	94%	92%	88%
Surgical Care Improvement Project				
Appropriate Beta Blocker Usage	245	98%	98%	98%
Appropriate VTP Within 24 Hours	444	96%	98%	98%
Controlled Postoperative Blood Glucose	173	99%	97%	97%
Perioperative Temperature Management	572	100%	100%	100%
Prophylactic Antibiotic Selection	359	99%	99%	99%
Prophylactic Antibiotic Selection (Outpatient)	116	84%	98%	98%
Prophylactic Antibiotic Stopped	347	97%	98%	98%
Prophylactic Antibiotic Timing	359	99%	99%	99%
Prophylactic Antibiotic Timing (Outpatient)	119	94%	97%	98%
Urinary Catheter Removal	344	89%	97%	97%
Survey of Patients' Hospital Experiences				
Area Around Room 'Always' Quiet at Night	300+	54%	58%	61%
Doctors 'Always' Communicated Well	300+	79%	80%	82%
Home Recovery Information Given	300+	84%	87%	85%
Hospital Given 9 or 10 on 10 Point Scale	300+	64%	72%	71%
Meds 'Always' Explained Before Given	300+	58%	64%	64%
Nurses 'Always' Communicated Well	300+	77%	81%	79%
Pain 'Always' Well Controlled	300+	71%	71%	71%
Room and Bathroom 'Always' Clean	300+	74%	75%	73%
Timely Help 'Always' Received	300+	60%	70%	68%
Would Definitely Recommend Hospital	300+	60%	71%	71%
Use of Medical Imaging				
Cardiac Imaging Stress Test before Surgery	574	6.4%	5.4%	5.3%
Combination Abdominal CT Scan	1,006	3.1%	7.1%	10.5%
Combination Brain/Sinus CT Scan	844	3.2%	2.8%	2.7%
Combination Chest CT Scan	485	3.1%	1.7%	2.7%
Follow-up Mammogram/Ultrasound	1,130	7.0%	8.7%	8.8%
Lumbar Spine MRI for Low Back Pain	79	32.9%	34.7%	37.2%

Trinity Medical Center East & Trinity Medical Center West

380 Summit Avenue
Steubenville, OH 43952
Phone: 740-283-7000
Fax: 740-283-7104
URL: www.trinityhealth.com
Type: Acute Care Hospitals
Emergency Services: Yes
Ownership: Voluntary non-profit - Other
Beds: 401

Key Personnel:
Radiology. . . . . Frank Hamilton
Quality Assurance . . . . Susan McLamara
Operating Room. . . . . Emily Milich-Fransic
Chief of Medical Staff . . . . A Reddy, MD
Emergency Room . . . . David Sarcon

Measure	Cases	This Hosp.	State Avg.	U.S. Avg.
Blood Clot Prevention and Treatment				
Anticoagulation Overlap Therapy[2]	58	98%	93%	93%
ICU Venous Thromboembolism Prophylaxis[2]	74	86%	93%	92%
Incidence of Potentially Preventable VTE[1,2]	-	-	6%	10%
UFH with Dosages/Platelet Monitoring[2]	57	100%	98%	97%
Venous Thromboembolism Prophylaxis[2]	415	80%	88%	85%
Warfarin Therapy Discharge Instructions[2]	32	97%	79%	75%
Chest Pain/Possible Heart Attack Care				
Aspirin Given Within 24 Hours of Arrival[1,3]	-	-	97%	96%
Fibrinolytic Meds Within 30 Min. of Arrival[3,7]	-	-	44%	58%
Average Time to ECG (minutes)[1,3]	-	-	6	7
Average Time to Transfer (minutes)[3,7]	-	-	58	60
Children's Asthma Care				
Received Home Management Plan of Care	-	-	85%	88%
Received Reliever Medication	-	-	100%	100%
Received Systemic Corticosteroids	-	-	100%	100%
Emergency Department				
Admittance Decision Time (minutes)[2]	907	79	90	98
Head CT Results Within 45 Min. of Arrival	20	25%	63%	57%
Patients Who Left ER Before Being Seen	48,285	1%	2%	2%
Time from ER Arrival to Admit. (minutes)[2]	907	208	265	274
Time from ER Arrival to Discharge (minutes)	448	110	128	134
Time in ER Before Being Evaluated (minutes)	402	20	22	26
Time to Pain Meds for Fractures (minutes)	82	38	54	57
Heart Attack Care				
Aspirin Given at Discharge	269	100%	99%	99%
Fibrinolytic Meds Within 30 Min. of Arrival[7]	-	-	80%	54%
PCI Within 90 Minutes of Arrival	30	93%	97%	96%
Statin Prescribed at Discharge	268	99%	98%	98%
Heart Failure Care				
ACE Inhibitor or ARB for LVSD	136	97%	97%	97%
Discharge Instructions Given	327	97%	96%	94%
Evaluation of LVS Function	491	100%	100%	99%
Medicare Spending				
Medicare Spending per Patient (ratio)	-	1.17	1.01	0.98
Pneumonia Care				
Appropriate Initial Antibiotic Given	217	94%	96%	95%
Blood Culture Timing	338	99%	98%	98%
Pregnancy and Delivery Care				
Newborn Deliveries Scheduled Early	38	5%	5%	6%
Preventive Care				
Immunization for Influenza[2]	606	94%	93%	90%
Immunization for Pneumonia[2]	845	93%	94%	92%
Stroke Care				
Anticoagulation Therapy for Atrial Fibrillation	12	92%	95%	95%
Antithrombotic Therapy Timing	91	99%	98%	98%
Assessed for Rehabilitation	81	88%	98%	97%
Discharged on Antithrombotic Therapy	80	100%	99%	99%
Discharged on Statin Medication	62	84%	95%	94%
Thrombolytic Therapy Timing[1]	-	-	65%	66%
Venous Thromboembolism Prophylaxis	95	84%	95%	94%
Written Stroke Educational Materials Given	45	44%	92%	88%
Surgical Care Improvement Project				
Appropriate Beta Blocker Usage	224	99%	98%	98%
Appropriate VTP Within 24 Hours	374	97%	98%	98%
Controlled Postoperative Blood Glucose	101	95%	97%	97%
Perioperative Temperature Management	468	100%	100%	100%
Prophylactic Antibiotic Selection	383	98%	99%	99%
Prophylactic Antibiotic Selection (Outpatient)	264	98%	98%	98%
Prophylactic Antibiotic Stopped	372	97%	98%	98%
Prophylactic Antibiotic Timing	384	100%	99%	99%
Prophylactic Antibiotic Timing (Outpatient)	265	98%	97%	98%
Urinary Catheter Removal	312	98%	97%	97%
Survey of Patients' Hospital Experiences				
Area Around Room 'Always' Quiet at Night	300+	52%	58%	61%
Doctors 'Always' Communicated Well	300+	77%	80%	82%
Home Recovery Information Given	300+	88%	87%	85%
Hospital Given 9 or 10 on 10 Point Scale	300+	69%	72%	71%
Meds 'Always' Explained Before Given	300+	63%	64%	64%
Nurses 'Always' Communicated Well	300+	79%	81%	79%
Pain 'Always' Well Controlled	300+	70%	71%	71%
Room and Bathroom 'Always' Clean	300+	72%	75%	73%
Timely Help 'Always' Received	300+	64%	70%	68%
Would Definitely Recommend Hospital	300+	70%	71%	71%
Use of Medical Imaging				
Cardiac Imaging Stress Test before Surgery	558	7.5%	5.4%	5.3%
Combination Abdominal CT Scan	683	14.9%	7.1%	10.5%
Combination Brain/Sinus CT Scan	718	3.1%	2.8%	2.7%
Combination Chest CT Scan	436	5.5%	1.7%	2.7%
Follow-up Mammogram/Ultrasound	1,101	8.6%	8.7%	8.8%
Lumbar Spine MRI for Low Back Pain	156	30.8%	34.7%	37.2%

Flower Hospital

5200 Harroun Road
Sylvania, OH 43560
Phone: 419-824-1444
URL: www.promedica.org
Type: Acute Care Hospitals
Emergency Services: Yes
Ownership: Voluntary non-profit - Private
Beds: 279

Measure	Cases	This Hosp.	State Avg.	U.S. Avg.
Blood Clot Prevention and Treatment				
Anticoagulation Overlap Therapy[2]	48	98%	93%	93%
ICU Venous Thromboembolism Prophylaxis[2]	77	100%	93%	92%
Incidence of Potentially Preventable VTE[1,2]	-	-	6%	10%
UFH with Dosages/Platelet Monitoring[2]	34	100%	98%	97%
Venous Thromboembolism Prophylaxis[2]	341	91%	88%	85%
Warfarin Therapy Discharge Instructions[2]	32	66%	79%	75%
Chest Pain/Possible Heart Attack Care				
Aspirin Given Within 24 Hours of Arrival	50	98%	97%	96%
Fibrinolytic Meds Within 30 Min. of Arrival[7]	-	-	44%	58%
Average Time to ECG (minutes)	53	5	6	7
Average Time to Transfer (minutes)	13	36	58	60
Children's Asthma Care				
Received Home Management Plan of Care	-	-	85%	88%
Received Reliever Medication	-	-	100%	100%
Received Systemic Corticosteroids	-	-	100%	100%
Emergency Department				
Admittance Decision Time (minutes)[2]	721	81	90	98
Head CT Results Within 45 Min. of Arrival[1]	-	-	63%	57%
Patients Who Left ER Before Being Seen	33,970	1%	2%	2%
Time from ER Arrival to Admit. (minutes)[2]	721	247	265	274
Time from ER Arrival to Discharge (minutes)	403	129	128	134
Time in ER Before Being Evaluated (minutes)	421	16	22	26
Time to Pain Meds for Fractures (minutes)	147	55	54	57
Heart Attack Care				
Aspirin Given at Discharge	24	100%	99%	99%
Fibrinolytic Meds Within 30 Min. of Arrival[7]	-	-	80%	54%
PCI Within 90 Minutes of Arrival[7]	-	-	97%	96%
Statin Prescribed at Discharge	20	100%	98%	98%
Heart Failure Care				
ACE Inhibitor or ARB for LVSD	26	100%	97%	97%
Discharge Instructions Given	125	98%	96%	94%
Evaluation of LVS Function	184	100%	100%	99%
Medicare Spending				
Medicare Spending per Patient (ratio)	-	1.06	1.01	0.98
Pneumonia Care				
Appropriate Initial Antibiotic Given	125	98%	96%	95%
Blood Culture Timing	192	99%	98%	98%
Pregnancy and Delivery Care				
Newborn Deliveries Scheduled Early[2]	24	0%	5%	6%
Preventive Care				
Immunization for Influenza[2]	548	99%	93%	90%
Immunization for Pneumonia[2]	716	99%	94%	92%
Stroke Care				
Anticoagulation Therapy for Atrial Fibrillation[1]	-	-	95%	95%
Antithrombotic Therapy Timing	69	96%	98%	98%
Assessed for Rehabilitation	77	96%	98%	97%
Discharged on Antithrombotic Therapy	73	100%	99%	99%
Discharged on Statin Medication	58	98%	95%	94%
Thrombolytic Therapy Timing[1]	-	-	65%	66%
Venous Thromboembolism Prophylaxis	78	99%	95%	94%
Written Stroke Educational Materials Given	37	97%	92%	88%
Surgical Care Improvement Project				
Appropriate Beta Blocker Usage[2]	146	99%	98%	98%
Appropriate VTP Within 24 Hours[2]	445	98%	98%	98%
Controlled Postoperative Blood Glucose[2,7]	-	-	97%	97%
Perioperative Temperature Management[2]	473	100%	100%	100%
Prophylactic Antibiotic Selection[2]	321	98%	99%	99%
Prophylactic Antibiotic Selection (Outpatient)	131	98%	98%	98%
Prophylactic Antibiotic Stopped[2]	305	97%	98%	98%
Prophylactic Antibiotic Timing[2]	321	99%	99%	99%
Prophylactic Antibiotic Timing (Outpatient)	131	92%	97%	98%
Urinary Catheter Removal[2]	259	100%	97%	97%
Survey of Patients' Hospital Experiences				
Area Around Room 'Always' Quiet at Night	300+	53%	58%	61%
Doctors 'Always' Communicated Well	300+	79%	80%	82%
Home Recovery Information Given	300+	89%	87%	85%
Hospital Given 9 or 10 on 10 Point Scale	300+	75%	72%	71%
Meds 'Always' Explained Before Given	300+	62%	64%	64%
Nurses 'Always' Communicated Well	300+	79%	81%	79%
Pain 'Always' Well Controlled	300+	71%	71%	71%
Room and Bathroom 'Always' Clean	300+	71%	75%	73%
Timely Help 'Always' Received	300+	66%	70%	68%

NOTE: Hospital profiles are in alphabetical order by state, then city, then hospital within the city; Rankings exclude hospitals with less than 25 cases except for patient surveys which excludes hospitals with less than 100 cases; (a) 100-299 cases; (1) The number of cases/patients is too few to report; (2) Data submitted were based on a sample of cases/patients; (3) Results are based on a shorter time period than required; (4) Data suppressed by CMS for one or more quarters; (5) Results are not available for this reporting period; (6) Fewer than 100 patients completed the HCAHPS survey; (7) No cases met the criteria for this measure; (8) The lower limit of the confidence interval cannot be calculated if the number of observed infections equals zero; (9) No data are available from the state/territory for this reporting period; (10) The scores shown reflect fewer than 50 completed surveys; (11) There were discrepancies in the data collection process; (12) This measure does not apply to this hospital for this reporting period; (13) Results cannot be calculated for this reporting period; (14) The results for this state are combined with nearby states to protect confidentiality; Please refer to the User's Guide for a full explanation of data.

Measure	Cases	This Hosp.	State Avg.	U.S. Avg.
Would Definitely Recommend Hospital	300+	76%	71%	71%
Use of Medical Imaging				
Cardiac Imaging Stress Test before Surgery	129	9.3%	5.4%	5.3%
Combination Abdominal CT Scan	576	2.4%	7.1%	10.5%
Combination Brain/Sinus CT Scan	424	1.7%	2.8%	2.7%
Combination Chest CT Scan	463	1.5%	1.7%	2.7%
Follow-up Mammogram/Ultrasound	754	9.8%	8.7%	8.8%
Lumbar Spine MRI for Low Back Pain	86	38.4%	34.7%	37.2%

Mercy Tiffin Hospital

45 Saint Lawrence Drive
Tiffin, OH 44883
Phone: 419-455-7000
Fax: 419-448-3181
Type: Acute Care Hospitals
Emergency Services: Yes
Ownership: Voluntary non-profit - Private
Beds: 105

Key Personnel:

Chief of Medical Staff.......... James Anthony, MD, MRO
Radiology.................. Jorge Cepeda
CEO/President.............. Adam Dittman
Operating Room............. Linda Hayman, RN
Pediatric Ambulatory Care...... Prasad Kakaiala, MD
Pediatric In-Patient Care....... Prasad Kakaiala, MD
Infection Control............. Susan Weithman
Quality Assurance............ Anne Zimmerman

Measure	Cases	This Hosp.	State Avg.	U.S. Avg.
Blood Clot Prevention and Treatment				
Anticoagulation Overlap Therapy[1,2]	-	-	93%	93%
ICU Venous Thromboembolism Prophylaxis[2]	13	100%	93%	92%
Incidence of Potentially Preventable VTE[2,7]	-	-	6%	10%
UFH with Dosages/Platelet Monitoring[1,2]	-	-	98%	97%
Venous Thromboembolism Prophylaxis[2]	111	95%	88%	85%
Warfarin Therapy Discharge Instructions[1,2]	-	-	79%	75%
Chest Pain/Possible Heart Attack Care				
Aspirin Given Within 24 Hours of Arrival	85	99%	97%	96%
Fibrinolytic Meds Within 30 Min. of Arrival[1]	-	-	44%	58%
Average Time to ECG (minutes)	91	7	6	7
Average Time to Transfer (minutes)	23	171	58	60
Children's Asthma Care				
Received Home Management Plan of Care	-	-	85%	88%
Received Reliever Medication	-	-	100%	100%
Received Systemic Corticosteroids	-	-	100%	100%
Emergency Department				
Admittance Decision Time (minutes)[2]	262	41	90	98
Head CT Results Within 45 Min. of Arrival	16	31%	63%	57%
Patients Who Left ER Before Being Seen	17,659	0%	2%	2%
Time from ER Arrival to Admit. (minutes)[2]	267	238	265	274
Time from ER Arrival to Discharge (minutes)	409	127	128	134
Time in ER Before Being Evaluated (minutes)	432	20	22	26
Time to Pain Meds for Fractures (minutes)	80	60	54	57
Heart Attack Care				
Aspirin Given at Discharge[1]	-	-	99%	99%
Fibrinolytic Meds Within 30 Min. of Arrival[7]	-	-	80%	54%
PCI Within 90 Minutes of Arrival[7]	-	-	97%	96%
Statin Prescribed at Discharge[1]	-	-	98%	98%
Heart Failure Care				
ACE Inhibitor or ARB for LVSD[1]	-	-	97%	97%
Discharge Instructions Given	43	100%	96%	94%
Evaluation of LVS Function	61	100%	100%	99%
Medicare Spending				
Medicare Spending per Patient (ratio)	-	0.87	1.01	0.98
Pneumonia Care				
Appropriate Initial Antibiotic Given	70	94%	96%	95%
Blood Culture Timing	107	96%	98%	98%
Pregnancy and Delivery Care				
Newborn Deliveries Scheduled Early[2]	30	7%	5%	6%
Preventive Care				
Immunization for Influenza[2]	258	94%	93%	90%
Immunization for Pneumonia[2]	309	94%	94%	92%
Stroke Care				
Anticoagulation Therapy for Atrial Fibrillation[1]	-	-	95%	95%
Antithrombotic Therapy Timing	16	100%	98%	98%
Assessed for Rehabilitation	18	94%	98%	97%
Discharged on Antithrombotic Therapy	18	89%	99%	99%
Discharged on Statin Medication	14	64%	95%	94%
Thrombolytic Therapy Timing[1]	-	-	65%	66%
Venous Thromboembolism Prophylaxis	16	75%	95%	94%
Written Stroke Educational Materials Given	11	100%	92%	88%
Surgical Care Improvement Project				
Appropriate Beta Blocker Usage	41	98%	98%	98%
Appropriate VTP Within 24 Hours	148	97%	98%	98%
Controlled Postoperative Blood Glucose[7]	-	-	97%	97%
Perioperative Temperature Management	164	99%	100%	100%
Prophylactic Antibiotic Selection	139	97%	99%	99%
Prophylactic Antibiotic Selection (Outpatient)	35	74%	98%	98%
Prophylactic Antibiotic Stopped	135	99%	98%	98%
Prophylactic Antibiotic Timing	139	96%	99%	99%
Prophylactic Antibiotic Timing (Outpatient)	18	94%	97%	98%
Urinary Catheter Removal	26	92%	97%	97%
Survey of Patients' Hospital Experiences				
Area Around Room 'Always' Quiet at Night	300+	62%	58%	61%
Doctors 'Always' Communicated Well	300+	80%	80%	82%
Home Recovery Information Given	300+	83%	87%	85%
Hospital Given 9 or 10 on 10 Point Scale	300+	73%	72%	71%
Meds 'Always' Explained Before Given	300+	65%	64%	64%
Nurses 'Always' Communicated Well	300+	79%	81%	79%
Pain 'Always' Well Controlled	300+	70%	71%	71%
Room and Bathroom 'Always' Clean	300+	81%	75%	73%
Timely Help 'Always' Received	300+	69%	70%	68%
Would Definitely Recommend Hospital	300+	67%	71%	71%
Use of Medical Imaging				
Cardiac Imaging Stress Test before Surgery	198	2.0%	5.4%	5.3%
Combination Abdominal CT Scan	357	32.8%	7.1%	10.5%
Combination Brain/Sinus CT Scan[1]	-	-	2.8%	2.7%
Combination Chest CT Scan	204	7.4%	1.7%	2.7%
Follow-up Mammogram/Ultrasound	541	3.9%	8.7%	8.8%
Lumbar Spine MRI for Low Back Pain[1]	-	-	34.7%	37.2%

Mercy Saint Anne Hospital

3404 Sylvania Avenue
Toledo, OH 43623
Phone: 419-407-2663
Fax: 419-251-2104
URL: www.mercyweb.org
Type: Acute Care Hospitals
Emergency Services: Yes
Ownership: Voluntary non-profit - Church
Beds: 88

Key Personnel:

Cardiology................. Frank Abbati, RN
Anesthesiology.............. Samuel Agubosim, MD
Surgery................... Mohammad Ahmed
Hemotology Center........... Adnan Alkhalili, RN
Radiology.................. Raluca Avram
Radiology.................. David R Cervantes, MD
CEO/President.............. Karen Connors
Quality Assurance............ Deb Nicotra

Measure	Cases	This Hosp.	State Avg.	U.S. Avg.
Blood Clot Prevention and Treatment				
Anticoagulation Overlap Therapy[2]	60	87%	93%	93%
ICU Venous Thromboembolism Prophylaxis[2]	111	98%	93%	92%
Incidence of Potentially Preventable VTE[1,2]	-	-	6%	10%
UFH with Dosages/Platelet Monitoring[2]	50	100%	98%	97%
Venous Thromboembolism Prophylaxis[2]	340	86%	88%	85%
Warfarin Therapy Discharge Instructions[2]	55	96%	79%	75%
Chest Pain/Possible Heart Attack Care				
Aspirin Given Within 24 Hours of Arrival	42	100%	97%	96%
Fibrinolytic Meds Within 30 Min. of Arrival[7]	-	-	44%	58%
Average Time to ECG (minutes)	44	8	6	7
Average Time to Transfer (minutes)	11	57	58	60
Children's Asthma Care				
Received Home Management Plan of Care	-	-	85%	88%
Received Reliever Medication	-	-	100%	100%
Received Systemic Corticosteroids	-	-	100%	100%
Emergency Department				
Admittance Decision Time (minutes)[2]	642	71	90	98
Head CT Results Within 45 Min. of Arrival[1]	-	-	63%	57%
Patients Who Left ER Before Being Seen	42,599	1%	2%	2%
Time from ER Arrival to Admit. (minutes)[2]	650	252	265	274
Time from ER Arrival to Discharge (minutes)	401	111	128	134
Time in ER Before Being Evaluated (minutes)	413	29	22	26
Time to Pain Meds for Fractures (minutes)	69	45	54	57
Heart Attack Care				
Aspirin Given at Discharge	23	96%	99%	99%
Fibrinolytic Meds Within 30 Min. of Arrival[7]	-	-	80%	54%
PCI Within 90 Minutes of Arrival[7]	-	-	97%	96%
Statin Prescribed at Discharge	17	94%	98%	98%
Heart Failure Care				
ACE Inhibitor or ARB for LVSD	51	90%	97%	97%
Discharge Instructions Given	137	99%	96%	94%
Evaluation of LVS Function	181	100%	100%	99%
Medicare Spending				
Medicare Spending per Patient (ratio)	-	1.04	1.01	0.98
Pneumonia Care				
Appropriate Initial Antibiotic Given	119	96%	96%	95%
Blood Culture Timing	205	99%	98%	98%
Pregnancy and Delivery Care				
Newborn Deliveries Scheduled Early[7]	-	-	5%	6%
Preventive Care				
Immunization for Influenza[2]	441	93%	93%	90%
Immunization for Pneumonia[2]	650	90%	94%	92%
Stroke Care				
Anticoagulation Therapy for Atrial Fibrillation[1]	-	-	95%	95%
Antithrombotic Therapy Timing	42	100%	98%	98%
Assessed for Rehabilitation	43	98%	98%	97%
Discharged on Antithrombotic Therapy	37	100%	99%	99%
Discharged on Statin Medication	38	92%	95%	94%
Thrombolytic Therapy Timing[7]	-	-	65%	66%
Venous Thromboembolism Prophylaxis	44	82%	95%	94%
Written Stroke Educational Materials Given	19	63%	92%	88%
Surgical Care Improvement Project				
Appropriate Beta Blocker Usage[2]	64	97%	98%	98%
Appropriate VTP Within 24 Hours[2]	242	98%	98%	98%
Controlled Postoperative Blood Glucose[2,7]	-	-	97%	97%
Perioperative Temperature Management[2]	269	100%	100%	100%
Prophylactic Antibiotic Selection[2]	160	99%	99%	99%
Prophylactic Antibiotic Selection (Outpatient)	86	99%	98%	98%
Prophylactic Antibiotic Stopped[2]	154	99%	98%	98%
Prophylactic Antibiotic Timing[2]	160	100%	99%	99%
Prophylactic Antibiotic Timing (Outpatient)	86	99%	97%	98%
Urinary Catheter Removal[2]	164	100%	97%	97%
Survey of Patients' Hospital Experiences				
Area Around Room 'Always' Quiet at Night	300+	62%	58%	61%
Doctors 'Always' Communicated Well	300+	79%	80%	82%
Home Recovery Information Given	300+	88%	87%	85%
Hospital Given 9 or 10 on 10 Point Scale	300+	77%	72%	71%
Meds 'Always' Explained Before Given	300+	62%	64%	64%
Nurses 'Always' Communicated Well	300+	82%	81%	79%
Pain 'Always' Well Controlled	300+	70%	71%	71%
Room and Bathroom 'Always' Clean	300+	76%	75%	73%
Timely Help 'Always' Received	300+	70%	70%	68%
Would Definitely Recommend Hospital	300+	79%	71%	71%
Use of Medical Imaging				
Cardiac Imaging Stress Test before Surgery	104	8.7%	5.4%	5.3%
Combination Abdominal CT Scan	641	1.9%	7.1%	10.5%
Combination Brain/Sinus CT Scan	468	1.7%	2.8%	2.7%
Combination Chest CT Scan	451	0.9%	1.7%	2.7%
Follow-up Mammogram/Ultrasound	1,334	8.5%	8.7%	8.8%
Lumbar Spine MRI for Low Back Pain	93	35.5%	34.7%	37.2%

Mercy Saint Vincent Medical Center

2213 Cherry Street
Toledo, OH 43608
Phone: 419-251-3232
Fax: 419-242-9806
URL: www.mhsnr.org
Type: Acute Care Hospitals
Emergency Services: Yes
Ownership: Voluntary non-profit - Church
Beds: 588

Key Personnel:

Chief of Medical Staff.......... Robert Nawarre, MD
CEO/President.............. Jeffrey Peterson

Measure	Cases	This Hosp.	State Avg.	U.S. Avg.
Blood Clot Prevention and Treatment				
Anticoagulation Overlap Therapy[2]	134	97%	93%	93%
ICU Venous Thromboembolism Prophylaxis[2]	86	97%	93%	92%
Incidence of Potentially Preventable VTE[2]	27	7%	6%	10%
UFH with Dosages/Platelet Monitoring[2]	85	100%	98%	97%
Venous Thromboembolism Prophylaxis[2]	314	87%	88%	85%
Warfarin Therapy Discharge Instructions[2]	102	91%	79%	75%

NOTE: Hospital profiles are in alphabetical order by state, then city, then hospital within the city; Rankings exclude hospitals with less than 25 cases except for patient surveys which excludes hospitals with less than 100 cases; (a) 100-299 cases; (1) The number of cases/patients is too few to report; (2) Data submitted were based on a sample of cases/patients; (3) Results are based on a shorter time period than required; (4) Data suppressed by CMS for one or more quarters; (5) Results are not available for this reporting period; (6) Fewer than 100 patients completed the HCAHPS survey; (7) No cases met the criteria for this measure; (8) The lower limit of the confidence interval cannot be calculated if the number of observed infections equals zero; (9) No data are available from the state/territory for this reporting period; (10) The scores shown reflect fewer than 50 completed surveys; (11) There were discrepancies in the data collection process; (12) This measure does not apply to this hospital for this reporting period; (13) Results cannot be calculated for this reporting period; (14) The results for this state are combined with nearby states to protect confidentiality; Please refer to the User's Guide for a full explanation of data.

Measure	Cases	This Hosp.	State Avg.	U.S. Avg.
Chest Pain/Possible Heart Attack Care				
Aspirin Given Within 24 Hours of Arrival[5]	-	-	97%	96%
Fibrinolytic Meds Within 30 Min. of Arrival[5]	-	-	44%	58%
Average Time to ECG (minutes)[5]	-	-	6	7
Average Time to Transfer (minutes)[5]	-	-	58	60
Children's Asthma Care				
Received Home Management Plan of Care	-	-	85%	88%
Received Reliever Medication	-	-	100%	100%
Received Systemic Corticosteroids	-	-	100%	100%
Emergency Department				
Admittance Decision Time (minutes)[2]	569	137	90	98
Head CT Results Within 45 Min. of Arrival[5]	-	-	63%	57%
Patients Who Left ER Before Being Seen	68,188	3%	2%	2%
Time from ER Arrival to Admit. (minutes)[2]	597	303	265	274
Time from ER Arrival to Discharge (minutes)	360	180	128	134
Time in ER Before Being Evaluated (minutes)	407	37	22	26
Time to Pain Meds for Fractures (minutes)	132	58	54	57
Heart Attack Care				
Aspirin Given at Discharge	624	100%	99%	99%
Fibrinolytic Meds Within 30 Min. of Arrival[7]	-	-	80%	54%
PCI Within 90 Minutes of Arrival	58	93%	97%	96%
Statin Prescribed at Discharge	625	100%	98%	98%
Heart Failure Care				
ACE Inhibitor or ARB for LVSD	244	100%	97%	97%
Discharge Instructions Given	421	100%	96%	94%
Evaluation of LVS Function	522	100%	100%	99%
Medicare Spending				
Medicare Spending per Patient (ratio)	-	1.03	1.01	0.98
Pneumonia Care				
Appropriate Initial Antibiotic Given	88	99%	96%	95%
Blood Culture Timing	186	98%	98%	98%
Pregnancy and Delivery Care				
Newborn Deliveries Scheduled Early	68	6%	5%	6%
Preventive Care				
Immunization for Influenza[2]	581	96%	93%	90%
Immunization for Pneumonia[2]	672	93%	94%	92%
Stroke Care				
Anticoagulation Therapy for Atrial Fibrillation	15	93%	95%	95%
Antithrombotic Therapy Timing	156	98%	98%	98%
Assessed for Rehabilitation	230	100%	98%	97%
Discharged on Antithrombotic Therapy	167	100%	99%	99%
Discharged on Statin Medication	137	99%	95%	94%
Thrombolytic Therapy Timing	17	76%	65%	66%
Venous Thromboembolism Prophylaxis	273	97%	95%	94%
Written Stroke Educational Materials Given	107	100%	92%	88%
Surgical Care Improvement Project				
Appropriate Beta Blocker Usage[2]	293	96%	98%	98%
Appropriate VTP Within 24 Hours[2]	260	96%	98%	98%
Controlled Postoperative Blood Glucose[2]	234	94%	97%	97%
Perioperative Temperature Management[2]	486	100%	100%	100%
Prophylactic Antibiotic Selection[2]	441	98%	99%	99%
Prophylactic Antibiotic Selection (Outpatient)	635	98%	98%	98%
Prophylactic Antibiotic Stopped[2]	431	100%	98%	98%
Prophylactic Antibiotic Timing[2]	442	99%	99%	99%
Prophylactic Antibiotic Timing (Outpatient)	652	96%	97%	98%
Urinary Catheter Removal[2]	338	97%	97%	97%
Survey of Patients' Hospital Experiences				
Area Around Room 'Always' Quiet at Night	300+	57%	58%	61%
Doctors 'Always' Communicated Well	300+	75%	80%	82%
Home Recovery Information Given	300+	87%	87%	85%
Hospital Given 9 or 10 on 10 Point Scale	300+	72%	72%	71%
Meds 'Always' Explained Before Given	300+	63%	64%	64%
Nurses 'Always' Communicated Well	300+	78%	81%	79%
Pain 'Always' Well Controlled	300+	69%	71%	71%
Room and Bathroom 'Always' Clean	300+	74%	75%	73%
Timely Help 'Always' Received	300+	67%	70%	68%
Would Definitely Recommend Hospital	300+	73%	71%	71%
Use of Medical Imaging				
Cardiac Imaging Stress Test before Surgery	388	4.1%	5.4%	5.3%
Combination Abdominal CT Scan	414	1.0%	7.1%	10.5%
Combination Brain/Sinus CT Scan	471	1.9%	2.8%	2.7%
Combination Chest CT Scan	318	0.3%	1.7%	2.7%
Follow-up Mammogram/Ultrasound	414	15.7%	8.7%	8.8%
Lumbar Spine MRI for Low Back Pain	71	36.6%	34.7%	37.2%

The Toledo Hospital

2142 North Cove Boulevard
Toledo, OH 43606
Phone: 419-291-7463
Fax: 419-469-3791
URL: www.promedica.org
Type: Acute Care Hospitals
Emergency Services: Yes
Ownership: Voluntary non-profit - Private
Beds: 794
Key Personnel:
CEO/President. . . . . Barbara Steele

Measure	Cases	This Hosp.	State Avg.	U.S. Avg.
Blood Clot Prevention and Treatment				
Anticoagulation Overlap Therapy[2]	143	82%	93%	93%
ICU Venous Thromboembolism Prophylaxis[2]	140	81%	93%	92%
Incidence of Potentially Preventable VTE[2]	46	2%	6%	10%
UFH with Dosages/Platelet Monitoring[2]	150	99%	98%	97%
Venous Thromboembolism Prophylaxis[2]	270	75%	88%	85%
Warfarin Therapy Discharge Instructions[2]	89	19%	79%	75%
Chest Pain/Possible Heart Attack Care				
Aspirin Given Within 24 Hours of Arrival[1,3]	-	-	97%	96%
Fibrinolytic Meds Within 30 Min. of Arrival[5]	-	-	44%	58%
Average Time to ECG (minutes)[1,3]	-	-	6	7
Average Time to Transfer (minutes)[5]	-	-	58	60
Children's Asthma Care				
Received Home Management Plan of Care	115	98%	85%	88%
Received Reliever Medication	116	100%	100%	100%
Received Systemic Corticosteroids	116	100%	100%	100%
Emergency Department				
Admittance Decision Time (minutes)[2]	441	88	90	98
Head CT Results Within 45 Min. of Arrival[5]	-	-	63%	57%
Patients Who Left ER Before Being Seen	91,991	2%	2%	2%
Time from ER Arrival to Admit. (minutes)[2]	456	273	265	274
Time from ER Arrival to Discharge (minutes)	383	106	128	134
Time in ER Before Being Evaluated (minutes)	336	27	22	26
Time to Pain Meds for Fractures (minutes)	217	54	54	57
Heart Attack Care				
Aspirin Given at Discharge[2]	310	100%	99%	99%
Fibrinolytic Meds Within 30 Min. of Arrival[2,7]	-	-	80%	54%
PCI Within 90 Minutes of Arrival[2]	28	96%	97%	96%
Statin Prescribed at Discharge[2]	299	99%	98%	98%
Heart Failure Care				
ACE Inhibitor or ARB for LVSD[2]	76	95%	97%	97%
Discharge Instructions Given[2]	214	81%	96%	94%
Evaluation of LVS Function[2]	289	100%	100%	99%
Medicare Spending				
Medicare Spending per Patient (ratio)	-	1.00	1.01	0.98
Pneumonia Care				
Appropriate Initial Antibiotic Given[2]	63	92%	96%	95%
Blood Culture Timing[2]	102	97%	98%	98%
Pregnancy and Delivery Care				
Newborn Deliveries Scheduled Early[2]	61	11%	5%	6%
Preventive Care				
Immunization for Influenza[2]	508	78%	93%	90%
Immunization for Pneumonia[2]	563	80%	94%	92%
Stroke Care				
Anticoagulation Therapy for Atrial Fibrillation[2]	19	89%	95%	95%
Antithrombotic Therapy Timing[2]	80	99%	98%	98%
Assessed for Rehabilitation[2]	106	97%	98%	97%
Discharged on Antithrombotic Therapy[2]	81	99%	99%	99%
Discharged on Statin Medication[2]	67	94%	95%	94%
Thrombolytic Therapy Timing[1,2]	-	-	65%	66%
Venous Thromboembolism Prophylaxis[2]	115	94%	95%	94%
Written Stroke Educational Materials Given[2]	46	78%	92%	88%
Surgical Care Improvement Project				
Appropriate Beta Blocker Usage[2]	308	97%	98%	98%
Appropriate VTP Within 24 Hours[2]	391	98%	98%	98%
Controlled Postoperative Blood Glucose[2]	157	97%	97%	97%
Perioperative Temperature Management[2]	554	100%	100%	100%
Prophylactic Antibiotic Selection[2]	513	98%	99%	99%
Prophylactic Antibiotic Selection (Outpatient)	608	97%	98%	98%
Prophylactic Antibiotic Stopped[2]	509	97%	98%	98%
Prophylactic Antibiotic Timing[2]	514	99%	99%	99%
Prophylactic Antibiotic Timing (Outpatient)	627	93%	97%	98%
Urinary Catheter Removal[2]	427	98%	97%	97%
Survey of Patients' Hospital Experiences				
Area Around Room 'Always' Quiet at Night	300+	57%	58%	61%
Doctors 'Always' Communicated Well	300+	78%	80%	82%
Home Recovery Information Given	300+	89%	87%	85%
Hospital Given 9 or 10 on 10 Point Scale	300+	70%	72%	71%
Meds 'Always' Explained Before Given	300+	60%	64%	64%
Nurses 'Always' Communicated Well	300+	77%	81%	79%
Pain 'Always' Well Controlled	300+	69%	71%	71%
Room and Bathroom 'Always' Clean	300+	67%	75%	73%
Timely Help 'Always' Received	300+	63%	70%	68%
Would Definitely Recommend Hospital	300+	73%	71%	71%
Use of Medical Imaging				
Cardiac Imaging Stress Test before Surgery	1,276	4.5%	5.4%	5.3%
Combination Abdominal CT Scan	832	3.5%	7.1%	10.5%
Combination Brain/Sinus CT Scan	690	1.6%	2.8%	2.7%
Combination Chest CT Scan	459	1.7%	1.7%	2.7%
Follow-up Mammogram/Ultrasound	2,265	8.5%	8.7%	8.8%
Lumbar Spine MRI for Low Back Pain	123	33.3%	34.7%	37.2%

University of Toledo Medical Center

3000 Arlington Avenue
Toledo, OH 43699
Phone: 419-383-3407
Fax: 419-383-2800
E-mail: utmc.webmaster@utoledo.edu
URL: www.utmc.utoledo.edu
Type: Acute Care Hospitals
Emergency Services: Yes
Ownership: Government - State
Beds: 319
Key Personnel:
Operating Room. . . . . Connie Ashbaugh, RN
CEO/President. . . . . Lloyd Jacobs
Chief of Medical Staff . . . . Daniel Morrissett, MD
Emergency Room . . . . Diane Ness
Pediatric Ambulatory Care . . . . . . Mark Puczynski, MD
Pediatric In-Patient Care . . . . Mark Puczynski, MD
Quality Assurance . . . . Mary Shapiro
Radiology. . . . . Lee S Woldenberg, MD

Measure	Cases	This Hosp.	State Avg.	U.S. Avg.
Blood Clot Prevention and Treatment				
Anticoagulation Overlap Therapy[2]	81	95%	93%	93%
ICU Venous Thromboembolism Prophylaxis[2]	82	99%	93%	92%
Incidence of Potentially Preventable VTE[2]	38	5%	6%	10%
UFH with Dosages/Platelet Monitoring[2]	94	100%	98%	97%
Venous Thromboembolism Prophylaxis[2]	322	89%	88%	85%
Warfarin Therapy Discharge Instructions[2]	46	91%	79%	75%
Chest Pain/Possible Heart Attack Care				
Aspirin Given Within 24 Hours of Arrival[5]	-	-	97%	96%
Fibrinolytic Meds Within 30 Min. of Arrival[5]	-	-	44%	58%
Average Time to ECG (minutes)[5]	-	-	6	7
Average Time to Transfer (minutes)[5]	-	-	58	60
Children's Asthma Care				
Received Home Management Plan of Care	-	-	85%	88%
Received Reliever Medication	-	-	100%	100%
Received Systemic Corticosteroids	-	-	100%	100%
Emergency Department				
Admittance Decision Time (minutes)[2]	614	93	90	98
Head CT Results Within 45 Min. of Arrival[5]	-	-	63%	57%
Patients Who Left ER Before Being Seen	27,073	2%	2%	2%
Time from ER Arrival to Admit. (minutes)[2]	619	327	265	274
Time from ER Arrival to Discharge (minutes)	433	126	128	134
Time in ER Before Being Evaluated (minutes)	443	47	22	26
Time to Pain Meds for Fractures (minutes)	20	70	54	57
Heart Attack Care				
Aspirin Given at Discharge[2]	209	99%	99%	99%
Fibrinolytic Meds Within 30 Min. of Arrival[2,7]	-	-	80%	54%
PCI Within 90 Minutes of Arrival[2]	23	100%	97%	96%
Statin Prescribed at Discharge[2]	201	100%	98%	98%
Heart Failure Care				
ACE Inhibitor or ARB for LVSD[2]	81	96%	97%	97%
Discharge Instructions Given[2]	224	93%	96%	94%
Evaluation of LVS Function[2]	281	100%	100%	99%
Medicare Spending				
Medicare Spending per Patient (ratio)	-	1.04	1.01	0.98
Pneumonia Care				

NOTE: Hospital profiles are in alphabetical order by state, then city, then hospital within the city; Rankings exclude hospitals with less than 25 cases except for patient surveys which excludes hospitals with less than 100 cases; (a) 100-299 cases; (1) The number of cases/patients is too few to report; (2) Data submitted were based on a sample of cases/patients; (3) Results are based on a shorter time period than required; (4) Data suppressed by CMS for one or more quarters; (5) Results are not available for this reporting period; (6) Fewer than 100 patients completed the HCAHPS survey; (7) No cases met the criteria for this measure; (8) The lower limit of the confidence interval cannot be calculated if the number of observed infections equals zero; (9) No data are available from the state/territory for this reporting period; (10) The scores shown reflect fewer than 50 completed surveys; (11) There were discrepancies in the data collection process; (12) This measure does not apply to this hospital for this reporting period; (13) Results cannot be calculated for this reporting period; (14) The results for this state are combined with nearby states to protect confidentiality; Please refer to the User's Guide for a full explanation of data.

Measure	Cases	This Hosp.	State Avg.	U.S. Avg.
Appropriate Initial Antibiotic Given[2]	38	82%	96%	95%
Blood Culture Timing[2]	100	94%	98%	98%
Pregnancy and Delivery Care				
Newborn Deliveries Scheduled Early[7]	-	-	5%	6%
Preventive Care				
Immunization for Influenza[2]	597	77%	93%	90%
Immunization for Pneumonia[2]	723	75%	94%	92%
Stroke Care				
Anticoagulation Therapy for Atrial Fibrillation[2]	13	92%	95%	95%
Antithrombotic Therapy Timing[2]	77	94%	98%	98%
Assessed for Rehabilitation[2]	101	98%	98%	97%
Discharged on Antithrombotic Therapy[2]	91	99%	99%	99%
Discharged on Statin Medication[2]	70	94%	95%	94%
Thrombolytic Therapy Timing[2]	17	12%	65%	66%
Venous Thromboembolism Prophylaxis[2]	113	91%	95%	94%
Written Stroke Educational Materials Given[2]	51	86%	92%	88%
Surgical Care Improvement Project				
Appropriate Beta Blocker Usage[2]	220	99%	98%	98%
Appropriate VTP Within 24 Hours[2]	273	97%	98%	98%
Controlled Postoperative Blood Glucose[2]	86	98%	97%	97%
Perioperative Temperature Management[2]	370	100%	100%	100%
Prophylactic Antibiotic Selection[2]	310	97%	99%	99%
Prophylactic Antibiotic Selection (Outpatient)	253	95%	98%	98%
Prophylactic Antibiotic Stopped[2]	287	99%	98%	98%
Prophylactic Antibiotic Timing[2]	312	99%	99%	99%
Prophylactic Antibiotic Timing (Outpatient)	237	98%	97%	98%
Urinary Catheter Removal[2]	281	96%	97%	97%
Survey of Patients' Hospital Experiences				
Area Around Room 'Always' Quiet at Night	300+	53%	58%	61%
Doctors 'Always' Communicated Well	300+	71%	80%	82%
Home Recovery Information Given	300+	81%	87%	85%
Hospital Given 9 or 10 on 10 Point Scale	300+	58%	72%	71%
Meds 'Always' Explained Before Given	300+	58%	64%	64%
Nurses 'Always' Communicated Well	300+	76%	81%	79%
Pain 'Always' Well Controlled	300+	66%	71%	71%
Room and Bathroom 'Always' Clean	300+	65%	75%	73%
Timely Help 'Always' Received	300+	54%	70%	68%
Would Definitely Recommend Hospital	300+	59%	71%	71%
Use of Medical Imaging				
Cardiac Imaging Stress Test before Surgery	233	5.6%	5.4%	5.3%
Combination Abdominal CT Scan	538	11.9%	7.1%	10.5%
Combination Brain/Sinus CT Scan	521	1.5%	2.8%	2.7%
Combination Chest CT Scan	302	0.0%	1.7%	2.7%
Follow-up Mammogram/Ultrasound	477	14.3%	8.7%	8.8%
Lumbar Spine MRI for Low Back Pain	164	39.6%	34.7%	37.2%

Upper Valley Medical Center

3130 North County Road 25a
Troy, OH 45373
Phone: 937-440-7853
Fax: 937-440-7739
E-mail: bwilson@uvmc.com
URL: www.uvmc.com
Type: Acute Care Hospitals
Emergency Services: Yes
Ownership: Voluntary non-profit - Private
Beds: 128

Key Personnel:

Chief of Medical Staff. . . . . Sayed Ali
Radiology. . . . . Diane Anderson
CEO/President. . . . . David J Meckstroth
Emergency Room . . . . Dee Mullen
Quality Assurance . . . . Tony White

Measure	Cases	This Hosp.	State Avg.	U.S. Avg.
Blood Clot Prevention and Treatment				
Anticoagulation Overlap Therapy[2]	70	91%	93%	93%
ICU Venous Thromboembolism Prophylaxis[2]	70	100%	93%	92%
Incidence of Potentially Preventable VTE[1,2]	-	-	6%	10%
UFH with Dosages/Platelet Monitoring[2]	27	100%	98%	97%
Venous Thromboembolism Prophylaxis[2]	360	94%	88%	85%
Warfarin Therapy Discharge Instructions[2]	60	100%	79%	75%
Chest Pain/Possible Heart Attack Care				
Aspirin Given Within 24 Hours of Arrival	74	100%	97%	96%
Fibrinolytic Meds Within 30 Min. of Arrival[7]	-	-	44%	58%
Average Time to ECG (minutes)	76	4	6	7
Average Time to Transfer (minutes)	38	64	58	60
Children's Asthma Care				
Received Home Management Plan of Care	-	-	85%	88%
Received Reliever Medication	-	-	100%	100%
Received Systemic Corticosteroids	-	-	100%	100%
Emergency Department				
Admittance Decision Time (minutes)[2]	781	133	90	98
Head CT Results Within 45 Min. of Arrival	22	73%	63%	57%
Patients Who Left ER Before Being Seen	44,042	3%	2%	2%
Time from ER Arrival to Admit. (minutes)[2]	787	263	265	274
Time from ER Arrival to Discharge (minutes)	409	176	128	134
Time in ER Before Being Evaluated (minutes)	442	36	22	26
Time to Pain Meds for Fractures (minutes)	118	65	54	57
Heart Attack Care				
Aspirin Given at Discharge	58	97%	99%	99%
Fibrinolytic Meds Within 30 Min. of Arrival[7]	-	-	80%	54%
PCI Within 90 Minutes of Arrival[7]	-	-	97%	96%
Statin Prescribed at Discharge	49	98%	98%	98%
Heart Failure Care				
ACE Inhibitor or ARB for LVSD	78	100%	97%	97%
Discharge Instructions Given	178	97%	96%	94%
Evaluation of LVS Function	229	100%	100%	99%
Medicare Spending				
Medicare Spending per Patient (ratio)	-	1.03	1.01	0.98
Pneumonia Care				
Appropriate Initial Antibiotic Given[2]	106	99%	96%	95%
Blood Culture Timing[2]	180	99%	98%	98%
Pregnancy and Delivery Care				
Newborn Deliveries Scheduled Early	52	2%	5%	6%
Preventive Care				
Immunization for Influenza[2]	574	100%	93%	90%
Immunization for Pneumonia[2]	762	99%	94%	92%
Stroke Care				
Anticoagulation Therapy for Atrial Fibrillation[1]	-	-	95%	95%
Antithrombotic Therapy Timing	73	100%	98%	98%
Assessed for Rehabilitation	70	99%	98%	97%
Discharged on Antithrombotic Therapy	68	99%	99%	99%
Discharged on Statin Medication	54	100%	95%	94%
Thrombolytic Therapy Timing[7]	-	-	65%	66%
Venous Thromboembolism Prophylaxis	70	97%	95%	94%
Written Stroke Educational Materials Given	33	94%	92%	88%
Surgical Care Improvement Project				
Appropriate Beta Blocker Usage	63	100%	98%	98%
Appropriate VTP Within 24 Hours	263	98%	98%	98%
Controlled Postoperative Blood Glucose[7]	-	-	97%	97%
Perioperative Temperature Management	291	100%	100%	100%
Prophylactic Antibiotic Selection	166	100%	99%	99%
Prophylactic Antibiotic Selection (Outpatient)	118	98%	98%	98%
Prophylactic Antibiotic Stopped	159	99%	98%	98%
Prophylactic Antibiotic Timing	166	99%	99%	99%
Prophylactic Antibiotic Timing (Outpatient)	118	99%	97%	98%
Urinary Catheter Removal	86	95%	97%	97%
Survey of Patients' Hospital Experiences				
Area Around Room 'Always' Quiet at Night[11]	300+	54%	58%	61%
Doctors 'Always' Communicated Well[11]	300+	80%	80%	82%
Home Recovery Information Given[11]	300+	92%	87%	85%
Hospital Given 9 or 10 on 10 Point Scale[11]	300+	70%	72%	71%
Meds 'Always' Explained Before Given[11]	300+	67%	64%	64%
Nurses 'Always' Communicated Well[11]	300+	81%	81%	79%
Pain 'Always' Well Controlled[11]	300+	73%	71%	71%
Room and Bathroom 'Always' Clean[11]	300+	74%	75%	73%
Timely Help 'Always' Received[11]	300+	73%	70%	68%
Would Definitely Recommend Hospital[11]	300+	64%	71%	71%
Use of Medical Imaging				
Cardiac Imaging Stress Test before Surgery	421	3.3%	5.4%	5.3%
Combination Abdominal CT Scan	770	7.9%	7.1%	10.5%
Combination Brain/Sinus CT Scan	789	2.0%	2.8%	2.7%
Combination Chest CT Scan	611	3.9%	1.7%	2.7%
Follow-up Mammogram/Ultrasound	1,605	7.0%	8.7%	8.8%
Lumbar Spine MRI for Low Back Pain	68	17.6%	34.7%	37.2%

Wyandot Memorial Hospital

885 North Sandusky Avenue
Upper Sandusky, OH 43351
Phone: 419-294-4991
Fax: 419-294-2233
URL: www.wyandotmemorial.com
Type: Critical Access Hospitals
Emergency Services: Yes
Ownership: Govt - Hospital Dist/Auth
Beds: 45

Key Personnel:

CEO . . . . Joseph A D'Ettorre
Cardiac Laboratory. . . . . Russ Merrin
Coronary Care . . . . Russ Merrin, BS, CMT
Operating Room. . . . . LuAnn Montz, RN
Infection Control. . . . . Valerie Schalk, RN
Chief of Medical Staff. . . . . Mary Anne Schwenning, MD
Quality Assurance . . . . Vicki Underwood

Measure	Cases	This Hosp.	State Avg.	U.S. Avg.
Blood Clot Prevention and Treatment				
Anticoagulation Overlap Therapy[5]	-	-	93%	93%
ICU Venous Thromboembolism Prophylaxis[5]	-	-	93%	92%
Incidence of Potentially Preventable VTE[5]	-	-	6%	10%
UFH with Dosages/Platelet Monitoring[5]	-	-	98%	97%
Venous Thromboembolism Prophylaxis[5]	-	-	88%	85%
Warfarin Therapy Discharge Instructions[5]	-	-	79%	75%
Chest Pain/Possible Heart Attack Care				
Aspirin Given Within 24 Hours of Arrival	-	-	97%	96%
Fibrinolytic Meds Within 30 Min. of Arrival	-	-	44%	58%
Average Time to ECG (minutes)	-	-	6	7
Average Time to Transfer (minutes)	-	-	58	60
Children's Asthma Care				
Received Home Management Plan of Care	-	-	85%	88%
Received Reliever Medication	-	-	100%	100%
Received Systemic Corticosteroids	-	-	100%	100%
Emergency Department				
Admittance Decision Time (minutes)[5]	-	-	90	98
Head CT Results Within 45 Min. of Arrival	-	-	63%	57%
Patients Who Left ER Before Being Seen	-	-	2%	2%
Time from ER Arrival to Admit. (minutes)[5]	-	-	265	274
Time from ER Arrival to Discharge (minutes)	-	-	128	134
Time in ER Before Being Evaluated (minutes)	-	-	22	26
Time to Pain Meds for Fractures (minutes)	-	-	54	57
Heart Attack Care				
Aspirin Given at Discharge[1]	-	-	99%	99%
Fibrinolytic Meds Within 30 Min. of Arrival[7]	-	-	80%	54%
PCI Within 90 Minutes of Arrival[7]	-	-	97%	96%
Statin Prescribed at Discharge[1]	-	-	98%	98%
Heart Failure Care				
ACE Inhibitor or ARB for LVSD[1]	-	-	97%	97%
Discharge Instructions Given[1]	-	-	96%	94%
Evaluation of LVS Function	18	78%	100%	99%
Medicare Spending				
Medicare Spending per Patient (ratio)	-	-	1.01	0.98
Pneumonia Care				
Appropriate Initial Antibiotic Given	28	82%	96%	95%
Blood Culture Timing	26	92%	98%	98%
Pregnancy and Delivery Care				
Newborn Deliveries Scheduled Early[5]	-	-	5%	6%
Preventive Care				
Immunization for Influenza[5]	-	-	93%	90%
Immunization for Pneumonia[5]	-	-	94%	92%
Stroke Care				
Anticoagulation Therapy for Atrial Fibrillation[2,7]	-	-	95%	95%
Antithrombotic Therapy Timing[1,2]	-	-	98%	98%
Assessed for Rehabilitation[1,2]	-	-	98%	97%
Discharged on Antithrombotic Therapy[1,2]	-	-	99%	99%
Discharged on Statin Medication[1,2]	-	-	95%	94%
Thrombolytic Therapy Timing[1,2]	-	-	65%	66%
Venous Thromboembolism Prophylaxis[1,2]	-	-	95%	94%
Written Stroke Educational Materials Given[1,2]	-	-	92%	88%
Surgical Care Improvement Project				
Appropriate Beta Blocker Usage	15	73%	98%	98%
Appropriate VTP Within 24 Hours	33	97%	98%	98%
Controlled Postoperative Blood Glucose[7]	-	-	97%	97%
Perioperative Temperature Management	46	100%	100%	100%
Prophylactic Antibiotic Selection	41	95%	99%	99%
Prophylactic Antibiotic Selection (Outpatient)	-	-	98%	98%

NOTE: Hospital profiles are in alphabetical order by state, then city, then hospital within the city; Rankings exclude hospitals with less than 25 cases except for patient surveys which excludes hospitals with less than 100 cases; (a) 100-299 cases; (1) The number of cases/patients is too few to report; (2) Data submitted were based on a sample of cases/patients; (3) Results are based on a shorter time period than required; (4) Data suppressed by CMS for one or more quarters; (5) Results are not available for this reporting period; (6) Fewer than 100 patients completed the HCAHPS survey; (7) No cases met the criteria for this measure; (8) The lower limit of the confidence interval cannot be calculated if the number of observed infections equals zero; (9) No data are available from the state/territory for this reporting period; (10) The scores shown reflect fewer than 50 completed surveys; (11) There were discrepancies in the data collection process; (12) This measure does not apply to this hospital for this reporting period; (13) Results cannot be calculated for this reporting period; (14) The results for this state are combined with nearby states to protect confidentiality; Please refer to the User's Guide for a full explanation of data.

Measure	Cases	This Hosp.	State Avg.	U.S. Avg.
Prophylactic Antibiotic Stopped	41	78%	98%	98%
Prophylactic Antibiotic Timing	41	78%	99%	99%
Prophylactic Antibiotic Timing (Outpatient)	-	-	97%	98%
Urinary Catheter Removal	30	80%	97%	97%
Survey of Patients' Hospital Experiences				
Area Around Room 'Always' Quiet at Night	(a)	55%	58%	61%
Doctors 'Always' Communicated Well	(a)	71%	80%	82%
Home Recovery Information Given	(a)	84%	87%	85%
Hospital Given 9 or 10 on 10 Point Scale	(a)	69%	72%	71%
Meds 'Always' Explained Before Given	(a)	60%	64%	64%
Nurses 'Always' Communicated Well	(a)	74%	81%	79%
Pain 'Always' Well Controlled	(a)	70%	71%	71%
Room and Bathroom 'Always' Clean	(a)	78%	75%	73%
Timely Help 'Always' Received	(a)	70%	70%	68%
Would Definitely Recommend Hospital	(a)	68%	71%	71%
Use of Medical Imaging				
Cardiac Imaging Stress Test before Surgery	-	-	5.4%	5.3%
Combination Abdominal CT Scan	-	-	7.1%	10.5%
Combination Brain/Sinus CT Scan	-	-	2.8%	2.7%
Combination Chest CT Scan	-	-	1.7%	2.7%
Follow-up Mammogram/Ultrasound	-	-	8.7%	8.8%
Lumbar Spine MRI for Low Back Pain	-	-	34.7%	37.2%

Mercy Memorial Hospital

904 Scioto Street
Urbana, OH 43078
Phone: 937-653-5231
Fax: 513-390-5554
Type: Critical Access Hospitals
Emergency Services: Yes
Ownership: Voluntary non-profit - Private
Beds: 73
Key Personnel:
President .... Paul Hiltz

Measure	Cases	This Hosp.	State Avg.	U.S. Avg.
Blood Clot Prevention and Treatment				
Anticoagulation Overlap Therapy[2]	11	100%	93%	93%
ICU Venous Thromboembolism Prophylaxis[2]	18	94%	93%	92%
Incidence of Potentially Preventable VTE[1,2]	-	-	6%	10%
UFH with Dosages/Platelet Monitoring[1,2]	-	-	98%	97%
Venous Thromboembolism Prophylaxis[2]	87	97%	88%	85%
Warfarin Therapy Discharge Instructions[2]	11	91%	79%	75%
Chest Pain/Possible Heart Attack Care				
Aspirin Given Within 24 Hours of Arrival[5]	-	-	97%	96%
Fibrinolytic Meds Within 30 Min. of Arrival[5]	-	-	44%	58%
Average Time to ECG (minutes)[5]	-	-	6	7
Average Time to Transfer (minutes)[5]	-	-	58	60
Children's Asthma Care				
Received Home Management Plan of Care	-	-	85%	88%
Received Reliever Medication	-	-	100%	100%
Received Systemic Corticosteroids	-	-	100%	100%
Emergency Department				
Admittance Decision Time (minutes)[2]	622	55	90	98
Head CT Results Within 45 Min. of Arrival[5]	-	-	63%	57%
Patients Who Left ER Before Being Seen	17,443	2%	2%	2%
Time from ER Arrival to Admit. (minutes)[2]	623	221	265	274
Time from ER Arrival to Discharge (minutes)[5]	-	-	128	134
Time in ER Before Being Evaluated (minutes)[5]	-	-	22	26
Time to Pain Meds for Fractures (minutes)[5]	-	-	54	57
Heart Attack Care				
Aspirin Given at Discharge[1]	-	-	99%	99%
Fibrinolytic Meds Within 30 Min. of Arrival[7]	-	-	80%	54%
PCI Within 90 Minutes of Arrival[7]	-	-	97%	96%
Statin Prescribed at Discharge[1]	-	-	98%	98%
Heart Failure Care				
ACE Inhibitor or ARB for LVSD	18	100%	97%	97%
Discharge Instructions Given	35	100%	96%	94%
Evaluation of LVS Function	46	100%	100%	99%
Medicare Spending				
Medicare Spending per Patient (ratio)	-	-	1.01	0.98
Pneumonia Care				
Appropriate Initial Antibiotic Given	28	100%	96%	95%
Blood Culture Timing	55	93%	98%	98%
Pregnancy and Delivery Care				
Newborn Deliveries Scheduled Early[7]	-	-	5%	6%
Preventive Care				
Immunization for Influenza[2]	324	94%	93%	90%
Immunization for Pneumonia[2]	493	94%	94%	92%
Stroke Care				
Anticoagulation Therapy for Atrial Fibrillation[7]	-	-	95%	95%
Antithrombotic Therapy Timing[1]	-	-	98%	98%
Assessed for Rehabilitation[1]	-	-	98%	97%
Discharged on Antithrombotic Therapy[1]	-	-	99%	99%
Discharged on Statin Medication[1]	-	-	95%	94%
Thrombolytic Therapy Timing[1]	-	-	65%	66%
Venous Thromboembolism Prophylaxis[1]	-	-	95%	94%
Written Stroke Educational Materials Given[1]	-	-	92%	88%
Surgical Care Improvement Project				
Appropriate Beta Blocker Usage	15	100%	98%	98%
Appropriate VTP Within 24 Hours	50	98%	98%	98%
Controlled Postoperative Blood Glucose[7]	-	-	97%	97%
Perioperative Temperature Management	51	100%	100%	100%
Prophylactic Antibiotic Selection	47	100%	99%	99%
Prophylactic Antibiotic Selection (Outpatient)[5]	-	-	98%	98%
Prophylactic Antibiotic Stopped	45	100%	98%	98%
Prophylactic Antibiotic Timing	47	98%	99%	99%
Prophylactic Antibiotic Timing (Outpatient)[5]	-	-	97%	98%
Urinary Catheter Removal	47	100%	97%	97%
Survey of Patients' Hospital Experiences				
Area Around Room 'Always' Quiet at Night	(a)	46%	58%	61%
Doctors 'Always' Communicated Well	(a)	76%	80%	82%
Home Recovery Information Given	(a)	86%	87%	85%
Hospital Given 9 or 10 on 10 Point Scale	(a)	68%	72%	71%
Meds 'Always' Explained Before Given	(a)	62%	64%	64%
Nurses 'Always' Communicated Well	(a)	81%	81%	79%
Pain 'Always' Well Controlled	(a)	68%	71%	71%
Room and Bathroom 'Always' Clean	(a)	80%	75%	73%
Timely Help 'Always' Received	(a)	74%	70%	68%
Would Definitely Recommend Hospital	(a)	64%	71%	71%
Use of Medical Imaging				
Cardiac Imaging Stress Test before Surgery	96	4.2%	5.4%	5.3%
Combination Abdominal CT Scan	318	3.5%	7.1%	10.5%
Combination Brain/Sinus CT Scan[1]	-	-	2.8%	2.7%
Combination Chest CT Scan	168	3.6%	1.7%	2.7%
Follow-up Mammogram/Ultrasound	287	4.5%	8.7%	8.8%
Lumbar Spine MRI for Low Back Pain[1]	-	-	34.7%	37.2%

Van Wert County Hospital

1250 S Washington Street
Van Wert, OH 45891
Phone: 419-238-8627
Fax: 419-238-2409
URL: www.vanwerthospital.org
Type: Acute Care Hospitals
Emergency Services: Yes
Ownership: Voluntary non-profit - Private
Beds: 100
Key Personnel:
Radiology.............................. Ashni Behal
Emergency Room .... Kathy Fischer
Infection Control.............. Linner Kelly
Chair/CEO.................. Barb Kohnen
CEO/President.............. Mark Minick
Operating Room.............. Brenda Wobler

Measure	Cases	This Hosp.	State Avg.	U.S. Avg.
Blood Clot Prevention and Treatment				
Anticoagulation Overlap Therapy[2]	12	58%	93%	93%
ICU Venous Thromboembolism Prophylaxis[2]	17	100%	93%	92%
Incidence of Potentially Preventable VTE[1,2]	-	-	6%	10%
UFH with Dosages/Platelet Monitoring[1,2]	-	-	98%	97%
Venous Thromboembolism Prophylaxis[2]	85	91%	88%	85%
Warfarin Therapy Discharge Instructions[2]	12	83%	79%	75%
Chest Pain/Possible Heart Attack Care				
Aspirin Given Within 24 Hours of Arrival	77	100%	97%	96%
Fibrinolytic Meds Within 30 Min. of Arrival[1]	-	-	44%	58%
Average Time to ECG (minutes)	80	9	6	7
Average Time to Transfer (minutes)[1]	-	-	58	60
Children's Asthma Care				
Received Home Management Plan of Care	-	-	85%	88%
Received Reliever Medication	-	-	100%	100%
Received Systemic Corticosteroids	-	-	100%	100%
Emergency Department				
Admittance Decision Time (minutes)[2]	258	78	90	98
Head CT Results Within 45 Min. of Arrival	14	43%	63%	57%
Patients Who Left ER Before Being Seen	16,847	0%	2%	2%
Time from ER Arrival to Admit. (minutes)[2]	386	203	265	274
Time from ER Arrival to Discharge (minutes)	365	91	128	134
Time in ER Before Being Evaluated (minutes)	326	18	22	26
Time to Pain Meds for Fractures (minutes)	82	51	54	57
Heart Attack Care				
Aspirin Given at Discharge[1]	-	-	99%	99%
Fibrinolytic Meds Within 30 Min. of Arrival[7]	-	-	80%	54%
PCI Within 90 Minutes of Arrival[7]	-	-	97%	96%
Statin Prescribed at Discharge[1]	-	-	98%	98%
Heart Failure Care				
ACE Inhibitor or ARB for LVSD[1]	-	-	97%	97%
Discharge Instructions Given	14	79%	96%	94%
Evaluation of LVS Function	18	94%	100%	99%
Medicare Spending				
Medicare Spending per Patient (ratio)	-	0.96	1.01	0.98
Pneumonia Care				
Appropriate Initial Antibiotic Given	53	98%	96%	95%
Blood Culture Timing	29	93%	98%	98%
Pregnancy and Delivery Care				
Newborn Deliveries Scheduled Early[1]	-	-	5%	6%
Preventive Care				
Immunization for Influenza[2]	264	79%	93%	90%
Immunization for Pneumonia[2]	373	89%	94%	92%
Stroke Care				
Anticoagulation Therapy for Atrial Fibrillation[1]	-	-	95%	95%
Antithrombotic Therapy Timing[1]	-	-	98%	98%
Assessed for Rehabilitation[1]	-	-	98%	97%
Discharged on Antithrombotic Therapy[1]	-	-	99%	99%
Discharged on Statin Medication[1]	-	-	95%	94%
Thrombolytic Therapy Timing[1]	-	-	65%	66%
Venous Thromboembolism Prophylaxis[1]	-	-	95%	94%
Written Stroke Educational Materials Given[1]	-	-	92%	88%
Surgical Care Improvement Project				
Appropriate Beta Blocker Usage	47	87%	98%	98%
Appropriate VTP Within 24 Hours	80	82%	98%	98%
Controlled Postoperative Blood Glucose[7]	-	-	97%	97%
Perioperative Temperature Management	130	98%	100%	100%
Prophylactic Antibiotic Selection	42	98%	99%	99%
Prophylactic Antibiotic Selection (Outpatient)	16	100%	98%	98%
Prophylactic Antibiotic Stopped	39	95%	98%	98%
Prophylactic Antibiotic Timing	42	93%	99%	99%
Prophylactic Antibiotic Timing (Outpatient)	16	100%	97%	98%
Urinary Catheter Removal	55	98%	97%	97%
Survey of Patients' Hospital Experiences				
Area Around Room 'Always' Quiet at Night	300+	58%	58%	61%
Doctors 'Always' Communicated Well	300+	80%	80%	82%
Home Recovery Information Given	300+	86%	87%	85%
Hospital Given 9 or 10 on 10 Point Scale	300+	70%	72%	71%
Meds 'Always' Explained Before Given	300+	58%	64%	64%
Nurses 'Always' Communicated Well	300+	80%	81%	79%
Pain 'Always' Well Controlled	300+	69%	71%	71%
Room and Bathroom 'Always' Clean	300+	76%	75%	73%
Timely Help 'Always' Received	300+	74%	70%	68%
Would Definitely Recommend Hospital	300+	63%	71%	71%
Use of Medical Imaging				
Cardiac Imaging Stress Test before Surgery	287	5.2%	5.4%	5.3%
Combination Abdominal CT Scan	314	13.1%	7.1%	10.5%
Combination Brain/Sinus CT Scan[1]	-	-	2.8%	2.7%
Combination Chest CT Scan	156	7.1%	1.7%	2.7%
Follow-up Mammogram/Ultrasound	340	5.3%	8.7%	8.8%
Lumbar Spine MRI for Low Back Pain[1]	-	-	34.7%	37.2%

Summa Wadsworth - Rittman Hospital

195 Wadsworth Road
Wadsworth, OH 44281
Phone: 330-331-1000
Fax: 330-336-0107
E-mail: prwrh@bright.net
URL: www.wrhospital.com
Type: Acute Care Hospitals
Emergency Services: Yes
Ownership: Voluntary non-profit - Private
Beds: 113
Key Personnel:
Emergency Room .... Jay Carter
Radiology.................. Norman Crocker
Chief of Medical Staff.......... Jeffrey S Morris
CEO/President.............. James Pope

NOTE: Hospital profiles are in alphabetical order by state, then city, then hospital within the city; Rankings exclude hospitals with less than 25 cases except for patient surveys which excludes hospitals with less than 100 cases; (a) 100-299 cases; (1) The number of cases/patients is too few to report; (2) Data submitted were based on a sample of cases/patients; (3) Results are based on a shorter time period than required; (4) Data suppressed by CMS for one or more quarters; (5) Results are not available for this reporting period; (6) Fewer than 100 patients completed the HCAHPS survey; (7) No cases met the criteria for this measure; (8) The lower limit of the confidence interval cannot be calculated if the number of observed infections equals zero; (9) No data are available from the state/territory for this reporting period; (10) The scores shown reflect fewer than 50 completed surveys; (11) There were discrepancies in the data collection process; (12) This measure does not apply to this hospital for this reporting period; (13) Results cannot be calculated for this reporting period; (14) The results for this state are combined with nearby states to protect confidentiality; Please refer to the User's Guide for a full explanation of data.

Measure	Cases	This Hosp.	State Avg.	U.S. Avg.
Blood Clot Prevention and Treatment				
Anticoagulation Overlap Therapy[2]	15	73%	93%	93%
ICU Venous Thromboembolism Prophylaxis[2]	69	84%	93%	92%
Incidence of Potentially Preventable VTE[1,2]	-	-	6%	10%
UFH with Dosages/Platelet Monitoring[1,2]	-	-	98%	97%
Venous Thromboembolism Prophylaxis[2]	227	78%	88%	85%
Warfarin Therapy Discharge Instructions[1,2]	-	-	79%	75%
Chest Pain/Possible Heart Attack Care				
Aspirin Given Within 24 Hours of Arrival	68	100%	97%	96%
Fibrinolytic Meds Within 30 Min. of Arrival[7]	-	-	44%	58%
Average Time to ECG (minutes)	71	5	6	7
Average Time to Transfer (minutes)[1]	-	-	58	60
Children's Asthma Care				
Received Home Management Plan of Care	-	-	85%	88%
Received Reliever Medication	-	-	100%	100%
Received Systemic Corticosteroids	-	-	100%	100%
Emergency Department				
Admittance Decision Time (minutes)[2]	155	104	90	98
Head CT Results Within 45 Min. of Arrival[1]	-	-	63%	57%
Patients Who Left ER Before Being Seen	18,661	1%	2%	2%
Time from ER Arrival to Admit. (minutes)[2]	442	262	265	274
Time from ER Arrival to Discharge (minutes)	354	116	128	134
Time in ER Before Being Evaluated (minutes)	336	16	22	26
Time to Pain Meds for Fractures (minutes)	77	46	54	57
Heart Attack Care				
Aspirin Given at Discharge[1]	-	-	99%	99%
Fibrinolytic Meds Within 30 Min. of Arrival[7]	-	-	80%	54%
PCI Within 90 Minutes of Arrival[7]	-	-	97%	96%
Statin Prescribed at Discharge[1]	-	-	98%	98%
Heart Failure Care				
ACE Inhibitor or ARB for LVSD	20	100%	97%	97%
Discharge Instructions Given	66	100%	96%	94%
Evaluation of LVS Function	89	100%	100%	99%
Medicare Spending				
Medicare Spending per Patient (ratio)	-	1.06	1.01	0.98
Pneumonia Care				
Appropriate Initial Antibiotic Given	120	98%	96%	95%
Blood Culture Timing	171	98%	98%	98%
Pregnancy and Delivery Care				
Newborn Deliveries Scheduled Early[7]	-	-	5%	6%
Preventive Care				
Immunization for Influenza[2]	304	100%	93%	90%
Immunization for Pneumonia[2]	478	99%	94%	92%
Stroke Care				
Anticoagulation Therapy for Atrial Fibrillation[3,7]	-	-	95%	95%
Antithrombotic Therapy Timing[3]	11	100%	98%	98%
Assessed for Rehabilitation[3]	11	100%	98%	97%
Discharged on Antithrombotic Therapy[1,3]	-	-	99%	99%
Discharged on Statin Medication[1,3]	-	-	95%	94%
Thrombolytic Therapy Timing[1,3]	-	-	65%	66%
Venous Thromboembolism Prophylaxis[3]	11	82%	95%	94%
Written Stroke Educational Materials Given[1,3]	-	-	92%	88%
Surgical Care Improvement Project				
Appropriate Beta Blocker Usage	33	100%	98%	98%
Appropriate VTP Within 24 Hours	123	99%	98%	98%
Controlled Postoperative Blood Glucose[7]	-	-	97%	97%
Perioperative Temperature Management	134	100%	100%	100%
Prophylactic Antibiotic Selection	103	100%	99%	99%
Prophylactic Antibiotic Selection (Outpatient)	97	98%	98%	98%
Prophylactic Antibiotic Stopped	103	93%	98%	98%
Prophylactic Antibiotic Timing	103	100%	99%	99%
Prophylactic Antibiotic Timing (Outpatient)	98	99%	97%	98%
Urinary Catheter Removal	22	100%	97%	97%
Survey of Patients' Hospital Experiences				
Area Around Room 'Always' Quiet at Night	300+	40%	58%	61%
Doctors 'Always' Communicated Well	300+	75%	80%	82%
Home Recovery Information Given	300+	86%	87%	85%
Hospital Given 9 or 10 on 10 Point Scale	300+	59%	72%	71%
Meds 'Always' Explained Before Given	300+	59%	64%	64%
Nurses 'Always' Communicated Well	300+	74%	81%	79%
Pain 'Always' Well Controlled	300+	66%	71%	71%
Room and Bathroom 'Always' Clean	300+	71%	75%	73%
Timely Help 'Always' Received	300+	58%	70%	68%
Would Definitely Recommend Hospital	300+	61%	71%	71%
Use of Medical Imaging				
Cardiac Imaging Stress Test before Surgery	149	8.7%	5.4%	5.3%
Combination Abdominal CT Scan	314	3.8%	7.1%	10.5%
Combination Brain/Sinus CT Scan[1]	-	-	2.8%	2.7%
Combination Chest CT Scan	123	0.0%	1.7%	2.7%
Follow-up Mammogram/Ultrasound	566	1.4%	8.7%	8.8%
Lumbar Spine MRI for Low Back Pain[1]	-	-	34.7%	37.2%

Saint Joseph Health Center

667 Eastland Ave Se
Warren, OH 44481
Phone: 330-841-4000
Type: Acute Care Hospitals
Emergency Services: Yes
Ownership: Voluntary non-profit - Other
Beds: 165

Key Personnel:
CEO/President. . . . . Elizabeth Buller
Chairman/CEO . . . . Ellen Malcolmson
Chief of Medical Staff . . . . Dr. Ted Rogovein, MD

Measure	Cases	This Hosp.	State Avg.	U.S. Avg.
Blood Clot Prevention and Treatment				
Anticoagulation Overlap Therapy[2]	68	66%	93%	93%
ICU Venous Thromboembolism Prophylaxis[2]	76	84%	93%	92%
Incidence of Potentially Preventable VTE[1,2]	-	-	6%	10%
UFH with Dosages/Platelet Monitoring[2]	42	100%	98%	97%
Venous Thromboembolism Prophylaxis[2]	354	70%	88%	85%
Warfarin Therapy Discharge Instructions[2]	42	93%	79%	75%
Chest Pain/Possible Heart Attack Care				
Aspirin Given Within 24 Hours of Arrival	96	94%	97%	96%
Fibrinolytic Meds Within 30 Min. of Arrival[7]	-	-	44%	58%
Average Time to ECG (minutes)	98	10	6	7
Average Time to Transfer (minutes)	26	64	58	60
Children's Asthma Care				
Received Home Management Plan of Care	-	-	85%	88%
Received Reliever Medication	-	-	100%	100%
Received Systemic Corticosteroids	-	-	100%	100%
Emergency Department				
Admittance Decision Time (minutes)[2]	790	114	90	98
Head CT Results Within 45 Min. of Arrival	29	55%	63%	57%
Patients Who Left ER Before Being Seen	72,980	2%	2%	2%
Time from ER Arrival to Admit. (minutes)[2]	792	320	265	274
Time from ER Arrival to Discharge (minutes)	390	114	128	134
Time in ER Before Being Evaluated (minutes)	423	25	22	26
Time to Pain Meds for Fractures (minutes)	166	46	54	57
Heart Attack Care				
Aspirin Given at Discharge	29	93%	99%	99%
Fibrinolytic Meds Within 30 Min. of Arrival[7]	-	-	80%	54%
PCI Within 90 Minutes of Arrival[7]	-	-	97%	96%
Statin Prescribed at Discharge	29	83%	98%	98%
Heart Failure Care				
ACE Inhibitor or ARB for LVSD[2]	56	98%	97%	97%
Discharge Instructions Given[2]	212	100%	96%	94%
Evaluation of LVS Function[2]	291	100%	100%	99%
Medicare Spending				
Medicare Spending per Patient (ratio)	-	1.06	1.01	0.98
Pneumonia Care				
Appropriate Initial Antibiotic Given[2]	55	96%	96%	95%
Blood Culture Timing[2]	171	98%	98%	98%
Pregnancy and Delivery Care				
Newborn Deliveries Scheduled Early	102	9%	5%	6%
Preventive Care				
Immunization for Influenza[2]	570	95%	93%	90%
Immunization for Pneumonia[2]	786	96%	94%	92%
Stroke Care				
Anticoagulation Therapy for Atrial Fibrillation[2]	11	100%	95%	95%
Antithrombotic Therapy Timing[2]	98	98%	98%	98%
Assessed for Rehabilitation[2]	98	98%	98%	97%
Discharged on Antithrombotic Therapy[2]	94	99%	99%	99%
Discharged on Statin Medication[2]	71	87%	95%	94%
Thrombolytic Therapy Timing[2,7]	-	-	65%	66%
Venous Thromboembolism Prophylaxis[2]	95	88%	95%	94%
Written Stroke Educational Materials Given[2]	52	100%	92%	88%
Surgical Care Improvement Project				
Appropriate Beta Blocker Usage[2]	119	96%	98%	98%
Appropriate VTP Within 24 Hours[2]	369	98%	98%	98%
Controlled Postoperative Blood Glucose[2,7]	-	-	97%	97%
Perioperative Temperature Management[2]	399	100%	100%	100%
Prophylactic Antibiotic Selection[2]	244	100%	99%	99%
Prophylactic Antibiotic Selection (Outpatient)	298	97%	98%	98%
Prophylactic Antibiotic Stopped[2]	237	100%	98%	98%
Prophylactic Antibiotic Timing[2]	244	100%	99%	99%
Prophylactic Antibiotic Timing (Outpatient)	302	94%	97%	98%
Urinary Catheter Removal[2]	265	95%	97%	97%
Survey of Patients' Hospital Experiences				
Area Around Room 'Always' Quiet at Night	300+	50%	58%	61%
Doctors 'Always' Communicated Well	300+	79%	80%	82%
Home Recovery Information Given	300+	88%	87%	85%
Hospital Given 9 or 10 on 10 Point Scale	300+	71%	72%	71%
Meds 'Always' Explained Before Given	300+	59%	64%	64%
Nurses 'Always' Communicated Well	300+	79%	81%	79%
Pain 'Always' Well Controlled	300+	70%	71%	71%
Room and Bathroom 'Always' Clean	300+	66%	75%	73%
Timely Help 'Always' Received	300+	64%	70%	68%
Would Definitely Recommend Hospital	300+	77%	71%	71%
Use of Medical Imaging				
Cardiac Imaging Stress Test before Surgery	192	4.7%	5.4%	5.3%
Combination Abdominal CT Scan	711	26.4%	7.1%	10.5%
Combination Brain/Sinus CT Scan	828	4.3%	2.8%	2.7%
Combination Chest CT Scan	491	1.4%	1.7%	2.7%
Follow-up Mammogram/Ultrasound	641	9.2%	8.7%	8.8%
Lumbar Spine MRI for Low Back Pain	92	31.5%	34.7%	37.2%

Trumbull Memorial Hospital

1350 East Market Street
Warren, OH 44482
Phone: 330-841-9011
Fax: 330-841-9281
URL: www.trumhosp.org
Type: Acute Care Hospitals
Emergency Services: Yes
Ownership: Proprietary
Beds: 350

Key Personnel:
Radiology. . . . . Thomas Groner, MD
CEO/President. . . . . N Kristopher Hoce
Intensive Care Unit. . . . . Martha Laurie, RN
Operating Room. . . . . Claudia Maksimoff, RN
Anesthesiology. . . . . Rickie Monroe, MD
Chief of Medical Staff. . . . . Yogesh Sheth, MD
Emergency Room . . . . JM Sudimack, MD

Measure	Cases	This Hosp.	State Avg.	U.S. Avg.
Blood Clot Prevention and Treatment				
Anticoagulation Overlap Therapy[2]	72	89%	93%	93%
ICU Venous Thromboembolism Prophylaxis[2]	147	92%	93%	92%
Incidence of Potentially Preventable VTE[1,2]	-	-	6%	10%
UFH with Dosages/Platelet Monitoring[2]	54	94%	98%	97%
Venous Thromboembolism Prophylaxis[2]	416	89%	88%	85%
Warfarin Therapy Discharge Instructions[2]	55	64%	79%	75%
Chest Pain/Possible Heart Attack Care				
Aspirin Given Within 24 Hours of Arrival	11	100%	97%	96%
Fibrinolytic Meds Within 30 Min. of Arrival[3,7]	-	-	44%	58%
Average Time to ECG (minutes)	11	7	6	7
Average Time to Transfer (minutes)[1,3]	-	-	58	60
Children's Asthma Care				
Received Home Management Plan of Care	-	-	85%	88%
Received Reliever Medication	-	-	100%	100%
Received Systemic Corticosteroids	-	-	100%	100%
Emergency Department				
Admittance Decision Time (minutes)[2]	787	122	90	98
Head CT Results Within 45 Min. of Arrival	31	74%	63%	57%
Patients Who Left ER Before Being Seen	40,141	4%	2%	2%
Time from ER Arrival to Admit. (minutes)[2]	825	331	265	274
Time from ER Arrival to Discharge (minutes)	355	160	128	134
Time in ER Before Being Evaluated (minutes)	418	18	22	26
Time to Pain Meds for Fractures (minutes)	56	74	54	57
Heart Attack Care				
Aspirin Given at Discharge	176	100%	99%	99%
Fibrinolytic Meds Within 30 Min. of Arrival[7]	-	-	80%	54%
PCI Within 90 Minutes of Arrival	31	94%	97%	96%
Statin Prescribed at Discharge	163	99%	98%	98%

NOTE: Hospital profiles are in alphabetical order by state, then city, then hospital within the city; Rankings exclude hospitals with less than 25 cases except for patient surveys which excludes hospitals with less than 100 cases; (a) 100-299 cases; (1) The number of cases/patients is too few to report; (2) Data submitted were based on a sample of cases/patients; (3) Results are based on a shorter time period than required; (4) Data suppressed by CMS for one or more quarters; (5) Results are not available for this reporting period; (6) Fewer than 100 patients completed the HCAHPS survey; (7) No cases met the criteria for this measure; (8) The lower limit of the confidence interval cannot be calculated if the number of observed infections equals zero; (9) No data are available from the state/territory for this reporting period; (10) The scores shown reflect fewer than 50 completed surveys; (11) There were discrepancies in the data collection process; (12) This measure does not apply to this hospital for this reporting period; (13) Results cannot be calculated for this reporting period; (14) The results for this state are combined with nearby states to protect confidentiality; Please refer to the User's Guide for a full explanation of data.

Measure	Cases	This Hosp.	State Avg.	U.S. Avg.
Heart Failure Care				
ACE Inhibitor or ARB for LVSD	107	93%	97%	97%
Discharge Instructions Given	358	83%	96%	94%
Evaluation of LVS Function	446	100%	100%	99%
Medicare Spending				
Medicare Spending per Patient (ratio)	-	1.02	1.01	0.98
Pneumonia Care				
Appropriate Initial Antibiotic Given	177	98%	96%	95%
Blood Culture Timing	265	99%	98%	98%
Pregnancy and Delivery Care				
Newborn Deliveries Scheduled Early[2]	41	2%	5%	6%
Preventive Care				
Immunization for Influenza[2]	628	99%	93%	90%
Immunization for Pneumonia[2]	863	99%	94%	92%
Stroke Care				
Anticoagulation Therapy for Atrial Fibrillation	18	100%	95%	95%
Antithrombotic Therapy Timing	81	99%	98%	98%
Assessed for Rehabilitation	87	98%	98%	97%
Discharged on Antithrombotic Therapy	83	99%	99%	99%
Discharged on Statin Medication	58	97%	95%	94%
Thrombolytic Therapy Timing[1]	-	-	65%	66%
Venous Thromboembolism Prophylaxis	91	95%	95%	94%
Written Stroke Educational Materials Given	51	90%	92%	88%
Surgical Care Improvement Project				
Appropriate Beta Blocker Usage	247	95%	98%	98%
Appropriate VTP Within 24 Hours	523	97%	98%	98%
Controlled Postoperative Blood Glucose	74	100%	97%	97%
Perioperative Temperature Management	587	100%	100%	100%
Prophylactic Antibiotic Selection	450	99%	99%	99%
Prophylactic Antibiotic Selection (Outpatient)	310	97%	98%	98%
Prophylactic Antibiotic Stopped	431	98%	98%	98%
Prophylactic Antibiotic Timing	450	100%	99%	99%
Prophylactic Antibiotic Timing (Outpatient)	310	99%	97%	98%
Urinary Catheter Removal	242	93%	97%	97%
Survey of Patients' Hospital Experiences				
Area Around Room 'Always' Quiet at Night	300+	51%	58%	61%
Doctors 'Always' Communicated Well	300+	77%	80%	82%
Home Recovery Information Given	300+	86%	87%	85%
Hospital Given 9 or 10 on 10 Point Scale	300+	58%	72%	71%
Meds 'Always' Explained Before Given	300+	58%	64%	64%
Nurses 'Always' Communicated Well	300+	73%	81%	79%
Pain 'Always' Well Controlled	300+	65%	71%	71%
Room and Bathroom 'Always' Clean	300+	58%	75%	73%
Timely Help 'Always' Received	300+	59%	70%	68%
Would Definitely Recommend Hospital	300+	56%	71%	71%
Use of Medical Imaging				
Cardiac Imaging Stress Test before Surgery	201	4.5%	5.4%	5.3%
Combination Abdominal CT Scan	740	2.4%	7.1%	10.5%
Combination Brain/Sinus CT Scan	620	4.7%	2.8%	2.7%
Combination Chest CT Scan	587	1.4%	1.7%	2.7%
Follow-up Mammogram/Ultrasound	1,729	11.6%	8.7%	8.8%
Lumbar Spine MRI for Low Back Pain	122	32.0%	34.7%	37.2%

South Pointe Hospital

20000 Harvard Road
Warrensville Heights, OH 44122
Phone: 216-491-6000
Fax: 216-491-7260
URL: www.southpointehospital.org
Type: Acute Care Hospitals
Emergency Services: Yes
Ownership: Voluntary non-profit - Other
Beds: 232

Key Personnel:
Emergency Room . . . . Jonathan Klein
CEO/President. . . . . Beverly Lozar
Cardiac Laboratory. . . . . Mark Pace
Chief of Medical Staff . . . . Charles Webb

Measure	Cases	This Hosp.	State Avg.	U.S. Avg.
Blood Clot Prevention and Treatment				
Anticoagulation Overlap Therapy[2]	102	87%	93%	93%
ICU Venous Thromboembolism Prophylaxis[2]	120	97%	93%	92%
Incidence of Potentially Preventable VTE[2]	16	0%	6%	10%
UFH with Dosages/Platelet Monitoring[2]	104	100%	98%	97%
Venous Thromboembolism Prophylaxis[2]	336	97%	88%	85%
Warfarin Therapy Discharge Instructions[2]	65	65%	79%	75%
Chest Pain/Possible Heart Attack Care				
Aspirin Given Within 24 Hours of Arrival	98	96%	97%	96%
Fibrinolytic Meds Within 30 Min. of Arrival[7]	-	-	44%	58%
Average Time to ECG (minutes)	102	6	6	7
Average Time to Transfer (minutes)[1]	-	-	58	60
Children's Asthma Care				
Received Home Management Plan of Care	-	-	85%	88%
Received Reliever Medication	-	-	100%	100%
Received Systemic Corticosteroids	-	-	100%	100%
Emergency Department				
Admittance Decision Time (minutes)[2]	685	97	90	98
Head CT Results Within 45 Min. of Arrival	14	50%	63%	57%
Patients Who Left ER Before Being Seen	40,231	1%	2%	2%
Time from ER Arrival to Admit. (minutes)[2]	695	250	265	274
Time from ER Arrival to Discharge (minutes)	390	105	128	134
Time in ER Before Being Evaluated (minutes)	443	17	22	26
Time to Pain Meds for Fractures (minutes)	88	48	54	57
Heart Attack Care				
Aspirin Given at Discharge	13	100%	99%	99%
Fibrinolytic Meds Within 30 Min. of Arrival[7]	-	-	80%	54%
PCI Within 90 Minutes of Arrival[7]	-	-	97%	96%
Statin Prescribed at Discharge	16	81%	98%	98%
Heart Failure Care				
ACE Inhibitor or ARB for LVSD	99	100%	97%	97%
Discharge Instructions Given	259	99%	96%	94%
Evaluation of LVS Function	327	100%	100%	99%
Medicare Spending				
Medicare Spending per Patient (ratio)	-	1.07	1.01	0.98
Pneumonia Care				
Appropriate Initial Antibiotic Given	108	100%	96%	95%
Blood Culture Timing	122	96%	98%	98%
Pregnancy and Delivery Care				
Newborn Deliveries Scheduled Early[7]	-	-	5%	6%
Preventive Care				
Immunization for Influenza[2]	606	94%	93%	90%
Immunization for Pneumonia[2]	1,011	94%	94%	92%
Stroke Care				
Anticoagulation Therapy for Atrial Fibrillation[1]	-	-	95%	95%
Antithrombotic Therapy Timing	62	100%	98%	98%
Assessed for Rehabilitation	70	100%	98%	97%
Discharged on Antithrombotic Therapy	66	100%	99%	99%
Discharged on Statin Medication	41	98%	95%	94%
Thrombolytic Therapy Timing[1]	-	-	65%	66%
Venous Thromboembolism Prophylaxis	70	100%	95%	94%
Written Stroke Educational Materials Given	37	100%	92%	88%
Surgical Care Improvement Project				
Appropriate Beta Blocker Usage	137	99%	98%	98%
Appropriate VTP Within 24 Hours	280	97%	98%	98%
Controlled Postoperative Blood Glucose[7]	-	-	97%	97%
Perioperative Temperature Management	371	100%	100%	100%
Prophylactic Antibiotic Selection	227	99%	99%	99%
Prophylactic Antibiotic Selection (Outpatient)	74	100%	98%	98%
Prophylactic Antibiotic Stopped	226	97%	98%	98%
Prophylactic Antibiotic Timing	227	100%	99%	99%
Prophylactic Antibiotic Timing (Outpatient)	77	96%	97%	98%
Urinary Catheter Removal	295	99%	97%	97%
Survey of Patients' Hospital Experiences				
Area Around Room 'Always' Quiet at Night	300+	57%	58%	61%
Doctors 'Always' Communicated Well	300+	80%	80%	82%
Home Recovery Information Given	300+	86%	87%	85%
Hospital Given 9 or 10 on 10 Point Scale	300+	70%	72%	71%
Meds 'Always' Explained Before Given	300+	63%	64%	64%
Nurses 'Always' Communicated Well	300+	80%	81%	79%
Pain 'Always' Well Controlled	300+	73%	71%	71%
Room and Bathroom 'Always' Clean	300+	76%	75%	73%
Timely Help 'Always' Received	300+	63%	70%	68%
Would Definitely Recommend Hospital	300+	68%	71%	71%
Use of Medical Imaging				
Cardiac Imaging Stress Test before Surgery	67	9.0%	5.4%	5.3%
Combination Abdominal CT Scan	572	4.0%	7.1%	10.5%
Combination Brain/Sinus CT Scan	676	4.0%	2.8%	2.7%
Combination Chest CT Scan	421	3.1%	1.7%	2.7%
Follow-up Mammogram/Ultrasound	836	10.6%	8.7%	8.8%
Lumbar Spine MRI for Low Back Pain	64	21.9%	34.7%	37.2%

Fayette County Memorial Hospital

1430 Columbus Avenue
Washington Ch, OH 43160
Phone: 740-333-1210
Fax: 740-333-2998
E-mail: brenda_hughes@fcmh.org
Type: Critical Access Hospitals
Emergency Services: Yes
Ownership: Government - Local
Beds: 70

Key Personnel:
CEO/President. . . . . Lyndon Christman
Infection Control. . . . . Lin Glass, RN
Quality Assurance . . . . Lin Glass, NR
Operating Room. . . . . Pam Melvin, RN
Radiology. . . . . Steven R Mustric
Chief of Medical Staff . . . . Dale Reno, DO

Measure	Cases	This Hosp.	State Avg.	U.S. Avg.
Blood Clot Prevention and Treatment				
Anticoagulation Overlap Therapy[1]	-	-	93%	93%
ICU Venous Thromboembolism Prophylaxis	154	96%	93%	92%
Incidence of Potentially Preventable VTE[7]	-	-	6%	10%
UFH with Dosages/Platelet Monitoring[1]	-	-	98%	97%
Venous Thromboembolism Prophylaxis	396	91%	88%	85%
Warfarin Therapy Discharge Instructions[1]	-	-	79%	75%
Chest Pain/Possible Heart Attack Care				
Aspirin Given Within 24 Hours of Arrival	79	90%	97%	96%
Fibrinolytic Meds Within 30 Min. of Arrival[7]	-	-	44%	58%
Average Time to ECG (minutes)	82	6	6	7
Average Time to Transfer (minutes)[1]	-	-	58	60
Children's Asthma Care				
Received Home Management Plan of Care	-	-	85%	88%
Received Reliever Medication	-	-	100%	100%
Received Systemic Corticosteroids	-	-	100%	100%
Emergency Department				
Admittance Decision Time (minutes)[5]	-	-	90	98
Head CT Results Within 45 Min. of Arrival[1,3]	-	-	63%	57%
Patients Who Left ER Before Being Seen[5]	-	-	2%	2%
Time from ER Arrival to Admit. (minutes)[5]	-	-	265	274
Time from ER Arrival to Discharge (minutes)[5]	-	-	128	134
Time in ER Before Being Evaluated (minutes)[5]	-	-	22	26
Time to Pain Meds for Fractures (minutes)[5]	-	-	54	57
Heart Attack Care				
Aspirin Given at Discharge[5]	-	-	99%	99%
Fibrinolytic Meds Within 30 Min. of Arrival[5]	-	-	80%	54%
PCI Within 90 Minutes of Arrival[5]	-	-	97%	96%
Statin Prescribed at Discharge[5]	-	-	98%	98%
Heart Failure Care				
ACE Inhibitor or ARB for LVSD[1]	-	-	97%	97%
Discharge Instructions Given	29	97%	96%	94%
Evaluation of LVS Function	41	98%	100%	99%
Medicare Spending				
Medicare Spending per Patient (ratio)	-	-	1.01	0.98
Pneumonia Care				
Appropriate Initial Antibiotic Given	44	100%	96%	95%
Blood Culture Timing	67	99%	98%	98%
Pregnancy and Delivery Care				
Newborn Deliveries Scheduled Early[5]	-	-	5%	6%
Preventive Care				
Immunization for Influenza	524	62%	93%	90%
Immunization for Pneumonia	790	75%	94%	92%
Stroke Care				
Anticoagulation Therapy for Atrial Fibrillation[7]	-	-	95%	95%
Antithrombotic Therapy Timing[1]	-	-	98%	98%
Assessed for Rehabilitation[1]	-	-	98%	97%
Discharged on Antithrombotic Therapy[1]	-	-	99%	99%
Discharged on Statin Medication[1]	-	-	95%	94%
Thrombolytic Therapy Timing[7]	-	-	65%	66%
Venous Thromboembolism Prophylaxis[1]	-	-	95%	94%
Written Stroke Educational Materials Given[7]	-	-	92%	88%
Surgical Care Improvement Project				
Appropriate Beta Blocker Usage[1]	-	-	98%	98%
Appropriate VTP Within 24 Hours	17	100%	98%	98%
Controlled Postoperative Blood Glucose[3,7]	-	-	97%	97%
Perioperative Temperature Management	20	100%	100%	100%
Prophylactic Antibiotic Selection[1]	-	-	99%	99%

NOTE: Hospital profiles are in alphabetical order by state, then city, then hospital within the city; Rankings exclude hospitals with less than 25 cases except for patient surveys which excludes hospitals with less than 100 cases; (a) 100-299 cases; (1) The number of cases/patients is too few to report; (2) Data submitted were based on a sample of cases/patients; (3) Results are based on a shorter time period than required; (4) Data suppressed by CMS for one or more quarters; (5) Results are not available for this reporting period; (6) Fewer than 100 patients completed the HCAHPS survey; (7) No cases met the criteria for this measure; (8) The lower limit of the confidence interval cannot be calculated if the number of observed infections equals zero; (9) No data are available from the state/territory for this reporting period; (10) The scores shown reflect fewer than 50 completed surveys; (11) There were discrepancies in the data collection process; (12) This measure does not apply to this hospital for this reporting period; (13) Results cannot be calculated for this reporting period; (14) The results for this state are combined with nearby states to protect confidentiality; Please refer to the User's Guide for a full explanation of data.

Measure	Cases	This Hosp.	State Avg.	U.S. Avg.
Prophylactic Antibiotic Selection (Outpatient)[1,3]	-	-	98%	98%
Prophylactic Antibiotic Stopped[1]	-	-	98%	98%
Prophylactic Antibiotic Timing[1]	-	-	99%	99%
Prophylactic Antibiotic Timing (Outpatient)[1,3]	-	-	97%	98%
Urinary Catheter Removal	12	92%	97%	97%
Survey of Patients' Hospital Experiences				
Area Around Room 'Always' Quiet at Night	(a)	52%	58%	61%
Doctors 'Always' Communicated Well	(a)	86%	80%	82%
Home Recovery Information Given	(a)	90%	87%	85%
Hospital Given 9 or 10 on 10 Point Scale	(a)	68%	72%	71%
Meds 'Always' Explained Before Given	(a)	71%	64%	64%
Nurses 'Always' Communicated Well	(a)	84%	81%	79%
Pain 'Always' Well Controlled	(a)	73%	71%	71%
Room and Bathroom 'Always' Clean	(a)	83%	75%	73%
Timely Help 'Always' Received	(a)	75%	70%	68%
Would Definitely Recommend Hospital	(a)	67%	71%	71%
Use of Medical Imaging				
Cardiac Imaging Stress Test before Surgery	75	6.7%	5.4%	5.3%
Combination Abdominal CT Scan	366	3.3%	7.1%	10.5%
Combination Brain/Sinus CT Scan[1]	-	-	2.8%	2.7%
Combination Chest CT Scan	152	0.7%	1.7%	2.7%
Follow-up Mammogram/Ultrasound	214	8.9%	8.7%	8.8%
Lumbar Spine MRI for Low Back Pain[1]	-	-	34.7%	37.2%

Fulton County Health Center

725 South Shoop Avenue
Wauseon, OH 43567
Phone: 419-335-2015
Fax: 419-330-2602
Type: Critical Access Hospitals
Emergency Services: Yes
Ownership: Voluntary non-profit - Private
Beds: 119

Key Personnel:
CEO/President. . . . . Dean Beck, MD
Chief of Medical Staff. . . . . Jana Bourn
Radiology. . . . . John Patrick Ewonus

Measure	Cases	This Hosp.	State Avg.	U.S. Avg.
Blood Clot Prevention and Treatment				
Anticoagulation Overlap Therapy[5]	-	-	93%	93%
ICU Venous Thromboembolism Prophylaxis[5]	-	-	93%	92%
Incidence of Potentially Preventable VTE[5]	-	-	6%	10%
UFH with Dosages/Platelet Monitoring[5]	-	-	98%	97%
Venous Thromboembolism Prophylaxis[5]	-	-	88%	85%
Warfarin Therapy Discharge Instructions[5]	-	-	79%	75%
Chest Pain/Possible Heart Attack Care				
Aspirin Given Within 24 Hours of Arrival	105	95%	97%	96%
Fibrinolytic Meds Within 30 Min. of Arrival[7]	-	-	44%	58%
Average Time to ECG (minutes)	109	8	6	7
Average Time to Transfer (minutes)[1]	-	-	58	60
Children's Asthma Care				
Received Home Management Plan of Care	-	-	85%	88%
Received Reliever Medication	-	-	100%	100%
Received Systemic Corticosteroids	-	-	100%	100%
Emergency Department				
Admittance Decision Time (minutes)[2]	136	62	90	98
Head CT Results Within 45 Min. of Arrival	20	40%	63%	57%
Patients Who Left ER Before Being Seen	16,733	0%	2%	2%
Time from ER Arrival to Admit. (minutes)[2]	138	194	265	274
Time from ER Arrival to Discharge (minutes)	341	107	128	134
Time in ER Before Being Evaluated (minutes)	378	16	22	26
Time to Pain Meds for Fractures (minutes)	70	50	54	57
Heart Attack Care				
Aspirin Given at Discharge[5]	-	-	99%	99%
Fibrinolytic Meds Within 30 Min. of Arrival[5]	-	-	80%	54%
PCI Within 90 Minutes of Arrival[5]	-	-	97%	96%
Statin Prescribed at Discharge[5]	-	-	98%	98%
Heart Failure Care				
ACE Inhibitor or ARB for LVSD[1]	-	-	97%	97%
Discharge Instructions Given	18	94%	96%	94%
Evaluation of LVS Function	24	92%	100%	99%
Medicare Spending				
Medicare Spending per Patient (ratio)	-	-	1.01	0.98
Pneumonia Care				
Appropriate Initial Antibiotic Given	34	88%	96%	95%
Blood Culture Timing	48	88%	98%	98%
Pregnancy and Delivery Care				
Newborn Deliveries Scheduled Early[2,3]	11	9%	5%	6%
Preventive Care				
Immunization for Influenza[2]	246	89%	93%	90%
Immunization for Pneumonia[2]	280	86%	94%	92%
Stroke Care				
Anticoagulation Therapy for Atrial Fibrillation[5]	-	-	95%	95%
Antithrombotic Therapy Timing[5]	-	-	98%	98%
Assessed for Rehabilitation[5]	-	-	98%	97%
Discharged on Antithrombotic Therapy[5]	-	-	99%	99%
Discharged on Statin Medication[5]	-	-	95%	94%
Thrombolytic Therapy Timing[5]	-	-	65%	66%
Venous Thromboembolism Prophylaxis[5]	-	-	95%	94%
Written Stroke Educational Materials Given[5]	-	-	92%	88%
Surgical Care Improvement Project				
Appropriate Beta Blocker Usage[2]	99	98%	98%	98%
Appropriate VTP Within 24 Hours[2]	237	100%	98%	98%
Controlled Postoperative Blood Glucose[2,7]	-	-	97%	97%
Perioperative Temperature Management[2]	260	100%	100%	100%
Prophylactic Antibiotic Selection[2]	216	99%	99%	99%
Prophylactic Antibiotic Selection (Outpatient)	97	98%	98%	98%
Prophylactic Antibiotic Stopped[2]	215	96%	98%	98%
Prophylactic Antibiotic Timing[2]	216	100%	99%	99%
Prophylactic Antibiotic Timing (Outpatient)	94	98%	97%	98%
Urinary Catheter Removal[2]	31	77%	97%	97%
Survey of Patients' Hospital Experiences				
Area Around Room 'Always' Quiet at Night	300+	54%	58%	61%
Doctors 'Always' Communicated Well	300+	82%	80%	82%
Home Recovery Information Given	300+	84%	87%	85%
Hospital Given 9 or 10 on 10 Point Scale	300+	77%	72%	71%
Meds 'Always' Explained Before Given	300+	63%	64%	64%
Nurses 'Always' Communicated Well	300+	76%	81%	79%
Pain 'Always' Well Controlled	300+	73%	71%	71%
Room and Bathroom 'Always' Clean	300+	80%	75%	73%
Timely Help 'Always' Received	300+	73%	70%	68%
Would Definitely Recommend Hospital	300+	75%	71%	71%
Use of Medical Imaging				
Cardiac Imaging Stress Test before Surgery	280	5.0%	5.4%	5.3%
Combination Abdominal CT Scan	443	6.1%	7.1%	10.5%
Combination Brain/Sinus CT Scan[1]	-	-	2.8%	2.7%
Combination Chest CT Scan	166	4.2%	1.7%	2.7%
Follow-up Mammogram/Ultrasound	655	4.6%	8.7%	8.8%
Lumbar Spine MRI for Low Back Pain	51	37.3%	34.7%	37.2%

Pike Community Hospital

100 Dawn Lane
Waverly, OH 45690
Phone: 740-947-2186
Fax: 740-947-6538
E-mail: pch1@bright.net
URL: www.adena.org
Type: Critical Access Hospitals
Emergency Services: Yes
Ownership: Voluntary non-profit - Private
Beds: 63

Key Personnel:
Operating Room. . . . . Pam Brown
Quality Assurance . . . . John Kovacic
Emergency Room . . . . Nikki McKee, RN
Infection Control. . . . . Angela Pelphrey, RN
Chief of Medical Staff. . . . . David Roddy, MD
CEO/President. . . . . Richard E Sobota

Measure	Cases	This Hosp.	State Avg.	U.S. Avg.
Blood Clot Prevention and Treatment				
Anticoagulation Overlap Therapy[5]	-	-	93%	93%
ICU Venous Thromboembolism Prophylaxis[5]	-	-	93%	92%
Incidence of Potentially Preventable VTE[5]	-	-	6%	10%
UFH with Dosages/Platelet Monitoring[5]	-	-	98%	97%
Venous Thromboembolism Prophylaxis[5]	-	-	88%	85%
Warfarin Therapy Discharge Instructions[5]	-	-	79%	75%
Chest Pain/Possible Heart Attack Care				
Aspirin Given Within 24 Hours of Arrival	-	-	97%	96%
Fibrinolytic Meds Within 30 Min. of Arrival	-	-	44%	58%
Average Time to ECG (minutes)	-	-	6	7
Average Time to Transfer (minutes)	-	-	58	60
Children's Asthma Care				
Received Home Management Plan of Care	-	-	85%	88%
Received Reliever Medication	-	-	100%	100%
Received Systemic Corticosteroids	-	-	100%	100%
Emergency Department				
Admittance Decision Time (minutes)[5]	-	-	90	98
Head CT Results Within 45 Min. of Arrival	-	-	63%	57%
Patients Who Left ER Before Being Seen	-	-	2%	2%
Time from ER Arrival to Admit. (minutes)[5]	-	-	265	274
Time from ER Arrival to Discharge (minutes)	-	-	128	134
Time in ER Before Being Evaluated (minutes)	-	-	22	26
Time to Pain Meds for Fractures (minutes)	-	-	54	57
Heart Attack Care				
Aspirin Given at Discharge[5]	-	-	99%	99%
Fibrinolytic Meds Within 30 Min. of Arrival[5]	-	-	80%	54%
PCI Within 90 Minutes of Arrival[5]	-	-	97%	96%
Statin Prescribed at Discharge[5]	-	-	98%	98%
Heart Failure Care				
ACE Inhibitor or ARB for LVSD[1,3]	-	-	97%	97%
Discharge Instructions Given[1,3]	-	-	96%	94%
Evaluation of LVS Function[3]	12	58%	100%	99%
Medicare Spending				
Medicare Spending per Patient (ratio)	-	-	1.01	0.98
Pneumonia Care				
Appropriate Initial Antibiotic Given[3]	24	92%	96%	95%
Blood Culture Timing[3]	38	74%	98%	98%
Pregnancy and Delivery Care				
Newborn Deliveries Scheduled Early[5]	-	-	5%	6%
Preventive Care				
Immunization for Influenza[5]	-	-	93%	90%
Immunization for Pneumonia[5]	-	-	94%	92%
Stroke Care				
Anticoagulation Therapy for Atrial Fibrillation[5]	-	-	95%	95%
Antithrombotic Therapy Timing[5]	-	-	98%	98%
Assessed for Rehabilitation[5]	-	-	98%	97%
Discharged on Antithrombotic Therapy[5]	-	-	99%	99%
Discharged on Statin Medication[5]	-	-	95%	94%
Thrombolytic Therapy Timing[5]	-	-	65%	66%
Venous Thromboembolism Prophylaxis[5]	-	-	95%	94%
Written Stroke Educational Materials Given[5]	-	-	92%	88%
Surgical Care Improvement Project				
Appropriate Beta Blocker Usage[5]	-	-	98%	98%
Appropriate VTP Within 24 Hours[5]	-	-	98%	98%
Controlled Postoperative Blood Glucose[5]	-	-	97%	97%
Perioperative Temperature Management[5]	-	-	100%	100%
Prophylactic Antibiotic Selection[5]	-	-	99%	99%
Prophylactic Antibiotic Selection (Outpatient)	-	-	98%	98%
Prophylactic Antibiotic Stopped[5]	-	-	98%	98%
Prophylactic Antibiotic Timing[5]	-	-	99%	99%
Prophylactic Antibiotic Timing (Outpatient)	-	-	97%	98%
Urinary Catheter Removal[5]	-	-	97%	97%
Survey of Patients' Hospital Experiences				
Area Around Room 'Always' Quiet at Night	(a)	47%	58%	61%
Doctors 'Always' Communicated Well	(a)	82%	80%	82%
Home Recovery Information Given	(a)	79%	87%	85%
Hospital Given 9 or 10 on 10 Point Scale	(a)	53%	72%	71%
Meds 'Always' Explained Before Given	(a)	58%	64%	64%
Nurses 'Always' Communicated Well	(a)	77%	81%	79%
Pain 'Always' Well Controlled	(a)	63%	71%	71%
Room and Bathroom 'Always' Clean	(a)	75%	75%	73%
Timely Help 'Always' Received	(a)	60%	70%	68%
Would Definitely Recommend Hospital	(a)	58%	71%	71%
Use of Medical Imaging				
Cardiac Imaging Stress Test before Surgery	-	-	5.4%	5.3%
Combination Abdominal CT Scan	-	-	7.1%	10.5%
Combination Brain/Sinus CT Scan	-	-	2.8%	2.7%
Combination Chest CT Scan	-	-	1.7%	2.7%
Follow-up Mammogram/Ultrasound	-	-	8.7%	8.8%
Lumbar Spine MRI for Low Back Pain	-	-	34.7%	37.2%

West Chester Hospital

7700 University Drive
West Chester, OH 45069
Phone: 513-298-3000
URL: www.westchesterhospital.uchealth.com
Type: Acute Care Hospitals
Emergency Services: Yes
Ownership: Voluntary non-profit - Private

Key Personnel:
Cardiology . . . . Mohamed Effat, MD

NOTE: Hospital profiles are in alphabetical order by state, then city, then hospital within the city; Rankings exclude hospitals with less than 25 cases except for patient surveys which excludes hospitals with less than 100 cases; (a) 100-299 cases; (1) The number of cases/patients is too few to report; (2) Data submitted were based on a sample of cases/patients; (3) Results are based on a shorter time period than required; (4) Data suppressed by CMS for one or more quarters; (5) Results are not available for this reporting period; (6) Fewer than 100 patients completed the HCAHPS survey; (7) No cases met the criteria for this measure; (8) The lower limit of the confidence interval cannot be calculated if the number of observed infections equals zero; (9) No data are available from the state/territory for this reporting period; (10) The scores shown reflect fewer than 50 completed surveys; (11) There were discrepancies in the data collection process; (12) This measure does not apply to this hospital for this reporting period; (13) Results cannot be calculated for this reporting period; (14) The results for this state are combined with nearby states to protect confidentiality; Please refer to the User's Guide for a full explanation of data.

President/CEO. . . . . Kevin Joseph, MD
Emergency Room . . . . Elizabeth Leenellet, MD
Radiology. . . . . Tom Nogueira, MD
Pulmonology . . . . Daniel Tanase, MD

Measure	Cases	This Hosp.	State Avg.	U.S. Avg.
Blood Clot Prevention and Treatment				
Anticoagulation Overlap Therapy[2]	79	91%	93%	93%
ICU Venous Thromboembolism Prophylaxis[2]	92	96%	93%	92%
Incidence of Potentially Preventable VTE[2]	11	9%	6%	10%
UFH with Dosages/Platelet Monitoring[2]	66	100%	98%	97%
Venous Thromboembolism Prophylaxis[2]	284	93%	88%	85%
Warfarin Therapy Discharge Instructions[2]	60	65%	79%	75%
Chest Pain/Possible Heart Attack Care				
Aspirin Given Within 24 Hours of Arrival[1,3]	-	-	97%	96%
Fibrinolytic Meds Within 30 Min. of Arrival[3,7]	-	-	44%	58%
Average Time to ECG (minutes)[1,3]	-	-	6	7
Average Time to Transfer (minutes)[3,7]	-	-	58	60
Children's Asthma Care				
Received Home Management Plan of Care	-	-	85%	88%
Received Reliever Medication	-	-	100%	100%
Received Systemic Corticosteroids	-	-	100%	100%
Emergency Department				
Admittance Decision Time (minutes)[2]	741	75	90	98
Head CT Results Within 45 Min. of Arrival[1]	-	-	63%	57%
Patients Who Left ER Before Being Seen	33,830	0%	2%	2%
Time from ER Arrival to Admit. (minutes)[2]	745	226	265	274
Time from ER Arrival to Discharge (minutes)	392	135	128	134
Time in ER Before Being Evaluated (minutes)	418	10	22	26
Time to Pain Meds for Fractures (minutes)	67	38	54	57
Heart Attack Care				
Aspirin Given at Discharge	216	98%	99%	99%
Fibrinolytic Meds Within 30 Min. of Arrival[7]	-	-	80%	54%
PCI Within 90 Minutes of Arrival	28	96%	97%	96%
Statin Prescribed at Discharge	206	96%	98%	98%
Heart Failure Care				
ACE Inhibitor or ARB for LVSD	59	95%	97%	97%
Discharge Instructions Given	186	86%	96%	94%
Evaluation of LVS Function	256	99%	100%	99%
Medicare Spending				
Medicare Spending per Patient (ratio)	-	1.01	1.01	0.98
Pneumonia Care				
Appropriate Initial Antibiotic Given	146	97%	96%	95%
Blood Culture Timing	260	98%	98%	98%
Pregnancy and Delivery Care				
Newborn Deliveries Scheduled Early[7]	-	-	5%	6%
Preventive Care				
Immunization for Influenza[2]	638	94%	93%	90%
Immunization for Pneumonia[2]	834	95%	94%	92%
Stroke Care				
Anticoagulation Therapy for Atrial Fibrillation[1]	-	-	95%	95%
Antithrombotic Therapy Timing	70	99%	98%	98%
Assessed for Rehabilitation	81	95%	98%	97%
Discharged on Antithrombotic Therapy	78	99%	99%	99%
Discharged on Statin Medication	66	100%	95%	94%
Thrombolytic Therapy Timing[1]	-	-	65%	66%
Venous Thromboembolism Prophylaxis	80	95%	95%	94%
Written Stroke Educational Materials Given	39	62%	92%	88%
Surgical Care Improvement Project				
Appropriate Beta Blocker Usage	299	98%	98%	98%
Appropriate VTP Within 24 Hours	999	98%	98%	98%
Controlled Postoperative Blood Glucose[7]	-	-	97%	97%
Perioperative Temperature Management	1,158	100%	100%	100%
Prophylactic Antibiotic Selection	858	99%	99%	99%
Prophylactic Antibiotic Selection (Outpatient)	260	96%	98%	98%
Prophylactic Antibiotic Stopped	852	98%	98%	98%
Prophylactic Antibiotic Timing	860	97%	99%	99%
Prophylactic Antibiotic Timing (Outpatient)	263	96%	97%	98%
Urinary Catheter Removal	815	98%	97%	97%
Survey of Patients' Hospital Experiences				
Area Around Room 'Always' Quiet at Night	300+	70%	58%	61%
Doctors 'Always' Communicated Well	300+	82%	80%	82%
Home Recovery Information Given	300+	86%	87%	85%
Hospital Given 9 or 10 on 10 Point Scale	300+	79%	72%	71%
Meds 'Always' Explained Before Given	300+	64%	64%	64%
Nurses 'Always' Communicated Well	300+	82%	81%	79%
Pain 'Always' Well Controlled	300+	73%	71%	71%
Room and Bathroom 'Always' Clean	300+	74%	75%	73%
Timely Help 'Always' Received	300+	66%	70%	68%
Would Definitely Recommend Hospital	300+	83%	71%	71%
Use of Medical Imaging				
Cardiac Imaging Stress Test before Surgery	270	4.8%	5.4%	5.3%
Combination Abdominal CT Scan	391	7.9%	7.1%	10.5%
Combination Brain/Sinus CT Scan[1]	-	-	2.8%	2.7%
Combination Chest CT Scan	235	1.3%	1.7%	2.7%
Follow-up Mammogram/Ultrasound	214	12.6%	8.7%	8.8%
Lumbar Spine MRI for Low Back Pain	74	29.7%	34.7%	37.2%

Mount Carmel Saint Ann's

500 South Cleveland Avenue
Westerville, OH 43081
Phone: 614-898-4000
Fax: 614-898-8668
URL: www.mchs.com
Type: Acute Care Hospitals
Emergency Services: Yes
Ownership: Voluntary non-profit - Church
Beds: 180

Key Personnel:
Radiology. Guillermo A Arbona
CEO/President. . . . . Joseph Calvaruso
Operating Room. . . . . Pam Evans
Pediatric Ambulatory Care . . . . . . Steve Lindner, MD
Pediatric In-Patient Care . . . . Steve Lindner, MD
Quality Assurance . . . . Judy Marshall
Chief of Medical Staff. . . . . Frank Orth
Infection Control. . . . . Barbara Shaw

Measure	Cases	This Hosp.	State Avg.	U.S. Avg.
Blood Clot Prevention and Treatment				
Anticoagulation Overlap Therapy[2]	103	97%	93%	93%
ICU Venous Thromboembolism Prophylaxis[2]	40	98%	93%	92%
Incidence of Potentially Preventable VTE[2]	18	17%	6%	10%
UFH with Dosages/Platelet Monitoring[2]	87	100%	98%	97%
Venous Thromboembolism Prophylaxis[2]	328	75%	88%	85%
Warfarin Therapy Discharge Instructions[2]	73	66%	79%	75%
Chest Pain/Possible Heart Attack Care				
Aspirin Given Within 24 Hours of Arrival[1]	-	-	97%	96%
Fibrinolytic Meds Within 30 Min. of Arrival[7]	-	-	44%	58%
Average Time to ECG (minutes)[1]	-	-	6	7
Average Time to Transfer (minutes)[7]	-	-	58	60
Children's Asthma Care				
Received Home Management Plan of Care	-	-	85%	88%
Received Reliever Medication	-	-	100%	100%
Received Systemic Corticosteroids	-	-	100%	100%
Emergency Department				
Admittance Decision Time (minutes)[2]	314	87	90	98
Head CT Results Within 45 Min. of Arrival	16	50%	63%	57%
Patients Who Left ER Before Being Seen	35,332	1%	2%	2%
Time from ER Arrival to Admit. (minutes)[2]	314	266	265	274
Time from ER Arrival to Discharge (minutes)	355	165	128	134
Time in ER Before Being Evaluated (minutes)	388	18	22	26
Time to Pain Meds for Fractures (minutes)	102	62	54	57
Heart Attack Care				
Aspirin Given at Discharge	169	98%	99%	99%
Fibrinolytic Meds Within 30 Min. of Arrival[7]	-	-	80%	54%
PCI Within 90 Minutes of Arrival	42	98%	97%	96%
Statin Prescribed at Discharge	161	96%	98%	98%
Heart Failure Care				
ACE Inhibitor or ARB for LVSD[2]	78	100%	97%	97%
Discharge Instructions Given[2]	196	97%	96%	94%
Evaluation of LVS Function[2]	265	100%	100%	99%
Medicare Spending				
Medicare Spending per Patient (ratio)	-	1.02	1.01	0.98
Pneumonia Care				
Appropriate Initial Antibiotic Given[2]	100	96%	96%	95%
Blood Culture Timing[2]	128	98%	98%	98%
Pregnancy and Delivery Care				
Newborn Deliveries Scheduled Early[2]	93	4%	5%	6%
Preventive Care				
Immunization for Influenza[2]	462	90%	93%	90%
Immunization for Pneumonia[2]	444	80%	94%	92%
Stroke Care				
Anticoagulation Therapy for Atrial Fibrillation[1,2]	-	-	95%	95%
Antithrombotic Therapy Timing[2]	63	95%	98%	98%
Assessed for Rehabilitation[2]	78	96%	98%	97%
Discharged on Antithrombotic Therapy[2]	75	99%	99%	99%
Discharged on Statin Medication[2]	57	95%	95%	94%
Thrombolytic Therapy Timing[1,2]	-	-	65%	66%
Venous Thromboembolism Prophylaxis[2]	72	85%	95%	94%
Written Stroke Educational Materials Given[2]	44	84%	92%	88%
Surgical Care Improvement Project				
Appropriate Beta Blocker Usage[2]	179	99%	98%	98%
Appropriate VTP Within 24 Hours[2]	321	97%	98%	98%
Controlled Postoperative Blood Glucose[2,7]	-	-	97%	97%
Perioperative Temperature Management[2]	488	100%	100%	100%
Prophylactic Antibiotic Selection[2]	333	99%	99%	99%
Prophylactic Antibiotic Selection (Outpatient)	281	99%	98%	98%
Prophylactic Antibiotic Stopped[2]	323	96%	98%	98%
Prophylactic Antibiotic Timing[2]	335	100%	99%	99%
Prophylactic Antibiotic Timing (Outpatient)	283	99%	97%	98%
Urinary Catheter Removal[2]	293	95%	97%	97%
Survey of Patients' Hospital Experiences				
Area Around Room 'Always' Quiet at Night	300+	54%	58%	61%
Doctors 'Always' Communicated Well	300+	76%	80%	82%
Home Recovery Information Given	300+	87%	87%	85%
Hospital Given 9 or 10 on 10 Point Scale	300+	69%	72%	71%
Meds 'Always' Explained Before Given	300+	56%	64%	64%
Nurses 'Always' Communicated Well	300+	75%	81%	79%
Pain 'Always' Well Controlled	300+	68%	71%	71%
Room and Bathroom 'Always' Clean	300+	65%	75%	73%
Timely Help 'Always' Received	300+	60%	70%	68%
Would Definitely Recommend Hospital	300+	70%	71%	71%
Use of Medical Imaging				
Cardiac Imaging Stress Test before Surgery	421	5.7%	5.4%	5.3%
Combination Abdominal CT Scan	743	3.2%	7.1%	10.5%
Combination Brain/Sinus CT Scan	715	3.4%	2.8%	2.7%
Combination Chest CT Scan	265	0.8%	1.7%	2.7%
Follow-up Mammogram/Ultrasound	1,312	5.6%	8.7%	8.8%
Lumbar Spine MRI for Low Back Pain	55	49.1%	34.7%	37.2%

Saint John Medical Center

29000 Center Ridge Road
Westlake, OH 44145
Phone: 440-835-8000
Fax: 440-827-5283
URL: www.sjws.net
Type: Acute Care Hospitals
Emergency Services: Yes
Ownership: Voluntary non-profit - Private
Beds: 200

Key Personnel:
Emergency Room . . . . Leslie Bush
Pediatric Ambulatory Care . . . . . . Ararind DePauly
Pediatric In-Patient Care . . . . Ararind DePauly
Cardiac Laboratory. . . . . Naim Farhat, MD
Radiology. . . . . Robert Konstan, MD
Operating Room. . . . . Adnan Mourany
Chief of Medical Staff . . . . James Myers, MD
President/CEO. . . . . William A. Young, Jr

Measure	Cases	This Hosp.	State Avg.	U.S. Avg.
Blood Clot Prevention and Treatment				
Anticoagulation Overlap Therapy[2]	71	87%	93%	93%
ICU Venous Thromboembolism Prophylaxis[2]	92	93%	93%	92%
Incidence of Potentially Preventable VTE[1,2]	-	-	6%	10%
UFH with Dosages/Platelet Monitoring[2]	34	100%	98%	97%
Venous Thromboembolism Prophylaxis[2]	288	85%	88%	85%
Warfarin Therapy Discharge Instructions[2]	42	76%	79%	75%
Chest Pain/Possible Heart Attack Care				
Aspirin Given Within 24 Hours of Arrival[1]	-	-	97%	96%
Fibrinolytic Meds Within 30 Min. of Arrival[3,7]	-	-	44%	58%
Average Time to ECG (minutes)[1]	-	-	6	7
Average Time to Transfer (minutes)[3,7]	-	-	58	60
Children's Asthma Care				
Received Home Management Plan of Care	34	62%	85%	88%
Received Reliever Medication	35	100%	100%	100%
Received Systemic Corticosteroids	35	100%	100%	100%
Emergency Department				
Admittance Decision Time (minutes)[2]	721	101	90	98
Head CT Results Within 45 Min. of Arrival	16	75%	63%	57%

NOTE: Hospital profiles are in alphabetical order by state, then city, then hospital within the city; Rankings exclude hospitals with less than 25 cases except for patient surveys which excludes hospitals with less than 100 cases; (a) 100-299 cases; (1) The number of cases/patients is too few to report; (2) Data submitted were based on a sample of cases/patients; (3) Results are based on a shorter time period than required; (4) Data suppressed by CMS for one or more quarters; (5) Results are not available for this reporting period; (6) Fewer than 100 patients completed the HCAHPS survey; (7) No cases met the criteria for this measure; (8) The lower limit of the confidence interval cannot be calculated if the number of observed infections equals zero; (9) No data are available from the state/territory for this reporting period; (10) The scores shown reflect fewer than 50 completed surveys; (11) There were discrepancies in the data collection process; (12) This measure does not apply to this hospital for this reporting period; (13) Results cannot be calculated for this reporting period; (14) The results for this state are combined with nearby states to protect confidentiality; Please refer to the User's Guide for a full explanation of data.

Patients Who Left ER Before Being Seen	37,893	1%	2%	2%
Time from ER Arrival to Admit. (minutes)[2]	766	256	265	274
Time from ER Arrival to Discharge (minutes)	356	136	128	134
Time in ER Before Being Evaluated (minutes)	404	17	22	26
Time to Pain Meds for Fractures (minutes)	133	54	54	57
Heart Attack Care				
Aspirin Given at Discharge[2]	227	100%	99%	99%
Fibrinolytic Meds Within 30 Min. of Arrival[2,7]	-	-	80%	54%
PCI Within 90 Minutes of Arrival[2]	38	100%	97%	96%
Statin Prescribed at Discharge[2]	219	100%	98%	98%
Heart Failure Care				
ACE Inhibitor or ARB for LVSD[2]	62	97%	97%	97%
Discharge Instructions Given[2]	190	87%	96%	94%
Evaluation of LVS Function[2]	268	99%	100%	99%
Medicare Spending				
Medicare Spending per Patient (ratio)	-	1.02	1.01	0.98
Pneumonia Care				
Appropriate Initial Antibiotic Given[2]	77	99%	96%	95%
Blood Culture Timing[2]	169	100%	98%	98%
Pregnancy and Delivery Care				
Newborn Deliveries Scheduled Early[2]	28	4%	5%	6%
Preventive Care				
Immunization for Influenza[2]	575	85%	93%	90%
Immunization for Pneumonia[2]	768	89%	94%	92%
Stroke Care				
Anticoagulation Therapy for Atrial Fibrillation[2]	18	100%	95%	95%
Antithrombotic Therapy Timing[2]	104	100%	98%	98%
Assessed for Rehabilitation[2]	110	100%	98%	97%
Discharged on Antithrombotic Therapy[2]	103	100%	99%	99%
Discharged on Statin Medication[2]	83	99%	95%	94%
Thrombolytic Therapy Timing[1,2]	-	-	65%	66%
Venous Thromboembolism Prophylaxis[2]	105	98%	95%	94%
Written Stroke Educational Materials Given[2]	61	95%	92%	88%
Surgical Care Improvement Project				
Appropriate Beta Blocker Usage[2]	162	99%	98%	98%
Appropriate VTP Within 24 Hours[2]	411	99%	98%	98%
Controlled Postoperative Blood Glucose[2]	33	100%	97%	97%
Perioperative Temperature Management[2]	440	100%	100%	100%
Prophylactic Antibiotic Selection[2]	297	96%	99%	99%
Prophylactic Antibiotic Selection (Outpatient)	256	98%	98%	98%
Prophylactic Antibiotic Stopped[2]	288	98%	98%	98%
Prophylactic Antibiotic Timing[2]	298	98%	99%	99%
Prophylactic Antibiotic Timing (Outpatient)	258	99%	97%	98%
Urinary Catheter Removal[2]	339	99%	97%	97%
Survey of Patients' Hospital Experiences				
Area Around Room 'Always' Quiet at Night	300+	54%	58%	61%
Doctors 'Always' Communicated Well	300+	75%	80%	82%
Home Recovery Information Given	300+	86%	87%	85%
Hospital Given 9 or 10 on 10 Point Scale	300+	72%	72%	71%
Meds 'Always' Explained Before Given	300+	61%	64%	64%
Nurses 'Always' Communicated Well	300+	77%	81%	79%
Pain 'Always' Well Controlled	300+	68%	71%	71%
Room and Bathroom 'Always' Clean	300+	68%	75%	73%
Timely Help 'Always' Received	300+	63%	70%	68%
Would Definitely Recommend Hospital	300+	73%	71%	71%
Use of Medical Imaging				
Cardiac Imaging Stress Test before Surgery	88	8.0%	5.4%	5.3%
Combination Abdominal CT Scan	624	7.9%	7.1%	10.5%
Combination Brain/Sinus CT Scan	670	3.9%	2.8%	2.7%
Combination Chest CT Scan	451	0.7%	1.7%	2.7%
Follow-up Mammogram/Ultrasound	602	11.6%	8.7%	8.8%
Lumbar Spine MRI for Low Back Pain[1]	-	-	34.7%	37.2%

Mercy Willard Hospital

1100 Neal Zick Road
Willard, OH 44890
Phone: 419-964-5000
URL: www.mercyweb.org/mercy_willard.aspx
Type: Critical Access Hospitals
Emergency Services: Yes
Ownership: Voluntary non-profit - Other
Beds: 25
Key Personnel:
CEO/President. . . . . Lynn Detterman

Measure	Cases	This Hosp.	State Avg.	U.S. Avg.
Blood Clot Prevention and Treatment				
Anticoagulation Overlap Therapy[1,2]	-	-	93%	93%
ICU Venous Thromboembolism Prophylaxis[2,7]	-	-	93%	92%
Incidence of Potentially Preventable VTE[2,7]	-	-	6%	10%
UFH with Dosages/Platelet Monitoring[2,7]	-	-	98%	97%
Venous Thromboembolism Prophylaxis[2]	94	94%	88%	85%
Warfarin Therapy Discharge Instructions[1,2]	-	-	79%	75%
Chest Pain/Possible Heart Attack Care				
Aspirin Given Within 24 Hours of Arrival[5]	-	-	97%	96%
Fibrinolytic Meds Within 30 Min. of Arrival[5]	-	-	44%	58%
Average Time to ECG (minutes)[5]	-	-	6	7
Average Time to Transfer (minutes)[5]	-	-	58	60
Children's Asthma Care				
Received Home Management Plan of Care	-	-	85%	88%
Received Reliever Medication	-	-	100%	100%
Received Systemic Corticosteroids	-	-	100%	100%
Emergency Department				
Admittance Decision Time (minutes)[2]	402	35	90	98
Head CT Results Within 45 Min. of Arrival[5]	-	-	63%	57%
Patients Who Left ER Before Being Seen[5]	-	-	2%	2%
Time from ER Arrival to Admit. (minutes)[2]	433	211	265	274
Time from ER Arrival to Discharge (minutes)[5]	-	-	128	134
Time in ER Before Being Evaluated (minutes)[5]	-	-	22	26
Time to Pain Meds for Fractures (minutes)[5]	-	-	54	57
Heart Attack Care				
Aspirin Given at Discharge[1,3]	-	-	99%	99%
Fibrinolytic Meds Within 30 Min. of Arrival[3,7]	-	-	80%	54%
PCI Within 90 Minutes of Arrival[3,7]	-	-	97%	96%
Statin Prescribed at Discharge[3,7]	-	-	98%	98%
Heart Failure Care				
ACE Inhibitor or ARB for LVSD[1]	-	-	97%	97%
Discharge Instructions Given	13	92%	96%	94%
Evaluation of LVS Function	23	91%	100%	99%
Medicare Spending				
Medicare Spending per Patient (ratio)	-	-	1.01	0.98
Pneumonia Care				
Appropriate Initial Antibiotic Given	32	88%	96%	95%
Blood Culture Timing	36	97%	98%	98%
Pregnancy and Delivery Care				
Newborn Deliveries Scheduled Early[3,7]	-	-	5%	6%
Preventive Care				
Immunization for Influenza[2]	273	90%	93%	90%
Immunization for Pneumonia[2]	434	91%	94%	92%
Stroke Care				
Anticoagulation Therapy for Atrial Fibrillation[1,3]	-	-	95%	95%
Antithrombotic Therapy Timing[3,7]	-	-	98%	98%
Assessed for Rehabilitation[1,3]	-	-	98%	97%
Discharged on Antithrombotic Therapy[1,3]	-	-	99%	99%
Discharged on Statin Medication[1,3]	-	-	95%	94%
Thrombolytic Therapy Timing[1,3]	-	-	65%	66%
Venous Thromboembolism Prophylaxis[1,3]	-	-	95%	94%
Written Stroke Educational Materials Given[3,7]	-	-	92%	88%
Surgical Care Improvement Project				
Appropriate Beta Blocker Usage	22	100%	98%	98%
Appropriate VTP Within 24 Hours	62	100%	98%	98%
Controlled Postoperative Blood Glucose[7]	-	-	97%	97%
Perioperative Temperature Management	62	100%	100%	100%
Prophylactic Antibiotic Selection	46	91%	99%	99%
Prophylactic Antibiotic Selection (Outpatient)[5]	-	-	98%	98%
Prophylactic Antibiotic Stopped	46	100%	98%	98%
Prophylactic Antibiotic Timing	46	96%	99%	99%
Prophylactic Antibiotic Timing (Outpatient)[5]	-	-	97%	98%
Urinary Catheter Removal	44	93%	97%	97%
Survey of Patients' Hospital Experiences				
Area Around Room 'Always' Quiet at Night	(a)	74%	58%	61%
Doctors 'Always' Communicated Well	(a)	90%	80%	82%
Home Recovery Information Given	(a)	88%	87%	85%
Hospital Given 9 or 10 on 10 Point Scale	(a)	87%	72%	71%
Meds 'Always' Explained Before Given	(a)	64%	64%	64%
Nurses 'Always' Communicated Well	(a)	89%	81%	79%
Pain 'Always' Well Controlled	(a)	82%	71%	71%
Room and Bathroom 'Always' Clean	(a)	88%	75%	73%
Timely Help 'Always' Received	(a)	81%	70%	68%
Would Definitely Recommend Hospital	(a)	83%	71%	71%
Use of Medical Imaging				
Cardiac Imaging Stress Test before Surgery	144	4.2%	5.4%	5.3%
Combination Abdominal CT Scan	187	3.7%	7.1%	10.5%
Combination Brain/Sinus CT Scan	176	0.6%	2.8%	2.7%
Combination Chest CT Scan	138	2.2%	1.7%	2.7%
Follow-up Mammogram/Ultrasound	281	19.9%	8.7%	8.8%
Lumbar Spine MRI for Low Back Pain[1]	-	-	34.7%	37.2%

Clinton Memorial Hospital

610 West Main Street
Wilmington, OH 45177
Phone: 937-382-6611
Fax: 937-382-9278
E-mail: clintonmemorialhospital@in-touch.net
Type: Acute Care Hospitals
Emergency Services: Yes
Ownership: Government - Local
Beds: 150
Key Personnel:
Radiology. Richard L Conti
CEO/President. . . . . Tim Crowley
Chairman/CEO . . . . Marcy Hawley
Chief of Medical Staff. . . . . Dr. Rajiv Patel

Measure	Cases	This Hosp.	State Avg.	U.S. Avg.
Blood Clot Prevention and Treatment				
Anticoagulation Overlap Therapy[2]	26	100%	93%	93%
ICU Venous Thromboembolism Prophylaxis[2]	47	98%	93%	92%
Incidence of Potentially Preventable VTE[1,2]	-	-	6%	10%
UFH with Dosages/Platelet Monitoring[1,2]	-	-	98%	97%
Venous Thromboembolism Prophylaxis[2]	243	87%	88%	85%
Warfarin Therapy Discharge Instructions[2]	21	67%	79%	75%
Chest Pain/Possible Heart Attack Care				
Aspirin Given Within 24 Hours of Arrival	80	100%	97%	96%
Fibrinolytic Meds Within 30 Min. of Arrival[1]	-	-	44%	58%
Average Time to ECG (minutes)	82	6	6	7
Average Time to Transfer (minutes)[1]	-	-	58	60
Children's Asthma Care				
Received Home Management Plan of Care	-	-	85%	88%
Received Reliever Medication	-	-	100%	100%
Received Systemic Corticosteroids	-	-	100%	100%
Emergency Department				
Admittance Decision Time (minutes)[2]	674	90	90	98
Head CT Results Within 45 Min. of Arrival	11	64%	63%	57%
Patients Who Left ER Before Being Seen	33,630	2%	2%	2%
Time from ER Arrival to Admit. (minutes)[2]	674	231	265	274
Time from ER Arrival to Discharge (minutes)	351	111	128	134
Time in ER Before Being Evaluated (minutes)	397	19	22	26
Time to Pain Meds for Fractures (minutes)	116	65	54	57
Heart Attack Care				
Aspirin Given at Discharge[1]	-	-	99%	99%
Fibrinolytic Meds Within 30 Min. of Arrival[7]	-	-	80%	54%
PCI Within 90 Minutes of Arrival[7]	-	-	97%	96%
Statin Prescribed at Discharge[1]	-	-	98%	98%
Heart Failure Care				
ACE Inhibitor or ARB for LVSD	28	96%	97%	97%
Discharge Instructions Given	93	90%	96%	94%
Evaluation of LVS Function	112	98%	100%	99%
Medicare Spending				
Medicare Spending per Patient (ratio)	-	0.94	1.01	0.98
Pneumonia Care				
Appropriate Initial Antibiotic Given	74	97%	96%	95%
Blood Culture Timing	124	98%	98%	98%
Pregnancy and Delivery Care				
Newborn Deliveries Scheduled Early	52	0%	5%	6%
Preventive Care				
Immunization for Influenza[2]	599	86%	93%	90%
Immunization for Pneumonia[2]	691	89%	94%	92%
Stroke Care				
Anticoagulation Therapy for Atrial Fibrillation[1]	-	-	95%	95%
Antithrombotic Therapy Timing	31	100%	98%	98%
Assessed for Rehabilitation	30	100%	98%	97%
Discharged on Antithrombotic Therapy	30	100%	99%	99%
Discharged on Statin Medication	22	100%	95%	94%
Thrombolytic Therapy Timing[1]	-	-	65%	66%
Venous Thromboembolism Prophylaxis	28	96%	95%	94%
Written Stroke Educational Materials Given	15	67%	92%	88%

NOTE: Hospital profiles are in alphabetical order by state, then city, then hospital within the city; Rankings exclude hospitals with less than 25 cases except for patient surveys which excludes hospitals with less than 100 cases; (a) 100-299 cases; (1) The number of cases/patients is too few to report; (2) Data submitted were based on a sample of cases/patients; (3) Results are based on a shorter time period than required; (4) Data suppressed by CMS for one or more quarters; (5) Results are not available for this reporting period; (6) Fewer than 100 patients completed the HCAHPS survey; (7) No cases met the criteria for this measure; (8) The lower limit of the confidence interval cannot be calculated if the number of observed infections equals zero; (9) No data are available from the state/territory for this reporting period; (10) The scores shown reflect fewer than 50 completed surveys; (11) There were discrepancies in the data collection process; (12) This measure does not apply to this hospital for this reporting period; (13) Results cannot be calculated for this reporting period; (14) The results for this state are combined with nearby states to protect confidentiality; Please refer to the User's Guide for a full explanation of data.

Measure	Cases	This Hosp.	State Avg.	U.S. Avg.
Surgical Care Improvement Project				
Appropriate Beta Blocker Usage	46	96%	98%	98%
Appropriate VTP Within 24 Hours	124	93%	98%	98%
Controlled Postoperative Blood Glucose[7]	-	-	97%	97%
Perioperative Temperature Management	149	100%	100%	100%
Prophylactic Antibiotic Selection	69	99%	99%	99%
Prophylactic Antibiotic Selection (Outpatient)	100	89%	98%	98%
Prophylactic Antibiotic Stopped	66	92%	98%	98%
Prophylactic Antibiotic Timing	72	100%	99%	99%
Prophylactic Antibiotic Timing (Outpatient)	103	97%	97%	98%
Urinary Catheter Removal	102	96%	97%	97%
Survey of Patients' Hospital Experiences				
Area Around Room 'Always' Quiet at Night	300+	58%	58%	61%
Doctors 'Always' Communicated Well	300+	78%	80%	82%
Home Recovery Information Given	300+	85%	87%	85%
Hospital Given 9 or 10 on 10 Point Scale	300+	60%	72%	71%
Meds 'Always' Explained Before Given	300+	56%	64%	64%
Nurses 'Always' Communicated Well	300+	75%	81%	79%
Pain 'Always' Well Controlled	300+	65%	71%	71%
Room and Bathroom 'Always' Clean	300+	76%	75%	73%
Timely Help 'Always' Received	300+	58%	70%	68%
Would Definitely Recommend Hospital	300+	60%	71%	71%
Use of Medical Imaging				
Cardiac Imaging Stress Test before Surgery	229	5.7%	5.4%	5.3%
Combination Abdominal CT Scan	545	12.8%	7.1%	10.5%
Combination Brain/Sinus CT Scan[1]	-	-	2.8%	2.7%
Combination Chest CT Scan	320	7.5%	1.7%	2.7%
Follow-up Mammogram/Ultrasound	835	5.6%	8.7%	8.8%
Lumbar Spine MRI for Low Back Pain	108	39.8%	34.7%	37.2%

Wooster Community Hospital

1761 Beall Avenue
Wooster, OH 44691
Phone: 330-263-8100
Fax: 330-263-8497
URL: www.woosterhospital.org
Type: Acute Care Hospitals
Emergency Services: Yes
Ownership: Government - Local
Beds: 130

Key Personnel:
Radiology.................. Brian A Aronson
Cardiac Laboratory............ Joel Chupp
Emergency Room .... William Elliott, MD
Chief of Medical Staff.......... Timothy Playl
CEO/President............... Bill Sheron
Quality Assurance .... Kathy Sisseroim

Measure	Cases	This Hosp.	State Avg.	U.S. Avg.
Blood Clot Prevention and Treatment				
Anticoagulation Overlap Therapy[2]	47	96%	93%	93%
ICU Venous Thromboembolism Prophylaxis[2]	51	96%	93%	92%
Incidence of Potentially Preventable VTE[1,2]	-	-	6%	10%
UFH with Dosages/Platelet Monitoring[2]	38	100%	98%	97%
Venous Thromboembolism Prophylaxis[2]	297	89%	88%	85%
Warfarin Therapy Discharge Instructions[2]	36	47%	79%	75%
Chest Pain/Possible Heart Attack Care				
Aspirin Given Within 24 Hours of Arrival	222	100%	97%	96%
Fibrinolytic Meds Within 30 Min. of Arrival[7]	-	-	44%	58%
Average Time to ECG (minutes)	229	5	6	7
Average Time to Transfer (minutes)	30	30	58	60
Children's Asthma Care				
Received Home Management Plan of Care	-	-	85%	88%
Received Reliever Medication	-	-	100%	100%
Received Systemic Corticosteroids	-	-	100%	100%
Emergency Department				
Admittance Decision Time (minutes)[2]	485	70	90	98
Head CT Results Within 45 Min. of Arrival	16	75%	63%	57%
Patients Who Left ER Before Being Seen	33,064	1%	2%	2%
Time from ER Arrival to Admit. (minutes)[2]	491	221	265	274
Time from ER Arrival to Discharge (minutes)	371	116	128	134
Time in ER Before Being Evaluated (minutes)	416	12	22	26
Time to Pain Meds for Fractures (minutes)	143	41	54	57
Heart Attack Care				
Aspirin Given at Discharge	19	89%	99%	99%
Fibrinolytic Meds Within 30 Min. of Arrival[7]	-	-	80%	54%
PCI Within 90 Minutes of Arrival[7]	-	-	97%	96%
Statin Prescribed at Discharge	17	88%	98%	98%
Heart Failure Care				
ACE Inhibitor or ARB for LVSD	43	93%	97%	97%
Discharge Instructions Given	120	93%	96%	94%
Evaluation of LVS Function	155	99%	100%	99%
Medicare Spending				
Medicare Spending per Patient (ratio)	-	0.95	1.01	0.98
Pneumonia Care				
Appropriate Initial Antibiotic Given	122	98%	96%	95%
Blood Culture Timing	189	97%	98%	98%
Pregnancy and Delivery Care				
Newborn Deliveries Scheduled Early[2]	35	3%	5%	6%
Preventive Care				
Immunization for Influenza[2]	480	98%	93%	90%
Immunization for Pneumonia[2]	578	96%	94%	92%
Stroke Care				
Anticoagulation Therapy for Atrial Fibrillation	13	92%	95%	95%
Antithrombotic Therapy Timing	62	100%	98%	98%
Assessed for Rehabilitation	63	98%	98%	97%
Discharged on Antithrombotic Therapy	62	100%	99%	99%
Discharged on Statin Medication	52	96%	95%	94%
Thrombolytic Therapy Timing[1]	-	-	65%	66%
Venous Thromboembolism Prophylaxis	63	98%	95%	94%
Written Stroke Educational Materials Given	28	100%	92%	88%
Surgical Care Improvement Project				
Appropriate Beta Blocker Usage	139	96%	98%	98%
Appropriate VTP Within 24 Hours	376	98%	98%	98%
Controlled Postoperative Blood Glucose[7]	-	-	97%	97%
Perioperative Temperature Management	434	100%	100%	100%
Prophylactic Antibiotic Selection	336	99%	99%	99%
Prophylactic Antibiotic Selection (Outpatient)	211	97%	98%	98%
Prophylactic Antibiotic Stopped	333	99%	98%	98%
Prophylactic Antibiotic Timing	337	98%	99%	99%
Prophylactic Antibiotic Timing (Outpatient)	212	98%	97%	98%
Urinary Catheter Removal	56	93%	97%	97%
Survey of Patients' Hospital Experiences				
Area Around Room 'Always' Quiet at Night	300+	65%	58%	61%
Doctors 'Always' Communicated Well	300+	81%	80%	82%
Home Recovery Information Given	300+	89%	87%	85%
Hospital Given 9 or 10 on 10 Point Scale	300+	79%	72%	71%
Meds 'Always' Explained Before Given	300+	65%	64%	64%
Nurses 'Always' Communicated Well	300+	82%	81%	79%
Pain 'Always' Well Controlled	300+	73%	71%	71%
Room and Bathroom 'Always' Clean	300+	79%	75%	73%
Timely Help 'Always' Received	300+	72%	70%	68%
Would Definitely Recommend Hospital	300+	79%	71%	71%
Use of Medical Imaging				
Cardiac Imaging Stress Test before Surgery	388	6.2%	5.4%	5.3%
Combination Abdominal CT Scan	511	1.4%	7.1%	10.5%
Combination Brain/Sinus CT Scan	523	1.7%	2.8%	2.7%
Combination Chest CT Scan	390	0.0%	1.7%	2.7%
Follow-up Mammogram/Ultrasound	659	5.5%	8.7%	8.8%
Lumbar Spine MRI for Low Back Pain[1]	-	-	34.7%	37.2%

Greene Memorial Hospital

1141 North Monroe Drive
Xenia, OH 45385
Phone: 937-352-2000
Fax: 937-376-6983
URL: www.ketteringhealth.org/greene
Type: Acute Care Hospitals
Emergency Services: Yes
Ownership: Voluntary non-profit - Private
Beds: 231

Key Personnel:
Radiology..................... David Brown, MD
Quality Assurance .... Sheila Harris
Operating Room............... Bonnie Hoagland, RN
Chief of Medical Staff.......... Craig Hurak
CEO/President............... Fred Manchur
Emergency Room .... Shanda Zaharako

Measure	Cases	This Hosp.	State Avg.	U.S. Avg.
Blood Clot Prevention and Treatment				
Anticoagulation Overlap Therapy[2]	19	100%	93%	93%
ICU Venous Thromboembolism Prophylaxis[2]	55	100%	93%	92%
Incidence of Potentially Preventable VTE[1,2]	-	-	6%	10%
UFH with Dosages/Platelet Monitoring[1,2]	-	-	98%	97%
Venous Thromboembolism Prophylaxis[2]	264	98%	88%	85%
Warfarin Therapy Discharge Instructions[1,2]	-	-	79%	75%
Chest Pain/Possible Heart Attack Care				
Aspirin Given Within 24 Hours of Arrival	17	100%	97%	96%
Fibrinolytic Meds Within 30 Min. of Arrival[7]	-	-	44%	58%
Average Time to ECG (minutes)	17	5	6	7
Average Time to Transfer (minutes)[1]	-	-	58	60
Children's Asthma Care				
Received Home Management Plan of Care	-	-	85%	88%
Received Reliever Medication	-	-	100%	100%
Received Systemic Corticosteroids	-	-	100%	100%
Emergency Department				
Admittance Decision Time (minutes)[2]	474	130	90	98
Head CT Results Within 45 Min. of Arrival[1]	-	-	63%	57%
Patients Who Left ER Before Being Seen	26,096	1%	2%	2%
Time from ER Arrival to Admit. (minutes)[2]	477	277	265	274
Time from ER Arrival to Discharge (minutes)	419	142	128	134
Time in ER Before Being Evaluated (minutes)	451	15	22	26
Time to Pain Meds for Fractures (minutes)	47	65	54	57
Heart Attack Care				
Aspirin Given at Discharge	14	100%	99%	99%
Fibrinolytic Meds Within 30 Min. of Arrival[7]	-	-	80%	54%
PCI Within 90 Minutes of Arrival[7]	-	-	97%	96%
Statin Prescribed at Discharge	11	100%	98%	98%
Heart Failure Care				
ACE Inhibitor or ARB for LVSD	33	100%	97%	97%
Discharge Instructions Given	113	99%	96%	94%
Evaluation of LVS Function	137	100%	100%	99%
Medicare Spending				
Medicare Spending per Patient (ratio)	-	0.97	1.01	0.98
Pneumonia Care				
Appropriate Initial Antibiotic Given	93	100%	96%	95%
Blood Culture Timing	131	100%	98%	98%
Pregnancy and Delivery Care				
Newborn Deliveries Scheduled Early[7]	-	-	5%	6%
Preventive Care				
Immunization for Influenza[2]	329	98%	93%	90%
Immunization for Pneumonia[2]	493	98%	94%	92%
Stroke Care				
Anticoagulation Therapy for Atrial Fibrillation[1]	-	-	95%	95%
Antithrombotic Therapy Timing	32	100%	98%	98%
Assessed for Rehabilitation	34	100%	98%	97%
Discharged on Antithrombotic Therapy	32	100%	99%	99%
Discharged on Statin Medication	19	100%	95%	94%
Thrombolytic Therapy Timing[7]	-	-	65%	66%
Venous Thromboembolism Prophylaxis	34	100%	95%	94%
Written Stroke Educational Materials Given	18	100%	92%	88%
Surgical Care Improvement Project				
Appropriate Beta Blocker Usage	39	100%	98%	98%
Appropriate VTP Within 24 Hours	112	99%	98%	98%
Controlled Postoperative Blood Glucose[7]	-	-	97%	97%
Perioperative Temperature Management	117	100%	100%	100%
Prophylactic Antibiotic Selection	75	100%	99%	99%
Prophylactic Antibiotic Selection (Outpatient)[1,3]	-	-	98%	98%
Prophylactic Antibiotic Stopped	74	99%	98%	98%
Prophylactic Antibiotic Timing	75	99%	99%	99%
Prophylactic Antibiotic Timing (Outpatient)[1,3]	-	-	97%	98%
Urinary Catheter Removal	101	98%	97%	97%
Survey of Patients' Hospital Experiences				
Area Around Room 'Always' Quiet at Night	300+	53%	58%	61%
Doctors 'Always' Communicated Well	300+	74%	80%	82%
Home Recovery Information Given	300+	84%	87%	85%
Hospital Given 9 or 10 on 10 Point Scale	300+	63%	72%	71%
Meds 'Always' Explained Before Given	300+	59%	64%	64%
Nurses 'Always' Communicated Well	300+	78%	81%	79%
Pain 'Always' Well Controlled	300+	65%	71%	71%
Room and Bathroom 'Always' Clean	300+	71%	75%	73%
Timely Help 'Always' Received	300+	61%	70%	68%
Would Definitely Recommend Hospital	300+	62%	71%	71%
Use of Medical Imaging				
Cardiac Imaging Stress Test before Surgery	122	3.3%	5.4%	5.3%
Combination Abdominal CT Scan	342	6.4%	7.1%	10.5%
Combination Brain/Sinus CT Scan[1]	-	-	2.8%	2.7%
Combination Chest CT Scan	139	2.9%	1.7%	2.7%
Follow-up Mammogram/Ultrasound	485	6.2%	8.7%	8.8%

NOTE: Hospital profiles are in alphabetical order by state, then city, then hospital within the city; Rankings exclude hospitals with less than 25 cases except for patient surveys which excludes hospitals with less than 100 cases; (a) 100-299 cases; (1) The number of cases/patients is too few to report; (2) Data submitted were based on a sample of cases/patients; (3) Results are based on a shorter time period than required; (4) Data suppressed by CMS for one or more quarters; (5) Results are not available for this reporting period; (6) Fewer than 100 patients completed the HCAHPS survey; (7) No cases met the criteria for this measure; (8) The lower limit of the confidence interval cannot be calculated if the number of observed infections equals zero; (9) No data are available from the state/territory for this reporting period; (10) The scores shown reflect fewer than 50 completed surveys; (11) There were discrepancies in the data collection process; (12) This measure does not apply to this hospital for this reporting period; (13) Results cannot be calculated for this reporting period; (14) The results for this state are combined with nearby states to protect confidentiality; Please refer to the User's Guide for a full explanation of data.

Measure	Cases	This Hosp.	State Avg.	U.S. Avg.
Lumbar Spine MRI for Low Back Pain[1]	-	-	34.7%	37.2%

Northside Medical Center

500 Gypsy Lane
Youngstown, OH 44501
Type: Acute Care Hospitals
Ownership: Proprietary
Phone: 330-884-1000
Fax: 330-884-3740
Emergency Services: Yes
Beds: 830

Key Personnel:

Patient Relations . . . . Marta Cimino
CEO/President. . . . . Kris Hoce
Operating Room. . . . . Sandy Johnson-Prater
Quality Assurance . . . . Mike am Keating
Anesthesiology. . . . . V Perni, MD
Chief of Medical Staff . . . . Robert Sinsheimer, MD
Emergency Room . . . . Craig Soltis, MD
Radiology. . . . . S Vibanker, MD

Measure	Cases	This Hosp.	State Avg.	U.S. Avg.
Blood Clot Prevention and Treatment				
Anticoagulation Overlap Therapy[2]	53	100%	93%	93%
ICU Venous Thromboembolism Prophylaxis[2]	91	97%	93%	92%
Incidence of Potentially Preventable VTE[2]	12	8%	6%	10%
UFH with Dosages/Platelet Monitoring[2]	43	100%	98%	97%
Venous Thromboembolism Prophylaxis[2]	415	90%	88%	85%
Warfarin Therapy Discharge Instructions[2]	37	97%	79%	75%
Chest Pain/Possible Heart Attack Care				
Aspirin Given Within 24 Hours of Arrival[1,3]	-	-	97%	96%
Fibrinolytic Meds Within 30 Min. of Arrival[3,7]	-	-	44%	58%
Average Time to ECG (minutes)[1,3]	-	-	6	7
Average Time to Transfer (minutes)[1,3]	-	-	58	60
Children's Asthma Care				
Received Home Management Plan of Care	-	-	85%	88%
Received Reliever Medication	-	-	100%	100%
Received Systemic Corticosteroids	-	-	100%	100%
Emergency Department				
Admittance Decision Time (minutes)[2]	691	130	90	98
Head CT Results Within 45 Min. of Arrival[1]	-	-	63%	57%
Patients Who Left ER Before Being Seen	30,448	1%	2%	2%
Time from ER Arrival to Admit. (minutes)[2]	693	315	265	274
Time from ER Arrival to Discharge (minutes)	381	131	128	134
Time in ER Before Being Evaluated (minutes)	421	16	22	26
Time to Pain Meds for Fractures (minutes)	67	48	54	57
Heart Attack Care				
Aspirin Given at Discharge	182	100%	99%	99%
Fibrinolytic Meds Within 30 Min. of Arrival[7]	-	-	80%	54%
PCI Within 90 Minutes of Arrival	16	94%	97%	96%
Statin Prescribed at Discharge	178	99%	98%	98%
Heart Failure Care				
ACE Inhibitor or ARB for LVSD	81	100%	97%	97%
Discharge Instructions Given	213	98%	96%	94%
Evaluation of LVS Function	291	100%	100%	99%
Medicare Spending				
Medicare Spending per Patient (ratio)	-	1.01	1.01	0.98
Pneumonia Care				
Appropriate Initial Antibiotic Given	114	98%	96%	95%
Blood Culture Timing	217	98%	98%	98%
Pregnancy and Delivery Care				
Newborn Deliveries Scheduled Early[2]	46	2%	5%	6%
Preventive Care				
Immunization for Influenza[2]	593	98%	93%	90%
Immunization for Pneumonia[2]	809	98%	94%	92%
Stroke Care				
Anticoagulation Therapy for Atrial Fibrillation[1]	-	-	95%	95%
Antithrombotic Therapy Timing	75	100%	98%	98%
Assessed for Rehabilitation	77	100%	98%	97%
Discharged on Antithrombotic Therapy	76	100%	99%	99%
Discharged on Statin Medication	66	98%	95%	94%
Thrombolytic Therapy Timing[1]	-	-	65%	66%
Venous Thromboembolism Prophylaxis	79	92%	95%	94%
Written Stroke Educational Materials Given	42	79%	92%	88%
Surgical Care Improvement Project				
Appropriate Beta Blocker Usage	279	99%	98%	98%
Appropriate VTP Within 24 Hours	648	98%	98%	98%
Controlled Postoperative Blood Glucose	74	95%	97%	97%
Perioperative Temperature Management	708	100%	100%	100%
Prophylactic Antibiotic Selection	621	99%	99%	99%
Prophylactic Antibiotic Selection (Outpatient)	142	100%	98%	98%
Prophylactic Antibiotic Stopped	610	98%	98%	98%
Prophylactic Antibiotic Timing	621	100%	99%	99%
Prophylactic Antibiotic Timing (Outpatient)	143	99%	97%	98%
Urinary Catheter Removal	344	97%	97%	97%
Survey of Patients' Hospital Experiences				
Area Around Room 'Always' Quiet at Night	300+	50%	58%	61%
Doctors 'Always' Communicated Well	300+	80%	80%	82%
Home Recovery Information Given	300+	86%	87%	85%
Hospital Given 9 or 10 on 10 Point Scale	300+	63%	72%	71%
Meds 'Always' Explained Before Given	300+	60%	64%	64%
Nurses 'Always' Communicated Well	300+	77%	81%	79%
Pain 'Always' Well Controlled	300+	67%	71%	71%
Room and Bathroom 'Always' Clean	300+	63%	75%	73%
Timely Help 'Always' Received	300+	61%	70%	68%
Would Definitely Recommend Hospital	300+	63%	71%	71%
Use of Medical Imaging				
Cardiac Imaging Stress Test before Surgery	164	7.3%	5.4%	5.3%
Combination Abdominal CT Scan	410	2.4%	7.1%	10.5%
Combination Brain/Sinus CT Scan[1]	-	-	2.8%	2.7%
Combination Chest CT Scan	207	0.0%	1.7%	2.7%
Follow-up Mammogram/Ultrasound	660	9.1%	8.7%	8.8%
Lumbar Spine MRI for Low Back Pain[1]	-	-	34.7%	37.2%

Saint Elizabeth Health Center

1044 Belmont Avenue
Youngstown, OH 44501
URL: www.hmhs.org
Type: Acute Care Hospitals
Ownership: Voluntary non-profit - Church
Phone: 330-746-7211
Fax: 330-480-2617
Emergency Services: Yes
Beds: 350

Key Personnel:

Chief of Medical Staff. . . . . Ken Heaps
Quality Assurance . . . . Mike Keating
Radiology. . . . . Ken Lavin
Coronary Care . . . . Lisa Parish
Pediatric Ambulatory Care . . . . . . Elenna Rossi, MD
Pediatric In-Patient Care . . . . Elenna Rossi, MD
CEO/President. . . . . Robert Shroder
Operating Room. . . . . Pat Stedman

Measure	Cases	This Hosp.	State Avg.	U.S. Avg.
Blood Clot Prevention and Treatment				
Anticoagulation Overlap Therapy[2]	123	80%	93%	93%
ICU Venous Thromboembolism Prophylaxis[2]	97	87%	93%	92%
Incidence of Potentially Preventable VTE[2]	34	3%	6%	10%
UFH with Dosages/Platelet Monitoring[2]	65	100%	98%	97%
Venous Thromboembolism Prophylaxis[2]	330	75%	88%	85%
Warfarin Therapy Discharge Instructions[2]	91	85%	79%	75%
Chest Pain/Possible Heart Attack Care				
Aspirin Given Within 24 Hours of Arrival[1,3]	-	-	97%	96%
Fibrinolytic Meds Within 30 Min. of Arrival[3,7]	-	-	44%	58%
Average Time to ECG (minutes)[1,3]	-	-	6	7
Average Time to Transfer (minutes)[3,7]	-	-	58	60
Children's Asthma Care				
Received Home Management Plan of Care	-	-	85%	88%
Received Reliever Medication	-	-	100%	100%
Received Systemic Corticosteroids	-	-	100%	100%
Emergency Department				
Admittance Decision Time (minutes)[2]	630	158	90	98
Head CT Results Within 45 Min. of Arrival[1]	-	-	63%	57%
Patients Who Left ER Before Being Seen	76,635	1%	2%	2%
Time from ER Arrival to Admit. (minutes)[2]	651	336	265	274
Time from ER Arrival to Discharge (minutes)	356	132	128	134
Time in ER Before Being Evaluated (minutes)	418	19	22	26
Time to Pain Meds for Fractures (minutes)	187	59	54	57
Heart Attack Care				
Aspirin Given at Discharge	537	99%	99%	99%
Fibrinolytic Meds Within 30 Min. of Arrival[7]	-	-	80%	54%
PCI Within 90 Minutes of Arrival	73	100%	97%	96%
Statin Prescribed at Discharge	534	97%	98%	98%
Heart Failure Care				
ACE Inhibitor or ARB for LVSD[2]	82	98%	97%	97%
Discharge Instructions Given[2]	229	100%	96%	94%
Evaluation of LVS Function[2]	293	100%	100%	99%
Medicare Spending				
Medicare Spending per Patient (ratio)	-	1.06	1.01	0.98
Pneumonia Care				
Appropriate Initial Antibiotic Given[2]	40	98%	96%	95%
Blood Culture Timing[2]	128	96%	98%	98%
Pregnancy and Delivery Care				
Newborn Deliveries Scheduled Early	150	1%	5%	6%
Preventive Care				
Immunization for Influenza[2]	577	85%	93%	90%
Immunization for Pneumonia[2]	768	85%	94%	92%
Stroke Care				
Anticoagulation Therapy for Atrial Fibrillation[2]	11	91%	95%	95%
Antithrombotic Therapy Timing[2]	101	91%	98%	98%
Assessed for Rehabilitation[2]	128	99%	98%	97%
Discharged on Antithrombotic Therapy[2]	105	97%	99%	99%
Discharged on Statin Medication[2]	88	93%	95%	94%
Thrombolytic Therapy Timing[1,2]	-	-	65%	66%
Venous Thromboembolism Prophylaxis[2]	125	91%	95%	94%
Written Stroke Educational Materials Given[2]	53	79%	92%	88%
Surgical Care Improvement Project				
Appropriate Beta Blocker Usage[2]	148	97%	98%	98%
Appropriate VTP Within 24 Hours[2]	382	97%	98%	98%
Controlled Postoperative Blood Glucose[2]	141	92%	97%	97%
Perioperative Temperature Management[2]	470	100%	100%	100%
Prophylactic Antibiotic Selection[2]	420	100%	99%	99%
Prophylactic Antibiotic Selection (Outpatient)	512	98%	98%	98%
Prophylactic Antibiotic Stopped[2]	410	98%	98%	98%
Prophylactic Antibiotic Timing[2]	421	99%	99%	99%
Prophylactic Antibiotic Timing (Outpatient)	514	97%	97%	98%
Urinary Catheter Removal[2]	347	93%	97%	97%
Survey of Patients' Hospital Experiences				
Area Around Room 'Always' Quiet at Night	300+	47%	58%	61%
Doctors 'Always' Communicated Well	300+	78%	80%	82%
Home Recovery Information Given	300+	81%	87%	85%
Hospital Given 9 or 10 on 10 Point Scale	300+	65%	72%	71%
Meds 'Always' Explained Before Given	300+	60%	64%	64%
Nurses 'Always' Communicated Well	300+	77%	81%	79%
Pain 'Always' Well Controlled	300+	68%	71%	71%
Room and Bathroom 'Always' Clean	300+	61%	75%	73%
Timely Help 'Always' Received	300+	62%	70%	68%
Would Definitely Recommend Hospital	300+	69%	71%	71%
Use of Medical Imaging				
Cardiac Imaging Stress Test before Surgery	1,187	4.8%	5.4%	5.3%
Combination Abdominal CT Scan	782	5.5%	7.1%	10.5%
Combination Brain/Sinus CT Scan	823	5.3%	2.8%	2.7%
Combination Chest CT Scan	412	7.3%	1.7%	2.7%
Follow-up Mammogram/Ultrasound	460	7.6%	8.7%	8.8%
Lumbar Spine MRI for Low Back Pain	54	38.9%	34.7%	37.2%

Surgical Hospital at Southwoods

7630 Southern Blvd
Youngstown, OH 44512
URL: www.surgeryatsouthwoods.com
Type: Acute Care Hospitals
Ownership: Voluntary non-profit - Private
Phone: 330-758-1954
Emergency Services: No

Measure	Cases	This Hosp.	State Avg.	U.S. Avg.
Blood Clot Prevention and Treatment				
Anticoagulation Overlap Therapy[1]	-	-	93%	93%
ICU Venous Thromboembolism Prophylaxis[7]	-	-	93%	92%
Incidence of Potentially Preventable VTE[1]	-	-	6%	10%
UFH with Dosages/Platelet Monitoring[1]	-	-	98%	97%
Venous Thromboembolism Prophylaxis	156	100%	88%	85%
Warfarin Therapy Discharge Instructions[1]	-	-	79%	75%
Chest Pain/Possible Heart Attack Care				
Aspirin Given Within 24 Hours of Arrival[5]	-	-	97%	96%
Fibrinolytic Meds Within 30 Min. of Arrival[5]	-	-	44%	58%
Average Time to ECG (minutes)[5]	-	-	6	7
Average Time to Transfer (minutes)[5]	-	-	58	60
Children's Asthma Care				
Received Home Management Plan of Care	-	-	85%	88%
Received Reliever Medication	-	-	100%	100%
Received Systemic Corticosteroids	-	-	100%	100%

NOTE: Hospital profiles are in alphabetical order by state, then city, then hospital within the city; Rankings exclude hospitals with less than 25 cases except for patient surveys which excludes hospitals with less than 100 cases; (a) 100-299 cases; (1) The number of cases/patients is too few to report; (2) Data submitted were based on a sample of cases/patients; (3) Results are based on a shorter time period than required; (4) Data suppressed by CMS for one or more quarters; (5) Results are not available for this reporting period; (6) Fewer than 100 patients completed the HCAHPS survey; (7) No cases met the criteria for this measure; (8) The lower limit of the confidence interval cannot be calculated if the number of observed infections equals zero; (9) No data are available from the state/territory for this reporting period; (10) The scores shown reflect fewer than 50 completed surveys; (11) There were discrepancies in the data collection process; (12) This measure does not apply to this hospital for this reporting period; (13) Results cannot be calculated for this reporting period; (14) The results for this state are combined with nearby states to protect confidentiality; Please refer to the User's Guide for a full explanation of data.

Emergency Department				
Admittance Decision Time (minutes)[7]	-	-	90	98
Head CT Results Within 45 Min. of Arrival[5]	-	-	63%	57%
Patients Who Left ER Before Being Seen[5]	-	-	2%	2%
Time from ER Arrival to Admit. (minutes)[7]	-	-	265	274
Time from ER Arrival to Discharge (minutes)[5]	-	-	128	134
Time in ER Before Being Evaluated (minutes)[5]	-	-	22	26
Time to Pain Meds for Fractures (minutes)[5]	-	-	54	57
Heart Attack Care				
Aspirin Given at Discharge[5]	-	-	99%	99%
Fibrinolytic Meds Within 30 Min. of Arrival[5]	-	-	80%	54%
PCI Within 90 Minutes of Arrival[5]	-	-	97%	96%
Statin Prescribed at Discharge[5]	-	-	98%	98%
Heart Failure Care				
ACE Inhibitor or ARB for LVSD[5]	-	-	97%	97%
Discharge Instructions Given[5]	-	-	96%	94%
Evaluation of LVS Function[5]	-	-	100%	99%
Medicare Spending				
Medicare Spending per Patient (ratio)	-	1.00	1.01	0.98
Pneumonia Care				
Appropriate Initial Antibiotic Given[5]	-	-	96%	95%
Blood Culture Timing[5]	-	-	98%	98%
Pregnancy and Delivery Care				
Newborn Deliveries Scheduled Early[7]	-	-	5%	6%
Preventive Care				
Immunization for Influenza	499	99%	93%	90%
Immunization for Pneumonia	502	99%	94%	92%
Stroke Care				
Anticoagulation Therapy for Atrial Fibrillation[5]	-	-	95%	95%
Antithrombotic Therapy Timing[5]	-	-	98%	98%
Assessed for Rehabilitation[5]	-	-	98%	97%
Discharged on Antithrombotic Therapy[5]	-	-	99%	99%
Discharged on Statin Medication[5]	-	-	95%	94%
Thrombolytic Therapy Timing[5]	-	-	65%	66%
Venous Thromboembolism Prophylaxis[5]	-	-	95%	94%
Written Stroke Educational Materials Given[5]	-	-	92%	88%
Surgical Care Improvement Project				
Appropriate Beta Blocker Usage	140	99%	98%	98%
Appropriate VTP Within 24 Hours	559	99%	98%	98%
Controlled Postoperative Blood Glucose[7]	-	-	97%	97%
Perioperative Temperature Management	594	100%	100%	100%
Prophylactic Antibiotic Selection	564	99%	99%	99%
Prophylactic Antibiotic Selection (Outpatient)	181	100%	98%	98%
Prophylactic Antibiotic Stopped	561	100%	98%	98%
Prophylactic Antibiotic Timing	564	100%	99%	99%
Prophylactic Antibiotic Timing (Outpatient)	181	99%	97%	98%
Urinary Catheter Removal	285	100%	97%	97%
Survey of Patients' Hospital Experiences				
Area Around Room 'Always' Quiet at Night	300+	84%	58%	61%
Doctors 'Always' Communicated Well	300+	91%	80%	82%
Home Recovery Information Given	300+	92%	87%	85%
Hospital Given 9 or 10 on 10 Point Scale	300+	95%	72%	71%
Meds 'Always' Explained Before Given	300+	79%	64%	64%
Nurses 'Always' Communicated Well	300+	95%	81%	79%
Pain 'Always' Well Controlled	300+	87%	71%	71%
Room and Bathroom 'Always' Clean	300+	90%	75%	73%
Timely Help 'Always' Received	300+	91%	70%	68%
Would Definitely Recommend Hospital	300+	96%	71%	71%
Use of Medical Imaging				
Cardiac Imaging Stress Test before Surgery[7]	-	-	5.4%	5.3%
Combination Abdominal CT Scan	106	12.3%	7.1%	10.5%
Combination Brain/Sinus CT Scan[1]	-	-	2.8%	2.7%
Combination Chest CT Scan	45	0.0%	1.7%	2.7%
Follow-up Mammogram/Ultrasound	117	4.3%	8.7%	8.8%
Lumbar Spine MRI for Low Back Pain[1]	-	-	34.7%	37.2%

Genesis Healthcare System

2951 Maple Avenue
Zanesville, OH 43701
Phone: 740-454-5000
Fax: 740-454-4781
URL: www.genesishcs.org
Type: Acute Care Hospitals
Emergency Services: Yes
Ownership: Voluntary non-profit - Private
Beds: 352

Key Personnel:

Emergency Room . . . . Bradley Allen
Radiology. Shane Backu
Infection Control. . . . . Kathy Blair
Operating Room. . . . . Firas Eladoumikdachi
Quality Assurance . . . . Mike Greene
CEO/President. . . . . Matthew Perry
Chief of Medical Staff . . . . Dan Scheerer, MD

Measure	Cases	This Hosp.	State Avg.	U.S. Avg.
Blood Clot Prevention and Treatment				
Anticoagulation Overlap Therapy[2]	77	88%	93%	93%
ICU Venous Thromboembolism Prophylaxis[2]	54	85%	93%	92%
Incidence of Potentially Preventable VTE[2]	12	17%	6%	10%
UFH with Dosages/Platelet Monitoring[2]	46	100%	98%	97%
Venous Thromboembolism Prophylaxis[2]	329	81%	88%	85%
Warfarin Therapy Discharge Instructions[2]	61	82%	79%	75%
Chest Pain/Possible Heart Attack Care				
Aspirin Given Within 24 Hours of Arrival[5]	-	-	97%	96%
Fibrinolytic Meds Within 30 Min. of Arrival[5]	-	-	44%	58%
Average Time to ECG (minutes)[5]	-	-	6	7
Average Time to Transfer (minutes)[5]	-	-	58	60
Children's Asthma Care				
Received Home Management Plan of Care	-	-	85%	88%
Received Reliever Medication	-	-	100%	100%
Received Systemic Corticosteroids	-	-	100%	100%
Emergency Department				
Admittance Decision Time (minutes)[2]	618	80	90	98
Head CT Results Within 45 Min. of Arrival	65	52%	63%	57%
Patients Who Left ER Before Being Seen	71,746	1%	2%	2%
Time from ER Arrival to Admit. (minutes)[2]	624	238	265	274
Time from ER Arrival to Discharge (minutes)	352	136	128	134
Time in ER Before Being Evaluated (minutes)	384	21	22	26
Time to Pain Meds for Fractures (minutes)	214	64	54	57
Heart Attack Care				
Aspirin Given at Discharge	429	99%	99%	99%
Fibrinolytic Meds Within 30 Min. of Arrival[7]	-	-	80%	54%
PCI Within 90 Minutes of Arrival	60	98%	97%	96%
Statin Prescribed at Discharge	415	98%	98%	98%
Heart Failure Care				
ACE Inhibitor or ARB for LVSD	107	91%	97%	97%
Discharge Instructions Given	328	100%	96%	94%
Evaluation of LVS Function	410	100%	100%	99%
Medicare Spending				
Medicare Spending per Patient (ratio)	-	0.94	1.01	0.98
Pneumonia Care				
Appropriate Initial Antibiotic Given	260	98%	96%	95%
Blood Culture Timing	361	100%	98%	98%
Pregnancy and Delivery Care				
Newborn Deliveries Scheduled Early[2]	37	11%	5%	6%
Preventive Care				
Immunization for Influenza[2]	540	84%	93%	90%
Immunization for Pneumonia[2]	702	92%	94%	92%
Stroke Care				
Anticoagulation Therapy for Atrial Fibrillation[1,2]	-	-	95%	95%
Antithrombotic Therapy Timing[2]	51	98%	98%	98%
Assessed for Rehabilitation[2]	70	96%	98%	97%
Discharged on Antithrombotic Therapy[2]	56	100%	99%	99%
Discharged on Statin Medication[2]	44	95%	95%	94%
Thrombolytic Therapy Timing[2,7]	-	-	65%	66%
Venous Thromboembolism Prophylaxis[2]	72	88%	95%	94%
Written Stroke Educational Materials Given[2]	41	100%	92%	88%
Surgical Care Improvement Project				
Appropriate Beta Blocker Usage[2]	223	97%	98%	98%
Appropriate VTP Within 24 Hours[2]	315	96%	98%	98%
Controlled Postoperative Blood Glucose[2]	97	100%	97%	97%
Perioperative Temperature Management[2]	430	99%	100%	100%
Prophylactic Antibiotic Selection[2]	379	99%	99%	99%
Prophylactic Antibiotic Selection (Outpatient)	346	96%	98%	98%
Prophylactic Antibiotic Stopped[2]	368	95%	98%	98%
Prophylactic Antibiotic Timing[2]	381	98%	99%	99%
Prophylactic Antibiotic Timing (Outpatient)	354	96%	97%	98%
Urinary Catheter Removal[2]	201	95%	97%	97%
Survey of Patients' Hospital Experiences				
Area Around Room 'Always' Quiet at Night	300+	48%	58%	61%
Doctors 'Always' Communicated Well	300+	73%	80%	82%
Home Recovery Information Given	300+	86%	87%	85%
Hospital Given 9 or 10 on 10 Point Scale	300+	62%	72%	71%
Meds 'Always' Explained Before Given	300+	58%	64%	64%
Nurses 'Always' Communicated Well	300+	76%	81%	79%
Pain 'Always' Well Controlled	300+	66%	71%	71%
Room and Bathroom 'Always' Clean	300+	70%	75%	73%
Timely Help 'Always' Received	300+	66%	70%	68%
Would Definitely Recommend Hospital	300+	65%	71%	71%
Use of Medical Imaging				
Cardiac Imaging Stress Test before Surgery	482	5.2%	5.4%	5.3%
Combination Abdominal CT Scan	1,552	6.3%	7.1%	10.5%
Combination Brain/Sinus CT Scan	1,065	3.9%	2.8%	2.7%
Combination Chest CT Scan	1,532	0.4%	1.7%	2.7%
Follow-up Mammogram/Ultrasound	3,053	9.5%	8.7%	8.8%
Lumbar Spine MRI for Low Back Pain	281	37.0%	34.7%	37.2%

NOTE: Hospital profiles are in alphabetical order by state, then city, then hospital within the city; Rankings exclude hospitals with less than 25 cases except for patient surveys which excludes hospitals with less than 100 cases; (a) 100-299 cases; (1) The number of cases/patients is too few to report; (2) Data submitted were based on a sample of cases/patients; (3) Results are based on a shorter time period than required; (4) Data suppressed by CMS for one or more quarters; (5) Results are not available for this reporting period; (6) Fewer than 100 patients completed the HCAHPS survey; (7) No cases met the criteria for this measure; (8) The lower limit of the confidence interval cannot be calculated if the number of observed infections equals zero; (9) No data are available from the state/territory for this reporting period; (10) The scores shown reflect fewer than 50 completed surveys; (11) There were discrepancies in the data collection process; (12) This measure does not apply to this hospital for this reporting period; (13) Results cannot be calculated for this reporting period; (14) The results for this state are combined with nearby states to protect confidentiality; Please refer to the User's Guide for a full explanation of data.

Blood Clot Prevention and Treatment

Anticoagulation Overlap Therapy

Hospital Name	City	Rate	Cases
Aria Health[2]	Philadelphia	100%	216
Einstein Medical Center Montgomery[2]	East Norriton	100%	43
Geisinger - Community Medical Center[2]	Scranton	100%	87
Heritage Valley Beaver[2]	Beaver	100%	108
Heritage Valley Sewickley[2]	Sewickley	100%	59
Lansdale Hospital[2]	Lansdale	100%	45
Mercy Suburban Hospital[2]	Norristown	100%	35
Nazareth Hospital[2]	Philadelphia	100%	73
Penn Highlands Dubois[2]	Dubois	100%	44
Penn Hosp of the Univ of PA Hlth Sys[2]	Philadelphia	100%	74
Reading Hospital[2]	Reading	100%	331
Roxborough Memorial Hospital[2]	Philadelphia	100%	29
Saint Mary Medical Center[2]	Langhorne	100%	181
UPMC East[2]	Monroeville	100%	94
UPMC Mckeesport[2]	Mc Keesport	100%	44
UPMC Mercy[2]	Pittsburgh	100%	161
UPMC Northwest[2]	Seneca	100%	78
UPMC Passavant[2]	Pittsburgh	100%	180
The Washington Hospital[2]	Washington	100%	76
Western Pennsylvania Hospital[2]	Pittsburgh	100%	33
Williamsport Regional Medical Center[2]	Williamsport	100%	73
York Hospital[2]	York	100%	271
Albert Einstein Medical Center[2]	Philadelphia	99%	151
Butler Memorial Hospital[2]	Butler	99%	86
Chestnut Hill Hospital[2]	Philadelphia	99%	99
Regional Hospital of Scranton[2]	Scranton	99%	69
UPMC Horizon	Greenville	99%	67
UPMC Presbyterian Shadyside[2]	Pittsburgh	99%	554
UPMC Saint Margaret[2]	Pittsburgh	99%	139
Chambersburg Hospital	Chambersburg	98%	119
Crozer Chester Medical Center[2]	Upland	98%	154
Delaware County Memorial Hospital[2]	Drexel Hill	98%	60
Easton Hospital[2]	Easton	98%	59
Evangelical Community Hospital	Lewisburg	98%	60
Lancaster General Hospital[2]	Lancaster	98%	298
Mercy Fitzgerald Hospital[2]	Darby	98%	181
Penn Presbyterian Medical Center[2]	Philadelphia	98%	108
Pottstown Memorial Medical Center[2]	Pottstown	98%	57
Saint Clair Memorial Hospital[2]	Pittsburgh	98%	159
Saint Luke's Hospital Bethlehem[2]	Bethlehem	98%	141
Saint Vincent Hospital[2]	Erie	98%	61
Geisinger Medical Center[2]	Danville	97%	163
Grand View Hospital[2]	Sellersville	97%	76
Holy Redeemer Hospital & Medical Center[2]	Meadowbrook	97%	59
Lancaster Regional Medical Center[2]	Lancaster	97%	32
Magee Womens Hosp of UPMC Health Sys[2]	Pittsburgh	97%	35
Main Line Hospital Paoli[2]	Paoli	97%	103
Phoenixville Hospital[2]	Phoenixville	97%	33
Saint Luke's Hospital - Anderson Campus[2]	Easton	97%	60
Schuylkill Med Ctr-East Norwegian St[2]	Pottsville	97%	39
UPMC Hamot[2]	Erie	97%	142
Acmh Hospital[2]	Kittanning	96%	45
Chester County Hospital[2]	West Chester	96%	80
Lehigh Valley Hospital[2]	Allentown	96%	244
Main Line Hospital Lankenau[2]	Wynnewood	96%	93
Milton S Hershey Medical Center[2]	Hershey	96%	152
Saint Luke's Miners Memorial Hospital[2]	Coaldale	96%	27
Saint Luke's Quakertown Hospital[2]	Quakertown	96%	26
Sharon Regional Health System[2]	Sharon	96%	48
Waynesboro Hospital	Waynesboro	96%	25
Allegheny General Hospital[2]	Pittsburgh	95%	199
Geisinger Wyoming Valley Medical Center[2]	Wilkes Barre	95%	106
Hospital of Univ of Pennsylvania[2]	Philadelphia	95%	233
Lehigh Valley Hospital - Muhlenberg[2]	Bethlehem	95%	130
Riddle Memorial Hospital[2]	Media	95%	59
Excela Health Frick Hospital[2]	Mount Pleasant	94%	31
Schuylkill Med Ctr-S Jackson St[2]	Pottsville	94%	50
Gettysburg Hospital[2]	Gettysburg	93%	72
Abington Memorial Hospital[2]	Abington	92%	212
Doylestown Hospital[2]	Doylestown	92%	85
Ephrata Community Hospital[2]	Ephrata	92%	63
Jefferson Regional Medical Center[2]	Pittsburgh	92%	160
Pocono Medical Center[2]	E Stroudsburg	92%	107
Grove City Medical Center[2]	Grove City	91%	35
Hahnemann University Hospital[2]	Philadelphia	91%	92
Memorial Hospital[2]	York	91%	86
Moses Taylor Hospital[2]	Scranton	91%	32
Ohio Valley General Hospital[2]	Mckees Rocks	91%	33
Temple University Hospital[2]	Philadelphia	91%	152
Conemaugh Valley Memorial Hospital[2]	Johnstown	90%	146
Pinnacle Health Hospitals[2]	Harrisburg	90%	210
Thomas Jefferson University Hospital[2]	Philadelphia	90%	189
Good Samaritan Hospital[2]	Lebanon	89%	95
Uniontown Hospital[2]	Uniontown	89%	46
Excela Health Latrobe Hospital[2]	Latrobe	88%	32
Hanover Hospital[2]	Hanover	88%	52
Wilkes-Barre General Hospital[2]	Wilkes-Barre	88%	123
Monongahela Valley Hospital[2]	Monongahela	87%	69
Mount Nittany Medical Center[2]	State College	87%	127
Penn Highlands Clearfield[2]	Clearfield	87%	30
Holy Spirit Hospital[2]	Camp Hill	86%	148
Lewistown Hospital[2]	Lewistown	86%	42
Excela Health Westmoreland Hospital[2]	Greensburg	85%	115
Main Line Hospital Bryn Mawr Campus[2]	Bryn Mawr	84%	98
Forbes Regional Hospital[2]	Monroeville	83%	109
Robert Packer Hospital[2]	Sayre	83%	83
UPMC Altoona[2]	Altoona	83%	180
Alle Kiski Medical Center[2]	Natrona	81%	43
Brandywine Hospital[2]	Coatesville	81%	37
Jameson Memorial Hospital[2]	New Castle	81%	67
Jeanes Hospital[2]	Philadelphia	80%	49
Lehigh Valley Hospital - Hazleton[2]	Hazleton	80%	25
Meadville Medical Center[2]	Meadville	71%	41
Saint Joseph Medical Center[2]	Reading	69%	74
Penn Highlands Elk[2]	Saint Marys	67%	27
Indiana Regional Medical Center[2]	Indiana	53%	57

ICU Venous Thromboembolism Prophylaxis

Hospital Name	City	Rate	Cases
Canonsburg General Hospital[2]	Canonsburg	100%	62
Conemaugh Valley Memorial Hospital[2]	Johnstown	100%	48
Easton Hospital[2]	Easton	100%	93
Excela Health Latrobe Hospital[2]	Latrobe	100%	91
Geisinger Medical Center[2]	Danville	100%	81
Grand View Hospital[2]	Sellersville	100%	75
Heritage Valley Beaver[2]	Beaver	100%	63
Heritage Valley Sewickley[2]	Sewickley	100%	89
Hospital of Univ of Pennsylvania[2]	Philadelphia	100%	123
Lock Haven Hospital[2]	Lock Haven	100%	64
Main Line Hospital Paoli[2]	Paoli	100%	40
Mercy Suburban Hospital[2]	Norristown	100%	74
Millcreek Community Hospital[2]	Erie	100%	34
Roxborough Memorial Hospital[2]	Philadelphia	100%	58
Saint Mary Medical Center[2]	Langhorne	100%	60
UPMC Horizon	Greenville	100%	548
UPMC Mckeesport[2]	Mc Keesport	100%	119
UPMC Saint Margaret[2]	Pittsburgh	100%	57
The Washington Hospital[2]	Washington	100%	52
Aria Health[2]	Philadelphia	99%	77
Chestnut Hill Hospital[2]	Philadelphia	99%	85
Hanover Hospital[2]	Hanover	99%	119
Lehigh Valley Hospital[2]	Allentown	99%	182
Mercy Fitzgerald Hospital[2]	Darby	99%	149
Penn Presbyterian Medical Center[2]	Philadelphia	99%	86
Penn Hosp of the Univ of PA Hlth Sys[2]	Philadelphia	99%	160
Reading Hospital[2]	Reading	99%	72
Saint Clair Memorial Hospital[2]	Pittsburgh	99%	73
Tyler Memorial Hospital[2]	Tunkhannock	99%	79
UPMC East[2]	Monroeville	99%	75
UPMC Hamot[2]	Erie	99%	125
York Hospital[2]	York	99%	77
Albert Einstein Medical Center[2]	Philadelphia	98%	93
Carlisle Regional Medical Center[2]	Carlisle	98%	40
Doylestown Hospital[2]	Doylestown	98%	58
Kane Community Hospital[2]	Kane	98%	62
Lancaster General Hospital[2]	Lancaster	98%	318
Lancaster Regional Medical Center[2]	Lancaster	98%	50
Lansdale Hospital[2]	Lansdale	98%	95
Meadville Medical Center[2]	Meadville	98%	122
Monongahela Valley Hospital[2]	Monongahela	98%	192
Nazareth Hospital[2]	Philadelphia	98%	59
Penn Highlands Clearfield[2]	Clearfield	98%	47
Penn Highlands Dubois[2]	Dubois	98%	147
Phoenixville Hospital[2]	Phoenixville	98%	115
Regional Hospital of Scranton[2]	Scranton	98%	109
Saint Joseph Medical Center[2]	Reading	98%	124
Saint Luke's Hospital Bethlehem[2]	Bethlehem	98%	123
UPMC Mercy[2]	Pittsburgh	98%	124
UPMC Passavant[2]	Pittsburgh	98%	91
UPMC Presbyterian Shadyside[2]	Pittsburgh	98%	105
Cancer Treatment Centers of America[2]	Philadelphia	97%	37
Crozer Chester Medical Center[2]	Upland	97%	63
Excela Health Frick Hospital[2]	Mount Pleasant	97%	67
Hahnemann University Hospital[2]	Philadelphia	97%	76
Heart of Lancaster Reg Med Ctr[2]	Lititz	97%	34
Riddle Memorial Hospital[2]	Media	97%	59
Waynesboro Hospital	Waynesboro	97%	243
Butler Memorial Hospital[2]	Butler	96%	181
Geisinger - Community Medical Center[2]	Scranton	96%	72
Grove City Medical Center[2]	Grove City	96%	26
Holy Spirit Hospital[2]	Camp Hill	96%	68
Lewistown Hospital[2]	Lewistown	96%	72
Moses Taylor Hospital[2]	Scranton	96%	57
Saint Luke's Hospital - Anderson Campus[2]	Easton	96%	53
Chambersburg Hospital	Chambersburg	95%	903
Evangelical Community Hospital	Lewisburg	95%	472
Excela Health Westmoreland Hospital[2]	Greensburg	95%	78
Geisinger Wyoming Valley Medical Center[2]	Wilkes Barre	95%	61
Main Line Hospital Lankenau[2]	Wynnewood	95%	79
Saint Vincent Hospital[2]	Erie	95%	259
Sunbury Community Hospital[2]	Sunbury	95%	38
UPMC Northwest[2]	Seneca	95%	37
Ephrata Community Hospital[2]	Ephrata	94%	83
Good Samaritan Hospital[2]	Lebanon	94%	100
Holy Redeemer Hospital & Medical Center[2]	Meadowbrook	94%	81
Lehigh Valley Hospital - Muhlenberg[2]	Bethlehem	94%	70
Main Line Hospital Bryn Mawr Campus[2]	Bryn Mawr	94%	68
Memorial Hospital Towanda[2]	Towanda	94%	35
Robert Packer Hospital[2]	Sayre	94%	109
Uniontown Hospital[2]	Uniontown	94%	78
Williamsport Regional Medical Center[2]	Williamsport	94%	109
Acmh Hospital[2]	Kittanning	93%	70
Alle Kiski Medical Center[2]	Natrona	93%	67
Einstein Medical Center Montgomery[2]	East Norriton	93%	74
Gettysburg Hospital[2]	Gettysburg	93%	72
Temple University Hospital[2]	Philadelphia	93%	113
Thomas Jefferson University Hospital[2]	Philadelphia	93%	142
Bradford Regional Medical Center[2]	Bradford	92%	26
Jennersville Regional Hospital[2]	West Grove	92%	49
Milton S Hershey Medical Center[2]	Hershey	92%	90
Pocono Medical Center[2]	E Stroudsburg	92%	106
Sacred Heart Hospital[2]	Allentown	92%	140
Brandywine Hospital[2]	Coatesville	91%	80
Highlands Hospital[2]	Connellsville	91%	35
Pinnacle Health Hospitals[2]	Harrisburg	91%	182
Pottstown Memorial Medical Center[2]	Pottstown	91%	98
Allegheny General Hospital[2]	Pittsburgh	90%	165
Berwick Hospital Center[2]	Berwick	90%	99
Saint Luke's Quakertown Hospital[2]	Quakertown	90%	41
Schuylkill Med Ctr-S Jackson St[2]	Pottsville	90%	90
Wayne Memorial Hospital[2]	Honesdale	90%	31
Abington Memorial Hospital[2]	Abington	89%	64
Miners Medical Center[2]	Hastings	89%	45
Schuylkill Med Ctr-East Norwegian St[2]	Pottsville	89%	66
Gnaden Huetten Memorial Hospital[2]	Lehighton	88%	56
J C Blair Memorial Hospital[2]	Huntingdon	88%	33
Jefferson Regional Medical Center[2]	Pittsburgh	88%	74
Warren General Hospital[2]	Warren	88%	41
Wilkes-Barre General Hospital[2]	Wilkes-Barre	88%	108
Mount Nittany Medical Center[2]	State College	87%	30
Sharon Regional Health System[2]	Sharon	87%	111
Southwest Regional Medical Center[2]	Waynesburg	87%	38
Forbes Regional Hospital[2]	Monroeville	85%	75
Memorial Hospital[2]	York	85%	109
Somerset Hospital[2]	Somerset	84%	89
Saint Joseph's Hospital[2]	Philadelphia	83%	66
UPMC Altoona[2]	Altoona	83%	81
Lower Bucks Hospital[2]	Bristol	82%	109
Penn Highlands Elk[2]	Saint Marys	82%	50
Western Pennsylvania Hospital[2]	Pittsburgh	82%	83
Titusville Hospital[2]	Titusville	81%	26
Soldiers & Sailors Memorial Hospital[2]	Wellsboro	80%	40
Jameson Memorial Hospital[2]	New Castle	77%	82
Windber Hospital[2]	Windber	76%	34
Palmerton Hospital[2]	Palmerton	74%	31
Ohio Valley General Hospital[2]	Mckees Rocks	72%	65
Lehigh Valley Hospital - Hazleton[2]	Hazleton	71%	51
Jeanes Hospital[2]	Philadelphia	67%	118
Clarion Hospital[2]	Clarion	65%	37
Ellwood City Hospital[2]	Ellwood City	54%	39
Geisinger - Bloomsburg Hospital[2]	Bloomsburg	54%	26
Indiana Regional Medical Center[2]	Indiana	47%	55

Incidence of Potentially Preventable VTE

Hospital Name	City	Rate	Cases
Geisinger Wyoming Valley Medical Center[2]	Wilkes Barre	0%	31
Lancaster General Hospital[2]	Lancaster	0%	57
Penn Hosp of the Univ of PA Hlth Sys[2]	Philadelphia	0%	35
Saint Clair Memorial Hospital[2]	Pittsburgh	0%	36
Saint Luke's Hospital Bethlehem[2]	Bethlehem	0%	33
UPMC Saint Margaret[2]	Pittsburgh	0%	25
UPMC Presbyterian Shadyside[2]	Pittsburgh	1%	247
Allegheny General Hospital[2]	Pittsburgh	2%	88
Crozer Chester Medical Center[2]	Upland	2%	44
Mercy Fitzgerald Hospital[2]	Darby	2%	46
Milton S Hershey Medical Center[2]	Hershey	2%	50
Thomas Jefferson University Hospital[2]	Philadelphia	2%	61
Hospital of Univ of Pennsylvania[2]	Philadelphia	3%	126
Saint Mary Medical Center[2]	Langhorne	3%	35
UPMC Hamot[2]	Erie	3%	30
UPMC Passavant[2]	Pittsburgh	3%	33
Abington Memorial Hospital[2]	Abington	4%	52
Geisinger Medical Center[2]	Danville	4%	48
Main Line Hospital Paoli[2]	Paoli	5%	37
Lehigh Valley Hospital[2]	Allentown	6%	62
Magee Womens Hosp of UPMC Health Sys[2]	Pittsburgh	6%	34
UPMC Mercy[2]	Pittsburgh	6%	53
Aria Health[2]	Philadelphia	7%	85

NOTE: Hospital profiles are in alphabetical order by state, then city, then hospital within the city; Rankings exclude hospitals with less than 25 cases except for patient surveys which excludes hospitals with less than 100 cases; (a) 100-299 cases; (1) The number of cases/patients is too few to report; (2) Data submitted were based on a sample of cases/patients; (3) Results are based on a shorter time period than required; (4) Data suppressed by CMS for one or more quarters; (5) Results are not available for this reporting period; (6) Fewer than 100 patients completed the HCAHPS survey; (7) No cases met the criteria for this measure; (8) The lower limit of the confidence interval cannot be calculated if the number of observed infections equals zero; (9) No data are available from the state/territory for this reporting period; (10) The scores shown reflect fewer than 50 completed surveys; (11) There were discrepancies in the data collection process; (12) This measure does not apply to this hospital for this reporting period; (13) Results cannot be calculated for this reporting period; (14) The results for this state are combined with nearby states to protect confidentiality; Please refer to the User's Guide for a full explanation of data.

Hospital Name	City	Rate	Cases
Reading Hospital[2]	Reading	7%	30
Temple University Hospital[2]	Philadelphia	8%	60
Hahnemann University Hospital[2]	Philadelphia	9%	32
Chambersburg Hospital	Chambersburg	10%	29
Riddle Memorial Hospital[2]	Media	12%	26
Conemaugh Valley Memorial Hospital[2]	Johnstown	15%	46
York Hospital[2]	York	15%	39
Albert Einstein Medical Center[2]	Philadelphia	17%	41
Pinnacle Health Hospitals[2]	Harrisburg	17%	41
UPMC Altoona[2]	Altoona	18%	33
Forbes Regional Hospital[2]	Monroeville	24%	38
Wilkes-Barre General Hospital[2]	Wilkes-Barre	38%	37
Jefferson Regional Medical Center[2]	Pittsburgh	44%	32

UFH with Dosages/Platelet Count Monitoring

Hospital Name	City	Rate	Cases
Abington Memorial Hospital[2]	Abington	100%	279
Acmh Hospital[2]	Kittanning	100%	32
Albert Einstein Medical Center[2]	Philadelphia	100%	113
Alle Kiski Medical Center[2]	Natrona	100%	53
Allegheny General Hospital[2]	Pittsburgh	100%	216
Aria Health[2]	Philadelphia	100%	151
Brandywine Hospital[2]	Coatesville	100%	40
Butler Memorial Hospital[2]	Butler	100%	88
Chambersburg Hospital	Chambersburg	100%	49
Chestnut Hill Hospital[2]	Philadelphia	100%	89
Conemaugh Valley Memorial Hospital[2]	Johnstown	100%	140
Crozer Chester Medical Center[2]	Upland	100%	114
Delaware County Memorial Hospital[2]	Drexel Hill	100%	41
Doylestown Hospital[2]	Doylestown	100%	44
Easton Hospital[2]	Easton	100%	47
Ephrata Community Hospital[2]	Ephrata	100%	67
Excela Health Frick Hospital[2]	Mount Pleasant	100%	28
Excela Health Latrobe Hospital[2]	Latrobe	100%	37
Excela Health Westmoreland Hospital[2]	Greensburg	100%	130
Forbes Regional Hospital[2]	Monroeville	100%	108
Geisinger - Community Medical Center[2]	Scranton	100%	91
Geisinger Medical Center[2]	Danville	100%	113
Geisinger Wyoming Valley Medical Center[2]	Wilkes Barre	100%	51
Grand View Hospital[2]	Sellersville	100%	34
Grove City Medical Center[2]	Grove City	100%	36
Hanover Hospital[2]	Hanover	100%	50
Heritage Valley Beaver[2]	Beaver	100%	104
Heritage Valley Sewickley[2]	Sewickley	100%	62
Holy Redeemer Hospital & Medical Center[2]	Meadowbrook	100%	61
Holy Spirit Hospital[2]	Camp Hill	100%	42
Hospital of Univ of Pennsylvania[2]	Philadelphia	100%	222
Jameson Memorial Hospital[2]	New Castle	100%	28
Jeanes Hospital[2]	Philadelphia	100%	47
Lancaster General Hospital[2]	Lancaster	100%	237
Lansdale Hospital[2]	Lansdale	100%	33
Lower Bucks Hospital[2]	Bristol	100%	28
Magee Womens Hosp of UPMC Health Sys[2]	Pittsburgh	100%	50
Main Line Hospital Paoli[2]	Paoli	100%	36
Meadville Medical Center[2]	Meadville	100%	38
Mercy Suburban Hospital[2]	Norristown	100%	39
Monongahela Valley Hospital[2]	Monongahela	100%	44
Moses Taylor Hospital[2]	Scranton	100%	29
Nazareth Hospital[2]	Philadelphia	100%	71
Penn Presbyterian Medical Center[2]	Philadelphia	100%	105
Penn Hosp of the Univ of PA Hlth Sys[2]	Philadelphia	100%	60
Pottstown Memorial Medical Center[2]	Pottstown	100%	67
Reading Hospital[2]	Reading	100%	248
Regional Hospital of Scranton[2]	Scranton	100%	72
Riddle Memorial Hospital[2]	Media	100%	64
Saint Clair Memorial Hospital[2]	Pittsburgh	100%	156
Saint Joseph Medical Center[2]	Reading	100%	75
Saint Luke's Hospital - Anderson Campus[2]	Easton	100%	43
Saint Mary Medical Center[2]	Langhorne	100%	260
Saint Vincent Hospital[2]	Erie	100%	60
Schuylkill Med Ctr-S Jackson St[2]	Pottsville	100%	28
Sharon Regional Health System[2]	Sharon	100%	48
Somerset Hospital[2]	Somerset	100%	25
Uniontown Hospital[2]	Uniontown	100%	30
UPMC East[2]	Monroeville	100%	87
UPMC Hamot[2]	Erie	100%	183
UPMC Horizon	Greenville	100%	62
UPMC Mckeesport[2]	Mc Keesport	100%	43
UPMC Mercy[2]	Pittsburgh	100%	140
UPMC Passavant[2]	Pittsburgh	100%	125
UPMC Presbyterian Shadyside[2]	Pittsburgh	100%	634
UPMC Saint Margaret[2]	Pittsburgh	100%	127
The Washington Hospital[2]	Washington	100%	84
Western Pennsylvania Hospital[2]	Pittsburgh	100%	47
Wilkes-Barre General Hospital[2]	Wilkes-Barre	100%	105
York Hospital[2]	York	100%	199
Jefferson Regional Medical Center[2]	Pittsburgh	99%	160
Memorial Hospital[2]	York	99%	68
Mercy Fitzgerald Hospital[2]	Darby	99%	156
Milton S Hershey Medical Center[2]	Hershey	99%	139
Pinnacle Health Hospitals[2]	Harrisburg	99%	139
Pocono Medical Center[2]	E Stroudsburg	99%	76
Saint Luke's Hospital Bethlehem[2]	Bethlehem	99%	98
UPMC Altoona[2]	Altoona	99%	79
Chester County Hospital[2]	West Chester	98%	59
Good Samaritan Hospital[2]	Lebanon	98%	46
Indiana Regional Medical Center[2]	Indiana	98%	56
Mount Nittany Medical Center[2]	State College	98%	122
Gettysburg Hospital[2]	Gettysburg	97%	34
Main Line Hospital Bryn Mawr Campus[2]	Bryn Mawr	97%	35
Main Line Hospital Lankenau[2]	Wynnewood	97%	107
Lehigh Valley Hospital - Muhlenberg[2]	Bethlehem	91%	128
Lehigh Valley Hospital[2]	Allentown	89%	260
Robert Packer Hospital[2]	Sayre	89%	37
Thomas Jefferson University Hospital[2]	Philadelphia	86%	168
Williamsport Regional Medical Center[2]	Williamsport	84%	31
Hahnemann University Hospital[2]	Philadelphia	67%	83
Temple University Hospital[2]	Philadelphia	60%	139

Venous Thromboembolism Prophylaxis

Hospital Name	City	Rate	Cases
Bucks County Specialty Hospital[2]	Bensalem	100%	31
Heritage Valley Sewickley[2]	Sewickley	100%	320
Hospital of Univ of Pennsylvania[2]	Philadelphia	100%	296
Mercy Suburban Hospital[2]	Norristown	100%	347
Mid - Valley Hospital[2]	Peckville	100%	174
Oss Orthopaedic Hospital[2]	York	100%	53
Physician's Care Surgical Hospital[2]	Royersford	100%	58
Surgical Specialty Ctr at Coord Hlth[2]	Allentown	100%	40
Tyler Memorial Hospital[2]	Tunkhannock	100%	325
UPMC Horizon	Greenville	100%	2295
Delaware County Memorial Hospital[2]	Drexel Hill	99%	409
Excela Health Frick Hospital[2]	Mount Pleasant	99%	370
Lewistown Hospital[2]	Lewistown	99%	368
Lock Haven Hospital[2]	Lock Haven	99%	260
Penn Presbyterian Medical Center[2]	Philadelphia	99%	283
Canonsburg General Hospital[2]	Canonsburg	98%	308
Chestnut Hill Hospital[2]	Philadelphia	98%	486
Doylestown Hospital[2]	Doylestown	98%	408
Evangelical Community Hospital	Lewisburg	98%	1849
Excela Health Latrobe Hospital[2]	Latrobe	98%	356
Heart of Lancaster Reg Med Ctr[2]	Lititz	98%	167
Monongahela Valley Hospital[2]	Monongahela	98%	694
Nazareth Hospital[2]	Philadelphia	98%	364
Saint Joseph Medical Center[2]	Reading	98%	712
Waynesboro Hospital	Waynesboro	98%	993
Easton Hospital[2]	Easton	97%	514
Lancaster General Hospital[2]	Lancaster	97%	2350
Lehigh Valley Hospital[2]	Allentown	97%	303
Main Line Hospital Lankenau[2]	Wynnewood	97%	346
UPMC Mercy[2]	Pittsburgh	97%	346
Bradford Regional Medical Center[2]	Bradford	96%	241
Hanover Hospital[2]	Hanover	96%	373
Penn Highlands Dubois[2]	Dubois	96%	207
Roxborough Memorial Hospital[2]	Philadelphia	96%	337
Sunbury Community Hospital[2]	Sunbury	96%	248
UPMC Mckeesport[2]	Mc Keesport	96%	384
UPMC Northwest[2]	Seneca	96%	524
Grove City Medical Center[2]	Grove City	95%	144
Heritage Valley Beaver[2]	Beaver	95%	370
Main Line Hospital Bryn Mawr Campus[2]	Bryn Mawr	95%	272
Mercy Fitzgerald Hospital[2]	Darby	95%	702
Moses Taylor Hospital[2]	Scranton	95%	408
Penn Hosp of the Univ of PA Hlth Sys[2]	Philadelphia	95%	267
Saint Luke's Hospital Bethlehem[2]	Bethlehem	95%	521
Uniontown Hospital[2]	Uniontown	95%	344
Carlisle Regional Medical Center[2]	Carlisle	94%	305
Grand View Hospital[2]	Sellersville	94%	311
Kane Community Hospital[2]	Kane	94%	214
Reading Hospital[2]	Reading	94%	365
Saint Luke's Hospital - Anderson Campus[2]	Easton	94%	345
Saint Luke's Quakertown Hospital[2]	Quakertown	94%	211
Surgical Institute of Reading[2]	Wyomissing	94%	50
UPMC Bedford Memorial[2]	Everett	94%	220
UPMC Hamot[2]	Erie	94%	425
UPMC Presbyterian Shadyside[2]	Pittsburgh	94%	412
Chambersburg Hospital	Chambersburg	93%	4293
J C Blair Memorial Hospital[2]	Huntingdon	93%	106
Lansdale Hospital[2]	Lansdale	93%	283
Lehigh Valley Hospital - Muhlenberg[2]	Bethlehem	93%	404
Magee Womens Hosp of UPMC Health Sys[2]	Pittsburgh	93%	368
Meadville Medical Center[2]	Meadville	93%	572
Pinnacle Health Hospitals[2]	Harrisburg	93%	536
Albert Einstein Medical Center[2]	Philadelphia	92%	334
Aria Health[2]	Philadelphia	92%	232
Butler Memorial Hospital[2]	Butler	92%	553
Crozer Chester Medical Center[2]	Upland	92%	330
Geisinger Medical Center[2]	Danville	92%	399
Gettysburg Hospital[2]	Gettysburg	92%	305
Millcreek Community Hospital[2]	Erie	92%	152
UPMC East[2]	Monroeville	92%	479
The Washington Hospital[2]	Washington	92%	366
Wayne Memorial Hospital[2]	Honesdale	92%	244
Conemaugh Valley Memorial Hospital[2]	Johnstown	91%	410
Ephrata Community Hospital[2]	Ephrata	91%	314
Good Samaritan Hospital[2]	Lebanon	91%	322
Jennersville Regional Hospital[2]	West Grove	91%	321
Lancaster Regional Medical Center[2]	Lancaster	91%	298
Schuylkill Med Ctr-S Jackson St[2]	Pottsville	91%	333
UPMC Saint Margaret[2]	Pittsburgh	91%	740
Acmh Hospital[2]	Kittanning	90%	308
Allegheny General Hospital[2]	Pittsburgh	90%	377
Main Line Hospital Paoli[2]	Paoli	90%	341
Phoenixville Hospital[2]	Phoenixville	90%	402
Pocono Medical Center[2]	E Stroudsburg	90%	441
Saint Luke's Miners Memorial Hospital[2]	Coaldale	90%	163
Southwest Regional Medical Center[2]	Waynesburg	90%	185
Warren General Hospital[2]	Warren	90%	186
Williamsport Regional Medical Center[2]	Williamsport	90%	353
Geisinger - Community Medical Center[2]	Scranton	89%	467
Mount Nittany Medical Center[2]	State College	89%	322
Riddle Memorial Hospital[2]	Media	89%	395
Schuylkill Med Ctr-East Norwegian St[2]	Pottsville	89%	350
UPMC Passavant[2]	Pittsburgh	89%	444
Alle Kiski Medical Center[2]	Natrona	88%	358
Saint Clair Memorial Hospital[2]	Pittsburgh	88%	296
Saint Vincent Hospital[2]	Erie	88%	719
York Hospital[2]	York	88%	361
Abington Memorial Hospital[2]	Abington	87%	309
Hahnemann University Hospital[2]	Philadelphia	87%	348
Holy Redeemer Hospital & Medical Center[2]	Meadowbrook	87%	324
Penn Highlands Clearfield[2]	Clearfield	87%	164
Pottstown Memorial Medical Center[2]	Pottstown	87%	509
Thomas Jefferson University Hospital[2]	Philadelphia	87%	639
Geisinger Wyoming Valley Medical Center[2]	Wilkes Barre	86%	415
Robert Packer Hospital[2]	Sayre	86%	383
Sacred Heart Hospital[2]	Allentown	86%	833
Sharon Regional Health System[2]	Sharon	86%	677
Temple University Hospital[2]	Philadelphia	86%	288
Excela Health Westmoreland Hospital[2]	Greensburg	85%	365
Saint Mary Medical Center[2]	Langhorne	85%	350
Milton S Hershey Medical Center[2]	Hershey	84%	318
Somerset Hospital[2]	Somerset	83%	280
Charles Cole Memorial Hospital[2,3]	Coudersport	82%	97
Holy Spirit Hospital[2]	Camp Hill	82%	363
Berwick Hospital Center[2]	Berwick	81%	246
Einstein Medical Center Montgomery[2]	East Norriton	81%	351
Memorial Hospital[2]	York	80%	370
Memorial Hospital Towanda[2]	Towanda	80%	79
Brandywine Hospital[2]	Coatesville	79%	414
Chester County Hospital[2]	West Chester	79%	393
Jeanes Hospital[2]	Philadelphia	79%	353
Cancer Treatment Centers of America[2]	Philadelphia	78%	158
Miners Medical Center[2]	Hastings	77%	243
Regional Hospital of Scranton[2]	Scranton	76%	540
Troy Community Hospital[2,3]	Troy	76%	59
Gnaden Huetten Memorial Hospital[2]	Lehighton	75%	228
Nason Hospital[2]	Roaring Spring	75%	118
Western Pennsylvania Hospital[2]	Pittsburgh	74%	435
Palmerton Hospital[2]	Palmerton	73%	124
Wilkes-Barre General Hospital[2]	Wilkes-Barre	73%	535
Jefferson Regional Medical Center[2]	Pittsburgh	72%	360
Lower Bucks Hospital[2]	Bristol	71%	301
Ohio Valley General Hospital[2]	Mckees Rocks	71%	283
Soldiers & Sailors Memorial Hospital[2]	Wellsboro	71%	143
Jameson Memorial Hospital[2]	New Castle	69%	424
Penn Highlands Elk[2]	Saint Marys	69%	285
Windber Hospital[2]	Windber	68%	104
Saint Joseph's Hospital[2]	Philadelphia	64%	259
UPMC Altoona[2]	Altoona	64%	300
Forbes Regional Hospital[2]	Monroeville	63%	440
Titusville Hospital[2]	Titusville	63%	190
Highlands Hospital[2]	Connellsville	62%	138
Lehigh Valley Hospital - Hazleton[2]	Hazleton	61%	394
Geisinger - Bloomsburg Hospital[2]	Bloomsburg	58%	180
Indiana Regional Medical Center[2]	Indiana	56%	380
Punxsutawney Area Hospital[2]	Punxsutawney	56%	114
Clarion Hospital[2]	Clarion	55%	178
Ellwood City Hospital[2]	Ellwood City	37%	144
Kensington Hospital	Philadelphia	0%	66

Warfarin Therapy Discharge Instructions

Hospital Name	City	Rate	Cases
Alle Kiski Medical Center[2]	Natrona	100%	30
Doylestown Hospital[2]	Doylestown	100%	64
Heritage Valley Beaver[2]	Beaver	100%	64
Heritage Valley Sewickley[2]	Sewickley	100%	38
Lewistown Hospital[2]	Lewistown	100%	33
Magee Womens Hosp of UPMC Health Sys[2]	Pittsburgh	100%	25
Meadville Medical Center[2]	Meadville	100%	30
Milton S Hershey Medical Center[2]	Hershey	100%	122
Nazareth Hospital[2]	Philadelphia	100%	48
Penn Highlands Clearfield[2]	Clearfield	100%	26

NOTE: Hospital profiles are in alphabetical order by state, then city, then hospital within the city; Rankings exclude hospitals with less than 25 cases except for patient surveys which excludes hospitals with less than 100 cases; (a) 100-299 cases; (1) The number of cases/patients is too few to report; (2) Data submitted were based on a sample of cases/patients; (3) Results are based on a shorter time period than required; (4) Data suppressed by CMS for one or more quarters; (5) Results are not available for this reporting period; (6) Fewer than 100 patients completed the HCAHPS survey; (7) No cases met the criteria for this measure; (8) The lower limit of the confidence interval cannot be calculated if the number of observed infections equals zero; (9) No data are available from the state/territory for this reporting period; (10) The scores shown reflect fewer than 50 completed surveys; (11) There were discrepancies in the data collection process; (12) This measure does not apply to this hospital for this reporting period; (13) Results cannot be calculated for this reporting period; (14) The results for this state are combined with nearby states to protect confidentiality; Please refer to the User's Guide for a full explanation of data.

Hospital Name	City	Rate	Cases
Penn Highlands Dubois[2]	Dubois	100%	33
Saint Clair Memorial Hospital[2]	Pittsburgh	100%	116
Saint Vincent Hospital[2]	Erie	100%	35
Sharon Regional Health System[2]	Sharon	100%	35
Uniontown Hospital[2]	Uniontown	100%	28
UPMC East[2]	Monroeville	100%	66
UPMC Hamot[2]	Erie	100%	84
UPMC Horizon	Greenville	100%	57
UPMC Mckeesport[2]	Mc Keesport	100%	27
UPMC Mercy[2]	Pittsburgh	100%	106
UPMC Northwest[2]	Seneca	100%	66
UPMC Passavant[2]	Pittsburgh	100%	129
UPMC Presbyterian Shadyside[2]	Pittsburgh	100%	345
UPMC Saint Margaret[2]	Pittsburgh	100%	97
Aria Health[2]	Philadelphia	99%	139
Butler Memorial Hospital[2]	Butler	99%	67
Chestnut Hill Hospital[2]	Philadelphia	98%	60
Gettysburg Hospital[2]	Gettysburg	98%	57
Monongahela Valley Hospital[2]	Monongahela	98%	54
Thomas Jefferson University Hospital[2]	Philadelphia	98%	115
Grand View Hospital[2]	Sellersville	97%	67
Excela Health Latrobe Hospital[2]	Latrobe	96%	25
Lancaster General Hospital[2]	Lancaster	96%	248
Schuylkill Med Ctr-S Jackson St[2]	Pottsville	96%	27
The Washington Hospital[2]	Washington	96%	45
Williamsport Regional Medical Center[2]	Williamsport	96%	52
York Hospital[2]	York	96%	196
Evangelical Community Hospital	Lewisburg	95%	43
Holy Redeemer Hospital & Medical Center[2]	Meadowbrook	95%	39
Acmh Hospital[2]	Kittanning	93%	30
Good Samaritan Hospital[2]	Lebanon	93%	72
Lancaster Regional Medical Center[2]	Lancaster	93%	27
Lansdale Hospital[2]	Lansdale	93%	29
Reading Hospital[2]	Reading	93%	236
Crozer Chester Medical Center[2]	Upland	92%	84
Delaware County Memorial Hospital[2]	Drexel Hill	92%	48
Ephrata Community Hospital[2]	Ephrata	92%	38
Western Pennsylvania Hospital[2]	Pittsburgh	92%	26
Geisinger Medical Center[2]	Danville	91%	111
Pottstown Memorial Medical Center[2]	Pottstown	90%	40
Easton Hospital[2]	Easton	89%	37
Saint Mary Medical Center[2]	Langhorne	89%	101
Abington Memorial Hospital[2]	Abington	88%	151
Chambersburg Hospital	Chambersburg	88%	86
Penn Presbyterian Medical Center[2]	Philadelphia	88%	67
Penn Hosp of the Univ of PA Hlth Sys[2]	Philadelphia	87%	54
Saint Luke's Hospital Bethlehem[2]	Bethlehem	81%	104
Conemaugh Valley Memorial Hospital[2]	Johnstown	80%	93
Geisinger - Community Medical Center[2]	Scranton	80%	65
Einstein Medical Center Montgomery[2]	East Norriton	79%	29
Saint Joseph Medical Center[2]	Reading	79%	63
Pinnacle Health Hospitals[2]	Harrisburg	77%	162
Allegheny General Hospital[2]	Pittsburgh	76%	127
Geisinger Wyoming Valley Medical Center[2]	Wilkes Barre	73%	59
Mercy Fitzgerald Hospital[2]	Darby	73%	117
Excela Health Westmoreland Hospital[2]	Greensburg	72%	80
Jameson Memorial Hospital[2]	New Castle	71%	41
Lehigh Valley Hospital[2]	Allentown	66%	153
Holy Spirit Hospital[2]	Camp Hill	65%	122
Regional Hospital of Scranton[2]	Scranton	65%	46
Saint Luke's Hospital - Anderson Campus[2]	Easton	64%	58
Lehigh Valley Hospital - Muhlenberg[2]	Bethlehem	63%	102
Robert Packer Hospital[2]	Sayre	63%	63
Hahnemann University Hospital[2]	Philadelphia	58%	79
Wilkes-Barre General Hospital[2]	Wilkes-Barre	56%	72
Albert Einstein Medical Center[2]	Philadelphia	55%	105
Hanover Hospital[2]	Hanover	55%	33
Riddle Memorial Hospital[2]	Media	54%	35
Forbes Regional Hospital[2]	Monroeville	42%	80
Main Line Hospital Lankenau[2]	Wynnewood	42%	57
Temple University Hospital[2]	Philadelphia	42%	112
Main Line Hospital Paoli[2]	Paoli	34%	71
Main Line Hospital Bryn Mawr Campus[2]	Bryn Mawr	33%	57
Jefferson Regional Medical Center[2]	Pittsburgh	32%	104
UPMC Altoona[2]	Altoona	25%	115
Mount Nittany Medical Center[2]	State College	24%	99
Memorial Hospital[2]	York	23%	71
Indiana Regional Medical Center[2]	Indiana	18%	45
Pocono Medical Center[2]	E Stroudsburg	18%	77
Chester County Hospital[2]	West Chester	16%	57
Hospital of Univ of Pennsylvania[2]	Philadelphia	10%	153
Jeanes Hospital[2]	Philadelphia	9%	35

Chest Pain/Possible Heart Attack Care

Aspirin Given Within 24 Hours of Arrival

Hospital Name	City	Rate	Cases
Bradford Regional Medical Center	Bradford	100%	68
Butler Memorial Hospital	Butler	100%	31
Charles Cole Memorial Hospital	Coudersport	100%	65
Excela Health Frick Hospital	Mount Pleasant	100%	28
Grand View Hospital	Sellersville	100%	55
Heart of Lancaster Reg Med Ctr	Lititz	100%	26
Heritage Valley Sewickley	Sewickley	100%	46
Memorial Hospital Towanda	Towanda	100%	31
Nason Hospital	Roaring Spring	100%	35
Penn Highlands Elk	Saint Marys	100%	49
Pottstown Memorial Medical Center	Pottstown	100%	88
Schuylkill Med Ctr-East Norwegian St	Pottsville	100%	106
Somerset Hospital	Somerset	100%	27
Sunbury Community Hospital	Sunbury	100%	37
Titusville Hospital	Titusville	100%	83
Tyler Memorial Hospital	Tunkhannock	100%	30
UPMC East[3]	Monroeville	100%	32
UPMC Saint Margaret	Pittsburgh	100%	118
Wayne Memorial Hospital	Honesdale	100%	56
Western Pennsylvania Hospital[3]	Pittsburgh	100%	34
Alle Kiski Medical Center	Natrona	99%	135
Canonsburg General Hospital	Canonsburg	99%	67
Chestnut Hill Hospital	Philadelphia	99%	82
Excela Health Latrobe Hospital	Latrobe	99%	91
UPMC Northwest	Seneca	99%	148
Carlisle Regional Medical Center	Carlisle	98%	63
Highlands Hospital	Connellsville	98%	47
Indiana Regional Medical Center	Indiana	98%	160
Lansdale Hospital	Lansdale	98%	43
Penn Highlands Clearfield	Clearfield	98%	120
Ephrata Community Hospital	Ephrata	97%	58
Hanover Hospital	Hanover	97%	90
Ohio Valley General Hospital	Mckees Rocks	97%	30
Soldiers & Sailors Memorial Hospital	Wellsboro	97%	101
Waynesboro Hospital	Waynesboro	97%	62
Clarion Hospital	Clarion	96%	55
Corry Memorial Hospital	Corry	96%	27
Gnaden Huetten Memorial Hospital	Lehighton	96%	54
Jameson Memorial Hospital	New Castle	96%	47
Lehigh Valley Hospital - Hazleton	Hazleton	96%	191
Muncy Valley Hospital	Muncy	96%	76
Penn Highlands Brookville	Brookville	96%	72
Southwest Regional Medical Center	Waynesburg	96%	69
UPMC Bedford Memorial	Everett	96%	85
UPMC Horizon	Greenville	96%	109
Warren General Hospital	Warren	96%	170
Delaware County Memorial Hospital	Drexel Hill	95%	43
Ellwood City Hospital	Ellwood City	95%	57
Grove City Medical Center	Grove City	95%	43
Schuylkill Med Ctr-S Jackson St	Pottsville	95%	61
J C Blair Memorial Hospital	Huntingdon	94%	134
Lewistown Hospital	Lewistown	94%	90
Geisinger - Bloomsburg Hospital	Bloomsburg	93%	42
Mercy Suburban Hospital	Norristown	93%	28
Windber Hospital	Windber	91%	32
Acmh Hospital	Kittanning	90%	29
Fulton County Medical Center	Mcconnellsburg	88%	41
Punxsutawney Area Hospital	Punxsutawney	88%	34
Miners Medical Center	Hastings	84%	74

Average Time to ECG (minutes)

Hospital Name	City	Min.	Cases
Ephrata Community Hospital	Ephrata	4	58
Heart of Lancaster Reg Med Ctr	Lititz	4	26
UPMC Bedford Memorial	Everett	4	89
Alle Kiski Medical Center	Natrona	5	145
Penn Highlands Brookville	Brookville	5	71
Southwest Regional Medical Center	Waynesburg	5	69
Titusville Hospital	Titusville	5	89
Bradford Regional Medical Center	Bradford	6	67
Canonsburg General Hospital	Canonsburg	6	68
Chestnut Hill Hospital	Philadelphia	6	85
Ellwood City Hospital	Ellwood City	6	58
Excela Health Frick Hospital	Mount Pleasant	6	29
Excela Health Latrobe Hospital	Latrobe	6	96
Wayne Memorial Hospital	Honesdale	6	57
Butler Memorial Hospital	Butler	7	31
Delaware County Memorial Hospital	Drexel Hill	7	44
Fulton County Medical Center	Mcconnellsburg	7	39
Gnaden Huetten Memorial Hospital	Lehighton	7	56
Grand View Hospital	Sellersville	7	55
Indiana Regional Medical Center	Indiana	7	163
Muncy Valley Hospital	Muncy	7	80
UPMC Northwest	Seneca	7	153
UPMC Saint Margaret	Pittsburgh	7	122
Acmh Hospital	Kittanning	8	29
Geisinger - Bloomsburg Hospital	Bloomsburg	8	43
Jennersville Regional Hospital	West Grove	8	25
Memorial Hospital Towanda	Towanda	8	31
Nason Hospital	Roaring Spring	8	35
Penn Highlands Elk	Saint Marys	8	54
Waynesboro Hospital	Waynesboro	8	65
Windber Hospital	Windber	8	33
Grove City Medical Center	Grove City	9	45
Hanover Hospital	Hanover	9	95
Heritage Valley Sewickley	Sewickley	9	44
Lansdale Hospital	Lansdale	9	45
Lewistown Hospital	Lewistown	9	91
UPMC East[3]	Monroeville	9	34
Charles Cole Memorial Hospital	Coudersport	10	67
Corry Memorial Hospital	Corry	10	27
Highlands Hospital	Connellsville	10	47
Punxsutawney Area Hospital	Punxsutawney	10	28
UPMC Horizon	Greenville	10	114
J C Blair Memorial Hospital	Huntingdon	11	144
Soldiers & Sailors Memorial Hospital	Wellsboro	11	107
Sunbury Community Hospital	Sunbury	11	42
Tyler Memorial Hospital	Tunkhannock	11	35
Western Pennsylvania Hospital[3]	Pittsburgh	11	33
Carlisle Regional Medical Center	Carlisle	12	64
Jameson Memorial Hospital	New Castle	12	48
Ohio Valley General Hospital	Mckees Rocks	12	29
Schuylkill Med Ctr-East Norwegian St	Pottsville	12	110
Warren General Hospital	Warren	12	176
Lehigh Valley Hospital - Hazleton	Hazleton	13	196
Schuylkill Med Ctr-S Jackson St	Pottsville	13	63
Clarion Hospital	Clarion	14	56
Somerset Hospital	Somerset	14	28
Mercy Suburban Hospital	Norristown	15	32
Pottstown Memorial Medical Center	Pottstown	15	89
Miners Medical Center	Hastings	17	76
Penn Highlands Clearfield	Clearfield	18	121

Average Time to Transfer (minutes)

Hospital Name	City	Min.	Cases
UPMC Saint Margaret	Pittsburgh	49	25
Chestnut Hill Hospital	Philadelphia	55	31
Alle Kiski Medical Center	Natrona	56	30
UPMC Horizon	Greenville	83	29

Children's Asthma Care

Received Home Management Plan of Care

Hospital Name	City	Rate	Cases
Children's Hospital of Philadelphia[2]	Philadelphia	91%	757
Children's Hospital of Pittsburgh of UPMC[2]	Pittsburgh	57%	337

Received Reliever Medication

Hospital Name	City	Rate	Cases
Children's Hospital of Philadelphia[2]	Philadelphia	100%	757
Children's Hospital of Pittsburgh of UPMC[2]	Pittsburgh	100%	341

Received Systemic Corticosteroids

Hospital Name	City	Rate	Cases
Children's Hospital of Philadelphia[2]	Philadelphia	100%	755
Children's Hospital of Pittsburgh of UPMC[2]	Pittsburgh	100%	341

Emergency Department

Admittance Decision Time (minutes)

Hospital Name	City	Min.	Cases
Barnes-Kasson County Hospital[2,3]	Susquehanna	25	363
Nason Hospital[2]	Roaring Spring	35	231
Western Pennsylvania Hospital[2]	Pittsburgh	38	104
Geisinger - Bloomsburg Hospital[2]	Bloomsburg	40	801
Miners Medical Center	Hastings	40	325
Schuylkill Med Ctr-S Jackson St[2]	Pottsville	40	513
Tyler Memorial Hospital[2]	Tunkhannock	45	212
Acmh Hospital[2]	Kittanning	46	96
Grove City Medical Center[2]	Grove City	46	315
UPMC Bedford Memorial[2]	Everett	49	358
Kane Community Hospital[2]	Kane	50	500
Memorial Hospital Towanda[2]	Towanda	50	291
Monongahela Valley Hospital[2]	Monongahela	50	917
Somerset Hospital[2]	Somerset	50	230
Charles Cole Memorial Hospital[2]	Coudersport	51	226
Excela Health Frick Hospital[2]	Mount Pleasant	52	716
Punxsutawney Area Hospital[2]	Punxsutawney	52	304
Tyrone Hospital[2]	Tyrone	53	374
Lewistown Hospital[2]	Lewistown	54	558
Heritage Valley Sewickley[2]	Sewickley	56	422
Indiana Regional Medical Center[2]	Indiana	56	498
Jameson Memorial Hospital[2]	New Castle	56	684
Titusville Hospital[2]	Titusville	58	572
Troy Community Hospital[2,3]	Troy	58	213
Butler Memorial Hospital[2]	Butler	59	262
UPMC Horizon[2]	Greenville	59	560
Schuylkill Med Ctr-East Norwegian St[2]	Pottsville	60	541
Southwest Regional Medical Center[2]	Waynesburg	60	387
UPMC Mckeesport[2]	Mc Keesport	60	849
Ohio Valley General Hospital[2]	Mckees Rocks	61	349
Saint Luke's Miners Memorial Hospital[2]	Coaldale	61	463

NOTE: Hospital profiles are in alphabetical order by state, then city, then hospital within the city; Rankings exclude hospitals with less than 25 cases except for patient surveys which excludes hospitals with less than 100 cases; (a) 100-299 cases; (1) The number of cases/patients is too few to report; (2) Data submitted were based on a sample of cases/patients; (3) Results are based on a shorter time period than required; (4) Data suppressed by CMS for one or more quarters; (5) Results are not available for this reporting period; (6) Fewer than 100 patients completed the HCAHPS survey; (7) No cases met the criteria for this measure; (8) The lower limit of the confidence interval cannot be calculated if the number of observed infections equals zero; (9) No data are available from the state/territory for this reporting period; (10) The scores shown reflect fewer than 50 completed surveys; (11) There were discrepancies in the data collection process; (12) This measure does not apply to this hospital for this reporting period; (13) Results cannot be calculated for this reporting period; (14) The results for this state are combined with nearby states to protect confidentiality; Please refer to the User's Guide for a full explanation of data.

Uniontown Hospital[2]	Uniontown	63	675
Excela Health Latrobe Hospital[2]	Latrobe	64	1096
Magee Womens Hosp of UPMC Health Sys[2]	Pittsburgh	64	96
Ellwood City Hospital[2]	Ellwood City	65	444
Gettysburg Hospital[2]	Gettysburg	65	435
Meadville Medical Center[2]	Meadville	65	1013
Palmerton Hospital[2]	Palmerton	65	293
Bradford Regional Medical Center[2]	Bradford	66	350
Windber Hospital[2]	Windber	66	175
Sunbury Community Hospital[2]	Sunbury	67	359
Penn Highlands Clearfield[2]	Clearfield	69	419
Canonsburg General Hospital[2]	Canonsburg	70	450
Clarion Hospital[2]	Clarion	70	335
Mid - Valley Hospital[2]	Peckville	70	128
Warren General Hospital[2]	Warren	70	185
Lock Haven Hospital[2]	Lock Haven	71	448
Sharon Regional Health System[2]	Sharon	73	213
Gnaden Huetten Memorial Hospital[2]	Lehighton	74	280
UPMC Altoona[2]	Altoona	74	868
Highlands Hospital[2]	Connellsville	75	417
J C Blair Memorial Hospital[2]	Huntingdon	76	145
UPMC Northwest[2]	Seneca	76	544
Heritage Valley Beaver[2]	Beaver	77	470
Millcreek Community Hospital[2]	Erie	77	215
UPMC East[2,3]	Monroeville	77	615
UPMC Passavant[2]	Pittsburgh	77	273
Conemaugh Valley Memorial Hospital[2]	Johnstown	78	639
Heart of Lancaster Reg Med Ctr[2]	Lititz	78	243
Penn Highlands Elk[2]	Saint Marys	78	435
Ephrata Community Hospital[2]	Ephrata	81	507
Lancaster General Hospital[2]	Lancaster	81	601
The Washington Hospital[2]	Washington	82	607
Saint Luke's Quakertown Hospital[2]	Quakertown	84	420
UPMC Hamot[2]	Erie	84	553
Williamsport Regional Medical Center[2]	Williamsport	84	303
Saint Luke's Hospital - Anderson Campus[2]	Easton	88	852
UPMC Presbyterian Shadyside[2]	Pittsburgh	88	460
Brandywine Hospital[2]	Coatesville	89	865
Excela Health Westmoreland Hospital[2]	Greensburg	89	870
Chester County Hospital[2]	West Chester	90	442
Roxborough Memorial Hospital[2]	Philadelphia	93	863
Easton Hospital[2]	Easton	94	800
Jennersville Regional Hospital[2]	West Grove	94	583
UPMC Saint Margaret[2]	Pittsburgh	94	671
Alle Kiski Medical Center[2]	Natrona	96	422
UPMC Mercy[2]	Pittsburgh	96	629
York Hospital[2]	York	96	338
Saint Clair Memorial Hospital[2]	Pittsburgh	97	578
Lansdale Hospital[2]	Lansdale	98	768
Chestnut Hill Hospital[2]	Philadelphia	99	1179
Jersey Shore Hospital[3]	Jersey Shore	100	262
Pinnacle Health Hospitals[2]	Harrisburg	100	611
Saint Luke's Hospital Bethlehem[2]	Bethlehem	101	982
Lehigh Valley Hospital - Hazleton[2]	Hazleton	103	597
Penn Highlands Dubois[2]	Dubois	103	416
Lower Bucks Hospital[2]	Bristol	104	791
Moses Taylor Hospital[2]	Scranton	105	461
Berwick Hospital Center[2]	Berwick	107	469
Soldiers & Sailors Memorial Hospital[2]	Wellsboro	108	247
Abington Memorial Hospital[2]	Abington	109	571
Temple University Hospital[2]	Philadelphia	109	594
Grand View Hospital[2]	Sellersville	113	633
Jeanes Hospital[2]	Philadelphia	113	960
Pottstown Memorial Medical Center[2]	Pottstown	115	943
Regional Hospital of Scranton[2]	Scranton	115	197
Carlisle Regional Medical Center[2]	Carlisle	116	516
Lehigh Valley Hospital - Muhlenberg[2]	Bethlehem	119	1028
Saint Joseph's Hospital[2]	Philadelphia	120	559
Waynesboro Hospital[2]	Waynesboro	123	471
Milton S Hershey Medical Center[2]	Hershey	124	571
Phoenixville Hospital[2]	Phoenixville	125	787
Saint Vincent Hospital[2]	Erie	128	1026
Allegheny General Hospital[2]	Pittsburgh	130	492
Forbes Regional Hospital[2]	Monroeville	130	547
Lehigh Valley Hospital[2]	Allentown	131	590
Hanover Hospital[2]	Hanover	133	808
Wilkes-Barre General Hospital[2]	Wilkes-Barre	133	930
Lancaster Regional Medical Center[2]	Lancaster	135	379
Saint Mary Medical Center[2]	Langhorne	137	732
Evangelical Community Hospital[2]	Lewisburg	138	638
Hahnemann University Hospital[2]	Philadelphia	139	585
Reading Hospital[2]	Reading	142	691
Chambersburg Hospital[2]	Chambersburg	144	675
Riddle Memorial Hospital[2]	Media	144	716
Penn Presbyterian Medical Center[2]	Philadelphia	145	706
Aria Health[2]	Philadelphia	148	715
Holy Spirit Hospital[2]	Camp Hill	148	417
Sacred Heart Hospital[2]	Allentown	152	757
Saint Joseph Medical Center[2]	Reading	152	588
Doylestown Hospital[2]	Doylestown	157	840
Jefferson Regional Medical Center[2]	Pittsburgh	157	613
Main Line Hospital Paoli[2]	Paoli	161	638
Einstein Medical Center Montgomery[2,3]	East Norriton	162	436
Holy Redeemer Hospital & Medical Center[2]	Meadowbrook	164	490
Hospital of Univ of Pennsylvania[2]	Philadelphia	165	332
Delaware County Memorial Hospital[2]	Drexel Hill	170	540
Main Line Hospital Lankenau[2]	Wynnewood	173	546
Good Samaritan Hospital[2]	Lebanon	175	403
Thomas Jefferson University Hospital[2]	Philadelphia	178	1380
Albert Einstein Medical Center[2]	Philadelphia	182	768
Pocono Medical Center[2]	E Stroudsburg	182	1018
Penn Hosp of the Univ of PA Hlth Sys[2]	Philadelphia	186	358
Mercy Fitzgerald Hospital[2]	Darby	194	2208
Crozer Chester Medical Center[2]	Upland	195	630
Nazareth Hospital[2]	Philadelphia	196	1080
Mount Nittany Medical Center[2]	State College	198	548
Mercy Suburban Hospital[2]	Norristown	204	802
Wayne Memorial Hospital[2]	Honesdale	212	380
Main Line Hospital Bryn Mawr Campus[2]	Bryn Mawr	214	556
Geisinger Medical Center[2]	Danville	220	680
Memorial Hospital[2]	York	220	737
Robert Packer Hospital[2]	Sayre	230	552
Geisinger Wyoming Valley Medical Center[2]	Wilkes Barre	288	766
Geisinger - Community Medical Center[2]	Scranton	300	1272

Head CT Results Within 45 Minutes of Arrival

Hospital Name	City	Rate	Cases
Mercy Suburban Hospital	Norristown	94%	36
Brandywine Hospital	Coatesville	90%	29
Chestnut Hill Hospital	Philadelphia	85%	26
Evangelical Community Hospital	Lewisburg	79%	33
Chester County Hospital	West Chester	76%	34
Lehigh Valley Hospital - Hazleton	Hazleton	72%	25
UPMC Passavant	Pittsburgh	70%	27
Aria Health	Philadelphia	68%	25
Hanover Hospital	Hanover	64%	25
Butler Memorial Hospital	Butler	63%	27
Doylestown Hospital	Doylestown	63%	30
UPMC Altoona	Altoona	33%	36

Patients Who Left ER Before Being Seen

Hospital Name	City	Rate	Cases
Abington Memorial Hospital	Abington	0%	105817
Barnes-Kasson County Hospital	Susquehanna	0%	3759
Berwick Hospital Center	Berwick	0%	12765
Bradford Regional Medical Center	Bradford	0%	21177
Butler Memorial Hospital	Butler	0%	46788
Delaware County Memorial Hospital	Drexel Hill	0%	40452
Doylestown Hospital	Doylestown	0%	45748
Einstein Medical Center Montgomery	East Norriton	0%	8987
Excela Health Frick Hospital	Mount Pleasant	0%	25694
Excela Health Latrobe Hospital	Latrobe	0%	35201
Fulton County Medical Center	Mcconnellsburg	0%	9746
Geisinger Medical Center	Danville	0%	49726
Grove City Medical Center	Grove City	0%	16970
Heritage Valley Beaver	Beaver	0%	50201
Heritage Valley Sewickley	Sewickley	0%	33437
Indiana Regional Medical Center	Indiana	0%	44489
J C Blair Memorial Hospital	Huntingdon	0%	17289
Kane Community Hospital	Kane	0%	6857
Lansdale Hospital	Lansdale	0%	27630
Lehigh Valley Hospital - Muhlenberg	Bethlehem	0%	58155
Lock Haven Hospital	Lock Haven	0%	12146
Main Line Hospital Bryn Mawr Campus	Bryn Mawr	0%	47825
Main Line Hospital Paoli	Paoli	0%	41520
Meyersdale Community Hospital	Myersdale	0%	4287
Miners Medical Center	Hastings	0%	10044
Mount Nittany Medical Center	State College	0%	49449
Penn Highlands Brookville	Brookville	0%	9622
Penn Highlands Elk	Saint Marys	0%	17355
Phoenixville Hospital	Phoenixville	0%	27985
Punxsutawney Area Hospital	Punxsutawney	0%	15798
Roxborough Memorial Hospital	Philadelphia	0%	20020
Saint Clair Memorial Hospital	Pittsburgh	0%	64774
Saint Mary Medical Center	Langhorne	0%	71261
Soldiers & Sailors Memorial Hospital	Wellsboro	0%	18627
Tyrone Hospital	Tyrone	0%	7829
Uniontown Hospital	Uniontown	0%	55589
UPMC Bedford Memorial	Everett	0%	16903
UPMC East	Monroeville	0%	17914
UPMC Northwest	Seneca	0%	32101
UPMC Presbyterian Shadyside	Pittsburgh	0%	107344
UPMC Saint Margaret	Pittsburgh	0%	40321
Wayne Memorial Hospital	Honesdale	0%	21908
Western Pennsylvania Hospital	Pittsburgh	0%	17515
Acmh Hospital	Kittanning	1%	25833
Alle Kiski Medical Center	Natrona	1%	37318
Allegheny General Hospital	Pittsburgh	1%	51023
Brandywine Hospital	Coatesville	1%	29188
Bucktail Medical Center	Renovo	1%	2113
Canonsburg General Hospital	Canonsburg	1%	21014
Carlisle Regional Medical Center	Carlisle	1%	28091
Chambersburg Hospital	Chambersburg	1%	56808
Chestnut Hill Hospital	Philadelphia	1%	32723
Clarion Hospital	Clarion	1%	18389
Corry Memorial Hospital	Corry	1%	10290
Crozer Chester Medical Center	Upland	1%	96669
Easton Hospital	Easton	1%	33381
Ellwood City Hospital	Ellwood City	1%	14644
Endless Mountains Health Systems	Montrose	1%	4500
Ephrata Community Hospital	Ephrata	1%	23353
Evangelical Community Hospital	Lewisburg	1%	33148
Excela Health Westmoreland Hospital	Greensburg	1%	59279
Forbes Regional Hospital	Monroeville	1%	25054
Geisinger - Community Medical Center	Scranton	1%	36296
Geisinger Wyoming Valley Medical Center	Wilkes Barre	1%	39944
Gnaden Huetten Memorial Hospital	Lehighton	1%	19558
Grand View Hospital	Sellersville	1%	35459
Heart of Lancaster Reg Med Ctr	Lititz	1%	13914
Highlands Hospital	Connellsville	1%	14068
Holy Redeemer Hospital & Medical Center	Meadowbrook	1%	30823
Holy Spirit Hospital	Camp Hill	1%	53674
Jefferson Regional Medical Center	Pittsburgh	1%	52791
Jennersville Regional Hospital	West Grove	1%	15486
Jersey Shore Hospital	Jersey Shore	1%	14100
Lancaster General Hospital	Lancaster	1%	107347
Lancaster Regional Medical Center	Lancaster	1%	23162
Lehigh Valley Hospital	Allentown	1%	89026
Lower Bucks Hospital	Bristol	1%	29978
Magee Womens Hosp of UPMC Health Sys	Pittsburgh	1%	22946
Main Line Hospital Lankenau	Wynnewood	1%	52716
Meadville Medical Center	Meadville	1%	32665
Mercy Suburban Hospital	Norristown	1%	25350
Mid - Valley Hospital	Peckville	1%	9735
Milton S Hershey Medical Center	Hershey	1%	64929
Monongahela Valley Hospital	Monongahela	1%	34604
Moses Taylor Hospital	Scranton	1%	32490
Muncy Valley Hospital	Muncy	1%	16028
Palmerton Hospital	Palmerton	1%	11521
Penn Highlands Clearfield	Clearfield	1%	25935
Penn Highlands Dubois	Dubois	1%	32692
Pottstown Memorial Medical Center	Pottstown	1%	43956
Reading Hospital	Reading	1%	133565
Riddle Memorial Hospital	Media	1%	32814
Sacred Heart Hospital	Allentown	1%	33121
Saint Luke's Hospital - Anderson Campus	Easton	1%	27198
Saint Luke's Hospital Bethlehem	Bethlehem	1%	108309
Saint Luke's Miners Memorial Hospital	Coaldale	1%	14494
Saint Luke's Quakertown Hospital	Quakertown	1%	15983
Saint Vincent Hospital	Erie	1%	65489
Schuylkill Med Ctr-East Norwegian St	Pottsville	1%	21669
Schuylkill Med Ctr-S Jackson St	Pottsville	1%	32957
Sharon Regional Health System	Sharon	1%	38822
Southwest Regional Medical Center	Waynesburg	1%	22463
Sunbury Community Hospital	Sunbury	1%	10923
Titusville Hospital	Titusville	1%	12097
Troy Community Hospital	Troy	1%	7186
Tyler Memorial Hospital	Tunkhannock	1%	8686
UPMC Altoona	Altoona	1%	59315
UPMC Hamot	Erie	1%	78477
UPMC Horizon	Greenville	1%	37254
UPMC Mckeesport	Mc Keesport	1%	41188
UPMC Mercy	Pittsburgh	1%	73045
UPMC Passavant	Pittsburgh	1%	60151
Warren General Hospital	Warren	1%	20835
The Washington Hospital	Washington	1%	48577
Waynesboro Hospital	Waynesboro	1%	11975
Windber Hospital	Windber	1%	11860
Charles Cole Memorial Hospital	Coudersport	2%	10135
Chester County Hospital	West Chester	2%	42390
Conemaugh Valley Memorial Hospital	Johnstown	2%	68109
Gettysburg Hospital	Gettysburg	2%	23150
Good Samaritan Hospital	Lebanon	2%	55049
Hahnemann University Hospital	Philadelphia	2%	47475
Hanover Hospital	Hanover	2%	31358
Jameson Memorial Hospital	New Castle	2%	35712
Lewistown Hospital	Lewistown	2%	33206
Memorial Hospital	York	2%	36443
Memorial Hospital Towanda	Towanda	2%	11376
Mercy Fitzgerald Hospital	Darby	2%	86942
Millcreek Community Hospital	Erie	2%	16459
Nason Hospital	Roaring Spring	2%	13692
Nazareth Hospital	Philadelphia	2%	45289
Ohio Valley General Hospital	Mckees Rocks	2%	20463
Penn Presbyterian Medical Center	Philadelphia	2%	38723
Penn Hosp of the Univ of PA Hlth Sys	Philadelphia	2%	34469
Pinnacle Health Hospitals	Harrisburg	2%	111929
Robert Packer Hospital	Sayre	2%	30332
Saint Joseph Medical Center	Reading	2%	41647
Wilkes-Barre General Hospital	Wilkes-Barre	2%	58906
Williamsport Regional Medical Center	Williamsport	2%	22877
York Hospital	York	2%	56691

NOTE: Hospital profiles are in alphabetical order by state, then city, then hospital within the city; Rankings exclude hospitals with less than 25 cases except for patient surveys which excludes hospitals with less than 100 cases; (a) 100-299 cases; (1) The number of cases/patients is too few to report; (2) Data submitted were based on a sample of cases/patients; (3) Results are based on a shorter time period than required; (4) Data suppressed by CMS for one or more quarters; (5) Results are not available for this reporting period; (6) Fewer than 100 patients completed the HCAHPS survey; (7) No cases met the criteria for this measure; (8) The lower limit of the confidence interval cannot be calculated if the number of observed infections equals zero; (9) No data are available from the state/territory for this reporting period; (10) The scores shown reflect fewer than 50 completed surveys; (11) There were discrepancies in the data collection process; (12) This measure does not apply to this hospital for this reporting period; (13) Results cannot be calculated for this reporting period; (14) The results for this state are combined with nearby states to protect confidentiality; Please refer to the User's Guide for a full explanation of data.

Albert Einstein Medical Center	Philadelphia	3%	122140
Geisinger - Bloomsburg Hospital	Bloomsburg	3%	13018
Lehigh Valley Hospital - Hazleton	Hazleton	3%	31397
Regional Hospital of Scranton	Scranton	3%	29689
Saint Joseph's Hospital	Philadelphia	3%	16715
Somerset Hospital	Somerset	3%	9350
Hospital of Univ of Pennsylvania	Philadelphia	4%	67086
Jeanes Hospital	Philadelphia	4%	36027
Pocono Medical Center	E Stroudsburg	4%	82215
Thomas Jefferson University Hospital	Philadelphia	4%	107129
Aria Health	Philadelphia	6%	113457
Temple University Hospital	Philadelphia	6%	151270

Time from ER Arrival to Being Admitted (minutes)

Hospital Name	City	Min.	Cases
Barnes-Kasson County Hospital[2,3]	Susquehanna	131	363
Miners Medical Center	Hastings	165	343
Kane Community Hospital[2]	Kane	170	523
Punxsutawney Area Hospital[2]	Punxsutawney	172	316
Grove City Medical Center[2]	Grove City	180	316
Western Pennsylvania Hospital[2]	Pittsburgh	183	125
Butler Memorial Hospital[2]	Butler	185	441
Millcreek Community Hospital[2]	Erie	185	221
UPMC Bedford Memorial[2]	Everett	188	379
Highlands Hospital[2]	Connellsville	193	420
UPMC Mckeesport[2]	Mc Keesport	193	908
Geisinger - Bloomsburg Hospital[2]	Bloomsburg	197	821
UPMC Northwest[2]	Seneca	198	565
Titusville Hospital[2]	Titusville	205	581
Southwest Regional Medical Center[2]	Waynesburg	207	394
Ellwood City Hospital[2]	Ellwood City	208	444
Memorial Hospital Towanda[2]	Towanda	208	299
Nason Hospital[2]	Roaring Spring	209	239
UPMC Horizon[2]	Greenville	210	587
Excela Health Frick Hospital[2]	Mount Pleasant	211	717
Schuylkill Med Ctr-S Jackson St[2]	Pottsville	211	556
UPMC East[2,3]	Monroeville	211	628
Indiana Regional Medical Center[2]	Indiana	212	498
Windber Hospital[2]	Windber	213	210
Lewistown Hospital[2]	Lewistown	214	576
Magee Womens Hosp of UPMC Health Sys[2]	Pittsburgh	215	98
Schuylkill Med Ctr-East Norwegian St[2]	Pottsville	215	610
Tyrone Hospital[2]	Tyrone	216	374
Palmerton Hospital[2]	Palmerton	218	309
Clarion Hospital[2]	Clarion	219	335
UPMC Hamot[2]	Erie	219	563
Monongahela Valley Hospital[2]	Monongahela	221	1032
UPMC Passavant[2]	Pittsburgh	221	283
UPMC Saint Margaret[2]	Pittsburgh	221	676
Acmh Hospital[2]	Kittanning	222	99
Saint Clair Memorial Hospital[2]	Pittsburgh	222	613
UPMC Mercy[2]	Pittsburgh	224	640
UPMC Presbyterian Shadyside[2]	Pittsburgh	225	481
Excela Health Latrobe Hospital[2]	Latrobe	230	1098
Lancaster General Hospital[2]	Lancaster	230	624
Somerset Hospital[2]	Somerset	230	257
Sharon Regional Health System[2]	Sharon	232	710
Soldiers & Sailors Memorial Hospital[2]	Wellsboro	234	251
Charles Cole Memorial Hospital[2]	Coudersport	235	227
Berwick Hospital Center[2]	Berwick	236	496
Heritage Valley Sewickley[2]	Sewickley	237	427
Jameson Memorial Hospital[2]	New Castle	237	685
Tyler Memorial Hospital[2]	Tunkhannock	237	213
UPMC Altoona[2]	Altoona	237	901
J C Blair Memorial Hospital[2]	Huntingdon	240	330
Meadville Medical Center[2]	Meadville	240	1116
Conemaugh Valley Memorial Hospital[2]	Johnstown	242	662
Penn Highlands Elk[2]	Saint Marys	243	482
Pinnacle Health Hospitals[2]	Harrisburg	244	611
Gnaden Huetten Memorial Hospital[2]	Lehighton	245	281
Saint Luke's Quakertown Hospital[2]	Quakertown	245	426
Mid - Valley Hospital[2]	Peckville	246	264
Saint Luke's Miners Memorial Hospital[2]	Coaldale	246	467
Bradford Regional Medical Center[2]	Bradford	248	350
Roxborough Memorial Hospital[2]	Philadelphia	250	863
Penn Highlands Dubois[2]	Dubois	252	416
Canonsburg General Hospital[2]	Canonsburg	254	456
Ohio Valley General Hospital[2]	Mckees Rocks	254	422
Uniontown Hospital[2]	Uniontown	254	692
Sunbury Community Hospital[2]	Sunbury	255	364
Grand View Hospital[2]	Sellersville	256	640
Brandywine Hospital[2]	Coatesville	257	884
Lock Haven Hospital[2]	Lock Haven	257	451
Troy Community Hospital[2,3]	Troy	257	213
Chestnut Hill Hospital[2]	Philadelphia	258	1179
Phoenixville Hospital[2]	Phoenixville	258	805
The Washington Hospital[2]	Washington	258	607
Saint Luke's Hospital - Anderson Campus[2]	Easton	259	857
Alle Kiski Medical Center[2]	Natrona	260	669
Heritage Valley Beaver[2]	Beaver	260	550
Heart of Lancaster Reg Med Ctr[2]	Lititz	261	243
Penn Highlands Clearfield[2]	Clearfield	262	438
Saint Luke's Hospital Bethlehem[2]	Bethlehem	262	1003
Lansdale Hospital[2]	Lansdale	263	796
Jennersville Regional Hospital[2]	West Grove	265	583
Jersey Shore Hospital[3]	Jersey Shore	265	312
Excela Health Westmoreland Hospital[2]	Greensburg	266	876
Waynesboro Hospital[2]	Waynesboro	266	476
Easton Hospital[2]	Easton	268	827
Jefferson Regional Medical Center[2]	Pittsburgh	270	616
Lehigh Valley Hospital - Hazleton[2]	Hazleton	272	641
Lower Bucks Hospital[2]	Bristol	273	796
Pottstown Memorial Medical Center[2]	Pottstown	274	948
Williamsport Regional Medical Center[2]	Williamsport	280	570
Abington Memorial Hospital[2]	Abington	283	599
Saint Vincent Hospital[2]	Erie	284	1037
Evangelical Community Hospital[2]	Lewisburg	286	638
Gettysburg Hospital[2]	Gettysburg	291	682
Carlisle Regional Medical Center[2]	Carlisle	294	518
Allegheny General Hospital[2]	Pittsburgh	295	546
Chambersburg Hospital[2]	Chambersburg	295	689
Moses Taylor Hospital[2]	Scranton	295	523
Jeanes Hospital[2]	Philadelphia	298	960
Warren General Hospital[2]	Warren	299	275
Mount Nittany Medical Center[2]	State College	302	587
Chester County Hospital[2]	West Chester	304	553
Sacred Heart Hospital[2]	Allentown	304	757
Saint Mary Medical Center[2]	Langhorne	304	732
Lancaster Regional Medical Center[2]	Lancaster	307	379
Forbes Regional Hospital[2]	Monroeville	310	628
Lehigh Valley Hospital - Muhlenberg[2]	Bethlehem	313	1030
Ephrata Community Hospital[2]	Ephrata	314	599
Main Line Hospital Paoli[2]	Paoli	316	638
Wilkes-Barre General Hospital[2]	Wilkes-Barre	320	983
Riddle Memorial Hospital[2]	Media	322	716
Regional Hospital of Scranton[2]	Scranton	325	223
Penn Presbyterian Medical Center[2]	Philadelphia	326	732
Temple University Hospital[2]	Philadelphia	329	594
Lehigh Valley Hospital[2]	Allentown	332	595
Hahnemann University Hospital[2]	Philadelphia	334	590
Pocono Medical Center[2]	E Stroudsburg	339	1019
York Hospital[2]	York	343	604
Doylestown Hospital[2]	Doylestown	349	841
Main Line Hospital Lankenau[2]	Wynnewood	350	546
Einstein Medical Center Montgomery[2,3]	East Norriton	354	442
Hanover Hospital[2]	Hanover	356	809
Mercy Suburban Hospital[2]	Norristown	356	805
Wayne Memorial Hospital[2]	Honesdale	356	397
Saint Joseph's Hospital[2]	Philadelphia	361	561
Holy Redeemer Hospital & Medical Center[2]	Meadowbrook	362	492
Reading Hospital[2]	Reading	368	701
Delaware County Memorial Hospital[2]	Drexel Hill	370	540
Geisinger Medical Center[2]	Danville	372	691
Albert Einstein Medical Center[2]	Philadelphia	374	774
Nazareth Hospital[2]	Philadelphia	374	1080
Main Line Hospital Bryn Mawr Campus[2]	Bryn Mawr	377	560
Mercy Fitzgerald Hospital[2]	Darby	386	2209
Aria Health[2]	Philadelphia	390	718
Crozer Chester Medical Center[2]	Upland	391	645
Milton S Hershey Medical Center[2]	Hershey	393	579
Holy Spirit Hospital[2]	Camp Hill	399	523
Good Samaritan Hospital[2]	Lebanon	406	549
Memorial Hospital[2]	York	407	739
Penn Hosp of the Univ of PA Hlth Sys[2]	Philadelphia	408	368
Thomas Jefferson University Hospital[2]	Philadelphia	410	1383
Hospital of Univ of Pennsylvania[2]	Philadelphia	418	337
Saint Joseph Medical Center[2]	Reading	426	739
Robert Packer Hospital[2]	Sayre	444	558
Geisinger - Community Medical Center[2]	Scranton	464	1285
Geisinger Wyoming Valley Medical Center[2]	Wilkes Barre	471	773

Time from ER Arrival to Discharge (minutes)

Hospital Name	City	Min.	Cases
Kane Community Hospital	Kane	72	571
Sacred Heart Hospital	Allentown	76	6935
Highlands Hospital	Connellsville	77	327
Miners Medical Center	Hastings	80	237
Tyrone Hospital	Tyrone	81	1218
Nason Hospital	Roaring Spring	87	378
Millcreek Community Hospital	Erie	88	289
Punxsutawney Area Hospital	Punxsutawney	88	377
Troy Community Hospital[3]	Troy	90	263
Schuylkill Med Ctr-S Jackson St	Pottsville	91	345
Palmerton Hospital	Palmerton	92	334
Ellwood City Hospital	Ellwood City	94	408
Grove City Medical Center	Grove City	95	362
Lower Bucks Hospital	Bristol	96	354
Soldiers & Sailors Memorial Hospital	Wellsboro	96	328
UPMC Bedford Memorial	Everett	96	552
UPMC Northwest	Seneca	97	541
Schuylkill Med Ctr-East Norwegian St	Pottsville	98	358
Easton Hospital	Easton	100	370
Southwest Regional Medical Center	Waynesburg	101	361
Acmh Hospital	Kittanning	102	439
Berwick Hospital Center	Berwick	102	386
Indiana Regional Medical Center	Indiana	103	338
Waynesboro Hospital	Waynesboro	103	364
Excela Health Frick Hospital	Mount Pleasant	104	460
Gnaden Huetten Memorial Hospital	Lehighton	105	343
Meadville Medical Center	Meadville	105	2176
Mid - Valley Hospital	Peckville	105	393
Titusville Hospital	Titusville	105	401
Lock Haven Hospital	Lock Haven	109	388
Sunbury Community Hospital	Sunbury	109	382
Tyler Memorial Hospital	Tunkhannock	110	361
Brandywine Hospital	Coatesville	111	384
Lancaster Regional Medical Center	Lancaster	112	495
Western Pennsylvania Hospital	Pittsburgh	112	401
Bradford Regional Medical Center	Bradford	113	608
Butler Memorial Hospital	Butler	113	302
Sharon Regional Health System	Sharon	113	1366
UPMC Horizon	Greenville	114	552
Saint Luke's Quakertown Hospital	Quakertown	115	354
Pocono Medical Center	E Stroudsburg	116	577
Excela Health Latrobe Hospital	Latrobe	118	441
Penn Highlands Dubois	Dubois	119	339
Alle Kiski Medical Center	Natrona	120	455
Saint Vincent Hospital	Erie	121	561
Heritage Valley Sewickley	Sewickley	123	392
Windber Hospital	Windber	123	335
Geisinger - Bloomsburg Hospital	Bloomsburg	124	337
Saint Luke's Miners Memorial Hospital	Coaldale	124	354
UPMC Altoona	Altoona	124	1523
Penn Highlands Elk	Saint Marys	126	452
Phoenixville Hospital	Phoenixville	126	397
Ohio Valley General Hospital	Mckees Rocks	127	339
UPMC East[3]	Monroeville	127	435
Chambersburg Hospital	Chambersburg	128	334
Conemaugh Valley Memorial Hospital	Johnstown	128	1192
J C Blair Memorial Hospital	Huntingdon	128	352
Roxborough Memorial Hospital	Philadelphia	128	396
Saint Luke's Hospital Bethlehem	Bethlehem	128	718
Einstein Medical Center Montgomery[3]	East Norriton	129	270
Heritage Valley Beaver	Beaver	129	395
Lancaster General Hospital	Lancaster	129	384
Clarion Hospital	Clarion	130	324
Saint Mary Medical Center	Langhorne	130	378
Canonsburg General Hospital	Canonsburg	131	453
Pottstown Memorial Medical Center	Pottstown	131	353
Uniontown Hospital	Uniontown	131	341
UPMC Mckeesport	Mc Keesport	132	527
UPMC Mercy	Pittsburgh	132	488
Chestnut Hill Hospital	Philadelphia	133	373
Jameson Memorial Hospital	New Castle	133	354
Memorial Hospital Towanda	Towanda	133	221
Nazareth Hospital	Philadelphia	134	344
Penn Highlands Clearfield	Clearfield	134	372
Saint Clair Memorial Hospital	Pittsburgh	135	302
Saint Luke's Hospital - Anderson Campus	Easton	136	360
Heart of Lancaster Reg Med Ctr	Lititz	138	388
Jennersville Regional Hospital	West Grove	138	370
Lansdale Hospital	Lansdale	138	370
UPMC Hamot	Erie	138	570
Grand View Hospital	Sellersville	139	592
Evangelical Community Hospital	Lewisburg	140	395
Mercy Fitzgerald Hospital	Darby	140	732
Regional Hospital of Scranton	Scranton	140	347
Carlisle Regional Medical Center	Carlisle	141	365
Lehigh Valley Hospital - Hazleton	Hazleton	141	435
Somerset Hospital	Somerset	141	401
Hahnemann University Hospital	Philadelphia	143	353
Lehigh Valley Hospital - Muhlenberg	Bethlehem	143	347
Main Line Hospital Paoli	Paoli	143	367
Excela Health Westmoreland Hospital	Greensburg	144	475
Monongahela Valley Hospital	Monongahela	144	663
Abington Memorial Hospital	Abington	145	389
Doylestown Hospital	Doylestown	145	361
Riddle Memorial Hospital	Media	145	369
Mercy Suburban Hospital	Norristown	146	359
Pinnacle Health Hospitals	Harrisburg	146	721
Crozer Chester Medical Center	Upland	148	405
Gettysburg Hospital	Gettysburg	148	361
Williamsport Regional Medical Center	Williamsport	148	544
Ephrata Community Hospital	Ephrata	149	408
UPMC Presbyterian Shadyside	Pittsburgh	149	528
The Washington Hospital	Washington	149	404
Magee Womens Hosp of UPMC Health Sys	Pittsburgh	151	589
Mount Nittany Medical Center	State College	151	357
UPMC Passavant	Pittsburgh	151	536
Wilkes-Barre General Hospital	Wilkes-Barre	153	355
Geisinger Medical Center	Danville	154	710
Penn Presbyterian Medical Center	Philadelphia	154	1311
Robert Packer Hospital	Sayre	155	553

NOTE: Hospital profiles are in alphabetical order by state, then city, then hospital within the city; Rankings exclude hospitals with less than 25 cases except for patient surveys which excludes hospitals with less than 100 cases; (a) 100-299 cases; (1) The number of cases/patients is too few to report; (2) Data submitted were based on a sample of cases/patients; (3) Results are based on a shorter time period than required; (4) Data suppressed by CMS for one or more quarters; (5) Results are not available for this reporting period; (6) Fewer than 100 patients completed the HCAHPS survey; (7) No cases met the criteria for this measure; (8) The lower limit of the confidence interval cannot be calculated if the number of observed infections equals zero; (9) No data are available from the state/territory for this reporting period; (10) The scores shown reflect fewer than 50 completed surveys; (11) There were discrepancies in the data collection process; (12) This measure does not apply to this hospital for this reporting period; (13) Results cannot be calculated for this reporting period; (14) The results for this state are combined with nearby states to protect confidentiality; Please refer to the User's Guide for a full explanation of data.

Hospital Name	City	Min.	Cases
Temple University Hospital	Philadelphia	155	347
Hanover Hospital	Hanover	156	808
Lewistown Hospital	Lewistown	156	336
Charles Cole Memorial Hospital	Coudersport	157	376
Jefferson Regional Medical Center	Pittsburgh	157	329
Main Line Hospital Bryn Mawr Campus	Bryn Mawr	157	362
Memorial Hospital	York	158	409
UPMC Saint Margaret	Pittsburgh	159	545
Chester County Hospital	West Chester	160	392
Lehigh Valley Hospital	Allentown	160	366
York Hospital	York	161	337
Good Samaritan Hospital	Lebanon	162	360
Wayne Memorial Hospital	Honesdale	164	359
Albert Einstein Medical Center	Philadelphia	166	549
Moses Taylor Hospital	Scranton	166	392
Forbes Regional Hospital	Monroeville	167	404
Warren General Hospital	Warren	167	321
Jeanes Hospital	Philadelphia	172	328
Delaware County Memorial Hospital	Drexel Hill	177	339
Geisinger - Community Medical Center	Scranton	179	673
Holy Spirit Hospital	Camp Hill	180	341
Allegheny General Hospital	Pittsburgh	182	421
Aria Health	Philadelphia	183	322
Main Line Hospital Lankenau	Wynnewood	185	371
Penn Hosp of the Univ of PA Hlth Sys	Philadelphia	192	488
Holy Redeemer Hospital & Medical Center	Meadowbrook	194	274
Milton S Hershey Medical Center	Hershey	194	461
Hospital of Univ of Pennsylvania	Philadelphia	195	343
Saint Joseph Medical Center	Reading	195	661
Thomas Jefferson University Hospital	Philadelphia	195	689
Saint Joseph's Hospital	Philadelphia	200	325
Reading Hospital	Reading	213	1226
Geisinger Wyoming Valley Medical Center	Wilkes Barre	226	664

Time in ER Before Being Evaluated (minutes)

Hospital Name	City	Min.	Cases
Grove City Medical Center	Grove City	0	386
Miners Medical Center	Hastings	5	371
Excela Health Frick Hospital	Mount Pleasant	8	504
UPMC East[3]	Monroeville	9	468
Penn Highlands Dubois	Dubois	10	380
Abington Memorial Hospital	Abington	11	417
UPMC Altoona	Altoona	12	1785
UPMC Northwest	Seneca	12	626
UPMC Presbyterian Shadyside	Pittsburgh	12	620
Butler Memorial Hospital	Butler	13	382
Excela Health Westmoreland Hospital	Greensburg	13	534
Lock Haven Hospital	Lock Haven	14	424
Soldiers & Sailors Memorial Hospital	Wellsboro	14	392
UPMC Mercy	Pittsburgh	14	623
Alle Kiski Medical Center	Natrona	15	502
Excela Health Latrobe Hospital	Latrobe	15	512
Kane Community Hospital	Kane	15	603
Nason Hospital	Roaring Spring	15	387
UPMC Bedford Memorial	Everett	15	623
Acmh Hospital	Kittanning	16	469
Lancaster General Hospital	Lancaster	16	414
Troy Community Hospital[3]	Troy	16	273
Western Pennsylvania Hospital	Pittsburgh	16	419
Memorial Hospital	York	17	443
Saint Mary Medical Center	Langhorne	17	423
Canonsburg General Hospital	Canonsburg	18	494
Saint Clair Memorial Hospital	Pittsburgh	18	376
Brandywine Hospital	Coatesville	19	422
Lancaster Regional Medical Center	Lancaster	19	548
Lansdale Hospital	Lansdale	19	408
Magee Womens Hosp of UPMC Health Sys	Pittsburgh	19	619
Punxsutawney Area Hospital	Punxsutawney	19	414
Riddle Memorial Hospital	Media	19	383
Sunbury Community Hospital	Sunbury	19	419
Tyrone Hospital	Tyrone	19	1316
Ellwood City Hospital	Ellwood City	20	413
Heart of Lancaster Reg Med Ctr	Lititz	20	403
Indiana Regional Medical Center	Indiana	20	377
Lehigh Valley Hospital - Muhlenberg	Bethlehem	20	377
Memorial Hospital Towanda	Towanda	20	241
Mid - Valley Hospital	Peckville	20	403
UPMC Horizon	Greenville	20	621
UPMC Passavant	Pittsburgh	20	623
Heritage Valley Sewickley	Sewickley	21	329
Milton S Hershey Medical Center	Hershey	21	491
Mount Nittany Medical Center	State College	21	233
Pottstown Memorial Medical Center	Pottstown	21	418
UPMC Mckeesport	Mc Keesport	21	621
UPMC Saint Margaret	Pittsburgh	21	618
Geisinger Medical Center	Danville	22	765
Heritage Valley Beaver	Beaver	22	335
Main Line Hospital Paoli	Paoli	22	383
Waynesboro Hospital	Waynesboro	22	375
Easton Hospital	Easton	23	415
Meadville Medical Center	Meadville	23	2297
Mercy Suburban Hospital	Norristown	23	406
Tyler Memorial Hospital	Tunkhannock	23	419
Berwick Hospital Center	Berwick	24	418
Highlands Hospital	Connellsville	24	377
Sharon Regional Health System	Sharon	24	1166
Chestnut Hill Hospital	Philadelphia	25	420
Conemaugh Valley Memorial Hospital	Johnstown	25	1306
Saint Vincent Hospital	Erie	25	569
Southwest Regional Medical Center	Waynesburg	25	414
Doylestown Hospital	Doylestown	26	384
Millcreek Community Hospital	Erie	26	385
Monongahela Valley Hospital	Monongahela	26	791
Sacred Heart Hospital	Allentown	26	7596
Saint Luke's Miners Memorial Hospital	Coaldale	26	373
Lewistown Hospital	Lewistown	27	380
Main Line Hospital Bryn Mawr Campus	Bryn Mawr	27	375
Roxborough Memorial Hospital	Philadelphia	27	417
Chester County Hospital	West Chester	28	412
Jennersville Regional Hospital	West Grove	28	411
Phoenixville Hospital	Phoenixville	28	421
Saint Luke's Quakertown Hospital	Quakertown	28	373
Bradford Regional Medical Center	Bradford	29	648
Lower Bucks Hospital	Bristol	29	402
Palmerton Hospital	Palmerton	29	368
UPMC Hamot	Erie	29	603
Carlisle Regional Medical Center	Carlisle	30	404
Chambersburg Hospital	Chambersburg	30	349
Penn Highlands Elk	Saint Marys	30	507
Regional Hospital of Scranton	Scranton	30	393
Uniontown Hospital	Uniontown	30	385
Hahnemann University Hospital	Philadelphia	31	403
The Washington Hospital	Washington	31	448
Evangelical Community Hospital	Lewisburg	32	414
Geisinger - Community Medical Center	Scranton	32	764
Gnaden Huetten Memorial Hospital	Lehighton	32	377
Windber Hospital	Windber	32	371
Grand View Hospital	Sellersville	33	640
Penn Hosp of the Univ of PA Hlth Sys	Philadelphia	33	143
Schuylkill Med Ctr-East Norwegian St	Pottsville	33	377
Lehigh Valley Hospital	Allentown	34	380
Titusville Hospital	Titusville	34	411
Hanover Hospital	Hanover	35	861
Jefferson Regional Medical Center	Pittsburgh	35	265
Mercy Fitzgerald Hospital	Darby	35	812
Wayne Memorial Hospital	Honesdale	35	388
Geisinger - Bloomsburg Hospital	Bloomsburg	36	368
Saint Luke's Hospital Bethlehem	Bethlehem	37	755
Geisinger Wyoming Valley Medical Center	Wilkes Barre	39	730
J C Blair Memorial Hospital	Huntingdon	39	324
Schuylkill Med Ctr-S Jackson St	Pottsville	39	361
Ohio Valley General Hospital	Mckees Rocks	40	353
Thomas Jefferson University Hospital	Philadelphia	40	699
Einstein Medical Center Montgomery[3]	East Norriton	41	294
Saint Luke's Hospital - Anderson Campus	Easton	41	382
Somerset Hospital	Somerset	41	416
Gettysburg Hospital	Gettysburg	42	383
Nazareth Hospital	Philadelphia	42	405
Allegheny General Hospital	Pittsburgh	43	481
Forbes Regional Hospital	Monroeville	44	461
Holy Spirit Hospital	Camp Hill	44	397
Robert Packer Hospital	Sayre	44	595
Warren General Hospital	Warren	44	356
Williamsport Regional Medical Center	Williamsport	44	503
Main Line Hospital Lankenau	Wynnewood	45	383
Moses Taylor Hospital	Scranton	45	386
Ephrata Community Hospital	Ephrata	46	426
Albert Einstein Medical Center	Philadelphia	48	535
Clarion Hospital	Clarion	48	382
Good Samaritan Hospital	Lebanon	48	371
Jameson Memorial Hospital	New Castle	48	379
Charles Cole Memorial Hospital	Coudersport	49	416
Pinnacle Health Hospitals	Harrisburg	50	690
Temple University Hospital	Philadelphia	50	365
Wilkes-Barre General Hospital	Wilkes-Barre	51	374
York Hospital	York	51	385
Penn Highlands Clearfield	Clearfield	55	285
Reading Hospital	Reading	57	1473
Saint Joseph Medical Center	Reading	57	619
Jeanes Hospital	Philadelphia	59	363
Lehigh Valley Hospital - Hazleton	Hazleton	60	438
Holy Redeemer Hospital & Medical Center	Meadowbrook	65	373
Hospital of Univ of Pennsylvania	Philadelphia	66	289
Penn Presbyterian Medical Center	Philadelphia	67	949
Saint Joseph's Hospital	Philadelphia	69	356
Aria Health	Philadelphia	74	345
Delaware County Memorial Hospital	Drexel Hill	78	320
Crozer Chester Medical Center	Upland	81	356

Time to Pain Meds for Bone Fractures (minutes)

Hospital Name	City	Min.	Cases
Excela Health Frick Hospital	Mount Pleasant	24	84
UPMC Northwest	Seneca	31	104
Grand View Hospital	Sellersville	36	176
Butler Memorial Hospital	Butler	37	117
Heart of Lancaster Reg Med Ctr	Lititz	38	72
UPMC Mercy	Pittsburgh	38	88
UPMC Bedford Memorial	Everett	39	54
Lehigh Valley Hospital - Muhlenberg	Bethlehem	40	161
Brandywine Hospital	Coatesville	41	98
Penn Highlands Dubois	Dubois	41	138
Meadville Medical Center	Meadville	43	117
Jameson Memorial Hospital	New Castle	44	95
Sharon Regional Health System	Sharon	44	82
Soldiers & Sailors Memorial Hospital	Wellsboro	44	64
Abington Memorial Hospital	Abington	45	221
Canonsburg General Hospital	Canonsburg	45	43
Easton Hospital	Easton	46	58
Einstein Medical Center Montgomery[3]	East Norriton	46	70
Evangelical Community Hospital	Lewisburg	46	152
Geisinger Wyoming Valley Medical Center	Wilkes Barre	46	146
Chester County Hospital	West Chester	47	147
Forbes Regional Hospital	Monroeville	47	71
Southwest Regional Medical Center	Waynesburg	47	35
Lock Haven Hospital	Lock Haven	48	50
Saint Luke's Miners Memorial Hospital	Coaldale	48	28
Acmh Hospital	Kittanning	49	79
Excela Health Westmoreland Hospital	Greensburg	49	143
Riddle Memorial Hospital	Media	49	71
UPMC Presbyterian Shadyside	Pittsburgh	49	74
Windber Hospital	Windber	49	27
Geisinger Medical Center	Danville	50	162
Heritage Valley Sewickley	Sewickley	50	78
Hospital of Univ of Pennsylvania	Philadelphia	50	39
Jennersville Regional Hospital	West Grove	50	104
Lansdale Hospital	Lansdale	50	80
Mid - Valley Hospital	Peckville	50	29
Saint Luke's Quakertown Hospital	Quakertown	50	42
Saint Mary Medical Center	Langhorne	50	379
Excela Health Latrobe Hospital	Latrobe	51	96
Phoenixville Hospital	Phoenixville	51	80
Hahnemann University Hospital	Philadelphia	52	36
Lancaster General Hospital	Lancaster	52	159
Sacred Heart Hospital	Allentown	52	44
Saint Clair Memorial Hospital	Pittsburgh	52	153
Waynesboro Hospital	Waynesboro	52	62
Highlands Hospital	Connellsville	53	41
Indiana Regional Medical Center	Indiana	53	65
Mount Nittany Medical Center	State College	53	140
Saint Vincent Hospital	Erie	53	193
Alle Kiski Medical Center	Natrona	54	68
Conemaugh Valley Memorial Hospital	Johnstown	54	153
Doylestown Hospital	Doylestown	54	175
Ellwood City Hospital	Ellwood City	54	43
Gettysburg Hospital	Gettysburg	54	113
Heritage Valley Beaver	Beaver	54	119
Penn Highlands Elk	Saint Marys	54	56
UPMC Hamot	Erie	54	203
Albert Einstein Medical Center	Philadelphia	55	143
Grove City Medical Center	Grove City	55	94
Lehigh Valley Hospital	Allentown	55	324
Tyler Memorial Hospital	Tunkhannock	55	51
Carlisle Regional Medical Center	Carlisle	56	78
Delaware County Memorial Hospital	Drexel Hill	56	114
Lancaster Regional Medical Center	Lancaster	56	41
UPMC Saint Margaret	Pittsburgh	57	75
Chambersburg Hospital	Chambersburg	58	120
Main Line Hospital Bryn Mawr Campus	Bryn Mawr	58	252
Pocono Medical Center	E Stroudsburg	58	392
Punxsutawney Area Hospital	Punxsutawney	58	67
Uniontown Hospital	Uniontown	58	82
Chestnut Hill Hospital	Philadelphia	59	136
Memorial Hospital	York	59	109
Penn Highlands Clearfield	Clearfield	59	63
Pinnacle Health Hospitals	Harrisburg	59	277
Titusville Hospital	Titusville	59	49
Crozer Chester Medical Center	Upland	60	254
The Washington Hospital	Washington	60	99
Robert Packer Hospital	Sayre	61	70
Saint Luke's Hospital Bethlehem	Bethlehem	61	137
UPMC Altoona	Altoona	61	218
UPMC Horizon	Greenville	61	141
Wilkes-Barre General Hospital	Wilkes-Barre	61	113
Ephrata Community Hospital	Ephrata	62	116
Gnaden Huetten Memorial Hospital	Lehighton	62	79
Mercy Suburban Hospital	Norristown	62	56
Nason Hospital	Roaring Spring	62	71
Lower Bucks Hospital	Bristol	63	43
Main Line Hospital Paoli	Paoli	63	142
Saint Luke's Hospital - Anderson Campus	Easton	63	101
Somerset Hospital	Somerset	63	101
Charles Cole Memorial Hospital	Coudersport	64	63
Schuylkill Med Ctr-East Norwegian St	Pottsville	64	52

NOTE: Hospital profiles are in alphabetical order by state, then city, then hospital within the city; Rankings exclude hospitals with less than 25 cases except for patient surveys which excludes hospitals with less than 100 cases; (a) 100-299 cases; (1) The number of cases/patients is too few to report; (2) Data submitted were based on a sample of cases/patients; (3) Results are based on a shorter time period than required; (4) Data suppressed by CMS for one or more quarters; (5) Results are not available for this reporting period; (6) Fewer than 100 patients completed the HCAHPS survey; (7) No cases met the criteria for this measure; (8) The lower limit of the confidence interval cannot be calculated if the number of observed infections equals zero; (9) No data are available from the state/territory for this reporting period; (10) The scores shown reflect fewer than 50 completed surveys; (11) There were discrepancies in the data collection process; (12) This measure does not apply to this hospital for this reporting period; (13) Results cannot be calculated for this reporting period; (14) The results for this state are combined with nearby states to protect confidentiality; Please refer to the User's Guide for a full explanation of data.

UPMC Passavant	Pittsburgh	64	191
J C Blair Memorial Hospital	Huntingdon	65	71
Jefferson Regional Medical Center	Pittsburgh	65	91
Palmerton Hospital	Palmerton	65	48
UPMC East[3]	Monroeville	65	77
Bradford Regional Medical Center	Bradford	66	52
Lewistown Hospital	Lewistown	66	52
Temple University Hospital	Philadelphia	66	93
Wayne Memorial Hospital	Honesdale	66	91
Pottstown Memorial Medical Center	Pottstown	67	124
Sunbury Community Hospital	Sunbury	67	42
Geisinger - Bloomsburg Hospital	Bloomsburg	68	81
York Hospital	York	68	121
Berwick Hospital Center	Berwick	69	54
Penn Hosp of the Univ of PA Hlth Sys	Philadelphia	69	25
Holy Spirit Hospital	Camp Hill	70	213
Mercy Fitzgerald Hospital	Darby	71	88
Milton S Hershey Medical Center	Hershey	71	243
Regional Hospital of Scranton	Scranton	71	42
Schuylkill Med Ctr-S Jackson St	Pottsville	72	109
Thomas Jefferson University Hospital	Philadelphia	72	185
Good Samaritan Hospital	Lebanon	73	98
Geisinger - Community Medical Center	Scranton	74	130
Hanover Hospital	Hanover	74	140
Millcreek Community Hospital	Erie	74	34
Nazareth Hospital	Philadelphia	76	134
Main Line Hospital Lankenau	Wynnewood	77	52
Moses Taylor Hospital	Scranton	77	71
UPMC Mckeesport	Mc Keesport	78	76
Jeanes Hospital	Philadelphia	80	104
Lehigh Valley Hospital - Hazleton	Hazleton	81	116
Holy Redeemer Hospital & Medical Center	Meadowbrook	83	138
Reading Hospital	Reading	83	321
Warren General Hospital	Warren	83	123
Monongahela Valley Hospital	Monongahela	84	91
Aria Health	Philadelphia	85	191
Williamsport Regional Medical Center	Williamsport	86	178
Saint Joseph's Hospital	Philadelphia	89	34
Allegheny General Hospital	Pittsburgh	90	71
Saint Joseph Medical Center	Reading	93	163
Clarion Hospital	Clarion	94	40
Penn Presbyterian Medical Center	Philadelphia	102	47

Heart Attack Care

Aspirin Given at Discharge

Hospital Name	City	Rate	Cases
Abington Memorial Hospital	Abington	100%	367
Allegheny General Hospital	Pittsburgh	100%	503
Butler Memorial Hospital	Butler	100%	302
Chester County Hospital	West Chester	100%	202
Doylestown Hospital	Doylestown	100%	305
Easton Hospital	Easton	100%	166
Einstein Medical Center Montgomery[3]	East Norriton	100%	179
Geisinger - Community Medical Center	Scranton	100%	218
Geisinger Medical Center	Danville	100%	637
Geisinger Wyoming Valley Medical Center	Wilkes Barre	100%	193
Good Samaritan Hospital	Lebanon	100%	203
Grand View Hospital	Sellersville	100%	39
Hanover Hospital	Hanover	100%	57
Heritage Valley Beaver	Beaver	100%	359
Holy Spirit Hospital	Camp Hill	100%	322
Hospital of Univ of Pennsylvania	Philadelphia	100%	212
Indiana Regional Medical Center	Indiana	100%	55
Jameson Memorial Hospital	New Castle	100%	76
Lancaster Regional Medical Center	Lancaster	100%	67
Lansdale Hospital	Lansdale	100%	41
Lehigh Valley Hospital	Allentown	100%	913
Lehigh Valley Hospital - Hazleton	Hazleton	100%	47
Lehigh Valley Hospital - Muhlenberg	Bethlehem	100%	247
Main Line Hospital Bryn Mawr Campus	Bryn Mawr	100%	208
Main Line Hospital Lankenau	Wynnewood	100%	276
Main Line Hospital Paoli	Paoli	100%	178
Memorial Hospital	York	100%	118
Mercy Fitzgerald Hospital	Darby	100%	144
Milton S Hershey Medical Center	Hershey	100%	396
Monongahela Valley Hospital	Monongahela	100%	155
Nazareth Hospital	Philadelphia	100%	169
Penn Highlands Dubois	Dubois	100%	268
Penn Presbyterian Medical Center[2]	Philadelphia	100%	306
Penn Hosp of the Univ of PA Hlth Sys	Philadelphia	100%	105
Pinnacle Health Hospitals	Harrisburg	100%	619
Pocono Medical Center	E Stroudsburg	100%	260
Pottstown Memorial Medical Center	Pottstown	100%	30
Reading Hospital	Reading	100%	429
Saint Clair Memorial Hospital	Pittsburgh	100%	244
Saint Joseph Medical Center	Reading	100%	137
Saint Luke's Hospital - Anderson Campus	Easton	100%	64
Saint Luke's Hospital Bethlehem	Bethlehem	100%	354
Saint Mary Medical Center	Langhorne	100%	499
Saint Vincent Hospital	Erie	100%	427
Sharon Regional Health System	Sharon	100%	130
Somerset Hospital	Somerset	100%	53
Temple University Hospital	Philadelphia	100%	311
Thomas Jefferson University Hospital	Philadelphia	100%	245
Uniontown Hospital	Uniontown	100%	158
UPMC East[3]	Monroeville	100%	63
UPMC Hamot	Erie	100%	706
UPMC Mckeesport	Mc Keesport	100%	161
UPMC Mercy	Pittsburgh	100%	346
UPMC Passavant	Pittsburgh	100%	412
UPMC Presbyterian Shadyside	Pittsburgh	100%	1069
VA Pittsburgh Healthcare System	Pittsburgh	100%	74
The Washington Hospital	Washington	100%	358
Western Pennsylvania Hospital	Pittsburgh	100%	69
Williamsport Regional Medical Center	Williamsport	100%	352
York Hospital	York	100%	683
Acmh Hospital	Kittanning	99%	96
Albert Einstein Medical Center	Philadelphia	99%	287
Alle Kiski Medical Center	Natrona	99%	96
Aria Health	Philadelphia	99%	509
Brandywine Hospital	Coatesville	99%	125
Conemaugh Valley Memorial Hospital	Johnstown	99%	580
Crozer Chester Medical Center	Upland	99%	364
Evangelical Community Hospital[2]	Lewisburg	99%	132
Excela Health Westmoreland Hospital	Greensburg	99%	562
Hahnemann University Hospital	Philadelphia	99%	206
Jeanes Hospital	Philadelphia	99%	162
Jefferson Regional Medical Center	Pittsburgh	99%	274
Lancaster General Hospital	Lancaster	99%	730
Meadville Medical Center	Meadville	99%	70
Phoenixville Hospital	Phoenixville	99%	259
Riddle Memorial Hospital	Media	99%	111
Robert Packer Hospital	Sayre	99%	466
UPMC Altoona	Altoona	99%	628
Wilkes-Barre General Hospital	Wilkes-Barre	99%	311
Chambersburg Hospital[2]	Chambersburg	98%	222
Excela Health Frick Hospital	Mount Pleasant	98%	44
Lewistown Hospital	Lewistown	98%	51
Mount Nittany Medical Center	State College	98%	129
Regional Hospital of Scranton	Scranton	98%	430
UPMC Saint Margaret	Pittsburgh	98%	89
Forbes Regional Hospital	Monroeville	97%	237
Holy Redeemer Hospital & Medical Center	Meadowbrook	97%	125
Roxborough Memorial Hospital	Philadelphia	97%	31
Chestnut Hill Hospital	Philadelphia	96%	25
Excela Health Latrobe Hospital	Latrobe	96%	70
Lower Bucks Hospital	Bristol	95%	73
Schuylkill Med Ctr-East Norwegian St	Pottsville	94%	36
Berwick Hospital Center	Berwick	93%	28
Schuylkill Med Ctr-S Jackson St	Pottsville	92%	39

PCI Within 90 Minutes of Arrival

Hospital Name	City	Rate	Cases
Albert Einstein Medical Center	Philadelphia	100%	36
Easton Hospital	Easton	100%	36
Geisinger Medical Center	Danville	100%	46
Geisinger Wyoming Valley Medical Center	Wilkes Barre	100%	44
Main Line Hospital Bryn Mawr Campus	Bryn Mawr	100%	33
Main Line Hospital Lankenau	Wynnewood	100%	31
Main Line Hospital Paoli	Paoli	100%	37
Pinnacle Health Hospitals	Harrisburg	100%	94
Pocono Medical Center	E Stroudsburg	100%	78
Reading Hospital	Reading	100%	108
Saint Clair Memorial Hospital	Pittsburgh	100%	58
Saint Joseph Medical Center	Reading	100%	31
Saint Luke's Hospital Bethlehem	Bethlehem	100%	56
Saint Mary Medical Center	Langhorne	100%	65
Temple University Hospital	Philadelphia	100%	39
UPMC Hamot	Erie	100%	76
UPMC Mercy	Pittsburgh	100%	36
UPMC Passavant	Pittsburgh	100%	55
UPMC Presbyterian Shadyside	Pittsburgh	100%	63
The Washington Hospital	Washington	100%	45
Heritage Valley Beaver	Beaver	99%	72
Lehigh Valley Hospital	Allentown	99%	123
Crozer Chester Medical Center	Upland	98%	48
Doylestown Hospital	Doylestown	98%	59
Forbes Regional Hospital	Monroeville	98%	63
Lehigh Valley Hospital - Muhlenberg	Bethlehem	98%	61
Wilkes-Barre General Hospital	Wilkes-Barre	98%	64
Williamsport Regional Medical Center	Williamsport	98%	44
York Hospital	York	98%	134
Allegheny General Hospital	Pittsburgh	97%	71
Butler Memorial Hospital	Butler	97%	35
Holy Spirit Hospital	Camp Hill	97%	67
Memorial Hospital	York	97%	32
Penn Highlands Dubois	Dubois	97%	30
Saint Vincent Hospital	Erie	97%	65
Sharon Regional Health System	Sharon	97%	38
Uniontown Hospital	Uniontown	97%	39
UPMC Mckeesport	Mc Keesport	97%	30
Abington Memorial Hospital	Abington	96%	78
Geisinger - Community Medical Center	Scranton	96%	54
Regional Hospital of Scranton	Scranton	96%	55
Good Samaritan Hospital	Lebanon	95%	56
Jefferson Regional Medical Center	Pittsburgh	95%	62
Milton S Hershey Medical Center	Hershey	95%	57
Mount Nittany Medical Center	State College	95%	38
Einstein Medical Center Montgomery[3]	East Norriton	94%	31
UPMC Altoona	Altoona	94%	103
Conemaugh Valley Memorial Hospital	Johnstown	92%	49
Phoenixville Hospital	Phoenixville	92%	38
Aria Health	Philadelphia	90%	51
Lancaster General Hospital	Lancaster	90%	135
Excela Health Westmoreland Hospital	Greensburg	89%	71
Robert Packer Hospital	Sayre	88%	34
Acmh Hospital	Kittanning	85%	26

Statin Prescribed at Discharge

Hospital Name	City	Rate	Cases
Albert Einstein Medical Center	Philadelphia	100%	289
Allegheny General Hospital	Pittsburgh	100%	480
Aria Health	Philadelphia	100%	498
Brandywine Hospital	Coatesville	100%	121
Doylestown Hospital	Doylestown	100%	281
Evangelical Community Hospital[2]	Lewisburg	100%	129
Excela Health Frick Hospital	Mount Pleasant	100%	41
Geisinger - Community Medical Center	Scranton	100%	227
Geisinger Medical Center	Danville	100%	625
Good Samaritan Hospital	Lebanon	100%	194
Grand View Hospital	Sellersville	100%	36
Hospital of Univ of Pennsylvania	Philadelphia	100%	207
Jameson Memorial Hospital	New Castle	100%	68
Lancaster Regional Medical Center	Lancaster	100%	66
Lansdale Hospital	Lansdale	100%	34
Lehigh Valley Hospital - Hazleton	Hazleton	100%	47
Main Line Hospital Bryn Mawr Campus	Bryn Mawr	100%	209
Main Line Hospital Lankenau	Wynnewood	100%	271
Main Line Hospital Paoli	Paoli	100%	171
Mercy Fitzgerald Hospital	Darby	100%	143
Penn Highlands Dubois	Dubois	100%	257
Penn Presbyterian Medical Center[2]	Philadelphia	100%	299
Penn Hosp of the Univ of PA Hlth Sys	Philadelphia	100%	107
Reading Hospital	Reading	100%	413
Riddle Memorial Hospital	Media	100%	117
Roxborough Memorial Hospital	Philadelphia	100%	29
Saint Joseph Medical Center	Reading	100%	125
Saint Luke's Hospital - Anderson Campus	Easton	100%	63
Saint Luke's Hospital Bethlehem	Bethlehem	100%	351
Saint Mary Medical Center	Langhorne	100%	442
Sharon Regional Health System	Sharon	100%	129
Somerset Hospital	Somerset	100%	49
Thomas Jefferson University Hospital	Philadelphia	100%	247
Uniontown Hospital	Uniontown	100%	147
UPMC East[3]	Monroeville	100%	56
UPMC Mckeesport	Mc Keesport	100%	149
UPMC Mercy	Pittsburgh	100%	320
UPMC Passavant	Pittsburgh	100%	407
UPMC Presbyterian Shadyside	Pittsburgh	100%	1006
The Washington Hospital	Washington	100%	344
Williamsport Regional Medical Center	Williamsport	100%	343
Acmh Hospital	Kittanning	99%	92
Alle Kiski Medical Center	Natrona	99%	96
Butler Memorial Hospital	Butler	99%	280
Chester County Hospital	West Chester	99%	196
Crozer Chester Medical Center	Upland	99%	363
Easton Hospital	Easton	99%	158
Einstein Medical Center Montgomery[3]	East Norriton	99%	174
Geisinger Wyoming Valley Medical Center	Wilkes Barre	99%	187
Heritage Valley Beaver	Beaver	99%	332
Holy Spirit Hospital	Camp Hill	99%	311
Lehigh Valley Hospital	Allentown	99%	874
Milton S Hershey Medical Center	Hershey	99%	392
Monongahela Valley Hospital	Monongahela	99%	150
Phoenixville Hospital	Phoenixville	99%	256
Pinnacle Health Hospitals	Harrisburg	99%	608
Saint Clair Memorial Hospital	Pittsburgh	99%	233
Temple University Hospital	Philadelphia	99%	303
UPMC Hamot	Erie	99%	694
VA Pittsburgh Healthcare System	Pittsburgh	99%	74
Western Pennsylvania Hospital	Pittsburgh	99%	68
York Hospital	York	99%	687
Abington Memorial Hospital	Abington	98%	365
Conemaugh Valley Memorial Hospital	Johnstown	98%	547
Hahnemann University Hospital	Philadelphia	98%	214
Holy Redeemer Hospital & Medical Center	Meadowbrook	98%	120
Jefferson Regional Medical Center	Pittsburgh	98%	270
Lancaster General Hospital	Lancaster	98%	700
Lehigh Valley Hospital - Muhlenberg	Bethlehem	98%	239
Mount Nittany Medical Center	State College	98%	129
Pocono Medical Center	E Stroudsburg	98%	253

NOTE: Hospital profiles are in alphabetical order by state, then city, then hospital within the city; Rankings exclude hospitals with less than 25 cases except for patient surveys which excludes hospitals with less than 100 cases; (a) 100-299 cases; (1) The number of cases/patients is too few to report; (2) Data submitted were based on a sample of cases/patients; (3) Results are based on a shorter time period than required; (4) Data suppressed by CMS for one or more quarters; (5) Results are not available for this reporting period; (6) Fewer than 100 patients completed the HCAHPS survey; (7) No cases met the criteria for this measure; (8) The lower limit of the confidence interval cannot be calculated if the number of observed infections equals zero; (9) No data are available from the state/territory for this reporting period; (10) The scores shown reflect fewer than 50 completed surveys; (11) There were discrepancies in the data collection process; (12) This measure does not apply to this hospital for this reporting period; (13) Results cannot be calculated for this reporting period; (14) The results for this state are combined with nearby states to protect confidentiality; Please refer to the User's Guide for a full explanation of data.

Robert Packer Hospital	Sayre	98%	447
Saint Vincent Hospital	Erie	98%	410
Excela Health Latrobe Hospital	Latrobe	97%	67
Excela Health Westmoreland Hospital	Greensburg	97%	548
Forbes Regional Hospital	Monroeville	97%	237
Nazareth Hospital	Philadelphia	97%	153
UPMC Altoona	Altoona	97%	582
Wilkes-Barre General Hospital	Wilkes-Barre	97%	293
Meadville Medical Center	Meadville	96%	73
Regional Hospital of Scranton	Scranton	96%	419
UPMC Horizon	Greenville	96%	27
Hanover Hospital	Hanover	95%	61
Jeanes Hospital	Philadelphia	95%	149
Memorial Hospital	York	95%	110
UPMC Saint Margaret	Pittsburgh	95%	80
Chambersburg Hospital[2]	Chambersburg	94%	222
Lower Bucks Hospital	Bristol	94%	70
Lewistown Hospital	Lewistown	93%	57
Schuylkill Med Ctr-S Jackson St	Pottsville	91%	35
Indiana Regional Medical Center	Indiana	86%	50
Pottstown Memorial Medical Center	Pottstown	78%	27
Berwick Hospital Center	Berwick	76%	25
Schuylkill Med Ctr-East Norwegian St	Pottsville	76%	34

Heart Failure Care

ACE Inhibitor or ARB for LVSD

Hospital Name	City	Rate	Cases
Acmh Hospital	Kittanning	100%	34
Allegheny General Hospital	Pittsburgh	100%	232
Butler Memorial Hospital	Butler	100%	98
Chester County Hospital	West Chester	100%	79
Chestnut Hill Hospital	Philadelphia	100%	103
Delaware County Memorial Hospital	Drexel Hill	100%	29
Doylestown Hospital	Doylestown	100%	119
Evangelical Community Hospital	Lewisburg	100%	35
Geisinger Wyoming Valley Medical Center	Wilkes Barre	100%	106
Good Samaritan Hospital	Lebanon	100%	54
Hanover Hospital	Hanover	100%	54
Heritage Valley Beaver[2]	Beaver	100%	70
Heritage Valley Sewickley	Sewickley	100%	42
Hospital of Univ of Pennsylvania[2]	Philadelphia	100%	358
Lehigh Valley Hospital - Hazleton	Hazleton	100%	45
Lehigh Valley Hospital - Muhlenberg	Bethlehem	100%	115
Main Line Hospital Bryn Mawr Campus	Bryn Mawr	100%	81
Main Line Hospital Lankenau	Wynnewood	100%	223
Memorial Hospital	York	100%	49
Mercy Fitzgerald Hospital	Darby	100%	279
Mercy Suburban Hospital	Norristown	100%	45
Milton S Hershey Medical Center	Hershey	100%	148
Moses Taylor Hospital	Scranton	100%	25
Nazareth Hospital	Philadelphia	100%	44
Penn Presbyterian Medical Center[2]	Philadelphia	100%	132
Penn Hosp of the Univ of PA Hlth Sys	Philadelphia	100%	104
Pinnacle Health Hospitals	Harrisburg	100%	195
Pottstown Memorial Medical Center	Pottstown	100%	62
Reading Hospital	Reading	100%	165
Riddle Memorial Hospital	Media	100%	58
Saint Joseph Medical Center	Reading	100%	50
Saint Luke's Hospital - Anderson Campus	Easton	100%	55
Saint Mary Medical Center	Langhorne	100%	155
Temple University Hospital	Philadelphia	100%	457
UPMC East[3]	Monroeville	100%	30
UPMC Horizon	Greenville	100%	43
UPMC Mckeesport	Mc Keesport	100%	81
UPMC Northwest	Seneca	100%	30
UPMC Passavant	Pittsburgh	100%	142
The Washington Hospital	Washington	100%	117
Wilkes Barre VA Medical Center	Wilkes-Barre	100%	28
Williamsport Regional Medical Center	Williamsport	100%	87
Abington Memorial Hospital	Abington	99%	245
Brandywine Hospital	Coatesville	99%	81
Crozer Chester Medical Center	Upland	99%	226
Holy Spirit Hospital	Camp Hill	99%	134
Lehigh Valley Hospital	Allentown	99%	238
Monongahela Valley Hospital	Monongahela	99%	71
Penn Highlands Dubois	Dubois	99%	81
Phoenixville Hospital	Phoenixville	99%	79
Pocono Medical Center	E Stroudsburg	99%	115
Saint Clair Memorial Hospital	Pittsburgh	99%	131
Saint Luke's Hospital Bethlehem	Bethlehem	99%	125
Thomas Jefferson University Hospital	Philadelphia	99%	312
UPMC Mercy	Pittsburgh	99%	142
UPMC Presbyterian Shadyside	Pittsburgh	99%	422
VA Pittsburgh Healthcare System	Pittsburgh	99%	92
Alle Kiski Medical Center	Natrona	98%	52
Grand View Hospital	Sellersville	98%	43
Hahnemann University Hospital	Philadelphia	98%	257
Main Line Hospital Paoli	Paoli	98%	60
Schuylkill Med Ctr-East Norwegian St	Pottsville	98%	40
Uniontown Hospital	Uniontown	98%	62
UPMC Hamot	Erie	98%	141
Ephrata Community Hospital	Ephrata	97%	35
Geisinger - Community Medical Center	Scranton	97%	98
Lancaster General Hospital	Lancaster	97%	207
Lansdale Hospital[2]	Lansdale	97%	62
Ohio Valley General Hospital	Mckees Rocks	97%	37
Saint Vincent Hospital	Erie	97%	102
Schuylkill Med Ctr-S Jackson St	Pottsville	97%	34
Wilkes-Barre General Hospital	Wilkes-Barre	97%	127
Albert Einstein Medical Center[2]	Philadelphia	96%	139
Aria Health	Philadelphia	96%	256
Geisinger Medical Center	Danville	96%	160
Lewistown Hospital	Lewistown	96%	54
Robert Packer Hospital	Sayre	96%	136
Somerset Hospital	Somerset	96%	27
UPMC Saint Margaret	Pittsburgh	96%	91
York Hospital	York	96%	217
Einstein Medical Center Montgomery[2,3]	East Norriton	95%	66
Jeanes Hospital	Philadelphia	95%	113
Meadville Medical Center	Meadville	95%	41
Roxborough Memorial Hospital	Philadelphia	95%	40
Easton Hospital	Easton	94%	81
UPMC Altoona	Altoona	94%	129
Conemaugh Valley Memorial Hospital	Johnstown	93%	180
Gettysburg Hospital	Gettysburg	93%	46
J C Blair Memorial Hospital	Huntingdon	93%	28
Mount Nittany Medical Center	State College	93%	56
Excela Health Latrobe Hospital	Latrobe	92%	40
Forbes Regional Hospital	Monroeville	92%	120
Holy Redeemer Hospital & Medical Center	Meadowbrook	92%	39
Jefferson Regional Medical Center	Pittsburgh	92%	155
Lebanon VA Medical Center	Lebanon	92%	25
Lower Bucks Hospital	Bristol	92%	60
Regional Hospital of Scranton	Scranton	92%	144
Chambersburg Hospital	Chambersburg	91%	87
Excela Health Westmoreland Hospital	Greensburg	89%	150
Jameson Memorial Hospital	New Castle	89%	64
Sacred Heart Hospital	Allentown	89%	27
Indiana Regional Medical Center	Indiana	88%	69
Excela Health Frick Hospital	Mount Pleasant	87%	31
Philadelphia VA Medical Center	Philadelphia	87%	107
Sharon Regional Health System	Sharon	86%	42
Jennersville Regional Hospital	West Grove	80%	25
Saint Joseph's Hospital	Philadelphia	79%	42
Ellwood City Hospital[2]	Ellwood City	78%	46

Discharge Instructions Given

Hospital Name	City	Rate	Cases
Albert Einstein Medical Center[2]	Philadelphia	100%	246
Bradford Regional Medical Center	Bradford	100%	49
Charles Cole Memorial Hospital	Coudersport	100%	25
Delaware County Memorial Hospital	Drexel Hill	100%	145
Einstein Medical Center Montgomery[2,3]	East Norriton	100%	179
Erie VA Medical Center	Erie	100%	29
Geisinger Medical Center	Danville	100%	620
Grove City Medical Center	Grove City	100%	40
Hanover Hospital	Hanover	100%	176
Holy Redeemer Hospital & Medical Center	Meadowbrook	100%	214
Holy Spirit Hospital	Camp Hill	100%	415
Hospital of Univ of Pennsylvania[2]	Philadelphia	100%	642
James E. Van Zandt VA Med Ctr-Altoona	Altoona	100%	40
Jeanes Hospital	Philadelphia	100%	286
Lancaster General Hospital	Lancaster	100%	816
Lansdale Hospital[2]	Lansdale	100%	162
Magee Womens Hosp of UPMC Health Sys	Pittsburgh	100%	65
Main Line Hospital Paoli	Paoli	100%	189
Memorial Hospital	York	100%	111
Mercy Fitzgerald Hospital	Darby	100%	499
Mercy Suburban Hospital	Norristown	100%	96
Nazareth Hospital	Philadelphia	100%	224
Penn Presbyterian Medical Center[2]	Philadelphia	100%	293
Pinnacle Health Hospitals	Harrisburg	100%	611
Saint Luke's Miners Memorial Hospital	Coaldale	100%	68
Saint Luke's Quakertown Hospital	Quakertown	100%	76
Saint Mary Medical Center	Langhorne	100%	409
Somerset Hospital	Somerset	100%	76
Titusville Hospital	Titusville	100%	35
UPMC Hamot	Erie	100%	374
UPMC Mckeesport	Mc Keesport	100%	283
UPMC Mercy	Pittsburgh	100%	299
UPMC Northwest	Seneca	100%	106
Williamsport Regional Medical Center	Williamsport	100%	239
Evangelical Community Hospital	Lewisburg	99%	106
Heritage Valley Beaver[2]	Beaver	99%	248
Jennersville Regional Hospital	West Grove	99%	85
Lehigh Valley Hospital - Hazleton	Hazleton	99%	193
Main Line Hospital Lankenau	Wynnewood	99%	533
Milton S Hershey Medical Center	Hershey	99%	460
Penn Hosp of the Univ of PA Hlth Sys	Philadelphia	99%	319
Phoenixville Hospital	Phoenixville	99%	147
Reading Hospital	Reading	99%	715
Roxborough Memorial Hospital	Philadelphia	99%	134
Saint Clair Memorial Hospital	Pittsburgh	99%	396
Thomas Jefferson University Hospital	Philadelphia	99%	840
Uniontown Hospital	Uniontown	99%	233
UPMC East[3]	Monroeville	99%	131
UPMC Horizon	Greenville	99%	165
Warren General Hospital	Warren	99%	67
Berwick Hospital Center	Berwick	98%	50
Butler Memorial Hospital	Butler	98%	202
Chester County Hospital	West Chester	98%	255
Chestnut Hill Hospital	Philadelphia	98%	180
Clarion Hospital	Clarion	98%	41
Crozer Chester Medical Center	Upland	98%	511
Doylestown Hospital	Doylestown	98%	357
Geisinger Wyoming Valley Medical Center	Wilkes Barre	98%	329
Gettysburg Hospital	Gettysburg	98%	133
Hahnemann University Hospital	Philadelphia	98%	493
Lehigh Valley Hospital - Muhlenberg	Bethlehem	98%	460
Millcreek Community Hospital	Erie	98%	58
Monongahela Valley Hospital	Monongahela	98%	259
Penn Highlands Dubois	Dubois	98%	209
Pottstown Memorial Medical Center	Pottstown	98%	168
Riddle Memorial Hospital	Media	98%	179
Saint Joseph Medical Center	Reading	98%	298
Saint Luke's Hospital Bethlehem	Bethlehem	98%	437
Schuylkill Med Ctr-S Jackson St	Pottsville	98%	122
Soldiers & Sailors Memorial Hospital	Wellsboro	98%	58
UPMC Presbyterian Shadyside	Pittsburgh	98%	1090
The Washington Hospital	Washington	98%	363
Wilkes-Barre General Hospital	Wilkes-Barre	98%	326
Allegheny General Hospital	Pittsburgh	97%	521
Barnes-Kasson County Hospital[2]	Susquehanna	97%	32
Easton Hospital	Easton	97%	259
Ellwood City Hospital[2]	Ellwood City	97%	90
Ephrata Community Hospital	Ephrata	97%	106
Excela Health Frick Hospital	Mount Pleasant	97%	124
Main Line Hospital Bryn Mawr Campus	Bryn Mawr	97%	262
Sacred Heart Hospital	Allentown	97%	98
Saint Luke's Hospital - Anderson Campus	Easton	97%	183
Temple University Hospital	Philadelphia	97%	993
Tyler Memorial Hospital	Tunkhannock	97%	30
UPMC Passavant	Pittsburgh	97%	409
VA Pittsburgh Healthcare System	Pittsburgh	97%	269
Aria Health	Philadelphia	96%	588
Brandywine Hospital	Coatesville	96%	212
Grand View Hospital	Sellersville	96%	178
Heritage Valley Sewickley	Sewickley	96%	135
Lehigh Valley Hospital	Allentown	96%	811
Nason Hospital	Roaring Spring	96%	46
Schuylkill Med Ctr-East Norwegian St	Pottsville	96%	145
York Hospital	York	96%	639
Abington Memorial Hospital	Abington	95%	570
Indiana Regional Medical Center	Indiana	95%	166
Pocono Medical Center	E Stroudsburg	95%	311
UPMC Altoona	Altoona	95%	376
UPMC Saint Margaret	Pittsburgh	95%	380
Waynesboro Hospital	Waynesboro	95%	91
Excela Health Latrobe Hospital	Latrobe	94%	187
Lewistown Hospital	Lewistown	94%	176
Lock Haven Hospital	Lock Haven	94%	53
Mount Nittany Medical Center	State College	94%	241
Palmerton Hospital	Palmerton	94%	62
Philadelphia VA Medical Center	Philadelphia	94%	219
Lancaster Regional Medical Center	Lancaster	92%	99
Lebanon VA Medical Center	Lebanon	92%	51
Moses Taylor Hospital	Scranton	92%	99
Conemaugh Valley Memorial Hospital	Johnstown	91%	620
Geisinger - Community Medical Center	Scranton	91%	283
Penn Highlands Clearfield	Clearfield	91%	53
Wilkes Barre VA Medical Center	Wilkes-Barre	91%	89
Geisinger - Bloomsburg Hospital	Bloomsburg	90%	52
Regional Hospital of Scranton	Scranton	90%	376
Wayne Memorial Hospital	Honesdale	90%	59
Chambersburg Hospital	Chambersburg	89%	356
Good Samaritan Hospital	Lebanon	89%	135
Heart of Lancaster Reg Med Ctr	Lititz	89%	35
Robert Packer Hospital	Sayre	89%	344
Sharon Regional Health System	Sharon	89%	189
Acmh Hospital	Kittanning	88%	104
Alle Kiski Medical Center	Natrona	88%	255
Excela Health Westmoreland Hospital	Greensburg	88%	438
Highlands Hospital	Connellsville	88%	57
Kane Community Hospital	Kane	88%	41
UPMC Bedford Memorial	Everett	88%	41
Corry Memorial Hospital	Corry	87%	30
Forbes Regional Hospital	Monroeville	87%	333
J C Blair Memorial Hospital	Huntingdon	87%	78
Penn Highlands Elk	Saint Marys	87%	106
Saint Vincent Hospital	Erie	87%	342
Sunbury Community Hospital	Sunbury	87%	31

NOTE: Hospital profiles are in alphabetical order by state, then city, then hospital within the city; Rankings exclude hospitals with less than 25 cases except for patient surveys which excludes hospitals with less than 100 cases; (a) 100-299 cases; (1) The number of cases/patients is too few to report; (2) Data submitted were based on a sample of cases/patients; (3) Results are based on a shorter time period than required; (4) Data suppressed by CMS for one or more quarters; (5) Results are not available for this reporting period; (6) Fewer than 100 patients completed the HCAHPS survey; (7) No cases met the criteria for this measure; (8) The lower limit of the confidence interval cannot be calculated if the number of observed infections equals zero; (9) No data are available from the state/territory for this reporting period; (10) The scores shown reflect fewer than 50 completed surveys; (11) There were discrepancies in the data collection process; (12) This measure does not apply to this hospital for this reporting period; (13) Results cannot be calculated for this reporting period; (14) The results for this state are combined with nearby states to protect confidentiality; Please refer to the User's Guide for a full explanation of data.

Hospital Name	City	Rate	Cases
Canonsburg General Hospital	Canonsburg	86%	73
Gnaden Huetten Memorial Hospital	Lehighton	86%	63
Carlisle Regional Medical Center	Carlisle	85%	73
Jefferson Regional Medical Center	Pittsburgh	85%	441
Lower Bucks Hospital	Bristol	84%	146
Western Pennsylvania Hospital	Pittsburgh	84%	64
Punxsutawney Area Hospital	Punxsutawney	83%	41
Jameson Memorial Hospital	New Castle	82%	192
Windber Hospital	Windber	82%	50
Ohio Valley General Hospital	Mckees Rocks	74%	97
Meadville Medical Center	Meadville	71%	126
Southwest Regional Medical Center	Waynesburg	64%	78
Saint Joseph's Hospital	Philadelphia	58%	115
Jersey Shore Hospital	Jersey Shore	55%	60
Miners Medical Center	Hastings	52%	29

Evaluation of LVS Function

Hospital Name	City	Rate	Cases
Abington Memorial Hospital	Abington	100%	803
Acmh Hospital	Kittanning	100%	139
Albert Einstein Medical Center[2]	Philadelphia	100%	328
Alle Kiski Medical Center	Natrona	100%	353
Allegheny General Hospital	Pittsburgh	100%	649
Aria Health	Philadelphia	100%	736
Berwick Hospital Center	Berwick	100%	72
Brandywine Hospital	Coatesville	100%	282
Butler Memorial Hospital	Butler	100%	266
Canonsburg General Hospital	Canonsburg	100%	98
Carlisle Regional Medical Center	Carlisle	100%	105
Chambersburg Hospital	Chambersburg	100%	424
Chester County Hospital	West Chester	100%	336
Chestnut Hill Hospital	Philadelphia	100%	281
Conemaugh Valley Memorial Hospital	Johnstown	100%	822
Crozer Chester Medical Center	Upland	100%	663
Delaware County Memorial Hospital	Drexel Hill	100%	191
Doylestown Hospital	Doylestown	100%	466
Easton Hospital	Easton	100%	339
Einstein Medical Center Montgomery[2,3]	East Norriton	100%	222
Ephrata Community Hospital	Ephrata	100%	152
Evangelical Community Hospital	Lewisburg	100%	131
Excela Health Latrobe Hospital	Latrobe	100%	244
Excela Health Westmoreland Hospital	Greensburg	100%	595
Forbes Regional Hospital	Monroeville	100%	455
Fulton County Medical Center	Mcconnellsburg	100%	27
Geisinger - Community Medical Center	Scranton	100%	359
Geisinger Medical Center	Danville	100%	791
Geisinger Wyoming Valley Medical Center	Wilkes Barre	100%	428
Good Samaritan Hospital	Lebanon	100%	196
Grand View Hospital	Sellersville	100%	230
Grove City Medical Center	Grove City	100%	79
Hahnemann University Hospital	Philadelphia	100%	540
Hanover Hospital	Hanover	100%	233
Heart of Lancaster Reg Med Ctr	Lititz	100%	54
Heritage Valley Beaver[2]	Beaver	100%	326
Heritage Valley Sewickley	Sewickley	100%	200
Highlands Hospital	Connellsville	100%	64
Holy Redeemer Hospital & Medical Center	Meadowbrook	100%	333
Holy Spirit Hospital	Camp Hill	100%	558
Hospital of Univ of Pennsylvania[2]	Philadelphia	100%	728
Indiana Regional Medical Center	Indiana	100%	220
J C Blair Memorial Hospital	Huntingdon	100%	102
James E. Van Zandt VA Med Ctr-Altoona	Altoona	100%	46
Jennersville Regional Hospital	West Grove	100%	115
Kane Community Hospital	Kane	100%	58
Lancaster General Hospital	Lancaster	100%	974
Lancaster Regional Medical Center	Lancaster	100%	122
Lansdale Hospital[2]	Lansdale	100%	241
Lebanon VA Medical Center	Lebanon	100%	66
Lehigh Valley Hospital	Allentown	100%	1033
Lehigh Valley Hospital - Hazleton	Hazleton	100%	287
Lehigh Valley Hospital - Muhlenberg	Bethlehem	100%	556
Lewistown Hospital	Lewistown	100%	246
Lock Haven Hospital	Lock Haven	100%	78
Lower Bucks Hospital	Bristol	100%	166
Magee Womens Hosp of UPMC Health Sys	Pittsburgh	100%	91
Main Line Hospital Bryn Mawr Campus	Bryn Mawr	100%	374
Main Line Hospital Lankenau	Wynnewood	100%	723
Main Line Hospital Paoli	Paoli	100%	267
Meadville Medical Center	Meadville	100%	185
Memorial Hospital Towanda	Towanda	100%	30
Mercy Fitzgerald Hospital	Darby	100%	584
Mercy Suburban Hospital	Norristown	100%	139
Mid - Valley Hospital	Peckville	100%	34
Milton S Hershey Medical Center	Hershey	100%	559
Monongahela Valley Hospital	Monongahela	100%	302
Moses Taylor Hospital	Scranton	100%	162
Mount Nittany Medical Center	State College	100%	299
Nason Hospital	Roaring Spring	100%	73
Nazareth Hospital	Philadelphia	100%	369
Ohio Valley General Hospital	Mckees Rocks	100%	143
Penn Highlands Dubois	Dubois	100%	252
Penn Highlands Elk	Saint Marys	100%	150
Penn Presbyterian Medical Center[2]	Philadelphia	100%	341
Penn Hosp of the Univ of PA Hlth Sys	Philadelphia	100%	358
Philadelphia VA Medical Center	Philadelphia	100%	235
Phoenixville Hospital	Phoenixville	100%	209
Pinnacle Health Hospitals	Harrisburg	100%	804
Pocono Medical Center	E Stroudsburg	100%	401
Pottstown Memorial Medical Center	Pottstown	100%	226
Punxsutawney Area Hospital	Punxsutawney	100%	49
Reading Hospital	Reading	100%	915
Riddle Memorial Hospital	Media	100%	268
Robert Packer Hospital	Sayre	100%	428
Roxborough Memorial Hospital	Philadelphia	100%	164
Saint Clair Memorial Hospital	Pittsburgh	100%	582
Saint Joseph Medical Center	Reading	100%	357
Saint Luke's Hospital - Anderson Campus	Easton	100%	237
Saint Luke's Hospital Bethlehem	Bethlehem	100%	568
Saint Luke's Miners Memorial Hospital	Coaldale	100%	94
Saint Luke's Quakertown Hospital	Quakertown	100%	114
Saint Mary Medical Center	Langhorne	100%	520
Saint Vincent Hospital	Erie	100%	452
Schuylkill Med Ctr-East Norwegian St	Pottsville	100%	239
Schuylkill Med Ctr-S Jackson St	Pottsville	100%	162
Sharon Regional Health System	Sharon	100%	232
Southwest Regional Medical Center	Waynesburg	100%	110
Sunbury Community Hospital	Sunbury	100%	56
Temple University Hospital	Philadelphia	100%	1077
Thomas Jefferson University Hospital	Philadelphia	100%	992
Titusville Hospital	Titusville	100%	42
Tyrone Hospital	Tyrone	100%	30
Uniontown Hospital	Uniontown	100%	330
UPMC Altoona	Altoona	100%	508
UPMC Bedford Memorial	Everett	100%	56
UPMC East[3]	Monroeville	100%	175
UPMC Hamot	Erie	100%	526
UPMC Horizon	Greenville	100%	208
UPMC Mckeesport	Mc Keesport	100%	398
UPMC Mercy	Pittsburgh	100%	408
UPMC Northwest	Seneca	100%	151
UPMC Passavant	Pittsburgh	100%	589
UPMC Presbyterian Shadyside	Pittsburgh	100%	1368
UPMC Saint Margaret	Pittsburgh	100%	543
VA Pittsburgh Healthcare System	Pittsburgh	100%	309
The Washington Hospital	Washington	100%	491
Waynesboro Hospital	Waynesboro	100%	103
Western Pennsylvania Hospital	Pittsburgh	100%	79
Wilkes Barre VA Medical Center	Wilkes-Barre	100%	104
Wilkes-Barre General Hospital	Wilkes-Barre	100%	513
Williamsport Regional Medical Center	Williamsport	100%	289
Windber Hospital	Windber	100%	63
York Hospital	York	100%	818
Excela Health Frick Hospital	Mount Pleasant	99%	146
Gnaden Huetten Memorial Hospital	Lehighton	99%	87
Jeanes Hospital	Philadelphia	99%	370
Jefferson Regional Medical Center	Pittsburgh	99%	546
Memorial Hospital	York	99%	136
Millcreek Community Hospital	Erie	99%	93
Penn Highlands Clearfield	Clearfield	99%	78
Regional Hospital of Scranton	Scranton	99%	530
Bradford Regional Medical Center	Bradford	98%	63
Gettysburg Hospital	Gettysburg	98%	183
Jameson Memorial Hospital	New Castle	98%	252
Sacred Heart Hospital	Allentown	98%	153
Somerset Hospital	Somerset	98%	103
Wayne Memorial Hospital	Honesdale	98%	87
Erie VA Medical Center	Erie	97%	32
Soldiers & Sailors Memorial Hospital	Wellsboro	97%	72
Tyler Memorial Hospital	Tunkhannock	97%	38
Barnes-Kasson County Hospital[2]	Susquehanna	96%	47
Ellwood City Hospital[2]	Ellwood City	96%	112
Warren General Hospital	Warren	96%	97
Charles Cole Memorial Hospital	Coudersport	95%	38
Clarion Hospital	Clarion	95%	55
Jersey Shore Hospital	Jersey Shore	93%	60
Troy Community Hospital[2]	Troy	93%	30
Geisinger - Bloomsburg Hospital	Bloomsburg	90%	70
Corry Memorial Hospital	Corry	89%	47
Palmerton Hospital	Palmerton	88%	76
Saint Joseph's Hospital	Philadelphia	84%	132
Miners Medical Center	Hastings	71%	38

Medicare Spending

Medicare Spending per Patient (ratio)

Hospital Name	City	Ratio	Cases
Valley Forge Medical Center & Hospital	Norristown	0.68	-
Eagleville Hospital	Eagleville	0.81	-
Wellspan Surgery & Rehab Hosp	York	0.85	-
Titusville Hospital	Titusville	0.87	-
Waynesboro Hospital	Waynesboro	0.87	-
Lock Haven Hospital	Lock Haven	0.89	-
Oss Orthopaedic Hospital	York	0.89	-
Bucks County Specialty Hospital	Bensalem	0.90	-
Memorial Hospital Towanda	Towanda	0.90	-
Kane Community Hospital	Kane	0.91	-
Robert Packer Hospital	Sayre	0.91	-
Chambersburg Hospital	Chambersburg	0.93	-
Evangelical Community Hospital	Lewisburg	0.93	-
Punxsutawney Area Hospital	Punxsutawney	0.93	-
Saint Luke's Quakertown Hospital	Quakertown	0.93	-
UPMC Horizon	Greenville	0.93	-
Bradford Regional Medical Center	Bradford	0.94	-
Penn Highlands Dubois	Dubois	0.94	-
Penn Highlands Elk	Saint Marys	0.94	-
UPMC Northwest	Seneca	0.94	-
Magee Womens Hosp of UPMC Health Sys	Pittsburgh	0.95	-
Tyler Memorial Hospital	Tunkhannock	0.95	-
Ellwood City Hospital	Ellwood City	0.96	-
Meadville Medical Center	Meadville	0.96	-
Berwick Hospital Center	Berwick	0.97	-
Gettysburg Hospital	Gettysburg	0.97	-
Hanover Hospital	Hanover	0.97	-
Lansdale Hospital	Lansdale	0.97	-
Lehigh Valley Hospital	Allentown	0.97	-
Monongahela Valley Hospital	Monongahela	0.97	-
Warren General Hospital	Warren	0.97	-
Windber Hospital	Windber	0.97	-
Clarion Hospital	Clarion	0.98	-
Lancaster General Hospital	Lancaster	0.98	-
Lehigh Valley Hospital - Muhlenberg	Bethlehem	0.98	-
Memorial Hospital	York	0.98	-
Milton S Hershey Medical Center	Hershey	0.98	-
Penn Highlands Clearfield	Clearfield	0.98	-
Riddle Memorial Hospital	Media	0.98	-
Saint Vincent Hospital	Erie	0.98	-
Soldiers & Sailors Memorial Hospital	Wellsboro	0.98	-
Surgical Institute of Reading	Wyomissing	0.98	-
UPMC Bedford Memorial	Everett	0.98	-
Conemaugh Valley Memorial Hospital	Johnstown	0.99	-
Ephrata Community Hospital	Ephrata	0.99	-
Grand View Hospital	Sellersville	0.99	-
Millcreek Community Hospital	Erie	0.99	-
Miners Medical Center	Hastings	0.99	-
Mount Nittany Medical Center	State College	0.99	-
Penn Presbyterian Medical Center	Philadelphia	0.99	-
Sharon Regional Health System	Sharon	0.99	-
Somerset Hospital	Somerset	0.99	-
Williamsport Regional Medical Center	Williamsport	0.99	-
Abington Memorial Hospital	Abington	1.00	-
Chester County Hospital	West Chester	1.00	-
Doylestown Hospital	Doylestown	1.00	-
Good Samaritan Hospital	Lebanon	1.00	-
Heart of Lancaster Reg Med Ctr	Lititz	1.00	-
Highlands Hospital	Connellsville	1.00	-
Saint Luke's Hospital Bethlehem	Bethlehem	1.00	-
Southwest Regional Medical Center	Waynesburg	1.00	-
UPMC East	Monroeville	1.00	-
Acmh Hospital	Kittanning	1.01	-
Coordinated Health Orthopedic Hospital	Bethlehem	1.01	-
Easton Hospital	Easton	1.01	-
Edgewood Surgical Hospital	Transfer	1.01	-
Excela Health Latrobe Hospital	Latrobe	1.01	-
J C Blair Memorial Hospital	Huntingdon	1.01	-
Main Line Hospital Lankenau	Wynnewood	1.01	-
Palmerton Hospital	Palmerton	1.01	-
Saint Joseph Medical Center	Reading	1.01	-
Surgical Specialty Ctr at Coord Hlth	Allentown	1.01	-
Thomas Jefferson University Hospital	Philadelphia	1.01	-
UPMC Presbyterian Shadyside	Pittsburgh	1.01	-
York Hospital	York	1.01	-
Canonsburg General Hospital	Canonsburg	1.02	-
Excela Health Frick Hospital	Mount Pleasant	1.02	-
Geisinger - Bloomsburg Hospital	Bloomsburg	1.02	-
Hospital of Univ of Pennsylvania	Philadelphia	1.02	-
Jennersville Regional Hospital	West Grove	1.02	-
Penn Hosp of the Univ of PA Hlth Sys	Philadelphia	1.02	-
Sacred Heart Hospital	Allentown	1.02	-
Saint Luke's Miners Memorial Hospital	Coaldale	1.02	-
Saint Mary Medical Center	Langhorne	1.02	-
Temple University Hospital	Philadelphia	1.02	-
Uniontown Hospital	Uniontown	1.02	-
Western Pennsylvania Hospital	Pittsburgh	1.02	-
Brandywine Hospital	Coatesville	1.03	-
Butler Memorial Hospital	Butler	1.03	-
Carlisle Regional Medical Center	Carlisle	1.03	-
Grove City Medical Center	Grove City	1.03	-
Hahnemann University Hospital	Philadelphia	1.03	-
Indiana Regional Medical Center	Indiana	1.03	-
Lewistown Hospital	Lewistown	1.03	-
Pocono Medical Center	E Stroudsburg	1.03	-
Reading Hospital	Reading	1.03	-

NOTE: Hospital profiles are in alphabetical order by state, then city, then hospital within the city; Rankings exclude hospitals with less than 25 cases except for patient surveys which excludes hospitals with less than 100 cases; (a) 100-299 cases; (1) The number of cases/patients is too few to report; (2) Data submitted were based on a sample of cases/patients; (3) Results are based on a shorter time period than required; (4) Data suppressed by CMS for one or more quarters; (5) Results are not available for this reporting period; (6) Fewer than 100 patients completed the HCAHPS survey; (7) No cases met the criteria for this measure; (8) The lower limit of the confidence interval cannot be calculated if the number of observed infections equals zero; (9) No data are available from the state/territory for this reporting period; (10) The scores shown reflect fewer than 50 completed surveys; (11) There were discrepancies in the data collection process; (12) This measure does not apply to this hospital for this reporting period; (13) Results cannot be calculated for this reporting period; (14) The results for this state are combined with nearby states to protect confidentiality; Please refer to the User's Guide for a full explanation of data.

UPMC Passavant	Pittsburgh	1.03	-
The Washington Hospital	Washington	1.03	-
Aria Health	Philadelphia	1.04	-
Einstein Medical Center Montgomery	East Norriton	1.04	-
Geisinger Medical Center	Danville	1.04	-
Heritage Valley Beaver	Beaver	1.04	-
Lehigh Valley Hospital - Hazleton	Hazleton	1.04	-
Phoenixville Hospital	Phoenixville	1.04	-
Saint Clair Memorial Hospital	Pittsburgh	1.04	-
Saint Luke's Hospital - Anderson Campus	Easton	1.04	-
Schuylkill Med Ctr-S Jackson St	Pottsville	1.04	-
Wayne Memorial Hospital	Honesdale	1.04	-
Chestnut Hill Hospital	Philadelphia	1.05	-
Gnaden Huetten Memorial Hospital	Lehighton	1.05	-
Holy Redeemer Hospital & Medical Center	Meadowbrook	1.05	-
Lancaster Regional Medical Center	Lancaster	1.05	-
Main Line Hospital Bryn Mawr Campus	Bryn Mawr	1.05	-
Mercy Fitzgerald Hospital	Darby	1.05	-
Pinnacle Health Hospitals	Harrisburg	1.05	-
Saint Joseph's Hospital	Philadelphia	1.05	-
Schuylkill Med Ctr-East Norwegian St	Pottsville	1.05	-
UPMC Hamot	Erie	1.05	-
Allegheny General Hospital	Pittsburgh	1.06	-
Jameson Memorial Hospital	New Castle	1.06	-
Main Line Hospital Paoli	Paoli	1.06	-
Nazareth Hospital	Philadelphia	1.06	-
Regional Hospital of Scranton	Scranton	1.06	-
Sunbury Community Hospital	Sunbury	1.06	-
UPMC Mckeesport	Mc Keesport	1.06	-
Albert Einstein Medical Center	Philadelphia	1.07	-
Crozer Chester Medical Center	Upland	1.07	-
Holy Spirit Hospital	Camp Hill	1.07	-
Pottstown Memorial Medical Center	Pottstown	1.07	-
UPMC Saint Margaret	Pittsburgh	1.07	-
Advanced Surgical Hospital	Washington	1.08	-
Excela Health Westmoreland Hospital	Greensburg	1.08	-
Heritage Valley Sewickley	Sewickley	1.08	-
Jefferson Regional Medical Center	Pittsburgh	1.08	-
Mercy Suburban Hospital	Norristown	1.08	-
Jeanes Hospital	Philadelphia	1.09	-
Alle Kiski Medical Center	Natrona	1.10	-
Geisinger - Community Medical Center	Scranton	1.10	-
Lower Bucks Hospital	Bristol	1.10	-
UPMC Altoona	Altoona	1.10	-
UPMC Mercy	Pittsburgh	1.10	-
Nason Hospital	Roaring Spring	1.11	-
Delaware County Memorial Hospital	Drexel Hill	1.12	-
Forbes Regional Hospital	Monroeville	1.12	-
Roxborough Memorial Hospital	Philadelphia	1.12	-
Moses Taylor Hospital	Scranton	1.14	-
Geisinger Wyoming Valley Medical Center	Wilkes Barre	1.15	-
Wilkes-Barre General Hospital	Wilkes-Barre	1.21	-
Ohio Valley General Hospital	Mckees Rocks	1.28	-
Cancer Treatment Centers of America	Philadelphia	1.29	-

Pneumonia Care

Appropriate Initial Antibiotic Given

Hospital Name	City	Rate	Cases
Allegheny General Hospital	Pittsburgh	100%	58
Carlisle Regional Medical Center	Carlisle	100%	74
Excela Health Latrobe Hospital	Latrobe	100%	138
Gettysburg Hospital	Gettysburg	100%	119
Heart of Lancaster Reg Med Ctr	Lititz	100%	50
Lancaster Regional Medical Center	Lancaster	100%	53
Lansdale Hospital[2]	Lansdale	100%	88
Lehigh Valley Hospital - Hazleton	Hazleton	100%	144
Lock Haven Hospital	Lock Haven	100%	54
Memorial Hospital Towanda[2]	Towanda	100%	60
Mercy Suburban Hospital	Norristown	100%	45
Muncy Valley Hospital	Muncy	100%	31
Penn Presbyterian Medical Center[2]	Philadelphia	100%	57
Phoenixville Hospital	Phoenixville	100%	88
Roxborough Memorial Hospital	Philadelphia	100%	59
Saint Clair Memorial Hospital	Pittsburgh	100%	298
Saint Joseph Medical Center	Reading	100%	119
Saint Luke's Quakertown Hospital	Quakertown	100%	66
Saint Vincent Hospital	Erie	100%	129
Soldiers & Sailors Memorial Hospital	Wellsboro	100%	75
Sunbury Community Hospital	Sunbury	100%	52
UPMC Mckeesport	Mc Keesport	100%	124
VA Pittsburgh Healthcare System	Pittsburgh	100%	69
Western Pennsylvania Hospital	Pittsburgh	100%	30
Williamsport Regional Medical Center	Williamsport	100%	126
Albert Einstein Medical Center	Philadelphia	99%	112
Excela Health Frick Hospital	Mount Pleasant	99%	80
Geisinger Medical Center	Danville	99%	225
Grand View Hospital	Sellersville	99%	149
Holy Spirit Hospital	Camp Hill	99%	420
Mercy Fitzgerald Hospital	Darby	99%	154
Nazareth Hospital	Philadelphia	99%	145
Penn Hosp of the Univ of PA Hlth Sys	Philadelphia	99%	67
Pinnacle Health Hospitals	Harrisburg	99%	303
UPMC Horizon	Greenville	99%	156
UPMC Mercy	Pittsburgh	99%	188
UPMC Presbyterian Shadyside	Pittsburgh	99%	219
York Hospital	York	99%	309
Brandywine Hospital	Coatesville	98%	135
Butler Memorial Hospital	Butler	98%	174
Crozer Chester Medical Center	Upland	98%	247
Delaware County Memorial Hospital	Drexel Hill	98%	125
Easton Hospital	Easton	98%	138
Geisinger Wyoming Valley Medical Center	Wilkes Barre	98%	149
Hanover Hospital	Hanover	98%	120
Heritage Valley Sewickley[2]	Sewickley	98%	101
Hospital of Univ of Pennsylvania	Philadelphia	98%	57
Main Line Hospital Lankenau	Wynnewood	98%	123
Milton S Hershey Medical Center	Hershey	98%	128
Ohio Valley General Hospital	Mckees Rocks	98%	85
Penn Highlands Dubois	Dubois	98%	80
Penn Highlands Elk	Saint Marys	98%	58
Pottstown Memorial Medical Center	Pottstown	98%	105
Reading Hospital	Reading	98%	433
Sacred Heart Hospital	Allentown	98%	62
Saint Luke's Hospital - Anderson Campus	Easton	98%	136
Saint Luke's Miners Memorial Hospital	Coaldale	98%	65
Saint Mary Medical Center	Langhorne	98%	294
Temple University Hospital	Philadelphia	98%	180
UPMC Bedford Memorial	Everett	98%	64
UPMC Northwest	Seneca	98%	95
Windber Hospital	Windber	98%	57
Abington Memorial Hospital	Abington	97%	254
Acmh Hospital	Kittanning	97%	110
Aria Health	Philadelphia	97%	406
Doylestown Hospital	Doylestown	97%	236
Ephrata Community Hospital	Ephrata	97%	129
Excela Health Westmoreland Hospital	Greensburg	97%	275
Fulton County Medical Center	Mcconnellsburg	97%	38
Geisinger - Community Medical Center	Scranton	97%	150
Holy Redeemer Hospital & Medical Center	Meadowbrook	97%	115
Jennersville Regional Hospital	West Grove	97%	116
Lancaster General Hospital	Lancaster	97%	346
Main Line Hospital Bryn Mawr Campus	Bryn Mawr	97%	112
Memorial Hospital	York	97%	67
Monongahela Valley Hospital	Monongahela	97%	151
Moses Taylor Hospital	Scranton	97%	92
Penn Highlands Clearfield	Clearfield	97%	68
Sharon Regional Health System	Sharon	97%	148
Thomas Jefferson University Hospital	Philadelphia	97%	223
Titusville Hospital	Titusville	97%	58
Tyler Memorial Hospital	Tunkhannock	97%	70
Uniontown Hospital[2]	Uniontown	97%	146
UPMC East[3]	Monroeville	97%	116
UPMC Saint Margaret	Pittsburgh	97%	178
The Washington Hospital	Washington	97%	213
Wayne Memorial Hospital	Honesdale	97%	90
Waynesboro Hospital	Waynesboro	97%	89
Alle Kiski Medical Center	Natrona	96%	122
Charles Cole Memorial Hospital	Coudersport	96%	45
Evangelical Community Hospital	Lewisburg	96%	119
Good Samaritan Hospital	Lebanon	96%	141
Grove City Medical Center	Grove City	96%	70
Hahnemann University Hospital	Philadelphia	96%	94
James E. Van Zandt VA Med Ctr-Altoona	Altoona	96%	25
Lebanon VA Medical Center	Lebanon	96%	27
Saint Luke's Hospital Bethlehem	Bethlehem	96%	236
Southwest Regional Medical Center	Waynesburg	96%	93
UPMC Hamot	Erie	96%	264
UPMC Passavant	Pittsburgh	96%	209
Wilkes Barre VA Medical Center	Wilkes-Barre	96%	50
Wilkes-Barre General Hospital	Wilkes-Barre	96%	247
Jeanes Hospital[2]	Philadelphia	95%	152
Lehigh Valley Hospital	Allentown	95%	332
Lehigh Valley Hospital - Muhlenberg	Bethlehem	95%	177
Meadville Medical Center	Meadville	95%	111
Palmerton Hospital	Palmerton	95%	41
Riddle Memorial Hospital	Media	95%	174
Robert Packer Hospital	Sayre	95%	105
Schuylkill Med Ctr-East Norwegian St	Pottsville	95%	105
Schuylkill Med Ctr-S Jackson St	Pottsville	95%	98
UPMC Altoona	Altoona	95%	303
Chambersburg Hospital[2]	Chambersburg	94%	81
Conemaugh Valley Memorial Hospital	Johnstown	94%	260
Einstein Medical Center Montgomery[3]	East Norriton	94%	70
Heritage Valley Beaver[2]	Beaver	94%	114
Lower Bucks Hospital	Bristol	94%	53
Magee Womens Hosp of UPMC Health Sys	Pittsburgh	94%	34
Main Line Hospital Paoli	Paoli	94%	113
Berwick Hospital Center	Berwick	93%	44
Canonsburg General Hospital	Canonsburg	93%	61
Chester County Hospital	West Chester	93%	170
Forbes Regional Hospital	Monroeville	93%	155
J C Blair Memorial Hospital	Huntingdon	93%	74
Jefferson Regional Medical Center	Pittsburgh	93%	229
Mount Nittany Medical Center	State College	93%	133
Nason Hospital	Roaring Spring	93%	84
Pocono Medical Center	E Stroudsburg	93%	192
Warren General Hospital	Warren	93%	81
Chestnut Hill Hospital	Philadelphia	92%	92
Geisinger - Bloomsburg Hospital	Bloomsburg	92%	73
Indiana Regional Medical Center	Indiana	92%	107
Corry Memorial Hospital	Corry	91%	35
Clarion Hospital	Clarion	90%	39
Lewistown Hospital	Lewistown	90%	143
Highlands Hospital	Connellsville	89%	55
Jameson Memorial Hospital	New Castle	89%	206
Philadelphia VA Medical Center	Philadelphia	89%	36
Barnes-Kasson County Hospital[2]	Susquehanna	88%	42
Bradford Regional Medical Center	Bradford	88%	97
Gnaden Huetten Memorial Hospital	Lehighton	88%	43
Punxsutawney Area Hospital	Punxsutawney	88%	43
Somerset Hospital	Somerset	88%	60
Millcreek Community Hospital	Erie	87%	31
Miners Medical Center	Hastings	86%	29
Jersey Shore Hospital	Jersey Shore	85%	54
Regional Hospital of Scranton	Scranton	85%	124
Penn Highlands Brookville	Brookville	84%	25
Ellwood City Hospital	Ellwood City	80%	41
Troy Community Hospital[2]	Troy	79%	28
Kane Community Hospital	Kane	75%	32
Saint Joseph's Hospital	Philadelphia	70%	37

Blood Culture Timing

Hospital Name	City	Rate	Cases
Alle Kiski Medical Center	Natrona	100%	121
Allegheny General Hospital	Pittsburgh	100%	36
Berwick Hospital Center	Berwick	100%	76
Charles Cole Memorial Hospital	Coudersport	100%	68
Corry Memorial Hospital	Corry	100%	53
Delaware County Memorial Hospital	Drexel Hill	100%	179
Excela Health Latrobe Hospital	Latrobe	100%	260
Excela Health Westmoreland Hospital	Greensburg	100%	511
Gnaden Huetten Memorial Hospital	Lehighton	100%	88
Grand View Hospital	Sellersville	100%	278
Hanover Hospital	Hanover	100%	212
Heart of Lancaster Reg Med Ctr	Lititz	100%	76
Holy Spirit Hospital	Camp Hill	100%	664
Kane Community Hospital	Kane	100%	63
Lancaster Regional Medical Center	Lancaster	100%	75
Lock Haven Hospital	Lock Haven	100%	67
Magee Womens Hosp of UPMC Health Sys	Pittsburgh	100%	33
Main Line Hospital Bryn Mawr Campus	Bryn Mawr	100%	250
Mercy Fitzgerald Hospital	Darby	100%	371
Moses Taylor Hospital	Scranton	100%	201
Penn Highlands Brookville	Brookville	100%	38
Pottstown Memorial Medical Center	Pottstown	100%	263
Roxborough Memorial Hospital	Philadelphia	100%	152
Saint Luke's Hospital Bethlehem	Bethlehem	100%	422
Saint Luke's Miners Memorial Hospital	Coaldale	100%	94
Saint Luke's Quakertown Hospital	Quakertown	100%	86
Saint Mary Medical Center	Langhorne	100%	494
Schuylkill Med Ctr-East Norwegian St	Pottsville	100%	175
Temple University Hospital	Philadelphia	100%	235
Tyrone Hospital	Tyrone	100%	33
UPMC Bedford Memorial	Everett	100%	88
UPMC Horizon	Greenville	100%	246
UPMC Mckeesport	Mc Keesport	100%	238
UPMC Northwest	Seneca	100%	184
UPMC Presbyterian Shadyside	Pittsburgh	100%	431
UPMC Saint Margaret	Pittsburgh	100%	216
VA Pittsburgh Healthcare System	Pittsburgh	100%	215
The Washington Hospital	Washington	100%	339
Western Pennsylvania Hospital	Pittsburgh	100%	50
Williamsport Regional Medical Center	Williamsport	100%	214
Windber Hospital	Windber	100%	67
Abington Memorial Hospital	Abington	99%	558
Bradford Regional Medical Center	Bradford	99%	148
Chester County Hospital	West Chester	99%	362
Conemaugh Valley Memorial Hospital	Johnstown	99%	397
Doylestown Hospital	Doylestown	99%	479
Easton Hospital	Easton	99%	247
Evangelical Community Hospital	Lewisburg	99%	217
Forbes Regional Hospital	Monroeville	99%	211
Geisinger Medical Center	Danville	99%	171
Geisinger Wyoming Valley Medical Center	Wilkes Barre	99%	185
Grove City Medical Center	Grove City	99%	110
Hahnemann University Hospital	Philadelphia	99%	232
Heritage Valley Sewickley[2]	Sewickley	99%	191
Highlands Hospital	Connellsville	99%	67
Hospital of Univ of Pennsylvania	Philadelphia	99%	205
Indiana Regional Medical Center	Indiana	99%	162
J C Blair Memorial Hospital	Huntingdon	99%	100

NOTE: Hospital profiles are in alphabetical order by state, then city, then hospital within the city; Rankings exclude hospitals with less than 25 cases except for patient surveys which excludes hospitals with less than 100 cases; (a) 100-299 cases; (1) The number of cases/patients is too few to report; (2) Data submitted were based on a sample of cases/patients; (3) Results are based on a shorter time period than required; (4) Data suppressed by CMS for one or more quarters; (5) Results are not available for this reporting period; (6) Fewer than 100 patients completed the HCAHPS survey; (7) No cases met the criteria for this measure; (8) The lower limit of the confidence interval cannot be calculated if the number of observed infections equals zero; (9) No data are available from the state/territory for this reporting period; (10) The scores shown reflect fewer than 50 completed surveys; (11) There were discrepancies in the data collection process; (12) This measure does not apply to this hospital for this reporting period; (13) Results cannot be calculated for this reporting period; (14) The results for this state are combined with nearby states to protect confidentiality; Please refer to the User's Guide for a full explanation of data.

Jennersville Regional Hospital	West Grove	99%	179
Lancaster General Hospital	Lancaster	99%	623
Lansdale Hospital[2]	Lansdale	99%	153
Lehigh Valley Hospital - Hazleton	Hazleton	99%	221
Memorial Hospital	York	99%	175
Monongahela Valley Hospital	Monongahela	99%	203
Penn Highlands Elk	Saint Marys	99%	145
Penn Presbyterian Medical Center[2]	Philadelphia	99%	120
Penn Hosp of the Univ of PA Hlth Sys	Philadelphia	99%	143
Phoenixville Hospital	Phoenixville	99%	190
Pinnacle Health Hospitals	Harrisburg	99%	493
Pocono Medical Center	E Stroudsburg	99%	339
Reading Hospital	Reading	99%	1119
Sacred Heart Hospital	Allentown	99%	96
Saint Clair Memorial Hospital	Pittsburgh	99%	253
Saint Luke's Hospital - Anderson Campus	Easton	99%	210
Soldiers & Sailors Memorial Hospital	Wellsboro	99%	133
Southwest Regional Medical Center	Waynesburg	99%	132
Sunbury Community Hospital	Sunbury	99%	68
Tyler Memorial Hospital	Tunkhannock	99%	92
UPMC Altoona	Altoona	99%	496
UPMC East[3]	Monroeville	99%	138
UPMC Mercy	Pittsburgh	99%	145
UPMC Passavant	Pittsburgh	99%	343
Wayne Memorial Hospital	Honesdale	99%	151
Waynesboro Hospital	Waynesboro	99%	136
Acmh Hospital	Kittanning	98%	162
Aria Health	Philadelphia	98%	850
Brandywine Hospital	Coatesville	98%	247
Canonsburg General Hospital	Canonsburg	98%	101
Chambersburg Hospital[2]	Chambersburg	98%	141
Crozer Chester Medical Center	Upland	98%	485
Einstein Medical Center Montgomery[3]	East Norriton	98%	48
Excela Health Frick Hospital	Mount Pleasant	98%	167
Geisinger - Community Medical Center	Scranton	98%	249
Gettysburg Hospital	Gettysburg	98%	208
Good Samaritan Hospital	Lebanon	98%	235
Holy Redeemer Hospital & Medical Center	Meadowbrook	98%	259
Jameson Memorial Hospital	New Castle	98%	360
Lebanon VA Medical Center	Lebanon	98%	51
Lewistown Hospital	Lewistown	98%	247
Lower Bucks Hospital	Bristol	98%	80
Main Line Hospital Lankenau	Wynnewood	98%	313
Main Line Hospital Paoli	Paoli	98%	164
Memorial Hospital Towanda[2]	Towanda	98%	89
Mercy Suburban Hospital	Norristown	98%	107
Milton S Hershey Medical Center	Hershey	98%	382
Nazareth Hospital	Philadelphia	98%	265
Ohio Valley General Hospital	Mckees Rocks	98%	103
Palmerton Hospital	Palmerton	98%	60
Penn Highlands Clearfield	Clearfield	98%	108
Penn Highlands Dubois	Dubois	98%	156
Riddle Memorial Hospital	Media	98%	241
Schuylkill Med Ctr-S Jackson St	Pottsville	98%	196
Thomas Jefferson University Hospital	Philadelphia	98%	502
Uniontown Hospital[2]	Uniontown	98%	253
UPMC Hamot	Erie	98%	465
Warren General Hospital	Warren	98%	127
Wilkes-Barre General Hospital	Wilkes-Barre	98%	406
Butler Memorial Hospital	Butler	97%	235
Carlisle Regional Medical Center	Carlisle	97%	124
Chestnut Hill Hospital	Philadelphia	97%	182
Fulton County Medical Center	Mcconnellsburg	97%	37
Geisinger - Bloomsburg Hospital	Bloomsburg	97%	103
James E. Van Zandt VA Med Ctr-Altoona	Altoona	97%	33
Lehigh Valley Hospital	Allentown	97%	703
Lehigh Valley Hospital - Muhlenberg	Bethlehem	97%	324
Millcreek Community Hospital	Erie	97%	32
Muncy Valley Hospital	Muncy	97%	37
Nason Hospital	Roaring Spring	97%	86
Philadelphia VA Medical Center	Philadelphia	97%	58
Saint Vincent Hospital	Erie	97%	218
Sharon Regional Health System	Sharon	97%	223
Wilkes Barre VA Medical Center	Wilkes-Barre	97%	79
Albert Einstein Medical Center	Philadelphia	96%	198
Ephrata Community Hospital	Ephrata	96%	202
Heritage Valley Beaver[2]	Beaver	96%	189
Meadville Medical Center	Meadville	96%	168
Mid - Valley Hospital	Peckville	96%	28
Mount Nittany Medical Center	State College	96%	165
Punxsutawney Area Hospital	Punxsutawney	96%	49
Regional Hospital of Scranton	Scranton	96%	249
Saint Joseph Medical Center	Reading	96%	235
Titusville Hospital	Titusville	96%	71
York Hospital	York	96%	398
Clarion Hospital	Clarion	95%	76
Jeanes Hospital[2]	Philadelphia	95%	169
Ellwood City Hospital	Ellwood City	93%	45
Robert Packer Hospital	Sayre	93%	212
Somerset Hospital	Somerset	93%	144
Saint Joseph's Hospital	Philadelphia	90%	72
Miners Medical Center	Hastings	89%	45
Jefferson Regional Medical Center	Pittsburgh	87%	267
Jersey Shore Hospital	Jersey Shore	87%	52
Troy Community Hospital[2]	Troy	84%	38

Pregnancy and Delivery Care

Newborns whose Deliveries were Scheduled Early

Hospital Name	City	Rate	Cases
Abington Memorial Hospital[2]	Abington	0%	79
Albert Einstein Medical Center[2]	Philadelphia	0%	43
Bradford Regional Medical Center[2]	Bradford	0%	26
Excela Health Westmoreland Hospital[2]	Greensburg	0%	145
Geisinger Medical Center[2]	Danville	0%	113
Geisinger Wyoming Valley Medical Center[2]	Wilkes Barre	0%	86
Gettysburg Hospital[2]	Gettysburg	0%	47
Good Samaritan Hospital[2]	Lebanon	0%	32
Hahnemann University Hospital[2]	Philadelphia	0%	38
Indiana Regional Medical Center[2]	Indiana	0%	57
Jennersville Regional Hospital[2]	West Grove	0%	35
Lehigh Valley Hospital	Allentown	0%	680
Magee Womens Hosp of UPMC Health Sys[2]	Pittsburgh	0%	105
Main Line Hospital Paoli[2]	Paoli	0%	33
Meadville Medical Center[2]	Meadville	0%	44
Millcreek Community Hospital	Erie	0%	36
Milton S Hershey Medical Center[2]	Hershey	0%	67
Moses Taylor Hospital[2]	Scranton	0%	51
Pinnacle Health Hospitals[2]	Harrisburg	0%	47
Reading Hospital[2]	Reading	0%	48
Robert Packer Hospital	Sayre	0%	47
Sacred Heart Hospital	Allentown	0%	41
Saint Luke's Hospital Bethlehem	Bethlehem	0%	221
UPMC Bedford Memorial[2]	Everett	0%	38
UPMC Hamot[2]	Erie	0%	183
UPMC Mercy[2]	Pittsburgh	0%	105
UPMC Northwest[2]	Seneca	0%	48
Wayne Memorial Hospital[2]	Honesdale	0%	26
Wilkes-Barre General Hospital[2]	Wilkes-Barre	0%	28
York Hospital[2]	York	0%	36
Heritage Valley Sewickley[2]	Sewickley	1%	85
Hospital of Univ of Pennsylvania[2]	Philadelphia	1%	72
Thomas Jefferson University Hospital	Philadelphia	1%	301
Western Pennsylvania Hospital[2]	Pittsburgh	1%	217
Holy Redeemer Hospital & Medical Center[2]	Meadowbrook	2%	229
Mount Nittany Medical Center[2]	State College	2%	110
Penn Highlands Dubois	Dubois	2%	64
Temple University Hospital[2]	Philadelphia	2%	41
Uniontown Hospital[2]	Uniontown	2%	105
Einstein Medical Center Montgomery[2]	East Norriton	3%	34
Grand View Hospital	Sellersville	3%	105
Nason Hospital[2]	Roaring Spring	3%	31
Phoenixville Hospital[2]	Phoenixville	3%	33
Saint Joseph Medical Center[2]	Reading	3%	35
Saint Mary Medical Center[2]	Langhorne	3%	35
The Washington Hospital	Washington	3%	116
Williamsport Regional Medical Center[2]	Williamsport	3%	34
Conemaugh Valley Memorial Hospital	Johnstown	4%	127
Penn Hosp of the Univ of PA Hlth Sys[2]	Philadelphia	4%	239
Forbes Regional Hospital	Monroeville	5%	91
Lancaster General Hospital[2]	Lancaster	5%	184
Heart of Lancaster Reg Med Ctr	Lititz	6%	48
Pocono Medical Center[2]	E Stroudsburg	6%	68
Schuylkill Med Ctr-S Jackson St[2]	Pottsville	6%	102
Memorial Hospital[2]	York	7%	29
Hanover Hospital[2]	Hanover	8%	39
Butler Memorial Hospital[2]	Butler	9%	87
Pottstown Memorial Medical Center[2]	Pottstown	9%	33
Saint Vincent Hospital	Erie	9%	76
Chester County Hospital[2]	West Chester	10%	49
Lewistown Hospital[2]	Lewistown	11%	47
UPMC Horizon[2]	Greenville	11%	66
Carlisle Regional Medical Center	Carlisle	12%	33
Doylestown Hospital[2]	Doylestown	12%	26
Saint Clair Memorial Hospital[2]	Pittsburgh	14%	36
Sharon Regional Health System	Sharon	14%	56
J C Blair Memorial Hospital	Huntingdon	20%	30
Lehigh Valley Hospital - Hazleton[2]	Hazleton	20%	106
Main Line Hospital Lankenau[2]	Wynnewood	21%	28
UPMC Altoona	Altoona	21%	129
Penn Highlands Elk	Saint Marys	25%	32
Evangelical Community Hospital[2]	Lewisburg	27%	44
Somerset Hospital	Somerset	43%	58
Jameson Memorial Hospital	New Castle	47%	66

Preventive Care

Immunization for Influenza

Hospital Name	City	Rate	Cases
Lehigh Valley Hospital - Hazleton[2]	Hazleton	100%	566
Moses Taylor Hospital[2]	Scranton	100%	532
Saint Luke's Miners Memorial Hospital[2]	Coaldale	100%	289
Tyrone Hospital	Tyrone	100%	285
UPMC East[2,3]	Monroeville	100%	342
The Washington Hospital[2]	Washington	100%	575
Butler Memorial Hospital[2]	Butler	99%	550
Carlisle Regional Medical Center[2]	Carlisle	99%	431
Charles Cole Memorial Hospital[2]	Coudersport	99%	395
Delaware County Memorial Hospital[2]	Drexel Hill	99%	504
Heart of Lancaster Reg Med Ctr[2]	Lititz	99%	256
Lancaster Regional Medical Center[2]	Lancaster	99%	434
Lehigh Valley Hospital - Muhlenberg[2]	Bethlehem	99%	590
Lock Haven Hospital[2]	Lock Haven	99%	289
Mid - Valley Hospital[2]	Peckville	99%	174
Penn Highlands Clearfield[2]	Clearfield	99%	271
Pottstown Memorial Medical Center[2]	Pottstown	99%	649
Roxborough Memorial Hospital[2]	Philadelphia	99%	451
Soldiers & Sailors Memorial Hospital[2]	Wellsboro	99%	257
Tyler Memorial Hospital[2]	Tunkhannock	99%	343
UPMC Presbyterian Shadyside[2]	Pittsburgh	99%	703
Berwick Hospital Center[2]	Berwick	98%	398
Ephrata Community Hospital[2]	Ephrata	98%	516
Excela Health Frick Hospital[2]	Mount Pleasant	98%	415
Geisinger - Community Medical Center[2]	Scranton	98%	786
Grand View Hospital[2]	Sellersville	98%	564
Hahnemann University Hospital[2]	Philadelphia	98%	578
Heritage Valley Beaver[2]	Beaver	98%	563
Heritage Valley Sewickley[2]	Sewickley	98%	561
James E. Van Zandt VA Med Ctr-Altoona[2,3]	Altoona	98%	140
Memorial Hospital[2]	York	98%	527
Milton S Hershey Medical Center[2]	Hershey	98%	615
Temple University Hospital[2]	Philadelphia	98%	535
Thomas Jefferson University Hospital[2]	Philadelphia	98%	1135
UPMC Bedford Memorial[2]	Everett	98%	347
UPMC Horizon[2]	Greenville	98%	651
UPMC Northwest[2]	Seneca	98%	620
Waynesboro Hospital[2]	Waynesboro	98%	321
Acmh Hospital[2]	Kittanning	97%	550
Barnes-Kasson County Hospital[2,3]	Susquehanna	97%	163
Chestnut Hill Hospital[2]	Philadelphia	97%	668
Hanover Hospital[2]	Hanover	97%	511
Lansdale Hospital[2]	Lansdale	97%	547
Penn Highlands Dubois[2]	Dubois	97%	512
Phoenixville Hospital[2]	Phoenixville	97%	609
Southwest Regional Medical Center[2]	Waynesburg	97%	292
UPMC Mercy[2]	Pittsburgh	97%	637
UPMC Passavant[2]	Pittsburgh	97%	717
UPMC Saint Margaret[2]	Pittsburgh	97%	717
York Hospital[2]	York	97%	518
Advanced Surgical Hospital	Washington	96%	241
Canonsburg General Hospital[2]	Canonsburg	96%	351
Coatesville VA Medical Center[2,3]	Coatesville	96%	139
Crozer Chester Medical Center[2]	Upland	96%	539
Doylestown Hospital[2]	Doylestown	96%	580
Easton Hospital[2]	Easton	96%	647
Excela Health Latrobe Hospital[2]	Latrobe	96%	766
Gettysburg Hospital[2]	Gettysburg	96%	457
Indiana Regional Medical Center[2]	Indiana	96%	534
Jennersville Regional Hospital[2]	West Grove	96%	338
Lehigh Valley Hospital[2]	Allentown	96%	546
Mercy Suburban Hospital[2]	Norristown	96%	434
Millcreek Community Hospital[2]	Erie	96%	418
Saint Luke's Hospital - Anderson Campus[2]	Easton	96%	490
Sunbury Community Hospital[2]	Sunbury	96%	334
UPMC Mckeesport[2]	Mc Keesport	96%	709
Wellspan Surgery & Rehab Hosp[2]	York	96%	232
Williamsport Regional Medical Center[2]	Williamsport	96%	591
Albert Einstein Medical Center[2]	Philadelphia	95%	639
Brandywine Hospital[2]	Coatesville	95%	665
Einstein Medical Center Montgomery[2,3]	East Norriton	95%	255
Erie VA Medical Center[2,3]	Erie	95%	128
Meadville Medical Center[2]	Meadville	95%	1060
Pinnacle Health Hospitals[2]	Harrisburg	95%	629
Reading Hospital[2]	Reading	95%	545
Sacred Heart Hospital[2]	Allentown	95%	1177
Saint Joseph Medical Center[2]	Reading	95%	552
Saint Luke's Quakertown Hospital[2]	Quakertown	95%	311
Wayne Memorial Hospital[2]	Honesdale	95%	298
Geisinger Wyoming Valley Medical Center[2]	Wilkes Barre	94%	649
Jameson Memorial Hospital[2]	New Castle	94%	539
Saint Luke's Hospital Bethlehem[2]	Bethlehem	94%	1074
Schuylkill Med Ctr-S Jackson St[2]	Pottsville	94%	442
Uniontown Hospital[2]	Uniontown	94%	491
UPMC Altoona[2]	Altoona	94%	1077
Valley Forge Medical Center & Hospital[2]	Norristown	94%	380
Chambersburg Hospital[2]	Chambersburg	93%	519
Edgewood Surgical Hospital	Transfer	93%	46
Geisinger Medical Center[2]	Danville	93%	678
Lancaster General Hospital[2]	Lancaster	93%	550
Lower Bucks Hospital[2]	Bristol	93%	441
Magee Womens Hosp of UPMC Health Sys[2]	Pittsburgh	93%	471
Memorial Hospital Towanda[2]	Towanda	93%	255

NOTE: Hospital profiles are in alphabetical order by state, then city, then hospital within the city; Rankings exclude hospitals with less than 25 cases except for patient surveys which excludes hospitals with less than 100 cases; (a) 100-299 cases; (1) The number of cases/patients is too few to report; (2) Data submitted were based on a sample of cases/patients; (3) Results are based on a shorter time period than required; (4) Data suppressed by CMS for one or more quarters; (5) Results are not available for this reporting period; (6) Fewer than 100 patients completed the HCAHPS survey; (7) No cases met the criteria for this measure; (8) The lower limit of the confidence interval cannot be calculated if the number of observed infections equals zero; (9) No data are available from the state/territory for this reporting period; (10) The scores shown reflect fewer than 50 completed surveys; (11) There were discrepancies in the data collection process; (12) This measure does not apply to this hospital for this reporting period; (13) Results cannot be calculated for this reporting period; (14) The results for this state are combined with nearby states to protect confidentiality; Please refer to the User's Guide for a full explanation of data.

Hospital Name	City	Rate	Cases
Mercy Fitzgerald Hospital[2]	Darby	93%	1212
Monongahela Valley Hospital[2]	Monongahela	93%	862
Nazareth Hospital[2]	Philadelphia	93%	602
Schuylkill Med Ctr-East Norwegian St[2]	Pottsville	93%	376
Titusville Hospital[2]	Titusville	93%	537
Troy Community Hospital[2,3]	Troy	93%	30
Chester County Hospital[2]	West Chester	92%	560
Conemaugh Valley Memorial Hospital[2]	Johnstown	92%	585
Ellwood City Hospital[2]	Ellwood City	92%	296
J C Blair Memorial Hospital[2]	Huntingdon	92%	278
Jeanes Hospital[2]	Philadelphia	92%	592
Pocono Medical Center[2]	E Stroudsburg	92%	662
Regional Hospital of Scranton[2]	Scranton	92%	673
Robert Packer Hospital[2]	Sayre	92%	656
Saint Clair Memorial Hospital[2]	Pittsburgh	92%	540
UPMC Hamot[2]	Erie	92%	608
Warren General Hospital[2]	Warren	92%	334
Highlands Hospital[2]	Connellsville	91%	278
Holy Redeemer Hospital & Medical Center[2]	Meadowbrook	91%	482
Penn Hosp of the Univ of PA Hlth Sys[2]	Philadelphia	91%	518
Surgical Institute of Reading[2]	Wyomissing	91%	197
Alle Kiski Medical Center[2]	Natrona	90%	646
Clarion Hospital[2]	Clarion	90%	262
Grove City Medical Center[2]	Grove City	90%	261
Main Line Hospital Paoli[2]	Paoli	90%	542
Ohio Valley General Hospital[2]	Mckees Rocks	90%	315
Oss Orthopaedic Hospital[2]	York	89%	394
Abington Memorial Hospital[2]	Abington	88%	548
Aria Health[2]	Philadelphia	88%	584
Excela Health Westmoreland Hospital[2]	Greensburg	88%	762
Jefferson Regional Medical Center[2]	Pittsburgh	88%	592
Lewistown Hospital[2]	Lewistown	88%	477
Punxsutawney Area Hospital[2]	Punxsutawney	88%	263
Wilkes-Barre General Hospital[2]	Wilkes-Barre	88%	672
Bradford Regional Medical Center[2]	Bradford	87%	308
Bucks County Specialty Hospital[2]	Bensalem	87%	311
Penn Highlands Elk[2]	Saint Marys	87%	278
Western Pennsylvania Hospital[2]	Pittsburgh	87%	438
Penn Presbyterian Medical Center[2]	Philadelphia	86%	962
Riddle Memorial Hospital[2]	Media	86%	550
Good Samaritan Hospital[2]	Lebanon	84%	541
Main Line Hospital Bryn Mawr Campus[2]	Bryn Mawr	84%	546
Evangelical Community Hospital[2]	Lewisburg	83%	510
Hospital of Univ of Pennsylvania[2]	Philadelphia	83%	527
Forbes Regional Hospital[2]	Monroeville	82%	605
Holy Spirit Hospital[2]	Camp Hill	82%	577
Nason Hospital[2]	Roaring Spring	82%	247
Palmerton Hospital[2]	Palmerton	82%	290
Geisinger - Bloomsburg Hospital[2]	Bloomsburg	81%	1081
Coordinated Health Orthopedic Hospital[2]	Bethlehem	79%	368
Main Line Hospital Lankenau[2]	Wynnewood	79%	545
Windber Hospital[2]	Windber	79%	249
Gnaden Huetten Memorial Hospital[2]	Lehighton	78%	333
Allegheny General Hospital[2]	Pittsburgh	75%	638
Miners Medical Center[2]	Hastings	74%	254
Kane Community Hospital[2]	Kane	73%	359
Cancer Treatment Centers of America[2]	Philadelphia	69%	276
Mount Nittany Medical Center[2]	State College	69%	528
Physician's Care Surgical Hospital[2]	Royersford	66%	126
Saint Joseph's Hospital[2]	Philadelphia	65%	342
Somerset Hospital[2]	Somerset	65%	314
Saint Vincent Hospital[2]	Erie	62%	1055
Surgical Specialty Ctr at Coord Hlth[2]	Allentown	59%	390
Saint Mary Medical Center[2]	Langhorne	58%	589
Sharon Regional Health System[2]	Sharon	58%	561
Eagleville Hospital[2]	Eagleville	55%	419
Kensington Hospital[2]	Philadelphia	2%	47

Immunization for Pneumonia

Hospital Name	City	Rate	Cases
Berwick Hospital Center[2]	Berwick	100%	515
Jennersville Regional Hospital[2]	West Grove	100%	449
Lehigh Valley Hospital - Hazleton[2]	Hazleton	100%	811
Mid - Valley Hospital[2]	Peckville	100%	259
Saint Luke's Miners Memorial Hospital[2]	Coaldale	100%	459
Tyrone Hospital[2]	Tyrone	100%	429
UPMC East[2,3]	Monroeville	100%	769
Wayne Memorial Hospital[2]	Honesdale	100%	405
Charles Cole Memorial Hospital[2]	Coudersport	99%	444
Delaware County Memorial Hospital[2]	Drexel Hill	99%	546
Hanover Hospital[2]	Hanover	99%	751
Heart of Lancaster Reg Med Ctr[2]	Lititz	99%	241
James E. Van Zandt VA Med Ctr-Altoona[2,3]	Altoona	99%	344
Lock Haven Hospital[2]	Lock Haven	99%	389
Millcreek Community Hospital[2]	Erie	99%	368
Moses Taylor Hospital[2]	Scranton	99%	518
Pottstown Memorial Medical Center[2]	Pottstown	99%	889
Roxborough Memorial Hospital[2]	Philadelphia	99%	689
Temple University Hospital[2]	Philadelphia	99%	627
Tyler Memorial Hospital[2]	Tunkhannock	99%	544
UPMC Presbyterian Shadyside[2]	Pittsburgh	99%	925
The Washington Hospital[2]	Washington	99%	744
Waynesboro Hospital[2]	Waynesboro	99%	422
Advanced Surgical Hospital	Washington	98%	321
Butler Memorial Hospital[2]	Butler	98%	702
Carlisle Regional Medical Center[2]	Carlisle	98%	548
Ephrata Community Hospital[2]	Ephrata	98%	647
Excela Health Frick Hospital[2]	Mount Pleasant	98%	691
Grand View Hospital[2]	Sellersville	98%	659
Heritage Valley Sewickley[2]	Sewickley	98%	681
Phoenixville Hospital[2]	Phoenixville	98%	780
Saint Clair Memorial Hospital[2]	Pittsburgh	98%	720
Titusville Hospital[2]	Titusville	98%	760
UPMC Horizon[2]	Greenville	98%	834
UPMC Northwest[2]	Seneca	98%	853
Easton Hospital[2]	Easton	97%	998
Geisinger - Community Medical Center[2]	Scranton	97%	1305
Geisinger Wyoming Valley Medical Center[2]	Wilkes Barre	97%	810
Heritage Valley Beaver[2]	Beaver	97%	752
Lancaster Regional Medical Center[2]	Lancaster	97%	527
Meadville Medical Center[2]	Meadville	97%	1254
Mercy Suburban Hospital[2]	Norristown	97%	654
Penn Highlands Clearfield[2]	Clearfield	97%	387
Penn Highlands Dubois[2]	Dubois	97%	595
UPMC Bedford Memorial[2]	Everett	97%	444
UPMC Mckeesport[2]	Mc Keesport	97%	1015
UPMC Saint Margaret[2]	Pittsburgh	97%	1108
Williamsport Regional Medical Center[2]	Williamsport	97%	791
Acmh Hospital[2]	Kittanning	96%	619
Alle Kiski Medical Center[2]	Natrona	96%	1023
Brandywine Hospital[2]	Coatesville	96%	861
Chambersburg Hospital[2]	Chambersburg	96%	731
Coatesville VA Medical Center[2,3]	Coatesville	96%	155
Conemaugh Valley Memorial Hospital[2]	Johnstown	96%	728
Geisinger Medical Center[2]	Danville	96%	807
Indiana Regional Medical Center[2]	Indiana	96%	747
Lansdale Hospital[2]	Lansdale	96%	834
Lewistown Hospital[2]	Lewistown	96%	672
Lower Bucks Hospital[2]	Bristol	96%	529
Memorial Hospital[2]	York	96%	694
Monongahela Valley Hospital[2]	Monongahela	96%	1338
Penn Highlands Elk[2]	Saint Marys	96%	487
Pinnacle Health Hospitals[2]	Harrisburg	96%	830
Robert Packer Hospital[2]	Sayre	96%	902
Schuylkill Med Ctr-East Norwegian St[2]	Pottsville	96%	639
Sunbury Community Hospital[2]	Sunbury	96%	459
Thomas Jefferson University Hospital[2]	Philadelphia	96%	1494
UPMC Altoona[2]	Altoona	96%	1369
UPMC Mercy[2]	Pittsburgh	96%	748
Crozer Chester Medical Center[2]	Upland	95%	657
Ellwood City Hospital[2]	Ellwood City	95%	422
Erie VA Medical Center[2,3]	Erie	95%	306
Lehigh Valley Hospital - Muhlenberg[2]	Bethlehem	95%	921
Sacred Heart Hospital[2]	Allentown	95%	973
Saint Joseph Medical Center[2]	Reading	95%	746
Saint Luke's Quakertown Hospital[2]	Quakertown	95%	437
Soldiers & Sailors Memorial Hospital[2]	Wellsboro	95%	301
Southwest Regional Medical Center[2]	Waynesburg	95%	455
UPMC Passavant[2]	Pittsburgh	95%	1017
York Hospital[2]	York	95%	660
Chester County Hospital[2]	West Chester	94%	618
Chestnut Hill Hospital[2]	Philadelphia	94%	1049
Gettysburg Hospital[2]	Gettysburg	94%	618
Hahnemann University Hospital[2]	Philadelphia	94%	649
Memorial Hospital Towanda[2]	Towanda	94%	309
Saint Luke's Hospital - Anderson Campus[2]	Easton	94%	772
UPMC Hamot[2]	Erie	94%	745
Cancer Treatment Centers of America[2]	Philadelphia	93%	183
Canonsburg General Hospital[2]	Canonsburg	93%	541
Grove City Medical Center[2]	Grove City	93%	386
Jameson Memorial Hospital[2]	New Castle	93%	754
Main Line Hospital Paoli[2]	Paoli	93%	646
Reading Hospital[2]	Reading	93%	690
Regional Hospital of Scranton[2]	Scranton	93%	1079
Saint Luke's Hospital Bethlehem[2]	Bethlehem	93%	1373
Schuylkill Med Ctr-S Jackson St[2]	Pottsville	93%	557
Troy Community Hospital[2,3]	Troy	93%	158
Uniontown Hospital[2]	Uniontown	93%	700
Doylestown Hospital[2]	Doylestown	92%	822
Excela Health Latrobe Hospital[2]	Latrobe	92%	1113
Gnaden Huetten Memorial Hospital[2]	Lehighton	92%	421
Ohio Valley General Hospital[2]	Mckees Rocks	92%	490
Oss Orthopaedic Hospital[2]	York	92%	465
Excela Health Westmoreland Hospital[2]	Greensburg	91%	1001
Lancaster General Hospital[2]	Lancaster	91%	698
Pocono Medical Center[2]	E Stroudsburg	91%	907
Warren General Hospital[2]	Warren	91%	348
Abington Memorial Hospital[2]	Abington	90%	637
Clarion Hospital[2]	Clarion	90%	375
Evangelical Community Hospital[2]	Lewisburg	90%	640
Jeanes Hospital[2]	Philadelphia	90%	844
Jefferson Regional Medical Center[2]	Pittsburgh	90%	952
Lehigh Valley Hospital[2]	Allentown	90%	668
Mercy Fitzgerald Hospital[2]	Darby	90%	1778
Punxsutawney Area Hospital[2]	Punxsutawney	90%	386
Somerset Hospital[2]	Somerset	90%	392
Albert Einstein Medical Center[2]	Philadelphia	89%	765
Milton S Hershey Medical Center[2]	Hershey	89%	596
Nazareth Hospital[2]	Philadelphia	89%	903
Palmerton Hospital[2]	Palmerton	89%	454
Wilkes-Barre General Hospital[2]	Wilkes-Barre	89%	969
J C Blair Memorial Hospital[2]	Huntingdon	88%	297
Wellspan Surgery & Rehab Hosp[2]	York	88%	292
Bradford Regional Medical Center[2]	Bradford	87%	363
Good Samaritan Hospital[2]	Lebanon	86%	702
Einstein Medical Center Montgomery[2,3]	East Norriton	85%	437
Holy Redeemer Hospital & Medical Center[2]	Meadowbrook	84%	524
Saint Mary Medical Center[2]	Langhorne	84%	743
Aria Health[2]	Philadelphia	83%	832
Magee Womens Hosp of UPMC Health Sys[2]	Pittsburgh	83%	249
Main Line Hospital Bryn Mawr Campus[2]	Bryn Mawr	83%	704
Penn Hosp of the Univ of PA Hlth Sys[2]	Philadelphia	83%	523
Highlands Hospital[2]	Connellsville	82%	399
Kane Community Hospital[2]	Kane	82%	549
Main Line Hospital Lankenau[2]	Wynnewood	82%	714
Nason Hospital[2]	Roaring Spring	82%	282
Penn Presbyterian Medical Center[2]	Philadelphia	82%	1158
Surgical Institute of Reading[2]	Wyomissing	82%	213
Windber Hospital[2]	Windber	82%	369
Barnes-Kasson County Hospital[2,3]	Susquehanna	81%	297
Edgewood Surgical Hospital	Transfer	81%	69
Mount Nittany Medical Center[2]	State College	81%	680
Riddle Memorial Hospital[2]	Media	81%	778
Valley Forge Medical Center & Hospital[2]	Norristown	81%	68
Holy Spirit Hospital[2]	Camp Hill	80%	796
Allegheny General Hospital[2]	Pittsburgh	79%	857
Saint Joseph's Hospital[2]	Philadelphia	79%	496
Hospital of Univ of Pennsylvania[2]	Philadelphia	78%	509
Saint Vincent Hospital[2]	Erie	78%	1425
Forbes Regional Hospital[2]	Monroeville	73%	856
Miners Medical Center[2]	Hastings	73%	372
Western Pennsylvania Hospital[2]	Pittsburgh	72%	312
Bucks County Specialty Hospital[2]	Bensalem	71%	288
Sharon Regional Health System[2]	Sharon	71%	826
Geisinger - Bloomsburg Hospital[2]	Bloomsburg	63%	1169
Physician's Care Surgical Hospital[2]	Royersford	59%	142
Coordinated Health Orthopedic Hospital[2]	Bethlehem	58%	413
Eagleville Hospital[2]	Eagleville	48%	199
Surgical Specialty Ctr at Coord Hlth[2]	Allentown	47%	369
Kensington Hospital[2]	Philadelphia	0%	38

Stroke Care

Anticoagulation Therapy for Atrial Fibrillation

Hospital Name	City	Rate	Cases
Allegheny General Hospital	Pittsburgh	100%	81
Geisinger - Community Medical Center	Scranton	100%	38
Hospital of Univ of Pennsylvania	Philadelphia	100%	39
Lehigh Valley Hospital	Allentown	100%	78
Main Line Hospital Bryn Mawr Campus	Bryn Mawr	100%	28
Saint Clair Memorial Hospital	Pittsburgh	100%	26
Saint Luke's Hospital Bethlehem	Bethlehem	100%	50
Saint Mary Medical Center	Langhorne	100%	42
Temple University Hospital	Philadelphia	100%	26
UPMC Altoona	Altoona	100%	41
UPMC Mercy	Pittsburgh	100%	73
UPMC Saint Margaret	Pittsburgh	100%	27
UPMC Presbyterian Shadyside	Pittsburgh	99%	153
York Hospital	York	99%	74
Doylestown Hospital	Doylestown	98%	44
Lancaster General Hospital	Lancaster	98%	94
UPMC Hamot	Erie	98%	40
Milton S Hershey Medical Center	Hershey	97%	59
The Washington Hospital	Washington	97%	31
Geisinger Medical Center	Danville	96%	49
Saint Vincent Hospital	Erie	95%	43
Aria Health	Philadelphia	94%	35
Conemaugh Valley Memorial Hospital	Johnstown	94%	35
Pinnacle Health Hospitals	Harrisburg	91%	57
Forbes Regional Hospital	Monroeville	90%	49
Reading Hospital	Reading	89%	38
Pocono Medical Center	E Stroudsburg	86%	29
Wilkes-Barre General Hospital	Wilkes-Barre	86%	35
Chambersburg Hospital	Chambersburg	82%	33

Antithrombotic Therapy Timing

Hospital Name	City	Rate	Cases
Abington Memorial Hospital[2]	Abington	100%	80
Acmh Hospital	Kittanning	100%	43
Butler Memorial Hospital	Butler	100%	132
Carlisle Regional Medical Center	Carlisle	100%	38
Chestnut Hill Hospital	Philadelphia	100%	100

NOTE: Hospital profiles are in alphabetical order by state, then city, then hospital within the city; Rankings exclude hospitals with less than 25 cases except for patient surveys which excludes hospitals with less than 100 cases; (a) 100-299 cases; (1) The number of cases/patients is too few to report; (2) Data submitted were based on a sample of cases/patients; (3) Results are based on a shorter time period than required; (4) Data suppressed by CMS for one or more quarters; (5) Results are not available for this reporting period; (6) Fewer than 100 patients completed the HCAHPS survey; (7) No cases met the criteria for this measure; (8) The lower limit of the confidence interval cannot be calculated if the number of observed infections equals zero; (9) No data are available from the state/territory for this reporting period; (10) The scores shown reflect fewer than 50 completed surveys; (11) There were discrepancies in the data collection process; (12) This measure does not apply to this hospital for this reporting period; (13) Results cannot be calculated for this reporting period; (14) The results for this state are combined with nearby states to protect confidentiality; Please refer to the User's Guide for a full explanation of data.

Hospital Name	City	Rate	Cases
Crozer Chester Medical Center	Upland	100%	251
Doylestown Hospital	Doylestown	100%	140
Ephrata Community Hospital	Ephrata	100%	67
Evangelical Community Hospital	Lewisburg	100%	66
Excela Health Latrobe Hospital	Latrobe	100%	38
Geisinger - Community Medical Center	Scranton	100%	174
Geisinger Medical Center	Danville	100%	256
Gettysburg Hospital	Gettysburg	100%	56
Gnaden Huetten Memorial Hospital	Lehighton	100%	27
Good Samaritan Hospital	Lebanon	100%	60
Hanover Hospital	Hanover	100%	89
Heritage Valley Beaver	Beaver	100%	121
Jeanes Hospital	Philadelphia	100%	84
Jennersville Regional Hospital	West Grove	100%	26
Lansdale Hospital	Lansdale	100%	65
Lehigh Valley Hospital	Allentown	100%	367
Lehigh Valley Hospital - Muhlenberg	Bethlehem	100%	108
Lewistown Hospital	Lewistown	100%	53
Main Line Hospital Bryn Mawr Campus	Bryn Mawr	100%	154
Main Line Hospital Lankenau	Wynnewood	100%	154
Mercy Fitzgerald Hospital	Darby	100%	193
Mercy Suburban Hospital	Norristown	100%	54
Nazareth Hospital	Philadelphia	100%	178
Penn Highlands Dubois	Dubois	100%	50
Penn Presbyterian Medical Center	Philadelphia	100%	91
Phoenixville Hospital	Phoenixville	100%	37
Pottstown Memorial Medical Center	Pottstown	100%	104
Riddle Memorial Hospital	Media	100%	109
Roxborough Memorial Hospital	Philadelphia	100%	29
Sacred Heart Hospital	Allentown	100%	31
Saint Clair Memorial Hospital	Pittsburgh	100%	148
Saint Joseph Medical Center	Reading	100%	93
Saint Luke's Hospital - Anderson Campus	Easton	100%	49
Schuylkill Med Ctr-East Norwegian St	Pottsville	100%	53
Temple University Hospital	Philadelphia	100%	256
UPMC East	Monroeville	100%	50
UPMC Horizon	Greenville	100%	60
UPMC Mckeesport	Mc Keesport	100%	72
UPMC Mercy	Pittsburgh	100%	201
UPMC Northwest	Seneca	100%	60
UPMC Saint Margaret	Pittsburgh	100%	145
Wayne Memorial Hospital	Honesdale	100%	30
Waynesboro Hospital	Waynesboro	100%	33
Williamsport Regional Medical Center	Williamsport	100%	135
Albert Einstein Medical Center[2]	Philadelphia	99%	110
Aria Health	Philadelphia	99%	259
Chester County Hospital	West Chester	99%	105
Delaware County Memorial Hospital	Drexel Hill	99%	74
Einstein Medical Center Montgomery[2]	East Norriton	99%	80
Grand View Hospital	Sellersville	99%	80
Heritage Valley Sewickley	Sewickley	99%	71
Holy Spirit Hospital	Camp Hill	99%	137
Lancaster General Hospital	Lancaster	99%	382
Main Line Hospital Paoli	Paoli	99%	141
Moses Taylor Hospital	Scranton	99%	81
Reading Hospital	Reading	99%	304
Saint Luke's Hospital Bethlehem	Bethlehem	99%	208
UPMC Hamot	Erie	99%	180
UPMC Passavant	Pittsburgh	99%	133
Brandywine Hospital	Coatesville	98%	54
Chambersburg Hospital	Chambersburg	98%	161
Conemaugh Valley Memorial Hospital	Johnstown	98%	226
Hospital of Univ of Pennsylvania	Philadelphia	98%	187
Jefferson Regional Medical Center[2]	Pittsburgh	98%	82
Lower Bucks Hospital	Bristol	98%	42
Memorial Hospital	York	98%	44
Milton S Hershey Medical Center	Hershey	98%	260
Monongahela Valley Hospital	Monongahela	98%	83
Robert Packer Hospital	Sayre	98%	116
Saint Mary Medical Center	Langhorne	98%	213
Saint Vincent Hospital	Erie	98%	209
Thomas Jefferson University Hospital[2]	Philadelphia	98%	114
Uniontown Hospital	Uniontown	98%	59
UPMC Altoona	Altoona	98%	256
The Washington Hospital	Washington	98%	131
Wilkes-Barre General Hospital	Wilkes-Barre	98%	149
York Hospital	York	98%	263
Allegheny General Hospital	Pittsburgh	97%	296
Easton Hospital	Easton	97%	65
Excela Health Frick Hospital	Mount Pleasant	97%	36
Geisinger Wyoming Valley Medical Center	Wilkes Barre	97%	165
Hahnemann University Hospital	Philadelphia	97%	96
Mount Nittany Medical Center	State College	97%	86
Penn Hosp of the Univ of PA Hlth Sys	Philadelphia	97%	62
Pocono Medical Center	E Stroudsburg	97%	153
Saint Luke's Quakertown Hospital	Quakertown	97%	37
Excela Health Westmoreland Hospital	Greensburg	96%	114
Indiana Regional Medical Center	Indiana	96%	74
Pinnacle Health Hospitals	Harrisburg	96%	295
Schuylkill Med Ctr-S Jackson St	Pottsville	96%	28
Holy Redeemer Hospital & Medical Center[2]	Meadowbrook	95%	75
Lehigh Valley Hospital - Hazleton	Hazleton	95%	74
Meadville Medical Center	Meadville	95%	73
UPMC Presbyterian Shadyside	Pittsburgh	95%	612
Alle Kiski Medical Center	Natrona	94%	72
Sharon Regional Health System	Sharon	94%	72
Regional Hospital of Scranton	Scranton	93%	101
Forbes Regional Hospital	Monroeville	91%	185
Jameson Memorial Hospital	New Castle	91%	74
Lancaster Regional Medical Center	Lancaster	89%	28

Assessed for Rehabilitation

Hospital Name	City	Rate	Cases
Abington Memorial Hospital[2]	Abington	100%	117
Albert Einstein Medical Center[2]	Philadelphia	100%	136
Butler Memorial Hospital	Butler	100%	141
Easton Hospital	Easton	100%	70
Ephrata Community Hospital	Ephrata	100%	76
Excela Health Latrobe Hospital	Latrobe	100%	42
Geisinger - Community Medical Center	Scranton	100%	216
Grand View Hospital	Sellersville	100%	86
Hahnemann University Hospital	Philadelphia	100%	106
Heritage Valley Sewickley	Sewickley	100%	68
Hospital of Univ of Pennsylvania	Philadelphia	100%	296
Lehigh Valley Hospital	Allentown	100%	588
Lehigh Valley Hospital - Muhlenberg	Bethlehem	100%	118
Main Line Hospital Lankenau	Wynnewood	100%	174
Main Line Hospital Paoli	Paoli	100%	166
Mercy Suburban Hospital	Norristown	100%	48
Milton S Hershey Medical Center	Hershey	100%	417
Moses Taylor Hospital	Scranton	100%	85
Phoenixville Hospital	Phoenixville	100%	37
Reading Hospital	Reading	100%	378
Riddle Memorial Hospital	Media	100%	132
Roxborough Memorial Hospital	Philadelphia	100%	32
Sacred Heart Hospital	Allentown	100%	32
Saint Clair Memorial Hospital	Pittsburgh	100%	158
UPMC Altoona	Altoona	100%	296
UPMC East	Monroeville	100%	55
UPMC Mercy	Pittsburgh	100%	311
UPMC Northwest	Seneca	100%	66
UPMC Passavant	Pittsburgh	100%	145
Wayne Memorial Hospital	Honesdale	100%	35
Waynesboro Hospital	Waynesboro	100%	39
Western Pennsylvania Hospital	Pittsburgh	100%	26
Williamsport Regional Medical Center	Williamsport	100%	147
Allegheny General Hospital	Pittsburgh	99%	537
Aria Health	Philadelphia	99%	263
Delaware County Memorial Hospital	Drexel Hill	99%	77
Doylestown Hospital	Doylestown	99%	159
Geisinger Wyoming Valley Medical Center	Wilkes Barre	99%	201
Holy Spirit Hospital	Camp Hill	99%	158
Main Line Hospital Bryn Mawr Campus	Bryn Mawr	99%	192
Mercy Fitzgerald Hospital	Darby	99%	209
Penn Presbyterian Medical Center	Philadelphia	99%	99
Pinnacle Health Hospitals	Harrisburg	99%	364
Saint Luke's Hospital Bethlehem	Bethlehem	99%	251
Saint Mary Medical Center	Langhorne	99%	261
Temple University Hospital	Philadelphia	99%	395
UPMC Hamot	Erie	99%	302
UPMC Mckeesport	Mc Keesport	99%	78
UPMC Presbyterian Shadyside	Pittsburgh	99%	1151
UPMC Saint Margaret	Pittsburgh	99%	157
York Hospital	York	99%	410
Acmh Hospital	Kittanning	98%	47
Chester County Hospital	West Chester	98%	98
Conemaugh Valley Memorial Hospital	Johnstown	98%	253
Crozer Chester Medical Center	Upland	98%	312
Evangelical Community Hospital	Lewisburg	98%	91
Geisinger Medical Center	Danville	98%	381
Gettysburg Hospital	Gettysburg	98%	59
Good Samaritan Hospital	Lebanon	98%	63
Jeanes Hospital	Philadelphia	98%	86
Lancaster General Hospital	Lancaster	98%	462
Monongahela Valley Hospital	Monongahela	98%	90
Nazareth Hospital	Philadelphia	98%	190
Saint Luke's Hospital - Anderson Campus	Easton	98%	49
Schuylkill Med Ctr-East Norwegian St	Pottsville	98%	51
Thomas Jefferson University Hospital[2]	Philadelphia	98%	193
The Washington Hospital	Washington	98%	146
Chestnut Hill Hospital	Philadelphia	97%	100
Excela Health Frick Hospital	Mount Pleasant	97%	37
Hanover Hospital	Hanover	97%	95
Lansdale Hospital	Lansdale	97%	70
Pottstown Memorial Medical Center	Pottstown	97%	106
Saint Luke's Quakertown Hospital	Quakertown	97%	39
Saint Vincent Hospital	Erie	97%	265
Einstein Medical Center Montgomery[2]	East Norriton	96%	80
Forbes Regional Hospital	Monroeville	96%	202
Gnaden Huetten Memorial Hospital	Lehighton	96%	27
Indiana Regional Medical Center	Indiana	96%	67
Jefferson Regional Medical Center[2]	Pittsburgh	96%	85
Memorial Hospital	York	96%	48
Penn Hosp of the Univ of PA Hlth Sys	Philadelphia	96%	81
Saint Joseph Medical Center	Reading	96%	100
Soldiers & Sailors Memorial Hospital	Wellsboro	96%	25
Uniontown Hospital	Uniontown	96%	53
Wilkes-Barre General Hospital	Wilkes-Barre	96%	195
Brandywine Hospital	Coatesville	95%	61
Jameson Memorial Hospital	New Castle	95%	81
Penn Highlands Dubois	Dubois	95%	59
Regional Hospital of Scranton	Scranton	95%	98
Alle Kiski Medical Center	Natrona	94%	69
Excela Health Westmoreland Hospital	Greensburg	94%	126
Holy Redeemer Hospital & Medical Center[2]	Meadowbrook	94%	79
Lancaster Regional Medical Center	Lancaster	94%	33
UPMC Horizon	Greenville	94%	65
Heritage Valley Beaver	Beaver	93%	117
Meadville Medical Center	Meadville	93%	76
Mount Nittany Medical Center	State College	93%	104
Pocono Medical Center	E Stroudsburg	93%	160
Carlisle Regional Medical Center	Carlisle	92%	40
Lehigh Valley Hospital - Hazleton	Hazleton	92%	73
Schuylkill Med Ctr-S Jackson St	Pottsville	92%	38
Lewistown Hospital	Lewistown	91%	58
Sharon Regional Health System	Sharon	91%	76
Chambersburg Hospital	Chambersburg	90%	190
Lower Bucks Hospital	Bristol	90%	40
Jennersville Regional Hospital	West Grove	89%	28
Robert Packer Hospital	Sayre	87%	137

Discharged on Antithrombotic Therapy

Hospital Name	City	Rate	Cases
Abington Memorial Hospital[2]	Abington	100%	100
Acmh Hospital	Kittanning	100%	44
Albert Einstein Medical Center[2]	Philadelphia	100%	114
Alle Kiski Medical Center	Natrona	100%	68
Aria Health	Philadelphia	100%	242
Carlisle Regional Medical Center	Carlisle	100%	39
Chestnut Hill Hospital	Philadelphia	100%	99
Conemaugh Valley Memorial Hospital	Johnstown	100%	218
Crozer Chester Medical Center	Upland	100%	274
Doylestown Hospital	Doylestown	100%	157
Easton Hospital	Easton	100%	68
Ephrata Community Hospital	Ephrata	100%	69
Evangelical Community Hospital	Lewisburg	100%	87
Excela Health Frick Hospital	Mount Pleasant	100%	36
Excela Health Latrobe Hospital	Latrobe	100%	38
Geisinger Wyoming Valley Medical Center	Wilkes Barre	100%	175
Gettysburg Hospital	Gettysburg	100%	57
Good Samaritan Hospital	Lebanon	100%	60
Hahnemann University Hospital	Philadelphia	100%	94
Hanover Hospital	Hanover	100%	90
Heritage Valley Beaver	Beaver	100%	113
Holy Spirit Hospital	Camp Hill	100%	143
Hospital of Univ of Pennsylvania	Philadelphia	100%	224
Jeanes Hospital	Philadelphia	100%	84
Jefferson Regional Medical Center[2]	Pittsburgh	100%	79
Lancaster General Hospital	Lancaster	100%	412
Lansdale Hospital	Lansdale	100%	66
Lehigh Valley Hospital	Allentown	100%	451
Lehigh Valley Hospital - Muhlenberg	Bethlehem	100%	116
Lewistown Hospital	Lewistown	100%	55
Main Line Hospital Bryn Mawr Campus	Bryn Mawr	100%	169
Main Line Hospital Lankenau	Wynnewood	100%	158
Main Line Hospital Paoli	Paoli	100%	144
Memorial Hospital	York	100%	47
Mercy Fitzgerald Hospital	Darby	100%	176
Mercy Suburban Hospital	Norristown	100%	48
Milton S Hershey Medical Center	Hershey	100%	298
Monongahela Valley Hospital	Monongahela	100%	85
Nazareth Hospital	Philadelphia	100%	177
Penn Highlands Dubois	Dubois	100%	59
Penn Presbyterian Medical Center	Philadelphia	100%	96
Penn Hosp of the Univ of PA Hlth Sys	Philadelphia	100%	72
Pinnacle Health Hospitals	Harrisburg	100%	334
Regional Hospital of Scranton	Scranton	100%	90
Riddle Memorial Hospital	Media	100%	115
Roxborough Memorial Hospital	Philadelphia	100%	31
Sacred Heart Hospital	Allentown	100%	32
Saint Clair Memorial Hospital	Pittsburgh	100%	155
Saint Joseph Medical Center	Reading	100%	95
Saint Luke's Hospital - Anderson Campus	Easton	100%	48
Saint Luke's Hospital Bethlehem	Bethlehem	100%	210
Saint Luke's Quakertown Hospital	Quakertown	100%	39
Saint Mary Medical Center	Langhorne	100%	221
Saint Vincent Hospital	Erie	100%	232
Schuylkill Med Ctr-East Norwegian St	Pottsville	100%	49
Soldiers & Sailors Memorial Hospital	Wellsboro	100%	25
Temple University Hospital	Philadelphia	100%	324
Thomas Jefferson University Hospital[2]	Philadelphia	100%	143
Uniontown Hospital	Uniontown	100%	53
UPMC Altoona	Altoona	100%	263

NOTE: Hospital profiles are in alphabetical order by state, then city, then hospital within the city; Rankings exclude hospitals with less than 25 cases except for patient surveys which excludes hospitals with less than 100 cases; (a) 100-299 cases; (1) The number of cases/patients is too few to report; (2) Data submitted were based on a sample of cases/patients; (3) Results are based on a shorter time period than required; (4) Data suppressed by CMS for one or more quarters; (5) Results are not available for this reporting period; (6) Fewer than 100 patients completed the HCAHPS survey; (7) No cases met the criteria for this measure; (8) The lower limit of the confidence interval cannot be calculated if the number of observed infections equals zero; (9) No data are available from the state/territory for this reporting period; (10) The scores shown reflect fewer than 50 completed surveys; (11) There were discrepancies in the data collection process; (12) This measure does not apply to this hospital for this reporting period; (13) Results cannot be calculated for this reporting period; (14) The results for this state are combined with nearby states to protect confidentiality; Please refer to the User's Guide for a full explanation of data.

Hospital Name	City	Rate	Cases
UPMC East	Monroeville	100%	54
UPMC Hamot	Erie	100%	255
UPMC Horizon	Greenville	100%	62
UPMC Mckeesport	Mc Keesport	100%	72
UPMC Mercy	Pittsburgh	100%	265
UPMC Passavant	Pittsburgh	100%	138
UPMC Presbyterian Shadyside	Pittsburgh	100%	838
UPMC Saint Margaret	Pittsburgh	100%	148
The Washington Hospital	Washington	100%	141
Waynesboro Hospital	Waynesboro	100%	36
Western Pennsylvania Hospital	Pittsburgh	100%	26
York Hospital	York	100%	346
Allegheny General Hospital	Pittsburgh	99%	391
Butler Memorial Hospital	Butler	99%	133
Chester County Hospital	West Chester	99%	98
Delaware County Memorial Hospital	Drexel Hill	99%	76
Einstein Medical Center Montgomery[2]	East Norriton	99%	74
Geisinger - Community Medical Center	Scranton	99%	181
Geisinger Medical Center	Danville	99%	280
Grand View Hospital	Sellersville	99%	84
Heritage Valley Sewickley	Sewickley	99%	67
Holy Redeemer Hospital & Medical Center[2]	Meadowbrook	99%	75
Indiana Regional Medical Center	Indiana	99%	67
Meadville Medical Center	Meadville	99%	73
Pottstown Memorial Medical Center	Pottstown	99%	98
Wilkes-Barre General Hospital	Wilkes-Barre	99%	168
Chambersburg Hospital	Chambersburg	98%	173
Excela Health Westmoreland Hospital	Greensburg	98%	115
Moses Taylor Hospital	Scranton	98%	82
Mount Nittany Medical Center	State College	98%	100
Pocono Medical Center	E Stroudsburg	98%	156
Robert Packer Hospital	Sayre	98%	122
UPMC Northwest	Seneca	98%	64
Williamsport Regional Medical Center	Williamsport	98%	133
Forbes Regional Hospital	Monroeville	97%	179
Lancaster Regional Medical Center	Lancaster	97%	32
Lehigh Valley Hospital - Hazleton	Hazleton	97%	70
Lower Bucks Hospital	Bristol	97%	39
Reading Hospital	Reading	97%	329
Schuylkill Med Ctr-S Jackson St	Pottsville	97%	35
Gnaden Huetten Memorial Hospital	Lehighton	96%	26
Jameson Memorial Hospital	New Castle	96%	79
Sharon Regional Health System	Sharon	94%	72
Wayne Memorial Hospital	Honesdale	94%	34
Brandywine Hospital	Coatesville	93%	57
Jennersville Regional Hospital	West Grove	93%	27
Phoenixville Hospital	Phoenixville	92%	36

Discharged on Statin Medication

Hospital Name	City	Rate	Cases
Albert Einstein Medical Center[2]	Philadelphia	100%	96
Excela Health Latrobe Hospital	Latrobe	100%	29
Main Line Hospital Bryn Mawr Campus	Bryn Mawr	100%	143
Main Line Hospital Lankenau	Wynnewood	100%	138
Main Line Hospital Paoli	Paoli	100%	108
Mercy Fitzgerald Hospital	Darby	100%	144
Mercy Suburban Hospital	Norristown	100%	41
Milton S Hershey Medical Center	Hershey	100%	230
Penn Highlands Dubois	Dubois	100%	41
Penn Hosp of the Univ of PA Hlth Sys	Philadelphia	100%	61
Riddle Memorial Hospital	Media	100%	97
Saint Clair Memorial Hospital	Pittsburgh	100%	111
Saint Vincent Hospital	Erie	100%	175
UPMC East	Monroeville	100%	43
UPMC Northwest	Seneca	100%	40
UPMC Saint Margaret	Pittsburgh	100%	107
Waynesboro Hospital	Waynesboro	100%	25
Doylestown Hospital	Doylestown	100%	112
Geisinger - Community Medical Center	Scranton	99%	142
Hanover Hospital	Hanover	99%	77
Hospital of Univ of Pennsylvania	Philadelphia	99%	171
Lehigh Valley Hospital	Allentown	99%	331
Penn Presbyterian Medical Center	Philadelphia	99%	85
Saint Luke's Hospital Bethlehem	Bethlehem	99%	173
Saint Mary Medical Center	Langhorne	99%	149
UPMC Mercy	Pittsburgh	99%	192
Butler Memorial Hospital	Butler	98%	105
Crozer Chester Medical Center	Upland	98%	215
Easton Hospital	Easton	98%	54
Geisinger Medical Center	Danville	98%	236
Lansdale Hospital	Lansdale	98%	59
Moses Taylor Hospital	Scranton	98%	57
Saint Luke's Hospital - Anderson Campus	Easton	98%	41
Temple University Hospital	Philadelphia	98%	247
Thomas Jefferson University Hospital[2]	Philadelphia	98%	104
UPMC Hamot	Erie	98%	202
UPMC Mckeesport	Mc Keesport	98%	48
Williamsport Regional Medical Center	Williamsport	98%	101
Aria Health	Philadelphia	97%	192
Grand View Hospital	Sellersville	97%	64
Hahnemann University Hospital	Philadelphia	97%	71
Lancaster General Hospital	Lancaster	97%	317
Nazareth Hospital	Philadelphia	97%	152
Pinnacle Health Hospitals	Harrisburg	97%	268
Saint Joseph Medical Center	Reading	97%	74
Saint Luke's Quakertown Hospital	Quakertown	97%	30
York Hospital	York	97%	297
Abington Memorial Hospital[2]	Abington	96%	76
Chester County Hospital	West Chester	96%	79
Delaware County Memorial Hospital	Drexel Hill	96%	45
Einstein Medical Center Montgomery[2]	East Norriton	96%	69
Excela Health Frick Hospital	Mount Pleasant	96%	28
Good Samaritan Hospital	Lebanon	96%	53
Lehigh Valley Hospital - Hazleton	Hazleton	96%	48
Lehigh Valley Hospital - Muhlenberg	Bethlehem	96%	89
UPMC Presbyterian Shadyside	Pittsburgh	96%	651
Allegheny General Hospital	Pittsburgh	95%	286
Conemaugh Valley Memorial Hospital	Johnstown	95%	179
Ephrata Community Hospital	Ephrata	95%	58
Evangelical Community Hospital	Lewisburg	95%	76
Forbes Regional Hospital	Monroeville	95%	147
Geisinger Wyoming Valley Medical Center	Wilkes Barre	95%	147
Holy Spirit Hospital	Camp Hill	95%	112
Monongahela Valley Hospital	Monongahela	95%	62
Uniontown Hospital	Uniontown	95%	40
UPMC Altoona	Altoona	95%	202
UPMC Horizon	Greenville	95%	40
UPMC Passavant	Pittsburgh	95%	99
Chestnut Hill Hospital	Philadelphia	94%	70
Gettysburg Hospital	Gettysburg	94%	49
Heritage Valley Sewickley	Sewickley	94%	50
Holy Redeemer Hospital & Medical Center[2]	Meadowbrook	94%	62
Jeanes Hospital	Philadelphia	94%	64
Robert Packer Hospital	Sayre	94%	98
The Washington Hospital	Washington	94%	107
Jefferson Regional Medical Center[2]	Pittsburgh	93%	68
Memorial Hospital	York	93%	41
Pottstown Memorial Medical Center	Pottstown	93%	85
Reading Hospital	Reading	93%	288
Wayne Memorial Hospital	Honesdale	93%	27
Acmh Hospital	Kittanning	92%	36
Excela Health Westmoreland Hospital	Greensburg	91%	95
Regional Hospital of Scranton	Scranton	91%	67
Lewistown Hospital	Lewistown	90%	48
Wilkes-Barre General Hospital	Wilkes-Barre	90%	143
Alle Kiski Medical Center	Natrona	89%	54
Heritage Valley Beaver	Beaver	89%	91
Meadville Medical Center	Meadville	89%	56
Chambersburg Hospital	Chambersburg	87%	148
Lower Bucks Hospital	Bristol	85%	33
Pocono Medical Center	E Stroudsburg	84%	124
Carlisle Regional Medical Center	Carlisle	83%	30
Mount Nittany Medical Center	State College	82%	80
Brandywine Hospital	Coatesville	81%	52
Lancaster Regional Medical Center	Lancaster	81%	27
Phoenixville Hospital	Phoenixville	77%	30
Schuylkill Med Ctr-East Norwegian St	Pottsville	75%	44
Sharon Regional Health System	Sharon	70%	64
Jameson Memorial Hospital	New Castle	64%	73
Schuylkill Med Ctr-S Jackson St	Pottsville	63%	35
Indiana Regional Medical Center	Indiana	57%	60

Thrombolytic Therapy Timing

Hospital Name	City	Rate	Cases
UPMC Mercy	Pittsburgh	100%	40
UPMC Presbyterian Shadyside	Pittsburgh	100%	33
Lehigh Valley Hospital	Allentown	97%	33
Reading Hospital	Reading	93%	29
Milton S Hershey Medical Center	Hershey	92%	36
Allegheny General Hospital	Pittsburgh	91%	43
UPMC Hamot	Erie	89%	27
York Hospital	York	83%	42
Pinnacle Health Hospitals	Harrisburg	77%	39

Venous Thromboembolism (VTE) Prophylaxis

Hospital Name	City	Rate	Cases
Easton Hospital	Easton	100%	68
Excela Health Frick Hospital	Mount Pleasant	100%	38
Excela Health Latrobe Hospital	Latrobe	100%	45
Hahnemann University Hospital	Philadelphia	100%	122
Heritage Valley Sewickley	Sewickley	100%	76
Lancaster General Hospital	Lancaster	100%	454
Lehigh Valley Hospital	Allentown	100%	602
Main Line Hospital Lankenau	Wynnewood	100%	175
Main Line Hospital Paoli	Paoli	100%	169
Mercy Suburban Hospital	Norristown	100%	51
Thomas Jefferson University Hospital[2]	Philadelphia	100%	211
UPMC East	Monroeville	100%	53
Wayne Memorial Hospital	Honesdale	100%	30
Waynesboro Hospital	Waynesboro	100%	38
Doylestown Hospital	Doylestown	99%	156
Evangelical Community Hospital	Lewisburg	99%	69
Grand View Hospital	Sellersville	99%	87
Milton S Hershey Medical Center	Hershey	99%	461
Penn Presbyterian Medical Center	Philadelphia	99%	103
Saint Clair Memorial Hospital	Pittsburgh	99%	153
Saint Joseph Medical Center	Reading	99%	92
Saint Mary Medical Center	Langhorne	99%	271
UPMC Mckeesport	Mc Keesport	99%	80
UPMC Mercy	Pittsburgh	99%	326
UPMC Presbyterian Shadyside	Pittsburgh	99%	1178
Acmh Hospital	Kittanning	98%	47
Aria Health	Philadelphia	98%	281
Butler Memorial Hospital	Butler	98%	149
Chester County Hospital	West Chester	98%	100
Hospital of Univ of Pennsylvania	Philadelphia	98%	309
Jeanes Hospital	Philadelphia	98%	85
Lehigh Valley Hospital - Muhlenberg	Bethlehem	98%	120
Lewistown Hospital	Lewistown	98%	51
Mercy Fitzgerald Hospital	Darby	98%	221
Monongahela Valley Hospital	Monongahela	98%	94
Moses Taylor Hospital	Scranton	98%	83
Nazareth Hospital	Philadelphia	98%	192
Penn Highlands Dubois	Dubois	98%	52
Saint Luke's Hospital - Anderson Campus	Easton	98%	47
Saint Luke's Hospital Bethlehem	Bethlehem	98%	282
Temple University Hospital	Philadelphia	98%	370
UPMC Hamot	Erie	98%	265
UPMC Horizon	Greenville	98%	63
Conemaugh Valley Memorial Hospital	Johnstown	97%	279
Geisinger - Community Medical Center	Scranton	97%	233
Hanover Hospital	Hanover	97%	93
Penn Hosp of the Univ of PA Hlth Sys	Philadelphia	97%	77
Phoenixville Hospital	Phoenixville	97%	37
Roxborough Memorial Hospital	Philadelphia	97%	34
Sacred Heart Hospital	Allentown	97%	32
Saint Luke's Quakertown Hospital	Quakertown	97%	37
UPMC Northwest	Seneca	97%	62
UPMC Passavant	Pittsburgh	97%	144
UPMC Saint Margaret	Pittsburgh	97%	163
Williamsport Regional Medical Center	Williamsport	97%	164
Allegheny General Hospital	Pittsburgh	96%	595
Ephrata Community Hospital	Ephrata	96%	70
Geisinger Medical Center	Danville	96%	396
Gettysburg Hospital	Gettysburg	96%	56
Holy Redeemer Hospital & Medical Center[2]	Meadowbrook	96%	83
Main Line Hospital Bryn Mawr Campus	Bryn Mawr	96%	194
Riddle Memorial Hospital	Media	96%	134
Saint Vincent Hospital	Erie	96%	261
York Hospital	York	96%	401
Albert Einstein Medical Center[2]	Philadelphia	95%	147
Carlisle Regional Medical Center	Carlisle	95%	37
Chestnut Hill Hospital	Philadelphia	95%	101
Crozer Chester Medical Center	Upland	95%	310
Delaware County Memorial Hospital	Drexel Hill	95%	80
Good Samaritan Hospital	Lebanon	95%	63
Reading Hospital	Reading	95%	381
Uniontown Hospital	Uniontown	95%	59
UPMC Altoona	Altoona	95%	297
Forbes Regional Hospital	Monroeville	94%	221
Meadville Medical Center	Meadville	94%	78
Abington Memorial Hospital[2]	Abington	93%	113
Heritage Valley Beaver	Beaver	93%	127
Jennersville Regional Hospital	West Grove	93%	29
Lancaster Regional Medical Center	Lancaster	93%	30
Chambersburg Hospital	Chambersburg	92%	180
Gnaden Huetten Memorial Hospital	Lehighton	92%	26
Holy Spirit Hospital	Camp Hill	92%	165
Western Pennsylvania Hospital	Pittsburgh	92%	26
The Washington Hospital	Washington	91%	144
Excela Health Westmoreland Hospital	Greensburg	90%	131
Mount Nittany Medical Center	State College	90%	97
Pinnacle Health Hospitals	Harrisburg	90%	373
Pottstown Memorial Medical Center	Pottstown	90%	119
Schuylkill Med Ctr-East Norwegian St	Pottsville	88%	59
Schuylkill Med Ctr-S Jackson St	Pottsville	88%	40
Wilkes-Barre General Hospital	Wilkes-Barre	88%	202
Lansdale Hospital	Lansdale	87%	75
Geisinger Wyoming Valley Medical Center	Wilkes Barre	86%	210
Robert Packer Hospital	Sayre	85%	140
Alle Kiski Medical Center	Natrona	84%	73
Brandywine Hospital	Coatesville	84%	62
Memorial Hospital	York	83%	47
Regional Hospital of Scranton	Scranton	81%	109
Pocono Medical Center	E Stroudsburg	80%	153
Einstein Medical Center Montgomery[2]	East Norriton	79%	89
Jefferson Regional Medical Center[2]	Pittsburgh	79%	87
Somerset Hospital	Somerset	78%	27
Lehigh Valley Hospital - Hazleton	Hazleton	75%	75
Jameson Memorial Hospital	New Castle	72%	80
Lower Bucks Hospital	Bristol	67%	45
Sharon Regional Health System	Sharon	67%	70

NOTE: Hospital profiles are in alphabetical order by state, then city, then hospital within the city; Rankings exclude hospitals with less than 25 cases except for patient surveys which excludes hospitals with less than 100 cases; (a) 100-299 cases; (1) The number of cases/patients is too few to report; (2) Data submitted were based on a sample of cases/patients; (3) Results are based on a shorter time period than required; (4) Data suppressed by CMS for one or more quarters; (5) Results are not available for this reporting period; (6) Fewer than 100 patients completed the HCAHPS survey; (7) No cases met the criteria for this measure; (8) The lower limit of the confidence interval cannot be calculated if the number of observed infections equals zero; (9) No data are available from the state/territory for this reporting period; (10) The scores shown reflect fewer than 50 completed surveys; (11) There were discrepancies in the data collection process; (12) This measure does not apply to this hospital for this reporting period; (13) Results cannot be calculated for this reporting period; (14) The results for this state are combined with nearby states to protect confidentiality; Please refer to the User's Guide for a full explanation of data.

Indiana Regional Medical Center	Indiana	66%	73

Written Stroke Educational Materials Given

Hospital Name	City	Rate	Cases
Albert Einstein Medical Center[2]	Philadelphia	100%	47
Doylestown Hospital	Doylestown	100%	91
Ephrata Community Hospital	Ephrata	100%	37
Hahnemann University Hospital	Philadelphia	100%	60
Heritage Valley Beaver	Beaver	100%	54
Heritage Valley Sewickley	Sewickley	100%	28
Holy Spirit Hospital	Camp Hill	100%	86
Memorial Hospital	York	100%	31
Mercy Fitzgerald Hospital	Darby	100%	126
Penn Highlands Dubois	Dubois	100%	34
Saint Clair Memorial Hospital	Pittsburgh	100%	85
Saint Mary Medical Center	Langhorne	100%	122
Thomas Jefferson University Hospital[2]	Philadelphia	100%	75
Uniontown Hospital	Uniontown	100%	29
UPMC Altoona	Altoona	100%	115
UPMC East	Monroeville	100%	37
UPMC Hamot	Erie	100%	157
UPMC Horizon	Greenville	100%	39
UPMC Mckeesport	Mc Keesport	100%	29
UPMC Northwest	Seneca	100%	39
UPMC Passavant	Pittsburgh	100%	60
Butler Memorial Hospital	Butler	99%	77
Geisinger - Community Medical Center	Scranton	99%	103
Main Line Hospital Paoli	Paoli	99%	67
Pocono Medical Center	E Stroudsburg	99%	97
Aria Health	Philadelphia	98%	134
Chester County Hospital	West Chester	98%	51
Hanover Hospital	Hanover	98%	51
Holy Redeemer Hospital & Medical Center[2]	Meadowbrook	98%	41
Main Line Hospital Bryn Mawr Campus	Bryn Mawr	98%	86
Riddle Memorial Hospital	Media	98%	66
Temple University Hospital	Philadelphia	98%	200
UPMC Saint Margaret	Pittsburgh	98%	82
Jefferson Regional Medical Center[2]	Pittsburgh	97%	37
Lehigh Valley Hospital - Muhlenberg	Bethlehem	97%	66
Moses Taylor Hospital	Scranton	97%	34
Nazareth Hospital	Philadelphia	97%	77
Grand View Hospital	Sellersville	96%	48
Lehigh Valley Hospital	Allentown	96%	295
Pinnacle Health Hospitals	Harrisburg	96%	195
Saint Luke's Hospital Bethlehem	Bethlehem	96%	120
UPMC Presbyterian Shadyside	Pittsburgh	96%	541
Williamsport Regional Medical Center	Williamsport	96%	80
Penn Hosp of the Univ of PA Hlth Sys	Philadelphia	95%	41
Geisinger Medical Center	Danville	94%	178
Lancaster General Hospital	Lancaster	94%	237
Main Line Hospital Lankenau	Wynnewood	94%	79
Crozer Chester Medical Center	Upland	93%	165
Delaware County Memorial Hospital	Drexel Hill	93%	43
Penn Presbyterian Medical Center	Philadelphia	93%	43
York Hospital	York	93%	196
Chestnut Hill Hospital	Philadelphia	92%	48
Monongahela Valley Hospital	Monongahela	92%	39
Sharon Regional Health System	Sharon	92%	38
The Washington Hospital	Washington	92%	66
Waynesboro Hospital	Waynesboro	92%	25
Hospital of Univ of Pennsylvania	Philadelphia	91%	142
Jeanes Hospital	Philadelphia	91%	46
Saint Luke's Hospital - Anderson Campus	Easton	91%	35
UPMC Mercy	Pittsburgh	91%	119
Conemaugh Valley Memorial Hospital	Johnstown	89%	127
Easton Hospital	Easton	89%	37
Milton S Hershey Medical Center	Hershey	88%	208
Reading Hospital	Reading	88%	177
Saint Vincent Hospital	Erie	87%	137
Regional Hospital of Scranton	Scranton	86%	56
Brandywine Hospital	Coatesville	85%	26
Forbes Regional Hospital	Monroeville	85%	95
Gettysburg Hospital	Gettysburg	85%	34
Allegheny General Hospital	Pittsburgh	84%	231
Saint Joseph Medical Center	Reading	84%	61
Lewistown Hospital	Lewistown	83%	29
Alle Kiski Medical Center	Natrona	82%	33
Geisinger Wyoming Valley Medical Center	Wilkes Barre	81%	101
Chambersburg Hospital	Chambersburg	77%	128
Lehigh Valley Hospital - Hazleton	Hazleton	77%	30
Pottstown Memorial Medical Center	Pottstown	76%	38
Wilkes-Barre General Hospital	Wilkes-Barre	75%	80
Good Samaritan Hospital	Lebanon	74%	27
Evangelical Community Hospital	Lewisburg	71%	56
Mount Nittany Medical Center	State College	69%	61
Excela Health Westmoreland Hospital	Greensburg	60%	55
Meadville Medical Center	Meadville	45%	33
Robert Packer Hospital	Sayre	43%	83
Abington Memorial Hospital[2]	Abington	42%	57
Jameson Memorial Hospital	New Castle	41%	39
Einstein Medical Center Montgomery[2]	East Norriton	31%	52
Lower Bucks Hospital	Bristol	31%	26

Surgical Care Improvement Project

Appropriate Beta Blocker Usage

Hospital Name	City	Rate	Cases
Charles Cole Memorial Hospital	Coudersport	100%	59
Chester County Hospital	West Chester	100%	309
Coordinated Health Orthopedic Hospital[2]	Bethlehem	100%	59
Edgewood Surgical Hospital	Transfer	100%	33
Geisinger Wyoming Valley Medical Center[2]	Wilkes Barre	100%	348
Good Samaritan Hospital[2]	Lebanon	100%	214
Grand View Hospital[2]	Sellersville	100%	142
Hanover Hospital	Hanover	100%	152
Hospital of Univ of Pennsylvania[2]	Philadelphia	100%	464
Jeanes Hospital	Philadelphia	100%	205
Lancaster Regional Medical Center	Lancaster	100%	200
Lehigh Valley Hospital - Hazleton	Hazleton	100%	110
Lower Bucks Hospital	Bristol	100%	26
Magee Womens Hosp of UPMC Health Sys	Pittsburgh	100%	454
Main Line Hospital Bryn Mawr Campus[2]	Bryn Mawr	100%	424
Main Line Hospital Lankenau[2]	Wynnewood	100%	517
Main Line Hospital Paoli[2]	Paoli	100%	262
Memorial Hospital	York	100%	56
Mercy Suburban Hospital	Norristown	100%	74
Oss Orthopaedic Hospital[2]	York	100%	89
Penn Highlands Elk	Saint Marys	100%	48
Pottstown Memorial Medical Center	Pottstown	100%	118
Reading Hospital[2]	Reading	100%	656
Saint Joseph Medical Center[2]	Reading	100%	237
Saint Luke's Hospital Bethlehem[2]	Bethlehem	100%	569
Saint Luke's Miners Memorial Hospital	Coaldale	100%	41
Saint Luke's Quakertown Hospital	Quakertown	100%	31
Saint Mary Medical Center	Langhorne	100%	575
Somerset Hospital	Somerset	100%	38
Southwest Regional Medical Center	Waynesburg	100%	28
Sunbury Community Hospital	Sunbury	100%	40
Temple University Hospital[2]	Philadelphia	100%	406
Titusville Hospital	Titusville	100%	36
Tyrone Hospital	Tyrone	100%	40
UPMC East[3]	Monroeville	100%	90
UPMC Horizon	Greenville	100%	234
UPMC Mercy	Pittsburgh	100%	473
UPMC Northwest	Seneca	100%	81
UPMC Passavant	Pittsburgh	100%	702
UPMC Presbyterian Shadyside	Pittsburgh	100%	2556
UPMC Saint Margaret	Pittsburgh	100%	546
The Washington Hospital	Washington	100%	291
Wellspan Surgery & Rehab Hosp[2]	York	100%	85
Wilkes Barre VA Medical Center[2]	Wilkes-Barre	100%	26
Williamsport Regional Medical Center[2]	Williamsport	100%	422
Acmh Hospital	Kittanning	99%	100
Advanced Surgical Hospital	Washington	99%	99
Aria Health	Philadelphia	99%	457
Butler Memorial Hospital	Butler	99%	450
Crozer Chester Medical Center[2]	Upland	99%	285
Einstein Medical Center Montgomery[2,3]	East Norriton	99%	147
Ephrata Community Hospital	Ephrata	99%	166
Forbes Regional Hospital[2]	Monroeville	99%	345
Geisinger - Community Medical Center[2]	Scranton	99%	277
Geisinger Medical Center[2]	Danville	99%	345
Gettysburg Hospital	Gettysburg	99%	101
Heritage Valley Beaver[2]	Beaver	99%	244
Holy Redeemer Hospital & Medical Center	Meadowbrook	99%	287
Milton S Hershey Medical Center[2]	Hershey	99%	553
Penn Presbyterian Medical Center[2]	Philadelphia	99%	745
Penn Hosp of the Univ of PA Hlth Sys[2]	Philadelphia	99%	202
Pinnacle Health Hospitals[2]	Harrisburg	99%	1132
Saint Vincent Hospital	Erie	99%	518
Schuylkill Med Ctr-S Jackson St	Pottsville	99%	87
Thomas Jefferson University Hospital[2]	Philadelphia	99%	779
UPMC Hamot[2]	Erie	99%	654
UPMC Mckeesport	Mc Keesport	99%	73
Western Pennsylvania Hospital	Pittsburgh	99%	98
York Hospital[2]	York	99%	518
Alle Kiski Medical Center	Natrona	98%	160
Allegheny General Hospital	Pittsburgh	98%	885
Brandywine Hospital	Coatesville	98%	129
Clarion Hospital	Clarion	98%	44
Conemaugh Valley Memorial Hospital	Johnstown	98%	640
Delaware County Memorial Hospital[2]	Drexel Hill	98%	148
Doylestown Hospital[2]	Doylestown	98%	322
Excela Health Latrobe Hospital	Latrobe	98%	134
Excela Health Westmoreland Hospital	Greensburg	98%	435
Holy Spirit Hospital[2]	Camp Hill	98%	389
Lancaster General Hospital[2]	Lancaster	98%	944
Lehigh Valley Hospital	Allentown	98%	1286
Lehigh Valley Hospital - Muhlenberg	Bethlehem	98%	223
Mount Nittany Medical Center	State College	98%	512
Nazareth Hospital	Philadelphia	98%	170
Ohio Valley General Hospital	Mckees Rocks	98%	60
Penn Highlands Dubois	Dubois	98%	199
Phoenixville Hospital	Phoenixville	98%	163
Robert Packer Hospital	Sayre	98%	577
Uniontown Hospital	Uniontown	98%	209
Waynesboro Hospital	Waynesboro	98%	48
Wilkes-Barre General Hospital	Wilkes-Barre	98%	491
Abington Memorial Hospital[2]	Abington	97%	219
Berwick Hospital Center	Berwick	97%	36
Carlisle Regional Medical Center	Carlisle	97%	157
Chambersburg Hospital[2]	Chambersburg	97%	239
Evangelical Community Hospital[2]	Lewisburg	97%	122
Jefferson Regional Medical Center	Pittsburgh	97%	643
Meadville Medical Center[2]	Meadville	97%	262
Mercy Fitzgerald Hospital	Darby	97%	211
Nason Hospital	Roaring Spring	97%	59
Penn Highlands Clearfield	Clearfield	97%	61
Pocono Medical Center	E Stroudsburg	97%	205
Regional Hospital of Scranton	Scranton	97%	402
Saint Clair Memorial Hospital	Pittsburgh	97%	500
Wayne Memorial Hospital	Honesdale	97%	74
Windber Hospital	Windber	97%	33
Cancer Treatment Centers of America	Philadelphia	96%	27
Grove City Medical Center	Grove City	96%	25
Heart of Lancaster Reg Med Ctr	Lititz	96%	25
Indiana Regional Medical Center	Indiana	96%	98
Lebanon VA Medical Center[2]	Lebanon	96%	57
Monongahela Valley Hospital	Monongahela	96%	180
Moses Taylor Hospital	Scranton	96%	133
Riddle Memorial Hospital[2]	Media	96%	257
Sacred Heart Hospital	Allentown	96%	74
Saint Luke's Hospital - Anderson Campus[2]	Easton	96%	28
UPMC Altoona	Altoona	96%	534
Easton Hospital	Easton	95%	236
Hahnemann University Hospital[2]	Philadelphia	95%	144
Heritage Valley Sewickley[2]	Sewickley	95%	94
Jameson Memorial Hospital	New Castle	95%	124
Sharon Regional Health System	Sharon	95%	187
Chestnut Hill Hospital	Philadelphia	94%	36
Gnaden Huetten Memorial Hospital	Lehighton	94%	34
Lansdale Hospital[2]	Lansdale	94%	85
Palmerton Hospital	Palmerton	94%	32
UPMC Bedford Memorial	Everett	94%	33
Canonsburg General Hospital	Canonsburg	93%	106
Punxsutawney Area Hospital	Punxsutawney	93%	28
Schuylkill Med Ctr-East Norwegian St	Pottsville	93%	72
VA Pittsburgh Healthcare System[2]	Pittsburgh	93%	270
Warren General Hospital	Warren	93%	45
Albert Einstein Medical Center[2]	Philadelphia	92%	245
Lewistown Hospital	Lewistown	92%	61
Geisinger - Bloomsburg Hospital	Bloomsburg	91%	58
Physician's Care Surgical Hospital[2]	Royersford	91%	32
Jennersville Regional Hospital	West Grove	88%	25
Philadelphia VA Medical Center[2]	Philadelphia	84%	32
Soldiers & Sailors Memorial Hospital	Wellsboro	84%	32
Surgical Institute of Reading[2]	Wyomissing	84%	99
J C Blair Memorial Hospital	Huntingdon	81%	31
Bradford Regional Medical Center	Bradford	79%	39

Appropriate VTP Within 24 Hours

Hospital Name	City	Rate	Cases
Advanced Surgical Hospital	Washington	100%	400
Bucks County Specialty Hospital[2]	Bensalem	100%	69
Butler Memorial Hospital	Butler	100%	769
Charles Cole Memorial Hospital	Coudersport	100%	252
Chester County Hospital	West Chester	100%	659
Coordinated Health Orthopedic Hospital[2]	Bethlehem	100%	200
Edgewood Surgical Hospital	Transfer	100%	110
Grand View Hospital[2]	Sellersville	100%	336
Holy Spirit Hospital[2]	Camp Hill	100%	726
Hospital of Univ of Pennsylvania[2]	Philadelphia	100%	478
Jeanes Hospital	Philadelphia	100%	431
Lancaster General Hospital[2]	Lancaster	100%	1774
Lancaster Regional Medical Center	Lancaster	100%	499
Lehigh Valley Hospital - Hazleton	Hazleton	100%	229
Main Line Hospital Lankenau[2]	Wynnewood	100%	779
Main Line Hospital Paoli[2]	Paoli	100%	738
Mercy Suburban Hospital	Norristown	100%	204
Milton S Hershey Medical Center[2]	Hershey	100%	989
Nason Hospital	Roaring Spring	100%	192
Oss Orthopaedic Hospital[2]	York	100%	298
Penn Presbyterian Medical Center[2]	Philadelphia	100%	1490
Penn Hosp of the Univ of PA Hlth Sys[2]	Philadelphia	100%	413
Philadelphia VA Medical Center[2]	Philadelphia	100%	63
Pinnacle Health Hospitals[2]	Harrisburg	100%	2656
Reading Hospital[2]	Reading	100%	1203
Roxborough Memorial Hospital	Philadelphia	100%	80
Saint Joseph Medical Center[2]	Reading	100%	346
Saint Vincent Hospital	Erie	100%	950
Somerset Hospital	Somerset	100%	148
Sunbury Community Hospital	Sunbury	100%	54

NOTE: Hospital profiles are in alphabetical order by state, then city, then hospital within the city; Rankings exclude hospitals with less than 25 cases except for patient surveys which excludes hospitals with less than 100 cases; (a) 100-299 cases; (1) The number of cases/patients is too few to report; (2) Data submitted were based on a sample of cases/patients; (3) Results are based on a shorter time period than required; (4) Data suppressed by CMS for one or more quarters; (5) Results are not available for this reporting period; (6) Fewer than 100 patients completed the HCAHPS survey; (7) No cases met the criteria for this measure; (8) The lower limit of the confidence interval cannot be calculated if the number of observed infections equals zero; (9) No data are available from the state/territory for this reporting period; (10) The scores shown reflect fewer than 50 completed surveys; (11) There were discrepancies in the data collection process; (12) This measure does not apply to this hospital for this reporting period; (13) Results cannot be calculated for this reporting period; (14) The results for this state are combined with nearby states to protect confidentiality; Please refer to the User's Guide for a full explanation of data.

Hospital Name	City	Rate	Cases
Surgical Specialty Ctr at Coord Hlth[2]	Allentown	100%	164
Temple University Hospital[2]	Philadelphia	100%	627
Thomas Jefferson University Hospital[2]	Philadelphia	100%	1890
Tyrone Hospital	Tyrone	100%	90
UPMC East[3]	Monroeville	100%	330
UPMC Horizon	Greenville	100%	542
UPMC Mercy	Pittsburgh	100%	1120
UPMC Presbyterian Shadyside	Pittsburgh	100%	5172
UPMC Saint Margaret	Pittsburgh	100%	1387
Wellspan Surgery & Rehab Hosp[2]	York	100%	268
Williamsport Regional Medical Center[2]	Williamsport	100%	989
Windber Hospital	Windber	100%	100
Abington Memorial Hospital[2]	Abington	99%	401
Albert Einstein Medical Center[2]	Philadelphia	99%	484
Aria Health	Philadelphia	99%	1171
Carlisle Regional Medical Center	Carlisle	99%	451
Chambersburg Hospital[2]	Chambersburg	99%	635
Chestnut Hill Hospital	Philadelphia	99%	195
Conemaugh Valley Memorial Hospital	Johnstown	99%	1054
Crozer Chester Medical Center[2]	Upland	99%	678
Delaware County Memorial Hospital[2]	Drexel Hill	99%	437
Easton Hospital	Easton	99%	482
Ephrata Community Hospital	Ephrata	99%	480
Excela Health Latrobe Hospital	Latrobe	99%	426
Excela Health Westmoreland Hospital	Greensburg	99%	959
Geisinger - Community Medical Center[2]	Scranton	99%	356
Gettysburg Hospital	Gettysburg	99%	345
Hahnemann University Hospital[2]	Philadelphia	99%	388
Hanover Hospital	Hanover	99%	415
Heart of Lancaster Reg Med Ctr	Lititz	99%	86
Holy Redeemer Hospital & Medical Center	Meadowbrook	99%	692
Indiana Regional Medical Center	Indiana	99%	296
Lansdale Hospital[2]	Lansdale	99%	272
Lebanon VA Medical Center[2]	Lebanon	99%	158
Magee Womens Hosp of UPMC Health Sys	Pittsburgh	99%	1784
Main Line Hospital Bryn Mawr Campus[2]	Bryn Mawr	99%	1262
Mercy Fitzgerald Hospital	Darby	99%	473
Millcreek Community Hospital	Erie	99%	108
Moses Taylor Hospital	Scranton	99%	425
Nazareth Hospital	Philadelphia	99%	375
Penn Highlands Clearfield	Clearfield	99%	163
Pottstown Memorial Medical Center	Pottstown	99%	398
Riddle Memorial Hospital[2]	Media	99%	965
Robert Packer Hospital	Sayre	99%	1095
Saint Clair Memorial Hospital	Pittsburgh	99%	1325
Saint Luke's Hospital Bethlehem[2]	Bethlehem	99%	1068
Saint Luke's Miners Memorial Hospital	Coaldale	99%	129
Saint Luke's Quakertown Hospital	Quakertown	99%	97
Schuylkill Med Ctr-S Jackson St	Pottsville	99%	192
Titusville Hospital	Titusville	99%	98
UPMC Altoona	Altoona	99%	980
UPMC Hamot[2]	Erie	99%	1027
UPMC Northwest	Seneca	99%	234
UPMC Passavant	Pittsburgh	99%	1825
Warren General Hospital	Warren	99%	162
The Washington Hospital	Washington	99%	518
Western Pennsylvania Hospital	Pittsburgh	99%	388
York Hospital[2]	York	99%	684
Acmh Hospital	Kittanning	98%	295
Alle Kiski Medical Center	Natrona	98%	351
Allegheny General Hospital	Pittsburgh	98%	1613
Canonsburg General Hospital	Canonsburg	98%	307
Excela Health Frick Hospital	Mount Pleasant	98%	55
Forbes Regional Hospital[2]	Monroeville	98%	562
Geisinger Medical Center[2]	Danville	98%	480
Heritage Valley Sewickley[2]	Sewickley	98%	361
Jameson Memorial Hospital	New Castle	98%	381
Jennersville Regional Hospital	West Grove	98%	80
Lehigh Valley Hospital	Allentown	98%	2810
Lehigh Valley Hospital - Muhlenberg	Bethlehem	98%	483
Meadville Medical Center[2]	Meadville	98%	622
Mount Nittany Medical Center	State College	98%	1451
Penn Highlands Dubois	Dubois	98%	321
Phoenixville Hospital	Phoenixville	98%	282
Punxsutawney Area Hospital	Punxsutawney	98%	86
Regional Hospital of Scranton	Scranton	98%	716
Sacred Heart Hospital	Allentown	98%	245
Saint Mary Medical Center	Langhorne	98%	1029
Sharon Regional Health System	Sharon	98%	455
Surgical Institute of Reading[2]	Wyomissing	98%	414
Uniontown Hospital	Uniontown	98%	588
UPMC Bedford Memorial	Everett	98%	113
VA Pittsburgh Healthcare System[2]	Pittsburgh	98%	297
Berwick Hospital Center	Berwick	97%	109
Bradford Regional Medical Center	Bradford	97%	149
Doylestown Hospital[2]	Doylestown	97%	658
Einstein Medical Center Montgomery[2,3]	East Norriton	97%	225
Geisinger - Bloomsburg Hospital	Bloomsburg	97%	186
Geisinger Wyoming Valley Medical Center[2]	Wilkes Barre	97%	492
Lower Bucks Hospital	Bristol	97%	65
Ohio Valley General Hospital	Mckees Rocks	97%	174
Palmerton Hospital	Palmerton	97%	93
Penn Highlands Elk	Saint Marys	97%	119
Pocono Medical Center	E Stroudsburg	97%	417
Schuylkill Med Ctr-East Norwegian St	Pottsville	97%	174
Southwest Regional Medical Center	Waynesburg	97%	78
Wayne Memorial Hospital	Honesdale	97%	255
Waynesboro Hospital	Waynesboro	97%	114
Wilkes Barre VA Medical Center[2]	Wilkes-Barre	97%	67
Wilkes-Barre General Hospital	Wilkes-Barre	97%	947
Brandywine Hospital	Coatesville	96%	207
Evangelical Community Hospital[2]	Lewisburg	96%	404
Good Samaritan Hospital[2]	Lebanon	96%	272
Grove City Medical Center	Grove City	96%	84
Lewistown Hospital	Lewistown	96%	168
Memorial Hospital	York	96%	217
UPMC Mckeesport	Mc Keesport	96%	210
Ellwood City Hospital[2]	Ellwood City	95%	77
Highlands Hospital	Connellsville	95%	37
Jefferson Regional Medical Center	Pittsburgh	95%	1113
Monongahela Valley Hospital	Monongahela	95%	485
Cancer Treatment Centers of America	Philadelphia	94%	156
Heritage Valley Beaver[2]	Beaver	94%	376
Saint Luke's Hospital - Anderson Campus[2]	Easton	93%	81
Soldiers & Sailors Memorial Hospital	Wellsboro	93%	137
Gnaden Huetten Memorial Hospital	Lehighton	92%	96
J C Blair Memorial Hospital	Huntingdon	91%	65
Jersey Shore Hospital	Jersey Shore	91%	35
Physician's Care Surgical Hospital[2]	Royersford	91%	167
Clarion Hospital	Clarion	90%	135
Saint Joseph's Hospital	Philadelphia	86%	43

Controlled Postoperative Blood Glucose

Hospital Name	City	Rate	Cases
Good Samaritan Hospital[2]	Lebanon	100%	135
Main Line Hospital Paoli[2]	Paoli	100%	42
Pinnacle Health Hospitals[2]	Harrisburg	100%	445
Saint Clair Memorial Hospital	Pittsburgh	100%	120
Abington Memorial Hospital[2]	Abington	99%	160
Butler Memorial Hospital	Butler	99%	334
Doylestown Hospital[2]	Doylestown	99%	192
Easton Hospital	Easton	99%	82
Excela Health Westmoreland Hospital	Greensburg	99%	154
Geisinger - Community Medical Center[2]	Scranton	99%	160
Heritage Valley Beaver[2]	Beaver	99%	147
Jefferson Regional Medical Center	Pittsburgh	99%	254
Lehigh Valley Hospital	Allentown	99%	549
Main Line Hospital Lankenau[2]	Wynnewood	99%	446
Penn Highlands Dubois	Dubois	99%	88
Reading Hospital[2]	Reading	99%	180
Saint Joseph Medical Center[2]	Reading	99%	130
Saint Luke's Hospital Bethlehem[2]	Bethlehem	99%	254
Saint Mary Medical Center	Langhorne	99%	240
Temple University Hospital[2]	Philadelphia	99%	239
UPMC Mercy	Pittsburgh	99%	158
UPMC Passavant	Pittsburgh	99%	208
Wilkes-Barre General Hospital	Wilkes-Barre	99%	192
York Hospital[2]	York	99%	395
Brandywine Hospital	Coatesville	98%	61
Conemaugh Valley Memorial Hospital	Johnstown	98%	211
Einstein Medical Center Montgomery[2,3]	East Norriton	98%	99
Forbes Regional Hospital[2]	Monroeville	98%	184
Hospital of Univ of Pennsylvania[2]	Philadelphia	98%	342
Lancaster General Hospital[2]	Lancaster	98%	294
Penn Hosp of the Univ of PA Hlth Sys[2]	Philadelphia	98%	124
Phoenixville Hospital	Phoenixville	98%	88
Pocono Medical Center	E Stroudsburg	98%	124
Thomas Jefferson University Hospital[2]	Philadelphia	98%	194
Aria Health	Philadelphia	97%	145
Holy Spirit Hospital[2]	Camp Hill	97%	181
Jeanes Hospital	Philadelphia	97%	72
Lehigh Valley Hospital - Muhlenberg	Bethlehem	97%	88
Saint Vincent Hospital	Erie	97%	314
UPMC Presbyterian Shadyside	Pittsburgh	97%	919
The Washington Hospital	Washington	97%	126
Williamsport Regional Medical Center[2]	Williamsport	97%	97
Allegheny General Hospital	Pittsburgh	96%	476
Main Line Hospital Bryn Mawr Campus[2]	Bryn Mawr	96%	70
Mercy Fitzgerald Hospital	Darby	96%	48
Penn Presbyterian Medical Center[2]	Philadelphia	96%	392
Regional Hospital of Scranton	Scranton	96%	209
UPMC Hamot[2]	Erie	96%	324
VA Pittsburgh Healthcare System[2]	Pittsburgh	96%	165
Albert Einstein Medical Center[2]	Philadelphia	95%	149
Chester County Hospital	West Chester	95%	96
Geisinger Medical Center[2]	Danville	95%	190
Geisinger Wyoming Valley Medical Center[2]	Wilkes Barre	95%	132
Hahnemann University Hospital[2]	Philadelphia	95%	61
Milton S Hershey Medical Center[2]	Hershey	95%	367
Robert Packer Hospital	Sayre	95%	200
UPMC Altoona	Altoona	95%	196
Lancaster Regional Medical Center	Lancaster	92%	52
Sharon Regional Health System	Sharon	90%	51
Crozer Chester Medical Center[2]	Upland	88%	103

Perioperative Temperature Management

Hospital Name	City	Rate	Cases
Abington Memorial Hospital[2]	Abington	100%	528
Acmh Hospital	Kittanning	100%	480
Advanced Surgical Hospital	Washington	100%	418
Albert Einstein Medical Center[2]	Philadelphia	100%	605
Alle Kiski Medical Center	Natrona	100%	393
Aria Health	Philadelphia	100%	1360
Berwick Hospital Center	Berwick	100%	134
Bradford Regional Medical Center	Bradford	100%	159
Brandywine Hospital	Coatesville	100%	238
Bucks County Specialty Hospital[2]	Bensalem	100%	150
Butler Memorial Hospital	Butler	100%	918
Cancer Treatment Centers of America	Philadelphia	100%	162
Carlisle Regional Medical Center	Carlisle	100%	528
Chambersburg Hospital[2]	Chambersburg	100%	746
Charles Cole Memorial Hospital	Coudersport	100%	274
Chester County Hospital	West Chester	100%	865
Chestnut Hill Hospital	Philadelphia	100%	274
Clarion Hospital	Clarion	100%	149
Coordinated Health Orthopedic Hospital[2]	Bethlehem	100%	211
Crozer Chester Medical Center[2]	Upland	100%	848
Delaware County Memorial Hospital[2]	Drexel Hill	100%	484
Doylestown Hospital[2]	Doylestown	100%	817
Einstein Medical Center Montgomery[2,3]	East Norriton	100%	283
Ephrata Community Hospital	Ephrata	100%	584
Evangelical Community Hospital[2]	Lewisburg	100%	464
Excela Health Frick Hospital	Mount Pleasant	100%	61
Excela Health Latrobe Hospital	Latrobe	100%	484
Excela Health Westmoreland Hospital	Greensburg	100%	1097
Forbes Regional Hospital[2]	Monroeville	100%	706
Geisinger - Bloomsburg Hospital	Bloomsburg	100%	205
Geisinger - Community Medical Center[2]	Scranton	100%	476
Gettysburg Hospital	Gettysburg	100%	379
Gnaden Huetten Memorial Hospital	Lehighton	100%	110
Good Samaritan Hospital[2]	Lebanon	100%	414
Grand View Hospital[2]	Sellersville	100%	412
Grove City Medical Center	Grove City	100%	93
Hahnemann University Hospital[2]	Philadelphia	100%	503
Hanover Hospital	Hanover	100%	474
Heart of Lancaster Reg Med Ctr	Lititz	100%	102
Heritage Valley Beaver[2]	Beaver	100%	525
Heritage Valley Sewickley[2]	Sewickley	100%	423
Highlands Hospital	Connellsville	100%	44
Holy Redeemer Hospital & Medical Center	Meadowbrook	100%	818
Holy Spirit Hospital[2]	Camp Hill	100%	866
Hospital of Univ of Pennsylvania[2]	Philadelphia	100%	654
Indiana Regional Medical Center	Indiana	100%	337
J C Blair Memorial Hospital	Huntingdon	100%	81
Jameson Memorial Hospital	New Castle	100%	417
Jeanes Hospital	Philadelphia	100%	503
Jennersville Regional Hospital	West Grove	100%	99
Jersey Shore Hospital	Jersey Shore	100%	41
Kane Community Hospital	Kane	100%	28
Lancaster General Hospital[2]	Lancaster	100%	2154
Lancaster Regional Medical Center	Lancaster	100%	611
Lansdale Hospital[2]	Lansdale	100%	306
Lebanon VA Medical Center[2]	Lebanon	100%	205
Lehigh Valley Hospital	Allentown	100%	3320
Lehigh Valley Hospital - Hazleton	Hazleton	100%	276
Lehigh Valley Hospital - Muhlenberg	Bethlehem	100%	550
Lewistown Hospital	Lewistown	100%	191
Lower Bucks Hospital	Bristol	100%	78
Magee Womens Hosp of UPMC Health Sys	Pittsburgh	100%	2094
Main Line Hospital Bryn Mawr Campus[2]	Bryn Mawr	100%	1470
Main Line Hospital Lankenau[2]	Wynnewood	100%	1270
Main Line Hospital Paoli[2]	Paoli	100%	934
Meadville Medical Center[2]	Meadville	100%	754
Memorial Hospital	York	100%	243
Mercy Fitzgerald Hospital	Darby	100%	553
Mercy Suburban Hospital	Norristown	100%	236
Millcreek Community Hospital	Erie	100%	121
Milton S Hershey Medical Center[2]	Hershey	100%	1230
Monongahela Valley Hospital	Monongahela	100%	589
Mount Nittany Medical Center	State College	100%	1618
Nason Hospital	Roaring Spring	100%	227
Nazareth Hospital	Philadelphia	100%	428
Ohio Valley General Hospital	Mckees Rocks	100%	197
Oss Orthopaedic Hospital[2]	York	100%	314
Penn Highlands Clearfield	Clearfield	100%	219
Penn Highlands Dubois	Dubois	100%	361
Penn Highlands Elk	Saint Marys	100%	138
Penn Presbyterian Medical Center[2]	Philadelphia	100%	1978
Penn Hosp of the Univ of PA Hlth Sys[2]	Philadelphia	100%	500
Phoenixville Hospital	Phoenixville	100%	393
Pinnacle Health Hospitals[2]	Harrisburg	100%	3003
Pocono Medical Center	E Stroudsburg	100%	523
Pottstown Memorial Medical Center	Pottstown	100%	438

NOTE: Hospital profiles are in alphabetical order by state, then city, then hospital within the city; Rankings exclude hospitals with less than 25 cases except for patient surveys which excludes hospitals with less than 100 cases; (a) 100-299 cases; (1) The number of cases/patients is too few to report; (2) Data submitted were based on a sample of cases/patients; (3) Results are based on a shorter time period than required; (4) Data suppressed by CMS for one or more quarters; (5) Results are not available for this reporting period; (6) Fewer than 100 patients completed the HCAHPS survey; (7) No cases met the criteria for this measure; (8) The lower limit of the confidence interval cannot be calculated if the number of observed infections equals zero; (9) No data are available from the state/territory for this reporting period; (10) The scores shown reflect fewer than 50 completed surveys; (11) There were discrepancies in the data collection process; (12) This measure does not apply to this hospital for this reporting period; (13) Results cannot be calculated for this reporting period; (14) The results for this state are combined with nearby states to protect confidentiality; Please refer to the User's Guide for a full explanation of data.

Hospital Name	City	Rate	Cases
Punxsutawney Area Hospital	Punxsutawney	100%	99
Reading Hospital[2]	Reading	100%	1488
Regional Hospital of Scranton	Scranton	100%	824
Riddle Memorial Hospital[2]	Media	100%	1037
Robert Packer Hospital	Sayre	100%	1330
Roxborough Memorial Hospital	Philadelphia	100%	83
Sacred Heart Hospital	Allentown	100%	279
Saint Clair Memorial Hospital	Pittsburgh	100%	1562
Saint Joseph Medical Center[2]	Reading	100%	414
Saint Luke's Hospital Bethlehem[2]	Bethlehem	100%	1295
Saint Luke's Miners Memorial Hospital	Coaldale	100%	141
Saint Luke's Quakertown Hospital	Quakertown	100%	108
Saint Mary Medical Center	Langhorne	100%	1414
Saint Vincent Hospital	Erie	100%	1106
Schuylkill Med Ctr-East Norwegian St	Pottsville	100%	205
Schuylkill Med Ctr-S Jackson St	Pottsville	100%	243
Sharon Regional Health System	Sharon	100%	521
Soldiers & Sailors Memorial Hospital	Wellsboro	100%	147
Somerset Hospital	Somerset	100%	181
Sunbury Community Hospital	Sunbury	100%	90
Surgical Specialty Ctr at Coord Hlth[2]	Allentown	100%	167
Temple University Hospital[2]	Philadelphia	100%	869
Thomas Jefferson University Hospital[2]	Philadelphia	100%	2700
Titusville Hospital	Titusville	100%	102
Tyrone Hospital	Tyrone	100%	122
Uniontown Hospital	Uniontown	100%	665
UPMC Altoona	Altoona	100%	1316
UPMC Bedford Memorial	Everett	100%	125
UPMC East[3]	Monroeville	100%	359
UPMC Hamot[2]	Erie	100%	1309
UPMC Horizon	Greenville	100%	662
UPMC Mckeesport	Mc Keesport	100%	269
UPMC Mercy	Pittsburgh	100%	1334
UPMC Passavant	Pittsburgh	100%	2060
UPMC Presbyterian Shadyside	Pittsburgh	100%	6520
UPMC Saint Margaret	Pittsburgh	100%	1565
VA Pittsburgh Healthcare System[2]	Pittsburgh	100%	399
The Washington Hospital	Washington	100%	686
Wayne Memorial Hospital	Honesdale	100%	275
Waynesboro Hospital	Waynesboro	100%	152
Wellspan Surgery & Rehab Hosp[2]	York	100%	302
Western Pennsylvania Hospital	Pittsburgh	100%	441
Wilkes-Barre General Hospital	Wilkes-Barre	100%	1086
Williamsport Regional Medical Center[2]	Williamsport	100%	1142
Windber Hospital	Windber	100%	137
York Hospital[2]	York	100%	956
Allegheny General Hospital	Pittsburgh	99%	1991
Canonsburg General Hospital	Canonsburg	99%	335
Conemaugh Valley Memorial Hospital	Johnstown	99%	1370
Easton Hospital	Easton	99%	556
Geisinger Medical Center[2]	Danville	99%	748
Geisinger Wyoming Valley Medical Center[2]	Wilkes Barre	99%	629
Jefferson Regional Medical Center	Pittsburgh	99%	1319
Palmerton Hospital	Palmerton	99%	100
Saint Luke's Hospital - Anderson Campus[2]	Easton	99%	91
Southwest Regional Medical Center	Waynesburg	99%	79
Surgical Institute of Reading[2]	Wyomissing	99%	419
UPMC Northwest	Seneca	99%	313
Warren General Hospital	Warren	99%	185
Moses Taylor Hospital	Scranton	98%	486
Physician's Care Surgical Hospital[2]	Royersford	98%	204
Wilkes Barre VA Medical Center[2]	Wilkes-Barre	97%	71
Ellwood City Hospital[2]	Ellwood City	96%	98
Edgewood Surgical Hospital	Transfer	93%	110
Philadelphia VA Medical Center[2]	Philadelphia	93%	90
Saint Joseph's Hospital	Philadelphia	80%	50

Prophylactic Antibiotic Selection

Hospital Name	City	Rate	Cases
Acmh Hospital	Kittanning	100%	350
Advanced Surgical Hospital	Washington	100%	384
Albert Einstein Medical Center[2]	Philadelphia	100%	487
Alle Kiski Medical Center	Natrona	100%	282
Bucks County Specialty Hospital[2]	Bensalem	100%	148
Butler Memorial Hospital	Butler	100%	977
Carlisle Regional Medical Center	Carlisle	100%	402
Chambersburg Hospital[2]	Chambersburg	100%	556
Chester County Hospital	West Chester	100%	628
Chestnut Hill Hospital	Philadelphia	100%	120
Conemaugh Valley Memorial Hospital	Johnstown	100%	960
Edgewood Surgical Hospital	Transfer	100%	102
Endless Mountains Health Systems	Montrose	100%	97
Excela Health Frick Hospital	Mount Pleasant	100%	27
Forbes Regional Hospital[2]	Monroeville	100%	609
Geisinger - Community Medical Center[2]	Scranton	100%	435
Geisinger Medical Center[2]	Danville	100%	561
Gettysburg Hospital	Gettysburg	100%	293
Good Samaritan Hospital[2]	Lebanon	100%	318
Grand View Hospital[2]	Sellersville	100%	272
Grove City Medical Center	Grove City	100%	76
Heart of Lancaster Reg Med Ctr	Lititz	100%	52
Indiana Regional Medical Center	Indiana	100%	244
Jennersville Regional Hospital	West Grove	100%	31
Lancaster Regional Medical Center	Lancaster	100%	447
Lansdale Hospital[2]	Lansdale	100%	213
Lehigh Valley Hospital	Allentown	100%	2297
Magee Womens Hosp of UPMC Health Sys	Pittsburgh	100%	1485
Main Line Hospital Bryn Mawr Campus[2]	Bryn Mawr	100%	1321
Main Line Hospital Lankenau[2]	Wynnewood	100%	1249
Memorial Hospital	York	100%	156
Milton S Hershey Medical Center[2]	Hershey	100%	1077
Nazareth Hospital	Philadelphia	100%	251
Oss Orthopaedic Hospital[2]	York	100%	230
Penn Highlands Dubois	Dubois	100%	330
Penn Presbyterian Medical Center[2]	Philadelphia	100%	1511
Philadelphia VA Medical Center	Philadelphia	100%	37
Pinnacle Health Hospitals[2]	Harrisburg	100%	2764
Punxsutawney Area Hospital	Punxsutawney	100%	62
Reading Hospital[2]	Reading	100%	1258
Riddle Memorial Hospital[2]	Media	100%	849
Roxborough Memorial Hospital	Philadelphia	100%	52
Sacred Heart Hospital	Allentown	100%	198
Saint Luke's Hospital - Anderson Campus[2]	Easton	100%	36
Saint Luke's Hospital Bethlehem[2]	Bethlehem	100%	1182
Saint Luke's Miners Memorial Hospital	Coaldale	100%	108
UPMC Bedford Memorial	Everett	100%	79
UPMC East[3]	Monroeville	100%	280
UPMC Hamot[2]	Erie	100%	1127
UPMC Horizon	Greenville	100%	478
UPMC Northwest	Seneca	100%	223
UPMC Passavant	Pittsburgh	100%	1253
UPMC Presbyterian Shadyside	Pittsburgh	100%	2754
UPMC Saint Margaret	Pittsburgh	100%	1150
VA Pittsburgh Healthcare System	Pittsburgh	100%	414
Wellspan Surgery & Rehab Hosp[2]	York	100%	217
Williamsport Regional Medical Center[2]	Williamsport	100%	953
York Hospital[2]	York	100%	833
Allegheny General Hospital	Pittsburgh	99%	1217
Aria Health	Philadelphia	99%	909
Charles Cole Memorial Hospital	Coudersport	99%	221
Coordinated Health Orthopedic Hospital[2]	Bethlehem	99%	145
Crozer Chester Medical Center[2]	Upland	99%	718
Doylestown Hospital[2]	Doylestown	99%	735
Easton Hospital	Easton	99%	416
Einstein Medical Center Montgomery[2,3]	East Norriton	99%	273
Ephrata Community Hospital	Ephrata	99%	397
Excela Health Latrobe Hospital	Latrobe	99%	347
Excela Health Westmoreland Hospital	Greensburg	99%	998
Geisinger Wyoming Valley Medical Center[2]	Wilkes Barre	99%	469
Hahnemann University Hospital[2]	Philadelphia	99%	429
Hanover Hospital	Hanover	99%	362
Heritage Valley Sewickley[2]	Sewickley	99%	274
Holy Redeemer Hospital & Medical Center	Meadowbrook	99%	621
Holy Spirit Hospital[2]	Camp Hill	99%	822
Hospital of Univ of Pennsylvania[2]	Philadelphia	99%	574
Jameson Memorial Hospital	New Castle	99%	313
Jeanes Hospital	Philadelphia	99%	439
Lancaster General Hospital[2]	Lancaster	99%	1702
Lehigh Valley Hospital - Hazleton	Hazleton	99%	131
Lehigh Valley Hospital - Muhlenberg	Bethlehem	99%	368
Main Line Hospital Paoli[2]	Paoli	99%	729
Meadville Medical Center[2]	Meadville	99%	614
Mercy Suburban Hospital	Norristown	99%	124
Moses Taylor Hospital	Scranton	99%	325
Mount Nittany Medical Center	State College	99%	1250
Nason Hospital	Roaring Spring	99%	180
Penn Highlands Clearfield	Clearfield	99%	154
Penn Hosp of the Univ of PA Hlth Sys[2]	Philadelphia	99%	412
Physician's Care Surgical Hospital[2]	Royersford	99%	189
Pottstown Memorial Medical Center	Pottstown	99%	288
Regional Hospital of Scranton	Scranton	99%	743
Robert Packer Hospital	Sayre	99%	891
Saint Clair Memorial Hospital	Pittsburgh	99%	1150
Saint Joseph Medical Center[2]	Reading	99%	385
Saint Mary Medical Center	Langhorne	99%	1012
Saint Vincent Hospital	Erie	99%	958
Schuylkill Med Ctr-S Jackson St	Pottsville	99%	147
Surgical Institute of Reading[2]	Wyomissing	99%	392
Temple University Hospital[2]	Philadelphia	99%	804
Thomas Jefferson University Hospital[2]	Philadelphia	99%	2364
Uniontown Hospital	Uniontown	99%	444
UPMC Mckeesport	Mc Keesport	99%	186
The Washington Hospital	Washington	99%	549
Waynesboro Hospital	Waynesboro	99%	107
Western Pennsylvania Hospital	Pittsburgh	99%	279
Windber Hospital	Windber	99%	94
Abington Memorial Hospital[2]	Abington	98%	520
Bradford Regional Medical Center	Bradford	98%	115
Brandywine Hospital	Coatesville	98%	198
Evangelical Community Hospital[2]	Lewisburg	98%	317
Geisinger - Bloomsburg Hospital	Bloomsburg	98%	157
Jefferson Regional Medical Center	Pittsburgh	98%	1102
Lower Bucks Hospital	Bristol	98%	45
Mercy Fitzgerald Hospital	Darby	98%	277
Monongahela Valley Hospital	Monongahela	98%	384
Ohio Valley General Hospital	Mckees Rocks	98%	130
Penn Highlands Elk	Saint Marys	98%	101
Phoenixville Hospital	Phoenixville	98%	266
Saint Luke's Quakertown Hospital	Quakertown	98%	66
Schuylkill Med Ctr-East Norwegian St	Pottsville	98%	129
Sharon Regional Health System	Sharon	98%	421
Tyrone Hospital	Tyrone	98%	112
UPMC Altoona	Altoona	98%	1049
UPMC Mercy	Pittsburgh	98%	760
Wilkes Barre VA Medical Center	Wilkes-Barre	98%	53
Wilkes-Barre General Hospital	Wilkes-Barre	98%	841
Delaware County Memorial Hospital[2]	Drexel Hill	97%	333
Pocono Medical Center	E Stroudsburg	97%	396
Soldiers & Sailors Memorial Hospital	Wellsboro	97%	103
Surgical Specialty Ctr at Coord Hlth[2]	Allentown	97%	141
Warren General Hospital	Warren	97%	147
Wayne Memorial Hospital	Honesdale	97%	175
Clarion Hospital	Clarion	96%	114
Gnaden Huetten Memorial Hospital	Lehighton	96%	72
Heritage Valley Beaver[2]	Beaver	96%	480
Lewistown Hospital	Lewistown	96%	125
Millcreek Community Hospital	Erie	96%	95
Southwest Regional Medical Center	Waynesburg	96%	46
Berwick Hospital Center	Berwick	95%	103
Canonsburg General Hospital	Canonsburg	95%	202
J C Blair Memorial Hospital	Huntingdon	95%	62
Lebanon VA Medical Center	Lebanon	95%	160
Palmerton Hospital	Palmerton	95%	74
Cancer Treatment Centers of America	Philadelphia	92%	49
Ellwood City Hospital[2]	Ellwood City	92%	75
Somerset Hospital	Somerset	92%	133
Jersey Shore Hospital	Jersey Shore	85%	33
Titusville Hospital	Titusville	73%	71

Prophylactic Antibiotic Selection (Outpatient)

Hospital Name	City	Rate	Cases
Berwick Hospital Center	Berwick	100%	33
Bucks County Specialty Hospital	Bensalem	100%	97
Coordinated Health Orthopedic Hospital	Bethlehem	100%	37
Good Samaritan Hospital	Lebanon	100%	418
Grove City Medical Center	Grove City	100%	89
Heart of Lancaster Reg Med Ctr	Lititz	100%	260
Jennersville Regional Hospital	West Grove	100%	55
Lancaster Regional Medical Center	Lancaster	100%	218
Lansdale Hospital	Lansdale	100%	83
Magee Womens Hosp of UPMC Health Sys	Pittsburgh	100%	661
Nazareth Hospital	Philadelphia	100%	88
Oss Orthopaedic Hospital	York	100%	291
Penn Highlands Clearfield	Clearfield	100%	67
Pinnacle Health Hospitals	Harrisburg	100%	1331
Saint Luke's Hospital - Anderson Campus	Easton	100%	60
Saint Luke's Quakertown Hospital	Quakertown	100%	31
Sharon Regional Health System	Sharon	100%	127
UPMC East[3]	Monroeville	100%	45
UPMC Passavant	Pittsburgh	100%	614
UPMC Presbyterian Shadyside	Pittsburgh	100%	1066
Wellspan Surgery & Rehab Hosp	York	100%	119
Williamsport Regional Medical Center	Williamsport	100%	592
Windber Hospital	Windber	100%	39
Butler Memorial Hospital	Butler	99%	368
Chester County Hospital	West Chester	99%	308
Geisinger Medical Center	Danville	99%	909
Geisinger Wyoming Valley Medical Center	Wilkes Barre	99%	656
Gettysburg Hospital	Gettysburg	99%	103
Holy Spirit Hospital	Camp Hill	99%	602
Indiana Regional Medical Center	Indiana	99%	165
Lehigh Valley Hospital - Muhlenberg	Bethlehem	99%	347
Monongahela Valley Hospital	Monongahela	99%	68
Penn Highlands Dubois	Dubois	99%	238
Reading Hospital	Reading	99%	949
Saint Joseph Medical Center	Reading	99%	315
Saint Luke's Hospital Bethlehem	Bethlehem	99%	737
Saint Mary Medical Center	Langhorne	99%	354
Saint Vincent Hospital	Erie	99%	321
Surgical Specialty Ctr at Coord Hlth	Allentown	99%	82
Temple University Hospital	Philadelphia	99%	361
UPMC Altoona	Altoona	99%	874
UPMC Hamot	Erie	99%	786
UPMC Mercy	Pittsburgh	99%	385
UPMC Northwest	Seneca	99%	168
UPMC Saint Margaret	Pittsburgh	99%	230
The Washington Hospital	Washington	99%	245
Western Pennsylvania Hospital	Pittsburgh	99%	340
Acmh Hospital	Kittanning	98%	50
Albert Einstein Medical Center	Philadelphia	98%	312
Alle Kiski Medical Center	Natrona	98%	253
Allegheny General Hospital	Pittsburgh	98%	648
Carlisle Regional Medical Center	Carlisle	98%	207

NOTE: Hospital profiles are in alphabetical order by state, then city, then hospital within the city; Rankings exclude hospitals with less than 25 cases except for patient surveys which excludes hospitals with less than 100 cases; (a) 100-299 cases; (1) The number of cases/patients is too few to report; (2) Data submitted were based on a sample of cases/patients; (3) Results are based on a shorter time period than required; (4) Data suppressed by CMS for one or more quarters; (5) Results are not available for this reporting period; (6) Fewer than 100 patients completed the HCAHPS survey; (7) No cases met the criteria for this measure; (8) The lower limit of the confidence interval cannot be calculated if the number of observed infections equals zero; (9) No data are available from the state/territory for this reporting period; (10) The scores shown reflect fewer than 50 completed surveys; (11) There were discrepancies in the data collection process; (12) This measure does not apply to this hospital for this reporting period; (13) Results cannot be calculated for this reporting period; (14) The results for this state are combined with nearby states to protect confidentiality; Please refer to the User's Guide for a full explanation of data.

Hospital Name	City	Rate	Cases
Chambersburg Hospital	Chambersburg	98%	395
Conemaugh Valley Memorial Hospital	Johnstown	98%	431
Doylestown Hospital	Doylestown	98%	329
Ephrata Community Hospital	Ephrata	98%	262
Evangelical Community Hospital	Lewisburg	98%	246
Excela Health Westmoreland Hospital	Greensburg	98%	209
Forbes Regional Hospital	Monroeville	98%	384
Geisinger - Community Medical Center	Scranton	98%	441
Grand View Hospital	Sellersville	98%	123
Hahnemann University Hospital	Philadelphia	98%	421
Hanover Hospital	Hanover	98%	122
Heritage Valley Beaver	Beaver	98%	185
Lancaster General Hospital	Lancaster	98%	1368
Lehigh Valley Hospital	Allentown	98%	1038
Main Line Hospital Lankenau	Wynnewood	98%	352
Mercy Suburban Hospital	Norristown	98%	64
Milton S Hershey Medical Center	Hershey	98%	1060
Phoenixville Hospital	Phoenixville	98%	129
Pocono Medical Center	E Stroudsburg	98%	315
Robert Packer Hospital	Sayre	98%	565
Uniontown Hospital	Uniontown	98%	193
UPMC Horizon	Greenville	98%	225
Wilkes-Barre General Hospital	Wilkes-Barre	98%	534
York Hospital	York	98%	674
Aria Health	Philadelphia	97%	143
Brandywine Hospital	Coatesville	97%	113
Crozer Chester Medical Center	Upland	97%	379
Easton Hospital	Easton	97%	248
Einstein Medical Center Montgomery[3]	East Norriton	97%	175
Excela Health Latrobe Hospital	Latrobe	97%	285
Gnaden Huetten Memorial Hospital	Lehighton	97%	72
Lewistown Hospital	Lewistown	97%	94
Meadville Medical Center	Meadville	97%	202
Memorial Hospital	York	97%	172
Moses Taylor Hospital	Scranton	97%	98
Mount Nittany Medical Center	State College	97%	296
Riddle Memorial Hospital	Media	97%	140
Saint Clair Memorial Hospital	Pittsburgh	97%	379
Soldiers & Sailors Memorial Hospital	Wellsboro	97%	38
Surgical Institute of Reading	Wyomissing	97%	177
UPMC Bedford Memorial	Everett	97%	39
Chestnut Hill Hospital	Philadelphia	96%	47
Heritage Valley Sewickley	Sewickley	96%	83
Jefferson Regional Medical Center	Pittsburgh	96%	328
Main Line Hospital Paoli	Paoli	96%	203
Penn Hosp of the Univ of PA Hlth Sys	Philadelphia	96%	428
Regional Hospital of Scranton	Scranton	96%	394
Thomas Jefferson University Hospital	Philadelphia	96%	460
J C Blair Memorial Hospital	Huntingdon	95%	63
Penn Highlands Elk	Saint Marys	95%	110
Punxsutawney Area Hospital	Punxsutawney	95%	41
Delaware County Memorial Hospital	Drexel Hill	94%	51
Sacred Heart Hospital	Allentown	94%	34
Wayne Memorial Hospital	Honesdale	94%	34
Abington Memorial Hospital	Abington	93%	423
Main Line Hospital Bryn Mawr Campus	Bryn Mawr	93%	268
Ohio Valley General Hospital	Mckees Rocks	93%	56
Pottstown Memorial Medical Center	Pottstown	93%	90
Warren General Hospital	Warren	93%	29
Hospital of Univ of Pennsylvania	Philadelphia	92%	667
Jeanes Hospital	Philadelphia	92%	112
Schuylkill Med Ctr-S Jackson St	Pottsville	92%	201
Sunbury Community Hospital	Sunbury	92%	37
Penn Presbyterian Medical Center	Philadelphia	91%	309
Jameson Memorial Hospital	New Castle	89%	124
Mercy Fitzgerald Hospital	Darby	88%	81
Lehigh Valley Hospital - Hazleton	Hazleton	87%	54
UPMC Mckeesport	Mc Keesport	85%	61
Penn Highlands Brookville	Brookville	78%	27
Holy Redeemer Hospital & Medical Center	Meadowbrook	76%	71
Somerset Hospital	Somerset	57%	37
Clarion Hospital	Clarion	51%	68

Prophylactic Antibiotic Stopped

Hospital Name	City	Rate	Cases
Advanced Surgical Hospital	Washington	100%	383
Aria Health	Philadelphia	100%	881
Bucks County Specialty Hospital[2]	Bensalem	100%	148
Chestnut Hill Hospital	Philadelphia	100%	119
Coordinated Health Orthopedic Hospital[2]	Bethlehem	100%	145
Doylestown Hospital[2]	Doylestown	100%	721
Edgewood Surgical Hospital	Transfer	100%	102
Endless Mountains Health Systems	Montrose	100%	97
Gettysburg Hospital	Gettysburg	100%	288
Hanover Hospital	Hanover	100%	355
Holy Redeemer Hospital & Medical Center	Meadowbrook	100%	616
Hospital of Univ of Pennsylvania[2]	Philadelphia	100%	527
Lehigh Valley Hospital	Allentown	100%	2265
Lower Bucks Hospital	Bristol	100%	45
Main Line Hospital Bryn Mawr Campus[2]	Bryn Mawr	100%	1308
Main Line Hospital Lankenau[2]	Wynnewood	100%	1218
Main Line Hospital Paoli[2]	Paoli	100%	674
Nazareth Hospital	Philadelphia	100%	243
Oss Orthopaedic Hospital[2]	York	100%	228
Penn Highlands Dubois	Dubois	100%	321
Physician's Care Surgical Hospital[2]	Royersford	100%	188
Pottstown Memorial Medical Center	Pottstown	100%	270
Punxsutawney Area Hospital	Punxsutawney	100%	60
Roxborough Memorial Hospital	Philadelphia	100%	50
Saint Luke's Hospital - Anderson Campus[2]	Easton	100%	34
Saint Luke's Quakertown Hospital	Quakertown	100%	65
Saint Vincent Hospital	Erie	100%	943
Soldiers & Sailors Memorial Hospital	Wellsboro	100%	103
Surgical Institute of Reading[2]	Wyomissing	100%	392
Titusville Hospital	Titusville	100%	64
Tyrone Hospital	Tyrone	100%	112
UPMC East[3]	Monroeville	100%	276
Wellspan Surgery & Rehab Hosp[2]	York	100%	217
York Hospital[2]	York	100%	774
Abington Memorial Hospital[2]	Abington	99%	512
Butler Memorial Hospital	Butler	99%	934
Carlisle Regional Medical Center	Carlisle	99%	394
Charles Cole Memorial Hospital	Coudersport	99%	221
Chester County Hospital	West Chester	99%	612
Conemaugh Valley Memorial Hospital	Johnstown	99%	947
Crozer Chester Medical Center[2]	Upland	99%	708
Easton Hospital	Easton	99%	406
Geisinger - Bloomsburg Hospital	Bloomsburg	99%	155
Geisinger - Community Medical Center[2]	Scranton	99%	425
Good Samaritan Hospital[2]	Lebanon	99%	304
Grand View Hospital[2]	Sellersville	99%	263
Grove City Medical Center	Grove City	99%	72
Heritage Valley Beaver[2]	Beaver	99%	471
Holy Spirit Hospital[2]	Camp Hill	99%	786
Lancaster Regional Medical Center	Lancaster	99%	432
Lehigh Valley Hospital - Hazleton	Hazleton	99%	113
Magee Womens Hosp of UPMC Health Sys	Pittsburgh	99%	1477
Meadville Medical Center[2]	Meadville	99%	610
Mercy Suburban Hospital	Norristown	99%	123
Millcreek Community Hospital	Erie	99%	87
Mount Nittany Medical Center	State College	99%	1230
Penn Highlands Elk	Saint Marys	99%	98
Penn Presbyterian Medical Center[2]	Philadelphia	99%	1472
Phoenixville Hospital	Phoenixville	99%	255
Pinnacle Health Hospitals[2]	Harrisburg	99%	2698
Reading Hospital[2]	Reading	99%	1241
Regional Hospital of Scranton	Scranton	99%	727
Riddle Memorial Hospital[2]	Media	99%	834
Sacred Heart Hospital	Allentown	99%	194
Saint Clair Memorial Hospital	Pittsburgh	99%	1134
Saint Joseph Medical Center[2]	Reading	99%	380
Saint Luke's Hospital Bethlehem[2]	Bethlehem	99%	1150
Saint Luke's Miners Memorial Hospital	Coaldale	99%	107
Saint Mary Medical Center	Langhorne	99%	999
Somerset Hospital	Somerset	99%	124
Surgical Specialty Ctr at Coord Hlth[2]	Allentown	99%	141
Temple University Hospital[2]	Philadelphia	99%	750
Thomas Jefferson University Hospital[2]	Philadelphia	99%	2339
UPMC Horizon	Greenville	99%	470
UPMC Mckeesport	Mc Keesport	99%	182
UPMC Northwest	Seneca	99%	221
UPMC Passavant	Pittsburgh	99%	1225
UPMC Presbyterian Shadyside	Pittsburgh	99%	2698
UPMC Saint Margaret	Pittsburgh	99%	1128
The Washington Hospital	Washington	99%	529
Waynesboro Hospital	Waynesboro	99%	102
Williamsport Regional Medical Center[2]	Williamsport	99%	939
Windber Hospital	Windber	99%	90
Acmh Hospital	Kittanning	98%	348
Berwick Hospital Center	Berwick	98%	102
Excela Health Latrobe Hospital	Latrobe	98%	343
Forbes Regional Hospital[2]	Monroeville	98%	598
Geisinger Medical Center[2]	Danville	98%	554
Geisinger Wyoming Valley Medical Center[2]	Wilkes Barre	98%	457
Heart of Lancaster Reg Med Ctr	Lititz	98%	51
Heritage Valley Sewickley[2]	Sewickley	98%	266
Jeanes Hospital	Philadelphia	98%	430
Lancaster General Hospital[2]	Lancaster	98%	1670
Lansdale Hospital[2]	Lansdale	98%	207
Mercy Fitzgerald Hospital	Darby	98%	269
Monongahela Valley Hospital	Monongahela	98%	375
Nason Hospital	Roaring Spring	98%	177
Pocono Medical Center	E Stroudsburg	98%	378
Robert Packer Hospital	Sayre	98%	883
Southwest Regional Medical Center	Waynesburg	98%	43
UPMC Mercy	Pittsburgh	98%	745
Warren General Hospital	Warren	98%	140
Western Pennsylvania Hospital	Pittsburgh	98%	274
Wilkes-Barre General Hospital	Wilkes-Barre	98%	826
Albert Einstein Medical Center[2]	Philadelphia	97%	483
Alle Kiski Medical Center	Natrona	97%	269
Allegheny General Hospital	Pittsburgh	97%	1187
Bradford Regional Medical Center	Bradford	97%	114
Einstein Medical Center Montgomery[2,3]	East Norriton	97%	269
Ephrata Community Hospital	Ephrata	97%	375
Evangelical Community Hospital[2]	Lewisburg	97%	316
Excela Health Westmoreland Hospital	Greensburg	97%	987
Gnaden Huetten Memorial Hospital	Lehighton	97%	64
Indiana Regional Medical Center	Indiana	97%	236
Jameson Memorial Hospital	New Castle	97%	304
Jefferson Regional Medical Center	Pittsburgh	97%	1084
Jennersville Regional Hospital	West Grove	97%	30
Lebanon VA Medical Center	Lebanon	97%	159
Memorial Hospital	York	97%	152
Milton S Hershey Medical Center[2]	Hershey	97%	1038
Moses Taylor Hospital	Scranton	97%	316
Palmerton Hospital	Palmerton	97%	72
Penn Highlands Clearfield	Clearfield	97%	154
Uniontown Hospital	Uniontown	97%	428
UPMC Altoona	Altoona	97%	1028
Brandywine Hospital	Coatesville	96%	197
Delaware County Memorial Hospital[2]	Drexel Hill	96%	327
Hahnemann University Hospital[2]	Philadelphia	96%	420
Lehigh Valley Hospital - Muhlenberg	Bethlehem	96%	359
Ohio Valley General Hospital	Mckees Rocks	96%	127
Schuylkill Med Ctr-S Jackson St	Pottsville	96%	145
UPMC Bedford Memorial	Everett	96%	77
UPMC Hamot[2]	Erie	96%	1114
VA Pittsburgh Healthcare System	Pittsburgh	96%	399
Wilkes Barre VA Medical Center	Wilkes-Barre	96%	51
Canonsburg General Hospital	Canonsburg	95%	198
Sharon Regional Health System	Sharon	95%	414
Chambersburg Hospital[2]	Chambersburg	94%	539
Penn Hosp of the Univ of PA Hlth Sys[2]	Philadelphia	94%	402
Wayne Memorial Hospital	Honesdale	94%	173
Lewistown Hospital	Lewistown	93%	119
Clarion Hospital	Clarion	92%	112
J C Blair Memorial Hospital	Huntingdon	92%	62
Schuylkill Med Ctr-East Norwegian St	Pottsville	92%	123
Jersey Shore Hospital	Jersey Shore	91%	33
Cancer Treatment Centers of America	Philadelphia	89%	38
Ellwood City Hospital[2]	Ellwood City	88%	75
Philadelphia VA Medical Center	Philadelphia	83%	35

Prophylactic Antibiotic Timing

Hospital Name	City	Rate	Cases
Advanced Surgical Hospital	Washington	100%	384
Albert Einstein Medical Center[2]	Philadelphia	100%	487
Alle Kiski Medical Center	Natrona	100%	282
Brandywine Hospital	Coatesville	100%	199
Bucks County Specialty Hospital[2]	Bensalem	100%	148
Carlisle Regional Medical Center	Carlisle	100%	403
Chambersburg Hospital[2]	Chambersburg	100%	556
Chester County Hospital	West Chester	100%	628
Delaware County Memorial Hospital[2]	Drexel Hill	100%	333
Doylestown Hospital[2]	Doylestown	100%	737
Excela Health Frick Hospital	Mount Pleasant	100%	27
Excela Health Latrobe Hospital	Latrobe	100%	347
Excela Health Westmoreland Hospital	Greensburg	100%	998
Forbes Regional Hospital[2]	Monroeville	100%	609
Gettysburg Hospital	Gettysburg	100%	295
Grand View Hospital[2]	Sellersville	100%	272
Heart of Lancaster Reg Med Ctr	Lititz	100%	52
Holy Redeemer Hospital & Medical Center	Meadowbrook	100%	621
Holy Spirit Hospital[2]	Camp Hill	100%	822
Hospital of Univ of Pennsylvania[2]	Philadelphia	100%	576
Indiana Regional Medical Center	Indiana	100%	244
Jeanes Hospital	Philadelphia	100%	440
Jennersville Regional Hospital	West Grove	100%	31
Lancaster Regional Medical Center	Lancaster	100%	448
Lansdale Hospital[2]	Lansdale	100%	213
Lehigh Valley Hospital	Allentown	100%	2298
Lewistown Hospital	Lewistown	100%	125
Magee Womens Hosp of UPMC Health Sys	Pittsburgh	100%	1480
Main Line Hospital Bryn Mawr Campus[2]	Bryn Mawr	100%	1323
Main Line Hospital Lankenau[2]	Wynnewood	100%	1248
Main Line Hospital Paoli[2]	Paoli	100%	729
Mercy Fitzgerald Hospital	Darby	100%	278
Mercy Suburban Hospital	Norristown	100%	125
Monongahela Valley Hospital	Monongahela	100%	385
Nazareth Hospital	Philadelphia	100%	252
Palmerton Hospital	Palmerton	100%	74
Penn Highlands Dubois	Dubois	100%	330
Pinnacle Health Hospitals[2]	Harrisburg	100%	2764
Punxsutawney Area Hospital	Punxsutawney	100%	62
Reading Hospital[2]	Reading	100%	1259
Regional Hospital of Scranton	Scranton	100%	744
Roxborough Memorial Hospital	Philadelphia	100%	52
Saint Clair Memorial Hospital	Pittsburgh	100%	1150
Saint Luke's Hospital - Anderson Campus[2]	Easton	100%	36
Saint Luke's Hospital Bethlehem[2]	Bethlehem	100%	1184
Saint Luke's Miners Memorial Hospital	Coaldale	100%	108
Saint Luke's Quakertown Hospital	Quakertown	100%	66

NOTE: Hospital profiles are in alphabetical order by state, then city, then hospital within the city; Rankings exclude hospitals with less than 25 cases except for patient surveys which excludes hospitals with less than 100 cases; (a) 100-299 cases; (1) The number of cases/patients is too few to report; (2) Data submitted were based on a sample of cases/patients; (3) Results are based on a shorter time period than required; (4) Data suppressed by CMS for one or more quarters; (5) Results are not available for this reporting period; (6) Fewer than 100 patients completed the HCAHPS survey; (7) No cases met the criteria for this measure; (8) The lower limit of the confidence interval cannot be calculated if the number of observed infections equals zero; (9) No data are available from the state/territory for this reporting period; (10) The scores shown reflect fewer than 50 completed surveys; (11) There were discrepancies in the data collection process; (12) This measure does not apply to this hospital for this reporting period; (13) Results cannot be calculated for this reporting period; (14) The results for this state are combined with nearby states to protect confidentiality; Please refer to the User's Guide for a full explanation of data.

Saint Mary Medical Center	Langhorne	100%	1012
Sharon Regional Health System	Sharon	100%	421
Southwest Regional Medical Center	Waynesburg	100%	46
Temple University Hospital[2]	Philadelphia	100%	804
Thomas Jefferson University Hospital[2]	Philadelphia	100%	2364
Tyrone Hospital	Tyrone	100%	112
UPMC Bedford Memorial	Everett	100%	79
UPMC East[3]	Monroeville	100%	280
UPMC Hamot[2]	Erie	100%	1128
UPMC Horizon	Greenville	100%	478
UPMC Mckeesport	Mc Keesport	100%	186
UPMC Presbyterian Shadyside	Pittsburgh	100%	2755
UPMC Saint Margaret	Pittsburgh	100%	1150
The Washington Hospital	Washington	100%	549
Wellspan Surgery & Rehab Hosp[2]	York	100%	217
Western Pennsylvania Hospital	Pittsburgh	100%	278
York Hospital[2]	York	100%	833
Abington Memorial Hospital[2]	Abington	99%	521
Acmh Hospital	Kittanning	99%	350
Allegheny General Hospital	Pittsburgh	99%	1218
Aria Health	Philadelphia	99%	910
Berwick Hospital Center	Berwick	99%	104
Butler Memorial Hospital	Butler	99%	977
Charles Cole Memorial Hospital	Coudersport	99%	221
Conemaugh Valley Memorial Hospital	Johnstown	99%	961
Coordinated Health Orthopedic Hospital[2]	Bethlehem	99%	145
Einstein Medical Center Montgomery[2,3]	East Norriton	99%	273
Geisinger - Bloomsburg Hospital	Bloomsburg	99%	158
Geisinger - Community Medical Center[2]	Scranton	99%	435
Geisinger Medical Center[2]	Danville	99%	561
Gnaden Huetten Memorial Hospital	Lehighton	99%	73
Good Samaritan Hospital[2]	Lebanon	99%	318
Heritage Valley Beaver[2]	Beaver	99%	481
Heritage Valley Sewickley[2]	Sewickley	99%	274
Jameson Memorial Hospital	New Castle	99%	313
Jefferson Regional Medical Center	Pittsburgh	99%	1102
Memorial Hospital	York	99%	156
Milton S Hershey Medical Center[2]	Hershey	99%	1078
Moses Taylor Hospital	Scranton	99%	325
Mount Nittany Medical Center	State College	99%	1251
Nason Hospital	Roaring Spring	99%	180
Oss Orthopaedic Hospital[2]	York	99%	230
Penn Highlands Clearfield	Clearfield	99%	154
Penn Highlands Elk	Saint Marys	99%	101
Penn Presbyterian Medical Center[2]	Philadelphia	99%	1514
Phoenixville Hospital	Phoenixville	99%	267
Pocono Medical Center	E Stroudsburg	99%	398
Pottstown Memorial Medical Center	Pottstown	99%	288
Riddle Memorial Hospital[2]	Media	99%	849
Robert Packer Hospital	Sayre	99%	891
Sacred Heart Hospital	Allentown	99%	199
Saint Joseph Medical Center[2]	Reading	99%	388
Saint Vincent Hospital	Erie	99%	958
Schuylkill Med Ctr-East Norwegian St	Pottsville	99%	129
Schuylkill Med Ctr-S Jackson St	Pottsville	99%	147
Uniontown Hospital	Uniontown	99%	444
UPMC Altoona	Altoona	99%	1049
UPMC Mercy	Pittsburgh	99%	763
UPMC Passavant	Pittsburgh	99%	1253
Wayne Memorial Hospital	Honesdale	99%	175
Wilkes-Barre General Hospital	Wilkes-Barre	99%	841
Williamsport Regional Medical Center[2]	Williamsport	99%	955
Chestnut Hill Hospital	Philadelphia	98%	120
Crozer Chester Medical Center[2]	Upland	98%	719
Easton Hospital	Easton	98%	418
Ephrata Community Hospital	Ephrata	98%	397
Evangelical Community Hospital[2]	Lewisburg	98%	317
Hanover Hospital	Hanover	98%	363
J C Blair Memorial Hospital	Huntingdon	98%	62
Lancaster General Hospital[2]	Lancaster	98%	1702
Lehigh Valley Hospital - Hazleton	Hazleton	98%	131
Lehigh Valley Hospital - Muhlenberg	Bethlehem	98%	368
Lower Bucks Hospital	Bristol	98%	45
Millcreek Community Hospital	Erie	98%	95
Penn Hosp of the Univ of PA Hlth Sys[2]	Philadelphia	98%	413
Soldiers & Sailors Memorial Hospital	Wellsboro	98%	105
Somerset Hospital	Somerset	98%	133
UPMC Northwest	Seneca	98%	224
VA Pittsburgh Healthcare System	Pittsburgh	98%	414
Wilkes Barre VA Medical Center	Wilkes-Barre	98%	53
Clarion Hospital	Clarion	97%	114
Geisinger Wyoming Valley Medical Center[2]	Wilkes Barre	97%	472
Hahnemann University Hospital[2]	Philadelphia	97%	431
Lebanon VA Medical Center	Lebanon	97%	160
Meadville Medical Center[2]	Meadville	97%	614
Ohio Valley General Hospital	Mckees Rocks	97%	130
Surgical Institute of Reading[2]	Wyomissing	97%	392
Surgical Specialty Ctr at Coord Hlth[2]	Allentown	97%	141
Warren General Hospital	Warren	97%	147
Waynesboro Hospital	Waynesboro	97%	107
Windber Hospital	Windber	97%	94
Bradford Regional Medical Center	Bradford	96%	115
Edgewood Surgical Hospital	Transfer	96%	102
Grove City Medical Center	Grove City	96%	76
Physician's Care Surgical Hospital[2]	Royersford	96%	190
Canonsburg General Hospital	Canonsburg	95%	202
Philadelphia VA Medical Center	Philadelphia	95%	37
Titusville Hospital	Titusville	94%	71
Ellwood City Hospital[2]	Ellwood City	92%	75
Jersey Shore Hospital	Jersey Shore	91%	33
Cancer Treatment Centers of America	Philadelphia	86%	49
Endless Mountains Health Systems	Montrose	85%	97

Prophylactic Antibiotic Timing (Outpatient)

Hospital Name	City	Rate	Cases
Acmh Hospital	Kittanning	100%	49
Berwick Hospital Center	Berwick	100%	33
Bucks County Specialty Hospital	Bensalem	100%	97
Chester County Hospital	West Chester	100%	308
Chestnut Hill Hospital	Philadelphia	100%	47
Einstein Medical Center Montgomery[3]	East Norriton	100%	175
Ephrata Community Hospital	Ephrata	100%	262
Heart of Lancaster Reg Med Ctr	Lititz	100%	260
Holy Spirit Hospital	Camp Hill	100%	602
Lansdale Hospital	Lansdale	100%	83
Magee Womens Hosp of UPMC Health Sys	Pittsburgh	100%	661
Nazareth Hospital	Philadelphia	100%	88
Penn Highlands Clearfield	Clearfield	100%	67
Pinnacle Health Hospitals	Harrisburg	100%	1331
Pocono Medical Center	E Stroudsburg	100%	315
Saint Joseph Medical Center	Reading	100%	308
Saint Luke's Quakertown Hospital	Quakertown	100%	31
Sharon Regional Health System	Sharon	100%	127
Somerset Hospital	Somerset	100%	37
Sunbury Community Hospital	Sunbury	100%	33
Surgical Specialty Ctr at Coord Hlth	Allentown	100%	82
UPMC Bedford Memorial	Everett	100%	39
UPMC East[3]	Monroeville	100%	45
UPMC Passavant	Pittsburgh	100%	613
Warren General Hospital	Warren	100%	29
The Washington Hospital	Washington	100%	232
Western Pennsylvania Hospital	Pittsburgh	100%	340
Alle Kiski Medical Center	Natrona	99%	196
Allegheny General Hospital	Pittsburgh	99%	648
Aria Health	Philadelphia	99%	145
Butler Memorial Hospital	Butler	99%	369
Carlisle Regional Medical Center	Carlisle	99%	196
Chambersburg Hospital	Chambersburg	99%	397
Conemaugh Valley Memorial Hospital	Johnstown	99%	432
Excela Health Latrobe Hospital	Latrobe	99%	286
Excela Health Westmoreland Hospital	Greensburg	99%	210
Forbes Regional Hospital	Monroeville	99%	387
Good Samaritan Hospital	Lebanon	99%	419
Grove City Medical Center	Grove City	99%	89
Hahnemann University Hospital	Philadelphia	99%	408
Heritage Valley Beaver	Beaver	99%	185
Indiana Regional Medical Center	Indiana	99%	115
Lancaster Regional Medical Center	Lancaster	99%	218
Lehigh Valley Hospital	Allentown	99%	1041
Milton S Hershey Medical Center	Hershey	99%	1060
Moses Taylor Hospital	Scranton	99%	98
Oss Orthopaedic Hospital	York	99%	291
Penn Highlands Dubois	Dubois	99%	162
Reading Hospital	Reading	99%	933
Riddle Memorial Hospital	Media	99%	142
Robert Packer Hospital	Sayre	99%	567
Saint Clair Memorial Hospital	Pittsburgh	99%	360
Saint Luke's Hospital Bethlehem	Bethlehem	99%	710
Saint Mary Medical Center	Langhorne	99%	355
Temple University Hospital	Philadelphia	99%	362
Thomas Jefferson University Hospital	Philadelphia	99%	460
Uniontown Hospital	Uniontown	99%	194
UPMC Altoona	Altoona	99%	882
UPMC Hamot	Erie	99%	793
UPMC Mercy	Pittsburgh	99%	384
UPMC Presbyterian Shadyside	Pittsburgh	99%	1042
UPMC Saint Margaret	Pittsburgh	99%	231
Wellspan Surgery & Rehab Hosp	York	99%	119
Abington Memorial Hospital	Abington	98%	423
Albert Einstein Medical Center	Philadelphia	98%	314
Crozer Chester Medical Center	Upland	98%	366
Doylestown Hospital	Doylestown	98%	332
Easton Hospital	Easton	98%	251
Geisinger - Community Medical Center	Scranton	98%	444
Gettysburg Hospital	Gettysburg	98%	104
Grand View Hospital	Sellersville	98%	123
Hanover Hospital	Hanover	98%	123
Jeanes Hospital	Philadelphia	98%	95
Jefferson Regional Medical Center	Pittsburgh	98%	332
Main Line Hospital Bryn Mawr Campus	Bryn Mawr	98%	269
Mercy Suburban Hospital	Norristown	98%	65
Pottstown Memorial Medical Center	Pottstown	98%	91
Saint Vincent Hospital	Erie	98%	325
Surgical Institute of Reading	Wyomissing	98%	177
UPMC Horizon	Greenville	98%	226
Williamsport Regional Medical Center	Williamsport	98%	590
Windber Hospital	Windber	98%	40
Brandywine Hospital	Coatesville	97%	116
Evangelical Community Hospital	Lewisburg	97%	250
Geisinger Wyoming Valley Medical Center	Wilkes Barre	97%	508
Jameson Memorial Hospital	New Castle	97%	121
Lehigh Valley Hospital - Muhlenberg	Bethlehem	97%	355
Penn Presbyterian Medical Center	Philadelphia	97%	318
Penn Hosp of the Univ of PA Hlth Sys	Philadelphia	97%	429
Sacred Heart Hospital	Allentown	97%	34
Saint Luke's Hospital - Anderson Campus	Easton	97%	61
Schuylkill Med Ctr-S Jackson St	Pottsville	97%	203
Soldiers & Sailors Memorial Hospital	Wellsboro	97%	38
Wilkes-Barre General Hospital	Wilkes-Barre	97%	545
York Hospital	York	97%	684
Lancaster General Hospital	Lancaster	96%	1370
Monongahela Valley Hospital	Monongahela	96%	67
Penn Highlands Elk	Saint Marys	96%	114
Regional Hospital of Scranton	Scranton	96%	404
UPMC Northwest	Seneca	96%	83
Coordinated Health Orthopedic Hospital	Bethlehem	95%	37
Geisinger Medical Center	Danville	95%	779
Gnaden Huetten Memorial Hospital	Lehighton	95%	55
Main Line Hospital Lankenau	Wynnewood	95%	360
Main Line Hospital Paoli	Paoli	95%	208
Ohio Valley General Hospital	Mckees Rocks	95%	56
Phoenixville Hospital	Phoenixville	95%	129
Heritage Valley Sewickley	Sewickley	94%	84
Hospital of Univ of Pennsylvania	Philadelphia	94%	631
Lewistown Hospital	Lewistown	94%	100
Meadville Medical Center	Meadville	94%	192
Mount Nittany Medical Center	State College	94%	299
Wayne Memorial Hospital	Honesdale	94%	34
Clarion Hospital	Clarion	93%	68
J C Blair Memorial Hospital	Huntingdon	92%	64
Delaware County Memorial Hospital	Drexel Hill	91%	53
Lehigh Valley Hospital - Hazleton	Hazleton	91%	56
UPMC Mckeesport	Mc Keesport	91%	65
Mercy Fitzgerald Hospital	Darby	90%	67
Memorial Hospital	York	89%	178
Holy Redeemer Hospital & Medical Center	Meadowbrook	82%	85
Punxsutawney Area Hospital	Punxsutawney	77%	26
Palmerton Hospital	Palmerton	53%	30

Urinary Catheter Removal

Hospital Name	City	Rate	Cases
Advanced Surgical Hospital	Washington	100%	195
Aria Health	Philadelphia	100%	1139
Bucks County Specialty Hospital[2]	Bensalem	100%	26
Butler Memorial Hospital	Butler	100%	461
Charles Cole Memorial Hospital	Coudersport	100%	218
Chester County Hospital	West Chester	100%	597
Chestnut Hill Hospital	Philadelphia	100%	108
Evangelical Community Hospital[2]	Lewisburg	100%	390
Good Samaritan Hospital[2]	Lebanon	100%	277
Grand View Hospital[2]	Sellersville	100%	64
Heart of Lancaster Reg Med Ctr	Lititz	100%	65
Highlands Hospital	Connellsville	100%	32
Hospital of Univ of Pennsylvania[2]	Philadelphia	100%	463
Jersey Shore Hospital	Jersey Shore	100%	38
Lancaster Regional Medical Center	Lancaster	100%	434
Lehigh Valley Hospital - Hazleton	Hazleton	100%	104
Lewistown Hospital	Lewistown	100%	99
Magee Womens Hosp of UPMC Health Sys	Pittsburgh	100%	1289
Main Line Hospital Paoli[2]	Paoli	100%	384
Memorial Hospital	York	100%	95
Mercy Suburban Hospital	Norristown	100%	68
Milton S Hershey Medical Center[2]	Hershey	100%	978
Oss Orthopaedic Hospital[2]	York	100%	106
Penn Presbyterian Medical Center[2]	Philadelphia	100%	1395
Physician's Care Surgical Hospital[2]	Royersford	100%	119
Pinnacle Health Hospitals[2]	Harrisburg	100%	1303
Roxborough Memorial Hospital	Philadelphia	100%	65
Saint Clair Memorial Hospital	Pittsburgh	100%	542
Saint Joseph Medical Center[2]	Reading	100%	328
Saint Luke's Hospital - Anderson Campus[2]	Easton	100%	57
Saint Luke's Hospital Bethlehem[2]	Bethlehem	100%	1110
Saint Luke's Miners Memorial Hospital	Coaldale	100%	115
Saint Mary Medical Center	Langhorne	100%	997
Somerset Hospital	Somerset	100%	70
Sunbury Community Hospital	Sunbury	100%	77
Temple University Hospital[2]	Philadelphia	100%	435
UPMC Bedford Memorial	Everett	100%	42
UPMC East[3]	Monroeville	100%	246
UPMC Mckeesport	Mc Keesport	100%	90
UPMC Mercy	Pittsburgh	100%	713
UPMC Presbyterian Shadyside	Pittsburgh	100%	4191
UPMC Saint Margaret	Pittsburgh	100%	1249

NOTE: Hospital profiles are in alphabetical order by state, then city, then hospital within the city; Rankings exclude hospitals with less than 25 cases except for patient surveys which excludes hospitals with less than 100 cases; (a) 100-299 cases; (1) The number of cases/patients is too few to report; (2) Data submitted were based on a sample of cases/patients; (3) Results are based on a shorter time period than required; (4) Data suppressed by CMS for one or more quarters; (5) Results are not available for this reporting period; (6) Fewer than 100 patients completed the HCAHPS survey; (7) No cases met the criteria for this measure; (8) The lower limit of the confidence interval cannot be calculated if the number of observed infections equals zero; (9) No data are available from the state/territory for this reporting period; (10) The scores shown reflect fewer than 50 completed surveys; (11) There were discrepancies in the data collection process; (12) This measure does not apply to this hospital for this reporting period; (13) Results cannot be calculated for this reporting period; (14) The results for this state are combined with nearby states to protect confidentiality; Please refer to the User's Guide for a full explanation of data.

Hospital Name	City	Rate	Cases
VA Pittsburgh Healthcare System[2]	Pittsburgh	100%	401
The Washington Hospital	Washington	100%	285
Waynesboro Hospital	Waynesboro	100%	51
Western Pennsylvania Hospital	Pittsburgh	100%	180
Wilkes-Barre General Hospital	Wilkes-Barre	100%	730
Williamsport Regional Medical Center[2]	Williamsport	100%	839
Abington Memorial Hospital[2]	Abington	99%	282
Albert Einstein Medical Center[2]	Philadelphia	99%	472
Allegheny General Hospital	Pittsburgh	99%	1805
Crozer Chester Medical Center[2]	Upland	99%	628
Geisinger Medical Center[2]	Danville	99%	367
Hanover Hospital	Hanover	99%	359
Holy Redeemer Hospital & Medical Center	Meadowbrook	99%	560
Indiana Regional Medical Center	Indiana	99%	222
Lancaster General Hospital[2]	Lancaster	99%	1821
Lebanon VA Medical Center[2]	Lebanon	99%	101
Lehigh Valley Hospital	Allentown	99%	1999
Main Line Hospital Bryn Mawr Campus[2]	Bryn Mawr	99%	186
Main Line Hospital Lankenau[2]	Wynnewood	99%	688
Mercy Fitzgerald Hospital	Darby	99%	338
Moses Taylor Hospital	Scranton	99%	272
Nazareth Hospital	Philadelphia	99%	271
Penn Highlands Dubois	Dubois	99%	268
Penn Highlands Elk	Saint Marys	99%	78
Penn Hosp of the Univ of PA Hlth Sys[2]	Philadelphia	99%	382
Pottstown Memorial Medical Center	Pottstown	99%	345
Reading Hospital[2]	Reading	99%	1147
Riddle Memorial Hospital[2]	Media	99%	904
Sacred Heart Hospital	Allentown	99%	74
Saint Vincent Hospital	Erie	99%	1075
Surgical Institute of Reading[2]	Wyomissing	99%	395
UPMC Hamot[2]	Erie	99%	1062
UPMC Northwest	Seneca	99%	128
UPMC Passavant	Pittsburgh	99%	1014
York Hospital[2]	York	99%	703
Acmh Hospital	Kittanning	98%	192
Carlisle Regional Medical Center	Carlisle	98%	91
Delaware County Memorial Hospital[2]	Drexel Hill	98%	313
Doylestown Hospital[2]	Doylestown	98%	678
Easton Hospital	Easton	98%	311
Ephrata Community Hospital	Ephrata	98%	480
Excela Health Westmoreland Hospital	Greensburg	98%	881
Geisinger Wyoming Valley Medical Center[2]	Wilkes Barre	98%	476
Gettysburg Hospital	Gettysburg	98%	104
Gnaden Huetten Memorial Hospital	Lehighton	98%	86
Grove City Medical Center	Grove City	98%	63
Hahnemann University Hospital[2]	Philadelphia	98%	325
Heritage Valley Beaver[2]	Beaver	98%	403
Holy Spirit Hospital[2]	Camp Hill	98%	495
Jeanes Hospital	Philadelphia	98%	294
Jennersville Regional Hospital	West Grove	98%	66
Lower Bucks Hospital	Bristol	98%	57
Palmerton Hospital	Palmerton	98%	83
Pocono Medical Center	E Stroudsburg	98%	426
Punxsutawney Area Hospital	Punxsutawney	98%	52
UPMC Horizon	Greenville	98%	125
Wayne Memorial Hospital	Honesdale	98%	192
Wilkes Barre VA Medical Center[2]	Wilkes-Barre	98%	57
Conemaugh Valley Memorial Hospital	Johnstown	97%	459
Excela Health Latrobe Hospital	Latrobe	97%	205
Forbes Regional Hospital[2]	Monroeville	97%	669
Geisinger - Bloomsburg Hospital	Bloomsburg	97%	103
Jameson Memorial Hospital	New Castle	97%	145
Lehigh Valley Hospital - Muhlenberg	Bethlehem	97%	281
Meadville Medical Center[2]	Meadville	97%	580
Millcreek Community Hospital	Erie	97%	33
Monongahela Valley Hospital	Monongahela	97%	176
Phoenixville Hospital	Phoenixville	97%	202
Saint Luke's Quakertown Hospital	Quakertown	97%	38
Soldiers & Sailors Memorial Hospital	Wellsboro	97%	97
Surgical Specialty Ctr at Coord Hlth[2]	Allentown	97%	153
Alle Kiski Medical Center	Natrona	96%	322
Chambersburg Hospital[2]	Chambersburg	96%	566
Einstein Medical Center Montgomery[2,3]	East Norriton	96%	134
Heritage Valley Sewickley[2]	Sewickley	96%	257
Schuylkill Med Ctr-East Norwegian St	Pottsville	96%	127
Sharon Regional Health System	Sharon	96%	296
Southwest Regional Medical Center	Waynesburg	96%	55
Thomas Jefferson University Hospital[2]	Philadelphia	96%	734
Titusville Hospital	Titusville	96%	51
Warren General Hospital	Warren	96%	90
Windber Hospital	Windber	96%	56
Excela Health Frick Hospital	Mount Pleasant	95%	38
Geisinger - Community Medical Center[2]	Scranton	95%	295
Jefferson Regional Medical Center	Pittsburgh	95%	1065
Robert Packer Hospital	Sayre	95%	329
Schuylkill Med Ctr-S Jackson St	Pottsville	95%	102
Uniontown Hospital	Uniontown	95%	254
Brandywine Hospital	Coatesville	94%	178
Clarion Hospital	Clarion	94%	124
Nason Hospital	Roaring Spring	94%	35
Canonsburg General Hospital	Canonsburg	93%	74
Coordinated Health Orthopedic Hospital[2]	Bethlehem	93%	181
Penn Highlands Clearfield	Clearfield	93%	76
Mount Nittany Medical Center	State College	92%	595
Ohio Valley General Hospital	Mckees Rocks	91%	64
Cancer Treatment Centers of America	Philadelphia	89%	53
UPMC Altoona	Altoona	88%	284
Lansdale Hospital[2]	Lansdale	87%	55
Berwick Hospital Center	Berwick	86%	37
Ellwood City Hospital[2]	Ellwood City	86%	29
Regional Hospital of Scranton	Scranton	85%	162
Philadelphia VA Medical Center[2]	Philadelphia	80%	60
J C Blair Memorial Hospital	Huntingdon	54%	28

Survey of Patients' Hospital Experiences

Area Around Room 'Always' Quiet at Night

Hospital Name	City	Rate	Cases
Physician's Care Surgical Hospital	Royersford	87%	300+
Advanced Surgical Hospital	Washington	86%	(a)
Bucks County Specialty Hospital	Bensalem	84%	300+
Surgical Specialty Ctr at Coord Hlth	Allentown	84%	300+
Surgical Institute of Reading	Wyomissing	82%	(a)
Oss Orthopaedic Hospital	York	80%	300+
Wellspan Surgery & Rehab Hosp	York	79%	(a)
Coordinated Health Orthopedic Hospital	Bethlehem	78%	300+
Mid - Valley Hospital	Peckville	71%	(a)
Titusville Hospital	Titusville	68%	300+
Corry Memorial Hospital	Corry	66%	(a)
Sacred Heart Hospital	Allentown	66%	300+
Tyrone Hospital	Tyrone	65%	(a)
Ellwood City Hospital	Ellwood City	64%	300+
Lansdale Hospital	Lansdale	64%	300+
Monongahela Valley Hospital	Monongahela	64%	300+
J C Blair Memorial Hospital	Huntingdon	62%	300+
Western Pennsylvania Hospital	Pittsburgh	62%	300+
Lock Haven Hospital	Lock Haven	61%	(a)
Phoenixville Hospital	Phoenixville	61%	300+
UPMC Bedford Memorial	Everett	61%	300+
UPMC East	Monroeville	61%	300+
Einstein Medical Center Montgomery	East Norriton	60%	300+
Jersey Shore Hospital	Jersey Shore	60%	(a)
Chambersburg Hospital	Chambersburg	58%	300+
Hahnemann University Hospital	Philadelphia	58%	300+
Penn Highlands Dubois	Dubois	58%	300+
Saint Luke's Miners Memorial Hospital	Coaldale	58%	300+
Delaware County Memorial Hospital	Drexel Hill	57%	300+
Excela Health Frick Hospital	Mount Pleasant	57%	300+
Heritage Valley Sewickley	Sewickley	57%	300+
Jennersville Regional Hospital	West Grove	57%	300+
Saint Joseph's Hospital	Philadelphia	57%	(a)
Saint Luke's Quakertown Hospital	Quakertown	57%	300+
Albert Einstein Medical Center	Philadelphia	56%	300+
Berwick Hospital Center	Berwick	56%	300+
Brandywine Hospital	Coatesville	56%	300+
Cancer Treatment Centers of America	Philadelphia	56%	(a)
Charles Cole Memorial Hospital	Coudersport	56%	300+
Chester County Hospital	West Chester	56%	300+
Easton Hospital	Easton	56%	300+
Geisinger - Bloomsburg Hospital	Bloomsburg	56%	300+
Heart of Lancaster Reg Med Ctr	Lititz	56%	300+
Main Line Hospital Lankenau	Wynnewood	56%	300+
Memorial Hospital Towanda	Towanda	56%	300+
Nason Hospital	Roaring Spring	56%	300+
Penn Highlands Elk	Saint Marys	56%	300+
Regional Hospital of Scranton	Scranton	56%	300+
Roxborough Memorial Hospital	Philadelphia	56%	(a)
Uniontown Hospital	Uniontown	56%	300+
UPMC Mckeesport	Mc Keesport	56%	300+
Carlisle Regional Medical Center	Carlisle	55%	300+
Chestnut Hill Hospital	Philadelphia	55%	300+
Excela Health Latrobe Hospital	Latrobe	55%	300+
Jefferson Regional Medical Center	Pittsburgh	55%	300+
Penn Presbyterian Medical Center	Philadelphia	55%	300+
Geisinger - Community Medical Center	Scranton	54%	300+
Gnaden Huetten Memorial Hospital	Lehighton	54%	300+
Grand View Hospital	Sellersville	54%	300+
Main Line Hospital Paoli	Paoli	54%	300+
Millcreek Community Hospital	Erie	54%	(a)
Muncy Valley Hospital	Muncy	54%	(a)
Riddle Memorial Hospital	Media	54%	300+
The Washington Hospital	Washington	54%	300+
Williamsport Regional Medical Center	Williamsport	54%	300+
Clarion Hospital	Clarion	53%	300+
Doylestown Hospital	Doylestown	53%	300+
Magee Womens Hosp of UPMC Health Sys	Pittsburgh	53%	300+
Mercy Fitzgerald Hospital	Darby	53%	300+
Mount Nittany Medical Center	State College	53%	300+
Palmerton Hospital	Palmerton	53%	300+
Pocono Medical Center	E Stroudsburg	53%	300+
Punxsutawney Area Hospital	Punxsutawney	53%	300+
Saint Joseph Medical Center	Reading	53%	300+
Saint Luke's Hospital - Anderson Campus	Easton	53%	300+
Saint Vincent Hospital	Erie	53%	300+
Schuylkill Med Ctr-S Jackson St	Pottsville	53%	300+
Temple University Hospital	Philadelphia	53%	300+
Thomas Jefferson University Hospital	Philadelphia	53%	300+
Waynesboro Hospital	Waynesboro	53%	300+
Canonsburg General Hospital	Canonsburg	52%	300+
Fulton County Medical Center	Mcconnellsburg	52%	(a)
Geisinger Medical Center	Danville	52%	300+
Gettysburg Hospital	Gettysburg	52%	300+
Hanover Hospital	Hanover	52%	300+
Holy Redeemer Hospital & Medical Center	Meadowbrook	52%	300+
Kane Community Hospital	Kane	52%	(a)
Main Line Hospital Bryn Mawr Campus	Bryn Mawr	52%	300+
Meadville Medical Center	Meadville	52%	300+
Moses Taylor Hospital	Scranton	52%	300+
Tyler Memorial Hospital	Tunkhannock	52%	300+
UPMC Altoona	Altoona	52%	300+
UPMC Mercy	Pittsburgh	52%	300+
Wayne Memorial Hospital	Honesdale	52%	300+
Windber Hospital	Windber	52%	300+
Barnes-Kasson County Hospital	Susquehanna	51%	(a)
Lancaster Regional Medical Center	Lancaster	51%	300+
Lehigh Valley Hospital - Muhlenberg	Bethlehem	51%	300+
Memorial Hospital	York	51%	300+
Ohio Valley General Hospital	Mckees Rocks	51%	300+
Penn Hosp of the Univ of PA Hlth Sys	Philadelphia	51%	300+
Soldiers & Sailors Memorial Hospital	Wellsboro	51%	300+
UPMC Presbyterian Shadyside	Pittsburgh	51%	300+
Wilkes-Barre General Hospital	Wilkes-Barre	51%	300+
Butler Memorial Hospital	Butler	50%	300+
Good Samaritan Hospital	Lebanon	50%	300+
Indiana Regional Medical Center	Indiana	50%	300+
Pinnacle Health Hospitals	Harrisburg	50%	300+
Saint Luke's Hospital Bethlehem	Bethlehem	50%	300+
UPMC Horizon	Greenville	50%	300+
UPMC Passavant	Pittsburgh	50%	300+
Warren General Hospital	Warren	50%	300+
Geisinger Wyoming Valley Medical Center	Wilkes Barre	49%	300+
Holy Spirit Hospital	Camp Hill	49%	300+
Nazareth Hospital	Philadelphia	49%	300+
Saint Mary Medical Center	Langhorne	49%	300+
Schuylkill Med Ctr-East Norwegian St	Pottsville	49%	300+
Southwest Regional Medical Center	Waynesburg	49%	300+
Sunbury Community Hospital	Sunbury	49%	(a)
UPMC Northwest	Seneca	49%	300+
Abington Memorial Hospital	Abington	48%	300+
Conemaugh Valley Memorial Hospital	Johnstown	48%	300+
Crozer Chester Medical Center	Upland	48%	300+
Lancaster General Hospital	Lancaster	48%	300+
Milton S Hershey Medical Center	Hershey	48%	300+
Penn Highlands Clearfield	Clearfield	48%	300+
Pottstown Memorial Medical Center	Pottstown	48%	300+
Sharon Regional Health System	Sharon	48%	300+
Alle Kiski Medical Center	Natrona	47%	300+
Excela Health Westmoreland Hospital	Greensburg	47%	300+
Grove City Medical Center	Grove City	47%	300+
Hospital of Univ of Pennsylvania	Philadelphia	47%	300+
Jeanes Hospital	Philadelphia	47%	300+
Lewistown Hospital	Lewistown	47%	300+
Allegheny General Hospital	Pittsburgh	46%	300+
Endless Mountains Health Systems	Montrose	46%	300+
Evangelical Community Hospital	Lewisburg	46%	300+
Jameson Memorial Hospital	New Castle	46%	300+
Lehigh Valley Hospital	Allentown	46%	300+
Lehigh Valley Hospital - Hazleton	Hazleton	46%	300+
Lower Bucks Hospital	Bristol	46%	(a)
Robert Packer Hospital	Sayre	46%	300+
UPMC Hamot	Erie	46%	300+
Acmh Hospital	Kittanning	45%	300+
Aria Health	Philadelphia	45%	300+
Ephrata Community Hospital	Ephrata	45%	300+
Saint Clair Memorial Hospital	Pittsburgh	45%	300+
Forbes Regional Hospital	Monroeville	44%	300+
Mercy Suburban Hospital	Norristown	44%	300+
Reading Hospital	Reading	44%	300+
Bradford Regional Medical Center	Bradford	43%	300+
Heritage Valley Beaver	Beaver	43%	(a)
Somerset Hospital	Somerset	43%	300+
UPMC Saint Margaret	Pittsburgh	43%	300+
York Hospital	York	42%	300+
Troy Community Hospital	Troy	41%	(a)
Highlands Hospital	Connellsville	40%	300+

Doctors 'Always' Communicated Well

Hospital Name	City	Rate	Cases
Advanced Surgical Hospital	Washington	91%	(a)
Physician's Care Surgical Hospital	Royersford	91%	300+
Mid - Valley Hospital	Peckville	90%	(a)

NOTE: Hospital profiles are in alphabetical order by state, then city, then hospital within the city; Rankings exclude hospitals with less than 25 cases except for patient surveys which excludes hospitals with less than 100 cases; (a) 100-299 cases; (1) The number of cases/patients is too few to report; (2) Data submitted were based on a sample of cases/patients; (3) Results are based on a shorter time period than required; (4) Data suppressed by CMS for one or more quarters; (5) Results are not available for this reporting period; (6) Fewer than 100 patients completed the HCAHPS survey; (7) No cases met the criteria for this measure; (8) The lower limit of the confidence interval cannot be calculated if the number of observed infections equals zero; (9) No data are available from the state/territory for this reporting period; (10) The scores shown reflect fewer than 50 completed surveys; (11) There were discrepancies in the data collection process; (12) This measure does not apply to this hospital for this reporting period; (13) Results cannot be calculated for this reporting period; (14) The results for this state are combined with nearby states to protect confidentiality; Please refer to the User's Guide for a full explanation of data.

Oss Orthopaedic Hospital	York	89%	300+
Surgical Institute of Reading	Wyomissing	89%	(a)
Wellspan Surgery & Rehab Hosp	York	89%	(a)
Cancer Treatment Centers of America	Philadelphia	88%	(a)
Fulton County Medical Center	Mcconnellsburg	88%	(a)
Tyler Memorial Hospital	Tunkhannock	88%	300+
Jersey Shore Hospital	Jersey Shore	87%	(a)
Saint Luke's Miners Memorial Hospital	Coaldale	87%	300+
Soldiers & Sailors Memorial Hospital	Wellsboro	87%	300+
Surgical Specialty Ctr at Coord Hlth	Allentown	87%	300+
Barnes-Kasson County Hospital	Susquehanna	86%	(a)
Coordinated Health Orthopedic Hospital	Bethlehem	86%	300+
Monongahela Valley Hospital	Monongahela	86%	300+
Muncy Valley Hospital	Muncy	86%	(a)
Titusville Hospital	Titusville	86%	300+
Highlands Hospital	Connellsville	85%	300+
Kane Community Hospital	Kane	85%	(a)
Penn Highlands Dubois	Dubois	85%	300+
Tyrone Hospital	Tyrone	85%	(a)
Bucks County Specialty Hospital	Bensalem	84%	300+
Canonsburg General Hospital	Canonsburg	84%	300+
Lansdale Hospital	Lansdale	84%	300+
Meadville Medical Center	Meadville	84%	300+
Endless Mountains Health Systems	Montrose	83%	300+
Evangelical Community Hospital	Lewisburg	83%	300+
Hanover Hospital	Hanover	83%	300+
Memorial Hospital Towanda	Towanda	83%	300+
Nason Hospital	Roaring Spring	83%	300+
Regional Hospital of Scranton	Scranton	83%	300+
Southwest Regional Medical Center	Waynesburg	83%	300+
Windber Hospital	Windber	83%	300+
Acmh Hospital	Kittanning	82%	300+
Berwick Hospital Center	Berwick	82%	300+
Carlisle Regional Medical Center	Carlisle	82%	300+
Charles Cole Memorial Hospital	Coudersport	82%	300+
Doylestown Hospital	Doylestown	82%	300+
Easton Hospital	Easton	82%	300+
Heritage Valley Sewickley	Sewickley	82%	300+
Lock Haven Hospital	Lock Haven	82%	(a)
Main Line Hospital Lankenau	Wynnewood	82%	300+
Schuylkill Med Ctr-S Jackson St	Pottsville	82%	300+
Sunbury Community Hospital	Sunbury	82%	(a)
Albert Einstein Medical Center	Philadelphia	81%	300+
Chester County Hospital	West Chester	81%	300+
Ellwood City Hospital	Ellwood City	81%	300+
Geisinger Wyoming Valley Medical Center	Wilkes Barre	81%	300+
Grove City Medical Center	Grove City	81%	300+
Hahnemann University Hospital	Philadelphia	81%	300+
Indiana Regional Medical Center	Indiana	81%	300+
J C Blair Memorial Hospital	Huntingdon	81%	300+
Moses Taylor Hospital	Scranton	81%	300+
Mount Nittany Medical Center	State College	81%	300+
Penn Highlands Clearfield	Clearfield	81%	300+
Penn Presbyterian Medical Center	Philadelphia	81%	300+
Riddle Memorial Hospital	Media	81%	300+
Saint Clair Memorial Hospital	Pittsburgh	81%	300+
Saint Luke's Hospital - Anderson Campus	Easton	81%	300+
Troy Community Hospital	Troy	81%	(a)
Wayne Memorial Hospital	Honesdale	81%	300+
Alle Kiski Medical Center	Natrona	80%	300+
Butler Memorial Hospital	Butler	80%	300+
Chestnut Hill Hospital	Philadelphia	80%	300+
Clarion Hospital	Clarion	80%	300+
Corry Memorial Hospital	Corry	80%	(a)
Excela Health Frick Hospital	Mount Pleasant	80%	300+
Excela Health Latrobe Hospital	Latrobe	80%	300+
Excela Health Westmoreland Hospital	Greensburg	80%	300+
Geisinger - Bloomsburg Hospital	Bloomsburg	80%	300+
Gettysburg Hospital	Gettysburg	80%	300+
Heart of Lancaster Reg Med Ctr	Lititz	80%	300+
Jefferson Regional Medical Center	Pittsburgh	80%	300+
Millcreek Community Hospital	Erie	80%	(a)
Sacred Heart Hospital	Allentown	80%	300+
Saint Luke's Quakertown Hospital	Quakertown	80%	300+
Uniontown Hospital	Uniontown	80%	300+
UPMC Altoona	Altoona	80%	300+
UPMC Bedford Memorial	Everett	80%	300+
UPMC Saint Margaret	Pittsburgh	80%	300+
The Washington Hospital	Washington	80%	300+
Waynesboro Hospital	Waynesboro	80%	300+
Western Pennsylvania Hospital	Pittsburgh	80%	300+
Wilkes-Barre General Hospital	Wilkes-Barre	80%	300+
Abington Memorial Hospital	Abington	79%	300+
Allegheny General Hospital	Pittsburgh	79%	300+
Bradford Regional Medical Center	Bradford	79%	300+
Geisinger Medical Center	Danville	79%	300+
Good Samaritan Hospital	Lebanon	79%	300+
Hospital of Univ of Pennsylvania	Philadelphia	79%	300+
Lancaster Regional Medical Center	Lancaster	79%	300+
Lehigh Valley Hospital - Hazleton	Hazleton	79%	300+
Magee Womens Hosp of UPMC Health Sys	Pittsburgh	79%	300+
Phoenixville Hospital	Phoenixville	79%	300+
Punxsutawney Area Hospital	Punxsutawney	79%	300+
Roxborough Memorial Hospital	Philadelphia	79%	(a)
Saint Vincent Hospital	Erie	79%	300+
Schuylkill Med Ctr-East Norwegian St	Pottsville	79%	300+
Sharon Regional Health System	Sharon	79%	300+
Temple University Hospital	Philadelphia	79%	300+
Thomas Jefferson University Hospital	Philadelphia	79%	300+
UPMC Passavant	Pittsburgh	79%	300+
UPMC Presbyterian Shadyside	Pittsburgh	79%	300+
Warren General Hospital	Warren	79%	300+
Williamsport Regional Medical Center	Williamsport	79%	300+
Brandywine Hospital	Coatesville	78%	300+
Holy Redeemer Hospital & Medical Center	Meadowbrook	78%	300+
Lehigh Valley Hospital - Muhlenberg	Bethlehem	78%	300+
Main Line Hospital Bryn Mawr Campus	Bryn Mawr	78%	300+
Main Line Hospital Paoli	Paoli	78%	300+
Milton S Hershey Medical Center	Hershey	78%	300+
Penn Highlands Elk	Saint Marys	78%	300+
Pocono Medical Center	E Stroudsburg	78%	300+
Saint Joseph Medical Center	Reading	78%	300+
UPMC Mckeesport	Mc Keesport	78%	300+
UPMC Northwest	Seneca	78%	300+
Conemaugh Valley Memorial Hospital	Johnstown	77%	300+
Delaware County Memorial Hospital	Drexel Hill	77%	300+
Geisinger - Community Medical Center	Scranton	77%	300+
Heritage Valley Beaver	Beaver	77%	(a)
Jameson Memorial Hospital	New Castle	77%	300+
Lehigh Valley Hospital	Allentown	77%	300+
Mercy Suburban Hospital	Norristown	77%	300+
Pinnacle Health Hospitals	Harrisburg	77%	300+
Saint Mary Medical Center	Langhorne	77%	300+
Forbes Regional Hospital	Monroeville	76%	300+
Grand View Hospital	Sellersville	76%	300+
Holy Spirit Hospital	Camp Hill	76%	300+
Jeanes Hospital	Philadelphia	76%	300+
Ohio Valley General Hospital	Mckees Rocks	76%	300+
Palmerton Hospital	Palmerton	76%	300+
Penn Hosp of the Univ of PA Hlth Sys	Philadelphia	76%	300+
Robert Packer Hospital	Sayre	76%	300+
Saint Luke's Hospital Bethlehem	Bethlehem	76%	300+
UPMC Hamot	Erie	76%	300+
UPMC Horizon	Greenville	76%	300+
UPMC Mercy	Pittsburgh	76%	300+
Ephrata Community Hospital	Ephrata	75%	300+
Gnaden Huetten Memorial Hospital	Lehighton	75%	300+
Lancaster General Hospital	Lancaster	75%	300+
Lewistown Hospital	Lewistown	75%	300+
Memorial Hospital	York	75%	300+
Mercy Fitzgerald Hospital	Darby	75%	300+
Pottstown Memorial Medical Center	Pottstown	75%	300+
Reading Hospital	Reading	75%	300+
Somerset Hospital	Somerset	75%	300+
UPMC East	Monroeville	75%	300+
Aria Health	Philadelphia	74%	300+
Crozer Chester Medical Center	Upland	74%	300+
Einstein Medical Center Montgomery	East Norriton	74%	300+
Jennersville Regional Hospital	West Grove	74%	300+
Chambersburg Hospital	Chambersburg	73%	300+
York Hospital	York	73%	300+
Saint Joseph's Hospital	Philadelphia	72%	(a)
Nazareth Hospital	Philadelphia	66%	300+
Lower Bucks Hospital	Bristol	64%	(a)

Home Recovery Information Given

Hospital Name	City	Rate	Cases
Advanced Surgical Hospital	Washington	94%	(a)
Oss Orthopaedic Hospital	York	94%	300+
Surgical Institute of Reading	Wyomissing	94%	(a)
Wellspan Surgery & Rehab Hosp	York	94%	(a)
Coordinated Health Orthopedic Hospital	Bethlehem	93%	300+
Physician's Care Surgical Hospital	Royersford	93%	300+
Surgical Specialty Ctr at Coord Hlth	Allentown	93%	300+
Cancer Treatment Centers of America	Philadelphia	92%	(a)
Excela Health Frick Hospital	Mount Pleasant	92%	300+
Punxsutawney Area Hospital	Punxsutawney	92%	300+
Ephrata Community Hospital	Ephrata	91%	300+
Bucks County Specialty Hospital	Bensalem	90%	300+
Hospital of Univ of Pennsylvania	Philadelphia	90%	300+
Saint Luke's Miners Memorial Hospital	Coaldale	90%	300+
Uniontown Hospital	Uniontown	90%	300+
Butler Memorial Hospital	Butler	89%	300+
Easton Hospital	Easton	89%	300+
Geisinger Medical Center	Danville	89%	300+
Grand View Hospital	Sellersville	89%	300+
Indiana Regional Medical Center	Indiana	89%	300+
Jefferson Regional Medical Center	Pittsburgh	89%	300+
Lewistown Hospital	Lewistown	89%	300+
Moses Taylor Hospital	Scranton	89%	300+
Penn Highlands Clearfield	Clearfield	89%	300+
Penn Highlands Dubois	Dubois	89%	300+
Pinnacle Health Hospitals	Harrisburg	89%	300+
Saint Luke's Quakertown Hospital	Quakertown	89%	300+
Tyler Memorial Hospital	Tunkhannock	89%	300+
Wayne Memorial Hospital	Honesdale	89%	300+
Charles Cole Memorial Hospital	Coudersport	88%	300+
Doylestown Hospital	Doylestown	88%	300+
Ellwood City Hospital	Ellwood City	88%	300+
Excela Health Latrobe Hospital	Latrobe	88%	300+
Good Samaritan Hospital	Lebanon	88%	300+
Grove City Medical Center	Grove City	88%	300+
Lancaster Regional Medical Center	Lancaster	88%	300+
Lehigh Valley Hospital - Muhlenberg	Bethlehem	88%	300+
Lock Haven Hospital	Lock Haven	88%	(a)
Mid - Valley Hospital	Peckville	88%	(a)
Milton S Hershey Medical Center	Hershey	88%	300+
Palmerton Hospital	Palmerton	88%	300+
Penn Highlands Elk	Saint Marys	88%	300+
Reading Hospital	Reading	88%	300+
Saint Joseph Medical Center	Reading	88%	300+
Titusville Hospital	Titusville	88%	300+
Tyrone Hospital	Tyrone	88%	(a)
UPMC Passavant	Pittsburgh	88%	300+
UPMC Presbyterian Shadyside	Pittsburgh	88%	300+
UPMC Saint Margaret	Pittsburgh	88%	300+
The Washington Hospital	Washington	88%	300+
Brandywine Hospital	Coatesville	87%	300+
Carlisle Regional Medical Center	Carlisle	87%	300+
Clarion Hospital	Clarion	87%	300+
Evangelical Community Hospital	Lewisburg	87%	300+
Geisinger Wyoming Valley Medical Center	Wilkes Barre	87%	300+
Heart of Lancaster Reg Med Ctr	Lititz	87%	300+
J C Blair Memorial Hospital	Huntingdon	87%	300+
Jameson Memorial Hospital	New Castle	87%	300+
Lehigh Valley Hospital	Allentown	87%	300+
Meadville Medical Center	Meadville	87%	300+
Mount Nittany Medical Center	State College	87%	300+
Nason Hospital	Roaring Spring	87%	300+
Penn Presbyterian Medical Center	Philadelphia	87%	300+
Phoenixville Hospital	Phoenixville	87%	300+
Somerset Hospital	Somerset	87%	300+
Sunbury Community Hospital	Sunbury	87%	(a)
Williamsport Regional Medical Center	Williamsport	87%	300+
Allegheny General Hospital	Pittsburgh	86%	300+
Chester County Hospital	West Chester	86%	300+
Gnaden Huetten Memorial Hospital	Lehighton	86%	300+
Hanover Hospital	Hanover	86%	300+
Holy Spirit Hospital	Camp Hill	86%	300+
Lancaster General Hospital	Lancaster	86%	300+
Main Line Hospital Lankenau	Wynnewood	86%	300+
Main Line Hospital Paoli	Paoli	86%	300+
Monongahela Valley Hospital	Monongahela	86%	300+
Pottstown Memorial Medical Center	Pottstown	86%	300+
Roxborough Memorial Hospital	Philadelphia	86%	(a)
Sacred Heart Hospital	Allentown	86%	300+
Saint Clair Memorial Hospital	Pittsburgh	86%	300+
Saint Luke's Hospital - Anderson Campus	Easton	86%	300+
Saint Mary Medical Center	Langhorne	86%	300+
Thomas Jefferson University Hospital	Philadelphia	86%	300+
UPMC East	Monroeville	86%	300+
UPMC Hamot	Erie	86%	300+
UPMC Horizon	Greenville	86%	300+
UPMC Mercy	Pittsburgh	86%	300+
UPMC Northwest	Seneca	86%	300+
Western Pennsylvania Hospital	Pittsburgh	86%	300+
Abington Memorial Hospital	Abington	85%	300+
Acmh Hospital	Kittanning	85%	300+
Alle Kiski Medical Center	Natrona	85%	300+
Endless Mountains Health Systems	Montrose	85%	300+
Excela Health Westmoreland Hospital	Greensburg	85%	300+
Geisinger - Bloomsburg Hospital	Bloomsburg	85%	300+
Gettysburg Hospital	Gettysburg	85%	300+
Holy Redeemer Hospital & Medical Center	Meadowbrook	85%	300+
Kane Community Hospital	Kane	85%	(a)
Lansdale Hospital	Lansdale	85%	300+
Magee Womens Hosp of UPMC Health Sys	Pittsburgh	85%	300+
Main Line Hospital Bryn Mawr Campus	Bryn Mawr	85%	300+
Memorial Hospital	York	85%	300+
Mercy Fitzgerald Hospital	Darby	85%	300+
Penn Hosp of the Univ of PA Hlth Sys	Philadelphia	85%	300+
Riddle Memorial Hospital	Media	85%	300+
Saint Luke's Hospital Bethlehem	Bethlehem	85%	300+
Saint Vincent Hospital	Erie	85%	300+
Sharon Regional Health System	Sharon	85%	300+
Soldiers & Sailors Memorial Hospital	Wellsboro	85%	300+
UPMC Mckeesport	Mc Keesport	85%	300+
Warren General Hospital	Warren	85%	300+
Waynesboro Hospital	Waynesboro	85%	300+
York Hospital	York	85%	300+
Aria Health	Philadelphia	84%	300+
Berwick Hospital Center	Berwick	84%	300+
Conemaugh Valley Memorial Hospital	Johnstown	84%	300+

NOTE: Hospital profiles are in alphabetical order by state, then city, then hospital within the city; Rankings exclude hospitals with less than 25 cases except for patient surveys which excludes hospitals with less than 100 cases; (a) 100-299 cases; (1) The number of cases/patients is too few to report; (2) Data submitted were based on a sample of cases/patients; (3) Results are based on a shorter time period than required; (4) Data suppressed by CMS for one or more quarters; (5) Results are not available for this reporting period; (6) Fewer than 100 patients completed the HCAHPS survey; (7) No cases met the criteria for this measure; (8) The lower limit of the confidence interval cannot be calculated if the number of observed infections equals zero; (9) No data are available from the state/territory for this reporting period; (10) The scores shown reflect fewer than 50 completed surveys; (11) There were discrepancies in the data collection process; (12) This measure does not apply to this hospital for this reporting period; (13) Results cannot be calculated for this reporting period; (14) The results for this state are combined with nearby states to protect confidentiality; Please refer to the User's Guide for a full explanation of data.

Hospital Name	City	Rate	Cases
Delaware County Memorial Hospital	Drexel Hill	84%	300+
Forbes Regional Hospital	Monroeville	84%	300+
Fulton County Medical Center	Mcconnellsburg	84%	(a)
Jersey Shore Hospital	Jersey Shore	84%	(a)
Memorial Hospital Towanda	Towanda	84%	300+
Mercy Suburban Hospital	Norristown	84%	300+
Nazareth Hospital	Philadelphia	84%	300+
Ohio Valley General Hospital	Mckees Rocks	84%	300+
Schuylkill Med Ctr-East Norwegian St	Pottsville	84%	300+
Troy Community Hospital	Troy	84%	(a)
UPMC Altoona	Altoona	84%	300+
UPMC Bedford Memorial	Everett	84%	300+
Albert Einstein Medical Center	Philadelphia	83%	300+
Barnes-Kasson County Hospital	Susquehanna	83%	(a)
Chestnut Hill Hospital	Philadelphia	83%	300+
Corry Memorial Hospital	Corry	83%	(a)
Geisinger - Community Medical Center	Scranton	83%	300+
Heritage Valley Sewickley	Sewickley	83%	300+
Lehigh Valley Hospital - Hazleton	Hazleton	83%	300+
Muncy Valley Hospital	Muncy	83%	(a)
Pocono Medical Center	E Stroudsburg	83%	300+
Regional Hospital of Scranton	Scranton	83%	300+
Robert Packer Hospital	Sayre	83%	300+
Temple University Hospital	Philadelphia	83%	300+
Windber Hospital	Windber	83%	300+
Bradford Regional Medical Center	Bradford	82%	300+
Crozer Chester Medical Center	Upland	82%	300+
Einstein Medical Center Montgomery	East Norriton	82%	300+
Heritage Valley Beaver	Beaver	82%	(a)
Highlands Hospital	Connellsville	82%	300+
Jennersville Regional Hospital	West Grove	82%	300+
Millcreek Community Hospital	Erie	82%	(a)
Wilkes-Barre General Hospital	Wilkes-Barre	82%	300+
Canonsburg General Hospital	Canonsburg	81%	300+
Hahnemann University Hospital	Philadelphia	81%	300+
Schuylkill Med Ctr-S Jackson St	Pottsville	81%	300+
Chambersburg Hospital	Chambersburg	80%	300+
Jeanes Hospital	Philadelphia	80%	300+
Lower Bucks Hospital	Bristol	80%	(a)
Southwest Regional Medical Center	Waynesburg	80%	300+
Saint Joseph's Hospital	Philadelphia	72%	(a)

Hospital Given 9 or 10 on 10 Point Scale

Hospital Name	City	Rate	Cases
Advanced Surgical Hospital	Washington	94%	(a)
Physician's Care Surgical Hospital	Royersford	94%	300+
Surgical Institute of Reading	Wyomissing	92%	(a)
Wellspan Surgery & Rehab Hosp	York	92%	(a)
Oss Orthopaedic Hospital	York	91%	300+
Surgical Specialty Ctr at Coord Hlth	Allentown	89%	300+
Bucks County Specialty Hospital	Bensalem	87%	300+
Cancer Treatment Centers of America	Philadelphia	87%	(a)
Coordinated Health Orthopedic Hospital	Bethlehem	83%	300+
Doylestown Hospital	Doylestown	83%	300+
Mid - Valley Hospital	Peckville	83%	(a)
Muncy Valley Hospital	Muncy	83%	(a)
Main Line Hospital Paoli	Paoli	82%	300+
Titusville Hospital	Titusville	80%	300+
Tyrone Hospital	Tyrone	80%	(a)
Saint Clair Memorial Hospital	Pittsburgh	79%	300+
Saint Luke's Hospital - Anderson Campus	Easton	79%	300+
Fulton County Medical Center	Mcconnellsburg	77%	(a)
Main Line Hospital Bryn Mawr Campus	Bryn Mawr	77%	300+
Main Line Hospital Lankenau	Wynnewood	77%	300+
Penn Highlands Dubois	Dubois	77%	300+
Saint Mary Medical Center	Langhorne	77%	300+
Jersey Shore Hospital	Jersey Shore	76%	(a)
Milton S Hershey Medical Center	Hershey	76%	300+
Waynesboro Hospital	Waynesboro	76%	300+
Geisinger Medical Center	Danville	75%	300+
Hospital of Univ of Pennsylvania	Philadelphia	75%	300+
Lehigh Valley Hospital - Muhlenberg	Bethlehem	75%	300+
Monongahela Valley Hospital	Monongahela	75%	300+
Mount Nittany Medical Center	State College	75%	300+
Saint Luke's Miners Memorial Hospital	Coaldale	75%	300+
Evangelical Community Hospital	Lewisburg	74%	300+
Lehigh Valley Hospital	Allentown	74%	300+
Saint Joseph Medical Center	Reading	74%	300+
Thomas Jefferson University Hospital	Philadelphia	74%	300+
Chester County Hospital	West Chester	73%	300+
Corry Memorial Hospital	Corry	73%	(a)
Heart of Lancaster Reg Med Ctr	Lititz	73%	300+
Jefferson Regional Medical Center	Pittsburgh	73%	300+
Lansdale Hospital	Lansdale	73%	300+
Nason Hospital	Roaring Spring	73%	300+
Phoenixville Hospital	Phoenixville	73%	300+
Tyler Memorial Hospital	Tunkhannock	73%	300+
UPMC East	Monroeville	73%	300+
Einstein Medical Center Montgomery	East Norriton	72%	300+
Grand View Hospital	Sellersville	72%	300+
Memorial Hospital Towanda	Towanda	72%	300+
Penn Presbyterian Medical Center	Philadelphia	72%	300+
Saint Luke's Hospital Bethlehem	Bethlehem	72%	300+
Saint Luke's Quakertown Hospital	Quakertown	72%	300+
Windber Hospital	Windber	72%	300+
Abington Memorial Hospital	Abington	71%	300+
Ellwood City Hospital	Ellwood City	71%	300+
Excela Health Frick Hospital	Mount Pleasant	71%	300+
Geisinger Wyoming Valley Medical Center	Wilkes Barre	71%	300+
Kane Community Hospital	Kane	71%	(a)
Lancaster General Hospital	Lancaster	71%	300+
Soldiers & Sailors Memorial Hospital	Wellsboro	71%	300+
UPMC Passavant	Pittsburgh	71%	300+
Good Samaritan Hospital	Lebanon	70%	300+
Holy Redeemer Hospital & Medical Center	Meadowbrook	70%	300+
Holy Spirit Hospital	Camp Hill	70%	300+
Indiana Regional Medical Center	Indiana	70%	300+
Magee Womens Hosp of UPMC Health Sys	Pittsburgh	70%	300+
Pinnacle Health Hospitals	Harrisburg	70%	300+
Riddle Memorial Hospital	Media	70%	300+
Robert Packer Hospital	Sayre	70%	300+
UPMC Altoona	Altoona	70%	300+
UPMC Hamot	Erie	70%	300+
Williamsport Regional Medical Center	Williamsport	70%	300+
Butler Memorial Hospital	Butler	69%	300+
Canonsburg General Hospital	Canonsburg	69%	300+
Gettysburg Hospital	Gettysburg	69%	300+
Lancaster Regional Medical Center	Lancaster	69%	300+
Ohio Valley General Hospital	Mckees Rocks	69%	300+
Saint Vincent Hospital	Erie	69%	300+
Sunbury Community Hospital	Sunbury	69%	(a)
UPMC Presbyterian Shadyside	Pittsburgh	69%	300+
Acmh Hospital	Kittanning	68%	300+
Chestnut Hill Hospital	Philadelphia	68%	300+
Clarion Hospital	Clarion	68%	300+
Meadville Medical Center	Meadville	68%	300+
Somerset Hospital	Somerset	68%	300+
Troy Community Hospital	Troy	68%	(a)
UPMC Saint Margaret	Pittsburgh	68%	300+
Chambersburg Hospital	Chambersburg	67%	300+
Conemaugh Valley Memorial Hospital	Johnstown	67%	300+
Ephrata Community Hospital	Ephrata	67%	300+
Excela Health Latrobe Hospital	Latrobe	67%	300+
Hanover Hospital	Hanover	67%	300+
Heritage Valley Sewickley	Sewickley	67%	300+
Millcreek Community Hospital	Erie	67%	(a)
Moses Taylor Hospital	Scranton	67%	300+
Punxsutawney Area Hospital	Punxsutawney	67%	300+
Western Pennsylvania Hospital	Pittsburgh	67%	300+
York Hospital	York	67%	300+
Charles Cole Memorial Hospital	Coudersport	66%	300+
Easton Hospital	Easton	66%	300+
Hahnemann University Hospital	Philadelphia	66%	300+
J C Blair Memorial Hospital	Huntingdon	66%	300+
Jeanes Hospital	Philadelphia	66%	300+
Memorial Hospital	York	66%	300+
Pocono Medical Center	E Stroudsburg	66%	300+
Schuylkill Med Ctr-East Norwegian St	Pottsville	66%	300+
Temple University Hospital	Philadelphia	66%	300+
The Washington Hospital	Washington	66%	300+
Allegheny General Hospital	Pittsburgh	65%	300+
Brandywine Hospital	Coatesville	65%	300+
Endless Mountains Health Systems	Montrose	65%	300+
Forbes Regional Hospital	Monroeville	65%	300+
Geisinger - Bloomsburg Hospital	Bloomsburg	65%	300+
Jennersville Regional Hospital	West Grove	65%	300+
Penn Highlands Elk	Saint Marys	65%	300+
Penn Hosp of the Univ of PA Hlth Sys	Philadelphia	65%	300+
Reading Hospital	Reading	65%	300+
Regional Hospital of Scranton	Scranton	65%	300+
Sacred Heart Hospital	Allentown	65%	300+
UPMC Bedford Memorial	Everett	65%	300+
Wayne Memorial Hospital	Honesdale	65%	300+
Alle Kiski Medical Center	Natrona	64%	300+
Sharon Regional Health System	Sharon	64%	300+
UPMC Mckeesport	Mc Keesport	64%	300+
Wilkes-Barre General Hospital	Wilkes-Barre	64%	300+
Aria Health	Philadelphia	63%	300+
Berwick Hospital Center	Berwick	63%	300+
Grove City Medical Center	Grove City	63%	300+
Schuylkill Med Ctr-S Jackson St	Pottsville	63%	300+
Uniontown Hospital	Uniontown	63%	300+
UPMC Mercy	Pittsburgh	63%	300+
Bradford Regional Medical Center	Bradford	62%	300+
Carlisle Regional Medical Center	Carlisle	62%	300+
UPMC Horizon	Greenville	62%	300+
UPMC Northwest	Seneca	62%	300+
Warren General Hospital	Warren	62%	300+
Albert Einstein Medical Center	Philadelphia	61%	300+
Delaware County Memorial Hospital	Drexel Hill	61%	300+
Excela Health Westmoreland Hospital	Greensburg	61%	300+
Heritage Valley Beaver	Beaver	61%	(a)
Highlands Hospital	Connellsville	61%	300+
Palmerton Hospital	Palmerton	60%	300+
Barnes-Kasson County Hospital	Susquehanna	59%	(a)
Lock Haven Hospital	Lock Haven	59%	(a)
Roxborough Memorial Hospital	Philadelphia	59%	(a)
Geisinger - Community Medical Center	Scranton	58%	300+
Gnaden Huetten Memorial Hospital	Lehighton	58%	300+
Lewistown Hospital	Lewistown	58%	300+
Jameson Memorial Hospital	New Castle	57%	300+
Mercy Suburban Hospital	Norristown	57%	300+
Nazareth Hospital	Philadelphia	57%	300+
Mercy Fitzgerald Hospital	Darby	56%	300+
Pottstown Memorial Medical Center	Pottstown	56%	300+
Crozer Chester Medical Center	Upland	55%	300+
Penn Highlands Clearfield	Clearfield	55%	300+
Lower Bucks Hospital	Bristol	54%	(a)
Southwest Regional Medical Center	Waynesburg	54%	300+
Lehigh Valley Hospital - Hazleton	Hazleton	53%	300+
Saint Joseph's Hospital	Philadelphia	47%	(a)

Meds 'Always' Explained Before Given

Hospital Name	City	Rate	Cases
Advanced Surgical Hospital	Washington	81%	(a)
Physician's Care Surgical Hospital	Royersford	76%	300+
Surgical Institute of Reading	Wyomissing	76%	(a)
Oss Orthopaedic Hospital	York	74%	300+
Wellspan Surgery & Rehab Hosp	York	74%	(a)
Cancer Treatment Centers of America	Philadelphia	73%	(a)
Surgical Specialty Ctr at Coord Hlth	Allentown	73%	300+
Bucks County Specialty Hospital	Bensalem	72%	300+
Mid - Valley Hospital	Peckville	72%	(a)
Kane Community Hospital	Kane	71%	(a)
Muncy Valley Hospital	Muncy	71%	(a)
Titusville Hospital	Titusville	70%	300+
Tyrone Hospital	Tyrone	70%	(a)
Coordinated Health Orthopedic Hospital	Bethlehem	69%	300+
Excela Health Frick Hospital	Mount Pleasant	69%	300+
Penn Highlands Dubois	Dubois	69%	300+
Saint Clair Memorial Hospital	Pittsburgh	69%	300+
Saint Luke's Miners Memorial Hospital	Coaldale	69%	300+
Soldiers & Sailors Memorial Hospital	Wellsboro	69%	300+
Highlands Hospital	Connellsville	68%	300+
Lansdale Hospital	Lansdale	68%	300+
Monongahela Valley Hospital	Monongahela	68%	300+
Hahnemann University Hospital	Philadelphia	67%	300+
Lock Haven Hospital	Lock Haven	67%	(a)
Mount Nittany Medical Center	State College	67%	300+
Troy Community Hospital	Troy	67%	(a)
Chester County Hospital	West Chester	66%	300+
Clarion Hospital	Clarion	66%	300+
Pinnacle Health Hospitals	Harrisburg	66%	300+
Saint Luke's Quakertown Hospital	Quakertown	66%	300+
Saint Mary Medical Center	Langhorne	66%	300+
Tyler Memorial Hospital	Tunkhannock	66%	300+
Waynesboro Hospital	Waynesboro	66%	300+
Abington Memorial Hospital	Abington	65%	300+
Charles Cole Memorial Hospital	Coudersport	65%	300+
Chestnut Hill Hospital	Philadelphia	65%	300+
Doylestown Hospital	Doylestown	65%	300+
Good Samaritan Hospital	Lebanon	65%	300+
Hospital of Univ of Pennsylvania	Philadelphia	65%	300+
Jersey Shore Hospital	Jersey Shore	65%	(a)
Main Line Hospital Lankenau	Wynnewood	65%	300+
Meadville Medical Center	Meadville	65%	300+
Penn Presbyterian Medical Center	Philadelphia	65%	300+
Riddle Memorial Hospital	Media	65%	300+
Saint Luke's Hospital - Anderson Campus	Easton	65%	300+
Berwick Hospital Center	Berwick	64%	300+
Canonsburg General Hospital	Canonsburg	64%	300+
Easton Hospital	Easton	64%	300+
Endless Mountains Health Systems	Montrose	64%	300+
Fulton County Medical Center	Mcconnellsburg	64%	(a)
Indiana Regional Medical Center	Indiana	64%	300+
Penn Highlands Elk	Saint Marys	64%	300+
Schuylkill Med Ctr-S Jackson St	Pottsville	64%	300+
Thomas Jefferson University Hospital	Philadelphia	64%	300+
Uniontown Hospital	Uniontown	64%	300+
UPMC Bedford Memorial	Everett	64%	300+
Windber Hospital	Windber	64%	300+
Conemaugh Valley Memorial Hospital	Johnstown	63%	300+
Evangelical Community Hospital	Lewisburg	63%	300+
Geisinger Medical Center	Danville	63%	300+
Heritage Valley Sewickley	Sewickley	63%	300+
J C Blair Memorial Hospital	Huntingdon	63%	300+
Lehigh Valley Hospital - Muhlenberg	Bethlehem	63%	300+
Main Line Hospital Bryn Mawr Campus	Bryn Mawr	63%	300+
Main Line Hospital Paoli	Paoli	63%	300+
Milton S Hershey Medical Center	Hershey	63%	300+
Nason Hospital	Roaring Spring	63%	300+
Phoenixville Hospital	Phoenixville	63%	300+
Sunbury Community Hospital	Sunbury	63%	(a)

NOTE: Hospital profiles are in alphabetical order by state, then city, then hospital within the city; Rankings exclude hospitals with less than 25 cases except for patient surveys which excludes hospitals with less than 100 cases; (a) 100-299 cases; (1) The number of cases/patients is too few to report; (2) Data submitted were based on a sample of cases/patients; (3) Results are based on a shorter time period than required; (4) Data suppressed by CMS for one or more quarters; (5) Results are not available for this reporting period; (6) Fewer than 100 patients completed the HCAHPS survey; (7) No cases met the criteria for this measure; (8) The lower limit of the confidence interval cannot be calculated if the number of observed infections equals zero; (9) No data are available from the state/territory for this reporting period; (10) The scores shown reflect fewer than 50 completed surveys; (11) There were discrepancies in the data collection process; (12) This measure does not apply to this hospital for this reporting period; (13) Results cannot be calculated for this reporting period; (14) The results for this state are combined with nearby states to protect confidentiality; Please refer to the User's Guide for a full explanation of data.

UPMC Saint Margaret	Pittsburgh	63%	300+
Western Pennsylvania Hospital	Pittsburgh	63%	300+
Acmh Hospital	Kittanning	62%	300+
Alle Kiski Medical Center	Natrona	62%	300+
Butler Memorial Hospital	Butler	62%	300+
Ellwood City Hospital	Ellwood City	62%	300+
Excela Health Westmoreland Hospital	Greensburg	62%	300+
Geisinger Wyoming Valley Medical Center	Wilkes Barre	62%	300+
Holy Spirit Hospital	Camp Hill	62%	300+
Lehigh Valley Hospital	Allentown	62%	300+
Memorial Hospital	York	62%	300+
UPMC Mckeesport	Mc Keesport	62%	300+
Wayne Memorial Hospital	Honesdale	62%	300+
Williamsport Regional Medical Center	Williamsport	62%	300+
Albert Einstein Medical Center	Philadelphia	61%	300+
Carlisle Regional Medical Center	Carlisle	61%	300+
Chambersburg Hospital	Chambersburg	61%	300+
Corry Memorial Hospital	Corry	61%	(a)
Excela Health Latrobe Hospital	Latrobe	61%	300+
Grove City Medical Center	Grove City	61%	300+
Hanover Hospital	Hanover	61%	300+
Jameson Memorial Hospital	New Castle	61%	300+
Jefferson Regional Medical Center	Pittsburgh	61%	300+
Magee Womens Hosp of UPMC Health Sys	Pittsburgh	61%	300+
Memorial Hospital Towanda	Towanda	61%	300+
Mercy Suburban Hospital	Norristown	61%	300+
Punxsutawney Area Hospital	Punxsutawney	61%	300+
Regional Hospital of Scranton	Scranton	61%	300+
Saint Joseph Medical Center	Reading	61%	300+
Saint Luke's Hospital Bethlehem	Bethlehem	61%	300+
Saint Vincent Hospital	Erie	61%	300+
UPMC Presbyterian Shadyside	Pittsburgh	61%	300+
Wilkes-Barre General Hospital	Wilkes-Barre	61%	300+
Barnes-Kasson County Hospital	Susquehanna	60%	(a)
Brandywine Hospital	Coatesville	60%	300+
Gettysburg Hospital	Gettysburg	60%	300+
Jeanes Hospital	Philadelphia	60%	300+
Lancaster Regional Medical Center	Lancaster	60%	300+
Moses Taylor Hospital	Scranton	60%	300+
Pocono Medical Center	E Stroudsburg	60%	300+
Robert Packer Hospital	Sayre	60%	300+
Roxborough Memorial Hospital	Philadelphia	60%	(a)
Schuylkill Med Ctr-East Norwegian St	Pottsville	60%	300+
Sharon Regional Health System	Sharon	60%	300+
Somerset Hospital	Somerset	60%	300+
Southwest Regional Medical Center	Waynesburg	60%	300+
Temple University Hospital	Philadelphia	60%	300+
UPMC East	Monroeville	60%	300+
The Washington Hospital	Washington	60%	300+
Aria Health	Philadelphia	59%	300+
Bradford Regional Medical Center	Bradford	59%	300+
Einstein Medical Center Montgomery	East Norriton	59%	300+
Geisinger - Bloomsburg Hospital	Bloomsburg	59%	300+
Geisinger - Community Medical Center	Scranton	59%	300+
Grand View Hospital	Sellersville	59%	300+
Holy Redeemer Hospital & Medical Center	Meadowbrook	59%	300+
Ohio Valley General Hospital	Mckees Rocks	59%	300+
Penn Hosp of the Univ of PA Hlth Sys	Philadelphia	59%	300+
Sacred Heart Hospital	Allentown	59%	300+
UPMC Northwest	Seneca	59%	300+
UPMC Passavant	Pittsburgh	59%	300+
Warren General Hospital	Warren	59%	300+
Allegheny General Hospital	Pittsburgh	58%	300+
Delaware County Memorial Hospital	Drexel Hill	58%	300+
Forbes Regional Hospital	Monroeville	58%	300+
Heart of Lancaster Reg Med Ctr	Lititz	58%	300+
Lancaster General Hospital	Lancaster	58%	300+
Lewistown Hospital	Lewistown	58%	300+
Mercy Fitzgerald Hospital	Darby	58%	300+
Pottstown Memorial Medical Center	Pottstown	58%	300+
UPMC Hamot	Erie	58%	300+
UPMC Horizon	Greenville	58%	300+
Crozer Chester Medical Center	Upland	57%	300+
Gnaden Huetten Memorial Hospital	Lehighton	57%	300+
Millcreek Community Hospital	Erie	57%	(a)
Penn Highlands Clearfield	Clearfield	57%	300+
Reading Hospital	Reading	57%	300+
UPMC Altoona	Altoona	57%	300+
UPMC Mercy	Pittsburgh	57%	300+
Ephrata Community Hospital	Ephrata	55%	300+
Jennersville Regional Hospital	West Grove	55%	300+
Palmerton Hospital	Palmerton	55%	300+
Saint Joseph's Hospital	Philadelphia	54%	(a)
York Hospital	York	54%	300+
Lehigh Valley Hospital - Hazleton	Hazleton	52%	300+
Nazareth Hospital	Philadelphia	51%	300+
Heritage Valley Beaver	Beaver	50%	(a)
Lower Bucks Hospital	Bristol	50%	(a)

Nurses 'Always' Communicated Well

Hospital Name	City	Rate	Cases
Advanced Surgical Hospital	Washington	96%	(a)
Physician's Care Surgical Hospital	Royersford	96%	300+
Surgical Institute of Reading	Wyomissing	94%	(a)
Wellspan Surgery & Rehab Hosp	York	94%	(a)
Bucks County Specialty Hospital	Bensalem	90%	300+
Oss Orthopaedic Hospital	York	90%	300+
Lansdale Hospital	Lansdale	88%	300+
Mid - Valley Hospital	Peckville	88%	(a)
Doylestown Hospital	Doylestown	86%	300+
Monongahela Valley Hospital	Monongahela	86%	300+
Surgical Specialty Ctr at Coord Hlth	Allentown	86%	300+
Cancer Treatment Centers of America	Philadelphia	85%	(a)
Coordinated Health Orthopedic Hospital	Bethlehem	85%	300+
Excela Health Frick Hospital	Mount Pleasant	85%	300+
Fulton County Medical Center	Mcconnellsburg	85%	(a)
Muncy Valley Hospital	Muncy	85%	(a)
Riddle Memorial Hospital	Media	85%	300+
Saint Clair Memorial Hospital	Pittsburgh	85%	300+
Tyrone Hospital	Tyrone	85%	(a)
Penn Highlands Dubois	Dubois	84%	300+
Chester County Hospital	West Chester	83%	300+
J C Blair Memorial Hospital	Huntingdon	83%	300+
Jersey Shore Hospital	Jersey Shore	83%	(a)
Main Line Hospital Bryn Mawr Campus	Bryn Mawr	83%	300+
Main Line Hospital Paoli	Paoli	83%	300+
Meadville Medical Center	Meadville	83%	300+
Mount Nittany Medical Center	State College	83%	300+
Saint Luke's Hospital - Anderson Campus	Easton	83%	300+
Saint Luke's Miners Memorial Hospital	Coaldale	83%	300+
Soldiers & Sailors Memorial Hospital	Wellsboro	83%	300+
Titusville Hospital	Titusville	83%	300+
Tyler Memorial Hospital	Tunkhannock	83%	300+
Windber Hospital	Windber	83%	300+
Acmh Hospital	Kittanning	82%	300+
Geisinger - Bloomsburg Hospital	Bloomsburg	82%	300+
Good Samaritan Hospital	Lebanon	82%	300+
Indiana Regional Medical Center	Indiana	82%	300+
Kane Community Hospital	Kane	82%	(a)
Saint Luke's Quakertown Hospital	Quakertown	82%	300+
Easton Hospital	Easton	81%	300+
Ellwood City Hospital	Ellwood City	81%	300+
Endless Mountains Health Systems	Montrose	81%	300+
Evangelical Community Hospital	Lewisburg	81%	300+
Geisinger Medical Center	Danville	81%	300+
Grand View Hospital	Sellersville	81%	300+
Heritage Valley Sewickley	Sewickley	81%	300+
Memorial Hospital Towanda	Towanda	81%	300+
Phoenixville Hospital	Phoenixville	81%	300+
Pinnacle Health Hospitals	Harrisburg	81%	300+
Saint Mary Medical Center	Langhorne	81%	300+
Schuylkill Med Ctr-S Jackson St	Pottsville	81%	300+
UPMC Bedford Memorial	Everett	81%	300+
Waynesboro Hospital	Waynesboro	81%	300+
Abington Memorial Hospital	Abington	80%	300+
Conemaugh Valley Memorial Hospital	Johnstown	80%	300+
Geisinger Wyoming Valley Medical Center	Wilkes Barre	80%	300+
Hanover Hospital	Hanover	80%	300+
Hospital of Univ of Pennsylvania	Philadelphia	80%	300+
Jefferson Regional Medical Center	Pittsburgh	80%	300+
Lehigh Valley Hospital	Allentown	80%	300+
Lehigh Valley Hospital - Muhlenberg	Bethlehem	80%	300+
Main Line Hospital Lankenau	Wynnewood	80%	300+
Milton S Hershey Medical Center	Hershey	80%	300+
Penn Presbyterian Medical Center	Philadelphia	80%	300+
Punxsutawney Area Hospital	Punxsutawney	80%	300+
Robert Packer Hospital	Sayre	80%	300+
Thomas Jefferson University Hospital	Philadelphia	80%	300+
UPMC Altoona	Altoona	80%	300+
The Washington Hospital	Washington	80%	300+
Wayne Memorial Hospital	Honesdale	80%	300+
Barnes-Kasson County Hospital	Susquehanna	79%	(a)
Butler Memorial Hospital	Butler	79%	300+
Canonsburg General Hospital	Canonsburg	79%	300+
Carlisle Regional Medical Center	Carlisle	79%	300+
Charles Cole Memorial Hospital	Coudersport	79%	300+
Clarion Hospital	Clarion	79%	300+
Gettysburg Hospital	Gettysburg	79%	300+
Highlands Hospital	Connellsville	79%	300+
Holy Spirit Hospital	Camp Hill	79%	300+
Lock Haven Hospital	Lock Haven	79%	(a)
Nason Hospital	Roaring Spring	79%	300+
Pocono Medical Center	E Stroudsburg	79%	300+
Schuylkill Med Ctr-East Norwegian St	Pottsville	79%	300+
Somerset Hospital	Somerset	79%	300+
Troy Community Hospital	Troy	79%	(a)
UPMC East	Monroeville	79%	300+
Albert Einstein Medical Center	Philadelphia	78%	300+
Berwick Hospital Center	Berwick	78%	300+
Bradford Regional Medical Center	Bradford	78%	300+
Corry Memorial Hospital	Corry	78%	(a)
Einstein Medical Center Montgomery	East Norriton	78%	300+
Ephrata Community Hospital	Ephrata	78%	300+
Excela Health Latrobe Hospital	Latrobe	78%	300+
Hahnemann University Hospital	Philadelphia	78%	300+
Heart of Lancaster Reg Med Ctr	Lititz	78%	300+
Holy Redeemer Hospital & Medical Center	Meadowbrook	78%	300+
Penn Highlands Elk	Saint Marys	78%	300+
Sharon Regional Health System	Sharon	78%	300+
Southwest Regional Medical Center	Waynesburg	78%	300+
UPMC Passavant	Pittsburgh	78%	300+
UPMC Presbyterian Shadyside	Pittsburgh	78%	300+
Warren General Hospital	Warren	78%	300+
Wilkes-Barre General Hospital	Wilkes-Barre	78%	300+
Williamsport Regional Medical Center	Williamsport	78%	300+
Aria Health	Philadelphia	77%	300+
Brandywine Hospital	Coatesville	77%	300+
Chambersburg Hospital	Chambersburg	77%	300+
Chestnut Hill Hospital	Philadelphia	77%	300+
Delaware County Memorial Hospital	Drexel Hill	77%	300+
Forbes Regional Hospital	Monroeville	77%	300+
Lancaster General Hospital	Lancaster	77%	300+
Lancaster Regional Medical Center	Lancaster	77%	300+
Lewistown Hospital	Lewistown	77%	300+
Moses Taylor Hospital	Scranton	77%	300+
Sacred Heart Hospital	Allentown	77%	300+
Saint Joseph Medical Center	Reading	77%	300+
Saint Vincent Hospital	Erie	77%	300+
Sunbury Community Hospital	Sunbury	77%	(a)
Uniontown Hospital	Uniontown	77%	300+
UPMC Mckeesport	Mc Keesport	77%	300+
UPMC Saint Margaret	Pittsburgh	77%	300+
Western Pennsylvania Hospital	Pittsburgh	77%	300+
Excela Health Westmoreland Hospital	Greensburg	76%	300+
Geisinger - Community Medical Center	Scranton	76%	300+
Grove City Medical Center	Grove City	76%	300+
Jameson Memorial Hospital	New Castle	76%	300+
Magee Womens Hosp of UPMC Health Sys	Pittsburgh	76%	300+
Memorial Hospital	York	76%	300+
Reading Hospital	Reading	76%	300+
Regional Hospital of Scranton	Scranton	76%	300+
Saint Luke's Hospital Bethlehem	Bethlehem	76%	300+
UPMC Hamot	Erie	76%	300+
Alle Kiski Medical Center	Natrona	75%	300+
Allegheny General Hospital	Pittsburgh	75%	300+
Mercy Fitzgerald Hospital	Darby	75%	300+
Ohio Valley General Hospital	Mckees Rocks	75%	300+
Palmerton Hospital	Palmerton	75%	300+
Pottstown Memorial Medical Center	Pottstown	75%	300+
York Hospital	York	75%	300+
Gnaden Huetten Memorial Hospital	Lehighton	74%	300+
Heritage Valley Beaver	Beaver	74%	(a)
Jeanes Hospital	Philadelphia	74%	300+
Jennersville Regional Hospital	West Grove	74%	300+
Lehigh Valley Hospital - Hazleton	Hazleton	74%	300+
Mercy Suburban Hospital	Norristown	74%	300+
Millcreek Community Hospital	Erie	74%	(a)
Roxborough Memorial Hospital	Philadelphia	74%	(a)
UPMC Mercy	Pittsburgh	74%	300+
UPMC Northwest	Seneca	74%	300+
Penn Highlands Clearfield	Clearfield	73%	300+
Temple University Hospital	Philadelphia	73%	300+
Nazareth Hospital	Philadelphia	72%	300+
Penn Hosp of the Univ of PA Hlth Sys	Philadelphia	72%	300+
UPMC Horizon	Greenville	72%	300+
Crozer Chester Medical Center	Upland	71%	300+
Lower Bucks Hospital	Bristol	69%	(a)
Saint Joseph's Hospital	Philadelphia	64%	(a)

Pain 'Always' Well Controlled

Hospital Name	City	Rate	Cases
Mid - Valley Hospital	Peckville	86%	(a)
Surgical Institute of Reading	Wyomissing	85%	(a)
Physician's Care Surgical Hospital	Royersford	84%	300+
Advanced Surgical Hospital	Washington	83%	(a)
Wellspan Surgery & Rehab Hosp	York	81%	(a)
Bucks County Specialty Hospital	Bensalem	79%	300+
Fulton County Medical Center	Mcconnellsburg	79%	(a)
Tyler Memorial Hospital	Tunkhannock	79%	300+
Doylestown Hospital	Doylestown	78%	300+
Oss Orthopaedic Hospital	York	78%	300+
Saint Luke's Miners Memorial Hospital	Coaldale	78%	300+
Penn Highlands Dubois	Dubois	77%	300+
Surgical Specialty Ctr at Coord Hlth	Allentown	77%	300+
Coordinated Health Orthopedic Hospital	Bethlehem	76%	300+
Monongahela Valley Hospital	Monongahela	76%	300+
Titusville Hospital	Titusville	76%	300+
Chester County Hospital	West Chester	75%	300+
Endless Mountains Health Systems	Montrose	75%	300+
Lansdale Hospital	Lansdale	75%	300+

NOTE: Hospital profiles are in alphabetical order by state, then city, then hospital within the city; Rankings exclude hospitals with less than 25 cases except for patient surveys which excludes hospitals with less than 100 cases; (a) 100-299 cases; (1) The number of cases/patients is too few to report; (2) Data submitted were based on a sample of cases/patients; (3) Results are based on a shorter time period than required; (4) Data suppressed by CMS for one or more quarters; (5) Results are not available for this reporting period; (6) Fewer than 100 patients completed the HCAHPS survey; (7) No cases met the criteria for this measure; (8) The lower limit of the confidence interval cannot be calculated if the number of observed infections equals zero; (9) No data are available from the state/territory for this reporting period; (10) The scores shown reflect fewer than 50 completed surveys; (11) There were discrepancies in the data collection process; (12) This measure does not apply to this hospital for this reporting period; (13) Results cannot be calculated for this reporting period; (14) The results for this state are combined with nearby states to protect confidentiality; Please refer to the User's Guide for a full explanation of data.

Meadville Medical Center	Meadville	75%	300+
Riddle Memorial Hospital	Media	75%	300+
Saint Clair Memorial Hospital	Pittsburgh	75%	300+
Saint Luke's Hospital - Anderson Campus	Easton	75%	300+
Tyrone Hospital	Tyrone	75%	(a)
Cancer Treatment Centers of America	Philadelphia	74%	(a)
Carlisle Regional Medical Center	Carlisle	74%	300+
Excela Health Frick Hospital	Mount Pleasant	74%	300+
Lock Haven Hospital	Lock Haven	74%	(a)
Main Line Hospital Paoli	Paoli	74%	300+
Memorial Hospital Towanda	Towanda	74%	300+
Soldiers & Sailors Memorial Hospital	Wellsboro	74%	300+
Easton Hospital	Easton	73%	300+
Good Samaritan Hospital	Lebanon	73%	300+
Grand View Hospital	Sellersville	73%	300+
Berwick Hospital Center	Berwick	72%	300+
Chambersburg Hospital	Chambersburg	72%	300+
Chestnut Hill Hospital	Philadelphia	72%	300+
Corry Memorial Hospital	Corry	72%	(a)
Ellwood City Hospital	Ellwood City	72%	300+
Forbes Regional Hospital	Monroeville	72%	300+
Geisinger Wyoming Valley Medical Center	Wilkes Barre	72%	300+
Heritage Valley Sewickley	Sewickley	72%	300+
Indiana Regional Medical Center	Indiana	72%	300+
J C Blair Memorial Hospital	Huntingdon	72%	300+
Main Line Hospital Bryn Mawr Campus	Bryn Mawr	72%	300+
Main Line Hospital Lankenau	Wynnewood	72%	300+
Mount Nittany Medical Center	State College	72%	300+
Saint Mary Medical Center	Langhorne	72%	300+
Schuylkill Med Ctr-East Norwegian St	Pottsville	72%	300+
Schuylkill Med Ctr-S Jackson St	Pottsville	72%	300+
The Washington Hospital	Washington	72%	300+
Waynesboro Hospital	Waynesboro	72%	300+
Windber Hospital	Windber	72%	300+
Acmh Hospital	Kittanning	71%	300+
Brandywine Hospital	Coatesville	71%	300+
Canonsburg General Hospital	Canonsburg	71%	300+
Charles Cole Memorial Hospital	Coudersport	71%	300+
Delaware County Memorial Hospital	Drexel Hill	71%	300+
Evangelical Community Hospital	Lewisburg	71%	300+
Excela Health Latrobe Hospital	Latrobe	71%	300+
Geisinger - Bloomsburg Hospital	Bloomsburg	71%	300+
Gettysburg Hospital	Gettysburg	71%	300+
Hahnemann University Hospital	Philadelphia	71%	300+
Heart of Lancaster Reg Med Ctr	Lititz	71%	300+
Memorial Hospital	York	71%	300+
Phoenixville Hospital	Phoenixville	71%	300+
Saint Luke's Hospital Bethlehem	Bethlehem	71%	300+
Saint Luke's Quakertown Hospital	Quakertown	71%	300+
Thomas Jefferson University Hospital	Philadelphia	71%	300+
UPMC East	Monroeville	71%	300+
Williamsport Regional Medical Center	Williamsport	71%	300+
Abington Memorial Hospital	Abington	70%	300+
Bradford Regional Medical Center	Bradford	70%	300+
Butler Memorial Hospital	Butler	70%	300+
Clarion Hospital	Clarion	70%	300+
Conemaugh Valley Memorial Hospital	Johnstown	70%	300+
Excela Health Westmoreland Hospital	Greensburg	70%	300+
Geisinger Medical Center	Danville	70%	300+
Hospital of Univ of Pennsylvania	Philadelphia	70%	300+
Jersey Shore Hospital	Jersey Shore	70%	(a)
Lancaster Regional Medical Center	Lancaster	70%	300+
Lehigh Valley Hospital - Muhlenberg	Bethlehem	70%	300+
Lewistown Hospital	Lewistown	70%	300+
Penn Presbyterian Medical Center	Philadelphia	70%	300+
Regional Hospital of Scranton	Scranton	70%	300+
Troy Community Hospital	Troy	70%	(a)
UPMC Mckeesport	Mc Keesport	70%	300+
Wilkes-Barre General Hospital	Wilkes-Barre	70%	300+
Ephrata Community Hospital	Ephrata	69%	300+
Holy Spirit Hospital	Camp Hill	69%	300+
Jeanes Hospital	Philadelphia	69%	300+
Kane Community Hospital	Kane	69%	(a)
Lehigh Valley Hospital	Allentown	69%	300+
Millcreek Community Hospital	Erie	69%	(a)
Milton S Hershey Medical Center	Hershey	69%	300+
Moses Taylor Hospital	Scranton	69%	300+
Muncy Valley Hospital	Muncy	69%	(a)
Pocono Medical Center	E Stroudsburg	69%	300+
Punxsutawney Area Hospital	Punxsutawney	69%	300+
Robert Packer Hospital	Sayre	69%	300+
Roxborough Memorial Hospital	Philadelphia	69%	(a)
Sacred Heart Hospital	Allentown	69%	300+
Saint Joseph Medical Center	Reading	69%	300+
Sharon Regional Health System	Sharon	69%	300+
Uniontown Hospital	Uniontown	69%	300+
UPMC Passavant	Pittsburgh	69%	300+
Wayne Memorial Hospital	Honesdale	69%	300+
Western Pennsylvania Hospital	Pittsburgh	69%	300+
Alle Kiski Medical Center	Natrona	68%	300+
Jefferson Regional Medical Center	Pittsburgh	68%	300+
Magee Womens Hosp of UPMC Health Sys	Pittsburgh	68%	300+
Nason Hospital	Roaring Spring	68%	300+
Penn Highlands Elk	Saint Marys	68%	300+
Pinnacle Health Hospitals	Harrisburg	68%	300+
Reading Hospital	Reading	68%	300+
Saint Vincent Hospital	Erie	68%	300+
Sunbury Community Hospital	Sunbury	68%	(a)
UPMC Altoona	Altoona	68%	300+
UPMC Bedford Memorial	Everett	68%	300+
UPMC Horizon	Greenville	68%	300+
UPMC Presbyterian Shadyside	Pittsburgh	68%	300+
Warren General Hospital	Warren	68%	300+
Albert Einstein Medical Center	Philadelphia	67%	300+
Allegheny General Hospital	Pittsburgh	67%	300+
Geisinger - Community Medical Center	Scranton	67%	300+
Hanover Hospital	Hanover	67%	300+
Heritage Valley Beaver	Beaver	67%	(a)
Holy Redeemer Hospital & Medical Center	Meadowbrook	67%	300+
Somerset Hospital	Somerset	67%	300+
Temple University Hospital	Philadelphia	67%	300+
UPMC Hamot	Erie	67%	300+
Aria Health	Philadelphia	66%	300+
Barnes-Kasson County Hospital	Susquehanna	66%	(a)
Einstein Medical Center Montgomery	East Norriton	66%	300+
Gnaden Huetten Memorial Hospital	Lehighton	66%	300+
Jennersville Regional Hospital	West Grove	66%	300+
UPMC Saint Margaret	Pittsburgh	66%	300+
York Hospital	York	66%	300+
Grove City Medical Center	Grove City	65%	300+
Highlands Hospital	Connellsville	65%	300+
Lancaster General Hospital	Lancaster	65%	300+
Southwest Regional Medical Center	Waynesburg	65%	300+
UPMC Mercy	Pittsburgh	65%	300+
Jameson Memorial Hospital	New Castle	64%	300+
Mercy Suburban Hospital	Norristown	64%	300+
Penn Hosp of the Univ of PA Hlth Sys	Philadelphia	64%	300+
Pottstown Memorial Medical Center	Pottstown	64%	300+
Lehigh Valley Hospital - Hazleton	Hazleton	63%	300+
Lower Bucks Hospital	Bristol	63%	(a)
Ohio Valley General Hospital	Mckees Rocks	63%	300+
Palmerton Hospital	Palmerton	63%	300+
UPMC Northwest	Seneca	63%	300+
Crozer Chester Medical Center	Upland	62%	300+
Mercy Fitzgerald Hospital	Darby	62%	300+
Penn Highlands Clearfield	Clearfield	62%	300+
Nazareth Hospital	Philadelphia	61%	300+
Saint Joseph's Hospital	Philadelphia	54%	(a)

Room and Bathroom 'Always' Clean

Hospital Name	City	Rate	Cases
Advanced Surgical Hospital	Washington	91%	(a)
Muncy Valley Hospital	Muncy	89%	(a)
Physician's Care Surgical Hospital	Royersford	89%	300+
Surgical Institute of Reading	Wyomissing	89%	(a)
Bucks County Specialty Hospital	Bensalem	87%	300+
Oss Orthopaedic Hospital	York	87%	300+
Soldiers & Sailors Memorial Hospital	Wellsboro	87%	300+
Tyrone Hospital	Tyrone	87%	(a)
Wellspan Surgery & Rehab Hosp	York	87%	(a)
Memorial Hospital Towanda	Towanda	86%	300+
Surgical Specialty Ctr at Coord Hlth	Allentown	85%	300+
Coordinated Health Orthopedic Hospital	Bethlehem	84%	300+
Kane Community Hospital	Kane	84%	(a)
Mid - Valley Hospital	Peckville	84%	(a)
Sunbury Community Hospital	Sunbury	84%	(a)
UPMC Bedford Memorial	Everett	84%	300+
Monongahela Valley Hospital	Monongahela	83%	300+
Nason Hospital	Roaring Spring	83%	300+
Hanover Hospital	Hanover	82%	300+
Titusville Hospital	Titusville	82%	300+
Troy Community Hospital	Troy	82%	(a)
Chambersburg Hospital	Chambersburg	81%	300+
Corry Memorial Hospital	Corry	81%	(a)
J C Blair Memorial Hospital	Huntingdon	81%	300+
Jersey Shore Hospital	Jersey Shore	81%	(a)
Mount Nittany Medical Center	State College	81%	300+
Fulton County Medical Center	Mcconnellsburg	80%	(a)
Good Samaritan Hospital	Lebanon	80%	300+
Lancaster Regional Medical Center	Lancaster	80%	300+
Meadville Medical Center	Meadville	80%	300+
Saint Luke's Quakertown Hospital	Quakertown	80%	300+
Cancer Treatment Centers of America	Philadelphia	79%	(a)
Excela Health Frick Hospital	Mount Pleasant	79%	300+
Heart of Lancaster Reg Med Ctr	Lititz	79%	300+
Barnes-Kasson County Hospital	Susquehanna	78%	(a)
Robert Packer Hospital	Sayre	78%	300+
Saint Luke's Hospital - Anderson Campus	Easton	78%	300+
Windber Hospital	Windber	78%	300+
Conemaugh Valley Memorial Hospital	Johnstown	77%	300+
Doylestown Hospital	Doylestown	77%	300+
Indiana Regional Medical Center	Indiana	77%	300+
Lansdale Hospital	Lansdale	77%	300+
Lehigh Valley Hospital - Hazleton	Hazleton	77%	300+
Pocono Medical Center	E Stroudsburg	77%	300+
The Washington Hospital	Washington	77%	300+
Carlisle Regional Medical Center	Carlisle	76%	300+
Charles Cole Memorial Hospital	Coudersport	76%	300+
Geisinger Medical Center	Danville	76%	300+
Gettysburg Hospital	Gettysburg	76%	300+
Grand View Hospital	Sellersville	76%	300+
Penn Highlands Dubois	Dubois	76%	300+
Saint Luke's Miners Memorial Hospital	Coaldale	76%	300+
Schuylkill Med Ctr-S Jackson St	Pottsville	76%	300+
Somerset Hospital	Somerset	76%	300+
Williamsport Regional Medical Center	Williamsport	76%	300+
Alle Kiski Medical Center	Natrona	75%	300+
Ellwood City Hospital	Ellwood City	75%	300+
Grove City Medical Center	Grove City	75%	300+
Jameson Memorial Hospital	New Castle	75%	300+
Lehigh Valley Hospital - Muhlenberg	Bethlehem	75%	300+
Schuylkill Med Ctr-East Norwegian St	Pottsville	75%	300+
Tyler Memorial Hospital	Tunkhannock	75%	300+
UPMC Altoona	Altoona	75%	300+
Wayne Memorial Hospital	Honesdale	75%	300+
Brandywine Hospital	Coatesville	74%	300+
Chester County Hospital	West Chester	74%	300+
Einstein Medical Center Montgomery	East Norriton	74%	300+
Endless Mountains Health Systems	Montrose	74%	300+
Geisinger Wyoming Valley Medical Center	Wilkes Barre	74%	300+
Penn Highlands Elk	Saint Marys	74%	300+
Phoenixville Hospital	Phoenixville	74%	300+
Waynesboro Hospital	Waynesboro	74%	300+
Evangelical Community Hospital	Lewisburg	73%	300+
Jefferson Regional Medical Center	Pittsburgh	73%	300+
Lewistown Hospital	Lewistown	73%	300+
Palmerton Hospital	Palmerton	73%	300+
Penn Highlands Clearfield	Clearfield	73%	300+
Canonsburg General Hospital	Canonsburg	72%	300+
Clarion Hospital	Clarion	72%	300+
Geisinger - Bloomsburg Hospital	Bloomsburg	72%	300+
Ohio Valley General Hospital	Mckees Rocks	72%	300+
UPMC East	Monroeville	72%	300+
UPMC Horizon	Greenville	72%	300+
Gnaden Huetten Memorial Hospital	Lehighton	71%	300+
Highlands Hospital	Connellsville	71%	300+
Lock Haven Hospital	Lock Haven	71%	(a)
Saint Luke's Hospital Bethlehem	Bethlehem	71%	300+
Acmh Hospital	Kittanning	70%	300+
Bradford Regional Medical Center	Bradford	70%	300+
Easton Hospital	Easton	70%	300+
Geisinger - Community Medical Center	Scranton	70%	300+
Holy Spirit Hospital	Camp Hill	70%	300+
Lancaster General Hospital	Lancaster	70%	300+
Main Line Hospital Bryn Mawr Campus	Bryn Mawr	70%	300+
Pinnacle Health Hospitals	Harrisburg	70%	300+
Punxsutawney Area Hospital	Punxsutawney	70%	300+
Regional Hospital of Scranton	Scranton	70%	300+
Riddle Memorial Hospital	Media	70%	300+
Saint Clair Memorial Hospital	Pittsburgh	70%	300+
UPMC Mckeesport	Mc Keesport	70%	300+
UPMC Northwest	Seneca	70%	300+
York Hospital	York	70%	300+
Allegheny General Hospital	Pittsburgh	69%	300+
Berwick Hospital Center	Berwick	69%	300+
Ephrata Community Hospital	Ephrata	69%	300+
Main Line Hospital Paoli	Paoli	69%	300+
Milton S Hershey Medical Center	Hershey	69%	300+
Roxborough Memorial Hospital	Philadelphia	69%	(a)
Saint Mary Medical Center	Langhorne	69%	300+
Holy Redeemer Hospital & Medical Center	Meadowbrook	68%	300+
Hospital of Univ of Pennsylvania	Philadelphia	68%	300+
Jennersville Regional Hospital	West Grove	68%	300+
Lower Bucks Hospital	Bristol	68%	(a)
Main Line Hospital Lankenau	Wynnewood	68%	300+
Memorial Hospital	York	68%	300+
Mercy Fitzgerald Hospital	Darby	68%	300+
Penn Presbyterian Medical Center	Philadelphia	68%	300+
Penn Hosp of the Univ of PA Hlth Sys	Philadelphia	68%	300+
Sacred Heart Hospital	Allentown	68%	300+
Saint Joseph Medical Center	Reading	68%	300+
UPMC Hamot	Erie	68%	300+
Wilkes-Barre General Hospital	Wilkes-Barre	68%	300+
Aria Health	Philadelphia	67%	300+
Southwest Regional Medical Center	Waynesburg	67%	300+
Temple University Hospital	Philadelphia	67%	300+
Uniontown Hospital	Uniontown	67%	300+
UPMC Passavant	Pittsburgh	67%	300+
Warren General Hospital	Warren	67%	300+
Chestnut Hill Hospital	Philadelphia	66%	300+
Excela Health Latrobe Hospital	Latrobe	66%	300+
Heritage Valley Sewickley	Sewickley	66%	300+
Lehigh Valley Hospital	Allentown	66%	300+

NOTE: Hospital profiles are in alphabetical order by state, then city, then hospital within the city; Rankings exclude hospitals with less than 25 cases except for patient surveys which excludes hospitals with less than 100 cases; (a) 100-299 cases; (1) The number of cases/patients is too few to report; (2) Data submitted were based on a sample of cases/patients; (3) Results are based on a shorter time period than required; (4) Data suppressed by CMS for one or more quarters; (5) Results are not available for this reporting period; (6) Fewer than 100 patients completed the HCAHPS survey; (7) No cases met the criteria for this measure; (8) The lower limit of the confidence interval cannot be calculated if the number of observed infections equals zero; (9) No data are available from the state/territory for this reporting period; (10) The scores shown reflect fewer than 50 completed surveys; (11) There were discrepancies in the data collection process; (12) This measure does not apply to this hospital for this reporting period; (13) Results cannot be calculated for this reporting period; (14) The results for this state are combined with nearby states to protect confidentiality; Please refer to the User's Guide for a full explanation of data.

Saint Vincent Hospital	Erie	66%	300+
Sharon Regional Health System	Sharon	66%	300+
Butler Memorial Hospital	Butler	65%	300+
Excela Health Westmoreland Hospital	Greensburg	65%	300+
Jeanes Hospital	Philadelphia	65%	300+
Moses Taylor Hospital	Scranton	65%	300+
Nazareth Hospital	Philadelphia	65%	300+
Saint Joseph's Hospital	Philadelphia	65%	(a)
Thomas Jefferson University Hospital	Philadelphia	65%	300+
Western Pennsylvania Hospital	Pittsburgh	65%	300+
Hahnemann University Hospital	Philadelphia	64%	300+
Magee Womens Hosp of UPMC Health Sys	Pittsburgh	64%	300+
Millcreek Community Hospital	Erie	64%	(a)
Abington Memorial Hospital	Abington	63%	300+
Pottstown Memorial Medical Center	Pottstown	63%	300+
Reading Hospital	Reading	63%	300+
UPMC Mercy	Pittsburgh	63%	300+
Albert Einstein Medical Center	Philadelphia	62%	300+
Heritage Valley Beaver	Beaver	62%	(a)
UPMC Saint Margaret	Pittsburgh	62%	300+
Delaware County Memorial Hospital	Drexel Hill	61%	300+
Forbes Regional Hospital	Monroeville	61%	300+
UPMC Presbyterian Shadyside	Pittsburgh	61%	300+
Crozer Chester Medical Center	Upland	59%	300+
Mercy Suburban Hospital	Norristown	57%	300+

Timely Help 'Always' Received

Hospital Name	City	Rate	Cases
Advanced Surgical Hospital	Washington	95%	(a)
Physician's Care Surgical Hospital	Royersford	95%	300+
Surgical Institute of Reading	Wyomissing	93%	(a)
Wellspan Surgery & Rehab Hosp	York	91%	(a)
Bucks County Specialty Hospital	Bensalem	88%	300+
Surgical Specialty Ctr at Coord Hlth	Allentown	88%	300+
Mid - Valley Hospital	Peckville	85%	(a)
Tyrone Hospital	Tyrone	85%	(a)
Coordinated Health Orthopedic Hospital	Bethlehem	80%	300+
Oss Orthopaedic Hospital	York	79%	300+
Doylestown Hospital	Doylestown	78%	300+
Endless Mountains Health Systems	Montrose	78%	300+
Fulton County Medical Center	Mcconnellsburg	78%	(a)
Geisinger - Bloomsburg Hospital	Bloomsburg	77%	300+
Titusville Hospital	Titusville	77%	300+
Tyler Memorial Hospital	Tunkhannock	77%	300+
Charles Cole Memorial Hospital	Coudersport	76%	300+
J C Blair Memorial Hospital	Huntingdon	76%	300+
Monongahela Valley Hospital	Monongahela	76%	300+
Penn Highlands Dubois	Dubois	76%	300+
Chester County Hospital	West Chester	75%	300+
Lansdale Hospital	Lansdale	75%	300+
Memorial Hospital Towanda	Towanda	75%	300+
Excela Health Frick Hospital	Mount Pleasant	74%	300+
Muncy Valley Hospital	Muncy	74%	(a)
Saint Clair Memorial Hospital	Pittsburgh	74%	300+
Acmh Hospital	Kittanning	73%	300+
Evangelical Community Hospital	Lewisburg	73%	300+
Schuylkill Med Ctr-East Norwegian St	Pottsville	73%	300+
Schuylkill Med Ctr-S Jackson St	Pottsville	73%	300+
Soldiers & Sailors Memorial Hospital	Wellsboro	73%	300+
Kane Community Hospital	Kane	72%	(a)
Meadville Medical Center	Meadville	72%	300+
Mount Nittany Medical Center	State College	72%	300+
Riddle Memorial Hospital	Media	72%	300+
Barnes-Kasson County Hospital	Susquehanna	71%	(a)
Ephrata Community Hospital	Ephrata	71%	300+
Excela Health Latrobe Hospital	Latrobe	71%	300+
Saint Luke's Hospital - Anderson Campus	Easton	71%	300+
Thomas Jefferson University Hospital	Philadelphia	71%	300+
Waynesboro Hospital	Waynesboro	71%	300+
Cancer Treatment Centers of America	Philadelphia	70%	(a)
Corry Memorial Hospital	Corry	70%	(a)
Geisinger Medical Center	Danville	70%	300+
Heart of Lancaster Reg Med Ctr	Lititz	70%	300+
Jefferson Regional Medical Center	Pittsburgh	70%	300+
Saint Luke's Miners Memorial Hospital	Coaldale	70%	300+
UPMC Bedford Memorial	Everett	70%	300+
Windber Hospital	Windber	70%	300+
Bradford Regional Medical Center	Bradford	69%	300+
Conemaugh Valley Memorial Hospital	Johnstown	69%	300+
Ellwood City Hospital	Ellwood City	69%	300+
Good Samaritan Hospital	Lebanon	69%	300+
Hanover Hospital	Hanover	69%	300+
Lancaster Regional Medical Center	Lancaster	69%	300+
Millcreek Community Hospital	Erie	69%	(a)
Saint Luke's Quakertown Hospital	Quakertown	69%	300+
Saint Mary Medical Center	Langhorne	69%	300+
Berwick Hospital Center	Berwick	68%	300+
Canonsburg General Hospital	Canonsburg	68%	300+
Carlisle Regional Medical Center	Carlisle	68%	300+
Forbes Regional Hospital	Monroeville	68%	300+
Geisinger Wyoming Valley Medical Center	Wilkes Barre	68%	300+
Gettysburg Hospital	Gettysburg	68%	300+
Main Line Hospital Bryn Mawr Campus	Bryn Mawr	68%	300+
Milton S Hershey Medical Center	Hershey	68%	300+
Robert Packer Hospital	Sayre	68%	300+
Sunbury Community Hospital	Sunbury	68%	(a)
Wayne Memorial Hospital	Honesdale	68%	300+
Indiana Regional Medical Center	Indiana	67%	300+
Jersey Shore Hospital	Jersey Shore	67%	(a)
Lehigh Valley Hospital	Allentown	67%	300+
Main Line Hospital Paoli	Paoli	67%	300+
Punxsutawney Area Hospital	Punxsutawney	67%	300+
UPMC East	Monroeville	67%	300+
UPMC Hamot	Erie	67%	300+
The Washington Hospital	Washington	67%	300+
Brandywine Hospital	Coatesville	66%	300+
Chambersburg Hospital	Chambersburg	66%	300+
Grand View Hospital	Sellersville	66%	300+
Nason Hospital	Roaring Spring	66%	300+
Penn Presbyterian Medical Center	Philadelphia	66%	300+
Saint Vincent Hospital	Erie	66%	300+
Sharon Regional Health System	Sharon	66%	300+
Heritage Valley Sewickley	Sewickley	65%	300+
Highlands Hospital	Connellsville	65%	300+
Lock Haven Hospital	Lock Haven	65%	(a)
Main Line Hospital Lankenau	Wynnewood	65%	300+
Nazareth Hospital	Philadelphia	65%	300+
Penn Highlands Elk	Saint Marys	65%	300+
Phoenixville Hospital	Phoenixville	65%	300+
Pinnacle Health Hospitals	Harrisburg	65%	300+
Pocono Medical Center	E Stroudsburg	65%	300+
Saint Luke's Hospital Bethlehem	Bethlehem	65%	300+
Somerset Hospital	Somerset	65%	300+
UPMC Mckeesport	Mc Keesport	65%	300+
Aria Health	Philadelphia	64%	300+
Clarion Hospital	Clarion	64%	300+
Excela Health Westmoreland Hospital	Greensburg	64%	300+
Hospital of Univ of Pennsylvania	Philadelphia	64%	300+
UPMC Altoona	Altoona	64%	300+
Warren General Hospital	Warren	64%	300+
Western Pennsylvania Hospital	Pittsburgh	64%	300+
Abington Memorial Hospital	Abington	63%	300+
Alle Kiski Medical Center	Natrona	63%	300+
Einstein Medical Center Montgomery	East Norriton	63%	300+
Holy Redeemer Hospital & Medical Center	Meadowbrook	63%	300+
Jeanes Hospital	Philadelphia	63%	300+
Sacred Heart Hospital	Allentown	63%	300+
Uniontown Hospital	Uniontown	63%	300+
Wilkes-Barre General Hospital	Wilkes-Barre	63%	300+
Albert Einstein Medical Center	Philadelphia	62%	300+
Easton Hospital	Easton	62%	300+
Geisinger - Community Medical Center	Scranton	62%	300+
Holy Spirit Hospital	Camp Hill	62%	300+
Lancaster General Hospital	Lancaster	62%	300+
Lehigh Valley Hospital - Muhlenberg	Bethlehem	62%	300+
Lewistown Hospital	Lewistown	62%	300+
Magee Womens Hosp of UPMC Health Sys	Pittsburgh	62%	300+
Palmerton Hospital	Palmerton	62%	300+
Regional Hospital of Scranton	Scranton	62%	300+
Southwest Regional Medical Center	Waynesburg	62%	300+
Delaware County Memorial Hospital	Drexel Hill	61%	300+
Hahnemann University Hospital	Philadelphia	61%	300+
Moses Taylor Hospital	Scranton	61%	300+
Ohio Valley General Hospital	Mckees Rocks	61%	300+
Penn Highlands Clearfield	Clearfield	61%	300+
UPMC Northwest	Seneca	61%	300+
UPMC Presbyterian Shadyside	Pittsburgh	61%	300+
Williamsport Regional Medical Center	Williamsport	61%	300+
Butler Memorial Hospital	Butler	60%	300+
Gnaden Huetten Memorial Hospital	Lehighton	60%	300+
Saint Joseph Medical Center	Reading	60%	300+
UPMC Horizon	Greenville	60%	300+
UPMC Passavant	Pittsburgh	60%	300+
York Hospital	York	60%	300+
Jennersville Regional Hospital	West Grove	59%	300+
Lehigh Valley Hospital - Hazleton	Hazleton	59%	300+
Memorial Hospital	York	59%	300+
UPMC Mercy	Pittsburgh	59%	300+
Heritage Valley Beaver	Beaver	58%	(a)
Lower Bucks Hospital	Bristol	57%	(a)
Reading Hospital	Reading	57%	300+
UPMC Saint Margaret	Pittsburgh	57%	300+
Chestnut Hill Hospital	Philadelphia	56%	300+
Penn Hosp of the Univ of PA Hlth Sys	Philadelphia	56%	300+
Roxborough Memorial Hospital	Philadelphia	56%	(a)
Temple University Hospital	Philadelphia	56%	300+
Crozer Chester Medical Center	Upland	55%	300+
Mercy Fitzgerald Hospital	Darby	55%	300+
Pottstown Memorial Medical Center	Pottstown	55%	300+
Grove City Medical Center	Grove City	54%	300+
Jameson Memorial Hospital	New Castle	54%	300+
Mercy Suburban Hospital	Norristown	54%	300+
Allegheny General Hospital	Pittsburgh	53%	300+
Troy Community Hospital	Troy	53%	(a)
Saint Joseph's Hospital	Philadelphia	45%	(a)

Would Definitely Recommend Hospital

Hospital Name	City	Rate	Cases
Advanced Surgical Hospital	Washington	95%	(a)
Surgical Institute of Reading	Wyomissing	95%	(a)
Physician's Care Surgical Hospital	Royersford	94%	300+
Wellspan Surgery & Rehab Hosp	York	94%	(a)
Cancer Treatment Centers of America	Philadelphia	93%	(a)
Oss Orthopaedic Hospital	York	93%	300+
Bucks County Specialty Hospital	Bensalem	90%	300+
Surgical Specialty Ctr at Coord Hlth	Allentown	88%	300+
Doylestown Hospital	Doylestown	87%	300+
Main Line Hospital Paoli	Paoli	86%	300+
Coordinated Health Orthopedic Hospital	Bethlehem	84%	300+
Saint Luke's Hospital - Anderson Campus	Easton	84%	300+
Main Line Hospital Bryn Mawr Campus	Bryn Mawr	82%	300+
Main Line Hospital Lankenau	Wynnewood	82%	300+
Saint Clair Memorial Hospital	Pittsburgh	82%	300+
Mid - Valley Hospital	Peckville	81%	(a)
Chester County Hospital	West Chester	80%	300+
Hospital of Univ of Pennsylvania	Philadelphia	80%	300+
Milton S Hershey Medical Center	Hershey	80%	300+
Saint Mary Medical Center	Langhorne	80%	300+
Tyrone Hospital	Tyrone	80%	(a)
Lehigh Valley Hospital	Allentown	79%	300+
Saint Joseph Medical Center	Reading	79%	300+
Einstein Medical Center Montgomery	East Norriton	78%	300+
Evangelical Community Hospital	Lewisburg	78%	300+
Lehigh Valley Hospital - Muhlenberg	Bethlehem	78%	300+
Titusville Hospital	Titusville	78%	300+
Abington Memorial Hospital	Abington	77%	300+
Geisinger Medical Center	Danville	77%	300+
Grand View Hospital	Sellersville	77%	300+
Lancaster General Hospital	Lancaster	77%	300+
Thomas Jefferson University Hospital	Philadelphia	77%	300+
Geisinger Wyoming Valley Medical Center	Wilkes Barre	76%	300+
Mount Nittany Medical Center	State College	76%	300+
Muncy Valley Hospital	Muncy	76%	(a)
Nason Hospital	Roaring Spring	76%	300+
Penn Highlands Dubois	Dubois	76%	300+
Pinnacle Health Hospitals	Harrisburg	76%	300+
Windber Hospital	Windber	76%	300+
Heart of Lancaster Reg Med Ctr	Lititz	75%	300+
Lansdale Hospital	Lansdale	75%	300+
Magee Womens Hosp of UPMC Health Sys	Pittsburgh	75%	300+
Phoenixville Hospital	Phoenixville	75%	300+
Riddle Memorial Hospital	Media	75%	300+
UPMC East	Monroeville	75%	300+
Jersey Shore Hospital	Jersey Shore	74%	(a)
Waynesboro Hospital	Waynesboro	74%	300+
Canonsburg General Hospital	Canonsburg	73%	300+
Ellwood City Hospital	Ellwood City	73%	300+
Heritage Valley Sewickley	Sewickley	73%	300+
Jefferson Regional Medical Center	Pittsburgh	73%	300+
Kane Community Hospital	Kane	73%	(a)
Lancaster Regional Medical Center	Lancaster	73%	300+
Penn Presbyterian Medical Center	Philadelphia	73%	300+
Saint Luke's Hospital Bethlehem	Bethlehem	73%	300+
Saint Luke's Miners Memorial Hospital	Coaldale	73%	300+
UPMC Hamot	Erie	73%	300+
Western Pennsylvania Hospital	Pittsburgh	73%	300+
Butler Memorial Hospital	Butler	72%	300+
Fulton County Medical Center	Mcconnellsburg	72%	(a)
Holy Redeemer Hospital & Medical Center	Meadowbrook	72%	300+
Holy Spirit Hospital	Camp Hill	72%	300+
Robert Packer Hospital	Sayre	72%	300+
Saint Vincent Hospital	Erie	72%	300+
Soldiers & Sailors Memorial Hospital	Wellsboro	72%	300+
UPMC Passavant	Pittsburgh	72%	300+
UPMC Presbyterian Shadyside	Pittsburgh	72%	300+
UPMC Saint Margaret	Pittsburgh	72%	300+
Memorial Hospital	York	71%	300+
Monongahela Valley Hospital	Monongahela	71%	300+
Penn Hosp of the Univ of PA Hlth Sys	Philadelphia	71%	300+
Saint Luke's Quakertown Hospital	Quakertown	71%	300+
Excela Health Frick Hospital	Mount Pleasant	70%	300+
Forbes Regional Hospital	Monroeville	70%	300+
Indiana Regional Medical Center	Indiana	70%	300+
Moses Taylor Hospital	Scranton	70%	300+
York Hospital	York	70%	300+
Ephrata Community Hospital	Ephrata	69%	300+
Gettysburg Hospital	Gettysburg	69%	300+
Good Samaritan Hospital	Lebanon	69%	300+
Meadville Medical Center	Meadville	69%	300+
Millcreek Community Hospital	Erie	69%	(a)
Troy Community Hospital	Troy	69%	(a)
Tyler Memorial Hospital	Tunkhannock	69%	300+
Williamsport Regional Medical Center	Williamsport	69%	300+

NOTE: Hospital profiles are in alphabetical order by state, then city, then hospital within the city; Rankings exclude hospitals with less than 25 cases except for patient surveys which excludes hospitals with less than 100 cases; (a) 100-299 cases; (1) The number of cases/patients is too few to report; (2) Data submitted were based on a sample of cases/patients; (3) Results are based on a shorter time period than required; (4) Data suppressed by CMS for one or more quarters; (5) Results are not available for this reporting period; (6) Fewer than 100 patients completed the HCAHPS survey; (7) No cases met the criteria for this measure; (8) The lower limit of the confidence interval cannot be calculated if the number of observed infections equals zero; (9) No data are available from the state/territory for this reporting period; (10) The scores shown reflect fewer than 50 completed surveys; (11) There were discrepancies in the data collection process; (12) This measure does not apply to this hospital for this reporting period; (13) Results cannot be calculated for this reporting period; (14) The results for this state are combined with nearby states to protect confidentiality; Please refer to the User's Guide for a full explanation of data.

Hospital Name	City	Rate	Cases
Allegheny General Hospital	Pittsburgh	68%	300+
Clarion Hospital	Clarion	68%	300+
Easton Hospital	Easton	68%	300+
Geisinger - Bloomsburg Hospital	Bloomsburg	68%	300+
Hahnemann University Hospital	Philadelphia	68%	300+
Memorial Hospital Towanda	Towanda	68%	300+
Regional Hospital of Scranton	Scranton	68%	300+
Sunbury Community Hospital	Sunbury	68%	(a)
The Washington Hospital	Washington	68%	300+
Wayne Memorial Hospital	Honesdale	68%	300+
Excela Health Latrobe Hospital	Latrobe	67%	300+
Hanover Hospital	Hanover	67%	300+
Chambersburg Hospital	Chambersburg	66%	300+
Chestnut Hill Hospital	Philadelphia	66%	300+
Jeanes Hospital	Philadelphia	66%	300+
Pocono Medical Center	E Stroudsburg	66%	300+
UPMC Altoona	Altoona	66%	300+
Wilkes-Barre General Hospital	Wilkes-Barre	66%	300+
Acmh Hospital	Kittanning	65%	300+
Conemaugh Valley Memorial Hospital	Johnstown	65%	300+
Reading Hospital	Reading	65%	300+
Temple University Hospital	Philadelphia	65%	300+
Corry Memorial Hospital	Corry	64%	(a)
UPMC Mercy	Pittsburgh	64%	300+
Aria Health	Philadelphia	63%	300+
Brandywine Hospital	Coatesville	63%	300+
Delaware County Memorial Hospital	Drexel Hill	63%	300+
Sacred Heart Hospital	Allentown	63%	300+
Sharon Regional Health System	Sharon	63%	300+
Warren General Hospital	Warren	63%	300+
Alle Kiski Medical Center	Natrona	62%	300+
Berwick Hospital Center	Berwick	62%	300+
Charles Cole Memorial Hospital	Coudersport	62%	300+
Endless Mountains Health Systems	Montrose	62%	300+
Ohio Valley General Hospital	Mckees Rocks	62%	300+
Punxsutawney Area Hospital	Punxsutawney	62%	300+
Albert Einstein Medical Center	Philadelphia	61%	300+
Geisinger - Community Medical Center	Scranton	61%	300+
Grove City Medical Center	Grove City	61%	300+
Jennersville Regional Hospital	West Grove	61%	300+
Palmerton Hospital	Palmerton	61%	300+
Roxborough Memorial Hospital	Philadelphia	61%	(a)
Schuylkill Med Ctr-East Norwegian St	Pottsville	61%	300+
UPMC Horizon	Greenville	61%	300+
UPMC Mckeesport	Mc Keesport	61%	300+
Excela Health Westmoreland Hospital	Greensburg	60%	300+
Gnaden Huetten Memorial Hospital	Lehighton	60%	300+
Heritage Valley Beaver	Beaver	60%	(a)
Highlands Hospital	Connellsville	60%	300+
UPMC Bedford Memorial	Everett	60%	300+
J C Blair Memorial Hospital	Huntingdon	59%	300+
Nazareth Hospital	Philadelphia	59%	300+
Schuylkill Med Ctr-S Jackson St	Pottsville	59%	300+
Somerset Hospital	Somerset	59%	300+
Uniontown Hospital	Uniontown	59%	300+
Mercy Suburban Hospital	Norristown	58%	300+
UPMC Northwest	Seneca	58%	300+
Carlisle Regional Medical Center	Carlisle	57%	300+
Lower Bucks Hospital	Bristol	57%	(a)
Penn Highlands Elk	Saint Marys	56%	300+
Barnes-Kasson County Hospital	Susquehanna	55%	(a)
Bradford Regional Medical Center	Bradford	54%	300+
Crozer Chester Medical Center	Upland	54%	300+
Lock Haven Hospital	Lock Haven	54%	(a)
Mercy Fitzgerald Hospital	Darby	54%	300+
Pottstown Memorial Medical Center	Pottstown	54%	300+
Lewistown Hospital	Lewistown	52%	300+
Southwest Regional Medical Center	Waynesburg	52%	300+
Jameson Memorial Hospital	New Castle	51%	300+
Lehigh Valley Hospital - Hazleton	Hazleton	50%	300+
Penn Highlands Clearfield	Clearfield	48%	300+
Saint Joseph's Hospital	Philadelphia	40%	(a)

Use of Medical Imaging

Cardiac Imaging Stress Test before OP Surgery

Hospital Name	City	Rate	Cases
Charles Cole Memorial Hospital	Coudersport	1.3%	156
Tyler Memorial Hospital	Tunkhannock	1.7%	59
Penn Highlands Brookville	Brookville	1.8%	109
Barnes-Kasson County Hospital	Susquehanna	1.9%	54
Fulton County Medical Center	Mcconnellsburg	2.8%	145
UPMC Hamot	Erie	3.0%	724
Williamsport Regional Medical Center	Williamsport	3.0%	593
Lancaster General Hospital	Lancaster	3.1%	1742
Sharon Regional Health System	Sharon	3.1%	816
Geisinger Wyoming Valley Medical Center	Wilkes Barre	3.2%	505
Heart of Lancaster Reg Med Ctr	Lititz	3.3%	60
Penn Highlands Elk	Saint Marys	3.4%	292
Pinnacle Health Hospitals	Harrisburg	3.4%	1867
Chestnut Hill Hospital	Philadelphia	3.5%	86
Palmerton Hospital	Palmerton	3.5%	86
Saint Luke's Miners Memorial Hospital	Coaldale	3.6%	140
Saint Joseph Medical Center	Reading	3.7%	82
Saint Luke's Quakertown Hospital	Quakertown	3.9%	154
Bradford Regional Medical Center	Bradford	4.0%	201
Ephrata Community Hospital	Ephrata	4.0%	273
Penn Highlands Clearfield	Clearfield	4.0%	100
Brandywine Hospital	Coatesville	4.1%	343
Jersey Shore Hospital	Jersey Shore	4.1%	49
Southwest Regional Medical Center	Waynesburg	4.1%	147
Ellwood City Hospital	Ellwood City	4.2%	119
Holy Redeemer Hospital & Medical Center	Meadowbrook	4.2%	401
Meyersdale Community Hospital	Myersdale	4.2%	48
Mount Nittany Medical Center	State College	4.2%	96
Penn Highlands Dubois	Dubois	4.2%	457
Wilkes-Barre General Hospital	Wilkes-Barre	4.2%	1238
Einstein Medical Center Montgomery	East Norriton	4.3%	46
Hanover Hospital	Hanover	4.3%	438
Milton S Hershey Medical Center	Hershey	4.3%	564
Troy Community Hospital	Troy	4.3%	47
Saint Vincent Hospital	Erie	4.4%	895
Chester County Hospital	West Chester	4.5%	178
Punxsutawney Area Hospital	Punxsutawney	4.5%	88
Soldiers & Sailors Memorial Hospital	Wellsboro	4.5%	267
Surgical Specialty Ctr at Coord Hlth	Allentown	4.5%	269
Alle Kiski Medical Center	Natrona	4.6%	173
Meadville Medical Center	Meadville	4.6%	502
York Hospital	York	4.6%	1874
Excela Health Frick Hospital	Mount Pleasant	4.7%	149
Lehigh Valley Hospital - Muhlenberg	Bethlehem	4.7%	1228
Moses Taylor Hospital	Scranton	4.7%	106
Carlisle Regional Medical Center	Carlisle	4.8%	147
Good Samaritan Hospital	Lebanon	4.8%	897
Penn Presbyterian Medical Center	Philadelphia	4.8%	421
Gnaden Huetten Memorial Hospital	Lehighton	4.9%	406
Main Line Hospital Lankenau	Wynnewood	4.9%	849
Reading Hospital	Reading	4.9%	466
Robert Packer Hospital	Sayre	4.9%	223
The Washington Hospital	Washington	4.9%	448
Allegheny General Hospital	Pittsburgh	5.0%	221
Crozer Chester Medical Center	Upland	5.0%	724
Holy Spirit Hospital	Camp Hill	5.0%	776
Chambersburg Hospital	Chambersburg	5.1%	802
Grand View Hospital	Sellersville	5.1%	495
Conemaugh Valley Memorial Hospital	Johnstown	5.2%	519
Hospital of Univ of Pennsylvania	Philadelphia	5.2%	852
Saint Luke's Hospital - Anderson Campus	Easton	5.2%	308
Butler Memorial Hospital	Butler	5.3%	490
Jennersville Regional Hospital	West Grove	5.3%	114
Saint Luke's Hospital Bethlehem	Bethlehem	5.3%	952
Canonsburg General Hospital	Canonsburg	5.4%	92
Geisinger Medical Center	Danville	5.4%	629
J C Blair Memorial Hospital	Huntingdon	5.4%	259
Lehigh Valley Hospital - Hazleton	Hazleton	5.4%	336
Mercy Fitzgerald Hospital	Darby	5.4%	129
Mercy Suburban Hospital	Norristown	5.4%	56
UPMC Horizon	Greenville	5.4%	423
Main Line Hospital Paoli	Paoli	5.5%	200
Sunbury Community Hospital	Sunbury	5.5%	55
UPMC Altoona	Altoona	5.5%	600
Gettysburg Hospital	Gettysburg	5.7%	422
Grove City Medical Center	Grove City	5.7%	158
Doylestown Hospital	Doylestown	5.8%	968
Somerset Hospital	Somerset	5.8%	139
Excela Health Westmoreland Hospital	Greensburg	5.9%	306
Ohio Valley General Hospital	Mckees Rocks	6.0%	100
Saint Mary Medical Center	Langhorne	6.1%	792
Aria Health	Philadelphia	6.2%	434
Lancaster Regional Medical Center	Lancaster	6.2%	65
Temple University Hospital	Philadelphia	6.2%	631
Highlands Hospital	Connellsville	6.3%	79
Waynesboro Hospital	Waynesboro	6.3%	159
Albert Einstein Medical Center	Philadelphia	6.4%	343
Abington Memorial Hospital	Abington	6.5%	979
Schuylkill Med Ctr-S Jackson St	Pottsville	6.5%	62
UPMC Bedford Memorial	Everett	6.5%	170
UPMC Saint Margaret	Pittsburgh	6.5%	232
Lehigh Valley Hospital	Allentown	6.6%	1122
Memorial Hospital Towanda	Towanda	6.7%	89
UPMC Passavant	Pittsburgh	6.8%	309
Hahnemann University Hospital	Philadelphia	6.9%	144
Saint Clair Memorial Hospital	Pittsburgh	6.9%	349
Evangelical Community Hospital	Lewisburg	7.0%	429
Heritage Valley Beaver	Beaver	7.0%	114
Warren General Hospital	Warren	7.0%	313
Geisinger - Community Medical Center	Scranton	7.1%	184
Memorial Hospital	York	7.2%	500
UPMC Presbyterian Shadyside	Pittsburgh	7.2%	680
Main Line Hospital Bryn Mawr Campus	Bryn Mawr	7.3%	193
Wayne Memorial Hospital	Honesdale	7.4%	229
Indiana Regional Medical Center	Indiana	7.5%	226
Nazareth Hospital	Philadelphia	7.5%	305
Titusville Hospital	Titusville	7.5%	67
Thomas Jefferson University Hospital	Philadelphia	7.7%	913
Corry Memorial Hospital	Corry	7.8%	64
Excela Health Latrobe Hospital	Latrobe	7.8%	141
Forbes Regional Hospital	Monroeville	7.8%	153
Lewistown Hospital	Lewistown	7.8%	386
Pocono Medical Center	E Stroudsburg	7.8%	566
Sacred Heart Hospital	Allentown	7.8%	206
UPMC Mckeesport	Mc Keesport	7.8%	90
Riddle Memorial Hospital	Media	7.9%	151
Uniontown Hospital	Uniontown	7.9%	191
Easton Hospital	Easton	8.0%	174
Jefferson Regional Medical Center	Pittsburgh	8.0%	427
Monongahela Valley Hospital	Monongahela	8.0%	125
Jeanes Hospital	Philadelphia	8.2%	293
Kane Community Hospital	Kane	8.2%	73
UPMC Northwest	Seneca	8.4%	250
Jameson Memorial Hospital	New Castle	8.5%	82
Phoenixville Hospital	Phoenixville	8.6%	139
UPMC Mercy	Pittsburgh	8.6%	314
Western Pennsylvania Hospital	Pittsburgh	9.1%	88
Regional Hospital of Scranton	Scranton	9.6%	135
Heritage Valley Sewickley	Sewickley	10.0%	80
Clarion Hospital	Clarion	10.2%	196
Acmh Hospital	Kittanning	11.0%	109
Pottstown Memorial Medical Center	Pottstown	11.0%	127
Magee Womens Hosp of UPMC Health Sys	Pittsburgh	11.8%	68
Penn Hosp of the Univ of PA Hlth Sys	Philadelphia	13.2%	106
UPMC East	Monroeville	13.3%	113

Combination Abdominal CT Scan

Hospital Name	City	Rate	Cases
Miners Medical Center	Hastings	0.0%	142
Saint Joseph's Hospital	Philadelphia	0.0%	66
Windber Hospital	Windber	0.5%	208
Conemaugh Valley Memorial Hospital	Johnstown	1.0%	630
Meyersdale Community Hospital	Myersdale	2.1%	94
Tyrone Hospital	Tyrone	2.1%	146
Lehigh Valley Hospital	Allentown	2.2%	1195
Lewistown Hospital	Lewistown	2.2%	742
Saint Luke's Miners Memorial Hospital	Coaldale	2.3%	442
Aria Health	Philadelphia	2.4%	1744
Magee Womens Hosp of UPMC Health Sys	Pittsburgh	2.4%	536
Penn Presbyterian Medical Center	Philadelphia	2.5%	317
Troy Community Hospital	Troy	2.5%	240
Schuylkill Med Ctr-East Norwegian St	Pottsville	3.0%	436
Meadville Medical Center	Meadville	3.2%	862
Memorial Hospital Towanda	Towanda	3.3%	269
J C Blair Memorial Hospital	Huntingdon	3.4%	293
Schuylkill Med Ctr-S Jackson St	Pottsville	3.4%	622
UPMC Mercy	Pittsburgh	3.7%	460
Excela Health Latrobe Hospital	Latrobe	4.0%	424
Geisinger - Community Medical Center	Scranton	4.0%	721
Endless Mountains Health Systems	Montrose	4.2%	95
Nazareth Hospital	Philadelphia	4.2%	448
Warren General Hospital	Warren	4.2%	525
Holy Redeemer Hospital & Medical Center	Meadowbrook	4.4%	619
Forbes Regional Hospital	Monroeville	4.5%	446
Lock Haven Hospital	Lock Haven	4.5%	242
Saint Luke's Quakertown Hospital	Quakertown	4.6%	452
Saint Luke's Hospital Bethlehem	Bethlehem	4.9%	2232
Sunbury Community Hospital	Sunbury	4.9%	183
Abington Memorial Hospital	Abington	5.1%	2604
Waynesboro Hospital	Waynesboro	5.1%	415
UPMC East	Monroeville	5.2%	252
Saint Clair Memorial Hospital	Pittsburgh	5.4%	886
Saint Luke's Hospital - Anderson Campus	Easton	5.4%	734
UPMC Bedford Memorial	Everett	5.4%	312
Heritage Valley Sewickley	Sewickley	5.7%	318
Hahnemann University Hospital	Philadelphia	5.8%	344
Pocono Medical Center	E Stroudsburg	5.9%	1614
Brandywine Hospital	Coatesville	6.1%	490
Lower Bucks Hospital	Bristol	6.1%	296
Williamsport Regional Medical Center	Williamsport	6.1%	1187
Charles Cole Memorial Hospital	Coudersport	6.5%	322
Geisinger Wyoming Valley Medical Center	Wilkes Barre	6.5%	1488
Acmh Hospital	Kittanning	6.8%	308
Chestnut Hill Hospital	Philadelphia	6.8%	512
Heritage Valley Beaver	Beaver	6.8%	675
Lancaster General Hospital	Lancaster	6.8%	2484
Lansdale Hospital	Lansdale	6.8%	621
Mount Nittany Medical Center	State College	6.8%	721
UPMC Northwest	Seneca	6.8%	996
Chester County Hospital	West Chester	6.9%	1355
Reading Hospital	Reading	7.0%	3069
Heart of Lancaster Reg Med Ctr	Lititz	7.1%	182
Ohio Valley General Hospital	Mckees Rocks	7.1%	140
Western Pennsylvania Hospital	Pittsburgh	7.1%	211
Grand View Hospital	Sellersville	7.2%	964

NOTE: Hospital profiles are in alphabetical order by state, then city, then hospital within the city; Rankings exclude hospitals with less than 25 cases except for patient surveys which excludes hospitals with less than 100 cases; (a) 100-299 cases; (1) The number of cases/patients is too few to report; (2) Data submitted were based on a sample of cases/patients; (3) Results are based on a shorter time period than required; (4) Data suppressed by CMS for one or more quarters; (5) Results are not available for this reporting period; (6) Fewer than 100 patients completed the HCAHPS survey; (7) No cases met the criteria for this measure; (8) The lower limit of the confidence interval cannot be calculated if the number of observed infections equals zero; (9) No data are available from the state/territory for this reporting period; (10) The scores shown reflect fewer than 50 completed surveys; (11) There were discrepancies in the data collection process; (12) This measure does not apply to this hospital for this reporting period; (13) Results cannot be calculated for this reporting period; (14) The results for this state are combined with nearby states to protect confidentiality; Please refer to the User's Guide for a full explanation of data.

Mercy Fitzgerald Hospital	Darby	7.3%	588
Riddle Memorial Hospital	Media	7.4%	848
Robert Packer Hospital	Sayre	7.5%	1287
Einstein Medical Center Montgomery	East Norriton	7.6%	408
Jersey Shore Hospital	Jersey Shore	7.6%	394
Easton Hospital	Easton	7.7%	853
Lehigh Valley Hospital - Muhlenberg	Bethlehem	7.7%	1489
UPMC Hamot	Erie	7.7%	1227
York Hospital	York	7.8%	2120
Hanover Hospital	Hanover	7.9%	820
Albert Einstein Medical Center	Philadelphia	8.1%	849
Sacred Heart Hospital	Allentown	8.1%	333
Crozer Chester Medical Center	Upland	8.2%	1666
Palmerton Hospital	Palmerton	8.3%	253
Titusville Hospital	Titusville	8.5%	270
Jeanes Hospital	Philadelphia	8.6%	648
Chambersburg Hospital	Chambersburg	8.7%	1283
Mercy Suburban Hospital	Norristown	8.7%	449
Saint Mary Medical Center	Langhorne	8.7%	1568
Penn Highlands Dubois	Dubois	8.9%	1071
Regional Hospital of Scranton	Scranton	8.9%	807
Excela Health Frick Hospital	Mount Pleasant	9.3%	248
Nason Hospital	Roaring Spring	9.3%	183
Penn Hosp of the Univ of PA Hlth Sys	Philadelphia	9.3%	881
UPMC Mckeesport	Mc Keesport	9.5%	304
Muncy Valley Hospital	Muncy	10.1%	407
Punxsutawney Area Hospital	Punxsutawney	10.3%	234
Saint Vincent Hospital	Erie	10.3%	857
The Washington Hospital	Washington	10.3%	379
UPMC Altoona	Altoona	10.4%	1313
Carlisle Regional Medical Center	Carlisle	10.5%	673
Geisinger Medical Center	Danville	10.7%	1884
Hospital of Univ of Pennsylvania	Philadelphia	10.7%	2448
Main Line Hospital Lankenau	Wynnewood	10.7%	1336
Evangelical Community Hospital	Lewisburg	10.9%	946
UPMC Horizon	Greenville	11.0%	729
UPMC Saint Margaret	Pittsburgh	11.3%	637
Butler Memorial Hospital	Butler	11.4%	770
Lehigh Valley Hospital - Hazleton	Hazleton	11.4%	755
Roxborough Memorial Hospital	Philadelphia	11.4%	158
Excela Health Westmoreland Hospital	Greensburg	11.6%	612
Main Line Hospital Paoli	Paoli	11.6%	1581
Jennersville Regional Hospital	West Grove	11.8%	364
Lancaster Regional Medical Center	Lancaster	11.8%	330
Moses Taylor Hospital	Scranton	12.7%	495
Thomas Jefferson University Hospital	Philadelphia	12.9%	1443
Doylestown Hospital	Doylestown	13.3%	1162
Main Line Hospital Bryn Mawr Campus	Bryn Mawr	13.7%	1026
Gnaden Huetten Memorial Hospital	Lehighton	14.2%	422
Uniontown Hospital	Uniontown	14.3%	920
UPMC Presbyterian Shadyside	Pittsburgh	14.3%	2936
Jefferson Regional Medical Center	Pittsburgh	14.9%	679
UPMC Passavant	Pittsburgh	15.2%	939
Berwick Hospital Center	Berwick	15.5%	193
Tyler Memorial Hospital	Tunkhannock	15.5%	206
Milton S Hershey Medical Center	Hershey	15.9%	2299
Barnes-Kasson County Hospital	Susquehanna	17.0%	141
Temple University Hospital	Philadelphia	17.8%	928
Millcreek Community Hospital	Erie	17.9%	112
Bradford Regional Medical Center	Bradford	18.3%	437
Geisinger - Bloomsburg Hospital	Bloomsburg	18.4%	239
Alle Kiski Medical Center	Natrona	18.6%	441
Wayne Memorial Hospital	Honesdale	18.8%	719
Holy Spirit Hospital	Camp Hill	19.1%	1079
Memorial Hospital	York	19.5%	687
Pinnacle Health Hospitals	Harrisburg	19.6%	1764
Ellwood City Hospital	Ellwood City	19.8%	106
Fulton County Medical Center	Mcconnellsburg	19.9%	241
Penn Highlands Brookville	Brookville	20.4%	421
Southwest Regional Medical Center	Waynesburg	20.4%	206
Grove City Medical Center	Grove City	20.6%	315
Phoenixville Hospital	Phoenixville	21.1%	564
Ephrata Community Hospital	Ephrata	21.2%	586
Gettysburg Hospital	Gettysburg	21.6%	597
Monongahela Valley Hospital	Monongahela	22.3%	385
Jameson Memorial Hospital	New Castle	24.2%	405
Pottstown Memorial Medical Center	Pottstown	24.3%	959
Somerset Hospital	Somerset	25.8%	318
Clarion Hospital	Clarion	27.0%	404
Indiana Regional Medical Center	Indiana	28.1%	352
Allegheny General Hospital	Pittsburgh	30.3%	659
Good Samaritan Hospital	Lebanon	32.4%	1099
Sharon Regional Health System	Sharon	32.9%	662
Highlands Hospital	Connellsville	33.0%	109
Wilkes-Barre General Hospital	Wilkes-Barre	34.1%	2185
Delaware County Memorial Hospital	Drexel Hill	35.0%	719
Mid - Valley Hospital	Peckville	36.7%	109
Kane Community Hospital	Kane	44.0%	207
Corry Memorial Hospital	Corry	49.3%	217
Canonsburg General Hospital	Canonsburg	51.1%	229
Soldiers & Sailors Memorial Hospital	Wellsboro	51.4%	449
Cancer Treatment Centers of America	Philadelphia	54.1%	375
Penn Highlands Elk	Saint Marys	55.9%	558
Penn Highlands Clearfield	Clearfield	57.1%	674
Saint Joseph Medical Center	Reading	67.4%	625

Combination Brain/Sinus CT Scan

Hospital Name	City	Rate	Cases
Penn Hosp of the Univ of PA Hlth Sys	Philadelphia	0.0%	307
Roxborough Memorial Hospital	Philadelphia	0.6%	160
Main Line Hospital Bryn Mawr Campus	Bryn Mawr	0.7%	1129
Good Samaritan Hospital	Lebanon	1.0%	934
Grand View Hospital	Sellersville	1.0%	733
Lancaster Regional Medical Center	Lancaster	1.2%	249
Butler Memorial Hospital	Butler	1.3%	699
Saint Luke's Quakertown Hospital	Quakertown	1.3%	318
Heritage Valley Beaver	Beaver	1.4%	588
Riddle Memorial Hospital	Media	1.4%	732
Soldiers & Sailors Memorial Hospital	Wellsboro	1.5%	404
J C Blair Memorial Hospital	Huntingdon	1.6%	321
Main Line Hospital Lankenau	Wynnewood	1.6%	1068
Lansdale Hospital	Lansdale	1.7%	660
Chambersburg Hospital	Chambersburg	1.8%	955
Meadville Medical Center	Meadville	1.8%	777
Saint Clair Memorial Hospital	Pittsburgh	1.8%	793
UPMC Hamot	Erie	1.9%	958
Crozer Chester Medical Center	Upland	2.0%	1194
Ephrata Community Hospital	Ephrata	2.0%	601
Doylestown Hospital	Doylestown	2.1%	861
Excela Health Westmoreland Hospital	Greensburg	2.1%	624
Milton S Hershey Medical Center	Hershey	2.1%	720
Alle Kiski Medical Center	Natrona	2.2%	404
Lehigh Valley Hospital - Hazleton	Hazleton	2.2%	732
Main Line Hospital Paoli	Paoli	2.2%	1154
Saint Vincent Hospital	Erie	2.2%	871
Temple University Hospital	Philadelphia	2.2%	715
Holy Redeemer Hospital & Medical Center	Meadowbrook	2.3%	574
York Hospital	York	2.3%	1557
Albert Einstein Medical Center	Philadelphia	2.5%	885
Reading Hospital	Reading	2.5%	2284
Saint Luke's Hospital Bethlehem	Bethlehem	2.5%	1511
Penn Highlands Elk	Saint Marys	2.6%	579
Pottstown Memorial Medical Center	Pottstown	2.6%	775
Sharon Regional Health System	Sharon	2.6%	572
Abington Memorial Hospital	Abington	2.7%	1826
Carlisle Regional Medical Center	Carlisle	2.7%	625
Chester County Hospital	West Chester	2.7%	884
Hanover Hospital	Hanover	2.7%	637
Pinnacle Health Hospitals	Harrisburg	2.7%	1057
Wayne Memorial Hospital	Honesdale	2.8%	603
Lehigh Valley Hospital - Muhlenberg	Bethlehem	2.9%	1116
Saint Joseph Medical Center	Reading	2.9%	719
Geisinger Medical Center	Danville	3.0%	1036
Conemaugh Valley Memorial Hospital	Johnstown	3.1%	674
Geisinger - Community Medical Center	Scranton	3.1%	736
Penn Highlands Dubois	Dubois	3.1%	700
Chestnut Hill Hospital	Philadelphia	3.2%	729
Mount Nittany Medical Center	State College	3.2%	722
Wilkes-Barre General Hospital	Wilkes-Barre	3.2%	1643
Lancaster General Hospital	Lancaster	3.3%	2373
Evangelical Community Hospital	Lewisburg	3.5%	779
Holy Spirit Hospital	Camp Hill	3.6%	1118
Saint Mary Medical Center	Langhorne	3.6%	1162
UPMC Passavant	Pittsburgh	3.6%	721
Pocono Medical Center	E Stroudsburg	3.9%	1070
UPMC Horizon	Greenville	3.9%	663
Aria Health	Philadelphia	4.0%	1386
Lehigh Valley Hospital	Allentown	4.0%	1312
Lewistown Hospital	Lewistown	4.0%	835
Thomas Jefferson University Hospital	Philadelphia	4.0%	1234
UPMC Presbyterian Shadyside	Pittsburgh	4.0%	928
UPMC Altoona	Altoona	4.1%	1128
Easton Hospital	Easton	4.3%	598
Memorial Hospital	York	4.3%	485
Jefferson Regional Medical Center	Pittsburgh	4.4%	595
UPMC Northwest	Seneca	4.4%	710
Geisinger Wyoming Valley Medical Center	Wilkes Barre	4.5%	910
Phoenixville Hospital	Phoenixville	4.7%	486
Acmh Hospital	Kittanning	4.8%	251
Memorial Hospital Towanda	Towanda	4.8%	210
Mercy Fitzgerald Hospital	Darby	4.9%	551
Brandywine Hospital	Coatesville	5.0%	583
Waynesboro Hospital	Waynesboro	5.1%	353
Penn Highlands Clearfield	Clearfield	5.2%	578
Mercy Suburban Hospital	Norristown	5.3%	438
UPMC Saint Margaret	Pittsburgh	5.3%	434
Bradford Regional Medical Center	Bradford	5.5%	397
Schuylkill Med Ctr-S Jackson St	Pottsville	5.7%	596
Lock Haven Hospital	Lock Haven	5.9%	219
Nazareth Hospital	Philadelphia	5.9%	577
Sacred Heart Hospital	Allentown	6.2%	276
Somerset Hospital	Somerset	6.3%	270
Berwick Hospital Center	Berwick	6.4%	235
Fulton County Medical Center	Mcconnellsburg	6.6%	273
Clarion Hospital	Clarion	6.7%	417
UPMC Mercy	Pittsburgh	6.7%	451
Monongahela Valley Hospital	Monongahela	7.4%	353
Ohio Valley General Hospital	Mckees Rocks	7.4%	176
Geisinger - Bloomsburg Hospital	Bloomsburg	7.6%	251
Heart of Lancaster Reg Med Ctr	Lititz	7.7%	195

Combination Chest CT Scan

Hospital Name	City	Rate	Cases
Brandywine Hospital	Coatesville	0.0%	302
Corry Memorial Hospital	Corry	0.0%	101
Crozer Chester Medical Center	Upland	0.0%	1190
Delaware County Memorial Hospital	Drexel Hill	0.0%	500
Forbes Regional Hospital	Monroeville	0.0%	204
Geisinger Wyoming Valley Medical Center	Wilkes Barre	0.0%	1381
Gettysburg Hospital	Gettysburg	0.0%	427
Grove City Medical Center	Grove City	0.0%	166
Heritage Valley Sewickley	Sewickley	0.0%	201
Indiana Regional Medical Center	Indiana	0.0%	233
Lewistown Hospital	Lewistown	0.0%	625
Lower Bucks Hospital	Bristol	0.0%	199
Magee Womens Hosp of UPMC Health Sys	Pittsburgh	0.0%	462
Memorial Hospital Towanda	Towanda	0.0%	121
Miners Medical Center	Hastings	0.0%	68
Mount Nittany Medical Center	State College	0.0%	367
Nazareth Hospital	Philadelphia	0.0%	325
Ohio Valley General Hospital	Mckees Rocks	0.0%	80
Penn Highlands Elk	Saint Marys	0.0%	253
Penn Presbyterian Medical Center	Philadelphia	0.0%	315
Saint Clair Memorial Hospital	Pittsburgh	0.0%	568
Schuylkill Med Ctr-East Norwegian St	Pottsville	0.0%	189
Sharon Regional Health System	Sharon	0.0%	441
Titusville Hospital	Titusville	0.0%	151
Tyler Memorial Hospital	Tunkhannock	0.0%	98
Tyrone Hospital	Tyrone	0.0%	50
Uniontown Hospital	Uniontown	0.0%	420
UPMC Mercy	Pittsburgh	0.0%	285
UPMC Saint Margaret	Pittsburgh	0.0%	509
Warren General Hospital	Warren	0.0%	277
The Washington Hospital	Washington	0.0%	361
Western Pennsylvania Hospital	Pittsburgh	0.0%	120
Windber Hospital	Windber	0.0%	120
Chester County Hospital	West Chester	0.1%	1034
Doylestown Hospital	Doylestown	0.1%	802
Hospital of Univ of Pennsylvania	Philadelphia	0.1%	3972
Penn Hosp of the Univ of PA Hlth Sys	Philadelphia	0.1%	833
Aria Health	Philadelphia	0.2%	1224
Holy Redeemer Hospital & Medical Center	Meadowbrook	0.2%	513
Jefferson Regional Medical Center	Pittsburgh	0.2%	438
Milton S Hershey Medical Center	Hershey	0.2%	2378
Riddle Memorial Hospital	Media	0.2%	573
Robert Packer Hospital	Sayre	0.2%	1044
UPMC Horizon	Greenville	0.2%	453
York Hospital	York	0.2%	2519
Saint Luke's Quakertown Hospital	Quakertown	0.3%	308
Saint Vincent Hospital	Erie	0.3%	380
Schuylkill Med Ctr-S Jackson St	Pottsville	0.3%	293
UPMC Presbyterian Shadyside	Pittsburgh	0.3%	3430
Wilkes-Barre General Hospital	Wilkes-Barre	0.3%	1435
Conemaugh Valley Memorial Hospital	Johnstown	0.4%	279
Lehigh Valley Hospital - Hazleton	Hazleton	0.4%	469
UPMC Hamot	Erie	0.4%	472
Cancer Treatment Centers of America	Philadelphia	0.5%	437
Carlisle Regional Medical Center	Carlisle	0.5%	414
Easton Hospital	Easton	0.5%	428
Holy Spirit Hospital	Camp Hill	0.5%	613
Jennersville Regional Hospital	West Grove	0.5%	214
Soldiers & Sailors Memorial Hospital	Wellsboro	0.5%	221
UPMC Passavant	Pittsburgh	0.5%	777
Monongahela Valley Hospital	Monongahela	0.6%	169
Alle Kiski Medical Center	Natrona	0.7%	292
Grand View Hospital	Sellersville	0.7%	845
Hahnemann University Hospital	Philadelphia	0.7%	275
Chambersburg Hospital	Chambersburg	0.8%	664
Lansdale Hospital	Lansdale	0.8%	494
Meadville Medical Center	Meadville	0.8%	512
Pinnacle Health Hospitals	Harrisburg	0.8%	1281
Williamsport Regional Medical Center	Williamsport	0.8%	610
Chestnut Hill Hospital	Philadelphia	0.9%	339
Jeanes Hospital	Philadelphia	0.9%	331
Saint Luke's Miners Memorial Hospital	Coaldale	0.9%	328
Troy Community Hospital	Troy	0.9%	111
Saint Luke's Hospital - Anderson Campus	Easton	1.0%	693
Heritage Valley Beaver	Beaver	1.1%	447
J C Blair Memorial Hospital	Huntingdon	1.1%	181
Abington Memorial Hospital	Abington	1.2%	2216
Good Samaritan Hospital	Lebanon	1.2%	500
Thomas Jefferson University Hospital	Philadelphia	1.2%	1105
Geisinger Medical Center	Danville	1.3%	1779

NOTE: Hospital profiles are in alphabetical order by state, then city, then hospital within the city; Rankings exclude hospitals with less than 25 cases except for patient surveys which excludes hospitals with less than 100 cases; (a) 100-299 cases; (1) The number of cases/patients is too few to report; (2) Data submitted were based on a sample of cases/patients; (3) Results are based on a shorter time period than required; (4) Data suppressed by CMS for one or more quarters; (5) Results are not available for this reporting period; (6) Fewer than 100 patients completed the HCAHPS survey; (7) No cases met the criteria for this measure; (8) The lower limit of the confidence interval cannot be calculated if the number of observed infections equals zero; (9) No data are available from the state/territory for this reporting period; (10) The scores shown reflect fewer than 50 completed surveys; (11) There were discrepancies in the data collection process; (12) This measure does not apply to this hospital for this reporting period; (13) Results cannot be calculated for this reporting period; (14) The results for this state are combined with nearby states to protect confidentiality; Please refer to the User's Guide for a full explanation of data.

Punxsutawney Area Hospital	Punxsutawney	1.4%	72
Saint Luke's Hospital Bethlehem	Bethlehem	1.4%	2063
UPMC Northwest	Seneca	1.4%	714
Waynesboro Hospital	Waynesboro	1.4%	220
Einstein Medical Center Montgomery	East Norriton	1.6%	315
Ellwood City Hospital	Ellwood City	1.6%	62
Jersey Shore Hospital	Jersey Shore	1.7%	172
Excela Health Latrobe Hospital	Latrobe	1.8%	328
Roxborough Memorial Hospital	Philadelphia	1.8%	114
UPMC East	Monroeville	1.8%	56
Acmh Hospital	Kittanning	2.2%	179
Canonsburg General Hospital	Canonsburg	2.3%	132
Lancaster General Hospital	Lancaster	2.3%	2554
Mercy Fitzgerald Hospital	Darby	2.3%	353
Nason Hospital	Roaring Spring	2.4%	84
Penn Highlands Dubois	Dubois	2.4%	595
Saint Joseph Medical Center	Reading	2.4%	422
Hanover Hospital	Hanover	2.5%	555
Heart of Lancaster Reg Med Ctr	Lititz	2.7%	75
Pocono Medical Center	E Stroudsburg	2.7%	731
UPMC Altoona	Altoona	2.8%	1046
Jameson Memorial Hospital	New Castle	2.9%	313
Reading Hospital	Reading	3.0%	3441
Temple University Hospital	Philadelphia	3.0%	905
UPMC Bedford Memorial	Everett	3.2%	126
Sacred Heart Hospital	Allentown	3.3%	245
Main Line Hospital Bryn Mawr Campus	Bryn Mawr	3.4%	1144
Lehigh Valley Hospital - Muhlenberg	Bethlehem	3.7%	1197
Main Line Hospital Paoli	Paoli	3.7%	1276
Mercy Suburban Hospital	Norristown	3.8%	213
Lancaster Regional Medical Center	Lancaster	3.9%	281
Albert Einstein Medical Center	Philadelphia	4.0%	623
Surgical Specialty Ctr at Coord Hlth	Allentown	4.2%	48
Moses Taylor Hospital	Scranton	4.3%	301
Pottstown Memorial Medical Center	Pottstown	4.4%	517
Allegheny General Hospital	Pittsburgh	4.6%	585
UPMC Mckeesport	Mc Keesport	4.7%	236
Excela Health Frick Hospital	Mount Pleasant	4.9%	185
Main Line Hospital Lankenau	Wynnewood	5.0%	1295
Lock Haven Hospital	Lock Haven	5.1%	59
Geisinger - Community Medical Center	Scranton	5.4%	370
Butler Memorial Hospital	Butler	5.6%	519
Penn Highlands Clearfield	Clearfield	5.7%	227
Regional Hospital of Scranton	Scranton	5.8%	538
Fulton County Medical Center	Mcconnellsburg	5.9%	85
Charles Cole Memorial Hospital	Coudersport	6.2%	307
Excela Health Westmoreland Hospital	Greensburg	6.5%	520
Evangelical Community Hospital	Lewisburg	6.8%	500
Saint Mary Medical Center	Langhorne	7.1%	996
Sunbury Community Hospital	Sunbury	7.4%	81
Lehigh Valley Hospital	Allentown	7.5%	772
Ephrata Community Hospital	Ephrata	8.2%	524
Clarion Hospital	Clarion	8.6%	162
Phoenixville Hospital	Phoenixville	9.3%	493
Palmerton Hospital	Palmerton	9.8%	164
Wayne Memorial Hospital	Honesdale	11.0%	465
Gnaden Huetten Memorial Hospital	Lehighton	11.8%	314
Muncy Valley Hospital	Muncy	12.8%	156
Berwick Hospital Center	Berwick	13.0%	69
Penn Highlands Brookville	Brookville	15.3%	150
Somerset Hospital	Somerset	20.1%	154
Southwest Regional Medical Center	Waynesburg	22.7%	110
Bradford Regional Medical Center	Bradford	25.2%	218
Geisinger - Bloomsburg Hospital	Bloomsburg	42.0%	50
Memorial Hospital	York	44.2%	224
Kane Community Hospital	Kane	48.4%	124

Follow-up Mammogram/Ultrasound

A follow-up rate near zero may indicate missed cancer; a rate higher than 14% may mean there is unnecessary follow up.

Hospital Name	City	Rate	Cases
Titusville Hospital	Titusville	1.2%	502
Clarion Hospital	Clarion	2.1%	719
Corry Memorial Hospital	Corry	2.3%	387
Millcreek Community Hospital	Erie	2.6%	114
Warren General Hospital	Warren	3.0%	919
Schuylkill Med Ctr-East Norwegian St	Pottsville	3.4%	525
Penn Highlands Brookville	Brookville	3.6%	277
UPMC Bedford Memorial	Everett	3.7%	519
Lehigh Valley Hospital - Hazleton	Hazleton	4.2%	1436
Penn Highlands Dubois	Dubois	4.2%	1758
Saint Mary Medical Center	Langhorne	4.2%	2348
Indiana Regional Medical Center	Indiana	4.3%	673
Uniontown Hospital	Uniontown	4.5%	785
Good Samaritan Hospital	Lebanon	4.6%	2432
Phoenixville Hospital	Phoenixville	4.7%	1616
Penn Highlands Clearfield	Clearfield	4.9%	717
Hahnemann University Hospital	Philadelphia	5.1%	549
Saint Luke's Miners Memorial Hospital	Coaldale	5.2%	463
Saint Vincent Hospital	Erie	5.2%	1335
J C Blair Memorial Hospital	Huntingdon	5.3%	848
Muncy Valley Hospital	Muncy	5.5%	434
Albert Einstein Medical Center	Philadelphia	5.6%	2805
Wayne Memorial Hospital	Honesdale	5.6%	1190
Meadville Medical Center	Meadville	5.7%	1500
Saint Luke's Quakertown Hospital	Quakertown	5.7%	715
Charles Cole Memorial Hospital	Coudersport	5.9%	404
Holy Redeemer Hospital & Medical Center	Meadowbrook	5.9%	1568
Lehigh Valley Hospital	Allentown	6.0%	4045
Wilkes-Barre General Hospital	Wilkes-Barre	6.1%	3695
Punxsutawney Area Hospital	Punxsutawney	6.2%	292
Canonsburg General Hospital	Canonsburg	6.3%	191
Delaware County Memorial Hospital	Drexel Hill	6.3%	930
UPMC Horizon	Greenville	6.5%	1187
Temple University Hospital	Philadelphia	6.6%	1619
Abington Memorial Hospital	Abington	6.7%	4395
Windber Hospital	Windber	6.8%	526
Gnaden Huetten Memorial Hospital	Lehighton	6.9%	824
Lehigh Valley Hospital - Muhlenberg	Bethlehem	6.9%	1955
Schuylkill Med Ctr-S Jackson St	Pottsville	7.0%	1429
Hospital of Univ of Pennsylvania	Philadelphia	7.1%	3324
Meyersdale Community Hospital	Myersdale	7.2%	139
Jersey Shore Hospital	Jersey Shore	7.3%	288
Palmerton Hospital	Palmerton	7.3%	288
Pottstown Memorial Medical Center	Pottstown	7.3%	1531
Somerset Hospital	Somerset	7.4%	337
Heart of Lancaster Reg Med Ctr	Lititz	7.5%	253
Milton S Hershey Medical Center	Hershey	7.5%	1425
Chestnut Hill Hospital	Philadelphia	7.6%	1963
Sacred Heart Hospital	Allentown	7.6%	1137
The Washington Hospital	Washington	7.7%	802
Barnes-Kasson County Hospital	Susquehanna	7.8%	128
Heritage Valley Sewickley	Sewickley	7.8%	218
Geisinger Wyoming Valley Medical Center	Wilkes Barre	7.9%	1503
Reading Hospital	Reading	8.0%	4251
Excela Health Latrobe Hospital	Latrobe	8.1%	617
Lock Haven Hospital	Lock Haven	8.1%	185
Memorial Hospital Towanda	Towanda	8.1%	358
Nason Hospital	Roaring Spring	8.1%	332
Conemaugh Valley Memorial Hospital	Johnstown	8.2%	1139
Saint Joseph Medical Center	Reading	8.3%	1415
Excela Health Frick Hospital	Mount Pleasant	8.4%	287
York Hospital	York	8.5%	5869
Lancaster General Hospital	Lancaster	8.6%	6214
Aria Health	Philadelphia	8.7%	1516
Crozer Chester Medical Center	Upland	8.8%	3275
Heritage Valley Beaver	Beaver	8.8%	1301
Jefferson Regional Medical Center	Pittsburgh	8.8%	521
Chambersburg Hospital	Chambersburg	8.9%	2715
Geisinger - Bloomsburg Hospital	Bloomsburg	8.9%	418
Lansdale Hospital	Lansdale	8.9%	1129
Doylestown Hospital	Doylestown	9.0%	3061
Penn Hosp of the Univ of PA Hlth Sys	Philadelphia	9.0%	1779
Sharon Regional Health System	Sharon	9.0%	980
Magee Womens Hosp of UPMC Health Sys	Pittsburgh	9.1%	4802
Bradford Regional Medical Center	Bradford	9.2%	819
Pinnacle Health Hospitals	Harrisburg	9.2%	4462
Chester County Hospital	West Chester	9.3%	2696
Excela Health Westmoreland Hospital	Greensburg	9.3%	1015
Mount Nittany Medical Center	State College	9.3%	1647
Saint Luke's Hospital - Anderson Campus	Easton	9.3%	257
Lower Bucks Hospital	Bristol	9.4%	657
Surgical Specialty Ctr at Coord Hlth	Allentown	9.5%	452
Fulton County Medical Center	Mcconnellsburg	9.6%	282
Lancaster Regional Medical Center	Lancaster	9.7%	1321
Penn Presbyterian Medical Center	Philadelphia	9.7%	236
Saint Clair Memorial Hospital	Pittsburgh	9.9%	543
Soldiers & Sailors Memorial Hospital	Wellsboro	9.9%	871
Holy Spirit Hospital	Camp Hill	10.0%	2039
UPMC Northwest	Seneca	10.0%	1426
Brandywine Hospital	Coatesville	10.1%	736
Ephrata Community Hospital	Ephrata	10.1%	1458
Regional Hospital of Scranton	Scranton	10.1%	673
Thomas Jefferson University Hospital	Philadelphia	10.2%	4978
Einstein Medical Center Montgomery	East Norriton	10.3%	755
UPMC Mckeesport	Mc Keesport	10.4%	433
Hanover Hospital	Hanover	10.5%	1062
Geisinger - Community Medical Center	Scranton	10.6%	786
Highlands Hospital	Connellsville	10.7%	168
UPMC Hamot	Erie	10.7%	1693
Mercy Fitzgerald Hospital	Darby	10.8%	1263
Miners Medical Center	Hastings	10.8%	120
Sunbury Community Hospital	Sunbury	10.9%	384
Berwick Hospital Center	Berwick	11.0%	464
Gettysburg Hospital	Gettysburg	11.0%	1440
Grove City Medical Center	Grove City	11.0%	408
Carlisle Regional Medical Center	Carlisle	11.1%	541
Grand View Hospital	Sellersville	11.2%	2468
UPMC Mercy	Pittsburgh	11.2%	357
Lewistown Hospital	Lewistown	11.4%	1061
Acmh Hospital	Kittanning	11.5%	488
Mercy Suburban Hospital	Norristown	11.5%	672
Saint Luke's Hospital Bethlehem	Bethlehem	11.5%	4386
Jennersville Regional Hospital	West Grove	11.8%	483
Pocono Medical Center	E Stroudsburg	11.8%	601
Roxborough Memorial Hospital	Philadelphia	11.8%	380
Riddle Memorial Hospital	Media	12.1%	1105
Main Line Hospital Bryn Mawr Campus	Bryn Mawr	12.2%	2123
Jeanes Hospital	Philadelphia	12.3%	1115
Main Line Hospital Paoli	Paoli	12.3%	2497
Forbes Regional Hospital	Monroeville	12.5%	343
Troy Community Hospital	Troy	12.5%	401
Butler Memorial Hospital	Butler	12.6%	1061
Monongahela Valley Hospital	Monongahela	12.6%	422
Memorial Hospital	York	12.7%	693
Geisinger Medical Center	Danville	12.8%	2641
Allegheny General Hospital	Pittsburgh	13.0%	660
Easton Hospital	Easton	13.0%	1602
Waynesboro Hospital	Waynesboro	13.0%	923
Ellwood City Hospital	Ellwood City	13.3%	180
Nazareth Hospital	Philadelphia	13.3%	443
Western Pennsylvania Hospital	Pittsburgh	13.4%	441
Moses Taylor Hospital	Scranton	13.6%	726
Evangelical Community Hospital	Lewisburg	13.8%	2010
Robert Packer Hospital	Sayre	13.8%	1621
Alle Kiski Medical Center	Natrona	14.2%	656
Tyrone Hospital	Tyrone	14.9%	114
Ohio Valley General Hospital	Mckees Rocks	15.1%	205
Penn Highlands Elk	Saint Marys	15.4%	1032
UPMC Altoona	Altoona	16.2%	1068
Main Line Hospital Lankenau	Wynnewood	17.2%	2698
Tyler Memorial Hospital	Tunkhannock	19.2%	182
Southwest Regional Medical Center	Waynesburg	19.6%	194
Jameson Memorial Hospital	New Castle	22.7%	432
Kane Community Hospital	Kane	42.9%	294

Lumbar Spine MRI for Low Back Pain

Hospital Name	City	Rate	Cases
Excela Health Westmoreland Hospital	Greensburg	25.0%	60
Milton S Hershey Medical Center	Hershey	25.7%	179
Hanover Hospital	Hanover	26.8%	123
Mercy Suburban Hospital	Norristown	27.3%	55
Mercy Fitzgerald Hospital	Darby	27.8%	90
UPMC Horizon	Greenville	28.2%	117
Edgewood Surgical Hospital	Transfer	28.6%	56
Nazareth Hospital	Philadelphia	29.2%	96
Brandywine Hospital	Coatesville	29.5%	95
Temple University Hospital	Philadelphia	29.6%	81
Gettysburg Hospital	Gettysburg	29.8%	114
Oss Orthopaedic Hospital	York	29.8%	272
Geisinger Medical Center	Danville	30.0%	267
Mount Nittany Medical Center	State College	30.0%	70
Holy Spirit Hospital	Camp Hill	30.1%	163
Surgical Specialty Ctr at Coord Hlth	Allentown	30.1%	302
Meadville Medical Center	Meadville	30.4%	161
Lewistown Hospital	Lewistown	30.5%	131
UPMC Hamot	Erie	31.0%	171
UPMC Passavant	Pittsburgh	31.1%	90
UPMC Altoona	Altoona	31.5%	143
Sharon Regional Health System	Sharon	32.3%	127
Lehigh Valley Hospital - Muhlenberg	Bethlehem	32.5%	77
Grand View Hospital	Sellersville	32.6%	141
Saint Luke's Hospital - Anderson Campus	Easton	33.1%	127
Chestnut Hill Hospital	Philadelphia	33.3%	75
Gnaden Huetten Memorial Hospital	Lehighton	33.3%	72
Williamsport Regional Medical Center	Williamsport	33.3%	123
York Hospital	York	33.7%	279
Hospital of Univ of Pennsylvania	Philadelphia	33.8%	317
Wilkes-Barre General Hospital	Wilkes-Barre	33.8%	219
Hahnemann University Hospital	Philadelphia	33.9%	62
Lower Bucks Hospital	Bristol	33.9%	59
Butler Memorial Hospital	Butler	34.2%	152
Wayne Memorial Hospital	Honesdale	34.2%	76
Doylestown Hospital	Doylestown	34.5%	171
Phoenixville Hospital	Phoenixville	34.8%	164
Chester County Hospital	West Chester	34.9%	152
Jefferson Regional Medical Center	Pittsburgh	35.0%	120
Acmh Hospital	Kittanning	35.1%	74
Chambersburg Hospital	Chambersburg	35.1%	245
Saint Clair Memorial Hospital	Pittsburgh	35.1%	94
Penn Highlands Elk	Saint Marys	35.2%	128
Crozer Chester Medical Center	Upland	35.4%	285
Schuylkill Med Ctr-S Jackson St	Pottsville	35.4%	147
Saint Vincent Hospital	Erie	35.5%	203
Ephrata Community Hospital	Ephrata	35.6%	132
Penn Highlands Dubois	Dubois	35.6%	160
Thomas Jefferson University Hospital	Philadelphia	35.9%	156
Soldiers & Sailors Memorial Hospital	Wellsboro	36.1%	83
Uniontown Hospital	Uniontown	36.4%	66
Main Line Hospital Lankenau	Wynnewood	36.7%	166
Saint Luke's Quakertown Hospital	Quakertown	36.8%	68
UPMC Presbyterian Shadyside	Pittsburgh	37.7%	204
Evangelical Community Hospital	Lewisburg	37.8%	98

NOTE: Hospital profiles are in alphabetical order by state, then city, then hospital within the city; Rankings exclude hospitals with less than 25 cases except for patient surveys which excludes hospitals with less than 100 cases; (a) 100-299 cases; (1) The number of cases/patients is too few to report; (2) Data submitted were based on a sample of cases/patients; (3) Results are based on a shorter time period than required; (4) Data suppressed by CMS for one or more quarters; (5) Results are not available for this reporting period; (6) Fewer than 100 patients completed the HCAHPS survey; (7) No cases met the criteria for this measure; (8) The lower limit of the confidence interval cannot be calculated if the number of observed infections equals zero; (9) No data are available from the state/territory for this reporting period; (10) The scores shown reflect fewer than 50 completed surveys; (11) There were discrepancies in the data collection process; (12) This measure does not apply to this hospital for this reporting period; (13) Results cannot be calculated for this reporting period; (14) The results for this state are combined with nearby states to protect confidentiality; Please refer to the User's Guide for a full explanation of data.

Somerset Hospital	Somerset	37.8%	45
Pinnacle Health Hospitals	Harrisburg	38.0%	418
Geisinger Wyoming Valley Medical Center	Wilkes Barre	38.3%	141
Saint Luke's Hospital Bethlehem	Bethlehem	38.4%	292
Saint Mary Medical Center	Langhorne	38.5%	351
The Washington Hospital	Washington	38.7%	62
Clarion Hospital	Clarion	38.9%	54
Allegheny General Hospital	Pittsburgh	39.2%	51
Abington Memorial Hospital	Abington	39.6%	227
Warren General Hospital	Warren	39.6%	101
Pottstown Memorial Medical Center	Pottstown	40.0%	190
Riddle Memorial Hospital	Media	40.0%	110
Reading Hospital	Reading	40.1%	262
Heritage Valley Beaver	Beaver	40.3%	77
Robert Packer Hospital	Sayre	40.3%	134
UPMC Saint Margaret	Pittsburgh	40.6%	101
UPMC Northwest	Seneca	41.1%	190
Lancaster Regional Medical Center	Lancaster	41.7%	144
Jameson Memorial Hospital	New Castle	41.9%	74
Monongahela Valley Hospital	Monongahela	42.0%	88
Titusville Hospital	Titusville	42.1%	38
Penn Highlands Clearfield	Clearfield	42.2%	45
Regional Hospital of Scranton	Scranton	42.3%	52
Bradford Regional Medical Center	Bradford	43.2%	74
Waynesboro Hospital	Waynesboro	43.6%	39
Memorial Hospital Towanda	Towanda	44.2%	43
Albert Einstein Medical Center	Philadelphia	44.8%	145
Lehigh Valley Hospital - Hazleton	Hazleton	45.1%	102
Saint Joseph Medical Center	Reading	45.1%	113
Sacred Heart Hospital	Allentown	45.3%	64
Geisinger - Community Medical Center	Scranton	45.7%	46
Pocono Medical Center	E Stroudsburg	45.9%	37
Lansdale Hospital	Lansdale	47.5%	59
Easton Hospital	Easton	49.2%	61
UPMC Mercy	Pittsburgh	50.0%	48
Alle Kiski Medical Center	Natrona	52.2%	46
Heritage Valley Sewickley	Sewickley	55.6%	36
Charles Cole Memorial Hospital	Coudersport	61.4%	44

NOTE: Hospital profiles are in alphabetical order by state, then city, then hospital within the city; Rankings exclude hospitals with less than 25 cases except for patient surveys which excludes hospitals with less than 100 cases; (a) 100-299 cases; (1) The number of cases/patients is too few to report; (2) Data submitted were based on a sample of cases/patients; (3) Results are based on a shorter time period than required; (4) Data suppressed by CMS for one or more quarters; (5) Results are not available for this reporting period; (6) Fewer than 100 patients completed the HCAHPS survey; (7) No cases met the criteria for this measure; (8) The lower limit of the confidence interval cannot be calculated if the number of observed infections equals zero; (9) No data are available from the state/territory for this reporting period; (10) The scores shown reflect fewer than 50 completed surveys; (11) There were discrepancies in the data collection process; (12) This measure does not apply to this hospital for this reporting period; (13) Results cannot be calculated for this reporting period; (14) The results for this state are combined with nearby states to protect confidentiality; Please refer to the User's Guide for a full explanation of data.

Abington Memorial Hospital

1200 Old York Road
Abington, PA 19001
Phone: 215-481-2000
Fax: 215-481-3619
URL: www.amh.org
Type: Acute Care Hospitals
Emergency Services: Yes
Ownership: Voluntary non-profit - Private
Beds: 508

Key Personnel:
Radiology. . . . . John Breckenridge, MD
Pediatric Ambulatory Care . . . . . . Joseph Cirotti, MD
Pediatric In-Patient Care . . . . Joseph Cirotti, MD
Operating Room. . . . . Teresa Howard
Chief of Medical Staff. . . . . Jack Kelly, MD
CEO/President. . . . . Laurence M. Merlis
Quality Assurance . . . . Tony Simek
Infection Control. . . . . Beth Stunn

Measure	Cases	This Hosp.	State Avg.	U.S. Avg.
Blood Clot Prevention and Treatment				
Anticoagulation Overlap Therapy[2]	212	92%	94%	93%
ICU Venous Thromboembolism Prophylaxis[2]	64	89%	94%	92%
Incidence of Potentially Preventable VTE[2]	52	4%	8%	10%
UFH with Dosages/Platelet Monitoring[2]	279	100%	98%	97%
Venous Thromboembolism Prophylaxis[2]	309	87%	90%	85%
Warfarin Therapy Discharge Instructions[2]	151	88%	78%	75%
Chest Pain/Possible Heart Attack Care				
Aspirin Given Within 24 Hours of Arrival[1,3]	-	-	97%	96%
Fibrinolytic Meds Within 30 Min. of Arrival[5]	-	-	44%	58%
Average Time to ECG (minutes)[1,3]	-	-	9	7
Average Time to Transfer (minutes)[5]	-	-	64	60
Children's Asthma Care				
Received Home Management Plan of Care	-	-	-	88%
Received Reliever Medication	-	-	-	100%
Received Systemic Corticosteroids	-	-	-	100%
Emergency Department				
Admittance Decision Time (minutes)[2]	571	109	104	98
Head CT Results Within 45 Min. of Arrival[1,3]	-	-	60%	57%
Patients Who Left ER Before Being Seen	>100k	0%	1%	2%
Time from ER Arrival to Admit. (minutes)[2]	599	283	276	274
Time from ER Arrival to Discharge (minutes)	389	145	125	134
Time in ER Before Being Evaluated (minutes)	417	11	26	26
Time to Pain Meds for Fractures (minutes)	221	45	58	57
Heart Attack Care				
Aspirin Given at Discharge	367	100%	99%	99%
Fibrinolytic Meds Within 30 Min. of Arrival[7]	-	-	40%	54%
PCI Within 90 Minutes of Arrival	78	96%	97%	96%
Statin Prescribed at Discharge	365	98%	99%	98%
Heart Failure Care				
ACE Inhibitor or ARB for LVSD	245	99%	97%	97%
Discharge Instructions Given	570	95%	96%	94%
Evaluation of LVS Function	803	100%	100%	99%
Medicare Spending				
Medicare Spending per Patient (ratio)	-	1.00	1.01	0.98
Pneumonia Care				
Appropriate Initial Antibiotic Given	254	97%	96%	95%
Blood Culture Timing	558	99%	98%	98%
Pregnancy and Delivery Care				
Newborn Deliveries Scheduled Early[2]	79	0%	4%	6%
Preventive Care				
Immunization for Influenza[2]	548	88%	91%	90%
Immunization for Pneumonia[2]	637	90%	92%	92%
Stroke Care				
Anticoagulation Therapy for Atrial Fibrillation[2]	18	83%	96%	95%
Antithrombotic Therapy Timing[2]	80	100%	98%	98%
Assessed for Rehabilitation[2]	117	100%	98%	97%
Discharged on Antithrombotic Therapy[2]	100	100%	99%	99%
Discharged on Statin Medication[2]	76	96%	95%	94%
Thrombolytic Therapy Timing[2]	11	73%	72%	66%
Venous Thromboembolism Prophylaxis[2]	113	93%	95%	94%
Written Stroke Educational Materials Given[2]	57	42%	90%	88%
Surgical Care Improvement Project				
Appropriate Beta Blocker Usage[2]	219	97%	98%	98%
Appropriate VTP Within 24 Hours[2]	401	99%	99%	98%
Controlled Postoperative Blood Glucose[2]	160	99%	98%	97%
Perioperative Temperature Management[2]	528	100%	100%	100%
Prophylactic Antibiotic Selection[2]	520	98%	99%	99%
Prophylactic Antibiotic Selection (Outpatient)	423	93%	98%	98%
Prophylactic Antibiotic Stopped[2]	512	99%	98%	98%
Prophylactic Antibiotic Timing[2]	521	99%	99%	99%
Prophylactic Antibiotic Timing (Outpatient)	423	98%	98%	98%
Urinary Catheter Removal[2]	282	99%	99%	97%
Survey of Patients' Hospital Experiences				
Area Around Room 'Always' Quiet at Night	300+	48%	54%	61%
Doctors 'Always' Communicated Well	300+	79%	80%	82%
Home Recovery Information Given	300+	85%	86%	85%
Hospital Given 9 or 10 on 10 Point Scale	300+	71%	69%	71%
Meds 'Always' Explained Before Given	300+	65%	63%	64%
Nurses 'Always' Communicated Well	300+	80%	79%	79%
Pain 'Always' Well Controlled	300+	70%	70%	71%
Room and Bathroom 'Always' Clean	300+	63%	73%	73%
Timely Help 'Always' Received	300+	63%	67%	68%
Would Definitely Recommend Hospital	300+	77%	70%	71%
Use of Medical Imaging				
Cardiac Imaging Stress Test before Surgery	979	6.5%	5.4%	5.3%
Combination Abdominal CT Scan	2,604	5.1%	12.2%	10.5%
Combination Brain/Sinus CT Scan	1,826	2.7%	3.1%	2.7%
Combination Chest CT Scan	2,216	1.2%	2.1%	2.7%
Follow-up Mammogram/Ultrasound	4,395	6.7%	9%	8.8%
Lumbar Spine MRI for Low Back Pain	227	39.6%	35.8%	37.2%

Lehigh Valley Hospital

1200 South Cedar Crest Boulvard
Allentown, PA 18105
Phone: 610-402-2273
Fax: 610-402-7523
URL: www.lvhhn.org
Type: Acute Care Hospitals
Emergency Services: Yes
Ownership: Voluntary non-profit - Private
Beds: 800

Key Personnel:
Infection Control. . . . . Terry Lynn Burger
Pediatrics. . . . . Nathan Hagstrom, MD
Operating Room. . . . . Brian Leader
Surgery . . . . Michael Pasquale, MD
Quality Assurance . . . . Georgene Saliba
Radiology. . . . . Sheila Sferrella
CEO/President. . . . . Elliot J Sussman, MD
Chief of Medical Staff. . . . . Thomas Whalen, MD

Measure	Cases	This Hosp.	State Avg.	U.S. Avg.
Blood Clot Prevention and Treatment				
Anticoagulation Overlap Therapy[2]	244	96%	94%	93%
ICU Venous Thromboembolism Prophylaxis[2]	182	99%	94%	92%
Incidence of Potentially Preventable VTE[2]	62	6%	8%	10%
UFH with Dosages/Platelet Monitoring[2]	260	89%	98%	97%
Venous Thromboembolism Prophylaxis[2]	303	97%	90%	85%
Warfarin Therapy Discharge Instructions[2]	153	66%	78%	75%
Chest Pain/Possible Heart Attack Care				
Aspirin Given Within 24 Hours of Arrival[1]	-	-	97%	96%
Fibrinolytic Meds Within 30 Min. of Arrival[5]	-	-	44%	58%
Average Time to ECG (minutes)[1]	-	-	9	7
Average Time to Transfer (minutes)[5]	-	-	64	60
Children's Asthma Care				
Received Home Management Plan of Care	-	-	-	88%
Received Reliever Medication	-	-	-	100%
Received Systemic Corticosteroids	-	-	-	100%
Emergency Department				
Admittance Decision Time (minutes)[2]	590	131	104	98
Head CT Results Within 45 Min. of Arrival[1]	-	-	60%	57%
Patients Who Left ER Before Being Seen	89,026	1%	1%	2%
Time from ER Arrival to Admit. (minutes)[2]	595	332	276	274
Time from ER Arrival to Discharge (minutes)	366	160	125	134
Time in ER Before Being Evaluated (minutes)	380	34	26	26
Time to Pain Meds for Fractures (minutes)	324	55	58	57
Heart Attack Care				
Aspirin Given at Discharge	913	100%	99%	99%
Fibrinolytic Meds Within 30 Min. of Arrival[7]	-	-	40%	54%
PCI Within 90 Minutes of Arrival	123	99%	97%	96%
Statin Prescribed at Discharge	874	99%	99%	98%
Heart Failure Care				
ACE Inhibitor or ARB for LVSD	238	99%	97%	97%
Discharge Instructions Given	811	96%	96%	94%
Evaluation of LVS Function	1,033	100%	100%	99%
Medicare Spending				
Medicare Spending per Patient (ratio)	-	0.97	1.01	0.98
Pneumonia Care				
Appropriate Initial Antibiotic Given	332	95%	96%	95%
Blood Culture Timing	703	97%	98%	98%
Pregnancy and Delivery Care				
Newborn Deliveries Scheduled Early	680	0%	4%	6%
Preventive Care				
Immunization for Influenza[2]	546	96%	91%	90%
Immunization for Pneumonia[2]	668	90%	92%	92%
Stroke Care				
Anticoagulation Therapy for Atrial Fibrillation	78	100%	96%	95%
Antithrombotic Therapy Timing	367	100%	98%	98%
Assessed for Rehabilitation	588	100%	98%	97%
Discharged on Antithrombotic Therapy	451	100%	99%	99%
Discharged on Statin Medication	331	99%	95%	94%
Thrombolytic Therapy Timing	33	97%	72%	66%
Venous Thromboembolism Prophylaxis	602	100%	95%	94%
Written Stroke Educational Materials Given	295	96%	90%	88%
Surgical Care Improvement Project				
Appropriate Beta Blocker Usage	1,286	98%	98%	98%
Appropriate VTP Within 24 Hours	2,810	98%	99%	98%
Controlled Postoperative Blood Glucose	549	99%	98%	97%
Perioperative Temperature Management	3,320	100%	100%	100%
Prophylactic Antibiotic Selection	2,297	100%	99%	99%
Prophylactic Antibiotic Selection (Outpatient)	1,038	98%	98%	98%
Prophylactic Antibiotic Stopped	2,265	100%	98%	98%
Prophylactic Antibiotic Timing	2,298	100%	99%	99%
Prophylactic Antibiotic Timing (Outpatient)	1,041	99%	98%	98%
Urinary Catheter Removal	1,999	99%	99%	97%
Survey of Patients' Hospital Experiences				
Area Around Room 'Always' Quiet at Night	300+	46%	54%	61%
Doctors 'Always' Communicated Well	300+	77%	80%	82%
Home Recovery Information Given	300+	87%	86%	85%
Hospital Given 9 or 10 on 10 Point Scale	300+	74%	69%	71%
Meds 'Always' Explained Before Given	300+	62%	63%	64%
Nurses 'Always' Communicated Well	300+	80%	79%	79%
Pain 'Always' Well Controlled	300+	69%	70%	71%
Room and Bathroom 'Always' Clean	300+	66%	73%	73%
Timely Help 'Always' Received	300+	67%	67%	68%
Would Definitely Recommend Hospital	300+	79%	70%	71%
Use of Medical Imaging				
Cardiac Imaging Stress Test before Surgery	1,122	6.6%	5.4%	5.3%
Combination Abdominal CT Scan	1,195	2.2%	12.2%	10.5%
Combination Brain/Sinus CT Scan	1,312	4.0%	3.1%	2.7%
Combination Chest CT Scan	772	7.5%	2.1%	2.7%
Follow-up Mammogram/Ultrasound	4,045	6.0%	9%	8.8%
Lumbar Spine MRI for Low Back Pain[1]	-	-	35.8%	37.2%

Sacred Heart Hospital

421 Chew Street
Allentown, PA 18102
Phone: 610-776-4900
Fax: 610-776-4559
E-mail: csodl@shh.org
URL: www.shh.org
Type: Acute Care Hospitals
Emergency Services: Yes
Ownership: Voluntary non-profit - Private
Beds: 243

Key Personnel:
Operating Room. . . . . Ronald W Ambe, RN
Radiology. . . . . Jeffrey Blinder
Infection Control. . . . . Mary Pavone
Chief of Medical Staff. . . . . Mary Roth, MD
Cardiac Laboratory. . . . . Sarrokh Sader
CEO/President. . . . . Frank Sparandero
Quality Assurance . . . . Lucia Williams

Measure	Cases	This Hosp.	State Avg.	U.S. Avg.
Blood Clot Prevention and Treatment				
Anticoagulation Overlap Therapy[2]	18	72%	94%	93%
ICU Venous Thromboembolism Prophylaxis[2]	140	92%	94%	92%
Incidence of Potentially Preventable VTE[1,2]	-	-	8%	10%
UFH with Dosages/Platelet Monitoring[2]	16	100%	98%	97%
Venous Thromboembolism Prophylaxis[2]	833	86%	90%	85%
Warfarin Therapy Discharge Instructions[1,2]	-	-	78%	75%
Chest Pain/Possible Heart Attack Care				
Aspirin Given Within 24 Hours of Arrival	19	95%	97%	96%
Fibrinolytic Meds Within 30 Min. of Arrival[7]	-	-	44%	58%

NOTE: Hospital profiles are in alphabetical order by state, then city, then hospital within the city; Rankings exclude hospitals with less than 25 cases except for patient surveys which excludes hospitals with less than 100 cases; (a) 100-299 cases; (1) The number of cases/patients is too few to report; (2) Data submitted were based on a sample of cases/patients; (3) Results are based on a shorter time period than required; (4) Data suppressed by CMS for one or more quarters; (5) Results are not available for this reporting period; (6) Fewer than 100 patients completed the HCAHPS survey; (7) No cases met the criteria for this measure; (8) The lower limit of the confidence interval cannot be calculated if the number of observed infections equals zero; (9) No data are available from the state/territory for this reporting period; (10) The scores shown reflect fewer than 50 completed surveys; (11) There were discrepancies in the data collection process; (12) This measure does not apply to this hospital for this reporting period; (13) Results cannot be calculated for this reporting period; (14) The results for this state are combined with nearby states to protect confidentiality; Please refer to the User's Guide for a full explanation of data.

Measure	Cases	This Hosp.	State Avg.	U.S. Avg.
Average Time to ECG (minutes)	19	13	9	7
Average Time to Transfer (minutes)[1]	-	-	64	60
Children's Asthma Care				
Received Home Management Plan of Care	-	-	-	88%
Received Reliever Medication	-	-	-	100%
Received Systemic Corticosteroids	-	-	-	100%
Emergency Department				
Admittance Decision Time (minutes)[2]	757	152	104	98
Head CT Results Within 45 Min. of Arrival[1]	-	-	60%	57%
Patients Who Left ER Before Being Seen	33,121	1%	1%	2%
Time from ER Arrival to Admit. (minutes)[2]	757	304	276	274
Time from ER Arrival to Discharge (minutes)	6,935	76	125	134
Time in ER Before Being Evaluated (minutes)	7,596	26	26	26
Time to Pain Meds for Fractures (minutes)	44	52	58	57
Heart Attack Care				
Aspirin Given at Discharge	19	100%	99%	99%
Fibrinolytic Meds Within 30 Min. of Arrival[7]	-	-	40%	54%
PCI Within 90 Minutes of Arrival[7]	-	-	97%	96%
Statin Prescribed at Discharge	19	84%	99%	98%
Heart Failure Care				
ACE Inhibitor or ARB for LVSD	27	89%	97%	97%
Discharge Instructions Given	98	97%	96%	94%
Evaluation of LVS Function	153	98%	100%	99%
Medicare Spending				
Medicare Spending per Patient (ratio)	-	1.02	1.01	0.98
Pneumonia Care				
Appropriate Initial Antibiotic Given	62	98%	96%	95%
Blood Culture Timing	96	99%	98%	98%
Pregnancy and Delivery Care				
Newborn Deliveries Scheduled Early	41	0%	4%	6%
Preventive Care				
Immunization for Influenza[2]	1,177	95%	91%	90%
Immunization for Pneumonia[2]	973	95%	92%	92%
Stroke Care				
Anticoagulation Therapy for Atrial Fibrillation[1]	-	-	96%	95%
Antithrombotic Therapy Timing	31	100%	98%	98%
Assessed for Rehabilitation	32	100%	98%	97%
Discharged on Antithrombotic Therapy	32	100%	99%	99%
Discharged on Statin Medication	24	88%	95%	94%
Thrombolytic Therapy Timing[1]	-	-	72%	66%
Venous Thromboembolism Prophylaxis	32	97%	95%	94%
Written Stroke Educational Materials Given	12	92%	90%	88%
Surgical Care Improvement Project				
Appropriate Beta Blocker Usage	74	96%	98%	98%
Appropriate VTP Within 24 Hours	245	98%	99%	98%
Controlled Postoperative Blood Glucose[7]	-	-	98%	97%
Perioperative Temperature Management	279	100%	100%	100%
Prophylactic Antibiotic Selection	198	100%	99%	99%
Prophylactic Antibiotic Selection (Outpatient)	34	94%	98%	98%
Prophylactic Antibiotic Stopped	194	99%	98%	98%
Prophylactic Antibiotic Timing	199	99%	99%	99%
Prophylactic Antibiotic Timing (Outpatient)	34	97%	98%	98%
Urinary Catheter Removal	74	99%	99%	97%
Survey of Patients' Hospital Experiences				
Area Around Room 'Always' Quiet at Night	300+	66%	54%	61%
Doctors 'Always' Communicated Well	300+	80%	80%	82%
Home Recovery Information Given	300+	86%	86%	85%
Hospital Given 9 or 10 on 10 Point Scale	300+	65%	69%	71%
Meds 'Always' Explained Before Given	300+	59%	63%	64%
Nurses 'Always' Communicated Well	300+	77%	79%	79%
Pain 'Always' Well Controlled	300+	69%	70%	71%
Room and Bathroom 'Always' Clean	300+	68%	73%	73%
Timely Help 'Always' Received	300+	63%	67%	68%
Would Definitely Recommend Hospital	300+	63%	70%	71%
Use of Medical Imaging				
Cardiac Imaging Stress Test before Surgery	206	7.8%	5.4%	5.3%
Combination Abdominal CT Scan	333	8.1%	12.2%	10.5%
Combination Brain/Sinus CT Scan	276	6.2%	3.1%	2.7%
Combination Chest CT Scan	245	3.3%	2.1%	2.7%
Follow-up Mammogram/Ultrasound	1,137	7.6%	9%	8.8%
Lumbar Spine MRI for Low Back Pain	64	45.3%	35.8%	37.2%

Surgical Specialty Center at Coordinated Health

1503 Cedar Crest Boulevard
Allentown, PA 18104
Phone: 610-871-9110
URL: www.coordinatedhealth.com
Type: Acute Care Hospitals
Emergency Services: No
Ownership: Physician

Measure	Cases	This Hosp.	State Avg.	U.S. Avg.
Blood Clot Prevention and Treatment				
Anticoagulation Overlap Therapy[2,7]	-	-	94%	93%
ICU Venous Thromboembolism Prophylaxis[2,7]	-	-	94%	92%
Incidence of Potentially Preventable VTE[2,7]	-	-	8%	10%
UFH with Dosages/Platelet Monitoring[2,7]	-	-	98%	97%
Venous Thromboembolism Prophylaxis[2]	40	100%	90%	85%
Warfarin Therapy Discharge Instructions[2,7]	-	-	78%	75%
Chest Pain/Possible Heart Attack Care				
Aspirin Given Within 24 Hours of Arrival[5]	-	-	97%	96%
Fibrinolytic Meds Within 30 Min. of Arrival[5]	-	-	44%	58%
Average Time to ECG (minutes)[5]	-	-	9	7
Average Time to Transfer (minutes)[5]	-	-	64	60
Children's Asthma Care				
Received Home Management Plan of Care	-	-	-	88%
Received Reliever Medication	-	-	-	100%
Received Systemic Corticosteroids	-	-	-	100%
Emergency Department				
Admittance Decision Time (minutes)[2,7]	-	-	104	98
Head CT Results Within 45 Min. of Arrival[5]	-	-	60%	57%
Patients Who Left ER Before Being Seen[5]	-	-	1%	2%
Time from ER Arrival to Admit. (minutes)[2,7]	-	-	276	274
Time from ER Arrival to Discharge (minutes)[5]	-	-	125	134
Time in ER Before Being Evaluated (minutes)[5]	-	-	26	26
Time to Pain Meds for Fractures (minutes)[5]	-	-	58	57
Heart Attack Care				
Aspirin Given at Discharge[5]	-	-	99%	99%
Fibrinolytic Meds Within 30 Min. of Arrival[5]	-	-	40%	54%
PCI Within 90 Minutes of Arrival[5]	-	-	97%	96%
Statin Prescribed at Discharge[5]	-	-	99%	98%
Heart Failure Care				
ACE Inhibitor or ARB for LVSD[5]	-	-	97%	97%
Discharge Instructions Given[5]	-	-	96%	94%
Evaluation of LVS Function[5]	-	-	100%	99%
Medicare Spending				
Medicare Spending per Patient (ratio)	-	1.01	1.01	0.98
Pneumonia Care				
Appropriate Initial Antibiotic Given[5]	-	-	96%	95%
Blood Culture Timing[5]	-	-	98%	98%
Pregnancy and Delivery Care				
Newborn Deliveries Scheduled Early[7]	-	-	4%	6%
Preventive Care				
Immunization for Influenza[2]	390	59%	91%	90%
Immunization for Pneumonia[2]	369	47%	92%	92%
Stroke Care				
Anticoagulation Therapy for Atrial Fibrillation[5]	-	-	96%	95%
Antithrombotic Therapy Timing[5]	-	-	98%	98%
Assessed for Rehabilitation[5]	-	-	98%	97%
Discharged on Antithrombotic Therapy[5]	-	-	99%	99%
Discharged on Statin Medication[5]	-	-	95%	94%
Thrombolytic Therapy Timing[5]	-	-	72%	66%
Venous Thromboembolism Prophylaxis[5]	-	-	95%	94%
Written Stroke Educational Materials Given[5]	-	-	90%	88%
Surgical Care Improvement Project				
Appropriate Beta Blocker Usage[2]	17	100%	98%	98%
Appropriate VTP Within 24 Hours[2]	164	100%	99%	98%
Controlled Postoperative Blood Glucose[2,7]	-	-	98%	97%
Perioperative Temperature Management[2]	167	100%	100%	100%
Prophylactic Antibiotic Selection[2]	141	97%	99%	99%
Prophylactic Antibiotic Selection (Outpatient)	82	99%	98%	98%
Prophylactic Antibiotic Stopped[2]	141	99%	98%	98%
Prophylactic Antibiotic Timing[2]	141	97%	99%	99%
Prophylactic Antibiotic Timing (Outpatient)	82	100%	98%	98%
Urinary Catheter Removal[2]	153	97%	99%	97%
Survey of Patients' Hospital Experiences				
Area Around Room 'Always' Quiet at Night	300+	84%	54%	61%
Doctors 'Always' Communicated Well	300+	87%	80%	82%
Home Recovery Information Given	300+	93%	86%	85%
Hospital Given 9 or 10 on 10 Point Scale	300+	89%	69%	71%
Meds 'Always' Explained Before Given	300+	73%	63%	64%
Nurses 'Always' Communicated Well	300+	86%	79%	79%
Pain 'Always' Well Controlled	300+	77%	70%	71%
Room and Bathroom 'Always' Clean	300+	85%	73%	73%
Timely Help 'Always' Received	300+	88%	67%	68%
Would Definitely Recommend Hospital	300+	88%	70%	71%
Use of Medical Imaging				
Cardiac Imaging Stress Test before Surgery	269	4.5%	5.4%	5.3%
Combination Abdominal CT Scan[1]	-	-	12.2%	10.5%
Combination Brain/Sinus CT Scan[1]	-	-	3.1%	2.7%
Combination Chest CT Scan	48	4.2%	2.1%	2.7%
Follow-up Mammogram/Ultrasound	452	9.5%	9%	8.8%
Lumbar Spine MRI for Low Back Pain	302	30.1%	35.8%	37.2%

James E. Van Zandt VA Medical Center - Altoona

2907 Pleasant Valley Boulevard
Altoona, PA 16602
Phone: 814-943-8164
Fax: 814-940-7898
URL: www.va.gov
Type: Acute Care - VA
Emergency Services: No
Ownership: Government Federal
Beds: 68
Key Personnel:
Infection Control. . . . . Jennifer Fouse
Chief of Medical Staff. . . . . Santha Kurian, MD

Measure	Cases	This Hosp.	State Avg.	U.S. Avg.
Blood Clot Prevention and Treatment				
Anticoagulation Overlap Therapy	-	-	94%	93%
ICU Venous Thromboembolism Prophylaxis	-	-	94%	92%
Incidence of Potentially Preventable VTE	-	-	8%	10%
UFH with Dosages/Platelet Monitoring	-	-	98%	97%
Venous Thromboembolism Prophylaxis	-	-	90%	85%
Warfarin Therapy Discharge Instructions	-	-	78%	75%
Chest Pain/Possible Heart Attack Care				
Aspirin Given Within 24 Hours of Arrival	-	-	97%	96%
Fibrinolytic Meds Within 30 Min. of Arrival	-	-	44%	58%
Average Time to ECG (minutes)	-	-	9	7
Average Time to Transfer (minutes)	-	-	64	60
Children's Asthma Care				
Received Home Management Plan of Care	-	-	-	88%
Received Reliever Medication	-	-	-	100%
Received Systemic Corticosteroids	-	-	-	100%
Emergency Department				
Admittance Decision Time (minutes)	-	-	104	98
Head CT Results Within 45 Min. of Arrival	-	-	60%	57%
Patients Who Left ER Before Being Seen	-	-	1%	2%
Time from ER Arrival to Admit. (minutes)	-	-	276	274
Time from ER Arrival to Discharge (minutes)	-	-	125	134
Time in ER Before Being Evaluated (minutes)	-	-	26	26
Time to Pain Meds for Fractures (minutes)	-	-	58	57
Heart Attack Care				
Aspirin Given at Discharge[1]	-	-	99%	99%
Fibrinolytic Meds Within 30 Min. of Arrival[5]	-	-	40%	54%
PCI Within 90 Minutes of Arrival[5]	-	-	97%	96%
Statin Prescribed at Discharge[1]	-	-	99%	98%
Heart Failure Care				
ACE Inhibitor or ARB for LVSD[1]	18	100%	97%	97%
Discharge Instructions Given	40	100%	96%	94%
Evaluation of LVS Function	46	100%	100%	99%
Medicare Spending				
Medicare Spending per Patient (ratio)	-	-	1.01	0.98
Pneumonia Care				
Appropriate Initial Antibiotic Given	25	96%	96%	95%
Blood Culture Timing	33	97%	98%	98%
Pregnancy and Delivery Care				
Newborn Deliveries Scheduled Early	-	-	4%	6%
Preventive Care				
Immunization for Influenza[2,3]	140	98%	91%	90%
Immunization for Pneumonia[2,3]	344	99%	92%	92%
Stroke Care				
Anticoagulation Therapy for Atrial Fibrillation	-	-	96%	95%
Antithrombotic Therapy Timing	-	-	98%	98%

NOTE: Hospital profiles are in alphabetical order by state, then city, then hospital within the city; Rankings exclude hospitals with less than 25 cases except for patient surveys which excludes hospitals with less than 100 cases; (a) 100-299 cases; (1) The number of cases/patients is too few to report; (2) Data submitted were based on a sample of cases/patients; (3) Results are based on a shorter time period than required; (4) Data suppressed by CMS for one or more quarters; (5) Results are not available for this reporting period; (6) Fewer than 100 patients completed the HCAHPS survey; (7) No cases met the criteria for this measure; (8) The lower limit of the confidence interval cannot be calculated if the number of observed infections equals zero; (9) No data are available from the state/territory for this reporting period; (10) The scores shown reflect fewer than 50 completed surveys; (11) There were discrepancies in the data collection process; (12) This measure does not apply to this hospital for this reporting period; (13) Results cannot be calculated for this reporting period; (14) The results for this state are combined with nearby states to protect confidentiality; Please refer to the User's Guide for a full explanation of data.

Measure	Cases	This Hosp.	State Avg.	U.S. Avg.
Assessed for Rehabilitation	-	-	98%	97%
Discharged on Antithrombotic Therapy	-	-	99%	99%
Discharged on Statin Medication	-	-	95%	94%
Thrombolytic Therapy Timing	-	-	72%	66%
Venous Thromboembolism Prophylaxis	-	-	95%	94%
Written Stroke Educational Materials Given	-	-	90%	88%
Surgical Care Improvement Project				
Appropriate Beta Blocker Usage[5]	-	-	98%	98%
Appropriate VTP Within 24 Hours[5]	-	-	99%	98%
Controlled Postoperative Blood Glucose[5]	-	-	98%	97%
Perioperative Temperature Management[5]	-	-	100%	100%
Prophylactic Antibiotic Selection[5]	-	-	99%	99%
Prophylactic Antibiotic Selection (Outpatient)	-	-	98%	98%
Prophylactic Antibiotic Stopped[5]	-	-	98%	98%
Prophylactic Antibiotic Timing[5]	-	-	99%	99%
Prophylactic Antibiotic Timing (Outpatient)	-	-	98%	98%
Urinary Catheter Removal[5]	-	-	99%	97%
Survey of Patients' Hospital Experiences				
Area Around Room 'Always' Quiet at Night	-	-	54%	61%
Doctors 'Always' Communicated Well	-	-	80%	82%
Home Recovery Information Given	-	-	86%	85%
Hospital Given 9 or 10 on 10 Point Scale	-	-	69%	71%
Meds 'Always' Explained Before Given	-	-	63%	64%
Nurses 'Always' Communicated Well	-	-	79%	79%
Pain 'Always' Well Controlled	-	-	70%	71%
Room and Bathroom 'Always' Clean	-	-	73%	73%
Timely Help 'Always' Received	-	-	67%	68%
Would Definitely Recommend Hospital	-	-	70%	71%
Use of Medical Imaging				
Cardiac Imaging Stress Test before Surgery	-	-	5.4%	5.3%
Combination Abdominal CT Scan	-	-	12.2%	10.5%
Combination Brain/Sinus CT Scan	-	-	3.1%	2.7%
Combination Chest CT Scan	-	-	2.1%	2.7%
Follow-up Mammogram/Ultrasound	-	-	9%	8.8%
Lumbar Spine MRI for Low Back Pain	-	-	35.8%	37.2%

UPMC Altoona

620 Howard Avenue
Altoona, PA 16601
Phone: 814-889-2011
Fax: 814-949-3115
E-mail: info@altoonaregional.org
URL: www.altoonaregional.org
Type: Acute Care Hospitals
Emergency Services: Yes
Ownership: Voluntary non-profit - Private
Beds: 470

Key Personnel:

Infection Control. . . . . Margaret Adams
Chief of Medical Staff. . . . . Linnane R. Batzel, MD, MBA
Radiology. . . . . Michael Corso
Quality Assurance . . . . Kathy J Mecklen
CEO/President. . . . . Jerry Murray
Pediatric Ambulatory Care . . . . . . Sharon Roscia, RN
Operating Room. . . . . Jan Schachtner, RN

Measure	Cases	This Hosp.	State Avg.	U.S. Avg.
Blood Clot Prevention and Treatment				
Anticoagulation Overlap Therapy[2]	180	83%	94%	93%
ICU Venous Thromboembolism Prophylaxis[2]	81	83%	94%	92%
Incidence of Potentially Preventable VTE[2]	33	18%	8%	10%
UFH with Dosages/Platelet Monitoring[2]	79	99%	98%	97%
Venous Thromboembolism Prophylaxis[2]	300	64%	90%	85%
Warfarin Therapy Discharge Instructions[2]	115	25%	78%	75%
Chest Pain/Possible Heart Attack Care				
Aspirin Given Within 24 Hours of Arrival[5]	-	-	97%	96%
Fibrinolytic Meds Within 30 Min. of Arrival[5]	-	-	44%	58%
Average Time to ECG (minutes)[5]	-	-	9	7
Average Time to Transfer (minutes)[5]	-	-	64	60
Children's Asthma Care				
Received Home Management Plan of Care	-	-	-	88%
Received Reliever Medication	-	-	-	100%
Received Systemic Corticosteroids	-	-	-	100%
Emergency Department				
Admittance Decision Time (minutes)[2]	868	74	104	98
Head CT Results Within 45 Min. of Arrival	36	33%	60%	57%
Patients Who Left ER Before Being Seen	59,315	1%	1%	2%
Time from ER Arrival to Admit. (minutes)[2]	901	237	276	274
Time from ER Arrival to Discharge (minutes)	1,523	124	125	134
Time in ER Before Being Evaluated (minutes)	1,785	12	26	26
Time to Pain Meds for Fractures (minutes)	218	61	58	57
Heart Attack Care				
Aspirin Given at Discharge	628	99%	99%	99%
Fibrinolytic Meds Within 30 Min. of Arrival[7]	-	-	40%	54%
PCI Within 90 Minutes of Arrival	103	94%	97%	96%
Statin Prescribed at Discharge	582	97%	99%	98%
Heart Failure Care				
ACE Inhibitor or ARB for LVSD	129	94%	97%	97%
Discharge Instructions Given	376	95%	96%	94%
Evaluation of LVS Function	508	100%	100%	99%
Medicare Spending				
Medicare Spending per Patient (ratio)	-	1.10	1.01	0.98
Pneumonia Care				
Appropriate Initial Antibiotic Given	303	95%	96%	95%
Blood Culture Timing	496	99%	98%	98%
Pregnancy and Delivery Care				
Newborn Deliveries Scheduled Early	129	21%	4%	6%
Preventive Care				
Immunization for Influenza[2]	1,077	94%	91%	90%
Immunization for Pneumonia[2]	1,369	96%	92%	92%
Stroke Care				
Anticoagulation Therapy for Atrial Fibrillation	41	100%	96%	95%
Antithrombotic Therapy Timing	256	98%	98%	98%
Assessed for Rehabilitation	296	100%	98%	97%
Discharged on Antithrombotic Therapy	263	100%	99%	99%
Discharged on Statin Medication	202	95%	95%	94%
Thrombolytic Therapy Timing	17	94%	72%	66%
Venous Thromboembolism Prophylaxis	297	95%	95%	94%
Written Stroke Educational Materials Given	115	100%	90%	88%
Surgical Care Improvement Project				
Appropriate Beta Blocker Usage	534	96%	98%	98%
Appropriate VTP Within 24 Hours	980	99%	99%	98%
Controlled Postoperative Blood Glucose	196	95%	98%	97%
Perioperative Temperature Management	1,316	100%	100%	100%
Prophylactic Antibiotic Selection	1,049	98%	99%	99%
Prophylactic Antibiotic Selection (Outpatient)	874	99%	98%	98%
Prophylactic Antibiotic Stopped	1,028	97%	98%	98%
Prophylactic Antibiotic Timing	1,049	99%	99%	99%
Prophylactic Antibiotic Timing (Outpatient)	882	99%	98%	98%
Urinary Catheter Removal	284	88%	99%	97%
Survey of Patients' Hospital Experiences				
Area Around Room 'Always' Quiet at Night	300+	52%	54%	61%
Doctors 'Always' Communicated Well	300+	80%	80%	82%
Home Recovery Information Given	300+	84%	86%	85%
Hospital Given 9 or 10 on 10 Point Scale	300+	70%	69%	71%
Meds 'Always' Explained Before Given	300+	57%	63%	64%
Nurses 'Always' Communicated Well	300+	80%	79%	79%
Pain 'Always' Well Controlled	300+	68%	70%	71%
Room and Bathroom 'Always' Clean	300+	75%	73%	73%
Timely Help 'Always' Received	300+	64%	67%	68%
Would Definitely Recommend Hospital	300+	66%	70%	71%
Use of Medical Imaging				
Cardiac Imaging Stress Test before Surgery	600	5.5%	5.4%	5.3%
Combination Abdominal CT Scan	1,313	10.4%	12.2%	10.5%
Combination Brain/Sinus CT Scan	1,128	4.1%	3.1%	2.7%
Combination Chest CT Scan	1,046	2.8%	2.1%	2.7%
Follow-up Mammogram/Ultrasound	1,068	16.2%	9%	8.8%
Lumbar Spine MRI for Low Back Pain	143	31.5%	35.8%	37.2%

Heritage Valley Beaver

1000 Dutch Ridge Road
Beaver, PA 15009
Phone: 412-728-7000
Fax: 724-773-8210
URL: www.heritagevalley.org
Type: Acute Care Hospitals
Emergency Services: Yes
Ownership: Voluntary non-profit - Private
Beds: 358

Key Personnel:

Cardiac Laboratory. . . . . Rhonda Beltz
Infection Control. . . . . Bruce Chamovitz, MD
Chief of Medical Staff. . . . . John T. Cinicola, MD
Quality Assurance . . . . Debbie Grady
Pediatric Ambulatory Care . . . . . . Krishana Kasi, MD
Pediatric In-Patient Care . . . . Krishana Kasi, MD
Radiology. . . . . Roland McGraner
CEO/President. . . . . Norman Mitry

Measure	Cases	This Hosp.	State Avg.	U.S. Avg.
Blood Clot Prevention and Treatment				
Anticoagulation Overlap Therapy[2]	108	100%	94%	93%
ICU Venous Thromboembolism Prophylaxis[2]	63	100%	94%	92%
Incidence of Potentially Preventable VTE[2]	18	0%	8%	10%
UFH with Dosages/Platelet Monitoring[2]	104	100%	98%	97%
Venous Thromboembolism Prophylaxis[2]	370	95%	90%	85%
Warfarin Therapy Discharge Instructions[2]	64	100%	78%	75%
Chest Pain/Possible Heart Attack Care				
Aspirin Given Within 24 Hours of Arrival[1]	-	-	97%	96%
Fibrinolytic Meds Within 30 Min. of Arrival[5]	-	-	44%	58%
Average Time to ECG (minutes)[1]	-	-	9	7
Average Time to Transfer (minutes)[5]	-	-	64	60
Children's Asthma Care				
Received Home Management Plan of Care	-	-	-	88%
Received Reliever Medication	-	-	-	100%
Received Systemic Corticosteroids	-	-	-	100%
Emergency Department				
Admittance Decision Time (minutes)[2]	470	77	104	98
Head CT Results Within 45 Min. of Arrival	24	79%	60%	57%
Patients Who Left ER Before Being Seen	50,201	0%	1%	2%
Time from ER Arrival to Admit. (minutes)[2]	550	260	276	274
Time from ER Arrival to Discharge (minutes)	395	129	125	134
Time in ER Before Being Evaluated (minutes)	335	22	26	26
Time to Pain Meds for Fractures (minutes)	119	54	58	57
Heart Attack Care				
Aspirin Given at Discharge	359	100%	99%	99%
Fibrinolytic Meds Within 30 Min. of Arrival[7]	-	-	40%	54%
PCI Within 90 Minutes of Arrival	72	99%	97%	96%
Statin Prescribed at Discharge	332	99%	99%	98%
Heart Failure Care				
ACE Inhibitor or ARB for LVSD[2]	70	100%	97%	97%
Discharge Instructions Given[2]	248	99%	96%	94%
Evaluation of LVS Function[2]	326	100%	100%	99%
Medicare Spending				
Medicare Spending per Patient (ratio)	-	1.04	1.01	0.98
Pneumonia Care				
Appropriate Initial Antibiotic Given[2]	114	94%	96%	95%
Blood Culture Timing[2]	189	96%	98%	98%
Pregnancy and Delivery Care				
Newborn Deliveries Scheduled Early[2]	21	0%	4%	6%
Preventive Care				
Immunization for Influenza[2]	563	98%	91%	90%
Immunization for Pneumonia[2]	752	97%	92%	92%
Stroke Care				
Anticoagulation Therapy for Atrial Fibrillation	16	100%	96%	95%
Antithrombotic Therapy Timing	121	100%	98%	98%
Assessed for Rehabilitation	117	93%	98%	97%
Discharged on Antithrombotic Therapy	113	100%	99%	99%
Discharged on Statin Medication	91	89%	95%	94%
Thrombolytic Therapy Timing[1]	-	-	72%	66%
Venous Thromboembolism Prophylaxis	127	93%	95%	94%
Written Stroke Educational Materials Given	54	100%	90%	88%
Surgical Care Improvement Project				
Appropriate Beta Blocker Usage[2]	244	99%	98%	98%
Appropriate VTP Within 24 Hours[2]	376	94%	99%	98%
Controlled Postoperative Blood Glucose[2]	147	99%	98%	97%
Perioperative Temperature Management[2]	525	100%	100%	100%
Prophylactic Antibiotic Selection[2]	480	96%	99%	99%
Prophylactic Antibiotic Selection (Outpatient)	185	98%	98%	98%
Prophylactic Antibiotic Stopped[2]	471	99%	98%	98%
Prophylactic Antibiotic Timing[2]	481	99%	99%	99%
Prophylactic Antibiotic Timing (Outpatient)	185	99%	98%	98%
Urinary Catheter Removal[2]	403	98%	99%	97%
Survey of Patients' Hospital Experiences				
Area Around Room 'Always' Quiet at Night	(a)	43%	54%	61%
Doctors 'Always' Communicated Well	(a)	77%	80%	82%
Home Recovery Information Given	(a)	82%	86%	85%
Hospital Given 9 or 10 on 10 Point Scale	(a)	61%	69%	71%
Meds 'Always' Explained Before Given	(a)	50%	63%	64%
Nurses 'Always' Communicated Well	(a)	74%	79%	79%
Pain 'Always' Well Controlled	(a)	67%	70%	71%

NOTE: Hospital profiles are in alphabetical order by state, then city, then hospital within the city; Rankings exclude hospitals with less than 25 cases except for patient surveys which excludes hospitals with less than 100 cases; (a) 100-299 cases; (1) The number of cases/patients is too few to report; (2) Data submitted were based on a sample of cases/patients; (3) Results are based on a shorter time period than required; (4) Data suppressed by CMS for one or more quarters; (5) Results are not available for this reporting period; (6) Fewer than 100 patients completed the HCAHPS survey; (7) No cases met the criteria for this measure; (8) The lower limit of the confidence interval cannot be calculated if the number of observed infections equals zero; (9) No data are available from the state/territory for this reporting period; (10) The scores shown reflect fewer than 50 completed surveys; (11) There were discrepancies in the data collection process; (12) This measure does not apply to this hospital for this reporting period; (13) Results cannot be calculated for this reporting period; (14) The results for this state are combined with nearby states to protect confidentiality; Please refer to the User's Guide for a full explanation of data.

Measure	Cases	This Hosp.	State Avg.	U.S. Avg.
Room and Bathroom 'Always' Clean	(a)	62%	73%	73%
Timely Help 'Always' Received	(a)	58%	67%	68%
Would Definitely Recommend Hospital	(a)	60%	70%	71%
Use of Medical Imaging				
Cardiac Imaging Stress Test before Surgery	114	7.0%	5.4%	5.3%
Combination Abdominal CT Scan	675	6.8%	12.2%	10.5%
Combination Brain/Sinus CT Scan	588	1.4%	3.1%	2.7%
Combination Chest CT Scan	447	1.1%	2.1%	2.7%
Follow-up Mammogram/Ultrasound	1,301	8.8%	9%	8.8%
Lumbar Spine MRI for Low Back Pain	77	40.3%	35.8%	37.2%

Bucks County Specialty Hospital

3300 Tillman Drive
Bensalem, PA 19020
Phone: 215-244-7400
URL: www.bcshospital.com
Type: Acute Care Hospitals
Emergency Services: No
Ownership: Proprietary

Measure	Cases	This Hosp.	State Avg.	U.S. Avg.
Blood Clot Prevention and Treatment				
Anticoagulation Overlap Therapy[2,7]	-	-	94%	93%
ICU Venous Thromboembolism Prophylaxis[2,7]	-	-	94%	92%
Incidence of Potentially Preventable VTE[2,7]	-	-	8%	10%
UFH with Dosages/Platelet Monitoring[2,7]	-	-	98%	97%
Venous Thromboembolism Prophylaxis[2]	31	100%	90%	85%
Warfarin Therapy Discharge Instructions[2,7]	-	-	78%	75%
Chest Pain/Possible Heart Attack Care				
Aspirin Given Within 24 Hours of Arrival[5]	-	-	97%	96%
Fibrinolytic Meds Within 30 Min. of Arrival[5]	-	-	44%	58%
Average Time to ECG (minutes)[5]	-	-	9	7
Average Time to Transfer (minutes)[5]	-	-	64	60
Children's Asthma Care				
Received Home Management Plan of Care	-	-	-	88%
Received Reliever Medication	-	-	-	100%
Received Systemic Corticosteroids	-	-	-	100%
Emergency Department				
Admittance Decision Time (minutes)[2,7]	-	-	104	98
Head CT Results Within 45 Min. of Arrival[5]	-	-	60%	57%
Patients Who Left ER Before Being Seen[5]	-	-	1%	2%
Time from ER Arrival to Admit. (minutes)[2,7]	-	-	276	274
Time from ER Arrival to Discharge (minutes)[5]	-	-	125	134
Time in ER Before Being Evaluated (minutes)[5]	-	-	26	26
Time to Pain Meds for Fractures (minutes)[5]	-	-	58	57
Heart Attack Care				
Aspirin Given at Discharge[5]	-	-	99%	99%
Fibrinolytic Meds Within 30 Min. of Arrival[5]	-	-	40%	54%
PCI Within 90 Minutes of Arrival[5]	-	-	97%	96%
Statin Prescribed at Discharge[5]	-	-	99%	98%
Heart Failure Care				
ACE Inhibitor or ARB for LVSD[5]	-	-	97%	97%
Discharge Instructions Given[5]	-	-	96%	94%
Evaluation of LVS Function[5]	-	-	100%	99%
Medicare Spending				
Medicare Spending per Patient (ratio)	-	0.90	1.01	0.98
Pneumonia Care				
Appropriate Initial Antibiotic Given[5]	-	-	96%	95%
Blood Culture Timing[5]	-	-	98%	98%
Pregnancy and Delivery Care				
Newborn Deliveries Scheduled Early[7]	-	-	4%	6%
Preventive Care				
Immunization for Influenza[2]	311	87%	91%	90%
Immunization for Pneumonia[2]	288	71%	92%	92%
Stroke Care				
Anticoagulation Therapy for Atrial Fibrillation[5]	-	-	96%	95%
Antithrombotic Therapy Timing[5]	-	-	98%	98%
Assessed for Rehabilitation[5]	-	-	98%	97%
Discharged on Antithrombotic Therapy[5]	-	-	99%	99%
Discharged on Statin Medication[5]	-	-	95%	94%
Thrombolytic Therapy Timing[5]	-	-	72%	66%
Venous Thromboembolism Prophylaxis[5]	-	-	95%	94%
Written Stroke Educational Materials Given[5]	-	-	90%	88%
Surgical Care Improvement Project				
Appropriate Beta Blocker Usage[2]	21	100%	98%	98%
Appropriate VTP Within 24 Hours[2]	69	100%	99%	98%
Controlled Postoperative Blood Glucose[2,7]	-	-	98%	97%
Perioperative Temperature Management[2]	150	100%	100%	100%
Prophylactic Antibiotic Selection[2]	148	100%	99%	99%
Prophylactic Antibiotic Selection (Outpatient)	97	100%	98%	98%
Prophylactic Antibiotic Stopped[2]	148	100%	98%	98%
Prophylactic Antibiotic Timing[2]	148	100%	99%	99%
Prophylactic Antibiotic Timing (Outpatient)	97	100%	98%	98%
Urinary Catheter Removal[2]	26	100%	99%	97%
Survey of Patients' Hospital Experiences				
Area Around Room 'Always' Quiet at Night	300+	84%	54%	61%
Doctors 'Always' Communicated Well	300+	84%	80%	82%
Home Recovery Information Given	300+	90%	86%	85%
Hospital Given 9 or 10 on 10 Point Scale	300+	87%	69%	71%
Meds 'Always' Explained Before Given	300+	72%	63%	64%
Nurses 'Always' Communicated Well	300+	90%	79%	79%
Pain 'Always' Well Controlled	300+	79%	70%	71%
Room and Bathroom 'Always' Clean	300+	87%	73%	73%
Timely Help 'Always' Received	300+	88%	67%	68%
Would Definitely Recommend Hospital	300+	90%	70%	71%
Use of Medical Imaging				
Cardiac Imaging Stress Test before Surgery[7]	-	-	5.4%	5.3%
Combination Abdominal CT Scan[7]	-	-	12.2%	10.5%
Combination Brain/Sinus CT Scan[7]	-	-	3.1%	2.7%
Combination Chest CT Scan[7]	-	-	2.1%	2.7%
Follow-up Mammogram/Ultrasound[7]	-	-	9%	8.8%
Lumbar Spine MRI for Low Back Pain[7]	-	-	35.8%	37.2%

Berwick Hospital Center

701 East 16th Street
Berwick, PA 18603
Phone: 570-759-5000
Fax: 570-759-3473
URL: www.berwick-hospital.com
Type: Acute Care Hospitals
Emergency Services: Yes
Ownership: Proprietary
Beds: 130

Key Personnel:
Quality Assurance . . . . Megan Benson
CEO/President. . . . . Donald Henderson
Chief of Medical Staff. . . . . Michael Kenny

Measure	Cases	This Hosp.	State Avg.	U.S. Avg.
Blood Clot Prevention and Treatment				
Anticoagulation Overlap Therapy[2]	13	85%	94%	93%
ICU Venous Thromboembolism Prophylaxis[2]	99	90%	94%	92%
Incidence of Potentially Preventable VTE[1,2]	-	-	8%	10%
UFH with Dosages/Platelet Monitoring[1,2]	-	-	98%	97%
Venous Thromboembolism Prophylaxis[2]	246	81%	90%	85%
Warfarin Therapy Discharge Instructions[2]	13	62%	78%	75%
Chest Pain/Possible Heart Attack Care				
Aspirin Given Within 24 Hours of Arrival	24	96%	97%	96%
Fibrinolytic Meds Within 30 Min. of Arrival[7]	-	-	44%	58%
Average Time to ECG (minutes)	24	4	9	7
Average Time to Transfer (minutes)[1]	-	-	64	60
Children's Asthma Care				
Received Home Management Plan of Care	-	-	-	88%
Received Reliever Medication	-	-	-	100%
Received Systemic Corticosteroids	-	-	-	100%
Emergency Department				
Admittance Decision Time (minutes)[2]	469	107	104	98
Head CT Results Within 45 Min. of Arrival[1]	-	-	60%	57%
Patients Who Left ER Before Being Seen	12,765	0%	1%	2%
Time from ER Arrival to Admit. (minutes)[2]	496	236	276	274
Time from ER Arrival to Discharge (minutes)	386	102	125	134
Time in ER Before Being Evaluated (minutes)	418	24	26	26
Time to Pain Meds for Fractures (minutes)	54	69	58	57
Heart Attack Care				
Aspirin Given at Discharge	28	93%	99%	99%
Fibrinolytic Meds Within 30 Min. of Arrival[7]	-	-	40%	54%
PCI Within 90 Minutes of Arrival[7]	-	-	97%	96%
Statin Prescribed at Discharge	25	76%	99%	98%
Heart Failure Care				
ACE Inhibitor or ARB for LVSD	13	92%	97%	97%
Discharge Instructions Given	50	98%	96%	94%
Evaluation of LVS Function	72	100%	100%	99%
Medicare Spending				
Medicare Spending per Patient (ratio)	-	0.97	1.01	0.98
Pneumonia Care				
Appropriate Initial Antibiotic Given	44	93%	96%	95%
Blood Culture Timing	76	100%	98%	98%
Pregnancy and Delivery Care				
Newborn Deliveries Scheduled Early[1,2]	-	-	4%	6%
Preventive Care				
Immunization for Influenza[2]	398	98%	91%	90%
Immunization for Pneumonia[2]	515	100%	92%	92%
Stroke Care				
Anticoagulation Therapy for Atrial Fibrillation[1]	-	-	96%	95%
Antithrombotic Therapy Timing	20	90%	98%	98%
Assessed for Rehabilitation	17	88%	98%	97%
Discharged on Antithrombotic Therapy	17	88%	99%	99%
Discharged on Statin Medication	14	79%	95%	94%
Thrombolytic Therapy Timing[1]	-	-	72%	66%
Venous Thromboembolism Prophylaxis	21	57%	95%	94%
Written Stroke Educational Materials Given[1]	-	-	90%	88%
Surgical Care Improvement Project				
Appropriate Beta Blocker Usage	36	97%	98%	98%
Appropriate VTP Within 24 Hours	109	97%	99%	98%
Controlled Postoperative Blood Glucose[7]	-	-	98%	97%
Perioperative Temperature Management	134	100%	100%	100%
Prophylactic Antibiotic Selection	103	95%	99%	99%
Prophylactic Antibiotic Selection (Outpatient)	33	100%	98%	98%
Prophylactic Antibiotic Stopped	102	98%	98%	98%
Prophylactic Antibiotic Timing	104	99%	99%	99%
Prophylactic Antibiotic Timing (Outpatient)	33	100%	98%	98%
Urinary Catheter Removal	37	86%	99%	97%
Survey of Patients' Hospital Experiences				
Area Around Room 'Always' Quiet at Night	300+	56%	54%	61%
Doctors 'Always' Communicated Well	300+	82%	80%	82%
Home Recovery Information Given	300+	84%	86%	85%
Hospital Given 9 or 10 on 10 Point Scale	300+	63%	69%	71%
Meds 'Always' Explained Before Given	300+	64%	63%	64%
Nurses 'Always' Communicated Well	300+	78%	79%	79%
Pain 'Always' Well Controlled	300+	72%	70%	71%
Room and Bathroom 'Always' Clean	300+	69%	73%	73%
Timely Help 'Always' Received	300+	68%	67%	68%
Would Definitely Recommend Hospital	300+	62%	70%	71%
Use of Medical Imaging				
Cardiac Imaging Stress Test before Surgery[1]	-	-	5.4%	5.3%
Combination Abdominal CT Scan	193	15.5%	12.2%	10.5%
Combination Brain/Sinus CT Scan	235	6.4%	3.1%	2.7%
Combination Chest CT Scan	69	13.0%	2.1%	2.7%
Follow-up Mammogram/Ultrasound	464	11.0%	9%	8.8%
Lumbar Spine MRI for Low Back Pain[1]	-	-	35.8%	37.2%

Coordinated Health Orthopedic Hospital

2310 Highland Avenue
Bethlehem, PA 18017
Phone: 610-691-4300
URL: www.coordinatedhealth.com
Type: Acute Care Hospitals
Emergency Services: No
Ownership: Proprietary

Key Personnel:
Anesthesiology. . . . . Sunita Arora, MD
CEO/President. . . . . Emil J Dilorio, MD
Cardiology. . . . . Stephen Ksiazek, MD
Radiology. . . . . Ada Kumar, MD

Measure	Cases	This Hosp.	State Avg.	U.S. Avg.
Blood Clot Prevention and Treatment				
Anticoagulation Overlap Therapy[2,7]	-	-	94%	93%
ICU Venous Thromboembolism Prophylaxis[2,7]	-	-	94%	92%
Incidence of Potentially Preventable VTE[2,7]	-	-	8%	10%
UFH with Dosages/Platelet Monitoring[2,7]	-	-	98%	97%
Venous Thromboembolism Prophylaxis[2]	16	100%	90%	85%
Warfarin Therapy Discharge Instructions[2,7]	-	-	78%	75%
Chest Pain/Possible Heart Attack Care				
Aspirin Given Within 24 Hours of Arrival[5]	-	-	97%	96%
Fibrinolytic Meds Within 30 Min. of Arrival[5]	-	-	44%	58%
Average Time to ECG (minutes)[5]	-	-	9	7
Average Time to Transfer (minutes)[5]	-	-	64	60
Children's Asthma Care				

NOTE: Hospital profiles are in alphabetical order by state, then city, then hospital within the city; Rankings exclude hospitals with less than 25 cases except for patient surveys which excludes hospitals with less than 100 cases; (a) 100-299 cases; (1) The number of cases/patients is too few to report; (2) Data submitted were based on a sample of cases/patients; (3) Results are based on a shorter time period than required; (4) Data suppressed by CMS for one or more quarters; (5) Results are not available for this reporting period; (6) Fewer than 100 patients completed the HCAHPS survey; (7) No cases met the criteria for this measure; (8) The lower limit of the confidence interval cannot be calculated if the number of observed infections equals zero; (9) No data are available from the state/territory for this reporting period; (10) The scores shown reflect fewer than 50 completed surveys; (11) There were discrepancies in the data collection process; (12) This measure does not apply to this hospital for this reporting period; (13) Results cannot be calculated for this reporting period; (14) The results for this state are combined with nearby states to protect confidentiality; Please refer to the User's Guide for a full explanation of data.

Measure	Cases	This Hosp.	State Avg.	U.S. Avg.
Received Home Management Plan of Care	-	-	-	88%
Received Reliever Medication	-	-	-	100%
Received Systemic Corticosteroids	-	-	-	100%
Emergency Department				
Admittance Decision Time (minutes)[2,7]	-	-	104	98
Head CT Results Within 45 Min. of Arrival[5]	-	-	60%	57%
Patients Who Left ER Before Being Seen[5]	-	-	1%	2%
Time from ER Arrival to Admit. (minutes)[2,7]	-	-	276	274
Time from ER Arrival to Discharge (minutes)[5]	-	-	125	134
Time in ER Before Being Evaluated (minutes)[5]	-	-	26	26
Time to Pain Meds for Fractures (minutes)[5]	-	-	58	57
Heart Attack Care				
Aspirin Given at Discharge[5]	-	-	99%	99%
Fibrinolytic Meds Within 30 Min. of Arrival[5]	-	-	40%	54%
PCI Within 90 Minutes of Arrival[5]	-	-	97%	96%
Statin Prescribed at Discharge[5]	-	-	99%	98%
Heart Failure Care				
ACE Inhibitor or ARB for LVSD[5]	-	-	97%	97%
Discharge Instructions Given[5]	-	-	96%	94%
Evaluation of LVS Function[5]	-	-	100%	99%
Medicare Spending				
Medicare Spending per Patient (ratio)	-	1.01	1.01	0.98
Pneumonia Care				
Appropriate Initial Antibiotic Given[5]	-	-	96%	95%
Blood Culture Timing[5]	-	-	98%	98%
Pregnancy and Delivery Care				
Newborn Deliveries Scheduled Early[7]	-	-	4%	6%
Preventive Care				
Immunization for Influenza[2]	368	79%	91%	90%
Immunization for Pneumonia[2]	413	58%	92%	92%
Stroke Care				
Anticoagulation Therapy for Atrial Fibrillation[5]	-	-	96%	95%
Antithrombotic Therapy Timing[5]	-	-	98%	98%
Assessed for Rehabilitation[5]	-	-	98%	97%
Discharged on Antithrombotic Therapy[5]	-	-	99%	99%
Discharged on Statin Medication[5]	-	-	95%	94%
Thrombolytic Therapy Timing[5]	-	-	72%	66%
Venous Thromboembolism Prophylaxis[5]	-	-	95%	94%
Written Stroke Educational Materials Given[5]	-	-	90%	88%
Surgical Care Improvement Project				
Appropriate Beta Blocker Usage[2]	59	100%	98%	98%
Appropriate VTP Within 24 Hours[2]	200	100%	99%	98%
Controlled Postoperative Blood Glucose[2,7]	-	-	98%	97%
Perioperative Temperature Management[2]	211	100%	100%	100%
Prophylactic Antibiotic Selection[2]	145	99%	99%	99%
Prophylactic Antibiotic Selection (Outpatient)	37	100%	98%	98%
Prophylactic Antibiotic Stopped[2]	145	100%	98%	98%
Prophylactic Antibiotic Timing[2]	145	99%	99%	99%
Prophylactic Antibiotic Timing (Outpatient)	37	95%	98%	98%
Urinary Catheter Removal[2]	181	93%	99%	97%
Survey of Patients' Hospital Experiences				
Area Around Room 'Always' Quiet at Night	300+	78%	54%	61%
Doctors 'Always' Communicated Well	300+	86%	80%	82%
Home Recovery Information Given	300+	93%	86%	85%
Hospital Given 9 or 10 on 10 Point Scale	300+	83%	69%	71%
Meds 'Always' Explained Before Given	300+	69%	63%	64%
Nurses 'Always' Communicated Well	300+	85%	79%	79%
Pain 'Always' Well Controlled	300+	76%	70%	71%
Room and Bathroom 'Always' Clean	300+	84%	73%	73%
Timely Help 'Always' Received	300+	80%	67%	68%
Would Definitely Recommend Hospital	300+	84%	70%	71%
Use of Medical Imaging				
Cardiac Imaging Stress Test before Surgery[7]	-	-	5.4%	5.3%
Combination Abdominal CT Scan[7]	-	-	12.2%	10.5%
Combination Brain/Sinus CT Scan[7]	-	-	3.1%	2.7%
Combination Chest CT Scan[7]	-	-	2.1%	2.7%
Follow-up Mammogram/Ultrasound[7]	-	-	9%	8.8%
Lumbar Spine MRI for Low Back Pain[7]	-	-	35.8%	37.2%

Lehigh Valley Hospital - Muhlenberg

2545 Schoenersville Road — Phone: 610-402-2273
Bethlehem, PA 18017 — Fax: 610-402-7523
URL: www.lvhn.org
Type: Acute Care Hospitals — Emergency Services: Yes
Ownership: Voluntary non-profit - Other — Beds: 148

Key Personnel:
Infection Control. . . . . Terry Burger, RN
Chief of Medical Staff. . . . . Linda L Lapos, MD
Quality Assurance . . . . Sue Lawrence
CEO/President. . . . . Elliot J Sussman
Pediatric Ambulatory Care . . . . John Van Brakle, MD
Pediatric In-Patient Care . . . . John Van Brakle, MD
Operating Room. . . . . Thomas V Whalen

Measure	Cases	This Hosp.	State Avg.	U.S. Avg.
Blood Clot Prevention and Treatment				
Anticoagulation Overlap Therapy[2]	130	95%	94%	93%
ICU Venous Thromboembolism Prophylaxis[2]	70	94%	94%	92%
Incidence of Potentially Preventable VTE[2]	12	8%	8%	10%
UFH with Dosages/Platelet Monitoring[2]	128	91%	98%	97%
Venous Thromboembolism Prophylaxis[2]	404	93%	90%	85%
Warfarin Therapy Discharge Instructions[2]	102	63%	78%	75%
Chest Pain/Possible Heart Attack Care				
Aspirin Given Within 24 Hours of Arrival[1,3]	-	-	97%	96%
Fibrinolytic Meds Within 30 Min. of Arrival[3,7]	-	-	44%	58%
Average Time to ECG (minutes)[1,3]	-	-	9	7
Average Time to Transfer (minutes)[3,7]	-	-	64	60
Children's Asthma Care				
Received Home Management Plan of Care	-	-	-	88%
Received Reliever Medication	-	-	-	100%
Received Systemic Corticosteroids	-	-	-	100%
Emergency Department				
Admittance Decision Time (minutes)[2]	1,028	119	104	98
Head CT Results Within 45 Min. of Arrival	17	47%	60%	57%
Patients Who Left ER Before Being Seen	58,155	0%	1%	2%
Time from ER Arrival to Admit. (minutes)[2]	1,030	313	276	274
Time from ER Arrival to Discharge (minutes)	347	143	125	134
Time in ER Before Being Evaluated (minutes)	377	20	26	26
Time to Pain Meds for Fractures (minutes)	161	40	58	57
Heart Attack Care				
Aspirin Given at Discharge	247	100%	99%	99%
Fibrinolytic Meds Within 30 Min. of Arrival[7]	-	-	40%	54%
PCI Within 90 Minutes of Arrival	61	98%	97%	96%
Statin Prescribed at Discharge	239	98%	99%	98%
Heart Failure Care				
ACE Inhibitor or ARB for LVSD	115	100%	97%	97%
Discharge Instructions Given	460	98%	96%	94%
Evaluation of LVS Function	556	100%	100%	99%
Medicare Spending				
Medicare Spending per Patient (ratio)	-	0.98	1.01	0.98
Pneumonia Care				
Appropriate Initial Antibiotic Given	177	95%	96%	95%
Blood Culture Timing	324	97%	98%	98%
Pregnancy and Delivery Care				
Newborn Deliveries Scheduled Early[7]	-	-	4%	6%
Preventive Care				
Immunization for Influenza[2]	590	99%	91%	90%
Immunization for Pneumonia[2]	921	95%	92%	92%
Stroke Care				
Anticoagulation Therapy for Atrial Fibrillation	18	100%	96%	95%
Antithrombotic Therapy Timing	108	100%	98%	98%
Assessed for Rehabilitation	118	100%	98%	97%
Discharged on Antithrombotic Therapy	116	100%	99%	99%
Discharged on Statin Medication	89	96%	95%	94%
Thrombolytic Therapy Timing[1]	-	-	72%	66%
Venous Thromboembolism Prophylaxis	120	98%	95%	94%
Written Stroke Educational Materials Given	66	97%	90%	88%
Surgical Care Improvement Project				
Appropriate Beta Blocker Usage	223	98%	98%	98%
Appropriate VTP Within 24 Hours	483	98%	99%	98%
Controlled Postoperative Blood Glucose	88	97%	98%	97%
Perioperative Temperature Management	550	100%	100%	100%
Prophylactic Antibiotic Selection	368	99%	99%	99%
Prophylactic Antibiotic Selection (Outpatient)	347	99%	98%	98%
Prophylactic Antibiotic Stopped	359	96%	98%	98%
Prophylactic Antibiotic Timing	368	98%	99%	99%
Prophylactic Antibiotic Timing (Outpatient)	355	97%	98%	98%
Urinary Catheter Removal	281	97%	99%	97%
Survey of Patients' Hospital Experiences				
Area Around Room 'Always' Quiet at Night	300+	51%	54%	61%
Doctors 'Always' Communicated Well	300+	78%	80%	82%
Home Recovery Information Given	300+	88%	86%	85%
Hospital Given 9 or 10 on 10 Point Scale	300+	75%	69%	71%
Meds 'Always' Explained Before Given	300+	63%	63%	64%
Nurses 'Always' Communicated Well	300+	80%	79%	79%
Pain 'Always' Well Controlled	300+	70%	70%	71%
Room and Bathroom 'Always' Clean	300+	75%	73%	73%
Timely Help 'Always' Received	300+	62%	67%	68%
Would Definitely Recommend Hospital	300+	78%	70%	71%
Use of Medical Imaging				
Cardiac Imaging Stress Test before Surgery	1,228	4.7%	5.4%	5.3%
Combination Abdominal CT Scan	1,489	7.7%	12.2%	10.5%
Combination Brain/Sinus CT Scan	1,116	2.9%	3.1%	2.7%
Combination Chest CT Scan	1,197	3.7%	2.1%	2.7%
Follow-up Mammogram/Ultrasound	1,955	6.9%	9%	8.8%
Lumbar Spine MRI for Low Back Pain	77	32.5%	35.8%	37.2%

Saint Luke's Hospital Bethlehem

801 Ostrum Street — Phone: 610-954-4000
Bethlehem, PA 18015 — Fax: 610-954-4979
URL: www.slhn-lehighvalley.org
Type: Acute Care Hospitals — Emergency Services: Yes
Ownership: Voluntary non-profit - Private — Beds: 436

Key Personnel:
President/CEO. . . . . Richard A. Anderson
Chief of Medical Staff . . . . James A Cowan, MD
Infection Control. . . . . Jeffrey A Jahre, MD
Operating Room. . . . . Patricia A Krenn, RN
Quality Assurance . . . . Janice Rader
Pediatric Ambulatory Care . . . . . . Stanley Stein, MD
Pediatric In-Patient Care . . . . Stanley Stein, MD
Radiology. . . . . G Edward Streubert, MD

Measure	Cases	This Hosp.	State Avg.	U.S. Avg.
Blood Clot Prevention and Treatment				
Anticoagulation Overlap Therapy[2]	141	98%	94%	93%
ICU Venous Thromboembolism Prophylaxis[2]	123	98%	94%	92%
Incidence of Potentially Preventable VTE[2]	33	0%	8%	10%
UFH with Dosages/Platelet Monitoring[2]	98	99%	98%	97%
Venous Thromboembolism Prophylaxis[2]	521	95%	90%	85%
Warfarin Therapy Discharge Instructions[2]	104	81%	78%	75%
Chest Pain/Possible Heart Attack Care				
Aspirin Given Within 24 Hours of Arrival[5]	-	-	97%	96%
Fibrinolytic Meds Within 30 Min. of Arrival[5]	-	-	44%	58%
Average Time to ECG (minutes)[5]	-	-	9	7
Average Time to Transfer (minutes)[5]	-	-	64	60
Children's Asthma Care				
Received Home Management Plan of Care	-	-	-	88%
Received Reliever Medication	-	-	-	100%
Received Systemic Corticosteroids	-	-	-	100%
Emergency Department				
Admittance Decision Time (minutes)[2]	982	101	104	98
Head CT Results Within 45 Min. of Arrival[1]	-	-	60%	57%
Patients Who Left ER Before Being Seen	>100k	1%	1%	2%
Time from ER Arrival to Admit. (minutes)[2]	1,003	262	276	274
Time from ER Arrival to Discharge (minutes)	718	128	125	134
Time in ER Before Being Evaluated (minutes)	755	37	26	26
Time to Pain Meds for Fractures (minutes)	137	61	58	57
Heart Attack Care				
Aspirin Given at Discharge	354	100%	99%	99%
Fibrinolytic Meds Within 30 Min. of Arrival[7]	-	-	40%	54%
PCI Within 90 Minutes of Arrival	56	100%	97%	96%
Statin Prescribed at Discharge	351	100%	99%	98%
Heart Failure Care				
ACE Inhibitor or ARB for LVSD	125	99%	97%	97%
Discharge Instructions Given	437	98%	96%	94%
Evaluation of LVS Function	568	100%	100%	99%
Medicare Spending				
Medicare Spending per Patient (ratio)	-	1.00	1.01	0.98

NOTE: Hospital profiles are in alphabetical order by state, then city, then hospital within the city; Rankings exclude hospitals with less than 25 cases except for patient surveys which excludes hospitals with less than 100 cases; (a) 100-299 cases; (1) The number of cases/patients is too few to report; (2) Data submitted were based on a sample of cases/patients; (3) Results are based on a shorter time period than required; (4) Data suppressed by CMS for one or more quarters; (5) Results are not available for this reporting period; (6) Fewer than 100 patients completed the HCAHPS survey; (7) No cases met the criteria for this measure; (8) The lower limit of the confidence interval cannot be calculated if the number of observed infections equals zero; (9) No data are available from the state/territory for this reporting period; (10) The scores shown reflect fewer than 50 completed surveys; (11) There were discrepancies in the data collection process; (12) This measure does not apply to this hospital for this reporting period; (13) Results cannot be calculated for this reporting period; (14) The results for this state are combined with nearby states to protect confidentiality; Please refer to the User's Guide for a full explanation of data.

Measure	Cases	This Hosp.	State Avg.	U.S. Avg.
Pneumonia Care				
Appropriate Initial Antibiotic Given	236	96%	96%	95%
Blood Culture Timing	422	100%	98%	98%
Pregnancy and Delivery Care				
Newborn Deliveries Scheduled Early	221	0%	4%	6%
Preventive Care				
Immunization for Influenza[2]	1,074	94%	91%	90%
Immunization for Pneumonia[2]	1,373	93%	92%	92%
Stroke Care				
Anticoagulation Therapy for Atrial Fibrillation	50	100%	96%	95%
Antithrombotic Therapy Timing	208	99%	98%	98%
Assessed for Rehabilitation	251	99%	98%	97%
Discharged on Antithrombotic Therapy	210	100%	99%	99%
Discharged on Statin Medication	173	99%	95%	94%
Thrombolytic Therapy Timing	22	95%	72%	66%
Venous Thromboembolism Prophylaxis	282	98%	95%	94%
Written Stroke Educational Materials Given	120	96%	90%	88%
Surgical Care Improvement Project				
Appropriate Beta Blocker Usage[2]	569	100%	98%	98%
Appropriate VTP Within 24 Hours[2]	1,068	99%	99%	98%
Controlled Postoperative Blood Glucose[2]	254	99%	98%	97%
Perioperative Temperature Management[2]	1,295	100%	100%	100%
Prophylactic Antibiotic Selection[2]	1,182	100%	99%	99%
Prophylactic Antibiotic Selection (Outpatient)	737	99%	98%	98%
Prophylactic Antibiotic Stopped[2]	1,150	99%	98%	98%
Prophylactic Antibiotic Timing[2]	1,184	100%	99%	99%
Prophylactic Antibiotic Timing (Outpatient)	710	99%	98%	98%
Urinary Catheter Removal[2]	1,110	100%	99%	97%
Survey of Patients' Hospital Experiences				
Area Around Room 'Always' Quiet at Night	300+	50%	54%	61%
Doctors 'Always' Communicated Well	300+	76%	80%	82%
Home Recovery Information Given	300+	85%	86%	85%
Hospital Given 9 or 10 on 10 Point Scale	300+	72%	69%	71%
Meds 'Always' Explained Before Given	300+	61%	63%	64%
Nurses 'Always' Communicated Well	300+	76%	79%	79%
Pain 'Always' Well Controlled	300+	71%	70%	71%
Room and Bathroom 'Always' Clean	300+	71%	73%	73%
Timely Help 'Always' Received	300+	65%	67%	68%
Would Definitely Recommend Hospital	300+	73%	70%	71%
Use of Medical Imaging				
Cardiac Imaging Stress Test before Surgery	952	5.3%	5.4%	5.3%
Combination Abdominal CT Scan	2,232	4.9%	12.2%	10.5%
Combination Brain/Sinus CT Scan	1,511	2.5%	3.1%	2.7%
Combination Chest CT Scan	2,063	1.4%	2.1%	2.7%
Follow-up Mammogram/Ultrasound	4,386	11.5%	9%	8.8%
Lumbar Spine MRI for Low Back Pain	292	38.4%	35.8%	37.2%

Geisinger - Bloomsburg Hospital

549 East Fair Street
Bloomsburg, PA 17815
Phone: 570-387-2100
Fax: 570-387-2434
E-mail: tbhadmin@sunlink.net
URL: www.tbhonline.org
Type: Acute Care Hospitals
Emergency Services: Yes
Ownership: Voluntary non-profit - Private
Beds: 117

Key Personnel:
Chief of Medical Staff . . . . Paul A Saloky, DO
CEO/President. . . . . Glenn Steele, Jr. MD

Measure	Cases	This Hosp.	State Avg.	U.S. Avg.
Blood Clot Prevention and Treatment				
Anticoagulation Overlap Therapy[2]	13	85%	94%	93%
ICU Venous Thromboembolism Prophylaxis[2]	26	54%	94%	92%
Incidence of Potentially Preventable VTE[1,2]	-	-	8%	10%
UFH with Dosages/Platelet Monitoring[1,2]	-	-	98%	97%
Venous Thromboembolism Prophylaxis[2]	180	58%	90%	85%
Warfarin Therapy Discharge Instructions[2]	12	50%	78%	75%
Chest Pain/Possible Heart Attack Care				
Aspirin Given Within 24 Hours of Arrival	42	93%	97%	96%
Fibrinolytic Meds Within 30 Min. of Arrival[7]	-	-	44%	58%
Average Time to ECG (minutes)	43	8	9	7
Average Time to Transfer (minutes)	18	58	64	60
Children's Asthma Care				
Received Home Management Plan of Care	-	-	-	88%
Received Reliever Medication	-	-	-	100%
Received Systemic Corticosteroids	-	-	-	100%
Emergency Department				
Admittance Decision Time (minutes)[2]	801	40	104	98
Head CT Results Within 45 Min. of Arrival	12	25%	60%	57%
Patients Who Left ER Before Being Seen	13,018	3%	1%	2%
Time from ER Arrival to Admit. (minutes)[2]	821	197	276	274
Time from ER Arrival to Discharge (minutes)	337	124	125	134
Time in ER Before Being Evaluated (minutes)	368	36	26	26
Time to Pain Meds for Fractures (minutes)	81	68	58	57
Heart Attack Care				
Aspirin Given at Discharge[1,3]	-	-	99%	99%
Fibrinolytic Meds Within 30 Min. of Arrival[3,7]	-	-	40%	54%
PCI Within 90 Minutes of Arrival[3,7]	-	-	97%	96%
Statin Prescribed at Discharge[1,3]	-	-	99%	98%
Heart Failure Care				
ACE Inhibitor or ARB for LVSD	15	100%	97%	97%
Discharge Instructions Given	52	90%	96%	94%
Evaluation of LVS Function	70	90%	100%	99%
Medicare Spending				
Medicare Spending per Patient (ratio)	-	1.02	1.01	0.98
Pneumonia Care				
Appropriate Initial Antibiotic Given	73	92%	96%	95%
Blood Culture Timing	103	97%	98%	98%
Pregnancy and Delivery Care				
Newborn Deliveries Scheduled Early[2]	19	0%	4%	6%
Preventive Care				
Immunization for Influenza[2]	1,081	81%	91%	90%
Immunization for Pneumonia[2]	1,169	63%	92%	92%
Stroke Care				
Anticoagulation Therapy for Atrial Fibrillation[1,3]	-	-	96%	95%
Antithrombotic Therapy Timing[1,3]	-	-	98%	98%
Assessed for Rehabilitation[1,3]	-	-	98%	97%
Discharged on Antithrombotic Therapy[1,3]	-	-	99%	99%
Discharged on Statin Medication[1,3]	-	-	95%	94%
Thrombolytic Therapy Timing[1,3]	-	-	72%	66%
Venous Thromboembolism Prophylaxis[1,3]	-	-	95%	94%
Written Stroke Educational Materials Given[1,3]	-	-	90%	88%
Surgical Care Improvement Project				
Appropriate Beta Blocker Usage	58	91%	98%	98%
Appropriate VTP Within 24 Hours	186	97%	99%	98%
Controlled Postoperative Blood Glucose[7]	-	-	98%	97%
Perioperative Temperature Management	205	100%	100%	100%
Prophylactic Antibiotic Selection	157	98%	99%	99%
Prophylactic Antibiotic Selection (Outpatient)	19	95%	98%	98%
Prophylactic Antibiotic Stopped	155	99%	98%	98%
Prophylactic Antibiotic Timing	158	99%	99%	99%
Prophylactic Antibiotic Timing (Outpatient)	20	90%	98%	98%
Urinary Catheter Removal	103	97%	99%	97%
Survey of Patients' Hospital Experiences				
Area Around Room 'Always' Quiet at Night	300+	56%	54%	61%
Doctors 'Always' Communicated Well	300+	80%	80%	82%
Home Recovery Information Given	300+	85%	86%	85%
Hospital Given 9 or 10 on 10 Point Scale	300+	65%	69%	71%
Meds 'Always' Explained Before Given	300+	59%	63%	64%
Nurses 'Always' Communicated Well	300+	82%	79%	79%
Pain 'Always' Well Controlled	300+	71%	70%	71%
Room and Bathroom 'Always' Clean	300+	72%	73%	73%
Timely Help 'Always' Received	300+	77%	67%	68%
Would Definitely Recommend Hospital	300+	68%	70%	71%
Use of Medical Imaging				
Cardiac Imaging Stress Test before Surgery[1]	-	-	5.4%	5.3%
Combination Abdominal CT Scan	239	18.4%	12.2%	10.5%
Combination Brain/Sinus CT Scan	251	7.6%	3.1%	2.7%
Combination Chest CT Scan	50	42.0%	2.1%	2.7%
Follow-up Mammogram/Ultrasound	418	8.9%	9%	8.8%
Lumbar Spine MRI for Low Back Pain[1]	-	-	35.8%	37.2%

Bradford Regional Medical Center

116 Interstate Parkway
Bradford, PA 16701
Phone: 814-368-4143
Fax: 814-368-5722
E-mail: webdirector@brmc.org
URL: www.bfdmed.org
Type: Acute Care Hospitals
Emergency Services: Yes
Ownership: Voluntary non-profit - Private
Beds: 127

Key Personnel:
CEO/President. . . . . Timothy J. Finan
Operating Room. . . . . Luis C Gonzalez, MD
Quality Assurance . . . . Gayle Gronemeir, RN
Radiology. . . . . G Michael Maresca, MD
Infection Control. . . . . Teri O'Brien, RN
Pediatric Ambulatory Care . . . . . . Anil Pradhan, MD
Pediatric In-Patient Care . . . . Anil Pradhan, MD
Chief of Medical Staff . . . . Peter Vaccaro, MD

Measure	Cases	This Hosp.	State Avg.	U.S. Avg.
Blood Clot Prevention and Treatment				
Anticoagulation Overlap Therapy[2]	20	80%	94%	93%
ICU Venous Thromboembolism Prophylaxis[2]	26	92%	94%	92%
Incidence of Potentially Preventable VTE[2,7]	-	-	8%	10%
UFH with Dosages/Platelet Monitoring[1,2]	-	-	98%	97%
Venous Thromboembolism Prophylaxis[2]	241	96%	90%	85%
Warfarin Therapy Discharge Instructions[2]	17	88%	78%	75%
Chest Pain/Possible Heart Attack Care				
Aspirin Given Within 24 Hours of Arrival	68	100%	97%	96%
Fibrinolytic Meds Within 30 Min. of Arrival[1]	-	-	44%	58%
Average Time to ECG (minutes)	67	6	9	7
Average Time to Transfer (minutes)[1]	-	-	64	60
Children's Asthma Care				
Received Home Management Plan of Care	-	-	-	88%
Received Reliever Medication	-	-	-	100%
Received Systemic Corticosteroids	-	-	-	100%
Emergency Department				
Admittance Decision Time (minutes)[2]	350	66	104	98
Head CT Results Within 45 Min. of Arrival	11	45%	60%	57%
Patients Who Left ER Before Being Seen	21,177	0%	1%	2%
Time from ER Arrival to Admit. (minutes)[2]	350	248	276	274
Time from ER Arrival to Discharge (minutes)	608	113	125	134
Time in ER Before Being Evaluated (minutes)	648	29	26	26
Time to Pain Meds for Fractures (minutes)	52	66	58	57
Heart Attack Care				
Aspirin Given at Discharge	17	94%	99%	99%
Fibrinolytic Meds Within 30 Min. of Arrival[7]	-	-	40%	54%
PCI Within 90 Minutes of Arrival[7]	-	-	97%	96%
Statin Prescribed at Discharge	17	71%	99%	98%
Heart Failure Care				
ACE Inhibitor or ARB for LVSD	21	100%	97%	97%
Discharge Instructions Given	49	100%	96%	94%
Evaluation of LVS Function	63	98%	100%	99%
Medicare Spending				
Medicare Spending per Patient (ratio)	-	0.94	1.01	0.98
Pneumonia Care				
Appropriate Initial Antibiotic Given	97	88%	96%	95%
Blood Culture Timing	148	99%	98%	98%
Pregnancy and Delivery Care				
Newborn Deliveries Scheduled Early[2]	26	0%	4%	6%
Preventive Care				
Immunization for Influenza[2]	308	87%	91%	90%
Immunization for Pneumonia[2]	363	87%	92%	92%
Stroke Care				
Anticoagulation Therapy for Atrial Fibrillation[1]	-	-	96%	95%
Antithrombotic Therapy Timing[1]	-	-	98%	98%
Assessed for Rehabilitation[1]	-	-	98%	97%
Discharged on Antithrombotic Therapy[1]	-	-	99%	99%
Discharged on Statin Medication[1]	-	-	95%	94%
Thrombolytic Therapy Timing[7]	-	-	72%	66%
Venous Thromboembolism Prophylaxis[1]	-	-	95%	94%
Written Stroke Educational Materials Given[7]	-	-	90%	88%
Surgical Care Improvement Project				
Appropriate Beta Blocker Usage	39	79%	98%	98%
Appropriate VTP Within 24 Hours	149	97%	99%	98%
Controlled Postoperative Blood Glucose[7]	-	-	98%	97%
Perioperative Temperature Management	159	100%	100%	100%

NOTE: Hospital profiles are in alphabetical order by state, then city, then hospital within the city; Rankings exclude hospitals with less than 25 cases except for patient surveys which excludes hospitals with less than 100 cases; (a) 100-299 cases; (1) The number of cases/patients is too few to report; (2) Data submitted were based on a sample of cases/patients; (3) Results are based on a shorter time period than required; (4) Data suppressed by CMS for one or more quarters; (5) Results are not available for this reporting period; (6) Fewer than 100 patients completed the HCAHPS survey; (7) No cases met the criteria for this measure; (8) The lower limit of the confidence interval cannot be calculated if the number of observed infections equals zero; (9) No data are available from the state/territory for this reporting period; (10) The scores shown reflect fewer than 50 completed surveys; (11) There were discrepancies in the data collection process; (12) This measure does not apply to this hospital for this reporting period; (13) Results cannot be calculated for this reporting period; (14) The results for this state are combined with nearby states to protect confidentiality; Please refer to the User's Guide for a full explanation of data.

Measure	Cases	This Hosp.	State Avg.	U.S. Avg.
Prophylactic Antibiotic Selection	115	98%	99%	99%
Prophylactic Antibiotic Selection (Outpatient)	23	83%	98%	98%
Prophylactic Antibiotic Stopped	114	97%	98%	98%
Prophylactic Antibiotic Timing	115	96%	99%	99%
Prophylactic Antibiotic Timing (Outpatient)	23	96%	98%	98%
Urinary Catheter Removal	24	79%	99%	97%
Survey of Patients' Hospital Experiences				
Area Around Room 'Always' Quiet at Night	300+	43%	54%	61%
Doctors 'Always' Communicated Well	300+	79%	80%	82%
Home Recovery Information Given	300+	82%	86%	85%
Hospital Given 9 or 10 on 10 Point Scale	300+	62%	69%	71%
Meds 'Always' Explained Before Given	300+	59%	63%	64%
Nurses 'Always' Communicated Well	300+	78%	79%	79%
Pain 'Always' Well Controlled	300+	70%	70%	71%
Room and Bathroom 'Always' Clean	300+	70%	73%	73%
Timely Help 'Always' Received	300+	69%	67%	68%
Would Definitely Recommend Hospital	300+	54%	70%	71%
Use of Medical Imaging				
Cardiac Imaging Stress Test before Surgery	201	4.0%	5.4%	5.3%
Combination Abdominal CT Scan	437	18.3%	12.2%	10.5%
Combination Brain/Sinus CT Scan	397	5.5%	3.1%	2.7%
Combination Chest CT Scan	218	25.2%	2.1%	2.7%
Follow-up Mammogram/Ultrasound	819	9.2%	9%	8.8%
Lumbar Spine MRI for Low Back Pain	74	43.2%	35.8%	37.2%

Lower Bucks Hospital

501 Bath Road
Bristol, PA 19007
Phone: 215-785-9200
Fax: 215-785-9172
E-mail: lowerbuckshospital@lowerbuckshospital.org
URL: www.lowerbuckshospital.org
Type: Acute Care Hospitals
Emergency Services: Yes
Ownership: Proprietary
Beds: 150

Key Personnel:

CEO . . . . Peter Adamo
CEO/President. . . . . Nathan Bosk
Chief of Medical Staff. . . . . Bruce Dershaw, MD
Quality Assurance . . . . Carol Evans
Pediatric In-Patient Care . . . . Gerry Green, DO
Radiology. . . . . Frederick Kraus, MD
Emergency Room . . . . Jennie Lutz, RN
Chairman/CEO . . . . Dr Prem Reddy, MD,FACC, FCCP

Measure	Cases	This Hosp.	State Avg.	U.S. Avg.
Blood Clot Prevention and Treatment				
Anticoagulation Overlap Therapy[2]	21	86%	94%	93%
ICU Venous Thromboembolism Prophylaxis[2]	109	82%	94%	92%
Incidence of Potentially Preventable VTE[1,2]	-	-	8%	10%
UFH with Dosages/Platelet Monitoring[2]	28	100%	98%	97%
Venous Thromboembolism Prophylaxis[2]	301	71%	90%	85%
Warfarin Therapy Discharge Instructions[2]	17	35%	78%	75%
Chest Pain/Possible Heart Attack Care				
Aspirin Given Within 24 Hours of Arrival[3,7]	-	-	97%	96%
Fibrinolytic Meds Within 30 Min. of Arrival[5]	-	-	44%	58%
Average Time to ECG (minutes)[3,7]	-	-	9	7
Average Time to Transfer (minutes)[5]	-	-	64	60
Children's Asthma Care				
Received Home Management Plan of Care	-	-	-	88%
Received Reliever Medication	-	-	-	100%
Received Systemic Corticosteroids	-	-	-	100%
Emergency Department				
Admittance Decision Time (minutes)[2]	791	104	104	98
Head CT Results Within 45 Min. of Arrival[1]	-	-	60%	57%
Patients Who Left ER Before Being Seen	29,978	1%	1%	2%
Time from ER Arrival to Admit. (minutes)[2]	796	273	276	274
Time from ER Arrival to Discharge (minutes)	354	96	125	134
Time in ER Before Being Evaluated (minutes)	402	29	26	26
Time to Pain Meds for Fractures (minutes)	43	63	58	57
Heart Attack Care				
Aspirin Given at Discharge	73	95%	99%	99%
Fibrinolytic Meds Within 30 Min. of Arrival[7]	-	-	40%	54%
PCI Within 90 Minutes of Arrival	14	64%	97%	96%
Statin Prescribed at Discharge	70	94%	99%	98%
Heart Failure Care				
ACE Inhibitor or ARB for LVSD	60	92%	97%	97%
Discharge Instructions Given	146	84%	96%	94%
Evaluation of LVS Function	166	100%	100%	99%
Medicare Spending				
Medicare Spending per Patient (ratio)	-	1.10	1.01	0.98
Pneumonia Care				
Appropriate Initial Antibiotic Given	53	94%	96%	95%
Blood Culture Timing	80	98%	98%	98%
Pregnancy and Delivery Care				
Newborn Deliveries Scheduled Early[7]	-	-	4%	6%
Preventive Care				
Immunization for Influenza[2]	441	93%	91%	90%
Immunization for Pneumonia[2]	529	96%	92%	92%
Stroke Care				
Anticoagulation Therapy for Atrial Fibrillation[1]	-	-	96%	95%
Antithrombotic Therapy Timing	42	98%	98%	98%
Assessed for Rehabilitation	40	90%	98%	97%
Discharged on Antithrombotic Therapy	39	97%	99%	99%
Discharged on Statin Medication	33	85%	95%	94%
Thrombolytic Therapy Timing[1]	-	-	72%	66%
Venous Thromboembolism Prophylaxis	45	67%	95%	94%
Written Stroke Educational Materials Given	26	31%	90%	88%
Surgical Care Improvement Project				
Appropriate Beta Blocker Usage	26	100%	98%	98%
Appropriate VTP Within 24 Hours	65	97%	99%	98%
Controlled Postoperative Blood Glucose[1]	-	-	98%	97%
Perioperative Temperature Management	78	100%	100%	100%
Prophylactic Antibiotic Selection	45	98%	99%	99%
Prophylactic Antibiotic Selection (Outpatient)	24	100%	98%	98%
Prophylactic Antibiotic Stopped	45	100%	98%	98%
Prophylactic Antibiotic Timing	45	98%	99%	99%
Prophylactic Antibiotic Timing (Outpatient)	23	100%	98%	98%
Urinary Catheter Removal	57	98%	99%	97%
Survey of Patients' Hospital Experiences				
Area Around Room 'Always' Quiet at Night	(a)	46%	54%	61%
Doctors 'Always' Communicated Well	(a)	64%	80%	82%
Home Recovery Information Given	(a)	80%	86%	85%
Hospital Given 9 or 10 on 10 Point Scale	(a)	54%	69%	71%
Meds 'Always' Explained Before Given	(a)	50%	63%	64%
Nurses 'Always' Communicated Well	(a)	69%	79%	79%
Pain 'Always' Well Controlled	(a)	63%	70%	71%
Room and Bathroom 'Always' Clean	(a)	68%	73%	73%
Timely Help 'Always' Received	(a)	57%	67%	68%
Would Definitely Recommend Hospital	(a)	57%	70%	71%
Use of Medical Imaging				
Cardiac Imaging Stress Test before Surgery[1]	-	-	5.4%	5.3%
Combination Abdominal CT Scan	296	6.1%	12.2%	10.5%
Combination Brain/Sinus CT Scan[1]	-	-	3.1%	2.7%
Combination Chest CT Scan	199	0.0%	2.1%	2.7%
Follow-up Mammogram/Ultrasound	657	9.4%	9%	8.8%
Lumbar Spine MRI for Low Back Pain	59	33.9%	35.8%	37.2%

Penn Highlands Brookville

100 Hospital Road
Brookville, PA 15825
Phone: 814-849-2312
Fax: 814-849-4841
URL: www.brookvillehospital.org
Type: Critical Access Hospitals
Emergency Services: Yes
Ownership: Voluntary non-profit - Private
Beds: 63

Key Personnel:

Infection Control. . . . . Patricia Abell, RN
Intensive Care Unit. . . . . David Buchanan, RN
Operating Room. . . . . Richard Bucheit, RN
Quality Assurance . . . . Tere Byerly
Emergency Room . . . . Paul E Harvey, MD
Chief of Medical Staff. . . . . Joseph Prusakowski, DO
CEO/President. . . . . John Sutika
Anesthesiology. . . . . Emerson Turnbull, CRNA

Measure	Cases	This Hosp.	State Avg.	U.S. Avg.
Blood Clot Prevention and Treatment				
Anticoagulation Overlap Therapy[5]	-	-	94%	93%
ICU Venous Thromboembolism Prophylaxis[5]	-	-	94%	92%
Incidence of Potentially Preventable VTE[5]	-	-	8%	10%
UFH with Dosages/Platelet Monitoring[5]	-	-	98%	97%
Venous Thromboembolism Prophylaxis[5]	-	-	90%	85%
Warfarin Therapy Discharge Instructions[5]	-	-	78%	75%
Chest Pain/Possible Heart Attack Care				
Aspirin Given Within 24 Hours of Arrival	72	96%	97%	96%
Fibrinolytic Meds Within 30 Min. of Arrival[1]	-	-	44%	58%
Average Time to ECG (minutes)	71	5	9	7
Average Time to Transfer (minutes)[1]	-	-	64	60
Children's Asthma Care				
Received Home Management Plan of Care	-	-	-	88%
Received Reliever Medication	-	-	-	100%
Received Systemic Corticosteroids	-	-	-	100%
Emergency Department				
Admittance Decision Time (minutes)[5]	-	-	104	98
Head CT Results Within 45 Min. of Arrival[5]	-	-	60%	57%
Patients Who Left ER Before Being Seen	9,622	0%	1%	2%
Time from ER Arrival to Admit. (minutes)[5]	-	-	276	274
Time from ER Arrival to Discharge (minutes)[5]	-	-	125	134
Time in ER Before Being Evaluated (minutes)[5]	-	-	26	26
Time to Pain Meds for Fractures (minutes)[5]	-	-	58	57
Heart Attack Care				
Aspirin Given at Discharge[1]	-	-	99%	99%
Fibrinolytic Meds Within 30 Min. of Arrival[7]	-	-	40%	54%
PCI Within 90 Minutes of Arrival[7]	-	-	97%	96%
Statin Prescribed at Discharge[1]	-	-	99%	98%
Heart Failure Care				
ACE Inhibitor or ARB for LVSD[1]	-	-	97%	97%
Discharge Instructions Given[1]	-	-	96%	94%
Evaluation of LVS Function	12	100%	100%	99%
Medicare Spending				
Medicare Spending per Patient (ratio)	-	-	1.01	0.98
Pneumonia Care				
Appropriate Initial Antibiotic Given	25	84%	96%	95%
Blood Culture Timing	38	100%	98%	98%
Pregnancy and Delivery Care				
Newborn Deliveries Scheduled Early[3,7]	-	-	4%	6%
Preventive Care				
Immunization for Influenza[5]	-	-	91%	90%
Immunization for Pneumonia[5]	-	-	92%	92%
Stroke Care				
Anticoagulation Therapy for Atrial Fibrillation[5]	-	-	96%	95%
Antithrombotic Therapy Timing[5]	-	-	98%	98%
Assessed for Rehabilitation[5]	-	-	98%	97%
Discharged on Antithrombotic Therapy[5]	-	-	99%	99%
Discharged on Statin Medication[5]	-	-	95%	94%
Thrombolytic Therapy Timing[5]	-	-	72%	66%
Venous Thromboembolism Prophylaxis[5]	-	-	95%	94%
Written Stroke Educational Materials Given[5]	-	-	90%	88%
Surgical Care Improvement Project				
Appropriate Beta Blocker Usage[1]	-	-	98%	98%
Appropriate VTP Within 24 Hours	13	100%	99%	98%
Controlled Postoperative Blood Glucose[7]	-	-	98%	97%
Perioperative Temperature Management	13	100%	100%	100%
Prophylactic Antibiotic Selection[1]	-	-	99%	99%
Prophylactic Antibiotic Selection (Outpatient)	27	78%	98%	98%
Prophylactic Antibiotic Stopped[1]	-	-	98%	98%
Prophylactic Antibiotic Timing[1]	-	-	99%	99%
Prophylactic Antibiotic Timing (Outpatient)	20	35%	98%	98%
Urinary Catheter Removal[1]	-	-	99%	97%
Survey of Patients' Hospital Experiences				
Area Around Room 'Always' Quiet at Night[5]	-	-	54%	61%
Doctors 'Always' Communicated Well[5]	-	-	80%	82%
Home Recovery Information Given[5]	-	-	86%	85%
Hospital Given 9 or 10 on 10 Point Scale[5]	-	-	69%	71%
Meds 'Always' Explained Before Given[5]	-	-	63%	64%
Nurses 'Always' Communicated Well[5]	-	-	79%	79%
Pain 'Always' Well Controlled[5]	-	-	70%	71%
Room and Bathroom 'Always' Clean[5]	-	-	73%	73%
Timely Help 'Always' Received[5]	-	-	67%	68%
Would Definitely Recommend Hospital[5]	-	-	70%	71%
Use of Medical Imaging				
Cardiac Imaging Stress Test before Surgery	109	1.8%	5.4%	5.3%
Combination Abdominal CT Scan	421	20.4%	12.2%	10.5%
Combination Brain/Sinus CT Scan[1]	-	-	3.1%	2.7%
Combination Chest CT Scan	150	15.3%	2.1%	2.7%
Follow-up Mammogram/Ultrasound	277	3.6%	9%	8.8%

NOTE: Hospital profiles are in alphabetical order by state, then city, then hospital within the city; Rankings exclude hospitals with less than 25 cases except for patient surveys which excludes hospitals with less than 100 cases; (a) 100-299 cases; (1) The number of cases/patients is too few to report; (2) Data submitted were based on a sample of cases/patients; (3) Results are based on a shorter time period than required; (4) Data suppressed by CMS for one or more quarters; (5) Results are not available for this reporting period; (6) Fewer than 100 patients completed the HCAHPS survey; (7) No cases met the criteria for this measure; (8) The lower limit of the confidence interval cannot be calculated if the number of observed infections equals zero; (9) No data are available from the state/territory for this reporting period; (10) The scores shown reflect fewer than 50 completed surveys; (11) There were discrepancies in the data collection process; (12) This measure does not apply to this hospital for this reporting period; (13) Results cannot be calculated for this reporting period; (14) The results for this state are combined with nearby states to protect confidentiality; Please refer to the User's Guide for a full explanation of data.

Lumbar Spine MRI for Low Back Pain[1]	-	-	35.8%	37.2%

Main Line Hospital Bryn Mawr Campus

130 South Bryn Mawr Ave
Bryn Mawr, PA 19010
Phone: 610-526-3000
Fax: 610-526-3068
URL: www.mainlinehealth.org
Type: Acute Care Hospitals
Emergency Services: Yes
Ownership: Voluntary non-profit - Private
Beds: 307

Key Personnel:
CEO/President.............. Andrea Gilbert
Infection Control............. Patti McBride, RN
Chief of Medical Staff.......... James L McCabe, Jr, MD
Quality Assurance .... Lee Patrick
Radiology.................. Emma L Simpson, MD
Pediatric In-Patient Care .... Robert L Stavis, MD

Measure	Cases	This Hosp.	State Avg.	U.S. Avg.
Blood Clot Prevention and Treatment				
Anticoagulation Overlap Therapy[2]	98	84%	94%	93%
ICU Venous Thromboembolism Prophylaxis[2]	68	94%	94%	92%
Incidence of Potentially Preventable VTE[2]	23	22%	8%	10%
UFH with Dosages/Platelet Monitoring[2]	35	97%	98%	97%
Venous Thromboembolism Prophylaxis[2]	272	95%	90%	85%
Warfarin Therapy Discharge Instructions[2]	57	33%	78%	75%
Chest Pain/Possible Heart Attack Care				
Aspirin Given Within 24 Hours of Arrival[1,3]	-	-	97%	96%
Fibrinolytic Meds Within 30 Min. of Arrival[5]	-	-	44%	58%
Average Time to ECG (minutes)[1,3]	-	-	9	7
Average Time to Transfer (minutes)[5]	-	-	64	60
Children's Asthma Care				
Received Home Management Plan of Care	-	-	-	88%
Received Reliever Medication	-	-	-	100%
Received Systemic Corticosteroids	-	-	-	100%
Emergency Department				
Admittance Decision Time (minutes)[2]	556	214	104	98
Head CT Results Within 45 Min. of Arrival[1]	-	-	60%	57%
Patients Who Left ER Before Being Seen	47,825	0%	1%	2%
Time from ER Arrival to Admit. (minutes)[2]	560	377	276	274
Time from ER Arrival to Discharge (minutes)	362	157	125	134
Time in ER Before Being Evaluated (minutes)	375	27	26	26
Time to Pain Meds for Fractures (minutes)	252	58	58	57
Heart Attack Care				
Aspirin Given at Discharge	208	100%	99%	99%
Fibrinolytic Meds Within 30 Min. of Arrival[7]	-	-	40%	54%
PCI Within 90 Minutes of Arrival	33	100%	97%	96%
Statin Prescribed at Discharge	209	100%	99%	98%
Heart Failure Care				
ACE Inhibitor or ARB for LVSD	81	100%	97%	97%
Discharge Instructions Given	262	97%	96%	94%
Evaluation of LVS Function	374	100%	100%	99%
Medicare Spending				
Medicare Spending per Patient (ratio)	-	1.05	1.01	0.98
Pneumonia Care				
Appropriate Initial Antibiotic Given	112	97%	96%	95%
Blood Culture Timing	250	100%	98%	98%
Pregnancy and Delivery Care				
Newborn Deliveries Scheduled Early[2]	21	0%	4%	6%
Preventive Care				
Immunization for Influenza[2]	546	84%	91%	90%
Immunization for Pneumonia[2]	704	83%	92%	92%
Stroke Care				
Anticoagulation Therapy for Atrial Fibrillation	28	100%	96%	95%
Antithrombotic Therapy Timing	154	100%	98%	98%
Assessed for Rehabilitation	192	99%	98%	97%
Discharged on Antithrombotic Therapy	169	100%	99%	99%
Discharged on Statin Medication	143	100%	95%	94%
Thrombolytic Therapy Timing	15	87%	72%	66%
Venous Thromboembolism Prophylaxis	194	96%	95%	94%
Written Stroke Educational Materials Given	86	98%	90%	88%
Surgical Care Improvement Project				
Appropriate Beta Blocker Usage[2]	424	100%	98%	98%
Appropriate VTP Within 24 Hours[2]	1,262	99%	99%	98%
Controlled Postoperative Blood Glucose[2]	70	96%	98%	97%
Perioperative Temperature Management[2]	1,470	100%	100%	100%
Prophylactic Antibiotic Selection[2]	1,321	100%	99%	99%
Prophylactic Antibiotic Selection (Outpatient)	268	93%	98%	98%
Prophylactic Antibiotic Stopped[2]	1,308	100%	98%	98%
Prophylactic Antibiotic Timing[2]	1,323	100%	99%	99%
Prophylactic Antibiotic Timing (Outpatient)	269	98%	98%	98%
Urinary Catheter Removal[2]	186	99%	99%	97%
Survey of Patients' Hospital Experiences				
Area Around Room 'Always' Quiet at Night	300+	52%	54%	61%
Doctors 'Always' Communicated Well	300+	78%	80%	82%
Home Recovery Information Given	300+	85%	86%	85%
Hospital Given 9 or 10 on 10 Point Scale	300+	77%	69%	71%
Meds 'Always' Explained Before Given	300+	63%	63%	64%
Nurses 'Always' Communicated Well	300+	83%	79%	79%
Pain 'Always' Well Controlled	300+	72%	70%	71%
Room and Bathroom 'Always' Clean	300+	70%	73%	73%
Timely Help 'Always' Received	300+	68%	67%	68%
Would Definitely Recommend Hospital	300+	82%	70%	71%
Use of Medical Imaging				
Cardiac Imaging Stress Test before Surgery	193	7.3%	5.4%	5.3%
Combination Abdominal CT Scan	1,026	13.7%	12.2%	10.5%
Combination Brain/Sinus CT Scan	1,129	0.7%	3.1%	2.7%
Combination Chest CT Scan	1,144	3.4%	2.1%	2.7%
Follow-up Mammogram/Ultrasound	2,123	12.2%	9%	8.8%
Lumbar Spine MRI for Low Back Pain[1]	-	-	35.8%	37.2%

Butler Memorial Hospital

One Hospital Way
Butler, PA 16001
Phone: 724-283-6666
Fax: 724-477-3607
URL: www.butlerhealthsystem.org
Type: Acute Care Hospitals
Emergency Services: Yes
Ownership: Voluntary non-profit - Private
Beds: 268

Key Personnel:
Pediatric In-Patient Care .... William Ashbaugh
Radiology.................. James W Backstrom
Quality Assurance .... Mark Edwards
Chief of Medical Staff.......... A Thomas McGill, MD
Cardiac Laboratory............ Margie McLaughlin
Infection Control............. Sharon Stephens
CEO/President.............. Joseph Stewart

Measure	Cases	This Hosp.	State Avg.	U.S. Avg.
Blood Clot Prevention and Treatment				
Anticoagulation Overlap Therapy[2]	86	99%	94%	93%
ICU Venous Thromboembolism Prophylaxis[2]	181	96%	94%	92%
Incidence of Potentially Preventable VTE[1,2]	-	-	8%	10%
UFH with Dosages/Platelet Monitoring[2]	88	100%	98%	97%
Venous Thromboembolism Prophylaxis[2]	553	92%	90%	85%
Warfarin Therapy Discharge Instructions[2]	67	99%	78%	75%
Chest Pain/Possible Heart Attack Care				
Aspirin Given Within 24 Hours of Arrival	31	100%	97%	96%
Fibrinolytic Meds Within 30 Min. of Arrival[3,7]	-	-	44%	58%
Average Time to ECG (minutes)	31	7	9	7
Average Time to Transfer (minutes)[1,3]	-	-	64	60
Children's Asthma Care				
Received Home Management Plan of Care	-	-	-	88%
Received Reliever Medication	-	-	-	100%
Received Systemic Corticosteroids	-	-	-	100%
Emergency Department				
Admittance Decision Time (minutes)[2]	262	59	104	98
Head CT Results Within 45 Min. of Arrival	27	63%	60%	57%
Patients Who Left ER Before Being Seen	46,788	0%	1%	2%
Time from ER Arrival to Admit. (minutes)[2]	441	185	276	274
Time from ER Arrival to Discharge (minutes)	302	113	125	134
Time in ER Before Being Evaluated (minutes)	382	13	26	26
Time to Pain Meds for Fractures (minutes)	117	37	58	57
Heart Attack Care				
Aspirin Given at Discharge	302	100%	99%	99%
Fibrinolytic Meds Within 30 Min. of Arrival[7]	-	-	40%	54%
PCI Within 90 Minutes of Arrival	35	97%	97%	96%
Statin Prescribed at Discharge	280	99%	99%	98%
Heart Failure Care				
ACE Inhibitor or ARB for LVSD	98	100%	97%	97%
Discharge Instructions Given	202	98%	96%	94%
Evaluation of LVS Function	266	100%	100%	99%
Medicare Spending				
Medicare Spending per Patient (ratio)	-	1.03	1.01	0.98
Pneumonia Care				
Appropriate Initial Antibiotic Given	174	98%	96%	95%
Blood Culture Timing	235	97%	98%	98%
Pregnancy and Delivery Care				
Newborn Deliveries Scheduled Early[2]	87	9%	4%	6%
Preventive Care				
Immunization for Influenza[2]	550	99%	91%	90%
Immunization for Pneumonia[2]	702	98%	92%	92%
Stroke Care				
Anticoagulation Therapy for Atrial Fibrillation	23	100%	96%	95%
Antithrombotic Therapy Timing	132	100%	98%	98%
Assessed for Rehabilitation	141	100%	98%	97%
Discharged on Antithrombotic Therapy	133	99%	99%	99%
Discharged on Statin Medication	105	98%	95%	94%
Thrombolytic Therapy Timing[1]	-	-	72%	66%
Venous Thromboembolism Prophylaxis	149	98%	95%	94%
Written Stroke Educational Materials Given	77	99%	90%	88%
Surgical Care Improvement Project				
Appropriate Beta Blocker Usage	450	99%	98%	98%
Appropriate VTP Within 24 Hours	769	100%	99%	98%
Controlled Postoperative Blood Glucose	334	99%	98%	97%
Perioperative Temperature Management	918	100%	100%	100%
Prophylactic Antibiotic Selection	977	100%	99%	99%
Prophylactic Antibiotic Selection (Outpatient)	368	99%	98%	98%
Prophylactic Antibiotic Stopped	934	99%	98%	98%
Prophylactic Antibiotic Timing	977	99%	99%	99%
Prophylactic Antibiotic Timing (Outpatient)	369	99%	98%	98%
Urinary Catheter Removal	461	100%	99%	97%
Survey of Patients' Hospital Experiences				
Area Around Room 'Always' Quiet at Night	300+	50%	54%	61%
Doctors 'Always' Communicated Well	300+	80%	80%	82%
Home Recovery Information Given	300+	89%	86%	85%
Hospital Given 9 or 10 on 10 Point Scale	300+	69%	69%	71%
Meds 'Always' Explained Before Given	300+	62%	63%	64%
Nurses 'Always' Communicated Well	300+	79%	79%	79%
Pain 'Always' Well Controlled	300+	70%	70%	71%
Room and Bathroom 'Always' Clean	300+	65%	73%	73%
Timely Help 'Always' Received	300+	60%	67%	68%
Would Definitely Recommend Hospital	300+	72%	70%	71%
Use of Medical Imaging				
Cardiac Imaging Stress Test before Surgery	490	5.3%	5.4%	5.3%
Combination Abdominal CT Scan	770	11.4%	12.2%	10.5%
Combination Brain/Sinus CT Scan	699	1.3%	3.1%	2.7%
Combination Chest CT Scan	519	5.6%	2.1%	2.7%
Follow-up Mammogram/Ultrasound	1,061	12.6%	9%	8.8%
Lumbar Spine MRI for Low Back Pain	152	34.2%	35.8%	37.2%

Holy Spirit Hospital

503 North 21st Street
Camp Hill, PA 17011
Phone: 717-763-2100
Fax: 717-763-2183
E-mail: info@hsh.org
URL: www.hsh.org
Type: Acute Care Hospitals
Emergency Services: Yes
Ownership: Voluntary non-profit - Private
Beds: 332

Key Personnel:
Emergency Room .... Ramesh Arora, MD
Patient Relations .... Mary Buhrman
Quality Assurance .... Franchesca Charney, RN
Cardiac Laboratory............ Chirstine Erdman
Radiology.................. Ken Gable
CEO/President.............. Romaine Niemeyer, SCC
Chief of Medical Staff.......... Joseph Torchia, MD
Infection Control............. Joseph Torchia, MD

Measure	Cases	This Hosp.	State Avg.	U.S. Avg.
Blood Clot Prevention and Treatment				
Anticoagulation Overlap Therapy[2]	148	86%	94%	93%
ICU Venous Thromboembolism Prophylaxis[2]	68	96%	94%	92%
Incidence of Potentially Preventable VTE[2]	15	13%	8%	10%
UFH with Dosages/Platelet Monitoring[2]	42	100%	98%	97%
Venous Thromboembolism Prophylaxis[2]	363	82%	90%	85%
Warfarin Therapy Discharge Instructions[2]	122	65%	78%	75%
Chest Pain/Possible Heart Attack Care				
Aspirin Given Within 24 Hours of Arrival[1,3]	-	-	97%	96%
Fibrinolytic Meds Within 30 Min. of Arrival[3,7]	-	-	44%	58%

NOTE: Hospital profiles are in alphabetical order by state, then city, then hospital within the city; Rankings exclude hospitals with less than 25 cases except for patient surveys which excludes hospitals with less than 100 cases; (a) 100-299 cases; (1) The number of cases/patients is too few to report; (2) Data submitted were based on a sample of cases/patients; (3) Results are based on a shorter time period than required; (4) Data suppressed by CMS for one or more quarters; (5) Results are not available for this reporting period; (6) Fewer than 100 patients completed the HCAHPS survey; (7) No cases met the criteria for this measure; (8) The lower limit of the confidence interval cannot be calculated if the number of observed infections equals zero; (9) No data are available from the state/territory for this reporting period; (10) The scores shown reflect fewer than 50 completed surveys; (11) There were discrepancies in the data collection process; (12) This measure does not apply to this hospital for this reporting period; (13) Results cannot be calculated for this reporting period; (14) The results for this state are combined with nearby states to protect confidentiality; Please refer to the User's Guide for a full explanation of data.

Average Time to ECG (minutes)[1,3]	-	-	9	7
Average Time to Transfer (minutes)[3,7]	-	-	64	60
Children's Asthma Care				
Received Home Management Plan of Care	-	-	-	88%
Received Reliever Medication	-	-	-	100%
Received Systemic Corticosteroids	-	-	-	100%
Emergency Department				
Admittance Decision Time (minutes)[2]	417	148	104	98
Head CT Results Within 45 Min. of Arrival[1]	-	-	60%	57%
Patients Who Left ER Before Being Seen	53,674	1%	1%	2%
Time from ER Arrival to Admit. (minutes)[2]	523	399	276	274
Time from ER Arrival to Discharge (minutes)	341	180	125	134
Time in ER Before Being Evaluated (minutes)	397	44	26	26
Time to Pain Meds for Fractures (minutes)	213	70	58	57
Heart Attack Care				
Aspirin Given at Discharge	322	100%	99%	99%
Fibrinolytic Meds Within 30 Min. of Arrival[7]	-	-	40%	54%
PCI Within 90 Minutes of Arrival	67	97%	97%	96%
Statin Prescribed at Discharge	311	99%	99%	98%
Heart Failure Care				
ACE Inhibitor or ARB for LVSD	134	99%	97%	97%
Discharge Instructions Given	415	100%	96%	94%
Evaluation of LVS Function	558	100%	100%	99%
Medicare Spending				
Medicare Spending per Patient (ratio)	-	1.07	1.01	0.98
Pneumonia Care				
Appropriate Initial Antibiotic Given	420	99%	96%	95%
Blood Culture Timing	664	100%	98%	98%
Pregnancy and Delivery Care				
Newborn Deliveries Scheduled Early[2]	24	0%	4%	6%
Preventive Care				
Immunization for Influenza[2]	577	82%	91%	90%
Immunization for Pneumonia[2]	796	80%	92%	92%
Stroke Care				
Anticoagulation Therapy for Atrial Fibrillation	21	100%	96%	95%
Antithrombotic Therapy Timing	137	99%	98%	98%
Assessed for Rehabilitation	158	99%	98%	97%
Discharged on Antithrombotic Therapy	143	100%	99%	99%
Discharged on Statin Medication	112	95%	95%	94%
Thrombolytic Therapy Timing	14	93%	72%	66%
Venous Thromboembolism Prophylaxis	165	92%	95%	94%
Written Stroke Educational Materials Given	86	100%	90%	88%
Surgical Care Improvement Project				
Appropriate Beta Blocker Usage[2]	389	98%	98%	98%
Appropriate VTP Within 24 Hours[2]	726	100%	99%	98%
Controlled Postoperative Blood Glucose[2]	181	97%	98%	97%
Perioperative Temperature Management[2]	866	100%	100%	100%
Prophylactic Antibiotic Selection[2]	822	99%	99%	99%
Prophylactic Antibiotic Selection (Outpatient)	602	99%	98%	98%
Prophylactic Antibiotic Stopped[2]	786	99%	98%	98%
Prophylactic Antibiotic Timing[2]	822	100%	99%	99%
Prophylactic Antibiotic Timing (Outpatient)	602	100%	98%	98%
Urinary Catheter Removal[2]	495	98%	99%	97%
Survey of Patients' Hospital Experiences				
Area Around Room 'Always' Quiet at Night	300+	49%	54%	61%
Doctors 'Always' Communicated Well	300+	76%	80%	82%
Home Recovery Information Given	300+	86%	86%	85%
Hospital Given 9 or 10 on 10 Point Scale	300+	70%	69%	71%
Meds 'Always' Explained Before Given	300+	62%	63%	64%
Nurses 'Always' Communicated Well	300+	79%	79%	79%
Pain 'Always' Well Controlled	300+	69%	70%	71%
Room and Bathroom 'Always' Clean	300+	70%	73%	73%
Timely Help 'Always' Received	300+	62%	67%	68%
Would Definitely Recommend Hospital	300+	72%	70%	71%
Use of Medical Imaging				
Cardiac Imaging Stress Test before Surgery	776	5.0%	5.4%	5.3%
Combination Abdominal CT Scan	1,079	19.1%	12.2%	10.5%
Combination Brain/Sinus CT Scan	1,118	3.6%	3.1%	2.7%
Combination Chest CT Scan	613	0.5%	2.1%	2.7%
Follow-up Mammogram/Ultrasound	2,039	10.0%	9%	8.8%
Lumbar Spine MRI for Low Back Pain	163	30.1%	35.8%	37.2%

Canonsburg General Hospital

100 Medical Boulevard
Canonsburg, PA 15317
URL: www.wpahs.org/cgh
Type: Acute Care Hospitals
Ownership: Voluntary non-profit - Private
Phone: 724-873-5892
Fax: 724-873-5876
Emergency Services: Yes
Beds: 120

Key Personnel:
Chief of Medical Staff. . . . . Thomas Corkery, DO
Quality Assurance . . . . Kathy Hayes
Emergency Room . . . . Jan Mandik
CEO/President. . . . . Jane Sarra

Measure	Cases	This Hosp.	State Avg.	U.S. Avg.
Blood Clot Prevention and Treatment				
Anticoagulation Overlap Therapy[2]	14	93%	94%	93%
ICU Venous Thromboembolism Prophylaxis[2]	62	100%	94%	92%
Incidence of Potentially Preventable VTE[2,7]	-	-	8%	10%
UFH with Dosages/Platelet Monitoring[2]	18	100%	98%	97%
Venous Thromboembolism Prophylaxis[2]	308	98%	90%	85%
Warfarin Therapy Discharge Instructions[1,2]	-	-	78%	75%
Chest Pain/Possible Heart Attack Care				
Aspirin Given Within 24 Hours of Arrival	67	99%	97%	96%
Fibrinolytic Meds Within 30 Min. of Arrival[7]	-	-	44%	58%
Average Time to ECG (minutes)	68	6	9	7
Average Time to Transfer (minutes)	13	60	64	60
Children's Asthma Care				
Received Home Management Plan of Care	-	-	-	88%
Received Reliever Medication	-	-	-	100%
Received Systemic Corticosteroids	-	-	-	100%
Emergency Department				
Admittance Decision Time (minutes)[2]	450	70	104	98
Head CT Results Within 45 Min. of Arrival	17	29%	60%	57%
Patients Who Left ER Before Being Seen	21,014	1%	1%	2%
Time from ER Arrival to Admit. (minutes)[2]	456	254	276	274
Time from ER Arrival to Discharge (minutes)	453	131	125	134
Time in ER Before Being Evaluated (minutes)	494	18	26	26
Time to Pain Meds for Fractures (minutes)	43	45	58	57
Heart Attack Care				
Aspirin Given at Discharge[1]	-	-	99%	99%
Fibrinolytic Meds Within 30 Min. of Arrival[7]	-	-	40%	54%
PCI Within 90 Minutes of Arrival[7]	-	-	97%	96%
Statin Prescribed at Discharge[1]	-	-	99%	98%
Heart Failure Care				
ACE Inhibitor or ARB for LVSD	18	94%	97%	97%
Discharge Instructions Given	73	86%	96%	94%
Evaluation of LVS Function	98	100%	100%	99%
Medicare Spending				
Medicare Spending per Patient (ratio)	-	1.02	1.01	0.98
Pneumonia Care				
Appropriate Initial Antibiotic Given	61	93%	96%	95%
Blood Culture Timing	101	98%	98%	98%
Pregnancy and Delivery Care				
Newborn Deliveries Scheduled Early[7]	-	-	4%	6%
Preventive Care				
Immunization for Influenza[2]	351	96%	91%	90%
Immunization for Pneumonia[2]	541	93%	92%	92%
Stroke Care				
Anticoagulation Therapy for Atrial Fibrillation[1]	-	-	96%	95%
Antithrombotic Therapy Timing	17	94%	98%	98%
Assessed for Rehabilitation	17	100%	98%	97%
Discharged on Antithrombotic Therapy	15	100%	99%	99%
Discharged on Statin Medication	15	67%	95%	94%
Thrombolytic Therapy Timing[1]	-	-	72%	66%
Venous Thromboembolism Prophylaxis	18	78%	95%	94%
Written Stroke Educational Materials Given[1]	-	-	90%	88%
Surgical Care Improvement Project				
Appropriate Beta Blocker Usage	106	93%	98%	98%
Appropriate VTP Within 24 Hours	307	98%	99%	98%
Controlled Postoperative Blood Glucose[7]	-	-	98%	97%
Perioperative Temperature Management	335	99%	100%	100%
Prophylactic Antibiotic Selection	202	95%	99%	99%
Prophylactic Antibiotic Selection (Outpatient)	22	95%	98%	98%
Prophylactic Antibiotic Stopped	198	95%	98%	98%
Prophylactic Antibiotic Timing	202	95%	99%	99%
Prophylactic Antibiotic Timing (Outpatient)	22	100%	98%	98%
Urinary Catheter Removal	74	93%	99%	97%
Survey of Patients' Hospital Experiences				
Area Around Room 'Always' Quiet at Night	300+	52%	54%	61%
Doctors 'Always' Communicated Well	300+	84%	80%	82%
Home Recovery Information Given	300+	81%	86%	85%
Hospital Given 9 or 10 on 10 Point Scale	300+	69%	69%	71%
Meds 'Always' Explained Before Given	300+	64%	63%	64%
Nurses 'Always' Communicated Well	300+	79%	79%	79%
Pain 'Always' Well Controlled	300+	71%	70%	71%
Room and Bathroom 'Always' Clean	300+	72%	73%	73%
Timely Help 'Always' Received	300+	68%	67%	68%
Would Definitely Recommend Hospital	300+	73%	70%	71%
Use of Medical Imaging				
Cardiac Imaging Stress Test before Surgery	92	5.4%	5.4%	5.3%
Combination Abdominal CT Scan	229	51.1%	12.2%	10.5%
Combination Brain/Sinus CT Scan[1]	-	-	3.1%	2.7%
Combination Chest CT Scan	132	2.3%	2.1%	2.7%
Follow-up Mammogram/Ultrasound	191	6.3%	9%	8.8%
Lumbar Spine MRI for Low Back Pain[1]	-	-	35.8%	37.2%

Carlisle Regional Medical Center

361 Alexander Spring Road
Carlisle, PA 17015
E-mail: livelifewell@crmcpa.hma-corp.com
URL: www.carlislermc.com
Type: Acute Care Hospitals
Ownership: Proprietary
Phone: 717-249-1212
Fax: 717-960-3256
Emergency Services: Yes
Beds: 200

Key Personnel:
Chief of Medical Staff. . . . . Joseph T Acri
Operating Room. . . . . David Bryant
Radiology. . . . . Dennis M Burton
Quality Assurance . . . . Georgina Laughman
CEO . . . . Rich Newell
Pediatric In-Patient Care . . . . Deb Raubenstine

Measure	Cases	This Hosp.	State Avg.	U.S. Avg.
Blood Clot Prevention and Treatment				
Anticoagulation Overlap Therapy[2]	22	91%	94%	93%
ICU Venous Thromboembolism Prophylaxis[2]	40	98%	94%	92%
Incidence of Potentially Preventable VTE[1,2]	-	-	8%	10%
UFH with Dosages/Platelet Monitoring[1,2]	-	-	98%	97%
Venous Thromboembolism Prophylaxis[2]	305	94%	90%	85%
Warfarin Therapy Discharge Instructions[2]	14	71%	78%	75%
Chest Pain/Possible Heart Attack Care				
Aspirin Given Within 24 Hours of Arrival	63	98%	97%	96%
Fibrinolytic Meds Within 30 Min. of Arrival[7]	-	-	44%	58%
Average Time to ECG (minutes)	64	12	9	7
Average Time to Transfer (minutes)	17	78	64	60
Children's Asthma Care				
Received Home Management Plan of Care	-	-	-	88%
Received Reliever Medication	-	-	-	100%
Received Systemic Corticosteroids	-	-	-	100%
Emergency Department				
Admittance Decision Time (minutes)[2]	516	116	104	98
Head CT Results Within 45 Min. of Arrival[1]	-	-	60%	57%
Patients Who Left ER Before Being Seen	28,091	1%	1%	2%
Time from ER Arrival to Admit. (minutes)[2]	518	294	276	274
Time from ER Arrival to Discharge (minutes)	365	141	125	134
Time in ER Before Being Evaluated (minutes)	404	30	26	26
Time to Pain Meds for Fractures (minutes)	78	56	58	57
Heart Attack Care				
Aspirin Given at Discharge[1]	-	-	99%	99%
Fibrinolytic Meds Within 30 Min. of Arrival[7]	-	-	40%	54%
PCI Within 90 Minutes of Arrival[7]	-	-	97%	96%
Statin Prescribed at Discharge[1]	-	-	99%	98%
Heart Failure Care				
ACE Inhibitor or ARB for LVSD	18	100%	97%	97%
Discharge Instructions Given	73	85%	96%	94%
Evaluation of LVS Function	105	100%	100%	99%
Medicare Spending				
Medicare Spending per Patient (ratio)	-	1.03	1.01	0.98
Pneumonia Care				
Appropriate Initial Antibiotic Given	74	100%	96%	95%
Blood Culture Timing	124	97%	98%	98%

NOTE: Hospital profiles are in alphabetical order by state, then city, then hospital within the city; Rankings exclude hospitals with less than 25 cases except for patient surveys which excludes hospitals with less than 100 cases; (a) 100-299 cases; (1) The number of cases/patients is too few to report; (2) Data submitted were based on a sample of cases/patients; (3) Results are based on a shorter time period than required; (4) Data suppressed by CMS for one or more quarters; (5) Results are not available for this reporting period; (6) Fewer than 100 patients completed the HCAHPS survey; (7) No cases met the criteria for this measure; (8) The lower limit of the confidence interval cannot be calculated if the number of observed infections equals zero; (9) No data are available from the state/territory for this reporting period; (10) The scores shown reflect fewer than 50 completed surveys; (11) There were discrepancies in the data collection process; (12) This measure does not apply to this hospital for this reporting period; (13) Results cannot be calculated for this reporting period; (14) The results for this state are combined with nearby states to protect confidentiality; Please refer to the User's Guide for a full explanation of data.

Measure	Cases	This Hosp.	State Avg.	U.S. Avg.
Pregnancy and Delivery Care				
Newborn Deliveries Scheduled Early	33	12%	4%	6%
Preventive Care				
Immunization for Influenza[2]	431	99%	91%	90%
Immunization for Pneumonia[2]	548	98%	92%	92%
Stroke Care				
Anticoagulation Therapy for Atrial Fibrillation[1]	-	-	96%	95%
Antithrombotic Therapy Timing	38	100%	98%	98%
Assessed for Rehabilitation	40	92%	98%	97%
Discharged on Antithrombotic Therapy	39	100%	99%	99%
Discharged on Statin Medication	30	83%	95%	94%
Thrombolytic Therapy Timing[1]	-	-	72%	66%
Venous Thromboembolism Prophylaxis	37	95%	95%	94%
Written Stroke Educational Materials Given	16	69%	90%	88%
Surgical Care Improvement Project				
Appropriate Beta Blocker Usage	157	97%	98%	98%
Appropriate VTP Within 24 Hours	451	99%	99%	98%
Controlled Postoperative Blood Glucose[7]	-	-	98%	97%
Perioperative Temperature Management	528	100%	100%	100%
Prophylactic Antibiotic Selection	402	100%	99%	99%
Prophylactic Antibiotic Selection (Outpatient)	207	98%	98%	98%
Prophylactic Antibiotic Stopped	394	99%	98%	98%
Prophylactic Antibiotic Timing	403	100%	99%	99%
Prophylactic Antibiotic Timing (Outpatient)	196	99%	98%	98%
Urinary Catheter Removal	91	98%	99%	97%
Survey of Patients' Hospital Experiences				
Area Around Room 'Always' Quiet at Night	300+	55%	54%	61%
Doctors 'Always' Communicated Well	300+	82%	80%	82%
Home Recovery Information Given	300+	87%	86%	85%
Hospital Given 9 or 10 on 10 Point Scale	300+	62%	69%	71%
Meds 'Always' Explained Before Given	300+	61%	63%	64%
Nurses 'Always' Communicated Well	300+	79%	79%	79%
Pain 'Always' Well Controlled	300+	74%	70%	71%
Room and Bathroom 'Always' Clean	300+	76%	73%	73%
Timely Help 'Always' Received	300+	68%	67%	68%
Would Definitely Recommend Hospital	300+	57%	70%	71%
Use of Medical Imaging				
Cardiac Imaging Stress Test before Surgery	147	4.8%	5.4%	5.3%
Combination Abdominal CT Scan	673	10.5%	12.2%	10.5%
Combination Brain/Sinus CT Scan	625	2.7%	3.1%	2.7%
Combination Chest CT Scan	414	0.5%	2.1%	2.7%
Follow-up Mammogram/Ultrasound	541	11.1%	9%	8.8%
Lumbar Spine MRI for Low Back Pain[1]	-	-	35.8%	37.2%

Chambersburg Hospital

112 North Seventh Street
Chambersburg, PA 17201
Phone: 717-267-3000
Fax: 717-267-7920
URL: www.summithealth.org
Type: Acute Care Hospitals
Emergency Services: Yes
Ownership: Voluntary non-profit - Other
Beds: 248

Key Personnel:
Emergency Room . . . . James Agnew, RN
Radiology. Amir R Batouli, MD
Operating Room. . . . . Stephen Lindsay Carter, RN
Quality Assurance . . . . Patricia Goulding, RN
Pediatric Ambulatory Care . . . . . . Carolyn Kent, RN
Chief of Medical Staff. . . . . Mark A Swatrz, MD

Measure	Cases	This Hosp.	State Avg.	U.S. Avg.
Blood Clot Prevention and Treatment				
Anticoagulation Overlap Therapy	119	98%	94%	93%
ICU Venous Thromboembolism Prophylaxis	903	95%	94%	92%
Incidence of Potentially Preventable VTE	29	10%	8%	10%
UFH with Dosages/Platelet Monitoring	49	100%	98%	97%
Venous Thromboembolism Prophylaxis	4,293	93%	90%	85%
Warfarin Therapy Discharge Instructions	86	88%	78%	75%
Chest Pain/Possible Heart Attack Care				
Aspirin Given Within 24 Hours of Arrival	20	95%	97%	96%
Fibrinolytic Meds Within 30 Min. of Arrival[3,7]	-	-	44%	58%
Average Time to ECG (minutes)	20	2	9	7
Average Time to Transfer (minutes)[3,7]	-	-	64	60
Children's Asthma Care				
Received Home Management Plan of Care	-	-	-	88%
Received Reliever Medication	-	-	-	100%
Received Systemic Corticosteroids	-	-	-	100%
Emergency Department				
Admittance Decision Time (minutes)[2]	675	144	104	98
Head CT Results Within 45 Min. of Arrival[1]	-	-	60%	57%
Patients Who Left ER Before Being Seen	56,808	1%	1%	2%
Time from ER Arrival to Admit. (minutes)[2]	689	295	276	274
Time from ER Arrival to Discharge (minutes)	334	128	125	134
Time in ER Before Being Evaluated (minutes)	349	30	26	26
Time to Pain Meds for Fractures (minutes)	120	58	58	57
Heart Attack Care				
Aspirin Given at Discharge[2]	222	98%	99%	99%
Fibrinolytic Meds Within 30 Min. of Arrival[2,7]	-	-	40%	54%
PCI Within 90 Minutes of Arrival[2]	23	100%	97%	96%
Statin Prescribed at Discharge[2]	222	94%	99%	98%
Heart Failure Care				
ACE Inhibitor or ARB for LVSD	87	91%	97%	97%
Discharge Instructions Given	356	89%	96%	94%
Evaluation of LVS Function	424	100%	100%	99%
Medicare Spending				
Medicare Spending per Patient (ratio)	-	0.93	1.01	0.98
Pneumonia Care				
Appropriate Initial Antibiotic Given[2]	81	94%	96%	95%
Blood Culture Timing[2]	141	98%	98%	98%
Pregnancy and Delivery Care				
Newborn Deliveries Scheduled Early[2]	20	0%	4%	6%
Preventive Care				
Immunization for Influenza[2]	519	93%	91%	90%
Immunization for Pneumonia[2]	731	96%	92%	92%
Stroke Care				
Anticoagulation Therapy for Atrial Fibrillation	33	82%	96%	95%
Antithrombotic Therapy Timing	161	98%	98%	98%
Assessed for Rehabilitation	190	90%	98%	97%
Discharged on Antithrombotic Therapy	173	98%	99%	99%
Discharged on Statin Medication	148	87%	95%	94%
Thrombolytic Therapy Timing	11	55%	72%	66%
Venous Thromboembolism Prophylaxis	180	92%	95%	94%
Written Stroke Educational Materials Given	128	77%	90%	88%
Surgical Care Improvement Project				
Appropriate Beta Blocker Usage[2]	239	97%	98%	98%
Appropriate VTP Within 24 Hours[2]	635	99%	99%	98%
Controlled Postoperative Blood Glucose[2,7]	-	-	98%	97%
Perioperative Temperature Management[2]	746	100%	100%	100%
Prophylactic Antibiotic Selection[2]	556	100%	99%	99%
Prophylactic Antibiotic Selection (Outpatient)	395	98%	98%	98%
Prophylactic Antibiotic Stopped[2]	539	94%	98%	98%
Prophylactic Antibiotic Timing[2]	556	100%	99%	99%
Prophylactic Antibiotic Timing (Outpatient)	397	99%	98%	98%
Urinary Catheter Removal[2]	566	96%	99%	97%
Survey of Patients' Hospital Experiences				
Area Around Room 'Always' Quiet at Night	300+	58%	54%	61%
Doctors 'Always' Communicated Well	300+	73%	80%	82%
Home Recovery Information Given	300+	80%	86%	85%
Hospital Given 9 or 10 on 10 Point Scale	300+	67%	69%	71%
Meds 'Always' Explained Before Given	300+	61%	63%	64%
Nurses 'Always' Communicated Well	300+	77%	79%	79%
Pain 'Always' Well Controlled	300+	72%	70%	71%
Room and Bathroom 'Always' Clean	300+	81%	73%	73%
Timely Help 'Always' Received	300+	66%	67%	68%
Would Definitely Recommend Hospital	300+	66%	70%	71%
Use of Medical Imaging				
Cardiac Imaging Stress Test before Surgery	802	5.1%	5.4%	5.3%
Combination Abdominal CT Scan	1,283	8.7%	12.2%	10.5%
Combination Brain/Sinus CT Scan	955	1.8%	3.1%	2.7%
Combination Chest CT Scan	664	0.8%	2.1%	2.7%
Follow-up Mammogram/Ultrasound	2,715	8.9%	9%	8.8%
Lumbar Spine MRI for Low Back Pain	245	35.1%	35.8%	37.2%

Clarion Hospital

271 Perkins Road
Clarion, PA 16214
Phone: 814-226-9500
Fax: 814-226-1224
URL: www.clarionhospital.org
Type: Acute Care Hospitals
Emergency Services: Yes
Ownership: Voluntary non-profit - Other
Beds: 96

Key Personnel:
Operating Room. . . . . Connie Aaron, RN
Anesthesiology. . . . . Ronald Buckley, D.O.
Emergency Room . . . . Arthur Dortort, DO
Quality Assurance . . . . Paul Edder
Chief of Medical Staff. . . . . John Meyers

Measure	Cases	This Hosp.	State Avg.	U.S. Avg.
Blood Clot Prevention and Treatment				
Anticoagulation Overlap Therapy[2]	24	38%	94%	93%
ICU Venous Thromboembolism Prophylaxis[2]	37	65%	94%	92%
Incidence of Potentially Preventable VTE[1,2]	-	-	8%	10%
UFH with Dosages/Platelet Monitoring[2]	17	53%	98%	97%
Venous Thromboembolism Prophylaxis[2]	178	55%	90%	85%
Warfarin Therapy Discharge Instructions[2]	16	69%	78%	75%
Chest Pain/Possible Heart Attack Care				
Aspirin Given Within 24 Hours of Arrival	55	96%	97%	96%
Fibrinolytic Meds Within 30 Min. of Arrival[1]	-	-	44%	58%
Average Time to ECG (minutes)	56	14	9	7
Average Time to Transfer (minutes)	15	61	64	60
Children's Asthma Care				
Received Home Management Plan of Care	-	-	-	88%
Received Reliever Medication	-	-	-	100%
Received Systemic Corticosteroids	-	-	-	100%
Emergency Department				
Admittance Decision Time (minutes)[2]	335	70	104	98
Head CT Results Within 45 Min. of Arrival	11	36%	60%	57%
Patients Who Left ER Before Being Seen	18,389	1%	1%	2%
Time from ER Arrival to Admit. (minutes)[2]	335	219	276	274
Time from ER Arrival to Discharge (minutes)	324	130	125	134
Time in ER Before Being Evaluated (minutes)	382	48	26	26
Time to Pain Meds for Fractures (minutes)	40	94	58	57
Heart Attack Care				
Aspirin Given at Discharge	14	93%	99%	99%
Fibrinolytic Meds Within 30 Min. of Arrival[7]	-	-	40%	54%
PCI Within 90 Minutes of Arrival[7]	-	-	97%	96%
Statin Prescribed at Discharge	14	64%	99%	98%
Heart Failure Care				
ACE Inhibitor or ARB for LVSD[1]	-	-	97%	97%
Discharge Instructions Given	41	98%	96%	94%
Evaluation of LVS Function	55	95%	100%	99%
Medicare Spending				
Medicare Spending per Patient (ratio)	-	0.98	1.01	0.98
Pneumonia Care				
Appropriate Initial Antibiotic Given	39	90%	96%	95%
Blood Culture Timing	76	95%	98%	98%
Pregnancy and Delivery Care				
Newborn Deliveries Scheduled Early[2]	11	27%	4%	6%
Preventive Care				
Immunization for Influenza[2]	262	90%	91%	90%
Immunization for Pneumonia[2]	375	90%	92%	92%
Stroke Care				
Anticoagulation Therapy for Atrial Fibrillation[1,2]	-	-	96%	95%
Antithrombotic Therapy Timing[2]	12	83%	98%	98%
Assessed for Rehabilitation[2]	13	85%	98%	97%
Discharged on Antithrombotic Therapy[2]	13	77%	99%	99%
Discharged on Statin Medication[2]	13	69%	95%	94%
Thrombolytic Therapy Timing[1,2]	-	-	72%	66%
Venous Thromboembolism Prophylaxis[2]	12	33%	95%	94%
Written Stroke Educational Materials Given[1,2]	-	-	90%	88%
Surgical Care Improvement Project				
Appropriate Beta Blocker Usage	44	98%	98%	98%
Appropriate VTP Within 24 Hours	135	90%	99%	98%
Controlled Postoperative Blood Glucose[7]	-	-	98%	97%
Perioperative Temperature Management	149	100%	100%	100%
Prophylactic Antibiotic Selection	114	96%	99%	99%
Prophylactic Antibiotic Selection (Outpatient)	68	51%	98%	98%
Prophylactic Antibiotic Stopped	112	92%	98%	98%
Prophylactic Antibiotic Timing	114	97%	99%	99%
Prophylactic Antibiotic Timing (Outpatient)	68	93%	98%	98%
Urinary Catheter Removal	124	94%	99%	97%
Survey of Patients' Hospital Experiences				
Area Around Room 'Always' Quiet at Night	300+	53%	54%	61%
Doctors 'Always' Communicated Well	300+	80%	80%	82%
Home Recovery Information Given	300+	87%	86%	85%

NOTE: Hospital profiles are in alphabetical order by state, then city, then hospital within the city; Rankings exclude hospitals with less than 25 cases except for patient surveys which excludes hospitals with less than 100 cases; (a) 100-299 cases; (1) The number of cases/patients is too few to report; (2) Data submitted were based on a sample of cases/patients; (3) Results are based on a shorter time period than required; (4) Data suppressed by CMS for one or more quarters; (5) Results are not available for this reporting period; (6) Fewer than 100 patients completed the HCAHPS survey; (7) No cases met the criteria for this measure; (8) The lower limit of the confidence interval cannot be calculated if the number of observed infections equals zero; (9) No data are available from the state/territory for this reporting period; (10) The scores shown reflect fewer than 50 completed surveys; (11) There were discrepancies in the data collection process; (12) This measure does not apply to this hospital for this reporting period; (13) Results cannot be calculated for this reporting period; (14) The results for this state are combined with nearby states to protect confidentiality; Please refer to the User's Guide for a full explanation of data.

Measure	Cases	This Hosp.	State Avg.	U.S. Avg.
Hospital Given 9 or 10 on 10 Point Scale	300+	68%	69%	71%
Meds 'Always' Explained Before Given	300+	66%	63%	64%
Nurses 'Always' Communicated Well	300+	79%	79%	79%
Pain 'Always' Well Controlled	300+	70%	70%	71%
Room and Bathroom 'Always' Clean	300+	72%	73%	73%
Timely Help 'Always' Received	300+	64%	67%	68%
Would Definitely Recommend Hospital	300+	68%	70%	71%
Use of Medical Imaging				
Cardiac Imaging Stress Test before Surgery	196	10.2%	5.4%	5.3%
Combination Abdominal CT Scan	404	27.0%	12.2%	10.5%
Combination Brain/Sinus CT Scan	417	6.7%	3.1%	2.7%
Combination Chest CT Scan	162	8.6%	2.1%	2.7%
Follow-up Mammogram/Ultrasound	719	2.1%	9%	8.8%
Lumbar Spine MRI for Low Back Pain	54	38.9%	35.8%	37.2%

Penn Highlands Clearfield

809 Turnpike Ave
Clearfield, PA 16830
Phone: 814-765-5341
Fax: 814-768-2445
E-mail: info@clearfieldhosp.org
URL: www.clearfieldhosp.org
Type: Acute Care Hospitals
Emergency Services: Yes
Ownership: Voluntary non-profit - Other
Beds: 83

Key Personnel:
Anesthesiology. . . . . Richard C Bedger Jr
Pediatrics. . . . . Linda Cindric
CEO/President. . . . . David J McConnell
Pulmonology . . . . Wayne Saxton

Measure	Cases	This Hosp.	State Avg.	U.S. Avg.
Blood Clot Prevention and Treatment				
Anticoagulation Overlap Therapy[2]	30	87%	94%	93%
ICU Venous Thromboembolism Prophylaxis[2]	47	98%	94%	92%
Incidence of Potentially Preventable VTE[1,2]	-	-	8%	10%
UFH with Dosages/Platelet Monitoring[1,2]	-	-	98%	97%
Venous Thromboembolism Prophylaxis[2]	164	87%	90%	85%
Warfarin Therapy Discharge Instructions[2]	26	100%	78%	75%
Chest Pain/Possible Heart Attack Care				
Aspirin Given Within 24 Hours of Arrival	120	98%	97%	96%
Fibrinolytic Meds Within 30 Min. of Arrival[1]	-	-	44%	58%
Average Time to ECG (minutes)	121	18	9	7
Average Time to Transfer (minutes)[1]	-	-	64	60
Children's Asthma Care				
Received Home Management Plan of Care	-	-	-	88%
Received Reliever Medication	-	-	-	100%
Received Systemic Corticosteroids	-	-	-	100%
Emergency Department				
Admittance Decision Time (minutes)[2]	419	69	104	98
Head CT Results Within 45 Min. of Arrival	11	9%	60%	57%
Patients Who Left ER Before Being Seen	25,935	1%	1%	2%
Time from ER Arrival to Admit. (minutes)[2]	438	262	276	274
Time from ER Arrival to Discharge (minutes)	372	134	125	134
Time in ER Before Being Evaluated (minutes)	285	55	26	26
Time to Pain Meds for Fractures (minutes)	63	59	58	57
Heart Attack Care				
Aspirin Given at Discharge[1]	-	-	99%	99%
Fibrinolytic Meds Within 30 Min. of Arrival[7]	-	-	40%	54%
PCI Within 90 Minutes of Arrival[7]	-	-	97%	96%
Statin Prescribed at Discharge[1]	-	-	99%	98%
Heart Failure Care				
ACE Inhibitor or ARB for LVSD	13	62%	97%	97%
Discharge Instructions Given	53	91%	96%	94%
Evaluation of LVS Function	78	99%	100%	99%
Medicare Spending				
Medicare Spending per Patient (ratio)	-	0.98	1.01	0.98
Pneumonia Care				
Appropriate Initial Antibiotic Given	68	97%	96%	95%
Blood Culture Timing	108	98%	98%	98%
Pregnancy and Delivery Care				
Newborn Deliveries Scheduled Early	18	6%	4%	6%
Preventive Care				
Immunization for Influenza[2]	271	99%	91%	90%
Immunization for Pneumonia[2]	387	97%	92%	92%
Stroke Care				
Anticoagulation Therapy for Atrial Fibrillation[1]	-	-	96%	95%
Antithrombotic Therapy Timing	18	100%	98%	98%
Assessed for Rehabilitation	18	94%	98%	97%
Discharged on Antithrombotic Therapy	18	94%	99%	99%
Discharged on Statin Medication	16	69%	95%	94%
Thrombolytic Therapy Timing[1]	-	-	72%	66%
Venous Thromboembolism Prophylaxis	18	89%	95%	94%
Written Stroke Educational Materials Given	11	45%	90%	88%
Surgical Care Improvement Project				
Appropriate Beta Blocker Usage	61	97%	98%	98%
Appropriate VTP Within 24 Hours	163	99%	99%	98%
Controlled Postoperative Blood Glucose[7]	-	-	98%	97%
Perioperative Temperature Management	219	100%	100%	100%
Prophylactic Antibiotic Selection	154	99%	99%	99%
Prophylactic Antibiotic Selection (Outpatient)	67	100%	98%	98%
Prophylactic Antibiotic Stopped	154	97%	98%	98%
Prophylactic Antibiotic Timing	154	99%	99%	99%
Prophylactic Antibiotic Timing (Outpatient)	67	100%	98%	98%
Urinary Catheter Removal	76	93%	99%	97%
Survey of Patients' Hospital Experiences				
Area Around Room 'Always' Quiet at Night	300+	48%	54%	61%
Doctors 'Always' Communicated Well	300+	81%	80%	82%
Home Recovery Information Given	300+	89%	86%	85%
Hospital Given 9 or 10 on 10 Point Scale	300+	55%	69%	71%
Meds 'Always' Explained Before Given	300+	57%	63%	64%
Nurses 'Always' Communicated Well	300+	73%	79%	79%
Pain 'Always' Well Controlled	300+	62%	70%	71%
Room and Bathroom 'Always' Clean	300+	73%	73%	73%
Timely Help 'Always' Received	300+	61%	67%	68%
Would Definitely Recommend Hospital	300+	48%	70%	71%
Use of Medical Imaging				
Cardiac Imaging Stress Test before Surgery	100	4.0%	5.4%	5.3%
Combination Abdominal CT Scan	674	57.1%	12.2%	10.5%
Combination Brain/Sinus CT Scan	578	5.2%	3.1%	2.7%
Combination Chest CT Scan	227	5.7%	2.1%	2.7%
Follow-up Mammogram/Ultrasound	717	4.9%	9%	8.8%
Lumbar Spine MRI for Low Back Pain	45	42.2%	35.8%	37.2%

Saint Luke's Miners Memorial Hospital

360 W Ruddle Street
Coaldale, PA 18218
Phone: 570-645-2131
Fax: 570-645-2121
URL: www.slhn-lehighvalley.org
Type: Acute Care Hospitals
Emergency Services: Yes
Ownership: Voluntary non-profit - Private
Beds: 61

Key Personnel:
Operating Room. . . . . Atul K Amin, RN
Radiology. . . . . James D Bohri, MD
CEO/President. . . . . William J Crossin
Chief of Medical Staff. . . . . Arthur Kennedy, MD
Quality Assurance . . . . Gail Marek
Infection Control. . . . . Kathy Matika, RN BSN
Anesthesiology. . . . . Smita Mody, MD
Emergency Room . . . . Eric Rodish, MD

Measure	Cases	This Hosp.	State Avg.	U.S. Avg.
Blood Clot Prevention and Treatment				
Anticoagulation Overlap Therapy[2]	27	96%	94%	93%
ICU Venous Thromboembolism Prophylaxis[2]	23	100%	94%	92%
Incidence of Potentially Preventable VTE[1,2]	-	-	8%	10%
UFH with Dosages/Platelet Monitoring[2]	11	100%	98%	97%
Venous Thromboembolism Prophylaxis[2]	163	90%	90%	85%
Warfarin Therapy Discharge Instructions[2]	21	71%	78%	75%
Chest Pain/Possible Heart Attack Care				
Aspirin Given Within 24 Hours of Arrival[3,7]	-	-	97%	96%
Fibrinolytic Meds Within 30 Min. of Arrival[5]	-	-	44%	58%
Average Time to ECG (minutes)[3,7]	-	-	9	7
Average Time to Transfer (minutes)[5]	-	-	64	60
Children's Asthma Care				
Received Home Management Plan of Care	-	-	-	88%
Received Reliever Medication	-	-	-	100%
Received Systemic Corticosteroids	-	-	-	100%
Emergency Department				
Admittance Decision Time (minutes)[2]	463	61	104	98
Head CT Results Within 45 Min. of Arrival[1]	-	-	60%	57%
Patients Who Left ER Before Being Seen	14,494	1%	1%	2%
Time from ER Arrival to Admit. (minutes)[2]	467	246	276	274
Time from ER Arrival to Discharge (minutes)	354	124	125	134
Time in ER Before Being Evaluated (minutes)	373	26	26	26
Time to Pain Meds for Fractures (minutes)	28	48	58	57
Heart Attack Care				
Aspirin Given at Discharge[1]	-	-	99%	99%
Fibrinolytic Meds Within 30 Min. of Arrival[7]	-	-	40%	54%
PCI Within 90 Minutes of Arrival[7]	-	-	97%	96%
Statin Prescribed at Discharge[1]	-	-	99%	98%
Heart Failure Care				
ACE Inhibitor or ARB for LVSD	13	100%	97%	97%
Discharge Instructions Given	68	100%	96%	94%
Evaluation of LVS Function	94	100%	100%	99%
Medicare Spending				
Medicare Spending per Patient (ratio)	-	1.02	1.01	0.98
Pneumonia Care				
Appropriate Initial Antibiotic Given	65	98%	96%	95%
Blood Culture Timing	94	100%	98%	98%
Pregnancy and Delivery Care				
Newborn Deliveries Scheduled Early[7]	-	-	4%	6%
Preventive Care				
Immunization for Influenza[2]	289	100%	91%	90%
Immunization for Pneumonia[2]	459	100%	92%	92%
Stroke Care				
Anticoagulation Therapy for Atrial Fibrillation[1]	-	-	96%	95%
Antithrombotic Therapy Timing	15	100%	98%	98%
Assessed for Rehabilitation	17	100%	98%	97%
Discharged on Antithrombotic Therapy	17	100%	99%	99%
Discharged on Statin Medication	14	100%	95%	94%
Thrombolytic Therapy Timing[7]	-	-	72%	66%
Venous Thromboembolism Prophylaxis	14	100%	95%	94%
Written Stroke Educational Materials Given	11	91%	90%	88%
Surgical Care Improvement Project				
Appropriate Beta Blocker Usage	41	100%	98%	98%
Appropriate VTP Within 24 Hours	129	99%	99%	98%
Controlled Postoperative Blood Glucose[7]	-	-	98%	97%
Perioperative Temperature Management	141	100%	100%	100%
Prophylactic Antibiotic Selection	108	100%	99%	99%
Prophylactic Antibiotic Selection (Outpatient)[1,3]	-	-	98%	98%
Prophylactic Antibiotic Stopped	107	99%	98%	98%
Prophylactic Antibiotic Timing	108	100%	99%	99%
Prophylactic Antibiotic Timing (Outpatient)[1,3]	-	-	98%	98%
Urinary Catheter Removal	115	100%	99%	97%
Survey of Patients' Hospital Experiences				
Area Around Room 'Always' Quiet at Night	300+	58%	54%	61%
Doctors 'Always' Communicated Well	300+	87%	80%	82%
Home Recovery Information Given	300+	90%	86%	85%
Hospital Given 9 or 10 on 10 Point Scale	300+	75%	69%	71%
Meds 'Always' Explained Before Given	300+	69%	63%	64%
Nurses 'Always' Communicated Well	300+	83%	79%	79%
Pain 'Always' Well Controlled	300+	78%	70%	71%
Room and Bathroom 'Always' Clean	300+	76%	73%	73%
Timely Help 'Always' Received	300+	70%	67%	68%
Would Definitely Recommend Hospital	300+	73%	70%	71%
Use of Medical Imaging				
Cardiac Imaging Stress Test before Surgery	140	3.6%	5.4%	5.3%
Combination Abdominal CT Scan	442	2.3%	12.2%	10.5%
Combination Brain/Sinus CT Scan[1]	-	-	3.1%	2.7%
Combination Chest CT Scan	328	0.9%	2.1%	2.7%
Follow-up Mammogram/Ultrasound	463	5.2%	9%	8.8%
Lumbar Spine MRI for Low Back Pain[1]	-	-	35.8%	37.2%

Brandywine Hospital

201 Reeceville Road
Coatesville, PA 19320
Phone: 610-383-8000
Fax: 610-383-8233
URL: www.brandywinehospital.com
Type: Acute Care Hospitals
Emergency Services: Yes
Ownership: Proprietary
Beds: 168

Key Personnel:
Radiology. . . . . Ronald Adelman, MD
Pediatric In-Patient Care . . . . F D'Urso, MD
Quality Assurance . . . . Kathy Zoph Herling
CEO/President. . . . . Marion McGowan
Chief of Medical Staff . . . . Robert Satriale, MD

Measure	Cases	This Hosp.	State Avg.	U.S. Avg.
Blood Clot Prevention and Treatment				

NOTE: Hospital profiles are in alphabetical order by state, then city, then hospital within the city; Rankings exclude hospitals with less than 25 cases except for patient surveys which excludes hospitals with less than 100 cases; (a) 100-299 cases; (1) The number of cases/patients is too few to report; (2) Data submitted were based on a sample of cases/patients; (3) Results are based on a shorter time period than required; (4) Data suppressed by CMS for one or more quarters; (5) Results are not available for this reporting period; (6) Fewer than 100 patients completed the HCAHPS survey; (7) No cases met the criteria for this measure; (8) The lower limit of the confidence interval cannot be calculated if the number of observed infections equals zero; (9) No data are available from the state/territory for this reporting period; (10) The scores shown reflect fewer than 50 completed surveys; (11) There were discrepancies in the data collection process; (12) This measure does not apply to this hospital for this reporting period; (13) Results cannot be calculated for this reporting period; (14) The results for this state are combined with nearby states to protect confidentiality; Please refer to the User's Guide for a full explanation of data.

Measure	Cases	This Hosp.	State Avg.	U.S. Avg.
Anticoagulation Overlap Therapy[2]	37	81%	94%	93%
ICU Venous Thromboembolism Prophylaxis[2]	80	91%	94%	92%
Incidence of Potentially Preventable VTE[1,2]	-	-	8%	10%
UFH with Dosages/Platelet Monitoring[2]	40	100%	98%	97%
Venous Thromboembolism Prophylaxis[2]	414	79%	90%	85%
Warfarin Therapy Discharge Instructions[2]	21	52%	78%	75%
Chest Pain/Possible Heart Attack Care				
Aspirin Given Within 24 Hours of Arrival	17	100%	97%	96%
Fibrinolytic Meds Within 30 Min. of Arrival[3,7]	-	-	44%	58%
Average Time to ECG (minutes)	19	8	9	7
Average Time to Transfer (minutes)[1,3]	-	-	64	60
Children's Asthma Care				
Received Home Management Plan of Care	-	-	-	88%
Received Reliever Medication	-	-	-	100%
Received Systemic Corticosteroids	-	-	-	100%
Emergency Department				
Admittance Decision Time (minutes)[2]	865	89	104	98
Head CT Results Within 45 Min. of Arrival	29	90%	60%	57%
Patients Who Left ER Before Being Seen	29,188	1%	1%	2%
Time from ER Arrival to Admit. (minutes)[2]	884	257	276	274
Time from ER Arrival to Discharge (minutes)	384	111	125	134
Time in ER Before Being Evaluated (minutes)	422	19	26	26
Time to Pain Meds for Fractures (minutes)	98	41	58	57
Heart Attack Care				
Aspirin Given at Discharge	125	99%	99%	99%
Fibrinolytic Meds Within 30 Min. of Arrival[7]	-	-	40%	54%
PCI Within 90 Minutes of Arrival	18	100%	97%	96%
Statin Prescribed at Discharge	121	100%	99%	98%
Heart Failure Care				
ACE Inhibitor or ARB for LVSD	81	99%	97%	97%
Discharge Instructions Given	212	96%	96%	94%
Evaluation of LVS Function	282	100%	100%	99%
Medicare Spending				
Medicare Spending per Patient (ratio)	-	1.03	1.01	0.98
Pneumonia Care				
Appropriate Initial Antibiotic Given	135	98%	96%	95%
Blood Culture Timing	247	98%	98%	98%
Pregnancy and Delivery Care				
Newborn Deliveries Scheduled Early[2,7]	-	-	4%	6%
Preventive Care				
Immunization for Influenza[2]	665	95%	91%	90%
Immunization for Pneumonia[2]	861	96%	92%	92%
Stroke Care				
Anticoagulation Therapy for Atrial Fibrillation	11	91%	96%	95%
Antithrombotic Therapy Timing	54	98%	98%	98%
Assessed for Rehabilitation	61	95%	98%	97%
Discharged on Antithrombotic Therapy	57	93%	99%	99%
Discharged on Statin Medication	52	81%	95%	94%
Thrombolytic Therapy Timing[1]	-	-	72%	66%
Venous Thromboembolism Prophylaxis	62	84%	95%	94%
Written Stroke Educational Materials Given	26	85%	90%	88%
Surgical Care Improvement Project				
Appropriate Beta Blocker Usage	129	98%	98%	98%
Appropriate VTP Within 24 Hours	207	96%	99%	98%
Controlled Postoperative Blood Glucose	61	98%	98%	97%
Perioperative Temperature Management	238	100%	100%	100%
Prophylactic Antibiotic Selection	198	98%	99%	99%
Prophylactic Antibiotic Selection (Outpatient)	113	97%	98%	98%
Prophylactic Antibiotic Stopped	197	96%	98%	98%
Prophylactic Antibiotic Timing	199	100%	99%	99%
Prophylactic Antibiotic Timing (Outpatient)	116	97%	98%	98%
Urinary Catheter Removal	178	94%	99%	97%
Survey of Patients' Hospital Experiences				
Area Around Room 'Always' Quiet at Night	300+	56%	54%	61%
Doctors 'Always' Communicated Well	300+	78%	80%	82%
Home Recovery Information Given	300+	87%	86%	85%
Hospital Given 9 or 10 on 10 Point Scale	300+	65%	69%	71%
Meds 'Always' Explained Before Given	300+	60%	63%	64%
Nurses 'Always' Communicated Well	300+	77%	79%	79%
Pain 'Always' Well Controlled	300+	71%	70%	71%
Room and Bathroom 'Always' Clean	300+	74%	73%	73%
Timely Help 'Always' Received	300+	66%	67%	68%
Would Definitely Recommend Hospital	300+	63%	70%	71%
Use of Medical Imaging				
Cardiac Imaging Stress Test before Surgery	343	4.1%	5.4%	5.3%
Combination Abdominal CT Scan	490	6.1%	12.2%	10.5%
Combination Brain/Sinus CT Scan	583	5.0%	3.1%	2.7%
Combination Chest CT Scan	302	0.0%	2.1%	2.7%
Follow-up Mammogram/Ultrasound	736	10.1%	9%	8.8%
Lumbar Spine MRI for Low Back Pain	95	29.5%	35.8%	37.2%

Coatesville VA Medical Center

1400 Black Horse Hill Road
Coatesville, PA 19320
Phone: 610-384-7711
Fax: 610-383-0207
Type: Acute Care - VA
Emergency Services: No
Ownership: Government Federal
Key Personnel:
Quality Assurance . . . . JoAnn Reny, RN
Chief of Medical Staff . . . . Jose D. Riojas

Measure	Cases	This Hosp.	State Avg.	U.S. Avg.
Blood Clot Prevention and Treatment				
Anticoagulation Overlap Therapy	-	-	94%	93%
ICU Venous Thromboembolism Prophylaxis	-	-	94%	92%
Incidence of Potentially Preventable VTE	-	-	8%	10%
UFH with Dosages/Platelet Monitoring	-	-	98%	97%
Venous Thromboembolism Prophylaxis	-	-	90%	85%
Warfarin Therapy Discharge Instructions	-	-	78%	75%
Chest Pain/Possible Heart Attack Care				
Aspirin Given Within 24 Hours of Arrival	-	-	97%	96%
Fibrinolytic Meds Within 30 Min. of Arrival	-	-	44%	58%
Average Time to ECG (minutes)	-	-	9	7
Average Time to Transfer (minutes)	-	-	64	60
Children's Asthma Care				
Received Home Management Plan of Care	-	-	-	88%
Received Reliever Medication	-	-	-	100%
Received Systemic Corticosteroids	-	-	-	100%
Emergency Department				
Admittance Decision Time (minutes)	-	-	104	98
Head CT Results Within 45 Min. of Arrival	-	-	60%	57%
Patients Who Left ER Before Being Seen	-	-	1%	2%
Time from ER Arrival to Admit. (minutes)	-	-	276	274
Time from ER Arrival to Discharge (minutes)	-	-	125	134
Time in ER Before Being Evaluated (minutes)	-	-	26	26
Time to Pain Meds for Fractures (minutes)	-	-	58	57
Heart Attack Care				
Aspirin Given at Discharge[5]	-	-	99%	99%
Fibrinolytic Meds Within 30 Min. of Arrival[5]	-	-	40%	54%
PCI Within 90 Minutes of Arrival[5]	-	-	97%	96%
Statin Prescribed at Discharge[5]	-	-	99%	98%
Heart Failure Care				
ACE Inhibitor or ARB for LVSD[5]	-	-	97%	97%
Discharge Instructions Given[5]	-	-	96%	94%
Evaluation of LVS Function[5]	-	-	100%	99%
Medicare Spending				
Medicare Spending per Patient (ratio)	-	-	1.01	0.98
Pneumonia Care				
Appropriate Initial Antibiotic Given[5]	-	-	96%	95%
Blood Culture Timing[5]	-	-	98%	98%
Pregnancy and Delivery Care				
Newborn Deliveries Scheduled Early	-	-	4%	6%
Preventive Care				
Immunization for Influenza[2,3]	139	96%	91%	90%
Immunization for Pneumonia[2,3]	155	96%	92%	92%
Stroke Care				
Anticoagulation Therapy for Atrial Fibrillation	-	-	96%	95%
Antithrombotic Therapy Timing	-	-	98%	98%
Assessed for Rehabilitation	-	-	98%	97%
Discharged on Antithrombotic Therapy	-	-	99%	99%
Discharged on Statin Medication	-	-	95%	94%
Thrombolytic Therapy Timing	-	-	72%	66%
Venous Thromboembolism Prophylaxis	-	-	95%	94%
Written Stroke Educational Materials Given	-	-	90%	88%
Surgical Care Improvement Project				
Appropriate Beta Blocker Usage[5]	-	-	98%	98%
Appropriate VTP Within 24 Hours[5]	-	-	99%	98%
Controlled Postoperative Blood Glucose[5]	-	-	98%	97%
Perioperative Temperature Management[5]	-	-	100%	100%
Prophylactic Antibiotic Selection[5]	-	-	99%	99%
Prophylactic Antibiotic Selection (Outpatient)	-	-	98%	98%
Prophylactic Antibiotic Stopped[5]	-	-	98%	98%
Prophylactic Antibiotic Timing[5]	-	-	99%	99%
Prophylactic Antibiotic Timing (Outpatient)	-	-	98%	98%
Urinary Catheter Removal[5]	-	-	99%	97%
Survey of Patients' Hospital Experiences				
Area Around Room 'Always' Quiet at Night	-	-	54%	61%
Doctors 'Always' Communicated Well	-	-	80%	82%
Home Recovery Information Given	-	-	86%	85%
Hospital Given 9 or 10 on 10 Point Scale	-	-	69%	71%
Meds 'Always' Explained Before Given	-	-	63%	64%
Nurses 'Always' Communicated Well	-	-	79%	79%
Pain 'Always' Well Controlled	-	-	70%	71%
Room and Bathroom 'Always' Clean	-	-	73%	73%
Timely Help 'Always' Received	-	-	67%	68%
Would Definitely Recommend Hospital	-	-	70%	71%
Use of Medical Imaging				
Cardiac Imaging Stress Test before Surgery	-	-	5.4%	5.3%
Combination Abdominal CT Scan	-	-	12.2%	10.5%
Combination Brain/Sinus CT Scan	-	-	3.1%	2.7%
Combination Chest CT Scan	-	-	2.1%	2.7%
Follow-up Mammogram/Ultrasound	-	-	9%	8.8%
Lumbar Spine MRI for Low Back Pain	-	-	35.8%	37.2%

Highlands Hospital

401 East Murphy Avenue
Connellsville, PA 15425
Phone: 724-628-1500
Fax: 724-626-2334
E-mail: webmaster@highlandshospital.org
URL: www.highlandshospital.org
Type: Acute Care Hospitals
Emergency Services: Yes
Ownership: Voluntary non-profit - Private
Beds: 87
Key Personnel:
CEO/President . . . . Michelle Cuttingham
Chief of Medical Staff . . . . Albert Enany, MD
Quality Assurance . . . . Barbra Morrison
Emergency Room . . . . Peter Stevenson

Measure	Cases	This Hosp.	State Avg.	U.S. Avg.
Blood Clot Prevention and Treatment				
Anticoagulation Overlap Therapy[2]	11	45%	94%	93%
ICU Venous Thromboembolism Prophylaxis[2]	35	91%	94%	92%
Incidence of Potentially Preventable VTE[1,2]	-	-	8%	10%
UFH with Dosages/Platelet Monitoring[2]	12	92%	98%	97%
Venous Thromboembolism Prophylaxis[2]	138	62%	90%	85%
Warfarin Therapy Discharge Instructions[2]	12	67%	78%	75%
Chest Pain/Possible Heart Attack Care				
Aspirin Given Within 24 Hours of Arrival	47	98%	97%	96%
Fibrinolytic Meds Within 30 Min. of Arrival[7]	-	-	44%	58%
Average Time to ECG (minutes)	47	10	9	7
Average Time to Transfer (minutes)[1]	-	-	64	60
Children's Asthma Care				
Received Home Management Plan of Care	-	-	-	88%
Received Reliever Medication	-	-	-	100%
Received Systemic Corticosteroids	-	-	-	100%
Emergency Department				
Admittance Decision Time (minutes)[2]	417	75	104	98
Head CT Results Within 45 Min. of Arrival[1]	-	-	60%	57%
Patients Who Left ER Before Being Seen	14,068	1%	1%	2%
Time from ER Arrival to Admit. (minutes)[2]	420	193	276	274
Time from ER Arrival to Discharge (minutes)	327	77	125	134
Time in ER Before Being Evaluated (minutes)	377	24	26	26
Time to Pain Meds for Fractures (minutes)	41	53	58	57
Heart Attack Care				
Aspirin Given at Discharge[1]	-	-	99%	99%
Fibrinolytic Meds Within 30 Min. of Arrival[7]	-	-	40%	54%
PCI Within 90 Minutes of Arrival[7]	-	-	97%	96%
Statin Prescribed at Discharge[1]	-	-	99%	98%
Heart Failure Care				
ACE Inhibitor or ARB for LVSD	16	88%	97%	97%
Discharge Instructions Given	57	88%	96%	94%
Evaluation of LVS Function	64	100%	100%	99%

NOTE: Hospital profiles are in alphabetical order by state, then city, then hospital within the city; Rankings exclude hospitals with less than 25 cases except for patient surveys which excludes hospitals with less than 100 cases; (a) 100-299 cases; (1) The number of cases/patients is too few to report; (2) Data submitted were based on a sample of cases/patients; (3) Results are based on a shorter time period than required; (4) Data suppressed by CMS for one or more quarters; (5) Results are not available for this reporting period; (6) Fewer than 100 patients completed the HCAHPS survey; (7) No cases met the criteria for this measure; (8) The lower limit of the confidence interval cannot be calculated if the number of observed infections equals zero; (9) No data are available from the state/territory for this reporting period; (10) The scores shown reflect fewer than 50 completed surveys; (11) There were discrepancies in the data collection process; (12) This measure does not apply to this hospital for this reporting period; (13) Results cannot be calculated for this reporting period; (14) The results for this state are combined with nearby states to protect confidentiality; Please refer to the User's Guide for a full explanation of data.

Medicare Spending				
Medicare Spending per Patient (ratio)	-	1.00	1.01	0.98
Pneumonia Care				
Appropriate Initial Antibiotic Given	55	89%	96%	95%
Blood Culture Timing	67	99%	98%	98%
Pregnancy and Delivery Care				
Newborn Deliveries Scheduled Early[7]	-	-	4%	6%
Preventive Care				
Immunization for Influenza[2]	278	91%	91%	90%
Immunization for Pneumonia[2]	399	82%	92%	92%
Stroke Care				
Anticoagulation Therapy for Atrial Fibrillation[1,3]	-	-	96%	95%
Antithrombotic Therapy Timing[1,3]	-	-	98%	98%
Assessed for Rehabilitation[1,3]	-	-	98%	97%
Discharged on Antithrombotic Therapy[1,3]	-	-	99%	99%
Discharged on Statin Medication[1,3]	-	-	95%	94%
Thrombolytic Therapy Timing[3,7]	-	-	72%	66%
Venous Thromboembolism Prophylaxis[1,3]	-	-	95%	94%
Written Stroke Educational Materials Given[3,7]	-	-	90%	88%
Surgical Care Improvement Project				
Appropriate Beta Blocker Usage	16	94%	98%	98%
Appropriate VTP Within 24 Hours	37	95%	99%	98%
Controlled Postoperative Blood Glucose[7]	-	-	98%	97%
Perioperative Temperature Management	44	100%	100%	100%
Prophylactic Antibiotic Selection	15	93%	99%	99%
Prophylactic Antibiotic Selection (Outpatient)[1,3]	-	-	98%	98%
Prophylactic Antibiotic Stopped	15	87%	98%	98%
Prophylactic Antibiotic Timing	16	94%	99%	99%
Prophylactic Antibiotic Timing (Outpatient)[1,3]	-	-	98%	98%
Urinary Catheter Removal	32	100%	99%	97%
Survey of Patients' Hospital Experiences				
Area Around Room 'Always' Quiet at Night	300+	40%	54%	61%
Doctors 'Always' Communicated Well	300+	85%	80%	82%
Home Recovery Information Given	300+	82%	86%	85%
Hospital Given 9 or 10 on 10 Point Scale	300+	61%	69%	71%
Meds 'Always' Explained Before Given	300+	68%	63%	64%
Nurses 'Always' Communicated Well	300+	79%	79%	79%
Pain 'Always' Well Controlled	300+	65%	70%	71%
Room and Bathroom 'Always' Clean	300+	71%	73%	73%
Timely Help 'Always' Received	300+	65%	67%	68%
Would Definitely Recommend Hospital	300+	60%	70%	71%
Use of Medical Imaging				
Cardiac Imaging Stress Test before Surgery	79	6.3%	5.4%	5.3%
Combination Abdominal CT Scan	109	33.0%	12.2%	10.5%
Combination Brain/Sinus CT Scan[1]	-	-	3.1%	2.7%
Combination Chest CT Scan[1]	-	-	2.1%	2.7%
Follow-up Mammogram/Ultrasound	168	10.7%	9%	8.8%
Lumbar Spine MRI for Low Back Pain[1]	-	-	35.8%	37.2%

Corry Memorial Hospital

965 Shamrock Lane
Corry, PA 16407
E-mail: info@corryhospital.org
URL: www.corryhospital.org
Type: Critical Access Hospitals
Ownership: Govt - Hospital Dist/Auth
Phone: 814-664-4641
Fax: 814-664-7967
Emergency Services: Yes
Beds: 55

Key Personnel:
Chief of Medical Staff. . . . . John E Balmer
Radiology. Paul A McGeehan
CEO/President. . . . . Barbara D Nichols, RN

Measure	Cases	This Hosp.	State Avg.	U.S. Avg.
Blood Clot Prevention and Treatment				
Anticoagulation Overlap Therapy[5]	-	-	94%	93%
ICU Venous Thromboembolism Prophylaxis[5]	-	-	94%	92%
Incidence of Potentially Preventable VTE[5]	-	-	8%	10%
UFH with Dosages/Platelet Monitoring[5]	-	-	98%	97%
Venous Thromboembolism Prophylaxis[5]	-	-	90%	85%
Warfarin Therapy Discharge Instructions[5]	-	-	78%	75%
Chest Pain/Possible Heart Attack Care				
Aspirin Given Within 24 Hours of Arrival	27	96%	97%	96%
Fibrinolytic Meds Within 30 Min. of Arrival[7]	-	-	44%	58%
Average Time to ECG (minutes)	27	10	9	7
Average Time to Transfer (minutes)[1]	-	-	64	60
Children's Asthma Care				
Received Home Management Plan of Care	-	-	-	88%
Received Reliever Medication	-	-	-	100%
Received Systemic Corticosteroids	-	-	-	100%
Emergency Department				
Admittance Decision Time (minutes)[5]	-	-	104	98
Head CT Results Within 45 Min. of Arrival[5]	-	-	60%	57%
Patients Who Left ER Before Being Seen	10,290	1%	1%	2%
Time from ER Arrival to Admit. (minutes)[5]	-	-	276	274
Time from ER Arrival to Discharge (minutes)[5]	-	-	125	134
Time in ER Before Being Evaluated (minutes)[5]	-	-	26	26
Time to Pain Meds for Fractures (minutes)[5]	-	-	58	57
Heart Attack Care				
Aspirin Given at Discharge[1,3]	-	-	99%	99%
Fibrinolytic Meds Within 30 Min. of Arrival[3,7]	-	-	40%	54%
PCI Within 90 Minutes of Arrival[3,7]	-	-	97%	96%
Statin Prescribed at Discharge[1,3]	-	-	99%	98%
Heart Failure Care				
ACE Inhibitor or ARB for LVSD[1]	-	-	97%	97%
Discharge Instructions Given	30	87%	96%	94%
Evaluation of LVS Function	47	89%	100%	99%
Medicare Spending				
Medicare Spending per Patient (ratio)	-	-	1.01	0.98
Pneumonia Care				
Appropriate Initial Antibiotic Given	35	91%	96%	95%
Blood Culture Timing	53	100%	98%	98%
Pregnancy and Delivery Care				
Newborn Deliveries Scheduled Early[5]	-	-	4%	6%
Preventive Care				
Immunization for Influenza[5]	-	-	91%	90%
Immunization for Pneumonia[5]	-	-	92%	92%
Stroke Care				
Anticoagulation Therapy for Atrial Fibrillation[5]	-	-	96%	95%
Antithrombotic Therapy Timing[5]	-	-	98%	98%
Assessed for Rehabilitation[5]	-	-	98%	97%
Discharged on Antithrombotic Therapy[5]	-	-	99%	99%
Discharged on Statin Medication[5]	-	-	95%	94%
Thrombolytic Therapy Timing[5]	-	-	72%	66%
Venous Thromboembolism Prophylaxis[5]	-	-	95%	94%
Written Stroke Educational Materials Given[5]	-	-	90%	88%
Surgical Care Improvement Project				
Appropriate Beta Blocker Usage[5]	-	-	98%	98%
Appropriate VTP Within 24 Hours[5]	-	-	99%	98%
Controlled Postoperative Blood Glucose[5]	-	-	98%	97%
Perioperative Temperature Management[5]	-	-	100%	100%
Prophylactic Antibiotic Selection[5]	-	-	99%	99%
Prophylactic Antibiotic Selection (Outpatient)[1,3]	-	-	98%	98%
Prophylactic Antibiotic Stopped[5]	-	-	98%	98%
Prophylactic Antibiotic Timing[5]	-	-	99%	99%
Prophylactic Antibiotic Timing (Outpatient)[1,3]	-	-	98%	98%
Urinary Catheter Removal[5]	-	-	99%	97%
Survey of Patients' Hospital Experiences				
Area Around Room 'Always' Quiet at Night	(a)	66%	54%	61%
Doctors 'Always' Communicated Well	(a)	80%	80%	82%
Home Recovery Information Given	(a)	83%	86%	85%
Hospital Given 9 or 10 on 10 Point Scale	(a)	73%	69%	71%
Meds 'Always' Explained Before Given	(a)	61%	63%	64%
Nurses 'Always' Communicated Well	(a)	78%	79%	79%
Pain 'Always' Well Controlled	(a)	72%	70%	71%
Room and Bathroom 'Always' Clean	(a)	81%	73%	73%
Timely Help 'Always' Received	(a)	70%	67%	68%
Would Definitely Recommend Hospital	(a)	64%	70%	71%
Use of Medical Imaging				
Cardiac Imaging Stress Test before Surgery	64	7.8%	5.4%	5.3%
Combination Abdominal CT Scan	217	49.3%	12.2%	10.5%
Combination Brain/Sinus CT Scan[1]	-	-	3.1%	2.7%
Combination Chest CT Scan	101	0.0%	2.1%	2.7%
Follow-up Mammogram/Ultrasound	387	2.3%	9%	8.8%
Lumbar Spine MRI for Low Back Pain[1]	-	-	35.8%	37.2%

Charles Cole Memorial Hospital

1001 East Second Street
Coudersport, PA 16915
URL: www.charlescolehospital.com
Type: Critical Access Hospitals
Ownership: Voluntary non-profit - Other
Phone: 814-274-9301
Fax: 814-274-0884
Emergency Services: Yes
Beds: 140

Key Personnel:
Emergency Room . . . . Michael Lettieri
CEO/President. . . . . Ed Pitchford
Anesthesiology. . . . . David Tonkin, MD

Measure	Cases	This Hosp.	State Avg.	U.S. Avg.
Blood Clot Prevention and Treatment				
Anticoagulation Overlap Therapy[2,3]	11	100%	94%	93%
ICU Venous Thromboembolism Prophylaxis[2,3]	21	95%	94%	92%
Incidence of Potentially Preventable VTE[2,3]	-	-	8%	10%
UFH with Dosages/Platelet Monitoring[1,2]	-	-	98%	97%
Venous Thromboembolism Prophylaxis[2,3]	97	82%	90%	85%
Warfarin Therapy Discharge Instructions[1,2]	-	-	78%	75%
Chest Pain/Possible Heart Attack Care				
Aspirin Given Within 24 Hours of Arrival	65	100%	97%	96%
Fibrinolytic Meds Within 30 Min. of Arrival[1]	-	-	44%	58%
Average Time to ECG (minutes)	67	10	9	7
Average Time to Transfer (minutes)[1]	-	-	64	60
Children's Asthma Care				
Received Home Management Plan of Care	-	-	-	88%
Received Reliever Medication	-	-	-	100%
Received Systemic Corticosteroids	-	-	-	100%
Emergency Department				
Admittance Decision Time (minutes)[2]	226	51	104	98
Head CT Results Within 45 Min. of Arrival[1]	-	-	60%	57%
Patients Who Left ER Before Being Seen	10,135	2%	1%	2%
Time from ER Arrival to Admit. (minutes)[2]	227	235	276	274
Time from ER Arrival to Discharge (minutes)	376	157	125	134
Time in ER Before Being Evaluated (minutes)	416	49	26	26
Time to Pain Meds for Fractures (minutes)	63	64	58	57
Heart Attack Care				
Aspirin Given at Discharge[1]	-	-	99%	99%
Fibrinolytic Meds Within 30 Min. of Arrival[7]	-	-	40%	54%
PCI Within 90 Minutes of Arrival[7]	-	-	97%	96%
Statin Prescribed at Discharge	11	100%	99%	98%
Heart Failure Care				
ACE Inhibitor or ARB for LVSD	16	94%	97%	97%
Discharge Instructions Given	25	100%	96%	94%
Evaluation of LVS Function	38	95%	100%	99%
Medicare Spending				
Medicare Spending per Patient (ratio)	-	-	1.01	0.98
Pneumonia Care				
Appropriate Initial Antibiotic Given	45	96%	96%	95%
Blood Culture Timing	68	100%	98%	98%
Pregnancy and Delivery Care				
Newborn Deliveries Scheduled Early[1,3]	-	-	4%	6%
Preventive Care				
Immunization for Influenza[2]	395	99%	91%	90%
Immunization for Pneumonia[2]	444	99%	92%	92%
Stroke Care				
Anticoagulation Therapy for Atrial Fibrillation[1,3]	-	-	96%	95%
Antithrombotic Therapy Timing[1,3]	-	-	98%	98%
Assessed for Rehabilitation[1,3]	-	-	98%	97%
Discharged on Antithrombotic Therapy[1,3]	-	-	99%	99%
Discharged on Statin Medication[1,3]	-	-	95%	94%
Thrombolytic Therapy Timing[3,7]	-	-	72%	66%
Venous Thromboembolism Prophylaxis[3]	11	100%	95%	94%
Written Stroke Educational Materials Given[3,7]	-	-	90%	88%
Surgical Care Improvement Project				
Appropriate Beta Blocker Usage	59	100%	98%	98%
Appropriate VTP Within 24 Hours	252	100%	99%	98%
Controlled Postoperative Blood Glucose[7]	-	-	98%	97%
Perioperative Temperature Management	274	100%	100%	100%
Prophylactic Antibiotic Selection	221	99%	99%	99%
Prophylactic Antibiotic Selection (Outpatient)	23	96%	98%	98%
Prophylactic Antibiotic Stopped	221	99%	98%	98%
Prophylactic Antibiotic Timing	221	99%	99%	99%
Prophylactic Antibiotic Timing (Outpatient)	23	96%	98%	98%

NOTE: Hospital profiles are in alphabetical order by state, then city, then hospital within the city; Rankings exclude hospitals with less than 25 cases except for patient surveys which excludes hospitals with less than 100 cases; (a) 100-299 cases; (1) The number of cases/patients is too few to report; (2) Data submitted were based on a sample of cases/patients; (3) Results are based on a shorter time period than required; (4) Data suppressed by CMS for one or more quarters; (5) Results are not available for this reporting period; (6) Fewer than 100 patients completed the HCAHPS survey; (7) No cases met the criteria for this measure; (8) The lower limit of the confidence interval cannot be calculated if the number of observed infections equals zero; (9) No data are available from the state/territory for this reporting period; (10) The scores shown reflect fewer than 50 completed surveys; (11) There were discrepancies in the data collection process; (12) This measure does not apply to this hospital for this reporting period; (13) Results cannot be calculated for this reporting period; (14) The results for this state are combined with nearby states to protect confidentiality; Please refer to the User's Guide for a full explanation of data.

Urinary Catheter Removal	218	100%	99%	97%
Survey of Patients' Hospital Experiences				
Area Around Room 'Always' Quiet at Night	300+	56%	54%	61%
Doctors 'Always' Communicated Well	300+	82%	80%	82%
Home Recovery Information Given	300+	88%	86%	85%
Hospital Given 9 or 10 on 10 Point Scale	300+	66%	69%	71%
Meds 'Always' Explained Before Given	300+	65%	63%	64%
Nurses 'Always' Communicated Well	300+	79%	79%	79%
Pain 'Always' Well Controlled	300+	71%	70%	71%
Room and Bathroom 'Always' Clean	300+	76%	73%	73%
Timely Help 'Always' Received	300+	76%	67%	68%
Would Definitely Recommend Hospital	300+	62%	70%	71%
Use of Medical Imaging				
Cardiac Imaging Stress Test before Surgery	156	1.3%	5.4%	5.3%
Combination Abdominal CT Scan	322	6.5%	12.2%	10.5%
Combination Brain/Sinus CT Scan[1]	-	-	3.1%	2.7%
Combination Chest CT Scan	307	6.2%	2.1%	2.7%
Follow-up Mammogram/Ultrasound	404	5.9%	9%	8.8%
Lumbar Spine MRI for Low Back Pain	44	61.4%	35.8%	37.2%

Geisinger Medical Center

100 North Academy Avenue
Danville, PA 17822
URL: www.geisinger.org
Type: Acute Care Hospitals
Ownership: Voluntary non-profit - Private

Phone: 570-271-6211
Fax: 570-271-5060
Emergency Services: Yes
Beds: 403

Key Personnel:
Chief of Medical Staff.......... Albert Bothe, Jr., MD, FACS
Infection Control.............. James E Bross, MD
Quality Assurance .... Chuck Miller
Radiology.................. Joseph Rosen
Pediatric In-Patient Care .... Michael Ryan
Emergency Room .... John Skiendzielewski
Operating Room.............. Susan Sneider
CEO/President............... Glenn D. Steele, Jr., MD, PhD

Measure	Cases	This Hosp.	State Avg.	U.S. Avg.
Blood Clot Prevention and Treatment				
Anticoagulation Overlap Therapy[2]	163	97%	94%	93%
ICU Venous Thromboembolism Prophylaxis[2]	81	100%	94%	92%
Incidence of Potentially Preventable VTE[2]	48	4%	8%	10%
UFH with Dosages/Platelet Monitoring[2]	113	100%	98%	97%
Venous Thromboembolism Prophylaxis[2]	399	92%	90%	85%
Warfarin Therapy Discharge Instructions[2]	111	91%	78%	75%
Chest Pain/Possible Heart Attack Care				
Aspirin Given Within 24 Hours of Arrival[5]	-	-	97%	96%
Fibrinolytic Meds Within 30 Min. of Arrival[5]	-	-	44%	58%
Average Time to ECG (minutes)[5]	-	-	9	7
Average Time to Transfer (minutes)[5]	-	-	64	60
Children's Asthma Care				
Received Home Management Plan of Care	-	-	-	88%
Received Reliever Medication	-	-	-	100%
Received Systemic Corticosteroids	-	-	-	100%
Emergency Department				
Admittance Decision Time (minutes)[2]	680	220	104	98
Head CT Results Within 45 Min. of Arrival[1]	-	-	60%	57%
Patients Who Left ER Before Being Seen	49,726	0%	1%	2%
Time from ER Arrival to Admit. (minutes)[2]	691	372	276	274
Time from ER Arrival to Discharge (minutes)	710	154	125	134
Time in ER Before Being Evaluated (minutes)	765	22	26	26
Time to Pain Meds for Fractures (minutes)	162	50	58	57
Heart Attack Care				
Aspirin Given at Discharge	637	100%	99%	99%
Fibrinolytic Meds Within 30 Min. of Arrival[7]	-	-	40%	54%
PCI Within 90 Minutes of Arrival	46	100%	97%	96%
Statin Prescribed at Discharge	625	100%	99%	98%
Heart Failure Care				
ACE Inhibitor or ARB for LVSD	160	96%	97%	97%
Discharge Instructions Given	620	100%	96%	94%
Evaluation of LVS Function	791	100%	100%	99%
Medicare Spending				
Medicare Spending per Patient (ratio)	-	1.04	1.01	0.98
Pneumonia Care				
Appropriate Initial Antibiotic Given	225	99%	96%	95%
Blood Culture Timing	171	99%	98%	98%
Pregnancy and Delivery Care				
Newborn Deliveries Scheduled Early[2]	113	0%	4%	6%
Preventive Care				
Immunization for Influenza[2]	678	93%	91%	90%
Immunization for Pneumonia[2]	807	96%	92%	92%
Stroke Care				
Anticoagulation Therapy for Atrial Fibrillation	49	96%	96%	95%
Antithrombotic Therapy Timing	256	100%	98%	98%
Assessed for Rehabilitation	381	98%	98%	97%
Discharged on Antithrombotic Therapy	280	99%	99%	99%
Discharged on Statin Medication	236	98%	95%	94%
Thrombolytic Therapy Timing	21	76%	72%	66%
Venous Thromboembolism Prophylaxis	396	96%	95%	94%
Written Stroke Educational Materials Given	178	94%	90%	88%
Surgical Care Improvement Project				
Appropriate Beta Blocker Usage[2]	345	99%	98%	98%
Appropriate VTP Within 24 Hours[2]	480	98%	99%	98%
Controlled Postoperative Blood Glucose[2]	190	95%	98%	97%
Perioperative Temperature Management[2]	748	99%	100%	100%
Prophylactic Antibiotic Selection[2]	561	100%	99%	99%
Prophylactic Antibiotic Selection (Outpatient)	909	99%	98%	98%
Prophylactic Antibiotic Stopped[2]	554	98%	98%	98%
Prophylactic Antibiotic Timing[2]	561	99%	99%	99%
Prophylactic Antibiotic Timing (Outpatient)	779	95%	98%	98%
Urinary Catheter Removal[2]	367	99%	99%	97%
Survey of Patients' Hospital Experiences				
Area Around Room 'Always' Quiet at Night	300+	52%	54%	61%
Doctors 'Always' Communicated Well	300+	79%	80%	82%
Home Recovery Information Given	300+	89%	86%	85%
Hospital Given 9 or 10 on 10 Point Scale	300+	75%	69%	71%
Meds 'Always' Explained Before Given	300+	63%	63%	64%
Nurses 'Always' Communicated Well	300+	81%	79%	79%
Pain 'Always' Well Controlled	300+	70%	70%	71%
Room and Bathroom 'Always' Clean	300+	76%	73%	73%
Timely Help 'Always' Received	300+	70%	67%	68%
Would Definitely Recommend Hospital	300+	77%	70%	71%
Use of Medical Imaging				
Cardiac Imaging Stress Test before Surgery	629	5.4%	5.4%	5.3%
Combination Abdominal CT Scan	1,884	10.7%	12.2%	10.5%
Combination Brain/Sinus CT Scan	1,036	3.0%	3.1%	2.7%
Combination Chest CT Scan	1,779	1.3%	2.1%	2.7%
Follow-up Mammogram/Ultrasound	2,641	12.8%	9%	8.8%
Lumbar Spine MRI for Low Back Pain	267	30.0%	35.8%	37.2%

Mercy Fitzgerald Hospital

Lansdowne & Baily Rds
Darby, PA 19023
E-mail: info@mercyhealth.org
URL: www.mercyhealth.org
Type: Acute Care Hospitals
Ownership: Voluntary non-profit - Other

Phone: 215-237-4000
Fax: 610-237-4202
Emergency Services: Yes
Beds: 218

Key Personnel:
Chief of Medical Staff.......... Sharon Carney, MD
CEO/President............... Brian Finestein
Quality Assurance .... Mary Stein

Measure	Cases	This Hosp.	State Avg.	U.S. Avg.
Blood Clot Prevention and Treatment				
Anticoagulation Overlap Therapy[2]	181	98%	94%	93%
ICU Venous Thromboembolism Prophylaxis[2]	149	99%	94%	92%
Incidence of Potentially Preventable VTE[2]	46	2%	8%	10%
UFH with Dosages/Platelet Monitoring[2]	156	99%	98%	97%
Venous Thromboembolism Prophylaxis[2]	702	95%	90%	85%
Warfarin Therapy Discharge Instructions[2]	117	73%	78%	75%
Chest Pain/Possible Heart Attack Care				
Aspirin Given Within 24 Hours of Arrival[1]	-	-	97%	96%
Fibrinolytic Meds Within 30 Min. of Arrival[3,7]	-	-	44%	58%
Average Time to ECG (minutes)[1]	-	-	9	7
Average Time to Transfer (minutes)[3,7]	-	-	64	60
Children's Asthma Care				
Received Home Management Plan of Care	-	-	-	88%
Received Reliever Medication	-	-	-	100%
Received Systemic Corticosteroids	-	-	-	100%
Emergency Department				
Admittance Decision Time (minutes)[2]	2,208	194	104	98
Head CT Results Within 45 Min. of Arrival	16	56%	60%	57%
Patients Who Left ER Before Being Seen	86,942	2%	1%	2%
Time from ER Arrival to Admit. (minutes)[2]	2,209	386	276	274
Time from ER Arrival to Discharge (minutes)	732	140	125	134
Time in ER Before Being Evaluated (minutes)	812	35	26	26
Time to Pain Meds for Fractures (minutes)	88	71	58	57
Heart Attack Care				
Aspirin Given at Discharge	144	100%	99%	99%
Fibrinolytic Meds Within 30 Min. of Arrival[7]	-	-	40%	54%
PCI Within 90 Minutes of Arrival	15	93%	97%	96%
Statin Prescribed at Discharge	143	100%	99%	98%
Heart Failure Care				
ACE Inhibitor or ARB for LVSD	279	100%	97%	97%
Discharge Instructions Given	499	100%	96%	94%
Evaluation of LVS Function	584	100%	100%	99%
Medicare Spending				
Medicare Spending per Patient (ratio)	-	1.05	1.01	0.98
Pneumonia Care				
Appropriate Initial Antibiotic Given	154	99%	96%	95%
Blood Culture Timing	371	100%	98%	98%
Pregnancy and Delivery Care				
Newborn Deliveries Scheduled Early[7]	-	-	4%	6%
Preventive Care				
Immunization for Influenza[2]	1,212	93%	91%	90%
Immunization for Pneumonia[2]	1,778	90%	92%	92%
Stroke Care				
Anticoagulation Therapy for Atrial Fibrillation[1]	-	-	96%	95%
Antithrombotic Therapy Timing	193	100%	98%	98%
Assessed for Rehabilitation	209	99%	98%	97%
Discharged on Antithrombotic Therapy	176	100%	99%	99%
Discharged on Statin Medication	144	100%	95%	94%
Thrombolytic Therapy Timing[1]	-	-	72%	66%
Venous Thromboembolism Prophylaxis	221	98%	95%	94%
Written Stroke Educational Materials Given	126	100%	90%	88%
Surgical Care Improvement Project				
Appropriate Beta Blocker Usage	211	97%	98%	98%
Appropriate VTP Within 24 Hours	473	99%	99%	98%
Controlled Postoperative Blood Glucose	48	96%	98%	97%
Perioperative Temperature Management	553	100%	100%	100%
Prophylactic Antibiotic Selection	277	98%	99%	99%
Prophylactic Antibiotic Selection (Outpatient)	81	88%	98%	98%
Prophylactic Antibiotic Stopped	269	98%	98%	98%
Prophylactic Antibiotic Timing	278	100%	99%	99%
Prophylactic Antibiotic Timing (Outpatient)	67	90%	98%	98%
Urinary Catheter Removal	338	99%	99%	97%
Survey of Patients' Hospital Experiences				
Area Around Room 'Always' Quiet at Night	300+	53%	54%	61%
Doctors 'Always' Communicated Well	300+	75%	80%	82%
Home Recovery Information Given	300+	85%	86%	85%
Hospital Given 9 or 10 on 10 Point Scale	300+	56%	69%	71%
Meds 'Always' Explained Before Given	300+	58%	63%	64%
Nurses 'Always' Communicated Well	300+	75%	79%	79%
Pain 'Always' Well Controlled	300+	62%	70%	71%
Room and Bathroom 'Always' Clean	300+	68%	73%	73%
Timely Help 'Always' Received	300+	55%	67%	68%
Would Definitely Recommend Hospital	300+	54%	70%	71%
Use of Medical Imaging				
Cardiac Imaging Stress Test before Surgery	129	5.4%	5.4%	5.3%
Combination Abdominal CT Scan	588	7.3%	12.2%	10.5%
Combination Brain/Sinus CT Scan	551	4.9%	3.1%	2.7%
Combination Chest CT Scan	353	2.3%	2.1%	2.7%
Follow-up Mammogram/Ultrasound	1,263	10.8%	9%	8.8%
Lumbar Spine MRI for Low Back Pain	90	27.8%	35.8%	37.2%

Doylestown Hospital

595 West State St
Doylestown, PA 18901
URL: www.dh.org
Type: Acute Care Hospitals
Ownership: Voluntary non-profit - Private

Phone: 215-345-2200
Fax: 215-345-2827
Emergency Services: Yes
Beds: 165

Key Personnel:
Radiology.................. Linda Barnhurst
CEO/President.............. James Brexler

NOTE: Hospital profiles are in alphabetical order by state, then city, then hospital within the city; Rankings exclude hospitals with less than 25 cases except for patient surveys which excludes hospitals with less than 100 cases; (a) 100-299 cases; (1) The number of cases/patients is too few to report; (2) Data submitted were based on a sample of cases/patients; (3) Results are based on a shorter time period than required; (4) Data suppressed by CMS for one or more quarters; (5) Results are not available for this reporting period; (6) Fewer than 100 patients completed the HCAHPS survey; (7) No cases met the criteria for this measure; (8) The lower limit of the confidence interval cannot be calculated if the number of observed infections equals zero; (9) No data are available from the state/territory for this reporting period; (10) The scores shown reflect fewer than 50 completed surveys; (11) There were discrepancies in the data collection process; (12) This measure does not apply to this hospital for this reporting period; (13) Results cannot be calculated for this reporting period; (14) The results for this state are combined with nearby states to protect confidentiality; Please refer to the User's Guide for a full explanation of data.

Chairman/CEO .... Carolyn Della-Rodolfa
Chief of Medical Staff.......... Scott S Levy
Cardiac Laboratory............ Dave Martens

Measure	Cases	This Hosp.	State Avg.	U.S. Avg.
Blood Clot Prevention and Treatment				
Anticoagulation Overlap Therapy[2]	85	92%	94%	93%
ICU Venous Thromboembolism Prophylaxis[2]	58	98%	94%	92%
Incidence of Potentially Preventable VTE[1,2]	-	-	8%	10%
UFH with Dosages/Platelet Monitoring[2]	44	100%	98%	97%
Venous Thromboembolism Prophylaxis[2]	408	98%	90%	85%
Warfarin Therapy Discharge Instructions[2]	64	100%	78%	75%
Chest Pain/Possible Heart Attack Care				
Aspirin Given Within 24 Hours of Arrival[1,3]	-	-	97%	96%
Fibrinolytic Meds Within 30 Min. of Arrival[5]	-	-	44%	58%
Average Time to ECG (minutes)[1,3]	-	-	9	7
Average Time to Transfer (minutes)[5]	-	-	64	60
Children's Asthma Care				
Received Home Management Plan of Care	-	-	-	88%
Received Reliever Medication	-	-	-	100%
Received Systemic Corticosteroids	-	-	-	100%
Emergency Department				
Admittance Decision Time (minutes)[2]	840	157	104	98
Head CT Results Within 45 Min. of Arrival	30	63%	60%	57%
Patients Who Left ER Before Being Seen	45,748	0%	1%	2%
Time from ER Arrival to Admit. (minutes)[2]	841	349	276	274
Time from ER Arrival to Discharge (minutes)	361	145	125	134
Time in ER Before Being Evaluated (minutes)	384	26	26	26
Time to Pain Meds for Fractures (minutes)	175	54	58	57
Heart Attack Care				
Aspirin Given at Discharge	305	100%	99%	99%
Fibrinolytic Meds Within 30 Min. of Arrival[7]	-	-	40%	54%
PCI Within 90 Minutes of Arrival	59	98%	97%	96%
Statin Prescribed at Discharge	281	100%	99%	98%
Heart Failure Care				
ACE Inhibitor or ARB for LVSD	119	100%	97%	97%
Discharge Instructions Given	357	98%	96%	94%
Evaluation of LVS Function	466	100%	100%	99%
Medicare Spending				
Medicare Spending per Patient (ratio)	-	1.00	1.01	0.98
Pneumonia Care				
Appropriate Initial Antibiotic Given	236	97%	96%	95%
Blood Culture Timing	479	99%	98%	98%
Pregnancy and Delivery Care				
Newborn Deliveries Scheduled Early[2]	26	12%	4%	6%
Preventive Care				
Immunization for Influenza[2]	580	96%	91%	90%
Immunization for Pneumonia[2]	822	92%	92%	92%
Stroke Care				
Anticoagulation Therapy for Atrial Fibrillation	44	98%	96%	95%
Antithrombotic Therapy Timing	140	100%	98%	98%
Assessed for Rehabilitation	159	99%	98%	97%
Discharged on Antithrombotic Therapy	157	100%	99%	99%
Discharged on Statin Medication	112	99%	95%	94%
Thrombolytic Therapy Timing	15	93%	72%	66%
Venous Thromboembolism Prophylaxis	156	99%	95%	94%
Written Stroke Educational Materials Given	91	100%	90%	88%
Surgical Care Improvement Project				
Appropriate Beta Blocker Usage[2]	322	98%	98%	98%
Appropriate VTP Within 24 Hours[2]	658	97%	99%	98%
Controlled Postoperative Blood Glucose[2]	192	99%	98%	97%
Perioperative Temperature Management[2]	817	100%	100%	100%
Prophylactic Antibiotic Selection[2]	735	99%	99%	99%
Prophylactic Antibiotic Selection (Outpatient)	329	98%	98%	98%
Prophylactic Antibiotic Stopped[2]	721	100%	98%	98%
Prophylactic Antibiotic Timing[2]	737	100%	99%	99%
Prophylactic Antibiotic Timing (Outpatient)	332	98%	98%	98%
Urinary Catheter Removal[2]	678	98%	99%	97%
Survey of Patients' Hospital Experiences				
Area Around Room 'Always' Quiet at Night	300+	53%	54%	61%
Doctors 'Always' Communicated Well	300+	82%	80%	82%
Home Recovery Information Given	300+	88%	86%	85%
Hospital Given 9 or 10 on 10 Point Scale	300+	83%	69%	71%
Meds 'Always' Explained Before Given	300+	65%	63%	64%
Nurses 'Always' Communicated Well	300+	86%	79%	79%
Pain 'Always' Well Controlled	300+	78%	70%	71%
Room and Bathroom 'Always' Clean	300+	77%	73%	73%
Timely Help 'Always' Received	300+	78%	67%	68%
Would Definitely Recommend Hospital	300+	87%	70%	71%
Use of Medical Imaging				
Cardiac Imaging Stress Test before Surgery	968	5.8%	5.4%	5.3%
Combination Abdominal CT Scan	1,162	13.3%	12.2%	10.5%
Combination Brain/Sinus CT Scan	861	2.1%	3.1%	2.7%
Combination Chest CT Scan	802	0.1%	2.1%	2.7%
Follow-up Mammogram/Ultrasound	3,061	9.0%	9%	8.8%
Lumbar Spine MRI for Low Back Pain	171	34.5%	35.8%	37.2%

Delaware County Memorial Hospital

501 North Lansdowne Ave
Drexel Hill, PA 19026
Phone: 215-284-8100
Fax: 610-284-8993
URL: www.crozer.org
Type: Acute Care Hospitals
Emergency Services: Yes
Ownership: Voluntary non-profit - Private
Beds: 247

Key Personnel:
Radiology.................... Thomas A DiLiberto, DO
Operating Room.............. Seth A Malin, RN
Chief of Medical Staff.......... Lawrence Mayer, MD
Quality Assurance .... Joan Meighan
Pediatric In-Patient Care .... David Pollack, MD
Emergency Room .... John Reilley, MD
President/CEO................ Joan K Richards

Measure	Cases	This Hosp.	State Avg.	U.S. Avg.
Blood Clot Prevention and Treatment				
Anticoagulation Overlap Therapy[2]	60	98%	94%	93%
ICU Venous Thromboembolism Prophylaxis[2]	23	100%	94%	92%
Incidence of Potentially Preventable VTE[1,2]	-	-	8%	10%
UFH with Dosages/Platelet Monitoring[2]	41	100%	98%	97%
Venous Thromboembolism Prophylaxis[2]	409	99%	90%	85%
Warfarin Therapy Discharge Instructions[2]	48	92%	78%	75%
Chest Pain/Possible Heart Attack Care				
Aspirin Given Within 24 Hours of Arrival	43	95%	97%	96%
Fibrinolytic Meds Within 30 Min. of Arrival[7]	-	-	44%	58%
Average Time to ECG (minutes)	44	7	9	7
Average Time to Transfer (minutes)	17	36	64	60
Children's Asthma Care				
Received Home Management Plan of Care	-	-	-	88%
Received Reliever Medication	-	-	-	100%
Received Systemic Corticosteroids	-	-	-	100%
Emergency Department				
Admittance Decision Time (minutes)[2]	540	170	104	98
Head CT Results Within 45 Min. of Arrival	14	86%	60%	57%
Patients Who Left ER Before Being Seen	40,452	0%	1%	2%
Time from ER Arrival to Admit. (minutes)[2]	540	370	276	274
Time from ER Arrival to Discharge (minutes)	339	177	125	134
Time in ER Before Being Evaluated (minutes)	320	78	26	26
Time to Pain Meds for Fractures (minutes)	114	56	58	57
Heart Attack Care				
Aspirin Given at Discharge	22	100%	99%	99%
Fibrinolytic Meds Within 30 Min. of Arrival[7]	-	-	40%	54%
PCI Within 90 Minutes of Arrival[7]	-	-	97%	96%
Statin Prescribed at Discharge	17	100%	99%	98%
Heart Failure Care				
ACE Inhibitor or ARB for LVSD	29	100%	97%	97%
Discharge Instructions Given	145	100%	96%	94%
Evaluation of LVS Function	191	100%	100%	99%
Medicare Spending				
Medicare Spending per Patient (ratio)	-	1.12	1.01	0.98
Pneumonia Care				
Appropriate Initial Antibiotic Given	125	98%	96%	95%
Blood Culture Timing	179	100%	98%	98%
Pregnancy and Delivery Care				
Newborn Deliveries Scheduled Early[2]	18	0%	4%	6%
Preventive Care				
Immunization for Influenza[2]	504	99%	91%	90%
Immunization for Pneumonia[2]	546	99%	92%	92%
Stroke Care				
Anticoagulation Therapy for Atrial Fibrillation[1]	-	-	96%	95%
Antithrombotic Therapy Timing	74	99%	98%	98%
Assessed for Rehabilitation	77	99%	98%	97%
Discharged on Antithrombotic Therapy	76	99%	99%	99%
Discharged on Statin Medication	45	96%	95%	94%
Thrombolytic Therapy Timing[1]	-	-	72%	66%
Venous Thromboembolism Prophylaxis	80	95%	95%	94%
Written Stroke Educational Materials Given	43	93%	90%	88%
Surgical Care Improvement Project				
Appropriate Beta Blocker Usage[2]	148	98%	98%	98%
Appropriate VTP Within 24 Hours[2]	437	99%	99%	98%
Controlled Postoperative Blood Glucose[2,7]	-	-	98%	97%
Perioperative Temperature Management[2]	484	100%	100%	100%
Prophylactic Antibiotic Selection[2]	333	97%	99%	99%
Prophylactic Antibiotic Selection (Outpatient)	51	94%	98%	98%
Prophylactic Antibiotic Stopped[2]	327	96%	98%	98%
Prophylactic Antibiotic Timing[2]	333	100%	99%	99%
Prophylactic Antibiotic Timing (Outpatient)	53	91%	98%	98%
Urinary Catheter Removal[2]	313	98%	99%	97%
Survey of Patients' Hospital Experiences				
Area Around Room 'Always' Quiet at Night	300+	57%	54%	61%
Doctors 'Always' Communicated Well	300+	77%	80%	82%
Home Recovery Information Given	300+	84%	86%	85%
Hospital Given 9 or 10 on 10 Point Scale	300+	61%	69%	71%
Meds 'Always' Explained Before Given	300+	58%	63%	64%
Nurses 'Always' Communicated Well	300+	77%	79%	79%
Pain 'Always' Well Controlled	300+	71%	70%	71%
Room and Bathroom 'Always' Clean	300+	61%	73%	73%
Timely Help 'Always' Received	300+	61%	67%	68%
Would Definitely Recommend Hospital	300+	63%	70%	71%
Use of Medical Imaging				
Cardiac Imaging Stress Test before Surgery[1]	-	-	5.4%	5.3%
Combination Abdominal CT Scan	719	35.0%	12.2%	10.5%
Combination Brain/Sinus CT Scan[1]	-	-	3.1%	2.7%
Combination Chest CT Scan	500	0.0%	2.1%	2.7%
Follow-up Mammogram/Ultrasound	930	6.3%	9%	8.8%
Lumbar Spine MRI for Low Back Pain[1]	-	-	35.8%	37.2%

Penn Highlands Dubois

100 Hospital Avenue
Dubois, PA 15801
Phone: 814-371-2200
Fax: 814-375-3342
URL: www.drmc.org
Type: Acute Care Hospitals
Emergency Services: Yes
Ownership: Voluntary non-profit - Other
Beds: 214

Key Personnel:
Infection Control.............. Carole Berger
Emergency Room .... Russell E Cameron
Hemotology Center .... Rose Campbell
CEO/President................ Raymond Graeca
Radiology.................... George M Kosco
Intensive Care Unit............ Jean Matsko
Operating Room.............. Mary Ann Nicometo

Measure	Cases	This Hosp.	State Avg.	U.S. Avg.
Blood Clot Prevention and Treatment				
Anticoagulation Overlap Therapy[2]	44	100%	94%	93%
ICU Venous Thromboembolism Prophylaxis[2]	147	98%	94%	92%
Incidence of Potentially Preventable VTE[1,2]	-	-	8%	10%
UFH with Dosages/Platelet Monitoring[2]	21	100%	98%	97%
Venous Thromboembolism Prophylaxis[2]	207	96%	90%	85%
Warfarin Therapy Discharge Instructions[2]	33	100%	78%	75%
Chest Pain/Possible Heart Attack Care				
Aspirin Given Within 24 Hours of Arrival[1,3]	-	-	97%	96%
Fibrinolytic Meds Within 30 Min. of Arrival[5]	-	-	44%	58%
Average Time to ECG (minutes)[1,3]	-	-	9	7
Average Time to Transfer (minutes)[5]	-	-	64	60
Children's Asthma Care				
Received Home Management Plan of Care	-	-	-	88%
Received Reliever Medication	-	-	-	100%
Received Systemic Corticosteroids	-	-	-	100%
Emergency Department				
Admittance Decision Time (minutes)[2]	416	103	104	98
Head CT Results Within 45 Min. of Arrival[1]	-	-	60%	57%
Patients Who Left ER Before Being Seen	32,692	1%	1%	2%
Time from ER Arrival to Admit. (minutes)[2]	416	252	276	274
Time from ER Arrival to Discharge (minutes)	339	119	125	134

NOTE: Hospital profiles are in alphabetical order by state, then city, then hospital within the city; Rankings exclude hospitals with less than 25 cases except for patient surveys which excludes hospitals with less than 100 cases; (a) 100-299 cases; (1) The number of cases/patients is too few to report; (2) Data submitted were based on a sample of cases/patients; (3) Results are based on a shorter time period than required; (4) Data suppressed by CMS for one or more quarters; (5) Results are not available for this reporting period; (6) Fewer than 100 patients completed the HCAHPS survey; (7) No cases met the criteria for this measure; (8) The lower limit of the confidence interval cannot be calculated if the number of observed infections equals zero; (9) No data are available from the state/territory for this reporting period; (10) The scores shown reflect fewer than 50 completed surveys; (11) There were discrepancies in the data collection process; (12) This measure does not apply to this hospital for this reporting period; (13) Results cannot be calculated for this reporting period; (14) The results for this state are combined with nearby states to protect confidentiality; Please refer to the User's Guide for a full explanation of data.

Measure	Cases	This Hosp.	State Avg.	U.S. Avg.
Time in ER Before Being Evaluated (minutes)	380	10	26	26
Time to Pain Meds for Fractures (minutes)	138	41	58	57
Heart Attack Care				
Aspirin Given at Discharge	268	100%	99%	99%
Fibrinolytic Meds Within 30 Min. of Arrival[1]	-	-	40%	54%
PCI Within 90 Minutes of Arrival	30	97%	97%	96%
Statin Prescribed at Discharge	257	100%	99%	98%
Heart Failure Care				
ACE Inhibitor or ARB for LVSD	81	99%	97%	97%
Discharge Instructions Given	209	98%	96%	94%
Evaluation of LVS Function	252	100%	100%	99%
Medicare Spending				
Medicare Spending per Patient (ratio)	-	0.94	1.01	0.98
Pneumonia Care				
Appropriate Initial Antibiotic Given	80	98%	96%	95%
Blood Culture Timing	156	98%	98%	98%
Pregnancy and Delivery Care				
Newborn Deliveries Scheduled Early	64	2%	4%	6%
Preventive Care				
Immunization for Influenza[2]	512	97%	91%	90%
Immunization for Pneumonia[2]	595	97%	92%	92%
Stroke Care				
Anticoagulation Therapy for Atrial Fibrillation	11	91%	96%	95%
Antithrombotic Therapy Timing	50	100%	98%	98%
Assessed for Rehabilitation	59	95%	98%	97%
Discharged on Antithrombotic Therapy	59	100%	99%	99%
Discharged on Statin Medication	41	100%	95%	94%
Thrombolytic Therapy Timing[1]	-	-	72%	66%
Venous Thromboembolism Prophylaxis	52	98%	95%	94%
Written Stroke Educational Materials Given	34	100%	90%	88%
Surgical Care Improvement Project				
Appropriate Beta Blocker Usage	199	98%	98%	98%
Appropriate VTP Within 24 Hours	321	98%	99%	98%
Controlled Postoperative Blood Glucose	88	99%	98%	97%
Perioperative Temperature Management	361	100%	100%	100%
Prophylactic Antibiotic Selection	330	100%	99%	99%
Prophylactic Antibiotic Selection (Outpatient)	238	99%	98%	98%
Prophylactic Antibiotic Stopped	321	100%	98%	98%
Prophylactic Antibiotic Timing	330	100%	99%	99%
Prophylactic Antibiotic Timing (Outpatient)	162	99%	98%	98%
Urinary Catheter Removal	268	99%	99%	97%
Survey of Patients' Hospital Experiences				
Area Around Room 'Always' Quiet at Night	300+	58%	54%	61%
Doctors 'Always' Communicated Well	300+	85%	80%	82%
Home Recovery Information Given	300+	89%	86%	85%
Hospital Given 9 or 10 on 10 Point Scale	300+	77%	69%	71%
Meds 'Always' Explained Before Given	300+	69%	63%	64%
Nurses 'Always' Communicated Well	300+	84%	79%	79%
Pain 'Always' Well Controlled	300+	77%	70%	71%
Room and Bathroom 'Always' Clean	300+	76%	73%	73%
Timely Help 'Always' Received	300+	76%	67%	68%
Would Definitely Recommend Hospital	300+	76%	70%	71%
Use of Medical Imaging				
Cardiac Imaging Stress Test before Surgery	457	4.2%	5.4%	5.3%
Combination Abdominal CT Scan	1,071	8.9%	12.2%	10.5%
Combination Brain/Sinus CT Scan	700	3.1%	3.1%	2.7%
Combination Chest CT Scan	595	2.4%	2.1%	2.7%
Follow-up Mammogram/Ultrasound	1,758	4.2%	9%	8.8%
Lumbar Spine MRI for Low Back Pain	160	35.6%	35.8%	37.2%

Eagleville Hospital

100 Eagleville Rd — Phone: 215-539-6000
Eagleville, PA 19408 — Fax: 610-539-8319
URL: www.eaglevillehospital.org
Type: Acute Care Hospitals — Emergency Services: No
Ownership: Voluntary non-profit - Private — Beds: 350

Key Personnel:
CEO/President.............. Maureen King Pollock
Chair/CEO.................. Jon A. Shapiro, MD

Measure	Cases	This Hosp.	State Avg.	U.S. Avg.
Blood Clot Prevention and Treatment				
Anticoagulation Overlap Therapy[2,7]	-	-	94%	93%
ICU Venous Thromboembolism Prophylaxis[2,7]	-	-	94%	92%
Incidence of Potentially Preventable VTE[1,2]	-	-	8%	10%
UFH with Dosages/Platelet Monitoring[2,7]	-	-	98%	97%
Venous Thromboembolism Prophylaxis[2,7]	-	-	90%	85%
Warfarin Therapy Discharge Instructions[2,7]	-	-	78%	75%
Chest Pain/Possible Heart Attack Care				
Aspirin Given Within 24 Hours of Arrival[5]	-	-	97%	96%
Fibrinolytic Meds Within 30 Min. of Arrival[5]	-	-	44%	58%
Average Time to ECG (minutes)[5]	-	-	9	7
Average Time to Transfer (minutes)[5]	-	-	64	60
Children's Asthma Care				
Received Home Management Plan of Care	-	-	-	88%
Received Reliever Medication	-	-	-	100%
Received Systemic Corticosteroids	-	-	-	100%
Emergency Department				
Admittance Decision Time (minutes)[2,7]	-	-	104	98
Head CT Results Within 45 Min. of Arrival[5]	-	-	60%	57%
Patients Who Left ER Before Being Seen[5]	-	-	1%	2%
Time from ER Arrival to Admit. (minutes)[2,7]	-	-	276	274
Time from ER Arrival to Discharge (minutes)[5]	-	-	125	134
Time in ER Before Being Evaluated (minutes)[5]	-	-	26	26
Time to Pain Meds for Fractures (minutes)[5]	-	-	58	57
Heart Attack Care				
Aspirin Given at Discharge[5]	-	-	99%	99%
Fibrinolytic Meds Within 30 Min. of Arrival[5]	-	-	40%	54%
PCI Within 90 Minutes of Arrival[5]	-	-	97%	96%
Statin Prescribed at Discharge[5]	-	-	99%	98%
Heart Failure Care				
ACE Inhibitor or ARB for LVSD[5]	-	-	97%	97%
Discharge Instructions Given[5]	-	-	96%	94%
Evaluation of LVS Function[5]	-	-	100%	99%
Medicare Spending				
Medicare Spending per Patient (ratio)	-	0.81	1.01	0.98
Pneumonia Care				
Appropriate Initial Antibiotic Given[5]	-	-	96%	95%
Blood Culture Timing[5]	-	-	98%	98%
Pregnancy and Delivery Care				
Newborn Deliveries Scheduled Early[7]	-	-	4%	6%
Preventive Care				
Immunization for Influenza[2]	419	55%	91%	90%
Immunization for Pneumonia[2]	199	48%	92%	92%
Stroke Care				
Anticoagulation Therapy for Atrial Fibrillation[5]	-	-	96%	95%
Antithrombotic Therapy Timing[5]	-	-	98%	98%
Assessed for Rehabilitation[5]	-	-	98%	97%
Discharged on Antithrombotic Therapy[5]	-	-	99%	99%
Discharged on Statin Medication[5]	-	-	95%	94%
Thrombolytic Therapy Timing[5]	-	-	72%	66%
Venous Thromboembolism Prophylaxis[5]	-	-	95%	94%
Written Stroke Educational Materials Given[5]	-	-	90%	88%
Surgical Care Improvement Project				
Appropriate Beta Blocker Usage[5]	-	-	98%	98%
Appropriate VTP Within 24 Hours[5]	-	-	99%	98%
Controlled Postoperative Blood Glucose[5]	-	-	98%	97%
Perioperative Temperature Management[5]	-	-	100%	100%
Prophylactic Antibiotic Selection[5]	-	-	99%	99%
Prophylactic Antibiotic Selection (Outpatient)[5]	-	-	98%	98%
Prophylactic Antibiotic Stopped[5]	-	-	98%	98%
Prophylactic Antibiotic Timing[5]	-	-	99%	99%
Prophylactic Antibiotic Timing (Outpatient)[5]	-	-	98%	98%
Urinary Catheter Removal[5]	-	-	99%	97%
Survey of Patients' Hospital Experiences				
Area Around Room 'Always' Quiet at Night[1]	-	-	54%	61%
Doctors 'Always' Communicated Well[1]	-	-	80%	82%
Home Recovery Information Given[1]	-	-	86%	85%
Hospital Given 9 or 10 on 10 Point Scale[1]	-	-	69%	71%
Meds 'Always' Explained Before Given[1]	-	-	63%	64%
Nurses 'Always' Communicated Well[1]	-	-	79%	79%
Pain 'Always' Well Controlled[1]	-	-	70%	71%
Room and Bathroom 'Always' Clean[1]	-	-	73%	73%
Timely Help 'Always' Received[1]	-	-	67%	68%
Would Definitely Recommend Hospital[1]	-	-	70%	71%
Use of Medical Imaging				
Cardiac Imaging Stress Test before Surgery[7]	-	-	5.4%	5.3%
Combination Abdominal CT Scan[7]	-	-	12.2%	10.5%
Combination Brain/Sinus CT Scan[7]	-	-	3.1%	2.7%
Combination Chest CT Scan[7]	-	-	2.1%	2.7%
Follow-up Mammogram/Ultrasound[7]	-	-	9%	8.8%
Lumbar Spine MRI for Low Back Pain[7]	-	-	35.8%	37.2%

Einstein Medical Center Montgomery

559 West Germantown Pike — Phone: 484-662-1000
East Norriton, PA 19403
Type: Acute Care Hospitals — Emergency Services: Yes
Ownership: Voluntary non-profit - Private

Measure	Cases	This Hosp.	State Avg.	U.S. Avg.
Blood Clot Prevention and Treatment				
Anticoagulation Overlap Therapy[2]	43	100%	94%	93%
ICU Venous Thromboembolism Prophylaxis[2]	74	93%	94%	92%
Incidence of Potentially Preventable VTE[1,2]	-	-	8%	10%
UFH with Dosages/Platelet Monitoring[2]	24	100%	98%	97%
Venous Thromboembolism Prophylaxis[2]	351	81%	90%	85%
Warfarin Therapy Discharge Instructions[2]	29	79%	78%	75%
Chest Pain/Possible Heart Attack Care				
Aspirin Given Within 24 Hours of Arrival[1,3]	-	-	97%	96%
Fibrinolytic Meds Within 30 Min. of Arrival[3,7]	-	-	44%	58%
Average Time to ECG (minutes)[1,3]	-	-	9	7
Average Time to Transfer (minutes)[3,7]	-	-	64	60
Children's Asthma Care				
Received Home Management Plan of Care	-	-	-	88%
Received Reliever Medication	-	-	-	100%
Received Systemic Corticosteroids	-	-	-	100%
Emergency Department				
Admittance Decision Time (minutes)[2,3]	436	162	104	98
Head CT Results Within 45 Min. of Arrival[1,3]	-	-	60%	57%
Patients Who Left ER Before Being Seen	8,987	0%	1%	2%
Time from ER Arrival to Admit. (minutes)[2,3]	442	354	276	274
Time from ER Arrival to Discharge (minutes)[3]	270	129	125	134
Time in ER Before Being Evaluated (minutes)[3]	294	41	26	26
Time to Pain Meds for Fractures (minutes)[3]	70	46	58	57
Heart Attack Care				
Aspirin Given at Discharge[3]	179	100%	99%	99%
Fibrinolytic Meds Within 30 Min. of Arrival[3,7]	-	-	40%	54%
PCI Within 90 Minutes of Arrival[3]	31	94%	97%	96%
Statin Prescribed at Discharge[3]	174	99%	99%	98%
Heart Failure Care				
ACE Inhibitor or ARB for LVSD[2,3]	66	95%	97%	97%
Discharge Instructions Given[2,3]	179	100%	96%	94%
Evaluation of LVS Function[2,3]	222	100%	100%	99%
Medicare Spending				
Medicare Spending per Patient (ratio)	-	1.04	1.01	0.98
Pneumonia Care				
Appropriate Initial Antibiotic Given[3]	70	94%	96%	95%
Blood Culture Timing[3]	48	98%	98%	98%
Pregnancy and Delivery Care				
Newborn Deliveries Scheduled Early[2]	34	3%	4%	6%
Preventive Care				
Immunization for Influenza[2,3]	255	95%	91%	90%
Immunization for Pneumonia[2,3]	437	85%	92%	92%
Stroke Care				
Anticoagulation Therapy for Atrial Fibrillation[1,2]	-	-	96%	95%
Antithrombotic Therapy Timing[2]	80	99%	98%	98%
Assessed for Rehabilitation[2]	80	96%	98%	97%
Discharged on Antithrombotic Therapy[2]	74	99%	99%	99%
Discharged on Statin Medication[2]	69	96%	95%	94%
Thrombolytic Therapy Timing[1,2]	-	-	72%	66%
Venous Thromboembolism Prophylaxis[2]	89	79%	95%	94%
Written Stroke Educational Materials Given[2]	52	31%	90%	88%
Surgical Care Improvement Project				
Appropriate Beta Blocker Usage[2,3]	147	99%	98%	98%
Appropriate VTP Within 24 Hours[2,3]	225	97%	99%	98%
Controlled Postoperative Blood Glucose[2,3]	99	98%	98%	97%
Perioperative Temperature Management[2,3]	283	100%	100%	100%
Prophylactic Antibiotic Selection[2,3]	273	99%	99%	99%
Prophylactic Antibiotic Selection (Outpatient)[3]	175	97%	98%	98%

NOTE: Hospital profiles are in alphabetical order by state, then city, then hospital within the city; Rankings exclude hospitals with less than 25 cases except for patient surveys which excludes hospitals with less than 100 cases; (a) 100-299 cases; (1) The number of cases/patients is too few to report; (2) Data submitted were based on a sample of cases/patients; (3) Results are based on a shorter time period than required; (4) Data suppressed by CMS for one or more quarters; (5) Results are not available for this reporting period; (6) Fewer than 100 patients completed the HCAHPS survey; (7) No cases met the criteria for this measure; (8) The lower limit of the confidence interval cannot be calculated if the number of observed infections equals zero; (9) No data are available from the state/territory for this reporting period; (10) The scores shown reflect fewer than 50 completed surveys; (11) There were discrepancies in the data collection process; (12) This measure does not apply to this hospital for this reporting period; (13) Results cannot be calculated for this reporting period; (14) The results for this state are combined with nearby states to protect confidentiality; Please refer to the User's Guide for a full explanation of data.

Measure	Cases	This Hosp.	State Avg.	U.S. Avg.
Prophylactic Antibiotic Stopped[2,3]	269	97%	98%	98%
Prophylactic Antibiotic Timing[2,3]	273	99%	99%	99%
Prophylactic Antibiotic Timing (Outpatient)[3]	175	100%	98%	98%
Urinary Catheter Removal[2,3]	134	96%	99%	97%
Survey of Patients' Hospital Experiences				
Area Around Room 'Always' Quiet at Night	300+	60%	54%	61%
Doctors 'Always' Communicated Well	300+	74%	80%	82%
Home Recovery Information Given	300+	82%	86%	85%
Hospital Given 9 or 10 on 10 Point Scale	300+	72%	69%	71%
Meds 'Always' Explained Before Given	300+	59%	63%	64%
Nurses 'Always' Communicated Well	300+	78%	79%	79%
Pain 'Always' Well Controlled	300+	66%	70%	71%
Room and Bathroom 'Always' Clean	300+	74%	73%	73%
Timely Help 'Always' Received	300+	63%	67%	68%
Would Definitely Recommend Hospital	300+	78%	70%	71%
Use of Medical Imaging				
Cardiac Imaging Stress Test before Surgery	46	4.3%	5.4%	5.3%
Combination Abdominal CT Scan	408	7.6%	12.2%	10.5%
Combination Brain/Sinus CT Scan[1]	-	-	3.1%	2.7%
Combination Chest CT Scan	315	1.6%	2.1%	2.7%
Follow-up Mammogram/Ultrasound	755	10.3%	9%	8.8%
Lumbar Spine MRI for Low Back Pain[1]	-	-	35.8%	37.2%

Pocono Medical Center

206 East Brown Street
East Stroudsburg, PA 18301
Phone: 570-476-3348
Fax: 570-476-3604
E-mail: feedback@pmchealthsystem.org
URL: www.poconohealthsystem.org
Type: Acute Care Hospitals
Emergency Services: Yes
Ownership: Voluntary non-profit - Private
Beds: 192

Key Personnel:

Radiology. . . . . Dana Burke, MD
Quality Assurance . . . . Eileen Caden
Chief of Medical Staff . . . . Howard Davis, MD
Cardiac Laboratory. . . . . Georganne DeGavany
Pediatric Ambulatory Care . . . . . . Arthur Dixon, MD
Pediatric In-Patient Care . . . . Arthur Dixon, MD
Operating Room. . . . . Thomas Gerold
President/CEO. . . . . Jeffrey E. Snyder

Measure	Cases	This Hosp.	State Avg.	U.S. Avg.
Blood Clot Prevention and Treatment				
Anticoagulation Overlap Therapy[2]	107	92%	94%	93%
ICU Venous Thromboembolism Prophylaxis[2]	106	92%	94%	92%
Incidence of Potentially Preventable VTE[2]	13	46%	8%	10%
UFH with Dosages/Platelet Monitoring[2]	76	99%	98%	97%
Venous Thromboembolism Prophylaxis[2]	441	90%	90%	85%
Warfarin Therapy Discharge Instructions[2]	77	18%	78%	75%
Chest Pain/Possible Heart Attack Care				
Aspirin Given Within 24 Hours of Arrival[1]	-	-	97%	96%
Fibrinolytic Meds Within 30 Min. of Arrival[3,7]	-	-	44%	58%
Average Time to ECG (minutes)[1]	-	-	9	7
Average Time to Transfer (minutes)[3,7]	-	-	64	60
Children's Asthma Care				
Received Home Management Plan of Care	-	-	-	88%
Received Reliever Medication	-	-	-	100%
Received Systemic Corticosteroids	-	-	-	100%
Emergency Department				
Admittance Decision Time (minutes)[2]	1,018	182	104	98
Head CT Results Within 45 Min. of Arrival[1]	-	-	60%	57%
Patients Who Left ER Before Being Seen	82,215	4%	1%	2%
Time from ER Arrival to Admit. (minutes)[2]	1,019	339	276	274
Time from ER Arrival to Discharge (minutes)	577	116	125	134
Time in ER Before Being Evaluated (minutes)[1]	-	-	26	26
Time to Pain Meds for Fractures (minutes)	392	58	58	57
Heart Attack Care				
Aspirin Given at Discharge	260	100%	99%	99%
Fibrinolytic Meds Within 30 Min. of Arrival[7]	-	-	40%	54%
PCI Within 90 Minutes of Arrival	78	100%	97%	96%
Statin Prescribed at Discharge	253	98%	99%	98%
Heart Failure Care				
ACE Inhibitor or ARB for LVSD	115	99%	97%	97%
Discharge Instructions Given	311	95%	96%	94%
Evaluation of LVS Function	401	100%	100%	99%
Medicare Spending				
Medicare Spending per Patient (ratio)	-	1.03	1.01	0.98
Pneumonia Care				
Appropriate Initial Antibiotic Given	192	93%	96%	95%
Blood Culture Timing	339	99%	98%	98%
Pregnancy and Delivery Care				
Newborn Deliveries Scheduled Early[2]	68	6%	4%	6%
Preventive Care				
Immunization for Influenza[2]	662	92%	91%	90%
Immunization for Pneumonia[2]	907	91%	92%	92%
Stroke Care				
Anticoagulation Therapy for Atrial Fibrillation	29	86%	96%	95%
Antithrombotic Therapy Timing	153	97%	98%	98%
Assessed for Rehabilitation	160	93%	98%	97%
Discharged on Antithrombotic Therapy	156	98%	99%	99%
Discharged on Statin Medication	124	84%	95%	94%
Thrombolytic Therapy Timing[1]	-	-	72%	66%
Venous Thromboembolism Prophylaxis	153	80%	95%	94%
Written Stroke Educational Materials Given	97	99%	90%	88%
Surgical Care Improvement Project				
Appropriate Beta Blocker Usage	205	97%	98%	98%
Appropriate VTP Within 24 Hours	417	97%	99%	98%
Controlled Postoperative Blood Glucose	124	98%	98%	97%
Perioperative Temperature Management	523	100%	100%	100%
Prophylactic Antibiotic Selection	396	97%	99%	99%
Prophylactic Antibiotic Selection (Outpatient)	315	98%	98%	98%
Prophylactic Antibiotic Stopped	378	98%	98%	98%
Prophylactic Antibiotic Timing	398	99%	99%	99%
Prophylactic Antibiotic Timing (Outpatient)	315	100%	98%	98%
Urinary Catheter Removal	426	98%	99%	97%
Survey of Patients' Hospital Experiences				
Area Around Room 'Always' Quiet at Night	300+	53%	54%	61%
Doctors 'Always' Communicated Well	300+	78%	80%	82%
Home Recovery Information Given	300+	83%	86%	85%
Hospital Given 9 or 10 on 10 Point Scale	300+	66%	69%	71%
Meds 'Always' Explained Before Given	300+	60%	63%	64%
Nurses 'Always' Communicated Well	300+	79%	79%	79%
Pain 'Always' Well Controlled	300+	69%	70%	71%
Room and Bathroom 'Always' Clean	300+	77%	73%	73%
Timely Help 'Always' Received	300+	65%	67%	68%
Would Definitely Recommend Hospital	300+	66%	70%	71%
Use of Medical Imaging				
Cardiac Imaging Stress Test before Surgery	566	7.8%	5.4%	5.3%
Combination Abdominal CT Scan	1,614	5.9%	12.2%	10.5%
Combination Brain/Sinus CT Scan	1,070	3.9%	3.1%	2.7%
Combination Chest CT Scan	731	2.7%	2.1%	2.7%
Follow-up Mammogram/Ultrasound	601	11.8%	9%	8.8%
Lumbar Spine MRI for Low Back Pain	37	45.9%	35.8%	37.2%

Easton Hospital

250 South 21st Street
Easton, PA 18042
Phone: 610-250-4076
Fax: 610-250-4078
URL: www.easton-hospital.com
Type: Acute Care Hospitals
Emergency Services: Yes
Ownership: Proprietary
Beds: 233

Key Personnel:

CEO/President. . . . . Roy Boyd
Anesthesiology. . . . . Michael Feldman, MD
Operating Room. . . . . Dave Kasprzak
Infection Control. . . . . Lisa Knaak
Pediatric In-Patient Care . . . . Prem K Marlapudi, MD
Quality Assurance . . . . Tara Reid
Emergency Room . . . . Robert N Slade, MD
Radiology. . . . . Charmaine Wallaesa

Measure	Cases	This Hosp.	State Avg.	U.S. Avg.
Blood Clot Prevention and Treatment				
Anticoagulation Overlap Therapy[2]	59	98%	94%	93%
ICU Venous Thromboembolism Prophylaxis[2]	93	100%	94%	92%
Incidence of Potentially Preventable VTE[2]	12	8%	8%	10%
UFH with Dosages/Platelet Monitoring[2]	47	100%	98%	97%
Venous Thromboembolism Prophylaxis[2]	514	97%	90%	85%
Warfarin Therapy Discharge Instructions[2]	37	89%	78%	75%
Chest Pain/Possible Heart Attack Care				
Aspirin Given Within 24 Hours of Arrival[1,3]	-	-	97%	96%
Fibrinolytic Meds Within 30 Min. of Arrival[5]	-	-	44%	58%
Average Time to ECG (minutes)[1,3]	-	-	9	7
Average Time to Transfer (minutes)[5]	-	-	64	60
Children's Asthma Care				
Received Home Management Plan of Care	-	-	-	88%
Received Reliever Medication	-	-	-	100%
Received Systemic Corticosteroids	-	-	-	100%
Emergency Department				
Admittance Decision Time (minutes)[2]	800	94	104	98
Head CT Results Within 45 Min. of Arrival[1]	-	-	60%	57%
Patients Who Left ER Before Being Seen	33,381	1%	1%	2%
Time from ER Arrival to Admit. (minutes)[2]	827	268	276	274
Time from ER Arrival to Discharge (minutes)	370	100	125	134
Time in ER Before Being Evaluated (minutes)	415	23	26	26
Time to Pain Meds for Fractures (minutes)	58	46	58	57
Heart Attack Care				
Aspirin Given at Discharge	166	100%	99%	99%
Fibrinolytic Meds Within 30 Min. of Arrival[7]	-	-	40%	54%
PCI Within 90 Minutes of Arrival	36	100%	97%	96%
Statin Prescribed at Discharge	158	99%	99%	98%
Heart Failure Care				
ACE Inhibitor or ARB for LVSD	81	94%	97%	97%
Discharge Instructions Given	259	97%	96%	94%
Evaluation of LVS Function	339	100%	100%	99%
Medicare Spending				
Medicare Spending per Patient (ratio)	-	1.01	1.01	0.98
Pneumonia Care				
Appropriate Initial Antibiotic Given	138	98%	96%	95%
Blood Culture Timing	247	99%	98%	98%
Pregnancy and Delivery Care				
Newborn Deliveries Scheduled Early[2]	22	5%	4%	6%
Preventive Care				
Immunization for Influenza[2]	647	96%	91%	90%
Immunization for Pneumonia[2]	998	97%	92%	92%
Stroke Care				
Anticoagulation Therapy for Atrial Fibrillation	16	100%	96%	95%
Antithrombotic Therapy Timing	65	97%	98%	98%
Assessed for Rehabilitation	70	100%	98%	97%
Discharged on Antithrombotic Therapy	68	100%	99%	99%
Discharged on Statin Medication	54	98%	95%	94%
Thrombolytic Therapy Timing[7]	-	-	72%	66%
Venous Thromboembolism Prophylaxis	68	100%	95%	94%
Written Stroke Educational Materials Given	37	89%	90%	88%
Surgical Care Improvement Project				
Appropriate Beta Blocker Usage	236	95%	98%	98%
Appropriate VTP Within 24 Hours	482	99%	99%	98%
Controlled Postoperative Blood Glucose	82	99%	98%	97%
Perioperative Temperature Management	556	99%	100%	100%
Prophylactic Antibiotic Selection	416	99%	99%	99%
Prophylactic Antibiotic Selection (Outpatient)	248	97%	98%	98%
Prophylactic Antibiotic Stopped	406	99%	98%	98%
Prophylactic Antibiotic Timing	418	98%	99%	99%
Prophylactic Antibiotic Timing (Outpatient)	251	98%	98%	98%
Urinary Catheter Removal	311	98%	99%	97%
Survey of Patients' Hospital Experiences				
Area Around Room 'Always' Quiet at Night	300+	56%	54%	61%
Doctors 'Always' Communicated Well	300+	82%	80%	82%
Home Recovery Information Given	300+	89%	86%	85%
Hospital Given 9 or 10 on 10 Point Scale	300+	66%	69%	71%
Meds 'Always' Explained Before Given	300+	64%	63%	64%
Nurses 'Always' Communicated Well	300+	81%	79%	79%
Pain 'Always' Well Controlled	300+	73%	70%	71%
Room and Bathroom 'Always' Clean	300+	70%	73%	73%
Timely Help 'Always' Received	300+	62%	67%	68%
Would Definitely Recommend Hospital	300+	68%	70%	71%
Use of Medical Imaging				
Cardiac Imaging Stress Test before Surgery	174	8.0%	5.4%	5.3%
Combination Abdominal CT Scan	853	7.7%	12.2%	10.5%
Combination Brain/Sinus CT Scan	598	4.3%	3.1%	2.7%
Combination Chest CT Scan	428	0.5%	2.1%	2.7%
Follow-up Mammogram/Ultrasound	1,602	13.0%	9%	8.8%
Lumbar Spine MRI for Low Back Pain	61	49.2%	35.8%	37.2%

NOTE: Hospital profiles are in alphabetical order by state, then city, then hospital within the city; Rankings exclude hospitals with less than 25 cases except for patient surveys which excludes hospitals with less than 100 cases; (a) 100-299 cases; (1) The number of cases/patients is too few to report; (2) Data submitted were based on a sample of cases/patients; (3) Results are based on a shorter time period than required; (4) Data suppressed by CMS for one or more quarters; (5) Results are not available for this reporting period; (6) Fewer than 100 patients completed the HCAHPS survey; (7) No cases met the criteria for this measure; (8) The lower limit of the confidence interval cannot be calculated if the number of observed infections equals zero; (9) No data are available from the state/territory for this reporting period; (10) The scores shown reflect fewer than 50 completed surveys; (11) There were discrepancies in the data collection process; (12) This measure does not apply to this hospital for this reporting period; (13) Results cannot be calculated for this reporting period; (14) The results for this state are combined with nearby states to protect confidentiality; Please refer to the User's Guide for a full explanation of data.

Saint Luke's Hospital - Anderson Campus

1872 Riverside Circle Phone: 610-954-3850
Easton, PA 18045
Type: Acute Care Hospitals Emergency Services: Yes
Ownership: Voluntary non-profit - Private

Measure	Cases	This Hosp.	State Avg.	U.S. Avg.
Blood Clot Prevention and Treatment				
Anticoagulation Overlap Therapy[2]	60	97%	94%	93%
ICU Venous Thromboembolism Prophylaxis[2]	53	96%	94%	92%
Incidence of Potentially Preventable VTE[1,2]	-	-	8%	10%
UFH with Dosages/Platelet Monitoring[2]	43	100%	98%	97%
Venous Thromboembolism Prophylaxis[2]	345	94%	90%	85%
Warfarin Therapy Discharge Instructions[2]	44	64%	78%	75%
Chest Pain/Possible Heart Attack Care				
Aspirin Given Within 24 Hours of Arrival[1,3]	-	-	97%	96%
Fibrinolytic Meds Within 30 Min. of Arrival[3,7]	-	-	44%	58%
Average Time to ECG (minutes)[1,3]	-	-	9	7
Average Time to Transfer (minutes)[1,3]	-	-	64	60
Children's Asthma Care				
Received Home Management Plan of Care	-	-	-	88%
Received Reliever Medication	-	-	-	100%
Received Systemic Corticosteroids	-	-	-	100%
Emergency Department				
Admittance Decision Time (minutes)[2]	852	88	104	98
Head CT Results Within 45 Min. of Arrival[1]	-	-	60%	57%
Patients Who Left ER Before Being Seen	27,198	1%	1%	2%
Time from ER Arrival to Admit. (minutes)[2]	857	259	276	274
Time from ER Arrival to Discharge (minutes)	360	136	125	134
Time in ER Before Being Evaluated (minutes)	382	41	26	26
Time to Pain Meds for Fractures (minutes)	101	63	58	57
Heart Attack Care				
Aspirin Given at Discharge	64	100%	99%	99%
Fibrinolytic Meds Within 30 Min. of Arrival[7]	-	-	40%	54%
PCI Within 90 Minutes of Arrival	13	100%	97%	96%
Statin Prescribed at Discharge	63	100%	99%	98%
Heart Failure Care				
ACE Inhibitor or ARB for LVSD	55	100%	97%	97%
Discharge Instructions Given	183	97%	96%	94%
Evaluation of LVS Function	237	100%	100%	99%
Medicare Spending				
Medicare Spending per Patient (ratio)	-	1.04	1.01	0.98
Pneumonia Care				
Appropriate Initial Antibiotic Given	136	98%	96%	95%
Blood Culture Timing	210	99%	98%	98%
Pregnancy and Delivery Care				
Newborn Deliveries Scheduled Early[7]	-	-	4%	6%
Preventive Care				
Immunization for Influenza[2]	490	96%	91%	90%
Immunization for Pneumonia[2]	772	94%	92%	92%
Stroke Care				
Anticoagulation Therapy for Atrial Fibrillation[1]	-	-	96%	95%
Antithrombotic Therapy Timing	49	100%	98%	98%
Assessed for Rehabilitation	49	98%	98%	97%
Discharged on Antithrombotic Therapy	48	100%	99%	99%
Discharged on Statin Medication	41	98%	95%	94%
Thrombolytic Therapy Timing[7]	-	-	72%	66%
Venous Thromboembolism Prophylaxis	47	98%	95%	94%
Written Stroke Educational Materials Given	35	91%	90%	88%
Surgical Care Improvement Project				
Appropriate Beta Blocker Usage[2]	28	96%	98%	98%
Appropriate VTP Within 24 Hours[2]	81	93%	99%	98%
Controlled Postoperative Blood Glucose[2,7]	-	-	98%	97%
Perioperative Temperature Management[2]	91	99%	100%	100%
Prophylactic Antibiotic Selection[2]	36	100%	99%	99%
Prophylactic Antibiotic Selection (Outpatient)	60	100%	98%	98%
Prophylactic Antibiotic Stopped[2]	34	100%	98%	98%
Prophylactic Antibiotic Timing[2]	36	100%	99%	99%
Prophylactic Antibiotic Timing (Outpatient)	61	97%	98%	98%
Urinary Catheter Removal[2]	57	100%	99%	97%
Survey of Patients' Hospital Experiences				
Area Around Room 'Always' Quiet at Night	300+	53%	54%	61%
Doctors 'Always' Communicated Well	300+	81%	80%	82%
Home Recovery Information Given	300+	86%	86%	85%
Hospital Given 9 or 10 on 10 Point Scale	300+	79%	69%	71%
Meds 'Always' Explained Before Given	300+	65%	63%	64%
Nurses 'Always' Communicated Well	300+	83%	79%	79%
Pain 'Always' Well Controlled	300+	75%	70%	71%
Room and Bathroom 'Always' Clean	300+	78%	73%	73%
Timely Help 'Always' Received	300+	71%	67%	68%
Would Definitely Recommend Hospital	300+	84%	70%	71%
Use of Medical Imaging				
Cardiac Imaging Stress Test before Surgery	308	5.2%	5.4%	5.3%
Combination Abdominal CT Scan	734	5.4%	12.2%	10.5%
Combination Brain/Sinus CT Scan[1]	-	-	3.1%	2.7%
Combination Chest CT Scan	693	1.0%	2.1%	2.7%
Follow-up Mammogram/Ultrasound	257	9.3%	9%	8.8%
Lumbar Spine MRI for Low Back Pain	127	33.1%	35.8%	37.2%

Ellwood City Hospital

724 Pershing Street Phone: 724-752-0081
Ellwood City, PA 16117 Fax: 724-752-0966
URL: www.echospital.org
Type: Acute Care Hospitals Emergency Services: Yes
Ownership: Voluntary non-profit - Other Beds: 95

Key Personnel:
Pulmonology . . . . Alagar Ravi
Radiology. . . . . Herzig Richard
CEO/President. . . . . Herbert S Skuba
Cardiology . . . . Pinto Thomas
Chief of Medical Staff. . . . . Peter Volpe

Measure	Cases	This Hosp.	State Avg.	U.S. Avg.
Blood Clot Prevention and Treatment				
Anticoagulation Overlap Therapy[2]	24	46%	94%	93%
ICU Venous Thromboembolism Prophylaxis[2]	39	54%	94%	92%
Incidence of Potentially Preventable VTE[1,2]	-	-	8%	10%
UFH with Dosages/Platelet Monitoring[2]	20	80%	98%	97%
Venous Thromboembolism Prophylaxis[2]	144	37%	90%	85%
Warfarin Therapy Discharge Instructions[2]	16	81%	78%	75%
Chest Pain/Possible Heart Attack Care				
Aspirin Given Within 24 Hours of Arrival	57	95%	97%	96%
Fibrinolytic Meds Within 30 Min. of Arrival[7]	-	-	44%	58%
Average Time to ECG (minutes)	58	6	9	7
Average Time to Transfer (minutes)	18	65	64	60
Children's Asthma Care				
Received Home Management Plan of Care	-	-	-	88%
Received Reliever Medication	-	-	-	100%
Received Systemic Corticosteroids	-	-	-	100%
Emergency Department				
Admittance Decision Time (minutes)[2]	444	65	104	98
Head CT Results Within 45 Min. of Arrival[1]	-	-	60%	57%
Patients Who Left ER Before Being Seen	14,644	1%	1%	2%
Time from ER Arrival to Admit. (minutes)[2]	444	208	276	274
Time from ER Arrival to Discharge (minutes)	408	94	125	134
Time in ER Before Being Evaluated (minutes)	413	20	26	26
Time to Pain Meds for Fractures (minutes)	43	54	58	57
Heart Attack Care				
Aspirin Given at Discharge[7]	-	-	99%	99%
Fibrinolytic Meds Within 30 Min. of Arrival[7]	-	-	40%	54%
PCI Within 90 Minutes of Arrival[7]	-	-	97%	96%
Statin Prescribed at Discharge[7]	-	-	99%	98%
Heart Failure Care				
ACE Inhibitor or ARB for LVSD[2]	46	78%	97%	97%
Discharge Instructions Given[2]	90	97%	96%	94%
Evaluation of LVS Function[2]	112	96%	100%	99%
Medicare Spending				
Medicare Spending per Patient (ratio)	-	0.96	1.01	0.98
Pneumonia Care				
Appropriate Initial Antibiotic Given	41	80%	96%	95%
Blood Culture Timing	45	93%	98%	98%
Pregnancy and Delivery Care				
Newborn Deliveries Scheduled Early[2]	20	0%	4%	6%
Preventive Care				
Immunization for Influenza[2]	296	92%	91%	90%
Immunization for Pneumonia[2]	422	95%	92%	92%
Stroke Care				
Anticoagulation Therapy for Atrial Fibrillation[1]	-	-	96%	95%
Antithrombotic Therapy Timing	22	100%	98%	98%
Assessed for Rehabilitation	18	56%	98%	97%
Discharged on Antithrombotic Therapy	18	94%	99%	99%
Discharged on Statin Medication	18	72%	95%	94%
Thrombolytic Therapy Timing[1]	-	-	72%	66%
Venous Thromboembolism Prophylaxis	22	82%	95%	94%
Written Stroke Educational Materials Given	13	54%	90%	88%
Surgical Care Improvement Project				
Appropriate Beta Blocker Usage[2]	23	96%	98%	98%
Appropriate VTP Within 24 Hours[2]	77	95%	99%	98%
Controlled Postoperative Blood Glucose[2,7]	-	-	98%	97%
Perioperative Temperature Management[2]	98	96%	100%	100%
Prophylactic Antibiotic Selection[2]	75	92%	99%	99%
Prophylactic Antibiotic Selection (Outpatient)	21	90%	98%	98%
Prophylactic Antibiotic Stopped[2]	75	88%	98%	98%
Prophylactic Antibiotic Timing[2]	75	92%	99%	99%
Prophylactic Antibiotic Timing (Outpatient)	21	100%	98%	98%
Urinary Catheter Removal[2]	29	86%	99%	97%
Survey of Patients' Hospital Experiences				
Area Around Room 'Always' Quiet at Night	300+	64%	54%	61%
Doctors 'Always' Communicated Well	300+	81%	80%	82%
Home Recovery Information Given	300+	88%	86%	85%
Hospital Given 9 or 10 on 10 Point Scale	300+	71%	69%	71%
Meds 'Always' Explained Before Given	300+	62%	63%	64%
Nurses 'Always' Communicated Well	300+	81%	79%	79%
Pain 'Always' Well Controlled	300+	72%	70%	71%
Room and Bathroom 'Always' Clean	300+	75%	73%	73%
Timely Help 'Always' Received	300+	69%	67%	68%
Would Definitely Recommend Hospital	300+	73%	70%	71%
Use of Medical Imaging				
Cardiac Imaging Stress Test before Surgery	119	4.2%	5.4%	5.3%
Combination Abdominal CT Scan	106	19.8%	12.2%	10.5%
Combination Brain/Sinus CT Scan[1]	-	-	3.1%	2.7%
Combination Chest CT Scan	62	1.6%	2.1%	2.7%
Follow-up Mammogram/Ultrasound	180	13.3%	9%	8.8%
Lumbar Spine MRI for Low Back Pain[1]	-	-	35.8%	37.2%

Ephrata Community Hospital

169 Martin Avenue Phone: 717-733-0311
Ephrata, PA 17522 Fax: 717-733-0876
URL: www.ephratahospital.org
Type: Acute Care Hospitals Emergency Services: Yes
Ownership: Voluntary non-profit - Other Beds: 133

Key Personnel:
Chief of Medical Staff. . . . . Christopher Hager
CEO/President. . . . . John M. Porter, Jr.

Measure	Cases	This Hosp.	State Avg.	U.S. Avg.
Blood Clot Prevention and Treatment				
Anticoagulation Overlap Therapy[2]	63	92%	94%	93%
ICU Venous Thromboembolism Prophylaxis[2]	83	94%	94%	92%
Incidence of Potentially Preventable VTE[1,2]	-	-	8%	10%
UFH with Dosages/Platelet Monitoring[2]	67	100%	98%	97%
Venous Thromboembolism Prophylaxis[2]	314	91%	90%	85%
Warfarin Therapy Discharge Instructions[2]	38	92%	78%	75%
Chest Pain/Possible Heart Attack Care				
Aspirin Given Within 24 Hours of Arrival	58	97%	97%	96%
Fibrinolytic Meds Within 30 Min. of Arrival[7]	-	-	44%	58%
Average Time to ECG (minutes)	58	4	9	7
Average Time to Transfer (minutes)	12	50	64	60
Children's Asthma Care				
Received Home Management Plan of Care	-	-	-	88%
Received Reliever Medication	-	-	-	100%
Received Systemic Corticosteroids	-	-	-	100%
Emergency Department				
Admittance Decision Time (minutes)[2]	507	81	104	98
Head CT Results Within 45 Min. of Arrival[1]	-	-	60%	57%
Patients Who Left ER Before Being Seen	23,353	1%	1%	2%
Time from ER Arrival to Admit. (minutes)[2]	599	314	276	274
Time from ER Arrival to Discharge (minutes)	408	149	125	134
Time in ER Before Being Evaluated (minutes)	426	46	26	26
Time to Pain Meds for Fractures (minutes)	116	62	58	57
Heart Attack Care				
Aspirin Given at Discharge	18	94%	99%	99%

NOTE: Hospital profiles are in alphabetical order by state, then city, then hospital within the city; Rankings exclude hospitals with less than 25 cases except for patient surveys which excludes hospitals with less than 100 cases; (a) 100-299 cases; (1) The number of cases/patients is too few to report; (2) Data submitted were based on a sample of cases/patients; (3) Results are based on a shorter time period than required; (4) Data suppressed by CMS for one or more quarters; (5) Results are not available for this reporting period; (6) Fewer than 100 patients completed the HCAHPS survey; (7) No cases met the criteria for this measure; (8) The lower limit of the confidence interval cannot be calculated if the number of observed infections equals zero; (9) No data are available from the state/territory for this reporting period; (10) The scores shown reflect fewer than 50 completed surveys; (11) There were discrepancies in the data collection process; (12) This measure does not apply to this hospital for this reporting period; (13) Results cannot be calculated for this reporting period; (14) The results for this state are combined with nearby states to protect confidentiality; Please refer to the User's Guide for a full explanation of data.

Measure	Cases	This Hosp.	State Avg.	U.S. Avg.
Fibrinolytic Meds Within 30 Min. of Arrival[7]	-	-	40%	54%
PCI Within 90 Minutes of Arrival[7]	-	-	97%	96%
Statin Prescribed at Discharge	17	82%	99%	98%
Heart Failure Care				
ACE Inhibitor or ARB for LVSD	35	97%	97%	97%
Discharge Instructions Given	106	97%	96%	94%
Evaluation of LVS Function	152	100%	100%	99%
Medicare Spending				
Medicare Spending per Patient (ratio)	-	0.99	1.01	0.98
Pneumonia Care				
Appropriate Initial Antibiotic Given	129	97%	96%	95%
Blood Culture Timing	202	96%	98%	98%
Pregnancy and Delivery Care				
Newborn Deliveries Scheduled Early[2]	23	4%	4%	6%
Preventive Care				
Immunization for Influenza[2]	516	98%	91%	90%
Immunization for Pneumonia[2]	647	98%	92%	92%
Stroke Care				
Anticoagulation Therapy for Atrial Fibrillation	16	94%	96%	95%
Antithrombotic Therapy Timing	67	100%	98%	98%
Assessed for Rehabilitation	76	100%	98%	97%
Discharged on Antithrombotic Therapy	69	100%	99%	99%
Discharged on Statin Medication	58	95%	95%	94%
Thrombolytic Therapy Timing[1]	-	-	72%	66%
Venous Thromboembolism Prophylaxis	70	96%	95%	94%
Written Stroke Educational Materials Given	37	100%	90%	88%
Surgical Care Improvement Project				
Appropriate Beta Blocker Usage	166	99%	98%	98%
Appropriate VTP Within 24 Hours	480	99%	99%	98%
Controlled Postoperative Blood Glucose[7]	-	-	98%	97%
Perioperative Temperature Management	584	100%	100%	100%
Prophylactic Antibiotic Selection	397	99%	99%	99%
Prophylactic Antibiotic Selection (Outpatient)	262	98%	98%	98%
Prophylactic Antibiotic Stopped	375	97%	98%	98%
Prophylactic Antibiotic Timing	397	98%	99%	99%
Prophylactic Antibiotic Timing (Outpatient)	262	100%	98%	98%
Urinary Catheter Removal	480	98%	99%	97%
Survey of Patients' Hospital Experiences				
Area Around Room 'Always' Quiet at Night	300+	45%	54%	61%
Doctors 'Always' Communicated Well	300+	75%	80%	82%
Home Recovery Information Given	300+	91%	86%	85%
Hospital Given 9 or 10 on 10 Point Scale	300+	67%	69%	71%
Meds 'Always' Explained Before Given	300+	55%	63%	64%
Nurses 'Always' Communicated Well	300+	78%	79%	79%
Pain 'Always' Well Controlled	300+	69%	70%	71%
Room and Bathroom 'Always' Clean	300+	69%	73%	73%
Timely Help 'Always' Received	300+	71%	67%	68%
Would Definitely Recommend Hospital	300+	69%	70%	71%
Use of Medical Imaging				
Cardiac Imaging Stress Test before Surgery	273	4.0%	5.4%	5.3%
Combination Abdominal CT Scan	586	21.2%	12.2%	10.5%
Combination Brain/Sinus CT Scan	601	2.0%	3.1%	2.7%
Combination Chest CT Scan	524	8.2%	2.1%	2.7%
Follow-up Mammogram/Ultrasound	1,458	10.1%	9%	8.8%
Lumbar Spine MRI for Low Back Pain	132	35.6%	35.8%	37.2%

Erie VA Medical Center

135 East 38th Street
Erie, PA 16504
Phone: 814-860-2576
Fax: 814-860-2135
Type: Acute Care - VA
Emergency Services: No
Ownership: Government Federal
Beds: 81

Key Personnel:
Chief of Medical Staff.......... Anthony Behm, DO
Operating Room.............. Prabhu Negi, MD
Quality Assurance .... Beth Thornton

Measure	Cases	This Hosp.	State Avg.	U.S. Avg.
Blood Clot Prevention and Treatment				
Anticoagulation Overlap Therapy	-	-	94%	93%
ICU Venous Thromboembolism Prophylaxis	-	-	94%	92%
Incidence of Potentially Preventable VTE	-	-	8%	10%
UFH with Dosages/Platelet Monitoring	-	-	98%	97%
Venous Thromboembolism Prophylaxis	-	-	90%	85%
Warfarin Therapy Discharge Instructions	-	-	78%	75%
Chest Pain/Possible Heart Attack Care				
Aspirin Given Within 24 Hours of Arrival	-	-	97%	96%
Fibrinolytic Meds Within 30 Min. of Arrival	-	-	44%	58%
Average Time to ECG (minutes)	-	-	9	7
Average Time to Transfer (minutes)	-	-	64	60
Children's Asthma Care				
Received Home Management Plan of Care	-	-	-	88%
Received Reliever Medication	-	-	-	100%
Received Systemic Corticosteroids	-	-	-	100%
Emergency Department				
Admittance Decision Time (minutes)	-	-	104	98
Head CT Results Within 45 Min. of Arrival	-	-	60%	57%
Patients Who Left ER Before Being Seen	-	-	1%	2%
Time from ER Arrival to Admit. (minutes)	-	-	276	274
Time from ER Arrival to Discharge (minutes)	-	-	125	134
Time in ER Before Being Evaluated (minutes)	-	-	26	26
Time to Pain Meds for Fractures (minutes)	-	-	58	57
Heart Attack Care				
Aspirin Given at Discharge[5]	-	-	99%	99%
Fibrinolytic Meds Within 30 Min. of Arrival[5]	-	-	40%	54%
PCI Within 90 Minutes of Arrival[5]	-	-	97%	96%
Statin Prescribed at Discharge[5]	-	-	99%	98%
Heart Failure Care				
ACE Inhibitor or ARB for LVSD[1]	12	92%	97%	97%
Discharge Instructions Given	29	100%	96%	94%
Evaluation of LVS Function	32	97%	100%	99%
Medicare Spending				
Medicare Spending per Patient (ratio)	-	-	1.01	0.98
Pneumonia Care				
Appropriate Initial Antibiotic Given[1]	21	100%	96%	95%
Blood Culture Timing[1]	-	-	98%	98%
Pregnancy and Delivery Care				
Newborn Deliveries Scheduled Early	-	-	4%	6%
Preventive Care				
Immunization for Influenza[2,3]	128	95%	91%	90%
Immunization for Pneumonia[2,3]	306	95%	92%	92%
Stroke Care				
Anticoagulation Therapy for Atrial Fibrillation	-	-	96%	95%
Antithrombotic Therapy Timing	-	-	98%	98%
Assessed for Rehabilitation	-	-	98%	97%
Discharged on Antithrombotic Therapy	-	-	99%	99%
Discharged on Statin Medication	-	-	95%	94%
Thrombolytic Therapy Timing	-	-	72%	66%
Venous Thromboembolism Prophylaxis	-	-	95%	94%
Written Stroke Educational Materials Given	-	-	90%	88%
Surgical Care Improvement Project				
Appropriate Beta Blocker Usage[5]	-	-	98%	98%
Appropriate VTP Within 24 Hours[5]	-	-	99%	98%
Controlled Postoperative Blood Glucose[5]	-	-	98%	97%
Perioperative Temperature Management[5]	-	-	100%	100%
Prophylactic Antibiotic Selection[5]	-	-	99%	99%
Prophylactic Antibiotic Selection (Outpatient)	-	-	98%	98%
Prophylactic Antibiotic Stopped[5]	-	-	98%	98%
Prophylactic Antibiotic Timing[5]	-	-	99%	99%
Prophylactic Antibiotic Timing (Outpatient)	-	-	98%	98%
Urinary Catheter Removal[5]	-	-	99%	97%
Survey of Patients' Hospital Experiences				
Area Around Room 'Always' Quiet at Night	-	-	54%	61%
Doctors 'Always' Communicated Well	-	-	80%	82%
Home Recovery Information Given	-	-	86%	85%
Hospital Given 9 or 10 on 10 Point Scale	-	-	69%	71%
Meds 'Always' Explained Before Given	-	-	63%	64%
Nurses 'Always' Communicated Well	-	-	79%	79%
Pain 'Always' Well Controlled	-	-	70%	71%
Room and Bathroom 'Always' Clean	-	-	73%	73%
Timely Help 'Always' Received	-	-	67%	68%
Would Definitely Recommend Hospital	-	-	70%	71%
Use of Medical Imaging				
Cardiac Imaging Stress Test before Surgery	-	-	5.4%	5.3%
Combination Abdominal CT Scan	-	-	12.2%	10.5%
Combination Brain/Sinus CT Scan	-	-	3.1%	2.7%
Combination Chest CT Scan	-	-	2.1%	2.7%
Follow-up Mammogram/Ultrasound	-	-	9%	8.8%
Lumbar Spine MRI for Low Back Pain	-	-	35.8%	37.2%

Millcreek Community Hospital

5515 Peach Street
Erie, PA 16509
Phone: 814-864-4031
Fax: 814-868-8142
URL: www.millcreekcommunityhospital.com
Type: Acute Care Hospitals
Emergency Services: Yes
Ownership: Voluntary non-profit - Church
Beds: 200

Key Personnel:
Emergency Room .... Dennis Augustini
CEO/President.............. Mary L Eckert
Cardiac Laboratory........... Wiliam A Esper

Measure	Cases	This Hosp.	State Avg.	U.S. Avg.
Blood Clot Prevention and Treatment				
Anticoagulation Overlap Therapy[1,2]	-	-	94%	93%
ICU Venous Thromboembolism Prophylaxis[2]	34	100%	94%	92%
Incidence of Potentially Preventable VTE[2,7]	-	-	8%	10%
UFH with Dosages/Platelet Monitoring[1,2]	-	-	98%	97%
Venous Thromboembolism Prophylaxis[2]	152	92%	90%	85%
Warfarin Therapy Discharge Instructions[1,2]	-	-	78%	75%
Chest Pain/Possible Heart Attack Care				
Aspirin Given Within 24 Hours of Arrival[1,3]	-	-	97%	96%
Fibrinolytic Meds Within 30 Min. of Arrival[3,7]	-	-	44%	58%
Average Time to ECG (minutes)[1,3]	-	-	9	7
Average Time to Transfer (minutes)[1,3]	-	-	64	60
Children's Asthma Care				
Received Home Management Plan of Care	-	-	-	88%
Received Reliever Medication	-	-	-	100%
Received Systemic Corticosteroids	-	-	-	100%
Emergency Department				
Admittance Decision Time (minutes)[2]	215	77	104	98
Head CT Results Within 45 Min. of Arrival[1,3]	-	-	60%	57%
Patients Who Left ER Before Being Seen	16,459	2%	1%	2%
Time from ER Arrival to Admit. (minutes)[2]	221	185	276	274
Time from ER Arrival to Discharge (minutes)	289	88	125	134
Time in ER Before Being Evaluated (minutes)	385	26	26	26
Time to Pain Meds for Fractures (minutes)	34	74	58	57
Heart Attack Care				
Aspirin Given at Discharge[1]	-	-	99%	99%
Fibrinolytic Meds Within 30 Min. of Arrival[7]	-	-	40%	54%
PCI Within 90 Minutes of Arrival[7]	-	-	97%	96%
Statin Prescribed at Discharge[1]	-	-	99%	98%
Heart Failure Care				
ACE Inhibitor or ARB for LVSD	14	100%	97%	97%
Discharge Instructions Given	58	98%	96%	94%
Evaluation of LVS Function	93	99%	100%	99%
Medicare Spending				
Medicare Spending per Patient (ratio)	-	0.99	1.01	0.98
Pneumonia Care				
Appropriate Initial Antibiotic Given	31	87%	96%	95%
Blood Culture Timing	32	97%	98%	98%
Pregnancy and Delivery Care				
Newborn Deliveries Scheduled Early	36	0%	4%	6%
Preventive Care				
Immunization for Influenza[2]	418	96%	91%	90%
Immunization for Pneumonia[2]	368	99%	92%	92%
Stroke Care				
Anticoagulation Therapy for Atrial Fibrillation[1]	-	-	96%	95%
Antithrombotic Therapy Timing	11	100%	98%	98%
Assessed for Rehabilitation	13	100%	98%	97%
Discharged on Antithrombotic Therapy	11	100%	99%	99%
Discharged on Statin Medication[1]	-	-	95%	94%
Thrombolytic Therapy Timing[1]	-	-	72%	66%
Venous Thromboembolism Prophylaxis	13	100%	95%	94%
Written Stroke Educational Materials Given[1]	-	-	90%	88%
Surgical Care Improvement Project				
Appropriate Beta Blocker Usage	19	100%	98%	98%
Appropriate VTP Within 24 Hours	108	99%	99%	98%
Controlled Postoperative Blood Glucose[7]	-	-	98%	97%
Perioperative Temperature Management	121	100%	100%	100%
Prophylactic Antibiotic Selection	95	96%	99%	99%
Prophylactic Antibiotic Selection (Outpatient)[1]	-	-	98%	98%

NOTE: Hospital profiles are in alphabetical order by state, then city, then hospital within the city; Rankings exclude hospitals with less than 25 cases except for patient surveys which excludes hospitals with less than 100 cases; (a) 100-299 cases; (1) The number of cases/patients is too few to report; (2) Data submitted were based on a sample of cases/patients; (3) Results are based on a shorter time period than required; (4) Data suppressed by CMS for one or more quarters; (5) Results are not available for this reporting period; (6) Fewer than 100 patients completed the HCAHPS survey; (7) No cases met the criteria for this measure; (8) The lower limit of the confidence interval cannot be calculated if the number of observed infections equals zero; (9) No data are available from the state/territory for this reporting period; (10) The scores shown reflect fewer than 50 completed surveys; (11) There were discrepancies in the data collection process; (12) This measure does not apply to this hospital for this reporting period; (13) Results cannot be calculated for this reporting period; (14) The results for this state are combined with nearby states to protect confidentiality; Please refer to the User's Guide for a full explanation of data.

Measure	Cases	This Hosp.	State Avg.	U.S. Avg.
Prophylactic Antibiotic Stopped	87	99%	98%	98%
Prophylactic Antibiotic Timing	95	98%	99%	99%
Prophylactic Antibiotic Timing (Outpatient)	11	82%	98%	98%
Urinary Catheter Removal	33	97%	99%	97%
Survey of Patients' Hospital Experiences				
Area Around Room 'Always' Quiet at Night	(a)	54%	54%	61%
Doctors 'Always' Communicated Well	(a)	80%	80%	82%
Home Recovery Information Given	(a)	82%	86%	85%
Hospital Given 9 or 10 on 10 Point Scale	(a)	67%	69%	71%
Meds 'Always' Explained Before Given	(a)	57%	63%	64%
Nurses 'Always' Communicated Well	(a)	74%	79%	79%
Pain 'Always' Well Controlled	(a)	69%	70%	71%
Room and Bathroom 'Always' Clean	(a)	64%	73%	73%
Timely Help 'Always' Received	(a)	69%	67%	68%
Would Definitely Recommend Hospital	(a)	69%	70%	71%
Use of Medical Imaging				
Cardiac Imaging Stress Test before Surgery[1]	-	-	5.4%	5.3%
Combination Abdominal CT Scan	112	17.9%	12.2%	10.5%
Combination Brain/Sinus CT Scan[1]	-	-	3.1%	2.7%
Combination Chest CT Scan[1]	-	-	2.1%	2.7%
Follow-up Mammogram/Ultrasound	114	2.6%	9%	8.8%
Lumbar Spine MRI for Low Back Pain[1]	-	-	35.8%	37.2%

Saint Vincent Hospital

232 West 25th Street
Erie, PA 16544
URL: www.svhs.org
Type: Acute Care Hospitals
Ownership: Voluntary non-profit - Private
Phone: 814-452-5000
Fax: 814-455-1675
Emergency Services: Yes
Beds: 490

Key Personnel:
Quality Assurance .... Bonnie Baughman
Pediatric Ambulatory Care ...... Cynthia Bowers
Pediatric In-Patient Care .... Cynthia Bowers
Chief of Medical Staff.......... Tony G. Farah, MD, FACC, FSCAI
Radiology.................. Richard S Kocan, MD
Operating Room.............. Veronica Maras, RN
Infection Control.............. Nancy Weissfox
CEO/President............... Scott Whalen, PhD, FACHE

Measure	Cases	This Hosp.	State Avg.	U.S. Avg.
Blood Clot Prevention and Treatment				
Anticoagulation Overlap Therapy[2]	61	98%	94%	93%
ICU Venous Thromboembolism Prophylaxis[2]	259	95%	94%	92%
Incidence of Potentially Preventable VTE[2]	13	15%	8%	10%
UFH with Dosages/Platelet Monitoring[2]	60	100%	98%	97%
Venous Thromboembolism Prophylaxis[2]	719	88%	90%	85%
Warfarin Therapy Discharge Instructions[2]	35	100%	78%	75%
Chest Pain/Possible Heart Attack Care				
Aspirin Given Within 24 Hours of Arrival[1]	-	-	97%	96%
Fibrinolytic Meds Within 30 Min. of Arrival[5]	-	-	44%	58%
Average Time to ECG (minutes)[1]	-	-	9	7
Average Time to Transfer (minutes)[5]	-	-	64	60
Children's Asthma Care				
Received Home Management Plan of Care	-	-	-	88%
Received Reliever Medication	-	-	-	100%
Received Systemic Corticosteroids	-	-	-	100%
Emergency Department				
Admittance Decision Time (minutes)[2]	1,026	128	104	98
Head CT Results Within 45 Min. of Arrival	13	69%	60%	57%
Patients Who Left ER Before Being Seen	65,489	1%	1%	2%
Time from ER Arrival to Admit. (minutes)[2]	1,037	284	276	274
Time from ER Arrival to Discharge (minutes)	561	121	125	134
Time in ER Before Being Evaluated (minutes)	569	25	26	26
Time to Pain Meds for Fractures (minutes)	193	53	58	57
Heart Attack Care				
Aspirin Given at Discharge	427	100%	99%	99%
Fibrinolytic Meds Within 30 Min. of Arrival[7]	-	-	40%	54%
PCI Within 90 Minutes of Arrival	65	97%	97%	96%
Statin Prescribed at Discharge	410	98%	99%	98%
Heart Failure Care				
ACE Inhibitor or ARB for LVSD	102	97%	97%	97%
Discharge Instructions Given	342	87%	96%	94%
Evaluation of LVS Function	452	100%	100%	99%
Medicare Spending				
Medicare Spending per Patient (ratio)	-	0.98	1.01	0.98
Pneumonia Care				
Appropriate Initial Antibiotic Given	129	100%	96%	95%
Blood Culture Timing	218	97%	98%	98%
Pregnancy and Delivery Care				
Newborn Deliveries Scheduled Early	76	9%	4%	6%
Preventive Care				
Immunization for Influenza[2]	1,055	62%	91%	90%
Immunization for Pneumonia[2]	1,425	78%	92%	92%
Stroke Care				
Anticoagulation Therapy for Atrial Fibrillation	43	95%	96%	95%
Antithrombotic Therapy Timing	209	98%	98%	98%
Assessed for Rehabilitation	265	97%	98%	97%
Discharged on Antithrombotic Therapy	232	100%	99%	99%
Discharged on Statin Medication	175	100%	95%	94%
Thrombolytic Therapy Timing	12	83%	72%	66%
Venous Thromboembolism Prophylaxis	261	96%	95%	94%
Written Stroke Educational Materials Given	137	87%	90%	88%
Surgical Care Improvement Project				
Appropriate Beta Blocker Usage	518	99%	98%	98%
Appropriate VTP Within 24 Hours	950	100%	99%	98%
Controlled Postoperative Blood Glucose	314	97%	98%	97%
Perioperative Temperature Management	1,106	100%	100%	100%
Prophylactic Antibiotic Selection	958	99%	99%	99%
Prophylactic Antibiotic Selection (Outpatient)	321	99%	98%	98%
Prophylactic Antibiotic Stopped	943	100%	98%	98%
Prophylactic Antibiotic Timing	958	99%	99%	99%
Prophylactic Antibiotic Timing (Outpatient)	325	98%	98%	98%
Urinary Catheter Removal	1,075	99%	99%	97%
Survey of Patients' Hospital Experiences				
Area Around Room 'Always' Quiet at Night	300+	53%	54%	61%
Doctors 'Always' Communicated Well	300+	79%	80%	82%
Home Recovery Information Given	300+	85%	86%	85%
Hospital Given 9 or 10 on 10 Point Scale	300+	69%	69%	71%
Meds 'Always' Explained Before Given	300+	61%	63%	64%
Nurses 'Always' Communicated Well	300+	77%	79%	79%
Pain 'Always' Well Controlled	300+	68%	70%	71%
Room and Bathroom 'Always' Clean	300+	66%	73%	73%
Timely Help 'Always' Received	300+	66%	67%	68%
Would Definitely Recommend Hospital	300+	72%	70%	71%
Use of Medical Imaging				
Cardiac Imaging Stress Test before Surgery	895	4.4%	5.4%	5.3%
Combination Abdominal CT Scan	857	10.3%	12.2%	10.5%
Combination Brain/Sinus CT Scan	871	2.2%	3.1%	2.7%
Combination Chest CT Scan	380	0.3%	2.1%	2.7%
Follow-up Mammogram/Ultrasound	1,335	5.2%	9%	8.8%
Lumbar Spine MRI for Low Back Pain	203	35.5%	35.8%	37.2%

UPMC Hamot

201 State Street
Erie, PA 16550
E-mail: info@hamot.org
URL: www.hamot.org
Type: Acute Care Hospitals
Ownership: Voluntary non-profit - Private
Phone: 814-877-6000
Fax: 814-877-7590
Emergency Services: Yes
Beds: 380

Key Personnel:
Pediatric Ambulatory Care ...... Robert Burns, MD
Chief of Medical Staff.......... Peter L. Depowski, MD, FCAP
CEO/President............... V. James Fiorenzo
Quality Assurance .... Paul Huckno
Operating Room.............. Mary Ellen Stoddart
Infection Control.............. Lee P VanVoris, MD
Radiology.................. Richard Willion
Pediatric In-Patient Care .... Ronald F Zieziula, MD

Measure	Cases	This Hosp.	State Avg.	U.S. Avg.
Blood Clot Prevention and Treatment				
Anticoagulation Overlap Therapy[2]	142	97%	94%	93%
ICU Venous Thromboembolism Prophylaxis[2]	125	99%	94%	92%
Incidence of Potentially Preventable VTE[2]	30	3%	8%	10%
UFH with Dosages/Platelet Monitoring[2]	183	100%	98%	97%
Venous Thromboembolism Prophylaxis[2]	425	94%	90%	85%
Warfarin Therapy Discharge Instructions[2]	84	100%	78%	75%
Chest Pain/Possible Heart Attack Care				
Aspirin Given Within 24 Hours of Arrival[3,7]	-	-	97%	96%
Fibrinolytic Meds Within 30 Min. of Arrival[5]	-	-	44%	58%
Average Time to ECG (minutes)[3,7]	-	-	9	7
Average Time to Transfer (minutes)[5]	-	-	64	60
Children's Asthma Care				
Received Home Management Plan of Care	-	-	-	88%
Received Reliever Medication	-	-	-	100%
Received Systemic Corticosteroids	-	-	-	100%
Emergency Department				
Admittance Decision Time (minutes)[2]	553	84	104	98
Head CT Results Within 45 Min. of Arrival[1]	-	-	60%	57%
Patients Who Left ER Before Being Seen	78,477	1%	1%	2%
Time from ER Arrival to Admit. (minutes)[2]	563	219	276	274
Time from ER Arrival to Discharge (minutes)	570	138	125	134
Time in ER Before Being Evaluated (minutes)	603	29	26	26
Time to Pain Meds for Fractures (minutes)	203	54	58	57
Heart Attack Care				
Aspirin Given at Discharge	706	100%	99%	99%
Fibrinolytic Meds Within 30 Min. of Arrival[7]	-	-	40%	54%
PCI Within 90 Minutes of Arrival	76	100%	97%	96%
Statin Prescribed at Discharge	694	99%	99%	98%
Heart Failure Care				
ACE Inhibitor or ARB for LVSD	141	98%	97%	97%
Discharge Instructions Given	374	100%	96%	94%
Evaluation of LVS Function	526	100%	100%	99%
Medicare Spending				
Medicare Spending per Patient (ratio)	-	1.05	1.01	0.98
Pneumonia Care				
Appropriate Initial Antibiotic Given	264	96%	96%	95%
Blood Culture Timing	465	98%	98%	98%
Pregnancy and Delivery Care				
Newborn Deliveries Scheduled Early[2]	183	0%	4%	6%
Preventive Care				
Immunization for Influenza[2]	608	92%	91%	90%
Immunization for Pneumonia[2]	745	94%	92%	92%
Stroke Care				
Anticoagulation Therapy for Atrial Fibrillation	40	98%	96%	95%
Antithrombotic Therapy Timing	180	99%	98%	98%
Assessed for Rehabilitation	302	99%	98%	97%
Discharged on Antithrombotic Therapy	255	100%	99%	99%
Discharged on Statin Medication	202	98%	95%	94%
Thrombolytic Therapy Timing	27	89%	72%	66%
Venous Thromboembolism Prophylaxis	265	98%	95%	94%
Written Stroke Educational Materials Given	157	100%	90%	88%
Surgical Care Improvement Project				
Appropriate Beta Blocker Usage[2]	654	99%	98%	98%
Appropriate VTP Within 24 Hours[2]	1,027	99%	99%	98%
Controlled Postoperative Blood Glucose[2]	324	96%	98%	97%
Perioperative Temperature Management[2]	1,309	100%	100%	100%
Prophylactic Antibiotic Selection[2]	1,127	100%	99%	99%
Prophylactic Antibiotic Selection (Outpatient)	786	99%	98%	98%
Prophylactic Antibiotic Stopped[2]	1,114	96%	98%	98%
Prophylactic Antibiotic Timing[2]	1,128	100%	99%	99%
Prophylactic Antibiotic Timing (Outpatient)	793	99%	98%	98%
Urinary Catheter Removal[2]	1,062	99%	99%	97%
Survey of Patients' Hospital Experiences				
Area Around Room 'Always' Quiet at Night	300+	46%	54%	61%
Doctors 'Always' Communicated Well	300+	76%	80%	82%
Home Recovery Information Given	300+	86%	86%	85%
Hospital Given 9 or 10 on 10 Point Scale	300+	70%	69%	71%
Meds 'Always' Explained Before Given	300+	58%	63%	64%
Nurses 'Always' Communicated Well	300+	76%	79%	79%
Pain 'Always' Well Controlled	300+	67%	70%	71%
Room and Bathroom 'Always' Clean	300+	68%	73%	73%
Timely Help 'Always' Received	300+	67%	67%	68%
Would Definitely Recommend Hospital	300+	73%	70%	71%
Use of Medical Imaging				
Cardiac Imaging Stress Test before Surgery	724	3.0%	5.4%	5.3%
Combination Abdominal CT Scan	1,227	7.7%	12.2%	10.5%
Combination Brain/Sinus CT Scan	958	1.9%	3.1%	2.7%
Combination Chest CT Scan	472	0.4%	2.1%	2.7%
Follow-up Mammogram/Ultrasound	1,693	10.7%	9%	8.8%
Lumbar Spine MRI for Low Back Pain	171	31.0%	35.8%	37.2%

NOTE: Hospital profiles are in alphabetical order by state, then city, then hospital within the city; Rankings exclude hospitals with less than 25 cases except for patient surveys which excludes hospitals with less than 100 cases; (a) 100-299 cases; (1) The number of cases/patients is too few to report; (2) Data submitted were based on a sample of cases/patients; (3) Results are based on a shorter time period than required; (4) Data suppressed by CMS for one or more quarters; (5) Results are not available for this reporting period; (6) Fewer than 100 patients completed the HCAHPS survey; (7) No cases met the criteria for this measure; (8) The lower limit of the confidence interval cannot be calculated if the number of observed infections equals zero; (9) No data are available from the state/territory for this reporting period; (10) The scores shown reflect fewer than 50 completed surveys; (11) There were discrepancies in the data collection process; (12) This measure does not apply to this hospital for this reporting period; (13) Results cannot be calculated for this reporting period; (14) The results for this state are combined with nearby states to protect confidentiality; Please refer to the User's Guide for a full explanation of data.

UPMC Bedford Memorial

10455 Lincoln Highway
Everett, PA 15537
URL: www.upmc.com
Type: Acute Care Hospitals
Ownership: Voluntary non-profit - Other

Phone: 814-623-6161
Fax: 814-624-4313
Emergency Services: Yes
Beds: 49

Key Personnel:
Operating Room. . . . . Anne Allendorfer
Radiology. . . . . Thomas Anderson
Pediatric In-Patient Care . . . . Barbara Antinora
Chief of Medical Staff. . . . . David Farber, MD
Infection Control. . . . . Beth Hullihen, RN
Coronary Care . . . . Kathleen Quinn
CEO/President. . . . . Roger P Winn
Quality Assurance . . . . Sherrill Wylie, RN

Measure	Cases	This Hosp.	State Avg.	U.S. Avg.
Blood Clot Prevention and Treatment				
Anticoagulation Overlap Therapy[2]	17	94%	94%	93%
ICU Venous Thromboembolism Prophylaxis[2]	23	100%	94%	92%
Incidence of Potentially Preventable VTE[1,2]	-	-	8%	10%
UFH with Dosages/Platelet Monitoring[2,7]	-	-	98%	97%
Venous Thromboembolism Prophylaxis[2]	220	94%	90%	85%
Warfarin Therapy Discharge Instructions[1,2]	-	-	78%	75%
Chest Pain/Possible Heart Attack Care				
Aspirin Given Within 24 Hours of Arrival	85	96%	97%	96%
Fibrinolytic Meds Within 30 Min. of Arrival[1]	-	-	44%	58%
Average Time to ECG (minutes)	89	4	9	7
Average Time to Transfer (minutes)	16	100	64	60
Children's Asthma Care				
Received Home Management Plan of Care	-	-	-	88%
Received Reliever Medication	-	-	-	100%
Received Systemic Corticosteroids	-	-	-	100%
Emergency Department				
Admittance Decision Time (minutes)[2]	358	49	104	98
Head CT Results Within 45 Min. of Arrival[1]	-	-	60%	57%
Patients Who Left ER Before Being Seen	16,903	0%	1%	2%
Time from ER Arrival to Admit. (minutes)[2]	379	188	276	274
Time from ER Arrival to Discharge (minutes)	552	96	125	134
Time in ER Before Being Evaluated (minutes)	623	15	26	26
Time to Pain Meds for Fractures (minutes)	54	39	58	57
Heart Attack Care				
Aspirin Given at Discharge[1]	-	-	99%	99%
Fibrinolytic Meds Within 30 Min. of Arrival[7]	-	-	40%	54%
PCI Within 90 Minutes of Arrival[7]	-	-	97%	96%
Statin Prescribed at Discharge[1]	-	-	99%	98%
Heart Failure Care				
ACE Inhibitor or ARB for LVSD	16	100%	97%	97%
Discharge Instructions Given	41	88%	96%	94%
Evaluation of LVS Function	56	100%	100%	99%
Medicare Spending				
Medicare Spending per Patient (ratio)	-	0.98	1.01	0.98
Pneumonia Care				
Appropriate Initial Antibiotic Given	64	98%	96%	95%
Blood Culture Timing	88	100%	98%	98%
Pregnancy and Delivery Care				
Newborn Deliveries Scheduled Early[2]	38	0%	4%	6%
Preventive Care				
Immunization for Influenza[2]	347	98%	91%	90%
Immunization for Pneumonia[2]	444	97%	92%	92%
Stroke Care				
Anticoagulation Therapy for Atrial Fibrillation[7]	-	-	96%	95%
Antithrombotic Therapy Timing	12	100%	98%	98%
Assessed for Rehabilitation[1]	-	-	98%	97%
Discharged on Antithrombotic Therapy[1]	-	-	99%	99%
Discharged on Statin Medication[1]	-	-	95%	94%
Thrombolytic Therapy Timing[7]	-	-	72%	66%
Venous Thromboembolism Prophylaxis[1]	-	-	95%	94%
Written Stroke Educational Materials Given[1]	-	-	90%	88%
Surgical Care Improvement Project				
Appropriate Beta Blocker Usage	33	94%	98%	98%
Appropriate VTP Within 24 Hours	113	98%	99%	98%
Controlled Postoperative Blood Glucose[7]	-	-	98%	97%
Perioperative Temperature Management	125	100%	100%	100%
Prophylactic Antibiotic Selection	79	100%	99%	99%
Prophylactic Antibiotic Selection (Outpatient)	39	97%	98%	98%
Prophylactic Antibiotic Stopped	77	96%	98%	98%
Prophylactic Antibiotic Timing	79	100%	99%	99%
Prophylactic Antibiotic Timing (Outpatient)	39	100%	98%	98%
Urinary Catheter Removal	42	100%	99%	97%
Survey of Patients' Hospital Experiences				
Area Around Room 'Always' Quiet at Night	300+	61%	54%	61%
Doctors 'Always' Communicated Well	300+	80%	80%	82%
Home Recovery Information Given	300+	84%	86%	85%
Hospital Given 9 or 10 on 10 Point Scale	300+	65%	69%	71%
Meds 'Always' Explained Before Given	300+	64%	63%	64%
Nurses 'Always' Communicated Well	300+	81%	79%	79%
Pain 'Always' Well Controlled	300+	68%	70%	71%
Room and Bathroom 'Always' Clean	300+	84%	73%	73%
Timely Help 'Always' Received	300+	70%	67%	68%
Would Definitely Recommend Hospital	300+	60%	70%	71%
Use of Medical Imaging				
Cardiac Imaging Stress Test before Surgery	170	6.5%	5.4%	5.3%
Combination Abdominal CT Scan	312	5.4%	12.2%	10.5%
Combination Brain/Sinus CT Scan[1]	-	-	3.1%	2.7%
Combination Chest CT Scan	126	3.2%	2.1%	2.7%
Follow-up Mammogram/Ultrasound	519	3.7%	9%	8.8%
Lumbar Spine MRI for Low Back Pain[1]	-	-	35.8%	37.2%

Gettysburg Hospital

147 Gettys Street
Gettysburg, PA 17325
URL: www.wellspan.org
Type: Acute Care Hospitals
Ownership: Voluntary non-profit - Other

Phone: 717-334-2121
Fax: 717-337-4162
Emergency Services: Yes
Beds: 76

Key Personnel:
Cardiology . . . . Rodney Canosa
Quality Assurance . . . . Tom Lawler
Radiology. . . . . Cynthia Shi
Anesthesiology. . . . . Filip Trojanowaski

Measure	Cases	This Hosp.	State Avg.	U.S. Avg.
Blood Clot Prevention and Treatment				
Anticoagulation Overlap Therapy[2]	72	93%	94%	93%
ICU Venous Thromboembolism Prophylaxis[2]	72	93%	94%	92%
Incidence of Potentially Preventable VTE[1,2]	-	-	8%	10%
UFH with Dosages/Platelet Monitoring[2]	34	97%	98%	97%
Venous Thromboembolism Prophylaxis[2]	305	92%	90%	85%
Warfarin Therapy Discharge Instructions[2]	57	98%	78%	75%
Chest Pain/Possible Heart Attack Care				
Aspirin Given Within 24 Hours of Arrival[1]	-	-	97%	96%
Fibrinolytic Meds Within 30 Min. of Arrival[3,7]	-	-	44%	58%
Average Time to ECG (minutes)[1]	-	-	9	7
Average Time to Transfer (minutes)[1,3]	-	-	64	60
Children's Asthma Care				
Received Home Management Plan of Care	-	-	-	88%
Received Reliever Medication	-	-	-	100%
Received Systemic Corticosteroids	-	-	-	100%
Emergency Department				
Admittance Decision Time (minutes)[2]	435	65	104	98
Head CT Results Within 45 Min. of Arrival[1]	-	-	60%	57%
Patients Who Left ER Before Being Seen	23,150	2%	1%	2%
Time from ER Arrival to Admit. (minutes)[2]	682	291	276	274
Time from ER Arrival to Discharge (minutes)	361	148	125	134
Time in ER Before Being Evaluated (minutes)	383	42	26	26
Time to Pain Meds for Fractures (minutes)	113	54	58	57
Heart Attack Care				
Aspirin Given at Discharge	19	100%	99%	99%
Fibrinolytic Meds Within 30 Min. of Arrival[7]	-	-	40%	54%
PCI Within 90 Minutes of Arrival[7]	-	-	97%	96%
Statin Prescribed at Discharge	20	100%	99%	98%
Heart Failure Care				
ACE Inhibitor or ARB for LVSD	46	93%	97%	97%
Discharge Instructions Given	133	98%	96%	94%
Evaluation of LVS Function	183	98%	100%	99%
Medicare Spending				
Medicare Spending per Patient (ratio)	-	0.97	1.01	0.98
Pneumonia Care				
Appropriate Initial Antibiotic Given	119	100%	96%	95%
Blood Culture Timing	208	98%	98%	98%
Pregnancy and Delivery Care				
Newborn Deliveries Scheduled Early[2]	47	0%	4%	6%
Preventive Care				
Immunization for Influenza[2]	457	96%	91%	90%
Immunization for Pneumonia[2]	618	94%	92%	92%
Stroke Care				
Anticoagulation Therapy for Atrial Fibrillation[1]	-	-	96%	95%
Antithrombotic Therapy Timing	56	100%	98%	98%
Assessed for Rehabilitation	59	98%	98%	97%
Discharged on Antithrombotic Therapy	57	100%	99%	99%
Discharged on Statin Medication	49	94%	95%	94%
Thrombolytic Therapy Timing[1]	-	-	72%	66%
Venous Thromboembolism Prophylaxis	56	96%	95%	94%
Written Stroke Educational Materials Given	34	85%	90%	88%
Surgical Care Improvement Project				
Appropriate Beta Blocker Usage	101	99%	98%	98%
Appropriate VTP Within 24 Hours	345	99%	99%	98%
Controlled Postoperative Blood Glucose[7]	-	-	98%	97%
Perioperative Temperature Management	379	100%	100%	100%
Prophylactic Antibiotic Selection	293	100%	99%	99%
Prophylactic Antibiotic Selection (Outpatient)	103	99%	98%	98%
Prophylactic Antibiotic Stopped	288	100%	98%	98%
Prophylactic Antibiotic Timing	295	100%	99%	99%
Prophylactic Antibiotic Timing (Outpatient)	104	98%	98%	98%
Urinary Catheter Removal	104	98%	99%	97%
Survey of Patients' Hospital Experiences				
Area Around Room 'Always' Quiet at Night	300+	52%	54%	61%
Doctors 'Always' Communicated Well	300+	80%	80%	82%
Home Recovery Information Given	300+	85%	86%	85%
Hospital Given 9 or 10 on 10 Point Scale	300+	69%	69%	71%
Meds 'Always' Explained Before Given	300+	60%	63%	64%
Nurses 'Always' Communicated Well	300+	79%	79%	79%
Pain 'Always' Well Controlled	300+	71%	70%	71%
Room and Bathroom 'Always' Clean	300+	76%	73%	73%
Timely Help 'Always' Received	300+	68%	67%	68%
Would Definitely Recommend Hospital	300+	69%	70%	71%
Use of Medical Imaging				
Cardiac Imaging Stress Test before Surgery	422	5.7%	5.4%	5.3%
Combination Abdominal CT Scan	597	21.6%	12.2%	10.5%
Combination Brain/Sinus CT Scan[1]	-	-	3.1%	2.7%
Combination Chest CT Scan	427	0.0%	2.1%	2.7%
Follow-up Mammogram/Ultrasound	1,440	11.0%	9%	8.8%
Lumbar Spine MRI for Low Back Pain	114	29.8%	35.8%	37.2%

Excela Health Westmoreland Hospital

532 West Pittsburgh Street
Greensburg, PA 15601
URL: www.westmoreland.org
Type: Acute Care Hospitals
Ownership: Voluntary non-profit - Other

Phone: 412-832-5050
Fax: 724-832-4313
Emergency Services: Yes
Beds: 302

Key Personnel:
Infection Control. . . . . Lisa D'Amilo, RN
Intensive Care Unit. . . . . Pam Donovan
Chief of Medical Staff. . . . . Carol J. Fox, MD
Radiology. . . . . Sam Raneri
CEO . . . . Robert J. Rogalski, Esq.
Quality Assurance . . . . Al Rosatti
Operating Room. . . . . Maryann Singley
Emergency Room . . . . Robert Whipkey, MD

Measure	Cases	This Hosp.	State Avg.	U.S. Avg.
Blood Clot Prevention and Treatment				
Anticoagulation Overlap Therapy[2]	115	85%	94%	93%
ICU Venous Thromboembolism Prophylaxis[2]	78	95%	94%	92%
Incidence of Potentially Preventable VTE[2]	11	45%	8%	10%
UFH with Dosages/Platelet Monitoring[2]	130	100%	98%	97%
Venous Thromboembolism Prophylaxis[2]	365	85%	90%	85%
Warfarin Therapy Discharge Instructions[2]	80	72%	78%	75%
Chest Pain/Possible Heart Attack Care				
Aspirin Given Within 24 Hours of Arrival	13	100%	97%	96%
Fibrinolytic Meds Within 30 Min. of Arrival[7]	-	-	44%	58%
Average Time to ECG (minutes)	14	7	9	7
Average Time to Transfer (minutes)[7]	-	-	64	60
Children's Asthma Care				

NOTE: Hospital profiles are in alphabetical order by state, then city, then hospital within the city; Rankings exclude hospitals with less than 25 cases except for patient surveys which excludes hospitals with less than 100 cases; (a) 100-299 cases; (1) The number of cases/patients is too few to report; (2) Data submitted were based on a sample of cases/patients; (3) Results are based on a shorter time period than required; (4) Data suppressed by CMS for one or more quarters; (5) Results are not available for this reporting period; (6) Fewer than 100 patients completed the HCAHPS survey; (7) No cases met the criteria for this measure; (8) The lower limit of the confidence interval cannot be calculated if the number of observed infections equals zero; (9) No data are available from the state/territory for this reporting period; (10) The scores shown reflect fewer than 50 completed surveys; (11) There were discrepancies in the data collection process; (12) This measure does not apply to this hospital for this reporting period; (13) Results cannot be calculated for this reporting period; (14) The results for this state are combined with nearby states to protect confidentiality; Please refer to the User's Guide for a full explanation of data.

Measure	Cases	This Hosp.	State Avg.	U.S. Avg.
Received Home Management Plan of Care	-	-	-	88%
Received Reliever Medication	-	-	-	100%
Received Systemic Corticosteroids	-	-	-	100%
Emergency Department				
Admittance Decision Time (minutes)[2]	870	89	104	98
Head CT Results Within 45 Min. of Arrival	15	40%	60%	57%
Patients Who Left ER Before Being Seen	59,279	1%	1%	2%
Time from ER Arrival to Admit. (minutes)[2]	876	266	276	274
Time from ER Arrival to Discharge (minutes)	475	144	125	134
Time in ER Before Being Evaluated (minutes)	534	13	26	26
Time to Pain Meds for Fractures (minutes)	143	49	58	57
Heart Attack Care				
Aspirin Given at Discharge	562	99%	99%	99%
Fibrinolytic Meds Within 30 Min. of Arrival[7]	-	-	40%	54%
PCI Within 90 Minutes of Arrival	71	89%	97%	96%
Statin Prescribed at Discharge	548	97%	99%	98%
Heart Failure Care				
ACE Inhibitor or ARB for LVSD	150	89%	97%	97%
Discharge Instructions Given	438	88%	96%	94%
Evaluation of LVS Function	595	100%	100%	99%
Medicare Spending				
Medicare Spending per Patient (ratio)	-	1.08	1.01	0.98
Pneumonia Care				
Appropriate Initial Antibiotic Given	275	97%	96%	95%
Blood Culture Timing	511	100%	98%	98%
Pregnancy and Delivery Care				
Newborn Deliveries Scheduled Early[2]	145	0%	4%	6%
Preventive Care				
Immunization for Influenza[2]	762	88%	91%	90%
Immunization for Pneumonia[2]	1,001	91%	92%	92%
Stroke Care				
Anticoagulation Therapy for Atrial Fibrillation	14	93%	96%	95%
Antithrombotic Therapy Timing	114	96%	98%	98%
Assessed for Rehabilitation	126	94%	98%	97%
Discharged on Antithrombotic Therapy	115	98%	99%	99%
Discharged on Statin Medication	95	91%	95%	94%
Thrombolytic Therapy Timing[1]	-	-	72%	66%
Venous Thromboembolism Prophylaxis	131	90%	95%	94%
Written Stroke Educational Materials Given	55	60%	90%	88%
Surgical Care Improvement Project				
Appropriate Beta Blocker Usage	435	98%	98%	98%
Appropriate VTP Within 24 Hours	959	99%	99%	98%
Controlled Postoperative Blood Glucose	154	99%	98%	97%
Perioperative Temperature Management	1,097	100%	100%	100%
Prophylactic Antibiotic Selection	998	99%	99%	99%
Prophylactic Antibiotic Selection (Outpatient)	209	98%	98%	98%
Prophylactic Antibiotic Stopped	987	97%	98%	98%
Prophylactic Antibiotic Timing	998	100%	99%	99%
Prophylactic Antibiotic Timing (Outpatient)	210	99%	98%	98%
Urinary Catheter Removal	881	98%	99%	97%
Survey of Patients' Hospital Experiences				
Area Around Room 'Always' Quiet at Night	300+	47%	54%	61%
Doctors 'Always' Communicated Well	300+	80%	80%	82%
Home Recovery Information Given	300+	85%	86%	85%
Hospital Given 9 or 10 on 10 Point Scale	300+	61%	69%	71%
Meds 'Always' Explained Before Given	300+	62%	63%	64%
Nurses 'Always' Communicated Well	300+	76%	79%	79%
Pain 'Always' Well Controlled	300+	70%	70%	71%
Room and Bathroom 'Always' Clean	300+	65%	73%	73%
Timely Help 'Always' Received	300+	64%	67%	68%
Would Definitely Recommend Hospital	300+	60%	70%	71%
Use of Medical Imaging				
Cardiac Imaging Stress Test before Surgery	306	5.9%	5.4%	5.3%
Combination Abdominal CT Scan	612	11.6%	12.2%	10.5%
Combination Brain/Sinus CT Scan	624	2.1%	3.1%	2.7%
Combination Chest CT Scan	520	6.5%	2.1%	2.7%
Follow-up Mammogram/Ultrasound	1,015	9.3%	9%	8.8%
Lumbar Spine MRI for Low Back Pain	60	25.0%	35.8%	37.2%

UPMC Horizon

110 North Main Street
Greenville, PA 16125
URL: www.upmc.com
Type: Acute Care Hospitals
Ownership: Voluntary non-profit - Private
Phone: 724-588-2100
Fax: 724-983-8877
Emergency Services: Yes
Beds: 218

Key Personnel:
Infection Control. . . . . Donna Carl, RN
Patient Relations . . . . Paula Cica
Chief of Medical Staff . . . . Robert Cindberg
Hemotology Center . . . . Sharon Larson
Emergency Room . . . . Joseph Noga
Intensive Care Unit. . . . . Elaine Owen, RN
CEO/President. . . . . Jeffrey A Romoff
Operating Room. . . . . Debbie Schuster

Measure	Cases	This Hosp.	State Avg.	U.S. Avg.
Blood Clot Prevention and Treatment				
Anticoagulation Overlap Therapy	67	99%	94%	93%
ICU Venous Thromboembolism Prophylaxis	548	100%	94%	92%
Incidence of Potentially Preventable VTE	11	0%	8%	10%
UFH with Dosages/Platelet Monitoring	62	100%	98%	97%
Venous Thromboembolism Prophylaxis	2,295	100%	90%	85%
Warfarin Therapy Discharge Instructions	57	100%	78%	75%
Chest Pain/Possible Heart Attack Care				
Aspirin Given Within 24 Hours of Arrival	109	96%	97%	96%
Fibrinolytic Meds Within 30 Min. of Arrival[1]	-	-	44%	58%
Average Time to ECG (minutes)	114	10	9	7
Average Time to Transfer (minutes)	29	83	64	60
Children's Asthma Care				
Received Home Management Plan of Care	-	-	-	88%
Received Reliever Medication	-	-	-	100%
Received Systemic Corticosteroids	-	-	-	100%
Emergency Department				
Admittance Decision Time (minutes)[2]	560	59	104	98
Head CT Results Within 45 Min. of Arrival[1]	-	-	60%	57%
Patients Who Left ER Before Being Seen	37,254	1%	1%	2%
Time from ER Arrival to Admit. (minutes)[2]	587	210	276	274
Time from ER Arrival to Discharge (minutes)	552	114	125	134
Time in ER Before Being Evaluated (minutes)	621	20	26	26
Time to Pain Meds for Fractures (minutes)	141	61	58	57
Heart Attack Care				
Aspirin Given at Discharge	24	96%	99%	99%
Fibrinolytic Meds Within 30 Min. of Arrival[7]	-	-	40%	54%
PCI Within 90 Minutes of Arrival[7]	-	-	97%	96%
Statin Prescribed at Discharge	27	96%	99%	98%
Heart Failure Care				
ACE Inhibitor or ARB for LVSD	43	100%	97%	97%
Discharge Instructions Given	165	99%	96%	94%
Evaluation of LVS Function	208	100%	100%	99%
Medicare Spending				
Medicare Spending per Patient (ratio)	-	0.93	1.01	0.98
Pneumonia Care				
Appropriate Initial Antibiotic Given	156	99%	96%	95%
Blood Culture Timing	246	100%	98%	98%
Pregnancy and Delivery Care				
Newborn Deliveries Scheduled Early[2]	66	11%	4%	6%
Preventive Care				
Immunization for Influenza[2]	651	98%	91%	90%
Immunization for Pneumonia[2]	834	98%	92%	92%
Stroke Care				
Anticoagulation Therapy for Atrial Fibrillation	17	94%	96%	95%
Antithrombotic Therapy Timing	60	100%	98%	98%
Assessed for Rehabilitation	65	94%	98%	97%
Discharged on Antithrombotic Therapy	62	100%	99%	99%
Discharged on Statin Medication	40	95%	95%	94%
Thrombolytic Therapy Timing[1]	-	-	72%	66%
Venous Thromboembolism Prophylaxis	63	98%	95%	94%
Written Stroke Educational Materials Given	39	100%	90%	88%
Surgical Care Improvement Project				
Appropriate Beta Blocker Usage	234	100%	98%	98%
Appropriate VTP Within 24 Hours	542	100%	99%	98%
Controlled Postoperative Blood Glucose[7]	-	-	98%	97%
Perioperative Temperature Management	662	100%	100%	100%
Prophylactic Antibiotic Selection	478	100%	99%	99%
Prophylactic Antibiotic Selection (Outpatient)	225	98%	98%	98%
Prophylactic Antibiotic Stopped	470	99%	98%	98%
Prophylactic Antibiotic Timing	478	100%	99%	99%
Prophylactic Antibiotic Timing (Outpatient)	226	98%	98%	98%
Urinary Catheter Removal	125	98%	99%	97%
Survey of Patients' Hospital Experiences				
Area Around Room 'Always' Quiet at Night	300+	50%	54%	61%
Doctors 'Always' Communicated Well	300+	76%	80%	82%
Home Recovery Information Given	300+	86%	86%	85%
Hospital Given 9 or 10 on 10 Point Scale	300+	62%	69%	71%
Meds 'Always' Explained Before Given	300+	58%	63%	64%
Nurses 'Always' Communicated Well	300+	72%	79%	79%
Pain 'Always' Well Controlled	300+	68%	70%	71%
Room and Bathroom 'Always' Clean	300+	72%	73%	73%
Timely Help 'Always' Received	300+	60%	67%	68%
Would Definitely Recommend Hospital	300+	61%	70%	71%
Use of Medical Imaging				
Cardiac Imaging Stress Test before Surgery	423	5.4%	5.4%	5.3%
Combination Abdominal CT Scan	729	11.0%	12.2%	10.5%
Combination Brain/Sinus CT Scan	663	3.9%	3.1%	2.7%
Combination Chest CT Scan	453	0.2%	2.1%	2.7%
Follow-up Mammogram/Ultrasound	1,187	6.5%	9%	8.8%
Lumbar Spine MRI for Low Back Pain	117	28.2%	35.8%	37.2%

Grove City Medical Center

631 North Broad Street Ext.
Grove City, PA 16127
E-mail: ushcommrelations@uchpa.org
URL: www.uchpa.org
Type: Acute Care Hospitals
Ownership: Voluntary non-profit - Private
Phone: 724-450-7000
Fax: 724-450-7179
Emergency Services: Yes
Beds: 95

Key Personnel:
Emergency Room . . . . Tony Bono, RN
Quality Assurance . . . . Bev Jack
Patient Relations . . . . Rob Jackson
CEO/President. . . . . Robert Jackson
Radiology. . . . . Gilbert Lawrence, MD
Intensive Care Unit. . . . . Sue Lee
Infection Control. . . . . Donna Leffler
Chief of Medical Staff . . . . S Sawardekar

Measure	Cases	This Hosp.	State Avg.	U.S. Avg.
Blood Clot Prevention and Treatment				
Anticoagulation Overlap Therapy[2]	35	91%	94%	93%
ICU Venous Thromboembolism Prophylaxis[2]	26	96%	94%	92%
Incidence of Potentially Preventable VTE[1,2]	-	-	8%	10%
UFH with Dosages/Platelet Monitoring[2]	36	100%	98%	97%
Venous Thromboembolism Prophylaxis[2]	144	95%	90%	85%
Warfarin Therapy Discharge Instructions[2]	24	100%	78%	75%
Chest Pain/Possible Heart Attack Care				
Aspirin Given Within 24 Hours of Arrival	43	95%	97%	96%
Fibrinolytic Meds Within 30 Min. of Arrival[7]	-	-	44%	58%
Average Time to ECG (minutes)	45	9	9	7
Average Time to Transfer (minutes)[1]	-	-	64	60
Children's Asthma Care				
Received Home Management Plan of Care	-	-	-	88%
Received Reliever Medication	-	-	-	100%
Received Systemic Corticosteroids	-	-	-	100%
Emergency Department				
Admittance Decision Time (minutes)[2]	315	46	104	98
Head CT Results Within 45 Min. of Arrival[1]	-	-	60%	57%
Patients Who Left ER Before Being Seen	16,970	0%	1%	2%
Time from ER Arrival to Admit. (minutes)[2]	316	180	276	274
Time from ER Arrival to Discharge (minutes)	362	95	125	134
Time in ER Before Being Evaluated (minutes)	386	0	26	26
Time to Pain Meds for Fractures (minutes)	94	55	58	57
Heart Attack Care				
Aspirin Given at Discharge[1,3]	-	-	99%	99%
Fibrinolytic Meds Within 30 Min. of Arrival[3,7]	-	-	40%	54%
PCI Within 90 Minutes of Arrival[3,7]	-	-	97%	96%
Statin Prescribed at Discharge[1,3]	-	-	99%	98%
Heart Failure Care				
ACE Inhibitor or ARB for LVSD	13	69%	97%	97%
Discharge Instructions Given	40	100%	96%	94%
Evaluation of LVS Function	79	100%	100%	99%

NOTE: Hospital profiles are in alphabetical order by state, then city, then hospital within the city; Rankings exclude hospitals with less than 25 cases except for patient surveys which excludes hospitals with less than 100 cases; (a) 100-299 cases; (1) The number of cases/patients is too few to report; (2) Data submitted were based on a sample of cases/patients; (3) Results are based on a shorter time period than required; (4) Data suppressed by CMS for one or more quarters; (5) Results are not available for this reporting period; (6) Fewer than 100 patients completed the HCAHPS survey; (7) No cases met the criteria for this measure; (8) The lower limit of the confidence interval cannot be calculated if the number of observed infections equals zero; (9) No data are available from the state/territory for this reporting period; (10) The scores shown reflect fewer than 50 completed surveys; (11) There were discrepancies in the data collection process; (12) This measure does not apply to this hospital for this reporting period; (13) Results cannot be calculated for this reporting period; (14) The results for this state are combined with nearby states to protect confidentiality; Please refer to the User's Guide for a full explanation of data.

Measure	Cases	This Hosp.	State Avg.	U.S. Avg.
Medicare Spending				
Medicare Spending per Patient (ratio)	-	1.03	1.01	0.98
Pneumonia Care				
Appropriate Initial Antibiotic Given	70	96%	96%	95%
Blood Culture Timing	110	99%	98%	98%
Pregnancy and Delivery Care				
Newborn Deliveries Scheduled Early	16	25%	4%	6%
Preventive Care				
Immunization for Influenza[2]	261	90%	91%	90%
Immunization for Pneumonia[2]	386	93%	92%	92%
Stroke Care				
Anticoagulation Therapy for Atrial Fibrillation[1]	-	-	96%	95%
Antithrombotic Therapy Timing	14	100%	98%	98%
Assessed for Rehabilitation	13	92%	98%	97%
Discharged on Antithrombotic Therapy	11	100%	99%	99%
Discharged on Statin Medication[1]	-	-	95%	94%
Thrombolytic Therapy Timing[1]	-	-	72%	66%
Venous Thromboembolism Prophylaxis	14	93%	95%	94%
Written Stroke Educational Materials Given[1]	-	-	90%	88%
Surgical Care Improvement Project				
Appropriate Beta Blocker Usage	25	96%	98%	98%
Appropriate VTP Within 24 Hours	84	96%	99%	98%
Controlled Postoperative Blood Glucose[7]	-	-	98%	97%
Perioperative Temperature Management	93	100%	100%	100%
Prophylactic Antibiotic Selection	76	100%	99%	99%
Prophylactic Antibiotic Selection (Outpatient)	89	100%	98%	98%
Prophylactic Antibiotic Stopped	72	99%	98%	98%
Prophylactic Antibiotic Timing	76	96%	99%	99%
Prophylactic Antibiotic Timing (Outpatient)	89	99%	98%	98%
Urinary Catheter Removal	63	98%	99%	97%
Survey of Patients' Hospital Experiences				
Area Around Room 'Always' Quiet at Night	300+	47%	54%	61%
Doctors 'Always' Communicated Well	300+	81%	80%	82%
Home Recovery Information Given	300+	88%	86%	85%
Hospital Given 9 or 10 on 10 Point Scale	300+	63%	69%	71%
Meds 'Always' Explained Before Given	300+	61%	63%	64%
Nurses 'Always' Communicated Well	300+	76%	79%	79%
Pain 'Always' Well Controlled	300+	65%	70%	71%
Room and Bathroom 'Always' Clean	300+	75%	73%	73%
Timely Help 'Always' Received	300+	54%	67%	68%
Would Definitely Recommend Hospital	300+	61%	70%	71%
Use of Medical Imaging				
Cardiac Imaging Stress Test before Surgery	158	5.7%	5.4%	5.3%
Combination Abdominal CT Scan	315	20.6%	12.2%	10.5%
Combination Brain/Sinus CT Scan[1]	-	-	3.1%	2.7%
Combination Chest CT Scan	166	0.0%	2.1%	2.7%
Follow-up Mammogram/Ultrasound	408	11.0%	9%	8.8%
Lumbar Spine MRI for Low Back Pain[1]	-	-	35.8%	37.2%

Hanover Hospital

300 Highland Ave
Hanover, PA 17331
Phone: 717-637-3711
Fax: 717-633-2217
URL: www.hanoverhospital.org
Type: Acute Care Hospitals
Emergency Services: Yes
Ownership: Voluntary non-profit - Private
Beds: 117
Key Personnel:
Radiology. . . . . Alicia M Cartagena
Quality Assurance . . . . Gary Grant
Infection Control. . . . . Jennifer Laughman
Chief of Medical Staff. . . . . John Lunsford, Jr, MD
Emergency Room . . . . David Pittman , MSN, RN
Operating Room. . . . . Connie Robinson
CEO/President. . . . . James E. Wissler
Patient Relations . . . . Laurie Wolf

Measure	Cases	This Hosp.	State Avg.	U.S. Avg.
Blood Clot Prevention and Treatment				
Anticoagulation Overlap Therapy[2]	52	88%	94%	93%
ICU Venous Thromboembolism Prophylaxis[2]	119	99%	94%	92%
Incidence of Potentially Preventable VTE[1,2]	-	-	8%	10%
UFH with Dosages/Platelet Monitoring[2]	50	100%	98%	97%
Venous Thromboembolism Prophylaxis[2]	373	96%	90%	85%
Warfarin Therapy Discharge Instructions[2]	33	55%	78%	75%
Chest Pain/Possible Heart Attack Care				
Aspirin Given Within 24 Hours of Arrival	90	97%	97%	96%
Fibrinolytic Meds Within 30 Min. of Arrival[7]	-	-	44%	58%
Average Time to ECG (minutes)	95	9	9	7
Average Time to Transfer (minutes)	20	56	64	60
Children's Asthma Care				
Received Home Management Plan of Care	-	-	-	88%
Received Reliever Medication	-	-	-	100%
Received Systemic Corticosteroids	-	-	-	100%
Emergency Department				
Admittance Decision Time (minutes)[2]	808	133	104	98
Head CT Results Within 45 Min. of Arrival	25	64%	60%	57%
Patients Who Left ER Before Being Seen	31,358	2%	1%	2%
Time from ER Arrival to Admit. (minutes)[2]	809	356	276	274
Time from ER Arrival to Discharge (minutes)	808	156	125	134
Time in ER Before Being Evaluated (minutes)	861	35	26	26
Time to Pain Meds for Fractures (minutes)	140	74	58	57
Heart Attack Care				
Aspirin Given at Discharge	57	100%	99%	99%
Fibrinolytic Meds Within 30 Min. of Arrival[7]	-	-	40%	54%
PCI Within 90 Minutes of Arrival[7]	-	-	97%	96%
Statin Prescribed at Discharge	61	95%	99%	98%
Heart Failure Care				
ACE Inhibitor or ARB for LVSD	54	100%	97%	97%
Discharge Instructions Given	176	100%	96%	94%
Evaluation of LVS Function	233	100%	100%	99%
Medicare Spending				
Medicare Spending per Patient (ratio)	-	0.97	1.01	0.98
Pneumonia Care				
Appropriate Initial Antibiotic Given	120	98%	96%	95%
Blood Culture Timing	212	100%	98%	98%
Pregnancy and Delivery Care				
Newborn Deliveries Scheduled Early[2]	39	8%	4%	6%
Preventive Care				
Immunization for Influenza[2]	511	97%	91%	90%
Immunization for Pneumonia[2]	751	99%	92%	92%
Stroke Care				
Anticoagulation Therapy for Atrial Fibrillation	17	100%	96%	95%
Antithrombotic Therapy Timing	89	100%	98%	98%
Assessed for Rehabilitation	95	97%	98%	97%
Discharged on Antithrombotic Therapy	90	100%	99%	99%
Discharged on Statin Medication	77	99%	95%	94%
Thrombolytic Therapy Timing[1]	-	-	72%	66%
Venous Thromboembolism Prophylaxis	93	97%	95%	94%
Written Stroke Educational Materials Given	51	98%	90%	88%
Surgical Care Improvement Project				
Appropriate Beta Blocker Usage	152	100%	98%	98%
Appropriate VTP Within 24 Hours	415	99%	99%	98%
Controlled Postoperative Blood Glucose[7]	-	-	98%	97%
Perioperative Temperature Management	474	100%	100%	100%
Prophylactic Antibiotic Selection	362	99%	99%	99%
Prophylactic Antibiotic Selection (Outpatient)	122	98%	98%	98%
Prophylactic Antibiotic Stopped	355	100%	98%	98%
Prophylactic Antibiotic Timing	363	98%	99%	99%
Prophylactic Antibiotic Timing (Outpatient)	123	98%	98%	98%
Urinary Catheter Removal	359	99%	99%	97%
Survey of Patients' Hospital Experiences				
Area Around Room 'Always' Quiet at Night	300+	52%	54%	61%
Doctors 'Always' Communicated Well	300+	83%	80%	82%
Home Recovery Information Given	300+	86%	86%	85%
Hospital Given 9 or 10 on 10 Point Scale	300+	67%	69%	71%
Meds 'Always' Explained Before Given	300+	61%	63%	64%
Nurses 'Always' Communicated Well	300+	80%	79%	79%
Pain 'Always' Well Controlled	300+	67%	70%	71%
Room and Bathroom 'Always' Clean	300+	82%	73%	73%
Timely Help 'Always' Received	300+	69%	67%	68%
Would Definitely Recommend Hospital	300+	67%	70%	71%
Use of Medical Imaging				
Cardiac Imaging Stress Test before Surgery	438	4.3%	5.4%	5.3%
Combination Abdominal CT Scan	820	7.9%	12.2%	10.5%
Combination Brain/Sinus CT Scan	637	2.7%	3.1%	2.7%
Combination Chest CT Scan	555	2.5%	2.1%	2.7%
Follow-up Mammogram/Ultrasound	1,062	10.5%	9%	8.8%
Lumbar Spine MRI for Low Back Pain	123	26.8%	35.8%	37.2%

Pinnacle Health Hospitals

409 South Second Street
Harrisburg, PA 17105
Phone: 717-782-5181
URL: www.pinnaclehealth.org
Type: Acute Care Hospitals
Emergency Services: Yes
Ownership: Voluntary non-profit - Other
Key Personnel:
CEO/President. . . . . Michael A. Young, FACHE

Measure	Cases	This Hosp.	State Avg.	U.S. Avg.
Blood Clot Prevention and Treatment				
Anticoagulation Overlap Therapy[2]	210	90%	94%	93%
ICU Venous Thromboembolism Prophylaxis[2]	182	91%	94%	92%
Incidence of Potentially Preventable VTE[2]	41	17%	8%	10%
UFH with Dosages/Platelet Monitoring[2]	139	99%	98%	97%
Venous Thromboembolism Prophylaxis[2]	536	93%	90%	85%
Warfarin Therapy Discharge Instructions[2]	162	77%	78%	75%
Chest Pain/Possible Heart Attack Care				
Aspirin Given Within 24 Hours of Arrival[5]	-	-	97%	96%
Fibrinolytic Meds Within 30 Min. of Arrival[5]	-	-	44%	58%
Average Time to ECG (minutes)[5]	-	-	9	7
Average Time to Transfer (minutes)[5]	-	-	64	60
Children's Asthma Care				
Received Home Management Plan of Care	-	-	-	88%
Received Reliever Medication	-	-	-	100%
Received Systemic Corticosteroids	-	-	-	100%
Emergency Department				
Admittance Decision Time (minutes)[2]	611	100	104	98
Head CT Results Within 45 Min. of Arrival	11	27%	60%	57%
Patients Who Left ER Before Being Seen	>100k	2%	1%	2%
Time from ER Arrival to Admit. (minutes)[2]	611	244	276	274
Time from ER Arrival to Discharge (minutes)	721	146	125	134
Time in ER Before Being Evaluated (minutes)	690	50	26	26
Time to Pain Meds for Fractures (minutes)	277	59	58	57
Heart Attack Care				
Aspirin Given at Discharge	619	100%	99%	99%
Fibrinolytic Meds Within 30 Min. of Arrival[7]	-	-	40%	54%
PCI Within 90 Minutes of Arrival	94	100%	97%	96%
Statin Prescribed at Discharge	608	99%	99%	98%
Heart Failure Care				
ACE Inhibitor or ARB for LVSD	195	100%	97%	97%
Discharge Instructions Given	611	100%	96%	94%
Evaluation of LVS Function	804	100%	100%	99%
Medicare Spending				
Medicare Spending per Patient (ratio)	-	1.05	1.01	0.98
Pneumonia Care				
Appropriate Initial Antibiotic Given	303	99%	96%	95%
Blood Culture Timing	493	99%	98%	98%
Pregnancy and Delivery Care				
Newborn Deliveries Scheduled Early[2]	47	0%	4%	6%
Preventive Care				
Immunization for Influenza[2]	629	95%	91%	90%
Immunization for Pneumonia[2]	830	96%	92%	92%
Stroke Care				
Anticoagulation Therapy for Atrial Fibrillation	57	91%	96%	95%
Antithrombotic Therapy Timing	295	96%	98%	98%
Assessed for Rehabilitation	364	99%	98%	97%
Discharged on Antithrombotic Therapy	334	100%	99%	99%
Discharged on Statin Medication	268	97%	95%	94%
Thrombolytic Therapy Timing	39	77%	72%	66%
Venous Thromboembolism Prophylaxis	373	90%	95%	94%
Written Stroke Educational Materials Given	195	96%	90%	88%
Surgical Care Improvement Project				
Appropriate Beta Blocker Usage[2]	1,132	99%	98%	98%
Appropriate VTP Within 24 Hours[2]	2,656	100%	99%	98%
Controlled Postoperative Blood Glucose[2]	445	100%	98%	97%
Perioperative Temperature Management[2]	3,003	100%	100%	100%
Prophylactic Antibiotic Selection[2]	2,764	100%	99%	99%
Prophylactic Antibiotic Selection (Outpatient)	1,331	100%	98%	98%
Prophylactic Antibiotic Stopped[2]	2,698	99%	98%	98%
Prophylactic Antibiotic Timing[2]	2,764	100%	99%	99%
Prophylactic Antibiotic Timing (Outpatient)	1,331	100%	98%	98%
Urinary Catheter Removal[2]	1,303	100%	99%	97%
Survey of Patients' Hospital Experiences				

NOTE: Hospital profiles are in alphabetical order by state, then city, then hospital within the city; Rankings exclude hospitals with less than 25 cases except for patient surveys which excludes hospitals with less than 100 cases; (a) 100-299 cases; (1) The number of cases/patients is too few to report; (2) Data submitted were based on a sample of cases/patients; (3) Results are based on a shorter time period than required; (4) Data suppressed by CMS for one or more quarters; (5) Results are not available for this reporting period; (6) Fewer than 100 patients completed the HCAHPS survey; (7) No cases met the criteria for this measure; (8) The lower limit of the confidence interval cannot be calculated if the number of observed infections equals zero; (9) No data are available from the state/territory for this reporting period; (10) The scores shown reflect fewer than 50 completed surveys; (11) There were discrepancies in the data collection process; (12) This measure does not apply to this hospital for this reporting period; (13) Results cannot be calculated for this reporting period; (14) The results for this state are combined with nearby states to protect confidentiality; Please refer to the User's Guide for a full explanation of data.

Area Around Room 'Always' Quiet at Night	300+	50%	54%	61%
Doctors 'Always' Communicated Well	300+	77%	80%	82%
Home Recovery Information Given	300+	89%	86%	85%
Hospital Given 9 or 10 on 10 Point Scale	300+	70%	69%	71%
Meds 'Always' Explained Before Given	300+	66%	63%	64%
Nurses 'Always' Communicated Well	300+	81%	79%	79%
Pain 'Always' Well Controlled	300+	68%	70%	71%
Room and Bathroom 'Always' Clean	300+	70%	73%	73%
Timely Help 'Always' Received	300+	65%	67%	68%
Would Definitely Recommend Hospital	300+	76%	70%	71%
Use of Medical Imaging				
Cardiac Imaging Stress Test before Surgery	1,867	3.4%	5.4%	5.3%
Combination Abdominal CT Scan	1,764	19.6%	12.2%	10.5%
Combination Brain/Sinus CT Scan	1,057	2.7%	3.1%	2.7%
Combination Chest CT Scan	1,281	0.8%	2.1%	2.7%
Follow-up Mammogram/Ultrasound	4,462	9.2%	9%	8.8%
Lumbar Spine MRI for Low Back Pain	418	38.0%	35.8%	37.2%

Miners Medical Center

290 Haida Avenue
Hastings, PA 16646
Phone: 814-247-3100
Fax: 814-247-3119
URL: www.minershosp.org
Type: Acute Care Hospitals
Emergency Services: Yes
Ownership: Voluntary non-profit - Private
Beds: 30

Key Personnel:
Radiology. Vallabhaneni Babu
Chief of Medical Staff. . . . . John Crawford
CEO/President. . . . . Steve Tucker

Measure	Cases	This Hosp.	State Avg.	U.S. Avg.
Blood Clot Prevention and Treatment				
Anticoagulation Overlap Therapy[2,7]	-	-	94%	93%
ICU Venous Thromboembolism Prophylaxis[2]	45	89%	94%	92%
Incidence of Potentially Preventable VTE[2,7]	-	-	8%	10%
UFH with Dosages/Platelet Monitoring[2,7]	-	-	98%	97%
Venous Thromboembolism Prophylaxis[2]	243	77%	90%	85%
Warfarin Therapy Discharge Instructions[2,7]	-	-	78%	75%
Chest Pain/Possible Heart Attack Care				
Aspirin Given Within 24 Hours of Arrival	74	84%	97%	96%
Fibrinolytic Meds Within 30 Min. of Arrival[7]	-	-	44%	58%
Average Time to ECG (minutes)	76	17	9	7
Average Time to Transfer (minutes)[1]	-	-	64	60
Children's Asthma Care				
Received Home Management Plan of Care	-	-	-	88%
Received Reliever Medication	-	-	-	100%
Received Systemic Corticosteroids	-	-	-	100%
Emergency Department				
Admittance Decision Time (minutes)	325	40	104	98
Head CT Results Within 45 Min. of Arrival[1,3]	-	-	60%	57%
Patients Who Left ER Before Being Seen	10,044	0%	1%	2%
Time from ER Arrival to Admit. (minutes)	343	165	276	274
Time from ER Arrival to Discharge (minutes)	237	80	125	134
Time in ER Before Being Evaluated (minutes)	371	5	26	26
Time to Pain Meds for Fractures (minutes)[1]	-	-	58	57
Heart Attack Care				
Aspirin Given at Discharge[1]	-	-	99%	99%
Fibrinolytic Meds Within 30 Min. of Arrival[7]	-	-	40%	54%
PCI Within 90 Minutes of Arrival[7]	-	-	97%	96%
Statin Prescribed at Discharge[1]	-	-	99%	98%
Heart Failure Care				
ACE Inhibitor or ARB for LVSD[1]	-	-	97%	97%
Discharge Instructions Given	29	52%	96%	94%
Evaluation of LVS Function	38	71%	100%	99%
Medicare Spending				
Medicare Spending per Patient (ratio)	-	0.99	1.01	0.98
Pneumonia Care				
Appropriate Initial Antibiotic Given	29	86%	96%	95%
Blood Culture Timing	45	89%	98%	98%
Pregnancy and Delivery Care				
Newborn Deliveries Scheduled Early[7]	-	-	4%	6%
Preventive Care				
Immunization for Influenza[2]	254	74%	91%	90%
Immunization for Pneumonia[2]	372	73%	92%	92%
Stroke Care				
Anticoagulation Therapy for Atrial Fibrillation[1,3]	-	-	96%	95%
Antithrombotic Therapy Timing[1,3]	-	-	98%	98%
Assessed for Rehabilitation[1,3]	-	-	98%	97%
Discharged on Antithrombotic Therapy[1,3]	-	-	99%	99%
Discharged on Statin Medication[1,3]	-	-	95%	94%
Thrombolytic Therapy Timing[1,3]	-	-	72%	66%
Venous Thromboembolism Prophylaxis[1,3]	-	-	95%	94%
Written Stroke Educational Materials Given[1,3]	-	-	90%	88%
Surgical Care Improvement Project				
Appropriate Beta Blocker Usage[1,3]	-	-	98%	98%
Appropriate VTP Within 24 Hours[3]	11	82%	99%	98%
Controlled Postoperative Blood Glucose[3,7]	-	-	98%	97%
Perioperative Temperature Management[3]	12	83%	100%	100%
Prophylactic Antibiotic Selection[3]	11	100%	99%	99%
Prophylactic Antibiotic Selection (Outpatient)[1]	-	-	98%	98%
Prophylactic Antibiotic Stopped[3]	11	100%	98%	98%
Prophylactic Antibiotic Timing[3]	11	91%	99%	99%
Prophylactic Antibiotic Timing (Outpatient)[1]	-	-	98%	98%
Urinary Catheter Removal[1,3]	-	-	99%	97%
Survey of Patients' Hospital Experiences				
Area Around Room 'Always' Quiet at Night[6]	<100	62%	54%	61%
Doctors 'Always' Communicated Well[6]	<100	91%	80%	82%
Home Recovery Information Given[6]	<100	87%	86%	85%
Hospital Given 9 or 10 on 10 Point Scale[6]	<100	66%	69%	71%
Meds 'Always' Explained Before Given[6]	<100	69%	63%	64%
Nurses 'Always' Communicated Well[6]	<100	77%	79%	79%
Pain 'Always' Well Controlled[6]	<100	72%	70%	71%
Room and Bathroom 'Always' Clean[6]	<100	76%	73%	73%
Timely Help 'Always' Received[6]	<100	80%	67%	68%
Would Definitely Recommend Hospital[6]	<100	73%	70%	71%
Use of Medical Imaging				
Cardiac Imaging Stress Test before Surgery[1]	-	-	5.4%	5.3%
Combination Abdominal CT Scan	142	0.0%	12.2%	10.5%
Combination Brain/Sinus CT Scan[1]	-	-	3.1%	2.7%
Combination Chest CT Scan	68	0.0%	2.1%	2.7%
Follow-up Mammogram/Ultrasound	120	10.8%	9%	8.8%
Lumbar Spine MRI for Low Back Pain[1]	-	-	35.8%	37.2%

Lehigh Valley Hospital - Hazleton

700 East Broad Street
Hazleton, PA 18201
Phone: 570-501-4000
Fax: 570-501-6203
URL: www.ghha.org
Type: Acute Care Hospitals
Emergency Services: Yes
Ownership: Voluntary non-profit - Other
Beds: 160

Key Personnel:
Quality Assurance . . . . Andrea Andrews
Radiology. . . . . Orest B Boyko
CEO/President. . . . . James D Edwards
Patient Relations . . . . Sue Farley
Operating Room. . . . . Kathy Guida
Infection Control. . . . . Edna Reis
Emergency Room . . . . Paul Tayoun, DO
Chief of Medical Staff. . . . . Anthony Valente, MD

Measure	Cases	This Hosp.	State Avg.	U.S. Avg.
Blood Clot Prevention and Treatment				
Anticoagulation Overlap Therapy[2]	25	80%	94%	93%
ICU Venous Thromboembolism Prophylaxis[2]	51	71%	94%	92%
Incidence of Potentially Preventable VTE[1,2]	-	-	8%	10%
UFH with Dosages/Platelet Monitoring[2]	19	47%	98%	97%
Venous Thromboembolism Prophylaxis[2]	394	61%	90%	85%
Warfarin Therapy Discharge Instructions[2]	14	71%	78%	75%
Chest Pain/Possible Heart Attack Care				
Aspirin Given Within 24 Hours of Arrival	191	96%	97%	96%
Fibrinolytic Meds Within 30 Min. of Arrival[7]	-	-	44%	58%
Average Time to ECG (minutes)	196	13	9	7
Average Time to Transfer (minutes)	15	68	64	60
Children's Asthma Care				
Received Home Management Plan of Care	-	-	-	88%
Received Reliever Medication	-	-	-	100%
Received Systemic Corticosteroids	-	-	-	100%
Emergency Department				
Admittance Decision Time (minutes)[2]	597	103	104	98
Head CT Results Within 45 Min. of Arrival	25	72%	60%	57%
Patients Who Left ER Before Being Seen	31,397	3%	1%	2%
Time from ER Arrival to Admit. (minutes)[2]	641	272	276	274
Time from ER Arrival to Discharge (minutes)	435	141	125	134
Time in ER Before Being Evaluated (minutes)	438	60	26	26
Time to Pain Meds for Fractures (minutes)	116	81	58	57
Heart Attack Care				
Aspirin Given at Discharge	47	100%	99%	99%
Fibrinolytic Meds Within 30 Min. of Arrival[7]	-	-	40%	54%
PCI Within 90 Minutes of Arrival[7]	-	-	97%	96%
Statin Prescribed at Discharge	47	100%	99%	98%
Heart Failure Care				
ACE Inhibitor or ARB for LVSD	45	100%	97%	97%
Discharge Instructions Given	193	99%	96%	94%
Evaluation of LVS Function	287	100%	100%	99%
Medicare Spending				
Medicare Spending per Patient (ratio)	-	1.04	1.01	0.98
Pneumonia Care				
Appropriate Initial Antibiotic Given	144	100%	96%	95%
Blood Culture Timing	221	99%	98%	98%
Pregnancy and Delivery Care				
Newborn Deliveries Scheduled Early[2]	106	20%	4%	6%
Preventive Care				
Immunization for Influenza[2]	566	100%	91%	90%
Immunization for Pneumonia[2]	811	100%	92%	92%
Stroke Care				
Anticoagulation Therapy for Atrial Fibrillation	14	93%	96%	95%
Antithrombotic Therapy Timing	74	95%	98%	98%
Assessed for Rehabilitation	73	92%	98%	97%
Discharged on Antithrombotic Therapy	70	97%	99%	99%
Discharged on Statin Medication	48	96%	95%	94%
Thrombolytic Therapy Timing[1]	-	-	72%	66%
Venous Thromboembolism Prophylaxis	75	75%	95%	94%
Written Stroke Educational Materials Given	30	77%	90%	88%
Surgical Care Improvement Project				
Appropriate Beta Blocker Usage	110	100%	98%	98%
Appropriate VTP Within 24 Hours	229	100%	99%	98%
Controlled Postoperative Blood Glucose[7]	-	-	98%	97%
Perioperative Temperature Management	276	100%	100%	100%
Prophylactic Antibiotic Selection	131	99%	99%	99%
Prophylactic Antibiotic Selection (Outpatient)	54	87%	98%	98%
Prophylactic Antibiotic Stopped	113	99%	98%	98%
Prophylactic Antibiotic Timing	131	98%	99%	99%
Prophylactic Antibiotic Timing (Outpatient)	56	91%	98%	98%
Urinary Catheter Removal	104	100%	99%	97%
Survey of Patients' Hospital Experiences				
Area Around Room 'Always' Quiet at Night	300+	46%	54%	61%
Doctors 'Always' Communicated Well	300+	79%	80%	82%
Home Recovery Information Given	300+	83%	86%	85%
Hospital Given 9 or 10 on 10 Point Scale	300+	53%	69%	71%
Meds 'Always' Explained Before Given	300+	52%	63%	64%
Nurses 'Always' Communicated Well	300+	74%	79%	79%
Pain 'Always' Well Controlled	300+	63%	70%	71%
Room and Bathroom 'Always' Clean	300+	77%	73%	73%
Timely Help 'Always' Received	300+	59%	67%	68%
Would Definitely Recommend Hospital	300+	50%	70%	71%
Use of Medical Imaging				
Cardiac Imaging Stress Test before Surgery	336	5.4%	5.4%	5.3%
Combination Abdominal CT Scan	755	11.4%	12.2%	10.5%
Combination Brain/Sinus CT Scan	732	2.2%	3.1%	2.7%
Combination Chest CT Scan	469	0.4%	2.1%	2.7%
Follow-up Mammogram/Ultrasound	1,436	4.2%	9%	8.8%
Lumbar Spine MRI for Low Back Pain	102	45.1%	35.8%	37.2%

Milton S Hershey Medical Center

500 University Drive
Hershey, PA 17033
Phone: 717-531-8521
Fax: 717-531-4162
URL: www.hmc.psu.edu
Type: Acute Care Hospitals
Emergency Services: Yes
Ownership: Voluntary non-profit - Other
Beds: 504

Key Personnel:
Surgery . . . . Peter Dillon, MD
Administrator . . . . Linda Duncan
Chief of Medical Staff. . . . . Carol Freer, MD
CEO/President. . . . . A. Craig Hillemeier, MD
Anesthesiology. . . . . Berend Mets, M.B., Ch.B., FR
Radiology. . . . . Timothy J. Mosher, MD

NOTE: Hospital profiles are in alphabetical order by state, then city, then hospital within the city; Rankings exclude hospitals with less than 25 cases except for patient surveys which excludes hospitals with less than 100 cases; (a) 100-299 cases; (1) The number of cases/patients is too few to report; (2) Data submitted were based on a sample of cases/patients; (3) Results are based on a shorter time period than required; (4) Data suppressed by CMS for one or more quarters; (5) Results are not available for this reporting period; (6) Fewer than 100 patients completed the HCAHPS survey; (7) No cases met the criteria for this measure; (8) The lower limit of the confidence interval cannot be calculated if the number of observed infections equals zero; (9) No data are available from the state/territory for this reporting period; (10) The scores shown reflect fewer than 50 completed surveys; (11) There were discrepancies in the data collection process; (12) This measure does not apply to this hospital for this reporting period; (13) Results cannot be calculated for this reporting period; (14) The results for this state are combined with nearby states to protect confidentiality; Please refer to the User's Guide for a full explanation of data.

Cardiac Laboratory. . . . . Gerald Neccareli
Emergency Room . . . . Susan Promes, M.D., MBA, FACE

Measure	Cases	This Hosp.	State Avg.	U.S. Avg.
Blood Clot Prevention and Treatment				
Anticoagulation Overlap Therapy[2]	152	96%	94%	93%
ICU Venous Thromboembolism Prophylaxis[2]	90	92%	94%	92%
Incidence of Potentially Preventable VTE[2]	50	2%	8%	10%
UFH with Dosages/Platelet Monitoring[2]	139	99%	98%	97%
Venous Thromboembolism Prophylaxis[2]	318	84%	90%	85%
Warfarin Therapy Discharge Instructions[2]	122	100%	78%	75%
Chest Pain/Possible Heart Attack Care				
Aspirin Given Within 24 Hours of Arrival[5]	-	-	97%	96%
Fibrinolytic Meds Within 30 Min. of Arrival[5]	-	-	44%	58%
Average Time to ECG (minutes)[5]	-	-	9	7
Average Time to Transfer (minutes)[5]	-	-	64	60
Children's Asthma Care				
Received Home Management Plan of Care	-	-	-	88%
Received Reliever Medication	-	-	-	100%
Received Systemic Corticosteroids	-	-	-	100%
Emergency Department				
Admittance Decision Time (minutes)[2]	571	124	104	98
Head CT Results Within 45 Min. of Arrival[1]	-	-	60%	57%
Patients Who Left ER Before Being Seen	64,929	1%	1%	2%
Time from ER Arrival to Admit. (minutes)[2]	579	393	276	274
Time from ER Arrival to Discharge (minutes)	461	194	125	134
Time in ER Before Being Evaluated (minutes)	491	21	26	26
Time to Pain Meds for Fractures (minutes)	243	71	58	57
Heart Attack Care				
Aspirin Given at Discharge	396	100%	99%	99%
Fibrinolytic Meds Within 30 Min. of Arrival[7]	-	-	40%	54%
PCI Within 90 Minutes of Arrival	57	95%	97%	96%
Statin Prescribed at Discharge	392	99%	99%	98%
Heart Failure Care				
ACE Inhibitor or ARB for LVSD	148	100%	97%	97%
Discharge Instructions Given	460	99%	96%	94%
Evaluation of LVS Function	559	100%	100%	99%
Medicare Spending				
Medicare Spending per Patient (ratio)	-	0.98	1.01	0.98
Pneumonia Care				
Appropriate Initial Antibiotic Given	128	98%	96%	95%
Blood Culture Timing	382	98%	98%	98%
Pregnancy and Delivery Care				
Newborn Deliveries Scheduled Early[2]	67	0%	4%	6%
Preventive Care				
Immunization for Influenza[2]	615	98%	91%	90%
Immunization for Pneumonia[2]	596	89%	92%	92%
Stroke Care				
Anticoagulation Therapy for Atrial Fibrillation	59	97%	96%	95%
Antithrombotic Therapy Timing	260	98%	98%	98%
Assessed for Rehabilitation	417	100%	98%	97%
Discharged on Antithrombotic Therapy	298	100%	99%	99%
Discharged on Statin Medication	230	100%	95%	94%
Thrombolytic Therapy Timing	36	92%	72%	66%
Venous Thromboembolism Prophylaxis	461	99%	95%	94%
Written Stroke Educational Materials Given	208	88%	90%	88%
Surgical Care Improvement Project				
Appropriate Beta Blocker Usage[2]	553	99%	98%	98%
Appropriate VTP Within 24 Hours[2]	989	100%	99%	98%
Controlled Postoperative Blood Glucose[2]	367	95%	98%	97%
Perioperative Temperature Management[2]	1,230	100%	100%	100%
Prophylactic Antibiotic Selection[2]	1,077	100%	99%	99%
Prophylactic Antibiotic Selection (Outpatient)	1,060	98%	98%	98%
Prophylactic Antibiotic Stopped[2]	1,038	97%	98%	98%
Prophylactic Antibiotic Timing[2]	1,078	99%	99%	99%
Prophylactic Antibiotic Timing (Outpatient)	1,060	99%	98%	98%
Urinary Catheter Removal[2]	978	100%	99%	97%
Survey of Patients' Hospital Experiences				
Area Around Room 'Always' Quiet at Night	300+	48%	54%	61%
Doctors 'Always' Communicated Well	300+	78%	80%	82%
Home Recovery Information Given	300+	88%	86%	85%
Hospital Given 9 or 10 on 10 Point Scale	300+	76%	69%	71%
Meds 'Always' Explained Before Given	300+	63%	63%	64%
Nurses 'Always' Communicated Well	300+	80%	79%	79%
Pain 'Always' Well Controlled	300+	69%	70%	71%
Room and Bathroom 'Always' Clean	300+	69%	73%	73%
Timely Help 'Always' Received	300+	68%	67%	68%
Would Definitely Recommend Hospital	300+	80%	70%	71%
Use of Medical Imaging				
Cardiac Imaging Stress Test before Surgery	564	4.3%	5.4%	5.3%
Combination Abdominal CT Scan	2,299	15.9%	12.2%	10.5%
Combination Brain/Sinus CT Scan	720	2.1%	3.1%	2.7%
Combination Chest CT Scan	2,378	0.2%	2.1%	2.7%
Follow-up Mammogram/Ultrasound	1,425	7.5%	9%	8.8%
Lumbar Spine MRI for Low Back Pain	179	25.7%	35.8%	37.2%

Wayne Memorial Hospital

601 Park Street
Honesdale, PA 18431
Phone: 570-253-8100
Fax: 570-253-8397
URL: www.wmh.org
Type: Acute Care Hospitals
Emergency Services: Yes
Ownership: Voluntary non-profit - Private
Beds: 95

Key Personnel:

Anesthesiology. . . . . RA Achecar, MD
Emergency Room . . . . Donna Eget, MD
CEO/President. . . . . David Hoff, FACHE
Intensive Care Unit. . . . . Lisa Kinzinger
Quality Assurance . . . . Marilyn Swendsen
Infection Control. . . . . Cinda Tietjen
Chief of Medical Staff. . . . . George Tietjen, MD

Measure	Cases	This Hosp.	State Avg.	U.S. Avg.
Blood Clot Prevention and Treatment				
Anticoagulation Overlap Therapy[2]	14	86%	94%	93%
ICU Venous Thromboembolism Prophylaxis[2]	31	90%	94%	92%
Incidence of Potentially Preventable VTE[2,7]	-	-	8%	10%
UFH with Dosages/Platelet Monitoring[2]	11	91%	98%	97%
Venous Thromboembolism Prophylaxis[2]	244	92%	90%	85%
Warfarin Therapy Discharge Instructions[2]	11	100%	78%	75%
Chest Pain/Possible Heart Attack Care				
Aspirin Given Within 24 Hours of Arrival	56	100%	97%	96%
Fibrinolytic Meds Within 30 Min. of Arrival[7]	-	-	44%	58%
Average Time to ECG (minutes)	57	6	9	7
Average Time to Transfer (minutes)[1]	-	-	64	60
Children's Asthma Care				
Received Home Management Plan of Care	-	-	-	88%
Received Reliever Medication	-	-	-	100%
Received Systemic Corticosteroids	-	-	-	100%
Emergency Department				
Admittance Decision Time (minutes)[2]	380	212	104	98
Head CT Results Within 45 Min. of Arrival[1]	-	-	60%	57%
Patients Who Left ER Before Being Seen	21,908	0%	1%	2%
Time from ER Arrival to Admit. (minutes)[2]	397	356	276	274
Time from ER Arrival to Discharge (minutes)	359	164	125	134
Time in ER Before Being Evaluated (minutes)	388	35	26	26
Time to Pain Meds for Fractures (minutes)	91	66	58	57
Heart Attack Care				
Aspirin Given at Discharge	12	100%	99%	99%
Fibrinolytic Meds Within 30 Min. of Arrival[7]	-	-	40%	54%
PCI Within 90 Minutes of Arrival[7]	-	-	97%	96%
Statin Prescribed at Discharge	12	100%	99%	98%
Heart Failure Care				
ACE Inhibitor or ARB for LVSD	19	100%	97%	97%
Discharge Instructions Given	59	90%	96%	94%
Evaluation of LVS Function	87	98%	100%	99%
Medicare Spending				
Medicare Spending per Patient (ratio)	-	1.04	1.01	0.98
Pneumonia Care				
Appropriate Initial Antibiotic Given	90	97%	96%	95%
Blood Culture Timing	151	99%	98%	98%
Pregnancy and Delivery Care				
Newborn Deliveries Scheduled Early[2]	26	0%	4%	6%
Preventive Care				
Immunization for Influenza[2]	298	95%	91%	90%
Immunization for Pneumonia[2]	405	100%	92%	92%
Stroke Care				
Anticoagulation Therapy for Atrial Fibrillation[1]	-	-	96%	95%
Antithrombotic Therapy Timing	30	100%	98%	98%
Assessed for Rehabilitation	35	100%	98%	97%
Discharged on Antithrombotic Therapy	34	94%	99%	99%
Discharged on Statin Medication	27	93%	95%	94%
Thrombolytic Therapy Timing[1]	-	-	72%	66%
Venous Thromboembolism Prophylaxis	30	100%	95%	94%
Written Stroke Educational Materials Given	23	78%	90%	88%
Surgical Care Improvement Project				
Appropriate Beta Blocker Usage	74	97%	98%	98%
Appropriate VTP Within 24 Hours	255	97%	99%	98%
Controlled Postoperative Blood Glucose[7]	-	-	98%	97%
Perioperative Temperature Management	275	100%	100%	100%
Prophylactic Antibiotic Selection	175	97%	99%	99%
Prophylactic Antibiotic Selection (Outpatient)	34	94%	98%	98%
Prophylactic Antibiotic Stopped	173	94%	98%	98%
Prophylactic Antibiotic Timing	175	99%	99%	99%
Prophylactic Antibiotic Timing (Outpatient)	34	94%	98%	98%
Urinary Catheter Removal	192	98%	99%	97%
Survey of Patients' Hospital Experiences				
Area Around Room 'Always' Quiet at Night	300+	52%	54%	61%
Doctors 'Always' Communicated Well	300+	81%	80%	82%
Home Recovery Information Given	300+	89%	86%	85%
Hospital Given 9 or 10 on 10 Point Scale	300+	65%	69%	71%
Meds 'Always' Explained Before Given	300+	62%	63%	64%
Nurses 'Always' Communicated Well	300+	80%	79%	79%
Pain 'Always' Well Controlled	300+	69%	70%	71%
Room and Bathroom 'Always' Clean	300+	75%	73%	73%
Timely Help 'Always' Received	300+	68%	67%	68%
Would Definitely Recommend Hospital	300+	68%	70%	71%
Use of Medical Imaging				
Cardiac Imaging Stress Test before Surgery	229	7.4%	5.4%	5.3%
Combination Abdominal CT Scan	719	18.8%	12.2%	10.5%
Combination Brain/Sinus CT Scan	603	2.8%	3.1%	2.7%
Combination Chest CT Scan	465	11.0%	2.1%	2.7%
Follow-up Mammogram/Ultrasound	1,190	5.6%	9%	8.8%
Lumbar Spine MRI for Low Back Pain	76	34.2%	35.8%	37.2%

J C Blair Memorial Hospital

1225 Warm Springs Ave
Huntingdon, PA 16652
Phone: 814-643-2290
Fax: 814-643-8813
URL: www.jcblair.org
Type: Acute Care Hospitals
Emergency Services: Yes
Ownership: Voluntary non-profit - Private
Beds: 104

Key Personnel:

Operating Room. . . . . Leigh Bizak, RN
Infection Control. . . . . Bethany Brown
Radiology. . . . . Larry Garman
CEO . . . . Lisa Mallon, ACHE
Coronary Care. . . . . Don McCauley
Pediatric Ambulatory Care . . . . . . Rita Notestine
Chief of Medical Staff. . . . . Christopher J Patitsas, MD
Quality Assurance . . . . Marlene Pierce

Measure	Cases	This Hosp.	State Avg.	U.S. Avg.
Blood Clot Prevention and Treatment				
Anticoagulation Overlap Therapy[2]	14	64%	94%	93%
ICU Venous Thromboembolism Prophylaxis[2]	33	88%	94%	92%
Incidence of Potentially Preventable VTE[1,2]	-	-	8%	10%
UFH with Dosages/Platelet Monitoring[1,2]	-	-	98%	97%
Venous Thromboembolism Prophylaxis[2]	106	93%	90%	85%
Warfarin Therapy Discharge Instructions[1,2]	-	-	78%	75%
Chest Pain/Possible Heart Attack Care				
Aspirin Given Within 24 Hours of Arrival	134	94%	97%	96%
Fibrinolytic Meds Within 30 Min. of Arrival[1]	-	-	44%	58%
Average Time to ECG (minutes)	144	11	9	7
Average Time to Transfer (minutes)[1]	-	-	64	60
Children's Asthma Care				
Received Home Management Plan of Care	-	-	-	88%
Received Reliever Medication	-	-	-	100%
Received Systemic Corticosteroids	-	-	-	100%
Emergency Department				
Admittance Decision Time (minutes)[2]	145	76	104	98
Head CT Results Within 45 Min. of Arrival[1]	-	-	60%	57%
Patients Who Left ER Before Being Seen	17,289	0%	1%	2%
Time from ER Arrival to Admit. (minutes)[2]	330	240	276	274
Time from ER Arrival to Discharge (minutes)	352	128	125	134

NOTE: Hospital profiles are in alphabetical order by state, then city, then hospital within the city; Rankings exclude hospitals with less than 25 cases except for patient surveys which excludes hospitals with less than 100 cases; (a) 100-299 cases; (1) The number of cases/patients is too few to report; (2) Data submitted were based on a sample of cases/patients; (3) Results are based on a shorter time period than required; (4) Data suppressed by CMS for one or more quarters; (5) Results are not available for this reporting period; (6) Fewer than 100 patients completed the HCAHPS survey; (7) No cases met the criteria for this measure; (8) The lower limit of the confidence interval cannot be calculated if the number of observed infections equals zero; (9) No data are available from the state/territory for this reporting period; (10) The scores shown reflect fewer than 50 completed surveys; (11) There were discrepancies in the data collection process; (12) This measure does not apply to this hospital for this reporting period; (13) Results cannot be calculated for this reporting period; (14) The results for this state are combined with nearby states to protect confidentiality; Please refer to the User's Guide for a full explanation of data.

Time in ER Before Being Evaluated (minutes)	324	39	26	26
Time to Pain Meds for Fractures (minutes)	71	65	58	57
Heart Attack Care				
Aspirin Given at Discharge[1]	-	-	99%	99%
Fibrinolytic Meds Within 30 Min. of Arrival[7]	-	-	40%	54%
PCI Within 90 Minutes of Arrival[7]	-	-	97%	96%
Statin Prescribed at Discharge[1]	-	-	99%	98%
Heart Failure Care				
ACE Inhibitor or ARB for LVSD	28	93%	97%	97%
Discharge Instructions Given	78	87%	96%	94%
Evaluation of LVS Function	102	100%	100%	99%
Medicare Spending				
Medicare Spending per Patient (ratio)	-	1.01	1.01	0.98
Pneumonia Care				
Appropriate Initial Antibiotic Given	74	93%	96%	95%
Blood Culture Timing	100	99%	98%	98%
Pregnancy and Delivery Care				
Newborn Deliveries Scheduled Early	30	20%	4%	6%
Preventive Care				
Immunization for Influenza[2]	278	92%	91%	90%
Immunization for Pneumonia[2]	297	88%	92%	92%
Stroke Care				
Anticoagulation Therapy for Atrial Fibrillation[1]	-	-	96%	95%
Antithrombotic Therapy Timing[1]	-	-	98%	98%
Assessed for Rehabilitation[1]	-	-	98%	97%
Discharged on Antithrombotic Therapy[1]	-	-	99%	99%
Discharged on Statin Medication[1]	-	-	95%	94%
Thrombolytic Therapy Timing[7]	-	-	72%	66%
Venous Thromboembolism Prophylaxis[1]	-	-	95%	94%
Written Stroke Educational Materials Given[1]	-	-	90%	88%
Surgical Care Improvement Project				
Appropriate Beta Blocker Usage	31	81%	98%	98%
Appropriate VTP Within 24 Hours	65	91%	99%	98%
Controlled Postoperative Blood Glucose[7]	-	-	98%	97%
Perioperative Temperature Management	81	100%	100%	100%
Prophylactic Antibiotic Selection	62	95%	99%	99%
Prophylactic Antibiotic Selection (Outpatient)	63	95%	98%	98%
Prophylactic Antibiotic Stopped	62	92%	98%	98%
Prophylactic Antibiotic Timing	62	98%	99%	99%
Prophylactic Antibiotic Timing (Outpatient)	64	92%	98%	98%
Urinary Catheter Removal	28	54%	99%	97%
Survey of Patients' Hospital Experiences				
Area Around Room 'Always' Quiet at Night	300+	62%	54%	61%
Doctors 'Always' Communicated Well	300+	81%	80%	82%
Home Recovery Information Given	300+	87%	86%	85%
Hospital Given 9 or 10 on 10 Point Scale	300+	66%	69%	71%
Meds 'Always' Explained Before Given	300+	63%	63%	64%
Nurses 'Always' Communicated Well	300+	83%	79%	79%
Pain 'Always' Well Controlled	300+	72%	70%	71%
Room and Bathroom 'Always' Clean	300+	81%	73%	73%
Timely Help 'Always' Received	300+	76%	67%	68%
Would Definitely Recommend Hospital	300+	59%	70%	71%
Use of Medical Imaging				
Cardiac Imaging Stress Test before Surgery	259	5.4%	5.4%	5.3%
Combination Abdominal CT Scan	293	3.4%	12.2%	10.5%
Combination Brain/Sinus CT Scan	321	1.6%	3.1%	2.7%
Combination Chest CT Scan	181	1.1%	2.1%	2.7%
Follow-up Mammogram/Ultrasound	848	5.3%	9%	8.8%
Lumbar Spine MRI for Low Back Pain[1]	-	-	35.8%	37.2%

Indiana Regional Medical Center

835 Hospital Road, PO Box 788
Indiana, PA 15701
Phone: 724-357-7000
Fax: 724-357-7449
E-mail: info@indianarmc.org
URL: www.indianarmc.org
Type: Acute Care Hospitals
Emergency Services: Yes
Ownership: Voluntary non-profit - Private
Beds: 162

Key Personnel:
Cardiac Laboratory. . . . . Lancy Brunetto
Chief of Medical Staff. . . . . Bruce A Bush, MD
Operating Room. . . . . Loraine George, RN
Quality Assurance . . . . Virginia Hostetter
Infection Control. . . . . David McDevitt, RN
Pediatric In-Patient Care . . . . Deborah Mikolic, RN
Radiology. . . . . Frank Simone, MD
CEO/President. . . . . Stephen A Wolfe

Measure	Cases	This Hosp.	State Avg.	U.S. Avg.
Blood Clot Prevention and Treatment				
Anticoagulation Overlap Therapy[2]	57	53%	94%	93%
ICU Venous Thromboembolism Prophylaxis[2]	55	47%	94%	92%
Incidence of Potentially Preventable VTE[2]	11	36%	8%	10%
UFH with Dosages/Platelet Monitoring[2]	56	98%	98%	97%
Venous Thromboembolism Prophylaxis[2]	380	56%	90%	85%
Warfarin Therapy Discharge Instructions[2]	45	18%	78%	75%
Chest Pain/Possible Heart Attack Care				
Aspirin Given Within 24 Hours of Arrival	160	98%	97%	96%
Fibrinolytic Meds Within 30 Min. of Arrival[1]	-	-	44%	58%
Average Time to ECG (minutes)	163	7	9	7
Average Time to Transfer (minutes)	23	85	64	60
Children's Asthma Care				
Received Home Management Plan of Care	-	-	-	88%
Received Reliever Medication	-	-	-	100%
Received Systemic Corticosteroids	-	-	-	100%
Emergency Department				
Admittance Decision Time (minutes)[2]	498	56	104	98
Head CT Results Within 45 Min. of Arrival	20	25%	60%	57%
Patients Who Left ER Before Being Seen	44,489	0%	1%	2%
Time from ER Arrival to Admit. (minutes)[2]	498	212	276	274
Time from ER Arrival to Discharge (minutes)	338	103	125	134
Time in ER Before Being Evaluated (minutes)	377	20	26	26
Time to Pain Meds for Fractures (minutes)	65	53	58	57
Heart Attack Care				
Aspirin Given at Discharge	55	100%	99%	99%
Fibrinolytic Meds Within 30 Min. of Arrival[7]	-	-	40%	54%
PCI Within 90 Minutes of Arrival[7]	-	-	97%	96%
Statin Prescribed at Discharge	50	86%	99%	98%
Heart Failure Care				
ACE Inhibitor or ARB for LVSD	69	88%	97%	97%
Discharge Instructions Given	166	95%	96%	94%
Evaluation of LVS Function	220	100%	100%	99%
Medicare Spending				
Medicare Spending per Patient (ratio)	-	1.03	1.01	0.98
Pneumonia Care				
Appropriate Initial Antibiotic Given	107	92%	96%	95%
Blood Culture Timing	162	99%	98%	98%
Pregnancy and Delivery Care				
Newborn Deliveries Scheduled Early[2]	57	0%	4%	6%
Preventive Care				
Immunization for Influenza[2]	534	96%	91%	90%
Immunization for Pneumonia[2]	747	96%	92%	92%
Stroke Care				
Anticoagulation Therapy for Atrial Fibrillation	11	64%	96%	95%
Antithrombotic Therapy Timing	74	96%	98%	98%
Assessed for Rehabilitation	67	96%	98%	97%
Discharged on Antithrombotic Therapy	67	99%	99%	99%
Discharged on Statin Medication	60	57%	95%	94%
Thrombolytic Therapy Timing	12	0%	72%	66%
Venous Thromboembolism Prophylaxis	73	66%	95%	94%
Written Stroke Educational Materials Given	23	9%	90%	88%
Surgical Care Improvement Project				
Appropriate Beta Blocker Usage	98	96%	98%	98%
Appropriate VTP Within 24 Hours	296	99%	99%	98%
Controlled Postoperative Blood Glucose[7]	-	-	98%	97%
Perioperative Temperature Management	337	100%	100%	100%
Prophylactic Antibiotic Selection	244	100%	99%	99%
Prophylactic Antibiotic Selection (Outpatient)	165	99%	98%	98%
Prophylactic Antibiotic Stopped	236	97%	98%	98%
Prophylactic Antibiotic Timing	244	100%	99%	99%
Prophylactic Antibiotic Timing (Outpatient)	115	99%	98%	98%
Urinary Catheter Removal	222	99%	99%	97%
Survey of Patients' Hospital Experiences				
Area Around Room 'Always' Quiet at Night	300+	50%	54%	61%
Doctors 'Always' Communicated Well	300+	81%	80%	82%
Home Recovery Information Given	300+	89%	86%	85%
Hospital Given 9 or 10 on 10 Point Scale	300+	70%	69%	71%
Meds 'Always' Explained Before Given	300+	64%	63%	64%
Nurses 'Always' Communicated Well	300+	82%	79%	79%
Pain 'Always' Well Controlled	300+	72%	70%	71%
Room and Bathroom 'Always' Clean	300+	77%	73%	73%
Timely Help 'Always' Received	300+	67%	67%	68%
Would Definitely Recommend Hospital	300+	70%	70%	71%
Use of Medical Imaging				
Cardiac Imaging Stress Test before Surgery	226	7.5%	5.4%	5.3%
Combination Abdominal CT Scan	352	28.1%	12.2%	10.5%
Combination Brain/Sinus CT Scan[1]	-	-	3.1%	2.7%
Combination Chest CT Scan	233	0.0%	2.1%	2.7%
Follow-up Mammogram/Ultrasound	673	4.3%	9%	8.8%
Lumbar Spine MRI for Low Back Pain[1]	-	-	35.8%	37.2%

Jersey Shore Hospital

1020 Thompson Street
Jersey Shore, PA 17740
Phone: 570-398-0100
Fax: 570-398-4412
URL: www.jsh.org
Type: Critical Access Hospitals
Emergency Services: Yes
Ownership: Voluntary non-profit - Private
Beds: 49

Key Personnel:
Chairman/CEO . . . . Richard Beatty, D.M.D
Chief of Medical Staff . . . . John Hunter
Emergency Room . . . . Barbara Kozlowski, RN
Operating Room. . . . . Barbara Kozlowski, RN
CEO/President. . . . . David A. Shannon
Radiology. . . . . Ed Sowul, RT, RDMS
Quality Assurance . . . . Samantha Weaver, RN, MSN

Measure	Cases	This Hosp.	State Avg.	U.S. Avg.
Blood Clot Prevention and Treatment				
Anticoagulation Overlap Therapy[1,3]	-	-	94%	93%
ICU Venous Thromboembolism Prophylaxis[3,7]	-	-	94%	92%
Incidence of Potentially Preventable VTE[3,7]	-	-	8%	10%
UFH with Dosages/Platelet Monitoring[1,3]	-	-	98%	97%
Venous Thromboembolism Prophylaxis[1,3]	-	-	90%	85%
Warfarin Therapy Discharge Instructions[1,3]	-	-	78%	75%
Chest Pain/Possible Heart Attack Care				
Aspirin Given Within 24 Hours of Arrival[5]	-	-	97%	96%
Fibrinolytic Meds Within 30 Min. of Arrival[5]	-	-	44%	58%
Average Time to ECG (minutes)[5]	-	-	9	7
Average Time to Transfer (minutes)[5]	-	-	64	60
Children's Asthma Care				
Received Home Management Plan of Care	-	-	-	88%
Received Reliever Medication	-	-	-	100%
Received Systemic Corticosteroids	-	-	-	100%
Emergency Department				
Admittance Decision Time (minutes)[3]	262	100	104	98
Head CT Results Within 45 Min. of Arrival[5]	-	-	60%	57%
Patients Who Left ER Before Being Seen	14,100	1%	1%	2%
Time from ER Arrival to Admit. (minutes)[3]	312	265	276	274
Time from ER Arrival to Discharge (minutes)[5]	-	-	125	134
Time in ER Before Being Evaluated (minutes)[5]	-	-	26	26
Time to Pain Meds for Fractures (minutes)[5]	-	-	58	57
Heart Attack Care				
Aspirin Given at Discharge[1,3]	-	-	99%	99%
Fibrinolytic Meds Within 30 Min. of Arrival[3,7]	-	-	40%	54%
PCI Within 90 Minutes of Arrival[3,7]	-	-	97%	96%
Statin Prescribed at Discharge[1,3]	-	-	99%	98%
Heart Failure Care				
ACE Inhibitor or ARB for LVSD[1]	-	-	97%	97%
Discharge Instructions Given	60	55%	96%	94%
Evaluation of LVS Function	60	93%	100%	99%
Medicare Spending				
Medicare Spending per Patient (ratio)	-	-	1.01	0.98
Pneumonia Care				
Appropriate Initial Antibiotic Given	54	85%	96%	95%
Blood Culture Timing	52	87%	98%	98%
Pregnancy and Delivery Care				
Newborn Deliveries Scheduled Early[5]	-	-	4%	6%
Preventive Care				
Immunization for Influenza[5]	-	-	91%	90%
Immunization for Pneumonia[5]	-	-	92%	92%
Stroke Care				
Anticoagulation Therapy for Atrial Fibrillation[1,3]	-	-	96%	95%
Antithrombotic Therapy Timing[1,3]	-	-	98%	98%
Assessed for Rehabilitation[1,3]	-	-	98%	97%
Discharged on Antithrombotic Therapy[1,3]	-	-	99%	99%

NOTE: Hospital profiles are in alphabetical order by state, then city, then hospital within the city; Rankings exclude hospitals with less than 25 cases except for patient surveys which excludes hospitals with less than 100 cases; (a) 100-299 cases; (1) The number of cases/patients is too few to report; (2) Data submitted were based on a sample of cases/patients; (3) Results are based on a shorter time period than required; (4) Data suppressed by CMS for one or more quarters; (5) Results are not available for this reporting period; (6) Fewer than 100 patients completed the HCAHPS survey; (7) No cases met the criteria for this measure; (8) The lower limit of the confidence interval cannot be calculated if the number of observed infections equals zero; (9) No data are available from the state/territory for this reporting period; (10) The scores shown reflect fewer than 50 completed surveys; (11) There were discrepancies in the data collection process; (12) This measure does not apply to this hospital for this reporting period; (13) Results cannot be calculated for this reporting period; (14) The results for this state are combined with nearby states to protect confidentiality; Please refer to the User's Guide for a full explanation of data.

Measure	Cases	This Hosp.	State Avg.	U.S. Avg.
Discharged on Statin Medication[1,3]	-	-	95%	94%
Thrombolytic Therapy Timing[1,3]	-	-	72%	66%
Venous Thromboembolism Prophylaxis[1,3]	-	-	95%	94%
Written Stroke Educational Materials Given[1,3]	-	-	90%	88%
Surgical Care Improvement Project				
Appropriate Beta Blocker Usage	16	100%	98%	98%
Appropriate VTP Within 24 Hours	35	91%	99%	98%
Controlled Postoperative Blood Glucose[7]	-	-	98%	97%
Perioperative Temperature Management	41	100%	100%	100%
Prophylactic Antibiotic Selection	33	85%	99%	99%
Prophylactic Antibiotic Selection (Outpatient)[5]	-	-	98%	98%
Prophylactic Antibiotic Stopped	33	91%	98%	98%
Prophylactic Antibiotic Timing	33	91%	99%	99%
Prophylactic Antibiotic Timing (Outpatient)[5]	-	-	98%	98%
Urinary Catheter Removal	38	100%	99%	97%
Survey of Patients' Hospital Experiences				
Area Around Room 'Always' Quiet at Night	(a)	60%	54%	61%
Doctors 'Always' Communicated Well	(a)	87%	80%	82%
Home Recovery Information Given	(a)	84%	86%	85%
Hospital Given 9 or 10 on 10 Point Scale	(a)	76%	69%	71%
Meds 'Always' Explained Before Given	(a)	65%	63%	64%
Nurses 'Always' Communicated Well	(a)	83%	79%	79%
Pain 'Always' Well Controlled	(a)	70%	70%	71%
Room and Bathroom 'Always' Clean	(a)	81%	73%	73%
Timely Help 'Always' Received	(a)	67%	67%	68%
Would Definitely Recommend Hospital	(a)	74%	70%	71%
Use of Medical Imaging				
Cardiac Imaging Stress Test before Surgery	49	4.1%	5.4%	5.3%
Combination Abdominal CT Scan	394	7.6%	12.2%	10.5%
Combination Brain/Sinus CT Scan[1]	-	-	3.1%	2.7%
Combination Chest CT Scan	172	1.7%	2.1%	2.7%
Follow-up Mammogram/Ultrasound	288	7.3%	9%	8.8%
Lumbar Spine MRI for Low Back Pain[1]	-	-	35.8%	37.2%

Conemaugh Valley Memorial Hospital

1086 Franklin Street
Johnstown, PA 15905
Phone: 814-534-9000
Fax: 814-534-3486
URL: www.conemaugh.org
Type: Acute Care Hospitals
Emergency Services: Yes
Ownership: Voluntary non-profit - Private
Beds: 474

Key Personnel:
Radiology. . . . . Jonathan Abrahms
Cardiac Laboratory. . . . . Samir A Hadeed, MD
Operating Room. . . . . Thomas S Helling, MD
Chief of Medical Staff. . . . . Adib N Khouzami, MD
Quality Assurance . . . . Karen Leoffler
Pediatric Ambulatory Care . . . . . . Matthew Masiello, MD
Infection Control. . . . . Louis A Schenfeld
CEO/President. . . . . Steven E Tucker

Measure	Cases	This Hosp.	State Avg.	U.S. Avg.
Blood Clot Prevention and Treatment				
Anticoagulation Overlap Therapy[2]	146	90%	94%	93%
ICU Venous Thromboembolism Prophylaxis[2]	48	100%	94%	92%
Incidence of Potentially Preventable VTE[2]	46	15%	8%	10%
UFH with Dosages/Platelet Monitoring[2]	140	100%	98%	97%
Venous Thromboembolism Prophylaxis[2]	410	91%	90%	85%
Warfarin Therapy Discharge Instructions[2]	93	80%	78%	75%
Chest Pain/Possible Heart Attack Care				
Aspirin Given Within 24 Hours of Arrival[1,3]	-	-	97%	96%
Fibrinolytic Meds Within 30 Min. of Arrival[3,7]	-	-	44%	58%
Average Time to ECG (minutes)[1,3]	-	-	9	7
Average Time to Transfer (minutes)[3,7]	-	-	64	60
Children's Asthma Care				
Received Home Management Plan of Care	-	-	-	88%
Received Reliever Medication	-	-	-	100%
Received Systemic Corticosteroids	-	-	-	100%
Emergency Department				
Admittance Decision Time (minutes)[2]	639	78	104	98
Head CT Results Within 45 Min. of Arrival[1]	-	-	60%	57%
Patients Who Left ER Before Being Seen	68,109	2%	1%	2%
Time from ER Arrival to Admit. (minutes)[2]	662	242	276	274
Time from ER Arrival to Discharge (minutes)	1,192	128	125	134
Time in ER Before Being Evaluated (minutes)	1,306	25	26	26
Time to Pain Meds for Fractures (minutes)	153	54	58	57
Heart Attack Care				
Aspirin Given at Discharge	580	99%	99%	99%
Fibrinolytic Meds Within 30 Min. of Arrival[7]	-	-	40%	54%
PCI Within 90 Minutes of Arrival	49	92%	97%	96%
Statin Prescribed at Discharge	547	98%	99%	98%
Heart Failure Care				
ACE Inhibitor or ARB for LVSD	180	93%	97%	97%
Discharge Instructions Given	620	91%	96%	94%
Evaluation of LVS Function	822	100%	100%	99%
Medicare Spending				
Medicare Spending per Patient (ratio)	-	0.99	1.01	0.98
Pneumonia Care				
Appropriate Initial Antibiotic Given	260	94%	96%	95%
Blood Culture Timing	397	99%	98%	98%
Pregnancy and Delivery Care				
Newborn Deliveries Scheduled Early	127	4%	4%	6%
Preventive Care				
Immunization for Influenza[2]	585	92%	91%	90%
Immunization for Pneumonia[2]	728	96%	92%	92%
Stroke Care				
Anticoagulation Therapy for Atrial Fibrillation	35	94%	96%	95%
Antithrombotic Therapy Timing	226	98%	98%	98%
Assessed for Rehabilitation	253	98%	98%	97%
Discharged on Antithrombotic Therapy	218	100%	99%	99%
Discharged on Statin Medication	179	95%	95%	94%
Thrombolytic Therapy Timing[1]	-	-	72%	66%
Venous Thromboembolism Prophylaxis	279	97%	95%	94%
Written Stroke Educational Materials Given	127	89%	90%	88%
Surgical Care Improvement Project				
Appropriate Beta Blocker Usage	640	98%	98%	98%
Appropriate VTP Within 24 Hours	1,054	99%	99%	98%
Controlled Postoperative Blood Glucose	211	98%	98%	97%
Perioperative Temperature Management	1,370	99%	100%	100%
Prophylactic Antibiotic Selection	960	100%	99%	99%
Prophylactic Antibiotic Selection (Outpatient)	431	98%	98%	98%
Prophylactic Antibiotic Stopped	947	99%	98%	98%
Prophylactic Antibiotic Timing	961	99%	99%	99%
Prophylactic Antibiotic Timing (Outpatient)	432	99%	98%	98%
Urinary Catheter Removal	459	97%	99%	97%
Survey of Patients' Hospital Experiences				
Area Around Room 'Always' Quiet at Night	300+	48%	54%	61%
Doctors 'Always' Communicated Well	300+	77%	80%	82%
Home Recovery Information Given	300+	84%	86%	85%
Hospital Given 9 or 10 on 10 Point Scale	300+	67%	69%	71%
Meds 'Always' Explained Before Given	300+	63%	63%	64%
Nurses 'Always' Communicated Well	300+	80%	79%	79%
Pain 'Always' Well Controlled	300+	70%	70%	71%
Room and Bathroom 'Always' Clean	300+	77%	73%	73%
Timely Help 'Always' Received	300+	69%	67%	68%
Would Definitely Recommend Hospital	300+	65%	70%	71%
Use of Medical Imaging				
Cardiac Imaging Stress Test before Surgery	519	5.2%	5.4%	5.3%
Combination Abdominal CT Scan	630	1.0%	12.2%	10.5%
Combination Brain/Sinus CT Scan	674	3.1%	3.1%	2.7%
Combination Chest CT Scan	279	0.4%	2.1%	2.7%
Follow-up Mammogram/Ultrasound	1,139	8.2%	9%	8.8%
Lumbar Spine MRI for Low Back Pain[1]	-	-	35.8%	37.2%

Kane Community Hospital

4372 Route 6
Kane, PA 16735
Phone: 814-837-8585
Fax: 814-837-7992
E-mail: info@kanehosp.com
URL: www.kanehosp.com
Type: Acute Care Hospitals
Emergency Services: Yes
Ownership: Voluntary non-profit - Private
Beds: 31

Key Personnel:
Infection Control. . . . . Pam Bray
Operating Room. . . . . K Joseph
Chief of Medical Staff. . . . . Linda Rettger, MD
CEO . . . . J Gary Rhodes
Radiology. . . . . Jamil Sarfraz, MD

Measure	Cases	This Hosp.	State Avg.	U.S. Avg.
Blood Clot Prevention and Treatment				
Anticoagulation Overlap Therapy[2]	14	71%	94%	93%
ICU Venous Thromboembolism Prophylaxis[2]	62	98%	94%	92%
Incidence of Potentially Preventable VTE[2,7]	-	-	8%	10%
UFH with Dosages/Platelet Monitoring[2]	13	100%	98%	97%
Venous Thromboembolism Prophylaxis[2]	214	94%	90%	85%
Warfarin Therapy Discharge Instructions[1,2]	-	-	78%	75%
Chest Pain/Possible Heart Attack Care				
Aspirin Given Within 24 Hours of Arrival[1,3]	-	-	97%	96%
Fibrinolytic Meds Within 30 Min. of Arrival[5]	-	-	44%	58%
Average Time to ECG (minutes)[1,3]	-	-	9	7
Average Time to Transfer (minutes)[5]	-	-	64	60
Children's Asthma Care				
Received Home Management Plan of Care	-	-	-	88%
Received Reliever Medication	-	-	-	100%
Received Systemic Corticosteroids	-	-	-	100%
Emergency Department				
Admittance Decision Time (minutes)[2]	500	50	104	98
Head CT Results Within 45 Min. of Arrival[1,3]	-	-	60%	57%
Patients Who Left ER Before Being Seen	6,857	0%	1%	2%
Time from ER Arrival to Admit. (minutes)[2]	523	170	276	274
Time from ER Arrival to Discharge (minutes)	571	72	125	134
Time in ER Before Being Evaluated (minutes)	603	15	26	26
Time to Pain Meds for Fractures (minutes)[1]	-	-	58	57
Heart Attack Care				
Aspirin Given at Discharge[1,3]	-	-	99%	99%
Fibrinolytic Meds Within 30 Min. of Arrival[3,7]	-	-	40%	54%
PCI Within 90 Minutes of Arrival[3,7]	-	-	97%	96%
Statin Prescribed at Discharge[1,3]	-	-	99%	98%
Heart Failure Care				
ACE Inhibitor or ARB for LVSD[1]	-	-	97%	97%
Discharge Instructions Given	41	88%	96%	94%
Evaluation of LVS Function	58	100%	100%	99%
Medicare Spending				
Medicare Spending per Patient (ratio)	-	0.91	1.01	0.98
Pneumonia Care				
Appropriate Initial Antibiotic Given	32	75%	96%	95%
Blood Culture Timing	63	100%	98%	98%
Pregnancy and Delivery Care				
Newborn Deliveries Scheduled Early[7]	-	-	4%	6%
Preventive Care				
Immunization for Influenza[2]	359	73%	91%	90%
Immunization for Pneumonia[2]	549	82%	92%	92%
Stroke Care				
Anticoagulation Therapy for Atrial Fibrillation[1]	-	-	96%	95%
Antithrombotic Therapy Timing	13	77%	98%	98%
Assessed for Rehabilitation	13	77%	98%	97%
Discharged on Antithrombotic Therapy	13	77%	99%	99%
Discharged on Statin Medication	11	36%	95%	94%
Thrombolytic Therapy Timing[7]	-	-	72%	66%
Venous Thromboembolism Prophylaxis	14	93%	95%	94%
Written Stroke Educational Materials Given[1]	-	-	90%	88%
Surgical Care Improvement Project				
Appropriate Beta Blocker Usage[1]	-	-	98%	98%
Appropriate VTP Within 24 Hours	24	100%	99%	98%
Controlled Postoperative Blood Glucose[7]	-	-	98%	97%
Perioperative Temperature Management	28	100%	100%	100%
Prophylactic Antibiotic Selection	17	100%	99%	99%
Prophylactic Antibiotic Selection (Outpatient)[5]	-	-	98%	98%
Prophylactic Antibiotic Stopped	15	53%	98%	98%
Prophylactic Antibiotic Timing	17	100%	99%	99%
Prophylactic Antibiotic Timing (Outpatient)[5]	-	-	98%	98%
Urinary Catheter Removal	24	100%	99%	97%
Survey of Patients' Hospital Experiences				
Area Around Room 'Always' Quiet at Night	(a)	52%	54%	61%
Doctors 'Always' Communicated Well	(a)	85%	80%	82%
Home Recovery Information Given	(a)	85%	86%	85%
Hospital Given 9 or 10 on 10 Point Scale	(a)	71%	69%	71%
Meds 'Always' Explained Before Given	(a)	71%	63%	64%
Nurses 'Always' Communicated Well	(a)	82%	79%	79%
Pain 'Always' Well Controlled	(a)	69%	70%	71%
Room and Bathroom 'Always' Clean	(a)	84%	73%	73%
Timely Help 'Always' Received	(a)	72%	67%	68%
Would Definitely Recommend Hospital	(a)	73%	70%	71%

NOTE: Hospital profiles are in alphabetical order by state, then city, then hospital within the city; Rankings exclude hospitals with less than 25 cases except for patient surveys which excludes hospitals with less than 100 cases; (a) 100-299 cases; (1) The number of cases/patients is too few to report; (2) Data submitted were based on a sample of cases/patients; (3) Results are based on a shorter time period than required; (4) Data suppressed by CMS for one or more quarters; (5) Results are not available for this reporting period; (6) Fewer than 100 patients completed the HCAHPS survey; (7) No cases met the criteria for this measure; (8) The lower limit of the confidence interval cannot be calculated if the number of observed infections equals zero; (9) No data are available from the state/territory for this reporting period; (10) The scores shown reflect fewer than 50 completed surveys; (11) There were discrepancies in the data collection process; (12) This measure does not apply to this hospital for this reporting period; (13) Results cannot be calculated for this reporting period; (14) The results for this state are combined with nearby states to protect confidentiality; Please refer to the User's Guide for a full explanation of data.

Use of Medical Imaging				
Cardiac Imaging Stress Test before Surgery	73	8.2%	5.4%	5.3%
Combination Abdominal CT Scan	207	44.0%	12.2%	10.5%
Combination Brain/Sinus CT Scan[1]	-	-	3.1%	2.7%
Combination Chest CT Scan	124	48.4%	2.1%	2.7%
Follow-up Mammogram/Ultrasound	294	42.9%	9%	8.8%
Lumbar Spine MRI for Low Back Pain[1]	-	-	35.8%	37.2%

Acmh Hospital

One Nolte Drive
Kittanning, PA 16201
Phone: 724-543-8404
Fax: 724-543-8704
E-mail: comrel@acmh.org
URL: www.acmh.org
Type: Acute Care Hospitals
Emergency Services: Yes
Ownership: Voluntary non-profit - Private
Beds: 177

Key Personnel:
Chief of Medical Staff . . . . Harold Altman, MD
Radiology . . . . Donley Charles
CEO/President . . . . John Lewis

Measure	Cases	This Hosp.	State Avg.	U.S. Avg.
Blood Clot Prevention and Treatment				
Anticoagulation Overlap Therapy[2]	45	96%	94%	93%
ICU Venous Thromboembolism Prophylaxis[2]	70	93%	94%	92%
Incidence of Potentially Preventable VTE[1,2]	-	-	8%	10%
UFH with Dosages/Platelet Monitoring[2]	32	100%	98%	97%
Venous Thromboembolism Prophylaxis[2]	308	90%	90%	85%
Warfarin Therapy Discharge Instructions[2]	30	93%	78%	75%
Chest Pain/Possible Heart Attack Care				
Aspirin Given Within 24 Hours of Arrival	29	90%	97%	96%
Fibrinolytic Meds Within 30 Min. of Arrival[7]	-	-	44%	58%
Average Time to ECG (minutes)	29	8	9	7
Average Time to Transfer (minutes)[1]	-	-	64	60
Children's Asthma Care				
Received Home Management Plan of Care	-	-	-	88%
Received Reliever Medication	-	-	-	100%
Received Systemic Corticosteroids	-	-	-	100%
Emergency Department				
Admittance Decision Time (minutes)[2]	96	46	104	98
Head CT Results Within 45 Min. of Arrival	13	77%	60%	57%
Patients Who Left ER Before Being Seen	25,833	1%	1%	2%
Time from ER Arrival to Admit. (minutes)[2]	99	222	276	274
Time from ER Arrival to Discharge (minutes)	439	102	125	134
Time in ER Before Being Evaluated (minutes)	469	16	26	26
Time to Pain Meds for Fractures (minutes)	79	49	58	57
Heart Attack Care				
Aspirin Given at Discharge	96	99%	99%	99%
Fibrinolytic Meds Within 30 Min. of Arrival[7]	-	-	40%	54%
PCI Within 90 Minutes of Arrival	26	85%	97%	96%
Statin Prescribed at Discharge	92	99%	99%	98%
Heart Failure Care				
ACE Inhibitor or ARB for LVSD	34	100%	97%	97%
Discharge Instructions Given	104	88%	96%	94%
Evaluation of LVS Function	139	100%	100%	99%
Medicare Spending				
Medicare Spending per Patient (ratio)	-	1.01	1.01	0.98
Pneumonia Care				
Appropriate Initial Antibiotic Given	110	97%	96%	95%
Blood Culture Timing	162	98%	98%	98%
Pregnancy and Delivery Care				
Newborn Deliveries Scheduled Early[2]	21	10%	4%	6%
Preventive Care				
Immunization for Influenza[2]	550	97%	91%	90%
Immunization for Pneumonia[2]	619	96%	92%	92%
Stroke Care				
Anticoagulation Therapy for Atrial Fibrillation[1]	-	-	96%	95%
Antithrombotic Therapy Timing	43	100%	98%	98%
Assessed for Rehabilitation	47	98%	98%	97%
Discharged on Antithrombotic Therapy	44	100%	99%	99%
Discharged on Statin Medication	36	92%	95%	94%
Thrombolytic Therapy Timing[1]	-	-	72%	66%
Venous Thromboembolism Prophylaxis	47	98%	95%	94%
Written Stroke Educational Materials Given	22	73%	90%	88%
Surgical Care Improvement Project				
Appropriate Beta Blocker Usage	100	99%	98%	98%
Appropriate VTP Within 24 Hours	295	98%	99%	98%
Controlled Postoperative Blood Glucose[7]	-	-	98%	97%
Perioperative Temperature Management	480	100%	100%	100%
Prophylactic Antibiotic Selection	350	100%	99%	99%
Prophylactic Antibiotic Selection (Outpatient)	50	98%	98%	98%
Prophylactic Antibiotic Stopped	348	98%	98%	98%
Prophylactic Antibiotic Timing	350	99%	99%	99%
Prophylactic Antibiotic Timing (Outpatient)	49	100%	98%	98%
Urinary Catheter Removal	192	98%	99%	97%
Survey of Patients' Hospital Experiences				
Area Around Room 'Always' Quiet at Night	300+	45%	54%	61%
Doctors 'Always' Communicated Well	300+	82%	80%	82%
Home Recovery Information Given	300+	85%	86%	85%
Hospital Given 9 or 10 on 10 Point Scale	300+	68%	69%	71%
Meds 'Always' Explained Before Given	300+	62%	63%	64%
Nurses 'Always' Communicated Well	300+	82%	79%	79%
Pain 'Always' Well Controlled	300+	71%	70%	71%
Room and Bathroom 'Always' Clean	300+	70%	73%	73%
Timely Help 'Always' Received	300+	73%	67%	68%
Would Definitely Recommend Hospital	300+	65%	70%	71%
Use of Medical Imaging				
Cardiac Imaging Stress Test before Surgery	109	11.0%	5.4%	5.3%
Combination Abdominal CT Scan	308	6.8%	12.2%	10.5%
Combination Brain/Sinus CT Scan	251	4.8%	3.1%	2.7%
Combination Chest CT Scan	179	2.2%	2.1%	2.7%
Follow-up Mammogram/Ultrasound	488	11.5%	9%	8.8%
Lumbar Spine MRI for Low Back Pain	74	35.1%	35.8%	37.2%

Lancaster General Hospital

555 North Duke Street
Lancaster, PA 17604
Phone: 717-299-5511
E-mail: info@lancastergeneral.org
URL: www.lancastergeneral.org
Type: Acute Care Hospitals
Emergency Services: Yes
Ownership: Voluntary non-profit - Other
Beds: 640

Key Personnel:
CEO/President . . . . Thomas E Beeman, Ph.D., FACHE
President . . . . Jay Bucher
Chief of Medical Staff . . . . Lee M. Duke, II, MD
Ambulatory Care . . . . André W Renna

Measure	Cases	This Hosp.	State Avg.	U.S. Avg.
Blood Clot Prevention and Treatment				
Anticoagulation Overlap Therapy[2]	298	98%	94%	93%
ICU Venous Thromboembolism Prophylaxis[2]	318	98%	94%	92%
Incidence of Potentially Preventable VTE[2]	57	0%	8%	10%
UFH with Dosages/Platelet Monitoring[2]	237	100%	98%	97%
Venous Thromboembolism Prophylaxis[2]	2,350	97%	90%	85%
Warfarin Therapy Discharge Instructions[2]	248	96%	78%	75%
Chest Pain/Possible Heart Attack Care				
Aspirin Given Within 24 Hours of Arrival[3,7]	-	-	97%	96%
Fibrinolytic Meds Within 30 Min. of Arrival[5]	-	-	44%	58%
Average Time to ECG (minutes)[3,7]	-	-	9	7
Average Time to Transfer (minutes)[5]	-	-	64	60
Children's Asthma Care				
Received Home Management Plan of Care	-	-	-	88%
Received Reliever Medication	-	-	-	100%
Received Systemic Corticosteroids	-	-	-	100%
Emergency Department				
Admittance Decision Time (minutes)[2]	601	81	104	98
Head CT Results Within 45 Min. of Arrival[1]	-	-	60%	57%
Patients Who Left ER Before Being Seen	>100k	1%	1%	2%
Time from ER Arrival to Admit. (minutes)[2]	624	230	276	274
Time from ER Arrival to Discharge (minutes)	384	129	125	134
Time in ER Before Being Evaluated (minutes)	414	16	26	26
Time to Pain Meds for Fractures (minutes)	159	52	58	57
Heart Attack Care				
Aspirin Given at Discharge	730	99%	99%	99%
Fibrinolytic Meds Within 30 Min. of Arrival[7]	-	-	40%	54%
PCI Within 90 Minutes of Arrival	135	90%	97%	96%
Statin Prescribed at Discharge	700	98%	99%	98%
Heart Failure Care				
ACE Inhibitor or ARB for LVSD	207	97%	97%	97%
Discharge Instructions Given	816	100%	96%	94%
Evaluation of LVS Function	974	100%	100%	99%
Medicare Spending				
Medicare Spending per Patient (ratio)	-	0.98	1.01	0.98
Pneumonia Care				
Appropriate Initial Antibiotic Given	346	97%	96%	95%
Blood Culture Timing	623	99%	98%	98%
Pregnancy and Delivery Care				
Newborn Deliveries Scheduled Early[2]	184	5%	4%	6%
Preventive Care				
Immunization for Influenza[2]	550	93%	91%	90%
Immunization for Pneumonia[2]	698	91%	92%	92%
Stroke Care				
Anticoagulation Therapy for Atrial Fibrillation	94	98%	96%	95%
Antithrombotic Therapy Timing	382	99%	98%	98%
Assessed for Rehabilitation	462	98%	98%	97%
Discharged on Antithrombotic Therapy	412	100%	99%	99%
Discharged on Statin Medication	317	97%	95%	94%
Thrombolytic Therapy Timing	17	65%	72%	66%
Venous Thromboembolism Prophylaxis	454	100%	95%	94%
Written Stroke Educational Materials Given	237	94%	90%	88%
Surgical Care Improvement Project				
Appropriate Beta Blocker Usage[2]	944	98%	98%	98%
Appropriate VTP Within 24 Hours[2]	1,774	100%	99%	98%
Controlled Postoperative Blood Glucose[2]	294	98%	98%	97%
Perioperative Temperature Management[2]	2,154	100%	100%	100%
Prophylactic Antibiotic Selection[2]	1,702	99%	99%	99%
Prophylactic Antibiotic Selection (Outpatient)	1,368	98%	98%	98%
Prophylactic Antibiotic Stopped[2]	1,670	98%	98%	98%
Prophylactic Antibiotic Timing[2]	1,702	98%	99%	99%
Prophylactic Antibiotic Timing (Outpatient)	1,370	96%	98%	98%
Urinary Catheter Removal[2]	1,821	99%	99%	97%
Survey of Patients' Hospital Experiences				
Area Around Room 'Always' Quiet at Night	300+	48%	54%	61%
Doctors 'Always' Communicated Well	300+	75%	80%	82%
Home Recovery Information Given	300+	86%	86%	85%
Hospital Given 9 or 10 on 10 Point Scale	300+	71%	69%	71%
Meds 'Always' Explained Before Given	300+	58%	63%	64%
Nurses 'Always' Communicated Well	300+	77%	79%	79%
Pain 'Always' Well Controlled	300+	65%	70%	71%
Room and Bathroom 'Always' Clean	300+	70%	73%	73%
Timely Help 'Always' Received	300+	62%	67%	68%
Would Definitely Recommend Hospital	300+	77%	70%	71%
Use of Medical Imaging				
Cardiac Imaging Stress Test before Surgery	1,742	3.1%	5.4%	5.3%
Combination Abdominal CT Scan	2,484	6.8%	12.2%	10.5%
Combination Brain/Sinus CT Scan	2,373	3.3%	3.1%	2.7%
Combination Chest CT Scan	2,554	2.3%	2.1%	2.7%
Follow-up Mammogram/Ultrasound	6,214	8.6%	9%	8.8%
Lumbar Spine MRI for Low Back Pain[1]	-	-	35.8%	37.2%

Lancaster Regional Medical Center

250 College Avenue
Lancaster, PA 17604
Phone: 717-291-8123
URL: www.lancasterregional.com
Type: Acute Care Hospitals
Emergency Services: Yes
Ownership: Proprietary

Key Personnel:
CEO . . . . Bob Moore, FACHE
Emergency Room . . . . Cindy Sapp

Measure	Cases	This Hosp.	State Avg.	U.S. Avg.
Blood Clot Prevention and Treatment				
Anticoagulation Overlap Therapy[2]	32	97%	94%	93%
ICU Venous Thromboembolism Prophylaxis[2]	50	98%	94%	92%
Incidence of Potentially Preventable VTE[1,2]	-	-	8%	10%
UFH with Dosages/Platelet Monitoring[2]	19	100%	98%	97%
Venous Thromboembolism Prophylaxis[2]	298	91%	90%	85%
Warfarin Therapy Discharge Instructions[2]	27	93%	78%	75%
Chest Pain/Possible Heart Attack Care				
Aspirin Given Within 24 Hours of Arrival[1,3]	-	-	97%	96%
Fibrinolytic Meds Within 30 Min. of Arrival[5]	-	-	44%	58%
Average Time to ECG (minutes)[1,3]	-	-	9	7
Average Time to Transfer (minutes)[5]	-	-	64	60

NOTE: Hospital profiles are in alphabetical order by state, then city, then hospital within the city; Rankings exclude hospitals with less than 25 cases except for patient surveys which excludes hospitals with less than 100 cases; (a) 100-299 cases; (1) The number of cases/patients is too few to report; (2) Data submitted were based on a sample of cases/patients; (3) Results are based on a shorter time period than required; (4) Data suppressed by CMS for one or more quarters; (5) Results are not available for this reporting period; (6) Fewer than 100 patients completed the HCAHPS survey; (7) No cases met the criteria for this measure; (8) The lower limit of the confidence interval cannot be calculated if the number of observed infections equals zero; (9) No data are available from the state/territory for this reporting period; (10) The scores shown reflect fewer than 50 completed surveys; (11) There were discrepancies in the data collection process; (12) This measure does not apply to this hospital for this reporting period; (13) Results cannot be calculated for this reporting period; (14) The results for this state are combined with nearby states to protect confidentiality; Please refer to the User's Guide for a full explanation of data.

Children's Asthma Care				
Received Home Management Plan of Care	-	-	-	88%
Received Reliever Medication	-	-	-	100%
Received Systemic Corticosteroids	-	-	-	100%
Emergency Department				
Admittance Decision Time (minutes)[2]	379	135	104	98
Head CT Results Within 45 Min. of Arrival[3,7]	-	-	60%	57%
Patients Who Left ER Before Being Seen	23,162	1%	1%	2%
Time from ER Arrival to Admit. (minutes)[2]	379	307	276	274
Time from ER Arrival to Discharge (minutes)	495	112	125	134
Time in ER Before Being Evaluated (minutes)	548	19	26	26
Time to Pain Meds for Fractures (minutes)	41	56	58	57
Heart Attack Care				
Aspirin Given at Discharge	67	100%	99%	99%
Fibrinolytic Meds Within 30 Min. of Arrival[7]	-	-	40%	54%
PCI Within 90 Minutes of Arrival[1]	-	-	97%	96%
Statin Prescribed at Discharge	66	100%	99%	98%
Heart Failure Care				
ACE Inhibitor or ARB for LVSD	21	100%	97%	97%
Discharge Instructions Given	99	92%	96%	94%
Evaluation of LVS Function	122	100%	100%	99%
Medicare Spending				
Medicare Spending per Patient (ratio)	-	1.05	1.01	0.98
Pneumonia Care				
Appropriate Initial Antibiotic Given	53	100%	96%	95%
Blood Culture Timing	75	100%	98%	98%
Pregnancy and Delivery Care				
Newborn Deliveries Scheduled Early[7]	-	-	4%	6%
Preventive Care				
Immunization for Influenza[2]	434	99%	91%	90%
Immunization for Pneumonia[2]	527	97%	92%	92%
Stroke Care				
Anticoagulation Therapy for Atrial Fibrillation[1]	-	-	96%	95%
Antithrombotic Therapy Timing	28	89%	98%	98%
Assessed for Rehabilitation	33	94%	98%	97%
Discharged on Antithrombotic Therapy	32	97%	99%	99%
Discharged on Statin Medication	27	81%	95%	94%
Thrombolytic Therapy Timing[7]	-	-	72%	66%
Venous Thromboembolism Prophylaxis	30	93%	95%	94%
Written Stroke Educational Materials Given	18	94%	90%	88%
Surgical Care Improvement Project				
Appropriate Beta Blocker Usage	200	100%	98%	98%
Appropriate VTP Within 24 Hours	499	100%	99%	98%
Controlled Postoperative Blood Glucose	52	92%	98%	97%
Perioperative Temperature Management	611	100%	100%	100%
Prophylactic Antibiotic Selection	447	100%	99%	99%
Prophylactic Antibiotic Selection (Outpatient)	218	100%	98%	98%
Prophylactic Antibiotic Stopped	432	99%	98%	98%
Prophylactic Antibiotic Timing	448	100%	99%	99%
Prophylactic Antibiotic Timing (Outpatient)	218	99%	98%	98%
Urinary Catheter Removal	434	100%	99%	97%
Survey of Patients' Hospital Experiences				
Area Around Room 'Always' Quiet at Night	300+	51%	54%	61%
Doctors 'Always' Communicated Well	300+	79%	80%	82%
Home Recovery Information Given	300+	88%	86%	85%
Hospital Given 9 or 10 on 10 Point Scale	300+	69%	69%	71%
Meds 'Always' Explained Before Given	300+	60%	63%	64%
Nurses 'Always' Communicated Well	300+	77%	79%	79%
Pain 'Always' Well Controlled	300+	70%	70%	71%
Room and Bathroom 'Always' Clean	300+	80%	73%	73%
Timely Help 'Always' Received	300+	69%	67%	68%
Would Definitely Recommend Hospital	300+	73%	70%	71%
Use of Medical Imaging				
Cardiac Imaging Stress Test before Surgery	65	6.2%	5.4%	5.3%
Combination Abdominal CT Scan	330	11.8%	12.2%	10.5%
Combination Brain/Sinus CT Scan	249	1.2%	3.1%	2.7%
Combination Chest CT Scan	281	3.9%	2.1%	2.7%
Follow-up Mammogram/Ultrasound	1,321	9.7%	9%	8.8%
Lumbar Spine MRI for Low Back Pain	144	41.7%	35.8%	37.2%

Saint Mary Medical Center

Langhorne - Newtown Rd
Langhorne, PA 19047
URL: www.stmaryhealthcare.org
Type: Acute Care Hospitals
Ownership: Voluntary non-profit - Church
Phone: 215-750-2003
Fax: 215-710-5190
Emergency Services: Yes
Beds: 373

Key Personnel:
Chief of Medical Staff.......... Deirdre Donaghy, MD
Operating Room.............. Teri Grisi, RN
Pediatric Ambulatory Care...... Prem Marlapudi
Pediatric In-Patient Care....... Prem Marlapudi
Radiology.................. Suzanne Monte, MD
Quality Assurance............ Deb Taonne, RN
Emergency Room............. Sid Vail, MD
CEO/President............... Gregory T Wozniak

Measure	Cases	This Hosp.	State Avg.	U.S. Avg.
Blood Clot Prevention and Treatment				
Anticoagulation Overlap Therapy[2]	181	100%	94%	93%
ICU Venous Thromboembolism Prophylaxis[2]	60	100%	94%	92%
Incidence of Potentially Preventable VTE[2]	35	3%	8%	10%
UFH with Dosages/Platelet Monitoring[2]	260	100%	98%	97%
Venous Thromboembolism Prophylaxis[2]	350	85%	90%	85%
Warfarin Therapy Discharge Instructions[2]	101	89%	78%	75%
Chest Pain/Possible Heart Attack Care				
Aspirin Given Within 24 Hours of Arrival[1,3]	-	-	97%	96%
Fibrinolytic Meds Within 30 Min. of Arrival[5]	-	-	44%	58%
Average Time to ECG (minutes)[1,3]	-	-	9	7
Average Time to Transfer (minutes)[5]	-	-	64	60
Children's Asthma Care				
Received Home Management Plan of Care	-	-	-	88%
Received Reliever Medication	-	-	-	100%
Received Systemic Corticosteroids	-	-	-	100%
Emergency Department				
Admittance Decision Time (minutes)[2]	732	137	104	98
Head CT Results Within 45 Min. of Arrival[1]	-	-	60%	57%
Patients Who Left ER Before Being Seen	71,261	0%	1%	2%
Time from ER Arrival to Admit. (minutes)[2]	732	304	276	274
Time from ER Arrival to Discharge (minutes)	378	130	125	134
Time in ER Before Being Evaluated (minutes)	423	17	26	26
Time to Pain Meds for Fractures (minutes)	379	50	58	57
Heart Attack Care				
Aspirin Given at Discharge	499	100%	99%	99%
Fibrinolytic Meds Within 30 Min. of Arrival[7]	-	-	40%	54%
PCI Within 90 Minutes of Arrival	65	100%	97%	96%
Statin Prescribed at Discharge	442	100%	99%	98%
Heart Failure Care				
ACE Inhibitor or ARB for LVSD	155	100%	97%	97%
Discharge Instructions Given	409	100%	96%	94%
Evaluation of LVS Function	520	100%	100%	99%
Medicare Spending				
Medicare Spending per Patient (ratio)	-	1.02	1.01	0.98
Pneumonia Care				
Appropriate Initial Antibiotic Given	294	98%	96%	95%
Blood Culture Timing	494	100%	98%	98%
Pregnancy and Delivery Care				
Newborn Deliveries Scheduled Early[2]	35	3%	4%	6%
Preventive Care				
Immunization for Influenza[2]	589	58%	91%	90%
Immunization for Pneumonia[2]	743	84%	92%	92%
Stroke Care				
Anticoagulation Therapy for Atrial Fibrillation	42	100%	96%	95%
Antithrombotic Therapy Timing	213	98%	98%	98%
Assessed for Rehabilitation	261	99%	98%	97%
Discharged on Antithrombotic Therapy	221	100%	99%	99%
Discharged on Statin Medication	149	99%	95%	94%
Thrombolytic Therapy Timing	23	96%	72%	66%
Venous Thromboembolism Prophylaxis	271	99%	95%	94%
Written Stroke Educational Materials Given	122	100%	90%	88%
Surgical Care Improvement Project				
Appropriate Beta Blocker Usage	575	100%	98%	98%
Appropriate VTP Within 24 Hours	1,029	98%	99%	98%
Controlled Postoperative Blood Glucose	240	99%	98%	97%
Perioperative Temperature Management	1,414	100%	100%	100%
Prophylactic Antibiotic Selection	1,012	99%	99%	99%
Prophylactic Antibiotic Selection (Outpatient)	354	99%	98%	98%
Prophylactic Antibiotic Stopped	999	99%	98%	98%
Prophylactic Antibiotic Timing	1,012	100%	99%	99%
Prophylactic Antibiotic Timing (Outpatient)	355	99%	98%	98%
Urinary Catheter Removal	997	100%	99%	97%
Survey of Patients' Hospital Experiences				
Area Around Room 'Always' Quiet at Night	300+	49%	54%	61%
Doctors 'Always' Communicated Well	300+	77%	80%	82%
Home Recovery Information Given	300+	86%	86%	85%
Hospital Given 9 or 10 on 10 Point Scale	300+	77%	69%	71%
Meds 'Always' Explained Before Given	300+	66%	63%	64%
Nurses 'Always' Communicated Well	300+	81%	79%	79%
Pain 'Always' Well Controlled	300+	72%	70%	71%
Room and Bathroom 'Always' Clean	300+	69%	73%	73%
Timely Help 'Always' Received	300+	69%	67%	68%
Would Definitely Recommend Hospital	300+	80%	70%	71%
Use of Medical Imaging				
Cardiac Imaging Stress Test before Surgery	792	6.1%	5.4%	5.3%
Combination Abdominal CT Scan	1,568	8.7%	12.2%	10.5%
Combination Brain/Sinus CT Scan	1,162	3.6%	3.1%	2.7%
Combination Chest CT Scan	996	7.1%	2.1%	2.7%
Follow-up Mammogram/Ultrasound	2,348	4.2%	9%	8.8%
Lumbar Spine MRI for Low Back Pain	351	38.5%	35.8%	37.2%

Lansdale Hospital

100 Medical Campus Drive
Lansdale, PA 19446
URL: www.cmmc-uhs.com
Type: Acute Care Hospitals
Ownership: Voluntary non-profit - Other
Phone: 215-368-2100
Fax: 215-361-4933
Emergency Services: Yes
Beds: 125

Key Personnel:
Radiology.................. Ronald Adelman
CEO/President.............. Gary Candia
Chief of Medical Staff......... Colleen Christian, MD
Infection Control............ Mary Doherty, RN
Quality Assurance........... Suzanne Lion
Anesthesiology............. Jay Mergaman, MD

Measure	Cases	This Hosp.	State Avg.	U.S. Avg.
Blood Clot Prevention and Treatment				
Anticoagulation Overlap Therapy[2]	45	100%	94%	93%
ICU Venous Thromboembolism Prophylaxis[2]	95	98%	94%	92%
Incidence of Potentially Preventable VTE[1,2]	-	-	8%	10%
UFH with Dosages/Platelet Monitoring[2]	33	100%	98%	97%
Venous Thromboembolism Prophylaxis[2]	283	93%	90%	85%
Warfarin Therapy Discharge Instructions[2]	29	93%	78%	75%
Chest Pain/Possible Heart Attack Care				
Aspirin Given Within 24 Hours of Arrival	43	98%	97%	96%
Fibrinolytic Meds Within 30 Min. of Arrival[7]	-	-	44%	58%
Average Time to ECG (minutes)	45	9	9	7
Average Time to Transfer (minutes)	22	69	64	60
Children's Asthma Care				
Received Home Management Plan of Care	-	-	-	88%
Received Reliever Medication	-	-	-	100%
Received Systemic Corticosteroids	-	-	-	100%
Emergency Department				
Admittance Decision Time (minutes)[2]	768	98	104	98
Head CT Results Within 45 Min. of Arrival	16	62%	60%	57%
Patients Who Left ER Before Being Seen	27,630	0%	1%	2%
Time from ER Arrival to Admit. (minutes)[2]	796	263	276	274
Time from ER Arrival to Discharge (minutes)	370	138	125	134
Time in ER Before Being Evaluated (minutes)	408	19	26	26
Time to Pain Meds for Fractures (minutes)	80	50	58	57
Heart Attack Care				
Aspirin Given at Discharge	41	100%	99%	99%
Fibrinolytic Meds Within 30 Min. of Arrival[7]	-	-	40%	54%
PCI Within 90 Minutes of Arrival[7]	-	-	97%	96%
Statin Prescribed at Discharge	34	100%	99%	98%
Heart Failure Care				
ACE Inhibitor or ARB for LVSD[2]	62	97%	97%	97%
Discharge Instructions Given[2]	162	100%	96%	94%
Evaluation of LVS Function[2]	241	100%	100%	99%
Medicare Spending				
Medicare Spending per Patient (ratio)	-	0.97	1.01	0.98
Pneumonia Care				

NOTE: Hospital profiles are in alphabetical order by state, then city, then hospital within the city; Rankings exclude hospitals with less than 25 cases except for patient surveys which excludes hospitals with less than 100 cases; (a) 100-299 cases; (1) The number of cases/patients is too few to report; (2) Data submitted were based on a sample of cases/patients; (3) Results are based on a shorter time period than required; (4) Data suppressed by CMS for one or more quarters; (5) Results are not available for this reporting period; (6) Fewer than 100 patients completed the HCAHPS survey; (7) No cases met the criteria for this measure; (8) The lower limit of the confidence interval cannot be calculated if the number of observed infections equals zero; (9) No data are available from the state/territory for this reporting period; (10) The scores shown reflect fewer than 50 completed surveys; (11) There were discrepancies in the data collection process; (12) This measure does not apply to this hospital for this reporting period; (13) Results cannot be calculated for this reporting period; (14) The results for this state are combined with nearby states to protect confidentiality; Please refer to the User's Guide for a full explanation of data.

Measure	Cases	This Hosp.	State Avg.	U.S. Avg.
Appropriate Initial Antibiotic Given[2]	88	100%	96%	95%
Blood Culture Timing[2]	153	99%	98%	98%
Pregnancy and Delivery Care				
Newborn Deliveries Scheduled Early[7]	-	-	4%	6%
Preventive Care				
Immunization for Influenza[2]	547	97%	91%	90%
Immunization for Pneumonia[2]	834	96%	92%	92%
Stroke Care				
Anticoagulation Therapy for Atrial Fibrillation	17	94%	96%	95%
Antithrombotic Therapy Timing	65	100%	98%	98%
Assessed for Rehabilitation	70	97%	98%	97%
Discharged on Antithrombotic Therapy	66	100%	99%	99%
Discharged on Statin Medication	59	98%	95%	94%
Thrombolytic Therapy Timing[1]	-	-	72%	66%
Venous Thromboembolism Prophylaxis	75	87%	95%	94%
Written Stroke Educational Materials Given	24	58%	90%	88%
Surgical Care Improvement Project				
Appropriate Beta Blocker Usage[2]	85	94%	98%	98%
Appropriate VTP Within 24 Hours[2]	272	99%	99%	98%
Controlled Postoperative Blood Glucose[2,7]	-	-	98%	97%
Perioperative Temperature Management[2]	306	100%	100%	100%
Prophylactic Antibiotic Selection[2]	213	100%	99%	99%
Prophylactic Antibiotic Selection (Outpatient)	83	100%	98%	98%
Prophylactic Antibiotic Stopped[2]	207	98%	98%	98%
Prophylactic Antibiotic Timing[2]	213	100%	99%	99%
Prophylactic Antibiotic Timing (Outpatient)	83	100%	98%	98%
Urinary Catheter Removal[2]	55	87%	99%	97%
Survey of Patients' Hospital Experiences				
Area Around Room 'Always' Quiet at Night	300+	64%	54%	61%
Doctors 'Always' Communicated Well	300+	84%	80%	82%
Home Recovery Information Given	300+	85%	86%	85%
Hospital Given 9 or 10 on 10 Point Scale	300+	73%	69%	71%
Meds 'Always' Explained Before Given	300+	68%	63%	64%
Nurses 'Always' Communicated Well	300+	88%	79%	79%
Pain 'Always' Well Controlled	300+	75%	70%	71%
Room and Bathroom 'Always' Clean	300+	77%	73%	73%
Timely Help 'Always' Received	300+	75%	67%	68%
Would Definitely Recommend Hospital	300+	75%	70%	71%
Use of Medical Imaging				
Cardiac Imaging Stress Test before Surgery[1]	-	-	5.4%	5.3%
Combination Abdominal CT Scan	621	6.8%	12.2%	10.5%
Combination Brain/Sinus CT Scan	660	1.7%	3.1%	2.7%
Combination Chest CT Scan	494	0.8%	2.1%	2.7%
Follow-up Mammogram/Ultrasound	1,129	8.9%	9%	8.8%
Lumbar Spine MRI for Low Back Pain	59	47.5%	35.8%	37.2%

Excela Health Latrobe Hospital

One Mellon Way
Latrobe, PA 15650
URL: www.excelahealth.org
Type: Acute Care Hospitals
Ownership: Voluntary non-profit - Other

Phone: 724-537-1000
Emergency Services: Yes

Measure	Cases	This Hosp.	State Avg.	U.S. Avg.
Blood Clot Prevention and Treatment				
Anticoagulation Overlap Therapy[2]	32	88%	94%	93%
ICU Venous Thromboembolism Prophylaxis[2]	91	100%	94%	92%
Incidence of Potentially Preventable VTE[1,2]	-	-	8%	10%
UFH with Dosages/Platelet Monitoring[2]	37	100%	98%	97%
Venous Thromboembolism Prophylaxis[2]	356	98%	90%	85%
Warfarin Therapy Discharge Instructions[2]	25	96%	78%	75%
Chest Pain/Possible Heart Attack Care				
Aspirin Given Within 24 Hours of Arrival	91	99%	97%	96%
Fibrinolytic Meds Within 30 Min. of Arrival[7]	-	-	44%	58%
Average Time to ECG (minutes)	96	6	9	7
Average Time to Transfer (minutes)	22	52	64	60
Children's Asthma Care				
Received Home Management Plan of Care	-	-	-	88%
Received Reliever Medication	-	-	-	100%
Received Systemic Corticosteroids	-	-	-	100%
Emergency Department				
Admittance Decision Time (minutes)[2]	1,096	64	104	98
Head CT Results Within 45 Min. of Arrival	16	69%	60%	57%
Patients Who Left ER Before Being Seen	35,201	0%	1%	2%
Time from ER Arrival to Admit. (minutes)[2]	1,098	230	276	274
Time from ER Arrival to Discharge (minutes)	441	118	125	134
Time in ER Before Being Evaluated (minutes)	512	15	26	26
Time to Pain Meds for Fractures (minutes)	96	51	58	57
Heart Attack Care				
Aspirin Given at Discharge	70	96%	99%	99%
Fibrinolytic Meds Within 30 Min. of Arrival[7]	-	-	40%	54%
PCI Within 90 Minutes of Arrival[7]	-	-	97%	96%
Statin Prescribed at Discharge	67	97%	99%	98%
Heart Failure Care				
ACE Inhibitor or ARB for LVSD	40	92%	97%	97%
Discharge Instructions Given	187	94%	96%	94%
Evaluation of LVS Function	244	100%	100%	99%
Medicare Spending				
Medicare Spending per Patient (ratio)	-	1.01	1.01	0.98
Pneumonia Care				
Appropriate Initial Antibiotic Given	138	100%	96%	95%
Blood Culture Timing	260	100%	98%	98%
Pregnancy and Delivery Care				
Newborn Deliveries Scheduled Early[7]	-	-	4%	6%
Preventive Care				
Immunization for Influenza[2]	766	96%	91%	90%
Immunization for Pneumonia[2]	1,113	92%	92%	92%
Stroke Care				
Anticoagulation Therapy for Atrial Fibrillation[1]	-	-	96%	95%
Antithrombotic Therapy Timing	38	100%	98%	98%
Assessed for Rehabilitation	42	100%	98%	97%
Discharged on Antithrombotic Therapy	38	100%	99%	99%
Discharged on Statin Medication	29	100%	95%	94%
Thrombolytic Therapy Timing[1]	-	-	72%	66%
Venous Thromboembolism Prophylaxis	45	100%	95%	94%
Written Stroke Educational Materials Given	23	96%	90%	88%
Surgical Care Improvement Project				
Appropriate Beta Blocker Usage	134	98%	98%	98%
Appropriate VTP Within 24 Hours	426	99%	99%	98%
Controlled Postoperative Blood Glucose[7]	-	-	98%	97%
Perioperative Temperature Management	484	100%	100%	100%
Prophylactic Antibiotic Selection	347	99%	99%	99%
Prophylactic Antibiotic Selection (Outpatient)	285	97%	98%	98%
Prophylactic Antibiotic Stopped	343	98%	98%	98%
Prophylactic Antibiotic Timing	347	100%	99%	99%
Prophylactic Antibiotic Timing (Outpatient)	286	99%	98%	98%
Urinary Catheter Removal	205	97%	99%	97%
Survey of Patients' Hospital Experiences				
Area Around Room 'Always' Quiet at Night	300+	55%	54%	61%
Doctors 'Always' Communicated Well	300+	80%	80%	82%
Home Recovery Information Given	300+	88%	86%	85%
Hospital Given 9 or 10 on 10 Point Scale	300+	67%	69%	71%
Meds 'Always' Explained Before Given	300+	61%	63%	64%
Nurses 'Always' Communicated Well	300+	78%	79%	79%
Pain 'Always' Well Controlled	300+	71%	70%	71%
Room and Bathroom 'Always' Clean	300+	66%	73%	73%
Timely Help 'Always' Received	300+	71%	67%	68%
Would Definitely Recommend Hospital	300+	67%	70%	71%
Use of Medical Imaging				
Cardiac Imaging Stress Test before Surgery	141	7.8%	5.4%	5.3%
Combination Abdominal CT Scan	424	4.0%	12.2%	10.5%
Combination Brain/Sinus CT Scan[1]	-	-	3.1%	2.7%
Combination Chest CT Scan	328	1.8%	2.1%	2.7%
Follow-up Mammogram/Ultrasound	617	8.1%	9%	8.8%
Lumbar Spine MRI for Low Back Pain[1]	-	-	35.8%	37.2%

Good Samaritan Hospital

Fourth & Walnut Streets
Lebanon, PA 17042
URL: www.gshleb.org
Type: Acute Care Hospitals
Ownership: Voluntary non-profit - Other

Phone: 717-270-7500
Emergency Services: Yes

Measure	Cases	This Hosp.	State Avg.	U.S. Avg.
Blood Clot Prevention and Treatment				
Anticoagulation Overlap Therapy[2]	95	89%	94%	93%
ICU Venous Thromboembolism Prophylaxis[2]	100	94%	94%	92%
Incidence of Potentially Preventable VTE[2]	16	0%	8%	10%
UFH with Dosages/Platelet Monitoring[2]	46	98%	98%	97%
Venous Thromboembolism Prophylaxis[2]	322	91%	90%	85%
Warfarin Therapy Discharge Instructions[2]	72	93%	78%	75%
Chest Pain/Possible Heart Attack Care				
Aspirin Given Within 24 Hours of Arrival[1]	-	-	97%	96%
Fibrinolytic Meds Within 30 Min. of Arrival[3,7]	-	-	44%	58%
Average Time to ECG (minutes)[1]	-	-	9	7
Average Time to Transfer (minutes)[1,3]	-	-	64	60
Children's Asthma Care				
Received Home Management Plan of Care	-	-	-	88%
Received Reliever Medication	-	-	-	100%
Received Systemic Corticosteroids	-	-	-	100%
Emergency Department				
Admittance Decision Time (minutes)[2]	403	175	104	98
Head CT Results Within 45 Min. of Arrival[1]	-	-	60%	57%
Patients Who Left ER Before Being Seen	55,049	2%	1%	2%
Time from ER Arrival to Admit. (minutes)[2]	549	406	276	274
Time from ER Arrival to Discharge (minutes)	360	162	125	134
Time in ER Before Being Evaluated (minutes)	371	48	26	26
Time to Pain Meds for Fractures (minutes)	98	73	58	57
Heart Attack Care				
Aspirin Given at Discharge	203	100%	99%	99%
Fibrinolytic Meds Within 30 Min. of Arrival[7]	-	-	40%	54%
PCI Within 90 Minutes of Arrival	56	95%	97%	96%
Statin Prescribed at Discharge	194	100%	99%	98%
Heart Failure Care				
ACE Inhibitor or ARB for LVSD	54	100%	97%	97%
Discharge Instructions Given	135	89%	96%	94%
Evaluation of LVS Function	196	100%	100%	99%
Medicare Spending				
Medicare Spending per Patient (ratio)	-	1.00	1.01	0.98
Pneumonia Care				
Appropriate Initial Antibiotic Given	141	96%	96%	95%
Blood Culture Timing	235	98%	98%	98%
Pregnancy and Delivery Care				
Newborn Deliveries Scheduled Early[2]	32	0%	4%	6%
Preventive Care				
Immunization for Influenza[2]	541	84%	91%	90%
Immunization for Pneumonia[2]	702	86%	92%	92%
Stroke Care				
Anticoagulation Therapy for Atrial Fibrillation[1]	-	-	96%	95%
Antithrombotic Therapy Timing	60	100%	98%	98%
Assessed for Rehabilitation	63	98%	98%	97%
Discharged on Antithrombotic Therapy	60	100%	99%	99%
Discharged on Statin Medication	53	96%	95%	94%
Thrombolytic Therapy Timing[1]	-	-	72%	66%
Venous Thromboembolism Prophylaxis	63	95%	95%	94%
Written Stroke Educational Materials Given	27	74%	90%	88%
Surgical Care Improvement Project				
Appropriate Beta Blocker Usage[2]	214	100%	98%	98%
Appropriate VTP Within 24 Hours[2]	272	96%	99%	98%
Controlled Postoperative Blood Glucose[2]	135	100%	98%	97%
Perioperative Temperature Management[2]	414	100%	100%	100%
Prophylactic Antibiotic Selection[2]	318	100%	99%	99%
Prophylactic Antibiotic Selection (Outpatient)	418	100%	98%	98%
Prophylactic Antibiotic Stopped[2]	304	99%	98%	98%
Prophylactic Antibiotic Timing[2]	318	99%	99%	99%
Prophylactic Antibiotic Timing (Outpatient)	419	99%	98%	98%
Urinary Catheter Removal[2]	277	100%	99%	97%
Survey of Patients' Hospital Experiences				
Area Around Room 'Always' Quiet at Night	300+	50%	54%	61%
Doctors 'Always' Communicated Well	300+	79%	80%	82%
Home Recovery Information Given	300+	88%	86%	85%
Hospital Given 9 or 10 on 10 Point Scale	300+	70%	69%	71%
Meds 'Always' Explained Before Given	300+	65%	63%	64%
Nurses 'Always' Communicated Well	300+	82%	79%	79%
Pain 'Always' Well Controlled	300+	73%	70%	71%
Room and Bathroom 'Always' Clean	300+	80%	73%	73%
Timely Help 'Always' Received	300+	69%	67%	68%
Would Definitely Recommend Hospital	300+	69%	70%	71%

NOTE: Hospital profiles are in alphabetical order by state, then city, then hospital within the city; Rankings exclude hospitals with less than 25 cases except for patient surveys which excludes hospitals with less than 100 cases; (a) 100-299 cases; (1) The number of cases/patients is too few to report; (2) Data submitted were based on a sample of cases/patients; (3) Results are based on a shorter time period than required; (4) Data suppressed by CMS for one or more quarters; (5) Results are not available for this reporting period; (6) Fewer than 100 patients completed the HCAHPS survey; (7) No cases met the criteria for this measure; (8) The lower limit of the confidence interval cannot be calculated if the number of observed infections equals zero; (9) No data are available from the state/territory for this reporting period; (10) The scores shown reflect fewer than 50 completed surveys; (11) There were discrepancies in the data collection process; (12) This measure does not apply to this hospital for this reporting period; (13) Results cannot be calculated for this reporting period; (14) The results for this state are combined with nearby states to protect confidentiality; Please refer to the User's Guide for a full explanation of data.

Use of Medical Imaging				
Cardiac Imaging Stress Test before Surgery	897	4.8%	5.4%	5.3%
Combination Abdominal CT Scan	1,099	32.4%	12.2%	10.5%
Combination Brain/Sinus CT Scan	934	1.0%	3.1%	2.7%
Combination Chest CT Scan	500	1.2%	2.1%	2.7%
Follow-up Mammogram/Ultrasound	2,432	4.6%	9%	8.8%
Lumbar Spine MRI for Low Back Pain[1]	-	-	35.8%	37.2%

Lebanon VA Medical Center

1700 South Lincoln Avenue
Lebanon, PA 17042
Phone: 717-228-5901
URL: www.lebanon.va.gov
Type: Acute Care - VA
Emergency Services: No
Ownership: Government Federal
Beds: 248

Measure	Cases	This Hosp.	State Avg.	U.S. Avg.
Blood Clot Prevention and Treatment				
Anticoagulation Overlap Therapy	-	-	94%	93%
ICU Venous Thromboembolism Prophylaxis	-	-	94%	92%
Incidence of Potentially Preventable VTE	-	-	8%	10%
UFH with Dosages/Platelet Monitoring	-	-	98%	97%
Venous Thromboembolism Prophylaxis	-	-	90%	85%
Warfarin Therapy Discharge Instructions	-	-	78%	75%
Chest Pain/Possible Heart Attack Care				
Aspirin Given Within 24 Hours of Arrival	-	-	97%	96%
Fibrinolytic Meds Within 30 Min. of Arrival	-	-	44%	58%
Average Time to ECG (minutes)	-	-	9	7
Average Time to Transfer (minutes)	-	-	64	60
Children's Asthma Care				
Received Home Management Plan of Care	-	-	-	88%
Received Reliever Medication	-	-	-	100%
Received Systemic Corticosteroids	-	-	-	100%
Emergency Department				
Admittance Decision Time (minutes)	-	-	104	98
Head CT Results Within 45 Min. of Arrival	-	-	60%	57%
Patients Who Left ER Before Being Seen	-	-	1%	2%
Time from ER Arrival to Admit. (minutes)	-	-	276	274
Time from ER Arrival to Discharge (minutes)	-	-	125	134
Time in ER Before Being Evaluated (minutes)	-	-	26	26
Time to Pain Meds for Fractures (minutes)	-	-	58	57
Heart Attack Care				
Aspirin Given at Discharge[5]	-	-	99%	99%
Fibrinolytic Meds Within 30 Min. of Arrival[5]	-	-	40%	54%
PCI Within 90 Minutes of Arrival[5]	-	-	97%	96%
Statin Prescribed at Discharge[5]	-	-	99%	98%
Heart Failure Care				
ACE Inhibitor or ARB for LVSD	25	92%	97%	97%
Discharge Instructions Given	51	92%	96%	94%
Evaluation of LVS Function	66	100%	100%	99%
Medicare Spending				
Medicare Spending per Patient (ratio)	-	-	1.01	0.98
Pneumonia Care				
Appropriate Initial Antibiotic Given	27	96%	96%	95%
Blood Culture Timing	51	98%	98%	98%
Pregnancy and Delivery Care				
Newborn Deliveries Scheduled Early	-	-	4%	6%
Preventive Care				
Immunization for Influenza[5]	-	-	91%	90%
Immunization for Pneumonia[5]	-	-	92%	92%
Stroke Care				
Anticoagulation Therapy for Atrial Fibrillation	-	-	96%	95%
Antithrombotic Therapy Timing	-	-	98%	98%
Assessed for Rehabilitation	-	-	98%	97%
Discharged on Antithrombotic Therapy	-	-	99%	99%
Discharged on Statin Medication	-	-	95%	94%
Thrombolytic Therapy Timing	-	-	72%	66%
Venous Thromboembolism Prophylaxis	-	-	95%	94%
Written Stroke Educational Materials Given	-	-	90%	88%
Surgical Care Improvement Project				
Appropriate Beta Blocker Usage[2]	57	96%	98%	98%
Appropriate VTP Within 24 Hours[2]	158	99%	99%	98%
Controlled Postoperative Blood Glucose[5]	-	-	98%	97%
Perioperative Temperature Management[2]	205	100%	100%	100%
Prophylactic Antibiotic Selection	160	95%	99%	99%
Prophylactic Antibiotic Selection (Outpatient)	-	-	98%	98%
Prophylactic Antibiotic Stopped	159	97%	98%	98%
Prophylactic Antibiotic Timing	160	97%	99%	99%
Prophylactic Antibiotic Timing (Outpatient)	-	-	98%	98%
Urinary Catheter Removal[2]	101	99%	99%	97%
Survey of Patients' Hospital Experiences				
Area Around Room 'Always' Quiet at Night	-	-	54%	61%
Doctors 'Always' Communicated Well	-	-	80%	82%
Home Recovery Information Given	-	-	86%	85%
Hospital Given 9 or 10 on 10 Point Scale	-	-	69%	71%
Meds 'Always' Explained Before Given	-	-	63%	64%
Nurses 'Always' Communicated Well	-	-	79%	79%
Pain 'Always' Well Controlled	-	-	70%	71%
Room and Bathroom 'Always' Clean	-	-	73%	73%
Timely Help 'Always' Received	-	-	67%	68%
Would Definitely Recommend Hospital	-	-	70%	71%
Use of Medical Imaging				
Cardiac Imaging Stress Test before Surgery	-	-	5.4%	5.3%
Combination Abdominal CT Scan	-	-	12.2%	10.5%
Combination Brain/Sinus CT Scan	-	-	3.1%	2.7%
Combination Chest CT Scan	-	-	2.1%	2.7%
Follow-up Mammogram/Ultrasound	-	-	9%	8.8%
Lumbar Spine MRI for Low Back Pain	-	-	35.8%	37.2%

Gnaden Huetten Memorial Hospital

211 North 12th Street
Lehighton, PA 18235
Phone: 607-377-1300
Fax: 610-377-7920
URL: www.bluemountainhealthsystem.org/services.asp
Type: Acute Care Hospitals
Emergency Services: Yes
Ownership: Voluntary non-profit - Private
Beds: 202

Key Personnel:
Anesthesiology. . . . . George Chmiel
President/CEO . . . . Andrew E. Harris
Ambulatory Care . . . . Joseph Lendvay

Measure	Cases	This Hosp.	State Avg.	U.S. Avg.
Blood Clot Prevention and Treatment				
Anticoagulation Overlap Therapy[2]	18	44%	94%	93%
ICU Venous Thromboembolism Prophylaxis[2]	56	88%	94%	92%
Incidence of Potentially Preventable VTE[2,7]	-	-	8%	10%
UFH with Dosages/Platelet Monitoring[1,2]	-	-	98%	97%
Venous Thromboembolism Prophylaxis[2]	228	75%	90%	85%
Warfarin Therapy Discharge Instructions[2]	13	23%	78%	75%
Chest Pain/Possible Heart Attack Care				
Aspirin Given Within 24 Hours of Arrival	54	96%	97%	96%
Fibrinolytic Meds Within 30 Min. of Arrival[7]	-	-	44%	58%
Average Time to ECG (minutes)	56	7	9	7
Average Time to Transfer (minutes)	16	50	64	60
Children's Asthma Care				
Received Home Management Plan of Care	-	-	-	88%
Received Reliever Medication	-	-	-	100%
Received Systemic Corticosteroids	-	-	-	100%
Emergency Department				
Admittance Decision Time (minutes)[2]	280	74	104	98
Head CT Results Within 45 Min. of Arrival[1]	-	-	60%	57%
Patients Who Left ER Before Being Seen	19,558	1%	1%	2%
Time from ER Arrival to Admit. (minutes)[2]	281	245	276	274
Time from ER Arrival to Discharge (minutes)	343	105	125	134
Time in ER Before Being Evaluated (minutes)	377	32	26	26
Time to Pain Meds for Fractures (minutes)	79	62	58	57
Heart Attack Care				
Aspirin Given at Discharge	13	100%	99%	99%
Fibrinolytic Meds Within 30 Min. of Arrival[7]	-	-	40%	54%
PCI Within 90 Minutes of Arrival[7]	-	-	97%	96%
Statin Prescribed at Discharge	12	83%	99%	98%
Heart Failure Care				
ACE Inhibitor or ARB for LVSD	22	100%	97%	97%
Discharge Instructions Given	63	86%	96%	94%
Evaluation of LVS Function	87	99%	100%	99%
Medicare Spending				
Medicare Spending per Patient (ratio)	-	1.05	1.01	0.98
Pneumonia Care				
Appropriate Initial Antibiotic Given	43	88%	96%	95%
Blood Culture Timing	88	100%	98%	98%
Pregnancy and Delivery Care				
Newborn Deliveries Scheduled Early[7]	-	-	4%	6%
Preventive Care				
Immunization for Influenza[2]	333	78%	91%	90%
Immunization for Pneumonia[2]	421	92%	92%	92%
Stroke Care				
Anticoagulation Therapy for Atrial Fibrillation[1]	-	-	96%	95%
Antithrombotic Therapy Timing	27	100%	98%	98%
Assessed for Rehabilitation	27	96%	98%	97%
Discharged on Antithrombotic Therapy	26	96%	99%	99%
Discharged on Statin Medication	22	55%	95%	94%
Thrombolytic Therapy Timing[1]	-	-	72%	66%
Venous Thromboembolism Prophylaxis	26	92%	95%	94%
Written Stroke Educational Materials Given	17	0%	90%	88%
Surgical Care Improvement Project				
Appropriate Beta Blocker Usage	34	94%	98%	98%
Appropriate VTP Within 24 Hours	96	92%	99%	98%
Controlled Postoperative Blood Glucose[7]	-	-	98%	97%
Perioperative Temperature Management	110	100%	100%	100%
Prophylactic Antibiotic Selection	72	96%	99%	99%
Prophylactic Antibiotic Selection (Outpatient)	72	97%	98%	98%
Prophylactic Antibiotic Stopped	64	97%	98%	98%
Prophylactic Antibiotic Timing	73	99%	99%	99%
Prophylactic Antibiotic Timing (Outpatient)	55	95%	98%	98%
Urinary Catheter Removal	86	98%	99%	97%
Survey of Patients' Hospital Experiences				
Area Around Room 'Always' Quiet at Night	300+	54%	54%	61%
Doctors 'Always' Communicated Well	300+	75%	80%	82%
Home Recovery Information Given	300+	86%	86%	85%
Hospital Given 9 or 10 on 10 Point Scale	300+	58%	69%	71%
Meds 'Always' Explained Before Given	300+	57%	63%	64%
Nurses 'Always' Communicated Well	300+	74%	79%	79%
Pain 'Always' Well Controlled	300+	66%	70%	71%
Room and Bathroom 'Always' Clean	300+	71%	73%	73%
Timely Help 'Always' Received	300+	60%	67%	68%
Would Definitely Recommend Hospital	300+	60%	70%	71%
Use of Medical Imaging				
Cardiac Imaging Stress Test before Surgery	406	4.9%	5.4%	5.3%
Combination Abdominal CT Scan	422	14.2%	12.2%	10.5%
Combination Brain/Sinus CT Scan[1]	-	-	3.1%	2.7%
Combination Chest CT Scan	314	11.8%	2.1%	2.7%
Follow-up Mammogram/Ultrasound	824	6.9%	9%	8.8%
Lumbar Spine MRI for Low Back Pain	72	33.3%	35.8%	37.2%

Evangelical Community Hospital

One Hospital Drive
Lewisburg, PA 17837
Phone: 570-522-2200
Fax: 570-522-2868
E-mail: information@evanhospital.com
URL: www.evanhospital.com
Type: Acute Care Hospitals
Emergency Services: Yes
Ownership: Voluntary non-profit - Other
Beds: 134

Key Personnel:
Patient Relations . . . . Angela Brouse
Quality Assurance . . . . Leigh Donecker
Chief of Medical Staff. . . . . J Lawrence Ginsburg, MD
Radiology. . . . . Naval Kant
Pediatric In-Patient Care . . . . Ruth Nolan
CEO/President. . . . . Michael N O'Keefe
Infection Control. . . . . Tamara Persina, RN
Emergency Room . . . . Darlene Rowe, RN

Measure	Cases	This Hosp.	State Avg.	U.S. Avg.
Blood Clot Prevention and Treatment				
Anticoagulation Overlap Therapy	60	98%	94%	93%
ICU Venous Thromboembolism Prophylaxis	472	95%	94%	92%
Incidence of Potentially Preventable VTE[1]	-	-	8%	10%
UFH with Dosages/Platelet Monitoring[1]	-	-	98%	97%
Venous Thromboembolism Prophylaxis	1,849	98%	90%	85%
Warfarin Therapy Discharge Instructions	43	95%	78%	75%
Chest Pain/Possible Heart Attack Care				
Aspirin Given Within 24 Hours of Arrival[1]	-	-	97%	96%
Fibrinolytic Meds Within 30 Min. of Arrival[3,7]	-	-	44%	58%
Average Time to ECG (minutes)[1]	-	-	9	7
Average Time to Transfer (minutes)[1,3]	-	-	64	60

NOTE: Hospital profiles are in alphabetical order by state, then city, then hospital within the city; Rankings exclude hospitals with less than 25 cases except for patient surveys which excludes hospitals with less than 100 cases; (a) 100-299 cases; (1) The number of cases/patients is too few to report; (2) Data submitted were based on a sample of cases/patients; (3) Results are based on a shorter time period than required; (4) Data suppressed by CMS for one or more quarters; (5) Results are not available for this reporting period; (6) Fewer than 100 patients completed the HCAHPS survey; (7) No cases met the criteria for this measure; (8) The lower limit of the confidence interval cannot be calculated if the number of observed infections equals zero; (9) No data are available from the state/territory for this reporting period; (10) The scores shown reflect fewer than 50 completed surveys; (11) There were discrepancies in the data collection process; (12) This measure does not apply to this hospital for this reporting period; (13) Results cannot be calculated for this reporting period; (14) The results for this state are combined with nearby states to protect confidentiality; Please refer to the User's Guide for a full explanation of data.

Children's Asthma Care				
Received Home Management Plan of Care	-	-	-	88%
Received Reliever Medication	-	-	-	100%
Received Systemic Corticosteroids	-	-	-	100%
Emergency Department				
Admittance Decision Time (minutes)[2]	638	138	104	98
Head CT Results Within 45 Min. of Arrival	33	79%	60%	57%
Patients Who Left ER Before Being Seen	33,148	1%	1%	2%
Time from ER Arrival to Admit. (minutes)[2]	638	286	276	274
Time from ER Arrival to Discharge (minutes)	395	140	125	134
Time in ER Before Being Evaluated (minutes)	414	32	26	26
Time to Pain Meds for Fractures (minutes)	152	46	58	57
Heart Attack Care				
Aspirin Given at Discharge[2]	132	99%	99%	99%
Fibrinolytic Meds Within 30 Min. of Arrival[1,2]	-	-	40%	54%
PCI Within 90 Minutes of Arrival[1,2]	-	-	97%	96%
Statin Prescribed at Discharge[2]	129	100%	99%	98%
Heart Failure Care				
ACE Inhibitor or ARB for LVSD	35	100%	97%	97%
Discharge Instructions Given	106	99%	96%	94%
Evaluation of LVS Function	131	100%	100%	99%
Medicare Spending				
Medicare Spending per Patient (ratio)	-	0.93	1.01	0.98
Pneumonia Care				
Appropriate Initial Antibiotic Given	119	96%	96%	95%
Blood Culture Timing	217	99%	98%	98%
Pregnancy and Delivery Care				
Newborn Deliveries Scheduled Early[2]	44	27%	4%	6%
Preventive Care				
Immunization for Influenza[2]	510	83%	91%	90%
Immunization for Pneumonia[2]	640	90%	92%	92%
Stroke Care				
Anticoagulation Therapy for Atrial Fibrillation	16	100%	96%	95%
Antithrombotic Therapy Timing	66	100%	98%	98%
Assessed for Rehabilitation	91	98%	98%	97%
Discharged on Antithrombotic Therapy	87	100%	99%	99%
Discharged on Statin Medication	76	95%	95%	94%
Thrombolytic Therapy Timing[1]	-	-	72%	66%
Venous Thromboembolism Prophylaxis	69	99%	95%	94%
Written Stroke Educational Materials Given	56	71%	90%	88%
Surgical Care Improvement Project				
Appropriate Beta Blocker Usage[2]	122	97%	98%	98%
Appropriate VTP Within 24 Hours[2]	404	96%	99%	98%
Controlled Postoperative Blood Glucose[2,7]	-	-	98%	97%
Perioperative Temperature Management[2]	464	100%	100%	100%
Prophylactic Antibiotic Selection[2]	317	98%	99%	99%
Prophylactic Antibiotic Selection (Outpatient)	246	98%	98%	98%
Prophylactic Antibiotic Stopped[2]	316	97%	98%	98%
Prophylactic Antibiotic Timing[2]	317	98%	99%	99%
Prophylactic Antibiotic Timing (Outpatient)	250	97%	98%	98%
Urinary Catheter Removal[2]	390	100%	99%	97%
Survey of Patients' Hospital Experiences				
Area Around Room 'Always' Quiet at Night	300+	46%	54%	61%
Doctors 'Always' Communicated Well	300+	83%	80%	82%
Home Recovery Information Given	300+	87%	86%	85%
Hospital Given 9 or 10 on 10 Point Scale	300+	74%	69%	71%
Meds 'Always' Explained Before Given	300+	63%	63%	64%
Nurses 'Always' Communicated Well	300+	81%	79%	79%
Pain 'Always' Well Controlled	300+	71%	70%	71%
Room and Bathroom 'Always' Clean	300+	73%	73%	73%
Timely Help 'Always' Received	300+	73%	67%	68%
Would Definitely Recommend Hospital	300+	78%	70%	71%
Use of Medical Imaging				
Cardiac Imaging Stress Test before Surgery	429	7.0%	5.4%	5.3%
Combination Abdominal CT Scan	946	10.9%	12.2%	10.5%
Combination Brain/Sinus CT Scan	779	3.5%	3.1%	2.7%
Combination Chest CT Scan	500	6.8%	2.1%	2.7%
Follow-up Mammogram/Ultrasound	2,010	13.8%	9%	8.8%
Lumbar Spine MRI for Low Back Pain	98	37.8%	35.8%	37.2%

Lewistown Hospital

400 Highland Avenue
Lewistown, PA 17044
URL: www.lewistownhospital.org
Type: Acute Care Hospitals
Ownership: Voluntary non-profit - Other

Phone: 717-248-5411
Fax: 717-242-7245
Emergency Services: Yes
Beds: 139

Key Personnel:
Operating Room. . . . . G Scott Anderson
Coronary Care . . . . Pamela Benson
Chief of Medical Staff. . . . . Gurpreet S Bhalla, MD
Pediatric Ambulatory Care . . . . . . Paul Brahmakulam, MD
Radiology. . . . . Jerome Derdel, MD
Infection Control. . . . . Linda Flanagan
CEO/President. . . . . Kay A Hamilton, RN MS
Quality Assurance . . . . Judi Olnick

Measure	Cases	This Hosp.	State Avg.	U.S. Avg.
Blood Clot Prevention and Treatment				
Anticoagulation Overlap Therapy[2]	42	86%	94%	93%
ICU Venous Thromboembolism Prophylaxis[2]	72	96%	94%	92%
Incidence of Potentially Preventable VTE[1,2]	-	-	8%	10%
UFH with Dosages/Platelet Monitoring[2]	14	100%	98%	97%
Venous Thromboembolism Prophylaxis[2]	368	99%	90%	85%
Warfarin Therapy Discharge Instructions[2]	33	100%	78%	75%
Chest Pain/Possible Heart Attack Care				
Aspirin Given Within 24 Hours of Arrival	90	94%	97%	96%
Fibrinolytic Meds Within 30 Min. of Arrival[1]	-	-	44%	58%
Average Time to ECG (minutes)	91	9	9	7
Average Time to Transfer (minutes)	16	82	64	60
Children's Asthma Care				
Received Home Management Plan of Care	-	-	-	88%
Received Reliever Medication	-	-	-	100%
Received Systemic Corticosteroids	-	-	-	100%
Emergency Department				
Admittance Decision Time (minutes)[2]	558	54	104	98
Head CT Results Within 45 Min. of Arrival	20	40%	60%	57%
Patients Who Left ER Before Being Seen	33,206	2%	1%	2%
Time from ER Arrival to Admit. (minutes)[2]	576	214	276	274
Time from ER Arrival to Discharge (minutes)	336	156	125	134
Time in ER Before Being Evaluated (minutes)	380	27	26	26
Time to Pain Meds for Fractures (minutes)	52	66	58	57
Heart Attack Care				
Aspirin Given at Discharge	51	98%	99%	99%
Fibrinolytic Meds Within 30 Min. of Arrival[7]	-	-	40%	54%
PCI Within 90 Minutes of Arrival[7]	-	-	97%	96%
Statin Prescribed at Discharge	57	93%	99%	98%
Heart Failure Care				
ACE Inhibitor or ARB for LVSD	54	96%	97%	97%
Discharge Instructions Given	176	94%	96%	94%
Evaluation of LVS Function	246	100%	100%	99%
Medicare Spending				
Medicare Spending per Patient (ratio)	-	1.03	1.01	0.98
Pneumonia Care				
Appropriate Initial Antibiotic Given	143	90%	96%	95%
Blood Culture Timing	247	98%	98%	98%
Pregnancy and Delivery Care				
Newborn Deliveries Scheduled Early[2]	47	11%	4%	6%
Preventive Care				
Immunization for Influenza[2]	477	88%	91%	90%
Immunization for Pneumonia[2]	672	96%	92%	92%
Stroke Care				
Anticoagulation Therapy for Atrial Fibrillation[1]	-	-	96%	95%
Antithrombotic Therapy Timing	53	100%	98%	98%
Assessed for Rehabilitation	58	91%	98%	97%
Discharged on Antithrombotic Therapy	55	100%	99%	99%
Discharged on Statin Medication	48	90%	95%	94%
Thrombolytic Therapy Timing[1]	-	-	72%	66%
Venous Thromboembolism Prophylaxis	51	98%	95%	94%
Written Stroke Educational Materials Given	29	83%	90%	88%
Surgical Care Improvement Project				
Appropriate Beta Blocker Usage	61	92%	98%	98%
Appropriate VTP Within 24 Hours	168	96%	99%	98%
Controlled Postoperative Blood Glucose[7]	-	-	98%	97%
Perioperative Temperature Management	191	100%	100%	100%
Prophylactic Antibiotic Selection	125	96%	99%	99%
Prophylactic Antibiotic Selection (Outpatient)	94	97%	98%	98%
Prophylactic Antibiotic Stopped	119	93%	98%	98%
Prophylactic Antibiotic Timing	125	100%	99%	99%
Prophylactic Antibiotic Timing (Outpatient)	100	94%	98%	98%
Urinary Catheter Removal	99	100%	99%	97%
Survey of Patients' Hospital Experiences				
Area Around Room 'Always' Quiet at Night	300+	47%	54%	61%
Doctors 'Always' Communicated Well	300+	75%	80%	82%
Home Recovery Information Given	300+	89%	86%	85%
Hospital Given 9 or 10 on 10 Point Scale	300+	58%	69%	71%
Meds 'Always' Explained Before Given	300+	58%	63%	64%
Nurses 'Always' Communicated Well	300+	77%	79%	79%
Pain 'Always' Well Controlled	300+	70%	70%	71%
Room and Bathroom 'Always' Clean	300+	73%	73%	73%
Timely Help 'Always' Received	300+	62%	67%	68%
Would Definitely Recommend Hospital	300+	52%	70%	71%
Use of Medical Imaging				
Cardiac Imaging Stress Test before Surgery	386	7.8%	5.4%	5.3%
Combination Abdominal CT Scan	742	2.2%	12.2%	10.5%
Combination Brain/Sinus CT Scan	835	4.0%	3.1%	2.7%
Combination Chest CT Scan	625	0.0%	2.1%	2.7%
Follow-up Mammogram/Ultrasound	1,061	11.4%	9%	8.8%
Lumbar Spine MRI for Low Back Pain	131	30.5%	35.8%	37.2%

Heart of Lancaster Regional Medical Center

1500 Highlands Drive
Lititz, PA 17543
URL: www.heartoflancaster.com
Type: Acute Care Hospitals
Ownership: Proprietary

Phone: 717-625-5000
Fax: 717-625-5619
Emergency Services: Yes
Beds: 154

Key Personnel:
Radiology. . . . . Alan R Alexander
CEO/President. . . . . Lee Christenson
Chief of Medical Staff . . . . Peter Pityk
Anesthesiology. . . . . Terry Prager, CRNA
Administrator . . . . Deborah Willwerth, RN,MSN

Measure	Cases	This Hosp.	State Avg.	U.S. Avg.
Blood Clot Prevention and Treatment				
Anticoagulation Overlap Therapy[2]	17	100%	94%	93%
ICU Venous Thromboembolism Prophylaxis[2]	34	97%	94%	92%
Incidence of Potentially Preventable VTE[2,7]	-	-	8%	10%
UFH with Dosages/Platelet Monitoring[2]	11	100%	98%	97%
Venous Thromboembolism Prophylaxis[2]	167	98%	90%	85%
Warfarin Therapy Discharge Instructions[2]	13	100%	78%	75%
Chest Pain/Possible Heart Attack Care				
Aspirin Given Within 24 Hours of Arrival	26	100%	97%	96%
Fibrinolytic Meds Within 30 Min. of Arrival[7]	-	-	44%	58%
Average Time to ECG (minutes)	26	4	9	7
Average Time to Transfer (minutes)	13	49	64	60
Children's Asthma Care				
Received Home Management Plan of Care	-	-	-	88%
Received Reliever Medication	-	-	-	100%
Received Systemic Corticosteroids	-	-	-	100%
Emergency Department				
Admittance Decision Time (minutes)[2]	243	78	104	98
Head CT Results Within 45 Min. of Arrival[3,7]	-	-	60%	57%
Patients Who Left ER Before Being Seen	13,914	1%	1%	2%
Time from ER Arrival to Admit. (minutes)[2]	243	261	276	274
Time from ER Arrival to Discharge (minutes)	388	138	125	134
Time in ER Before Being Evaluated (minutes)	403	20	26	26
Time to Pain Meds for Fractures (minutes)	72	38	58	57
Heart Attack Care				
Aspirin Given at Discharge[1]	-	-	99%	99%
Fibrinolytic Meds Within 30 Min. of Arrival[7]	-	-	40%	54%
PCI Within 90 Minutes of Arrival[7]	-	-	97%	96%
Statin Prescribed at Discharge[1]	-	-	99%	98%
Heart Failure Care				
ACE Inhibitor or ARB for LVSD	14	100%	97%	97%
Discharge Instructions Given	35	89%	96%	94%
Evaluation of LVS Function	54	100%	100%	99%
Medicare Spending				
Medicare Spending per Patient (ratio)	-	1.00	1.01	0.98
Pneumonia Care				

NOTE: Hospital profiles are in alphabetical order by state, then city, then hospital within the city; Rankings exclude hospitals with less than 25 cases except for patient surveys which excludes hospitals with less than 100 cases; (a) 100-299 cases; (1) The number of cases/patients is too few to report; (2) Data submitted were based on a sample of cases/patients; (3) Results are based on a shorter time period than required; (4) Data suppressed by CMS for one or more quarters; (5) Results are not available for this reporting period; (6) Fewer than 100 patients completed the HCAHPS survey; (7) No cases met the criteria for this measure; (8) The lower limit of the confidence interval cannot be calculated if the number of observed infections equals zero; (9) No data are available from the state/territory for this reporting period; (10) The scores shown reflect fewer than 50 completed surveys; (11) There were discrepancies in the data collection process; (12) This measure does not apply to this hospital for this reporting period; (13) Results cannot be calculated for this reporting period; (14) The results for this state are combined with nearby states to protect confidentiality; Please refer to the User's Guide for a full explanation of data.

Measure	Cases	This Hosp.	State Avg.	U.S. Avg.
Appropriate Initial Antibiotic Given	50	100%	96%	95%
Blood Culture Timing	76	100%	98%	98%
Pregnancy and Delivery Care				
Newborn Deliveries Scheduled Early	48	6%	4%	6%
Preventive Care				
Immunization for Influenza[2]	256	99%	91%	90%
Immunization for Pneumonia[2]	241	99%	92%	92%
Stroke Care				
Anticoagulation Therapy for Atrial Fibrillation[1]	-	-	96%	95%
Antithrombotic Therapy Timing	24	100%	98%	98%
Assessed for Rehabilitation	22	100%	98%	97%
Discharged on Antithrombotic Therapy	22	100%	99%	99%
Discharged on Statin Medication	18	100%	95%	94%
Thrombolytic Therapy Timing[7]	-	-	72%	66%
Venous Thromboembolism Prophylaxis	23	96%	95%	94%
Written Stroke Educational Materials Given	12	75%	90%	88%
Surgical Care Improvement Project				
Appropriate Beta Blocker Usage	25	96%	98%	98%
Appropriate VTP Within 24 Hours	86	99%	99%	98%
Controlled Postoperative Blood Glucose[7]	-	-	98%	97%
Perioperative Temperature Management	102	100%	100%	100%
Prophylactic Antibiotic Selection	52	100%	99%	99%
Prophylactic Antibiotic Selection (Outpatient)	260	100%	98%	98%
Prophylactic Antibiotic Stopped	51	98%	98%	98%
Prophylactic Antibiotic Timing	52	100%	99%	99%
Prophylactic Antibiotic Timing (Outpatient)	260	100%	98%	98%
Urinary Catheter Removal	65	100%	99%	97%
Survey of Patients' Hospital Experiences				
Area Around Room 'Always' Quiet at Night	300+	56%	54%	61%
Doctors 'Always' Communicated Well	300+	80%	80%	82%
Home Recovery Information Given	300+	87%	86%	85%
Hospital Given 9 or 10 on 10 Point Scale	300+	73%	69%	71%
Meds 'Always' Explained Before Given	300+	58%	63%	64%
Nurses 'Always' Communicated Well	300+	78%	79%	79%
Pain 'Always' Well Controlled	300+	71%	70%	71%
Room and Bathroom 'Always' Clean	300+	79%	73%	73%
Timely Help 'Always' Received	300+	70%	67%	68%
Would Definitely Recommend Hospital	300+	75%	70%	71%
Use of Medical Imaging				
Cardiac Imaging Stress Test before Surgery	60	3.3%	5.4%	5.3%
Combination Abdominal CT Scan	182	7.1%	12.2%	10.5%
Combination Brain/Sinus CT Scan	195	7.7%	3.1%	2.7%
Combination Chest CT Scan	75	2.7%	2.1%	2.7%
Follow-up Mammogram/Ultrasound	253	7.5%	9%	8.8%
Lumbar Spine MRI for Low Back Pain[1]	-	-	35.8%	37.2%

Lock Haven Hospital

24 Cree Drive
Lock Haven, PA 17745
Phone: 570-893-5000
Fax: 570-893-5172
URL: www.lockhavenhospital.com
Type: Acute Care Hospitals
Emergency Services: Yes
Ownership: Proprietary
Beds: 260

Key Personnel:

Chief of Medical Staff.......... Keith Adams, MD
Pediatric Ambulatory Care ...... P Bhatt, MD
Pediatric In-Patient Care .... P Bhatt, MD
Infection Control.............. Nancry Bolze
Radiology.................... Cyndy Bower
Operating Room............... Sue Counsil
Quality Assurance .... Michelle Polk
CEO/President................ Gary Rhoads

Measure	Cases	This Hosp.	State Avg.	U.S. Avg.
Blood Clot Prevention and Treatment				
Anticoagulation Overlap Therapy[1,2]	-	-	94%	93%
ICU Venous Thromboembolism Prophylaxis[2]	64	100%	94%	92%
Incidence of Potentially Preventable VTE[1,2]	-	-	8%	10%
UFH with Dosages/Platelet Monitoring[1,2]	-	-	98%	97%
Venous Thromboembolism Prophylaxis[2]	260	99%	90%	85%
Warfarin Therapy Discharge Instructions[1,2]	-	-	78%	75%
Chest Pain/Possible Heart Attack Care				
Aspirin Given Within 24 Hours of Arrival	19	100%	97%	96%
Fibrinolytic Meds Within 30 Min. of Arrival[1]	-	-	44%	58%
Average Time to ECG (minutes)	22	10	9	7
Average Time to Transfer (minutes)[1]	-	-	64	60
Children's Asthma Care				
Received Home Management Plan of Care	-	-	-	88%
Received Reliever Medication	-	-	-	100%
Received Systemic Corticosteroids	-	-	-	100%
Emergency Department				
Admittance Decision Time (minutes)[2]	448	71	104	98
Head CT Results Within 45 Min. of Arrival[1]	-	-	60%	57%
Patients Who Left ER Before Being Seen	12,146	0%	1%	2%
Time from ER Arrival to Admit. (minutes)[2]	451	257	276	274
Time from ER Arrival to Discharge (minutes)	388	109	125	134
Time in ER Before Being Evaluated (minutes)	424	14	26	26
Time to Pain Meds for Fractures (minutes)	50	48	58	57
Heart Attack Care				
Aspirin Given at Discharge	16	100%	99%	99%
Fibrinolytic Meds Within 30 Min. of Arrival[7]	-	-	40%	54%
PCI Within 90 Minutes of Arrival[7]	-	-	97%	96%
Statin Prescribed at Discharge	13	100%	99%	98%
Heart Failure Care				
ACE Inhibitor or ARB for LVSD	16	94%	97%	97%
Discharge Instructions Given	53	94%	96%	94%
Evaluation of LVS Function	78	100%	100%	99%
Medicare Spending				
Medicare Spending per Patient (ratio)	-	0.89	1.01	0.98
Pneumonia Care				
Appropriate Initial Antibiotic Given	54	100%	96%	95%
Blood Culture Timing	67	100%	98%	98%
Pregnancy and Delivery Care				
Newborn Deliveries Scheduled Early[1,2]	-	-	4%	6%
Preventive Care				
Immunization for Influenza[2]	289	99%	91%	90%
Immunization for Pneumonia[2]	389	99%	92%	92%
Stroke Care				
Anticoagulation Therapy for Atrial Fibrillation[1]	-	-	96%	95%
Antithrombotic Therapy Timing	16	100%	98%	98%
Assessed for Rehabilitation	14	100%	98%	97%
Discharged on Antithrombotic Therapy[1]	-	-	99%	99%
Discharged on Statin Medication	12	100%	95%	94%
Thrombolytic Therapy Timing[7]	-	-	72%	66%
Venous Thromboembolism Prophylaxis	18	100%	95%	94%
Written Stroke Educational Materials Given[1]	-	-	90%	88%
Surgical Care Improvement Project				
Appropriate Beta Blocker Usage[1]	-	-	98%	98%
Appropriate VTP Within 24 Hours	13	100%	99%	98%
Controlled Postoperative Blood Glucose[7]	-	-	98%	97%
Perioperative Temperature Management[1]	-	-	100%	100%
Prophylactic Antibiotic Selection[1]	-	-	99%	99%
Prophylactic Antibiotic Selection (Outpatient)	17	76%	98%	98%
Prophylactic Antibiotic Stopped[1]	-	-	98%	98%
Prophylactic Antibiotic Timing[1]	-	-	99%	99%
Prophylactic Antibiotic Timing (Outpatient)	16	81%	98%	98%
Urinary Catheter Removal[1]	-	-	99%	97%
Survey of Patients' Hospital Experiences				
Area Around Room 'Always' Quiet at Night	(a)	61%	54%	61%
Doctors 'Always' Communicated Well	(a)	82%	80%	82%
Home Recovery Information Given	(a)	88%	86%	85%
Hospital Given 9 or 10 on 10 Point Scale	(a)	59%	69%	71%
Meds 'Always' Explained Before Given	(a)	67%	63%	64%
Nurses 'Always' Communicated Well	(a)	79%	79%	79%
Pain 'Always' Well Controlled	(a)	74%	70%	71%
Room and Bathroom 'Always' Clean	(a)	71%	73%	73%
Timely Help 'Always' Received	(a)	65%	67%	68%
Would Definitely Recommend Hospital	(a)	54%	70%	71%
Use of Medical Imaging				
Cardiac Imaging Stress Test before Surgery[1]	-	-	5.4%	5.3%
Combination Abdominal CT Scan	242	4.5%	12.2%	10.5%
Combination Brain/Sinus CT Scan	219	5.9%	3.1%	2.7%
Combination Chest CT Scan	59	5.1%	2.1%	2.7%
Follow-up Mammogram/Ultrasound	185	8.1%	9%	8.8%
Lumbar Spine MRI for Low Back Pain[1]	-	-	35.8%	37.2%

UPMC Mckeesport

1500 Fifth Avenue
Mc Keesport, PA 15132
Phone: 412-664-2000
Fax: 412-664-2925
URL: www.selectmedicalcorp.com
Type: Acute Care Hospitals
Emergency Services: Yes
Ownership: Voluntary non-profit - Private
Beds: 30

Key Personnel:

Chief of Medical Staff.......... Mehboob K Chaudhry
President/CEO................ David S. Chernow
Quality Assurance .... Joseph Ferraro
Pediatric In-Patient Care .... LJ Silberman, MD

Measure	Cases	This Hosp.	State Avg.	U.S. Avg.
Blood Clot Prevention and Treatment				
Anticoagulation Overlap Therapy[2]	44	100%	94%	93%
ICU Venous Thromboembolism Prophylaxis[2]	119	100%	94%	92%
Incidence of Potentially Preventable VTE[1,2]	-	-	8%	10%
UFH with Dosages/Platelet Monitoring[2]	43	100%	98%	97%
Venous Thromboembolism Prophylaxis[2]	384	96%	90%	85%
Warfarin Therapy Discharge Instructions[2]	27	100%	78%	75%
Chest Pain/Possible Heart Attack Care				
Aspirin Given Within 24 Hours of Arrival[1]	-	-	97%	96%
Fibrinolytic Meds Within 30 Min. of Arrival[3,7]	-	-	44%	58%
Average Time to ECG (minutes)[1]	-	-	9	7
Average Time to Transfer (minutes)[3,7]	-	-	64	60
Children's Asthma Care				
Received Home Management Plan of Care	-	-	-	88%
Received Reliever Medication	-	-	-	100%
Received Systemic Corticosteroids	-	-	-	100%
Emergency Department				
Admittance Decision Time (minutes)[2]	849	60	104	98
Head CT Results Within 45 Min. of Arrival[1]	-	-	60%	57%
Patients Who Left ER Before Being Seen	41,188	1%	1%	2%
Time from ER Arrival to Admit. (minutes)[2]	908	193	276	274
Time from ER Arrival to Discharge (minutes)	527	132	125	134
Time in ER Before Being Evaluated (minutes)	621	21	26	26
Time to Pain Meds for Fractures (minutes)	76	78	58	57
Heart Attack Care				
Aspirin Given at Discharge	161	100%	99%	99%
Fibrinolytic Meds Within 30 Min. of Arrival[7]	-	-	40%	54%
PCI Within 90 Minutes of Arrival	30	97%	97%	96%
Statin Prescribed at Discharge	149	100%	99%	98%
Heart Failure Care				
ACE Inhibitor or ARB for LVSD	81	100%	97%	97%
Discharge Instructions Given	283	100%	96%	94%
Evaluation of LVS Function	398	100%	100%	99%
Medicare Spending				
Medicare Spending per Patient (ratio)	-	1.06	1.01	0.98
Pneumonia Care				
Appropriate Initial Antibiotic Given	124	100%	96%	95%
Blood Culture Timing	238	100%	98%	98%
Pregnancy and Delivery Care				
Newborn Deliveries Scheduled Early[7]	-	-	4%	6%
Preventive Care				
Immunization for Influenza[2]	709	96%	91%	90%
Immunization for Pneumonia[2]	1,015	97%	92%	92%
Stroke Care				
Anticoagulation Therapy for Atrial Fibrillation	12	92%	96%	95%
Antithrombotic Therapy Timing	72	100%	98%	98%
Assessed for Rehabilitation	78	99%	98%	97%
Discharged on Antithrombotic Therapy	72	100%	99%	99%
Discharged on Statin Medication	48	98%	95%	94%
Thrombolytic Therapy Timing[1]	-	-	72%	66%
Venous Thromboembolism Prophylaxis	80	99%	95%	94%
Written Stroke Educational Materials Given	29	100%	90%	88%
Surgical Care Improvement Project				
Appropriate Beta Blocker Usage	73	99%	98%	98%
Appropriate VTP Within 24 Hours	210	96%	99%	98%
Controlled Postoperative Blood Glucose[7]	-	-	98%	97%
Perioperative Temperature Management	269	100%	100%	100%
Prophylactic Antibiotic Selection	186	99%	99%	99%
Prophylactic Antibiotic Selection (Outpatient)	61	85%	98%	98%
Prophylactic Antibiotic Stopped	182	99%	98%	98%
Prophylactic Antibiotic Timing	186	100%	99%	99%

NOTE: Hospital profiles are in alphabetical order by state, then city, then hospital within the city; Rankings exclude hospitals with less than 25 cases except for patient surveys which excludes hospitals with less than 100 cases; (a) 100-299 cases; (1) The number of cases/patients is too few to report; (2) Data submitted were based on a sample of cases/patients; (3) Results are based on a shorter time period than required; (4) Data suppressed by CMS for one or more quarters; (5) Results are not available for this reporting period; (6) Fewer than 100 patients completed the HCAHPS survey; (7) No cases met the criteria for this measure; (8) The lower limit of the confidence interval cannot be calculated if the number of observed infections equals zero; (9) No data are available from the state/territory for this reporting period; (10) The scores shown reflect fewer than 50 completed surveys; (11) There were discrepancies in the data collection process; (12) This measure does not apply to this hospital for this reporting period; (13) Results cannot be calculated for this reporting period; (14) The results for this state are combined with nearby states to protect confidentiality; Please refer to the User's Guide for a full explanation of data.

Measure	Cases	This Hosp.	State Avg.	U.S. Avg.
Prophylactic Antibiotic Timing (Outpatient)	65	91%	98%	98%
Urinary Catheter Removal	90	100%	99%	97%
Survey of Patients' Hospital Experiences				
Area Around Room 'Always' Quiet at Night	300+	56%	54%	61%
Doctors 'Always' Communicated Well	300+	78%	80%	82%
Home Recovery Information Given	300+	85%	86%	85%
Hospital Given 9 or 10 on 10 Point Scale	300+	64%	69%	71%
Meds 'Always' Explained Before Given	300+	62%	63%	64%
Nurses 'Always' Communicated Well	300+	77%	79%	79%
Pain 'Always' Well Controlled	300+	70%	70%	71%
Room and Bathroom 'Always' Clean	300+	70%	73%	73%
Timely Help 'Always' Received	300+	65%	67%	68%
Would Definitely Recommend Hospital	300+	61%	70%	71%
Use of Medical Imaging				
Cardiac Imaging Stress Test before Surgery	90	7.8%	5.4%	5.3%
Combination Abdominal CT Scan	304	9.5%	12.2%	10.5%
Combination Brain/Sinus CT Scan[1]	-	-	3.1%	2.7%
Combination Chest CT Scan	236	4.7%	2.1%	2.7%
Follow-up Mammogram/Ultrasound	433	10.4%	9%	8.8%
Lumbar Spine MRI for Low Back Pain[1]	-	-	35.8%	37.2%

Fulton County Medical Center

214 Peach Orchard Road
Mcconnellsburg, PA 17233
Phone: 717-485-3155
Fax: 717-485-5605
E-mail: marketing@fcmc-pa.org
URL: www.fcmcpa.org

Type: Critical Access Hospitals
Emergency Services: Yes
Ownership: Voluntary non-profit - Private
Beds: 82

Key Personnel:

Coronary Care . . . . Sherri Fisher
Operating Room. . . . . Cherry Hale
CEO/President. . . . . Jason Hawkins
Cardiac Laboratory. . . . . Kim Hsrnish
Chief of Medical Staff. . . . . Sharon Martin, MD
Infection Control. . . . . Barbara Weller

Measure	Cases	This Hosp.	State Avg.	U.S. Avg.
Blood Clot Prevention and Treatment				
Anticoagulation Overlap Therapy[5]	-	-	94%	93%
ICU Venous Thromboembolism Prophylaxis[5]	-	-	94%	92%
Incidence of Potentially Preventable VTE[5]	-	-	8%	10%
UFH with Dosages/Platelet Monitoring[5]	-	-	98%	97%
Venous Thromboembolism Prophylaxis[5]	-	-	90%	85%
Warfarin Therapy Discharge Instructions[5]	-	-	78%	75%
Chest Pain/Possible Heart Attack Care				
Aspirin Given Within 24 Hours of Arrival	41	88%	97%	96%
Fibrinolytic Meds Within 30 Min. of Arrival[3,7]	-	-	44%	58%
Average Time to ECG (minutes)	39	7	9	7
Average Time to Transfer (minutes)[1,3]	-	-	64	60
Children's Asthma Care				
Received Home Management Plan of Care	-	-	-	88%
Received Reliever Medication	-	-	-	100%
Received Systemic Corticosteroids	-	-	-	100%
Emergency Department				
Admittance Decision Time (minutes)[5]	-	-	104	98
Head CT Results Within 45 Min. of Arrival[5]	-	-	60%	57%
Patients Who Left ER Before Being Seen	9,746	0%	1%	2%
Time from ER Arrival to Admit. (minutes)[5]	-	-	276	274
Time from ER Arrival to Discharge (minutes)[5]	-	-	125	134
Time in ER Before Being Evaluated (minutes)[5]	-	-	26	26
Time to Pain Meds for Fractures (minutes)[5]	-	-	58	57
Heart Attack Care				
Aspirin Given at Discharge[3,7]	-	-	99%	99%
Fibrinolytic Meds Within 30 Min. of Arrival[3,7]	-	-	40%	54%
PCI Within 90 Minutes of Arrival[3,7]	-	-	97%	96%
Statin Prescribed at Discharge[3,7]	-	-	99%	98%
Heart Failure Care				
ACE Inhibitor or ARB for LVSD[1]	-	-	97%	97%
Discharge Instructions Given	21	71%	96%	94%
Evaluation of LVS Function	27	100%	100%	99%
Medicare Spending				
Medicare Spending per Patient (ratio)	-	-	1.01	0.98
Pneumonia Care				
Appropriate Initial Antibiotic Given	38	97%	96%	95%
Blood Culture Timing	37	97%	98%	98%
Pregnancy and Delivery Care				
Newborn Deliveries Scheduled Early[3,7]	-	-	4%	6%
Preventive Care				
Immunization for Influenza[5]	-	-	91%	90%
Immunization for Pneumonia[5]	-	-	92%	92%
Stroke Care				
Anticoagulation Therapy for Atrial Fibrillation[5]	-	-	96%	95%
Antithrombotic Therapy Timing[5]	-	-	98%	98%
Assessed for Rehabilitation[5]	-	-	98%	97%
Discharged on Antithrombotic Therapy[5]	-	-	99%	99%
Discharged on Statin Medication[5]	-	-	95%	94%
Thrombolytic Therapy Timing[5]	-	-	72%	66%
Venous Thromboembolism Prophylaxis[5]	-	-	95%	94%
Written Stroke Educational Materials Given[5]	-	-	90%	88%
Surgical Care Improvement Project				
Appropriate Beta Blocker Usage[5]	-	-	98%	98%
Appropriate VTP Within 24 Hours[5]	-	-	99%	98%
Controlled Postoperative Blood Glucose[5]	-	-	98%	97%
Perioperative Temperature Management[5]	-	-	100%	100%
Prophylactic Antibiotic Selection[5]	-	-	99%	99%
Prophylactic Antibiotic Selection (Outpatient)[5]	-	-	98%	98%
Prophylactic Antibiotic Stopped[5]	-	-	98%	98%
Prophylactic Antibiotic Timing[5]	-	-	99%	99%
Prophylactic Antibiotic Timing (Outpatient)[5]	-	-	98%	98%
Urinary Catheter Removal[5]	-	-	99%	97%
Survey of Patients' Hospital Experiences				
Area Around Room 'Always' Quiet at Night	(a)	52%	54%	61%
Doctors 'Always' Communicated Well	(a)	88%	80%	82%
Home Recovery Information Given	(a)	84%	86%	85%
Hospital Given 9 or 10 on 10 Point Scale	(a)	77%	69%	71%
Meds 'Always' Explained Before Given	(a)	64%	63%	64%
Nurses 'Always' Communicated Well	(a)	85%	79%	79%
Pain 'Always' Well Controlled	(a)	79%	70%	71%
Room and Bathroom 'Always' Clean	(a)	80%	73%	73%
Timely Help 'Always' Received	(a)	78%	67%	68%
Would Definitely Recommend Hospital	(a)	72%	70%	71%
Use of Medical Imaging				
Cardiac Imaging Stress Test before Surgery	145	2.8%	5.4%	5.3%
Combination Abdominal CT Scan	241	19.9%	12.2%	10.5%
Combination Brain/Sinus CT Scan	273	6.6%	3.1%	2.7%
Combination Chest CT Scan	85	5.9%	2.1%	2.7%
Follow-up Mammogram/Ultrasound	282	9.6%	9%	8.8%
Lumbar Spine MRI for Low Back Pain[1]	-	-	35.8%	37.2%

Ohio Valley General Hospital

25 Heckel Road
Mckees Rocks, PA 15136
Phone: 412-777-6161
Fax: 412-777-6189
URL: www.ohiovalleyhospital.org

Type: Acute Care Hospitals
Emergency Services: Yes
Ownership: Voluntary non-profit - Private
Beds: 119

Key Personnel:

Chief of Medical Staff. . . . . Roberta L Bashore
Emergency Room . . . . William Held
CEO/President. . . . . David W. Scott, FACHE

Measure	Cases	This Hosp.	State Avg.	U.S. Avg.
Blood Clot Prevention and Treatment				
Anticoagulation Overlap Therapy[2]	33	91%	94%	93%
ICU Venous Thromboembolism Prophylaxis[2]	65	72%	94%	92%
Incidence of Potentially Preventable VTE[1,2]	-	-	8%	10%
UFH with Dosages/Platelet Monitoring[2]	17	100%	98%	97%
Venous Thromboembolism Prophylaxis[2]	283	71%	90%	85%
Warfarin Therapy Discharge Instructions[2]	19	21%	78%	75%
Chest Pain/Possible Heart Attack Care				
Aspirin Given Within 24 Hours of Arrival	30	97%	97%	96%
Fibrinolytic Meds Within 30 Min. of Arrival[7]	-	-	44%	58%
Average Time to ECG (minutes)	29	12	9	7
Average Time to Transfer (minutes)[1]	-	-	64	60
Children's Asthma Care				
Received Home Management Plan of Care	-	-	-	88%
Received Reliever Medication	-	-	-	100%
Received Systemic Corticosteroids	-	-	-	100%
Emergency Department				
Admittance Decision Time (minutes)[2]	349	61	104	98
Head CT Results Within 45 Min. of Arrival[1]	-	-	60%	57%
Patients Who Left ER Before Being Seen	20,463	2%	1%	2%
Time from ER Arrival to Admit. (minutes)[2]	422	254	276	274
Time from ER Arrival to Discharge (minutes)	339	127	125	134
Time in ER Before Being Evaluated (minutes)	353	40	26	26
Time to Pain Meds for Fractures (minutes)	18	70	58	57
Heart Attack Care				
Aspirin Given at Discharge	11	100%	99%	99%
Fibrinolytic Meds Within 30 Min. of Arrival[7]	-	-	40%	54%
PCI Within 90 Minutes of Arrival[7]	-	-	97%	96%
Statin Prescribed at Discharge	12	92%	99%	98%
Heart Failure Care				
ACE Inhibitor or ARB for LVSD	37	97%	97%	97%
Discharge Instructions Given	97	74%	96%	94%
Evaluation of LVS Function	143	100%	100%	99%
Medicare Spending				
Medicare Spending per Patient (ratio)	-	1.28	1.01	0.98
Pneumonia Care				
Appropriate Initial Antibiotic Given	85	98%	96%	95%
Blood Culture Timing	103	98%	98%	98%
Pregnancy and Delivery Care				
Newborn Deliveries Scheduled Early[7]	-	-	4%	6%
Preventive Care				
Immunization for Influenza[2]	315	90%	91%	90%
Immunization for Pneumonia[2]	490	92%	92%	92%
Stroke Care				
Anticoagulation Therapy for Atrial Fibrillation[1]	-	-	96%	95%
Antithrombotic Therapy Timing	20	100%	98%	98%
Assessed for Rehabilitation	20	100%	98%	97%
Discharged on Antithrombotic Therapy	19	100%	99%	99%
Discharged on Statin Medication	17	76%	95%	94%
Thrombolytic Therapy Timing[1]	-	-	72%	66%
Venous Thromboembolism Prophylaxis	22	64%	95%	94%
Written Stroke Educational Materials Given[1]	-	-	90%	88%
Surgical Care Improvement Project				
Appropriate Beta Blocker Usage	60	98%	98%	98%
Appropriate VTP Within 24 Hours	174	97%	99%	98%
Controlled Postoperative Blood Glucose[7]	-	-	98%	97%
Perioperative Temperature Management	197	100%	100%	100%
Prophylactic Antibiotic Selection	130	98%	99%	99%
Prophylactic Antibiotic Selection (Outpatient)	56	93%	98%	98%
Prophylactic Antibiotic Stopped	127	96%	98%	98%
Prophylactic Antibiotic Timing	130	97%	99%	99%
Prophylactic Antibiotic Timing (Outpatient)	56	95%	98%	98%
Urinary Catheter Removal	64	91%	99%	97%
Survey of Patients' Hospital Experiences				
Area Around Room 'Always' Quiet at Night	300+	51%	54%	61%
Doctors 'Always' Communicated Well	300+	76%	80%	82%
Home Recovery Information Given	300+	84%	86%	85%
Hospital Given 9 or 10 on 10 Point Scale	300+	69%	69%	71%
Meds 'Always' Explained Before Given	300+	59%	63%	64%
Nurses 'Always' Communicated Well	300+	75%	79%	79%
Pain 'Always' Well Controlled	300+	63%	70%	71%
Room and Bathroom 'Always' Clean	300+	72%	73%	73%
Timely Help 'Always' Received	300+	61%	67%	68%
Would Definitely Recommend Hospital	300+	62%	70%	71%
Use of Medical Imaging				
Cardiac Imaging Stress Test before Surgery	100	6.0%	5.4%	5.3%
Combination Abdominal CT Scan	140	7.1%	12.2%	10.5%
Combination Brain/Sinus CT Scan	176	7.4%	3.1%	2.7%
Combination Chest CT Scan	80	0.0%	2.1%	2.7%
Follow-up Mammogram/Ultrasound	205	15.1%	9%	8.8%
Lumbar Spine MRI for Low Back Pain[1]	-	-	35.8%	37.2%

Holy Redeemer Hospital & Medical Center

1648 Huntingdon Pike
Meadowbrook, PA 19046
Phone: 215-947-3000
Fax: 215-938-3232
E-mail: inforef@holyredeemer.com
URL: www.holyredeemer.com

Type: Acute Care Hospitals
Emergency Services: Yes
Ownership: Voluntary non-profit - Church
Beds: 249

Key Personnel:

Operating Room. . . . . Donna M Angotti, RN
Pediatric Ambulatory Care . . . . . . L Stewart Barbera, MD

NOTE: Hospital profiles are in alphabetical order by state, then city, then hospital within the city; Rankings exclude hospitals with less than 25 cases except for patient surveys which excludes hospitals with less than 100 cases; (a) 100-299 cases; (1) The number of cases/patients is too few to report; (2) Data submitted were based on a sample of cases/patients; (3) Results are based on a shorter time period than required; (4) Data suppressed by CMS for one or more quarters; (5) Results are not available for this reporting period; (6) Fewer than 100 patients completed the HCAHPS survey; (7) No cases met the criteria for this measure; (8) The lower limit of the confidence interval cannot be calculated if the number of observed infections equals zero; (9) No data are available from the state/territory for this reporting period; (10) The scores shown reflect fewer than 50 completed surveys; (11) There were discrepancies in the data collection process; (12) This measure does not apply to this hospital for this reporting period; (13) Results cannot be calculated for this reporting period; (14) The results for this state are combined with nearby states to protect confidentiality; Please refer to the User's Guide for a full explanation of data.

Pediatric In-Patient Care . . . . L Stewart Barbera, MD
Chief of Medical Staff. . . . . William Gibbons, MD
CEO/President. . . . . Mark T Jones
Quality Assurance . . . . Debra Shank

Measure	Cases	This Hosp.	State Avg.	U.S. Avg.
Blood Clot Prevention and Treatment				
Anticoagulation Overlap Therapy[2]	59	97%	94%	93%
ICU Venous Thromboembolism Prophylaxis[2]	81	94%	94%	92%
Incidence of Potentially Preventable VTE[2]	20	10%	8%	10%
UFH with Dosages/Platelet Monitoring[2]	61	100%	98%	97%
Venous Thromboembolism Prophylaxis[2]	324	87%	90%	85%
Warfarin Therapy Discharge Instructions[2]	39	95%	78%	75%
Chest Pain/Possible Heart Attack Care				
Aspirin Given Within 24 Hours of Arrival[1]	-	-	97%	96%
Fibrinolytic Meds Within 30 Min. of Arrival[3,7]	-	-	44%	58%
Average Time to ECG (minutes)[1]	-	-	9	7
Average Time to Transfer (minutes)[3,7]	-	-	64	60
Children's Asthma Care				
Received Home Management Plan of Care	-	-	-	88%
Received Reliever Medication	-	-	-	100%
Received Systemic Corticosteroids	-	-	-	100%
Emergency Department				
Admittance Decision Time (minutes)[2]	490	164	104	98
Head CT Results Within 45 Min. of Arrival[1]	-	-	60%	57%
Patients Who Left ER Before Being Seen	30,823	1%	1%	2%
Time from ER Arrival to Admit. (minutes)[2]	492	362	276	274
Time from ER Arrival to Discharge (minutes)	274	194	125	134
Time in ER Before Being Evaluated (minutes)	373	65	26	26
Time to Pain Meds for Fractures (minutes)	138	83	58	57
Heart Attack Care				
Aspirin Given at Discharge	125	97%	99%	99%
Fibrinolytic Meds Within 30 Min. of Arrival[7]	-	-	40%	54%
PCI Within 90 Minutes of Arrival	22	91%	97%	96%
Statin Prescribed at Discharge	120	98%	99%	98%
Heart Failure Care				
ACE Inhibitor or ARB for LVSD	39	92%	97%	97%
Discharge Instructions Given	214	100%	96%	94%
Evaluation of LVS Function	333	100%	100%	99%
Medicare Spending				
Medicare Spending per Patient (ratio)	-	1.05	1.01	0.98
Pneumonia Care				
Appropriate Initial Antibiotic Given	115	97%	96%	95%
Blood Culture Timing	259	98%	98%	98%
Pregnancy and Delivery Care				
Newborn Deliveries Scheduled Early[2]	229	2%	4%	6%
Preventive Care				
Immunization for Influenza[2]	482	91%	91%	90%
Immunization for Pneumonia[2]	524	84%	92%	92%
Stroke Care				
Anticoagulation Therapy for Atrial Fibrillation[2]	17	94%	96%	95%
Antithrombotic Therapy Timing[2]	75	95%	98%	98%
Assessed for Rehabilitation[2]	79	94%	98%	97%
Discharged on Antithrombotic Therapy[2]	75	99%	99%	99%
Discharged on Statin Medication[2]	62	94%	95%	94%
Thrombolytic Therapy Timing[1,2]	-	-	72%	66%
Venous Thromboembolism Prophylaxis[2]	83	96%	95%	94%
Written Stroke Educational Materials Given[2]	41	98%	90%	88%
Surgical Care Improvement Project				
Appropriate Beta Blocker Usage	287	99%	98%	98%
Appropriate VTP Within 24 Hours	692	99%	99%	98%
Controlled Postoperative Blood Glucose[7]	-	-	98%	97%
Perioperative Temperature Management	818	100%	100%	100%
Prophylactic Antibiotic Selection	621	99%	99%	99%
Prophylactic Antibiotic Selection (Outpatient)	71	76%	98%	98%
Prophylactic Antibiotic Stopped	616	100%	98%	98%
Prophylactic Antibiotic Timing	621	100%	99%	99%
Prophylactic Antibiotic Timing (Outpatient)	85	82%	98%	98%
Urinary Catheter Removal	560	99%	99%	97%
Survey of Patients' Hospital Experiences				
Area Around Room 'Always' Quiet at Night	300+	52%	54%	61%
Doctors 'Always' Communicated Well	300+	78%	80%	82%
Home Recovery Information Given	300+	85%	86%	85%
Hospital Given 9 or 10 on 10 Point Scale	300+	70%	69%	71%
Meds 'Always' Explained Before Given	300+	59%	63%	64%
Nurses 'Always' Communicated Well	300+	78%	79%	79%
Pain 'Always' Well Controlled	300+	67%	70%	71%
Room and Bathroom 'Always' Clean	300+	68%	73%	73%
Timely Help 'Always' Received	300+	63%	67%	68%
Would Definitely Recommend Hospital	300+	72%	70%	71%
Use of Medical Imaging				
Cardiac Imaging Stress Test before Surgery	401	4.2%	5.4%	5.3%
Combination Abdominal CT Scan	619	4.4%	12.2%	10.5%
Combination Brain/Sinus CT Scan	574	2.3%	3.1%	2.7%
Combination Chest CT Scan	513	0.2%	2.1%	2.7%
Follow-up Mammogram/Ultrasound	1,568	5.9%	9%	8.8%
Lumbar Spine MRI for Low Back Pain[7]	-	-	35.8%	37.2%

Meadville Medical Center

751 Liberty Street
Meadville, PA 16335
URL: www.mmchs.org
Type: Acute Care Hospitals
Ownership: Voluntary non-profit - Other
Phone: 814-333-5000
Fax: 814-333-9456
Emergency Services: Yes
Beds: 277

Key Personnel:
Quality Assurance . . . . Connie Brady
Chief of Medical Staff. . . . . Denise Johnson, MD
Emergency Room . . . . Peter Lultschik, MD
CEO/President. . . . . Philip Pandolph
Chairman/CEO . . . . Mark Stevens

Measure	Cases	This Hosp.	State Avg.	U.S. Avg.
Blood Clot Prevention and Treatment				
Anticoagulation Overlap Therapy[2]	41	71%	94%	93%
ICU Venous Thromboembolism Prophylaxis[2]	122	98%	94%	92%
Incidence of Potentially Preventable VTE[1,2]	-	-	8%	10%
UFH with Dosages/Platelet Monitoring[2]	38	100%	98%	97%
Venous Thromboembolism Prophylaxis[2]	572	93%	90%	85%
Warfarin Therapy Discharge Instructions[2]	30	100%	78%	75%
Chest Pain/Possible Heart Attack Care				
Aspirin Given Within 24 Hours of Arrival	23	100%	97%	96%
Fibrinolytic Meds Within 30 Min. of Arrival[3,7]	-	-	44%	58%
Average Time to ECG (minutes)	24	10	9	7
Average Time to Transfer (minutes)[1,3]	-	-	64	60
Children's Asthma Care				
Received Home Management Plan of Care	-	-	-	88%
Received Reliever Medication	-	-	-	100%
Received Systemic Corticosteroids	-	-	-	100%
Emergency Department				
Admittance Decision Time (minutes)[2]	1,013	65	104	98
Head CT Results Within 45 Min. of Arrival[1]	-	-	60%	57%
Patients Who Left ER Before Being Seen	32,665	1%	1%	2%
Time from ER Arrival to Admit. (minutes)[2]	1,116	240	276	274
Time from ER Arrival to Discharge (minutes)	2,176	105	125	134
Time in ER Before Being Evaluated (minutes)	2,297	23	26	26
Time to Pain Meds for Fractures (minutes)	117	43	58	57
Heart Attack Care				
Aspirin Given at Discharge	70	99%	99%	99%
Fibrinolytic Meds Within 30 Min. of Arrival[7]	-	-	40%	54%
PCI Within 90 Minutes of Arrival	21	86%	97%	96%
Statin Prescribed at Discharge	73	96%	99%	98%
Heart Failure Care				
ACE Inhibitor or ARB for LVSD	41	95%	97%	97%
Discharge Instructions Given	126	71%	96%	94%
Evaluation of LVS Function	185	100%	100%	99%
Medicare Spending				
Medicare Spending per Patient (ratio)	-	0.96	1.01	0.98
Pneumonia Care				
Appropriate Initial Antibiotic Given	111	95%	96%	95%
Blood Culture Timing	168	96%	98%	98%
Pregnancy and Delivery Care				
Newborn Deliveries Scheduled Early[2]	44	0%	4%	6%
Preventive Care				
Immunization for Influenza[2]	1,060	95%	91%	90%
Immunization for Pneumonia[2]	1,254	97%	92%	92%
Stroke Care				
Anticoagulation Therapy for Atrial Fibrillation	14	100%	96%	95%
Antithrombotic Therapy Timing	73	95%	98%	98%
Assessed for Rehabilitation	76	93%	98%	97%
Discharged on Antithrombotic Therapy	73	99%	99%	99%
Discharged on Statin Medication	56	89%	95%	94%
Thrombolytic Therapy Timing[1]	-	-	72%	66%
Venous Thromboembolism Prophylaxis	78	94%	95%	94%
Written Stroke Educational Materials Given	33	45%	90%	88%
Surgical Care Improvement Project				
Appropriate Beta Blocker Usage[2]	262	97%	98%	98%
Appropriate VTP Within 24 Hours[2]	622	98%	99%	98%
Controlled Postoperative Blood Glucose[2,7]	-	-	98%	97%
Perioperative Temperature Management[2]	754	100%	100%	100%
Prophylactic Antibiotic Selection[2]	614	99%	99%	99%
Prophylactic Antibiotic Selection (Outpatient)	202	97%	98%	98%
Prophylactic Antibiotic Stopped[2]	610	99%	98%	98%
Prophylactic Antibiotic Timing[2]	614	97%	99%	99%
Prophylactic Antibiotic Timing (Outpatient)	192	94%	98%	98%
Urinary Catheter Removal[2]	580	97%	99%	97%
Survey of Patients' Hospital Experiences				
Area Around Room 'Always' Quiet at Night	300+	52%	54%	61%
Doctors 'Always' Communicated Well	300+	84%	80%	82%
Home Recovery Information Given	300+	87%	86%	85%
Hospital Given 9 or 10 on 10 Point Scale	300+	68%	69%	71%
Meds 'Always' Explained Before Given	300+	65%	63%	64%
Nurses 'Always' Communicated Well	300+	83%	79%	79%
Pain 'Always' Well Controlled	300+	75%	70%	71%
Room and Bathroom 'Always' Clean	300+	80%	73%	73%
Timely Help 'Always' Received	300+	72%	67%	68%
Would Definitely Recommend Hospital	300+	69%	70%	71%
Use of Medical Imaging				
Cardiac Imaging Stress Test before Surgery	502	4.6%	5.4%	5.3%
Combination Abdominal CT Scan	862	3.2%	12.2%	10.5%
Combination Brain/Sinus CT Scan	777	1.8%	3.1%	2.7%
Combination Chest CT Scan	512	0.8%	2.1%	2.7%
Follow-up Mammogram/Ultrasound	1,500	5.7%	9%	8.8%
Lumbar Spine MRI for Low Back Pain	161	30.4%	35.8%	37.2%

Riddle Memorial Hospital

1068 West Baltimore Pike
Media, PA 19063
URL: www.riddlehospital.org
Type: Acute Care Hospitals
Ownership: Voluntary non-profit - Private
Phone: 610-566-9400
Fax: 610-891-3592
Emergency Services: Yes
Beds: 248

Key Personnel:
Operating Room. . . . . William H Ayers, RN
Infection Control. . . . . Carolyn Bingeman
Patient Relations . . . . Cathy Boyer
Emergency Room . . . . Louise Hummel, RN
Chief of Medical Staff. . . . . George Lieb, MD
President . . . . Gary L. Perecko
Intensive Care Unit. . . . . Marianne Schwalbe
Quality Assurance . . . . Janet Webb

Measure	Cases	This Hosp.	State Avg.	U.S. Avg.
Blood Clot Prevention and Treatment				
Anticoagulation Overlap Therapy[2]	59	95%	94%	93%
ICU Venous Thromboembolism Prophylaxis[2]	59	97%	94%	92%
Incidence of Potentially Preventable VTE[2]	26	12%	8%	10%
UFH with Dosages/Platelet Monitoring[2]	64	100%	98%	97%
Venous Thromboembolism Prophylaxis[2]	395	89%	90%	85%
Warfarin Therapy Discharge Instructions[2]	35	54%	78%	75%
Chest Pain/Possible Heart Attack Care				
Aspirin Given Within 24 Hours of Arrival[3,7]	-	-	97%	96%
Fibrinolytic Meds Within 30 Min. of Arrival[5]	-	-	44%	58%
Average Time to ECG (minutes)[3,7]	-	-	9	7
Average Time to Transfer (minutes)[5]	-	-	64	60
Children's Asthma Care				
Received Home Management Plan of Care	-	-	-	88%
Received Reliever Medication	-	-	-	100%
Received Systemic Corticosteroids	-	-	-	100%
Emergency Department				
Admittance Decision Time (minutes)[2]	716	144	104	98
Head CT Results Within 45 Min. of Arrival[1]	-	-	60%	57%
Patients Who Left ER Before Being Seen	32,814	1%	1%	2%
Time from ER Arrival to Admit. (minutes)[2]	716	322	276	274
Time from ER Arrival to Discharge (minutes)	369	145	125	134

NOTE: Hospital profiles are in alphabetical order by state, then city, then hospital within the city; Rankings exclude hospitals with less than 25 cases except for patient surveys which excludes hospitals with less than 100 cases; (a) 100-299 cases; (1) The number of cases/patients is too few to report; (2) Data submitted were based on a sample of cases/patients; (3) Results are based on a shorter time period than required; (4) Data suppressed by CMS for one or more quarters; (5) Results are not available for this reporting period; (6) Fewer than 100 patients completed the HCAHPS survey; (7) No cases met the criteria for this measure; (8) The lower limit of the confidence interval cannot be calculated if the number of observed infections equals zero; (9) No data are available from the state/territory for this reporting period; (10) The scores shown reflect fewer than 50 completed surveys; (11) There were discrepancies in the data collection process; (12) This measure does not apply to this hospital for this reporting period; (13) Results cannot be calculated for this reporting period; (14) The results for this state are combined with nearby states to protect confidentiality; Please refer to the User's Guide for a full explanation of data.

Measure	Cases	This Hosp.	State Avg.	U.S. Avg.
Time in ER Before Being Evaluated (minutes)	383	19	26	26
Time to Pain Meds for Fractures (minutes)	71	49	58	57
Heart Attack Care				
Aspirin Given at Discharge	111	99%	99%	99%
Fibrinolytic Meds Within 30 Min. of Arrival[7]	-	-	40%	54%
PCI Within 90 Minutes of Arrival	24	100%	97%	96%
Statin Prescribed at Discharge	117	100%	99%	98%
Heart Failure Care				
ACE Inhibitor or ARB for LVSD	58	100%	97%	97%
Discharge Instructions Given	179	98%	96%	94%
Evaluation of LVS Function	268	100%	100%	99%
Medicare Spending				
Medicare Spending per Patient (ratio)	-	0.98	1.01	0.98
Pneumonia Care				
Appropriate Initial Antibiotic Given	174	95%	96%	95%
Blood Culture Timing	241	98%	98%	98%
Pregnancy and Delivery Care				
Newborn Deliveries Scheduled Early[2]	17	0%	4%	6%
Preventive Care				
Immunization for Influenza[2]	550	86%	91%	90%
Immunization for Pneumonia[2]	778	81%	92%	92%
Stroke Care				
Anticoagulation Therapy for Atrial Fibrillation	23	100%	96%	95%
Antithrombotic Therapy Timing	109	100%	98%	98%
Assessed for Rehabilitation	132	100%	98%	97%
Discharged on Antithrombotic Therapy	115	100%	99%	99%
Discharged on Statin Medication	97	100%	95%	94%
Thrombolytic Therapy Timing	11	91%	72%	66%
Venous Thromboembolism Prophylaxis	134	96%	95%	94%
Written Stroke Educational Materials Given	66	98%	90%	88%
Surgical Care Improvement Project				
Appropriate Beta Blocker Usage[2]	257	96%	98%	98%
Appropriate VTP Within 24 Hours[2]	965	99%	99%	98%
Controlled Postoperative Blood Glucose[2,7]	-	-	98%	97%
Perioperative Temperature Management[2]	1,037	100%	100%	100%
Prophylactic Antibiotic Selection[2]	849	100%	99%	99%
Prophylactic Antibiotic Selection (Outpatient)	140	97%	98%	98%
Prophylactic Antibiotic Stopped[2]	834	99%	98%	98%
Prophylactic Antibiotic Timing[2]	849	99%	99%	99%
Prophylactic Antibiotic Timing (Outpatient)	142	99%	98%	98%
Urinary Catheter Removal[2]	904	99%	99%	97%
Survey of Patients' Hospital Experiences				
Area Around Room 'Always' Quiet at Night	300+	54%	54%	61%
Doctors 'Always' Communicated Well	300+	81%	80%	82%
Home Recovery Information Given	300+	85%	86%	85%
Hospital Given 9 or 10 on 10 Point Scale	300+	70%	69%	71%
Meds 'Always' Explained Before Given	300+	65%	63%	64%
Nurses 'Always' Communicated Well	300+	85%	79%	79%
Pain 'Always' Well Controlled	300+	75%	70%	71%
Room and Bathroom 'Always' Clean	300+	70%	73%	73%
Timely Help 'Always' Received	300+	72%	67%	68%
Would Definitely Recommend Hospital	300+	75%	70%	71%
Use of Medical Imaging				
Cardiac Imaging Stress Test before Surgery	151	7.9%	5.4%	5.3%
Combination Abdominal CT Scan	848	7.4%	12.2%	10.5%
Combination Brain/Sinus CT Scan	732	1.4%	3.1%	2.7%
Combination Chest CT Scan	573	0.2%	2.1%	2.7%
Follow-up Mammogram/Ultrasound	1,105	12.1%	9%	8.8%
Lumbar Spine MRI for Low Back Pain	110	40.0%	35.8%	37.2%

Monongahela Valley Hospital

1163 Country Club Road
Monongahela, PA 15063
E-mail: mail@monvalleyhospital.com
URL: www.monvalleyhospital.com
Type: Acute Care Hospitals
Ownership: Voluntary non-profit - Private

Phone: 724-258-1000
Fax: 724-258-1884
Emergency Services: Yes
Beds: 226

Key Personnel:
Quality Assurance . . . . Diane Cooper, RN
President/CEO. . . . . Louis J Panza, Jr
Operating Room. . . . . Fernand N Parent, RN
Radiology. . . . . Douglas Wilson

Measure	Cases	This Hosp.	State Avg.	U.S. Avg.
Blood Clot Prevention and Treatment				
Anticoagulation Overlap Therapy[2]	69	87%	94%	93%
ICU Venous Thromboembolism Prophylaxis[2]	192	98%	94%	92%
Incidence of Potentially Preventable VTE[1,2]	-	-	8%	10%
UFH with Dosages/Platelet Monitoring[2]	44	100%	98%	97%
Venous Thromboembolism Prophylaxis[2]	694	98%	90%	85%
Warfarin Therapy Discharge Instructions[2]	54	98%	78%	75%
Chest Pain/Possible Heart Attack Care				
Aspirin Given Within 24 Hours of Arrival	22	100%	97%	96%
Fibrinolytic Meds Within 30 Min. of Arrival[3,7]	-	-	44%	58%
Average Time to ECG (minutes)	24	9	9	7
Average Time to Transfer (minutes)[1,3]	-	-	64	60
Children's Asthma Care				
Received Home Management Plan of Care	-	-	-	88%
Received Reliever Medication	-	-	-	100%
Received Systemic Corticosteroids	-	-	-	100%
Emergency Department				
Admittance Decision Time (minutes)[2]	917	50	104	98
Head CT Results Within 45 Min. of Arrival[1]	-	-	60%	57%
Patients Who Left ER Before Being Seen	34,604	1%	1%	2%
Time from ER Arrival to Admit. (minutes)[2]	1,032	221	276	274
Time from ER Arrival to Discharge (minutes)	663	144	125	134
Time in ER Before Being Evaluated (minutes)	791	26	26	26
Time to Pain Meds for Fractures (minutes)	91	84	58	57
Heart Attack Care				
Aspirin Given at Discharge	155	100%	99%	99%
Fibrinolytic Meds Within 30 Min. of Arrival[7]	-	-	40%	54%
PCI Within 90 Minutes of Arrival	18	89%	97%	96%
Statin Prescribed at Discharge	150	99%	99%	98%
Heart Failure Care				
ACE Inhibitor or ARB for LVSD	71	99%	97%	97%
Discharge Instructions Given	259	98%	96%	94%
Evaluation of LVS Function	302	100%	100%	99%
Medicare Spending				
Medicare Spending per Patient (ratio)	-	0.97	1.01	0.98
Pneumonia Care				
Appropriate Initial Antibiotic Given	151	97%	96%	95%
Blood Culture Timing	203	99%	98%	98%
Pregnancy and Delivery Care				
Newborn Deliveries Scheduled Early[7]	-	-	4%	6%
Preventive Care				
Immunization for Influenza[2]	862	93%	91%	90%
Immunization for Pneumonia[2]	1,338	96%	92%	92%
Stroke Care				
Anticoagulation Therapy for Atrial Fibrillation	17	100%	96%	95%
Antithrombotic Therapy Timing	83	98%	98%	98%
Assessed for Rehabilitation	90	98%	98%	97%
Discharged on Antithrombotic Therapy	85	100%	99%	99%
Discharged on Statin Medication	62	95%	95%	94%
Thrombolytic Therapy Timing[1]	-	-	72%	66%
Venous Thromboembolism Prophylaxis	94	98%	95%	94%
Written Stroke Educational Materials Given	39	92%	90%	88%
Surgical Care Improvement Project				
Appropriate Beta Blocker Usage	180	96%	98%	98%
Appropriate VTP Within 24 Hours	485	95%	99%	98%
Controlled Postoperative Blood Glucose[7]	-	-	98%	97%
Perioperative Temperature Management	589	100%	100%	100%
Prophylactic Antibiotic Selection	384	98%	99%	99%
Prophylactic Antibiotic Selection (Outpatient)	68	99%	98%	98%
Prophylactic Antibiotic Stopped	375	98%	98%	98%
Prophylactic Antibiotic Timing	385	100%	99%	99%
Prophylactic Antibiotic Timing (Outpatient)	67	96%	98%	98%
Urinary Catheter Removal	176	97%	99%	97%
Survey of Patients' Hospital Experiences				
Area Around Room 'Always' Quiet at Night	300+	64%	54%	61%
Doctors 'Always' Communicated Well	300+	86%	80%	82%
Home Recovery Information Given	300+	86%	86%	85%
Hospital Given 9 or 10 on 10 Point Scale	300+	75%	69%	71%
Meds 'Always' Explained Before Given	300+	68%	63%	64%
Nurses 'Always' Communicated Well	300+	86%	79%	79%
Pain 'Always' Well Controlled	300+	76%	70%	71%
Room and Bathroom 'Always' Clean	300+	83%	73%	73%
Timely Help 'Always' Received	300+	76%	67%	68%
Would Definitely Recommend Hospital	300+	71%	70%	71%
Use of Medical Imaging				
Cardiac Imaging Stress Test before Surgery	125	8.0%	5.4%	5.3%
Combination Abdominal CT Scan	385	22.3%	12.2%	10.5%
Combination Brain/Sinus CT Scan	353	7.4%	3.1%	2.7%
Combination Chest CT Scan	169	0.6%	2.1%	2.7%
Follow-up Mammogram/Ultrasound	422	12.6%	9%	8.8%
Lumbar Spine MRI for Low Back Pain	88	42.0%	35.8%	37.2%

Forbes Regional Hospital

2570 Haymaker Rd
Monroeville, PA 15146
URL: www.wpahs.org
Type: Acute Care Hospitals
Ownership: Voluntary non-profit - Other

Phone: 412-858-2000
Fax: 412-858-2532
Emergency Services: Yes
Beds: 340

Key Personnel:
Patient Relations . . . . Jaye Faher
Emergency Room . . . . Angela Henzler
CEO/President. . . . . Reese Jackson
Quality Assurance . . . . Ann Mitchell
Chief of Medical Staff . . . . Mark Rubino, MD

Measure	Cases	This Hosp.	State Avg.	U.S. Avg.
Blood Clot Prevention and Treatment				
Anticoagulation Overlap Therapy[2]	109	83%	94%	93%
ICU Venous Thromboembolism Prophylaxis[2]	75	85%	94%	92%
Incidence of Potentially Preventable VTE[2]	38	24%	8%	10%
UFH with Dosages/Platelet Monitoring[2]	108	100%	98%	97%
Venous Thromboembolism Prophylaxis[2]	440	63%	90%	85%
Warfarin Therapy Discharge Instructions[2]	80	42%	78%	75%
Chest Pain/Possible Heart Attack Care				
Aspirin Given Within 24 Hours of Arrival[3]	13	100%	97%	96%
Fibrinolytic Meds Within 30 Min. of Arrival[3,7]	-	-	44%	58%
Average Time to ECG (minutes)[3]	13	10	9	7
Average Time to Transfer (minutes)[3,7]	-	-	64	60
Children's Asthma Care				
Received Home Management Plan of Care	-	-	-	88%
Received Reliever Medication	-	-	-	100%
Received Systemic Corticosteroids	-	-	-	100%
Emergency Department				
Admittance Decision Time (minutes)[2]	547	130	104	98
Head CT Results Within 45 Min. of Arrival	22	68%	60%	57%
Patients Who Left ER Before Being Seen	25,054	1%	1%	2%
Time from ER Arrival to Admit. (minutes)[2]	628	310	276	274
Time from ER Arrival to Discharge (minutes)	404	167	125	134
Time in ER Before Being Evaluated (minutes)	461	44	26	26
Time to Pain Meds for Fractures (minutes)	71	47	58	57
Heart Attack Care				
Aspirin Given at Discharge	237	97%	99%	99%
Fibrinolytic Meds Within 30 Min. of Arrival[7]	-	-	40%	54%
PCI Within 90 Minutes of Arrival	63	98%	97%	96%
Statin Prescribed at Discharge	237	97%	99%	98%
Heart Failure Care				
ACE Inhibitor or ARB for LVSD	120	92%	97%	97%
Discharge Instructions Given	333	87%	96%	94%
Evaluation of LVS Function	455	100%	100%	99%
Medicare Spending				
Medicare Spending per Patient (ratio)	-	1.12	1.01	0.98
Pneumonia Care				
Appropriate Initial Antibiotic Given	155	93%	96%	95%
Blood Culture Timing	211	99%	98%	98%
Pregnancy and Delivery Care				
Newborn Deliveries Scheduled Early	91	5%	4%	6%
Preventive Care				
Immunization for Influenza[2]	605	82%	91%	90%
Immunization for Pneumonia[2]	856	73%	92%	92%
Stroke Care				
Anticoagulation Therapy for Atrial Fibrillation	49	90%	96%	95%
Antithrombotic Therapy Timing	185	91%	98%	98%
Assessed for Rehabilitation	202	96%	98%	97%
Discharged on Antithrombotic Therapy	179	97%	99%	99%
Discharged on Statin Medication	147	95%	95%	94%
Thrombolytic Therapy Timing	16	75%	72%	66%
Venous Thromboembolism Prophylaxis	221	94%	95%	94%
Written Stroke Educational Materials Given	95	85%	90%	88%

NOTE: Hospital profiles are in alphabetical order by state, then city, then hospital within the city; Rankings exclude hospitals with less than 25 cases except for patient surveys which excludes hospitals with less than 100 cases; (a) 100-299 cases; (1) The number of cases/patients is too few to report; (2) Data submitted were based on a sample of cases/patients; (3) Results are based on a shorter time period than required; (4) Data suppressed by CMS for one or more quarters; (5) Results are not available for this reporting period; (6) Fewer than 100 patients completed the HCAHPS survey; (7) No cases met the criteria for this measure; (8) The lower limit of the confidence interval cannot be calculated if the number of observed infections equals zero; (9) No data are available from the state/territory for this reporting period; (10) The scores shown reflect fewer than 50 completed surveys; (11) There were discrepancies in the data collection process; (12) This measure does not apply to this hospital for this reporting period; (13) Results cannot be calculated for this reporting period; (14) The results for this state are combined with nearby states to protect confidentiality; Please refer to the User's Guide for a full explanation of data.

Surgical Care Improvement Project				
Appropriate Beta Blocker Usage[2]	345	99%	98%	98%
Appropriate VTP Within 24 Hours[2]	562	98%	99%	98%
Controlled Postoperative Blood Glucose[2]	184	98%	98%	97%
Perioperative Temperature Management[2]	706	100%	100%	100%
Prophylactic Antibiotic Selection[2]	609	100%	99%	99%
Prophylactic Antibiotic Selection (Outpatient)	384	98%	98%	98%
Prophylactic Antibiotic Stopped[2]	598	98%	98%	98%
Prophylactic Antibiotic Timing[2]	609	100%	99%	99%
Prophylactic Antibiotic Timing (Outpatient)	387	99%	98%	98%
Urinary Catheter Removal[2]	669	97%	99%	97%
Survey of Patients' Hospital Experiences				
Area Around Room 'Always' Quiet at Night	300+	44%	54%	61%
Doctors 'Always' Communicated Well	300+	76%	80%	82%
Home Recovery Information Given	300+	84%	86%	85%
Hospital Given 9 or 10 on 10 Point Scale	300+	65%	69%	71%
Meds 'Always' Explained Before Given	300+	58%	63%	64%
Nurses 'Always' Communicated Well	300+	77%	79%	79%
Pain 'Always' Well Controlled	300+	72%	70%	71%
Room and Bathroom 'Always' Clean	300+	61%	73%	73%
Timely Help 'Always' Received	300+	68%	67%	68%
Would Definitely Recommend Hospital	300+	70%	70%	71%
Use of Medical Imaging				
Cardiac Imaging Stress Test before Surgery	153	7.8%	5.4%	5.3%
Combination Abdominal CT Scan	446	4.5%	12.2%	10.5%
Combination Brain/Sinus CT Scan[1]	-	-	3.1%	2.7%
Combination Chest CT Scan	204	0.0%	2.1%	2.7%
Follow-up Mammogram/Ultrasound	343	12.5%	9%	8.8%
Lumbar Spine MRI for Low Back Pain[1]	-	-	35.8%	37.2%

UPMC East

2775 Mosside Boulevard
Monroeville, PA 15146
URL: www.upmc.com
Type: Acute Care Hospitals
Ownership: Voluntary non-profit - Private
Phone: 412-357-3000
Emergency Services: Yes

Measure	Cases	This Hosp.	State Avg.	U.S. Avg.
Blood Clot Prevention and Treatment				
Anticoagulation Overlap Therapy[2]	94	100%	94%	93%
ICU Venous Thromboembolism Prophylaxis[2]	75	99%	94%	92%
Incidence of Potentially Preventable VTE[2]	14	0%	8%	10%
UFH with Dosages/Platelet Monitoring[2]	87	100%	98%	97%
Venous Thromboembolism Prophylaxis[2]	479	92%	90%	85%
Warfarin Therapy Discharge Instructions[2]	66	100%	78%	75%
Chest Pain/Possible Heart Attack Care				
Aspirin Given Within 24 Hours of Arrival[3]	32	100%	97%	96%
Fibrinolytic Meds Within 30 Min. of Arrival[3,7]	-	-	44%	58%
Average Time to ECG (minutes)[3]	34	9	9	7
Average Time to Transfer (minutes)[3,7]	-	-	64	60
Children's Asthma Care				
Received Home Management Plan of Care	-	-	-	88%
Received Reliever Medication	-	-	-	100%
Received Systemic Corticosteroids	-	-	-	100%
Emergency Department				
Admittance Decision Time (minutes)[2,3]	615	77	104	98
Head CT Results Within 45 Min. of Arrival[1,3]	-	-	60%	57%
Patients Who Left ER Before Being Seen	17,914	0%	1%	2%
Time from ER Arrival to Admit. (minutes)[2,3]	628	211	276	274
Time from ER Arrival to Discharge (minutes)[3]	435	127	125	134
Time in ER Before Being Evaluated (minutes)[3]	468	9	26	26
Time to Pain Meds for Fractures (minutes)[3]	77	65	58	57
Heart Attack Care				
Aspirin Given at Discharge[3]	63	100%	99%	99%
Fibrinolytic Meds Within 30 Min. of Arrival[3,7]	-	-	40%	54%
PCI Within 90 Minutes of Arrival[3]	14	93%	97%	96%
Statin Prescribed at Discharge[3]	56	100%	99%	98%
Heart Failure Care				
ACE Inhibitor or ARB for LVSD[3]	30	100%	97%	97%
Discharge Instructions Given[3]	131	99%	96%	94%
Evaluation of LVS Function[3]	175	100%	100%	99%
Medicare Spending				
Medicare Spending per Patient (ratio)	-	1.00	1.01	0.98
Pneumonia Care				
Appropriate Initial Antibiotic Given[3]	116	97%	96%	95%
Blood Culture Timing[3]	138	99%	98%	98%
Pregnancy and Delivery Care				
Newborn Deliveries Scheduled Early[7]	-	-	4%	6%
Preventive Care				
Immunization for Influenza[2,3]	342	100%	91%	90%
Immunization for Pneumonia[2,3]	769	100%	92%	92%
Stroke Care				
Anticoagulation Therapy for Atrial Fibrillation[1]	-	-	96%	95%
Antithrombotic Therapy Timing	50	100%	98%	98%
Assessed for Rehabilitation	55	100%	98%	97%
Discharged on Antithrombotic Therapy	54	100%	99%	99%
Discharged on Statin Medication	43	100%	95%	94%
Thrombolytic Therapy Timing[1]	-	-	72%	66%
Venous Thromboembolism Prophylaxis	53	100%	95%	94%
Written Stroke Educational Materials Given	37	100%	90%	88%
Surgical Care Improvement Project				
Appropriate Beta Blocker Usage[3]	90	100%	98%	98%
Appropriate VTP Within 24 Hours[3]	330	100%	99%	98%
Controlled Postoperative Blood Glucose[3,7]	-	-	98%	97%
Perioperative Temperature Management[3]	359	100%	100%	100%
Prophylactic Antibiotic Selection[3]	280	100%	99%	99%
Prophylactic Antibiotic Selection (Outpatient)[3]	45	100%	98%	98%
Prophylactic Antibiotic Stopped[3]	276	100%	98%	98%
Prophylactic Antibiotic Timing[3]	280	100%	99%	99%
Prophylactic Antibiotic Timing (Outpatient)[3]	45	100%	98%	98%
Urinary Catheter Removal[3]	246	100%	99%	97%
Survey of Patients' Hospital Experiences				
Area Around Room 'Always' Quiet at Night	300+	61%	54%	61%
Doctors 'Always' Communicated Well	300+	75%	80%	82%
Home Recovery Information Given	300+	86%	86%	85%
Hospital Given 9 or 10 on 10 Point Scale	300+	73%	69%	71%
Meds 'Always' Explained Before Given	300+	60%	63%	64%
Nurses 'Always' Communicated Well	300+	79%	79%	79%
Pain 'Always' Well Controlled	300+	71%	70%	71%
Room and Bathroom 'Always' Clean	300+	72%	73%	73%
Timely Help 'Always' Received	300+	67%	67%	68%
Would Definitely Recommend Hospital	300+	75%	70%	71%
Use of Medical Imaging				
Cardiac Imaging Stress Test before Surgery	113	13.3%	5.4%	5.3%
Combination Abdominal CT Scan	252	5.2%	12.2%	10.5%
Combination Brain/Sinus CT Scan[1]	-	-	3.1%	2.7%
Combination Chest CT Scan	56	1.8%	2.1%	2.7%
Follow-up Mammogram/Ultrasound[7]	-	-	9%	8.8%
Lumbar Spine MRI for Low Back Pain[1]	-	-	35.8%	37.2%

Endless Mountains Health Systems

100 Hospital Drive
Montrose, PA 18801
E-mail: emhsweb@hotmail.com
URL: www.endlesscare.org
Type: Critical Access Hospitals
Ownership: Voluntary non-profit - Private
Phone: 570-278-3801
Fax: 570-278-3648
Emergency Services: Yes
Beds: 22

Key Personnel:
Intensive Care Unit. . . . . Ann Marie Baldwin
Operating Room. . . . . David J Bertsch, RN
Quality Assurance . . . . Rex Catlin
CEO/President. . . . . Rexford O Catlin
Emergency Room . . . . Ihab Dana, MD
Radiology. . . . . Paul Shaderowfs, MD
Chief of Medical Staff . . . . Joseph Speicher, DO
Infection Control. . . . . Joseph Speicher, DO

Measure	Cases	This Hosp.	State Avg.	U.S. Avg.
Blood Clot Prevention and Treatment				
Anticoagulation Overlap Therapy[5]	-	-	94%	93%
ICU Venous Thromboembolism Prophylaxis[5]	-	-	94%	92%
Incidence of Potentially Preventable VTE[5]	-	-	8%	10%
UFH with Dosages/Platelet Monitoring[5]	-	-	98%	97%
Venous Thromboembolism Prophylaxis[5]	-	-	90%	85%
Warfarin Therapy Discharge Instructions[5]	-	-	78%	75%
Chest Pain/Possible Heart Attack Care				
Aspirin Given Within 24 Hours of Arrival[5]	-	-	97%	96%
Fibrinolytic Meds Within 30 Min. of Arrival[5]	-	-	44%	58%
Average Time to ECG (minutes)[5]	-	-	9	7
Average Time to Transfer (minutes)[5]	-	-	64	60
Children's Asthma Care				
Received Home Management Plan of Care	-	-	-	88%
Received Reliever Medication	-	-	-	100%
Received Systemic Corticosteroids	-	-	-	100%
Emergency Department				
Admittance Decision Time (minutes)[5]	-	-	104	98
Head CT Results Within 45 Min. of Arrival[5]	-	-	60%	57%
Patients Who Left ER Before Being Seen	4,500	1%	1%	2%
Time from ER Arrival to Admit. (minutes)[5]	-	-	276	274
Time from ER Arrival to Discharge (minutes)[5]	-	-	125	134
Time in ER Before Being Evaluated (minutes)[5]	-	-	26	26
Time to Pain Meds for Fractures (minutes)[5]	-	-	58	57
Heart Attack Care				
Aspirin Given at Discharge[1]	-	-	99%	99%
Fibrinolytic Meds Within 30 Min. of Arrival[7]	-	-	40%	54%
PCI Within 90 Minutes of Arrival[7]	-	-	97%	96%
Statin Prescribed at Discharge[1]	-	-	99%	98%
Heart Failure Care				
ACE Inhibitor or ARB for LVSD[1]	-	-	97%	97%
Discharge Instructions Given	12	58%	96%	94%
Evaluation of LVS Function	16	75%	100%	99%
Medicare Spending				
Medicare Spending per Patient (ratio)	-	-	1.01	0.98
Pneumonia Care				
Appropriate Initial Antibiotic Given	16	88%	96%	95%
Blood Culture Timing[1]	-	-	98%	98%
Pregnancy and Delivery Care				
Newborn Deliveries Scheduled Early[5]	-	-	4%	6%
Preventive Care				
Immunization for Influenza[5]	-	-	91%	90%
Immunization for Pneumonia[5]	-	-	92%	92%
Stroke Care				
Anticoagulation Therapy for Atrial Fibrillation[5]	-	-	96%	95%
Antithrombotic Therapy Timing[5]	-	-	98%	98%
Assessed for Rehabilitation[5]	-	-	98%	97%
Discharged on Antithrombotic Therapy[5]	-	-	99%	99%
Discharged on Statin Medication[5]	-	-	95%	94%
Thrombolytic Therapy Timing[5]	-	-	72%	66%
Venous Thromboembolism Prophylaxis[5]	-	-	95%	94%
Written Stroke Educational Materials Given[5]	-	-	90%	88%
Surgical Care Improvement Project				
Appropriate Beta Blocker Usage[1,3]	-	-	98%	98%
Appropriate VTP Within 24 Hours[3]	20	95%	99%	98%
Controlled Postoperative Blood Glucose[3,7]	-	-	98%	97%
Perioperative Temperature Management[3]	20	100%	100%	100%
Prophylactic Antibiotic Selection	97	100%	99%	99%
Prophylactic Antibiotic Selection (Outpatient)[5]	-	-	98%	98%
Prophylactic Antibiotic Stopped	97	100%	98%	98%
Prophylactic Antibiotic Timing	97	85%	99%	99%
Prophylactic Antibiotic Timing (Outpatient)[5]	-	-	98%	98%
Urinary Catheter Removal[3]	20	100%	99%	97%
Survey of Patients' Hospital Experiences				
Area Around Room 'Always' Quiet at Night	300+	46%	54%	61%
Doctors 'Always' Communicated Well	300+	83%	80%	82%
Home Recovery Information Given	300+	85%	86%	85%
Hospital Given 9 or 10 on 10 Point Scale	300+	65%	69%	71%
Meds 'Always' Explained Before Given	300+	64%	63%	64%
Nurses 'Always' Communicated Well	300+	81%	79%	79%
Pain 'Always' Well Controlled	300+	75%	70%	71%
Room and Bathroom 'Always' Clean	300+	74%	73%	73%
Timely Help 'Always' Received	300+	78%	67%	68%
Would Definitely Recommend Hospital	300+	62%	70%	71%
Use of Medical Imaging				
Cardiac Imaging Stress Test before Surgery[7]	-	-	5.4%	5.3%
Combination Abdominal CT Scan	95	4.2%	12.2%	10.5%
Combination Brain/Sinus CT Scan[1]	-	-	3.1%	2.7%
Combination Chest CT Scan[1]	-	-	2.1%	2.7%
Follow-up Mammogram/Ultrasound[7]	-	-	9%	8.8%
Lumbar Spine MRI for Low Back Pain[7]	-	-	35.8%	37.2%

NOTE: Hospital profiles are in alphabetical order by state, then city, then hospital within the city; Rankings exclude hospitals with less than 25 cases except for patient surveys which excludes hospitals with less than 100 cases; (a) 100-299 cases; (1) The number of cases/patients is too few to report; (2) Data submitted were based on a sample of cases/patients; (3) Results are based on a shorter time period than required; (4) Data suppressed by CMS for one or more quarters; (5) Results are not available for this reporting period; (6) Fewer than 100 patients completed the HCAHPS survey; (7) No cases met the criteria for this measure; (8) The lower limit of the confidence interval cannot be calculated if the number of observed infections equals zero; (9) No data are available from the state/territory for this reporting period; (10) The scores shown reflect fewer than 50 completed surveys; (11) There were discrepancies in the data collection process; (12) This measure does not apply to this hospital for this reporting period; (13) Results cannot be calculated for this reporting period; (14) The results for this state are combined with nearby states to protect confidentiality; Please refer to the User's Guide for a full explanation of data.

Excela Health Frick Hospital

508 South Church Street
Mount Pleasant, PA 15666
URL: www.excelahealth.org
Type: Acute Care Hospitals
Ownership: Voluntary non-profit - Other

Phone: 724-547-1500
Fax: 724-547-1131
Emergency Services: Yes
Beds: 171

Key Personnel:

Radiology. . . . . Matthew Banks
Chair/CEO . . . . James R. Breisinger
Chief of Medical Staff . . . . Carol J. Fox, MD
Operating Room. . . . . Melissa Kaufman
Surgery . . . . Sam Raneri
CEO . . . . Robert J. Rogalski, ESQ
Quality Assurance . . . . Al Rosatti
CEO/President. . . . . Joseph Teluso

Measure	Cases	This Hosp.	State Avg.	U.S. Avg.
Blood Clot Prevention and Treatment				
Anticoagulation Overlap Therapy[2]	31	94%	94%	93%
ICU Venous Thromboembolism Prophylaxis[2]	67	97%	94%	92%
Incidence of Potentially Preventable VTE[1,2]	-	-	8%	10%
UFH with Dosages/Platelet Monitoring[2]	28	100%	98%	97%
Venous Thromboembolism Prophylaxis[2]	370	99%	90%	85%
Warfarin Therapy Discharge Instructions[2]	18	100%	78%	75%
Chest Pain/Possible Heart Attack Care				
Aspirin Given Within 24 Hours of Arrival	28	100%	97%	96%
Fibrinolytic Meds Within 30 Min. of Arrival[7]	-	-	44%	58%
Average Time to ECG (minutes)	29	6	9	7
Average Time to Transfer (minutes)[1]	-	-	64	60
Children's Asthma Care				
Received Home Management Plan of Care	-	-	-	88%
Received Reliever Medication	-	-	-	100%
Received Systemic Corticosteroids	-	-	-	100%
Emergency Department				
Admittance Decision Time (minutes)[2]	716	52	104	98
Head CT Results Within 45 Min. of Arrival[1]	-	-	60%	57%
Patients Who Left ER Before Being Seen	25,694	0%	1%	2%
Time from ER Arrival to Admit. (minutes)[2]	717	211	276	274
Time from ER Arrival to Discharge (minutes)	460	104	125	134
Time in ER Before Being Evaluated (minutes)	504	8	26	26
Time to Pain Meds for Fractures (minutes)	84	24	58	57
Heart Attack Care				
Aspirin Given at Discharge	44	98%	99%	99%
Fibrinolytic Meds Within 30 Min. of Arrival[7]	-	-	40%	54%
PCI Within 90 Minutes of Arrival[7]	-	-	97%	96%
Statin Prescribed at Discharge	41	100%	99%	98%
Heart Failure Care				
ACE Inhibitor or ARB for LVSD	31	87%	97%	97%
Discharge Instructions Given	124	97%	96%	94%
Evaluation of LVS Function	146	99%	100%	99%
Medicare Spending				
Medicare Spending per Patient (ratio)	-	1.02	1.01	0.98
Pneumonia Care				
Appropriate Initial Antibiotic Given	80	99%	96%	95%
Blood Culture Timing	167	98%	98%	98%
Pregnancy and Delivery Care				
Newborn Deliveries Scheduled Early[7]	-	-	4%	6%
Preventive Care				
Immunization for Influenza[2]	415	98%	91%	90%
Immunization for Pneumonia[2]	691	98%	92%	92%
Stroke Care				
Anticoagulation Therapy for Atrial Fibrillation[1]	-	-	96%	95%
Antithrombotic Therapy Timing	36	97%	98%	98%
Assessed for Rehabilitation	37	97%	98%	97%
Discharged on Antithrombotic Therapy	36	100%	99%	99%
Discharged on Statin Medication	28	96%	95%	94%
Thrombolytic Therapy Timing[7]	-	-	72%	66%
Venous Thromboembolism Prophylaxis	38	100%	95%	94%
Written Stroke Educational Materials Given	22	86%	90%	88%
Surgical Care Improvement Project				
Appropriate Beta Blocker Usage	23	96%	98%	98%
Appropriate VTP Within 24 Hours	55	98%	99%	98%
Controlled Postoperative Blood Glucose[7]	-	-	98%	97%
Perioperative Temperature Management	61	100%	100%	100%
Prophylactic Antibiotic Selection	27	100%	99%	99%
Prophylactic Antibiotic Selection (Outpatient)	15	93%	98%	98%
Prophylactic Antibiotic Stopped	24	83%	98%	98%
Prophylactic Antibiotic Timing	27	100%	99%	99%
Prophylactic Antibiotic Timing (Outpatient)	15	100%	98%	98%
Urinary Catheter Removal	38	95%	99%	97%
Survey of Patients' Hospital Experiences				
Area Around Room 'Always' Quiet at Night	300+	57%	54%	61%
Doctors 'Always' Communicated Well	300+	80%	80%	82%
Home Recovery Information Given	300+	92%	86%	85%
Hospital Given 9 or 10 on 10 Point Scale	300+	71%	69%	71%
Meds 'Always' Explained Before Given	300+	69%	63%	64%
Nurses 'Always' Communicated Well	300+	85%	79%	79%
Pain 'Always' Well Controlled	300+	74%	70%	71%
Room and Bathroom 'Always' Clean	300+	79%	73%	73%
Timely Help 'Always' Received	300+	74%	67%	68%
Would Definitely Recommend Hospital	300+	70%	70%	71%
Use of Medical Imaging				
Cardiac Imaging Stress Test before Surgery	149	4.7%	5.4%	5.3%
Combination Abdominal CT Scan	248	9.3%	12.2%	10.5%
Combination Brain/Sinus CT Scan[1]	-	-	3.1%	2.7%
Combination Chest CT Scan	185	4.9%	2.1%	2.7%
Follow-up Mammogram/Ultrasound	287	8.4%	9%	8.8%
Lumbar Spine MRI for Low Back Pain[1]	-	-	35.8%	37.2%

Muncy Valley Hospital

215 East Water Street
Muncy, PA 17756
URL: www.shscares.org
Type: Critical Access Hospitals
Ownership: Voluntary non-profit - Private

Phone: 570-546-8282
Fax: 570-546-8009
Emergency Services: Yes
Beds: 139

Key Personnel:

Emergency Room . . . . Mark Beyer, MD
CEO/President. . . . . Steven P Johnson
Chief of Medical Staff . . . . Timothy A Mannello
Quality Assurance . . . . Robert C Wallace

Measure	Cases	This Hosp.	State Avg.	U.S. Avg.
Blood Clot Prevention and Treatment				
Anticoagulation Overlap Therapy[5]	-	-	94%	93%
ICU Venous Thromboembolism Prophylaxis[5]	-	-	94%	92%
Incidence of Potentially Preventable VTE[5]	-	-	8%	10%
UFH with Dosages/Platelet Monitoring[5]	-	-	98%	97%
Venous Thromboembolism Prophylaxis[5]	-	-	90%	85%
Warfarin Therapy Discharge Instructions[5]	-	-	78%	75%
Chest Pain/Possible Heart Attack Care				
Aspirin Given Within 24 Hours of Arrival	76	96%	97%	96%
Fibrinolytic Meds Within 30 Min. of Arrival[7]	-	-	44%	58%
Average Time to ECG (minutes)	80	7	9	7
Average Time to Transfer (minutes)[1]	-	-	64	60
Children's Asthma Care				
Received Home Management Plan of Care	-	-	-	88%
Received Reliever Medication	-	-	-	100%
Received Systemic Corticosteroids	-	-	-	100%
Emergency Department				
Admittance Decision Time (minutes)[5]	-	-	104	98
Head CT Results Within 45 Min. of Arrival[5]	-	-	60%	57%
Patients Who Left ER Before Being Seen	16,028	1%	1%	2%
Time from ER Arrival to Admit. (minutes)[5]	-	-	276	274
Time from ER Arrival to Discharge (minutes)[5]	-	-	125	134
Time in ER Before Being Evaluated (minutes)[5]	-	-	26	26
Time to Pain Meds for Fractures (minutes)[5]	-	-	58	57
Heart Attack Care				
Aspirin Given at Discharge[1,3]	-	-	99%	99%
Fibrinolytic Meds Within 30 Min. of Arrival[3,7]	-	-	40%	54%
PCI Within 90 Minutes of Arrival[3,7]	-	-	97%	96%
Statin Prescribed at Discharge[1,3]	-	-	99%	98%
Heart Failure Care				
ACE Inhibitor or ARB for LVSD[1]	-	-	97%	97%
Discharge Instructions Given	13	100%	96%	94%
Evaluation of LVS Function	19	100%	100%	99%
Medicare Spending				
Medicare Spending per Patient (ratio)	-	-	1.01	0.98
Pneumonia Care				
Appropriate Initial Antibiotic Given	31	100%	96%	95%
Blood Culture Timing	37	97%	98%	98%
Pregnancy and Delivery Care				
Newborn Deliveries Scheduled Early[3,7]	-	-	4%	6%
Preventive Care				
Immunization for Influenza[5]	-	-	91%	90%
Immunization for Pneumonia[5]	-	-	92%	92%
Stroke Care				
Anticoagulation Therapy for Atrial Fibrillation[5]	-	-	96%	95%
Antithrombotic Therapy Timing[5]	-	-	98%	98%
Assessed for Rehabilitation[5]	-	-	98%	97%
Discharged on Antithrombotic Therapy[5]	-	-	99%	99%
Discharged on Statin Medication[5]	-	-	95%	94%
Thrombolytic Therapy Timing[5]	-	-	72%	66%
Venous Thromboembolism Prophylaxis[5]	-	-	95%	94%
Written Stroke Educational Materials Given[5]	-	-	90%	88%
Surgical Care Improvement Project				
Appropriate Beta Blocker Usage[1]	-	-	98%	98%
Appropriate VTP Within 24 Hours	11	100%	99%	98%
Controlled Postoperative Blood Glucose[7]	-	-	98%	97%
Perioperative Temperature Management	11	100%	100%	100%
Prophylactic Antibiotic Selection[1]	-	-	99%	99%
Prophylactic Antibiotic Selection (Outpatient)[1,3]	-	-	98%	98%
Prophylactic Antibiotic Stopped[1]	-	-	98%	98%
Prophylactic Antibiotic Timing[1]	-	-	99%	99%
Prophylactic Antibiotic Timing (Outpatient)[1,3]	-	-	98%	98%
Urinary Catheter Removal[1]	-	-	99%	97%
Survey of Patients' Hospital Experiences				
Area Around Room 'Always' Quiet at Night	(a)	54%	54%	61%
Doctors 'Always' Communicated Well	(a)	86%	80%	82%
Home Recovery Information Given	(a)	83%	86%	85%
Hospital Given 9 or 10 on 10 Point Scale	(a)	83%	69%	71%
Meds 'Always' Explained Before Given	(a)	71%	63%	64%
Nurses 'Always' Communicated Well	(a)	85%	79%	79%
Pain 'Always' Well Controlled	(a)	69%	70%	71%
Room and Bathroom 'Always' Clean	(a)	89%	73%	73%
Timely Help 'Always' Received	(a)	74%	67%	68%
Would Definitely Recommend Hospital	(a)	76%	70%	71%
Use of Medical Imaging				
Cardiac Imaging Stress Test before Surgery[1]	-	-	5.4%	5.3%
Combination Abdominal CT Scan	407	10.1%	12.2%	10.5%
Combination Brain/Sinus CT Scan[1]	-	-	3.1%	2.7%
Combination Chest CT Scan	156	12.8%	2.1%	2.7%
Follow-up Mammogram/Ultrasound	434	5.5%	9%	8.8%
Lumbar Spine MRI for Low Back Pain[7]	-	-	35.8%	37.2%

Meyersdale Community Hospital

200 Hospital Drive
Myersdale, PA 15552
Type: Critical Access Hospitals
Ownership: Government - Local

Phone: 814-634-5911
Emergency Services: Yes

Measure	Cases	This Hosp.	State Avg.	U.S. Avg.
Blood Clot Prevention and Treatment				
Anticoagulation Overlap Therapy[5]	-	-	94%	93%
ICU Venous Thromboembolism Prophylaxis[5]	-	-	94%	92%
Incidence of Potentially Preventable VTE[5]	-	-	8%	10%
UFH with Dosages/Platelet Monitoring[5]	-	-	98%	97%
Venous Thromboembolism Prophylaxis[5]	-	-	90%	85%
Warfarin Therapy Discharge Instructions[5]	-	-	78%	75%
Chest Pain/Possible Heart Attack Care				
Aspirin Given Within 24 Hours of Arrival[1,3]	-	-	97%	96%
Fibrinolytic Meds Within 30 Min. of Arrival[3,7]	-	-	44%	58%
Average Time to ECG (minutes)[1,3]	-	-	9	7
Average Time to Transfer (minutes)[1,3]	-	-	64	60
Children's Asthma Care				
Received Home Management Plan of Care	-	-	-	88%
Received Reliever Medication	-	-	-	100%
Received Systemic Corticosteroids	-	-	-	100%
Emergency Department				
Admittance Decision Time (minutes)[5]	-	-	104	98
Head CT Results Within 45 Min. of Arrival[5]	-	-	60%	57%
Patients Who Left ER Before Being Seen	4,287	0%	1%	2%
Time from ER Arrival to Admit. (minutes)[5]	-	-	276	274

NOTE: Hospital profiles are in alphabetical order by state, then city, then hospital within the city; Rankings exclude hospitals with less than 25 cases except for patient surveys which excludes hospitals with less than 100 cases; (a) 100-299 cases; (1) The number of cases/patients is too few to report; (2) Data submitted were based on a sample of cases/patients; (3) Results are based on a shorter time period than required; (4) Data suppressed by CMS for one or more quarters; (5) Results are not available for this reporting period; (6) Fewer than 100 patients completed the HCAHPS survey; (7) No cases met the criteria for this measure; (8) The lower limit of the confidence interval cannot be calculated if the number of observed infections equals zero; (9) No data are available from the state/territory for this reporting period; (10) The scores shown reflect fewer than 50 completed surveys; (11) There were discrepancies in the data collection process; (12) This measure does not apply to this hospital for this reporting period; (13) Results cannot be calculated for this reporting period; (14) The results for this state are combined with nearby states to protect confidentiality; Please refer to the User's Guide for a full explanation of data.

Measure	Cases	This Hosp.	State Avg.	U.S. Avg.
Time from ER Arrival to Discharge (minutes)[5]	-	-	125	134
Time in ER Before Being Evaluated (minutes)[5]	-	-	26	26
Time to Pain Meds for Fractures (minutes)[5]	-	-	58	57
Heart Attack Care				
Aspirin Given at Discharge[1,3]	-	-	99%	99%
Fibrinolytic Meds Within 30 Min. of Arrival[3,7]	-	-	40%	54%
PCI Within 90 Minutes of Arrival[3,7]	-	-	97%	96%
Statin Prescribed at Discharge[1,3]	-	-	99%	98%
Heart Failure Care				
ACE Inhibitor or ARB for LVSD[1]	-	-	97%	97%
Discharge Instructions Given	12	92%	96%	94%
Evaluation of LVS Function	18	83%	100%	99%
Medicare Spending				
Medicare Spending per Patient (ratio)		-	1.01	0.98
Pneumonia Care				
Appropriate Initial Antibiotic Given[1]	-	-	96%	95%
Blood Culture Timing	18	94%	98%	98%
Pregnancy and Delivery Care				
Newborn Deliveries Scheduled Early[5]	-	-	4%	6%
Preventive Care				
Immunization for Influenza[5]	-	-	91%	90%
Immunization for Pneumonia[5]	-	-	92%	92%
Stroke Care				
Anticoagulation Therapy for Atrial Fibrillation[5]	-	-	96%	95%
Antithrombotic Therapy Timing[5]	-	-	98%	98%
Assessed for Rehabilitation[5]	-	-	98%	97%
Discharged on Antithrombotic Therapy[5]	-	-	99%	99%
Discharged on Statin Medication[5]	-	-	95%	94%
Thrombolytic Therapy Timing[5]	-	-	72%	66%
Venous Thromboembolism Prophylaxis[5]	-	-	95%	94%
Written Stroke Educational Materials Given[5]	-	-	90%	88%
Surgical Care Improvement Project				
Appropriate Beta Blocker Usage[5]	-	-	98%	98%
Appropriate VTP Within 24 Hours[5]	-	-	99%	98%
Controlled Postoperative Blood Glucose[5]	-	-	98%	97%
Perioperative Temperature Management[5]	-	-	100%	100%
Prophylactic Antibiotic Selection[5]	-	-	99%	99%
Prophylactic Antibiotic Selection (Outpatient)[5]	-	-	98%	98%
Prophylactic Antibiotic Stopped[5]	-	-	98%	98%
Prophylactic Antibiotic Timing[5]	-	-	99%	99%
Prophylactic Antibiotic Timing (Outpatient)[5]	-	-	98%	98%
Urinary Catheter Removal[5]	-	-	99%	97%
Survey of Patients' Hospital Experiences				
Area Around Room 'Always' Quiet at Night[6]	<100	47%	54%	61%
Doctors 'Always' Communicated Well[6]	<100	88%	80%	82%
Home Recovery Information Given[6]	<100	91%	86%	85%
Hospital Given 9 or 10 on 10 Point Scale[6]	<100	73%	69%	71%
Meds 'Always' Explained Before Given[6]	<100	63%	63%	64%
Nurses 'Always' Communicated Well[6]	<100	82%	79%	79%
Pain 'Always' Well Controlled[6]	<100	73%	70%	71%
Room and Bathroom 'Always' Clean[6]	<100	90%	73%	73%
Timely Help 'Always' Received[6]	<100	75%	67%	68%
Would Definitely Recommend Hospital[6]	<100	71%	70%	71%
Use of Medical Imaging				
Cardiac Imaging Stress Test before Surgery	48	4.2%	5.4%	5.3%
Combination Abdominal CT Scan	94	2.1%	12.2%	10.5%
Combination Brain/Sinus CT Scan[1]	-	-	3.1%	2.7%
Combination Chest CT Scan[1]	-	-	2.1%	2.7%
Follow-up Mammogram/Ultrasound	139	7.2%	9%	8.8%
Lumbar Spine MRI for Low Back Pain[1]	-	-	35.8%	37.2%

Alle Kiski Medical Center

1301 Carlisle St
Natrona, PA 15065
URL: www.wpahs.org
Type: Acute Care Hospitals
Ownership: Voluntary non-profit - Other
Phone: 412-224-5100
Fax: 724-226-7490
Emergency Services: Yes
Beds: 260

Key Personnel:
CEO/President. . . . . Ned Laubacher
Chief of Medical Staff . . . . Mohan M Patel, MD
Ambulatory Care . . . . Jeff Polana
Anesthesiology. . . . . Fred Weniger

Measure	Cases	This Hosp.	State Avg.	U.S. Avg.
Blood Clot Prevention and Treatment				
Anticoagulation Overlap Therapy[2]	43	81%	94%	93%
ICU Venous Thromboembolism Prophylaxis[2]	67	93%	94%	92%
Incidence of Potentially Preventable VTE[1,2]	-	-	8%	10%
UFH with Dosages/Platelet Monitoring[2]	53	100%	98%	97%
Venous Thromboembolism Prophylaxis[2]	358	88%	90%	85%
Warfarin Therapy Discharge Instructions[2]	30	100%	78%	75%
Chest Pain/Possible Heart Attack Care				
Aspirin Given Within 24 Hours of Arrival	135	99%	97%	96%
Fibrinolytic Meds Within 30 Min. of Arrival[7]	-	-	44%	58%
Average Time to ECG (minutes)	145	5	9	7
Average Time to Transfer (minutes)	30	56	64	60
Children's Asthma Care				
Received Home Management Plan of Care	-	-	-	88%
Received Reliever Medication	-	-	-	100%
Received Systemic Corticosteroids	-	-	-	100%
Emergency Department				
Admittance Decision Time (minutes)[2]	422	96	104	98
Head CT Results Within 45 Min. of Arrival	15	100%	60%	57%
Patients Who Left ER Before Being Seen	37,318	1%	1%	2%
Time from ER Arrival to Admit. (minutes)[2]	669	260	276	274
Time from ER Arrival to Discharge (minutes)	455	120	125	134
Time in ER Before Being Evaluated (minutes)	502	15	26	26
Time to Pain Meds for Fractures (minutes)	68	54	58	57
Heart Attack Care				
Aspirin Given at Discharge	96	99%	99%	99%
Fibrinolytic Meds Within 30 Min. of Arrival[7]	-	-	40%	54%
PCI Within 90 Minutes of Arrival[7]	-	-	97%	96%
Statin Prescribed at Discharge	96	99%	99%	98%
Heart Failure Care				
ACE Inhibitor or ARB for LVSD	52	98%	97%	97%
Discharge Instructions Given	255	88%	96%	94%
Evaluation of LVS Function	353	100%	100%	99%
Medicare Spending				
Medicare Spending per Patient (ratio)	-	1.10	1.01	0.98
Pneumonia Care				
Appropriate Initial Antibiotic Given	122	96%	96%	95%
Blood Culture Timing	121	100%	98%	98%
Pregnancy and Delivery Care				
Newborn Deliveries Scheduled Early[7]	-	-	4%	6%
Preventive Care				
Immunization for Influenza[2]	646	90%	91%	90%
Immunization for Pneumonia[2]	1,023	96%	92%	92%
Stroke Care				
Anticoagulation Therapy for Atrial Fibrillation	13	77%	96%	95%
Antithrombotic Therapy Timing	72	94%	98%	98%
Assessed for Rehabilitation	69	94%	98%	97%
Discharged on Antithrombotic Therapy	68	100%	99%	99%
Discharged on Statin Medication	54	89%	95%	94%
Thrombolytic Therapy Timing[1]	-	-	72%	66%
Venous Thromboembolism Prophylaxis	73	84%	95%	94%
Written Stroke Educational Materials Given	33	82%	90%	88%
Surgical Care Improvement Project				
Appropriate Beta Blocker Usage	160	98%	98%	98%
Appropriate VTP Within 24 Hours	351	98%	99%	98%
Controlled Postoperative Blood Glucose[7]	-	-	98%	97%
Perioperative Temperature Management	393	100%	100%	100%
Prophylactic Antibiotic Selection	282	100%	99%	99%
Prophylactic Antibiotic Selection (Outpatient)	253	98%	98%	98%
Prophylactic Antibiotic Stopped	269	97%	98%	98%
Prophylactic Antibiotic Timing	282	100%	99%	99%
Prophylactic Antibiotic Timing (Outpatient)	196	99%	98%	98%
Urinary Catheter Removal	322	96%	99%	97%
Survey of Patients' Hospital Experiences				
Area Around Room 'Always' Quiet at Night	300+	47%	54%	61%
Doctors 'Always' Communicated Well	300+	80%	80%	82%
Home Recovery Information Given	300+	85%	86%	85%
Hospital Given 9 or 10 on 10 Point Scale	300+	64%	69%	71%
Meds 'Always' Explained Before Given	300+	62%	63%	64%
Nurses 'Always' Communicated Well	300+	75%	79%	79%
Pain 'Always' Well Controlled	300+	68%	70%	71%
Room and Bathroom 'Always' Clean	300+	75%	73%	73%
Timely Help 'Always' Received	300+	63%	67%	68%
Would Definitely Recommend Hospital	300+	62%	70%	71%
Use of Medical Imaging				
Cardiac Imaging Stress Test before Surgery	173	4.6%	5.4%	5.3%
Combination Abdominal CT Scan	441	18.6%	12.2%	10.5%
Combination Brain/Sinus CT Scan	404	2.2%	3.1%	2.7%
Combination Chest CT Scan	292	0.7%	2.1%	2.7%
Follow-up Mammogram/Ultrasound	656	14.2%	9%	8.8%
Lumbar Spine MRI for Low Back Pain	46	52.2%	35.8%	37.2%

Jameson Memorial Hospital

1211 Wilmington Avenue
New Castle, PA 16105
Type: Acute Care Hospitals
Ownership: Voluntary non-profit - Other
Phone: 724-658-9001
Fax: 724-656-4142
Emergency Services: Yes
Beds: 230

Key Personnel:
President/CEO. . . . . Douglas Danko, MD
President . . . . Robert Mc Gann
Quality Assurance . . . . Holly Hampe
Radiology. . . . . Julian Proctor
Emergency Room . . . . Richard Wadas

Measure	Cases	This Hosp.	State Avg.	U.S. Avg.
Blood Clot Prevention and Treatment				
Anticoagulation Overlap Therapy[2]	67	81%	94%	93%
ICU Venous Thromboembolism Prophylaxis[2]	82	77%	94%	92%
Incidence of Potentially Preventable VTE[2]	22	27%	8%	10%
UFH with Dosages/Platelet Monitoring[2]	64	100%	98%	97%
Venous Thromboembolism Prophylaxis[2]	424	69%	90%	85%
Warfarin Therapy Discharge Instructions[2]	41	71%	78%	75%
Chest Pain/Possible Heart Attack Care				
Aspirin Given Within 24 Hours of Arrival	47	96%	97%	96%
Fibrinolytic Meds Within 30 Min. of Arrival[7]	-	-	44%	58%
Average Time to ECG (minutes)	48	12	9	7
Average Time to Transfer (minutes)	21	122	64	60
Children's Asthma Care				
Received Home Management Plan of Care	-	-	-	88%
Received Reliever Medication	-	-	-	100%
Received Systemic Corticosteroids	-	-	-	100%
Emergency Department				
Admittance Decision Time (minutes)[2]	684	56	104	98
Head CT Results Within 45 Min. of Arrival	14	64%	60%	57%
Patients Who Left ER Before Being Seen	35,712	2%	1%	2%
Time from ER Arrival to Admit. (minutes)[2]	685	237	276	274
Time from ER Arrival to Discharge (minutes)	354	133	125	134
Time in ER Before Being Evaluated (minutes)	379	48	26	26
Time to Pain Meds for Fractures (minutes)	95	44	58	57
Heart Attack Care				
Aspirin Given at Discharge	76	100%	99%	99%
Fibrinolytic Meds Within 30 Min. of Arrival[7]	-	-	40%	54%
PCI Within 90 Minutes of Arrival[1]	-	-	97%	96%
Statin Prescribed at Discharge	68	100%	99%	98%
Heart Failure Care				
ACE Inhibitor or ARB for LVSD	64	89%	97%	97%
Discharge Instructions Given	192	82%	96%	94%
Evaluation of LVS Function	252	98%	100%	99%
Medicare Spending				
Medicare Spending per Patient (ratio)	-	1.06	1.01	0.98
Pneumonia Care				
Appropriate Initial Antibiotic Given	206	89%	96%	95%
Blood Culture Timing	360	98%	98%	98%
Pregnancy and Delivery Care				
Newborn Deliveries Scheduled Early	66	47%	4%	6%
Preventive Care				
Immunization for Influenza[2]	539	94%	91%	90%
Immunization for Pneumonia[2]	754	93%	92%	92%
Stroke Care				
Anticoagulation Therapy for Atrial Fibrillation	13	92%	96%	95%
Antithrombotic Therapy Timing	74	91%	98%	98%
Assessed for Rehabilitation	81	95%	98%	97%
Discharged on Antithrombotic Therapy	79	96%	99%	99%
Discharged on Statin Medication	73	64%	95%	94%
Thrombolytic Therapy Timing[1]	-	-	72%	66%
Venous Thromboembolism Prophylaxis	80	72%	95%	94%

NOTE: Hospital profiles are in alphabetical order by state, then city, then hospital within the city; Rankings exclude hospitals with less than 25 cases except for patient surveys which excludes hospitals with less than 100 cases; (a) 100-299 cases; (1) The number of cases/patients is too few to report; (2) Data submitted were based on a sample of cases/patients; (3) Results are based on a shorter time period than required; (4) Data suppressed by CMS for one or more quarters; (5) Results are not available for this reporting period; (6) Fewer than 100 patients completed the HCAHPS survey; (7) No cases met the criteria for this measure; (8) The lower limit of the confidence interval cannot be calculated if the number of observed infections equals zero; (9) No data are available from the state/territory for this reporting period; (10) The scores shown reflect fewer than 50 completed surveys; (11) There were discrepancies in the data collection process; (12) This measure does not apply to this hospital for this reporting period; (13) Results cannot be calculated for this reporting period; (14) The results for this state are combined with nearby states to protect confidentiality; Please refer to the User's Guide for a full explanation of data.

Measure	Cases	This Hosp.	State Avg.	U.S. Avg.
Written Stroke Educational Materials Given	39	41%	90%	88%
Surgical Care Improvement Project				
Appropriate Beta Blocker Usage	124	95%	98%	98%
Appropriate VTP Within 24 Hours	381	98%	99%	98%
Controlled Postoperative Blood Glucose[7]	-	-	98%	97%
Perioperative Temperature Management	417	100%	100%	100%
Prophylactic Antibiotic Selection	313	99%	99%	99%
Prophylactic Antibiotic Selection (Outpatient)	124	89%	98%	98%
Prophylactic Antibiotic Stopped	304	97%	98%	98%
Prophylactic Antibiotic Timing	313	99%	99%	99%
Prophylactic Antibiotic Timing (Outpatient)	121	97%	98%	98%
Urinary Catheter Removal	145	97%	99%	97%
Survey of Patients' Hospital Experiences				
Area Around Room 'Always' Quiet at Night	300+	46%	54%	61%
Doctors 'Always' Communicated Well	300+	77%	80%	82%
Home Recovery Information Given	300+	87%	86%	85%
Hospital Given 9 or 10 on 10 Point Scale	300+	57%	69%	71%
Meds 'Always' Explained Before Given	300+	61%	63%	64%
Nurses 'Always' Communicated Well	300+	76%	79%	79%
Pain 'Always' Well Controlled	300+	64%	70%	71%
Room and Bathroom 'Always' Clean	300+	75%	73%	73%
Timely Help 'Always' Received	300+	54%	67%	68%
Would Definitely Recommend Hospital	300+	51%	70%	71%
Use of Medical Imaging				
Cardiac Imaging Stress Test before Surgery	82	8.5%	5.4%	5.3%
Combination Abdominal CT Scan	405	24.2%	12.2%	10.5%
Combination Brain/Sinus CT Scan[1]	-	-	3.1%	2.7%
Combination Chest CT Scan	313	2.9%	2.1%	2.7%
Follow-up Mammogram/Ultrasound	432	22.7%	9%	8.8%
Lumbar Spine MRI for Low Back Pain	74	41.9%	35.8%	37.2%

Mercy Suburban Hospital

2701 Dekalb Pike
Norristown, PA 19401
URL: www.mercyhealth.org
Type: Acute Care Hospitals
Ownership: Voluntary non-profit - Church
Phone: 215-278-2000
Fax: 610-272-4642
Emergency Services: Yes
Beds: 140

Key Personnel:
Operating Room. . . . . Marc Alpert, RN
Radiology. . . . . David M Bolden, DO
Infection Control. . . . . Cyndy Darcy, RN
Chief of Medical Staff. . . . . Joseph Koehler, DO
Emergency Room . . . . Patrick Moran
Quality Assurance . . . . Susan Paparella, RN
Chairman/CEO . . . . Kent T. Peterson

Measure	Cases	This Hosp.	State Avg.	U.S. Avg.
Blood Clot Prevention and Treatment				
Anticoagulation Overlap Therapy[2]	35	100%	94%	93%
ICU Venous Thromboembolism Prophylaxis[2]	74	100%	94%	92%
Incidence of Potentially Preventable VTE[2]	11	0%	8%	10%
UFH with Dosages/Platelet Monitoring[2]	39	100%	98%	97%
Venous Thromboembolism Prophylaxis[2]	347	100%	90%	85%
Warfarin Therapy Discharge Instructions[2]	17	100%	78%	75%
Chest Pain/Possible Heart Attack Care				
Aspirin Given Within 24 Hours of Arrival	28	93%	97%	96%
Fibrinolytic Meds Within 30 Min. of Arrival[7]	-	-	44%	58%
Average Time to ECG (minutes)	32	15	9	7
Average Time to Transfer (minutes)[7]	-	-	64	60
Children's Asthma Care				
Received Home Management Plan of Care	-	-	-	88%
Received Reliever Medication	-	-	-	100%
Received Systemic Corticosteroids	-	-	-	100%
Emergency Department				
Admittance Decision Time (minutes)[2]	802	204	104	98
Head CT Results Within 45 Min. of Arrival	36	94%	60%	57%
Patients Who Left ER Before Being Seen	25,350	1%	1%	2%
Time from ER Arrival to Admit. (minutes)[2]	805	356	276	274
Time from ER Arrival to Discharge (minutes)	359	146	125	134
Time in ER Before Being Evaluated (minutes)	406	23	26	26
Time to Pain Meds for Fractures (minutes)	56	62	58	57
Heart Attack Care				
Aspirin Given at Discharge	17	100%	99%	99%
Fibrinolytic Meds Within 30 Min. of Arrival[7]	-	-	40%	54%
PCI Within 90 Minutes of Arrival[7]	-	-	97%	96%
Statin Prescribed at Discharge	18	94%	99%	98%
Heart Failure Care				
ACE Inhibitor or ARB for LVSD	45	100%	97%	97%
Discharge Instructions Given	96	100%	96%	94%
Evaluation of LVS Function	139	100%	100%	99%
Medicare Spending				
Medicare Spending per Patient (ratio)	-	1.08	1.01	0.98
Pneumonia Care				
Appropriate Initial Antibiotic Given	45	100%	96%	95%
Blood Culture Timing	107	98%	98%	98%
Pregnancy and Delivery Care				
Newborn Deliveries Scheduled Early[7]	-	-	4%	6%
Preventive Care				
Immunization for Influenza[2]	434	96%	91%	90%
Immunization for Pneumonia[2]	654	97%	92%	92%
Stroke Care				
Anticoagulation Therapy for Atrial Fibrillation[1]	-	-	96%	95%
Antithrombotic Therapy Timing	54	100%	98%	98%
Assessed for Rehabilitation	48	100%	98%	97%
Discharged on Antithrombotic Therapy	48	100%	99%	99%
Discharged on Statin Medication	41	100%	95%	94%
Thrombolytic Therapy Timing[7]	-	-	72%	66%
Venous Thromboembolism Prophylaxis	51	100%	95%	94%
Written Stroke Educational Materials Given	13	100%	90%	88%
Surgical Care Improvement Project				
Appropriate Beta Blocker Usage	74	100%	98%	98%
Appropriate VTP Within 24 Hours	204	100%	99%	98%
Controlled Postoperative Blood Glucose[7]	-	-	98%	97%
Perioperative Temperature Management	236	100%	100%	100%
Prophylactic Antibiotic Selection	124	99%	99%	99%
Prophylactic Antibiotic Selection (Outpatient)	64	98%	98%	98%
Prophylactic Antibiotic Stopped	123	99%	98%	98%
Prophylactic Antibiotic Timing	125	100%	99%	99%
Prophylactic Antibiotic Timing (Outpatient)	65	98%	98%	98%
Urinary Catheter Removal	68	100%	99%	97%
Survey of Patients' Hospital Experiences				
Area Around Room 'Always' Quiet at Night	300+	44%	54%	61%
Doctors 'Always' Communicated Well	300+	77%	80%	82%
Home Recovery Information Given	300+	84%	86%	85%
Hospital Given 9 or 10 on 10 Point Scale	300+	57%	69%	71%
Meds 'Always' Explained Before Given	300+	61%	63%	64%
Nurses 'Always' Communicated Well	300+	74%	79%	79%
Pain 'Always' Well Controlled	300+	64%	70%	71%
Room and Bathroom 'Always' Clean	300+	57%	73%	73%
Timely Help 'Always' Received	300+	54%	67%	68%
Would Definitely Recommend Hospital	300+	58%	70%	71%
Use of Medical Imaging				
Cardiac Imaging Stress Test before Surgery	56	5.4%	5.4%	5.3%
Combination Abdominal CT Scan	449	8.7%	12.2%	10.5%
Combination Brain/Sinus CT Scan	438	5.3%	3.1%	2.7%
Combination Chest CT Scan	213	3.8%	2.1%	2.7%
Follow-up Mammogram/Ultrasound	672	11.5%	9%	8.8%
Lumbar Spine MRI for Low Back Pain	55	27.3%	35.8%	37.2%

Valley Forge Medical Center & Hospital

1033 W Germantown Pike
Norristown, PA 19401
E-mail: gslocum@vfmc.net
URL: www.vfmc.net
Type: Acute Care Hospitals
Ownership: Proprietary
Phone: 215-539-8500
Fax: 610-539-0910
Emergency Services: No
Beds: 78

Key Personnel:
CEO/President. . . . . Marian Colcher, MSW
Chief of Medical Staff . . . . Robert E Colcher, MD
Quality Assurance . . . . Frederick Jakes
Patient Relations . . . . Maureen King

Measure	Cases	This Hosp.	State Avg.	U.S. Avg.
Blood Clot Prevention and Treatment				
Anticoagulation Overlap Therapy[2,7]	-	-	94%	93%
ICU Venous Thromboembolism Prophylaxis[2,7]	-	-	94%	92%
Incidence of Potentially Preventable VTE[2,7]	-	-	8%	10%
UFH with Dosages/Platelet Monitoring[2,7]	-	-	98%	97%
Venous Thromboembolism Prophylaxis[2,7]	-	-	90%	85%
Warfarin Therapy Discharge Instructions[2,7]	-	-	78%	75%
Chest Pain/Possible Heart Attack Care				
Aspirin Given Within 24 Hours of Arrival[5]	-	-	97%	96%
Fibrinolytic Meds Within 30 Min. of Arrival[5]	-	-	44%	58%
Average Time to ECG (minutes)[5]	-	-	9	7
Average Time to Transfer (minutes)[5]	-	-	64	60
Children's Asthma Care				
Received Home Management Plan of Care	-	-	-	88%
Received Reliever Medication	-	-	-	100%
Received Systemic Corticosteroids	-	-	-	100%
Emergency Department				
Admittance Decision Time (minutes)[2,7]	-	-	104	98
Head CT Results Within 45 Min. of Arrival[5]	-	-	60%	57%
Patients Who Left ER Before Being Seen[5]	-	-	1%	2%
Time from ER Arrival to Admit. (minutes)[2,7]	-	-	276	274
Time from ER Arrival to Discharge (minutes)[5]	-	-	125	134
Time in ER Before Being Evaluated (minutes)[5]	-	-	26	26
Time to Pain Meds for Fractures (minutes)[5]	-	-	58	57
Heart Attack Care				
Aspirin Given at Discharge[5]	-	-	99%	99%
Fibrinolytic Meds Within 30 Min. of Arrival[5]	-	-	40%	54%
PCI Within 90 Minutes of Arrival[5]	-	-	97%	96%
Statin Prescribed at Discharge[5]	-	-	99%	98%
Heart Failure Care				
ACE Inhibitor or ARB for LVSD[5]	-	-	97%	97%
Discharge Instructions Given[5]	-	-	96%	94%
Evaluation of LVS Function[5]	-	-	100%	99%
Medicare Spending				
Medicare Spending per Patient (ratio)	-	0.68	1.01	0.98
Pneumonia Care				
Appropriate Initial Antibiotic Given[5]	-	-	96%	95%
Blood Culture Timing[5]	-	-	98%	98%
Pregnancy and Delivery Care				
Newborn Deliveries Scheduled Early[7]	-	-	4%	6%
Preventive Care				
Immunization for Influenza[2]	380	94%	91%	90%
Immunization for Pneumonia[2]	68	81%	92%	92%
Stroke Care				
Anticoagulation Therapy for Atrial Fibrillation[5]	-	-	96%	95%
Antithrombotic Therapy Timing[5]	-	-	98%	98%
Assessed for Rehabilitation[5]	-	-	98%	97%
Discharged on Antithrombotic Therapy[5]	-	-	99%	99%
Discharged on Statin Medication[5]	-	-	95%	94%
Thrombolytic Therapy Timing[5]	-	-	72%	66%
Venous Thromboembolism Prophylaxis[5]	-	-	95%	94%
Written Stroke Educational Materials Given[5]	-	-	90%	88%
Surgical Care Improvement Project				
Appropriate Beta Blocker Usage[5]	-	-	98%	98%
Appropriate VTP Within 24 Hours[5]	-	-	99%	98%
Controlled Postoperative Blood Glucose[5]	-	-	98%	97%
Perioperative Temperature Management[5]	-	-	100%	100%
Prophylactic Antibiotic Selection[5]	-	-	99%	99%
Prophylactic Antibiotic Selection (Outpatient)[5]	-	-	98%	98%
Prophylactic Antibiotic Stopped[5]	-	-	98%	98%
Prophylactic Antibiotic Timing[5]	-	-	99%	99%
Prophylactic Antibiotic Timing (Outpatient)[5]	-	-	98%	98%
Urinary Catheter Removal[5]	-	-	99%	97%
Survey of Patients' Hospital Experiences				
Area Around Room 'Always' Quiet at Night[1]	-	-	54%	61%
Doctors 'Always' Communicated Well[1]	-	-	80%	82%
Home Recovery Information Given[1]	-	-	86%	85%
Hospital Given 9 or 10 on 10 Point Scale[1]	-	-	69%	71%
Meds 'Always' Explained Before Given[1]	-	-	63%	64%
Nurses 'Always' Communicated Well[1]	-	-	79%	79%
Pain 'Always' Well Controlled[1]	-	-	70%	71%
Room and Bathroom 'Always' Clean[1]	-	-	73%	73%
Timely Help 'Always' Received[1]	-	-	67%	68%
Would Definitely Recommend Hospital[1]	-	-	70%	71%
Use of Medical Imaging				
Cardiac Imaging Stress Test before Surgery[7]	-	-	5.4%	5.3%
Combination Abdominal CT Scan[7]	-	-	12.2%	10.5%
Combination Brain/Sinus CT Scan[7]	-	-	3.1%	2.7%

NOTE: Hospital profiles are in alphabetical order by state, then city, then hospital within the city; Rankings exclude hospitals with less than 25 cases except for patient surveys which excludes hospitals with less than 100 cases; (a) 100-299 cases; (1) The number of cases/patients is too few to report; (2) Data submitted were based on a sample of cases/patients; (3) Results are based on a shorter time period than required; (4) Data suppressed by CMS for one or more quarters; (5) Results are not available for this reporting period; (6) Fewer than 100 patients completed the HCAHPS survey; (7) No cases met the criteria for this measure; (8) The lower limit of the confidence interval cannot be calculated if the number of observed infections equals zero; (9) No data are available from the state/territory for this reporting period; (10) The scores shown reflect fewer than 50 completed surveys; (11) There were discrepancies in the data collection process; (12) This measure does not apply to this hospital for this reporting period; (13) Results cannot be calculated for this reporting period; (14) The results for this state are combined with nearby states to protect confidentiality; Please refer to the User's Guide for a full explanation of data.

Combination Chest CT Scan[7]	-	-	2.1%	2.7%
Follow-up Mammogram/Ultrasound[7]	-	-	9%	8.8%
Lumbar Spine MRI for Low Back Pain[7]	-	-	35.8%	37.2%

Palmerton Hospital

135 Lafayette Avenue
Palmerton, PA 18071
Phone: 610-826-3141
Fax: 610-826-1282
URL: www.palmertonhospital.com
Type: Acute Care Hospitals
Emergency Services: Yes
Ownership: Voluntary non-profit - Other
Beds: 70

Key Personnel:
Pediatric In-Patient Care . . . . Nancy Andreas, RN
Patient Relations . . . . Dana Beisel
Radiology. . . . . Edie Berger
Operating Room. . . . . Betty Ann Flyte, RN
Quality Assurance . . . . Susanne Garszczynski, PhD
CEO/President. . . . . Richard Hager
Infection Control. . . . . Doreen Harleman, RN
Chief of Medical Staff. . . . . Thomas Tachousky, MD

Measure	Cases	This Hosp.	State Avg.	U.S. Avg.
Blood Clot Prevention and Treatment				
Anticoagulation Overlap Therapy[1,2]	-	-	94%	93%
ICU Venous Thromboembolism Prophylaxis[2]	31	74%	94%	92%
Incidence of Potentially Preventable VTE[1,2]	-	-	8%	10%
UFH with Dosages/Platelet Monitoring[1,2]	-	-	98%	97%
Venous Thromboembolism Prophylaxis[2]	124	73%	90%	85%
Warfarin Therapy Discharge Instructions[1,2]	-	-	78%	75%
Chest Pain/Possible Heart Attack Care				
Aspirin Given Within 24 Hours of Arrival	21	100%	97%	96%
Fibrinolytic Meds Within 30 Min. of Arrival[3,7]	-	-	44%	58%
Average Time to ECG (minutes)	21	6	9	7
Average Time to Transfer (minutes)[1,3]	-	-	64	60
Children's Asthma Care				
Received Home Management Plan of Care	-	-	-	88%
Received Reliever Medication	-	-	-	100%
Received Systemic Corticosteroids	-	-	-	100%
Emergency Department				
Admittance Decision Time (minutes)[2]	293	65	104	98
Head CT Results Within 45 Min. of Arrival[1,3]	-	-	60%	57%
Patients Who Left ER Before Being Seen	11,521	1%	1%	2%
Time from ER Arrival to Admit. (minutes)[2]	309	218	276	274
Time from ER Arrival to Discharge (minutes)	334	92	125	134
Time in ER Before Being Evaluated (minutes)	368	29	26	26
Time to Pain Meds for Fractures (minutes)	48	65	58	57
Heart Attack Care				
Aspirin Given at Discharge[1]	-	-	99%	99%
Fibrinolytic Meds Within 30 Min. of Arrival[7]	-	-	40%	54%
PCI Within 90 Minutes of Arrival[7]	-	-	97%	96%
Statin Prescribed at Discharge[1]	-	-	99%	98%
Heart Failure Care				
ACE Inhibitor or ARB for LVSD[1]	-	-	97%	97%
Discharge Instructions Given	62	94%	96%	94%
Evaluation of LVS Function	76	88%	100%	99%
Medicare Spending				
Medicare Spending per Patient (ratio)	-	1.01	1.01	0.98
Pneumonia Care				
Appropriate Initial Antibiotic Given	41	95%	96%	95%
Blood Culture Timing	60	98%	98%	98%
Pregnancy and Delivery Care				
Newborn Deliveries Scheduled Early[7]	-	-	4%	6%
Preventive Care				
Immunization for Influenza[2]	290	82%	91%	90%
Immunization for Pneumonia[2]	454	89%	92%	92%
Stroke Care				
Anticoagulation Therapy for Atrial Fibrillation[1]	-	-	96%	95%
Antithrombotic Therapy Timing	18	100%	98%	98%
Assessed for Rehabilitation	20	95%	98%	97%
Discharged on Antithrombotic Therapy	20	100%	99%	99%
Discharged on Statin Medication	17	94%	95%	94%
Thrombolytic Therapy Timing[1]	-	-	72%	66%
Venous Thromboembolism Prophylaxis	19	89%	95%	94%
Written Stroke Educational Materials Given	14	29%	90%	88%
Surgical Care Improvement Project				
Appropriate Beta Blocker Usage	32	94%	98%	98%
Appropriate VTP Within 24 Hours	93	97%	99%	98%
Controlled Postoperative Blood Glucose[7]	-	-	98%	97%
Perioperative Temperature Management	100	99%	100%	100%
Prophylactic Antibiotic Selection	74	95%	99%	99%
Prophylactic Antibiotic Selection (Outpatient)	16	100%	98%	98%
Prophylactic Antibiotic Stopped	72	97%	98%	98%
Prophylactic Antibiotic Timing	74	100%	99%	99%
Prophylactic Antibiotic Timing (Outpatient)	30	53%	98%	98%
Urinary Catheter Removal	83	98%	99%	97%
Survey of Patients' Hospital Experiences				
Area Around Room 'Always' Quiet at Night	300+	53%	54%	61%
Doctors 'Always' Communicated Well	300+	76%	80%	82%
Home Recovery Information Given	300+	88%	86%	85%
Hospital Given 9 or 10 on 10 Point Scale	300+	60%	69%	71%
Meds 'Always' Explained Before Given	300+	55%	63%	64%
Nurses 'Always' Communicated Well	300+	75%	79%	79%
Pain 'Always' Well Controlled	300+	63%	70%	71%
Room and Bathroom 'Always' Clean	300+	73%	73%	73%
Timely Help 'Always' Received	300+	62%	67%	68%
Would Definitely Recommend Hospital	300+	61%	70%	71%
Use of Medical Imaging				
Cardiac Imaging Stress Test before Surgery	86	3.5%	5.4%	5.3%
Combination Abdominal CT Scan	253	8.3%	12.2%	10.5%
Combination Brain/Sinus CT Scan[1]	-	-	3.1%	2.7%
Combination Chest CT Scan	164	9.8%	2.1%	2.7%
Follow-up Mammogram/Ultrasound	288	7.3%	9%	8.8%
Lumbar Spine MRI for Low Back Pain[7]	-	-	35.8%	37.2%

Main Line Hospital Paoli

255 West Lancaster Avenue
Paoli, PA 19301
Phone: 610-648-1000
Fax: 610-526-4047
URL: www.mainlinehealth.org
Type: Acute Care Hospitals
Emergency Services: Yes
Ownership: Voluntary non-profit - Private
Beds: 208

Key Personnel:
Emergency Room . . . . Donald J Armstrong, MD
Operating Room. . . . . William M Dellevigne
CEO/President. . . . . Barbara Tachovsky, RN, MS
Infection Control. . . . . David Trevino, MD

Measure	Cases	This Hosp.	State Avg.	U.S. Avg.
Blood Clot Prevention and Treatment				
Anticoagulation Overlap Therapy[2]	103	97%	94%	93%
ICU Venous Thromboembolism Prophylaxis[2]	40	100%	94%	92%
Incidence of Potentially Preventable VTE[2]	37	5%	8%	10%
UFH with Dosages/Platelet Monitoring[2]	36	100%	98%	97%
Venous Thromboembolism Prophylaxis[2]	341	90%	90%	85%
Warfarin Therapy Discharge Instructions[2]	71	34%	78%	75%
Chest Pain/Possible Heart Attack Care				
Aspirin Given Within 24 Hours of Arrival[3,7]	-	-	97%	96%
Fibrinolytic Meds Within 30 Min. of Arrival[5]	-	-	44%	58%
Average Time to ECG (minutes)[3,7]	-	-	9	7
Average Time to Transfer (minutes)[5]	-	-	64	60
Children's Asthma Care				
Received Home Management Plan of Care	-	-	-	88%
Received Reliever Medication	-	-	-	100%
Received Systemic Corticosteroids	-	-	-	100%
Emergency Department				
Admittance Decision Time (minutes)[2]	638	161	104	98
Head CT Results Within 45 Min. of Arrival[1]	-	-	60%	57%
Patients Who Left ER Before Being Seen	41,520	0%	1%	2%
Time from ER Arrival to Admit. (minutes)[2]	638	316	276	274
Time from ER Arrival to Discharge (minutes)	367	143	125	134
Time in ER Before Being Evaluated (minutes)	383	22	26	26
Time to Pain Meds for Fractures (minutes)	142	63	58	57
Heart Attack Care				
Aspirin Given at Discharge	178	100%	99%	99%
Fibrinolytic Meds Within 30 Min. of Arrival[7]	-	-	40%	54%
PCI Within 90 Minutes of Arrival	37	100%	97%	96%
Statin Prescribed at Discharge	171	100%	99%	98%
Heart Failure Care				
ACE Inhibitor or ARB for LVSD	60	98%	97%	97%
Discharge Instructions Given	189	100%	96%	94%
Evaluation of LVS Function	267	100%	100%	99%
Medicare Spending				
Medicare Spending per Patient (ratio)	-	1.06	1.01	0.98
Pneumonia Care				
Appropriate Initial Antibiotic Given	113	94%	96%	95%
Blood Culture Timing	164	98%	98%	98%
Pregnancy and Delivery Care				
Newborn Deliveries Scheduled Early[2]	33	0%	4%	6%
Preventive Care				
Immunization for Influenza[2]	542	90%	91%	90%
Immunization for Pneumonia[2]	646	93%	92%	92%
Stroke Care				
Anticoagulation Therapy for Atrial Fibrillation	21	100%	96%	95%
Antithrombotic Therapy Timing	141	99%	98%	98%
Assessed for Rehabilitation	166	100%	98%	97%
Discharged on Antithrombotic Therapy	144	100%	99%	99%
Discharged on Statin Medication	108	100%	95%	94%
Thrombolytic Therapy Timing[1]	-	-	72%	66%
Venous Thromboembolism Prophylaxis	169	100%	95%	94%
Written Stroke Educational Materials Given	67	99%	90%	88%
Surgical Care Improvement Project				
Appropriate Beta Blocker Usage[2]	262	100%	98%	98%
Appropriate VTP Within 24 Hours[2]	738	100%	99%	98%
Controlled Postoperative Blood Glucose[2]	42	100%	98%	97%
Perioperative Temperature Management[2]	934	100%	100%	100%
Prophylactic Antibiotic Selection[2]	729	99%	99%	99%
Prophylactic Antibiotic Selection (Outpatient)	203	96%	98%	98%
Prophylactic Antibiotic Stopped[2]	674	100%	98%	98%
Prophylactic Antibiotic Timing[2]	729	100%	99%	99%
Prophylactic Antibiotic Timing (Outpatient)	208	95%	98%	98%
Urinary Catheter Removal[2]	384	100%	99%	97%
Survey of Patients' Hospital Experiences				
Area Around Room 'Always' Quiet at Night	300+	54%	54%	61%
Doctors 'Always' Communicated Well	300+	78%	80%	82%
Home Recovery Information Given	300+	86%	86%	85%
Hospital Given 9 or 10 on 10 Point Scale	300+	82%	69%	71%
Meds 'Always' Explained Before Given	300+	63%	63%	64%
Nurses 'Always' Communicated Well	300+	83%	79%	79%
Pain 'Always' Well Controlled	300+	74%	70%	71%
Room and Bathroom 'Always' Clean	300+	69%	73%	73%
Timely Help 'Always' Received	300+	67%	67%	68%
Would Definitely Recommend Hospital	300+	86%	70%	71%
Use of Medical Imaging				
Cardiac Imaging Stress Test before Surgery	200	5.5%	5.4%	5.3%
Combination Abdominal CT Scan	1,581	11.6%	12.2%	10.5%
Combination Brain/Sinus CT Scan	1,154	2.2%	3.1%	2.7%
Combination Chest CT Scan	1,276	3.7%	2.1%	2.7%
Follow-up Mammogram/Ultrasound	2,497	12.3%	9%	8.8%
Lumbar Spine MRI for Low Back Pain[1]	-	-	35.8%	37.2%

Mid - Valley Hospital

1400 Main Street
Peckville, PA 18452
Phone: 570-383-5000
Fax: 570-383-5504
Type: Critical Access Hospitals
Emergency Services: Yes
Ownership: Proprietary
Beds: 25

Key Personnel:
Patient Relations . . . . Rebecca Christoph
CEO . . . . Michael D. Billing
Cardiac Laboratory. . . . . W David Filvatatrick
Emergency Room . . . . Frank Schell, MD
Quality Assurance . . . . Katie Sunday

Measure	Cases	This Hosp.	State Avg.	U.S. Avg.
Blood Clot Prevention and Treatment				
Anticoagulation Overlap Therapy[1,2]	-	-	94%	93%
ICU Venous Thromboembolism Prophylaxis[2,7]	-	-	94%	92%
Incidence of Potentially Preventable VTE[2,7]	-	-	8%	10%
UFH with Dosages/Platelet Monitoring[1,2]	-	-	98%	97%
Venous Thromboembolism Prophylaxis[2]	174	100%	90%	85%
Warfarin Therapy Discharge Instructions[2,7]	-	-	78%	75%
Chest Pain/Possible Heart Attack Care				
Aspirin Given Within 24 Hours of Arrival	15	100%	97%	96%
Fibrinolytic Meds Within 30 Min. of Arrival[7]	-	-	44%	58%
Average Time to ECG (minutes)	15	10	9	7
Average Time to Transfer (minutes)[1]	-	-	64	60

NOTE: Hospital profiles are in alphabetical order by state, then city, then hospital within the city; Rankings exclude hospitals with less than 25 cases except for patient surveys which excludes hospitals with less than 100 cases; (a) 100-299 cases; (1) The number of cases/patients is too few to report; (2) Data submitted were based on a sample of cases/patients; (3) Results are based on a shorter time period than required; (4) Data suppressed by CMS for one or more quarters; (5) Results are not available for this reporting period; (6) Fewer than 100 patients completed the HCAHPS survey; (7) No cases met the criteria for this measure; (8) The lower limit of the confidence interval cannot be calculated if the number of observed infections equals zero; (9) No data are available from the state/territory for this reporting period; (10) The scores shown reflect fewer than 50 completed surveys; (11) There were discrepancies in the data collection process; (12) This measure does not apply to this hospital for this reporting period; (13) Results cannot be calculated for this reporting period; (14) The results for this state are combined with nearby states to protect confidentiality; Please refer to the User's Guide for a full explanation of data.

Measure	Cases	This Hosp.	State Avg.	U.S. Avg.
Children's Asthma Care				
Received Home Management Plan of Care	-	-	-	88%
Received Reliever Medication	-	-	-	100%
Received Systemic Corticosteroids	-	-	-	100%
Emergency Department				
Admittance Decision Time (minutes)[2]	128	70	104	98
Head CT Results Within 45 Min. of Arrival[1,3]	-	-	60%	57%
Patients Who Left ER Before Being Seen	9,735	1%	1%	2%
Time from ER Arrival to Admit. (minutes)[2]	264	246	276	274
Time from ER Arrival to Discharge (minutes)	393	105	125	134
Time in ER Before Being Evaluated (minutes)	403	20	26	26
Time to Pain Meds for Fractures (minutes)	29	50	58	57
Heart Attack Care				
Aspirin Given at Discharge[1,3]	-	-	99%	99%
Fibrinolytic Meds Within 30 Min. of Arrival[3,7]	-	-	40%	54%
PCI Within 90 Minutes of Arrival[3,7]	-	-	97%	96%
Statin Prescribed at Discharge[1,3]	-	-	99%	98%
Heart Failure Care				
ACE Inhibitor or ARB for LVSD[1]	-	-	97%	97%
Discharge Instructions Given	20	100%	96%	94%
Evaluation of LVS Function	34	100%	100%	99%
Medicare Spending				
Medicare Spending per Patient (ratio)	-	-	1.01	0.98
Pneumonia Care				
Appropriate Initial Antibiotic Given	18	100%	96%	95%
Blood Culture Timing	28	96%	98%	98%
Pregnancy and Delivery Care				
Newborn Deliveries Scheduled Early[3,7]	-	-	4%	6%
Preventive Care				
Immunization for Influenza[2]	174	99%	91%	90%
Immunization for Pneumonia[2]	259	100%	92%	92%
Stroke Care				
Anticoagulation Therapy for Atrial Fibrillation[3,7]	-	-	96%	95%
Antithrombotic Therapy Timing[1,3]	-	-	98%	98%
Assessed for Rehabilitation[1,3]	-	-	98%	97%
Discharged on Antithrombotic Therapy[1,3]	-	-	99%	99%
Discharged on Statin Medication[1,3]	-	-	95%	94%
Thrombolytic Therapy Timing[3,7]	-	-	72%	66%
Venous Thromboembolism Prophylaxis[1,3]	-	-	95%	94%
Written Stroke Educational Materials Given[1,3]	-	-	90%	88%
Surgical Care Improvement Project				
Appropriate Beta Blocker Usage[5]	-	-	98%	98%
Appropriate VTP Within 24 Hours[5]	-	-	99%	98%
Controlled Postoperative Blood Glucose[5]	-	-	98%	97%
Perioperative Temperature Management[5]	-	-	100%	100%
Prophylactic Antibiotic Selection[5]	-	-	99%	99%
Prophylactic Antibiotic Selection (Outpatient)[5]	-	-	98%	98%
Prophylactic Antibiotic Stopped[5]	-	-	98%	98%
Prophylactic Antibiotic Timing[5]	-	-	99%	99%
Prophylactic Antibiotic Timing (Outpatient)[5]	-	-	98%	98%
Urinary Catheter Removal[5]	-	-	99%	97%
Survey of Patients' Hospital Experiences				
Area Around Room 'Always' Quiet at Night	(a)	71%	54%	61%
Doctors 'Always' Communicated Well	(a)	90%	80%	82%
Home Recovery Information Given	(a)	88%	86%	85%
Hospital Given 9 or 10 on 10 Point Scale	(a)	83%	69%	71%
Meds 'Always' Explained Before Given	(a)	72%	63%	64%
Nurses 'Always' Communicated Well	(a)	88%	79%	79%
Pain 'Always' Well Controlled	(a)	86%	70%	71%
Room and Bathroom 'Always' Clean	(a)	84%	73%	73%
Timely Help 'Always' Received	(a)	85%	67%	68%
Would Definitely Recommend Hospital	(a)	81%	70%	71%
Use of Medical Imaging				
Cardiac Imaging Stress Test before Surgery[1]	-	-	5.4%	5.3%
Combination Abdominal CT Scan	109	36.7%	12.2%	10.5%
Combination Brain/Sinus CT Scan[1]	-	-	3.1%	2.7%
Combination Chest CT Scan[1]	-	-	2.1%	2.7%
Follow-up Mammogram/Ultrasound[7]	-	-	9%	8.8%
Lumbar Spine MRI for Low Back Pain[7]	-	-	35.8%	37.2%

Albert Einstein Medical Center

5501 Old York Road
Philadelphia, PA 19141
URL: www.einstein.edu
Type: Acute Care Hospitals
Ownership: Voluntary non-profit - Other
Phone: 215-456-6090
Fax: 215-456-6242
Emergency Services: Yes
Beds: 1,200

Key Personnel:
Pediatric In-Patient Care . . . . Allan Arbeter, MD
Operating Room. . . . . Cathy Costello
Infection Control . . . . Robert Fisher, MD
CEO/President. . . . . Barry Freedman
Chief of Medical Staff. . . . . Leonard Greenberg, MD
Emergency Room . . . . Patty Lynch
Quality Assurance . . . . Sara Potter
Radiology. . . . . Henrietta Rosenburg, MD

Measure	Cases	This Hosp.	State Avg.	U.S. Avg.
Blood Clot Prevention and Treatment				
Anticoagulation Overlap Therapy[2]	151	99%	94%	93%
ICU Venous Thromboembolism Prophylaxis[2]	93	98%	94%	92%
Incidence of Potentially Preventable VTE[2]	41	17%	8%	10%
UFH with Dosages/Platelet Monitoring[2]	113	100%	98%	97%
Venous Thromboembolism Prophylaxis[2]	334	92%	90%	85%
Warfarin Therapy Discharge Instructions[2]	105	55%	78%	75%
Chest Pain/Possible Heart Attack Care				
Aspirin Given Within 24 Hours of Arrival[5]	-	-	97%	96%
Fibrinolytic Meds Within 30 Min. of Arrival[5]	-	-	44%	58%
Average Time to ECG (minutes)[5]	-	-	9	7
Average Time to Transfer (minutes)[5]	-	-	64	60
Children's Asthma Care				
Received Home Management Plan of Care	-	-	-	88%
Received Reliever Medication	-	-	-	100%
Received Systemic Corticosteroids	-	-	-	100%
Emergency Department				
Admittance Decision Time (minutes)[2]	768	182	104	98
Head CT Results Within 45 Min. of Arrival[3,7]	-	-	60%	57%
Patients Who Left ER Before Being Seen	>100k	3%	1%	2%
Time from ER Arrival to Admit. (minutes)[2]	774	374	276	274
Time from ER Arrival to Discharge (minutes)	549	166	125	134
Time in ER Before Being Evaluated (minutes)	535	48	26	26
Time to Pain Meds for Fractures (minutes)	143	55	58	57
Heart Attack Care				
Aspirin Given at Discharge	287	99%	99%	99%
Fibrinolytic Meds Within 30 Min. of Arrival[7]	-	-	40%	54%
PCI Within 90 Minutes of Arrival	36	100%	97%	96%
Statin Prescribed at Discharge	289	100%	99%	98%
Heart Failure Care				
ACE Inhibitor or ARB for LVSD[2]	139	96%	97%	97%
Discharge Instructions Given[2]	246	100%	96%	94%
Evaluation of LVS Function[2]	328	100%	100%	99%
Medicare Spending				
Medicare Spending per Patient (ratio)	-	1.07	1.01	0.98
Pneumonia Care				
Appropriate Initial Antibiotic Given	112	99%	96%	95%
Blood Culture Timing	198	96%	98%	98%
Pregnancy and Delivery Care				
Newborn Deliveries Scheduled Early[2]	43	0%	4%	6%
Preventive Care				
Immunization for Influenza[2]	639	95%	91%	90%
Immunization for Pneumonia[2]	765	89%	92%	92%
Stroke Care				
Anticoagulation Therapy for Atrial Fibrillation[1,2]	-	-	96%	95%
Antithrombotic Therapy Timing[2]	110	99%	98%	98%
Assessed for Rehabilitation[2]	136	100%	98%	97%
Discharged on Antithrombotic Therapy[2]	114	100%	99%	99%
Discharged on Statin Medication[2]	96	100%	95%	94%
Thrombolytic Therapy Timing[1,2]	-	-	72%	66%
Venous Thromboembolism Prophylaxis[2]	147	95%	95%	94%
Written Stroke Educational Materials Given[2]	47	100%	90%	88%
Surgical Care Improvement Project				
Appropriate Beta Blocker Usage[2]	245	92%	98%	98%
Appropriate VTP Within 24 Hours[2]	484	99%	99%	98%
Controlled Postoperative Blood Glucose[2]	149	95%	98%	97%
Perioperative Temperature Management[2]	605	100%	100%	100%
Prophylactic Antibiotic Selection[2]	487	100%	99%	99%
Prophylactic Antibiotic Selection (Outpatient)	312	98%	98%	98%
Prophylactic Antibiotic Stopped[2]	483	97%	98%	98%
Prophylactic Antibiotic Timing[2]	487	100%	99%	99%
Prophylactic Antibiotic Timing (Outpatient)	314	98%	98%	98%
Urinary Catheter Removal[2]	472	99%	99%	97%
Survey of Patients' Hospital Experiences				
Area Around Room 'Always' Quiet at Night	300+	56%	54%	61%
Doctors 'Always' Communicated Well	300+	81%	80%	82%
Home Recovery Information Given	300+	83%	86%	85%
Hospital Given 9 or 10 on 10 Point Scale	300+	61%	69%	71%
Meds 'Always' Explained Before Given	300+	61%	63%	64%
Nurses 'Always' Communicated Well	300+	78%	79%	79%
Pain 'Always' Well Controlled	300+	67%	70%	71%
Room and Bathroom 'Always' Clean	300+	62%	73%	73%
Timely Help 'Always' Received	300+	62%	67%	68%
Would Definitely Recommend Hospital	300+	61%	70%	71%
Use of Medical Imaging				
Cardiac Imaging Stress Test before Surgery	343	6.4%	5.4%	5.3%
Combination Abdominal CT Scan	849	8.1%	12.2%	10.5%
Combination Brain/Sinus CT Scan	885	2.5%	3.1%	2.7%
Combination Chest CT Scan	623	4.0%	2.1%	2.7%
Follow-up Mammogram/Ultrasound	2,805	5.6%	9%	8.8%
Lumbar Spine MRI for Low Back Pain	145	44.8%	35.8%	37.2%

Aria Health

10800 Knights Road
Philadelphia, PA 19114
URL: www.ariahealth.com
Type: Acute Care Hospitals
Ownership: Voluntary non-profit - Private
Phone: 215-612-4129
Emergency Services: Yes
Beds: 252

Key Personnel:
Radiology. . . . . Ronald Adelman, MD
Cardiology . . . . Khalid Almuti, MD
Emergency Room . . . . Jeffrey D Anderson, MD
Pediatrics. . . . . Barbara Gold, MD

Measure	Cases	This Hosp.	State Avg.	U.S. Avg.
Blood Clot Prevention and Treatment				
Anticoagulation Overlap Therapy[2]	216	100%	94%	93%
ICU Venous Thromboembolism Prophylaxis[2]	77	99%	94%	92%
Incidence of Potentially Preventable VTE[2]	85	7%	8%	10%
UFH with Dosages/Platelet Monitoring[2]	151	100%	98%	97%
Venous Thromboembolism Prophylaxis[2]	232	92%	90%	85%
Warfarin Therapy Discharge Instructions[2]	139	99%	78%	75%
Chest Pain/Possible Heart Attack Care				
Aspirin Given Within 24 Hours of Arrival[1]	-	-	97%	96%
Fibrinolytic Meds Within 30 Min. of Arrival[3,7]	-	-	44%	58%
Average Time to ECG (minutes)[1]	-	-	9	7
Average Time to Transfer (minutes)[3,7]	-	-	64	60
Children's Asthma Care				
Received Home Management Plan of Care	-	-	-	88%
Received Reliever Medication	-	-	-	100%
Received Systemic Corticosteroids	-	-	-	100%
Emergency Department				
Admittance Decision Time (minutes)[2]	715	148	104	98
Head CT Results Within 45 Min. of Arrival	25	68%	60%	57%
Patients Who Left ER Before Being Seen	>100k	6%	1%	2%
Time from ER Arrival to Admit. (minutes)[2]	718	390	276	274
Time from ER Arrival to Discharge (minutes)	322	183	125	134
Time in ER Before Being Evaluated (minutes)	345	74	26	26
Time to Pain Meds for Fractures (minutes)	191	85	58	57
Heart Attack Care				
Aspirin Given at Discharge	509	99%	99%	99%
Fibrinolytic Meds Within 30 Min. of Arrival[1]	-	-	40%	54%
PCI Within 90 Minutes of Arrival	51	90%	97%	96%
Statin Prescribed at Discharge	498	100%	99%	98%
Heart Failure Care				
ACE Inhibitor or ARB for LVSD	256	96%	97%	97%
Discharge Instructions Given	588	96%	96%	94%
Evaluation of LVS Function	736	100%	100%	99%
Medicare Spending				
Medicare Spending per Patient (ratio)	-	1.04	1.01	0.98
Pneumonia Care				
Appropriate Initial Antibiotic Given	406	97%	96%	95%

NOTE: Hospital profiles are in alphabetical order by state, then city, then hospital within the city; Rankings exclude hospitals with less than 25 cases except for patient surveys which excludes hospitals with less than 100 cases; (a) 100-299 cases; (1) The number of cases/patients is too few to report; (2) Data submitted were based on a sample of cases/patients; (3) Results are based on a shorter time period than required; (4) Data suppressed by CMS for one or more quarters; (5) Results are not available for this reporting period; (6) Fewer than 100 patients completed the HCAHPS survey; (7) No cases met the criteria for this measure; (8) The lower limit of the confidence interval cannot be calculated if the number of observed infections equals zero; (9) No data are available from the state/territory for this reporting period; (10) The scores shown reflect fewer than 50 completed surveys; (11) There were discrepancies in the data collection process; (12) This measure does not apply to this hospital for this reporting period; (13) Results cannot be calculated for this reporting period; (14) The results for this state are combined with nearby states to protect confidentiality; Please refer to the User's Guide for a full explanation of data.

Measure	Cases	This Hosp.	State Avg.	U.S. Avg.
Blood Culture Timing	850	98%	98%	98%
Pregnancy and Delivery Care				
Newborn Deliveries Scheduled Early[7]	-	-	4%	6%
Preventive Care				
Immunization for Influenza[2]	584	88%	91%	90%
Immunization for Pneumonia[2]	832	83%	92%	92%
Stroke Care				
Anticoagulation Therapy for Atrial Fibrillation	35	94%	96%	95%
Antithrombotic Therapy Timing	259	99%	98%	98%
Assessed for Rehabilitation	263	99%	98%	97%
Discharged on Antithrombotic Therapy	242	100%	99%	99%
Discharged on Statin Medication	192	97%	95%	94%
Thrombolytic Therapy Timing	12	92%	72%	66%
Venous Thromboembolism Prophylaxis	281	98%	95%	94%
Written Stroke Educational Materials Given	134	98%	90%	88%
Surgical Care Improvement Project				
Appropriate Beta Blocker Usage	457	99%	98%	98%
Appropriate VTP Within 24 Hours	1,171	99%	99%	98%
Controlled Postoperative Blood Glucose	145	97%	98%	97%
Perioperative Temperature Management	1,360	100%	100%	100%
Prophylactic Antibiotic Selection	909	99%	99%	99%
Prophylactic Antibiotic Selection (Outpatient)	143	97%	98%	98%
Prophylactic Antibiotic Stopped	881	100%	98%	98%
Prophylactic Antibiotic Timing	910	99%	99%	99%
Prophylactic Antibiotic Timing (Outpatient)	145	99%	98%	98%
Urinary Catheter Removal	1,139	100%	99%	97%
Survey of Patients' Hospital Experiences				
Area Around Room 'Always' Quiet at Night	300+	45%	54%	61%
Doctors 'Always' Communicated Well	300+	74%	80%	82%
Home Recovery Information Given	300+	84%	86%	85%
Hospital Given 9 or 10 on 10 Point Scale	300+	63%	69%	71%
Meds 'Always' Explained Before Given	300+	59%	63%	64%
Nurses 'Always' Communicated Well	300+	77%	79%	79%
Pain 'Always' Well Controlled	300+	66%	70%	71%
Room and Bathroom 'Always' Clean	300+	67%	73%	73%
Timely Help 'Always' Received	300+	64%	67%	68%
Would Definitely Recommend Hospital	300+	63%	70%	71%
Use of Medical Imaging				
Cardiac Imaging Stress Test before Surgery	434	6.2%	5.4%	5.3%
Combination Abdominal CT Scan	1,744	2.4%	12.2%	10.5%
Combination Brain/Sinus CT Scan	1,386	4.0%	3.1%	2.7%
Combination Chest CT Scan	1,224	0.2%	2.1%	2.7%
Follow-up Mammogram/Ultrasound	1,516	8.7%	9%	8.8%
Lumbar Spine MRI for Low Back Pain[1]	-	-	35.8%	37.2%

Cancer Treatment Centers of America

1331 East Wyoming Avenue
Philadelphia, PA 19124
URL: www.cancercenter.com
Phone: 215-744-6728
Fax: 215-537-7899
Type: Acute Care Hospitals
Emergency Services: No
Ownership: Voluntary non-profit - Private
Beds: 22

Key Personnel:
CEO/President. . . . . Robert Amon
Emergency Room . . . . Carol Behrle, RN
Pediatric In-Patient Care . . . . Stewart Cooler, MD
Operating Room. . . . . Lynn Frechette, RN
Chief of Medical Staff . . . . Holly Leppert, DO
Quality Assurance . . . . Sandra Sacks

Measure	Cases	This Hosp.	State Avg.	U.S. Avg.
Blood Clot Prevention and Treatment				
Anticoagulation Overlap Therapy[1,2]	-	-	94%	93%
ICU Venous Thromboembolism Prophylaxis[2]	37	97%	94%	92%
Incidence of Potentially Preventable VTE[2]	11	9%	8%	10%
UFH with Dosages/Platelet Monitoring[2]	11	100%	98%	97%
Venous Thromboembolism Prophylaxis[2]	158	78%	90%	85%
Warfarin Therapy Discharge Instructions[1,2]	-	-	78%	75%
Chest Pain/Possible Heart Attack Care				
Aspirin Given Within 24 Hours of Arrival[5]	-	-	97%	96%
Fibrinolytic Meds Within 30 Min. of Arrival[5]	-	-	44%	58%
Average Time to ECG (minutes)[5]	-	-	9	7
Average Time to Transfer (minutes)[5]	-	-	64	60
Children's Asthma Care				
Received Home Management Plan of Care	-	-	-	88%
Received Reliever Medication	-	-	-	100%
Received Systemic Corticosteroids	-	-	-	100%
Emergency Department				
Admittance Decision Time (minutes)[2,7]	-	-	104	98
Head CT Results Within 45 Min. of Arrival[5]	-	-	60%	57%
Patients Who Left ER Before Being Seen[5]	-	-	1%	2%
Time from ER Arrival to Admit. (minutes)[2,7]	-	-	276	274
Time from ER Arrival to Discharge (minutes)[5]	-	-	125	134
Time in ER Before Being Evaluated (minutes)[5]	-	-	26	26
Time to Pain Meds for Fractures (minutes)[5]	-	-	58	57
Heart Attack Care				
Aspirin Given at Discharge[1,3]	-	-	99%	99%
Fibrinolytic Meds Within 30 Min. of Arrival[3,7]	-	-	40%	54%
PCI Within 90 Minutes of Arrival[3,7]	-	-	97%	96%
Statin Prescribed at Discharge[1,3]	-	-	99%	98%
Heart Failure Care				
ACE Inhibitor or ARB for LVSD[1]	-	-	97%	97%
Discharge Instructions Given[1]	-	-	96%	94%
Evaluation of LVS Function[1]	-	-	100%	99%
Medicare Spending				
Medicare Spending per Patient (ratio)	-	1.29	1.01	0.98
Pneumonia Care				
Appropriate Initial Antibiotic Given[7]	-	-	96%	95%
Blood Culture Timing[7]	-	-	98%	98%
Pregnancy and Delivery Care				
Newborn Deliveries Scheduled Early[7]	-	-	4%	6%
Preventive Care				
Immunization for Influenza[2]	276	69%	91%	90%
Immunization for Pneumonia[2]	183	93%	92%	92%
Stroke Care				
Anticoagulation Therapy for Atrial Fibrillation[3,7]	-	-	96%	95%
Antithrombotic Therapy Timing[3,7]	-	-	98%	98%
Assessed for Rehabilitation[1,3]	-	-	98%	97%
Discharged on Antithrombotic Therapy[1,3]	-	-	99%	99%
Discharged on Statin Medication[1,3]	-	-	95%	94%
Thrombolytic Therapy Timing[3,7]	-	-	72%	66%
Venous Thromboembolism Prophylaxis[1,3]	-	-	95%	94%
Written Stroke Educational Materials Given[1,3]	-	-	90%	88%
Surgical Care Improvement Project				
Appropriate Beta Blocker Usage	27	96%	98%	98%
Appropriate VTP Within 24 Hours	156	94%	99%	98%
Controlled Postoperative Blood Glucose[7]	-	-	98%	97%
Perioperative Temperature Management	162	100%	100%	100%
Prophylactic Antibiotic Selection	49	92%	99%	99%
Prophylactic Antibiotic Selection (Outpatient)	16	94%	98%	98%
Prophylactic Antibiotic Stopped	38	89%	98%	98%
Prophylactic Antibiotic Timing	49	86%	99%	99%
Prophylactic Antibiotic Timing (Outpatient)	17	94%	98%	98%
Urinary Catheter Removal	53	89%	99%	97%
Survey of Patients' Hospital Experiences				
Area Around Room 'Always' Quiet at Night	(a)	56%	54%	61%
Doctors 'Always' Communicated Well	(a)	88%	80%	82%
Home Recovery Information Given	(a)	92%	86%	85%
Hospital Given 9 or 10 on 10 Point Scale	(a)	87%	69%	71%
Meds 'Always' Explained Before Given	(a)	73%	63%	64%
Nurses 'Always' Communicated Well	(a)	85%	79%	79%
Pain 'Always' Well Controlled	(a)	74%	70%	71%
Room and Bathroom 'Always' Clean	(a)	79%	73%	73%
Timely Help 'Always' Received	(a)	70%	67%	68%
Would Definitely Recommend Hospital	(a)	93%	70%	71%
Use of Medical Imaging				
Cardiac Imaging Stress Test before Surgery[7]	-	-	5.4%	5.3%
Combination Abdominal CT Scan	375	54.1%	12.2%	10.5%
Combination Brain/Sinus CT Scan[7]	-	-	3.1%	2.7%
Combination Chest CT Scan	437	0.5%	2.1%	2.7%
Follow-up Mammogram/Ultrasound[1]	-	-	9%	8.8%
Lumbar Spine MRI for Low Back Pain[7]	-	-	35.8%	37.2%

Chestnut Hill Hospital

8835 Germantown Ave
Philadelphia, PA 19118
URL: www.chh.org
Phone: 215-248-8200
Fax: 215-248-8053
Type: Acute Care Hospitals
Emergency Services: Yes
Ownership: Proprietary
Beds: 200

Key Personnel:
Radiology. . . . . Kevin Byrne
Quality Assurance . . . . James Danihel
Emergency Room . . . . Ann Mary Pata
Chief of Medical Staff . . . . John Scanlon
CEO/President. . . . . Brooks Turkel

Measure	Cases	This Hosp.	State Avg.	U.S. Avg.
Blood Clot Prevention and Treatment				
Anticoagulation Overlap Therapy[2]	99	99%	94%	93%
ICU Venous Thromboembolism Prophylaxis[2]	85	99%	94%	92%
Incidence of Potentially Preventable VTE[2]	14	21%	8%	10%
UFH with Dosages/Platelet Monitoring[2]	89	100%	98%	97%
Venous Thromboembolism Prophylaxis[2]	486	98%	90%	85%
Warfarin Therapy Discharge Instructions[2]	60	98%	78%	75%
Chest Pain/Possible Heart Attack Care				
Aspirin Given Within 24 Hours of Arrival	82	99%	97%	96%
Fibrinolytic Meds Within 30 Min. of Arrival[1]	-	-	44%	58%
Average Time to ECG (minutes)	85	6	9	7
Average Time to Transfer (minutes)	31	55	64	60
Children's Asthma Care				
Received Home Management Plan of Care	-	-	-	88%
Received Reliever Medication	-	-	-	100%
Received Systemic Corticosteroids	-	-	-	100%
Emergency Department				
Admittance Decision Time (minutes)[2]	1,179	99	104	98
Head CT Results Within 45 Min. of Arrival	26	85%	60%	57%
Patients Who Left ER Before Being Seen	32,723	1%	1%	2%
Time from ER Arrival to Admit. (minutes)[2]	1,179	258	276	274
Time from ER Arrival to Discharge (minutes)	373	133	125	134
Time in ER Before Being Evaluated (minutes)	420	25	26	26
Time to Pain Meds for Fractures (minutes)	136	59	58	57
Heart Attack Care				
Aspirin Given at Discharge	25	96%	99%	99%
Fibrinolytic Meds Within 30 Min. of Arrival[7]	-	-	40%	54%
PCI Within 90 Minutes of Arrival[7]	-	-	97%	96%
Statin Prescribed at Discharge	22	91%	99%	98%
Heart Failure Care				
ACE Inhibitor or ARB for LVSD	103	100%	97%	97%
Discharge Instructions Given	180	98%	96%	94%
Evaluation of LVS Function	281	100%	100%	99%
Medicare Spending				
Medicare Spending per Patient (ratio)	-	1.05	1.01	0.98
Pneumonia Care				
Appropriate Initial Antibiotic Given	92	92%	96%	95%
Blood Culture Timing	182	97%	98%	98%
Pregnancy and Delivery Care				
Newborn Deliveries Scheduled Early[2,7]	-	-	4%	6%
Preventive Care				
Immunization for Influenza[2]	668	97%	91%	90%
Immunization for Pneumonia[2]	1,049	94%	92%	92%
Stroke Care				
Anticoagulation Therapy for Atrial Fibrillation[1]	-	-	96%	95%
Antithrombotic Therapy Timing	100	100%	98%	98%
Assessed for Rehabilitation	100	97%	98%	97%
Discharged on Antithrombotic Therapy	99	100%	99%	99%
Discharged on Statin Medication	70	94%	95%	94%
Thrombolytic Therapy Timing[7]	-	-	72%	66%
Venous Thromboembolism Prophylaxis	101	95%	95%	94%
Written Stroke Educational Materials Given	48	92%	90%	88%
Surgical Care Improvement Project				
Appropriate Beta Blocker Usage	36	94%	98%	98%
Appropriate VTP Within 24 Hours	195	99%	99%	98%
Controlled Postoperative Blood Glucose[7]	-	-	98%	97%
Perioperative Temperature Management	274	100%	100%	100%
Prophylactic Antibiotic Selection	120	100%	99%	99%
Prophylactic Antibiotic Selection (Outpatient)	47	96%	98%	98%
Prophylactic Antibiotic Stopped	119	100%	98%	98%

NOTE: Hospital profiles are in alphabetical order by state, then city, then hospital within the city; Rankings exclude hospitals with less than 25 cases except for patient surveys which excludes hospitals with less than 100 cases; (a) 100-299 cases; (1) The number of cases/patients is too few to report; (2) Data submitted were based on a sample of cases/patients; (3) Results are based on a shorter time period than required; (4) Data suppressed by CMS for one or more quarters; (5) Results are not available for this reporting period; (6) Fewer than 100 patients completed the HCAHPS survey; (7) No cases met the criteria for this measure; (8) The lower limit of the confidence interval cannot be calculated if the number of observed infections equals zero; (9) No data are available from the state/territory for this reporting period; (10) The scores shown reflect fewer than 50 completed surveys; (11) There were discrepancies in the data collection process; (12) This measure does not apply to this hospital for this reporting period; (13) Results cannot be calculated for this reporting period; (14) The results for this state are combined with nearby states to protect confidentiality; Please refer to the User's Guide for a full explanation of data.

Measure	Cases	This Hosp.	State Avg.	U.S. Avg.
Prophylactic Antibiotic Timing	120	98%	99%	99%
Prophylactic Antibiotic Timing (Outpatient)	47	100%	98%	98%
Urinary Catheter Removal	108	100%	99%	97%
Survey of Patients' Hospital Experiences				
Area Around Room 'Always' Quiet at Night	300+	55%	54%	61%
Doctors 'Always' Communicated Well	300+	80%	80%	82%
Home Recovery Information Given	300+	83%	86%	85%
Hospital Given 9 or 10 on 10 Point Scale	300+	68%	69%	71%
Meds 'Always' Explained Before Given	300+	65%	63%	64%
Nurses 'Always' Communicated Well	300+	77%	79%	79%
Pain 'Always' Well Controlled	300+	72%	70%	71%
Room and Bathroom 'Always' Clean	300+	66%	73%	73%
Timely Help 'Always' Received	300+	56%	67%	68%
Would Definitely Recommend Hospital	300+	66%	70%	71%
Use of Medical Imaging				
Cardiac Imaging Stress Test before Surgery	86	3.5%	5.4%	5.3%
Combination Abdominal CT Scan	512	6.8%	12.2%	10.5%
Combination Brain/Sinus CT Scan	729	3.2%	3.1%	2.7%
Combination Chest CT Scan	339	0.9%	2.1%	2.7%
Follow-up Mammogram/Ultrasound	1,963	7.6%	9%	8.8%
Lumbar Spine MRI for Low Back Pain	75	33.3%	35.8%	37.2%

Children's Hospital of Philadelphia

34th Saint & Civic Center Blvd
Philadelphia, PA 19104
Phone: 215-590-3745
Fax: 215-860-4090
URL: www.chop.edu
Type: Childrens
Emergency Services: Yes
Ownership: Voluntary non-profit - Private
Beds: 430

Key Personnel:
Radiology.................... Kenneth E Fellows, Jr, DM
CEO/President................ Edmond Notebaert

Measure	Cases	This Hosp.	State Avg.	U.S. Avg.
Blood Clot Prevention and Treatment				
Anticoagulation Overlap Therapy[5]	-	-	94%	93%
ICU Venous Thromboembolism Prophylaxis[5]	-	-	94%	92%
Incidence of Potentially Preventable VTE[5]	-	-	8%	10%
UFH with Dosages/Platelet Monitoring[5]	-	-	98%	97%
Venous Thromboembolism Prophylaxis[5]	-	-	90%	85%
Warfarin Therapy Discharge Instructions[5]	-	-	78%	75%
Chest Pain/Possible Heart Attack Care				
Aspirin Given Within 24 Hours of Arrival	-	-	97%	96%
Fibrinolytic Meds Within 30 Min. of Arrival	-	-	44%	58%
Average Time to ECG (minutes)	-	-	9	7
Average Time to Transfer (minutes)	-	-	64	60
Children's Asthma Care				
Received Home Management Plan of Care[2]	757	91%	-	88%
Received Reliever Medication[2]	757	100%	-	100%
Received Systemic Corticosteroids[2]	755	100%	-	100%
Emergency Department				
Admittance Decision Time (minutes)[5]	-	-	104	98
Head CT Results Within 45 Min. of Arrival	-	-	60%	57%
Patients Who Left ER Before Being Seen	-	-	1%	2%
Time from ER Arrival to Admit. (minutes)[5]	-	-	276	274
Time from ER Arrival to Discharge (minutes)	-	-	125	134
Time in ER Before Being Evaluated (minutes)	-	-	26	26
Time to Pain Meds for Fractures (minutes)	-	-	58	57
Heart Attack Care				
Aspirin Given at Discharge[5]	-	-	99%	99%
Fibrinolytic Meds Within 30 Min. of Arrival[5]	-	-	40%	54%
PCI Within 90 Minutes of Arrival[5]	-	-	97%	96%
Statin Prescribed at Discharge[5]	-	-	99%	98%
Heart Failure Care				
ACE Inhibitor or ARB for LVSD[5]	-	-	97%	97%
Discharge Instructions Given[5]	-	-	96%	94%
Evaluation of LVS Function[5]	-	-	100%	99%
Medicare Spending				
Medicare Spending per Patient (ratio)	-	-	1.01	0.98
Pneumonia Care				
Appropriate Initial Antibiotic Given[5]	-	-	96%	95%
Blood Culture Timing[5]	-	-	98%	98%
Pregnancy and Delivery Care				
Newborn Deliveries Scheduled Early[5]	-	-	4%	6%
Preventive Care				
Immunization for Influenza[5]	-	-	91%	90%
Immunization for Pneumonia[5]	-	-	92%	92%
Stroke Care				
Anticoagulation Therapy for Atrial Fibrillation[5]	-	-	96%	95%
Antithrombotic Therapy Timing[5]	-	-	98%	98%
Assessed for Rehabilitation[5]	-	-	98%	97%
Discharged on Antithrombotic Therapy[5]	-	-	99%	99%
Discharged on Statin Medication[5]	-	-	95%	94%
Thrombolytic Therapy Timing[5]	-	-	72%	66%
Venous Thromboembolism Prophylaxis[5]	-	-	95%	94%
Written Stroke Educational Materials Given[5]	-	-	90%	88%
Surgical Care Improvement Project				
Appropriate Beta Blocker Usage[5]	-	-	98%	98%
Appropriate VTP Within 24 Hours[5]	-	-	99%	98%
Controlled Postoperative Blood Glucose[5]	-	-	98%	97%
Perioperative Temperature Management[5]	-	-	100%	100%
Prophylactic Antibiotic Selection[5]	-	-	99%	99%
Prophylactic Antibiotic Selection (Outpatient)	-	-	98%	98%
Prophylactic Antibiotic Stopped[5]	-	-	98%	98%
Prophylactic Antibiotic Timing[5]	-	-	99%	99%
Prophylactic Antibiotic Timing (Outpatient)	-	-	98%	98%
Urinary Catheter Removal[5]	-	-	99%	97%
Survey of Patients' Hospital Experiences				
Area Around Room 'Always' Quiet at Night[5]	-	-	54%	61%
Doctors 'Always' Communicated Well[5]	-	-	80%	82%
Home Recovery Information Given[5]	-	-	86%	85%
Hospital Given 9 or 10 on 10 Point Scale[5]	-	-	69%	71%
Meds 'Always' Explained Before Given[5]	-	-	63%	64%
Nurses 'Always' Communicated Well[5]	-	-	79%	79%
Pain 'Always' Well Controlled[5]	-	-	70%	71%
Room and Bathroom 'Always' Clean[5]	-	-	73%	73%
Timely Help 'Always' Received[5]	-	-	67%	68%
Would Definitely Recommend Hospital[5]	-	-	70%	71%
Use of Medical Imaging				
Cardiac Imaging Stress Test before Surgery	-	-	5.4%	5.3%
Combination Abdominal CT Scan	-	-	12.2%	10.5%
Combination Brain/Sinus CT Scan	-	-	3.1%	2.7%
Combination Chest CT Scan	-	-	2.1%	2.7%
Follow-up Mammogram/Ultrasound	-	-	9%	8.8%
Lumbar Spine MRI for Low Back Pain	-	-	35.8%	37.2%

Hahnemann University Hospital

230 North Broad Street
Philadelphia, PA 19102
Phone: 215-762-7000
Fax: 215-762-8109
URL: www.hahnemannhospital.com
Type: Acute Care Hospitals
Emergency Services: Yes
Ownership: Proprietary
Beds: 540

Key Personnel:
Infection Control............... Kathy Arias
Pediatric In-Patient Care .... James DeMarco
Chief of Medical Staff .... Jeffrey Glassroth
CEO/President.............. Michael Halter, FACHE
Quality Assurance .... Doug McCusker
Emergency Room .... Phillip Mead, MD
Radiology.................... Charles Mulhern
Operating Room............... Patty Robertson

Measure	Cases	This Hosp.	State Avg.	U.S. Avg.
Blood Clot Prevention and Treatment				
Anticoagulation Overlap Therapy[2]	92	91%	94%	93%
ICU Venous Thromboembolism Prophylaxis[2]	76	97%	94%	92%
Incidence of Potentially Preventable VTE[2]	32	9%	8%	10%
UFH with Dosages/Platelet Monitoring[2]	83	67%	98%	97%
Venous Thromboembolism Prophylaxis[2]	348	87%	90%	85%
Warfarin Therapy Discharge Instructions[2]	79	58%	78%	75%
Chest Pain/Possible Heart Attack Care				
Aspirin Given Within 24 Hours of Arrival[3,7]	-	-	97%	96%
Fibrinolytic Meds Within 30 Min. of Arrival[5]	-	-	44%	58%
Average Time to ECG (minutes)[3,7]	-	-	9	7
Average Time to Transfer (minutes)[5]	-	-	64	60
Children's Asthma Care				
Received Home Management Plan of Care	-	-	-	88%
Received Reliever Medication	-	-	-	100%
Received Systemic Corticosteroids	-	-	-	100%
Emergency Department				
Admittance Decision Time (minutes)[2]	585	139	104	98
Head CT Results Within 45 Min. of Arrival[1]	-	-	60%	57%
Patients Who Left ER Before Being Seen	47,475	2%	1%	2%
Time from ER Arrival to Admit. (minutes)[2]	590	334	276	274
Time from ER Arrival to Discharge (minutes)	353	143	125	134
Time in ER Before Being Evaluated (minutes)	403	31	26	26
Time to Pain Meds for Fractures (minutes)	36	52	58	57
Heart Attack Care				
Aspirin Given at Discharge	206	99%	99%	99%
Fibrinolytic Meds Within 30 Min. of Arrival[7]	-	-	40%	54%
PCI Within 90 Minutes of Arrival	15	100%	97%	96%
Statin Prescribed at Discharge	214	98%	99%	98%
Heart Failure Care				
ACE Inhibitor or ARB for LVSD	257	98%	97%	97%
Discharge Instructions Given	493	98%	96%	94%
Evaluation of LVS Function	540	100%	100%	99%
Medicare Spending				
Medicare Spending per Patient (ratio)	-	1.03	1.01	0.98
Pneumonia Care				
Appropriate Initial Antibiotic Given	94	96%	96%	95%
Blood Culture Timing	232	99%	98%	98%
Pregnancy and Delivery Care				
Newborn Deliveries Scheduled Early[2]	38	0%	4%	6%
Preventive Care				
Immunization for Influenza[2]	578	98%	91%	90%
Immunization for Pneumonia[2]	649	94%	92%	92%
Stroke Care				
Anticoagulation Therapy for Atrial Fibrillation	11	100%	96%	95%
Antithrombotic Therapy Timing	96	97%	98%	98%
Assessed for Rehabilitation	106	100%	98%	97%
Discharged on Antithrombotic Therapy	94	100%	99%	99%
Discharged on Statin Medication	71	97%	95%	94%
Thrombolytic Therapy Timing[1]	-	-	72%	66%
Venous Thromboembolism Prophylaxis	122	100%	95%	94%
Written Stroke Educational Materials Given	60	100%	90%	88%
Surgical Care Improvement Project				
Appropriate Beta Blocker Usage[2]	144	95%	98%	98%
Appropriate VTP Within 24 Hours[2]	388	99%	99%	98%
Controlled Postoperative Blood Glucose[2]	61	95%	98%	97%
Perioperative Temperature Management[2]	503	100%	100%	100%
Prophylactic Antibiotic Selection[2]	429	99%	99%	99%
Prophylactic Antibiotic Selection (Outpatient)	421	98%	98%	98%
Prophylactic Antibiotic Stopped[2]	420	96%	98%	98%
Prophylactic Antibiotic Timing[2]	431	97%	99%	99%
Prophylactic Antibiotic Timing (Outpatient)	408	99%	98%	98%
Urinary Catheter Removal[2]	325	98%	99%	97%
Survey of Patients' Hospital Experiences				
Area Around Room 'Always' Quiet at Night	300+	58%	54%	61%
Doctors 'Always' Communicated Well	300+	81%	80%	82%
Home Recovery Information Given	300+	81%	86%	85%
Hospital Given 9 or 10 on 10 Point Scale	300+	66%	69%	71%
Meds 'Always' Explained Before Given	300+	67%	63%	64%
Nurses 'Always' Communicated Well	300+	78%	79%	79%
Pain 'Always' Well Controlled	300+	71%	70%	71%
Room and Bathroom 'Always' Clean	300+	64%	73%	73%
Timely Help 'Always' Received	300+	61%	67%	68%
Would Definitely Recommend Hospital	300+	68%	70%	71%
Use of Medical Imaging				
Cardiac Imaging Stress Test before Surgery	144	6.9%	5.4%	5.3%
Combination Abdominal CT Scan	344	5.8%	12.2%	10.5%
Combination Brain/Sinus CT Scan[1]	-	-	3.1%	2.7%
Combination Chest CT Scan	275	0.7%	2.1%	2.7%
Follow-up Mammogram/Ultrasound	549	5.1%	9%	8.8%
Lumbar Spine MRI for Low Back Pain	62	33.9%	35.8%	37.2%

Hospital of Univ of Pennsylvania

34th & Spruce Sts
Philadelphia, PA 19104
Phone: 215-662-3227
Fax: 215-349-5864
URL: www.upenn.edu
Type: Acute Care Hospitals
Emergency Services: Yes
Ownership: Voluntary non-profit - Private
Beds: 725

Key Personnel:
Emergency Room .... William Baxt, MD
Radiology.................... R Nick Bryan, MD

NOTE: Hospital profiles are in alphabetical order by state, then city, then hospital within the city; Rankings exclude hospitals with less than 25 cases except for patient surveys which excludes hospitals with less than 100 cases; (a) 100-299 cases; (1) The number of cases/patients is too few to report; (2) Data submitted were based on a sample of cases/patients; (3) Results are based on a shorter time period than required; (4) Data suppressed by CMS for one or more quarters; (5) Results are not available for this reporting period; (6) Fewer than 100 patients completed the HCAHPS survey; (7) No cases met the criteria for this measure; (8) The lower limit of the confidence interval cannot be calculated if the number of observed infections equals zero; (9) No data are available from the state/territory for this reporting period; (10) The scores shown reflect fewer than 50 completed surveys; (11) There were discrepancies in the data collection process; (12) This measure does not apply to this hospital for this reporting period; (13) Results cannot be calculated for this reporting period; (14) The results for this state are combined with nearby states to protect confidentiality; Please refer to the User's Guide for a full explanation of data.

Infection Control. . . . . Harvey Friedman, MD
Chief of Medical Staff. . . . . Stanley Goldfarb, MD
President . . . . Amy Gutmann
CEO/President. . . . . Robert D Marlin
Operating Room. . . . . Noreen McHugh, RN
Quality Assurance . . . . Mary Ellen Nepps

Measure	Cases	This Hosp.	State Avg.	U.S. Avg.
Blood Clot Prevention and Treatment				
Anticoagulation Overlap Therapy[2]	233	95%	94%	93%
ICU Venous Thromboembolism Prophylaxis[2]	123	100%	94%	92%
Incidence of Potentially Preventable VTE[2]	126	3%	8%	10%
UFH with Dosages/Platelet Monitoring[2]	222	100%	98%	97%
Venous Thromboembolism Prophylaxis[2]	296	100%	90%	85%
Warfarin Therapy Discharge Instructions[2]	153	10%	78%	75%
Chest Pain/Possible Heart Attack Care				
Aspirin Given Within 24 Hours of Arrival[5]	-	-	97%	96%
Fibrinolytic Meds Within 30 Min. of Arrival[5]	-	-	44%	58%
Average Time to ECG (minutes)[5]	-	-	9	7
Average Time to Transfer (minutes)[5]	-	-	64	60
Children's Asthma Care				
Received Home Management Plan of Care	-	-	-	88%
Received Reliever Medication	-	-	-	100%
Received Systemic Corticosteroids	-	-	-	100%
Emergency Department				
Admittance Decision Time (minutes)[2]	332	165	104	98
Head CT Results Within 45 Min. of Arrival[1,3]	-	-	60%	57%
Patients Who Left ER Before Being Seen	67,086	4%	1%	2%
Time from ER Arrival to Admit. (minutes)[2]	337	418	276	274
Time from ER Arrival to Discharge (minutes)	343	195	125	134
Time in ER Before Being Evaluated (minutes)	289	66	26	26
Time to Pain Meds for Fractures (minutes)	39	50	58	57
Heart Attack Care				
Aspirin Given at Discharge	212	100%	99%	99%
Fibrinolytic Meds Within 30 Min. of Arrival[7]	-	-	40%	54%
PCI Within 90 Minutes of Arrival	18	100%	97%	96%
Statin Prescribed at Discharge	207	100%	99%	98%
Heart Failure Care				
ACE Inhibitor or ARB for LVSD[2]	358	100%	97%	97%
Discharge Instructions Given[2]	642	100%	96%	94%
Evaluation of LVS Function[2]	728	100%	100%	99%
Medicare Spending				
Medicare Spending per Patient (ratio)	-	1.02	1.01	0.98
Pneumonia Care				
Appropriate Initial Antibiotic Given	57	98%	96%	95%
Blood Culture Timing	205	99%	98%	98%
Pregnancy and Delivery Care				
Newborn Deliveries Scheduled Early[2]	72	1%	4%	6%
Preventive Care				
Immunization for Influenza[2]	527	83%	91%	90%
Immunization for Pneumonia[2]	509	78%	92%	92%
Stroke Care				
Anticoagulation Therapy for Atrial Fibrillation	39	100%	96%	95%
Antithrombotic Therapy Timing	187	98%	98%	98%
Assessed for Rehabilitation	296	100%	98%	97%
Discharged on Antithrombotic Therapy	224	100%	99%	99%
Discharged on Statin Medication	171	99%	95%	94%
Thrombolytic Therapy Timing	18	83%	72%	66%
Venous Thromboembolism Prophylaxis	309	98%	95%	94%
Written Stroke Educational Materials Given	142	91%	90%	88%
Surgical Care Improvement Project				
Appropriate Beta Blocker Usage[2]	464	100%	98%	98%
Appropriate VTP Within 24 Hours[2]	478	100%	99%	98%
Controlled Postoperative Blood Glucose[2]	342	98%	98%	97%
Perioperative Temperature Management[2]	654	100%	100%	100%
Prophylactic Antibiotic Selection[2]	574	99%	99%	99%
Prophylactic Antibiotic Selection (Outpatient)	667	92%	98%	98%
Prophylactic Antibiotic Stopped[2]	527	100%	98%	98%
Prophylactic Antibiotic Timing[2]	576	100%	99%	99%
Prophylactic Antibiotic Timing (Outpatient)	631	94%	98%	98%
Urinary Catheter Removal[2]	463	100%	99%	97%
Survey of Patients' Hospital Experiences				
Area Around Room 'Always' Quiet at Night	300+	47%	54%	61%
Doctors 'Always' Communicated Well	300+	79%	80%	82%
Home Recovery Information Given	300+	90%	86%	85%
Hospital Given 9 or 10 on 10 Point Scale	300+	75%	69%	71%
Meds 'Always' Explained Before Given	300+	65%	63%	64%
Nurses 'Always' Communicated Well	300+	80%	79%	79%
Pain 'Always' Well Controlled	300+	70%	70%	71%
Room and Bathroom 'Always' Clean	300+	68%	73%	73%
Timely Help 'Always' Received	300+	64%	67%	68%
Would Definitely Recommend Hospital	300+	80%	70%	71%
Use of Medical Imaging				
Cardiac Imaging Stress Test before Surgery	852	5.2%	5.4%	5.3%
Combination Abdominal CT Scan	2,448	10.7%	12.2%	10.5%
Combination Brain/Sinus CT Scan[1]	-	-	3.1%	2.7%
Combination Chest CT Scan	3,972	0.1%	2.1%	2.7%
Follow-up Mammogram/Ultrasound	3,324	7.1%	9%	8.8%
Lumbar Spine MRI for Low Back Pain	317	33.8%	35.8%	37.2%

Jeanes Hospital

7600 Central Avenue
Philadelphia, PA 19111
Phone: 215-728-2000
Fax: 215-728-3345
E-mail: information.jeanes@tuhs.temple.edu
URL: www.jeanes.com
Type: Acute Care Hospitals
Emergency Services: Yes
Ownership: Voluntary non-profit - Private
Beds: 197

Key Personnel:
Emergency Room . . . . Lawrence Albert
Operating Room. . . . . Carole Campbell
Quality Assurance . . . . Deborah Dunaj
President/CEO. . . . . Linda J. Grass
Anesthesiology. . . . . Subash Reddy, MD
Chief of Medical Staff. . . . . Joel Weissman
Infection Control. . . . . Simone Woodwell
Patient Relations . . . . Sally Ziska

Measure	Cases	This Hosp.	State Avg.	U.S. Avg.
Blood Clot Prevention and Treatment				
Anticoagulation Overlap Therapy[2]	49	80%	94%	93%
ICU Venous Thromboembolism Prophylaxis[2]	118	67%	94%	92%
Incidence of Potentially Preventable VTE[2]	18	17%	8%	10%
UFH with Dosages/Platelet Monitoring[2]	47	100%	98%	97%
Venous Thromboembolism Prophylaxis[2]	353	79%	90%	85%
Warfarin Therapy Discharge Instructions[2]	35	9%	78%	75%
Chest Pain/Possible Heart Attack Care				
Aspirin Given Within 24 Hours of Arrival[1,3]	-	-	97%	96%
Fibrinolytic Meds Within 30 Min. of Arrival[5]	-	-	44%	58%
Average Time to ECG (minutes)[1,3]	-	-	9	7
Average Time to Transfer (minutes)[5]	-	-	64	60
Children's Asthma Care				
Received Home Management Plan of Care	-	-	-	88%
Received Reliever Medication	-	-	-	100%
Received Systemic Corticosteroids	-	-	-	100%
Emergency Department				
Admittance Decision Time (minutes)[2]	960	113	104	98
Head CT Results Within 45 Min. of Arrival	19	32%	60%	57%
Patients Who Left ER Before Being Seen	36,027	4%	1%	2%
Time from ER Arrival to Admit. (minutes)[2]	960	298	276	274
Time from ER Arrival to Discharge (minutes)	328	172	125	134
Time in ER Before Being Evaluated (minutes)	363	59	26	26
Time to Pain Meds for Fractures (minutes)	104	80	58	57
Heart Attack Care				
Aspirin Given at Discharge	162	99%	99%	99%
Fibrinolytic Meds Within 30 Min. of Arrival[7]	-	-	40%	54%
PCI Within 90 Minutes of Arrival	18	100%	97%	96%
Statin Prescribed at Discharge	149	95%	99%	98%
Heart Failure Care				
ACE Inhibitor or ARB for LVSD	113	95%	97%	97%
Discharge Instructions Given	286	100%	96%	94%
Evaluation of LVS Function	370	99%	100%	99%
Medicare Spending				
Medicare Spending per Patient (ratio)	-	1.09	1.01	0.98
Pneumonia Care				
Appropriate Initial Antibiotic Given[2]	152	95%	96%	95%
Blood Culture Timing[2]	169	95%	98%	98%
Pregnancy and Delivery Care				
Newborn Deliveries Scheduled Early[7]	-	-	4%	6%
Preventive Care				
Immunization for Influenza[2]	592	92%	91%	90%
Immunization for Pneumonia[2]	844	90%	92%	92%
Stroke Care				
Anticoagulation Therapy for Atrial Fibrillation[1]	-	-	96%	95%
Antithrombotic Therapy Timing	84	100%	98%	98%
Assessed for Rehabilitation	86	98%	98%	97%
Discharged on Antithrombotic Therapy	84	100%	99%	99%
Discharged on Statin Medication	64	94%	95%	94%
Thrombolytic Therapy Timing[1]	-	-	72%	66%
Venous Thromboembolism Prophylaxis	85	98%	95%	94%
Written Stroke Educational Materials Given	46	91%	90%	88%
Surgical Care Improvement Project				
Appropriate Beta Blocker Usage	205	100%	98%	98%
Appropriate VTP Within 24 Hours	431	100%	99%	98%
Controlled Postoperative Blood Glucose	72	97%	98%	97%
Perioperative Temperature Management	503	100%	100%	100%
Prophylactic Antibiotic Selection	439	99%	99%	99%
Prophylactic Antibiotic Selection (Outpatient)	112	92%	98%	98%
Prophylactic Antibiotic Stopped	430	98%	98%	98%
Prophylactic Antibiotic Timing	440	100%	99%	99%
Prophylactic Antibiotic Timing (Outpatient)	95	98%	98%	98%
Urinary Catheter Removal	294	98%	99%	97%
Survey of Patients' Hospital Experiences				
Area Around Room 'Always' Quiet at Night	300+	47%	54%	61%
Doctors 'Always' Communicated Well	300+	76%	80%	82%
Home Recovery Information Given	300+	80%	86%	85%
Hospital Given 9 or 10 on 10 Point Scale	300+	66%	69%	71%
Meds 'Always' Explained Before Given	300+	60%	63%	64%
Nurses 'Always' Communicated Well	300+	74%	79%	79%
Pain 'Always' Well Controlled	300+	69%	70%	71%
Room and Bathroom 'Always' Clean	300+	65%	73%	73%
Timely Help 'Always' Received	300+	63%	67%	68%
Would Definitely Recommend Hospital	300+	66%	70%	71%
Use of Medical Imaging				
Cardiac Imaging Stress Test before Surgery	293	8.2%	5.4%	5.3%
Combination Abdominal CT Scan	648	8.6%	12.2%	10.5%
Combination Brain/Sinus CT Scan[1]	-	-	3.1%	2.7%
Combination Chest CT Scan	331	0.9%	2.1%	2.7%
Follow-up Mammogram/Ultrasound	1,115	12.3%	9%	8.8%
Lumbar Spine MRI for Low Back Pain[1]	-	-	35.8%	37.2%

Kensington Hospital

136 W Diamond Street
Philadelphia, PA 19122
Phone: 215-426-8100
Fax: 215-291-6030
Type: Acute Care Hospitals
Emergency Services: No
Ownership: Voluntary non-profit - Other
Beds: 45

Key Personnel:
Infection Control. . . . . Judy Arentzen
Operating Room. . . . . Bill Mihal

Measure	Cases	This Hosp.	State Avg.	U.S. Avg.
Blood Clot Prevention and Treatment				
Anticoagulation Overlap Therapy[7]	-	-	94%	93%
ICU Venous Thromboembolism Prophylaxis[7]	-	-	94%	92%
Incidence of Potentially Preventable VTE[7]	-	-	8%	10%
UFH with Dosages/Platelet Monitoring[7]	-	-	98%	97%
Venous Thromboembolism Prophylaxis	66	0%	90%	85%
Warfarin Therapy Discharge Instructions[7]	-	-	78%	75%
Chest Pain/Possible Heart Attack Care				
Aspirin Given Within 24 Hours of Arrival[5]	-	-	97%	96%
Fibrinolytic Meds Within 30 Min. of Arrival[5]	-	-	44%	58%
Average Time to ECG (minutes)[5]	-	-	9	7
Average Time to Transfer (minutes)[5]	-	-	64	60
Children's Asthma Care				
Received Home Management Plan of Care	-	-	-	88%
Received Reliever Medication	-	-	-	100%
Received Systemic Corticosteroids	-	-	-	100%
Emergency Department				
Admittance Decision Time (minutes)[2,7]	-	-	104	98
Head CT Results Within 45 Min. of Arrival[5]	-	-	60%	57%
Patients Who Left ER Before Being Seen[5]	-	-	1%	2%
Time from ER Arrival to Admit. (minutes)[2,7]	-	-	276	274
Time from ER Arrival to Discharge (minutes)[5]	-	-	125	134
Time in ER Before Being Evaluated (minutes)[5]	-	-	26	26

NOTE: Hospital profiles are in alphabetical order by state, then city, then hospital within the city; Rankings exclude hospitals with less than 25 cases except for patient surveys which excludes hospitals with less than 100 cases; (a) 100-299 cases; (1) The number of cases/patients is too few to report; (2) Data submitted were based on a sample of cases/patients; (3) Results are based on a shorter time period than required; (4) Data suppressed by CMS for one or more quarters; (5) Results are not available for this reporting period; (6) Fewer than 100 patients completed the HCAHPS survey; (7) No cases met the criteria for this measure; (8) The lower limit of the confidence interval cannot be calculated if the number of observed infections equals zero; (9) No data are available from the state/territory for this reporting period; (10) The scores shown reflect fewer than 50 completed surveys; (11) There were discrepancies in the data collection process; (12) This measure does not apply to this hospital for this reporting period; (13) Results cannot be calculated for this reporting period; (14) The results for this state are combined with nearby states to protect confidentiality; Please refer to the User's Guide for a full explanation of data.

Measure	Cases	This Hosp.	State Avg.	U.S. Avg.
Time to Pain Meds for Fractures (minutes)[5]	-	-	58	57
Heart Attack Care				
Aspirin Given at Discharge[5]	-	-	99%	99%
Fibrinolytic Meds Within 30 Min. of Arrival[5]	-	-	40%	54%
PCI Within 90 Minutes of Arrival[5]	-	-	97%	96%
Statin Prescribed at Discharge[5]	-	-	99%	98%
Heart Failure Care				
ACE Inhibitor or ARB for LVSD[5]	-	-	97%	97%
Discharge Instructions Given[5]	-	-	96%	94%
Evaluation of LVS Function[5]	-	-	100%	99%
Medicare Spending				
Medicare Spending per Patient (ratio)[1]	-	-	1.01	0.98
Pneumonia Care				
Appropriate Initial Antibiotic Given[5]	-	-	96%	95%
Blood Culture Timing[5]	-	-	98%	98%
Pregnancy and Delivery Care				
Newborn Deliveries Scheduled Early[2,7]	-	-	4%	6%
Preventive Care				
Immunization for Influenza[2]	47	2%	91%	90%
Immunization for Pneumonia[2]	38	0%	92%	92%
Stroke Care				
Anticoagulation Therapy for Atrial Fibrillation[5]	-	-	96%	95%
Antithrombotic Therapy Timing[5]	-	-	98%	98%
Assessed for Rehabilitation[5]	-	-	98%	97%
Discharged on Antithrombotic Therapy[5]	-	-	99%	99%
Discharged on Statin Medication[5]	-	-	95%	94%
Thrombolytic Therapy Timing[5]	-	-	72%	66%
Venous Thromboembolism Prophylaxis[5]	-	-	95%	94%
Written Stroke Educational Materials Given[5]	-	-	90%	88%
Surgical Care Improvement Project				
Appropriate Beta Blocker Usage[5]	-	-	98%	98%
Appropriate VTP Within 24 Hours[5]	-	-	99%	98%
Controlled Postoperative Blood Glucose[5]	-	-	98%	97%
Perioperative Temperature Management[5]	-	-	100%	100%
Prophylactic Antibiotic Selection[5]	-	-	99%	99%
Prophylactic Antibiotic Selection (Outpatient)[5]	-	-	98%	98%
Prophylactic Antibiotic Stopped[5]	-	-	98%	98%
Prophylactic Antibiotic Timing[5]	-	-	99%	99%
Prophylactic Antibiotic Timing (Outpatient)[5]	-	-	98%	98%
Urinary Catheter Removal[5]	-	-	99%	97%
Survey of Patients' Hospital Experiences				
Area Around Room 'Always' Quiet at Night[10]	<100	61%	54%	61%
Doctors 'Always' Communicated Well[10]	<100	54%	80%	82%
Home Recovery Information Given[10]	<100	39%	86%	85%
Hospital Given 9 or 10 on 10 Point Scale[10]	<100	10%	69%	71%
Meds 'Always' Explained Before Given[10]	<100	30%	63%	64%
Nurses 'Always' Communicated Well[10]	<100	45%	79%	79%
Pain 'Always' Well Controlled[10]	<100	7%	70%	71%
Room and Bathroom 'Always' Clean[10]	<100	82%	73%	73%
Timely Help 'Always' Received[10]	<100	68%	67%	68%
Would Definitely Recommend Hospital[10]	<100	49%	70%	71%
Use of Medical Imaging				
Cardiac Imaging Stress Test before Surgery[7]	-	-	5.4%	5.3%
Combination Abdominal CT Scan[7]	-	-	12.2%	10.5%
Combination Brain/Sinus CT Scan[7]	-	-	3.1%	2.7%
Combination Chest CT Scan[7]	-	-	2.1%	2.7%
Follow-up Mammogram/Ultrasound[7]	-	-	9%	8.8%
Lumbar Spine MRI for Low Back Pain[7]	-	-	35.8%	37.2%

Nazareth Hospital

2601 Holme Ave
Philadelphia, PA 19152
E-mail: info@nazarethhospital.org
URL: www.nazarethhospital.org
Type: Acute Care Hospitals
Ownership: Voluntary non-profit - Church
Phone: 215-335-6000
Fax: 215-335-6668
Emergency Services: Yes
Beds: 347

Key Personnel:
Quality Assurance . . . . Nancy Anderson
CEO/President. . . . . Pat DeAngelis
Chief of Medical Staff . . . . George Duber, MD
Emergency Room . . . . Trisha Harbison
Operating Room. . . . . Sandra Larson
Radiology. . . . . Donald Ostrum, MD

Measure	Cases	This Hosp.	State Avg.	U.S. Avg.
Blood Clot Prevention and Treatment				
Anticoagulation Overlap Therapy[2]	73	100%	94%	93%
ICU Venous Thromboembolism Prophylaxis[2]	59	98%	94%	92%
Incidence of Potentially Preventable VTE[1,2]	-	-	8%	10%
UFH with Dosages/Platelet Monitoring[2]	71	100%	98%	97%
Venous Thromboembolism Prophylaxis[2]	364	98%	90%	85%
Warfarin Therapy Discharge Instructions[2]	48	100%	78%	75%
Chest Pain/Possible Heart Attack Care				
Aspirin Given Within 24 Hours of Arrival[5]	-	-	97%	96%
Fibrinolytic Meds Within 30 Min. of Arrival[5]	-	-	44%	58%
Average Time to ECG (minutes)[5]	-	-	9	7
Average Time to Transfer (minutes)[5]	-	-	64	60
Children's Asthma Care				
Received Home Management Plan of Care	-	-	-	88%
Received Reliever Medication	-	-	-	100%
Received Systemic Corticosteroids	-	-	-	100%
Emergency Department				
Admittance Decision Time (minutes)[2]	1,080	196	104	98
Head CT Results Within 45 Min. of Arrival	17	82%	60%	57%
Patients Who Left ER Before Being Seen	45,289	2%	1%	2%
Time from ER Arrival to Admit. (minutes)[2]	1,080	374	276	274
Time from ER Arrival to Discharge (minutes)	344	134	125	134
Time in ER Before Being Evaluated (minutes)	405	42	26	26
Time to Pain Meds for Fractures (minutes)	134	76	58	57
Heart Attack Care				
Aspirin Given at Discharge	169	100%	99%	99%
Fibrinolytic Meds Within 30 Min. of Arrival[7]	-	-	40%	54%
PCI Within 90 Minutes of Arrival	18	67%	97%	96%
Statin Prescribed at Discharge	153	97%	99%	98%
Heart Failure Care				
ACE Inhibitor or ARB for LVSD	44	100%	97%	97%
Discharge Instructions Given	224	100%	96%	94%
Evaluation of LVS Function	369	100%	100%	99%
Medicare Spending				
Medicare Spending per Patient (ratio)	-	1.06	1.01	0.98
Pneumonia Care				
Appropriate Initial Antibiotic Given	145	99%	96%	95%
Blood Culture Timing	265	98%	98%	98%
Pregnancy and Delivery Care				
Newborn Deliveries Scheduled Early[7]	-	-	4%	6%
Preventive Care				
Immunization for Influenza[2]	602	93%	91%	90%
Immunization for Pneumonia[2]	903	89%	92%	92%
Stroke Care				
Anticoagulation Therapy for Atrial Fibrillation	14	93%	96%	95%
Antithrombotic Therapy Timing	178	100%	98%	98%
Assessed for Rehabilitation	190	98%	98%	97%
Discharged on Antithrombotic Therapy	177	100%	99%	99%
Discharged on Statin Medication	152	97%	95%	94%
Thrombolytic Therapy Timing[1]	-	-	72%	66%
Venous Thromboembolism Prophylaxis	192	98%	95%	94%
Written Stroke Educational Materials Given	77	97%	90%	88%
Surgical Care Improvement Project				
Appropriate Beta Blocker Usage	170	98%	98%	98%
Appropriate VTP Within 24 Hours	375	99%	99%	98%
Controlled Postoperative Blood Glucose[7]	-	-	98%	97%
Perioperative Temperature Management	428	100%	100%	100%
Prophylactic Antibiotic Selection	251	100%	99%	99%
Prophylactic Antibiotic Selection (Outpatient)	88	100%	98%	98%
Prophylactic Antibiotic Stopped	243	100%	98%	98%
Prophylactic Antibiotic Timing	252	100%	99%	99%
Prophylactic Antibiotic Timing (Outpatient)	88	100%	98%	98%
Urinary Catheter Removal	271	99%	99%	97%
Survey of Patients' Hospital Experiences				
Area Around Room 'Always' Quiet at Night	300+	49%	54%	61%
Doctors 'Always' Communicated Well	300+	66%	80%	82%
Home Recovery Information Given	300+	84%	86%	85%
Hospital Given 9 or 10 on 10 Point Scale	300+	57%	69%	71%
Meds 'Always' Explained Before Given	300+	51%	63%	64%
Nurses 'Always' Communicated Well	300+	72%	79%	79%
Pain 'Always' Well Controlled	300+	61%	70%	71%
Room and Bathroom 'Always' Clean	300+	65%	73%	73%
Timely Help 'Always' Received	300+	65%	67%	68%
Would Definitely Recommend Hospital	300+	59%	70%	71%
Use of Medical Imaging				
Cardiac Imaging Stress Test before Surgery	305	7.5%	5.4%	5.3%
Combination Abdominal CT Scan	448	4.2%	12.2%	10.5%
Combination Brain/Sinus CT Scan	577	5.9%	3.1%	2.7%
Combination Chest CT Scan	325	0.0%	2.1%	2.7%
Follow-up Mammogram/Ultrasound	443	13.3%	9%	8.8%
Lumbar Spine MRI for Low Back Pain	96	29.2%	35.8%	37.2%

Penn Presbyterian Medical Center

51 North 39th Street
Philadelphia, PA 19104
URL: www.pennhealth.com
Type: Acute Care Hospitals
Ownership: Voluntary non-profit - Other
Phone: 215-662-8000
Fax: 215-662-8936
Emergency Services: Yes
Beds: 344

Key Personnel:
Radiology. . . . . David Freiman, MD
Chief of Medical Staff . . . . Lawrence Gavin, MD
Operating Room. . . . . Barbara Schock
Emergency Room . . . . Cheryl Ann Smaller
Quality Assurance . . . . Rhoda Vaflor
CEO/President. . . . . Michele Volpe

Measure	Cases	This Hosp.	State Avg.	U.S. Avg.
Blood Clot Prevention and Treatment				
Anticoagulation Overlap Therapy[2]	108	98%	94%	93%
ICU Venous Thromboembolism Prophylaxis[2]	86	99%	94%	92%
Incidence of Potentially Preventable VTE[2]	11	0%	8%	10%
UFH with Dosages/Platelet Monitoring[2]	105	100%	98%	97%
Venous Thromboembolism Prophylaxis[2]	283	99%	90%	85%
Warfarin Therapy Discharge Instructions[2]	67	88%	78%	75%
Chest Pain/Possible Heart Attack Care				
Aspirin Given Within 24 Hours of Arrival[5]	-	-	97%	96%
Fibrinolytic Meds Within 30 Min. of Arrival[5]	-	-	44%	58%
Average Time to ECG (minutes)[5]	-	-	9	7
Average Time to Transfer (minutes)[5]	-	-	64	60
Children's Asthma Care				
Received Home Management Plan of Care	-	-	-	88%
Received Reliever Medication	-	-	-	100%
Received Systemic Corticosteroids	-	-	-	100%
Emergency Department				
Admittance Decision Time (minutes)[2]	706	145	104	98
Head CT Results Within 45 Min. of Arrival[1,3]	-	-	60%	57%
Patients Who Left ER Before Being Seen	38,723	2%	1%	2%
Time from ER Arrival to Admit. (minutes)[2]	732	326	276	274
Time from ER Arrival to Discharge (minutes)	1,311	154	125	134
Time in ER Before Being Evaluated (minutes)	949	67	26	26
Time to Pain Meds for Fractures (minutes)	47	102	58	57
Heart Attack Care				
Aspirin Given at Discharge[2]	306	100%	99%	99%
Fibrinolytic Meds Within 30 Min. of Arrival[2,7]	-	-	40%	54%
PCI Within 90 Minutes of Arrival[2,7]	-	-	97%	96%
Statin Prescribed at Discharge[2]	299	100%	99%	98%
Heart Failure Care				
ACE Inhibitor or ARB for LVSD[2]	132	100%	97%	97%
Discharge Instructions Given[2]	293	100%	96%	94%
Evaluation of LVS Function[2]	341	100%	100%	99%
Medicare Spending				
Medicare Spending per Patient (ratio)	-	0.99	1.01	0.98
Pneumonia Care				
Appropriate Initial Antibiotic Given[2]	57	100%	96%	95%
Blood Culture Timing[2]	120	99%	98%	98%
Pregnancy and Delivery Care				
Newborn Deliveries Scheduled Early[7]	-	-	4%	6%
Preventive Care				
Immunization for Influenza[2]	962	86%	91%	90%
Immunization for Pneumonia[2]	1,158	82%	92%	92%
Stroke Care				
Anticoagulation Therapy for Atrial Fibrillation[1]	-	-	96%	95%
Antithrombotic Therapy Timing	91	100%	98%	98%
Assessed for Rehabilitation	99	99%	98%	97%
Discharged on Antithrombotic Therapy	96	100%	99%	99%
Discharged on Statin Medication	85	99%	95%	94%
Thrombolytic Therapy Timing[1]	-	-	72%	66%

NOTE: Hospital profiles are in alphabetical order by state, then city, then hospital within the city; Rankings exclude hospitals with less than 25 cases except for patient surveys which excludes hospitals with less than 100 cases; (a) 100-299 cases; (1) The number of cases/patients is too few to report; (2) Data submitted were based on a sample of cases/patients; (3) Results are based on a shorter time period than required; (4) Data suppressed by CMS for one or more quarters; (5) Results are not available for this reporting period; (6) Fewer than 100 patients completed the HCAHPS survey; (7) No cases met the criteria for this measure; (8) The lower limit of the confidence interval cannot be calculated if the number of observed infections equals zero; (9) No data are available from the state/territory for this reporting period; (10) The scores shown reflect fewer than 50 completed surveys; (11) There were discrepancies in the data collection process; (12) This measure does not apply to this hospital for this reporting period; (13) Results cannot be calculated for this reporting period; (14) The results for this state are combined with nearby states to protect confidentiality; Please refer to the User's Guide for a full explanation of data.

Measure	Cases	This Hosp.	State Avg.	U.S. Avg.
Venous Thromboembolism Prophylaxis	103	99%	95%	94%
Written Stroke Educational Materials Given	43	93%	90%	88%
Surgical Care Improvement Project				
Appropriate Beta Blocker Usage[2]	745	99%	98%	98%
Appropriate VTP Within 24 Hours[2]	1,490	100%	99%	98%
Controlled Postoperative Blood Glucose[2]	392	96%	98%	97%
Perioperative Temperature Management[2]	1,978	100%	100%	100%
Prophylactic Antibiotic Selection[2]	1,511	100%	99%	99%
Prophylactic Antibiotic Selection (Outpatient)	309	91%	98%	98%
Prophylactic Antibiotic Stopped[2]	1,472	99%	98%	98%
Prophylactic Antibiotic Timing[2]	1,514	99%	99%	99%
Prophylactic Antibiotic Timing (Outpatient)	318	97%	98%	98%
Urinary Catheter Removal[2]	1,395	100%	99%	97%
Survey of Patients' Hospital Experiences				
Area Around Room 'Always' Quiet at Night	300+	55%	54%	61%
Doctors 'Always' Communicated Well	300+	81%	80%	82%
Home Recovery Information Given	300+	87%	86%	85%
Hospital Given 9 or 10 on 10 Point Scale	300+	72%	69%	71%
Meds 'Always' Explained Before Given	300+	65%	63%	64%
Nurses 'Always' Communicated Well	300+	80%	79%	79%
Pain 'Always' Well Controlled	300+	70%	70%	71%
Room and Bathroom 'Always' Clean	300+	68%	73%	73%
Timely Help 'Always' Received	300+	66%	67%	68%
Would Definitely Recommend Hospital	300+	73%	70%	71%
Use of Medical Imaging				
Cardiac Imaging Stress Test before Surgery	421	4.8%	5.4%	5.3%
Combination Abdominal CT Scan	317	2.5%	12.2%	10.5%
Combination Brain/Sinus CT Scan[1]	-	-	3.1%	2.7%
Combination Chest CT Scan	315	0.0%	2.1%	2.7%
Follow-up Mammogram/Ultrasound	236	9.7%	9%	8.8%
Lumbar Spine MRI for Low Back Pain[1]	-	-	35.8%	37.2%

Pennsylvania Hospital of the Univ of PA Health Sys

800 Spruce Street
Philadelphia, PA 19107
Phone: 215-829-3000
Fax: 215-349-8312
URL: www.pennmedicine.org/pahosp
Type: Acute Care Hospitals
Emergency Services: Yes
Ownership: Voluntary non-profit - Private
Beds: 520

Key Personnel:
Infection Control. . . . . Jessica Bunson
Anesthesiology. . . . . Jason Cwik, MD
Cardiac Laboratory. . . . . Howard C Herman, MD
Intensive Care Unit. . . . . Francis Kempf, MD
Radiology. . . . . Harold I Litt, MD, PhD
Hemotology Center . . . . David M Mintzer, MD
Emergency Room . . . . Kathleen Nasci, MD
Chief of Medical Staff. . . . . Charles Wolf, MD

Measure	Cases	This Hosp.	State Avg.	U.S. Avg.
Blood Clot Prevention and Treatment				
Anticoagulation Overlap Therapy[2]	74	100%	94%	93%
ICU Venous Thromboembolism Prophylaxis[2]	160	99%	94%	92%
Incidence of Potentially Preventable VTE[2]	35	0%	8%	10%
UFH with Dosages/Platelet Monitoring[2]	60	100%	98%	97%
Venous Thromboembolism Prophylaxis[2]	267	95%	90%	85%
Warfarin Therapy Discharge Instructions[2]	54	87%	78%	75%
Chest Pain/Possible Heart Attack Care				
Aspirin Given Within 24 Hours of Arrival[5]	-	-	97%	96%
Fibrinolytic Meds Within 30 Min. of Arrival[5]	-	-	44%	58%
Average Time to ECG (minutes)[5]	-	-	9	7
Average Time to Transfer (minutes)[5]	-	-	64	60
Children's Asthma Care				
Received Home Management Plan of Care	-	-	-	88%
Received Reliever Medication	-	-	-	100%
Received Systemic Corticosteroids	-	-	-	100%
Emergency Department				
Admittance Decision Time (minutes)[2]	358	186	104	98
Head CT Results Within 45 Min. of Arrival[1]	-	-	60%	57%
Patients Who Left ER Before Being Seen	34,469	2%	1%	2%
Time from ER Arrival to Admit. (minutes)[2]	368	408	276	274
Time from ER Arrival to Discharge (minutes)	488	192	125	134
Time in ER Before Being Evaluated (minutes)	143	33	26	26
Time to Pain Meds for Fractures (minutes)	25	69	58	57
Heart Attack Care				
Aspirin Given at Discharge	105	100%	99%	99%
Fibrinolytic Meds Within 30 Min. of Arrival[7]	-	-	40%	54%
PCI Within 90 Minutes of Arrival	12	92%	97%	96%
Statin Prescribed at Discharge	107	100%	99%	98%
Heart Failure Care				
ACE Inhibitor or ARB for LVSD	104	100%	97%	97%
Discharge Instructions Given	319	99%	96%	94%
Evaluation of LVS Function	358	100%	100%	99%
Medicare Spending				
Medicare Spending per Patient (ratio)	-	1.02	1.01	0.98
Pneumonia Care				
Appropriate Initial Antibiotic Given	67	99%	96%	95%
Blood Culture Timing	143	99%	98%	98%
Pregnancy and Delivery Care				
Newborn Deliveries Scheduled Early[2]	239	4%	4%	6%
Preventive Care				
Immunization for Influenza[2]	518	91%	91%	90%
Immunization for Pneumonia[2]	523	83%	92%	92%
Stroke Care				
Anticoagulation Therapy for Atrial Fibrillation	11	100%	96%	95%
Antithrombotic Therapy Timing	62	97%	98%	98%
Assessed for Rehabilitation	81	96%	98%	97%
Discharged on Antithrombotic Therapy	72	100%	99%	99%
Discharged on Statin Medication	61	100%	95%	94%
Thrombolytic Therapy Timing[1]	-	-	72%	66%
Venous Thromboembolism Prophylaxis	77	97%	95%	94%
Written Stroke Educational Materials Given	41	95%	90%	88%
Surgical Care Improvement Project				
Appropriate Beta Blocker Usage[2]	202	99%	98%	98%
Appropriate VTP Within 24 Hours[2]	413	100%	99%	98%
Controlled Postoperative Blood Glucose[2]	124	98%	98%	97%
Perioperative Temperature Management[2]	500	100%	100%	100%
Prophylactic Antibiotic Selection[2]	412	99%	99%	99%
Prophylactic Antibiotic Selection (Outpatient)	428	96%	98%	98%
Prophylactic Antibiotic Stopped[2]	402	94%	98%	98%
Prophylactic Antibiotic Timing[2]	413	98%	99%	99%
Prophylactic Antibiotic Timing (Outpatient)	429	97%	98%	98%
Urinary Catheter Removal[2]	382	99%	99%	97%
Survey of Patients' Hospital Experiences				
Area Around Room 'Always' Quiet at Night	300+	51%	54%	61%
Doctors 'Always' Communicated Well	300+	76%	80%	82%
Home Recovery Information Given	300+	85%	86%	85%
Hospital Given 9 or 10 on 10 Point Scale	300+	65%	69%	71%
Meds 'Always' Explained Before Given	300+	59%	63%	64%
Nurses 'Always' Communicated Well	300+	72%	79%	79%
Pain 'Always' Well Controlled	300+	64%	70%	71%
Room and Bathroom 'Always' Clean	300+	68%	73%	73%
Timely Help 'Always' Received	300+	56%	67%	68%
Would Definitely Recommend Hospital	300+	71%	70%	71%
Use of Medical Imaging				
Cardiac Imaging Stress Test before Surgery	106	13.2%	5.4%	5.3%
Combination Abdominal CT Scan	881	9.3%	12.2%	10.5%
Combination Brain/Sinus CT Scan	307	0.0%	3.1%	2.7%
Combination Chest CT Scan	833	0.1%	2.1%	2.7%
Follow-up Mammogram/Ultrasound	1,779	9.0%	9%	8.8%
Lumbar Spine MRI for Low Back Pain[1]	-	-	35.8%	37.2%

Philadelphia VA Medical Center

University & Woodland Avenu
Philadelphia, PA 19104
Phone: 215-823-5857
Fax: 215-823-6054
URL: www.philadelphia.va.gov
Type: Acute Care - VA
Emergency Services: No
Ownership: Government Federal
Beds: 675

Key Personnel:
Emergency Room . . . . J Abraham, MD
Quality Assurance . . . . Rosemary Campbell, RN
CEO/President. . . . . Richard S Citron, FACHE
Chief of Medical Staff. . . . . Peter R McCombs, MD
Radiology. . . . . M Scanlon, MD

Measure	Cases	This Hosp.	State Avg.	U.S. Avg.
Blood Clot Prevention and Treatment				
Anticoagulation Overlap Therapy	-	-	94%	93%
ICU Venous Thromboembolism Prophylaxis	-	-	94%	92%
Incidence of Potentially Preventable VTE	-	-	8%	10%
UFH with Dosages/Platelet Monitoring	-	-	98%	97%
Venous Thromboembolism Prophylaxis	-	-	90%	85%
Warfarin Therapy Discharge Instructions	-	-	78%	75%
Chest Pain/Possible Heart Attack Care				
Aspirin Given Within 24 Hours of Arrival	-	-	97%	96%
Fibrinolytic Meds Within 30 Min. of Arrival	-	-	44%	58%
Average Time to ECG (minutes)	-	-	9	7
Average Time to Transfer (minutes)	-	-	64	60
Children's Asthma Care				
Received Home Management Plan of Care	-	-	-	88%
Received Reliever Medication	-	-	-	100%
Received Systemic Corticosteroids	-	-	-	100%
Emergency Department				
Admittance Decision Time (minutes)	-	-	104	98
Head CT Results Within 45 Min. of Arrival	-	-	60%	57%
Patients Who Left ER Before Being Seen	-	-	1%	2%
Time from ER Arrival to Admit. (minutes)	-	-	276	274
Time from ER Arrival to Discharge (minutes)	-	-	125	134
Time in ER Before Being Evaluated (minutes)	-	-	26	26
Time to Pain Meds for Fractures (minutes)	-	-	58	57
Heart Attack Care				
Aspirin Given at Discharge[5]	-	-	99%	99%
Fibrinolytic Meds Within 30 Min. of Arrival[5]	-	-	40%	54%
PCI Within 90 Minutes of Arrival[5]	-	-	97%	96%
Statin Prescribed at Discharge[5]	-	-	99%	98%
Heart Failure Care				
ACE Inhibitor or ARB for LVSD	107	87%	97%	97%
Discharge Instructions Given	219	94%	96%	94%
Evaluation of LVS Function	235	100%	100%	99%
Medicare Spending				
Medicare Spending per Patient (ratio)	-	-	1.01	0.98
Pneumonia Care				
Appropriate Initial Antibiotic Given	36	89%	96%	95%
Blood Culture Timing	58	97%	98%	98%
Pregnancy and Delivery Care				
Newborn Deliveries Scheduled Early	-	-	4%	6%
Preventive Care				
Immunization for Influenza[5]	-	-	91%	90%
Immunization for Pneumonia[5]	-	-	92%	92%
Stroke Care				
Anticoagulation Therapy for Atrial Fibrillation	-	-	96%	95%
Antithrombotic Therapy Timing	-	-	98%	98%
Assessed for Rehabilitation	-	-	98%	97%
Discharged on Antithrombotic Therapy	-	-	99%	99%
Discharged on Statin Medication	-	-	95%	94%
Thrombolytic Therapy Timing	-	-	72%	66%
Venous Thromboembolism Prophylaxis	-	-	95%	94%
Written Stroke Educational Materials Given	-	-	90%	88%
Surgical Care Improvement Project				
Appropriate Beta Blocker Usage[2]	32	84%	98%	98%
Appropriate VTP Within 24 Hours[2]	63	100%	99%	98%
Controlled Postoperative Blood Glucose[5]	-	-	98%	97%
Perioperative Temperature Management[2]	90	93%	100%	100%
Prophylactic Antibiotic Selection	37	100%	99%	99%
Prophylactic Antibiotic Selection (Outpatient)	-	-	98%	98%
Prophylactic Antibiotic Stopped	35	83%	98%	98%
Prophylactic Antibiotic Timing	37	95%	99%	99%
Prophylactic Antibiotic Timing (Outpatient)	-	-	98%	98%
Urinary Catheter Removal[2]	60	80%	99%	97%
Survey of Patients' Hospital Experiences				
Area Around Room 'Always' Quiet at Night	-	-	54%	61%
Doctors 'Always' Communicated Well	-	-	80%	82%
Home Recovery Information Given	-	-	86%	85%
Hospital Given 9 or 10 on 10 Point Scale	-	-	69%	71%
Meds 'Always' Explained Before Given	-	-	63%	64%
Nurses 'Always' Communicated Well	-	-	79%	79%
Pain 'Always' Well Controlled	-	-	70%	71%
Room and Bathroom 'Always' Clean	-	-	73%	73%
Timely Help 'Always' Received	-	-	67%	68%
Would Definitely Recommend Hospital	-	-	70%	71%
Use of Medical Imaging				
Cardiac Imaging Stress Test before Surgery	-	-	5.4%	5.3%

NOTE: Hospital profiles are in alphabetical order by state, then city, then hospital within the city; Rankings exclude hospitals with less than 25 cases except for patient surveys which excludes hospitals with less than 100 cases; (a) 100-299 cases; (1) The number of cases/patients is too few to report; (2) Data submitted were based on a sample of cases/patients; (3) Results are based on a shorter time period than required; (4) Data suppressed by CMS for one or more quarters; (5) Results are not available for this reporting period; (6) Fewer than 100 patients completed the HCAHPS survey; (7) No cases met the criteria for this measure; (8) The lower limit of the confidence interval cannot be calculated if the number of observed infections equals zero; (9) No data are available from the state/territory for this reporting period; (10) The scores shown reflect fewer than 50 completed surveys; (11) There were discrepancies in the data collection process; (12) This measure does not apply to this hospital for this reporting period; (13) Results cannot be calculated for this reporting period; (14) The results for this state are combined with nearby states to protect confidentiality; Please refer to the User's Guide for a full explanation of data.

Combination Abdominal CT Scan	-	-	12.2%	10.5%
Combination Brain/Sinus CT Scan	-	-	3.1%	2.7%
Combination Chest CT Scan	-	-	2.1%	2.7%
Follow-up Mammogram/Ultrasound	-	-	9%	8.8%
Lumbar Spine MRI for Low Back Pain	-	-	35.8%	37.2%

Roxborough Memorial Hospital

5800 Ridge Ave
Philadelphia, PA 19128
URL: www.roxboroughmemorial.com
Phone: 215-483-9900
Fax: 215-487-4221
Type: Acute Care Hospitals
Emergency Services: Yes
Ownership: Proprietary
Beds: 165

Key Personnel:
CEO . . . . Peter Adamo
Pediatric Ambulatory Care . . . . . . Charlene Brock, MD
Pediatric In-Patient Care . . . . Charlene Brock, MD
Emergency Room . . . . Robert Cameron, MD
CEO/President. . . . . John J Donnelly, Jr
Radiology. . . . . Laurie Gutstein, MD
Quality Assurance . . . . Kathleen Phillips
Chairman/CEO . . . . Prem Reddy

Measure	Cases	This Hosp.	State Avg.	U.S. Avg.
Blood Clot Prevention and Treatment				
Anticoagulation Overlap Therapy[2]	29	100%	94%	93%
ICU Venous Thromboembolism Prophylaxis[2]	58	100%	94%	92%
Incidence of Potentially Preventable VTE[1,2]	-	-	8%	10%
UFH with Dosages/Platelet Monitoring[2]	23	100%	98%	97%
Venous Thromboembolism Prophylaxis[2]	337	96%	90%	85%
Warfarin Therapy Discharge Instructions[2]	11	82%	78%	75%
Chest Pain/Possible Heart Attack Care				
Aspirin Given Within 24 Hours of Arrival[1,3]	-	-	97%	96%
Fibrinolytic Meds Within 30 Min. of Arrival[3,7]	-	-	44%	58%
Average Time to ECG (minutes)[1,3]	-	-	9	7
Average Time to Transfer (minutes)[1,3]	-	-	64	60
Children's Asthma Care				
Received Home Management Plan of Care	-	-	-	88%
Received Reliever Medication	-	-	-	100%
Received Systemic Corticosteroids	-	-	-	100%
Emergency Department				
Admittance Decision Time (minutes)[2]	863	93	104	98
Head CT Results Within 45 Min. of Arrival[1]	-	-	60%	57%
Patients Who Left ER Before Being Seen	20,020	0%	1%	2%
Time from ER Arrival to Admit. (minutes)[2]	863	250	276	274
Time from ER Arrival to Discharge (minutes)	396	128	125	134
Time in ER Before Being Evaluated (minutes)	417	27	26	26
Time to Pain Meds for Fractures (minutes)	13	95	58	57
Heart Attack Care				
Aspirin Given at Discharge	31	97%	99%	99%
Fibrinolytic Meds Within 30 Min. of Arrival[7]	-	-	40%	54%
PCI Within 90 Minutes of Arrival[7]	-	-	97%	96%
Statin Prescribed at Discharge	29	100%	99%	98%
Heart Failure Care				
ACE Inhibitor or ARB for LVSD	40	95%	97%	97%
Discharge Instructions Given	134	99%	96%	94%
Evaluation of LVS Function	164	100%	100%	99%
Medicare Spending				
Medicare Spending per Patient (ratio)	-	1.12	1.01	0.98
Pneumonia Care				
Appropriate Initial Antibiotic Given	59	100%	96%	95%
Blood Culture Timing	152	100%	98%	98%
Pregnancy and Delivery Care				
Newborn Deliveries Scheduled Early[7]	-	-	4%	6%
Preventive Care				
Immunization for Influenza[2]	451	99%	91%	90%
Immunization for Pneumonia[2]	689	99%	92%	92%
Stroke Care				
Anticoagulation Therapy for Atrial Fibrillation[7]	-	-	96%	95%
Antithrombotic Therapy Timing	29	100%	98%	98%
Assessed for Rehabilitation	32	100%	98%	97%
Discharged on Antithrombotic Therapy	31	100%	99%	99%
Discharged on Statin Medication	24	100%	95%	94%
Thrombolytic Therapy Timing[1]	-	-	72%	66%
Venous Thromboembolism Prophylaxis	34	97%	95%	94%
Written Stroke Educational Materials Given	14	100%	90%	88%
Surgical Care Improvement Project				
Appropriate Beta Blocker Usage	21	100%	98%	98%
Appropriate VTP Within 24 Hours	80	100%	99%	98%
Controlled Postoperative Blood Glucose[7]	-	-	98%	97%
Perioperative Temperature Management	83	100%	100%	100%
Prophylactic Antibiotic Selection	52	100%	99%	99%
Prophylactic Antibiotic Selection (Outpatient)[5]	-	-	98%	98%
Prophylactic Antibiotic Stopped	50	100%	98%	98%
Prophylactic Antibiotic Timing	52	100%	99%	99%
Prophylactic Antibiotic Timing (Outpatient)[5]	-	-	98%	98%
Urinary Catheter Removal	65	100%	99%	97%
Survey of Patients' Hospital Experiences				
Area Around Room 'Always' Quiet at Night	(a)	56%	54%	61%
Doctors 'Always' Communicated Well	(a)	79%	80%	82%
Home Recovery Information Given	(a)	86%	86%	85%
Hospital Given 9 or 10 on 10 Point Scale	(a)	59%	69%	71%
Meds 'Always' Explained Before Given	(a)	60%	63%	64%
Nurses 'Always' Communicated Well	(a)	74%	79%	79%
Pain 'Always' Well Controlled	(a)	69%	70%	71%
Room and Bathroom 'Always' Clean	(a)	69%	73%	73%
Timely Help 'Always' Received	(a)	56%	67%	68%
Would Definitely Recommend Hospital	(a)	61%	70%	71%
Use of Medical Imaging				
Cardiac Imaging Stress Test before Surgery[7]	-	-	5.4%	5.3%
Combination Abdominal CT Scan	158	11.4%	12.2%	10.5%
Combination Brain/Sinus CT Scan	160	0.6%	3.1%	2.7%
Combination Chest CT Scan	114	1.8%	2.1%	2.7%
Follow-up Mammogram/Ultrasound	380	11.8%	9%	8.8%
Lumbar Spine MRI for Low Back Pain[1]	-	-	35.8%	37.2%

Saint Joseph's Hospital

1600 West Girard Avenue
Philadelphia, PA 19130
URL: www.nphs.com
Phone: 215-787-2000
Fax: 215-787-2195
Type: Acute Care Hospitals
Emergency Services: Yes
Ownership: Voluntary non-profit - Private
Beds: 146

Key Personnel:
Operating Room. . . . . Jackie Dixon
Emergency Room . . . . H Greene
Quality Assurance . . . . Wilda Seymour
Chief of Medical Staff . . . . Shailendra Vaidya, MD
CEO/President. . . . . George J Walmsley

Measure	Cases	This Hosp.	State Avg.	U.S. Avg.
Blood Clot Prevention and Treatment				
Anticoagulation Overlap Therapy[2]	13	62%	94%	93%
ICU Venous Thromboembolism Prophylaxis[2]	66	83%	94%	92%
Incidence of Potentially Preventable VTE[1,2]	-	-	8%	10%
UFH with Dosages/Platelet Monitoring[2]	11	82%	98%	97%
Venous Thromboembolism Prophylaxis[2]	259	64%	90%	85%
Warfarin Therapy Discharge Instructions[1,2]	-	-	78%	75%
Chest Pain/Possible Heart Attack Care				
Aspirin Given Within 24 Hours of Arrival[5]	-	-	97%	96%
Fibrinolytic Meds Within 30 Min. of Arrival[5]	-	-	44%	58%
Average Time to ECG (minutes)[5]	-	-	9	7
Average Time to Transfer (minutes)[5]	-	-	64	60
Children's Asthma Care				
Received Home Management Plan of Care	-	-	-	88%
Received Reliever Medication	-	-	-	100%
Received Systemic Corticosteroids	-	-	-	100%
Emergency Department				
Admittance Decision Time (minutes)[2]	559	120	104	98
Head CT Results Within 45 Min. of Arrival	11	9%	60%	57%
Patients Who Left ER Before Being Seen	16,715	3%	1%	2%
Time from ER Arrival to Admit. (minutes)[2]	561	361	276	274
Time from ER Arrival to Discharge (minutes)	325	200	125	134
Time in ER Before Being Evaluated (minutes)	356	69	26	26
Time to Pain Meds for Fractures (minutes)	34	89	58	57
Heart Attack Care				
Aspirin Given at Discharge[1]	-	-	99%	99%
Fibrinolytic Meds Within 30 Min. of Arrival[7]	-	-	40%	54%
PCI Within 90 Minutes of Arrival[7]	-	-	97%	96%
Statin Prescribed at Discharge[1]	-	-	99%	98%
Heart Failure Care				
ACE Inhibitor or ARB for LVSD	42	79%	97%	97%
Discharge Instructions Given	115	58%	96%	94%
Evaluation of LVS Function	132	84%	100%	99%
Medicare Spending				
Medicare Spending per Patient (ratio)	-	1.05	1.01	0.98
Pneumonia Care				
Appropriate Initial Antibiotic Given	37	70%	96%	95%
Blood Culture Timing	72	90%	98%	98%
Pregnancy and Delivery Care				
Newborn Deliveries Scheduled Early[7]	-	-	4%	6%
Preventive Care				
Immunization for Influenza[2]	342	65%	91%	90%
Immunization for Pneumonia[2]	496	79%	92%	92%
Stroke Care				
Anticoagulation Therapy for Atrial Fibrillation[7]	-	-	96%	95%
Antithrombotic Therapy Timing[1]	-	-	98%	98%
Assessed for Rehabilitation[1]	-	-	98%	97%
Discharged on Antithrombotic Therapy[1]	-	-	99%	99%
Discharged on Statin Medication[1]	-	-	95%	94%
Thrombolytic Therapy Timing[1]	-	-	72%	66%
Venous Thromboembolism Prophylaxis	12	58%	95%	94%
Written Stroke Educational Materials Given[1]	-	-	90%	88%
Surgical Care Improvement Project				
Appropriate Beta Blocker Usage	12	25%	98%	98%
Appropriate VTP Within 24 Hours	43	86%	99%	98%
Controlled Postoperative Blood Glucose[7]	-	-	98%	97%
Perioperative Temperature Management	50	80%	100%	100%
Prophylactic Antibiotic Selection	15	80%	99%	99%
Prophylactic Antibiotic Selection (Outpatient)[1,3]	-	-	98%	98%
Prophylactic Antibiotic Stopped	15	67%	98%	98%
Prophylactic Antibiotic Timing	15	80%	99%	99%
Prophylactic Antibiotic Timing (Outpatient)[1,3]	-	-	98%	98%
Urinary Catheter Removal	19	63%	99%	97%
Survey of Patients' Hospital Experiences				
Area Around Room 'Always' Quiet at Night	(a)	57%	54%	61%
Doctors 'Always' Communicated Well	(a)	72%	80%	82%
Home Recovery Information Given	(a)	72%	86%	85%
Hospital Given 9 or 10 on 10 Point Scale	(a)	47%	69%	71%
Meds 'Always' Explained Before Given	(a)	54%	63%	64%
Nurses 'Always' Communicated Well	(a)	64%	79%	79%
Pain 'Always' Well Controlled	(a)	54%	70%	71%
Room and Bathroom 'Always' Clean	(a)	65%	73%	73%
Timely Help 'Always' Received	(a)	45%	67%	68%
Would Definitely Recommend Hospital	(a)	40%	70%	71%
Use of Medical Imaging				
Cardiac Imaging Stress Test before Surgery[1]	-	-	5.4%	5.3%
Combination Abdominal CT Scan	66	0.0%	12.2%	10.5%
Combination Brain/Sinus CT Scan[1]	-	-	3.1%	2.7%
Combination Chest CT Scan[1]	-	-	2.1%	2.7%
Follow-up Mammogram/Ultrasound[1]	-	-	9%	8.8%
Lumbar Spine MRI for Low Back Pain[7]	-	-	35.8%	37.2%

Temple University Hospital

3401 North Broad Street
Philadelphia, PA 19140
URL: www.tuh.templehealth.org
Phone: 215-707-2000
Fax: 215-707-8012
Type: Acute Care Hospitals
Emergency Services: Yes
Ownership: Voluntary non-profit - Private
Beds: 514

Key Personnel:
Pediatric Ambulatory Care . . . . . . Stephen Aronoff
Pediatric In-Patient Care . . . . Stephen Aronoff
Chief of Medical Staff . . . . Sidney Cohen
Radiology. . . . . Robert A Gatenby
President/CEO. . . . . John Kastanis, FACHE
Quality Assurance . . . . Janet Leach
Operating Room. . . . . Marsha Reddin, RN
Infection Control. . . . . Keith St John

Measure	Cases	This Hosp.	State Avg.	U.S. Avg.
Blood Clot Prevention and Treatment				
Anticoagulation Overlap Therapy[2]	152	91%	94%	93%
ICU Venous Thromboembolism Prophylaxis[2]	113	93%	94%	92%
Incidence of Potentially Preventable VTE[2]	60	8%	8%	10%
UFH with Dosages/Platelet Monitoring[2]	139	60%	98%	97%
Venous Thromboembolism Prophylaxis[2]	288	86%	90%	85%

NOTE: Hospital profiles are in alphabetical order by state, then city, then hospital within the city; Rankings exclude hospitals with less than 25 cases except for patient surveys which excludes hospitals with less than 100 cases; (a) 100-299 cases; (1) The number of cases/patients is too few to report; (2) Data submitted were based on a sample of cases/patients; (3) Results are based on a shorter time period than required; (4) Data suppressed by CMS for one or more quarters; (5) Results are not available for this reporting period; (6) Fewer than 100 patients completed the HCAHPS survey; (7) No cases met the criteria for this measure; (8) The lower limit of the confidence interval cannot be calculated if the number of observed infections equals zero; (9) No data are available from the state/territory for this reporting period; (10) The scores shown reflect fewer than 50 completed surveys; (11) There were discrepancies in the data collection process; (12) This measure does not apply to this hospital for this reporting period; (13) Results cannot be calculated for this reporting period; (14) The results for this state are combined with nearby states to protect confidentiality; Please refer to the User's Guide for a full explanation of data.

Warfarin Therapy Discharge Instructions[2]	112	42%	78%	75%
Chest Pain/Possible Heart Attack Care				
Aspirin Given Within 24 Hours of Arrival[5]	-	-	97%	96%
Fibrinolytic Meds Within 30 Min. of Arrival[5]	-	-	44%	58%
Average Time to ECG (minutes)[5]	-	-	9	7
Average Time to Transfer (minutes)[5]	-	-	64	60
Children's Asthma Care				
Received Home Management Plan of Care	-	-	-	88%
Received Reliever Medication	-	-	-	100%
Received Systemic Corticosteroids	-	-	-	100%
Emergency Department				
Admittance Decision Time (minutes)[2]	594	109	104	98
Head CT Results Within 45 Min. of Arrival[1,3]	-	-	60%	57%
Patients Who Left ER Before Being Seen	>100k	6%	1%	2%
Time from ER Arrival to Admit. (minutes)[2]	594	329	276	274
Time from ER Arrival to Discharge (minutes)	347	155	125	134
Time in ER Before Being Evaluated (minutes)	365	50	26	26
Time to Pain Meds for Fractures (minutes)	93	66	58	57
Heart Attack Care				
Aspirin Given at Discharge	311	100%	99%	99%
Fibrinolytic Meds Within 30 Min. of Arrival[7]	-	-	40%	54%
PCI Within 90 Minutes of Arrival	39	100%	97%	96%
Statin Prescribed at Discharge	303	99%	99%	98%
Heart Failure Care				
ACE Inhibitor or ARB for LVSD	457	100%	97%	97%
Discharge Instructions Given	993	97%	96%	94%
Evaluation of LVS Function	1,077	100%	100%	99%
Medicare Spending				
Medicare Spending per Patient (ratio)	-	1.02	1.01	0.98
Pneumonia Care				
Appropriate Initial Antibiotic Given	180	98%	96%	95%
Blood Culture Timing	235	100%	98%	98%
Pregnancy and Delivery Care				
Newborn Deliveries Scheduled Early[2]	41	2%	4%	6%
Preventive Care				
Immunization for Influenza[2]	535	98%	91%	90%
Immunization for Pneumonia[2]	627	99%	92%	92%
Stroke Care				
Anticoagulation Therapy for Atrial Fibrillation	26	100%	96%	95%
Antithrombotic Therapy Timing	256	100%	98%	98%
Assessed for Rehabilitation	395	99%	98%	97%
Discharged on Antithrombotic Therapy	324	100%	99%	99%
Discharged on Statin Medication	247	98%	95%	94%
Thrombolytic Therapy Timing	19	100%	72%	66%
Venous Thromboembolism Prophylaxis	370	98%	95%	94%
Written Stroke Educational Materials Given	200	98%	90%	88%
Surgical Care Improvement Project				
Appropriate Beta Blocker Usage[2]	406	100%	98%	98%
Appropriate VTP Within 24 Hours[2]	627	100%	99%	98%
Controlled Postoperative Blood Glucose[2]	239	99%	98%	97%
Perioperative Temperature Management[2]	869	100%	100%	100%
Prophylactic Antibiotic Selection[2]	804	99%	99%	99%
Prophylactic Antibiotic Selection (Outpatient)	361	99%	98%	98%
Prophylactic Antibiotic Stopped[2]	750	99%	98%	98%
Prophylactic Antibiotic Timing[2]	804	100%	99%	99%
Prophylactic Antibiotic Timing (Outpatient)	362	99%	98%	98%
Urinary Catheter Removal[2]	435	100%	99%	97%
Survey of Patients' Hospital Experiences				
Area Around Room 'Always' Quiet at Night	300+	53%	54%	61%
Doctors 'Always' Communicated Well	300+	79%	80%	82%
Home Recovery Information Given	300+	83%	86%	85%
Hospital Given 9 or 10 on 10 Point Scale	300+	66%	69%	71%
Meds 'Always' Explained Before Given	300+	60%	63%	64%
Nurses 'Always' Communicated Well	300+	73%	79%	79%
Pain 'Always' Well Controlled	300+	67%	70%	71%
Room and Bathroom 'Always' Clean	300+	67%	73%	73%
Timely Help 'Always' Received	300+	56%	67%	68%
Would Definitely Recommend Hospital	300+	65%	70%	71%
Use of Medical Imaging				
Cardiac Imaging Stress Test before Surgery	631	6.2%	5.4%	5.3%
Combination Abdominal CT Scan	928	17.8%	12.2%	10.5%
Combination Brain/Sinus CT Scan	715	2.2%	3.1%	2.7%
Combination Chest CT Scan	905	3.0%	2.1%	2.7%
Follow-up Mammogram/Ultrasound	1,619	6.6%	9%	8.8%
Lumbar Spine MRI for Low Back Pain	81	29.6%	35.8%	37.2%

Thomas Jefferson University Hospital

111 South 11th Street
Philadelphia, PA 19107
Phone: 215-955-6000
Fax: 215-955-2197
URL: www.jeffersonhospital.org
Type: Acute Care Hospitals
Emergency Services: Yes
Ownership: Voluntary non-profit - Private
Beds: 957

Key Personnel:
CEO/President. . . . . Thomas J Lewis
Chief of Medical Staff. . . . . Geno Merli, MD, FACP

Measure	Cases	This Hosp.	State Avg.	U.S. Avg.
Blood Clot Prevention and Treatment				
Anticoagulation Overlap Therapy[2]	189	90%	94%	93%
ICU Venous Thromboembolism Prophylaxis[2]	142	93%	94%	92%
Incidence of Potentially Preventable VTE[2]	61	2%	8%	10%
UFH with Dosages/Platelet Monitoring[2]	168	86%	98%	97%
Venous Thromboembolism Prophylaxis[2]	639	87%	90%	85%
Warfarin Therapy Discharge Instructions[2]	115	98%	78%	75%
Chest Pain/Possible Heart Attack Care				
Aspirin Given Within 24 Hours of Arrival[1,3]	-	-	97%	96%
Fibrinolytic Meds Within 30 Min. of Arrival[5]	-	-	44%	58%
Average Time to ECG (minutes)[3]	12	12	9	7
Average Time to Transfer (minutes)[5]	-	-	64	60
Children's Asthma Care				
Received Home Management Plan of Care	-	-	-	88%
Received Reliever Medication	-	-	-	100%
Received Systemic Corticosteroids	-	-	-	100%
Emergency Department				
Admittance Decision Time (minutes)[2]	1,380	178	104	98
Head CT Results Within 45 Min. of Arrival	14	50%	60%	57%
Patients Who Left ER Before Being Seen	>100k	4%	1%	2%
Time from ER Arrival to Admit. (minutes)[2]	1,383	410	276	274
Time from ER Arrival to Discharge (minutes)	689	195	125	134
Time in ER Before Being Evaluated (minutes)	699	40	26	26
Time to Pain Meds for Fractures (minutes)	185	72	58	57
Heart Attack Care				
Aspirin Given at Discharge	245	100%	99%	99%
Fibrinolytic Meds Within 30 Min. of Arrival[7]	-	-	40%	54%
PCI Within 90 Minutes of Arrival	13	100%	97%	96%
Statin Prescribed at Discharge	247	100%	99%	98%
Heart Failure Care				
ACE Inhibitor or ARB for LVSD	312	99%	97%	97%
Discharge Instructions Given	840	99%	96%	94%
Evaluation of LVS Function	992	100%	100%	99%
Medicare Spending				
Medicare Spending per Patient (ratio)	-	1.01	1.01	0.98
Pneumonia Care				
Appropriate Initial Antibiotic Given	223	97%	96%	95%
Blood Culture Timing	502	98%	98%	98%
Pregnancy and Delivery Care				
Newborn Deliveries Scheduled Early	301	1%	4%	6%
Preventive Care				
Immunization for Influenza[2]	1,135	98%	91%	90%
Immunization for Pneumonia[2]	1,494	96%	92%	92%
Stroke Care				
Anticoagulation Therapy for Atrial Fibrillation[2]	14	100%	96%	95%
Antithrombotic Therapy Timing[2]	114	98%	98%	98%
Assessed for Rehabilitation[2]	193	98%	98%	97%
Discharged on Antithrombotic Therapy[2]	143	100%	99%	99%
Discharged on Statin Medication[2]	104	98%	95%	94%
Thrombolytic Therapy Timing[1,2]	-	-	72%	66%
Venous Thromboembolism Prophylaxis[2]	211	100%	95%	94%
Written Stroke Educational Materials Given[2]	75	100%	90%	88%
Surgical Care Improvement Project				
Appropriate Beta Blocker Usage[2]	779	99%	98%	98%
Appropriate VTP Within 24 Hours[2]	1,890	100%	99%	98%
Controlled Postoperative Blood Glucose[2]	194	98%	98%	97%
Perioperative Temperature Management[2]	2,700	100%	100%	100%
Prophylactic Antibiotic Selection[2]	2,364	99%	99%	99%
Prophylactic Antibiotic Selection (Outpatient)	460	96%	98%	98%
Prophylactic Antibiotic Stopped[2]	2,339	99%	98%	98%
Prophylactic Antibiotic Timing[2]	2,364	100%	99%	99%
Prophylactic Antibiotic Timing (Outpatient)	460	99%	98%	98%
Urinary Catheter Removal[2]	734	96%	99%	97%
Survey of Patients' Hospital Experiences				
Area Around Room 'Always' Quiet at Night	300+	53%	54%	61%
Doctors 'Always' Communicated Well	300+	79%	80%	82%
Home Recovery Information Given	300+	86%	86%	85%
Hospital Given 9 or 10 on 10 Point Scale	300+	74%	69%	71%
Meds 'Always' Explained Before Given	300+	64%	63%	64%
Nurses 'Always' Communicated Well	300+	80%	79%	79%
Pain 'Always' Well Controlled	300+	71%	70%	71%
Room and Bathroom 'Always' Clean	300+	65%	73%	73%
Timely Help 'Always' Received	300+	71%	67%	68%
Would Definitely Recommend Hospital	300+	77%	70%	71%
Use of Medical Imaging				
Cardiac Imaging Stress Test before Surgery	913	7.7%	5.4%	5.3%
Combination Abdominal CT Scan	1,443	12.9%	12.2%	10.5%
Combination Brain/Sinus CT Scan	1,234	4.0%	3.1%	2.7%
Combination Chest CT Scan	1,105	1.2%	2.1%	2.7%
Follow-up Mammogram/Ultrasound	4,978	10.2%	9%	8.8%
Lumbar Spine MRI for Low Back Pain	156	35.9%	35.8%	37.2%

Phoenixville Hospital

140 Nutt Road
Phoenixville, PA 19460
Phone: 610-983-1000
Fax: 610-983-1488
URL: www.pennhealth.com
Type: Acute Care Hospitals
Emergency Services: Yes
Ownership: Proprietary
Beds: 106

Key Personnel:
Radiology. . . . . Geoffrey A Agrons, MD
Quality Assurance . . . . Sue Detwiler, RN
Chief of Medical Staff. . . . . Joel W Eisner, MD
Infection Control. . . . . Carolyn Peterson
CEO/President. . . . . Mark B Real, MD
Pediatric Ambulatory Care . . . . . . Maurice Rozwat, MD
Pediatric In-Patient Care . . . . Maurice Rozwat, MD
Operating Room. . . . . Barbara Shaffer

Measure	Cases	This Hosp.	State Avg.	U.S. Avg.
Blood Clot Prevention and Treatment				
Anticoagulation Overlap Therapy[2]	33	97%	94%	93%
ICU Venous Thromboembolism Prophylaxis[2]	115	98%	94%	92%
Incidence of Potentially Preventable VTE[1,2]	-	-	8%	10%
UFH with Dosages/Platelet Monitoring[2]	13	100%	98%	97%
Venous Thromboembolism Prophylaxis[2]	402	90%	90%	85%
Warfarin Therapy Discharge Instructions[2]	19	47%	78%	75%
Chest Pain/Possible Heart Attack Care				
Aspirin Given Within 24 Hours of Arrival[1,3]	-	-	97%	96%
Fibrinolytic Meds Within 30 Min. of Arrival[5]	-	-	44%	58%
Average Time to ECG (minutes)[1,3]	-	-	9	7
Average Time to Transfer (minutes)[5]	-	-	64	60
Children's Asthma Care				
Received Home Management Plan of Care	-	-	-	88%
Received Reliever Medication	-	-	-	100%
Received Systemic Corticosteroids	-	-	-	100%
Emergency Department				
Admittance Decision Time (minutes)[2]	787	125	104	98
Head CT Results Within 45 Min. of Arrival	11	73%	60%	57%
Patients Who Left ER Before Being Seen	27,985	0%	1%	2%
Time from ER Arrival to Admit. (minutes)[2]	805	258	276	274
Time from ER Arrival to Discharge (minutes)	397	126	125	134
Time in ER Before Being Evaluated (minutes)	421	28	26	26
Time to Pain Meds for Fractures (minutes)	80	51	58	57
Heart Attack Care				
Aspirin Given at Discharge	259	99%	99%	99%
Fibrinolytic Meds Within 30 Min. of Arrival[7]	-	-	40%	54%
PCI Within 90 Minutes of Arrival	38	92%	97%	96%
Statin Prescribed at Discharge	256	99%	99%	98%
Heart Failure Care				
ACE Inhibitor or ARB for LVSD	79	99%	97%	97%
Discharge Instructions Given	147	99%	96%	94%
Evaluation of LVS Function	209	100%	100%	99%
Medicare Spending				
Medicare Spending per Patient (ratio)	-	1.04	1.01	0.98

NOTE: Hospital profiles are in alphabetical order by state, then city, then hospital within the city; Rankings exclude hospitals with less than 25 cases except for patient surveys which excludes hospitals with less than 100 cases; (a) 100-299 cases; (1) The number of cases/patients is too few to report; (2) Data submitted were based on a sample of cases/patients; (3) Results are based on a shorter time period than required; (4) Data suppressed by CMS for one or more quarters; (5) Results are not available for this reporting period; (6) Fewer than 100 patients completed the HCAHPS survey; (7) No cases met the criteria for this measure; (8) The lower limit of the confidence interval cannot be calculated if the number of observed infections equals zero; (9) No data are available from the state/territory for this reporting period; (10) The scores shown reflect fewer than 50 completed surveys; (11) There were discrepancies in the data collection process; (12) This measure does not apply to this hospital for this reporting period; (13) Results cannot be calculated for this reporting period; (14) The results for this state are combined with nearby states to protect confidentiality; Please refer to the User's Guide for a full explanation of data.

Measure	Cases	This Hosp.	State Avg.	U.S. Avg.
Pneumonia Care				
Appropriate Initial Antibiotic Given	88	100%	96%	95%
Blood Culture Timing	190	99%	98%	98%
Pregnancy and Delivery Care				
Newborn Deliveries Scheduled Early[2]	33	3%	4%	6%
Preventive Care				
Immunization for Influenza[2]	609	97%	91%	90%
Immunization for Pneumonia[2]	780	98%	92%	92%
Stroke Care				
Anticoagulation Therapy for Atrial Fibrillation[1]	-	-	96%	95%
Antithrombotic Therapy Timing	37	100%	98%	98%
Assessed for Rehabilitation	37	100%	98%	97%
Discharged on Antithrombotic Therapy	36	92%	99%	99%
Discharged on Statin Medication	30	77%	95%	94%
Thrombolytic Therapy Timing[7]	-	-	72%	66%
Venous Thromboembolism Prophylaxis	37	97%	95%	94%
Written Stroke Educational Materials Given	19	58%	90%	88%
Surgical Care Improvement Project				
Appropriate Beta Blocker Usage	163	98%	98%	98%
Appropriate VTP Within 24 Hours	282	98%	99%	98%
Controlled Postoperative Blood Glucose	88	98%	98%	97%
Perioperative Temperature Management	393	100%	100%	100%
Prophylactic Antibiotic Selection	266	98%	99%	99%
Prophylactic Antibiotic Selection (Outpatient)	129	98%	98%	98%
Prophylactic Antibiotic Stopped	255	99%	98%	98%
Prophylactic Antibiotic Timing	267	99%	99%	99%
Prophylactic Antibiotic Timing (Outpatient)	129	95%	98%	98%
Urinary Catheter Removal	202	97%	99%	97%
Survey of Patients' Hospital Experiences				
Area Around Room 'Always' Quiet at Night	300+	61%	54%	61%
Doctors 'Always' Communicated Well	300+	79%	80%	82%
Home Recovery Information Given	300+	87%	86%	85%
Hospital Given 9 or 10 on 10 Point Scale	300+	73%	69%	71%
Meds 'Always' Explained Before Given	300+	63%	63%	64%
Nurses 'Always' Communicated Well	300+	81%	79%	79%
Pain 'Always' Well Controlled	300+	71%	70%	71%
Room and Bathroom 'Always' Clean	300+	74%	73%	73%
Timely Help 'Always' Received	300+	65%	67%	68%
Would Definitely Recommend Hospital	300+	75%	70%	71%
Use of Medical Imaging				
Cardiac Imaging Stress Test before Surgery	139	8.6%	5.4%	5.3%
Combination Abdominal CT Scan	564	21.1%	12.2%	10.5%
Combination Brain/Sinus CT Scan	486	4.7%	3.1%	2.7%
Combination Chest CT Scan	493	9.3%	2.1%	2.7%
Follow-up Mammogram/Ultrasound	1,616	4.7%	9%	8.8%
Lumbar Spine MRI for Low Back Pain	164	34.8%	35.8%	37.2%

Allegheny General Hospital

320 East North Avenue
Pittsburgh, PA 15212
Phone: 412-359-3131
Fax: 412-359-3888
URL: www.allhealth.edu
Type: Acute Care Hospitals
Emergency Services: Yes
Ownership: Voluntary non-profit - Other
Beds: 755

Key Personnel:
Operating Room. . . . . Vicky Butler, RN
Quality Assurance . . . . Kathleen Engelmeier
Chief of Medical Staff. . . . . Tony G. Farah, MD, FACC, FSCAI
Pediatric Ambulatory Care . . . . . . Mary Goessler, MD
Pediatric In-Patient Care . . . . Mary Goessler, MD
CEO/President. . . . . Michael Harlovic
Infection Control. . . . . Cheryl Herbert
Radiology. . . . . David Parda, MD

Measure	Cases	This Hosp.	State Avg.	U.S. Avg.
Blood Clot Prevention and Treatment				
Anticoagulation Overlap Therapy[2]	199	95%	94%	93%
ICU Venous Thromboembolism Prophylaxis[2]	165	90%	94%	92%
Incidence of Potentially Preventable VTE[2]	88	2%	8%	10%
UFH with Dosages/Platelet Monitoring[2]	216	100%	98%	97%
Venous Thromboembolism Prophylaxis[2]	377	90%	90%	85%
Warfarin Therapy Discharge Instructions[2]	127	76%	78%	75%
Chest Pain/Possible Heart Attack Care				
Aspirin Given Within 24 Hours of Arrival[1]	-	-	97%	96%
Fibrinolytic Meds Within 30 Min. of Arrival[5]	-	-	44%	58%
Average Time to ECG (minutes)[1]	-	-	9	7
Average Time to Transfer (minutes)[5]	-	-	64	60
Children's Asthma Care				
Received Home Management Plan of Care	-	-	-	88%
Received Reliever Medication	-	-	-	100%
Received Systemic Corticosteroids	-	-	-	100%
Emergency Department				
Admittance Decision Time (minutes)[2]	492	130	104	98
Head CT Results Within 45 Min. of Arrival[1]	-	-	60%	57%
Patients Who Left ER Before Being Seen	51,023	1%	1%	2%
Time from ER Arrival to Admit. (minutes)[2]	546	295	276	274
Time from ER Arrival to Discharge (minutes)	421	182	125	134
Time in ER Before Being Evaluated (minutes)	481	43	26	26
Time to Pain Meds for Fractures (minutes)	71	90	58	57
Heart Attack Care				
Aspirin Given at Discharge	503	100%	99%	99%
Fibrinolytic Meds Within 30 Min. of Arrival[1]	-	-	40%	54%
PCI Within 90 Minutes of Arrival	71	97%	97%	96%
Statin Prescribed at Discharge	480	100%	99%	98%
Heart Failure Care				
ACE Inhibitor or ARB for LVSD	232	100%	97%	97%
Discharge Instructions Given	521	97%	96%	94%
Evaluation of LVS Function	649	100%	100%	99%
Medicare Spending				
Medicare Spending per Patient (ratio)	-	1.06	1.01	0.98
Pneumonia Care				
Appropriate Initial Antibiotic Given	58	100%	96%	95%
Blood Culture Timing	36	100%	98%	98%
Pregnancy and Delivery Care				
Newborn Deliveries Scheduled Early[7]	-	-	4%	6%
Preventive Care				
Immunization for Influenza[2]	638	75%	91%	90%
Immunization for Pneumonia[2]	857	79%	92%	92%
Stroke Care				
Anticoagulation Therapy for Atrial Fibrillation	81	100%	96%	95%
Antithrombotic Therapy Timing	296	97%	98%	98%
Assessed for Rehabilitation	537	99%	98%	97%
Discharged on Antithrombotic Therapy	391	99%	99%	99%
Discharged on Statin Medication	286	95%	95%	94%
Thrombolytic Therapy Timing	43	91%	72%	66%
Venous Thromboembolism Prophylaxis	595	96%	95%	94%
Written Stroke Educational Materials Given	231	84%	90%	88%
Surgical Care Improvement Project				
Appropriate Beta Blocker Usage	885	98%	98%	98%
Appropriate VTP Within 24 Hours	1,613	98%	99%	98%
Controlled Postoperative Blood Glucose	476	96%	98%	97%
Perioperative Temperature Management	1,991	99%	100%	100%
Prophylactic Antibiotic Selection	1,217	99%	99%	99%
Prophylactic Antibiotic Selection (Outpatient)	648	98%	98%	98%
Prophylactic Antibiotic Stopped	1,187	97%	98%	98%
Prophylactic Antibiotic Timing	1,218	99%	99%	99%
Prophylactic Antibiotic Timing (Outpatient)	648	99%	98%	98%
Urinary Catheter Removal	1,805	99%	99%	97%
Survey of Patients' Hospital Experiences				
Area Around Room 'Always' Quiet at Night	300+	46%	54%	61%
Doctors 'Always' Communicated Well	300+	79%	80%	82%
Home Recovery Information Given	300+	86%	86%	85%
Hospital Given 9 or 10 on 10 Point Scale	300+	65%	69%	71%
Meds 'Always' Explained Before Given	300+	58%	63%	64%
Nurses 'Always' Communicated Well	300+	75%	79%	79%
Pain 'Always' Well Controlled	300+	67%	70%	71%
Room and Bathroom 'Always' Clean	300+	69%	73%	73%
Timely Help 'Always' Received	300+	53%	67%	68%
Would Definitely Recommend Hospital	300+	68%	70%	71%
Use of Medical Imaging				
Cardiac Imaging Stress Test before Surgery	221	5.0%	5.4%	5.3%
Combination Abdominal CT Scan	659	30.3%	12.2%	10.5%
Combination Brain/Sinus CT Scan[1]	-	-	3.1%	2.7%
Combination Chest CT Scan	585	4.6%	2.1%	2.7%
Follow-up Mammogram/Ultrasound	660	13.0%	9%	8.8%
Lumbar Spine MRI for Low Back Pain	51	39.2%	35.8%	37.2%

Children's Hospital of Pittsburgh of UPMC

4401 Penn Avenue
Pittsburgh, PA 15224
Phone: 412-692-5325
Fax: 412-692-5800
URL: www.chp.edu
Type: Childrens
Emergency Services: Yes
Ownership: Voluntary non-profit - Other
Beds: 260

Key Personnel:
Quality Assurance . . . . Karen Calhoon
Chief of Medical Staff. . . . . Steven G Docimo, MD
Infection Control. . . . . Adrian Farley, RN
Radiology. . . . . Charles Finz, MD
CEO/President. . . . . Christopher A Gessner
Pediatric In-Patient Care . . . . George K Gittes, MD
Operating Room. . . . . Diane Hupp, RN
Pediatric Ambulatory Care . . . . . . David H Perlmutter, MD

Measure	Cases	This Hosp.	State Avg.	U.S. Avg.
Blood Clot Prevention and Treatment				
Anticoagulation Overlap Therapy[5]	-	-	94%	93%
ICU Venous Thromboembolism Prophylaxis[5]	-	-	94%	92%
Incidence of Potentially Preventable VTE[5]	-	-	8%	10%
UFH with Dosages/Platelet Monitoring[5]	-	-	98%	97%
Venous Thromboembolism Prophylaxis[5]	-	-	90%	85%
Warfarin Therapy Discharge Instructions[5]	-	-	78%	75%
Chest Pain/Possible Heart Attack Care				
Aspirin Given Within 24 Hours of Arrival	-	-	97%	96%
Fibrinolytic Meds Within 30 Min. of Arrival	-	-	44%	58%
Average Time to ECG (minutes)	-	-	9	7
Average Time to Transfer (minutes)	-	-	64	60
Children's Asthma Care				
Received Home Management Plan of Care[2]	337	57%	-	88%
Received Reliever Medication[2]	341	100%	-	100%
Received Systemic Corticosteroids[2]	341	100%	-	100%
Emergency Department				
Admittance Decision Time (minutes)[5]	-	-	104	98
Head CT Results Within 45 Min. of Arrival	-	-	60%	57%
Patients Who Left ER Before Being Seen	-	-	1%	2%
Time from ER Arrival to Admit. (minutes)[5]	-	-	276	274
Time from ER Arrival to Discharge (minutes)	-	-	125	134
Time in ER Before Being Evaluated (minutes)	-	-	26	26
Time to Pain Meds for Fractures (minutes)	-	-	58	57
Heart Attack Care				
Aspirin Given at Discharge[5]	-	-	99%	99%
Fibrinolytic Meds Within 30 Min. of Arrival[5]	-	-	40%	54%
PCI Within 90 Minutes of Arrival[5]	-	-	97%	96%
Statin Prescribed at Discharge[5]	-	-	99%	98%
Heart Failure Care				
ACE Inhibitor or ARB for LVSD[5]	-	-	97%	97%
Discharge Instructions Given[5]	-	-	96%	94%
Evaluation of LVS Function[5]	-	-	100%	99%
Medicare Spending				
Medicare Spending per Patient (ratio)	-	-	1.01	0.98
Pneumonia Care				
Appropriate Initial Antibiotic Given[5]	-	-	96%	95%
Blood Culture Timing[5]	-	-	98%	98%
Pregnancy and Delivery Care				
Newborn Deliveries Scheduled Early[5]	-	-	4%	6%
Preventive Care				
Immunization for Influenza[5]	-	-	91%	90%
Immunization for Pneumonia[5]	-	-	92%	92%
Stroke Care				
Anticoagulation Therapy for Atrial Fibrillation[5]	-	-	96%	95%
Antithrombotic Therapy Timing[5]	-	-	98%	98%
Assessed for Rehabilitation[5]	-	-	98%	97%
Discharged on Antithrombotic Therapy[5]	-	-	99%	99%
Discharged on Statin Medication[5]	-	-	95%	94%
Thrombolytic Therapy Timing[5]	-	-	72%	66%
Venous Thromboembolism Prophylaxis[5]	-	-	95%	94%
Written Stroke Educational Materials Given[5]	-	-	90%	88%
Surgical Care Improvement Project				
Appropriate Beta Blocker Usage[5]	-	-	98%	98%
Appropriate VTP Within 24 Hours[5]	-	-	99%	98%
Controlled Postoperative Blood Glucose[5]	-	-	98%	97%
Perioperative Temperature Management[5]	-	-	100%	100%
Prophylactic Antibiotic Selection[5]	-	-	99%	99%

NOTE: Hospital profiles are in alphabetical order by state, then city, then hospital within the city; Rankings exclude hospitals with less than 25 cases except for patient surveys which excludes hospitals with less than 100 cases; (a) 100-299 cases; (1) The number of cases/patients is too few to report; (2) Data submitted were based on a sample of cases/patients; (3) Results are based on a shorter time period than required; (4) Data suppressed by CMS for one or more quarters; (5) Results are not available for this reporting period; (6) Fewer than 100 patients completed the HCAHPS survey; (7) No cases met the criteria for this measure; (8) The lower limit of the confidence interval cannot be calculated if the number of observed infections equals zero; (9) No data are available from the state/territory for this reporting period; (10) The scores shown reflect fewer than 50 completed surveys; (11) There were discrepancies in the data collection process; (12) This measure does not apply to this hospital for this reporting period; (13) Results cannot be calculated for this reporting period; (14) The results for this state are combined with nearby states to protect confidentiality; Please refer to the User's Guide for a full explanation of data.

Measure	Cases	This Hosp.	State Avg.	U.S. Avg.
Prophylactic Antibiotic Selection (Outpatient)	-	-	98%	98%
Prophylactic Antibiotic Stopped[5]	-	-	98%	98%
Prophylactic Antibiotic Timing[5]	-	-	99%	99%
Prophylactic Antibiotic Timing (Outpatient)	-	-	98%	98%
Urinary Catheter Removal[5]	-	-	99%	97%
Survey of Patients' Hospital Experiences				
Area Around Room 'Always' Quiet at Night[5]	-	-	54%	61%
Doctors 'Always' Communicated Well[5]	-	-	80%	82%
Home Recovery Information Given[5]	-	-	86%	85%
Hospital Given 9 or 10 on 10 Point Scale[5]	-	-	69%	71%
Meds 'Always' Explained Before Given[5]	-	-	63%	64%
Nurses 'Always' Communicated Well[5]	-	-	79%	79%
Pain 'Always' Well Controlled[5]	-	-	70%	71%
Room and Bathroom 'Always' Clean[5]	-	-	73%	73%
Timely Help 'Always' Received[5]	-	-	67%	68%
Would Definitely Recommend Hospital[5]	-	-	70%	71%
Use of Medical Imaging				
Cardiac Imaging Stress Test before Surgery	-	-	5.4%	5.3%
Combination Abdominal CT Scan	-	-	12.2%	10.5%
Combination Brain/Sinus CT Scan	-	-	3.1%	2.7%
Combination Chest CT Scan	-	-	2.1%	2.7%
Follow-up Mammogram/Ultrasound	-	-	9%	8.8%
Lumbar Spine MRI for Low Back Pain	-	-	35.8%	37.2%

Jefferson Regional Medical Center

565 Coal Valley Rd
Pittsburgh, PA 15236
URL: www.jeffersonregional.com
Type: Acute Care Hospitals
Ownership: Voluntary non-profit - Private

Phone: 412-469-5000
Fax: 412-469-2495
Emergency Services: Yes
Beds: 390

Key Personnel:
Chief of Medical Staff.......... Richard F. Collins, Jr, MD
Intensive Care Unit............ Jewell Coulter
CEO/President................ John J. Dempster
Anesthesiology............... Robert A. Gregg, MD
Quality Assurance .... Edward Guzik
Radiology.................. Kate Labuskes
Surgery.................... Mark L. Lesh, MD

Measure	Cases	This Hosp.	State Avg.	U.S. Avg.
Blood Clot Prevention and Treatment				
Anticoagulation Overlap Therapy[2]	160	92%	94%	93%
ICU Venous Thromboembolism Prophylaxis[2]	74	88%	94%	92%
Incidence of Potentially Preventable VTE[2]	32	44%	8%	10%
UFH with Dosages/Platelet Monitoring[2]	160	99%	98%	97%
Venous Thromboembolism Prophylaxis[2]	360	72%	90%	85%
Warfarin Therapy Discharge Instructions[2]	104	32%	78%	75%
Chest Pain/Possible Heart Attack Care				
Aspirin Given Within 24 Hours of Arrival[1]	-	-	97%	96%
Fibrinolytic Meds Within 30 Min. of Arrival[5]	-	-	44%	58%
Average Time to ECG (minutes)[1]	-	-	9	7
Average Time to Transfer (minutes)[5]	-	-	64	60
Children's Asthma Care				
Received Home Management Plan of Care	-	-	-	88%
Received Reliever Medication	-	-	-	100%
Received Systemic Corticosteroids	-	-	-	100%
Emergency Department				
Admittance Decision Time (minutes)[2]	613	157	104	98
Head CT Results Within 45 Min. of Arrival[1]	-	-	60%	57%
Patients Who Left ER Before Being Seen	52,791	1%	1%	2%
Time from ER Arrival to Admit. (minutes)[2]	616	270	276	274
Time from ER Arrival to Discharge (minutes)	329	157	125	134
Time in ER Before Being Evaluated (minutes)	265	35	26	26
Time to Pain Meds for Fractures (minutes)	91	65	58	57
Heart Attack Care				
Aspirin Given at Discharge	274	99%	99%	99%
Fibrinolytic Meds Within 30 Min. of Arrival[7]	-	-	40%	54%
PCI Within 90 Minutes of Arrival	62	95%	97%	96%
Statin Prescribed at Discharge	270	98%	99%	98%
Heart Failure Care				
ACE Inhibitor or ARB for LVSD	155	92%	97%	97%
Discharge Instructions Given	441	85%	96%	94%
Evaluation of LVS Function	546	99%	100%	99%
Medicare Spending				
Medicare Spending per Patient (ratio)	-	1.08	1.01	0.98
Pneumonia Care				
Appropriate Initial Antibiotic Given	229	93%	96%	95%
Blood Culture Timing	267	87%	98%	98%
Pregnancy and Delivery Care				
Newborn Deliveries Scheduled Early[7]	-	-	4%	6%
Preventive Care				
Immunization for Influenza[2]	592	88%	91%	90%
Immunization for Pneumonia[2]	952	90%	92%	92%
Stroke Care				
Anticoagulation Therapy for Atrial Fibrillation[2]	19	100%	96%	95%
Antithrombotic Therapy Timing[2]	82	98%	98%	98%
Assessed for Rehabilitation[2]	85	96%	98%	97%
Discharged on Antithrombotic Therapy[2]	79	100%	99%	99%
Discharged on Statin Medication[2]	68	93%	95%	94%
Thrombolytic Therapy Timing[1,2]	-	-	72%	66%
Venous Thromboembolism Prophylaxis[2]	87	79%	95%	94%
Written Stroke Educational Materials Given[2]	37	97%	90%	88%
Surgical Care Improvement Project				
Appropriate Beta Blocker Usage	643	97%	98%	98%
Appropriate VTP Within 24 Hours	1,113	95%	99%	98%
Controlled Postoperative Blood Glucose	254	99%	98%	97%
Perioperative Temperature Management	1,319	99%	100%	100%
Prophylactic Antibiotic Selection	1,102	98%	99%	99%
Prophylactic Antibiotic Selection (Outpatient)	328	96%	98%	98%
Prophylactic Antibiotic Stopped	1,084	97%	98%	98%
Prophylactic Antibiotic Timing	1,102	99%	99%	99%
Prophylactic Antibiotic Timing (Outpatient)	332	98%	98%	98%
Urinary Catheter Removal	1,065	95%	99%	97%
Survey of Patients' Hospital Experiences				
Area Around Room 'Always' Quiet at Night	300+	55%	54%	61%
Doctors 'Always' Communicated Well	300+	80%	80%	82%
Home Recovery Information Given	300+	89%	86%	85%
Hospital Given 9 or 10 on 10 Point Scale	300+	73%	69%	71%
Meds 'Always' Explained Before Given	300+	61%	63%	64%
Nurses 'Always' Communicated Well	300+	80%	79%	79%
Pain 'Always' Well Controlled	300+	68%	70%	71%
Room and Bathroom 'Always' Clean	300+	73%	73%	73%
Timely Help 'Always' Received	300+	70%	67%	68%
Would Definitely Recommend Hospital	300+	73%	70%	71%
Use of Medical Imaging				
Cardiac Imaging Stress Test before Surgery	427	8.0%	5.4%	5.3%
Combination Abdominal CT Scan	679	14.9%	12.2%	10.5%
Combination Brain/Sinus CT Scan	595	4.4%	3.1%	2.7%
Combination Chest CT Scan	438	0.2%	2.1%	2.7%
Follow-up Mammogram/Ultrasound	521	8.8%	9%	8.8%
Lumbar Spine MRI for Low Back Pain	120	35.0%	35.8%	37.2%

Magee Womens Hospital of UPMC Health System

300 Halket Street
Pittsburgh, PA 15213
E-mail: upmcweb@upmc.edu
URL: www.magee.edu
Type: Acute Care Hospitals
Ownership: Voluntary non-profit - Other

Phone: 412-641-4010
Fax: 412-641-4343
Emergency Services: Yes
Beds: 287

Key Personnel:
Chief of Medical Staff.......... Jerome H Aarons, MD
Pediatric In-Patient Care .... Sherin Devaskar, MD
Intensive Care Unit............ Herbert Jacob, MD
Operating Room.............. Linda Pechin
Anesthesiology............... Sivam Ramanathan, MD
Quality Assurance .... Sandra Read-Triebsch
Emergency Room .... Carol Simmons, MD
Radiology.................. Jules J Sumkin, DO

Measure	Cases	This Hosp.	State Avg.	U.S. Avg.
Blood Clot Prevention and Treatment				
Anticoagulation Overlap Therapy[2]	35	97%	94%	93%
ICU Venous Thromboembolism Prophylaxis[2]	22	100%	94%	92%
Incidence of Potentially Preventable VTE[2]	34	6%	8%	10%
UFH with Dosages/Platelet Monitoring[2]	50	100%	98%	97%
Venous Thromboembolism Prophylaxis[2]	368	93%	90%	85%
Warfarin Therapy Discharge Instructions[2]	25	100%	78%	75%
Chest Pain/Possible Heart Attack Care				
Aspirin Given Within 24 Hours of Arrival[1,3]	-	-	97%	96%
Fibrinolytic Meds Within 30 Min. of Arrival[3,7]	-	-	44%	58%
Average Time to ECG (minutes)[1,3]	-	-	9	7
Average Time to Transfer (minutes)[3,7]	-	-	64	60
Children's Asthma Care				
Received Home Management Plan of Care	-	-	-	88%
Received Reliever Medication	-	-	-	100%
Received Systemic Corticosteroids	-	-	-	100%
Emergency Department				
Admittance Decision Time (minutes)[2]	96	64	104	98
Head CT Results Within 45 Min. of Arrival[3,7]	-	-	60%	57%
Patients Who Left ER Before Being Seen	22,946	1%	1%	2%
Time from ER Arrival to Admit. (minutes)[2]	98	215	276	274
Time from ER Arrival to Discharge (minutes)	589	151	125	134
Time in ER Before Being Evaluated (minutes)	619	19	26	26
Time to Pain Meds for Fractures (minutes)[1]	-	-	58	57
Heart Attack Care				
Aspirin Given at Discharge[1]	-	-	99%	99%
Fibrinolytic Meds Within 30 Min. of Arrival[7]	-	-	40%	54%
PCI Within 90 Minutes of Arrival[7]	-	-	97%	96%
Statin Prescribed at Discharge[1]	-	-	99%	98%
Heart Failure Care				
ACE Inhibitor or ARB for LVSD	19	100%	97%	97%
Discharge Instructions Given	65	100%	96%	94%
Evaluation of LVS Function	91	100%	100%	99%
Medicare Spending				
Medicare Spending per Patient (ratio)	-	0.95	1.01	0.98
Pneumonia Care				
Appropriate Initial Antibiotic Given	34	94%	96%	95%
Blood Culture Timing	33	100%	98%	98%
Pregnancy and Delivery Care				
Newborn Deliveries Scheduled Early[2]	105	0%	4%	6%
Preventive Care				
Immunization for Influenza[2]	471	93%	91%	90%
Immunization for Pneumonia[2]	249	83%	92%	92%
Stroke Care				
Anticoagulation Therapy for Atrial Fibrillation[1]	-	-	96%	95%
Antithrombotic Therapy Timing	12	100%	98%	98%
Assessed for Rehabilitation	19	100%	98%	97%
Discharged on Antithrombotic Therapy	17	100%	99%	99%
Discharged on Statin Medication[1]	-	-	95%	94%
Thrombolytic Therapy Timing[7]	-	-	72%	66%
Venous Thromboembolism Prophylaxis	19	100%	95%	94%
Written Stroke Educational Materials Given	12	100%	90%	88%
Surgical Care Improvement Project				
Appropriate Beta Blocker Usage	454	100%	98%	98%
Appropriate VTP Within 24 Hours	1,784	99%	99%	98%
Controlled Postoperative Blood Glucose[7]	-	-	98%	97%
Perioperative Temperature Management	2,094	100%	100%	100%
Prophylactic Antibiotic Selection	1,485	100%	99%	99%
Prophylactic Antibiotic Selection (Outpatient)	661	100%	98%	98%
Prophylactic Antibiotic Stopped	1,477	99%	98%	98%
Prophylactic Antibiotic Timing	1,480	100%	99%	99%
Prophylactic Antibiotic Timing (Outpatient)	661	100%	98%	98%
Urinary Catheter Removal	1,289	100%	99%	97%
Survey of Patients' Hospital Experiences				
Area Around Room 'Always' Quiet at Night	300+	53%	54%	61%
Doctors 'Always' Communicated Well	300+	79%	80%	82%
Home Recovery Information Given	300+	85%	86%	85%
Hospital Given 9 or 10 on 10 Point Scale	300+	70%	69%	71%
Meds 'Always' Explained Before Given	300+	61%	63%	64%
Nurses 'Always' Communicated Well	300+	76%	79%	79%
Pain 'Always' Well Controlled	300+	68%	70%	71%
Room and Bathroom 'Always' Clean	300+	64%	73%	73%
Timely Help 'Always' Received	300+	62%	67%	68%
Would Definitely Recommend Hospital	300+	75%	70%	71%
Use of Medical Imaging				
Cardiac Imaging Stress Test before Surgery	68	11.8%	5.4%	5.3%
Combination Abdominal CT Scan	536	2.4%	12.2%	10.5%
Combination Brain/Sinus CT Scan[1]	-	-	3.1%	2.7%
Combination Chest CT Scan	462	0.0%	2.1%	2.7%
Follow-up Mammogram/Ultrasound	4,802	9.1%	9%	8.8%
Lumbar Spine MRI for Low Back Pain[1]	-	-	35.8%	37.2%

NOTE: Hospital profiles are in alphabetical order by state, then city, then hospital within the city; Rankings exclude hospitals with less than 25 cases except for patient surveys which excludes hospitals with less than 100 cases; (a) 100-299 cases; (1) The number of cases/patients is too few to report; (2) Data submitted were based on a sample of cases/patients; (3) Results are based on a shorter time period than required; (4) Data suppressed by CMS for one or more quarters; (5) Results are not available for this reporting period; (6) Fewer than 100 patients completed the HCAHPS survey; (7) No cases met the criteria for this measure; (8) The lower limit of the confidence interval cannot be calculated if the number of observed infections equals zero; (9) No data are available from the state/territory for this reporting period; (10) The scores shown reflect fewer than 50 completed surveys; (11) There were discrepancies in the data collection process; (12) This measure does not apply to this hospital for this reporting period; (13) Results cannot be calculated for this reporting period; (14) The results for this state are combined with nearby states to protect confidentiality; Please refer to the User's Guide for a full explanation of data.

Saint Clair Memorial Hospital

1000 Bower Hill Road
Pittsburgh, PA 15243
Phone: 412-942-6209
Fax: 412-572-6561
URL: www.stclair.org
Type: Acute Care Hospitals
Emergency Services: Yes
Ownership: Voluntary non-profit - Private
Beds: 314

Key Personnel:
Operating Room. . . . . James M. Collins
Emergency Room . . . . Karen Klein, RN
Quality Assurance . . . . Linda Lattner
Radiology. . . . . Donald P Orr, MD
Pediatric Ambulatory Care . . . . . . Charles Silverstein, MD
Pediatric In-Patient Care . . . . Charles Silverstein, MD
Chief of Medical Staff. . . . . G. Alan Yeasted, MD

Measure	Cases	This Hosp.	State Avg.	U.S. Avg.
Blood Clot Prevention and Treatment				
Anticoagulation Overlap Therapy[2]	159	98%	94%	93%
ICU Venous Thromboembolism Prophylaxis[2]	73	99%	94%	92%
Incidence of Potentially Preventable VTE[2]	36	0%	8%	10%
UFH with Dosages/Platelet Monitoring[2]	156	100%	98%	97%
Venous Thromboembolism Prophylaxis[2]	296	88%	90%	85%
Warfarin Therapy Discharge Instructions[2]	116	100%	78%	75%
Chest Pain/Possible Heart Attack Care				
Aspirin Given Within 24 Hours of Arrival[3,7]	-	-	97%	96%
Fibrinolytic Meds Within 30 Min. of Arrival[5]	-	-	44%	58%
Average Time to ECG (minutes)[3,7]	-	-	9	7
Average Time to Transfer (minutes)[5]	-	-	64	60
Children's Asthma Care				
Received Home Management Plan of Care	-	-	-	88%
Received Reliever Medication	-	-	-	100%
Received Systemic Corticosteroids	-	-	-	100%
Emergency Department				
Admittance Decision Time (minutes)[2]	578	97	104	98
Head CT Results Within 45 Min. of Arrival	15	80%	60%	57%
Patients Who Left ER Before Being Seen	64,774	0%	1%	2%
Time from ER Arrival to Admit. (minutes)[2]	613	222	276	274
Time from ER Arrival to Discharge (minutes)	302	135	125	134
Time in ER Before Being Evaluated (minutes)	376	18	26	26
Time to Pain Meds for Fractures (minutes)	153	52	58	57
Heart Attack Care				
Aspirin Given at Discharge	244	100%	99%	99%
Fibrinolytic Meds Within 30 Min. of Arrival[7]	-	-	40%	54%
PCI Within 90 Minutes of Arrival	58	100%	97%	96%
Statin Prescribed at Discharge	233	99%	99%	98%
Heart Failure Care				
ACE Inhibitor or ARB for LVSD	131	99%	97%	97%
Discharge Instructions Given	396	99%	96%	94%
Evaluation of LVS Function	582	100%	100%	99%
Medicare Spending				
Medicare Spending per Patient (ratio)	-	1.04	1.01	0.98
Pneumonia Care				
Appropriate Initial Antibiotic Given	298	100%	96%	95%
Blood Culture Timing	253	99%	98%	98%
Pregnancy and Delivery Care				
Newborn Deliveries Scheduled Early[2]	36	14%	4%	6%
Preventive Care				
Immunization for Influenza[2]	540	92%	91%	90%
Immunization for Pneumonia[2]	720	98%	92%	92%
Stroke Care				
Anticoagulation Therapy for Atrial Fibrillation	26	100%	96%	95%
Antithrombotic Therapy Timing	148	100%	98%	98%
Assessed for Rehabilitation	158	100%	98%	97%
Discharged on Antithrombotic Therapy	155	100%	99%	99%
Discharged on Statin Medication	111	100%	95%	94%
Thrombolytic Therapy Timing[1]	-	-	72%	66%
Venous Thromboembolism Prophylaxis	153	99%	95%	94%
Written Stroke Educational Materials Given	85	100%	90%	88%
Surgical Care Improvement Project				
Appropriate Beta Blocker Usage	500	97%	98%	98%
Appropriate VTP Within 24 Hours	1,325	99%	99%	98%
Controlled Postoperative Blood Glucose	120	100%	98%	97%
Perioperative Temperature Management	1,562	100%	100%	100%
Prophylactic Antibiotic Selection	1,150	99%	99%	99%
Prophylactic Antibiotic Selection (Outpatient)	379	97%	98%	98%
Prophylactic Antibiotic Stopped	1,134	99%	98%	98%
Prophylactic Antibiotic Timing	1,150	100%	99%	99%
Prophylactic Antibiotic Timing (Outpatient)	360	99%	98%	98%
Urinary Catheter Removal	542	100%	99%	97%
Survey of Patients' Hospital Experiences				
Area Around Room 'Always' Quiet at Night	300+	45%	54%	61%
Doctors 'Always' Communicated Well	300+	81%	80%	82%
Home Recovery Information Given	300+	86%	86%	85%
Hospital Given 9 or 10 on 10 Point Scale	300+	79%	69%	71%
Meds 'Always' Explained Before Given	300+	69%	63%	64%
Nurses 'Always' Communicated Well	300+	85%	79%	79%
Pain 'Always' Well Controlled	300+	75%	70%	71%
Room and Bathroom 'Always' Clean	300+	70%	73%	73%
Timely Help 'Always' Received	300+	74%	67%	68%
Would Definitely Recommend Hospital	300+	82%	70%	71%
Use of Medical Imaging				
Cardiac Imaging Stress Test before Surgery	349	6.9%	5.4%	5.3%
Combination Abdominal CT Scan	886	5.4%	12.2%	10.5%
Combination Brain/Sinus CT Scan	793	1.8%	3.1%	2.7%
Combination Chest CT Scan	568	0.0%	2.1%	2.7%
Follow-up Mammogram/Ultrasound	543	9.9%	9%	8.8%
Lumbar Spine MRI for Low Back Pain	94	35.1%	35.8%	37.2%

UPMC Mercy

1400 Locust Street
Pittsburgh, PA 15219
Phone: 412-232-8111
Fax: 412-232-7408
URL: www.upmc.com/hospitalsfacilities/mercy/pages/default.aspx
Type: Acute Care Hospitals
Emergency Services: Yes
Ownership: Voluntary non-profit - Other
Beds: 416

Key Personnel:
Pediatric In-Patient Care . . . . Bradley J Bradford, MD
Chief of Medical Staff. . . . . John Brungo, MD
CEO/President. . . . . Kenneth A Eshak
Infection Control. . . . . Sharon Krystofiak
Radiology. . . . . Sylvia Lesic
Quality Assurance . . . . Mary Menegazzi
Operating Room. . . . . Claudia Osburn

Measure	Cases	This Hosp.	State Avg.	U.S. Avg.
Blood Clot Prevention and Treatment				
Anticoagulation Overlap Therapy[2]	161	100%	94%	93%
ICU Venous Thromboembolism Prophylaxis[2]	124	98%	94%	92%
Incidence of Potentially Preventable VTE[2]	53	6%	8%	10%
UFH with Dosages/Platelet Monitoring[2]	140	100%	98%	97%
Venous Thromboembolism Prophylaxis[2]	346	97%	90%	85%
Warfarin Therapy Discharge Instructions[2]	106	100%	78%	75%
Chest Pain/Possible Heart Attack Care				
Aspirin Given Within 24 Hours of Arrival[1,3]	-	-	97%	96%
Fibrinolytic Meds Within 30 Min. of Arrival[5]	-	-	44%	58%
Average Time to ECG (minutes)[1,3]	-	-	9	7
Average Time to Transfer (minutes)[5]	-	-	64	60
Children's Asthma Care				
Received Home Management Plan of Care	-	-	-	88%
Received Reliever Medication	-	-	-	100%
Received Systemic Corticosteroids	-	-	-	100%
Emergency Department				
Admittance Decision Time (minutes)[2]	629	96	104	98
Head CT Results Within 45 Min. of Arrival[1]	-	-	60%	57%
Patients Who Left ER Before Being Seen	73,045	1%	1%	2%
Time from ER Arrival to Admit. (minutes)[2]	640	224	276	274
Time from ER Arrival to Discharge (minutes)	488	132	125	134
Time in ER Before Being Evaluated (minutes)	623	14	26	26
Time to Pain Meds for Fractures (minutes)	88	38	58	57
Heart Attack Care				
Aspirin Given at Discharge	346	100%	99%	99%
Fibrinolytic Meds Within 30 Min. of Arrival[7]	-	-	40%	54%
PCI Within 90 Minutes of Arrival	36	100%	97%	96%
Statin Prescribed at Discharge	320	100%	99%	98%
Heart Failure Care				
ACE Inhibitor or ARB for LVSD	142	99%	97%	97%
Discharge Instructions Given	299	100%	96%	94%
Evaluation of LVS Function	408	100%	100%	99%
Medicare Spending				
Medicare Spending per Patient (ratio)	-	1.10	1.01	0.98
Pneumonia Care				
Appropriate Initial Antibiotic Given	188	99%	96%	95%
Blood Culture Timing	145	99%	98%	98%
Pregnancy and Delivery Care				
Newborn Deliveries Scheduled Early[2]	105	0%	4%	6%
Preventive Care				
Immunization for Influenza[2]	637	97%	91%	90%
Immunization for Pneumonia[2]	748	96%	92%	92%
Stroke Care				
Anticoagulation Therapy for Atrial Fibrillation	73	100%	96%	95%
Antithrombotic Therapy Timing	201	100%	98%	98%
Assessed for Rehabilitation	311	100%	98%	97%
Discharged on Antithrombotic Therapy	265	100%	99%	99%
Discharged on Statin Medication	192	99%	95%	94%
Thrombolytic Therapy Timing	40	100%	72%	66%
Venous Thromboembolism Prophylaxis	326	99%	95%	94%
Written Stroke Educational Materials Given	119	91%	90%	88%
Surgical Care Improvement Project				
Appropriate Beta Blocker Usage	473	100%	98%	98%
Appropriate VTP Within 24 Hours	1,120	100%	99%	98%
Controlled Postoperative Blood Glucose	158	99%	98%	97%
Perioperative Temperature Management	1,334	100%	100%	100%
Prophylactic Antibiotic Selection	760	98%	99%	99%
Prophylactic Antibiotic Selection (Outpatient)	385	99%	98%	98%
Prophylactic Antibiotic Stopped	745	98%	98%	98%
Prophylactic Antibiotic Timing	763	99%	99%	99%
Prophylactic Antibiotic Timing (Outpatient)	384	99%	98%	98%
Urinary Catheter Removal	713	100%	99%	97%
Survey of Patients' Hospital Experiences				
Area Around Room 'Always' Quiet at Night	300+	52%	54%	61%
Doctors 'Always' Communicated Well	300+	76%	80%	82%
Home Recovery Information Given	300+	86%	86%	85%
Hospital Given 9 or 10 on 10 Point Scale	300+	63%	69%	71%
Meds 'Always' Explained Before Given	300+	57%	63%	64%
Nurses 'Always' Communicated Well	300+	74%	79%	79%
Pain 'Always' Well Controlled	300+	65%	70%	71%
Room and Bathroom 'Always' Clean	300+	63%	73%	73%
Timely Help 'Always' Received	300+	59%	67%	68%
Would Definitely Recommend Hospital	300+	64%	70%	71%
Use of Medical Imaging				
Cardiac Imaging Stress Test before Surgery	314	8.6%	5.4%	5.3%
Combination Abdominal CT Scan	460	3.7%	12.2%	10.5%
Combination Brain/Sinus CT Scan	451	6.7%	3.1%	2.7%
Combination Chest CT Scan	285	0.0%	2.1%	2.7%
Follow-up Mammogram/Ultrasound	357	11.2%	9%	8.8%
Lumbar Spine MRI for Low Back Pain	48	50.0%	35.8%	37.2%

UPMC Passavant

9100 Babcock Boulevard
Pittsburgh, PA 15237
Phone: 412-367-6700
Fax: 412-367-6527
URL: www.passavant.upmc.com
Type: Acute Care Hospitals
Emergency Services: Yes
Ownership: Voluntary non-profit - Private
Beds: 272

Key Personnel:
CEO/President. . . . . Raymond Beck
Radiology. . . . . Robert A Erbstein, MD
Emergency Room . . . . William Kristin, MD
Pediatric Ambulatory Care . . . . . . Howard K Scott
Pediatric In-Patient Care . . . . Howard K Scott
Chief of Medical Staff. . . . . Thomas Shcauble, MD
Quality Assurance . . . . Connie Susich

Measure	Cases	This Hosp.	State Avg.	U.S. Avg.
Blood Clot Prevention and Treatment				
Anticoagulation Overlap Therapy[2]	180	100%	94%	93%
ICU Venous Thromboembolism Prophylaxis[2]	91	98%	94%	92%
Incidence of Potentially Preventable VTE[2]	33	3%	8%	10%
UFH with Dosages/Platelet Monitoring[2]	125	100%	98%	97%
Venous Thromboembolism Prophylaxis[2]	444	89%	90%	85%
Warfarin Therapy Discharge Instructions[2]	129	100%	78%	75%
Chest Pain/Possible Heart Attack Care				
Aspirin Given Within 24 Hours of Arrival	17	94%	97%	96%
Fibrinolytic Meds Within 30 Min. of Arrival[3,7]	-	-	44%	58%
Average Time to ECG (minutes)	17	6	9	7
Average Time to Transfer (minutes)[1,3]	-	-	64	60
Children's Asthma Care				

NOTE: Hospital profiles are in alphabetical order by state, then city, then hospital within the city; Rankings exclude hospitals with less than 25 cases except for patient surveys which excludes hospitals with less than 100 cases; (a) 100-299 cases; (1) The number of cases/patients is too few to report; (2) Data submitted were based on a sample of cases/patients; (3) Results are based on a shorter time period than required; (4) Data suppressed by CMS for one or more quarters; (5) Results are not available for this reporting period; (6) Fewer than 100 patients completed the HCAHPS survey; (7) No cases met the criteria for this measure; (8) The lower limit of the confidence interval cannot be calculated if the number of observed infections equals zero; (9) No data are available from the state/territory for this reporting period; (10) The scores shown reflect fewer than 50 completed surveys; (11) There were discrepancies in the data collection process; (12) This measure does not apply to this hospital for this reporting period; (13) Results cannot be calculated for this reporting period; (14) The results for this state are combined with nearby states to protect confidentiality; Please refer to the User's Guide for a full explanation of data.

Measure	Cases	This Hosp.	State Avg.	U.S. Avg.
Received Home Management Plan of Care	-	-	-	88%
Received Reliever Medication	-	-	-	100%
Received Systemic Corticosteroids	-	-	-	100%
Emergency Department				
Admittance Decision Time (minutes)[2]	273	77	104	98
Head CT Results Within 45 Min. of Arrival	27	70%	60%	57%
Patients Who Left ER Before Being Seen	60,151	1%	1%	2%
Time from ER Arrival to Admit. (minutes)[2]	283	221	276	274
Time from ER Arrival to Discharge (minutes)	536	151	125	134
Time in ER Before Being Evaluated (minutes)	623	20	26	26
Time to Pain Meds for Fractures (minutes)	191	64	58	57
Heart Attack Care				
Aspirin Given at Discharge	412	100%	99%	99%
Fibrinolytic Meds Within 30 Min. of Arrival[7]	-	-	40%	54%
PCI Within 90 Minutes of Arrival	55	100%	97%	96%
Statin Prescribed at Discharge	407	100%	99%	98%
Heart Failure Care				
ACE Inhibitor or ARB for LVSD	142	100%	97%	97%
Discharge Instructions Given	409	97%	96%	94%
Evaluation of LVS Function	589	100%	100%	99%
Medicare Spending				
Medicare Spending per Patient (ratio)	-	1.03	1.01	0.98
Pneumonia Care				
Appropriate Initial Antibiotic Given	209	96%	96%	95%
Blood Culture Timing	343	99%	98%	98%
Pregnancy and Delivery Care				
Newborn Deliveries Scheduled Early[2,7]	-	-	4%	6%
Preventive Care				
Immunization for Influenza[2]	717	97%	91%	90%
Immunization for Pneumonia[2]	1,017	95%	92%	92%
Stroke Care				
Anticoagulation Therapy for Atrial Fibrillation	22	100%	96%	95%
Antithrombotic Therapy Timing	133	99%	98%	98%
Assessed for Rehabilitation	145	100%	98%	97%
Discharged on Antithrombotic Therapy	138	100%	99%	99%
Discharged on Statin Medication	99	95%	95%	94%
Thrombolytic Therapy Timing[1]	-	-	72%	66%
Venous Thromboembolism Prophylaxis	144	97%	95%	94%
Written Stroke Educational Materials Given	60	100%	90%	88%
Surgical Care Improvement Project				
Appropriate Beta Blocker Usage	702	100%	98%	98%
Appropriate VTP Within 24 Hours	1,825	99%	99%	98%
Controlled Postoperative Blood Glucose	208	99%	98%	97%
Perioperative Temperature Management	2,060	100%	100%	100%
Prophylactic Antibiotic Selection	1,253	100%	99%	99%
Prophylactic Antibiotic Selection (Outpatient)	614	100%	98%	98%
Prophylactic Antibiotic Stopped	1,225	99%	98%	98%
Prophylactic Antibiotic Timing	1,253	99%	99%	99%
Prophylactic Antibiotic Timing (Outpatient)	613	100%	98%	98%
Urinary Catheter Removal	1,014	99%	99%	97%
Survey of Patients' Hospital Experiences				
Area Around Room 'Always' Quiet at Night	300+	50%	54%	61%
Doctors 'Always' Communicated Well	300+	79%	80%	82%
Home Recovery Information Given	300+	88%	86%	85%
Hospital Given 9 or 10 on 10 Point Scale	300+	71%	69%	71%
Meds 'Always' Explained Before Given	300+	59%	63%	64%
Nurses 'Always' Communicated Well	300+	78%	79%	79%
Pain 'Always' Well Controlled	300+	69%	70%	71%
Room and Bathroom 'Always' Clean	300+	67%	73%	73%
Timely Help 'Always' Received	300+	60%	67%	68%
Would Definitely Recommend Hospital	300+	72%	70%	71%
Use of Medical Imaging				
Cardiac Imaging Stress Test before Surgery	309	6.8%	5.4%	5.3%
Combination Abdominal CT Scan	939	15.2%	12.2%	10.5%
Combination Brain/Sinus CT Scan	721	3.6%	3.1%	2.7%
Combination Chest CT Scan	777	0.5%	2.1%	2.7%
Follow-up Mammogram/Ultrasound[7]	-	-	9%	8.8%
Lumbar Spine MRI for Low Back Pain	90	31.1%	35.8%	37.2%

UPMC Presbyterian Shadyside

200 Lothrop Street
Pittsburgh, PA 15213
URL: www.upmc.edu
Phone: 412-647-8788
Fax: 412-647-4881
Type: Acute Care Hospitals
Ownership: Voluntary non-profit - Private
Emergency Services: Yes
Beds: 1,227

Key Personnel:
Hemotology Center . . . . Ronald Herberman, MD
Quality Assurance . . . . April Lana Forf
Emergency Room . . . . Andrew B Peitzman, MD
Intensive Care Unit. . . . . Jorge Rakela, MD
CEO/President. . . . . Jeffrey Romoff
Radiology. . . . . Jules H Sumkin, MD
Chief of Medical Staff . . . . Edward Wing, MD
Anesthesiology. . . . . Peter Winters, MD

Measure	Cases	This Hosp.	State Avg.	U.S. Avg.
Blood Clot Prevention and Treatment				
Anticoagulation Overlap Therapy[2]	554	99%	94%	93%
ICU Venous Thromboembolism Prophylaxis[2]	105	98%	94%	92%
Incidence of Potentially Preventable VTE[2]	247	1%	8%	10%
UFH with Dosages/Platelet Monitoring[2]	634	100%	98%	97%
Venous Thromboembolism Prophylaxis[2]	412	94%	90%	85%
Warfarin Therapy Discharge Instructions[2]	345	100%	78%	75%
Chest Pain/Possible Heart Attack Care				
Aspirin Given Within 24 Hours of Arrival[1,3]	-	-	97%	96%
Fibrinolytic Meds Within 30 Min. of Arrival[5]	-	-	44%	58%
Average Time to ECG (minutes)[1,3]	-	-	9	7
Average Time to Transfer (minutes)[5]	-	-	64	60
Children's Asthma Care				
Received Home Management Plan of Care	-	-	-	88%
Received Reliever Medication	-	-	-	100%
Received Systemic Corticosteroids	-	-	-	100%
Emergency Department				
Admittance Decision Time (minutes)[2]	460	88	104	98
Head CT Results Within 45 Min. of Arrival[1]	-	-	60%	57%
Patients Who Left ER Before Being Seen	>100k	0%	1%	2%
Time from ER Arrival to Admit. (minutes)[2]	481	225	276	274
Time from ER Arrival to Discharge (minutes)	528	149	125	134
Time in ER Before Being Evaluated (minutes)	620	12	26	26
Time to Pain Meds for Fractures (minutes)	74	49	58	57
Heart Attack Care				
Aspirin Given at Discharge	1,069	100%	99%	99%
Fibrinolytic Meds Within 30 Min. of Arrival[7]	-	-	40%	54%
PCI Within 90 Minutes of Arrival	63	100%	97%	96%
Statin Prescribed at Discharge	1,006	100%	99%	98%
Heart Failure Care				
ACE Inhibitor or ARB for LVSD	422	99%	97%	97%
Discharge Instructions Given	1,090	98%	96%	94%
Evaluation of LVS Function	1,368	100%	100%	99%
Medicare Spending				
Medicare Spending per Patient (ratio)	-	1.01	1.01	0.98
Pneumonia Care				
Appropriate Initial Antibiotic Given	219	99%	96%	95%
Blood Culture Timing	431	100%	98%	98%
Pregnancy and Delivery Care				
Newborn Deliveries Scheduled Early[7]	-	-	4%	6%
Preventive Care				
Immunization for Influenza[2]	703	99%	91%	90%
Immunization for Pneumonia[2]	925	99%	92%	92%
Stroke Care				
Anticoagulation Therapy for Atrial Fibrillation	153	99%	96%	95%
Antithrombotic Therapy Timing	612	95%	98%	98%
Assessed for Rehabilitation	1,151	99%	98%	97%
Discharged on Antithrombotic Therapy	838	100%	99%	99%
Discharged on Statin Medication	651	96%	95%	94%
Thrombolytic Therapy Timing	33	100%	72%	66%
Venous Thromboembolism Prophylaxis	1,178	99%	95%	94%
Written Stroke Educational Materials Given	541	96%	90%	88%
Surgical Care Improvement Project				
Appropriate Beta Blocker Usage	2,556	100%	98%	98%
Appropriate VTP Within 24 Hours	5,172	100%	99%	98%
Controlled Postoperative Blood Glucose	919	97%	98%	97%
Perioperative Temperature Management	6,520	100%	100%	100%
Prophylactic Antibiotic Selection	2,754	100%	99%	99%
Prophylactic Antibiotic Selection (Outpatient)	1,066	100%	98%	98%
Prophylactic Antibiotic Stopped	2,698	99%	98%	98%
Prophylactic Antibiotic Timing	2,755	100%	99%	99%
Prophylactic Antibiotic Timing (Outpatient)	1,042	99%	98%	98%
Urinary Catheter Removal	4,191	100%	99%	97%
Survey of Patients' Hospital Experiences				
Area Around Room 'Always' Quiet at Night	300+	51%	54%	61%
Doctors 'Always' Communicated Well	300+	79%	80%	82%
Home Recovery Information Given	300+	88%	86%	85%
Hospital Given 9 or 10 on 10 Point Scale	300+	69%	69%	71%
Meds 'Always' Explained Before Given	300+	61%	63%	64%
Nurses 'Always' Communicated Well	300+	78%	79%	79%
Pain 'Always' Well Controlled	300+	68%	70%	71%
Room and Bathroom 'Always' Clean	300+	61%	73%	73%
Timely Help 'Always' Received	300+	61%	67%	68%
Would Definitely Recommend Hospital	300+	72%	70%	71%
Use of Medical Imaging				
Cardiac Imaging Stress Test before Surgery	680	7.2%	5.4%	5.3%
Combination Abdominal CT Scan	2,936	14.3%	12.2%	10.5%
Combination Brain/Sinus CT Scan	928	4.0%	3.1%	2.7%
Combination Chest CT Scan	3,430	0.3%	2.1%	2.7%
Follow-up Mammogram/Ultrasound[7]	-	-	9%	8.8%
Lumbar Spine MRI for Low Back Pain	204	37.7%	35.8%	37.2%

UPMC Saint Margaret

815 Freeport Road
Pittsburgh, PA 15215
URL: www.stmargaret.upmc.com
Phone: 412-784-4000
Fax: 412-784-4788
Type: Acute Care Hospitals
Ownership: Voluntary non-profit - Private
Emergency Services: Yes
Beds: 250

Key Personnel:
Operating Room. . . . . M Cook, RN
Cardiac Laboratory. . . . . Jean Culhane
Radiology. . . . . Bill Simmons
CEO/President. . . . . Richard E Sobehart

Measure	Cases	This Hosp.	State Avg.	U.S. Avg.
Blood Clot Prevention and Treatment				
Anticoagulation Overlap Therapy[2]	139	99%	94%	93%
ICU Venous Thromboembolism Prophylaxis[2]	57	100%	94%	92%
Incidence of Potentially Preventable VTE[2]	25	0%	8%	10%
UFH with Dosages/Platelet Monitoring[2]	127	100%	98%	97%
Venous Thromboembolism Prophylaxis[2]	740	91%	90%	85%
Warfarin Therapy Discharge Instructions[2]	97	100%	78%	75%
Chest Pain/Possible Heart Attack Care				
Aspirin Given Within 24 Hours of Arrival	118	100%	97%	96%
Fibrinolytic Meds Within 30 Min. of Arrival[1]	-	-	44%	58%
Average Time to ECG (minutes)	122	7	9	7
Average Time to Transfer (minutes)	25	49	64	60
Children's Asthma Care				
Received Home Management Plan of Care	-	-	-	88%
Received Reliever Medication	-	-	-	100%
Received Systemic Corticosteroids	-	-	-	100%
Emergency Department				
Admittance Decision Time (minutes)[2]	671	94	104	98
Head CT Results Within 45 Min. of Arrival	16	88%	60%	57%
Patients Who Left ER Before Being Seen	40,321	0%	1%	2%
Time from ER Arrival to Admit. (minutes)[2]	676	221	276	274
Time from ER Arrival to Discharge (minutes)	545	159	125	134
Time in ER Before Being Evaluated (minutes)	618	21	26	26
Time to Pain Meds for Fractures (minutes)	75	57	58	57
Heart Attack Care				
Aspirin Given at Discharge	89	98%	99%	99%
Fibrinolytic Meds Within 30 Min. of Arrival[7]	-	-	40%	54%
PCI Within 90 Minutes of Arrival[7]	-	-	97%	96%
Statin Prescribed at Discharge	80	95%	99%	98%
Heart Failure Care				
ACE Inhibitor or ARB for LVSD	91	96%	97%	97%
Discharge Instructions Given	380	95%	96%	94%
Evaluation of LVS Function	543	100%	100%	99%
Medicare Spending				
Medicare Spending per Patient (ratio)	-	1.07	1.01	0.98
Pneumonia Care				
Appropriate Initial Antibiotic Given	178	97%	96%	95%

NOTE: Hospital profiles are in alphabetical order by state, then city, then hospital within the city; Rankings exclude hospitals with less than 25 cases except for patient surveys which excludes hospitals with less than 100 cases; (a) 100-299 cases; (1) The number of cases/patients is too few to report; (2) Data submitted were based on a sample of cases/patients; (3) Results are based on a shorter time period than required; (4) Data suppressed by CMS for one or more quarters; (5) Results are not available for this reporting period; (6) Fewer than 100 patients completed the HCAHPS survey; (7) No cases met the criteria for this measure; (8) The lower limit of the confidence interval cannot be calculated if the number of observed infections equals zero; (9) No data are available from the state/territory for this reporting period; (10) The scores shown reflect fewer than 50 completed surveys; (11) There were discrepancies in the data collection process; (12) This measure does not apply to this hospital for this reporting period; (13) Results cannot be calculated for this reporting period; (14) The results for this state are combined with nearby states to protect confidentiality; Please refer to the User's Guide for a full explanation of data.

Measure	Cases	This Hosp.	State Avg.	U.S. Avg.
Blood Culture Timing	216	100%	98%	98%
Pregnancy and Delivery Care				
Newborn Deliveries Scheduled Early[7]	-	-	4%	6%
Preventive Care				
Immunization for Influenza[2]	717	97%	91%	90%
Immunization for Pneumonia[2]	1,108	97%	92%	92%
Stroke Care				
Anticoagulation Therapy for Atrial Fibrillation	27	100%	96%	95%
Antithrombotic Therapy Timing	145	100%	98%	98%
Assessed for Rehabilitation	157	99%	98%	97%
Discharged on Antithrombotic Therapy	148	100%	99%	99%
Discharged on Statin Medication	107	100%	95%	94%
Thrombolytic Therapy Timing[1]	-	-	72%	66%
Venous Thromboembolism Prophylaxis	163	97%	95%	94%
Written Stroke Educational Materials Given	82	98%	90%	88%
Surgical Care Improvement Project				
Appropriate Beta Blocker Usage	546	100%	98%	98%
Appropriate VTP Within 24 Hours	1,387	100%	99%	98%
Controlled Postoperative Blood Glucose[7]	-	-	98%	97%
Perioperative Temperature Management	1,565	100%	100%	100%
Prophylactic Antibiotic Selection	1,150	100%	99%	99%
Prophylactic Antibiotic Selection (Outpatient)	230	99%	98%	98%
Prophylactic Antibiotic Stopped	1,128	99%	98%	98%
Prophylactic Antibiotic Timing	1,150	100%	99%	99%
Prophylactic Antibiotic Timing (Outpatient)	231	99%	98%	98%
Urinary Catheter Removal	1,249	100%	99%	97%
Survey of Patients' Hospital Experiences				
Area Around Room 'Always' Quiet at Night	300+	43%	54%	61%
Doctors 'Always' Communicated Well	300+	80%	80%	82%
Home Recovery Information Given	300+	88%	86%	85%
Hospital Given 9 or 10 on 10 Point Scale	300+	68%	69%	71%
Meds 'Always' Explained Before Given	300+	63%	63%	64%
Nurses 'Always' Communicated Well	300+	77%	79%	79%
Pain 'Always' Well Controlled	300+	66%	70%	71%
Room and Bathroom 'Always' Clean	300+	62%	73%	73%
Timely Help 'Always' Received	300+	57%	67%	68%
Would Definitely Recommend Hospital	300+	72%	70%	71%
Use of Medical Imaging				
Cardiac Imaging Stress Test before Surgery	232	6.5%	5.4%	5.3%
Combination Abdominal CT Scan	637	11.3%	12.2%	10.5%
Combination Brain/Sinus CT Scan	434	5.3%	3.1%	2.7%
Combination Chest CT Scan	509	0.0%	2.1%	2.7%
Follow-up Mammogram/Ultrasound[7]	-	-	9%	8.8%
Lumbar Spine MRI for Low Back Pain	101	40.6%	35.8%	37.2%

VA Pittsburgh Healthcare System

University Drive C
Pittsburgh, PA 15240
Phone: 412-688-6100
Fax: 412-688-6121
URL: www.pittsburg.va.gov
Type: Acute Care - VA
Emergency Services: No
Ownership: Government Federal
Beds: 146

Key Personnel:
Anesthesiology. . . . . Richard J Bjerke, MD
CEO/President. . . . . Terry Gerick Wolf, FACHE
Radiology. . . . . B Kart, MD
Infection Control. . . . . Robert Muder
Quality Assurance . . . . Barbara Reichbaum, RN
Intensive Care Unit. . . . . Paul Rogers, MD
Chief of Medical Staff. . . . . Ali Sonel, MD
Operating Room. . . . . Mark Wilson, MD, PhD

Measure	Cases	This Hosp.	State Avg.	U.S. Avg.
Blood Clot Prevention and Treatment				
Anticoagulation Overlap Therapy	-	-	94%	93%
ICU Venous Thromboembolism Prophylaxis	-	-	94%	92%
Incidence of Potentially Preventable VTE	-	-	8%	10%
UFH with Dosages/Platelet Monitoring	-	-	98%	97%
Venous Thromboembolism Prophylaxis	-	-	90%	85%
Warfarin Therapy Discharge Instructions	-	-	78%	75%
Chest Pain/Possible Heart Attack Care				
Aspirin Given Within 24 Hours of Arrival	-	-	97%	96%
Fibrinolytic Meds Within 30 Min. of Arrival	-	-	44%	58%
Average Time to ECG (minutes)	-	-	9	7
Average Time to Transfer (minutes)	-	-	64	60
Children's Asthma Care				
Received Home Management Plan of Care	-	-	-	88%
Received Reliever Medication	-	-	-	100%
Received Systemic Corticosteroids	-	-	-	100%
Emergency Department				
Admittance Decision Time (minutes)	-	-	104	98
Head CT Results Within 45 Min. of Arrival	-	-	60%	57%
Patients Who Left ER Before Being Seen	-	-	1%	2%
Time from ER Arrival to Admit. (minutes)	-	-	276	274
Time from ER Arrival to Discharge (minutes)	-	-	125	134
Time in ER Before Being Evaluated (minutes)	-	-	26	26
Time to Pain Meds for Fractures (minutes)	-	-	58	57
Heart Attack Care				
Aspirin Given at Discharge	74	100%	99%	99%
Fibrinolytic Meds Within 30 Min. of Arrival[5]	-	-	40%	54%
PCI Within 90 Minutes of Arrival[1]	12	83%	97%	96%
Statin Prescribed at Discharge	74	99%	99%	98%
Heart Failure Care				
ACE Inhibitor or ARB for LVSD	92	99%	97%	97%
Discharge Instructions Given	269	97%	96%	94%
Evaluation of LVS Function	309	100%	100%	99%
Medicare Spending				
Medicare Spending per Patient (ratio)	-	-	1.01	0.98
Pneumonia Care				
Appropriate Initial Antibiotic Given	69	100%	96%	95%
Blood Culture Timing	215	100%	98%	98%
Pregnancy and Delivery Care				
Newborn Deliveries Scheduled Early	-	-	4%	6%
Preventive Care				
Immunization for Influenza[5]	-	-	91%	90%
Immunization for Pneumonia[5]	-	-	92%	92%
Stroke Care				
Anticoagulation Therapy for Atrial Fibrillation	-	-	96%	95%
Antithrombotic Therapy Timing	-	-	98%	98%
Assessed for Rehabilitation	-	-	98%	97%
Discharged on Antithrombotic Therapy	-	-	99%	99%
Discharged on Statin Medication	-	-	95%	94%
Thrombolytic Therapy Timing	-	-	72%	66%
Venous Thromboembolism Prophylaxis	-	-	95%	94%
Written Stroke Educational Materials Given	-	-	90%	88%
Surgical Care Improvement Project				
Appropriate Beta Blocker Usage[2]	270	93%	98%	98%
Appropriate VTP Within 24 Hours[2]	297	98%	99%	98%
Controlled Postoperative Blood Glucose[2]	165	96%	98%	97%
Perioperative Temperature Management[2]	399	100%	100%	100%
Prophylactic Antibiotic Selection	414	100%	99%	99%
Prophylactic Antibiotic Selection (Outpatient)	-	-	98%	98%
Prophylactic Antibiotic Stopped	399	96%	98%	98%
Prophylactic Antibiotic Timing	414	98%	99%	99%
Prophylactic Antibiotic Timing (Outpatient)	-	-	98%	98%
Urinary Catheter Removal[2]	401	100%	99%	97%
Survey of Patients' Hospital Experiences				
Area Around Room 'Always' Quiet at Night	-	-	54%	61%
Doctors 'Always' Communicated Well	-	-	80%	82%
Home Recovery Information Given	-	-	86%	85%
Hospital Given 9 or 10 on 10 Point Scale	-	-	69%	71%
Meds 'Always' Explained Before Given	-	-	63%	64%
Nurses 'Always' Communicated Well	-	-	79%	79%
Pain 'Always' Well Controlled	-	-	70%	71%
Room and Bathroom 'Always' Clean	-	-	73%	73%
Timely Help 'Always' Received	-	-	67%	68%
Would Definitely Recommend Hospital	-	-	70%	71%
Use of Medical Imaging				
Cardiac Imaging Stress Test before Surgery	-	-	5.4%	5.3%
Combination Abdominal CT Scan	-	-	12.2%	10.5%
Combination Brain/Sinus CT Scan	-	-	3.1%	2.7%
Combination Chest CT Scan	-	-	2.1%	2.7%
Follow-up Mammogram/Ultrasound	-	-	9%	8.8%
Lumbar Spine MRI for Low Back Pain	-	-	35.8%	37.2%

Western Pennsylvania Hospital

4800 Friendship Avenue
Pittsburgh, PA 15224
Phone: 412-578-5000
Fax: 412-578-1296
URL: www.wpahs.org/wph/contact/index.html
Type: Acute Care Hospitals
Emergency Services: Yes
Ownership: Voluntary non-profit - Private
Beds: 542

Key Personnel:
Emergency Room . . . . Thomas Campbell, MD
Operating Room. . . . . Philip F Caushaj, MD
Chief of Medical Staff . . . . William Goldfarb, MD
Cardiac Laboratory. . . . . Alan H Gradman, MD
Radiology. . . . . Paul Kiproff, MD
Pediatric In-Patient Care . . . . . . Alan Lamtzy, MD
CEO/President. . . . . Duke Rupert
Infection Control. . . . . David L Weinbaum, MD

Measure	Cases	This Hosp.	State Avg.	U.S. Avg.
Blood Clot Prevention and Treatment				
Anticoagulation Overlap Therapy[2]	33	100%	94%	93%
ICU Venous Thromboembolism Prophylaxis[2]	83	82%	94%	92%
Incidence of Potentially Preventable VTE[2]	19	32%	8%	10%
UFH with Dosages/Platelet Monitoring[2]	47	100%	98%	97%
Venous Thromboembolism Prophylaxis[2]	435	74%	90%	85%
Warfarin Therapy Discharge Instructions[2]	26	92%	78%	75%
Chest Pain/Possible Heart Attack Care				
Aspirin Given Within 24 Hours of Arrival[3]	34	100%	97%	96%
Fibrinolytic Meds Within 30 Min. of Arrival[3,7]	-	-	44%	58%
Average Time to ECG (minutes)[3]	33	11	9	7
Average Time to Transfer (minutes)[1,3]	-	-	64	60
Children's Asthma Care				
Received Home Management Plan of Care	-	-	-	88%
Received Reliever Medication	-	-	-	100%
Received Systemic Corticosteroids	-	-	-	100%
Emergency Department				
Admittance Decision Time (minutes)[2]	104	38	104	98
Head CT Results Within 45 Min. of Arrival[1]	-	-	60%	57%
Patients Who Left ER Before Being Seen	17,515	0%	1%	2%
Time from ER Arrival to Admit. (minutes)[2]	125	183	276	274
Time from ER Arrival to Discharge (minutes)	401	112	125	134
Time in ER Before Being Evaluated (minutes)	419	16	26	26
Time to Pain Meds for Fractures (minutes)[1]	-	-	58	57
Heart Attack Care				
Aspirin Given at Discharge	69	100%	99%	99%
Fibrinolytic Meds Within 30 Min. of Arrival[7]	-	-	40%	54%
PCI Within 90 Minutes of Arrival[1]	-	-	97%	96%
Statin Prescribed at Discharge	68	99%	99%	98%
Heart Failure Care				
ACE Inhibitor or ARB for LVSD	20	100%	97%	97%
Discharge Instructions Given	64	84%	96%	94%
Evaluation of LVS Function	79	100%	100%	99%
Medicare Spending				
Medicare Spending per Patient (ratio)	-	1.02	1.01	0.98
Pneumonia Care				
Appropriate Initial Antibiotic Given	30	100%	96%	95%
Blood Culture Timing	50	100%	98%	98%
Pregnancy and Delivery Care				
Newborn Deliveries Scheduled Early[2]	217	1%	4%	6%
Preventive Care				
Immunization for Influenza[2]	438	87%	91%	90%
Immunization for Pneumonia[2]	312	72%	92%	92%
Stroke Care				
Anticoagulation Therapy for Atrial Fibrillation[1]	-	-	96%	95%
Antithrombotic Therapy Timing	24	100%	98%	98%
Assessed for Rehabilitation	26	100%	98%	97%
Discharged on Antithrombotic Therapy	26	100%	99%	99%
Discharged on Statin Medication	21	100%	95%	94%
Thrombolytic Therapy Timing[1]	-	-	72%	66%
Venous Thromboembolism Prophylaxis	26	92%	95%	94%
Written Stroke Educational Materials Given[1]	-	-	90%	88%
Surgical Care Improvement Project				
Appropriate Beta Blocker Usage	98	99%	98%	98%
Appropriate VTP Within 24 Hours	388	99%	99%	98%
Controlled Postoperative Blood Glucose	19	100%	98%	97%
Perioperative Temperature Management	441	100%	100%	100%
Prophylactic Antibiotic Selection	279	99%	99%	99%

NOTE: Hospital profiles are in alphabetical order by state, then city, then hospital within the city; Rankings exclude hospitals with less than 25 cases except for patient surveys which excludes hospitals with less than 100 cases; (a) 100-299 cases; (1) The number of cases/patients is too few to report; (2) Data submitted were based on a sample of cases/patients; (3) Results are based on a shorter time period than required; (4) Data suppressed by CMS for one or more quarters; (5) Results are not available for this reporting period; (6) Fewer than 100 patients completed the HCAHPS survey; (7) No cases met the criteria for this measure; (8) The lower limit of the confidence interval cannot be calculated if the number of observed infections equals zero; (9) No data are available from the state/territory for this reporting period; (10) The scores shown reflect fewer than 50 completed surveys; (11) There were discrepancies in the data collection process; (12) This measure does not apply to this hospital for this reporting period; (13) Results cannot be calculated for this reporting period; (14) The results for this state are combined with nearby states to protect confidentiality; Please refer to the User's Guide for a full explanation of data.

Measure	Cases	This Hosp.	State Avg.	U.S. Avg.
Prophylactic Antibiotic Selection (Outpatient)	340	99%	98%	98%
Prophylactic Antibiotic Stopped	274	98%	98%	98%
Prophylactic Antibiotic Timing	278	100%	99%	99%
Prophylactic Antibiotic Timing (Outpatient)	340	100%	98%	98%
Urinary Catheter Removal	180	100%	99%	97%
Survey of Patients' Hospital Experiences				
Area Around Room 'Always' Quiet at Night	300+	62%	54%	61%
Doctors 'Always' Communicated Well	300+	80%	80%	82%
Home Recovery Information Given	300+	86%	86%	85%
Hospital Given 9 or 10 on 10 Point Scale	300+	67%	69%	71%
Meds 'Always' Explained Before Given	300+	63%	63%	64%
Nurses 'Always' Communicated Well	300+	77%	79%	79%
Pain 'Always' Well Controlled	300+	69%	70%	71%
Room and Bathroom 'Always' Clean	300+	65%	73%	73%
Timely Help 'Always' Received	300+	64%	67%	68%
Would Definitely Recommend Hospital	300+	73%	70%	71%
Use of Medical Imaging				
Cardiac Imaging Stress Test before Surgery	88	9.1%	5.4%	5.3%
Combination Abdominal CT Scan	211	7.1%	12.2%	10.5%
Combination Brain/Sinus CT Scan[1]	-	-	3.1%	2.7%
Combination Chest CT Scan	120	0.0%	2.1%	2.7%
Follow-up Mammogram/Ultrasound	441	13.4%	9%	8.8%
Lumbar Spine MRI for Low Back Pain[1]	-	-	35.8%	37.2%

Pottstown Memorial Medical Center

1600 East High Street & Armand Hammer Blvd
Phone: 610-327-7000
Pottstown, PA 19464
Fax: 610-327-7432
URL: www.pmmctr.org
Type: Acute Care Hospitals
Emergency Services: Yes
Ownership: Proprietary
Beds: 299

Key Personnel:

Operating Room. . . . . Cindy Iannelli
Infection Control. . . . . Elizabeth Jabbs
CEO/President. . . . . John Kirby
Patient Relations . . . . Karen Reifsnyder
Chief of Medical Staff . . . . Richard F Saylor, MD
Emergency Room . . . . Marvin Silverman, DO
Radiology. . . . . Stephen Whitmoyer
Quality Assurance . . . . Nancy Yocom

Measure	Cases	This Hosp.	State Avg.	U.S. Avg.
Blood Clot Prevention and Treatment				
Anticoagulation Overlap Therapy[2]	57	98%	94%	93%
ICU Venous Thromboembolism Prophylaxis[2]	98	91%	94%	92%
Incidence of Potentially Preventable VTE[2]	16	6%	8%	10%
UFH with Dosages/Platelet Monitoring[2]	67	100%	98%	97%
Venous Thromboembolism Prophylaxis[2]	509	87%	90%	85%
Warfarin Therapy Discharge Instructions[2]	40	90%	78%	75%
Chest Pain/Possible Heart Attack Care				
Aspirin Given Within 24 Hours of Arrival	88	100%	97%	96%
Fibrinolytic Meds Within 30 Min. of Arrival[7]	-	-	44%	58%
Average Time to ECG (minutes)	89	15	9	7
Average Time to Transfer (minutes)	19	57	64	60
Children's Asthma Care				
Received Home Management Plan of Care	-	-	-	88%
Received Reliever Medication	-	-	-	100%
Received Systemic Corticosteroids	-	-	-	100%
Emergency Department				
Admittance Decision Time (minutes)[2]	943	115	104	98
Head CT Results Within 45 Min. of Arrival[1]	-	-	60%	57%
Patients Who Left ER Before Being Seen	43,956	1%	1%	2%
Time from ER Arrival to Admit. (minutes)[2]	948	274	276	274
Time from ER Arrival to Discharge (minutes)	353	131	125	134
Time in ER Before Being Evaluated (minutes)	418	21	26	26
Time to Pain Meds for Fractures (minutes)	124	67	58	57
Heart Attack Care				
Aspirin Given at Discharge	30	100%	99%	99%
Fibrinolytic Meds Within 30 Min. of Arrival[7]	-	-	40%	54%
PCI Within 90 Minutes of Arrival[7]	-	-	97%	96%
Statin Prescribed at Discharge	27	78%	99%	98%
Heart Failure Care				
ACE Inhibitor or ARB for LVSD	62	100%	97%	97%
Discharge Instructions Given	168	98%	96%	94%
Evaluation of LVS Function	226	100%	100%	99%
Medicare Spending				
Medicare Spending per Patient (ratio)	-	1.07	1.01	0.98
Pneumonia Care				
Appropriate Initial Antibiotic Given	105	98%	96%	95%
Blood Culture Timing	263	100%	98%	98%
Pregnancy and Delivery Care				
Newborn Deliveries Scheduled Early[2]	33	9%	4%	6%
Preventive Care				
Immunization for Influenza[2]	649	99%	91%	90%
Immunization for Pneumonia[2]	889	99%	92%	92%
Stroke Care				
Anticoagulation Therapy for Atrial Fibrillation	21	100%	96%	95%
Antithrombotic Therapy Timing	104	100%	98%	98%
Assessed for Rehabilitation	106	97%	98%	97%
Discharged on Antithrombotic Therapy	98	99%	99%	99%
Discharged on Statin Medication	85	93%	95%	94%
Thrombolytic Therapy Timing[1]	-	-	72%	66%
Venous Thromboembolism Prophylaxis	119	90%	95%	94%
Written Stroke Educational Materials Given	38	76%	90%	88%
Surgical Care Improvement Project				
Appropriate Beta Blocker Usage	118	100%	98%	98%
Appropriate VTP Within 24 Hours	398	99%	99%	98%
Controlled Postoperative Blood Glucose[7]	-	-	98%	97%
Perioperative Temperature Management	438	100%	100%	100%
Prophylactic Antibiotic Selection	288	99%	99%	99%
Prophylactic Antibiotic Selection (Outpatient)	90	93%	98%	98%
Prophylactic Antibiotic Stopped	270	100%	98%	98%
Prophylactic Antibiotic Timing	288	99%	99%	99%
Prophylactic Antibiotic Timing (Outpatient)	91	98%	98%	98%
Urinary Catheter Removal	345	99%	99%	97%
Survey of Patients' Hospital Experiences				
Area Around Room 'Always' Quiet at Night	300+	48%	54%	61%
Doctors 'Always' Communicated Well	300+	75%	80%	82%
Home Recovery Information Given	300+	86%	86%	85%
Hospital Given 9 or 10 on 10 Point Scale	300+	56%	69%	71%
Meds 'Always' Explained Before Given	300+	58%	63%	64%
Nurses 'Always' Communicated Well	300+	75%	79%	79%
Pain 'Always' Well Controlled	300+	64%	70%	71%
Room and Bathroom 'Always' Clean	300+	63%	73%	73%
Timely Help 'Always' Received	300+	55%	67%	68%
Would Definitely Recommend Hospital	300+	54%	70%	71%
Use of Medical Imaging				
Cardiac Imaging Stress Test before Surgery	127	11.0%	5.4%	5.3%
Combination Abdominal CT Scan	959	24.3%	12.2%	10.5%
Combination Brain/Sinus CT Scan	775	2.6%	3.1%	2.7%
Combination Chest CT Scan	517	4.4%	2.1%	2.7%
Follow-up Mammogram/Ultrasound	1,531	7.3%	9%	8.8%
Lumbar Spine MRI for Low Back Pain	190	40.0%	35.8%	37.2%

Schuylkill Medical Center - East Norwegian Street

700 East Norwegian Street
Phone: 570-621-4000
Pottsville, PA 17901
Fax: 570-621-4775
URL: www.schuylkillhealth.com
Type: Acute Care Hospitals
Emergency Services: Yes
Ownership: Voluntary non-profit - Church
Beds: 221

Key Personnel:

Quality Assurance . . . . Patricia Baldwin
CEO/President. . . . . Peter U Bergmann
Coronary Care. . . . . Cynthia Cappel
Infection Control. . . . . Susan Light
Chief of Medical Staff. . . . . Thomas McLaughlin, MD
Operating Room. . . . . Rose Ann Mucci
Pediatric In-Patient Care . . . . Carol Rowan, RN

Measure	Cases	This Hosp.	State Avg.	U.S. Avg.
Blood Clot Prevention and Treatment				
Anticoagulation Overlap Therapy[2]	39	97%	94%	93%
ICU Venous Thromboembolism Prophylaxis[2]	66	89%	94%	92%
Incidence of Potentially Preventable VTE[1,2]	-	-	8%	10%
UFH with Dosages/Platelet Monitoring[2]	13	100%	98%	97%
Venous Thromboembolism Prophylaxis[2]	350	89%	90%	85%
Warfarin Therapy Discharge Instructions[2]	20	95%	78%	75%
Chest Pain/Possible Heart Attack Care				
Aspirin Given Within 24 Hours of Arrival	106	100%	97%	96%
Fibrinolytic Meds Within 30 Min. of Arrival[7]	-	-	44%	58%
Average Time to ECG (minutes)	110	12	9	7
Average Time to Transfer (minutes)	14	66	64	60
Children's Asthma Care				
Received Home Management Plan of Care	-	-	-	88%
Received Reliever Medication	-	-	-	100%
Received Systemic Corticosteroids	-	-	-	100%
Emergency Department				
Admittance Decision Time (minutes)[2]	541	60	104	98
Head CT Results Within 45 Min. of Arrival[1]	-	-	60%	57%
Patients Who Left ER Before Being Seen	21,669	1%	1%	2%
Time from ER Arrival to Admit. (minutes)[2]	610	215	276	274
Time from ER Arrival to Discharge (minutes)	358	98	125	134
Time in ER Before Being Evaluated (minutes)	377	33	26	26
Time to Pain Meds for Fractures (minutes)	52	64	58	57
Heart Attack Care				
Aspirin Given at Discharge	36	94%	99%	99%
Fibrinolytic Meds Within 30 Min. of Arrival[7]	-	-	40%	54%
PCI Within 90 Minutes of Arrival[7]	-	-	97%	96%
Statin Prescribed at Discharge	34	76%	99%	98%
Heart Failure Care				
ACE Inhibitor or ARB for LVSD	40	98%	97%	97%
Discharge Instructions Given	145	96%	96%	94%
Evaluation of LVS Function	239	100%	100%	99%
Medicare Spending				
Medicare Spending per Patient (ratio)	-	1.05	1.01	0.98
Pneumonia Care				
Appropriate Initial Antibiotic Given	105	95%	96%	95%
Blood Culture Timing	175	100%	98%	98%
Pregnancy and Delivery Care				
Newborn Deliveries Scheduled Early[7]	-	-	4%	6%
Preventive Care				
Immunization for Influenza[2]	376	93%	91%	90%
Immunization for Pneumonia[2]	639	96%	92%	92%
Stroke Care				
Anticoagulation Therapy for Atrial Fibrillation	12	100%	96%	95%
Antithrombotic Therapy Timing	53	100%	98%	98%
Assessed for Rehabilitation	51	98%	98%	97%
Discharged on Antithrombotic Therapy	49	100%	99%	99%
Discharged on Statin Medication	44	75%	95%	94%
Thrombolytic Therapy Timing[1]	-	-	72%	66%
Venous Thromboembolism Prophylaxis	59	88%	95%	94%
Written Stroke Educational Materials Given	15	67%	90%	88%
Surgical Care Improvement Project				
Appropriate Beta Blocker Usage	72	93%	98%	98%
Appropriate VTP Within 24 Hours	174	97%	99%	98%
Controlled Postoperative Blood Glucose[7]	-	-	98%	97%
Perioperative Temperature Management	205	100%	100%	100%
Prophylactic Antibiotic Selection	129	98%	99%	99%
Prophylactic Antibiotic Selection (Outpatient)[1]	-	-	98%	98%
Prophylactic Antibiotic Stopped	123	92%	98%	98%
Prophylactic Antibiotic Timing	129	99%	99%	99%
Prophylactic Antibiotic Timing (Outpatient)[1]	-	-	98%	98%
Urinary Catheter Removal	127	96%	99%	97%
Survey of Patients' Hospital Experiences				
Area Around Room 'Always' Quiet at Night	300+	49%	54%	61%
Doctors 'Always' Communicated Well	300+	79%	80%	82%
Home Recovery Information Given	300+	84%	86%	85%
Hospital Given 9 or 10 on 10 Point Scale	300+	66%	69%	71%
Meds 'Always' Explained Before Given	300+	60%	63%	64%
Nurses 'Always' Communicated Well	300+	79%	79%	79%
Pain 'Always' Well Controlled	300+	72%	70%	71%
Room and Bathroom 'Always' Clean	300+	75%	73%	73%
Timely Help 'Always' Received	300+	73%	67%	68%
Would Definitely Recommend Hospital	300+	61%	70%	71%
Use of Medical Imaging				
Cardiac Imaging Stress Test before Surgery[1]	-	-	5.4%	5.3%
Combination Abdominal CT Scan	436	3.0%	12.2%	10.5%
Combination Brain/Sinus CT Scan[1]	-	-	3.1%	2.7%
Combination Chest CT Scan	189	0.0%	2.1%	2.7%
Follow-up Mammogram/Ultrasound	525	3.4%	9%	8.8%
Lumbar Spine MRI for Low Back Pain[7]	-	-	35.8%	37.2%

NOTE: Hospital profiles are in alphabetical order by state, then city, then hospital within the city; Rankings exclude hospitals with less than 25 cases except for patient surveys which excludes hospitals with less than 100 cases; (a) 100-299 cases; (1) The number of cases/patients is too few to report; (2) Data submitted were based on a sample of cases/patients; (3) Results are based on a shorter time period than required; (4) Data suppressed by CMS for one or more quarters; (5) Results are not available for this reporting period; (6) Fewer than 100 patients completed the HCAHPS survey; (7) No cases met the criteria for this measure; (8) The lower limit of the confidence interval cannot be calculated if the number of observed infections equals zero; (9) No data are available from the state/territory for this reporting period; (10) The scores shown reflect fewer than 50 completed surveys; (11) There were discrepancies in the data collection process; (12) This measure does not apply to this hospital for this reporting period; (13) Results cannot be calculated for this reporting period; (14) The results for this state are combined with nearby states to protect confidentiality; Please refer to the User's Guide for a full explanation of data.

Schuylkill Medical Center - South Jackson Street

420 South Jackson Street Phone: 570-621-5000
Pottsville, PA 17901
URL: www.pottsvillehospital.com
Type: Acute Care Hospitals Emergency Services: Yes
Ownership: Voluntary non-profit - Private Beds: 200
Key Personnel:
CEO/President. . . . . John E Simodejka
Administrator . . . . Cathy Sophy, RN

Measure	Cases	This Hosp.	State Avg.	U.S. Avg.
Blood Clot Prevention and Treatment				
Anticoagulation Overlap Therapy[2]	50	94%	94%	93%
ICU Venous Thromboembolism Prophylaxis[2]	90	90%	94%	92%
Incidence of Potentially Preventable VTE[1,2]	-	-	8%	10%
UFH with Dosages/Platelet Monitoring[2]	28	100%	98%	97%
Venous Thromboembolism Prophylaxis[2]	333	91%	90%	85%
Warfarin Therapy Discharge Instructions[2]	27	96%	78%	75%
Chest Pain/Possible Heart Attack Care				
Aspirin Given Within 24 Hours of Arrival	61	95%	97%	96%
Fibrinolytic Meds Within 30 Min. of Arrival[7]	-	-	44%	58%
Average Time to ECG (minutes)	63	13	9	7
Average Time to Transfer (minutes)	11	49	64	60
Children's Asthma Care				
Received Home Management Plan of Care	-	-	-	88%
Received Reliever Medication	-	-	-	100%
Received Systemic Corticosteroids	-	-	-	100%
Emergency Department				
Admittance Decision Time (minutes)[2]	513	40	104	98
Head CT Results Within 45 Min. of Arrival[1]	-	-	60%	57%
Patients Who Left ER Before Being Seen	32,957	1%	1%	2%
Time from ER Arrival to Admit. (minutes)[2]	556	211	276	274
Time from ER Arrival to Discharge (minutes)	345	91	125	134
Time in ER Before Being Evaluated (minutes)	361	39	26	26
Time to Pain Meds for Fractures (minutes)	109	72	58	57
Heart Attack Care				
Aspirin Given at Discharge	39	92%	99%	99%
Fibrinolytic Meds Within 30 Min. of Arrival[7]	-	-	40%	54%
PCI Within 90 Minutes of Arrival[7]	-	-	97%	96%
Statin Prescribed at Discharge	35	91%	99%	98%
Heart Failure Care				
ACE Inhibitor or ARB for LVSD	34	97%	97%	97%
Discharge Instructions Given	122	98%	96%	94%
Evaluation of LVS Function	162	100%	100%	99%
Medicare Spending				
Medicare Spending per Patient (ratio)	-	1.04	1.01	0.98
Pneumonia Care				
Appropriate Initial Antibiotic Given	98	95%	96%	95%
Blood Culture Timing	196	98%	98%	98%
Pregnancy and Delivery Care				
Newborn Deliveries Scheduled Early[2]	102	6%	4%	6%
Preventive Care				
Immunization for Influenza[2]	442	94%	91%	90%
Immunization for Pneumonia[2]	557	93%	92%	92%
Stroke Care				
Anticoagulation Therapy for Atrial Fibrillation	11	91%	96%	95%
Antithrombotic Therapy Timing	28	96%	98%	98%
Assessed for Rehabilitation	38	92%	98%	97%
Discharged on Antithrombotic Therapy	35	97%	99%	99%
Discharged on Statin Medication	35	63%	95%	94%
Thrombolytic Therapy Timing[7]	-	-	72%	66%
Venous Thromboembolism Prophylaxis	40	88%	95%	94%
Written Stroke Educational Materials Given	12	92%	90%	88%
Surgical Care Improvement Project				
Appropriate Beta Blocker Usage	87	99%	98%	98%
Appropriate VTP Within 24 Hours	192	99%	99%	98%
Controlled Postoperative Blood Glucose[7]	-	-	98%	97%
Perioperative Temperature Management	243	100%	100%	100%
Prophylactic Antibiotic Selection	147	99%	99%	99%
Prophylactic Antibiotic Selection (Outpatient)	201	92%	98%	98%
Prophylactic Antibiotic Stopped	145	96%	98%	98%
Prophylactic Antibiotic Timing	147	99%	99%	99%
Prophylactic Antibiotic Timing (Outpatient)	203	97%	98%	98%
Urinary Catheter Removal	102	95%	99%	97%
Survey of Patients' Hospital Experiences				
Area Around Room 'Always' Quiet at Night	300+	53%	54%	61%
Doctors 'Always' Communicated Well	300+	82%	80%	82%
Home Recovery Information Given	300+	81%	86%	85%
Hospital Given 9 or 10 on 10 Point Scale	300+	63%	69%	71%
Meds 'Always' Explained Before Given	300+	64%	63%	64%
Nurses 'Always' Communicated Well	300+	81%	79%	79%
Pain 'Always' Well Controlled	300+	72%	70%	71%
Room and Bathroom 'Always' Clean	300+	76%	73%	73%
Timely Help 'Always' Received	300+	73%	67%	68%
Would Definitely Recommend Hospital	300+	59%	70%	71%
Use of Medical Imaging				
Cardiac Imaging Stress Test before Surgery	62	6.5%	5.4%	5.3%
Combination Abdominal CT Scan	622	3.4%	12.2%	10.5%
Combination Brain/Sinus CT Scan	596	5.7%	3.1%	2.7%
Combination Chest CT Scan	293	0.3%	2.1%	2.7%
Follow-up Mammogram/Ultrasound	1,429	7.0%	9%	8.8%
Lumbar Spine MRI for Low Back Pain	147	35.4%	35.8%	37.2%

Punxsutawney Area Hospital

81 Hillcrest Drive Phone: 814-938-1800
Punxsutawney, PA 15767 Fax: 814-938-1630
URL: www.pah.org
Type: Acute Care Hospitals Emergency Services: Yes
Ownership: Voluntary non-profit - Private Beds: 55
Key Personnel:
Intensive Care Unit. . . . . Shirley Brothers
Infection Control. . . . . Kathleen Crowell
Quality Assurance . . . . Kathleen Crowell
Radiology. . . . . Richard Foster, MD
Chief of Medical Staff . . . . Nancy Meehan
Emergency Room . . . . Earl Morgan, MD
Operating Room. . . . . Pat Parrish

Measure	Cases	This Hosp.	State Avg.	U.S. Avg.
Blood Clot Prevention and Treatment				
Anticoagulation Overlap Therapy[2]	17	76%	94%	93%
ICU Venous Thromboembolism Prophylaxis[2]	23	87%	94%	92%
Incidence of Potentially Preventable VTE[1,2]	-	-	8%	10%
UFH with Dosages/Platelet Monitoring[2]	11	100%	98%	97%
Venous Thromboembolism Prophylaxis[2]	114	56%	90%	85%
Warfarin Therapy Discharge Instructions[2]	11	100%	78%	75%
Chest Pain/Possible Heart Attack Care				
Aspirin Given Within 24 Hours of Arrival	34	88%	97%	96%
Fibrinolytic Meds Within 30 Min. of Arrival[1]	-	-	44%	58%
Average Time to ECG (minutes)	28	10	9	7
Average Time to Transfer (minutes)[1]	-	-	64	60
Children's Asthma Care				
Received Home Management Plan of Care	-	-	-	88%
Received Reliever Medication	-	-	-	100%
Received Systemic Corticosteroids	-	-	-	100%
Emergency Department				
Admittance Decision Time (minutes)[2]	304	52	104	98
Head CT Results Within 45 Min. of Arrival	12	42%	60%	57%
Patients Who Left ER Before Being Seen	15,798	0%	1%	2%
Time from ER Arrival to Admit. (minutes)[2]	316	172	276	274
Time from ER Arrival to Discharge (minutes)	377	88	125	134
Time in ER Before Being Evaluated (minutes)	414	19	26	26
Time to Pain Meds for Fractures (minutes)	67	58	58	57
Heart Attack Care				
Aspirin Given at Discharge[1]	-	-	99%	99%
Fibrinolytic Meds Within 30 Min. of Arrival[7]	-	-	40%	54%
PCI Within 90 Minutes of Arrival[7]	-	-	97%	96%
Statin Prescribed at Discharge[1]	-	-	99%	98%
Heart Failure Care				
ACE Inhibitor or ARB for LVSD	12	92%	97%	97%
Discharge Instructions Given	41	83%	96%	94%
Evaluation of LVS Function	49	100%	100%	99%
Medicare Spending				
Medicare Spending per Patient (ratio)	-	0.93	1.01	0.98
Pneumonia Care				
Appropriate Initial Antibiotic Given	43	88%	96%	95%
Blood Culture Timing	49	96%	98%	98%
Pregnancy and Delivery Care				
Newborn Deliveries Scheduled Early	17	12%	4%	6%
Preventive Care				
Immunization for Influenza[2]	263	88%	91%	90%
Immunization for Pneumonia[2]	386	90%	92%	92%
Stroke Care				
Anticoagulation Therapy for Atrial Fibrillation[1]	-	-	96%	95%
Antithrombotic Therapy Timing[1]	-	-	98%	98%
Assessed for Rehabilitation	12	100%	98%	97%
Discharged on Antithrombotic Therapy	11	100%	99%	99%
Discharged on Statin Medication[1]	-	-	95%	94%
Thrombolytic Therapy Timing[1]	-	-	72%	66%
Venous Thromboembolism Prophylaxis[1]	-	-	95%	94%
Written Stroke Educational Materials Given	11	100%	90%	88%
Surgical Care Improvement Project				
Appropriate Beta Blocker Usage	28	93%	98%	98%
Appropriate VTP Within 24 Hours	86	98%	99%	98%
Controlled Postoperative Blood Glucose[7]	-	-	98%	97%
Perioperative Temperature Management	99	100%	100%	100%
Prophylactic Antibiotic Selection	62	100%	99%	99%
Prophylactic Antibiotic Selection (Outpatient)	41	95%	98%	98%
Prophylactic Antibiotic Stopped	60	100%	98%	98%
Prophylactic Antibiotic Timing	62	100%	99%	99%
Prophylactic Antibiotic Timing (Outpatient)	26	77%	98%	98%
Urinary Catheter Removal	52	98%	99%	97%
Survey of Patients' Hospital Experiences				
Area Around Room 'Always' Quiet at Night	300+	53%	54%	61%
Doctors 'Always' Communicated Well	300+	79%	80%	82%
Home Recovery Information Given	300+	92%	86%	85%
Hospital Given 9 or 10 on 10 Point Scale	300+	67%	69%	71%
Meds 'Always' Explained Before Given	300+	61%	63%	64%
Nurses 'Always' Communicated Well	300+	80%	79%	79%
Pain 'Always' Well Controlled	300+	69%	70%	71%
Room and Bathroom 'Always' Clean	300+	70%	73%	73%
Timely Help 'Always' Received	300+	67%	67%	68%
Would Definitely Recommend Hospital	300+	62%	70%	71%
Use of Medical Imaging				
Cardiac Imaging Stress Test before Surgery	88	4.5%	5.4%	5.3%
Combination Abdominal CT Scan	234	10.3%	12.2%	10.5%
Combination Brain/Sinus CT Scan[1]	-	-	3.1%	2.7%
Combination Chest CT Scan	72	1.4%	2.1%	2.7%
Follow-up Mammogram/Ultrasound	292	6.2%	9%	8.8%
Lumbar Spine MRI for Low Back Pain[1]	-	-	35.8%	37.2%

Saint Luke's Quakertown Hospital

1021 Park Avenue Phone: 215-538-4500
Quakertown, PA 18951 Fax: 215-529-5294
URL: www.slhn-lehighvalley.com
Type: Acute Care Hospitals Emergency Services: Yes
Ownership: Voluntary non-profit - Private Beds: 89
Key Personnel:
Anesthesiology. . . . . Mitshell Baker
Radiology. . . . . James Bohri
Radiology. . . . . James D Bohri
Imaging . . . . Joseph Bucich
Pulmonology . . . . Mark Dovey
Chief of Medical Staff . . . . Thomas Filipowitz, MD
CEO/President. . . . . Edward Nawrocki
Anesthesiology. . . . . Farooq QUERESHI, MD

Measure	Cases	This Hosp.	State Avg.	U.S. Avg.
Blood Clot Prevention and Treatment				
Anticoagulation Overlap Therapy[2]	26	96%	94%	93%
ICU Venous Thromboembolism Prophylaxis[2]	41	90%	94%	92%
Incidence of Potentially Preventable VTE[1,2]	-	-	8%	10%
UFH with Dosages/Platelet Monitoring[1,2]	-	-	98%	97%
Venous Thromboembolism Prophylaxis[2]	211	94%	90%	85%
Warfarin Therapy Discharge Instructions[2]	20	70%	78%	75%
Chest Pain/Possible Heart Attack Care				
Aspirin Given Within 24 Hours of Arrival[1,3]	-	-	97%	96%
Fibrinolytic Meds Within 30 Min. of Arrival[3,7]	-	-	44%	58%
Average Time to ECG (minutes)[1,3]	-	-	9	7
Average Time to Transfer (minutes)[3,7]	-	-	64	60
Children's Asthma Care				
Received Home Management Plan of Care	-	-	-	88%
Received Reliever Medication	-	-	-	100%
Received Systemic Corticosteroids	-	-	-	100%

NOTE: Hospital profiles are in alphabetical order by state, then city, then hospital within the city; Rankings exclude hospitals with less than 25 cases except for patient surveys which excludes hospitals with less than 100 cases; (a) 100-299 cases; (1) The number of cases/patients is too few to report; (2) Data submitted were based on a sample of cases/patients; (3) Results are based on a shorter time period than required; (4) Data suppressed by CMS for one or more quarters; (5) Results are not available for this reporting period; (6) Fewer than 100 patients completed the HCAHPS survey; (7) No cases met the criteria for this measure; (8) The lower limit of the confidence interval cannot be calculated if the number of observed infections equals zero; (9) No data are available from the state/territory for this reporting period; (10) The scores shown reflect fewer than 50 completed surveys; (11) There were discrepancies in the data collection process; (12) This measure does not apply to this hospital for this reporting period; (13) Results cannot be calculated for this reporting period; (14) The results for this state are combined with nearby states to protect confidentiality; Please refer to the User's Guide for a full explanation of data.

Emergency Department				
Admittance Decision Time (minutes)[2]	420	84	104	98
Head CT Results Within 45 Min. of Arrival[1]	-	-	60%	57%
Patients Who Left ER Before Being Seen	15,983	1%	1%	2%
Time from ER Arrival to Admit. (minutes)[2]	426	245	276	274
Time from ER Arrival to Discharge (minutes)	354	115	125	134
Time in ER Before Being Evaluated (minutes)	373	28	26	26
Time to Pain Meds for Fractures (minutes)	42	50	58	57
Heart Attack Care				
Aspirin Given at Discharge[1]	-	-	99%	99%
Fibrinolytic Meds Within 30 Min. of Arrival[7]	-	-	40%	54%
PCI Within 90 Minutes of Arrival[7]	-	-	97%	96%
Statin Prescribed at Discharge[1]	-	-	99%	98%
Heart Failure Care				
ACE Inhibitor or ARB for LVSD	20	100%	97%	97%
Discharge Instructions Given	76	100%	96%	94%
Evaluation of LVS Function	114	100%	100%	99%
Medicare Spending				
Medicare Spending per Patient (ratio)	-	0.93	1.01	0.98
Pneumonia Care				
Appropriate Initial Antibiotic Given	66	100%	96%	95%
Blood Culture Timing	86	100%	98%	98%
Pregnancy and Delivery Care				
Newborn Deliveries Scheduled Early[7]	-	-	4%	6%
Preventive Care				
Immunization for Influenza[2]	311	95%	91%	90%
Immunization for Pneumonia[2]	437	95%	92%	92%
Stroke Care				
Anticoagulation Therapy for Atrial Fibrillation[1]	-	-	96%	95%
Antithrombotic Therapy Timing	37	97%	98%	98%
Assessed for Rehabilitation	39	97%	98%	97%
Discharged on Antithrombotic Therapy	39	100%	99%	99%
Discharged on Statin Medication	30	97%	95%	94%
Thrombolytic Therapy Timing[7]	-	-	72%	66%
Venous Thromboembolism Prophylaxis	37	97%	95%	94%
Written Stroke Educational Materials Given	18	100%	90%	88%
Surgical Care Improvement Project				
Appropriate Beta Blocker Usage	31	100%	98%	98%
Appropriate VTP Within 24 Hours	97	99%	99%	98%
Controlled Postoperative Blood Glucose[7]	-	-	98%	97%
Perioperative Temperature Management	108	100%	100%	100%
Prophylactic Antibiotic Selection	66	98%	99%	99%
Prophylactic Antibiotic Selection (Outpatient)	31	100%	98%	98%
Prophylactic Antibiotic Stopped	65	100%	98%	98%
Prophylactic Antibiotic Timing	66	100%	99%	99%
Prophylactic Antibiotic Timing (Outpatient)	31	100%	98%	98%
Urinary Catheter Removal	38	97%	99%	97%
Survey of Patients' Hospital Experiences				
Area Around Room 'Always' Quiet at Night	300+	57%	54%	61%
Doctors 'Always' Communicated Well	300+	80%	80%	82%
Home Recovery Information Given	300+	89%	86%	85%
Hospital Given 9 or 10 on 10 Point Scale	300+	72%	69%	71%
Meds 'Always' Explained Before Given	300+	66%	63%	64%
Nurses 'Always' Communicated Well	300+	82%	79%	79%
Pain 'Always' Well Controlled	300+	71%	70%	71%
Room and Bathroom 'Always' Clean	300+	80%	73%	73%
Timely Help 'Always' Received	300+	69%	67%	68%
Would Definitely Recommend Hospital	300+	71%	70%	71%
Use of Medical Imaging				
Cardiac Imaging Stress Test before Surgery	154	3.9%	5.4%	5.3%
Combination Abdominal CT Scan	452	4.6%	12.2%	10.5%
Combination Brain/Sinus CT Scan	318	1.3%	3.1%	2.7%
Combination Chest CT Scan	308	0.3%	2.1%	2.7%
Follow-up Mammogram/Ultrasound	715	5.7%	9%	8.8%
Lumbar Spine MRI for Low Back Pain	68	36.8%	35.8%	37.2%

Reading Hospital

Sixth Avenue & Spruce St
Reading, PA 19603
Phone: 610-988-8000
Fax: 610-988-5192
E-mail: info@readinghospital.org
URL: www.readinghospital.org
Type: Acute Care Hospitals
Emergency Services: Yes
Ownership: Voluntary non-profit - Other
Beds: 804

Key Personnel:
Infection Control . . . . Kenneth J DeBenedictis, MD
Quality Assurance . . . . Debra Levengood
Chief of Medical Staff . . . . Gerald Malick, MD
Anesthesiology. . . . . Francis Plucinsley, MD
Emergency Room . . . . Kristen Sandel
CEO/President. . . . . Scott R Wolfe
Radiology. . . . . Albert Yuen

Measure	Cases	This Hosp.	State Avg.	U.S. Avg.
Blood Clot Prevention and Treatment				
Anticoagulation Overlap Therapy[2]	331	100%	94%	93%
ICU Venous Thromboembolism Prophylaxis[2]	72	99%	94%	92%
Incidence of Potentially Preventable VTE[2]	30	7%	8%	10%
UFH with Dosages/Platelet Monitoring[2]	248	100%	98%	97%
Venous Thromboembolism Prophylaxis[2]	365	94%	90%	85%
Warfarin Therapy Discharge Instructions[2]	236	93%	78%	75%
Chest Pain/Possible Heart Attack Care				
Aspirin Given Within 24 Hours of Arrival[1,3]	-	-	97%	96%
Fibrinolytic Meds Within 30 Min. of Arrival[3,7]	-	-	44%	58%
Average Time to ECG (minutes)[1,3]	-	-	9	7
Average Time to Transfer (minutes)[3,7]	-	-	64	60
Children's Asthma Care				
Received Home Management Plan of Care	-	-	-	88%
Received Reliever Medication	-	-	-	100%
Received Systemic Corticosteroids	-	-	-	100%
Emergency Department				
Admittance Decision Time (minutes)[2]	691	142	104	98
Head CT Results Within 45 Min. of Arrival	12	58%	60%	57%
Patients Who Left ER Before Being Seen	>100k	1%	1%	2%
Time from ER Arrival to Admit. (minutes)[2]	701	368	276	274
Time from ER Arrival to Discharge (minutes)	1,226	213	125	134
Time in ER Before Being Evaluated (minutes)	1,473	57	26	26
Time to Pain Meds for Fractures (minutes)	321	83	58	57
Heart Attack Care				
Aspirin Given at Discharge	429	100%	99%	99%
Fibrinolytic Meds Within 30 Min. of Arrival[7]	-	-	40%	54%
PCI Within 90 Minutes of Arrival	108	100%	97%	96%
Statin Prescribed at Discharge	413	100%	99%	98%
Heart Failure Care				
ACE Inhibitor or ARB for LVSD	165	100%	97%	97%
Discharge Instructions Given	715	99%	96%	94%
Evaluation of LVS Function	915	100%	100%	99%
Medicare Spending				
Medicare Spending per Patient (ratio)	-	1.03	1.01	0.98
Pneumonia Care				
Appropriate Initial Antibiotic Given	433	98%	96%	95%
Blood Culture Timing	1,119	99%	98%	98%
Pregnancy and Delivery Care				
Newborn Deliveries Scheduled Early[2]	48	0%	4%	6%
Preventive Care				
Immunization for Influenza[2]	545	95%	91%	90%
Immunization for Pneumonia[2]	690	93%	92%	92%
Stroke Care				
Anticoagulation Therapy for Atrial Fibrillation	38	89%	96%	95%
Antithrombotic Therapy Timing	304	99%	98%	98%
Assessed for Rehabilitation	378	100%	98%	97%
Discharged on Antithrombotic Therapy	329	97%	99%	99%
Discharged on Statin Medication	288	93%	95%	94%
Thrombolytic Therapy Timing	29	93%	72%	66%
Venous Thromboembolism Prophylaxis	381	95%	95%	94%
Written Stroke Educational Materials Given	177	88%	90%	88%
Surgical Care Improvement Project				
Appropriate Beta Blocker Usage[2]	656	100%	98%	98%
Appropriate VTP Within 24 Hours[2]	1,203	100%	99%	98%
Controlled Postoperative Blood Glucose[2]	180	99%	98%	97%
Perioperative Temperature Management[2]	1,488	100%	100%	100%
Prophylactic Antibiotic Selection[2]	1,258	100%	99%	99%
Prophylactic Antibiotic Selection (Outpatient)	949	99%	98%	98%
Prophylactic Antibiotic Stopped[2]	1,241	99%	98%	98%
Prophylactic Antibiotic Timing[2]	1,259	100%	99%	99%
Prophylactic Antibiotic Timing (Outpatient)	933	99%	98%	98%
Urinary Catheter Removal[2]	1,147	99%	99%	97%
Survey of Patients' Hospital Experiences				
Area Around Room 'Always' Quiet at Night	300+	44%	54%	61%
Doctors 'Always' Communicated Well	300+	75%	80%	82%
Home Recovery Information Given	300+	88%	86%	85%
Hospital Given 9 or 10 on 10 Point Scale	300+	65%	69%	71%
Meds 'Always' Explained Before Given	300+	57%	63%	64%
Nurses 'Always' Communicated Well	300+	76%	79%	79%
Pain 'Always' Well Controlled	300+	68%	70%	71%
Room and Bathroom 'Always' Clean	300+	63%	73%	73%
Timely Help 'Always' Received	300+	57%	67%	68%
Would Definitely Recommend Hospital	300+	65%	70%	71%
Use of Medical Imaging				
Cardiac Imaging Stress Test before Surgery	466	4.9%	5.4%	5.3%
Combination Abdominal CT Scan	3,069	7.0%	12.2%	10.5%
Combination Brain/Sinus CT Scan	2,284	2.5%	3.1%	2.7%
Combination Chest CT Scan	3,441	3.0%	2.1%	2.7%
Follow-up Mammogram/Ultrasound	4,251	8.0%	9%	8.8%
Lumbar Spine MRI for Low Back Pain	262	40.1%	35.8%	37.2%

Saint Joseph Medical Center

2500 Bernville Road
Reading, PA 19605
Phone: 610-378-2300
Fax: 610-378-2706
URL: www.sjmcberks.org
Type: Acute Care Hospitals
Emergency Services: Yes
Ownership: Voluntary non-profit - Church
Beds: 220

Key Personnel:
Quality Assurance . . . . Loretta Boyd, RN
Radiology. . . . . Steven R Chmielewski, MD
Chief of Medical Staff . . . . Howard Davis, MD
Pediatric Ambulatory Care . . . . . . Mary Ann Mancano, MD
Pediatric In-Patient Care . . . . . . Mary Ann Mancano, MD
Operating Room. . . . . Cyndie Miller, RN
President/CEO. . . . . John Morahan
Emergency Room . . . . Ann Tranqualto, RN

Measure	Cases	This Hosp.	State Avg.	U.S. Avg.
Blood Clot Prevention and Treatment				
Anticoagulation Overlap Therapy[2]	74	69%	94%	93%
ICU Venous Thromboembolism Prophylaxis[2]	124	98%	94%	92%
Incidence of Potentially Preventable VTE[1,2]	-	-	8%	10%
UFH with Dosages/Platelet Monitoring[2]	75	100%	98%	97%
Venous Thromboembolism Prophylaxis[2]	712	98%	90%	85%
Warfarin Therapy Discharge Instructions[2]	63	79%	78%	75%
Chest Pain/Possible Heart Attack Care				
Aspirin Given Within 24 Hours of Arrival[5]	-	-	97%	96%
Fibrinolytic Meds Within 30 Min. of Arrival[5]	-	-	44%	58%
Average Time to ECG (minutes)[5]	-	-	9	7
Average Time to Transfer (minutes)[5]	-	-	64	60
Children's Asthma Care				
Received Home Management Plan of Care	-	-	-	88%
Received Reliever Medication	-	-	-	100%
Received Systemic Corticosteroids	-	-	-	100%
Emergency Department				
Admittance Decision Time (minutes)[2]	588	152	104	98
Head CT Results Within 45 Min. of Arrival	20	40%	60%	57%
Patients Who Left ER Before Being Seen	41,647	2%	1%	2%
Time from ER Arrival to Admit. (minutes)[2]	739	426	276	274
Time from ER Arrival to Discharge (minutes)	661	195	125	134
Time in ER Before Being Evaluated (minutes)	619	57	26	26
Time to Pain Meds for Fractures (minutes)	163	93	58	57
Heart Attack Care				
Aspirin Given at Discharge	137	100%	99%	99%
Fibrinolytic Meds Within 30 Min. of Arrival[7]	-	-	40%	54%
PCI Within 90 Minutes of Arrival	31	100%	97%	96%
Statin Prescribed at Discharge	125	100%	99%	98%
Heart Failure Care				
ACE Inhibitor or ARB for LVSD	50	100%	97%	97%
Discharge Instructions Given	298	98%	96%	94%
Evaluation of LVS Function	357	100%	100%	99%
Medicare Spending				

NOTE: Hospital profiles are in alphabetical order by state, then city, then hospital within the city; Rankings exclude hospitals with less than 25 cases except for patient surveys which excludes hospitals with less than 100 cases; (a) 100-299 cases; (1) The number of cases/patients is too few to report; (2) Data submitted were based on a sample of cases/patients; (3) Results are based on a shorter time period than required; (4) Data suppressed by CMS for one or more quarters; (5) Results are not available for this reporting period; (6) Fewer than 100 patients completed the HCAHPS survey; (7) No cases met the criteria for this measure; (8) The lower limit of the confidence interval cannot be calculated if the number of observed infections equals zero; (9) No data are available from the state/territory for this reporting period; (10) The scores shown reflect fewer than 50 completed surveys; (11) There were discrepancies in the data collection process; (12) This measure does not apply to this hospital for this reporting period; (13) Results cannot be calculated for this reporting period; (14) The results for this state are combined with nearby states to protect confidentiality; Please refer to the User's Guide for a full explanation of data.

Measure	Cases	This Hosp.	State Avg.	U.S. Avg.
Medicare Spending per Patient (ratio)	-	1.01	1.01	0.98
Pneumonia Care				
Appropriate Initial Antibiotic Given	119	100%	96%	95%
Blood Culture Timing	235	96%	98%	98%
Pregnancy and Delivery Care				
Newborn Deliveries Scheduled Early[2]	35	3%	4%	6%
Preventive Care				
Immunization for Influenza[2]	552	95%	91%	90%
Immunization for Pneumonia[2]	746	95%	92%	92%
Stroke Care				
Anticoagulation Therapy for Atrial Fibrillation[1]	-	-	96%	95%
Antithrombotic Therapy Timing	93	100%	98%	98%
Assessed for Rehabilitation	100	96%	98%	97%
Discharged on Antithrombotic Therapy	95	100%	99%	99%
Discharged on Statin Medication	74	97%	95%	94%
Thrombolytic Therapy Timing	21	19%	72%	66%
Venous Thromboembolism Prophylaxis	92	99%	95%	94%
Written Stroke Educational Materials Given	61	84%	90%	88%
Surgical Care Improvement Project				
Appropriate Beta Blocker Usage[2]	237	100%	98%	98%
Appropriate VTP Within 24 Hours[2]	346	100%	99%	98%
Controlled Postoperative Blood Glucose[2]	130	99%	98%	97%
Perioperative Temperature Management[2]	414	100%	100%	100%
Prophylactic Antibiotic Selection[2]	385	99%	99%	99%
Prophylactic Antibiotic Selection (Outpatient)	315	99%	98%	98%
Prophylactic Antibiotic Stopped[2]	380	99%	98%	98%
Prophylactic Antibiotic Timing[2]	388	99%	99%	99%
Prophylactic Antibiotic Timing (Outpatient)	308	100%	98%	98%
Urinary Catheter Removal[2]	328	100%	99%	97%
Survey of Patients' Hospital Experiences				
Area Around Room 'Always' Quiet at Night	300+	53%	54%	61%
Doctors 'Always' Communicated Well	300+	78%	80%	82%
Home Recovery Information Given	300+	88%	86%	85%
Hospital Given 9 or 10 on 10 Point Scale	300+	74%	69%	71%
Meds 'Always' Explained Before Given	300+	61%	63%	64%
Nurses 'Always' Communicated Well	300+	77%	79%	79%
Pain 'Always' Well Controlled	300+	69%	70%	71%
Room and Bathroom 'Always' Clean	300+	68%	73%	73%
Timely Help 'Always' Received	300+	60%	67%	68%
Would Definitely Recommend Hospital	300+	79%	70%	71%
Use of Medical Imaging				
Cardiac Imaging Stress Test before Surgery	82	3.7%	5.4%	5.3%
Combination Abdominal CT Scan	625	67.4%	12.2%	10.5%
Combination Brain/Sinus CT Scan	719	2.9%	3.1%	2.7%
Combination Chest CT Scan	422	2.4%	2.1%	2.7%
Follow-up Mammogram/Ultrasound	1,415	8.3%	9%	8.8%
Lumbar Spine MRI for Low Back Pain	113	45.1%	35.8%	37.2%

Bucktail Medical Center

1001 Pine Street
Renovo, PA 17764
Phone: 570-923-1000
Type: Critical Access Hospitals
Emergency Services: Yes
Ownership: Voluntary non-profit - Private

Measure	Cases	This Hosp.	State Avg.	U.S. Avg.
Blood Clot Prevention and Treatment				
Anticoagulation Overlap Therapy[5]	-	-	94%	93%
ICU Venous Thromboembolism Prophylaxis[5]	-	-	94%	92%
Incidence of Potentially Preventable VTE[5]	-	-	8%	10%
UFH with Dosages/Platelet Monitoring[5]	-	-	98%	97%
Venous Thromboembolism Prophylaxis[5]	-	-	90%	85%
Warfarin Therapy Discharge Instructions[5]	-	-	78%	75%
Chest Pain/Possible Heart Attack Care				
Aspirin Given Within 24 Hours of Arrival[3]	15	100%	97%	96%
Fibrinolytic Meds Within 30 Min. of Arrival[3,7]	-	-	44%	58%
Average Time to ECG (minutes)[3]	16	12	9	7
Average Time to Transfer (minutes)[1,3]	-	-	64	60
Children's Asthma Care				
Received Home Management Plan of Care	-	-	-	88%
Received Reliever Medication	-	-	-	100%
Received Systemic Corticosteroids	-	-	-	100%
Emergency Department				
Admittance Decision Time (minutes)[5]	-	-	104	98
Head CT Results Within 45 Min. of Arrival[3,7]	-	-	60%	57%
Patients Who Left ER Before Being Seen	2,113	1%	1%	2%
Time from ER Arrival to Admit. (minutes)[5]	-	-	276	274
Time from ER Arrival to Discharge (minutes)[5]	-	-	125	134
Time in ER Before Being Evaluated (minutes)[5]	-	-	26	26
Time to Pain Meds for Fractures (minutes)[5]	-	-	58	57
Heart Attack Care				
Aspirin Given at Discharge[1,3]	-	-	99%	99%
Fibrinolytic Meds Within 30 Min. of Arrival[3,7]	-	-	40%	54%
PCI Within 90 Minutes of Arrival[3,7]	-	-	97%	96%
Statin Prescribed at Discharge[1,3]	-	-	99%	98%
Heart Failure Care				
ACE Inhibitor or ARB for LVSD[3,7]	-	-	97%	97%
Discharge Instructions Given[3,7]	-	-	96%	94%
Evaluation of LVS Function[1,3]	-	-	100%	99%
Medicare Spending				
Medicare Spending per Patient (ratio)	-	-	1.01	0.98
Pneumonia Care				
Appropriate Initial Antibiotic Given[1,2]	-	-	96%	95%
Blood Culture Timing[1,2]	-	-	98%	98%
Pregnancy and Delivery Care				
Newborn Deliveries Scheduled Early[2,3]	-	-	4%	6%
Preventive Care				
Immunization for Influenza[5]	-	-	91%	90%
Immunization for Pneumonia[5]	-	-	92%	92%
Stroke Care				
Anticoagulation Therapy for Atrial Fibrillation[5]	-	-	96%	95%
Antithrombotic Therapy Timing[5]	-	-	98%	98%
Assessed for Rehabilitation[5]	-	-	98%	97%
Discharged on Antithrombotic Therapy[5]	-	-	99%	99%
Discharged on Statin Medication[5]	-	-	95%	94%
Thrombolytic Therapy Timing[5]	-	-	72%	66%
Venous Thromboembolism Prophylaxis[5]	-	-	95%	94%
Written Stroke Educational Materials Given[5]	-	-	90%	88%
Surgical Care Improvement Project				
Appropriate Beta Blocker Usage[5]	-	-	98%	98%
Appropriate VTP Within 24 Hours[5]	-	-	99%	98%
Controlled Postoperative Blood Glucose[5]	-	-	98%	97%
Perioperative Temperature Management[5]	-	-	100%	100%
Prophylactic Antibiotic Selection[5]	-	-	99%	99%
Prophylactic Antibiotic Selection (Outpatient)[5]	-	-	98%	98%
Prophylactic Antibiotic Stopped[5]	-	-	98%	98%
Prophylactic Antibiotic Timing[5]	-	-	99%	99%
Prophylactic Antibiotic Timing (Outpatient)[5]	-	-	98%	98%
Urinary Catheter Removal[5]	-	-	99%	97%
Survey of Patients' Hospital Experiences				
Area Around Room 'Always' Quiet at Night[10]	<100	65%	54%	61%
Doctors 'Always' Communicated Well[10]	<100	84%	80%	82%
Home Recovery Information Given[10]	<100	85%	86%	85%
Hospital Given 9 or 10 on 10 Point Scale[10]	<100	82%	69%	71%
Meds 'Always' Explained Before Given[10]	<100	84%	63%	64%
Nurses 'Always' Communicated Well[10]	<100	87%	79%	79%
Pain 'Always' Well Controlled[10]	<100	88%	70%	71%
Room and Bathroom 'Always' Clean[10]	<100	100%	73%	73%
Timely Help 'Always' Received[10]	<100	84%	67%	68%
Would Definitely Recommend Hospital[10]	<100	87%	70%	71%
Use of Medical Imaging				
Cardiac Imaging Stress Test before Surgery[7]	-	-	5.4%	5.3%
Combination Abdominal CT Scan[7]	-	-	12.2%	10.5%
Combination Brain/Sinus CT Scan[7]	-	-	3.1%	2.7%
Combination Chest CT Scan[7]	-	-	2.1%	2.7%
Follow-up Mammogram/Ultrasound[7]	-	-	9%	8.8%
Lumbar Spine MRI for Low Back Pain[7]	-	-	35.8%	37.2%

Nason Hospital

105 Nason Drive
Roaring Spring, PA 16673
Phone: 814-224-2141
Fax: 814-224-6236
URL: www.nasonhospital.com
Type: Acute Care Hospitals
Emergency Services: Yes
Ownership: Voluntary non-profit - Private
Beds: 40

Key Personnel:

Operating Room. . . . . Howard M Black, RN
Pediatric Ambulatory Care . . . . . . Joseph Castel, MD
Pediatric In-Patient Care . . . . Joseph Castel, MD
CEO/President. . . . . Garrett W Hoover, MA, MHA
Infection Control. . . . . Janice Kanode, RN
Chief of Medical Staff . . . . Darron Locke, MD
Radiology. . . . . Francis X Pessolano
Quality Assurance . . . . Faith Shea

Measure	Cases	This Hosp.	State Avg.	U.S. Avg.
Blood Clot Prevention and Treatment				
Anticoagulation Overlap Therapy[2]	17	88%	94%	93%
ICU Venous Thromboembolism Prophylaxis[2]	19	79%	94%	92%
Incidence of Potentially Preventable VTE[1,2]	-	-	8%	10%
UFH with Dosages/Platelet Monitoring[1,2]	-	-	98%	97%
Venous Thromboembolism Prophylaxis[2]	118	75%	90%	85%
Warfarin Therapy Discharge Instructions[2]	15	93%	78%	75%
Chest Pain/Possible Heart Attack Care				
Aspirin Given Within 24 Hours of Arrival	35	100%	97%	96%
Fibrinolytic Meds Within 30 Min. of Arrival[1]	-	-	44%	58%
Average Time to ECG (minutes)	35	8	9	7
Average Time to Transfer (minutes)[7]	-	-	64	60
Children's Asthma Care				
Received Home Management Plan of Care	-	-	-	88%
Received Reliever Medication	-	-	-	100%
Received Systemic Corticosteroids	-	-	-	100%
Emergency Department				
Admittance Decision Time (minutes)[2]	231	35	104	98
Head CT Results Within 45 Min. of Arrival[7]	-	-	60%	57%
Patients Who Left ER Before Being Seen	13,692	2%	1%	2%
Time from ER Arrival to Admit. (minutes)[2]	239	209	276	274
Time from ER Arrival to Discharge (minutes)	378	87	125	134
Time in ER Before Being Evaluated (minutes)	387	15	26	26
Time to Pain Meds for Fractures (minutes)	71	62	58	57
Heart Attack Care				
Aspirin Given at Discharge[1]	-	-	99%	99%
Fibrinolytic Meds Within 30 Min. of Arrival[7]	-	-	40%	54%
PCI Within 90 Minutes of Arrival[7]	-	-	97%	96%
Statin Prescribed at Discharge[1]	-	-	99%	98%
Heart Failure Care				
ACE Inhibitor or ARB for LVSD	11	73%	97%	97%
Discharge Instructions Given	46	96%	96%	94%
Evaluation of LVS Function	73	100%	100%	99%
Medicare Spending				
Medicare Spending per Patient (ratio)	-	1.11	1.01	0.98
Pneumonia Care				
Appropriate Initial Antibiotic Given	84	93%	96%	95%
Blood Culture Timing	86	97%	98%	98%
Pregnancy and Delivery Care				
Newborn Deliveries Scheduled Early[2]	31	3%	4%	6%
Preventive Care				
Immunization for Influenza[2]	247	82%	91%	90%
Immunization for Pneumonia[2]	282	82%	92%	92%
Stroke Care				
Anticoagulation Therapy for Atrial Fibrillation[1]	-	-	96%	95%
Antithrombotic Therapy Timing[1]	-	-	98%	98%
Assessed for Rehabilitation[1]	-	-	98%	97%
Discharged on Antithrombotic Therapy[1]	-	-	99%	99%
Discharged on Statin Medication[1]	-	-	95%	94%
Thrombolytic Therapy Timing[7]	-	-	72%	66%
Venous Thromboembolism Prophylaxis[1]	-	-	95%	94%
Written Stroke Educational Materials Given[1]	-	-	90%	88%
Surgical Care Improvement Project				
Appropriate Beta Blocker Usage	59	97%	98%	98%
Appropriate VTP Within 24 Hours	192	100%	99%	98%
Controlled Postoperative Blood Glucose[7]	-	-	98%	97%
Perioperative Temperature Management	227	100%	100%	100%
Prophylactic Antibiotic Selection	180	99%	99%	99%
Prophylactic Antibiotic Selection (Outpatient)	18	100%	98%	98%
Prophylactic Antibiotic Stopped	177	98%	98%	98%
Prophylactic Antibiotic Timing	180	99%	99%	99%
Prophylactic Antibiotic Timing (Outpatient)	19	95%	98%	98%
Urinary Catheter Removal	35	94%	99%	97%
Survey of Patients' Hospital Experiences				
Area Around Room 'Always' Quiet at Night	300+	56%	54%	61%
Doctors 'Always' Communicated Well	300+	83%	80%	82%

NOTE: Hospital profiles are in alphabetical order by state, then city, then hospital within the city; Rankings exclude hospitals with less than 25 cases except for patient surveys which excludes hospitals with less than 100 cases; (a) 100-299 cases; (1) The number of cases/patients is too few to report; (2) Data submitted were based on a sample of cases/patients; (3) Results are based on a shorter time period than required; (4) Data suppressed by CMS for one or more quarters; (5) Results are not available for this reporting period; (6) Fewer than 100 patients completed the HCAHPS survey; (7) No cases met the criteria for this measure; (8) The lower limit of the confidence interval cannot be calculated if the number of observed infections equals zero; (9) No data are available from the state/territory for this reporting period; (10) The scores shown reflect fewer than 50 completed surveys; (11) There were discrepancies in the data collection process; (12) This measure does not apply to this hospital for this reporting period; (13) Results cannot be calculated for this reporting period; (14) The results for this state are combined with nearby states to protect confidentiality; Please refer to the User's Guide for a full explanation of data.

Measure	Cases	This Hosp.	State Avg.	U.S. Avg.
Home Recovery Information Given	300+	87%	86%	85%
Hospital Given 9 or 10 on 10 Point Scale	300+	73%	69%	71%
Meds 'Always' Explained Before Given	300+	63%	63%	64%
Nurses 'Always' Communicated Well	300+	79%	79%	79%
Pain 'Always' Well Controlled	300+	68%	70%	71%
Room and Bathroom 'Always' Clean	300+	83%	73%	73%
Timely Help 'Always' Received	300+	66%	67%	68%
Would Definitely Recommend Hospital	300+	76%	70%	71%
Use of Medical Imaging				
Cardiac Imaging Stress Test before Surgery[1]	-	-	5.4%	5.3%
Combination Abdominal CT Scan	183	9.3%	12.2%	10.5%
Combination Brain/Sinus CT Scan[1]	-	-	3.1%	2.7%
Combination Chest CT Scan	84	2.4%	2.1%	2.7%
Follow-up Mammogram/Ultrasound	332	8.1%	9%	8.8%
Lumbar Spine MRI for Low Back Pain[1]	-	-	35.8%	37.2%

Physician's Care Surgical Hospital

454 Enterprise Drive
Royersford, PA 19468
Phone: 610-495-4793
URL: www.phycarehospital.com
Type: Acute Care Hospitals
Emergency Services: No
Ownership: Proprietary

Measure	Cases	This Hosp.	State Avg.	U.S. Avg.
Blood Clot Prevention and Treatment				
Anticoagulation Overlap Therapy[2,7]	-	-	94%	93%
ICU Venous Thromboembolism Prophylaxis[2,7]	-	-	94%	92%
Incidence of Potentially Preventable VTE[2,7]	-	-	8%	10%
UFH with Dosages/Platelet Monitoring[2,7]	-	-	98%	97%
Venous Thromboembolism Prophylaxis[2]	58	100%	90%	85%
Warfarin Therapy Discharge Instructions[2,7]	-	-	78%	75%
Chest Pain/Possible Heart Attack Care				
Aspirin Given Within 24 Hours of Arrival[5]	-	-	97%	96%
Fibrinolytic Meds Within 30 Min. of Arrival[5]	-	-	44%	58%
Average Time to ECG (minutes)[5]	-	-	9	7
Average Time to Transfer (minutes)[5]	-	-	64	60
Children's Asthma Care				
Received Home Management Plan of Care	-	-	-	88%
Received Reliever Medication	-	-	-	100%
Received Systemic Corticosteroids	-	-	-	100%
Emergency Department				
Admittance Decision Time (minutes)[2,7]	-	-	104	98
Head CT Results Within 45 Min. of Arrival[5]	-	-	60%	57%
Patients Who Left ER Before Being Seen[5]	-	-	1%	2%
Time from ER Arrival to Admit. (minutes)[2,7]	-	-	276	274
Time from ER Arrival to Discharge (minutes)[5]	-	-	125	134
Time in ER Before Being Evaluated (minutes)[5]	-	-	26	26
Time to Pain Meds for Fractures (minutes)[5]	-	-	58	57
Heart Attack Care				
Aspirin Given at Discharge[5]	-	-	99%	99%
Fibrinolytic Meds Within 30 Min. of Arrival[5]	-	-	40%	54%
PCI Within 90 Minutes of Arrival[5]	-	-	97%	96%
Statin Prescribed at Discharge[5]	-	-	99%	98%
Heart Failure Care				
ACE Inhibitor or ARB for LVSD[5]	-	-	97%	97%
Discharge Instructions Given[5]	-	-	96%	94%
Evaluation of LVS Function[5]	-	-	100%	99%
Medicare Spending				
Medicare Spending per Patient (ratio)[1]	-	-	1.01	0.98
Pneumonia Care				
Appropriate Initial Antibiotic Given[5]	-	-	96%	95%
Blood Culture Timing[5]	-	-	98%	98%
Pregnancy and Delivery Care				
Newborn Deliveries Scheduled Early[7]	-	-	4%	6%
Preventive Care				
Immunization for Influenza[2]	126	66%	91%	90%
Immunization for Pneumonia[2]	142	59%	92%	92%
Stroke Care				
Anticoagulation Therapy for Atrial Fibrillation[5]	-	-	96%	95%
Antithrombotic Therapy Timing[5]	-	-	98%	98%
Assessed for Rehabilitation[5]	-	-	98%	97%
Discharged on Antithrombotic Therapy[5]	-	-	99%	99%
Discharged on Statin Medication[5]	-	-	95%	94%
Thrombolytic Therapy Timing[5]	-	-	72%	66%
Venous Thromboembolism Prophylaxis[5]	-	-	95%	94%
Written Stroke Educational Materials Given[5]	-	-	90%	88%
Surgical Care Improvement Project				
Appropriate Beta Blocker Usage[2]	32	91%	98%	98%
Appropriate VTP Within 24 Hours[2]	167	91%	99%	98%
Controlled Postoperative Blood Glucose[2,7]	-	-	98%	97%
Perioperative Temperature Management[2]	204	98%	100%	100%
Prophylactic Antibiotic Selection[2]	189	99%	99%	99%
Prophylactic Antibiotic Selection (Outpatient)[5]	-	-	98%	98%
Prophylactic Antibiotic Stopped[2]	188	100%	98%	98%
Prophylactic Antibiotic Timing[2]	190	96%	99%	99%
Prophylactic Antibiotic Timing (Outpatient)[5]	-	-	98%	98%
Urinary Catheter Removal[2]	119	100%	99%	97%
Survey of Patients' Hospital Experiences				
Area Around Room 'Always' Quiet at Night	300+	87%	54%	61%
Doctors 'Always' Communicated Well	300+	91%	80%	82%
Home Recovery Information Given	300+	93%	86%	85%
Hospital Given 9 or 10 on 10 Point Scale	300+	94%	69%	71%
Meds 'Always' Explained Before Given	300+	76%	63%	64%
Nurses 'Always' Communicated Well	300+	96%	79%	79%
Pain 'Always' Well Controlled	300+	84%	70%	71%
Room and Bathroom 'Always' Clean	300+	89%	73%	73%
Timely Help 'Always' Received	300+	95%	67%	68%
Would Definitely Recommend Hospital	300+	94%	70%	71%
Use of Medical Imaging				
Cardiac Imaging Stress Test before Surgery[7]	-	-	5.4%	5.3%
Combination Abdominal CT Scan[7]	-	-	12.2%	10.5%
Combination Brain/Sinus CT Scan[7]	-	-	3.1%	2.7%
Combination Chest CT Scan[7]	-	-	2.1%	2.7%
Follow-up Mammogram/Ultrasound[7]	-	-	9%	8.8%
Lumbar Spine MRI for Low Back Pain[7]	-	-	35.8%	37.2%

Penn Highlands Elk

763 Johnsonburg Road
Saint Marys, PA 15857
Phone: 814-788-8000
Fax: 814-788-8046
URL: www.elkregional.org
Type: Acute Care Hospitals
Emergency Services: Yes
Ownership: Voluntary non-profit - Private
Beds: 87

Key Personnel:
CEO/President. . . . . Greg Bauer, NHA/CHE
Radiology. . . . . Richard Bolden
Chief of Medical Staff. . . . . David Caruso
Emergency Room . . . . Jayant L Patankar, MD
Operating Room. . . . . Kaye Schneider
Quality Assurance . . . . Kathy Wonderly, RN

Measure	Cases	This Hosp.	State Avg.	U.S. Avg.
Blood Clot Prevention and Treatment				
Anticoagulation Overlap Therapy[2]	27	67%	94%	93%
ICU Venous Thromboembolism Prophylaxis[2]	50	82%	94%	92%
Incidence of Potentially Preventable VTE[1,2]	-	-	8%	10%
UFH with Dosages/Platelet Monitoring[2]	16	100%	98%	97%
Venous Thromboembolism Prophylaxis[2]	285	69%	90%	85%
Warfarin Therapy Discharge Instructions[2]	19	58%	78%	75%
Chest Pain/Possible Heart Attack Care				
Aspirin Given Within 24 Hours of Arrival	49	100%	97%	96%
Fibrinolytic Meds Within 30 Min. of Arrival[1]	-	-	44%	58%
Average Time to ECG (minutes)	54	8	9	7
Average Time to Transfer (minutes)[1]	-	-	64	60
Children's Asthma Care				
Received Home Management Plan of Care	-	-	-	88%
Received Reliever Medication	-	-	-	100%
Received Systemic Corticosteroids	-	-	-	100%
Emergency Department				
Admittance Decision Time (minutes)[2]	435	78	104	98
Head CT Results Within 45 Min. of Arrival	20	35%	60%	57%
Patients Who Left ER Before Being Seen	17,355	0%	1%	2%
Time from ER Arrival to Admit. (minutes)[2]	482	243	276	274
Time from ER Arrival to Discharge (minutes)	452	126	125	134
Time in ER Before Being Evaluated (minutes)	507	30	26	26
Time to Pain Meds for Fractures (minutes)	56	54	58	57
Heart Attack Care				
Aspirin Given at Discharge[1]	-	-	99%	99%
Fibrinolytic Meds Within 30 Min. of Arrival[7]	-	-	40%	54%
PCI Within 90 Minutes of Arrival[7]	-	-	97%	96%
Statin Prescribed at Discharge[1]	-	-	99%	98%
Heart Failure Care				
ACE Inhibitor or ARB for LVSD	18	83%	97%	97%
Discharge Instructions Given	106	87%	96%	94%
Evaluation of LVS Function	150	100%	100%	99%
Medicare Spending				
Medicare Spending per Patient (ratio)	-	0.94	1.01	0.98
Pneumonia Care				
Appropriate Initial Antibiotic Given	58	98%	96%	95%
Blood Culture Timing	145	99%	98%	98%
Pregnancy and Delivery Care				
Newborn Deliveries Scheduled Early	32	25%	4%	6%
Preventive Care				
Immunization for Influenza[2]	278	87%	91%	90%
Immunization for Pneumonia[2]	487	96%	92%	92%
Stroke Care				
Anticoagulation Therapy for Atrial Fibrillation[1]	-	-	96%	95%
Antithrombotic Therapy Timing	17	94%	98%	98%
Assessed for Rehabilitation	19	100%	98%	97%
Discharged on Antithrombotic Therapy	18	89%	99%	99%
Discharged on Statin Medication	15	67%	95%	94%
Thrombolytic Therapy Timing[1]	-	-	72%	66%
Venous Thromboembolism Prophylaxis	24	83%	95%	94%
Written Stroke Educational Materials Given[1]	-	-	90%	88%
Surgical Care Improvement Project				
Appropriate Beta Blocker Usage	48	100%	98%	98%
Appropriate VTP Within 24 Hours	119	97%	99%	98%
Controlled Postoperative Blood Glucose[7]	-	-	98%	97%
Perioperative Temperature Management	138	100%	100%	100%
Prophylactic Antibiotic Selection	101	98%	99%	99%
Prophylactic Antibiotic Selection (Outpatient)	110	95%	98%	98%
Prophylactic Antibiotic Stopped	98	99%	98%	98%
Prophylactic Antibiotic Timing	101	99%	99%	99%
Prophylactic Antibiotic Timing (Outpatient)	114	96%	98%	98%
Urinary Catheter Removal	78	99%	99%	97%
Survey of Patients' Hospital Experiences				
Area Around Room 'Always' Quiet at Night	300+	56%	54%	61%
Doctors 'Always' Communicated Well	300+	78%	80%	82%
Home Recovery Information Given	300+	88%	86%	85%
Hospital Given 9 or 10 on 10 Point Scale	300+	65%	69%	71%
Meds 'Always' Explained Before Given	300+	64%	63%	64%
Nurses 'Always' Communicated Well	300+	78%	79%	79%
Pain 'Always' Well Controlled	300+	68%	70%	71%
Room and Bathroom 'Always' Clean	300+	74%	73%	73%
Timely Help 'Always' Received	300+	65%	67%	68%
Would Definitely Recommend Hospital	300+	56%	70%	71%
Use of Medical Imaging				
Cardiac Imaging Stress Test before Surgery	292	3.4%	5.4%	5.3%
Combination Abdominal CT Scan	558	55.9%	12.2%	10.5%
Combination Brain/Sinus CT Scan	579	2.6%	3.1%	2.7%
Combination Chest CT Scan	253	0.0%	2.1%	2.7%
Follow-up Mammogram/Ultrasound	1,032	15.4%	9%	8.8%
Lumbar Spine MRI for Low Back Pain	128	35.2%	35.8%	37.2%

Robert Packer Hospital

One Guthrie Square
Sayre, PA 18840
Phone: 570-888-6666
Fax: 570-882-5152
URL: www.guthrie.org
Type: Acute Care Hospitals
Emergency Services: Yes
Ownership: Voluntary non-profit - Other
Beds: 238

Key Personnel:
CEO/President. . . . . Marie Droege
Quality Assurance . . . . Theresa Godrich
Intensive Care Unit. . . . . Lisa Jarvis
Emergency Room . . . . Edward Jones
Infection Control. . . . . Allen Kilbourne
Chief of Medical Staff . . . . Ferrol J Lee, MD
Pediatric In-Patient Care . . . . Gerry Terwilliger, MD

Measure	Cases	This Hosp.	State Avg.	U.S. Avg.
Blood Clot Prevention and Treatment				
Anticoagulation Overlap Therapy[2]	83	83%	94%	93%
ICU Venous Thromboembolism Prophylaxis[2]	109	94%	94%	92%
Incidence of Potentially Preventable VTE[1,2]	-	-	8%	10%

NOTE: Hospital profiles are in alphabetical order by state, then city, then hospital within the city; Rankings exclude hospitals with less than 25 cases except for patient surveys which excludes hospitals with less than 100 cases; (a) 100-299 cases; (1) The number of cases/patients is too few to report; (2) Data submitted were based on a sample of cases/patients; (3) Results are based on a shorter time period than required; (4) Data suppressed by CMS for one or more quarters; (5) Results are not available for this reporting period; (6) Fewer than 100 patients completed the HCAHPS survey; (7) No cases met the criteria for this measure; (8) The lower limit of the confidence interval cannot be calculated if the number of observed infections equals zero; (9) No data are available from the state/territory for this reporting period; (10) The scores shown reflect fewer than 50 completed surveys; (11) There were discrepancies in the data collection process; (12) This measure does not apply to this hospital for this reporting period; (13) Results cannot be calculated for this reporting period; (14) The results for this state are combined with nearby states to protect confidentiality; Please refer to the User's Guide for a full explanation of data.

Measure	Cases	This Hosp.	State Avg.	U.S. Avg.
UFH with Dosages/Platelet Monitoring[2]	37	89%	98%	97%
Venous Thromboembolism Prophylaxis[2]	383	86%	90%	85%
Warfarin Therapy Discharge Instructions[2]	63	63%	78%	75%
Chest Pain/Possible Heart Attack Care				
Aspirin Given Within 24 Hours of Arrival[3,7]	-	-	97%	96%
Fibrinolytic Meds Within 30 Min. of Arrival[5]	-	-	44%	58%
Average Time to ECG (minutes)[3,7]	-	-	9	7
Average Time to Transfer (minutes)[5]	-	-	64	60
Children's Asthma Care				
Received Home Management Plan of Care	-	-	-	88%
Received Reliever Medication	-	-	-	100%
Received Systemic Corticosteroids	-	-	-	100%
Emergency Department				
Admittance Decision Time (minutes)[2]	552	230	104	98
Head CT Results Within 45 Min. of Arrival[1,3]	-	-	60%	57%
Patients Who Left ER Before Being Seen	30,332	2%	1%	2%
Time from ER Arrival to Admit. (minutes)[2]	558	444	276	274
Time from ER Arrival to Discharge (minutes)	553	155	125	134
Time in ER Before Being Evaluated (minutes)	595	44	26	26
Time to Pain Meds for Fractures (minutes)	70	61	58	57
Heart Attack Care				
Aspirin Given at Discharge	466	99%	99%	99%
Fibrinolytic Meds Within 30 Min. of Arrival[7]	-	-	40%	54%
PCI Within 90 Minutes of Arrival	34	88%	97%	96%
Statin Prescribed at Discharge	447	98%	99%	98%
Heart Failure Care				
ACE Inhibitor or ARB for LVSD	136	96%	97%	97%
Discharge Instructions Given	344	89%	96%	94%
Evaluation of LVS Function	428	100%	100%	99%
Medicare Spending				
Medicare Spending per Patient (ratio)		0.91	1.01	0.98
Pneumonia Care				
Appropriate Initial Antibiotic Given	105	95%	96%	95%
Blood Culture Timing	212	93%	98%	98%
Pregnancy and Delivery Care				
Newborn Deliveries Scheduled Early	47	0%	4%	6%
Preventive Care				
Immunization for Influenza[2]	656	92%	91%	90%
Immunization for Pneumonia[2]	902	96%	92%	92%
Stroke Care				
Anticoagulation Therapy for Atrial Fibrillation	22	64%	96%	95%
Antithrombotic Therapy Timing	116	98%	98%	98%
Assessed for Rehabilitation	137	87%	98%	97%
Discharged on Antithrombotic Therapy	122	98%	99%	99%
Discharged on Statin Medication	98	94%	95%	94%
Thrombolytic Therapy Timing	11	36%	72%	66%
Venous Thromboembolism Prophylaxis	140	85%	95%	94%
Written Stroke Educational Materials Given	83	43%	90%	88%
Surgical Care Improvement Project				
Appropriate Beta Blocker Usage	577	98%	98%	98%
Appropriate VTP Within 24 Hours	1,095	99%	99%	98%
Controlled Postoperative Blood Glucose	200	95%	98%	97%
Perioperative Temperature Management	1,330	100%	100%	100%
Prophylactic Antibiotic Selection	891	99%	99%	99%
Prophylactic Antibiotic Selection (Outpatient)	565	98%	98%	98%
Prophylactic Antibiotic Stopped	883	98%	98%	98%
Prophylactic Antibiotic Timing	891	99%	99%	99%
Prophylactic Antibiotic Timing (Outpatient)	567	99%	98%	98%
Urinary Catheter Removal	329	95%	99%	97%
Survey of Patients' Hospital Experiences				
Area Around Room 'Always' Quiet at Night	300+	46%	54%	61%
Doctors 'Always' Communicated Well	300+	76%	80%	82%
Home Recovery Information Given	300+	83%	86%	85%
Hospital Given 9 or 10 on 10 Point Scale	300+	70%	69%	71%
Meds 'Always' Explained Before Given	300+	60%	63%	64%
Nurses 'Always' Communicated Well	300+	80%	79%	79%
Pain 'Always' Well Controlled	300+	69%	70%	71%
Room and Bathroom 'Always' Clean	300+	78%	73%	73%
Timely Help 'Always' Received	300+	68%	67%	68%
Would Definitely Recommend Hospital	300+	72%	70%	71%
Use of Medical Imaging				
Cardiac Imaging Stress Test before Surgery	223	4.9%	5.4%	5.3%
Combination Abdominal CT Scan	1,287	7.5%	12.2%	10.5%
Combination Brain/Sinus CT Scan[1]	-	-	3.1%	2.7%
Combination Chest CT Scan	1,044	0.2%	2.1%	2.7%
Follow-up Mammogram/Ultrasound	1,621	13.8%	9%	8.8%
Lumbar Spine MRI for Low Back Pain	134	40.3%	35.8%	37.2%

Geisinger - Community Medical Center

1822 Mulberry Street
Scranton, PA 18510
URL: www.cmchealthsys.org
Type: Acute Care Hospitals
Ownership: Voluntary non-profit - Private
Phone: 570-969-8240
Fax: 570-969-7191
Emergency Services: Yes
Beds: 299

Key Personnel:
Infection Control. . . . . Trina Augustine
Operating Room. . . . . John Delmar
Quality Assurance . . . . Marge Gallagher, RN
CEO/President. . . . . C Richard Hartman, MD
Cardiac Laboratory. . . . . Chaufe Huang, MD
Radiology. . . . . Burton Marks, DO
Coronary Care . . . . Si Ramakrishna, MD
Chief of Medical Staff. . . . . Vincent Ross, MD

Measure	Cases	This Hosp.	State Avg.	U.S. Avg.
Blood Clot Prevention and Treatment				
Anticoagulation Overlap Therapy[2]	87	100%	94%	93%
ICU Venous Thromboembolism Prophylaxis[2]	72	96%	94%	92%
Incidence of Potentially Preventable VTE[1,2]	-	-	8%	10%
UFH with Dosages/Platelet Monitoring[2]	91	100%	98%	97%
Venous Thromboembolism Prophylaxis[2]	467	89%	90%	85%
Warfarin Therapy Discharge Instructions[2]	65	80%	78%	75%
Chest Pain/Possible Heart Attack Care				
Aspirin Given Within 24 Hours of Arrival[3,7]	-	-	97%	96%
Fibrinolytic Meds Within 30 Min. of Arrival[5]	-	-	44%	58%
Average Time to ECG (minutes)[3,7]	-	-	9	7
Average Time to Transfer (minutes)[5]	-	-	64	60
Children's Asthma Care				
Received Home Management Plan of Care	-	-	-	88%
Received Reliever Medication	-	-	-	100%
Received Systemic Corticosteroids	-	-	-	100%
Emergency Department				
Admittance Decision Time (minutes)[2]	1,272	300	104	98
Head CT Results Within 45 Min. of Arrival[1]	-	-	60%	57%
Patients Who Left ER Before Being Seen	36,296	1%	1%	2%
Time from ER Arrival to Admit. (minutes)[2]	1,285	464	276	274
Time from ER Arrival to Discharge (minutes)	673	179	125	134
Time in ER Before Being Evaluated (minutes)	764	32	26	26
Time to Pain Meds for Fractures (minutes)	130	74	58	57
Heart Attack Care				
Aspirin Given at Discharge	218	100%	99%	99%
Fibrinolytic Meds Within 30 Min. of Arrival[7]	-	-	40%	54%
PCI Within 90 Minutes of Arrival	54	96%	97%	96%
Statin Prescribed at Discharge	227	100%	99%	98%
Heart Failure Care				
ACE Inhibitor or ARB for LVSD	98	97%	97%	97%
Discharge Instructions Given	283	91%	96%	94%
Evaluation of LVS Function	359	100%	100%	99%
Medicare Spending				
Medicare Spending per Patient (ratio)	-	1.10	1.01	0.98
Pneumonia Care				
Appropriate Initial Antibiotic Given	150	97%	96%	95%
Blood Culture Timing	249	98%	98%	98%
Pregnancy and Delivery Care				
Newborn Deliveries Scheduled Early[7]	-	-	4%	6%
Preventive Care				
Immunization for Influenza[2]	786	98%	91%	90%
Immunization for Pneumonia[2]	1,305	97%	92%	92%
Stroke Care				
Anticoagulation Therapy for Atrial Fibrillation	38	100%	96%	95%
Antithrombotic Therapy Timing	174	100%	98%	98%
Assessed for Rehabilitation	216	100%	98%	97%
Discharged on Antithrombotic Therapy	181	99%	99%	99%
Discharged on Statin Medication	142	99%	95%	94%
Thrombolytic Therapy Timing	19	84%	72%	66%
Venous Thromboembolism Prophylaxis	233	97%	95%	94%
Written Stroke Educational Materials Given	103	99%	90%	88%
Surgical Care Improvement Project				
Appropriate Beta Blocker Usage[2]	277	99%	98%	98%
Appropriate VTP Within 24 Hours[2]	356	99%	99%	98%
Controlled Postoperative Blood Glucose[2]	160	99%	98%	97%
Perioperative Temperature Management[2]	476	100%	100%	100%
Prophylactic Antibiotic Selection[2]	435	100%	99%	99%
Prophylactic Antibiotic Selection (Outpatient)	441	98%	98%	98%
Prophylactic Antibiotic Stopped[2]	425	99%	98%	98%
Prophylactic Antibiotic Timing[2]	435	99%	99%	99%
Prophylactic Antibiotic Timing (Outpatient)	444	98%	98%	98%
Urinary Catheter Removal[2]	295	95%	99%	97%
Survey of Patients' Hospital Experiences				
Area Around Room 'Always' Quiet at Night	300+	54%	54%	61%
Doctors 'Always' Communicated Well	300+	77%	80%	82%
Home Recovery Information Given	300+	83%	86%	85%
Hospital Given 9 or 10 on 10 Point Scale	300+	58%	69%	71%
Meds 'Always' Explained Before Given	300+	59%	63%	64%
Nurses 'Always' Communicated Well	300+	76%	79%	79%
Pain 'Always' Well Controlled	300+	67%	70%	71%
Room and Bathroom 'Always' Clean	300+	70%	73%	73%
Timely Help 'Always' Received	300+	62%	67%	68%
Would Definitely Recommend Hospital	300+	61%	70%	71%
Use of Medical Imaging				
Cardiac Imaging Stress Test before Surgery	184	7.1%	5.4%	5.3%
Combination Abdominal CT Scan	721	4.0%	12.2%	10.5%
Combination Brain/Sinus CT Scan	736	3.1%	3.1%	2.7%
Combination Chest CT Scan	370	5.4%	2.1%	2.7%
Follow-up Mammogram/Ultrasound	786	10.6%	9%	8.8%
Lumbar Spine MRI for Low Back Pain	46	45.7%	35.8%	37.2%

Moses Taylor Hospital

700 Quincy Avenue
Scranton, PA 18510
E-mail: mediaser@mth.org
URL: www.mth.org
Type: Acute Care Hospitals
Ownership: Voluntary non-profit - Private
Phone: 570-340-2100
Fax: 570-969-2629
Emergency Services: Yes
Beds: 224

Key Personnel:
CEO/President. . . . . Harold E Anderson
Pediatric Ambulatory Care . . . . . . Stanley Blondek, MD
Pediatric In-Patient Care . . . . Stanley Blondek, MD
Chief of Medical Staff. . . . . Carmen A Brutico Jr, MD
Operating Room. . . . . Terence A Cochran, RN
Quality Assurance . . . . Pam Maidlatesi, RN
Infection Control. . . . . Alice McDonald, RN

Measure	Cases	This Hosp.	State Avg.	U.S. Avg.
Blood Clot Prevention and Treatment				
Anticoagulation Overlap Therapy[2]	32	91%	94%	93%
ICU Venous Thromboembolism Prophylaxis[2]	57	96%	94%	92%
Incidence of Potentially Preventable VTE[1,2]	-	-	8%	10%
UFH with Dosages/Platelet Monitoring[2]	29	100%	98%	97%
Venous Thromboembolism Prophylaxis[2]	408	95%	90%	85%
Warfarin Therapy Discharge Instructions[2]	22	95%	78%	75%
Chest Pain/Possible Heart Attack Care				
Aspirin Given Within 24 Hours of Arrival	23	100%	97%	96%
Fibrinolytic Meds Within 30 Min. of Arrival[7]	-	-	44%	58%
Average Time to ECG (minutes)	23	9	9	7
Average Time to Transfer (minutes)[1]	-	-	64	60
Children's Asthma Care				
Received Home Management Plan of Care	-	-	-	88%
Received Reliever Medication	-	-	-	100%
Received Systemic Corticosteroids	-	-	-	100%
Emergency Department				
Admittance Decision Time (minutes)[2]	461	105	104	98
Head CT Results Within 45 Min. of Arrival[1]	-	-	60%	57%
Patients Who Left ER Before Being Seen	32,490	1%	1%	2%
Time from ER Arrival to Admit. (minutes)[2]	523	295	276	274
Time from ER Arrival to Discharge (minutes)	392	166	125	134
Time in ER Before Being Evaluated (minutes)	386	45	26	26
Time to Pain Meds for Fractures (minutes)	71	77	58	57
Heart Attack Care				
Aspirin Given at Discharge[1]	-	-	99%	99%
Fibrinolytic Meds Within 30 Min. of Arrival[7]	-	-	40%	54%
PCI Within 90 Minutes of Arrival[7]	-	-	97%	96%

NOTE: Hospital profiles are in alphabetical order by state, then city, then hospital within the city; Rankings exclude hospitals with less than 25 cases except for patient surveys which excludes hospitals with less than 100 cases; (a) 100-299 cases; (1) The number of cases/patients is too few to report; (2) Data submitted were based on a sample of cases/patients; (3) Results are based on a shorter time period than required; (4) Data suppressed by CMS for one or more quarters; (5) Results are not available for this reporting period; (6) Fewer than 100 patients completed the HCAHPS survey; (7) No cases met the criteria for this measure; (8) The lower limit of the confidence interval cannot be calculated if the number of observed infections equals zero; (9) No data are available from the state/territory for this reporting period; (10) The scores shown reflect fewer than 50 completed surveys; (11) There were discrepancies in the data collection process; (12) This measure does not apply to this hospital for this reporting period; (13) Results cannot be calculated for this reporting period; (14) The results for this state are combined with nearby states to protect confidentiality; Please refer to the User's Guide for a full explanation of data.

Measure	Cases	This Hosp.	State Avg.	U.S. Avg.
Statin Prescribed at Discharge[1]	-	-	99%	98%
Heart Failure Care				
ACE Inhibitor or ARB for LVSD	25	100%	97%	97%
Discharge Instructions Given	99	92%	96%	94%
Evaluation of LVS Function	162	100%	100%	99%
Medicare Spending				
Medicare Spending per Patient (ratio)	-	1.14	1.01	0.98
Pneumonia Care				
Appropriate Initial Antibiotic Given	92	97%	96%	95%
Blood Culture Timing	201	100%	98%	98%
Pregnancy and Delivery Care				
Newborn Deliveries Scheduled Early[2]	51	0%	4%	6%
Preventive Care				
Immunization for Influenza[2]	532	100%	91%	90%
Immunization for Pneumonia[2]	518	99%	92%	92%
Stroke Care				
Anticoagulation Therapy for Atrial Fibrillation	22	100%	96%	95%
Antithrombotic Therapy Timing	81	99%	98%	98%
Assessed for Rehabilitation	85	100%	98%	97%
Discharged on Antithrombotic Therapy	82	98%	99%	99%
Discharged on Statin Medication	57	98%	95%	94%
Thrombolytic Therapy Timing[1]	-	-	72%	66%
Venous Thromboembolism Prophylaxis	83	98%	95%	94%
Written Stroke Educational Materials Given	34	97%	90%	88%
Surgical Care Improvement Project				
Appropriate Beta Blocker Usage	133	96%	98%	98%
Appropriate VTP Within 24 Hours	425	99%	99%	98%
Controlled Postoperative Blood Glucose[7]	-	-	98%	97%
Perioperative Temperature Management	486	98%	100%	100%
Prophylactic Antibiotic Selection	325	99%	99%	99%
Prophylactic Antibiotic Selection (Outpatient)	98	97%	98%	98%
Prophylactic Antibiotic Stopped	316	97%	98%	98%
Prophylactic Antibiotic Timing	325	99%	99%	99%
Prophylactic Antibiotic Timing (Outpatient)	98	99%	98%	98%
Urinary Catheter Removal	272	99%	99%	97%
Survey of Patients' Hospital Experiences				
Area Around Room 'Always' Quiet at Night	300+	52%	54%	61%
Doctors 'Always' Communicated Well	300+	81%	80%	82%
Home Recovery Information Given	300+	89%	86%	85%
Hospital Given 9 or 10 on 10 Point Scale	300+	67%	69%	71%
Meds 'Always' Explained Before Given	300+	60%	63%	64%
Nurses 'Always' Communicated Well	300+	77%	79%	79%
Pain 'Always' Well Controlled	300+	69%	70%	71%
Room and Bathroom 'Always' Clean	300+	65%	73%	73%
Timely Help 'Always' Received	300+	61%	67%	68%
Would Definitely Recommend Hospital	300+	70%	70%	71%
Use of Medical Imaging				
Cardiac Imaging Stress Test before Surgery	106	4.7%	5.4%	5.3%
Combination Abdominal CT Scan	495	12.7%	12.2%	10.5%
Combination Brain/Sinus CT Scan[1]	-	-	3.1%	2.7%
Combination Chest CT Scan	301	4.3%	2.1%	2.7%
Follow-up Mammogram/Ultrasound	726	13.6%	9%	8.8%
Lumbar Spine MRI for Low Back Pain[1]	-	-	35.8%	37.2%

Regional Hospital of Scranton

746 Jefferson Avenue
Scranton, PA 18501
Phone: 570-348-7100
Fax: 570-348-7639
URL: www.mercyhealthpartners.com
Type: Acute Care Hospitals
Emergency Services: Yes
Ownership: Voluntary non-profit - Church
Beds: 373

Key Personnel:

CEO/President. . . . . John Nespoli

Measure	Cases	This Hosp.	State Avg.	U.S. Avg.
Blood Clot Prevention and Treatment				
Anticoagulation Overlap Therapy[2]	69	99%	94%	93%
ICU Venous Thromboembolism Prophylaxis[2]	109	98%	94%	92%
Incidence of Potentially Preventable VTE[2]	12	25%	8%	10%
UFH with Dosages/Platelet Monitoring[2]	72	100%	98%	97%
Venous Thromboembolism Prophylaxis[2]	540	76%	90%	85%
Warfarin Therapy Discharge Instructions[2]	46	65%	78%	75%
Chest Pain/Possible Heart Attack Care				
Aspirin Given Within 24 Hours of Arrival[5]	-	-	97%	96%
Fibrinolytic Meds Within 30 Min. of Arrival[5]	-	-	44%	58%
Average Time to ECG (minutes)[5]	-	-	9	7
Average Time to Transfer (minutes)[5]	-	-	64	60
Children's Asthma Care				
Received Home Management Plan of Care	-	-	-	88%
Received Reliever Medication	-	-	-	100%
Received Systemic Corticosteroids	-	-	-	100%
Emergency Department				
Admittance Decision Time (minutes)[2]	197	115	104	98
Head CT Results Within 45 Min. of Arrival[1]	-	-	60%	57%
Patients Who Left ER Before Being Seen	29,689	3%	1%	2%
Time from ER Arrival to Admit. (minutes)[2]	223	325	276	274
Time from ER Arrival to Discharge (minutes)	347	140	125	134
Time in ER Before Being Evaluated (minutes)	393	30	26	26
Time to Pain Meds for Fractures (minutes)	42	71	58	57
Heart Attack Care				
Aspirin Given at Discharge	430	98%	99%	99%
Fibrinolytic Meds Within 30 Min. of Arrival[7]	-	-	40%	54%
PCI Within 90 Minutes of Arrival	55	96%	97%	96%
Statin Prescribed at Discharge	419	96%	99%	98%
Heart Failure Care				
ACE Inhibitor or ARB for LVSD	144	92%	97%	97%
Discharge Instructions Given	376	90%	96%	94%
Evaluation of LVS Function	530	99%	100%	99%
Medicare Spending				
Medicare Spending per Patient (ratio)	-	1.06	1.01	0.98
Pneumonia Care				
Appropriate Initial Antibiotic Given	124	85%	96%	95%
Blood Culture Timing	249	96%	98%	98%
Pregnancy and Delivery Care				
Newborn Deliveries Scheduled Early[7]	-	-	4%	6%
Preventive Care				
Immunization for Influenza[2]	673	92%	91%	90%
Immunization for Pneumonia[2]	1,079	93%	92%	92%
Stroke Care				
Anticoagulation Therapy for Atrial Fibrillation	14	93%	96%	95%
Antithrombotic Therapy Timing	101	93%	98%	98%
Assessed for Rehabilitation	98	95%	98%	97%
Discharged on Antithrombotic Therapy	90	100%	99%	99%
Discharged on Statin Medication	67	91%	95%	94%
Thrombolytic Therapy Timing	15	0%	72%	66%
Venous Thromboembolism Prophylaxis	109	81%	95%	94%
Written Stroke Educational Materials Given	56	86%	90%	88%
Surgical Care Improvement Project				
Appropriate Beta Blocker Usage	402	97%	98%	98%
Appropriate VTP Within 24 Hours	716	98%	99%	98%
Controlled Postoperative Blood Glucose	209	96%	98%	97%
Perioperative Temperature Management	824	100%	100%	100%
Prophylactic Antibiotic Selection	743	99%	99%	99%
Prophylactic Antibiotic Selection (Outpatient)	394	96%	98%	98%
Prophylactic Antibiotic Stopped	727	99%	98%	98%
Prophylactic Antibiotic Timing	744	100%	99%	99%
Prophylactic Antibiotic Timing (Outpatient)	404	96%	98%	98%
Urinary Catheter Removal	162	85%	99%	97%
Survey of Patients' Hospital Experiences				
Area Around Room 'Always' Quiet at Night	300+	56%	54%	61%
Doctors 'Always' Communicated Well	300+	83%	80%	82%
Home Recovery Information Given	300+	83%	86%	85%
Hospital Given 9 or 10 on 10 Point Scale	300+	65%	69%	71%
Meds 'Always' Explained Before Given	300+	61%	63%	64%
Nurses 'Always' Communicated Well	300+	76%	79%	79%
Pain 'Always' Well Controlled	300+	70%	70%	71%
Room and Bathroom 'Always' Clean	300+	70%	73%	73%
Timely Help 'Always' Received	300+	62%	67%	68%
Would Definitely Recommend Hospital	300+	68%	70%	71%
Use of Medical Imaging				
Cardiac Imaging Stress Test before Surgery	135	9.6%	5.4%	5.3%
Combination Abdominal CT Scan	807	8.9%	12.2%	10.5%
Combination Brain/Sinus CT Scan[1]	-	-	3.1%	2.7%
Combination Chest CT Scan	538	5.8%	2.1%	2.7%
Follow-up Mammogram/Ultrasound	673	10.1%	9%	8.8%
Lumbar Spine MRI for Low Back Pain	52	42.3%	35.8%	37.2%

Grand View Hospital

700 Lawn Avenue
Sellersville, PA 18960
Phone: 215-453-4615
Fax: 215-453-9151
E-mail: info@gvh.org
URL: www.gvh.org
Type: Acute Care Hospitals
Emergency Services: Yes
Ownership: Voluntary non-profit - Other
Beds: 198

Key Personnel:

Pediatric In-Patient Care . . . . Andrew Chu, MD
Pediatric Ambulatory Care . . . . . . Marie Clarke
CEO/President. . . . . Stuart H Fine
Chief of Medical Staff . . . . Anthony Foderaro, MD
Radiology. . . . . Anthony E Foderaro
Infection Control. . . . . Dean Miller
Coronary Care . . . . Teresa Shoultes
Quality Assurance . . . . Kathleen Slagel

Measure	Cases	This Hosp.	State Avg.	U.S. Avg.
Blood Clot Prevention and Treatment				
Anticoagulation Overlap Therapy[2]	76	97%	94%	93%
ICU Venous Thromboembolism Prophylaxis[2]	75	100%	94%	92%
Incidence of Potentially Preventable VTE[2]	11	0%	8%	10%
UFH with Dosages/Platelet Monitoring[2]	34	100%	98%	97%
Venous Thromboembolism Prophylaxis[2]	311	94%	90%	85%
Warfarin Therapy Discharge Instructions[2]	67	97%	78%	75%
Chest Pain/Possible Heart Attack Care				
Aspirin Given Within 24 Hours of Arrival	55	100%	97%	96%
Fibrinolytic Meds Within 30 Min. of Arrival[7]	-	-	44%	58%
Average Time to ECG (minutes)	55	7	9	7
Average Time to Transfer (minutes)	20	32	64	60
Children's Asthma Care				
Received Home Management Plan of Care	-	-	-	88%
Received Reliever Medication	-	-	-	100%
Received Systemic Corticosteroids	-	-	-	100%
Emergency Department				
Admittance Decision Time (minutes)[2]	633	113	104	98
Head CT Results Within 45 Min. of Arrival[1]	-	-	60%	57%
Patients Who Left ER Before Being Seen	35,459	1%	1%	2%
Time from ER Arrival to Admit. (minutes)[2]	640	256	276	274
Time from ER Arrival to Discharge (minutes)	592	139	125	134
Time in ER Before Being Evaluated (minutes)	640	33	26	26
Time to Pain Meds for Fractures (minutes)	176	36	58	57
Heart Attack Care				
Aspirin Given at Discharge	39	100%	99%	99%
Fibrinolytic Meds Within 30 Min. of Arrival[7]	-	-	40%	54%
PCI Within 90 Minutes of Arrival[1]	-	-	97%	96%
Statin Prescribed at Discharge	36	100%	99%	98%
Heart Failure Care				
ACE Inhibitor or ARB for LVSD	43	98%	97%	97%
Discharge Instructions Given	178	96%	96%	94%
Evaluation of LVS Function	230	100%	100%	99%
Medicare Spending				
Medicare Spending per Patient (ratio)	-	0.99	1.01	0.98
Pneumonia Care				
Appropriate Initial Antibiotic Given	149	99%	96%	95%
Blood Culture Timing	278	100%	98%	98%
Pregnancy and Delivery Care				
Newborn Deliveries Scheduled Early	105	3%	4%	6%
Preventive Care				
Immunization for Influenza[2]	564	98%	91%	90%
Immunization for Pneumonia[2]	659	98%	92%	92%
Stroke Care				
Anticoagulation Therapy for Atrial Fibrillation	17	100%	96%	95%
Antithrombotic Therapy Timing	80	99%	98%	98%
Assessed for Rehabilitation	86	100%	98%	97%
Discharged on Antithrombotic Therapy	84	99%	99%	99%
Discharged on Statin Medication	64	97%	95%	94%
Thrombolytic Therapy Timing[1]	-	-	72%	66%
Venous Thromboembolism Prophylaxis	87	99%	95%	94%
Written Stroke Educational Materials Given	48	96%	90%	88%
Surgical Care Improvement Project				
Appropriate Beta Blocker Usage[2]	142	100%	98%	98%
Appropriate VTP Within 24 Hours[2]	336	100%	99%	98%
Controlled Postoperative Blood Glucose[2,7]	-	-	98%	97%
Perioperative Temperature Management[2]	412	100%	100%	100%

NOTE: Hospital profiles are in alphabetical order by state, then city, then hospital within the city; Rankings exclude hospitals with less than 25 cases except for patient surveys which excludes hospitals with less than 100 cases; (a) 100-299 cases; (1) The number of cases/patients is too few to report; (2) Data submitted were based on a sample of cases/patients; (3) Results are based on a shorter time period than required; (4) Data suppressed by CMS for one or more quarters; (5) Results are not available for this reporting period; (6) Fewer than 100 patients completed the HCAHPS survey; (7) No cases met the criteria for this measure; (8) The lower limit of the confidence interval cannot be calculated if the number of observed infections equals zero; (9) No data are available from the state/territory for this reporting period; (10) The scores shown reflect fewer than 50 completed surveys; (11) There were discrepancies in the data collection process; (12) This measure does not apply to this hospital for this reporting period; (13) Results cannot be calculated for this reporting period; (14) The results for this state are combined with nearby states to protect confidentiality; Please refer to the User's Guide for a full explanation of data.

Prophylactic Antibiotic Selection[2]	272	100%	99%	99%
Prophylactic Antibiotic Selection (Outpatient)	123	98%	98%	98%
Prophylactic Antibiotic Stopped[2]	263	99%	98%	98%
Prophylactic Antibiotic Timing[2]	272	100%	99%	99%
Prophylactic Antibiotic Timing (Outpatient)	123	98%	98%	98%
Urinary Catheter Removal[2]	64	100%	99%	97%
Survey of Patients' Hospital Experiences				
Area Around Room 'Always' Quiet at Night	300+	54%	54%	61%
Doctors 'Always' Communicated Well	300+	76%	80%	82%
Home Recovery Information Given	300+	89%	86%	85%
Hospital Given 9 or 10 on 10 Point Scale	300+	72%	69%	71%
Meds 'Always' Explained Before Given	300+	59%	63%	64%
Nurses 'Always' Communicated Well	300+	81%	79%	79%
Pain 'Always' Well Controlled	300+	73%	70%	71%
Room and Bathroom 'Always' Clean	300+	76%	73%	73%
Timely Help 'Always' Received	300+	66%	67%	68%
Would Definitely Recommend Hospital	300+	77%	70%	71%
Use of Medical Imaging				
Cardiac Imaging Stress Test before Surgery	495	5.1%	5.4%	5.3%
Combination Abdominal CT Scan	964	7.2%	12.2%	10.5%
Combination Brain/Sinus CT Scan	733	1.0%	3.1%	2.7%
Combination Chest CT Scan	845	0.7%	2.1%	2.7%
Follow-up Mammogram/Ultrasound	2,468	11.2%	9%	8.8%
Lumbar Spine MRI for Low Back Pain	141	32.6%	35.8%	37.2%

UPMC Northwest

100 Fairfield Drive
Seneca, PA 16346
URL: www.northwest.upmc.com
Type: Acute Care Hospitals
Ownership: Voluntary non-profit - Other

Phone: 814-676-7600
Emergency Services: Yes

Key Personnel:
CEO/President. . . . . David P Gibbons
Infection Control. . . . . Karen Latshaw

Measure	Cases	This Hosp.	State Avg.	U.S. Avg.
Blood Clot Prevention and Treatment				
Anticoagulation Overlap Therapy[2]	78	100%	94%	93%
ICU Venous Thromboembolism Prophylaxis[2]	37	95%	94%	92%
Incidence of Potentially Preventable VTE[1,2]	-	-	8%	10%
UFH with Dosages/Platelet Monitoring[2]	21	100%	98%	97%
Venous Thromboembolism Prophylaxis[2]	524	96%	90%	85%
Warfarin Therapy Discharge Instructions[2]	66	100%	78%	75%
Chest Pain/Possible Heart Attack Care				
Aspirin Given Within 24 Hours of Arrival	148	99%	97%	96%
Fibrinolytic Meds Within 30 Min. of Arrival[1]	-	-	44%	58%
Average Time to ECG (minutes)	153	7	9	7
Average Time to Transfer (minutes)	21	44	64	60
Children's Asthma Care				
Received Home Management Plan of Care	-	-	-	88%
Received Reliever Medication	-	-	-	100%
Received Systemic Corticosteroids	-	-	-	100%
Emergency Department				
Admittance Decision Time (minutes)[2]	544	76	104	98
Head CT Results Within 45 Min. of Arrival	21	67%	60%	57%
Patients Who Left ER Before Being Seen	32,101	0%	1%	2%
Time from ER Arrival to Admit. (minutes)[2]	565	198	276	274
Time from ER Arrival to Discharge (minutes)	541	97	125	134
Time in ER Before Being Evaluated (minutes)	626	12	26	26
Time to Pain Meds for Fractures (minutes)	104	31	58	57
Heart Attack Care				
Aspirin Given at Discharge	19	95%	99%	99%
Fibrinolytic Meds Within 30 Min. of Arrival[7]	-	-	40%	54%
PCI Within 90 Minutes of Arrival[7]	-	-	97%	96%
Statin Prescribed at Discharge	14	86%	99%	98%
Heart Failure Care				
ACE Inhibitor or ARB for LVSD	30	100%	97%	97%
Discharge Instructions Given	106	100%	96%	94%
Evaluation of LVS Function	151	100%	100%	99%
Medicare Spending				
Medicare Spending per Patient (ratio)	-	0.94	1.01	0.98
Pneumonia Care				
Appropriate Initial Antibiotic Given	95	98%	96%	95%
Blood Culture Timing	184	100%	98%	98%
Pregnancy and Delivery Care				
Newborn Deliveries Scheduled Early[2]	48	0%	4%	6%
Preventive Care				
Immunization for Influenza[2]	620	98%	91%	90%
Immunization for Pneumonia[2]	853	98%	92%	92%
Stroke Care				
Anticoagulation Therapy for Atrial Fibrillation[1]	-	-	96%	95%
Antithrombotic Therapy Timing	60	100%	98%	98%
Assessed for Rehabilitation	66	100%	98%	97%
Discharged on Antithrombotic Therapy	64	98%	99%	99%
Discharged on Statin Medication	40	100%	95%	94%
Thrombolytic Therapy Timing[1]	-	-	72%	66%
Venous Thromboembolism Prophylaxis	62	97%	95%	94%
Written Stroke Educational Materials Given	39	100%	90%	88%
Surgical Care Improvement Project				
Appropriate Beta Blocker Usage	81	100%	98%	98%
Appropriate VTP Within 24 Hours	234	99%	99%	98%
Controlled Postoperative Blood Glucose[7]	-	-	98%	97%
Perioperative Temperature Management	313	99%	100%	100%
Prophylactic Antibiotic Selection	223	100%	99%	99%
Prophylactic Antibiotic Selection (Outpatient)	168	99%	98%	98%
Prophylactic Antibiotic Stopped	221	99%	98%	98%
Prophylactic Antibiotic Timing	224	98%	99%	99%
Prophylactic Antibiotic Timing (Outpatient)	83	96%	98%	98%
Urinary Catheter Removal	128	99%	99%	97%
Survey of Patients' Hospital Experiences				
Area Around Room 'Always' Quiet at Night	300+	49%	54%	61%
Doctors 'Always' Communicated Well	300+	78%	80%	82%
Home Recovery Information Given	300+	86%	86%	85%
Hospital Given 9 or 10 on 10 Point Scale	300+	62%	69%	71%
Meds 'Always' Explained Before Given	300+	59%	63%	64%
Nurses 'Always' Communicated Well	300+	74%	79%	79%
Pain 'Always' Well Controlled	300+	63%	70%	71%
Room and Bathroom 'Always' Clean	300+	70%	73%	73%
Timely Help 'Always' Received	300+	61%	67%	68%
Would Definitely Recommend Hospital	300+	58%	70%	71%
Use of Medical Imaging				
Cardiac Imaging Stress Test before Surgery	250	8.4%	5.4%	5.3%
Combination Abdominal CT Scan	996	6.8%	12.2%	10.5%
Combination Brain/Sinus CT Scan	710	4.4%	3.1%	2.7%
Combination Chest CT Scan	714	1.4%	2.1%	2.7%
Follow-up Mammogram/Ultrasound	1,426	10.0%	9%	8.8%
Lumbar Spine MRI for Low Back Pain	190	41.1%	35.8%	37.2%

Heritage Valley Sewickley

720 Blackburn Road
Sewickley, PA 15143
URL: www.heritagevalley.org
Type: Acute Care Hospitals
Ownership: Voluntary non-profit - Private

Phone: 412-741-6600
Fax: 412-749-7400
Emergency Services: Yes
Beds: 221

Key Personnel:
Chief of Medical Staff. . . . . John T. Cinicola, MD
Operating Room. . . . . Michael D Felix
Emergency Room . . . . Lind Honyk
President/CEO. . . . . Norman S Mitry
Pediatric Ambulatory Care . . . . . . Thom J Roberts
Pediatric In-Patient Care . . . . Thom J Roberts
Quality Assurance . . . . Catherine Williams

Measure	Cases	This Hosp.	State Avg.	U.S. Avg.
Blood Clot Prevention and Treatment				
Anticoagulation Overlap Therapy[2]	59	100%	94%	93%
ICU Venous Thromboembolism Prophylaxis[2]	89	100%	94%	92%
Incidence of Potentially Preventable VTE[2]	12	0%	8%	10%
UFH with Dosages/Platelet Monitoring[2]	62	100%	98%	97%
Venous Thromboembolism Prophylaxis[2]	320	100%	90%	85%
Warfarin Therapy Discharge Instructions[2]	38	100%	78%	75%
Chest Pain/Possible Heart Attack Care				
Aspirin Given Within 24 Hours of Arrival	46	100%	97%	96%
Fibrinolytic Meds Within 30 Min. of Arrival[7]	-	-	44%	58%
Average Time to ECG (minutes)	44	9	9	7
Average Time to Transfer (minutes)	18	56	64	60
Children's Asthma Care				
Received Home Management Plan of Care	-	-	-	88%
Received Reliever Medication	-	-	-	100%
Received Systemic Corticosteroids	-	-	-	100%
Emergency Department				
Admittance Decision Time (minutes)[2]	422	56	104	98
Head CT Results Within 45 Min. of Arrival[1]	-	-	60%	57%
Patients Who Left ER Before Being Seen	33,437	0%	1%	2%
Time from ER Arrival to Admit. (minutes)[2]	427	237	276	274
Time from ER Arrival to Discharge (minutes)	392	123	125	134
Time in ER Before Being Evaluated (minutes)	329	21	26	26
Time to Pain Meds for Fractures (minutes)	78	50	58	57
Heart Attack Care				
Aspirin Given at Discharge	24	100%	99%	99%
Fibrinolytic Meds Within 30 Min. of Arrival[7]	-	-	40%	54%
PCI Within 90 Minutes of Arrival[7]	-	-	97%	96%
Statin Prescribed at Discharge	18	94%	99%	98%
Heart Failure Care				
ACE Inhibitor or ARB for LVSD	42	100%	97%	97%
Discharge Instructions Given	135	96%	96%	94%
Evaluation of LVS Function	200	100%	100%	99%
Medicare Spending				
Medicare Spending per Patient (ratio)	-	1.08	1.01	0.98
Pneumonia Care				
Appropriate Initial Antibiotic Given[2]	101	98%	96%	95%
Blood Culture Timing[2]	191	99%	98%	98%
Pregnancy and Delivery Care				
Newborn Deliveries Scheduled Early[2]	85	1%	4%	6%
Preventive Care				
Immunization for Influenza[2]	561	98%	91%	90%
Immunization for Pneumonia[2]	681	98%	92%	92%
Stroke Care				
Anticoagulation Therapy for Atrial Fibrillation[1]	-	-	96%	95%
Antithrombotic Therapy Timing	71	99%	98%	98%
Assessed for Rehabilitation	68	100%	98%	97%
Discharged on Antithrombotic Therapy	67	99%	99%	99%
Discharged on Statin Medication	50	94%	95%	94%
Thrombolytic Therapy Timing[7]	-	-	72%	66%
Venous Thromboembolism Prophylaxis	76	100%	95%	94%
Written Stroke Educational Materials Given	28	100%	90%	88%
Surgical Care Improvement Project				
Appropriate Beta Blocker Usage[2]	94	95%	98%	98%
Appropriate VTP Within 24 Hours[2]	361	98%	99%	98%
Controlled Postoperative Blood Glucose[2,7]	-	-	98%	97%
Perioperative Temperature Management[2]	423	100%	100%	100%
Prophylactic Antibiotic Selection[2]	274	99%	99%	99%
Prophylactic Antibiotic Selection (Outpatient)	83	96%	98%	98%
Prophylactic Antibiotic Stopped[2]	266	98%	98%	98%
Prophylactic Antibiotic Timing[2]	274	99%	99%	99%
Prophylactic Antibiotic Timing (Outpatient)	84	94%	98%	98%
Urinary Catheter Removal[2]	257	96%	99%	97%
Survey of Patients' Hospital Experiences				
Area Around Room 'Always' Quiet at Night	300+	57%	54%	61%
Doctors 'Always' Communicated Well	300+	82%	80%	82%
Home Recovery Information Given	300+	83%	86%	85%
Hospital Given 9 or 10 on 10 Point Scale	300+	67%	69%	71%
Meds 'Always' Explained Before Given	300+	63%	63%	64%
Nurses 'Always' Communicated Well	300+	81%	79%	79%
Pain 'Always' Well Controlled	300+	72%	70%	71%
Room and Bathroom 'Always' Clean	300+	66%	73%	73%
Timely Help 'Always' Received	300+	65%	67%	68%
Would Definitely Recommend Hospital	300+	73%	70%	71%
Use of Medical Imaging				
Cardiac Imaging Stress Test before Surgery	80	10.0%	5.4%	5.3%
Combination Abdominal CT Scan	318	5.7%	12.2%	10.5%
Combination Brain/Sinus CT Scan[1]	-	-	3.1%	2.7%
Combination Chest CT Scan	201	0.0%	2.1%	2.7%
Follow-up Mammogram/Ultrasound	218	7.8%	9%	8.8%
Lumbar Spine MRI for Low Back Pain	36	55.6%	35.8%	37.2%

NOTE: Hospital profiles are in alphabetical order by state, then city, then hospital within the city; Rankings exclude hospitals with less than 25 cases except for patient surveys which excludes hospitals with less than 100 cases; (a) 100-299 cases; (1) The number of cases/patients is too few to report; (2) Data submitted were based on a sample of cases/patients; (3) Results are based on a shorter time period than required; (4) Data suppressed by CMS for one or more quarters; (5) Results are not available for this reporting period; (6) Fewer than 100 patients completed the HCAHPS survey; (7) No cases met the criteria for this measure; (8) The lower limit of the confidence interval cannot be calculated if the number of observed infections equals zero; (9) No data are available from the state/territory for this reporting period; (10) The scores shown reflect fewer than 50 completed surveys; (11) There were discrepancies in the data collection process; (12) This measure does not apply to this hospital for this reporting period; (13) Results cannot be calculated for this reporting period; (14) The results for this state are combined with nearby states to protect confidentiality; Please refer to the User's Guide for a full explanation of data.

Sharon Regional Health System

740 East State Street
Sharon, PA 16146
Phone: 724-983-3800
Fax: 724-983-3896
E-mail: info@srhs.org
URL: www.sharonregional.com
Type: Acute Care Hospitals
Emergency Services: Yes
Ownership: Voluntary non-profit - Other
Beds: 240

Key Personnel:
Coronary Care . . . . Mary Jane Altham, RN
Operating Room. . . . . Michelle Aurin
Radiology. . . . . Arlene B Baratz
Quality Assurance . . . . Ginny Catterson
Chief of Medical Staff. . . . . Matthew D Crago
Infection Control. . . . . Sally Tice, RN
CEO/President. . . . . John A Zidansek

Measure	Cases	This Hosp.	State Avg.	U.S. Avg.
Blood Clot Prevention and Treatment				
Anticoagulation Overlap Therapy[2]	48	96%	94%	93%
ICU Venous Thromboembolism Prophylaxis[2]	111	87%	94%	92%
Incidence of Potentially Preventable VTE[1,2]	-	-	8%	10%
UFH with Dosages/Platelet Monitoring[2]	48	100%	98%	97%
Venous Thromboembolism Prophylaxis[2]	677	86%	90%	85%
Warfarin Therapy Discharge Instructions[2]	35	100%	78%	75%
Chest Pain/Possible Heart Attack Care				
Aspirin Given Within 24 Hours of Arrival[1]	-	-	97%	96%
Fibrinolytic Meds Within 30 Min. of Arrival[3,7]	-	-	44%	58%
Average Time to ECG (minutes)[1]	-	-	9	7
Average Time to Transfer (minutes)[3,7]	-	-	64	60
Children's Asthma Care				
Received Home Management Plan of Care	-	-	-	88%
Received Reliever Medication	-	-	-	100%
Received Systemic Corticosteroids	-	-	-	100%
Emergency Department				
Admittance Decision Time (minutes)[2]	213	73	104	98
Head CT Results Within 45 Min. of Arrival	17	88%	60%	57%
Patients Who Left ER Before Being Seen	38,822	1%	1%	2%
Time from ER Arrival to Admit. (minutes)[2]	710	232	276	274
Time from ER Arrival to Discharge (minutes)	1,366	113	125	134
Time in ER Before Being Evaluated (minutes)	1,166	24	26	26
Time to Pain Meds for Fractures (minutes)	82	44	58	57
Heart Attack Care				
Aspirin Given at Discharge	130	100%	99%	99%
Fibrinolytic Meds Within 30 Min. of Arrival[7]	-	-	40%	54%
PCI Within 90 Minutes of Arrival	38	97%	97%	96%
Statin Prescribed at Discharge	129	100%	99%	98%
Heart Failure Care				
ACE Inhibitor or ARB for LVSD	42	86%	97%	97%
Discharge Instructions Given	189	89%	96%	94%
Evaluation of LVS Function	232	100%	100%	99%
Medicare Spending				
Medicare Spending per Patient (ratio)	-	0.99	1.01	0.98
Pneumonia Care				
Appropriate Initial Antibiotic Given	148	97%	96%	95%
Blood Culture Timing	223	97%	98%	98%
Pregnancy and Delivery Care				
Newborn Deliveries Scheduled Early	56	14%	4%	6%
Preventive Care				
Immunization for Influenza[2]	561	58%	91%	90%
Immunization for Pneumonia[2]	826	71%	92%	92%
Stroke Care				
Anticoagulation Therapy for Atrial Fibrillation[1]	-	-	96%	95%
Antithrombotic Therapy Timing	72	94%	98%	98%
Assessed for Rehabilitation	76	91%	98%	97%
Discharged on Antithrombotic Therapy	72	94%	99%	99%
Discharged on Statin Medication	64	70%	95%	94%
Thrombolytic Therapy Timing[7]	-	-	72%	66%
Venous Thromboembolism Prophylaxis	70	67%	95%	94%
Written Stroke Educational Materials Given	38	92%	90%	88%
Surgical Care Improvement Project				
Appropriate Beta Blocker Usage	187	95%	98%	98%
Appropriate VTP Within 24 Hours	455	98%	99%	98%
Controlled Postoperative Blood Glucose	51	90%	98%	97%
Perioperative Temperature Management	521	100%	100%	100%
Prophylactic Antibiotic Selection	421	98%	99%	99%
Prophylactic Antibiotic Selection (Outpatient)	127	100%	98%	98%
Prophylactic Antibiotic Stopped	414	95%	98%	98%
Prophylactic Antibiotic Timing	421	100%	99%	99%
Prophylactic Antibiotic Timing (Outpatient)	127	100%	98%	98%
Urinary Catheter Removal	296	96%	99%	97%
Survey of Patients' Hospital Experiences				
Area Around Room 'Always' Quiet at Night	300+	48%	54%	61%
Doctors 'Always' Communicated Well	300+	79%	80%	82%
Home Recovery Information Given	300+	85%	86%	85%
Hospital Given 9 or 10 on 10 Point Scale	300+	64%	69%	71%
Meds 'Always' Explained Before Given	300+	60%	63%	64%
Nurses 'Always' Communicated Well	300+	78%	79%	79%
Pain 'Always' Well Controlled	300+	69%	70%	71%
Room and Bathroom 'Always' Clean	300+	66%	73%	73%
Timely Help 'Always' Received	300+	66%	67%	68%
Would Definitely Recommend Hospital	300+	63%	70%	71%
Use of Medical Imaging				
Cardiac Imaging Stress Test before Surgery	816	3.1%	5.4%	5.3%
Combination Abdominal CT Scan	662	32.9%	12.2%	10.5%
Combination Brain/Sinus CT Scan	572	2.6%	3.1%	2.7%
Combination Chest CT Scan	441	0.0%	2.1%	2.7%
Follow-up Mammogram/Ultrasound	980	9.0%	9%	8.8%
Lumbar Spine MRI for Low Back Pain	127	32.3%	35.8%	37.2%

Somerset Hospital

225 South Center Avenue
Somerset, PA 15501
Phone: 814-443-5000
Fax: 814-443-4937
E-mail: admin@schol.com
URL: www.somersethospital.com
Type: Acute Care Hospitals
Emergency Services: Yes
Ownership: Voluntary non-profit - Private
Beds: 167

Key Personnel:
Chief of Medical Staff. . . . . Wassim Abosamra
Radiology. . . . . Thomas M Anderson, Jr
Intensive Care Unit. . . . . M Boyce, RN
CEO/President. . . . . Michael J Farrell
Infection Control. . . . . Erika Marker
Emergency Room . . . . Shomendra K Moitra, MD
Quality Assurance . . . . Pam Ream
Operating Room. . . . . Donna Zimmera

Measure	Cases	This Hosp.	State Avg.	U.S. Avg.
Blood Clot Prevention and Treatment				
Anticoagulation Overlap Therapy[2]	17	59%	94%	93%
ICU Venous Thromboembolism Prophylaxis[2]	89	84%	94%	92%
Incidence of Potentially Preventable VTE[1,2]	-	-	8%	10%
UFH with Dosages/Platelet Monitoring[2]	25	100%	98%	97%
Venous Thromboembolism Prophylaxis[2]	280	83%	90%	85%
Warfarin Therapy Discharge Instructions[2]	17	100%	78%	75%
Chest Pain/Possible Heart Attack Care				
Aspirin Given Within 24 Hours of Arrival	27	100%	97%	96%
Fibrinolytic Meds Within 30 Min. of Arrival[1]	-	-	44%	58%
Average Time to ECG (minutes)	28	14	9	7
Average Time to Transfer (minutes)[1]	-	-	64	60
Children's Asthma Care				
Received Home Management Plan of Care	-	-	-	88%
Received Reliever Medication	-	-	-	100%
Received Systemic Corticosteroids	-	-	-	100%
Emergency Department				
Admittance Decision Time (minutes)[2]	230	50	104	98
Head CT Results Within 45 Min. of Arrival[1]	-	-	60%	57%
Patients Who Left ER Before Being Seen	9,350	3%	1%	2%
Time from ER Arrival to Admit. (minutes)[2]	257	230	276	274
Time from ER Arrival to Discharge (minutes)	401	141	125	134
Time in ER Before Being Evaluated (minutes)	416	41	26	26
Time to Pain Meds for Fractures (minutes)	101	63	58	57
Heart Attack Care				
Aspirin Given at Discharge	53	100%	99%	99%
Fibrinolytic Meds Within 30 Min. of Arrival[7]	-	-	40%	54%
PCI Within 90 Minutes of Arrival[1]	-	-	97%	96%
Statin Prescribed at Discharge	49	100%	99%	98%
Heart Failure Care				
ACE Inhibitor or ARB for LVSD	27	96%	97%	97%
Discharge Instructions Given	76	100%	96%	94%
Evaluation of LVS Function	103	98%	100%	99%
Medicare Spending				
Medicare Spending per Patient (ratio)	-	0.99	1.01	0.98
Pneumonia Care				
Appropriate Initial Antibiotic Given	60	88%	96%	95%
Blood Culture Timing	144	93%	98%	98%
Pregnancy and Delivery Care				
Newborn Deliveries Scheduled Early	58	43%	4%	6%
Preventive Care				
Immunization for Influenza[2]	314	65%	91%	90%
Immunization for Pneumonia[2]	392	90%	92%	92%
Stroke Care				
Anticoagulation Therapy for Atrial Fibrillation[1]	-	-	96%	95%
Antithrombotic Therapy Timing	23	100%	98%	98%
Assessed for Rehabilitation	23	91%	98%	97%
Discharged on Antithrombotic Therapy	21	90%	99%	99%
Discharged on Statin Medication	21	90%	95%	94%
Thrombolytic Therapy Timing[1]	-	-	72%	66%
Venous Thromboembolism Prophylaxis	27	78%	95%	94%
Written Stroke Educational Materials Given	14	100%	90%	88%
Surgical Care Improvement Project				
Appropriate Beta Blocker Usage	38	100%	98%	98%
Appropriate VTP Within 24 Hours	148	100%	99%	98%
Controlled Postoperative Blood Glucose[7]	-	-	98%	97%
Perioperative Temperature Management	181	100%	100%	100%
Prophylactic Antibiotic Selection	133	92%	99%	99%
Prophylactic Antibiotic Selection (Outpatient)	37	57%	98%	98%
Prophylactic Antibiotic Stopped	124	99%	98%	98%
Prophylactic Antibiotic Timing	133	98%	99%	99%
Prophylactic Antibiotic Timing (Outpatient)	37	100%	98%	98%
Urinary Catheter Removal	70	100%	99%	97%
Survey of Patients' Hospital Experiences				
Area Around Room 'Always' Quiet at Night	300+	43%	54%	61%
Doctors 'Always' Communicated Well	300+	75%	80%	82%
Home Recovery Information Given	300+	87%	86%	85%
Hospital Given 9 or 10 on 10 Point Scale	300+	68%	69%	71%
Meds 'Always' Explained Before Given	300+	60%	63%	64%
Nurses 'Always' Communicated Well	300+	79%	79%	79%
Pain 'Always' Well Controlled	300+	67%	70%	71%
Room and Bathroom 'Always' Clean	300+	76%	73%	73%
Timely Help 'Always' Received	300+	65%	67%	68%
Would Definitely Recommend Hospital	300+	59%	70%	71%
Use of Medical Imaging				
Cardiac Imaging Stress Test before Surgery	139	5.8%	5.4%	5.3%
Combination Abdominal CT Scan	318	25.8%	12.2%	10.5%
Combination Brain/Sinus CT Scan	270	6.3%	3.1%	2.7%
Combination Chest CT Scan	154	20.1%	2.1%	2.7%
Follow-up Mammogram/Ultrasound	337	7.4%	9%	8.8%
Lumbar Spine MRI for Low Back Pain	45	37.8%	35.8%	37.2%

Mount Nittany Medical Center

1800 East Park Ave
State College, PA 16803
Phone: 814-231-7000
Fax: 814-234-6100
E-mail: info@mountnittany.org
URL: www.mountnittany.org
Type: Acute Care Hospitals
Emergency Services: Yes
Ownership: Voluntary non-profit - Other
Beds: 201

Key Personnel:
President/CEO. . . . . Steve Brown, FACHE
Coronary Care . . . . Jeffrey Eaton, MD
Radiology. . . . . Ari Geselowitz, MD
Operating Room. . . . . James S Martin, MD
Quality Assurance . . . . Gail Miller
Chief of Medical Staff. . . . . Wayne J. Sebastianelli, MD
Infection Control. . . . . Marlene Stetson, RN
Pediatric In-Patient Care . . . . . . Tracy Trudel, MD

Measure	Cases	This Hosp.	State Avg.	U.S. Avg.
Blood Clot Prevention and Treatment				
Anticoagulation Overlap Therapy[2]	127	87%	94%	93%
ICU Venous Thromboembolism Prophylaxis[2]	30	87%	94%	92%
Incidence of Potentially Preventable VTE[2]	11	27%	8%	10%
UFH with Dosages/Platelet Monitoring[2]	122	98%	98%	97%
Venous Thromboembolism Prophylaxis[2]	322	89%	90%	85%
Warfarin Therapy Discharge Instructions[2]	99	24%	78%	75%
Chest Pain/Possible Heart Attack Care				

NOTE: Hospital profiles are in alphabetical order by state, then city, then hospital within the city; Rankings exclude hospitals with less than 25 cases except for patient surveys which excludes hospitals with less than 100 cases; (a) 100-299 cases; (1) The number of cases/patients is too few to report; (2) Data submitted were based on a sample of cases/patients; (3) Results are based on a shorter time period than required; (4) Data suppressed by CMS for one or more quarters; (5) Results are not available for this reporting period; (6) Fewer than 100 patients completed the HCAHPS survey; (7) No cases met the criteria for this measure; (8) The lower limit of the confidence interval cannot be calculated if the number of observed infections equals zero; (9) No data are available from the state/territory for this reporting period; (10) The scores shown reflect fewer than 50 completed surveys; (11) There were discrepancies in the data collection process; (12) This measure does not apply to this hospital for this reporting period; (13) Results cannot be calculated for this reporting period; (14) The results for this state are combined with nearby states to protect confidentiality; Please refer to the User's Guide for a full explanation of data.

Measure	Cases	This Hosp.	State Avg.	U.S. Avg.
Aspirin Given Within 24 Hours of Arrival[3]	11	100%	97%	96%
Fibrinolytic Meds Within 30 Min. of Arrival[3,7]	-	-	44%	58%
Average Time to ECG (minutes)[3]	11	5	9	7
Average Time to Transfer (minutes)[3,7]	-	-	64	60
Children's Asthma Care				
Received Home Management Plan of Care	-	-	-	88%
Received Reliever Medication	-	-	-	100%
Received Systemic Corticosteroids	-	-	-	100%
Emergency Department				
Admittance Decision Time (minutes)[2]	548	198	104	98
Head CT Results Within 45 Min. of Arrival	16	69%	60%	57%
Patients Who Left ER Before Being Seen	49,449	0%	1%	2%
Time from ER Arrival to Admit. (minutes)[2]	587	302	276	274
Time from ER Arrival to Discharge (minutes)	357	151	125	134
Time in ER Before Being Evaluated (minutes)	233	21	26	26
Time to Pain Meds for Fractures (minutes)	140	53	58	57
Heart Attack Care				
Aspirin Given at Discharge	129	98%	99%	99%
Fibrinolytic Meds Within 30 Min. of Arrival[7]	-	-	40%	54%
PCI Within 90 Minutes of Arrival	38	95%	97%	96%
Statin Prescribed at Discharge	129	98%	99%	98%
Heart Failure Care				
ACE Inhibitor or ARB for LVSD	56	93%	97%	97%
Discharge Instructions Given	241	94%	96%	94%
Evaluation of LVS Function	299	100%	100%	99%
Medicare Spending				
Medicare Spending per Patient (ratio)	-	0.99	1.01	0.98
Pneumonia Care				
Appropriate Initial Antibiotic Given	133	93%	96%	95%
Blood Culture Timing	165	96%	98%	98%
Pregnancy and Delivery Care				
Newborn Deliveries Scheduled Early[2]	110	2%	4%	6%
Preventive Care				
Immunization for Influenza[2]	528	69%	91%	90%
Immunization for Pneumonia[2]	680	81%	92%	92%
Stroke Care				
Anticoagulation Therapy for Atrial Fibrillation	16	88%	96%	95%
Antithrombotic Therapy Timing	86	97%	98%	98%
Assessed for Rehabilitation	104	93%	98%	97%
Discharged on Antithrombotic Therapy	100	98%	99%	99%
Discharged on Statin Medication	80	82%	95%	94%
Thrombolytic Therapy Timing	12	58%	72%	66%
Venous Thromboembolism Prophylaxis	97	90%	95%	94%
Written Stroke Educational Materials Given	61	69%	90%	88%
Surgical Care Improvement Project				
Appropriate Beta Blocker Usage	512	98%	98%	98%
Appropriate VTP Within 24 Hours	1,451	98%	99%	98%
Controlled Postoperative Blood Glucose[7]	-	-	98%	97%
Perioperative Temperature Management	1,618	100%	100%	100%
Prophylactic Antibiotic Selection	1,250	99%	99%	99%
Prophylactic Antibiotic Selection (Outpatient)	296	97%	98%	98%
Prophylactic Antibiotic Stopped	1,230	99%	98%	98%
Prophylactic Antibiotic Timing	1,251	99%	99%	99%
Prophylactic Antibiotic Timing (Outpatient)	299	94%	98%	98%
Urinary Catheter Removal	595	92%	99%	97%
Survey of Patients' Hospital Experiences				
Area Around Room 'Always' Quiet at Night	300+	53%	54%	61%
Doctors 'Always' Communicated Well	300+	81%	80%	82%
Home Recovery Information Given	300+	87%	86%	85%
Hospital Given 9 or 10 on 10 Point Scale	300+	75%	69%	71%
Meds 'Always' Explained Before Given	300+	67%	63%	64%
Nurses 'Always' Communicated Well	300+	83%	79%	79%
Pain 'Always' Well Controlled	300+	72%	70%	71%
Room and Bathroom 'Always' Clean	300+	81%	73%	73%
Timely Help 'Always' Received	300+	72%	67%	68%
Would Definitely Recommend Hospital	300+	76%	70%	71%
Use of Medical Imaging				
Cardiac Imaging Stress Test before Surgery	96	4.2%	5.4%	5.3%
Combination Abdominal CT Scan	721	6.8%	12.2%	10.5%
Combination Brain/Sinus CT Scan	722	3.2%	3.1%	2.7%
Combination Chest CT Scan	367	0.0%	2.1%	2.7%
Follow-up Mammogram/Ultrasound	1,647	9.3%	9%	8.8%
Lumbar Spine MRI for Low Back Pain	70	30.0%	35.8%	37.2%

Sunbury Community Hospital

350 North 11th Street
Sunbury, PA 17801
URL: www.schopc.org
Type: Acute Care Hospitals
Ownership: Proprietary

Phone: 570-286-3333
Fax: 570-286-3576

Emergency Services: Yes
Beds: 123

Key Personnel:
Operating Room. . . . . Brian A Batman, MD
Quality Assurance . . . . Liz Bendas, RN
Emergency Room . . . . Frederick Burke, RN, BSN
Anesthesiology. . . . . Francisco A Furtado, MD
Chief of Medical Staff . . . . John C Ninos, MD
CEO/President. . . . . R Clifford Park

Measure	Cases	This Hosp.	State Avg.	U.S. Avg.
Blood Clot Prevention and Treatment				
Anticoagulation Overlap Therapy[2]	13	100%	94%	93%
ICU Venous Thromboembolism Prophylaxis[2]	38	95%	94%	92%
Incidence of Potentially Preventable VTE[1,2]	-	-	8%	10%
UFH with Dosages/Platelet Monitoring[1,2]	-	-	98%	97%
Venous Thromboembolism Prophylaxis[2]	248	96%	90%	85%
Warfarin Therapy Discharge Instructions[1,2]	-	-	78%	75%
Chest Pain/Possible Heart Attack Care				
Aspirin Given Within 24 Hours of Arrival	37	100%	97%	96%
Fibrinolytic Meds Within 30 Min. of Arrival[1]	-	-	44%	58%
Average Time to ECG (minutes)	42	11	9	7
Average Time to Transfer (minutes)[1]	-	-	64	60
Children's Asthma Care				
Received Home Management Plan of Care	-	-	-	88%
Received Reliever Medication	-	-	-	100%
Received Systemic Corticosteroids	-	-	-	100%
Emergency Department				
Admittance Decision Time (minutes)[2]	359	67	104	98
Head CT Results Within 45 Min. of Arrival[1]	-	-	60%	57%
Patients Who Left ER Before Being Seen	10,923	1%	1%	2%
Time from ER Arrival to Admit. (minutes)[2]	364	255	276	274
Time from ER Arrival to Discharge (minutes)	382	109	125	134
Time in ER Before Being Evaluated (minutes)	419	19	26	26
Time to Pain Meds for Fractures (minutes)	42	67	58	57
Heart Attack Care				
Aspirin Given at Discharge[1]	-	-	99%	99%
Fibrinolytic Meds Within 30 Min. of Arrival[7]	-	-	40%	54%
PCI Within 90 Minutes of Arrival[7]	-	-	97%	96%
Statin Prescribed at Discharge[1]	-	-	99%	98%
Heart Failure Care				
ACE Inhibitor or ARB for LVSD[1]	-	-	97%	97%
Discharge Instructions Given	31	87%	96%	94%
Evaluation of LVS Function	56	100%	100%	99%
Medicare Spending				
Medicare Spending per Patient (ratio)	-	1.06	1.01	0.98
Pneumonia Care				
Appropriate Initial Antibiotic Given	52	100%	96%	95%
Blood Culture Timing	68	99%	98%	98%
Pregnancy and Delivery Care				
Newborn Deliveries Scheduled Early[2,7]	-	-	4%	6%
Preventive Care				
Immunization for Influenza[2]	334	96%	91%	90%
Immunization for Pneumonia[2]	459	96%	92%	92%
Stroke Care				
Anticoagulation Therapy for Atrial Fibrillation[1]	-	-	96%	95%
Antithrombotic Therapy Timing[1]	-	-	98%	98%
Assessed for Rehabilitation[1]	-	-	98%	97%
Discharged on Antithrombotic Therapy[1]	-	-	99%	99%
Discharged on Statin Medication[1]	-	-	95%	94%
Thrombolytic Therapy Timing[7]	-	-	72%	66%
Venous Thromboembolism Prophylaxis[1]	-	-	95%	94%
Written Stroke Educational Materials Given[1]	-	-	90%	88%
Surgical Care Improvement Project				
Appropriate Beta Blocker Usage	40	100%	98%	98%
Appropriate VTP Within 24 Hours	54	100%	99%	98%
Controlled Postoperative Blood Glucose[7]	-	-	98%	97%
Perioperative Temperature Management	90	100%	100%	100%
Prophylactic Antibiotic Selection	11	100%	99%	99%
Prophylactic Antibiotic Selection (Outpatient)	37	92%	98%	98%
Prophylactic Antibiotic Stopped	11	91%	98%	98%
Prophylactic Antibiotic Timing	11	100%	99%	99%
Prophylactic Antibiotic Timing (Outpatient)	33	100%	98%	98%
Urinary Catheter Removal	77	100%	99%	97%
Survey of Patients' Hospital Experiences				
Area Around Room 'Always' Quiet at Night	(a)	49%	54%	61%
Doctors 'Always' Communicated Well	(a)	82%	80%	82%
Home Recovery Information Given	(a)	87%	86%	85%
Hospital Given 9 or 10 on 10 Point Scale	(a)	69%	69%	71%
Meds 'Always' Explained Before Given	(a)	63%	63%	64%
Nurses 'Always' Communicated Well	(a)	77%	79%	79%
Pain 'Always' Well Controlled	(a)	68%	70%	71%
Room and Bathroom 'Always' Clean	(a)	84%	73%	73%
Timely Help 'Always' Received	(a)	68%	67%	68%
Would Definitely Recommend Hospital	(a)	68%	70%	71%
Use of Medical Imaging				
Cardiac Imaging Stress Test before Surgery	55	5.5%	5.4%	5.3%
Combination Abdominal CT Scan	183	4.9%	12.2%	10.5%
Combination Brain/Sinus CT Scan[1]	-	-	3.1%	2.7%
Combination Chest CT Scan	81	7.4%	2.1%	2.7%
Follow-up Mammogram/Ultrasound	384	10.9%	9%	8.8%
Lumbar Spine MRI for Low Back Pain[1]	-	-	35.8%	37.2%

Barnes-Kasson County Hospital

2872 Turnpike Street
Susquehanna, PA 18847
Type: Critical Access Hospitals
Ownership: Voluntary non-profit - Private

Phone: 570-853-3135
Emergency Services: Yes

Measure	Cases	This Hosp.	State Avg.	U.S. Avg.
Blood Clot Prevention and Treatment				
Anticoagulation Overlap Therapy[5]	-	-	94%	93%
ICU Venous Thromboembolism Prophylaxis[5]	-	-	94%	92%
Incidence of Potentially Preventable VTE[5]	-	-	8%	10%
UFH with Dosages/Platelet Monitoring[5]	-	-	98%	97%
Venous Thromboembolism Prophylaxis[5]	-	-	90%	85%
Warfarin Therapy Discharge Instructions[5]	-	-	78%	75%
Chest Pain/Possible Heart Attack Care				
Aspirin Given Within 24 Hours of Arrival[5]	-	-	97%	96%
Fibrinolytic Meds Within 30 Min. of Arrival[5]	-	-	44%	58%
Average Time to ECG (minutes)[5]	-	-	9	7
Average Time to Transfer (minutes)[5]	-	-	64	60
Children's Asthma Care				
Received Home Management Plan of Care	-	-	-	88%
Received Reliever Medication	-	-	-	100%
Received Systemic Corticosteroids	-	-	-	100%
Emergency Department				
Admittance Decision Time (minutes)[2,3]	363	25	104	98
Head CT Results Within 45 Min. of Arrival[5]	-	-	60%	57%
Patients Who Left ER Before Being Seen	3,759	0%	1%	2%
Time from ER Arrival to Admit. (minutes)[2,3]	363	131	276	274
Time from ER Arrival to Discharge (minutes)[5]	-	-	125	134
Time in ER Before Being Evaluated (minutes)[5]	-	-	26	26
Time to Pain Meds for Fractures (minutes)[5]	-	-	58	57
Heart Attack Care				
Aspirin Given at Discharge[5]	-	-	99%	99%
Fibrinolytic Meds Within 30 Min. of Arrival[5]	-	-	40%	54%
PCI Within 90 Minutes of Arrival[5]	-	-	97%	96%
Statin Prescribed at Discharge[5]	-	-	99%	98%
Heart Failure Care				
ACE Inhibitor or ARB for LVSD[2]	20	65%	97%	97%
Discharge Instructions Given[2]	32	97%	96%	94%
Evaluation of LVS Function[2]	47	96%	100%	99%
Medicare Spending				
Medicare Spending per Patient (ratio)	-	-	1.01	0.98
Pneumonia Care				
Appropriate Initial Antibiotic Given[2]	42	88%	96%	95%
Blood Culture Timing[2]	21	71%	98%	98%
Pregnancy and Delivery Care				
Newborn Deliveries Scheduled Early[5]	-	-	4%	6%
Preventive Care				
Immunization for Influenza[2,3]	163	97%	91%	90%

NOTE: Hospital profiles are in alphabetical order by state, then city, then hospital within the city; Rankings exclude hospitals with less than 25 cases except for patient surveys which excludes hospitals with less than 100 cases; (a) 100-299 cases; (1) The number of cases/patients is too few to report; (2) Data submitted were based on a sample of cases/patients; (3) Results are based on a shorter time period than required; (4) Data suppressed by CMS for one or more quarters; (5) Results are not available for this reporting period; (6) Fewer than 100 patients completed the HCAHPS survey; (7) No cases met the criteria for this measure; (8) The lower limit of the confidence interval cannot be calculated if the number of observed infections equals zero; (9) No data are available from the state/territory for this reporting period; (10) The scores shown reflect fewer than 50 completed surveys; (11) There were discrepancies in the data collection process; (12) This measure does not apply to this hospital for this reporting period; (13) Results cannot be calculated for this reporting period; (14) The results for this state are combined with nearby states to protect confidentiality; Please refer to the User's Guide for a full explanation of data.

Measure	Cases	This Hosp.	State Avg.	U.S. Avg.
Immunization for Pneumonia[2,3]	297	81%	92%	92%
Stroke Care				
Anticoagulation Therapy for Atrial Fibrillation[5]	-	-	96%	95%
Antithrombotic Therapy Timing[5]	-	-	98%	98%
Assessed for Rehabilitation[5]	-	-	98%	97%
Discharged on Antithrombotic Therapy[5]	-	-	99%	99%
Discharged on Statin Medication[5]	-	-	95%	94%
Thrombolytic Therapy Timing[5]	-	-	72%	66%
Venous Thromboembolism Prophylaxis[5]	-	-	95%	94%
Written Stroke Educational Materials Given[5]	-	-	90%	88%
Surgical Care Improvement Project				
Appropriate Beta Blocker Usage[5]	-	-	98%	98%
Appropriate VTP Within 24 Hours[5]	-	-	99%	98%
Controlled Postoperative Blood Glucose[5]	-	-	98%	97%
Perioperative Temperature Management[5]	-	-	100%	100%
Prophylactic Antibiotic Selection[5]	-	-	99%	99%
Prophylactic Antibiotic Selection (Outpatient)[5]	-	-	98%	98%
Prophylactic Antibiotic Stopped[5]	-	-	98%	98%
Prophylactic Antibiotic Timing[5]	-	-	99%	99%
Prophylactic Antibiotic Timing (Outpatient)[5]	-	-	98%	98%
Urinary Catheter Removal[5]	-	-	99%	97%
Survey of Patients' Hospital Experiences				
Area Around Room 'Always' Quiet at Night	(a)	51%	54%	61%
Doctors 'Always' Communicated Well	(a)	86%	80%	82%
Home Recovery Information Given	(a)	83%	86%	85%
Hospital Given 9 or 10 on 10 Point Scale	(a)	59%	69%	71%
Meds 'Always' Explained Before Given	(a)	60%	63%	64%
Nurses 'Always' Communicated Well	(a)	79%	79%	79%
Pain 'Always' Well Controlled	(a)	66%	70%	71%
Room and Bathroom 'Always' Clean	(a)	78%	73%	73%
Timely Help 'Always' Received	(a)	71%	67%	68%
Would Definitely Recommend Hospital	(a)	55%	70%	71%
Use of Medical Imaging				
Cardiac Imaging Stress Test before Surgery	54	1.9%	5.4%	5.3%
Combination Abdominal CT Scan	141	17.0%	12.2%	10.5%
Combination Brain/Sinus CT Scan[1]	-	-	3.1%	2.7%
Combination Chest CT Scan[1]	-	-	2.1%	2.7%
Follow-up Mammogram/Ultrasound	128	7.8%	9%	8.8%
Lumbar Spine MRI for Low Back Pain[1]	-	-	35.8%	37.2%

Titusville Hospital

406 West Oak Street
Titusville, PA 16354
Phone: 814-827-1851
Fax: 814-827-3099
URL: www.titusvillehospital.org
Type: Acute Care Hospitals
Emergency Services: Yes
Ownership: Voluntary non-profit - Private
Beds: 95

Key Personnel:

Infection Control. . . . . Brenda Burnett
Operating Room. . . . . Anil Dutt, RN
Quality Assurance . . . . Linda Harris
Chief of Medical Staff. . . . . Terri See

Measure	Cases	This Hosp.	State Avg.	U.S. Avg.
Blood Clot Prevention and Treatment				
Anticoagulation Overlap Therapy[1,2]	-	-	94%	93%
ICU Venous Thromboembolism Prophylaxis[2]	26	81%	94%	92%
Incidence of Potentially Preventable VTE[2,7]	-	-	8%	10%
UFH with Dosages/Platelet Monitoring[1,2]	-	-	98%	97%
Venous Thromboembolism Prophylaxis[2]	190	63%	90%	85%
Warfarin Therapy Discharge Instructions[1,2]	-	-	78%	75%
Chest Pain/Possible Heart Attack Care				
Aspirin Given Within 24 Hours of Arrival	83	100%	97%	96%
Fibrinolytic Meds Within 30 Min. of Arrival[1]	-	-	44%	58%
Average Time to ECG (minutes)	89	5	9	7
Average Time to Transfer (minutes)[1]	-	-	64	60
Children's Asthma Care				
Received Home Management Plan of Care	-	-	-	88%
Received Reliever Medication	-	-	-	100%
Received Systemic Corticosteroids	-	-	-	100%
Emergency Department				
Admittance Decision Time (minutes)[2]	572	58	104	98
Head CT Results Within 45 Min. of Arrival[1]	-	-	60%	57%
Patients Who Left ER Before Being Seen	12,097	1%	1%	2%
Time from ER Arrival to Admit. (minutes)[2]	581	205	276	274
Time from ER Arrival to Discharge (minutes)	401	105	125	134
Time in ER Before Being Evaluated (minutes)	411	34	26	26
Time to Pain Meds for Fractures (minutes)	49	59	58	57
Heart Attack Care				
Aspirin Given at Discharge[1]	-	-	99%	99%
Fibrinolytic Meds Within 30 Min. of Arrival[7]	-	-	40%	54%
PCI Within 90 Minutes of Arrival[7]	-	-	97%	96%
Statin Prescribed at Discharge[1]	-	-	99%	98%
Heart Failure Care				
ACE Inhibitor or ARB for LVSD	19	100%	97%	97%
Discharge Instructions Given	35	100%	96%	94%
Evaluation of LVS Function	42	100%	100%	99%
Medicare Spending				
Medicare Spending per Patient (ratio)	-	0.87	1.01	0.98
Pneumonia Care				
Appropriate Initial Antibiotic Given	58	97%	96%	95%
Blood Culture Timing	71	96%	98%	98%
Pregnancy and Delivery Care				
Newborn Deliveries Scheduled Early	16	0%	4%	6%
Preventive Care				
Immunization for Influenza[2]	537	93%	91%	90%
Immunization for Pneumonia[2]	760	98%	92%	92%
Stroke Care				
Anticoagulation Therapy for Atrial Fibrillation[7]	-	-	96%	95%
Antithrombotic Therapy Timing[1]	-	-	98%	98%
Assessed for Rehabilitation[1]	-	-	98%	97%
Discharged on Antithrombotic Therapy[1]	-	-	99%	99%
Discharged on Statin Medication[1]	-	-	95%	94%
Thrombolytic Therapy Timing[7]	-	-	72%	66%
Venous Thromboembolism Prophylaxis[1]	-	-	95%	94%
Written Stroke Educational Materials Given[1]	-	-	90%	88%
Surgical Care Improvement Project				
Appropriate Beta Blocker Usage	36	100%	98%	98%
Appropriate VTP Within 24 Hours	98	99%	99%	98%
Controlled Postoperative Blood Glucose[7]	-	-	98%	97%
Perioperative Temperature Management	102	100%	100%	100%
Prophylactic Antibiotic Selection	71	73%	99%	99%
Prophylactic Antibiotic Selection (Outpatient)	14	14%	98%	98%
Prophylactic Antibiotic Stopped	64	100%	98%	98%
Prophylactic Antibiotic Timing	71	94%	99%	99%
Prophylactic Antibiotic Timing (Outpatient)	16	88%	98%	98%
Urinary Catheter Removal	51	96%	99%	97%
Survey of Patients' Hospital Experiences				
Area Around Room 'Always' Quiet at Night	300+	68%	54%	61%
Doctors 'Always' Communicated Well	300+	86%	80%	82%
Home Recovery Information Given	300+	88%	86%	85%
Hospital Given 9 or 10 on 10 Point Scale	300+	80%	69%	71%
Meds 'Always' Explained Before Given	300+	70%	63%	64%
Nurses 'Always' Communicated Well	300+	83%	79%	79%
Pain 'Always' Well Controlled	300+	76%	70%	71%
Room and Bathroom 'Always' Clean	300+	82%	73%	73%
Timely Help 'Always' Received	300+	77%	67%	68%
Would Definitely Recommend Hospital	300+	78%	70%	71%
Use of Medical Imaging				
Cardiac Imaging Stress Test before Surgery	67	7.5%	5.4%	5.3%
Combination Abdominal CT Scan	270	8.5%	12.2%	10.5%
Combination Brain/Sinus CT Scan[1]	-	-	3.1%	2.7%
Combination Chest CT Scan	151	0.0%	2.1%	2.7%
Follow-up Mammogram/Ultrasound	502	1.2%	9%	8.8%
Lumbar Spine MRI for Low Back Pain	38	42.1%	35.8%	37.2%

Memorial Hospital Towanda

91 Hospital Drive
Towanda, PA 18848
Phone: 570-265-2191
Fax: 570-265-5763
E-mail: memhosp@epix.net
URL: www.memorialhospital.org
Type: Acute Care Hospitals
Emergency Services: Yes
Ownership: Voluntary non-profit - Private
Beds: 94

Key Personnel:

Emergency Room . . . . Anthony Anzalone
CEO/President. . . . . Gary A Baker
Chief of Medical Staff . . . . Stephen Becker, MD
Quality Assurance . . . . Anita Bennett
Operating Room. . . . . Caroline Brown, RN
Patient Relations . . . . Lynn Dibble
Surgery . . . . Geeta Krishnan
Radiology. . . . . Dave Sickler

Measure	Cases	This Hosp.	State Avg.	U.S. Avg.
Blood Clot Prevention and Treatment				
Anticoagulation Overlap Therapy[1,2]	-	-	94%	93%
ICU Venous Thromboembolism Prophylaxis[2]	35	94%	94%	92%
Incidence of Potentially Preventable VTE[1,2]	-	-	8%	10%
UFH with Dosages/Platelet Monitoring[1,2]	-	-	98%	97%
Venous Thromboembolism Prophylaxis[2]	79	80%	90%	85%
Warfarin Therapy Discharge Instructions[1,2]	-	-	78%	75%
Chest Pain/Possible Heart Attack Care				
Aspirin Given Within 24 Hours of Arrival	31	100%	97%	96%
Fibrinolytic Meds Within 30 Min. of Arrival[7]	-	-	44%	58%
Average Time to ECG (minutes)	31	8	9	7
Average Time to Transfer (minutes)[1]	-	-	64	60
Children's Asthma Care				
Received Home Management Plan of Care	-	-	-	88%
Received Reliever Medication	-	-	-	100%
Received Systemic Corticosteroids	-	-	-	100%
Emergency Department				
Admittance Decision Time (minutes)[2]	291	50	104	98
Head CT Results Within 45 Min. of Arrival[1,3]	-	-	60%	57%
Patients Who Left ER Before Being Seen	11,376	2%	1%	2%
Time from ER Arrival to Admit. (minutes)[2]	299	208	276	274
Time from ER Arrival to Discharge (minutes)	221	133	125	134
Time in ER Before Being Evaluated (minutes)	241	20	26	26
Time to Pain Meds for Fractures (minutes)	13	45	58	57
Heart Attack Care				
Aspirin Given at Discharge[1]	-	-	99%	99%
Fibrinolytic Meds Within 30 Min. of Arrival[7]	-	-	40%	54%
PCI Within 90 Minutes of Arrival[7]	-	-	97%	96%
Statin Prescribed at Discharge[1]	-	-	99%	98%
Heart Failure Care				
ACE Inhibitor or ARB for LVSD[1]	-	-	97%	97%
Discharge Instructions Given	24	100%	96%	94%
Evaluation of LVS Function	30	100%	100%	99%
Medicare Spending				
Medicare Spending per Patient (ratio)	-	0.90	1.01	0.98
Pneumonia Care				
Appropriate Initial Antibiotic Given[2]	60	100%	96%	95%
Blood Culture Timing[2]	89	98%	98%	98%
Pregnancy and Delivery Care				
Newborn Deliveries Scheduled Early[2]	18	6%	4%	6%
Preventive Care				
Immunization for Influenza[2]	255	93%	91%	90%
Immunization for Pneumonia[2]	309	94%	92%	92%
Stroke Care				
Anticoagulation Therapy for Atrial Fibrillation[7]	-	-	96%	95%
Antithrombotic Therapy Timing[1]	-	-	98%	98%
Assessed for Rehabilitation[1]	-	-	98%	97%
Discharged on Antithrombotic Therapy[1]	-	-	99%	99%
Discharged on Statin Medication[1]	-	-	95%	94%
Thrombolytic Therapy Timing[7]	-	-	72%	66%
Venous Thromboembolism Prophylaxis[1]	-	-	95%	94%
Written Stroke Educational Materials Given[1]	-	-	90%	88%
Surgical Care Improvement Project				
Appropriate Beta Blocker Usage[1]	-	-	98%	98%
Appropriate VTP Within 24 Hours	21	100%	99%	98%
Controlled Postoperative Blood Glucose[7]	-	-	98%	97%
Perioperative Temperature Management	20	100%	100%	100%
Prophylactic Antibiotic Selection[1]	-	-	99%	99%
Prophylactic Antibiotic Selection (Outpatient)[1]	-	-	98%	98%
Prophylactic Antibiotic Stopped[1]	-	-	98%	98%
Prophylactic Antibiotic Timing[1]	-	-	99%	99%
Prophylactic Antibiotic Timing (Outpatient)[1]	-	-	98%	98%
Urinary Catheter Removal[1]	-	-	99%	97%
Survey of Patients' Hospital Experiences				
Area Around Room 'Always' Quiet at Night	300+	56%	54%	61%
Doctors 'Always' Communicated Well	300+	83%	80%	82%
Home Recovery Information Given	300+	84%	86%	85%
Hospital Given 9 or 10 on 10 Point Scale	300+	72%	69%	71%
Meds 'Always' Explained Before Given	300+	61%	63%	64%

NOTE: Hospital profiles are in alphabetical order by state, then city, then hospital within the city; Rankings exclude hospitals with less than 25 cases except for patient surveys which excludes hospitals with less than 100 cases; (a) 100-299 cases; (1) The number of cases/patients is too few to report; (2) Data submitted were based on a sample of cases/patients; (3) Results are based on a shorter time period than required; (4) Data suppressed by CMS for one or more quarters; (5) Results are not available for this reporting period; (6) Fewer than 100 patients completed the HCAHPS survey; (7) No cases met the criteria for this measure; (8) The lower limit of the confidence interval cannot be calculated if the number of observed infections equals zero; (9) No data are available from the state/territory for this reporting period; (10) The scores shown reflect fewer than 50 completed surveys; (11) There were discrepancies in the data collection process; (12) This measure does not apply to this hospital for this reporting period; (13) Results cannot be calculated for this reporting period; (14) The results for this state are combined with nearby states to protect confidentiality; Please refer to the User's Guide for a full explanation of data.

Nurses 'Always' Communicated Well	300+	81%	79%	79%
Pain 'Always' Well Controlled	300+	74%	70%	71%
Room and Bathroom 'Always' Clean	300+	86%	73%	73%
Timely Help 'Always' Received	300+	75%	67%	68%
Would Definitely Recommend Hospital	300+	68%	70%	71%
Use of Medical Imaging				
Cardiac Imaging Stress Test before Surgery	89	6.7%	5.4%	5.3%
Combination Abdominal CT Scan	269	3.3%	12.2%	10.5%
Combination Brain/Sinus CT Scan	210	4.8%	3.1%	2.7%
Combination Chest CT Scan	121	0.0%	2.1%	2.7%
Follow-up Mammogram/Ultrasound	358	8.1%	9%	8.8%
Lumbar Spine MRI for Low Back Pain	43	44.2%	35.8%	37.2%

Edgewood Surgical Hospital

239 Edgewood Drive Extension
Transfer, PA 16154
Phone: 724-646-0400
Fax: 724-646-0413
E-mail: mailbox@edgewoodsurgical.com
URL: www.edgewoodsurgical.com
Type: Acute Care Hospitals
Emergency Services: No
Ownership: Physician

Key Personnel:
Anesthesiology. . . . . Anthony J. Candella Jr., D.O.
Cardiology . . . . Pradeep Kumar, M.D., FACC, FAC
CEO/President. . . . . Anthony J Puorro FACHE

Measure	Cases	This Hosp.	State Avg.	U.S. Avg.
Blood Clot Prevention and Treatment				
Anticoagulation Overlap Therapy[7]	-	-	94%	93%
ICU Venous Thromboembolism Prophylaxis[7]	-	-	94%	92%
Incidence of Potentially Preventable VTE[7]	-	-	8%	10%
UFH with Dosages/Platelet Monitoring[7]	-	-	98%	97%
Venous Thromboembolism Prophylaxis[7]	-	-	90%	85%
Warfarin Therapy Discharge Instructions[7]	-	-	78%	75%
Chest Pain/Possible Heart Attack Care				
Aspirin Given Within 24 Hours of Arrival[5]	-	-	97%	96%
Fibrinolytic Meds Within 30 Min. of Arrival[5]	-	-	44%	58%
Average Time to ECG (minutes)[5]	-	-	9	7
Average Time to Transfer (minutes)[5]	-	-	64	60
Children's Asthma Care				
Received Home Management Plan of Care	-	-	-	88%
Received Reliever Medication	-	-	-	100%
Received Systemic Corticosteroids	-	-	-	100%
Emergency Department				
Admittance Decision Time (minutes)[2,7]	-	-	104	98
Head CT Results Within 45 Min. of Arrival[5]	-	-	60%	57%
Patients Who Left ER Before Being Seen[5]	-	-	1%	2%
Time from ER Arrival to Admit. (minutes)[2,7]	-	-	276	274
Time from ER Arrival to Discharge (minutes)[5]	-	-	125	134
Time in ER Before Being Evaluated (minutes)[5]	-	-	26	26
Time to Pain Meds for Fractures (minutes)[5]	-	-	58	57
Heart Attack Care				
Aspirin Given at Discharge[5]	-	-	99%	99%
Fibrinolytic Meds Within 30 Min. of Arrival[5]	-	-	40%	54%
PCI Within 90 Minutes of Arrival[5]	-	-	97%	96%
Statin Prescribed at Discharge[5]	-	-	99%	98%
Heart Failure Care				
ACE Inhibitor or ARB for LVSD[5]	-	-	97%	97%
Discharge Instructions Given[5]	-	-	96%	94%
Evaluation of LVS Function[5]	-	-	100%	99%
Medicare Spending				
Medicare Spending per Patient (ratio)	-	1.01	1.01	0.98
Pneumonia Care				
Appropriate Initial Antibiotic Given[5]	-	-	96%	95%
Blood Culture Timing[5]	-	-	98%	98%
Pregnancy and Delivery Care				
Newborn Deliveries Scheduled Early[7]	-	-	4%	6%
Preventive Care				
Immunization for Influenza	46	93%	91%	90%
Immunization for Pneumonia	69	81%	92%	92%
Stroke Care				
Anticoagulation Therapy for Atrial Fibrillation[5]	-	-	96%	95%
Antithrombotic Therapy Timing[5]	-	-	98%	98%
Assessed for Rehabilitation[5]	-	-	98%	97%
Discharged on Antithrombotic Therapy[5]	-	-	99%	99%
Discharged on Statin Medication[5]	-	-	95%	94%
Thrombolytic Therapy Timing[5]	-	-	72%	66%
Venous Thromboembolism Prophylaxis[5]	-	-	95%	94%
Written Stroke Educational Materials Given[5]	-	-	90%	88%
Surgical Care Improvement Project				
Appropriate Beta Blocker Usage	33	100%	98%	98%
Appropriate VTP Within 24 Hours	110	100%	99%	98%
Controlled Postoperative Blood Glucose[7]	-	-	98%	97%
Perioperative Temperature Management	110	93%	100%	100%
Prophylactic Antibiotic Selection	102	100%	99%	99%
Prophylactic Antibiotic Selection (Outpatient)[5]	-	-	98%	98%
Prophylactic Antibiotic Stopped	102	100%	98%	98%
Prophylactic Antibiotic Timing	102	96%	99%	99%
Prophylactic Antibiotic Timing (Outpatient)[5]	-	-	98%	98%
Urinary Catheter Removal	14	100%	99%	97%
Survey of Patients' Hospital Experiences				
Area Around Room 'Always' Quiet at Night[6]	<100	86%	54%	61%
Doctors 'Always' Communicated Well[6]	<100	90%	80%	82%
Home Recovery Information Given[6]	<100	94%	86%	85%
Hospital Given 9 or 10 on 10 Point Scale[6]	<100	95%	69%	71%
Meds 'Always' Explained Before Given[6]	<100	82%	63%	64%
Nurses 'Always' Communicated Well[6]	<100	93%	79%	79%
Pain 'Always' Well Controlled[6]	<100	84%	70%	71%
Room and Bathroom 'Always' Clean[6]	<100	85%	73%	73%
Timely Help 'Always' Received[6]	<100	93%	67%	68%
Would Definitely Recommend Hospital[6]	<100	92%	70%	71%
Use of Medical Imaging				
Cardiac Imaging Stress Test before Surgery[7]	-	-	5.4%	5.3%
Combination Abdominal CT Scan[7]	-	-	12.2%	10.5%
Combination Brain/Sinus CT Scan[7]	-	-	3.1%	2.7%
Combination Chest CT Scan[7]	-	-	2.1%	2.7%
Follow-up Mammogram/Ultrasound[7]	-	-	9%	8.8%
Lumbar Spine MRI for Low Back Pain	56	28.6%	35.8%	37.2%

Troy Community Hospital

275 Guthrie Drive
Troy, PA 16947
Phone: 570-297-2121
Fax: 570-297-3970
Type: Critical Access Hospitals
Emergency Services: Yes
Ownership: Voluntary non-profit - Private
Beds: 32

Key Personnel:
Emergency Room . . . . George P Abraham, MD
Infection Control. . . . . Sheila Angove, BSN
President . . . . Frederick J Bloom, MD
Operating Room. . . . . Mark O Connell, RN
Quality Assurance . . . . Joan Delovich
Chief of Medical Staff . . . . Vance Good, MD
Patient Relations . . . . Beverly Jackson, RN
President/CEO. . . . . Joseph A. Scopelliti, MD

Measure	Cases	This Hosp.	State Avg.	U.S. Avg.
Blood Clot Prevention and Treatment				
Anticoagulation Overlap Therapy[2,3]	-	-	94%	93%
ICU Venous Thromboembolism Prophylaxis[2,3]	-	-	94%	92%
Incidence of Potentially Preventable VTE[2,3]	-	-	8%	10%
UFH with Dosages/Platelet Monitoring[2,3]	-	-	98%	97%
Venous Thromboembolism Prophylaxis[2,3]	59	76%	90%	85%
Warfarin Therapy Discharge Instructions[2,3]	-	-	78%	75%
Chest Pain/Possible Heart Attack Care				
Aspirin Given Within 24 Hours of Arrival[3]	17	100%	97%	96%
Fibrinolytic Meds Within 30 Min. of Arrival[3,7]	-	-	44%	58%
Average Time to ECG (minutes)[3]	17	5	9	7
Average Time to Transfer (minutes)[1,3]	-	-	64	60
Children's Asthma Care				
Received Home Management Plan of Care	-	-	-	88%
Received Reliever Medication	-	-	-	100%
Received Systemic Corticosteroids	-	-	-	100%
Emergency Department				
Admittance Decision Time (minutes)[2,3]	213	58	104	98
Head CT Results Within 45 Min. of Arrival[3,7]	-	-	60%	57%
Patients Who Left ER Before Being Seen	7,186	1%	1%	2%
Time from ER Arrival to Admit. (minutes)[2,3]	213	257	276	274
Time from ER Arrival to Discharge (minutes)[3]	263	90	125	134
Time in ER Before Being Evaluated (minutes)[3]	273	16	26	26
Time to Pain Meds for Fractures (minutes)[5]	-	-	58	57
Heart Attack Care				
Aspirin Given at Discharge[1,2]	-	-	99%	99%
Fibrinolytic Meds Within 30 Min. of Arrival[2,3]	-	-	40%	54%
PCI Within 90 Minutes of Arrival[2,3]	-	-	97%	96%
Statin Prescribed at Discharge[1,2]	-	-	99%	98%
Heart Failure Care				
ACE Inhibitor or ARB for LVSD[2]	12	92%	97%	97%
Discharge Instructions Given[2]	20	85%	96%	94%
Evaluation of LVS Function[2]	30	93%	100%	99%
Medicare Spending				
Medicare Spending per Patient (ratio)	-	-	1.01	0.98
Pneumonia Care				
Appropriate Initial Antibiotic Given[2]	28	79%	96%	95%
Blood Culture Timing[2]	38	84%	98%	98%
Pregnancy and Delivery Care				
Newborn Deliveries Scheduled Early[5]	-	-	4%	6%
Preventive Care				
Immunization for Influenza[2,3]	30	93%	91%	90%
Immunization for Pneumonia[2,3]	158	93%	92%	92%
Stroke Care				
Anticoagulation Therapy for Atrial Fibrillation[2,3]	-	-	96%	95%
Antithrombotic Therapy Timing[1,2]	-	-	98%	98%
Assessed for Rehabilitation[1,2]	-	-	98%	97%
Discharged on Antithrombotic Therapy[1,2]	-	-	99%	99%
Discharged on Statin Medication[1,2]	-	-	95%	94%
Thrombolytic Therapy Timing[2,3]	-	-	72%	66%
Venous Thromboembolism Prophylaxis[1,2]	-	-	95%	94%
Written Stroke Educational Materials Given[2,3]	-	-	90%	88%
Surgical Care Improvement Project				
Appropriate Beta Blocker Usage[5]	-	-	98%	98%
Appropriate VTP Within 24 Hours[5]	-	-	99%	98%
Controlled Postoperative Blood Glucose[5]	-	-	98%	97%
Perioperative Temperature Management[5]	-	-	100%	100%
Prophylactic Antibiotic Selection[5]	-	-	99%	99%
Prophylactic Antibiotic Selection (Outpatient)[5]	-	-	98%	98%
Prophylactic Antibiotic Stopped[5]	-	-	98%	98%
Prophylactic Antibiotic Timing[5]	-	-	99%	99%
Prophylactic Antibiotic Timing (Outpatient)[5]	-	-	98%	98%
Urinary Catheter Removal[5]	-	-	99%	97%
Survey of Patients' Hospital Experiences				
Area Around Room 'Always' Quiet at Night	(a)	41%	54%	61%
Doctors 'Always' Communicated Well	(a)	81%	80%	82%
Home Recovery Information Given	(a)	84%	86%	85%
Hospital Given 9 or 10 on 10 Point Scale	(a)	68%	69%	71%
Meds 'Always' Explained Before Given	(a)	67%	63%	64%
Nurses 'Always' Communicated Well	(a)	79%	79%	79%
Pain 'Always' Well Controlled	(a)	70%	70%	71%
Room and Bathroom 'Always' Clean	(a)	82%	73%	73%
Timely Help 'Always' Received	(a)	53%	67%	68%
Would Definitely Recommend Hospital	(a)	69%	70%	71%
Use of Medical Imaging				
Cardiac Imaging Stress Test before Surgery	47	4.3%	5.4%	5.3%
Combination Abdominal CT Scan	240	2.5%	12.2%	10.5%
Combination Brain/Sinus CT Scan[1]	-	-	3.1%	2.7%
Combination Chest CT Scan	111	0.9%	2.1%	2.7%
Follow-up Mammogram/Ultrasound	401	12.5%	9%	8.8%
Lumbar Spine MRI for Low Back Pain[1]	-	-	35.8%	37.2%

Tyler Memorial Hospital

5950 State Route 6 West
Tunkhannock, PA 18657
Phone: 570-836-2161
Fax: 570-836-7057
E-mail: mercytyler@health-partners.org
URL: www.tylerhospital.com
Type: Acute Care Hospitals
Emergency Services: Yes
Ownership: Voluntary non-profit - Other
Beds: 58

Key Personnel:
Cardiac Laboratory. . . . . Joyce Enders
CEO/President. . . . . Denise Gleski
Operating Room. . . . . Robert Glicini
Radiology. . . . . Ian A Kellman, MD
Infection Control. . . . . Kathy Ritter
Quality Assurance . . . . Kathy Ritter
Chief of Medical Staff . . . . Pamela A Shields, CPCS

Measure	Cases	This Hosp.	State Avg.	U.S. Avg.
Blood Clot Prevention and Treatment				

NOTE: Hospital profiles are in alphabetical order by state, then city, then hospital within the city; Rankings exclude hospitals with less than 25 cases except for patient surveys which excludes hospitals with less than 100 cases; (a) 100-299 cases; (1) The number of cases/patients is too few to report; (2) Data submitted were based on a sample of cases/patients; (3) Results are based on a shorter time period than required; (4) Data suppressed by CMS for one or more quarters; (5) Results are not available for this reporting period; (6) Fewer than 100 patients completed the HCAHPS survey; (7) No cases met the criteria for this measure; (8) The lower limit of the confidence interval cannot be calculated if the number of observed infections equals zero; (9) No data are available from the state/territory for this reporting period; (10) The scores shown reflect fewer than 50 completed surveys; (11) There were discrepancies in the data collection process; (12) This measure does not apply to this hospital for this reporting period; (13) Results cannot be calculated for this reporting period; (14) The results for this state are combined with nearby states to protect confidentiality; Please refer to the User's Guide for a full explanation of data.

Measure	Cases	This Hosp.	State Avg.	U.S. Avg.
Anticoagulation Overlap Therapy[1,2]	-	-	94%	93%
ICU Venous Thromboembolism Prophylaxis[2]	79	99%	94%	92%
Incidence of Potentially Preventable VTE[1,2]	-	-	8%	10%
UFH with Dosages/Platelet Monitoring[1,2]	-	-	98%	97%
Venous Thromboembolism Prophylaxis[2]	325	100%	90%	85%
Warfarin Therapy Discharge Instructions[1,2]	-	-	78%	75%
Chest Pain/Possible Heart Attack Care				
Aspirin Given Within 24 Hours of Arrival	30	100%	97%	96%
Fibrinolytic Meds Within 30 Min. of Arrival[7]	-	-	44%	58%
Average Time to ECG (minutes)	35	11	9	7
Average Time to Transfer (minutes)[1]	-	-	64	60
Children's Asthma Care				
Received Home Management Plan of Care	-	-	-	88%
Received Reliever Medication	-	-	-	100%
Received Systemic Corticosteroids	-	-	-	100%
Emergency Department				
Admittance Decision Time (minutes)[2]	212	45	104	98
Head CT Results Within 45 Min. of Arrival[1]	-	-	60%	57%
Patients Who Left ER Before Being Seen	8,686	1%	1%	2%
Time from ER Arrival to Admit. (minutes)[2]	213	237	276	274
Time from ER Arrival to Discharge (minutes)	361	110	125	134
Time in ER Before Being Evaluated (minutes)	419	23	26	26
Time to Pain Meds for Fractures (minutes)	51	55	58	57
Heart Attack Care				
Aspirin Given at Discharge[1,3]	-	-	99%	99%
Fibrinolytic Meds Within 30 Min. of Arrival[3,7]	-	-	40%	54%
PCI Within 90 Minutes of Arrival[3,7]	-	-	97%	96%
Statin Prescribed at Discharge[1,3]	-	-	99%	98%
Heart Failure Care				
ACE Inhibitor or ARB for LVSD[1]	-	-	97%	97%
Discharge Instructions Given	30	97%	96%	94%
Evaluation of LVS Function	38	97%	100%	99%
Medicare Spending				
Medicare Spending per Patient (ratio)	-	0.95	1.01	0.98
Pneumonia Care				
Appropriate Initial Antibiotic Given	70	97%	96%	95%
Blood Culture Timing	92	99%	98%	98%
Pregnancy and Delivery Care				
Newborn Deliveries Scheduled Early[7]	-	-	4%	6%
Preventive Care				
Immunization for Influenza[2]	343	99%	91%	90%
Immunization for Pneumonia[2]	544	99%	92%	92%
Stroke Care				
Anticoagulation Therapy for Atrial Fibrillation[3,7]	-	-	96%	95%
Antithrombotic Therapy Timing[1,3]	-	-	98%	98%
Assessed for Rehabilitation[1,3]	-	-	98%	97%
Discharged on Antithrombotic Therapy[1,3]	-	-	99%	99%
Discharged on Statin Medication[1,3]	-	-	95%	94%
Thrombolytic Therapy Timing[3,7]	-	-	72%	66%
Venous Thromboembolism Prophylaxis[1,3]	-	-	95%	94%
Written Stroke Educational Materials Given[1,3]	-	-	90%	88%
Surgical Care Improvement Project				
Appropriate Beta Blocker Usage[1]	-	-	98%	98%
Appropriate VTP Within 24 Hours[1]	-	-	99%	98%
Controlled Postoperative Blood Glucose[7]	-	-	98%	97%
Perioperative Temperature Management[1]	-	-	100%	100%
Prophylactic Antibiotic Selection[1]	-	-	99%	99%
Prophylactic Antibiotic Selection (Outpatient)[5]	-	-	98%	98%
Prophylactic Antibiotic Stopped[1]	-	-	98%	98%
Prophylactic Antibiotic Timing[1]	-	-	99%	99%
Prophylactic Antibiotic Timing (Outpatient)[5]	-	-	98%	98%
Urinary Catheter Removal[1]	-	-	99%	97%
Survey of Patients' Hospital Experiences				
Area Around Room 'Always' Quiet at Night	300+	52%	54%	61%
Doctors 'Always' Communicated Well	300+	88%	80%	82%
Home Recovery Information Given	300+	89%	86%	85%
Hospital Given 9 or 10 on 10 Point Scale	300+	73%	69%	71%
Meds 'Always' Explained Before Given	300+	66%	63%	64%
Nurses 'Always' Communicated Well	300+	83%	79%	79%
Pain 'Always' Well Controlled	300+	79%	70%	71%
Room and Bathroom 'Always' Clean	300+	75%	73%	73%
Timely Help 'Always' Received	300+	77%	67%	68%
Would Definitely Recommend Hospital	300+	69%	70%	71%
Use of Medical Imaging				
Cardiac Imaging Stress Test before Surgery	59	1.7%	5.4%	5.3%
Combination Abdominal CT Scan	206	15.5%	12.2%	10.5%
Combination Brain/Sinus CT Scan[1]	-	-	3.1%	2.7%
Combination Chest CT Scan	98	0.0%	2.1%	2.7%
Follow-up Mammogram/Ultrasound	182	19.2%	9%	8.8%
Lumbar Spine MRI for Low Back Pain[1]	-	-	35.8%	37.2%

Tyrone Hospital

221 Hospital Drive
Tyrone, PA 16686
Phone: 814-684-1255
URL: www.tyronehospital.org
Type: Critical Access Hospitals
Emergency Services: Yes
Ownership: Voluntary non-profit - Private

Measure	Cases	This Hosp.	State Avg.	U.S. Avg.
Blood Clot Prevention and Treatment				
Anticoagulation Overlap Therapy[1,3]	-	-	94%	93%
ICU Venous Thromboembolism Prophylaxis[3,7]	-	-	94%	92%
Incidence of Potentially Preventable VTE[3,7]	-	-	8%	10%
UFH with Dosages/Platelet Monitoring[3,7]	-	-	98%	97%
Venous Thromboembolism Prophylaxis[3,7]	-	-	90%	85%
Warfarin Therapy Discharge Instructions[3,7]	-	-	78%	75%
Chest Pain/Possible Heart Attack Care				
Aspirin Given Within 24 Hours of Arrival	17	88%	97%	96%
Fibrinolytic Meds Within 30 Min. of Arrival[7]	-	-	44%	58%
Average Time to ECG (minutes)	20	12	9	7
Average Time to Transfer (minutes)[1]	-	-	64	60
Children's Asthma Care				
Received Home Management Plan of Care	-	-	-	88%
Received Reliever Medication	-	-	-	100%
Received Systemic Corticosteroids	-	-	-	100%
Emergency Department				
Admittance Decision Time (minutes)[2]	374	53	104	98
Head CT Results Within 45 Min. of Arrival[5]	-	-	60%	57%
Patients Who Left ER Before Being Seen	7,829	0%	1%	2%
Time from ER Arrival to Admit. (minutes)[2]	374	216	276	274
Time from ER Arrival to Discharge (minutes)	1,218	81	125	134
Time in ER Before Being Evaluated (minutes)	1,316	19	26	26
Time to Pain Meds for Fractures (minutes)[5]	-	-	58	57
Heart Attack Care				
Aspirin Given at Discharge[1]	-	-	99%	99%
Fibrinolytic Meds Within 30 Min. of Arrival[7]	-	-	40%	54%
PCI Within 90 Minutes of Arrival[7]	-	-	97%	96%
Statin Prescribed at Discharge[1]	-	-	99%	98%
Heart Failure Care				
ACE Inhibitor or ARB for LVSD[1]	-	-	97%	97%
Discharge Instructions Given	19	100%	96%	94%
Evaluation of LVS Function	30	100%	100%	99%
Medicare Spending				
Medicare Spending per Patient (ratio)	-	-	1.01	0.98
Pneumonia Care				
Appropriate Initial Antibiotic Given	22	91%	96%	95%
Blood Culture Timing	33	100%	98%	98%
Pregnancy and Delivery Care				
Newborn Deliveries Scheduled Early[5]	-	-	4%	6%
Preventive Care				
Immunization for Influenza	285	100%	91%	90%
Immunization for Pneumonia[2]	429	100%	92%	92%
Stroke Care				
Anticoagulation Therapy for Atrial Fibrillation[5]	-	-	96%	95%
Antithrombotic Therapy Timing[5]	-	-	98%	98%
Assessed for Rehabilitation[5]	-	-	98%	97%
Discharged on Antithrombotic Therapy[5]	-	-	99%	99%
Discharged on Statin Medication[5]	-	-	95%	94%
Thrombolytic Therapy Timing[5]	-	-	72%	66%
Venous Thromboembolism Prophylaxis[5]	-	-	95%	94%
Written Stroke Educational Materials Given[5]	-	-	90%	88%
Surgical Care Improvement Project				
Appropriate Beta Blocker Usage	40	100%	98%	98%
Appropriate VTP Within 24 Hours	90	100%	99%	98%
Controlled Postoperative Blood Glucose[7]	-	-	98%	97%
Perioperative Temperature Management	122	100%	100%	100%
Prophylactic Antibiotic Selection	112	98%	99%	99%
Prophylactic Antibiotic Selection (Outpatient)[1,3]	-	-	98%	98%
Prophylactic Antibiotic Stopped	112	100%	98%	98%
Prophylactic Antibiotic Timing	112	100%	99%	99%
Prophylactic Antibiotic Timing (Outpatient)[1,3]	-	-	98%	98%
Urinary Catheter Removal[1]	-	-	99%	97%
Survey of Patients' Hospital Experiences				
Area Around Room 'Always' Quiet at Night	(a)	65%	54%	61%
Doctors 'Always' Communicated Well	(a)	85%	80%	82%
Home Recovery Information Given	(a)	88%	86%	85%
Hospital Given 9 or 10 on 10 Point Scale	(a)	80%	69%	71%
Meds 'Always' Explained Before Given	(a)	70%	63%	64%
Nurses 'Always' Communicated Well	(a)	85%	79%	79%
Pain 'Always' Well Controlled	(a)	75%	70%	71%
Room and Bathroom 'Always' Clean	(a)	87%	73%	73%
Timely Help 'Always' Received	(a)	85%	67%	68%
Would Definitely Recommend Hospital	(a)	80%	70%	71%
Use of Medical Imaging				
Cardiac Imaging Stress Test before Surgery[7]	-	-	5.4%	5.3%
Combination Abdominal CT Scan	146	2.1%	12.2%	10.5%
Combination Brain/Sinus CT Scan[1]	-	-	3.1%	2.7%
Combination Chest CT Scan	50	0.0%	2.1%	2.7%
Follow-up Mammogram/Ultrasound	114	14.9%	9%	8.8%
Lumbar Spine MRI for Low Back Pain[1]	-	-	35.8%	37.2%

Uniontown Hospital

500 West Berkeley Street
Uniontown, PA 15401
Phone: 724-430-5000
Fax: 724-430-3342
URL: www.uniontownhospital.com
Type: Acute Care Hospitals
Emergency Services: Yes
Ownership: Voluntary non-profit - Other
Beds: 209

Key Personnel:

Operating Room. . . . . Brandon M Ball
Pediatric In-Patient Care . . . . Mani Balu, MD
Emergency Room . . . . Cataldo Corrado
Quality Assurance . . . . Jan Curry
CEO . . . . Steve Handy
Chief of Medical Staff . . . . Danette Minehart
Cardiac Laboratory. . . . . Kris Shiley
Radiology. . . . . Judith Taylor, MD

Measure	Cases	This Hosp.	State Avg.	U.S. Avg.
Blood Clot Prevention and Treatment				
Anticoagulation Overlap Therapy[2]	46	89%	94%	93%
ICU Venous Thromboembolism Prophylaxis[2]	78	94%	94%	92%
Incidence of Potentially Preventable VTE[1,2]	-	-	8%	10%
UFH with Dosages/Platelet Monitoring[2]	30	100%	98%	97%
Venous Thromboembolism Prophylaxis[2]	344	95%	90%	85%
Warfarin Therapy Discharge Instructions[2]	28	100%	78%	75%
Chest Pain/Possible Heart Attack Care				
Aspirin Given Within 24 Hours of Arrival	18	94%	97%	96%
Fibrinolytic Meds Within 30 Min. of Arrival[3,7]	-	-	44%	58%
Average Time to ECG (minutes)	18	20	9	7
Average Time to Transfer (minutes)[1,3]	-	-	64	60
Children's Asthma Care				
Received Home Management Plan of Care	-	-	-	88%
Received Reliever Medication	-	-	-	100%
Received Systemic Corticosteroids	-	-	-	100%
Emergency Department				
Admittance Decision Time (minutes)[2]	675	63	104	98
Head CT Results Within 45 Min. of Arrival	12	58%	60%	57%
Patients Who Left ER Before Being Seen	55,589	0%	1%	2%
Time from ER Arrival to Admit. (minutes)[2]	692	254	276	274
Time from ER Arrival to Discharge (minutes)	341	131	125	134
Time in ER Before Being Evaluated (minutes)	385	30	26	26
Time to Pain Meds for Fractures (minutes)	82	58	58	57
Heart Attack Care				
Aspirin Given at Discharge	158	100%	99%	99%
Fibrinolytic Meds Within 30 Min. of Arrival[7]	-	-	40%	54%
PCI Within 90 Minutes of Arrival	39	97%	97%	96%
Statin Prescribed at Discharge	147	100%	99%	98%
Heart Failure Care				
ACE Inhibitor or ARB for LVSD	62	98%	97%	97%
Discharge Instructions Given	233	99%	96%	94%

NOTE: Hospital profiles are in alphabetical order by state, then city, then hospital within the city; Rankings exclude hospitals with less than 25 cases except for patient surveys which excludes hospitals with less than 100 cases; (a) 100-299 cases; (1) The number of cases/patients is too few to report; (2) Data submitted were based on a sample of cases/patients; (3) Results are based on a shorter time period than required; (4) Data suppressed by CMS for one or more quarters; (5) Results are not available for this reporting period; (6) Fewer than 100 patients completed the HCAHPS survey; (7) No cases met the criteria for this measure; (8) The lower limit of the confidence interval cannot be calculated if the number of observed infections equals zero; (9) No data are available from the state/territory for this reporting period; (10) The scores shown reflect fewer than 50 completed surveys; (11) There were discrepancies in the data collection process; (12) This measure does not apply to this hospital for this reporting period; (13) Results cannot be calculated for this reporting period; (14) The results for this state are combined with nearby states to protect confidentiality; Please refer to the User's Guide for a full explanation of data.

Measure	Cases	This Hosp.	State Avg.	U.S. Avg.
Evaluation of LVS Function	330	100%	100%	99%
Medicare Spending				
Medicare Spending per Patient (ratio)	-	1.02	1.01	0.98
Pneumonia Care				
Appropriate Initial Antibiotic Given[2]	146	97%	96%	95%
Blood Culture Timing[2]	253	98%	98%	98%
Pregnancy and Delivery Care				
Newborn Deliveries Scheduled Early[2]	105	2%	4%	6%
Preventive Care				
Immunization for Influenza[2]	491	94%	91%	90%
Immunization for Pneumonia[2]	700	93%	92%	92%
Stroke Care				
Anticoagulation Therapy for Atrial Fibrillation[1]	-	-	96%	95%
Antithrombotic Therapy Timing	59	98%	98%	98%
Assessed for Rehabilitation	53	96%	98%	97%
Discharged on Antithrombotic Therapy	53	100%	99%	99%
Discharged on Statin Medication	40	95%	95%	94%
Thrombolytic Therapy Timing[1]	-	-	72%	66%
Venous Thromboembolism Prophylaxis	59	95%	95%	94%
Written Stroke Educational Materials Given	29	100%	90%	88%
Surgical Care Improvement Project				
Appropriate Beta Blocker Usage	209	98%	98%	98%
Appropriate VTP Within 24 Hours	588	98%	99%	98%
Controlled Postoperative Blood Glucose[7]	-	-	98%	97%
Perioperative Temperature Management	665	100%	100%	100%
Prophylactic Antibiotic Selection	444	99%	99%	99%
Prophylactic Antibiotic Selection (Outpatient)	193	98%	98%	98%
Prophylactic Antibiotic Stopped	428	97%	98%	98%
Prophylactic Antibiotic Timing	444	99%	99%	99%
Prophylactic Antibiotic Timing (Outpatient)	194	99%	98%	98%
Urinary Catheter Removal	254	95%	99%	97%
Survey of Patients' Hospital Experiences				
Area Around Room 'Always' Quiet at Night	300+	56%	54%	61%
Doctors 'Always' Communicated Well	300+	80%	80%	82%
Home Recovery Information Given	300+	90%	86%	85%
Hospital Given 9 or 10 on 10 Point Scale	300+	63%	69%	71%
Meds 'Always' Explained Before Given	300+	64%	63%	64%
Nurses 'Always' Communicated Well	300+	77%	79%	79%
Pain 'Always' Well Controlled	300+	69%	70%	71%
Room and Bathroom 'Always' Clean	300+	67%	73%	73%
Timely Help 'Always' Received	300+	63%	67%	68%
Would Definitely Recommend Hospital	300+	59%	70%	71%
Use of Medical Imaging				
Cardiac Imaging Stress Test before Surgery	191	7.9%	5.4%	5.3%
Combination Abdominal CT Scan	920	14.3%	12.2%	10.5%
Combination Brain/Sinus CT Scan[1]	-	-	3.1%	2.7%
Combination Chest CT Scan	420	0.0%	2.1%	2.7%
Follow-up Mammogram/Ultrasound	785	4.5%	9%	8.8%
Lumbar Spine MRI for Low Back Pain	66	36.4%	35.8%	37.2%

Crozer Chester Medical Center

One Medical Center Boulevard
Upland, PA 19013
URL: www.crozer.org
Type: Acute Care Hospitals
Ownership: Voluntary non-profit - Other
Phone: 610-447-2000
Fax: 610-447-2234
Emergency Services: Yes
Beds: 422

Key Personnel:
Pediatric Ambulatory Care . . . . . . Gerald Kolsky, MD
Pediatric In-Patient Care . . . . Gerald Kolsky, MD
Quality Assurance . . . . Linda Ramsey
CEO/President. . . . . Joan K. Richards
Infection Control. . . . . Sally Ryan, RN
Radiology. . . . . Joseph R Stock, MD
Operating Room. . . . . Diane Wolk, RN
Chief of Medical Staff. . . . . Paul Woolf, MD

Measure	Cases	This Hosp.	State Avg.	U.S. Avg.
Blood Clot Prevention and Treatment				
Anticoagulation Overlap Therapy[2]	154	98%	94%	93%
ICU Venous Thromboembolism Prophylaxis[2]	63	97%	94%	92%
Incidence of Potentially Preventable VTE[2]	44	2%	8%	10%
UFH with Dosages/Platelet Monitoring[2]	114	100%	98%	97%
Venous Thromboembolism Prophylaxis[2]	330	92%	90%	85%
Warfarin Therapy Discharge Instructions[2]	84	92%	78%	75%
Chest Pain/Possible Heart Attack Care				
Aspirin Given Within 24 Hours of Arrival[1,3]	-	-	97%	96%
Fibrinolytic Meds Within 30 Min. of Arrival[3,7]	-	-	44%	58%
Average Time to ECG (minutes)[1,3]	-	-	9	7
Average Time to Transfer (minutes)[3,7]	-	-	64	60
Children's Asthma Care				
Received Home Management Plan of Care	-	-	-	88%
Received Reliever Medication	-	-	-	100%
Received Systemic Corticosteroids	-	-	-	100%
Emergency Department				
Admittance Decision Time (minutes)[2]	630	195	104	98
Head CT Results Within 45 Min. of Arrival[1]	-	-	60%	57%
Patients Who Left ER Before Being Seen	96,669	1%	1%	2%
Time from ER Arrival to Admit. (minutes)[2]	645	391	276	274
Time from ER Arrival to Discharge (minutes)	405	148	125	134
Time in ER Before Being Evaluated (minutes)	356	81	26	26
Time to Pain Meds for Fractures (minutes)	254	60	58	57
Heart Attack Care				
Aspirin Given at Discharge	364	99%	99%	99%
Fibrinolytic Meds Within 30 Min. of Arrival[7]	-	-	40%	54%
PCI Within 90 Minutes of Arrival	48	98%	97%	96%
Statin Prescribed at Discharge	363	99%	99%	98%
Heart Failure Care				
ACE Inhibitor or ARB for LVSD	226	99%	97%	97%
Discharge Instructions Given	511	98%	96%	94%
Evaluation of LVS Function	663	100%	100%	99%
Medicare Spending				
Medicare Spending per Patient (ratio)	-	1.07	1.01	0.98
Pneumonia Care				
Appropriate Initial Antibiotic Given	247	98%	96%	95%
Blood Culture Timing	485	98%	98%	98%
Pregnancy and Delivery Care				
Newborn Deliveries Scheduled Early[2]	12	0%	4%	6%
Preventive Care				
Immunization for Influenza[2]	539	96%	91%	90%
Immunization for Pneumonia[2]	657	95%	92%	92%
Stroke Care				
Anticoagulation Therapy for Atrial Fibrillation	23	96%	96%	95%
Antithrombotic Therapy Timing	251	100%	98%	98%
Assessed for Rehabilitation	312	98%	98%	97%
Discharged on Antithrombotic Therapy	274	100%	99%	99%
Discharged on Statin Medication	215	98%	95%	94%
Thrombolytic Therapy Timing	16	62%	72%	66%
Venous Thromboembolism Prophylaxis	310	95%	95%	94%
Written Stroke Educational Materials Given	165	93%	90%	88%
Surgical Care Improvement Project				
Appropriate Beta Blocker Usage[2]	285	99%	98%	98%
Appropriate VTP Within 24 Hours[2]	678	99%	99%	98%
Controlled Postoperative Blood Glucose[2]	103	88%	98%	97%
Perioperative Temperature Management[2]	848	100%	100%	100%
Prophylactic Antibiotic Selection[2]	718	99%	99%	99%
Prophylactic Antibiotic Selection (Outpatient)	379	97%	98%	98%
Prophylactic Antibiotic Stopped[2]	708	99%	98%	98%
Prophylactic Antibiotic Timing[2]	719	98%	99%	99%
Prophylactic Antibiotic Timing (Outpatient)	366	98%	98%	98%
Urinary Catheter Removal[2]	628	99%	99%	97%
Survey of Patients' Hospital Experiences				
Area Around Room 'Always' Quiet at Night	300+	48%	54%	61%
Doctors 'Always' Communicated Well	300+	74%	80%	82%
Home Recovery Information Given	300+	82%	86%	85%
Hospital Given 9 or 10 on 10 Point Scale	300+	55%	69%	71%
Meds 'Always' Explained Before Given	300+	57%	63%	64%
Nurses 'Always' Communicated Well	300+	71%	79%	79%
Pain 'Always' Well Controlled	300+	62%	70%	71%
Room and Bathroom 'Always' Clean	300+	59%	73%	73%
Timely Help 'Always' Received	300+	55%	67%	68%
Would Definitely Recommend Hospital	300+	54%	70%	71%
Use of Medical Imaging				
Cardiac Imaging Stress Test before Surgery	724	5.0%	5.4%	5.3%
Combination Abdominal CT Scan	1,666	8.2%	12.2%	10.5%
Combination Brain/Sinus CT Scan	1,194	2.0%	3.1%	2.7%
Combination Chest CT Scan	1,190	0.0%	2.1%	2.7%
Follow-up Mammogram/Ultrasound	3,275	8.8%	9%	8.8%
Lumbar Spine MRI for Low Back Pain	285	35.4%	35.8%	37.2%

Warren General Hospital

Two Crescent Park West
Warren, PA 16365
Type: Acute Care Hospitals
Ownership: Voluntary non-profit - Private
Phone: 814-723-3300
Fax: 814-723-2248
Emergency Services: Yes
Beds: 89

Key Personnel:
Anesthesiology. . . . . Niaz Ahmed, MD
Radiology. . . . . Julius Berta, MD
Pediatric Ambulatory Care . . . . . . David McConnell, Jr, MD
Pediatric In-Patient Care . . . . David McConnell, Jr, MD
CEO/President. . . . . John P Papalia

Measure	Cases	This Hosp.	State Avg.	U.S. Avg.
Blood Clot Prevention and Treatment				
Anticoagulation Overlap Therapy[2]	17	76%	94%	93%
ICU Venous Thromboembolism Prophylaxis[2]	41	88%	94%	92%
Incidence of Potentially Preventable VTE[1,2]	-	-	8%	10%
UFH with Dosages/Platelet Monitoring[2]	11	82%	98%	97%
Venous Thromboembolism Prophylaxis[2]	186	90%	90%	85%
Warfarin Therapy Discharge Instructions[2]	11	82%	78%	75%
Chest Pain/Possible Heart Attack Care				
Aspirin Given Within 24 Hours of Arrival	170	96%	97%	96%
Fibrinolytic Meds Within 30 Min. of Arrival[1]	-	-	44%	58%
Average Time to ECG (minutes)	176	12	9	7
Average Time to Transfer (minutes)[1]	-	-	64	60
Children's Asthma Care				
Received Home Management Plan of Care	-	-	-	88%
Received Reliever Medication	-	-	-	100%
Received Systemic Corticosteroids	-	-	-	100%
Emergency Department				
Admittance Decision Time (minutes)[2]	185	70	104	98
Head CT Results Within 45 Min. of Arrival	15	60%	60%	57%
Patients Who Left ER Before Being Seen	20,835	1%	1%	2%
Time from ER Arrival to Admit. (minutes)[2]	275	299	276	274
Time from ER Arrival to Discharge (minutes)	321	167	125	134
Time in ER Before Being Evaluated (minutes)	356	44	26	26
Time to Pain Meds for Fractures (minutes)	123	83	58	57
Heart Attack Care				
Aspirin Given at Discharge[1]	-	-	99%	99%
Fibrinolytic Meds Within 30 Min. of Arrival[7]	-	-	40%	54%
PCI Within 90 Minutes of Arrival[7]	-	-	97%	96%
Statin Prescribed at Discharge[1]	-	-	99%	98%
Heart Failure Care				
ACE Inhibitor or ARB for LVSD	14	79%	97%	97%
Discharge Instructions Given	67	99%	96%	94%
Evaluation of LVS Function	97	96%	100%	99%
Medicare Spending				
Medicare Spending per Patient (ratio)	-	0.97	1.01	0.98
Pneumonia Care				
Appropriate Initial Antibiotic Given	81	93%	96%	95%
Blood Culture Timing	127	98%	98%	98%
Pregnancy and Delivery Care				
Newborn Deliveries Scheduled Early[2]	20	5%	4%	6%
Preventive Care				
Immunization for Influenza[2]	334	92%	91%	90%
Immunization for Pneumonia[2]	348	91%	92%	92%
Stroke Care				
Anticoagulation Therapy for Atrial Fibrillation[1,3]	-	-	96%	95%
Antithrombotic Therapy Timing[3]	13	92%	98%	98%
Assessed for Rehabilitation[3]	16	94%	98%	97%
Discharged on Antithrombotic Therapy[3]	14	93%	99%	99%
Discharged on Statin Medication[3]	13	77%	95%	94%
Thrombolytic Therapy Timing[1,3]	-	-	72%	66%
Venous Thromboembolism Prophylaxis[3]	13	92%	95%	94%
Written Stroke Educational Materials Given[1,3]	-	-	90%	88%
Surgical Care Improvement Project				
Appropriate Beta Blocker Usage	45	93%	98%	98%
Appropriate VTP Within 24 Hours	162	99%	99%	98%
Controlled Postoperative Blood Glucose[7]	-	-	98%	97%
Perioperative Temperature Management	185	99%	100%	100%
Prophylactic Antibiotic Selection	147	97%	99%	99%
Prophylactic Antibiotic Selection (Outpatient)	29	93%	98%	98%

NOTE: Hospital profiles are in alphabetical order by state, then city, then hospital within the city; Rankings exclude hospitals with less than 25 cases except for patient surveys which excludes hospitals with less than 100 cases; (a) 100-299 cases; (1) The number of cases/patients is too few to report; (2) Data submitted were based on a sample of cases/patients; (3) Results are based on a shorter time period than required; (4) Data suppressed by CMS for one or more quarters; (5) Results are not available for this reporting period; (6) Fewer than 100 patients completed the HCAHPS survey; (7) No cases met the criteria for this measure; (8) The lower limit of the confidence interval cannot be calculated if the number of observed infections equals zero; (9) No data are available from the state/territory for this reporting period; (10) The scores shown reflect fewer than 50 completed surveys; (11) There were discrepancies in the data collection process; (12) This measure does not apply to this hospital for this reporting period; (13) Results cannot be calculated for this reporting period; (14) The results for this state are combined with nearby states to protect confidentiality; Please refer to the User's Guide for a full explanation of data.

Measure	Cases	This Hosp.	State Avg.	U.S. Avg.
Prophylactic Antibiotic Stopped	140	98%	98%	98%
Prophylactic Antibiotic Timing	147	97%	99%	99%
Prophylactic Antibiotic Timing (Outpatient)	29	100%	98%	98%
Urinary Catheter Removal	90	96%	99%	97%
Survey of Patients' Hospital Experiences				
Area Around Room 'Always' Quiet at Night	300+	50%	54%	61%
Doctors 'Always' Communicated Well	300+	79%	80%	82%
Home Recovery Information Given	300+	85%	86%	85%
Hospital Given 9 or 10 on 10 Point Scale	300+	62%	69%	71%
Meds 'Always' Explained Before Given	300+	59%	63%	64%
Nurses 'Always' Communicated Well	300+	78%	79%	79%
Pain 'Always' Well Controlled	300+	68%	70%	71%
Room and Bathroom 'Always' Clean	300+	67%	73%	73%
Timely Help 'Always' Received	300+	64%	67%	68%
Would Definitely Recommend Hospital	300+	63%	70%	71%
Use of Medical Imaging				
Cardiac Imaging Stress Test before Surgery	313	7.0%	5.4%	5.3%
Combination Abdominal CT Scan	525	4.2%	12.2%	10.5%
Combination Brain/Sinus CT Scan[1]	-	-	3.1%	2.7%
Combination Chest CT Scan	277	0.0%	2.1%	2.7%
Follow-up Mammogram/Ultrasound	919	3.0%	9%	8.8%
Lumbar Spine MRI for Low Back Pain	101	39.6%	35.8%	37.2%

Advanced Surgical Hospital

100 Trich Drive
Washington, PA 15301
Phone: 724-884-0710
URL: www.ashospital.net
Type: Acute Care Hospitals
Emergency Services: No
Ownership: Proprietary
Beds: 14
Key Personnel:
Anesthesiology. . . . . Bryan Matusic, DO
CEO . . . . Lloyd Scarrow

Measure	Cases	This Hosp.	State Avg.	U.S. Avg.
Blood Clot Prevention and Treatment				
Anticoagulation Overlap Therapy[7]	-	-	94%	93%
ICU Venous Thromboembolism Prophylaxis[7]	-	-	94%	92%
Incidence of Potentially Preventable VTE[7]	-	-	8%	10%
UFH with Dosages/Platelet Monitoring[7]	-	-	98%	97%
Venous Thromboembolism Prophylaxis[1]	-	-	90%	85%
Warfarin Therapy Discharge Instructions[7]	-	-	78%	75%
Chest Pain/Possible Heart Attack Care				
Aspirin Given Within 24 Hours of Arrival[3,7]	-	-	97%	96%
Fibrinolytic Meds Within 30 Min. of Arrival[5]	-	-	44%	58%
Average Time to ECG (minutes)[3,7]	-	-	9	7
Average Time to Transfer (minutes)[5]	-	-	64	60
Children's Asthma Care				
Received Home Management Plan of Care	-	-	-	88%
Received Reliever Medication	-	-	-	100%
Received Systemic Corticosteroids	-	-	-	100%
Emergency Department				
Admittance Decision Time (minutes)[7]	-	-	104	98
Head CT Results Within 45 Min. of Arrival[5]	-	-	60%	57%
Patients Who Left ER Before Being Seen[1]	-	-	1%	2%
Time from ER Arrival to Admit. (minutes)[7]	-	-	276	274
Time from ER Arrival to Discharge (minutes)	12	90	125	134
Time in ER Before Being Evaluated (minutes)	15	35	26	26
Time to Pain Meds for Fractures (minutes)[3,7]	-	-	58	57
Heart Attack Care				
Aspirin Given at Discharge[5]	-	-	99%	99%
Fibrinolytic Meds Within 30 Min. of Arrival[5]	-	-	40%	54%
PCI Within 90 Minutes of Arrival[5]	-	-	97%	96%
Statin Prescribed at Discharge[5]	-	-	99%	98%
Heart Failure Care				
ACE Inhibitor or ARB for LVSD[5]	-	-	97%	97%
Discharge Instructions Given[5]	-	-	96%	94%
Evaluation of LVS Function[5]	-	-	100%	99%
Medicare Spending				
Medicare Spending per Patient (ratio)	-	1.08	1.01	0.98
Pneumonia Care				
Appropriate Initial Antibiotic Given[5]	-	-	96%	95%
Blood Culture Timing[5]	-	-	98%	98%
Pregnancy and Delivery Care				
Newborn Deliveries Scheduled Early[7]	-	-	4%	6%
Preventive Care				
Immunization for Influenza	241	96%	91%	90%
Immunization for Pneumonia	321	98%	92%	92%
Stroke Care				
Anticoagulation Therapy for Atrial Fibrillation[5]	-	-	96%	95%
Antithrombotic Therapy Timing[5]	-	-	98%	98%
Assessed for Rehabilitation[5]	-	-	98%	97%
Discharged on Antithrombotic Therapy[5]	-	-	99%	99%
Discharged on Statin Medication[5]	-	-	95%	94%
Thrombolytic Therapy Timing[5]	-	-	72%	66%
Venous Thromboembolism Prophylaxis[5]	-	-	95%	94%
Written Stroke Educational Materials Given[5]	-	-	90%	88%
Surgical Care Improvement Project				
Appropriate Beta Blocker Usage	99	99%	98%	98%
Appropriate VTP Within 24 Hours	400	100%	99%	98%
Controlled Postoperative Blood Glucose[7]	-	-	98%	97%
Perioperative Temperature Management	418	100%	100%	100%
Prophylactic Antibiotic Selection	384	100%	99%	99%
Prophylactic Antibiotic Selection (Outpatient)[1,3]	-	-	98%	98%
Prophylactic Antibiotic Stopped	383	100%	98%	98%
Prophylactic Antibiotic Timing	384	100%	99%	99%
Prophylactic Antibiotic Timing (Outpatient)[1,3]	-	-	98%	98%
Urinary Catheter Removal	195	100%	99%	97%
Survey of Patients' Hospital Experiences				
Area Around Room 'Always' Quiet at Night	(a)	86%	54%	61%
Doctors 'Always' Communicated Well	(a)	91%	80%	82%
Home Recovery Information Given	(a)	94%	86%	85%
Hospital Given 9 or 10 on 10 Point Scale	(a)	94%	69%	71%
Meds 'Always' Explained Before Given	(a)	81%	63%	64%
Nurses 'Always' Communicated Well	(a)	96%	79%	79%
Pain 'Always' Well Controlled	(a)	83%	70%	71%
Room and Bathroom 'Always' Clean	(a)	91%	73%	73%
Timely Help 'Always' Received	(a)	95%	67%	68%
Would Definitely Recommend Hospital	(a)	95%	70%	71%
Use of Medical Imaging				
Cardiac Imaging Stress Test before Surgery[7]	-	-	5.4%	5.3%
Combination Abdominal CT Scan[7]	-	-	12.2%	10.5%
Combination Brain/Sinus CT Scan[7]	-	-	3.1%	2.7%
Combination Chest CT Scan[7]	-	-	2.1%	2.7%
Follow-up Mammogram/Ultrasound[7]	-	-	9%	8.8%
Lumbar Spine MRI for Low Back Pain[1]	-	-	35.8%	37.2%

The Washington Hospital

155 Wilson Avenue
Washington, PA 15301
Phone: 724-225-7000
Fax: 724-223-3784
E-mail: info@washingtonhospital.org
URL: www.washingtonhospital.org
Type: Acute Care Hospitals
Emergency Services: Yes
Ownership: Government - Local
Beds: 239
Key Personnel:
Quality Assurance . . . . Colleen C Allison
Radiology. . . . . Giovanna M Aracri
Chief of Medical Staff. . . . . Dennis P Brown, MD
Operating Room. . . . . Kathy Hearn
CEO/President. . . . . Telford W Thomas
Pediatric Ambulatory Care . . . . . . Paul M Wodlinger, MD
Pediatric In-Patient Care . . . . Paul M Wodlinger, MD

Measure	Cases	This Hosp.	State Avg.	U.S. Avg.
Blood Clot Prevention and Treatment				
Anticoagulation Overlap Therapy[2]	76	100%	94%	93%
ICU Venous Thromboembolism Prophylaxis[2]	52	100%	94%	92%
Incidence of Potentially Preventable VTE[2]	20	0%	8%	10%
UFH with Dosages/Platelet Monitoring[2]	84	100%	98%	97%
Venous Thromboembolism Prophylaxis[2]	366	92%	90%	85%
Warfarin Therapy Discharge Instructions[2]	45	96%	78%	75%
Chest Pain/Possible Heart Attack Care				
Aspirin Given Within 24 Hours of Arrival[1,3]	-	-	97%	96%
Fibrinolytic Meds Within 30 Min. of Arrival[5]	-	-	44%	58%
Average Time to ECG (minutes)[1,3]	-	-	9	7
Average Time to Transfer (minutes)[5]	-	-	64	60
Children's Asthma Care				
Received Home Management Plan of Care	-	-	-	88%
Received Reliever Medication	-	-	-	100%
Received Systemic Corticosteroids	-	-	-	100%
Emergency Department				
Admittance Decision Time (minutes)[2]	607	82	104	98
Head CT Results Within 45 Min. of Arrival	15	80%	60%	57%
Patients Who Left ER Before Being Seen	48,577	1%	1%	2%
Time from ER Arrival to Admit. (minutes)[2]	607	258	276	274
Time from ER Arrival to Discharge (minutes)	404	149	125	134
Time in ER Before Being Evaluated (minutes)	448	31	26	26
Time to Pain Meds for Fractures (minutes)	99	60	58	57
Heart Attack Care				
Aspirin Given at Discharge	358	100%	99%	99%
Fibrinolytic Meds Within 30 Min. of Arrival[7]	-	-	40%	54%
PCI Within 90 Minutes of Arrival	45	100%	97%	96%
Statin Prescribed at Discharge	344	100%	99%	98%
Heart Failure Care				
ACE Inhibitor or ARB for LVSD	117	100%	97%	97%
Discharge Instructions Given	363	98%	96%	94%
Evaluation of LVS Function	491	100%	100%	99%
Medicare Spending				
Medicare Spending per Patient (ratio)	-	1.03	1.01	0.98
Pneumonia Care				
Appropriate Initial Antibiotic Given	213	97%	96%	95%
Blood Culture Timing	339	100%	98%	98%
Pregnancy and Delivery Care				
Newborn Deliveries Scheduled Early	116	3%	4%	6%
Preventive Care				
Immunization for Influenza[2]	575	100%	91%	90%
Immunization for Pneumonia[2]	744	99%	92%	92%
Stroke Care				
Anticoagulation Therapy for Atrial Fibrillation	31	97%	96%	95%
Antithrombotic Therapy Timing	131	98%	98%	98%
Assessed for Rehabilitation	146	98%	98%	97%
Discharged on Antithrombotic Therapy	141	100%	99%	99%
Discharged on Statin Medication	107	94%	95%	94%
Thrombolytic Therapy Timing[1]	-	-	72%	66%
Venous Thromboembolism Prophylaxis	144	91%	95%	94%
Written Stroke Educational Materials Given	66	92%	90%	88%
Surgical Care Improvement Project				
Appropriate Beta Blocker Usage	291	100%	98%	98%
Appropriate VTP Within 24 Hours	518	99%	99%	98%
Controlled Postoperative Blood Glucose	126	97%	98%	97%
Perioperative Temperature Management	686	100%	100%	100%
Prophylactic Antibiotic Selection	549	99%	99%	99%
Prophylactic Antibiotic Selection (Outpatient)	245	99%	98%	98%
Prophylactic Antibiotic Stopped	529	99%	98%	98%
Prophylactic Antibiotic Timing	549	100%	99%	99%
Prophylactic Antibiotic Timing (Outpatient)	232	100%	98%	98%
Urinary Catheter Removal	285	100%	99%	97%
Survey of Patients' Hospital Experiences				
Area Around Room 'Always' Quiet at Night	300+	54%	54%	61%
Doctors 'Always' Communicated Well	300+	80%	80%	82%
Home Recovery Information Given	300+	88%	86%	85%
Hospital Given 9 or 10 on 10 Point Scale	300+	66%	69%	71%
Meds 'Always' Explained Before Given	300+	60%	63%	64%
Nurses 'Always' Communicated Well	300+	80%	79%	79%
Pain 'Always' Well Controlled	300+	72%	70%	71%
Room and Bathroom 'Always' Clean	300+	77%	73%	73%
Timely Help 'Always' Received	300+	67%	67%	68%
Would Definitely Recommend Hospital	300+	68%	70%	71%
Use of Medical Imaging				
Cardiac Imaging Stress Test before Surgery	448	4.9%	5.4%	5.3%
Combination Abdominal CT Scan	379	10.3%	12.2%	10.5%
Combination Brain/Sinus CT Scan[1]	-	-	3.1%	2.7%
Combination Chest CT Scan	361	0.0%	2.1%	2.7%
Follow-up Mammogram/Ultrasound	802	7.7%	9%	8.8%
Lumbar Spine MRI for Low Back Pain	62	38.7%	35.8%	37.2%

Waynesboro Hospital

501 East Main St
Waynesboro, PA 17268
Phone: 717-765-4000
Fax: 717-765-3431
URL: www.summithealth.org
Type: Acute Care Hospitals
Emergency Services: Yes
Ownership: Voluntary non-profit - Other
Beds: 64
Key Personnel:
Emergency Room . . . . Thomas E Anderson, DO

NOTE: Hospital profiles are in alphabetical order by state, then city, then hospital within the city; Rankings exclude hospitals with less than 25 cases except for patient surveys which excludes hospitals with less than 100 cases; (a) 100-299 cases; (1) The number of cases/patients is too few to report; (2) Data submitted were based on a sample of cases/patients; (3) Results are based on a shorter time period than required; (4) Data suppressed by CMS for one or more quarters; (5) Results are not available for this reporting period; (6) Fewer than 100 patients completed the HCAHPS survey; (7) No cases met the criteria for this measure; (8) The lower limit of the confidence interval cannot be calculated if the number of observed infections equals zero; (9) No data are available from the state/territory for this reporting period; (10) The scores shown reflect fewer than 50 completed surveys; (11) There were discrepancies in the data collection process; (12) This measure does not apply to this hospital for this reporting period; (13) Results cannot be calculated for this reporting period; (14) The results for this state are combined with nearby states to protect confidentiality; Please refer to the User's Guide for a full explanation of data.

Operating Room. . . . . Christopher S Andrews
Radiology. . . . . Amir R Batouli
Intensive Care Unit. . . . . Karen Clark
Quality Assurance . . . . Debra Davis, RN
CEO/President. . . . . Norman B Epstein
Chief of Medical Staff . . . . Shannsul M Hag, MD
Infection Control. . . . . Mary McDonald, RN

Measure	Cases	This Hosp.	State Avg.	U.S. Avg.
Blood Clot Prevention and Treatment				
Anticoagulation Overlap Therapy	25	96%	94%	93%
ICU Venous Thromboembolism Prophylaxis	243	97%	94%	92%
Incidence of Potentially Preventable VTE[1]	-	-	8%	10%
UFH with Dosages/Platelet Monitoring	16	100%	98%	97%
Venous Thromboembolism Prophylaxis	993	98%	90%	85%
Warfarin Therapy Discharge Instructions	23	91%	78%	75%
Chest Pain/Possible Heart Attack Care				
Aspirin Given Within 24 Hours of Arrival	62	97%	97%	96%
Fibrinolytic Meds Within 30 Min. of Arrival[7]	-	-	44%	58%
Average Time to ECG (minutes)	65	8	9	7
Average Time to Transfer (minutes)	20	76	64	60
Children's Asthma Care				
Received Home Management Plan of Care	-	-	-	88%
Received Reliever Medication	-	-	-	100%
Received Systemic Corticosteroids	-	-	-	100%
Emergency Department				
Admittance Decision Time (minutes)[2]	471	123	104	98
Head CT Results Within 45 Min. of Arrival[1]	-	-	60%	57%
Patients Who Left ER Before Being Seen	11,975	1%	1%	2%
Time from ER Arrival to Admit. (minutes)[2]	476	266	276	274
Time from ER Arrival to Discharge (minutes)	364	103	125	134
Time in ER Before Being Evaluated (minutes)	375	22	26	26
Time to Pain Meds for Fractures (minutes)	62	52	58	57
Heart Attack Care				
Aspirin Given at Discharge	18	100%	99%	99%
Fibrinolytic Meds Within 30 Min. of Arrival[7]	-	-	40%	54%
PCI Within 90 Minutes of Arrival[7]	-	-	97%	96%
Statin Prescribed at Discharge	18	100%	99%	98%
Heart Failure Care				
ACE Inhibitor or ARB for LVSD	21	100%	97%	97%
Discharge Instructions Given	91	95%	96%	94%
Evaluation of LVS Function	103	100%	100%	99%
Medicare Spending				
Medicare Spending per Patient (ratio)	-	0.87	1.01	0.98
Pneumonia Care				
Appropriate Initial Antibiotic Given	89	97%	96%	95%
Blood Culture Timing	136	99%	98%	98%
Pregnancy and Delivery Care				
Newborn Deliveries Scheduled Early[2]	20	5%	4%	6%
Preventive Care				
Immunization for Influenza[2]	321	98%	91%	90%
Immunization for Pneumonia[2]	422	99%	92%	92%
Stroke Care				
Anticoagulation Therapy for Atrial Fibrillation[1]	-	-	96%	95%
Antithrombotic Therapy Timing	33	100%	98%	98%
Assessed for Rehabilitation	39	100%	98%	97%
Discharged on Antithrombotic Therapy	36	100%	99%	99%
Discharged on Statin Medication	25	100%	95%	94%
Thrombolytic Therapy Timing[1]	-	-	72%	66%
Venous Thromboembolism Prophylaxis	38	100%	95%	94%
Written Stroke Educational Materials Given	25	92%	90%	88%
Surgical Care Improvement Project				
Appropriate Beta Blocker Usage	48	98%	98%	98%
Appropriate VTP Within 24 Hours	114	97%	99%	98%
Controlled Postoperative Blood Glucose[7]	-	-	98%	97%
Perioperative Temperature Management	152	100%	100%	100%
Prophylactic Antibiotic Selection	107	99%	99%	99%
Prophylactic Antibiotic Selection (Outpatient)	18	100%	98%	98%
Prophylactic Antibiotic Stopped	102	99%	98%	98%
Prophylactic Antibiotic Timing	107	97%	99%	99%
Prophylactic Antibiotic Timing (Outpatient)	18	100%	98%	98%
Urinary Catheter Removal	51	100%	99%	97%
Survey of Patients' Hospital Experiences				
Area Around Room 'Always' Quiet at Night	300+	53%	54%	61%
Doctors 'Always' Communicated Well	300+	80%	80%	82%
Home Recovery Information Given	300+	85%	86%	85%
Hospital Given 9 or 10 on 10 Point Scale	300+	76%	69%	71%
Meds 'Always' Explained Before Given	300+	66%	63%	64%
Nurses 'Always' Communicated Well	300+	81%	79%	79%
Pain 'Always' Well Controlled	300+	72%	70%	71%
Room and Bathroom 'Always' Clean	300+	74%	73%	73%
Timely Help 'Always' Received	300+	71%	67%	68%
Would Definitely Recommend Hospital	300+	74%	70%	71%
Use of Medical Imaging				
Cardiac Imaging Stress Test before Surgery	159	6.3%	5.4%	5.3%
Combination Abdominal CT Scan	415	5.1%	12.2%	10.5%
Combination Brain/Sinus CT Scan	353	5.1%	3.1%	2.7%
Combination Chest CT Scan	220	1.4%	2.1%	2.7%
Follow-up Mammogram/Ultrasound	923	13.0%	9%	8.8%
Lumbar Spine MRI for Low Back Pain	39	43.6%	35.8%	37.2%

Southwest Regional Medical Center

350 Bonar Avenue
Waynesburg, PA 15370
Phone: 724-627-2602
Fax: 724-627-7639
E-mail: jeggleston@gcmhcare.com
URL: www.gcmhcare.com
Type: Acute Care Hospitals
Emergency Services: Yes
Ownership: Proprietary
Beds: 54
Key Personnel:
Pediatric In-Patient Care . . . . Daniel Church, MD
Quality Assurance . . . . Deanna Cunningham, RN, BA, MSSL
Infection Control. . . . . Mary Lee Headlee, RN
Chief of Medical Staff . . . . Bernard Imrich, MD
Pediatric Ambulatory Care . . . . . . Satish Kumar, MD
CEO/President. . . . . Raoul M Walsh
Coronary Care . . . . Barbara Walters
Operating Room. . . . . Billy Wood, RN

Measure	Cases	This Hosp.	State Avg.	U.S. Avg.
Blood Clot Prevention and Treatment				
Anticoagulation Overlap Therapy[1,2]	-	-	94%	93%
ICU Venous Thromboembolism Prophylaxis[2]	38	87%	94%	92%
Incidence of Potentially Preventable VTE[1,2]	-	-	8%	10%
UFH with Dosages/Platelet Monitoring[1,2]	-	-	98%	97%
Venous Thromboembolism Prophylaxis[2]	185	90%	90%	85%
Warfarin Therapy Discharge Instructions[1,2]	-	-	78%	75%
Chest Pain/Possible Heart Attack Care				
Aspirin Given Within 24 Hours of Arrival	69	96%	97%	96%
Fibrinolytic Meds Within 30 Min. of Arrival[7]	-	-	44%	58%
Average Time to ECG (minutes)	69	5	9	7
Average Time to Transfer (minutes)	12	60	64	60
Children's Asthma Care				
Received Home Management Plan of Care	-	-	-	88%
Received Reliever Medication	-	-	-	100%
Received Systemic Corticosteroids	-	-	-	100%
Emergency Department				
Admittance Decision Time (minutes)[2]	387	60	104	98
Head CT Results Within 45 Min. of Arrival[1]	-	-	60%	57%
Patients Who Left ER Before Being Seen	22,463	1%	1%	2%
Time from ER Arrival to Admit. (minutes)[2]	394	207	276	274
Time from ER Arrival to Discharge (minutes)	361	101	125	134
Time in ER Before Being Evaluated (minutes)	414	25	26	26
Time to Pain Meds for Fractures (minutes)	35	47	58	57
Heart Attack Care				
Aspirin Given at Discharge	13	85%	99%	99%
Fibrinolytic Meds Within 30 Min. of Arrival[7]	-	-	40%	54%
PCI Within 90 Minutes of Arrival[7]	-	-	97%	96%
Statin Prescribed at Discharge	12	92%	99%	98%
Heart Failure Care				
ACE Inhibitor or ARB for LVSD	23	100%	97%	97%
Discharge Instructions Given	78	64%	96%	94%
Evaluation of LVS Function	110	100%	100%	99%
Medicare Spending				
Medicare Spending per Patient (ratio)	-	1.00	1.01	0.98
Pneumonia Care				
Appropriate Initial Antibiotic Given	93	96%	96%	95%
Blood Culture Timing	132	99%	98%	98%
Pregnancy and Delivery Care				
Newborn Deliveries Scheduled Early[7]	-	-	4%	6%
Preventive Care				
Immunization for Influenza[2]	292	97%	91%	90%
Immunization for Pneumonia[2]	455	95%	92%	92%
Stroke Care				
Anticoagulation Therapy for Atrial Fibrillation[3,7]	-	-	96%	95%
Antithrombotic Therapy Timing[1,3]	-	-	98%	98%
Assessed for Rehabilitation[1,3]	-	-	98%	97%
Discharged on Antithrombotic Therapy[1,3]	-	-	99%	99%
Discharged on Statin Medication[1,3]	-	-	95%	94%
Thrombolytic Therapy Timing[3,7]	-	-	72%	66%
Venous Thromboembolism Prophylaxis[1,3]	-	-	95%	94%
Written Stroke Educational Materials Given[1,3]	-	-	90%	88%
Surgical Care Improvement Project				
Appropriate Beta Blocker Usage	28	100%	98%	98%
Appropriate VTP Within 24 Hours	78	97%	99%	98%
Controlled Postoperative Blood Glucose[7]	-	-	98%	97%
Perioperative Temperature Management	79	99%	100%	100%
Prophylactic Antibiotic Selection	46	96%	99%	99%
Prophylactic Antibiotic Selection (Outpatient)	13	100%	98%	98%
Prophylactic Antibiotic Stopped	43	98%	98%	98%
Prophylactic Antibiotic Timing	46	100%	99%	99%
Prophylactic Antibiotic Timing (Outpatient)	13	92%	98%	98%
Urinary Catheter Removal	55	96%	99%	97%
Survey of Patients' Hospital Experiences				
Area Around Room 'Always' Quiet at Night	300+	49%	54%	61%
Doctors 'Always' Communicated Well	300+	83%	80%	82%
Home Recovery Information Given	300+	80%	86%	85%
Hospital Given 9 or 10 on 10 Point Scale	300+	54%	69%	71%
Meds 'Always' Explained Before Given	300+	60%	63%	64%
Nurses 'Always' Communicated Well	300+	78%	79%	79%
Pain 'Always' Well Controlled	300+	65%	70%	71%
Room and Bathroom 'Always' Clean	300+	67%	73%	73%
Timely Help 'Always' Received	300+	62%	67%	68%
Would Definitely Recommend Hospital	300+	52%	70%	71%
Use of Medical Imaging				
Cardiac Imaging Stress Test before Surgery	147	4.1%	5.4%	5.3%
Combination Abdominal CT Scan	206	20.4%	12.2%	10.5%
Combination Brain/Sinus CT Scan[1]	-	-	3.1%	2.7%
Combination Chest CT Scan	110	22.7%	2.1%	2.7%
Follow-up Mammogram/Ultrasound	194	19.6%	9%	8.8%
Lumbar Spine MRI for Low Back Pain[1]	-	-	35.8%	37.2%

Soldiers & Sailors Memorial Hospital

32-36 Central Avenue
Wellsboro, PA 16901
Phone: 570-724-1631
Fax: 570-724-7235
URL: www.laurelhs.org
Type: Acute Care Hospitals
Emergency Services: Yes
Ownership: Voluntary non-profit - Other
Beds: 103
Key Personnel:
Radiology. . . . . Enrico J Doganiero
Quality Assurance . . . . Judy Feil
Emergency Room . . . . Susan Held, Dir
President/CEO. . . . . Steve A. Kramer
Chief of Medical Staff . . . . Anthony Nespola, MD

Measure	Cases	This Hosp.	State Avg.	U.S. Avg.
Blood Clot Prevention and Treatment				
Anticoagulation Overlap Therapy[2]	19	84%	94%	93%
ICU Venous Thromboembolism Prophylaxis[2]	40	80%	94%	92%
Incidence of Potentially Preventable VTE[1,2]	-	-	8%	10%
UFH with Dosages/Platelet Monitoring[1,2]	-	-	98%	97%
Venous Thromboembolism Prophylaxis[2]	143	71%	90%	85%
Warfarin Therapy Discharge Instructions[2]	16	94%	78%	75%
Chest Pain/Possible Heart Attack Care				
Aspirin Given Within 24 Hours of Arrival	101	97%	97%	96%
Fibrinolytic Meds Within 30 Min. of Arrival[7]	-	-	44%	58%
Average Time to ECG (minutes)	107	11	9	7
Average Time to Transfer (minutes)[7]	-	-	64	60
Children's Asthma Care				
Received Home Management Plan of Care	-	-	-	88%
Received Reliever Medication	-	-	-	100%
Received Systemic Corticosteroids	-	-	-	100%
Emergency Department				
Admittance Decision Time (minutes)[2]	247	108	104	98

NOTE: Hospital profiles are in alphabetical order by state, then city, then hospital within the city; Rankings exclude hospitals with less than 25 cases except for patient surveys which excludes hospitals with less than 100 cases; (a) 100-299 cases; (1) The number of cases/patients is too few to report; (2) Data submitted were based on a sample of cases/patients; (3) Results are based on a shorter time period than required; (4) Data suppressed by CMS for one or more quarters; (5) Results are not available for this reporting period; (6) Fewer than 100 patients completed the HCAHPS survey; (7) No cases met the criteria for this measure; (8) The lower limit of the confidence interval cannot be calculated if the number of observed infections equals zero; (9) No data are available from the state/territory for this reporting period; (10) The scores shown reflect fewer than 50 completed surveys; (11) There were discrepancies in the data collection process; (12) This measure does not apply to this hospital for this reporting period; (13) Results cannot be calculated for this reporting period; (14) The results for this state are combined with nearby states to protect confidentiality; Please refer to the User's Guide for a full explanation of data.

Measure	Cases	This Hosp.	State Avg.	U.S. Avg.
Head CT Results Within 45 Min. of Arrival[1]	-	-	60%	57%
Patients Who Left ER Before Being Seen	18,627	0%	1%	2%
Time from ER Arrival to Admit. (minutes)[2]	251	234	276	274
Time from ER Arrival to Discharge (minutes)	328	96	125	134
Time in ER Before Being Evaluated (minutes)	392	14	26	26
Time to Pain Meds for Fractures (minutes)	64	44	58	57
Heart Attack Care				
Aspirin Given at Discharge	22	95%	99%	99%
Fibrinolytic Meds Within 30 Min. of Arrival[7]	-	-	40%	54%
PCI Within 90 Minutes of Arrival[7]	-	-	97%	96%
Statin Prescribed at Discharge	21	90%	99%	98%
Heart Failure Care				
ACE Inhibitor or ARB for LVSD	19	100%	97%	97%
Discharge Instructions Given	58	98%	96%	94%
Evaluation of LVS Function	72	97%	100%	99%
Medicare Spending				
Medicare Spending per Patient (ratio)	-	0.98	1.01	0.98
Pneumonia Care				
Appropriate Initial Antibiotic Given	75	100%	96%	95%
Blood Culture Timing	133	99%	98%	98%
Pregnancy and Delivery Care				
Newborn Deliveries Scheduled Early[2]	23	9%	4%	6%
Preventive Care				
Immunization for Influenza[2]	257	99%	91%	90%
Immunization for Pneumonia[2]	301	95%	92%	92%
Stroke Care				
Anticoagulation Therapy for Atrial Fibrillation[1]	-	-	96%	95%
Antithrombotic Therapy Timing	23	87%	98%	98%
Assessed for Rehabilitation	25	96%	98%	97%
Discharged on Antithrombotic Therapy	25	100%	99%	99%
Discharged on Statin Medication	24	75%	95%	94%
Thrombolytic Therapy Timing[7]	-	-	72%	66%
Venous Thromboembolism Prophylaxis	22	95%	95%	94%
Written Stroke Educational Materials Given	18	89%	90%	88%
Surgical Care Improvement Project				
Appropriate Beta Blocker Usage	32	84%	98%	98%
Appropriate VTP Within 24 Hours	137	93%	99%	98%
Controlled Postoperative Blood Glucose[7]	-	-	98%	97%
Perioperative Temperature Management	147	100%	100%	100%
Prophylactic Antibiotic Selection	103	97%	99%	99%
Prophylactic Antibiotic Selection (Outpatient)	38	97%	98%	98%
Prophylactic Antibiotic Stopped	103	100%	98%	98%
Prophylactic Antibiotic Timing	105	98%	99%	99%
Prophylactic Antibiotic Timing (Outpatient)	38	97%	98%	98%
Urinary Catheter Removal	97	97%	99%	97%
Survey of Patients' Hospital Experiences				
Area Around Room 'Always' Quiet at Night	300+	51%	54%	61%
Doctors 'Always' Communicated Well	300+	87%	80%	82%
Home Recovery Information Given	300+	85%	86%	85%
Hospital Given 9 or 10 on 10 Point Scale	300+	71%	69%	71%
Meds 'Always' Explained Before Given	300+	69%	63%	64%
Nurses 'Always' Communicated Well	300+	83%	79%	79%
Pain 'Always' Well Controlled	300+	74%	70%	71%
Room and Bathroom 'Always' Clean	300+	87%	73%	73%
Timely Help 'Always' Received	300+	73%	67%	68%
Would Definitely Recommend Hospital	300+	72%	70%	71%
Use of Medical Imaging				
Cardiac Imaging Stress Test before Surgery	267	4.5%	5.4%	5.3%
Combination Abdominal CT Scan	449	51.4%	12.2%	10.5%
Combination Brain/Sinus CT Scan	404	1.5%	3.1%	2.7%
Combination Chest CT Scan	221	0.5%	2.1%	2.7%
Follow-up Mammogram/Ultrasound	871	9.9%	9%	8.8%
Lumbar Spine MRI for Low Back Pain	83	36.1%	35.8%	37.2%

Chester County Hospital

701 East Marshall Street
West Chester, PA 19380
Phone: 610-431-5000
Fax: 610-430-2956
URL: www.cchosp.com
Type: Acute Care Hospitals
Emergency Services: Yes
Ownership: Voluntary non-profit - Private
Beds: 261

Key Personnel:

Radiology. . . . . William J Barry
CEO/President. . . . . Michael J. Duncan
Emergency Room . . . . Donna Froio
Quality Assurance . . . . Virginia Handler
Chief of Medical Staff. . . . . Azam Husain, MD
Pediatric Ambulatory Care . . . . . . Neil Pennington, MD
Pediatric In-Patient Care . . . . Neil Pennington, MD
Operating Room. . . . . Shirl Portwood

Measure	Cases	This Hosp.	State Avg.	U.S. Avg.
Blood Clot Prevention and Treatment				
Anticoagulation Overlap Therapy[2]	80	96%	94%	93%
ICU Venous Thromboembolism Prophylaxis[2]	22	100%	94%	92%
Incidence of Potentially Preventable VTE[2]	14	7%	8%	10%
UFH with Dosages/Platelet Monitoring[2]	59	98%	98%	97%
Venous Thromboembolism Prophylaxis[2]	393	79%	90%	85%
Warfarin Therapy Discharge Instructions[2]	57	16%	78%	75%
Chest Pain/Possible Heart Attack Care				
Aspirin Given Within 24 Hours of Arrival[5]	-	-	97%	96%
Fibrinolytic Meds Within 30 Min. of Arrival[5]	-	-	44%	58%
Average Time to ECG (minutes)[5]	-	-	9	7
Average Time to Transfer (minutes)[5]	-	-	64	60
Children's Asthma Care				
Received Home Management Plan of Care	-	-	-	88%
Received Reliever Medication	-	-	-	100%
Received Systemic Corticosteroids	-	-	-	100%
Emergency Department				
Admittance Decision Time (minutes)[2]	442	90	104	98
Head CT Results Within 45 Min. of Arrival	34	76%	60%	57%
Patients Who Left ER Before Being Seen	42,390	2%	1%	2%
Time from ER Arrival to Admit. (minutes)[2]	553	304	276	274
Time from ER Arrival to Discharge (minutes)	392	160	125	134
Time in ER Before Being Evaluated (minutes)	412	28	26	26
Time to Pain Meds for Fractures (minutes)	147	47	58	57
Heart Attack Care				
Aspirin Given at Discharge	202	100%	99%	99%
Fibrinolytic Meds Within 30 Min. of Arrival[7]	-	-	40%	54%
PCI Within 90 Minutes of Arrival	22	100%	97%	96%
Statin Prescribed at Discharge	196	99%	99%	98%
Heart Failure Care				
ACE Inhibitor or ARB for LVSD	79	100%	97%	97%
Discharge Instructions Given	255	98%	96%	94%
Evaluation of LVS Function	336	100%	100%	99%
Medicare Spending				
Medicare Spending per Patient (ratio)	-	1.00	1.01	0.98
Pneumonia Care				
Appropriate Initial Antibiotic Given	170	93%	96%	95%
Blood Culture Timing	362	99%	98%	98%
Pregnancy and Delivery Care				
Newborn Deliveries Scheduled Early[2]	49	10%	4%	6%
Preventive Care				
Immunization for Influenza[2]	560	92%	91%	90%
Immunization for Pneumonia[2]	618	94%	92%	92%
Stroke Care				
Anticoagulation Therapy for Atrial Fibrillation	18	100%	96%	95%
Antithrombotic Therapy Timing	105	99%	98%	98%
Assessed for Rehabilitation	98	98%	98%	97%
Discharged on Antithrombotic Therapy	98	99%	99%	99%
Discharged on Statin Medication	79	96%	95%	94%
Thrombolytic Therapy Timing[1]	-	-	72%	66%
Venous Thromboembolism Prophylaxis	100	98%	95%	94%
Written Stroke Educational Materials Given	51	98%	90%	88%
Surgical Care Improvement Project				
Appropriate Beta Blocker Usage	309	100%	98%	98%
Appropriate VTP Within 24 Hours	659	100%	99%	98%
Controlled Postoperative Blood Glucose	96	95%	98%	97%
Perioperative Temperature Management	865	100%	100%	100%
Prophylactic Antibiotic Selection	628	100%	99%	99%
Prophylactic Antibiotic Selection (Outpatient)	308	99%	98%	98%
Prophylactic Antibiotic Stopped	612	99%	98%	98%
Prophylactic Antibiotic Timing	628	100%	99%	99%
Prophylactic Antibiotic Timing (Outpatient)	308	100%	98%	98%
Urinary Catheter Removal	597	100%	99%	97%
Survey of Patients' Hospital Experiences				
Area Around Room 'Always' Quiet at Night	300+	56%	54%	61%
Doctors 'Always' Communicated Well	300+	81%	80%	82%
Home Recovery Information Given	300+	86%	86%	85%
Hospital Given 9 or 10 on 10 Point Scale	300+	73%	69%	71%
Meds 'Always' Explained Before Given	300+	66%	63%	64%
Nurses 'Always' Communicated Well	300+	83%	79%	79%
Pain 'Always' Well Controlled	300+	75%	70%	71%
Room and Bathroom 'Always' Clean	300+	74%	73%	73%
Timely Help 'Always' Received	300+	75%	67%	68%
Would Definitely Recommend Hospital	300+	80%	70%	71%
Use of Medical Imaging				
Cardiac Imaging Stress Test before Surgery	178	4.5%	5.4%	5.3%
Combination Abdominal CT Scan	1,355	6.9%	12.2%	10.5%
Combination Brain/Sinus CT Scan	884	2.7%	3.1%	2.7%
Combination Chest CT Scan	1,034	0.1%	2.1%	2.7%
Follow-up Mammogram/Ultrasound	2,696	9.3%	9%	8.8%
Lumbar Spine MRI for Low Back Pain	152	34.9%	35.8%	37.2%

Jennersville Regional Hospital

1015 West Baltimore Pike
West Grove, PA 19390
Phone: 610-869-1000
Fax: 610-869-1362
URL: www.jennersville.com
Type: Acute Care Hospitals
Emergency Services: Yes
Ownership: Proprietary
Beds: 64

Key Personnel:

Operating Room. . . . . Elaine Cook
CEO/President. . . . . Scott Phillips

Measure	Cases	This Hosp.	State Avg.	U.S. Avg.
Blood Clot Prevention and Treatment				
Anticoagulation Overlap Therapy[2]	13	92%	94%	93%
ICU Venous Thromboembolism Prophylaxis[2]	49	92%	94%	92%
Incidence of Potentially Preventable VTE[1,2]	-	-	8%	10%
UFH with Dosages/Platelet Monitoring[1,2]	-	-	98%	97%
Venous Thromboembolism Prophylaxis[2]	321	91%	90%	85%
Warfarin Therapy Discharge Instructions[1,2]	-	-	78%	75%
Chest Pain/Possible Heart Attack Care				
Aspirin Given Within 24 Hours of Arrival	24	92%	97%	96%
Fibrinolytic Meds Within 30 Min. of Arrival[1]	-	-	44%	58%
Average Time to ECG (minutes)	25	8	9	7
Average Time to Transfer (minutes)[1]	-	-	64	60
Children's Asthma Care				
Received Home Management Plan of Care	-	-	-	88%
Received Reliever Medication	-	-	-	100%
Received Systemic Corticosteroids	-	-	-	100%
Emergency Department				
Admittance Decision Time (minutes)[2]	583	94	104	98
Head CT Results Within 45 Min. of Arrival[1]	-	-	60%	57%
Patients Who Left ER Before Being Seen	15,486	1%	1%	2%
Time from ER Arrival to Admit. (minutes)[2]	583	265	276	274
Time from ER Arrival to Discharge (minutes)	370	138	125	134
Time in ER Before Being Evaluated (minutes)	411	28	26	26
Time to Pain Meds for Fractures (minutes)	104	50	58	57
Heart Attack Care				
Aspirin Given at Discharge[1]	-	-	99%	99%
Fibrinolytic Meds Within 30 Min. of Arrival[1]	-	-	40%	54%
PCI Within 90 Minutes of Arrival[7]	-	-	97%	96%
Statin Prescribed at Discharge[1]	-	-	99%	98%
Heart Failure Care				
ACE Inhibitor or ARB for LVSD	25	80%	97%	97%
Discharge Instructions Given	85	99%	96%	94%
Evaluation of LVS Function	115	100%	100%	99%
Medicare Spending				
Medicare Spending per Patient (ratio)	-	1.02	1.01	0.98
Pneumonia Care				
Appropriate Initial Antibiotic Given	116	97%	96%	95%
Blood Culture Timing	179	99%	98%	98%
Pregnancy and Delivery Care				
Newborn Deliveries Scheduled Early[2]	35	0%	4%	6%
Preventive Care				
Immunization for Influenza[2]	338	96%	91%	90%
Immunization for Pneumonia[2]	449	100%	92%	92%
Stroke Care				
Anticoagulation Therapy for Atrial Fibrillation[1]	-	-	96%	95%
Antithrombotic Therapy Timing	26	100%	98%	98%
Assessed for Rehabilitation	28	89%	98%	97%

NOTE: Hospital profiles are in alphabetical order by state, then city, then hospital within the city; Rankings exclude hospitals with less than 25 cases except for patient surveys which excludes hospitals with less than 100 cases; (a) 100-299 cases; (1) The number of cases/patients is too few to report; (2) Data submitted were based on a sample of cases/patients; (3) Results are based on a shorter time period than required; (4) Data suppressed by CMS for one or more quarters; (5) Results are not available for this reporting period; (6) Fewer than 100 patients completed the HCAHPS survey; (7) No cases met the criteria for this measure; (8) The lower limit of the confidence interval cannot be calculated if the number of observed infections equals zero; (9) No data are available from the state/territory for this reporting period; (10) The scores shown reflect fewer than 50 completed surveys; (11) There were discrepancies in the data collection process; (12) This measure does not apply to this hospital for this reporting period; (13) Results cannot be calculated for this reporting period; (14) The results for this state are combined with nearby states to protect confidentiality; Please refer to the User's Guide for a full explanation of data.

Discharged on Antithrombotic Therapy	27	93%	99%	99%
Discharged on Statin Medication	23	91%	95%	94%
Thrombolytic Therapy Timing[7]	-	-	72%	66%
Venous Thromboembolism Prophylaxis	29	93%	95%	94%
Written Stroke Educational Materials Given	17	100%	90%	88%
Surgical Care Improvement Project				
Appropriate Beta Blocker Usage	25	88%	98%	98%
Appropriate VTP Within 24 Hours	80	98%	99%	98%
Controlled Postoperative Blood Glucose[7]	-	-	98%	97%
Perioperative Temperature Management	99	100%	100%	100%
Prophylactic Antibiotic Selection	31	100%	99%	99%
Prophylactic Antibiotic Selection (Outpatient)	55	100%	98%	98%
Prophylactic Antibiotic Stopped	30	97%	98%	98%
Prophylactic Antibiotic Timing	31	100%	99%	99%
Prophylactic Antibiotic Timing (Outpatient)	16	100%	98%	98%
Urinary Catheter Removal	66	98%	99%	97%
Survey of Patients' Hospital Experiences				
Area Around Room 'Always' Quiet at Night	300+	57%	54%	61%
Doctors 'Always' Communicated Well	300+	74%	80%	82%
Home Recovery Information Given	300+	82%	86%	85%
Hospital Given 9 or 10 on 10 Point Scale	300+	65%	69%	71%
Meds 'Always' Explained Before Given	300+	55%	63%	64%
Nurses 'Always' Communicated Well	300+	74%	79%	79%
Pain 'Always' Well Controlled	300+	66%	70%	71%
Room and Bathroom 'Always' Clean	300+	68%	73%	73%
Timely Help 'Always' Received	300+	59%	67%	68%
Would Definitely Recommend Hospital	300+	61%	70%	71%
Use of Medical Imaging				
Cardiac Imaging Stress Test before Surgery	114	5.3%	5.4%	5.3%
Combination Abdominal CT Scan	364	11.8%	12.2%	10.5%
Combination Brain/Sinus CT Scan[1]	-	-	3.1%	2.7%
Combination Chest CT Scan	214	0.5%	2.1%	2.7%
Follow-up Mammogram/Ultrasound	483	11.8%	9%	8.8%
Lumbar Spine MRI for Low Back Pain[1]	-	-	35.8%	37.2%

Geisinger Wyoming Valley Medical Center

1000 East Mountain Boulevard
Wilkes Barre, PA 18711
URL: www.geisinger.org
Type: Acute Care Hospitals
Ownership: Voluntary non-profit - Private
Phone: 570-826-7300
Fax: 570-819-5545
Emergency Services: Yes
Beds: 177

Key Personnel:
Radiology. . . . . John Arthur Baxter, MD
Chief of Medical Staff. . . . . Howard R Grant
Operating Room. . . . . Rosalie King, RN
Pediatric In-Patient Care . . . . Janis Maksimak, MD
Quality Assurance . . . . Pat McCulloch, RN
CEO/President. . . . . Glenn Steele, Jr, MD

Measure	Cases	This Hosp.	State Avg.	U.S. Avg.
Blood Clot Prevention and Treatment				
Anticoagulation Overlap Therapy[2]	106	95%	94%	93%
ICU Venous Thromboembolism Prophylaxis[2]	61	95%	94%	92%
Incidence of Potentially Preventable VTE[2]	31	0%	8%	10%
UFH with Dosages/Platelet Monitoring[2]	51	100%	98%	97%
Venous Thromboembolism Prophylaxis[2]	415	86%	90%	85%
Warfarin Therapy Discharge Instructions[2]	59	73%	78%	75%
Chest Pain/Possible Heart Attack Care				
Aspirin Given Within 24 Hours of Arrival[5]	-	-	97%	96%
Fibrinolytic Meds Within 30 Min. of Arrival[5]	-	-	44%	58%
Average Time to ECG (minutes)[5]	-	-	9	7
Average Time to Transfer (minutes)[5]	-	-	64	60
Children's Asthma Care				
Received Home Management Plan of Care	-	-	-	88%
Received Reliever Medication	-	-	-	100%
Received Systemic Corticosteroids	-	-	-	100%
Emergency Department				
Admittance Decision Time (minutes)[2]	766	288	104	98
Head CT Results Within 45 Min. of Arrival[1]	-	-	60%	57%
Patients Who Left ER Before Being Seen	39,944	1%	1%	2%
Time from ER Arrival to Admit. (minutes)[2]	773	471	276	274
Time from ER Arrival to Discharge (minutes)	664	226	125	134
Time in ER Before Being Evaluated (minutes)	730	39	26	26
Time to Pain Meds for Fractures (minutes)	146	46	58	57
Heart Attack Care				
Aspirin Given at Discharge	193	100%	99%	99%
Fibrinolytic Meds Within 30 Min. of Arrival[7]	-	-	40%	54%
PCI Within 90 Minutes of Arrival	44	100%	97%	96%
Statin Prescribed at Discharge	187	99%	99%	98%
Heart Failure Care				
ACE Inhibitor or ARB for LVSD	106	100%	97%	97%
Discharge Instructions Given	329	98%	96%	94%
Evaluation of LVS Function	428	100%	100%	99%
Medicare Spending				
Medicare Spending per Patient (ratio)	-	1.15	1.01	0.98
Pneumonia Care				
Appropriate Initial Antibiotic Given	149	98%	96%	95%
Blood Culture Timing	185	99%	98%	98%
Pregnancy and Delivery Care				
Newborn Deliveries Scheduled Early[2]	86	0%	4%	6%
Preventive Care				
Immunization for Influenza[2]	649	94%	91%	90%
Immunization for Pneumonia[2]	810	97%	92%	92%
Stroke Care				
Anticoagulation Therapy for Atrial Fibrillation	23	96%	96%	95%
Antithrombotic Therapy Timing	165	97%	98%	98%
Assessed for Rehabilitation	201	99%	98%	97%
Discharged on Antithrombotic Therapy	175	100%	99%	99%
Discharged on Statin Medication	147	95%	95%	94%
Thrombolytic Therapy Timing	23	57%	72%	66%
Venous Thromboembolism Prophylaxis	210	86%	95%	94%
Written Stroke Educational Materials Given	101	81%	90%	88%
Surgical Care Improvement Project				
Appropriate Beta Blocker Usage[2]	348	100%	98%	98%
Appropriate VTP Within 24 Hours[2]	492	97%	99%	98%
Controlled Postoperative Blood Glucose[2]	132	95%	98%	97%
Perioperative Temperature Management[2]	629	99%	100%	100%
Prophylactic Antibiotic Selection[2]	469	99%	99%	99%
Prophylactic Antibiotic Selection (Outpatient)	656	99%	98%	98%
Prophylactic Antibiotic Stopped[2]	457	98%	98%	98%
Prophylactic Antibiotic Timing[2]	472	97%	99%	99%
Prophylactic Antibiotic Timing (Outpatient)	508	97%	98%	98%
Urinary Catheter Removal[2]	476	98%	99%	97%
Survey of Patients' Hospital Experiences				
Area Around Room 'Always' Quiet at Night	300+	49%	54%	61%
Doctors 'Always' Communicated Well	300+	81%	80%	82%
Home Recovery Information Given	300+	87%	86%	85%
Hospital Given 9 or 10 on 10 Point Scale	300+	71%	69%	71%
Meds 'Always' Explained Before Given	300+	62%	63%	64%
Nurses 'Always' Communicated Well	300+	80%	79%	79%
Pain 'Always' Well Controlled	300+	72%	70%	71%
Room and Bathroom 'Always' Clean	300+	74%	73%	73%
Timely Help 'Always' Received	300+	68%	67%	68%
Would Definitely Recommend Hospital	300+	76%	70%	71%
Use of Medical Imaging				
Cardiac Imaging Stress Test before Surgery	505	3.2%	5.4%	5.3%
Combination Abdominal CT Scan	1,488	6.5%	12.2%	10.5%
Combination Brain/Sinus CT Scan	910	4.5%	3.1%	2.7%
Combination Chest CT Scan	1,381	0.0%	2.1%	2.7%
Follow-up Mammogram/Ultrasound	1,503	7.9%	9%	8.8%
Lumbar Spine MRI for Low Back Pain	141	38.3%	35.8%	37.2%

Wilkes Barre VA Medical Center

1111 East End Boulevard
Wilkes-Barre, PA 18711
URL: www.va.gov
Type: Acute Care - VA
Ownership: Government Federal
Phone: 570-824-3521
Fax: 570-821-7264
Emergency Services: No
Beds: 111

Key Personnel:
Infection Control. . . . . Patricia Baldwin, RN
Anesthesiology. . . . . Mufti Basta, MD
Quality Assurance . . . . Yvonne Bohlander, RN
Chief of Medical Staff. . . . . William K Grossman, MD
CEO/President. . . . . Roland E Moore

Measure	Cases	This Hosp.	State Avg.	U.S. Avg.
Blood Clot Prevention and Treatment				
Anticoagulation Overlap Therapy	-	-	94%	93%
ICU Venous Thromboembolism Prophylaxis	-	-	94%	92%
Incidence of Potentially Preventable VTE	-	-	8%	10%
UFH with Dosages/Platelet Monitoring	-	-	98%	97%
Venous Thromboembolism Prophylaxis	-	-	90%	85%
Warfarin Therapy Discharge Instructions	-	-	78%	75%
Chest Pain/Possible Heart Attack Care				
Aspirin Given Within 24 Hours of Arrival	-	-	97%	96%
Fibrinolytic Meds Within 30 Min. of Arrival	-	-	44%	58%
Average Time to ECG (minutes)	-	-	9	7
Average Time to Transfer (minutes)	-	-	64	60
Children's Asthma Care				
Received Home Management Plan of Care	-	-	-	88%
Received Reliever Medication	-	-	-	100%
Received Systemic Corticosteroids	-	-	-	100%
Emergency Department				
Admittance Decision Time (minutes)	-	-	104	98
Head CT Results Within 45 Min. of Arrival	-	-	60%	57%
Patients Who Left ER Before Being Seen	-	-	1%	2%
Time from ER Arrival to Admit. (minutes)	-	-	276	274
Time from ER Arrival to Discharge (minutes)	-	-	125	134
Time in ER Before Being Evaluated (minutes)	-	-	26	26
Time to Pain Meds for Fractures (minutes)	-	-	58	57
Heart Attack Care				
Aspirin Given at Discharge[1]	15	100%	99%	99%
Fibrinolytic Meds Within 30 Min. of Arrival[5]	-	-	40%	54%
PCI Within 90 Minutes of Arrival[5]	-	-	97%	96%
Statin Prescribed at Discharge[1]	14	100%	99%	98%
Heart Failure Care				
ACE Inhibitor or ARB for LVSD	28	100%	97%	97%
Discharge Instructions Given	89	91%	96%	94%
Evaluation of LVS Function	104	100%	100%	99%
Medicare Spending				
Medicare Spending per Patient (ratio)	-	-	1.01	0.98
Pneumonia Care				
Appropriate Initial Antibiotic Given	50	96%	96%	95%
Blood Culture Timing	79	97%	98%	98%
Pregnancy and Delivery Care				
Newborn Deliveries Scheduled Early	-	-	4%	6%
Preventive Care				
Immunization for Influenza[5]	-	-	91%	90%
Immunization for Pneumonia[5]	-	-	92%	92%
Stroke Care				
Anticoagulation Therapy for Atrial Fibrillation	-	-	96%	95%
Antithrombotic Therapy Timing	-	-	98%	98%
Assessed for Rehabilitation	-	-	98%	97%
Discharged on Antithrombotic Therapy	-	-	99%	99%
Discharged on Statin Medication	-	-	95%	94%
Thrombolytic Therapy Timing	-	-	72%	66%
Venous Thromboembolism Prophylaxis	-	-	95%	94%
Written Stroke Educational Materials Given	-	-	90%	88%
Surgical Care Improvement Project				
Appropriate Beta Blocker Usage[2]	26	100%	98%	98%
Appropriate VTP Within 24 Hours[2]	67	97%	99%	98%
Controlled Postoperative Blood Glucose[5]	-	-	98%	97%
Perioperative Temperature Management[2]	71	97%	100%	100%
Prophylactic Antibiotic Selection	53	98%	99%	99%
Prophylactic Antibiotic Selection (Outpatient)	-	-	98%	98%
Prophylactic Antibiotic Stopped	51	96%	98%	98%
Prophylactic Antibiotic Timing	53	98%	99%	99%
Prophylactic Antibiotic Timing (Outpatient)	-	-	98%	98%
Urinary Catheter Removal[2]	57	98%	99%	97%
Survey of Patients' Hospital Experiences				
Area Around Room 'Always' Quiet at Night	-	-	54%	61%
Doctors 'Always' Communicated Well	-	-	80%	82%
Home Recovery Information Given	-	-	86%	85%
Hospital Given 9 or 10 on 10 Point Scale	-	-	69%	71%
Meds 'Always' Explained Before Given	-	-	63%	64%
Nurses 'Always' Communicated Well	-	-	79%	79%
Pain 'Always' Well Controlled	-	-	70%	71%
Room and Bathroom 'Always' Clean	-	-	73%	73%
Timely Help 'Always' Received	-	-	67%	68%
Would Definitely Recommend Hospital	-	-	70%	71%
Use of Medical Imaging				

NOTE: Hospital profiles are in alphabetical order by state, then city, then hospital within the city; Rankings exclude hospitals with less than 25 cases except for patient surveys which excludes hospitals with less than 100 cases; (a) 100-299 cases; (1) The number of cases/patients is too few to report; (2) Data submitted were based on a sample of cases/patients; (3) Results are based on a shorter time period than required; (4) Data suppressed by CMS for one or more quarters; (5) Results are not available for this reporting period; (6) Fewer than 100 patients completed the HCAHPS survey; (7) No cases met the criteria for this measure; (8) The lower limit of the confidence interval cannot be calculated if the number of observed infections equals zero; (9) No data are available from the state/territory for this reporting period; (10) The scores shown reflect fewer than 50 completed surveys; (11) There were discrepancies in the data collection process; (12) This measure does not apply to this hospital for this reporting period; (13) Results cannot be calculated for this reporting period; (14) The results for this state are combined with nearby states to protect confidentiality; Please refer to the User's Guide for a full explanation of data.

Cardiac Imaging Stress Test before Surgery	-	-	5.4%	5.3%
Combination Abdominal CT Scan	-	-	12.2%	10.5%
Combination Brain/Sinus CT Scan	-	-	3.1%	2.7%
Combination Chest CT Scan	-	-	2.1%	2.7%
Follow-up Mammogram/Ultrasound	-	-	9%	8.8%
Lumbar Spine MRI for Low Back Pain	-	-	35.8%	37.2%

Wilkes-Barre General Hospital

575 North River Street
Wilkes-Barre, PA 18764
Phone: 570-829-8111
Fax: 570-552-7410
URL: www.wvhcs.org
Type: Acute Care Hospitals
Emergency Services: Yes
Ownership: Voluntary non-profit - Private
Beds: 519

Key Personnel:
Infection Control. . . . . Nancy Alonzo
Chief of Medical Staff. . . . . Robert Brown
Pediatric Ambulatory Care . . . . . . Michael Imbrogno, MD
Pediatric In-Patient Care . . . . Michael Imbrogno, MD
Emergency Room . . . . Cynthia Liskof, MD
Quality Assurance . . . . Gwen Michaels
Radiology. . . . . N Shah, MD
CEO/President. . . . . Ron Stern

Measure	Cases	This Hosp.	State Avg.	U.S. Avg.
Blood Clot Prevention and Treatment				
Anticoagulation Overlap Therapy[2]	123	88%	94%	93%
ICU Venous Thromboembolism Prophylaxis[2]	108	88%	94%	92%
Incidence of Potentially Preventable VTE[2]	37	38%	8%	10%
UFH with Dosages/Platelet Monitoring[2]	105	100%	98%	97%
Venous Thromboembolism Prophylaxis[2]	535	73%	90%	85%
Warfarin Therapy Discharge Instructions[2]	72	56%	78%	75%
Chest Pain/Possible Heart Attack Care				
Aspirin Given Within 24 Hours of Arrival[5]	-	-	97%	96%
Fibrinolytic Meds Within 30 Min. of Arrival[5]	-	-	44%	58%
Average Time to ECG (minutes)[5]	-	-	9	7
Average Time to Transfer (minutes)[5]	-	-	64	60
Children's Asthma Care				
Received Home Management Plan of Care	-	-	-	88%
Received Reliever Medication	-	-	-	100%
Received Systemic Corticosteroids	-	-	-	100%
Emergency Department				
Admittance Decision Time (minutes)[2]	930	133	104	98
Head CT Results Within 45 Min. of Arrival[1]	-	-	60%	57%
Patients Who Left ER Before Being Seen	58,906	2%	1%	2%
Time from ER Arrival to Admit. (minutes)[2]	983	320	276	274
Time from ER Arrival to Discharge (minutes)	355	153	125	134
Time in ER Before Being Evaluated (minutes)	374	51	26	26
Time to Pain Meds for Fractures (minutes)	113	61	58	57
Heart Attack Care				
Aspirin Given at Discharge	311	99%	99%	99%
Fibrinolytic Meds Within 30 Min. of Arrival[7]	-	-	40%	54%
PCI Within 90 Minutes of Arrival	64	98%	97%	96%
Statin Prescribed at Discharge	293	97%	99%	98%
Heart Failure Care				
ACE Inhibitor or ARB for LVSD	127	97%	97%	97%
Discharge Instructions Given	326	98%	96%	94%
Evaluation of LVS Function	513	100%	100%	99%
Medicare Spending				
Medicare Spending per Patient (ratio)	-	1.21	1.01	0.98
Pneumonia Care				
Appropriate Initial Antibiotic Given	247	96%	96%	95%
Blood Culture Timing	406	98%	98%	98%
Pregnancy and Delivery Care				
Newborn Deliveries Scheduled Early[2]	28	0%	4%	6%
Preventive Care				
Immunization for Influenza[2]	672	88%	91%	90%
Immunization for Pneumonia[2]	969	89%	92%	92%
Stroke Care				
Anticoagulation Therapy for Atrial Fibrillation	35	86%	96%	95%
Antithrombotic Therapy Timing	149	98%	98%	98%
Assessed for Rehabilitation	195	96%	98%	97%
Discharged on Antithrombotic Therapy	168	99%	99%	99%
Discharged on Statin Medication	143	90%	95%	94%
Thrombolytic Therapy Timing[1]	-	-	72%	66%
Venous Thromboembolism Prophylaxis	202	88%	95%	94%
Written Stroke Educational Materials Given	80	75%	90%	88%
Surgical Care Improvement Project				
Appropriate Beta Blocker Usage	491	98%	98%	98%
Appropriate VTP Within 24 Hours	947	97%	99%	98%
Controlled Postoperative Blood Glucose	192	99%	98%	97%
Perioperative Temperature Management	1,086	100%	100%	100%
Prophylactic Antibiotic Selection	841	98%	99%	99%
Prophylactic Antibiotic Selection (Outpatient)	534	98%	98%	98%
Prophylactic Antibiotic Stopped	826	98%	98%	98%
Prophylactic Antibiotic Timing	841	99%	99%	99%
Prophylactic Antibiotic Timing (Outpatient)	545	97%	98%	98%
Urinary Catheter Removal	730	100%	99%	97%
Survey of Patients' Hospital Experiences				
Area Around Room 'Always' Quiet at Night	300+	51%	54%	61%
Doctors 'Always' Communicated Well	300+	80%	80%	82%
Home Recovery Information Given	300+	82%	86%	85%
Hospital Given 9 or 10 on 10 Point Scale	300+	64%	69%	71%
Meds 'Always' Explained Before Given	300+	61%	63%	64%
Nurses 'Always' Communicated Well	300+	78%	79%	79%
Pain 'Always' Well Controlled	300+	70%	70%	71%
Room and Bathroom 'Always' Clean	300+	68%	73%	73%
Timely Help 'Always' Received	300+	63%	67%	68%
Would Definitely Recommend Hospital	300+	66%	70%	71%
Use of Medical Imaging				
Cardiac Imaging Stress Test before Surgery	1,238	4.2%	5.4%	5.3%
Combination Abdominal CT Scan	2,185	34.1%	12.2%	10.5%
Combination Brain/Sinus CT Scan	1,643	3.2%	3.1%	2.7%
Combination Chest CT Scan	1,435	0.3%	2.1%	2.7%
Follow-up Mammogram/Ultrasound	3,695	6.1%	9%	8.8%
Lumbar Spine MRI for Low Back Pain	219	33.8%	35.8%	37.2%

Williamsport Regional Medical Center

700 High Street
Williamsport, PA 17701
Phone: 570-321-1000
URL: www.susquehannahealth.org
Type: Acute Care Hospitals
Emergency Services: Yes
Ownership: Voluntary non-profit - Other

Key Personnel:
CEO/President. . . . . Steven P Johnson

Measure	Cases	This Hosp.	State Avg.	U.S. Avg.
Blood Clot Prevention and Treatment				
Anticoagulation Overlap Therapy[2]	73	100%	94%	93%
ICU Venous Thromboembolism Prophylaxis[2]	109	94%	94%	92%
Incidence of Potentially Preventable VTE[1,2]	-	-	8%	10%
UFH with Dosages/Platelet Monitoring[2]	31	84%	98%	97%
Venous Thromboembolism Prophylaxis[2]	353	90%	90%	85%
Warfarin Therapy Discharge Instructions[2]	52	96%	78%	75%
Chest Pain/Possible Heart Attack Care				
Aspirin Given Within 24 Hours of Arrival[1,3]	-	-	97%	96%
Fibrinolytic Meds Within 30 Min. of Arrival[5]	-	-	44%	58%
Average Time to ECG (minutes)[1,3]	-	-	9	7
Average Time to Transfer (minutes)[5]	-	-	64	60
Children's Asthma Care				
Received Home Management Plan of Care	-	-	-	88%
Received Reliever Medication	-	-	-	100%
Received Systemic Corticosteroids	-	-	-	100%
Emergency Department				
Admittance Decision Time (minutes)[2]	303	84	104	98
Head CT Results Within 45 Min. of Arrival[1]	-	-	60%	57%
Patients Who Left ER Before Being Seen	22,877	2%	1%	2%
Time from ER Arrival to Admit. (minutes)[2]	570	280	276	274
Time from ER Arrival to Discharge (minutes)	544	148	125	134
Time in ER Before Being Evaluated (minutes)	503	44	26	26
Time to Pain Meds for Fractures (minutes)	178	86	58	57
Heart Attack Care				
Aspirin Given at Discharge	352	100%	99%	99%
Fibrinolytic Meds Within 30 Min. of Arrival[7]	-	-	40%	54%
PCI Within 90 Minutes of Arrival	44	98%	97%	96%
Statin Prescribed at Discharge	343	100%	99%	98%
Heart Failure Care				
ACE Inhibitor or ARB for LVSD	87	100%	97%	97%
Discharge Instructions Given	239	100%	96%	94%
Evaluation of LVS Function	289	100%	100%	99%
Medicare Spending				
Medicare Spending per Patient (ratio)	-	0.99	1.01	0.98
Pneumonia Care				
Appropriate Initial Antibiotic Given	126	100%	96%	95%
Blood Culture Timing	214	100%	98%	98%
Pregnancy and Delivery Care				
Newborn Deliveries Scheduled Early[2]	34	3%	4%	6%
Preventive Care				
Immunization for Influenza[2]	591	96%	91%	90%
Immunization for Pneumonia[2]	791	97%	92%	92%
Stroke Care				
Anticoagulation Therapy for Atrial Fibrillation	21	100%	96%	95%
Antithrombotic Therapy Timing	135	100%	98%	98%
Assessed for Rehabilitation	147	100%	98%	97%
Discharged on Antithrombotic Therapy	133	98%	99%	99%
Discharged on Statin Medication	101	98%	95%	94%
Thrombolytic Therapy Timing[1]	-	-	72%	66%
Venous Thromboembolism Prophylaxis	164	97%	95%	94%
Written Stroke Educational Materials Given	80	96%	90%	88%
Surgical Care Improvement Project				
Appropriate Beta Blocker Usage[2]	422	100%	98%	98%
Appropriate VTP Within 24 Hours[2]	989	100%	99%	98%
Controlled Postoperative Blood Glucose[2]	97	97%	98%	97%
Perioperative Temperature Management[2]	1,142	100%	100%	100%
Prophylactic Antibiotic Selection[2]	953	100%	99%	99%
Prophylactic Antibiotic Selection (Outpatient)	592	100%	98%	98%
Prophylactic Antibiotic Stopped[2]	939	99%	98%	98%
Prophylactic Antibiotic Timing[2]	955	99%	99%	99%
Prophylactic Antibiotic Timing (Outpatient)	590	98%	98%	98%
Urinary Catheter Removal[2]	839	100%	99%	97%
Survey of Patients' Hospital Experiences				
Area Around Room 'Always' Quiet at Night	300+	54%	54%	61%
Doctors 'Always' Communicated Well	300+	79%	80%	82%
Home Recovery Information Given	300+	87%	86%	85%
Hospital Given 9 or 10 on 10 Point Scale	300+	70%	69%	71%
Meds 'Always' Explained Before Given	300+	62%	63%	64%
Nurses 'Always' Communicated Well	300+	78%	79%	79%
Pain 'Always' Well Controlled	300+	71%	70%	71%
Room and Bathroom 'Always' Clean	300+	76%	73%	73%
Timely Help 'Always' Received	300+	61%	67%	68%
Would Definitely Recommend Hospital	300+	69%	70%	71%
Use of Medical Imaging				
Cardiac Imaging Stress Test before Surgery	593	3.0%	5.4%	5.3%
Combination Abdominal CT Scan	1,187	6.1%	12.2%	10.5%
Combination Brain/Sinus CT Scan[1]	-	-	3.1%	2.7%
Combination Chest CT Scan	610	0.8%	2.1%	2.7%
Follow-up Mammogram/Ultrasound[7]	-	-	9%	8.8%
Lumbar Spine MRI for Low Back Pain	123	33.3%	35.8%	37.2%

Windber Hospital

600 Somerset Avenue
Windber, PA 15963
Phone: 814-467-3000
Fax: 814-467-3451
E-mail: info@windbercare.com
URL: www.windbercare.com
Type: Acute Care Hospitals
Emergency Services: Yes
Ownership: Voluntary non-profit - Private
Beds: 82

Key Personnel:
Radiology. . . . . Jonathan Abraha, MD
Pediatric In-Patient Care . . . . Masood Boroumand, MD
Emergency Room . . . . James Eckenrod, MD
Anesthesiology. . . . . Libang Fu, RN
Chief of Medical Staff. . . . . Jerry L Gray, MD
Anesthesiology. . . . . John Johnson, RN
Cardiology . . . . Gorgi Kozeski, RN
Intensive Care Unit. . . . . Chris Spinos, RN

Measure	Cases	This Hosp.	State Avg.	U.S. Avg.
Blood Clot Prevention and Treatment				
Anticoagulation Overlap Therapy[2]	17	76%	94%	93%
ICU Venous Thromboembolism Prophylaxis[2]	34	76%	94%	92%
Incidence of Potentially Preventable VTE[1,2]	-	-	8%	10%
UFH with Dosages/Platelet Monitoring[1,2]	-	-	98%	97%
Venous Thromboembolism Prophylaxis[2]	104	68%	90%	85%
Warfarin Therapy Discharge Instructions[2]	12	67%	78%	75%
Chest Pain/Possible Heart Attack Care				

NOTE: Hospital profiles are in alphabetical order by state, then city, then hospital within the city; Rankings exclude hospitals with less than 25 cases except for patient surveys which excludes hospitals with less than 100 cases; (a) 100-299 cases; (1) The number of cases/patients is too few to report; (2) Data submitted were based on a sample of cases/patients; (3) Results are based on a shorter time period than required; (4) Data suppressed by CMS for one or more quarters; (5) Results are not available for this reporting period; (6) Fewer than 100 patients completed the HCAHPS survey; (7) No cases met the criteria for this measure; (8) The lower limit of the confidence interval cannot be calculated if the number of observed infections equals zero; (9) No data are available from the state/territory for this reporting period; (10) The scores shown reflect fewer than 50 completed surveys; (11) There were discrepancies in the data collection process; (12) This measure does not apply to this hospital for this reporting period; (13) Results cannot be calculated for this reporting period; (14) The results for this state are combined with nearby states to protect confidentiality; Please refer to the User's Guide for a full explanation of data.

Measure	Cases	This Hosp.	State Avg.	U.S. Avg.
Aspirin Given Within 24 Hours of Arrival	32	91%	97%	96%
Fibrinolytic Meds Within 30 Min. of Arrival[7]	-	-	44%	58%
Average Time to ECG (minutes)	33	8	9	7
Average Time to Transfer (minutes)[1]	-	-	64	60
Children's Asthma Care				
Received Home Management Plan of Care	-	-	-	88%
Received Reliever Medication	-	-	-	100%
Received Systemic Corticosteroids	-	-	-	100%
Emergency Department				
Admittance Decision Time (minutes)[2]	175	66	104	98
Head CT Results Within 45 Min. of Arrival[1]	-	-	60%	57%
Patients Who Left ER Before Being Seen	11,860	1%	1%	2%
Time from ER Arrival to Admit. (minutes)[2]	210	213	276	274
Time from ER Arrival to Discharge (minutes)	335	123	125	134
Time in ER Before Being Evaluated (minutes)	371	32	26	26
Time to Pain Meds for Fractures (minutes)	27	49	58	57
Heart Attack Care				
Aspirin Given at Discharge[1]	-	-	99%	99%
Fibrinolytic Meds Within 30 Min. of Arrival[7]	-	-	40%	54%
PCI Within 90 Minutes of Arrival[7]	-	-	97%	96%
Statin Prescribed at Discharge[1]	-	-	99%	98%
Heart Failure Care				
ACE Inhibitor or ARB for LVSD	12	83%	97%	97%
Discharge Instructions Given	50	82%	96%	94%
Evaluation of LVS Function	63	100%	100%	99%
Medicare Spending				
Medicare Spending per Patient (ratio)	-	0.97	1.01	0.98
Pneumonia Care				
Appropriate Initial Antibiotic Given	57	98%	96%	95%
Blood Culture Timing	67	100%	98%	98%
Pregnancy and Delivery Care				
Newborn Deliveries Scheduled Early[1]	-	-	4%	6%
Preventive Care				
Immunization for Influenza[2]	249	79%	91%	90%
Immunization for Pneumonia[2]	369	82%	92%	92%
Stroke Care				
Anticoagulation Therapy for Atrial Fibrillation[1]	-	-	96%	95%
Antithrombotic Therapy Timing[1]	-	-	98%	98%
Assessed for Rehabilitation[1]	-	-	98%	97%
Discharged on Antithrombotic Therapy[1]	-	-	99%	99%
Discharged on Statin Medication[1]	-	-	95%	94%
Thrombolytic Therapy Timing[7]	-	-	72%	66%
Venous Thromboembolism Prophylaxis[1]	-	-	95%	94%
Written Stroke Educational Materials Given[1]	-	-	90%	88%
Surgical Care Improvement Project				
Appropriate Beta Blocker Usage	33	97%	98%	98%
Appropriate VTP Within 24 Hours	100	100%	99%	98%
Controlled Postoperative Blood Glucose[7]	-	-	98%	97%
Perioperative Temperature Management	137	100%	100%	100%
Prophylactic Antibiotic Selection	94	99%	99%	99%
Prophylactic Antibiotic Selection (Outpatient)	39	100%	98%	98%
Prophylactic Antibiotic Stopped	90	99%	98%	98%
Prophylactic Antibiotic Timing	94	97%	99%	99%
Prophylactic Antibiotic Timing (Outpatient)	40	98%	98%	98%
Urinary Catheter Removal	56	96%	99%	97%
Survey of Patients' Hospital Experiences				
Area Around Room 'Always' Quiet at Night	300+	52%	54%	61%
Doctors 'Always' Communicated Well	300+	83%	80%	82%
Home Recovery Information Given	300+	83%	86%	85%
Hospital Given 9 or 10 on 10 Point Scale	300+	72%	69%	71%
Meds 'Always' Explained Before Given	300+	64%	63%	64%
Nurses 'Always' Communicated Well	300+	83%	79%	79%
Pain 'Always' Well Controlled	300+	72%	70%	71%
Room and Bathroom 'Always' Clean	300+	78%	73%	73%
Timely Help 'Always' Received	300+	70%	67%	68%
Would Definitely Recommend Hospital	300+	76%	70%	71%
Use of Medical Imaging				
Cardiac Imaging Stress Test before Surgery[1]	-	-	5.4%	5.3%
Combination Abdominal CT Scan	208	0.5%	12.2%	10.5%
Combination Brain/Sinus CT Scan[1]	-	-	3.1%	2.7%
Combination Chest CT Scan	120	0.0%	2.1%	2.7%
Follow-up Mammogram/Ultrasound	526	6.8%	9%	8.8%
Lumbar Spine MRI for Low Back Pain[1]	-	-	35.8%	37.2%

Main Line Hospital Lankenau

100 Lancaster Ave
Wynnewood, PA 19096
Phone: 610-645-2000
Fax: 610-645-8007
URL: www.mainlinehealth.org/lh
Type: Acute Care Hospitals
Emergency Services: Yes
Ownership: Voluntary non-profit - Private
Beds: 341

Key Personnel:

Quality Assurance . . . . Joan Anders
CEO/President. . . . . Phil Robinson

Measure	Cases	This Hosp.	State Avg.	U.S. Avg.
Blood Clot Prevention and Treatment				
Anticoagulation Overlap Therapy[2]	93	96%	94%	93%
ICU Venous Thromboembolism Prophylaxis[2]	79	95%	94%	92%
Incidence of Potentially Preventable VTE[2]	12	8%	8%	10%
UFH with Dosages/Platelet Monitoring[2]	107	97%	98%	97%
Venous Thromboembolism Prophylaxis[2]	346	97%	90%	85%
Warfarin Therapy Discharge Instructions[2]	57	42%	78%	75%
Chest Pain/Possible Heart Attack Care				
Aspirin Given Within 24 Hours of Arrival[1,3]	-	-	97%	96%
Fibrinolytic Meds Within 30 Min. of Arrival[5]	-	-	44%	58%
Average Time to ECG (minutes)[1,3]	-	-	9	7
Average Time to Transfer (minutes)[5]	-	-	64	60
Children's Asthma Care				
Received Home Management Plan of Care	-	-	-	88%
Received Reliever Medication	-	-	-	100%
Received Systemic Corticosteroids	-	-	-	100%
Emergency Department				
Admittance Decision Time (minutes)[2]	546	173	104	98
Head CT Results Within 45 Min. of Arrival[1]	-	-	60%	57%
Patients Who Left ER Before Being Seen	52,716	1%	1%	2%
Time from ER Arrival to Admit. (minutes)[2]	546	350	276	274
Time from ER Arrival to Discharge (minutes)	371	185	125	134
Time in ER Before Being Evaluated (minutes)	383	45	26	26
Time to Pain Meds for Fractures (minutes)	52	77	58	57
Heart Attack Care				
Aspirin Given at Discharge	276	100%	99%	99%
Fibrinolytic Meds Within 30 Min. of Arrival[7]	-	-	40%	54%
PCI Within 90 Minutes of Arrival	31	100%	97%	96%
Statin Prescribed at Discharge	271	100%	99%	98%
Heart Failure Care				
ACE Inhibitor or ARB for LVSD	223	100%	97%	97%
Discharge Instructions Given	533	99%	96%	94%
Evaluation of LVS Function	723	100%	100%	99%
Medicare Spending				
Medicare Spending per Patient (ratio)	-	1.01	1.01	0.98
Pneumonia Care				
Appropriate Initial Antibiotic Given	123	98%	96%	95%
Blood Culture Timing	313	98%	98%	98%
Pregnancy and Delivery Care				
Newborn Deliveries Scheduled Early[2]	28	21%	4%	6%
Preventive Care				
Immunization for Influenza[2]	545	79%	91%	90%
Immunization for Pneumonia[2]	714	82%	92%	92%
Stroke Care				
Anticoagulation Therapy for Atrial Fibrillation	22	100%	96%	95%
Antithrombotic Therapy Timing	154	100%	98%	98%
Assessed for Rehabilitation	174	100%	98%	97%
Discharged on Antithrombotic Therapy	158	100%	99%	99%
Discharged on Statin Medication	138	100%	95%	94%
Thrombolytic Therapy Timing[1]	-	-	72%	66%
Venous Thromboembolism Prophylaxis	175	100%	95%	94%
Written Stroke Educational Materials Given	79	94%	90%	88%
Surgical Care Improvement Project				
Appropriate Beta Blocker Usage[2]	517	100%	98%	98%
Appropriate VTP Within 24 Hours[2]	779	100%	99%	98%
Controlled Postoperative Blood Glucose[2]	446	99%	98%	97%
Perioperative Temperature Management[2]	1,270	100%	100%	100%
Prophylactic Antibiotic Selection[2]	1,249	100%	99%	99%
Prophylactic Antibiotic Selection (Outpatient)	352	98%	98%	98%
Prophylactic Antibiotic Stopped[2]	1,218	100%	98%	98%
Prophylactic Antibiotic Timing[2]	1,248	100%	99%	99%
Prophylactic Antibiotic Timing (Outpatient)	360	95%	98%	98%
Urinary Catheter Removal[2]	688	99%	99%	97%
Survey of Patients' Hospital Experiences				
Area Around Room 'Always' Quiet at Night	300+	56%	54%	61%
Doctors 'Always' Communicated Well	300+	82%	80%	82%
Home Recovery Information Given	300+	86%	86%	85%
Hospital Given 9 or 10 on 10 Point Scale	300+	77%	69%	71%
Meds 'Always' Explained Before Given	300+	65%	63%	64%
Nurses 'Always' Communicated Well	300+	80%	79%	79%
Pain 'Always' Well Controlled	300+	72%	70%	71%
Room and Bathroom 'Always' Clean	300+	68%	73%	73%
Timely Help 'Always' Received	300+	65%	67%	68%
Would Definitely Recommend Hospital	300+	82%	70%	71%
Use of Medical Imaging				
Cardiac Imaging Stress Test before Surgery	849	4.9%	5.4%	5.3%
Combination Abdominal CT Scan	1,336	10.7%	12.2%	10.5%
Combination Brain/Sinus CT Scan	1,068	1.6%	3.1%	2.7%
Combination Chest CT Scan	1,295	5.0%	2.1%	2.7%
Follow-up Mammogram/Ultrasound	2,698	17.2%	9%	8.8%
Lumbar Spine MRI for Low Back Pain	166	36.7%	35.8%	37.2%

Surgical Institute of Reading

2752 Century Boulevard
Wyomissing, PA 19610
Phone: 717-999-9999
URL: www.sireading.com
Type: Acute Care Hospitals
Emergency Services: No
Ownership: Proprietary

Key Personnel:

Administrator . . . . Deborah Beissel

Measure	Cases	This Hosp.	State Avg.	U.S. Avg.
Blood Clot Prevention and Treatment				
Anticoagulation Overlap Therapy[2,7]	-	-	94%	93%
ICU Venous Thromboembolism Prophylaxis[2,7]	-	-	94%	92%
Incidence of Potentially Preventable VTE[2,7]	-	-	8%	10%
UFH with Dosages/Platelet Monitoring[2,7]	-	-	98%	97%
Venous Thromboembolism Prophylaxis[2]	50	94%	90%	85%
Warfarin Therapy Discharge Instructions[2,7]	-	-	78%	75%
Chest Pain/Possible Heart Attack Care				
Aspirin Given Within 24 Hours of Arrival[5]	-	-	97%	96%
Fibrinolytic Meds Within 30 Min. of Arrival[5]	-	-	44%	58%
Average Time to ECG (minutes)[5]	-	-	9	7
Average Time to Transfer (minutes)[5]	-	-	64	60
Children's Asthma Care				
Received Home Management Plan of Care	-	-	-	88%
Received Reliever Medication	-	-	-	100%
Received Systemic Corticosteroids	-	-	-	100%
Emergency Department				
Admittance Decision Time (minutes)[2,7]	-	-	104	98
Head CT Results Within 45 Min. of Arrival[5]	-	-	60%	57%
Patients Who Left ER Before Being Seen[5]	-	-	1%	2%
Time from ER Arrival to Admit. (minutes)[2,7]	-	-	276	274
Time from ER Arrival to Discharge (minutes)[5]	-	-	125	134
Time in ER Before Being Evaluated (minutes)[5]	-	-	26	26
Time to Pain Meds for Fractures (minutes)[5]	-	-	58	57
Heart Attack Care				
Aspirin Given at Discharge[5]	-	-	99%	99%
Fibrinolytic Meds Within 30 Min. of Arrival[5]	-	-	40%	54%
PCI Within 90 Minutes of Arrival[5]	-	-	97%	96%
Statin Prescribed at Discharge[5]	-	-	99%	98%
Heart Failure Care				
ACE Inhibitor or ARB for LVSD[5]	-	-	97%	97%
Discharge Instructions Given[5]	-	-	96%	94%
Evaluation of LVS Function[5]	-	-	100%	99%
Medicare Spending				
Medicare Spending per Patient (ratio)	-	0.98	1.01	0.98
Pneumonia Care				
Appropriate Initial Antibiotic Given[5]	-	-	96%	95%
Blood Culture Timing[5]	-	-	98%	98%
Pregnancy and Delivery Care				
Newborn Deliveries Scheduled Early[7]	-	-	4%	6%
Preventive Care				
Immunization for Influenza[2]	197	91%	91%	90%
Immunization for Pneumonia[2]	213	82%	92%	92%

NOTE: Hospital profiles are in alphabetical order by state, then city, then hospital within the city; Rankings exclude hospitals with less than 25 cases except for patient surveys which excludes hospitals with less than 100 cases; (a) 100-299 cases; (1) The number of cases/patients is too few to report; (2) Data submitted were based on a sample of cases/patients; (3) Results are based on a shorter time period than required; (4) Data suppressed by CMS for one or more quarters; (5) Results are not available for this reporting period; (6) Fewer than 100 patients completed the HCAHPS survey; (7) No cases met the criteria for this measure; (8) The lower limit of the confidence interval cannot be calculated if the number of observed infections equals zero; (9) No data are available from the state/territory for this reporting period; (10) The scores shown reflect fewer than 50 completed surveys; (11) There were discrepancies in the data collection process; (12) This measure does not apply to this hospital for this reporting period; (13) Results cannot be calculated for this reporting period; (14) The results for this state are combined with nearby states to protect confidentiality; Please refer to the User's Guide for a full explanation of data.

Measure	Cases	This Hosp.	State Avg.	U.S. Avg.
Stroke Care				
Anticoagulation Therapy for Atrial Fibrillation[5]	-	-	96%	95%
Antithrombotic Therapy Timing[5]	-	-	98%	98%
Assessed for Rehabilitation[5]	-	-	98%	97%
Discharged on Antithrombotic Therapy[5]	-	-	99%	99%
Discharged on Statin Medication[5]	-	-	95%	94%
Thrombolytic Therapy Timing[5]	-	-	72%	66%
Venous Thromboembolism Prophylaxis[5]	-	-	95%	94%
Written Stroke Educational Materials Given[5]	-	-	90%	88%
Surgical Care Improvement Project				
Appropriate Beta Blocker Usage[2]	99	84%	98%	98%
Appropriate VTP Within 24 Hours[2]	414	98%	99%	98%
Controlled Postoperative Blood Glucose[2,7]	-	-	98%	97%
Perioperative Temperature Management[2]	419	99%	100%	100%
Prophylactic Antibiotic Selection[2]	392	99%	99%	99%
Prophylactic Antibiotic Selection (Outpatient)	177	97%	98%	98%
Prophylactic Antibiotic Stopped[2]	392	100%	98%	98%
Prophylactic Antibiotic Timing[2]	392	97%	99%	99%
Prophylactic Antibiotic Timing (Outpatient)	177	98%	98%	98%
Urinary Catheter Removal[2]	395	99%	99%	97%
Survey of Patients' Hospital Experiences				
Area Around Room 'Always' Quiet at Night	(a)	82%	54%	61%
Doctors 'Always' Communicated Well	(a)	89%	80%	82%
Home Recovery Information Given	(a)	94%	86%	85%
Hospital Given 9 or 10 on 10 Point Scale	(a)	92%	69%	71%
Meds 'Always' Explained Before Given	(a)	76%	63%	64%
Nurses 'Always' Communicated Well	(a)	94%	79%	79%
Pain 'Always' Well Controlled	(a)	85%	70%	71%
Room and Bathroom 'Always' Clean	(a)	89%	73%	73%
Timely Help 'Always' Received	(a)	93%	67%	68%
Would Definitely Recommend Hospital	(a)	95%	70%	71%
Use of Medical Imaging				
Cardiac Imaging Stress Test before Surgery[7]	-	-	5.4%	5.3%
Combination Abdominal CT Scan[1]	-	-	12.2%	10.5%
Combination Brain/Sinus CT Scan[1]	-	-	3.1%	2.7%
Combination Chest CT Scan[1]	-	-	2.1%	2.7%
Follow-up Mammogram/Ultrasound[7]	-	-	9%	8.8%
Lumbar Spine MRI for Low Back Pain[7]	-	-	35.8%	37.2%

Memorial Hospital

325 South Belmont Street
York, PA 17403
Phone: 717-843-8623
Fax: 717-849-5329
URL: www.mhyork.org
Type: Acute Care Hospitals
Emergency Services: Yes
Ownership: Voluntary non-profit - Private
Beds: 100

Key Personnel:

CEO/President. . . . . Sally J Dixon
Pediatric Ambulatory Care . . . . . . Philip Eppley, DO
Pediatric In-Patient Care . . . . Philip Eppley, DO
Infection Control. . . . . Carol Harvey, RN
Operating Room. . . . . Sandy Kimbrell, RN
Cardiac Laboratory. . . . . Jeanne Long
Quality Assurance . . . . Susan Nelson
Chief of Medical Staff. . . . . Hugh E Palmer, DO

Measure	Cases	This Hosp.	State Avg.	U.S. Avg.
Blood Clot Prevention and Treatment				
Anticoagulation Overlap Therapy[2]	86	91%	94%	93%
ICU Venous Thromboembolism Prophylaxis[2]	109	85%	94%	92%
Incidence of Potentially Preventable VTE[1,2]	-	-	8%	10%
UFH with Dosages/Platelet Monitoring[2]	68	99%	98%	97%
Venous Thromboembolism Prophylaxis[2]	370	80%	90%	85%
Warfarin Therapy Discharge Instructions[2]	71	23%	78%	75%
Chest Pain/Possible Heart Attack Care				
Aspirin Given Within 24 Hours of Arrival[1,3]	-	-	97%	96%
Fibrinolytic Meds Within 30 Min. of Arrival[3,7]	-	-	44%	58%
Average Time to ECG (minutes)[1,3]	-	-	9	7
Average Time to Transfer (minutes)[1,3]	-	-	64	60
Children's Asthma Care				
Received Home Management Plan of Care	-	-	-	88%
Received Reliever Medication	-	-	-	100%
Received Systemic Corticosteroids	-	-	-	100%
Emergency Department				
Admittance Decision Time (minutes)[2]	737	220	104	98
Head CT Results Within 45 Min. of Arrival[1]	-	-	60%	57%
Patients Who Left ER Before Being Seen	36,443	2%	1%	2%
Time from ER Arrival to Admit. (minutes)[2]	739	407	276	274
Time from ER Arrival to Discharge (minutes)	409	158	125	134
Time in ER Before Being Evaluated (minutes)	443	17	26	26
Time to Pain Meds for Fractures (minutes)	109	59	58	57
Heart Attack Care				
Aspirin Given at Discharge	118	100%	99%	99%
Fibrinolytic Meds Within 30 Min. of Arrival[7]	-	-	40%	54%
PCI Within 90 Minutes of Arrival	32	97%	97%	96%
Statin Prescribed at Discharge	110	95%	99%	98%
Heart Failure Care				
ACE Inhibitor or ARB for LVSD	49	100%	97%	97%
Discharge Instructions Given	111	100%	96%	94%
Evaluation of LVS Function	136	99%	100%	99%
Medicare Spending				
Medicare Spending per Patient (ratio)	-	0.98	1.01	0.98
Pneumonia Care				
Appropriate Initial Antibiotic Given	67	97%	96%	95%
Blood Culture Timing	175	99%	98%	98%
Pregnancy and Delivery Care				
Newborn Deliveries Scheduled Early[2]	29	7%	4%	6%
Preventive Care				
Immunization for Influenza[2]	527	98%	91%	90%
Immunization for Pneumonia[2]	694	96%	92%	92%
Stroke Care				
Anticoagulation Therapy for Atrial Fibrillation[1]	-	-	96%	95%
Antithrombotic Therapy Timing	44	98%	98%	98%
Assessed for Rehabilitation	48	96%	98%	97%
Discharged on Antithrombotic Therapy	47	100%	99%	99%
Discharged on Statin Medication	41	93%	95%	94%
Thrombolytic Therapy Timing[1]	-	-	72%	66%
Venous Thromboembolism Prophylaxis	47	83%	95%	94%
Written Stroke Educational Materials Given	31	100%	90%	88%
Surgical Care Improvement Project				
Appropriate Beta Blocker Usage	56	100%	98%	98%
Appropriate VTP Within 24 Hours	217	96%	99%	98%
Controlled Postoperative Blood Glucose[7]	-	-	98%	97%
Perioperative Temperature Management	243	100%	100%	100%
Prophylactic Antibiotic Selection	156	100%	99%	99%
Prophylactic Antibiotic Selection (Outpatient)	172	97%	98%	98%
Prophylactic Antibiotic Stopped	152	97%	98%	98%
Prophylactic Antibiotic Timing	156	99%	99%	99%
Prophylactic Antibiotic Timing (Outpatient)	178	89%	98%	98%
Urinary Catheter Removal	95	100%	99%	97%
Survey of Patients' Hospital Experiences				
Area Around Room 'Always' Quiet at Night	300+	51%	54%	61%
Doctors 'Always' Communicated Well	300+	75%	80%	82%
Home Recovery Information Given	300+	85%	86%	85%
Hospital Given 9 or 10 on 10 Point Scale	300+	66%	69%	71%
Meds 'Always' Explained Before Given	300+	62%	63%	64%
Nurses 'Always' Communicated Well	300+	76%	79%	79%
Pain 'Always' Well Controlled	300+	71%	70%	71%
Room and Bathroom 'Always' Clean	300+	68%	73%	73%
Timely Help 'Always' Received	300+	59%	67%	68%
Would Definitely Recommend Hospital	300+	71%	70%	71%
Use of Medical Imaging				
Cardiac Imaging Stress Test before Surgery	500	7.2%	5.4%	5.3%
Combination Abdominal CT Scan	687	19.5%	12.2%	10.5%
Combination Brain/Sinus CT Scan	485	4.3%	3.1%	2.7%
Combination Chest CT Scan	224	44.2%	2.1%	2.7%
Follow-up Mammogram/Ultrasound	693	12.7%	9%	8.8%
Lumbar Spine MRI for Low Back Pain[1]	-	-	35.8%	37.2%

Oss Orthopaedic Hospital

1861 Powder Mill Rd
York, PA 17402
Phone: 717-718-2000
URL: www.osshealth.com
Type: Acute Care Hospitals
Emergency Services: No
Ownership: Proprietary

Measure	Cases	This Hosp.	State Avg.	U.S. Avg.
Blood Clot Prevention and Treatment				
Anticoagulation Overlap Therapy[2,7]	-	-	94%	93%
ICU Venous Thromboembolism Prophylaxis[2,7]	-	-	94%	92%
Incidence of Potentially Preventable VTE[1,2]	-	-	8%	10%
UFH with Dosages/Platelet Monitoring[2,7]	-	-	98%	97%
Venous Thromboembolism Prophylaxis[2]	53	100%	90%	85%
Warfarin Therapy Discharge Instructions[2,7]	-	-	78%	75%
Chest Pain/Possible Heart Attack Care				
Aspirin Given Within 24 Hours of Arrival[5]	-	-	97%	96%
Fibrinolytic Meds Within 30 Min. of Arrival[5]	-	-	44%	58%
Average Time to ECG (minutes)[5]	-	-	9	7
Average Time to Transfer (minutes)[5]	-	-	64	60
Children's Asthma Care				
Received Home Management Plan of Care	-	-	-	88%
Received Reliever Medication	-	-	-	100%
Received Systemic Corticosteroids	-	-	-	100%
Emergency Department				
Admittance Decision Time (minutes)[2,7]	-	-	104	98
Head CT Results Within 45 Min. of Arrival[5]	-	-	60%	57%
Patients Who Left ER Before Being Seen[5]	-	-	1%	2%
Time from ER Arrival to Admit. (minutes)[2,7]	-	-	276	274
Time from ER Arrival to Discharge (minutes)[5]	-	-	125	134
Time in ER Before Being Evaluated (minutes)[5]	-	-	26	26
Time to Pain Meds for Fractures (minutes)[5]	-	-	58	57
Heart Attack Care				
Aspirin Given at Discharge[5]	-	-	99%	99%
Fibrinolytic Meds Within 30 Min. of Arrival[5]	-	-	40%	54%
PCI Within 90 Minutes of Arrival[5]	-	-	97%	96%
Statin Prescribed at Discharge[5]	-	-	99%	98%
Heart Failure Care				
ACE Inhibitor or ARB for LVSD[5]	-	-	97%	97%
Discharge Instructions Given[5]	-	-	96%	94%
Evaluation of LVS Function[5]	-	-	100%	99%
Medicare Spending				
Medicare Spending per Patient (ratio)	-	0.89	1.01	0.98
Pneumonia Care				
Appropriate Initial Antibiotic Given[5]	-	-	96%	95%
Blood Culture Timing[5]	-	-	98%	98%
Pregnancy and Delivery Care				
Newborn Deliveries Scheduled Early[7]	-	-	4%	6%
Preventive Care				
Immunization for Influenza[2]	394	89%	91%	90%
Immunization for Pneumonia[2]	465	92%	92%	92%
Stroke Care				
Anticoagulation Therapy for Atrial Fibrillation[5]	-	-	96%	95%
Antithrombotic Therapy Timing[5]	-	-	98%	98%
Assessed for Rehabilitation[5]	-	-	98%	97%
Discharged on Antithrombotic Therapy[5]	-	-	99%	99%
Discharged on Statin Medication[5]	-	-	95%	94%
Thrombolytic Therapy Timing[5]	-	-	72%	66%
Venous Thromboembolism Prophylaxis[5]	-	-	95%	94%
Written Stroke Educational Materials Given[5]	-	-	90%	88%
Surgical Care Improvement Project				
Appropriate Beta Blocker Usage[2]	89	100%	98%	98%
Appropriate VTP Within 24 Hours[2]	298	100%	99%	98%
Controlled Postoperative Blood Glucose[2,7]	-	-	98%	97%
Perioperative Temperature Management[2]	314	100%	100%	100%
Prophylactic Antibiotic Selection[2]	230	100%	99%	99%
Prophylactic Antibiotic Selection (Outpatient)	291	100%	98%	98%
Prophylactic Antibiotic Stopped[2]	228	100%	98%	98%
Prophylactic Antibiotic Timing[2]	230	99%	99%	99%
Prophylactic Antibiotic Timing (Outpatient)	291	99%	98%	98%
Urinary Catheter Removal[2]	106	100%	99%	97%
Survey of Patients' Hospital Experiences				
Area Around Room 'Always' Quiet at Night	300+	80%	54%	61%
Doctors 'Always' Communicated Well	300+	89%	80%	82%
Home Recovery Information Given	300+	94%	86%	85%
Hospital Given 9 or 10 on 10 Point Scale	300+	91%	69%	71%
Meds 'Always' Explained Before Given	300+	74%	63%	64%
Nurses 'Always' Communicated Well	300+	90%	79%	79%
Pain 'Always' Well Controlled	300+	78%	70%	71%
Room and Bathroom 'Always' Clean	300+	87%	73%	73%
Timely Help 'Always' Received	300+	79%	67%	68%
Would Definitely Recommend Hospital	300+	93%	70%	71%

NOTE: Hospital profiles are in alphabetical order by state, then city, then hospital within the city; Rankings exclude hospitals with less than 25 cases except for patient surveys which excludes hospitals with less than 100 cases; (a) 100-299 cases; (1) The number of cases/patients is too few to report; (2) Data submitted were based on a sample of cases/patients; (3) Results are based on a shorter time period than required; (4) Data suppressed by CMS for one or more quarters; (5) Results are not available for this reporting period; (6) Fewer than 100 patients completed the HCAHPS survey; (7) No cases met the criteria for this measure; (8) The lower limit of the confidence interval cannot be calculated if the number of observed infections equals zero; (9) No data are available from the state/territory for this reporting period; (10) The scores shown reflect fewer than 50 completed surveys; (11) There were discrepancies in the data collection process; (12) This measure does not apply to this hospital for this reporting period; (13) Results cannot be calculated for this reporting period; (14) The results for this state are combined with nearby states to protect confidentiality; Please refer to the User's Guide for a full explanation of data.

Use of Medical Imaging				
Cardiac Imaging Stress Test before Surgery[7]	-	-	5.4%	5.3%
Combination Abdominal CT Scan[1]	-	-	12.2%	10.5%
Combination Brain/Sinus CT Scan[7]	-	-	3.1%	2.7%
Combination Chest CT Scan[1]	-	-	2.1%	2.7%
Follow-up Mammogram/Ultrasound[7]	-	-	9%	8.8%
Lumbar Spine MRI for Low Back Pain	272	29.8%	35.8%	37.2%

Wellspan Surgery & Rehabilitation Hospital

55 Monument Road
York, PA 17403
Phone: 717-812-6100
URL: www.wellspan.org
Type: Acute Care Hospitals
Emergency Services: No
Ownership: Voluntary non-profit - Private

Measure	Cases	This Hosp.	State Avg.	U.S. Avg.
Blood Clot Prevention and Treatment				
Anticoagulation Overlap Therapy[2,7]	-	-	94%	93%
ICU Venous Thromboembolism Prophylaxis[2,7]	-	-	94%	92%
Incidence of Potentially Preventable VTE[2,7]	-	-	8%	10%
UFH with Dosages/Platelet Monitoring[2,7]	-	-	98%	97%
Venous Thromboembolism Prophylaxis[2]	22	100%	90%	85%
Warfarin Therapy Discharge Instructions[2,7]	-	-	78%	75%
Chest Pain/Possible Heart Attack Care				
Aspirin Given Within 24 Hours of Arrival[5]	-	-	97%	96%
Fibrinolytic Meds Within 30 Min. of Arrival[5]	-	-	44%	58%
Average Time to ECG (minutes)[5]	-	-	9	7
Average Time to Transfer (minutes)[5]	-	-	64	60
Children's Asthma Care				
Received Home Management Plan of Care	-	-	-	88%
Received Reliever Medication	-	-	-	100%
Received Systemic Corticosteroids	-	-	-	100%
Emergency Department				
Admittance Decision Time (minutes)[2,7]	-	-	104	98
Head CT Results Within 45 Min. of Arrival[5]	-	-	60%	57%
Patients Who Left ER Before Being Seen[5]	-	-	1%	2%
Time from ER Arrival to Admit. (minutes)[2,7]	-	-	276	274
Time from ER Arrival to Discharge (minutes)[5]	-	-	125	134
Time in ER Before Being Evaluated (minutes)[5]	-	-	26	26
Time to Pain Meds for Fractures (minutes)[5]	-	-	58	57
Heart Attack Care				
Aspirin Given at Discharge[5]	-	-	99%	99%
Fibrinolytic Meds Within 30 Min. of Arrival[5]	-	-	40%	54%
PCI Within 90 Minutes of Arrival[5]	-	-	97%	96%
Statin Prescribed at Discharge[5]	-	-	99%	98%
Heart Failure Care				
ACE Inhibitor or ARB for LVSD[5]	-	-	97%	97%
Discharge Instructions Given[5]	-	-	96%	94%
Evaluation of LVS Function[5]	-	-	100%	99%
Medicare Spending				
Medicare Spending per Patient (ratio)	-	0.85	1.01	0.98
Pneumonia Care				
Appropriate Initial Antibiotic Given[5]	-	-	96%	95%
Blood Culture Timing[5]	-	-	98%	98%
Pregnancy and Delivery Care				
Newborn Deliveries Scheduled Early[7]	-	-	4%	6%
Preventive Care				
Immunization for Influenza[2]	232	96%	91%	90%
Immunization for Pneumonia[2]	292	88%	92%	92%
Stroke Care				
Anticoagulation Therapy for Atrial Fibrillation[5]	-	-	96%	95%
Antithrombotic Therapy Timing[5]	-	-	98%	98%
Assessed for Rehabilitation[5]	-	-	98%	97%
Discharged on Antithrombotic Therapy[5]	-	-	99%	99%
Discharged on Statin Medication[5]	-	-	95%	94%
Thrombolytic Therapy Timing[5]	-	-	72%	66%
Venous Thromboembolism Prophylaxis[5]	-	-	95%	94%
Written Stroke Educational Materials Given[5]	-	-	90%	88%
Surgical Care Improvement Project				
Appropriate Beta Blocker Usage[2]	85	100%	98%	98%
Appropriate VTP Within 24 Hours[2]	268	100%	99%	98%
Controlled Postoperative Blood Glucose[2,7]	-	-	98%	97%
Perioperative Temperature Management[2]	302	100%	100%	100%
Prophylactic Antibiotic Selection[2]	217	100%	99%	99%
Prophylactic Antibiotic Selection (Outpatient)	119	100%	98%	98%
Prophylactic Antibiotic Stopped[2]	217	100%	98%	98%
Prophylactic Antibiotic Timing[2]	217	100%	99%	99%
Prophylactic Antibiotic Timing (Outpatient)	119	99%	98%	98%
Urinary Catheter Removal[2]	17	100%	99%	97%
Survey of Patients' Hospital Experiences				
Area Around Room 'Always' Quiet at Night	(a)	79%	54%	61%
Doctors 'Always' Communicated Well	(a)	89%	80%	82%
Home Recovery Information Given	(a)	94%	86%	85%
Hospital Given 9 or 10 on 10 Point Scale	(a)	92%	69%	71%
Meds 'Always' Explained Before Given	(a)	74%	63%	64%
Nurses 'Always' Communicated Well	(a)	94%	79%	79%
Pain 'Always' Well Controlled	(a)	81%	70%	71%
Room and Bathroom 'Always' Clean	(a)	87%	73%	73%
Timely Help 'Always' Received	(a)	91%	67%	68%
Would Definitely Recommend Hospital	(a)	94%	70%	71%
Use of Medical Imaging				
Cardiac Imaging Stress Test before Surgery[7]	-	-	5.4%	5.3%
Combination Abdominal CT Scan[7]	-	-	12.2%	10.5%
Combination Brain/Sinus CT Scan[7]	-	-	3.1%	2.7%
Combination Chest CT Scan[1]	-	-	2.1%	2.7%
Follow-up Mammogram/Ultrasound[7]	-	-	9%	8.8%
Lumbar Spine MRI for Low Back Pain[7]	-	-	35.8%	37.2%

York Hospital

1001 South George Street
York, PA 17403
Phone: 717-851-2345
Fax: 717-851-3100
URL: www.wellspan.org
Type: Acute Care Hospitals
Emergency Services: Yes
Ownership: Voluntary non-profit - Private
Beds: 466

Key Personnel:

Chief of Medical Staff. . . . . John H McConville, MD
Infection Control. . . . . John H McConville, MD
Operating Room. . . . . Dawn E Noll, RN
CEO/President. . . . . Keith D. Noll
Pediatric In-Patient Care . . . . David Turkewitz, MD

Measure	Cases	This Hosp.	State Avg.	U.S. Avg.
Blood Clot Prevention and Treatment				
Anticoagulation Overlap Therapy[2]	271	100%	94%	93%
ICU Venous Thromboembolism Prophylaxis[2]	77	99%	94%	92%
Incidence of Potentially Preventable VTE[2]	39	15%	8%	10%
UFH with Dosages/Platelet Monitoring[2]	199	100%	98%	97%
Venous Thromboembolism Prophylaxis[2]	361	88%	90%	85%
Warfarin Therapy Discharge Instructions[2]	196	96%	78%	75%
Chest Pain/Possible Heart Attack Care				
Aspirin Given Within 24 Hours of Arrival[3,7]	-	-	97%	96%
Fibrinolytic Meds Within 30 Min. of Arrival[5]	-	-	44%	58%
Average Time to ECG (minutes)[3,7]	-	-	9	7
Average Time to Transfer (minutes)[5]	-	-	64	60
Children's Asthma Care				
Received Home Management Plan of Care	-	-	-	88%
Received Reliever Medication	-	-	-	100%
Received Systemic Corticosteroids	-	-	-	100%
Emergency Department				
Admittance Decision Time (minutes)[2]	338	96	104	98
Head CT Results Within 45 Min. of Arrival[1]	-	-	60%	57%
Patients Who Left ER Before Being Seen	56,691	2%	1%	2%
Time from ER Arrival to Admit. (minutes)[2]	604	343	276	274
Time from ER Arrival to Discharge (minutes)	337	161	125	134
Time in ER Before Being Evaluated (minutes)	385	51	26	26
Time to Pain Meds for Fractures (minutes)	121	68	58	57
Heart Attack Care				
Aspirin Given at Discharge	683	100%	99%	99%
Fibrinolytic Meds Within 30 Min. of Arrival[7]	-	-	40%	54%
PCI Within 90 Minutes of Arrival	134	98%	97%	96%
Statin Prescribed at Discharge	687	99%	99%	98%
Heart Failure Care				
ACE Inhibitor or ARB for LVSD	217	96%	97%	97%
Discharge Instructions Given	639	96%	96%	94%
Evaluation of LVS Function	818	100%	100%	99%
Medicare Spending				
Medicare Spending per Patient (ratio)	-	1.01	1.01	0.98
Pneumonia Care				
Appropriate Initial Antibiotic Given	309	99%	96%	95%
Blood Culture Timing	398	96%	98%	98%
Pregnancy and Delivery Care				
Newborn Deliveries Scheduled Early[2]	36	0%	4%	6%
Preventive Care				
Immunization for Influenza[2]	518	97%	91%	90%
Immunization for Pneumonia[2]	660	95%	92%	92%
Stroke Care				
Anticoagulation Therapy for Atrial Fibrillation	74	99%	96%	95%
Antithrombotic Therapy Timing	263	98%	98%	98%
Assessed for Rehabilitation	410	99%	98%	97%
Discharged on Antithrombotic Therapy	346	100%	99%	99%
Discharged on Statin Medication	297	97%	95%	94%
Thrombolytic Therapy Timing	42	83%	72%	66%
Venous Thromboembolism Prophylaxis	401	96%	95%	94%
Written Stroke Educational Materials Given	196	93%	90%	88%
Surgical Care Improvement Project				
Appropriate Beta Blocker Usage[2]	518	99%	98%	98%
Appropriate VTP Within 24 Hours[2]	684	99%	99%	98%
Controlled Postoperative Blood Glucose[2]	395	99%	98%	97%
Perioperative Temperature Management[2]	956	100%	100%	100%
Prophylactic Antibiotic Selection[2]	833	100%	99%	99%
Prophylactic Antibiotic Selection (Outpatient)	674	98%	98%	98%
Prophylactic Antibiotic Stopped[2]	774	100%	98%	98%
Prophylactic Antibiotic Timing[2]	833	100%	99%	99%
Prophylactic Antibiotic Timing (Outpatient)	684	97%	98%	98%
Urinary Catheter Removal[2]	703	99%	99%	97%
Survey of Patients' Hospital Experiences				
Area Around Room 'Always' Quiet at Night	300+	42%	54%	61%
Doctors 'Always' Communicated Well	300+	73%	80%	82%
Home Recovery Information Given	300+	85%	86%	85%
Hospital Given 9 or 10 on 10 Point Scale	300+	67%	69%	71%
Meds 'Always' Explained Before Given	300+	54%	63%	64%
Nurses 'Always' Communicated Well	300+	75%	79%	79%
Pain 'Always' Well Controlled	300+	66%	70%	71%
Room and Bathroom 'Always' Clean	300+	70%	73%	73%
Timely Help 'Always' Received	300+	60%	67%	68%
Would Definitely Recommend Hospital	300+	70%	70%	71%
Use of Medical Imaging				
Cardiac Imaging Stress Test before Surgery	1,874	4.6%	5.4%	5.3%
Combination Abdominal CT Scan	2,120	7.8%	12.2%	10.5%
Combination Brain/Sinus CT Scan	1,557	2.3%	3.1%	2.7%
Combination Chest CT Scan	2,519	0.2%	2.1%	2.7%
Follow-up Mammogram/Ultrasound	5,869	8.5%	9%	8.8%
Lumbar Spine MRI for Low Back Pain	279	33.7%	35.8%	37.2%

NOTE: Hospital profiles are in alphabetical order by state, then city, then hospital within the city; Rankings exclude hospitals with less than 25 cases except for patient surveys which excludes hospitals with less than 100 cases; (a) 100-299 cases; (1) The number of cases/patients is too few to report; (2) Data submitted were based on a sample of cases/patients; (3) Results are based on a shorter time period than required; (4) Data suppressed by CMS for one or more quarters; (5) Results are not available for this reporting period; (6) Fewer than 100 patients completed the HCAHPS survey; (7) No cases met the criteria for this measure; (8) The lower limit of the confidence interval cannot be calculated if the number of observed infections equals zero; (9) No data are available from the state/territory for this reporting period; (10) The scores shown reflect fewer than 50 completed surveys; (11) There were discrepancies in the data collection process; (12) This measure does not apply to this hospital for this reporting period; (13) Results cannot be calculated for this reporting period; (14) The results for this state are combined with nearby states to protect confidentiality; Please refer to the User's Guide for a full explanation of data.

Blood Clot Prevention and Treatment

Anticoagulation Overlap Therapy

Hospital Name	City	Rate	Cases
Landmark Medical Center[2]	Woonsocket	100%	42
Miriam Hospital[2]	Providence	100%	131
Rhode Island Hospital[2]	Providence	99%	183
Newport Hospital[2]	Newport	97%	39
South County Hospital[2]	Wakefield	97%	30
Westerly Hospital[2]	Westerly	96%	28
Kent County Memorial Hospital[2]	Warwick	94%	117
Memorial Hospital of Rhode Island[2]	Pawtucket	94%	47
Saint Joseph Health Services of RI[2]	N Providence	94%	71

ICU Venous Thromboembolism Prophylaxis

Hospital Name	City	Rate	Cases
Kent County Memorial Hospital[2]	Warwick	97%	35
Memorial Hospital of Rhode Island[2]	Pawtucket	97%	77
Newport Hospital[2]	Newport	94%	85
Westerly Hospital[2]	Westerly	94%	47
Rhode Island Hospital[2]	Providence	90%	88
Miriam Hospital[2]	Providence	89%	71
Landmark Medical Center[2]	Woonsocket	87%	47
Saint Joseph Health Services of RI[2]	N Providence	87%	39
South County Hospital[2]	Wakefield	85%	47

Incidence of Potentially Preventable VTE

Hospital Name	City	Rate	Cases
Rhode Island Hospital[2]	Providence	5%	40

UFH with Dosages/Platelet Count Monitoring

Hospital Name	City	Rate	Cases
Kent County Memorial Hospital[2]	Warwick	100%	99
Landmark Medical Center[2]	Woonsocket	100%	41
Memorial Hospital of Rhode Island[2]	Pawtucket	100%	42
Miriam Hospital[2]	Providence	100%	92
Saint Joseph Health Services of RI[2]	N Providence	100%	45
Rhode Island Hospital[2]	Providence	99%	144

Venous Thromboembolism Prophylaxis

Hospital Name	City	Rate	Cases
Memorial Hospital of Rhode Island[2]	Pawtucket	94%	335
Miriam Hospital[2]	Providence	93%	357
Westerly Hospital[2]	Westerly	91%	295
Newport Hospital[2]	Newport	88%	279
Rhode Island Hospital[2]	Providence	88%	319
Roger Williams Medical Center[2]	Providence	84%	265
Landmark Medical Center[2]	Woonsocket	82%	408
Kent County Memorial Hospital[2]	Warwick	78%	319
South County Hospital[2]	Wakefield	78%	230
Women & Infants Hospital of Rhode Island[2]	Providence	76%	140
Saint Joseph Health Services of RI[2]	N Providence	74%	363

Warfarin Therapy Discharge Instructions

Hospital Name	City	Rate	Cases
Miriam Hospital[2]	Providence	85%	98
Landmark Medical Center[2]	Woonsocket	79%	34
Newport Hospital[2]	Newport	79%	34
Saint Joseph Health Services of RI[2]	N Providence	76%	45
Memorial Hospital of Rhode Island[2]	Pawtucket	62%	37
Kent County Memorial Hospital[2]	Warwick	52%	85
Rhode Island Hospital[2]	Providence	28%	123

Chest Pain/Possible Heart Attack Care

Aspirin Given Within 24 Hours of Arrival

Hospital Name	City	Rate	Cases
Newport Hospital	Newport	100%	81
Westerly Hospital	Westerly	100%	59
Kent County Memorial Hospital	Warwick	99%	147
South County Hospital	Wakefield	94%	33
Saint Joseph Health Services of RI	N Providence	88%	50

Average Time to ECG (minutes)

Hospital Name	City	Min.	Cases
Newport Hospital	Newport	6	83
Westerly Hospital	Westerly	9	60
Kent County Memorial Hospital	Warwick	10	151
Saint Joseph Health Services of RI	N Providence	14	52

Children's Asthma Care

No hospitals met the 25 case threshold.

Emergency Department

Admittance Decision Time (minutes)

Hospital Name	City	Min.	Cases
Women & Infants Hospital of Rhode Island[2]	Providence	58	427
Westerly Hospital[2]	Westerly	84	351
Miriam Hospital[2]	Providence	99	752
Newport Hospital[2]	Newport	102	409
South County Hospital[2]	Wakefield	103	335
Roger Williams Medical Center[2]	Providence	115	508
Rhode Island Hospital[2]	Providence	117	795
Memorial Hospital of Rhode Island[2]	Pawtucket	126	748
Landmark Medical Center[2]	Woonsocket	128	956
Saint Joseph Health Services of RI[2]	N Providence	146	673
Kent County Memorial Hospital[2]	Warwick	172	694

Patients Who Left ER Before Being Seen

Hospital Name	City	Rate	Cases
Kent County Memorial Hospital	Warwick	1%	70105
South County Hospital	Wakefield	1%	26958
Westerly Hospital	Westerly	1%	23229
Landmark Medical Center	Woonsocket	2%	40589
Memorial Hospital of Rhode Island	Pawtucket	2%	34408
Miriam Hospital	Providence	2%	60035
Saint Joseph Health Services of RI	N Providence	2%	25871
Women & Infants Hospital of Rhode Island	Providence	2%	28753
Newport Hospital	Newport	3%	31947
Roger Williams Medical Center	Providence	3%	26087
Rhode Island Hospital	Providence	4%	159584

Time from ER Arrival to Being Admitted (minutes)

Hospital Name	City	Min.	Cases
Women & Infants Hospital of Rhode Island[2]	Providence	141	429
Newport Hospital[2]	Newport	284	412
Miriam Hospital[2]	Providence	312	752
Westerly Hospital[2]	Westerly	312	388
South County Hospital[2]	Wakefield	324	354
Memorial Hospital of Rhode Island[2]	Pawtucket	326	748
Roger Williams Medical Center[2]	Providence	346	508
Landmark Medical Center[2]	Woonsocket	348	962
Kent County Memorial Hospital[2]	Warwick	357	697
Rhode Island Hospital[2]	Providence	388	795
Saint Joseph Health Services of RI[2]	N Providence	390	679

Time from ER Arrival to Discharge (minutes)

Hospital Name	City	Min.	Cases
Landmark Medical Center	Woonsocket	116	1516
Westerly Hospital	Westerly	116	320
Kent County Memorial Hospital	Warwick	146	321
Newport Hospital	Newport	146	359
South County Hospital	Wakefield	151	404
Memorial Hospital of Rhode Island	Pawtucket	166	386
Saint Joseph Health Services of RI	N Providence	170	396
Women & Infants Hospital of Rhode Island	Providence	171	381
Roger Williams Medical Center	Providence	185	339
Miriam Hospital	Providence	207	541
Rhode Island Hospital	Providence	246	347

Time in ER Before Being Evaluated (minutes)

Hospital Name	City	Min.	Cases
South County Hospital	Wakefield	25	448
Saint Joseph Health Services of RI	N Providence	26	473
Kent County Memorial Hospital	Warwick	27	189
Landmark Medical Center	Woonsocket	29	1727
Women & Infants Hospital of Rhode Island	Providence	29	406
Memorial Hospital of Rhode Island	Pawtucket	31	455
Westerly Hospital	Westerly	35	350
Newport Hospital	Newport	53	402
Miriam Hospital	Providence	57	644
Roger Williams Medical Center	Providence	71	401
Rhode Island Hospital	Providence	86	402

Time to Pain Meds for Bone Fractures (minutes)

Hospital Name	City	Min.	Cases
Rhode Island Hospital	Providence	40	338
Kent County Memorial Hospital	Warwick	49	157
Landmark Medical Center	Woonsocket	51	82
Westerly Hospital	Westerly	53	45
South County Hospital	Wakefield	58	174
Newport Hospital	Newport	59	115
Miriam Hospital	Providence	71	81
Memorial Hospital of Rhode Island	Pawtucket	72	32
Roger Williams Medical Center	Providence	78	44
Saint Joseph Health Services of RI	N Providence	84	80

Heart Attack Care

Aspirin Given at Discharge

Hospital Name	City	Rate	Cases
Landmark Medical Center	Woonsocket	100%	167
Miriam Hospital	Providence	100%	494
Rhode Island Hospital	Providence	100%	720
Saint Joseph Health Services of RI	N Providence	100%	29
Westerly Hospital	Westerly	100%	28
Kent County Memorial Hospital[2]	Warwick	99%	139
Memorial Hospital of Rhode Island	Pawtucket	97%	30
Roger Williams Medical Center	Providence	97%	63

PCI Within 90 Minutes of Arrival

Hospital Name	City	Rate	Cases
Miriam Hospital	Providence	98%	88
Rhode Island Hospital	Providence	98%	104
Landmark Medical Center	Woonsocket	97%	32

Statin Prescribed at Discharge

Hospital Name	City	Rate	Cases
Rhode Island Hospital	Providence	100%	695
Miriam Hospital	Providence	99%	484
Landmark Medical Center	Woonsocket	95%	152
Memorial Hospital of Rhode Island	Pawtucket	93%	27
Kent County Memorial Hospital[2]	Warwick	86%	141
Westerly Hospital	Westerly	81%	27
Roger Williams Medical Center	Providence	78%	58

Heart Failure Care

ACE Inhibitor or ARB for LVSD

Hospital Name	City	Rate	Cases
Newport Hospital	Newport	100%	35
Rhode Island Hospital[2]	Providence	100%	86
Miriam Hospital[2]	Providence	99%	140
Providence VA Medical Center	Providence	97%	30
Saint Joseph Health Services of RI	N Providence	97%	32
Westerly Hospital	Westerly	97%	29
Landmark Medical Center	Woonsocket	96%	45
South County Hospital	Wakefield	93%	28
Memorial Hospital of Rhode Island	Pawtucket	86%	50
Kent County Memorial Hospital	Warwick	83%	94

Discharge Instructions Given

Hospital Name	City	Rate	Cases
Roger Williams Medical Center	Providence	100%	62
Memorial Hospital of Rhode Island	Pawtucket	98%	147
Providence VA Medical Center	Providence	98%	106
South County Hospital	Wakefield	98%	103
Saint Joseph Health Services of RI	N Providence	97%	147
Landmark Medical Center	Woonsocket	96%	180
Newport Hospital	Newport	96%	94
Miriam Hospital[2]	Providence	92%	406
Rhode Island Hospital[2]	Providence	87%	233
Kent County Memorial Hospital	Warwick	84%	296
Westerly Hospital	Westerly	79%	92

Evaluation of LVS Function

Hospital Name	City	Rate	Cases
Kent County Memorial Hospital	Warwick	100%	420
Landmark Medical Center	Woonsocket	100%	257
Miriam Hospital[2]	Providence	100%	541
Newport Hospital	Newport	100%	139
Providence VA Medical Center	Providence	100%	126
Rhode Island Hospital[2]	Providence	100%	291
South County Hospital	Wakefield	100%	133
Westerly Hospital	Westerly	100%	131
Memorial Hospital of Rhode Island	Pawtucket	99%	198
Saint Joseph Health Services of RI	N Providence	99%	257
Roger Williams Medical Center	Providence	97%	112

Medicare Spending

Medicare Spending per Patient (ratio)

Hospital Name	City	Ratio	Cases
South County Hospital	Wakefield	0.92	-
Rhode Island Hospital	Providence	0.99	-
Westerly Hospital	Westerly	1.00	-
Women & Infants Hospital of Rhode Island	Providence	1.00	-
Newport Hospital	Newport	1.01	-
Memorial Hospital of Rhode Island	Pawtucket	1.02	-
Miriam Hospital	Providence	1.02	-
Roger Williams Medical Center	Providence	1.02	-
Kent County Memorial Hospital	Warwick	1.06	-
Landmark Medical Center	Woonsocket	1.06	-
Saint Joseph Health Services of RI	N Providence	1.08	-

NOTE: Hospital profiles are in alphabetical order by state, then city, then hospital within the city; Rankings exclude hospitals with less than 25 cases except for patient surveys which excludes hospitals with less than 100 cases; (a) 100-299 cases; (1) The number of cases/patients is too few to report; (2) Data submitted were based on a sample of cases/patients; (3) Results are based on a shorter time period than required; (4) Data suppressed by CMS for one or more quarters; (5) Results are not available for this reporting period; (6) Fewer than 100 patients completed the HCAHPS survey; (7) No cases met the criteria for this measure; (8) The lower limit of the confidence interval cannot be calculated if the number of observed infections equals zero; (9) No data are available from the state/territory for this reporting period; (10) The scores shown reflect fewer than 50 completed surveys; (11) There were discrepancies in the data collection process; (12) This measure does not apply to this hospital for this reporting period; (13) Results cannot be calculated for this reporting period; (14) The results for this state are combined with nearby states to protect confidentiality; Please refer to the User's Guide for a full explanation of data.

Pneumonia Care

Appropriate Initial Antibiotic Given

Hospital Name	City	Rate	Cases
Providence VA Medical Center	Providence	100%	49
South County Hospital	Wakefield	100%	51
Landmark Medical Center	Woonsocket	99%	133
Miriam Hospital[2]	Providence	99%	152
Roger Williams Medical Center	Providence	99%	67
Newport Hospital	Newport	98%	89
Rhode Island Hospital[2]	Providence	98%	56
Saint Joseph Health Services of RI	N Providence	94%	89
Westerly Hospital	Westerly	94%	71
Kent County Memorial Hospital[2]	Warwick	93%	103
Memorial Hospital of Rhode Island[2]	Pawtucket	93%	67

Blood Culture Timing

Hospital Name	City	Rate	Cases
Newport Hospital	Newport	99%	138
Miriam Hospital[2]	Providence	98%	288
Landmark Medical Center	Woonsocket	97%	146
Providence VA Medical Center	Providence	97%	98
South County Hospital	Wakefield	97%	120
Memorial Hospital of Rhode Island[2]	Pawtucket	96%	118
Rhode Island Hospital[2]	Providence	96%	144
Roger Williams Medical Center	Providence	96%	136
Westerly Hospital	Westerly	96%	108
Saint Joseph Health Services of RI	N Providence	94%	146
Kent County Memorial Hospital[2]	Warwick	93%	214

Pregnancy and Delivery Care

Newborns whose Deliveries were Scheduled Early

Hospital Name	City	Rate	Cases
Kent County Memorial Hospital	Warwick	1%	129
Women & Infants Hospital of Rhode Island[2]	Providence	1%	100
Newport Hospital	Newport	23%	47

Preventive Care

Immunization for Influenza

Hospital Name	City	Rate	Cases
Landmark Medical Center[2]	Woonsocket	96%	551
Memorial Hospital of Rhode Island[2]	Pawtucket	96%	535
Kent County Memorial Hospital[2]	Warwick	95%	557
South County Hospital[2]	Wakefield	94%	486
Newport Hospital[2]	Newport	93%	358
Women & Infants Hospital of Rhode Island[2]	Providence	91%	333
Saint Joseph Health Services of RI[2]	N Providence	90%	601
Westerly Hospital[2]	Westerly	87%	303
Miriam Hospital[2]	Providence	84%	616
Roger Williams Medical Center[2]	Providence	72%	613
Rhode Island Hospital[2]	Providence	67%	574

Immunization for Pneumonia

Hospital Name	City	Rate	Cases
Kent County Memorial Hospital[2]	Warwick	97%	727
Memorial Hospital of Rhode Island[2]	Pawtucket	97%	672
South County Hospital[2]	Wakefield	97%	680
Landmark Medical Center[2]	Woonsocket	95%	866
Newport Hospital[2]	Newport	94%	436
Saint Joseph Health Services of RI[2]	N Providence	92%	724
Westerly Hospital[2]	Westerly	86%	458
Miriam Hospital[2]	Providence	83%	955
Rhode Island Hospital[2]	Providence	71%	645
Women & Infants Hospital of Rhode Island[2]	Providence	62%	80
Roger Williams Medical Center[2]	Providence	53%	752

Stroke Care

Anticoagulation Therapy for Atrial Fibrillation

Hospital Name	City	Rate	Cases
Miriam Hospital	Providence	97%	38
Rhode Island Hospital	Providence	95%	56
Kent County Memorial Hospital	Warwick	92%	26

Antithrombotic Therapy Timing

Hospital Name	City	Rate	Cases
Landmark Medical Center	Woonsocket	100%	59
Memorial Hospital of Rhode Island	Pawtucket	100%	39
Roger Williams Medical Center	Providence	100%	30
Westerly Hospital	Westerly	100%	26
Kent County Memorial Hospital	Warwick	99%	128
Miriam Hospital	Providence	99%	185
Newport Hospital	Newport	98%	56
South County Hospital	Wakefield	98%	47
Rhode Island Hospital	Providence	96%	235

Assessed for Rehabilitation

Hospital Name	City	Rate	Cases
Kent County Memorial Hospital	Warwick	100%	150
Memorial Hospital of Rhode Island	Pawtucket	100%	42
Miriam Hospital	Providence	100%	209
South County Hospital	Wakefield	100%	56
Landmark Medical Center	Woonsocket	97%	59
Newport Hospital	Newport	97%	61
Westerly Hospital	Westerly	96%	26
Rhode Island Hospital	Providence	94%	504
Roger Williams Medical Center	Providence	92%	38

Discharged on Antithrombotic Therapy

Hospital Name	City	Rate	Cases
Kent County Memorial Hospital	Warwick	100%	148
Miriam Hospital	Providence	100%	203
Rhode Island Hospital	Providence	100%	357
Roger Williams Medical Center	Providence	100%	36
South County Hospital	Wakefield	100%	52
Westerly Hospital	Westerly	100%	26
Memorial Hospital of Rhode Island	Pawtucket	98%	42
Newport Hospital	Newport	98%	59
Landmark Medical Center	Woonsocket	97%	59

Discharged on Statin Medication

Hospital Name	City	Rate	Cases
Memorial Hospital of Rhode Island	Pawtucket	100%	31
Miriam Hospital	Providence	99%	172
Newport Hospital	Newport	98%	47
Rhode Island Hospital	Providence	97%	289
South County Hospital	Wakefield	97%	39
Roger Williams Medical Center	Providence	96%	28
Kent County Memorial Hospital	Warwick	94%	115
Landmark Medical Center	Woonsocket	88%	41

Thrombolytic Therapy Timing

Hospital Name	City	Rate	Cases
Miriam Hospital	Providence	88%	33
Rhode Island Hospital	Providence	87%	54

Venous Thromboembolism (VTE) Prophylaxis

Hospital Name	City	Rate	Cases
Memorial Hospital of Rhode Island	Pawtucket	100%	42
Miriam Hospital	Providence	98%	191
Rhode Island Hospital	Providence	96%	489
South County Hospital	Wakefield	94%	49
Kent County Memorial Hospital	Warwick	93%	153
Newport Hospital	Newport	93%	61
Landmark Medical Center	Woonsocket	92%	64
Roger Williams Medical Center	Providence	92%	36
Westerly Hospital	Westerly	88%	25

Written Stroke Educational Materials Given

Hospital Name	City	Rate	Cases
Newport Hospital	Newport	100%	34
Kent County Memorial Hospital	Warwick	97%	76
South County Hospital	Wakefield	96%	26
Miriam Hospital	Providence	94%	99
Rhode Island Hospital	Providence	92%	261
Landmark Medical Center	Woonsocket	80%	25
Memorial Hospital of Rhode Island	Pawtucket	71%	28

Surgical Care Improvement Project

Appropriate Beta Blocker Usage

Hospital Name	City	Rate	Cases
Kent County Memorial Hospital[2]	Warwick	99%	183
Newport Hospital	Newport	99%	84
Rhode Island Hospital[2]	Providence	99%	299
Saint Joseph Health Services of RI[2]	N Providence	99%	105
Landmark Medical Center	Woonsocket	98%	83
Memorial Hospital of Rhode Island	Pawtucket	98%	57
Miriam Hospital[2]	Providence	98%	399
Providence VA Medical Center[2]	Providence	98%	43
Roger Williams Medical Center	Providence	97%	146
South County Hospital[2]	Wakefield	97%	73
Westerly Hospital	Westerly	97%	64

Appropriate VTP Within 24 Hours

Hospital Name	City	Rate	Cases
Providence VA Medical Center[2]	Providence	100%	90
Memorial Hospital of Rhode Island	Pawtucket	99%	195
Miriam Hospital[2]	Providence	99%	1132
Rhode Island Hospital[2]	Providence	99%	366
South County Hospital[2]	Wakefield	99%	310
Saint Joseph Health Services of RI[2]	N Providence	98%	348
Women & Infants Hospital of Rhode Island[2]	Providence	98%	166
Roger Williams Medical Center	Providence	97%	471
Kent County Memorial Hospital[2]	Warwick	96%	512
Landmark Medical Center	Woonsocket	96%	164
Newport Hospital	Newport	96%	244
Westerly Hospital	Westerly	95%	163

Controlled Postoperative Blood Glucose

Hospital Name	City	Rate	Cases
Rhode Island Hospital[2]	Providence	98%	162

Perioperative Temperature Management

Hospital Name	City	Rate	Cases
Kent County Memorial Hospital[2]	Warwick	100%	569
Landmark Medical Center	Woonsocket	100%	221
Memorial Hospital of Rhode Island	Pawtucket	100%	229
Miriam Hospital[2]	Providence	100%	1268
Newport Hospital	Newport	100%	264
Providence VA Medical Center[2]	Providence	100%	106
Rhode Island Hospital[2]	Providence	100%	493
Roger Williams Medical Center	Providence	100%	499
South County Hospital[2]	Wakefield	100%	378
Westerly Hospital	Westerly	100%	189
Women & Infants Hospital of Rhode Island[2]	Providence	100%	218
Saint Joseph Health Services of RI[2]	N Providence	98%	362

Prophylactic Antibiotic Selection

Hospital Name	City	Rate	Cases
Newport Hospital	Newport	100%	174
Providence VA Medical Center	Providence	100%	62
Westerly Hospital	Westerly	100%	131
Landmark Medical Center	Woonsocket	99%	123
Miriam Hospital[2]	Providence	99%	835
Rhode Island Hospital[2]	Providence	99%	425
Roger Williams Medical Center	Providence	99%	280
Kent County Memorial Hospital[2]	Warwick	98%	358
Saint Joseph Health Services of RI[2]	N Providence	98%	222
South County Hospital[2]	Wakefield	98%	257
Women & Infants Hospital of Rhode Island[2]	Providence	98%	107
Memorial Hospital of Rhode Island	Pawtucket	97%	135

Prophylactic Antibiotic Selection (Outpatient)

Hospital Name	City	Rate	Cases
Landmark Medical Center	Woonsocket	100%	84
Memorial Hospital of Rhode Island	Pawtucket	100%	86
Rhode Island Hospital	Providence	100%	483
Westerly Hospital	Westerly	100%	61
Miriam Hospital	Providence	99%	290
Roger Williams Medical Center	Providence	99%	70
Women & Infants Hospital of Rhode Island	Providence	99%	712
Saint Joseph Health Services of RI	N Providence	97%	315
South County Hospital	Wakefield	96%	84
Newport Hospital	Newport	95%	59
Kent County Memorial Hospital	Warwick	92%	246

Prophylactic Antibiotic Stopped

Hospital Name	City	Rate	Cases
Providence VA Medical Center	Providence	100%	60
Roger Williams Medical Center	Providence	100%	276
Saint Joseph Health Services of RI[2]	N Providence	100%	221
Memorial Hospital of Rhode Island	Pawtucket	99%	130
Miriam Hospital[2]	Providence	99%	825
Rhode Island Hospital[2]	Providence	99%	408
South County Hospital[2]	Wakefield	99%	256
Newport Hospital	Newport	98%	171
Westerly Hospital	Westerly	98%	126
Women & Infants Hospital of Rhode Island[2]	Providence	98%	107
Landmark Medical Center	Woonsocket	97%	114
Kent County Memorial Hospital[2]	Warwick	96%	349

Prophylactic Antibiotic Timing

Hospital Name	City	Rate	Cases
Providence VA Medical Center	Providence	100%	62
Rhode Island Hospital[2]	Providence	100%	428
Roger Williams Medical Center	Providence	100%	280
Saint Joseph Health Services of RI[2]	N Providence	100%	223
Westerly Hospital	Westerly	100%	131
Landmark Medical Center	Woonsocket	99%	124
Memorial Hospital of Rhode Island	Pawtucket	99%	135
Miriam Hospital[2]	Providence	99%	837
Newport Hospital	Newport	99%	174
South County Hospital[2]	Wakefield	99%	257
Women & Infants Hospital of Rhode Island[2]	Providence	99%	107
Kent County Memorial Hospital[2]	Warwick	96%	358

Prophylactic Antibiotic Timing (Outpatient)

Hospital Name	City	Rate	Cases
Newport Hospital	Newport	100%	59
Women & Infants Hospital of Rhode Island	Providence	100%	713

NOTE: Hospital profiles are in alphabetical order by state, then city, then hospital within the city; Rankings exclude hospitals with less than 25 cases except for patient surveys which excludes hospitals with less than 100 cases; (a) 100-299 cases; (1) The number of cases/patients is too few to report; (2) Data submitted were based on a sample of cases/patients; (3) Results are based on a shorter time period than required; (4) Data suppressed by CMS for one or more quarters; (5) Results are not available for this reporting period; (6) Fewer than 100 patients completed the HCAHPS survey; (7) No cases met the criteria for this measure; (8) The lower limit of the confidence interval cannot be calculated if the number of observed infections equals zero; (9) No data are available from the state/territory for this reporting period; (10) The scores shown reflect fewer than 50 completed surveys; (11) There were discrepancies in the data collection process; (12) This measure does not apply to this hospital for this reporting period; (13) Results cannot be calculated for this reporting period; (14) The results for this state are combined with nearby states to protect confidentiality; Please refer to the User's Guide for a full explanation of data.

Hospital Name	City	Rate	Cases
Landmark Medical Center	Woonsocket	99%	85
Rhode Island Hospital	Providence	99%	440
Saint Joseph Health Services of RI	N Providence	98%	317
Westerly Hospital	Westerly	98%	61
Memorial Hospital of Rhode Island	Pawtucket	97%	86
Miriam Hospital	Providence	95%	297
South County Hospital	Wakefield	94%	82
Kent County Memorial Hospital	Warwick	90%	252
Roger Williams Medical Center	Providence	88%	75

Urinary Catheter Removal

Hospital Name	City	Rate	Cases
Newport Hospital	Newport	100%	60
Providence VA Medical Center[2]	Providence	100%	73
Miriam Hospital[2]	Providence	99%	820
Roger Williams Medical Center	Providence	99%	255
Westerly Hospital	Westerly	99%	152
Memorial Hospital of Rhode Island	Pawtucket	98%	130
Saint Joseph Health Services of RI[2]	N Providence	98%	205
South County Hospital[2]	Wakefield	98%	257
Landmark Medical Center	Woonsocket	97%	95
Rhode Island Hospital[2]	Providence	95%	389
Kent County Memorial Hospital[2]	Warwick	93%	412

Survey of Patients' Hospital Experiences

Area Around Room 'Always' Quiet at Night

Hospital Name	City	Rate	Cases
South County Hospital	Wakefield	66%	300+
Newport Hospital	Newport	59%	300+
Roger Williams Medical Center	Providence	59%	300+
Saint Joseph Health Services of RI	N Providence	58%	300+
Westerly Hospital	Westerly	54%	300+
Women & Infants Hospital of Rhode Island	Providence	54%	300+
Memorial Hospital of Rhode Island	Pawtucket	53%	300+
Kent County Memorial Hospital	Warwick	52%	300+
Rhode Island Hospital	Providence	49%	300+
Miriam Hospital	Providence	47%	300+
Landmark Medical Center	Woonsocket	42%	300+

Doctors 'Always' Communicated Well

Hospital Name	City	Rate	Cases
South County Hospital	Wakefield	87%	300+
Westerly Hospital	Westerly	84%	300+
Memorial Hospital of Rhode Island	Pawtucket	83%	300+
Miriam Hospital	Providence	81%	300+
Kent County Memorial Hospital	Warwick	80%	300+
Newport Hospital	Newport	79%	300+
Rhode Island Hospital	Providence	79%	300+
Roger Williams Medical Center	Providence	79%	300+
Saint Joseph Health Services of RI	N Providence	79%	300+
Women & Infants Hospital of Rhode Island	Providence	78%	300+
Landmark Medical Center	Woonsocket	73%	300+

Home Recovery Information Given

Hospital Name	City	Rate	Cases
South County Hospital	Wakefield	92%	300+
Miriam Hospital	Providence	89%	300+
Saint Joseph Health Services of RI	N Providence	89%	300+
Roger Williams Medical Center	Providence	87%	300+
Newport Hospital	Newport	86%	300+
Rhode Island Hospital	Providence	86%	300+
Memorial Hospital of Rhode Island	Pawtucket	83%	300+
Westerly Hospital	Westerly	83%	300+
Kent County Memorial Hospital	Warwick	82%	300+
Landmark Medical Center	Woonsocket	81%	300+
Women & Infants Hospital of Rhode Island	Providence	81%	300+

Hospital Given 9 or 10 on 10 Point Scale

Hospital Name	City	Rate	Cases
South County Hospital	Wakefield	84%	300+
Miriam Hospital	Providence	76%	300+
Women & Infants Hospital of Rhode Island	Providence	74%	300+
Newport Hospital	Newport	72%	300+
Westerly Hospital	Westerly	70%	300+
Kent County Memorial Hospital	Warwick	67%	300+
Memorial Hospital of Rhode Island	Pawtucket	67%	300+
Rhode Island Hospital	Providence	67%	300+
Saint Joseph Health Services of RI	N Providence	67%	300+
Roger Williams Medical Center	Providence	66%	300+
Landmark Medical Center	Woonsocket	54%	300+

Meds 'Always' Explained Before Given

Hospital Name	City	Rate	Cases
South County Hospital	Wakefield	70%	300+
Westerly Hospital	Westerly	66%	300+
Saint Joseph Health Services of RI	N Providence	65%	300+
Miriam Hospital	Providence	64%	300+
Memorial Hospital of Rhode Island	Pawtucket	62%	300+
Roger Williams Medical Center	Providence	60%	300+
Newport Hospital	Newport	59%	300+
Rhode Island Hospital	Providence	59%	300+
Women & Infants Hospital of Rhode Island	Providence	59%	300+
Kent County Memorial Hospital	Warwick	58%	300+
Landmark Medical Center	Woonsocket	54%	300+

Nurses 'Always' Communicated Well

Hospital Name	City	Rate	Cases
South County Hospital	Wakefield	86%	300+
Miriam Hospital	Providence	82%	300+
Newport Hospital	Newport	82%	300+
Saint Joseph Health Services of RI	N Providence	81%	300+
Kent County Memorial Hospital	Warwick	80%	300+
Memorial Hospital of Rhode Island	Pawtucket	79%	300+
Westerly Hospital	Westerly	79%	300+
Roger Williams Medical Center	Providence	78%	300+
Women & Infants Hospital of Rhode Island	Providence	77%	300+
Rhode Island Hospital	Providence	76%	300+
Landmark Medical Center	Woonsocket	74%	300+

Pain 'Always' Well Controlled

Hospital Name	City	Rate	Cases
South County Hospital	Wakefield	78%	300+
Saint Joseph Health Services of RI	N Providence	74%	300+
Roger Williams Medical Center	Providence	73%	300+
Women & Infants Hospital of Rhode Island	Providence	73%	300+
Miriam Hospital	Providence	72%	300+
Newport Hospital	Newport	72%	300+
Memorial Hospital of Rhode Island	Pawtucket	71%	300+
Westerly Hospital	Westerly	70%	300+
Kent County Memorial Hospital	Warwick	68%	300+
Rhode Island Hospital	Providence	68%	300+
Landmark Medical Center	Woonsocket	67%	300+

Room and Bathroom 'Always' Clean

Hospital Name	City	Rate	Cases
Westerly Hospital	Westerly	80%	300+
Memorial Hospital of Rhode Island	Pawtucket	77%	300+
Newport Hospital	Newport	77%	300+
South County Hospital	Wakefield	77%	300+
Roger Williams Medical Center	Providence	76%	300+
Miriam Hospital	Providence	75%	300+
Rhode Island Hospital	Providence	74%	300+
Kent County Memorial Hospital	Warwick	69%	300+
Landmark Medical Center	Woonsocket	68%	300+
Saint Joseph Health Services of RI	N Providence	68%	300+
Women & Infants Hospital of Rhode Island	Providence	66%	300+

Timely Help 'Always' Received

Hospital Name	City	Rate	Cases
South County Hospital	Wakefield	78%	300+
Saint Joseph Health Services of RI	N Providence	70%	300+
Roger Williams Medical Center	Providence	69%	300+
Kent County Memorial Hospital	Warwick	68%	300+
Memorial Hospital of Rhode Island	Pawtucket	68%	300+
Newport Hospital	Newport	68%	300+
Westerly Hospital	Westerly	64%	300+
Miriam Hospital	Providence	63%	300+
Women & Infants Hospital of Rhode Island	Providence	63%	300+
Landmark Medical Center	Woonsocket	62%	300+
Rhode Island Hospital	Providence	62%	300+

Would Definitely Recommend Hospital

Hospital Name	City	Rate	Cases
South County Hospital	Wakefield	86%	300+
Miriam Hospital	Providence	83%	300+
Women & Infants Hospital of Rhode Island	Providence	80%	300+
Newport Hospital	Newport	72%	300+
Rhode Island Hospital	Providence	72%	300+
Westerly Hospital	Westerly	72%	300+
Memorial Hospital of Rhode Island	Pawtucket	71%	300+
Roger Williams Medical Center	Providence	69%	300+
Kent County Memorial Hospital	Warwick	68%	300+
Saint Joseph Health Services of RI	N Providence	65%	300+
Landmark Medical Center	Woonsocket	57%	300+

Use of Medical Imaging

Cardiac Imaging Stress Test before OP Surgery

Hospital Name	City	Rate	Cases
Westerly Hospital	Westerly	3.5%	86
Miriam Hospital	Providence	3.8%	609
Rhode Island Hospital	Providence	4.9%	367
South County Hospital	Wakefield	5.3%	131
Kent County Memorial Hospital	Warwick	5.8%	274
Memorial Hospital of Rhode Island	Pawtucket	5.9%	219
Landmark Medical Center	Woonsocket	7.4%	108
Newport Hospital	Newport	9.4%	85

Combination Abdominal CT Scan

Hospital Name	City	Rate	Cases
Women & Infants Hospital of Rhode Island	Providence	1.2%	341
Landmark Medical Center	Woonsocket	2.8%	469
Rhode Island Hospital	Providence	2.9%	1797
Miriam Hospital	Providence	3.3%	1704
Memorial Hospital of Rhode Island	Pawtucket	3.8%	449
Newport Hospital	Newport	5.5%	637
South County Hospital	Wakefield	5.5%	512
Kent County Memorial Hospital	Warwick	5.6%	944
Saint Joseph Health Services of RI	N Providence	8.4%	406
Westerly Hospital	Westerly	8.5%	543
Roger Williams Medical Center	Providence	10.6%	387

Combination Brain/Sinus CT Scan

Hospital Name	City	Rate	Cases
Roger Williams Medical Center	Providence	1.6%	430
Westerly Hospital	Westerly	2.0%	494
Landmark Medical Center	Woonsocket	2.7%	524
South County Hospital	Wakefield	2.7%	673
Kent County Memorial Hospital	Warwick	3.5%	1388
Miriam Hospital	Providence	3.7%	1304
Saint Joseph Health Services of RI	N Providence	3.8%	446
Memorial Hospital of Rhode Island	Pawtucket	4.2%	471
Rhode Island Hospital	Providence	6.1%	1838

Combination Chest CT Scan

Hospital Name	City	Rate	Cases
Memorial Hospital of Rhode Island	Pawtucket	0.0%	325
Miriam Hospital	Providence	0.0%	1242
Westerly Hospital	Westerly	0.0%	449
Women & Infants Hospital of Rhode Island	Providence	0.0%	320
Landmark Medical Center	Woonsocket	0.9%	228
Saint Joseph Health Services of RI	N Providence	0.9%	211
Kent County Memorial Hospital	Warwick	1.4%	498
Roger Williams Medical Center	Providence	1.9%	308
South County Hospital	Wakefield	1.9%	311
Rhode Island Hospital	Providence	2.0%	1633
Newport Hospital	Newport	24.7%	430

Follow-up Mammogram/Ultrasound

A follow-up rate near zero may indicate missed cancer; a rate higher than 14% may mean there is unnecessary follow up.

Hospital Name	City	Rate	Cases
Roger Williams Medical Center	Providence	4.5%	223
Rhode Island Hospital	Providence	5.0%	1726
Landmark Medical Center	Woonsocket	5.8%	633
Women & Infants Hospital of Rhode Island	Providence	6.4%	987
Newport Hospital	Newport	6.6%	1124
Miriam Hospital	Providence	7.2%	763
Westerly Hospital	Westerly	7.9%	891
South County Hospital	Wakefield	8.8%	1104
Kent County Memorial Hospital	Warwick	10.1%	1398
Memorial Hospital of Rhode Island	Pawtucket	14.6%	398
Saint Joseph Health Services of RI	N Providence	21.6%	310

Lumbar Spine MRI for Low Back Pain

Hospital Name	City	Rate	Cases
Westerly Hospital	Westerly	24.8%	109
South County Hospital	Wakefield	30.3%	89
Newport Hospital	Newport	31.6%	114
Kent County Memorial Hospital	Warwick	38.7%	75
Rhode Island Hospital	Providence	39.4%	71

NOTE: Hospital profiles are in alphabetical order by state, then city, then hospital within the city; Rankings exclude hospitals with less than 25 cases except for patient surveys which excludes hospitals with less than 100 cases; (a) 100-299 cases; (1) The number of cases/patients is too few to report; (2) Data submitted were based on a sample of cases/patients; (3) Results are based on a shorter time period than required; (4) Data suppressed by CMS for one or more quarters; (5) Results are not available for this reporting period; (6) Fewer than 100 patients completed the HCAHPS survey; (7) No cases met the criteria for this measure; (8) The lower limit of the confidence interval cannot be calculated if the number of observed infections equals zero; (9) No data are available from the state/territory for this reporting period; (10) The scores shown reflect fewer than 50 completed surveys; (11) There were discrepancies in the data collection process; (12) This measure does not apply to this hospital for this reporting period; (13) Results cannot be calculated for this reporting period; (14) The results for this state are combined with nearby states to protect confidentiality; Please refer to the User's Guide for a full explanation of data.

Newport Hospital

Friendship Street
Newport, RI 02840
Phone: 401-846-6400
Fax: 401-845-1089
URL: www.newporthospital.org
Type: Acute Care Hospitals
Emergency Services: Yes
Ownership: Voluntary non-profit - Private
Beds: 129

Key Personnel:
CEO/President. . . . . Timothy J. Babineau, MD
Operating Room. . . . . Mark A Billington
President . . . . Crista Durand
Pediatric In-Patient Care . . . . Keivan Ettefagh, MD
Radiology. . . . . Donald B Fletcher
Chief of Medical Staff . . . . Thomas McGue, MD
Quality Assurance . . . . Ann Travis, RN
Emergency Room . . . . Benjamin Walker, MD

Measure	Cases	This Hosp.	State Avg.	U.S. Avg.
Blood Clot Prevention and Treatment				
Anticoagulation Overlap Therapy[2]	39	97%	97%	93%
ICU Venous Thromboembolism Prophylaxis[2]	85	94%	92%	92%
Incidence of Potentially Preventable VTE[1,2]	-	-	10%	10%
UFH with Dosages/Platelet Monitoring[2]	21	100%	99%	97%
Venous Thromboembolism Prophylaxis[2]	279	88%	85%	85%
Warfarin Therapy Discharge Instructions[2]	34	79%	61%	75%
Chest Pain/Possible Heart Attack Care				
Aspirin Given Within 24 Hours of Arrival	81	100%	97%	96%
Fibrinolytic Meds Within 30 Min. of Arrival[7]	-	-	100%	58%
Average Time to ECG (minutes)	83	6	10	7
Average Time to Transfer (minutes)	19	63	67	60
Children's Asthma Care				
Received Home Management Plan of Care	-	-	-	88%
Received Reliever Medication	-	-	-	100%
Received Systemic Corticosteroids	-	-	-	100%
Emergency Department				
Admittance Decision Time (minutes)[2]	409	102	115	98
Head CT Results Within 45 Min. of Arrival[1]	-	-	53%	57%
Patients Who Left ER Before Being Seen	31,947	3%	2%	2%
Time from ER Arrival to Admit. (minutes)[2]	412	284	334	274
Time from ER Arrival to Discharge (minutes)	359	146	152	134
Time in ER Before Being Evaluated (minutes)	402	53	37	26
Time to Pain Meds for Fractures (minutes)	115	59	54	57
Heart Attack Care				
Aspirin Given at Discharge	19	100%	100%	99%
Fibrinolytic Meds Within 30 Min. of Arrival[7]	-	-	-	54%
PCI Within 90 Minutes of Arrival[7]	-	-	98%	96%
Statin Prescribed at Discharge	19	89%	96%	98%
Heart Failure Care				
ACE Inhibitor or ARB for LVSD	35	100%	95%	97%
Discharge Instructions Given	94	96%	91%	94%
Evaluation of LVS Function	139	100%	100%	99%
Medicare Spending				
Medicare Spending per Patient (ratio)	-	1.01	1.02	0.98
Pneumonia Care				
Appropriate Initial Antibiotic Given	89	98%	97%	95%
Blood Culture Timing	138	99%	96%	98%
Pregnancy and Delivery Care				
Newborn Deliveries Scheduled Early	47	23%	4%	6%
Preventive Care				
Immunization for Influenza[2]	358	93%	87%	90%
Immunization for Pneumonia[2]	436	94%	86%	92%
Stroke Care				
Anticoagulation Therapy for Atrial Fibrillation	16	94%	94%	95%
Antithrombotic Therapy Timing	56	98%	98%	98%
Assessed for Rehabilitation	61	97%	97%	97%
Discharged on Antithrombotic Therapy	59	98%	100%	99%
Discharged on Statin Medication	47	98%	97%	94%
Thrombolytic Therapy Timing[1]	-	-	81%	66%
Venous Thromboembolism Prophylaxis	61	93%	95%	94%
Written Stroke Educational Materials Given	34	100%	90%	88%
Surgical Care Improvement Project				
Appropriate Beta Blocker Usage	84	99%	98%	98%
Appropriate VTP Within 24 Hours	244	96%	98%	98%
Controlled Postoperative Blood Glucose[7]	-	-	98%	97%
Perioperative Temperature Management	264	100%	100%	100%
Prophylactic Antibiotic Selection	174	100%	99%	99%
Prophylactic Antibiotic Selection (Outpatient)	59	95%	98%	98%
Prophylactic Antibiotic Stopped	171	98%	99%	98%
Prophylactic Antibiotic Timing	174	99%	99%	99%
Prophylactic Antibiotic Timing (Outpatient)	59	100%	97%	98%
Urinary Catheter Removal	60	100%	97%	97%
Survey of Patients' Hospital Experiences				
Area Around Room 'Always' Quiet at Night	300+	59%	54%	61%
Doctors 'Always' Communicated Well	300+	79%	80%	82%
Home Recovery Information Given	300+	86%	85%	85%
Hospital Given 9 or 10 on 10 Point Scale	300+	72%	69%	71%
Meds 'Always' Explained Before Given	300+	59%	61%	64%
Nurses 'Always' Communicated Well	300+	82%	79%	79%
Pain 'Always' Well Controlled	300+	72%	71%	71%
Room and Bathroom 'Always' Clean	300+	77%	73%	73%
Timely Help 'Always' Received	300+	68%	67%	68%
Would Definitely Recommend Hospital	300+	72%	72%	71%
Use of Medical Imaging				
Cardiac Imaging Stress Test before Surgery	85	9.4%	5.1%	5.3%
Combination Abdominal CT Scan	637	5.5%	4.6%	10.5%
Combination Brain/Sinus CT Scan[1]	-	-	3.9%	2.7%
Combination Chest CT Scan	430	24.7%	2.7%	2.7%
Follow-up Mammogram/Ultrasound	1,124	6.6%	7.9%	8.8%
Lumbar Spine MRI for Low Back Pain	114	31.6%	30.6%	37.2%

Saint Joseph Health Services of RI

200 High Service Avenue
North Providence, RI 02904
Phone: 401-456-3000
Fax: 401-456-3028
URL: www.fatimahospital.com
Type: Acute Care Hospitals
Emergency Services: Yes
Ownership: Voluntary non-profit - Private
Beds: 386

Key Personnel:
Quality Assurance . . . . Bruce Campbell
Radiology. . . . . Denise Driscoll
Infection Control. . . . . Marlene Fishman
CEO/President. . . . . Thomas C. Hughes
Operating Room. . . . . Kathy Squillante
Pediatric Ambulatory Care . . . . . . Alfred Toselli, MD
Pediatric In-Patient Care . . . . Alfred Toselli, MD

Measure	Cases	This Hosp.	State Avg.	U.S. Avg.
Blood Clot Prevention and Treatment				
Anticoagulation Overlap Therapy[2]	71	94%	97%	93%
ICU Venous Thromboembolism Prophylaxis[2]	39	87%	92%	92%
Incidence of Potentially Preventable VTE[2]	16	19%	10%	10%
UFH with Dosages/Platelet Monitoring[2]	45	100%	99%	97%
Venous Thromboembolism Prophylaxis[2]	363	74%	85%	85%
Warfarin Therapy Discharge Instructions[2]	45	76%	61%	75%
Chest Pain/Possible Heart Attack Care				
Aspirin Given Within 24 Hours of Arrival	50	88%	97%	96%
Fibrinolytic Meds Within 30 Min. of Arrival[7]	-	-	100%	58%
Average Time to ECG (minutes)	52	14	10	7
Average Time to Transfer (minutes)[1]	-	-	67	60
Children's Asthma Care				
Received Home Management Plan of Care	-	-	-	88%
Received Reliever Medication	-	-	-	100%
Received Systemic Corticosteroids	-	-	-	100%
Emergency Department				
Admittance Decision Time (minutes)[2]	673	146	115	98
Head CT Results Within 45 Min. of Arrival[1]	-	-	53%	57%
Patients Who Left ER Before Being Seen	25,871	2%	2%	2%
Time from ER Arrival to Admit. (minutes)[2]	679	390	334	274
Time from ER Arrival to Discharge (minutes)	396	170	152	134
Time in ER Before Being Evaluated (minutes)	473	26	37	26
Time to Pain Meds for Fractures (minutes)	80	84	54	57
Heart Attack Care				
Aspirin Given at Discharge	29	100%	100%	99%
Fibrinolytic Meds Within 30 Min. of Arrival[7]	-	-	-	54%
PCI Within 90 Minutes of Arrival[7]	-	-	98%	96%
Statin Prescribed at Discharge	23	83%	96%	98%
Heart Failure Care				
ACE Inhibitor or ARB for LVSD	32	97%	95%	97%
Discharge Instructions Given	147	97%	91%	94%
Evaluation of LVS Function	257	99%	100%	99%
Medicare Spending				
Medicare Spending per Patient (ratio)	-	1.08	1.02	0.98
Pneumonia Care				
Appropriate Initial Antibiotic Given	89	94%	97%	95%
Blood Culture Timing	146	94%	96%	98%
Pregnancy and Delivery Care				
Newborn Deliveries Scheduled Early[7]	-	-	4%	6%
Preventive Care				
Immunization for Influenza[2]	601	90%	87%	90%
Immunization for Pneumonia[2]	724	92%	86%	92%
Stroke Care				
Anticoagulation Therapy for Atrial Fibrillation[1,2]	-	-	94%	95%
Antithrombotic Therapy Timing[2]	18	94%	98%	98%
Assessed for Rehabilitation[2]	22	95%	97%	97%
Discharged on Antithrombotic Therapy[2]	19	100%	100%	99%
Discharged on Statin Medication[2]	18	94%	97%	94%
Thrombolytic Therapy Timing[1,2]	-	-	81%	66%
Venous Thromboembolism Prophylaxis[2]	23	74%	95%	94%
Written Stroke Educational Materials Given[1,2]	-	-	90%	88%
Surgical Care Improvement Project				
Appropriate Beta Blocker Usage[2]	105	99%	98%	98%
Appropriate VTP Within 24 Hours[2]	348	98%	98%	98%
Controlled Postoperative Blood Glucose[2,7]	-	-	98%	97%
Perioperative Temperature Management[2]	362	98%	100%	100%
Prophylactic Antibiotic Selection[2]	222	98%	99%	99%
Prophylactic Antibiotic Selection (Outpatient)	315	97%	98%	98%
Prophylactic Antibiotic Stopped[2]	221	100%	99%	98%
Prophylactic Antibiotic Timing[2]	223	100%	99%	99%
Prophylactic Antibiotic Timing (Outpatient)	317	98%	97%	98%
Urinary Catheter Removal[2]	205	98%	97%	97%
Survey of Patients' Hospital Experiences				
Area Around Room 'Always' Quiet at Night	300+	58%	54%	61%
Doctors 'Always' Communicated Well	300+	79%	80%	82%
Home Recovery Information Given	300+	89%	85%	85%
Hospital Given 9 or 10 on 10 Point Scale	300+	67%	69%	71%
Meds 'Always' Explained Before Given	300+	65%	61%	64%
Nurses 'Always' Communicated Well	300+	81%	79%	79%
Pain 'Always' Well Controlled	300+	74%	71%	71%
Room and Bathroom 'Always' Clean	300+	68%	73%	73%
Timely Help 'Always' Received	300+	70%	67%	68%
Would Definitely Recommend Hospital	300+	65%	72%	71%
Use of Medical Imaging				
Cardiac Imaging Stress Test before Surgery[1]	-	-	5.1%	5.3%
Combination Abdominal CT Scan	406	8.4%	4.6%	10.5%
Combination Brain/Sinus CT Scan	446	3.8%	3.9%	2.7%
Combination Chest CT Scan	211	0.9%	2.7%	2.7%
Follow-up Mammogram/Ultrasound	310	21.6%	7.9%	8.8%
Lumbar Spine MRI for Low Back Pain[1]	-	-	30.6%	37.2%

Memorial Hospital of Rhode Island

111 Brewster Street
Pawtucket, RI 02860
Phone: 401-729-2000
Fax: 401-729-3054
URL: www.mhriweb.org
Type: Acute Care Hospitals
Emergency Services: Yes
Ownership: Voluntary non-profit - Private
Beds: 294

Key Personnel:
Pediatric Ambulatory Care . . . . . . Louise Kiessling, MD
Pediatric In-Patient Care . . . . Louise Kiessling, MD
CEO/President. . . . . Edward Schottland
Chair/CEO . . . . George W. Shuster

Measure	Cases	This Hosp.	State Avg.	U.S. Avg.
Blood Clot Prevention and Treatment				
Anticoagulation Overlap Therapy[2]	47	94%	97%	93%
ICU Venous Thromboembolism Prophylaxis[2]	77	97%	92%	92%
Incidence of Potentially Preventable VTE[1,2]	-	-	10%	10%
UFH with Dosages/Platelet Monitoring[2]	42	100%	99%	97%
Venous Thromboembolism Prophylaxis[2]	335	94%	85%	85%
Warfarin Therapy Discharge Instructions[2]	37	62%	61%	75%
Chest Pain/Possible Heart Attack Care				
Aspirin Given Within 24 Hours of Arrival	23	96%	97%	96%
Fibrinolytic Meds Within 30 Min. of Arrival[7]	-	-	100%	58%
Average Time to ECG (minutes)	23	15	10	7
Average Time to Transfer (minutes)[1]	-	-	67	60
Children's Asthma Care				
Received Home Management Plan of Care	-	-	-	88%

NOTE: Hospital profiles are in alphabetical order by state, then city, then hospital within the city; Rankings exclude hospitals with less than 25 cases except for patient surveys which excludes hospitals with less than 100 cases; (a) 100-299 cases; (1) The number of cases/patients is too few to report; (2) Data submitted were based on a sample of cases/patients; (3) Results are based on a shorter time period than required; (4) Data suppressed by CMS for one or more quarters; (5) Results are not available for this reporting period; (6) Fewer than 100 patients completed the HCAHPS survey; (7) No cases met the criteria for this measure; (8) The lower limit of the confidence interval cannot be calculated if the number of observed infections equals zero; (9) No data are available from the state/territory for this reporting period; (10) The scores shown reflect fewer than 50 completed surveys; (11) There were discrepancies in the data collection process; (12) This measure does not apply to this hospital for this reporting period; (13) Results cannot be calculated for this reporting period; (14) The results for this state are combined with nearby states to protect confidentiality; Please refer to the User's Guide for a full explanation of data.

Measure	Cases	This Hosp.	State Avg.	U.S. Avg.
Received Reliever Medication	-	-	-	100%
Received Systemic Corticosteroids	-	-	-	100%
Emergency Department				
Admittance Decision Time (minutes)[2]	748	126	115	98
Head CT Results Within 45 Min. of Arrival[1]	-	-	53%	57%
Patients Who Left ER Before Being Seen	34,408	2%	2%	2%
Time from ER Arrival to Admit. (minutes)[2]	748	326	334	274
Time from ER Arrival to Discharge (minutes)	386	166	152	134
Time in ER Before Being Evaluated (minutes)	455	31	37	26
Time to Pain Meds for Fractures (minutes)	32	72	54	57
Heart Attack Care				
Aspirin Given at Discharge	30	97%	100%	99%
Fibrinolytic Meds Within 30 Min. of Arrival[7]	-	-	-	54%
PCI Within 90 Minutes of Arrival[7]	-	-	98%	96%
Statin Prescribed at Discharge	27	93%	96%	98%
Heart Failure Care				
ACE Inhibitor or ARB for LVSD	50	86%	95%	97%
Discharge Instructions Given	147	98%	91%	94%
Evaluation of LVS Function	198	99%	100%	99%
Medicare Spending				
Medicare Spending per Patient (ratio)	-	1.02	1.02	0.98
Pneumonia Care				
Appropriate Initial Antibiotic Given[2]	67	93%	97%	95%
Blood Culture Timing[2]	118	96%	96%	98%
Pregnancy and Delivery Care				
Newborn Deliveries Scheduled Early[2]	17	0%	4%	6%
Preventive Care				
Immunization for Influenza[2]	535	96%	87%	90%
Immunization for Pneumonia[2]	672	97%	86%	92%
Stroke Care				
Anticoagulation Therapy for Atrial Fibrillation[1]	-	-	94%	95%
Antithrombotic Therapy Timing	39	100%	98%	98%
Assessed for Rehabilitation	42	100%	97%	97%
Discharged on Antithrombotic Therapy	42	98%	100%	99%
Discharged on Statin Medication	31	100%	97%	94%
Thrombolytic Therapy Timing[1]	-	-	81%	66%
Venous Thromboembolism Prophylaxis	42	100%	95%	94%
Written Stroke Educational Materials Given	28	71%	90%	88%
Surgical Care Improvement Project				
Appropriate Beta Blocker Usage	57	98%	98%	98%
Appropriate VTP Within 24 Hours	195	99%	98%	98%
Controlled Postoperative Blood Glucose[7]	-	-	98%	97%
Perioperative Temperature Management	229	100%	100%	100%
Prophylactic Antibiotic Selection	135	97%	99%	99%
Prophylactic Antibiotic Selection (Outpatient)	86	100%	98%	98%
Prophylactic Antibiotic Stopped	130	99%	99%	98%
Prophylactic Antibiotic Timing	135	99%	99%	99%
Prophylactic Antibiotic Timing (Outpatient)	86	97%	97%	98%
Urinary Catheter Removal	130	98%	97%	97%
Survey of Patients' Hospital Experiences				
Area Around Room 'Always' Quiet at Night	300+	53%	54%	61%
Doctors 'Always' Communicated Well	300+	83%	80%	82%
Home Recovery Information Given	300+	83%	85%	85%
Hospital Given 9 or 10 on 10 Point Scale	300+	67%	69%	71%
Meds 'Always' Explained Before Given	300+	62%	61%	64%
Nurses 'Always' Communicated Well	300+	79%	79%	79%
Pain 'Always' Well Controlled	300+	71%	71%	71%
Room and Bathroom 'Always' Clean	300+	77%	73%	73%
Timely Help 'Always' Received	300+	68%	67%	68%
Would Definitely Recommend Hospital	300+	71%	72%	71%
Use of Medical Imaging				
Cardiac Imaging Stress Test before Surgery	219	5.9%	5.1%	5.3%
Combination Abdominal CT Scan	449	3.8%	4.6%	10.5%
Combination Brain/Sinus CT Scan	471	4.2%	3.9%	2.7%
Combination Chest CT Scan	325	0.0%	2.7%	2.7%
Follow-up Mammogram/Ultrasound	398	14.6%	7.9%	8.8%
Lumbar Spine MRI for Low Back Pain[1]	-	-	30.6%	37.2%

Miriam Hospital

164 Summit Avenue
Providence, RI 02906
Phone: 401-793-2500
Fax: 401-793-2923
URL: www.lifespan.org/partners/tmh
Type: Acute Care Hospitals
Emergency Services: Yes
Ownership: Voluntary non-profit - Private
Beds: 247

Key Personnel:
President . . . . Arthur J. Sampson, MD
Chief of Medical Staff . . . . Thomas F. Tracy, MD

Measure	Cases	This Hosp.	State Avg.	U.S. Avg.
Blood Clot Prevention and Treatment				
Anticoagulation Overlap Therapy[2]	131	100%	97%	93%
ICU Venous Thromboembolism Prophylaxis[2]	71	89%	92%	92%
Incidence of Potentially Preventable VTE[2]	19	11%	10%	10%
UFH with Dosages/Platelet Monitoring[2]	92	100%	99%	97%
Venous Thromboembolism Prophylaxis[2]	357	93%	85%	85%
Warfarin Therapy Discharge Instructions[2]	98	85%	61%	75%
Chest Pain/Possible Heart Attack Care				
Aspirin Given Within 24 Hours of Arrival[1,3]	-	-	97%	96%
Fibrinolytic Meds Within 30 Min. of Arrival[5]	-	-	100%	58%
Average Time to ECG (minutes)[1,3]	-	-	10	7
Average Time to Transfer (minutes)[5]	-	-	67	60
Children's Asthma Care				
Received Home Management Plan of Care	-	-	-	88%
Received Reliever Medication	-	-	-	100%
Received Systemic Corticosteroids	-	-	-	100%
Emergency Department				
Admittance Decision Time (minutes)[2]	752	99	115	98
Head CT Results Within 45 Min. of Arrival	20	40%	53%	57%
Patients Who Left ER Before Being Seen	60,035	2%	2%	2%
Time from ER Arrival to Admit. (minutes)[2]	752	312	334	274
Time from ER Arrival to Discharge (minutes)	541	207	152	134
Time in ER Before Being Evaluated (minutes)	644	57	37	26
Time to Pain Meds for Fractures (minutes)	81	71	54	57
Heart Attack Care				
Aspirin Given at Discharge	494	100%	100%	99%
Fibrinolytic Meds Within 30 Min. of Arrival[7]	-	-	-	54%
PCI Within 90 Minutes of Arrival	88	98%	98%	96%
Statin Prescribed at Discharge	484	99%	96%	98%
Heart Failure Care				
ACE Inhibitor or ARB for LVSD[2]	140	99%	95%	97%
Discharge Instructions Given[2]	406	92%	91%	94%
Evaluation of LVS Function[2]	541	100%	100%	99%
Medicare Spending				
Medicare Spending per Patient (ratio)	-	1.02	1.02	0.98
Pneumonia Care				
Appropriate Initial Antibiotic Given[2]	152	99%	97%	95%
Blood Culture Timing[2]	288	98%	96%	98%
Pregnancy and Delivery Care				
Newborn Deliveries Scheduled Early[7]	-	-	4%	6%
Preventive Care				
Immunization for Influenza[2]	616	84%	87%	90%
Immunization for Pneumonia[2]	955	83%	86%	92%
Stroke Care				
Anticoagulation Therapy for Atrial Fibrillation	38	97%	94%	95%
Antithrombotic Therapy Timing	185	99%	98%	98%
Assessed for Rehabilitation	209	100%	97%	97%
Discharged on Antithrombotic Therapy	203	100%	100%	99%
Discharged on Statin Medication	172	99%	97%	94%
Thrombolytic Therapy Timing	33	88%	81%	66%
Venous Thromboembolism Prophylaxis	191	98%	95%	94%
Written Stroke Educational Materials Given	99	94%	90%	88%
Surgical Care Improvement Project				
Appropriate Beta Blocker Usage[2]	399	98%	98%	98%
Appropriate VTP Within 24 Hours[2]	1,132	99%	98%	98%
Controlled Postoperative Blood Glucose[2,7]	-	-	98%	97%
Perioperative Temperature Management[2]	1,268	100%	100%	100%
Prophylactic Antibiotic Selection[2]	835	99%	99%	99%
Prophylactic Antibiotic Selection (Outpatient)	290	99%	98%	98%
Prophylactic Antibiotic Stopped[2]	825	99%	99%	98%
Prophylactic Antibiotic Timing[2]	837	99%	99%	99%
Prophylactic Antibiotic Timing (Outpatient)	297	95%	97%	98%
Urinary Catheter Removal[2]	820	99%	97%	97%
Survey of Patients' Hospital Experiences				
Area Around Room 'Always' Quiet at Night	300+	47%	54%	61%
Doctors 'Always' Communicated Well	300+	81%	80%	82%
Home Recovery Information Given	300+	89%	85%	85%
Hospital Given 9 or 10 on 10 Point Scale	300+	76%	69%	71%
Meds 'Always' Explained Before Given	300+	64%	61%	64%
Nurses 'Always' Communicated Well	300+	82%	79%	79%
Pain 'Always' Well Controlled	300+	72%	71%	71%
Room and Bathroom 'Always' Clean	300+	75%	73%	73%
Timely Help 'Always' Received	300+	63%	67%	68%
Would Definitely Recommend Hospital	300+	83%	72%	71%
Use of Medical Imaging				
Cardiac Imaging Stress Test before Surgery	609	3.8%	5.1%	5.3%
Combination Abdominal CT Scan	1,704	3.3%	4.6%	10.5%
Combination Brain/Sinus CT Scan	1,304	3.7%	3.9%	2.7%
Combination Chest CT Scan	1,242	0.0%	2.7%	2.7%
Follow-up Mammogram/Ultrasound	763	7.2%	7.9%	8.8%
Lumbar Spine MRI for Low Back Pain[1]	-	-	30.6%	37.2%

Providence VA Medical Center

830 Chalkstone Avenue
Providence, RI 02908
Phone: 401-457-3042
Fax: 401-457-3370
URL: www.visn1.med.va.gov/providence
Type: Acute Care - VA
Emergency Services: No
Ownership: Government Federal
Beds: 73

Key Personnel:
Patient Relations . . . . Deborah A Clickner, MEd RN
Chief of Medical Staff . . . . Gregory M Gillette
Emergency Room . . . . Satish Sharma, MD

Measure	Cases	This Hosp.	State Avg.	U.S. Avg.
Blood Clot Prevention and Treatment				
Anticoagulation Overlap Therapy	-	-	97%	93%
ICU Venous Thromboembolism Prophylaxis	-	-	92%	92%
Incidence of Potentially Preventable VTE	-	-	10%	10%
UFH with Dosages/Platelet Monitoring	-	-	99%	97%
Venous Thromboembolism Prophylaxis	-	-	85%	85%
Warfarin Therapy Discharge Instructions	-	-	61%	75%
Chest Pain/Possible Heart Attack Care				
Aspirin Given Within 24 Hours of Arrival	-	-	97%	96%
Fibrinolytic Meds Within 30 Min. of Arrival	-	-	100%	58%
Average Time to ECG (minutes)	-	-	10	7
Average Time to Transfer (minutes)	-	-	67	60
Children's Asthma Care				
Received Home Management Plan of Care	-	-	-	88%
Received Reliever Medication	-	-	-	100%
Received Systemic Corticosteroids	-	-	-	100%
Emergency Department				
Admittance Decision Time (minutes)	-	-	115	98
Head CT Results Within 45 Min. of Arrival	-	-	53%	57%
Patients Who Left ER Before Being Seen	-	-	2%	2%
Time from ER Arrival to Admit. (minutes)	-	-	334	274
Time from ER Arrival to Discharge (minutes)	-	-	152	134
Time in ER Before Being Evaluated (minutes)	-	-	37	26
Time to Pain Meds for Fractures (minutes)	-	-	54	57
Heart Attack Care				
Aspirin Given at Discharge[5]	-	-	100%	99%
Fibrinolytic Meds Within 30 Min. of Arrival[5]	-	-	-	54%
PCI Within 90 Minutes of Arrival[5]	-	-	98%	96%
Statin Prescribed at Discharge[5]	-	-	96%	98%
Heart Failure Care				
ACE Inhibitor or ARB for LVSD	30	97%	95%	97%
Discharge Instructions Given	106	98%	91%	94%
Evaluation of LVS Function	126	100%	100%	99%
Medicare Spending				
Medicare Spending per Patient (ratio)	-	-	1.02	0.98
Pneumonia Care				
Appropriate Initial Antibiotic Given	49	100%	97%	95%
Blood Culture Timing	98	97%	96%	98%
Pregnancy and Delivery Care				
Newborn Deliveries Scheduled Early	-	-	4%	6%
Preventive Care				
Immunization for Influenza[5]	-	-	87%	90%
Immunization for Pneumonia[5]	-	-	86%	92%

NOTE: Hospital profiles are in alphabetical order by state, then city, then hospital within the city; Rankings exclude hospitals with less than 25 cases except for patient surveys which excludes hospitals with less than 100 cases; (a) 100-299 cases; (1) The number of cases/patients is too few to report; (2) Data submitted were based on a sample of cases/patients; (3) Results are based on a shorter time period than required; (4) Data suppressed by CMS for one or more quarters; (5) Results are not available for this reporting period; (6) Fewer than 100 patients completed the HCAHPS survey; (7) No cases met the criteria for this measure; (8) The lower limit of the confidence interval cannot be calculated if the number of observed infections equals zero; (9) No data are available from the state/territory for this reporting period; (10) The scores shown reflect fewer than 50 completed surveys; (11) There were discrepancies in the data collection process; (12) This measure does not apply to this hospital for this reporting period; (13) Results cannot be calculated for this reporting period; (14) The results for this state are combined with nearby states to protect confidentiality; Please refer to the User's Guide for a full explanation of data.

Measure	Cases	This Hosp.	State Avg.	U.S. Avg.
Stroke Care				
Anticoagulation Therapy for Atrial Fibrillation	-	-	94%	95%
Antithrombotic Therapy Timing	-	-	98%	98%
Assessed for Rehabilitation	-	-	97%	97%
Discharged on Antithrombotic Therapy	-	-	100%	99%
Discharged on Statin Medication	-	-	97%	94%
Thrombolytic Therapy Timing	-	-	81%	66%
Venous Thromboembolism Prophylaxis	-	-	95%	94%
Written Stroke Educational Materials Given	-	-	90%	88%
Surgical Care Improvement Project				
Appropriate Beta Blocker Usage[2]	43	98%	98%	98%
Appropriate VTP Within 24 Hours[2]	90	100%	98%	98%
Controlled Postoperative Blood Glucose[5]	-	-	98%	97%
Perioperative Temperature Management[2]	106	100%	100%	100%
Prophylactic Antibiotic Selection	62	100%	99%	99%
Prophylactic Antibiotic Selection (Outpatient)	-	-	98%	98%
Prophylactic Antibiotic Stopped	60	100%	99%	98%
Prophylactic Antibiotic Timing	62	100%	99%	99%
Prophylactic Antibiotic Timing (Outpatient)	-	-	97%	98%
Urinary Catheter Removal[2]	73	100%	97%	97%
Survey of Patients' Hospital Experiences				
Area Around Room 'Always' Quiet at Night	-	-	54%	61%
Doctors 'Always' Communicated Well	-	-	80%	82%
Home Recovery Information Given	-	-	85%	85%
Hospital Given 9 or 10 on 10 Point Scale	-	-	69%	71%
Meds 'Always' Explained Before Given	-	-	61%	64%
Nurses 'Always' Communicated Well	-	-	79%	79%
Pain 'Always' Well Controlled	-	-	71%	71%
Room and Bathroom 'Always' Clean	-	-	73%	73%
Timely Help 'Always' Received	-	-	67%	68%
Would Definitely Recommend Hospital	-	-	72%	71%
Use of Medical Imaging				
Cardiac Imaging Stress Test before Surgery	-	-	5.1%	5.3%
Combination Abdominal CT Scan	-	-	4.6%	10.5%
Combination Brain/Sinus CT Scan	-	-	3.9%	2.7%
Combination Chest CT Scan	-	-	2.7%	2.7%
Follow-up Mammogram/Ultrasound	-	-	7.9%	8.8%
Lumbar Spine MRI for Low Back Pain	-	-	30.6%	37.2%

Rhode Island Hospital

593 Eddy Street
Providence, RI 02902
URL: www.rhodeislandhospital.org
Type: Acute Care Hospitals
Ownership: Voluntary non-profit - Private
Phone: 401-444-4000
Fax: 401-444-4218
Emergency Services: Yes
Beds: 719

Key Personnel:
CEO/President. . . . . Timothy J Babineau, MD
Radiology. . . . . John Cronan, MD
Quality Assurance . . . . Joan Flynn
Emergency Room . . . . Frantz Gibbs, MD
Chief of Medical Staff . . . . Martha Mainiero, MD
Coronary Care . . . . George McKendall, MD
Operating Room. . . . . Barbara Riley, RN

Measure	Cases	This Hosp.	State Avg.	U.S. Avg.
Blood Clot Prevention and Treatment				
Anticoagulation Overlap Therapy[2]	183	99%	97%	93%
ICU Venous Thromboembolism Prophylaxis[2]	88	90%	92%	92%
Incidence of Potentially Preventable VTE[2]	40	5%	10%	10%
UFH with Dosages/Platelet Monitoring[2]	144	99%	99%	97%
Venous Thromboembolism Prophylaxis[2]	319	88%	85%	85%
Warfarin Therapy Discharge Instructions[2]	123	28%	61%	75%
Chest Pain/Possible Heart Attack Care				
Aspirin Given Within 24 Hours of Arrival[5]	-	-	97%	96%
Fibrinolytic Meds Within 30 Min. of Arrival[5]	-	-	100%	58%
Average Time to ECG (minutes)[5]	-	-	10	7
Average Time to Transfer (minutes)[5]	-	-	67	60
Children's Asthma Care				
Received Home Management Plan of Care	-	-	-	88%
Received Reliever Medication	-	-	-	100%
Received Systemic Corticosteroids	-	-	-	100%
Emergency Department				
Admittance Decision Time (minutes)[2]	795	117	115	98
Head CT Results Within 45 Min. of Arrival[7]	-	-	53%	57%
Patients Who Left ER Before Being Seen	>100k	4%	2%	2%
Time from ER Arrival to Admit. (minutes)[2]	795	388	334	274
Time from ER Arrival to Discharge (minutes)	347	246	152	134
Time in ER Before Being Evaluated (minutes)	402	86	37	26
Time to Pain Meds for Fractures (minutes)	338	40	54	57
Heart Attack Care				
Aspirin Given at Discharge	720	100%	100%	99%
Fibrinolytic Meds Within 30 Min. of Arrival[7]	-	-	-	54%
PCI Within 90 Minutes of Arrival	104	98%	98%	96%
Statin Prescribed at Discharge	695	100%	96%	98%
Heart Failure Care				
ACE Inhibitor or ARB for LVSD[2]	86	100%	95%	97%
Discharge Instructions Given[2]	233	87%	91%	94%
Evaluation of LVS Function[2]	291	100%	100%	99%
Medicare Spending				
Medicare Spending per Patient (ratio)	-	0.99	1.02	0.98
Pneumonia Care				
Appropriate Initial Antibiotic Given[2]	56	98%	97%	95%
Blood Culture Timing[2]	144	96%	96%	98%
Pregnancy and Delivery Care				
Newborn Deliveries Scheduled Early[7]	-	-	4%	6%
Preventive Care				
Immunization for Influenza[2]	574	67%	87%	90%
Immunization for Pneumonia[2]	645	71%	86%	92%
Stroke Care				
Anticoagulation Therapy for Atrial Fibrillation	56	95%	94%	95%
Antithrombotic Therapy Timing	235	96%	98%	98%
Assessed for Rehabilitation	504	94%	97%	97%
Discharged on Antithrombotic Therapy	357	100%	100%	99%
Discharged on Statin Medication	289	97%	97%	94%
Thrombolytic Therapy Timing	54	87%	81%	66%
Venous Thromboembolism Prophylaxis	489	96%	95%	94%
Written Stroke Educational Materials Given	261	92%	90%	88%
Surgical Care Improvement Project				
Appropriate Beta Blocker Usage[2]	299	99%	98%	98%
Appropriate VTP Within 24 Hours[2]	366	99%	98%	98%
Controlled Postoperative Blood Glucose[2]	162	98%	98%	97%
Perioperative Temperature Management[2]	493	100%	100%	100%
Prophylactic Antibiotic Selection[2]	425	99%	99%	99%
Prophylactic Antibiotic Selection (Outpatient)	483	100%	98%	98%
Prophylactic Antibiotic Stopped[2]	408	99%	99%	98%
Prophylactic Antibiotic Timing[2]	428	100%	99%	99%
Prophylactic Antibiotic Timing (Outpatient)	440	99%	97%	98%
Urinary Catheter Removal[2]	389	95%	97%	97%
Survey of Patients' Hospital Experiences				
Area Around Room 'Always' Quiet at Night	300+	49%	54%	61%
Doctors 'Always' Communicated Well	300+	79%	80%	82%
Home Recovery Information Given	300+	86%	85%	85%
Hospital Given 9 or 10 on 10 Point Scale	300+	67%	69%	71%
Meds 'Always' Explained Before Given	300+	59%	61%	64%
Nurses 'Always' Communicated Well	300+	76%	79%	79%
Pain 'Always' Well Controlled	300+	68%	71%	71%
Room and Bathroom 'Always' Clean	300+	74%	73%	73%
Timely Help 'Always' Received	300+	62%	67%	68%
Would Definitely Recommend Hospital	300+	72%	72%	71%
Use of Medical Imaging				
Cardiac Imaging Stress Test before Surgery	367	4.9%	5.1%	5.3%
Combination Abdominal CT Scan	1,797	2.9%	4.6%	10.5%
Combination Brain/Sinus CT Scan	1,838	6.1%	3.9%	2.7%
Combination Chest CT Scan	1,633	2.0%	2.7%	2.7%
Follow-up Mammogram/Ultrasound	1,726	5.0%	7.9%	8.8%
Lumbar Spine MRI for Low Back Pain	71	39.4%	30.6%	37.2%

Roger Williams Medical Center

825 Chalkstone Avenue
Providence, RI 02908
URL: www.rwmc.com
Type: Acute Care Hospitals
Ownership: Voluntary non-profit - Private
Phone: 401-456-2000
Fax: 401-456-2029
Emergency Services: Yes
Beds: 238

Key Personnel:
Emergency Room . . . . Michael Bonitati
Chief of Medical Staff. . . . . Thomas Dennucci
Quality Assurance . . . . Joyce Hackley
CEO/President. . . . . Robert A Urciuoli

Measure	Cases	This Hosp.	State Avg.	U.S. Avg.
Blood Clot Prevention and Treatment				
Anticoagulation Overlap Therapy[2]	23	83%	97%	93%
ICU Venous Thromboembolism Prophylaxis[2]	20	95%	92%	92%
Incidence of Potentially Preventable VTE[1,2]	-	-	10%	10%
UFH with Dosages/Platelet Monitoring[2]	19	95%	99%	97%
Venous Thromboembolism Prophylaxis[2]	265	84%	85%	85%
Warfarin Therapy Discharge Instructions[2]	16	50%	61%	75%
Chest Pain/Possible Heart Attack Care				
Aspirin Given Within 24 Hours of Arrival	13	92%	97%	96%
Fibrinolytic Meds Within 30 Min. of Arrival[7]	-	-	100%	58%
Average Time to ECG (minutes)	14	16	10	7
Average Time to Transfer (minutes)[1]	-	-	67	60
Children's Asthma Care				
Received Home Management Plan of Care	-	-	-	88%
Received Reliever Medication	-	-	-	100%
Received Systemic Corticosteroids	-	-	-	100%
Emergency Department				
Admittance Decision Time (minutes)[2]	508	115	115	98
Head CT Results Within 45 Min. of Arrival[1]	-	-	53%	57%
Patients Who Left ER Before Being Seen	26,087	3%	2%	2%
Time from ER Arrival to Admit. (minutes)[2]	508	346	334	274
Time from ER Arrival to Discharge (minutes)	339	185	152	134
Time in ER Before Being Evaluated (minutes)	401	71	37	26
Time to Pain Meds for Fractures (minutes)	44	78	54	57
Heart Attack Care				
Aspirin Given at Discharge	63	97%	100%	99%
Fibrinolytic Meds Within 30 Min. of Arrival[7]	-	-	-	54%
PCI Within 90 Minutes of Arrival[7]	-	-	98%	96%
Statin Prescribed at Discharge	58	78%	96%	98%
Heart Failure Care				
ACE Inhibitor or ARB for LVSD	22	100%	95%	97%
Discharge Instructions Given	62	100%	91%	94%
Evaluation of LVS Function	112	97%	100%	99%
Medicare Spending				
Medicare Spending per Patient (ratio)	-	1.02	1.02	0.98
Pneumonia Care				
Appropriate Initial Antibiotic Given	67	99%	97%	95%
Blood Culture Timing	136	96%	96%	98%
Pregnancy and Delivery Care				
Newborn Deliveries Scheduled Early[7]	-	-	4%	6%
Preventive Care				
Immunization for Influenza[2]	613	72%	87%	90%
Immunization for Pneumonia[2]	752	53%	86%	92%
Stroke Care				
Anticoagulation Therapy for Atrial Fibrillation	14	93%	94%	95%
Antithrombotic Therapy Timing	30	100%	98%	98%
Assessed for Rehabilitation	38	92%	97%	97%
Discharged on Antithrombotic Therapy	36	100%	100%	99%
Discharged on Statin Medication	28	96%	97%	94%
Thrombolytic Therapy Timing[1]	-	-	81%	66%
Venous Thromboembolism Prophylaxis	36	92%	95%	94%
Written Stroke Educational Materials Given	13	69%	90%	88%
Surgical Care Improvement Project				
Appropriate Beta Blocker Usage	146	97%	98%	98%
Appropriate VTP Within 24 Hours	471	97%	98%	98%
Controlled Postoperative Blood Glucose[7]	-	-	98%	97%
Perioperative Temperature Management	499	100%	100%	100%
Prophylactic Antibiotic Selection	280	99%	99%	99%
Prophylactic Antibiotic Selection (Outpatient)	70	99%	98%	98%
Prophylactic Antibiotic Stopped	276	100%	99%	98%
Prophylactic Antibiotic Timing	280	100%	99%	99%
Prophylactic Antibiotic Timing (Outpatient)	75	88%	97%	98%
Urinary Catheter Removal	255	99%	97%	97%
Survey of Patients' Hospital Experiences				
Area Around Room 'Always' Quiet at Night	300+	59%	54%	61%
Doctors 'Always' Communicated Well	300+	79%	80%	82%
Home Recovery Information Given	300+	87%	85%	85%
Hospital Given 9 or 10 on 10 Point Scale	300+	66%	69%	71%
Meds 'Always' Explained Before Given	300+	60%	61%	64%
Nurses 'Always' Communicated Well	300+	78%	79%	79%
Pain 'Always' Well Controlled	300+	73%	71%	71%

NOTE: Hospital profiles are in alphabetical order by state, then city, then hospital within the city; Rankings exclude hospitals with less than 25 cases except for patient surveys which excludes hospitals with less than 100 cases; (a) 100-299 cases; (1) The number of cases/patients is too few to report; (2) Data submitted were based on a sample of cases/patients; (3) Results are based on a shorter time period than required; (4) Data suppressed by CMS for one or more quarters; (5) Results are not available for this reporting period; (6) Fewer than 100 patients completed the HCAHPS survey; (7) No cases met the criteria for this measure; (8) The lower limit of the confidence interval cannot be calculated if the number of observed infections equals zero; (9) No data are available from the state/territory for this reporting period; (10) The scores shown reflect fewer than 50 completed surveys; (11) There were discrepancies in the data collection process; (12) This measure does not apply to this hospital for this reporting period; (13) Results cannot be calculated for this reporting period; (14) The results for this state are combined with nearby states to protect confidentiality; Please refer to the User's Guide for a full explanation of data.

Measure	Cases	This Hosp.	State Avg.	U.S. Avg.
Room and Bathroom 'Always' Clean	300+	76%	73%	73%
Timely Help 'Always' Received	300+	69%	67%	68%
Would Definitely Recommend Hospital	300+	69%	72%	71%
Use of Medical Imaging				
Cardiac Imaging Stress Test before Surgery[1]	-	-	5.1%	5.3%
Combination Abdominal CT Scan	387	10.6%	4.6%	10.5%
Combination Brain/Sinus CT Scan	430	1.6%	3.9%	2.7%
Combination Chest CT Scan	308	1.9%	2.7%	2.7%
Follow-up Mammogram/Ultrasound	223	4.5%	7.9%	8.8%
Lumbar Spine MRI for Low Back Pain[1]	-	-	30.6%	37.2%

Women & Infants Hospital of Rhode Island

101 Dudley Street
Providence, RI 02905
Phone: 401-274-1100
Fax: 401-453-7666
E-mail: mkernan@wihri.org
URL: www.womenandinfants.com
Type: Acute Care Hospitals
Emergency Services: Yes
Ownership: Voluntary non-profit - Private
Beds: 137

Key Personnel:
Radiology.................... Michael Atalay, MD
Anesthesiology.............. Kue Choi, MD
Quality Assurance .... Deborah L Gard
Patient Relations .... Paula Gillette, RN
CEO/President................ Dennis D. Keefe
Infection Control.............. Fatima Muriel
Pediatric In-Patient Care .... James Padbury, MD
Chief of Medical Staff.......... Karen Rosene-Montell, MD

Measure	Cases	This Hosp.	State Avg.	U.S. Avg.
Blood Clot Prevention and Treatment				
Anticoagulation Overlap Therapy[1,2]	-	-	97%	93%
ICU Venous Thromboembolism Prophylaxis[2,7]	-	-	92%	92%
Incidence of Potentially Preventable VTE[1,2]	-	-	10%	10%
UFH with Dosages/Platelet Monitoring[1,2]	-	-	99%	97%
Venous Thromboembolism Prophylaxis[2]	140	76%	85%	85%
Warfarin Therapy Discharge Instructions[1,2]	-	-	61%	75%
Chest Pain/Possible Heart Attack Care				
Aspirin Given Within 24 Hours of Arrival[1]	-	-	97%	96%
Fibrinolytic Meds Within 30 Min. of Arrival[5]	-	-	100%	58%
Average Time to ECG (minutes)[1]	-	-	10	7
Average Time to Transfer (minutes)[5]	-	-	67	60
Children's Asthma Care				
Received Home Management Plan of Care	-	-	-	88%
Received Reliever Medication	-	-	-	100%
Received Systemic Corticosteroids	-	-	-	100%
Emergency Department				
Admittance Decision Time (minutes)[2]	427	58	115	98
Head CT Results Within 45 Min. of Arrival[5]	-	-	53%	57%
Patients Who Left ER Before Being Seen	28,753	2%	2%	2%
Time from ER Arrival to Admit. (minutes)[2]	429	141	334	274
Time from ER Arrival to Discharge (minutes)	381	171	152	134
Time in ER Before Being Evaluated (minutes)	406	29	37	26
Time to Pain Meds for Fractures (minutes)[5]	-	-	54	57
Heart Attack Care				
Aspirin Given at Discharge[5]	-	-	100%	99%
Fibrinolytic Meds Within 30 Min. of Arrival[5]	-	-	-	54%
PCI Within 90 Minutes of Arrival[5]	-	-	98%	96%
Statin Prescribed at Discharge[5]	-	-	96%	98%
Heart Failure Care				
ACE Inhibitor or ARB for LVSD[3,7]	-	-	95%	97%
Discharge Instructions Given[1,3]	-	-	91%	94%
Evaluation of LVS Function[1,3]	-	-	100%	99%
Medicare Spending				
Medicare Spending per Patient (ratio)	-	1.00	1.02	0.98
Pneumonia Care				
Appropriate Initial Antibiotic Given[7]	-	-	97%	95%
Blood Culture Timing[1]	-	-	96%	98%
Pregnancy and Delivery Care				
Newborn Deliveries Scheduled Early[2]	100	1%	4%	6%
Preventive Care				
Immunization for Influenza[2]	333	91%	87%	90%
Immunization for Pneumonia[2]	80	62%	86%	92%
Stroke Care				
Anticoagulation Therapy for Atrial Fibrillation[5]	-	-	94%	95%
Antithrombotic Therapy Timing[5]	-	-	98%	98%
Assessed for Rehabilitation[5]	-	-	97%	97%
Discharged on Antithrombotic Therapy[5]	-	-	100%	99%
Discharged on Statin Medication[5]	-	-	97%	94%
Thrombolytic Therapy Timing[5]	-	-	81%	66%
Venous Thromboembolism Prophylaxis[5]	-	-	95%	94%
Written Stroke Educational Materials Given[5]	-	-	90%	88%
Surgical Care Improvement Project				
Appropriate Beta Blocker Usage[2]	23	100%	98%	98%
Appropriate VTP Within 24 Hours[2]	166	98%	98%	98%
Controlled Postoperative Blood Glucose[2,7]	-	-	98%	97%
Perioperative Temperature Management[2]	218	100%	100%	100%
Prophylactic Antibiotic Selection[2]	107	98%	99%	99%
Prophylactic Antibiotic Selection (Outpatient)	712	99%	98%	98%
Prophylactic Antibiotic Stopped[2]	107	98%	99%	98%
Prophylactic Antibiotic Timing[2]	107	99%	99%	99%
Prophylactic Antibiotic Timing (Outpatient)	713	100%	97%	98%
Urinary Catheter Removal[1,2]	-	-	97%	97%
Survey of Patients' Hospital Experiences				
Area Around Room 'Always' Quiet at Night	300+	54%	54%	61%
Doctors 'Always' Communicated Well	300+	78%	80%	82%
Home Recovery Information Given	300+	81%	85%	85%
Hospital Given 9 or 10 on 10 Point Scale	300+	74%	69%	71%
Meds 'Always' Explained Before Given	300+	59%	61%	64%
Nurses 'Always' Communicated Well	300+	77%	79%	79%
Pain 'Always' Well Controlled	300+	73%	71%	71%
Room and Bathroom 'Always' Clean	300+	66%	73%	73%
Timely Help 'Always' Received	300+	63%	67%	68%
Would Definitely Recommend Hospital	300+	80%	72%	71%
Use of Medical Imaging				
Cardiac Imaging Stress Test before Surgery[7]	-	-	5.1%	5.3%
Combination Abdominal CT Scan	341	1.2%	4.6%	10.5%
Combination Brain/Sinus CT Scan[1]	-	-	3.9%	2.7%
Combination Chest CT Scan	320	0.0%	2.7%	2.7%
Follow-up Mammogram/Ultrasound	987	6.4%	7.9%	8.8%
Lumbar Spine MRI for Low Back Pain[1]	-	-	30.6%	37.2%

South County Hospital

100 Kenyon Ave
Wakefield, RI 02879
Phone: 401-782-8000
Fax: 401-783-6330
E-mail: info@schospital.com
URL: www.schospital.com
Type: Acute Care Hospitals
Emergency Services: Yes
Ownership: Voluntary non-profit - Private
Beds: 100

Key Personnel:
Chief of Medical Staff.......... Richard A Black, MD
Infection Control.............. Lee Ann Buenn
CEO/President................ Louis R Giancola
Quality Assurance .... Debra Keaney
Chair/CEO.................... Eve T. Keenan, RN
Patient Relations .... Barbara Seagrave
Radiology.................... Jeffrey E Silverstein
Cardiac Laboratory............. Sherri Zinno

Measure	Cases	This Hosp.	State Avg.	U.S. Avg.
Blood Clot Prevention and Treatment				
Anticoagulation Overlap Therapy[2]	30	97%	97%	93%
ICU Venous Thromboembolism Prophylaxis[2]	47	85%	92%	92%
Incidence of Potentially Preventable VTE[1,2]	-	-	10%	10%
UFH with Dosages/Platelet Monitoring[1,2]	-	-	99%	97%
Venous Thromboembolism Prophylaxis[2]	230	78%	85%	85%
Warfarin Therapy Discharge Instructions[2]	24	96%	61%	75%
Chest Pain/Possible Heart Attack Care				
Aspirin Given Within 24 Hours of Arrival	33	94%	97%	96%
Fibrinolytic Meds Within 30 Min. of Arrival[1]	-	-	100%	58%
Average Time to ECG (minutes)	22	7	10	7
Average Time to Transfer (minutes)[1]	-	-	67	60
Children's Asthma Care				
Received Home Management Plan of Care	-	-	-	88%
Received Reliever Medication	-	-	-	100%
Received Systemic Corticosteroids	-	-	-	100%
Emergency Department				
Admittance Decision Time (minutes)[2]	335	103	115	98
Head CT Results Within 45 Min. of Arrival	23	57%	53%	57%
Patients Who Left ER Before Being Seen	26,958	1%	2%	2%
Time from ER Arrival to Admit. (minutes)[2]	354	324	334	274
Time from ER Arrival to Discharge (minutes)	404	151	152	134
Time in ER Before Being Evaluated (minutes)	448	25	37	26
Time to Pain Meds for Fractures (minutes)	174	58	54	57
Heart Attack Care				
Aspirin Given at Discharge	24	100%	100%	99%
Fibrinolytic Meds Within 30 Min. of Arrival[7]	-	-	-	54%
PCI Within 90 Minutes of Arrival[7]	-	-	98%	96%
Statin Prescribed at Discharge	24	96%	96%	98%
Heart Failure Care				
ACE Inhibitor or ARB for LVSD	28	93%	95%	97%
Discharge Instructions Given	103	98%	91%	94%
Evaluation of LVS Function	133	100%	100%	99%
Medicare Spending				
Medicare Spending per Patient (ratio)	-	0.92	1.02	0.98
Pneumonia Care				
Appropriate Initial Antibiotic Given	51	100%	97%	95%
Blood Culture Timing	120	97%	96%	98%
Pregnancy and Delivery Care				
Newborn Deliveries Scheduled Early[2]	14	0%	4%	6%
Preventive Care				
Immunization for Influenza[2]	486	94%	87%	90%
Immunization for Pneumonia[2]	680	97%	86%	92%
Stroke Care				
Anticoagulation Therapy for Atrial Fibrillation	11	100%	94%	95%
Antithrombotic Therapy Timing	47	98%	98%	98%
Assessed for Rehabilitation	56	100%	97%	97%
Discharged on Antithrombotic Therapy	52	100%	100%	99%
Discharged on Statin Medication	39	97%	97%	94%
Thrombolytic Therapy Timing	11	36%	81%	66%
Venous Thromboembolism Prophylaxis	49	94%	95%	94%
Written Stroke Educational Materials Given	26	96%	90%	88%
Surgical Care Improvement Project				
Appropriate Beta Blocker Usage[2]	73	97%	98%	98%
Appropriate VTP Within 24 Hours[2]	310	99%	98%	98%
Controlled Postoperative Blood Glucose[2,7]	-	-	98%	97%
Perioperative Temperature Management[2]	378	100%	100%	100%
Prophylactic Antibiotic Selection[2]	257	98%	99%	99%
Prophylactic Antibiotic Selection (Outpatient)	84	96%	98%	98%
Prophylactic Antibiotic Stopped[2]	256	99%	99%	98%
Prophylactic Antibiotic Timing[2]	257	99%	99%	99%
Prophylactic Antibiotic Timing (Outpatient)	82	94%	97%	98%
Urinary Catheter Removal[2]	257	98%	97%	97%
Survey of Patients' Hospital Experiences				
Area Around Room 'Always' Quiet at Night	300+	66%	54%	61%
Doctors 'Always' Communicated Well	300+	87%	80%	82%
Home Recovery Information Given	300+	92%	85%	85%
Hospital Given 9 or 10 on 10 Point Scale	300+	84%	69%	71%
Meds 'Always' Explained Before Given	300+	70%	61%	64%
Nurses 'Always' Communicated Well	300+	86%	79%	79%
Pain 'Always' Well Controlled	300+	78%	71%	71%
Room and Bathroom 'Always' Clean	300+	77%	73%	73%
Timely Help 'Always' Received	300+	78%	67%	68%
Would Definitely Recommend Hospital	300+	86%	72%	71%
Use of Medical Imaging				
Cardiac Imaging Stress Test before Surgery	131	5.3%	5.1%	5.3%
Combination Abdominal CT Scan	512	5.5%	4.6%	10.5%
Combination Brain/Sinus CT Scan	673	2.7%	3.9%	2.7%
Combination Chest CT Scan	311	1.9%	2.7%	2.7%
Follow-up Mammogram/Ultrasound	1,104	8.8%	7.9%	8.8%
Lumbar Spine MRI for Low Back Pain	89	30.3%	30.6%	37.2%

Kent County Memorial Hospital

455 Toll Gate Rd
Warwick, RI 02886
Phone: 401-737-7000
Fax: 401-736-1000
E-mail: info@kentri.org
URL: www.kentri.org
Type: Acute Care Hospitals
Emergency Services: Yes
Ownership: Voluntary non-profit - Private
Beds: 359

Key Personnel:
CEO/President................ Michael Dacey, MD, MS, FACP
Patient Relations .... Mary Ann Glynn, RN, MBA
Chair/CEO.................... George W. Shuster
Chief of Medical Staff.......... Joseph W. Spinale, DO, FACC, FASNC

NOTE: Hospital profiles are in alphabetical order by state, then city, then hospital within the city; Rankings exclude hospitals with less than 25 cases except for patient surveys which excludes hospitals with less than 100 cases; (a) 100-299 cases; (1) The number of cases/patients is too few to report; (2) Data submitted were based on a sample of cases/patients; (3) Results are based on a shorter time period than required; (4) Data suppressed by CMS for one or more quarters; (5) Results are not available for this reporting period; (6) Fewer than 100 patients completed the HCAHPS survey; (7) No cases met the criteria for this measure; (8) The lower limit of the confidence interval cannot be calculated if the number of observed infections equals zero; (9) No data are available from the state/territory for this reporting period; (10) The scores shown reflect fewer than 50 completed surveys; (11) There were discrepancies in the data collection process; (12) This measure does not apply to this hospital for this reporting period; (13) Results cannot be calculated for this reporting period; (14) The results for this state are combined with nearby states to protect confidentiality; Please refer to the User's Guide for a full explanation of data.

Measure	Cases	This Hosp.	State Avg.	U.S. Avg.
Blood Clot Prevention and Treatment				
Anticoagulation Overlap Therapy[2]	117	94%	97%	93%
ICU Venous Thromboembolism Prophylaxis[2]	35	97%	92%	92%
Incidence of Potentially Preventable VTE[2]	14	14%	10%	10%
UFH with Dosages/Platelet Monitoring[2]	99	100%	99%	97%
Venous Thromboembolism Prophylaxis[2]	319	78%	85%	85%
Warfarin Therapy Discharge Instructions[2]	85	52%	61%	75%
Chest Pain/Possible Heart Attack Care				
Aspirin Given Within 24 Hours of Arrival	147	99%	97%	96%
Fibrinolytic Meds Within 30 Min. of Arrival[7]	-	-	100%	58%
Average Time to ECG (minutes)	151	10	10	7
Average Time to Transfer (minutes)	21	60	67	60
Children's Asthma Care				
Received Home Management Plan of Care	-	-	-	88%
Received Reliever Medication	-	-	-	100%
Received Systemic Corticosteroids	-	-	-	100%
Emergency Department				
Admittance Decision Time (minutes)[2]	694	172	115	98
Head CT Results Within 45 Min. of Arrival	16	44%	53%	57%
Patients Who Left ER Before Being Seen	70,105	1%	2%	2%
Time from ER Arrival to Admit. (minutes)[2]	697	357	334	274
Time from ER Arrival to Discharge (minutes)	321	146	152	134
Time in ER Before Being Evaluated (minutes)	189	27	37	26
Time to Pain Meds for Fractures (minutes)	157	49	54	57
Heart Attack Care				
Aspirin Given at Discharge[2]	139	99%	100%	99%
Fibrinolytic Meds Within 30 Min. of Arrival[2,7]	-	-	-	54%
PCI Within 90 Minutes of Arrival[2,7]	-	-	98%	96%
Statin Prescribed at Discharge[2]	141	86%	96%	98%
Heart Failure Care				
ACE Inhibitor or ARB for LVSD	94	83%	95%	97%
Discharge Instructions Given	296	84%	91%	94%
Evaluation of LVS Function	420	100%	100%	99%
Medicare Spending				
Medicare Spending per Patient (ratio)	-	1.06	1.02	0.98
Pneumonia Care				
Appropriate Initial Antibiotic Given[2]	103	93%	97%	95%
Blood Culture Timing[2]	214	93%	96%	98%
Pregnancy and Delivery Care				
Newborn Deliveries Scheduled Early	129	1%	4%	6%
Preventive Care				
Immunization for Influenza[2]	557	95%	87%	90%
Immunization for Pneumonia[2]	727	97%	86%	92%
Stroke Care				
Anticoagulation Therapy for Atrial Fibrillation	26	92%	94%	95%
Antithrombotic Therapy Timing	128	99%	98%	98%
Assessed for Rehabilitation	150	100%	97%	97%
Discharged on Antithrombotic Therapy	148	100%	100%	99%
Discharged on Statin Medication	115	94%	97%	94%
Thrombolytic Therapy Timing	21	100%	81%	66%
Venous Thromboembolism Prophylaxis	153	93%	95%	94%
Written Stroke Educational Materials Given	76	97%	90%	88%
Surgical Care Improvement Project				
Appropriate Beta Blocker Usage[2]	183	99%	98%	98%
Appropriate VTP Within 24 Hours[2]	512	96%	98%	98%
Controlled Postoperative Blood Glucose[2,7]	-	-	98%	97%
Perioperative Temperature Management[2]	569	100%	100%	100%
Prophylactic Antibiotic Selection[2]	358	98%	99%	99%
Prophylactic Antibiotic Selection (Outpatient)	246	92%	98%	98%
Prophylactic Antibiotic Stopped[2]	349	96%	99%	98%
Prophylactic Antibiotic Timing[2]	358	96%	99%	99%
Prophylactic Antibiotic Timing (Outpatient)	252	90%	97%	98%
Urinary Catheter Removal[2]	412	93%	97%	97%
Survey of Patients' Hospital Experiences				
Area Around Room 'Always' Quiet at Night	300+	52%	54%	61%
Doctors 'Always' Communicated Well	300+	80%	80%	82%
Home Recovery Information Given	300+	82%	85%	85%
Hospital Given 9 or 10 on 10 Point Scale	300+	67%	69%	71%
Meds 'Always' Explained Before Given	300+	58%	61%	64%
Nurses 'Always' Communicated Well	300+	80%	79%	79%
Pain 'Always' Well Controlled	300+	68%	71%	71%
Room and Bathroom 'Always' Clean	300+	69%	73%	73%
Timely Help 'Always' Received	300+	68%	67%	68%
Would Definitely Recommend Hospital	300+	68%	72%	71%
Use of Medical Imaging				
Cardiac Imaging Stress Test before Surgery	274	5.8%	5.1%	5.3%
Combination Abdominal CT Scan	944	5.6%	4.6%	10.5%
Combination Brain/Sinus CT Scan	1,388	3.5%	3.9%	2.7%
Combination Chest CT Scan	498	1.4%	2.7%	2.7%
Follow-up Mammogram/Ultrasound	1,398	10.1%	7.9%	8.8%
Lumbar Spine MRI for Low Back Pain	75	38.7%	30.6%	37.2%

Westerly Hospital

25 Wells Street
Westerly, RI 02891
Type: Acute Care Hospitals
Ownership: Voluntary non-profit - Private
Phone: 401-596-6000
Fax: 401-348-3714
Emergency Services: Yes
Beds: 125

Key Personnel:
CEO/President . . . . Bruce D. Cummings
Chairman/CEO . . . . Stephen Greene, CPA

Measure	Cases	This Hosp.	State Avg.	U.S. Avg.
Blood Clot Prevention and Treatment				
Anticoagulation Overlap Therapy[2]	28	96%	97%	93%
ICU Venous Thromboembolism Prophylaxis[2]	47	94%	92%	92%
Incidence of Potentially Preventable VTE[1,2]	-	-	10%	10%
UFH with Dosages/Platelet Monitoring[2]	14	100%	99%	97%
Venous Thromboembolism Prophylaxis[2]	295	91%	85%	85%
Warfarin Therapy Discharge Instructions[2]	20	65%	61%	75%
Chest Pain/Possible Heart Attack Care				
Aspirin Given Within 24 Hours of Arrival	59	100%	97%	96%
Fibrinolytic Meds Within 30 Min. of Arrival[1]	-	-	100%	58%
Average Time to ECG (minutes)	60	9	10	7
Average Time to Transfer (minutes)[1]	-	-	67	60
Children's Asthma Care				
Received Home Management Plan of Care	-	-	-	88%
Received Reliever Medication	-	-	-	100%
Received Systemic Corticosteroids	-	-	-	100%
Emergency Department				
Admittance Decision Time (minutes)[2]	351	84	115	98
Head CT Results Within 45 Min. of Arrival[1]	-	-	53%	57%
Patients Who Left ER Before Being Seen	23,229	1%	2%	2%
Time from ER Arrival to Admit. (minutes)[2]	388	312	334	274
Time from ER Arrival to Discharge (minutes)	320	116	152	134
Time in ER Before Being Evaluated (minutes)	350	35	37	26
Time to Pain Meds for Fractures (minutes)	45	53	54	57
Heart Attack Care				
Aspirin Given at Discharge	28	100%	100%	99%
Fibrinolytic Meds Within 30 Min. of Arrival[7]	-	-	-	54%
PCI Within 90 Minutes of Arrival[7]	-	-	98%	96%
Statin Prescribed at Discharge	27	81%	96%	98%
Heart Failure Care				
ACE Inhibitor or ARB for LVSD	29	97%	95%	97%
Discharge Instructions Given	92	79%	91%	94%
Evaluation of LVS Function	131	100%	100%	99%
Medicare Spending				
Medicare Spending per Patient (ratio)	-	1.00	1.02	0.98
Pneumonia Care				
Appropriate Initial Antibiotic Given	71	94%	97%	95%
Blood Culture Timing	108	96%	96%	98%
Pregnancy and Delivery Care				
Newborn Deliveries Scheduled Early	15	7%	4%	6%
Preventive Care				
Immunization for Influenza[2]	303	87%	87%	90%
Immunization for Pneumonia[2]	458	86%	86%	92%
Stroke Care				
Anticoagulation Therapy for Atrial Fibrillation[1]	-	-	94%	95%
Antithrombotic Therapy Timing	26	100%	98%	98%
Assessed for Rehabilitation	26	96%	97%	97%
Discharged on Antithrombotic Therapy	26	100%	100%	99%
Discharged on Statin Medication	21	95%	97%	94%
Thrombolytic Therapy Timing[7]	-	-	81%	66%
Venous Thromboembolism Prophylaxis	25	88%	95%	94%
Written Stroke Educational Materials Given	15	33%	90%	88%
Surgical Care Improvement Project				
Appropriate Beta Blocker Usage	64	97%	98%	98%
Appropriate VTP Within 24 Hours	163	95%	98%	98%
Controlled Postoperative Blood Glucose[7]	-	-	98%	97%
Perioperative Temperature Management	189	100%	100%	100%
Prophylactic Antibiotic Selection	131	100%	99%	99%
Prophylactic Antibiotic Selection (Outpatient)	61	100%	98%	98%
Prophylactic Antibiotic Stopped	126	98%	99%	98%
Prophylactic Antibiotic Timing	131	100%	99%	99%
Prophylactic Antibiotic Timing (Outpatient)	61	98%	97%	98%
Urinary Catheter Removal	152	99%	97%	97%
Survey of Patients' Hospital Experiences				
Area Around Room 'Always' Quiet at Night	300+	54%	54%	61%
Doctors 'Always' Communicated Well	300+	84%	80%	82%
Home Recovery Information Given	300+	83%	85%	85%
Hospital Given 9 or 10 on 10 Point Scale	300+	70%	69%	71%
Meds 'Always' Explained Before Given	300+	66%	61%	64%
Nurses 'Always' Communicated Well	300+	79%	79%	79%
Pain 'Always' Well Controlled	300+	70%	71%	71%
Room and Bathroom 'Always' Clean	300+	80%	73%	73%
Timely Help 'Always' Received	300+	64%	67%	68%
Would Definitely Recommend Hospital	300+	72%	72%	71%
Use of Medical Imaging				
Cardiac Imaging Stress Test before Surgery	86	3.5%	5.1%	5.3%
Combination Abdominal CT Scan	543	8.5%	4.6%	10.5%
Combination Brain/Sinus CT Scan	494	2.0%	3.9%	2.7%
Combination Chest CT Scan	449	0.0%	2.7%	2.7%
Follow-up Mammogram/Ultrasound	891	7.9%	7.9%	8.8%
Lumbar Spine MRI for Low Back Pain	109	24.8%	30.6%	37.2%

Landmark Medical Center

115 Cass Ave
Woonsocket, RI 02895
URL: www.landmarkmedical.org
Type: Acute Care Hospitals
Ownership: Voluntary non-profit - Private
Phone: 401-769-4100
Fax: 401-767-1674
Emergency Services: Yes
Beds: 233

Key Personnel:
Chief of Medical Staff . . . . Edward Anderson
Coronary Care . . . . Patricia Bibeault, RN
Radiology . . . . Vincent A DeCesaris
CEO/President . . . . Gary J Gaube
Quality Assurance . . . . Linda Kissick
Infection Control . . . . Isabelle Reis, RN
Pediatric Ambulatory Care . . . . . . Richard Smith, MD
Pediatric In-Patient Care . . . . Richard Smith, MD

Measure	Cases	This Hosp.	State Avg.	U.S. Avg.
Blood Clot Prevention and Treatment				
Anticoagulation Overlap Therapy[2]	42	100%	97%	93%
ICU Venous Thromboembolism Prophylaxis[2]	47	87%	92%	92%
Incidence of Potentially Preventable VTE[1,2]	-	-	10%	10%
UFH with Dosages/Platelet Monitoring[2]	41	100%	99%	97%
Venous Thromboembolism Prophylaxis[2]	408	82%	85%	85%
Warfarin Therapy Discharge Instructions[2]	34	79%	61%	75%
Chest Pain/Possible Heart Attack Care				
Aspirin Given Within 24 Hours of Arrival[1]	-	-	97%	96%
Fibrinolytic Meds Within 30 Min. of Arrival[3,7]	-	-	100%	58%
Average Time to ECG (minutes)	11	2	10	7
Average Time to Transfer (minutes)[3,7]	-	-	67	60
Children's Asthma Care				
Received Home Management Plan of Care	-	-	-	88%
Received Reliever Medication	-	-	-	100%
Received Systemic Corticosteroids	-	-	-	100%
Emergency Department				
Admittance Decision Time (minutes)[2]	956	128	115	98
Head CT Results Within 45 Min. of Arrival[1]	-	-	53%	57%
Patients Who Left ER Before Being Seen	40,589	2%	2%	2%
Time from ER Arrival to Admit. (minutes)[2]	962	348	334	274
Time from ER Arrival to Discharge (minutes)	1,516	116	152	134
Time in ER Before Being Evaluated (minutes)	1,727	29	37	26
Time to Pain Meds for Fractures (minutes)	82	51	54	57
Heart Attack Care				
Aspirin Given at Discharge	167	100%	100%	99%
Fibrinolytic Meds Within 30 Min. of Arrival[7]	-	-	-	54%
PCI Within 90 Minutes of Arrival	32	97%	98%	96%
Statin Prescribed at Discharge	152	95%	96%	98%

NOTE: Hospital profiles are in alphabetical order by state, then city, then hospital within the city; Rankings exclude hospitals with less than 25 cases except for patient surveys which excludes hospitals with less than 100 cases; (a) 100-299 cases; (1) The number of cases/patients is too few to report; (2) Data submitted were based on a sample of cases/patients; (3) Results are based on a shorter time period than required; (4) Data suppressed by CMS for one or more quarters; (5) Results are not available for this reporting period; (6) Fewer than 100 patients completed the HCAHPS survey; (7) No cases met the criteria for this measure; (8) The lower limit of the confidence interval cannot be calculated if the number of observed infections equals zero; (9) No data are available from the state/territory for this reporting period; (10) The scores shown reflect fewer than 50 completed surveys; (11) There were discrepancies in the data collection process; (12) This measure does not apply to this hospital for this reporting period; (13) Results cannot be calculated for this reporting period; (14) The results for this state are combined with nearby states to protect confidentiality; Please refer to the User's Guide for a full explanation of data.

Heart Failure Care				
ACE Inhibitor or ARB for LVSD	45	96%	95%	97%
Discharge Instructions Given	180	96%	91%	94%
Evaluation of LVS Function	257	100%	100%	99%
Medicare Spending				
Medicare Spending per Patient (ratio)	-	1.06	1.02	0.98
Pneumonia Care				
Appropriate Initial Antibiotic Given	133	99%	97%	95%
Blood Culture Timing	146	97%	96%	98%
Pregnancy and Delivery Care				
Newborn Deliveries Scheduled Early	19	0%	4%	6%
Preventive Care				
Immunization for Influenza[2]	551	96%	87%	90%
Immunization for Pneumonia[2]	866	95%	86%	92%
Stroke Care				
Anticoagulation Therapy for Atrial Fibrillation	13	100%	94%	95%
Antithrombotic Therapy Timing	59	100%	98%	98%
Assessed for Rehabilitation	59	97%	97%	97%
Discharged on Antithrombotic Therapy	59	97%	100%	99%
Discharged on Statin Medication	41	88%	97%	94%
Thrombolytic Therapy Timing[1]	-	-	81%	66%
Venous Thromboembolism Prophylaxis	64	92%	95%	94%
Written Stroke Educational Materials Given	25	80%	90%	88%
Surgical Care Improvement Project				
Appropriate Beta Blocker Usage	83	98%	98%	98%
Appropriate VTP Within 24 Hours	164	96%	98%	98%
Controlled Postoperative Blood Glucose[7]	-	-	98%	97%
Perioperative Temperature Management	221	100%	100%	100%
Prophylactic Antibiotic Selection	123	99%	99%	99%
Prophylactic Antibiotic Selection (Outpatient)	84	100%	98%	98%
Prophylactic Antibiotic Stopped	114	97%	99%	98%
Prophylactic Antibiotic Timing	124	99%	99%	99%
Prophylactic Antibiotic Timing (Outpatient)	85	99%	97%	98%
Urinary Catheter Removal	95	97%	97%	97%
Survey of Patients' Hospital Experiences				
Area Around Room 'Always' Quiet at Night	300+	42%	54%	61%
Doctors 'Always' Communicated Well	300+	73%	80%	82%
Home Recovery Information Given	300+	81%	85%	85%
Hospital Given 9 or 10 on 10 Point Scale	300+	54%	69%	71%
Meds 'Always' Explained Before Given	300+	54%	61%	64%
Nurses 'Always' Communicated Well	300+	74%	79%	79%
Pain 'Always' Well Controlled	300+	67%	71%	71%
Room and Bathroom 'Always' Clean	300+	68%	73%	73%
Timely Help 'Always' Received	300+	62%	67%	68%
Would Definitely Recommend Hospital	300+	57%	72%	71%
Use of Medical Imaging				
Cardiac Imaging Stress Test before Surgery	108	7.4%	5.1%	5.3%
Combination Abdominal CT Scan	469	2.8%	4.6%	10.5%
Combination Brain/Sinus CT Scan	524	2.7%	3.9%	2.7%
Combination Chest CT Scan	228	0.9%	2.7%	2.7%
Follow-up Mammogram/Ultrasound	633	5.8%	7.9%	8.8%
Lumbar Spine MRI for Low Back Pain[1]	-	-	30.6%	37.2%

NOTE: Hospital profiles are in alphabetical order by state, then city, then hospital within the city; Rankings exclude hospitals with less than 25 cases except for patient surveys which excludes hospitals with less than 100 cases; (a) 100-299 cases; (1) The number of cases/patients is too few to report; (2) Data submitted were based on a sample of cases/patients; (3) Results are based on a shorter time period than required; (4) Data suppressed by CMS for one or more quarters; (5) Results are not available for this reporting period; (6) Fewer than 100 patients completed the HCAHPS survey; (7) No cases met the criteria for this measure; (8) The lower limit of the confidence interval cannot be calculated if the number of observed infections equals zero; (9) No data are available from the state/territory for this reporting period; (10) The scores shown reflect fewer than 50 completed surveys; (11) There were discrepancies in the data collection process; (12) This measure does not apply to this hospital for this reporting period; (13) Results cannot be calculated for this reporting period; (14) The results for this state are combined with nearby states to protect confidentiality; Please refer to the User's Guide for a full explanation of data.

Blood Clot Prevention and Treatment

Anticoagulation Overlap Therapy

Hospital Name	City	Rate	Cases
Blount Memorial Hospital[2]	Maryville	100%	71
Dyersburg Regional Medical Center[2]	Dyersburg	100%	25
Fort Sanders Regional Medical Center[2]	Knoxville	100%	77
Laughlin Memorial Hospital[2]	Greeneville	100%	25
Leconte Medical Center[2]	Sevierville	100%	33
Methodist Medical Center of Oak Ridge[2]	Oak Ridge	100%	58
Morristown Hamblen Hospital Association[2]	Morristown	100%	37
Northcrest Medical Center[2]	Springfield	100%	35
Sumner Regional Medical Center[2]	Gallatin	100%	53
Tristar Hendersonville Medical Center[2]	Hendersonville	100%	63
Tristar Stonecrest Medical Center[2]	Smyrna	100%	29
Vanderbilt University Hospital[2]	Nashville	100%	195
Baptist Memorial Hospital[2]	Memphis	99%	277
Parkwest Medical Center[2]	Knoxville	99%	108
Regional Hospital of Jackson[2]	Jackson	99%	72
Tristar Skyline Medical Center[2]	Nashville	99%	81
Cumberland Medical Center[2]	Crossville	98%	56
Tristar Summit Medical Center[2]	Hermitage	98%	83
Wellmont Bristol Regional Medical Center[2]	Bristol	98%	97
Parkridge Medical Center[2]	Chattanooga	97%	94
Regional Medical Center at Memphis[2]	Memphis	97%	60
Skyridge Medical Center[2]	Cleveland	97%	73
Southern Tennessee Medical Center[2]	Winchester	97%	39
Tristar Horizon Medical Center[2]	Dickson	97%	35
Tristar Southern Hills Medical Center[2]	Nashville	97%	36
University Medical Center[2]	Lebanon	97%	33
Gateway Medical Center[2]	Clarksville	96%	50
Johnson City Medical Center[2]	Johnson City	96%	188
Maury Regional Hospital[2]	Columbia	96%	92
Saint Francis Hospital[2]	Memphis	96%	75
Takoma Regional Hospital[2]	Greeneville	96%	28
Franklin Woods Community Hospital[2]	Johnson City	95%	41
Saint Francis Bartlett Medical Center[2]	Bartlett	95%	81
University of Tn Memorial Hospital[2]	Knoxville	94%	196
Starr Regional Medical Center Athens[2]	Athens	93%	29
Methodist Healthcare Memphis Hospitals[2]	Memphis	92%	477
Saint Thomas Midtown Hospital[2]	Nashville	91%	114
Tristar Centennial Medical Center[2]	Nashville	91%	94
Jackson - Madison County General Hospital[2]	Jackson	90%	239
Wellmont Holston Valley Medical Center[2]	Kingsport	90%	137
Cookeville Regional Medical Center[2]	Cookeville	88%	154
Erlanger Medical Center[2]	Chattanooga	88%	142
Indian Path Medical Center[2]	Kingsport	88%	51
Williamson Medical Center[2]	Franklin	88%	68
Saint Thomas West Hospital[2]	Nashville	84%	165
Tennova Healthcare[2]	Knoxville	83%	114
Memorial Healthcare System[2]	Chattanooga	77%	149
Saint Thomas Rutherford Hospital[2]	Murfreesboro	73%	113

ICU Venous Thromboembolism Prophylaxis

Hospital Name	City	Rate	Cases
Fort Loudoun Medical Center[2]	Lenoir City	100%	49
Fort Sanders Regional Medical Center[2]	Knoxville	100%	74
Hillside Hospital[2]	Pulaski	100%	35
Lakeway Regional Hospital[2]	Morristown	100%	91
Leconte Medical Center[2]	Sevierville	100%	73
Livingston Regional Hospital[2]	Livingston	100%	47
Parkridge Medical Center[2]	Chattanooga	100%	121
Parkwest Medical Center[2]	Knoxville	100%	30
Starr Regional Medical Center Athens[2]	Athens	100%	50
Northcrest Medical Center[2]	Springfield	99%	78
Regional Hospital of Jackson[2]	Jackson	99%	138
Tristar Skyline Medical Center[2]	Nashville	99%	162
University of Tn Memorial Hospital[2]	Knoxville	99%	148
Baptist Memorial Hospital Union City[2]	Union City	98%	49
Cookeville Regional Medical Center[2]	Cookeville	98%	115
Dyersburg Regional Medical Center[2]	Dyersburg	98%	89
Laughlin Memorial Hospital[2]	Greeneville	98%	41
Morristown Hamblen Hospital Association[2]	Morristown	98%	47
Saint Francis Hospital[2]	Memphis	98%	87
Takoma Regional Hospital[2]	Greeneville	98%	63
Tristar Southern Hills Medical Center[2]	Nashville	98%	157
Maury Regional Hospital[2]	Columbia	97%	93
Roane Medical Center[2]	Harriman	97%	61
Skyridge Medical Center[2]	Cleveland	97%	107
Tristar Horizon Medical Center[2]	Dickson	97%	87
Tristar Summit Medical Center[2]	Hermitage	97%	68
Gateway Medical Center[2]	Clarksville	96%	51
Heritage Medical Center[2]	Shelbyville	96%	101
Sweetwater Hospital Association[2]	Sweetwater	96%	46
Tristar Stonecrest Medical Center[2]	Smyrna	96%	114
Volunteer Community Hospital[2]	Martin	96%	57
Blount Memorial Hospital[2]	Maryville	94%	72
Methodist Healthcare Memphis Hospitals[2]	Memphis	94%	106
Tristar Centennial Medical Center[2]	Nashville	94%	97
Tristar Hendersonville Medical Center[2]	Hendersonville	94%	142
Baptist Memorial Hospital[2]	Memphis	93%	168
Saint Francis Bartlett Medical Center[2]	Bartlett	93%	69
Sumner Regional Medical Center[2]	Gallatin	93%	112
Franklin Woods Community Hospital[2]	Johnson City	92%	39
Johnson City Medical Center[2]	Johnson City	92%	97
Williamson Medical Center[2]	Franklin	92%	95
Cumberland Medical Center[2]	Crossville	90%	90
Saint Thomas Midtown Hospital[2]	Nashville	90%	58
Vanderbilt University Hospital[2]	Nashville	90%	175
Harton Regional Medical Center[2]	Tullahoma	89%	57
Lincoln Medical Center[2]	Fayetteville	89%	38
Tennova Healthcare-Jefferson Mem Hosp[2]	Jefferson City	89%	38
Claiborne County Hospital[2]	Tazewell	88%	100
Crockett Hospital[2]	Lawrenceburg	88%	41
Jackson - Madison County General Hospital[2]	Jackson	88%	109
Tennova Healthcare-Newport Med Ctr[2]	Newport	88%	65
Baptist Memorial Hospital Tipton	Covington	87%	95
Sycamore Shoals Hospital[2]	Elizabethton	87%	67
Indian Path Medical Center[2]	Kingsport	86%	80
Southern Tennessee Medical Center[2]	Winchester	86%	93
Tennova Healthcare-Lafollett Med Ctr[2]	La Follette	86%	56
Henry County Medical Center[2]	Paris	85%	54
Erlanger Medical Center[2]	Chattanooga	84%	157
Saint Thomas West Hospital[2]	Nashville	84%	114
Highlands Medical Center[2]	Sparta	83%	29
Saint Thomas Rutherford Hospital[2]	Murfreesboro	83%	92
Tennova Healthcare[2]	Knoxville	83%	94
Metro Nashville General Hospital[2]	Nashville	82%	147
River Park Hospital[2]	Mc Minnville	82%	80
Wellmont Holston Valley Medical Center[2]	Kingsport	81%	91
Methodist Medical Center of Oak Ridge[2]	Oak Ridge	77%	74
Regional Medical Center at Memphis[2]	Memphis	77%	223
Starr Regional Medical Center Etowah[2,3]	Etowah	73%	37
Memorial Healthcare System[2]	Chattanooga	72%	183
University Medical Center[2]	Lebanon	71%	75
Delta Medical Center[2]	Memphis	69%	49
Wellmont Hawkins County Memorial Hospital[2]	Rogersville	69%	42
Stones River Hosp & Dekalb Comm Hosp[2]	Smithville	56%	61

Incidence of Potentially Preventable VTE

Hospital Name	City	Rate	Cases
Blount Memorial Hospital[2]	Maryville	0%	26
University of Tn Memorial Hospital[2]	Knoxville	0%	71
Johnson City Medical Center[2]	Johnson City	1%	74
Regional Medical Center at Memphis[2]	Memphis	6%	31
Baptist Memorial Hospital[2]	Memphis	7%	72
Methodist Healthcare Memphis Hospitals[2]	Memphis	7%	91
Parkwest Medical Center[2]	Knoxville	8%	26
Saint Thomas West Hospital[2]	Nashville	9%	44
Vanderbilt University Hospital[2]	Nashville	9%	57
Jackson - Madison County General Hospital[2]	Jackson	12%	50
Tristar Skyline Medical Center[2]	Nashville	14%	29
Wellmont Holston Valley Medical Center[2]	Kingsport	15%	46
Memorial Healthcare System[2]	Chattanooga	24%	34
Erlanger Medical Center[2]	Chattanooga	57%	30

UFH with Dosages/Platelet Count Monitoring

Hospital Name	City	Rate	Cases
Baptist Memorial Hospital[2]	Memphis	100%	274
Cookeville Regional Medical Center[2]	Cookeville	100%	92
Fort Sanders Regional Medical Center[2]	Knoxville	100%	27
Memorial Healthcare System[2]	Chattanooga	100%	150
Methodist Healthcare Memphis Hospitals[2]	Memphis	100%	398
Parkridge Medical Center[2]	Chattanooga	100%	89
Parkwest Medical Center[2]	Knoxville	100%	32
Regional Hospital of Jackson[2]	Jackson	100%	64
Regional Medical Center at Memphis[2]	Memphis	100%	43
Saint Francis Bartlett Medical Center[2]	Bartlett	100%	75
Saint Francis Hospital[2]	Memphis	100%	42
Saint Thomas West Hospital[2]	Nashville	100%	90
Southern Tennessee Medical Center[2]	Winchester	100%	29
Tennova Healthcare-Lafollett Med Ctr[2]	La Follette	100%	25
Tristar Skyline Medical Center[2]	Nashville	100%	25
University of Tn Memorial Hospital[2]	Knoxville	100%	112
Vanderbilt University Hospital[2]	Nashville	100%	163
Wellmont Bristol Regional Medical Center[2]	Bristol	100%	42
Wellmont Holston Valley Medical Center[2]	Kingsport	100%	96
Jackson - Madison County General Hospital[2]	Jackson	99%	223
Johnson City Medical Center[2]	Johnson City	99%	82
Skyridge Medical Center[2]	Cleveland	98%	63
Tennova Healthcare[2]	Knoxville	98%	44
Tristar Centennial Medical Center[2]	Nashville	98%	64
Indian Path Medical Center[2]	Kingsport	96%	25
Erlanger Medical Center[2]	Chattanooga	93%	147

Venous Thromboembolism Prophylaxis

Hospital Name	City	Rate	Cases
Henderson County Community Hospital[2]	Lexington	100%	303
Livingston Regional Hospital[2]	Livingston	100%	241
Saint Thomas Hospital for Spinal Surgery[2]	Nashville	100%	26
United Regional Medical Center[2]	Manchester	100%	125
Dyersburg Regional Medical Center[2]	Dyersburg	99%	288
Fort Loudoun Medical Center[2]	Lenoir City	99%	186
Leconte Medical Center[2]	Sevierville	99%	295
Fort Sanders Regional Medical Center[2]	Knoxville	98%	414
McNairy Regional Hospital[2]	Selmer	98%	304
Regional Hospital of Jackson[2]	Jackson	98%	394
Starr Regional Medical Center Athens[2]	Athens	98%	204
Tristar Skyline Medical Center[2]	Nashville	98%	297
University of Tn Memorial Hospital[2]	Knoxville	98%	341
Volunteer Community Hospital[2]	Martin	98%	161
Baptist Memorial Hospital Huntingdon	Huntingdon	97%	246
McKenzie Regional Hospital[2]	Mc Kenzie	97%	191
Morristown Hamblen Hospital Association[2]	Morristown	97%	402
Tennova Healthcare-Jefferson Mem Hosp[2]	Jefferson City	97%	177
Tristar Horizon Medical Center[2]	Dickson	97%	359
Blount Memorial Hospital[2]	Maryville	96%	369
Tristar Stonecrest Medical Center[2]	Smyrna	96%	272
Heritage Medical Center[2]	Shelbyville	95%	224
Northcrest Medical Center[2]	Springfield	95%	259
Sumner Regional Medical Center[2]	Gallatin	95%	295
Tristar Summit Medical Center[2]	Hermitage	95%	320
Hillside Hospital[2]	Pulaski	94%	105
Saint Francis Hospital[2]	Memphis	94%	343
Skyridge Medical Center[2]	Cleveland	94%	330
Takoma Regional Hospital[2]	Greeneville	94%	131
Crockett Hospital[2]	Lawrenceburg	93%	153
Parkridge Medical Center[2]	Chattanooga	93%	319
Parkwest Medical Center[2]	Knoxville	93%	307
Roane Medical Center[2]	Harriman	93%	329
Baptist Memorial Hospital Union City[2]	Union City	92%	204
Vanderbilt University Hospital[2]	Nashville	92%	309
Gateway Medical Center[2]	Clarksville	91%	387
Lakeway Regional Hospital[2]	Morristown	91%	223
Laughlin Memorial Hospital[2]	Greeneville	91%	277
Methodist Healthcare Memphis Hospitals[2]	Memphis	90%	318
Saint Francis Bartlett Medical Center[2]	Bartlett	89%	386
Indian Path Medical Center[2]	Kingsport	88%	337
Maury Regional Hospital[2]	Columbia	88%	313
Methodist Medical Center of Oak Ridge[2]	Oak Ridge	88%	395
Sweetwater Hospital Association[2]	Sweetwater	88%	180
Henry County Medical Center[2]	Paris	87%	255
Methodist Healthcare Fayette Hospital[2]	Somerville	87%	79
Tristar Ashland City Medical Center[2]	Ashland City	87%	54
Wellmont Bristol Regional Medical Center[2]	Bristol	87%	359
Baptist Memorial Hospital[2]	Memphis	86%	611
Southern Tennessee Medical Center[2]	Winchester	86%	349
Tristar Hendersonville Medical Center[2]	Hendersonville	86%	277
Tristar Southern Hills Medical Center[2]	Nashville	86%	250
Riverview Regional Medical Center[2]	Carthage	85%	105
Lincoln Medical Center[2]	Fayetteville	84%	126
Regional Medical Center at Memphis[2]	Memphis	84%	571
Tennova Healthcare-Newport Med Ctr[2]	Newport	84%	188
Cookeville Regional Medical Center[2]	Cookeville	83%	322
Cumberland Medical Center[2]	Crossville	83%	382
Franklin Woods Community Hospital[2]	Johnson City	83%	312
Tristar Centennial Medical Center[2]	Nashville	83%	358
Wayne Medical Center	Waynesboro	83%	281
Jackson - Madison County General Hospital[2]	Jackson	82%	349
River Park Hospital[2]	Mc Minnville	82%	201
Saint Thomas Rutherford Hospital[2]	Murfreesboro	82%	328
Wellmont Holston Valley Medical Center[2]	Kingsport	82%	301
Haywood Park Community Hospital[2]	Brownsville	81%	134
Jellico Community Hospital[2]	Jellico	81%	100
Tennova Healthcare[2]	Knoxville	81%	300
Williamson Medical Center[2]	Franklin	81%	285
Grandview Medical Center[2]	Jasper	80%	164
Johnson City Medical Center[2]	Johnson City	80%	351
Sycamore Shoals Hospital[2]	Elizabethton	80%	262
Memorial Healthcare System[2]	Chattanooga	78%	732
Claiborne County Hospital[2]	Tazewell	77%	254
Saint Thomas Midtown Hospital[2]	Nashville	77%	333
Erlanger Medical Center[2]	Chattanooga	76%	313
Saint Thomas West Hospital[2]	Nashville	76%	267
Metro Nashville General Hospital[2]	Nashville	74%	253
Wellmont Hawkins County Memorial Hospital[2]	Rogersville	73%	289
Tennova Healthcare-Lafollett Med Ctr[2]	La Follette	72%	216
Delta Medical Center[2]	Memphis	70%	186
Baptist Memorial Hospital Tipton	Covington	64%	385
Starr Regional Medical Center Etowah[2,3]	Etowah	64%	107
Hardin Medical Center[2]	Savannah	60%	171
Harton Regional Medical Center[2]	Tullahoma	60%	392
Highlands Medical Center[2]	Sparta	60%	102
University Medical Center[2]	Lebanon	56%	352
Jamestown Regional Medical Center[2]	Jamestown	54%	185
Stones River Hosp & Dekalb Comm Hosp[2]	Woodbury	50%	278
Milan General Hospital[2]	Milan	49%	86
Stones River Hosp & Dekalb Comm Hosp[2]	Smithville	48%	287
Bolivar General Hospital[2]	Bolivar	46%	87
Cumberland River Hospital[2]	Celina	40%	134
Decatur County General Hospital[2]	Parsons	35%	322

NOTE: Hospital profiles are in alphabetical order by state, then city, then hospital within the city; Rankings exclude hospitals with less than 25 cases except for patient surveys which excludes hospitals with less than 100 cases; (a) 100-299 cases; (1) The number of cases/patients is too few to report; (2) Data submitted were based on a sample of cases/patients; (3) Results are based on a shorter time period than required; (4) Data suppressed by CMS for one or more quarters; (5) Results are not available for this reporting period; (6) Fewer than 100 patients completed the HCAHPS survey; (7) No cases met the criteria for this measure; (8) The lower limit of the confidence interval cannot be calculated if the number of observed infections equals zero; (9) No data are available from the state/territory for this reporting period; (10) The scores shown reflect fewer than 50 completed surveys; (11) There were discrepancies in the data collection process; (12) This measure does not apply to this hospital for this reporting period; (13) Results cannot be calculated for this reporting period; (14) The results for this state are combined with nearby states to protect confidentiality; Please refer to the User's Guide for a full explanation of data.

Hospital Name	City	Rate	Cases
Unicoi County Memorial Hospital[2]	Erwin	32%	113
Perry Community Hospital[2]	Linden	9%	244

Warfarin Therapy Discharge Instructions

Hospital Name	City	Rate	Cases
Leconte Medical Center[2]	Sevierville	100%	25
Morristown Hamblen Hospital Association[2]	Morristown	100%	31
Northcrest Medical Center[2]	Springfield	100%	26
Saint Francis Bartlett Medical Center[2]	Bartlett	100%	57
Saint Francis Hospital[2]	Memphis	100%	68
Skyridge Medical Center[2]	Cleveland	100%	56
Starr Regional Medical Center Athens[2]	Athens	100%	27
Sumner Regional Medical Center[2]	Gallatin	100%	39
Tristar Skyline Medical Center[2]	Nashville	100%	58
Vanderbilt University Hospital[2]	Nashville	100%	154
Wellmont Bristol Regional Medical Center[2]	Bristol	100%	82
Cumberland Medical Center[2]	Crossville	98%	49
Fort Sanders Regional Medical Center[2]	Knoxville	98%	64
Jackson - Madison County General Hospital[2]	Jackson	98%	172
Regional Hospital of Jackson[2]	Jackson	98%	52
Tristar Hendersonville Medical Center[2]	Hendersonville	98%	50
Parkwest Medical Center[2]	Knoxville	97%	76
Southern Tennessee Medical Center[2]	Winchester	97%	30
Methodist Medical Center of Oak Ridge[2]	Oak Ridge	96%	45
Tristar Centennial Medical Center[2]	Nashville	95%	74
Gateway Medical Center[2]	Clarksville	94%	35
Williamson Medical Center[2]	Franklin	93%	41
Parkridge Medical Center[2]	Chattanooga	92%	79
Tennova Healthcare[2]	Knoxville	92%	83
Tristar Summit Medical Center[2]	Hermitage	92%	65
Tristar Southern Hills Medical Center[2]	Nashville	90%	31
Erlanger Medical Center[2]	Chattanooga	87%	79
University of Tn Memorial Hospital[2]	Knoxville	87%	123
Tristar Horizon Medical Center[2]	Dickson	84%	25
Baptist Memorial Hospital[2]	Memphis	83%	196
Regional Medical Center at Memphis[2]	Memphis	83%	48
Blount Memorial Hospital[2]	Maryville	82%	44
Saint Thomas Rutherford Hospital[2]	Murfreesboro	79%	94
Saint Thomas West Hospital[2]	Nashville	74%	132
Saint Thomas Midtown Hospital[2]	Nashville	71%	92
Wellmont Holston Valley Medical Center[2]	Kingsport	61%	100
Methodist Healthcare Memphis Hospitals[2]	Memphis	58%	384
Franklin Woods Community Hospital[2]	Johnson City	50%	34
University Medical Center[2]	Lebanon	48%	29
Memorial Healthcare System[2]	Chattanooga	36%	115
Johnson City Medical Center[2]	Johnson City	26%	126
Cookeville Regional Medical Center[2]	Cookeville	21%	112
Maury Regional Hospital[2]	Columbia	16%	69
Indian Path Medical Center[2]	Kingsport	9%	34

Chest Pain/Possible Heart Attack Care

Aspirin Given Within 24 Hours of Arrival

Hospital Name	City	Rate	Cases
Baptist Memorial Hospital Union City	Union City	100%	177
Henderson County Community Hospital	Lexington	100%	58
Heritage Medical Center	Shelbyville	100%	77
Johnson County Community Hospital	Mountain City	100%	73
Laughlin Memorial Hospital	Greeneville	100%	39
Milan General Hospital	Milan	100%	98
Northcrest Medical Center	Springfield	100%	29
Parkridge Medical Center	Chattanooga	100%	30
Rhea Medical Center	Dayton	100%	29
Saint Thomas Rutherford Hospital	Murfreesboro	100%	32
Skyridge Medical Center	Cleveland	100%	78
Sumner Regional Medical Center	Gallatin	100%	34
Tristar Ashland City Medical Center	Ashland City	100%	51
Tristar Hendersonville Medical Center	Hendersonville	100%	25
Tristar Stonecrest Medical Center	Smyrna	100%	52
Franklin Woods Community Hospital	Johnson City	99%	101
Hardin Medical Center	Savannah	99%	205
Haywood Park Community Hospital	Brownsville	99%	87
Tennova Healthcare-Lafollett Med Ctr	La Follette	99%	93
Tennova Healthcare-Newport Med Ctr	Newport	99%	127
Volunteer Community Hospital	Martin	99%	191
Cumberland Medical Center	Crossville	98%	149
Dyersburg Regional Medical Center	Dyersburg	98%	248
Gateway Medical Center	Clarksville	98%	44
Gibson General Hospital[3]	Trenton	98%	42
Harton Regional Medical Center	Tullahoma	98%	54
Leconte Medical Center	Sevierville	98%	99
McKenzie Regional Hospital	Mc Kenzie	98%	122
McNairy Regional Hospital	Selmer	98%	91
River Park Hospital	Mc Minnville	98%	110
Saint Francis Bartlett Medical Center	Bartlett	98%	48
Starr Regional Medical Center Athens	Athens	98%	123
Takoma Regional Hospital	Greeneville	98%	88
Tristar Horizon Medical Center	Dickson	98%	126
Wellmont Hawkins County Memorial Hospital	Rogersville	98%	49
Bolivar General Hospital	Bolivar	97%	108
Henry County Medical Center	Paris	97%	205
Hillside Hospital	Pulaski	97%	69
Jamestown Regional Medical Center	Jamestown	97%	63
Lincoln Medical Center	Fayetteville	97%	76
Methodist Healthcare Fayette Hospital	Somerville	97%	62
Riverview Regional Medical Center	Carthage	97%	62
Southern Tennessee Medical Center	Winchester	97%	92
Sycamore Shoals Hospital	Elizabethton	97%	137
Tennova Healthcare-Jefferson Mem Hosp	Jefferson City	97%	97
Unicoi County Memorial Hospital	Erwin	97%	34
Jellico Community Hospital	Jellico	96%	27
Livingston Regional Hospital	Livingston	96%	48
Crockett Hospital	Lawrenceburg	95%	166
Fort Loudoun Medical Center	Lenoir City	95%	39
Macon County General Hospital	Lafayette	95%	57
Baptist Memorial Hospital Huntingdon	Huntingdon	94%	81
Lauderdale Community Hospital	Ripley	94%	68
Memorial Healthcare System	Chattanooga	94%	34
Stones River Hosp & Dekalb Comm Hosp	Smithville	93%	70
University Medical Center	Lebanon	93%	61
Williamson Medical Center	Franklin	93%	27
Roane Medical Center	Harriman	92%	66
Humboldt General Hospital[3]	Humboldt	91%	45
Sweetwater Hospital Association	Sweetwater	91%	70
Baptist Memorial Hospital Tipton	Covington	90%	168
Grandview Medical Center	Jasper	90%	49
Marshall Medical Center	Lewisburg	90%	68
Claibome County Hospital	Tazewell	89%	72
Lakeway Regional Hospital	Morristown	88%	25
Highlands Medical Center	Sparta	85%	46
Decatur County General Hospital	Parsons	84%	57
Wayne Medical Center	Waynesboro	82%	38
Medical Center of Manchester	Manchester	80%	44
Perry Community Hospital	Linden	71%	49

Average Time to ECG (minutes)

Hospital Name	City	Min.	Cases
Henderson County Community Hospital	Lexington	0	62
Dyersburg Regional Medical Center	Dyersburg	2	254
Livingston Regional Hospital	Livingston	2	50
Skyridge Medical Center	Cleveland	2	79
Franklin Woods Community Hospital	Johnson City	3	109
Harton Regional Medical Center	Tullahoma	3	56
Lakeway Regional Hospital	Morristown	3	25
Parkridge Medical Center	Chattanooga	3	34
River Park Hospital	Mc Minnville	3	112
Sycamore Shoals Hospital	Elizabethton	3	143
Unicoi County Memorial Hospital	Erwin	3	34
Bolivar General Hospital	Bolivar	4	116
Crockett Hospital	Lawrenceburg	4	171
Gibson General Hospital[3]	Trenton	4	43
Heritage Medical Center	Shelbyville	4	83
Lincoln Medical Center	Fayetteville	4	81
McKenzie Regional Hospital	Mc Kenzie	4	129
Methodist Healthcare Fayette Hospital	Somerville	4	64
Starr Regional Medical Center Athens	Athens	4	126
Tristar Hendersonville Medical Center	Hendersonville	4	25
Tristar Stonecrest Medical Center	Smyrna	4	54
Baptist Memorial Hospital Union City	Union City	5	192
Gateway Medical Center	Clarksville	5	46
Henry County Medical Center	Paris	5	207
Perry Community Hospital	Linden	5	51
Rhea Medical Center	Dayton	5	30
Stones River Hosp & Dekalb Comm Hosp	Smithville	5	75
University Medical Center	Lebanon	5	67
Volunteer Community Hospital	Martin	5	208
Hillside Hospital	Pulaski	6	77
Humboldt General Hospital[3]	Humboldt	6	48
McNairy Regional Hospital	Selmer	6	93
Memorial Healthcare System	Chattanooga	6	35
Milan General Hospital	Milan	6	102
Riverview Regional Medical Center	Carthage	6	64
Saint Francis Bartlett Medical Center	Bartlett	6	47
Saint Thomas Rutherford Hospital	Murfreesboro	6	31
Southern Tennessee Medical Center	Winchester	6	93
Tennova Healthcare-Newport Med Ctr	Newport	6	136
Tristar Ashland City Medical Center	Ashland City	6	53
Tristar Horizon Medical Center	Dickson	6	132
Cumberland Medical Center	Crossville	7	156
Fort Loudoun Medical Center	Lenoir City	7	41
Highlands Medical Center	Sparta	7	47
Jamestown Regional Medical Center	Jamestown	7	87
Johnson County Community Hospital	Mountain City	7	76
Laughlin Memorial Hospital	Greeneville	7	41
Starr Regional Medical Center Etowah	Etowah	7	25
Sumner Regional Medical Center	Gallatin	7	35
Tennova Healthcare-Jefferson Mem Hosp	Jefferson City	7	98
Tennova Healthcare-Lafollett Med Ctr	La Follette	7	98
Wellmont Hawkins County Memorial Hospital	Rogersville	7	51
Williamson Medical Center	Franklin	7	27
Baptist Memorial Hospital Huntingdon	Huntingdon	8	84
Claibome County Hospital	Tazewell	8	77
Hardin Medical Center	Savannah	9	216
Haywood Park Community Hospital	Brownsville	9	89
Lauderdale Community Hospital	Ripley	9	69
Northcrest Medical Center	Springfield	9	31
Leconte Medical Center	Sevierville	10	101
Macon County General Hospital	Lafayette	10	66
Roane Medical Center	Harriman	10	68
Takoma Regional Hospital	Greeneville	10	93
Wayne Medical Center	Waynesboro	10	39
Marshall Medical Center	Lewisburg	11	73
Baptist Memorial Hospital Tipton	Covington	12	174
Decatur County General Hospital	Parsons	12	59
Grandview Medical Center	Jasper	12	50
Jellico Community Hospital	Jellico	12	27
Sweetwater Hospital Association	Sweetwater	13	70
Medical Center of Manchester	Manchester	28	46

Average Time to Transfer (minutes)

Hospital Name	City	Min.	Cases
Tristar Horizon Medical Center	Dickson	23	26
Skyridge Medical Center	Cleveland	30	28
Leconte Medical Center	Sevierville	46	30

Children's Asthma Care

Received Home Management Plan of Care

Hospital Name	City	Rate	Cases
Johnson City Medical Center[2]	Johnson City	94%	69
Methodist Healthcare Memphis Hospitals[2]	Memphis	89%	352
Erlanger Medical Center	Chattanooga	68%	28

Received Reliever Medication

Hospital Name	City	Rate	Cases
Erlanger Medical Center	Chattanooga	100%	28
Johnson City Medical Center[2]	Johnson City	100%	69
Methodist Healthcare Memphis Hospitals[2]	Memphis	100%	352

Received Systemic Corticosteroids

Hospital Name	City	Rate	Cases
Erlanger Medical Center	Chattanooga	100%	28
Johnson City Medical Center[2]	Johnson City	100%	68
Methodist Healthcare Memphis Hospitals[2]	Memphis	100%	352

Emergency Department

Admittance Decision Time (minutes)

Hospital Name	City	Min.	Cases
Perry Community Hospital[2]	Linden	0	222
Cumberland River Hospital	Celina	25	247
Riverview Regional Medical Center[2]	Carthage	28	445
Henderson County Community Hospital[2]	Lexington	34	426
Grandview Medical Center[2]	Jasper	36	469
McKenzie Regional Hospital[2]	Mc Kenzie	37	259
Jellico Community Hospital[2]	Jellico	40	310
Methodist Healthcare Fayette Hospital[2]	Somerville	43	39
Stones River Hosp & Dekalb Comm Hosp[2]	Woodbury	44	309
Laughlin Memorial Hospital[2]	Greeneville	45	444
Tristar Ashland City Medical Center[2]	Ashland City	45	57
Livingston Regional Hospital[2]	Livingston	48	164
Haywood Park Community Hospital[2]	Brownsville	49	171
Decatur County General Hospital[2]	Parsons	50	428
Stones River Hosp & Dekalb Comm Hosp[2]	Smithville	50	312
Cumberland Medical Center[2]	Crossville	51	514
Starr Regional Medical Center Etowah[2,3]	Etowah	51	249
Sycamore Shoals Hospital[2]	Elizabethton	51	363
Hillside Hospital[2]	Pulaski	53	290
Regional Hospital of Jackson[2]	Jackson	54	767
Dyersburg Regional Medical Center[2]	Dyersburg	55	481
Lincoln Medical Center[2]	Fayetteville	56	286
Southern Tennessee Medical Center[2]	Winchester	56	444
Sumner Regional Medical Center[2]	Gallatin	57	532
Jamestown Regional Medical Center[2]	Jamestown	59	308
Baptist Memorial Hospital Huntingdon[2]	Huntingdon	61	187
Franklin Woods Community Hospital[2]	Johnson City	61	272
Northcrest Medical Center[2]	Springfield	61	340
University Medical Center[2]	Lebanon	61	449
Henry County Medical Center[2]	Paris	62	304
Tennova Healthcare-Jefferson Mem Hosp[2]	Jefferson City	62	529
River Park Hospital[2]	Mc Minnville	63	409
Tennova Healthcare-Lafollett Med Ctr[2]	La Follette	63	493
Crockett Hospital[2]	Lawrenceburg	64	220
Hardin Medical Center[2]	Savannah	65	324
Lakeway Regional Hospital[2]	Morristown	65	462
Methodist Healthcare Memphis Hospitals[2]	Memphis	65	591
Unicoi County Memorial Hospital[2]	Erwin	65	321
United Regional Medical Center[2]	Manchester	66	264
Tennova Healthcare-Newport Med Ctr[2]	Newport	67	530

NOTE: Hospital profiles are in alphabetical order by state, then city, then hospital within the city; Rankings exclude hospitals with less than 25 cases except for patient surveys which excludes hospitals with less than 100 cases; (a) 100-299 cases; (1) The number of cases/patients is too few to report; (2) Data submitted were based on a sample of cases/patients; (3) Results are based on a shorter time period than required; (4) Data suppressed by CMS for one or more quarters; (5) Results are not available for this reporting period; (6) Fewer than 100 patients completed the HCAHPS survey; (7) No cases met the criteria for this measure; (8) The lower limit of the confidence interval cannot be calculated if the number of observed infections equals zero; (9) No data are available from the state/territory for this reporting period; (10) The scores shown reflect fewer than 50 completed surveys; (11) There were discrepancies in the data collection process; (12) This measure does not apply to this hospital for this reporting period; (13) Results cannot be calculated for this reporting period; (14) The results for this state are combined with nearby states to protect confidentiality; Please refer to the User's Guide for a full explanation of data.

Metro Nashville General Hospital[2]	Nashville	68	231
Saint Thomas West Hospital[2]	Nashville	68	381
Baptist Memorial Hospital Union City[2]	Union City	69	244
Sweetwater Hospital Association[2]	Sweetwater	69	335
Highlands Medical Center[2]	Sparta	70	425
Starr Regional Medical Center Athens[2]	Athens	70	265
Wayne Medical Center	Waynesboro	70	194
Harton Regional Medical Center[2]	Tullahoma	71	459
Saint Thomas Midtown Hospital[2]	Nashville	71	355
Wellmont Hawkins County Memorial Hospital[2]	Rogersville	71	477
Baptist Memorial Hospital Tipton[2]	Covington	72	218
Tristar Horizon Medical Center[2]	Dickson	72	600
McNairy Regional Hospital[2]	Selmer	75	370
Tristar Stonecrest Medical Center[2]	Smyrna	76	389
Tristar Hendersonville Medical Center[2]	Hendersonville	77	677
Tristar Summit Medical Center[2]	Hermitage	80	777
Takoma Regional Hospital[2]	Greeneville	81	295
Heritage Medical Center[2]	Shelbyville	82	486
Milan General Hospital	Milan	85	66
Volunteer Community Hospital[2]	Martin	86	279
Maury Regional Hospital[2]	Columbia	87	437
Roane Medical Center[2]	Harriman	87	343
Saint Thomas Rutherford Hospital[2]	Murfreesboro	88	546
Williamson Medical Center[2]	Franklin	90	481
Jackson - Madison County General Hospital[2]	Jackson	92	480
Bolivar General Hospital	Bolivar	93	189
Cookeville Regional Medical Center[2]	Cookeville	94	487
Baptist Memorial Hospital[2]	Memphis	95	960
Claiborne County Hospital[2]	Tazewell	95	484
Morristown Hamblen Hospital Association[2]	Morristown	96	765
Delta Medical Center[2]	Memphis	100	319
Tristar Centennial Medical Center[2]	Nashville	101	414
Tristar Southern Hills Medical Center[2]	Nashville	103	537
Tristar Skyline Medical Center[2]	Nashville	105	716
Blount Memorial Hospital[2]	Maryville	106	788
Johnson City Medical Center[2]	Johnson City	106	338
Saint Francis Bartlett Medical Center[2]	Bartlett	107	791
Parkridge Medical Center[2]	Chattanooga	108	536
University of Tn Memorial Hospital[2]	Knoxville	111	137
Leconte Medical Center[2]	Sevierville	115	548
Fort Loudoun Medical Center[2]	Lenoir City	121	523
Vanderbilt University Hospital[2]	Nashville	121	257
Memorial Healthcare System[2]	Chattanooga	122	1202
Wellmont Bristol Regional Medical Center[2]	Bristol	122	589
Saint Francis Hospital[2]	Memphis	131	1180
Skyridge Medical Center[2]	Cleveland	132	736
Indian Path Medical Center[2]	Kingsport	137	374
Regional Medical Center at Memphis[2]	Memphis	137	879
Gateway Medical Center[2]	Clarksville	138	587
Parkwest Medical Center[2]	Knoxville	146	445
Methodist Medical Center of Oak Ridge[2]	Oak Ridge	147	780
Erlanger Medical Center[2]	Chattanooga	150	392
Fort Sanders Regional Medical Center[2]	Knoxville	161	616
Tennova Healthcare[2]	Knoxville	161	700
Wellmont Holston Valley Medical Center[2]	Kingsport	206	605

Head CT Results Within 45 Minutes of Arrival

Hospital Name	City	Rate	Cases
Gateway Medical Center	Clarksville	80%	25
Skyridge Medical Center	Cleveland	55%	38
Methodist Healthcare Memphis Hospitals	Memphis	41%	27
Tennova Healthcare	Knoxville	26%	27

Patients Who Left ER Before Being Seen

Hospital Name	City	Rate	Cases
Fort Loudoun Medical Center	Lenoir City	0%	21672
Johnson County Community Hospital	Mountain City	0%	10947
Williamson Medical Center	Franklin	0%	38750
Baptist Memorial Hospital	Memphis	1%	79761
Baptist Memorial Hospital Union City	Union City	1%	18843
Copper Basin Medical Center	Copperhill	1%	6427
Crockett Hospital	Lawrenceburg	1%	14603
Cumberland Medical Center	Crossville	1%	34949
Cumberland River Hospital	Celina	1%	4567
Fort Sanders Regional Medical Center	Knoxville	1%	51582
Franklin Woods Community Hospital	Johnson City	1%	26515
Gibson General Hospital	Trenton	1%	7355
Haywood Park Community Hospital	Brownsville	1%	6230
Henderson County Community Hospital	Lexington	1%	10575
Heritage Medical Center	Shelbyville	1%	20802
Highlands Medical Center	Sparta	1%	12629
Humboldt General Hospital	Humboldt	1%	9956
Indian Path Medical Center	Kingsport	1%	36020
Jamestown Regional Medical Center	Jamestown	1%	10600
Laughlin Memorial Hospital	Greeneville	1%	28170
Maury Regional Hospital	Columbia	1%	49938
McKenzie Regional Hospital	Mc Kenzie	1%	6676
McNairy Regional Hospital	Selmer	1%	11367
Northcrest Medical Center	Springfield	1%	30133
Regional Medical Center at Memphis	Memphis	1%	31239
Riverview Regional Medical Center	Carthage	1%	8895
Saint Thomas West Hospital	Nashville	1%	34039
Southern Tennessee Medical Center	Winchester	1%	18436
Stones River Hosp & Dekalb Comm Hosp	Smithville	1%	9729
Sumner Regional Medical Center	Gallatin	1%	37850
Sycamore Shoals Hospital	Elizabethton	1%	23715
Tennova Healthcare-Jefferson Mem Hosp	Jefferson City	1%	25327
Tennova Healthcare-Lafollett Med Ctr	La Follette	1%	21985
Tennova Healthcare-Newport Med Ctr	Newport	1%	34828
Tristar Ashland City Medical Center	Ashland City	1%	11762
Tristar Hendersonville Medical Center	Hendersonville	1%	31282
Tristar Horizon Medical Center	Dickson	1%	37794
Tristar Skyline Medical Center	Nashville	1%	54976
Tristar Southern Hills Medical Center	Nashville	1%	40711
Tristar Stonecrest Medical Center	Smyrna	1%	47094
Tristar Summit Medical Center	Hermitage	1%	51504
Unicoi County Memorial Hospital	Erwin	1%	7282
University of Tn Memorial Hospital	Knoxville	1%	80433
Volunteer Community Hospital	Martin	1%	11485
Wellmont Holston Valley Medical Center	Kingsport	1%	62964
Baptist Memorial Hospital Huntingdon	Huntingdon	2%	7805
Baptist Memorial Hospital Tipton	Covington	2%	21655
Blount Memorial Hospital	Maryville	2%	54697
Claiborne County Hospital	Tazewell	2%	14697
Decatur County General Hospital	Parsons	2%	5382
Delta Medical Center	Memphis	2%	27279
Dyersburg Regional Medical Center	Dyersburg	2%	27493
Grandview Medical Center	Jasper	2%	18364
Hardin Medical Center	Savannah	2%	19234
Harton Regional Medical Center	Tullahoma	2%	27618
Hillside Hospital	Pulaski	2%	11549
Jellico Community Hospital	Jellico	2%	6005
Lincoln Medical Center	Fayetteville	2%	18328
Livingston Regional Hospital	Livingston	2%	12487
Methodist Healthcare Fayette Hospital	Somerville	2%	8129
Methodist Medical Center of Oak Ridge	Oak Ridge	2%	44459
Parkridge Medical Center	Chattanooga	2%	76341
Parkwest Medical Center	Knoxville	2%	49422
Perry Community Hospital	Linden	2%	4534
Regional Hospital of Jackson	Jackson	2%	23708
River Park Hospital	Mc Minnville	2%	24636
Saint Thomas Midtown Hospital	Nashville	2%	52828
Starr Regional Medical Center Athens	Athens	2%	33015
Stones River Hosp & Dekalb Comm Hosp	Woodbury	2%	6390
Sweetwater Hospital Association	Sweetwater	2%	24711
Takoma Regional Hospital	Greeneville	2%	21539
Tennova Healthcare	Knoxville	2%	103147
Tristar Centennial Medical Center	Nashville	2%	32312
University Medical Center	Lebanon	2%	29656
Vanderbilt University Hospital	Nashville	2%	121750
Wayne Medical Center	Waynesboro	2%	3911
Wellmont Hawkins County Memorial Hospital	Rogersville	2%	18223
Cookeville Regional Medical Center	Cookeville	3%	50553
Henry County Medical Center	Paris	3%	19373
Johnson City Medical Center	Johnson City	3%	53187
Marshall Medical Center	Lewisburg	3%	13993
Memorial Healthcare System	Chattanooga	3%	58322
Methodist Healthcare Memphis Hospitals	Memphis	3%	337004
Morristown Hamblen Hospital Association	Morristown	3%	40009
Roane Medical Center	Harriman	3%	21231
Saint Francis Bartlett Medical Center	Bartlett	3%	36561
Saint Thomas Rutherford Hospital	Murfreesboro	3%	78924
Skyridge Medical Center	Cleveland	3%	57228
Starr Regional Medical Center Etowah	Etowah	3%	13431
Wellmont Bristol Regional Medical Center	Bristol	3%	64536
Bolivar General Hospital	Bolivar	4%	9900
Erlanger Medical Center	Chattanooga	4%	109897
Gateway Medical Center	Clarksville	4%	66288
Jackson - Madison County General Hospital	Jackson	4%	85854
Metro Nashville General Hospital	Nashville	4%	37577
Milan General Hospital	Milan	4%	8041
Saint Francis Hospital	Memphis	4%	42317
Leconte Medical Center	Sevierville	5%	54577
Lakeway Regional Hospital	Morristown	6%	15635

Time from ER Arrival to Being Admitted (minutes)

Hospital Name	City	Min.	Cases
Cumberland River Hospital	Celina	118	285
Henderson County Community Hospital[2]	Lexington	141	427
McKenzie Regional Hospital[2]	Mc Kenzie	146	260
Perry Community Hospital[2]	Linden	155	273
Riverview Regional Medical Center[2]	Carthage	155	445
Decatur County General Hospital[2]	Parsons	161	441
Livingston Regional Hospital[2]	Livingston	164	164
Tristar Ashland City Medical Center[2]	Ashland City	166	60
Regional Hospital of Jackson[2]	Jackson	173	775
Laughlin Memorial Hospital[2]	Greeneville	180	444
Stones River Hosp & Dekalb Comm Hosp[2]	Woodbury	180	309
Haywood Park Community Hospital[2]	Brownsville	183	179
Jamestown Regional Medical Center[2]	Jamestown	183	314
Stones River Hosp & Dekalb Comm Hosp[2]	Smithville	185	312
Cumberland Medical Center[2]	Crossville	190	517
Hillside Hospital[2]	Pulaski	192	293
Southern Tennessee Medical Center[2]	Winchester	192	444
Jellico Community Hospital[2]	Jellico	197	324
Saint Thomas Midtown Hospital[2]	Nashville	199	360
Tennova Healthcare-Lafollett Med Ctr[2]	La Follette	200	496
Harton Regional Medical Center[2]	Tullahoma	201	459
Dyersburg Regional Medical Center[2]	Dyersburg	202	487
Tristar Hendersonville Medical Center[2]	Hendersonville	203	682
University Medical Center[2]	Lebanon	206	460
Starr Regional Medical Center Etowah[2,3]	Etowah	207	255
Saint Thomas West Hospital[2]	Nashville	208	395
Sycamore Shoals Hospital[2]	Elizabethton	214	419
United Regional Medical Center[2]	Manchester	214	276
Henry County Medical Center[2]	Paris	215	323
Wellmont Hawkins County Memorial Hospital[2]	Rogersville	215	481
Baptist Memorial Hospital Huntingdon[2]	Huntingdon	219	206
Heritage Medical Center[2]	Shelbyville	219	494
Starr Regional Medical Center Athens[2]	Athens	219	265
Saint Thomas Rutherford Hospital[2]	Murfreesboro	220	557
Tennova Healthcare-Newport Med Ctr[2]	Newport	220	534
Volunteer Community Hospital[2]	Martin	220	284
Tennova Healthcare-Jefferson Mem Hosp[2]	Jefferson City	221	543
Sumner Regional Medical Center[2]	Gallatin	222	534
Crockett Hospital[2]	Lawrenceburg	223	226
River Park Hospital[2]	Mc Minnville	223	413
Grandview Medical Center[2]	Jasper	224	475
Baptist Memorial Hospital Union City[2]	Union City	226	252
McNairy Regional Hospital[2]	Selmer	226	377
Unicoi County Memorial Hospital[2]	Erwin	226	332
Wayne Medical Center	Waynesboro	227	344
Lincoln Medical Center[2]	Fayetteville	228	286
Highlands Medical Center[2]	Sparta	229	427
Tristar Horizon Medical Center[2]	Dickson	229	601
Tristar Southern Hills Medical Center[2]	Nashville	229	566
Hardin Medical Center[2]	Savannah	230	328
Tristar Stonecrest Medical Center[2]	Smyrna	232	469
Metro Nashville General Hospital[2]	Nashville	233	233
Tristar Summit Medical Center[2]	Hermitage	233	778
Tristar Centennial Medical Center[2]	Nashville	236	422
Tristar Skyline Medical Center[2]	Nashville	236	716
Franklin Woods Community Hospital[2]	Johnson City	237	371
Methodist Healthcare Fayette Hospital[2]	Somerville	240	55
Claiborne County Hospital[2]	Tazewell	242	502
Johnson City Medical Center[2]	Johnson City	242	418
Maury Regional Hospital[2]	Columbia	244	439
Milan General Hospital	Milan	250	84
Williamson Medical Center[2]	Franklin	250	485
Northcrest Medical Center[2]	Springfield	252	343
Parkridge Medical Center[2]	Chattanooga	255	537
Lakeway Regional Hospital[2]	Morristown	257	465
Takoma Regional Hospital[2]	Greeneville	257	320
Bolivar General Hospital	Bolivar	262	189
Baptist Memorial Hospital Tipton[2]	Covington	266	226
Jackson - Madison County General Hospital[2]	Jackson	266	522
Gateway Medical Center[2]	Clarksville	268	601
Tennova Healthcare[2]	Knoxville	268	736
Cookeville Regional Medical Center[2]	Cookeville	271	487
Fort Loudoun Medical Center[2]	Lenoir City	272	533
Indian Path Medical Center[2]	Kingsport	272	452
Sweetwater Hospital Association[2]	Sweetwater	275	337
Morristown Hamblen Hospital Association[2]	Morristown	276	765
Methodist Healthcare Memphis Hospitals[2]	Memphis	278	624
University of Tn Memorial Hospital[2]	Knoxville	279	261
Wellmont Bristol Regional Medical Center[2]	Bristol	282	602
Delta Medical Center[2]	Memphis	292	320
Erlanger Medical Center[2]	Chattanooga	292	396
Memorial Healthcare System[2]	Chattanooga	293	1204
Baptist Memorial Hospital[2]	Memphis	298	1027
Roane Medical Center[2]	Harriman	299	531
Leconte Medical Center[2]	Sevierville	312	562
Blount Memorial Hospital[2]	Maryville	313	857
Fort Sanders Regional Medical Center[2]	Knoxville	313	617
Skyridge Medical Center[2]	Cleveland	316	747
Methodist Medical Center of Oak Ridge[2]	Oak Ridge	329	797
Parkwest Medical Center[2]	Knoxville	337	454
Saint Francis Hospital[2]	Memphis	338	1180
Regional Medical Center at Memphis[2]	Memphis	354	969
Vanderbilt University Hospital[2]	Nashville	361	295
Saint Francis Bartlett Medical Center[2]	Bartlett	364	818
Wellmont Holston Valley Medical Center[2]	Kingsport	371	627

Time from ER Arrival to Discharge (minutes)

Hospital Name	City	Min.	Cases
Haywood Park Community Hospital	Brownsville	63	321
Cumberland River Hospital	Celina	72	312
Henderson County Community Hospital	Lexington	76	352
Tristar Ashland City Medical Center	Ashland City	79	394
Starr Regional Medical Center Athens	Athens	81	403
McKenzie Regional Hospital	Mc Kenzie	82	309
Decatur County General Hospital	Parsons	86	323

NOTE: Hospital profiles are in alphabetical order by state, then city, then hospital within the city; Rankings exclude hospitals with less than 25 cases except for patient surveys which excludes hospitals with less than 100 cases; (a) 100-299 cases; (1) The number of cases/patients is too few to report; (2) Data submitted were based on a sample of cases/patients; (3) Results are based on a shorter time period than required; (4) Data suppressed by CMS for one or more quarters; (5) Results are not available for this reporting period; (6) Fewer than 100 patients completed the HCAHPS survey; (7) No cases met the criteria for this measure; (8) The lower limit of the confidence interval cannot be calculated if the number of observed infections equals zero; (9) No data are available from the state/territory for this reporting period; (10) The scores shown reflect fewer than 50 completed surveys; (11) There were discrepancies in the data collection process; (12) This measure does not apply to this hospital for this reporting period; (13) Results cannot be calculated for this reporting period; (14) The results for this state are combined with nearby states to protect confidentiality; Please refer to the User's Guide for a full explanation of data.

Stones River Hosp & Dekalb Comm Hosp	Woodbury	89	365
Humboldt General Hospital[3]	Humboldt	91	289
Jamestown Regional Medical Center	Jamestown	92	798
Johnson County Community Hospital	Mountain City	94	350
Livingston Regional Hospital	Livingston	97	381
Stones River Hosp & Dekalb Comm Hosp	Smithville	97	305
Perry Community Hospital	Linden	100	628
Tennova Healthcare-Newport Med Ctr	Newport	103	1254
Methodist Healthcare Fayette Hospital	Somerville	104	382
Volunteer Community Hospital	Martin	105	346
Crockett Hospital	Lawrenceburg	106	392
Tennova Healthcare-Lafollett Med Ctr	La Follette	106	1350
Laughlin Memorial Hospital	Greeneville	108	364
Highlands Medical Center	Sparta	109	395
Wellmont Hawkins County Memorial Hospital	Rogersville	109	346
Cumberland Medical Center	Crossville	110	355
Harton Regional Medical Center	Tullahoma	111	422
Parkridge Medical Center	Chattanooga	111	491
Erlanger Medical Center	Chattanooga	112	374
Regional Hospital of Jackson	Jackson	113	381
Riverview Regional Medical Center	Carthage	113	382
Starr Regional Medical Center Etowah	Etowah	113	355
Indian Path Medical Center	Kingsport	114	356
Gibson General Hospital[3]	Trenton	115	275
Baptist Memorial Hospital Union City	Union City	116	341
Heritage Medical Center	Shelbyville	116	382
McNairy Regional Hospital	Selmer	116	353
Hillside Hospital	Pulaski	117	366
Takoma Regional Hospital	Greeneville	118	334
Tristar Hendersonville Medical Center	Hendersonville	118	415
Tennova Healthcare-Jefferson Mem Hosp	Jefferson City	119	1563
Claiborne County Hospital	Tazewell	120	364
Northcrest Medical Center	Springfield	121	357
Tristar Horizon Medical Center	Dickson	121	414
Franklin Woods Community Hospital	Johnson City	122	348
Unicoi County Memorial Hospital	Erwin	122	396
Southern Tennessee Medical Center	Winchester	123	372
Baptist Memorial Hospital Huntingdon	Huntingdon	124	225
Bolivar General Hospital	Bolivar	124	362
Sycamore Shoals Hospital	Elizabethton	124	307
Tristar Southern Hills Medical Center	Nashville	124	427
Metro Nashville General Hospital	Nashville	126	336
Tristar Stonecrest Medical Center	Smyrna	127	435
Baptist Memorial Hospital Tipton	Covington	129	390
Milan General Hospital	Milan	129	375
Dyersburg Regional Medical Center	Dyersburg	130	346
United Regional Medical Center	Manchester	130	334
Delta Medical Center	Memphis	131	337
Sweetwater Hospital Association	Sweetwater	132	1433
Tristar Centennial Medical Center	Nashville	132	474
University Medical Center	Lebanon	133	586
Henry County Medical Center	Paris	135	435
Tennova Healthcare	Knoxville	135	1597
Tristar Skyline Medical Center	Nashville	136	448
Wayne Medical Center	Waynesboro	136	1276
Grandview Medical Center	Jasper	137	441
Johnson City Medical Center	Johnson City	138	321
Lakeway Regional Hospital	Morristown	138	358
River Park Hospital	Mc Minnville	138	351
Fort Sanders Regional Medical Center	Knoxville	140	405
Hardin Medical Center	Savannah	140	329
Gateway Medical Center	Clarksville	142	376
Jellico Community Hospital	Jellico	142	328
Methodist Medical Center of Oak Ridge	Oak Ridge	144	409
Cookeville Regional Medical Center	Cookeville	145	373
Fort Loudoun Medical Center	Lenoir City	146	392
Roane Medical Center	Harriman	149	394
Tristar Summit Medical Center	Hermitage	152	498
Methodist Healthcare Memphis Hospitals	Memphis	155	416
Lincoln Medical Center	Fayetteville	157	358
Saint Thomas West Hospital	Nashville	158	348
Williamson Medical Center	Franklin	159	363
Sumner Regional Medical Center	Gallatin	161	422
Saint Thomas Rutherford Hospital	Murfreesboro	162	344
Morristown Hamblen Hospital Association	Morristown	166	388
Wellmont Holston Valley Medical Center	Kingsport	166	354
Baptist Memorial Hospital	Memphis	170	697
Memorial Healthcare System	Chattanooga	170	699
Skyridge Medical Center	Cleveland	170	384
Saint Thomas Midtown Hospital	Nashville	171	373
Leconte Medical Center	Sevierville	174	398
Wellmont Bristol Regional Medical Center	Bristol	175	351
Blount Memorial Hospital	Maryville	176	385
Maury Regional Hospital	Columbia	179	391
Parkwest Medical Center	Knoxville	188	414
University of Tn Memorial Hospital	Knoxville	196	350
Jackson - Madison County General Hospital	Jackson	203	375
Vanderbilt University Hospital	Nashville	209	326
Saint Francis Bartlett Medical Center	Bartlett	211	462
Saint Francis Hospital	Memphis	254	409
Regional Medical Center at Memphis	Memphis	305	2172

Time in ER Before Being Evaluated (minutes)

Hospital Name	City	Min.	Cases
Livingston Regional Hospital	Livingston	8	443
Tristar Centennial Medical Center	Nashville	9	522
Perry Community Hospital	Linden	10	720
Riverview Regional Medical Center	Carthage	12	430
Tristar Ashland City Medical Center	Ashland City	12	431
Crockett Hospital	Lawrenceburg	13	351
Parkridge Medical Center	Chattanooga	13	536
Starr Regional Medical Center Athens	Athens	13	430
Sumner Regional Medical Center	Gallatin	13	498
Tristar Stonecrest Medical Center	Smyrna	13	483
Hillside Hospital	Pulaski	14	459
Tennova Healthcare-Newport Med Ctr	Newport	14	1360
Tristar Hendersonville Medical Center	Hendersonville	14	450
Tristar Southern Hills Medical Center	Nashville	14	489
Tristar Summit Medical Center	Hermitage	14	514
Jamestown Regional Medical Center	Jamestown	15	935
McKenzie Regional Hospital	Mc Kenzie	15	423
Tristar Skyline Medical Center	Nashville	15	529
Decatur County General Hospital	Parsons	16	353
Henderson County Community Hospital	Lexington	16	434
McNairy Regional Hospital	Selmer	16	419
Sycamore Shoals Hospital	Elizabethton	16	357
Tristar Horizon Medical Center	Dickson	17	472
Methodist Healthcare Fayette Hospital	Somerville	18	434
Northcrest Medical Center	Springfield	18	391
Maury Regional Hospital	Columbia	20	427
Tennova Healthcare-Lafollett Med Ctr	La Follette	20	1455
Claiborne County Hospital	Tazewell	21	365
Milan General Hospital	Milan	21	403
Stones River Hosp & Dekalb Comm Hosp	Smithville	21	378
Stones River Hosp & Dekalb Comm Hosp	Woodbury	21	383
Unicoi County Memorial Hospital	Erwin	21	410
Baptist Memorial Hospital Huntingdon	Huntingdon	22	379
Heritage Medical Center	Shelbyville	22	414
Indian Path Medical Center	Kingsport	22	366
Southern Tennessee Medical Center	Winchester	22	430
Tennova Healthcare	Knoxville	22	1705
Humboldt General Hospital[3]	Humboldt	23	299
Saint Thomas West Hospital	Nashville	23	389
Tennova Healthcare-Jefferson Mem Hosp	Jefferson City	23	1682
Cookeville Regional Medical Center	Cookeville	24	426
Haywood Park Community Hospital	Brownsville	24	420
Wayne Medical Center	Waynesboro	24	1568
Cumberland Medical Center	Crossville	25	383
Cumberland River Hospital	Celina	25	350
Johnson City Medical Center	Johnson City	25	373
Highlands Medical Center	Sparta	26	428
River Park Hospital	Mc Minnville	26	421
Takoma Regional Hospital	Greeneville	26	327
Harton Regional Medical Center	Tullahoma	27	461
Baptist Memorial Hospital Union City	Union City	28	378
Hardin Medical Center	Savannah	28	373
Gibson General Hospital[3]	Trenton	29	293
Lincoln Medical Center	Fayetteville	29	400
Saint Thomas Midtown Hospital	Nashville	29	392
Starr Regional Medical Center Etowah	Etowah	29	343
University Medical Center	Lebanon	29	645
Wellmont Hawkins County Memorial Hospital	Rogersville	29	373
Baptist Memorial Hospital	Memphis	30	783
Gateway Medical Center	Clarksville	30	408
Lakeway Regional Hospital	Morristown	30	404
Memorial Healthcare System	Chattanooga	30	590
Regional Hospital of Jackson	Jackson	31	396
Fort Sanders Regional Medical Center	Knoxville	32	410
Sweetwater Hospital Association	Sweetwater	32	1567
Fort Loudoun Medical Center	Lenoir City	33	429
Franklin Woods Community Hospital	Johnson City	34	278
Johnson County Community Hospital	Mountain City	34	195
Saint Thomas Rutherford Hospital	Murfreesboro	34	374
Volunteer Community Hospital	Martin	34	419
Blount Memorial Hospital	Maryville	35	395
Dyersburg Regional Medical Center	Dyersburg	35	414
Metro Nashville General Hospital	Nashville	35	370
Roane Medical Center	Harriman	35	436
Baptist Memorial Hospital Tipton	Covington	36	415
Laughlin Memorial Hospital	Greeneville	36	382
Methodist Medical Center of Oak Ridge	Oak Ridge	36	447
University of Tn Memorial Hospital	Knoxville	37	377
United Regional Medical Center	Manchester	38	391
Henry County Medical Center	Paris	39	485
Skyridge Medical Center	Cleveland	39	410
Grandview Medical Center	Jasper	40	475
Parkwest Medical Center	Knoxville	40	456
Bolivar General Hospital	Bolivar	41	414
Morristown Hamblen Hospital Association	Morristown	41	425
Erlanger Medical Center	Chattanooga	42	384
Saint Francis Hospital	Memphis	43	427
Williamson Medical Center	Franklin	43	354
Jackson - Madison County General Hospital	Jackson	44	414
Jellico Community Hospital	Jellico	44	362
Leconte Medical Center	Sevierville	48	435
Regional Medical Center at Memphis	Memphis	50	2299
Wellmont Bristol Regional Medical Center	Bristol	56	377
Wellmont Holston Valley Medical Center	Kingsport	56	376
Saint Francis Bartlett Medical Center	Bartlett	57	477
Delta Medical Center	Memphis	58	362
Methodist Healthcare Memphis Hospitals	Memphis	61	434
Vanderbilt University Hospital	Nashville	96	98

Time to Pain Meds for Bone Fractures (minutes)

Hospital Name	City	Min.	Cases
Livingston Regional Hospital	Livingston	18	52
Dyersburg Regional Medical Center	Dyersburg	26	154
Hillside Hospital	Pulaski	27	33
Riverview Regional Medical Center	Carthage	34	47
Sumner Regional Medical Center	Gallatin	34	136
Tristar Centennial Medical Center	Nashville	36	73
Tristar Horizon Medical Center	Dickson	37	147
Southern Tennessee Medical Center	Winchester	38	91
Tennova Healthcare-Newport Med Ctr	Newport	38	111
Tristar Stonecrest Medical Center	Smyrna	39	181
Roane Medical Center	Harriman	40	53
Tristar Hendersonville Medical Center	Hendersonville	40	152
Tristar Ashland City Medical Center	Ashland City	43	27
Harton Regional Medical Center	Tullahoma	44	96
Tristar Skyline Medical Center	Nashville	44	163
Henderson County Community Hospital	Lexington	45	38
Sycamore Shoals Hospital	Elizabethton	45	77
Tristar Southern Hills Medical Center	Nashville	45	98
University Medical Center	Lebanon	46	128
Crockett Hospital	Lawrenceburg	48	90
McNairy Regional Hospital	Selmer	48	28
Tristar Summit Medical Center	Hermitage	48	170
Erlanger Medical Center	Chattanooga	49	295
Northcrest Medical Center	Springfield	49	127
Tennova Healthcare-Jefferson Mem Hosp	Jefferson City	49	103
Claiborne County Hospital	Tazewell	50	71
Cumberland Medical Center	Crossville	50	56
Jamestown Regional Medical Center	Jamestown	50	70
Vanderbilt University Hospital	Nashville	50	372
Wayne Medical Center	Waynesboro	50	26
United Regional Medical Center	Manchester	51	31
Johnson City Medical Center	Johnson City	52	189
Saint Thomas Midtown Hospital	Nashville	53	93
Stones River Hosp & Dekalb Comm Hosp	Smithville	53	50
Tennova Healthcare-Lafollett Med Ctr	La Follette	53	94
Cookeville Regional Medical Center	Cookeville	54	138
Gateway Medical Center	Clarksville	54	264
Parkwest Medical Center	Knoxville	54	78
Starr Regional Medical Center Athens	Athens	54	89
Johnson County Community Hospital	Mountain City	55	33
Regional Hospital of Jackson	Jackson	56	69
Franklin Woods Community Hospital	Johnson City	57	73
Lakeway Regional Hospital	Morristown	57	41
Parkridge Medical Center	Chattanooga	58	140
Morristown Hamblen Hospital Association	Morristown	60	90
Saint Thomas Rutherford Hospital	Murfreesboro	60	238
Wellmont Hawkins County Memorial Hospital	Rogersville	60	61
Blount Memorial Hospital	Maryville	62	222
Bolivar General Hospital	Bolivar	62	30
Fort Loudoun Medical Center	Lenoir City	62	55
Jackson - Madison County General Hospital	Jackson	62	153
Lincoln Medical Center	Fayetteville	62	98
River Park Hospital	Mc Minnville	62	94
Saint Thomas West Hospital	Nashville	62	65
Takoma Regional Hospital	Greeneville	62	74
Tennova Healthcare	Knoxville	62	450
Indian Path Medical Center	Kingsport	63	60
Heritage Medical Center	Shelbyville	64	78
Starr Regional Medical Center Etowah	Etowah	64	31
Maury Regional Hospital	Columbia	65	202
Highlands Medical Center	Sparta	67	57
Leconte Medical Center	Sevierville	67	176
Hardin Medical Center	Savannah	68	89
Laughlin Memorial Hospital	Greeneville	68	104
Stones River Hosp & Dekalb Comm Hosp	Woodbury	68	26
Sweetwater Hospital Association	Sweetwater	68	64
Williamson Medical Center	Franklin	68	194
Baptist Memorial Hospital Huntingdon	Huntingdon	70	36
Memorial Healthcare System	Chattanooga	70	214
Baptist Memorial Hospital	Memphis	71	249
Methodist Medical Center of Oak Ridge	Oak Ridge	71	54
Wellmont Bristol Regional Medical Center	Bristol	71	147
Baptist Memorial Hospital Union City	Union City	72	76
Fort Sanders Regional Medical Center	Knoxville	72	129
Volunteer Community Hospital	Martin	72	37
Grandview Medical Center	Jasper	78	54
Jellico Community Hospital	Jellico	78	44
Henry County Medical Center	Paris	80	77

NOTE: Hospital profiles are in alphabetical order by state, then city, then hospital within the city; Rankings exclude hospitals with less than 25 cases except for patient surveys which excludes hospitals with less than 100 cases; (a) 100-299 cases; (1) The number of cases/patients is too few to report; (2) Data submitted were based on a sample of cases/patients; (3) Results are based on a shorter time period than required; (4) Data suppressed by CMS for one or more quarters; (5) Results are not available for this reporting period; (6) Fewer than 100 patients completed the HCAHPS survey; (7) No cases met the criteria for this measure; (8) The lower limit of the confidence interval cannot be calculated if the number of observed infections equals zero; (9) No data are available from the state/territory for this reporting period; (10) The scores shown reflect fewer than 50 completed surveys; (11) There were discrepancies in the data collection process; (12) This measure does not apply to this hospital for this reporting period; (13) Results cannot be calculated for this reporting period; (14) The results for this state are combined with nearby states to protect confidentiality; Please refer to the User's Guide for a full explanation of data.

University of Tn Memorial Hospital	Knoxville	80	301
Metro Nashville General Hospital	Nashville	82	63
Baptist Memorial Hospital Tipton	Covington	83	93
Saint Francis Hospital	Memphis	84	45
Saint Francis Bartlett Medical Center	Bartlett	86	122
Wellmont Holston Valley Medical Center	Kingsport	92	238
Skyridge Medical Center	Cleveland	94	295
Delta Medical Center	Memphis	96	46
Methodist Healthcare Memphis Hospitals	Memphis	99	444
Regional Medical Center at Memphis	Memphis	126	122

Heart Attack Care

Aspirin Given at Discharge

Hospital Name	City	Rate	Cases
Baptist Memorial Hospital	Memphis	100%	643
Cookeville Regional Medical Center	Cookeville	100%	510
Erlanger Medical Center	Chattanooga	100%	385
Fort Sanders Regional Medical Center[2]	Knoxville	100%	214
Gateway Medical Center	Clarksville	100%	167
Jackson - Madison County General Hospital	Jackson	100%	1162
Laughlin Memorial Hospital	Greeneville	100%	48
Leconte Medical Center	Sevierville	100%	31
Memphis VA Medical Center	Memphis	100%	46
Methodist Healthcare Memphis Hospitals[2]	Memphis	100%	619
Methodist Medical Center of Oak Ridge[2]	Oak Ridge	100%	242
Metro Nashville General Hospital[2]	Nashville	100%	28
Morristown Hamblen Hospital Association[2]	Morristown	100%	146
Mountain Home VA Medical Center	Mountain Home	100%	83
Northcrest Medical Center	Springfield	100%	48
Parkridge Medical Center	Chattanooga	100%	253
Parkwest Medical Center[2]	Knoxville	100%	338
Regional Hospital of Jackson	Jackson	100%	420
Saint Francis Hospital	Memphis	100%	273
Sumner Regional Medical Center	Gallatin	100%	111
Tristar Centennial Medical Center[2]	Nashville	100%	449
Tristar Hendersonville Medical Center	Hendersonville	100%	49
Tristar Horizon Medical Center	Dickson	100%	42
Tristar Skyline Medical Center	Nashville	100%	132
Tristar Stonecrest Medical Center[2]	Smyrna	100%	50
Tristar Summit Medical Center[2]	Hermitage	100%	152
University of Tn Memorial Hospital[2]	Knoxville	100%	303
Wellmont Bristol Regional Medical Center[2]	Bristol	100%	262
Blount Memorial Hospital	Maryville	99%	194
Indian Path Medical Center[2]	Kingsport	99%	149
Johnson City Medical Center[2]	Johnson City	99%	288
Maury Regional Hospital	Columbia	99%	317
Memorial Healthcare System[2]	Chattanooga	99%	332
Saint Thomas Rutherford Hospital	Murfreesboro	99%	227
Saint Thomas West Hospital	Nashville	99%	1318
Tennova Healthcare	Knoxville	99%	551
Tristar Southern Hills Medical Center	Nashville	99%	100
VA Middle Tennessee Healthcare System	Nashville	99%	119
Saint Thomas Midtown Hospital	Nashville	98%	250
Vanderbilt University Hospital[2]	Nashville	98%	376
Wellmont Holston Valley Medical Center[2]	Kingsport	98%	261
Harton Regional Medical Center	Tullahoma	96%	56
Cumberland Medical Center	Crossville	94%	31
University Medical Center	Lebanon	94%	34
Saint Francis Bartlett Medical Center	Bartlett	93%	27
Williamson Medical Center	Franklin	92%	110
Skyridge Medical Center	Cleveland	91%	35

PCI Within 90 Minutes of Arrival

Hospital Name	City	Rate	Cases
Baptist Memorial Hospital	Memphis	100%	44
Cookeville Regional Medical Center	Cookeville	100%	60
Fort Sanders Regional Medical Center[2]	Knoxville	100%	42
Johnson City Medical Center[2]	Johnson City	100%	27
Memorial Healthcare System[2]	Chattanooga	100%	40
Tristar Skyline Medical Center	Nashville	100%	41
Wellmont Bristol Regional Medical Center[2]	Bristol	100%	32
Wellmont Holston Valley Medical Center[2]	Kingsport	100%	30
Blount Memorial Hospital	Maryville	99%	68
Erlanger Medical Center	Chattanooga	99%	71
Saint Thomas West Hospital	Nashville	99%	67
Gateway Medical Center	Clarksville	98%	43
Jackson - Madison County General Hospital	Jackson	98%	92
Maury Regional Hospital	Columbia	98%	51
Methodist Medical Center of Oak Ridge[2]	Oak Ridge	98%	54
Parkwest Medical Center[2]	Knoxville	98%	44
Saint Thomas Rutherford Hospital	Murfreesboro	98%	45
Tristar Summit Medical Center[2]	Hermitage	98%	56
University of Tn Memorial Hospital[2]	Knoxville	98%	53
Methodist Healthcare Memphis Hospitals[2]	Memphis	96%	81
Saint Francis Hospital	Memphis	95%	40
Saint Thomas Midtown Hospital	Nashville	93%	28
Tennova Healthcare	Knoxville	93%	71
Williamson Medical Center	Franklin	81%	42

Statin Prescribed at Discharge

Hospital Name	City	Rate	Cases
Baptist Memorial Hospital	Memphis	100%	586
Fort Sanders Regional Medical Center[2]	Knoxville	100%	202
Gateway Medical Center	Clarksville	100%	167
Jackson - Madison County General Hospital	Jackson	100%	1164
Johnson City Medical Center[2]	Johnson City	100%	279
Leconte Medical Center	Sevierville	100%	33
Memphis VA Medical Center	Memphis	100%	45
Methodist Healthcare Memphis Hospitals[2]	Memphis	100%	596
Methodist Medical Center of Oak Ridge[2]	Oak Ridge	100%	245
Metro Nashville General Hospital[2]	Nashville	100%	28
Mountain Home VA Medical Center	Mountain Home	100%	79
Northcrest Medical Center	Springfield	100%	43
Parkwest Medical Center[2]	Knoxville	100%	332
Saint Francis Bartlett Medical Center	Bartlett	100%	26
Saint Francis Hospital	Memphis	100%	275
Sumner Regional Medical Center	Gallatin	100%	114
Tristar Centennial Medical Center[2]	Nashville	100%	437
Tristar Hendersonville Medical Center	Hendersonville	100%	46
Tristar Skyline Medical Center	Nashville	100%	126
Tristar Stonecrest Medical Center[2]	Smyrna	100%	49
Wellmont Bristol Regional Medical Center[2]	Bristol	100%	255
Wellmont Holston Valley Medical Center[2]	Kingsport	100%	260
Erlanger Medical Center	Chattanooga	99%	389
Maury Regional Hospital	Columbia	99%	314
Memorial Healthcare System[2]	Chattanooga	99%	340
Morristown Hamblen Hospital Association[2]	Morristown	99%	159
Parkridge Medical Center	Chattanooga	99%	245
Regional Hospital of Jackson	Jackson	99%	378
Tristar Southern Hills Medical Center	Nashville	99%	95
Tristar Summit Medical Center[2]	Hermitage	99%	153
VA Middle Tennessee Healthcare System	Nashville	99%	115
Cookeville Regional Medical Center	Cookeville	98%	491
Harton Regional Medical Center	Tullahoma	98%	56
Indian Path Medical Center[2]	Kingsport	98%	147
Laughlin Memorial Hospital	Greeneville	98%	45
Saint Thomas West Hospital	Nashville	98%	1260
Tennova Healthcare	Knoxville	98%	527
University of Tn Memorial Hospital[2]	Knoxville	98%	302
Vanderbilt University Hospital[2]	Nashville	98%	350
Blount Memorial Hospital	Maryville	97%	194
Cumberland Medical Center	Crossville	97%	32
Saint Thomas Rutherford Hospital	Murfreesboro	97%	239
Skyridge Medical Center	Cleveland	97%	35
Tristar Horizon Medical Center	Dickson	97%	39
Williamson Medical Center	Franklin	97%	107
Saint Thomas Midtown Hospital	Nashville	95%	241
University Medical Center	Lebanon	94%	32

Heart Failure Care

ACE Inhibitor or ARB for LVSD

Hospital Name	City	Rate	Cases
Baptist Memorial Hospital	Memphis	100%	369
Baptist Memorial Hospital Union City	Union City	100%	25
Erlanger Medical Center	Chattanooga	100%	136
Fort Sanders Regional Medical Center[2]	Knoxville	100%	60
Harton Regional Medical Center	Tullahoma	100%	43
Jackson - Madison County General Hospital	Jackson	100%	379
Laughlin Memorial Hospital	Greeneville	100%	35
Leconte Medical Center	Sevierville	100%	25
Methodist Healthcare Memphis Hospitals[2]	Memphis	100%	281
Methodist Medical Center of Oak Ridge[2]	Oak Ridge	100%	55
Northcrest Medical Center	Springfield	100%	39
Saint Francis Bartlett Medical Center	Bartlett	100%	46
Saint Francis Hospital	Memphis	100%	221
Sumner Regional Medical Center	Gallatin	100%	40
Tristar Centennial Medical Center[2]	Nashville	100%	170
Tristar Hendersonville Medical Center	Hendersonville	100%	41
Tristar Horizon Medical Center	Dickson	100%	41
Tristar Southern Hills Medical Center	Nashville	100%	35
Tristar Stonecrest Medical Center[2]	Smyrna	100%	31
Tristar Summit Medical Center[2]	Hermitage	100%	75
University of Tn Memorial Hospital[2]	Knoxville	100%	109
Wellmont Bristol Regional Medical Center[2]	Bristol	100%	69
Memphis VA Medical Center	Memphis	99%	135
Regional Hospital of Jackson	Jackson	99%	105
Wellmont Holston Valley Medical Center[2]	Kingsport	99%	71
Parkridge Medical Center	Chattanooga	98%	93
Tristar Skyline Medical Center	Nashville	98%	58
VA Middle Tennessee Healthcare System	Nashville	98%	159
Delta Medical Center	Memphis	97%	38
Johnson City Medical Center[2]	Johnson City	97%	105
Maury Regional Hospital	Columbia	97%	94
Morristown Hamblen Hospital Association[2]	Morristown	97%	37
Mountain Home VA Medical Center	Mountain Home	97%	70
Parkwest Medical Center[2]	Knoxville	97%	67
River Park Hospital	Mc Minnville	97%	31
Vanderbilt University Hospital[2]	Nashville	97%	107
Metro Nashville General Hospital[2]	Nashville	95%	85
Regional Medical Center at Memphis	Memphis	95%	73
Saint Thomas Midtown Hospital	Nashville	95%	246
Saint Thomas Rutherford Hospital	Murfreesboro	95%	127
Saint Thomas West Hospital	Nashville	95%	335
Williamson Medical Center	Franklin	95%	55
Blount Memorial Hospital[2]	Maryville	94%	70
Gateway Medical Center	Clarksville	94%	89
Memorial Healthcare System[2]	Chattanooga	94%	116
Skyridge Medical Center	Cleveland	94%	82
Tennova Healthcare	Knoxville	94%	160
Tennova Healthcare-Lafollett Med Ctr	La Follette	93%	27
Southern Tennessee Medical Center	Winchester	92%	49
Indian Path Medical Center[2]	Kingsport	89%	45
Cumberland Medical Center	Crossville	86%	57
Cookeville Regional Medical Center	Cookeville	84%	108

Discharge Instructions Given

Hospital Name	City	Rate	Cases
Baptist Memorial Hospital Tipton	Covington	100%	37
Fort Loudoun Medical Center	Lenoir City	100%	69
Fort Sanders Regional Medical Center[2]	Knoxville	100%	177
Gateway Medical Center	Clarksville	100%	167
Heritage Medical Center	Shelbyville	100%	60
Lakeway Regional Hospital	Morristown	100%	51
Laughlin Memorial Hospital	Greeneville	100%	119
Livingston Regional Hospital	Livingston	100%	47
Memphis VA Medical Center	Memphis	100%	300
Methodist Medical Center of Oak Ridge[2]	Oak Ridge	100%	225
Northcrest Medical Center	Springfield	100%	72
Parkwest Medical Center[2]	Knoxville	100%	248
Riverview Regional Medical Center	Carthage	100%	35
Roane Medical Center[2]	Harriman	100%	53
Sumner Regional Medical Center	Gallatin	100%	122
Tristar Hendersonville Medical Center	Hendersonville	100%	120
Tristar Skyline Medical Center	Nashville	100%	208
Tristar Southern Hills Medical Center	Nashville	100%	120
Tristar Summit Medical Center[2]	Hermitage	100%	192
United Regional Medical Center[2]	Manchester	100%	31
Wellmont Bristol Regional Medical Center[2]	Bristol	100%	218
Wellmont Holston Valley Medical Center[2]	Kingsport	100%	223
Dyersburg Regional Medical Center	Dyersburg	99%	87
Methodist Healthcare Memphis Hospitals[2]	Memphis	99%	687
Morristown Hamblen Hospital Association[2]	Morristown	99%	126
Saint Francis Hospital	Memphis	99%	533
Henry County Medical Center	Paris	98%	53
Lincoln Medical Center	Fayetteville	98%	44
Maury Regional Hospital	Columbia	98%	254
Starr Regional Medical Center Athens	Athens	98%	46
Tristar Stonecrest Medical Center[2]	Smyrna	98%	109
Parkridge Medical Center	Chattanooga	97%	274
Saint Francis Bartlett Medical Center	Bartlett	97%	154
Takoma Regional Hospital[2]	Greeneville	97%	37
Tristar Horizon Medical Center	Dickson	97%	168
Baptist Memorial Hospital	Memphis	96%	1165
Jellico Community Hospital[2]	Jellico	96%	51
Perry Community Hospital[2]	Linden	96%	25
Skyridge Medical Center	Cleveland	96%	194
Stones River Hosp & Dekalb Comm Hosp	Smithville	96%	48
Vanderbilt University Hospital[2]	Nashville	96%	314
Jamestown Regional Medical Center	Jamestown	95%	95
Regional Hospital of Jackson	Jackson	95%	236
Tristar Centennial Medical Center[2]	Nashville	95%	389
University of Tn Memorial Hospital[2]	Knoxville	95%	256
Baptist Memorial Hospital Union City	Union City	94%	64
Jackson - Madison County General Hospital	Jackson	94%	897
Mountain Home VA Medical Center	Mountain Home	94%	191
Saint Thomas Midtown Hospital	Nashville	94%	600
VA Middle Tennessee Healthcare System	Nashville	94%	469
Harton Regional Medical Center	Tullahoma	93%	100
Southern Tennessee Medical Center	Winchester	93%	147
Sycamore Shoals Hospital[2]	Elizabethton	93%	55
Tennova Healthcare	Knoxville	93%	512
University Medical Center	Lebanon	93%	71
Volunteer Community Hospital	Martin	93%	29
Wellmont Hawkins County Memorial Hospital	Rogersville	93%	30
Saint Thomas Rutherford Hospital	Murfreesboro	91%	379
Cumberland Medical Center	Crossville	90%	161
Delta Medical Center	Memphis	90%	87
Leconte Medical Center	Sevierville	90%	84
Saint Thomas West Hospital	Nashville	89%	864
Williamson Medical Center	Franklin	89%	129
Blount Memorial Hospital[2]	Maryville	87%	212
Indian Path Medical Center[2]	Kingsport	87%	111
Tennova Healthcare-Jefferson Mem Hosp	Jefferson City	87%	75
River Park Hospital	Mc Minnville	86%	143
Tennova Healthcare-Newport Med Ctr	Newport	86%	86
Erlanger Medical Center	Chattanooga	85%	282
Starr Regional Medical Center Etowah[3]	Etowah	84%	43
Crockett Hospital	Lawrenceburg	82%	39
Regional Medical Center at Memphis	Memphis	81%	125

NOTE: Hospital profiles are in alphabetical order by state, then city, then hospital within the city; Rankings exclude hospitals with less than 25 cases except for patient surveys which excludes hospitals with less than 100 cases; (a) 100-299 cases; (1) The number of cases/patients is too few to report; (2) Data submitted were based on a sample of cases/patients; (3) Results are based on a shorter time period than required; (4) Data suppressed by CMS for one or more quarters; (5) Results are not available for this reporting period; (6) Fewer than 100 patients completed the HCAHPS survey; (7) No cases met the criteria for this measure; (8) The lower limit of the confidence interval cannot be calculated if the number of observed infections equals zero; (9) No data are available from the state/territory for this reporting period; (10) The scores shown reflect fewer than 50 completed surveys; (11) There were discrepancies in the data collection process; (12) This measure does not apply to this hospital for this reporting period; (13) Results cannot be calculated for this reporting period; (14) The results for this state are combined with nearby states to protect confidentiality; Please refer to the User's Guide for a full explanation of data.

Hospital Name	City	Rate	Cases
Tennova Healthcare-Lafollett Med Ctr	La Follette	80%	98
Memorial Healthcare System[2]	Chattanooga	78%	376
Claiborne County Hospital[2]	Tazewell	77%	39
Johnson City Medical Center[2]	Johnson City	77%	240
Metro Nashville General Hospital[2]	Nashville	76%	148
Cookeville Regional Medical Center	Cookeville	72%	269
Grandview Medical Center	Jasper	72%	36
Sweetwater Hospital Association	Sweetwater	72%	60
Franklin Woods Community Hospital[2]	Johnson City	70%	33

Evaluation of LVS Function

Hospital Name	City	Rate	Cases
Baptist Memorial Hospital	Memphis	100%	1342
Baptist Memorial Hospital Huntingdon	Huntingdon	100%	26
Baptist Memorial Hospital Tipton	Covington	100%	44
Baptist Memorial Hospital Union City	Union City	100%	90
Blount Memorial Hospital[2]	Maryville	100%	267
Crockett Hospital	Lawrenceburg	100%	52
Dyersburg Regional Medical Center	Dyersburg	100%	131
Erlanger Medical Center	Chattanooga	100%	331
Fort Loudoun Medical Center	Lenoir City	100%	75
Fort Sanders Regional Medical Center[2]	Knoxville	100%	224
Franklin Woods Community Hospital[2]	Johnson City	100%	47
Gateway Medical Center	Clarksville	100%	194
Harton Regional Medical Center	Tullahoma	100%	122
Henderson County Community Hospital	Lexington	100%	33
Henry County Medical Center	Paris	100%	71
Heritage Medical Center	Shelbyville	100%	69
Hillside Hospital	Pulaski	100%	31
Indian Path Medical Center[2]	Kingsport	100%	143
Jackson - Madison County General Hospital	Jackson	100%	1123
Johnson City Medical Center[2]	Johnson City	100%	295
Livingston Regional Hospital	Livingston	100%	64
Maury Regional Hospital	Columbia	100%	333
McKenzie Regional Hospital	Mc Kenzie	100%	27
Memorial Healthcare System[2]	Chattanooga	100%	438
Memphis VA Medical Center	Memphis	100%	307
Methodist Healthcare Memphis Hospitals[2]	Memphis	100%	795
Methodist Medical Center of Oak Ridge[2]	Oak Ridge	100%	285
Morristown Hamblen Hospital Association[2]	Morristown	100%	103
Mountain Home VA Medical Center	Mountain Home	100%	215
Northcrest Medical Center	Springfield	100%	85
Parkridge Medical Center	Chattanooga	100%	317
Parkwest Medical Center[2]	Knoxville	100%	311
Regional Hospital of Jackson	Jackson	100%	287
Regional Medical Center at Memphis	Memphis	100%	133
Riverview Regional Medical Center	Carthage	100%	44
Roane Medical Center[2]	Harriman	100%	58
Saint Francis Bartlett Medical Center	Bartlett	100%	189
Saint Francis Hospital	Memphis	100%	617
Saint Thomas Midtown Hospital	Nashville	100%	660
Saint Thomas Rutherford Hospital	Murfreesboro	100%	468
Skyridge Medical Center	Cleveland	100%	236
Stones River Hosp & Dekalb Comm Hosp	Smithville	100%	70
Sumner Regional Medical Center	Gallatin	100%	147
Sycamore Shoals Hospital[2]	Elizabethton	100%	86
Tennova Healthcare	Knoxville	100%	608
Tennova Healthcare-Jefferson Mem Hosp	Jefferson City	100%	92
Tennova Healthcare-Lafollett Med Ctr	La Follette	100%	138
Tennova Healthcare-Newport Med Ctr	Newport	100%	100
Tristar Centennial Medical Center[2]	Nashville	100%	459
Tristar Hendersonville Medical Center	Hendersonville	100%	152
Tristar Horizon Medical Center	Dickson	100%	209
Tristar Skyline Medical Center	Nashville	100%	235
Tristar Southern Hills Medical Center	Nashville	100%	135
Tristar Stonecrest Medical Center[2]	Smyrna	100%	135
Tristar Summit Medical Center[2]	Hermitage	100%	246
University Medical Center	Lebanon	100%	102
University of Tn Memorial Hospital[2]	Knoxville	100%	298
Vanderbilt University Hospital[2]	Nashville	100%	362
Wellmont Bristol Regional Medical Center[2]	Bristol	100%	268
Wellmont Hawkins County Memorial Hospital	Rogersville	100%	32
Cookeville Regional Medical Center	Cookeville	99%	332
Cumberland Medical Center	Crossville	99%	201
Jellico Community Hospital[2]	Jellico	99%	67
Laughlin Memorial Hospital	Greeneville	99%	145
Leconte Medical Center	Sevierville	99%	100
River Park Hospital	Mc Minnville	99%	184
Saint Thomas West Hospital	Nashville	99%	981
VA Middle Tennessee Healthcare System	Nashville	99%	500
Wellmont Holston Valley Medical Center[2]	Kingsport	99%	277
Williamson Medical Center	Franklin	99%	169
Jamestown Regional Medical Center	Jamestown	98%	121
Lakeway Regional Hospital	Morristown	98%	61
Lincoln Medical Center	Fayetteville	98%	61
Starr Regional Medical Center Athens	Athens	98%	54
Takoma Regional Hospital[2]	Greeneville	98%	45
Volunteer Community Hospital	Martin	98%	41
Rhea Medical Center	Dayton	97%	30
Stones River Hosp & Dekalb Comm Hosp	Woodbury	97%	35
Unicoi County Memorial Hospital	Erwin	97%	29
Delta Medical Center	Memphis	96%	89
Metro Nashville General Hospital[2]	Nashville	96%	137
Claiborne County Hospital[2]	Tazewell	95%	57
Southern Tennessee Medical Center	Winchester	95%	169
Highlands Medical Center[2]	Sparta	94%	32
Grandview Medical Center	Jasper	93%	54
Sweetwater Hospital Association	Sweetwater	92%	72
United Regional Medical Center[2]	Manchester	92%	37
Starr Regional Medical Center Etowah[3]	Etowah	90%	50
Wayne Medical Center	Waynesboro	81%	27
Cumberland River Hospital	Celina	55%	29
Perry Community Hospital[2]	Linden	0%	44

Medicare Spending

Medicare Spending per Patient (ratio)

Hospital Name	City	Ratio	Cases
Wayne Medical Center	Waynesboro	0.73	-
United Regional Medical Center	Manchester	0.86	-
Fort Loudoun Medical Center	Lenoir City	0.87	-
Jellico Community Hospital	Jellico	0.89	-
Saint Thomas Hospital for Spinal Surgery	Nashville	0.89	-
Leconte Medical Center	Sevierville	0.90	-
Cumberland Medical Center	Crossville	0.91	-
Metro Nashville General Hospital	Nashville	0.91	-
Stones River Hosp & Dekalb Comm Hosp	Smithville	0.91	-
Hardin Medical Center	Savannah	0.92	-
Tennova Healthcare-Newport Med Ctr	Newport	0.92	-
Wellmont Hawkins County Memorial Hospital	Rogersville	0.93	-
Cumberland River Hospital	Celina	0.94	-
Laughlin Memorial Hospital	Greeneville	0.95	-
Methodist Medical Center of Oak Ridge	Oak Ridge	0.95	-
Takoma Regional Hospital	Greeneville	0.96	-
Tennova Healthcare	Knoxville	0.96	-
University of Tn Memorial Hospital	Knoxville	0.96	-
Blount Memorial Hospital	Maryville	0.97	-
Claiborne County Hospital	Tazewell	0.97	-
Cookeville Regional Medical Center	Cookeville	0.97	-
Crockett Hospital	Lawrenceburg	0.97	-
Memorial Healthcare System	Chattanooga	0.97	-
Northcrest Medical Center	Springfield	0.97	-
Parkwest Medical Center	Knoxville	0.97	-
River Park Hospital	Mc Minnville	0.97	-
Saint Thomas West Hospital	Nashville	0.97	-
Tennova Healthcare-Lafollett Med Ctr	La Follette	0.97	-
Unicoi County Memorial Hospital	Erwin	0.97	-
Baptist Memorial Hospital Tipton	Covington	0.98	-
Fort Sanders Regional Medical Center	Knoxville	0.98	-
Franklin Woods Community Hospital	Johnson City	0.98	-
Grandview Medical Center	Jasper	0.98	-
Jamestown Regional Medical Center	Jamestown	0.98	-
Saint Thomas Rutherford Hospital	Murfreesboro	0.98	-
Vanderbilt University Hospital	Nashville	0.98	-
Maury Regional Hospital	Columbia	0.99	-
McNairy Regional Hospital	Selmer	0.99	-
Southern Tennessee Medical Center	Winchester	0.99	-
Baptist Memorial Hospital	Memphis	1.00	-
Haywood Park Community Hospital	Brownsville	1.00	-
Highlands Medical Center	Sparta	1.00	-
Indian Path Medical Center	Kingsport	1.00	-
Jackson - Madison County General Hospital	Jackson	1.00	-
Parkridge Medical Center	Chattanooga	1.00	-
Regional Medical Center at Memphis	Memphis	1.00	-
Sweetwater Hospital Association	Sweetwater	1.00	-
Wellmont Holston Valley Medical Center	Kingsport	1.00	-
Harton Regional Medical Center	Tullahoma	1.01	-
Hillside Hospital	Pulaski	1.01	-
Lakeway Regional Hospital	Morristown	1.01	-
Methodist Healthcare Memphis Hospitals	Memphis	1.01	-
Morristown Hamblen Hospital Association	Morristown	1.01	-
Regional Hospital of Jackson	Jackson	1.01	-
Roane Medical Center	Harriman	1.01	-
Saint Thomas Midtown Hospital	Nashville	1.01	-
Tristar Centennial Medical Center	Nashville	1.01	-
Tristar Summit Medical Center	Hermitage	1.01	-
Bolivar General Hospital	Bolivar	1.02	-
Henry County Medical Center	Paris	1.02	-
Johnson City Medical Center	Johnson City	1.02	-
Skyridge Medical Center	Cleveland	1.02	-
Tristar Hendersonville Medical Center	Hendersonville	1.02	-
Decatur County General Hospital	Parsons	1.03	-
Erlanger Medical Center	Chattanooga	1.03	-
Gateway Medical Center	Clarksville	1.03	-
Milan General Hospital	Milan	1.03	-
Tennova Healthcare-Jefferson Mem Hosp	Jefferson City	1.03	-
Tristar Horizon Medical Center	Dickson	1.03	-
Wellmont Bristol Regional Medical Center	Bristol	1.03	-
Dyersburg Regional Medical Center	Dyersburg	1.04	-
Heritage Medical Center	Shelbyville	1.04	-
Livingston Regional Hospital	Livingston	1.04	-
Tristar Stonecrest Medical Center	Smyrna	1.04	-
Baptist Memorial Hospital Huntingdon	Huntingdon	1.05	-
Henderson County Community Hospital	Lexington	1.05	-
Saint Francis Bartlett Medical Center	Bartlett	1.05	-
Tristar Skyline Medical Center	Nashville	1.05	-
University Medical Center	Lebanon	1.05	-
McKenzie Regional Hospital	Mc Kenzie	1.06	-
Methodist Healthcare Fayette Hospital	Somerville	1.06	-
Saint Francis Hospital	Memphis	1.06	-
Starr Regional Medical Center Athens	Athens	1.06	-
Tristar Southern Hills Medical Center	Nashville	1.06	-
Williamson Medical Center	Franklin	1.06	-
Baptist Memorial Hospital Union City	Union City	1.08	-
Delta Medical Center	Memphis	1.08	-
Lincoln Medical Center	Fayetteville	1.08	-
Sumner Regional Medical Center	Gallatin	1.08	-
Sycamore Shoals Hospital	Elizabethton	1.08	-
Perry Community Hospital	Linden	1.09	-
Volunteer Community Hospital	Martin	1.11	-
Stones River Hosp & Dekalb Comm Hosp	Woodbury	1.13	-

Pneumonia Care

Appropriate Initial Antibiotic Given

Hospital Name	City	Rate	Cases
Baptist Memorial Hospital Huntingdon	Huntingdon	100%	27
Baptist Memorial Hospital Tipton	Covington	100%	50
Baptist Memorial Hospital Union City	Union City	100%	38
Blount Memorial Hospital[2]	Maryville	100%	101
Henderson County Community Hospital	Lexington	100%	27
McKenzie Regional Hospital	Mc Kenzie	100%	36
Memorial Healthcare System[2]	Chattanooga	100%	189
Methodist Medical Center of Oak Ridge[2]	Oak Ridge	100%	102
Mountain Home VA Medical Center	Mountain Home	100%	86
Regional Hospital of Jackson	Jackson	100%	47
Stones River Hosp & Dekalb Comm Hosp	Smithville	100%	95
Takoma Regional Hospital[2]	Greeneville	100%	78
Tristar Hendersonville Medical Center	Hendersonville	100%	139
Tristar Southern Hills Medical Center	Nashville	100%	100
Tristar Stonecrest Medical Center[2]	Smyrna	100%	116
Baptist Memorial Hospital	Memphis	99%	412
Henry County Medical Center	Paris	99%	88
Indian Path Medical Center[2]	Kingsport	99%	83
Leconte Medical Center[2]	Sevierville	99%	138
Morristown Hamblen Hospital Association[2]	Morristown	99%	145
Northcrest Medical Center[2]	Springfield	99%	137
Saint Francis Hospital	Memphis	99%	147
Starr Regional Medical Center Athens	Athens	99%	83
Cookeville Regional Medical Center	Cookeville	98%	253
Cumberland Medical Center	Crossville	98%	170
Dyersburg Regional Medical Center	Dyersburg	98%	61
Harton Regional Medical Center	Tullahoma	98%	114
Methodist Healthcare Memphis Hospitals[2]	Memphis	98%	164
Parkwest Medical Center[2]	Knoxville	98%	113
Sycamore Shoals Hospital[2]	Elizabethton	98%	84
Tennova Healthcare-Jefferson Mem Hosp	Jefferson City	98%	104
Tristar Horizon Medical Center	Dickson	98%	130
Tristar Summit Medical Center[2]	Hermitage	98%	89
VA Middle Tennessee Healthcare System	Nashville	98%	125
Fort Sanders Regional Medical Center[2]	Knoxville	97%	106
Heritage Medical Center	Shelbyville	97%	62
Johnson City Medical Center[2]	Johnson City	97%	68
Lakeway Regional Hospital	Morristown	97%	69
Maury Regional Hospital[2]	Columbia	97%	73
McNairy Regional Hospital	Selmer	97%	38
Memphis VA Medical Center	Memphis	97%	74
Parkridge Medical Center	Chattanooga	97%	203
Riverview Regional Medical Center	Carthage	97%	66
Roane Medical Center[2]	Harriman	97%	87
Southern Tennessee Medical Center	Winchester	97%	119
Sumner Regional Medical Center	Gallatin	97%	219
Tristar Centennial Medical Center[2]	Nashville	97%	76
Wellmont Bristol Regional Medical Center[2]	Bristol	97%	77
Fort Loudoun Medical Center[2]	Lenoir City	96%	76
Jamestown Regional Medical Center	Jamestown	96%	71
Laughlin Memorial Hospital	Greeneville	96%	155
Skyridge Medical Center	Cleveland	96%	169
Tennova Healthcare-Lafollett Med Ctr	La Follette	96%	104
Crockett Hospital	Lawrenceburg	95%	129
Gateway Medical Center	Clarksville	95%	259
Livingston Regional Hospital	Livingston	95%	155
Saint Francis Bartlett Medical Center[2]	Bartlett	95%	133
Saint Thomas West Hospital	Nashville	95%	198
Sweetwater Hospital Association	Sweetwater	95%	127
University Medical Center	Lebanon	95%	139
Volunteer Community Hospital	Martin	95%	41
Saint Thomas Rutherford Hospital	Murfreesboro	94%	309
Tennova Healthcare	Knoxville	94%	468
Tennova Healthcare-Newport Med Ctr	Newport	94%	108
University of Tn Memorial Hospital[2]	Knoxville	94%	68

NOTE: Hospital profiles are in alphabetical order by state, then city, then hospital within the city; Rankings exclude hospitals with less than 25 cases except for patient surveys which excludes hospitals with less than 100 cases; (a) 100-299 cases; (1) The number of cases/patients is too few to report; (2) Data submitted were based on a sample of cases/patients; (3) Results are based on a shorter time period than required; (4) Data suppressed by CMS for one or more quarters; (5) Results are not available for this reporting period; (6) Fewer than 100 patients completed the HCAHPS survey; (7) No cases met the criteria for this measure; (8) The lower limit of the confidence interval cannot be calculated if the number of observed infections equals zero; (9) No data are available from the state/territory for this reporting period; (10) The scores shown reflect fewer than 50 completed surveys; (11) There were discrepancies in the data collection process; (12) This measure does not apply to this hospital for this reporting period; (13) Results cannot be calculated for this reporting period; (14) The results for this state are combined with nearby states to protect confidentiality; Please refer to the User's Guide for a full explanation of data.

Hospital Name	City	Rate	Cases
Erlanger Medical Center	Chattanooga	93%	118
Hillside Hospital	Pulaski	93%	56
Macon County General Hospital	Lafayette	93%	30
Rhea Medical Center	Dayton	93%	103
Saint Thomas Midtown Hospital	Nashville	93%	191
Tristar Skyline Medical Center[2]	Nashville	93%	76
Franklin Woods Community Hospital[2]	Johnson City	92%	117
Williamson Medical Center	Franklin	92%	113
Hardin Medical Center	Savannah	91%	89
Wellmont Hawkins County Memorial Hospital	Rogersville	91%	98
Jackson - Madison County General Hospital[2]	Jackson	90%	88
Wellmont Holston Valley Medical Center[2]	Kingsport	90%	62
Grandview Medical Center	Jasper	89%	94
Highlands Medical Center[2]	Sparta	89%	100
Marshall Medical Center	Lewisburg	89%	27
Metro Nashville General Hospital[2]	Nashville	89%	27
Regional Medical Center at Memphis	Memphis	89%	37
Stones River Hosp & Dekalb Comm Hosp	Woodbury	89%	44
Decatur County General Hospital	Parsons	88%	26
Unicoi County Memorial Hospital	Erwin	88%	41
River Park Hospital	Mc Minnville	87%	116
Lincoln Medical Center	Fayetteville	86%	71
United Regional Medical Center[2]	Manchester	86%	132
Claiborne County Hospital[2]	Tazewell	85%	47
Vanderbilt University Hospital[2]	Nashville	85%	34
Jellico Community Hospital[2]	Jellico	83%	66
Starr Regional Medical Center Etowah[3]	Etowah	80%	44
Wayne Medical Center	Waynesboro	79%	43
Perry Community Hospital[2]	Linden	50%	26

Blood Culture Timing

Hospital Name	City	Rate	Cases
Baptist Memorial Hospital	Memphis	100%	638
Baptist Memorial Hospital Huntingdon	Huntingdon	100%	29
Baptist Memorial Hospital Union City	Union City	100%	76
Decatur County General Hospital	Parsons	100%	38
Fort Sanders Regional Medical Center[2]	Knoxville	100%	178
Henderson County Community Hospital	Lexington	100%	45
Henry County Medical Center	Paris	100%	111
Heritage Medical Center	Shelbyville	100%	101
Highlands Medical Center[2]	Sparta	100%	99
Jamestown Regional Medical Center	Jamestown	100%	66
Jellico Community Hospital[2]	Jellico	100%	138
Lauderdale Community Hospital	Ripley	100%	26
Livingston Regional Hospital	Livingston	100%	204
McKenzie Regional Hospital	Mc Kenzie	100%	42
Memorial Healthcare System[2]	Chattanooga	100%	342
Methodist Medical Center of Oak Ridge[2]	Oak Ridge	100%	78
Morristown Hamblen Hospital Association[2]	Morristown	100%	213
Mountain Home VA Medical Center	Mountain Home	100%	222
Northcrest Medical Center[2]	Springfield	100%	297
Parkridge Medical Center	Chattanooga	100%	312
Regional Hospital of Jackson	Jackson	100%	108
Riverview Regional Medical Center	Carthage	100%	94
Skyridge Medical Center	Cleveland	100%	302
Sumner Regional Medical Center	Gallatin	100%	246
Takoma Regional Hospital[2]	Greeneville	100%	135
Tristar Hendersonville Medical Center	Hendersonville	100%	212
Tristar Horizon Medical Center	Dickson	100%	204
Tristar Southern Hills Medical Center	Nashville	100%	97
Tristar Stonecrest Medical Center[2]	Smyrna	100%	213
Trousdale Medical Center	Hartsville	100%	25
Claiborne County Hospital[2]	Tazewell	99%	132
Crockett Hospital	Lawrenceburg	99%	147
Dyersburg Regional Medical Center	Dyersburg	99%	104
Erlanger Medical Center	Chattanooga	99%	158
Gateway Medical Center	Clarksville	99%	305
Harton Regional Medical Center	Tullahoma	99%	148
Jackson - Madison County General Hospital[2]	Jackson	99%	193
Lakeway Regional Hospital	Morristown	99%	100
Leconte Medical Center[2]	Sevierville	99%	190
Methodist Healthcare Memphis Hospitals[2]	Memphis	99%	252
Parkwest Medical Center[2]	Knoxville	99%	169
Roane Medical Center[2]	Harriman	99%	139
Saint Francis Hospital	Memphis	99%	201
Saint Thomas Midtown Hospital	Nashville	99%	237
Stones River Hosp & Dekalb Comm Hosp	Smithville	99%	108
Sweetwater Hospital Association	Sweetwater	99%	207
Tennova Healthcare-Jefferson Mem Hosp	Jefferson City	99%	161
Tennova Healthcare-Newport Med Ctr	Newport	99%	240
Tristar Skyline Medical Center[2]	Nashville	99%	174
Tristar Summit Medical Center[2]	Hermitage	99%	160
University Medical Center	Lebanon	99%	217
VA Middle Tennessee Healthcare System	Nashville	99%	217
Wellmont Holston Valley Medical Center[2]	Kingsport	99%	109
Cookeville Regional Medical Center	Cookeville	98%	471
Cumberland Medical Center	Crossville	98%	292
Grandview Medical Center	Jasper	98%	89
Hardin Medical Center	Savannah	98%	131
Johnson City Medical Center[2]	Johnson City	98%	131
River Park Hospital	Mc Minnville	98%	152
Saint Francis Bartlett Medical Center[2]	Bartlett	98%	170
Southern Tennessee Medical Center	Winchester	98%	174
Starr Regional Medical Center Athens	Athens	98%	115
Stones River Hosp & Dekalb Comm Hosp	Woodbury	98%	53
Sycamore Shoals Hospital[2]	Elizabethton	98%	121
Tennova Healthcare-Lafollett Med Ctr	La Follette	98%	216
Tristar Centennial Medical Center[2]	Nashville	98%	88
University of Tn Memorial Hospital[2]	Knoxville	98%	132
Wellmont Bristol Regional Medical Center[2]	Bristol	98%	124
Wellmont Hawkins County Memorial Hospital	Rogersville	98%	143
Williamson Medical Center	Franklin	98%	136
Blount Memorial Hospital[2]	Maryville	97%	163
Delta Medical Center	Memphis	97%	31
Fort Loudoun Medical Center[2]	Lenoir City	97%	115
Laughlin Memorial Hospital	Greeneville	97%	260
Lincoln Medical Center	Fayetteville	97%	145
Maury Regional Hospital[2]	Columbia	97%	150
McNairy Regional Hospital	Selmer	97%	30
Rhea Medical Center	Dayton	97%	109
Saint Thomas West Hospital	Nashville	97%	334
Tennova Healthcare	Knoxville	97%	746
Baptist Memorial Hospital Tipton	Covington	96%	57
Franklin Woods Community Hospital[2]	Johnson City	96%	148
Hillside Hospital	Pulaski	96%	78
Indian Path Medical Center[2]	Kingsport	96%	130
Memphis VA Medical Center	Memphis	96%	238
Metro Nashville General Hospital[2]	Nashville	96%	45
Regional Medical Center at Memphis	Memphis	96%	82
Saint Thomas Rutherford Hospital	Murfreesboro	96%	340
Volunteer Community Hospital	Martin	96%	52
Wayne Medical Center	Waynesboro	96%	45
Marshall Medical Center	Lewisburg	94%	36
United Regional Medical Center[2]	Manchester	94%	99
Vanderbilt University Hospital[2]	Nashville	94%	93
Macon County General Hospital	Lafayette	92%	49
Starr Regional Medical Center Etowah[3]	Etowah	92%	63
Unicoi County Memorial Hospital	Erwin	67%	55

Pregnancy and Delivery Care

Newborns whose Deliveries were Scheduled Early

Hospital Name	City	Rate	Cases
Dyersburg Regional Medical Center[2]	Dyersburg	0%	30
Fort Sanders Regional Medical Center[2]	Knoxville	0%	30
Methodist Medical Center of Oak Ridge	Oak Ridge	0%	29
Northcrest Medical Center	Springfield	0%	59
Tristar Horizon Medical Center[2]	Dickson	0%	33
University of Tn Memorial Hospital[2]	Knoxville	0%	34
Morristown Hamblen Hospital Association	Morristown	1%	138
Parkridge Medical Center	Chattanooga	1%	154
Vanderbilt University Hospital	Nashville	2%	207
Blount Memorial Hospital[2]	Maryville	3%	35
Jackson - Madison County General Hospital	Jackson	3%	248
Parkwest Medical Center[2]	Knoxville	3%	148
Takoma Regional Hospital[2]	Greeneville	3%	34
Volunteer Community Hospital[2]	Martin	3%	32
Williamson Medical Center[2]	Franklin	3%	32
Baptist Memorial Hospital[2]	Memphis	4%	123
Cumberland Medical Center[2]	Crossville	4%	27
Gateway Medical Center[2]	Clarksville	4%	73
Henry County Medical Center[2]	Paris	4%	28
Methodist Healthcare Memphis Hospitals[2]	Memphis	4%	91
Regional Hospital of Jackson[2]	Jackson	4%	28
Skyridge Medical Center[2]	Cleveland	4%	46
Tennova Healthcare	Knoxville	4%	184
Tristar Summit Medical Center[2]	Hermitage	4%	47
Leconte Medical Center	Sevierville	5%	205
Saint Thomas Midtown Hospital[2]	Nashville	5%	112
Tristar Stonecrest Medical Center[2]	Smyrna	5%	43
Livingston Regional Hospital[2]	Livingston	6%	31
Regional Medical Center at Memphis[2]	Memphis	6%	48
Sumner Regional Medical Center[2]	Gallatin	6%	36
Tristar Centennial Medical Center[2]	Nashville	6%	48
Baptist Memorial Hospital Union City[2]	Union City	7%	28
Harton Regional Medical Center[2]	Tullahoma	7%	46
Wellmont Bristol Regional Medical Center[2]	Bristol	7%	43
Crockett Hospital[2]	Lawrenceburg	8%	26
Saint Thomas Rutherford Hospital[2]	Murfreesboro	8%	60
Southern Tennessee Medical Center[2]	Winchester	10%	40
River Park Hospital[2]	Mc Minnville	12%	41
Cookeville Regional Medical Center	Cookeville	13%	119
Erlanger Medical Center	Chattanooga	13%	635
Laughlin Memorial Hospital[2]	Greeneville	13%	39
University Medical Center	Lebanon	15%	84
Starr Regional Medical Center Athens[2]	Athens	17%	35
Saint Francis Bartlett Medical Center[2]	Bartlett	26%	27

Preventive Care

Immunization for Influenza

Hospital Name	City	Rate	Cases
Baptist Memorial Hospital Huntingdon[2]	Huntingdon	100%	231
Dyersburg Regional Medical Center[2]	Dyersburg	100%	424
Henderson County Community Hospital[2]	Lexington	100%	311
Heritage Medical Center[2]	Shelbyville	100%	331
Hillside Hospital[2]	Pulaski	100%	264
Livingston Regional Hospital[2]	Livingston	100%	261
McNairy Regional Hospital[2]	Selmer	100%	283
Methodist Healthcare Fayette Hospital[2]	Somerville	100%	64
Regional Hospital of Jackson[2]	Jackson	100%	623
Stones River Hosp & Dekalb Comm Hosp[2]	Smithville	100%	282
Takoma Regional Hospital[2]	Greeneville	100%	246
Tristar Ashland City Medical Center[2]	Ashland City	100%	46
Fort Loudoun Medical Center[2]	Lenoir City	99%	346
Gateway Medical Center[2]	Clarksville	99%	568
Haywood Park Community Hospital[2]	Brownsville	99%	183
Jamestown Regional Medical Center[2]	Jamestown	99%	289
Maury Regional Hospital[2]	Columbia	99%	556
McKenzie Regional Hospital[2]	Mc Kenzie	99%	360
Riverview Regional Medical Center[2]	Carthage	99%	274
Saint Francis Hospital[2]	Memphis	99%	1674
Sumner Regional Medical Center[2]	Gallatin	99%	518
Tristar Southern Hills Medical Center[2]	Nashville	99%	438
University Medical Center[2]	Lebanon	99%	590
Volunteer Community Hospital[2]	Martin	99%	276
Bolivar General Hospital	Bolivar	98%	99
Crockett Hospital[2]	Lawrenceburg	98%	268
Indian Path Medical Center[2]	Kingsport	98%	540
Lakeway Regional Hospital[2]	Morristown	98%	303
Laughlin Memorial Hospital[2]	Greeneville	98%	345
Leconte Medical Center[2]	Sevierville	98%	442
Lincoln Medical Center[2]	Fayetteville	98%	284
Memorial Healthcare System[2]	Chattanooga	98%	840
Methodist Healthcare Memphis Hospitals[2]	Memphis	98%	521
Northcrest Medical Center[2]	Springfield	98%	336
Southern Tennessee Medical Center[2]	Winchester	98%	420
Tennova Healthcare-Jefferson Mem Hosp[2]	Jefferson City	98%	328
Tennova Healthcare-Lafollett Med Ctr[2]	La Follette	98%	282
Tennova Healthcare-Newport Med Ctr[2]	Newport	98%	350
Tristar Horizon Medical Center[2]	Dickson	98%	430
Wellmont Bristol Regional Medical Center[2]	Bristol	98%	553
Wellmont Hawkins County Memorial Hospital[2]	Rogersville	98%	289
Baptist Memorial Hospital Union City[2]	Union City	97%	274
Blount Memorial Hospital[2]	Maryville	97%	580
Harton Regional Medical Center[2]	Tullahoma	97%	497
Jackson - Madison County General Hospital[2]	Jackson	97%	548
Starr Regional Medical Center Athens[2]	Athens	97%	272
Sycamore Shoals Hospital[2]	Elizabethton	97%	312
Tristar Stonecrest Medical Center[2]	Smyrna	97%	504
Franklin Woods Community Hospital[2]	Johnson City	96%	453
Saint Thomas West Hospital[2]	Nashville	96%	621
Skyridge Medical Center[2]	Cleveland	96%	625
Stones River Hosp & Dekalb Comm Hosp[2]	Woodbury	96%	239
Tennova Healthcare[2]	Knoxville	96%	725
Tristar Centennial Medical Center[2]	Nashville	96%	618
Tristar Skyline Medical Center[2]	Nashville	96%	602
University of Tn Memorial Hospital[2]	Knoxville	96%	567
Wellmont Holston Valley Medical Center[2]	Kingsport	96%	543
Baptist Memorial Hospital[2]	Memphis	95%	1284
Baptist Memorial Hospital Tipton[2]	Covington	95%	265
Parkridge Medical Center[2]	Chattanooga	95%	583
Henry County Medical Center[2]	Paris	94%	373
Johnson City Medical Center[2]	Johnson City	94%	577
Milan General Hospital	Milan	94%	108
Tristar Summit Medical Center[2]	Hermitage	94%	537
Williamson Medical Center[2]	Franklin	94%	530
Delta Medical Center[2]	Memphis	93%	280
Fort Sanders Regional Medical Center[2]	Knoxville	93%	588
Jellico Community Hospital[2]	Jellico	93%	257
Methodist Medical Center of Oak Ridge[2]	Oak Ridge	93%	658
Morristown Hamblen Hospital Association[2]	Morristown	93%	605
Vanderbilt University Hospital[2]	Nashville	93%	549
Hardin Medical Center[2]	Savannah	92%	230
Parkwest Medical Center[2]	Knoxville	92%	658
River Park Hospital[2]	Mc Minnville	92%	343
Sweetwater Hospital Association[2]	Sweetwater	91%	302
Wayne Medical Center	Waynesboro	91%	272
Highlands Medical Center[2]	Sparta	90%	326
Roane Medical Center[2]	Harriman	90%	299
Grandview Medical Center[2]	Jasper	89%	298
Saint Francis Bartlett Medical Center[2]	Bartlett	89%	589
Saint Thomas Rutherford Hospital[2]	Murfreesboro	89%	528
Decatur County General Hospital[2]	Parsons	88%	250
Erlanger Medical Center[2]	Chattanooga	88%	482
Saint Thomas Hospital for Spinal Surgery[2]	Nashville	84%	321
United Regional Medical Center[2]	Manchester	84%	304
Saint Thomas Midtown Hospital[2]	Nashville	83%	510
Starr Regional Medical Center Etowah[2]	Etowah	83%	290

NOTE: Hospital profiles are in alphabetical order by state, then city, then hospital within the city; Rankings exclude hospitals with less than 25 cases except for patient surveys which excludes hospitals with less than 100 cases; (a) 100-299 cases; (1) The number of cases/patients is too few to report; (2) Data submitted were based on a sample of cases/patients; (3) Results are based on a shorter time period than required; (4) Data suppressed by CMS for one or more quarters; (5) Results are not available for this reporting period; (6) Fewer than 100 patients completed the HCAHPS survey; (7) No cases met the criteria for this measure; (8) The lower limit of the confidence interval cannot be calculated if the number of observed infections equals zero; (9) No data are available from the state/territory for this reporting period; (10) The scores shown reflect fewer than 50 completed surveys; (11) There were discrepancies in the data collection process; (12) This measure does not apply to this hospital for this reporting period; (13) Results cannot be calculated for this reporting period; (14) The results for this state are combined with nearby states to protect confidentiality; Please refer to the User's Guide for a full explanation of data.

Hospital Name	City	Rate	Cases
Claiborne County Hospital[2]	Tazewell	81%	283
Metro Nashville General Hospital[2]	Nashville	78%	343
Unicoi County Memorial Hospital[2]	Erwin	77%	298
Cumberland River Hospital	Celina	76%	243
Tristar Hendersonville Medical Center[2]	Hendersonville	76%	541
Cookeville Regional Medical Center[2]	Cookeville	72%	536
Cumberland Medical Center[2]	Crossville	71%	461
Regional Medical Center at Memphis[2]	Memphis	31%	616
Perry Community Hospital[2]	Linden	24%	314

Immunization for Pneumonia

Hospital Name	City	Rate	Cases
Baptist Memorial Hospital Huntingdon[2]	Huntingdon	100%	363
Dyersburg Regional Medical Center[2]	Dyersburg	100%	553
Henderson County Community Hospital[2]	Lexington	100%	423
Heritage Medical Center[2]	Shelbyville	100%	490
Jamestown Regional Medical Center[2]	Jamestown	100%	479
Lakeway Regional Hospital[2]	Morristown	100%	406
Livingston Regional Hospital[2]	Livingston	100%	318
McNairy Regional Hospital[2]	Selmer	100%	351
Northcrest Medical Center[2]	Springfield	100%	422
Regional Hospital of Jackson[2]	Jackson	100%	906
Stones River Hosp & Dekalb Comm Hosp[2]	Smithville	100%	475
Sumner Regional Medical Center[2]	Gallatin	100%	670
Tennova Healthcare-Newport Med Ctr[2]	Newport	100%	489
Volunteer Community Hospital[2]	Martin	100%	322
Wellmont Hawkins County Memorial Hospital[2]	Rogersville	100%	441
Bolivar General Hospital	Bolivar	99%	140
Gateway Medical Center[2]	Clarksville	99%	637
Hillside Hospital[2]	Pulaski	99%	326
Lincoln Medical Center[2]	Fayetteville	99%	342
Maury Regional Hospital[2]	Columbia	99%	724
McKenzie Regional Hospital[2]	Mc Kenzie	99%	329
Memorial Healthcare System[2]	Chattanooga	99%	1489
Riverview Regional Medical Center[2]	Carthage	99%	389
Takoma Regional Hospital[2]	Greeneville	99%	313
Tennova Healthcare-Jefferson Mem Hosp[2]	Jefferson City	99%	507
Tennova Healthcare-Lafollett Med Ctr[2]	La Follette	99%	485
Wellmont Bristol Regional Medical Center[2]	Bristol	99%	805
Wellmont Holston Valley Medical Center[2]	Kingsport	99%	780
Baptist Memorial Hospital[2]	Memphis	98%	1448
Harton Regional Medical Center[2]	Tullahoma	98%	582
Haywood Park Community Hospital[2]	Brownsville	98%	222
Methodist Healthcare Fayette Hospital[2]	Somerville	98%	113
Southern Tennessee Medical Center[2]	Winchester	98%	531
Tristar Horizon Medical Center[2]	Dickson	98%	634
Tristar Southern Hills Medical Center[2]	Nashville	98%	640
Tristar Stonecrest Medical Center[2]	Smyrna	98%	540
University Medical Center[2]	Lebanon	98%	629
Baptist Memorial Hospital Union City[2]	Union City	97%	357
Crockett Hospital[2]	Lawrenceburg	97%	335
Fort Loudoun Medical Center[2]	Lenoir City	97%	546
Indian Path Medical Center[2]	Kingsport	97%	717
Jackson - Madison County General Hospital[2]	Jackson	97%	748
Jellico Community Hospital[2]	Jellico	97%	340
Laughlin Memorial Hospital[2]	Greeneville	97%	461
Methodist Healthcare Memphis Hospitals[2]	Memphis	97%	585
Parkridge Medical Center[2]	Chattanooga	97%	772
River Park Hospital[2]	Mc Minnville	97%	446
Saint Francis Hospital[2]	Memphis	97%	1417
Starr Regional Medical Center Athens[2]	Athens	97%	304
Tristar Ashland City Medical Center[2]	Ashland City	97%	66
University of Tn Memorial Hospital[2]	Knoxville	97%	661
Baptist Memorial Hospital Tipton[2]	Covington	96%	231
Methodist Medical Center of Oak Ridge[2]	Oak Ridge	96%	927
Milan General Hospital	Milan	96%	161
Morristown Hamblen Hospital Association[2]	Morristown	96%	828
Tristar Skyline Medical Center[2]	Nashville	96%	964
Decatur County General Hospital[2]	Parsons	95%	403
Franklin Woods Community Hospital[2]	Johnson City	95%	487
Henry County Medical Center[2]	Paris	95%	507
Highlands Medical Center[2]	Sparta	95%	458
Leconte Medical Center[2]	Sevierville	95%	521
Saint Francis Bartlett Medical Center[2]	Bartlett	95%	722
Skyridge Medical Center[2]	Cleveland	95%	771
Stones River Hosp & Dekalb Comm Hosp[2]	Woodbury	95%	375
Sycamore Shoals Hospital[2]	Elizabethton	95%	508
Tennova Healthcare[2]	Knoxville	95%	953
Tristar Centennial Medical Center[2]	Nashville	95%	720
Blount Memorial Hospital[2]	Maryville	94%	773
Hardin Medical Center[2]	Savannah	94%	267
Sweetwater Hospital Association[2]	Sweetwater	94%	425
Wayne Medical Center	Waynesboro	94%	410
Roane Medical Center[2]	Harriman	93%	502
Williamson Medical Center[2]	Franklin	92%	586
Starr Regional Medical Center Etowah[2,3]	Etowah	91%	364
Tristar Summit Medical Center[2]	Hermitage	91%	708
Cumberland Medical Center[2]	Crossville	90%	648
Fort Sanders Regional Medical Center[2]	Knoxville	90%	777
Johnson City Medical Center[2]	Johnson City	90%	743
United Regional Medical Center[2]	Manchester	90%	399

Hospital Name	City	Rate	Cases
Grandview Medical Center[2]	Jasper	89%	423
Parkwest Medical Center[2]	Knoxville	89%	747
Saint Thomas Rutherford Hospital[2]	Murfreesboro	87%	632
Vanderbilt University Hospital[2]	Nashville	87%	459
Saint Thomas Hospital for Spinal Surgery[2]	Nashville	86%	341
Saint Thomas West Hospital[2]	Nashville	86%	984
Claiborne County Hospital[2]	Tazewell	85%	425
Metro Nashville General Hospital[2]	Nashville	85%	309
Tristar Hendersonville Medical Center[2]	Hendersonville	85%	685
Cookeville Regional Medical Center[2]	Cookeville	84%	776
Erlanger Medical Center[2]	Chattanooga	83%	448
Saint Thomas Midtown Hospital[2]	Nashville	77%	524
Delta Medical Center[2]	Memphis	76%	385
Cumberland River Hospital	Celina	71%	452
Unicoi County Memorial Hospital[2]	Erwin	57%	568
Regional Medical Center at Memphis[2]	Memphis	38%	317
Perry Community Hospital[2]	Linden	23%	561

Stroke Care

Anticoagulation Therapy for Atrial Fibrillation

Hospital Name	City	Rate	Cases
Saint Thomas West Hospital	Nashville	100%	44
University of Tn Memorial Hospital	Knoxville	100%	45
Vanderbilt University Hospital[2]	Nashville	100%	69
Fort Sanders Regional Medical Center	Knoxville	98%	45
Baptist Memorial Hospital	Memphis	97%	64
Parkwest Medical Center	Knoxville	97%	31
Tristar Skyline Medical Center	Nashville	97%	32
Jackson - Madison County General Hospital	Jackson	96%	54
Methodist Healthcare Memphis Hospitals[2]	Memphis	93%	29
Johnson City Medical Center	Johnson City	90%	52
Maury Regional Hospital	Columbia	88%	26
Erlanger Medical Center[2]	Chattanooga	87%	39
Tennova Healthcare	Knoxville	86%	36

Antithrombotic Therapy Timing

Hospital Name	City	Rate	Cases
Baptist Memorial Hospital Union City	Union City	100%	29
Blount Memorial Hospital[2]	Maryville	100%	89
Dyersburg Regional Medical Center	Dyersburg	100%	36
Fort Loudoun Medical Center	Lenoir City	100%	26
Fort Sanders Regional Medical Center	Knoxville	100%	258
Henry County Medical Center	Paris	100%	38
Leconte Medical Center	Sevierville	100%	50
Methodist Medical Center of Oak Ridge[2]	Oak Ridge	100%	89
Morristown Hamblen Hospital Association[2]	Morristown	100%	73
Parkridge Medical Center	Chattanooga	100%	56
Regional Hospital of Jackson	Jackson	100%	54
Southern Tennessee Medical Center	Winchester	100%	31
Tennova Healthcare-Jefferson Mem Hosp	Jefferson City	100%	29
Tennova Healthcare-Newport Med Ctr	Newport	100%	26
Tristar Horizon Medical Center	Dickson	100%	45
Tristar Southern Hills Medical Center	Nashville	100%	46
Tristar Stonecrest Medical Center[2]	Smyrna	100%	29
Tristar Summit Medical Center	Hermitage	100%	159
Wellmont Bristol Regional Medical Center	Bristol	100%	174
Maury Regional Hospital	Columbia	99%	147
Methodist Healthcare Memphis Hospitals[2]	Memphis	99%	402
Saint Thomas Rutherford Hospital	Murfreesboro	99%	144
Saint Thomas West Hospital	Nashville	99%	272
Vanderbilt University Hospital[2]	Nashville	99%	264
Baptist Memorial Hospital	Memphis	98%	397
Cookeville Regional Medical Center	Cookeville	98%	162
Cumberland Medical Center[2]	Crossville	98%	49
Gateway Medical Center	Clarksville	98%	88
Johnson City Medical Center	Johnson City	98%	228
Parkwest Medical Center	Knoxville	98%	155
Saint Francis Bartlett Medical Center	Bartlett	98%	60
Saint Francis Hospital	Memphis	98%	182
Sumner Regional Medical Center	Gallatin	98%	48
Tennova Healthcare	Knoxville	98%	210
Tristar Centennial Medical Center	Nashville	98%	137
Tristar Hendersonville Medical Center	Hendersonville	98%	60
Tristar Skyline Medical Center	Nashville	98%	287
Williamson Medical Center[2]	Franklin	98%	41
Jackson - Madison County General Hospital	Jackson	97%	411
Lakeway Regional Hospital	Morristown	97%	30
Memorial Healthcare System[2]	Chattanooga	97%	150
University of Tn Memorial Hospital	Knoxville	97%	228
Erlanger Medical Center[2]	Chattanooga	93%	155
Indian Path Medical Center	Kingsport	93%	45
Wellmont Holston Valley Medical Center[2]	Kingsport	93%	58
Harton Regional Medical Center	Tullahoma	92%	39
Regional Medical Center at Memphis	Memphis	89%	56
Laughlin Memorial Hospital[2]	Greeneville	84%	38
Saint Thomas Midtown Hospital	Nashville	78%	108

Assessed for Rehabilitation

Hospital Name	City	Rate	Cases
Baptist Memorial Hospital	Memphis	100%	518
Crockett Hospital	Lawrenceburg	100%	25
Fort Loudoun Medical Center	Lenoir City	100%	29
Laughlin Memorial Hospital[2]	Greeneville	100%	42
Methodist Healthcare Memphis Hospitals[2]	Memphis	100%	461
Methodist Medical Center of Oak Ridge[2]	Oak Ridge	100%	98
Morristown Hamblen Hospital Association[2]	Morristown	100%	76
Parkwest Medical Center	Knoxville	100%	188
Saint Francis Hospital	Memphis	100%	202
Southern Tennessee Medical Center	Winchester	100%	29
Sumner Regional Medical Center	Gallatin	100%	52
Tennova Healthcare-Jefferson Mem Hosp	Jefferson City	100%	29
Tennova Healthcare-Newport Med Ctr	Newport	100%	27
Tristar Hendersonville Medical Center	Hendersonville	100%	66
Tristar Horizon Medical Center	Dickson	100%	39
Tristar Skyline Medical Center	Nashville	100%	434
Tristar Southern Hills Medical Center	Nashville	100%	58
Tristar Stonecrest Medical Center[2]	Smyrna	100%	36
Tristar Summit Medical Center	Hermitage	100%	184
Wellmont Bristol Regional Medical Center	Bristol	100%	209
Blount Memorial Hospital[2]	Maryville	99%	102
Fort Sanders Regional Medical Center	Knoxville	99%	362
Maury Regional Hospital	Columbia	99%	177
Tristar Centennial Medical Center	Nashville	99%	177
University of Tn Memorial Hospital	Knoxville	99%	373
Cumberland Medical Center[2]	Crossville	98%	48
Leconte Medical Center	Sevierville	98%	63
Parkridge Medical Center	Chattanooga	98%	65
Regional Hospital of Jackson	Jackson	98%	56
Saint Thomas West Hospital	Nashville	98%	378
Wellmont Holston Valley Medical Center[2]	Kingsport	98%	80
Jackson - Madison County General Hospital	Jackson	97%	498
Regional Medical Center at Memphis	Memphis	97%	69
Saint Francis Bartlett Medical Center	Bartlett	97%	59
Tennova Healthcare	Knoxville	97%	232
Vanderbilt University Hospital[2]	Nashville	97%	478
Baptist Memorial Hospital Union City	Union City	96%	28
Erlanger Medical Center[2]	Chattanooga	96%	202
Gateway Medical Center	Clarksville	96%	89
Johnson City Medical Center	Johnson City	96%	296
Dyersburg Regional Medical Center	Dyersburg	95%	44
Indian Path Medical Center	Kingsport	94%	48
Henry County Medical Center	Paris	93%	43
Saint Thomas Rutherford Hospital	Murfreesboro	93%	174
Williamson Medical Center[2]	Franklin	93%	42
Saint Thomas Midtown Hospital	Nashville	89%	175
Harton Regional Medical Center	Tullahoma	88%	34
Cookeville Regional Medical Center	Cookeville	84%	171
Memorial Healthcare System[2]	Chattanooga	80%	164

Discharged on Antithrombotic Therapy

Hospital Name	City	Rate	Cases
Baptist Memorial Hospital Union City	Union City	100%	27
Blount Memorial Hospital[2]	Maryville	100%	99
Crockett Hospital	Lawrenceburg	100%	25
Dyersburg Regional Medical Center	Dyersburg	100%	42
Fort Sanders Regional Medical Center	Knoxville	100%	307
Henry County Medical Center	Paris	100%	43
Jackson - Madison County General Hospital	Jackson	100%	442
Laughlin Memorial Hospital[2]	Greeneville	100%	42
Methodist Healthcare Memphis Hospitals[2]	Memphis	100%	416
Methodist Medical Center of Oak Ridge[2]	Oak Ridge	100%	95
Morristown Hamblen Hospital Association[2]	Morristown	100%	45
Parkridge Medical Center	Chattanooga	100%	65
Parkwest Medical Center	Knoxville	100%	163
Regional Hospital of Jackson	Jackson	100%	53
Regional Medical Center at Memphis	Memphis	100%	60
Saint Francis Hospital	Memphis	100%	178
Saint Thomas West Hospital	Nashville	100%	309
Southern Tennessee Medical Center	Winchester	100%	26
Sumner Regional Medical Center	Gallatin	100%	49
Tennova Healthcare	Knoxville	100%	212
Tennova Healthcare-Jefferson Mem Hosp	Jefferson City	100%	29
Tennova Healthcare-Newport Med Ctr	Newport	100%	27
Tristar Centennial Medical Center	Nashville	100%	155
Tristar Hendersonville Medical Center	Hendersonville	100%	64
Tristar Horizon Medical Center	Dickson	100%	39
Tristar Skyline Medical Center	Nashville	100%	331
Tristar Stonecrest Medical Center[2]	Smyrna	100%	35
Tristar Summit Medical Center	Hermitage	100%	164
Wellmont Bristol Regional Medical Center	Bristol	100%	185
Baptist Memorial Hospital	Memphis	99%	420
Gateway Medical Center	Clarksville	99%	88
Maury Regional Hospital	Columbia	99%	163
Saint Thomas Rutherford Hospital	Murfreesboro	99%	163
University of Tn Memorial Hospital	Knoxville	99%	271
Vanderbilt University Hospital[2]	Nashville	99%	346
Cumberland Medical Center[2]	Crossville	98%	46

NOTE: Hospital profiles are in alphabetical order by state, then city, then hospital within the city; Rankings exclude hospitals with less than 25 cases except for patient surveys which excludes hospitals with less than 100 cases; (a) 100-299 cases; (1) The number of cases/patients is too few to report; (2) Data submitted were based on a sample of cases/patients; (3) Results are based on a shorter time period than required; (4) Data suppressed by CMS for one or more quarters; (5) Results are not available for this reporting period; (6) Fewer than 100 patients completed the HCAHPS survey; (7) No cases met the criteria for this measure; (8) The lower limit of the confidence interval cannot be calculated if the number of observed infections equals zero; (9) No data are available from the state/territory for this reporting period; (10) The scores shown reflect fewer than 50 completed surveys; (11) There were discrepancies in the data collection process; (12) This measure does not apply to this hospital for this reporting period; (13) Results cannot be calculated for this reporting period; (14) The results for this state are combined with nearby states to protect confidentiality; Please refer to the User's Guide for a full explanation of data.

Indian Path Medical Center	Kingsport	98%	44
Leconte Medical Center	Sevierville	98%	62
Saint Francis Bartlett Medical Center	Bartlett	98%	56
Tristar Southern Hills Medical Center	Nashville	98%	57
Cookeville Regional Medical Center	Cookeville	97%	155
Fort Loudoun Medical Center	Lenoir City	97%	29
Memorial Healthcare System[2]	Chattanooga	97%	160
Saint Thomas Midtown Hospital	Nashville	97%	137
Johnson City Medical Center	Johnson City	96%	234
Williamson Medical Center[2]	Franklin	95%	41
Harton Regional Medical Center	Tullahoma	94%	33
Wellmont Holston Valley Medical Center[2]	Kingsport	92%	65
Erlanger Medical Center[2]	Chattanooga	89%	158

Discharged on Statin Medication

Hospital Name	City	Rate	Cases
Dyersburg Regional Medical Center	Dyersburg	100%	35
Methodist Medical Center of Oak Ridge[2]	Oak Ridge	100%	58
Parkridge Medical Center	Chattanooga	100%	50
Sumner Regional Medical Center	Gallatin	100%	42
Tristar Centennial Medical Center	Nashville	100%	115
Tristar Hendersonville Medical Center	Hendersonville	100%	48
Tristar Horizon Medical Center	Dickson	100%	30
Tristar Southern Hills Medical Center	Nashville	100%	50
Tristar Stonecrest Medical Center[2]	Smyrna	100%	28
Baptist Memorial Hospital	Memphis	99%	317
Blount Memorial Hospital[2]	Maryville	99%	80
Methodist Healthcare Memphis Hospitals[2]	Memphis	99%	326
Saint Francis Hospital	Memphis	99%	141
Tristar Summit Medical Center	Hermitage	99%	109
Jackson - Madison County General Hospital	Jackson	98%	337
Leconte Medical Center	Sevierville	98%	45
Morristown Hamblen Hospital Association[2]	Morristown	98%	66
Saint Francis Bartlett Medical Center	Bartlett	98%	43
Wellmont Bristol Regional Medical Center	Bristol	98%	124
Fort Sanders Regional Medical Center	Knoxville	97%	225
Maury Regional Hospital	Columbia	97%	127
Regional Hospital of Jackson	Jackson	97%	36
Tristar Skyline Medical Center	Nashville	97%	249
University of Tn Memorial Hospital	Knoxville	97%	222
Parkwest Medical Center	Knoxville	96%	106
Laughlin Memorial Hospital[2]	Greeneville	95%	38
Saint Thomas West Hospital	Nashville	95%	237
Vanderbilt University Hospital[2]	Nashville	94%	273
Wellmont Holston Valley Medical Center[2]	Kingsport	94%	48
Gateway Medical Center	Clarksville	93%	67
Johnson City Medical Center	Johnson City	93%	183
Regional Medical Center at Memphis	Memphis	93%	46
Tennova Healthcare	Knoxville	92%	167
Indian Path Medical Center	Kingsport	89%	35
Erlanger Medical Center[2]	Chattanooga	88%	128
Memorial Healthcare System[2]	Chattanooga	86%	133
Saint Thomas Midtown Hospital	Nashville	86%	112
Cookeville Regional Medical Center	Cookeville	85%	124
Saint Thomas Rutherford Hospital	Murfreesboro	84%	112
Cumberland Medical Center[2]	Crossville	83%	35
Williamson Medical Center[2]	Franklin	80%	35
Henry County Medical Center	Paris	58%	40

Thrombolytic Therapy Timing

Hospital Name	City	Rate	Cases
University of Tn Memorial Hospital	Knoxville	97%	30
Baptist Memorial Hospital	Memphis	61%	36
Tennova Healthcare	Knoxville	28%	25
Memorial Healthcare System[2]	Chattanooga	6%	51

Venous Thromboembolism (VTE) Prophylaxis

Hospital Name	City	Rate	Cases
Baptist Memorial Hospital Union City	Union City	100%	30
Blount Memorial Hospital[2]	Maryville	100%	96
Dyersburg Regional Medical Center	Dyersburg	100%	35
Lakeway Regional Hospital	Morristown	100%	30
Morristown Hamblen Hospital Association[2]	Morristown	100%	76
Saint Francis Hospital	Memphis	100%	217
Southern Tennessee Medical Center	Winchester	100%	33
Tristar Horizon Medical Center	Dickson	100%	46
Tristar Skyline Medical Center	Nashville	100%	442
Tristar Stonecrest Medical Center[2]	Smyrna	100%	25
Wellmont Bristol Regional Medical Center	Bristol	100%	219
Methodist Healthcare Memphis Hospitals[2]	Memphis	99%	456
Methodist Medical Center of Oak Ridge[2]	Oak Ridge	99%	97
Tristar Centennial Medical Center	Nashville	99%	174
Cumberland Medical Center[2]	Crossville	98%	50
Leconte Medical Center	Sevierville	98%	49
Tristar Hendersonville Medical Center	Hendersonville	98%	60
Tristar Southern Hills Medical Center	Nashville	98%	56
University of Tn Memorial Hospital	Knoxville	98%	409
Fort Sanders Regional Medical Center	Knoxville	97%	378
Tennova Healthcare-Jefferson Mem Hosp	Jefferson City	97%	32
Maury Regional Hospital	Columbia	96%	167
Parkridge Medical Center	Chattanooga	96%	57
Parkwest Medical Center	Knoxville	96%	197
Sumner Regional Medical Center	Gallatin	96%	50
Tristar Summit Medical Center	Hermitage	96%	185
Baptist Memorial Hospital	Memphis	95%	561
Regional Hospital of Jackson	Jackson	95%	56
Jackson - Madison County General Hospital	Jackson	93%	512
Saint Thomas Rutherford Hospital	Murfreesboro	93%	153
Saint Francis Bartlett Medical Center	Bartlett	92%	61
Saint Thomas West Hospital	Nashville	92%	369
Johnson City Medical Center	Johnson City	91%	311
Harton Regional Medical Center	Tullahoma	90%	41
Cookeville Regional Medical Center	Cookeville	89%	182
Gateway Medical Center	Clarksville	89%	89
Vanderbilt University Hospital[2]	Nashville	88%	458
Tennova Healthcare	Knoxville	87%	231
Indian Path Medical Center	Kingsport	85%	48
Wellmont Holston Valley Medical Center[2]	Kingsport	84%	81
Erlanger Medical Center[2]	Chattanooga	83%	237
Memorial Healthcare System[2]	Chattanooga	83%	157
Regional Medical Center at Memphis	Memphis	82%	68
Laughlin Memorial Hospital[2]	Greeneville	81%	37
Saint Thomas Midtown Hospital	Nashville	80%	174
Williamson Medical Center[2]	Franklin	80%	41
Henry County Medical Center	Paris	76%	34

Written Stroke Educational Materials Given

Hospital Name	City	Rate	Cases
Fort Sanders Regional Medical Center	Knoxville	100%	207
Laughlin Memorial Hospital[2]	Greeneville	100%	28
Methodist Medical Center of Oak Ridge[2]	Oak Ridge	100%	64
Morristown Hamblen Hospital Association[2]	Morristown	100%	51
Sumner Regional Medical Center	Gallatin	100%	25
Wellmont Bristol Regional Medical Center	Bristol	100%	110
Parkwest Medical Center	Knoxville	99%	94
Saint Francis Hospital	Memphis	98%	112
University of Tn Memorial Hospital	Knoxville	98%	197
Blount Memorial Hospital[2]	Maryville	97%	62
Maury Regional Hospital	Columbia	97%	88
Saint Francis Bartlett Medical Center	Bartlett	97%	32
Baptist Memorial Hospital	Memphis	96%	299
Harton Regional Medical Center	Tullahoma	96%	27
Methodist Healthcare Memphis Hospitals[2]	Memphis	96%	303
Parkridge Medical Center	Chattanooga	96%	49
Tristar Skyline Medical Center	Nashville	96%	209
Tristar Southern Hills Medical Center	Nashville	94%	34
Tristar Summit Medical Center	Hermitage	94%	105
Tristar Centennial Medical Center	Nashville	93%	92
Saint Thomas West Hospital	Nashville	92%	221
Tristar Hendersonville Medical Center	Hendersonville	92%	39
Leconte Medical Center	Sevierville	88%	48
Dyersburg Regional Medical Center	Dyersburg	86%	28
Jackson - Madison County General Hospital	Jackson	86%	243
Saint Thomas Rutherford Hospital	Murfreesboro	86%	109
Williamson Medical Center[2]	Franklin	84%	25
Johnson City Medical Center	Johnson City	82%	158
Vanderbilt University Hospital[2]	Nashville	81%	268
Tennova Healthcare	Knoxville	80%	133
Gateway Medical Center	Clarksville	77%	57
Erlanger Medical Center[2]	Chattanooga	75%	115
Regional Hospital of Jackson	Jackson	72%	29
Saint Thomas Midtown Hospital	Nashville	70%	98
Cookeville Regional Medical Center	Cookeville	43%	105
Indian Path Medical Center	Kingsport	43%	30
Wellmont Holston Valley Medical Center[2]	Kingsport	30%	46
Memorial Healthcare System[2]	Chattanooga	12%	104
Regional Medical Center at Memphis	Memphis	6%	48

Surgical Care Improvement Project

Appropriate Beta Blocker Usage

Hospital Name	City	Rate	Cases
Baptist Memorial Hospital[2]	Memphis	100%	350
Baptist Memorial Hospital Union City	Union City	100%	35
Blount Memorial Hospital[2]	Maryville	100%	119
Fort Sanders Regional Medical Center[2]	Knoxville	100%	257
Henry County Medical Center	Paris	100%	146
Laughlin Memorial Hospital	Greeneville	100%	72
Methodist Medical Center of Oak Ridge[2]	Oak Ridge	100%	208
Morristown Hamblen Hospital Association[2]	Morristown	100%	105
Northcrest Medical Center[2]	Springfield	100%	63
Parkridge Medical Center[2]	Chattanooga	100%	206
Regional Hospital of Jackson	Jackson	100%	125
Skyridge Medical Center	Cleveland	100%	73
Southern Tennessee Medical Center	Winchester	100%	60
Sumner Regional Medical Center	Gallatin	100%	111
Tristar Horizon Medical Center	Dickson	100%	25
Tristar Southern Hills Medical Center	Nashville	100%	67
University of Tn Memorial Hospital[2]	Knoxville	100%	201
Wellmont Bristol Regional Medical Center[2]	Bristol	100%	176
Methodist Healthcare Memphis Hospitals[2]	Memphis	99%	616
Saint Francis Hospital[2]	Memphis	99%	356
Tristar Centennial Medical Center[2]	Nashville	99%	330
Tristar Skyline Medical Center[2]	Nashville	99%	146
Tristar Stonecrest Medical Center[2]	Smyrna	99%	73
Tristar Summit Medical Center[2]	Hermitage	99%	140
University Medical Center	Lebanon	99%	101
Vanderbilt University Hospital[2]	Nashville	99%	240
Cookeville Regional Medical Center	Cookeville	98%	492
Erlanger Medical Center[2]	Chattanooga	98%	134
Gateway Medical Center	Clarksville	98%	189
Indian Path Medical Center[2]	Kingsport	98%	96
Jackson - Madison County General Hospital[2]	Jackson	98%	592
Leconte Medical Center[2]	Sevierville	98%	57
Saint Thomas Midtown Hospital[2]	Nashville	98%	216
Saint Thomas West Hospital[2]	Nashville	98%	238
Tennova Healthcare	Knoxville	98%	868
Tristar Hendersonville Medical Center	Hendersonville	98%	103
Wellmont Holston Valley Medical Center[2]	Kingsport	98%	209
Johnson City Medical Center[2]	Johnson City	97%	226
Maury Regional Hospital[2]	Columbia	97%	164
Saint Thomas Rutherford Hospital[2]	Murfreesboro	97%	158
Sycamore Shoals Hospital[2]	Elizabethton	97%	35
Parkwest Medical Center[2]	Knoxville	96%	339
Saint Francis Bartlett Medical Center[2]	Bartlett	96%	113
Memphis VA Medical Center[2]	Memphis	94%	155
Mountain Home VA Medical Center[2]	Mountain Home	94%	86
VA Middle Tennessee Healthcare System[2]	Nashville	94%	104
Lakeway Regional Hospital	Morristown	92%	53
Memorial Healthcare System[2]	Chattanooga	92%	519
Harton Regional Medical Center	Tullahoma	91%	64
Regional Medical Center at Memphis	Memphis	91%	58
Williamson Medical Center[2]	Franklin	91%	104
Cumberland Medical Center[2]	Crossville	86%	109
Starr Regional Medical Center Athens	Athens	86%	28
Unicoi County Memorial Hospital	Erwin	77%	31
Metro Nashville General Hospital[2]	Nashville	75%	28

Appropriate VTP Within 24 Hours

Hospital Name	City	Rate	Cases
Baptist Memorial Hospital Tipton	Covington	100%	46
Baptist Memorial Hospital Union City	Union City	100%	132
Blount Memorial Hospital[2]	Maryville	100%	387
Dyersburg Regional Medical Center	Dyersburg	100%	67
Fort Loudoun Medical Center[2]	Lenoir City	100%	52
Franklin Woods Community Hospital[2]	Johnson City	100%	106
Henry County Medical Center	Paris	100%	416
Heritage Medical Center	Shelbyville	100%	28
Lakeway Regional Hospital	Morristown	100%	123
Livingston Regional Hospital	Livingston	100%	29
Maury Regional Hospital[2]	Columbia	100%	512
McKenzie Regional Hospital	Mc Kenzie	100%	34
Methodist Healthcare Memphis Hospitals[2]	Memphis	100%	1452
Milan General Hospital	Milan	100%	37
Morristown Hamblen Hospital Association[2]	Morristown	100%	308
Northcrest Medical Center[2]	Springfield	100%	206
Regional Hospital of Jackson	Jackson	100%	443
Saint Francis Hospital[2]	Memphis	100%	635
Southern Tennessee Medical Center	Winchester	100%	214
Stones River Hosp & Dekalb Comm Hosp	Smithville	100%	44
Sumner Regional Medical Center	Gallatin	100%	391
Sycamore Shoals Hospital[2]	Elizabethton	100%	126
VA Middle Tennessee Healthcare System[2]	Nashville	100%	136
Vanderbilt University Hospital[2]	Nashville	100%	411
Volunteer Community Hospital	Martin	100%	43
Baptist Memorial Hospital[2]	Memphis	99%	680
Fort Sanders Regional Medical Center[2]	Knoxville	99%	549
Gateway Medical Center	Clarksville	99%	503
Methodist Medical Center of Oak Ridge[2]	Oak Ridge	99%	487
Mountain Home VA Medical Center[2]	Mountain Home	99%	175
Parkridge Medical Center[2]	Chattanooga	99%	374
Parkwest Medical Center[2]	Knoxville	99%	619
Saint Thomas West Hospital[2]	Nashville	99%	474
Tristar Centennial Medical Center[2]	Nashville	99%	539
Tristar Hendersonville Medical Center	Hendersonville	99%	331
Tristar Stonecrest Medical Center[2]	Smyrna	99%	234
Tristar Summit Medical Center[2]	Hermitage	99%	399
University Medical Center	Lebanon	99%	324
Wellmont Bristol Regional Medical Center[2]	Bristol	99%	285
Erlanger Medical Center[2]	Chattanooga	98%	318
Indian Path Medical Center[2]	Kingsport	98%	306
Johnson City Medical Center[2]	Johnson City	98%	337
Memphis VA Medical Center[2]	Memphis	98%	263
Skyridge Medical Center	Cleveland	98%	263
Tennova Healthcare	Knoxville	98%	1987
Tennova Healthcare-Jefferson Mem Hosp	Jefferson City	98%	51
Tristar Horizon Medical Center	Dickson	98%	121
Tristar Skyline Medical Center[2]	Nashville	98%	368
Tristar Southern Hills Medical Center	Nashville	98%	268
University of Tn Memorial Hospital[2]	Knoxville	98%	396
Harton Regional Medical Center	Tullahoma	97%	184

NOTE: Hospital profiles are in alphabetical order by state, then city, then hospital within the city; Rankings exclude hospitals with less than 25 cases except for patient surveys which excludes hospitals with less than 100 cases; (a) 100-299 cases; (1) The number of cases/patients is too few to report; (2) Data submitted were based on a sample of cases/patients; (3) Results are based on a shorter time period than required; (4) Data suppressed by CMS for one or more quarters; (5) Results are not available for this reporting period; (6) Fewer than 100 patients completed the HCAHPS survey; (7) No cases met the criteria for this measure; (8) The lower limit of the confidence interval cannot be calculated if the number of observed infections equals zero; (9) No data are available from the state/territory for this reporting period; (10) The scores shown reflect fewer than 50 completed surveys; (11) There were discrepancies in the data collection process; (12) This measure does not apply to this hospital for this reporting period; (13) Results cannot be calculated for this reporting period; (14) The results for this state are combined with nearby states to protect confidentiality; Please refer to the User's Guide for a full explanation of data.

Hospital Name	City	Rate	Cases
Jackson - Madison County General Hospital[2]	Jackson	97%	1153
Memorial Healthcare System[2]	Chattanooga	97%	529
Regional Medical Center at Memphis	Memphis	97%	435
Saint Francis Bartlett Medical Center[2]	Bartlett	97%	267
Saint Thomas Midtown Hospital[2]	Nashville	97%	404
Unicoi County Memorial Hospital	Erwin	97%	92
Wellmont Holston Valley Medical Center[2]	Kingsport	97%	332
Crockett Hospital	Lawrenceburg	96%	28
Roane Medical Center[2]	Harriman	96%	55
Williamson Medical Center[2]	Franklin	96%	285
Cookeville Regional Medical Center	Cookeville	95%	828
Cumberland Medical Center[2]	Crossville	95%	239
Leconte Medical Center[2]	Sevierville	95%	193
Laughlin Memorial Hospital	Greeneville	94%	259
River Park Hospital	Mc Minnville	94%	82
Saint Thomas Rutherford Hospital[2]	Murfreesboro	94%	514
Starr Regional Medical Center Athens	Athens	94%	97
Lincoln Medical Center	Fayetteville	93%	75
Metro Nashville General Hospital[2]	Nashville	93%	162
Takoma Regional Hospital[2]	Greeneville	93%	70
Highlands Medical Center[2]	Sparta	92%	72
Delta Medical Center	Memphis	89%	71
Grandview Medical Center	Jasper	88%	33
Starr Regional Medical Center Etowah[3]	Etowah	88%	32
Hardin Medical Center	Savannah	87%	47
Sweetwater Hospital Association	Sweetwater	81%	59
Claiborne County Hospital[2]	Tazewell	78%	41

Controlled Postoperative Blood Glucose

Hospital Name	City	Rate	Cases
Saint Thomas Midtown Hospital[2]	Nashville	100%	132
Johnson City Medical Center[2]	Johnson City	99%	116
Saint Francis Hospital[2]	Memphis	99%	163
VA Middle Tennessee Healthcare System[2]	Nashville	99%	85
Fort Sanders Regional Medical Center[2]	Knoxville	98%	130
Gateway Medical Center	Clarksville	98%	53
Methodist Healthcare Memphis Hospitals[2]	Memphis	98%	195
Parkwest Medical Center[2]	Knoxville	98%	240
Methodist Medical Center of Oak Ridge[2]	Oak Ridge	97%	125
Parkridge Medical Center[2]	Chattanooga	97%	126
University of Tn Memorial Hospital[2]	Knoxville	97%	147
Vanderbilt University Hospital[2]	Nashville	97%	101
Maury Regional Hospital[2]	Columbia	96%	50
Saint Thomas West Hospital[2]	Nashville	96%	161
Wellmont Bristol Regional Medical Center[2]	Bristol	96%	97
Cookeville Regional Medical Center	Cookeville	95%	221
Tennova Healthcare	Knoxville	95%	281
Tristar Centennial Medical Center[2]	Nashville	95%	190
Wellmont Holston Valley Medical Center[2]	Kingsport	94%	125
Jackson - Madison County General Hospital[2]	Jackson	93%	376
Baptist Memorial Hospital[2]	Memphis	91%	141
Memorial Healthcare System[2]	Chattanooga	91%	595
Erlanger Medical Center[2]	Chattanooga	87%	94
Memphis VA Medical Center[2]	Memphis	87%	78

Perioperative Temperature Management

Hospital Name	City	Rate	Cases
Baptist Memorial Hospital[2]	Memphis	100%	887
Baptist Memorial Hospital Tipton	Covington	100%	56
Baptist Memorial Hospital Union City	Union City	100%	143
Blount Memorial Hospital[2]	Maryville	100%	479
Claiborne County Hospital[2]	Tazewell	100%	48
Cookeville Regional Medical Center	Cookeville	100%	1140
Crockett Hospital	Lawrenceburg	100%	32
Cumberland Medical Center[2]	Crossville	100%	266
Delta Medical Center	Memphis	100%	71
Dyersburg Regional Medical Center	Dyersburg	100%	80
Erlanger Medical Center[2]	Chattanooga	100%	405
Fort Loudoun Medical Center[2]	Lenoir City	100%	62
Fort Sanders Regional Medical Center[2]	Knoxville	100%	640
Franklin Woods Community Hospital[2]	Johnson City	100%	119
Gateway Medical Center	Clarksville	100%	581
Grandview Medical Center	Jasper	100%	35
Hardin Medical Center	Savannah	100%	48
Harton Regional Medical Center	Tullahoma	100%	231
Henry County Medical Center	Paris	100%	475
Heritage Medical Center	Shelbyville	100%	33
Highlands Medical Center[2]	Sparta	100%	118
Hillside Hospital	Pulaski	100%	27
Indian Path Medical Center[2]	Kingsport	100%	340
Jackson - Madison County General Hospital[2]	Jackson	100%	1357
Johnson City Medical Center[2]	Johnson City	100%	461
Lakeway Regional Hospital	Morristown	100%	135
Laughlin Memorial Hospital	Greeneville	100%	267
Leconte Medical Center[2]	Sevierville	100%	215
Lincoln Medical Center	Fayetteville	100%	79
Livingston Regional Hospital	Livingston	100%	30
Maury Regional Hospital[2]	Columbia	100%	569
McKenzie Regional Hospital	Mc Kenzie	100%	42
Memphis VA Medical Center[2]	Memphis	100%	391
Methodist Healthcare Memphis Hospitals[2]	Memphis	100%	1928
Methodist Medical Center of Oak Ridge[2]	Oak Ridge	100%	567
Metro Nashville General Hospital[2]	Nashville	100%	184
Milan General Hospital	Milan	100%	37
Morristown Hamblen Hospital Association[2]	Morristown	100%	333
Mountain Home VA Medical Center[2]	Mountain Home	100%	207
Northcrest Medical Center[2]	Springfield	100%	214
Parkridge Medical Center[2]	Chattanooga	100%	464
Parkwest Medical Center[2]	Knoxville	100%	778
Regional Hospital of Jackson	Jackson	100%	476
Regional Medical Center at Memphis	Memphis	100%	531
Rhea Medical Center	Dayton	100%	25
River Park Hospital	Mc Minnville	100%	97
Roane Medical Center[2]	Harriman	100%	58
Saint Francis Bartlett Medical Center[2]	Bartlett	100%	395
Saint Francis Hospital[2]	Memphis	100%	885
Saint Thomas Midtown Hospital[2]	Nashville	100%	524
Saint Thomas West Hospital[2]	Nashville	100%	619
Skyridge Medical Center	Cleveland	100%	292
Southern Tennessee Medical Center	Winchester	100%	229
Starr Regional Medical Center Athens	Athens	100%	122
Starr Regional Medical Center Etowah[3]	Etowah	100%	33
Stones River Hosp & Dekalb Comm Hosp	Smithville	100%	50
Sumner Regional Medical Center	Gallatin	100%	438
Sweetwater Hospital Association	Sweetwater	100%	70
Sycamore Shoals Hospital[2]	Elizabethton	100%	141
Tennova Healthcare	Knoxville	100%	2496
Tennova Healthcare-Jefferson Mem Hosp	Jefferson City	100%	53
Tristar Centennial Medical Center[2]	Nashville	100%	705
Tristar Hendersonville Medical Center	Hendersonville	100%	390
Tristar Horizon Medical Center	Dickson	100%	133
Tristar Skyline Medical Center[2]	Nashville	100%	451
Tristar Southern Hills Medical Center	Nashville	100%	299
Tristar Stonecrest Medical Center[2]	Smyrna	100%	284
Tristar Summit Medical Center[2]	Hermitage	100%	472
Unicoi County Memorial Hospital	Erwin	100%	97
University Medical Center	Lebanon	100%	367
University of Tn Memorial Hospital[2]	Knoxville	100%	522
VA Middle Tennessee Healthcare System[2]	Nashville	100%	240
Vanderbilt University Hospital[2]	Nashville	100%	645
Volunteer Community Hospital	Martin	100%	46
Wellmont Bristol Regional Medical Center[2]	Bristol	100%	419
Wellmont Holston Valley Medical Center[2]	Kingsport	100%	407
Williamson Medical Center[2]	Franklin	100%	339
Memorial Healthcare System[2]	Chattanooga	99%	715
Saint Thomas Rutherford Hospital[2]	Murfreesboro	99%	599
Takoma Regional Hospital[2]	Greeneville	99%	81

Prophylactic Antibiotic Selection

Hospital Name	City	Rate	Cases
Baptist Memorial Hospital Union City	Union City	100%	108
Delta Medical Center	Memphis	100%	53
Dyersburg Regional Medical Center	Dyersburg	100%	43
Fort Loudoun Medical Center[2]	Lenoir City	100%	25
Fort Sanders Regional Medical Center[2]	Knoxville	100%	540
Franklin Woods Community Hospital[2]	Johnson City	100%	30
Gateway Medical Center	Clarksville	100%	461
Hardin Medical Center	Savannah	100%	33
Henry County Medical Center	Paris	100%	358
Indian Path Medical Center[2]	Kingsport	100%	231
Lakeway Regional Hospital	Morristown	100%	103
Livingston Regional Hospital	Livingston	100%	26
Maury Regional Hospital[2]	Columbia	100%	451
Memorial Healthcare System[2]	Chattanooga	100%	1012
Methodist Medical Center of Oak Ridge[2]	Oak Ridge	100%	483
Morristown Hamblen Hospital Association[2]	Morristown	100%	260
Mountain Home VA Medical Center	Mountain Home	100%	111
Northcrest Medical Center[2]	Springfield	100%	148
Parkridge Medical Center[2]	Chattanooga	100%	397
Parkwest Medical Center[2]	Knoxville	100%	761
Regional Hospital of Jackson	Jackson	100%	314
Saint Francis Bartlett Medical Center[2]	Bartlett	100%	269
Saint Francis Hospital[2]	Memphis	100%	733
Saint Thomas West Hospital[2]	Nashville	100%	566
Southern Tennessee Medical Center	Winchester	100%	155
Stones River Hosp & Dekalb Comm Hosp	Smithville	100%	36
Sycamore Shoals Hospital[2]	Elizabethton	100%	111
Takoma Regional Hospital[2]	Greeneville	100%	39
Tennova Healthcare-Jefferson Mem Hosp	Jefferson City	100%	37
Tristar Centennial Medical Center[2]	Nashville	100%	587
Tristar Hendersonville Medical Center	Hendersonville	100%	255
Tristar Horizon Medical Center	Dickson	100%	76
Tristar Southern Hills Medical Center	Nashville	100%	172
Tristar Stonecrest Medical Center[2]	Smyrna	100%	176
Tristar Summit Medical Center[2]	Hermitage	100%	265
Unicoi County Memorial Hospital	Erwin	100%	84
VA Middle Tennessee Healthcare System	Nashville	100%	135
Volunteer Community Hospital	Martin	100%	29
Cookeville Regional Medical Center	Cookeville	99%	810
Erlanger Medical Center[2]	Chattanooga	99%	329
Jackson - Madison County General Hospital[2]	Jackson	99%	1234
Johnson City Medical Center[2]	Johnson City	99%	405
Laughlin Memorial Hospital	Greeneville	99%	204
Leconte Medical Center[2]	Sevierville	99%	147
Memphis VA Medical Center	Memphis	99%	251
Methodist Healthcare Memphis Hospitals[2]	Memphis	99%	1114
Regional Medical Center at Memphis	Memphis	99%	148
Starr Regional Medical Center Athens	Athens	99%	82
Sumner Regional Medical Center	Gallatin	99%	317
Tennova Healthcare	Knoxville	99%	1826
Tristar Skyline Medical Center[2]	Nashville	99%	257
Vanderbilt University Hospital[2]	Nashville	99%	373
Wellmont Holston Valley Medical Center[2]	Kingsport	99%	411
Baptist Memorial Hospital[2]	Memphis	98%	659
Blount Memorial Hospital[2]	Maryville	98%	318
Lincoln Medical Center	Fayetteville	98%	58
River Park Hospital	Mc Minnville	98%	54
Saint Thomas Midtown Hospital[2]	Nashville	98%	497
Saint Thomas Rutherford Hospital[2]	Murfreesboro	98%	433
Skyridge Medical Center	Cleveland	98%	177
University Medical Center	Lebanon	98%	252
University of Tn Memorial Hospital[2]	Knoxville	98%	476
Wellmont Bristol Regional Medical Center[2]	Bristol	98%	304
Cumberland Medical Center[2]	Crossville	97%	175
Williamson Medical Center[2]	Franklin	97%	233
Highlands Medical Center[2]	Sparta	96%	84
Baptist Memorial Hospital Tipton	Covington	95%	42
Harton Regional Medical Center	Tullahoma	95%	161
Metro Nashville General Hospital[2]	Nashville	89%	104
Sweetwater Hospital Association	Sweetwater	89%	28

Prophylactic Antibiotic Selection (Outpatient)

Hospital Name	City	Rate	Cases
Baptist Memorial Hospital	Memphis	100%	1267
Fort Sanders Regional Medical Center	Knoxville	100%	636
Highlands Medical Center	Sparta	100%	40
Lakeway Regional Hospital	Morristown	100%	85
Leconte Medical Center	Sevierville	100%	84
Methodist Medical Center of Oak Ridge	Oak Ridge	100%	449
Parkridge Medical Center	Chattanooga	100%	686
Regional Hospital of Jackson	Jackson	100%	236
River Park Hospital	Mc Minnville	100%	41
Saint Thomas Hospital for Spinal Surgery	Nashville	100%	833
Sumner Regional Medical Center	Gallatin	100%	108
Tristar Hendersonville Medical Center	Hendersonville	100%	236
Tristar Horizon Medical Center	Dickson	100%	54
Tristar Stonecrest Medical Center	Smyrna	100%	227
Volunteer Community Hospital	Martin	100%	65
Blount Memorial Hospital	Maryville	99%	144
Cookeville Regional Medical Center	Cookeville	99%	659
Dyersburg Regional Medical Center	Dyersburg	99%	68
Gateway Medical Center	Clarksville	99%	248
Harton Regional Medical Center	Tullahoma	99%	289
Maury Regional Hospital	Columbia	99%	427
Parkwest Medical Center	Knoxville	99%	883
Saint Francis Hospital	Memphis	99%	474
Tristar Centennial Medical Center	Nashville	99%	790
Tristar Southern Hills Medical Center	Nashville	99%	156
University Medical Center	Lebanon	99%	202
Vanderbilt University Hospital	Nashville	99%	966
Wellmont Bristol Regional Medical Center	Bristol	99%	440
Baptist Memorial Hospital Union City	Union City	98%	62
Erlanger Medical Center	Chattanooga	98%	686
Franklin Woods Community Hospital	Johnson City	98%	323
Indian Path Medical Center	Kingsport	98%	254
Johnson City Medical Center	Johnson City	98%	618
Memorial Healthcare System	Chattanooga	98%	872
Methodist Healthcare Memphis Hospitals	Memphis	98%	841
Morristown Hamblen Hospital Association	Morristown	98%	171
Saint Francis Bartlett Medical Center	Bartlett	98%	178
Saint Thomas West Hospital	Nashville	98%	521
Skyridge Medical Center	Cleveland	98%	226
Southern Tennessee Medical Center	Winchester	98%	165
Takoma Regional Hospital	Greeneville	98%	45
Tristar Skyline Medical Center	Nashville	98%	342
Tristar Summit Medical Center	Hermitage	98%	387
University of Tn Memorial Hospital	Knoxville	98%	910
Wellmont Holston Valley Medical Center	Kingsport	98%	661
Henry County Medical Center	Paris	97%	185
Jackson - Madison County General Hospital	Jackson	97%	696
Livingston Regional Hospital	Livingston	97%	34
Northcrest Medical Center	Springfield	97%	102
Tennova Healthcare	Knoxville	97%	1209
Williamson Medical Center	Franklin	97%	250
Sycamore Shoals Hospital	Elizabethton	96%	48
Metro Nashville General Hospital	Nashville	95%	41
Saint Thomas Midtown Hospital	Nashville	95%	665
Starr Regional Medical Center Athens	Athens	94%	63
United Regional Medical Center	Manchester	94%	84
Regional Medical Center at Memphis	Memphis	93%	56
Tennova Healthcare-Jefferson Mem Hosp	Jefferson City	93%	55
Delta Medical Center	Memphis	92%	25

NOTE: Hospital profiles are in alphabetical order by state, then city, then hospital within the city; Rankings exclude hospitals with less than 25 cases except for patient surveys which excludes hospitals with less than 100 cases; (a) 100-299 cases; (1) The number of cases/patients is too few to report; (2) Data submitted were based on a sample of cases/patients; (3) Results are based on a shorter time period than required; (4) Data suppressed by CMS for one or more quarters; (5) Results are not available for this reporting period; (6) Fewer than 100 patients completed the HCAHPS survey; (7) No cases met the criteria for this measure; (8) The lower limit of the confidence interval cannot be calculated if the number of observed infections equals zero; (9) No data are available from the state/territory for this reporting period; (10) The scores shown reflect fewer than 50 completed surveys; (11) There were discrepancies in the data collection process; (12) This measure does not apply to this hospital for this reporting period; (13) Results cannot be calculated for this reporting period; (14) The results for this state are combined with nearby states to protect confidentiality; Please refer to the User's Guide for a full explanation of data.

Saint Thomas Rutherford Hospital	Murfreesboro	91%	518
Laughlin Memorial Hospital	Greeneville	90%	111
Tennova Healthcare-Lafollett Med Ctr	La Follette	85%	48
Cumberland Medical Center	Crossville	78%	119
Starr Regional Medical Center Etowah	Etowah	59%	29

Prophylactic Antibiotic Stopped

Hospital Name	City	Rate	Cases
Baptist Memorial Hospital Union City	Union City	100%	102
Franklin Woods Community Hospital[2]	Johnson City	100%	29
Highlands Medical Center[2]	Sparta	100%	84
Laughlin Memorial Hospital	Greeneville	100%	198
Morristown Hamblen Hospital Association[2]	Morristown	100%	260
Mountain Home VA Medical Center	Mountain Home	100%	109
Northcrest Medical Center[2]	Springfield	100%	145
Saint Francis Hospital[2]	Memphis	100%	708
Tristar Hendersonville Medical Center	Hendersonville	100%	236
Tristar Summit Medical Center[2]	Hermitage	100%	251
Unicoi County Memorial Hospital	Erwin	100%	84
Volunteer Community Hospital	Martin	100%	27
Wellmont Holston Valley Medical Center[2]	Kingsport	100%	407
Blount Memorial Hospital[2]	Maryville	99%	306
Fort Sanders Regional Medical Center[2]	Knoxville	99%	533
Henry County Medical Center	Paris	99%	337
Indian Path Medical Center[2]	Kingsport	99%	222
Leconte Medical Center[2]	Sevierville	99%	140
Maury Regional Hospital[2]	Columbia	99%	442
Memorial Healthcare System[2]	Chattanooga	99%	997
Methodist Healthcare Memphis Hospitals[2]	Memphis	99%	1088
Parkwest Medical Center[2]	Knoxville	99%	739
Regional Hospital of Jackson	Jackson	99%	305
Saint Thomas West Hospital[2]	Nashville	99%	556
Sycamore Shoals Hospital[2]	Elizabethton	99%	109
Tristar Centennial Medical Center[2]	Nashville	99%	560
Tristar Horizon Medical Center	Dickson	99%	70
Wellmont Bristol Regional Medical Center[2]	Bristol	99%	292
Baptist Memorial Hospital[2]	Memphis	98%	636
Baptist Memorial Hospital Tipton	Covington	98%	41
Dyersburg Regional Medical Center	Dyersburg	98%	42
Methodist Medical Center of Oak Ridge[2]	Oak Ridge	98%	459
Parkridge Medical Center[2]	Chattanooga	98%	379
River Park Hospital	Mc Minnville	98%	51
Saint Francis Bartlett Medical Center[2]	Bartlett	98%	260
Saint Thomas Midtown Hospital[2]	Nashville	98%	491
Sumner Regional Medical Center	Gallatin	98%	311
Tennova Healthcare	Knoxville	98%	1773
Tristar Skyline Medical Center[2]	Nashville	98%	239
Tristar Southern Hills Medical Center	Nashville	98%	169
University Medical Center	Lebanon	98%	237
University of Tn Memorial Hospital[2]	Knoxville	98%	441
VA Middle Tennessee Healthcare System	Nashville	98%	128
Vanderbilt University Hospital[2]	Nashville	98%	365
Erlanger Medical Center[2]	Chattanooga	97%	310
Gateway Medical Center	Clarksville	97%	440
Hardin Medical Center	Savannah	97%	33
Harton Regional Medical Center	Tullahoma	97%	134
Memphis VA Medical Center	Memphis	97%	244
Tennova Healthcare-Jefferson Mem Hosp	Jefferson City	97%	36
Tristar Stonecrest Medical Center[2]	Smyrna	97%	172
Fort Loudoun Medical Center[2]	Lenoir City	96%	25
Jackson - Madison County General Hospital[2]	Jackson	96%	1197
Johnson City Medical Center[2]	Johnson City	96%	388
Lakeway Regional Hospital	Morristown	96%	96
Southern Tennessee Medical Center	Winchester	96%	150
Williamson Medical Center[2]	Franklin	96%	231
Starr Regional Medical Center Athens	Athens	95%	80
Takoma Regional Hospital[2]	Greeneville	95%	37
Cumberland Medical Center[2]	Crossville	94%	172
Lincoln Medical Center	Fayetteville	94%	50
Metro Nashville General Hospital[2]	Nashville	94%	104
Skyridge Medical Center	Cleveland	94%	173
Cookeville Regional Medical Center	Cookeville	93%	766
Regional Medical Center at Memphis	Memphis	92%	145
Saint Thomas Rutherford Hospital[2]	Murfreesboro	92%	424
Stones River Hosp & Dekalb Comm Hosp	Smithville	85%	33
Delta Medical Center	Memphis	84%	49

Prophylactic Antibiotic Timing

Hospital Name	City	Rate	Cases
Baptist Memorial Hospital Tipton	Covington	100%	42
Baptist Memorial Hospital Union City	Union City	100%	108
Blount Memorial Hospital[2]	Maryville	100%	318
Dyersburg Regional Medical Center	Dyersburg	100%	43
Franklin Woods Community Hospital[2]	Johnson City	100%	30
Henry County Medical Center	Paris	100%	358
Indian Path Medical Center[2]	Kingsport	100%	231
Laughlin Memorial Hospital	Greeneville	100%	204
Livingston Regional Hospital	Livingston	100%	26
Methodist Medical Center of Oak Ridge[2]	Oak Ridge	100%	486
Morristown Hamblen Hospital Association[2]	Morristown	100%	260
Northcrest Medical Center[2]	Springfield	100%	148
Parkwest Medical Center[2]	Knoxville	100%	761
Regional Hospital of Jackson	Jackson	100%	314
Saint Francis Bartlett Medical Center[2]	Bartlett	100%	269
Saint Thomas West Hospital[2]	Nashville	100%	567
Southern Tennessee Medical Center	Winchester	100%	155
Starr Regional Medical Center Athens	Athens	100%	82
Stones River Hosp & Dekalb Comm Hosp	Smithville	100%	36
Sumner Regional Medical Center	Gallatin	100%	317
Tennova Healthcare	Knoxville	100%	1828
Tristar Centennial Medical Center[2]	Nashville	100%	587
Tristar Horizon Medical Center	Dickson	100%	76
Tristar Skyline Medical Center[2]	Nashville	100%	257
Unicoi County Memorial Hospital	Erwin	100%	84
University Medical Center	Lebanon	100%	252
Volunteer Community Hospital	Martin	100%	29
Wellmont Bristol Regional Medical Center[2]	Bristol	100%	304
Baptist Memorial Hospital[2]	Memphis	99%	660
Fort Sanders Regional Medical Center[2]	Knoxville	99%	541
Gateway Medical Center	Clarksville	99%	461
Harton Regional Medical Center	Tullahoma	99%	161
Highlands Medical Center[2]	Sparta	99%	84
Jackson - Madison County General Hospital[2]	Jackson	99%	1235
Leconte Medical Center[2]	Sevierville	99%	147
Maury Regional Hospital[2]	Columbia	99%	451
Methodist Healthcare Memphis Hospitals[2]	Memphis	99%	1115
Parkridge Medical Center[2]	Chattanooga	99%	397
Regional Medical Center at Memphis	Memphis	99%	145
Saint Francis Hospital[2]	Memphis	99%	733
Saint Thomas Midtown Hospital[2]	Nashville	99%	498
Sycamore Shoals Hospital[2]	Elizabethton	99%	111
Tristar Southern Hills Medical Center	Nashville	99%	172
Tristar Stonecrest Medical Center[2]	Smyrna	99%	176
Tristar Summit Medical Center[2]	Hermitage	99%	265
University of Tn Memorial Hospital[2]	Knoxville	99%	476
VA Middle Tennessee Healthcare System	Nashville	99%	135
Vanderbilt University Hospital[2]	Nashville	99%	373
Wellmont Holston Valley Medical Center[2]	Kingsport	99%	411
Cookeville Regional Medical Center	Cookeville	98%	812
Johnson City Medical Center[2]	Johnson City	98%	405
Memorial Healthcare System[2]	Chattanooga	98%	1014
Mountain Home VA Medical Center	Mountain Home	98%	111
Saint Thomas Rutherford Hospital[2]	Murfreesboro	98%	436
Skyridge Medical Center	Cleveland	98%	177
Williamson Medical Center[2]	Franklin	98%	233
Lakeway Regional Hospital	Morristown	97%	104
Lincoln Medical Center	Fayetteville	97%	58
Takoma Regional Hospital[2]	Greeneville	97%	39
Tennova Healthcare-Jefferson Mem Hosp	Jefferson City	97%	37
Tristar Hendersonville Medical Center	Hendersonville	97%	255
Delta Medical Center	Memphis	96%	53
Erlanger Medical Center[2]	Chattanooga	96%	329
Fort Loudoun Medical Center[2]	Lenoir City	96%	25
Metro Nashville General Hospital[2]	Nashville	96%	104
Memphis VA Medical Center	Memphis	94%	252
River Park Hospital	Mc Minnville	94%	54
Hardin Medical Center	Savannah	91%	33
Cumberland Medical Center[2]	Crossville	90%	175
Sweetwater Hospital Association	Sweetwater	82%	28

Prophylactic Antibiotic Timing (Outpatient)

Hospital Name	City	Rate	Cases
Baptist Memorial Hospital	Memphis	100%	1268
Baptist Memorial Hospital Union City	Union City	100%	62
Dyersburg Regional Medical Center	Dyersburg	100%	68
Lakeway Regional Hospital	Morristown	100%	85
Leconte Medical Center	Sevierville	100%	84
Livingston Regional Hospital	Livingston	100%	34
Parkridge Medical Center	Chattanooga	100%	684
Regional Hospital of Jackson	Jackson	100%	236
Saint Thomas Hospital for Spinal Surgery	Nashville	100%	834
Skyridge Medical Center	Cleveland	100%	221
Tennova Healthcare-Jefferson Mem Hosp	Jefferson City	100%	55
Tristar Centennial Medical Center	Nashville	100%	790
Tristar Horizon Medical Center	Dickson	100%	54
Tristar Stonecrest Medical Center	Smyrna	100%	216
Tristar Summit Medical Center	Hermitage	100%	388
Volunteer Community Hospital	Martin	100%	65
Williamson Medical Center	Franklin	100%	250
Cookeville Regional Medical Center	Cookeville	99%	660
Fort Sanders Regional Medical Center	Knoxville	99%	637
Franklin Woods Community Hospital	Johnson City	99%	325
Gateway Medical Center	Clarksville	99%	248
Harton Regional Medical Center	Tullahoma	99%	292
Laughlin Memorial Hospital	Greeneville	99%	111
Maury Regional Hospital	Columbia	99%	427
Memorial Healthcare System	Chattanooga	99%	855
Methodist Healthcare Memphis Hospitals	Memphis	99%	841
Methodist Medical Center of Oak Ridge	Oak Ridge	99%	450
Parkwest Medical Center	Knoxville	99%	877
Saint Francis Hospital	Memphis	99%	477
Southern Tennessee Medical Center	Winchester	99%	164
Tristar Skyline Medical Center	Nashville	99%	342
Tristar Southern Hills Medical Center	Nashville	99%	157
Wellmont Bristol Regional Medical Center	Bristol	99%	441
Wellmont Holston Valley Medical Center	Kingsport	99%	659
Erlanger Medical Center	Chattanooga	98%	690
Jackson - Madison County General Hospital	Jackson	98%	697
Northcrest Medical Center	Springfield	98%	101
Saint Francis Bartlett Medical Center	Bartlett	98%	179
Saint Thomas West Hospital	Nashville	98%	521
Tennova Healthcare-Lafollett Med Ctr	La Follette	98%	48
Tristar Hendersonville Medical Center	Hendersonville	98%	237
University of Tn Memorial Hospital	Knoxville	98%	906
Indian Path Medical Center	Kingsport	97%	229
Johnson City Medical Center	Johnson City	97%	621
Morristown Hamblen Hospital Association	Morristown	97%	172
Saint Thomas Rutherford Hospital	Murfreesboro	97%	524
Starr Regional Medical Center Athens	Athens	97%	65
Sumner Regional Medical Center	Gallatin	97%	111
Tennova Healthcare	Knoxville	97%	1189
Vanderbilt University Hospital	Nashville	97%	755
Highlands Medical Center	Sparta	95%	41
University Medical Center	Lebanon	95%	211
Blount Memorial Hospital	Maryville	94%	145
Henry County Medical Center	Paris	94%	194
Saint Thomas Midtown Hospital	Nashville	94%	670
Metro Nashville General Hospital	Nashville	93%	42
Regional Medical Center at Memphis	Memphis	93%	58
River Park Hospital	Mc Minnville	93%	44
Takoma Regional Hospital	Greeneville	93%	46
Sycamore Shoals Hospital	Elizabethton	92%	52
Cumberland Medical Center	Crossville	90%	126
United Regional Medical Center	Manchester	87%	84
Delta Medical Center	Memphis	85%	26

Urinary Catheter Removal

Hospital Name	City	Rate	Cases
Baptist Memorial Hospital Union City	Union City	100%	70
Dyersburg Regional Medical Center	Dyersburg	100%	44
Fort Sanders Regional Medical Center[2]	Knoxville	100%	426
Henry County Medical Center	Paris	100%	70
Lakeway Regional Hospital	Morristown	100%	102
Laughlin Memorial Hospital	Greeneville	100%	211
Lincoln Medical Center	Fayetteville	100%	33
Methodist Healthcare Memphis Hospitals[2]	Memphis	100%	635
Morristown Hamblen Hospital Association[2]	Morristown	100%	256
Northcrest Medical Center[2]	Springfield	100%	184
Regional Hospital of Jackson	Jackson	100%	367
Saint Francis Bartlett Medical Center[2]	Bartlett	100%	96
Saint Francis Hospital[2]	Memphis	100%	457
Stones River Hosp & Dekalb Comm Hosp	Smithville	100%	38
Sumner Regional Medical Center	Gallatin	100%	282
Tristar Summit Medical Center[2]	Hermitage	100%	280
Baptist Memorial Hospital[2]	Memphis	99%	355
Blount Memorial Hospital[2]	Maryville	99%	287
Harton Regional Medical Center	Tullahoma	99%	115
Maury Regional Hospital[2]	Columbia	99%	387
Methodist Medical Center of Oak Ridge[2]	Oak Ridge	99%	302
Saint Thomas Midtown Hospital[2]	Nashville	99%	418
Tristar Centennial Medical Center[2]	Nashville	99%	513
Tristar Hendersonville Medical Center	Hendersonville	99%	251
Fort Loudoun Medical Center[2]	Lenoir City	98%	44
Mountain Home VA Medical Center[2]	Mountain Home	98%	135
Parkridge Medical Center[2]	Chattanooga	98%	231
Parkwest Medical Center[2]	Knoxville	98%	554
Regional Medical Center at Memphis	Memphis	98%	176
Roane Medical Center[2]	Harriman	98%	40
Saint Thomas West Hospital[2]	Nashville	98%	510
Southern Tennessee Medical Center	Winchester	98%	179
Takoma Regional Hospital[2]	Greeneville	98%	51
Tristar Stonecrest Medical Center[2]	Smyrna	98%	170
Gateway Medical Center	Clarksville	98%	442
Indian Path Medical Center[2]	Kingsport	97%	101
Tristar Horizon Medical Center	Dickson	97%	79
Tristar Skyline Medical Center[2]	Nashville	97%	316
Tristar Southern Hills Medical Center	Nashville	97%	198
Wellmont Bristol Regional Medical Center[2]	Bristol	97%	250
Franklin Woods Community Hospital[2]	Johnson City	96%	57
Johnson City Medical Center[2]	Johnson City	96%	401
Skyridge Medical Center	Cleveland	96%	134
Sycamore Shoals Hospital[2]	Elizabethton	96%	73
Tennova Healthcare	Knoxville	96%	1011
Vanderbilt University Hospital[2]	Nashville	96%	388
Jackson - Madison County General Hospital[2]	Jackson	95%	1247
University of Tn Memorial Hospital[2]	Knoxville	95%	429
Wellmont Holston Valley Medical Center[2]	Kingsport	95%	237
Leconte Medical Center[2]	Sevierville	94%	67
Tennova Healthcare-Jefferson Mem Hosp	Jefferson City	94%	36
University Medical Center	Lebanon	94%	234
Williamson Medical Center[2]	Franklin	94%	246
Cookeville Regional Medical Center	Cookeville	93%	828

NOTE: Hospital profiles are in alphabetical order by state, then city, then hospital within the city; Rankings exclude hospitals with less than 25 cases except for patient surveys which excludes hospitals with less than 100 cases; (a) 100-299 cases; (1) The number of cases/patients is too few to report; (2) Data submitted were based on a sample of cases/patients; (3) Results are based on a shorter time period than required; (4) Data suppressed by CMS for one or more quarters; (5) Results are not available for this reporting period; (6) Fewer than 100 patients completed the HCAHPS survey; (7) No cases met the criteria for this measure; (8) The lower limit of the confidence interval cannot be calculated if the number of observed infections equals zero; (9) No data are available from the state/territory for this reporting period; (10) The scores shown reflect fewer than 50 completed surveys; (11) There were discrepancies in the data collection process; (12) This measure does not apply to this hospital for this reporting period; (13) Results cannot be calculated for this reporting period; (14) The results for this state are combined with nearby states to protect confidentiality; Please refer to the User's Guide for a full explanation of data.

Erlanger Medical Center[2]	Chattanooga	93%	211
VA Middle Tennessee Healthcare System[2]	Nashville	93%	85
Starr Regional Medical Center Etowah[3]	Etowah	92%	25
Memorial Healthcare System[2]	Chattanooga	91%	833
Memphis VA Medical Center[2]	Memphis	91%	155
Metro Nashville General Hospital[2]	Nashville	91%	109
Saint Thomas Rutherford Hospital[2]	Murfreesboro	90%	449
Starr Regional Medical Center Athens	Athens	90%	62
River Park Hospital	Mc Minnville	88%	69
Hardin Medical Center	Savannah	87%	31
Cumberland Medical Center[2]	Crossville	83%	192
Highlands Medical Center[2]	Sparta	81%	36
Unicoi County Memorial Hospital	Erwin	80%	88

Survey of Patients' Hospital Experiences

Area Around Room 'Always' Quiet at Night

Hospital Name	City	Rate	Cases
Saint Thomas Hospital for Spinal Surgery	Nashville	82%	300+
Delta Medical Center	Memphis	77%	300+
McNairy Regional Hospital	Selmer	77%	(a)
Franklin Woods Community Hospital	Johnson City	76%	300+
United Regional Medical Center	Manchester	76%	(a)
Henry County Medical Center	Paris	73%	300+
Copper Basin Medical Center	Copperhill	72%	(a)
Hardin Medical Center	Savannah	72%	300+
Wellmont Hawkins County Memorial Hospital	Rogersville	72%	(a)
Jackson - Madison County General Hospital	Jackson	71%	300+
Regional Hospital of Jackson	Jackson	71%	300+
Riverview Regional Medical Center	Carthage	71%	(a)
Stones River Hosp & Dekalb Comm Hosp	Smithville	71%	(a)
Tristar Stonecrest Medical Center	Smyrna	71%	300+
Dyersburg Regional Medical Center	Dyersburg	70%	300+
Fort Loudoun Medical Center	Lenoir City	70%	300+
Henderson County Community Hospital	Lexington	70%	(a)
Memorial Healthcare System	Chattanooga	70%	300+
Methodist Healthcare Memphis Hospitals	Memphis	70%	300+
Parkwest Medical Center	Knoxville	70%	300+
Baptist Memorial Hospital Tipton	Covington	69%	(a)
Baptist Memorial Hospital Union City	Union City	69%	300+
Grandview Medical Center	Jasper	69%	(a)
Saint Francis Bartlett Medical Center	Bartlett	69%	300+
Starr Regional Medical Center Etowah	Etowah	69%	(a)
Sweetwater Hospital Association	Sweetwater	69%	300+
Heritage Medical Center	Shelbyville	68%	300+
Highlands Medical Center	Sparta	68%	(a)
Roane Medical Center	Harriman	68%	300+
Starr Regional Medical Center Athens	Athens	68%	300+
Tristar Southern Hills Medical Center	Nashville	68%	300+
Hillside Hospital	Pulaski	67%	(a)
Jamestown Regional Medical Center	Jamestown	67%	300+
McKenzie Regional Hospital	Mc Kenzie	67%	(a)
Methodist Medical Center of Oak Ridge	Oak Ridge	67%	300+
Saint Francis Hospital	Memphis	67%	300+
Sycamore Shoals Hospital	Elizabethton	67%	300+
Tristar Centennial Medical Center	Nashville	67%	300+
Tristar Horizon Medical Center	Dickson	67%	300+
University of Tn Memorial Hospital	Knoxville	67%	300+
Jellico Community Hospital[11]	Jellico	66%	(a)
Parkridge Medical Center	Chattanooga	66%	300+
Rhea Medical Center	Dayton	66%	(a)
River Park Hospital	Mc Minnville	66%	300+
Macon County General Hospital	Lafayette	65%	(a)
Tristar Skyline Medical Center	Nashville	65%	300+
Williamson Medical Center	Franklin	65%	300+
Baptist Memorial Hospital	Memphis	64%	300+
Laughlin Memorial Hospital	Greeneville	64%	300+
Lincoln Medical Center	Fayetteville	64%	(a)
Maury Regional Hospital	Columbia	64%	300+
Regional Medical Center at Memphis	Memphis	64%	300+
Skyridge Medical Center	Cleveland	64%	300+
Sumner Regional Medical Center	Gallatin	64%	300+
Tennova Healthcare	Knoxville	64%	300+
Tennova Healthcare-Newport Med Ctr	Newport	64%	300+
Tristar Summit Medical Center	Hermitage	64%	300+
Wellmont Bristol Regional Medical Center	Bristol	64%	300+
Fort Sanders Regional Medical Center	Knoxville	63%	300+
Metro Nashville General Hospital	Nashville	63%	300+
Saint Thomas Rutherford Hospital	Murfreesboro	63%	300+
Wayne Medical Center	Waynesboro	63%	(a)
Cookeville Regional Medical Center	Cookeville	62%	300+
Indian Path Medical Center	Kingsport	62%	300+
Lakeway Regional Hospital	Morristown	62%	300+
Leconte Medical Center	Sevierville	62%	300+
Southern Tennessee Medical Center	Winchester	62%	300+
Takoma Regional Hospital[11]	Greeneville	62%	300+
Tennova Healthcare-Jefferson Mem Hosp	Jefferson City	62%	300+
Unicoi County Memorial Hospital	Erwin	62%	(a)
Vanderbilt University Hospital	Nashville	62%	300+
Crockett Hospital	Lawrenceburg	61%	300+
Gateway Medical Center	Clarksville	61%	300+
Livingston Regional Hospital	Livingston	61%	300+
Saint Thomas West Hospital	Nashville	61%	300+
Morristown Hamblen Hospital Association	Morristown	60%	300+
Saint Thomas Midtown Hospital	Nashville	60%	300+
University Medical Center	Lebanon	60%	300+
Wellmont Holston Valley Medical Center	Kingsport	59%	300+
Claiborne County Hospital	Tazewell	58%	(a)
Cumberland Medical Center	Crossville	58%	300+
Harton Regional Medical Center	Tullahoma	58%	300+
Tristar Hendersonville Medical Center	Hendersonville	58%	300+
Erlanger Medical Center[11]	Chattanooga	57%	300+
Volunteer Community Hospital	Martin	56%	300+
Johnson City Medical Center	Johnson City	53%	300+
Tennova Healthcare-Lafollett Med Ctr	La Follette	52%	(a)
Blount Memorial Hospital	Maryville	51%	300+
Northcrest Medical Center	Springfield	51%	300+

Doctors 'Always' Communicated Well

Hospital Name	City	Rate	Cases
Copper Basin Medical Center	Copperhill	91%	(a)
Livingston Regional Hospital	Livingston	90%	300+
Jamestown Regional Medical Center	Jamestown	89%	300+
Jellico Community Hospital[11]	Jellico	89%	(a)
McNairy Regional Hospital	Selmer	89%	(a)
Stones River Hosp & Dekalb Comm Hosp	Smithville	89%	(a)
United Regional Medical Center	Manchester	89%	(a)
Hardin Medical Center	Savannah	88%	300+
Saint Thomas Hospital for Spinal Surgery	Nashville	88%	300+
Sweetwater Hospital Association	Sweetwater	88%	300+
Henderson County Community Hospital	Lexington	87%	(a)
Roane Medical Center	Harriman	87%	300+
Sycamore Shoals Hospital	Elizabethton	87%	300+
Wayne Medical Center	Waynesboro	87%	(a)
Wellmont Hawkins County Memorial Hospital	Rogersville	87%	(a)
Baptist Memorial Hospital Union City	Union City	86%	300+
Riverview Regional Medical Center	Carthage	86%	(a)
Starr Regional Medical Center Etowah	Etowah	86%	(a)
Williamson Medical Center	Franklin	86%	300+
Fort Loudoun Medical Center	Lenoir City	85%	300+
Highlands Medical Center	Sparta	85%	(a)
Laughlin Memorial Hospital	Greeneville	85%	300+
Saint Thomas Midtown Hospital	Nashville	85%	300+
Saint Thomas Rutherford Hospital	Murfreesboro	85%	300+
Volunteer Community Hospital	Martin	85%	300+
Baptist Memorial Hospital Tipton	Covington	84%	(a)
Claiborne County Hospital	Tazewell	84%	(a)
Hillside Hospital	Pulaski	84%	(a)
Maury Regional Hospital	Columbia	84%	300+
Memorial Healthcare System	Chattanooga	84%	300+
Parkwest Medical Center	Knoxville	84%	300+
Saint Thomas West Hospital	Nashville	84%	300+
Skyridge Medical Center	Cleveland	84%	300+
Starr Regional Medical Center Athens	Athens	84%	300+
Tristar Centennial Medical Center	Nashville	84%	300+
Unicoi County Memorial Hospital	Erwin	84%	(a)
Fort Sanders Regional Medical Center	Knoxville	83%	300+
Grandview Medical Center	Jasper	83%	(a)
Henry County Medical Center	Paris	83%	300+
Macon County General Hospital	Lafayette	83%	(a)
Methodist Medical Center of Oak Ridge	Oak Ridge	83%	300+
Saint Francis Hospital	Memphis	83%	300+
Vanderbilt University Hospital	Nashville	83%	300+
Wellmont Holston Valley Medical Center	Kingsport	83%	300+
Cookeville Regional Medical Center	Cookeville	82%	300+
Heritage Medical Center	Shelbyville	82%	300+
Indian Path Medical Center	Kingsport	82%	300+
Lakeway Regional Hospital	Morristown	82%	300+
Lincoln Medical Center	Fayetteville	82%	(a)
Metro Nashville General Hospital	Nashville	82%	300+
Parkridge Medical Center	Chattanooga	82%	300+
Regional Hospital of Jackson	Jackson	82%	300+
Southern Tennessee Medical Center	Winchester	82%	300+
University Medical Center	Lebanon	82%	300+
University of Tn Memorial Hospital	Knoxville	82%	300+
Wellmont Bristol Regional Medical Center	Bristol	82%	300+
Dyersburg Regional Medical Center	Dyersburg	81%	300+
Franklin Woods Community Hospital	Johnson City	81%	300+
Leconte Medical Center	Sevierville	81%	300+
McKenzie Regional Hospital	Mc Kenzie	81%	(a)
Methodist Healthcare Memphis Hospitals	Memphis	81%	300+
Morristown Hamblen Hospital Association	Morristown	81%	300+
Rhea Medical Center	Dayton	81%	(a)
Saint Francis Bartlett Medical Center	Bartlett	81%	300+
Tennova Healthcare	Knoxville	81%	300+
Tennova Healthcare-Jefferson Mem Hosp	Jefferson City	81%	300+
Tristar Horizon Medical Center	Dickson	81%	300+
Tristar Stonecrest Medical Center	Smyrna	81%	300+
Gateway Medical Center	Clarksville	80%	300+
Jackson - Madison County General Hospital	Jackson	80%	300+
Northcrest Medical Center	Springfield	80%	300+
Tristar Southern Hills Medical Center	Nashville	80%	300+
Blount Memorial Hospital	Maryville	79%	300+
Crockett Hospital	Lawrenceburg	79%	300+
Cumberland Medical Center	Crossville	79%	300+
Erlanger Medical Center[11]	Chattanooga	79%	300+
Harton Regional Medical Center	Tullahoma	79%	300+
Sumner Regional Medical Center	Gallatin	79%	300+
Tristar Skyline Medical Center	Nashville	79%	300+
Tristar Summit Medical Center	Hermitage	79%	300+
Baptist Memorial Hospital	Memphis	78%	300+
Regional Medical Center at Memphis	Memphis	78%	300+
Takoma Regional Hospital[11]	Greeneville	78%	300+
Tennova Healthcare-Newport Med Ctr	Newport	78%	300+
Johnson City Medical Center	Johnson City	77%	300+
River Park Hospital	Mc Minnville	77%	300+
Tristar Hendersonville Medical Center	Hendersonville	77%	300+
Tennova Healthcare-Lafollett Med Ctr	La Follette	76%	(a)
Delta Medical Center	Memphis	75%	300+

Home Recovery Information Given

Hospital Name	City	Rate	Cases
United Regional Medical Center	Manchester	98%	(a)
Jellico Community Hospital[11]	Jellico	90%	(a)
Baptist Memorial Hospital Union City	Union City	89%	300+
Cookeville Regional Medical Center	Cookeville	88%	300+
Fort Loudoun Medical Center	Lenoir City	88%	300+
Fort Sanders Regional Medical Center	Knoxville	88%	300+
Hardin Medical Center	Savannah	88%	300+
Memorial Healthcare System	Chattanooga	88%	300+
Parkwest Medical Center	Knoxville	88%	300+
Saint Thomas Hospital for Spinal Surgery	Nashville	88%	300+
Tristar Centennial Medical Center	Nashville	88%	300+
Vanderbilt University Hospital	Nashville	88%	300+
Copper Basin Medical Center	Copperhill	87%	(a)
Franklin Woods Community Hospital	Johnson City	87%	300+
Henderson County Community Hospital	Lexington	87%	(a)
Laughlin Memorial Hospital	Greeneville	87%	300+
McKenzie Regional Hospital	Mc Kenzie	87%	(a)
Methodist Medical Center of Oak Ridge	Oak Ridge	87%	300+
Morristown Hamblen Hospital Association	Morristown	87%	300+
Saint Thomas Rutherford Hospital	Murfreesboro	87%	300+
Starr Regional Medical Center Etowah	Etowah	87%	(a)
Takoma Regional Hospital[11]	Greeneville	87%	300+
Tristar Horizon Medical Center	Dickson	87%	300+
Tristar Stonecrest Medical Center	Smyrna	87%	300+
Tristar Summit Medical Center	Hermitage	87%	300+
University of Tn Memorial Hospital	Knoxville	87%	300+
Volunteer Community Hospital	Martin	87%	300+
Wellmont Hawkins County Memorial Hospital	Rogersville	87%	(a)
Dyersburg Regional Medical Center	Dyersburg	86%	300+
Indian Path Medical Center	Kingsport	86%	300+
Leconte Medical Center	Sevierville	86%	300+
Lincoln Medical Center	Fayetteville	86%	(a)
Methodist Healthcare Memphis Hospitals	Memphis	86%	300+
Parkridge Medical Center	Chattanooga	86%	300+
Roane Medical Center	Harriman	86%	300+
Saint Thomas West Hospital	Nashville	86%	300+
Southern Tennessee Medical Center	Winchester	86%	300+
Starr Regional Medical Center Athens	Athens	86%	300+
Sycamore Shoals Hospital	Elizabethton	86%	300+
Tristar Skyline Medical Center	Nashville	86%	300+
Henry County Medical Center	Paris	85%	300+
Heritage Medical Center	Shelbyville	85%	300+
Hillside Hospital	Pulaski	85%	(a)
Johnson City Medical Center	Johnson City	85%	300+
McNairy Regional Hospital	Selmer	85%	(a)
Metro Nashville General Hospital	Nashville	85%	300+
Regional Medical Center at Memphis	Memphis	85%	300+
Rhea Medical Center	Dayton	85%	(a)
Saint Francis Bartlett Medical Center	Bartlett	85%	300+
Skyridge Medical Center	Cleveland	85%	300+
Stones River Hosp & Dekalb Comm Hosp	Smithville	85%	(a)
Tristar Hendersonville Medical Center	Hendersonville	85%	300+
Claiborne County Hospital	Tazewell	84%	(a)
Crockett Hospital	Lawrenceburg	84%	300+
Lakeway Regional Hospital	Morristown	84%	300+
Macon County General Hospital	Lafayette	84%	(a)
Northcrest Medical Center	Springfield	84%	300+
Saint Thomas Midtown Hospital	Nashville	84%	300+
Sumner Regional Medical Center	Gallatin	84%	300+
Sweetwater Hospital Association	Sweetwater	84%	300+
Tristar Southern Hills Medical Center	Nashville	84%	300+
Wayne Medical Center	Waynesboro	84%	(a)
Blount Memorial Hospital	Maryville	83%	300+
Cumberland Medical Center	Crossville	83%	300+
Erlanger Medical Center[11]	Chattanooga	83%	300+
Highlands Medical Center	Sparta	83%	(a)
Maury Regional Hospital	Columbia	83%	300+
Regional Hospital of Jackson	Jackson	83%	300+
Riverview Regional Medical Center	Carthage	83%	(a)
Wellmont Bristol Regional Medical Center	Bristol	83%	300+

NOTE: Hospital profiles are in alphabetical order by state, then city, then hospital within the city; Rankings exclude hospitals with less than 25 cases except for patient surveys which excludes hospitals with less than 100 cases; (a) 100-299 cases; (1) The number of cases/patients is too few to report; (2) Data submitted were based on a sample of cases/patients; (3) Results are based on a shorter time period than required; (4) Data suppressed by CMS for one or more quarters; (5) Results are not available for this reporting period; (6) Fewer than 100 patients completed the HCAHPS survey; (7) No cases met the criteria for this measure; (8) The lower limit of the confidence interval cannot be calculated if the number of observed infections equals zero; (9) No data are available from the state/territory for this reporting period; (10) The scores shown reflect fewer than 50 completed surveys; (11) There were discrepancies in the data collection process; (12) This measure does not apply to this hospital for this reporting period; (13) Results cannot be calculated for this reporting period; (14) The results for this state are combined with nearby states to protect confidentiality; Please refer to the User's Guide for a full explanation of data.

Wellmont Holston Valley Medical Center	Kingsport	83%	300+
Baptist Memorial Hospital Tipton	Covington	82%	(a)
Gateway Medical Center	Clarksville	82%	300+
Livingston Regional Hospital	Livingston	82%	300+
River Park Hospital	Mc Minnville	82%	300+
Tennova Healthcare	Knoxville	82%	300+
Tennova Healthcare-Jefferson Mem Hosp	Jefferson City	82%	300+
Tennova Healthcare-Lafollett Med Ctr	La Follette	82%	(a)
University Medical Center	Lebanon	82%	300+
Williamson Medical Center	Franklin	82%	300+
Baptist Memorial Hospital	Memphis	81%	300+
Delta Medical Center	Memphis	81%	300+
Grandview Medical Center	Jasper	81%	(a)
Jackson - Madison County General Hospital	Jackson	81%	300+
Jamestown Regional Medical Center	Jamestown	81%	300+
Saint Francis Hospital	Memphis	81%	300+
Unicoi County Memorial Hospital	Erwin	81%	(a)
Harton Regional Medical Center	Tullahoma	80%	300+
Tennova Healthcare-Newport Med Ctr	Newport	79%	300+

Hospital Given 9 or 10 on 10 Point Scale

Hospital Name	City	Rate	Cases
Saint Thomas Hospital for Spinal Surgery	Nashville	87%	300+
University of Tn Memorial Hospital	Knoxville	81%	300+
Franklin Woods Community Hospital	Johnson City	80%	300+
Memorial Healthcare System	Chattanooga	80%	300+
Parkwest Medical Center	Knoxville	79%	300+
Vanderbilt University Hospital	Nashville	79%	300+
Copper Basin Medical Center	Copperhill	78%	(a)
Jellico Community Hospital[11]	Jellico	78%	(a)
Wellmont Hawkins County Memorial Hospital	Rogersville	78%	(a)
Williamson Medical Center	Franklin	78%	300+
Baptist Memorial Hospital Union City	Union City	77%	300+
Fort Sanders Regional Medical Center	Knoxville	77%	300+
Sycamore Shoals Hospital	Elizabethton	77%	300+
Laughlin Memorial Hospital	Greeneville	76%	300+
Tristar Centennial Medical Center	Nashville	76%	300+
Macon County General Hospital	Lafayette	75%	(a)
Maury Regional Hospital	Columbia	75%	300+
Saint Thomas West Hospital	Nashville	75%	300+
Cookeville Regional Medical Center	Cookeville	74%	300+
Hardin Medical Center	Savannah	74%	300+
Henderson County Community Hospital	Lexington	74%	(a)
Baptist Memorial Hospital	Memphis	73%	300+
Indian Path Medical Center	Kingsport	73%	300+
Jackson - Madison County General Hospital	Jackson	73%	300+
Leconte Medical Center	Sevierville	73%	300+
Methodist Healthcare Memphis Hospitals	Memphis	73%	300+
Methodist Medical Center of Oak Ridge	Oak Ridge	73%	300+
Sweetwater Hospital Association	Sweetwater	73%	300+
United Regional Medical Center	Manchester	73%	(a)
Parkridge Medical Center	Chattanooga	72%	300+
Regional Hospital of Jackson	Jackson	72%	300+
Saint Thomas Rutherford Hospital	Murfreesboro	72%	300+
Stones River Hosp & Dekalb Comm Hosp	Smithville	72%	(a)
Tristar Summit Medical Center	Hermitage	72%	300+
Wellmont Bristol Regional Medical Center	Bristol	72%	300+
Wellmont Holston Valley Medical Center	Kingsport	72%	300+
Highlands Medical Center	Sparta	71%	(a)
Riverview Regional Medical Center	Carthage	71%	(a)
Saint Thomas Midtown Hospital	Nashville	71%	300+
Takoma Regional Hospital[11]	Greeneville	71%	300+
Tristar Horizon Medical Center	Dickson	71%	300+
Tristar Stonecrest Medical Center	Smyrna	71%	300+
Henry County Medical Center	Paris	70%	300+
Rhea Medical Center	Dayton	70%	(a)
Fort Loudoun Medical Center	Lenoir City	69%	300+
Grandview Medical Center	Jasper	69%	(a)
McKenzie Regional Hospital	Mc Kenzie	69%	(a)
Saint Francis Hospital	Memphis	69%	300+
Volunteer Community Hospital	Martin	69%	300+
McNairy Regional Hospital	Selmer	68%	(a)
Metro Nashville General Hospital	Nashville	68%	300+
Saint Francis Bartlett Medical Center	Bartlett	68%	300+
Sumner Regional Medical Center	Gallatin	68%	300+
Tristar Southern Hills Medical Center	Nashville	68%	300+
Wayne Medical Center	Waynesboro	68%	(a)
Dyersburg Regional Medical Center	Dyersburg	67%	300+
Erlanger Medical Center[11]	Chattanooga	67%	300+
Heritage Medical Center	Shelbyville	67%	300+
Morristown Hamblen Hospital Association	Morristown	67%	300+
Northcrest Medical Center	Springfield	67%	300+
Tennova Healthcare-Jefferson Mem Hosp	Jefferson City	67%	300+
Tristar Skyline Medical Center	Nashville	67%	300+
Regional Medical Center at Memphis	Memphis	66%	300+
Starr Regional Medical Center Athens	Athens	66%	300+
Tennova Healthcare	Knoxville	66%	300+
Johnson City Medical Center	Johnson City	65%	300+
Roane Medical Center	Harriman	65%	300+
Starr Regional Medical Center Etowah	Etowah	65%	(a)
Hillside Hospital	Pulaski	64%	(a)
Livingston Regional Hospital	Livingston	64%	300+
Skyridge Medical Center	Cleveland	64%	300+
Southern Tennessee Medical Center	Winchester	64%	300+
Tristar Hendersonville Medical Center	Hendersonville	64%	300+
River Park Hospital	Mc Minnville	63%	300+
Unicoi County Memorial Hospital	Erwin	63%	(a)
Baptist Memorial Hospital Tipton	Covington	62%	(a)
Crockett Hospital	Lawrenceburg	62%	300+
Jamestown Regional Medical Center	Jamestown	62%	300+
Tennova Healthcare-Newport Med Ctr	Newport	62%	300+
Blount Memorial Hospital	Maryville	61%	300+
Cumberland Medical Center	Crossville	61%	300+
Lakeway Regional Hospital	Morristown	61%	300+
Gateway Medical Center	Clarksville	60%	300+
Lincoln Medical Center	Fayetteville	60%	(a)
Delta Medical Center	Memphis	59%	300+
Claiborne County Hospital	Tazewell	57%	(a)
Harton Regional Medical Center	Tullahoma	56%	300+
University Medical Center	Lebanon	52%	300+
Tennova Healthcare-Lafollett Med Ctr	La Follette	51%	(a)

Meds 'Always' Explained Before Given

Hospital Name	City	Rate	Cases
Henderson County Community Hospital	Lexington	78%	(a)
Saint Thomas Hospital for Spinal Surgery	Nashville	78%	300+
Baptist Memorial Hospital Tipton	Covington	76%	(a)
Copper Basin Medical Center	Copperhill	75%	(a)
Wellmont Hawkins County Memorial Hospital	Rogersville	74%	(a)
McNairy Regional Hospital	Selmer	73%	(a)
Sweetwater Hospital Association	Sweetwater	72%	300+
Fort Loudoun Medical Center	Lenoir City	70%	300+
Jellico Community Hospital[11]	Jellico	70%	(a)
Saint Thomas Rutherford Hospital	Murfreesboro	70%	300+
Baptist Memorial Hospital Union City	Union City	69%	300+
Fort Sanders Regional Medical Center	Knoxville	69%	300+
Hardin Medical Center	Savannah	69%	300+
Morristown Hamblen Hospital Association	Morristown	69%	300+
Riverview Regional Medical Center	Carthage	69%	(a)
Saint Thomas Midtown Hospital	Nashville	69%	300+
Laughlin Memorial Hospital	Greeneville	68%	300+
Maury Regional Hospital	Columbia	68%	300+
Saint Thomas West Hospital	Nashville	68%	300+
Unicoi County Memorial Hospital	Erwin	68%	(a)
Wayne Medical Center	Waynesboro	68%	(a)
Dyersburg Regional Medical Center	Dyersburg	67%	300+
Memorial Healthcare System	Chattanooga	67%	300+
Regional Hospital of Jackson	Jackson	67%	300+
Sycamore Shoals Hospital	Elizabethton	67%	300+
University of Tn Memorial Hospital	Knoxville	67%	300+
Cookeville Regional Medical Center	Cookeville	66%	300+
Parkwest Medical Center	Knoxville	66%	300+
Roane Medical Center	Harriman	66%	300+
Franklin Woods Community Hospital	Johnson City	65%	300+
Heritage Medical Center	Shelbyville	65%	300+
Leconte Medical Center	Sevierville	65%	300+
Macon County General Hospital	Lafayette	65%	(a)
McKenzie Regional Hospital	Mc Kenzie	65%	(a)
Methodist Healthcare Memphis Hospitals	Memphis	65%	300+
Methodist Medical Center of Oak Ridge	Oak Ridge	65%	300+
Starr Regional Medical Center Etowah	Etowah	65%	(a)
Gateway Medical Center	Clarksville	64%	300+
Henry County Medical Center	Paris	64%	300+
Livingston Regional Hospital	Livingston	64%	300+
Regional Medical Center at Memphis	Memphis	64%	300+
Skyridge Medical Center	Cleveland	64%	300+
Stones River Hosp & Dekalb Comm Hosp	Smithville	64%	(a)
Tristar Horizon Medical Center	Dickson	64%	300+
Tristar Summit Medical Center	Hermitage	64%	300+
United Regional Medical Center	Manchester	64%	(a)
Vanderbilt University Hospital	Nashville	64%	300+
Grandview Medical Center	Jasper	63%	(a)
Indian Path Medical Center	Kingsport	63%	300+
Jackson - Madison County General Hospital	Jackson	63%	300+
Lincoln Medical Center	Fayetteville	63%	(a)
Metro Nashville General Hospital	Nashville	63%	300+
Northcrest Medical Center	Springfield	63%	300+
Parkridge Medical Center	Chattanooga	63%	300+
Sumner Regional Medical Center	Gallatin	63%	300+
Tristar Centennial Medical Center	Nashville	63%	300+
Volunteer Community Hospital	Martin	63%	300+
Wellmont Holston Valley Medical Center	Kingsport	63%	300+
Highlands Medical Center	Sparta	62%	(a)
Hillside Hospital	Pulaski	62%	(a)
Tristar Skyline Medical Center	Nashville	62%	300+
Tristar Stonecrest Medical Center	Smyrna	62%	300+
Williamson Medical Center	Franklin	62%	300+
Blount Memorial Hospital	Maryville	61%	300+
Jamestown Regional Medical Center	Jamestown	61%	300+
Lakeway Regional Hospital	Morristown	61%	300+
Rhea Medical Center	Dayton	61%	(a)
Saint Francis Bartlett Medical Center	Bartlett	61%	300+
Southern Tennessee Medical Center	Winchester	61%	300+
Takoma Regional Hospital[11]	Greeneville	61%	300+
Tennova Healthcare	Knoxville	61%	300+
Tristar Southern Hills Medical Center	Nashville	61%	300+
Wellmont Bristol Regional Medical Center	Bristol	61%	300+
Crockett Hospital	Lawrenceburg	60%	300+
Johnson City Medical Center	Johnson City	60%	300+
Starr Regional Medical Center Athens	Athens	60%	300+
Tennova Healthcare-Jefferson Mem Hosp	Jefferson City	60%	300+
Erlanger Medical Center[11]	Chattanooga	59%	300+
River Park Hospital	Mc Minnville	59%	300+
Saint Francis Hospital	Memphis	59%	300+
Tennova Healthcare-Lafollett Med Ctr	La Follette	59%	(a)
Tennova Healthcare-Newport Med Ctr	Newport	59%	300+
Baptist Memorial Hospital	Memphis	58%	300+
Claiborne County Hospital	Tazewell	58%	(a)
Cumberland Medical Center	Crossville	58%	300+
Tristar Hendersonville Medical Center	Hendersonville	57%	300+
University Medical Center	Lebanon	56%	300+
Harton Regional Medical Center	Tullahoma	55%	300+
Delta Medical Center	Memphis	54%	300+

Nurses 'Always' Communicated Well

Hospital Name	City	Rate	Cases
Saint Thomas Hospital for Spinal Surgery	Nashville	89%	300+
Wellmont Hawkins County Memorial Hospital	Rogersville	89%	(a)
Henderson County Community Hospital	Lexington	88%	(a)
Copper Basin Medical Center	Copperhill	87%	(a)
Jellico Community Hospital[11]	Jellico	87%	(a)
United Regional Medical Center	Manchester	87%	(a)
Baptist Memorial Hospital Union City	Union City	85%	300+
Sycamore Shoals Hospital	Elizabethton	84%	300+
Laughlin Memorial Hospital	Greeneville	83%	300+
Fort Sanders Regional Medical Center	Knoxville	82%	300+
Hardin Medical Center	Savannah	82%	300+
Macon County General Hospital	Lafayette	82%	(a)
Maury Regional Hospital	Columbia	82%	300+
Memorial Healthcare System	Chattanooga	82%	300+
University of Tn Memorial Hospital	Knoxville	82%	300+
Wellmont Bristol Regional Medical Center	Bristol	82%	300+
Fort Loudoun Medical Center	Lenoir City	81%	300+
Franklin Woods Community Hospital	Johnson City	81%	300+
Indian Path Medical Center	Kingsport	81%	300+
Jackson - Madison County General Hospital	Jackson	81%	300+
Jamestown Regional Medical Center	Jamestown	81%	300+
McNairy Regional Hospital	Selmer	81%	(a)
Parkwest Medical Center	Knoxville	81%	300+
Riverview Regional Medical Center	Carthage	81%	(a)
Saint Thomas West Hospital	Nashville	81%	300+
Stones River Hosp & Dekalb Comm Hosp	Smithville	81%	(a)
Sweetwater Hospital Association	Sweetwater	81%	300+
Tristar Horizon Medical Center	Dickson	81%	300+
Vanderbilt University Hospital	Nashville	81%	300+
Wellmont Holston Valley Medical Center	Kingsport	81%	300+
Williamson Medical Center	Franklin	81%	300+
Baptist Memorial Hospital Tipton	Covington	80%	(a)
Cookeville Regional Medical Center	Cookeville	80%	300+
Dyersburg Regional Medical Center	Dyersburg	80%	300+
Methodist Healthcare Memphis Hospitals	Memphis	80%	300+
Methodist Medical Center of Oak Ridge	Oak Ridge	80%	300+
Saint Thomas Rutherford Hospital	Murfreesboro	80%	300+
Tristar Centennial Medical Center	Nashville	80%	300+
Volunteer Community Hospital	Martin	80%	300+
Wayne Medical Center	Waynesboro	80%	(a)
Highlands Medical Center	Sparta	79%	(a)
Leconte Medical Center	Sevierville	79%	300+
Morristown Hamblen Hospital Association	Morristown	79%	300+
Northcrest Medical Center	Springfield	79%	300+
Rhea Medical Center	Dayton	79%	(a)
Saint Thomas Midtown Hospital	Nashville	79%	300+
Tennova Healthcare-Jefferson Mem Hosp	Jefferson City	79%	300+
Henry County Medical Center	Paris	78%	300+
Livingston Regional Hospital	Livingston	78%	300+
Parkridge Medical Center	Chattanooga	78%	300+
Regional Hospital of Jackson	Jackson	78%	300+
Roane Medical Center	Harriman	78%	300+
Saint Francis Hospital	Memphis	78%	300+
Skyridge Medical Center	Cleveland	78%	300+
Takoma Regional Hospital[11]	Greeneville	78%	300+
Tennova Healthcare-Newport Med Ctr	Newport	78%	300+
Crockett Hospital	Lawrenceburg	77%	300+
Cumberland Medical Center	Crossville	77%	300+
Heritage Medical Center	Shelbyville	77%	300+
Hillside Hospital	Pulaski	77%	(a)
Johnson City Medical Center	Johnson City	77%	300+
Starr Regional Medical Center Athens	Athens	77%	300+
Starr Regional Medical Center Etowah	Etowah	77%	(a)
Sumner Regional Medical Center	Gallatin	77%	300+
Baptist Memorial Hospital	Memphis	76%	300+
Erlanger Medical Center[11]	Chattanooga	76%	300+
Grandview Medical Center	Jasper	76%	(a)

NOTE: Hospital profiles are in alphabetical order by state, then city, then hospital within the city; Rankings exclude hospitals with less than 25 cases except for patient surveys which excludes hospitals with less than 100 cases; (a) 100-299 cases; (1) The number of cases/patients is too few to report; (2) Data submitted were based on a sample of cases/patients; (3) Results are based on a shorter time period than required; (4) Data suppressed by CMS for one or more quarters; (5) Results are not available for this reporting period; (6) Fewer than 100 patients completed the HCAHPS survey; (7) No cases met the criteria for this measure; (8) The lower limit of the confidence interval cannot be calculated if the number of observed infections equals zero; (9) No data are available from the state/territory for this reporting period; (10) The scores shown reflect fewer than 50 completed surveys; (11) There were discrepancies in the data collection process; (12) This measure does not apply to this hospital for this reporting period; (13) Results cannot be calculated for this reporting period; (14) The results for this state are combined with nearby states to protect confidentiality; Please refer to the User's Guide for a full explanation of data.

Hospital Name	City	Rate	Cases
Regional Medical Center at Memphis	Memphis	76%	300+
Southern Tennessee Medical Center	Winchester	76%	300+
Tennova Healthcare	Knoxville	76%	300+
Tristar Southern Hills Medical Center	Nashville	76%	300+
Tristar Stonecrest Medical Center	Smyrna	76%	300+
Tristar Summit Medical Center	Hermitage	76%	300+
Lakeway Regional Hospital	Morristown	75%	300+
McKenzie Regional Hospital	Mc Kenzie	75%	(a)
River Park Hospital	Mc Minnville	75%	300+
Tristar Skyline Medical Center	Nashville	75%	300+
Blount Memorial Hospital	Maryville	74%	300+
Gateway Medical Center	Clarksville	74%	300+
Lincoln Medical Center	Fayetteville	74%	(a)
Saint Francis Bartlett Medical Center	Bartlett	74%	300+
Tristar Hendersonville Medical Center	Hendersonville	73%	300+
Unicoi County Memorial Hospital	Erwin	73%	(a)
Delta Medical Center	Memphis	72%	300+
Harton Regional Medical Center	Tullahoma	72%	300+
Metro Nashville General Hospital	Nashville	72%	300+
Claiborne County Hospital	Tazewell	71%	(a)
Tennova Healthcare-Lafollett Med Ctr	La Follette	71%	(a)
University Medical Center	Lebanon	69%	300+

Pain 'Always' Well Controlled

Hospital Name	City	Rate	Cases
United Regional Medical Center	Manchester	83%	(a)
Saint Thomas Hospital for Spinal Surgery	Nashville	81%	300+
Copper Basin Medical Center	Copperhill	80%	(a)
Henderson County Community Hospital	Lexington	78%	(a)
Macon County General Hospital	Lafayette	78%	(a)
Baptist Memorial Hospital Union City	Union City	76%	300+
Fort Sanders Regional Medical Center	Knoxville	76%	300+
Hardin Medical Center	Savannah	76%	300+
Henry County Medical Center	Paris	76%	300+
Sycamore Shoals Hospital	Elizabethton	76%	300+
Wellmont Hawkins County Memorial Hospital	Rogersville	76%	(a)
Grandview Medical Center	Jasper	75%	(a)
Riverview Regional Medical Center	Carthage	75%	(a)
Wayne Medical Center	Waynesboro	75%	(a)
Dyersburg Regional Medical Center	Dyersburg	74%	300+
Franklin Woods Community Hospital	Johnson City	74%	300+
Laughlin Memorial Hospital	Greeneville	74%	300+
McKenzie Regional Hospital	Mc Kenzie	74%	(a)
Memorial Healthcare System	Chattanooga	74%	300+
Stones River Hosp & Dekalb Comm Hosp	Smithville	74%	(a)
Tristar Horizon Medical Center	Dickson	74%	300+
Volunteer Community Hospital	Martin	74%	300+
Jellico Community Hospital[11]	Jellico	73%	(a)
Parkwest Medical Center	Knoxville	73%	300+
Saint Thomas West Hospital	Nashville	73%	300+
Sweetwater Hospital Association	Sweetwater	73%	300+
Takoma Regional Hospital[11]	Greeneville	73%	300+
University of Tn Memorial Hospital	Knoxville	73%	300+
Vanderbilt University Hospital	Nashville	73%	300+
Jackson - Madison County General Hospital	Jackson	72%	300+
McNairy Regional Hospital	Selmer	72%	(a)
Methodist Healthcare Memphis Hospitals	Memphis	72%	300+
Methodist Medical Center of Oak Ridge	Oak Ridge	72%	300+
Parkridge Medical Center	Chattanooga	72%	300+
Regional Hospital of Jackson	Jackson	72%	300+
Skyridge Medical Center	Cleveland	72%	300+
Starr Regional Medical Center Athens	Athens	72%	300+
Williamson Medical Center	Franklin	72%	300+
Fort Loudoun Medical Center	Lenoir City	71%	300+
Maury Regional Hospital	Columbia	71%	300+
Metro Nashville General Hospital	Nashville	71%	300+
Northcrest Medical Center	Springfield	71%	300+
Saint Francis Bartlett Medical Center	Bartlett	71%	300+
Saint Francis Hospital	Memphis	71%	300+
Saint Thomas Rutherford Hospital	Murfreesboro	71%	300+
Tristar Centennial Medical Center	Nashville	71%	300+
Wellmont Bristol Regional Medical Center	Bristol	71%	300+
Cookeville Regional Medical Center	Cookeville	70%	300+
Highlands Medical Center	Sparta	70%	(a)
Rhea Medical Center	Dayton	70%	(a)
Saint Thomas Midtown Hospital	Nashville	70%	300+
Sumner Regional Medical Center	Gallatin	70%	300+
Tristar Skyline Medical Center	Nashville	70%	300+
Tristar Stonecrest Medical Center	Smyrna	70%	300+
Wellmont Holston Valley Medical Center	Kingsport	70%	300+
Baptist Memorial Hospital	Memphis	69%	300+
Cumberland Medical Center	Crossville	69%	300+
Indian Path Medical Center	Kingsport	69%	300+
Jamestown Regional Medical Center	Jamestown	69%	300+
Leconte Medical Center	Sevierville	69%	300+
Lincoln Medical Center	Fayetteville	69%	(a)
Livingston Regional Hospital	Livingston	69%	300+
Tennova Healthcare	Knoxville	69%	300+
Tristar Southern Hills Medical Center	Nashville	69%	300+
Tristar Summit Medical Center	Hermitage	69%	300+
Baptist Memorial Hospital Tipton	Covington	68%	(a)
Regional Medical Center at Memphis	Memphis	68%	300+
River Park Hospital	Mc Minnville	68%	300+
Roane Medical Center	Harriman	68%	300+
Southern Tennessee Medical Center	Winchester	68%	300+
Tennova Healthcare-Jefferson Mem Hosp	Jefferson City	68%	300+
Crockett Hospital	Lawrenceburg	67%	300+
Erlanger Medical Center[11]	Chattanooga	67%	300+
Gateway Medical Center	Clarksville	67%	300+
Heritage Medical Center	Shelbyville	67%	300+
Johnson City Medical Center	Johnson City	67%	300+
Blount Memorial Hospital	Maryville	66%	300+
Hillside Hospital	Pulaski	66%	(a)
Lakeway Regional Hospital	Morristown	66%	300+
Tristar Hendersonville Medical Center	Hendersonville	66%	300+
Claiborne County Hospital	Tazewell	65%	(a)
Starr Regional Medical Center Etowah	Etowah	65%	(a)
Tennova Healthcare-Newport Med Ctr	Newport	65%	300+
Unicoi County Memorial Hospital	Erwin	65%	(a)
Delta Medical Center	Memphis	64%	300+
Morristown Hamblen Hospital Association	Morristown	64%	300+
University Medical Center	Lebanon	63%	300+
Harton Regional Medical Center	Tullahoma	61%	300+
Tennova Healthcare-Lafollett Med Ctr	La Follette	55%	(a)

Room and Bathroom 'Always' Clean

Hospital Name	City	Rate	Cases
Wellmont Hawkins County Memorial Hospital	Rogersville	87%	(a)
United Regional Medical Center	Manchester	86%	(a)
Baptist Memorial Hospital Union City	Union City	84%	300+
Jellico Community Hospital[11]	Jellico	84%	(a)
Saint Thomas Hospital for Spinal Surgery	Nashville	81%	300+
Macon County General Hospital	Lafayette	80%	(a)
Sweetwater Hospital Association	Sweetwater	79%	300+
Franklin Woods Community Hospital	Johnson City	78%	300+
Hardin Medical Center	Savannah	77%	300+
Laughlin Memorial Hospital	Greeneville	77%	300+
Tristar Horizon Medical Center	Dickson	77%	300+
Tristar Southern Hills Medical Center	Nashville	77%	300+
University of Tn Memorial Hospital	Knoxville	77%	300+
Volunteer Community Hospital	Martin	77%	300+
Copper Basin Medical Center	Copperhill	76%	(a)
Northcrest Medical Center	Springfield	76%	300+
Parkwest Medical Center	Knoxville	76%	300+
Sycamore Shoals Hospital	Elizabethton	76%	300+
Tristar Stonecrest Medical Center	Smyrna	76%	300+
Wayne Medical Center	Waynesboro	76%	(a)
Baptist Memorial Hospital Tipton	Covington	75%	(a)
Fort Sanders Regional Medical Center	Knoxville	75%	300+
Grandview Medical Center	Jasper	75%	(a)
Henry County Medical Center	Paris	75%	300+
Highlands Medical Center	Sparta	75%	(a)
McKenzie Regional Hospital	Mc Kenzie	75%	(a)
Tennova Healthcare-Lafollett Med Ctr	La Follette	75%	(a)
Unicoi County Memorial Hospital	Erwin	75%	(a)
Williamson Medical Center	Franklin	75%	300+
Delta Medical Center	Memphis	74%	300+
Henderson County Community Hospital	Lexington	74%	(a)
Jackson - Madison County General Hospital	Jackson	74%	300+
Maury Regional Hospital	Columbia	74%	300+
Memorial Healthcare System	Chattanooga	74%	300+
Methodist Medical Center of Oak Ridge	Oak Ridge	74%	300+
Takoma Regional Hospital[11]	Greeneville	74%	300+
Lincoln Medical Center	Fayetteville	73%	(a)
Roane Medical Center	Harriman	73%	300+
Tennova Healthcare-Newport Med Ctr	Newport	73%	300+
Heritage Medical Center	Shelbyville	72%	300+
Riverview Regional Medical Center	Carthage	72%	(a)
Stones River Hosp & Dekalb Comm Hosp	Smithville	72%	(a)
Wellmont Bristol Regional Medical Center	Bristol	72%	300+
Baptist Memorial Hospital	Memphis	71%	300+
Cumberland Medical Center	Crossville	71%	300+
Gateway Medical Center	Clarksville	71%	300+
Hillside Hospital	Pulaski	71%	(a)
Leconte Medical Center	Sevierville	71%	300+
McNairy Regional Hospital	Selmer	71%	(a)
Morristown Hamblen Hospital Association	Morristown	71%	300+
Rhea Medical Center	Dayton	71%	(a)
Tristar Summit Medical Center	Hermitage	71%	300+
Cookeville Regional Medical Center	Cookeville	70%	300+
Crockett Hospital	Lawrenceburg	70%	300+
Methodist Healthcare Memphis Hospitals	Memphis	70%	300+
Metro Nashville General Hospital	Nashville	70%	300+
Saint Thomas Rutherford Hospital	Murfreesboro	70%	300+
Tristar Centennial Medical Center	Nashville	70%	300+
Erlanger Medical Center[11]	Chattanooga	69%	300+
Fort Loudoun Medical Center	Lenoir City	69%	300+
Indian Path Medical Center	Kingsport	69%	300+
Lakeway Regional Hospital	Morristown	69%	300+
Blount Memorial Hospital	Maryville	68%	300+
Dyersburg Regional Medical Center	Dyersburg	68%	300+
Harton Regional Medical Center	Tullahoma	68%	300+
Livingston Regional Hospital	Livingston	68%	300+
Parkridge Medical Center	Chattanooga	68%	300+
Regional Hospital of Jackson	Jackson	68%	300+
River Park Hospital	Mc Minnville	68%	300+
Southern Tennessee Medical Center	Winchester	68%	300+
Starr Regional Medical Center Athens	Athens	68%	300+
Starr Regional Medical Center Etowah	Etowah	68%	(a)
Sumner Regional Medical Center	Gallatin	68%	300+
Tennova Healthcare-Jefferson Mem Hosp	Jefferson City	68%	300+
Tristar Hendersonville Medical Center	Hendersonville	68%	300+
Wellmont Holston Valley Medical Center	Kingsport	68%	300+
Tennova Healthcare	Knoxville	67%	300+
Tristar Skyline Medical Center	Nashville	67%	300+
Regional Medical Center at Memphis	Memphis	66%	300+
Saint Francis Hospital	Memphis	66%	300+
Skyridge Medical Center	Cleveland	66%	300+
Jamestown Regional Medical Center	Jamestown	65%	300+
Johnson City Medical Center	Johnson City	65%	300+
Saint Francis Bartlett Medical Center	Bartlett	65%	300+
University Medical Center	Lebanon	65%	300+
Vanderbilt University Hospital	Nashville	64%	300+
Claiborne County Hospital	Tazewell	63%	(a)
Saint Thomas Midtown Hospital	Nashville	61%	300+
Saint Thomas West Hospital	Nashville	60%	300+

Timely Help 'Always' Received

Hospital Name	City	Rate	Cases
United Regional Medical Center	Manchester	87%	(a)
Saint Thomas Hospital for Spinal Surgery	Nashville	84%	300+
Macon County General Hospital	Lafayette	82%	(a)
Baptist Memorial Hospital Union City	Union City	80%	300+
Henderson County Community Hospital	Lexington	80%	(a)
Sycamore Shoals Hospital	Elizabethton	79%	300+
Wellmont Hawkins County Memorial Hospital	Rogersville	79%	(a)
Baptist Memorial Hospital Tipton	Covington	74%	(a)
Jellico Community Hospital[11]	Jellico	74%	(a)
Highlands Medical Center	Sparta	73%	(a)
Laughlin Memorial Hospital	Greeneville	73%	300+
Stones River Hosp & Dekalb Comm Hosp	Smithville	73%	(a)
Hardin Medical Center	Savannah	72%	300+
Jamestown Regional Medical Center	Jamestown	72%	300+
Maury Regional Hospital	Columbia	72%	300+
Rhea Medical Center	Dayton	72%	(a)
Sweetwater Hospital Association	Sweetwater	72%	300+
Copper Basin Medical Center	Copperhill	71%	(a)
Dyersburg Regional Medical Center	Dyersburg	71%	300+
Grandview Medical Center	Jasper	71%	(a)
Unicoi County Memorial Hospital	Erwin	71%	(a)
Fort Sanders Regional Medical Center	Knoxville	70%	300+
Franklin Woods Community Hospital	Johnson City	70%	300+
Henry County Medical Center	Paris	69%	300+
Memorial Healthcare System	Chattanooga	69%	300+
Riverview Regional Medical Center	Carthage	69%	(a)
Roane Medical Center	Harriman	69%	300+
Tristar Horizon Medical Center	Dickson	69%	300+
Wayne Medical Center	Waynesboro	69%	(a)
Williamson Medical Center	Franklin	69%	300+
Cookeville Regional Medical Center	Cookeville	68%	300+
Hillside Hospital	Pulaski	68%	(a)
Jackson - Madison County General Hospital	Jackson	68%	300+
Methodist Medical Center of Oak Ridge	Oak Ridge	68%	300+
Takoma Regional Hospital[11]	Greeneville	68%	300+
Volunteer Community Hospital	Martin	68%	300+
McKenzie Regional Hospital	Mc Kenzie	67%	(a)
Sumner Regional Medical Center	Gallatin	67%	300+
Tristar Centennial Medical Center	Nashville	67%	300+
University of Tn Memorial Hospital	Knoxville	67%	300+
Vanderbilt University Hospital	Nashville	67%	300+
Crockett Hospital	Lawrenceburg	66%	300+
Northcrest Medical Center	Springfield	66%	300+
Parkwest Medical Center	Knoxville	66%	300+
Regional Hospital of Jackson	Jackson	66%	300+
Saint Francis Bartlett Medical Center	Bartlett	66%	300+
Starr Regional Medical Center Etowah	Etowah	66%	(a)
Indian Path Medical Center	Kingsport	65%	300+
Morristown Hamblen Hospital Association	Morristown	65%	300+
Parkridge Medical Center	Chattanooga	65%	300+
Saint Thomas West Hospital	Nashville	65%	300+
Wellmont Bristol Regional Medical Center	Bristol	65%	300+
Wellmont Holston Valley Medical Center	Kingsport	65%	300+
Cumberland Medical Center	Crossville	64%	300+
Heritage Medical Center	Shelbyville	64%	300+
Johnson City Medical Center	Johnson City	64%	300+
Leconte Medical Center	Sevierville	64%	300+
Livingston Regional Hospital	Livingston	64%	300+
McNairy Regional Hospital	Selmer	64%	(a)
Skyridge Medical Center	Cleveland	64%	300+
Erlanger Medical Center[11]	Chattanooga	63%	300+
Methodist Healthcare Memphis Hospitals	Memphis	63%	300+
Starr Regional Medical Center Athens	Athens	63%	300+
Tennova Healthcare-Newport Med Ctr	Newport	63%	300+

NOTE: Hospital profiles are in alphabetical order by state, then city, then hospital within the city; Rankings exclude hospitals with less than 25 cases except for patient surveys which excludes hospitals with less than 100 cases; (a) 100-299 cases; (1) The number of cases/patients is too few to report; (2) Data submitted were based on a sample of cases/patients; (3) Results are based on a shorter time period than required; (4) Data suppressed by CMS for one or more quarters; (5) Results are not available for this reporting period; (6) Fewer than 100 patients completed the HCAHPS survey; (7) No cases met the criteria for this measure; (8) The lower limit of the confidence interval cannot be calculated if the number of observed infections equals zero; (9) No data are available from the state/territory for this reporting period; (10) The scores shown reflect fewer than 50 completed surveys; (11) There were discrepancies in the data collection process; (12) This measure does not apply to this hospital for this reporting period; (13) Results cannot be calculated for this reporting period; (14) The results for this state are combined with nearby states to protect confidentiality; Please refer to the User's Guide for a full explanation of data.

Hospital Name	City	Rate	Cases
Lincoln Medical Center	Fayetteville	62%	(a)
Regional Medical Center at Memphis	Memphis	62%	300+
River Park Hospital	Mc Minnville	62%	300+
Saint Francis Hospital	Memphis	62%	300+
Saint Thomas Midtown Hospital	Nashville	62%	300+
Tennova Healthcare	Knoxville	62%	300+
Tennova Healthcare-Jefferson Mem Hosp	Jefferson City	62%	300+
Claiborne County Hospital	Tazewell	61%	(a)
Fort Loudoun Medical Center	Lenoir City	61%	300+
Lakeway Regional Hospital	Morristown	61%	300+
Saint Thomas Rutherford Hospital	Murfreesboro	61%	300+
Tristar Southern Hills Medical Center	Nashville	61%	300+
Tristar Stonecrest Medical Center	Smyrna	61%	300+
Gateway Medical Center	Clarksville	60%	300+
Tristar Skyline Medical Center	Nashville	60%	300+
Tristar Summit Medical Center	Hermitage	60%	300+
Metro Nashville General Hospital	Nashville	59%	300+
Tennova Healthcare-Lafollett Med Ctr	La Follette	59%	(a)
Tristar Hendersonville Medical Center	Hendersonville	59%	300+
Baptist Memorial Hospital	Memphis	58%	300+
Blount Memorial Hospital	Maryville	58%	300+
Delta Medical Center	Memphis	55%	300+
Harton Regional Medical Center	Tullahoma	55%	300+
Southern Tennessee Medical Center	Winchester	54%	300+
University Medical Center	Lebanon	51%	300+
Unicoi County Memorial Hospital	Erwin	66%	(a)
Northcrest Medical Center	Springfield	65%	300+
Volunteer Community Hospital	Martin	65%	300+
Blount Memorial Hospital	Maryville	64%	300+
Grandview Medical Center	Jasper	64%	(a)
Southern Tennessee Medical Center	Winchester	64%	300+
Tristar Southern Hills Medical Center	Nashville	64%	300+
Heritage Medical Center	Shelbyville	62%	300+
Baptist Memorial Hospital Tipton	Covington	61%	(a)
Cumberland Medical Center	Crossville	61%	300+
Dyersburg Regional Medical Center	Dyersburg	61%	300+
Skyridge Medical Center	Cleveland	61%	300+
Delta Medical Center	Memphis	60%	300+
Lincoln Medical Center	Fayetteville	60%	(a)
McNairy Regional Hospital	Selmer	60%	(a)
Gateway Medical Center	Clarksville	59%	300+
Jamestown Regional Medical Center	Jamestown	59%	300+
Hillside Hospital	Pulaski	58%	(a)
Crockett Hospital	Lawrenceburg	57%	300+
Tennova Healthcare-Newport Med Ctr	Newport	57%	300+
River Park Hospital	Mc Minnville	56%	300+
Wayne Medical Center	Waynesboro	56%	(a)
Claiborne County Hospital	Tazewell	55%	(a)
Harton Regional Medical Center	Tullahoma	55%	300+
University Medical Center	Lebanon	51%	300+
Tennova Healthcare-Lafollett Med Ctr	La Follette	48%	(a)

Would Definitely Recommend Hospital

Hospital Name	City	Rate	Cases
Saint Thomas Hospital for Spinal Surgery	Nashville	90%	300+
Saint Thomas West Hospital	Nashville	88%	300+
Copper Basin Medical Center	Copperhill	86%	(a)
University of Tn Memorial Hospital	Knoxville	85%	300+
Memorial Healthcare System	Chattanooga	83%	300+
Vanderbilt University Hospital	Nashville	83%	300+
Franklin Woods Community Hospital	Johnson City	82%	300+
Fort Sanders Regional Medical Center	Knoxville	81%	300+
Parkwest Medical Center	Knoxville	81%	300+
Williamson Medical Center	Franklin	80%	300+
Tristar Centennial Medical Center	Nashville	79%	300+
Wellmont Hawkins County Memorial Hospital	Rogersville	79%	(a)
Cookeville Regional Medical Center	Cookeville	78%	300+
Jellico Community Hospital[11]	Jellico	77%	(a)
Methodist Healthcare Memphis Hospitals	Memphis	77%	300+
Indian Path Medical Center	Kingsport	76%	300+
Saint Thomas Midtown Hospital	Nashville	76%	300+
Sycamore Shoals Hospital	Elizabethton	76%	300+
Baptist Memorial Hospital	Memphis	75%	300+
Jackson - Madison County General Hospital	Jackson	75%	300+
Maury Regional Hospital	Columbia	75%	300+
Methodist Medical Center of Oak Ridge	Oak Ridge	75%	300+
Saint Thomas Rutherford Hospital	Murfreesboro	75%	300+
Takoma Regional Hospital[11]	Greeneville	75%	300+
Wellmont Holston Valley Medical Center	Kingsport	75%	300+
Parkridge Medical Center	Chattanooga	74%	300+
Wellmont Bristol Regional Medical Center	Bristol	74%	300+
Erlanger Medical Center[11]	Chattanooga	73%	300+
Laughlin Memorial Hospital	Greeneville	73%	300+
Regional Hospital of Jackson	Jackson	73%	300+
Starr Regional Medical Center Etowah	Etowah	73%	(a)
Stones River Hosp & Dekalb Comm Hosp	Smithville	73%	(a)
Tristar Summit Medical Center	Hermitage	73%	300+
Henry County Medical Center	Paris	72%	300+
Leconte Medical Center	Sevierville	72%	300+
Macon County General Hospital	Lafayette	72%	(a)
Regional Medical Center at Memphis	Memphis	72%	300+
Tristar Stonecrest Medical Center	Smyrna	72%	300+
Fort Loudoun Medical Center	Lenoir City	71%	300+
Saint Francis Bartlett Medical Center	Bartlett	71%	300+
Saint Francis Hospital	Memphis	71%	300+
Sweetwater Hospital Association	Sweetwater	71%	300+
Baptist Memorial Hospital Union City	Union City	70%	300+
Highlands Medical Center	Sparta	70%	(a)
Hardin Medical Center	Savannah	69%	300+
Roane Medical Center	Harriman	69%	300+
Sumner Regional Medical Center	Gallatin	69%	300+
Tennova Healthcare	Knoxville	69%	300+
Tristar Hendersonville Medical Center	Hendersonville	69%	300+
Morristown Hamblen Hospital Association	Morristown	68%	300+
Rhea Medical Center	Dayton	68%	(a)
Riverview Regional Medical Center	Carthage	68%	(a)
Tristar Skyline Medical Center	Nashville	68%	300+
Henderson County Community Hospital	Lexington	67%	(a)
Livingston Regional Hospital	Livingston	67%	300+
Metro Nashville General Hospital	Nashville	67%	300+
United Regional Medical Center	Manchester	67%	(a)
Johnson City Medical Center	Johnson City	66%	300+
Lakeway Regional Hospital	Morristown	66%	300+
McKenzie Regional Hospital	Mc Kenzie	66%	(a)
Starr Regional Medical Center Athens	Athens	66%	300+
Tennova Healthcare-Jefferson Mem Hosp	Jefferson City	66%	300+
Tristar Horizon Medical Center	Dickson	66%	300+

Use of Medical Imaging

Cardiac Imaging Stress Test before OP Surgery

Hospital Name	City	Rate	Cases
Saint Francis Bartlett Medical Center	Bartlett	0.0%	105
Tristar Stonecrest Medical Center	Smyrna	0.0%	60
Franklin Woods Community Hospital	Johnson City	1.9%	53
Marshall Medical Center	Lewisburg	1.9%	52
Tennova Healthcare-Newport Med Ctr	Newport	1.9%	103
Grandview Medical Center	Jasper	2.1%	48
Hillside Hospital	Pulaski	2.2%	93
Johnson County Community Hospital	Mountain City	2.2%	92
Lincoln Medical Center	Fayetteville	2.8%	106
Williamson Medical Center	Franklin	3.0%	198
Saint Francis Hospital	Memphis	3.1%	225
Henry County Medical Center	Paris	3.5%	402
River Park Hospital	Mc Minnville	3.5%	231
Blount Memorial Hospital	Maryville	3.7%	574
Cumberland Medical Center	Crossville	3.8%	367
Erlanger Medical Center	Chattanooga	3.8%	664
Hardin Medical Center	Savannah	3.8%	261
Regional Medical Center at Memphis	Memphis	3.9%	127
Skyridge Medical Center	Cleveland	3.9%	76
Gateway Medical Center	Clarksville	4.0%	522
Sycamore Shoals Hospital	Elizabethton	4.1%	97
Rhea Medical Center	Dayton	4.2%	143
Methodist Healthcare Memphis Hospitals	Memphis	4.3%	2726
Roane Medical Center	Harriman	4.3%	185
Johnson City Medical Center	Johnson City	4.4%	1087
Saint Thomas Midtown Hospital	Nashville	4.4%	1135
Wellmont Holston Valley Medical Center	Kingsport	4.4%	1912
Jackson - Madison County General Hospital	Jackson	4.5%	750
Tennova Healthcare	Knoxville	4.6%	1642
Fort Sanders Regional Medical Center	Knoxville	4.7%	512
Harton Regional Medical Center	Tullahoma	4.7%	212
Saint Thomas Rutherford Hospital	Murfreesboro	4.7%	782
Cookeville Regional Medical Center	Cookeville	4.8%	1477
Dyersburg Regional Medical Center	Dyersburg	4.8%	227
Memorial Healthcare System	Chattanooga	4.8%	2902
Laughlin Memorial Hospital	Greeneville	4.9%	245
Saint Thomas West Hospital	Nashville	4.9%	2047
Baptist Memorial Hospital Union City	Union City	5.0%	121
Fort Loudoun Medical Center	Lenoir City	5.0%	298
Tennova Healthcare-Lafollett Med Ctr	La Follette	5.0%	141
Methodist Medical Center of Oak Ridge	Oak Ridge	5.2%	231
Leconte Medical Center	Sevierville	5.3%	397
Indian Path Medical Center	Kingsport	5.4%	147
Parkwest Medical Center	Knoxville	5.4%	1220
Wellmont Bristol Regional Medical Center	Bristol	5.4%	627
Baptist Memorial Hospital	Memphis	5.5%	2874
Copper Basin Medical Center	Copperhill	5.5%	55
Tennova Healthcare-Jefferson Mem Hosp	Jefferson City	5.5%	220
Regional Hospital of Jackson	Jackson	5.6%	179
Heritage Medical Center	Shelbyville	5.7%	174
Southern Tennessee Medical Center	Winchester	5.7%	175
Sumner Regional Medical Center	Gallatin	5.8%	206
Tristar Skyline Medical Center	Nashville	5.8%	103
Northcrest Medical Center	Springfield	5.9%	170
Vanderbilt University Hospital	Nashville	5.9%	1157
Starr Regional Medical Center Athens	Athens	6.1%	179
Livingston Regional Hospital	Livingston	6.6%	137
Tristar Horizon Medical Center	Dickson	6.8%	73
Crockett Hospital	Lawrenceburg	6.9%	130
Maury Regional Hospital	Columbia	7.0%	426
Takoma Regional Hospital	Greeneville	7.1%	112
Tristar Summit Medical Center	Hermitage	7.1%	99
Parkridge Medical Center	Chattanooga	7.7%	298
United Regional Medical Center	Manchester	8.6%	70
Tristar Centennial Medical Center	Nashville	10.4%	106
University Medical Center	Lebanon	12.2%	90

Combination Abdominal CT Scan

Hospital Name	City	Rate	Cases
Gibson General Hospital	Trenton	0.0%	84
Lauderdale Community Hospital	Ripley	0.5%	187
Milan General Hospital	Milan	0.6%	161
Hillside Hospital	Pulaski	0.7%	294
Saint Thomas Rutherford Hospital	Murfreesboro	0.8%	641
Southern Tennessee Medical Center	Winchester	0.9%	536
Bolivar General Hospital	Bolivar	1.0%	102
Haywood Park Community Hospital	Brownsville	1.6%	124
McKenzie Regional Hospital	Mc Kenzie	1.7%	60
Blount Memorial Hospital	Maryville	2.0%	986
McNairy Regional Hospital	Selmer	2.1%	192
Stones River Hosp & Dekalb Comm Hosp	Smithville	2.5%	240
Baptist Memorial Hospital	Memphis	2.7%	2052
Henderson County Community Hospital	Lexington	2.9%	170
Lincoln Medical Center	Fayetteville	3.1%	257
Methodist Healthcare Fayette Hospital	Somerville	3.2%	218
Claiborne County Hospital	Tazewell	3.3%	424
River Park Hospital	Mc Minnville	3.3%	363
Methodist Medical Center of Oak Ridge	Oak Ridge	3.7%	1148
Tennova Healthcare-Jefferson Mem Hosp	Jefferson City	3.7%	561
Tristar Stonecrest Medical Center	Smyrna	3.7%	352
Baptist Memorial Hospital Union City	Union City	3.8%	525
Tennova Healthcare	Knoxville	4.0%	1787
Tristar Horizon Medical Center	Dickson	4.0%	504
Saint Thomas Midtown Hospital	Nashville	4.1%	611
Hardin Medical Center	Savannah	4.2%	565
Jackson - Madison County General Hospital	Jackson	4.3%	1992
Regional Hospital of Jackson	Jackson	4.5%	314
Copper Basin Medical Center	Copperhill	4.8%	269
Macon County General Hospital	Lafayette	4.9%	123
Volunteer Community Hospital	Martin	4.9%	247
Stones River Hosp & Dekalb Comm Hosp	Woodbury	5.4%	56
Tristar Skyline Medical Center	Nashville	5.4%	634
Dyersburg Regional Medical Center	Dyersburg	5.5%	685
Humboldt General Hospital	Humboldt	5.5%	91
Saint Thomas West Hospital	Nashville	5.5%	921
University of Tn Memorial Hospital	Knoxville	5.6%	2406
Cumberland Medical Center	Crossville	5.8%	895
Laughlin Memorial Hospital	Greeneville	5.9%	798
Methodist Healthcare Memphis Hospitals	Memphis	6.0%	6797
Tristar Southern Hills Medical Center	Nashville	6.0%	381
Medical Center of Manchester	Manchester	6.1%	164
Fort Sanders Regional Medical Center	Knoxville	6.5%	827
Tennova Healthcare-Newport Med Ctr	Newport	6.5%	354
Jamestown Regional Medical Center	Jamestown	6.6%	213
Rhea Medical Center	Dayton	6.6%	424
Sumner Regional Medical Center	Gallatin	6.7%	631
Gateway Medical Center	Clarksville	6.8%	1040
Northcrest Medical Center	Springfield	7.2%	713
Tristar Centennial Medical Center	Nashville	7.3%	821
Lakeway Regional Hospital	Morristown	7.6%	224
Tristar Ashland City Medical Center	Ashland City	7.6%	79
Roane Medical Center	Harriman	7.9%	342
University Medical Center	Lebanon	8.1%	579
Sweetwater Hospital Association	Sweetwater	8.3%	375
Takoma Regional Hospital	Greeneville	8.3%	300
Maury Regional Hospital	Columbia	8.5%	1478
Regional Medical Center at Memphis	Memphis	8.5%	294
Wellmont Holston Valley Medical Center	Kingsport	8.6%	628
Leconte Medical Center	Sevierville	8.9%	903
Decatur County General Hospital	Parsons	9.2%	195
Skyridge Medical Center	Cleveland	9.2%	1077
Starr Regional Medical Center Etowah	Etowah	9.2%	207
Sycamore Shoals Hospital	Elizabethton	9.2%	448
Cookeville Regional Medical Center	Cookeville	9.3%	1442
Franklin Woods Community Hospital	Johnson City	9.4%	604
Johnson County Community Hospital	Mountain City	9.4%	181
Crockett Hospital	Lawrenceburg	9.5%	505
Riverview Regional Medical Center	Carthage	9.5%	168
Tristar Summit Medical Center	Hermitage	9.7%	802
Parkwest Medical Center	Knoxville	10.0%	1078
Wellmont Hawkins County Memorial Hospital	Rogersville	10.0%	239
Wellmont Bristol Regional Medical Center	Bristol	10.3%	1376
Saint Francis Bartlett Medical Center	Bartlett	10.5%	631
Saint Francis Hospital	Memphis	10.9%	598
Marshall Medical Center	Lewisburg	11.1%	108
Morristown Hamblen Hospital Association	Morristown	11.4%	568
Parkridge Medical Center	Chattanooga	11.6%	924
Fort Loudoun Medical Center	Lenoir City	11.7%	386
Williamson Medical Center	Franklin	11.7%	693
Heritage Medical Center	Shelbyville	11.9%	235

NOTE: Hospital profiles are in alphabetical order by state, then city, then hospital within the city; Rankings exclude hospitals with less than 25 cases except for patient surveys which excludes hospitals with less than 100 cases; (a) 100-299 cases; (1) The number of cases/patients is too few to report; (2) Data submitted were based on a sample of cases/patients; (3) Results are based on a shorter time period than required; (4) Data suppressed by CMS for one or more quarters; (5) Results are not available for this reporting period; (6) Fewer than 100 patients completed the HCAHPS survey; (7) No cases met the criteria for this measure; (8) The lower limit of the confidence interval cannot be calculated if the number of observed infections equals zero; (9) No data are available from the state/territory for this reporting period; (10) The scores shown reflect fewer than 50 completed surveys; (11) There were discrepancies in the data collection process; (12) This measure does not apply to this hospital for this reporting period; (13) Results cannot be calculated for this reporting period; (14) The results for this state are combined with nearby states to protect confidentiality; Please refer to the User's Guide for a full explanation of data.

Hospital Name	City	Rate	Cases
Tristar Hendersonville Medical Center	Hendersonville	11.9%	446
Johnson City Medical Center	Johnson City	12.0%	930
Wayne Medical Center	Waynesboro	12.2%	180
Tennova Healthcare-Lafollett Med Ctr	La Follette	13.2%	288
Metro Nashville General Hospital	Nashville	13.7%	73
United Regional Medical Center	Manchester	14.6%	96
Cumberland River Hospital	Celina	14.7%	68
Harton Regional Medical Center	Tullahoma	14.7%	484
Henry County Medical Center	Paris	15.5%	909
Baptist Memorial Hospital Huntingdon	Huntingdon	16.7%	150
Starr Regional Medical Center Athens	Athens	18.3%	448
Indian Path Medical Center	Kingsport	18.9%	487
Erlanger Medical Center	Chattanooga	19.4%	1028
Unicoi County Memorial Hospital	Erwin	19.4%	217
Livingston Regional Hospital	Livingston	20.7%	314
Highlands Medical Center	Sparta	21.2%	231
Memorial Healthcare System	Chattanooga	24.9%	3045
Vanderbilt University Hospital	Nashville	27.2%	3037
Grandview Medical Center	Jasper	27.4%	314
Jellico Community Hospital	Jellico	29.3%	164
Baptist Memorial Hospital Tipton	Covington	30.3%	756

Combination Brain/Sinus CT Scan

Hospital Name	City	Rate	Cases
Perry Community Hospital	Linden	0.0%	65
Tristar Ashland City Medical Center	Ashland City	0.0%	131
Baptist Memorial Hospital Tipton	Covington	0.3%	341
Tennova Healthcare-Jefferson Mem Hosp	Jefferson City	0.8%	479
Cumberland Medical Center	Crossville	0.9%	1146
Starr Regional Medical Center Etowah	Etowah	0.9%	231
Wellmont Hawkins County Memorial Hospital	Rogersville	1.0%	201
Decatur County General Hospital	Parsons	1.2%	246
Sumner Regional Medical Center	Gallatin	1.3%	381
Methodist Medical Center of Oak Ridge	Oak Ridge	1.5%	804
Baptist Memorial Hospital Union City	Union City	1.6%	490
Sweetwater Hospital Association	Sweetwater	1.9%	413
University of Tn Memorial Hospital	Knoxville	1.9%	1586
Erlanger Medical Center	Chattanooga	2.0%	1013
River Park Hospital	Mc Minnville	2.2%	459
Tristar Summit Medical Center	Hermitage	2.2%	549
Williamson Medical Center	Franklin	2.4%	712
Tristar Skyline Medical Center	Nashville	2.5%	825
Crockett Hospital	Lawrenceburg	2.6%	540
Saint Thomas Rutherford Hospital	Murfreesboro	2.6%	803
Wellmont Holston Valley Medical Center	Kingsport	2.6%	741
Cookeville Regional Medical Center	Cookeville	2.7%	1510
Maury Regional Hospital	Columbia	2.7%	1240
Vanderbilt University Hospital	Nashville	2.7%	592
Henry County Medical Center	Paris	2.8%	643
Baptist Memorial Hospital	Memphis	3.0%	2019
Fort Sanders Regional Medical Center	Knoxville	3.0%	734
Johnson City Medical Center	Johnson City	3.0%	888
Parkwest Medical Center	Knoxville	3.0%	1207
Saint Thomas West Hospital	Nashville	3.0%	795
Tristar Centennial Medical Center	Nashville	3.0%	667
Memorial Healthcare System	Chattanooga	3.1%	2192
Saint Francis Hospital	Memphis	3.1%	654
Tennova Healthcare	Knoxville	3.2%	1361
Gateway Medical Center	Clarksville	3.4%	1222
Wellmont Bristol Regional Medical Center	Bristol	3.5%	797
Methodist Healthcare Memphis Hospitals	Memphis	3.7%	3976
Parkridge Medical Center	Chattanooga	3.7%	804
Roane Medical Center	Harriman	3.8%	532
Southern Tennessee Medical Center	Winchester	3.8%	606
Heritage Medical Center	Shelbyville	4.0%	450
Starr Regional Medical Center Athens	Athens	4.0%	429
Jackson - Madison County General Hospital	Jackson	4.1%	1861
Morristown Hamblen Hospital Association	Morristown	4.3%	691
Franklin Woods Community Hospital	Johnson City	4.8%	372
Volunteer Community Hospital	Martin	4.8%	289
Blount Memorial Hospital	Maryville	4.9%	823
Skyridge Medical Center	Cleveland	4.9%	1039
Northcrest Medical Center	Springfield	5.0%	714
Medical Center of Manchester	Manchester	5.1%	235
Saint Francis Bartlett Medical Center	Bartlett	5.5%	542
Tristar Hendersonville Medical Center	Hendersonville	5.5%	457
Hardin Medical Center	Savannah	5.6%	588
Laughlin Memorial Hospital	Greeneville	5.8%	535
Livingston Regional Hospital	Livingston	5.8%	292
Leconte Medical Center	Sevierville	5.9%	632
Sycamore Shoals Hospital	Elizabethton	5.9%	406
Milan General Hospital	Milan	6.4%	249
Johnson County Community Hospital	Mountain City	6.8%	161
Delta Medical Center	Memphis	7.1%	99
Indian Path Medical Center	Kingsport	7.2%	390
Regional Medical Center at Memphis	Memphis	10.4%	364

Combination Chest CT Scan

Hospital Name	City	Rate	Cases
Hardin Medical Center	Savannah	0.0%	271
Hillside Hospital	Pulaski	0.0%	180
Johnson County Community Hospital	Mountain City	0.0%	96
Lakeway Regional Hospital	Morristown	0.0%	98
Lauderdale Community Hospital	Ripley	0.0%	95
Milan General Hospital	Milan	0.0%	59
Riverview Regional Medical Center	Carthage	0.0%	73
Saint Thomas Rutherford Hospital	Murfreesboro	0.0%	87
Sycamore Shoals Hospital	Elizabethton	0.0%	242
Tristar Skyline Medical Center	Nashville	0.0%	402
Unicoi County Memorial Hospital	Erwin	0.0%	86
Sumner Regional Medical Center	Gallatin	0.2%	547
Baptist Memorial Hospital Union City	Union City	0.3%	307
University of Tn Memorial Hospital	Knoxville	0.3%	2614
Wellmont Holston Valley Medical Center	Kingsport	0.3%	333
Blount Memorial Hospital	Maryville	0.4%	710
Methodist Medical Center of Oak Ridge	Oak Ridge	0.4%	739
Regional Hospital of Jackson	Jackson	0.4%	269
Southern Tennessee Medical Center	Winchester	0.4%	267
Jackson - Madison County General Hospital	Jackson	0.6%	1264
Tristar Southern Hills Medical Center	Nashville	0.6%	163
Baptist Memorial Hospital	Memphis	0.7%	1526
Saint Francis Hospital	Memphis	0.7%	281
Tristar Stonecrest Medical Center	Smyrna	0.7%	135
Tristar Horizon Medical Center	Dickson	0.9%	215
Tristar Summit Medical Center	Hermitage	0.9%	429
Crockett Hospital	Lawrenceburg	1.0%	391
Franklin Woods Community Hospital	Johnson City	1.0%	294
McNairy Regional Hospital	Selmer	1.1%	90
Claiborne County Hospital	Tazewell	1.2%	247
Vanderbilt University Hospital	Nashville	1.2%	2968
Tristar Hendersonville Medical Center	Hendersonville	1.3%	233
Dyersburg Regional Medical Center	Dyersburg	1.4%	348
Saint Thomas West Hospital	Nashville	1.4%	834
Henderson County Community Hospital	Lexington	1.7%	60
Indian Path Medical Center	Kingsport	1.8%	164
Saint Thomas Midtown Hospital	Nashville	1.8%	272
Tennova Healthcare	Knoxville	1.8%	1434
Methodist Healthcare Memphis Hospitals	Memphis	1.9%	5952
Johnson City Medical Center	Johnson City	2.0%	662
Tristar Centennial Medical Center	Nashville	2.1%	630
River Park Hospital	Mc Minnville	2.5%	201
Macon County General Hospital	Lafayette	2.8%	108
Laughlin Memorial Hospital	Greeneville	2.9%	547
Volunteer Community Hospital	Martin	2.9%	102
Baptist Memorial Hospital Tipton	Covington	3.1%	797
Methodist Healthcare Fayette Hospital	Somerville	3.1%	96
Saint Francis Bartlett Medical Center	Bartlett	3.1%	226
University Medical Center	Lebanon	3.3%	338
Cumberland Medical Center	Crossville	3.4%	882
Fort Loudoun Medical Center	Lenoir City	3.7%	410
Marshall Medical Center	Lewisburg	3.7%	107
Decatur County General Hospital	Parsons	3.8%	80
Stones River Hosp & Dekalb Comm Hosp	Smithville	4.0%	126
Livingston Regional Hospital	Livingston	4.1%	147
Tennova Healthcare-Jefferson Mem Hosp	Jefferson City	4.2%	309
Copper Basin Medical Center	Copperhill	4.3%	138
Parkwest Medical Center	Knoxville	4.5%	962
Fort Sanders Regional Medical Center	Knoxville	4.6%	740
Gateway Medical Center	Clarksville	4.6%	571
Takoma Regional Hospital	Greeneville	4.6%	174
Leconte Medical Center	Sevierville	4.7%	612
Maury Regional Hospital	Columbia	4.7%	1396
Tennova Healthcare-Newport Med Ctr	Newport	4.8%	189
Sweetwater Hospital Association	Sweetwater	4.9%	204
Memorial Healthcare System	Chattanooga	5.4%	1687
Wellmont Bristol Regional Medical Center	Bristol	5.4%	885
Parkridge Medical Center	Chattanooga	5.5%	310
Regional Medical Center at Memphis	Memphis	5.5%	271
Roane Medical Center	Harriman	6.1%	229
Wayne Medical Center	Waynesboro	6.2%	129
Cookeville Regional Medical Center	Cookeville	6.3%	1015
Williamson Medical Center	Franklin	8.1%	359
Erlanger Medical Center	Chattanooga	8.2%	984
Skyridge Medical Center	Cleveland	8.2%	685
Wellmont Hawkins County Memorial Hospital	Rogersville	8.2%	134
Jamestown Regional Medical Center	Jamestown	8.7%	126
Harton Regional Medical Center	Tullahoma	8.9%	257
Starr Regional Medical Center Athens	Athens	8.9%	190
Henry County Medical Center	Paris	9.1%	492
Highlands Medical Center	Sparta	9.1%	99
Northcrest Medical Center	Springfield	10.1%	367
Starr Regional Medical Center Etowah	Etowah	10.5%	105
Heritage Medical Center	Shelbyville	11.0%	173
Rhea Medical Center	Dayton	11.0%	155
Tennova Healthcare-Lafollett Med Ctr	La Follette	11.8%	186
Morristown Hamblen Hospital Association	Morristown	15.2%	276
Baptist Memorial Hospital Huntingdon	Huntingdon	25.4%	67
United Regional Medical Center	Manchester	26.2%	61
Lincoln Medical Center	Fayetteville	26.6%	169
Grandview Medical Center	Jasper	35.8%	106
Jellico Community Hospital	Jellico	36.1%	119

Follow-up Mammogram/Ultrasound

A follow-up rate near zero may indicate missed cancer; a rate higher than 14% may mean there is unnecessary follow up.

Hospital Name	City	Rate	Cases
Copper Basin Medical Center	Copperhill	2.1%	189
Indian Path Medical Center	Kingsport	3.4%	594
Memorial Healthcare System	Chattanooga	3.6%	5007
Erlanger Medical Center	Chattanooga	3.7%	2187
United Regional Medical Center	Manchester	3.8%	210
Metro Nashville General Hospital	Nashville	4.1%	73
Cumberland Medical Center	Crossville	4.2%	2264
Regional Hospital of Jackson	Jackson	4.3%	233
River Park Hospital	Mc Minnville	4.4%	797
Wellmont Holston Valley Medical Center	Kingsport	4.4%	1671
Gateway Medical Center	Clarksville	4.7%	1404
Wellmont Hawkins County Memorial Hospital	Rogersville	4.7%	274
Morristown Hamblen Hospital Association	Morristown	4.8%	670
Saint Thomas Midtown Hospital	Nashville	4.8%	2088
Skyridge Medical Center	Cleveland	4.9%	1097
Haywood Park Community Hospital	Brownsville	5.0%	278
Livingston Regional Hospital	Livingston	5.0%	398
Johnson County Community Hospital	Mountain City	5.3%	225
Roane Medical Center	Harriman	5.4%	390
Southern Tennessee Medical Center	Winchester	5.4%	1044
McNairy Regional Hospital	Selmer	5.5%	293
Unicoi County Memorial Hospital	Erwin	5.5%	308
Williamson Medical Center	Franklin	5.5%	914
Tristar Horizon Medical Center	Dickson	5.8%	709
Dyersburg Regional Medical Center	Dyersburg	6.1%	899
Fort Sanders Regional Medical Center	Knoxville	6.1%	684
University of Tn Memorial Hospital	Knoxville	6.1%	2152
Volunteer Community Hospital	Martin	6.1%	428
Baptist Memorial Hospital Huntingdon	Huntingdon	6.3%	239
Lauderdale Community Hospital	Ripley	6.7%	285
Lincoln Medical Center	Fayetteville	6.7%	509
Baptist Memorial Hospital Union City	Union City	7.0%	441
Maury Regional Hospital	Columbia	7.1%	2506
Sycamore Shoals Hospital	Elizabethton	7.1%	704
Saint Thomas West Hospital	Nashville	7.2%	1918
Rhea Medical Center	Dayton	7.3%	558
Wellmont Bristol Regional Medical Center	Bristol	7.3%	1295
Johnson City Medical Center	Johnson City	7.4%	3073
Lakeway Regional Hospital	Morristown	7.4%	122
Tristar Summit Medical Center	Hermitage	7.4%	1365
Decatur County General Hospital	Parsons	7.5%	281
Henry County Medical Center	Paris	7.5%	1038
Wayne Medical Center	Waynesboro	7.6%	172
Stones River Hosp & Dekalb Comm Hosp	Smithville	7.7%	286
Marshall Medical Center	Lewisburg	7.8%	370
Hillside Hospital	Pulaski	7.9%	570
Stones River Hosp & Dekalb Comm Hosp	Woodbury	7.9%	76
Sweetwater Hospital Association	Sweetwater	8.0%	225
Tennova Healthcare-Lafollett Med Ctr	La Follette	8.0%	326
Parkwest Medical Center	Knoxville	8.4%	1121
Riverview Regional Medical Center	Carthage	8.6%	163
Tristar Stonecrest Medical Center	Smyrna	8.6%	523
Cookeville Regional Medical Center	Cookeville	8.7%	1443
Milan General Hospital	Milan	8.7%	669
Parkridge Medical Center	Chattanooga	8.9%	587
Tristar Centennial Medical Center	Nashville	8.9%	1129
Starr Regional Medical Center Etowah	Etowah	9.1%	154
Fort Loudoun Medical Center	Lenoir City	9.2%	510
Baptist Memorial Hospital	Memphis	9.4%	3822
Crockett Hospital	Lawrenceburg	9.4%	762
Methodist Medical Center of Oak Ridge	Oak Ridge	9.4%	2572
Heritage Medical Center	Shelbyville	9.5%	623
Jackson - Madison County General Hospital	Jackson	9.6%	2127
Methodist Healthcare Memphis Hospitals	Memphis	9.9%	5444
Northcrest Medical Center	Springfield	10.0%	772
Saint Francis Hospital	Memphis	10.0%	1623
Claiborne County Hospital	Tazewell	10.2%	283
Methodist Healthcare Fayette Hospital	Somerville	10.3%	204
Regional Medical Center at Memphis	Memphis	10.4%	240
Tristar Hendersonville Medical Center	Hendersonville	10.5%	679
Highlands Medical Center	Sparta	10.7%	356
Tristar Skyline Medical Center	Nashville	10.8%	793
Saint Francis Bartlett Medical Center	Bartlett	11.0%	520
University Medical Center	Lebanon	11.1%	701
Vanderbilt University Hospital	Nashville	11.1%	144
Delta Medical Center	Memphis	11.2%	98
Takoma Regional Hospital	Greeneville	11.2%	463
Leconte Medical Center	Sevierville	11.3%	1217
Henderson County Community Hospital	Lexington	11.4%	166
Tennova Healthcare-Jefferson Mem Hosp	Jefferson City	11.6%	774
Starr Regional Medical Center Athens	Athens	11.7%	1017
Tristar Southern Hills Medical Center	Nashville	12.1%	530
Bolivar General Hospital	Bolivar	12.4%	178
Blount Memorial Hospital	Maryville	12.6%	1598
Laughlin Memorial Hospital	Greeneville	13.1%	1011
Grandview Medical Center	Jasper	13.2%	318

NOTE: Hospital profiles are in alphabetical order by state, then city, then hospital within the city; Rankings exclude hospitals with less than 25 cases except for patient surveys which excludes hospitals with less than 100 cases; (a) 100-299 cases; (1) The number of cases/patients is too few to report; (2) Data submitted were based on a sample of cases/patients; (3) Results are based on a shorter time period than required; (4) Data suppressed by CMS for one or more quarters; (5) Results are not available for this reporting period; (6) Fewer than 100 patients completed the HCAHPS survey; (7) No cases met the criteria for this measure; (8) The lower limit of the confidence interval cannot be calculated if the number of observed infections equals zero; (9) No data are available from the state/territory for this reporting period; (10) The scores shown reflect fewer than 50 completed surveys; (11) There were discrepancies in the data collection process; (12) This measure does not apply to this hospital for this reporting period; (13) Results cannot be calculated for this reporting period; (14) The results for this state are combined with nearby states to protect confidentiality; Please refer to the User's Guide for a full explanation of data.

Jamestown Regional Medical Center	Jamestown	13.4%	320
Hardin Medical Center	Savannah	13.7%	614
Tennova Healthcare	Knoxville	14.8%	2596
Baptist Memorial Hospital Tipton	Covington	15.7%	470
Sumner Regional Medical Center	Gallatin	16.2%	635
Tennova Healthcare-Newport Med Ctr	Newport	17.2%	448
Harton Regional Medical Center	Tullahoma	18.9%	1080
Macon County General Hospital	Lafayette	19.3%	192
Jellico Community Hospital	Jellico	21.3%	267

Lumbar Spine MRI for Low Back Pain

Hospital Name	City	Rate	Cases
United Regional Medical Center	Manchester	23.5%	149
Roane Medical Center	Harriman	24.7%	89
Rhea Medical Center	Dayton	27.5%	69
Sumner Regional Medical Center	Gallatin	27.7%	101
Tennova Healthcare	Knoxville	27.7%	256
Tristar Hendersonville Medical Center	Hendersonville	28.0%	82
Fort Sanders Regional Medical Center	Knoxville	29.8%	191
Morristown Hamblen Hospital Association	Morristown	30.1%	176
Henry County Medical Center	Paris	30.3%	152
Methodist Medical Center of Oak Ridge	Oak Ridge	31.0%	300
Tristar Horizon Medical Center	Dickson	31.1%	61
Maury Regional Hospital	Columbia	31.2%	215
Parkridge Medical Center	Chattanooga	31.3%	67
Tristar Skyline Medical Center	Nashville	31.6%	155
Williamson Medical Center	Franklin	31.6%	225
Saint Francis Hospital	Memphis	31.7%	189
Cookeville Regional Medical Center	Cookeville	31.9%	427
Lakeway Regional Hospital	Morristown	32.0%	122
Vanderbilt University Hospital	Nashville	32.1%	56
Gateway Medical Center	Clarksville	32.7%	113
Jackson - Madison County General Hospital	Jackson	32.7%	514
Harton Regional Medical Center	Tullahoma	33.1%	130
Crockett Hospital	Lawrenceburg	33.3%	81
Franklin Woods Community Hospital	Johnson City	33.6%	122
Tennova Healthcare-Jefferson Mem Hosp	Jefferson City	33.8%	80
Leconte Medical Center	Sevierville	34.6%	162
Tristar Centennial Medical Center	Nashville	35.4%	144
Parkwest Medical Center	Knoxville	35.6%	135
Methodist Healthcare Memphis Hospitals	Memphis	35.7%	392
Memorial Healthcare System	Chattanooga	35.8%	413
Johnson City Medical Center	Johnson City	35.9%	248
Southern Tennessee Medical Center	Winchester	36.0%	111
Heritage Medical Center	Shelbyville	36.1%	72
University of Tn Memorial Hospital	Knoxville	36.1%	252
Indian Path Medical Center	Kingsport	36.2%	94
Takoma Regional Hospital	Greeneville	37.0%	46
Dyersburg Regional Medical Center	Dyersburg	37.1%	124
Tristar Summit Medical Center	Hermitage	37.1%	143
Baptist Memorial Hospital	Memphis	37.2%	199
Fort Loudoun Medical Center	Lenoir City	37.5%	72
Livingston Regional Hospital	Livingston	38.6%	70
River Park Hospital	Mc Minnville	38.8%	85
Erlanger Medical Center	Chattanooga	39.0%	82
Saint Francis Bartlett Medical Center	Bartlett	39.0%	59
Starr Regional Medical Center Athens	Athens	39.0%	105
Highlands Medical Center	Sparta	39.2%	51
Saint Thomas West Hospital	Nashville	39.6%	111
Skyridge Medical Center	Cleveland	39.6%	255
Wellmont Bristol Regional Medical Center	Bristol	40.0%	365
Hardin Medical Center	Savannah	40.8%	76
Claiborne County Hospital	Tazewell	41.3%	92
Sweetwater Hospital Association	Sweetwater	41.7%	48
Baptist Memorial Hospital Union City	Union City	42.6%	115
Sycamore Shoals Hospital	Elizabethton	42.9%	84
University Medical Center	Lebanon	43.2%	44
Starr Regional Medical Center Etowah	Etowah	43.3%	60
Unicoi County Memorial Hospital	Erwin	43.9%	41
Cumberland Medical Center	Crossville	44.2%	308
Blount Memorial Hospital	Maryville	45.0%	189
Tennova Healthcare-Lafollett Med Ctr	La Follette	46.0%	87
Laughlin Memorial Hospital	Greeneville	46.7%	107
Tennova Healthcare-Newport Med Ctr	Newport	51.0%	51
Wellmont Hawkins County Memorial Hospital	Rogersville	63.8%	47

NOTE: Hospital profiles are in alphabetical order by state, then city, then hospital within the city; Rankings exclude hospitals with less than 25 cases except for patient surveys which excludes hospitals with less than 100 cases; (a) 100-299 cases; (1) The number of cases/patients is too few to report; (2) Data submitted were based on a sample of cases/patients; (3) Results are based on a shorter time period than required; (4) Data suppressed by CMS for one or more quarters; (5) Results are not available for this reporting period; (6) Fewer than 100 patients completed the HCAHPS survey; (7) No cases met the criteria for this measure; (8) The lower limit of the confidence interval cannot be calculated if the number of observed infections equals zero; (9) No data are available from the state/territory for this reporting period; (10) The scores shown reflect fewer than 50 completed surveys; (11) There were discrepancies in the data collection process; (12) This measure does not apply to this hospital for this reporting period; (13) Results cannot be calculated for this reporting period; (14) The results for this state are combined with nearby states to protect confidentiality; Please refer to the User's Guide for a full explanation of data.

Tristar Ashland City Medical Center

313 North Main St
Ashland City, TN 37015
Phone: 615-792-3030
URL: www.centennialashlandcity.com
Type: Critical Access Hospitals
Emergency Services: Yes
Ownership: Proprietary
Beds: 12
Key Personnel:
Administrator . . . . Darrell White, RN

Measure	Cases	This Hosp.	State Avg.	U.S. Avg.
Blood Clot Prevention and Treatment				
Anticoagulation Overlap Therapy[1,2]	-	-	92%	93%
ICU Venous Thromboembolism Prophylaxis[2,7]	-	-	90%	92%
Incidence of Potentially Preventable VTE[2,7]	-	-	10%	10%
UFH with Dosages/Platelet Monitoring[2,7]	-	-	99%	97%
Venous Thromboembolism Prophylaxis[2]	54	87%	83%	85%
Warfarin Therapy Discharge Instructions[1,2]	-	-	78%	75%
Chest Pain/Possible Heart Attack Care				
Aspirin Given Within 24 Hours of Arrival	51	100%	96%	96%
Fibrinolytic Meds Within 30 Min. of Arrival[7]	-	-	72%	58%
Average Time to ECG (minutes)	53	6	6	7
Average Time to Transfer (minutes)[1]	-	-	53	60
Children's Asthma Care				
Received Home Management Plan of Care	-	-	-	88%
Received Reliever Medication	-	-	-	100%
Received Systemic Corticosteroids	-	-	-	100%
Emergency Department				
Admittance Decision Time (minutes)[2]	57	45	82	98
Head CT Results Within 45 Min. of Arrival[1]	-	-	52%	57%
Patients Who Left ER Before Being Seen	11,762	1%	2%	2%
Time from ER Arrival to Admit. (minutes)[2]	60	166	243	274
Time from ER Arrival to Discharge (minutes)	394	79	131	134
Time in ER Before Being Evaluated (minutes)	431	12	25	26
Time to Pain Meds for Fractures (minutes)	27	43	60	57
Heart Attack Care				
Aspirin Given at Discharge[5]	-	-	99%	99%
Fibrinolytic Meds Within 30 Min. of Arrival[5]	-	-	33%	54%
PCI Within 90 Minutes of Arrival[5]	-	-	98%	96%
Statin Prescribed at Discharge[5]	-	-	99%	98%
Heart Failure Care				
ACE Inhibitor or ARB for LVSD[5]	-	-	97%	97%
Discharge Instructions Given[5]	-	-	93%	94%
Evaluation of LVS Function[5]	-	-	99%	99%
Medicare Spending				
Medicare Spending per Patient (ratio)	-	-	1	0.98
Pneumonia Care				
Appropriate Initial Antibiotic Given[1,2]	-	-	95%	95%
Blood Culture Timing[1,2]	-	-	98%	98%
Pregnancy and Delivery Care				
Newborn Deliveries Scheduled Early[2,7]	-	-	6%	6%
Preventive Care				
Immunization for Influenza[2]	46	100%	93%	90%
Immunization for Pneumonia[2]	66	97%	93%	92%
Stroke Care				
Anticoagulation Therapy for Atrial Fibrillation[5]	-	-	94%	95%
Antithrombotic Therapy Timing[5]	-	-	97%	98%
Assessed for Rehabilitation[5]	-	-	97%	97%
Discharged on Antithrombotic Therapy[5]	-	-	99%	99%
Discharged on Statin Medication[5]	-	-	94%	94%
Thrombolytic Therapy Timing[5]	-	-	57%	66%
Venous Thromboembolism Prophylaxis[5]	-	-	93%	94%
Written Stroke Educational Materials Given[5]	-	-	84%	88%
Surgical Care Improvement Project				
Appropriate Beta Blocker Usage[5]	-	-	97%	98%
Appropriate VTP Within 24 Hours[5]	-	-	98%	98%
Controlled Postoperative Blood Glucose[5]	-	-	95%	97%
Perioperative Temperature Management[5]	-	-	100%	100%
Prophylactic Antibiotic Selection[5]	-	-	99%	99%
Prophylactic Antibiotic Selection (Outpatient)[1,3]	-	-	98%	98%
Prophylactic Antibiotic Stopped[5]	-	-	98%	98%
Prophylactic Antibiotic Timing[5]	-	-	99%	99%
Prophylactic Antibiotic Timing (Outpatient)[1,3]	-	-	98%	98%
Urinary Catheter Removal[5]	-	-	96%	97%
Survey of Patients' Hospital Experiences				
Area Around Room 'Always' Quiet at Night[10]	<100	85%	67%	61%
Doctors 'Always' Communicated Well[10]	<100	97%	84%	82%
Home Recovery Information Given[10]	<100	89%	85%	85%
Hospital Given 9 or 10 on 10 Point Scale[10]	<100	82%	70%	71%
Meds 'Always' Explained Before Given[10]	<100	100%	66%	64%
Nurses 'Always' Communicated Well[10]	<100	89%	80%	79%
Pain 'Always' Well Controlled[10]	<100	71%	72%	71%
Room and Bathroom 'Always' Clean[10]	<100	79%	73%	73%
Timely Help 'Always' Received[10]	<100	89%	68%	68%
Would Definitely Recommend Hospital[10]	<100	88%	70%	71%
Use of Medical Imaging				
Cardiac Imaging Stress Test before Surgery[7]	-	-	4.8%	5.3%
Combination Abdominal CT Scan	79	7.6%	9.6%	10.5%
Combination Brain/Sinus CT Scan	131	0.0%	3.3%	2.7%
Combination Chest CT Scan[1]	-	-	3.4%	2.7%
Follow-up Mammogram/Ultrasound[1]	-	-	8.3%	8.8%
Lumbar Spine MRI for Low Back Pain[1]	-	-	35.3%	37.2%

Starr Regional Medical Center Athens

1114 W Madison Ave
Athens, TN 37371
Phone: 423-745-1411
Fax: 423-745-8630
URL: www.athensrmc.com
Type: Acute Care Hospitals
Emergency Services: Yes
Ownership: Proprietary
Beds: 118
Key Personnel:
Emergency Room . . . . Brett Atchley, MD
Chief of Medical Staff. . . . . Michael Hahn
Radiology. . . . . Douglas S Hayes, RT
CEO . . . . Mark Nichols
Cardiac Laboratory. . . . . Judy Parham
CEO/President. . . . . John Workman

Measure	Cases	This Hosp.	State Avg.	U.S. Avg.
Blood Clot Prevention and Treatment				
Anticoagulation Overlap Therapy[2]	29	93%	92%	93%
ICU Venous Thromboembolism Prophylaxis[2]	50	100%	90%	92%
Incidence of Potentially Preventable VTE[1,2]	-	-	10%	10%
UFH with Dosages/Platelet Monitoring[1,2]	-	-	99%	97%
Venous Thromboembolism Prophylaxis[2]	204	98%	83%	85%
Warfarin Therapy Discharge Instructions[2]	27	100%	78%	75%
Chest Pain/Possible Heart Attack Care				
Aspirin Given Within 24 Hours of Arrival	123	98%	96%	96%
Fibrinolytic Meds Within 30 Min. of Arrival[1]	-	-	72%	58%
Average Time to ECG (minutes)	126	4	6	7
Average Time to Transfer (minutes)[1]	-	-	53	60
Children's Asthma Care				
Received Home Management Plan of Care	-	-	-	88%
Received Reliever Medication	-	-	-	100%
Received Systemic Corticosteroids	-	-	-	100%
Emergency Department				
Admittance Decision Time (minutes)[2]	265	70	82	98
Head CT Results Within 45 Min. of Arrival[1]	-	-	52%	57%
Patients Who Left ER Before Being Seen	33,015	2%	2%	2%
Time from ER Arrival to Admit. (minutes)[2]	265	219	243	274
Time from ER Arrival to Discharge (minutes)	403	81	131	134
Time in ER Before Being Evaluated (minutes)	430	13	25	26
Time to Pain Meds for Fractures (minutes)	89	54	60	57
Heart Attack Care				
Aspirin Given at Discharge[1]	-	-	99%	99%
Fibrinolytic Meds Within 30 Min. of Arrival[7]	-	-	33%	54%
PCI Within 90 Minutes of Arrival[7]	-	-	98%	96%
Statin Prescribed at Discharge[1]	-	-	99%	98%
Heart Failure Care				
ACE Inhibitor or ARB for LVSD	19	100%	97%	97%
Discharge Instructions Given	46	98%	93%	94%
Evaluation of LVS Function	54	98%	99%	99%
Medicare Spending				
Medicare Spending per Patient (ratio)	-	1.06	1	0.98
Pneumonia Care				
Appropriate Initial Antibiotic Given	83	99%	95%	95%
Blood Culture Timing	115	98%	98%	98%
Pregnancy and Delivery Care				
Newborn Deliveries Scheduled Early[2]	35	17%	6%	6%
Preventive Care				
Immunization for Influenza[2]	272	97%	93%	90%
Immunization for Pneumonia[2]	304	97%	93%	92%
Stroke Care				
Anticoagulation Therapy for Atrial Fibrillation[7]	-	-	94%	95%
Antithrombotic Therapy Timing	14	86%	97%	98%
Assessed for Rehabilitation	11	100%	97%	97%
Discharged on Antithrombotic Therapy	11	100%	99%	99%
Discharged on Statin Medication	11	55%	94%	94%
Thrombolytic Therapy Timing[1]	-	-	57%	66%
Venous Thromboembolism Prophylaxis	13	77%	93%	94%
Written Stroke Educational Materials Given[1]	-	-	84%	88%
Surgical Care Improvement Project				
Appropriate Beta Blocker Usage	28	86%	97%	98%
Appropriate VTP Within 24 Hours	97	94%	98%	98%
Controlled Postoperative Blood Glucose[7]	-	-	95%	97%
Perioperative Temperature Management	122	100%	100%	100%
Prophylactic Antibiotic Selection	82	99%	99%	99%
Prophylactic Antibiotic Selection (Outpatient)	63	94%	98%	98%
Prophylactic Antibiotic Stopped	80	95%	98%	98%
Prophylactic Antibiotic Timing	82	100%	99%	99%
Prophylactic Antibiotic Timing (Outpatient)	65	97%	98%	98%
Urinary Catheter Removal	62	90%	96%	97%
Survey of Patients' Hospital Experiences				
Area Around Room 'Always' Quiet at Night	300+	68%	67%	61%
Doctors 'Always' Communicated Well	300+	84%	84%	82%
Home Recovery Information Given	300+	86%	85%	85%
Hospital Given 9 or 10 on 10 Point Scale	300+	66%	70%	71%
Meds 'Always' Explained Before Given	300+	60%	66%	64%
Nurses 'Always' Communicated Well	300+	77%	80%	79%
Pain 'Always' Well Controlled	300+	72%	72%	71%
Room and Bathroom 'Always' Clean	300+	68%	73%	73%
Timely Help 'Always' Received	300+	63%	68%	68%
Would Definitely Recommend Hospital	300+	66%	70%	71%
Use of Medical Imaging				
Cardiac Imaging Stress Test before Surgery	179	6.1%	4.8%	5.3%
Combination Abdominal CT Scan	448	18.3%	9.6%	10.5%
Combination Brain/Sinus CT Scan	429	4.0%	3.3%	2.7%
Combination Chest CT Scan	190	8.9%	3.4%	2.7%
Follow-up Mammogram/Ultrasound	1,017	11.7%	8.3%	8.8%
Lumbar Spine MRI for Low Back Pain	105	39.0%	35.3%	37.2%

Saint Francis Bartlett Medical Center

2986 Kate Bond Rd
Bartlett, TN 38133
Phone: 901-820-7050
Fax: 901-820-7051
URL: www.saintfrancisbartlett.com
Type: Acute Care Hospitals
Emergency Services: Yes
Ownership: Proprietary
Beds: 100
Key Personnel:
Chief of Medical Staff. . . . . Peter Lindy, MD
CEO/President. . . . . Kern Mullins
Emergency Room . . . . Clinton Price

Measure	Cases	This Hosp.	State Avg.	U.S. Avg.
Blood Clot Prevention and Treatment				
Anticoagulation Overlap Therapy[2]	81	95%	92%	93%
ICU Venous Thromboembolism Prophylaxis[2]	69	93%	90%	92%
Incidence of Potentially Preventable VTE[1,2]	-	-	10%	10%
UFH with Dosages/Platelet Monitoring[2]	75	100%	99%	97%
Venous Thromboembolism Prophylaxis[2]	386	89%	83%	85%
Warfarin Therapy Discharge Instructions[2]	57	100%	78%	75%
Chest Pain/Possible Heart Attack Care				
Aspirin Given Within 24 Hours of Arrival	48	98%	96%	96%
Fibrinolytic Meds Within 30 Min. of Arrival[7]	-	-	72%	58%
Average Time to ECG (minutes)	47	6	6	7
Average Time to Transfer (minutes)	18	36	53	60
Children's Asthma Care				
Received Home Management Plan of Care	-	-	-	88%
Received Reliever Medication	-	-	-	100%
Received Systemic Corticosteroids	-	-	-	100%
Emergency Department				
Admittance Decision Time (minutes)[2]	791	107	82	98
Head CT Results Within 45 Min. of Arrival[1]	-	-	52%	57%
Patients Who Left ER Before Being Seen	36,561	3%	2%	2%
Time from ER Arrival to Admit. (minutes)[2]	818	364	243	274
Time from ER Arrival to Discharge (minutes)	462	211	131	134

NOTE: Hospital profiles are in alphabetical order by state, then city, then hospital within the city; Rankings exclude hospitals with less than 25 cases except for patient surveys which excludes hospitals with less than 100 cases; (a) 100-299 cases; (1) The number of cases/patients is too few to report; (2) Data submitted were based on a sample of cases/patients; (3) Results are based on a shorter time period than required; (4) Data suppressed by CMS for one or more quarters; (5) Results are not available for this reporting period; (6) Fewer than 100 patients completed the HCAHPS survey; (7) No cases met the criteria for this measure; (8) The lower limit of the confidence interval cannot be calculated if the number of observed infections equals zero; (9) No data are available from the state/territory for this reporting period; (10) The scores shown reflect fewer than 50 completed surveys; (11) There were discrepancies in the data collection process; (12) This measure does not apply to this hospital for this reporting period; (13) Results cannot be calculated for this reporting period; (14) The results for this state are combined with nearby states to protect confidentiality; Please refer to the User's Guide for a full explanation of data.

Time in ER Before Being Evaluated (minutes)	477	57	25	26
Time to Pain Meds for Fractures (minutes)	122	86	60	57
Heart Attack Care				
Aspirin Given at Discharge	27	93%	99%	99%
Fibrinolytic Meds Within 30 Min. of Arrival[7]	-	-	33%	54%
PCI Within 90 Minutes of Arrival[7]	-	-	98%	96%
Statin Prescribed at Discharge	26	100%	99%	98%
Heart Failure Care				
ACE Inhibitor or ARB for LVSD	46	100%	97%	97%
Discharge Instructions Given	154	97%	93%	94%
Evaluation of LVS Function	189	100%	99%	99%
Medicare Spending				
Medicare Spending per Patient (ratio)	-	1.05	1	0.98
Pneumonia Care				
Appropriate Initial Antibiotic Given[2]	133	95%	95%	95%
Blood Culture Timing[2]	170	98%	98%	98%
Pregnancy and Delivery Care				
Newborn Deliveries Scheduled Early[2]	27	26%	6%	6%
Preventive Care				
Immunization for Influenza[2]	589	89%	93%	90%
Immunization for Pneumonia[2]	722	95%	93%	92%
Stroke Care				
Anticoagulation Therapy for Atrial Fibrillation[1]	-	-	94%	95%
Antithrombotic Therapy Timing	60	98%	97%	98%
Assessed for Rehabilitation	59	97%	97%	97%
Discharged on Antithrombotic Therapy	56	98%	99%	99%
Discharged on Statin Medication	43	98%	94%	94%
Thrombolytic Therapy Timing[1]	-	-	57%	66%
Venous Thromboembolism Prophylaxis	61	92%	93%	94%
Written Stroke Educational Materials Given	32	97%	84%	88%
Surgical Care Improvement Project				
Appropriate Beta Blocker Usage[2]	113	96%	97%	98%
Appropriate VTP Within 24 Hours[2]	267	97%	98%	98%
Controlled Postoperative Blood Glucose[2,7]	-	-	95%	97%
Perioperative Temperature Management[2]	395	100%	100%	100%
Prophylactic Antibiotic Selection[2]	269	100%	99%	99%
Prophylactic Antibiotic Selection (Outpatient)	178	98%	98%	98%
Prophylactic Antibiotic Stopped[2]	260	98%	98%	98%
Prophylactic Antibiotic Timing[2]	269	100%	99%	99%
Prophylactic Antibiotic Timing (Outpatient)	179	98%	98%	98%
Urinary Catheter Removal[2]	96	100%	96%	97%
Survey of Patients' Hospital Experiences				
Area Around Room 'Always' Quiet at Night	300+	69%	67%	61%
Doctors 'Always' Communicated Well	300+	81%	84%	82%
Home Recovery Information Given	300+	85%	85%	85%
Hospital Given 9 or 10 on 10 Point Scale	300+	68%	70%	71%
Meds 'Always' Explained Before Given	300+	61%	66%	64%
Nurses 'Always' Communicated Well	300+	74%	80%	79%
Pain 'Always' Well Controlled	300+	71%	72%	71%
Room and Bathroom 'Always' Clean	300+	65%	73%	73%
Timely Help 'Always' Received	300+	66%	68%	68%
Would Definitely Recommend Hospital	300+	71%	70%	71%
Use of Medical Imaging				
Cardiac Imaging Stress Test before Surgery	105	0.0%	4.8%	5.3%
Combination Abdominal CT Scan	631	10.5%	9.6%	10.5%
Combination Brain/Sinus CT Scan	542	5.5%	3.3%	2.7%
Combination Chest CT Scan	226	3.1%	3.4%	2.7%
Follow-up Mammogram/Ultrasound	520	11.0%	8.3%	8.8%
Lumbar Spine MRI for Low Back Pain	59	39.0%	35.3%	37.2%

Bolivar General Hospital

650 Nuckolls Road
Bolivar, TN 38008
URL: www.wth.net
Type: Acute Care Hospitals
Ownership: Govt - Hospital Dist/Auth

Phone: 731-658-3100
Fax: 731-658-2843

Emergency Services: Yes
Beds: 61

Key Personnel:
Radiology. . . . . Gregory Bruno
Chief of Medical Staff. . . . . Charles Frost
CEO/President. . . . . Ruby Kirby

Measure	Cases	This Hosp.	State Avg.	U.S. Avg.
Blood Clot Prevention and Treatment				
Anticoagulation Overlap Therapy[2,7]	-	-	92%	93%
ICU Venous Thromboembolism Prophylaxis[2,7]	-	-	90%	92%
Incidence of Potentially Preventable VTE[2,7]	-	-	10%	10%
UFH with Dosages/Platelet Monitoring[2,7]	-	-	99%	97%
Venous Thromboembolism Prophylaxis[2]	87	46%	83%	85%
Warfarin Therapy Discharge Instructions[2,7]	-	-	78%	75%
Chest Pain/Possible Heart Attack Care				
Aspirin Given Within 24 Hours of Arrival	108	97%	96%	96%
Fibrinolytic Meds Within 30 Min. of Arrival[1]	-	-	72%	58%
Average Time to ECG (minutes)	116	4	6	7
Average Time to Transfer (minutes)[1]	-	-	53	60
Children's Asthma Care				
Received Home Management Plan of Care	-	-	-	88%
Received Reliever Medication	-	-	-	100%
Received Systemic Corticosteroids	-	-	-	100%
Emergency Department				
Admittance Decision Time (minutes)	189	93	82	98
Head CT Results Within 45 Min. of Arrival[1]	-	-	52%	57%
Patients Who Left ER Before Being Seen	9,900	4%	2%	2%
Time from ER Arrival to Admit. (minutes)	189	262	243	274
Time from ER Arrival to Discharge (minutes)	362	124	131	134
Time in ER Before Being Evaluated (minutes)	414	41	25	26
Time to Pain Meds for Fractures (minutes)	30	62	60	57
Heart Attack Care				
Aspirin Given at Discharge[1,3]	-	-	99%	99%
Fibrinolytic Meds Within 30 Min. of Arrival[3,7]	-	-	33%	54%
PCI Within 90 Minutes of Arrival[3,7]	-	-	98%	96%
Statin Prescribed at Discharge[1,3]	-	-	99%	98%
Heart Failure Care				
ACE Inhibitor or ARB for LVSD[1]	-	-	97%	97%
Discharge Instructions Given	12	100%	93%	94%
Evaluation of LVS Function	11	100%	99%	99%
Medicare Spending				
Medicare Spending per Patient (ratio)	-	1.02	1	0.98
Pneumonia Care				
Appropriate Initial Antibiotic Given	12	67%	95%	95%
Blood Culture Timing	21	100%	98%	98%
Pregnancy and Delivery Care				
Newborn Deliveries Scheduled Early[7]	-	-	6%	6%
Preventive Care				
Immunization for Influenza	99	98%	93%	90%
Immunization for Pneumonia	140	99%	93%	92%
Stroke Care				
Anticoagulation Therapy for Atrial Fibrillation[3,7]	-	-	94%	95%
Antithrombotic Therapy Timing[1,3]	-	-	97%	98%
Assessed for Rehabilitation[1,3]	-	-	97%	97%
Discharged on Antithrombotic Therapy[1,3]	-	-	99%	99%
Discharged on Statin Medication[1,3]	-	-	94%	94%
Thrombolytic Therapy Timing[3,7]	-	-	57%	66%
Venous Thromboembolism Prophylaxis[1,3]	-	-	93%	94%
Written Stroke Educational Materials Given[3,7]	-	-	84%	88%
Surgical Care Improvement Project				
Appropriate Beta Blocker Usage[5]	-	-	97%	98%
Appropriate VTP Within 24 Hours[5]	-	-	98%	98%
Controlled Postoperative Blood Glucose[5]	-	-	95%	97%
Perioperative Temperature Management[5]	-	-	100%	100%
Prophylactic Antibiotic Selection[5]	-	-	99%	99%
Prophylactic Antibiotic Selection (Outpatient)[5]	-	-	98%	98%
Prophylactic Antibiotic Stopped[5]	-	-	98%	98%
Prophylactic Antibiotic Timing[5]	-	-	99%	99%
Prophylactic Antibiotic Timing (Outpatient)[5]	-	-	98%	98%
Urinary Catheter Removal[5]	-	-	96%	97%
Survey of Patients' Hospital Experiences				
Area Around Room 'Always' Quiet at Night[10]	<100	90%	67%	61%
Doctors 'Always' Communicated Well[10]	<100	88%	84%	82%
Home Recovery Information Given[10]	<100	93%	85%	85%
Hospital Given 9 or 10 on 10 Point Scale[10]	<100	72%	70%	71%
Meds 'Always' Explained Before Given[10]	<100	77%	66%	64%
Nurses 'Always' Communicated Well[10]	<100	93%	80%	79%
Pain 'Always' Well Controlled[10]	<100	88%	72%	71%
Room and Bathroom 'Always' Clean[10]	<100	97%	73%	73%
Timely Help 'Always' Received[10]	<100	93%	68%	68%
Would Definitely Recommend Hospital[10]	<100	69%	70%	71%
Use of Medical Imaging				
Cardiac Imaging Stress Test before Surgery[7]	-	-	4.8%	5.3%
Combination Abdominal CT Scan	102	1.0%	9.6%	10.5%
Combination Brain/Sinus CT Scan[1]	-	-	3.3%	2.7%
Combination Chest CT Scan[1]	-	-	3.4%	2.7%
Follow-up Mammogram/Ultrasound	178	12.4%	8.3%	8.8%
Lumbar Spine MRI for Low Back Pain[7]	-	-	35.3%	37.2%

Wellmont Bristol Regional Medical Center

One Medical Park Blvd
Bristol, TN 37620
URL: www.wellmont.org
Type: Acute Care Hospitals
Ownership: Govt - Hospital Dist/Auth

Phone: 423-844-1121
Fax: 423-844-4202

Emergency Services: Yes
Beds: 348

Key Personnel:
Anesthesiology. . . . . Dennis Aguirre, MD
CEO/President. . . . . Bart Hove
Chief of Medical Staff . . . . Gail Stanley, MD

Measure	Cases	This Hosp.	State Avg.	U.S. Avg.
Blood Clot Prevention and Treatment				
Anticoagulation Overlap Therapy[2]	97	98%	92%	93%
ICU Venous Thromboembolism Prophylaxis[2]	14	86%	90%	92%
Incidence of Potentially Preventable VTE[1,2]	-	-	10%	10%
UFH with Dosages/Platelet Monitoring[2]	42	100%	99%	97%
Venous Thromboembolism Prophylaxis[2]	359	87%	83%	85%
Warfarin Therapy Discharge Instructions[2]	82	100%	78%	75%
Chest Pain/Possible Heart Attack Care				
Aspirin Given Within 24 Hours of Arrival[3,7]	-	-	96%	96%
Fibrinolytic Meds Within 30 Min. of Arrival[5]	-	-	72%	58%
Average Time to ECG (minutes)[3,7]	-	-	6	7
Average Time to Transfer (minutes)[5]	-	-	53	60
Children's Asthma Care				
Received Home Management Plan of Care	-	-	-	88%
Received Reliever Medication	-	-	-	100%
Received Systemic Corticosteroids	-	-	-	100%
Emergency Department				
Admittance Decision Time (minutes)[2]	589	122	82	98
Head CT Results Within 45 Min. of Arrival[1]	-	-	52%	57%
Patients Who Left ER Before Being Seen	64,536	3%	2%	2%
Time from ER Arrival to Admit. (minutes)[2]	602	282	243	274
Time from ER Arrival to Discharge (minutes)	351	175	131	134
Time in ER Before Being Evaluated (minutes)	377	56	25	26
Time to Pain Meds for Fractures (minutes)	147	71	60	57
Heart Attack Care				
Aspirin Given at Discharge[2]	262	100%	99%	99%
Fibrinolytic Meds Within 30 Min. of Arrival[2,7]	-	-	33%	54%
PCI Within 90 Minutes of Arrival[2]	32	100%	98%	96%
Statin Prescribed at Discharge[2]	255	100%	99%	98%
Heart Failure Care				
ACE Inhibitor or ARB for LVSD[2]	69	100%	97%	97%
Discharge Instructions Given[2]	218	100%	93%	94%
Evaluation of LVS Function[2]	268	100%	99%	99%
Medicare Spending				
Medicare Spending per Patient (ratio)	-	1.03	1	0.98
Pneumonia Care				
Appropriate Initial Antibiotic Given[2]	77	97%	95%	95%
Blood Culture Timing[2]	124	98%	98%	98%
Pregnancy and Delivery Care				
Newborn Deliveries Scheduled Early[2]	43	7%	6%	6%
Preventive Care				
Immunization for Influenza[2]	553	98%	93%	90%
Immunization for Pneumonia[2]	805	99%	93%	92%
Stroke Care				
Anticoagulation Therapy for Atrial Fibrillation	19	100%	94%	95%
Antithrombotic Therapy Timing	174	100%	97%	98%
Assessed for Rehabilitation	209	100%	97%	97%
Discharged on Antithrombotic Therapy	185	100%	99%	99%
Discharged on Statin Medication	124	98%	94%	94%
Thrombolytic Therapy Timing[1]	-	-	57%	66%
Venous Thromboembolism Prophylaxis	219	100%	93%	94%
Written Stroke Educational Materials Given	110	100%	84%	88%
Surgical Care Improvement Project				
Appropriate Beta Blocker Usage[2]	176	100%	97%	98%

NOTE: Hospital profiles are in alphabetical order by state, then city, then hospital within the city; Rankings exclude hospitals with less than 25 cases except for patient surveys which excludes hospitals with less than 100 cases; (a) 100-299 cases; (1) The number of cases/patients is too few to report; (2) Data submitted were based on a sample of cases/patients; (3) Results are based on a shorter time period than required; (4) Data suppressed by CMS for one or more quarters; (5) Results are not available for this reporting period; (6) Fewer than 100 patients completed the HCAHPS survey; (7) No cases met the criteria for this measure; (8) The lower limit of the confidence interval cannot be calculated if the number of observed infections equals zero; (9) No data are available from the state/territory for this reporting period; (10) The scores shown reflect fewer than 50 completed surveys; (11) There were discrepancies in the data collection process; (12) This measure does not apply to this hospital for this reporting period; (13) Results cannot be calculated for this reporting period; (14) The results for this state are combined with nearby states to protect confidentiality; Please refer to the User's Guide for a full explanation of data.

Measure	Cases	This Hosp.	State Avg.	U.S. Avg.
Appropriate VTP Within 24 Hours[2]	285	99%	98%	98%
Controlled Postoperative Blood Glucose[2]	97	96%	95%	97%
Perioperative Temperature Management[2]	419	100%	100%	100%
Prophylactic Antibiotic Selection[2]	304	98%	99%	99%
Prophylactic Antibiotic Selection (Outpatient)	440	99%	98%	98%
Prophylactic Antibiotic Stopped[2]	292	99%	98%	98%
Prophylactic Antibiotic Timing[2]	304	100%	99%	99%
Prophylactic Antibiotic Timing (Outpatient)	441	99%	98%	98%
Urinary Catheter Removal[2]	250	97%	96%	97%
Survey of Patients' Hospital Experiences				
Area Around Room 'Always' Quiet at Night	300+	64%	67%	61%
Doctors 'Always' Communicated Well	300+	82%	84%	82%
Home Recovery Information Given	300+	83%	85%	85%
Hospital Given 9 or 10 on 10 Point Scale	300+	72%	70%	71%
Meds 'Always' Explained Before Given	300+	61%	66%	64%
Nurses 'Always' Communicated Well	300+	82%	80%	79%
Pain 'Always' Well Controlled	300+	71%	72%	71%
Room and Bathroom 'Always' Clean	300+	72%	73%	73%
Timely Help 'Always' Received	300+	65%	68%	68%
Would Definitely Recommend Hospital	300+	74%	70%	71%
Use of Medical Imaging				
Cardiac Imaging Stress Test before Surgery	627	5.4%	4.8%	5.3%
Combination Abdominal CT Scan	1,376	10.3%	9.6%	10.5%
Combination Brain/Sinus CT Scan	797	3.5%	3.3%	2.7%
Combination Chest CT Scan	885	5.4%	3.4%	2.7%
Follow-up Mammogram/Ultrasound	1,295	7.3%	8.3%	8.8%
Lumbar Spine MRI for Low Back Pain	365	40.0%	35.3%	37.2%

Haywood Park Community Hospital

2545 N Washington Ave
Brownsville, TN 38012
Phone: 731-772-4110
Fax: 731-772-9428
Type: Acute Care Hospitals
Emergency Services: Yes
Ownership: Proprietary
Beds: 62

Key Personnel:
CEO/President. . . . . Kim Anthony
Operating Room. . . . . Dr Percival
Radiology. . . . . Ann Tran
Infection Control. . . . . Hannah Vickers, RN

Measure	Cases	This Hosp.	State Avg.	U.S. Avg.
Blood Clot Prevention and Treatment				
Anticoagulation Overlap Therapy[2,7]	-	-	92%	93%
ICU Venous Thromboembolism Prophylaxis[2,7]	-	-	90%	92%
Incidence of Potentially Preventable VTE[2,7]	-	-	10%	10%
UFH with Dosages/Platelet Monitoring[2,7]	-	-	99%	97%
Venous Thromboembolism Prophylaxis[2]	134	81%	83%	85%
Warfarin Therapy Discharge Instructions[2,7]	-	-	78%	75%
Chest Pain/Possible Heart Attack Care				
Aspirin Given Within 24 Hours of Arrival	87	99%	96%	96%
Fibrinolytic Meds Within 30 Min. of Arrival[1]	-	-	72%	58%
Average Time to ECG (minutes)	89	9	6	7
Average Time to Transfer (minutes)[1]	-	-	53	60
Children's Asthma Care				
Received Home Management Plan of Care	-	-	-	88%
Received Reliever Medication	-	-	-	100%
Received Systemic Corticosteroids	-	-	-	100%
Emergency Department				
Admittance Decision Time (minutes)[2]	171	49	82	98
Head CT Results Within 45 Min. of Arrival[1]	-	-	52%	57%
Patients Who Left ER Before Being Seen	6,230	1%	2%	2%
Time from ER Arrival to Admit. (minutes)[2]	179	183	243	274
Time from ER Arrival to Discharge (minutes)	321	63	131	134
Time in ER Before Being Evaluated (minutes)	420	24	25	26
Time to Pain Meds for Fractures (minutes)	20	44	60	57
Heart Attack Care				
Aspirin Given at Discharge[1,3]	-	-	99%	99%
Fibrinolytic Meds Within 30 Min. of Arrival[3,7]	-	-	33%	54%
PCI Within 90 Minutes of Arrival[3,7]	-	-	98%	96%
Statin Prescribed at Discharge[1,3]	-	-	99%	98%
Heart Failure Care				
ACE Inhibitor or ARB for LVSD[1]	-	-	97%	97%
Discharge Instructions Given[1]	-	-	93%	94%
Evaluation of LVS Function[1]	-	-	99%	99%
Medicare Spending				
Medicare Spending per Patient (ratio)	-	1.00	1	0.98
Pneumonia Care				
Appropriate Initial Antibiotic Given	17	100%	95%	95%
Blood Culture Timing	21	100%	98%	98%
Pregnancy and Delivery Care				
Newborn Deliveries Scheduled Early[2,7]	-	-	6%	6%
Preventive Care				
Immunization for Influenza[2]	183	99%	93%	90%
Immunization for Pneumonia[2]	222	98%	93%	92%
Stroke Care				
Anticoagulation Therapy for Atrial Fibrillation[1,3]	-	-	94%	95%
Antithrombotic Therapy Timing[1,3]	-	-	97%	98%
Assessed for Rehabilitation[1,3]	-	-	97%	97%
Discharged on Antithrombotic Therapy[1,3]	-	-	99%	99%
Discharged on Statin Medication[1,3]	-	-	94%	94%
Thrombolytic Therapy Timing[3,7]	-	-	57%	66%
Venous Thromboembolism Prophylaxis[1,3]	-	-	93%	94%
Written Stroke Educational Materials Given[1,3]	-	-	84%	88%
Surgical Care Improvement Project				
Appropriate Beta Blocker Usage[5]	-	-	97%	98%
Appropriate VTP Within 24 Hours[5]	-	-	98%	98%
Controlled Postoperative Blood Glucose[5]	-	-	95%	97%
Perioperative Temperature Management[5]	-	-	100%	100%
Prophylactic Antibiotic Selection[5]	-	-	99%	99%
Prophylactic Antibiotic Selection (Outpatient)[5]	-	-	98%	98%
Prophylactic Antibiotic Stopped[5]	-	-	98%	98%
Prophylactic Antibiotic Timing[5]	-	-	99%	99%
Prophylactic Antibiotic Timing (Outpatient)[5]	-	-	98%	98%
Urinary Catheter Removal[5]	-	-	96%	97%
Survey of Patients' Hospital Experiences				
Area Around Room 'Always' Quiet at Night[6]	<100	91%	67%	61%
Doctors 'Always' Communicated Well[6]	<100	94%	84%	82%
Home Recovery Information Given[6]	<100	83%	85%	85%
Hospital Given 9 or 10 on 10 Point Scale[6]	<100	84%	70%	71%
Meds 'Always' Explained Before Given[6]	<100	69%	66%	64%
Nurses 'Always' Communicated Well[6]	<100	90%	80%	79%
Pain 'Always' Well Controlled[6]	<100	86%	72%	71%
Room and Bathroom 'Always' Clean[6]	<100	79%	73%	73%
Timely Help 'Always' Received[6]	<100	88%	68%	68%
Would Definitely Recommend Hospital[6]	<100	72%	70%	71%
Use of Medical Imaging				
Cardiac Imaging Stress Test before Surgery[7]	-	-	4.8%	5.3%
Combination Abdominal CT Scan	124	1.6%	9.6%	10.5%
Combination Brain/Sinus CT Scan[1]	-	-	3.3%	2.7%
Combination Chest CT Scan[1]	-	-	3.4%	2.7%
Follow-up Mammogram/Ultrasound	278	5.0%	8.3%	8.8%
Lumbar Spine MRI for Low Back Pain[1]	-	-	35.3%	37.2%

Camden General Hospital

175 Hospital Drive
Camden, TN 38320
Phone: 731-584-6135
Fax: 731-584-0124
URL: www.wth.net
Type: Critical Access Hospitals
Emergency Services: Yes
Ownership: Govt - Hospital Dist/Auth
Beds: 83

Key Personnel:
Anesthesiology. . . . . Alan Adama, DO
Anesthesiology. . . . . Charles Anderson
Cardiology . . . . John W Baker
Cardiology . . . . Christopher Cherry
Anesthesiology. . . . . Laura Ermenc
Cardiology . . . . Henry K Lui
CEO/President. . . . . Jim Moss

Measure	Cases	This Hosp.	State Avg.	U.S. Avg.
Blood Clot Prevention and Treatment				
Anticoagulation Overlap Therapy[5]	-	-	92%	93%
ICU Venous Thromboembolism Prophylaxis[5]	-	-	90%	92%
Incidence of Potentially Preventable VTE[5]	-	-	10%	10%
UFH with Dosages/Platelet Monitoring[5]	-	-	99%	97%
Venous Thromboembolism Prophylaxis[5]	-	-	83%	85%
Warfarin Therapy Discharge Instructions[5]	-	-	78%	75%
Chest Pain/Possible Heart Attack Care				
Aspirin Given Within 24 Hours of Arrival	-	-	96%	96%
Fibrinolytic Meds Within 30 Min. of Arrival	-	-	72%	58%
Average Time to ECG (minutes)	-	-	6	7
Average Time to Transfer (minutes)	-	-	53	60
Children's Asthma Care				
Received Home Management Plan of Care	-	-	-	88%
Received Reliever Medication	-	-	-	100%
Received Systemic Corticosteroids	-	-	-	100%
Emergency Department				
Admittance Decision Time (minutes)[5]	-	-	82	98
Head CT Results Within 45 Min. of Arrival	-	-	52%	57%
Patients Who Left ER Before Being Seen	-	-	2%	2%
Time from ER Arrival to Admit. (minutes)[5]	-	-	243	274
Time from ER Arrival to Discharge (minutes)	-	-	131	134
Time in ER Before Being Evaluated (minutes)	-	-	25	26
Time to Pain Meds for Fractures (minutes)	-	-	60	57
Heart Attack Care				
Aspirin Given at Discharge[5]	-	-	99%	99%
Fibrinolytic Meds Within 30 Min. of Arrival[5]	-	-	33%	54%
PCI Within 90 Minutes of Arrival[5]	-	-	98%	96%
Statin Prescribed at Discharge[5]	-	-	99%	98%
Heart Failure Care				
ACE Inhibitor or ARB for LVSD[5]	-	-	97%	97%
Discharge Instructions Given[5]	-	-	93%	94%
Evaluation of LVS Function[5]	-	-	99%	99%
Medicare Spending				
Medicare Spending per Patient (ratio)	-	-	1	0.98
Pneumonia Care				
Appropriate Initial Antibiotic Given	12	58%	95%	95%
Blood Culture Timing	24	96%	98%	98%
Pregnancy and Delivery Care				
Newborn Deliveries Scheduled Early[3,7]	-	-	6%	6%
Preventive Care				
Immunization for Influenza[5]	-	-	93%	90%
Immunization for Pneumonia[5]	-	-	93%	92%
Stroke Care				
Anticoagulation Therapy for Atrial Fibrillation[3,7]	-	-	94%	95%
Antithrombotic Therapy Timing[1,3]	-	-	97%	98%
Assessed for Rehabilitation[1,3]	-	-	97%	97%
Discharged on Antithrombotic Therapy[1,3]	-	-	99%	99%
Discharged on Statin Medication[1,3]	-	-	94%	94%
Thrombolytic Therapy Timing[1,3]	-	-	57%	66%
Venous Thromboembolism Prophylaxis[1,3]	-	-	93%	94%
Written Stroke Educational Materials Given[3,7]	-	-	84%	88%
Surgical Care Improvement Project				
Appropriate Beta Blocker Usage[5]	-	-	97%	98%
Appropriate VTP Within 24 Hours[5]	-	-	98%	98%
Controlled Postoperative Blood Glucose[5]	-	-	95%	97%
Perioperative Temperature Management[5]	-	-	100%	100%
Prophylactic Antibiotic Selection[5]	-	-	99%	99%
Prophylactic Antibiotic Selection (Outpatient)	-	-	98%	98%
Prophylactic Antibiotic Stopped[5]	-	-	98%	98%
Prophylactic Antibiotic Timing[5]	-	-	99%	99%
Prophylactic Antibiotic Timing (Outpatient)	-	-	98%	98%
Urinary Catheter Removal[5]	-	-	96%	97%
Survey of Patients' Hospital Experiences				
Area Around Room 'Always' Quiet at Night[10]	<100	81%	67%	61%
Doctors 'Always' Communicated Well[10]	<100	96%	84%	82%
Home Recovery Information Given[10]	<100	76%	85%	85%
Hospital Given 9 or 10 on 10 Point Scale[10]	<100	85%	70%	71%
Meds 'Always' Explained Before Given[10]	<100	50%	66%	64%
Nurses 'Always' Communicated Well[10]	<100	87%	80%	79%
Pain 'Always' Well Controlled[10]	<100	67%	72%	71%
Room and Bathroom 'Always' Clean[10]	<100	87%	73%	73%
Timely Help 'Always' Received[10]	<100	76%	68%	68%
Would Definitely Recommend Hospital[10]	<100	81%	70%	71%
Use of Medical Imaging				
Cardiac Imaging Stress Test before Surgery	-	-	4.8%	5.3%
Combination Abdominal CT Scan	-	-	9.6%	10.5%
Combination Brain/Sinus CT Scan	-	-	3.3%	2.7%
Combination Chest CT Scan	-	-	3.4%	2.7%
Follow-up Mammogram/Ultrasound	-	-	8.3%	8.8%
Lumbar Spine MRI for Low Back Pain	-	-	35.3%	37.2%

NOTE: Hospital profiles are in alphabetical order by state, then city, then hospital within the city; Rankings exclude hospitals with less than 25 cases except for patient surveys which excludes hospitals with less than 100 cases; (a) 100-299 cases; (1) The number of cases/patients is too few to report; (2) Data submitted were based on a sample of cases/patients; (3) Results are based on a shorter time period than required; (4) Data suppressed by CMS for one or more quarters; (5) Results are not available for this reporting period; (6) Fewer than 100 patients completed the HCAHPS survey; (7) No cases met the criteria for this measure; (8) The lower limit of the confidence interval cannot be calculated if the number of observed infections equals zero; (9) No data are available from the state/territory for this reporting period; (10) The scores shown reflect fewer than 50 completed surveys; (11) There were discrepancies in the data collection process; (12) This measure does not apply to this hospital for this reporting period; (13) Results cannot be calculated for this reporting period; (14) The results for this state are combined with nearby states to protect confidentiality; Please refer to the User's Guide for a full explanation of data.

Riverview Regional Medical Center

158 Hospital Drive
Carthage, TN 37030
Phone: 615-735-9815
URL: www.sumner.org
Type: Critical Access Hospitals
Emergency Services: Yes
Ownership: Proprietary
Beds: 25

Key Personnel:
Emergency Room . . . . Holly Bush, RN
Operating Room. . . . . Susie Dennis
Quality Assurance . . . . Marcie Mofield, RN
Chief of Medical Staff. . . . . Glenn Nabors
CEO/President. . . . . Ed Chip Sanford
Anesthesiology. . . . . Wayne Winfree, CRNA

Measure	Cases	This Hosp.	State Avg.	U.S. Avg.
Blood Clot Prevention and Treatment				
Anticoagulation Overlap Therapy[1,2]	-	-	92%	93%
ICU Venous Thromboembolism Prophylaxis[2]	14	93%	90%	92%
Incidence of Potentially Preventable VTE[1,2]	-	-	10%	10%
UFH with Dosages/Platelet Monitoring[2,7]	-	-	99%	97%
Venous Thromboembolism Prophylaxis[2]	105	85%	83%	85%
Warfarin Therapy Discharge Instructions[1,2]	-	-	78%	75%
Chest Pain/Possible Heart Attack Care				
Aspirin Given Within 24 Hours of Arrival	62	97%	96%	96%
Fibrinolytic Meds Within 30 Min. of Arrival	12	75%	72%	58%
Average Time to ECG (minutes)	64	6	6	7
Average Time to Transfer (minutes)[1]	-	-	53	60
Children's Asthma Care				
Received Home Management Plan of Care	-	-	-	88%
Received Reliever Medication	-	-	-	100%
Received Systemic Corticosteroids	-	-	-	100%
Emergency Department				
Admittance Decision Time (minutes)[2]	445	28	82	98
Head CT Results Within 45 Min. of Arrival[1]	-	-	52%	57%
Patients Who Left ER Before Being Seen	8,895	1%	2%	2%
Time from ER Arrival to Admit. (minutes)[2]	445	155	243	274
Time from ER Arrival to Discharge (minutes)	382	113	131	134
Time in ER Before Being Evaluated (minutes)	430	12	25	26
Time to Pain Meds for Fractures (minutes)	47	34	60	57
Heart Attack Care				
Aspirin Given at Discharge[1]	-	-	99%	99%
Fibrinolytic Meds Within 30 Min. of Arrival[1]	-	-	33%	54%
PCI Within 90 Minutes of Arrival[7]	-	-	98%	96%
Statin Prescribed at Discharge[1]	-	-	99%	98%
Heart Failure Care				
ACE Inhibitor or ARB for LVSD	13	100%	97%	97%
Discharge Instructions Given	35	100%	93%	94%
Evaluation of LVS Function	44	100%	99%	99%
Medicare Spending				
Medicare Spending per Patient (ratio)	-	-	1	0.98
Pneumonia Care				
Appropriate Initial Antibiotic Given	66	97%	95%	95%
Blood Culture Timing	94	100%	98%	98%
Pregnancy and Delivery Care				
Newborn Deliveries Scheduled Early[1,2]	-	-	6%	6%
Preventive Care				
Immunization for Influenza[2]	274	99%	93%	90%
Immunization for Pneumonia[2]	389	99%	93%	92%
Stroke Care				
Anticoagulation Therapy for Atrial Fibrillation[7]	-	-	94%	95%
Antithrombotic Therapy Timing[1]	-	-	97%	98%
Assessed for Rehabilitation[1]	-	-	97%	97%
Discharged on Antithrombotic Therapy[1]	-	-	99%	99%
Discharged on Statin Medication[1]	-	-	94%	94%
Thrombolytic Therapy Timing[7]	-	-	57%	66%
Venous Thromboembolism Prophylaxis[1]	-	-	93%	94%
Written Stroke Educational Materials Given[1]	-	-	84%	88%
Surgical Care Improvement Project				
Appropriate Beta Blocker Usage[1]	-	-	97%	98%
Appropriate VTP Within 24 Hours	11	91%	98%	98%
Controlled Postoperative Blood Glucose[7]	-	-	95%	97%
Perioperative Temperature Management	15	100%	100%	100%
Prophylactic Antibiotic Selection[1]	-	-	99%	99%
Prophylactic Antibiotic Selection (Outpatient)[1,3]	-	-	98%	98%
Prophylactic Antibiotic Stopped[1]	-	-	98%	98%
Prophylactic Antibiotic Timing[1]	-	-	99%	99%
Prophylactic Antibiotic Timing (Outpatient)[1,3]	-	-	98%	98%
Urinary Catheter Removal	13	100%	96%	97%
Survey of Patients' Hospital Experiences				
Area Around Room 'Always' Quiet at Night	(a)	71%	67%	61%
Doctors 'Always' Communicated Well	(a)	86%	84%	82%
Home Recovery Information Given	(a)	83%	85%	85%
Hospital Given 9 or 10 on 10 Point Scale	(a)	71%	70%	71%
Meds 'Always' Explained Before Given	(a)	69%	66%	64%
Nurses 'Always' Communicated Well	(a)	81%	80%	79%
Pain 'Always' Well Controlled	(a)	75%	72%	71%
Room and Bathroom 'Always' Clean	(a)	72%	73%	73%
Timely Help 'Always' Received	(a)	69%	68%	68%
Would Definitely Recommend Hospital	(a)	68%	70%	71%
Use of Medical Imaging				
Cardiac Imaging Stress Test before Surgery[1]	-	-	4.8%	5.3%
Combination Abdominal CT Scan	168	9.5%	9.6%	10.5%
Combination Brain/Sinus CT Scan[1]	-	-	3.3%	2.7%
Combination Chest CT Scan	73	0.0%	3.4%	2.7%
Follow-up Mammogram/Ultrasound	163	8.6%	8.3%	8.8%
Lumbar Spine MRI for Low Back Pain[1]	-	-	35.3%	37.2%

Cumberland River Hospital

100 Old Jefferson St
Celina, TN 38551
Phone: 931-243-3581
Fax: 931-243-5263
Type: Acute Care Hospitals
Emergency Services: Yes
Ownership: Physician
Beds: 26

Key Personnel:
Chief of Medical Staff. . . . . Kenneth Beaty
Radiology. . . . . Jim Hayes
CEO/President. . . . . Andrea McLerran

Measure	Cases	This Hosp.	State Avg.	U.S. Avg.
Blood Clot Prevention and Treatment				
Anticoagulation Overlap Therapy[1,2]	-	-	92%	93%
ICU Venous Thromboembolism Prophylaxis[2,7]	-	-	90%	92%
Incidence of Potentially Preventable VTE[2,7]	-	-	10%	10%
UFH with Dosages/Platelet Monitoring[2,7]	-	-	99%	97%
Venous Thromboembolism Prophylaxis[2]	134	40%	83%	85%
Warfarin Therapy Discharge Instructions[1,2]	-	-	78%	75%
Chest Pain/Possible Heart Attack Care				
Aspirin Given Within 24 Hours of Arrival[1,3]	-	-	96%	96%
Fibrinolytic Meds Within 30 Min. of Arrival[3,7]	-	-	72%	58%
Average Time to ECG (minutes)[1,3]	-	-	6	7
Average Time to Transfer (minutes)[3,7]	-	-	53	60
Children's Asthma Care				
Received Home Management Plan of Care	-	-	-	88%
Received Reliever Medication	-	-	-	100%
Received Systemic Corticosteroids	-	-	-	100%
Emergency Department				
Admittance Decision Time (minutes)	247	25	82	98
Head CT Results Within 45 Min. of Arrival[1]	-	-	52%	57%
Patients Who Left ER Before Being Seen	4,567	1%	2%	2%
Time from ER Arrival to Admit. (minutes)	285	118	243	274
Time from ER Arrival to Discharge (minutes)	312	72	131	134
Time in ER Before Being Evaluated (minutes)	350	25	25	26
Time to Pain Meds for Fractures (minutes)	11	35	60	57
Heart Attack Care				
Aspirin Given at Discharge[1]	-	-	99%	99%
Fibrinolytic Meds Within 30 Min. of Arrival[7]	-	-	33%	54%
PCI Within 90 Minutes of Arrival[7]	-	-	98%	96%
Statin Prescribed at Discharge[1]	-	-	99%	98%
Heart Failure Care				
ACE Inhibitor or ARB for LVSD[1]	-	-	97%	97%
Discharge Instructions Given	16	62%	93%	94%
Evaluation of LVS Function	29	55%	99%	99%
Medicare Spending				
Medicare Spending per Patient (ratio)	-	0.94	1	0.98
Pneumonia Care				
Appropriate Initial Antibiotic Given	23	91%	95%	95%
Blood Culture Timing[1]	-	-	98%	98%
Pregnancy and Delivery Care				
Newborn Deliveries Scheduled Early[7]	-	-	6%	6%
Preventive Care				
Immunization for Influenza	243	76%	93%	90%
Immunization for Pneumonia	452	71%	93%	92%
Stroke Care				
Anticoagulation Therapy for Atrial Fibrillation[7]	-	-	94%	95%
Antithrombotic Therapy Timing	13	92%	97%	98%
Assessed for Rehabilitation	13	92%	97%	97%
Discharged on Antithrombotic Therapy	11	91%	99%	99%
Discharged on Statin Medication[1]	-	-	94%	94%
Thrombolytic Therapy Timing[1]	-	-	57%	66%
Venous Thromboembolism Prophylaxis	17	47%	93%	94%
Written Stroke Educational Materials Given[1]	-	-	84%	88%
Surgical Care Improvement Project				
Appropriate Beta Blocker Usage[5]	-	-	97%	98%
Appropriate VTP Within 24 Hours[5]	-	-	98%	98%
Controlled Postoperative Blood Glucose[5]	-	-	95%	97%
Perioperative Temperature Management[5]	-	-	100%	100%
Prophylactic Antibiotic Selection[5]	-	-	99%	99%
Prophylactic Antibiotic Selection (Outpatient)[5]	-	-	98%	98%
Prophylactic Antibiotic Stopped[5]	-	-	98%	98%
Prophylactic Antibiotic Timing[5]	-	-	99%	99%
Prophylactic Antibiotic Timing (Outpatient)[5]	-	-	98%	98%
Urinary Catheter Removal[5]	-	-	96%	97%
Survey of Patients' Hospital Experiences				
Area Around Room 'Always' Quiet at Night[6]	<100	56%	67%	61%
Doctors 'Always' Communicated Well[6]	<100	88%	84%	82%
Home Recovery Information Given[6]	<100	82%	85%	85%
Hospital Given 9 or 10 on 10 Point Scale[6]	<100	58%	70%	71%
Meds 'Always' Explained Before Given[6]	<100	69%	66%	64%
Nurses 'Always' Communicated Well[6]	<100	80%	80%	79%
Pain 'Always' Well Controlled[6]	<100	75%	72%	71%
Room and Bathroom 'Always' Clean[6]	<100	79%	73%	73%
Timely Help 'Always' Received[6]	<100	68%	68%	68%
Would Definitely Recommend Hospital[6]	<100	68%	70%	71%
Use of Medical Imaging				
Cardiac Imaging Stress Test before Surgery[7]	-	-	4.8%	5.3%
Combination Abdominal CT Scan	68	14.7%	9.6%	10.5%
Combination Brain/Sinus CT Scan[1]	-	-	3.3%	2.7%
Combination Chest CT Scan[1]	-	-	3.4%	2.7%
Follow-up Mammogram/Ultrasound[7]	-	-	8.3%	8.8%
Lumbar Spine MRI for Low Back Pain[7]	-	-	35.3%	37.2%

Saint Thomas Hickman Hospital

135 East Swan Street
Centerville, TN 37033
Phone: 931-729-4271
Fax: 931-729-4612
Type: Critical Access Hospitals
Emergency Services: Yes
Ownership: Voluntary non-profit - Other
Beds: 25

Key Personnel:
CEO/President. . . . . Donna Bourdon
Chief of Medical Staff . . . . Sai Oh
Emergency Room . . . . Darlene Swart, RN

Measure	Cases	This Hosp.	State Avg.	U.S. Avg.
Blood Clot Prevention and Treatment				
Anticoagulation Overlap Therapy[5]	-	-	92%	93%
ICU Venous Thromboembolism Prophylaxis[5]	-	-	90%	92%
Incidence of Potentially Preventable VTE[5]	-	-	10%	10%
UFH with Dosages/Platelet Monitoring[5]	-	-	99%	97%
Venous Thromboembolism Prophylaxis[5]	-	-	83%	85%
Warfarin Therapy Discharge Instructions[5]	-	-	78%	75%
Chest Pain/Possible Heart Attack Care				
Aspirin Given Within 24 Hours of Arrival	-	-	96%	96%
Fibrinolytic Meds Within 30 Min. of Arrival	-	-	72%	58%
Average Time to ECG (minutes)	-	-	6	7
Average Time to Transfer (minutes)	-	-	53	60
Children's Asthma Care				
Received Home Management Plan of Care	-	-	-	88%
Received Reliever Medication	-	-	-	100%
Received Systemic Corticosteroids	-	-	-	100%
Emergency Department				
Admittance Decision Time (minutes)[5]	-	-	82	98
Head CT Results Within 45 Min. of Arrival	-	-	52%	57%
Patients Who Left ER Before Being Seen	-	-	2%	2%
Time from ER Arrival to Admit. (minutes)[5]	-	-	243	274
Time from ER Arrival to Discharge (minutes)	-	-	131	134

NOTE: Hospital profiles are in alphabetical order by state, then city, then hospital within the city; Rankings exclude hospitals with less than 25 cases except for patient surveys which excludes hospitals with less than 100 cases; (a) 100-299 cases; (1) The number of cases/patients is too few to report; (2) Data submitted were based on a sample of cases/patients; (3) Results are based on a shorter time period than required; (4) Data suppressed by CMS for one or more quarters; (5) Results are not available for this reporting period; (6) Fewer than 100 patients completed the HCAHPS survey; (7) No cases met the criteria for this measure; (8) The lower limit of the confidence interval cannot be calculated if the number of observed infections equals zero; (9) No data are available from the state/territory for this reporting period; (10) The scores shown reflect fewer than 50 completed surveys; (11) There were discrepancies in the data collection process; (12) This measure does not apply to this hospital for this reporting period; (13) Results cannot be calculated for this reporting period; (14) The results for this state are combined with nearby states to protect confidentiality; Please refer to the User's Guide for a full explanation of data.

Measure	Cases	This Hosp.	State Avg.	U.S. Avg.
Time in ER Before Being Evaluated (minutes)	-	-	25	26
Time to Pain Meds for Fractures (minutes)	-	-	60	57
Heart Attack Care				
Aspirin Given at Discharge[5]	-	-	99%	99%
Fibrinolytic Meds Within 30 Min. of Arrival[5]	-	-	33%	54%
PCI Within 90 Minutes of Arrival[5]	-	-	98%	96%
Statin Prescribed at Discharge[5]	-	-	99%	98%
Heart Failure Care				
ACE Inhibitor or ARB for LVSD[1,3]	-	-	97%	97%
Discharge Instructions Given[1,3]	-	-	93%	94%
Evaluation of LVS Function[1,3]	-	-	99%	99%
Medicare Spending				
Medicare Spending per Patient (ratio)	-	-	1	0.98
Pneumonia Care				
Appropriate Initial Antibiotic Given	12	58%	95%	95%
Blood Culture Timing	16	94%	98%	98%
Pregnancy and Delivery Care				
Newborn Deliveries Scheduled Early[5]	-	-	6%	6%
Preventive Care				
Immunization for Influenza[5]	-	-	93%	90%
Immunization for Pneumonia[5]	-	-	93%	92%
Stroke Care				
Anticoagulation Therapy for Atrial Fibrillation[5]	-	-	94%	95%
Antithrombotic Therapy Timing[5]	-	-	97%	98%
Assessed for Rehabilitation[5]	-	-	97%	97%
Discharged on Antithrombotic Therapy[5]	-	-	99%	99%
Discharged on Statin Medication[5]	-	-	94%	94%
Thrombolytic Therapy Timing[5]	-	-	57%	66%
Venous Thromboembolism Prophylaxis[5]	-	-	93%	94%
Written Stroke Educational Materials Given[5]	-	-	84%	88%
Surgical Care Improvement Project				
Appropriate Beta Blocker Usage[5]	-	-	97%	98%
Appropriate VTP Within 24 Hours[5]	-	-	98%	98%
Controlled Postoperative Blood Glucose[5]	-	-	95%	97%
Perioperative Temperature Management[5]	-	-	100%	100%
Prophylactic Antibiotic Selection[5]	-	-	99%	99%
Prophylactic Antibiotic Selection (Outpatient)	-	-	98%	98%
Prophylactic Antibiotic Stopped[5]	-	-	98%	98%
Prophylactic Antibiotic Timing[5]	-	-	99%	99%
Prophylactic Antibiotic Timing (Outpatient)	-	-	98%	98%
Urinary Catheter Removal[5]	-	-	96%	97%
Survey of Patients' Hospital Experiences				
Area Around Room 'Always' Quiet at Night[5]	-	-	67%	61%
Doctors 'Always' Communicated Well[5]	-	-	84%	82%
Home Recovery Information Given[5]	-	-	85%	85%
Hospital Given 9 or 10 on 10 Point Scale[5]	-	-	70%	71%
Meds 'Always' Explained Before Given[5]	-	-	66%	64%
Nurses 'Always' Communicated Well[5]	-	-	80%	79%
Pain 'Always' Well Controlled[5]	-	-	72%	71%
Room and Bathroom 'Always' Clean[5]	-	-	73%	73%
Timely Help 'Always' Received[5]	-	-	68%	68%
Would Definitely Recommend Hospital[5]	-	-	70%	71%
Use of Medical Imaging				
Cardiac Imaging Stress Test before Surgery	-	-	4.8%	5.3%
Combination Abdominal CT Scan	-	-	9.6%	10.5%
Combination Brain/Sinus CT Scan	-	-	3.3%	2.7%
Combination Chest CT Scan	-	-	3.4%	2.7%
Follow-up Mammogram/Ultrasound	-	-	8.3%	8.8%
Lumbar Spine MRI for Low Back Pain	-	-	35.3%	37.2%

Erlanger Medical Center

975 E 3rd St
Chattanooga, TN 37403
Phone: 423-778-7000
Fax: 423-778-7454
URL: www.erlanger.org
Type: Acute Care Hospitals
Emergency Services: Yes
Ownership: Govt - Hospital Dist/Auth
Beds: 819

Key Personnel:

Quality Assurance .... Mike Bettinger
Chief of Medical Staff .... Woods Blake, MD
CEO/President .... Jim Brexler
Infection Control .... Steve Hawkins, MD
Radiology .... Robert Phlegar, MD
Pediatric Ambulatory Care ...... Nita Shumaker, MD
Pediatric In-Patient Care .... Nita Shumaker, MD

Measure	Cases	This Hosp.	State Avg.	U.S. Avg.
Blood Clot Prevention and Treatment				
Anticoagulation Overlap Therapy[2]	142	88%	92%	93%
ICU Venous Thromboembolism Prophylaxis[2]	157	84%	90%	92%
Incidence of Potentially Preventable VTE[2]	30	57%	10%	10%
UFH with Dosages/Platelet Monitoring[2]	147	93%	99%	97%
Venous Thromboembolism Prophylaxis[2]	313	76%	83%	85%
Warfarin Therapy Discharge Instructions[2]	79	87%	78%	75%
Chest Pain/Possible Heart Attack Care				
Aspirin Given Within 24 Hours of Arrival	15	100%	96%	96%
Fibrinolytic Meds Within 30 Min. of Arrival[7]	-	-	72%	58%
Average Time to ECG (minutes)	16	6	6	7
Average Time to Transfer (minutes)[1]	-	-	53	60
Children's Asthma Care				
Received Home Management Plan of Care	28	68%	-	88%
Received Reliever Medication	28	100%	-	100%
Received Systemic Corticosteroids	28	100%	-	100%
Emergency Department				
Admittance Decision Time (minutes)[2]	392	150	82	98
Head CT Results Within 45 Min. of Arrival[1]	-	-	52%	57%
Patients Who Left ER Before Being Seen	>100k	4%	2%	2%
Time from ER Arrival to Admit. (minutes)[2]	396	292	243	274
Time from ER Arrival to Discharge (minutes)	374	112	131	134
Time in ER Before Being Evaluated (minutes)	364	42	25	26
Time to Pain Meds for Fractures (minutes)	295	49	60	57
Heart Attack Care				
Aspirin Given at Discharge	385	100%	99%	99%
Fibrinolytic Meds Within 30 Min. of Arrival[7]	-	-	33%	54%
PCI Within 90 Minutes of Arrival	71	99%	98%	96%
Statin Prescribed at Discharge	389	99%	99%	98%
Heart Failure Care				
ACE Inhibitor or ARB for LVSD	136	100%	97%	97%
Discharge Instructions Given	282	85%	93%	94%
Evaluation of LVS Function	331	100%	99%	99%
Medicare Spending				
Medicare Spending per Patient (ratio)	-	1.03	1	0.98
Pneumonia Care				
Appropriate Initial Antibiotic Given	118	93%	95%	95%
Blood Culture Timing	158	99%	98%	98%
Pregnancy and Delivery Care				
Newborn Deliveries Scheduled Early	635	13%	6%	6%
Preventive Care				
Immunization for Influenza[2]	482	88%	93%	90%
Immunization for Pneumonia[2]	448	83%	93%	92%
Stroke Care				
Anticoagulation Therapy for Atrial Fibrillation[2]	39	87%	94%	95%
Antithrombotic Therapy Timing[2]	155	93%	97%	98%
Assessed for Rehabilitation[2]	202	96%	97%	97%
Discharged on Antithrombotic Therapy[2]	158	89%	99%	99%
Discharged on Statin Medication[2]	128	88%	94%	94%
Thrombolytic Therapy Timing[1,2]	-	-	57%	66%
Venous Thromboembolism Prophylaxis[2]	237	83%	93%	94%
Written Stroke Educational Materials Given[2]	115	75%	84%	88%
Surgical Care Improvement Project				
Appropriate Beta Blocker Usage[2]	134	98%	97%	98%
Appropriate VTP Within 24 Hours[2]	318	98%	98%	98%
Controlled Postoperative Blood Glucose[2]	94	87%	95%	97%
Perioperative Temperature Management[2]	405	100%	100%	100%
Prophylactic Antibiotic Selection[2]	329	99%	99%	99%
Prophylactic Antibiotic Selection (Outpatient)	686	98%	98%	98%
Prophylactic Antibiotic Stopped[2]	310	97%	98%	98%
Prophylactic Antibiotic Timing[2]	329	96%	99%	99%
Prophylactic Antibiotic Timing (Outpatient)	690	98%	98%	98%
Urinary Catheter Removal[2]	211	93%	96%	97%
Survey of Patients' Hospital Experiences				
Area Around Room 'Always' Quiet at Night[11]	300+	57%	67%	61%
Doctors 'Always' Communicated Well[11]	300+	79%	84%	82%
Home Recovery Information Given[11]	300+	83%	85%	85%
Hospital Given 9 or 10 on 10 Point Scale[11]	300+	67%	70%	71%
Meds 'Always' Explained Before Given[11]	300+	59%	66%	64%
Nurses 'Always' Communicated Well[11]	300+	76%	80%	79%
Pain 'Always' Well Controlled[11]	300+	67%	72%	71%
Room and Bathroom 'Always' Clean[11]	300+	69%	73%	73%
Timely Help 'Always' Received[11]	300+	63%	68%	68%
Would Definitely Recommend Hospital[11]	300+	73%	70%	71%
Use of Medical Imaging				
Cardiac Imaging Stress Test before Surgery	664	3.8%	4.8%	5.3%
Combination Abdominal CT Scan	1,028	19.4%	9.6%	10.5%
Combination Brain/Sinus CT Scan	1,013	2.0%	3.3%	2.7%
Combination Chest CT Scan	984	8.2%	3.4%	2.7%
Follow-up Mammogram/Ultrasound	2,187	3.7%	8.3%	8.8%
Lumbar Spine MRI for Low Back Pain	82	39.0%	35.3%	37.2%

Memorial Healthcare System

2525 Desales Ave
Chattanooga, TN 37404
Phone: 423-495-2525
Fax: 423-495-6722
URL: www.memorial.org
Type: Acute Care Hospitals
Emergency Services: Yes
Ownership: Voluntary non-profit - Church
Beds: 322

Key Personnel:

Radiology .... Stan Casteel
Infection Control .... Gwen Davis
Quality Assurance .... Beverly Gordon
Cardiac Laboratory .... Laura Hartman, RN
CEO/President .... James M. Hobson
Chief of Medical Staff .... Kevin L. Lewis, MD
Emergency Room .... Runay Valentine

Measure	Cases	This Hosp.	State Avg.	U.S. Avg.
Blood Clot Prevention and Treatment				
Anticoagulation Overlap Therapy[2]	149	77%	92%	93%
ICU Venous Thromboembolism Prophylaxis[2]	183	72%	90%	92%
Incidence of Potentially Preventable VTE[2]	34	24%	10%	10%
UFH with Dosages/Platelet Monitoring[2]	150	100%	99%	97%
Venous Thromboembolism Prophylaxis[2]	732	78%	83%	85%
Warfarin Therapy Discharge Instructions[2]	115	36%	78%	75%
Chest Pain/Possible Heart Attack Care				
Aspirin Given Within 24 Hours of Arrival	34	94%	96%	96%
Fibrinolytic Meds Within 30 Min. of Arrival[7]	-	-	72%	58%
Average Time to ECG (minutes)	35	6	6	7
Average Time to Transfer (minutes)	11	41	53	60
Children's Asthma Care				
Received Home Management Plan of Care	-	-	-	88%
Received Reliever Medication	-	-	-	100%
Received Systemic Corticosteroids	-	-	-	100%
Emergency Department				
Admittance Decision Time (minutes)[2]	1,202	122	82	98
Head CT Results Within 45 Min. of Arrival[1]	-	-	52%	57%
Patients Who Left ER Before Being Seen	58,322	3%	2%	2%
Time from ER Arrival to Admit. (minutes)[2]	1,204	293	243	274
Time from ER Arrival to Discharge (minutes)	699	170	131	134
Time in ER Before Being Evaluated (minutes)	590	30	25	26
Time to Pain Meds for Fractures (minutes)	214	70	60	57
Heart Attack Care				
Aspirin Given at Discharge[2]	332	99%	99%	99%
Fibrinolytic Meds Within 30 Min. of Arrival[1,2]	-	-	33%	54%
PCI Within 90 Minutes of Arrival[2]	40	100%	98%	96%
Statin Prescribed at Discharge[2]	340	99%	99%	98%
Heart Failure Care				
ACE Inhibitor or ARB for LVSD[2]	116	94%	97%	97%
Discharge Instructions Given[2]	376	78%	93%	94%
Evaluation of LVS Function[2]	438	100%	99%	99%
Medicare Spending				
Medicare Spending per Patient (ratio)	-	0.97	1	0.98
Pneumonia Care				
Appropriate Initial Antibiotic Given[2]	189	100%	95%	95%
Blood Culture Timing[2]	342	100%	98%	98%
Pregnancy and Delivery Care				
Newborn Deliveries Scheduled Early[7]	-	-	6%	6%
Preventive Care				
Immunization for Influenza[2]	840	98%	93%	90%
Immunization for Pneumonia[2]	1,489	99%	93%	92%
Stroke Care				
Anticoagulation Therapy for Atrial Fibrillation[2]	20	80%	94%	95%
Antithrombotic Therapy Timing[2]	150	97%	97%	98%
Assessed for Rehabilitation[2]	164	80%	97%	97%
Discharged on Antithrombotic Therapy[2]	160	97%	99%	99%

NOTE: Hospital profiles are in alphabetical order by state, then city, then hospital within the city; Rankings exclude hospitals with less than 25 cases except for patient surveys which excludes hospitals with less than 100 cases; (a) 100-299 cases; (1) The number of cases/patients is too few to report; (2) Data submitted were based on a sample of cases/patients; (3) Results are based on a shorter time period than required; (4) Data suppressed by CMS for one or more quarters; (5) Results are not available for this reporting period; (6) Fewer than 100 patients completed the HCAHPS survey; (7) No cases met the criteria for this measure; (8) The lower limit of the confidence interval cannot be calculated if the number of observed infections equals zero; (9) No data are available from the state/territory for this reporting period; (10) The scores shown reflect fewer than 50 completed surveys; (11) There were discrepancies in the data collection process; (12) This measure does not apply to this hospital for this reporting period; (13) Results cannot be calculated for this reporting period; (14) The results for this state are combined with nearby states to protect confidentiality; Please refer to the User's Guide for a full explanation of data.

Measure	Cases	This Hosp.	State Avg.	U.S. Avg.
Discharged on Statin Medication[2]	133	86%	94%	94%
Thrombolytic Therapy Timing[2]	51	6%	57%	66%
Venous Thromboembolism Prophylaxis[2]	157	83%	93%	94%
Written Stroke Educational Materials Given[2]	104	12%	84%	88%
Surgical Care Improvement Project				
Appropriate Beta Blocker Usage[2]	519	92%	97%	98%
Appropriate VTP Within 24 Hours[2]	529	97%	98%	98%
Controlled Postoperative Blood Glucose[2]	595	91%	95%	97%
Perioperative Temperature Management[2]	715	99%	100%	100%
Prophylactic Antibiotic Selection[2]	1,012	100%	99%	99%
Prophylactic Antibiotic Selection (Outpatient)	872	98%	98%	98%
Prophylactic Antibiotic Stopped[2]	997	99%	98%	98%
Prophylactic Antibiotic Timing[2]	1,014	98%	99%	99%
Prophylactic Antibiotic Timing (Outpatient)	855	99%	98%	98%
Urinary Catheter Removal[2]	833	91%	96%	97%
Survey of Patients' Hospital Experiences				
Area Around Room 'Always' Quiet at Night	300+	70%	67%	61%
Doctors 'Always' Communicated Well	300+	84%	84%	82%
Home Recovery Information Given	300+	88%	85%	85%
Hospital Given 9 or 10 on 10 Point Scale	300+	80%	70%	71%
Meds 'Always' Explained Before Given	300+	67%	66%	64%
Nurses 'Always' Communicated Well	300+	82%	80%	79%
Pain 'Always' Well Controlled	300+	74%	72%	71%
Room and Bathroom 'Always' Clean	300+	74%	73%	73%
Timely Help 'Always' Received	300+	69%	68%	68%
Would Definitely Recommend Hospital	300+	83%	70%	71%
Use of Medical Imaging				
Cardiac Imaging Stress Test before Surgery	2,902	4.8%	4.8%	5.3%
Combination Abdominal CT Scan	3,045	24.9%	9.6%	10.5%
Combination Brain/Sinus CT Scan	2,192	3.1%	3.3%	2.7%
Combination Chest CT Scan	1,687	5.4%	3.4%	2.7%
Follow-up Mammogram/Ultrasound	5,007	3.6%	8.3%	8.8%
Lumbar Spine MRI for Low Back Pain	413	35.8%	35.3%	37.2%

Parkridge Medical Center

2333 Mccallie Ave
Chattanooga, TN 37404
URL: www.tristarhealth.com
Phone: 423-894-4220
Fax: 423-493-1208
Type: Acute Care Hospitals
Ownership: Proprietary
Emergency Services: Yes
Beds: 296

Key Personnel:
Chief of Medical Staff. . . . . Kirk Brody, MD
Radiology. . . . . Sharon Hobbs
Quality Assurance . . . . Judy Ketchersid
Patient Relations . . . . Sherry Maxwell
CEO/President. . . . . Darrell Moore
Operating Room. . . . . Adam Royer
Infection Control. . . . . Susan Schnell
Pediatric In-Patient Care . . . . Teresa C Walker

Measure	Cases	This Hosp.	State Avg.	U.S. Avg.
Blood Clot Prevention and Treatment				
Anticoagulation Overlap Therapy[2]	94	97%	92%	93%
ICU Venous Thromboembolism Prophylaxis[2]	121	100%	90%	92%
Incidence of Potentially Preventable VTE[2]	14	7%	10%	10%
UFH with Dosages/Platelet Monitoring[2]	89	100%	99%	97%
Venous Thromboembolism Prophylaxis[2]	319	93%	83%	85%
Warfarin Therapy Discharge Instructions[2]	79	92%	78%	75%
Chest Pain/Possible Heart Attack Care				
Aspirin Given Within 24 Hours of Arrival	30	100%	96%	96%
Fibrinolytic Meds Within 30 Min. of Arrival[7]	-	-	72%	58%
Average Time to ECG (minutes)	34	3	6	7
Average Time to Transfer (minutes)[1]	-	-	53	60
Children's Asthma Care				
Received Home Management Plan of Care	-	-	-	88%
Received Reliever Medication	-	-	-	100%
Received Systemic Corticosteroids	-	-	-	100%
Emergency Department				
Admittance Decision Time (minutes)[2]	536	108	82	98
Head CT Results Within 45 Min. of Arrival[1]	-	-	52%	57%
Patients Who Left ER Before Being Seen	76,341	2%	2%	2%
Time from ER Arrival to Admit. (minutes)[2]	537	255	243	274
Time from ER Arrival to Discharge (minutes)	491	111	131	134
Time in ER Before Being Evaluated (minutes)	536	13	25	26
Time to Pain Meds for Fractures (minutes)	140	58	60	57
Heart Attack Care				
Aspirin Given at Discharge	253	100%	99%	99%
Fibrinolytic Meds Within 30 Min. of Arrival[1]	-	-	33%	54%
PCI Within 90 Minutes of Arrival	20	100%	98%	96%
Statin Prescribed at Discharge	245	99%	99%	98%
Heart Failure Care				
ACE Inhibitor or ARB for LVSD	93	98%	97%	97%
Discharge Instructions Given	274	97%	93%	94%
Evaluation of LVS Function	317	100%	99%	99%
Medicare Spending				
Medicare Spending per Patient (ratio)	-	1.00	1	0.98
Pneumonia Care				
Appropriate Initial Antibiotic Given	203	97%	95%	95%
Blood Culture Timing	312	100%	98%	98%
Pregnancy and Delivery Care				
Newborn Deliveries Scheduled Early	154	1%	6%	6%
Preventive Care				
Immunization for Influenza[2]	583	95%	93%	90%
Immunization for Pneumonia[2]	772	97%	93%	92%
Stroke Care				
Anticoagulation Therapy for Atrial Fibrillation[1]	-	-	94%	95%
Antithrombotic Therapy Timing	56	100%	97%	98%
Assessed for Rehabilitation	65	98%	97%	97%
Discharged on Antithrombotic Therapy	65	100%	99%	99%
Discharged on Statin Medication	50	100%	94%	94%
Thrombolytic Therapy Timing[1]	-	-	57%	66%
Venous Thromboembolism Prophylaxis	57	96%	93%	94%
Written Stroke Educational Materials Given	49	96%	84%	88%
Surgical Care Improvement Project				
Appropriate Beta Blocker Usage[2]	206	100%	97%	98%
Appropriate VTP Within 24 Hours[2]	374	99%	98%	98%
Controlled Postoperative Blood Glucose[2]	126	97%	95%	97%
Perioperative Temperature Management[2]	464	100%	100%	100%
Prophylactic Antibiotic Selection[2]	397	100%	99%	99%
Prophylactic Antibiotic Selection (Outpatient)	686	100%	98%	98%
Prophylactic Antibiotic Stopped[2]	379	98%	98%	98%
Prophylactic Antibiotic Timing[2]	397	99%	99%	99%
Prophylactic Antibiotic Timing (Outpatient)	684	100%	98%	98%
Urinary Catheter Removal[2]	231	98%	96%	97%
Survey of Patients' Hospital Experiences				
Area Around Room 'Always' Quiet at Night	300+	66%	67%	61%
Doctors 'Always' Communicated Well	300+	82%	84%	82%
Home Recovery Information Given	300+	86%	85%	85%
Hospital Given 9 or 10 on 10 Point Scale	300+	72%	70%	71%
Meds 'Always' Explained Before Given	300+	63%	66%	64%
Nurses 'Always' Communicated Well	300+	78%	80%	79%
Pain 'Always' Well Controlled	300+	72%	72%	71%
Room and Bathroom 'Always' Clean	300+	68%	73%	73%
Timely Help 'Always' Received	300+	65%	68%	68%
Would Definitely Recommend Hospital	300+	74%	70%	71%
Use of Medical Imaging				
Cardiac Imaging Stress Test before Surgery	298	7.7%	4.8%	5.3%
Combination Abdominal CT Scan	924	11.6%	9.6%	10.5%
Combination Brain/Sinus CT Scan	804	3.7%	3.3%	2.7%
Combination Chest CT Scan	310	5.5%	3.4%	2.7%
Follow-up Mammogram/Ultrasound	587	8.9%	8.3%	8.8%
Lumbar Spine MRI for Low Back Pain	67	31.3%	35.3%	37.2%

Gateway Medical Center

651 Dunlop Lane
Clarksville, TN 37040
URL: www.todaysgateway.com
Phone: 931-502-1000
Type: Acute Care Hospitals
Ownership: Govt - Hospital Dist/Auth
Emergency Services: Yes
Beds: 270

Key Personnel:
President . . . . Angie Allen
Emergency . . . . Randy Likes
CEO . . . . Tim Puthoff
Radiology. . . . . Dan Stames

Measure	Cases	This Hosp.	State Avg.	U.S. Avg.
Blood Clot Prevention and Treatment				
Anticoagulation Overlap Therapy[2]	50	96%	92%	93%
ICU Venous Thromboembolism Prophylaxis[2]	51	96%	90%	92%
Incidence of Potentially Preventable VTE[1,2]	-	-	10%	10%
UFH with Dosages/Platelet Monitoring[1,2]	-	-	99%	97%
Venous Thromboembolism Prophylaxis[2]	387	91%	83%	85%
Warfarin Therapy Discharge Instructions[2]	35	94%	78%	75%
Chest Pain/Possible Heart Attack Care				
Aspirin Given Within 24 Hours of Arrival	44	98%	96%	96%
Fibrinolytic Meds Within 30 Min. of Arrival[7]	-	-	72%	58%
Average Time to ECG (minutes)	46	5	6	7
Average Time to Transfer (minutes)[7]	-	-	53	60
Children's Asthma Care				
Received Home Management Plan of Care	-	-	-	88%
Received Reliever Medication	-	-	-	100%
Received Systemic Corticosteroids	-	-	-	100%
Emergency Department				
Admittance Decision Time (minutes)[2]	587	138	82	98
Head CT Results Within 45 Min. of Arrival	25	80%	52%	57%
Patients Who Left ER Before Being Seen	66,288	4%	2%	2%
Time from ER Arrival to Admit. (minutes)[2]	601	268	243	274
Time from ER Arrival to Discharge (minutes)	376	142	131	134
Time in ER Before Being Evaluated (minutes)	408	30	25	26
Time to Pain Meds for Fractures (minutes)	264	54	60	57
Heart Attack Care				
Aspirin Given at Discharge	167	100%	99%	99%
Fibrinolytic Meds Within 30 Min. of Arrival[7]	-	-	33%	54%
PCI Within 90 Minutes of Arrival	43	98%	98%	96%
Statin Prescribed at Discharge	167	100%	99%	98%
Heart Failure Care				
ACE Inhibitor or ARB for LVSD	89	94%	97%	97%
Discharge Instructions Given	167	100%	93%	94%
Evaluation of LVS Function	194	100%	99%	99%
Medicare Spending				
Medicare Spending per Patient (ratio)	-	1.03	1	0.98
Pneumonia Care				
Appropriate Initial Antibiotic Given	259	95%	95%	95%
Blood Culture Timing	305	99%	98%	98%
Pregnancy and Delivery Care				
Newborn Deliveries Scheduled Early[2]	73	4%	6%	6%
Preventive Care				
Immunization for Influenza[2]	568	99%	93%	90%
Immunization for Pneumonia[2]	637	99%	93%	92%
Stroke Care				
Anticoagulation Therapy for Atrial Fibrillation[1]	-	-	94%	95%
Antithrombotic Therapy Timing	88	98%	97%	98%
Assessed for Rehabilitation	89	96%	97%	97%
Discharged on Antithrombotic Therapy	88	99%	99%	99%
Discharged on Statin Medication	67	93%	94%	94%
Thrombolytic Therapy Timing[7]	-	-	57%	66%
Venous Thromboembolism Prophylaxis	89	89%	93%	94%
Written Stroke Educational Materials Given	57	77%	84%	88%
Surgical Care Improvement Project				
Appropriate Beta Blocker Usage	189	98%	97%	98%
Appropriate VTP Within 24 Hours	503	99%	98%	98%
Controlled Postoperative Blood Glucose	53	98%	95%	97%
Perioperative Temperature Management	581	100%	100%	100%
Prophylactic Antibiotic Selection	461	100%	99%	99%
Prophylactic Antibiotic Selection (Outpatient)	248	99%	98%	98%
Prophylactic Antibiotic Stopped	440	97%	98%	98%
Prophylactic Antibiotic Timing	461	99%	99%	99%
Prophylactic Antibiotic Timing (Outpatient)	248	99%	98%	98%
Urinary Catheter Removal	442	97%	96%	97%
Survey of Patients' Hospital Experiences				
Area Around Room 'Always' Quiet at Night	300+	61%	67%	61%
Doctors 'Always' Communicated Well	300+	80%	84%	82%
Home Recovery Information Given	300+	82%	85%	85%
Hospital Given 9 or 10 on 10 Point Scale	300+	60%	70%	71%
Meds 'Always' Explained Before Given	300+	64%	66%	64%
Nurses 'Always' Communicated Well	300+	74%	80%	79%
Pain 'Always' Well Controlled	300+	67%	72%	71%
Room and Bathroom 'Always' Clean	300+	71%	73%	73%
Timely Help 'Always' Received	300+	60%	68%	68%
Would Definitely Recommend Hospital	300+	59%	70%	71%
Use of Medical Imaging				

NOTE: Hospital profiles are in alphabetical order by state, then city, then hospital within the city; Rankings exclude hospitals with less than 25 cases except for patient surveys which excludes hospitals with less than 100 cases; (a) 100-299 cases; (1) The number of cases/patients is too few to report; (2) Data submitted were based on a sample of cases/patients; (3) Results are based on a shorter time period than required; (4) Data suppressed by CMS for one or more quarters; (5) Results are not available for this reporting period; (6) Fewer than 100 patients completed the HCAHPS survey; (7) No cases met the criteria for this measure; (8) The lower limit of the confidence interval cannot be calculated if the number of observed infections equals zero; (9) No data are available from the state/territory for this reporting period; (10) The scores shown reflect fewer than 50 completed surveys; (11) There were discrepancies in the data collection process; (12) This measure does not apply to this hospital for this reporting period; (13) Results cannot be calculated for this reporting period; (14) The results for this state are combined with nearby states to protect confidentiality; Please refer to the User's Guide for a full explanation of data.

Cardiac Imaging Stress Test before Surgery	522	4.0%	4.8%	5.3%
Combination Abdominal CT Scan	1,040	6.8%	9.6%	10.5%
Combination Brain/Sinus CT Scan	1,222	3.4%	3.3%	2.7%
Combination Chest CT Scan	571	4.6%	3.4%	2.7%
Follow-up Mammogram/Ultrasound	1,404	4.7%	8.3%	8.8%
Lumbar Spine MRI for Low Back Pain	113	32.7%	35.3%	37.2%

Skyridge Medical Center

2305 Chambliss Ave Nw
Cleveland, TN 37311
Phone: 423-339-4132
URL: www.skyridgemedcenter.com
Type: Acute Care Hospitals
Emergency Services: Yes
Ownership: Proprietary
Key Personnel:
Emergency Room . . . . Stephen Heinz, MD
President/CEO. . . . . Maureen Tarrant

Measure	Cases	This Hosp.	State Avg.	U.S. Avg.
Blood Clot Prevention and Treatment				
Anticoagulation Overlap Therapy[2]	73	97%	92%	93%
ICU Venous Thromboembolism Prophylaxis[2]	107	97%	90%	92%
Incidence of Potentially Preventable VTE[1,2]	-	-	10%	10%
UFH with Dosages/Platelet Monitoring[2]	63	98%	99%	97%
Venous Thromboembolism Prophylaxis[2]	330	94%	83%	85%
Warfarin Therapy Discharge Instructions[2]	56	100%	78%	75%
Chest Pain/Possible Heart Attack Care				
Aspirin Given Within 24 Hours of Arrival	78	100%	96%	96%
Fibrinolytic Meds Within 30 Min. of Arrival[7]	-	-	72%	58%
Average Time to ECG (minutes)	79	2	6	7
Average Time to Transfer (minutes)	28	30	53	60
Children's Asthma Care				
Received Home Management Plan of Care	-	-	-	88%
Received Reliever Medication	-	-	-	100%
Received Systemic Corticosteroids	-	-	-	100%
Emergency Department				
Admittance Decision Time (minutes)[2]	736	132	82	98
Head CT Results Within 45 Min. of Arrival	38	55%	52%	57%
Patients Who Left ER Before Being Seen	57,228	3%	2%	2%
Time from ER Arrival to Admit. (minutes)[2]	747	316	243	274
Time from ER Arrival to Discharge (minutes)	384	170	131	134
Time in ER Before Being Evaluated (minutes)	410	39	25	26
Time to Pain Meds for Fractures (minutes)	295	94	60	57
Heart Attack Care				
Aspirin Given at Discharge	35	91%	99%	99%
Fibrinolytic Meds Within 30 Min. of Arrival[7]	-	-	33%	54%
PCI Within 90 Minutes of Arrival[7]	-	-	98%	96%
Statin Prescribed at Discharge	35	97%	99%	98%
Heart Failure Care				
ACE Inhibitor or ARB for LVSD	82	94%	97%	97%
Discharge Instructions Given	194	96%	93%	94%
Evaluation of LVS Function	236	100%	99%	99%
Medicare Spending				
Medicare Spending per Patient (ratio)	-	1.02	1	0.98
Pneumonia Care				
Appropriate Initial Antibiotic Given	169	96%	95%	95%
Blood Culture Timing	302	100%	98%	98%
Pregnancy and Delivery Care				
Newborn Deliveries Scheduled Early[2]	46	4%	6%	6%
Preventive Care				
Immunization for Influenza[2]	625	96%	93%	90%
Immunization for Pneumonia[2]	771	95%	93%	92%
Stroke Care				
Anticoagulation Therapy for Atrial Fibrillation[1]	-	-	94%	95%
Antithrombotic Therapy Timing[1]	-	-	97%	98%
Assessed for Rehabilitation[1]	-	-	97%	97%
Discharged on Antithrombotic Therapy[1]	-	-	99%	99%
Discharged on Statin Medication[1]	-	-	94%	94%
Thrombolytic Therapy Timing[1]	-	-	57%	66%
Venous Thromboembolism Prophylaxis[1]	-	-	93%	94%
Written Stroke Educational Materials Given[1]	-	-	84%	88%
Surgical Care Improvement Project				
Appropriate Beta Blocker Usage	73	100%	97%	98%
Appropriate VTP Within 24 Hours	263	98%	98%	98%
Controlled Postoperative Blood Glucose[7]	-	-	95%	97%
Perioperative Temperature Management	292	100%	100%	100%
Prophylactic Antibiotic Selection	177	98%	99%	99%
Prophylactic Antibiotic Selection (Outpatient)	226	98%	98%	98%
Prophylactic Antibiotic Stopped	173	94%	98%	98%
Prophylactic Antibiotic Timing	177	98%	99%	99%
Prophylactic Antibiotic Timing (Outpatient)	221	100%	98%	98%
Urinary Catheter Removal	134	96%	96%	97%
Survey of Patients' Hospital Experiences				
Area Around Room 'Always' Quiet at Night	300+	64%	67%	61%
Doctors 'Always' Communicated Well	300+	84%	84%	82%
Home Recovery Information Given	300+	85%	85%	85%
Hospital Given 9 or 10 on 10 Point Scale	300+	64%	70%	71%
Meds 'Always' Explained Before Given	300+	64%	66%	64%
Nurses 'Always' Communicated Well	300+	78%	80%	79%
Pain 'Always' Well Controlled	300+	72%	72%	71%
Room and Bathroom 'Always' Clean	300+	66%	73%	73%
Timely Help 'Always' Received	300+	64%	68%	68%
Would Definitely Recommend Hospital	300+	61%	70%	71%
Use of Medical Imaging				
Cardiac Imaging Stress Test before Surgery	76	3.9%	4.8%	5.3%
Combination Abdominal CT Scan	1,077	9.2%	9.6%	10.5%
Combination Brain/Sinus CT Scan	1,039	4.9%	3.3%	2.7%
Combination Chest CT Scan	685	8.2%	3.4%	2.7%
Follow-up Mammogram/Ultrasound	1,097	4.9%	8.3%	8.8%
Lumbar Spine MRI for Low Back Pain	255	39.6%	35.3%	37.2%

Maury Regional Hospital

1224 Trotwood Ave
Columbia, TN 38401
Phone: 931-381-1111
Fax: 931-380-4016
URL: www.maurgregional.com
Type: Acute Care Hospitals
Emergency Services: Yes
Ownership: Government - Local
Beds: 255
Key Personnel:
Infection Control. . . . . Roger Anderson
Patient Relations . . . . Cindy Fox
Chief of Medical Staff. . . . . Anthony D Khim
Anesthesiology. . . . . Jeff Kirkpatrick, MD
Operating Room. . . . . Stephen Noe
CEO/President. . . . . Robert Otwell
Quality Assurance . . . . Sue Parsons
Radiology. . . . . Terrie Stinson

Measure	Cases	This Hosp.	State Avg.	U.S. Avg.
Blood Clot Prevention and Treatment				
Anticoagulation Overlap Therapy[2]	92	96%	92%	93%
ICU Venous Thromboembolism Prophylaxis[2]	93	97%	90%	92%
Incidence of Potentially Preventable VTE[2]	14	7%	10%	10%
UFH with Dosages/Platelet Monitoring[2]	20	95%	99%	97%
Venous Thromboembolism Prophylaxis[2]	313	88%	83%	85%
Warfarin Therapy Discharge Instructions[2]	69	16%	78%	75%
Chest Pain/Possible Heart Attack Care				
Aspirin Given Within 24 Hours of Arrival[1]	-	-	96%	96%
Fibrinolytic Meds Within 30 Min. of Arrival[3,7]	-	-	72%	58%
Average Time to ECG (minutes)[1]	-	-	6	7
Average Time to Transfer (minutes)[3,7]	-	-	53	60
Children's Asthma Care				
Received Home Management Plan of Care	-	-	-	88%
Received Reliever Medication	-	-	-	100%
Received Systemic Corticosteroids	-	-	-	100%
Emergency Department				
Admittance Decision Time (minutes)[2]	437	87	82	98
Head CT Results Within 45 Min. of Arrival	17	65%	52%	57%
Patients Who Left ER Before Being Seen	49,938	1%	2%	2%
Time from ER Arrival to Admit. (minutes)[2]	439	244	243	274
Time from ER Arrival to Discharge (minutes)	391	179	131	134
Time in ER Before Being Evaluated (minutes)	427	20	25	26
Time to Pain Meds for Fractures (minutes)	202	65	60	57
Heart Attack Care				
Aspirin Given at Discharge	317	99%	99%	99%
Fibrinolytic Meds Within 30 Min. of Arrival[7]	-	-	33%	54%
PCI Within 90 Minutes of Arrival	51	98%	98%	96%
Statin Prescribed at Discharge	314	99%	99%	98%
Heart Failure Care				
ACE Inhibitor or ARB for LVSD	94	97%	97%	97%
Discharge Instructions Given	254	98%	93%	94%
Evaluation of LVS Function	333	100%	99%	99%
Medicare Spending				
Medicare Spending per Patient (ratio)	-	0.99	1	0.98
Pneumonia Care				
Appropriate Initial Antibiotic Given[2]	73	97%	95%	95%
Blood Culture Timing[2]	150	97%	98%	98%
Pregnancy and Delivery Care				
Newborn Deliveries Scheduled Early[2]	21	5%	6%	6%
Preventive Care				
Immunization for Influenza[2]	556	99%	93%	90%
Immunization for Pneumonia[2]	724	99%	93%	92%
Stroke Care				
Anticoagulation Therapy for Atrial Fibrillation	26	88%	94%	95%
Antithrombotic Therapy Timing	147	99%	97%	98%
Assessed for Rehabilitation	177	99%	97%	97%
Discharged on Antithrombotic Therapy	163	99%	99%	99%
Discharged on Statin Medication	127	97%	94%	94%
Thrombolytic Therapy Timing	19	68%	57%	66%
Venous Thromboembolism Prophylaxis	167	96%	93%	94%
Written Stroke Educational Materials Given	88	97%	84%	88%
Surgical Care Improvement Project				
Appropriate Beta Blocker Usage[2]	164	97%	97%	98%
Appropriate VTP Within 24 Hours[2]	512	100%	98%	98%
Controlled Postoperative Blood Glucose[2]	50	96%	95%	97%
Perioperative Temperature Management[2]	569	100%	100%	100%
Prophylactic Antibiotic Selection[2]	451	100%	99%	99%
Prophylactic Antibiotic Selection (Outpatient)	427	99%	98%	98%
Prophylactic Antibiotic Stopped[2]	442	99%	98%	98%
Prophylactic Antibiotic Timing[2]	451	99%	99%	99%
Prophylactic Antibiotic Timing (Outpatient)	427	99%	98%	98%
Urinary Catheter Removal[2]	387	99%	96%	97%
Survey of Patients' Hospital Experiences				
Area Around Room 'Always' Quiet at Night	300+	64%	67%	61%
Doctors 'Always' Communicated Well	300+	84%	84%	82%
Home Recovery Information Given	300+	83%	85%	85%
Hospital Given 9 or 10 on 10 Point Scale	300+	75%	70%	71%
Meds 'Always' Explained Before Given	300+	68%	66%	64%
Nurses 'Always' Communicated Well	300+	82%	80%	79%
Pain 'Always' Well Controlled	300+	71%	72%	71%
Room and Bathroom 'Always' Clean	300+	74%	73%	73%
Timely Help 'Always' Received	300+	72%	68%	68%
Would Definitely Recommend Hospital	300+	75%	70%	71%
Use of Medical Imaging				
Cardiac Imaging Stress Test before Surgery	426	7.0%	4.8%	5.3%
Combination Abdominal CT Scan	1,478	8.5%	9.6%	10.5%
Combination Brain/Sinus CT Scan	1,240	2.7%	3.3%	2.7%
Combination Chest CT Scan	1,396	4.7%	3.4%	2.7%
Follow-up Mammogram/Ultrasound	2,506	7.1%	8.3%	8.8%
Lumbar Spine MRI for Low Back Pain	215	31.2%	35.3%	37.2%

Cookeville Regional Medical Center

1 Medical Center Boulevard
Cookeville, TN 38501
Phone: 931-646-2000
Fax: 931-646-2635
URL: www.crmchealth.org
Type: Acute Care Hospitals
Emergency Services: Yes
Ownership: Government - Local
Beds: 247
Key Personnel:
Anesthesiology. . . . . Blake Butler, MD
Radiology. . . . . Ginny Charnock, MD
Chief of Medical Staff. . . . . Jeff Gleason
CEO . . . . Paul Korth

Measure	Cases	This Hosp.	State Avg.	U.S. Avg.
Blood Clot Prevention and Treatment				
Anticoagulation Overlap Therapy[2]	154	88%	92%	93%
ICU Venous Thromboembolism Prophylaxis[2]	115	98%	90%	92%
Incidence of Potentially Preventable VTE[2]	18	0%	10%	10%
UFH with Dosages/Platelet Monitoring[2]	92	100%	99%	97%
Venous Thromboembolism Prophylaxis[2]	322	83%	83%	85%
Warfarin Therapy Discharge Instructions[2]	112	21%	78%	75%
Chest Pain/Possible Heart Attack Care				
Aspirin Given Within 24 Hours of Arrival[1]	-	-	96%	96%
Fibrinolytic Meds Within 30 Min. of Arrival[3,7]	-	-	72%	58%
Average Time to ECG (minutes)[1]	-	-	6	7

NOTE: Hospital profiles are in alphabetical order by state, then city, then hospital within the city; Rankings exclude hospitals with less than 25 cases except for patient surveys which excludes hospitals with less than 100 cases; (a) 100-299 cases; (1) The number of cases/patients is too few to report; (2) Data submitted were based on a sample of cases/patients; (3) Results are based on a shorter time period than required; (4) Data suppressed by CMS for one or more quarters; (5) Results are not available for this reporting period; (6) Fewer than 100 patients completed the HCAHPS survey; (7) No cases met the criteria for this measure; (8) The lower limit of the confidence interval cannot be calculated if the number of observed infections equals zero; (9) No data are available from the state/territory for this reporting period; (10) The scores shown reflect fewer than 50 completed surveys; (11) There were discrepancies in the data collection process; (12) This measure does not apply to this hospital for this reporting period; (13) Results cannot be calculated for this reporting period; (14) The results for this state are combined with nearby states to protect confidentiality; Please refer to the User's Guide for a full explanation of data.

Measure	Cases	This Hosp.	State Avg.	U.S. Avg.
Average Time to Transfer (minutes)[3,7]	-	-	53	60
Children's Asthma Care				
Received Home Management Plan of Care	-	-	-	88%
Received Reliever Medication	-	-	-	100%
Received Systemic Corticosteroids	-	-	-	100%
Emergency Department				
Admittance Decision Time (minutes)[2]	487	94	82	98
Head CT Results Within 45 Min. of Arrival	14	29%	52%	57%
Patients Who Left ER Before Being Seen	50,553	3%	2%	2%
Time from ER Arrival to Admit. (minutes)[2]	487	271	243	274
Time from ER Arrival to Discharge (minutes)	373	145	131	134
Time in ER Before Being Evaluated (minutes)	426	24	25	26
Time to Pain Meds for Fractures (minutes)	138	54	60	57
Heart Attack Care				
Aspirin Given at Discharge	510	100%	99%	99%
Fibrinolytic Meds Within 30 Min. of Arrival[7]	-	-	33%	54%
PCI Within 90 Minutes of Arrival	60	100%	98%	96%
Statin Prescribed at Discharge	491	98%	99%	98%
Heart Failure Care				
ACE Inhibitor or ARB for LVSD	108	84%	97%	97%
Discharge Instructions Given	269	72%	93%	94%
Evaluation of LVS Function	332	99%	99%	99%
Medicare Spending				
Medicare Spending per Patient (ratio)	-	0.97	1	0.98
Pneumonia Care				
Appropriate Initial Antibiotic Given	253	98%	95%	95%
Blood Culture Timing	471	98%	98%	98%
Pregnancy and Delivery Care				
Newborn Deliveries Scheduled Early	119	13%	6%	6%
Preventive Care				
Immunization for Influenza[2]	536	72%	93%	90%
Immunization for Pneumonia[2]	776	84%	93%	92%
Stroke Care				
Anticoagulation Therapy for Atrial Fibrillation	18	94%	94%	95%
Antithrombotic Therapy Timing	162	98%	97%	98%
Assessed for Rehabilitation	171	84%	97%	97%
Discharged on Antithrombotic Therapy	155	97%	99%	99%
Discharged on Statin Medication	124	85%	94%	94%
Thrombolytic Therapy Timing	11	0%	57%	66%
Venous Thromboembolism Prophylaxis	182	89%	93%	94%
Written Stroke Educational Materials Given	105	43%	84%	88%
Surgical Care Improvement Project				
Appropriate Beta Blocker Usage	492	98%	97%	98%
Appropriate VTP Within 24 Hours	828	95%	98%	98%
Controlled Postoperative Blood Glucose	221	95%	95%	97%
Perioperative Temperature Management	1,140	100%	100%	100%
Prophylactic Antibiotic Selection	810	99%	99%	99%
Prophylactic Antibiotic Selection (Outpatient)	659	99%	98%	98%
Prophylactic Antibiotic Stopped	766	93%	98%	98%
Prophylactic Antibiotic Timing	812	98%	99%	99%
Prophylactic Antibiotic Timing (Outpatient)	660	99%	98%	98%
Urinary Catheter Removal	828	93%	96%	97%
Survey of Patients' Hospital Experiences				
Area Around Room 'Always' Quiet at Night	300+	62%	67%	61%
Doctors 'Always' Communicated Well	300+	82%	84%	82%
Home Recovery Information Given	300+	88%	85%	85%
Hospital Given 9 or 10 on 10 Point Scale	300+	74%	70%	71%
Meds 'Always' Explained Before Given	300+	66%	66%	64%
Nurses 'Always' Communicated Well	300+	80%	80%	79%
Pain 'Always' Well Controlled	300+	70%	72%	71%
Room and Bathroom 'Always' Clean	300+	70%	73%	73%
Timely Help 'Always' Received	300+	68%	68%	68%
Would Definitely Recommend Hospital	300+	78%	70%	71%
Use of Medical Imaging				
Cardiac Imaging Stress Test before Surgery	1,477	4.8%	4.8%	5.3%
Combination Abdominal CT Scan	1,442	9.3%	9.6%	10.5%
Combination Brain/Sinus CT Scan	1,510	2.7%	3.3%	2.7%
Combination Chest CT Scan	1,015	6.3%	3.4%	2.7%
Follow-up Mammogram/Ultrasound	1,443	8.7%	8.3%	8.8%
Lumbar Spine MRI for Low Back Pain	427	31.9%	35.3%	37.2%

Copper Basin Medical Center

Highway 68
Copperhill, TN 37317
Phone: 423-496-5511
Fax: 423-496-8171
Type: Critical Access Hospitals
Emergency Services: Yes
Ownership: Voluntary non-profit - Other
Beds: 44
Key Personnel:
Patient Relations . . . . Chris Cook
Infection Control. . . . . Nancy Gessling
CEO/President. . . . . David W Hyatt
Emergency Room . . . . Tonya Niz
Chief of Medical Staff. . . . . Allen S Uhlik, MD

Measure	Cases	This Hosp.	State Avg.	U.S. Avg.
Blood Clot Prevention and Treatment				
Anticoagulation Overlap Therapy[5]	-	-	92%	93%
ICU Venous Thromboembolism Prophylaxis[5]	-	-	90%	92%
Incidence of Potentially Preventable VTE[5]	-	-	10%	10%
UFH with Dosages/Platelet Monitoring[5]	-	-	99%	97%
Venous Thromboembolism Prophylaxis[5]	-	-	83%	85%
Warfarin Therapy Discharge Instructions[5]	-	-	78%	75%
Chest Pain/Possible Heart Attack Care				
Aspirin Given Within 24 Hours of Arrival	23	83%	96%	96%
Fibrinolytic Meds Within 30 Min. of Arrival[1,3]	-	-	72%	58%
Average Time to ECG (minutes)	24	14	6	7
Average Time to Transfer (minutes)[1,3]	-	-	53	60
Children's Asthma Care				
Received Home Management Plan of Care	-	-	-	88%
Received Reliever Medication	-	-	-	100%
Received Systemic Corticosteroids	-	-	-	100%
Emergency Department				
Admittance Decision Time (minutes)[5]	-	-	82	98
Head CT Results Within 45 Min. of Arrival[1]	-	-	52%	57%
Patients Who Left ER Before Being Seen	6,427	1%	2%	2%
Time from ER Arrival to Admit. (minutes)[5]	-	-	243	274
Time from ER Arrival to Discharge (minutes)[1,3]	-	-	131	134
Time in ER Before Being Evaluated (minutes)[3]	14	18	25	26
Time to Pain Meds for Fractures (minutes)[1]	-	-	60	57
Heart Attack Care				
Aspirin Given at Discharge[1,2]	-	-	99%	99%
Fibrinolytic Meds Within 30 Min. of Arrival[2,3]	-	-	33%	54%
PCI Within 90 Minutes of Arrival[2,3]	-	-	98%	96%
Statin Prescribed at Discharge[1,2]	-	-	99%	98%
Heart Failure Care				
ACE Inhibitor or ARB for LVSD[1,2]	-	-	97%	97%
Discharge Instructions Given[1,2]	-	-	93%	94%
Evaluation of LVS Function[1,2]	-	-	99%	99%
Medicare Spending				
Medicare Spending per Patient (ratio)	-	-	1	0.98
Pneumonia Care				
Appropriate Initial Antibiotic Given[2]	16	50%	95%	95%
Blood Culture Timing[2]	15	87%	98%	98%
Pregnancy and Delivery Care				
Newborn Deliveries Scheduled Early[5]	-	-	6%	6%
Preventive Care				
Immunization for Influenza[5]	-	-	93%	90%
Immunization for Pneumonia[5]	-	-	93%	92%
Stroke Care				
Anticoagulation Therapy for Atrial Fibrillation[5]	-	-	94%	95%
Antithrombotic Therapy Timing[5]	-	-	97%	98%
Assessed for Rehabilitation[5]	-	-	97%	97%
Discharged on Antithrombotic Therapy[5]	-	-	99%	99%
Discharged on Statin Medication[5]	-	-	94%	94%
Thrombolytic Therapy Timing[5]	-	-	57%	66%
Venous Thromboembolism Prophylaxis[5]	-	-	93%	94%
Written Stroke Educational Materials Given[5]	-	-	84%	88%
Surgical Care Improvement Project				
Appropriate Beta Blocker Usage[5]	-	-	97%	98%
Appropriate VTP Within 24 Hours[5]	-	-	98%	98%
Controlled Postoperative Blood Glucose[5]	-	-	95%	97%
Perioperative Temperature Management[5]	-	-	100%	100%
Prophylactic Antibiotic Selection[5]	-	-	99%	99%
Prophylactic Antibiotic Selection (Outpatient)[5]	-	-	98%	98%
Prophylactic Antibiotic Stopped[5]	-	-	98%	98%
Prophylactic Antibiotic Timing[5]	-	-	99%	99%
Prophylactic Antibiotic Timing (Outpatient)[5]	-	-	98%	98%
Urinary Catheter Removal[5]	-	-	96%	97%
Survey of Patients' Hospital Experiences				
Area Around Room 'Always' Quiet at Night	(a)	72%	67%	61%
Doctors 'Always' Communicated Well	(a)	91%	84%	82%
Home Recovery Information Given	(a)	87%	85%	85%
Hospital Given 9 or 10 on 10 Point Scale	(a)	78%	70%	71%
Meds 'Always' Explained Before Given	(a)	75%	66%	64%
Nurses 'Always' Communicated Well	(a)	87%	80%	79%
Pain 'Always' Well Controlled	(a)	80%	72%	71%
Room and Bathroom 'Always' Clean	(a)	76%	73%	73%
Timely Help 'Always' Received	(a)	71%	68%	68%
Would Definitely Recommend Hospital	(a)	86%	70%	71%
Use of Medical Imaging				
Cardiac Imaging Stress Test before Surgery	55	5.5%	4.8%	5.3%
Combination Abdominal CT Scan	269	4.8%	9.6%	10.5%
Combination Brain/Sinus CT Scan[1]	-	-	3.3%	2.7%
Combination Chest CT Scan	138	4.3%	3.4%	2.7%
Follow-up Mammogram/Ultrasound	189	2.1%	8.3%	8.8%
Lumbar Spine MRI for Low Back Pain[1]	-	-	35.3%	37.2%

Baptist Memorial Hospital Tipton

1995 Highway 51 S
Covington, TN 38019
Phone: 901-476-2621
Fax: 901-475-5504
URL: www.bmhcc.org
Type: Acute Care Hospitals
Emergency Services: Yes
Ownership: Voluntary non-profit - Church
Beds: 70
Key Personnel:
Radiology. . . . . James D Acker
CEO . . . . Sam Lynd

Measure	Cases	This Hosp.	State Avg.	U.S. Avg.
Blood Clot Prevention and Treatment				
Anticoagulation Overlap Therapy	13	100%	92%	93%
ICU Venous Thromboembolism Prophylaxis	95	87%	90%	92%
Incidence of Potentially Preventable VTE[7]	-	-	10%	10%
UFH with Dosages/Platelet Monitoring[1]	-	-	99%	97%
Venous Thromboembolism Prophylaxis	385	64%	83%	85%
Warfarin Therapy Discharge Instructions	11	100%	78%	75%
Chest Pain/Possible Heart Attack Care				
Aspirin Given Within 24 Hours of Arrival	168	90%	96%	96%
Fibrinolytic Meds Within 30 Min. of Arrival[1]	-	-	72%	58%
Average Time to ECG (minutes)	174	12	6	7
Average Time to Transfer (minutes)[1]	-	-	53	60
Children's Asthma Care				
Received Home Management Plan of Care	-	-	-	88%
Received Reliever Medication	-	-	-	100%
Received Systemic Corticosteroids	-	-	-	100%
Emergency Department				
Admittance Decision Time (minutes)[2]	218	72	82	98
Head CT Results Within 45 Min. of Arrival[1]	-	-	52%	57%
Patients Who Left ER Before Being Seen	21,655	2%	2%	2%
Time from ER Arrival to Admit. (minutes)[2]	226	266	243	274
Time from ER Arrival to Discharge (minutes)	390	129	131	134
Time in ER Before Being Evaluated (minutes)	415	36	25	26
Time to Pain Meds for Fractures (minutes)	93	83	60	57
Heart Attack Care				
Aspirin Given at Discharge[3,7]	-	-	99%	99%
Fibrinolytic Meds Within 30 Min. of Arrival[3,7]	-	-	33%	54%
PCI Within 90 Minutes of Arrival[3,7]	-	-	98%	96%
Statin Prescribed at Discharge[3,7]	-	-	99%	98%
Heart Failure Care				
ACE Inhibitor or ARB for LVSD[1]	-	-	97%	97%
Discharge Instructions Given	37	100%	93%	94%
Evaluation of LVS Function	44	100%	99%	99%
Medicare Spending				
Medicare Spending per Patient (ratio)	-	0.98	1	0.98
Pneumonia Care				
Appropriate Initial Antibiotic Given	50	100%	95%	95%
Blood Culture Timing	57	96%	98%	98%
Pregnancy and Delivery Care				
Newborn Deliveries Scheduled Early[2,7]	-	-	6%	6%
Preventive Care				
Immunization for Influenza[2]	265	95%	93%	90%

NOTE: Hospital profiles are in alphabetical order by state, then city, then hospital within the city; Rankings exclude hospitals with less than 25 cases except for patient surveys which excludes hospitals with less than 100 cases; (a) 100-299 cases; (1) The number of cases/patients is too few to report; (2) Data submitted were based on a sample of cases/patients; (3) Results are based on a shorter time period than required; (4) Data suppressed by CMS for one or more quarters; (5) Results are not available for this reporting period; (6) Fewer than 100 patients completed the HCAHPS survey; (7) No cases met the criteria for this measure; (8) The lower limit of the confidence interval cannot be calculated if the number of observed infections equals zero; (9) No data are available from the state/territory for this reporting period; (10) The scores shown reflect fewer than 50 completed surveys; (11) There were discrepancies in the data collection process; (12) This measure does not apply to this hospital for this reporting period; (13) Results cannot be calculated for this reporting period; (14) The results for this state are combined with nearby states to protect confidentiality; Please refer to the User's Guide for a full explanation of data.

Measure	Cases	This Hosp.	State Avg.	U.S. Avg.
Immunization for Pneumonia[2]	231	96%	93%	92%
Stroke Care				
Anticoagulation Therapy for Atrial Fibrillation[7]	-	-	94%	95%
Antithrombotic Therapy Timing[1]	-	-	97%	98%
Assessed for Rehabilitation[1]	-	-	97%	97%
Discharged on Antithrombotic Therapy[1]	-	-	99%	99%
Discharged on Statin Medication[1]	-	-	94%	94%
Thrombolytic Therapy Timing[7]	-	-	57%	66%
Venous Thromboembolism Prophylaxis[1]	-	-	93%	94%
Written Stroke Educational Materials Given[1]	-	-	84%	88%
Surgical Care Improvement Project				
Appropriate Beta Blocker Usage	11	100%	97%	98%
Appropriate VTP Within 24 Hours	46	100%	98%	98%
Controlled Postoperative Blood Glucose[7]	-	-	95%	97%
Perioperative Temperature Management	56	100%	100%	100%
Prophylactic Antibiotic Selection	42	95%	99%	99%
Prophylactic Antibiotic Selection (Outpatient)[1]	-	-	98%	98%
Prophylactic Antibiotic Stopped	41	98%	98%	98%
Prophylactic Antibiotic Timing	42	100%	99%	99%
Prophylactic Antibiotic Timing (Outpatient)[1]	-	-	98%	98%
Urinary Catheter Removal	23	100%	96%	97%
Survey of Patients' Hospital Experiences				
Area Around Room 'Always' Quiet at Night	(a)	69%	67%	61%
Doctors 'Always' Communicated Well	(a)	84%	84%	82%
Home Recovery Information Given	(a)	82%	85%	85%
Hospital Given 9 or 10 on 10 Point Scale	(a)	62%	70%	71%
Meds 'Always' Explained Before Given	(a)	76%	66%	64%
Nurses 'Always' Communicated Well	(a)	80%	80%	79%
Pain 'Always' Well Controlled	(a)	68%	72%	71%
Room and Bathroom 'Always' Clean	(a)	75%	73%	73%
Timely Help 'Always' Received	(a)	74%	68%	68%
Would Definitely Recommend Hospital	(a)	61%	70%	71%
Use of Medical Imaging				
Cardiac Imaging Stress Test before Surgery[1]	-	-	4.8%	5.3%
Combination Abdominal CT Scan	756	30.3%	9.6%	10.5%
Combination Brain/Sinus CT Scan	341	0.3%	3.3%	2.7%
Combination Chest CT Scan	797	3.1%	3.4%	2.7%
Follow-up Mammogram/Ultrasound	470	15.7%	8.3%	8.8%
Lumbar Spine MRI for Low Back Pain[1]	-	-	35.3%	37.2%

Cumberland Medical Center

421 S Main St
Crossville, TN 38555
Phone: 931-484-9511
Fax: 931-707-8150
E-mail: jmartin@cmchealthcare.org
URL: www.cmchealthcare.org
Type: Acute Care Hospitals
Emergency Services: Yes
Ownership: Voluntary non-profit - Private
Beds: 202

Key Personnel:
Radiology. . . . . Richard L Bilbrey, MD
CEO/President. . . . . Donna Franklin
Cardiac Laboratory. . . . . Dian Jones
Pediatric Ambulatory Care . . . . . . MH Koucheki, MD
Anesthesiology. . . . . Thomas LaSalle, DO
Emergency Room . . . . David McKinney
Chief of Medical Staff. . . . . Timothy Spitler

Measure	Cases	This Hosp.	State Avg.	U.S. Avg.
Blood Clot Prevention and Treatment				
Anticoagulation Overlap Therapy[2]	56	98%	92%	93%
ICU Venous Thromboembolism Prophylaxis[2]	90	90%	90%	92%
Incidence of Potentially Preventable VTE[2]	12	8%	10%	10%
UFH with Dosages/Platelet Monitoring[2]	23	100%	99%	97%
Venous Thromboembolism Prophylaxis[2]	382	83%	83%	85%
Warfarin Therapy Discharge Instructions[2]	49	98%	78%	75%
Chest Pain/Possible Heart Attack Care				
Aspirin Given Within 24 Hours of Arrival	149	98%	96%	96%
Fibrinolytic Meds Within 30 Min. of Arrival[1]	-	-	72%	58%
Average Time to ECG (minutes)	156	7	6	7
Average Time to Transfer (minutes)	12	38	53	60
Children's Asthma Care				
Received Home Management Plan of Care	-	-	-	88%
Received Reliever Medication	-	-	-	100%
Received Systemic Corticosteroids	-	-	-	100%
Emergency Department				
Admittance Decision Time (minutes)[2]	514	51	82	98
Head CT Results Within 45 Min. of Arrival	18	83%	52%	57%
Patients Who Left ER Before Being Seen	34,949	1%	2%	2%
Time from ER Arrival to Admit. (minutes)[2]	517	190	243	274
Time from ER Arrival to Discharge (minutes)	355	110	131	134
Time in ER Before Being Evaluated (minutes)	383	25	25	26
Time to Pain Meds for Fractures (minutes)	56	50	60	57
Heart Attack Care				
Aspirin Given at Discharge	31	94%	99%	99%
Fibrinolytic Meds Within 30 Min. of Arrival[7]	-	-	33%	54%
PCI Within 90 Minutes of Arrival[7]	-	-	98%	96%
Statin Prescribed at Discharge	32	97%	99%	98%
Heart Failure Care				
ACE Inhibitor or ARB for LVSD	57	86%	97%	97%
Discharge Instructions Given	161	90%	93%	94%
Evaluation of LVS Function	201	99%	99%	99%
Medicare Spending				
Medicare Spending per Patient (ratio)	-	0.91	1	0.98
Pneumonia Care				
Appropriate Initial Antibiotic Given	170	98%	95%	95%
Blood Culture Timing	292	98%	98%	98%
Pregnancy and Delivery Care				
Newborn Deliveries Scheduled Early[2]	27	4%	6%	6%
Preventive Care				
Immunization for Influenza[2]	461	71%	93%	90%
Immunization for Pneumonia[2]	648	90%	93%	92%
Stroke Care				
Anticoagulation Therapy for Atrial Fibrillation[1,2]	-	-	94%	95%
Antithrombotic Therapy Timing[2]	49	98%	97%	98%
Assessed for Rehabilitation[2]	48	98%	97%	97%
Discharged on Antithrombotic Therapy[2]	46	98%	99%	99%
Discharged on Statin Medication[2]	35	83%	94%	94%
Thrombolytic Therapy Timing[1,2]	-	-	57%	66%
Venous Thromboembolism Prophylaxis[2]	50	98%	93%	94%
Written Stroke Educational Materials Given[2]	24	50%	84%	88%
Surgical Care Improvement Project				
Appropriate Beta Blocker Usage[2]	109	86%	97%	98%
Appropriate VTP Within 24 Hours[2]	239	95%	98%	98%
Controlled Postoperative Blood Glucose[2,7]	-	-	95%	97%
Perioperative Temperature Management[2]	266	100%	100%	100%
Prophylactic Antibiotic Selection[2]	175	97%	99%	99%
Prophylactic Antibiotic Selection (Outpatient)	119	78%	98%	98%
Prophylactic Antibiotic Stopped[2]	172	94%	98%	98%
Prophylactic Antibiotic Timing[2]	175	90%	99%	99%
Prophylactic Antibiotic Timing (Outpatient)	126	90%	98%	98%
Urinary Catheter Removal[2]	192	83%	96%	97%
Survey of Patients' Hospital Experiences				
Area Around Room 'Always' Quiet at Night	300+	58%	67%	61%
Doctors 'Always' Communicated Well	300+	79%	84%	82%
Home Recovery Information Given	300+	83%	85%	85%
Hospital Given 9 or 10 on 10 Point Scale	300+	61%	70%	71%
Meds 'Always' Explained Before Given	300+	58%	66%	64%
Nurses 'Always' Communicated Well	300+	77%	80%	79%
Pain 'Always' Well Controlled	300+	69%	72%	71%
Room and Bathroom 'Always' Clean	300+	71%	73%	73%
Timely Help 'Always' Received	300+	64%	68%	68%
Would Definitely Recommend Hospital	300+	61%	70%	71%
Use of Medical Imaging				
Cardiac Imaging Stress Test before Surgery	367	3.8%	4.8%	5.3%
Combination Abdominal CT Scan	895	5.8%	9.6%	10.5%
Combination Brain/Sinus CT Scan	1,146	0.9%	3.3%	2.7%
Combination Chest CT Scan	882	3.4%	3.4%	2.7%
Follow-up Mammogram/Ultrasound	2,264	4.2%	8.3%	8.8%
Lumbar Spine MRI for Low Back Pain	308	44.2%	35.3%	37.2%

Rhea Medical Center

9400 Rhea County Highway
Dayton, TN 37321
Phone: 423-775-1121
Fax: 423-775-6621
Type: Critical Access Hospitals
Emergency Services: Yes
Ownership: Government - Local
Beds: 131

Key Personnel:
CEO/President. . . . . Kennedy Croom
Radiology. . . . . Roger Miller
Pediatrics. . . . . James Nelson
Cardiology . . . . J. Walter Sledge
Emergency Room . . . . John Staley, MD
Surgery . . . . Craig Swafford

Measure	Cases	This Hosp.	State Avg.	U.S. Avg.
Blood Clot Prevention and Treatment				
Anticoagulation Overlap Therapy[5]	-	-	92%	93%
ICU Venous Thromboembolism Prophylaxis[5]	-	-	90%	92%
Incidence of Potentially Preventable VTE[5]	-	-	10%	10%
UFH with Dosages/Platelet Monitoring[5]	-	-	99%	97%
Venous Thromboembolism Prophylaxis[5]	-	-	83%	85%
Warfarin Therapy Discharge Instructions[5]	-	-	78%	75%
Chest Pain/Possible Heart Attack Care				
Aspirin Given Within 24 Hours of Arrival	29	100%	96%	96%
Fibrinolytic Meds Within 30 Min. of Arrival[7]	-	-	72%	58%
Average Time to ECG (minutes)	30	5	6	7
Average Time to Transfer (minutes)[1]	-	-	53	60
Children's Asthma Care				
Received Home Management Plan of Care	-	-	-	88%
Received Reliever Medication	-	-	-	100%
Received Systemic Corticosteroids	-	-	-	100%
Emergency Department				
Admittance Decision Time (minutes)[5]	-	-	82	98
Head CT Results Within 45 Min. of Arrival[5]	-	-	52%	57%
Patients Who Left ER Before Being Seen[5]	-	-	2%	2%
Time from ER Arrival to Admit. (minutes)[5]	-	-	243	274
Time from ER Arrival to Discharge (minutes)[5]	-	-	131	134
Time in ER Before Being Evaluated (minutes)[5]	-	-	25	26
Time to Pain Meds for Fractures (minutes)[5]	-	-	60	57
Heart Attack Care				
Aspirin Given at Discharge[3,7]	-	-	99%	99%
Fibrinolytic Meds Within 30 Min. of Arrival[3,7]	-	-	33%	54%
PCI Within 90 Minutes of Arrival[3,7]	-	-	98%	96%
Statin Prescribed at Discharge[3,7]	-	-	99%	98%
Heart Failure Care				
ACE Inhibitor or ARB for LVSD[1]	-	-	97%	97%
Discharge Instructions Given	22	82%	93%	94%
Evaluation of LVS Function	30	97%	99%	99%
Medicare Spending				
Medicare Spending per Patient (ratio)	-	-	1	0.98
Pneumonia Care				
Appropriate Initial Antibiotic Given	103	93%	95%	95%
Blood Culture Timing	109	97%	98%	98%
Pregnancy and Delivery Care				
Newborn Deliveries Scheduled Early[5]	-	-	6%	6%
Preventive Care				
Immunization for Influenza[5]	-	-	93%	90%
Immunization for Pneumonia[5]	-	-	93%	92%
Stroke Care				
Anticoagulation Therapy for Atrial Fibrillation[5]	-	-	94%	95%
Antithrombotic Therapy Timing[5]	-	-	97%	98%
Assessed for Rehabilitation[5]	-	-	97%	97%
Discharged on Antithrombotic Therapy[5]	-	-	99%	99%
Discharged on Statin Medication[5]	-	-	94%	94%
Thrombolytic Therapy Timing[5]	-	-	57%	66%
Venous Thromboembolism Prophylaxis[5]	-	-	93%	94%
Written Stroke Educational Materials Given[5]	-	-	84%	88%
Surgical Care Improvement Project				
Appropriate Beta Blocker Usage[1]	-	-	97%	98%
Appropriate VTP Within 24 Hours	23	87%	98%	98%
Controlled Postoperative Blood Glucose[7]	-	-	95%	97%
Perioperative Temperature Management	25	100%	100%	100%
Prophylactic Antibiotic Selection	11	100%	99%	99%
Prophylactic Antibiotic Selection (Outpatient)[1,3]	-	-	98%	98%
Prophylactic Antibiotic Stopped	11	91%	98%	98%
Prophylactic Antibiotic Timing	11	100%	99%	99%
Prophylactic Antibiotic Timing (Outpatient)[1,3]	-	-	98%	98%
Urinary Catheter Removal	12	100%	96%	97%
Survey of Patients' Hospital Experiences				
Area Around Room 'Always' Quiet at Night	(a)	66%	67%	61%
Doctors 'Always' Communicated Well	(a)	81%	84%	82%
Home Recovery Information Given	(a)	85%	85%	85%
Hospital Given 9 or 10 on 10 Point Scale	(a)	70%	70%	71%
Meds 'Always' Explained Before Given	(a)	61%	66%	64%

NOTE: Hospital profiles are in alphabetical order by state, then city, then hospital within the city; Rankings exclude hospitals with less than 25 cases except for patient surveys which excludes hospitals with less than 100 cases; (a) 100-299 cases; (1) The number of cases/patients is too few to report; (2) Data submitted were based on a sample of cases/patients; (3) Results are based on a shorter time period than required; (4) Data suppressed by CMS for one or more quarters; (5) Results are not available for this reporting period; (6) Fewer than 100 patients completed the HCAHPS survey; (7) No cases met the criteria for this measure; (8) The lower limit of the confidence interval cannot be calculated if the number of observed infections equals zero; (9) No data are available from the state/territory for this reporting period; (10) The scores shown reflect fewer than 50 completed surveys; (11) There were discrepancies in the data collection process; (12) This measure does not apply to this hospital for this reporting period; (13) Results cannot be calculated for this reporting period; (14) The results for this state are combined with nearby states to protect confidentiality; Please refer to the User's Guide for a full explanation of data.

Nurses 'Always' Communicated Well	(a)	79%	80%	79%
Pain 'Always' Well Controlled	(a)	70%	72%	71%
Room and Bathroom 'Always' Clean	(a)	71%	73%	73%
Timely Help 'Always' Received	(a)	72%	68%	68%
Would Definitely Recommend Hospital	(a)	68%	70%	71%
Use of Medical Imaging				
Cardiac Imaging Stress Test before Surgery	143	4.2%	4.8%	5.3%
Combination Abdominal CT Scan	424	6.6%	9.6%	10.5%
Combination Brain/Sinus CT Scan[1]	-	-	3.3%	2.7%
Combination Chest CT Scan	155	11.0%	3.4%	2.7%
Follow-up Mammogram/Ultrasound	558	7.3%	8.3%	8.8%
Lumbar Spine MRI for Low Back Pain	69	27.5%	35.3%	37.2%

Tristar Horizon Medical Center

111 Highway 70 East
Dickson, TN 37055
Type: Acute Care Hospitals
Ownership: Proprietary
Phone: 615-446-0446
Fax: 615-441-2514
Emergency Services: Yes
Beds: 150

Key Personnel:
Radiology. . . . . John J Alarcon
Anesthesiology. . . . . Barry Brasfield, MD
Emergency Room . . . . Gina Bullington, RN
Infection Control. . . . . Donna Clark
Quality Assurance . . . . Tori Howk
CEO . . . . John A. Marshall
Chief of Medical Staff. . . . . Van Mills
Operating Room. . . . . Megan Weiss

Measure	Cases	This Hosp.	State Avg.	U.S. Avg.
Blood Clot Prevention and Treatment				
Anticoagulation Overlap Therapy[2]	35	97%	92%	93%
ICU Venous Thromboembolism Prophylaxis[2]	87	97%	90%	92%
Incidence of Potentially Preventable VTE[1,2]	-	-	10%	10%
UFH with Dosages/Platelet Monitoring[2]	11	100%	99%	97%
Venous Thromboembolism Prophylaxis[2]	359	97%	83%	85%
Warfarin Therapy Discharge Instructions[2]	25	84%	78%	75%
Chest Pain/Possible Heart Attack Care				
Aspirin Given Within 24 Hours of Arrival	126	98%	96%	96%
Fibrinolytic Meds Within 30 Min. of Arrival[7]	-	-	72%	58%
Average Time to ECG (minutes)	132	6	6	7
Average Time to Transfer (minutes)	26	23	53	60
Children's Asthma Care				
Received Home Management Plan of Care	-	-	-	88%
Received Reliever Medication	-	-	-	100%
Received Systemic Corticosteroids	-	-	-	100%
Emergency Department				
Admittance Decision Time (minutes)[2]	600	72	82	98
Head CT Results Within 45 Min. of Arrival	19	95%	52%	57%
Patients Who Left ER Before Being Seen	37,794	1%	2%	2%
Time from ER Arrival to Admit. (minutes)[2]	601	229	243	274
Time from ER Arrival to Discharge (minutes)	414	121	131	134
Time in ER Before Being Evaluated (minutes)	472	17	25	26
Time to Pain Meds for Fractures (minutes)	147	37	60	57
Heart Attack Care				
Aspirin Given at Discharge	42	100%	99%	99%
Fibrinolytic Meds Within 30 Min. of Arrival[7]	-	-	33%	54%
PCI Within 90 Minutes of Arrival[1]	-	-	98%	96%
Statin Prescribed at Discharge	39	97%	99%	98%
Heart Failure Care				
ACE Inhibitor or ARB for LVSD	41	100%	97%	97%
Discharge Instructions Given	168	97%	93%	94%
Evaluation of LVS Function	209	100%	99%	99%
Medicare Spending				
Medicare Spending per Patient (ratio)	-	1.03	1	0.98
Pneumonia Care				
Appropriate Initial Antibiotic Given	130	98%	95%	95%
Blood Culture Timing	204	100%	98%	98%
Pregnancy and Delivery Care				
Newborn Deliveries Scheduled Early[2]	33	0%	6%	6%
Preventive Care				
Immunization for Influenza[2]	430	98%	93%	90%
Immunization for Pneumonia[2]	634	98%	93%	92%
Stroke Care				
Anticoagulation Therapy for Atrial Fibrillation[1]	-	-	94%	95%
Antithrombotic Therapy Timing	45	100%	97%	98%
Assessed for Rehabilitation	39	100%	97%	97%
Discharged on Antithrombotic Therapy	39	100%	99%	99%
Discharged on Statin Medication	30	100%	94%	94%
Thrombolytic Therapy Timing[7]	-	-	57%	66%
Venous Thromboembolism Prophylaxis	46	100%	93%	94%
Written Stroke Educational Materials Given	18	94%	84%	88%
Surgical Care Improvement Project				
Appropriate Beta Blocker Usage	25	100%	97%	98%
Appropriate VTP Within 24 Hours	121	98%	98%	98%
Controlled Postoperative Blood Glucose[7]	-	-	95%	97%
Perioperative Temperature Management	133	100%	100%	100%
Prophylactic Antibiotic Selection	76	100%	99%	99%
Prophylactic Antibiotic Selection (Outpatient)	54	100%	98%	98%
Prophylactic Antibiotic Stopped	70	99%	98%	98%
Prophylactic Antibiotic Timing	76	100%	99%	99%
Prophylactic Antibiotic Timing (Outpatient)	54	100%	98%	98%
Urinary Catheter Removal	79	97%	96%	97%
Survey of Patients' Hospital Experiences				
Area Around Room 'Always' Quiet at Night	300+	67%	67%	61%
Doctors 'Always' Communicated Well	300+	81%	84%	82%
Home Recovery Information Given	300+	87%	85%	85%
Hospital Given 9 or 10 on 10 Point Scale	300+	71%	70%	71%
Meds 'Always' Explained Before Given	300+	64%	66%	64%
Nurses 'Always' Communicated Well	300+	81%	80%	79%
Pain 'Always' Well Controlled	300+	74%	72%	71%
Room and Bathroom 'Always' Clean	300+	77%	73%	73%
Timely Help 'Always' Received	300+	69%	68%	68%
Would Definitely Recommend Hospital	300+	66%	70%	71%
Use of Medical Imaging				
Cardiac Imaging Stress Test before Surgery	73	6.8%	4.8%	5.3%
Combination Abdominal CT Scan	504	4.0%	9.6%	10.5%
Combination Brain/Sinus CT Scan[1]	-	-	3.3%	2.7%
Combination Chest CT Scan	215	0.9%	3.4%	2.7%
Follow-up Mammogram/Ultrasound	709	5.8%	8.3%	8.8%
Lumbar Spine MRI for Low Back Pain	61	31.1%	35.3%	37.2%

Dyersburg Regional Medical Center

400 Tickle St
Dyersburg, TN 38024
URL: www.dyersburgregionalmc.com
Type: Acute Care Hospitals
Ownership: Proprietary
Phone: 731-285-2410
Emergency Services: Yes

Measure	Cases	This Hosp.	State Avg.	U.S. Avg.
Blood Clot Prevention and Treatment				
Anticoagulation Overlap Therapy[2]	25	100%	92%	93%
ICU Venous Thromboembolism Prophylaxis[2]	89	98%	90%	92%
Incidence of Potentially Preventable VTE[1,2]	-	-	10%	10%
UFH with Dosages/Platelet Monitoring[2]	17	100%	99%	97%
Venous Thromboembolism Prophylaxis[2]	288	99%	83%	85%
Warfarin Therapy Discharge Instructions[2]	15	100%	78%	75%
Chest Pain/Possible Heart Attack Care				
Aspirin Given Within 24 Hours of Arrival	248	98%	96%	96%
Fibrinolytic Meds Within 30 Min. of Arrival	12	83%	72%	58%
Average Time to ECG (minutes)	254	2	6	7
Average Time to Transfer (minutes)[1]	-	-	53	60
Children's Asthma Care				
Received Home Management Plan of Care	-	-	-	88%
Received Reliever Medication	-	-	-	100%
Received Systemic Corticosteroids	-	-	-	100%
Emergency Department				
Admittance Decision Time (minutes)[2]	481	55	82	98
Head CT Results Within 45 Min. of Arrival	19	63%	52%	57%
Patients Who Left ER Before Being Seen	27,493	2%	2%	2%
Time from ER Arrival to Admit. (minutes)[2]	487	202	243	274
Time from ER Arrival to Discharge (minutes)	346	130	131	134
Time in ER Before Being Evaluated (minutes)	414	35	25	26
Time to Pain Meds for Fractures (minutes)	154	26	60	57
Heart Attack Care				
Aspirin Given at Discharge	15	100%	99%	99%
Fibrinolytic Meds Within 30 Min. of Arrival[7]	-	-	33%	54%
PCI Within 90 Minutes of Arrival[7]	-	-	98%	96%
Statin Prescribed at Discharge	16	94%	99%	98%
Heart Failure Care				
ACE Inhibitor or ARB for LVSD	23	100%	97%	97%
Discharge Instructions Given	87	99%	93%	94%
Evaluation of LVS Function	131	100%	99%	99%
Medicare Spending				
Medicare Spending per Patient (ratio)	-	1.04	1	0.98
Pneumonia Care				
Appropriate Initial Antibiotic Given	61	98%	95%	95%
Blood Culture Timing	104	99%	98%	98%
Pregnancy and Delivery Care				
Newborn Deliveries Scheduled Early[2]	30	0%	6%	6%
Preventive Care				
Immunization for Influenza[2]	424	100%	93%	90%
Immunization for Pneumonia[2]	553	100%	93%	92%
Stroke Care				
Anticoagulation Therapy for Atrial Fibrillation[1]	-	-	94%	95%
Antithrombotic Therapy Timing	36	100%	97%	98%
Assessed for Rehabilitation	44	95%	97%	97%
Discharged on Antithrombotic Therapy	42	100%	99%	99%
Discharged on Statin Medication	35	100%	94%	94%
Thrombolytic Therapy Timing[7]	-	-	57%	66%
Venous Thromboembolism Prophylaxis	35	100%	93%	94%
Written Stroke Educational Materials Given	28	86%	84%	88%
Surgical Care Improvement Project				
Appropriate Beta Blocker Usage	16	100%	97%	98%
Appropriate VTP Within 24 Hours	67	100%	98%	98%
Controlled Postoperative Blood Glucose[7]	-	-	95%	97%
Perioperative Temperature Management	80	100%	100%	100%
Prophylactic Antibiotic Selection	43	100%	99%	99%
Prophylactic Antibiotic Selection (Outpatient)	68	99%	98%	98%
Prophylactic Antibiotic Stopped	42	98%	98%	98%
Prophylactic Antibiotic Timing	43	100%	99%	99%
Prophylactic Antibiotic Timing (Outpatient)	68	100%	98%	98%
Urinary Catheter Removal	44	100%	96%	97%
Survey of Patients' Hospital Experiences				
Area Around Room 'Always' Quiet at Night	300+	70%	67%	61%
Doctors 'Always' Communicated Well	300+	81%	84%	82%
Home Recovery Information Given	300+	86%	85%	85%
Hospital Given 9 or 10 on 10 Point Scale	300+	67%	70%	71%
Meds 'Always' Explained Before Given	300+	67%	66%	64%
Nurses 'Always' Communicated Well	300+	80%	80%	79%
Pain 'Always' Well Controlled	300+	74%	72%	71%
Room and Bathroom 'Always' Clean	300+	68%	73%	73%
Timely Help 'Always' Received	300+	71%	68%	68%
Would Definitely Recommend Hospital	300+	61%	70%	71%
Use of Medical Imaging				
Cardiac Imaging Stress Test before Surgery	227	4.8%	4.8%	5.3%
Combination Abdominal CT Scan	685	5.5%	9.6%	10.5%
Combination Brain/Sinus CT Scan[1]	-	-	3.3%	2.7%
Combination Chest CT Scan	348	1.4%	3.4%	2.7%
Follow-up Mammogram/Ultrasound	899	6.1%	8.3%	8.8%
Lumbar Spine MRI for Low Back Pain	124	37.1%	35.3%	37.2%

Sycamore Shoals Hospital

1501 West Elk Avenue
Elizabethton, TN 37643
URL: www.msha.com
Type: Acute Care Hospitals
Ownership: Voluntary non-profit - Private
Phone: 423-542-1300
Fax: 423-542-1439
Emergency Services: Yes
Beds: 121

Key Personnel:
Chair/CEO. . . . . Barbara Allen
Radiology. . . . . Vincent Becker
Chief of Medical Staff . . . . Elizabeth Clemens
CEO/President. . . . . Scott Williams

Measure	Cases	This Hosp.	State Avg.	U.S. Avg.
Blood Clot Prevention and Treatment				
Anticoagulation Overlap Therapy[2]	24	88%	92%	93%
ICU Venous Thromboembolism Prophylaxis[2]	67	87%	90%	92%
Incidence of Potentially Preventable VTE[2,7]	-	-	10%	10%
UFH with Dosages/Platelet Monitoring[1,2]	-	-	99%	97%
Venous Thromboembolism Prophylaxis[2]	262	80%	83%	85%
Warfarin Therapy Discharge Instructions[2]	19	74%	78%	75%
Chest Pain/Possible Heart Attack Care				

NOTE: Hospital profiles are in alphabetical order by state, then city, then hospital within the city; Rankings exclude hospitals with less than 25 cases except for patient surveys which excludes hospitals with less than 100 cases; (a) 100-299 cases; (1) The number of cases/patients is too few to report; (2) Data submitted were based on a sample of cases/patients; (3) Results are based on a shorter time period than required; (4) Data suppressed by CMS for one or more quarters; (5) Results are not available for this reporting period; (6) Fewer than 100 patients completed the HCAHPS survey; (7) No cases met the criteria for this measure; (8) The lower limit of the confidence interval cannot be calculated if the number of observed infections equals zero; (9) No data are available from the state/territory for this reporting period; (10) The scores shown reflect fewer than 50 completed surveys; (11) There were discrepancies in the data collection process; (12) This measure does not apply to this hospital for this reporting period; (13) Results cannot be calculated for this reporting period; (14) The results for this state are combined with nearby states to protect confidentiality; Please refer to the User's Guide for a full explanation of data.

Measure	Cases	This Hosp.	State Avg.	U.S. Avg.
Aspirin Given Within 24 Hours of Arrival	137	97%	96%	96%
Fibrinolytic Meds Within 30 Min. of Arrival[7]	-	-	72%	58%
Average Time to ECG (minutes)	143	3	6	7
Average Time to Transfer (minutes)	12	44	53	60
Children's Asthma Care				
Received Home Management Plan of Care	-	-	-	88%
Received Reliever Medication	-	-	-	100%
Received Systemic Corticosteroids	-	-	-	100%
Emergency Department				
Admittance Decision Time (minutes)[2]	363	51	82	98
Head CT Results Within 45 Min. of Arrival[1]	-	-	52%	57%
Patients Who Left ER Before Being Seen	23,715	1%	2%	2%
Time from ER Arrival to Admit. (minutes)[2]	419	214	243	274
Time from ER Arrival to Discharge (minutes)	307	124	131	134
Time in ER Before Being Evaluated (minutes)	357	16	25	26
Time to Pain Meds for Fractures (minutes)	77	45	60	57
Heart Attack Care				
Aspirin Given at Discharge[1,2]	-	-	99%	99%
Fibrinolytic Meds Within 30 Min. of Arrival[2,3]	-	-	33%	54%
PCI Within 90 Minutes of Arrival[2,3]	-	-	98%	96%
Statin Prescribed at Discharge[1,2]	-	-	99%	98%
Heart Failure Care				
ACE Inhibitor or ARB for LVSD[2]	22	100%	97%	97%
Discharge Instructions Given[2]	55	93%	93%	94%
Evaluation of LVS Function[2]	86	100%	99%	99%
Medicare Spending				
Medicare Spending per Patient (ratio)	-	1.08	1	0.98
Pneumonia Care				
Appropriate Initial Antibiotic Given[2]	84	98%	95%	95%
Blood Culture Timing[2]	121	98%	98%	98%
Pregnancy and Delivery Care				
Newborn Deliveries Scheduled Early[7]	-	-	6%	6%
Preventive Care				
Immunization for Influenza[2]	312	97%	93%	90%
Immunization for Pneumonia[2]	508	95%	93%	92%
Stroke Care				
Anticoagulation Therapy for Atrial Fibrillation[1]	-	-	94%	95%
Antithrombotic Therapy Timing	22	95%	97%	98%
Assessed for Rehabilitation	19	95%	97%	97%
Discharged on Antithrombotic Therapy	19	100%	99%	99%
Discharged on Statin Medication	16	69%	94%	94%
Thrombolytic Therapy Timing[1]	-	-	57%	66%
Venous Thromboembolism Prophylaxis	22	68%	93%	94%
Written Stroke Educational Materials Given[1]	-	-	84%	88%
Surgical Care Improvement Project				
Appropriate Beta Blocker Usage[2]	35	97%	97%	98%
Appropriate VTP Within 24 Hours[2]	126	100%	98%	98%
Controlled Postoperative Blood Glucose[2,7]	-	-	95%	97%
Perioperative Temperature Management[2]	141	100%	100%	100%
Prophylactic Antibiotic Selection[2]	111	100%	99%	99%
Prophylactic Antibiotic Selection (Outpatient)	48	96%	98%	98%
Prophylactic Antibiotic Stopped[2]	109	99%	98%	98%
Prophylactic Antibiotic Timing[2]	111	99%	99%	99%
Prophylactic Antibiotic Timing (Outpatient)	52	92%	98%	98%
Urinary Catheter Removal[2]	73	96%	96%	97%
Survey of Patients' Hospital Experiences				
Area Around Room 'Always' Quiet at Night	300+	67%	67%	61%
Doctors 'Always' Communicated Well	300+	87%	84%	82%
Home Recovery Information Given	300+	86%	85%	85%
Hospital Given 9 or 10 on 10 Point Scale	300+	77%	70%	71%
Meds 'Always' Explained Before Given	300+	67%	66%	64%
Nurses 'Always' Communicated Well	300+	84%	80%	79%
Pain 'Always' Well Controlled	300+	76%	72%	71%
Room and Bathroom 'Always' Clean	300+	76%	73%	73%
Timely Help 'Always' Received	300+	79%	68%	68%
Would Definitely Recommend Hospital	300+	76%	70%	71%
Use of Medical Imaging				
Cardiac Imaging Stress Test before Surgery	97	4.1%	4.8%	5.3%
Combination Abdominal CT Scan	448	9.2%	9.6%	10.5%
Combination Brain/Sinus CT Scan	406	5.9%	3.3%	2.7%
Combination Chest CT Scan	242	0.0%	3.4%	2.7%
Follow-up Mammogram/Ultrasound	704	7.1%	8.3%	8.8%
Lumbar Spine MRI for Low Back Pain	84	42.9%	35.3%	37.2%

Houston County Community Hospital

5001 East Main Street
Erin, TN 37061
Type: Acute Care Hospitals
Ownership: Government - Local
Phone: 931-289-4211
Emergency Services: Yes

Measure	Cases	This Hosp.	State Avg.	U.S. Avg.
Blood Clot Prevention and Treatment				
Anticoagulation Overlap Therapy[5]	-	-	92%	93%
ICU Venous Thromboembolism Prophylaxis[5]	-	-	90%	92%
Incidence of Potentially Preventable VTE[5]	-	-	10%	10%
UFH with Dosages/Platelet Monitoring[5]	-	-	99%	97%
Venous Thromboembolism Prophylaxis[5]	-	-	83%	85%
Warfarin Therapy Discharge Instructions[5]	-	-	78%	75%
Chest Pain/Possible Heart Attack Care				
Aspirin Given Within 24 Hours of Arrival[5]	-	-	96%	96%
Fibrinolytic Meds Within 30 Min. of Arrival[5]	-	-	72%	58%
Average Time to ECG (minutes)[5]	-	-	6	7
Average Time to Transfer (minutes)[5]	-	-	53	60
Children's Asthma Care				
Received Home Management Plan of Care	-	-	-	88%
Received Reliever Medication	-	-	-	100%
Received Systemic Corticosteroids	-	-	-	100%
Emergency Department				
Admittance Decision Time (minutes)[5]	-	-	82	98
Head CT Results Within 45 Min. of Arrival[5]	-	-	52%	57%
Patients Who Left ER Before Being Seen[5]	-	-	2%	2%
Time from ER Arrival to Admit. (minutes)[5]	-	-	243	274
Time from ER Arrival to Discharge (minutes)[5]	-	-	131	134
Time in ER Before Being Evaluated (minutes)[5]	-	-	25	26
Time to Pain Meds for Fractures (minutes)[5]	-	-	60	57
Heart Attack Care				
Aspirin Given at Discharge[5]	-	-	99%	99%
Fibrinolytic Meds Within 30 Min. of Arrival[5]	-	-	33%	54%
PCI Within 90 Minutes of Arrival[5]	-	-	98%	96%
Statin Prescribed at Discharge[5]	-	-	99%	98%
Heart Failure Care				
ACE Inhibitor or ARB for LVSD[5]	-	-	97%	97%
Discharge Instructions Given[5]	-	-	93%	94%
Evaluation of LVS Function[5]	-	-	99%	99%
Medicare Spending				
Medicare Spending per Patient (ratio)	-	-	1	0.98
Pneumonia Care				
Appropriate Initial Antibiotic Given[5]	-	-	95%	95%
Blood Culture Timing[5]	-	-	98%	98%
Pregnancy and Delivery Care				
Newborn Deliveries Scheduled Early[5]	-	-	6%	6%
Preventive Care				
Immunization for Influenza[5]	-	-	93%	90%
Immunization for Pneumonia[5]	-	-	93%	92%
Stroke Care				
Anticoagulation Therapy for Atrial Fibrillation[5]	-	-	94%	95%
Antithrombotic Therapy Timing[5]	-	-	97%	98%
Assessed for Rehabilitation[5]	-	-	97%	97%
Discharged on Antithrombotic Therapy[5]	-	-	99%	99%
Discharged on Statin Medication[5]	-	-	94%	94%
Thrombolytic Therapy Timing[5]	-	-	57%	66%
Venous Thromboembolism Prophylaxis[5]	-	-	93%	94%
Written Stroke Educational Materials Given[5]	-	-	84%	88%
Surgical Care Improvement Project				
Appropriate Beta Blocker Usage[5]	-	-	97%	98%
Appropriate VTP Within 24 Hours[5]	-	-	98%	98%
Controlled Postoperative Blood Glucose[5]	-	-	95%	97%
Perioperative Temperature Management[5]	-	-	100%	100%
Prophylactic Antibiotic Selection[5]	-	-	99%	99%
Prophylactic Antibiotic Selection (Outpatient)[5]	-	-	98%	98%
Prophylactic Antibiotic Stopped[5]	-	-	98%	98%
Prophylactic Antibiotic Timing[5]	-	-	99%	99%
Prophylactic Antibiotic Timing (Outpatient)[5]	-	-	98%	98%
Urinary Catheter Removal[5]	-	-	96%	97%
Survey of Patients' Hospital Experiences				
Area Around Room 'Always' Quiet at Night[5]	-	-	67%	61%
Doctors 'Always' Communicated Well[5]	-	-	84%	82%
Home Recovery Information Given[5]	-	-	85%	85%
Hospital Given 9 or 10 on 10 Point Scale[5]	-	-	70%	71%
Meds 'Always' Explained Before Given[5]	-	-	66%	64%
Nurses 'Always' Communicated Well[5]	-	-	80%	79%
Pain 'Always' Well Controlled[5]	-	-	72%	71%
Room and Bathroom 'Always' Clean[5]	-	-	73%	73%
Timely Help 'Always' Received[5]	-	-	68%	68%
Would Definitely Recommend Hospital[5]	-	-	70%	71%
Use of Medical Imaging				
Cardiac Imaging Stress Test before Surgery[7]	-	-	4.8%	5.3%
Combination Abdominal CT Scan[7]	-	-	9.6%	10.5%
Combination Brain/Sinus CT Scan[7]	-	-	3.3%	2.7%
Combination Chest CT Scan[7]	-	-	3.4%	2.7%
Follow-up Mammogram/Ultrasound[7]	-	-	8.3%	8.8%
Lumbar Spine MRI for Low Back Pain[7]	-	-	35.3%	37.2%

Unicoi County Memorial Hospital

Greenway Circle
Erwin, TN 37650
Type: Acute Care Hospitals
Ownership: Voluntary non-profit - Private
Phone: 423-743-3141
Fax: 423-743-2807
Emergency Services: Yes
Beds: 46

Key Personnel:
Chair/CEO. . . . . Barbara Allen
CEO/President. . . . . Alan Levine
Chief of Medical Staff . . . . Morris Seligman
Radiology. . . . . Michael Slemp

Measure	Cases	This Hosp.	State Avg.	U.S. Avg.
Blood Clot Prevention and Treatment				
Anticoagulation Overlap Therapy[2]	22	59%	92%	93%
ICU Venous Thromboembolism Prophylaxis[1,2]	-	-	90%	92%
Incidence of Potentially Preventable VTE[1,2]	-	-	10%	10%
UFH with Dosages/Platelet Monitoring[2,7]	-	-	99%	97%
Venous Thromboembolism Prophylaxis[2]	113	32%	83%	85%
Warfarin Therapy Discharge Instructions[2]	22	5%	78%	75%
Chest Pain/Possible Heart Attack Care				
Aspirin Given Within 24 Hours of Arrival	34	97%	96%	96%
Fibrinolytic Meds Within 30 Min. of Arrival[7]	-	-	72%	58%
Average Time to ECG (minutes)	34	3	6	7
Average Time to Transfer (minutes)[1]	-	-	53	60
Children's Asthma Care				
Received Home Management Plan of Care	-	-	-	88%
Received Reliever Medication	-	-	-	100%
Received Systemic Corticosteroids	-	-	-	100%
Emergency Department				
Admittance Decision Time (minutes)[2]	321	65	82	98
Head CT Results Within 45 Min. of Arrival[1,3]	-	-	52%	57%
Patients Who Left ER Before Being Seen	7,282	1%	2%	2%
Time from ER Arrival to Admit. (minutes)[2]	332	226	243	274
Time from ER Arrival to Discharge (minutes)	396	122	131	134
Time in ER Before Being Evaluated (minutes)	410	21	25	26
Time to Pain Meds for Fractures (minutes)[1]	-	-	60	57
Heart Attack Care				
Aspirin Given at Discharge[5]	-	-	99%	99%
Fibrinolytic Meds Within 30 Min. of Arrival[5]	-	-	33%	54%
PCI Within 90 Minutes of Arrival[5]	-	-	98%	96%
Statin Prescribed at Discharge[5]	-	-	99%	98%
Heart Failure Care				
ACE Inhibitor or ARB for LVSD	12	67%	97%	97%
Discharge Instructions Given	17	59%	93%	94%
Evaluation of LVS Function	29	97%	99%	99%
Medicare Spending				
Medicare Spending per Patient (ratio)	-	0.97	1	0.98
Pneumonia Care				
Appropriate Initial Antibiotic Given	41	88%	95%	95%
Blood Culture Timing	55	67%	98%	98%
Pregnancy and Delivery Care				
Newborn Deliveries Scheduled Early[7]	-	-	6%	6%
Preventive Care				
Immunization for Influenza[2]	298	77%	93%	90%
Immunization for Pneumonia[2]	568	57%	93%	92%
Stroke Care				

NOTE: Hospital profiles are in alphabetical order by state, then city, then hospital within the city; Rankings exclude hospitals with less than 25 cases except for patient surveys which excludes hospitals with less than 100 cases; (a) 100-299 cases; (1) The number of cases/patients is too few to report; (2) Data submitted were based on a sample of cases/patients; (3) Results are based on a shorter time period than required; (4) Data suppressed by CMS for one or more quarters; (5) Results are not available for this reporting period; (6) Fewer than 100 patients completed the HCAHPS survey; (7) No cases met the criteria for this measure; (8) The lower limit of the confidence interval cannot be calculated if the number of observed infections equals zero; (9) No data are available from the state/territory for this reporting period; (10) The scores shown reflect fewer than 50 completed surveys; (11) There were discrepancies in the data collection process; (12) This measure does not apply to this hospital for this reporting period; (13) Results cannot be calculated for this reporting period; (14) The results for this state are combined with nearby states to protect confidentiality; Please refer to the User's Guide for a full explanation of data.

Measure	Cases	This Hosp.	State Avg.	U.S. Avg.
Anticoagulation Therapy for Atrial Fibrillation[3,7]	-	-	94%	95%
Antithrombotic Therapy Timing[1,3]	-	-	97%	98%
Assessed for Rehabilitation[1,3]	-	-	97%	97%
Discharged on Antithrombotic Therapy[1,3]	-	-	99%	99%
Discharged on Statin Medication[1,3]	-	-	94%	94%
Thrombolytic Therapy Timing[3,7]	-	-	57%	66%
Venous Thromboembolism Prophylaxis[1,3]	-	-	93%	94%
Written Stroke Educational Materials Given[1,3]	-	-	84%	88%
Surgical Care Improvement Project				
Appropriate Beta Blocker Usage	31	77%	97%	98%
Appropriate VTP Within 24 Hours	92	97%	98%	98%
Controlled Postoperative Blood Glucose[7]	-	-	95%	97%
Perioperative Temperature Management	97	100%	100%	100%
Prophylactic Antibiotic Selection	84	100%	99%	99%
Prophylactic Antibiotic Selection (Outpatient)[1,3]	-	-	98%	98%
Prophylactic Antibiotic Stopped	84	100%	98%	98%
Prophylactic Antibiotic Timing	84	100%	99%	99%
Prophylactic Antibiotic Timing (Outpatient)[1,3]	-	-	98%	98%
Urinary Catheter Removal	88	80%	96%	97%
Survey of Patients' Hospital Experiences				
Area Around Room 'Always' Quiet at Night	(a)	62%	67%	61%
Doctors 'Always' Communicated Well	(a)	84%	84%	82%
Home Recovery Information Given	(a)	81%	85%	85%
Hospital Given 9 or 10 on 10 Point Scale	(a)	63%	70%	71%
Meds 'Always' Explained Before Given	(a)	68%	66%	64%
Nurses 'Always' Communicated Well	(a)	73%	80%	79%
Pain 'Always' Well Controlled	(a)	65%	72%	71%
Room and Bathroom 'Always' Clean	(a)	75%	73%	73%
Timely Help 'Always' Received	(a)	71%	68%	68%
Would Definitely Recommend Hospital	(a)	66%	70%	71%
Use of Medical Imaging				
Cardiac Imaging Stress Test before Surgery[7]	-	-	4.8%	5.3%
Combination Abdominal CT Scan	217	19.4%	9.6%	10.5%
Combination Brain/Sinus CT Scan[1]	-	-	3.3%	2.7%
Combination Chest CT Scan	86	0.0%	3.4%	2.7%
Follow-up Mammogram/Ultrasound	308	5.5%	8.3%	8.8%
Lumbar Spine MRI for Low Back Pain	41	43.9%	35.3%	37.2%

Starr Regional Medical Center Etowah

886 Highway 411 North
Etowah, TN 37331
Type: Acute Care Hospitals
Ownership: Govt - Hospital Dist/Auth
Phone: 423-263-3600
Fax: 423-263-3793
Emergency Services: Yes
Beds: 160

Key Personnel:
CEO/President. . . . . Steve Clapp
Radiology. . . . . Stephen Lemings, MD
CEO . . . . Mark Noichols
Emergency Room . . . . Rick Popp, MD
Hemotology Center . . . . Robert D Shumaker, MD

Measure	Cases	This Hosp.	State Avg.	U.S. Avg.
Blood Clot Prevention and Treatment				
Anticoagulation Overlap Therapy[1,2]	-	-	92%	93%
ICU Venous Thromboembolism Prophylaxis[2,3]	37	73%	90%	92%
Incidence of Potentially Preventable VTE[2,3]	-	-	10%	10%
UFH with Dosages/Platelet Monitoring[2,3]	-	-	99%	97%
Venous Thromboembolism Prophylaxis[2,3]	107	64%	83%	85%
Warfarin Therapy Discharge Instructions[1,2]	-	-	78%	75%
Chest Pain/Possible Heart Attack Care				
Aspirin Given Within 24 Hours of Arrival	23	83%	96%	96%
Fibrinolytic Meds Within 30 Min. of Arrival[1]	-	-	72%	58%
Average Time to ECG (minutes)	25	7	6	7
Average Time to Transfer (minutes)[1]	-	-	53	60
Children's Asthma Care				
Received Home Management Plan of Care	-	-	-	88%
Received Reliever Medication	-	-	-	100%
Received Systemic Corticosteroids	-	-	-	100%
Emergency Department				
Admittance Decision Time (minutes)[2,3]	249	51	82	98
Head CT Results Within 45 Min. of Arrival[3,7]	-	-	52%	57%
Patients Who Left ER Before Being Seen	13,431	3%	2%	2%
Time from ER Arrival to Admit. (minutes)[2,3]	255	207	243	274
Time from ER Arrival to Discharge (minutes)	355	113	131	134
Time in ER Before Being Evaluated (minutes)	343	29	25	26
Time to Pain Meds for Fractures (minutes)	31	64	60	57
Heart Attack Care				
Aspirin Given at Discharge[1,3]	-	-	99%	99%
Fibrinolytic Meds Within 30 Min. of Arrival[3,7]	-	-	33%	54%
PCI Within 90 Minutes of Arrival[3,7]	-	-	98%	96%
Statin Prescribed at Discharge[1,3]	-	-	99%	98%
Heart Failure Care				
ACE Inhibitor or ARB for LVSD[3]	22	91%	97%	97%
Discharge Instructions Given[3]	43	84%	93%	94%
Evaluation of LVS Function[3]	50	90%	99%	99%
Medicare Spending				
Medicare Spending per Patient (ratio)	-	-	1	0.98
Pneumonia Care				
Appropriate Initial Antibiotic Given[3]	44	80%	95%	95%
Blood Culture Timing[3]	63	92%	98%	98%
Pregnancy and Delivery Care				
Newborn Deliveries Scheduled Early[7]	-	-	6%	6%
Preventive Care				
Immunization for Influenza[2]	290	83%	93%	90%
Immunization for Pneumonia[2,3]	364	91%	93%	92%
Stroke Care				
Anticoagulation Therapy for Atrial Fibrillation[1,3]	-	-	94%	95%
Antithrombotic Therapy Timing[1,3]	-	-	97%	98%
Assessed for Rehabilitation[1,3]	-	-	97%	97%
Discharged on Antithrombotic Therapy[1,3]	-	-	99%	99%
Discharged on Statin Medication[1,3]	-	-	94%	94%
Thrombolytic Therapy Timing[1,3]	-	-	57%	66%
Venous Thromboembolism Prophylaxis[1,3]	-	-	93%	94%
Written Stroke Educational Materials Given[1,3]	-	-	84%	88%
Surgical Care Improvement Project				
Appropriate Beta Blocker Usage[1,3]	-	-	97%	98%
Appropriate VTP Within 24 Hours[3]	32	88%	98%	98%
Controlled Postoperative Blood Glucose[3,7]	-	-	95%	97%
Perioperative Temperature Management[3]	33	100%	100%	100%
Prophylactic Antibiotic Selection[3]	24	100%	99%	99%
Prophylactic Antibiotic Selection (Outpatient)	29	59%	98%	98%
Prophylactic Antibiotic Stopped[3]	24	88%	98%	98%
Prophylactic Antibiotic Timing[3]	24	92%	99%	99%
Prophylactic Antibiotic Timing (Outpatient)[1]	-	-	98%	98%
Urinary Catheter Removal[3]	25	92%	96%	97%
Survey of Patients' Hospital Experiences				
Area Around Room 'Always' Quiet at Night	(a)	69%	67%	61%
Doctors 'Always' Communicated Well	(a)	86%	84%	82%
Home Recovery Information Given	(a)	87%	85%	85%
Hospital Given 9 or 10 on 10 Point Scale	(a)	65%	70%	71%
Meds 'Always' Explained Before Given	(a)	65%	66%	64%
Nurses 'Always' Communicated Well	(a)	77%	80%	79%
Pain 'Always' Well Controlled	(a)	65%	72%	71%
Room and Bathroom 'Always' Clean	(a)	68%	73%	73%
Timely Help 'Always' Received	(a)	66%	68%	68%
Would Definitely Recommend Hospital	(a)	73%	70%	71%
Use of Medical Imaging				
Cardiac Imaging Stress Test before Surgery[1]	-	-	4.8%	5.3%
Combination Abdominal CT Scan	207	9.2%	9.6%	10.5%
Combination Brain/Sinus CT Scan	231	0.9%	3.3%	2.7%
Combination Chest CT Scan	105	10.5%	3.4%	2.7%
Follow-up Mammogram/Ultrasound	154	9.1%	8.3%	8.8%
Lumbar Spine MRI for Low Back Pain	60	43.3%	35.3%	37.2%

Lincoln Medical Center

106 Medical Center Blvd
Fayetteville, TN 37334
URL: www.lchealthsystems.com
Type: Acute Care Hospitals
Ownership: Government - Local
Phone: 931-438-1100
Fax: 931-438-7456
Emergency Services: Yes
Beds: 49

Key Personnel:
CEO/President. . . . . Gary Kendrick

Measure	Cases	This Hosp.	State Avg.	U.S. Avg.
Blood Clot Prevention and Treatment				
Anticoagulation Overlap Therapy[1,2]	-	-	92%	93%
ICU Venous Thromboembolism Prophylaxis[2]	38	89%	90%	92%
Incidence of Potentially Preventable VTE[2,7]	-	-	10%	10%
UFH with Dosages/Platelet Monitoring[1,2]	-	-	99%	97%
Venous Thromboembolism Prophylaxis[2]	126	84%	83%	85%
Warfarin Therapy Discharge Instructions[1,2]	-	-	78%	75%
Chest Pain/Possible Heart Attack Care				
Aspirin Given Within 24 Hours of Arrival	76	97%	96%	96%
Fibrinolytic Meds Within 30 Min. of Arrival[1]	-	-	72%	58%
Average Time to ECG (minutes)	81	4	6	7
Average Time to Transfer (minutes)[1]	-	-	53	60
Children's Asthma Care				
Received Home Management Plan of Care	-	-	-	88%
Received Reliever Medication	-	-	-	100%
Received Systemic Corticosteroids	-	-	-	100%
Emergency Department				
Admittance Decision Time (minutes)[2]	286	56	82	98
Head CT Results Within 45 Min. of Arrival	17	53%	52%	57%
Patients Who Left ER Before Being Seen	18,328	2%	2%	2%
Time from ER Arrival to Admit. (minutes)[2]	286	228	243	274
Time from ER Arrival to Discharge (minutes)	358	157	131	134
Time in ER Before Being Evaluated (minutes)	400	29	25	26
Time to Pain Meds for Fractures (minutes)	98	62	60	57
Heart Attack Care				
Aspirin Given at Discharge[1,3]	-	-	99%	99%
Fibrinolytic Meds Within 30 Min. of Arrival[3,7]	-	-	33%	54%
PCI Within 90 Minutes of Arrival[3,7]	-	-	98%	96%
Statin Prescribed at Discharge[1,3]	-	-	99%	98%
Heart Failure Care				
ACE Inhibitor or ARB for LVSD	16	100%	97%	97%
Discharge Instructions Given	44	98%	93%	94%
Evaluation of LVS Function	61	98%	99%	99%
Medicare Spending				
Medicare Spending per Patient (ratio)	-	1.08	1	0.98
Pneumonia Care				
Appropriate Initial Antibiotic Given	71	86%	95%	95%
Blood Culture Timing	145	97%	98%	98%
Pregnancy and Delivery Care				
Newborn Deliveries Scheduled Early	17	6%	6%	6%
Preventive Care				
Immunization for Influenza[2]	284	98%	93%	90%
Immunization for Pneumonia[2]	342	99%	93%	92%
Stroke Care				
Anticoagulation Therapy for Atrial Fibrillation[1]	-	-	94%	95%
Antithrombotic Therapy Timing	11	100%	97%	98%
Assessed for Rehabilitation[1]	-	-	97%	97%
Discharged on Antithrombotic Therapy[1]	-	-	99%	99%
Discharged on Statin Medication[1]	-	-	94%	94%
Thrombolytic Therapy Timing[7]	-	-	57%	66%
Venous Thromboembolism Prophylaxis	11	91%	93%	94%
Written Stroke Educational Materials Given[1]	-	-	84%	88%
Surgical Care Improvement Project				
Appropriate Beta Blocker Usage[1]	-	-	97%	98%
Appropriate VTP Within 24 Hours	75	93%	98%	98%
Controlled Postoperative Blood Glucose[7]	-	-	95%	97%
Perioperative Temperature Management	79	100%	100%	100%
Prophylactic Antibiotic Selection	58	98%	99%	99%
Prophylactic Antibiotic Selection (Outpatient)	16	94%	98%	98%
Prophylactic Antibiotic Stopped	50	94%	98%	98%
Prophylactic Antibiotic Timing	58	97%	99%	99%
Prophylactic Antibiotic Timing (Outpatient)	13	100%	98%	98%
Urinary Catheter Removal	33	100%	96%	97%
Survey of Patients' Hospital Experiences				
Area Around Room 'Always' Quiet at Night	(a)	64%	67%	61%
Doctors 'Always' Communicated Well	(a)	82%	84%	82%
Home Recovery Information Given	(a)	86%	85%	85%
Hospital Given 9 or 10 on 10 Point Scale	(a)	60%	70%	71%
Meds 'Always' Explained Before Given	(a)	63%	66%	64%
Nurses 'Always' Communicated Well	(a)	74%	80%	79%
Pain 'Always' Well Controlled	(a)	69%	72%	71%
Room and Bathroom 'Always' Clean	(a)	73%	73%	73%
Timely Help 'Always' Received	(a)	62%	68%	68%
Would Definitely Recommend Hospital	(a)	60%	70%	71%
Use of Medical Imaging				
Cardiac Imaging Stress Test before Surgery	106	2.8%	4.8%	5.3%
Combination Abdominal CT Scan	257	3.1%	9.6%	10.5%

NOTE: Hospital profiles are in alphabetical order by state, then city, then hospital within the city; Rankings exclude hospitals with less than 25 cases except for patient surveys which excludes hospitals with less than 100 cases; (a) 100-299 cases; (1) The number of cases/patients is too few to report; (2) Data submitted were based on a sample of cases/patients; (3) Results are based on a shorter time period than required; (4) Data suppressed by CMS for one or more quarters; (5) Results are not available for this reporting period; (6) Fewer than 100 patients completed the HCAHPS survey; (7) No cases met the criteria for this measure; (8) The lower limit of the confidence interval cannot be calculated if the number of observed infections equals zero; (9) No data are available from the state/territory for this reporting period; (10) The scores shown reflect fewer than 50 completed surveys; (11) There were discrepancies in the data collection process; (12) This measure does not apply to this hospital for this reporting period; (13) Results cannot be calculated for this reporting period; (14) The results for this state are combined with nearby states to protect confidentiality; Please refer to the User's Guide for a full explanation of data.

Measure	Cases	This Hosp.	State Avg.	U.S. Avg.
Combination Brain/Sinus CT Scan[1]	-	-	3.3%	2.7%
Combination Chest CT Scan	169	26.6%	3.4%	2.7%
Follow-up Mammogram/Ultrasound	509	6.7%	8.3%	8.8%
Lumbar Spine MRI for Low Back Pain[1]	-	-	35.3%	37.2%

Williamson Medical Center

4321 Carothers Parkway
Franklin, TN 37067
Phone: 615-435-5000
Fax: 615-435-5576
E-mail: information@wmed.org
URL: www.williamsonmedicalcenter.org
Type: Acute Care Hospitals
Emergency Services: Yes
Ownership: Govt - Hospital Dist/Auth
Beds: 185

Key Personnel:
Radiology.................... John Alarcon
Chief of Medical Staff.......... Starling C Evins, MD
CEO/President............... Dennis Miller, FACHE

Measure	Cases	This Hosp.	State Avg.	U.S. Avg.
Blood Clot Prevention and Treatment				
Anticoagulation Overlap Therapy[2]	68	88%	92%	93%
ICU Venous Thromboembolism Prophylaxis[2]	95	92%	90%	92%
Incidence of Potentially Preventable VTE[2]	11	9%	10%	10%
UFH with Dosages/Platelet Monitoring[2]	14	71%	99%	97%
Venous Thromboembolism Prophylaxis[2]	285	81%	83%	85%
Warfarin Therapy Discharge Instructions[2]	41	93%	78%	75%
Chest Pain/Possible Heart Attack Care				
Aspirin Given Within 24 Hours of Arrival	27	93%	96%	96%
Fibrinolytic Meds Within 30 Min. of Arrival[7]	-	-	72%	58%
Average Time to ECG (minutes)	27	7	6	7
Average Time to Transfer (minutes)[1]	-	-	53	60
Children's Asthma Care				
Received Home Management Plan of Care	-	-	-	88%
Received Reliever Medication	-	-	-	100%
Received Systemic Corticosteroids	-	-	-	100%
Emergency Department				
Admittance Decision Time (minutes)[2]	481	90	82	98
Head CT Results Within 45 Min. of Arrival	23	57%	52%	57%
Patients Who Left ER Before Being Seen	38,750	0%	2%	2%
Time from ER Arrival to Admit. (minutes)[2]	485	250	243	274
Time from ER Arrival to Discharge (minutes)	363	159	131	134
Time in ER Before Being Evaluated (minutes)	354	43	25	26
Time to Pain Meds for Fractures (minutes)	194	68	60	57
Heart Attack Care				
Aspirin Given at Discharge	110	92%	99%	99%
Fibrinolytic Meds Within 30 Min. of Arrival[7]	-	-	33%	54%
PCI Within 90 Minutes of Arrival	42	81%	98%	96%
Statin Prescribed at Discharge	107	97%	99%	98%
Heart Failure Care				
ACE Inhibitor or ARB for LVSD	55	95%	97%	97%
Discharge Instructions Given	129	89%	93%	94%
Evaluation of LVS Function	169	99%	99%	99%
Medicare Spending				
Medicare Spending per Patient (ratio)	-	1.06	1	0.98
Pneumonia Care				
Appropriate Initial Antibiotic Given	113	92%	95%	95%
Blood Culture Timing	136	98%	98%	98%
Pregnancy and Delivery Care				
Newborn Deliveries Scheduled Early[2]	32	3%	6%	6%
Preventive Care				
Immunization for Influenza[2]	530	94%	93%	90%
Immunization for Pneumonia[2]	586	92%	93%	92%
Stroke Care				
Anticoagulation Therapy for Atrial Fibrillation[1,2]	-	-	94%	95%
Antithrombotic Therapy Timing[2]	41	98%	97%	98%
Assessed for Rehabilitation[2]	42	93%	97%	97%
Discharged on Antithrombotic Therapy[2]	41	95%	99%	99%
Discharged on Statin Medication[2]	35	80%	94%	94%
Thrombolytic Therapy Timing[1,2]	-	-	57%	66%
Venous Thromboembolism Prophylaxis[2]	41	80%	93%	94%
Written Stroke Educational Materials Given[2]	25	84%	84%	88%
Surgical Care Improvement Project				
Appropriate Beta Blocker Usage[2]	104	91%	97%	98%
Appropriate VTP Within 24 Hours[2]	285	96%	98%	98%
Controlled Postoperative Blood Glucose[2,7]	-	-	95%	97%
Perioperative Temperature Management[2]	339	100%	100%	100%
Prophylactic Antibiotic Selection[2]	233	97%	99%	99%
Prophylactic Antibiotic Selection (Outpatient)	250	97%	98%	98%
Prophylactic Antibiotic Stopped[2]	231	96%	98%	98%
Prophylactic Antibiotic Timing[2]	233	98%	99%	99%
Prophylactic Antibiotic Timing (Outpatient)	250	100%	98%	98%
Urinary Catheter Removal[2]	246	94%	96%	97%
Survey of Patients' Hospital Experiences				
Area Around Room 'Always' Quiet at Night	300+	65%	67%	61%
Doctors 'Always' Communicated Well	300+	86%	84%	82%
Home Recovery Information Given	300+	82%	85%	85%
Hospital Given 9 or 10 on 10 Point Scale	300+	78%	70%	71%
Meds 'Always' Explained Before Given	300+	62%	66%	64%
Nurses 'Always' Communicated Well	300+	81%	80%	79%
Pain 'Always' Well Controlled	300+	72%	72%	71%
Room and Bathroom 'Always' Clean	300+	75%	73%	73%
Timely Help 'Always' Received	300+	69%	68%	68%
Would Definitely Recommend Hospital	300+	80%	70%	71%
Use of Medical Imaging				
Cardiac Imaging Stress Test before Surgery	198	3.0%	4.8%	5.3%
Combination Abdominal CT Scan	693	11.7%	9.6%	10.5%
Combination Brain/Sinus CT Scan	712	2.4%	3.3%	2.7%
Combination Chest CT Scan	359	8.1%	3.4%	2.7%
Follow-up Mammogram/Ultrasound	914	5.5%	8.3%	8.8%
Lumbar Spine MRI for Low Back Pain	225	31.6%	35.3%	37.2%

Sumner Regional Medical Center

555 Hartsville Pike
Gallatin, TN 37066
Phone: 615-452-4210
Fax: 615-451-6145
URL: www.mysumnermedical.com
Type: Acute Care Hospitals
Emergency Services: Yes
Ownership: Proprietary
Beds: 155

Key Personnel:
Anesthesiology............... Mark Carter, MD
Emergency Room .... James Robert Gill, MD
CEO .... Susan Peach, BSN, MBA
CEO/President............... William T Sugg

Measure	Cases	This Hosp.	State Avg.	U.S. Avg.
Blood Clot Prevention and Treatment				
Anticoagulation Overlap Therapy[2]	53	100%	92%	93%
ICU Venous Thromboembolism Prophylaxis[2]	112	93%	90%	92%
Incidence of Potentially Preventable VTE[2]	12	8%	10%	10%
UFH with Dosages/Platelet Monitoring[1,2]	-	-	99%	97%
Venous Thromboembolism Prophylaxis[2]	295	95%	83%	85%
Warfarin Therapy Discharge Instructions[2]	39	100%	78%	75%
Chest Pain/Possible Heart Attack Care				
Aspirin Given Within 24 Hours of Arrival	34	100%	96%	96%
Fibrinolytic Meds Within 30 Min. of Arrival[7]	-	-	72%	58%
Average Time to ECG (minutes)	35	7	6	7
Average Time to Transfer (minutes)[1]	-	-	53	60
Children's Asthma Care				
Received Home Management Plan of Care	-	-	-	88%
Received Reliever Medication	-	-	-	100%
Received Systemic Corticosteroids	-	-	-	100%
Emergency Department				
Admittance Decision Time (minutes)[2]	532	57	82	98
Head CT Results Within 45 Min. of Arrival[1]	-	-	52%	57%
Patients Who Left ER Before Being Seen	37,850	1%	2%	2%
Time from ER Arrival to Admit. (minutes)[2]	534	222	243	274
Time from ER Arrival to Discharge (minutes)	422	161	131	134
Time in ER Before Being Evaluated (minutes)	498	13	25	26
Time to Pain Meds for Fractures (minutes)	136	34	60	57
Heart Attack Care				
Aspirin Given at Discharge	111	100%	99%	99%
Fibrinolytic Meds Within 30 Min. of Arrival[7]	-	-	33%	54%
PCI Within 90 Minutes of Arrival	21	100%	98%	96%
Statin Prescribed at Discharge	114	100%	99%	98%
Heart Failure Care				
ACE Inhibitor or ARB for LVSD	40	100%	97%	97%
Discharge Instructions Given	122	100%	93%	94%
Evaluation of LVS Function	147	100%	99%	99%
Medicare Spending				
Medicare Spending per Patient (ratio)	-	1.08	1	0.98
Pneumonia Care				
Appropriate Initial Antibiotic Given	219	97%	95%	95%
Blood Culture Timing	246	100%	98%	98%
Pregnancy and Delivery Care				
Newborn Deliveries Scheduled Early[2]	36	6%	6%	6%
Preventive Care				
Immunization for Influenza[2]	518	99%	93%	90%
Immunization for Pneumonia[2]	670	100%	93%	92%
Stroke Care				
Anticoagulation Therapy for Atrial Fibrillation[1]	-	-	94%	95%
Antithrombotic Therapy Timing	48	98%	97%	98%
Assessed for Rehabilitation	52	100%	97%	97%
Discharged on Antithrombotic Therapy	49	100%	99%	99%
Discharged on Statin Medication	42	100%	94%	94%
Thrombolytic Therapy Timing[7]	-	-	57%	66%
Venous Thromboembolism Prophylaxis	50	96%	93%	94%
Written Stroke Educational Materials Given	25	100%	84%	88%
Surgical Care Improvement Project				
Appropriate Beta Blocker Usage	111	100%	97%	98%
Appropriate VTP Within 24 Hours	391	100%	98%	98%
Controlled Postoperative Blood Glucose[7]	-	-	95%	97%
Perioperative Temperature Management	438	100%	100%	100%
Prophylactic Antibiotic Selection	317	99%	99%	99%
Prophylactic Antibiotic Selection (Outpatient)	108	100%	98%	98%
Prophylactic Antibiotic Stopped	311	98%	98%	98%
Prophylactic Antibiotic Timing	317	100%	99%	99%
Prophylactic Antibiotic Timing (Outpatient)	111	97%	98%	98%
Urinary Catheter Removal	282	100%	96%	97%
Survey of Patients' Hospital Experiences				
Area Around Room 'Always' Quiet at Night	300+	64%	67%	61%
Doctors 'Always' Communicated Well	300+	79%	84%	82%
Home Recovery Information Given	300+	84%	85%	85%
Hospital Given 9 or 10 on 10 Point Scale	300+	68%	70%	71%
Meds 'Always' Explained Before Given	300+	63%	66%	64%
Nurses 'Always' Communicated Well	300+	77%	80%	79%
Pain 'Always' Well Controlled	300+	70%	72%	71%
Room and Bathroom 'Always' Clean	300+	68%	73%	73%
Timely Help 'Always' Received	300+	67%	68%	68%
Would Definitely Recommend Hospital	300+	69%	70%	71%
Use of Medical Imaging				
Cardiac Imaging Stress Test before Surgery	206	5.8%	4.8%	5.3%
Combination Abdominal CT Scan	631	6.7%	9.6%	10.5%
Combination Brain/Sinus CT Scan	381	1.3%	3.3%	2.7%
Combination Chest CT Scan	547	0.2%	3.4%	2.7%
Follow-up Mammogram/Ultrasound	635	16.2%	8.3%	8.8%
Lumbar Spine MRI for Low Back Pain	101	27.7%	35.3%	37.2%

Baptist Rehabilitation Germantown

2100 Exeter Road
Germantown, TN 38138
Phone: 901-757-1350
Fax: 901-226-4519
URL: www.bmhcc.org
Type: Acute Care Hospitals
Emergency Services: No
Ownership: Voluntary non-profit - Private
Beds: 60

Key Personnel:
Radiology.................... James D Acker
CEO .... Brian Hogan

Measure	Cases	This Hosp.	State Avg.	U.S. Avg.
Blood Clot Prevention and Treatment				
Anticoagulation Overlap Therapy[5]	-	-	92%	93%
ICU Venous Thromboembolism Prophylaxis[5]	-	-	90%	92%
Incidence of Potentially Preventable VTE[5]	-	-	10%	10%
UFH with Dosages/Platelet Monitoring[5]	-	-	99%	97%
Venous Thromboembolism Prophylaxis[5]	-	-	83%	85%
Warfarin Therapy Discharge Instructions[5]	-	-	78%	75%
Chest Pain/Possible Heart Attack Care				
Aspirin Given Within 24 Hours of Arrival	-	-	96%	96%
Fibrinolytic Meds Within 30 Min. of Arrival	-	-	72%	58%
Average Time to ECG (minutes)	-	-	6	7
Average Time to Transfer (minutes)	-	-	53	60
Children's Asthma Care				
Received Home Management Plan of Care	-	-	-	88%
Received Reliever Medication	-	-	-	100%
Received Systemic Corticosteroids	-	-	-	100%

NOTE: Hospital profiles are in alphabetical order by state, then city, then hospital within the city; Rankings exclude hospitals with less than 25 cases except for patient surveys which excludes hospitals with less than 100 cases; (a) 100-299 cases; (1) The number of cases/patients is too few to report; (2) Data submitted were based on a sample of cases/patients; (3) Results are based on a shorter time period than required; (4) Data suppressed by CMS for one or more quarters; (5) Results are not available for this reporting period; (6) Fewer than 100 patients completed the HCAHPS survey; (7) No cases met the criteria for this measure; (8) The lower limit of the confidence interval cannot be calculated if the number of observed infections equals zero; (9) No data are available from the state/territory for this reporting period; (10) The scores shown reflect fewer than 50 completed surveys; (11) There were discrepancies in the data collection process; (12) This measure does not apply to this hospital for this reporting period; (13) Results cannot be calculated for this reporting period; (14) The results for this state are combined with nearby states to protect confidentiality; Please refer to the User's Guide for a full explanation of data.

Measure	Cases	This Hosp.	State Avg.	U.S. Avg.
Emergency Department				
Admittance Decision Time (minutes)[5]	-	-	82	98
Head CT Results Within 45 Min. of Arrival	-	-	52%	57%
Patients Who Left ER Before Being Seen	-	-	2%	2%
Time from ER Arrival to Admit. (minutes)[5]	-	-	243	274
Time from ER Arrival to Discharge (minutes)	-	-	131	134
Time in ER Before Being Evaluated (minutes)	-	-	25	26
Time to Pain Meds for Fractures (minutes)	-	-	60	57
Heart Attack Care				
Aspirin Given at Discharge[5]	-	-	99%	99%
Fibrinolytic Meds Within 30 Min. of Arrival[5]	-	-	33%	54%
PCI Within 90 Minutes of Arrival[5]	-	-	98%	96%
Statin Prescribed at Discharge[5]	-	-	99%	98%
Heart Failure Care				
ACE Inhibitor or ARB for LVSD[5]	-	-	97%	97%
Discharge Instructions Given[5]	-	-	93%	94%
Evaluation of LVS Function[5]	-	-	99%	99%
Medicare Spending				
Medicare Spending per Patient (ratio)	-	-	1	0.98
Pneumonia Care				
Appropriate Initial Antibiotic Given[5]	-	-	95%	95%
Blood Culture Timing[5]	-	-	98%	98%
Pregnancy and Delivery Care				
Newborn Deliveries Scheduled Early[7]	-	-	6%	6%
Preventive Care				
Immunization for Influenza[5]	-	-	93%	90%
Immunization for Pneumonia[5]	-	-	93%	92%
Stroke Care				
Anticoagulation Therapy for Atrial Fibrillation[5]	-	-	94%	95%
Antithrombotic Therapy Timing[5]	-	-	97%	98%
Assessed for Rehabilitation[5]	-	-	97%	97%
Discharged on Antithrombotic Therapy[5]	-	-	99%	99%
Discharged on Statin Medication[5]	-	-	94%	94%
Thrombolytic Therapy Timing[5]	-	-	57%	66%
Venous Thromboembolism Prophylaxis[5]	-	-	93%	94%
Written Stroke Educational Materials Given[5]	-	-	84%	88%
Surgical Care Improvement Project				
Appropriate Beta Blocker Usage[5]	-	-	97%	98%
Appropriate VTP Within 24 Hours[5]	-	-	98%	98%
Controlled Postoperative Blood Glucose[5]	-	-	95%	97%
Perioperative Temperature Management[5]	-	-	100%	100%
Prophylactic Antibiotic Selection[5]	-	-	99%	99%
Prophylactic Antibiotic Selection (Outpatient)	-	-	98%	98%
Prophylactic Antibiotic Stopped[5]	-	-	98%	98%
Prophylactic Antibiotic Timing[5]	-	-	99%	99%
Prophylactic Antibiotic Timing (Outpatient)	-	-	98%	98%
Urinary Catheter Removal[5]	-	-	96%	97%
Survey of Patients' Hospital Experiences				
Area Around Room 'Always' Quiet at Night[1]	-	-	67%	61%
Doctors 'Always' Communicated Well[1]	-	-	84%	82%
Home Recovery Information Given[1]	-	-	85%	85%
Hospital Given 9 or 10 on 10 Point Scale[1]	-	-	70%	71%
Meds 'Always' Explained Before Given[1]	-	-	66%	64%
Nurses 'Always' Communicated Well[1]	-	-	80%	79%
Pain 'Always' Well Controlled[1]	-	-	72%	71%
Room and Bathroom 'Always' Clean[1]	-	-	73%	73%
Timely Help 'Always' Received[1]	-	-	68%	68%
Would Definitely Recommend Hospital[1]	-	-	70%	71%
Use of Medical Imaging				
Cardiac Imaging Stress Test before Surgery	-	-	4.8%	5.3%
Combination Abdominal CT Scan	-	-	9.6%	10.5%
Combination Brain/Sinus CT Scan	-	-	3.3%	2.7%
Combination Chest CT Scan	-	-	3.4%	2.7%
Follow-up Mammogram/Ultrasound	-	-	8.3%	8.8%
Lumbar Spine MRI for Low Back Pain	-	-	35.3%	37.2%

Laughlin Memorial Hospital

1420 Tusculum Blvd
Greeneville, TN 37745
Phone: 423-787-5000
Fax: 423-787-5083
Type: Acute Care Hospitals
Emergency Services: Yes
Ownership: Voluntary non-profit - Private
Beds: 230
Key Personnel:
Radiology. . . . . Phillip Marino
CEO/President. . . . . Charles H Whitefield

Measure	Cases	This Hosp.	State Avg.	U.S. Avg.
Blood Clot Prevention and Treatment				
Anticoagulation Overlap Therapy[2]	25	100%	92%	93%
ICU Venous Thromboembolism Prophylaxis[2]	41	98%	90%	92%
Incidence of Potentially Preventable VTE[1,2]	-	-	10%	10%
UFH with Dosages/Platelet Monitoring[1,2]	-	-	99%	97%
Venous Thromboembolism Prophylaxis[2]	277	91%	83%	85%
Warfarin Therapy Discharge Instructions[2]	22	100%	78%	75%
Chest Pain/Possible Heart Attack Care				
Aspirin Given Within 24 Hours of Arrival	39	100%	96%	96%
Fibrinolytic Meds Within 30 Min. of Arrival[7]	-	-	72%	58%
Average Time to ECG (minutes)	41	7	6	7
Average Time to Transfer (minutes)	19	37	53	60
Children's Asthma Care				
Received Home Management Plan of Care	-	-	-	88%
Received Reliever Medication	-	-	-	100%
Received Systemic Corticosteroids	-	-	-	100%
Emergency Department				
Admittance Decision Time (minutes)[2]	444	45	82	98
Head CT Results Within 45 Min. of Arrival[1]	-	-	52%	57%
Patients Who Left ER Before Being Seen	28,170	1%	2%	2%
Time from ER Arrival to Admit. (minutes)[2]	444	180	243	274
Time from ER Arrival to Discharge (minutes)	364	108	131	134
Time in ER Before Being Evaluated (minutes)	382	36	25	26
Time to Pain Meds for Fractures (minutes)	104	68	60	57
Heart Attack Care				
Aspirin Given at Discharge	48	100%	99%	99%
Fibrinolytic Meds Within 30 Min. of Arrival[7]	-	-	33%	54%
PCI Within 90 Minutes of Arrival[1]	-	-	98%	96%
Statin Prescribed at Discharge	45	98%	99%	98%
Heart Failure Care				
ACE Inhibitor or ARB for LVSD	35	100%	97%	97%
Discharge Instructions Given	119	100%	93%	94%
Evaluation of LVS Function	145	99%	99%	99%
Medicare Spending				
Medicare Spending per Patient (ratio)	-	0.95	1	0.98
Pneumonia Care				
Appropriate Initial Antibiotic Given	155	96%	95%	95%
Blood Culture Timing	260	97%	98%	98%
Pregnancy and Delivery Care				
Newborn Deliveries Scheduled Early[2]	39	13%	6%	6%
Preventive Care				
Immunization for Influenza[2]	345	98%	93%	90%
Immunization for Pneumonia[2]	461	97%	93%	92%
Stroke Care				
Anticoagulation Therapy for Atrial Fibrillation[1,2]	-	-	94%	95%
Antithrombotic Therapy Timing[2]	38	84%	97%	98%
Assessed for Rehabilitation[2]	42	100%	97%	97%
Discharged on Antithrombotic Therapy[2]	42	100%	99%	99%
Discharged on Statin Medication[2]	38	95%	94%	94%
Thrombolytic Therapy Timing[1,2]	-	-	57%	66%
Venous Thromboembolism Prophylaxis[2]	37	81%	93%	94%
Written Stroke Educational Materials Given[2]	28	100%	84%	88%
Surgical Care Improvement Project				
Appropriate Beta Blocker Usage	72	100%	97%	98%
Appropriate VTP Within 24 Hours	259	94%	98%	98%
Controlled Postoperative Blood Glucose[7]	-	-	95%	97%
Perioperative Temperature Management	267	100%	100%	100%
Prophylactic Antibiotic Selection	204	99%	99%	99%
Prophylactic Antibiotic Selection (Outpatient)	111	90%	98%	98%
Prophylactic Antibiotic Stopped	198	100%	98%	98%
Prophylactic Antibiotic Timing	204	100%	99%	99%
Prophylactic Antibiotic Timing (Outpatient)	111	99%	98%	98%
Urinary Catheter Removal	211	100%	96%	97%
Survey of Patients' Hospital Experiences				
Area Around Room 'Always' Quiet at Night	300+	64%	67%	61%
Doctors 'Always' Communicated Well	300+	85%	84%	82%
Home Recovery Information Given	300+	87%	85%	85%
Hospital Given 9 or 10 on 10 Point Scale	300+	76%	70%	71%
Meds 'Always' Explained Before Given	300+	68%	66%	64%
Nurses 'Always' Communicated Well	300+	83%	80%	79%
Pain 'Always' Well Controlled	300+	74%	72%	71%
Room and Bathroom 'Always' Clean	300+	77%	73%	73%
Timely Help 'Always' Received	300+	73%	68%	68%
Would Definitely Recommend Hospital	300+	73%	70%	71%
Use of Medical Imaging				
Cardiac Imaging Stress Test before Surgery	245	4.9%	4.8%	5.3%
Combination Abdominal CT Scan	798	5.9%	9.6%	10.5%
Combination Brain/Sinus CT Scan	535	5.8%	3.3%	2.7%
Combination Chest CT Scan	547	2.9%	3.4%	2.7%
Follow-up Mammogram/Ultrasound	1,011	13.1%	8.3%	8.8%
Lumbar Spine MRI for Low Back Pain	107	46.7%	35.3%	37.2%

Takoma Regional Hospital

401 Takoma Ave
Greeneville, TN 37743
Phone: 423-639-3151
Fax: 423-636-2374
URL: www.takoma.org
Type: Acute Care Hospitals
Emergency Services: Yes
Ownership: Voluntary non-profit - Private
Beds: 115
Key Personnel:
Operating Room. . . . . William Bridges
Coronary Care. . . . . Dwayne Covington
Chief of Medical Staff. . . . . Raymond Kohne, MD
Radiology. . . . . Raymond E Kohne
Infection Control. . . . . Peggy McCoy
Quality Assurance . . . . Karen Tilson
Pediatric Ambulatory Care . . . . . . Yvonne Waddell
CEO/President. . . . . Carlyle Walton

Measure	Cases	This Hosp.	State Avg.	U.S. Avg.
Blood Clot Prevention and Treatment				
Anticoagulation Overlap Therapy[2]	28	96%	92%	93%
ICU Venous Thromboembolism Prophylaxis[2]	63	98%	90%	92%
Incidence of Potentially Preventable VTE[1,2]	-	-	10%	10%
UFH with Dosages/Platelet Monitoring[1,2]	-	-	99%	97%
Venous Thromboembolism Prophylaxis[2]	131	94%	83%	85%
Warfarin Therapy Discharge Instructions[2]	21	100%	78%	75%
Chest Pain/Possible Heart Attack Care				
Aspirin Given Within 24 Hours of Arrival	88	98%	96%	96%
Fibrinolytic Meds Within 30 Min. of Arrival[1]	-	-	72%	58%
Average Time to ECG (minutes)	93	10	6	7
Average Time to Transfer (minutes)[1]	-	-	53	60
Children's Asthma Care				
Received Home Management Plan of Care	-	-	-	88%
Received Reliever Medication	-	-	-	100%
Received Systemic Corticosteroids	-	-	-	100%
Emergency Department				
Admittance Decision Time (minutes)[2]	295	81	82	98
Head CT Results Within 45 Min. of Arrival[1,3]	-	-	52%	57%
Patients Who Left ER Before Being Seen	21,539	2%	2%	2%
Time from ER Arrival to Admit. (minutes)[2]	320	257	243	274
Time from ER Arrival to Discharge (minutes)	334	118	131	134
Time in ER Before Being Evaluated (minutes)	327	26	25	26
Time to Pain Meds for Fractures (minutes)	74	62	60	57
Heart Attack Care				
Aspirin Given at Discharge[1,2]	-	-	99%	99%
Fibrinolytic Meds Within 30 Min. of Arrival[2,7]	-	-	33%	54%
PCI Within 90 Minutes of Arrival[2,7]	-	-	98%	96%
Statin Prescribed at Discharge[1,2]	-	-	99%	98%
Heart Failure Care				
ACE Inhibitor or ARB for LVSD[2]	18	94%	97%	97%
Discharge Instructions Given[2]	37	97%	93%	94%
Evaluation of LVS Function[2]	45	98%	99%	99%
Medicare Spending				
Medicare Spending per Patient (ratio)	-	0.96	1	0.98
Pneumonia Care				
Appropriate Initial Antibiotic Given[2]	78	100%	95%	95%
Blood Culture Timing[2]	135	100%	98%	98%
Pregnancy and Delivery Care				
Newborn Deliveries Scheduled Early[2]	34	3%	6%	6%
Preventive Care				
Immunization for Influenza[2]	246	100%	93%	90%
Immunization for Pneumonia[2]	313	99%	93%	92%
Stroke Care				
Anticoagulation Therapy for Atrial Fibrillation[1,2]	-	-	94%	95%
Antithrombotic Therapy Timing[2]	15	93%	97%	98%
Assessed for Rehabilitation[2]	14	86%	97%	97%

NOTE: Hospital profiles are in alphabetical order by state, then city, then hospital within the city; Rankings exclude hospitals with less than 25 cases except for patient surveys which excludes hospitals with less than 100 cases; (a) 100-299 cases; (1) The number of cases/patients is too few to report; (2) Data submitted were based on a sample of cases/patients; (3) Results are based on a shorter time period than required; (4) Data suppressed by CMS for one or more quarters; (5) Results are not available for this reporting period; (6) Fewer than 100 patients completed the HCAHPS survey; (7) No cases met the criteria for this measure; (8) The lower limit of the confidence interval cannot be calculated if the number of observed infections equals zero; (9) No data are available from the state/territory for this reporting period; (10) The scores shown reflect fewer than 50 completed surveys; (11) There were discrepancies in the data collection process; (12) This measure does not apply to this hospital for this reporting period; (13) Results cannot be calculated for this reporting period; (14) The results for this state are combined with nearby states to protect confidentiality; Please refer to the User's Guide for a full explanation of data.

Measure	Cases	This Hosp.	State Avg.	U.S. Avg.
Discharged on Antithrombotic Therapy[2]	13	92%	99%	99%
Discharged on Statin Medication[2]	14	64%	94%	94%
Thrombolytic Therapy Timing[2,7]	-	-	57%	66%
Venous Thromboembolism Prophylaxis[2]	16	100%	93%	94%
Written Stroke Educational Materials Given[1,2]	-	-	84%	88%
Surgical Care Improvement Project				
Appropriate Beta Blocker Usage[2]	24	75%	97%	98%
Appropriate VTP Within 24 Hours[2]	70	93%	98%	98%
Controlled Postoperative Blood Glucose[2,7]	-	-	95%	97%
Perioperative Temperature Management[2]	81	99%	100%	100%
Prophylactic Antibiotic Selection[2]	39	100%	99%	99%
Prophylactic Antibiotic Selection (Outpatient)	45	98%	98%	98%
Prophylactic Antibiotic Stopped[2]	37	95%	98%	98%
Prophylactic Antibiotic Timing[2]	39	97%	99%	99%
Prophylactic Antibiotic Timing (Outpatient)	46	93%	98%	98%
Urinary Catheter Removal[2]	51	98%	96%	97%
Survey of Patients' Hospital Experiences				
Area Around Room 'Always' Quiet at Night[11]	300+	62%	67%	61%
Doctors 'Always' Communicated Well[11]	300+	78%	84%	82%
Home Recovery Information Given[11]	300+	87%	85%	85%
Hospital Given 9 or 10 on 10 Point Scale[11]	300+	71%	70%	71%
Meds 'Always' Explained Before Given[11]	300+	61%	66%	64%
Nurses 'Always' Communicated Well[11]	300+	78%	80%	79%
Pain 'Always' Well Controlled[11]	300+	73%	72%	71%
Room and Bathroom 'Always' Clean[11]	300+	74%	73%	73%
Timely Help 'Always' Received[11]	300+	68%	68%	68%
Would Definitely Recommend Hospital[11]	300+	75%	70%	71%
Use of Medical Imaging				
Cardiac Imaging Stress Test before Surgery	112	7.1%	4.8%	5.3%
Combination Abdominal CT Scan	300	8.3%	9.6%	10.5%
Combination Brain/Sinus CT Scan[1]	-	-	3.3%	2.7%
Combination Chest CT Scan	174	4.6%	3.4%	2.7%
Follow-up Mammogram/Ultrasound	463	11.2%	8.3%	8.8%
Lumbar Spine MRI for Low Back Pain	46	37.0%	35.3%	37.2%

Roane Medical Center

8045 Roane Medical Center Drive
Harriman, TN 37748
URL: www.roanemedical.com
Phone: 865-316-1000
Fax: 865-882-4484
Type: Acute Care Hospitals
Ownership: Govt - Hospital Dist/Auth
Emergency Services: Yes
Beds: 85

Key Personnel:

Radiology. Steven Addonizio
CEO/President. . . . . Jim Gann

Measure	Cases	This Hosp.	State Avg.	U.S. Avg.
Blood Clot Prevention and Treatment				
Anticoagulation Overlap Therapy[2]	11	100%	92%	93%
ICU Venous Thromboembolism Prophylaxis[2]	61	97%	90%	92%
Incidence of Potentially Preventable VTE[2,7]	-	-	10%	10%
UFH with Dosages/Platelet Monitoring[1,2]	-	-	99%	97%
Venous Thromboembolism Prophylaxis[2]	329	93%	83%	85%
Warfarin Therapy Discharge Instructions[1,2]	-	-	78%	75%
Chest Pain/Possible Heart Attack Care				
Aspirin Given Within 24 Hours of Arrival	66	92%	96%	96%
Fibrinolytic Meds Within 30 Min. of Arrival[7]	-	-	72%	58%
Average Time to ECG (minutes)	68	10	6	7
Average Time to Transfer (minutes)	16	68	53	60
Children's Asthma Care				
Received Home Management Plan of Care	-	-	-	88%
Received Reliever Medication	-	-	-	100%
Received Systemic Corticosteroids	-	-	-	100%
Emergency Department				
Admittance Decision Time (minutes)[2]	343	87	82	98
Head CT Results Within 45 Min. of Arrival[1]	-	-	52%	57%
Patients Who Left ER Before Being Seen	21,231	3%	2%	2%
Time from ER Arrival to Admit. (minutes)[2]	531	299	243	274
Time from ER Arrival to Discharge (minutes)	394	149	131	134
Time in ER Before Being Evaluated (minutes)	436	35	25	26
Time to Pain Meds for Fractures (minutes)	53	40	60	57
Heart Attack Care				
Aspirin Given at Discharge[1,2]	-	-	99%	99%
Fibrinolytic Meds Within 30 Min. of Arrival[2,7]	-	-	33%	54%
PCI Within 90 Minutes of Arrival[2,7]	-	-	98%	96%
Statin Prescribed at Discharge[1,2]	-	-	99%	98%
Heart Failure Care				
ACE Inhibitor or ARB for LVSD[2]	11	82%	97%	97%
Discharge Instructions Given[2]	53	100%	93%	94%
Evaluation of LVS Function[2]	58	100%	99%	99%
Medicare Spending				
Medicare Spending per Patient (ratio)	-	1.01	1	0.98
Pneumonia Care				
Appropriate Initial Antibiotic Given[2]	87	97%	95%	95%
Blood Culture Timing[2]	139	99%	98%	98%
Pregnancy and Delivery Care				
Newborn Deliveries Scheduled Early[7]	-	-	6%	6%
Preventive Care				
Immunization for Influenza[2]	299	90%	93%	90%
Immunization for Pneumonia[2]	502	93%	93%	92%
Stroke Care				
Anticoagulation Therapy for Atrial Fibrillation[1,2]	-	-	94%	95%
Antithrombotic Therapy Timing[2]	16	100%	97%	98%
Assessed for Rehabilitation[2]	17	100%	97%	97%
Discharged on Antithrombotic Therapy[2]	14	100%	99%	99%
Discharged on Statin Medication[2]	12	92%	94%	94%
Thrombolytic Therapy Timing[2,7]	-	-	57%	66%
Venous Thromboembolism Prophylaxis[2]	19	100%	93%	94%
Written Stroke Educational Materials Given[2]	13	92%	84%	88%
Surgical Care Improvement Project				
Appropriate Beta Blocker Usage[2]	13	77%	97%	98%
Appropriate VTP Within 24 Hours[2]	55	96%	98%	98%
Controlled Postoperative Blood Glucose[2,7]	-	-	95%	97%
Perioperative Temperature Management[2]	58	100%	100%	100%
Prophylactic Antibiotic Selection[1,2]	-	-	99%	99%
Prophylactic Antibiotic Selection (Outpatient)[1,3]	-	-	98%	98%
Prophylactic Antibiotic Stopped[1,2]	-	-	98%	98%
Prophylactic Antibiotic Timing[1,2]	-	-	99%	99%
Prophylactic Antibiotic Timing (Outpatient)[1,3]	-	-	98%	98%
Urinary Catheter Removal[2]	40	98%	96%	97%
Survey of Patients' Hospital Experiences				
Area Around Room 'Always' Quiet at Night	300+	68%	67%	61%
Doctors 'Always' Communicated Well	300+	87%	84%	82%
Home Recovery Information Given	300+	86%	85%	85%
Hospital Given 9 or 10 on 10 Point Scale	300+	65%	70%	71%
Meds 'Always' Explained Before Given	300+	66%	66%	64%
Nurses 'Always' Communicated Well	300+	78%	80%	79%
Pain 'Always' Well Controlled	300+	68%	72%	71%
Room and Bathroom 'Always' Clean	300+	73%	73%	73%
Timely Help 'Always' Received	300+	69%	68%	68%
Would Definitely Recommend Hospital	300+	69%	70%	71%
Use of Medical Imaging				
Cardiac Imaging Stress Test before Surgery	185	4.3%	4.8%	5.3%
Combination Abdominal CT Scan	342	7.9%	9.6%	10.5%
Combination Brain/Sinus CT Scan	532	3.8%	3.3%	2.7%
Combination Chest CT Scan	229	6.1%	3.4%	2.7%
Follow-up Mammogram/Ultrasound	390	5.4%	8.3%	8.8%
Lumbar Spine MRI for Low Back Pain	89	24.7%	35.3%	37.2%

Trousdale Medical Center

500 Church Street
Hartsville, TN 37074
Phone: 615-374-2221
Fax: 615-374-2928
Type: Critical Access Hospitals
Ownership: Voluntary non-profit - Other
Emergency Services: Yes
Beds: 25

Key Personnel:

Radiology. Brent Frisbie
Administrator . . . . Rod Harkleroad, RN, MBA
Infection Control. . . . . Kim Kichy
Emergency Room . . . . Floyd Reid
Chief of Medical Staff. . . . . B T Samson
Quality Assurance . . . . Martha Stack

Measure	Cases	This Hosp.	State Avg.	U.S. Avg.
Blood Clot Prevention and Treatment				
Anticoagulation Overlap Therapy[5]	-	-	92%	93%
ICU Venous Thromboembolism Prophylaxis[5]	-	-	90%	92%
Incidence of Potentially Preventable VTE[5]	-	-	10%	10%
UFH with Dosages/Platelet Monitoring[5]	-	-	99%	97%
Venous Thromboembolism Prophylaxis[5]	-	-	83%	85%
Warfarin Therapy Discharge Instructions[5]	-	-	78%	75%
Chest Pain/Possible Heart Attack Care				
Aspirin Given Within 24 Hours of Arrival	-	-	96%	96%
Fibrinolytic Meds Within 30 Min. of Arrival	-	-	72%	58%
Average Time to ECG (minutes)	-	-	6	7
Average Time to Transfer (minutes)	-	-	53	60
Children's Asthma Care				
Received Home Management Plan of Care	-	-	-	88%
Received Reliever Medication	-	-	-	100%
Received Systemic Corticosteroids	-	-	-	100%
Emergency Department				
Admittance Decision Time (minutes)[5]	-	-	82	98
Head CT Results Within 45 Min. of Arrival	-	-	52%	57%
Patients Who Left ER Before Being Seen	-	-	2%	2%
Time from ER Arrival to Admit. (minutes)[5]	-	-	243	274
Time from ER Arrival to Discharge (minutes)	-	-	131	134
Time in ER Before Being Evaluated (minutes)	-	-	25	26
Time to Pain Meds for Fractures (minutes)	-	-	60	57
Heart Attack Care				
Aspirin Given at Discharge[3,7]	-	-	99%	99%
Fibrinolytic Meds Within 30 Min. of Arrival[3,7]	-	-	33%	54%
PCI Within 90 Minutes of Arrival[3,7]	-	-	98%	96%
Statin Prescribed at Discharge[3,7]	-	-	99%	98%
Heart Failure Care				
ACE Inhibitor or ARB for LVSD[1]	-	-	97%	97%
Discharge Instructions Given	14	86%	93%	94%
Evaluation of LVS Function	16	75%	99%	99%
Medicare Spending				
Medicare Spending per Patient (ratio)	-	-	1	0.98
Pneumonia Care				
Appropriate Initial Antibiotic Given	24	100%	95%	95%
Blood Culture Timing	25	100%	98%	98%
Pregnancy and Delivery Care				
Newborn Deliveries Scheduled Early[3,7]	-	-	6%	6%
Preventive Care				
Immunization for Influenza[5]	-	-	93%	90%
Immunization for Pneumonia[5]	-	-	93%	92%
Stroke Care				
Anticoagulation Therapy for Atrial Fibrillation[5]	-	-	94%	95%
Antithrombotic Therapy Timing[5]	-	-	97%	98%
Assessed for Rehabilitation[5]	-	-	97%	97%
Discharged on Antithrombotic Therapy[5]	-	-	99%	99%
Discharged on Statin Medication[5]	-	-	94%	94%
Thrombolytic Therapy Timing[5]	-	-	57%	66%
Venous Thromboembolism Prophylaxis[5]	-	-	93%	94%
Written Stroke Educational Materials Given[5]	-	-	84%	88%
Surgical Care Improvement Project				
Appropriate Beta Blocker Usage[5]	-	-	97%	98%
Appropriate VTP Within 24 Hours[5]	-	-	98%	98%
Controlled Postoperative Blood Glucose[5]	-	-	95%	97%
Perioperative Temperature Management[5]	-	-	100%	100%
Prophylactic Antibiotic Selection[5]	-	-	99%	99%
Prophylactic Antibiotic Selection (Outpatient)	-	-	98%	98%
Prophylactic Antibiotic Stopped[5]	-	-	98%	98%
Prophylactic Antibiotic Timing[5]	-	-	99%	99%
Prophylactic Antibiotic Timing (Outpatient)	-	-	98%	98%
Urinary Catheter Removal[5]	-	-	96%	97%
Survey of Patients' Hospital Experiences				
Area Around Room 'Always' Quiet at Night[6]	<100	76%	67%	61%
Doctors 'Always' Communicated Well[6]	<100	93%	84%	82%
Home Recovery Information Given[6]	<100	87%	85%	85%
Hospital Given 9 or 10 on 10 Point Scale[6]	<100	80%	70%	71%
Meds 'Always' Explained Before Given[6]	<100	71%	66%	64%
Nurses 'Always' Communicated Well[6]	<100	84%	80%	79%
Pain 'Always' Well Controlled[6]	<100	76%	72%	71%
Room and Bathroom 'Always' Clean[6]	<100	89%	73%	73%
Timely Help 'Always' Received[6]	<100	75%	68%	68%
Would Definitely Recommend Hospital[6]	<100	80%	70%	71%
Use of Medical Imaging				
Cardiac Imaging Stress Test before Surgery	-	-	4.8%	5.3%
Combination Abdominal CT Scan	-	-	9.6%	10.5%
Combination Brain/Sinus CT Scan	-	-	3.3%	2.7%

NOTE: Hospital profiles are in alphabetical order by state, then city, then hospital within the city; Rankings exclude hospitals with less than 25 cases except for patient surveys which excludes hospitals with less than 100 cases; (a) 100-299 cases; (1) The number of cases/patients is too few to report; (2) Data submitted were based on a sample of cases/patients; (3) Results are based on a shorter time period than required; (4) Data suppressed by CMS for one or more quarters; (5) Results are not available for this reporting period; (6) Fewer than 100 patients completed the HCAHPS survey; (7) No cases met the criteria for this measure; (8) The lower limit of the confidence interval cannot be calculated if the number of observed infections equals zero; (9) No data are available from the state/territory for this reporting period; (10) The scores shown reflect fewer than 50 completed surveys; (11) There were discrepancies in the data collection process; (12) This measure does not apply to this hospital for this reporting period; (13) Results cannot be calculated for this reporting period; (14) The results for this state are combined with nearby states to protect confidentiality; Please refer to the User's Guide for a full explanation of data.

Combination Chest CT Scan	-	-	3.4%	2.7%
Follow-up Mammogram/Ultrasound	-	-	8.3%	8.8%
Lumbar Spine MRI for Low Back Pain	-	-	35.3%	37.2%

Tristar Hendersonville Medical Center

355 New Shackle Island Rd
Hendersonville, TN 37075
Phone: 615-338-1000
Fax: 615-338-1101
URL: www.hendersonvillemedicalcenter.com
Type: Acute Care Hospitals
Emergency Services: Yes
Ownership: Voluntary non-profit - Other
Beds: 110

Key Personnel:
Radiology. . . . . John J Alarcon
CEO/President. . . . . Regina Bartlett
Operating Room. . . . . John Andrew Boskind
Chief of Medical Staff . . . . Tracy Callista, MD
Cardiac Laboratory. . . . . Jim Oliver
Infection Control. . . . . Debbie Smith
Quality Assurance . . . . Karen Stanley

Measure	Cases	This Hosp.	State Avg.	U.S. Avg.
Blood Clot Prevention and Treatment				
Anticoagulation Overlap Therapy[2]	63	100%	92%	93%
ICU Venous Thromboembolism Prophylaxis[2]	142	94%	90%	92%
Incidence of Potentially Preventable VTE[1,2]	-	-	10%	10%
UFH with Dosages/Platelet Monitoring[2]	19	100%	99%	97%
Venous Thromboembolism Prophylaxis[2]	277	86%	83%	85%
Warfarin Therapy Discharge Instructions[2]	50	98%	78%	75%
Chest Pain/Possible Heart Attack Care				
Aspirin Given Within 24 Hours of Arrival	25	100%	96%	96%
Fibrinolytic Meds Within 30 Min. of Arrival[3,7]	-	-	72%	58%
Average Time to ECG (minutes)	25	4	6	7
Average Time to Transfer (minutes)[1,3]	-	-	53	60
Children's Asthma Care				
Received Home Management Plan of Care	-	-	-	88%
Received Reliever Medication	-	-	-	100%
Received Systemic Corticosteroids	-	-	-	100%
Emergency Department				
Admittance Decision Time (minutes)[2]	677	77	82	98
Head CT Results Within 45 Min. of Arrival[1]	-	-	52%	57%
Patients Who Left ER Before Being Seen	31,282	1%	2%	2%
Time from ER Arrival to Admit. (minutes)[2]	682	203	243	274
Time from ER Arrival to Discharge (minutes)	415	118	131	134
Time in ER Before Being Evaluated (minutes)	450	14	25	26
Time to Pain Meds for Fractures (minutes)	152	40	60	57
Heart Attack Care				
Aspirin Given at Discharge	49	100%	99%	99%
Fibrinolytic Meds Within 30 Min. of Arrival[7]	-	-	33%	54%
PCI Within 90 Minutes of Arrival	13	100%	98%	96%
Statin Prescribed at Discharge	46	100%	99%	98%
Heart Failure Care				
ACE Inhibitor or ARB for LVSD	41	100%	97%	97%
Discharge Instructions Given	120	100%	93%	94%
Evaluation of LVS Function	152	100%	99%	99%
Medicare Spending				
Medicare Spending per Patient (ratio)	-	1.02	1	0.98
Pneumonia Care				
Appropriate Initial Antibiotic Given	139	100%	95%	95%
Blood Culture Timing	212	100%	98%	98%
Pregnancy and Delivery Care				
Newborn Deliveries Scheduled Early[2]	19	0%	6%	6%
Preventive Care				
Immunization for Influenza[2]	541	76%	93%	90%
Immunization for Pneumonia[2]	685	85%	93%	92%
Stroke Care				
Anticoagulation Therapy for Atrial Fibrillation[1]	-	-	94%	95%
Antithrombotic Therapy Timing	60	98%	97%	98%
Assessed for Rehabilitation	66	100%	97%	97%
Discharged on Antithrombotic Therapy	64	100%	99%	99%
Discharged on Statin Medication	48	100%	94%	94%
Thrombolytic Therapy Timing[7]	-	-	57%	66%
Venous Thromboembolism Prophylaxis	60	98%	93%	94%
Written Stroke Educational Materials Given	39	92%	84%	88%
Surgical Care Improvement Project				
Appropriate Beta Blocker Usage	103	98%	97%	98%
Appropriate VTP Within 24 Hours	331	99%	98%	98%
Controlled Postoperative Blood Glucose[7]	-	-	95%	97%
Perioperative Temperature Management	390	100%	100%	100%
Prophylactic Antibiotic Selection	255	100%	99%	99%
Prophylactic Antibiotic Selection (Outpatient)	236	100%	98%	98%
Prophylactic Antibiotic Stopped	236	100%	98%	98%
Prophylactic Antibiotic Timing	255	97%	99%	99%
Prophylactic Antibiotic Timing (Outpatient)	237	98%	98%	98%
Urinary Catheter Removal	251	99%	96%	97%
Survey of Patients' Hospital Experiences				
Area Around Room 'Always' Quiet at Night	300+	58%	67%	61%
Doctors 'Always' Communicated Well	300+	77%	84%	82%
Home Recovery Information Given	300+	85%	85%	85%
Hospital Given 9 or 10 on 10 Point Scale	300+	64%	70%	71%
Meds 'Always' Explained Before Given	300+	57%	66%	64%
Nurses 'Always' Communicated Well	300+	73%	80%	79%
Pain 'Always' Well Controlled	300+	66%	72%	71%
Room and Bathroom 'Always' Clean	300+	68%	73%	73%
Timely Help 'Always' Received	300+	59%	68%	68%
Would Definitely Recommend Hospital	300+	69%	70%	71%
Use of Medical Imaging				
Cardiac Imaging Stress Test before Surgery[1]	-	-	4.8%	5.3%
Combination Abdominal CT Scan	446	11.9%	9.6%	10.5%
Combination Brain/Sinus CT Scan	457	5.5%	3.3%	2.7%
Combination Chest CT Scan	233	1.3%	3.4%	2.7%
Follow-up Mammogram/Ultrasound	679	10.5%	8.3%	8.8%
Lumbar Spine MRI for Low Back Pain	82	28.0%	35.3%	37.2%

Tristar Summit Medical Center

5655 Frist Blvd
Hermitage, TN 37076
Phone: 615-316-3000
Fax: 615-316-3557
URL: www.summitmedctr.com
Type: Acute Care Hospitals
Emergency Services: Yes
Ownership: Proprietary
Beds: 204

Key Personnel:
Radiology. . . . . Lisa A Altieri, MD
Chief of Medical Staff . . . . Wendy Brandon
Operating Room. . . . . Stephanie Davis
Emergency Room . . . . Randy Farrar
Quality Assurance . . . . Patsy Parrell
CEO/President. . . . . Jeff Whitehorn

Measure	Cases	This Hosp.	State Avg.	U.S. Avg.
Blood Clot Prevention and Treatment				
Anticoagulation Overlap Therapy[2]	83	98%	92%	93%
ICU Venous Thromboembolism Prophylaxis[2]	68	97%	90%	92%
Incidence of Potentially Preventable VTE[2]	15	0%	10%	10%
UFH with Dosages/Platelet Monitoring[2]	14	100%	99%	97%
Venous Thromboembolism Prophylaxis[2]	320	95%	83%	85%
Warfarin Therapy Discharge Instructions[2]	65	92%	78%	75%
Chest Pain/Possible Heart Attack Care				
Aspirin Given Within 24 Hours of Arrival	18	100%	96%	96%
Fibrinolytic Meds Within 30 Min. of Arrival[3,7]	-	-	72%	58%
Average Time to ECG (minutes)	19	4	6	7
Average Time to Transfer (minutes)[3,7]	-	-	53	60
Children's Asthma Care				
Received Home Management Plan of Care	-	-	-	88%
Received Reliever Medication	-	-	-	100%
Received Systemic Corticosteroids	-	-	-	100%
Emergency Department				
Admittance Decision Time (minutes)[2]	777	80	82	98
Head CT Results Within 45 Min. of Arrival[1]	-	-	52%	57%
Patients Who Left ER Before Being Seen	51,504	1%	2%	2%
Time from ER Arrival to Admit. (minutes)[2]	778	233	243	274
Time from ER Arrival to Discharge (minutes)	498	152	131	134
Time in ER Before Being Evaluated (minutes)	514	14	25	26
Time to Pain Meds for Fractures (minutes)	170	48	60	57
Heart Attack Care				
Aspirin Given at Discharge[2]	152	100%	99%	99%
Fibrinolytic Meds Within 30 Min. of Arrival[2,7]	-	-	33%	54%
PCI Within 90 Minutes of Arrival[2]	56	98%	98%	96%
Statin Prescribed at Discharge[2]	153	99%	99%	98%
Heart Failure Care				
ACE Inhibitor or ARB for LVSD[2]	75	100%	97%	97%
Discharge Instructions Given[2]	192	100%	93%	94%
Evaluation of LVS Function[2]	246	100%	99%	99%
Medicare Spending				
Medicare Spending per Patient (ratio)	-	1.01	1	0.98
Pneumonia Care				
Appropriate Initial Antibiotic Given[2]	89	98%	95%	95%
Blood Culture Timing[2]	160	99%	98%	98%
Pregnancy and Delivery Care				
Newborn Deliveries Scheduled Early[2]	47	4%	6%	6%
Preventive Care				
Immunization for Influenza[2]	537	94%	93%	90%
Immunization for Pneumonia[2]	708	91%	93%	92%
Stroke Care				
Anticoagulation Therapy for Atrial Fibrillation	22	100%	94%	95%
Antithrombotic Therapy Timing	159	100%	97%	98%
Assessed for Rehabilitation	184	100%	97%	97%
Discharged on Antithrombotic Therapy	164	100%	99%	99%
Discharged on Statin Medication	109	99%	94%	94%
Thrombolytic Therapy Timing[1]	-	-	57%	66%
Venous Thromboembolism Prophylaxis	185	96%	93%	94%
Written Stroke Educational Materials Given	105	94%	84%	88%
Surgical Care Improvement Project				
Appropriate Beta Blocker Usage[2]	140	99%	97%	98%
Appropriate VTP Within 24 Hours[2]	399	99%	98%	98%
Controlled Postoperative Blood Glucose[2,7]	-	-	95%	97%
Perioperative Temperature Management[2]	472	100%	100%	100%
Prophylactic Antibiotic Selection[2]	265	100%	99%	99%
Prophylactic Antibiotic Selection (Outpatient)	387	98%	98%	98%
Prophylactic Antibiotic Stopped[2]	251	100%	98%	98%
Prophylactic Antibiotic Timing[2]	265	99%	99%	99%
Prophylactic Antibiotic Timing (Outpatient)	388	100%	98%	98%
Urinary Catheter Removal[2]	280	100%	96%	97%
Survey of Patients' Hospital Experiences				
Area Around Room 'Always' Quiet at Night	300+	64%	67%	61%
Doctors 'Always' Communicated Well	300+	79%	84%	82%
Home Recovery Information Given	300+	87%	85%	85%
Hospital Given 9 or 10 on 10 Point Scale	300+	72%	70%	71%
Meds 'Always' Explained Before Given	300+	64%	66%	64%
Nurses 'Always' Communicated Well	300+	76%	80%	79%
Pain 'Always' Well Controlled	300+	69%	72%	71%
Room and Bathroom 'Always' Clean	300+	71%	73%	73%
Timely Help 'Always' Received	300+	60%	68%	68%
Would Definitely Recommend Hospital	300+	73%	70%	71%
Use of Medical Imaging				
Cardiac Imaging Stress Test before Surgery	99	7.1%	4.8%	5.3%
Combination Abdominal CT Scan	802	9.7%	9.6%	10.5%
Combination Brain/Sinus CT Scan	549	2.2%	3.3%	2.7%
Combination Chest CT Scan	429	0.9%	3.4%	2.7%
Follow-up Mammogram/Ultrasound	1,365	7.4%	8.3%	8.8%
Lumbar Spine MRI for Low Back Pain	143	37.1%	35.3%	37.2%

Humboldt General Hospital

3525 Chere Carol Rd
Humboldt, TN 38343
Phone: 731-784-2321
Fax: 731-824-5569
Type: Acute Care Hospitals
Emergency Services: Yes
Ownership: Govt - Hospital Dist/Auth
Beds: 62

Key Personnel:
Emergency Room . . . . Renoda Crone
Operating Room. . . . . Linda Elmore
Radiology. . . . . Keith Garner
CEO/President. . . . . Bill Kail
Chief of Medical Staff . . . . Jennifer Utley
Infection Control. . . . . Della Yarbrough

Measure	Cases	This Hosp.	State Avg.	U.S. Avg.
Blood Clot Prevention and Treatment				
Anticoagulation Overlap Therapy	-	-	92%	93%
ICU Venous Thromboembolism Prophylaxis	-	-	90%	92%
Incidence of Potentially Preventable VTE	-	-	10%	10%
UFH with Dosages/Platelet Monitoring	-	-	99%	97%
Venous Thromboembolism Prophylaxis	-	-	83%	85%
Warfarin Therapy Discharge Instructions	-	-	78%	75%
Chest Pain/Possible Heart Attack Care				
Aspirin Given Within 24 Hours of Arrival[3]	45	91%	96%	96%
Fibrinolytic Meds Within 30 Min. of Arrival[3,7]	-	-	72%	58%
Average Time to ECG (minutes)[3]	48	6	6	7

NOTE: Hospital profiles are in alphabetical order by state, then city, then hospital within the city; Rankings exclude hospitals with less than 25 cases except for patient surveys which excludes hospitals with less than 100 cases; (a) 100-299 cases; (1) The number of cases/patients is too few to report; (2) Data submitted were based on a sample of cases/patients; (3) Results are based on a shorter time period than required; (4) Data suppressed by CMS for one or more quarters; (5) Results are not available for this reporting period; (6) Fewer than 100 patients completed the HCAHPS survey; (7) No cases met the criteria for this measure; (8) The lower limit of the confidence interval cannot be calculated if the number of observed infections equals zero; (9) No data are available from the state/territory for this reporting period; (10) The scores shown reflect fewer than 50 completed surveys; (11) There were discrepancies in the data collection process; (12) This measure does not apply to this hospital for this reporting period; (13) Results cannot be calculated for this reporting period; (14) The results for this state are combined with nearby states to protect confidentiality; Please refer to the User's Guide for a full explanation of data.

Measure	Cases	This Hosp.	State Avg.	U.S. Avg.
Average Time to Transfer (minutes)[1,3]	-	-	53	60
Children's Asthma Care				
Received Home Management Plan of Care	-	-	-	88%
Received Reliever Medication	-	-	-	100%
Received Systemic Corticosteroids	-	-	-	100%
Emergency Department				
Admittance Decision Time (minutes)	-	-	82	98
Head CT Results Within 45 Min. of Arrival[1,3]	-	-	52%	57%
Patients Who Left ER Before Being Seen	9,956	1%	2%	2%
Time from ER Arrival to Admit. (minutes)	-	-	243	274
Time from ER Arrival to Discharge (minutes)[3]	289	91	131	134
Time in ER Before Being Evaluated (minutes)[3]	299	23	25	26
Time to Pain Meds for Fractures (minutes)[3]	18	56	60	57
Heart Attack Care				
Aspirin Given at Discharge	-	-	99%	99%
Fibrinolytic Meds Within 30 Min. of Arrival	-	-	33%	54%
PCI Within 90 Minutes of Arrival	-	-	98%	96%
Statin Prescribed at Discharge	-	-	99%	98%
Heart Failure Care				
ACE Inhibitor or ARB for LVSD	-	-	97%	97%
Discharge Instructions Given	-	-	93%	94%
Evaluation of LVS Function	-	-	99%	99%
Medicare Spending				
Medicare Spending per Patient (ratio)	-	-	1	0.98
Pneumonia Care				
Appropriate Initial Antibiotic Given	-	-	95%	95%
Blood Culture Timing	-	-	98%	98%
Pregnancy and Delivery Care				
Newborn Deliveries Scheduled Early	-	-	6%	6%
Preventive Care				
Immunization for Influenza	-	-	93%	90%
Immunization for Pneumonia	-	-	93%	92%
Stroke Care				
Anticoagulation Therapy for Atrial Fibrillation	-	-	94%	95%
Antithrombotic Therapy Timing	-	-	97%	98%
Assessed for Rehabilitation	-	-	97%	97%
Discharged on Antithrombotic Therapy	-	-	99%	99%
Discharged on Statin Medication	-	-	94%	94%
Thrombolytic Therapy Timing	-	-	57%	66%
Venous Thromboembolism Prophylaxis	-	-	93%	94%
Written Stroke Educational Materials Given	-	-	84%	88%
Surgical Care Improvement Project				
Appropriate Beta Blocker Usage	-	-	97%	98%
Appropriate VTP Within 24 Hours	-	-	98%	98%
Controlled Postoperative Blood Glucose	-	-	95%	97%
Perioperative Temperature Management	-	-	100%	100%
Prophylactic Antibiotic Selection	-	-	99%	99%
Prophylactic Antibiotic Selection (Outpatient)[5]	-	-	98%	98%
Prophylactic Antibiotic Stopped	-	-	98%	98%
Prophylactic Antibiotic Timing	-	-	99%	99%
Prophylactic Antibiotic Timing (Outpatient)[5]	-	-	98%	98%
Urinary Catheter Removal	-	-	96%	97%
Survey of Patients' Hospital Experiences				
Area Around Room 'Always' Quiet at Night	-	-	67%	61%
Doctors 'Always' Communicated Well	-	-	84%	82%
Home Recovery Information Given	-	-	85%	85%
Hospital Given 9 or 10 on 10 Point Scale	-	-	70%	71%
Meds 'Always' Explained Before Given	-	-	66%	64%
Nurses 'Always' Communicated Well	-	-	80%	79%
Pain 'Always' Well Controlled	-	-	72%	71%
Room and Bathroom 'Always' Clean	-	-	73%	73%
Timely Help 'Always' Received	-	-	68%	68%
Would Definitely Recommend Hospital	-	-	70%	71%
Use of Medical Imaging				
Cardiac Imaging Stress Test before Surgery[7]	-	-	4.8%	5.3%
Combination Abdominal CT Scan	91	5.5%	9.6%	10.5%
Combination Brain/Sinus CT Scan[1]	-	-	3.3%	2.7%
Combination Chest CT Scan[1]	-	-	3.4%	2.7%
Follow-up Mammogram/Ultrasound[7]	-	-	8.3%	8.8%
Lumbar Spine MRI for Low Back Pain[7]	-	-	35.3%	37.2%

Baptist Memorial Hospital Huntingdon

631 Rb Wilson Dr
Huntingdon, TN 38344
URL: www.bmhcc.org
Type: Acute Care Hospitals
Ownership: Voluntary non-profit - Church
Phone: 731-986-4461
Fax: 731-986-7288
Emergency Services: Yes
Beds: 72

Key Personnel:
Radiology. Jacob Abraham
CEO/President. . . . . Paul DePriest, MD

Measure	Cases	This Hosp.	State Avg.	U.S. Avg.
Blood Clot Prevention and Treatment				
Anticoagulation Overlap Therapy[1]	-	-	92%	93%
ICU Venous Thromboembolism Prophylaxis	24	96%	90%	92%
Incidence of Potentially Preventable VTE[1]	-	-	10%	10%
UFH with Dosages/Platelet Monitoring[1]	-	-	99%	97%
Venous Thromboembolism Prophylaxis	246	97%	83%	85%
Warfarin Therapy Discharge Instructions[1]	-	-	78%	75%
Chest Pain/Possible Heart Attack Care				
Aspirin Given Within 24 Hours of Arrival	81	94%	96%	96%
Fibrinolytic Meds Within 30 Min. of Arrival[1]	-	-	72%	58%
Average Time to ECG (minutes)	84	8	6	7
Average Time to Transfer (minutes)[1]	-	-	53	60
Children's Asthma Care				
Received Home Management Plan of Care	-	-	-	88%
Received Reliever Medication	-	-	-	100%
Received Systemic Corticosteroids	-	-	-	100%
Emergency Department				
Admittance Decision Time (minutes)[2]	187	61	82	98
Head CT Results Within 45 Min. of Arrival[1]	-	-	52%	57%
Patients Who Left ER Before Being Seen	7,805	2%	2%	2%
Time from ER Arrival to Admit. (minutes)[2]	206	219	243	274
Time from ER Arrival to Discharge (minutes)	225	124	131	134
Time in ER Before Being Evaluated (minutes)	379	22	25	26
Time to Pain Meds for Fractures (minutes)	36	70	60	57
Heart Attack Care				
Aspirin Given at Discharge[1,3]	-	-	99%	99%
Fibrinolytic Meds Within 30 Min. of Arrival[3,7]	-	-	33%	54%
PCI Within 90 Minutes of Arrival[3,7]	-	-	98%	96%
Statin Prescribed at Discharge[1,3]	-	-	99%	98%
Heart Failure Care				
ACE Inhibitor or ARB for LVSD[1]	-	-	97%	97%
Discharge Instructions Given	16	100%	93%	94%
Evaluation of LVS Function	26	100%	99%	99%
Medicare Spending				
Medicare Spending per Patient (ratio)	-	1.05	1	0.98
Pneumonia Care				
Appropriate Initial Antibiotic Given	27	100%	95%	95%
Blood Culture Timing	29	100%	98%	98%
Pregnancy and Delivery Care				
Newborn Deliveries Scheduled Early[7]	-	-	6%	6%
Preventive Care				
Immunization for Influenza[2]	231	100%	93%	90%
Immunization for Pneumonia[2]	363	100%	93%	92%
Stroke Care				
Anticoagulation Therapy for Atrial Fibrillation[1]	-	-	94%	95%
Antithrombotic Therapy Timing	20	95%	97%	98%
Assessed for Rehabilitation	20	100%	97%	97%
Discharged on Antithrombotic Therapy	20	100%	99%	99%
Discharged on Statin Medication	16	75%	94%	94%
Thrombolytic Therapy Timing[7]	-	-	57%	66%
Venous Thromboembolism Prophylaxis	20	95%	93%	94%
Written Stroke Educational Materials Given[1]	-	-	84%	88%
Surgical Care Improvement Project				
Appropriate Beta Blocker Usage[1]	-	-	97%	98%
Appropriate VTP Within 24 Hours	15	93%	98%	98%
Controlled Postoperative Blood Glucose[7]	-	-	95%	97%
Perioperative Temperature Management	17	100%	100%	100%
Prophylactic Antibiotic Selection	11	100%	99%	99%
Prophylactic Antibiotic Selection (Outpatient)[1,3]	-	-	98%	98%
Prophylactic Antibiotic Stopped	11	100%	98%	98%
Prophylactic Antibiotic Timing	11	100%	99%	99%
Prophylactic Antibiotic Timing (Outpatient)[1,3]	-	-	98%	98%
Urinary Catheter Removal[1]	-	-	96%	97%
Survey of Patients' Hospital Experiences				
Area Around Room 'Always' Quiet at Night[6]	<100	79%	67%	61%
Doctors 'Always' Communicated Well[6]	<100	90%	84%	82%
Home Recovery Information Given[6]	<100	88%	85%	85%
Hospital Given 9 or 10 on 10 Point Scale[6]	<100	84%	70%	71%
Meds 'Always' Explained Before Given[6]	<100	74%	66%	64%
Nurses 'Always' Communicated Well[6]	<100	90%	80%	79%
Pain 'Always' Well Controlled[6]	<100	76%	72%	71%
Room and Bathroom 'Always' Clean[6]	<100	81%	73%	73%
Timely Help 'Always' Received[6]	<100	83%	68%	68%
Would Definitely Recommend Hospital[6]	<100	74%	70%	71%
Use of Medical Imaging				
Cardiac Imaging Stress Test before Surgery[1]	-	-	4.8%	5.3%
Combination Abdominal CT Scan	150	16.7%	9.6%	10.5%
Combination Brain/Sinus CT Scan[1]	-	-	3.3%	2.7%
Combination Chest CT Scan	67	25.4%	3.4%	2.7%
Follow-up Mammogram/Ultrasound	239	6.3%	8.3%	8.8%
Lumbar Spine MRI for Low Back Pain[1]	-	-	35.3%	37.2%

Jackson - Madison County General Hospital

620 Skyline Drive
Jackson, TN 38301
URL: www.wth.org
Type: Acute Care Hospitals
Ownership: Govt - Hospital Dist/Auth
Phone: 731-541-5000
Emergency Services: Yes

Key Personnel:
Infection Control. . . . . Ellena Henderson
CEO/President. . . . . Jim Moss
Hemotology Center . . . . Gina Myracle
Radiology. Kelly Yenawine

Measure	Cases	This Hosp.	State Avg.	U.S. Avg.
Blood Clot Prevention and Treatment				
Anticoagulation Overlap Therapy[2]	239	90%	92%	93%
ICU Venous Thromboembolism Prophylaxis[2]	109	88%	90%	92%
Incidence of Potentially Preventable VTE[2]	50	12%	10%	10%
UFH with Dosages/Platelet Monitoring[2]	223	99%	99%	97%
Venous Thromboembolism Prophylaxis[2]	349	82%	83%	85%
Warfarin Therapy Discharge Instructions[2]	172	98%	78%	75%
Chest Pain/Possible Heart Attack Care				
Aspirin Given Within 24 Hours of Arrival[3,7]	-	-	96%	96%
Fibrinolytic Meds Within 30 Min. of Arrival[5]	-	-	72%	58%
Average Time to ECG (minutes)[3,7]	-	-	6	7
Average Time to Transfer (minutes)[5]	-	-	53	60
Children's Asthma Care				
Received Home Management Plan of Care	-	-	-	88%
Received Reliever Medication	-	-	-	100%
Received Systemic Corticosteroids	-	-	-	100%
Emergency Department				
Admittance Decision Time (minutes)[2]	480	92	82	98
Head CT Results Within 45 Min. of Arrival	11	18%	52%	57%
Patients Who Left ER Before Being Seen	85,854	4%	2%	2%
Time from ER Arrival to Admit. (minutes)[2]	522	266	243	274
Time from ER Arrival to Discharge (minutes)	375	203	131	134
Time in ER Before Being Evaluated (minutes)	414	44	25	26
Time to Pain Meds for Fractures (minutes)	153	62	60	57
Heart Attack Care				
Aspirin Given at Discharge	1,162	100%	99%	99%
Fibrinolytic Meds Within 30 Min. of Arrival[7]	-	-	33%	54%
PCI Within 90 Minutes of Arrival	92	98%	98%	96%
Statin Prescribed at Discharge	1,164	100%	99%	98%
Heart Failure Care				
ACE Inhibitor or ARB for LVSD	379	100%	97%	97%
Discharge Instructions Given	897	94%	93%	94%
Evaluation of LVS Function	1,123	100%	99%	99%
Medicare Spending				
Medicare Spending per Patient (ratio)	-	1.00	1	0.98
Pneumonia Care				
Appropriate Initial Antibiotic Given[2]	88	90%	95%	95%
Blood Culture Timing[2]	193	99%	98%	98%
Pregnancy and Delivery Care				
Newborn Deliveries Scheduled Early	248	3%	6%	6%
Preventive Care				
Immunization for Influenza[2]	548	97%	93%	90%

NOTE: Hospital profiles are in alphabetical order by state, then city, then hospital within the city; Rankings exclude hospitals with less than 25 cases except for patient surveys which excludes hospitals with less than 100 cases; (a) 100-299 cases; (1) The number of cases/patients is too few to report; (2) Data submitted were based on a sample of cases/patients; (3) Results are based on a shorter time period than required; (4) Data suppressed by CMS for one or more quarters; (5) Results are not available for this reporting period; (6) Fewer than 100 patients completed the HCAHPS survey; (7) No cases met the criteria for this measure; (8) The lower limit of the confidence interval cannot be calculated if the number of observed infections equals zero; (9) No data are available from the state/territory for this reporting period; (10) The scores shown reflect fewer than 50 completed surveys; (11) There were discrepancies in the data collection process; (12) This measure does not apply to this hospital for this reporting period; (13) Results cannot be calculated for this reporting period; (14) The results for this state are combined with nearby states to protect confidentiality; Please refer to the User's Guide for a full explanation of data.

Measure	Cases	This Hosp.	State Avg.	U.S. Avg.
Immunization for Pneumonia[2]	748	97%	93%	92%
Stroke Care				
Anticoagulation Therapy for Atrial Fibrillation	54	96%	94%	95%
Antithrombotic Therapy Timing	411	97%	97%	98%
Assessed for Rehabilitation	498	97%	97%	97%
Discharged on Antithrombotic Therapy	442	100%	99%	99%
Discharged on Statin Medication	337	98%	94%	94%
Thrombolytic Therapy Timing	24	88%	57%	66%
Venous Thromboembolism Prophylaxis	512	93%	93%	94%
Written Stroke Educational Materials Given	243	86%	84%	88%
Surgical Care Improvement Project				
Appropriate Beta Blocker Usage[2]	592	98%	97%	98%
Appropriate VTP Within 24 Hours[2]	1,153	97%	98%	98%
Controlled Postoperative Blood Glucose[2]	376	93%	95%	97%
Perioperative Temperature Management[2]	1,357	100%	100%	100%
Prophylactic Antibiotic Selection[2]	1,234	99%	99%	99%
Prophylactic Antibiotic Selection (Outpatient)	696	97%	98%	98%
Prophylactic Antibiotic Stopped[2]	1,197	96%	98%	98%
Prophylactic Antibiotic Timing[2]	1,235	99%	99%	99%
Prophylactic Antibiotic Timing (Outpatient)	697	98%	98%	98%
Urinary Catheter Removal[2]	1,247	95%	96%	97%
Survey of Patients' Hospital Experiences				
Area Around Room 'Always' Quiet at Night	300+	71%	67%	61%
Doctors 'Always' Communicated Well	300+	80%	84%	82%
Home Recovery Information Given	300+	81%	85%	85%
Hospital Given 9 or 10 on 10 Point Scale	300+	73%	70%	71%
Meds 'Always' Explained Before Given	300+	63%	66%	64%
Nurses 'Always' Communicated Well	300+	81%	80%	79%
Pain 'Always' Well Controlled	300+	72%	72%	71%
Room and Bathroom 'Always' Clean	300+	74%	73%	73%
Timely Help 'Always' Received	300+	68%	68%	68%
Would Definitely Recommend Hospital	300+	75%	70%	71%
Use of Medical Imaging				
Cardiac Imaging Stress Test before Surgery	750	4.5%	4.8%	5.3%
Combination Abdominal CT Scan	1,992	4.3%	9.6%	10.5%
Combination Brain/Sinus CT Scan	1,861	4.1%	3.3%	2.7%
Combination Chest CT Scan	1,264	0.6%	3.4%	2.7%
Follow-up Mammogram/Ultrasound	2,127	9.6%	8.3%	8.8%
Lumbar Spine MRI for Low Back Pain	514	32.7%	35.3%	37.2%

Regional Hospital of Jackson

367 Hospital Blvd
Jackson, TN 38305
URL: www.regionalhospitaljackson.com
Type: Acute Care Hospitals
Ownership: Proprietary
Phone: 731-661-2000
Fax: 731-661-2257
Emergency Services: Yes
Beds: 98

Key Personnel:
Operating Room. . . . . Teresa Ayers
Cardiac Laboratory. . . . . Jorge Delgado
Infection Control. . . . . Jill Kilby
Chief of Medical Staff. . . . . Laurence Martin, MD
CEO/President. . . . . Tim Puthoff
Radiology. . . . . Gary Weiss

Measure	Cases	This Hosp.	State Avg.	U.S. Avg.
Blood Clot Prevention and Treatment				
Anticoagulation Overlap Therapy[2]	72	99%	92%	93%
ICU Venous Thromboembolism Prophylaxis[2]	138	99%	90%	92%
Incidence of Potentially Preventable VTE[1,2]	-	-	10%	10%
UFH with Dosages/Platelet Monitoring[2]	64	100%	99%	97%
Venous Thromboembolism Prophylaxis[2]	394	98%	83%	85%
Warfarin Therapy Discharge Instructions[2]	52	98%	78%	75%
Chest Pain/Possible Heart Attack Care				
Aspirin Given Within 24 Hours of Arrival[1,3]	-	-	96%	96%
Fibrinolytic Meds Within 30 Min. of Arrival[3,7]	-	-	72%	58%
Average Time to ECG (minutes)[1,3]	-	-	6	7
Average Time to Transfer (minutes)[3,7]	-	-	53	60
Children's Asthma Care				
Received Home Management Plan of Care	-	-	-	88%
Received Reliever Medication	-	-	-	100%
Received Systemic Corticosteroids	-	-	-	100%
Emergency Department				
Admittance Decision Time (minutes)[2]	767	54	82	98
Head CT Results Within 45 Min. of Arrival[1]	-	-	52%	57%
Patients Who Left ER Before Being Seen	23,708	2%	2%	2%
Time from ER Arrival to Admit. (minutes)[2]	775	173	243	274
Time from ER Arrival to Discharge (minutes)	381	113	131	134
Time in ER Before Being Evaluated (minutes)	396	31	25	26
Time to Pain Meds for Fractures (minutes)	69	56	60	57
Heart Attack Care				
Aspirin Given at Discharge	420	100%	99%	99%
Fibrinolytic Meds Within 30 Min. of Arrival[7]	-	-	33%	54%
PCI Within 90 Minutes of Arrival[1]	-	-	98%	96%
Statin Prescribed at Discharge	378	99%	99%	98%
Heart Failure Care				
ACE Inhibitor or ARB for LVSD	105	99%	97%	97%
Discharge Instructions Given	236	95%	93%	94%
Evaluation of LVS Function	287	100%	99%	99%
Medicare Spending				
Medicare Spending per Patient (ratio)	-	1.01	1	0.98
Pneumonia Care				
Appropriate Initial Antibiotic Given	47	100%	95%	95%
Blood Culture Timing	108	100%	98%	98%
Pregnancy and Delivery Care				
Newborn Deliveries Scheduled Early[2]	28	4%	6%	6%
Preventive Care				
Immunization for Influenza[2]	623	100%	93%	90%
Immunization for Pneumonia[2]	906	100%	93%	92%
Stroke Care				
Anticoagulation Therapy for Atrial Fibrillation[1]	-	-	94%	95%
Antithrombotic Therapy Timing	54	100%	97%	98%
Assessed for Rehabilitation	56	98%	97%	97%
Discharged on Antithrombotic Therapy	53	100%	99%	99%
Discharged on Statin Medication	36	97%	94%	94%
Thrombolytic Therapy Timing[7]	-	-	57%	66%
Venous Thromboembolism Prophylaxis	56	95%	93%	94%
Written Stroke Educational Materials Given	29	72%	84%	88%
Surgical Care Improvement Project				
Appropriate Beta Blocker Usage	125	100%	97%	98%
Appropriate VTP Within 24 Hours	443	100%	98%	98%
Controlled Postoperative Blood Glucose[7]	-	-	95%	97%
Perioperative Temperature Management	476	100%	100%	100%
Prophylactic Antibiotic Selection	314	100%	99%	99%
Prophylactic Antibiotic Selection (Outpatient)	236	100%	98%	98%
Prophylactic Antibiotic Stopped	305	99%	98%	98%
Prophylactic Antibiotic Timing	314	100%	99%	99%
Prophylactic Antibiotic Timing (Outpatient)	236	100%	98%	98%
Urinary Catheter Removal	367	100%	96%	97%
Survey of Patients' Hospital Experiences				
Area Around Room 'Always' Quiet at Night	300+	71%	67%	61%
Doctors 'Always' Communicated Well	300+	82%	84%	82%
Home Recovery Information Given	300+	83%	85%	85%
Hospital Given 9 or 10 on 10 Point Scale	300+	72%	70%	71%
Meds 'Always' Explained Before Given	300+	67%	66%	64%
Nurses 'Always' Communicated Well	300+	78%	80%	79%
Pain 'Always' Well Controlled	300+	72%	72%	71%
Room and Bathroom 'Always' Clean	300+	68%	73%	73%
Timely Help 'Always' Received	300+	66%	68%	68%
Would Definitely Recommend Hospital	300+	73%	70%	71%
Use of Medical Imaging				
Cardiac Imaging Stress Test before Surgery	179	5.6%	4.8%	5.3%
Combination Abdominal CT Scan	314	4.5%	9.6%	10.5%
Combination Brain/Sinus CT Scan[1]	-	-	3.3%	2.7%
Combination Chest CT Scan	269	0.4%	3.4%	2.7%
Follow-up Mammogram/Ultrasound	233	4.3%	8.3%	8.8%
Lumbar Spine MRI for Low Back Pain[1]	-	-	35.3%	37.2%

Jamestown Regional Medical Center

436 Central Avenue West
Jamestown, TN 38556
URL: www.jamestownregional.org
Type: Acute Care Hospitals
Ownership: Proprietary
Phone: 931-879-3352
Fax: 931-879-4896
Emergency Services: Yes
Beds: 85

Key Personnel:
Radiology. . . . . Alfonso C Findley
Emergency Room . . . . Scott Goecke
Ambulatory Care . . . . Sheila Krapp
Pediatrics. . . . . Myra QUANRUD
Radiology. . . . . Madhu Reddy
CEO/President. . . . . Martin I Richman
Radiology. . . . . Gary Wade, RN
Surgery . . . . Patrick Walter, MD

Measure	Cases	This Hosp.	State Avg.	U.S. Avg.
Blood Clot Prevention and Treatment				
Anticoagulation Overlap Therapy[2]	11	91%	92%	93%
ICU Venous Thromboembolism Prophylaxis[2,7]	-	-	90%	92%
Incidence of Potentially Preventable VTE[1,2]	-	-	10%	10%
UFH with Dosages/Platelet Monitoring[1,2]	-	-	99%	97%
Venous Thromboembolism Prophylaxis[2]	185	54%	83%	85%
Warfarin Therapy Discharge Instructions[1,2]	-	-	78%	75%
Chest Pain/Possible Heart Attack Care				
Aspirin Given Within 24 Hours of Arrival	63	97%	96%	96%
Fibrinolytic Meds Within 30 Min. of Arrival[1]	-	-	72%	58%
Average Time to ECG (minutes)	87	7	6	7
Average Time to Transfer (minutes)[7]	-	-	53	60
Children's Asthma Care				
Received Home Management Plan of Care	-	-	-	88%
Received Reliever Medication	-	-	-	100%
Received Systemic Corticosteroids	-	-	-	100%
Emergency Department				
Admittance Decision Time (minutes)[2]	308	59	82	98
Head CT Results Within 45 Min. of Arrival	12	67%	52%	57%
Patients Who Left ER Before Being Seen	10,600	1%	2%	2%
Time from ER Arrival to Admit. (minutes)[2]	314	183	243	274
Time from ER Arrival to Discharge (minutes)	798	92	131	134
Time in ER Before Being Evaluated (minutes)	935	15	25	26
Time to Pain Meds for Fractures (minutes)	70	50	60	57
Heart Attack Care				
Aspirin Given at Discharge[1,3]	-	-	99%	99%
Fibrinolytic Meds Within 30 Min. of Arrival[3,7]	-	-	33%	54%
PCI Within 90 Minutes of Arrival[3,7]	-	-	98%	96%
Statin Prescribed at Discharge[1,3]	-	-	99%	98%
Heart Failure Care				
ACE Inhibitor or ARB for LVSD	14	79%	97%	97%
Discharge Instructions Given	95	95%	93%	94%
Evaluation of LVS Function	121	98%	99%	99%
Medicare Spending				
Medicare Spending per Patient (ratio)	-	0.98	1	0.98
Pneumonia Care				
Appropriate Initial Antibiotic Given	71	96%	95%	95%
Blood Culture Timing	66	100%	98%	98%
Pregnancy and Delivery Care				
Newborn Deliveries Scheduled Early[7]	-	-	6%	6%
Preventive Care				
Immunization for Influenza[2]	289	99%	93%	90%
Immunization for Pneumonia[2]	479	100%	93%	92%
Stroke Care				
Anticoagulation Therapy for Atrial Fibrillation[1]	-	-	94%	95%
Antithrombotic Therapy Timing[1]	-	-	97%	98%
Assessed for Rehabilitation[1]	-	-	97%	97%
Discharged on Antithrombotic Therapy[1]	-	-	99%	99%
Discharged on Statin Medication[1]	-	-	94%	94%
Thrombolytic Therapy Timing[7]	-	-	57%	66%
Venous Thromboembolism Prophylaxis[1]	-	-	93%	94%
Written Stroke Educational Materials Given[1]	-	-	84%	88%
Surgical Care Improvement Project				
Appropriate Beta Blocker Usage[3,7]	-	-	97%	98%
Appropriate VTP Within 24 Hours[1,3]	-	-	98%	98%
Controlled Postoperative Blood Glucose[3,7]	-	-	95%	97%
Perioperative Temperature Management[1,3]	-	-	100%	100%
Prophylactic Antibiotic Selection[3,7]	-	-	99%	99%
Prophylactic Antibiotic Selection (Outpatient)[1,3]	-	-	98%	98%
Prophylactic Antibiotic Stopped[3,7]	-	-	98%	98%
Prophylactic Antibiotic Timing[3,7]	-	-	99%	99%
Prophylactic Antibiotic Timing (Outpatient)[1,3]	-	-	98%	98%
Urinary Catheter Removal[1,3]	-	-	96%	97%
Survey of Patients' Hospital Experiences				
Area Around Room 'Always' Quiet at Night	300+	67%	67%	61%
Doctors 'Always' Communicated Well	300+	89%	84%	82%
Home Recovery Information Given	300+	81%	85%	85%
Hospital Given 9 or 10 on 10 Point Scale	300+	62%	70%	71%
Meds 'Always' Explained Before Given	300+	61%	66%	64%

NOTE: Hospital profiles are in alphabetical order by state, then city, then hospital within the city; Rankings exclude hospitals with less than 25 cases except for patient surveys which excludes hospitals with less than 100 cases; (a) 100-299 cases; (1) The number of cases/patients is too few to report; (2) Data submitted were based on a sample of cases/patients; (3) Results are based on a shorter time period than required; (4) Data suppressed by CMS for one or more quarters; (5) Results are not available for this reporting period; (6) Fewer than 100 patients completed the HCAHPS survey; (7) No cases met the criteria for this measure; (8) The lower limit of the confidence interval cannot be calculated if the number of observed infections equals zero; (9) No data are available from the state/territory for this reporting period; (10) The scores shown reflect fewer than 50 completed surveys; (11) There were discrepancies in the data collection process; (12) This measure does not apply to this hospital for this reporting period; (13) Results cannot be calculated for this reporting period; (14) The results for this state are combined with nearby states to protect confidentiality; Please refer to the User's Guide for a full explanation of data.

Measure	Cases	This Hosp.	State Avg.	U.S. Avg.
Nurses 'Always' Communicated Well	300+	81%	80%	79%
Pain 'Always' Well Controlled	300+	69%	72%	71%
Room and Bathroom 'Always' Clean	300+	65%	73%	73%
Timely Help 'Always' Received	300+	72%	68%	68%
Would Definitely Recommend Hospital	300+	59%	70%	71%
Use of Medical Imaging				
Cardiac Imaging Stress Test before Surgery[1]	-	-	4.8%	5.3%
Combination Abdominal CT Scan	213	6.6%	9.6%	10.5%
Combination Brain/Sinus CT Scan[1]	-	-	3.3%	2.7%
Combination Chest CT Scan	126	8.7%	3.4%	2.7%
Follow-up Mammogram/Ultrasound	320	13.4%	8.3%	8.8%
Lumbar Spine MRI for Low Back Pain[7]	-	-	35.3%	37.2%

Grandview Medical Center

1000 Highway 28
Jasper, TN 37347
Phone: 423-837-9500
Fax: 423-837-9406
URL: www.grandviewhospital.com
Type: Acute Care Hospitals
Emergency Services: Yes
Ownership: Voluntary non-profit - Private
Beds: 100
Key Personnel:
Chief of Medical Staff.......... Charles Adcock
CEO/President............... Dan Aranda
Infection Control.............. Sue Headrick
Operating Room............... Conrad Manayan
Emergency Room .... Helen McGowan
Quality Assurance .... Holly Stewart

Measure	Cases	This Hosp.	State Avg.	U.S. Avg.
Blood Clot Prevention and Treatment				
Anticoagulation Overlap Therapy[2]	12	83%	92%	93%
ICU Venous Thromboembolism Prophylaxis[2]	18	83%	90%	92%
Incidence of Potentially Preventable VTE[2,7]	-	-	10%	10%
UFH with Dosages/Platelet Monitoring[1,2]	-	-	99%	97%
Venous Thromboembolism Prophylaxis[2]	164	80%	83%	85%
Warfarin Therapy Discharge Instructions[2]	11	82%	78%	75%
Chest Pain/Possible Heart Attack Care				
Aspirin Given Within 24 Hours of Arrival	49	90%	96%	96%
Fibrinolytic Meds Within 30 Min. of Arrival[1]	-	-	72%	58%
Average Time to ECG (minutes)	50	12	6	7
Average Time to Transfer (minutes)[1]	-	-	53	60
Children's Asthma Care				
Received Home Management Plan of Care	-	-	-	88%
Received Reliever Medication	-	-	-	100%
Received Systemic Corticosteroids	-	-	-	100%
Emergency Department				
Admittance Decision Time (minutes)[2]	469	36	82	98
Head CT Results Within 45 Min. of Arrival[1]	-	-	52%	57%
Patients Who Left ER Before Being Seen	18,364	2%	2%	2%
Time from ER Arrival to Admit. (minutes)[2]	475	224	243	274
Time from ER Arrival to Discharge (minutes)	441	137	131	134
Time in ER Before Being Evaluated (minutes)	475	40	25	26
Time to Pain Meds for Fractures (minutes)	54	78	60	57
Heart Attack Care				
Aspirin Given at Discharge[1]	-	-	99%	99%
Fibrinolytic Meds Within 30 Min. of Arrival[7]	-	-	33%	54%
PCI Within 90 Minutes of Arrival[7]	-	-	98%	96%
Statin Prescribed at Discharge[1]	-	-	99%	98%
Heart Failure Care				
ACE Inhibitor or ARB for LVSD	14	100%	97%	97%
Discharge Instructions Given	36	72%	93%	94%
Evaluation of LVS Function	54	93%	99%	99%
Medicare Spending				
Medicare Spending per Patient (ratio)	-	0.98	1	0.98
Pneumonia Care				
Appropriate Initial Antibiotic Given	94	89%	95%	95%
Blood Culture Timing	89	98%	98%	98%
Pregnancy and Delivery Care				
Newborn Deliveries Scheduled Early[2,7]	-	-	6%	6%
Preventive Care				
Immunization for Influenza[2]	298	89%	93%	90%
Immunization for Pneumonia[2]	423	89%	93%	92%
Stroke Care				
Anticoagulation Therapy for Atrial Fibrillation[7]	-	-	94%	95%
Antithrombotic Therapy Timing[1]	-	-	97%	98%
Assessed for Rehabilitation[1]	-	-	97%	97%
Discharged on Antithrombotic Therapy[1]	-	-	99%	99%
Discharged on Statin Medication[1]	-	-	94%	94%
Thrombolytic Therapy Timing[1]	-	-	57%	66%
Venous Thromboembolism Prophylaxis[1]	-	-	93%	94%
Written Stroke Educational Materials Given[1]	-	-	84%	88%
Surgical Care Improvement Project				
Appropriate Beta Blocker Usage[1]	-	-	97%	98%
Appropriate VTP Within 24 Hours	33	88%	98%	98%
Controlled Postoperative Blood Glucose[7]	-	-	95%	97%
Perioperative Temperature Management	35	100%	100%	100%
Prophylactic Antibiotic Selection[1]	-	-	99%	99%
Prophylactic Antibiotic Selection (Outpatient)[1,3]	-	-	98%	98%
Prophylactic Antibiotic Stopped[1]	-	-	98%	98%
Prophylactic Antibiotic Timing[1]	-	-	99%	99%
Prophylactic Antibiotic Timing (Outpatient)[1,3]	-	-	98%	98%
Urinary Catheter Removal	12	92%	96%	97%
Survey of Patients' Hospital Experiences				
Area Around Room 'Always' Quiet at Night	(a)	69%	67%	61%
Doctors 'Always' Communicated Well	(a)	83%	84%	82%
Home Recovery Information Given	(a)	81%	85%	85%
Hospital Given 9 or 10 on 10 Point Scale	(a)	69%	70%	71%
Meds 'Always' Explained Before Given	(a)	63%	66%	64%
Nurses 'Always' Communicated Well	(a)	76%	80%	79%
Pain 'Always' Well Controlled	(a)	75%	72%	71%
Room and Bathroom 'Always' Clean	(a)	75%	73%	73%
Timely Help 'Always' Received	(a)	71%	68%	68%
Would Definitely Recommend Hospital	(a)	64%	70%	71%
Use of Medical Imaging				
Cardiac Imaging Stress Test before Surgery	48	2.1%	4.8%	5.3%
Combination Abdominal CT Scan	314	27.4%	9.6%	10.5%
Combination Brain/Sinus CT Scan[1]	-	-	3.3%	2.7%
Combination Chest CT Scan	106	35.8%	3.4%	2.7%
Follow-up Mammogram/Ultrasound	318	13.2%	8.3%	8.8%
Lumbar Spine MRI for Low Back Pain[1]	-	-	35.3%	37.2%

Tennova Healthcare - Jefferson Memorial Hospital

110 Hospital Drive
Jefferson City, TN 37760
Phone: 865-471-2500
Fax: 865-471-2450
URL: www.stmaryshealth.com
Type: Acute Care Hospitals
Emergency Services: No
Ownership: Proprietary
Beds: 58
Key Personnel:
Radiology.................... Christopher Aikens
Chief of Medical Staff.......... Leann Byrd, MD
CEO/President............... Debra K London

Measure	Cases	This Hosp.	State Avg.	U.S. Avg.
Blood Clot Prevention and Treatment				
Anticoagulation Overlap Therapy[2]	23	91%	92%	93%
ICU Venous Thromboembolism Prophylaxis[2]	38	89%	90%	92%
Incidence of Potentially Preventable VTE[1,2]	-	-	10%	10%
UFH with Dosages/Platelet Monitoring[1,2]	-	-	99%	97%
Venous Thromboembolism Prophylaxis[2]	177	97%	83%	85%
Warfarin Therapy Discharge Instructions[2]	22	45%	78%	75%
Chest Pain/Possible Heart Attack Care				
Aspirin Given Within 24 Hours of Arrival	97	97%	96%	96%
Fibrinolytic Meds Within 30 Min. of Arrival[7]	-	-	72%	58%
Average Time to ECG (minutes)	98	7	6	7
Average Time to Transfer (minutes)[1]	-	-	53	60
Children's Asthma Care				
Received Home Management Plan of Care	-	-	-	88%
Received Reliever Medication	-	-	-	100%
Received Systemic Corticosteroids	-	-	-	100%
Emergency Department				
Admittance Decision Time (minutes)[2]	529	62	82	98
Head CT Results Within 45 Min. of Arrival	12	92%	52%	57%
Patients Who Left ER Before Being Seen	25,327	1%	2%	2%
Time from ER Arrival to Admit. (minutes)[2]	543	221	243	274
Time from ER Arrival to Discharge (minutes)	1,563	119	131	134
Time in ER Before Being Evaluated (minutes)	1,682	23	25	26
Time to Pain Meds for Fractures (minutes)	103	49	60	57
Heart Attack Care				
Aspirin Given at Discharge[1]	-	-	99%	99%
Fibrinolytic Meds Within 30 Min. of Arrival[7]	-	-	33%	54%
PCI Within 90 Minutes of Arrival[7]	-	-	98%	96%
Statin Prescribed at Discharge[1]	-	-	99%	98%
Heart Failure Care				
ACE Inhibitor or ARB for LVSD	24	96%	97%	97%
Discharge Instructions Given	75	87%	93%	94%
Evaluation of LVS Function	92	100%	99%	99%
Medicare Spending				
Medicare Spending per Patient (ratio)	-	1.03	1	0.98
Pneumonia Care				
Appropriate Initial Antibiotic Given	104	98%	95%	95%
Blood Culture Timing	161	99%	98%	98%
Pregnancy and Delivery Care				
Newborn Deliveries Scheduled Early[7]	-	-	6%	6%
Preventive Care				
Immunization for Influenza[2]	328	98%	93%	90%
Immunization for Pneumonia[2]	507	99%	93%	92%
Stroke Care				
Anticoagulation Therapy for Atrial Fibrillation[1]	-	-	94%	95%
Antithrombotic Therapy Timing	29	100%	97%	98%
Assessed for Rehabilitation	29	100%	97%	97%
Discharged on Antithrombotic Therapy	29	100%	99%	99%
Discharged on Statin Medication	23	91%	94%	94%
Thrombolytic Therapy Timing[1]	-	-	57%	66%
Venous Thromboembolism Prophylaxis	32	97%	93%	94%
Written Stroke Educational Materials Given	17	53%	84%	88%
Surgical Care Improvement Project				
Appropriate Beta Blocker Usage	15	87%	97%	98%
Appropriate VTP Within 24 Hours	51	98%	98%	98%
Controlled Postoperative Blood Glucose[7]	-	-	95%	97%
Perioperative Temperature Management	53	100%	100%	100%
Prophylactic Antibiotic Selection	37	100%	99%	99%
Prophylactic Antibiotic Selection (Outpatient)	55	93%	98%	98%
Prophylactic Antibiotic Stopped	36	97%	98%	98%
Prophylactic Antibiotic Timing	37	97%	99%	99%
Prophylactic Antibiotic Timing (Outpatient)	55	100%	98%	98%
Urinary Catheter Removal	36	94%	96%	97%
Survey of Patients' Hospital Experiences				
Area Around Room 'Always' Quiet at Night	300+	62%	67%	61%
Doctors 'Always' Communicated Well	300+	81%	84%	82%
Home Recovery Information Given	300+	82%	85%	85%
Hospital Given 9 or 10 on 10 Point Scale	300+	67%	70%	71%
Meds 'Always' Explained Before Given	300+	60%	66%	64%
Nurses 'Always' Communicated Well	300+	79%	80%	79%
Pain 'Always' Well Controlled	300+	68%	72%	71%
Room and Bathroom 'Always' Clean	300+	68%	73%	73%
Timely Help 'Always' Received	300+	62%	68%	68%
Would Definitely Recommend Hospital	300+	66%	70%	71%
Use of Medical Imaging				
Cardiac Imaging Stress Test before Surgery	220	5.5%	4.8%	5.3%
Combination Abdominal CT Scan	561	3.7%	9.6%	10.5%
Combination Brain/Sinus CT Scan	479	0.8%	3.3%	2.7%
Combination Chest CT Scan	309	4.2%	3.4%	2.7%
Follow-up Mammogram/Ultrasound	774	11.6%	8.3%	8.8%
Lumbar Spine MRI for Low Back Pain	80	33.8%	35.3%	37.2%

Jellico Community Hospital

188 Hospital Lane
Jellico, TN 37762
Phone: 423-784-7252
Fax: 423-784-1136
URL: www.jellicohospital.com
Type: Acute Care Hospitals
Emergency Services: Yes
Ownership: Voluntary non-profit - Church
Beds: 54
Key Personnel:
Radiology.................... Robert Anderson
Chief of Medical Staff.......... David Bosscher, MD
Quality Assurance .... Pam Hodge
Patient Relations .... Sharon Lewis
Infection Control.............. Judy McKiddy, RN
Operating Room............... Wilma Morgan
Intensive Care Unit............ Joyee Reese, RN
CEO/President............... Erik Wangsness

Measure	Cases	This Hosp.	State Avg.	U.S. Avg.
Blood Clot Prevention and Treatment				
Anticoagulation Overlap Therapy[1,2]	-	-	92%	93%
ICU Venous Thromboembolism Prophylaxis[2]	17	94%	90%	92%

NOTE: Hospital profiles are in alphabetical order by state, then city, then hospital within the city; Rankings exclude hospitals with less than 25 cases except for patient surveys which excludes hospitals with less than 100 cases; (a) 100-299 cases; (1) The number of cases/patients is too few to report; (2) Data submitted were based on a sample of cases/patients; (3) Results are based on a shorter time period than required; (4) Data suppressed by CMS for one or more quarters; (5) Results are not available for this reporting period; (6) Fewer than 100 patients completed the HCAHPS survey; (7) No cases met the criteria for this measure; (8) The lower limit of the confidence interval cannot be calculated if the number of observed infections equals zero; (9) No data are available from the state/territory for this reporting period; (10) The scores shown reflect fewer than 50 completed surveys; (11) There were discrepancies in the data collection process; (12) This measure does not apply to this hospital for this reporting period; (13) Results cannot be calculated for this reporting period; (14) The results for this state are combined with nearby states to protect confidentiality; Please refer to the User's Guide for a full explanation of data.

Incidence of Potentially Preventable VTE[2,7]	-	-	10%	10%
UFH with Dosages/Platelet Monitoring[1,2]	-	-	99%	97%
Venous Thromboembolism Prophylaxis[2]	100	81%	83%	85%
Warfarin Therapy Discharge Instructions[1,2]	-	-	78%	75%
Chest Pain/Possible Heart Attack Care				
Aspirin Given Within 24 Hours of Arrival	27	96%	96%	96%
Fibrinolytic Meds Within 30 Min. of Arrival[7]	-	-	72%	58%
Average Time to ECG (minutes)	27	12	6	7
Average Time to Transfer (minutes)[1]	-	-	53	60
Children's Asthma Care				
Received Home Management Plan of Care	-	-	-	88%
Received Reliever Medication	-	-	-	100%
Received Systemic Corticosteroids	-	-	-	100%
Emergency Department				
Admittance Decision Time (minutes)[2]	310	40	82	98
Head CT Results Within 45 Min. of Arrival[1,3]	-	-	52%	57%
Patients Who Left ER Before Being Seen	6,005	2%	2%	2%
Time from ER Arrival to Admit. (minutes)[2]	324	197	243	274
Time from ER Arrival to Discharge (minutes)	328	142	131	134
Time in ER Before Being Evaluated (minutes)	362	44	25	26
Time to Pain Meds for Fractures (minutes)	44	78	60	57
Heart Attack Care				
Aspirin Given at Discharge[1,2]	-	-	99%	99%
Fibrinolytic Meds Within 30 Min. of Arrival[2,3]	-	-	33%	54%
PCI Within 90 Minutes of Arrival[2,3]	-	-	98%	96%
Statin Prescribed at Discharge[1,2]	-	-	99%	98%
Heart Failure Care				
ACE Inhibitor or ARB for LVSD[2]	19	79%	97%	97%
Discharge Instructions Given[2]	51	96%	93%	94%
Evaluation of LVS Function[2]	67	99%	99%	99%
Medicare Spending				
Medicare Spending per Patient (ratio)	-	0.89	1	0.98
Pneumonia Care				
Appropriate Initial Antibiotic Given[2]	66	83%	95%	95%
Blood Culture Timing[2]	138	100%	98%	98%
Pregnancy and Delivery Care				
Newborn Deliveries Scheduled Early[2]	22	9%	6%	6%
Preventive Care				
Immunization for Influenza[2]	257	93%	93%	90%
Immunization for Pneumonia[2]	340	97%	93%	92%
Stroke Care				
Anticoagulation Therapy for Atrial Fibrillation[2,7]	-	-	94%	95%
Antithrombotic Therapy Timing[1,2]	-	-	97%	98%
Assessed for Rehabilitation[1,2]	-	-	97%	97%
Discharged on Antithrombotic Therapy[1,2]	-	-	99%	99%
Discharged on Statin Medication[1,2]	-	-	94%	94%
Thrombolytic Therapy Timing[2,7]	-	-	57%	66%
Venous Thromboembolism Prophylaxis[1,2]	-	-	93%	94%
Written Stroke Educational Materials Given[1,2]	-	-	84%	88%
Surgical Care Improvement Project				
Appropriate Beta Blocker Usage[1,2]	-	-	97%	98%
Appropriate VTP Within 24 Hours[2]	16	88%	98%	98%
Controlled Postoperative Blood Glucose[2,7]	-	-	95%	97%
Perioperative Temperature Management[2]	24	100%	100%	100%
Prophylactic Antibiotic Selection[2]	17	100%	99%	99%
Prophylactic Antibiotic Selection (Outpatient)	17	94%	98%	98%
Prophylactic Antibiotic Stopped[2]	16	100%	98%	98%
Prophylactic Antibiotic Timing[2]	17	100%	99%	99%
Prophylactic Antibiotic Timing (Outpatient)	18	83%	98%	98%
Urinary Catheter Removal[1,2]	-	-	96%	97%
Survey of Patients' Hospital Experiences				
Area Around Room 'Always' Quiet at Night[11]	(a)	66%	67%	61%
Doctors 'Always' Communicated Well[11]	(a)	89%	84%	82%
Home Recovery Information Given[11]	(a)	90%	85%	85%
Hospital Given 9 or 10 on 10 Point Scale[11]	(a)	78%	70%	71%
Meds 'Always' Explained Before Given[11]	(a)	70%	66%	64%
Nurses 'Always' Communicated Well[11]	(a)	87%	80%	79%
Pain 'Always' Well Controlled[11]	(a)	73%	72%	71%
Room and Bathroom 'Always' Clean[11]	(a)	84%	73%	73%
Timely Help 'Always' Received[11]	(a)	74%	68%	68%
Would Definitely Recommend Hospital[11]	(a)	77%	70%	71%
Use of Medical Imaging				
Cardiac Imaging Stress Test before Surgery[1]	-	-	4.8%	5.3%
Combination Abdominal CT Scan	164	29.3%	9.6%	10.5%
Combination Brain/Sinus CT Scan[1]	-	-	3.3%	2.7%
Combination Chest CT Scan	119	36.1%	3.4%	2.7%
Follow-up Mammogram/Ultrasound	267	21.3%	8.3%	8.8%
Lumbar Spine MRI for Low Back Pain[1]	-	-	35.3%	37.2%

Franklin Woods Community Hospital

300 Medical Tech Parkway
Johnson City, TN 37604
URL: www.msha.com
Phone: 423-302-1120
Fax: 423-854-5748
Type: Acute Care Hospitals
Ownership: Voluntary non-profit - Private
Emergency Services: Yes
Beds: 80

Key Personnel:
Emergency Room . . . . Atif Atyia
Chief of Medical Staff. . . . . T Hopson
CEO/President. . . . . Lindy White

Measure	Cases	This Hosp.	State Avg.	U.S. Avg.
Blood Clot Prevention and Treatment				
Anticoagulation Overlap Therapy[2]	41	95%	92%	93%
ICU Venous Thromboembolism Prophylaxis[2]	39	92%	90%	92%
Incidence of Potentially Preventable VTE[1,2]	-	-	10%	10%
UFH with Dosages/Platelet Monitoring[1,2]	-	-	99%	97%
Venous Thromboembolism Prophylaxis[2]	312	83%	83%	85%
Warfarin Therapy Discharge Instructions[2]	34	50%	78%	75%
Chest Pain/Possible Heart Attack Care				
Aspirin Given Within 24 Hours of Arrival	101	99%	96%	96%
Fibrinolytic Meds Within 30 Min. of Arrival[7]	-	-	72%	58%
Average Time to ECG (minutes)	109	3	6	7
Average Time to Transfer (minutes)[1]	-	-	53	60
Children's Asthma Care				
Received Home Management Plan of Care	-	-	-	88%
Received Reliever Medication	-	-	-	100%
Received Systemic Corticosteroids	-	-	-	100%
Emergency Department				
Admittance Decision Time (minutes)[2]	272	61	82	98
Head CT Results Within 45 Min. of Arrival[1]	-	-	52%	57%
Patients Who Left ER Before Being Seen	26,515	1%	2%	2%
Time from ER Arrival to Admit. (minutes)[2]	371	237	243	274
Time from ER Arrival to Discharge (minutes)	348	122	131	134
Time in ER Before Being Evaluated (minutes)	278	34	25	26
Time to Pain Meds for Fractures (minutes)	73	57	60	57
Heart Attack Care				
Aspirin Given at Discharge[1,3]	-	-	99%	99%
Fibrinolytic Meds Within 30 Min. of Arrival[3,7]	-	-	33%	54%
PCI Within 90 Minutes of Arrival[3,7]	-	-	98%	96%
Statin Prescribed at Discharge[1,3]	-	-	99%	98%
Heart Failure Care				
ACE Inhibitor or ARB for LVSD[2]	12	100%	97%	97%
Discharge Instructions Given[2]	33	70%	93%	94%
Evaluation of LVS Function[2]	47	100%	99%	99%
Medicare Spending				
Medicare Spending per Patient (ratio)	-	0.98	1	0.98
Pneumonia Care				
Appropriate Initial Antibiotic Given[2]	117	92%	95%	95%
Blood Culture Timing[2]	148	96%	98%	98%
Pregnancy and Delivery Care				
Newborn Deliveries Scheduled Early[2]	24	8%	6%	6%
Preventive Care				
Immunization for Influenza[2]	453	96%	93%	90%
Immunization for Pneumonia[2]	487	95%	93%	92%
Stroke Care				
Anticoagulation Therapy for Atrial Fibrillation[5]	-	-	94%	95%
Antithrombotic Therapy Timing[5]	-	-	97%	98%
Assessed for Rehabilitation[5]	-	-	97%	97%
Discharged on Antithrombotic Therapy[5]	-	-	99%	99%
Discharged on Statin Medication[5]	-	-	94%	94%
Thrombolytic Therapy Timing[5]	-	-	57%	66%
Venous Thromboembolism Prophylaxis[5]	-	-	93%	94%
Written Stroke Educational Materials Given[5]	-	-	84%	88%
Surgical Care Improvement Project				
Appropriate Beta Blocker Usage[2]	23	87%	97%	98%
Appropriate VTP Within 24 Hours[2]	106	100%	98%	98%
Controlled Postoperative Blood Glucose[2,7]	-	-	95%	97%
Perioperative Temperature Management[2]	119	100%	100%	100%
Prophylactic Antibiotic Selection[2]	30	100%	99%	99%
Prophylactic Antibiotic Selection (Outpatient)	323	98%	98%	98%
Prophylactic Antibiotic Stopped[2]	29	100%	98%	98%
Prophylactic Antibiotic Timing[2]	30	100%	99%	99%
Prophylactic Antibiotic Timing (Outpatient)	325	99%	98%	98%
Urinary Catheter Removal[2]	57	96%	96%	97%
Survey of Patients' Hospital Experiences				
Area Around Room 'Always' Quiet at Night	300+	76%	67%	61%
Doctors 'Always' Communicated Well	300+	81%	84%	82%
Home Recovery Information Given	300+	87%	85%	85%
Hospital Given 9 or 10 on 10 Point Scale	300+	80%	70%	71%
Meds 'Always' Explained Before Given	300+	65%	66%	64%
Nurses 'Always' Communicated Well	300+	81%	80%	79%
Pain 'Always' Well Controlled	300+	74%	72%	71%
Room and Bathroom 'Always' Clean	300+	78%	73%	73%
Timely Help 'Always' Received	300+	70%	68%	68%
Would Definitely Recommend Hospital	300+	82%	70%	71%
Use of Medical Imaging				
Cardiac Imaging Stress Test before Surgery	53	1.9%	4.8%	5.3%
Combination Abdominal CT Scan	604	9.4%	9.6%	10.5%
Combination Brain/Sinus CT Scan	372	4.8%	3.3%	2.7%
Combination Chest CT Scan	294	1.0%	3.4%	2.7%
Follow-up Mammogram/Ultrasound[7]	-	-	8.3%	8.8%
Lumbar Spine MRI for Low Back Pain	122	33.6%	35.3%	37.2%

Johnson City Medical Center

400 N State of Franklin Rd
Johnson City, TN 37604
URL: www.msha.com
Phone: 423-431-6111
Fax: 423-431-2910
Type: Acute Care Hospitals
Ownership: Voluntary non-profit - Private
Emergency Services: Yes
Beds: 488

Key Personnel:
Intensive Care Unit. . . . . Gayle Broyles
Emergency Room . . . . Candace Jennings
CEO/President. . . . . Alan Levine
Chief of Medical Staff. . . . . Kenneth Marshall, MD
Cardiac Laboratory. . . . . Sindy Salyer
Radiology. . . . . George Spence, MD
Patient Relations . . . . Tom Tull
Operating Room. . . . . Chris York

Measure	Cases	This Hosp.	State Avg.	U.S. Avg.
Blood Clot Prevention and Treatment				
Anticoagulation Overlap Therapy[2]	188	96%	92%	93%
ICU Venous Thromboembolism Prophylaxis[2]	97	92%	90%	92%
Incidence of Potentially Preventable VTE[2]	74	1%	10%	10%
UFH with Dosages/Platelet Monitoring[2]	82	99%	99%	97%
Venous Thromboembolism Prophylaxis[2]	351	80%	83%	85%
Warfarin Therapy Discharge Instructions[2]	126	26%	78%	75%
Chest Pain/Possible Heart Attack Care				
Aspirin Given Within 24 Hours of Arrival[1,3]	-	-	96%	96%
Fibrinolytic Meds Within 30 Min. of Arrival[5]	-	-	72%	58%
Average Time to ECG (minutes)[1,3]	-	-	6	7
Average Time to Transfer (minutes)[5]	-	-	53	60
Children's Asthma Care				
Received Home Management Plan of Care[2]	69	94%	-	88%
Received Reliever Medication[2]	69	100%	-	100%
Received Systemic Corticosteroids[2]	68	100%	-	100%
Emergency Department				
Admittance Decision Time (minutes)[2]	338	106	82	98
Head CT Results Within 45 Min. of Arrival[1]	-	-	52%	57%
Patients Who Left ER Before Being Seen	53,187	3%	2%	2%
Time from ER Arrival to Admit. (minutes)[2]	418	242	243	274
Time from ER Arrival to Discharge (minutes)	321	138	131	134
Time in ER Before Being Evaluated (minutes)	373	25	25	26
Time to Pain Meds for Fractures (minutes)	189	52	60	57
Heart Attack Care				
Aspirin Given at Discharge[2]	288	99%	99%	99%
Fibrinolytic Meds Within 30 Min. of Arrival[2,7]	-	-	33%	54%
PCI Within 90 Minutes of Arrival[2]	27	100%	98%	96%
Statin Prescribed at Discharge[2]	279	100%	99%	98%
Heart Failure Care				
ACE Inhibitor or ARB for LVSD[2]	105	97%	97%	97%

NOTE: Hospital profiles are in alphabetical order by state, then city, then hospital within the city; Rankings exclude hospitals with less than 25 cases except for patient surveys which excludes hospitals with less than 100 cases; (a) 100-299 cases; (1) The number of cases/patients is too few to report; (2) Data submitted were based on a sample of cases/patients; (3) Results are based on a shorter time period than required; (4) Data suppressed by CMS for one or more quarters; (5) Results are not available for this reporting period; (6) Fewer than 100 patients completed the HCAHPS survey; (7) No cases met the criteria for this measure; (8) The lower limit of the confidence interval cannot be calculated if the number of observed infections equals zero; (9) No data are available from the state/territory for this reporting period; (10) The scores shown reflect fewer than 50 completed surveys; (11) There were discrepancies in the data collection process; (12) This measure does not apply to this hospital for this reporting period; (13) Results cannot be calculated for this reporting period; (14) The results for this state are combined with nearby states to protect confidentiality; Please refer to the User's Guide for a full explanation of data.

Measure	Cases	This Hosp.	State Avg.	U.S. Avg.
Discharge Instructions Given[2]	240	77%	93%	94%
Evaluation of LVS Function[2]	295	100%	99%	99%
Medicare Spending				
Medicare Spending per Patient (ratio)	-	1.02	1	0.98
Pneumonia Care				
Appropriate Initial Antibiotic Given[2]	68	97%	95%	95%
Blood Culture Timing[2]	131	98%	98%	98%
Pregnancy and Delivery Care				
Newborn Deliveries Scheduled Early[2]	17	0%	6%	6%
Preventive Care				
Immunization for Influenza[2]	577	94%	93%	90%
Immunization for Pneumonia[2]	743	90%	93%	92%
Stroke Care				
Anticoagulation Therapy for Atrial Fibrillation	52	90%	94%	95%
Antithrombotic Therapy Timing	228	98%	97%	98%
Assessed for Rehabilitation	296	96%	97%	97%
Discharged on Antithrombotic Therapy	234	96%	99%	99%
Discharged on Statin Medication	183	93%	94%	94%
Thrombolytic Therapy Timing	15	73%	57%	66%
Venous Thromboembolism Prophylaxis	311	91%	93%	94%
Written Stroke Educational Materials Given	158	82%	84%	88%
Surgical Care Improvement Project				
Appropriate Beta Blocker Usage[2]	226	97%	97%	98%
Appropriate VTP Within 24 Hours[2]	337	98%	98%	98%
Controlled Postoperative Blood Glucose[2]	116	99%	95%	97%
Perioperative Temperature Management[2]	461	100%	100%	100%
Prophylactic Antibiotic Selection[2]	405	99%	99%	99%
Prophylactic Antibiotic Selection (Outpatient)	618	98%	98%	98%
Prophylactic Antibiotic Stopped[2]	388	96%	98%	98%
Prophylactic Antibiotic Timing[2]	405	98%	99%	99%
Prophylactic Antibiotic Timing (Outpatient)	621	97%	98%	98%
Urinary Catheter Removal[2]	401	96%	96%	97%
Survey of Patients' Hospital Experiences				
Area Around Room 'Always' Quiet at Night	300+	53%	67%	61%
Doctors 'Always' Communicated Well	300+	77%	84%	82%
Home Recovery Information Given	300+	85%	85%	85%
Hospital Given 9 or 10 on 10 Point Scale	300+	65%	70%	71%
Meds 'Always' Explained Before Given	300+	60%	66%	64%
Nurses 'Always' Communicated Well	300+	77%	80%	79%
Pain 'Always' Well Controlled	300+	67%	72%	71%
Room and Bathroom 'Always' Clean	300+	65%	73%	73%
Timely Help 'Always' Received	300+	64%	68%	68%
Would Definitely Recommend Hospital	300+	66%	70%	71%
Use of Medical Imaging				
Cardiac Imaging Stress Test before Surgery	1,087	4.4%	4.8%	5.3%
Combination Abdominal CT Scan	930	12.0%	9.6%	10.5%
Combination Brain/Sinus CT Scan	888	3.0%	3.3%	2.7%
Combination Chest CT Scan	662	2.0%	3.4%	2.7%
Follow-up Mammogram/Ultrasound	3,073	7.4%	8.3%	8.8%
Lumbar Spine MRI for Low Back Pain	248	35.9%	35.3%	37.2%

Indian Path Medical Center

2000 Brookside Dr
Kingsport, TN 37660
Phone: 423-431-1941
URL: www.msha.com
Type: Acute Care Hospitals
Emergency Services: Yes
Ownership: Voluntary non-profit - Private
Beds: 261

Key Personnel:
Hemotology Center . . . . Kyle Colvett, MD
Emergency Room . . . . EC Goulding, MD
CEO/President. . . . . Monty McLaurin

Measure	Cases	This Hosp.	State Avg.	U.S. Avg.
Blood Clot Prevention and Treatment				
Anticoagulation Overlap Therapy[2]	51	88%	92%	93%
ICU Venous Thromboembolism Prophylaxis[2]	80	86%	90%	92%
Incidence of Potentially Preventable VTE[1,2]	-	-	10%	10%
UFH with Dosages/Platelet Monitoring[2]	25	96%	99%	97%
Venous Thromboembolism Prophylaxis[2]	337	88%	83%	85%
Warfarin Therapy Discharge Instructions[2]	34	9%	78%	75%
Chest Pain/Possible Heart Attack Care				
Aspirin Given Within 24 Hours of Arrival	15	93%	96%	96%
Fibrinolytic Meds Within 30 Min. of Arrival[7]	-	-	72%	58%
Average Time to ECG (minutes)	16	4	6	7
Average Time to Transfer (minutes)[7]	-	-	53	60
Children's Asthma Care				
Received Home Management Plan of Care	-	-	-	88%
Received Reliever Medication	-	-	-	100%
Received Systemic Corticosteroids	-	-	-	100%
Emergency Department				
Admittance Decision Time (minutes)[2]	374	137	82	98
Head CT Results Within 45 Min. of Arrival[1]	-	-	52%	57%
Patients Who Left ER Before Being Seen	36,020	1%	2%	2%
Time from ER Arrival to Admit. (minutes)[2]	452	272	243	274
Time from ER Arrival to Discharge (minutes)	356	114	131	134
Time in ER Before Being Evaluated (minutes)	366	22	25	26
Time to Pain Meds for Fractures (minutes)	60	63	60	57
Heart Attack Care				
Aspirin Given at Discharge[2]	149	99%	99%	99%
Fibrinolytic Meds Within 30 Min. of Arrival[2,7]	-	-	33%	54%
PCI Within 90 Minutes of Arrival[2]	15	87%	98%	96%
Statin Prescribed at Discharge[2]	147	98%	99%	98%
Heart Failure Care				
ACE Inhibitor or ARB for LVSD[2]	45	89%	97%	97%
Discharge Instructions Given[2]	111	87%	93%	94%
Evaluation of LVS Function[2]	143	100%	99%	99%
Medicare Spending				
Medicare Spending per Patient (ratio)	-	1.00	1	0.98
Pneumonia Care				
Appropriate Initial Antibiotic Given[2]	83	99%	95%	95%
Blood Culture Timing[2]	130	96%	98%	98%
Pregnancy and Delivery Care				
Newborn Deliveries Scheduled Early[2]	24	8%	6%	6%
Preventive Care				
Immunization for Influenza[2]	540	98%	93%	90%
Immunization for Pneumonia[2]	717	97%	93%	92%
Stroke Care				
Anticoagulation Therapy for Atrial Fibrillation[1]	-	-	94%	95%
Antithrombotic Therapy Timing	45	93%	97%	98%
Assessed for Rehabilitation	48	94%	97%	97%
Discharged on Antithrombotic Therapy	44	98%	99%	99%
Discharged on Statin Medication	35	89%	94%	94%
Thrombolytic Therapy Timing[1]	-	-	57%	66%
Venous Thromboembolism Prophylaxis	48	85%	93%	94%
Written Stroke Educational Materials Given	30	43%	84%	88%
Surgical Care Improvement Project				
Appropriate Beta Blocker Usage[2]	96	98%	97%	98%
Appropriate VTP Within 24 Hours[2]	306	98%	98%	98%
Controlled Postoperative Blood Glucose[2,7]	-	-	95%	97%
Perioperative Temperature Management[2]	340	100%	100%	100%
Prophylactic Antibiotic Selection[2]	231	100%	99%	99%
Prophylactic Antibiotic Selection (Outpatient)	254	98%	98%	98%
Prophylactic Antibiotic Stopped[2]	222	99%	98%	98%
Prophylactic Antibiotic Timing[2]	231	100%	99%	99%
Prophylactic Antibiotic Timing (Outpatient)	229	97%	98%	98%
Urinary Catheter Removal[2]	101	97%	96%	97%
Survey of Patients' Hospital Experiences				
Area Around Room 'Always' Quiet at Night	300+	62%	67%	61%
Doctors 'Always' Communicated Well	300+	82%	84%	82%
Home Recovery Information Given	300+	86%	85%	85%
Hospital Given 9 or 10 on 10 Point Scale	300+	73%	70%	71%
Meds 'Always' Explained Before Given	300+	63%	66%	64%
Nurses 'Always' Communicated Well	300+	81%	80%	79%
Pain 'Always' Well Controlled	300+	69%	72%	71%
Room and Bathroom 'Always' Clean	300+	69%	73%	73%
Timely Help 'Always' Received	300+	65%	68%	68%
Would Definitely Recommend Hospital	300+	76%	70%	71%
Use of Medical Imaging				
Cardiac Imaging Stress Test before Surgery	147	5.4%	4.8%	5.3%
Combination Abdominal CT Scan	487	18.9%	9.6%	10.5%
Combination Brain/Sinus CT Scan	390	7.2%	3.3%	2.7%
Combination Chest CT Scan	164	1.8%	3.4%	2.7%
Follow-up Mammogram/Ultrasound	594	3.4%	8.3%	8.8%
Lumbar Spine MRI for Low Back Pain	94	36.2%	35.3%	37.2%

Wellmont Holston Valley Medical Center

130 West Ravine Road
Phone: 423-224-4000
Kingsport, TN 37662
Fax: 423-224-6419
URL: www.wellmont.org
Type: Acute Care Hospitals
Emergency Services: Yes
Ownership: Voluntary non-profit - Private
Beds: 540

Key Personnel:
CEO/President. . . . . Tim Attebery
Chief of Medical Staff. . . . . Dr. Daniel Carlson, MD
Infection Control. . . . . Eleanor Duncan
Pediatric Ambulatory Care . . . . . . Art Garrett, MD
Pediatric In-Patient Care . . . . Art Garrett, MD
Operating Room. . . . . Ilene Hess, RN
Quality Assurance . . . . Justine Hill
Radiology. . . . . Larry Westerfield, MD

Measure	Cases	This Hosp.	State Avg.	U.S. Avg.
Blood Clot Prevention and Treatment				
Anticoagulation Overlap Therapy[2]	137	90%	92%	93%
ICU Venous Thromboembolism Prophylaxis[2]	91	81%	90%	92%
Incidence of Potentially Preventable VTE[2]	46	15%	10%	10%
UFH with Dosages/Platelet Monitoring[2]	96	100%	99%	97%
Venous Thromboembolism Prophylaxis[2]	301	82%	83%	85%
Warfarin Therapy Discharge Instructions[2]	100	61%	78%	75%
Chest Pain/Possible Heart Attack Care				
Aspirin Given Within 24 Hours of Arrival[3,7]	-	-	96%	96%
Fibrinolytic Meds Within 30 Min. of Arrival[5]	-	-	72%	58%
Average Time to ECG (minutes)[3,7]	-	-	6	7
Average Time to Transfer (minutes)[5]	-	-	53	60
Children's Asthma Care				
Received Home Management Plan of Care	-	-	-	88%
Received Reliever Medication	-	-	-	100%
Received Systemic Corticosteroids	-	-	-	100%
Emergency Department				
Admittance Decision Time (minutes)[2]	605	206	82	98
Head CT Results Within 45 Min. of Arrival[1]	-	-	52%	57%
Patients Who Left ER Before Being Seen	62,964	1%	2%	2%
Time from ER Arrival to Admit. (minutes)[2]	627	371	243	274
Time from ER Arrival to Discharge (minutes)	354	166	131	134
Time in ER Before Being Evaluated (minutes)	376	56	25	26
Time to Pain Meds for Fractures (minutes)	238	92	60	57
Heart Attack Care				
Aspirin Given at Discharge[2]	261	98%	99%	99%
Fibrinolytic Meds Within 30 Min. of Arrival[2,7]	-	-	33%	54%
PCI Within 90 Minutes of Arrival[2]	30	100%	98%	96%
Statin Prescribed at Discharge[2]	260	100%	99%	98%
Heart Failure Care				
ACE Inhibitor or ARB for LVSD[2]	71	99%	97%	97%
Discharge Instructions Given[2]	223	100%	93%	94%
Evaluation of LVS Function[2]	277	99%	99%	99%
Medicare Spending				
Medicare Spending per Patient (ratio)	-	1.00	1	0.98
Pneumonia Care				
Appropriate Initial Antibiotic Given[2]	62	90%	95%	95%
Blood Culture Timing[2]	109	99%	98%	98%
Pregnancy and Delivery Care				
Newborn Deliveries Scheduled Early[2]	17	0%	6%	6%
Preventive Care				
Immunization for Influenza[2]	543	96%	93%	90%
Immunization for Pneumonia[2]	780	99%	93%	92%
Stroke Care				
Anticoagulation Therapy for Atrial Fibrillation[1,2]	-	-	94%	95%
Antithrombotic Therapy Timing[2]	58	93%	97%	98%
Assessed for Rehabilitation[2]	80	98%	97%	97%
Discharged on Antithrombotic Therapy[2]	65	92%	99%	99%
Discharged on Statin Medication[2]	48	94%	94%	94%
Thrombolytic Therapy Timing[1,2]	-	-	57%	66%
Venous Thromboembolism Prophylaxis[2]	81	84%	93%	94%
Written Stroke Educational Materials Given[2]	46	30%	84%	88%
Surgical Care Improvement Project				
Appropriate Beta Blocker Usage[2]	209	98%	97%	98%
Appropriate VTP Within 24 Hours[2]	332	97%	98%	98%
Controlled Postoperative Blood Glucose[2]	125	94%	95%	97%
Perioperative Temperature Management[2]	407	100%	100%	100%
Prophylactic Antibiotic Selection[2]	411	99%	99%	99%

NOTE: Hospital profiles are in alphabetical order by state, then city, then hospital within the city; Rankings exclude hospitals with less than 25 cases except for patient surveys which excludes hospitals with less than 100 cases; (a) 100-299 cases; (1) The number of cases/patients is too few to report; (2) Data submitted were based on a sample of cases/patients; (3) Results are based on a shorter time period than required; (4) Data suppressed by CMS for one or more quarters; (5) Results are not available for this reporting period; (6) Fewer than 100 patients completed the HCAHPS survey; (7) No cases met the criteria for this measure; (8) The lower limit of the confidence interval cannot be calculated if the number of observed infections equals zero; (9) No data are available from the state/territory for this reporting period; (10) The scores shown reflect fewer than 50 completed surveys; (11) There were discrepancies in the data collection process; (12) This measure does not apply to this hospital for this reporting period; (13) Results cannot be calculated for this reporting period; (14) The results for this state are combined with nearby states to protect confidentiality; Please refer to the User's Guide for a full explanation of data.

Prophylactic Antibiotic Selection (Outpatient)	661	98%	98%	98%
Prophylactic Antibiotic Stopped[2]	407	100%	98%	98%
Prophylactic Antibiotic Timing[2]	411	99%	99%	99%
Prophylactic Antibiotic Timing (Outpatient)	659	99%	98%	98%
Urinary Catheter Removal[2]	237	95%	96%	97%
Survey of Patients' Hospital Experiences				
Area Around Room 'Always' Quiet at Night	300+	59%	67%	61%
Doctors 'Always' Communicated Well	300+	83%	84%	82%
Home Recovery Information Given	300+	83%	85%	85%
Hospital Given 9 or 10 on 10 Point Scale	300+	72%	70%	71%
Meds 'Always' Explained Before Given	300+	63%	66%	64%
Nurses 'Always' Communicated Well	300+	81%	80%	79%
Pain 'Always' Well Controlled	300+	70%	72%	71%
Room and Bathroom 'Always' Clean	300+	68%	73%	73%
Timely Help 'Always' Received	300+	65%	68%	68%
Would Definitely Recommend Hospital	300+	75%	70%	71%
Use of Medical Imaging				
Cardiac Imaging Stress Test before Surgery	1,912	4.4%	4.8%	5.3%
Combination Abdominal CT Scan	628	8.6%	9.6%	10.5%
Combination Brain/Sinus CT Scan	741	2.6%	3.3%	2.7%
Combination Chest CT Scan	333	0.3%	3.4%	2.7%
Follow-up Mammogram/Ultrasound	1,671	4.4%	8.3%	8.8%
Lumbar Spine MRI for Low Back Pain[1]	-	-	35.3%	37.2%

Fort Sanders Regional Medical Center

1901 W Clinch Ave
Knoxville, TN 37916
Phone: 865-541-1101
Fax: 865-541-2840
URL: www.fsregional.com
Type: Acute Care Hospitals
Emergency Services: Yes
Ownership: Voluntary non-profit - Private
Beds: 541

Key Personnel:
Emergency Room . . . . Charles Adams, MD
Infection Control. . . . . John Adams, MD
Radiology. . . . . Steven J Addonizio
CEO/President. . . . . Keith N. Altshuler, FACHE
Chief of Medical Staff . . . . David Ayers
Anesthesiology. . . . . Wilson Beamer, MD

Measure	Cases	This Hosp.	State Avg.	U.S. Avg.
Blood Clot Prevention and Treatment				
Anticoagulation Overlap Therapy[2]	77	100%	92%	93%
ICU Venous Thromboembolism Prophylaxis[2]	74	100%	90%	92%
Incidence of Potentially Preventable VTE[2]	20	0%	10%	10%
UFH with Dosages/Platelet Monitoring[2]	27	100%	99%	97%
Venous Thromboembolism Prophylaxis[2]	414	98%	83%	85%
Warfarin Therapy Discharge Instructions[2]	64	98%	78%	75%
Chest Pain/Possible Heart Attack Care				
Aspirin Given Within 24 Hours of Arrival[5]	-	-	96%	96%
Fibrinolytic Meds Within 30 Min. of Arrival[5]	-	-	72%	58%
Average Time to ECG (minutes)[5]	-	-	6	7
Average Time to Transfer (minutes)[5]	-	-	53	60
Children's Asthma Care				
Received Home Management Plan of Care	-	-	-	88%
Received Reliever Medication	-	-	-	100%
Received Systemic Corticosteroids	-	-	-	100%
Emergency Department				
Admittance Decision Time (minutes)[2]	616	161	82	98
Head CT Results Within 45 Min. of Arrival[1,3]	-	-	52%	57%
Patients Who Left ER Before Being Seen	51,582	1%	2%	2%
Time from ER Arrival to Admit. (minutes)[2]	617	313	243	274
Time from ER Arrival to Discharge (minutes)	405	140	131	134
Time in ER Before Being Evaluated (minutes)	410	32	25	26
Time to Pain Meds for Fractures (minutes)	129	72	60	57
Heart Attack Care				
Aspirin Given at Discharge[2]	214	100%	99%	99%
Fibrinolytic Meds Within 30 Min. of Arrival[2,7]	-	-	33%	54%
PCI Within 90 Minutes of Arrival[2]	42	100%	98%	96%
Statin Prescribed at Discharge[2]	202	100%	99%	98%
Heart Failure Care				
ACE Inhibitor or ARB for LVSD[2]	60	100%	97%	97%
Discharge Instructions Given[2]	177	100%	93%	94%
Evaluation of LVS Function[2]	224	100%	99%	99%
Medicare Spending				
Medicare Spending per Patient (ratio)	-	0.98	1	0.98
Pneumonia Care				
Appropriate Initial Antibiotic Given[2]	106	97%	95%	95%
Blood Culture Timing[2]	178	100%	98%	98%
Pregnancy and Delivery Care				
Newborn Deliveries Scheduled Early[2]	30	0%	6%	6%
Preventive Care				
Immunization for Influenza[2]	588	93%	93%	90%
Immunization for Pneumonia[2]	777	90%	93%	92%
Stroke Care				
Anticoagulation Therapy for Atrial Fibrillation	45	98%	94%	95%
Antithrombotic Therapy Timing	258	100%	97%	98%
Assessed for Rehabilitation	362	99%	97%	97%
Discharged on Antithrombotic Therapy	307	100%	99%	99%
Discharged on Statin Medication	225	97%	94%	94%
Thrombolytic Therapy Timing	18	72%	57%	66%
Venous Thromboembolism Prophylaxis	378	97%	93%	94%
Written Stroke Educational Materials Given	207	100%	84%	88%
Surgical Care Improvement Project				
Appropriate Beta Blocker Usage[2]	257	100%	97%	98%
Appropriate VTP Within 24 Hours[2]	549	99%	98%	98%
Controlled Postoperative Blood Glucose[2]	130	98%	95%	97%
Perioperative Temperature Management[2]	640	100%	100%	100%
Prophylactic Antibiotic Selection[2]	540	100%	99%	99%
Prophylactic Antibiotic Selection (Outpatient)	636	100%	98%	98%
Prophylactic Antibiotic Stopped[2]	533	99%	98%	98%
Prophylactic Antibiotic Timing[2]	541	99%	99%	99%
Prophylactic Antibiotic Timing (Outpatient)	637	99%	98%	98%
Urinary Catheter Removal[2]	426	100%	96%	97%
Survey of Patients' Hospital Experiences				
Area Around Room 'Always' Quiet at Night	300+	63%	67%	61%
Doctors 'Always' Communicated Well	300+	83%	84%	82%
Home Recovery Information Given	300+	88%	85%	85%
Hospital Given 9 or 10 on 10 Point Scale	300+	77%	70%	71%
Meds 'Always' Explained Before Given	300+	69%	66%	64%
Nurses 'Always' Communicated Well	300+	82%	80%	79%
Pain 'Always' Well Controlled	300+	76%	72%	71%
Room and Bathroom 'Always' Clean	300+	75%	73%	73%
Timely Help 'Always' Received	300+	70%	68%	68%
Would Definitely Recommend Hospital	300+	81%	70%	71%
Use of Medical Imaging				
Cardiac Imaging Stress Test before Surgery	512	4.7%	4.8%	5.3%
Combination Abdominal CT Scan	827	6.5%	9.6%	10.5%
Combination Brain/Sinus CT Scan	734	3.0%	3.3%	2.7%
Combination Chest CT Scan	740	4.6%	3.4%	2.7%
Follow-up Mammogram/Ultrasound	684	6.1%	8.3%	8.8%
Lumbar Spine MRI for Low Back Pain	191	29.8%	35.3%	37.2%

Parkwest Medical Center

9352 Park West Blvd
Knoxville, TN 37923
Phone: 865-970-9800
Fax: 865-373-1012
URL: www.yesparkwest.com
Type: Acute Care Hospitals
Emergency Services: Yes
Ownership: Voluntary non-profit - Private
Beds: 414

Key Personnel:
Infection Control. . . . . Margaret Chambers, RN
Chief of Medical Staff . . . . Mitchell Dickson, MD
Operating Room. . . . . Brenda Ginn, RN
CEO/President. . . . . Rick Lassiter
Radiology. . . . . Jeffrey Roesch, MD
Quality Assurance . . . . Linda Tillman, RN
Cardiac Laboratory. . . . . Laura Zeletnac

Measure	Cases	This Hosp.	State Avg.	U.S. Avg.
Blood Clot Prevention and Treatment				
Anticoagulation Overlap Therapy[2]	108	99%	92%	93%
ICU Venous Thromboembolism Prophylaxis[2]	30	100%	90%	92%
Incidence of Potentially Preventable VTE[2]	26	8%	10%	10%
UFH with Dosages/Platelet Monitoring[2]	32	100%	99%	97%
Venous Thromboembolism Prophylaxis[2]	307	93%	83%	85%
Warfarin Therapy Discharge Instructions[2]	76	97%	78%	75%
Chest Pain/Possible Heart Attack Care				
Aspirin Given Within 24 Hours of Arrival[1,3]	-	-	96%	96%
Fibrinolytic Meds Within 30 Min. of Arrival[5]	-	-	72%	58%
Average Time to ECG (minutes)[1,3]	-	-	6	7
Average Time to Transfer (minutes)[5]	-	-	53	60
Children's Asthma Care				
Received Home Management Plan of Care	-	-	-	88%
Received Reliever Medication	-	-	-	100%
Received Systemic Corticosteroids	-	-	-	100%
Emergency Department				
Admittance Decision Time (minutes)[2]	445	146	82	98
Head CT Results Within 45 Min. of Arrival	18	44%	52%	57%
Patients Who Left ER Before Being Seen	49,422	2%	2%	2%
Time from ER Arrival to Admit. (minutes)[2]	454	337	243	274
Time from ER Arrival to Discharge (minutes)	414	188	131	134
Time in ER Before Being Evaluated (minutes)	456	40	25	26
Time to Pain Meds for Fractures (minutes)	78	54	60	57
Heart Attack Care				
Aspirin Given at Discharge[2]	338	100%	99%	99%
Fibrinolytic Meds Within 30 Min. of Arrival[1,2]	-	-	33%	54%
PCI Within 90 Minutes of Arrival[2]	44	98%	98%	96%
Statin Prescribed at Discharge[2]	332	100%	99%	98%
Heart Failure Care				
ACE Inhibitor or ARB for LVSD[2]	67	97%	97%	97%
Discharge Instructions Given[2]	248	100%	93%	94%
Evaluation of LVS Function[2]	311	100%	99%	99%
Medicare Spending				
Medicare Spending per Patient (ratio)	-	0.97	1	0.98
Pneumonia Care				
Appropriate Initial Antibiotic Given[2]	113	98%	95%	95%
Blood Culture Timing[2]	169	99%	98%	98%
Pregnancy and Delivery Care				
Newborn Deliveries Scheduled Early[2]	148	3%	6%	6%
Preventive Care				
Immunization for Influenza[2]	658	92%	93%	90%
Immunization for Pneumonia[2]	747	89%	93%	92%
Stroke Care				
Anticoagulation Therapy for Atrial Fibrillation	31	97%	94%	95%
Antithrombotic Therapy Timing	155	98%	97%	98%
Assessed for Rehabilitation	188	100%	97%	97%
Discharged on Antithrombotic Therapy	163	100%	99%	99%
Discharged on Statin Medication	106	96%	94%	94%
Thrombolytic Therapy Timing[1]	-	-	57%	66%
Venous Thromboembolism Prophylaxis	197	96%	93%	94%
Written Stroke Educational Materials Given	94	99%	84%	88%
Surgical Care Improvement Project				
Appropriate Beta Blocker Usage[2]	339	96%	97%	98%
Appropriate VTP Within 24 Hours[2]	619	99%	98%	98%
Controlled Postoperative Blood Glucose[2]	240	98%	95%	97%
Perioperative Temperature Management[2]	778	100%	100%	100%
Prophylactic Antibiotic Selection[2]	761	100%	99%	99%
Prophylactic Antibiotic Selection (Outpatient)	883	99%	98%	98%
Prophylactic Antibiotic Stopped[2]	739	99%	98%	98%
Prophylactic Antibiotic Timing[2]	761	100%	99%	99%
Prophylactic Antibiotic Timing (Outpatient)	877	99%	98%	98%
Urinary Catheter Removal[2]	554	98%	96%	97%
Survey of Patients' Hospital Experiences				
Area Around Room 'Always' Quiet at Night	300+	70%	67%	61%
Doctors 'Always' Communicated Well	300+	84%	84%	82%
Home Recovery Information Given	300+	88%	85%	85%
Hospital Given 9 or 10 on 10 Point Scale	300+	79%	70%	71%
Meds 'Always' Explained Before Given	300+	66%	66%	64%
Nurses 'Always' Communicated Well	300+	81%	80%	79%
Pain 'Always' Well Controlled	300+	73%	72%	71%
Room and Bathroom 'Always' Clean	300+	76%	73%	73%
Timely Help 'Always' Received	300+	66%	68%	68%
Would Definitely Recommend Hospital	300+	81%	70%	71%
Use of Medical Imaging				
Cardiac Imaging Stress Test before Surgery	1,220	5.4%	4.8%	5.3%
Combination Abdominal CT Scan	1,078	10.0%	9.6%	10.5%
Combination Brain/Sinus CT Scan	1,207	3.0%	3.3%	2.7%
Combination Chest CT Scan	962	4.5%	3.4%	2.7%
Follow-up Mammogram/Ultrasound	1,121	8.4%	8.3%	8.8%
Lumbar Spine MRI for Low Back Pain	135	35.6%	35.3%	37.2%

NOTE: Hospital profiles are in alphabetical order by state, then city, then hospital within the city; Rankings exclude hospitals with less than 25 cases except for patient surveys which excludes hospitals with less than 100 cases; (a) 100-299 cases; (1) The number of cases/patients is too few to report; (2) Data submitted were based on a sample of cases/patients; (3) Results are based on a shorter time period than required; (4) Data suppressed by CMS for one or more quarters; (5) Results are not available for this reporting period; (6) Fewer than 100 patients completed the HCAHPS survey; (7) No cases met the criteria for this measure; (8) The lower limit of the confidence interval cannot be calculated if the number of observed infections equals zero; (9) No data are available from the state/territory for this reporting period; (10) The scores shown reflect fewer than 50 completed surveys; (11) There were discrepancies in the data collection process; (12) This measure does not apply to this hospital for this reporting period; (13) Results cannot be calculated for this reporting period; (14) The results for this state are combined with nearby states to protect confidentiality; Please refer to the User's Guide for a full explanation of data.

Tennova Healthcare

900 East Oak Hill Avenue
Knoxville, TN 37917
URL: www.stmaryshealth.com
Type: Acute Care Hospitals
Ownership: Proprietary
Phone: 865-545-8000
Fax: 865-545-6732
Emergency Services: Yes
Beds: 506

Key Personnel:
Anesthesiology. . . . . Paul Baker
Infection Control. . . . . Stephanie Brooks
Intensive Care Unit. . . . . Doug Clark
Quality Assurance . . . . Carol Kortz
Radiology. . . . . William McKissick
Chief of Medical Staff. . . . . Joseph Minardo
Operating Room. . . . . Kathy Romero

Measure	Cases	This Hosp.	State Avg.	U.S. Avg.
Blood Clot Prevention and Treatment				
Anticoagulation Overlap Therapy[2]	114	83%	92%	93%
ICU Venous Thromboembolism Prophylaxis[2]	94	83%	90%	92%
Incidence of Potentially Preventable VTE[2]	24	21%	10%	10%
UFH with Dosages/Platelet Monitoring[2]	44	98%	99%	97%
Venous Thromboembolism Prophylaxis[2]	300	81%	83%	85%
Warfarin Therapy Discharge Instructions[2]	83	92%	78%	75%
Chest Pain/Possible Heart Attack Care				
Aspirin Given Within 24 Hours of Arrival	19	100%	96%	96%
Fibrinolytic Meds Within 30 Min. of Arrival[7]	-	-	72%	58%
Average Time to ECG (minutes)	18	6	6	7
Average Time to Transfer (minutes)[1]	-	-	53	60
Children's Asthma Care				
Received Home Management Plan of Care	-	-	-	88%
Received Reliever Medication	-	-	-	100%
Received Systemic Corticosteroids	-	-	-	100%
Emergency Department				
Admittance Decision Time (minutes)[2]	700	161	82	98
Head CT Results Within 45 Min. of Arrival	27	26%	52%	57%
Patients Who Left ER Before Being Seen	>100k	2%	2%	2%
Time from ER Arrival to Admit. (minutes)[2]	736	268	243	274
Time from ER Arrival to Discharge (minutes)	1,597	135	131	134
Time in ER Before Being Evaluated (minutes)	1,705	22	25	26
Time to Pain Meds for Fractures (minutes)	450	62	60	57
Heart Attack Care				
Aspirin Given at Discharge	551	99%	99%	99%
Fibrinolytic Meds Within 30 Min. of Arrival[7]	-	-	33%	54%
PCI Within 90 Minutes of Arrival	71	93%	98%	96%
Statin Prescribed at Discharge	527	98%	99%	98%
Heart Failure Care				
ACE Inhibitor or ARB for LVSD	160	94%	97%	97%
Discharge Instructions Given	512	93%	93%	94%
Evaluation of LVS Function	608	100%	99%	99%
Medicare Spending				
Medicare Spending per Patient (ratio)	-	0.96	1	0.98
Pneumonia Care				
Appropriate Initial Antibiotic Given	468	94%	95%	95%
Blood Culture Timing	746	97%	98%	98%
Pregnancy and Delivery Care				
Newborn Deliveries Scheduled Early	184	4%	6%	6%
Preventive Care				
Immunization for Influenza[2]	725	96%	93%	90%
Immunization for Pneumonia[2]	953	95%	93%	92%
Stroke Care				
Anticoagulation Therapy for Atrial Fibrillation	36	86%	94%	95%
Antithrombotic Therapy Timing	210	98%	97%	98%
Assessed for Rehabilitation	232	97%	97%	97%
Discharged on Antithrombotic Therapy	212	100%	99%	99%
Discharged on Statin Medication	167	92%	94%	94%
Thrombolytic Therapy Timing	25	28%	57%	66%
Venous Thromboembolism Prophylaxis	231	87%	93%	94%
Written Stroke Educational Materials Given	133	80%	84%	88%
Surgical Care Improvement Project				
Appropriate Beta Blocker Usage	868	98%	97%	98%
Appropriate VTP Within 24 Hours	1,987	98%	98%	98%
Controlled Postoperative Blood Glucose	281	95%	95%	97%
Perioperative Temperature Management	2,496	100%	100%	100%
Prophylactic Antibiotic Selection	1,826	99%	99%	99%
Prophylactic Antibiotic Selection (Outpatient)	1,209	97%	98%	98%
Prophylactic Antibiotic Stopped	1,773	98%	98%	98%
Prophylactic Antibiotic Timing	1,828	100%	99%	99%
Prophylactic Antibiotic Timing (Outpatient)	1,189	97%	98%	98%
Urinary Catheter Removal	1,011	96%	96%	97%
Survey of Patients' Hospital Experiences				
Area Around Room 'Always' Quiet at Night	300+	64%	67%	61%
Doctors 'Always' Communicated Well	300+	81%	84%	82%
Home Recovery Information Given	300+	82%	85%	85%
Hospital Given 9 or 10 on 10 Point Scale	300+	66%	70%	71%
Meds 'Always' Explained Before Given	300+	61%	66%	64%
Nurses 'Always' Communicated Well	300+	76%	80%	79%
Pain 'Always' Well Controlled	300+	69%	72%	71%
Room and Bathroom 'Always' Clean	300+	67%	73%	73%
Timely Help 'Always' Received	300+	62%	68%	68%
Would Definitely Recommend Hospital	300+	69%	70%	71%
Use of Medical Imaging				
Cardiac Imaging Stress Test before Surgery	1,642	4.6%	4.8%	5.3%
Combination Abdominal CT Scan	1,787	4.0%	9.6%	10.5%
Combination Brain/Sinus CT Scan	1,361	3.2%	3.3%	2.7%
Combination Chest CT Scan	1,434	1.8%	3.4%	2.7%
Follow-up Mammogram/Ultrasound	2,596	14.8%	8.3%	8.8%
Lumbar Spine MRI for Low Back Pain	256	27.7%	35.3%	37.2%

University of Tn Memorial Hospital

1924 Alcoa Highway
Knoxville, TN 37920
URL: www.utmedicalcenter.org
Type: Acute Care Hospitals
Ownership: Voluntary non-profit - Private
Phone: 865-544-9000
Fax: 865-670-6112
Emergency Services: Yes
Beds: 602

Key Personnel:
Radiology. . . . . James W Boyd
Chief of Medical Staff. . . . . Raymond Dideter
Infection Control. . . . . Eva Harris, RN
CEO/President. . . . . Joseph R. Landsman
Operating Room. . . . . Gregory J Mancini, RN
Pediatric Ambulatory Care . . . . . . Eddie Moore, MD
Pediatric In-Patient Care . . . . Eddie Moore, MD
Chairman/CEO . . . . William Rukeyser

Measure	Cases	This Hosp.	State Avg.	U.S. Avg.
Blood Clot Prevention and Treatment				
Anticoagulation Overlap Therapy[2]	196	94%	92%	93%
ICU Venous Thromboembolism Prophylaxis[2]	148	99%	90%	92%
Incidence of Potentially Preventable VTE[2]	71	0%	10%	10%
UFH with Dosages/Platelet Monitoring[2]	112	100%	99%	97%
Venous Thromboembolism Prophylaxis[2]	341	98%	83%	85%
Warfarin Therapy Discharge Instructions[2]	123	87%	78%	75%
Chest Pain/Possible Heart Attack Care				
Aspirin Given Within 24 Hours of Arrival[3,7]	-	-	96%	96%
Fibrinolytic Meds Within 30 Min. of Arrival[3,7]	-	-	72%	58%
Average Time to ECG (minutes)[1,3]	-	-	6	7
Average Time to Transfer (minutes)[3,7]	-	-	53	60
Children's Asthma Care				
Received Home Management Plan of Care	-	-	-	88%
Received Reliever Medication	-	-	-	100%
Received Systemic Corticosteroids	-	-	-	100%
Emergency Department				
Admittance Decision Time (minutes)[2]	137	111	82	98
Head CT Results Within 45 Min. of Arrival[1]	-	-	52%	57%
Patients Who Left ER Before Being Seen	80,433	1%	2%	2%
Time from ER Arrival to Admit. (minutes)[2]	261	279	243	274
Time from ER Arrival to Discharge (minutes)	350	196	131	134
Time in ER Before Being Evaluated (minutes)	377	37	25	26
Time to Pain Meds for Fractures (minutes)	301	80	60	57
Heart Attack Care				
Aspirin Given at Discharge[2]	303	100%	99%	99%
Fibrinolytic Meds Within 30 Min. of Arrival[2,7]	-	-	33%	54%
PCI Within 90 Minutes of Arrival[2]	53	98%	98%	96%
Statin Prescribed at Discharge[2]	302	98%	99%	98%
Heart Failure Care				
ACE Inhibitor or ARB for LVSD[2]	109	100%	97%	97%
Discharge Instructions Given[2]	256	95%	93%	94%
Evaluation of LVS Function[2]	298	100%	99%	99%
Medicare Spending				
Medicare Spending per Patient (ratio)	-	0.96	1	0.98
Pneumonia Care				
Appropriate Initial Antibiotic Given[2]	68	94%	95%	95%
Blood Culture Timing[2]	132	98%	98%	98%
Pregnancy and Delivery Care				
Newborn Deliveries Scheduled Early[2]	34	0%	6%	6%
Preventive Care				
Immunization for Influenza[2]	567	96%	93%	90%
Immunization for Pneumonia[2]	661	97%	93%	92%
Stroke Care				
Anticoagulation Therapy for Atrial Fibrillation	45	100%	94%	95%
Antithrombotic Therapy Timing	228	97%	97%	98%
Assessed for Rehabilitation	373	99%	97%	97%
Discharged on Antithrombotic Therapy	271	99%	99%	99%
Discharged on Statin Medication	222	97%	94%	94%
Thrombolytic Therapy Timing	30	97%	57%	66%
Venous Thromboembolism Prophylaxis	409	98%	93%	94%
Written Stroke Educational Materials Given	197	98%	84%	88%
Surgical Care Improvement Project				
Appropriate Beta Blocker Usage[2]	201	100%	97%	98%
Appropriate VTP Within 24 Hours[2]	396	98%	98%	98%
Controlled Postoperative Blood Glucose[2]	147	97%	95%	97%
Perioperative Temperature Management[2]	522	100%	100%	100%
Prophylactic Antibiotic Selection[2]	476	98%	99%	99%
Prophylactic Antibiotic Selection (Outpatient)	910	98%	98%	98%
Prophylactic Antibiotic Stopped[2]	441	98%	98%	98%
Prophylactic Antibiotic Timing[2]	476	99%	99%	99%
Prophylactic Antibiotic Timing (Outpatient)	906	98%	98%	98%
Urinary Catheter Removal[2]	429	95%	96%	97%
Survey of Patients' Hospital Experiences				
Area Around Room 'Always' Quiet at Night	300+	67%	67%	61%
Doctors 'Always' Communicated Well	300+	82%	84%	82%
Home Recovery Information Given	300+	87%	85%	85%
Hospital Given 9 or 10 on 10 Point Scale	300+	81%	70%	71%
Meds 'Always' Explained Before Given	300+	67%	66%	64%
Nurses 'Always' Communicated Well	300+	82%	80%	79%
Pain 'Always' Well Controlled	300+	73%	72%	71%
Room and Bathroom 'Always' Clean	300+	77%	73%	73%
Timely Help 'Always' Received	300+	67%	68%	68%
Would Definitely Recommend Hospital	300+	85%	70%	71%
Use of Medical Imaging				
Cardiac Imaging Stress Test before Surgery[1]	-	-	4.8%	5.3%
Combination Abdominal CT Scan	2,406	5.6%	9.6%	10.5%
Combination Brain/Sinus CT Scan	1,586	1.9%	3.3%	2.7%
Combination Chest CT Scan	2,614	0.3%	3.4%	2.7%
Follow-up Mammogram/Ultrasound	2,152	6.1%	8.3%	8.8%
Lumbar Spine MRI for Low Back Pain	252	36.1%	35.3%	37.2%

Tennova Healthcare - Lafollett Medical Center

923 East Central Avenue
La Follette, TN 37766
URL: www.stmaryshealth.com
Type: Acute Care Hospitals
Ownership: Voluntary non-profit - Church
Phone: 423-907-1200
Fax: 423-907-1164
Emergency Services: Yes
Beds: 164

Key Personnel:
Chief of Medical Staff . . . . Errol Britto
Radiology. . . . . Thomas Cohen

Measure	Cases	This Hosp.	State Avg.	U.S. Avg.
Blood Clot Prevention and Treatment				
Anticoagulation Overlap Therapy[2]	22	68%	92%	93%
ICU Venous Thromboembolism Prophylaxis[2]	56	86%	90%	92%
Incidence of Potentially Preventable VTE[1,2]	-	-	10%	10%
UFH with Dosages/Platelet Monitoring[2]	25	100%	99%	97%
Venous Thromboembolism Prophylaxis[2]	216	72%	83%	85%
Warfarin Therapy Discharge Instructions[2]	19	100%	78%	75%
Chest Pain/Possible Heart Attack Care				
Aspirin Given Within 24 Hours of Arrival	93	99%	96%	96%
Fibrinolytic Meds Within 30 Min. of Arrival[1]	-	-	72%	58%
Average Time to ECG (minutes)	98	7	6	7
Average Time to Transfer (minutes)[1]	-	-	53	60
Children's Asthma Care				
Received Home Management Plan of Care	-	-	-	88%
Received Reliever Medication	-	-	-	100%
Received Systemic Corticosteroids	-	-	-	100%

NOTE: Hospital profiles are in alphabetical order by state, then city, then hospital within the city; Rankings exclude hospitals with less than 25 cases except for patient surveys which excludes hospitals with less than 100 cases; (a) 100-299 cases; (1) The number of cases/patients is too few to report; (2) Data submitted were based on a sample of cases/patients; (3) Results are based on a shorter time period than required; (4) Data suppressed by CMS for one or more quarters; (5) Results are not available for this reporting period; (6) Fewer than 100 patients completed the HCAHPS survey; (7) No cases met the criteria for this measure; (8) The lower limit of the confidence interval cannot be calculated if the number of observed infections equals zero; (9) No data are available from the state/territory for this reporting period; (10) The scores shown reflect fewer than 50 completed surveys; (11) There were discrepancies in the data collection process; (12) This measure does not apply to this hospital for this reporting period; (13) Results cannot be calculated for this reporting period; (14) The results for this state are combined with nearby states to protect confidentiality; Please refer to the User's Guide for a full explanation of data.

Emergency Department				
Admittance Decision Time (minutes)[2]	493	63	82	98
Head CT Results Within 45 Min. of Arrival[1]	-	-	52%	57%
Patients Who Left ER Before Being Seen	21,985	1%	2%	2%
Time from ER Arrival to Admit. (minutes)[2]	496	200	243	274
Time from ER Arrival to Discharge (minutes)	1,350	106	131	134
Time in ER Before Being Evaluated (minutes)	1,455	20	25	26
Time to Pain Meds for Fractures (minutes)	94	53	60	57
Heart Attack Care				
Aspirin Given at Discharge[1]	-	-	99%	99%
Fibrinolytic Meds Within 30 Min. of Arrival[7]	-	-	33%	54%
PCI Within 90 Minutes of Arrival[7]	-	-	98%	96%
Statin Prescribed at Discharge[1]	-	-	99%	98%
Heart Failure Care				
ACE Inhibitor or ARB for LVSD	27	93%	97%	97%
Discharge Instructions Given	98	80%	93%	94%
Evaluation of LVS Function	138	100%	99%	99%
Medicare Spending				
Medicare Spending per Patient (ratio)	-	0.97	1	0.98
Pneumonia Care				
Appropriate Initial Antibiotic Given	104	96%	95%	95%
Blood Culture Timing	216	98%	98%	98%
Pregnancy and Delivery Care				
Newborn Deliveries Scheduled Early[7]	-	-	6%	6%
Preventive Care				
Immunization for Influenza[2]	282	98%	93%	90%
Immunization for Pneumonia[2]	485	99%	93%	92%
Stroke Care				
Anticoagulation Therapy for Atrial Fibrillation[1]	-	-	94%	95%
Antithrombotic Therapy Timing	17	88%	97%	98%
Assessed for Rehabilitation	15	100%	97%	97%
Discharged on Antithrombotic Therapy	14	100%	99%	99%
Discharged on Statin Medication	12	83%	94%	94%
Thrombolytic Therapy Timing[1]	-	-	57%	66%
Venous Thromboembolism Prophylaxis	19	68%	93%	94%
Written Stroke Educational Materials Given[1]	-	-	84%	88%
Surgical Care Improvement Project				
Appropriate Beta Blocker Usage[1]	-	-	97%	98%
Appropriate VTP Within 24 Hours[1]	-	-	98%	98%
Controlled Postoperative Blood Glucose[7]	-	-	95%	97%
Perioperative Temperature Management[1]	-	-	100%	100%
Prophylactic Antibiotic Selection[1]	-	-	99%	99%
Prophylactic Antibiotic Selection (Outpatient)	48	85%	98%	98%
Prophylactic Antibiotic Stopped[1]	-	-	98%	98%
Prophylactic Antibiotic Timing[1]	-	-	99%	99%
Prophylactic Antibiotic Timing (Outpatient)	48	98%	98%	98%
Urinary Catheter Removal[1]	-	-	96%	97%
Survey of Patients' Hospital Experiences				
Area Around Room 'Always' Quiet at Night	(a)	52%	67%	61%
Doctors 'Always' Communicated Well	(a)	76%	84%	82%
Home Recovery Information Given	(a)	82%	85%	85%
Hospital Given 9 or 10 on 10 Point Scale	(a)	51%	70%	71%
Meds 'Always' Explained Before Given	(a)	59%	66%	64%
Nurses 'Always' Communicated Well	(a)	71%	80%	79%
Pain 'Always' Well Controlled	(a)	55%	72%	71%
Room and Bathroom 'Always' Clean	(a)	75%	73%	73%
Timely Help 'Always' Received	(a)	59%	68%	68%
Would Definitely Recommend Hospital	(a)	48%	70%	71%
Use of Medical Imaging				
Cardiac Imaging Stress Test before Surgery	141	5.0%	4.8%	5.3%
Combination Abdominal CT Scan	288	13.2%	9.6%	10.5%
Combination Brain/Sinus CT Scan[1]	-	-	3.3%	2.7%
Combination Chest CT Scan	186	11.8%	3.4%	2.7%
Follow-up Mammogram/Ultrasound	326	8.0%	8.3%	8.8%
Lumbar Spine MRI for Low Back Pain	87	46.0%	35.3%	37.2%

Macon County General Hospital

204 Medical Drive
Lafayette, TN 37083
URL: www.mcgh.net
Phone: 615-666-2147
Fax: 615-666-7002
Type: Critical Access Hospitals
Ownership: Voluntary non-profit - Private
Emergency Services: Yes
Beds: 43

Key Personnel:
Radiology. . . . . Michael Hencey, MD
Emergency Room . . . . Hanna C Ilia, MD
Cardiology . . . . Jung Lee, MD
Surgery . . . . Thomas Taylor, MD
CEO/President. . . . . Dennis A Wolford
Infection Control. . . . . Dixie Wooten, LPN

Measure	Cases	This Hosp.	State Avg.	U.S. Avg.
Blood Clot Prevention and Treatment				
Anticoagulation Overlap Therapy[5]	-	-	92%	93%
ICU Venous Thromboembolism Prophylaxis[5]	-	-	90%	92%
Incidence of Potentially Preventable VTE[5]	-	-	10%	10%
UFH with Dosages/Platelet Monitoring[5]	-	-	99%	97%
Venous Thromboembolism Prophylaxis[5]	-	-	83%	85%
Warfarin Therapy Discharge Instructions[5]	-	-	78%	75%
Chest Pain/Possible Heart Attack Care				
Aspirin Given Within 24 Hours of Arrival	57	95%	96%	96%
Fibrinolytic Meds Within 30 Min. of Arrival[1]	-	-	72%	58%
Average Time to ECG (minutes)	66	10	6	7
Average Time to Transfer (minutes)[1]	-	-	53	60
Children's Asthma Care				
Received Home Management Plan of Care	-	-	-	88%
Received Reliever Medication	-	-	-	100%
Received Systemic Corticosteroids	-	-	-	100%
Emergency Department				
Admittance Decision Time (minutes)[5]	-	-	82	98
Head CT Results Within 45 Min. of Arrival[5]	-	-	52%	57%
Patients Who Left ER Before Being Seen[5]	-	-	2%	2%
Time from ER Arrival to Admit. (minutes)[5]	-	-	243	274
Time from ER Arrival to Discharge (minutes)[5]	-	-	131	134
Time in ER Before Being Evaluated (minutes)[5]	-	-	25	26
Time to Pain Meds for Fractures (minutes)[5]	-	-	60	57
Heart Attack Care				
Aspirin Given at Discharge[5]	-	-	99%	99%
Fibrinolytic Meds Within 30 Min. of Arrival[5]	-	-	33%	54%
PCI Within 90 Minutes of Arrival[5]	-	-	98%	96%
Statin Prescribed at Discharge[5]	-	-	99%	98%
Heart Failure Care				
ACE Inhibitor or ARB for LVSD[1]	-	-	97%	97%
Discharge Instructions Given	15	93%	93%	94%
Evaluation of LVS Function	22	95%	99%	99%
Medicare Spending				
Medicare Spending per Patient (ratio)	-	-	1	0.98
Pneumonia Care				
Appropriate Initial Antibiotic Given	30	93%	95%	95%
Blood Culture Timing	49	92%	98%	98%
Pregnancy and Delivery Care				
Newborn Deliveries Scheduled Early[5]	-	-	6%	6%
Preventive Care				
Immunization for Influenza[5]	-	-	93%	90%
Immunization for Pneumonia[5]	-	-	93%	92%
Stroke Care				
Anticoagulation Therapy for Atrial Fibrillation[5]	-	-	94%	95%
Antithrombotic Therapy Timing[5]	-	-	97%	98%
Assessed for Rehabilitation[5]	-	-	97%	97%
Discharged on Antithrombotic Therapy[5]	-	-	99%	99%
Discharged on Statin Medication[5]	-	-	94%	94%
Thrombolytic Therapy Timing[5]	-	-	57%	66%
Venous Thromboembolism Prophylaxis[5]	-	-	93%	94%
Written Stroke Educational Materials Given[5]	-	-	84%	88%
Surgical Care Improvement Project				
Appropriate Beta Blocker Usage[5]	-	-	97%	98%
Appropriate VTP Within 24 Hours[5]	-	-	98%	98%
Controlled Postoperative Blood Glucose[5]	-	-	95%	97%
Perioperative Temperature Management[5]	-	-	100%	100%
Prophylactic Antibiotic Selection[5]	-	-	99%	99%
Prophylactic Antibiotic Selection (Outpatient)[3,7]	-	-	98%	98%
Prophylactic Antibiotic Stopped[5]	-	-	98%	98%
Prophylactic Antibiotic Timing[5]	-	-	99%	99%
Prophylactic Antibiotic Timing (Outpatient)[1,3]	-	-	98%	98%
Urinary Catheter Removal[5]	-	-	96%	97%
Survey of Patients' Hospital Experiences				
Area Around Room 'Always' Quiet at Night	(a)	65%	67%	61%
Doctors 'Always' Communicated Well	(a)	83%	84%	82%
Home Recovery Information Given	(a)	84%	85%	85%
Hospital Given 9 or 10 on 10 Point Scale	(a)	75%	70%	71%
Meds 'Always' Explained Before Given	(a)	65%	66%	64%
Nurses 'Always' Communicated Well	(a)	82%	80%	79%
Pain 'Always' Well Controlled	(a)	78%	72%	71%
Room and Bathroom 'Always' Clean	(a)	80%	73%	73%
Timely Help 'Always' Received	(a)	82%	68%	68%
Would Definitely Recommend Hospital	(a)	72%	70%	71%
Use of Medical Imaging				
Cardiac Imaging Stress Test before Surgery[1]	-	-	4.8%	5.3%
Combination Abdominal CT Scan	123	4.9%	9.6%	10.5%
Combination Brain/Sinus CT Scan[1]	-	-	3.3%	2.7%
Combination Chest CT Scan	108	2.8%	3.4%	2.7%
Follow-up Mammogram/Ultrasound	192	19.3%	8.3%	8.8%
Lumbar Spine MRI for Low Back Pain[1]	-	-	35.3%	37.2%

Crockett Hospital

Hwy 43 S Box 847
Lawrenceburg, TN 38464
Phone: 931-762-6571
Fax: 931-766-3248
E-mail: robert.augustin@lifepointhospitals.com
URL: www.crocketthospital.com
Type: Acute Care Hospitals
Ownership: Proprietary
Emergency Services: Yes
Beds: 107

Key Personnel:
Radiology. . . . . William Wesley Brewer
CEO/President. . . . . Jack Buck
Chief of Medical Staff. . . . . Kimberly Goodemote

Measure	Cases	This Hosp.	State Avg.	U.S. Avg.
Blood Clot Prevention and Treatment				
Anticoagulation Overlap Therapy[2]	14	79%	92%	93%
ICU Venous Thromboembolism Prophylaxis[2]	41	88%	90%	92%
Incidence of Potentially Preventable VTE[1,2]	-	-	10%	10%
UFH with Dosages/Platelet Monitoring[2,7]	-	-	99%	97%
Venous Thromboembolism Prophylaxis[2]	153	93%	83%	85%
Warfarin Therapy Discharge Instructions[1,2]	-	-	78%	75%
Chest Pain/Possible Heart Attack Care				
Aspirin Given Within 24 Hours of Arrival	166	95%	96%	96%
Fibrinolytic Meds Within 30 Min. of Arrival[1]	-	-	72%	58%
Average Time to ECG (minutes)	171	4	6	7
Average Time to Transfer (minutes)	12	42	53	60
Children's Asthma Care				
Received Home Management Plan of Care	-	-	-	88%
Received Reliever Medication	-	-	-	100%
Received Systemic Corticosteroids	-	-	-	100%
Emergency Department				
Admittance Decision Time (minutes)[2]	220	64	82	98
Head CT Results Within 45 Min. of Arrival[1]	-	-	52%	57%
Patients Who Left ER Before Being Seen	14,603	1%	2%	2%
Time from ER Arrival to Admit. (minutes)[2]	226	223	243	274
Time from ER Arrival to Discharge (minutes)	392	106	131	134
Time in ER Before Being Evaluated (minutes)	351	13	25	26
Time to Pain Meds for Fractures (minutes)	90	48	60	57
Heart Attack Care				
Aspirin Given at Discharge[1,3]	-	-	99%	99%
Fibrinolytic Meds Within 30 Min. of Arrival[3,7]	-	-	33%	54%
PCI Within 90 Minutes of Arrival[3,7]	-	-	98%	96%
Statin Prescribed at Discharge[1,3]	-	-	99%	98%
Heart Failure Care				
ACE Inhibitor or ARB for LVSD[1]	-	-	97%	97%
Discharge Instructions Given	39	82%	93%	94%
Evaluation of LVS Function	52	100%	99%	99%
Medicare Spending				
Medicare Spending per Patient (ratio)	-	0.97	1	0.98
Pneumonia Care				
Appropriate Initial Antibiotic Given	129	95%	95%	95%
Blood Culture Timing	147	99%	98%	98%
Pregnancy and Delivery Care				
Newborn Deliveries Scheduled Early[2]	26	8%	6%	6%
Preventive Care				
Immunization for Influenza[2]	268	98%	93%	90%
Immunization for Pneumonia[2]	335	97%	93%	92%
Stroke Care				
Anticoagulation Therapy for Atrial Fibrillation[1]	-	-	94%	95%

NOTE: Hospital profiles are in alphabetical order by state, then city, then hospital within the city; Rankings exclude hospitals with less than 25 cases except for patient surveys which excludes hospitals with less than 100 cases; (a) 100-299 cases; (1) The number of cases/patients is too few to report; (2) Data submitted were based on a sample of cases/patients; (3) Results are based on a shorter time period than required; (4) Data suppressed by CMS for one or more quarters; (5) Results are not available for this reporting period; (6) Fewer than 100 patients completed the HCAHPS survey; (7) No cases met the criteria for this measure; (8) The lower limit of the confidence interval cannot be calculated if the number of observed infections equals zero; (9) No data are available from the state/territory for this reporting period; (10) The scores shown reflect fewer than 50 completed surveys; (11) There were discrepancies in the data collection process; (12) This measure does not apply to this hospital for this reporting period; (13) Results cannot be calculated for this reporting period; (14) The results for this state are combined with nearby states to protect confidentiality; Please refer to the User's Guide for a full explanation of data.

Measure	Cases	This Hosp.	State Avg.	U.S. Avg.
Antithrombotic Therapy Timing	24	100%	97%	98%
Assessed for Rehabilitation	25	100%	97%	97%
Discharged on Antithrombotic Therapy	25	100%	99%	99%
Discharged on Statin Medication	19	95%	94%	94%
Thrombolytic Therapy Timing[1]	-	-	57%	66%
Venous Thromboembolism Prophylaxis	22	95%	93%	94%
Written Stroke Educational Materials Given	11	64%	84%	88%
Surgical Care Improvement Project				
Appropriate Beta Blocker Usage	11	91%	97%	98%
Appropriate VTP Within 24 Hours	28	96%	98%	98%
Controlled Postoperative Blood Glucose[7]	-	-	95%	97%
Perioperative Temperature Management	32	100%	100%	100%
Prophylactic Antibiotic Selection	24	100%	99%	99%
Prophylactic Antibiotic Selection (Outpatient)[1,3]	-	-	98%	98%
Prophylactic Antibiotic Stopped	24	100%	98%	98%
Prophylactic Antibiotic Timing	24	100%	99%	99%
Prophylactic Antibiotic Timing (Outpatient)[1,3]	-	-	98%	98%
Urinary Catheter Removal	18	100%	96%	97%
Survey of Patients' Hospital Experiences				
Area Around Room 'Always' Quiet at Night	300+	61%	67%	61%
Doctors 'Always' Communicated Well	300+	79%	84%	82%
Home Recovery Information Given	300+	84%	85%	85%
Hospital Given 9 or 10 on 10 Point Scale	300+	62%	70%	71%
Meds 'Always' Explained Before Given	300+	60%	66%	64%
Nurses 'Always' Communicated Well	300+	77%	80%	79%
Pain 'Always' Well Controlled	300+	67%	72%	71%
Room and Bathroom 'Always' Clean	300+	70%	73%	73%
Timely Help 'Always' Received	300+	66%	68%	68%
Would Definitely Recommend Hospital	300+	57%	70%	71%
Use of Medical Imaging				
Cardiac Imaging Stress Test before Surgery	130	6.9%	4.8%	5.3%
Combination Abdominal CT Scan	505	9.5%	9.6%	10.5%
Combination Brain/Sinus CT Scan	540	2.6%	3.3%	2.7%
Combination Chest CT Scan	391	1.0%	3.4%	2.7%
Follow-up Mammogram/Ultrasound	762	9.4%	8.3%	8.8%
Lumbar Spine MRI for Low Back Pain	81	33.3%	35.3%	37.2%

University Medical Center

1411 Baddour Parkway
Lebanon, TN 37087
Phone: 615-444-8262
Fax: 615-443-2553
URL: www.universitymedicalcenter.com
Type: Acute Care Hospitals
Emergency Services: Yes
Ownership: Voluntary non-profit - Private
Beds: 257

Key Personnel:
CEO . . . . Matt Caldwell
Emergency Room . . . . Scott Giles, MD
Administrator . . . . Steve Simpson

Measure	Cases	This Hosp.	State Avg.	U.S. Avg.
Blood Clot Prevention and Treatment				
Anticoagulation Overlap Therapy[2]	33	97%	92%	93%
ICU Venous Thromboembolism Prophylaxis[2]	75	71%	90%	92%
Incidence of Potentially Preventable VTE[1,2]	-	-	10%	10%
UFH with Dosages/Platelet Monitoring[2]	14	100%	99%	97%
Venous Thromboembolism Prophylaxis[2]	352	56%	83%	85%
Warfarin Therapy Discharge Instructions[2]	29	48%	78%	75%
Chest Pain/Possible Heart Attack Care				
Aspirin Given Within 24 Hours of Arrival	61	93%	96%	96%
Fibrinolytic Meds Within 30 Min. of Arrival[7]	-	-	72%	58%
Average Time to ECG (minutes)	67	5	6	7
Average Time to Transfer (minutes)	13	69	53	60
Children's Asthma Care				
Received Home Management Plan of Care	-	-	-	88%
Received Reliever Medication	-	-	-	100%
Received Systemic Corticosteroids	-	-	-	100%
Emergency Department				
Admittance Decision Time (minutes)[2]	449	61	82	98
Head CT Results Within 45 Min. of Arrival[1]	-	-	52%	57%
Patients Who Left ER Before Being Seen	29,656	2%	2%	2%
Time from ER Arrival to Admit. (minutes)[2]	460	206	243	274
Time from ER Arrival to Discharge (minutes)	586	133	131	134
Time in ER Before Being Evaluated (minutes)	645	29	25	26
Time to Pain Meds for Fractures (minutes)	128	46	60	57
Heart Attack Care				
Aspirin Given at Discharge	34	94%	99%	99%
Fibrinolytic Meds Within 30 Min. of Arrival[7]	-	-	33%	54%
PCI Within 90 Minutes of Arrival[7]	-	-	98%	96%
Statin Prescribed at Discharge	32	94%	99%	98%
Heart Failure Care				
ACE Inhibitor or ARB for LVSD	21	100%	97%	97%
Discharge Instructions Given	71	93%	93%	94%
Evaluation of LVS Function	102	100%	99%	99%
Medicare Spending				
Medicare Spending per Patient (ratio)	-	1.05	1	0.98
Pneumonia Care				
Appropriate Initial Antibiotic Given	139	95%	95%	95%
Blood Culture Timing	217	99%	98%	98%
Pregnancy and Delivery Care				
Newborn Deliveries Scheduled Early	84	15%	6%	6%
Preventive Care				
Immunization for Influenza[2]	590	99%	93%	90%
Immunization for Pneumonia[2]	629	98%	93%	92%
Stroke Care				
Anticoagulation Therapy for Atrial Fibrillation[1]	-	-	94%	95%
Antithrombotic Therapy Timing	24	92%	97%	98%
Assessed for Rehabilitation	23	100%	97%	97%
Discharged on Antithrombotic Therapy	22	95%	99%	99%
Discharged on Statin Medication	17	88%	94%	94%
Thrombolytic Therapy Timing[7]	-	-	57%	66%
Venous Thromboembolism Prophylaxis	18	61%	93%	94%
Written Stroke Educational Materials Given	11	91%	84%	88%
Surgical Care Improvement Project				
Appropriate Beta Blocker Usage	101	99%	97%	98%
Appropriate VTP Within 24 Hours	324	99%	98%	98%
Controlled Postoperative Blood Glucose[7]	-	-	95%	97%
Perioperative Temperature Management	367	100%	100%	100%
Prophylactic Antibiotic Selection	252	98%	99%	99%
Prophylactic Antibiotic Selection (Outpatient)	202	99%	98%	98%
Prophylactic Antibiotic Stopped	237	98%	98%	98%
Prophylactic Antibiotic Timing	252	100%	99%	99%
Prophylactic Antibiotic Timing (Outpatient)	211	95%	98%	98%
Urinary Catheter Removal	234	94%	96%	97%
Survey of Patients' Hospital Experiences				
Area Around Room 'Always' Quiet at Night	300+	60%	67%	61%
Doctors 'Always' Communicated Well	300+	82%	84%	82%
Home Recovery Information Given	300+	82%	85%	85%
Hospital Given 9 or 10 on 10 Point Scale	300+	52%	70%	71%
Meds 'Always' Explained Before Given	300+	56%	66%	64%
Nurses 'Always' Communicated Well	300+	69%	80%	79%
Pain 'Always' Well Controlled	300+	63%	72%	71%
Room and Bathroom 'Always' Clean	300+	65%	73%	73%
Timely Help 'Always' Received	300+	51%	68%	68%
Would Definitely Recommend Hospital	300+	51%	70%	71%
Use of Medical Imaging				
Cardiac Imaging Stress Test before Surgery	90	12.2%	4.8%	5.3%
Combination Abdominal CT Scan	579	8.1%	9.6%	10.5%
Combination Brain/Sinus CT Scan[1]	-	-	3.3%	2.7%
Combination Chest CT Scan	338	3.3%	3.4%	2.7%
Follow-up Mammogram/Ultrasound	701	11.1%	8.3%	8.8%
Lumbar Spine MRI for Low Back Pain	44	43.2%	35.3%	37.2%

Fort Loudoun Medical Center

550 Fort Loudoun Medical Center Dr
Lenoir City, TN 37772
Phone: 865-271-6000
Fax: 865-271-6514
URL: www.fsloudon.com
Type: Acute Care Hospitals
Emergency Services: Yes
Ownership: Voluntary non-profit - Other
Beds: 50

Key Personnel:
Radiology. . . . . Steven J Addonizio
Operating Room. . . . . John Eason
CEO/President. . . . . Jeffrey Feike
Chief of Medical Staff. . . . . Steven Knight, MD
Infection Control. . . . . Connie Moore
Quality Assurance . . . . Connie Moore, RN

Measure	Cases	This Hosp.	State Avg.	U.S. Avg.
Blood Clot Prevention and Treatment				
Anticoagulation Overlap Therapy[2]	14	100%	92%	93%
ICU Venous Thromboembolism Prophylaxis[2]	49	100%	90%	92%
Incidence of Potentially Preventable VTE[1,2]	-	-	10%	10%
UFH with Dosages/Platelet Monitoring[1,2]	-	-	99%	97%
Venous Thromboembolism Prophylaxis[2]	186	99%	83%	85%
Warfarin Therapy Discharge Instructions[1,2]	-	-	78%	75%
Chest Pain/Possible Heart Attack Care				
Aspirin Given Within 24 Hours of Arrival	39	95%	96%	96%
Fibrinolytic Meds Within 30 Min. of Arrival[7]	-	-	72%	58%
Average Time to ECG (minutes)	41	7	6	7
Average Time to Transfer (minutes)[1]	-	-	53	60
Children's Asthma Care				
Received Home Management Plan of Care	-	-	-	88%
Received Reliever Medication	-	-	-	100%
Received Systemic Corticosteroids	-	-	-	100%
Emergency Department				
Admittance Decision Time (minutes)[2]	523	121	82	98
Head CT Results Within 45 Min. of Arrival[1]	-	-	52%	57%
Patients Who Left ER Before Being Seen	21,672	0%	2%	2%
Time from ER Arrival to Admit. (minutes)[2]	533	272	243	274
Time from ER Arrival to Discharge (minutes)	392	146	131	134
Time in ER Before Being Evaluated (minutes)	429	33	25	26
Time to Pain Meds for Fractures (minutes)	55	62	60	57
Heart Attack Care				
Aspirin Given at Discharge[1]	-	-	99%	99%
Fibrinolytic Meds Within 30 Min. of Arrival[7]	-	-	33%	54%
PCI Within 90 Minutes of Arrival[7]	-	-	98%	96%
Statin Prescribed at Discharge[1]	-	-	99%	98%
Heart Failure Care				
ACE Inhibitor or ARB for LVSD	21	95%	97%	97%
Discharge Instructions Given	69	100%	93%	94%
Evaluation of LVS Function	75	100%	99%	99%
Medicare Spending				
Medicare Spending per Patient (ratio)	-	0.87	1	0.98
Pneumonia Care				
Appropriate Initial Antibiotic Given[2]	76	96%	95%	95%
Blood Culture Timing[2]	115	97%	98%	98%
Pregnancy and Delivery Care				
Newborn Deliveries Scheduled Early[7]	-	-	6%	6%
Preventive Care				
Immunization for Influenza[2]	346	99%	93%	90%
Immunization for Pneumonia[2]	546	97%	93%	92%
Stroke Care				
Anticoagulation Therapy for Atrial Fibrillation[1]	-	-	94%	95%
Antithrombotic Therapy Timing	26	100%	97%	98%
Assessed for Rehabilitation	29	100%	97%	97%
Discharged on Antithrombotic Therapy	29	97%	99%	99%
Discharged on Statin Medication	19	100%	94%	94%
Thrombolytic Therapy Timing[7]	-	-	57%	66%
Venous Thromboembolism Prophylaxis	24	100%	93%	94%
Written Stroke Educational Materials Given	15	100%	84%	88%
Surgical Care Improvement Project				
Appropriate Beta Blocker Usage[2]	13	92%	97%	98%
Appropriate VTP Within 24 Hours[2]	52	100%	98%	98%
Controlled Postoperative Blood Glucose[2,7]	-	-	95%	97%
Perioperative Temperature Management[2]	62	100%	100%	100%
Prophylactic Antibiotic Selection[2]	25	100%	99%	99%
Prophylactic Antibiotic Selection (Outpatient)	19	100%	98%	98%
Prophylactic Antibiotic Stopped[2]	25	96%	98%	98%
Prophylactic Antibiotic Timing[2]	25	96%	99%	99%
Prophylactic Antibiotic Timing (Outpatient)	20	95%	98%	98%
Urinary Catheter Removal[2]	44	98%	96%	97%
Survey of Patients' Hospital Experiences				
Area Around Room 'Always' Quiet at Night	300+	70%	67%	61%
Doctors 'Always' Communicated Well	300+	85%	84%	82%
Home Recovery Information Given	300+	88%	85%	85%
Hospital Given 9 or 10 on 10 Point Scale	300+	69%	70%	71%
Meds 'Always' Explained Before Given	300+	70%	66%	64%
Nurses 'Always' Communicated Well	300+	81%	80%	79%
Pain 'Always' Well Controlled	300+	71%	72%	71%
Room and Bathroom 'Always' Clean	300+	69%	73%	73%
Timely Help 'Always' Received	300+	61%	68%	68%
Would Definitely Recommend Hospital	300+	71%	70%	71%
Use of Medical Imaging				

NOTE: Hospital profiles are in alphabetical order by state, then city, then hospital within the city; Rankings exclude hospitals with less than 25 cases except for patient surveys which excludes hospitals with less than 100 cases; (a) 100-299 cases; (1) The number of cases/patients is too few to report; (2) Data submitted were based on a sample of cases/patients; (3) Results are based on a shorter time period than required; (4) Data suppressed by CMS for one or more quarters; (5) Results are not available for this reporting period; (6) Fewer than 100 patients completed the HCAHPS survey; (7) No cases met the criteria for this measure; (8) The lower limit of the confidence interval cannot be calculated if the number of observed infections equals zero; (9) No data are available from the state/territory for this reporting period; (10) The scores shown reflect fewer than 50 completed surveys; (11) There were discrepancies in the data collection process; (12) This measure does not apply to this hospital for this reporting period; (13) Results cannot be calculated for this reporting period; (14) The results for this state are combined with nearby states to protect confidentiality; Please refer to the User's Guide for a full explanation of data.

Cardiac Imaging Stress Test before Surgery	298	5.0%	4.8%	5.3%
Combination Abdominal CT Scan	386	11.7%	9.6%	10.5%
Combination Brain/Sinus CT Scan[1]	-	-	3.3%	2.7%
Combination Chest CT Scan	410	3.7%	3.4%	2.7%
Follow-up Mammogram/Ultrasound	510	9.2%	8.3%	8.8%
Lumbar Spine MRI for Low Back Pain	72	37.5%	35.3%	37.2%

Marshall Medical Center

1080 North Ellington Parkway
Lewisburg, TN 37091
Phone: 931-359-6276
Fax: 931-359-9522
Type: Critical Access Hospitals
Emergency Services: Yes
Ownership: Govt - Hospital Dist/Auth
Beds: 119

Key Personnel:
Chief of Medical Staff.......... Jerry Arnold, MD
CEO/President............... Phyllis Brown
Radiology.................. Robert J Mahoney

Measure	Cases	This Hosp.	State Avg.	U.S. Avg.
Blood Clot Prevention and Treatment				
Anticoagulation Overlap Therapy[5]	-	-	92%	93%
ICU Venous Thromboembolism Prophylaxis[5]	-	-	90%	92%
Incidence of Potentially Preventable VTE[5]	-	-	10%	10%
UFH with Dosages/Platelet Monitoring[5]	-	-	99%	97%
Venous Thromboembolism Prophylaxis[5]	-	-	83%	85%
Warfarin Therapy Discharge Instructions[5]	-	-	78%	75%
Chest Pain/Possible Heart Attack Care				
Aspirin Given Within 24 Hours of Arrival	68	90%	96%	96%
Fibrinolytic Meds Within 30 Min. of Arrival[7]	-	-	72%	58%
Average Time to ECG (minutes)	73	11	6	7
Average Time to Transfer (minutes)[7]	-	-	53	60
Children's Asthma Care				
Received Home Management Plan of Care	-	-	-	88%
Received Reliever Medication	-	-	-	100%
Received Systemic Corticosteroids	-	-	-	100%
Emergency Department				
Admittance Decision Time (minutes)[5]	-	-	82	98
Head CT Results Within 45 Min. of Arrival[5]	-	-	52%	57%
Patients Who Left ER Before Being Seen	13,993	3%	2%	2%
Time from ER Arrival to Admit. (minutes)[5]	-	-	243	274
Time from ER Arrival to Discharge (minutes)[5]	-	-	131	134
Time in ER Before Being Evaluated (minutes)[5]	-	-	25	26
Time to Pain Meds for Fractures (minutes)[5]	-	-	60	57
Heart Attack Care				
Aspirin Given at Discharge[5]	-	-	99%	99%
Fibrinolytic Meds Within 30 Min. of Arrival[5]	-	-	33%	54%
PCI Within 90 Minutes of Arrival[5]	-	-	98%	96%
Statin Prescribed at Discharge[5]	-	-	99%	98%
Heart Failure Care				
ACE Inhibitor or ARB for LVSD[1]	-	-	97%	97%
Discharge Instructions Given[1]	-	-	93%	94%
Evaluation of LVS Function	11	100%	99%	99%
Medicare Spending				
Medicare Spending per Patient (ratio)	-	-	1	0.98
Pneumonia Care				
Appropriate Initial Antibiotic Given	27	89%	95%	95%
Blood Culture Timing	36	94%	98%	98%
Pregnancy and Delivery Care				
Newborn Deliveries Scheduled Early[5]	-	-	6%	6%
Preventive Care				
Immunization for Influenza[5]	-	-	93%	90%
Immunization for Pneumonia[5]	-	-	93%	92%
Stroke Care				
Anticoagulation Therapy for Atrial Fibrillation[5]	-	-	94%	95%
Antithrombotic Therapy Timing[5]	-	-	97%	98%
Assessed for Rehabilitation[5]	-	-	97%	97%
Discharged on Antithrombotic Therapy[5]	-	-	99%	99%
Discharged on Statin Medication[5]	-	-	94%	94%
Thrombolytic Therapy Timing[5]	-	-	57%	66%
Venous Thromboembolism Prophylaxis[5]	-	-	93%	94%
Written Stroke Educational Materials Given[5]	-	-	84%	88%
Surgical Care Improvement Project				
Appropriate Beta Blocker Usage[5]	-	-	97%	98%
Appropriate VTP Within 24 Hours[5]	-	-	98%	98%
Controlled Postoperative Blood Glucose[5]	-	-	95%	97%
Perioperative Temperature Management[5]	-	-	100%	100%
Prophylactic Antibiotic Selection[5]	-	-	99%	99%
Prophylactic Antibiotic Selection (Outpatient)[1,3]	-	-	98%	98%
Prophylactic Antibiotic Stopped[5]	-	-	98%	98%
Prophylactic Antibiotic Timing[5]	-	-	99%	99%
Prophylactic Antibiotic Timing (Outpatient)[1,3]	-	-	98%	98%
Urinary Catheter Removal[5]	-	-	96%	97%
Survey of Patients' Hospital Experiences				
Area Around Room 'Always' Quiet at Night[6]	<100	81%	67%	61%
Doctors 'Always' Communicated Well[6]	<100	87%	84%	82%
Home Recovery Information Given[6]	<100	83%	85%	85%
Hospital Given 9 or 10 on 10 Point Scale[6]	<100	72%	70%	71%
Meds 'Always' Explained Before Given[6]	<100	64%	66%	64%
Nurses 'Always' Communicated Well[6]	<100	84%	80%	79%
Pain 'Always' Well Controlled[6]	<100	74%	72%	71%
Room and Bathroom 'Always' Clean[6]	<100	75%	73%	73%
Timely Help 'Always' Received[6]	<100	86%	68%	68%
Would Definitely Recommend Hospital[6]	<100	64%	70%	71%
Use of Medical Imaging				
Cardiac Imaging Stress Test before Surgery	52	1.9%	4.8%	5.3%
Combination Abdominal CT Scan	108	11.1%	9.6%	10.5%
Combination Brain/Sinus CT Scan[1]	-	-	3.3%	2.7%
Combination Chest CT Scan	107	3.7%	3.4%	2.7%
Follow-up Mammogram/Ultrasound	370	7.8%	8.3%	8.8%
Lumbar Spine MRI for Low Back Pain[1]	-	-	35.3%	37.2%

Henderson County Community Hospital

200 W Church St
Lexington, TN 38351
Phone: 731-968-1801
Fax: 731-968-8113
URL: www.hendersoncchospital.com
Type: Acute Care Hospitals
Emergency Services: Yes
Ownership: Proprietary
Beds: 36

Key Personnel:
CEO/President.............. Holly Fowler
Chief of Medical Staff.......... Charles White, Jr
Emergency Room .... Joe Wilhite, MD

Measure	Cases	This Hosp.	State Avg.	U.S. Avg.
Blood Clot Prevention and Treatment				
Anticoagulation Overlap Therapy[1,2]	-	-	92%	93%
ICU Venous Thromboembolism Prophylaxis[2,7]	-	-	90%	92%
Incidence of Potentially Preventable VTE[1,2]	-	-	10%	10%
UFH with Dosages/Platelet Monitoring[1,2]	-	-	99%	97%
Venous Thromboembolism Prophylaxis[2]	303	100%	83%	85%
Warfarin Therapy Discharge Instructions[2,7]	-	-	78%	75%
Chest Pain/Possible Heart Attack Care				
Aspirin Given Within 24 Hours of Arrival	58	100%	96%	96%
Fibrinolytic Meds Within 30 Min. of Arrival[1]	-	-	72%	58%
Average Time to ECG (minutes)	62	0	6	7
Average Time to Transfer (minutes)[7]	-	-	53	60
Children's Asthma Care				
Received Home Management Plan of Care	-	-	-	88%
Received Reliever Medication	-	-	-	100%
Received Systemic Corticosteroids	-	-	-	100%
Emergency Department				
Admittance Decision Time (minutes)[2]	426	34	82	98
Head CT Results Within 45 Min. of Arrival[1]	-	-	52%	57%
Patients Who Left ER Before Being Seen	10,575	1%	2%	2%
Time from ER Arrival to Admit. (minutes)[2]	427	141	243	274
Time from ER Arrival to Discharge (minutes)	352	76	131	134
Time in ER Before Being Evaluated (minutes)	434	16	25	26
Time to Pain Meds for Fractures (minutes)	38	45	60	57
Heart Attack Care				
Aspirin Given at Discharge[1,3]	-	-	99%	99%
Fibrinolytic Meds Within 30 Min. of Arrival[3,7]	-	-	33%	54%
PCI Within 90 Minutes of Arrival[3,7]	-	-	98%	96%
Statin Prescribed at Discharge[1,3]	-	-	99%	98%
Heart Failure Care				
ACE Inhibitor or ARB for LVSD[1]	-	-	97%	97%
Discharge Instructions Given	23	96%	93%	94%
Evaluation of LVS Function	33	100%	99%	99%
Medicare Spending				
Medicare Spending per Patient (ratio)	-	1.05	1	0.98
Pneumonia Care				
Appropriate Initial Antibiotic Given	27	100%	95%	95%
Blood Culture Timing	45	100%	98%	98%
Pregnancy and Delivery Care				
Newborn Deliveries Scheduled Early[2,7]	-	-	6%	6%
Preventive Care				
Immunization for Influenza[2]	311	100%	93%	90%
Immunization for Pneumonia[2]	423	100%	93%	92%
Stroke Care				
Anticoagulation Therapy for Atrial Fibrillation[3,7]	-	-	94%	95%
Antithrombotic Therapy Timing[1,3]	-	-	97%	98%
Assessed for Rehabilitation[1,3]	-	-	97%	97%
Discharged on Antithrombotic Therapy[1,3]	-	-	99%	99%
Discharged on Statin Medication[1,3]	-	-	94%	94%
Thrombolytic Therapy Timing[1,3]	-	-	57%	66%
Venous Thromboembolism Prophylaxis[1,3]	-	-	93%	94%
Written Stroke Educational Materials Given[3,7]	-	-	84%	88%
Surgical Care Improvement Project				
Appropriate Beta Blocker Usage[1]	-	-	97%	98%
Appropriate VTP Within 24 Hours[1]	-	-	98%	98%
Controlled Postoperative Blood Glucose[7]	-	-	95%	97%
Perioperative Temperature Management[1]	-	-	100%	100%
Prophylactic Antibiotic Selection[1]	-	-	99%	99%
Prophylactic Antibiotic Selection (Outpatient)[1,3]	-	-	98%	98%
Prophylactic Antibiotic Stopped[1]	-	-	98%	98%
Prophylactic Antibiotic Timing[1]	-	-	99%	99%
Prophylactic Antibiotic Timing (Outpatient)[1,3]	-	-	98%	98%
Urinary Catheter Removal[1]	-	-	96%	97%
Survey of Patients' Hospital Experiences				
Area Around Room 'Always' Quiet at Night	(a)	70%	67%	61%
Doctors 'Always' Communicated Well	(a)	87%	84%	82%
Home Recovery Information Given	(a)	87%	85%	85%
Hospital Given 9 or 10 on 10 Point Scale	(a)	74%	70%	71%
Meds 'Always' Explained Before Given	(a)	78%	66%	64%
Nurses 'Always' Communicated Well	(a)	88%	80%	79%
Pain 'Always' Well Controlled	(a)	78%	72%	71%
Room and Bathroom 'Always' Clean	(a)	74%	73%	73%
Timely Help 'Always' Received	(a)	80%	68%	68%
Would Definitely Recommend Hospital	(a)	67%	70%	71%
Use of Medical Imaging				
Cardiac Imaging Stress Test before Surgery[1]	-	-	4.8%	5.3%
Combination Abdominal CT Scan	170	2.9%	9.6%	10.5%
Combination Brain/Sinus CT Scan[1]	-	-	3.3%	2.7%
Combination Chest CT Scan	60	1.7%	3.4%	2.7%
Follow-up Mammogram/Ultrasound	166	11.4%	8.3%	8.8%
Lumbar Spine MRI for Low Back Pain[1]	-	-	35.3%	37.2%

Perry Community Hospital

2718 Squirrel Hollow Drive
Linden, TN 37096
Phone: 931-589-2121
Fax: 931-589-3331
E-mail: pdbosp@mtcase.net
Type: Acute Care Hospitals
Emergency Services: Yes
Ownership: Proprietary
Beds: 53

Key Personnel:
Chief of Medical Staff.......... Andrew Averett, MD
Quality Assurance .... Brenda Stom
Emergency Room .... Leah Watkins, RN

Measure	Cases	This Hosp.	State Avg.	U.S. Avg.
Blood Clot Prevention and Treatment				
Anticoagulation Overlap Therapy[2,7]	-	-	92%	93%
ICU Venous Thromboembolism Prophylaxis[2,7]	-	-	90%	92%
Incidence of Potentially Preventable VTE[2,7]	-	-	10%	10%
UFH with Dosages/Platelet Monitoring[2,7]	-	-	99%	97%
Venous Thromboembolism Prophylaxis[2]	244	9%	83%	85%
Warfarin Therapy Discharge Instructions[2,7]	-	-	78%	75%
Chest Pain/Possible Heart Attack Care				
Aspirin Given Within 24 Hours of Arrival	49	71%	96%	96%
Fibrinolytic Meds Within 30 Min. of Arrival[1,3]	-	-	72%	58%
Average Time to ECG (minutes)	51	5	6	7
Average Time to Transfer (minutes)[1,3]	-	-	53	60
Children's Asthma Care				
Received Home Management Plan of Care	-	-	-	88%
Received Reliever Medication	-	-	-	100%
Received Systemic Corticosteroids	-	-	-	100%

NOTE: Hospital profiles are in alphabetical order by state, then city, then hospital within the city; Rankings exclude hospitals with less than 25 cases except for patient surveys which excludes hospitals with less than 100 cases; (a) 100-299 cases; (1) The number of cases/patients is too few to report; (2) Data submitted were based on a sample of cases/patients; (3) Results are based on a shorter time period than required; (4) Data suppressed by CMS for one or more quarters; (5) Results are not available for this reporting period; (6) Fewer than 100 patients completed the HCAHPS survey; (7) No cases met the criteria for this measure; (8) The lower limit of the confidence interval cannot be calculated if the number of observed infections equals zero; (9) No data are available from the state/territory for this reporting period; (10) The scores shown reflect fewer than 50 completed surveys; (11) There were discrepancies in the data collection process; (12) This measure does not apply to this hospital for this reporting period; (13) Results cannot be calculated for this reporting period; (14) The results for this state are combined with nearby states to protect confidentiality; Please refer to the User's Guide for a full explanation of data.

Measure	Cases	This Hosp.	State Avg.	U.S. Avg.
Emergency Department				
Admittance Decision Time (minutes)[2]	222	0	82	98
Head CT Results Within 45 Min. of Arrival[1]	-	-	52%	57%
Patients Who Left ER Before Being Seen	4,534	2%	2%	2%
Time from ER Arrival to Admit. (minutes)[2]	273	155	243	274
Time from ER Arrival to Discharge (minutes)	628	100	131	134
Time in ER Before Being Evaluated (minutes)	720	10	25	26
Time to Pain Meds for Fractures (minutes)	17	45	60	57
Heart Attack Care				
Aspirin Given at Discharge[1,2]	-	-	99%	99%
Fibrinolytic Meds Within 30 Min. of Arrival[1,2]	-	-	33%	54%
PCI Within 90 Minutes of Arrival[2,3]	-	-	98%	96%
Statin Prescribed at Discharge[1,2]	-	-	99%	98%
Heart Failure Care				
ACE Inhibitor or ARB for LVSD[2,7]	-	-	97%	97%
Discharge Instructions Given[2]	25	96%	93%	94%
Evaluation of LVS Function[2]	44	0%	99%	99%
Medicare Spending				
Medicare Spending per Patient (ratio)	-	1.09	1	0.98
Pneumonia Care				
Appropriate Initial Antibiotic Given[2]	26	50%	95%	95%
Blood Culture Timing[1,2]	-	-	98%	98%
Pregnancy and Delivery Care				
Newborn Deliveries Scheduled Early[2,7]	-	-	6%	6%
Preventive Care				
Immunization for Influenza[2]	314	24%	93%	90%
Immunization for Pneumonia[2]	561	23%	93%	92%
Stroke Care				
Anticoagulation Therapy for Atrial Fibrillation[5]	-	-	94%	95%
Antithrombotic Therapy Timing[5]	-	-	97%	98%
Assessed for Rehabilitation[5]	-	-	97%	97%
Discharged on Antithrombotic Therapy[5]	-	-	99%	99%
Discharged on Statin Medication[5]	-	-	94%	94%
Thrombolytic Therapy Timing[5]	-	-	57%	66%
Venous Thromboembolism Prophylaxis[5]	-	-	93%	94%
Written Stroke Educational Materials Given[5]	-	-	84%	88%
Surgical Care Improvement Project				
Appropriate Beta Blocker Usage[5]	-	-	97%	98%
Appropriate VTP Within 24 Hours[5]	-	-	98%	98%
Controlled Postoperative Blood Glucose[5]	-	-	95%	97%
Perioperative Temperature Management[5]	-	-	100%	100%
Prophylactic Antibiotic Selection[5]	-	-	99%	99%
Prophylactic Antibiotic Selection (Outpatient)[5]	-	-	98%	98%
Prophylactic Antibiotic Stopped[5]	-	-	98%	98%
Prophylactic Antibiotic Timing[5]	-	-	99%	99%
Prophylactic Antibiotic Timing (Outpatient)[5]	-	-	98%	98%
Urinary Catheter Removal[5]	-	-	96%	97%
Survey of Patients' Hospital Experiences				
Area Around Room 'Always' Quiet at Night[6]	<100	50%	67%	61%
Doctors 'Always' Communicated Well[6]	<100	77%	84%	82%
Home Recovery Information Given[6]	<100	86%	85%	85%
Hospital Given 9 or 10 on 10 Point Scale[6]	<100	52%	70%	71%
Meds 'Always' Explained Before Given[6]	<100	53%	66%	64%
Nurses 'Always' Communicated Well[6]	<100	72%	80%	79%
Pain 'Always' Well Controlled[6]	<100	63%	72%	71%
Room and Bathroom 'Always' Clean[6]	<100	57%	73%	73%
Timely Help 'Always' Received[6]	<100	62%	68%	68%
Would Definitely Recommend Hospital[6]	<100	67%	70%	71%
Use of Medical Imaging				
Cardiac Imaging Stress Test before Surgery[7]	-	-	4.8%	5.3%
Combination Abdominal CT Scan[1]	-	-	9.6%	10.5%
Combination Brain/Sinus CT Scan	65	0.0%	3.3%	2.7%
Combination Chest CT Scan[1]	-	-	3.4%	2.7%
Follow-up Mammogram/Ultrasound[7]	-	-	8.3%	8.8%
Lumbar Spine MRI for Low Back Pain[7]	-	-	35.3%	37.2%

Livingston Regional Hospital

315 Oak Saint Box 550 Phone: 931-823-5611
Livingston, TN 38570 Fax: 931-403-2334
URL: www.livingstonregionalhospital.com
Type: Acute Care Hospitals Emergency Services: Yes
Ownership: Voluntary non-profit - Other Beds: 114
Key Personnel:
Chief of Medical Staff.......... John Clough, MD
Pediatric Ambulatory Care...... Jessie Lee Copeland, MD
CEO...................... Joanne Fenton, MBA, BNS, FACHE
Emergency Room............ Richard Fields, MD
Radiology.................. Donald Huff, MD

Measure	Cases	This Hosp.	State Avg.	U.S. Avg.
Blood Clot Prevention and Treatment				
Anticoagulation Overlap Therapy[1,2]	-	-	92%	93%
ICU Venous Thromboembolism Prophylaxis[2]	47	100%	90%	92%
Incidence of Potentially Preventable VTE[1,2]	-	-	10%	10%
UFH with Dosages/Platelet Monitoring[1,2]	-	-	99%	97%
Venous Thromboembolism Prophylaxis[2]	241	100%	83%	85%
Warfarin Therapy Discharge Instructions[1,2]	-	-	78%	75%
Chest Pain/Possible Heart Attack Care				
Aspirin Given Within 24 Hours of Arrival	48	96%	96%	96%
Fibrinolytic Meds Within 30 Min. of Arrival[7]	-	-	72%	58%
Average Time to ECG (minutes)	50	2	6	7
Average Time to Transfer (minutes)[1]	-	-	53	60
Children's Asthma Care				
Received Home Management Plan of Care	-	-	-	88%
Received Reliever Medication	-	-	-	100%
Received Systemic Corticosteroids	-	-	-	100%
Emergency Department				
Admittance Decision Time (minutes)[2]	164	48	82	98
Head CT Results Within 45 Min. of Arrival[1]	-	-	52%	57%
Patients Who Left ER Before Being Seen	12,487	2%	2%	2%
Time from ER Arrival to Admit. (minutes)[2]	164	164	243	274
Time from ER Arrival to Discharge (minutes)	381	97	131	134
Time in ER Before Being Evaluated (minutes)	443	8	25	26
Time to Pain Meds for Fractures (minutes)	52	18	60	57
Heart Attack Care				
Aspirin Given at Discharge[1,3]	-	-	99%	99%
Fibrinolytic Meds Within 30 Min. of Arrival[3,7]	-	-	33%	54%
PCI Within 90 Minutes of Arrival[3,7]	-	-	98%	96%
Statin Prescribed at Discharge[1,3]	-	-	99%	98%
Heart Failure Care				
ACE Inhibitor or ARB for LVSD	13	100%	97%	97%
Discharge Instructions Given	47	100%	93%	94%
Evaluation of LVS Function	64	100%	99%	99%
Medicare Spending				
Medicare Spending per Patient (ratio)	-	1.04	1	0.98
Pneumonia Care				
Appropriate Initial Antibiotic Given	155	95%	95%	95%
Blood Culture Timing	204	100%	98%	98%
Pregnancy and Delivery Care				
Newborn Deliveries Scheduled Early[2]	31	6%	6%	6%
Preventive Care				
Immunization for Influenza[2]	261	100%	93%	90%
Immunization for Pneumonia[2]	318	100%	93%	92%
Stroke Care				
Anticoagulation Therapy for Atrial Fibrillation[7]	-	-	94%	95%
Antithrombotic Therapy Timing	17	94%	97%	98%
Assessed for Rehabilitation	17	100%	97%	97%
Discharged on Antithrombotic Therapy	16	100%	99%	99%
Discharged on Statin Medication	13	85%	94%	94%
Thrombolytic Therapy Timing[7]	-	-	57%	66%
Venous Thromboembolism Prophylaxis	16	88%	93%	94%
Written Stroke Educational Materials Given[1]	-	-	84%	88%
Surgical Care Improvement Project				
Appropriate Beta Blocker Usage[1]	-	-	97%	98%
Appropriate VTP Within 24 Hours	29	100%	98%	98%
Controlled Postoperative Blood Glucose[7]	-	-	95%	97%
Perioperative Temperature Management	30	100%	100%	100%
Prophylactic Antibiotic Selection	26	100%	99%	99%
Prophylactic Antibiotic Selection (Outpatient)	34	97%	98%	98%
Prophylactic Antibiotic Stopped	24	88%	98%	98%
Prophylactic Antibiotic Timing	26	100%	99%	99%
Prophylactic Antibiotic Timing (Outpatient)	34	100%	98%	98%
Urinary Catheter Removal	22	95%	96%	97%
Survey of Patients' Hospital Experiences				
Area Around Room 'Always' Quiet at Night	300+	61%	67%	61%
Doctors 'Always' Communicated Well	300+	90%	84%	82%
Home Recovery Information Given	300+	82%	85%	85%
Hospital Given 9 or 10 on 10 Point Scale	300+	64%	70%	71%
Meds 'Always' Explained Before Given	300+	64%	66%	64%
Nurses 'Always' Communicated Well	300+	78%	80%	79%
Pain 'Always' Well Controlled	300+	69%	72%	71%
Room and Bathroom 'Always' Clean	300+	68%	73%	73%
Timely Help 'Always' Received	300+	64%	68%	68%
Would Definitely Recommend Hospital	300+	67%	70%	71%
Use of Medical Imaging				
Cardiac Imaging Stress Test before Surgery	137	6.6%	4.8%	5.3%
Combination Abdominal CT Scan	314	20.7%	9.6%	10.5%
Combination Brain/Sinus CT Scan	292	5.8%	3.3%	2.7%
Combination Chest CT Scan	147	4.1%	3.4%	2.7%
Follow-up Mammogram/Ultrasound	398	5.0%	8.3%	8.8%
Lumbar Spine MRI for Low Back Pain	70	38.6%	35.3%	37.2%

Medical Center of Manchester

481 Interstate Drive Phone: 931-728-6354
Manchester, TN 37355 Fax: 931-728-5420
Type: Critical Access Hospitals Emergency Services: Yes
Ownership: Proprietary Beds: 49
Key Personnel:
Intensive Care Unit............ Brenda Ballard, RN
Chief of Medical Staff.......... AR Brandon, DO
Emergency Room............ Gina Brennan, RN
CEO/President.............. Robert J Couch
Infection Control............. Suzanne Knox, LPN
Operating Room.............. Lisa Winkler

Measure	Cases	This Hosp.	State Avg.	U.S. Avg.
Blood Clot Prevention and Treatment				
Anticoagulation Overlap Therapy[5]	-	-	92%	93%
ICU Venous Thromboembolism Prophylaxis[5]	-	-	90%	92%
Incidence of Potentially Preventable VTE[5]	-	-	10%	10%
UFH with Dosages/Platelet Monitoring[5]	-	-	99%	97%
Venous Thromboembolism Prophylaxis[5]	-	-	83%	85%
Warfarin Therapy Discharge Instructions[5]	-	-	78%	75%
Chest Pain/Possible Heart Attack Care				
Aspirin Given Within 24 Hours of Arrival	44	80%	96%	96%
Fibrinolytic Meds Within 30 Min. of Arrival[1]	-	-	72%	58%
Average Time to ECG (minutes)	46	28	6	7
Average Time to Transfer (minutes)[1]	-	-	53	60
Children's Asthma Care				
Received Home Management Plan of Care	-	-	-	88%
Received Reliever Medication	-	-	-	100%
Received Systemic Corticosteroids	-	-	-	100%
Emergency Department				
Admittance Decision Time (minutes)[5]	-	-	82	98
Head CT Results Within 45 Min. of Arrival[5]	-	-	52%	57%
Patients Who Left ER Before Being Seen[5]	-	-	2%	2%
Time from ER Arrival to Admit. (minutes)[5]	-	-	243	274
Time from ER Arrival to Discharge (minutes)[5]	-	-	131	134
Time in ER Before Being Evaluated (minutes)[5]	-	-	25	26
Time to Pain Meds for Fractures (minutes)[5]	-	-	60	57
Heart Attack Care				
Aspirin Given at Discharge[5]	-	-	99%	99%
Fibrinolytic Meds Within 30 Min. of Arrival[5]	-	-	33%	54%
PCI Within 90 Minutes of Arrival[5]	-	-	98%	96%
Statin Prescribed at Discharge[5]	-	-	99%	98%
Heart Failure Care				
ACE Inhibitor or ARB for LVSD[1]	-	-	97%	97%
Discharge Instructions Given	17	59%	93%	94%
Evaluation of LVS Function	21	33%	99%	99%
Medicare Spending				
Medicare Spending per Patient (ratio)	-	-	1	0.98
Pneumonia Care				
Appropriate Initial Antibiotic Given[1]	-	-	95%	95%
Blood Culture Timing[1]	-	-	98%	98%
Pregnancy and Delivery Care				
Newborn Deliveries Scheduled Early[5]	-	-	6%	6%
Preventive Care				
Immunization for Influenza[5]	-	-	93%	90%
Immunization for Pneumonia[5]	-	-	93%	92%
Stroke Care				
Anticoagulation Therapy for Atrial Fibrillation[5]	-	-	94%	95%

NOTE: Hospital profiles are in alphabetical order by state, then city, then hospital within the city; Rankings exclude hospitals with less than 25 cases except for patient surveys which excludes hospitals with less than 100 cases; (a) 100-299 cases; (1) The number of cases/patients is too few to report; (2) Data submitted were based on a sample of cases/patients; (3) Results are based on a shorter time period than required; (4) Data suppressed by CMS for one or more quarters; (5) Results are not available for this reporting period; (6) Fewer than 100 patients completed the HCAHPS survey; (7) No cases met the criteria for this measure; (8) The lower limit of the confidence interval cannot be calculated if the number of observed infections equals zero; (9) No data are available from the state/territory for this reporting period; (10) The scores shown reflect fewer than 50 completed surveys; (11) There were discrepancies in the data collection process; (12) This measure does not apply to this hospital for this reporting period; (13) Results cannot be calculated for this reporting period; (14) The results for this state are combined with nearby states to protect confidentiality; Please refer to the User's Guide for a full explanation of data.

Measure	Cases	This Hosp.	State Avg.	U.S. Avg.
Antithrombotic Therapy Timing[5]	-	-	97%	98%
Assessed for Rehabilitation[5]	-	-	97%	97%
Discharged on Antithrombotic Therapy[5]	-	-	99%	99%
Discharged on Statin Medication[5]	-	-	94%	94%
Thrombolytic Therapy Timing[5]	-	-	57%	66%
Venous Thromboembolism Prophylaxis[5]	-	-	93%	94%
Written Stroke Educational Materials Given[5]	-	-	84%	88%
Surgical Care Improvement Project				
Appropriate Beta Blocker Usage[5]	-	-	97%	98%
Appropriate VTP Within 24 Hours[5]	-	-	98%	98%
Controlled Postoperative Blood Glucose[5]	-	-	95%	97%
Perioperative Temperature Management[5]	-	-	100%	100%
Prophylactic Antibiotic Selection[5]	-	-	99%	99%
Prophylactic Antibiotic Selection (Outpatient)[5]	-	-	98%	98%
Prophylactic Antibiotic Stopped[5]	-	-	98%	98%
Prophylactic Antibiotic Timing[5]	-	-	99%	99%
Prophylactic Antibiotic Timing (Outpatient)[5]	-	-	98%	98%
Urinary Catheter Removal[5]	-	-	96%	97%
Survey of Patients' Hospital Experiences				
Area Around Room 'Always' Quiet at Night[5]	-	-	67%	61%
Doctors 'Always' Communicated Well[5]	-	-	84%	82%
Home Recovery Information Given[5]	-	-	85%	85%
Hospital Given 9 or 10 on 10 Point Scale[5]	-	-	70%	71%
Meds 'Always' Explained Before Given[5]	-	-	66%	64%
Nurses 'Always' Communicated Well[5]	-	-	80%	79%
Pain 'Always' Well Controlled[5]	-	-	72%	71%
Room and Bathroom 'Always' Clean[5]	-	-	73%	73%
Timely Help 'Always' Received[5]	-	-	68%	68%
Would Definitely Recommend Hospital[5]	-	-	70%	71%
Use of Medical Imaging				
Cardiac Imaging Stress Test before Surgery[1]	-	-	4.8%	5.3%
Combination Abdominal CT Scan	164	6.1%	9.6%	10.5%
Combination Brain/Sinus CT Scan	235	5.1%	3.3%	2.7%
Combination Chest CT Scan[1]	-	-	3.4%	2.7%
Follow-up Mammogram/Ultrasound[7]	-	-	8.3%	8.8%
Lumbar Spine MRI for Low Back Pain[1]	-	-	35.3%	37.2%

United Regional Medical Center

1001 Mcarthur St
Manchester, TN 37355
URL: www.urmchealthcare.com
Type: Acute Care Hospitals
Ownership: Proprietary
Phone: 931-728-3586
Fax: 931-728-6877
Emergency Services: Yes
Beds: 126

Key Personnel:

Quality Assurance . . . . Pam Adderson, RN
Chairman/CEO . . . . Glenn Davis, MD
Chief of Medical Staff . . . . Glenn Davis
CEO/President. . . . . Robert George
Emergency Room . . . . Richie Lupo
Radiology. . . . . Wendell McAbee
Operating Room. . . . . Councill C Rudolph
Infection Control. . . . . Virginia Smith, RN

Measure	Cases	This Hosp.	State Avg.	U.S. Avg.
Blood Clot Prevention and Treatment				
Anticoagulation Overlap Therapy[1,2]	-	-	92%	93%
ICU Venous Thromboembolism Prophylaxis[2,7]	-	-	90%	92%
Incidence of Potentially Preventable VTE[2,7]	-	-	10%	10%
UFH with Dosages/Platelet Monitoring[2,7]	-	-	99%	97%
Venous Thromboembolism Prophylaxis[2]	125	100%	83%	85%
Warfarin Therapy Discharge Instructions[1,2]	-	-	78%	75%
Chest Pain/Possible Heart Attack Care				
Aspirin Given Within 24 Hours of Arrival[3]	24	100%	96%	96%
Fibrinolytic Meds Within 30 Min. of Arrival[3,7]	-	-	72%	58%
Average Time to ECG (minutes)[3]	23	9	6	7
Average Time to Transfer (minutes)[1,3]	-	-	53	60
Children's Asthma Care				
Received Home Management Plan of Care	-	-	-	88%
Received Reliever Medication	-	-	-	100%
Received Systemic Corticosteroids	-	-	-	100%
Emergency Department				
Admittance Decision Time (minutes)[2]	264	66	82	98
Head CT Results Within 45 Min. of Arrival[5]	-	-	52%	57%
Patients Who Left ER Before Being Seen[5]	-	-	2%	2%
Time from ER Arrival to Admit. (minutes)[2]	276	214	243	274
Time from ER Arrival to Discharge (minutes)	334	130	131	134
Time in ER Before Being Evaluated (minutes)	391	38	25	26
Time to Pain Meds for Fractures (minutes)	31	51	60	57
Heart Attack Care				
Aspirin Given at Discharge[5]	-	-	99%	99%
Fibrinolytic Meds Within 30 Min. of Arrival[5]	-	-	33%	54%
PCI Within 90 Minutes of Arrival[5]	-	-	98%	96%
Statin Prescribed at Discharge[5]	-	-	99%	98%
Heart Failure Care				
ACE Inhibitor or ARB for LVSD[1,2]	-	-	97%	97%
Discharge Instructions Given[2]	31	100%	93%	94%
Evaluation of LVS Function[2]	37	92%	99%	99%
Medicare Spending				
Medicare Spending per Patient (ratio) *	-	0.86	1	0.98
Pneumonia Care				
Appropriate Initial Antibiotic Given[2]	132	86%	95%	95%
Blood Culture Timing[2]	99	94%	98%	98%
Pregnancy and Delivery Care				
Newborn Deliveries Scheduled Early[7]	-	-	6%	6%
Preventive Care				
Immunization for Influenza[2]	304	84%	93%	90%
Immunization for Pneumonia[2]	399	90%	93%	92%
Stroke Care				
Anticoagulation Therapy for Atrial Fibrillation[5]	-	-	94%	95%
Antithrombotic Therapy Timing[5]	-	-	97%	98%
Assessed for Rehabilitation[5]	-	-	97%	97%
Discharged on Antithrombotic Therapy[5]	-	-	99%	99%
Discharged on Statin Medication[5]	-	-	94%	94%
Thrombolytic Therapy Timing[5]	-	-	57%	66%
Venous Thromboembolism Prophylaxis[5]	-	-	93%	94%
Written Stroke Educational Materials Given[5]	-	-	84%	88%
Surgical Care Improvement Project				
Appropriate Beta Blocker Usage[1,3]	-	-	97%	98%
Appropriate VTP Within 24 Hours[1,3]	-	-	98%	98%
Controlled Postoperative Blood Glucose[3,7]	-	-	95%	97%
Perioperative Temperature Management[3]	11	100%	100%	100%
Prophylactic Antibiotic Selection[1,3]	-	-	99%	99%
Prophylactic Antibiotic Selection (Outpatient)	84	94%	98%	98%
Prophylactic Antibiotic Stopped[1,3]	-	-	98%	98%
Prophylactic Antibiotic Timing[1,3]	-	-	99%	99%
Prophylactic Antibiotic Timing (Outpatient)	84	87%	98%	98%
Urinary Catheter Removal[3,7]	-	-	96%	97%
Survey of Patients' Hospital Experiences				
Area Around Room 'Always' Quiet at Night	(a)	76%	67%	61%
Doctors 'Always' Communicated Well	(a)	89%	84%	82%
Home Recovery Information Given	(a)	98%	85%	85%
Hospital Given 9 or 10 on 10 Point Scale	(a)	73%	70%	71%
Meds 'Always' Explained Before Given	(a)	64%	66%	64%
Nurses 'Always' Communicated Well	(a)	87%	80%	79%
Pain 'Always' Well Controlled	(a)	83%	72%	71%
Room and Bathroom 'Always' Clean	(a)	86%	73%	73%
Timely Help 'Always' Received	(a)	87%	68%	68%
Would Definitely Recommend Hospital	(a)	67%	70%	71%
Use of Medical Imaging				
Cardiac Imaging Stress Test before Surgery	70	8.6%	4.8%	5.3%
Combination Abdominal CT Scan	96	14.6%	9.6%	10.5%
Combination Brain/Sinus CT Scan[1]	-	-	3.3%	2.7%
Combination Chest CT Scan	61	26.2%	3.4%	2.7%
Follow-up Mammogram/Ultrasound	210	3.8%	8.3%	8.8%
Lumbar Spine MRI for Low Back Pain	149	23.5%	35.3%	37.2%

Volunteer Community Hospital

161 Mount Pelia Rd
Martin, TN 38237
URL: www.chs.net
Type: Acute Care Hospitals
Ownership: Proprietary
Phone: 731-587-4261
Fax: 731-587-6142
Emergency Services: Yes
Beds: 65

Key Personnel:

Quality Assurance . . . . Lori Brown
Radiology. . . . . Michelle Melotti, MD
Chief of Medical Staff . . . . Cynthia Phillips
Operating Room. . . . . Michael Saridakis
Intensive Care Unit. . . . . Lois Shanks, RN
CEO/President. . . . . Steve Westenhofer
Emergency Room . . . . James A Whitlock, DO
Infection Control. . . . . Betty Wilson

Measure	Cases	This Hosp.	State Avg.	U.S. Avg.
Blood Clot Prevention and Treatment				
Anticoagulation Overlap Therapy[1,2]	-	-	92%	93%
ICU Venous Thromboembolism Prophylaxis[2]	57	96%	90%	92%
Incidence of Potentially Preventable VTE[2,7]	-	-	10%	10%
UFH with Dosages/Platelet Monitoring[1,2]	-	-	99%	97%
Venous Thromboembolism Prophylaxis[2]	161	98%	83%	85%
Warfarin Therapy Discharge Instructions[1,2]	-	-	78%	75%
Chest Pain/Possible Heart Attack Care				
Aspirin Given Within 24 Hours of Arrival	191	99%	96%	96%
Fibrinolytic Meds Within 30 Min. of Arrival[1]	-	-	72%	58%
Average Time to ECG (minutes)	208	5	6	7
Average Time to Transfer (minutes)[1]	-	-	53	60
Children's Asthma Care				
Received Home Management Plan of Care	-	-	-	88%
Received Reliever Medication	-	-	-	100%
Received Systemic Corticosteroids	-	-	-	100%
Emergency Department				
Admittance Decision Time (minutes)[2]	279	86	82	98
Head CT Results Within 45 Min. of Arrival[1,3]	-	-	52%	57%
Patients Who Left ER Before Being Seen	11,485	1%	2%	2%
Time from ER Arrival to Admit. (minutes)[2]	284	220	243	274
Time from ER Arrival to Discharge (minutes)	346	105	131	134
Time in ER Before Being Evaluated (minutes)	419	34	25	26
Time to Pain Meds for Fractures (minutes)	37	72	60	57
Heart Attack Care				
Aspirin Given at Discharge[1,3]	-	-	99%	99%
Fibrinolytic Meds Within 30 Min. of Arrival[3,7]	-	-	33%	54%
PCI Within 90 Minutes of Arrival[3,7]	-	-	98%	96%
Statin Prescribed at Discharge[1,3]	-	-	99%	98%
Heart Failure Care				
ACE Inhibitor or ARB for LVSD[1]	-	-	97%	97%
Discharge Instructions Given	29	93%	93%	94%
Evaluation of LVS Function	41	98%	99%	99%
Medicare Spending				
Medicare Spending per Patient (ratio)	-	1.11	1	0.98
Pneumonia Care				
Appropriate Initial Antibiotic Given	41	95%	95%	95%
Blood Culture Timing	52	96%	98%	98%
Pregnancy and Delivery Care				
Newborn Deliveries Scheduled Early[2]	32	3%	6%	6%
Preventive Care				
Immunization for Influenza[2]	276	99%	93%	90%
Immunization for Pneumonia[2]	322	100%	93%	92%
Stroke Care				
Anticoagulation Therapy for Atrial Fibrillation[1]	-	-	94%	95%
Antithrombotic Therapy Timing[1]	-	-	97%	98%
Assessed for Rehabilitation[1]	-	-	97%	97%
Discharged on Antithrombotic Therapy[1]	-	-	99%	99%
Discharged on Statin Medication[1]	-	-	94%	94%
Thrombolytic Therapy Timing[7]	-	-	57%	66%
Venous Thromboembolism Prophylaxis	11	91%	93%	94%
Written Stroke Educational Materials Given[1]	-	-	84%	88%
Surgical Care Improvement Project				
Appropriate Beta Blocker Usage[1]	-	-	97%	98%
Appropriate VTP Within 24 Hours	43	100%	98%	98%
Controlled Postoperative Blood Glucose[7]	-	-	95%	97%
Perioperative Temperature Management	46	100%	100%	100%
Prophylactic Antibiotic Selection	29	100%	99%	99%
Prophylactic Antibiotic Selection (Outpatient)	65	100%	98%	98%
Prophylactic Antibiotic Stopped	27	100%	98%	98%
Prophylactic Antibiotic Timing	29	100%	99%	99%
Prophylactic Antibiotic Timing (Outpatient)	65	100%	98%	98%
Urinary Catheter Removal	12	100%	96%	97%
Survey of Patients' Hospital Experiences				
Area Around Room 'Always' Quiet at Night	300+	56%	67%	61%
Doctors 'Always' Communicated Well	300+	85%	84%	82%
Home Recovery Information Given	300+	87%	85%	85%
Hospital Given 9 or 10 on 10 Point Scale	300+	69%	70%	71%
Meds 'Always' Explained Before Given	300+	63%	66%	64%

NOTE: Hospital profiles are in alphabetical order by state, then city, then hospital within the city; Rankings exclude hospitals with less than 25 cases except for patient surveys which excludes hospitals with less than 100 cases; (a) 100-299 cases; (1) The number of cases/patients is too few to report; (2) Data submitted were based on a sample of cases/patients; (3) Results are based on a shorter time period than required; (4) Data suppressed by CMS for one or more quarters; (5) Results are not available for this reporting period; (6) Fewer than 100 patients completed the HCAHPS survey; (7) No cases met the criteria for this measure; (8) The lower limit of the confidence interval cannot be calculated if the number of observed infections equals zero; (9) No data are available from the state/territory for this reporting period; (10) The scores shown reflect fewer than 50 completed surveys; (11) There were discrepancies in the data collection process; (12) This measure does not apply to this hospital for this reporting period; (13) Results cannot be calculated for this reporting period; (14) The results for this state are combined with nearby states to protect confidentiality; Please refer to the User's Guide for a full explanation of data.

Measure	Cases	This Hosp.	State Avg.	U.S. Avg.
Nurses 'Always' Communicated Well	300+	80%	80%	79%
Pain 'Always' Well Controlled	300+	74%	72%	71%
Room and Bathroom 'Always' Clean	300+	77%	73%	73%
Timely Help 'Always' Received	300+	68%	68%	68%
Would Definitely Recommend Hospital	300+	65%	70%	71%
Use of Medical Imaging				
Cardiac Imaging Stress Test before Surgery[1]	-	-	4.8%	5.3%
Combination Abdominal CT Scan	247	4.9%	9.6%	10.5%
Combination Brain/Sinus CT Scan	289	4.8%	3.3%	2.7%
Combination Chest CT Scan	102	2.9%	3.4%	2.7%
Follow-up Mammogram/Ultrasound	428	6.1%	8.3%	8.8%
Lumbar Spine MRI for Low Back Pain[1]	-	-	35.3%	37.2%

Blount Memorial Hospital

907 E Lamar Alexander Parkway
Maryville, TN 37804
Phone: 865-983-7211
Fax: 865-977-5550
URL: www.blountmemorial.org
Type: Acute Care Hospitals
Emergency Services: Yes
Ownership: Government - Local
Beds: 272

Key Personnel:
Chief of Medical Staff.......... Marvin Beard, MD
Radiology.................... Daniel Cotton, MD
CEO/President................ Don Heinemann
Emergency Room .... Shirley Hutton
Operating Room.............. Carolyn Phillips

Measure	Cases	This Hosp.	State Avg.	U.S. Avg.
Blood Clot Prevention and Treatment				
Anticoagulation Overlap Therapy[2]	71	100%	92%	93%
ICU Venous Thromboembolism Prophylaxis[2]	72	94%	90%	92%
Incidence of Potentially Preventable VTE[2]	26	0%	10%	10%
UFH with Dosages/Platelet Monitoring[2]	12	100%	99%	97%
Venous Thromboembolism Prophylaxis[2]	369	96%	83%	85%
Warfarin Therapy Discharge Instructions[2]	44	82%	78%	75%
Chest Pain/Possible Heart Attack Care				
Aspirin Given Within 24 Hours of Arrival[5]	-	-	96%	96%
Fibrinolytic Meds Within 30 Min. of Arrival[5]	-	-	72%	58%
Average Time to ECG (minutes)[5]	-	-	6	7
Average Time to Transfer (minutes)[5]	-	-	53	60
Children's Asthma Care				
Received Home Management Plan of Care	-	-	-	88%
Received Reliever Medication	-	-	-	100%
Received Systemic Corticosteroids	-	-	-	100%
Emergency Department				
Admittance Decision Time (minutes)[2]	788	106	82	98
Head CT Results Within 45 Min. of Arrival	11	73%	52%	57%
Patients Who Left ER Before Being Seen	54,697	2%	2%	2%
Time from ER Arrival to Admit. (minutes)[2]	857	313	243	274
Time from ER Arrival to Discharge (minutes)	385	176	131	134
Time in ER Before Being Evaluated (minutes)	395	35	25	26
Time to Pain Meds for Fractures (minutes)	222	62	60	57
Heart Attack Care				
Aspirin Given at Discharge	194	99%	99%	99%
Fibrinolytic Meds Within 30 Min. of Arrival[7]	-	-	33%	54%
PCI Within 90 Minutes of Arrival	68	99%	98%	96%
Statin Prescribed at Discharge	194	97%	99%	98%
Heart Failure Care				
ACE Inhibitor or ARB for LVSD[2]	70	94%	97%	97%
Discharge Instructions Given[2]	212	87%	93%	94%
Evaluation of LVS Function[2]	267	100%	99%	99%
Medicare Spending				
Medicare Spending per Patient (ratio)	-	0.97	1	0.98
Pneumonia Care				
Appropriate Initial Antibiotic Given[2]	101	100%	95%	95%
Blood Culture Timing[2]	163	97%	98%	98%
Pregnancy and Delivery Care				
Newborn Deliveries Scheduled Early[2]	35	3%	6%	6%
Preventive Care				
Immunization for Influenza[2]	580	97%	93%	90%
Immunization for Pneumonia[2]	773	94%	93%	92%
Stroke Care				
Anticoagulation Therapy for Atrial Fibrillation[2]	13	100%	94%	95%
Antithrombotic Therapy Timing[2]	89	100%	97%	98%
Assessed for Rehabilitation[2]	102	99%	97%	97%
Discharged on Antithrombotic Therapy[2]	99	100%	99%	99%
Discharged on Statin Medication[2]	80	99%	94%	94%
Thrombolytic Therapy Timing[2]	12	92%	57%	66%
Venous Thromboembolism Prophylaxis[2]	96	100%	93%	94%
Written Stroke Educational Materials Given[2]	62	97%	84%	88%
Surgical Care Improvement Project				
Appropriate Beta Blocker Usage[2]	119	100%	97%	98%
Appropriate VTP Within 24 Hours[2]	387	100%	98%	98%
Controlled Postoperative Blood Glucose[2,7]	-	-	95%	97%
Perioperative Temperature Management[2]	479	100%	100%	100%
Prophylactic Antibiotic Selection[2]	318	98%	99%	99%
Prophylactic Antibiotic Selection (Outpatient)	144	99%	98%	98%
Prophylactic Antibiotic Stopped[2]	306	99%	98%	98%
Prophylactic Antibiotic Timing[2]	318	100%	99%	99%
Prophylactic Antibiotic Timing (Outpatient)	145	94%	98%	98%
Urinary Catheter Removal[2]	287	99%	96%	97%
Survey of Patients' Hospital Experiences				
Area Around Room 'Always' Quiet at Night	300+	51%	67%	61%
Doctors 'Always' Communicated Well	300+	79%	84%	82%
Home Recovery Information Given	300+	83%	85%	85%
Hospital Given 9 or 10 on 10 Point Scale	300+	61%	70%	71%
Meds 'Always' Explained Before Given	300+	61%	66%	64%
Nurses 'Always' Communicated Well	300+	74%	80%	79%
Pain 'Always' Well Controlled	300+	66%	72%	71%
Room and Bathroom 'Always' Clean	300+	68%	73%	73%
Timely Help 'Always' Received	300+	58%	68%	68%
Would Definitely Recommend Hospital	300+	64%	70%	71%
Use of Medical Imaging				
Cardiac Imaging Stress Test before Surgery	574	3.7%	4.8%	5.3%
Combination Abdominal CT Scan	986	2.0%	9.6%	10.5%
Combination Brain/Sinus CT Scan	823	4.9%	3.3%	2.7%
Combination Chest CT Scan	710	0.4%	3.4%	2.7%
Follow-up Mammogram/Ultrasound	1,598	12.6%	8.3%	8.8%
Lumbar Spine MRI for Low Back Pain	189	45.0%	35.3%	37.2%

McKenzie Regional Hospital

161 Hospital Drive
Mc Kenzie, TN 38201
Phone: 731-352-5344
Fax: 731-352-2733
URL: www.mckenzieregionalhospital.com
Type: Acute Care Hospitals
Emergency Services: Yes
Ownership: Proprietary
Beds: 45

Key Personnel:
CEO/President............... Darrell Blaylock
Chief of Medical Staff.......... Terry Colotta, MD
Emergency Room .... Denna Jackson
Patient Relations .... Kim Ladd
Operating Room.............. Regina Lockaby
Radiology.................... Ricky Scott

Measure	Cases	This Hosp.	State Avg.	U.S. Avg.
Blood Clot Prevention and Treatment				
Anticoagulation Overlap Therapy[1,2]	-	-	92%	93%
ICU Venous Thromboembolism Prophylaxis[2,7]	-	-	90%	92%
Incidence of Potentially Preventable VTE[2,7]	-	-	10%	10%
UFH with Dosages/Platelet Monitoring[1,2]	-	-	99%	97%
Venous Thromboembolism Prophylaxis[2]	191	97%	83%	85%
Warfarin Therapy Discharge Instructions[1,2]	-	-	78%	75%
Chest Pain/Possible Heart Attack Care				
Aspirin Given Within 24 Hours of Arrival	122	98%	96%	96%
Fibrinolytic Meds Within 30 Min. of Arrival[1]	-	-	72%	58%
Average Time to ECG (minutes)	129	4	6	7
Average Time to Transfer (minutes)[7]	-	-	53	60
Children's Asthma Care				
Received Home Management Plan of Care	-	-	-	88%
Received Reliever Medication	-	-	-	100%
Received Systemic Corticosteroids	-	-	-	100%
Emergency Department				
Admittance Decision Time (minutes)[2]	259	37	82	98
Head CT Results Within 45 Min. of Arrival[1]	-	-	52%	57%
Patients Who Left ER Before Being Seen	6,676	1%	2%	2%
Time from ER Arrival to Admit. (minutes)[2]	260	146	243	274
Time from ER Arrival to Discharge (minutes)	309	82	131	134
Time in ER Before Being Evaluated (minutes)	423	15	25	26
Time to Pain Meds for Fractures (minutes)	24	48	60	57
Heart Attack Care				
Aspirin Given at Discharge[1,3]	-	-	99%	99%
Fibrinolytic Meds Within 30 Min. of Arrival[3,7]	-	-	33%	54%
PCI Within 90 Minutes of Arrival[3,7]	-	-	98%	96%
Statin Prescribed at Discharge[1,3]	-	-	99%	98%
Heart Failure Care				
ACE Inhibitor or ARB for LVSD[1]	-	-	97%	97%
Discharge Instructions Given	24	100%	93%	94%
Evaluation of LVS Function	27	100%	99%	99%
Medicare Spending				
Medicare Spending per Patient (ratio)	-	1.06	1	0.98
Pneumonia Care				
Appropriate Initial Antibiotic Given	36	100%	95%	95%
Blood Culture Timing	42	100%	98%	98%
Pregnancy and Delivery Care				
Newborn Deliveries Scheduled Early[1,2]	-	-	6%	6%
Preventive Care				
Immunization for Influenza[2]	360	99%	93%	90%
Immunization for Pneumonia[2]	329	99%	93%	92%
Stroke Care				
Anticoagulation Therapy for Atrial Fibrillation[1]	-	-	94%	95%
Antithrombotic Therapy Timing[1]	-	-	97%	98%
Assessed for Rehabilitation[1]	-	-	97%	97%
Discharged on Antithrombotic Therapy[1]	-	-	99%	99%
Discharged on Statin Medication[1]	-	-	94%	94%
Thrombolytic Therapy Timing[1]	-	-	57%	66%
Venous Thromboembolism Prophylaxis[1]	-	-	93%	94%
Written Stroke Educational Materials Given[1]	-	-	84%	88%
Surgical Care Improvement Project				
Appropriate Beta Blocker Usage[1]	-	-	97%	98%
Appropriate VTP Within 24 Hours	34	100%	98%	98%
Controlled Postoperative Blood Glucose[7]	-	-	95%	97%
Perioperative Temperature Management	42	100%	100%	100%
Prophylactic Antibiotic Selection	20	100%	99%	99%
Prophylactic Antibiotic Selection (Outpatient)[1]	-	-	98%	98%
Prophylactic Antibiotic Stopped	20	100%	98%	98%
Prophylactic Antibiotic Timing	21	95%	99%	99%
Prophylactic Antibiotic Timing (Outpatient)[1]	-	-	98%	98%
Urinary Catheter Removal[1]	-	-	96%	97%
Survey of Patients' Hospital Experiences				
Area Around Room 'Always' Quiet at Night	(a)	67%	67%	61%
Doctors 'Always' Communicated Well	(a)	81%	84%	82%
Home Recovery Information Given	(a)	87%	85%	85%
Hospital Given 9 or 10 on 10 Point Scale	(a)	69%	70%	71%
Meds 'Always' Explained Before Given	(a)	65%	66%	64%
Nurses 'Always' Communicated Well	(a)	75%	80%	79%
Pain 'Always' Well Controlled	(a)	74%	72%	71%
Room and Bathroom 'Always' Clean	(a)	75%	73%	73%
Timely Help 'Always' Received	(a)	67%	68%	68%
Would Definitely Recommend Hospital	(a)	66%	70%	71%
Use of Medical Imaging				
Cardiac Imaging Stress Test before Surgery[1]	-	-	4.8%	5.3%
Combination Abdominal CT Scan	60	1.7%	9.6%	10.5%
Combination Brain/Sinus CT Scan[1]	-	-	3.3%	2.7%
Combination Chest CT Scan[1]	-	-	3.4%	2.7%
Follow-up Mammogram/Ultrasound[1]	-	-	8.3%	8.8%
Lumbar Spine MRI for Low Back Pain[1]	-	-	35.3%	37.2%

River Park Hospital

1559 Sparta Street
Mc Minnville, TN 37110
Phone: 931-815-4101
Fax: 931-815-4638
URL: www.riverparkhospital.com
Type: Acute Care Hospitals
Emergency Services: Yes
Ownership: Proprietary
Beds: 127

Key Personnel:
Operating Room.............. William Bradfor Brock
Chief of Medical Staff.......... Timothy M Fisher, DO
Radiology.................... Wendell V McAbee, MD
CEO .... Tim McGill
CEO/President................ John R McLain
Pediatric Ambulatory Care ...... Jeffrey K McVey, DO
Patient Relations .... Elaine Neal

Measure	Cases	This Hosp.	State Avg.	U.S. Avg.
Blood Clot Prevention and Treatment				
Anticoagulation Overlap Therapy[2]	14	57%	92%	93%
ICU Venous Thromboembolism Prophylaxis[2]	80	82%	90%	92%

NOTE: Hospital profiles are in alphabetical order by state, then city, then hospital within the city; Rankings exclude hospitals with less than 25 cases except for patient surveys which excludes hospitals with less than 100 cases; (a) 100-299 cases; (1) The number of cases/patients is too few to report; (2) Data submitted were based on a sample of cases/patients; (3) Results are based on a shorter time period than required; (4) Data suppressed by CMS for one or more quarters; (5) Results are not available for this reporting period; (6) Fewer than 100 patients completed the HCAHPS survey; (7) No cases met the criteria for this measure; (8) The lower limit of the confidence interval cannot be calculated if the number of observed infections equals zero; (9) No data are available from the state/territory for this reporting period; (10) The scores shown reflect fewer than 50 completed surveys; (11) There were discrepancies in the data collection process; (12) This measure does not apply to this hospital for this reporting period; (13) Results cannot be calculated for this reporting period; (14) The results for this state are combined with nearby states to protect confidentiality; Please refer to the User's Guide for a full explanation of data.

Incidence of Potentially Preventable VTE[1,2]	-	-	10%	10%
UFH with Dosages/Platelet Monitoring[1,2]	-	-	99%	97%
Venous Thromboembolism Prophylaxis[2]	201	82%	83%	85%
Warfarin Therapy Discharge Instructions[1,2]	-	-	78%	75%
Chest Pain/Possible Heart Attack Care				
Aspirin Given Within 24 Hours of Arrival	110	98%	96%	96%
Fibrinolytic Meds Within 30 Min. of Arrival[1]	-	-	72%	58%
Average Time to ECG (minutes)	112	3	6	7
Average Time to Transfer (minutes)[1]	-	-	53	60
Children's Asthma Care				
Received Home Management Plan of Care	-	-	-	88%
Received Reliever Medication	-	-	-	100%
Received Systemic Corticosteroids	-	-	-	100%
Emergency Department				
Admittance Decision Time (minutes)[2]	409	63	82	98
Head CT Results Within 45 Min. of Arrival[1]	-	-	52%	57%
Patients Who Left ER Before Being Seen	24,636	2%	2%	2%
Time from ER Arrival to Admit. (minutes)[2]	413	223	243	274
Time from ER Arrival to Discharge (minutes)	351	138	131	134
Time in ER Before Being Evaluated (minutes)	421	26	25	26
Time to Pain Meds for Fractures (minutes)	94	62	60	57
Heart Attack Care				
Aspirin Given at Discharge[1]	-	-	99%	99%
Fibrinolytic Meds Within 30 Min. of Arrival[7]	-	-	33%	54%
PCI Within 90 Minutes of Arrival[7]	-	-	98%	96%
Statin Prescribed at Discharge[1]	-	-	99%	98%
Heart Failure Care				
ACE Inhibitor or ARB for LVSD	31	97%	97%	97%
Discharge Instructions Given	143	86%	93%	94%
Evaluation of LVS Function	184	99%	99%	99%
Medicare Spending				
Medicare Spending per Patient (ratio)	-	0.97	1	0.98
Pneumonia Care				
Appropriate Initial Antibiotic Given	116	87%	95%	95%
Blood Culture Timing	152	98%	98%	98%
Pregnancy and Delivery Care				
Newborn Deliveries Scheduled Early[2]	41	12%	6%	6%
Preventive Care				
Immunization for Influenza[2]	343	92%	93%	90%
Immunization for Pneumonia[2]	446	97%	93%	92%
Stroke Care				
Anticoagulation Therapy for Atrial Fibrillation[1]	-	-	94%	95%
Antithrombotic Therapy Timing	19	79%	97%	98%
Assessed for Rehabilitation	16	100%	97%	97%
Discharged on Antithrombotic Therapy	14	93%	99%	99%
Discharged on Statin Medication	13	62%	94%	94%
Thrombolytic Therapy Timing[1]	-	-	57%	66%
Venous Thromboembolism Prophylaxis	18	89%	93%	94%
Written Stroke Educational Materials Given[1]	-	-	84%	88%
Surgical Care Improvement Project				
Appropriate Beta Blocker Usage	17	71%	97%	98%
Appropriate VTP Within 24 Hours	82	94%	98%	98%
Controlled Postoperative Blood Glucose[7]	-	-	95%	97%
Perioperative Temperature Management	97	100%	100%	100%
Prophylactic Antibiotic Selection	54	98%	99%	99%
Prophylactic Antibiotic Selection (Outpatient)	41	100%	98%	98%
Prophylactic Antibiotic Stopped	51	98%	98%	98%
Prophylactic Antibiotic Timing	54	94%	99%	99%
Prophylactic Antibiotic Timing (Outpatient)	44	93%	98%	98%
Urinary Catheter Removal	69	88%	96%	97%
Survey of Patients' Hospital Experiences				
Area Around Room 'Always' Quiet at Night	300+	66%	67%	61%
Doctors 'Always' Communicated Well	300+	77%	84%	82%
Home Recovery Information Given	300+	82%	85%	85%
Hospital Given 9 or 10 on 10 Point Scale	300+	63%	70%	71%
Meds 'Always' Explained Before Given	300+	59%	66%	64%
Nurses 'Always' Communicated Well	300+	75%	80%	79%
Pain 'Always' Well Controlled	300+	68%	72%	71%
Room and Bathroom 'Always' Clean	300+	68%	73%	73%
Timely Help 'Always' Received	300+	62%	68%	68%
Would Definitely Recommend Hospital	300+	56%	70%	71%
Use of Medical Imaging				
Cardiac Imaging Stress Test before Surgery	231	3.5%	4.8%	5.3%
Combination Abdominal CT Scan	363	3.3%	9.6%	10.5%
Combination Brain/Sinus CT Scan	459	2.2%	3.3%	2.7%
Combination Chest CT Scan	201	2.5%	3.4%	2.7%
Follow-up Mammogram/Ultrasound	797	4.4%	8.3%	8.8%
Lumbar Spine MRI for Low Back Pain	85	38.8%	35.3%	37.2%

Baptist Memorial Hospital

6019 Walnut Grove Road
Memphis, TN 38120
E-mail: info.memphis@bmhcc.org
URL: www.bmhcc.org
Type: Acute Care Hospitals
Ownership: Voluntary non-profit - Private

Phone: 901-226-5000
Fax: 901-227-6149
Emergency Services: Yes
Beds: 706

Key Personnel:
Anesthesiology. . . . . James W. Bailey, MD
CEO/President. . . . . Dana Dye
Emergency Room . . . . William Falvey, MD
Infection Control. . . . . Katie Morrissette
Chief of Medical Staff . . . . Dr. Chris Patrick
Hemotology Center . . . . Ric Ransom
Radiology. . . . . Johnny Stanford
Operating Room. . . . . Martha Ullrich

Measure	Cases	This Hosp.	State Avg.	U.S. Avg.
Blood Clot Prevention and Treatment				
Anticoagulation Overlap Therapy[2]	277	99%	92%	93%
ICU Venous Thromboembolism Prophylaxis[2]	168	93%	90%	92%
Incidence of Potentially Preventable VTE[2]	72	7%	10%	10%
UFH with Dosages/Platelet Monitoring[2]	274	100%	99%	97%
Venous Thromboembolism Prophylaxis[2]	611	86%	83%	85%
Warfarin Therapy Discharge Instructions[2]	196	83%	78%	75%
Chest Pain/Possible Heart Attack Care				
Aspirin Given Within 24 Hours of Arrival[1]	-	-	96%	96%
Fibrinolytic Meds Within 30 Min. of Arrival[3,7]	-	-	72%	58%
Average Time to ECG (minutes)[1]	-	-	6	7
Average Time to Transfer (minutes)[3,7]	-	-	53	60
Children's Asthma Care				
Received Home Management Plan of Care	-	-	-	88%
Received Reliever Medication	-	-	-	100%
Received Systemic Corticosteroids	-	-	-	100%
Emergency Department				
Admittance Decision Time (minutes)[2]	960	95	82	98
Head CT Results Within 45 Min. of Arrival[1]	-	-	52%	57%
Patients Who Left ER Before Being Seen	79,761	1%	2%	2%
Time from ER Arrival to Admit. (minutes)[2]	1,027	298	243	274
Time from ER Arrival to Discharge (minutes)	697	170	131	134
Time in ER Before Being Evaluated (minutes)	783	30	25	26
Time to Pain Meds for Fractures (minutes)	249	71	60	57
Heart Attack Care				
Aspirin Given at Discharge	643	100%	99%	99%
Fibrinolytic Meds Within 30 Min. of Arrival[7]	-	-	33%	54%
PCI Within 90 Minutes of Arrival	44	100%	98%	96%
Statin Prescribed at Discharge	586	100%	99%	98%
Heart Failure Care				
ACE Inhibitor or ARB for LVSD	369	100%	97%	97%
Discharge Instructions Given	1,165	96%	93%	94%
Evaluation of LVS Function	1,342	100%	99%	99%
Medicare Spending				
Medicare Spending per Patient (ratio)	-	1.00	1	0.98
Pneumonia Care				
Appropriate Initial Antibiotic Given	412	99%	95%	95%
Blood Culture Timing	638	100%	98%	98%
Pregnancy and Delivery Care				
Newborn Deliveries Scheduled Early[2]	123	4%	6%	6%
Preventive Care				
Immunization for Influenza[2]	1,284	95%	93%	90%
Immunization for Pneumonia[2]	1,448	98%	93%	92%
Stroke Care				
Anticoagulation Therapy for Atrial Fibrillation	64	97%	94%	95%
Antithrombotic Therapy Timing	397	98%	97%	98%
Assessed for Rehabilitation	518	100%	97%	97%
Discharged on Antithrombotic Therapy	420	99%	99%	99%
Discharged on Statin Medication	317	99%	94%	94%
Thrombolytic Therapy Timing	36	61%	57%	66%
Venous Thromboembolism Prophylaxis	561	95%	93%	94%
Written Stroke Educational Materials Given	299	96%	84%	88%
Surgical Care Improvement Project				
Appropriate Beta Blocker Usage[2]	350	100%	97%	98%
Appropriate VTP Within 24 Hours[2]	680	99%	98%	98%
Controlled Postoperative Blood Glucose[2]	141	91%	95%	97%
Perioperative Temperature Management[2]	887	100%	100%	100%
Prophylactic Antibiotic Selection[2]	659	98%	99%	99%
Prophylactic Antibiotic Selection (Outpatient)	1,267	100%	98%	98%
Prophylactic Antibiotic Stopped[2]	636	98%	98%	98%
Prophylactic Antibiotic Timing[2]	660	99%	99%	99%
Prophylactic Antibiotic Timing (Outpatient)	1,268	100%	98%	98%
Urinary Catheter Removal[2]	355	99%	96%	97%
Survey of Patients' Hospital Experiences				
Area Around Room 'Always' Quiet at Night	300+	64%	67%	61%
Doctors 'Always' Communicated Well	300+	78%	84%	82%
Home Recovery Information Given	300+	81%	85%	85%
Hospital Given 9 or 10 on 10 Point Scale	300+	73%	70%	71%
Meds 'Always' Explained Before Given	300+	58%	66%	64%
Nurses 'Always' Communicated Well	300+	76%	80%	79%
Pain 'Always' Well Controlled	300+	69%	72%	71%
Room and Bathroom 'Always' Clean	300+	71%	73%	73%
Timely Help 'Always' Received	300+	58%	68%	68%
Would Definitely Recommend Hospital	300+	75%	70%	71%
Use of Medical Imaging				
Cardiac Imaging Stress Test before Surgery	2,874	5.5%	4.8%	5.3%
Combination Abdominal CT Scan	2,052	2.7%	9.6%	10.5%
Combination Brain/Sinus CT Scan	2,019	3.0%	3.3%	2.7%
Combination Chest CT Scan	1,526	0.7%	3.4%	2.7%
Follow-up Mammogram/Ultrasound	3,822	9.4%	8.3%	8.8%
Lumbar Spine MRI for Low Back Pain	199	37.2%	35.3%	37.2%

Delta Medical Center

3000 Getwell Rd
Memphis, TN 38118
URL: www.deltamedcenter.com
Type: Acute Care Hospitals
Ownership: Proprietary

Phone: 901-369-8100
Fax: 901-369-8503
Emergency Services: Yes
Beds: 243

Key Personnel:
Infection Control. . . . . Debbie Braddock
Operating Room. . . . . Hazel Collins
CEO/President. . . . . J Gene Faile
Emergency Room . . . . Rita Garner
Coronary Care . . . . Mary Hammons
Anesthesiology. . . . . Salwa Moustafa, MD
Quality Assurance . . . . Shayne Racheals
Chief of Medical Staff . . . . Gregory Vandevan

Measure	Cases	This Hosp.	State Avg.	U.S. Avg.
Blood Clot Prevention and Treatment				
Anticoagulation Overlap Therapy[2]	15	100%	92%	93%
ICU Venous Thromboembolism Prophylaxis[2]	49	69%	90%	92%
Incidence of Potentially Preventable VTE[1,2]	-	-	10%	10%
UFH with Dosages/Platelet Monitoring[2]	12	100%	99%	97%
Venous Thromboembolism Prophylaxis[2]	186	70%	83%	85%
Warfarin Therapy Discharge Instructions[2]	12	67%	78%	75%
Chest Pain/Possible Heart Attack Care				
Aspirin Given Within 24 Hours of Arrival[5]	-	-	96%	96%
Fibrinolytic Meds Within 30 Min. of Arrival[5]	-	-	72%	58%
Average Time to ECG (minutes)[5]	-	-	6	7
Average Time to Transfer (minutes)[5]	-	-	53	60
Children's Asthma Care				
Received Home Management Plan of Care	-	-	-	88%
Received Reliever Medication	-	-	-	100%
Received Systemic Corticosteroids	-	-	-	100%
Emergency Department				
Admittance Decision Time (minutes)[2]	319	100	82	98
Head CT Results Within 45 Min. of Arrival[1,3]	-	-	52%	57%
Patients Who Left ER Before Being Seen	27,279	2%	2%	2%
Time from ER Arrival to Admit. (minutes)[2]	320	292	243	274
Time from ER Arrival to Discharge (minutes)	337	131	131	134
Time in ER Before Being Evaluated (minutes)	362	58	25	26
Time to Pain Meds for Fractures (minutes)	46	96	60	57
Heart Attack Care				
Aspirin Given at Discharge[1,3]	-	-	99%	99%

NOTE: Hospital profiles are in alphabetical order by state, then city, then hospital within the city; Rankings exclude hospitals with less than 25 cases except for patient surveys which excludes hospitals with less than 100 cases; (a) 100-299 cases; (1) The number of cases/patients is too few to report; (2) Data submitted were based on a sample of cases/patients; (3) Results are based on a shorter time period than required; (4) Data suppressed by CMS for one or more quarters; (5) Results are not available for this reporting period; (6) Fewer than 100 patients completed the HCAHPS survey; (7) No cases met the criteria for this measure; (8) The lower limit of the confidence interval cannot be calculated if the number of observed infections equals zero; (9) No data are available from the state/territory for this reporting period; (10) The scores shown reflect fewer than 50 completed surveys; (11) There were discrepancies in the data collection process; (12) This measure does not apply to this hospital for this reporting period; (13) Results cannot be calculated for this reporting period; (14) The results for this state are combined with nearby states to protect confidentiality; Please refer to the User's Guide for a full explanation of data.

Measure	Cases	This Hosp.	State Avg.	U.S. Avg.
Fibrinolytic Meds Within 30 Min. of Arrival[3,7]	-	-	33%	54%
PCI Within 90 Minutes of Arrival[3,7]	-	-	98%	96%
Statin Prescribed at Discharge[1,3]	-	-	99%	98%
Heart Failure Care				
ACE Inhibitor or ARB for LVSD	38	97%	97%	97%
Discharge Instructions Given	87	90%	93%	94%
Evaluation of LVS Function	89	96%	99%	99%
Medicare Spending				
Medicare Spending per Patient (ratio)	-	1.08	1	0.98
Pneumonia Care				
Appropriate Initial Antibiotic Given	20	70%	95%	95%
Blood Culture Timing	31	97%	98%	98%
Pregnancy and Delivery Care				
Newborn Deliveries Scheduled Early[7]	-	-	6%	6%
Preventive Care				
Immunization for Influenza[2]	280	93%	93%	90%
Immunization for Pneumonia[2]	385	76%	93%	92%
Stroke Care				
Anticoagulation Therapy for Atrial Fibrillation[1]	-	-	94%	95%
Antithrombotic Therapy Timing[1]	-	-	97%	98%
Assessed for Rehabilitation[1]	-	-	97%	97%
Discharged on Antithrombotic Therapy[1]	-	-	99%	99%
Discharged on Statin Medication[1]	-	-	94%	94%
Thrombolytic Therapy Timing[1]	-	-	57%	66%
Venous Thromboembolism Prophylaxis[1]	-	-	93%	94%
Written Stroke Educational Materials Given[1]	-	-	84%	88%
Surgical Care Improvement Project				
Appropriate Beta Blocker Usage	19	79%	97%	98%
Appropriate VTP Within 24 Hours	71	89%	98%	98%
Controlled Postoperative Blood Glucose[7]	-	-	95%	97%
Perioperative Temperature Management	71	100%	100%	100%
Prophylactic Antibiotic Selection	53	100%	99%	99%
Prophylactic Antibiotic Selection (Outpatient)	25	92%	98%	98%
Prophylactic Antibiotic Stopped	49	84%	98%	98%
Prophylactic Antibiotic Timing	53	96%	99%	99%
Prophylactic Antibiotic Timing (Outpatient)	26	85%	98%	98%
Urinary Catheter Removal	22	95%	96%	97%
Survey of Patients' Hospital Experiences				
Area Around Room 'Always' Quiet at Night	300+	77%	67%	61%
Doctors 'Always' Communicated Well	300+	75%	84%	82%
Home Recovery Information Given	300+	81%	85%	85%
Hospital Given 9 or 10 on 10 Point Scale	300+	59%	70%	71%
Meds 'Always' Explained Before Given	300+	54%	66%	64%
Nurses 'Always' Communicated Well	300+	72%	80%	79%
Pain 'Always' Well Controlled	300+	64%	72%	71%
Room and Bathroom 'Always' Clean	300+	74%	73%	73%
Timely Help 'Always' Received	300+	55%	68%	68%
Would Definitely Recommend Hospital	300+	60%	70%	71%
Use of Medical Imaging				
Cardiac Imaging Stress Test before Surgery[1]	-	-	4.8%	5.3%
Combination Abdominal CT Scan[1]	-	-	9.6%	10.5%
Combination Brain/Sinus CT Scan	99	7.1%	3.3%	2.7%
Combination Chest CT Scan[1]	-	-	3.4%	2.7%
Follow-up Mammogram/Ultrasound	98	11.2%	8.3%	8.8%
Lumbar Spine MRI for Low Back Pain[1]	-	-	35.3%	37.2%

Memphis VA Medical Center

1030 Jefferson Avenue
Memphis, TN 38104
Phone: 901-577-7200
Fax: 901-577-7251
URL: www.va.gov/sta/guide/home.asp
Type: Acute Care - VA
Emergency Services: No
Ownership: Government Federal
Beds: 263

Key Personnel:

Quality Assurance . . . . Melinda Kincade
Chief of Medical Staff. . . . . Christopher Marino, MD
Cardiac Laboratory. . . . . K Ramanathan, MD
CEO/President. . . . . James L Robinson, III
Radiology. . . . . John R Ware, MD
Infection Control. . . . . Ellen W Whitnack, MD

Measure	Cases	This Hosp.	State Avg.	U.S. Avg.
Blood Clot Prevention and Treatment				
Anticoagulation Overlap Therapy	-	-	92%	93%
ICU Venous Thromboembolism Prophylaxis	-	-	90%	92%
Incidence of Potentially Preventable VTE	-	-	10%	10%
UFH with Dosages/Platelet Monitoring	-	-	99%	97%
Venous Thromboembolism Prophylaxis	-	-	83%	85%
Warfarin Therapy Discharge Instructions	-	-	78%	75%
Chest Pain/Possible Heart Attack Care				
Aspirin Given Within 24 Hours of Arrival	-	-	96%	96%
Fibrinolytic Meds Within 30 Min. of Arrival	-	-	72%	58%
Average Time to ECG (minutes)	-	-	6	7
Average Time to Transfer (minutes)	-	-	53	60
Children's Asthma Care				
Received Home Management Plan of Care	-	-	-	88%
Received Reliever Medication	-	-	-	100%
Received Systemic Corticosteroids	-	-	-	100%
Emergency Department				
Admittance Decision Time (minutes)	-	-	82	98
Head CT Results Within 45 Min. of Arrival	-	-	52%	57%
Patients Who Left ER Before Being Seen	-	-	2%	2%
Time from ER Arrival to Admit. (minutes)	-	-	243	274
Time from ER Arrival to Discharge (minutes)	-	-	131	134
Time in ER Before Being Evaluated (minutes)	-	-	25	26
Time to Pain Meds for Fractures (minutes)	-	-	60	57
Heart Attack Care				
Aspirin Given at Discharge	46	100%	99%	99%
Fibrinolytic Meds Within 30 Min. of Arrival[5]	-	-	33%	54%
PCI Within 90 Minutes of Arrival[1]	-	-	98%	96%
Statin Prescribed at Discharge	45	100%	99%	98%
Heart Failure Care				
ACE Inhibitor or ARB for LVSD	135	99%	97%	97%
Discharge Instructions Given	300	100%	93%	94%
Evaluation of LVS Function	307	100%	99%	99%
Medicare Spending				
Medicare Spending per Patient (ratio)	-	-	1	0.98
Pneumonia Care				
Appropriate Initial Antibiotic Given	74	97%	95%	95%
Blood Culture Timing	238	96%	98%	98%
Pregnancy and Delivery Care				
Newborn Deliveries Scheduled Early	-	-	6%	6%
Preventive Care				
Immunization for Influenza[5]	-	-	93%	90%
Immunization for Pneumonia[5]	-	-	93%	92%
Stroke Care				
Anticoagulation Therapy for Atrial Fibrillation	-	-	94%	95%
Antithrombotic Therapy Timing	-	-	97%	98%
Assessed for Rehabilitation	-	-	97%	97%
Discharged on Antithrombotic Therapy	-	-	99%	99%
Discharged on Statin Medication	-	-	94%	94%
Thrombolytic Therapy Timing	-	-	57%	66%
Venous Thromboembolism Prophylaxis	-	-	93%	94%
Written Stroke Educational Materials Given	-	-	84%	88%
Surgical Care Improvement Project				
Appropriate Beta Blocker Usage[2]	155	94%	97%	98%
Appropriate VTP Within 24 Hours[2]	263	98%	98%	98%
Controlled Postoperative Blood Glucose[2]	78	87%	95%	97%
Perioperative Temperature Management[2]	391	100%	100%	100%
Prophylactic Antibiotic Selection	251	99%	99%	99%
Prophylactic Antibiotic Selection (Outpatient)	-	-	98%	98%
Prophylactic Antibiotic Stopped	244	97%	98%	98%
Prophylactic Antibiotic Timing	252	94%	99%	99%
Prophylactic Antibiotic Timing (Outpatient)	-	-	98%	98%
Urinary Catheter Removal[2]	155	91%	96%	97%
Survey of Patients' Hospital Experiences				
Area Around Room 'Always' Quiet at Night	-	-	67%	61%
Doctors 'Always' Communicated Well	-	-	84%	82%
Home Recovery Information Given	-	-	85%	85%
Hospital Given 9 or 10 on 10 Point Scale	-	-	70%	71%
Meds 'Always' Explained Before Given	-	-	66%	64%
Nurses 'Always' Communicated Well	-	-	80%	79%
Pain 'Always' Well Controlled	-	-	72%	71%
Room and Bathroom 'Always' Clean	-	-	73%	73%
Timely Help 'Always' Received	-	-	68%	68%
Would Definitely Recommend Hospital	-	-	70%	71%
Use of Medical Imaging				
Cardiac Imaging Stress Test before Surgery	-	-	4.8%	5.3%
Combination Abdominal CT Scan	-	-	9.6%	10.5%
Combination Brain/Sinus CT Scan	-	-	3.3%	2.7%
Combination Chest CT Scan	-	-	3.4%	2.7%
Follow-up Mammogram/Ultrasound	-	-	8.3%	8.8%
Lumbar Spine MRI for Low Back Pain	-	-	35.3%	37.2%

Methodist Healthcare Memphis Hospitals

1265 Union Ave Suite 700
Memphis, TN 38104
Phone: 901-516-8274
Fax: 901-516-0528
URL: www.methodisthealth.org
Type: Acute Care Hospitals
Emergency Services: Yes
Ownership: Voluntary non-profit - Church
Beds: 693

Key Personnel:

Intensive Care Unit. . . . . Donna Brown
Quality Assurance . . . . Carl Cross
Hemotology Center . . . . Irving Fleming
Radiology. . . . . Davis Moser, MD
CEO/President. . . . . Gary Shorb
Infection Control. . . . . Bryan Simmons, MD
Emergency Room . . . . Ferrell Varner, Jr, DM
Operating Room. . . . . Bonnie Williams

Measure	Cases	This Hosp.	State Avg.	U.S. Avg.
Blood Clot Prevention and Treatment				
Anticoagulation Overlap Therapy[2]	477	92%	92%	93%
ICU Venous Thromboembolism Prophylaxis[2]	106	94%	90%	92%
Incidence of Potentially Preventable VTE[2]	91	7%	10%	10%
UFH with Dosages/Platelet Monitoring[2]	398	100%	99%	97%
Venous Thromboembolism Prophylaxis[2]	318	90%	83%	85%
Warfarin Therapy Discharge Instructions[2]	384	58%	78%	75%
Chest Pain/Possible Heart Attack Care				
Aspirin Given Within 24 Hours of Arrival[1]	-	-	96%	96%
Fibrinolytic Meds Within 30 Min. of Arrival[3,7]	-	-	72%	58%
Average Time to ECG (minutes)[1]	-	-	6	7
Average Time to Transfer (minutes)[3,7]	-	-	53	60
Children's Asthma Care				
Received Home Management Plan of Care[2]	352	89%	-	88%
Received Reliever Medication[2]	352	100%	-	100%
Received Systemic Corticosteroids[2]	352	100%	-	100%
Emergency Department				
Admittance Decision Time (minutes)[2]	591	65	82	98
Head CT Results Within 45 Min. of Arrival	27	41%	52%	57%
Patients Who Left ER Before Being Seen	>100k	3%	2%	2%
Time from ER Arrival to Admit. (minutes)[2]	624	278	243	274
Time from ER Arrival to Discharge (minutes)	416	155	131	134
Time in ER Before Being Evaluated (minutes)	434	61	25	26
Time to Pain Meds for Fractures (minutes)	444	99	60	57
Heart Attack Care				
Aspirin Given at Discharge[2]	619	100%	99%	99%
Fibrinolytic Meds Within 30 Min. of Arrival[2,7]	-	-	33%	54%
PCI Within 90 Minutes of Arrival[2]	81	96%	98%	96%
Statin Prescribed at Discharge[2]	596	100%	99%	98%
Heart Failure Care				
ACE Inhibitor or ARB for LVSD[2]	281	100%	97%	97%
Discharge Instructions Given[2]	687	99%	93%	94%
Evaluation of LVS Function[2]	795	100%	99%	99%
Medicare Spending				
Medicare Spending per Patient (ratio)	-	1.01	1	0.98
Pneumonia Care				
Appropriate Initial Antibiotic Given[2]	164	98%	95%	95%
Blood Culture Timing[2]	252	99%	98%	98%
Pregnancy and Delivery Care				
Newborn Deliveries Scheduled Early[2]	91	4%	6%	6%
Preventive Care				
Immunization for Influenza[2]	521	98%	93%	90%
Immunization for Pneumonia[2]	585	97%	93%	92%
Stroke Care				
Anticoagulation Therapy for Atrial Fibrillation[2]	29	93%	94%	95%
Antithrombotic Therapy Timing[2]	402	99%	97%	98%
Assessed for Rehabilitation[2]	461	100%	97%	97%
Discharged on Antithrombotic Therapy[2]	416	100%	99%	99%
Discharged on Statin Medication[2]	326	99%	94%	94%
Thrombolytic Therapy Timing[2]	11	73%	57%	66%
Venous Thromboembolism Prophylaxis[2]	456	99%	93%	94%
Written Stroke Educational Materials Given[2]	303	96%	84%	88%

NOTE: Hospital profiles are in alphabetical order by state, then city, then hospital within the city; Rankings exclude hospitals with less than 25 cases except for patient surveys which excludes hospitals with less than 100 cases; (a) 100-299 cases; (1) The number of cases/patients is too few to report; (2) Data submitted were based on a sample of cases/patients; (3) Results are based on a shorter time period than required; (4) Data suppressed by CMS for one or more quarters; (5) Results are not available for this reporting period; (6) Fewer than 100 patients completed the HCAHPS survey; (7) No cases met the criteria for this measure; (8) The lower limit of the confidence interval cannot be calculated if the number of observed infections equals zero; (9) No data are available from the state/territory for this reporting period; (10) The scores shown reflect fewer than 50 completed surveys; (11) There were discrepancies in the data collection process; (12) This measure does not apply to this hospital for this reporting period; (13) Results cannot be calculated for this reporting period; (14) The results for this state are combined with nearby states to protect confidentiality; Please refer to the User's Guide for a full explanation of data.

Measure	Cases	This Hosp.	State Avg.	U.S. Avg.
Surgical Care Improvement Project				
Appropriate Beta Blocker Usage[2]	616	99%	97%	98%
Appropriate VTP Within 24 Hours[2]	1,452	100%	98%	98%
Controlled Postoperative Blood Glucose[2]	195	98%	95%	97%
Perioperative Temperature Management[2]	1,928	100%	100%	100%
Prophylactic Antibiotic Selection[2]	1,114	99%	99%	99%
Prophylactic Antibiotic Selection (Outpatient)	841	98%	98%	98%
Prophylactic Antibiotic Stopped[2]	1,088	99%	98%	98%
Prophylactic Antibiotic Timing[2]	1,115	99%	99%	99%
Prophylactic Antibiotic Timing (Outpatient)	841	99%	98%	98%
Urinary Catheter Removal[2]	635	100%	96%	97%
Survey of Patients' Hospital Experiences				
Area Around Room 'Always' Quiet at Night	300+	70%	67%	61%
Doctors 'Always' Communicated Well	300+	81%	84%	82%
Home Recovery Information Given	300+	86%	85%	85%
Hospital Given 9 or 10 on 10 Point Scale	300+	73%	70%	71%
Meds 'Always' Explained Before Given	300+	65%	66%	64%
Nurses 'Always' Communicated Well	300+	80%	80%	79%
Pain 'Always' Well Controlled	300+	72%	72%	71%
Room and Bathroom 'Always' Clean	300+	70%	73%	73%
Timely Help 'Always' Received	300+	63%	68%	68%
Would Definitely Recommend Hospital	300+	77%	70%	71%
Use of Medical Imaging				
Cardiac Imaging Stress Test before Surgery	2,726	4.3%	4.8%	5.3%
Combination Abdominal CT Scan	6,797	6.0%	9.6%	10.5%
Combination Brain/Sinus CT Scan	3,976	3.7%	3.3%	2.7%
Combination Chest CT Scan	5,952	1.9%	3.4%	2.7%
Follow-up Mammogram/Ultrasound	5,444	9.9%	8.3%	8.8%
Lumbar Spine MRI for Low Back Pain	392	35.7%	35.3%	37.2%

Regional Medical Center at Memphis

877 Jefferson Avenue
Memphis, TN 38103
E-mail: ssnell@the-med.org
URL: www.the-med.org
Phone: 901-545-7928
Fax: 901-545-8649
Type: Acute Care Hospitals
Ownership: Govt - Hospital Dist/Auth
Emergency Services: Yes
Beds: 631

Key Personnel:
Quality Assurance .... Terri Adams
CEO/President .... Reginald W. Coopwood, MD
Operating Room .... Linda Duncan
Radiology .... Judy Perkins
Chief of Medical Staff .... Stuart Polly, MD
Infection Control .... Stuart Polly, MD
Cardiac Laboratory .... Brenda Theus

Measure	Cases	This Hosp.	State Avg.	U.S. Avg.
Blood Clot Prevention and Treatment				
Anticoagulation Overlap Therapy[2]	60	97%	92%	93%
ICU Venous Thromboembolism Prophylaxis[2]	223	77%	90%	92%
Incidence of Potentially Preventable VTE[2]	31	6%	10%	10%
UFH with Dosages/Platelet Monitoring[2]	43	100%	99%	97%
Venous Thromboembolism Prophylaxis[2]	571	84%	83%	85%
Warfarin Therapy Discharge Instructions[2]	48	83%	78%	75%
Chest Pain/Possible Heart Attack Care				
Aspirin Given Within 24 Hours of Arrival	18	100%	96%	96%
Fibrinolytic Meds Within 30 Min. of Arrival[7]	-	-	72%	58%
Average Time to ECG (minutes)	18	26	6	7
Average Time to Transfer (minutes)[1]	-	-	53	60
Children's Asthma Care				
Received Home Management Plan of Care	-	-	-	88%
Received Reliever Medication	-	-	-	100%
Received Systemic Corticosteroids	-	-	-	100%
Emergency Department				
Admittance Decision Time (minutes)[2]	879	137	82	98
Head CT Results Within 45 Min. of Arrival	11	0%	52%	57%
Patients Who Left ER Before Being Seen	31,239	1%	2%	2%
Time from ER Arrival to Admit. (minutes)[2]	969	354	243	274
Time from ER Arrival to Discharge (minutes)	2,172	305	131	134
Time in ER Before Being Evaluated (minutes)	2,299	50	25	26
Time to Pain Meds for Fractures (minutes)	122	126	60	57
Heart Attack Care				
Aspirin Given at Discharge	19	100%	99%	99%
Fibrinolytic Meds Within 30 Min. of Arrival[7]	-	-	33%	54%
PCI Within 90 Minutes of Arrival[7]	-	-	98%	96%
Statin Prescribed at Discharge	19	95%	99%	98%
Heart Failure Care				
ACE Inhibitor or ARB for LVSD	73	95%	97%	97%
Discharge Instructions Given	125	81%	93%	94%
Evaluation of LVS Function	133	100%	99%	99%
Medicare Spending				
Medicare Spending per Patient (ratio)	-	1.00	1	0.98
Pneumonia Care				
Appropriate Initial Antibiotic Given	37	89%	95%	95%
Blood Culture Timing	82	96%	98%	98%
Pregnancy and Delivery Care				
Newborn Deliveries Scheduled Early[2]	48	6%	6%	6%
Preventive Care				
Immunization for Influenza[2]	616	31%	93%	90%
Immunization for Pneumonia[2]	317	38%	93%	92%
Stroke Care				
Anticoagulation Therapy for Atrial Fibrillation[1]	-	-	94%	95%
Antithrombotic Therapy Timing	56	89%	97%	98%
Assessed for Rehabilitation	69	97%	97%	97%
Discharged on Antithrombotic Therapy	60	100%	99%	99%
Discharged on Statin Medication	46	93%	94%	94%
Thrombolytic Therapy Timing[1]	-	-	57%	66%
Venous Thromboembolism Prophylaxis	68	82%	93%	94%
Written Stroke Educational Materials Given	48	6%	84%	88%
Surgical Care Improvement Project				
Appropriate Beta Blocker Usage	58	91%	97%	98%
Appropriate VTP Within 24 Hours	435	97%	98%	98%
Controlled Postoperative Blood Glucose[1]	-	-	95%	97%
Perioperative Temperature Management	531	100%	100%	100%
Prophylactic Antibiotic Selection	148	99%	99%	99%
Prophylactic Antibiotic Selection (Outpatient)	56	93%	98%	98%
Prophylactic Antibiotic Stopped	145	92%	98%	98%
Prophylactic Antibiotic Timing	145	99%	99%	99%
Prophylactic Antibiotic Timing (Outpatient)	58	93%	98%	98%
Urinary Catheter Removal	176	98%	96%	97%
Survey of Patients' Hospital Experiences				
Area Around Room 'Always' Quiet at Night	300+	64%	67%	61%
Doctors 'Always' Communicated Well	300+	78%	84%	82%
Home Recovery Information Given	300+	85%	85%	85%
Hospital Given 9 or 10 on 10 Point Scale	300+	66%	70%	71%
Meds 'Always' Explained Before Given	300+	64%	66%	64%
Nurses 'Always' Communicated Well	300+	76%	80%	79%
Pain 'Always' Well Controlled	300+	68%	72%	71%
Room and Bathroom 'Always' Clean	300+	66%	73%	73%
Timely Help 'Always' Received	300+	62%	68%	68%
Would Definitely Recommend Hospital	300+	72%	70%	71%
Use of Medical Imaging				
Cardiac Imaging Stress Test before Surgery	127	3.9%	4.8%	5.3%
Combination Abdominal CT Scan	294	8.5%	9.6%	10.5%
Combination Brain/Sinus CT Scan	364	10.4%	3.3%	2.7%
Combination Chest CT Scan	271	5.5%	3.4%	2.7%
Follow-up Mammogram/Ultrasound	240	10.4%	8.3%	8.8%
Lumbar Spine MRI for Low Back Pain[1]	-	-	35.3%	37.2%

Saint Francis Hospital

5959 Park Ave
Memphis, TN 38119
URL: www.saintfrancishosp.com
Phone: 901-765-1000
Fax: 901-765-1799
Type: Acute Care Hospitals
Ownership: Proprietary
Emergency Services: Yes
Beds: 651

Key Personnel:
President/CEO .... David L. Archer
Emergency Room .... Jack Bandura, MD
Quality Assurance .... Tricia Caughley
Pediatric In-Patient Care .... Isaac John, MD
Chief of Medical Staff .... Robert Kraus, MD
Anesthesiology .... Kays Nawaf, MD
Radiology .... R Steven Roney, MD
Infection Control .... Mike Todai

Measure	Cases	This Hosp.	State Avg.	U.S. Avg.
Blood Clot Prevention and Treatment				
Anticoagulation Overlap Therapy[2]	75	96%	92%	93%
ICU Venous Thromboembolism Prophylaxis[2]	87	98%	90%	92%
Incidence of Potentially Preventable VTE[2]	13	0%	10%	10%
UFH with Dosages/Platelet Monitoring[2]	42	100%	99%	97%
Venous Thromboembolism Prophylaxis[2]	343	94%	83%	85%
Warfarin Therapy Discharge Instructions[2]	68	100%	78%	75%
Chest Pain/Possible Heart Attack Care				
Aspirin Given Within 24 Hours of Arrival[5]	-	-	96%	96%
Fibrinolytic Meds Within 30 Min. of Arrival[5]	-	-	72%	58%
Average Time to ECG (minutes)[5]	-	-	6	7
Average Time to Transfer (minutes)[5]	-	-	53	60
Children's Asthma Care				
Received Home Management Plan of Care	-	-	-	88%
Received Reliever Medication	-	-	-	100%
Received Systemic Corticosteroids	-	-	-	100%
Emergency Department				
Admittance Decision Time (minutes)[2]	1,180	131	82	98
Head CT Results Within 45 Min. of Arrival[1,3]	-	-	52%	57%
Patients Who Left ER Before Being Seen	42,317	4%	2%	2%
Time from ER Arrival to Admit. (minutes)[2]	1,180	338	243	274
Time from ER Arrival to Discharge (minutes)	409	254	131	134
Time in ER Before Being Evaluated (minutes)	427	43	25	26
Time to Pain Meds for Fractures (minutes)	45	84	60	57
Heart Attack Care				
Aspirin Given at Discharge	273	100%	99%	99%
Fibrinolytic Meds Within 30 Min. of Arrival[7]	-	-	33%	54%
PCI Within 90 Minutes of Arrival	40	95%	98%	96%
Statin Prescribed at Discharge	275	100%	99%	98%
Heart Failure Care				
ACE Inhibitor or ARB for LVSD	221	100%	97%	97%
Discharge Instructions Given	533	99%	93%	94%
Evaluation of LVS Function	617	100%	99%	99%
Medicare Spending				
Medicare Spending per Patient (ratio)	-	1.06	1	0.98
Pneumonia Care				
Appropriate Initial Antibiotic Given	147	99%	95%	95%
Blood Culture Timing	201	99%	98%	98%
Pregnancy and Delivery Care				
Newborn Deliveries Scheduled Early[2]	20	0%	6%	6%
Preventive Care				
Immunization for Influenza[2]	1,674	99%	93%	90%
Immunization for Pneumonia[2]	1,417	97%	93%	92%
Stroke Care				
Anticoagulation Therapy for Atrial Fibrillation	14	100%	94%	95%
Antithrombotic Therapy Timing	182	98%	97%	98%
Assessed for Rehabilitation	202	100%	97%	97%
Discharged on Antithrombotic Therapy	178	100%	99%	99%
Discharged on Statin Medication	141	99%	94%	94%
Thrombolytic Therapy Timing	12	100%	57%	66%
Venous Thromboembolism Prophylaxis	217	100%	93%	94%
Written Stroke Educational Materials Given	112	98%	84%	88%
Surgical Care Improvement Project				
Appropriate Beta Blocker Usage[2]	356	99%	97%	98%
Appropriate VTP Within 24 Hours[2]	635	100%	98%	98%
Controlled Postoperative Blood Glucose[2]	163	99%	95%	97%
Perioperative Temperature Management[2]	885	100%	100%	100%
Prophylactic Antibiotic Selection[2]	733	100%	99%	99%
Prophylactic Antibiotic Selection (Outpatient)	474	99%	98%	98%
Prophylactic Antibiotic Stopped[2]	708	100%	98%	98%
Prophylactic Antibiotic Timing[2]	733	99%	99%	99%
Prophylactic Antibiotic Timing (Outpatient)	477	99%	98%	98%
Urinary Catheter Removal[2]	457	100%	96%	97%
Survey of Patients' Hospital Experiences				
Area Around Room 'Always' Quiet at Night	300+	67%	67%	61%
Doctors 'Always' Communicated Well	300+	83%	84%	82%
Home Recovery Information Given	300+	81%	85%	85%
Hospital Given 9 or 10 on 10 Point Scale	300+	69%	70%	71%
Meds 'Always' Explained Before Given	300+	59%	66%	64%
Nurses 'Always' Communicated Well	300+	78%	80%	79%
Pain 'Always' Well Controlled	300+	71%	72%	71%
Room and Bathroom 'Always' Clean	300+	66%	73%	73%
Timely Help 'Always' Received	300+	62%	68%	68%
Would Definitely Recommend Hospital	300+	71%	70%	71%
Use of Medical Imaging				
Cardiac Imaging Stress Test before Surgery	225	3.1%	4.8%	5.3%

NOTE: Hospital profiles are in alphabetical order by state, then city, then hospital within the city; Rankings exclude hospitals with less than 25 cases except for patient surveys which excludes hospitals with less than 100 cases; (a) 100-299 cases; (1) The number of cases/patients is too few to report; (2) Data submitted were based on a sample of cases/patients; (3) Results are based on a shorter time period than required; (4) Data suppressed by CMS for one or more quarters; (5) Results are not available for this reporting period; (6) Fewer than 100 patients completed the HCAHPS survey; (7) No cases met the criteria for this measure; (8) The lower limit of the confidence interval cannot be calculated if the number of observed infections equals zero; (9) No data are available from the state/territory for this reporting period; (10) The scores shown reflect fewer than 50 completed surveys; (11) There were discrepancies in the data collection process; (12) This measure does not apply to this hospital for this reporting period; (13) Results cannot be calculated for this reporting period; (14) The results for this state are combined with nearby states to protect confidentiality; Please refer to the User's Guide for a full explanation of data.

Measure	Cases	This Hosp.	State Avg.	U.S. Avg.
Combination Abdominal CT Scan	598	10.9%	9.6%	10.5%
Combination Brain/Sinus CT Scan	654	3.1%	3.3%	2.7%
Combination Chest CT Scan	281	0.7%	3.4%	2.7%
Follow-up Mammogram/Ultrasound	1,623	10.0%	8.3%	8.8%
Lumbar Spine MRI for Low Back Pain	189	31.7%	35.3%	37.2%

Milan General Hospital

4039 Highland St
Milan, TN 38358
Type: Acute Care Hospitals
Ownership: Government - Local
Phone: 731-686-1591
Fax: 731-686-5129
Emergency Services: Yes
Beds: 72

Key Personnel:
Quality Assurance . . . . Jerry Barker
Operating Room. . . . . June Bolton
Infection Control. . . . . Sandra Isbell
Chief of Medical Staff. . . . . Kim Tozer, MD

Measure	Cases	This Hosp.	State Avg.	U.S. Avg.
Blood Clot Prevention and Treatment				
Anticoagulation Overlap Therapy[1,2]	-	-	92%	93%
ICU Venous Thromboembolism Prophylaxis[2]	14	86%	90%	92%
Incidence of Potentially Preventable VTE[2,7]	-	-	10%	10%
UFH with Dosages/Platelet Monitoring[2,7]	-	-	99%	97%
Venous Thromboembolism Prophylaxis[2]	86	49%	83%	85%
Warfarin Therapy Discharge Instructions[1,2]	-	-	78%	75%
Chest Pain/Possible Heart Attack Care				
Aspirin Given Within 24 Hours of Arrival	98	100%	96%	96%
Fibrinolytic Meds Within 30 Min. of Arrival[1]	-	-	72%	58%
Average Time to ECG (minutes)	102	6	6	7
Average Time to Transfer (minutes)[7]	-	-	53	60
Children's Asthma Care				
Received Home Management Plan of Care	-	-	-	88%
Received Reliever Medication	-	-	-	100%
Received Systemic Corticosteroids	-	-	-	100%
Emergency Department				
Admittance Decision Time (minutes)	66	85	82	98
Head CT Results Within 45 Min. of Arrival[1]	-	-	52%	57%
Patients Who Left ER Before Being Seen	8,041	4%	2%	2%
Time from ER Arrival to Admit. (minutes)	84	250	243	274
Time from ER Arrival to Discharge (minutes)	375	129	131	134
Time in ER Before Being Evaluated (minutes)	403	21	25	26
Time to Pain Meds for Fractures (minutes)	19	70	60	57
Heart Attack Care				
Aspirin Given at Discharge[1,3]	-	-	99%	99%
Fibrinolytic Meds Within 30 Min. of Arrival[3,7]	-	-	33%	54%
PCI Within 90 Minutes of Arrival[3,7]	-	-	98%	96%
Statin Prescribed at Discharge[1,3]	-	-	99%	98%
Heart Failure Care				
ACE Inhibitor or ARB for LVSD[1,3]	-	-	97%	97%
Discharge Instructions Given[1,3]	-	-	93%	94%
Evaluation of LVS Function[1,3]	-	-	99%	99%
Medicare Spending				
Medicare Spending per Patient (ratio)	-	1.03	1	0.98
Pneumonia Care				
Appropriate Initial Antibiotic Given[1]	-	-	95%	95%
Blood Culture Timing	14	79%	98%	98%
Pregnancy and Delivery Care				
Newborn Deliveries Scheduled Early[7]	-	-	6%	6%
Preventive Care				
Immunization for Influenza	108	94%	93%	90%
Immunization for Pneumonia	161	96%	93%	92%
Stroke Care				
Anticoagulation Therapy for Atrial Fibrillation[3,7]	-	-	94%	95%
Antithrombotic Therapy Timing[1,3]	-	-	97%	98%
Assessed for Rehabilitation[1,3]	-	-	97%	97%
Discharged on Antithrombotic Therapy[1,3]	-	-	99%	99%
Discharged on Statin Medication[1,3]	-	-	94%	94%
Thrombolytic Therapy Timing[3,7]	-	-	57%	66%
Venous Thromboembolism Prophylaxis[1,3]	-	-	93%	94%
Written Stroke Educational Materials Given[1,3]	-	-	84%	88%
Surgical Care Improvement Project				
Appropriate Beta Blocker Usage[1]	-	-	97%	98%
Appropriate VTP Within 24 Hours	37	100%	98%	98%
Controlled Postoperative Blood Glucose[7]	-	-	95%	97%
Perioperative Temperature Management	37	100%	100%	100%
Prophylactic Antibiotic Selection[1]	-	-	99%	99%
Prophylactic Antibiotic Selection (Outpatient)	11	100%	98%	98%
Prophylactic Antibiotic Stopped[1]	-	-	98%	98%
Prophylactic Antibiotic Timing[1]	-	-	99%	99%
Prophylactic Antibiotic Timing (Outpatient)	11	91%	98%	98%
Urinary Catheter Removal	19	100%	96%	97%
Survey of Patients' Hospital Experiences				
Area Around Room 'Always' Quiet at Night[10]	<100	83%	67%	61%
Doctors 'Always' Communicated Well[10]	<100	90%	84%	82%
Home Recovery Information Given[10]	<100	86%	85%	85%
Hospital Given 9 or 10 on 10 Point Scale[10]	<100	75%	70%	71%
Meds 'Always' Explained Before Given[10]	<100	76%	66%	64%
Nurses 'Always' Communicated Well[10]	<100	84%	80%	79%
Pain 'Always' Well Controlled[10]	<100	78%	72%	71%
Room and Bathroom 'Always' Clean[10]	<100	89%	73%	73%
Timely Help 'Always' Received[10]	<100	69%	68%	68%
Would Definitely Recommend Hospital[10]	<100	70%	70%	71%
Use of Medical Imaging				
Cardiac Imaging Stress Test before Surgery[7]	-	-	4.8%	5.3%
Combination Abdominal CT Scan	161	0.6%	9.6%	10.5%
Combination Brain/Sinus CT Scan	249	6.4%	3.3%	2.7%
Combination Chest CT Scan	59	0.0%	3.4%	2.7%
Follow-up Mammogram/Ultrasound	669	8.7%	8.3%	8.8%
Lumbar Spine MRI for Low Back Pain[7]	-	-	35.3%	37.2%

Lakeway Regional Hospital

726 Mcfarland St
Morristown, TN 37814
Type: Acute Care Hospitals
Ownership: Proprietary
Phone: 423-522-6000
Fax: 423-587-8548
Emergency Services: Yes
Beds: 135

Key Personnel:
Radiology. . . . . Michael Adler
Emergency Room . . . . Debbie Boyd
Chief of Medical Staff. . . . . Paul Cardall, MD
Operating Room. . . . . Pat Freeman
Intensive Care Unit. . . . . Anne Johnson, RN
Quality Assurance . . . . Kristen Kilgore, RN
CEO/President. . . . . Priscilla Mills
Infection Control. . . . . Eva Stinson, RN

Measure	Cases	This Hosp.	State Avg.	U.S. Avg.
Blood Clot Prevention and Treatment				
Anticoagulation Overlap Therapy[2]	17	100%	92%	93%
ICU Venous Thromboembolism Prophylaxis[2]	91	100%	90%	92%
Incidence of Potentially Preventable VTE[1,2]	-	-	10%	10%
UFH with Dosages/Platelet Monitoring[2]	11	100%	99%	97%
Venous Thromboembolism Prophylaxis[2]	223	91%	83%	85%
Warfarin Therapy Discharge Instructions[1,2]	-	-	78%	75%
Chest Pain/Possible Heart Attack Care				
Aspirin Given Within 24 Hours of Arrival	25	88%	96%	96%
Fibrinolytic Meds Within 30 Min. of Arrival[7]	-	-	72%	58%
Average Time to ECG (minutes)	25	3	6	7
Average Time to Transfer (minutes)[1]	-	-	53	60
Children's Asthma Care				
Received Home Management Plan of Care	-	-	-	88%
Received Reliever Medication	-	-	-	100%
Received Systemic Corticosteroids	-	-	-	100%
Emergency Department				
Admittance Decision Time (minutes)[2]	462	65	82	98
Head CT Results Within 45 Min. of Arrival[1]	-	-	52%	57%
Patients Who Left ER Before Being Seen	15,635	6%	2%	2%
Time from ER Arrival to Admit. (minutes)[2]	465	257	243	274
Time from ER Arrival to Discharge (minutes)	358	138	131	134
Time in ER Before Being Evaluated (minutes)	404	30	25	26
Time to Pain Meds for Fractures (minutes)	41	57	60	57
Heart Attack Care				
Aspirin Given at Discharge	12	100%	99%	99%
Fibrinolytic Meds Within 30 Min. of Arrival[7]	-	-	33%	54%
PCI Within 90 Minutes of Arrival[7]	-	-	98%	96%
Statin Prescribed at Discharge	15	100%	99%	98%
Heart Failure Care				
ACE Inhibitor or ARB for LVSD	11	100%	97%	97%
Discharge Instructions Given	51	100%	93%	94%
Evaluation of LVS Function	61	98%	99%	99%
Medicare Spending				
Medicare Spending per Patient (ratio)	-	1.01	1	0.98
Pneumonia Care				
Appropriate Initial Antibiotic Given	69	97%	95%	95%
Blood Culture Timing	100	99%	98%	98%
Pregnancy and Delivery Care				
Newborn Deliveries Scheduled Early[2]	22	18%	6%	6%
Preventive Care				
Immunization for Influenza[2]	303	98%	93%	90%
Immunization for Pneumonia[2]	406	100%	93%	92%
Stroke Care				
Anticoagulation Therapy for Atrial Fibrillation[1]	-	-	94%	95%
Antithrombotic Therapy Timing	30	97%	97%	98%
Assessed for Rehabilitation	22	100%	97%	97%
Discharged on Antithrombotic Therapy	22	100%	99%	99%
Discharged on Statin Medication	18	94%	94%	94%
Thrombolytic Therapy Timing[1]	-	-	57%	66%
Venous Thromboembolism Prophylaxis	30	100%	93%	94%
Written Stroke Educational Materials Given	12	100%	84%	88%
Surgical Care Improvement Project				
Appropriate Beta Blocker Usage	53	92%	97%	98%
Appropriate VTP Within 24 Hours	123	100%	98%	98%
Controlled Postoperative Blood Glucose[7]	-	-	95%	97%
Perioperative Temperature Management	135	100%	100%	100%
Prophylactic Antibiotic Selection	103	100%	99%	99%
Prophylactic Antibiotic Selection (Outpatient)	85	100%	98%	98%
Prophylactic Antibiotic Stopped	96	96%	98%	98%
Prophylactic Antibiotic Timing	104	97%	99%	99%
Prophylactic Antibiotic Timing (Outpatient)	85	100%	98%	98%
Urinary Catheter Removal	102	100%	96%	97%
Survey of Patients' Hospital Experiences				
Area Around Room 'Always' Quiet at Night	300+	62%	67%	61%
Doctors 'Always' Communicated Well	300+	82%	84%	82%
Home Recovery Information Given	300+	84%	85%	85%
Hospital Given 9 or 10 on 10 Point Scale	300+	61%	70%	71%
Meds 'Always' Explained Before Given	300+	61%	66%	64%
Nurses 'Always' Communicated Well	300+	75%	80%	79%
Pain 'Always' Well Controlled	300+	66%	72%	71%
Room and Bathroom 'Always' Clean	300+	69%	73%	73%
Timely Help 'Always' Received	300+	61%	68%	68%
Would Definitely Recommend Hospital	300+	66%	70%	71%
Use of Medical Imaging				
Cardiac Imaging Stress Test before Surgery[1]	-	-	4.8%	5.3%
Combination Abdominal CT Scan	224	7.6%	9.6%	10.5%
Combination Brain/Sinus CT Scan[1]	-	-	3.3%	2.7%
Combination Chest CT Scan	98	0.0%	3.4%	2.7%
Follow-up Mammogram/Ultrasound	122	7.4%	8.3%	8.8%
Lumbar Spine MRI for Low Back Pain	122	32.0%	35.3%	37.2%

Morristown Hamblen Hospital Association

908 W 4th North St
Morristown, TN 37814
URL: www.mhhs1.org
Type: Acute Care Hospitals
Ownership: Government - Local
Phone: 423-586-4231
Fax: 423-585-1271
Emergency Services: Yes
Beds: 155

Key Personnel:
Radiology. . . . . Stephen J Brown
Quality Assurance . . . . Rita Bunch
CEO/President. . . . . Richard L Clark
Operating Room. . . . . David Crawford
Anesthesiology. . . . . Mark Davenport, MD
Chief of Medical Staff. . . . . Sunil Ramaprasad, MD
Infection Control. . . . . Tarry Samsel
Emergency Room . . . . Cynthia Thompson, RN

Measure	Cases	This Hosp.	State Avg.	U.S. Avg.
Blood Clot Prevention and Treatment				
Anticoagulation Overlap Therapy[2]	37	100%	92%	93%
ICU Venous Thromboembolism Prophylaxis[2]	47	98%	90%	92%
Incidence of Potentially Preventable VTE[2,7]	-	-	10%	10%
UFH with Dosages/Platelet Monitoring[2]	18	100%	99%	97%
Venous Thromboembolism Prophylaxis[2]	402	97%	83%	85%
Warfarin Therapy Discharge Instructions[2]	31	100%	78%	75%
Chest Pain/Possible Heart Attack Care				
Aspirin Given Within 24 Hours of Arrival	11	100%	96%	96%

NOTE: Hospital profiles are in alphabetical order by state, then city, then hospital within the city; Rankings exclude hospitals with less than 25 cases except for patient surveys which excludes hospitals with less than 100 cases; (a) 100-299 cases; (1) The number of cases/patients is too few to report; (2) Data submitted were based on a sample of cases/patients; (3) Results are based on a shorter time period than required; (4) Data suppressed by CMS for one or more quarters; (5) Results are not available for this reporting period; (6) Fewer than 100 patients completed the HCAHPS survey; (7) No cases met the criteria for this measure; (8) The lower limit of the confidence interval cannot be calculated if the number of observed infections equals zero; (9) No data are available from the state/territory for this reporting period; (10) The scores shown reflect fewer than 50 completed surveys; (11) There were discrepancies in the data collection process; (12) This measure does not apply to this hospital for this reporting period; (13) Results cannot be calculated for this reporting period; (14) The results for this state are combined with nearby states to protect confidentiality; Please refer to the User's Guide for a full explanation of data.

Measure	Cases	This Hosp.	State Avg.	U.S. Avg.
Fibrinolytic Meds Within 30 Min. of Arrival[3,7]	-	-	72%	58%
Average Time to ECG (minutes)	12	11	6	7
Average Time to Transfer (minutes)[1,3]	-	-	53	60
Children's Asthma Care				
Received Home Management Plan of Care	-	-	-	88%
Received Reliever Medication	-	-	-	100%
Received Systemic Corticosteroids	-	-	-	100%
Emergency Department				
Admittance Decision Time (minutes)[2]	765	96	82	98
Head CT Results Within 45 Min. of Arrival	13	92%	52%	57%
Patients Who Left ER Before Being Seen	40,009	3%	2%	2%
Time from ER Arrival to Admit. (minutes)[2]	765	276	243	274
Time from ER Arrival to Discharge (minutes)	388	166	131	134
Time in ER Before Being Evaluated (minutes)	425	41	25	26
Time to Pain Meds for Fractures (minutes)	90	60	60	57
Heart Attack Care				
Aspirin Given at Discharge[2]	146	100%	99%	99%
Fibrinolytic Meds Within 30 Min. of Arrival[2,7]	-	-	33%	54%
PCI Within 90 Minutes of Arrival[2]	20	100%	98%	96%
Statin Prescribed at Discharge[2]	159	99%	99%	98%
Heart Failure Care				
ACE Inhibitor or ARB for LVSD[2]	37	97%	97%	97%
Discharge Instructions Given[2]	126	99%	93%	94%
Evaluation of LVS Function[2]	103	100%	99%	99%
Medicare Spending				
Medicare Spending per Patient (ratio)	-	1.01	1	0.98
Pneumonia Care				
Appropriate Initial Antibiotic Given[2]	145	99%	95%	95%
Blood Culture Timing[2]	213	100%	98%	98%
Pregnancy and Delivery Care				
Newborn Deliveries Scheduled Early	138	1%	6%	6%
Preventive Care				
Immunization for Influenza[2]	605	93%	93%	90%
Immunization for Pneumonia[2]	828	96%	93%	92%
Stroke Care				
Anticoagulation Therapy for Atrial Fibrillation[2]	11	100%	94%	95%
Antithrombotic Therapy Timing[2]	73	100%	97%	98%
Assessed for Rehabilitation[2]	76	100%	97%	97%
Discharged on Antithrombotic Therapy[2]	45	100%	99%	99%
Discharged on Statin Medication[2]	66	98%	94%	94%
Thrombolytic Therapy Timing[2,7]	-	-	57%	66%
Venous Thromboembolism Prophylaxis[2]	76	100%	93%	94%
Written Stroke Educational Materials Given[2]	51	100%	84%	88%
Surgical Care Improvement Project				
Appropriate Beta Blocker Usage[2]	105	100%	97%	98%
Appropriate VTP Within 24 Hours[2]	308	100%	98%	98%
Controlled Postoperative Blood Glucose[2,7]	-	-	95%	97%
Perioperative Temperature Management[2]	333	100%	100%	100%
Prophylactic Antibiotic Selection[2]	260	100%	99%	99%
Prophylactic Antibiotic Selection (Outpatient)	171	98%	98%	98%
Prophylactic Antibiotic Stopped[2]	260	100%	98%	98%
Prophylactic Antibiotic Timing[2]	260	100%	99%	99%
Prophylactic Antibiotic Timing (Outpatient)	172	97%	98%	98%
Urinary Catheter Removal[2]	256	100%	96%	97%
Survey of Patients' Hospital Experiences				
Area Around Room 'Always' Quiet at Night	300+	60%	67%	61%
Doctors 'Always' Communicated Well	300+	81%	84%	82%
Home Recovery Information Given	300+	87%	85%	85%
Hospital Given 9 or 10 on 10 Point Scale	300+	67%	70%	71%
Meds 'Always' Explained Before Given	300+	69%	66%	64%
Nurses 'Always' Communicated Well	300+	79%	80%	79%
Pain 'Always' Well Controlled	300+	64%	72%	71%
Room and Bathroom 'Always' Clean	300+	71%	73%	73%
Timely Help 'Always' Received	300+	65%	68%	68%
Would Definitely Recommend Hospital	300+	68%	70%	71%
Use of Medical Imaging				
Cardiac Imaging Stress Test before Surgery[1]	-	-	4.8%	5.3%
Combination Abdominal CT Scan	568	11.4%	9.6%	10.5%
Combination Brain/Sinus CT Scan	691	4.3%	3.3%	2.7%
Combination Chest CT Scan	276	15.2%	3.4%	2.7%
Follow-up Mammogram/Ultrasound	670	4.8%	8.3%	8.8%
Lumbar Spine MRI for Low Back Pain	176	30.1%	35.3%	37.2%

Johnson County Community Hospital

1901 S Shady St
Mountain City, TN 37683
URL: www.msha.com
Type: Critical Access Hospitals
Ownership: Voluntary non-profit - Private
Phone: 423-727-1110
Fax: 423-727-1105
Emergency Services: Yes
Beds: 2

Measure	Cases	This Hosp.	State Avg.	U.S. Avg.
Blood Clot Prevention and Treatment				
Anticoagulation Overlap Therapy	-	-	92%	93%
ICU Venous Thromboembolism Prophylaxis	-	-	90%	92%
Incidence of Potentially Preventable VTE	-	-	10%	10%
UFH with Dosages/Platelet Monitoring	-	-	99%	97%
Venous Thromboembolism Prophylaxis	-	-	83%	85%
Warfarin Therapy Discharge Instructions	-	-	78%	75%
Chest Pain/Possible Heart Attack Care				
Aspirin Given Within 24 Hours of Arrival	73	100%	96%	96%
Fibrinolytic Meds Within 30 Min. of Arrival[7]	-	-	72%	58%
Average Time to ECG (minutes)	76	7	6	7
Average Time to Transfer (minutes)[1]	-	-	53	60
Children's Asthma Care				
Received Home Management Plan of Care	-	-	-	88%
Received Reliever Medication	-	-	-	100%
Received Systemic Corticosteroids	-	-	-	100%
Emergency Department				
Admittance Decision Time (minutes)	-	-	82	98
Head CT Results Within 45 Min. of Arrival[1]	-	-	52%	57%
Patients Who Left ER Before Being Seen	10,947	0%	2%	2%
Time from ER Arrival to Admit. (minutes)	-	-	243	274
Time from ER Arrival to Discharge (minutes)	350	94	131	134
Time in ER Before Being Evaluated (minutes)	195	34	25	26
Time to Pain Meds for Fractures (minutes)	33	55	60	57
Heart Attack Care				
Aspirin Given at Discharge	-	-	99%	99%
Fibrinolytic Meds Within 30 Min. of Arrival	-	-	33%	54%
PCI Within 90 Minutes of Arrival	-	-	98%	96%
Statin Prescribed at Discharge	-	-	99%	98%
Heart Failure Care				
ACE Inhibitor or ARB for LVSD	-	-	97%	97%
Discharge Instructions Given	-	-	93%	94%
Evaluation of LVS Function	-	-	99%	99%
Medicare Spending				
Medicare Spending per Patient (ratio)	-	-	1	0.98
Pneumonia Care				
Appropriate Initial Antibiotic Given	-	-	95%	95%
Blood Culture Timing	-	-	98%	98%
Pregnancy and Delivery Care				
Newborn Deliveries Scheduled Early	-	-	6%	6%
Preventive Care				
Immunization for Influenza	-	-	93%	90%
Immunization for Pneumonia	-	-	93%	92%
Stroke Care				
Anticoagulation Therapy for Atrial Fibrillation	-	-	94%	95%
Antithrombotic Therapy Timing	-	-	97%	98%
Assessed for Rehabilitation	-	-	97%	97%
Discharged on Antithrombotic Therapy	-	-	99%	99%
Discharged on Statin Medication	-	-	94%	94%
Thrombolytic Therapy Timing	-	-	57%	66%
Venous Thromboembolism Prophylaxis	-	-	93%	94%
Written Stroke Educational Materials Given	-	-	84%	88%
Surgical Care Improvement Project				
Appropriate Beta Blocker Usage	-	-	97%	98%
Appropriate VTP Within 24 Hours	-	-	98%	98%
Controlled Postoperative Blood Glucose	-	-	95%	97%
Perioperative Temperature Management	-	-	100%	100%
Prophylactic Antibiotic Selection	-	-	99%	99%
Prophylactic Antibiotic Selection (Outpatient)[5]	-	-	98%	98%
Prophylactic Antibiotic Stopped	-	-	98%	98%
Prophylactic Antibiotic Timing	-	-	99%	99%
Prophylactic Antibiotic Timing (Outpatient)[5]	-	-	98%	98%
Urinary Catheter Removal	-	-	96%	97%
Survey of Patients' Hospital Experiences				
Area Around Room 'Always' Quiet at Night	-	-	67%	61%
Doctors 'Always' Communicated Well	-	-	84%	82%
Home Recovery Information Given	-	-	85%	85%
Hospital Given 9 or 10 on 10 Point Scale	-	-	70%	71%
Meds 'Always' Explained Before Given	-	-	66%	64%
Nurses 'Always' Communicated Well	-	-	80%	79%
Pain 'Always' Well Controlled	-	-	72%	71%
Room and Bathroom 'Always' Clean	-	-	73%	73%
Timely Help 'Always' Received	-	-	68%	68%
Would Definitely Recommend Hospital	-	-	70%	71%
Use of Medical Imaging				
Cardiac Imaging Stress Test before Surgery	92	2.2%	4.8%	5.3%
Combination Abdominal CT Scan	181	9.4%	9.6%	10.5%
Combination Brain/Sinus CT Scan	161	6.8%	3.3%	2.7%
Combination Chest CT Scan	96	0.0%	3.4%	2.7%
Follow-up Mammogram/Ultrasound	225	5.3%	8.3%	8.8%
Lumbar Spine MRI for Low Back Pain[1]	-	-	35.3%	37.2%

Mountain Home VA Medical Center

Sidney & Lamont Streets
Mountain Home, TN 37684
URL: www.mountainhome.va.gov
Type: Acute Care - VA
Ownership: Government Federal
Phone: 423-926-1171
Fax: 423-979-3572
Emergency Services: No
Beds: 199

Key Personnel:
CEO/President. . . . . Carl J Gerber, MD
Operating Room. . . . . Lori Hagen, RN
Chief of Medical Staff . . . . Richard M Jordan, MD
Radiology. . . . . Pradeep Kumar, MD
Quality Assurance . . . . Norma Swanson

Measure	Cases	This Hosp.	State Avg.	U.S. Avg.
Blood Clot Prevention and Treatment				
Anticoagulation Overlap Therapy	-	-	92%	93%
ICU Venous Thromboembolism Prophylaxis	-	-	90%	92%
Incidence of Potentially Preventable VTE	-	-	10%	10%
UFH with Dosages/Platelet Monitoring	-	-	99%	97%
Venous Thromboembolism Prophylaxis	-	-	83%	85%
Warfarin Therapy Discharge Instructions	-	-	78%	75%
Chest Pain/Possible Heart Attack Care				
Aspirin Given Within 24 Hours of Arrival	-	-	96%	96%
Fibrinolytic Meds Within 30 Min. of Arrival	-	-	72%	58%
Average Time to ECG (minutes)	-	-	6	7
Average Time to Transfer (minutes)	-	-	53	60
Children's Asthma Care				
Received Home Management Plan of Care	-	-	-	88%
Received Reliever Medication	-	-	-	100%
Received Systemic Corticosteroids	-	-	-	100%
Emergency Department				
Admittance Decision Time (minutes)	-	-	82	98
Head CT Results Within 45 Min. of Arrival	-	-	52%	57%
Patients Who Left ER Before Being Seen	-	-	2%	2%
Time from ER Arrival to Admit. (minutes)	-	-	243	274
Time from ER Arrival to Discharge (minutes)	-	-	131	134
Time in ER Before Being Evaluated (minutes)	-	-	25	26
Time to Pain Meds for Fractures (minutes)	-	-	60	57
Heart Attack Care				
Aspirin Given at Discharge	83	100%	99%	99%
Fibrinolytic Meds Within 30 Min. of Arrival[5]	-	-	33%	54%
PCI Within 90 Minutes of Arrival[1]	-	-	98%	96%
Statin Prescribed at Discharge	79	100%	99%	98%
Heart Failure Care				
ACE Inhibitor or ARB for LVSD	70	97%	97%	97%
Discharge Instructions Given	191	94%	93%	94%
Evaluation of LVS Function	215	100%	99%	99%
Medicare Spending				
Medicare Spending per Patient (ratio)	-	-	1	0.98
Pneumonia Care				
Appropriate Initial Antibiotic Given	86	100%	95%	95%
Blood Culture Timing	222	100%	98%	98%
Pregnancy and Delivery Care				
Newborn Deliveries Scheduled Early	-	-	6%	6%
Preventive Care				
Immunization for Influenza[5]	-	-	93%	90%
Immunization for Pneumonia[5]	-	-	93%	92%
Stroke Care				

NOTE: Hospital profiles are in alphabetical order by state, then city, then hospital within the city; Rankings exclude hospitals with less than 25 cases except for patient surveys which excludes hospitals with less than 100 cases; (a) 100-299 cases; (1) The number of cases/patients is too few to report; (2) Data submitted were based on a sample of cases/patients; (3) Results are based on a shorter time period than required; (4) Data suppressed by CMS for one or more quarters; (5) Results are not available for this reporting period; (6) Fewer than 100 patients completed the HCAHPS survey; (7) No cases met the criteria for this measure; (8) The lower limit of the confidence interval cannot be calculated if the number of observed infections equals zero; (9) No data are available from the state/territory for this reporting period; (10) The scores shown reflect fewer than 50 completed surveys; (11) There were discrepancies in the data collection process; (12) This measure does not apply to this hospital for this reporting period; (13) Results cannot be calculated for this reporting period; (14) The results for this state are combined with nearby states to protect confidentiality; Please refer to the User's Guide for a full explanation of data.

Measure	Cases	This Hosp.	State Avg.	U.S. Avg.
Anticoagulation Therapy for Atrial Fibrillation	-	-	94%	95%
Antithrombotic Therapy Timing	-	-	97%	98%
Assessed for Rehabilitation	-	-	97%	97%
Discharged on Antithrombotic Therapy	-	-	99%	99%
Discharged on Statin Medication	-	-	94%	94%
Thrombolytic Therapy Timing	-	-	57%	66%
Venous Thromboembolism Prophylaxis	-	-	93%	94%
Written Stroke Educational Materials Given	-	-	84%	88%
Surgical Care Improvement Project				
Appropriate Beta Blocker Usage[2]	86	94%	97%	98%
Appropriate VTP Within 24 Hours[2]	175	99%	98%	98%
Controlled Postoperative Blood Glucose[5]	-	-	95%	97%
Perioperative Temperature Management[2]	207	100%	100%	100%
Prophylactic Antibiotic Selection	111	100%	99%	99%
Prophylactic Antibiotic Selection (Outpatient)	-	-	98%	98%
Prophylactic Antibiotic Stopped	109	100%	98%	98%
Prophylactic Antibiotic Timing	111	98%	99%	99%
Prophylactic Antibiotic Timing (Outpatient)	-	-	98%	98%
Urinary Catheter Removal[2]	135	98%	96%	97%
Survey of Patients' Hospital Experiences				
Area Around Room 'Always' Quiet at Night	-	-	67%	61%
Doctors 'Always' Communicated Well	-	-	84%	82%
Home Recovery Information Given	-	-	85%	85%
Hospital Given 9 or 10 on 10 Point Scale	-	-	70%	71%
Meds 'Always' Explained Before Given	-	-	66%	64%
Nurses 'Always' Communicated Well	-	-	80%	79%
Pain 'Always' Well Controlled	-	-	72%	71%
Room and Bathroom 'Always' Clean	-	-	73%	73%
Timely Help 'Always' Received	-	-	68%	68%
Would Definitely Recommend Hospital	-	-	70%	71%
Use of Medical Imaging				
Cardiac Imaging Stress Test before Surgery	-	-	4.8%	5.3%
Combination Abdominal CT Scan	-	-	9.6%	10.5%
Combination Brain/Sinus CT Scan	-	-	3.3%	2.7%
Combination Chest CT Scan	-	-	3.4%	2.7%
Follow-up Mammogram/Ultrasound	-	-	8.3%	8.8%
Lumbar Spine MRI for Low Back Pain	-	-	35.3%	37.2%

Saint Thomas Rutherford Hospital

1700 Medical Center Parkway — Phone: 615-396-4100
Murfreesboro, TN 37129 — Fax: 615-396-4659
URL: www.mtmc.org
Type: Acute Care Hospitals — Emergency Services: Yes
Ownership: Voluntary non-profit - Church — Beds: 288

Key Personnel:
Chief of Medical Staff. . . . . Andy Brown, MD
Radiology. Eric Dame
Emergency Room . . . . Patty Dixon
Quality Assurance . . . . Retta Fann
CEO/President. . . . . Gordon B Ferguson
Operating Room. . . . . Bennie Porter, RN

Measure	Cases	This Hosp.	State Avg.	U.S. Avg.
Blood Clot Prevention and Treatment				
Anticoagulation Overlap Therapy[2]	113	73%	92%	93%
ICU Venous Thromboembolism Prophylaxis[2]	92	83%	90%	92%
Incidence of Potentially Preventable VTE[2]	19	5%	10%	10%
UFH with Dosages/Platelet Monitoring[2]	16	94%	99%	97%
Venous Thromboembolism Prophylaxis[2]	328	82%	83%	85%
Warfarin Therapy Discharge Instructions[2]	94	79%	78%	75%
Chest Pain/Possible Heart Attack Care				
Aspirin Given Within 24 Hours of Arrival	32	100%	96%	96%
Fibrinolytic Meds Within 30 Min. of Arrival[7]	-	-	72%	58%
Average Time to ECG (minutes)	31	6	6	7
Average Time to Transfer (minutes)[1]	-	-	53	60
Children's Asthma Care				
Received Home Management Plan of Care	-	-	-	88%
Received Reliever Medication	-	-	-	100%
Received Systemic Corticosteroids	-	-	-	100%
Emergency Department				
Admittance Decision Time (minutes)[2]	546	88	82	98
Head CT Results Within 45 Min. of Arrival	12	75%	52%	57%
Patients Who Left ER Before Being Seen	78,924	3%	2%	2%
Time from ER Arrival to Admit. (minutes)[2]	557	220	243	274
Time from ER Arrival to Discharge (minutes)	344	162	131	134
Time in ER Before Being Evaluated (minutes)	374	34	25	26
Time to Pain Meds for Fractures (minutes)	238	60	60	57
Heart Attack Care				
Aspirin Given at Discharge	227	99%	99%	99%
Fibrinolytic Meds Within 30 Min. of Arrival[7]	-	-	33%	54%
PCI Within 90 Minutes of Arrival	45	98%	98%	96%
Statin Prescribed at Discharge	239	97%	99%	98%
Heart Failure Care				
ACE Inhibitor or ARB for LVSD	127	95%	97%	97%
Discharge Instructions Given	379	91%	93%	94%
Evaluation of LVS Function	468	100%	99%	99%
Medicare Spending				
Medicare Spending per Patient (ratio)	-	0.98	1	0.98
Pneumonia Care				
Appropriate Initial Antibiotic Given	309	94%	95%	95%
Blood Culture Timing	340	96%	98%	98%
Pregnancy and Delivery Care				
Newborn Deliveries Scheduled Early[2]	60	8%	6%	6%
Preventive Care				
Immunization for Influenza[2]	528	89%	93%	90%
Immunization for Pneumonia[2]	632	87%	93%	92%
Stroke Care				
Anticoagulation Therapy for Atrial Fibrillation	14	100%	94%	95%
Antithrombotic Therapy Timing	144	99%	97%	98%
Assessed for Rehabilitation	174	93%	97%	97%
Discharged on Antithrombotic Therapy	163	99%	99%	99%
Discharged on Statin Medication	112	84%	94%	94%
Thrombolytic Therapy Timing	11	91%	57%	66%
Venous Thromboembolism Prophylaxis	153	93%	93%	94%
Written Stroke Educational Materials Given	109	86%	84%	88%
Surgical Care Improvement Project				
Appropriate Beta Blocker Usage[2]	158	97%	97%	98%
Appropriate VTP Within 24 Hours[2]	514	94%	98%	98%
Controlled Postoperative Blood Glucose[2,7]	-	-	95%	97%
Perioperative Temperature Management[2]	599	99%	100%	100%
Prophylactic Antibiotic Selection[2]	433	98%	99%	99%
Prophylactic Antibiotic Selection (Outpatient)	518	91%	98%	98%
Prophylactic Antibiotic Stopped[2]	424	92%	98%	98%
Prophylactic Antibiotic Timing[2]	436	98%	99%	99%
Prophylactic Antibiotic Timing (Outpatient)	524	97%	98%	98%
Urinary Catheter Removal[2]	449	90%	96%	97%
Survey of Patients' Hospital Experiences				
Area Around Room 'Always' Quiet at Night	300+	63%	67%	61%
Doctors 'Always' Communicated Well	300+	85%	84%	82%
Home Recovery Information Given	300+	87%	85%	85%
Hospital Given 9 or 10 on 10 Point Scale	300+	72%	70%	71%
Meds 'Always' Explained Before Given	300+	70%	66%	64%
Nurses 'Always' Communicated Well	300+	80%	80%	79%
Pain 'Always' Well Controlled	300+	71%	72%	71%
Room and Bathroom 'Always' Clean	300+	70%	73%	73%
Timely Help 'Always' Received	300+	61%	68%	68%
Would Definitely Recommend Hospital	300+	75%	70%	71%
Use of Medical Imaging				
Cardiac Imaging Stress Test before Surgery	782	4.7%	4.8%	5.3%
Combination Abdominal CT Scan	641	0.8%	9.6%	10.5%
Combination Brain/Sinus CT Scan	803	2.6%	3.3%	2.7%
Combination Chest CT Scan	87	0.0%	3.4%	2.7%
Follow-up Mammogram/Ultrasound[7]	-	-	8.3%	8.8%
Lumbar Spine MRI for Low Back Pain[1]	-	-	35.3%	37.2%

Trustpoint Hospital

1009 North Thompson Lane — Phone: 615-577-1111
Murfreesboro, TN 37129
Type: Acute Care Hospitals — Emergency Services: No
Ownership: Proprietary

Measure	Cases	This Hosp.	State Avg.	U.S. Avg.
Blood Clot Prevention and Treatment				
Anticoagulation Overlap Therapy[3,7]	-	-	92%	93%
ICU Venous Thromboembolism Prophylaxis[3,7]	-	-	90%	92%
Incidence of Potentially Preventable VTE[3,7]	-	-	10%	10%
UFH with Dosages/Platelet Monitoring[3,7]	-	-	99%	97%
Venous Thromboembolism Prophylaxis[3]	20	90%	83%	85%
Warfarin Therapy Discharge Instructions[3,7]	-	-	78%	75%
Chest Pain/Possible Heart Attack Care				
Aspirin Given Within 24 Hours of Arrival[5]	-	-	96%	96%
Fibrinolytic Meds Within 30 Min. of Arrival[5]	-	-	72%	58%
Average Time to ECG (minutes)[5]	-	-	6	7
Average Time to Transfer (minutes)[5]	-	-	53	60
Children's Asthma Care				
Received Home Management Plan of Care	-	-	-	88%
Received Reliever Medication	-	-	-	100%
Received Systemic Corticosteroids	-	-	-	100%
Emergency Department				
Admittance Decision Time (minutes)[3,7]	-	-	82	98
Head CT Results Within 45 Min. of Arrival[5]	-	-	52%	57%
Patients Who Left ER Before Being Seen[5]	-	-	2%	2%
Time from ER Arrival to Admit. (minutes)[3,7]	-	-	243	274
Time from ER Arrival to Discharge (minutes)[5]	-	-	131	134
Time in ER Before Being Evaluated (minutes)[5]	-	-	25	26
Time to Pain Meds for Fractures (minutes)[5]	-	-	60	57
Heart Attack Care				
Aspirin Given at Discharge[5]	-	-	99%	99%
Fibrinolytic Meds Within 30 Min. of Arrival[5]	-	-	33%	54%
PCI Within 90 Minutes of Arrival[5]	-	-	98%	96%
Statin Prescribed at Discharge[5]	-	-	99%	98%
Heart Failure Care				
ACE Inhibitor or ARB for LVSD[5]	-	-	97%	97%
Discharge Instructions Given[5]	-	-	93%	94%
Evaluation of LVS Function[5]	-	-	99%	99%
Medicare Spending				
Medicare Spending per Patient (ratio)	-	-	1	0.98
Pneumonia Care				
Appropriate Initial Antibiotic Given[5]	-	-	95%	95%
Blood Culture Timing[5]	-	-	98%	98%
Pregnancy and Delivery Care				
Newborn Deliveries Scheduled Early[3,7]	-	-	6%	6%
Preventive Care				
Immunization for Influenza[5]	-	-	93%	90%
Immunization for Pneumonia[3]	17	94%	93%	92%
Stroke Care				
Anticoagulation Therapy for Atrial Fibrillation[5]	-	-	94%	95%
Antithrombotic Therapy Timing[5]	-	-	97%	98%
Assessed for Rehabilitation[5]	-	-	97%	97%
Discharged on Antithrombotic Therapy[5]	-	-	99%	99%
Discharged on Statin Medication[5]	-	-	94%	94%
Thrombolytic Therapy Timing[5]	-	-	57%	66%
Venous Thromboembolism Prophylaxis[5]	-	-	93%	94%
Written Stroke Educational Materials Given[5]	-	-	84%	88%
Surgical Care Improvement Project				
Appropriate Beta Blocker Usage[5]	-	-	97%	98%
Appropriate VTP Within 24 Hours[5]	-	-	98%	98%
Controlled Postoperative Blood Glucose[5]	-	-	95%	97%
Perioperative Temperature Management[5]	-	-	100%	100%
Prophylactic Antibiotic Selection[5]	-	-	99%	99%
Prophylactic Antibiotic Selection (Outpatient)[5]	-	-	98%	98%
Prophylactic Antibiotic Stopped[5]	-	-	98%	98%
Prophylactic Antibiotic Timing[5]	-	-	99%	99%
Prophylactic Antibiotic Timing (Outpatient)[5]	-	-	98%	98%
Urinary Catheter Removal[5]	-	-	96%	97%
Survey of Patients' Hospital Experiences				
Area Around Room 'Always' Quiet at Night[1]	-	-	67%	61%
Doctors 'Always' Communicated Well[1]	-	-	84%	82%
Home Recovery Information Given[1]	-	-	85%	85%
Hospital Given 9 or 10 on 10 Point Scale[1]	-	-	70%	71%
Meds 'Always' Explained Before Given[1]	-	-	66%	64%
Nurses 'Always' Communicated Well[1]	-	-	80%	79%
Pain 'Always' Well Controlled[1]	-	-	72%	71%
Room and Bathroom 'Always' Clean[1]	-	-	73%	73%
Timely Help 'Always' Received[1]	-	-	68%	68%
Would Definitely Recommend Hospital[1]	-	-	70%	71%
Use of Medical Imaging				
Cardiac Imaging Stress Test before Surgery[7]	-	-	4.8%	5.3%
Combination Abdominal CT Scan[7]	-	-	9.6%	10.5%
Combination Brain/Sinus CT Scan[7]	-	-	3.3%	2.7%

NOTE: Hospital profiles are in alphabetical order by state, then city, then hospital within the city; Rankings exclude hospitals with less than 25 cases except for patient surveys which excludes hospitals with less than 100 cases; (a) 100-299 cases; (1) The number of cases/patients is too few to report; (2) Data submitted were based on a sample of cases/patients; (3) Results are based on a shorter time period than required; (4) Data suppressed by CMS for one or more quarters; (5) Results are not available for this reporting period; (6) Fewer than 100 patients completed the HCAHPS survey; (7) No cases met the criteria for this measure; (8) The lower limit of the confidence interval cannot be calculated if the number of observed infections equals zero; (9) No data are available from the state/territory for this reporting period; (10) The scores shown reflect fewer than 50 completed surveys; (11) There were discrepancies in the data collection process; (12) This measure does not apply to this hospital for this reporting period; (13) Results cannot be calculated for this reporting period; (14) The results for this state are combined with nearby states to protect confidentiality; Please refer to the User's Guide for a full explanation of data.

Measure	Cases	This Hosp.	State Avg.	U.S. Avg.
Combination Chest CT Scan[7]	-	-	3.4%	2.7%
Follow-up Mammogram/Ultrasound[7]	-	-	8.3%	8.8%
Lumbar Spine MRI for Low Back Pain[7]	-	-	35.3%	37.2%

Metro Nashville General Hospital

1818 Albion Street
Nashville, TN 37208
Type: Acute Care Hospitals
Ownership: Govt - Hospital Dist/Auth
Phone: 615-341-4490
Fax: 615-341-4493
Emergency Services: Yes
Beds: 150

Key Personnel:
CEO . . . . Robert M. Lonis, CPA
Chief of Medical Staff . . . . Chike Nzerue, MD
CEO/President. . . . . Roxane Spitzer, PHD

Measure	Cases	This Hosp.	State Avg.	U.S. Avg.
Blood Clot Prevention and Treatment				
Anticoagulation Overlap Therapy[2]	18	78%	92%	93%
ICU Venous Thromboembolism Prophylaxis[2]	147	82%	90%	92%
Incidence of Potentially Preventable VTE[1,2]	-	-	10%	10%
UFH with Dosages/Platelet Monitoring[1,2]	-	-	99%	97%
Venous Thromboembolism Prophylaxis[2]	253	74%	83%	85%
Warfarin Therapy Discharge Instructions[2]	15	53%	78%	75%
Chest Pain/Possible Heart Attack Care				
Aspirin Given Within 24 Hours of Arrival[1,3]	-	-	96%	96%
Fibrinolytic Meds Within 30 Min. of Arrival[3,7]	-	-	72%	58%
Average Time to ECG (minutes)[1,3]	-	-	6	7
Average Time to Transfer (minutes)[1,3]	-	-	53	60
Children's Asthma Care				
Received Home Management Plan of Care	-	-	-	88%
Received Reliever Medication	-	-	-	100%
Received Systemic Corticosteroids	-	-	-	100%
Emergency Department				
Admittance Decision Time (minutes)[2]	231	68	82	98
Head CT Results Within 45 Min. of Arrival[1]	-	-	52%	57%
Patients Who Left ER Before Being Seen	37,577	4%	2%	2%
Time from ER Arrival to Admit. (minutes)[2]	233	233	243	274
Time from ER Arrival to Discharge (minutes)	336	126	131	134
Time in ER Before Being Evaluated (minutes)	370	35	25	26
Time to Pain Meds for Fractures (minutes)	63	82	60	57
Heart Attack Care				
Aspirin Given at Discharge[2]	28	100%	99%	99%
Fibrinolytic Meds Within 30 Min. of Arrival[2,7]	-	-	33%	54%
PCI Within 90 Minutes of Arrival[2,7]	-	-	98%	96%
Statin Prescribed at Discharge[2]	28	100%	99%	98%
Heart Failure Care				
ACE Inhibitor or ARB for LVSD[2]	85	95%	97%	97%
Discharge Instructions Given[2]	148	76%	93%	94%
Evaluation of LVS Function[2]	137	96%	99%	99%
Medicare Spending				
Medicare Spending per Patient (ratio)	-	0.91	1	0.98
Pneumonia Care				
Appropriate Initial Antibiotic Given[2]	27	89%	95%	95%
Blood Culture Timing[2]	45	96%	98%	98%
Pregnancy and Delivery Care				
Newborn Deliveries Scheduled Early[2]	23	9%	6%	6%
Preventive Care				
Immunization for Influenza[2]	343	78%	93%	90%
Immunization for Pneumonia[2]	309	85%	93%	92%
Stroke Care				
Anticoagulation Therapy for Atrial Fibrillation[1,2]	-	-	94%	95%
Antithrombotic Therapy Timing[2]	20	95%	97%	98%
Assessed for Rehabilitation[2]	22	95%	97%	97%
Discharged on Antithrombotic Therapy[2]	19	100%	99%	99%
Discharged on Statin Medication[2]	19	89%	94%	94%
Thrombolytic Therapy Timing[1,2]	-	-	57%	66%
Venous Thromboembolism Prophylaxis[2]	24	75%	93%	94%
Written Stroke Educational Materials Given[2]	21	5%	84%	88%
Surgical Care Improvement Project				
Appropriate Beta Blocker Usage[2]	28	75%	97%	98%
Appropriate VTP Within 24 Hours[2]	162	93%	98%	98%
Controlled Postoperative Blood Glucose[2,7]	-	-	95%	97%
Perioperative Temperature Management[2]	184	100%	100%	100%
Prophylactic Antibiotic Selection[2]	104	89%	99%	99%
Prophylactic Antibiotic Selection (Outpatient)	41	95%	98%	98%
Prophylactic Antibiotic Stopped[2]	104	94%	98%	98%
Prophylactic Antibiotic Timing[2]	104	96%	99%	99%
Prophylactic Antibiotic Timing (Outpatient)	42	93%	98%	98%
Urinary Catheter Removal[2]	109	91%	96%	97%
Survey of Patients' Hospital Experiences				
Area Around Room 'Always' Quiet at Night	300+	63%	67%	61%
Doctors 'Always' Communicated Well	300+	82%	84%	82%
Home Recovery Information Given	300+	85%	85%	85%
Hospital Given 9 or 10 on 10 Point Scale	300+	68%	70%	71%
Meds 'Always' Explained Before Given	300+	63%	66%	64%
Nurses 'Always' Communicated Well	300+	72%	80%	79%
Pain 'Always' Well Controlled	300+	71%	72%	71%
Room and Bathroom 'Always' Clean	300+	70%	73%	73%
Timely Help 'Always' Received	300+	59%	68%	68%
Would Definitely Recommend Hospital	300+	67%	70%	71%
Use of Medical Imaging				
Cardiac Imaging Stress Test before Surgery[1]	-	-	4.8%	5.3%
Combination Abdominal CT Scan	73	13.7%	9.6%	10.5%
Combination Brain/Sinus CT Scan[1]	-	-	3.3%	2.7%
Combination Chest CT Scan[1]	-	-	3.4%	2.7%
Follow-up Mammogram/Ultrasound	73	4.1%	8.3%	8.8%
Lumbar Spine MRI for Low Back Pain[1]	-	-	35.3%	37.2%

Saint Thomas Hospital for Spinal Surgery

2011 Murphy Avenue
Nashville, TN 37203
URL: www.hospitalforspinalsurgery.com
Type: Acute Care Hospitals
Ownership: Voluntary non-profit - Other
Phone: 615-515-8200
Emergency Services: No
Beds: 18

Key Personnel:
CEO/President. . . . . Elissa Christiansen
Quality Assurance . . . . Stephanie Purtee
Administrator . . . . Kathy Watson

Measure	Cases	This Hosp.	State Avg.	U.S. Avg.
Blood Clot Prevention and Treatment				
Anticoagulation Overlap Therapy[2,7]	-	-	92%	93%
ICU Venous Thromboembolism Prophylaxis[2,7]	-	-	90%	92%
Incidence of Potentially Preventable VTE[2,7]	-	-	10%	10%
UFH with Dosages/Platelet Monitoring[2,7]	-	-	99%	97%
Venous Thromboembolism Prophylaxis[2]	26	100%	83%	85%
Warfarin Therapy Discharge Instructions[2,7]	-	-	78%	75%
Chest Pain/Possible Heart Attack Care				
Aspirin Given Within 24 Hours of Arrival[5]	-	-	96%	96%
Fibrinolytic Meds Within 30 Min. of Arrival[5]	-	-	72%	58%
Average Time to ECG (minutes)[5]	-	-	6	7
Average Time to Transfer (minutes)[5]	-	-	53	60
Children's Asthma Care				
Received Home Management Plan of Care	-	-	-	88%
Received Reliever Medication	-	-	-	100%
Received Systemic Corticosteroids	-	-	-	100%
Emergency Department				
Admittance Decision Time (minutes)[2,7]	-	-	82	98
Head CT Results Within 45 Min. of Arrival[5]	-	-	52%	57%
Patients Who Left ER Before Being Seen[5]	-	-	2%	2%
Time from ER Arrival to Admit. (minutes)[2,7]	-	-	243	274
Time from ER Arrival to Discharge (minutes)[5]	-	-	131	134
Time in ER Before Being Evaluated (minutes)[5]	-	-	25	26
Time to Pain Meds for Fractures (minutes)[5]	-	-	60	57
Heart Attack Care				
Aspirin Given at Discharge[5]	-	-	99%	99%
Fibrinolytic Meds Within 30 Min. of Arrival[5]	-	-	33%	54%
PCI Within 90 Minutes of Arrival[5]	-	-	98%	96%
Statin Prescribed at Discharge[5]	-	-	99%	98%
Heart Failure Care				
ACE Inhibitor or ARB for LVSD[5]	-	-	97%	97%
Discharge Instructions Given[5]	-	-	93%	94%
Evaluation of LVS Function[5]	-	-	99%	99%
Medicare Spending				
Medicare Spending per Patient (ratio)	-	0.89	1	0.98
Pneumonia Care				
Appropriate Initial Antibiotic Given[5]	-	-	95%	95%
Blood Culture Timing[5]	-	-	98%	98%
Pregnancy and Delivery Care				
Newborn Deliveries Scheduled Early[7]	-	-	6%	6%
Preventive Care				
Immunization for Influenza[2]	321	84%	93%	90%
Immunization for Pneumonia[2]	341	86%	93%	92%
Stroke Care				
Anticoagulation Therapy for Atrial Fibrillation[5]	-	-	94%	95%
Antithrombotic Therapy Timing[5]	-	-	97%	98%
Assessed for Rehabilitation[5]	-	-	97%	97%
Discharged on Antithrombotic Therapy[5]	-	-	99%	99%
Discharged on Statin Medication[5]	-	-	94%	94%
Thrombolytic Therapy Timing[5]	-	-	57%	66%
Venous Thromboembolism Prophylaxis[5]	-	-	93%	94%
Written Stroke Educational Materials Given[5]	-	-	84%	88%
Surgical Care Improvement Project				
Appropriate Beta Blocker Usage[5]	-	-	97%	98%
Appropriate VTP Within 24 Hours[5]	-	-	98%	98%
Controlled Postoperative Blood Glucose[5]	-	-	95%	97%
Perioperative Temperature Management[5]	-	-	100%	100%
Prophylactic Antibiotic Selection[5]	-	-	99%	99%
Prophylactic Antibiotic Selection (Outpatient)	833	100%	98%	98%
Prophylactic Antibiotic Stopped[5]	-	-	98%	98%
Prophylactic Antibiotic Timing[5]	-	-	99%	99%
Prophylactic Antibiotic Timing (Outpatient)	834	100%	98%	98%
Urinary Catheter Removal[5]	-	-	96%	97%
Survey of Patients' Hospital Experiences				
Area Around Room 'Always' Quiet at Night	300+	82%	67%	61%
Doctors 'Always' Communicated Well	300+	88%	84%	82%
Home Recovery Information Given	300+	88%	85%	85%
Hospital Given 9 or 10 on 10 Point Scale	300+	87%	70%	71%
Meds 'Always' Explained Before Given	300+	78%	66%	64%
Nurses 'Always' Communicated Well	300+	89%	80%	79%
Pain 'Always' Well Controlled	300+	81%	72%	71%
Room and Bathroom 'Always' Clean	300+	81%	73%	73%
Timely Help 'Always' Received	300+	84%	68%	68%
Would Definitely Recommend Hospital	300+	90%	70%	71%
Use of Medical Imaging				
Cardiac Imaging Stress Test before Surgery[7]	-	-	4.8%	5.3%
Combination Abdominal CT Scan[7]	-	-	9.6%	10.5%
Combination Brain/Sinus CT Scan[7]	-	-	3.3%	2.7%
Combination Chest CT Scan[7]	-	-	3.4%	2.7%
Follow-up Mammogram/Ultrasound[7]	-	-	8.3%	8.8%
Lumbar Spine MRI for Low Back Pain[7]	-	-	35.3%	37.2%

Saint Thomas Midtown Hospital

2000 Church St
Nashville, TN 37236
URL: www.baptisthospital.com
Type: Acute Care Hospitals
Ownership: Voluntary non-profit - Private
Phone: 615-284-5555
Fax: 615-284-8686
Emergency Services: Yes
Beds: 723

Key Personnel:
Quality Assurance . . . . Sue Carter, RN
Pediatric Ambulatory Care . . . . . . Ralph Greenbaum, MD
Pediatric In-Patient Care . . . . Ralph Greenbaum, MD
Radiology. . . . . Michael Seshul, MD
Chief of Medical Staff . . . . Geoffrey Smallwood, MD
Infection Control. . . . . Virginia Tankersly, RN
Operating Room. . . . . Perri Lynn White

Measure	Cases	This Hosp.	State Avg.	U.S. Avg.
Blood Clot Prevention and Treatment				
Anticoagulation Overlap Therapy[2]	114	91%	92%	93%
ICU Venous Thromboembolism Prophylaxis[2]	58	90%	90%	92%
Incidence of Potentially Preventable VTE[2]	22	18%	10%	10%
UFH with Dosages/Platelet Monitoring[2]	13	92%	99%	97%
Venous Thromboembolism Prophylaxis[2]	333	77%	83%	85%
Warfarin Therapy Discharge Instructions[2]	92	71%	78%	75%
Chest Pain/Possible Heart Attack Care				
Aspirin Given Within 24 Hours of Arrival[5]	-	-	96%	96%
Fibrinolytic Meds Within 30 Min. of Arrival[5]	-	-	72%	58%
Average Time to ECG (minutes)[5]	-	-	6	7
Average Time to Transfer (minutes)[5]	-	-	53	60
Children's Asthma Care				
Received Home Management Plan of Care	-	-	-	88%
Received Reliever Medication	-	-	-	100%
Received Systemic Corticosteroids	-	-	-	100%

NOTE: Hospital profiles are in alphabetical order by state, then city, then hospital within the city; Rankings exclude hospitals with less than 25 cases except for patient surveys which excludes hospitals with less than 100 cases; (a) 100-299 cases; (1) The number of cases/patients is too few to report; (2) Data submitted were based on a sample of cases/patients; (3) Results are based on a shorter time period than required; (4) Data suppressed by CMS for one or more quarters; (5) Results are not available for this reporting period; (6) Fewer than 100 patients completed the HCAHPS survey; (7) No cases met the criteria for this measure; (8) The lower limit of the confidence interval cannot be calculated if the number of observed infections equals zero; (9) No data are available from the state/territory for this reporting period; (10) The scores shown reflect fewer than 50 completed surveys; (11) There were discrepancies in the data collection process; (12) This measure does not apply to this hospital for this reporting period; (13) Results cannot be calculated for this reporting period; (14) The results for this state are combined with nearby states to protect confidentiality; Please refer to the User's Guide for a full explanation of data.

Measure	Cases	This Hosp.	State Avg.	U.S. Avg.
Emergency Department				
Admittance Decision Time (minutes)[2]	355	71	82	98
Head CT Results Within 45 Min. of Arrival[1]	-	-	52%	57%
Patients Who Left ER Before Being Seen	52,828	2%	2%	2%
Time from ER Arrival to Admit. (minutes)[2]	360	199	243	274
Time from ER Arrival to Discharge (minutes)	373	171	131	134
Time in ER Before Being Evaluated (minutes)	392	29	25	26
Time to Pain Meds for Fractures (minutes)	93	53	60	57
Heart Attack Care				
Aspirin Given at Discharge	250	98%	99%	99%
Fibrinolytic Meds Within 30 Min. of Arrival[7]	-	-	33%	54%
PCI Within 90 Minutes of Arrival	28	93%	98%	96%
Statin Prescribed at Discharge	241	95%	99%	98%
Heart Failure Care				
ACE Inhibitor or ARB for LVSD	246	95%	97%	97%
Discharge Instructions Given	600	94%	93%	94%
Evaluation of LVS Function	660	100%	99%	99%
Medicare Spending				
Medicare Spending per Patient (ratio)	-	1.01	1	0.98
Pneumonia Care				
Appropriate Initial Antibiotic Given	191	93%	95%	95%
Blood Culture Timing	237	99%	98%	98%
Pregnancy and Delivery Care				
Newborn Deliveries Scheduled Early[2]	112	5%	6%	6%
Preventive Care				
Immunization for Influenza[2]	510	83%	93%	90%
Immunization for Pneumonia[2]	524	77%	93%	92%
Stroke Care				
Anticoagulation Therapy for Atrial Fibrillation	14	93%	94%	95%
Antithrombotic Therapy Timing	108	78%	97%	98%
Assessed for Rehabilitation	175	89%	97%	97%
Discharged on Antithrombotic Therapy	137	97%	99%	99%
Discharged on Statin Medication	112	86%	94%	94%
Thrombolytic Therapy Timing	18	11%	57%	66%
Venous Thromboembolism Prophylaxis	174	80%	93%	94%
Written Stroke Educational Materials Given	98	70%	84%	88%
Surgical Care Improvement Project				
Appropriate Beta Blocker Usage[2]	216	98%	97%	98%
Appropriate VTP Within 24 Hours[2]	404	97%	98%	98%
Controlled Postoperative Blood Glucose[2]	132	100%	95%	97%
Perioperative Temperature Management[2]	524	100%	100%	100%
Prophylactic Antibiotic Selection[2]	497	98%	99%	99%
Prophylactic Antibiotic Selection (Outpatient)	665	95%	98%	98%
Prophylactic Antibiotic Stopped[2]	491	98%	98%	98%
Prophylactic Antibiotic Timing[2]	498	99%	99%	99%
Prophylactic Antibiotic Timing (Outpatient)	670	94%	98%	98%
Urinary Catheter Removal[2]	418	99%	96%	97%
Survey of Patients' Hospital Experiences				
Area Around Room 'Always' Quiet at Night	300+	60%	67%	61%
Doctors 'Always' Communicated Well	300+	85%	84%	82%
Home Recovery Information Given	300+	84%	85%	85%
Hospital Given 9 or 10 on 10 Point Scale	300+	71%	70%	71%
Meds 'Always' Explained Before Given	300+	69%	66%	64%
Nurses 'Always' Communicated Well	300+	79%	80%	79%
Pain 'Always' Well Controlled	300+	70%	72%	71%
Room and Bathroom 'Always' Clean	300+	61%	73%	73%
Timely Help 'Always' Received	300+	62%	68%	68%
Would Definitely Recommend Hospital	300+	76%	70%	71%
Use of Medical Imaging				
Cardiac Imaging Stress Test before Surgery	1,135	4.4%	4.8%	5.3%
Combination Abdominal CT Scan	611	4.1%	9.6%	10.5%
Combination Brain/Sinus CT Scan[1]	-	-	3.3%	2.7%
Combination Chest CT Scan	272	1.8%	3.4%	2.7%
Follow-up Mammogram/Ultrasound	2,088	4.8%	8.3%	8.8%
Lumbar Spine MRI for Low Back Pain[1]	-	-	35.3%	37.2%

Saint Thomas West Hospital

4220 Harding Rd, PO Box 380 Phone: 615-222-2111
Nashville, TN 37205 Fax: 615-222-4482
URL: www.stthomas.org
Type: Acute Care Hospitals Emergency Services: Yes
Ownership: Voluntary non-profit - Church Beds: 541

Key Personnel:

CEO/President. . . . . Thomas E Beeman
Emergency Room . . . . Kevin Bonner, MD
Chief of Medical Staff. . . . . John Johnson
Infection Control. . . . . Deanie Lancaster
Quality Assurance . . . . Linda Poteete
Hemotology Center . . . . Paul Rosenblatt, MD
Radiology. . . . . K James Schumacher, MD
Intensive Care Unit. . . . . CS Thomas, Jr, MD

Measure	Cases	This Hosp.	State Avg.	U.S. Avg.
Blood Clot Prevention and Treatment				
Anticoagulation Overlap Therapy[2]	165	84%	92%	93%
ICU Venous Thromboembolism Prophylaxis[2]	114	84%	90%	92%
Incidence of Potentially Preventable VTE[2]	44	9%	10%	10%
UFH with Dosages/Platelet Monitoring[2]	90	100%	99%	97%
Venous Thromboembolism Prophylaxis[2]	267	76%	83%	85%
Warfarin Therapy Discharge Instructions[2]	132	74%	78%	75%
Chest Pain/Possible Heart Attack Care				
Aspirin Given Within 24 Hours of Arrival[5]	-	-	96%	96%
Fibrinolytic Meds Within 30 Min. of Arrival[5]	-	-	72%	58%
Average Time to ECG (minutes)[5]	-	-	6	7
Average Time to Transfer (minutes)[5]	-	-	53	60
Children's Asthma Care				
Received Home Management Plan of Care	-	-	-	88%
Received Reliever Medication	-	-	-	100%
Received Systemic Corticosteroids	-	-	-	100%
Emergency Department				
Admittance Decision Time (minutes)[2]	381	68	82	98
Head CT Results Within 45 Min. of Arrival[1]	-	-	52%	57%
Patients Who Left ER Before Being Seen	34,039	1%	2%	2%
Time from ER Arrival to Admit. (minutes)[2]	395	208	243	274
Time from ER Arrival to Discharge (minutes)	348	158	131	134
Time in ER Before Being Evaluated (minutes)	389	23	25	26
Time to Pain Meds for Fractures (minutes)	65	62	60	57
Heart Attack Care				
Aspirin Given at Discharge	1,318	99%	99%	99%
Fibrinolytic Meds Within 30 Min. of Arrival[7]	-	-	33%	54%
PCI Within 90 Minutes of Arrival	67	99%	98%	96%
Statin Prescribed at Discharge	1,260	98%	99%	98%
Heart Failure Care				
ACE Inhibitor or ARB for LVSD	335	95%	97%	97%
Discharge Instructions Given	864	89%	93%	94%
Evaluation of LVS Function	981	99%	99%	99%
Medicare Spending				
Medicare Spending per Patient (ratio)	-	0.97	1	0.98
Pneumonia Care				
Appropriate Initial Antibiotic Given	198	95%	95%	95%
Blood Culture Timing	334	97%	98%	98%
Pregnancy and Delivery Care				
Newborn Deliveries Scheduled Early[2,7]	-	-	6%	6%
Preventive Care				
Immunization for Influenza[2]	621	96%	93%	90%
Immunization for Pneumonia[2]	984	86%	93%	92%
Stroke Care				
Anticoagulation Therapy for Atrial Fibrillation	44	100%	94%	95%
Antithrombotic Therapy Timing	272	99%	97%	98%
Assessed for Rehabilitation	378	98%	97%	97%
Discharged on Antithrombotic Therapy	309	100%	99%	99%
Discharged on Statin Medication	237	95%	94%	94%
Thrombolytic Therapy Timing	22	86%	57%	66%
Venous Thromboembolism Prophylaxis	369	92%	93%	94%
Written Stroke Educational Materials Given	221	92%	84%	88%
Surgical Care Improvement Project				
Appropriate Beta Blocker Usage[2]	238	98%	97%	98%
Appropriate VTP Within 24 Hours[2]	474	99%	98%	98%
Controlled Postoperative Blood Glucose[2]	161	96%	95%	97%
Perioperative Temperature Management[2]	619	100%	100%	100%
Prophylactic Antibiotic Selection[2]	566	100%	99%	99%
Prophylactic Antibiotic Selection (Outpatient)	521	98%	98%	98%
Prophylactic Antibiotic Stopped[2]	556	99%	98%	98%
Prophylactic Antibiotic Timing[2]	567	100%	99%	99%
Prophylactic Antibiotic Timing (Outpatient)	521	98%	98%	98%
Urinary Catheter Removal[2]	510	98%	96%	97%
Survey of Patients' Hospital Experiences				
Area Around Room 'Always' Quiet at Night	300+	61%	67%	61%
Doctors 'Always' Communicated Well	300+	84%	84%	82%
Home Recovery Information Given	300+	86%	85%	85%
Hospital Given 9 or 10 on 10 Point Scale	300+	75%	70%	71%
Meds 'Always' Explained Before Given	300+	68%	66%	64%
Nurses 'Always' Communicated Well	300+	81%	80%	79%
Pain 'Always' Well Controlled	300+	73%	72%	71%
Room and Bathroom 'Always' Clean	300+	60%	73%	73%
Timely Help 'Always' Received	300+	65%	68%	68%
Would Definitely Recommend Hospital	300+	88%	70%	71%
Use of Medical Imaging				
Cardiac Imaging Stress Test before Surgery	2,047	4.9%	4.8%	5.3%
Combination Abdominal CT Scan	921	5.5%	9.6%	10.5%
Combination Brain/Sinus CT Scan	795	3.0%	3.3%	2.7%
Combination Chest CT Scan	834	1.4%	3.4%	2.7%
Follow-up Mammogram/Ultrasound	1,918	7.2%	8.3%	8.8%
Lumbar Spine MRI for Low Back Pain	111	39.6%	35.3%	37.2%

Tristar Centennial Medical Center

2300 Patterson Street Phone: 615-342-1000
Nashville, TN 37203
Type: Acute Care Hospitals Emergency Services: Yes
Ownership: Proprietary

Key Personnel:

CEO/President. . . . . Thomas L Herron FACHE

Measure	Cases	This Hosp.	State Avg.	U.S. Avg.
Blood Clot Prevention and Treatment				
Anticoagulation Overlap Therapy[2]	94	91%	92%	93%
ICU Venous Thromboembolism Prophylaxis[2]	97	94%	90%	92%
Incidence of Potentially Preventable VTE[2]	14	0%	10%	10%
UFH with Dosages/Platelet Monitoring[2]	64	98%	99%	97%
Venous Thromboembolism Prophylaxis[2]	358	83%	83%	85%
Warfarin Therapy Discharge Instructions[2]	74	95%	78%	75%
Chest Pain/Possible Heart Attack Care				
Aspirin Given Within 24 Hours of Arrival	20	100%	96%	96%
Fibrinolytic Meds Within 30 Min. of Arrival[3,7]	-	-	72%	58%
Average Time to ECG (minutes)	22	6	6	7
Average Time to Transfer (minutes)[1,3]	-	-	53	60
Children's Asthma Care				
Received Home Management Plan of Care	-	-	-	88%
Received Reliever Medication	-	-	-	100%
Received Systemic Corticosteroids	-	-	-	100%
Emergency Department				
Admittance Decision Time (minutes)[2]	414	101	82	98
Head CT Results Within 45 Min. of Arrival[7]	-	-	52%	57%
Patients Who Left ER Before Being Seen	32,312	2%	2%	2%
Time from ER Arrival to Admit. (minutes)[2]	422	236	243	274
Time from ER Arrival to Discharge (minutes)	474	132	131	134
Time in ER Before Being Evaluated (minutes)	522	9	25	26
Time to Pain Meds for Fractures (minutes)	73	36	60	57
Heart Attack Care				
Aspirin Given at Discharge[2]	449	100%	99%	99%
Fibrinolytic Meds Within 30 Min. of Arrival[2,7]	-	-	33%	54%
PCI Within 90 Minutes of Arrival[2]	16	100%	98%	96%
Statin Prescribed at Discharge[2]	437	100%	99%	98%
Heart Failure Care				
ACE Inhibitor or ARB for LVSD[2]	170	100%	97%	97%
Discharge Instructions Given[2]	389	95%	93%	94%
Evaluation of LVS Function[2]	459	100%	99%	99%
Medicare Spending				
Medicare Spending per Patient (ratio)	-	1.01	1	0.98
Pneumonia Care				
Appropriate Initial Antibiotic Given[2]	76	97%	95%	95%
Blood Culture Timing[2]	88	98%	98%	98%
Pregnancy and Delivery Care				
Newborn Deliveries Scheduled Early[2]	48	6%	6%	6%
Preventive Care				
Immunization for Influenza[2]	618	96%	93%	90%
Immunization for Pneumonia[2]	720	95%	93%	92%
Stroke Care				
Anticoagulation Therapy for Atrial Fibrillation	20	100%	94%	95%
Antithrombotic Therapy Timing	137	98%	97%	98%
Assessed for Rehabilitation	177	99%	97%	97%
Discharged on Antithrombotic Therapy	155	100%	99%	99%

NOTE: Hospital profiles are in alphabetical order by state, then city, then hospital within the city; Rankings exclude hospitals with less than 25 cases except for patient surveys which excludes hospitals with less than 100 cases; (a) 100-299 cases; (1) The number of cases/patients is too few to report; (2) Data submitted were based on a sample of cases/patients; (3) Results are based on a shorter time period than required; (4) Data suppressed by CMS for one or more quarters; (5) Results are not available for this reporting period; (6) Fewer than 100 patients completed the HCAHPS survey; (7) No cases met the criteria for this measure; (8) The lower limit of the confidence interval cannot be calculated if the number of observed infections equals zero; (9) No data are available from the state/territory for this reporting period; (10) The scores shown reflect fewer than 50 completed surveys; (11) There were discrepancies in the data collection process; (12) This measure does not apply to this hospital for this reporting period; (13) Results cannot be calculated for this reporting period; (14) The results for this state are combined with nearby states to protect confidentiality; Please refer to the User's Guide for a full explanation of data.

Discharged on Statin Medication	115	100%	94%	94%
Thrombolytic Therapy Timing[1]	-	-	57%	66%
Venous Thromboembolism Prophylaxis	174	99%	93%	94%
Written Stroke Educational Materials Given	92	93%	84%	88%
Surgical Care Improvement Project				
Appropriate Beta Blocker Usage[2]	330	99%	97%	98%
Appropriate VTP Within 24 Hours[2]	539	99%	98%	98%
Controlled Postoperative Blood Glucose[2]	190	95%	95%	97%
Perioperative Temperature Management[2]	705	100%	100%	100%
Prophylactic Antibiotic Selection[2]	587	100%	99%	99%
Prophylactic Antibiotic Selection (Outpatient)	790	99%	98%	98%
Prophylactic Antibiotic Stopped[2]	560	99%	98%	98%
Prophylactic Antibiotic Timing[2]	587	100%	99%	99%
Prophylactic Antibiotic Timing (Outpatient)	790	100%	98%	98%
Urinary Catheter Removal[2]	513	99%	96%	97%
Survey of Patients' Hospital Experiences				
Area Around Room 'Always' Quiet at Night	300+	67%	67%	61%
Doctors 'Always' Communicated Well	300+	84%	84%	82%
Home Recovery Information Given	300+	88%	85%	85%
Hospital Given 9 or 10 on 10 Point Scale	300+	76%	70%	71%
Meds 'Always' Explained Before Given	300+	63%	66%	64%
Nurses 'Always' Communicated Well	300+	80%	80%	79%
Pain 'Always' Well Controlled	300+	71%	72%	71%
Room and Bathroom 'Always' Clean	300+	70%	73%	73%
Timely Help 'Always' Received	300+	67%	68%	68%
Would Definitely Recommend Hospital	300+	79%	70%	71%
Use of Medical Imaging				
Cardiac Imaging Stress Test before Surgery	106	10.4%	4.8%	5.3%
Combination Abdominal CT Scan	821	7.3%	9.6%	10.5%
Combination Brain/Sinus CT Scan	667	3.0%	3.3%	2.7%
Combination Chest CT Scan	630	2.1%	3.4%	2.7%
Follow-up Mammogram/Ultrasound	1,129	8.9%	8.3%	8.8%
Lumbar Spine MRI for Low Back Pain	144	35.4%	35.3%	37.2%

Tristar Skyline Medical Center

3441 Dickerson Pike
Nashville, TN 37207
URL: www.skylinemedicalcenter.com
Type: Acute Care Hospitals
Ownership: Voluntary non-profit - Private
Phone: 615-769-2000
Fax: 615-769-2211
Emergency Services: Yes
Beds: 196

Key Personnel:
CEO/President. . . . . Mike Garfield
Radiology. . . . . Rick Phillips, CRA

Measure	Cases	This Hosp.	State Avg.	U.S. Avg.
Blood Clot Prevention and Treatment				
Anticoagulation Overlap Therapy[2]	81	99%	92%	93%
ICU Venous Thromboembolism Prophylaxis[2]	162	99%	90%	92%
Incidence of Potentially Preventable VTE[2]	29	14%	10%	10%
UFH with Dosages/Platelet Monitoring[2]	25	100%	99%	97%
Venous Thromboembolism Prophylaxis[2]	297	98%	83%	85%
Warfarin Therapy Discharge Instructions[2]	58	100%	78%	75%
Chest Pain/Possible Heart Attack Care				
Aspirin Given Within 24 Hours of Arrival	19	100%	96%	96%
Fibrinolytic Meds Within 30 Min. of Arrival[7]	-	-	72%	58%
Average Time to ECG (minutes)	19	5	6	7
Average Time to Transfer (minutes)[7]	-	-	53	60
Children's Asthma Care				
Received Home Management Plan of Care	-	-	-	88%
Received Reliever Medication	-	-	-	100%
Received Systemic Corticosteroids	-	-	-	100%
Emergency Department				
Admittance Decision Time (minutes)[2]	716	105	82	98
Head CT Results Within 45 Min. of Arrival[1]	-	-	52%	57%
Patients Who Left ER Before Being Seen	54,976	1%	2%	2%
Time from ER Arrival to Admit. (minutes)[2]	716	236	243	274
Time from ER Arrival to Discharge (minutes)	448	136	131	134
Time in ER Before Being Evaluated (minutes)	529	15	25	26
Time to Pain Meds for Fractures (minutes)	163	44	60	57
Heart Attack Care				
Aspirin Given at Discharge	132	100%	99%	99%
Fibrinolytic Meds Within 30 Min. of Arrival[7]	-	-	33%	54%
PCI Within 90 Minutes of Arrival	41	100%	98%	96%
Statin Prescribed at Discharge	126	100%	99%	98%
Heart Failure Care				
ACE Inhibitor or ARB for LVSD	58	98%	97%	97%
Discharge Instructions Given	208	100%	93%	94%
Evaluation of LVS Function	235	100%	99%	99%
Medicare Spending				
Medicare Spending per Patient (ratio)	-	1.05	1	0.98
Pneumonia Care				
Appropriate Initial Antibiotic Given[2]	76	93%	95%	95%
Blood Culture Timing[2]	174	99%	98%	98%
Pregnancy and Delivery Care				
Newborn Deliveries Scheduled Early[2,7]	-	-	6%	6%
Preventive Care				
Immunization for Influenza[2]	602	96%	93%	90%
Immunization for Pneumonia[2]	964	96%	93%	92%
Stroke Care				
Anticoagulation Therapy for Atrial Fibrillation	32	97%	94%	95%
Antithrombotic Therapy Timing	287	98%	97%	98%
Assessed for Rehabilitation	434	100%	97%	97%
Discharged on Antithrombotic Therapy	331	100%	99%	99%
Discharged on Statin Medication	249	97%	94%	94%
Thrombolytic Therapy Timing	19	100%	57%	66%
Venous Thromboembolism Prophylaxis	442	100%	93%	94%
Written Stroke Educational Materials Given	209	96%	84%	88%
Surgical Care Improvement Project				
Appropriate Beta Blocker Usage[2]	146	99%	97%	98%
Appropriate VTP Within 24 Hours[2]	368	98%	98%	98%
Controlled Postoperative Blood Glucose[2,7]	-	-	95%	97%
Perioperative Temperature Management[2]	451	100%	100%	100%
Prophylactic Antibiotic Selection[2]	257	99%	99%	99%
Prophylactic Antibiotic Selection (Outpatient)	342	98%	98%	98%
Prophylactic Antibiotic Stopped[2]	239	98%	98%	98%
Prophylactic Antibiotic Timing[2]	257	100%	99%	99%
Prophylactic Antibiotic Timing (Outpatient)	342	99%	98%	98%
Urinary Catheter Removal[2]	316	97%	96%	97%
Survey of Patients' Hospital Experiences				
Area Around Room 'Always' Quiet at Night	300+	65%	67%	61%
Doctors 'Always' Communicated Well	300+	79%	84%	82%
Home Recovery Information Given	300+	86%	85%	85%
Hospital Given 9 or 10 on 10 Point Scale	300+	67%	70%	71%
Meds 'Always' Explained Before Given	300+	62%	66%	64%
Nurses 'Always' Communicated Well	300+	75%	80%	79%
Pain 'Always' Well Controlled	300+	70%	72%	71%
Room and Bathroom 'Always' Clean	300+	67%	73%	73%
Timely Help 'Always' Received	300+	60%	68%	68%
Would Definitely Recommend Hospital	300+	68%	70%	71%
Use of Medical Imaging				
Cardiac Imaging Stress Test before Surgery	103	5.8%	4.8%	5.3%
Combination Abdominal CT Scan	634	5.4%	9.6%	10.5%
Combination Brain/Sinus CT Scan	825	2.5%	3.3%	2.7%
Combination Chest CT Scan	402	0.0%	3.4%	2.7%
Follow-up Mammogram/Ultrasound	793	10.8%	8.3%	8.8%
Lumbar Spine MRI for Low Back Pain	155	31.6%	35.3%	37.2%

Tristar Southern Hills Medical Center

391 Wallace Rd
Nashville, TN 37211
URL: www.southernhills.com
Type: Acute Care Hospitals
Ownership: Proprietary
Phone: 615-781-4000
Fax: 615-781-4113
Emergency Services: Yes
Beds: 160

Key Personnel:
Operating Room. . . . . Suhail H Allos
Chief of Medical Staff. . . . . Robert Bishop, MD
Radiology. . . . . Christopher J Bodin
Intensive Care Unit. . . . . Darlene Cantrell
Infection Control. . . . . Jane Harris
Emergency Room . . . . Eric Morris, MD
CEO/President. . . . . Thomas H Ozburn

Measure	Cases	This Hosp.	State Avg.	U.S. Avg.
Blood Clot Prevention and Treatment				
Anticoagulation Overlap Therapy[2]	36	97%	92%	93%
ICU Venous Thromboembolism Prophylaxis[2]	157	98%	90%	92%
Incidence of Potentially Preventable VTE[1,2]	-	-	10%	10%
UFH with Dosages/Platelet Monitoring[2]	17	88%	99%	97%
Venous Thromboembolism Prophylaxis[2]	250	86%	83%	85%
Warfarin Therapy Discharge Instructions[2]	31	90%	78%	75%
Chest Pain/Possible Heart Attack Care				
Aspirin Given Within 24 Hours of Arrival	12	100%	96%	96%
Fibrinolytic Meds Within 30 Min. of Arrival[3,7]	-	-	72%	58%
Average Time to ECG (minutes)	13	4	6	7
Average Time to Transfer (minutes)[3,7]	-	-	53	60
Children's Asthma Care				
Received Home Management Plan of Care	-	-	-	88%
Received Reliever Medication	-	-	-	100%
Received Systemic Corticosteroids	-	-	-	100%
Emergency Department				
Admittance Decision Time (minutes)[2]	537	103	82	98
Head CT Results Within 45 Min. of Arrival	14	86%	52%	57%
Patients Who Left ER Before Being Seen	40,711	1%	2%	2%
Time from ER Arrival to Admit. (minutes)[2]	566	229	243	274
Time from ER Arrival to Discharge (minutes)	427	124	131	134
Time in ER Before Being Evaluated (minutes)	489	14	25	26
Time to Pain Meds for Fractures (minutes)	98	45	60	57
Heart Attack Care				
Aspirin Given at Discharge	100	99%	99%	99%
Fibrinolytic Meds Within 30 Min. of Arrival[7]	-	-	33%	54%
PCI Within 90 Minutes of Arrival	19	100%	98%	96%
Statin Prescribed at Discharge	95	99%	99%	98%
Heart Failure Care				
ACE Inhibitor or ARB for LVSD	35	100%	97%	97%
Discharge Instructions Given	120	100%	93%	94%
Evaluation of LVS Function	135	100%	99%	99%
Medicare Spending				
Medicare Spending per Patient (ratio)	-	1.06	1	0.98
Pneumonia Care				
Appropriate Initial Antibiotic Given	100	100%	95%	95%
Blood Culture Timing	97	100%	98%	98%
Pregnancy and Delivery Care				
Newborn Deliveries Scheduled Early[2,7]	-	-	6%	6%
Preventive Care				
Immunization for Influenza[2]	438	99%	93%	90%
Immunization for Pneumonia[2]	640	98%	93%	92%
Stroke Care				
Anticoagulation Therapy for Atrial Fibrillation[1]	-	-	94%	95%
Antithrombotic Therapy Timing	46	100%	97%	98%
Assessed for Rehabilitation	58	100%	97%	97%
Discharged on Antithrombotic Therapy	57	98%	99%	99%
Discharged on Statin Medication	50	100%	94%	94%
Thrombolytic Therapy Timing[1]	-	-	57%	66%
Venous Thromboembolism Prophylaxis	56	98%	93%	94%
Written Stroke Educational Materials Given	34	94%	84%	88%
Surgical Care Improvement Project				
Appropriate Beta Blocker Usage	67	100%	97%	98%
Appropriate VTP Within 24 Hours	268	98%	98%	98%
Controlled Postoperative Blood Glucose[7]	-	-	95%	97%
Perioperative Temperature Management	299	100%	100%	100%
Prophylactic Antibiotic Selection	172	100%	99%	99%
Prophylactic Antibiotic Selection (Outpatient)	156	99%	98%	98%
Prophylactic Antibiotic Stopped	169	98%	98%	98%
Prophylactic Antibiotic Timing	172	99%	99%	99%
Prophylactic Antibiotic Timing (Outpatient)	157	99%	98%	98%
Urinary Catheter Removal	198	97%	96%	97%
Survey of Patients' Hospital Experiences				
Area Around Room 'Always' Quiet at Night	300+	68%	67%	61%
Doctors 'Always' Communicated Well	300+	80%	84%	82%
Home Recovery Information Given	300+	84%	85%	85%
Hospital Given 9 or 10 on 10 Point Scale	300+	68%	70%	71%
Meds 'Always' Explained Before Given	300+	61%	66%	64%
Nurses 'Always' Communicated Well	300+	76%	80%	79%
Pain 'Always' Well Controlled	300+	69%	72%	71%
Room and Bathroom 'Always' Clean	300+	77%	73%	73%
Timely Help 'Always' Received	300+	61%	68%	68%
Would Definitely Recommend Hospital	300+	64%	70%	71%
Use of Medical Imaging				
Cardiac Imaging Stress Test before Surgery[1]	-	-	4.8%	5.3%
Combination Abdominal CT Scan	381	6.0%	9.6%	10.5%
Combination Brain/Sinus CT Scan[1]	-	-	3.3%	2.7%

NOTE: Hospital profiles are in alphabetical order by state, then city, then hospital within the city; Rankings exclude hospitals with less than 25 cases except for patient surveys which excludes hospitals with less than 100 cases; (a) 100-299 cases; (1) The number of cases/patients is too few to report; (2) Data submitted were based on a sample of cases/patients; (3) Results are based on a shorter time period than required; (4) Data suppressed by CMS for one or more quarters; (5) Results are not available for this reporting period; (6) Fewer than 100 patients completed the HCAHPS survey; (7) No cases met the criteria for this measure; (8) The lower limit of the confidence interval cannot be calculated if the number of observed infections equals zero; (9) No data are available from the state/territory for this reporting period; (10) The scores shown reflect fewer than 50 completed surveys; (11) There were discrepancies in the data collection process; (12) This measure does not apply to this hospital for this reporting period; (13) Results cannot be calculated for this reporting period; (14) The results for this state are combined with nearby states to protect confidentiality; Please refer to the User's Guide for a full explanation of data.

Combination Chest CT Scan	163	0.6%	3.4%	2.7%
Follow-up Mammogram/Ultrasound	530	12.1%	8.3%	8.8%
Lumbar Spine MRI for Low Back Pain[1]	-	-	35.3%	37.2%

VA Middle Tennessee Healthcare System

1310 24th Avenue South
Nashville, TN 37212
Phone: 615-327-5332
Fax: 615-321-6350
URL: www.tennesseevalley.va.gov
Type: Acute Care - VA
Emergency Services: No
Ownership: Government Federal
Beds: 238

Key Personnel:
Quality Assurance . . . . Dolores Kaplan, RN
Chief of Medical Staff. . . . . John H Newman, MD
CEO/President. . . . . David N Pannington

Measure	Cases	This Hosp.	State Avg.	U.S. Avg.
Blood Clot Prevention and Treatment				
Anticoagulation Overlap Therapy	-	-	92%	93%
ICU Venous Thromboembolism Prophylaxis	-	-	90%	92%
Incidence of Potentially Preventable VTE	-	-	10%	10%
UFH with Dosages/Platelet Monitoring	-	-	99%	97%
Venous Thromboembolism Prophylaxis	-	-	83%	85%
Warfarin Therapy Discharge Instructions	-	-	78%	75%
Chest Pain/Possible Heart Attack Care				
Aspirin Given Within 24 Hours of Arrival	-	-	96%	96%
Fibrinolytic Meds Within 30 Min. of Arrival	-	-	72%	58%
Average Time to ECG (minutes)	-	-	6	7
Average Time to Transfer (minutes)	-	-	53	60
Children's Asthma Care				
Received Home Management Plan of Care	-	-	-	88%
Received Reliever Medication	-	-	-	100%
Received Systemic Corticosteroids	-	-	-	100%
Emergency Department				
Admittance Decision Time (minutes)	-	-	82	98
Head CT Results Within 45 Min. of Arrival	-	-	52%	57%
Patients Who Left ER Before Being Seen	-	-	2%	2%
Time from ER Arrival to Admit. (minutes)	-	-	243	274
Time from ER Arrival to Discharge (minutes)	-	-	131	134
Time in ER Before Being Evaluated (minutes)	-	-	25	26
Time to Pain Meds for Fractures (minutes)	-	-	60	57
Heart Attack Care				
Aspirin Given at Discharge	119	99%	99%	99%
Fibrinolytic Meds Within 30 Min. of Arrival[5]	-	-	33%	54%
PCI Within 90 Minutes of Arrival[1]	-	-	98%	96%
Statin Prescribed at Discharge	115	99%	99%	98%
Heart Failure Care				
ACE Inhibitor or ARB for LVSD	159	98%	97%	97%
Discharge Instructions Given	469	94%	93%	94%
Evaluation of LVS Function	500	99%	99%	99%
Medicare Spending				
Medicare Spending per Patient (ratio)	-	-	1	0.98
Pneumonia Care				
Appropriate Initial Antibiotic Given	125	98%	95%	95%
Blood Culture Timing	217	99%	98%	98%
Pregnancy and Delivery Care				
Newborn Deliveries Scheduled Early	-	-	6%	6%
Preventive Care				
Immunization for Influenza[5]	-	-	93%	90%
Immunization for Pneumonia[5]	-	-	93%	92%
Stroke Care				
Anticoagulation Therapy for Atrial Fibrillation	-	-	94%	95%
Antithrombotic Therapy Timing	-	-	97%	98%
Assessed for Rehabilitation	-	-	97%	97%
Discharged on Antithrombotic Therapy	-	-	99%	99%
Discharged on Statin Medication	-	-	94%	94%
Thrombolytic Therapy Timing	-	-	57%	66%
Venous Thromboembolism Prophylaxis	-	-	93%	94%
Written Stroke Educational Materials Given	-	-	84%	88%
Surgical Care Improvement Project				
Appropriate Beta Blocker Usage[2]	104	94%	97%	98%
Appropriate VTP Within 24 Hours[2]	136	100%	98%	98%
Controlled Postoperative Blood Glucose[2]	85	99%	95%	97%
Perioperative Temperature Management[2]	240	100%	100%	100%
Prophylactic Antibiotic Selection	135	100%	99%	99%
Prophylactic Antibiotic Selection (Outpatient)	-	-	98%	98%
Prophylactic Antibiotic Stopped	128	98%	98%	98%
Prophylactic Antibiotic Timing	135	99%	99%	99%
Prophylactic Antibiotic Timing (Outpatient)	-	-	98%	98%
Urinary Catheter Removal[2]	85	93%	96%	97%
Survey of Patients' Hospital Experiences				
Area Around Room 'Always' Quiet at Night	-	-	67%	61%
Doctors 'Always' Communicated Well	-	-	84%	82%
Home Recovery Information Given	-	-	85%	85%
Hospital Given 9 or 10 on 10 Point Scale	-	-	70%	71%
Meds 'Always' Explained Before Given	-	-	66%	64%
Nurses 'Always' Communicated Well	-	-	80%	79%
Pain 'Always' Well Controlled	-	-	72%	71%
Room and Bathroom 'Always' Clean	-	-	73%	73%
Timely Help 'Always' Received	-	-	68%	68%
Would Definitely Recommend Hospital	-	-	70%	71%
Use of Medical Imaging				
Cardiac Imaging Stress Test before Surgery	-	-	4.8%	5.3%
Combination Abdominal CT Scan	-	-	9.6%	10.5%
Combination Brain/Sinus CT Scan	-	-	3.3%	2.7%
Combination Chest CT Scan	-	-	3.4%	2.7%
Follow-up Mammogram/Ultrasound	-	-	8.3%	8.8%
Lumbar Spine MRI for Low Back Pain	-	-	35.3%	37.2%

Vanderbilt University Hospital

1161 21st Avenue South
Nashville, TN 37232
Phone: 615-322-3454
Fax: 615-343-7317
URL: www.mc.vanderbilt.edu
Type: Acute Care Hospitals
Emergency Services: Yes
Ownership: Voluntary non-profit - Private
Beds: 705

Key Personnel:
CEO/President. . . . . Norman Burmy
Operating Room. . . . . Nancy Feistrizer
Pediatric Ambulatory Care . . . . . . Thomas Graham, MD
Radiology. . . . . Dennis Halahan, MD
Chief of Medical Staff. . . . . Allen B Kaiser, MD
Quality Assurance . . . . Paul Miles, MD
Infection Control. . . . . William Schaffner, MD
Pediatric In-Patient Care . . . . Terrell Smith

Measure	Cases	This Hosp.	State Avg.	U.S. Avg.
Blood Clot Prevention and Treatment				
Anticoagulation Overlap Therapy[2]	195	100%	92%	93%
ICU Venous Thromboembolism Prophylaxis[2]	175	90%	90%	92%
Incidence of Potentially Preventable VTE[2]	57	9%	10%	10%
UFH with Dosages/Platelet Monitoring[2]	163	100%	99%	97%
Venous Thromboembolism Prophylaxis[2]	309	92%	83%	85%
Warfarin Therapy Discharge Instructions[2]	154	100%	78%	75%
Chest Pain/Possible Heart Attack Care				
Aspirin Given Within 24 Hours of Arrival[5]	-	-	96%	96%
Fibrinolytic Meds Within 30 Min. of Arrival[5]	-	-	72%	58%
Average Time to ECG (minutes)[5]	-	-	6	7
Average Time to Transfer (minutes)[5]	-	-	53	60
Children's Asthma Care				
Received Home Management Plan of Care	-	-	-	88%
Received Reliever Medication	-	-	-	100%
Received Systemic Corticosteroids	-	-	-	100%
Emergency Department				
Admittance Decision Time (minutes)[2]	257	121	82	98
Head CT Results Within 45 Min. of Arrival[1]	-	-	52%	57%
Patients Who Left ER Before Being Seen	>100k	2%	2%	2%
Time from ER Arrival to Admit. (minutes)[2]	295	361	243	274
Time from ER Arrival to Discharge (minutes)	326	209	131	134
Time in ER Before Being Evaluated (minutes)	98	96	25	26
Time to Pain Meds for Fractures (minutes)	372	50	60	57
Heart Attack Care				
Aspirin Given at Discharge[2]	376	98%	99%	99%
Fibrinolytic Meds Within 30 Min. of Arrival[2,7]	-	-	33%	54%
PCI Within 90 Minutes of Arrival[2]	20	100%	98%	96%
Statin Prescribed at Discharge[2]	350	98%	99%	98%
Heart Failure Care				
ACE Inhibitor or ARB for LVSD[2]	107	97%	97%	97%
Discharge Instructions Given[2]	314	96%	93%	94%
Evaluation of LVS Function[2]	362	100%	99%	99%
Medicare Spending				
Medicare Spending per Patient (ratio)	-	0.98	1	0.98
Pneumonia Care				
Appropriate Initial Antibiotic Given[2]	34	85%	95%	95%
Blood Culture Timing[2]	93	94%	98%	98%
Pregnancy and Delivery Care				
Newborn Deliveries Scheduled Early	207	2%	6%	6%
Preventive Care				
Immunization for Influenza[2]	549	93%	93%	90%
Immunization for Pneumonia[2]	459	87%	93%	92%
Stroke Care				
Anticoagulation Therapy for Atrial Fibrillation[2]	69	100%	94%	95%
Antithrombotic Therapy Timing[2]	264	99%	97%	98%
Assessed for Rehabilitation[2]	478	97%	97%	97%
Discharged on Antithrombotic Therapy[2]	346	99%	99%	99%
Discharged on Statin Medication[2]	273	94%	94%	94%
Thrombolytic Therapy Timing[2]	13	100%	57%	66%
Venous Thromboembolism Prophylaxis[2]	458	88%	93%	94%
Written Stroke Educational Materials Given[2]	268	81%	84%	88%
Surgical Care Improvement Project				
Appropriate Beta Blocker Usage[2]	240	99%	97%	98%
Appropriate VTP Within 24 Hours[2]	411	100%	98%	98%
Controlled Postoperative Blood Glucose[2]	101	97%	95%	97%
Perioperative Temperature Management[2]	645	100%	100%	100%
Prophylactic Antibiotic Selection[2]	373	99%	99%	99%
Prophylactic Antibiotic Selection (Outpatient)	966	99%	98%	98%
Prophylactic Antibiotic Stopped[2]	365	98%	98%	98%
Prophylactic Antibiotic Timing[2]	373	99%	99%	99%
Prophylactic Antibiotic Timing (Outpatient)	755	97%	98%	98%
Urinary Catheter Removal[2]	388	96%	96%	97%
Survey of Patients' Hospital Experiences				
Area Around Room 'Always' Quiet at Night	300+	62%	67%	61%
Doctors 'Always' Communicated Well	300+	83%	84%	82%
Home Recovery Information Given	300+	88%	85%	85%
Hospital Given 9 or 10 on 10 Point Scale	300+	79%	70%	71%
Meds 'Always' Explained Before Given	300+	64%	66%	64%
Nurses 'Always' Communicated Well	300+	81%	80%	79%
Pain 'Always' Well Controlled	300+	73%	72%	71%
Room and Bathroom 'Always' Clean	300+	64%	73%	73%
Timely Help 'Always' Received	300+	67%	68%	68%
Would Definitely Recommend Hospital	300+	83%	70%	71%
Use of Medical Imaging				
Cardiac Imaging Stress Test before Surgery	1,157	5.9%	4.8%	5.3%
Combination Abdominal CT Scan	3,037	27.2%	9.6%	10.5%
Combination Brain/Sinus CT Scan	592	2.7%	3.3%	2.7%
Combination Chest CT Scan	2,968	1.2%	3.4%	2.7%
Follow-up Mammogram/Ultrasound	144	11.1%	8.3%	8.8%
Lumbar Spine MRI for Low Back Pain	56	32.1%	35.3%	37.2%

Tennova Healthcare - Newport Medical Center

435 2nd St
Newport, TN 37821
Phone: 423-625-2200
Fax: 423-625-2215
URL: www.baptistoneword.org
Type: Acute Care Hospitals
Emergency Services: Yes
Ownership: Voluntary non-profit - Church
Beds: 103

Key Personnel:
CEO/President. . . . . James Becker
Intensive Care Unit. . . . . Judy Henry, RN
Infection Control. . . . . Deanna Hill, RN
Operating Room. . . . . Sue Monroe, RN
Chief of Medical Staff. . . . . Tish Perkins
Quality Assurance . . . . Sherry Rolen, RN
Radiology. . . . . John Stallworth
Emergency Room . . . . Kenneth Tazil, MD

Measure	Cases	This Hosp.	State Avg.	U.S. Avg.
Blood Clot Prevention and Treatment				
Anticoagulation Overlap Therapy[2]	16	62%	92%	93%
ICU Venous Thromboembolism Prophylaxis[2]	65	88%	90%	92%
Incidence of Potentially Preventable VTE[1,2]	-	-	10%	10%
UFH with Dosages/Platelet Monitoring[1,2]	-	-	99%	97%
Venous Thromboembolism Prophylaxis[2]	188	84%	83%	85%
Warfarin Therapy Discharge Instructions[2]	13	69%	78%	75%
Chest Pain/Possible Heart Attack Care				
Aspirin Given Within 24 Hours of Arrival	127	99%	96%	96%
Fibrinolytic Meds Within 30 Min. of Arrival[1]	-	-	72%	58%

NOTE: Hospital profiles are in alphabetical order by state, then city, then hospital within the city; Rankings exclude hospitals with less than 25 cases except for patient surveys which excludes hospitals with less than 100 cases; (a) 100-299 cases; (1) The number of cases/patients is too few to report; (2) Data submitted were based on a sample of cases/patients; (3) Results are based on a shorter time period than required; (4) Data suppressed by CMS for one or more quarters; (5) Results are not available for this reporting period; (6) Fewer than 100 patients completed the HCAHPS survey; (7) No cases met the criteria for this measure; (8) The lower limit of the confidence interval cannot be calculated if the number of observed infections equals zero; (9) No data are available from the state/territory for this reporting period; (10) The scores shown reflect fewer than 50 completed surveys; (11) There were discrepancies in the data collection process; (12) This measure does not apply to this hospital for this reporting period; (13) Results cannot be calculated for this reporting period; (14) The results for this state are combined with nearby states to protect confidentiality; Please refer to the User's Guide for a full explanation of data.

Measure	Cases	This Hosp.	State Avg.	U.S. Avg.
Average Time to ECG (minutes)	136	6	6	7
Average Time to Transfer (minutes)[1]	-	-	53	60
Children's Asthma Care				
Received Home Management Plan of Care	-	-	-	88%
Received Reliever Medication	-	-	-	100%
Received Systemic Corticosteroids	-	-	-	100%
Emergency Department				
Admittance Decision Time (minutes)[2]	530	67	82	98
Head CT Results Within 45 Min. of Arrival	15	87%	52%	57%
Patients Who Left ER Before Being Seen	34,828	1%	2%	2%
Time from ER Arrival to Admit. (minutes)[2]	534	220	243	274
Time from ER Arrival to Discharge (minutes)	1,254	103	131	134
Time in ER Before Being Evaluated (minutes)	1,360	14	25	26
Time to Pain Meds for Fractures (minutes)	111	38	60	57
Heart Attack Care				
Aspirin Given at Discharge[1]	-	-	99%	99%
Fibrinolytic Meds Within 30 Min. of Arrival[7]	-	-	33%	54%
PCI Within 90 Minutes of Arrival[7]	-	-	98%	96%
Statin Prescribed at Discharge[1]	-	-	99%	98%
Heart Failure Care				
ACE Inhibitor or ARB for LVSD	24	92%	97%	97%
Discharge Instructions Given	86	86%	93%	94%
Evaluation of LVS Function	100	100%	99%	99%
Medicare Spending				
Medicare Spending per Patient (ratio)	-	0.92	1	0.98
Pneumonia Care				
Appropriate Initial Antibiotic Given	108	94%	95%	95%
Blood Culture Timing	240	99%	98%	98%
Pregnancy and Delivery Care				
Newborn Deliveries Scheduled Early	24	4%	6%	6%
Preventive Care				
Immunization for Influenza[2]	350	98%	93%	90%
Immunization for Pneumonia[2]	489	100%	93%	92%
Stroke Care				
Anticoagulation Therapy for Atrial Fibrillation[1]	-	-	94%	95%
Antithrombotic Therapy Timing	26	100%	97%	98%
Assessed for Rehabilitation	27	100%	97%	97%
Discharged on Antithrombotic Therapy	27	100%	99%	99%
Discharged on Statin Medication	18	94%	94%	94%
Thrombolytic Therapy Timing[1]	-	-	57%	66%
Venous Thromboembolism Prophylaxis	24	83%	93%	94%
Written Stroke Educational Materials Given	16	75%	84%	88%
Surgical Care Improvement Project				
Appropriate Beta Blocker Usage[7]	-	-	97%	98%
Appropriate VTP Within 24 Hours[1]	-	-	98%	98%
Controlled Postoperative Blood Glucose[7]	-	-	95%	97%
Perioperative Temperature Management[1]	-	-	100%	100%
Prophylactic Antibiotic Selection[7]	-	-	99%	99%
Prophylactic Antibiotic Selection (Outpatient)[3,7]	-	-	98%	98%
Prophylactic Antibiotic Stopped[7]	-	-	98%	98%
Prophylactic Antibiotic Timing[7]	-	-	99%	99%
Prophylactic Antibiotic Timing (Outpatient)[3,7]	-	-	98%	98%
Urinary Catheter Removal[1]	-	-	96%	97%
Survey of Patients' Hospital Experiences				
Area Around Room 'Always' Quiet at Night	300+	64%	67%	61%
Doctors 'Always' Communicated Well	300+	78%	84%	82%
Home Recovery Information Given	300+	79%	85%	85%
Hospital Given 9 or 10 on 10 Point Scale	300+	62%	70%	71%
Meds 'Always' Explained Before Given	300+	59%	66%	64%
Nurses 'Always' Communicated Well	300+	78%	80%	79%
Pain 'Always' Well Controlled	300+	65%	72%	71%
Room and Bathroom 'Always' Clean	300+	73%	73%	73%
Timely Help 'Always' Received	300+	63%	68%	68%
Would Definitely Recommend Hospital	300+	57%	70%	71%
Use of Medical Imaging				
Cardiac Imaging Stress Test before Surgery	103	1.9%	4.8%	5.3%
Combination Abdominal CT Scan	354	6.5%	9.6%	10.5%
Combination Brain/Sinus CT Scan[1]	-	-	3.3%	2.7%
Combination Chest CT Scan	189	4.8%	3.4%	2.7%
Follow-up Mammogram/Ultrasound	448	17.2%	8.3%	8.8%
Lumbar Spine MRI for Low Back Pain	51	51.0%	35.3%	37.2%

Methodist Medical Center of Oak Ridge

990 Oak Ridge Turnpike Box 529
Oak Ridge, TN 37830
Phone: 865-835-1000
Fax: 865-835-1795
URL: www.mmcoakridge.com
Type: Acute Care Hospitals
Emergency Services: Yes
Ownership: Voluntary non-profit - Private
Beds: 301

Key Personnel:
CEO/President . . . . Mike Belbeck, FACHE
Operating Room. . . . . Earlene Brewer
Cardiac Laboratory. . . . . Sue Harris, RN
Chief of Medical Staff . . . . Bill Molony, MD
Radiology. . . . . William Prater, MD
Quality Assurance . . . . Lee Young

Measure	Cases	This Hosp.	State Avg.	U.S. Avg.
Blood Clot Prevention and Treatment				
Anticoagulation Overlap Therapy[2]	58	100%	92%	93%
ICU Venous Thromboembolism Prophylaxis[2]	74	77%	90%	92%
Incidence of Potentially Preventable VTE[1,2]	-	-	10%	10%
UFH with Dosages/Platelet Monitoring[2]	24	100%	99%	97%
Venous Thromboembolism Prophylaxis[2]	395	88%	83%	85%
Warfarin Therapy Discharge Instructions[2]	45	96%	78%	75%
Chest Pain/Possible Heart Attack Care				
Aspirin Given Within 24 Hours of Arrival[1]	-	-	96%	96%
Fibrinolytic Meds Within 30 Min. of Arrival[5]	-	-	72%	58%
Average Time to ECG (minutes)[1]	-	-	6	7
Average Time to Transfer (minutes)[5]	-	-	53	60
Children's Asthma Care				
Received Home Management Plan of Care	-	-	-	88%
Received Reliever Medication	-	-	-	100%
Received Systemic Corticosteroids	-	-	-	100%
Emergency Department				
Admittance Decision Time (minutes)[2]	780	147	82	98
Head CT Results Within 45 Min. of Arrival	13	77%	52%	57%
Patients Who Left ER Before Being Seen	44,459	2%	2%	2%
Time from ER Arrival to Admit. (minutes)[2]	797	329	243	274
Time from ER Arrival to Discharge (minutes)	409	144	131	134
Time in ER Before Being Evaluated (minutes)	447	36	25	26
Time to Pain Meds for Fractures (minutes)	54	71	60	57
Heart Attack Care				
Aspirin Given at Discharge[2]	242	100%	99%	99%
Fibrinolytic Meds Within 30 Min. of Arrival[2,7]	-	-	33%	54%
PCI Within 90 Minutes of Arrival[2]	54	98%	98%	96%
Statin Prescribed at Discharge[2]	245	100%	99%	98%
Heart Failure Care				
ACE Inhibitor or ARB for LVSD[2]	55	100%	97%	97%
Discharge Instructions Given[2]	225	100%	93%	94%
Evaluation of LVS Function[2]	285	100%	99%	99%
Medicare Spending				
Medicare Spending per Patient (ratio)	-	0.95	1	0.98
Pneumonia Care				
Appropriate Initial Antibiotic Given[2]	102	100%	95%	95%
Blood Culture Timing[2]	78	100%	98%	98%
Pregnancy and Delivery Care				
Newborn Deliveries Scheduled Early	29	0%	6%	6%
Preventive Care				
Immunization for Influenza[2]	658	93%	93%	90%
Immunization for Pneumonia[2]	927	96%	93%	92%
Stroke Care				
Anticoagulation Therapy for Atrial Fibrillation[2]	18	100%	94%	95%
Antithrombotic Therapy Timing[2]	89	100%	97%	98%
Assessed for Rehabilitation[2]	98	100%	97%	97%
Discharged on Antithrombotic Therapy[2]	95	100%	99%	99%
Discharged on Statin Medication[2]	58	100%	94%	94%
Thrombolytic Therapy Timing[1,2]	-	-	57%	66%
Venous Thromboembolism Prophylaxis[2]	97	99%	93%	94%
Written Stroke Educational Materials Given[2]	64	100%	84%	88%
Surgical Care Improvement Project				
Appropriate Beta Blocker Usage[2]	208	100%	97%	98%
Appropriate VTP Within 24 Hours[2]	487	99%	98%	98%
Controlled Postoperative Blood Glucose[2]	125	97%	95%	97%
Perioperative Temperature Management[2]	567	100%	100%	100%
Prophylactic Antibiotic Selection[2]	483	100%	99%	99%
Prophylactic Antibiotic Selection (Outpatient)	449	100%	98%	98%
Prophylactic Antibiotic Stopped[2]	459	98%	98%	98%
Prophylactic Antibiotic Timing[2]	486	100%	99%	99%
Prophylactic Antibiotic Timing (Outpatient)	450	99%	98%	98%
Urinary Catheter Removal[2]	302	99%	96%	97%
Survey of Patients' Hospital Experiences				
Area Around Room 'Always' Quiet at Night	300+	67%	67%	61%
Doctors 'Always' Communicated Well	300+	83%	84%	82%
Home Recovery Information Given	300+	87%	85%	85%
Hospital Given 9 or 10 on 10 Point Scale	300+	73%	70%	71%
Meds 'Always' Explained Before Given	300+	65%	66%	64%
Nurses 'Always' Communicated Well	300+	80%	80%	79%
Pain 'Always' Well Controlled	300+	72%	72%	71%
Room and Bathroom 'Always' Clean	300+	74%	73%	73%
Timely Help 'Always' Received	300+	68%	68%	68%
Would Definitely Recommend Hospital	300+	75%	70%	71%
Use of Medical Imaging				
Cardiac Imaging Stress Test before Surgery	231	5.2%	4.8%	5.3%
Combination Abdominal CT Scan	1,148	3.7%	9.6%	10.5%
Combination Brain/Sinus CT Scan	804	1.5%	3.3%	2.7%
Combination Chest CT Scan	739	0.4%	3.4%	2.7%
Follow-up Mammogram/Ultrasound	2,572	9.4%	8.3%	8.8%
Lumbar Spine MRI for Low Back Pain	300	31.0%	35.3%	37.2%

Henry County Medical Center

301 Tyson Av
Paris, TN 38242
Phone: 731-642-1220
Fax: 731-642-9588
E-mail: hcmc@aeneas.net
URL: www.hcmc-tn.org
Type: Acute Care Hospitals
Emergency Services: Yes
Ownership: Govt - Hospital Dist/Auth
Beds: 142

Key Personnel:
Administrator . . . . Lisa Casteel
President . . . . Mike Garner
CEO/President. . . . . Thomas H Gee
Radiology. . . . . Robb Mitchell
Chief of Medical Staff . . . . Philip Nanney
Chairman/CEO . . . . Phil Wichlan

Measure	Cases	This Hosp.	State Avg.	U.S. Avg.
Blood Clot Prevention and Treatment				
Anticoagulation Overlap Therapy[2]	13	92%	92%	93%
ICU Venous Thromboembolism Prophylaxis[2]	54	85%	90%	92%
Incidence of Potentially Preventable VTE[2,7]	-	-	10%	10%
UFH with Dosages/Platelet Monitoring[1,2]	-	-	99%	97%
Venous Thromboembolism Prophylaxis[2]	255	87%	83%	85%
Warfarin Therapy Discharge Instructions[2]	11	100%	78%	75%
Chest Pain/Possible Heart Attack Care				
Aspirin Given Within 24 Hours of Arrival	205	97%	96%	96%
Fibrinolytic Meds Within 30 Min. of Arrival	18	72%	72%	58%
Average Time to ECG (minutes)	207	5	6	7
Average Time to Transfer (minutes)[7]	-	-	53	60
Children's Asthma Care				
Received Home Management Plan of Care	-	-	-	88%
Received Reliever Medication	-	-	-	100%
Received Systemic Corticosteroids	-	-	-	100%
Emergency Department				
Admittance Decision Time (minutes)[2]	304	62	82	98
Head CT Results Within 45 Min. of Arrival	22	55%	52%	57%
Patients Who Left ER Before Being Seen	19,373	3%	2%	2%
Time from ER Arrival to Admit. (minutes)[2]	323	215	243	274
Time from ER Arrival to Discharge (minutes)	435	135	131	134
Time in ER Before Being Evaluated (minutes)	485	39	25	26
Time to Pain Meds for Fractures (minutes)	77	80	60	57
Heart Attack Care				
Aspirin Given at Discharge	15	100%	99%	99%
Fibrinolytic Meds Within 30 Min. of Arrival[7]	-	-	33%	54%
PCI Within 90 Minutes of Arrival[7]	-	-	98%	96%
Statin Prescribed at Discharge	12	83%	99%	98%
Heart Failure Care				
ACE Inhibitor or ARB for LVSD	23	100%	97%	97%
Discharge Instructions Given	53	98%	93%	94%
Evaluation of LVS Function	71	100%	99%	99%
Medicare Spending				
Medicare Spending per Patient (ratio)	-	1.02	1	0.98
Pneumonia Care				
Appropriate Initial Antibiotic Given	88	99%	95%	95%

NOTE: Hospital profiles are in alphabetical order by state, then city, then hospital within the city; Rankings exclude hospitals with less than 25 cases except for patient surveys which excludes hospitals with less than 100 cases; (a) 100-299 cases; (1) The number of cases/patients is too few to report; (2) Data submitted were based on a sample of cases/patients; (3) Results are based on a shorter time period than required; (4) Data suppressed by CMS for one or more quarters; (5) Results are not available for this reporting period; (6) Fewer than 100 patients completed the HCAHPS survey; (7) No cases met the criteria for this measure; (8) The lower limit of the confidence interval cannot be calculated if the number of observed infections equals zero; (9) No data are available from the state/territory for this reporting period; (10) The scores shown reflect fewer than 50 completed surveys; (11) There were discrepancies in the data collection process; (12) This measure does not apply to this hospital for this reporting period; (13) Results cannot be calculated for this reporting period; (14) The results for this state are combined with nearby states to protect confidentiality; Please refer to the User's Guide for a full explanation of data.

Measure	Cases	This Hosp.	State Avg.	U.S. Avg.
Blood Culture Timing	111	100%	98%	98%
Pregnancy and Delivery Care				
Newborn Deliveries Scheduled Early[2]	28	4%	6%	6%
Preventive Care				
Immunization for Influenza[2]	373	94%	93%	90%
Immunization for Pneumonia[2]	507	95%	93%	92%
Stroke Care				
Anticoagulation Therapy for Atrial Fibrillation[1]	-	-	94%	95%
Antithrombotic Therapy Timing	38	100%	97%	98%
Assessed for Rehabilitation	43	93%	97%	97%
Discharged on Antithrombotic Therapy	43	100%	99%	99%
Discharged on Statin Medication	40	58%	94%	94%
Thrombolytic Therapy Timing[7]	-	-	57%	66%
Venous Thromboembolism Prophylaxis	34	76%	93%	94%
Written Stroke Educational Materials Given	20	50%	84%	88%
Surgical Care Improvement Project				
Appropriate Beta Blocker Usage	146	100%	97%	98%
Appropriate VTP Within 24 Hours	416	100%	98%	98%
Controlled Postoperative Blood Glucose[7]	-	-	95%	97%
Perioperative Temperature Management	475	100%	100%	100%
Prophylactic Antibiotic Selection	358	100%	99%	99%
Prophylactic Antibiotic Selection (Outpatient)	185	97%	98%	98%
Prophylactic Antibiotic Stopped	337	99%	98%	98%
Prophylactic Antibiotic Timing	358	100%	99%	99%
Prophylactic Antibiotic Timing (Outpatient)	194	94%	98%	98%
Urinary Catheter Removal	70	100%	96%	97%
Survey of Patients' Hospital Experiences				
Area Around Room 'Always' Quiet at Night	300+	73%	67%	61%
Doctors 'Always' Communicated Well	300+	83%	84%	82%
Home Recovery Information Given	300+	85%	85%	85%
Hospital Given 9 or 10 on 10 Point Scale	300+	70%	70%	71%
Meds 'Always' Explained Before Given	300+	64%	66%	64%
Nurses 'Always' Communicated Well	300+	78%	80%	79%
Pain 'Always' Well Controlled	300+	76%	72%	71%
Room and Bathroom 'Always' Clean	300+	75%	73%	73%
Timely Help 'Always' Received	300+	69%	68%	68%
Would Definitely Recommend Hospital	300+	72%	70%	71%
Use of Medical Imaging				
Cardiac Imaging Stress Test before Surgery	402	3.5%	4.8%	5.3%
Combination Abdominal CT Scan	909	15.5%	9.6%	10.5%
Combination Brain/Sinus CT Scan	643	2.8%	3.3%	2.7%
Combination Chest CT Scan	492	9.1%	3.4%	2.7%
Follow-up Mammogram/Ultrasound	1,038	7.5%	8.3%	8.8%
Lumbar Spine MRI for Low Back Pain	152	30.3%	35.3%	37.2%

Decatur County General Hospital

969 Tennessee Ave S
Parsons, TN 38363
Phone: 731-847-3031
Fax: 731-847-1122
E-mail: info@dcgh.org
URL: www.dcgh.org
Type: Acute Care Hospitals
Emergency Services: Yes
Ownership: Government - Local
Beds: 40

Key Personnel:
Operating Room. . . . . Charles Alderson
Chief of Medical Staff . . . . Thomas Hamilton
Emergency Room . . . . Thomas Hamilton, MD
Intensive Care Unit. . . . . Wanda Hamm
Radiology. . . . . Patrick Murphy, MD
Infection Control. . . . . Linda Quinn
Quality Assurance . . . . Sue Ringger, RN

Measure	Cases	This Hosp.	State Avg.	U.S. Avg.
Blood Clot Prevention and Treatment				
Anticoagulation Overlap Therapy[1,2]	-	-	92%	93%
ICU Venous Thromboembolism Prophylaxis[2,7]	-	-	90%	92%
Incidence of Potentially Preventable VTE[2,7]	-	-	10%	10%
UFH with Dosages/Platelet Monitoring[1,2]	-	-	99%	97%
Venous Thromboembolism Prophylaxis[2]	322	35%	83%	85%
Warfarin Therapy Discharge Instructions[1,2]	-	-	78%	75%
Chest Pain/Possible Heart Attack Care				
Aspirin Given Within 24 Hours of Arrival	57	84%	96%	96%
Fibrinolytic Meds Within 30 Min. of Arrival[1]	-	-	72%	58%
Average Time to ECG (minutes)	59	12	6	7
Average Time to Transfer (minutes)[7]	-	-	53	60
Children's Asthma Care				
Received Home Management Plan of Care	-	-	-	88%
Received Reliever Medication	-	-	-	100%
Received Systemic Corticosteroids	-	-	-	100%
Emergency Department				
Admittance Decision Time (minutes)[2]	428	50	82	98
Head CT Results Within 45 Min. of Arrival[1]	-	-	52%	57%
Patients Who Left ER Before Being Seen	5,382	2%	2%	2%
Time from ER Arrival to Admit. (minutes)[2]	441	161	243	274
Time from ER Arrival to Discharge (minutes)	323	86	131	134
Time in ER Before Being Evaluated (minutes)	353	16	25	26
Time to Pain Meds for Fractures (minutes)	15	55	60	57
Heart Attack Care				
Aspirin Given at Discharge[1]	-	-	99%	99%
Fibrinolytic Meds Within 30 Min. of Arrival[7]	-	-	33%	54%
PCI Within 90 Minutes of Arrival[7]	-	-	98%	96%
Statin Prescribed at Discharge[1]	-	-	99%	98%
Heart Failure Care				
ACE Inhibitor or ARB for LVSD[7]	-	-	97%	97%
Discharge Instructions Given	16	100%	93%	94%
Evaluation of LVS Function	23	87%	99%	99%
Medicare Spending				
Medicare Spending per Patient (ratio)	-	1.03	1	0.98
Pneumonia Care				
Appropriate Initial Antibiotic Given	26	88%	95%	95%
Blood Culture Timing	38	100%	98%	98%
Pregnancy and Delivery Care				
Newborn Deliveries Scheduled Early[7]	-	-	6%	6%
Preventive Care				
Immunization for Influenza[2]	250	88%	93%	90%
Immunization for Pneumonia[2]	403	95%	93%	92%
Stroke Care				
Anticoagulation Therapy for Atrial Fibrillation[2,3]	-	-	94%	95%
Antithrombotic Therapy Timing[1,2]	-	-	97%	98%
Assessed for Rehabilitation[1,2]	-	-	97%	97%
Discharged on Antithrombotic Therapy[1,2]	-	-	99%	99%
Discharged on Statin Medication[1,2]	-	-	94%	94%
Thrombolytic Therapy Timing[1,2]	-	-	57%	66%
Venous Thromboembolism Prophylaxis[1,2]	-	-	93%	94%
Written Stroke Educational Materials Given[2,3]	-	-	84%	88%
Surgical Care Improvement Project				
Appropriate Beta Blocker Usage[5]	-	-	97%	98%
Appropriate VTP Within 24 Hours[5]	-	-	98%	98%
Controlled Postoperative Blood Glucose[5]	-	-	95%	97%
Perioperative Temperature Management[5]	-	-	100%	100%
Prophylactic Antibiotic Selection[5]	-	-	99%	99%
Prophylactic Antibiotic Selection (Outpatient)[5]	-	-	98%	98%
Prophylactic Antibiotic Stopped[5]	-	-	98%	98%
Prophylactic Antibiotic Timing[5]	-	-	99%	99%
Prophylactic Antibiotic Timing (Outpatient)[5]	-	-	98%	98%
Urinary Catheter Removal[5]	-	-	96%	97%
Survey of Patients' Hospital Experiences				
Area Around Room 'Always' Quiet at Night[6]	<100	65%	67%	61%
Doctors 'Always' Communicated Well[6]	<100	83%	84%	82%
Home Recovery Information Given[6]	<100	82%	85%	85%
Hospital Given 9 or 10 on 10 Point Scale[6]	<100	64%	70%	71%
Meds 'Always' Explained Before Given[6]	<100	58%	66%	64%
Nurses 'Always' Communicated Well[6]	<100	75%	80%	79%
Pain 'Always' Well Controlled[6]	<100	67%	72%	71%
Room and Bathroom 'Always' Clean[6]	<100	69%	73%	73%
Timely Help 'Always' Received[6]	<100	64%	68%	68%
Would Definitely Recommend Hospital[6]	<100	65%	70%	71%
Use of Medical Imaging				
Cardiac Imaging Stress Test before Surgery[7]	-	-	4.8%	5.3%
Combination Abdominal CT Scan	195	9.2%	9.6%	10.5%
Combination Brain/Sinus CT Scan	246	1.2%	3.3%	2.7%
Combination Chest CT Scan	80	3.8%	3.4%	2.7%
Follow-up Mammogram/Ultrasound	281	7.5%	8.3%	8.8%
Lumbar Spine MRI for Low Back Pain[1]	-	-	35.3%	37.2%

Hillside Hospital

1265 E College St
Pulaski, TN 38478
Phone: 931-363-7531
Fax: 931-424-7520
URL: www.hillsidehospital.com
Type: Acute Care Hospitals
Emergency Services: Yes
Ownership: Proprietary
Beds: 95

Key Personnel:
Chief of Medical Staff . . . . Gigi Alejandrino, MD
Operating Room. . . . . Denida Cox
Emergency Room . . . . Miranda Danley
CEO/President. . . . . Donald Gavin
Quality Assurance . . . . Penni Patterson
Radiology. . . . . Richard Stults
Infection Control. . . . . Debbie Weaver

Measure	Cases	This Hosp.	State Avg.	U.S. Avg.
Blood Clot Prevention and Treatment				
Anticoagulation Overlap Therapy[1,2]	-	-	92%	93%
ICU Venous Thromboembolism Prophylaxis[2]	35	100%	90%	92%
Incidence of Potentially Preventable VTE[1,2]	-	-	10%	10%
UFH with Dosages/Platelet Monitoring[2,7]	-	-	99%	97%
Venous Thromboembolism Prophylaxis[2]	105	94%	83%	85%
Warfarin Therapy Discharge Instructions[1,2]	-	-	78%	75%
Chest Pain/Possible Heart Attack Care				
Aspirin Given Within 24 Hours of Arrival	69	97%	96%	96%
Fibrinolytic Meds Within 30 Min. of Arrival[1]	-	-	72%	58%
Average Time to ECG (minutes)	77	6	6	7
Average Time to Transfer (minutes)[1]	-	-	53	60
Children's Asthma Care				
Received Home Management Plan of Care	-	-	-	88%
Received Reliever Medication	-	-	-	100%
Received Systemic Corticosteroids	-	-	-	100%
Emergency Department				
Admittance Decision Time (minutes)[2]	290	53	82	98
Head CT Results Within 45 Min. of Arrival[1]	-	-	52%	57%
Patients Who Left ER Before Being Seen	11,549	2%	2%	2%
Time from ER Arrival to Admit. (minutes)[2]	293	192	243	274
Time from ER Arrival to Discharge (minutes)	366	117	131	134
Time in ER Before Being Evaluated (minutes)	459	14	25	26
Time to Pain Meds for Fractures (minutes)	33	27	60	57
Heart Attack Care				
Aspirin Given at Discharge[1]	-	-	99%	99%
Fibrinolytic Meds Within 30 Min. of Arrival[7]	-	-	33%	54%
PCI Within 90 Minutes of Arrival[7]	-	-	98%	96%
Statin Prescribed at Discharge[1]	-	-	99%	98%
Heart Failure Care				
ACE Inhibitor or ARB for LVSD[1]	-	-	97%	97%
Discharge Instructions Given	19	84%	93%	94%
Evaluation of LVS Function	31	100%	99%	99%
Medicare Spending				
Medicare Spending per Patient (ratio)	-	1.01	1	0.98
Pneumonia Care				
Appropriate Initial Antibiotic Given	56	93%	95%	95%
Blood Culture Timing	78	96%	98%	98%
Pregnancy and Delivery Care				
Newborn Deliveries Scheduled Early[2]	16	12%	6%	6%
Preventive Care				
Immunization for Influenza[2]	264	100%	93%	90%
Immunization for Pneumonia[2]	326	99%	93%	92%
Stroke Care				
Anticoagulation Therapy for Atrial Fibrillation[7]	-	-	94%	95%
Antithrombotic Therapy Timing[1]	-	-	97%	98%
Assessed for Rehabilitation[1]	-	-	97%	97%
Discharged on Antithrombotic Therapy[1]	-	-	99%	99%
Discharged on Statin Medication[1]	-	-	94%	94%
Thrombolytic Therapy Timing[1]	-	-	57%	66%
Venous Thromboembolism Prophylaxis[1]	-	-	93%	94%
Written Stroke Educational Materials Given[1]	-	-	84%	88%
Surgical Care Improvement Project				
Appropriate Beta Blocker Usage[1]	-	-	97%	98%
Appropriate VTP Within 24 Hours	24	100%	98%	98%
Controlled Postoperative Blood Glucose[7]	-	-	95%	97%
Perioperative Temperature Management	27	100%	100%	100%
Prophylactic Antibiotic Selection	16	100%	99%	99%
Prophylactic Antibiotic Selection (Outpatient)[1]	-	-	98%	98%

NOTE: Hospital profiles are in alphabetical order by state, then city, then hospital within the city; Rankings exclude hospitals with less than 25 cases except for patient surveys which excludes hospitals with less than 100 cases; (a) 100-299 cases; (1) The number of cases/patients is too few to report; (2) Data submitted were based on a sample of cases/patients; (3) Results are based on a shorter time period than required; (4) Data suppressed by CMS for one or more quarters; (5) Results are not available for this reporting period; (6) Fewer than 100 patients completed the HCAHPS survey; (7) No cases met the criteria for this measure; (8) The lower limit of the confidence interval cannot be calculated if the number of observed infections equals zero; (9) No data are available from the state/territory for this reporting period; (10) The scores shown reflect fewer than 50 completed surveys; (11) There were discrepancies in the data collection process; (12) This measure does not apply to this hospital for this reporting period; (13) Results cannot be calculated for this reporting period; (14) The results for this state are combined with nearby states to protect confidentiality; Please refer to the User's Guide for a full explanation of data.

Measure	Cases	This Hosp.	State Avg.	U.S. Avg.
Prophylactic Antibiotic Stopped	14	93%	98%	98%
Prophylactic Antibiotic Timing	16	100%	99%	99%
Prophylactic Antibiotic Timing (Outpatient)[1]	-	-	98%	98%
Urinary Catheter Removal	14	100%	96%	97%
Survey of Patients' Hospital Experiences				
Area Around Room 'Always' Quiet at Night	(a)	67%	67%	61%
Doctors 'Always' Communicated Well	(a)	84%	84%	82%
Home Recovery Information Given	(a)	85%	85%	85%
Hospital Given 9 or 10 on 10 Point Scale	(a)	64%	70%	71%
Meds 'Always' Explained Before Given	(a)	62%	66%	64%
Nurses 'Always' Communicated Well	(a)	77%	80%	79%
Pain 'Always' Well Controlled	(a)	66%	72%	71%
Room and Bathroom 'Always' Clean	(a)	71%	73%	73%
Timely Help 'Always' Received	(a)	68%	68%	68%
Would Definitely Recommend Hospital	(a)	58%	70%	71%
Use of Medical Imaging				
Cardiac Imaging Stress Test before Surgery	93	2.2%	4.8%	5.3%
Combination Abdominal CT Scan	294	0.7%	9.6%	10.5%
Combination Brain/Sinus CT Scan[1]	-	-	3.3%	2.7%
Combination Chest CT Scan	180	0.0%	3.4%	2.7%
Follow-up Mammogram/Ultrasound	570	7.9%	8.3%	8.8%
Lumbar Spine MRI for Low Back Pain[1]	-	-	35.3%	37.2%

Lauderdale Community Hospital

326 Asbury Avenue
Ripley, TN 38063
Phone: 731-221-2200
Fax: 731-221-2499
URL: www.lauderdalehospital.com
Type: Critical Access Hospitals
Ownership: Proprietary
Emergency Services: Yes
Beds: 25

Key Personnel:
Radiology. . . . . Billinda Baggett
Operating Room. . . . . Denise Blankenship, RN
Chief of Medical Staff . . . . Richard Guerrant, MD
Infection Control. . . . . Cynthia Kidd, RN
Quality Assurance . . . . Cheryl Manns
CEO . . . . Scott Tongate

Measure	Cases	This Hosp.	State Avg.	U.S. Avg.
Blood Clot Prevention and Treatment				
Anticoagulation Overlap Therapy[5]	-	-	92%	93%
ICU Venous Thromboembolism Prophylaxis[5]	-	-	90%	92%
Incidence of Potentially Preventable VTE[5]	-	-	10%	10%
UFH with Dosages/Platelet Monitoring[5]	-	-	99%	97%
Venous Thromboembolism Prophylaxis[5]	-	-	83%	85%
Warfarin Therapy Discharge Instructions[5]	-	-	78%	75%
Chest Pain/Possible Heart Attack Care				
Aspirin Given Within 24 Hours of Arrival	68	94%	96%	96%
Fibrinolytic Meds Within 30 Min. of Arrival[1]	-	-	72%	58%
Average Time to ECG (minutes)	69	9	6	7
Average Time to Transfer (minutes)[7]	-	-	53	60
Children's Asthma Care				
Received Home Management Plan of Care	-	-	-	88%
Received Reliever Medication	-	-	-	100%
Received Systemic Corticosteroids	-	-	-	100%
Emergency Department				
Admittance Decision Time (minutes)[5]	-	-	82	98
Head CT Results Within 45 Min. of Arrival[5]	-	-	52%	57%
Patients Who Left ER Before Being Seen[5]	-	-	2%	2%
Time from ER Arrival to Admit. (minutes)[5]	-	-	243	274
Time from ER Arrival to Discharge (minutes)[5]	-	-	131	134
Time in ER Before Being Evaluated (minutes)[5]	-	-	25	26
Time to Pain Meds for Fractures (minutes)[5]	-	-	60	57
Heart Attack Care				
Aspirin Given at Discharge[1,3]	-	-	99%	99%
Fibrinolytic Meds Within 30 Min. of Arrival[3,7]	-	-	33%	54%
PCI Within 90 Minutes of Arrival[5]	-	-	98%	96%
Statin Prescribed at Discharge[1,3]	-	-	99%	98%
Heart Failure Care				
ACE Inhibitor or ARB for LVSD[1]	-	-	97%	97%
Discharge Instructions Given	14	100%	93%	94%
Evaluation of LVS Function	19	74%	99%	99%
Medicare Spending				
Medicare Spending per Patient (ratio)	-	-	1	0.98
Pneumonia Care				
Appropriate Initial Antibiotic Given[1]	-	-	95%	95%
Blood Culture Timing	26	100%	98%	98%
Pregnancy and Delivery Care				
Newborn Deliveries Scheduled Early[5]	-	-	6%	6%
Preventive Care				
Immunization for Influenza[5]	-	-	93%	90%
Immunization for Pneumonia[5]	-	-	93%	92%
Stroke Care				
Anticoagulation Therapy for Atrial Fibrillation[5]	-	-	94%	95%
Antithrombotic Therapy Timing[5]	-	-	97%	98%
Assessed for Rehabilitation[5]	-	-	97%	97%
Discharged on Antithrombotic Therapy[5]	-	-	99%	99%
Discharged on Statin Medication[5]	-	-	94%	94%
Thrombolytic Therapy Timing[5]	-	-	57%	66%
Venous Thromboembolism Prophylaxis[5]	-	-	93%	94%
Written Stroke Educational Materials Given[5]	-	-	84%	88%
Surgical Care Improvement Project				
Appropriate Beta Blocker Usage[5]	-	-	97%	98%
Appropriate VTP Within 24 Hours[5]	-	-	98%	98%
Controlled Postoperative Blood Glucose[5]	-	-	95%	97%
Perioperative Temperature Management[5]	-	-	100%	100%
Prophylactic Antibiotic Selection[5]	-	-	99%	99%
Prophylactic Antibiotic Selection (Outpatient)[5]	-	-	98%	98%
Prophylactic Antibiotic Stopped[5]	-	-	98%	98%
Prophylactic Antibiotic Timing[5]	-	-	99%	99%
Prophylactic Antibiotic Timing (Outpatient)[5]	-	-	98%	98%
Urinary Catheter Removal[5]	-	-	96%	97%
Survey of Patients' Hospital Experiences				
Area Around Room 'Always' Quiet at Night[5]	-	-	67%	61%
Doctors 'Always' Communicated Well[5]	-	-	84%	82%
Home Recovery Information Given[5]	-	-	85%	85%
Hospital Given 9 or 10 on 10 Point Scale[5]	-	-	70%	71%
Meds 'Always' Explained Before Given[5]	-	-	66%	64%
Nurses 'Always' Communicated Well[5]	-	-	80%	79%
Pain 'Always' Well Controlled[5]	-	-	72%	71%
Room and Bathroom 'Always' Clean[5]	-	-	73%	73%
Timely Help 'Always' Received[5]	-	-	68%	68%
Would Definitely Recommend Hospital[5]	-	-	70%	71%
Use of Medical Imaging				
Cardiac Imaging Stress Test before Surgery[1]	-	-	4.8%	5.3%
Combination Abdominal CT Scan	187	0.5%	9.6%	10.5%
Combination Brain/Sinus CT Scan[1]	-	-	3.3%	2.7%
Combination Chest CT Scan	95	0.0%	3.4%	2.7%
Follow-up Mammogram/Ultrasound	285	6.7%	8.3%	8.8%
Lumbar Spine MRI for Low Back Pain[1]	-	-	35.3%	37.2%

Wellmont Hawkins County Memorial Hospital

851 Locust Street
Rogersville, TN 37857
Phone: 423-921-7000
Fax: 423-921-7022
Type: Acute Care Hospitals
Ownership: Voluntary non-profit - Private
Emergency Services: Yes
Beds: 50

Key Personnel:
Radiology. . . . . Anton Allen
Chief of Medical Staff . . . . Stephen Baumrucker, MD
Quality Assurance . . . . Mary Jo Fleenor
Operating Room. . . . . Charlene Presley, RN
Infection Control. . . . . Cathy Sandidge, RN

Measure	Cases	This Hosp.	State Avg.	U.S. Avg.
Blood Clot Prevention and Treatment				
Anticoagulation Overlap Therapy[1,2]	-	-	92%	93%
ICU Venous Thromboembolism Prophylaxis[2]	42	69%	90%	92%
Incidence of Potentially Preventable VTE[2,7]	-	-	10%	10%
UFH with Dosages/Platelet Monitoring[1,2]	-	-	99%	97%
Venous Thromboembolism Prophylaxis[2]	289	73%	83%	85%
Warfarin Therapy Discharge Instructions[1,2]	-	-	78%	75%
Chest Pain/Possible Heart Attack Care				
Aspirin Given Within 24 Hours of Arrival	49	98%	96%	96%
Fibrinolytic Meds Within 30 Min. of Arrival[7]	-	-	72%	58%
Average Time to ECG (minutes)	51	7	6	7
Average Time to Transfer (minutes)	12	52	53	60
Children's Asthma Care				
Received Home Management Plan of Care	-	-	-	88%
Received Reliever Medication	-	-	-	100%
Received Systemic Corticosteroids	-	-	-	100%
Emergency Department				
Admittance Decision Time (minutes)[2]	477	71	82	98
Head CT Results Within 45 Min. of Arrival	14	50%	52%	57%
Patients Who Left ER Before Being Seen	18,223	2%	2%	2%
Time from ER Arrival to Admit. (minutes)[2]	481	215	243	274
Time from ER Arrival to Discharge (minutes)	346	109	131	134
Time in ER Before Being Evaluated (minutes)	373	29	25	26
Time to Pain Meds for Fractures (minutes)	61	60	60	57
Heart Attack Care				
Aspirin Given at Discharge[1]	-	-	99%	99%
Fibrinolytic Meds Within 30 Min. of Arrival[7]	-	-	33%	54%
PCI Within 90 Minutes of Arrival[7]	-	-	98%	96%
Statin Prescribed at Discharge[1]	-	-	99%	98%
Heart Failure Care				
ACE Inhibitor or ARB for LVSD[1]	-	-	97%	97%
Discharge Instructions Given	30	93%	93%	94%
Evaluation of LVS Function	32	100%	99%	99%
Medicare Spending				
Medicare Spending per Patient (ratio)	-	0.93	1	0.98
Pneumonia Care				
Appropriate Initial Antibiotic Given	98	91%	95%	95%
Blood Culture Timing	143	98%	98%	98%
Pregnancy and Delivery Care				
Newborn Deliveries Scheduled Early[7]	-	-	6%	6%
Preventive Care				
Immunization for Influenza[2]	289	98%	93%	90%
Immunization for Pneumonia[2]	441	100%	93%	92%
Stroke Care				
Anticoagulation Therapy for Atrial Fibrillation[1]	-	-	94%	95%
Antithrombotic Therapy Timing	12	100%	97%	98%
Assessed for Rehabilitation	12	100%	97%	97%
Discharged on Antithrombotic Therapy	12	92%	99%	99%
Discharged on Statin Medication[1]	-	-	94%	94%
Thrombolytic Therapy Timing[1]	-	-	57%	66%
Venous Thromboembolism Prophylaxis[1]	-	-	93%	94%
Written Stroke Educational Materials Given[1]	-	-	84%	88%
Surgical Care Improvement Project				
Appropriate Beta Blocker Usage[1,2]	-	-	97%	98%
Appropriate VTP Within 24 Hours[2,3]	12	92%	98%	98%
Controlled Postoperative Blood Glucose[2,3]	-	-	95%	97%
Perioperative Temperature Management[2,3]	12	100%	100%	100%
Prophylactic Antibiotic Selection[1,2]	-	-	99%	99%
Prophylactic Antibiotic Selection (Outpatient)[3,7]	-	-	98%	98%
Prophylactic Antibiotic Stopped[1,2]	-	-	98%	98%
Prophylactic Antibiotic Timing[1,2]	-	-	99%	99%
Prophylactic Antibiotic Timing (Outpatient)[3,7]	-	-	98%	98%
Urinary Catheter Removal[2,3]	12	92%	96%	97%
Survey of Patients' Hospital Experiences				
Area Around Room 'Always' Quiet at Night	(a)	72%	67%	61%
Doctors 'Always' Communicated Well	(a)	87%	84%	82%
Home Recovery Information Given	(a)	87%	85%	85%
Hospital Given 9 or 10 on 10 Point Scale	(a)	78%	70%	71%
Meds 'Always' Explained Before Given	(a)	74%	66%	64%
Nurses 'Always' Communicated Well	(a)	89%	80%	79%
Pain 'Always' Well Controlled	(a)	76%	72%	71%
Room and Bathroom 'Always' Clean	(a)	87%	73%	73%
Timely Help 'Always' Received	(a)	79%	68%	68%
Would Definitely Recommend Hospital	(a)	79%	70%	71%
Use of Medical Imaging				
Cardiac Imaging Stress Test before Surgery[1]	-	-	4.8%	5.3%
Combination Abdominal CT Scan	239	10.0%	9.6%	10.5%
Combination Brain/Sinus CT Scan	201	1.0%	3.3%	2.7%
Combination Chest CT Scan	134	8.2%	3.4%	2.7%
Follow-up Mammogram/Ultrasound	274	4.7%	8.3%	8.8%
Lumbar Spine MRI for Low Back Pain	47	63.8%	35.3%	37.2%

Hardin Medical Center

935 Wayne Road
Savannah, TN 38372
Phone: 731-926-8121
Fax: 731-926-8080
Type: Acute Care Hospitals
Ownership: Government - Local
Emergency Services: Yes
Beds: 58

Key Personnel:
Intensive Care Unit. . . . . Carolyn Carpenter
Operating Room. . . . . Cindy Coleman

NOTE: Hospital profiles are in alphabetical order by state, then city, then hospital within the city; Rankings exclude hospitals with less than 25 cases except for patient surveys which excludes hospitals with less than 100 cases; (a) 100-299 cases; (1) The number of cases/patients is too few to report; (2) Data submitted were based on a sample of cases/patients; (3) Results are based on a shorter time period than required; (4) Data suppressed by CMS for one or more quarters; (5) Results are not available for this reporting period; (6) Fewer than 100 patients completed the HCAHPS survey; (7) No cases met the criteria for this measure; (8) The lower limit of the confidence interval cannot be calculated if the number of observed infections equals zero; (9) No data are available from the state/territory for this reporting period; (10) The scores shown reflect fewer than 50 completed surveys; (11) There were discrepancies in the data collection process; (12) This measure does not apply to this hospital for this reporting period; (13) Results cannot be calculated for this reporting period; (14) The results for this state are combined with nearby states to protect confidentiality; Please refer to the User's Guide for a full explanation of data.

Infection Control.............. Diane DeBerry
Quality Assurance .... Diane DeBerry
Hemotology Center .... Connie Hurt
CEO/President................ Nicholas P. Lewis
Emergency Room .... Suzanne Stricklin, RN
Chief of Medical Staff.......... Gilbert Thayer, M.D., FACOG

Measure	Cases	This Hosp.	State Avg.	U.S. Avg.
Blood Clot Prevention and Treatment				
Anticoagulation Overlap Therapy[2]	11	64%	92%	93%
ICU Venous Thromboembolism Prophylaxis[2,7]	-	-	90%	92%
Incidence of Potentially Preventable VTE[2,7]	-	-	10%	10%
UFH with Dosages/Platelet Monitoring[1,2]	-	-	99%	97%
Venous Thromboembolism Prophylaxis[2]	171	60%	83%	85%
Warfarin Therapy Discharge Instructions[1,2]	-	-	78%	75%
Chest Pain/Possible Heart Attack Care				
Aspirin Given Within 24 Hours of Arrival	205	99%	96%	96%
Fibrinolytic Meds Within 30 Min. of Arrival[1]	-	-	72%	58%
Average Time to ECG (minutes)	216	9	6	7
Average Time to Transfer (minutes)[1]	-	-	53	60
Children's Asthma Care				
Received Home Management Plan of Care	-	-	-	88%
Received Reliever Medication	-	-	-	100%
Received Systemic Corticosteroids	-	-	-	100%
Emergency Department				
Admittance Decision Time (minutes)[2]	324	65	82	98
Head CT Results Within 45 Min. of Arrival	17	47%	52%	57%
Patients Who Left ER Before Being Seen	19,234	2%	2%	2%
Time from ER Arrival to Admit. (minutes)[2]	328	230	243	274
Time from ER Arrival to Discharge (minutes)	329	140	131	134
Time in ER Before Being Evaluated (minutes)	373	28	25	26
Time to Pain Meds for Fractures (minutes)	89	68	60	57
Heart Attack Care				
Aspirin Given at Discharge[1]	-	-	99%	99%
Fibrinolytic Meds Within 30 Min. of Arrival[7]	-	-	33%	54%
PCI Within 90 Minutes of Arrival[7]	-	-	98%	96%
Statin Prescribed at Discharge[1]	-	-	99%	98%
Heart Failure Care				
ACE Inhibitor or ARB for LVSD[1]	-	-	97%	97%
Discharge Instructions Given[1]	-	-	93%	94%
Evaluation of LVS Function	18	100%	99%	99%
Medicare Spending				
Medicare Spending per Patient (ratio)	-	0.92	1	0.98
Pneumonia Care				
Appropriate Initial Antibiotic Given	89	91%	95%	95%
Blood Culture Timing	131	98%	98%	98%
Pregnancy and Delivery Care				
Newborn Deliveries Scheduled Early	13	8%	6%	6%
Preventive Care				
Immunization for Influenza[2]	230	92%	93%	90%
Immunization for Pneumonia[2]	267	94%	93%	92%
Stroke Care				
Anticoagulation Therapy for Atrial Fibrillation[1]	-	-	94%	95%
Antithrombotic Therapy Timing	16	88%	97%	98%
Assessed for Rehabilitation	15	73%	97%	97%
Discharged on Antithrombotic Therapy	15	87%	99%	99%
Discharged on Statin Medication	14	50%	94%	94%
Thrombolytic Therapy Timing[1]	-	-	57%	66%
Venous Thromboembolism Prophylaxis	14	79%	93%	94%
Written Stroke Educational Materials Given[1]	-	-	84%	88%
Surgical Care Improvement Project				
Appropriate Beta Blocker Usage	16	75%	97%	98%
Appropriate VTP Within 24 Hours	47	87%	98%	98%
Controlled Postoperative Blood Glucose[7]	-	-	95%	97%
Perioperative Temperature Management	48	100%	100%	100%
Prophylactic Antibiotic Selection	33	100%	99%	99%
Prophylactic Antibiotic Selection (Outpatient)[1]	-	-	98%	98%
Prophylactic Antibiotic Stopped	33	97%	98%	98%
Prophylactic Antibiotic Timing	33	91%	99%	99%
Prophylactic Antibiotic Timing (Outpatient)[1]	-	-	98%	98%
Urinary Catheter Removal	31	87%	96%	97%
Survey of Patients' Hospital Experiences				
Area Around Room 'Always' Quiet at Night	300+	72%	67%	61%
Doctors 'Always' Communicated Well	300+	88%	84%	82%
Home Recovery Information Given	300+	88%	85%	85%
Hospital Given 9 or 10 on 10 Point Scale	300+	74%	70%	71%
Meds 'Always' Explained Before Given	300+	69%	66%	64%
Nurses 'Always' Communicated Well	300+	82%	80%	79%
Pain 'Always' Well Controlled	300+	76%	72%	71%
Room and Bathroom 'Always' Clean	300+	77%	73%	73%
Timely Help 'Always' Received	300+	72%	68%	68%
Would Definitely Recommend Hospital	300+	69%	70%	71%
Use of Medical Imaging				
Cardiac Imaging Stress Test before Surgery	261	3.8%	4.8%	5.3%
Combination Abdominal CT Scan	565	4.2%	9.6%	10.5%
Combination Brain/Sinus CT Scan	588	5.6%	3.3%	2.7%
Combination Chest CT Scan	271	0.0%	3.4%	2.7%
Follow-up Mammogram/Ultrasound	614	13.7%	8.3%	8.8%
Lumbar Spine MRI for Low Back Pain	76	40.8%	35.3%	37.2%

McNairy Regional Hospital

705 E Poplar Ave
Selmer, TN 38375
Phone: 731-645-3221
URL: www.mcnairyregionalhospital.com
Type: Acute Care Hospitals
Emergency Services: Yes
Ownership: Proprietary
Beds: 45
Key Personnel:
Radiology.................... Bonnie Lancaster
Anesthesiology................ Jay Turner

Measure	Cases	This Hosp.	State Avg.	U.S. Avg.
Blood Clot Prevention and Treatment				
Anticoagulation Overlap Therapy[2,7]	-	-	92%	93%
ICU Venous Thromboembolism Prophylaxis[2,7]	-	-	90%	92%
Incidence of Potentially Preventable VTE[2,7]	-	-	10%	10%
UFH with Dosages/Platelet Monitoring[2,7]	-	-	99%	97%
Venous Thromboembolism Prophylaxis[2]	304	98%	83%	85%
Warfarin Therapy Discharge Instructions[2,7]	-	-	78%	75%
Chest Pain/Possible Heart Attack Care				
Aspirin Given Within 24 Hours of Arrival	91	98%	96%	96%
Fibrinolytic Meds Within 30 Min. of Arrival[1]	-	-	72%	58%
Average Time to ECG (minutes)	93	6	6	7
Average Time to Transfer (minutes)[7]	-	-	53	60
Children's Asthma Care				
Received Home Management Plan of Care	-	-	-	88%
Received Reliever Medication	-	-	-	100%
Received Systemic Corticosteroids	-	-	-	100%
Emergency Department				
Admittance Decision Time (minutes)[2]	370	75	82	98
Head CT Results Within 45 Min. of Arrival[1]	-	-	52%	57%
Patients Who Left ER Before Being Seen	11,367	1%	2%	2%
Time from ER Arrival to Admit. (minutes)[2]	377	226	243	274
Time from ER Arrival to Discharge (minutes)	353	116	131	134
Time in ER Before Being Evaluated (minutes)	419	16	25	26
Time to Pain Meds for Fractures (minutes)	28	48	60	57
Heart Attack Care				
Aspirin Given at Discharge[1]	-	-	99%	99%
Fibrinolytic Meds Within 30 Min. of Arrival[7]	-	-	33%	54%
PCI Within 90 Minutes of Arrival[7]	-	-	98%	96%
Statin Prescribed at Discharge[1]	-	-	99%	98%
Heart Failure Care				
ACE Inhibitor or ARB for LVSD[1]	-	-	97%	97%
Discharge Instructions Given	13	85%	93%	94%
Evaluation of LVS Function	23	100%	99%	99%
Medicare Spending				
Medicare Spending per Patient (ratio)	-	0.99	1	0.98
Pneumonia Care				
Appropriate Initial Antibiotic Given	38	97%	95%	95%
Blood Culture Timing	30	97%	98%	98%
Pregnancy and Delivery Care				
Newborn Deliveries Scheduled Early[1,2]	-	-	6%	6%
Preventive Care				
Immunization for Influenza[2]	283	100%	93%	90%
Immunization for Pneumonia[2]	351	100%	93%	92%
Stroke Care				
Anticoagulation Therapy for Atrial Fibrillation[3,7]	-	-	94%	95%
Antithrombotic Therapy Timing[1,3]	-	-	97%	98%
Assessed for Rehabilitation[1,3]	-	-	97%	97%
Discharged on Antithrombotic Therapy[1,3]	-	-	99%	99%
Discharged on Statin Medication[1,3]	-	-	94%	94%
Thrombolytic Therapy Timing[3,7]	-	-	57%	66%
Venous Thromboembolism Prophylaxis[1,3]	-	-	93%	94%
Written Stroke Educational Materials Given[1,3]	-	-	84%	88%
Surgical Care Improvement Project				
Appropriate Beta Blocker Usage[1,3]	-	-	97%	98%
Appropriate VTP Within 24 Hours[1,3]	-	-	98%	98%
Controlled Postoperative Blood Glucose[3,7]	-	-	95%	97%
Perioperative Temperature Management[3]	11	100%	100%	100%
Prophylactic Antibiotic Selection[1,3]	-	-	99%	99%
Prophylactic Antibiotic Selection (Outpatient)[3]	24	96%	98%	98%
Prophylactic Antibiotic Stopped[1,3]	-	-	98%	98%
Prophylactic Antibiotic Timing[1,3]	-	-	99%	99%
Prophylactic Antibiotic Timing (Outpatient)[3]	24	100%	98%	98%
Urinary Catheter Removal[1,3]	-	-	96%	97%
Survey of Patients' Hospital Experiences				
Area Around Room 'Always' Quiet at Night	(a)	77%	67%	61%
Doctors 'Always' Communicated Well	(a)	89%	84%	82%
Home Recovery Information Given	(a)	85%	85%	85%
Hospital Given 9 or 10 on 10 Point Scale	(a)	68%	70%	71%
Meds 'Always' Explained Before Given	(a)	73%	66%	64%
Nurses 'Always' Communicated Well	(a)	81%	80%	79%
Pain 'Always' Well Controlled	(a)	72%	72%	71%
Room and Bathroom 'Always' Clean	(a)	71%	73%	73%
Timely Help 'Always' Received	(a)	64%	68%	68%
Would Definitely Recommend Hospital	(a)	60%	70%	71%
Use of Medical Imaging				
Cardiac Imaging Stress Test before Surgery[1]	-	-	4.8%	5.3%
Combination Abdominal CT Scan	192	2.1%	9.6%	10.5%
Combination Brain/Sinus CT Scan[1]	-	-	3.3%	2.7%
Combination Chest CT Scan	90	1.1%	3.4%	2.7%
Follow-up Mammogram/Ultrasound	293	5.5%	8.3%	8.8%
Lumbar Spine MRI for Low Back Pain[1]	-	-	35.3%	37.2%

Leconte Medical Center

742 Middlecreek Road
Sevierville, TN 37862
Phone: 865-446-7500
URL: www.lecontemedicalcenter.com
Type: Acute Care Hospitals
Emergency Services: Yes
Ownership: Voluntary non-profit - Other
Key Personnel:
President/CEO................ Jenny Hanson, RN

Measure	Cases	This Hosp.	State Avg.	U.S. Avg.
Blood Clot Prevention and Treatment				
Anticoagulation Overlap Therapy[2]	33	100%	92%	93%
ICU Venous Thromboembolism Prophylaxis[2]	73	100%	90%	92%
Incidence of Potentially Preventable VTE[1,2]	-	-	10%	10%
UFH with Dosages/Platelet Monitoring[1,2]	-	-	99%	97%
Venous Thromboembolism Prophylaxis[2]	295	99%	83%	85%
Warfarin Therapy Discharge Instructions[2]	25	100%	78%	75%
Chest Pain/Possible Heart Attack Care				
Aspirin Given Within 24 Hours of Arrival	99	98%	96%	96%
Fibrinolytic Meds Within 30 Min. of Arrival[7]	-	-	72%	58%
Average Time to ECG (minutes)	101	10	6	7
Average Time to Transfer (minutes)	30	46	53	60
Children's Asthma Care				
Received Home Management Plan of Care	-	-	-	88%
Received Reliever Medication	-	-	-	100%
Received Systemic Corticosteroids	-	-	-	100%
Emergency Department				
Admittance Decision Time (minutes)[2]	548	115	82	98
Head CT Results Within 45 Min. of Arrival	18	44%	52%	57%
Patients Who Left ER Before Being Seen	54,577	5%	2%	2%
Time from ER Arrival to Admit. (minutes)[2]	562	312	243	274
Time from ER Arrival to Discharge (minutes)	398	174	131	134
Time in ER Before Being Evaluated (minutes)	435	48	25	26
Time to Pain Meds for Fractures (minutes)	176	67	60	57
Heart Attack Care				
Aspirin Given at Discharge	31	100%	99%	99%
Fibrinolytic Meds Within 30 Min. of Arrival[7]	-	-	33%	54%
PCI Within 90 Minutes of Arrival[7]	-	-	98%	96%
Statin Prescribed at Discharge	33	100%	99%	98%

NOTE: Hospital profiles are in alphabetical order by state, then city, then hospital within the city; Rankings exclude hospitals with less than 25 cases except for patient surveys which excludes hospitals with less than 100 cases; (a) 100-299 cases; (1) The number of cases/patients is too few to report; (2) Data submitted were based on a sample of cases/patients; (3) Results are based on a shorter time period than required; (4) Data suppressed by CMS for one or more quarters; (5) Results are not available for this reporting period; (6) Fewer than 100 patients completed the HCAHPS survey; (7) No cases met the criteria for this measure; (8) The lower limit of the confidence interval cannot be calculated if the number of observed infections equals zero; (9) No data are available from the state/territory for this reporting period; (10) The scores shown reflect fewer than 50 completed surveys; (11) There were discrepancies in the data collection process; (12) This measure does not apply to this hospital for this reporting period; (13) Results cannot be calculated for this reporting period; (14) The results for this state are combined with nearby states to protect confidentiality; Please refer to the User's Guide for a full explanation of data.

Measure	Cases	This Hosp.	State Avg.	U.S. Avg.
Heart Failure Care				
ACE Inhibitor or ARB for LVSD	25	100%	97%	97%
Discharge Instructions Given	84	90%	93%	94%
Evaluation of LVS Function	100	99%	99%	99%
Medicare Spending				
Medicare Spending per Patient (ratio)	-	0.90	1	0.98
Pneumonia Care				
Appropriate Initial Antibiotic Given[2]	138	99%	95%	95%
Blood Culture Timing[2]	190	99%	98%	98%
Pregnancy and Delivery Care				
Newborn Deliveries Scheduled Early	205	5%	6%	6%
Preventive Care				
Immunization for Influenza[2]	442	98%	93%	90%
Immunization for Pneumonia[2]	521	95%	93%	92%
Stroke Care				
Anticoagulation Therapy for Atrial Fibrillation[1]	-	-	94%	95%
Antithrombotic Therapy Timing	50	100%	97%	98%
Assessed for Rehabilitation	63	98%	97%	97%
Discharged on Antithrombotic Therapy	62	98%	99%	99%
Discharged on Statin Medication	45	98%	94%	94%
Thrombolytic Therapy Timing[1]	-	-	57%	66%
Venous Thromboembolism Prophylaxis	49	98%	93%	94%
Written Stroke Educational Materials Given	48	88%	84%	88%
Surgical Care Improvement Project				
Appropriate Beta Blocker Usage[2]	57	98%	97%	98%
Appropriate VTP Within 24 Hours[2]	193	95%	98%	98%
Controlled Postoperative Blood Glucose[2,7]	-	-	95%	97%
Perioperative Temperature Management[2]	215	100%	100%	100%
Prophylactic Antibiotic Selection[2]	147	99%	99%	99%
Prophylactic Antibiotic Selection (Outpatient)	84	100%	98%	98%
Prophylactic Antibiotic Stopped[2]	140	99%	98%	98%
Prophylactic Antibiotic Timing[2]	147	99%	99%	99%
Prophylactic Antibiotic Timing (Outpatient)	84	100%	98%	98%
Urinary Catheter Removal[2]	67	94%	96%	97%
Survey of Patients' Hospital Experiences				
Area Around Room 'Always' Quiet at Night	300+	62%	67%	61%
Doctors 'Always' Communicated Well	300+	81%	84%	82%
Home Recovery Information Given	300+	86%	85%	85%
Hospital Given 9 or 10 on 10 Point Scale	300+	73%	70%	71%
Meds 'Always' Explained Before Given	300+	65%	66%	64%
Nurses 'Always' Communicated Well	300+	79%	80%	79%
Pain 'Always' Well Controlled	300+	69%	72%	71%
Room and Bathroom 'Always' Clean	300+	71%	73%	73%
Timely Help 'Always' Received	300+	64%	68%	68%
Would Definitely Recommend Hospital	300+	72%	70%	71%
Use of Medical Imaging				
Cardiac Imaging Stress Test before Surgery	397	5.3%	4.8%	5.3%
Combination Abdominal CT Scan	903	8.9%	9.6%	10.5%
Combination Brain/Sinus CT Scan	632	5.9%	3.3%	2.7%
Combination Chest CT Scan	612	4.7%	3.4%	2.7%
Follow-up Mammogram/Ultrasound	1,217	11.3%	8.3%	8.8%
Lumbar Spine MRI for Low Back Pain	162	34.6%	35.3%	37.2%

Heritage Medical Center

2835 Hwy 231 N
Shelbyville, TN 37160
Phone: 931-685-5433
URL: www.heritagemedicalcenter.com
Type: Acute Care Hospitals
Emergency Services: Yes
Ownership: Proprietary

Measure	Cases	This Hosp.	State Avg.	U.S. Avg.
Blood Clot Prevention and Treatment				
Anticoagulation Overlap Therapy[2]	16	100%	92%	93%
ICU Venous Thromboembolism Prophylaxis[2]	101	96%	90%	92%
Incidence of Potentially Preventable VTE[1,2]	-	-	10%	10%
UFH with Dosages/Platelet Monitoring[1,2]	-	-	99%	97%
Venous Thromboembolism Prophylaxis[2]	224	95%	83%	85%
Warfarin Therapy Discharge Instructions[2]	13	100%	78%	75%
Chest Pain/Possible Heart Attack Care				
Aspirin Given Within 24 Hours of Arrival	77	100%	96%	96%
Fibrinolytic Meds Within 30 Min. of Arrival[1]	-	-	72%	58%
Average Time to ECG (minutes)	83	4	6	7
Average Time to Transfer (minutes)	21	46	53	60
Children's Asthma Care				
Received Home Management Plan of Care	-	-	-	88%
Received Reliever Medication	-	-	-	100%
Received Systemic Corticosteroids	-	-	-	100%
Emergency Department				
Admittance Decision Time (minutes)[2]	486	82	82	98
Head CT Results Within 45 Min. of Arrival[1]	-	-	52%	57%
Patients Who Left ER Before Being Seen	20,802	1%	2%	2%
Time from ER Arrival to Admit. (minutes)[2]	494	219	243	274
Time from ER Arrival to Discharge (minutes)	382	116	131	134
Time in ER Before Being Evaluated (minutes)	414	22	25	26
Time to Pain Meds for Fractures (minutes)	78	64	60	57
Heart Attack Care				
Aspirin Given at Discharge[1,3]	-	-	99%	99%
Fibrinolytic Meds Within 30 Min. of Arrival[3,7]	-	-	33%	54%
PCI Within 90 Minutes of Arrival[3,7]	-	-	98%	96%
Statin Prescribed at Discharge[1,3]	-	-	99%	98%
Heart Failure Care				
ACE Inhibitor or ARB for LVSD	18	100%	97%	97%
Discharge Instructions Given	60	100%	93%	94%
Evaluation of LVS Function	69	100%	99%	99%
Medicare Spending				
Medicare Spending per Patient (ratio)	-	1.04	1	0.98
Pneumonia Care				
Appropriate Initial Antibiotic Given	62	97%	95%	95%
Blood Culture Timing	101	100%	98%	98%
Pregnancy and Delivery Care				
Newborn Deliveries Scheduled Early[2,7]	-	-	6%	6%
Preventive Care				
Immunization for Influenza[2]	331	100%	93%	90%
Immunization for Pneumonia[2]	490	100%	93%	92%
Stroke Care				
Anticoagulation Therapy for Atrial Fibrillation[1]	-	-	94%	95%
Antithrombotic Therapy Timing	17	100%	97%	98%
Assessed for Rehabilitation	20	100%	97%	97%
Discharged on Antithrombotic Therapy	20	100%	99%	99%
Discharged on Statin Medication	12	100%	94%	94%
Thrombolytic Therapy Timing[7]	-	-	57%	66%
Venous Thromboembolism Prophylaxis	17	100%	93%	94%
Written Stroke Educational Materials Given	16	100%	84%	88%
Surgical Care Improvement Project				
Appropriate Beta Blocker Usage[1]	-	-	97%	98%
Appropriate VTP Within 24 Hours	28	100%	98%	98%
Controlled Postoperative Blood Glucose[7]	-	-	95%	97%
Perioperative Temperature Management	33	100%	100%	100%
Prophylactic Antibiotic Selection	12	100%	99%	99%
Prophylactic Antibiotic Selection (Outpatient)	16	100%	98%	98%
Prophylactic Antibiotic Stopped	12	100%	98%	98%
Prophylactic Antibiotic Timing	12	100%	99%	99%
Prophylactic Antibiotic Timing (Outpatient)	16	100%	98%	98%
Urinary Catheter Removal	13	100%	96%	97%
Survey of Patients' Hospital Experiences				
Area Around Room 'Always' Quiet at Night	300+	68%	67%	61%
Doctors 'Always' Communicated Well	300+	82%	84%	82%
Home Recovery Information Given	300+	85%	85%	85%
Hospital Given 9 or 10 on 10 Point Scale	300+	67%	70%	71%
Meds 'Always' Explained Before Given	300+	65%	66%	64%
Nurses 'Always' Communicated Well	300+	77%	80%	79%
Pain 'Always' Well Controlled	300+	67%	72%	71%
Room and Bathroom 'Always' Clean	300+	72%	73%	73%
Timely Help 'Always' Received	300+	64%	68%	68%
Would Definitely Recommend Hospital	300+	62%	70%	71%
Use of Medical Imaging				
Cardiac Imaging Stress Test before Surgery	174	5.7%	4.8%	5.3%
Combination Abdominal CT Scan	235	11.9%	9.6%	10.5%
Combination Brain/Sinus CT Scan	450	4.0%	3.3%	2.7%
Combination Chest CT Scan	173	11.0%	3.4%	2.7%
Follow-up Mammogram/Ultrasound	623	9.5%	8.3%	8.8%
Lumbar Spine MRI for Low Back Pain	72	36.1%	35.3%	37.2%

Stones River Hospital & Dekalb Community Hospital

520 W Main St
Smithville, TN 37166
Phone: 615-215-5000
Fax: 615-215-5604
URL: www.dekalb-hospital.com
Type: Acute Care Hospitals
Emergency Services: Yes
Ownership: Voluntary non-profit - Church
Beds: 71
Key Personnel:
CEO/President. . . . . Dennis Smock

Measure	Cases	This Hosp.	State Avg.	U.S. Avg.
Blood Clot Prevention and Treatment				
Anticoagulation Overlap Therapy[2]	11	64%	92%	93%
ICU Venous Thromboembolism Prophylaxis[2]	61	56%	90%	92%
Incidence of Potentially Preventable VTE[2,7]	-	-	10%	10%
UFH with Dosages/Platelet Monitoring[2,7]	-	-	99%	97%
Venous Thromboembolism Prophylaxis[2]	287	48%	83%	85%
Warfarin Therapy Discharge Instructions[1,2]	-	-	78%	75%
Chest Pain/Possible Heart Attack Care				
Aspirin Given Within 24 Hours of Arrival	70	93%	96%	96%
Fibrinolytic Meds Within 30 Min. of Arrival[1]	-	-	72%	58%
Average Time to ECG (minutes)	75	5	6	7
Average Time to Transfer (minutes)[1]	-	-	53	60
Children's Asthma Care				
Received Home Management Plan of Care	-	-	-	88%
Received Reliever Medication	-	-	-	100%
Received Systemic Corticosteroids	-	-	-	100%
Emergency Department				
Admittance Decision Time (minutes)[2]	312	50	82	98
Head CT Results Within 45 Min. of Arrival[1]	-	-	52%	57%
Patients Who Left ER Before Being Seen	9,729	1%	2%	2%
Time from ER Arrival to Admit. (minutes)[2]	312	185	243	274
Time from ER Arrival to Discharge (minutes)	305	97	131	134
Time in ER Before Being Evaluated (minutes)	378	21	25	26
Time to Pain Meds for Fractures (minutes)	50	53	60	57
Heart Attack Care				
Aspirin Given at Discharge[1,3]	-	-	99%	99%
Fibrinolytic Meds Within 30 Min. of Arrival[3,7]	-	-	33%	54%
PCI Within 90 Minutes of Arrival[3,7]	-	-	98%	96%
Statin Prescribed at Discharge[1,3]	-	-	99%	98%
Heart Failure Care				
ACE Inhibitor or ARB for LVSD	12	100%	97%	97%
Discharge Instructions Given	48	96%	93%	94%
Evaluation of LVS Function	70	100%	99%	99%
Medicare Spending				
Medicare Spending per Patient (ratio)	-	0.91	1	0.98
Pneumonia Care				
Appropriate Initial Antibiotic Given	95	100%	95%	95%
Blood Culture Timing	108	99%	98%	98%
Pregnancy and Delivery Care				
Newborn Deliveries Scheduled Early[7]	-	-	6%	6%
Preventive Care				
Immunization for Influenza[2]	282	100%	93%	90%
Immunization for Pneumonia[2]	475	100%	93%	92%
Stroke Care				
Anticoagulation Therapy for Atrial Fibrillation[1,2]	-	-	94%	95%
Antithrombotic Therapy Timing[1,2]	-	-	97%	98%
Assessed for Rehabilitation[1,2]	-	-	97%	97%
Discharged on Antithrombotic Therapy[1,2]	-	-	99%	99%
Discharged on Statin Medication[1,2]	-	-	94%	94%
Thrombolytic Therapy Timing[2,7]	-	-	57%	66%
Venous Thromboembolism Prophylaxis[1,2]	-	-	93%	94%
Written Stroke Educational Materials Given[2,7]	-	-	84%	88%
Surgical Care Improvement Project				
Appropriate Beta Blocker Usage	16	100%	97%	98%
Appropriate VTP Within 24 Hours	44	100%	98%	98%
Controlled Postoperative Blood Glucose[7]	-	-	95%	97%
Perioperative Temperature Management	50	100%	100%	100%
Prophylactic Antibiotic Selection	36	100%	99%	99%
Prophylactic Antibiotic Selection (Outpatient)[1,3]	-	-	98%	98%
Prophylactic Antibiotic Stopped	33	85%	98%	98%
Prophylactic Antibiotic Timing	36	100%	99%	99%
Prophylactic Antibiotic Timing (Outpatient)[1,3]	-	-	98%	98%
Urinary Catheter Removal	38	100%	96%	97%
Survey of Patients' Hospital Experiences				

NOTE: Hospital profiles are in alphabetical order by state, then city, then hospital within the city; Rankings exclude hospitals with less than 25 cases except for patient surveys which excludes hospitals with less than 100 cases; (a) 100-299 cases; (1) The number of cases/patients is too few to report; (2) Data submitted were based on a sample of cases/patients; (3) Results are based on a shorter time period than required; (4) Data suppressed by CMS for one or more quarters; (5) Results are not available for this reporting period; (6) Fewer than 100 patients completed the HCAHPS survey; (7) No cases met the criteria for this measure; (8) The lower limit of the confidence interval cannot be calculated if the number of observed infections equals zero; (9) No data are available from the state/territory for this reporting period; (10) The scores shown reflect fewer than 50 completed surveys; (11) There were discrepancies in the data collection process; (12) This measure does not apply to this hospital for this reporting period; (13) Results cannot be calculated for this reporting period; (14) The results for this state are combined with nearby states to protect confidentiality; Please refer to the User's Guide for a full explanation of data.

Measure	Cases	This Hosp.	State Avg.	U.S. Avg.
Area Around Room 'Always' Quiet at Night	(a)	71%	67%	61%
Doctors 'Always' Communicated Well	(a)	89%	84%	82%
Home Recovery Information Given	(a)	85%	85%	85%
Hospital Given 9 or 10 on 10 Point Scale	(a)	72%	70%	71%
Meds 'Always' Explained Before Given	(a)	64%	66%	64%
Nurses 'Always' Communicated Well	(a)	81%	80%	79%
Pain 'Always' Well Controlled	(a)	74%	72%	71%
Room and Bathroom 'Always' Clean	(a)	72%	73%	73%
Timely Help 'Always' Received	(a)	73%	68%	68%
Would Definitely Recommend Hospital	(a)	73%	70%	71%
Use of Medical Imaging				
Cardiac Imaging Stress Test before Surgery[1]	-	-	4.8%	5.3%
Combination Abdominal CT Scan	240	2.5%	9.6%	10.5%
Combination Brain/Sinus CT Scan[1]	-	-	3.3%	2.7%
Combination Chest CT Scan	126	4.0%	3.4%	2.7%
Follow-up Mammogram/Ultrasound	286	7.7%	8.3%	8.8%
Lumbar Spine MRI for Low Back Pain[1]	-	-	35.3%	37.2%

Tristar Stonecrest Medical Center

200 Stonecrest Boulevard — Phone: 615-768-2000
Smyrna, TN 37167 — Fax: 615-768-2203
URL: www.stonecrestmedical.com
Type: Acute Care Hospitals — Emergency Services: Yes
Ownership: Proprietary — Beds: 75

Key Personnel:
Radiology. . . . . Christopher J Bodin
Chief of Medical Staff. . . . . Anita Dhar
CEO/President. . . . . Neil A Heatherly, CHE

Measure	Cases	This Hosp.	State Avg.	U.S. Avg.
Blood Clot Prevention and Treatment				
Anticoagulation Overlap Therapy[2]	29	100%	92%	93%
ICU Venous Thromboembolism Prophylaxis[2]	114	96%	90%	92%
Incidence of Potentially Preventable VTE[1,2]	-	-	10%	10%
UFH with Dosages/Platelet Monitoring[1,2]	-	-	99%	97%
Venous Thromboembolism Prophylaxis[2]	272	96%	83%	85%
Warfarin Therapy Discharge Instructions[2]	24	100%	78%	75%
Chest Pain/Possible Heart Attack Care				
Aspirin Given Within 24 Hours of Arrival	52	100%	96%	96%
Fibrinolytic Meds Within 30 Min. of Arrival[7]	-	-	72%	58%
Average Time to ECG (minutes)	54	4	6	7
Average Time to Transfer (minutes)[1]	-	-	53	60
Children's Asthma Care				
Received Home Management Plan of Care	-	-	-	88%
Received Reliever Medication	-	-	-	100%
Received Systemic Corticosteroids	-	-	-	100%
Emergency Department				
Admittance Decision Time (minutes)[2]	389	76	82	98
Head CT Results Within 45 Min. of Arrival	13	85%	52%	57%
Patients Who Left ER Before Being Seen	47,094	1%	2%	2%
Time from ER Arrival to Admit. (minutes)[2]	469	232	243	274
Time from ER Arrival to Discharge (minutes)	435	127	131	134
Time in ER Before Being Evaluated (minutes)	483	13	25	26
Time to Pain Meds for Fractures (minutes)	181	39	60	57
Heart Attack Care				
Aspirin Given at Discharge[2]	50	100%	99%	99%
Fibrinolytic Meds Within 30 Min. of Arrival[1,2]	-	-	33%	54%
PCI Within 90 Minutes of Arrival[2]	11	100%	98%	96%
Statin Prescribed at Discharge[2]	49	100%	99%	98%
Heart Failure Care				
ACE Inhibitor or ARB for LVSD[2]	31	100%	97%	97%
Discharge Instructions Given[2]	109	98%	93%	94%
Evaluation of LVS Function[2]	135	100%	99%	99%
Medicare Spending				
Medicare Spending per Patient (ratio)	-	1.04	1	0.98
Pneumonia Care				
Appropriate Initial Antibiotic Given[2]	116	100%	95%	95%
Blood Culture Timing[2]	213	100%	98%	98%
Pregnancy and Delivery Care				
Newborn Deliveries Scheduled Early[2]	43	5%	6%	6%
Preventive Care				
Immunization for Influenza[2]	504	97%	93%	90%
Immunization for Pneumonia[2]	540	98%	93%	92%
Stroke Care				
Anticoagulation Therapy for Atrial Fibrillation[1,2]	-	-	94%	95%
Antithrombotic Therapy Timing[2]	29	100%	97%	98%
Assessed for Rehabilitation[2]	36	100%	97%	97%
Discharged on Antithrombotic Therapy[2]	35	100%	99%	99%
Discharged on Statin Medication[2]	28	100%	94%	94%
Thrombolytic Therapy Timing[2,7]	-	-	57%	66%
Venous Thromboembolism Prophylaxis[2]	25	100%	93%	94%
Written Stroke Educational Materials Given[2]	22	86%	84%	88%
Surgical Care Improvement Project				
Appropriate Beta Blocker Usage[2]	73	99%	97%	98%
Appropriate VTP Within 24 Hours[2]	234	99%	98%	98%
Controlled Postoperative Blood Glucose[2,7]	-	-	95%	97%
Perioperative Temperature Management[2]	284	100%	100%	100%
Prophylactic Antibiotic Selection[2]	176	100%	99%	99%
Prophylactic Antibiotic Selection (Outpatient)	227	100%	98%	98%
Prophylactic Antibiotic Stopped[2]	172	97%	98%	98%
Prophylactic Antibiotic Timing[2]	176	99%	99%	99%
Prophylactic Antibiotic Timing (Outpatient)	216	100%	98%	98%
Urinary Catheter Removal[2]	170	98%	96%	97%
Survey of Patients' Hospital Experiences				
Area Around Room 'Always' Quiet at Night	300+	71%	67%	61%
Doctors 'Always' Communicated Well	300+	81%	84%	82%
Home Recovery Information Given	300+	87%	85%	85%
Hospital Given 9 or 10 on 10 Point Scale	300+	71%	70%	71%
Meds 'Always' Explained Before Given	300+	62%	66%	64%
Nurses 'Always' Communicated Well	300+	76%	80%	79%
Pain 'Always' Well Controlled	300+	70%	72%	71%
Room and Bathroom 'Always' Clean	300+	76%	73%	73%
Timely Help 'Always' Received	300+	61%	68%	68%
Would Definitely Recommend Hospital	300+	72%	70%	71%
Use of Medical Imaging				
Cardiac Imaging Stress Test before Surgery	60	0.0%	4.8%	5.3%
Combination Abdominal CT Scan	352	3.7%	9.6%	10.5%
Combination Brain/Sinus CT Scan[1]	-	-	3.3%	2.7%
Combination Chest CT Scan	135	0.7%	3.4%	2.7%
Follow-up Mammogram/Ultrasound	523	8.6%	8.3%	8.8%
Lumbar Spine MRI for Low Back Pain[1]	-	-	35.3%	37.2%

Wellmont Hancock County Hospital

1517 Main Street Hwy 33 — Phone: 423-733-5001
Sneedville, TN 37869
URL: www.wellmont.org
Type: Critical Access Hospitals — Emergency Services: Yes
Ownership: Voluntary non-profit - Private

Key Personnel:
CEO/President. . . . . Fred Pelle
Chief of Medical Staff. . . . . John Short

Measure	Cases	This Hosp.	State Avg.	U.S. Avg.
Blood Clot Prevention and Treatment				
Anticoagulation Overlap Therapy[5]	-	-	92%	93%
ICU Venous Thromboembolism Prophylaxis[5]	-	-	90%	92%
Incidence of Potentially Preventable VTE[5]	-	-	10%	10%
UFH with Dosages/Platelet Monitoring[5]	-	-	99%	97%
Venous Thromboembolism Prophylaxis[5]	-	-	83%	85%
Warfarin Therapy Discharge Instructions[5]	-	-	78%	75%
Chest Pain/Possible Heart Attack Care				
Aspirin Given Within 24 Hours of Arrival	-	-	96%	96%
Fibrinolytic Meds Within 30 Min. of Arrival	-	-	72%	58%
Average Time to ECG (minutes)	-	-	6	7
Average Time to Transfer (minutes)	-	-	53	60
Children's Asthma Care				
Received Home Management Plan of Care	-	-	-	88%
Received Reliever Medication	-	-	-	100%
Received Systemic Corticosteroids	-	-	-	100%
Emergency Department				
Admittance Decision Time (minutes)[5]	-	-	82	98
Head CT Results Within 45 Min. of Arrival	-	-	52%	57%
Patients Who Left ER Before Being Seen	-	-	2%	2%
Time from ER Arrival to Admit. (minutes)[5]	-	-	243	274
Time from ER Arrival to Discharge (minutes)	-	-	131	134
Time in ER Before Being Evaluated (minutes)	-	-	25	26
Time to Pain Meds for Fractures (minutes)	-	-	60	57
Heart Attack Care				
Aspirin Given at Discharge[1,3]	-	-	99%	99%
Fibrinolytic Meds Within 30 Min. of Arrival[3,7]	-	-	33%	54%
PCI Within 90 Minutes of Arrival[3,7]	-	-	98%	96%
Statin Prescribed at Discharge[1,3]	-	-	99%	98%
Heart Failure Care				
ACE Inhibitor or ARB for LVSD[7]	-	-	97%	97%
Discharge Instructions Given[1]	-	-	93%	94%
Evaluation of LVS Function[1]	-	-	99%	99%
Medicare Spending				
Medicare Spending per Patient (ratio)	-	-	1	0.98
Pneumonia Care				
Appropriate Initial Antibiotic Given	18	78%	95%	95%
Blood Culture Timing	22	95%	98%	98%
Pregnancy and Delivery Care				
Newborn Deliveries Scheduled Early[7]	-	-	6%	6%
Preventive Care				
Immunization for Influenza[5]	-	-	93%	90%
Immunization for Pneumonia[5]	-	-	93%	92%
Stroke Care				
Anticoagulation Therapy for Atrial Fibrillation[5]	-	-	94%	95%
Antithrombotic Therapy Timing[5]	-	-	97%	98%
Assessed for Rehabilitation[5]	-	-	97%	97%
Discharged on Antithrombotic Therapy[5]	-	-	99%	99%
Discharged on Statin Medication[5]	-	-	94%	94%
Thrombolytic Therapy Timing[5]	-	-	57%	66%
Venous Thromboembolism Prophylaxis[5]	-	-	93%	94%
Written Stroke Educational Materials Given[5]	-	-	84%	88%
Surgical Care Improvement Project				
Appropriate Beta Blocker Usage[5]	-	-	97%	98%
Appropriate VTP Within 24 Hours[5]	-	-	98%	98%
Controlled Postoperative Blood Glucose[5]	-	-	95%	97%
Perioperative Temperature Management[5]	-	-	100%	100%
Prophylactic Antibiotic Selection[5]	-	-	99%	99%
Prophylactic Antibiotic Selection (Outpatient)	-	-	98%	98%
Prophylactic Antibiotic Stopped[5]	-	-	98%	98%
Prophylactic Antibiotic Timing[5]	-	-	99%	99%
Prophylactic Antibiotic Timing (Outpatient)	-	-	98%	98%
Urinary Catheter Removal[5]	-	-	96%	97%
Survey of Patients' Hospital Experiences				
Area Around Room 'Always' Quiet at Night[10]	<100	79%	67%	61%
Doctors 'Always' Communicated Well[10]	<100	93%	84%	82%
Home Recovery Information Given[10]	<100	96%	85%	85%
Hospital Given 9 or 10 on 10 Point Scale[10]	<100	96%	70%	71%
Meds 'Always' Explained Before Given[10]	<100	76%	66%	64%
Nurses 'Always' Communicated Well[10]	<100	92%	80%	79%
Pain 'Always' Well Controlled[10]	<100	78%	72%	71%
Room and Bathroom 'Always' Clean[10]	<100	96%	73%	73%
Timely Help 'Always' Received[10]	<100	84%	68%	68%
Would Definitely Recommend Hospital[10]	<100	93%	70%	71%
Use of Medical Imaging				
Cardiac Imaging Stress Test before Surgery	-	-	4.8%	5.3%
Combination Abdominal CT Scan	-	-	9.6%	10.5%
Combination Brain/Sinus CT Scan	-	-	3.3%	2.7%
Combination Chest CT Scan	-	-	3.4%	2.7%
Follow-up Mammogram/Ultrasound	-	-	8.3%	8.8%
Lumbar Spine MRI for Low Back Pain	-	-	35.3%	37.2%

Methodist Healthcare Fayette Hospital

214 Lakeview Rd — Phone: 901-516-4014
Somerville, TN 38068
Type: Acute Care Hospitals — Emergency Services: Yes
Ownership: Voluntary non-profit - Church

Key Personnel:
CEO/President. . . . . David Crislip

Measure	Cases	This Hosp.	State Avg.	U.S. Avg.
Blood Clot Prevention and Treatment				
Anticoagulation Overlap Therapy[1,2]	-	-	92%	93%
ICU Venous Thromboembolism Prophylaxis[2,7]	-	-	90%	92%
Incidence of Potentially Preventable VTE[2,7]	-	-	10%	10%
UFH with Dosages/Platelet Monitoring[2,7]	-	-	99%	97%
Venous Thromboembolism Prophylaxis[2]	79	87%	83%	85%
Warfarin Therapy Discharge Instructions[2,7]	-	-	78%	75%

NOTE: Hospital profiles are in alphabetical order by state, then city, then hospital within the city; Rankings exclude hospitals with less than 25 cases except for patient surveys which excludes hospitals with less than 100 cases; (a) 100-299 cases; (1) The number of cases/patients is too few to report; (2) Data submitted were based on a sample of cases/patients; (3) Results are based on a shorter time period than required; (4) Data suppressed by CMS for one or more quarters; (5) Results are not available for this reporting period; (6) Fewer than 100 patients completed the HCAHPS survey; (7) No cases met the criteria for this measure; (8) The lower limit of the confidence interval cannot be calculated if the number of observed infections equals zero; (9) No data are available from the state/territory for this reporting period; (10) The scores shown reflect fewer than 50 completed surveys; (11) There were discrepancies in the data collection process; (12) This measure does not apply to this hospital for this reporting period; (13) Results cannot be calculated for this reporting period; (14) The results for this state are combined with nearby states to protect confidentiality; Please refer to the User's Guide for a full explanation of data.

Measure	Cases	This Hosp.	State Avg.	U.S. Avg.
Chest Pain/Possible Heart Attack Care				
Aspirin Given Within 24 Hours of Arrival	62	97%	96%	96%
Fibrinolytic Meds Within 30 Min. of Arrival[1]	-	-	72%	58%
Average Time to ECG (minutes)	64	4	6	7
Average Time to Transfer (minutes)[1]	-	-	53	60
Children's Asthma Care				
Received Home Management Plan of Care	-	-	-	88%
Received Reliever Medication	-	-	-	100%
Received Systemic Corticosteroids	-	-	-	100%
Emergency Department				
Admittance Decision Time (minutes)[2]	39	43	82	98
Head CT Results Within 45 Min. of Arrival[1]	-	-	52%	57%
Patients Who Left ER Before Being Seen	8,129	2%	2%	2%
Time from ER Arrival to Admit. (minutes)[2]	55	240	243	274
Time from ER Arrival to Discharge (minutes)	382	104	131	134
Time in ER Before Being Evaluated (minutes)	434	18	25	26
Time to Pain Meds for Fractures (minutes)	22	60	60	57
Heart Attack Care				
Aspirin Given at Discharge[5]	-	-	99%	99%
Fibrinolytic Meds Within 30 Min. of Arrival[5]	-	-	33%	54%
PCI Within 90 Minutes of Arrival[5]	-	-	98%	96%
Statin Prescribed at Discharge[5]	-	-	99%	98%
Heart Failure Care				
ACE Inhibitor or ARB for LVSD[1,3]	-	-	97%	97%
Discharge Instructions Given[1,3]	-	-	93%	94%
Evaluation of LVS Function[1,3]	-	-	99%	99%
Medicare Spending				
Medicare Spending per Patient (ratio)	-	1.06	1	0.98
Pneumonia Care				
Appropriate Initial Antibiotic Given[1,3]	-	-	95%	95%
Blood Culture Timing[1,3]	-	-	98%	98%
Pregnancy and Delivery Care				
Newborn Deliveries Scheduled Early[7]	-	-	6%	6%
Preventive Care				
Immunization for Influenza[2]	64	100%	93%	90%
Immunization for Pneumonia[2]	113	98%	93%	92%
Stroke Care				
Anticoagulation Therapy for Atrial Fibrillation[5]	-	-	94%	95%
Antithrombotic Therapy Timing[5]	-	-	97%	98%
Assessed for Rehabilitation[5]	-	-	97%	97%
Discharged on Antithrombotic Therapy[5]	-	-	99%	99%
Discharged on Statin Medication[5]	-	-	94%	94%
Thrombolytic Therapy Timing[5]	-	-	57%	66%
Venous Thromboembolism Prophylaxis[5]	-	-	93%	94%
Written Stroke Educational Materials Given[5]	-	-	84%	88%
Surgical Care Improvement Project				
Appropriate Beta Blocker Usage[5]	-	-	97%	98%
Appropriate VTP Within 24 Hours[5]	-	-	98%	98%
Controlled Postoperative Blood Glucose[5]	-	-	95%	97%
Perioperative Temperature Management[5]	-	-	100%	100%
Prophylactic Antibiotic Selection[5]	-	-	99%	99%
Prophylactic Antibiotic Selection (Outpatient)[5]	-	-	98%	98%
Prophylactic Antibiotic Stopped[5]	-	-	98%	98%
Prophylactic Antibiotic Timing[5]	-	-	99%	99%
Prophylactic Antibiotic Timing (Outpatient)[5]	-	-	98%	98%
Urinary Catheter Removal[5]	-	-	96%	97%
Survey of Patients' Hospital Experiences				
Area Around Room 'Always' Quiet at Night[10]	<100	77%	67%	61%
Doctors 'Always' Communicated Well[10]	<100	96%	84%	82%
Home Recovery Information Given[10]	<100	76%	85%	85%
Hospital Given 9 or 10 on 10 Point Scale[10]	<100	78%	70%	71%
Meds 'Always' Explained Before Given[10]	<100	90%	66%	64%
Nurses 'Always' Communicated Well[10]	<100	92%	80%	79%
Pain 'Always' Well Controlled[10]	<100	91%	72%	71%
Room and Bathroom 'Always' Clean[10]	<100	69%	73%	73%
Timely Help 'Always' Received[10]	<100	90%	68%	68%
Would Definitely Recommend Hospital[10]	<100	79%	70%	71%
Use of Medical Imaging				
Cardiac Imaging Stress Test before Surgery[1]	-	-	4.8%	5.3%
Combination Abdominal CT Scan	218	3.2%	9.6%	10.5%
Combination Brain/Sinus CT Scan[1]	-	-	3.3%	2.7%
Combination Chest CT Scan	96	3.1%	3.4%	2.7%
Follow-up Mammogram/Ultrasound	204	10.3%	8.3%	8.8%
Lumbar Spine MRI for Low Back Pain[1]	-	-	35.3%	37.2%

Highlands Medical Center

401 Sewell Dr
Sparta, TN 38583
URL: www.whitecountyhospital.com
Type: Acute Care Hospitals
Ownership: Proprietary
Phone: 931-738-9211
Fax: 931-837-4133
Emergency Services: Yes
Beds: 60

Key Personnel:

Chief of Medical Staff. . . . . John Langloif
CEO/President. . . . . Bill Little
Chairman/CEO . . . . Craig Lynn
Radiology. . . . . Gary Militana, MD
Surgery. Kevin Purgiel, DO
Emergency Room . . . . Herbert Smith, RN
Cardiac Laboratory. . . . . Greg Williams

Measure	Cases	This Hosp.	State Avg.	U.S. Avg.
Blood Clot Prevention and Treatment				
Anticoagulation Overlap Therapy[1,2]	-	-	92%	93%
ICU Venous Thromboembolism Prophylaxis[2]	29	83%	90%	92%
Incidence of Potentially Preventable VTE[2,7]	-	-	10%	10%
UFH with Dosages/Platelet Monitoring[1,2]	-	-	99%	97%
Venous Thromboembolism Prophylaxis[2]	102	60%	83%	85%
Warfarin Therapy Discharge Instructions[1,2]	-	-	78%	75%
Chest Pain/Possible Heart Attack Care				
Aspirin Given Within 24 Hours of Arrival	46	85%	96%	96%
Fibrinolytic Meds Within 30 Min. of Arrival[1]	-	-	72%	58%
Average Time to ECG (minutes)	47	7	6	7
Average Time to Transfer (minutes)[1]	-	-	53	60
Children's Asthma Care				
Received Home Management Plan of Care	-	-	-	88%
Received Reliever Medication	-	-	-	100%
Received Systemic Corticosteroids	-	-	-	100%
Emergency Department				
Admittance Decision Time (minutes)[2]	425	70	82	98
Head CT Results Within 45 Min. of Arrival[1]	-	-	52%	57%
Patients Who Left ER Before Being Seen	12,629	1%	2%	2%
Time from ER Arrival to Admit. (minutes)[2]	427	229	243	274
Time from ER Arrival to Discharge (minutes)	395	109	131	134
Time in ER Before Being Evaluated (minutes)	428	26	25	26
Time to Pain Meds for Fractures (minutes)	57	67	60	57
Heart Attack Care				
Aspirin Given at Discharge[2]	15	67%	99%	99%
Fibrinolytic Meds Within 30 Min. of Arrival[2,7]	-	-	33%	54%
PCI Within 90 Minutes of Arrival[2,7]	-	-	98%	96%
Statin Prescribed at Discharge[2]	16	38%	99%	98%
Heart Failure Care				
ACE Inhibitor or ARB for LVSD[1,2]	-	-	97%	97%
Discharge Instructions Given[2]	24	100%	93%	94%
Evaluation of LVS Function[2]	32	94%	99%	99%
Medicare Spending				
Medicare Spending per Patient (ratio)	-	1.00	1	0.98
Pneumonia Care				
Appropriate Initial Antibiotic Given[2]	100	89%	95%	95%
Blood Culture Timing[2]	99	100%	98%	98%
Pregnancy and Delivery Care				
Newborn Deliveries Scheduled Early[2,7]	-	-	6%	6%
Preventive Care				
Immunization for Influenza[2]	326	90%	93%	90%
Immunization for Pneumonia[2]	458	95%	93%	92%
Stroke Care				
Anticoagulation Therapy for Atrial Fibrillation[1]	-	-	94%	95%
Antithrombotic Therapy Timing[1]	-	-	97%	98%
Assessed for Rehabilitation[1]	-	-	97%	97%
Discharged on Antithrombotic Therapy[1]	-	-	99%	99%
Discharged on Statin Medication[1]	-	-	94%	94%
Thrombolytic Therapy Timing[7]	-	-	57%	66%
Venous Thromboembolism Prophylaxis[1]	-	-	93%	94%
Written Stroke Educational Materials Given[1]	-	-	84%	88%
Surgical Care Improvement Project				
Appropriate Beta Blocker Usage[1,2]	-	-	97%	98%
Appropriate VTP Within 24 Hours[2]	72	92%	98%	98%
Controlled Postoperative Blood Glucose[2,7]	-	-	95%	97%
Perioperative Temperature Management[2]	118	100%	100%	100%
Prophylactic Antibiotic Selection[2]	84	96%	99%	99%
Prophylactic Antibiotic Selection (Outpatient)	40	100%	98%	98%
Prophylactic Antibiotic Stopped[2]	84	100%	98%	98%
Prophylactic Antibiotic Timing[2]	84	99%	99%	99%
Prophylactic Antibiotic Timing (Outpatient)	41	95%	98%	98%
Urinary Catheter Removal[2]	36	81%	96%	97%
Survey of Patients' Hospital Experiences				
Area Around Room 'Always' Quiet at Night	(a)	68%	67%	61%
Doctors 'Always' Communicated Well	(a)	85%	84%	82%
Home Recovery Information Given	(a)	83%	85%	85%
Hospital Given 9 or 10 on 10 Point Scale	(a)	71%	70%	71%
Meds 'Always' Explained Before Given	(a)	62%	66%	64%
Nurses 'Always' Communicated Well	(a)	79%	80%	79%
Pain 'Always' Well Controlled	(a)	70%	72%	71%
Room and Bathroom 'Always' Clean	(a)	75%	73%	73%
Timely Help 'Always' Received	(a)	73%	68%	68%
Would Definitely Recommend Hospital	(a)	70%	70%	71%
Use of Medical Imaging				
Cardiac Imaging Stress Test before Surgery[1]	-	-	4.8%	5.3%
Combination Abdominal CT Scan	231	21.2%	9.6%	10.5%
Combination Brain/Sinus CT Scan[1]	-	-	3.3%	2.7%
Combination Chest CT Scan	99	9.1%	3.4%	2.7%
Follow-up Mammogram/Ultrasound	356	10.7%	8.3%	8.8%
Lumbar Spine MRI for Low Back Pain	51	39.2%	35.3%	37.2%

Northcrest Medical Center

100 Northcrest Drive
Springfield, TN 37172
URL: www.northcrest.com
Type: Acute Care Hospitals
Ownership: Voluntary non-profit - Other
Phone: 615-384-2411
Fax: 615-384-1509
Emergency Services: Yes
Beds: 109

Key Personnel:

Radiology. . . . . Robert Stanton Amonette
Anesthesiology. . . . . Carol Cobb
Operating Room. . . . . Daniel Davis, RN
Chief of Medical Staff. . . . . Jeff Fosnes, MD
Quality Assurance . . . . Carol Harrison
Intensive Care Unit. . . . . Karen String, RN
Infection Control. . . . . Marylin Worsham, RN
Emergency Room . . . . Laura Zervas

Measure	Cases	This Hosp.	State Avg.	U.S. Avg.
Blood Clot Prevention and Treatment				
Anticoagulation Overlap Therapy[2]	35	100%	92%	93%
ICU Venous Thromboembolism Prophylaxis[2]	78	99%	90%	92%
Incidence of Potentially Preventable VTE[2,7]	-	-	10%	10%
UFH with Dosages/Platelet Monitoring[2]	11	100%	99%	97%
Venous Thromboembolism Prophylaxis[2]	259	95%	83%	85%
Warfarin Therapy Discharge Instructions[2]	26	100%	78%	75%
Chest Pain/Possible Heart Attack Care				
Aspirin Given Within 24 Hours of Arrival	29	100%	96%	96%
Fibrinolytic Meds Within 30 Min. of Arrival[7]	-	-	72%	58%
Average Time to ECG (minutes)	31	9	6	7
Average Time to Transfer (minutes)[1]	-	-	53	60
Children's Asthma Care				
Received Home Management Plan of Care	-	-	-	88%
Received Reliever Medication	-	-	-	100%
Received Systemic Corticosteroids	-	-	-	100%
Emergency Department				
Admittance Decision Time (minutes)[2]	340	61	82	98
Head CT Results Within 45 Min. of Arrival	11	55%	52%	57%
Patients Who Left ER Before Being Seen	30,133	1%	2%	2%
Time from ER Arrival to Admit. (minutes)[2]	343	252	243	274
Time from ER Arrival to Discharge (minutes)	357	121	131	134
Time in ER Before Being Evaluated (minutes)	391	18	25	26
Time to Pain Meds for Fractures (minutes)	127	49	60	57
Heart Attack Care				
Aspirin Given at Discharge	48	100%	99%	99%
Fibrinolytic Meds Within 30 Min. of Arrival[7]	-	-	33%	54%
PCI Within 90 Minutes of Arrival	13	100%	98%	96%
Statin Prescribed at Discharge	43	100%	99%	98%
Heart Failure Care				
ACE Inhibitor or ARB for LVSD	39	100%	97%	97%
Discharge Instructions Given	72	100%	93%	94%

NOTE: Hospital profiles are in alphabetical order by state, then city, then hospital within the city; Rankings exclude hospitals with less than 25 cases except for patient surveys which excludes hospitals with less than 100 cases; (a) 100-299 cases; (1) The number of cases/patients is too few to report; (2) Data submitted were based on a sample of cases/patients; (3) Results are based on a shorter time period than required; (4) Data suppressed by CMS for one or more quarters; (5) Results are not available for this reporting period; (6) Fewer than 100 patients completed the HCAHPS survey; (7) No cases met the criteria for this measure; (8) The lower limit of the confidence interval cannot be calculated if the number of observed infections equals zero; (9) No data are available from the state/territory for this reporting period; (10) The scores shown reflect fewer than 50 completed surveys; (11) There were discrepancies in the data collection process; (12) This measure does not apply to this hospital for this reporting period; (13) Results cannot be calculated for this reporting period; (14) The results for this state are combined with nearby states to protect confidentiality; Please refer to the User's Guide for a full explanation of data.

Measure	Cases	This Hosp.	State Avg.	U.S. Avg.
Evaluation of LVS Function	85	100%	99%	99%
Medicare Spending				
Medicare Spending per Patient (ratio)	-	0.97	1	0.98
Pneumonia Care				
Appropriate Initial Antibiotic Given[2]	137	99%	95%	95%
Blood Culture Timing[2]	297	100%	98%	98%
Pregnancy and Delivery Care				
Newborn Deliveries Scheduled Early	59	0%	6%	6%
Preventive Care				
Immunization for Influenza[2]	336	98%	93%	90%
Immunization for Pneumonia[2]	422	100%	93%	92%
Stroke Care				
Anticoagulation Therapy for Atrial Fibrillation[1]	-	-	94%	95%
Antithrombotic Therapy Timing	13	100%	97%	98%
Assessed for Rehabilitation	19	100%	97%	97%
Discharged on Antithrombotic Therapy	19	100%	99%	99%
Discharged on Statin Medication	11	100%	94%	94%
Thrombolytic Therapy Timing[7]	-	-	57%	66%
Venous Thromboembolism Prophylaxis	14	93%	93%	94%
Written Stroke Educational Materials Given[1]	-	-	84%	88%
Surgical Care Improvement Project				
Appropriate Beta Blocker Usage[2]	63	100%	97%	98%
Appropriate VTP Within 24 Hours[2]	206	100%	98%	98%
Controlled Postoperative Blood Glucose[2,7]	-	-	95%	97%
Perioperative Temperature Management[2]	214	100%	100%	100%
Prophylactic Antibiotic Selection[2]	148	100%	99%	99%
Prophylactic Antibiotic Selection (Outpatient)	102	97%	98%	98%
Prophylactic Antibiotic Stopped[2]	145	100%	98%	98%
Prophylactic Antibiotic Timing[2]	148	100%	99%	99%
Prophylactic Antibiotic Timing (Outpatient)	101	98%	98%	98%
Urinary Catheter Removal[2]	184	100%	96%	97%
Survey of Patients' Hospital Experiences				
Area Around Room 'Always' Quiet at Night	300+	51%	67%	61%
Doctors 'Always' Communicated Well	300+	80%	84%	82%
Home Recovery Information Given	300+	84%	85%	85%
Hospital Given 9 or 10 on 10 Point Scale	300+	67%	70%	71%
Meds 'Always' Explained Before Given	300+	63%	66%	64%
Nurses 'Always' Communicated Well	300+	79%	80%	79%
Pain 'Always' Well Controlled	300+	71%	72%	71%
Room and Bathroom 'Always' Clean	300+	76%	73%	73%
Timely Help 'Always' Received	300+	66%	68%	68%
Would Definitely Recommend Hospital	300+	65%	70%	71%
Use of Medical Imaging				
Cardiac Imaging Stress Test before Surgery	170	5.9%	4.8%	5.3%
Combination Abdominal CT Scan	713	7.2%	9.6%	10.5%
Combination Brain/Sinus CT Scan	714	5.0%	3.3%	2.7%
Combination Chest CT Scan	367	10.1%	3.4%	2.7%
Follow-up Mammogram/Ultrasound	772	10.0%	8.3%	8.8%
Lumbar Spine MRI for Low Back Pain[1]	-	-	35.3%	37.2%

Sweetwater Hospital Association

304 Wright St
Sweetwater, TN 37874
Phone: 865-213-8200
URL: www.sweetwaterhospital.org
Type: Acute Care Hospitals
Emergency Services: Yes
Ownership: Voluntary non-profit - Private
Beds: 59

Key Personnel:
CEO/President. . . . . Scott Bowman
Radiology. . . . . Bob Wilkins

Measure	Cases	This Hosp.	State Avg.	U.S. Avg.
Blood Clot Prevention and Treatment				
Anticoagulation Overlap Therapy[2]	11	73%	92%	93%
ICU Venous Thromboembolism Prophylaxis[2]	46	96%	90%	92%
Incidence of Potentially Preventable VTE[2,7]	-	-	10%	10%
UFH with Dosages/Platelet Monitoring[1,2]	-	-	99%	97%
Venous Thromboembolism Prophylaxis[2]	180	88%	83%	85%
Warfarin Therapy Discharge Instructions[1,2]	-	-	78%	75%
Chest Pain/Possible Heart Attack Care				
Aspirin Given Within 24 Hours of Arrival	70	91%	96%	96%
Fibrinolytic Meds Within 30 Min. of Arrival[7]	-	-	72%	58%
Average Time to ECG (minutes)	70	13	6	7
Average Time to Transfer (minutes)[1]	-	-	53	60
Children's Asthma Care				
Received Home Management Plan of Care	-	-	-	88%
Received Reliever Medication	-	-	-	100%
Received Systemic Corticosteroids	-	-	-	100%
Emergency Department				
Admittance Decision Time (minutes)[2]	335	69	82	98
Head CT Results Within 45 Min. of Arrival[1]	-	-	52%	57%
Patients Who Left ER Before Being Seen	24,711	2%	2%	2%
Time from ER Arrival to Admit. (minutes)[2]	337	275	243	274
Time from ER Arrival to Discharge (minutes)	1,433	132	131	134
Time in ER Before Being Evaluated (minutes)	1,567	32	25	26
Time to Pain Meds for Fractures (minutes)	64	68	60	57
Heart Attack Care				
Aspirin Given at Discharge[1]	-	-	99%	99%
Fibrinolytic Meds Within 30 Min. of Arrival[7]	-	-	33%	54%
PCI Within 90 Minutes of Arrival[7]	-	-	98%	96%
Statin Prescribed at Discharge[1]	-	-	99%	98%
Heart Failure Care				
ACE Inhibitor or ARB for LVSD	21	95%	97%	97%
Discharge Instructions Given	60	72%	93%	94%
Evaluation of LVS Function	72	92%	99%	99%
Medicare Spending				
Medicare Spending per Patient (ratio)	-	1.00	1	0.98
Pneumonia Care				
Appropriate Initial Antibiotic Given	127	95%	95%	95%
Blood Culture Timing	207	99%	98%	98%
Pregnancy and Delivery Care				
Newborn Deliveries Scheduled Early	16	0%	6%	6%
Preventive Care				
Immunization for Influenza[2]	302	91%	93%	90%
Immunization for Pneumonia[2]	425	94%	93%	92%
Stroke Care				
Anticoagulation Therapy for Atrial Fibrillation[1]	-	-	94%	95%
Antithrombotic Therapy Timing	16	88%	97%	98%
Assessed for Rehabilitation	19	74%	97%	97%
Discharged on Antithrombotic Therapy	19	84%	99%	99%
Discharged on Statin Medication	19	68%	94%	94%
Thrombolytic Therapy Timing[1]	-	-	57%	66%
Venous Thromboembolism Prophylaxis	18	61%	93%	94%
Written Stroke Educational Materials Given	13	54%	84%	88%
Surgical Care Improvement Project				
Appropriate Beta Blocker Usage	16	44%	97%	98%
Appropriate VTP Within 24 Hours	59	81%	98%	98%
Controlled Postoperative Blood Glucose[7]	-	-	95%	97%
Perioperative Temperature Management	70	100%	100%	100%
Prophylactic Antibiotic Selection	28	89%	99%	99%
Prophylactic Antibiotic Selection (Outpatient)	19	100%	98%	98%
Prophylactic Antibiotic Stopped	24	92%	98%	98%
Prophylactic Antibiotic Timing	28	82%	99%	99%
Prophylactic Antibiotic Timing (Outpatient)	19	89%	98%	98%
Urinary Catheter Removal	18	94%	96%	97%
Survey of Patients' Hospital Experiences				
Area Around Room 'Always' Quiet at Night	300+	69%	67%	61%
Doctors 'Always' Communicated Well	300+	88%	84%	82%
Home Recovery Information Given	300+	84%	85%	85%
Hospital Given 9 or 10 on 10 Point Scale	300+	73%	70%	71%
Meds 'Always' Explained Before Given	300+	72%	66%	64%
Nurses 'Always' Communicated Well	300+	81%	80%	79%
Pain 'Always' Well Controlled	300+	73%	72%	71%
Room and Bathroom 'Always' Clean	300+	79%	73%	73%
Timely Help 'Always' Received	300+	72%	68%	68%
Would Definitely Recommend Hospital	300+	71%	70%	71%
Use of Medical Imaging				
Cardiac Imaging Stress Test before Surgery[1]	-	-	4.8%	5.3%
Combination Abdominal CT Scan	375	8.3%	9.6%	10.5%
Combination Brain/Sinus CT Scan	413	1.9%	3.3%	2.7%
Combination Chest CT Scan	204	4.9%	3.4%	2.7%
Follow-up Mammogram/Ultrasound	225	8.0%	8.3%	8.8%
Lumbar Spine MRI for Low Back Pain	48	41.7%	35.3%	37.2%

Claiborne County Hospital

1850 Old Knoxville Highway
Tazewell, TN 37879
Phone: 423-626-4211
Fax: 423-626-9926
URL: www.claibornehospital.org
Type: Acute Care Hospitals
Emergency Services: Yes
Ownership: Government - Local
Beds: 85

Key Personnel:
Intensive Care Unit. . . . . Jackie Carpenter
Chief of Medical Staff . . . . Richard Clark
CEO/President. . . . . Michael Hutchins
Infection Control. . . . . Mary Moore, RN
Emergency Room . . . . Tim Runions
Operating Room. . . . . Nancy Steadman
Quality Assurance . . . . Linda Vanlandingham

Measure	Cases	This Hosp.	State Avg.	U.S. Avg.
Blood Clot Prevention and Treatment				
Anticoagulation Overlap Therapy[1,2]	-	-	92%	93%
ICU Venous Thromboembolism Prophylaxis[2]	100	88%	90%	92%
Incidence of Potentially Preventable VTE[1,2]	-	-	10%	10%
UFH with Dosages/Platelet Monitoring[1,2]	-	-	99%	97%
Venous Thromboembolism Prophylaxis[2]	254	77%	83%	85%
Warfarin Therapy Discharge Instructions[1,2]	-	-	78%	75%
Chest Pain/Possible Heart Attack Care				
Aspirin Given Within 24 Hours of Arrival	72	89%	96%	96%
Fibrinolytic Meds Within 30 Min. of Arrival[7]	-	-	72%	58%
Average Time to ECG (minutes)	77	8	6	7
Average Time to Transfer (minutes)	18	69	53	60
Children's Asthma Care				
Received Home Management Plan of Care	-	-	-	88%
Received Reliever Medication	-	-	-	100%
Received Systemic Corticosteroids	-	-	-	100%
Emergency Department				
Admittance Decision Time (minutes)[2]	484	95	82	98
Head CT Results Within 45 Min. of Arrival[1]	-	-	52%	57%
Patients Who Left ER Before Being Seen	14,697	2%	2%	2%
Time from ER Arrival to Admit. (minutes)[2]	502	242	243	274
Time from ER Arrival to Discharge (minutes)	364	120	131	134
Time in ER Before Being Evaluated (minutes)	365	21	25	26
Time to Pain Meds for Fractures (minutes)	71	50	60	57
Heart Attack Care				
Aspirin Given at Discharge[1,2]	-	-	99%	99%
Fibrinolytic Meds Within 30 Min. of Arrival[2,3]	-	-	33%	54%
PCI Within 90 Minutes of Arrival[2,3]	-	-	98%	96%
Statin Prescribed at Discharge[1,2]	-	-	99%	98%
Heart Failure Care				
ACE Inhibitor or ARB for LVSD[1,2]	-	-	97%	97%
Discharge Instructions Given[2]	39	77%	93%	94%
Evaluation of LVS Function[2]	57	95%	99%	99%
Medicare Spending				
Medicare Spending per Patient (ratio)	-	0.97	1	0.98
Pneumonia Care				
Appropriate Initial Antibiotic Given[2]	47	85%	95%	95%
Blood Culture Timing[2]	132	99%	98%	98%
Pregnancy and Delivery Care				
Newborn Deliveries Scheduled Early[2,7]	-	-	6%	6%
Preventive Care				
Immunization for Influenza[2]	283	81%	93%	90%
Immunization for Pneumonia[2]	425	85%	93%	92%
Stroke Care				
Anticoagulation Therapy for Atrial Fibrillation[1,2]	-	-	94%	95%
Antithrombotic Therapy Timing[2]	15	80%	97%	98%
Assessed for Rehabilitation[2]	19	100%	97%	97%
Discharged on Antithrombotic Therapy[2]	19	84%	99%	99%
Discharged on Statin Medication[2]	17	35%	94%	94%
Thrombolytic Therapy Timing[2,7]	-	-	57%	66%
Venous Thromboembolism Prophylaxis[2]	15	60%	93%	94%
Written Stroke Educational Materials Given[2]	13	46%	84%	88%
Surgical Care Improvement Project				
Appropriate Beta Blocker Usage[2]	12	100%	97%	98%
Appropriate VTP Within 24 Hours[2]	41	78%	98%	98%
Controlled Postoperative Blood Glucose[2,7]	-	-	95%	97%
Perioperative Temperature Management[2]	48	100%	100%	100%
Prophylactic Antibiotic Selection[1,2]	-	-	99%	99%
Prophylactic Antibiotic Selection (Outpatient)	19	95%	98%	98%

NOTE: Hospital profiles are in alphabetical order by state, then city, then hospital within the city; Rankings exclude hospitals with less than 25 cases except for patient surveys which excludes hospitals with less than 100 cases; (a) 100-299 cases; (1) The number of cases/patients is too few to report; (2) Data submitted were based on a sample of cases/patients; (3) Results are based on a shorter time period than required; (4) Data suppressed by CMS for one or more quarters; (5) Results are not available for this reporting period; (6) Fewer than 100 patients completed the HCAHPS survey; (7) No cases met the criteria for this measure; (8) The lower limit of the confidence interval cannot be calculated if the number of observed infections equals zero; (9) No data are available from the state/territory for this reporting period; (10) The scores shown reflect fewer than 50 completed surveys; (11) There were discrepancies in the data collection process; (12) This measure does not apply to this hospital for this reporting period; (13) Results cannot be calculated for this reporting period; (14) The results for this state are combined with nearby states to protect confidentiality; Please refer to the User's Guide for a full explanation of data.

Measure	Cases	This Hosp.	State Avg.	U.S. Avg.
Prophylactic Antibiotic Stopped[1,2]	-	-	98%	98%
Prophylactic Antibiotic Timing[1,2]	-	-	99%	99%
Prophylactic Antibiotic Timing (Outpatient)	20	95%	98%	98%
Urinary Catheter Removal[2]	23	48%	96%	97%
Survey of Patients' Hospital Experiences				
Area Around Room 'Always' Quiet at Night	(a)	58%	67%	61%
Doctors 'Always' Communicated Well	(a)	84%	84%	82%
Home Recovery Information Given	(a)	84%	85%	85%
Hospital Given 9 or 10 on 10 Point Scale	(a)	57%	70%	71%
Meds 'Always' Explained Before Given	(a)	58%	66%	64%
Nurses 'Always' Communicated Well	(a)	71%	80%	79%
Pain 'Always' Well Controlled	(a)	65%	72%	71%
Room and Bathroom 'Always' Clean	(a)	63%	73%	73%
Timely Help 'Always' Received	(a)	61%	68%	68%
Would Definitely Recommend Hospital	(a)	55%	70%	71%
Use of Medical Imaging				
Cardiac Imaging Stress Test before Surgery[1]	-	-	4.8%	5.3%
Combination Abdominal CT Scan	424	3.3%	9.6%	10.5%
Combination Brain/Sinus CT Scan[1]	-	-	3.3%	2.7%
Combination Chest CT Scan	247	1.2%	3.4%	2.7%
Follow-up Mammogram/Ultrasound	283	10.2%	8.3%	8.8%
Lumbar Spine MRI for Low Back Pain	92	41.3%	35.3%	37.2%

Gibson General Hospital

200 Hospital Dr
Trenton, TN 38382
Phone: 731-855-7900
Fax: 731-855-7570
URL: www.wth.net
Type: Acute Care Hospitals
Emergency Services: Yes
Ownership: Voluntary non-profit - Other
Beds: 100

Key Personnel:
Chief of Medical Staff.......... Ezekiel O Adetunji
Radiology.................... Gregory C Bruno
CEO/President............... Sherry Scruggs

Measure	Cases	This Hosp.	State Avg.	U.S. Avg.
Blood Clot Prevention and Treatment				
Anticoagulation Overlap Therapy	-	-	92%	93%
ICU Venous Thromboembolism Prophylaxis	-	-	90%	92%
Incidence of Potentially Preventable VTE	-	-	10%	10%
UFH with Dosages/Platelet Monitoring	-	-	99%	97%
Venous Thromboembolism Prophylaxis	-	-	83%	85%
Warfarin Therapy Discharge Instructions	-	-	78%	75%
Chest Pain/Possible Heart Attack Care				
Aspirin Given Within 24 Hours of Arrival[3]	42	98%	96%	96%
Fibrinolytic Meds Within 30 Min. of Arrival[1,3]	-	-	72%	58%
Average Time to ECG (minutes)[3]	43	4	6	7
Average Time to Transfer (minutes)[3,7]	-	-	53	60
Children's Asthma Care				
Received Home Management Plan of Care	-	-	-	88%
Received Reliever Medication	-	-	-	100%
Received Systemic Corticosteroids	-	-	-	100%
Emergency Department				
Admittance Decision Time (minutes)	-	-	82	98
Head CT Results Within 45 Min. of Arrival[1,3]	-	-	52%	57%
Patients Who Left ER Before Being Seen	7,355	1%	2%	2%
Time from ER Arrival to Admit. (minutes)	-	-	243	274
Time from ER Arrival to Discharge (minutes)[3]	275	115	131	134
Time in ER Before Being Evaluated (minutes)[3]	293	29	25	26
Time to Pain Meds for Fractures (minutes)[3]	22	100	60	57
Heart Attack Care				
Aspirin Given at Discharge	-	-	99%	99%
Fibrinolytic Meds Within 30 Min. of Arrival	-	-	33%	54%
PCI Within 90 Minutes of Arrival	-	-	98%	96%
Statin Prescribed at Discharge	-	-	99%	98%
Heart Failure Care				
ACE Inhibitor or ARB for LVSD	-	-	97%	97%
Discharge Instructions Given	-	-	93%	94%
Evaluation of LVS Function	-	-	99%	99%
Medicare Spending				
Medicare Spending per Patient (ratio)	-	-	1	0.98
Pneumonia Care				
Appropriate Initial Antibiotic Given	-	-	95%	95%
Blood Culture Timing	-	-	98%	98%
Pregnancy and Delivery Care				
Newborn Deliveries Scheduled Early	-	-	6%	6%
Preventive Care				
Immunization for Influenza	-	-	93%	90%
Immunization for Pneumonia	-	-	93%	92%
Stroke Care				
Anticoagulation Therapy for Atrial Fibrillation	-	-	94%	95%
Antithrombotic Therapy Timing	-	-	97%	98%
Assessed for Rehabilitation	-	-	97%	97%
Discharged on Antithrombotic Therapy	-	-	99%	99%
Discharged on Statin Medication	-	-	94%	94%
Thrombolytic Therapy Timing	-	-	57%	66%
Venous Thromboembolism Prophylaxis	-	-	93%	94%
Written Stroke Educational Materials Given	-	-	84%	88%
Surgical Care Improvement Project				
Appropriate Beta Blocker Usage	-	-	97%	98%
Appropriate VTP Within 24 Hours	-	-	98%	98%
Controlled Postoperative Blood Glucose	-	-	95%	97%
Perioperative Temperature Management	-	-	100%	100%
Prophylactic Antibiotic Selection	-	-	99%	99%
Prophylactic Antibiotic Selection (Outpatient)[3,7]	-	-	98%	98%
Prophylactic Antibiotic Stopped	-	-	98%	98%
Prophylactic Antibiotic Timing	-	-	99%	99%
Prophylactic Antibiotic Timing (Outpatient)[3,7]	-	-	98%	98%
Urinary Catheter Removal	-	-	96%	97%
Survey of Patients' Hospital Experiences				
Area Around Room 'Always' Quiet at Night	-	-	67%	61%
Doctors 'Always' Communicated Well	-	-	84%	82%
Home Recovery Information Given	-	-	85%	85%
Hospital Given 9 or 10 on 10 Point Scale	-	-	70%	71%
Meds 'Always' Explained Before Given	-	-	66%	64%
Nurses 'Always' Communicated Well	-	-	80%	79%
Pain 'Always' Well Controlled	-	-	72%	71%
Room and Bathroom 'Always' Clean	-	-	73%	73%
Timely Help 'Always' Received	-	-	68%	68%
Would Definitely Recommend Hospital	-	-	70%	71%
Use of Medical Imaging				
Cardiac Imaging Stress Test before Surgery[7]	-	-	4.8%	5.3%
Combination Abdominal CT Scan	84	0.0%	9.6%	10.5%
Combination Brain/Sinus CT Scan[1]	-	-	3.3%	2.7%
Combination Chest CT Scan[1]	-	-	3.4%	2.7%
Follow-up Mammogram/Ultrasound[7]	-	-	8.3%	8.8%
Lumbar Spine MRI for Low Back Pain[7]	-	-	35.3%	37.2%

Harton Regional Medical Center

1801 N Jackson Saint Box 460
Tullahoma, TN 37388
Phone: 931-393-3000
Fax: 931-455-4220
URL: www.hartonmedicalcenter.com
Type: Acute Care Hospitals
Emergency Services: Yes
Ownership: Voluntary non-profit - Other
Beds: 137

Key Personnel:
Radiology.................. Joel S Birdwell
Operating Room.............. Mark Blair
CEO/President............... Dwayne Blaylock
Chief of Medical Staff.......... J Denny Crabtree, MD
Quality Assurance............ Cindy Nadeau
CEO....................... Russ Spray

Measure	Cases	This Hosp.	State Avg.	U.S. Avg.
Blood Clot Prevention and Treatment				
Anticoagulation Overlap Therapy[2]	21	100%	92%	93%
ICU Venous Thromboembolism Prophylaxis[2]	57	89%	90%	92%
Incidence of Potentially Preventable VTE[2]	11	18%	10%	10%
UFH with Dosages/Platelet Monitoring[1,2]	-	-	99%	97%
Venous Thromboembolism Prophylaxis[2]	392	60%	83%	85%
Warfarin Therapy Discharge Instructions[2]	17	94%	78%	75%
Chest Pain/Possible Heart Attack Care				
Aspirin Given Within 24 Hours of Arrival	54	98%	96%	96%
Fibrinolytic Meds Within 30 Min. of Arrival[1]	-	-	72%	58%
Average Time to ECG (minutes)	56	3	6	7
Average Time to Transfer (minutes)[1]	-	-	53	60
Children's Asthma Care				
Received Home Management Plan of Care	-	-	-	88%
Received Reliever Medication	-	-	-	100%
Received Systemic Corticosteroids	-	-	-	100%
Emergency Department				
Admittance Decision Time (minutes)[2]	459	71	82	98
Head CT Results Within 45 Min. of Arrival[1]	-	-	52%	57%
Patients Who Left ER Before Being Seen	27,618	2%	2%	2%
Time from ER Arrival to Admit. (minutes)[2]	459	201	243	274
Time from ER Arrival to Discharge (minutes)	422	111	131	134
Time in ER Before Being Evaluated (minutes)	461	27	25	26
Time to Pain Meds for Fractures (minutes)	96	44	60	57
Heart Attack Care				
Aspirin Given at Discharge	56	96%	99%	99%
Fibrinolytic Meds Within 30 Min. of Arrival[1]	-	-	33%	54%
PCI Within 90 Minutes of Arrival	11	100%	98%	96%
Statin Prescribed at Discharge	56	98%	99%	98%
Heart Failure Care				
ACE Inhibitor or ARB for LVSD	43	100%	97%	97%
Discharge Instructions Given	100	93%	93%	94%
Evaluation of LVS Function	122	100%	99%	99%
Medicare Spending				
Medicare Spending per Patient (ratio)	-	1.01	1	0.98
Pneumonia Care				
Appropriate Initial Antibiotic Given	114	98%	95%	95%
Blood Culture Timing	148	99%	98%	98%
Pregnancy and Delivery Care				
Newborn Deliveries Scheduled Early[2]	46	7%	6%	6%
Preventive Care				
Immunization for Influenza[2]	497	97%	93%	90%
Immunization for Pneumonia[2]	582	98%	93%	92%
Stroke Care				
Anticoagulation Therapy for Atrial Fibrillation[1]	-	-	94%	95%
Antithrombotic Therapy Timing	39	92%	97%	98%
Assessed for Rehabilitation	34	88%	97%	97%
Discharged on Antithrombotic Therapy	33	94%	99%	99%
Discharged on Statin Medication	24	83%	94%	94%
Thrombolytic Therapy Timing[1]	-	-	57%	66%
Venous Thromboembolism Prophylaxis	41	90%	93%	94%
Written Stroke Educational Materials Given	27	96%	84%	88%
Surgical Care Improvement Project				
Appropriate Beta Blocker Usage	64	91%	97%	98%
Appropriate VTP Within 24 Hours	184	97%	98%	98%
Controlled Postoperative Blood Glucose[7]	-	-	95%	97%
Perioperative Temperature Management	231	100%	100%	100%
Prophylactic Antibiotic Selection	161	95%	99%	99%
Prophylactic Antibiotic Selection (Outpatient)	289	99%	98%	98%
Prophylactic Antibiotic Stopped	134	97%	98%	98%
Prophylactic Antibiotic Timing	161	99%	99%	99%
Prophylactic Antibiotic Timing (Outpatient)	292	99%	98%	98%
Urinary Catheter Removal	115	99%	96%	97%
Survey of Patients' Hospital Experiences				
Area Around Room 'Always' Quiet at Night	300+	58%	67%	61%
Doctors 'Always' Communicated Well	300+	79%	84%	82%
Home Recovery Information Given	300+	80%	85%	85%
Hospital Given 9 or 10 on 10 Point Scale	300+	56%	70%	71%
Meds 'Always' Explained Before Given	300+	55%	66%	64%
Nurses 'Always' Communicated Well	300+	72%	80%	79%
Pain 'Always' Well Controlled	300+	61%	72%	71%
Room and Bathroom 'Always' Clean	300+	68%	73%	73%
Timely Help 'Always' Received	300+	55%	68%	68%
Would Definitely Recommend Hospital	300+	55%	70%	71%
Use of Medical Imaging				
Cardiac Imaging Stress Test before Surgery	212	4.7%	4.8%	5.3%
Combination Abdominal CT Scan	484	14.7%	9.6%	10.5%
Combination Brain/Sinus CT Scan[1]	-	-	3.3%	2.7%
Combination Chest CT Scan	257	8.9%	3.4%	2.7%
Follow-up Mammogram/Ultrasound	1,080	18.9%	8.3%	8.8%
Lumbar Spine MRI for Low Back Pain	130	33.1%	35.3%	37.2%

Baptist Memorial Hospital Union City

1201 Bishop St, PO Box 310
Union City, TN 38261
Phone: 731-885-2410
Fax: 731-884-8603
E-mail: info.unioncity@bmhcc.org
URL: www.bmhcc.org
Type: Acute Care Hospitals
Emergency Services: Yes
Ownership: Voluntary non-profit - Private
Beds: 173

Key Personnel:
Administrator................ Barry Bondurant

NOTE: Hospital profiles are in alphabetical order by state, then city, then hospital within the city; Rankings exclude hospitals with less than 25 cases except for patient surveys which excludes hospitals with less than 100 cases; (a) 100-299 cases; (1) The number of cases/patients is too few to report; (2) Data submitted were based on a sample of cases/patients; (3) Results are based on a shorter time period than required; (4) Data suppressed by CMS for one or more quarters; (5) Results are not available for this reporting period; (6) Fewer than 100 patients completed the HCAHPS survey; (7) No cases met the criteria for this measure; (8) The lower limit of the confidence interval cannot be calculated if the number of observed infections equals zero; (9) No data are available from the state/territory for this reporting period; (10) The scores shown reflect fewer than 50 completed surveys; (11) There were discrepancies in the data collection process; (12) This measure does not apply to this hospital for this reporting period; (13) Results cannot be calculated for this reporting period; (14) The results for this state are combined with nearby states to protect confidentiality; Please refer to the User's Guide for a full explanation of data.

Cardiac Laboratory. . . . . James Hall, MD
CEO/President. . . . . Jason Little
Chief of Medical Staff. . . . . David StClair, MD

Measure	Cases	This Hosp.	State Avg.	U.S. Avg.
Blood Clot Prevention and Treatment				
Anticoagulation Overlap Therapy[2]	20	100%	92%	93%
ICU Venous Thromboembolism Prophylaxis[2]	49	98%	90%	92%
Incidence of Potentially Preventable VTE[1,2]	-	-	10%	10%
UFH with Dosages/Platelet Monitoring[2]	16	100%	99%	97%
Venous Thromboembolism Prophylaxis[2]	204	92%	83%	85%
Warfarin Therapy Discharge Instructions[2]	16	100%	78%	75%
Chest Pain/Possible Heart Attack Care				
Aspirin Given Within 24 Hours of Arrival	177	100%	96%	96%
Fibrinolytic Meds Within 30 Min. of Arrival	14	100%	72%	58%
Average Time to ECG (minutes)	192	5	6	7
Average Time to Transfer (minutes)[1]	-	-	53	60
Children's Asthma Care				
Received Home Management Plan of Care	-	-	-	88%
Received Reliever Medication	-	-	-	100%
Received Systemic Corticosteroids	-	-	-	100%
Emergency Department				
Admittance Decision Time (minutes)[2]	244	69	82	98
Head CT Results Within 45 Min. of Arrival[1]	-	-	52%	57%
Patients Who Left ER Before Being Seen	18,843	1%	2%	2%
Time from ER Arrival to Admit. (minutes)[2]	252	226	243	274
Time from ER Arrival to Discharge (minutes)	341	116	131	134
Time in ER Before Being Evaluated (minutes)	378	28	25	26
Time to Pain Meds for Fractures (minutes)	76	72	60	57
Heart Attack Care				
Aspirin Given at Discharge[1]	-	-	99%	99%
Fibrinolytic Meds Within 30 Min. of Arrival[1]	-	-	33%	54%
PCI Within 90 Minutes of Arrival[7]	-	-	98%	96%
Statin Prescribed at Discharge[1]	-	-	99%	98%
Heart Failure Care				
ACE Inhibitor or ARB for LVSD	25	100%	97%	97%
Discharge Instructions Given	64	94%	93%	94%
Evaluation of LVS Function	90	100%	99%	99%
Medicare Spending				
Medicare Spending per Patient (ratio)	-	1.08	1	0.98
Pneumonia Care				
Appropriate Initial Antibiotic Given	38	100%	95%	95%
Blood Culture Timing	76	100%	98%	98%
Pregnancy and Delivery Care				
Newborn Deliveries Scheduled Early[2]	28	7%	6%	6%
Preventive Care				
Immunization for Influenza[2]	274	97%	93%	90%
Immunization for Pneumonia[2]	357	97%	93%	92%
Stroke Care				
Anticoagulation Therapy for Atrial Fibrillation[7]	-	-	94%	95%
Antithrombotic Therapy Timing	29	100%	97%	98%
Assessed for Rehabilitation	28	96%	97%	97%
Discharged on Antithrombotic Therapy	27	100%	99%	99%
Discharged on Statin Medication	24	100%	94%	94%
Thrombolytic Therapy Timing[7]	-	-	57%	66%
Venous Thromboembolism Prophylaxis	30	100%	93%	94%
Written Stroke Educational Materials Given	11	73%	84%	88%
Surgical Care Improvement Project				
Appropriate Beta Blocker Usage	35	100%	97%	98%
Appropriate VTP Within 24 Hours	132	100%	98%	98%
Controlled Postoperative Blood Glucose[7]	-	-	95%	97%
Perioperative Temperature Management	143	100%	100%	100%
Prophylactic Antibiotic Selection	108	100%	99%	99%
Prophylactic Antibiotic Selection (Outpatient)	62	98%	98%	98%
Prophylactic Antibiotic Stopped	102	100%	98%	98%
Prophylactic Antibiotic Timing	108	100%	99%	99%
Prophylactic Antibiotic Timing (Outpatient)	62	100%	98%	98%
Urinary Catheter Removal	70	100%	96%	97%
Survey of Patients' Hospital Experiences				
Area Around Room 'Always' Quiet at Night	300+	69%	67%	61%
Doctors 'Always' Communicated Well	300+	86%	84%	82%
Home Recovery Information Given	300+	89%	85%	85%
Hospital Given 9 or 10 on 10 Point Scale	300+	77%	70%	71%
Meds 'Always' Explained Before Given	300+	69%	66%	64%
Nurses 'Always' Communicated Well	300+	85%	80%	79%
Pain 'Always' Well Controlled	300+	76%	72%	71%
Room and Bathroom 'Always' Clean	300+	84%	73%	73%
Timely Help 'Always' Received	300+	80%	68%	68%
Would Definitely Recommend Hospital	300+	70%	70%	71%
Use of Medical Imaging				
Cardiac Imaging Stress Test before Surgery	121	5.0%	4.8%	5.3%
Combination Abdominal CT Scan	525	3.8%	9.6%	10.5%
Combination Brain/Sinus CT Scan	490	1.6%	3.3%	2.7%
Combination Chest CT Scan	307	0.3%	3.4%	2.7%
Follow-up Mammogram/Ultrasound	441	7.0%	8.3%	8.8%
Lumbar Spine MRI for Low Back Pain	115	42.6%	35.3%	37.2%

Wayne Medical Center

103 J V Mangubat Dr
Waynesboro, TN 38485
Type: Acute Care Hospitals
Ownership: Voluntary non-profit - Other
Phone: 931-722-5411
Fax: 931-722-7170
Emergency Services: Yes
Beds: 80

Key Personnel:
Cardiac Laboratory. . . . . Dr Jaques Heibig
Operating Room. . . . . Tammy Howell, RN
Radiology. . . . . Hubert Langley, MD
Chief of Medical Staff. . . . . Dr David Magas
Infection Control. . . . . Dr John Olson
Quality Assurance . . . . Paula Petty, RN
CEO/President. . . . . Mike Sears

Measure	Cases	This Hosp.	State Avg.	U.S. Avg.
Blood Clot Prevention and Treatment				
Anticoagulation Overlap Therapy[1]	-	-	92%	93%
ICU Venous Thromboembolism Prophylaxis[7]	-	-	90%	92%
Incidence of Potentially Preventable VTE[1]	-	-	10%	10%
UFH with Dosages/Platelet Monitoring[7]	-	-	99%	97%
Venous Thromboembolism Prophylaxis	281	83%	83%	85%
Warfarin Therapy Discharge Instructions[1]	-	-	78%	75%
Chest Pain/Possible Heart Attack Care				
Aspirin Given Within 24 Hours of Arrival	38	82%	96%	96%
Fibrinolytic Meds Within 30 Min. of Arrival[7]	-	-	72%	58%
Average Time to ECG (minutes)	39	10	6	7
Average Time to Transfer (minutes)[1]	-	-	53	60
Children's Asthma Care				
Received Home Management Plan of Care	-	-	-	88%
Received Reliever Medication	-	-	-	100%
Received Systemic Corticosteroids	-	-	-	100%
Emergency Department				
Admittance Decision Time (minutes)	194	70	82	98
Head CT Results Within 45 Min. of Arrival[1]	-	-	52%	57%
Patients Who Left ER Before Being Seen	3,911	2%	2%	2%
Time from ER Arrival to Admit. (minutes)	344	227	243	274
Time from ER Arrival to Discharge (minutes)	1,276	136	131	134
Time in ER Before Being Evaluated (minutes)	1,568	24	25	26
Time to Pain Meds for Fractures (minutes)	26	50	60	57
Heart Attack Care				
Aspirin Given at Discharge[3,7]	-	-	99%	99%
Fibrinolytic Meds Within 30 Min. of Arrival[3,7]	-	-	33%	54%
PCI Within 90 Minutes of Arrival[3,7]	-	-	98%	96%
Statin Prescribed at Discharge[3,7]	-	-	99%	98%
Heart Failure Care				
ACE Inhibitor or ARB for LVSD[1]	-	-	97%	97%
Discharge Instructions Given	17	82%	93%	94%
Evaluation of LVS Function	27	81%	99%	99%
Medicare Spending				
Medicare Spending per Patient (ratio)	-	0.73	1	0.98
Pneumonia Care				
Appropriate Initial Antibiotic Given	43	79%	95%	95%
Blood Culture Timing	45	96%	98%	98%
Pregnancy and Delivery Care				
Newborn Deliveries Scheduled Early[7]	-	-	6%	6%
Preventive Care				
Immunization for Influenza	272	91%	93%	90%
Immunization for Pneumonia	410	94%	93%	92%
Stroke Care				
Anticoagulation Therapy for Atrial Fibrillation[3,7]	-	-	94%	95%
Antithrombotic Therapy Timing[1,3]	-	-	97%	98%
Assessed for Rehabilitation[1,3]	-	-	97%	97%
Discharged on Antithrombotic Therapy[1,3]	-	-	99%	99%
Discharged on Statin Medication[1,3]	-	-	94%	94%
Thrombolytic Therapy Timing[1,3]	-	-	57%	66%
Venous Thromboembolism Prophylaxis[3,7]	-	-	93%	94%
Written Stroke Educational Materials Given[1,3]	-	-	84%	88%
Surgical Care Improvement Project				
Appropriate Beta Blocker Usage[5]	-	-	97%	98%
Appropriate VTP Within 24 Hours[5]	-	-	98%	98%
Controlled Postoperative Blood Glucose[5]	-	-	95%	97%
Perioperative Temperature Management[5]	-	-	100%	100%
Prophylactic Antibiotic Selection[5]	-	-	99%	99%
Prophylactic Antibiotic Selection (Outpatient)[5]	-	-	98%	98%
Prophylactic Antibiotic Stopped[5]	-	-	98%	98%
Prophylactic Antibiotic Timing[5]	-	-	99%	99%
Prophylactic Antibiotic Timing (Outpatient)[5]	-	-	98%	98%
Urinary Catheter Removal[5]	-	-	96%	97%
Survey of Patients' Hospital Experiences				
Area Around Room 'Always' Quiet at Night	(a)	63%	67%	61%
Doctors 'Always' Communicated Well	(a)	87%	84%	82%
Home Recovery Information Given	(a)	84%	85%	85%
Hospital Given 9 or 10 on 10 Point Scale	(a)	68%	70%	71%
Meds 'Always' Explained Before Given	(a)	68%	66%	64%
Nurses 'Always' Communicated Well	(a)	80%	80%	79%
Pain 'Always' Well Controlled	(a)	75%	72%	71%
Room and Bathroom 'Always' Clean	(a)	76%	73%	73%
Timely Help 'Always' Received	(a)	69%	68%	68%
Would Definitely Recommend Hospital	(a)	56%	70%	71%
Use of Medical Imaging				
Cardiac Imaging Stress Test before Surgery[7]	-	-	4.8%	5.3%
Combination Abdominal CT Scan	180	12.2%	9.6%	10.5%
Combination Brain/Sinus CT Scan[1]	-	-	3.3%	2.7%
Combination Chest CT Scan	129	6.2%	3.4%	2.7%
Follow-up Mammogram/Ultrasound	172	7.6%	8.3%	8.8%
Lumbar Spine MRI for Low Back Pain[1]	-	-	35.3%	37.2%

Southern Tennessee Medical Center

185 Hospital Road
Winchester, TN 37398
URL: www.southerntennessee.com
Type: Acute Care Hospitals
Ownership: Proprietary
Phone: 931-967-8295
Fax: 931-967-4464
Emergency Services: Yes
Beds: 131

Key Personnel:
Chief of Medical Staff. . . . . Lia C Boyanton
Anesthesiology. . . . . Esme H Brown, MD
Radiology. . . . . Paul Ellis, MD
Hemotology Center . . . . Henry J Goolsby III, MD
CEO/President. . . . . Lenae King

Measure	Cases	This Hosp.	State Avg.	U.S. Avg.
Blood Clot Prevention and Treatment				
Anticoagulation Overlap Therapy[2]	39	97%	92%	93%
ICU Venous Thromboembolism Prophylaxis[2]	93	86%	90%	92%
Incidence of Potentially Preventable VTE[1,2]	-	-	10%	10%
UFH with Dosages/Platelet Monitoring[2]	29	100%	99%	97%
Venous Thromboembolism Prophylaxis[2]	349	86%	83%	85%
Warfarin Therapy Discharge Instructions[2]	30	97%	78%	75%
Chest Pain/Possible Heart Attack Care				
Aspirin Given Within 24 Hours of Arrival	92	97%	96%	96%
Fibrinolytic Meds Within 30 Min. of Arrival[1]	-	-	72%	58%
Average Time to ECG (minutes)	93	6	6	7
Average Time to Transfer (minutes)[1]	-	-	53	60
Children's Asthma Care				
Received Home Management Plan of Care	-	-	-	88%
Received Reliever Medication	-	-	-	100%
Received Systemic Corticosteroids	-	-	-	100%
Emergency Department				
Admittance Decision Time (minutes)[2]	444	56	82	98
Head CT Results Within 45 Min. of Arrival[1]	-	-	52%	57%
Patients Who Left ER Before Being Seen	18,436	1%	2%	2%
Time from ER Arrival to Admit. (minutes)[2]	444	192	243	274
Time from ER Arrival to Discharge (minutes)	372	123	131	134
Time in ER Before Being Evaluated (minutes)	430	22	25	26
Time to Pain Meds for Fractures (minutes)	91	38	60	57

NOTE: Hospital profiles are in alphabetical order by state, then city, then hospital within the city; Rankings exclude hospitals with less than 25 cases except for patient surveys which excludes hospitals with less than 100 cases; (a) 100-299 cases; (1) The number of cases/patients is too few to report; (2) Data submitted were based on a sample of cases/patients; (3) Results are based on a shorter time period than required; (4) Data suppressed by CMS for one or more quarters; (5) Results are not available for this reporting period; (6) Fewer than 100 patients completed the HCAHPS survey; (7) No cases met the criteria for this measure; (8) The lower limit of the confidence interval cannot be calculated if the number of observed infections equals zero; (9) No data are available from the state/territory for this reporting period; (10) The scores shown reflect fewer than 50 completed surveys; (11) There were discrepancies in the data collection process; (12) This measure does not apply to this hospital for this reporting period; (13) Results cannot be calculated for this reporting period; (14) The results for this state are combined with nearby states to protect confidentiality; Please refer to the User's Guide for a full explanation of data.

Measure	Cases	This Hosp.	State Avg.	U.S. Avg.
Heart Attack Care				
Aspirin Given at Discharge	19	100%	99%	99%
Fibrinolytic Meds Within 30 Min. of Arrival[7]	-	-	33%	54%
PCI Within 90 Minutes of Arrival[7]	-	-	98%	96%
Statin Prescribed at Discharge	20	95%	99%	98%
Heart Failure Care				
ACE Inhibitor or ARB for LVSD	49	92%	97%	97%
Discharge Instructions Given	147	93%	93%	94%
Evaluation of LVS Function	169	95%	99%	99%
Medicare Spending				
Medicare Spending per Patient (ratio)	-	0.99	1	0.98
Pneumonia Care				
Appropriate Initial Antibiotic Given	119	97%	95%	95%
Blood Culture Timing	174	98%	98%	98%
Pregnancy and Delivery Care				
Newborn Deliveries Scheduled Early[2]	40	10%	6%	6%
Preventive Care				
Immunization for Influenza[2]	420	98%	93%	90%
Immunization for Pneumonia[2]	531	98%	93%	92%
Stroke Care				
Anticoagulation Therapy for Atrial Fibrillation[1]	-	-	94%	95%
Antithrombotic Therapy Timing	31	100%	97%	98%
Assessed for Rehabilitation	29	100%	97%	97%
Discharged on Antithrombotic Therapy	26	100%	99%	99%
Discharged on Statin Medication	21	95%	94%	94%
Thrombolytic Therapy Timing[1]	-	-	57%	66%
Venous Thromboembolism Prophylaxis	33	100%	93%	94%
Written Stroke Educational Materials Given	11	91%	84%	88%
Surgical Care Improvement Project				
Appropriate Beta Blocker Usage	60	100%	97%	98%
Appropriate VTP Within 24 Hours	214	100%	98%	98%
Controlled Postoperative Blood Glucose[7]	-	-	95%	97%
Perioperative Temperature Management	229	100%	100%	100%
Prophylactic Antibiotic Selection	155	100%	99%	99%
Prophylactic Antibiotic Selection (Outpatient)	165	98%	98%	98%
Prophylactic Antibiotic Stopped	150	96%	98%	98%
Prophylactic Antibiotic Timing	155	100%	99%	99%
Prophylactic Antibiotic Timing (Outpatient)	164	99%	98%	98%
Urinary Catheter Removal	179	98%	96%	97%
Survey of Patients' Hospital Experiences				
Area Around Room 'Always' Quiet at Night	300+	62%	67%	61%
Doctors 'Always' Communicated Well	300+	82%	84%	82%
Home Recovery Information Given	300+	86%	85%	85%
Hospital Given 9 or 10 on 10 Point Scale	300+	64%	70%	71%
Meds 'Always' Explained Before Given	300+	61%	66%	64%
Nurses 'Always' Communicated Well	300+	76%	80%	79%
Pain 'Always' Well Controlled	300+	68%	72%	71%
Room and Bathroom 'Always' Clean	300+	68%	73%	73%
Timely Help 'Always' Received	300+	54%	68%	68%
Would Definitely Recommend Hospital	300+	64%	70%	71%
Use of Medical Imaging				
Cardiac Imaging Stress Test before Surgery	175	5.7%	4.8%	5.3%
Combination Abdominal CT Scan	536	0.9%	9.6%	10.5%
Combination Brain/Sinus CT Scan	606	3.8%	3.3%	2.7%
Combination Chest CT Scan	267	0.4%	3.4%	2.7%
Follow-up Mammogram/Ultrasound	1,044	5.4%	8.3%	8.8%
Lumbar Spine MRI for Low Back Pain	111	36.0%	35.3%	37.2%

Stones River Hospital & Dekalb Community Hospital

324 Doolittle Road
Woodbury, TN 37190
E-mail: info@srhtn.com
URL: www.stonesriverhospital.com
Phone: 615-563-4001
Fax: 615-563-7314
Type: Acute Care Hospitals
Ownership: Proprietary
Emergency Services: Yes
Beds: 55

Key Personnel:

Quality Assurance . . . . Pamela Anderson
CEO/President. . . . . Sue Conley
Radiology. . . . . Eric A Dame, MD
Operating Room. . . . . Jim Fedusenko
Infection Control. . . . . Vida King, RN
Chief of Medical Staff. . . . . Jeff Todd
Anesthesiology. . . . . Lloyd Trivett
Emergency Room . . . . Mark Weeks, MD

Measure	Cases	This Hosp.	State Avg.	U.S. Avg.
Blood Clot Prevention and Treatment				
Anticoagulation Overlap Therapy[1,2]	-	-	92%	93%
ICU Venous Thromboembolism Prophylaxis[2,7]	-	-	90%	92%
Incidence of Potentially Preventable VTE[2,7]	-	-	10%	10%
UFH with Dosages/Platelet Monitoring[1,2]	-	-	99%	97%
Venous Thromboembolism Prophylaxis[2]	278	50%	83%	85%
Warfarin Therapy Discharge Instructions[1,2]	-	-	78%	75%
Chest Pain/Possible Heart Attack Care				
Aspirin Given Within 24 Hours of Arrival[1,3]	-	-	96%	96%
Fibrinolytic Meds Within 30 Min. of Arrival[3,7]	-	-	72%	58%
Average Time to ECG (minutes)[1,3]	-	-	6	7
Average Time to Transfer (minutes)[3,7]	-	-	53	60
Children's Asthma Care				
Received Home Management Plan of Care	-	-	-	88%
Received Reliever Medication	-	-	-	100%
Received Systemic Corticosteroids	-	-	-	100%
Emergency Department				
Admittance Decision Time (minutes)[2]	309	44	82	98
Head CT Results Within 45 Min. of Arrival[1]	-	-	52%	57%
Patients Who Left ER Before Being Seen	6,390	2%	2%	2%
Time from ER Arrival to Admit. (minutes)[2]	309	180	243	274
Time from ER Arrival to Discharge (minutes)	365	89	131	134
Time in ER Before Being Evaluated (minutes)	383	21	25	26
Time to Pain Meds for Fractures (minutes)	26	68	60	57
Heart Attack Care				
Aspirin Given at Discharge[1,3]	-	-	99%	99%
Fibrinolytic Meds Within 30 Min. of Arrival[3,7]	-	-	33%	54%
PCI Within 90 Minutes of Arrival[3,7]	-	-	98%	96%
Statin Prescribed at Discharge[1,3]	-	-	99%	98%
Heart Failure Care				
ACE Inhibitor or ARB for LVSD[1]	-	-	97%	97%
Discharge Instructions Given	22	82%	93%	94%
Evaluation of LVS Function	35	97%	99%	99%
Medicare Spending				
Medicare Spending per Patient (ratio)	-	1.13	1	0.98
Pneumonia Care				
Appropriate Initial Antibiotic Given	44	89%	95%	95%
Blood Culture Timing	53	98%	98%	98%
Pregnancy and Delivery Care				
Newborn Deliveries Scheduled Early[7]	-	-	6%	6%
Preventive Care				
Immunization for Influenza[2]	239	96%	93%	90%
Immunization for Pneumonia[2]	375	95%	93%	92%
Stroke Care				
Anticoagulation Therapy for Atrial Fibrillation[1,2]	-	-	94%	95%
Antithrombotic Therapy Timing[1,2]	-	-	97%	98%
Assessed for Rehabilitation[1,2]	-	-	97%	97%
Discharged on Antithrombotic Therapy[1,2]	-	-	99%	99%
Discharged on Statin Medication[1,2]	-	-	94%	94%
Thrombolytic Therapy Timing[2,7]	-	-	57%	66%
Venous Thromboembolism Prophylaxis[1,2]	-	-	93%	94%
Written Stroke Educational Materials Given[1,2]	-	-	84%	88%
Surgical Care Improvement Project				
Appropriate Beta Blocker Usage[5]	-	-	97%	98%
Appropriate VTP Within 24 Hours[5]	-	-	98%	98%
Controlled Postoperative Blood Glucose[5]	-	-	95%	97%
Perioperative Temperature Management[5]	-	-	100%	100%
Prophylactic Antibiotic Selection[5]	-	-	99%	99%
Prophylactic Antibiotic Selection (Outpatient)[1,3]	-	-	98%	98%
Prophylactic Antibiotic Stopped[5]	-	-	98%	98%
Prophylactic Antibiotic Timing[5]	-	-	99%	99%
Prophylactic Antibiotic Timing (Outpatient)[1,3]	-	-	98%	98%
Urinary Catheter Removal[5]	-	-	96%	97%
Survey of Patients' Hospital Experiences				
Area Around Room 'Always' Quiet at Night[6]	<100	64%	67%	61%
Doctors 'Always' Communicated Well[6]	<100	91%	84%	82%
Home Recovery Information Given[6]	<100	86%	85%	85%
Hospital Given 9 or 10 on 10 Point Scale[6]	<100	62%	70%	71%
Meds 'Always' Explained Before Given[6]	<100	66%	66%	64%
Nurses 'Always' Communicated Well[6]	<100	79%	80%	79%
Pain 'Always' Well Controlled[6]	<100	67%	72%	71%
Room and Bathroom 'Always' Clean[6]	<100	75%	73%	73%
Timely Help 'Always' Received[6]	<100	63%	68%	68%
Would Definitely Recommend Hospital[6]	<100	69%	70%	71%
Use of Medical Imaging				
Cardiac Imaging Stress Test before Surgery[1]	-	-	4.8%	5.3%
Combination Abdominal CT Scan	56	5.4%	9.6%	10.5%
Combination Brain/Sinus CT Scan[1]	-	-	3.3%	2.7%
Combination Chest CT Scan[1]	-	-	3.4%	2.7%
Follow-up Mammogram/Ultrasound	76	7.9%	8.3%	8.8%
Lumbar Spine MRI for Low Back Pain[1]	-	-	35.3%	37.2%

NOTE: Hospital profiles are in alphabetical order by state, then city, then hospital within the city; Rankings exclude hospitals with less than 25 cases except for patient surveys which excludes hospitals with less than 100 cases; (a) 100-299 cases; (1) The number of cases/patients is too few to report; (2) Data submitted were based on a sample of cases/patients; (3) Results are based on a shorter time period than required; (4) Data suppressed by CMS for one or more quarters; (5) Results are not available for this reporting period; (6) Fewer than 100 patients completed the HCAHPS survey; (7) No cases met the criteria for this measure; (8) The lower limit of the confidence interval cannot be calculated if the number of observed infections equals zero; (9) No data are available from the state/territory for this reporting period; (10) The scores shown reflect fewer than 50 completed surveys; (11) There were discrepancies in the data collection process; (12) This measure does not apply to this hospital for this reporting period; (13) Results cannot be calculated for this reporting period; (14) The results for this state are combined with nearby states to protect confidentiality; Please refer to the User's Guide for a full explanation of data.

Blood Clot Prevention and Treatment

Anticoagulation Overlap Therapy

Hospital Name	City	Rate	Cases
Southwestern Vermont Medical Center[2]	Bennington	100%	40
Fletcher Allen Hospital of Vermont[2]	Burlington	99%	113
Rutland Regional Medical Center[2]	Rutland	97%	59

ICU Venous Thromboembolism Prophylaxis

Hospital Name	City	Rate	Cases
Central Vermont Medical Center[2]	Barre	98%	98
Southwestern Vermont Medical Center[2]	Bennington	96%	69
Brattleboro Memorial Hospital[2]	Brattleboro	90%	42
Fletcher Allen Hospital of Vermont[2]	Burlington	89%	107

Incidence of Potentially Preventable VTE

Hospital Name	City	Rate	Cases
Fletcher Allen Hospital of Vermont[2]	Burlington	4%	45

UFH with Dosages/Platelet Count Monitoring

Hospital Name	City	Rate	Cases
Fletcher Allen Hospital of Vermont[2]	Burlington	93%	103

Venous Thromboembolism Prophylaxis

Hospital Name	City	Rate	Cases
Northwestern Medical Center[2]	Saint Albans	95%	189
Fletcher Allen Hospital of Vermont[2]	Burlington	94%	281
Southwestern Vermont Medical Center[2]	Bennington	94%	318
Brattleboro Memorial Hospital[2]	Brattleboro	93%	119
Central Vermont Medical Center[2]	Barre	92%	204
Rutland Regional Medical Center[2]	Rutland	73%	338

Warfarin Therapy Discharge Instructions

Hospital Name	City	Rate	Cases
Southwestern Vermont Medical Center[2]	Bennington	96%	27
Rutland Regional Medical Center[2]	Rutland	92%	51
Fletcher Allen Hospital of Vermont[2]	Burlington	62%	95

Chest Pain/Possible Heart Attack Care

Aspirin Given Within 24 Hours of Arrival

Hospital Name	City	Rate	Cases
Central Vermont Medical Center	Barre	100%	149
Northwestern Medical Center	Saint Albans	99%	188
Southwestern Vermont Medical Center	Bennington	99%	143
Rutland Regional Medical Center	Rutland	98%	57
Brattleboro Memorial Hospital	Brattleboro	97%	77

Average Time to ECG (minutes)

Hospital Name	City	Min.	Cases
Northwestern Medical Center	Saint Albans	2	192
Central Vermont Medical Center	Barre	6	153
Southwestern Vermont Medical Center	Bennington	6	149
Rutland Regional Medical Center	Rutland	7	58
Brattleboro Memorial Hospital	Brattleboro	11	82

Average Time to Transfer (minutes)

Hospital Name	City	Min.	Cases
Central Vermont Medical Center	Barre	33	30

Children's Asthma Care

No hospitals met the 25 case threshold.

Emergency Department

Admittance Decision Time (minutes)

Hospital Name	City	Min.	Cases
Northwestern Medical Center[2]	Saint Albans	43	318
Brattleboro Memorial Hospital[2]	Brattleboro	85	306
Rutland Regional Medical Center[2]	Rutland	109	609
Central Vermont Medical Center[2]	Barre	134	242
Southwestern Vermont Medical Center[2]	Bennington	152	571
Fletcher Allen Hospital of Vermont[2]	Burlington	154	556

Patients Who Left ER Before Being Seen

Hospital Name	City	Rate	Cases
Central Vermont Medical Center	Barre	0%	26998
Northwestern Medical Center	Saint Albans	0%	29165
Brattleboro Memorial Hospital	Brattleboro	2%	13363
Fletcher Allen Hospital of Vermont	Burlington	2%	60048
Southwestern Vermont Medical Center	Bennington	2%	3056
Rutland Regional Medical Center	Rutland	4%	35073

Time from ER Arrival to Being Admitted (minutes)

Hospital Name	City	Min.	Cases
Northwestern Medical Center[2]	Saint Albans	205	318
Brattleboro Memorial Hospital[2]	Brattleboro	231	310
Central Vermont Medical Center[2]	Barre	271	248
Rutland Regional Medical Center[2]	Rutland	282	619
Southwestern Vermont Medical Center[2]	Bennington	306	576
Fletcher Allen Hospital of Vermont[2]	Burlington	363	556

Time from ER Arrival to Discharge (minutes)

Hospital Name	City	Min.	Cases
Northwestern Medical Center	Saint Albans	97	388
Central Vermont Medical Center	Barre	105	376
Brattleboro Memorial Hospital	Brattleboro	120	387
Rutland Regional Medical Center	Rutland	145	382
Fletcher Allen Hospital of Vermont	Burlington	166	1490
Southwestern Vermont Medical Center	Bennington	166	350

Time in ER Before Being Evaluated (minutes)

Hospital Name	City	Min.	Cases
Northwestern Medical Center	Saint Albans	18	410
Brattleboro Memorial Hospital	Brattleboro	26	435
Southwestern Vermont Medical Center	Bennington	26	391
Fletcher Allen Hospital of Vermont	Burlington	27	1591
Rutland Regional Medical Center	Rutland	42	413
Central Vermont Medical Center	Barre	62	86

Time to Pain Meds for Bone Fractures (minutes)

Hospital Name	City	Min.	Cases
Brattleboro Memorial Hospital	Brattleboro	40	72
Northwestern Medical Center	Saint Albans	46	86
Central Vermont Medical Center	Barre	52	82
Southwestern Vermont Medical Center	Bennington	72	125
Rutland Regional Medical Center	Rutland	74	99
Fletcher Allen Hospital of Vermont	Burlington	79	217

Heart Attack Care

Aspirin Given at Discharge

Hospital Name	City	Rate	Cases
Fletcher Allen Hospital of Vermont	Burlington	100%	897

PCI Within 90 Minutes of Arrival

Hospital Name	City	Rate	Cases
Fletcher Allen Hospital of Vermont	Burlington	98%	57

Statin Prescribed at Discharge

Hospital Name	City	Rate	Cases
Fletcher Allen Hospital of Vermont	Burlington	100%	863

Heart Failure Care

ACE Inhibitor or ARB for LVSD

Hospital Name	City	Rate	Cases
Rutland Regional Medical Center	Rutland	100%	43
Fletcher Allen Hospital of Vermont	Burlington	96%	143

Discharge Instructions Given

Hospital Name	City	Rate	Cases
Springfield Hospital	Springfield	100%	25
Fletcher Allen Hospital of Vermont	Burlington	99%	364
Porter Hospital	Middlebury	98%	45
Rutland Regional Medical Center	Rutland	97%	76
Northwestern Medical Center	Saint Albans	96%	27
White River Junction VA Medical Center	White River Jct	93%	44
Central Vermont Medical Center	Barre	92%	63
Southwestern Vermont Medical Center	Bennington	86%	87
Copley Hospital	Morrisville	70%	33
Northeastern Vermont Regional Hospital	Saint Johnsbury	70%	30

Evaluation of LVS Function

Hospital Name	City	Rate	Cases
Copley Hospital	Morrisville	100%	41
Fletcher Allen Hospital of Vermont	Burlington	100%	469
Gifford Medical Center	Randolph	100%	35
Mount Ascutney Hospital	Windsor	100%	26
North Country Hospital & Health Center	Newport	100%	40
Northwestern Medical Center	Saint Albans	100%	39
Rutland Regional Medical Center	Rutland	100%	90
Southwestern Vermont Medical Center	Bennington	100%	120
Springfield Hospital	Springfield	100%	36
White River Junction VA Medical Center	White River Jct	100%	53
Porter Hospital	Middlebury	98%	54
Brattleboro Memorial Hospital	Brattleboro	97%	29
Central Vermont Medical Center	Barre	97%	99
Northeastern Vermont Regional Hospital	Saint Johnsbury	95%	37

Medicare Spending

Medicare Spending per Patient (ratio)

Hospital Name	City	Ratio	Cases
Southwestern Vermont Medical Center	Bennington	0.90	-
Northwestern Medical Center	Saint Albans	0.94	-
Central Vermont Medical Center	Barre	0.95	-
Fletcher Allen Hospital of Vermont	Burlington	0.97	-
Rutland Regional Medical Center	Rutland	0.99	-
Brattleboro Memorial Hospital	Brattleboro	1.08	-

Pneumonia Care

Appropriate Initial Antibiotic Given

Hospital Name	City	Rate	Cases
Springfield Hospital	Springfield	100%	89
Central Vermont Medical Center	Barre	99%	95
Northwestern Medical Center	Saint Albans	99%	93
Brattleboro Memorial Hospital	Brattleboro	98%	46
Gifford Medical Center	Randolph	98%	43
Porter Hospital	Middlebury	98%	98
Northeastern Vermont Regional Hospital	Saint Johnsbury	97%	60
Southwestern Vermont Medical Center[2]	Bennington	97%	97
Rutland Regional Medical Center	Rutland	96%	122
Copley Hospital	Morrisville	94%	47
Fletcher Allen Hospital of Vermont	Burlington	94%	127
North Country Hospital & Health Center	Newport	94%	35

Blood Culture Timing

Hospital Name	City	Rate	Cases
Gifford Medical Center	Randolph	100%	40
North Country Hospital & Health Center	Newport	100%	69
Central Vermont Medical Center	Barre	99%	143
Northwestern Medical Center	Saint Albans	99%	122
Springfield Hospital	Springfield	99%	113
Brattleboro Memorial Hospital	Brattleboro	98%	66
Fletcher Allen Hospital of Vermont	Burlington	98%	203
Northeastern Vermont Regional Hospital	Saint Johnsbury	98%	63
Porter Hospital	Middlebury	98%	107
Rutland Regional Medical Center	Rutland	98%	126
Copley Hospital	Morrisville	96%	46
Southwestern Vermont Medical Center[2]	Bennington	96%	219
White River Junction VA Medical Center	White River Jct	96%	25

Pregnancy and Delivery Care

Newborns whose Deliveries were Scheduled Early

Hospital Name	City	Rate	Cases
Brattleboro Memorial Hospital[2]	Brattleboro	3%	34
Central Vermont Medical Center[2]	Barre	4%	26
Northwestern Medical Center	Saint Albans	6%	34
Southwestern Vermont Medical Center	Bennington	7%	30

Preventive Care

Immunization for Influenza

Hospital Name	City	Rate	Cases
Central Vermont Medical Center[2]	Barre	96%	306
Northwestern Medical Center[2]	Saint Albans	96%	257
Rutland Regional Medical Center[2]	Rutland	95%	527
Southwestern Vermont Medical Center[2]	Bennington	94%	406
Brattleboro Memorial Hospital[2]	Brattleboro	92%	272
Fletcher Allen Hospital of Vermont[2]	Burlington	87%	508

Immunization for Pneumonia

Hospital Name	City	Rate	Cases
Central Vermont Medical Center[2]	Barre	96%	391
Northwestern Medical Center[2]	Saint Albans	96%	280
Brattleboro Memorial Hospital[2]	Brattleboro	95%	281
Rutland Regional Medical Center[2]	Rutland	95%	728
Southwestern Vermont Medical Center[2]	Bennington	95%	547
Fletcher Allen Hospital of Vermont[2]	Burlington	92%	590

Stroke Care

Antithrombotic Therapy Timing

Hospital Name	City	Rate	Cases
Brattleboro Memorial Hospital	Brattleboro	100%	27
Southwestern Vermont Medical Center	Bennington	100%	28
Rutland Regional Medical Center	Rutland	98%	47
Fletcher Allen Hospital of Vermont[2]	Burlington	74%	50

Assessed for Rehabilitation

Hospital Name	City	Rate	Cases
Brattleboro Memorial Hospital	Brattleboro	100%	26
Fletcher Allen Hospital of Vermont[2]	Burlington	97%	97
Rutland Regional Medical Center	Rutland	94%	53

NOTE: Hospital profiles are in alphabetical order by state, then city, then hospital within the city; Rankings exclude hospitals with less than 25 cases except for patient surveys which excludes hospitals with less than 100 cases; (a) 100-299 cases; (1) The number of cases/patients is too few to report; (2) Data submitted were based on a sample of cases/patients; (3) Results are based on a shorter time period than required; (4) Data suppressed by CMS for one or more quarters; (5) Results are not available for this reporting period; (6) Fewer than 100 patients completed the HCAHPS survey; (7) No cases met the criteria for this measure; (8) The lower limit of the confidence interval cannot be calculated if the number of observed infections equals zero; (9) No data are available from the state/territory for this reporting period; (10) The scores shown reflect fewer than 50 completed surveys; (11) There were discrepancies in the data collection process; (12) This measure does not apply to this hospital for this reporting period; (13) Results cannot be calculated for this reporting period; (14) The results for this state are combined with nearby states to protect confidentiality; Please refer to the User's Guide for a full explanation of data.

Hospital Name	City	Rate	Cases
Southwestern Vermont Medical Center	Bennington	90%	30

Discharged on Antithrombotic Therapy

Hospital Name	City	Rate	Cases
Brattleboro Memorial Hospital	Brattleboro	100%	26
Fletcher Allen Hospital of Vermont[2]	Burlington	100%	77
Rutland Regional Medical Center	Rutland	100%	51
Southwestern Vermont Medical Center	Bennington	97%	29

Discharged on Statin Medication

Hospital Name	City	Rate	Cases
Fletcher Allen Hospital of Vermont[2]	Burlington	100%	60
Rutland Regional Medical Center	Rutland	73%	37

Venous Thromboembolism (VTE) Prophylaxis

Hospital Name	City	Rate	Cases
Brattleboro Memorial Hospital	Brattleboro	100%	27
Fletcher Allen Hospital of Vermont[2]	Burlington	99%	96
Southwestern Vermont Medical Center	Bennington	94%	31
Rutland Regional Medical Center	Rutland	67%	45

Written Stroke Educational Materials Given

Hospital Name	City	Rate	Cases
Fletcher Allen Hospital of Vermont[2]	Burlington	98%	54
Rutland Regional Medical Center	Rutland	82%	33

Surgical Care Improvement Project

Appropriate Beta Blocker Usage

Hospital Name	City	Rate	Cases
Porter Hospital[2]	Middlebury	100%	41
Brattleboro Memorial Hospital	Brattleboro	99%	72
Fletcher Allen Hospital of Vermont[2]	Burlington	99%	224
Central Vermont Medical Center	Barre	98%	49
Rutland Regional Medical Center[2]	Rutland	98%	168
Southwestern Vermont Medical Center[2]	Bennington	98%	59
White River Junction VA Medical Center[2]	White River Jct	98%	61
Copley Hospital	Morrisville	96%	50
Northwestern Medical Center	Saint Albans	95%	44
North Country Hospital & Health Center	Newport	90%	29

Appropriate VTP Within 24 Hours

Hospital Name	City	Rate	Cases
Brattleboro Memorial Hospital	Brattleboro	100%	223
Gifford Medical Center	Randolph	100%	53
Northeastern Vermont Regional Hospital[2]	Saint Johnsbury	100%	96
Porter Hospital[2]	Middlebury	100%	150
Springfield Hospital[2]	Springfield	100%	56
Fletcher Allen Hospital of Vermont[2]	Burlington	99%	316
Rutland Regional Medical Center[2]	Rutland	99%	467
Southwestern Vermont Medical Center[2]	Bennington	99%	210
White River Junction VA Medical Center[2]	White River Jct	99%	120
Northwestern Medical Center	Saint Albans	98%	150
Central Vermont Medical Center	Barre	97%	183
Copley Hospital	Morrisville	97%	188
North Country Hospital & Health Center	Newport	90%	82

Controlled Postoperative Blood Glucose

Hospital Name	City	Rate	Cases
Fletcher Allen Hospital of Vermont[2]	Burlington	94%	125

Perioperative Temperature Management

Hospital Name	City	Rate	Cases
Brattleboro Memorial Hospital	Brattleboro	100%	248
Central Vermont Medical Center	Barre	100%	196
Copley Hospital	Morrisville	100%	211
Fletcher Allen Hospital of Vermont[2]	Burlington	100%	424
Gifford Medical Center	Randolph	100%	58
North Country Hospital & Health Center	Newport	100%	96
Northeastern Vermont Regional Hospital[2]	Saint Johnsbury	100%	100
Rutland Regional Medical Center[2]	Rutland	100%	571
Southwestern Vermont Medical Center[2]	Bennington	100%	234
Springfield Hospital[2]	Springfield	100%	58
Northwestern Medical Center	Saint Albans	99%	184
Porter Hospital[2]	Middlebury	99%	167
White River Junction VA Medical Center[2]	White River Jct	99%	148

Prophylactic Antibiotic Selection

Hospital Name	City	Rate	Cases
Central Vermont Medical Center	Barre	100%	143
Gifford Medical Center	Randolph	100%	55
Southwestern Vermont Medical Center[2]	Bennington	100%	159
White River Junction VA Medical Center	White River Jct	100%	82
Brattleboro Memorial Hospital	Brattleboro	99%	194
Copley Hospital	Morrisville	99%	195
Fletcher Allen Hospital of Vermont[2]	Burlington	99%	402
North Country Hospital & Health Center	Newport	99%	73
Rutland Regional Medical Center[2]	Rutland	99%	436
Northwestern Medical Center	Saint Albans	98%	146
Porter Hospital[2]	Middlebury	98%	127
Springfield Hospital[2]	Springfield	97%	36
Northeastern Vermont Regional Hospital[2]	Saint Johnsbury	95%	88

Prophylactic Antibiotic Selection (Outpatient)

Hospital Name	City	Rate	Cases
Brattleboro Memorial Hospital	Brattleboro	100%	55
Southwestern Vermont Medical Center	Bennington	100%	112
Fletcher Allen Hospital of Vermont	Burlington	99%	959
Rutland Regional Medical Center	Rutland	99%	119
Central Vermont Medical Center	Barre	97%	69
Northwestern Medical Center	Saint Albans	93%	94

Prophylactic Antibiotic Stopped

Hospital Name	City	Rate	Cases
Brattleboro Memorial Hospital	Brattleboro	100%	188
Copley Hospital	Morrisville	100%	192
Fletcher Allen Hospital of Vermont[2]	Burlington	100%	397
Rutland Regional Medical Center[2]	Rutland	100%	428
Springfield Hospital[2]	Springfield	100%	36
Central Vermont Medical Center	Barre	99%	143
North Country Hospital & Health Center	Newport	99%	72
Porter Hospital[2]	Middlebury	99%	123
Southwestern Vermont Medical Center[2]	Bennington	99%	159
Northwestern Medical Center	Saint Albans	97%	143
Northeastern Vermont Regional Hospital[2]	Saint Johnsbury	95%	87
Gifford Medical Center	Randolph	94%	54
White River Junction VA Medical Center	White River Jct	94%	81

Prophylactic Antibiotic Timing

Hospital Name	City	Rate	Cases
North Country Hospital & Health Center	Newport	100%	73
Rutland Regional Medical Center[2]	Rutland	100%	437
Springfield Hospital[2]	Springfield	100%	36
White River Junction VA Medical Center	White River Jct	100%	82
Brattleboro Memorial Hospital	Brattleboro	99%	194
Northwestern Medical Center	Saint Albans	99%	146
Porter Hospital[2]	Middlebury	99%	128
Southwestern Vermont Medical Center[2]	Bennington	99%	159
Fletcher Allen Hospital of Vermont[2]	Burlington	98%	404
Central Vermont Medical Center	Barre	97%	143
Copley Hospital	Morrisville	97%	195
Northeastern Vermont Regional Hospital[2]	Saint Johnsbury	95%	88
Gifford Medical Center	Randolph	93%	55

Prophylactic Antibiotic Timing (Outpatient)

Hospital Name	City	Rate	Cases
Brattleboro Memorial Hospital	Brattleboro	100%	55
Northwestern Medical Center	Saint Albans	99%	95
Southwestern Vermont Medical Center	Bennington	99%	112
Fletcher Allen Hospital of Vermont	Burlington	97%	898
Central Vermont Medical Center	Barre	92%	62
Rutland Regional Medical Center	Rutland	90%	129

Urinary Catheter Removal

Hospital Name	City	Rate	Cases
Gifford Medical Center	Randolph	100%	51
Northeastern Vermont Regional Hospital[2]	Saint Johnsbury	100%	87
Southwestern Vermont Medical Center[2]	Bennington	100%	171
Springfield Hospital[2]	Springfield	100%	49
Brattleboro Memorial Hospital	Brattleboro	99%	98
Copley Hospital	Morrisville	99%	190
Rutland Regional Medical Center[2]	Rutland	99%	256
Central Vermont Medical Center	Barre	98%	151
White River Junction VA Medical Center[2]	White River Jct	97%	86
Fletcher Allen Hospital of Vermont[2]	Burlington	96%	335
Northwestern Medical Center	Saint Albans	96%	132
Porter Hospital[2]	Middlebury	96%	136
North Country Hospital & Health Center	Newport	70%	33

Survey of Patients' Hospital Experiences

Area Around Room 'Always' Quiet at Night

Hospital Name	City	Rate	Cases
Brattleboro Memorial Hospital	Brattleboro	61%	300+
Northeastern Vermont Regional Hospital	Saint Johnsbury	60%	300+
Copley Hospital	Morrisville	58%	300+
Central Vermont Medical Center	Barre	54%	300+
Gifford Medical Center	Randolph	54%	300+
North Country Hospital & Health Center	Newport	52%	300+
Northwestern Medical Center	Saint Albans	51%	300+
Porter Hospital	Middlebury	51%	300+
Springfield Hospital	Springfield	51%	300+
Rutland Regional Medical Center	Rutland	50%	300+
Southwestern Vermont Medical Center	Bennington	47%	300+
Fletcher Allen Hospital of Vermont	Burlington	40%	300+

Doctors 'Always' Communicated Well

Hospital Name	City	Rate	Cases
Copley Hospital	Morrisville	85%	300+
Northeastern Vermont Regional Hospital	Saint Johnsbury	84%	300+
North Country Hospital & Health Center	Newport	83%	300+
Rutland Regional Medical Center	Rutland	83%	300+
Porter Hospital	Middlebury	82%	300+
Southwestern Vermont Medical Center	Bennington	82%	300+
Gifford Medical Center	Randolph	80%	300+
Northwestern Medical Center	Saint Albans	80%	300+
Brattleboro Memorial Hospital	Brattleboro	79%	300+
Central Vermont Medical Center	Barre	79%	300+
Springfield Hospital	Springfield	79%	300+
Fletcher Allen Hospital of Vermont	Burlington	77%	300+

Home Recovery Information Given

Hospital Name	City	Rate	Cases
Central Vermont Medical Center	Barre	90%	300+
North Country Hospital & Health Center	Newport	90%	300+
Gifford Medical Center	Randolph	89%	300+
Northeastern Vermont Regional Hospital	Saint Johnsbury	89%	300+
Rutland Regional Medical Center	Rutland	89%	300+
Copley Hospital	Morrisville	88%	300+
Fletcher Allen Hospital of Vermont	Burlington	88%	300+
Porter Hospital	Middlebury	88%	300+
Southwestern Vermont Medical Center	Bennington	88%	300+
Brattleboro Memorial Hospital	Brattleboro	86%	300+
Northwestern Medical Center	Saint Albans	86%	300+
Springfield Hospital	Springfield	86%	300+

Hospital Given 9 or 10 on 10 Point Scale

Hospital Name	City	Rate	Cases
Copley Hospital	Morrisville	76%	300+
Southwestern Vermont Medical Center	Bennington	74%	300+
Northeastern Vermont Regional Hospital	Saint Johnsbury	73%	300+
Northwestern Medical Center	Saint Albans	72%	300+
Central Vermont Medical Center	Barre	71%	300+
Gifford Medical Center	Randolph	71%	300+
Rutland Regional Medical Center	Rutland	70%	300+
Porter Hospital	Middlebury	68%	300+
Brattleboro Memorial Hospital	Brattleboro	67%	300+
North Country Hospital & Health Center	Newport	67%	300+
Fletcher Allen Hospital of Vermont	Burlington	66%	300+
Springfield Hospital	Springfield	62%	300+

Meds 'Always' Explained Before Given

Hospital Name	City	Rate	Cases
Northeastern Vermont Regional Hospital	Saint Johnsbury	73%	300+
Southwestern Vermont Medical Center	Bennington	69%	300+
Copley Hospital	Morrisville	68%	300+
Rutland Regional Medical Center	Rutland	68%	300+
Porter Hospital	Middlebury	67%	300+
Central Vermont Medical Center	Barre	66%	300+
Brattleboro Memorial Hospital	Brattleboro	65%	300+
North Country Hospital & Health Center	Newport	65%	300+
Northwestern Medical Center	Saint Albans	65%	300+
Gifford Medical Center	Randolph	64%	300+
Fletcher Allen Hospital of Vermont	Burlington	61%	300+
Springfield Hospital	Springfield	61%	300+

Nurses 'Always' Communicated Well

Hospital Name	City	Rate	Cases
Rutland Regional Medical Center	Rutland	85%	300+
Copley Hospital	Morrisville	83%	300+
Southwestern Vermont Medical Center	Bennington	83%	300+
Central Vermont Medical Center	Barre	81%	300+
North Country Hospital & Health Center	Newport	80%	300+
Northeastern Vermont Regional Hospital	Saint Johnsbury	80%	300+
Porter Hospital	Middlebury	80%	300+
Brattleboro Memorial Hospital	Brattleboro	79%	300+
Fletcher Allen Hospital of Vermont	Burlington	78%	300+
Gifford Medical Center	Randolph	78%	300+
Northwestern Medical Center	Saint Albans	78%	300+
Springfield Hospital	Springfield	73%	300+

Pain 'Always' Well Controlled

Hospital Name	City	Rate	Cases
Rutland Regional Medical Center	Rutland	76%	300+
Central Vermont Medical Center	Barre	75%	300+
Copley Hospital	Morrisville	75%	300+
Southwestern Vermont Medical Center	Bennington	74%	300+
Brattleboro Memorial Hospital	Brattleboro	72%	300+
Northwestern Medical Center	Saint Albans	72%	300+
Fletcher Allen Hospital of Vermont	Burlington	69%	300+
Northeastern Vermont Regional Hospital	Saint Johnsbury	69%	300+
Porter Hospital	Middlebury	69%	300+

NOTE: Hospital profiles are in alphabetical order by state, then city, then hospital within the city; Rankings exclude hospitals with less than 25 cases except for patient surveys which excludes hospitals with less than 100 cases; (a) 100-299 cases; (1) The number of cases/patients is too few to report; (2) Data submitted were based on a sample of cases/patients; (3) Results are based on a shorter time period than required; (4) Data suppressed by CMS for one or more quarters; (5) Results are not available for this reporting period; (6) Fewer than 100 patients completed the HCAHPS survey; (7) No cases met the criteria for this measure; (8) The lower limit of the confidence interval cannot be calculated if the number of observed infections equals zero; (9) No data are available from the state/territory for this reporting period; (10) The scores shown reflect fewer than 50 completed surveys; (11) There were discrepancies in the data collection process; (12) This measure does not apply to this hospital for this reporting period; (13) Results cannot be calculated for this reporting period; (14) The results for this state are combined with nearby states to protect confidentiality; Please refer to the User's Guide for a full explanation of data.

North Country Hospital & Health Center	Newport	68%	300+
Gifford Medical Center	Randolph	65%	300+
Springfield Hospital	Springfield	62%	300+

Room and Bathroom 'Always' Clean

Hospital Name	City	Rate	Cases
Northeastern Vermont Regional Hospital	Saint Johnsbury	88%	300+
Central Vermont Medical Center	Barre	81%	300+
Copley Hospital	Morrisville	79%	300+
North Country Hospital & Health Center	Newport	78%	300+
Rutland Regional Medical Center	Rutland	78%	300+
Southwestern Vermont Medical Center	Bennington	78%	300+
Brattleboro Memorial Hospital	Brattleboro	77%	300+
Northwestern Medical Center	Saint Albans	76%	300+
Porter Hospital	Middlebury	74%	300+
Gifford Medical Center	Randolph	72%	300+
Springfield Hospital	Springfield	70%	300+
Fletcher Allen Hospital of Vermont	Burlington	67%	300+

Timely Help 'Always' Received

Hospital Name	City	Rate	Cases
Copley Hospital	Morrisville	76%	300+
Rutland Regional Medical Center	Rutland	75%	300+
North Country Hospital & Health Center	Newport	74%	300+
Southwestern Vermont Medical Center	Bennington	74%	300+
Brattleboro Memorial Hospital	Brattleboro	73%	300+
Northeastern Vermont Regional Hospital	Saint Johnsbury	72%	300+
Central Vermont Medical Center	Barre	70%	300+
Fletcher Allen Hospital of Vermont	Burlington	66%	300+
Northwestern Medical Center	Saint Albans	65%	300+
Gifford Medical Center	Randolph	64%	300+
Porter Hospital	Middlebury	64%	300+
Springfield Hospital	Springfield	60%	300+

Would Definitely Recommend Hospital

Hospital Name	City	Rate	Cases
Southwestern Vermont Medical Center	Bennington	79%	300+
Copley Hospital	Morrisville	77%	300+
Northwestern Medical Center	Saint Albans	76%	300+
Gifford Medical Center	Randolph	75%	300+
Fletcher Allen Hospital of Vermont	Burlington	74%	300+
Brattleboro Memorial Hospital	Brattleboro	70%	300+
Central Vermont Medical Center	Barre	70%	300+
Northeastern Vermont Regional Hospital	Saint Johnsbury	70%	300+
Porter Hospital	Middlebury	70%	300+
Rutland Regional Medical Center	Rutland	70%	300+
North Country Hospital & Health Center	Newport	68%	300+
Springfield Hospital	Springfield	62%	300+

Use of Medical Imaging

Cardiac Imaging Stress Test before OP Surgery

Hospital Name	City	Rate	Cases
Fletcher Allen Hospital of Vermont	Burlington	3.5%	797
Brattleboro Memorial Hospital	Brattleboro	4.1%	172
Central Vermont Medical Center	Barre	4.9%	347
Northwestern Medical Center	Saint Albans	5.3%	226
Southwestern Vermont Medical Center	Bennington	6.2%	454
Rutland Regional Medical Center	Rutland	6.4%	513

Combination Abdominal CT Scan

Hospital Name	City	Rate	Cases
Brattleboro Memorial Hospital	Brattleboro	3.6%	330
Fletcher Allen Hospital of Vermont	Burlington	4.5%	1719
Central Vermont Medical Center	Barre	4.6%	570
Rutland Regional Medical Center	Rutland	5.7%	752
Southwestern Vermont Medical Center	Bennington	7.3%	588
Northwestern Medical Center	Saint Albans	7.7%	659

Combination Brain/Sinus CT Scan

Hospital Name	City	Rate	Cases
Northwestern Medical Center	Saint Albans	0.7%	441
Fletcher Allen Hospital of Vermont	Burlington	1.5%	985
Southwestern Vermont Medical Center	Bennington	2.3%	518
Central Vermont Medical Center	Barre	2.4%	536
Rutland Regional Medical Center	Rutland	2.7%	699
Brattleboro Memorial Hospital	Brattleboro	4.8%	315

Combination Chest CT Scan

Hospital Name	City	Rate	Cases
Central Vermont Medical Center	Barre	0.0%	347
Northwestern Medical Center	Saint Albans	0.0%	347
Southwestern Vermont Medical Center	Bennington	0.0%	399
Fletcher Allen Hospital of Vermont	Burlington	0.3%	1733
Brattleboro Memorial Hospital	Brattleboro	0.5%	201
Rutland Regional Medical Center	Rutland	3.1%	605

Follow-up Mammogram/Ultrasound

A follow-up rate near zero may indicate missed cancer; a rate higher than 14% may mean there is unnecessary follow up.

Hospital Name	City	Rate	Cases
Rutland Regional Medical Center	Rutland	4.9%	2253
Central Vermont Medical Center	Barre	8.7%	1992
Brattleboro Memorial Hospital	Brattleboro	8.8%	1170
Southwestern Vermont Medical Center	Bennington	9.0%	1415
Northwestern Medical Center	Saint Albans	9.3%	1090
Fletcher Allen Hospital of Vermont	Burlington	9.8%	5214

Lumbar Spine MRI for Low Back Pain

Hospital Name	City	Rate	Cases
Fletcher Allen Hospital of Vermont	Burlington	21.1%	327
Rutland Regional Medical Center	Rutland	32.0%	175
Southwestern Vermont Medical Center	Bennington	40.9%	110
Northwestern Medical Center	Saint Albans	42.4%	125
Central Vermont Medical Center	Barre	43.8%	105

NOTE: Hospital profiles are in alphabetical order by state, then city, then hospital within the city; Rankings exclude hospitals with less than 25 cases except for patient surveys which excludes hospitals with less than 100 cases; (a) 100-299 cases; (1) The number of cases/patients is too few to report; (2) Data submitted were based on a sample of cases/patients; (3) Results are based on a shorter time period than required; (4) Data suppressed by CMS for one or more quarters; (5) Results are not available for this reporting period; (6) Fewer than 100 patients completed the HCAHPS survey; (7) No cases met the criteria for this measure; (8) The lower limit of the confidence interval cannot be calculated if the number of observed infections equals zero; (9) No data are available from the state/territory for this reporting period; (10) The scores shown reflect fewer than 50 completed surveys; (11) There were discrepancies in the data collection process; (12) This measure does not apply to this hospital for this reporting period; (13) Results cannot be calculated for this reporting period; (14) The results for this state are combined with nearby states to protect confidentiality; Please refer to the User's Guide for a full explanation of data.

Central Vermont Medical Center

Box 547 Phone: 802-371-4100
Barre, VT 05641 Fax: 802-371-4401
URL: www.cvmc.hitchcock.org
Type: Acute Care Hospitals Emergency Services: Yes
Ownership: Voluntary non-profit - Private Beds: 210

Key Personnel:
Infection Control.............. Jane Barranco
Quality Assurance .... Russell Davignon, MD
Chief of Medical Staff.......... Russle Davignon, DO
Pediatric Ambulatory Care ...... William Gaidys, MD
Pediatric In-Patient Care .... William Gaidys, MD
Radiology.................. Robert D Johnson, MD
Operating Room.............. Karin Morrow
CEO/President............... Judy Tarr

Measure	Cases	This Hosp.	State Avg.	U.S. Avg.
Blood Clot Prevention and Treatment				
Anticoagulation Overlap Therapy[2]	14	93%	98%	93%
ICU Venous Thromboembolism Prophylaxis[2]	98	98%	94%	92%
Incidence of Potentially Preventable VTE[2,7]	-	-	4%	10%
UFH with Dosages/Platelet Monitoring[1,2]	-	-	95%	97%
Venous Thromboembolism Prophylaxis[2]	204	92%	89%	85%
Warfarin Therapy Discharge Instructions[1,2]	-	-	78%	75%
Chest Pain/Possible Heart Attack Care				
Aspirin Given Within 24 Hours of Arrival	149	100%	98%	96%
Fibrinolytic Meds Within 30 Min. of Arrival[7]	-	-	79%	58%
Average Time to ECG (minutes)	153	6	6	7
Average Time to Transfer (minutes)	30	33	31	60
Children's Asthma Care				
Received Home Management Plan of Care	-	-	-	88%
Received Reliever Medication	-	-	-	100%
Received Systemic Corticosteroids	-	-	-	100%
Emergency Department				
Admittance Decision Time (minutes)[2]	242	134	114	98
Head CT Results Within 45 Min. of Arrival	16	38%	45%	57%
Patients Who Left ER Before Being Seen	26,998	0%	2%	2%
Time from ER Arrival to Admit. (minutes)[2]	248	271	279	274
Time from ER Arrival to Discharge (minutes)	376	105	136	134
Time in ER Before Being Evaluated (minutes)	86	62	27	26
Time to Pain Meds for Fractures (minutes)	82	52	61	57
Heart Attack Care				
Aspirin Given at Discharge[1]	-	-	100%	99%
Fibrinolytic Meds Within 30 Min. of Arrival[7]	-	-	-	54%
PCI Within 90 Minutes of Arrival[7]	-	-	98%	96%
Statin Prescribed at Discharge[1]	-	-	99%	98%
Heart Failure Care				
ACE Inhibitor or ARB for LVSD	22	100%	96%	97%
Discharge Instructions Given	63	92%	94%	94%
Evaluation of LVS Function	99	97%	99%	99%
Medicare Spending				
Medicare Spending per Patient (ratio)	-	0.95	1.01	0.98
Pneumonia Care				
Appropriate Initial Antibiotic Given	95	99%	97%	95%
Blood Culture Timing	143	99%	98%	98%
Pregnancy and Delivery Care				
Newborn Deliveries Scheduled Early[2]	26	4%	4%	6%
Preventive Care				
Immunization for Influenza[2]	306	96%	93%	90%
Immunization for Pneumonia[2]	391	96%	94%	92%
Stroke Care				
Anticoagulation Therapy for Atrial Fibrillation[1]	-	-	96%	95%
Antithrombotic Therapy Timing	23	96%	92%	98%
Assessed for Rehabilitation	24	100%	96%	97%
Discharged on Antithrombotic Therapy	23	100%	99%	99%
Discharged on Statin Medication	17	100%	93%	94%
Thrombolytic Therapy Timing[1]	-	-	70%	66%
Venous Thromboembolism Prophylaxis	23	100%	92%	94%
Written Stroke Educational Materials Given[1]	-	-	83%	88%
Surgical Care Improvement Project				
Appropriate Beta Blocker Usage	49	98%	98%	98%
Appropriate VTP Within 24 Hours	183	97%	98%	98%
Controlled Postoperative Blood Glucose[7]	-	-	94%	97%
Perioperative Temperature Management	196	100%	100%	100%
Prophylactic Antibiotic Selection	143	100%	99%	99%
Prophylactic Antibiotic Selection (Outpatient)	69	97%	99%	98%
Prophylactic Antibiotic Stopped	143	99%	99%	98%
Prophylactic Antibiotic Timing	143	97%	98%	99%
Prophylactic Antibiotic Timing (Outpatient)	62	92%	97%	98%
Urinary Catheter Removal	151	98%	97%	97%
Survey of Patients' Hospital Experiences				
Area Around Room 'Always' Quiet at Night	300+	54%	53%	61%
Doctors 'Always' Communicated Well	300+	79%	82%	82%
Home Recovery Information Given	300+	90%	88%	85%
Hospital Given 9 or 10 on 10 Point Scale	300+	71%	71%	71%
Meds 'Always' Explained Before Given	300+	66%	66%	64%
Nurses 'Always' Communicated Well	300+	81%	81%	79%
Pain 'Always' Well Controlled	300+	75%	70%	71%
Room and Bathroom 'Always' Clean	300+	81%	78%	73%
Timely Help 'Always' Received	300+	70%	69%	68%
Would Definitely Recommend Hospital	300+	70%	73%	71%
Use of Medical Imaging				
Cardiac Imaging Stress Test before Surgery	347	4.9%	5%	5.3%
Combination Abdominal CT Scan	570	4.6%	4.6%	10.5%
Combination Brain/Sinus CT Scan	536	2.4%	2%	2.7%
Combination Chest CT Scan	347	0.0%	0.8%	2.7%
Follow-up Mammogram/Ultrasound	1,992	8.7%	9.1%	8.8%
Lumbar Spine MRI for Low Back Pain	105	43.8%	32.1%	37.2%

Southwestern Vermont Medical Center

100 Hospital Drive Phone: 802-442-6361
Bennington, VT 05201 Fax: 802-442-8331
URL: www.svhealthcare.org
Type: Acute Care Hospitals Emergency Services: Yes
Ownership: Voluntary non-profit - Private Beds: 99

Key Personnel:
Emergency Room .... Christopher Barsotti
Radiology.................. Terrell L Coffield
Quality Assurance .... Patricia Hebert
Chief of Medical Staff.......... Robert Pezzulich, MD
CEO/President............... Harvey Yorke

Measure	Cases	This Hosp.	State Avg.	U.S. Avg.
Blood Clot Prevention and Treatment				
Anticoagulation Overlap Therapy[2]	40	100%	98%	93%
ICU Venous Thromboembolism Prophylaxis[2]	69	96%	94%	92%
Incidence of Potentially Preventable VTE[1,2]	-	-	4%	10%
UFH with Dosages/Platelet Monitoring[2,7]	-	-	95%	97%
Venous Thromboembolism Prophylaxis[2]	318	94%	89%	85%
Warfarin Therapy Discharge Instructions[2]	27	96%	78%	75%
Chest Pain/Possible Heart Attack Care				
Aspirin Given Within 24 Hours of Arrival	143	99%	98%	96%
Fibrinolytic Meds Within 30 Min. of Arrival[1]	-	-	79%	58%
Average Time to ECG (minutes)	149	6	6	7
Average Time to Transfer (minutes)[1]	-	-	31	60
Children's Asthma Care				
Received Home Management Plan of Care	-	-	-	88%
Received Reliever Medication	-	-	-	100%
Received Systemic Corticosteroids	-	-	-	100%
Emergency Department				
Admittance Decision Time (minutes)[2]	571	152	114	98
Head CT Results Within 45 Min. of Arrival	12	50%	45%	57%
Patients Who Left ER Before Being Seen	3,056	2%	2%	2%
Time from ER Arrival to Admit. (minutes)[2]	576	306	279	274
Time from ER Arrival to Discharge (minutes)	350	166	136	134
Time in ER Before Being Evaluated (minutes)	391	26	27	26
Time to Pain Meds for Fractures (minutes)	125	72	61	57
Heart Attack Care				
Aspirin Given at Discharge	19	100%	100%	99%
Fibrinolytic Meds Within 30 Min. of Arrival[7]	-	-	-	54%
PCI Within 90 Minutes of Arrival[7]	-	-	98%	96%
Statin Prescribed at Discharge	17	94%	99%	98%
Heart Failure Care				
ACE Inhibitor or ARB for LVSD	22	95%	96%	97%
Discharge Instructions Given	87	86%	94%	94%
Evaluation of LVS Function	120	100%	99%	99%
Medicare Spending				
Medicare Spending per Patient (ratio)	-	0.90	1.01	0.98
Pneumonia Care				
Appropriate Initial Antibiotic Given[2]	97	97%	97%	95%
Blood Culture Timing[2]	219	96%	98%	98%
Pregnancy and Delivery Care				
Newborn Deliveries Scheduled Early	30	7%	4%	6%
Preventive Care				
Immunization for Influenza[2]	406	94%	93%	90%
Immunization for Pneumonia[2]	547	95%	94%	92%
Stroke Care				
Anticoagulation Therapy for Atrial Fibrillation[1]	-	-	96%	95%
Antithrombotic Therapy Timing	28	100%	92%	98%
Assessed for Rehabilitation	30	90%	96%	97%
Discharged on Antithrombotic Therapy	29	97%	99%	99%
Discharged on Statin Medication	23	91%	93%	94%
Thrombolytic Therapy Timing[7]	-	-	70%	66%
Venous Thromboembolism Prophylaxis	31	94%	92%	94%
Written Stroke Educational Materials Given	15	27%	83%	88%
Surgical Care Improvement Project				
Appropriate Beta Blocker Usage[2]	59	98%	98%	98%
Appropriate VTP Within 24 Hours[2]	210	99%	98%	98%
Controlled Postoperative Blood Glucose[2,7]	-	-	94%	97%
Perioperative Temperature Management[2]	234	100%	100%	100%
Prophylactic Antibiotic Selection[2]	159	100%	99%	99%
Prophylactic Antibiotic Selection (Outpatient)	112	100%	99%	98%
Prophylactic Antibiotic Stopped[2]	159	99%	99%	98%
Prophylactic Antibiotic Timing[2]	159	99%	98%	99%
Prophylactic Antibiotic Timing (Outpatient)	112	99%	97%	98%
Urinary Catheter Removal[2]	171	100%	97%	97%
Survey of Patients' Hospital Experiences				
Area Around Room 'Always' Quiet at Night	300+	47%	53%	61%
Doctors 'Always' Communicated Well	300+	82%	82%	82%
Home Recovery Information Given	300+	88%	88%	85%
Hospital Given 9 or 10 on 10 Point Scale	300+	74%	71%	71%
Meds 'Always' Explained Before Given	300+	69%	66%	64%
Nurses 'Always' Communicated Well	300+	83%	81%	79%
Pain 'Always' Well Controlled	300+	74%	70%	71%
Room and Bathroom 'Always' Clean	300+	78%	78%	73%
Timely Help 'Always' Received	300+	74%	69%	68%
Would Definitely Recommend Hospital	300+	79%	73%	71%
Use of Medical Imaging				
Cardiac Imaging Stress Test before Surgery	454	6.2%	5%	5.3%
Combination Abdominal CT Scan	588	7.3%	4.6%	10.5%
Combination Brain/Sinus CT Scan	518	2.3%	2%	2.7%
Combination Chest CT Scan	399	0.0%	0.8%	2.7%
Follow-up Mammogram/Ultrasound	1,415	9.0%	9.1%	8.8%
Lumbar Spine MRI for Low Back Pain	110	40.9%	32.1%	37.2%

Brattleboro Memorial Hospital

17 Belmont Ave Phone: 802-257-0341
Brattleboro, VT 05301 Fax: 802-257-8822
E-mail: info@bmhvt.org
URL: www.bmhvt.org
Type: Acute Care Hospitals Emergency Services: Yes
Ownership: Voluntary non-profit - Private Beds: 47

Key Personnel:
Chief of Medical Staff.......... David Albright, MD
Quality Assurance .... Corinne Bristol, RN
Cardiology.................. Mark Burke, MD
Anesthesiology............... Michael Burrell, MD
Radiology.................. Edward F Elliott Jr
Surgery .... Gregory Gadowski, MD
CEO/President............... Michael O Rogers

Measure	Cases	This Hosp.	State Avg.	U.S. Avg.
Blood Clot Prevention and Treatment				
Anticoagulation Overlap Therapy[2]	15	100%	98%	93%
ICU Venous Thromboembolism Prophylaxis[2]	42	90%	94%	92%
Incidence of Potentially Preventable VTE[2,7]	-	-	4%	10%
UFH with Dosages/Platelet Monitoring[1,2]	-	-	95%	97%
Venous Thromboembolism Prophylaxis[2]	119	93%	89%	85%
Warfarin Therapy Discharge Instructions[2]	13	92%	78%	75%
Chest Pain/Possible Heart Attack Care				
Aspirin Given Within 24 Hours of Arrival	77	97%	98%	96%
Fibrinolytic Meds Within 30 Min. of Arrival	14	71%	79%	58%
Average Time to ECG (minutes)	82	11	6	7
Average Time to Transfer (minutes)[7]	-	-	31	60

NOTE: Hospital profiles are in alphabetical order by state, then city, then hospital within the city; Rankings exclude hospitals with less than 25 cases except for patient surveys which excludes hospitals with less than 100 cases; (a) 100-299 cases; (1) The number of cases/patients is too few to report; (2) Data submitted were based on a sample of cases/patients; (3) Results are based on a shorter time period than required; (4) Data suppressed by CMS for one or more quarters; (5) Results are not available for this reporting period; (6) Fewer than 100 patients completed the HCAHPS survey; (7) No cases met the criteria for this measure; (8) The lower limit of the confidence interval cannot be calculated if the number of observed infections equals zero; (9) No data are available from the state/territory for this reporting period; (10) The scores shown reflect fewer than 50 completed surveys; (11) There were discrepancies in the data collection process; (12) This measure does not apply to this hospital for this reporting period; (13) Results cannot be calculated for this reporting period; (14) The results for this state are combined with nearby states to protect confidentiality; Please refer to the User's Guide for a full explanation of data.

Measure	Cases	This Hosp.	State Avg.	U.S. Avg.
Children's Asthma Care				
Received Home Management Plan of Care	-	-	-	88%
Received Reliever Medication	-	-	-	100%
Received Systemic Corticosteroids	-	-	-	100%
Emergency Department				
Admittance Decision Time (minutes)[2]	306	85	114	98
Head CT Results Within 45 Min. of Arrival[1]	-	-	45%	57%
Patients Who Left ER Before Being Seen	13,363	2%	2%	2%
Time from ER Arrival to Admit. (minutes)[2]	310	231	279	274
Time from ER Arrival to Discharge (minutes)	387	120	136	134
Time in ER Before Being Evaluated (minutes)	435	26	27	26
Time to Pain Meds for Fractures (minutes)	72	40	61	57
Heart Attack Care				
Aspirin Given at Discharge[1]	-	-	100%	99%
Fibrinolytic Meds Within 30 Min. of Arrival[7]	-	-	-	54%
PCI Within 90 Minutes of Arrival[7]	-	-	98%	96%
Statin Prescribed at Discharge[1]	-	-	99%	98%
Heart Failure Care				
ACE Inhibitor or ARB for LVSD[1]	-	-	96%	97%
Discharge Instructions Given	22	91%	94%	94%
Evaluation of LVS Function	29	97%	99%	99%
Medicare Spending				
Medicare Spending per Patient (ratio)	-	1.08	1.01	0.98
Pneumonia Care				
Appropriate Initial Antibiotic Given	46	98%	97%	95%
Blood Culture Timing	66	98%	98%	98%
Pregnancy and Delivery Care				
Newborn Deliveries Scheduled Early[2]	34	3%	4%	6%
Preventive Care				
Immunization for Influenza[2]	272	92%	93%	90%
Immunization for Pneumonia[2]	281	95%	94%	92%
Stroke Care				
Anticoagulation Therapy for Atrial Fibrillation[1]	-	-	96%	95%
Antithrombotic Therapy Timing	27	100%	92%	98%
Assessed for Rehabilitation	26	100%	96%	97%
Discharged on Antithrombotic Therapy	26	100%	99%	99%
Discharged on Statin Medication	21	100%	93%	94%
Thrombolytic Therapy Timing[7]	-	-	70%	66%
Venous Thromboembolism Prophylaxis	27	100%	92%	94%
Written Stroke Educational Materials Given[1]	-	-	83%	88%
Surgical Care Improvement Project				
Appropriate Beta Blocker Usage	72	99%	98%	98%
Appropriate VTP Within 24 Hours	223	100%	98%	98%
Controlled Postoperative Blood Glucose[7]	-	-	94%	97%
Perioperative Temperature Management	248	100%	100%	100%
Prophylactic Antibiotic Selection	194	99%	99%	99%
Prophylactic Antibiotic Selection (Outpatient)	55	100%	99%	98%
Prophylactic Antibiotic Stopped	188	100%	99%	98%
Prophylactic Antibiotic Timing	194	99%	98%	99%
Prophylactic Antibiotic Timing (Outpatient)	55	100%	97%	98%
Urinary Catheter Removal	98	99%	97%	97%
Survey of Patients' Hospital Experiences				
Area Around Room 'Always' Quiet at Night	300+	61%	53%	61%
Doctors 'Always' Communicated Well	300+	79%	82%	82%
Home Recovery Information Given	300+	86%	88%	85%
Hospital Given 9 or 10 on 10 Point Scale	300+	67%	71%	71%
Meds 'Always' Explained Before Given	300+	65%	66%	64%
Nurses 'Always' Communicated Well	300+	79%	81%	79%
Pain 'Always' Well Controlled	300+	72%	70%	71%
Room and Bathroom 'Always' Clean	300+	77%	78%	73%
Timely Help 'Always' Received	300+	73%	69%	68%
Would Definitely Recommend Hospital	300+	70%	73%	71%
Use of Medical Imaging				
Cardiac Imaging Stress Test before Surgery	172	4.1%	5%	5.3%
Combination Abdominal CT Scan	330	3.6%	4.6%	10.5%
Combination Brain/Sinus CT Scan	315	4.8%	2%	2.7%
Combination Chest CT Scan	201	0.5%	0.8%	2.7%
Follow-up Mammogram/Ultrasound	1,170	8.8%	9.1%	8.8%
Lumbar Spine MRI for Low Back Pain[1]	-	-	32.1%	37.2%

Fletcher Allen Hospital of Vermont

111 Colchester Ave
Burlington, VT 05401
Phone: 802-847-0000
Fax: 802-847-5540
URL: www.fletcherallen.org
Type: Acute Care Hospitals
Emergency Services: Yes
Ownership: Voluntary non-profit - Other
Beds: 562

Key Personnel:
Radiology. . . . . Steve Braff
President/CEO. . . . . John R. Brumsted, MD
Emergency Room . . . . Ramsey Herrington, MD
Chief of Medical Staff . . . . Stephen Leffler, MD
Operating Room. . . . . Stephen Shackford, MD

Measure	Cases	This Hosp.	State Avg.	U.S. Avg.
Blood Clot Prevention and Treatment				
Anticoagulation Overlap Therapy[2]	113	99%	98%	93%
ICU Venous Thromboembolism Prophylaxis[2]	107	89%	94%	92%
Incidence of Potentially Preventable VTE[2]	45	4%	4%	10%
UFH with Dosages/Platelet Monitoring[2]	103	93%	95%	97%
Venous Thromboembolism Prophylaxis[2]	281	94%	89%	85%
Warfarin Therapy Discharge Instructions[2]	95	62%	78%	75%
Chest Pain/Possible Heart Attack Care				
Aspirin Given Within 24 Hours of Arrival[5]	-	-	98%	96%
Fibrinolytic Meds Within 30 Min. of Arrival[5]	-	-	79%	58%
Average Time to ECG (minutes)[5]	-	-	6	7
Average Time to Transfer (minutes)[5]	-	-	31	60
Children's Asthma Care				
Received Home Management Plan of Care	-	-	-	88%
Received Reliever Medication	-	-	-	100%
Received Systemic Corticosteroids	-	-	-	100%
Emergency Department				
Admittance Decision Time (minutes)[2]	556	154	114	98
Head CT Results Within 45 Min. of Arrival[7]	-	-	45%	57%
Patients Who Left ER Before Being Seen	60,048	2%	2%	2%
Time from ER Arrival to Admit. (minutes)[2]	556	363	279	274
Time from ER Arrival to Discharge (minutes)	1,490	166	136	134
Time in ER Before Being Evaluated (minutes)	1,591	27	27	26
Time to Pain Meds for Fractures (minutes)	217	79	61	57
Heart Attack Care				
Aspirin Given at Discharge	897	100%	100%	99%
Fibrinolytic Meds Within 30 Min. of Arrival[7]	-	-	-	54%
PCI Within 90 Minutes of Arrival	57	98%	98%	96%
Statin Prescribed at Discharge	863	100%	99%	98%
Heart Failure Care				
ACE Inhibitor or ARB for LVSD	143	96%	96%	97%
Discharge Instructions Given	364	99%	94%	94%
Evaluation of LVS Function	469	100%	99%	99%
Medicare Spending				
Medicare Spending per Patient (ratio)	-	0.97	1.01	0.98
Pneumonia Care				
Appropriate Initial Antibiotic Given	127	94%	97%	95%
Blood Culture Timing	203	98%	98%	98%
Pregnancy and Delivery Care				
Newborn Deliveries Scheduled Early[2]	17	0%	4%	6%
Preventive Care				
Immunization for Influenza[2]	508	87%	93%	90%
Immunization for Pneumonia[2]	590	92%	94%	92%
Stroke Care				
Anticoagulation Therapy for Atrial Fibrillation[2]	20	100%	96%	95%
Antithrombotic Therapy Timing[2]	50	74%	92%	98%
Assessed for Rehabilitation[2]	97	97%	96%	97%
Discharged on Antithrombotic Therapy[2]	77	100%	99%	99%
Discharged on Statin Medication[2]	60	100%	93%	94%
Thrombolytic Therapy Timing[1,2]	-	-	70%	66%
Venous Thromboembolism Prophylaxis[2]	96	99%	92%	94%
Written Stroke Educational Materials Given[2]	54	98%	83%	88%
Surgical Care Improvement Project				
Appropriate Beta Blocker Usage[2]	224	99%	98%	98%
Appropriate VTP Within 24 Hours[2]	316	99%	98%	98%
Controlled Postoperative Blood Glucose[2]	125	94%	94%	97%
Perioperative Temperature Management[2]	424	100%	100%	100%
Prophylactic Antibiotic Selection[2]	402	99%	99%	99%
Prophylactic Antibiotic Selection (Outpatient)	959	99%	99%	98%
Prophylactic Antibiotic Stopped[2]	397	100%	99%	98%
Prophylactic Antibiotic Timing[2]	404	98%	98%	99%
Prophylactic Antibiotic Timing (Outpatient)	898	97%	97%	98%
Urinary Catheter Removal[2]	335	96%	97%	97%
Survey of Patients' Hospital Experiences				
Area Around Room 'Always' Quiet at Night	300+	40%	53%	61%
Doctors 'Always' Communicated Well	300+	77%	82%	82%
Home Recovery Information Given	300+	88%	88%	85%
Hospital Given 9 or 10 on 10 Point Scale	300+	66%	71%	71%
Meds 'Always' Explained Before Given	300+	61%	66%	64%
Nurses 'Always' Communicated Well	300+	78%	81%	79%
Pain 'Always' Well Controlled	300+	69%	70%	71%
Room and Bathroom 'Always' Clean	300+	67%	78%	73%
Timely Help 'Always' Received	300+	66%	69%	68%
Would Definitely Recommend Hospital	300+	74%	73%	71%
Use of Medical Imaging				
Cardiac Imaging Stress Test before Surgery	797	3.5%	5%	5.3%
Combination Abdominal CT Scan	1,719	4.5%	4.6%	10.5%
Combination Brain/Sinus CT Scan	985	1.5%	2%	2.7%
Combination Chest CT Scan	1,733	0.3%	0.8%	2.7%
Follow-up Mammogram/Ultrasound	5,214	9.8%	9.1%	8.8%
Lumbar Spine MRI for Low Back Pain	327	21.1%	32.1%	37.2%

Porter Hospital

115 Porter Drive
Middlebury, VT 05753
Phone: 802-388-4701
Fax: 802-388-8859
URL: www.portermedical.org
Type: Critical Access Hospitals
Emergency Services: Yes
Ownership: Voluntary non-profit - Private
Beds: 45

Key Personnel:
Chief of Medical Staff . . . . Rebecca Adams, MD
Infection Control. . . . . Sheila Boise
Pediatric Ambulatory Care . . . . . . Johana Brakeley, MD
Pediatric In-Patient Care . . . . Johana Brakeley, MD
Radiology. . . . . C Wade Cobb
Quality Assurance . . . . Lyn Farr

Measure	Cases	This Hosp.	State Avg.	U.S. Avg.
Blood Clot Prevention and Treatment				
Anticoagulation Overlap Therapy[5]	-	-	98%	93%
ICU Venous Thromboembolism Prophylaxis[5]	-	-	94%	92%
Incidence of Potentially Preventable VTE[5]	-	-	4%	10%
UFH with Dosages/Platelet Monitoring[5]	-	-	95%	97%
Venous Thromboembolism Prophylaxis[5]	-	-	89%	85%
Warfarin Therapy Discharge Instructions[5]	-	-	78%	75%
Chest Pain/Possible Heart Attack Care				
Aspirin Given Within 24 Hours of Arrival	-	-	98%	96%
Fibrinolytic Meds Within 30 Min. of Arrival	-	-	79%	58%
Average Time to ECG (minutes)	-	-	6	7
Average Time to Transfer (minutes)	-	-	31	60
Children's Asthma Care				
Received Home Management Plan of Care	-	-	-	88%
Received Reliever Medication	-	-	-	100%
Received Systemic Corticosteroids	-	-	-	100%
Emergency Department				
Admittance Decision Time (minutes)[5]	-	-	114	98
Head CT Results Within 45 Min. of Arrival	-	-	45%	57%
Patients Who Left ER Before Being Seen	-	-	2%	2%
Time from ER Arrival to Admit. (minutes)[5]	-	-	279	274
Time from ER Arrival to Discharge (minutes)	-	-	136	134
Time in ER Before Being Evaluated (minutes)	-	-	27	26
Time to Pain Meds for Fractures (minutes)	-	-	61	57
Heart Attack Care				
Aspirin Given at Discharge[1,3]	-	-	100%	99%
Fibrinolytic Meds Within 30 Min. of Arrival[3,7]	-	-	-	54%
PCI Within 90 Minutes of Arrival[3,7]	-	-	98%	96%
Statin Prescribed at Discharge[1,3]	-	-	99%	98%
Heart Failure Care				
ACE Inhibitor or ARB for LVSD[1]	-	-	96%	97%
Discharge Instructions Given	45	98%	94%	94%
Evaluation of LVS Function	54	98%	99%	99%
Medicare Spending				
Medicare Spending per Patient (ratio)	-	-	1.01	0.98
Pneumonia Care				
Appropriate Initial Antibiotic Given	98	98%	97%	95%
Blood Culture Timing	107	98%	98%	98%

NOTE: Hospital profiles are in alphabetical order by state, then city, then hospital within the city; Rankings exclude hospitals with less than 25 cases except for patient surveys which excludes hospitals with less than 100 cases; (a) 100-299 cases; (1) The number of cases/patients is too few to report; (2) Data submitted were based on a sample of cases/patients; (3) Results are based on a shorter time period than required; (4) Data suppressed by CMS for one or more quarters; (5) Results are not available for this reporting period; (6) Fewer than 100 patients completed the HCAHPS survey; (7) No cases met the criteria for this measure; (8) The lower limit of the confidence interval cannot be calculated if the number of observed infections equals zero; (9) No data are available from the state/territory for this reporting period; (10) The scores shown reflect fewer than 50 completed surveys; (11) There were discrepancies in the data collection process; (12) This measure does not apply to this hospital for this reporting period; (13) Results cannot be calculated for this reporting period; (14) The results for this state are combined with nearby states to protect confidentiality; Please refer to the User's Guide for a full explanation of data.

Measure	Cases	This Hosp.	State Avg.	U.S. Avg.
Pregnancy and Delivery Care				
Newborn Deliveries Scheduled Early[5]	-	-	4%	6%
Preventive Care				
Immunization for Influenza[5]	-	-	93%	90%
Immunization for Pneumonia[5]	-	-	94%	92%
Stroke Care				
Anticoagulation Therapy for Atrial Fibrillation[5]	-	-	96%	95%
Antithrombotic Therapy Timing[5]	-	-	92%	98%
Assessed for Rehabilitation[5]	-	-	96%	97%
Discharged on Antithrombotic Therapy[5]	-	-	99%	99%
Discharged on Statin Medication[5]	-	-	93%	94%
Thrombolytic Therapy Timing[5]	-	-	70%	66%
Venous Thromboembolism Prophylaxis[5]	-	-	92%	94%
Written Stroke Educational Materials Given[5]	-	-	83%	88%
Surgical Care Improvement Project				
Appropriate Beta Blocker Usage[2]	41	100%	98%	98%
Appropriate VTP Within 24 Hours[2]	150	100%	98%	98%
Controlled Postoperative Blood Glucose[2,7]	-	-	94%	97%
Perioperative Temperature Management[2]	167	99%	100%	100%
Prophylactic Antibiotic Selection[2]	127	98%	99%	99%
Prophylactic Antibiotic Selection (Outpatient)	-	-	99%	98%
Prophylactic Antibiotic Stopped[2]	123	99%	99%	98%
Prophylactic Antibiotic Timing[2]	128	99%	98%	99%
Prophylactic Antibiotic Timing (Outpatient)	-	-	97%	98%
Urinary Catheter Removal[2]	136	96%	97%	97%
Survey of Patients' Hospital Experiences				
Area Around Room 'Always' Quiet at Night	300+	51%	53%	61%
Doctors 'Always' Communicated Well	300+	82%	82%	82%
Home Recovery Information Given	300+	88%	88%	85%
Hospital Given 9 or 10 on 10 Point Scale	300+	68%	71%	71%
Meds 'Always' Explained Before Given	300+	67%	66%	64%
Nurses 'Always' Communicated Well	300+	80%	81%	79%
Pain 'Always' Well Controlled	300+	69%	70%	71%
Room and Bathroom 'Always' Clean	300+	74%	78%	73%
Timely Help 'Always' Received	300+	64%	69%	68%
Would Definitely Recommend Hospital	300+	70%	73%	71%
Use of Medical Imaging				
Cardiac Imaging Stress Test before Surgery	-	-	5%	5.3%
Combination Abdominal CT Scan	-	-	4.6%	10.5%
Combination Brain/Sinus CT Scan	-	-	2%	2.7%
Combination Chest CT Scan	-	-	0.8%	2.7%
Follow-up Mammogram/Ultrasound	-	-	9.1%	8.8%
Lumbar Spine MRI for Low Back Pain	-	-	32.1%	37.2%

Copley Hospital

528 Washington Highway
Morrisville, VT 05661
Phone: 802-888-4231
Fax: 802-888-8223
E-mail: pwright@chsi.org
URL: www.copleyvt.org
Type: Critical Access Hospitals
Emergency Services: Yes
Ownership: Voluntary non-profit - Private
Beds: 53

Key Personnel:
Radiology. . . . . Richard Bennum
Quality Assurance . . . . Joseph Falworth
Operating Room. . . . . Patricia Jaqua
CEO/President. . . . . Melvyn Patashnick
Chief of Medical Staff. . . . . Joel Silverstein, MD
Infection Control. . . . . Carol Wood-Koob, RN

Measure	Cases	This Hosp.	State Avg.	U.S. Avg.
Blood Clot Prevention and Treatment				
Anticoagulation Overlap Therapy[5]	-	-	98%	93%
ICU Venous Thromboembolism Prophylaxis[5]	-	-	94%	92%
Incidence of Potentially Preventable VTE[5]	-	-	4%	10%
UFH with Dosages/Platelet Monitoring[5]	-	-	95%	97%
Venous Thromboembolism Prophylaxis[5]	-	-	89%	85%
Warfarin Therapy Discharge Instructions[5]	-	-	78%	75%
Chest Pain/Possible Heart Attack Care				
Aspirin Given Within 24 Hours of Arrival	-	-	98%	96%
Fibrinolytic Meds Within 30 Min. of Arrival	-	-	79%	58%
Average Time to ECG (minutes)	-	-	6	7
Average Time to Transfer (minutes)	-	-	31	60
Children's Asthma Care				
Received Home Management Plan of Care	-	-	-	88%
Received Reliever Medication	-	-	-	100%
Received Systemic Corticosteroids	-	-	-	100%
Emergency Department				
Admittance Decision Time (minutes)[5]	-	-	114	98
Head CT Results Within 45 Min. of Arrival	-	-	45%	57%
Patients Who Left ER Before Being Seen	-	-	2%	2%
Time from ER Arrival to Admit. (minutes)[5]	-	-	279	274
Time from ER Arrival to Discharge (minutes)	-	-	136	134
Time in ER Before Being Evaluated (minutes)	-	-	27	26
Time to Pain Meds for Fractures (minutes)	-	-	61	57
Heart Attack Care				
Aspirin Given at Discharge[1]	-	-	100%	99%
Fibrinolytic Meds Within 30 Min. of Arrival[7]	-	-	-	54%
PCI Within 90 Minutes of Arrival[7]	-	-	98%	96%
Statin Prescribed at Discharge[1]	-	-	99%	98%
Heart Failure Care				
ACE Inhibitor or ARB for LVSD[1]	-	-	96%	97%
Discharge Instructions Given	33	70%	94%	94%
Evaluation of LVS Function	41	100%	99%	99%
Medicare Spending				
Medicare Spending per Patient (ratio)	-	-	1.01	0.98
Pneumonia Care				
Appropriate Initial Antibiotic Given	47	94%	97%	95%
Blood Culture Timing	46	96%	98%	98%
Pregnancy and Delivery Care				
Newborn Deliveries Scheduled Early[5]	-	-	4%	6%
Preventive Care				
Immunization for Influenza[5]	-	-	93%	90%
Immunization for Pneumonia[5]	-	-	94%	92%
Stroke Care				
Anticoagulation Therapy for Atrial Fibrillation[5]	-	-	96%	95%
Antithrombotic Therapy Timing[5]	-	-	92%	98%
Assessed for Rehabilitation[5]	-	-	96%	97%
Discharged on Antithrombotic Therapy[5]	-	-	99%	99%
Discharged on Statin Medication[5]	-	-	93%	94%
Thrombolytic Therapy Timing[5]	-	-	70%	66%
Venous Thromboembolism Prophylaxis[5]	-	-	92%	94%
Written Stroke Educational Materials Given[5]	-	-	83%	88%
Surgical Care Improvement Project				
Appropriate Beta Blocker Usage	50	96%	98%	98%
Appropriate VTP Within 24 Hours	188	97%	98%	98%
Controlled Postoperative Blood Glucose[7]	-	-	94%	97%
Perioperative Temperature Management	211	100%	100%	100%
Prophylactic Antibiotic Selection	195	99%	99%	99%
Prophylactic Antibiotic Selection (Outpatient)	-	-	99%	98%
Prophylactic Antibiotic Stopped	192	100%	99%	98%
Prophylactic Antibiotic Timing	195	97%	98%	99%
Prophylactic Antibiotic Timing (Outpatient)	-	-	97%	98%
Urinary Catheter Removal	190	99%	97%	97%
Survey of Patients' Hospital Experiences				
Area Around Room 'Always' Quiet at Night	300+	58%	53%	61%
Doctors 'Always' Communicated Well	300+	85%	82%	82%
Home Recovery Information Given	300+	88%	88%	85%
Hospital Given 9 or 10 on 10 Point Scale	300+	76%	71%	71%
Meds 'Always' Explained Before Given	300+	68%	66%	64%
Nurses 'Always' Communicated Well	300+	83%	81%	79%
Pain 'Always' Well Controlled	300+	75%	70%	71%
Room and Bathroom 'Always' Clean	300+	79%	78%	73%
Timely Help 'Always' Received	300+	76%	69%	68%
Would Definitely Recommend Hospital	300+	77%	73%	71%
Use of Medical Imaging				
Cardiac Imaging Stress Test before Surgery	-	-	5%	5.3%
Combination Abdominal CT Scan	-	-	4.6%	10.5%
Combination Brain/Sinus CT Scan	-	-	2%	2.7%
Combination Chest CT Scan	-	-	0.8%	2.7%
Follow-up Mammogram/Ultrasound	-	-	9.1%	8.8%
Lumbar Spine MRI for Low Back Pain	-	-	32.1%	37.2%

North Country Hospital & Health Center

189 Prouty Drive
Newport, VT 05855
Phone: 802-334-7331
Fax: 802-334-4510
URL: www.nchsi.org
Type: Critical Access Hospitals
Emergency Services: Yes
Ownership: Voluntary non-profit - Private
Beds: 25

Key Personnel:
Intensive Care Unit. . . . . Chris Convard
Pediatric In-Patient Care . . . . Kathy Fabian, RN
CEO/President. . . . . Claudio Fort
Quality Assurance . . . . Stephen Halikas
Infection Control. . . . . Jean Holcomb
Emergency Room . . . . R Ron Holland, MD
Patient Relations . . . . Carol Loux
Radiology. . . . . Steven Perlin

Measure	Cases	This Hosp.	State Avg.	U.S. Avg.
Blood Clot Prevention and Treatment				
Anticoagulation Overlap Therapy[5]	-	-	98%	93%
ICU Venous Thromboembolism Prophylaxis[5]	-	-	94%	92%
Incidence of Potentially Preventable VTE[5]	-	-	4%	10%
UFH with Dosages/Platelet Monitoring[5]	-	-	95%	97%
Venous Thromboembolism Prophylaxis[5]	-	-	89%	85%
Warfarin Therapy Discharge Instructions[5]	-	-	78%	75%
Chest Pain/Possible Heart Attack Care				
Aspirin Given Within 24 Hours of Arrival	-	-	98%	96%
Fibrinolytic Meds Within 30 Min. of Arrival	-	-	79%	58%
Average Time to ECG (minutes)	-	-	6	7
Average Time to Transfer (minutes)	-	-	31	60
Children's Asthma Care				
Received Home Management Plan of Care	-	-	-	88%
Received Reliever Medication	-	-	-	100%
Received Systemic Corticosteroids	-	-	-	100%
Emergency Department				
Admittance Decision Time (minutes)[5]	-	-	114	98
Head CT Results Within 45 Min. of Arrival	-	-	45%	57%
Patients Who Left ER Before Being Seen	-	-	2%	2%
Time from ER Arrival to Admit. (minutes)[5]	-	-	279	274
Time from ER Arrival to Discharge (minutes)	-	-	136	134
Time in ER Before Being Evaluated (minutes)	-	-	27	26
Time to Pain Meds for Fractures (minutes)	-	-	61	57
Heart Attack Care				
Aspirin Given at Discharge[1]	-	-	100%	99%
Fibrinolytic Meds Within 30 Min. of Arrival[7]	-	-	-	54%
PCI Within 90 Minutes of Arrival[7]	-	-	98%	96%
Statin Prescribed at Discharge[1]	-	-	99%	98%
Heart Failure Care				
ACE Inhibitor or ARB for LVSD[1]	-	-	96%	97%
Discharge Instructions Given	24	96%	94%	94%
Evaluation of LVS Function	40	100%	99%	99%
Medicare Spending				
Medicare Spending per Patient (ratio)	-	-	1.01	0.98
Pneumonia Care				
Appropriate Initial Antibiotic Given	35	94%	97%	95%
Blood Culture Timing	69	100%	98%	98%
Pregnancy and Delivery Care				
Newborn Deliveries Scheduled Early[5]	-	-	4%	6%
Preventive Care				
Immunization for Influenza[5]	-	-	93%	90%
Immunization for Pneumonia[5]	-	-	94%	92%
Stroke Care				
Anticoagulation Therapy for Atrial Fibrillation[5]	-	-	96%	95%
Antithrombotic Therapy Timing[5]	-	-	92%	98%
Assessed for Rehabilitation[5]	-	-	96%	97%
Discharged on Antithrombotic Therapy[5]	-	-	99%	99%
Discharged on Statin Medication[5]	-	-	93%	94%
Thrombolytic Therapy Timing[5]	-	-	70%	66%
Venous Thromboembolism Prophylaxis[5]	-	-	92%	94%
Written Stroke Educational Materials Given[5]	-	-	83%	88%
Surgical Care Improvement Project				
Appropriate Beta Blocker Usage	29	90%	98%	98%
Appropriate VTP Within 24 Hours	82	90%	98%	98%
Controlled Postoperative Blood Glucose[7]	-	-	94%	97%
Perioperative Temperature Management	96	100%	100%	100%
Prophylactic Antibiotic Selection	73	99%	99%	99%

NOTE: Hospital profiles are in alphabetical order by state, then city, then hospital within the city; Rankings exclude hospitals with less than 25 cases except for patient surveys which excludes hospitals with less than 100 cases; (a) 100-299 cases; (1) The number of cases/patients is too few to report; (2) Data submitted were based on a sample of cases/patients; (3) Results are based on a shorter time period than required; (4) Data suppressed by CMS for one or more quarters; (5) Results are not available for this reporting period; (6) Fewer than 100 patients completed the HCAHPS survey; (7) No cases met the criteria for this measure; (8) The lower limit of the confidence interval cannot be calculated if the number of observed infections equals zero; (9) No data are available from the state/territory for this reporting period; (10) The scores shown reflect fewer than 50 completed surveys; (11) There were discrepancies in the data collection process; (12) This measure does not apply to this hospital for this reporting period; (13) Results cannot be calculated for this reporting period; (14) The results for this state are combined with nearby states to protect confidentiality; Please refer to the User's Guide for a full explanation of data.

Prophylactic Antibiotic Selection (Outpatient)	-	-	99%	98%
Prophylactic Antibiotic Stopped	72	99%	99%	98%
Prophylactic Antibiotic Timing	73	100%	98%	99%
Prophylactic Antibiotic Timing (Outpatient)	-	-	97%	98%
Urinary Catheter Removal	33	70%	97%	97%
Survey of Patients' Hospital Experiences				
Area Around Room 'Always' Quiet at Night	300+	52%	53%	61%
Doctors 'Always' Communicated Well	300+	83%	82%	82%
Home Recovery Information Given	300+	90%	88%	85%
Hospital Given 9 or 10 on 10 Point Scale	300+	67%	71%	71%
Meds 'Always' Explained Before Given	300+	65%	66%	64%
Nurses 'Always' Communicated Well	300+	80%	81%	79%
Pain 'Always' Well Controlled	300+	68%	70%	71%
Room and Bathroom 'Always' Clean	300+	78%	78%	73%
Timely Help 'Always' Received	300+	74%	69%	68%
Would Definitely Recommend Hospital	300+	68%	73%	71%
Use of Medical Imaging				
Cardiac Imaging Stress Test before Surgery	-	-	5%	5.3%
Combination Abdominal CT Scan	-	-	4.6%	10.5%
Combination Brain/Sinus CT Scan	-	-	2%	2.7%
Combination Chest CT Scan	-	-	0.8%	2.7%
Follow-up Mammogram/Ultrasound	-	-	9.1%	8.8%
Lumbar Spine MRI for Low Back Pain	-	-	32.1%	37.2%

Gifford Medical Center

44 South Main Street
Randolph, VT 05060
Phone: 802-728-4441
Fax: 802-728-4245
E-mail: info@giffordmed.org
URL: www.giffordmed.org
Type: Critical Access Hospitals
Emergency Services: Yes
Ownership: Voluntary non-profit - Other
Beds: 55

Key Personnel:
Chief of Medical Staff . . . . Louis DiNicola, MD
Emergency Room . . . . Larry Ermold
Chair/CEO . . . . Gus Meyer
Infection Control . . . . D Simpson, RN
Radiology . . . . Erin M Tsai
CEO/President . . . . Joseph Woodin

Measure	Cases	This Hosp.	State Avg.	U.S. Avg.
Blood Clot Prevention and Treatment				
Anticoagulation Overlap Therapy[5]	-	-	98%	93%
ICU Venous Thromboembolism Prophylaxis[5]	-	-	94%	92%
Incidence of Potentially Preventable VTE[5]	-	-	4%	10%
UFH with Dosages/Platelet Monitoring[5]	-	-	95%	97%
Venous Thromboembolism Prophylaxis[5]	-	-	89%	85%
Warfarin Therapy Discharge Instructions[5]	-	-	78%	75%
Chest Pain/Possible Heart Attack Care				
Aspirin Given Within 24 Hours of Arrival	-	-	98%	96%
Fibrinolytic Meds Within 30 Min. of Arrival	-	-	79%	58%
Average Time to ECG (minutes)	-	-	6	7
Average Time to Transfer (minutes)	-	-	31	60
Children's Asthma Care				
Received Home Management Plan of Care	-	-	-	88%
Received Reliever Medication	-	-	-	100%
Received Systemic Corticosteroids	-	-	-	100%
Emergency Department				
Admittance Decision Time (minutes)[5]	-	-	114	98
Head CT Results Within 45 Min. of Arrival	-	-	45%	57%
Patients Who Left ER Before Being Seen	-	-	2%	2%
Time from ER Arrival to Admit. (minutes)[5]	-	-	279	274
Time from ER Arrival to Discharge (minutes)	-	-	136	134
Time in ER Before Being Evaluated (minutes)	-	-	27	26
Time to Pain Meds for Fractures (minutes)	-	-	61	57
Heart Attack Care				
Aspirin Given at Discharge[1]	-	-	100%	99%
Fibrinolytic Meds Within 30 Min. of Arrival[7]	-	-	-	54%
PCI Within 90 Minutes of Arrival[7]	-	-	98%	96%
Statin Prescribed at Discharge[1]	-	-	99%	98%
Heart Failure Care				
ACE Inhibitor or ARB for LVSD[1]	-	-	96%	97%
Discharge Instructions Given	23	100%	94%	94%
Evaluation of LVS Function	35	100%	99%	99%
Medicare Spending				
Medicare Spending per Patient (ratio)	-	-	1.01	0.98
Pneumonia Care				
Appropriate Initial Antibiotic Given	43	98%	97%	95%
Blood Culture Timing	40	100%	98%	98%
Pregnancy and Delivery Care				
Newborn Deliveries Scheduled Early[5]	-	-	4%	6%
Preventive Care				
Immunization for Influenza[5]	-	-	93%	90%
Immunization for Pneumonia[5]	-	-	94%	92%
Stroke Care				
Anticoagulation Therapy for Atrial Fibrillation[5]	-	-	96%	95%
Antithrombotic Therapy Timing[5]	-	-	92%	98%
Assessed for Rehabilitation[5]	-	-	96%	97%
Discharged on Antithrombotic Therapy[5]	-	-	99%	99%
Discharged on Statin Medication[5]	-	-	93%	94%
Thrombolytic Therapy Timing[5]	-	-	70%	66%
Venous Thromboembolism Prophylaxis[5]	-	-	92%	94%
Written Stroke Educational Materials Given[5]	-	-	83%	88%
Surgical Care Improvement Project				
Appropriate Beta Blocker Usage	14	71%	98%	98%
Appropriate VTP Within 24 Hours	53	100%	98%	98%
Controlled Postoperative Blood Glucose[7]	-	-	94%	97%
Perioperative Temperature Management	58	100%	100%	100%
Prophylactic Antibiotic Selection	55	100%	99%	99%
Prophylactic Antibiotic Selection (Outpatient)	-	-	99%	98%
Prophylactic Antibiotic Stopped	54	94%	99%	98%
Prophylactic Antibiotic Timing	55	93%	98%	99%
Prophylactic Antibiotic Timing (Outpatient)	-	-	97%	98%
Urinary Catheter Removal	51	100%	97%	97%
Survey of Patients' Hospital Experiences				
Area Around Room 'Always' Quiet at Night	300+	54%	53%	61%
Doctors 'Always' Communicated Well	300+	80%	82%	82%
Home Recovery Information Given	300+	89%	88%	85%
Hospital Given 9 or 10 on 10 Point Scale	300+	71%	71%	71%
Meds 'Always' Explained Before Given	300+	64%	66%	64%
Nurses 'Always' Communicated Well	300+	78%	81%	79%
Pain 'Always' Well Controlled	300+	65%	70%	71%
Room and Bathroom 'Always' Clean	300+	72%	78%	73%
Timely Help 'Always' Received	300+	64%	69%	68%
Would Definitely Recommend Hospital	300+	75%	73%	71%
Use of Medical Imaging				
Cardiac Imaging Stress Test before Surgery	-	-	5%	5.3%
Combination Abdominal CT Scan	-	-	4.6%	10.5%
Combination Brain/Sinus CT Scan	-	-	2%	2.7%
Combination Chest CT Scan	-	-	0.8%	2.7%
Follow-up Mammogram/Ultrasound	-	-	9.1%	8.8%
Lumbar Spine MRI for Low Back Pain	-	-	32.1%	37.2%

Rutland Regional Medical Center

160 Allen St
Rutland, VT 05701
Phone: 802-775-7111
Fax: 802-747-6207
URL: www.rrmc.org
Type: Acute Care Hospitals
Emergency Services: Yes
Ownership: Voluntary non-profit - Other
Beds: 188

Key Personnel:
Radiology . . . . Jean-Christophe Bieb, MD
CEO/President . . . . Thomas W Huebner
Chief of Medical Staff . . . . Richard D Lovett, MD
Quality Assurance . . . . Linda McElhinney
Pediatric Ambulatory Care . . . . . . David Schneider, DO
Pediatric In-Patient Care . . . . David Schneider, DO
Operating Room . . . . Carol Welsh, RN

Measure	Cases	This Hosp.	State Avg.	U.S. Avg.
Blood Clot Prevention and Treatment				
Anticoagulation Overlap Therapy[2]	59	97%	98%	93%
ICU Venous Thromboembolism Prophylaxis[2]	22	100%	94%	92%
Incidence of Potentially Preventable VTE[1,2]	-	-	4%	10%
UFH with Dosages/Platelet Monitoring[2]	12	100%	95%	97%
Venous Thromboembolism Prophylaxis[2]	338	73%	89%	85%
Warfarin Therapy Discharge Instructions[2]	51	92%	78%	75%
Chest Pain/Possible Heart Attack Care				
Aspirin Given Within 24 Hours of Arrival	57	98%	98%	96%
Fibrinolytic Meds Within 30 Min. of Arrival	14	79%	79%	58%
Average Time to ECG (minutes)	58	7	6	7
Average Time to Transfer (minutes)[1]	-	-	31	60
Children's Asthma Care				
Received Home Management Plan of Care	-	-	-	88%
Received Reliever Medication	-	-	-	100%
Received Systemic Corticosteroids	-	-	-	100%
Emergency Department				
Admittance Decision Time (minutes)[2]	609	109	114	98
Head CT Results Within 45 Min. of Arrival	17	53%	45%	57%
Patients Who Left ER Before Being Seen	35,073	4%	2%	2%
Time from ER Arrival to Admit. (minutes)[2]	619	282	279	274
Time from ER Arrival to Discharge (minutes)	382	145	136	134
Time in ER Before Being Evaluated (minutes)	413	42	27	26
Time to Pain Meds for Fractures (minutes)	99	74	61	57
Heart Attack Care				
Aspirin Given at Discharge	24	100%	100%	99%
Fibrinolytic Meds Within 30 Min. of Arrival[7]	-	-	-	54%
PCI Within 90 Minutes of Arrival[7]	-	-	98%	96%
Statin Prescribed at Discharge	18	100%	99%	98%
Heart Failure Care				
ACE Inhibitor or ARB for LVSD	43	100%	96%	97%
Discharge Instructions Given	76	97%	94%	94%
Evaluation of LVS Function	90	100%	99%	99%
Medicare Spending				
Medicare Spending per Patient (ratio)	-	0.99	1.01	0.98
Pneumonia Care				
Appropriate Initial Antibiotic Given	122	96%	97%	95%
Blood Culture Timing	126	98%	98%	98%
Pregnancy and Delivery Care				
Newborn Deliveries Scheduled Early	18	0%	4%	6%
Preventive Care				
Immunization for Influenza[2]	527	95%	93%	90%
Immunization for Pneumonia[2]	728	95%	94%	92%
Stroke Care				
Anticoagulation Therapy for Atrial Fibrillation	11	91%	96%	95%
Antithrombotic Therapy Timing	47	98%	92%	98%
Assessed for Rehabilitation	53	94%	96%	97%
Discharged on Antithrombotic Therapy	51	100%	99%	99%
Discharged on Statin Medication	37	73%	93%	94%
Thrombolytic Therapy Timing[1]	-	-	70%	66%
Venous Thromboembolism Prophylaxis	45	67%	92%	94%
Written Stroke Educational Materials Given	33	82%	83%	88%
Surgical Care Improvement Project				
Appropriate Beta Blocker Usage[2]	168	98%	98%	98%
Appropriate VTP Within 24 Hours[2]	467	99%	98%	98%
Controlled Postoperative Blood Glucose[2,7]	-	-	94%	97%
Perioperative Temperature Management[2]	571	100%	100%	100%
Prophylactic Antibiotic Selection[2]	436	99%	99%	99%
Prophylactic Antibiotic Selection (Outpatient)	119	99%	99%	98%
Prophylactic Antibiotic Stopped[2]	428	100%	99%	98%
Prophylactic Antibiotic Timing[2]	437	100%	98%	99%
Prophylactic Antibiotic Timing (Outpatient)	129	90%	97%	98%
Urinary Catheter Removal[2]	256	99%	97%	97%
Survey of Patients' Hospital Experiences				
Area Around Room 'Always' Quiet at Night	300+	50%	53%	61%
Doctors 'Always' Communicated Well	300+	83%	82%	82%
Home Recovery Information Given	300+	89%	88%	85%
Hospital Given 9 or 10 on 10 Point Scale	300+	70%	71%	71%
Meds 'Always' Explained Before Given	300+	68%	66%	64%
Nurses 'Always' Communicated Well	300+	85%	81%	79%
Pain 'Always' Well Controlled	300+	76%	70%	71%
Room and Bathroom 'Always' Clean	300+	78%	78%	73%
Timely Help 'Always' Received	300+	75%	69%	68%
Would Definitely Recommend Hospital	300+	70%	73%	71%
Use of Medical Imaging				
Cardiac Imaging Stress Test before Surgery	513	6.4%	5%	5.3%
Combination Abdominal CT Scan	752	5.7%	4.6%	10.5%
Combination Brain/Sinus CT Scan	699	2.7%	2%	2.7%
Combination Chest CT Scan	605	3.1%	0.8%	2.7%
Follow-up Mammogram/Ultrasound	2,253	4.9%	9.1%	8.8%
Lumbar Spine MRI for Low Back Pain	175	32.0%	32.1%	37.2%

NOTE: Hospital profiles are in alphabetical order by state, then city, then hospital within the city; Rankings exclude hospitals with less than 25 cases except for patient surveys which excludes hospitals with less than 100 cases; (a) 100-299 cases; (1) The number of cases/patients is too few to report; (2) Data submitted were based on a sample of cases/patients; (3) Results are based on a shorter time period than required; (4) Data suppressed by CMS for one or more quarters; (5) Results are not available for this reporting period; (6) Fewer than 100 patients completed the HCAHPS survey; (7) No cases met the criteria for this measure; (8) The lower limit of the confidence interval cannot be calculated if the number of observed infections equals zero; (9) No data are available from the state/territory for this reporting period; (10) The scores shown reflect fewer than 50 completed surveys; (11) There were discrepancies in the data collection process; (12) This measure does not apply to this hospital for this reporting period; (13) Results cannot be calculated for this reporting period; (14) The results for this state are combined with nearby states to protect confidentiality; Please refer to the User's Guide for a full explanation of data.

Northwestern Medical Center

133 Fairfield Street
Saint Albans, VT 05478
Phone: 802-524-5911
Fax: 802-524-1238
E-mail: insights@nmcinc.org
URL: www.northwesternmedicalcenter.org
Type: Acute Care Hospitals
Emergency Services: Yes
Ownership: Voluntary non-profit - Other
Beds: 70

Key Personnel:

CEO . . . . Jill Berry Bowen
Quality Assurance . . . . Jane Catton
Chief of Medical Staff . . . . James Duncan
Radiology. . . . . Luis Gonzalez
Emergency Room . . . . Ed Haak, MD

Measure	Cases	This Hosp.	State Avg.	U.S. Avg.
Blood Clot Prevention and Treatment				
Anticoagulation Overlap Therapy[2]	13	100%	98%	93%
ICU Venous Thromboembolism Prophylaxis[2]	14	100%	94%	92%
Incidence of Potentially Preventable VTE[1,2]	-	-	4%	10%
UFH with Dosages/Platelet Monitoring[1,2]	-	-	95%	97%
Venous Thromboembolism Prophylaxis[2]	189	95%	89%	85%
Warfarin Therapy Discharge Instructions[2]	11	100%	78%	75%
Chest Pain/Possible Heart Attack Care				
Aspirin Given Within 24 Hours of Arrival	188	99%	98%	96%
Fibrinolytic Meds Within 30 Min. of Arrival[7]	-	-	79%	58%
Average Time to ECG (minutes)	192	2	6	7
Average Time to Transfer (minutes)	13	27	31	60
Children's Asthma Care				
Received Home Management Plan of Care	-	-	-	88%
Received Reliever Medication	-	-	-	100%
Received Systemic Corticosteroids	-	-	-	100%
Emergency Department				
Admittance Decision Time (minutes)[2]	318	43	114	98
Head CT Results Within 45 Min. of Arrival[1]	-	-	45%	57%
Patients Who Left ER Before Being Seen	29,165	0%	2%	2%
Time from ER Arrival to Admit. (minutes)[2]	318	205	279	274
Time from ER Arrival to Discharge (minutes)	388	97	136	134
Time in ER Before Being Evaluated (minutes)	410	18	27	26
Time to Pain Meds for Fractures (minutes)	86	46	61	57
Heart Attack Care				
Aspirin Given at Discharge[1]	-	-	100%	99%
Fibrinolytic Meds Within 30 Min. of Arrival[7]	-	-	-	54%
PCI Within 90 Minutes of Arrival[7]	-	-	98%	96%
Statin Prescribed at Discharge[1]	-	-	99%	98%
Heart Failure Care				
ACE Inhibitor or ARB for LVSD[1]	-	-	96%	97%
Discharge Instructions Given	27	96%	94%	94%
Evaluation of LVS Function	39	100%	99%	99%
Medicare Spending				
Medicare Spending per Patient (ratio)	-	0.94	1.01	0.98
Pneumonia Care				
Appropriate Initial Antibiotic Given	93	99%	97%	95%
Blood Culture Timing	122	99%	98%	98%
Pregnancy and Delivery Care				
Newborn Deliveries Scheduled Early	34	6%	4%	6%
Preventive Care				
Immunization for Influenza[2]	257	96%	93%	90%
Immunization for Pneumonia[2]	280	96%	94%	92%
Stroke Care				
Anticoagulation Therapy for Atrial Fibrillation[1]	-	-	96%	95%
Antithrombotic Therapy Timing	22	100%	92%	98%
Assessed for Rehabilitation	24	100%	96%	97%
Discharged on Antithrombotic Therapy	22	95%	99%	99%
Discharged on Statin Medication	15	100%	93%	94%
Thrombolytic Therapy Timing[1]	-	-	70%	66%
Venous Thromboembolism Prophylaxis	22	91%	92%	94%
Written Stroke Educational Materials Given[1]	-	-	83%	88%
Surgical Care Improvement Project				
Appropriate Beta Blocker Usage	44	95%	98%	98%
Appropriate VTP Within 24 Hours	150	98%	98%	98%
Controlled Postoperative Blood Glucose[7]	-	-	94%	97%
Perioperative Temperature Management	184	99%	100%	100%
Prophylactic Antibiotic Selection	146	98%	99%	99%
Prophylactic Antibiotic Selection (Outpatient)	94	93%	99%	98%
Prophylactic Antibiotic Stopped	143	97%	99%	98%
Prophylactic Antibiotic Timing	146	99%	98%	99%
Prophylactic Antibiotic Timing (Outpatient)	95	99%	97%	98%
Urinary Catheter Removal	132	96%	97%	97%
Survey of Patients' Hospital Experiences				
Area Around Room 'Always' Quiet at Night	300+	51%	53%	61%
Doctors 'Always' Communicated Well	300+	80%	82%	82%
Home Recovery Information Given	300+	86%	88%	85%
Hospital Given 9 or 10 on 10 Point Scale	300+	72%	71%	71%
Meds 'Always' Explained Before Given	300+	65%	66%	64%
Nurses 'Always' Communicated Well	300+	78%	81%	79%
Pain 'Always' Well Controlled	300+	72%	70%	71%
Room and Bathroom 'Always' Clean	300+	76%	78%	73%
Timely Help 'Always' Received	300+	65%	69%	68%
Would Definitely Recommend Hospital	300+	76%	73%	71%
Use of Medical Imaging				
Cardiac Imaging Stress Test before Surgery	226	5.3%	5%	5.3%
Combination Abdominal CT Scan	659	7.7%	4.6%	10.5%
Combination Brain/Sinus CT Scan	441	0.7%	2%	2.7%
Combination Chest CT Scan	347	0.0%	0.8%	2.7%
Follow-up Mammogram/Ultrasound	1,090	9.3%	9.1%	8.8%
Lumbar Spine MRI for Low Back Pain	125	42.4%	32.1%	37.2%

Northeastern Vermont Regional Hospital

1315 Hospital Drive
Saint Johnsbury, VT 05819
Phone: 802-748-7400
Fax: 802-748-7398
URL: www.nvrh.org
Type: Critical Access Hospitals
Emergency Services: Yes
Ownership: Voluntary non-profit - Private
Beds: 100

Key Personnel:

Emergency Room . . . . Stanley Baker
CEO/President. . . . . Paul Bengtson
Radiology. . . . . Richard Bennum
Cardiac Laboratory. . . . . Mark Heipzman
Chief of Medical Staff . . . . Craig Schein, MD
Infection Control. . . . . Colleen Sinon
Quality Assurance . . . . Colleen Sinon
Operating Room. . . . . Dolores Vieua

Measure	Cases	This Hosp.	State Avg.	U.S. Avg.
Blood Clot Prevention and Treatment				
Anticoagulation Overlap Therapy[5]	-	-	98%	93%
ICU Venous Thromboembolism Prophylaxis[5]	-	-	94%	92%
Incidence of Potentially Preventable VTE[5]	-	-	4%	10%
UFH with Dosages/Platelet Monitoring[5]	-	-	95%	97%
Venous Thromboembolism Prophylaxis[5]	-	-	89%	85%
Warfarin Therapy Discharge Instructions[5]	-	-	78%	75%
Chest Pain/Possible Heart Attack Care				
Aspirin Given Within 24 Hours of Arrival	-	-	98%	96%
Fibrinolytic Meds Within 30 Min. of Arrival	-	-	79%	58%
Average Time to ECG (minutes)	-	-	6	7
Average Time to Transfer (minutes)	-	-	31	60
Children's Asthma Care				
Received Home Management Plan of Care	-	-	-	88%
Received Reliever Medication	-	-	-	100%
Received Systemic Corticosteroids	-	-	-	100%
Emergency Department				
Admittance Decision Time (minutes)[5]	-	-	114	98
Head CT Results Within 45 Min. of Arrival	-	-	45%	57%
Patients Who Left ER Before Being Seen	-	-	2%	2%
Time from ER Arrival to Admit. (minutes)[5]	-	-	279	274
Time from ER Arrival to Discharge (minutes)	-	-	136	134
Time in ER Before Being Evaluated (minutes)	-	-	27	26
Time to Pain Meds for Fractures (minutes)	-	-	61	57
Heart Attack Care				
Aspirin Given at Discharge[1]	-	-	100%	99%
Fibrinolytic Meds Within 30 Min. of Arrival[7]	-	-	-	54%
PCI Within 90 Minutes of Arrival[7]	-	-	98%	96%
Statin Prescribed at Discharge[1]	-	-	99%	98%
Heart Failure Care				
ACE Inhibitor or ARB for LVSD	11	100%	96%	97%
Discharge Instructions Given	30	70%	94%	94%
Evaluation of LVS Function	37	95%	99%	99%
Medicare Spending				
Medicare Spending per Patient (ratio)	-	-	1.01	0.98
Pneumonia Care				
Appropriate Initial Antibiotic Given	60	97%	97%	95%
Blood Culture Timing	63	98%	98%	98%
Pregnancy and Delivery Care				
Newborn Deliveries Scheduled Early[5]	-	-	4%	6%
Preventive Care				
Immunization for Influenza[5]	-	-	93%	90%
Immunization for Pneumonia[5]	-	-	94%	92%
Stroke Care				
Anticoagulation Therapy for Atrial Fibrillation[5]	-	-	96%	95%
Antithrombotic Therapy Timing[5]	-	-	92%	98%
Assessed for Rehabilitation[5]	-	-	96%	97%
Discharged on Antithrombotic Therapy[5]	-	-	99%	99%
Discharged on Statin Medication[5]	-	-	93%	94%
Thrombolytic Therapy Timing[5]	-	-	70%	66%
Venous Thromboembolism Prophylaxis[5]	-	-	92%	94%
Written Stroke Educational Materials Given[5]	-	-	83%	88%
Surgical Care Improvement Project				
Appropriate Beta Blocker Usage[2]	14	100%	98%	98%
Appropriate VTP Within 24 Hours[2]	96	100%	98%	98%
Controlled Postoperative Blood Glucose[2,7]	-	-	94%	97%
Perioperative Temperature Management[2]	100	100%	100%	100%
Prophylactic Antibiotic Selection[2]	88	95%	99%	99%
Prophylactic Antibiotic Selection (Outpatient)	-	-	99%	98%
Prophylactic Antibiotic Stopped[2]	87	95%	99%	98%
Prophylactic Antibiotic Timing[2]	88	95%	98%	99%
Prophylactic Antibiotic Timing (Outpatient)	-	-	97%	98%
Urinary Catheter Removal[2]	87	100%	97%	97%
Survey of Patients' Hospital Experiences				
Area Around Room 'Always' Quiet at Night	300+	60%	53%	61%
Doctors 'Always' Communicated Well	300+	84%	82%	82%
Home Recovery Information Given	300+	89%	88%	85%
Hospital Given 9 or 10 on 10 Point Scale	300+	73%	71%	71%
Meds 'Always' Explained Before Given	300+	73%	66%	64%
Nurses 'Always' Communicated Well	300+	80%	81%	79%
Pain 'Always' Well Controlled	300+	69%	70%	71%
Room and Bathroom 'Always' Clean	300+	88%	78%	73%
Timely Help 'Always' Received	300+	72%	69%	68%
Would Definitely Recommend Hospital	300+	70%	73%	71%
Use of Medical Imaging				
Cardiac Imaging Stress Test before Surgery	-	-	5%	5.3%
Combination Abdominal CT Scan	-	-	4.6%	10.5%
Combination Brain/Sinus CT Scan	-	-	2%	2.7%
Combination Chest CT Scan	-	-	0.8%	2.7%
Follow-up Mammogram/Ultrasound	-	-	9.1%	8.8%
Lumbar Spine MRI for Low Back Pain	-	-	32.1%	37.2%

Springfield Hospital

PO Box 2003
Springfield, VT 05156
Phone: 802-885-2151
Fax: 802-885-3959
Type: Critical Access Hospitals
Emergency Services: Yes
Ownership: Voluntary non-profit - Private
Beds: 69

Key Personnel:

Radiology. . . . . Thomas E Brennan
Quality Assurance . . . . Pam Brown
Chief of Medical Staff . . . . Karen Clay, MD
CEO/President. . . . . Thomas Crawford
Infection Control. . . . . Becky Howe
Operating Room. . . . . Eric Warren, BSN

Measure	Cases	This Hosp.	State Avg.	U.S. Avg.
Blood Clot Prevention and Treatment				
Anticoagulation Overlap Therapy[5]	-	-	98%	93%
ICU Venous Thromboembolism Prophylaxis[5]	-	-	94%	92%
Incidence of Potentially Preventable VTE[5]	-	-	4%	10%
UFH with Dosages/Platelet Monitoring[5]	-	-	95%	97%
Venous Thromboembolism Prophylaxis[5]	-	-	89%	85%
Warfarin Therapy Discharge Instructions[5]	-	-	78%	75%
Chest Pain/Possible Heart Attack Care				
Aspirin Given Within 24 Hours of Arrival	-	-	98%	96%
Fibrinolytic Meds Within 30 Min. of Arrival	-	-	79%	58%
Average Time to ECG (minutes)	-	-	6	7
Average Time to Transfer (minutes)	-	-	31	60
Children's Asthma Care				
Received Home Management Plan of Care	-	-	-	88%

NOTE: Hospital profiles are in alphabetical order by state, then city, then hospital within the city; Rankings exclude hospitals with less than 25 cases except for patient surveys which excludes hospitals with less than 100 cases; (a) 100-299 cases; (1) The number of cases/patients is too few to report; (2) Data submitted were based on a sample of cases/patients; (3) Results are based on a shorter time period than required; (4) Data suppressed by CMS for one or more quarters; (5) Results are not available for this reporting period; (6) Fewer than 100 patients completed the HCAHPS survey; (7) No cases met the criteria for this measure; (8) The lower limit of the confidence interval cannot be calculated if the number of observed infections equals zero; (9) No data are available from the state/territory for this reporting period; (10) The scores shown reflect fewer than 50 completed surveys; (11) There were discrepancies in the data collection process; (12) This measure does not apply to this hospital for this reporting period; (13) Results cannot be calculated for this reporting period; (14) The results for this state are combined with nearby states to protect confidentiality; Please refer to the User's Guide for a full explanation of data.

Measure	Cases	This Hosp.	State Avg.	U.S. Avg.
Received Reliever Medication	-	-	-	100%
Received Systemic Corticosteroids	-	-	-	100%
Emergency Department				
Admittance Decision Time (minutes)[5]	-	-	114	98
Head CT Results Within 45 Min. of Arrival	-	-	45%	57%
Patients Who Left ER Before Being Seen	-	-	2%	2%
Time from ER Arrival to Admit. (minutes)[5]	-	-	279	274
Time from ER Arrival to Discharge (minutes)	-	-	136	134
Time in ER Before Being Evaluated (minutes)	-	-	27	26
Time to Pain Meds for Fractures (minutes)	-	-	61	57
Heart Attack Care				
Aspirin Given at Discharge[1]	-	-	100%	99%
Fibrinolytic Meds Within 30 Min. of Arrival[1]	-	-	-	54%
PCI Within 90 Minutes of Arrival[7]	-	-	98%	96%
Statin Prescribed at Discharge[1]	-	-	99%	98%
Heart Failure Care				
ACE Inhibitor or ARB for LVSD[1]	-	-	96%	97%
Discharge Instructions Given	25	100%	94%	94%
Evaluation of LVS Function	36	100%	99%	99%
Medicare Spending				
Medicare Spending per Patient (ratio)	-	-	1.01	0.98
Pneumonia Care				
Appropriate Initial Antibiotic Given	89	100%	97%	95%
Blood Culture Timing	113	99%	98%	98%
Pregnancy and Delivery Care				
Newborn Deliveries Scheduled Early[5]	-	-	4%	6%
Preventive Care				
Immunization for Influenza[5]	-	-	93%	90%
Immunization for Pneumonia[5]	-	-	94%	92%
Stroke Care				
Anticoagulation Therapy for Atrial Fibrillation[5]	-	-	96%	95%
Antithrombotic Therapy Timing[5]	-	-	92%	98%
Assessed for Rehabilitation[5]	-	-	96%	97%
Discharged on Antithrombotic Therapy[5]	-	-	99%	99%
Discharged on Statin Medication[5]	-	-	93%	94%
Thrombolytic Therapy Timing[5]	-	-	70%	66%
Venous Thromboembolism Prophylaxis[5]	-	-	92%	94%
Written Stroke Educational Materials Given[5]	-	-	83%	88%
Surgical Care Improvement Project				
Appropriate Beta Blocker Usage[2]	14	100%	98%	98%
Appropriate VTP Within 24 Hours[2]	56	100%	98%	98%
Controlled Postoperative Blood Glucose[2,7]	-	-	94%	97%
Perioperative Temperature Management[2]	58	100%	100%	100%
Prophylactic Antibiotic Selection[2]	36	97%	99%	99%
Prophylactic Antibiotic Selection (Outpatient)	-	-	99%	98%
Prophylactic Antibiotic Stopped[2]	36	100%	99%	98%
Prophylactic Antibiotic Timing[2]	36	100%	98%	99%
Prophylactic Antibiotic Timing (Outpatient)	-	-	97%	98%
Urinary Catheter Removal[2]	49	100%	97%	97%
Survey of Patients' Hospital Experiences				
Area Around Room 'Always' Quiet at Night	300+	51%	53%	61%
Doctors 'Always' Communicated Well	300+	79%	82%	82%
Home Recovery Information Given	300+	86%	88%	85%
Hospital Given 9 or 10 on 10 Point Scale	300+	62%	71%	71%
Meds 'Always' Explained Before Given	300+	61%	66%	64%
Nurses 'Always' Communicated Well	300+	73%	81%	79%
Pain 'Always' Well Controlled	300+	62%	70%	71%
Room and Bathroom 'Always' Clean	300+	70%	78%	73%
Timely Help 'Always' Received	300+	60%	69%	68%
Would Definitely Recommend Hospital	300+	62%	73%	71%
Use of Medical Imaging				
Cardiac Imaging Stress Test before Surgery	-	-	5%	5.3%
Combination Abdominal CT Scan	-	-	4.6%	10.5%
Combination Brain/Sinus CT Scan	-	-	2%	2.7%
Combination Chest CT Scan	-	-	0.8%	2.7%
Follow-up Mammogram/Ultrasound	-	-	9.1%	8.8%
Lumbar Spine MRI for Low Back Pain	-	-	32.1%	37.2%

Grace Cottage Hospital

PO Box 216
Townshend, VT 05353
Phone: 802-365-7920
Fax: 802-365-7031
E-mail: info@gracecottage.org
URL: www.gracecottage.org
Type: Critical Access Hospitals
Emergency Services: Yes
Ownership: Voluntary non-profit - Private
Beds: 19

Key Personnel:

Emergency Room . . . . Kimona Alin, MD
CEO/President. . . . . Michael Brant
Radiology. . . . . Edward Elliott
Pediatrics. . . . . Elizabeth Linder, MD
Quality Assurance . . . . Mary Morgan
Chief of Medical Staff . . . . Timothy Shafer

Measure	Cases	This Hosp.	State Avg.	U.S. Avg.
Blood Clot Prevention and Treatment				
Anticoagulation Overlap Therapy[5]	-	-	98%	93%
ICU Venous Thromboembolism Prophylaxis[5]	-	-	94%	92%
Incidence of Potentially Preventable VTE[5]	-	-	4%	10%
UFH with Dosages/Platelet Monitoring[5]	-	-	95%	97%
Venous Thromboembolism Prophylaxis[5]	-	-	89%	85%
Warfarin Therapy Discharge Instructions[5]	-	-	78%	75%
Chest Pain/Possible Heart Attack Care				
Aspirin Given Within 24 Hours of Arrival	-	-	98%	96%
Fibrinolytic Meds Within 30 Min. of Arrival	-	-	79%	58%
Average Time to ECG (minutes)	-	-	6	7
Average Time to Transfer (minutes)	-	-	31	60
Children's Asthma Care				
Received Home Management Plan of Care	-	-	-	88%
Received Reliever Medication	-	-	-	100%
Received Systemic Corticosteroids	-	-	-	100%
Emergency Department				
Admittance Decision Time (minutes)[5]	-	-	114	98
Head CT Results Within 45 Min. of Arrival	-	-	45%	57%
Patients Who Left ER Before Being Seen	-	-	2%	2%
Time from ER Arrival to Admit. (minutes)[5]	-	-	279	274
Time from ER Arrival to Discharge (minutes)	-	-	136	134
Time in ER Before Being Evaluated (minutes)	-	-	27	26
Time to Pain Meds for Fractures (minutes)	-	-	61	57
Heart Attack Care				
Aspirin Given at Discharge[5]	-	-	100%	99%
Fibrinolytic Meds Within 30 Min. of Arrival[5]	-	-	-	54%
PCI Within 90 Minutes of Arrival[5]	-	-	98%	96%
Statin Prescribed at Discharge[5]	-	-	99%	98%
Heart Failure Care				
ACE Inhibitor or ARB for LVSD[1]	-	-	96%	97%
Discharge Instructions Given[1]	-	-	94%	94%
Evaluation of LVS Function	11	91%	99%	99%
Medicare Spending				
Medicare Spending per Patient (ratio)	-	-	1.01	0.98
Pneumonia Care				
Appropriate Initial Antibiotic Given	14	100%	97%	95%
Blood Culture Timing	12	100%	98%	98%
Pregnancy and Delivery Care				
Newborn Deliveries Scheduled Early[5]	-	-	4%	6%
Preventive Care				
Immunization for Influenza[5]	-	-	93%	90%
Immunization for Pneumonia[5]	-	-	94%	92%
Stroke Care				
Anticoagulation Therapy for Atrial Fibrillation[5]	-	-	96%	95%
Antithrombotic Therapy Timing[5]	-	-	92%	98%
Assessed for Rehabilitation[5]	-	-	96%	97%
Discharged on Antithrombotic Therapy[5]	-	-	99%	99%
Discharged on Statin Medication[5]	-	-	93%	94%
Thrombolytic Therapy Timing[5]	-	-	70%	66%
Venous Thromboembolism Prophylaxis[5]	-	-	92%	94%
Written Stroke Educational Materials Given[5]	-	-	83%	88%
Surgical Care Improvement Project				
Appropriate Beta Blocker Usage[5]	-	-	98%	98%
Appropriate VTP Within 24 Hours[5]	-	-	98%	98%
Controlled Postoperative Blood Glucose[5]	-	-	94%	97%
Perioperative Temperature Management[5]	-	-	100%	100%
Prophylactic Antibiotic Selection[5]	-	-	99%	99%
Prophylactic Antibiotic Selection (Outpatient)	-	-	99%	98%
Prophylactic Antibiotic Stopped[5]	-	-	99%	98%
Prophylactic Antibiotic Timing[5]	-	-	98%	99%
Prophylactic Antibiotic Timing (Outpatient)	-	-	97%	98%
Urinary Catheter Removal[5]	-	-	97%	97%
Survey of Patients' Hospital Experiences				
Area Around Room 'Always' Quiet at Night[10]	<100	57%	53%	61%
Doctors 'Always' Communicated Well[10]	<100	95%	82%	82%
Home Recovery Information Given[10]	<100	89%	88%	85%
Hospital Given 9 or 10 on 10 Point Scale[10]	<100	83%	71%	71%
Meds 'Always' Explained Before Given[10]	<100	66%	66%	64%
Nurses 'Always' Communicated Well[10]	<100	90%	81%	79%
Pain 'Always' Well Controlled[10]	<100	64%	70%	71%
Room and Bathroom 'Always' Clean[10]	<100	79%	78%	73%
Timely Help 'Always' Received[10]	<100	69%	69%	68%
Would Definitely Recommend Hospital[10]	<100	74%	73%	71%
Use of Medical Imaging				
Cardiac Imaging Stress Test before Surgery	-	-	5%	5.3%
Combination Abdominal CT Scan	-	-	4.6%	10.5%
Combination Brain/Sinus CT Scan	-	-	2%	2.7%
Combination Chest CT Scan	-	-	0.8%	2.7%
Follow-up Mammogram/Ultrasound	-	-	9.1%	8.8%
Lumbar Spine MRI for Low Back Pain	-	-	32.1%	37.2%

White River Junction VA Medical Center

215 N. Main St.
White River Junction, VT 05009
Phone: 802-295-9363
Fax: 802-296-6354
E-mail: vhawrjwww@med.va.gov
URL: www.visn1.med.va.gov/wrj
Type: Acute Care - VA
Emergency Services: No
Ownership: Government Federal
Beds: 60

Key Personnel:

Intensive Care Unit. . . . . James Geiling, MD
Chief of Medical Staff . . . . M. Ganga Hematillake
Anesthesiology. . . . . Frederick Perkins, MD
Operating Room. . . . . Frank Pindyck, MD
Quality Assurance . . . . Joanne B Puckett, RN MeD
Infection Control. . . . . Laura Smith, RN

Measure	Cases	This Hosp.	State Avg.	U.S. Avg.
Blood Clot Prevention and Treatment				
Anticoagulation Overlap Therapy	-	-	98%	93%
ICU Venous Thromboembolism Prophylaxis	-	-	94%	92%
Incidence of Potentially Preventable VTE	-	-	4%	10%
UFH with Dosages/Platelet Monitoring	-	-	95%	97%
Venous Thromboembolism Prophylaxis	-	-	89%	85%
Warfarin Therapy Discharge Instructions	-	-	78%	75%
Chest Pain/Possible Heart Attack Care				
Aspirin Given Within 24 Hours of Arrival	-	-	98%	96%
Fibrinolytic Meds Within 30 Min. of Arrival	-	-	79%	58%
Average Time to ECG (minutes)	-	-	6	7
Average Time to Transfer (minutes)	-	-	31	60
Children's Asthma Care				
Received Home Management Plan of Care	-	-	-	88%
Received Reliever Medication	-	-	-	100%
Received Systemic Corticosteroids	-	-	-	100%
Emergency Department				
Admittance Decision Time (minutes)	-	-	114	98
Head CT Results Within 45 Min. of Arrival	-	-	45%	57%
Patients Who Left ER Before Being Seen	-	-	2%	2%
Time from ER Arrival to Admit. (minutes)	-	-	279	274
Time from ER Arrival to Discharge (minutes)	-	-	136	134
Time in ER Before Being Evaluated (minutes)	-	-	27	26
Time to Pain Meds for Fractures (minutes)	-	-	61	57
Heart Attack Care				
Aspirin Given at Discharge[1]	-	-	100%	99%
Fibrinolytic Meds Within 30 Min. of Arrival[5]	-	-	-	54%
PCI Within 90 Minutes of Arrival[5]	-	-	98%	96%
Statin Prescribed at Discharge[1]	-	-	99%	98%
Heart Failure Care				
ACE Inhibitor or ARB for LVSD[1]	17	88%	96%	97%
Discharge Instructions Given	44	93%	94%	94%
Evaluation of LVS Function	53	100%	99%	99%
Medicare Spending				
Medicare Spending per Patient (ratio)	-	-	1.01	0.98
Pneumonia Care				

NOTE: Hospital profiles are in alphabetical order by state, then city, then hospital within the city; Rankings exclude hospitals with less than 25 cases except for patient surveys which excludes hospitals with less than 100 cases; (a) 100-299 cases; (1) The number of cases/patients is too few to report; (2) Data submitted were based on a sample of cases/patients; (3) Results are based on a shorter time period than required; (4) Data suppressed by CMS for one or more quarters; (5) Results are not available for this reporting period; (6) Fewer than 100 patients completed the HCAHPS survey; (7) No cases met the criteria for this measure; (8) The lower limit of the confidence interval cannot be calculated if the number of observed infections equals zero; (9) No data are available from the state/territory for this reporting period; (10) The scores shown reflect fewer than 50 completed surveys; (11) There were discrepancies in the data collection process; (12) This measure does not apply to this hospital for this reporting period; (13) Results cannot be calculated for this reporting period; (14) The results for this state are combined with nearby states to protect confidentiality; Please refer to the User's Guide for a full explanation of data.

Measure	Cases	This Hosp.	State Avg.	U.S. Avg.
Appropriate Initial Antibiotic Given[1]	21	95%	97%	95%
Blood Culture Timing	25	96%	98%	98%
Pregnancy and Delivery Care				
Newborn Deliveries Scheduled Early	-	-	4%	6%
Preventive Care				
Immunization for Influenza[5]	-	-	93%	90%
Immunization for Pneumonia[5]	-	-	94%	92%
Stroke Care				
Anticoagulation Therapy for Atrial Fibrillation	-	-	96%	95%
Antithrombotic Therapy Timing	-	-	92%	98%
Assessed for Rehabilitation	-	-	96%	97%
Discharged on Antithrombotic Therapy	-	-	99%	99%
Discharged on Statin Medication	-	-	93%	94%
Thrombolytic Therapy Timing	-	-	70%	66%
Venous Thromboembolism Prophylaxis	-	-	92%	94%
Written Stroke Educational Materials Given	-	-	83%	88%
Surgical Care Improvement Project				
Appropriate Beta Blocker Usage[2]	61	98%	98%	98%
Appropriate VTP Within 24 Hours[2]	120	99%	98%	98%
Controlled Postoperative Blood Glucose[5]	-	-	94%	97%
Perioperative Temperature Management[2]	148	99%	100%	100%
Prophylactic Antibiotic Selection	82	100%	99%	99%
Prophylactic Antibiotic Selection (Outpatient)	-	-	99%	98%
Prophylactic Antibiotic Stopped	81	94%	99%	98%
Prophylactic Antibiotic Timing	82	100%	98%	99%
Prophylactic Antibiotic Timing (Outpatient)	-	-	97%	98%
Urinary Catheter Removal[2]	86	97%	97%	97%
Survey of Patients' Hospital Experiences				
Area Around Room 'Always' Quiet at Night	-	-	53%	61%
Doctors 'Always' Communicated Well	-	-	82%	82%
Home Recovery Information Given	-	-	88%	85%
Hospital Given 9 or 10 on 10 Point Scale	-	-	71%	71%
Meds 'Always' Explained Before Given	-	-	66%	64%
Nurses 'Always' Communicated Well	-	-	81%	79%
Pain 'Always' Well Controlled	-	-	70%	71%
Room and Bathroom 'Always' Clean	-	-	78%	73%
Timely Help 'Always' Received	-	-	69%	68%
Would Definitely Recommend Hospital	-	-	73%	71%
Use of Medical Imaging				
Cardiac Imaging Stress Test before Surgery	-	-	5%	5.3%
Combination Abdominal CT Scan	-	-	4.6%	10.5%
Combination Brain/Sinus CT Scan	-	-	2%	2.7%
Combination Chest CT Scan	-	-	0.8%	2.7%
Follow-up Mammogram/Ultrasound	-	-	9.1%	8.8%
Lumbar Spine MRI for Low Back Pain	-	-	32.1%	37.2%

Mount Ascutney Hospital

289 County Road
Windsor, VT 05089
URL: www.mtascutneyhospital.org
Type: Critical Access Hospitals
Ownership: Voluntary non-profit - Private
Phone: 802-674-6711
Fax: 802-674-7155
Emergency Services: Yes
Beds: 91

Key Personnel:

Quality Assurance . . . . Cheryl Briere
Infection Control. . . . . Mary Lou Campbell
Radiology. . . . . Robert M Friedlander, MD
Cardiac Laboratory. . . . . J Jones
Intensive Care Unit. . . . . William Palmer
Chief of Medical Staff. . . . . David Russo
CEO/President. . . . . Richard Slusky
Operating Room. . . . . Julie Weld, RN

Measure	Cases	This Hosp.	State Avg.	U.S. Avg.
Blood Clot Prevention and Treatment				
Anticoagulation Overlap Therapy[5]	-	-	98%	93%
ICU Venous Thromboembolism Prophylaxis[5]	-	-	94%	92%
Incidence of Potentially Preventable VTE[5]	-	-	4%	10%
UFH with Dosages/Platelet Monitoring[5]	-	-	95%	97%
Venous Thromboembolism Prophylaxis[5]	-	-	89%	85%
Warfarin Therapy Discharge Instructions[5]	-	-	78%	75%
Chest Pain/Possible Heart Attack Care				
Aspirin Given Within 24 Hours of Arrival	-	-	98%	96%
Fibrinolytic Meds Within 30 Min. of Arrival	-	-	79%	58%
Average Time to ECG (minutes)	-	-	6	7
Average Time to Transfer (minutes)	-	-	31	60
Children's Asthma Care				
Received Home Management Plan of Care	-	-	-	88%
Received Reliever Medication	-	-	-	100%
Received Systemic Corticosteroids	-	-	-	100%
Emergency Department				
Admittance Decision Time (minutes)[5]	-	-	114	98
Head CT Results Within 45 Min. of Arrival	-	-	45%	57%
Patients Who Left ER Before Being Seen	-	-	2%	2%
Time from ER Arrival to Admit. (minutes)[5]	-	-	279	274
Time from ER Arrival to Discharge (minutes)	-	-	136	134
Time in ER Before Being Evaluated (minutes)	-	-	27	26
Time to Pain Meds for Fractures (minutes)	-	-	61	57
Heart Attack Care				
Aspirin Given at Discharge[1,3]	-	-	100%	99%
Fibrinolytic Meds Within 30 Min. of Arrival[3,7]	-	-	-	54%
PCI Within 90 Minutes of Arrival[3,7]	-	-	98%	96%
Statin Prescribed at Discharge[1,3]	-	-	99%	98%
Heart Failure Care				
ACE Inhibitor or ARB for LVSD[1]	-	-	96%	97%
Discharge Instructions Given	12	75%	94%	94%
Evaluation of LVS Function	26	100%	99%	99%
Medicare Spending				
Medicare Spending per Patient (ratio)	-	-	1.01	0.98
Pneumonia Care				
Appropriate Initial Antibiotic Given	11	91%	97%	95%
Blood Culture Timing	21	95%	98%	98%
Pregnancy and Delivery Care				
Newborn Deliveries Scheduled Early[5]	-	-	4%	6%
Preventive Care				
Immunization for Influenza[5]	-	-	93%	90%
Immunization for Pneumonia[5]	-	-	94%	92%
Stroke Care				
Anticoagulation Therapy for Atrial Fibrillation[5]	-	-	96%	95%
Antithrombotic Therapy Timing[5]	-	-	92%	98%
Assessed for Rehabilitation[5]	-	-	96%	97%
Discharged on Antithrombotic Therapy[5]	-	-	99%	99%
Discharged on Statin Medication[5]	-	-	93%	94%
Thrombolytic Therapy Timing[5]	-	-	70%	66%
Venous Thromboembolism Prophylaxis[5]	-	-	92%	94%
Written Stroke Educational Materials Given[5]	-	-	83%	88%
Surgical Care Improvement Project				
Appropriate Beta Blocker Usage[3,7]	-	-	98%	98%
Appropriate VTP Within 24 Hours[1,3]	-	-	98%	98%
Controlled Postoperative Blood Glucose[3,7]	-	-	94%	97%
Perioperative Temperature Management[1,3]	-	-	100%	100%
Prophylactic Antibiotic Selection[3,7]	-	-	99%	99%
Prophylactic Antibiotic Selection (Outpatient)	-	-	99%	98%
Prophylactic Antibiotic Stopped[3,7]	-	-	99%	98%
Prophylactic Antibiotic Timing[3,7]	-	-	98%	99%
Prophylactic Antibiotic Timing (Outpatient)	-	-	97%	98%
Urinary Catheter Removal[1,3]	-	-	97%	97%
Survey of Patients' Hospital Experiences				
Area Around Room 'Always' Quiet at Night[6]	<100	55%	53%	61%
Doctors 'Always' Communicated Well[6]	<100	77%	82%	82%
Home Recovery Information Given[6]	<100	88%	88%	85%
Hospital Given 9 or 10 on 10 Point Scale[6]	<100	74%	71%	71%
Meds 'Always' Explained Before Given[6]	<100	65%	66%	64%
Nurses 'Always' Communicated Well[6]	<100	81%	81%	79%
Pain 'Always' Well Controlled[6]	<100	76%	70%	71%
Room and Bathroom 'Always' Clean[6]	<100	93%	78%	73%
Timely Help 'Always' Received[6]	<100	67%	69%	68%
Would Definitely Recommend Hospital[6]	<100	84%	73%	71%
Use of Medical Imaging				
Cardiac Imaging Stress Test before Surgery	-	-	5%	5.3%
Combination Abdominal CT Scan	-	-	4.6%	10.5%
Combination Brain/Sinus CT Scan	-	-	2%	2.7%
Combination Chest CT Scan	-	-	0.8%	2.7%
Follow-up Mammogram/Ultrasound	-	-	9.1%	8.8%
Lumbar Spine MRI for Low Back Pain	-	-	32.1%	37.2%

NOTE: Hospital profiles are in alphabetical order by state, then city, then hospital within the city; Rankings exclude hospitals with less than 25 cases except for patient surveys which excludes hospitals with less than 100 cases; (a) 100-299 cases; (1) The number of cases/patients is too few to report; (2) Data submitted were based on a sample of cases/patients; (3) Results are based on a shorter time period than required; (4) Data suppressed by CMS for one or more quarters; (5) Results are not available for this reporting period; (6) Fewer than 100 patients completed the HCAHPS survey; (7) No cases met the criteria for this measure; (8) The lower limit of the confidence interval cannot be calculated if the number of observed infections equals zero; (9) No data are available from the state/territory for this reporting period; (10) The scores shown reflect fewer than 50 completed surveys; (11) There were discrepancies in the data collection process; (12) This measure does not apply to this hospital for this reporting period; (13) Results cannot be calculated for this reporting period; (14) The results for this state are combined with nearby states to protect confidentiality; Please refer to the User's Guide for a full explanation of data.

Blood Clot Prevention and Treatment

Anticoagulation Overlap Therapy

Hospital Name	City	Rate	Cases
Bon Secours Mem Reg Med Ctr[2]	Mechanicsville	100%	90
Carilion New River Valley Medical Center[2]	Christiansburg	100%	54
Cjw Medical Center[2]	Richmond	100%	214
Culpeper Regional Hospital[2]	Culpeper	100%	29
John Randolph Medical Center[2]	Hopewell	100%	44
Lewisgale Medical Center[2]	Salem	100%	105
Mary Washington Hospital[2]	Fredericksburg	100%	154
Novant Health Prince William Med Ctr[2]	Manassas	100%	55
Reston Hospital Center[2]	Reston	100%	82
Riverside Walter Reed Hospital[2]	Gloucester	100%	28
Rockingham Memorial Hospital[2]	Harrisonburg	100%	109
Sentara Obici Hospital[2]	Suffolk	100%	56
Sentara Princess Anne Hospital[2]	Virginia Beach	100%	88
Spotsylvania Regional Medical Center[2]	Fredericksburg	100%	26
Stafford Hospital[2]	Stafford	100%	59
Twin County Regional Hospital[2]	Galax	100%	27
Centra Health[2]	Lynchburg	99%	153
Henrico Doctors' Hospital[2]	Richmond	99%	172
Inova Fairfax Hospital[2]	Falls Church	99%	245
Riverside Regional Medical Center[2]	Newport News	99%	85
Bon Secours Saint Marys Hospital[2]	Richmond	98%	98
Johnston Memorial Hospital[2]	Abingdon	98%	44
Mary Immaculate Hospital[2]	Newport News	98%	41
Bon Secours Saint Francis Medical Center[2]	Midlothian	97%	73
Fauquier Hospital[2]	Warrenton	97%	62
Inova Loudoun Hospital[2]	Leesburg	97%	102
Sentara Leigh Hospital[2]	Norfolk	97%	103
Carilion Roanoke Memorial Hospital[2]	Roanoke	96%	242
Inova Alexandria Hospital[2]	Alexandria	96%	102
Danville Regional Medical Center[2]	Danville	95%	91
Medical College of Virginia Hospitals[2]	Richmond	95%	167
Sentara Norfolk General Hospital[2]	Norfolk	94%	51
Bon Secours Maryview Medical Center[2]	Portsmouth	93%	41
Sentara Virginia Beach General Hospital[2]	Virginia Beach	93%	103
Virginia Hospital Center[2]	Arlington	93%	127
Augusta Health[2]	Fishersville	92%	80
Sentara Northern Virginia Medical Center[2]	Woodbridge	92%	64
Southside Community Hospital[2]	Farmville	92%	26
University of Virginia Medical Center[2]	Charlottesville	92%	109
Clinch Valley Medical Center[2]	Richlands	91%	35
Sentara Williamsburg Reg Med Ctr[2]	Williamsburg	91%	95
Mem Hosp of Martinsville & Henry Co[2]	Martinsville	90%	40
Sentara Careplex Hospital[2]	Hampton	90%	91
Martha Jefferson Hospital[2]	Charlottesville	89%	101
Southside Regional Medical Center[2]	Petersburg	88%	83
Winchester Medical Center[2]	Winchester	88%	155
Chesapeake General Hospital[2]	Chesapeake	87%	138
Inova Fair Oaks Hospital[2]	Fairfax	86%	77
Halifax Regional Hospital[2]	Halifax	85%	33
Wellmont Lonesome Pine Hospital[2]	Big Stone Gap	81%	27
Community Memorial Healthcenter[2]	South Hill	71%	34

ICU Venous Thromboembolism Prophylaxis

Hospital Name	City	Rate	Cases
Carilion Franklin Memorial Hospital[2]	Rocky Mount	100%	55
Henrico Doctors' Hospital[2]	Richmond	100%	97
Inova Fair Oaks Hospital[2]	Fairfax	100%	41
John Randolph Medical Center[2]	Hopewell	100%	89
Lewisgale Hospital Alleghany[2]	Low Moor	100%	52
Lewisgale Hospital Pulaski[2]	Pulaski	100%	61
Lewisgale Medical Center[2]	Salem	100%	105
Mary Immaculate Hospital[2]	Newport News	100%	53
Riverside Regional Medical Center[2]	Newport News	100%	155
Riverside Tappahannock Hospital[2]	Tappahannock	100%	92
Rockingham Memorial Hospital[2]	Harrisonburg	100%	30
Sentara Obici Hospital[2]	Suffolk	100%	60
Southampton Memorial Hospital[2]	Franklin	100%	58
Southern Virginia Regional Medical Center[2]	Emporia	100%	53
Spotsylvania Regional Medical Center[2]	Fredericksburg	100%	51
Virginia Hospital Center[2]	Arlington	100%	74
Wythe County Community Hospital[2]	Wytheville	100%	44
Clinch Valley Medical Center[2]	Richlands	99%	96
Community Memorial Healthcenter[2]	South Hill	99%	76
Fauquier Hospital[2]	Warrenton	99%	67
Bon Secours Mem Reg Med Ctr[2]	Mechanicsville	98%	66
Danville Regional Medical Center[2]	Danville	98%	85
Inova Alexandria Hospital[2]	Alexandria	98%	60
Lewisgale Hospital Montgomery[2]	Blacksburg	98%	48
Mary Washington Hospital[2]	Fredericksburg	98%	65
Norton Community Hospital[2]	Norton	98%	90
Reston Hospital Center[2]	Reston	98%	87
Sentara Leigh Hospital[2]	Norfolk	98%	50
Sentara Norfolk General Hospital[2]	Norfolk	98%	65
Stafford Hospital[2]	Stafford	98%	46
Warren Memorial Hospital[2]	Front Royal	98%	40
Cjw Medical Center[2]	Richmond	97%	159
Novant Health Prince William Med Ctr[2]	Manassas	97%	73
Sentara Careplex Hospital[2]	Hampton	97%	96
Bedford Memorial Hospital[2]	Bedford	96%	90
Bon Secours Richmond Community Hospital[2]	Richmond	96%	49
Riverside Walter Reed Hospital[2]	Gloucester	96%	125
Sentara Princess Anne Hospital[2]	Virginia Beach	96%	85
Sentara Williamsburg Reg Med Ctr[2]	Williamsburg	96%	74
Inova Loudoun Hospital[2]	Leesburg	95%	57
Sentara Northern Virginia Medical Center[2]	Woodbridge	95%	91
Bon Secours Depaul Medical Center[2]	Norfolk	94%	112
Bon Secours Saint Francis Medical Center[2]	Midlothian	94%	53
Bon Secours Saint Marys Hospital[2]	Richmond	94%	72
Buchanan General Hospital[2]	Grundy	94%	31
Medical College of Virginia Hospitals[2]	Richmond	94%	118
Carilion Roanoke Memorial Hospital[2]	Roanoke	93%	121
Inova Fairfax Hospital[2]	Falls Church	93%	85
Sentara Virginia Beach General Hospital[2]	Virginia Beach	93%	56
Southside Regional Medical Center[2]	Petersburg	93%	106
Halifax Regional Hospital[2]	Halifax	92%	110
Riverside Shore Memorial Hospital[2]	Nassawadox	92%	102
Twin County Regional Hospital[2]	Galax	92%	66
Rappahannock General Hospital[2]	Kilmarnock	91%	43
University of Virginia Medical Center[2]	Charlottesville	91%	111
Wellmont Lonesome Pine Hospital[2]	Big Stone Gap	90%	115
Inova Mount Vernon Hospital[2]	Alexandria	89%	38
Mem Hosp of Martinsville & Henry Co[2]	Martinsville	89%	128
Martha Jefferson Hospital[2]	Charlottesville	88%	52
Winchester Medical Center[2]	Winchester	88%	69
Culpeper Regional Hospital[2]	Culpeper	87%	38
Bon Secours Maryview Medical Center[2]	Portsmouth	85%	59
Southside Community Hospital[2]	Farmville	85%	86
Centra Health[2]	Lynchburg	84%	110
Chesapeake General Hospital[2]	Chesapeake	83%	77
Johnston Memorial Hospital[2]	Abingdon	83%	69
Carilion New River Valley Medical Center[2]	Christiansburg	81%	70
Russell County Medical Center[2]	Lebanon	78%	32

Incidence of Potentially Preventable VTE

Hospital Name	City	Rate	Cases
Cjw Medical Center[2]	Richmond	0%	34
Henrico Doctors' Hospital[2]	Richmond	0%	31
Lewisgale Medical Center[2]	Salem	0%	25
Mary Washington Hospital[2]	Fredericksburg	0%	33
Sentara Virginia Beach General Hospital[2]	Virginia Beach	0%	29
Carilion Roanoke Memorial Hospital[2]	Roanoke	6%	80
Inova Alexandria Hospital[2]	Alexandria	6%	35
Medical College of Virginia Hospitals[2]	Richmond	7%	70
University of Virginia Medical Center[2]	Charlottesville	8%	87
Inova Fairfax Hospital[2]	Falls Church	19%	69
Winchester Medical Center[2]	Winchester	24%	29

UFH with Dosages/Platelet Count Monitoring

Hospital Name	City	Rate	Cases
Bon Secours Saint Marys Hospital[2]	Richmond	100%	31
Carilion New River Valley Medical Center[2]	Christiansburg	100%	28
Carilion Roanoke Memorial Hospital[2]	Roanoke	100%	160
Chesapeake General Hospital[2]	Chesapeake	100%	83
Cjw Medical Center[2]	Richmond	100%	149
Clinch Valley Medical Center[2]	Richlands	100%	35
Community Memorial Healthcenter[2]	South Hill	100%	28
Danville Regional Medical Center[2]	Danville	100%	55
Henrico Doctors' Hospital[2]	Richmond	100%	69
Inova Alexandria Hospital[2]	Alexandria	100%	93
Inova Fairfax Hospital[2]	Falls Church	100%	144
John Randolph Medical Center[2]	Hopewell	100%	33
Lewisgale Medical Center[2]	Salem	100%	37
Martha Jefferson Hospital[2]	Charlottesville	100%	28
Mary Washington Hospital[2]	Fredericksburg	100%	53
Riverside Regional Medical Center[2]	Newport News	100%	26
Rockingham Memorial Hospital[2]	Harrisonburg	100%	75
Sentara Careplex Hospital[2]	Hampton	100%	62
Sentara Leigh Hospital[2]	Norfolk	100%	71
Sentara Northern Virginia Medical Center[2]	Woodbridge	100%	38
Sentara Obici Hospital[2]	Suffolk	100%	63
Sentara Virginia Beach General Hospital[2]	Virginia Beach	100%	129
Southside Regional Medical Center[2]	Petersburg	100%	64
Virginia Hospital Center[2]	Arlington	100%	69
Winchester Medical Center[2]	Winchester	100%	126
Medical College of Virginia Hospitals[2]	Richmond	99%	144
Sentara Princess Anne Hospital[2]	Virginia Beach	99%	81
Sentara Norfolk General Hospital[2]	Norfolk	98%	53
Sentara Williamsburg Reg Med Ctr[2]	Williamsburg	96%	50
Augusta Health[2]	Fishersville	95%	39
Reston Hospital Center[2]	Reston	93%	28
Bon Secours Maryview Medical Center[2]	Portsmouth	92%	36
University of Virginia Medical Center[2]	Charlottesville	88%	186

Venous Thromboembolism Prophylaxis

Hospital Name	City	Rate	Cases
John Randolph Medical Center[2]	Hopewell	100%	359
Lewisgale Hospital Pulaski[2]	Pulaski	100%	205
Mary Washington Hospital[2]	Fredericksburg	100%	365
Riverside Tappahannock Hospital[2]	Tappahannock	100%	234
Stafford Hospital[2]	Stafford	100%	312
Henrico Doctors' Hospital[2]	Richmond	99%	382
Lewisgale Hospital Alleghany[2]	Low Moor	99%	222
Lewisgale Hospital Montgomery[2]	Blacksburg	99%	324
Lewisgale Medical Center[2]	Salem	99%	305
Spotsylvania Regional Medical Center[2]	Fredericksburg	99%	339
Cjw Medical Center[2]	Richmond	98%	327
Mary Immaculate Hospital[2]	Newport News	98%	234
Reston Hospital Center[2]	Reston	98%	314
Riverside Walter Reed Hospital[2]	Gloucester	98%	291
Clinch Valley Medical Center[2]	Richlands	97%	380
Smyth County Community Hospital[2]	Marion	97%	134
Warren Memorial Hospital[2]	Front Royal	97%	143
Bon Secours Richmond Community Hospital[2]	Richmond	96%	78
Riverside Regional Medical Center[2]	Newport News	96%	427
Riverside Shore Memorial Hospital[2]	Nassawadox	96%	364
Rockingham Memorial Hospital[2]	Harrisonburg	96%	314
Southern Virginia Regional Medical Center[2]	Emporia	96%	344
Virginia Hospital Center[2]	Arlington	96%	304
Danville Regional Medical Center[2]	Danville	95%	371
Novant Health Prince William Med Ctr[2]	Manassas	95%	230
Bon Secours Saint Francis Medical Center[2]	Midlothian	94%	357
Norton Community Hospital[2]	Norton	94%	215
Sentara Leigh Hospital[2]	Norfolk	94%	349
Sentara Princess Anne Hospital[2]	Virginia Beach	94%	386
Wythe County Community Hospital[2]	Wytheville	94%	140
Bon Secours Mem Reg Med Ctr[2]	Mechanicsville	92%	369
Culpeper Regional Hospital[2]	Culpeper	92%	246
Rappahannock General Hospital[2]	Kilmarnock	92%	111
Sentara Careplex Hospital[2]	Hampton	92%	313
Sentara Norfolk General Hospital[2]	Norfolk	92%	376
Bon Secours Depaul Medical Center[2]	Norfolk	91%	313
Bon Secours Saint Marys Hospital[2]	Richmond	91%	315
Carilion New River Valley Medical Center[2]	Christiansburg	91%	357
Mem Hosp of Martinsville & Henry Co[2]	Martinsville	91%	311
Sentara Northern Virginia Medical Center[2]	Woodbridge	91%	354
Sentara Obici Hospital[2]	Suffolk	91%	379
Southampton Memorial Hospital[2]	Franklin	91%	218
Augusta Health[2]	Fishersville	90%	312
Bedford Memorial Hospital[2]	Bedford	90%	213
Inova Fair Oaks Hospital[2]	Fairfax	90%	318
Sentara Williamsburg Reg Med Ctr[2]	Williamsburg	90%	354
University of Virginia Medical Center[2]	Charlottesville	89%	281
Winchester Medical Center[2]	Winchester	89%	319
Community Memorial Healthcenter[2]	South Hill	88%	322
Fauquier Hospital[2]	Warrenton	88%	354
Carilion Roanoke Memorial Hospital[2]	Roanoke	87%	485
Carilion Tazewell Community Hospital[2]	Tazewell	87%	114
Inova Alexandria Hospital[2]	Alexandria	87%	354
Southside Regional Medical Center[2]	Petersburg	87%	420
Carilion Franklin Memorial Hospital[2]	Rocky Mount	86%	214
Inova Fairfax Hospital[2]	Falls Church	86%	322
Medical College of Virginia Hospitals[2]	Richmond	85%	338
Inova Loudoun Hospital[2]	Leesburg	84%	315
Halifax Regional Hospital[2]	Halifax	83%	344
Wellmont Lonesome Pine Hospital[2]	Big Stone Gap	83%	370
Centra Health[2]	Lynchburg	82%	315
Martha Jefferson Hospital[2]	Charlottesville	82%	321
Sentara Virginia Beach General Hospital[2]	Virginia Beach	82%	386
Bon Secours Maryview Medical Center[2]	Portsmouth	81%	275
Buchanan General Hospital[2]	Grundy	80%	108
Twin County Regional Hospital[2]	Galax	80%	216
Johnston Memorial Hospital[2]	Abingdon	79%	333
Chesapeake General Hospital[2]	Chesapeake	78%	380
Inova Mount Vernon Hospital[2]	Alexandria	77%	235
Southside Community Hospital[2]	Farmville	76%	345
Russell County Medical Center[2]	Lebanon	71%	170
Eastern State Hospital[2]	Williamsburg	11%	38

Warfarin Therapy Discharge Instructions

Hospital Name	City	Rate	Cases
Bon Secours Saint Marys Hospital[2]	Richmond	100%	66
Carilion New River Valley Medical Center[2]	Christiansburg	100%	51
Clinch Valley Medical Center[2]	Richlands	100%	28
Danville Regional Medical Center[2]	Danville	100%	55
Henrico Doctors' Hospital[2]	Richmond	100%	132
John Randolph Medical Center[2]	Hopewell	100%	37
Lewisgale Medical Center[2]	Salem	100%	64
Mary Immaculate Hospital[2]	Newport News	100%	29
Reston Hospital Center[2]	Reston	100%	62
Riverside Walter Reed Hospital[2]	Gloucester	100%	28
Sentara Norfolk General Hospital[2]	Norfolk	100%	41
Novant Health Prince William Med Ctr[2]	Manassas	98%	40
Rockingham Memorial Hospital[2]	Harrisonburg	98%	81
Sentara Careplex Hospital[2]	Hampton	98%	64
Bon Secours Maryview Medical Center[2]	Portsmouth	97%	32
Bon Secours Mem Reg Med Ctr[2]	Mechanicsville	97%	62
Sentara Leigh Hospital[2]	Norfolk	97%	77

NOTE: Hospital profiles are in alphabetical order by state, then city, then hospital within the city; Rankings exclude hospitals with less than 25 cases except for patient surveys which excludes hospitals with less than 100 cases; (a) 100-299 cases; (1) The number of cases/patients is too few to report; (2) Data submitted were based on a sample of cases/patients; (3) Results are based on a shorter time period than required; (4) Data suppressed by CMS for one or more quarters; (5) Results are not available for this reporting period; (6) Fewer than 100 patients completed the HCAHPS survey; (7) No cases met the criteria for this measure; (8) The lower limit of the confidence interval cannot be calculated if the number of observed infections equals zero; (9) No data are available from the state/territory for this reporting period; (10) The scores shown reflect fewer than 50 completed surveys; (11) There were discrepancies in the data collection process; (12) This measure does not apply to this hospital for this reporting period; (13) Results cannot be calculated for this reporting period; (14) The results for this state are combined with nearby states to protect confidentiality; Please refer to the User's Guide for a full explanation of data.

Sentara Obici Hospital[2]	Suffolk	97%	32
Bon Secours Saint Francis Medical Center[2]	Midlothian	96%	53
Cjw Medical Center[2]	Richmond	96%	167
Sentara Williamsburg Reg Med Ctr[2]	Williamsburg	96%	75
Sentara Northern Virginia Medical Center[2]	Woodbridge	95%	44
Fauquier Hospital[2]	Warrenton	94%	53
Sentara Virginia Beach General Hospital[2]	Virginia Beach	94%	64
Sentara Princess Anne Hospital[2]	Virginia Beach	93%	71
Mem Hosp of Martinsville & Henry Co[2]	Martinsville	92%	25
Carilion Roanoke Memorial Hospital[2]	Roanoke	90%	164
Southside Regional Medical Center[2]	Petersburg	88%	49
Inova Loudoun Hospital[2]	Leesburg	87%	86
Riverside Regional Medical Center[2]	Newport News	85%	72
Inova Alexandria Hospital[2]	Alexandria	78%	77
Winchester Medical Center[2]	Winchester	78%	138
Martha Jefferson Hospital[2]	Charlottesville	74%	74
Augusta Health[2]	Fishersville	73%	67
Inova Fair Oaks Hospital[2]	Fairfax	66%	59
Chesapeake General Hospital[2]	Chesapeake	65%	113
Virginia Hospital Center[2]	Arlington	61%	102
Medical College of Virginia Hospitals[2]	Richmond	60%	129
Inova Fairfax Hospital[2]	Falls Church	56%	174
Johnston Memorial Hospital[2]	Abingdon	52%	31
University of Virginia Medical Center[2]	Charlottesville	27%	89
Stafford Hospital[2]	Stafford	15%	48
Mary Washington Hospital[2]	Fredericksburg	11%	112
Centra Health[2]	Lynchburg	5%	115

Chest Pain/Possible Heart Attack Care

Aspirin Given Within 24 Hours of Arrival

Hospital Name	City	Rate	Cases
Clinch Valley Medical Center	Richlands	100%	55
Community Memorial Healthcenter	South Hill	100%	132
Inova Fair Oaks Hospital	Fairfax	100%	66
Inova Mount Vernon Hospital	Alexandria	100%	33
John Randolph Medical Center	Hopewell	100%	29
Johnston Memorial Hospital	Abingdon	100%	130
Lewisgale Hospital Alleghany	Low Moor	100%	67
Lewisgale Hospital Pulaski	Pulaski	100%	65
Mem Hosp of Martinsville & Henry Co	Martinsville	100%	51
Norton Community Hospital	Norton	100%	215
Rappahannock General Hospital	Kilmarnock	100%	86
Riverside Shore Memorial Hospital	Nassawadox	100%	26
Riverside Tappahannock Hospital	Tappahannock	100%	44
Sentara Obici Hospital	Suffolk	100%	53
Sentara Princess Anne Hospital	Virginia Beach	100%	35
Sentara Virginia Beach General Hospital	Virginia Beach	100%	37
Culpeper Regional Hospital	Culpeper	99%	147
Dickenson Community Hospital	Clintwood	99%	98
Buchanan General Hospital	Grundy	98%	108
Carilion Franklin Memorial Hospital	Rocky Mount	98%	97
Carilion New River Valley Medical Center	Christiansburg	98%	83
Riverside Walter Reed Hospital	Gloucester	98%	51
Russell County Medical Center	Lebanon	98%	46
Smyth County Community Hospital	Marion	98%	107
Southampton Memorial Hospital	Franklin	98%	50
Southern Virginia Regional Medical Center	Emporia	98%	49
Fauquier Hospital	Warrenton	97%	62
Inova Loudoun Hospital	Leesburg	97%	37
Twin County Regional Hospital	Galax	97%	123
Wythe County Community Hospital	Wytheville	97%	100
Carilion Tazewell Community Hospital	Tazewell	96%	70
Southside Community Hospital	Farmville	96%	118
Carilion Giles Community Hospital	Pearisburg	95%	58
Wellmont Lonesome Pine Hospital	Big Stone Gap	95%	62
Inova Alexandria Hospital	Alexandria	94%	33
Stafford Hospital	Stafford	94%	35
Inova Fairfax Hospital	Falls Church	93%	29
Bedford Memorial Hospital	Bedford	91%	53

Average Time to ECG (minutes)

Hospital Name	City	Min.	Cases
Johnston Memorial Hospital	Abingdon	0	134
John Randolph Medical Center	Hopewell	1	31
Community Memorial Healthcenter	South Hill	3	136
Lewisgale Hospital Pulaski	Pulaski	3	66
Buchanan General Hospital	Grundy	4	122
Dickenson Community Hospital	Clintwood	4	100
Riverside Shore Memorial Hospital	Nassawadox	4	27
Riverside Walter Reed Hospital	Gloucester	4	52
Smyth County Community Hospital	Marion	4	111
Inova Mount Vernon Hospital	Alexandria	5	34
Russell County Medical Center	Lebanon	5	48
Sentara Princess Anne Hospital	Virginia Beach	5	36
Southern Virginia Regional Medical Center	Emporia	5	50
Southside Community Hospital	Farmville	5	132
Inova Alexandria Hospital	Alexandria	6	35
Mem Hosp of Martinsville & Henry Co	Martinsville	6	52
Norton Community Hospital	Norton	6	227
Sentara Obici Hospital	Suffolk	6	52
Sentara Virginia Beach General Hospital	Virginia Beach	6	36
Southampton Memorial Hospital	Franklin	6	52
Wellmont Lonesome Pine Hospital	Big Stone Gap	6	68
Fauquier Hospital	Warrenton	7	65
Lewisgale Hospital Alleghany	Low Moor	7	71
Rappahannock General Hospital	Kilmarnock	7	92
Riverside Tappahannock Hospital	Tappahannock	7	44
Twin County Regional Hospital	Galax	7	123
Clinch Valley Medical Center	Richlands	8	60
Wythe County Community Hospital	Wytheville	8	102
Stafford Hospital	Stafford	9	36
Carilion Giles Community Hospital	Pearisburg	10	58
Inova Fair Oaks Hospital	Fairfax	10	66
Inova Loudoun Hospital	Leesburg	10	41
Bedford Memorial Hospital	Bedford	14	54
Inova Fairfax Hospital	Falls Church	14	29
Culpeper Regional Hospital	Culpeper	15	150
Carilion Franklin Memorial Hospital	Rocky Mount	17	107
Carilion New River Valley Medical Center	Christiansburg	21	85
Carilion Tazewell Community Hospital	Tazewell	29	62

Average Time to Transfer (minutes)

Hospital Name	City	Min.	Cases
Southern Virginia Regional Medical Center	Emporia	42	32

Children's Asthma Care

Received Home Management Plan of Care

Hospital Name	City	Rate	Cases
Centra Health	Lynchburg	97%	97
University of Virginia Medical Center[2]	Charlottesville	97%	39
Inova Fairfax Hospital[2]	Falls Church	95%	198
Mary Washington Hospital	Fredericksburg	70%	63

Received Reliever Medication

Hospital Name	City	Rate	Cases
Centra Health	Lynchburg	100%	101
Inova Fairfax Hospital[2]	Falls Church	100%	199
Mary Washington Hospital	Fredericksburg	100%	69
University of Virginia Medical Center	Charlottesville	100%	39

Received Systemic Corticosteroids

Hospital Name	City	Rate	Cases
Centra Health	Lynchburg	100%	101
Mary Washington Hospital	Fredericksburg	100%	69
University of Virginia Medical Center	Charlottesville	100%	39
Inova Fairfax Hospital[2]	Falls Church	99%	199

Emergency Department

Admittance Decision Time (minutes)

Hospital Name	City	Min.	Cases
Smyth County Community Hospital[2]	Marion	32	323
Culpeper Regional Hospital[2]	Culpeper	40	455
Wythe County Community Hospital[2]	Wytheville	42	374
Norton Community Hospital[2]	Norton	43	209
Carilion Tazewell Community Hospital[2]	Tazewell	44	476
Russell County Medical Center[2]	Lebanon	47	369
Buchanan General Hospital[2]	Grundy	50	396
John Randolph Medical Center[2]	Hopewell	50	852
Lewisgale Hospital Alleghany[2]	Low Moor	50	398
Lewisgale Hospital Montgomery[2]	Blacksburg	50	472
Wellmont Lonesome Pine Hospital[2]	Big Stone Gap	53	743
Clinch Valley Medical Center[2]	Richlands	54	479
Spotsylvania Regional Medical Center[2]	Fredericksburg	59	635
Lewisgale Medical Center[2]	Salem	61	697
Twin County Regional Hospital[2]	Galax	61	379
Bedford Memorial Hospital[2]	Bedford	67	576
Johnston Memorial Hospital[2]	Abingdon	68	604
Lewisgale Hospital Pulaski[2]	Pulaski	68	515
Southampton Memorial Hospital[2]	Franklin	70	412
Southern Virginia Regional Medical Center[2]	Emporia	72	578
Southside Community Hospital[2]	Farmville	73	684
Inova Fair Oaks Hospital[2]	Fairfax	74	408
Augusta Health[2]	Fishersville	77	603
Henrico Doctors' Hospital[2]	Richmond	82	683
Danville Regional Medical Center[2]	Danville	85	783
Page Memorial Hospital[2]	Luray	85	321
Stafford Hospital[2]	Stafford	85	539
Carilion Franklin Memorial Hospital[2]	Rocky Mount	87	447
Warren Memorial Hospital[2]	Front Royal	87	285
Community Memorial Healthcenter[2]	South Hill	88	549
Sentara Obici Hospital[2]	Suffolk	89	687
Mary Immaculate Hospital[2]	Newport News	92	458
Riverside Shore Memorial Hospital[2]	Nassawadox	92	495
Sentara Princess Anne Hospital[2]	Virginia Beach	95	649
Mary Washington Hospital[2]	Fredericksburg	97	647
University of Virginia Medical Center[2]	Charlottesville	101	477
Cjw Medical Center[2]	Richmond	102	848
Rappahannock General Hospital[2]	Kilmarnock	102	606
Virginia Hospital Center[2]	Arlington	102	398
Bon Secours Richmond Community Hospital[2]	Richmond	103	234
Halifax Regional Hospital[2]	Halifax	103	535
Reston Hospital Center[2]	Reston	103	479
Sentara Virginia Beach General Hospital[2]	Virginia Beach	103	918
Carilion Stonewall Jackson Hospital[2]	Lexington	107	375
Sentara Williamsburg Reg Med Ctr[2]	Williamsburg	107	777
Sentara Leigh Hospital[2]	Norfolk	109	715
Riverside Tappahannock Hospital[2]	Tappahannock	110	532
Inova Alexandria Hospital[2]	Alexandria	111	512
Carilion Giles Community Hospital[2]	Pearisburg	112	282
Riverside Regional Medical Center[2]	Newport News	112	608
Fauquier Hospital[2]	Warrenton	116	662
Riverside Walter Reed Hospital[2]	Gloucester	119	546
Chesapeake General Hospital[2]	Chesapeake	121	628
Inova Loudoun Hospital[2]	Leesburg	122	512
Inova Mount Vernon Hospital[2]	Alexandria	123	508
Bon Secours Saint Marys Hospital[2]	Richmond	124	607
Winchester Medical Center[2]	Winchester	124	428
Southside Regional Medical Center[2]	Petersburg	125	844
Sentara Careplex Hospital[2]	Hampton	126	912
Centra Health[2]	Lynchburg	127	650
Bon Secours Saint Francis Medical Center[2]	Midlothian	134	591
Inova Fairfax Hospital[2]	Falls Church	134	443
Bon Secours Depaul Medical Center[2]	Norfolk	137	633
Rockingham Memorial Hospital[2]	Harrisonburg	137	771
Sentara Norfolk General Hospital[2]	Norfolk	137	563
Martha Jefferson Hospital[2]	Charlottesville	141	591
Bon Secours Maryview Medical Center[2]	Portsmouth	146	466
Sentara Northern Virginia Medical Center[2]	Woodbridge	149	598
Carilion New River Valley Medical Center[2]	Christiansburg	163	567
Medical College of Virginia Hospitals[2]	Richmond	164	533
Carilion Roanoke Memorial Hospital[2]	Roanoke	173	370
Novant Health Prince William Med Ctr[2]	Manassas	173	454
Mem Hosp of Martinsville & Henry Co[2]	Martinsville	210	776
Bon Secours Mem Reg Med Ctr[2]	Mechanicsville	235	802

Head CT Results Within 45 Minutes of Arrival

Hospital Name	City	Rate	Cases
Rappahannock General Hospital	Kilmarnock	24%	42

Patients Who Left ER Before Being Seen

Hospital Name	City	Rate	Cases
Bon Secours Saint Francis Medical Center	Midlothian	0%	47167
Dickenson Community Hospital	Clintwood	0%	6949
Inova Alexandria Hospital	Alexandria	0%	109273
Inova Fair Oaks Hospital	Fairfax	0%	55831
Inova Loudoun Hospital	Leesburg	0%	68033
Page Memorial Hospital	Luray	0%	14412
Smyth County Community Hospital	Marion	0%	18053
Virginia Hospital Center	Arlington	0%	65368
Bon Secours Mem Reg Med Ctr	Mechanicsville	1%	77623
Bon Secours Saint Marys Hospital	Richmond	1%	43791
Buchanan General Hospital	Grundy	1%	10886
Chesapeake General Hospital	Chesapeake	1%	72634
Clinch Valley Medical Center	Richlands	1%	20100
Community Memorial Healthcenter	South Hill	1%	21372
Culpeper Regional Hospital	Culpeper	1%	31840
Fauquier Hospital	Warrenton	1%	35278
Halifax Regional Hospital	Halifax	1%	30553
Henrico Doctors' Hospital	Richmond	1%	79496
Inova Fairfax Hospital	Falls Church	1%	142794
John Randolph Medical Center	Hopewell	1%	36876
Johnston Memorial Hospital	Abingdon	1%	42676
Lewisgale Hospital Montgomery	Blacksburg	1%	26490
Lewisgale Hospital Pulaski	Pulaski	1%	18462
Martha Jefferson Hospital	Charlottesville	1%	52957
Norton Community Hospital	Norton	1%	22143
Novant Health Prince William Med Ctr	Manassas	1%	76126
Pioneer Health Services of Patrick County	Stuart	1%	5105
Reston Hospital Center	Reston	1%	44109
Riverside Tappahannock Hospital	Tappahannock	1%	19508
Riverside Walter Reed Hospital	Gloucester	1%	24503
Russell County Medical Center	Lebanon	1%	16006
Sentara Careplex Hospital	Hampton	1%	118707
Sentara Leigh Hospital	Norfolk	1%	66722
Sentara Obici Hospital	Suffolk	1%	74968
Sentara Princess Anne Hospital	Virginia Beach	1%	74620
Sentara Virginia Beach General Hospital	Virginia Beach	1%	82555
Sentara Williamsburg Reg Med Ctr	Williamsburg	1%	44104
Shenandoah Memorial Hospital	Woodstock	1%	18622
Southampton Memorial Hospital	Franklin	1%	14833
Southside Community Hospital	Farmville	1%	33232
Spotsylvania Regional Medical Center	Fredericksburg	1%	36598
Stafford Hospital	Stafford	1%	34283
Twin County Regional Hospital	Galax	1%	24689
Warren Memorial Hospital	Front Royal	1%	27241

NOTE: Hospital profiles are in alphabetical order by state, then city, then hospital within the city; Rankings exclude hospitals with less than 25 cases except for patient surveys which excludes hospitals with less than 100 cases; (a) 100-299 cases; (1) The number of cases/patients is too few to report; (2) Data submitted were based on a sample of cases/patients; (3) Results are based on a shorter time period than required; (4) Data suppressed by CMS for one or more quarters; (5) Results are not available for this reporting period; (6) Fewer than 100 patients completed the HCAHPS survey; (7) No cases met the criteria for this measure; (8) The lower limit of the confidence interval cannot be calculated if the number of observed infections equals zero; (9) No data are available from the state/territory for this reporting period; (10) The scores shown reflect fewer than 50 completed surveys; (11) There were discrepancies in the data collection process; (12) This measure does not apply to this hospital for this reporting period; (13) Results cannot be calculated for this reporting period; (14) The results for this state are combined with nearby states to protect confidentiality; Please refer to the User's Guide for a full explanation of data.

Winchester Medical Center	Winchester	1%	70046
Wythe County Community Hospital	Wytheville	1%	18356
Bedford Memorial Hospital	Bedford	2%	16626
Cjw Medical Center	Richmond	2%	127310
Inova Mount Vernon Hospital	Alexandria	2%	30461
Lewisgale Hospital Alleghany	Low Moor	2%	14786
Lewisgale Medical Center	Salem	2%	46189
Mary Immaculate Hospital	Newport News	2%	42518
Mem Hosp of Martinsville & Henry Co	Martinsville	2%	43332
Riverside Shore Memorial Hospital	Nassawadox	2%	16510
Rockingham Memorial Hospital	Harrisonburg	2%	75392
Sentara Norfolk General Hospital	Norfolk	2%	69401
Sentara Northern Virginia Medical Center	Woodbridge	2%	74293
Southern Virginia Regional Medical Center	Emporia	2%	13483
Southside Regional Medical Center	Petersburg	2%	60128
University of Virginia Medical Center	Charlottesville	2%	61779
Wellmont Lonesome Pine Hospital	Big Stone Gap	2%	28756
Augusta Health	Fishersville	3%	65455
Bon Secours Depaul Medical Center	Norfolk	3%	36578
Bon Secours Richmond Community Hospital	Richmond	3%	33699
Carilion Franklin Memorial Hospital	Rocky Mount	3%	25845
Carilion New River Valley Medical Center	Christiansburg	3%	34278
Mary Washington Hospital	Fredericksburg	3%	61802
Rappahannock General Hospital	Kilmarnock	3%	11749
Riverside Regional Medical Center	Newport News	3%	65747
Carilion Tazewell Community Hospital	Tazewell	4%	11661
Centra Health	Lynchburg	4%	99565
Bon Secours Maryview Medical Center	Portsmouth	5%	73653
Carilion Roanoke Memorial Hospital	Roanoke	5%	84761
Medical College of Virginia Hospitals	Richmond	7%	92231
Danville Regional Medical Center	Danville	8%	43244

Time from ER Arrival to Being Admitted (minutes)

Hospital Name	City	Min.	Cases
Smyth County Community Hospital[2]	Marion	168	368
Russell County Medical Center[2]	Lebanon	182	396
Wellmont Lonesome Pine Hospital[2]	Big Stone Gap	202	743
Wythe County Community Hospital[2]	Wytheville	204	375
Johnston Memorial Hospital[2]	Abingdon	210	698
Southern Virginia Regional Medical Center[2]	Emporia	210	578
Lewisgale Hospital Montgomery[2]	Blacksburg	211	477
Clinch Valley Medical Center[2]	Richlands	212	479
Lewisgale Hospital Alleghany[2]	Low Moor	213	398
Buchanan General Hospital[2]	Grundy	216	396
Twin County Regional Hospital[2]	Galax	223	380
Culpeper Regional Hospital[2]	Culpeper	225	455
Lewisgale Hospital Pulaski[2]	Pulaski	226	516
Southside Community Hospital[2]	Farmville	234	695
Lewisgale Medical Center[2]	Salem	236	697
Southampton Memorial Hospital[2]	Franklin	238	438
Spotsylvania Regional Medical Center[2]	Fredericksburg	240	635
Warren Memorial Hospital[2]	Front Royal	241	326
Norton Community Hospital[2]	Norton	242	328
Henrico Doctors' Hospital[2]	Richmond	243	686
Page Memorial Hospital[2]	Luray	243	333
John Randolph Medical Center[2]	Hopewell	244	852
Inova Fair Oaks Hospital[2]	Fairfax	245	408
Cjw Medical Center[2]	Richmond	253	848
Reston Hospital Center[2]	Reston	257	479
Stafford Hospital[2]	Stafford	257	540
Carilion Tazewell Community Hospital[2]	Tazewell	259	488
Bedford Memorial Hospital[2]	Bedford	260	606
Augusta Health[2]	Fishersville	262	612
Carilion Franklin Memorial Hospital[2]	Rocky Mount	264	452
Danville Regional Medical Center[2]	Danville	265	807
Mary Washington Hospital[2]	Fredericksburg	265	652
Community Memorial Healthcenter[2]	South Hill	267	580
Riverside Shore Memorial Hospital[2]	Nassawadox	267	505
Southside Regional Medical Center[2]	Petersburg	269	863
Virginia Hospital Center[2]	Arlington	272	404
Carilion Stonewall Jackson Hospital[2]	Lexington	274	468
Carilion Giles Community Hospital[2]	Pearisburg	276	350
Sentara Williamsburg Reg Med Ctr[2]	Williamsburg	283	777
Halifax Regional Hospital[2]	Halifax	285	538
Mary Immaculate Hospital[2]	Newport News	286	462
Rockingham Memorial Hospital[2]	Harrisonburg	289	772
Bon Secours Saint Francis Medical Center[2]	Midlothian	291	602
Inova Alexandria Hospital[2]	Alexandria	292	514
Inova Mount Vernon Hospital[2]	Alexandria	292	513
Riverside Walter Reed Hospital[2]	Gloucester	293	546
Sentara Obici Hospital[2]	Suffolk	294	691
Bon Secours Saint Marys Hospital[2]	Richmond	296	613
Riverside Tappahannock Hospital[2]	Tappahannock	298	533
Fauquier Hospital[2]	Warrenton	302	761
Inova Loudoun Hospital[2]	Leesburg	305	514
Rappahannock General Hospital[2]	Kilmarnock	309	621
Sentara Virginia Beach General Hospital[2]	Virginia Beach	312	918
Bon Secours Richmond Community Hospital[2]	Richmond	314	234
Sentara Princess Anne Hospital[2]	Virginia Beach	314	657
Centra Health[2]	Lynchburg	328	665
Riverside Regional Medical Center[2]	Newport News	328	609
Sentara Careplex Hospital[2]	Hampton	335	915
Inova Fairfax Hospital[2]	Falls Church	342	465
Martha Jefferson Hospital[2]	Charlottesville	342	593
Sentara Northern Virginia Medical Center[2]	Woodbridge	344	601
Mem Hosp of Martinsville & Henry Co[2]	Martinsville	346	777
Novant Health Prince William Med Ctr[2]	Manassas	352	454
Chesapeake General Hospital[2]	Chesapeake	355	661
Sentara Leigh Hospital[2]	Norfolk	355	717
Medical College of Virginia Hospitals[2]	Richmond	365	534
Bon Secours Depaul Medical Center[2]	Norfolk	367	641
University of Virginia Medical Center[2]	Charlottesville	369	477
Carilion New River Valley Medical Center[2]	Christiansburg	372	567
Winchester Medical Center[2]	Winchester	377	467
Sentara Norfolk General Hospital[2]	Norfolk	378	565
Bon Secours Maryview Medical Center[2]	Portsmouth	389	507
Carilion Roanoke Memorial Hospital[2]	Roanoke	396	377
Bon Secours Mem Reg Med Ctr[2]	Mechanicsville	423	805

Time from ER Arrival to Discharge (minutes)

Hospital Name	City	Min.	Cases
Dickenson Community Hospital	Clintwood	70	217
Smyth County Community Hospital	Marion	91	203
Lewisgale Hospital Alleghany	Low Moor	96	409
Russell County Medical Center	Lebanon	96	349
Southern Virginia Regional Medical Center	Emporia	99	390
John Randolph Medical Center	Hopewell	110	487
Lewisgale Hospital Pulaski	Pulaski	112	478
Twin County Regional Hospital	Galax	113	365
Johnston Memorial Hospital	Abingdon	116	374
Bon Secours Saint Francis Medical Center	Midlothian	117	396
Warren Memorial Hospital	Front Royal	117	334
Bon Secours Richmond Community Hospital	Richmond	121	358
Riverside Tappahannock Hospital	Tappahannock	122	359
Inova Alexandria Hospital	Alexandria	123	910
Mary Immaculate Hospital	Newport News	123	391
Spotsylvania Regional Medical Center	Fredericksburg	123	474
Culpeper Regional Hospital	Culpeper	124	335
Lewisgale Hospital Montgomery	Blacksburg	124	427
Novant Health Prince William Med Ctr	Manassas	124	487
Reston Hospital Center	Reston	125	437
Wellmont Lonesome Pine Hospital	Big Stone Gap	125	708
Community Memorial Healthcenter	South Hill	126	327
Wythe County Community Hospital	Wytheville	127	470
Rockingham Memorial Hospital	Harrisonburg	130	543
Southside Community Hospital	Farmville	130	387
Southampton Memorial Hospital	Franklin	131	396
Buchanan General Hospital	Grundy	132	1104
Halifax Regional Hospital	Halifax	132	386
Riverside Walter Reed Hospital	Gloucester	132	353
Bedford Memorial Hospital	Bedford	133	355
Henrico Doctors' Hospital	Richmond	134	499
Inova Mount Vernon Hospital	Alexandria	134	686
Norton Community Hospital	Norton	134	353
Inova Loudoun Hospital	Leesburg	136	777
Stafford Hospital	Stafford	136	395
Inova Fair Oaks Hospital	Fairfax	137	715
Cjw Medical Center	Richmond	138	498
Southside Regional Medical Center	Petersburg	138	366
Augusta Health	Fishersville	140	439
Clinch Valley Medical Center	Richlands	141	383
Inova Fairfax Hospital	Falls Church	144	862
Mem Hosp of Martinsville & Henry Co	Martinsville	146	425
Mary Washington Hospital	Fredericksburg	147	391
Bon Secours Saint Marys Hospital	Richmond	148	431
Carilion Franklin Memorial Hospital	Rocky Mount	148	332
Rappahannock General Hospital	Kilmarnock	151	331
Virginia Hospital Center	Arlington	152	421
Carilion Tazewell Community Hospital	Tazewell	158	323
Chesapeake General Hospital	Chesapeake	159	371
Carilion Giles Community Hospital	Pearisburg	160	344
Riverside Shore Memorial Hospital	Nassawadox	161	359
Martha Jefferson Hospital	Charlottesville	162	386
Sentara Obici Hospital	Suffolk	163	6172
Fauquier Hospital	Warrenton	169	380
Bon Secours Maryview Medical Center	Portsmouth	170	378
Lewisgale Medical Center	Salem	170	457
Sentara Northern Virginia Medical Center	Woodbridge	170	5753
Sentara Virginia Beach General Hospital	Virginia Beach	173	6423
Bon Secours Mem Reg Med Ctr	Mechanicsville	175	405
Sentara Careplex Hospital	Hampton	177	8023
Bon Secours Depaul Medical Center	Norfolk	182	372
Carilion New River Valley Medical Center	Christiansburg	185	382
University of Virginia Medical Center	Charlottesville	190	391
Riverside Regional Medical Center	Newport News	192	352
Sentara Princess Anne Hospital	Virginia Beach	195	5914
Winchester Medical Center	Winchester	196	330
Sentara Williamsburg Reg Med Ctr	Williamsburg	197	3348
Danville Regional Medical Center	Danville	199	426
Centra Health	Lynchburg	211	380
Carilion Roanoke Memorial Hospital	Roanoke	222	352
Sentara Leigh Hospital	Norfolk	226	3924
Sentara Norfolk General Hospital	Norfolk	229	5351
Medical College of Virginia Hospitals	Richmond	235	399

Time in ER Before Being Evaluated (minutes)

Hospital Name	City	Min.	Cases
Bon Secours Saint Francis Medical Center	Midlothian	9	421
Henrico Doctors' Hospital	Richmond	11	530
Reston Hospital Center	Reston	12	496
Cjw Medical Center	Richmond	13	548
John Randolph Medical Center	Hopewell	13	524
Clinch Valley Medical Center	Richlands	14	469
Lewisgale Hospital Pulaski	Pulaski	14	512
Lewisgale Medical Center	Salem	14	522
Bon Secours Mem Reg Med Ctr	Mechanicsville	15	414
Dickenson Community Hospital	Clintwood	15	228
Lewisgale Hospital Montgomery	Blacksburg	15	474
Smyth County Community Hospital	Marion	15	383
Twin County Regional Hospital	Galax	15	398
Spotsylvania Regional Medical Center	Fredericksburg	16	504
Inova Loudoun Hospital	Leesburg	17	821
Bon Secours Saint Marys Hospital	Richmond	18	460
Martha Jefferson Hospital	Charlottesville	18	408
Southern Virginia Regional Medical Center	Emporia	18	422
Community Memorial Healthcenter	South Hill	19	382
Mem Hosp of Martinsville & Henry Co	Martinsville	19	498
Novant Health Prince William Med Ctr	Manassas	19	518
Norton Community Hospital	Norton	20	360
Russell County Medical Center	Lebanon	20	388
Virginia Hospital Center	Arlington	20	445
Bon Secours Richmond Community Hospital	Richmond	21	384
Lewisgale Hospital Alleghany	Low Moor	21	460
Augusta Health	Fishersville	22	390
Buchanan General Hospital	Grundy	22	1325
Johnston Memorial Hospital	Abingdon	22	407
Mary Immaculate Hospital	Newport News	22	376
Stafford Hospital	Stafford	24	336
Wythe County Community Hospital	Wytheville	24	512
Warren Memorial Hospital	Front Royal	25	357
Southampton Memorial Hospital	Franklin	26	409
Halifax Regional Hospital	Halifax	27	399
Inova Alexandria Hospital	Alexandria	28	943
Inova Fair Oaks Hospital	Fairfax	29	735
Sentara Careplex Hospital	Hampton	29	8338
Chesapeake General Hospital	Chesapeake	30	338
Culpeper Regional Hospital	Culpeper	30	380
Riverside Shore Memorial Hospital	Nassawadox	30	400
Southside Regional Medical Center	Petersburg	30	416
Bon Secours Maryview Medical Center	Portsmouth	31	396
Rockingham Memorial Hospital	Harrisonburg	31	571
Fauquier Hospital	Warrenton	32	406
Mary Washington Hospital	Fredericksburg	32	297
Danville Regional Medical Center	Danville	33	460
Inova Fairfax Hospital	Falls Church	34	934
Inova Mount Vernon Hospital	Alexandria	34	735
Carilion Giles Community Hospital	Pearisburg	35	311
Rappahannock General Hospital	Kilmarnock	35	378
Sentara Obici Hospital	Suffolk	35	6497
University of Virginia Medical Center	Charlottesville	37	353
Bedford Memorial Hospital	Bedford	38	289
Sentara Williamsburg Reg Med Ctr	Williamsburg	38	3850
Riverside Tappahannock Hospital	Tappahannock	40	382
Sentara Northern Virginia Medical Center	Woodbridge	40	6828
Wellmont Lonesome Pine Hospital	Big Stone Gap	40	751
Bon Secours Depaul Medical Center	Norfolk	41	403
Carilion Tazewell Community Hospital	Tazewell	42	342
Sentara Virginia Beach General Hospital	Virginia Beach	43	6844
Carilion Franklin Memorial Hospital	Rocky Mount	45	312
Sentara Norfolk General Hospital	Norfolk	51	5484
Riverside Walter Reed Hospital	Gloucester	52	375
Southside Community Hospital	Farmville	56	377
Sentara Princess Anne Hospital	Virginia Beach	58	6184
Carilion Roanoke Memorial Hospital	Roanoke	60	313
Winchester Medical Center	Winchester	63	342
Carilion New River Valley Medical Center	Christiansburg	69	399
Sentara Leigh Hospital	Norfolk	71	3963
Medical College of Virginia Hospitals	Richmond	74	360
Riverside Regional Medical Center	Newport News	83	364
Centra Health	Lynchburg	88	384

Time to Pain Meds for Bone Fractures (minutes)

Hospital Name	City	Min.	Cases
Lewisgale Hospital Montgomery	Blacksburg	29	73
Lewisgale Hospital Alleghany	Low Moor	30	36
Lewisgale Hospital Pulaski	Pulaski	31	40
Henrico Doctors' Hospital	Richmond	33	120
Cjw Medical Center	Richmond	34	232
Lewisgale Medical Center	Salem	35	89
Reston Hospital Center	Reston	36	288
Spotsylvania Regional Medical Center	Fredericksburg	36	103
John Randolph Medical Center	Hopewell	37	92

NOTE: Hospital profiles are in alphabetical order by state, then city, then hospital within the city; Rankings exclude hospitals with less than 25 cases except for patient surveys which excludes hospitals with less than 100 cases; (a) 100-299 cases; (1) The number of cases/patients is too few to report; (2) Data submitted were based on a sample of cases/patients; (3) Results are based on a shorter time period than required; (4) Data suppressed by CMS for one or more quarters; (5) Results are not available for this reporting period; (6) Fewer than 100 patients completed the HCAHPS survey; (7) No cases met the criteria for this measure; (8) The lower limit of the confidence interval cannot be calculated if the number of observed infections equals zero; (9) No data are available from the state/territory for this reporting period; (10) The scores shown reflect fewer than 50 completed surveys; (11) There were discrepancies in the data collection process; (12) This measure does not apply to this hospital for this reporting period; (13) Results cannot be calculated for this reporting period; (14) The results for this state are combined with nearby states to protect confidentiality; Please refer to the User's Guide for a full explanation of data.

Hospital Name	City	Rate	Cases
Culpeper Regional Hospital	Culpeper	38	90
Southampton Memorial Hospital	Franklin	38	42
Virginia Hospital Center	Arlington	39	203
Buchanan General Hospital	Grundy	40	51
Southside Community Hospital	Farmville	40	78
Twin County Regional Hospital	Galax	40	82
Bon Secours Saint Marys Hospital	Richmond	44	250
Southern Virginia Regional Medical Center	Emporia	44	62
Clinch Valley Medical Center	Richlands	45	81
Inova Alexandria Hospital	Alexandria	45	246
Inova Fair Oaks Hospital	Fairfax	46	245
Johnston Memorial Hospital	Abingdon	46	108
Mem Hosp of Martinsville & Henry Co	Martinsville	46	145
Smyth County Community Hospital	Marion	46	57
Wythe County Community Hospital	Wytheville	46	114
Novant Health Prince William Med Ctr	Manassas	47	362
Russell County Medical Center	Lebanon	47	40
Community Memorial Healthcenter	South Hill	48	88
Bon Secours Saint Francis Medical Center	Midlothian	49	145
Inova Loudoun Hospital	Leesburg	50	221
Norton Community Hospital	Norton	50	57
Riverside Tappahannock Hospital	Tappahannock	52	75
Inova Fairfax Hospital	Falls Church	54	454
Inova Mount Vernon Hospital	Alexandria	55	127
Sentara Northern Virginia Medical Center	Woodbridge	55	241
Martha Jefferson Hospital	Charlottesville	56	205
Mary Immaculate Hospital	Newport News	56	82
Medical College of Virginia Hospitals	Richmond	56	152
Sentara Princess Anne Hospital	Virginia Beach	56	173
Sentara Virginia Beach General Hospital	Virginia Beach	56	192
Riverside Walter Reed Hospital	Gloucester	58	116
Rockingham Memorial Hospital	Harrisonburg	59	202
Stafford Hospital	Stafford	59	143
Danville Regional Medical Center	Danville	60	164
Mary Washington Hospital	Fredericksburg	60	270
Sentara Leigh Hospital	Norfolk	61	97
University of Virginia Medical Center	Charlottesville	61	117
Chesapeake General Hospital	Chesapeake	62	186
Riverside Shore Memorial Hospital	Nassawadox	62	36
Sentara Obici Hospital	Suffolk	62	118
Warren Memorial Hospital	Front Royal	62	45
Fauquier Hospital	Warrenton	63	153
Augusta Health	Fishersville	64	165
Carilion New River Valley Medical Center	Christiansburg	64	112
Centra Health	Lynchburg	64	164
Sentara Careplex Hospital	Hampton	65	146
Rappahannock General Hospital	Kilmarnock	67	68
Carilion Tazewell Community Hospital	Tazewell	69	43
Bon Secours Maryview Medical Center	Portsmouth	73	117
Bon Secours Mem Reg Med Ctr	Mechanicsville	73	238
Riverside Regional Medical Center	Newport News	73	170
Southside Regional Medical Center	Petersburg	73	155
Bon Secours Richmond Community Hospital	Richmond	74	37
Halifax Regional Hospital	Halifax	77	97
Carilion Giles Community Hospital	Pearisburg	78	68
Sentara Norfolk General Hospital	Norfolk	81	82
Sentara Williamsburg Reg Med Ctr	Williamsburg	83	107
Wellmont Lonesome Pine Hospital	Big Stone Gap	84	67
Carilion Franklin Memorial Hospital	Rocky Mount	86	110
Bedford Memorial Hospital	Bedford	90	74
Bon Secours Depaul Medical Center	Norfolk	92	101
Winchester Medical Center	Winchester	96	143
Carilion Roanoke Memorial Hospital	Roanoke	100	482

Heart Attack Care

Aspirin Given at Discharge

Hospital Name	City	Rate	Cases
Augusta Health	Fishersville	100%	222
Bon Secours Depaul Medical Center	Norfolk	100%	94
Bon Secours Maryview Medical Center	Portsmouth	100%	210
Bon Secours Mem Reg Med Ctr	Mechanicsville	100%	361
Centra Health	Lynchburg	100%	619
Cjw Medical Center[2]	Richmond	100%	300
Clinch Valley Medical Center	Richlands	100%	37
Danville Regional Medical Center	Danville	100%	139
Henrico Doctors' Hospital	Richmond	100%	296
Inova Alexandria Hospital	Alexandria	100%	229
Inova Loudoun Hospital	Leesburg	100%	206
John Randolph Medical Center	Hopewell	100%	38
Lewisgale Hospital Montgomery	Blacksburg	100%	93
Lewisgale Medical Center[2]	Salem	100%	303
Mary Immaculate Hospital	Newport News	100%	67
Mary Washington Hospital	Fredericksburg	100%	420
Mem Hosp of Martinsville & Henry Co	Martinsville	100%	73
Reston Hospital Center	Reston	100%	146
Richmond VA Medical Center	Richmond	100%	64
Riverside Regional Medical Center	Newport News	100%	418
Riverside Walter Reed Hospital	Gloucester	100%	28
Rockingham Memorial Hospital[2]	Harrisonburg	100%	261
Sentara Careplex Hospital	Hampton	100%	116
Sentara Leigh Hospital	Norfolk	100%	111
Sentara Norfolk General Hospital	Norfolk	100%	643
Sentara Obici Hospital	Suffolk	100%	55
Sentara Princess Anne Hospital	Virginia Beach	100%	57
Sentara Williamsburg Reg Med Ctr	Williamsburg	100%	103
Spotsylvania Regional Medical Center	Fredericksburg	100%	83
Stafford Hospital	Stafford	100%	25
Virginia Hospital Center	Arlington	100%	200
Wellmont Lonesome Pine Hospital	Big Stone Gap	100%	28
Winchester Medical Center[2]	Winchester	100%	298
Bon Secours Saint Francis Medical Center	Midlothian	99%	156
Bon Secours Saint Marys Hospital	Richmond	99%	206
Carilion Roanoke Memorial Hospital	Roanoke	99%	1120
Chesapeake General Hospital	Chesapeake	99%	223
Martha Jefferson Hospital	Charlottesville	99%	170
Medical College of Virginia Hospitals	Richmond	99%	385
Novant Health Prince William Med Ctr	Manassas	99%	167
Sentara Virginia Beach General Hospital	Virginia Beach	99%	291
Southside Regional Medical Center	Petersburg	99%	267
University of Virginia Medical Center[2]	Charlottesville	99%	339
Halifax Regional Hospital	Halifax	98%	82
Inova Fairfax Hospital[2]	Falls Church	98%	290
Sentara Northern Virginia Medical Center	Woodbridge	98%	106
Johnston Memorial Hospital[2]	Abingdon	97%	35
Salem VA Medical Center	Salem	97%	32

PCI Within 90 Minutes of Arrival

Hospital Name	City	Rate	Cases
Augusta Health	Fishersville	100%	67
Bon Secours Saint Francis Medical Center	Midlothian	100%	40
Cjw Medical Center[2]	Richmond	100%	39
Inova Alexandria Hospital	Alexandria	100%	30
Inova Loudoun Hospital	Leesburg	100%	42
Lewisgale Medical Center[2]	Salem	100%	35
Medical College of Virginia Hospitals	Richmond	100%	56
Rockingham Memorial Hospital[2]	Harrisonburg	100%	64
Sentara Careplex Hospital	Hampton	100%	43
Sentara Norfolk General Hospital	Norfolk	100%	42
Sentara Virginia Beach General Hospital	Virginia Beach	100%	41
Sentara Williamsburg Reg Med Ctr	Williamsburg	100%	35
Winchester Medical Center[2]	Winchester	100%	28
Chesapeake General Hospital	Chesapeake	98%	54
Inova Fairfax Hospital[2]	Falls Church	98%	52
Mary Washington Hospital	Fredericksburg	98%	50
Reston Hospital Center	Reston	98%	47
Riverside Regional Medical Center	Newport News	98%	60
Bon Secours Maryview Medical Center	Portsmouth	97%	29
Martha Jefferson Hospital	Charlottesville	97%	31
Sentara Leigh Hospital	Norfolk	97%	36
Bon Secours Mem Reg Med Ctr	Mechanicsville	96%	52
Bon Secours Saint Marys Hospital	Richmond	96%	46
Centra Health	Lynchburg	96%	104
Henrico Doctors' Hospital	Richmond	96%	54
Novant Health Prince William Med Ctr	Manassas	96%	51
Virginia Hospital Center	Arlington	95%	41
Carilion Roanoke Memorial Hospital	Roanoke	94%	127
University of Virginia Medical Center[2]	Charlottesville	93%	41
Southside Regional Medical Center	Petersburg	92%	48
Danville Regional Medical Center	Danville	81%	26

Statin Prescribed at Discharge

Hospital Name	City	Rate	Cases
Bon Secours Maryview Medical Center	Portsmouth	100%	207
Bon Secours Saint Francis Medical Center	Midlothian	100%	149
Cjw Medical Center[2]	Richmond	100%	284
Clinch Valley Medical Center	Richlands	100%	39
Danville Regional Medical Center	Danville	100%	134
Henrico Doctors' Hospital	Richmond	100%	304
Inova Alexandria Hospital	Alexandria	100%	226
John Randolph Medical Center	Hopewell	100%	39
Lewisgale Hospital Montgomery	Blacksburg	100%	91
Lewisgale Medical Center[2]	Salem	100%	291
Mary Washington Hospital	Fredericksburg	100%	408
Medical College of Virginia Hospitals	Richmond	100%	376
Novant Health Prince William Med Ctr	Manassas	100%	162
Reston Hospital Center	Reston	100%	136
Richmond VA Medical Center	Richmond	100%	60
Riverside Regional Medical Center	Newport News	100%	412
Riverside Walter Reed Hospital	Gloucester	100%	25
Rockingham Memorial Hospital[2]	Harrisonburg	100%	261
Salem VA Medical Center	Salem	100%	30
Sentara Careplex Hospital	Hampton	100%	116
Sentara Norfolk General Hospital	Norfolk	100%	637
Sentara Virginia Beach General Hospital	Virginia Beach	100%	288
Spotsylvania Regional Medical Center	Fredericksburg	100%	79
Virginia Hospital Center	Arlington	100%	190
Wellmont Lonesome Pine Hospital	Big Stone Gap	100%	26
Winchester Medical Center[2]	Winchester	100%	283
Augusta Health	Fishersville	99%	218
Bon Secours Depaul Medical Center	Norfolk	99%	90
Bon Secours Mem Reg Med Ctr	Mechanicsville	99%	350
Carilion Roanoke Memorial Hospital	Roanoke	99%	1060
Centra Health	Lynchburg	99%	615
Inova Fairfax Hospital[2]	Falls Church	99%	286
Inova Loudoun Hospital	Leesburg	99%	198
Martha Jefferson Hospital	Charlottesville	99%	175
Mary Immaculate Hospital	Newport News	99%	69
Sentara Leigh Hospital	Norfolk	99%	105
Sentara Williamsburg Reg Med Ctr	Williamsburg	99%	101
Southside Regional Medical Center	Petersburg	99%	255
University of Virginia Medical Center[2]	Charlottesville	99%	331
Bon Secours Saint Marys Hospital	Richmond	98%	197
Chesapeake General Hospital	Chesapeake	98%	220
Sentara Northern Virginia Medical Center	Woodbridge	98%	103
Sentara Obici Hospital	Suffolk	98%	50
Halifax Regional Hospital	Halifax	97%	73
Sentara Princess Anne Hospital	Virginia Beach	96%	48
Johnston Memorial Hospital[2]	Abingdon	94%	34
Mem Hosp of Martinsville & Henry Co	Martinsville	94%	72
Culpeper Regional Hospital	Culpeper	88%	26

Heart Failure Care

ACE Inhibitor or ARB for LVSD

Hospital Name	City	Rate	Cases
Augusta Health	Fishersville	100%	96
Bon Secours Maryview Medical Center	Portsmouth	100%	83
Bon Secours Mem Reg Med Ctr	Mechanicsville	100%	101
Bon Secours Richmond Community Hospital	Richmond	100%	25
Carilion New River Valley Medical Center	Christiansburg	100%	36
Cjw Medical Center[2]	Richmond	100%	192
Clinch Valley Medical Center	Richlands	100%	31
Community Memorial Healthcenter	South Hill	100%	41
Henrico Doctors' Hospital	Richmond	100%	163
Inova Alexandria Hospital[2]	Alexandria	100%	106
Inova Loudoun Hospital[2]	Leesburg	100%	62
John Randolph Medical Center	Hopewell	100%	68
Lewisgale Hospital Montgomery	Blacksburg	100%	35
Lewisgale Hospital Pulaski	Pulaski	100%	41
Lewisgale Medical Center[2]	Salem	100%	72
Martha Jefferson Hospital	Charlottesville	100%	78
Mary Immaculate Hospital	Newport News	100%	58
Mary Washington Hospital	Fredericksburg	100%	147
Novant Health Prince William Med Ctr	Manassas	100%	59
Reston Hospital Center	Reston	100%	40
Riverside Regional Medical Center	Newport News	100%	175
Riverside Shore Memorial Hospital	Nassawadox	100%	64
Riverside Walter Reed Hospital	Gloucester	100%	45
Rockingham Memorial Hospital[2]	Harrisonburg	100%	78
Salem VA Medical Center	Salem	100%	41
Sentara Norfolk General Hospital	Norfolk	100%	408
Sentara Northern Virginia Medical Center	Woodbridge	100%	92
Sentara Princess Anne Hospital	Virginia Beach	100%	99
Sentara Virginia Beach General Hospital	Virginia Beach	100%	129
Sentara Williamsburg Reg Med Ctr	Williamsburg	100%	78
Southampton Memorial Hospital	Franklin	100%	40
Spotsylvania Regional Medical Center	Fredericksburg	100%	35
Stafford Hospital	Stafford	100%	31
Winchester Medical Center[2]	Winchester	100%	103
Bon Secours Saint Francis Medical Center	Midlothian	99%	79
Bon Secours Saint Marys Hospital[2]	Richmond	99%	97
Danville Regional Medical Center[2]	Danville	99%	97
Southside Regional Medical Center	Petersburg	99%	241
Centra Health[2]	Lynchburg	98%	191
Halifax Regional Hospital	Halifax	98%	49
Mem Hosp of Martinsville & Henry Co	Martinsville	98%	66
Sentara Leigh Hospital	Norfolk	98%	158
University of Virginia Medical Center[2]	Charlottesville	98%	99
Chesapeake General Hospital[2]	Chesapeake	97%	116
Medical College of Virginia Hospitals	Richmond	97%	337
Richmond VA Medical Center	Richmond	97%	116
Sentara Obici Hospital	Suffolk	97%	108
Southern Virginia Regional Medical Center	Emporia	97%	70
Virginia Hospital Center	Arlington	97%	73
Sentara Careplex Hospital	Hampton	96%	106
Carilion Roanoke Memorial Hospital	Roanoke	95%	270
Culpeper Regional Hospital	Culpeper	95%	38
Inova Mount Vernon Hospital	Alexandria	95%	58
Johnston Memorial Hospital[2]	Abingdon	95%	44
Bon Secours Depaul Medical Center	Norfolk	93%	68
Inova Fairfax Hospital[2]	Falls Church	93%	104
Fauquier Hospital	Warrenton	91%	34
Wellmont Lonesome Pine Hospital	Big Stone Gap	90%	31
Southside Community Hospital	Farmville	88%	78

Discharge Instructions Given

Hospital Name	City	Rate	Cases
Bon Secours Maryview Medical Center	Portsmouth	100%	291
Bon Secours Mem Reg Med Ctr	Mechanicsville	100%	334

NOTE: Hospital profiles are in alphabetical order by state, then city, then hospital within the city; Rankings exclude hospitals with less than 25 cases except for patient surveys which excludes hospitals with less than 100 cases; (a) 100-299 cases; (1) The number of cases/patients is too few to report; (2) Data submitted were based on a sample of cases/patients; (3) Results are based on a shorter time period than required; (4) Data suppressed by CMS for one or more quarters; (5) Results are not available for this reporting period; (6) Fewer than 100 patients completed the HCAHPS survey; (7) No cases met the criteria for this measure; (8) The lower limit of the confidence interval cannot be calculated if the number of observed infections equals zero; (9) No data are available from the state/territory for this reporting period; (10) The scores shown reflect fewer than 50 completed surveys; (11) There were discrepancies in the data collection process; (12) This measure does not apply to this hospital for this reporting period; (13) Results cannot be calculated for this reporting period; (14) The results for this state are combined with nearby states to protect confidentiality; Please refer to the User's Guide for a full explanation of data.

Bon Secours Richmond Community Hospital	Richmond	100%	44
Bon Secours Saint Marys Hospital[2]	Richmond	100%	243
Carilion Franklin Memorial Hospital	Rocky Mount	100%	75
Carilion Giles Community Hospital	Pearisburg	100%	31
Clinch Valley Medical Center	Richlands	100%	134
Community Memorial Healthcenter	South Hill	100%	160
Hampton VA Medical Center	Hampton	100%	76
John Randolph Medical Center	Hopewell	100%	134
Lewisgale Medical Center[2]	Salem	100%	244
Norton Community Hospital[2]	Norton	100%	64
Reston Hospital Center	Reston	100%	211
Richmond VA Medical Center	Richmond	100%	286
Riverside Tappahannock Hospital	Tappahannock	100%	67
Sentara Leigh Hospital	Norfolk	100%	361
Sentara Norfolk General Hospital	Norfolk	100%	879
Smyth County Community Hospital[2]	Marion	100%	42
Spotsylvania Regional Medical Center	Fredericksburg	100%	94
Bon Secours Saint Francis Medical Center	Midlothian	99%	195
Mary Immaculate Hospital	Newport News	99%	173
Mary Washington Hospital	Fredericksburg	99%	401
Medical College of Virginia Hospitals	Richmond	99%	704
Riverside Regional Medical Center	Newport News	99%	422
Sentara Northern Virginia Medical Center	Woodbridge	99%	305
Sentara Virginia Beach General Hospital	Virginia Beach	99%	399
Sentara Williamsburg Reg Med Ctr	Williamsburg	99%	251
Southside Regional Medical Center	Petersburg	99%	484
Bedford Memorial Hospital	Bedford	98%	41
Carilion Roanoke Memorial Hospital	Roanoke	98%	692
Carilion Stonewall Jackson Hospital	Lexington	98%	54
Henrico Doctors' Hospital	Richmond	98%	417
Rappahannock General Hospital	Kilmarnock	98%	55
Riverside Shore Memorial Hospital	Nassawadox	98%	107
Sentara Careplex Hospital	Hampton	98%	321
Sentara Princess Anne Hospital	Virginia Beach	98%	298
Southern Virginia Regional Medical Center	Emporia	98%	150
Wythe County Community Hospital	Wytheville	98%	48
Bon Secours Depaul Medical Center	Norfolk	97%	175
Cjw Medical Center[2]	Richmond	97%	520
Danville Regional Medical Center[2]	Danville	97%	204
Lewisgale Hospital Montgomery	Blacksburg	97%	62
Riverside Walter Reed Hospital	Gloucester	97%	101
Salem VA Medical Center	Salem	97%	112
Stafford Hospital	Stafford	97%	95
University of Virginia Medical Center[2]	Charlottesville	97%	225
Virginia Hospital Center	Arlington	97%	176
Augusta Health	Fishersville	96%	299
Buchanan General Hospital	Grundy	96%	28
Carilion New River Valley Medical Center	Christiansburg	96%	162
Rockingham Memorial Hospital[2]	Harrisonburg	96%	287
Sentara Obici Hospital	Suffolk	95%	303
Warren Memorial Hospital	Front Royal	95%	57
Winchester Medical Center[2]	Winchester	94%	315
Johnston Memorial Hospital[2]	Abingdon	93%	132
Fauquier Hospital	Warrenton	92%	104
Inova Fair Oaks Hospital	Fairfax	92%	151
Inova Loudoun Hospital[2]	Leesburg	92%	219
Inova Mount Vernon Hospital	Alexandria	92%	170
Lewisgale Hospital Alleghany	Low Moor	92%	76
Lewisgale Hospital Pulaski	Pulaski	92%	64
Russell County Medical Center[2]	Lebanon	92%	60
Southampton Memorial Hospital	Franklin	92%	75
Chesapeake General Hospital[2]	Chesapeake	91%	257
Novant Health Prince William Med Ctr	Manassas	91%	137
Wellmont Lonesome Pine Hospital	Big Stone Gap	91%	98
Culpeper Regional Hospital	Culpeper	90%	124
Inova Alexandria Hospital[2]	Alexandria	90%	235
Martha Jefferson Hospital	Charlottesville	90%	210
Twin County Regional Hospital	Galax	90%	68
Halifax Regional Hospital	Halifax	88%	187
Shenandoah Memorial Hospital	Woodstock	81%	32
Mem Hosp of Martinsville & Henry Co	Martinsville	80%	189
Centra Health[2]	Lynchburg	76%	600
Southside Community Hospital	Farmville	70%	142
Inova Fairfax Hospital[2]	Falls Church	57%	249

Evaluation of LVS Function

Hospital Name	City	Rate	Cases
Augusta Health	Fishersville	100%	394
Bon Secours Maryview Medical Center	Portsmouth	100%	330
Bon Secours Mem Reg Med Ctr	Mechanicsville	100%	410
Bon Secours Richmond Community Hospital	Richmond	100%	56
Bon Secours Saint Francis Medical Center	Midlothian	100%	235
Bon Secours Saint Marys Hospital[2]	Richmond	100%	323
Buchanan General Hospital	Grundy	100%	34
Carilion Giles Community Hospital	Pearisburg	100%	41
Carilion New River Valley Medical Center	Christiansburg	100%	194
Carilion Stonewall Jackson Hospital	Lexington	100%	86
Carilion Tazewell Community Hospital	Tazewell	100%	33
Centra Health[2]	Lynchburg	100%	733
Chesapeake General Hospital[2]	Chesapeake	100%	320
Cjw Medical Center[2]	Richmond	100%	655
Clinch Valley Medical Center	Richlands	100%	146
Community Memorial Healthcenter	South Hill	100%	197
Danville Regional Medical Center[2]	Danville	100%	266
Fauquier Hospital	Warrenton	100%	127
Halifax Regional Hospital	Halifax	100%	237
Hampton VA Medical Center	Hampton	100%	84
Henrico Doctors' Hospital	Richmond	100%	508
Inova Fair Oaks Hospital	Fairfax	100%	177
Inova Loudoun Hospital[2]	Leesburg	100%	271
John Randolph Medical Center	Hopewell	100%	173
Lewisgale Hospital Alleghany	Low Moor	100%	100
Lewisgale Hospital Montgomery	Blacksburg	100%	86
Lewisgale Hospital Pulaski	Pulaski	100%	99
Lewisgale Medical Center[2]	Salem	100%	322
Martha Jefferson Hospital	Charlottesville	100%	257
Mary Immaculate Hospital	Newport News	100%	211
Mary Washington Hospital	Fredericksburg	100%	486
Medical College of Virginia Hospitals	Richmond	100%	761
Mem Hosp of Martinsville & Henry Co	Martinsville	100%	274
Norton Community Hospital[2]	Norton	100%	74
Novant Health Prince William Med Ctr	Manassas	100%	156
Reston Hospital Center	Reston	100%	263
Richmond VA Medical Center	Richmond	100%	309
Riverside Regional Medical Center	Newport News	100%	518
Riverside Shore Memorial Hospital	Nassawadox	100%	125
Riverside Tappahannock Hospital	Tappahannock	100%	86
Riverside Walter Reed Hospital	Gloucester	100%	129
Rockingham Memorial Hospital[2]	Harrisonburg	100%	355
Salem VA Medical Center	Salem	100%	136
Sentara Careplex Hospital	Hampton	100%	386
Sentara Leigh Hospital	Norfolk	100%	428
Sentara Norfolk General Hospital	Norfolk	100%	971
Sentara Northern Virginia Medical Center	Woodbridge	100%	355
Sentara Obici Hospital	Suffolk	100%	369
Sentara Princess Anne Hospital	Virginia Beach	100%	340
Sentara Virginia Beach General Hospital	Virginia Beach	100%	484
Sentara Williamsburg Reg Med Ctr	Williamsburg	100%	306
Shenandoah Memorial Hospital	Woodstock	100%	44
Smyth County Community Hospital[2]	Marion	100%	56
Southampton Memorial Hospital	Franklin	100%	90
Southern Virginia Regional Medical Center	Emporia	100%	169
Southside Community Hospital	Farmville	100%	187
Southside Regional Medical Center	Petersburg	100%	597
Spotsylvania Regional Medical Center	Fredericksburg	100%	108
Twin County Regional Hospital	Galax	100%	105
Virginia Hospital Center	Arlington	100%	232
Warren Memorial Hospital	Front Royal	100%	72
Wellmont Lonesome Pine Hospital	Big Stone Gap	100%	121
Winchester Medical Center[2]	Winchester	100%	360
Wythe County Community Hospital	Wytheville	100%	75
Bon Secours Depaul Medical Center	Norfolk	99%	211
Carilion Franklin Memorial Hospital	Rocky Mount	99%	93
Carilion Roanoke Memorial Hospital	Roanoke	99%	929
Culpeper Regional Hospital	Culpeper	99%	154
Inova Alexandria Hospital[2]	Alexandria	99%	290
Inova Mount Vernon Hospital	Alexandria	99%	193
Johnston Memorial Hospital[2]	Abingdon	99%	158
Stafford Hospital	Stafford	99%	102
University of Virginia Medical Center[2]	Charlottesville	99%	277
Bedford Memorial Hospital	Bedford	98%	59
Inova Fairfax Hospital[2]	Falls Church	98%	295
Rappahannock General Hospital	Kilmarnock	98%	66
Russell County Medical Center[2]	Lebanon	96%	69
Page Memorial Hospital	Luray	90%	31

Medicare Spending

Medicare Spending per Patient (ratio)

Hospital Name	City	Ratio	Cases
Eastern State Hospital	Williamsburg	0.66	-
Wellmont Lonesome Pine Hospital	Big Stone Gap	0.85	-
Riverside Walter Reed Hospital	Gloucester	0.86	-
Southampton Memorial Hospital	Franklin	0.87	-
Carilion Franklin Memorial Hospital	Rocky Mount	0.88	-
Clinch Valley Medical Center	Richlands	0.89	-
Halifax Regional Hospital	Halifax	0.89	-
Riverside Tappahannock Hospital	Tappahannock	0.89	-
Warren Memorial Hospital	Front Royal	0.89	-
Rappahannock General Hospital	Kilmarnock	0.90	-
Augusta Health	Fishersville	0.91	-
Riverside Shore Memorial Hospital	Nassawadox	0.91	-
Southern Virginia Regional Medical Center	Emporia	0.91	-
Bedford Memorial Hospital	Bedford	0.92	-
Rockingham Memorial Hospital	Harrisonburg	0.92	-
Community Memorial Healthcenter	South Hill	0.93	-
Culpeper Regional Hospital	Culpeper	0.93	-
Inova Mount Vernon Hospital	Alexandria	0.93	-
Lewisgale Hospital Alleghany	Low Moor	0.93	-
Russell County Medical Center	Lebanon	0.93	-
Spotsylvania Regional Medical Center	Fredericksburg	0.93	-
Johnston Memorial Hospital	Abingdon	0.94	-
Martha Jefferson Hospital	Charlottesville	0.94	-
Norton Community Hospital	Norton	0.94	-
Smyth County Community Hospital	Marion	0.94	-
Buchanan General Hospital	Grundy	0.95	-
Inova Fair Oaks Hospital	Fairfax	0.95	-
Lewisgale Hospital Montgomery	Blacksburg	0.95	-
Sentara Princess Anne Hospital	Virginia Beach	0.95	-
Sentara Williamsburg Reg Med Ctr	Williamsburg	0.95	-
Virginia Hospital Center	Arlington	0.95	-
Winchester Medical Center	Winchester	0.95	-
Bon Secours Mem Reg Med Ctr	Mechanicsville	0.96	-
Centra Health	Lynchburg	0.96	-
Mary Immaculate Hospital	Newport News	0.96	-
Stafford Hospital	Stafford	0.96	-
Carilion New River Valley Medical Center	Christiansburg	0.97	-
Carilion Roanoke Memorial Hospital	Roanoke	0.97	-
Sentara Obici Hospital	Suffolk	0.97	-
Sentara Virginia Beach General Hospital	Virginia Beach	0.97	-
Wythe County Community Hospital	Wytheville	0.97	-
Bon Secours Maryview Medical Center	Portsmouth	0.98	-
Inova Fairfax Hospital	Falls Church	0.98	-
Medical College of Virginia Hospitals	Richmond	0.98	-
Riverside Regional Medical Center	Newport News	0.98	-
Sentara Leigh Hospital	Norfolk	0.98	-
Sentara Norfolk General Hospital	Norfolk	0.98	-
Bon Secours Richmond Community Hospital	Richmond	0.99	-
Fauquier Hospital	Warrenton	0.99	-
Henrico Doctors' Hospital	Richmond	0.99	-
Lewisgale Hospital Pulaski	Pulaski	0.99	-
Reston Hospital Center	Reston	0.99	-
Sentara Careplex Hospital	Hampton	0.99	-
Bon Secours Saint Marys Hospital	Richmond	1.00	-
Chesapeake General Hospital	Chesapeake	1.00	-
Danville Regional Medical Center	Danville	1.00	-
Inova Alexandria Hospital	Alexandria	1.01	-
Mary Washington Hospital	Fredericksburg	1.01	-
Novant Health Prince William Med Ctr	Manassas	1.01	-
Southside Community Hospital	Farmville	1.01	-
Twin County Regional Hospital	Galax	1.01	-
University of Virginia Medical Center	Charlottesville	1.01	-
Bon Secours Depaul Medical Center	Norfolk	1.02	-
Cjw Medical Center	Richmond	1.02	-
Inova Loudoun Hospital	Leesburg	1.02	-
Mem Hosp of Martinsville & Henry Co	Martinsville	1.02	-
Bon Secours Saint Francis Medical Center	Midlothian	1.03	-
John Randolph Medical Center	Hopewell	1.03	-
Lewisgale Medical Center	Salem	1.03	-
Sentara Northern Virginia Medical Center	Woodbridge	1.04	-
Southside Regional Medical Center	Petersburg	1.06	-
Carilion Tazewell Community Hospital	Tazewell	1.08	-

Pneumonia Care

Appropriate Initial Antibiotic Given

Hospital Name	City	Rate	Cases
Bon Secours Mem Reg Med Ctr[2]	Mechanicsville	100%	180
Buchanan General Hospital	Grundy	100%	58
John Randolph Medical Center	Hopewell	100%	85
Lewisgale Hospital Montgomery	Blacksburg	100%	64
Lewisgale Medical Center	Salem	100%	178
Mary Washington Hospital[2]	Fredericksburg	100%	236
Reston Hospital Center	Reston	100%	103
Riverside Tappahannock Hospital	Tappahannock	100%	66
Sentara Northern Virginia Medical Center	Woodbridge	100%	137
Sentara Princess Anne Hospital	Virginia Beach	100%	162
Sentara Virginia Beach General Hospital	Virginia Beach	100%	180
Spotsylvania Regional Medical Center	Fredericksburg	100%	67
Stafford Hospital	Stafford	100%	86
Wythe County Community Hospital	Wytheville	100%	115
Augusta Health	Fishersville	99%	170
Clinch Valley Medical Center	Richlands	99%	80
Inova Alexandria Hospital[2]	Alexandria	99%	76
Lewisgale Hospital Pulaski	Pulaski	99%	67
Novant Health Prince William Med Ctr	Manassas	99%	92
Rockingham Memorial Hospital[2]	Harrisonburg	99%	143
Sentara Leigh Hospital	Norfolk	99%	157
Sentara Norfolk General Hospital	Norfolk	99%	120
Sentara Obici Hospital	Suffolk	99%	90
Virginia Hospital Center[2]	Arlington	99%	80
Bon Secours Maryview Medical Center	Portsmouth	98%	113
Cjw Medical Center[2]	Richmond	98%	218
Danville Regional Medical Center[2]	Danville	98%	88
Henrico Doctors' Hospital	Richmond	98%	150
Inova Fair Oaks Hospital[2]	Fairfax	98%	109
Mary Immaculate Hospital	Newport News	98%	121
Mem Hosp of Martinsville & Henry Co[2]	Martinsville	98%	87
Riverside Shore Memorial Hospital	Nassawadox	98%	63
Riverside Walter Reed Hospital	Gloucester	98%	113
Sentara Careplex Hospital	Hampton	98%	128

NOTE: Hospital profiles are in alphabetical order by state, then city, then hospital within the city; Rankings exclude hospitals with less than 25 cases except for patient surveys which excludes hospitals with less than 100 cases; (a) 100-299 cases; (1) The number of cases/patients is too few to report; (2) Data submitted were based on a sample of cases/patients; (3) Results are based on a shorter time period than required; (4) Data suppressed by CMS for one or more quarters; (5) Results are not available for this reporting period; (6) Fewer than 100 patients completed the HCAHPS survey; (7) No cases met the criteria for this measure; (8) The lower limit of the confidence interval cannot be calculated if the number of observed infections equals zero; (9) No data are available from the state/territory for this reporting period; (10) The scores shown reflect fewer than 50 completed surveys; (11) There were discrepancies in the data collection process; (12) This measure does not apply to this hospital for this reporting period; (13) Results cannot be calculated for this reporting period; (14) The results for this state are combined with nearby states to protect confidentiality; Please refer to the User's Guide for a full explanation of data.

Smyth County Community Hospital[2]	Marion	98%	48
Carilion Franklin Memorial Hospital	Rocky Mount	97%	88
Carilion Tazewell Community Hospital	Tazewell	97%	39
Centra Health[2]	Lynchburg	97%	190
Chesapeake General Hospital[2]	Chesapeake	97%	91
Inova Mount Vernon Hospital	Alexandria	97%	67
Lewisgale Hospital Alleghany	Low Moor	97%	77
Norton Community Hospital[2]	Norton	97%	64
Riverside Regional Medical Center	Newport News	97%	161
Warren Memorial Hospital	Front Royal	97%	64
Bon Secours Richmond Community Hospital	Richmond	96%	46
Carilion Stonewall Jackson Hospital	Lexington	96%	28
Community Memorial Healthcenter	South Hill	96%	54
Fauquier Hospital	Warrenton	96%	118
Inova Loudoun Hospital[2]	Leesburg	96%	77
Southside Regional Medical Center	Petersburg	96%	159
Winchester Medical Center[2]	Winchester	96%	98
Bon Secours Saint Marys Hospital[2]	Richmond	95%	81
Carilion New River Valley Medical Center	Christiansburg	95%	110
Carilion Roanoke Memorial Hospital	Roanoke	95%	237
Culpeper Regional Hospital	Culpeper	95%	87
Inova Fairfax Hospital[2]	Falls Church	95%	66
Shenandoah Memorial Hospital	Woodstock	95%	96
Bedford Memorial Hospital	Bedford	94%	66
Bon Secours Depaul Medical Center	Norfolk	94%	106
Bon Secours Saint Francis Medical Center	Midlothian	94%	126
Johnston Memorial Hospital[2]	Abingdon	94%	87
Salem VA Medical Center	Salem	94%	52
Martha Jefferson Hospital[2]	Charlottesville	93%	90
Medical College of Virginia Hospitals	Richmond	93%	109
Richmond VA Medical Center	Richmond	93%	58
Southside Community Hospital	Farmville	93%	96
Twin County Regional Hospital	Galax	93%	97
Halifax Regional Hospital	Halifax	92%	51
Russell County Medical Center[2]	Lebanon	92%	87
Southampton Memorial Hospital	Franklin	92%	37
Southern Virginia Regional Medical Center	Emporia	92%	128
Wellmont Lonesome Pine Hospital	Big Stone Gap	91%	98
Sentara Williamsburg Reg Med Ctr	Williamsburg	90%	135
University of Virginia Medical Center[2]	Charlottesville	87%	47
Carilion Giles Community Hospital	Pearisburg	86%	57
Pioneer Health Services of Patrick County	Stuart	84%	38
Rappahannock General Hospital	Kilmarnock	83%	47

Blood Culture Timing

Hospital Name	City	Rate	Cases
Bon Secours Mem Reg Med Ctr[2]	Mechanicsville	100%	284
Buchanan General Hospital	Grundy	100%	76
Cjw Medical Center[2]	Richmond	100%	382
Clinch Valley Medical Center	Richlands	100%	129
Henrico Doctors' Hospital	Richmond	100%	286
Lewisgale Hospital Alleghany	Low Moor	100%	107
Lewisgale Hospital Montgomery	Blacksburg	100%	102
Lewisgale Hospital Pulaski	Pulaski	100%	123
Lewisgale Medical Center	Salem	100%	311
Page Memorial Hospital	Luray	100%	25
Sentara Careplex Hospital	Hampton	100%	228
Smyth County Community Hospital[2]	Marion	100%	88
Spotsylvania Regional Medical Center	Fredericksburg	100%	96
Stafford Hospital	Stafford	100%	104
Twin County Regional Hospital	Galax	100%	204
Augusta Health	Fishersville	99%	330
Bon Secours Saint Marys Hospital[2]	Richmond	99%	154
Carilion Franklin Memorial Hospital	Rocky Mount	99%	133
Carilion New River Valley Medical Center	Christiansburg	99%	172
Centra Health[2]	Lynchburg	99%	279
Inova Fair Oaks Hospital[2]	Fairfax	99%	154
Inova Loudoun Hospital[2]	Leesburg	99%	106
John Randolph Medical Center	Hopewell	99%	133
Johnston Memorial Hospital[2]	Abingdon	99%	152
Mary Washington Hospital[2]	Fredericksburg	99%	323
Medical College of Virginia Hospitals	Richmond	99%	202
Novant Health Prince William Med Ctr	Manassas	99%	179
Reston Hospital Center	Reston	99%	167
Riverside Tappahannock Hospital	Tappahannock	99%	98
Riverside Walter Reed Hospital	Gloucester	99%	167
Rockingham Memorial Hospital[2]	Harrisonburg	99%	286
Salem VA Medical Center	Salem	99%	79
Sentara Leigh Hospital	Norfolk	99%	278
Sentara Norfolk General Hospital	Norfolk	99%	259
Sentara Northern Virginia Medical Center	Woodbridge	99%	233
Sentara Virginia Beach General Hospital	Virginia Beach	99%	404
Sentara Williamsburg Reg Med Ctr	Williamsburg	99%	181
Virginia Hospital Center[2]	Arlington	99%	123
Warren Memorial Hospital	Front Royal	99%	114
Wellmont Lonesome Pine Hospital	Big Stone Gap	99%	149
Bon Secours Richmond Community Hospital	Richmond	98%	66
Carilion Roanoke Memorial Hospital	Roanoke	98%	446
Inova Alexandria Hospital[2]	Alexandria	98%	108
Inova Mount Vernon Hospital	Alexandria	98%	91
Mary Immaculate Hospital	Newport News	98%	160
Mem Hosp of Martinsville & Henry Co[2]	Martinsville	98%	161
Riverside Regional Medical Center	Newport News	98%	237
Riverside Shore Memorial Hospital	Nassawadox	98%	118
Southern Virginia Regional Medical Center	Emporia	98%	132
Southside Community Hospital	Farmville	98%	169
Wythe County Community Hospital	Wytheville	98%	168
Bon Secours Saint Francis Medical Center	Midlothian	97%	229
Carilion Tazewell Community Hospital	Tazewell	97%	72
Community Memorial Healthcenter	South Hill	97%	119
Fauquier Hospital	Warrenton	97%	213
Hampton VA Medical Center	Hampton	97%	34
Russell County Medical Center[2]	Lebanon	97%	108
Sentara Obici Hospital	Suffolk	97%	177
Sentara Princess Anne Hospital	Virginia Beach	97%	312
Southside Regional Medical Center	Petersburg	97%	235
Bon Secours Depaul Medical Center	Norfolk	96%	179
Danville Regional Medical Center[2]	Danville	96%	131
Pioneer Health Services of Patrick County	Stuart	96%	45
Shenandoah Memorial Hospital	Woodstock	96%	153
Bedford Memorial Hospital	Bedford	95%	111
Carilion Stonewall Jackson Hospital	Lexington	95%	57
Chesapeake General Hospital[2]	Chesapeake	95%	133
Culpeper Regional Hospital	Culpeper	95%	194
Rappahannock General Hospital	Kilmarnock	95%	63
Southampton Memorial Hospital	Franklin	95%	75
Carilion Giles Community Hospital	Pearisburg	94%	67
Halifax Regional Hospital	Halifax	94%	71
Inova Fairfax Hospital[2]	Falls Church	94%	103
Richmond VA Medical Center	Richmond	94%	122
Winchester Medical Center[2]	Winchester	94%	154
Martha Jefferson Hospital[2]	Charlottesville	93%	181
University of Virginia Medical Center[2]	Charlottesville	92%	134
Norton Community Hospital[2]	Norton	91%	132
Bon Secours Maryview Medical Center	Portsmouth	89%	243

Pregnancy and Delivery Care

Newborns whose Deliveries were Scheduled Early

Hospital Name	City	Rate	Cases
Lewisgale Medical Center	Salem	0%	81
Novant Health Prince William Med Ctr[2]	Manassas	0%	41
Riverside Regional Medical Center[2]	Newport News	0%	56
Sentara Leigh Hospital	Norfolk	0%	178
Sentara Norfolk General Hospital	Norfolk	0%	130
Sentara Northern Virginia Medical Center	Woodbridge	0%	149
Sentara Obici Hospital	Suffolk	0%	128
Sentara Princess Anne Hospital	Virginia Beach	0%	178
Sentara Williamsburg Reg Med Ctr	Williamsburg	0%	76
Southampton Memorial Hospital[2]	Franklin	0%	28
Centra Health	Lynchburg	1%	192
Reston Hospital Center[2]	Reston	1%	72
Cjw Medical Center[2]	Richmond	2%	57
Wellmont Lonesome Pine Hospital	Big Stone Gap	2%	44
Bon Secours Saint Francis Medical Center[2]	Midlothian	3%	35
Carilion Roanoke Memorial Hospital	Roanoke	3%	224
Inova Alexandria Hospital[2]	Alexandria	3%	235
Lewisgale Hospital Montgomery	Blacksburg	3%	33
Rockingham Memorial Hospital[2]	Harrisonburg	3%	34
Clinch Valley Medical Center[2]	Richlands	4%	28
Fauquier Hospital	Warrenton	4%	70
Riverside Shore Memorial Hospital[2]	Nassawadox	4%	28
Southside Regional Medical Center[2]	Petersburg	4%	72
Spotsylvania Regional Medical Center	Fredericksburg	4%	49
Winchester Medical Center[2]	Winchester	4%	26
Henrico Doctors' Hospital[2]	Richmond	5%	76
Bon Secours Maryview Medical Center[2]	Portsmouth	6%	33
Danville Regional Medical Center[2]	Danville	6%	36
Chesapeake General Hospital	Chesapeake	7%	225
Inova Fair Oaks Hospital[2]	Fairfax	7%	251
Southside Community Hospital	Farmville	7%	57
Bon Secours Depaul Medical Center[2]	Norfolk	8%	26
Mem Hosp of Martinsville & Henry Co[2]	Martinsville	8%	40
Mary Washington Hospital	Fredericksburg	9%	239
Inova Fairfax Hospital[2]	Falls Church	10%	439
Inova Loudoun Hospital[2]	Leesburg	10%	135
Stafford Hospital	Stafford	10%	51
Virginia Hospital Center[2]	Arlington	10%	77
Culpeper Regional Hospital	Culpeper	11%	37
Bon Secours Mem Reg Med Ctr[2]	Mechanicsville	14%	29
Mary Immaculate Hospital[2]	Newport News	18%	38
Martha Jefferson Hospital[2]	Charlottesville	20%	25
Bon Secours Saint Marys Hospital[2]	Richmond	24%	58
Carilion New River Valley Medical Center	Christiansburg	27%	94
Halifax Regional Hospital	Halifax	27%	37

Preventive Care

Immunization for Influenza

Hospital Name	City	Rate	Cases
Henrico Doctors' Hospital[2]	Richmond	100%	622
John Randolph Medical Center[2]	Hopewell	100%	493
Lewisgale Medical Center[2]	Salem	100%	602
Southern Virginia Regional Medical Center[2]	Emporia	100%	304
Clinch Valley Medical Center[2]	Richlands	99%	448
Lewisgale Hospital Montgomery[2]	Blacksburg	99%	435
Reston Hospital Center[2]	Reston	99%	535
Riverside Tappahannock Hospital[2]	Tappahannock	99%	290
Smyth County Community Hospital[2]	Marion	99%	304
Southampton Memorial Hospital[2]	Franklin	99%	312
Wythe County Community Hospital[2]	Wytheville	99%	294
Cjw Medical Center[2]	Richmond	98%	657
Fauquier Hospital[2]	Warrenton	98%	536
Lewisgale Hospital Alleghany[2]	Low Moor	98%	319
Medical College of Virginia Hospitals[2]	Richmond	98%	547
Sentara Careplex Hospital[2]	Hampton	98%	603
Warren Memorial Hospital[2]	Front Royal	98%	258
Carilion Franklin Memorial Hospital[2]	Rocky Mount	97%	364
Carilion Stonewall Jackson Hospital[2]	Lexington	97%	284
Johnston Memorial Hospital[2]	Abingdon	97%	560
Lewisgale Hospital Pulaski[2]	Pulaski	97%	303
Mary Immaculate Hospital[2]	Newport News	97%	569
Mem Hosp of Martinsville & Henry Co[2]	Martinsville	97%	521
Russell County Medical Center[2]	Lebanon	97%	299
Spotsylvania Regional Medical Center[2]	Fredericksburg	97%	475
Virginia Hospital Center[2]	Arlington	97%	492
Bon Secours Mem Reg Med Ctr[2]	Mechanicsville	96%	568
Bon Secours Richmond Community Hospital[2]	Richmond	96%	294
Bon Secours Saint Marys Hospital[2]	Richmond	96%	578
Chesapeake General Hospital[2]	Chesapeake	96%	530
Shenandoah Memorial Hospital[2,3]	Woodstock	96%	140
Wellmont Lonesome Pine Hospital[2]	Big Stone Gap	96%	516
Carilion Giles Community Hospital[2]	Pearisburg	95%	277
Rappahannock General Hospital[2]	Kilmarnock	95%	456
Riverside Regional Medical Center[2]	Newport News	95%	488
Riverside Shore Memorial Hospital[2]	Nassawadox	95%	347
Rockingham Memorial Hospital[2]	Harrisonburg	95%	591
Sentara Virginia Beach General Hospital[2]	Virginia Beach	95%	594
Culpeper Regional Hospital[2]	Culpeper	94%	300
Inova Loudoun Hospital[2]	Leesburg	94%	464
Riverside Walter Reed Hospital[2]	Gloucester	94%	292
Sentara Williamsburg Reg Med Ctr[2]	Williamsburg	94%	542
Southside Regional Medical Center[2]	Petersburg	94%	608
Community Memorial Healthcenter[2]	South Hill	93%	334
Inova Alexandria Hospital[2]	Alexandria	93%	519
Inova Mount Vernon Hospital[2]	Alexandria	93%	592
Page Memorial Hospital[2]	Luray	93%	288
Bon Secours Saint Francis Medical Center[2]	Midlothian	92%	580
Twin County Regional Hospital[2]	Galax	92%	315
Carilion New River Valley Medical Center[2]	Christiansburg	91%	522
Carilion Tazewell Community Hospital[2]	Tazewell	91%	270
Inova Fair Oaks Hospital[2]	Fairfax	91%	462
Novant Health Prince William Med Ctr[2]	Manassas	91%	628
Sentara Leigh Hospital[2]	Norfolk	91%	554
Sentara Obici Hospital[2]	Suffolk	91%	534
Carilion Roanoke Memorial Hospital[2]	Roanoke	90%	537
Centra Health[2]	Lynchburg	90%	586
Danville Regional Medical Center[2]	Danville	90%	526
Sentara Princess Anne Hospital[2]	Virginia Beach	90%	489
Southside Community Hospital[2]	Farmville	90%	469
Winchester Medical Center[2]	Winchester	90%	515
Augusta Health[2]	Fishersville	89%	543
Inova Fairfax Hospital[2]	Falls Church	88%	480
Norton Community Hospital[2]	Norton	88%	376
Halifax Regional Hospital[2]	Halifax	86%	437
Martha Jefferson Hospital[2]	Charlottesville	84%	542
Mary Washington Hospital[2]	Fredericksburg	82%	544
Bedford Memorial Hospital[2]	Bedford	80%	473
Buchanan General Hospital[2]	Grundy	80%	283
Sentara Northern Virginia Medical Center[2]	Woodbridge	79%	516
Stafford Hospital[2]	Stafford	79%	360
Bon Secours Depaul Medical Center[2]	Norfolk	78%	556
Eastern State Hospital[2]	Williamsburg	76%	33
Sentara Norfolk General Hospital[2]	Norfolk	74%	527
Bon Secours Maryview Medical Center[2]	Portsmouth	73%	593
University of Virginia Medical Center[2]	Charlottesville	54%	533

Immunization for Pneumonia

Hospital Name	City	Rate	Cases
John Randolph Medical Center[2]	Hopewell	100%	717
Lewisgale Hospital Alleghany[2]	Low Moor	100%	523
Lewisgale Medical Center[2]	Salem	100%	832
Riverside Tappahannock Hospital[2]	Tappahannock	100%	477
Clinch Valley Medical Center[2]	Richlands	99%	554
Henrico Doctors' Hospital[2]	Richmond	99%	786
Lewisgale Hospital Montgomery[2]	Blacksburg	99%	551
Lewisgale Hospital Pulaski[2]	Pulaski	99%	491
Mem Hosp of Martinsville & Henry Co[2]	Martinsville	99%	741
Smyth County Community Hospital[2]	Marion	99%	471
Southampton Memorial Hospital[2]	Franklin	99%	406
Southern Virginia Regional Medical Center[2]	Emporia	99%	483
Spotsylvania Regional Medical Center[2]	Fredericksburg	99%	490

NOTE: Hospital profiles are in alphabetical order by state, then city, then hospital within the city; Rankings exclude hospitals with less than 25 cases except for patient surveys which excludes hospitals with less than 100 cases; (a) 100-299 cases; (1) The number of cases/patients is too few to report; (2) Data submitted were based on a sample of cases/patients; (3) Results are based on a shorter time period than required; (4) Data suppressed by CMS for one or more quarters; (5) Results are not available for this reporting period; (6) Fewer than 100 patients completed the HCAHPS survey; (7) No cases met the criteria for this measure; (8) The lower limit of the confidence interval cannot be calculated if the number of observed infections equals zero; (9) No data are available from the state/territory for this reporting period; (10) The scores shown reflect fewer than 50 completed surveys; (11) There were discrepancies in the data collection process; (12) This measure does not apply to this hospital for this reporting period; (13) Results cannot be calculated for this reporting period; (14) The results for this state are combined with nearby states to protect confidentiality; Please refer to the User's Guide for a full explanation of data.

Hospital Name	City	Rate	Cases
Warren Memorial Hospital[2]	Front Royal	99%	320
Wellmont Lonesome Pine Hospital[2]	Big Stone Gap	99%	695
Carilion Franklin Memorial Hospital[2]	Rocky Mount	98%	531
Cjw Medical Center[2]	Richmond	98%	788
Fauquier Hospital[2]	Warrenton	98%	659
Russell County Medical Center[2]	Lebanon	98%	468
Wythe County Community Hospital[2]	Wytheville	98%	364
Carilion Stonewall Jackson Hospital[2]	Lexington	97%	551
Rappahannock General Hospital[2]	Kilmarnock	97%	600
Reston Hospital Center[2]	Reston	97%	494
Riverside Shore Memorial Hospital[2]	Nassawadox	97%	445
Rockingham Memorial Hospital[2]	Harrisonburg	97%	720
Sentara Careplex Hospital[2]	Hampton	97%	891
Bon Secours Mem Reg Med Ctr[2]	Mechanicsville	96%	805
Bon Secours Saint Marys Hospital[2]	Richmond	96%	674
Carilion Giles Community Hospital[2]	Pearisburg	96%	495
Carilion New River Valley Medical Center[2]	Christiansburg	96%	616
Community Memorial Healthcenter[2]	South Hill	96%	515
Mary Immaculate Hospital[2]	Newport News	96%	639
Sentara Williamsburg Reg Med Ctr[2]	Williamsburg	96%	752
Southside Regional Medical Center[2]	Petersburg	96%	741
Twin County Regional Hospital[2]	Galax	96%	365
Carilion Tazewell Community Hospital[2]	Tazewell	95%	405
Culpeper Regional Hospital[2]	Culpeper	95%	399
Novant Health Prince William Med Ctr[2]	Manassas	95%	545
Riverside Regional Medical Center[2]	Newport News	95%	611
Sentara Obici Hospital[2]	Suffolk	95%	695
Southside Community Hospital[2]	Farmville	95%	615
Centra Health[2]	Lynchburg	94%	733
Danville Regional Medical Center[2]	Danville	94%	711
Johnston Memorial Hospital[2]	Abingdon	94%	760
Page Memorial Hospital[2]	Luray	94%	459
Riverside Walter Reed Hospital[2]	Gloucester	94%	470
Sentara Leigh Hospital[2]	Norfolk	94%	704
Shenandoah Memorial Hospital[2,3]	Woodstock	94%	335
Bon Secours Richmond Community Hospital[2]	Richmond	93%	300
Buchanan General Hospital[2]	Grundy	93%	409
Chesapeake General Hospital[2]	Chesapeake	93%	618
Inova Alexandria Hospital[2]	Alexandria	93%	510
Inova Loudoun Hospital[2]	Leesburg	93%	443
Martha Jefferson Hospital[2]	Charlottesville	93%	686
Sentara Princess Anne Hospital[2]	Virginia Beach	93%	557
Stafford Hospital[2]	Stafford	93%	374
Augusta Health[2]	Fishersville	92%	741
Carilion Roanoke Memorial Hospital[2]	Roanoke	92%	662
Inova Mount Vernon Hospital[2]	Alexandria	92%	752
Sentara Virginia Beach General Hospital[2]	Virginia Beach	92%	883
Inova Fair Oaks Hospital[2]	Fairfax	91%	368
Medical College of Virginia Hospitals[2]	Richmond	91%	562
Mary Washington Hospital[2]	Fredericksburg	90%	657
Virginia Hospital Center[2]	Arlington	90%	548
Winchester Medical Center[2]	Winchester	90%	691
Bon Secours Saint Francis Medical Center[2]	Midlothian	89%	640
Eastern State Hospital[2]	Williamsburg	89%	53
Bedford Memorial Hospital[2]	Bedford	88%	733
Halifax Regional Hospital[2]	Halifax	86%	582
Inova Fairfax Hospital[2]	Falls Church	85%	401
Norton Community Hospital[2]	Norton	84%	393
Bon Secours Depaul Medical Center[2]	Norfolk	82%	680
Sentara Northern Virginia Medical Center[2]	Woodbridge	80%	542
Sentara Norfolk General Hospital[2]	Norfolk	79%	625
Bon Secours Maryview Medical Center[2]	Portsmouth	71%	685
University of Virginia Medical Center[2]	Charlottesville	48%	579

Stroke Care

Anticoagulation Therapy for Atrial Fibrillation

Hospital Name	City	Rate	Cases
Bon Secours Mem Reg Med Ctr	Mechanicsville	100%	28
Cjw Medical Center[2]	Richmond	100%	36
Virginia Hospital Center	Arlington	100%	30
Carilion Roanoke Memorial Hospital	Roanoke	98%	43
Riverside Regional Medical Center	Newport News	97%	31
Sentara Virginia Beach General Hospital	Virginia Beach	96%	28
Mary Washington Hospital	Fredericksburg	93%	29
Winchester Medical Center	Winchester	93%	55
Bon Secours Maryview Medical Center	Portsmouth	88%	26

Antithrombotic Therapy Timing

Hospital Name	City	Rate	Cases
Bon Secours Depaul Medical Center	Norfolk	100%	83
Bon Secours Mem Reg Med Ctr	Mechanicsville	100%	237
Bon Secours Richmond Community Hospital	Richmond	100%	37
Carilion Roanoke Memorial Hospital	Roanoke	100%	360
Chesapeake General Hospital[2]	Chesapeake	100%	94
Cjw Medical Center[2]	Richmond	100%	245
Clinch Valley Medical Center	Richlands	100%	28
Community Memorial Healthcenter	South Hill	100%	54
Danville Regional Medical Center[2]	Danville	100%	104
Halifax Regional Hospital	Halifax	100%	61
Henrico Doctors' Hospital	Richmond	100%	151
Inova Fair Oaks Hospital	Fairfax	100%	62
Inova Fairfax Hospital[2]	Falls Church	100%	146
Inova Loudoun Hospital[2]	Leesburg	100%	105
Inova Mount Vernon Hospital	Alexandria	100%	63
John Randolph Medical Center[2]	Hopewell	100%	66
Johnston Memorial Hospital	Abingdon	100%	69
Lewisgale Hospital Alleghany[2]	Low Moor	100%	25
Lewisgale Hospital Montgomery	Blacksburg	100%	38
Lewisgale Hospital Pulaski[2]	Pulaski	100%	29
Lewisgale Medical Center	Salem	100%	176
Mary Immaculate Hospital	Newport News	100%	39
Mem Hosp of Martinsville & Henry Co	Martinsville	100%	78
Rappahannock General Hospital	Kilmarnock	100%	37
Reston Hospital Center	Reston	100%	109
Riverside Regional Medical Center	Newport News	100%	212
Sentara Careplex Hospital	Hampton	100%	191
Sentara Leigh Hospital	Norfolk	100%	172
Sentara Norfolk General Hospital	Norfolk	100%	226
Sentara Northern Virginia Medical Center	Woodbridge	100%	108
Sentara Obici Hospital	Suffolk	100%	136
Sentara Princess Anne Hospital	Virginia Beach	100%	104
Sentara Williamsburg Reg Med Ctr	Williamsburg	100%	133
Stafford Hospital	Stafford	100%	25
Virginia Hospital Center	Arlington	100%	172
Augusta Health[2]	Fishersville	99%	79
Bon Secours Saint Marys Hospital	Richmond	99%	163
Inova Alexandria Hospital[2]	Alexandria	99%	109
Rockingham Memorial Hospital	Harrisonburg	99%	118
Sentara Virginia Beach General Hospital	Virginia Beach	99%	174
Southside Regional Medical Center	Petersburg	99%	147
Winchester Medical Center	Winchester	99%	251
Bon Secours Saint Francis Medical Center	Midlothian	98%	63
Centra Health[2]	Lynchburg	98%	97
Mary Washington Hospital	Fredericksburg	98%	250
Novant Health Prince William Med Ctr	Manassas	98%	40
Riverside Walter Reed Hospital	Gloucester	98%	46
Twin County Regional Hospital	Galax	98%	43
University of Virginia Medical Center[2]	Charlottesville	98%	47
Bon Secours Maryview Medical Center	Portsmouth	97%	149
Carilion New River Valley Medical Center	Christiansburg	97%	65
Martha Jefferson Hospital	Charlottesville	97%	87
Medical College of Virginia Hospitals[2]	Richmond	97%	61
Fauquier Hospital	Warrenton	94%	52
Riverside Shore Memorial Hospital	Nassawadox	94%	36
Southampton Memorial Hospital	Franklin	93%	30
Southern Virginia Regional Medical Center	Emporia	92%	26
Southside Community Hospital	Farmville	91%	35

Assessed for Rehabilitation

Hospital Name	City	Rate	Cases
Bon Secours Depaul Medical Center	Norfolk	100%	124
Bon Secours Maryview Medical Center	Portsmouth	100%	155
Carilion Roanoke Memorial Hospital	Roanoke	100%	494
Cjw Medical Center[2]	Richmond	100%	296
Community Memorial Healthcenter	South Hill	100%	47
Henrico Doctors' Hospital	Richmond	100%	191
John Randolph Medical Center[2]	Hopewell	100%	59
Lewisgale Hospital Alleghany[2]	Low Moor	100%	26
Lewisgale Hospital Montgomery	Blacksburg	100%	34
Lewisgale Hospital Pulaski[2]	Pulaski	100%	32
Lewisgale Medical Center	Salem	100%	191
Mary Immaculate Hospital	Newport News	100%	41
Reston Hospital Center	Reston	100%	133
Riverside Walter Reed Hospital	Gloucester	100%	45
Sentara Careplex Hospital	Hampton	100%	203
Sentara Norfolk General Hospital	Norfolk	100%	334
Sentara Northern Virginia Medical Center	Woodbridge	100%	127
Sentara Obici Hospital	Suffolk	100%	146
Sentara Princess Anne Hospital	Virginia Beach	100%	114
Sentara Virginia Beach General Hospital	Virginia Beach	100%	206
Sentara Williamsburg Reg Med Ctr	Williamsburg	100%	139
Southampton Memorial Hospital	Franklin	100%	31
Southern Virginia Regional Medical Center	Emporia	100%	25
Spotsylvania Regional Medical Center[2]	Fredericksburg	100%	25
Twin County Regional Hospital	Galax	100%	50
University of Virginia Medical Center[2]	Charlottesville	100%	87
Winchester Medical Center	Winchester	100%	308
Bon Secours Saint Francis Medical Center	Midlothian	99%	75
Bon Secours Saint Marys Hospital	Richmond	99%	225
Carilion New River Valley Medical Center	Christiansburg	99%	67
Inova Fair Oaks Hospital	Fairfax	99%	68
Inova Loudoun Hospital[2]	Leesburg	99%	110
Martha Jefferson Hospital	Charlottesville	99%	136
Mem Hosp of Martinsville & Henry Co	Martinsville	99%	77
Riverside Regional Medical Center	Newport News	99%	312
Rockingham Memorial Hospital	Harrisonburg	99%	147
Sentara Leigh Hospital	Norfolk	99%	189
Virginia Hospital Center	Arlington	99%	217
Bon Secours Mem Reg Med Ctr	Mechanicsville	98%	267
Centra Health[2]	Lynchburg	98%	113
Danville Regional Medical Center[2]	Danville	98%	107
Fauquier Hospital	Warrenton	98%	54
Inova Fairfax Hospital[2]	Falls Church	98%	244
Inova Mount Vernon Hospital	Alexandria	98%	61
Novant Health Prince William Med Ctr	Manassas	98%	66
Southside Community Hospital	Farmville	98%	40
Augusta Health[2]	Fishersville	97%	107
Bon Secours Richmond Community Hospital	Richmond	97%	39
Chesapeake General Hospital[2]	Chesapeake	97%	87
Southside Regional Medical Center	Petersburg	97%	155
Stafford Hospital	Stafford	96%	26
Inova Alexandria Hospital[2]	Alexandria	95%	127
Mary Washington Hospital	Fredericksburg	95%	290
Medical College of Virginia Hospitals[2]	Richmond	95%	121
Riverside Shore Memorial Hospital	Nassawadox	94%	48
Johnston Memorial Hospital	Abingdon	92%	74
Rappahannock General Hospital	Kilmarnock	92%	39
Halifax Regional Hospital	Halifax	90%	67

Discharged on Antithrombotic Therapy

Hospital Name	City	Rate	Cases
Augusta Health[2]	Fishersville	100%	104
Bon Secours Mem Reg Med Ctr	Mechanicsville	100%	258
Bon Secours Richmond Community Hospital	Richmond	100%	38
Bon Secours Saint Francis Medical Center	Midlothian	100%	72
Carilion New River Valley Medical Center	Christiansburg	100%	66
Carilion Roanoke Memorial Hospital	Roanoke	100%	390
Centra Health[2]	Lynchburg	100%	100
Chesapeake General Hospital[2]	Chesapeake	100%	81
Cjw Medical Center[2]	Richmond	100%	260
Community Memorial Healthcenter	South Hill	100%	45
Fauquier Hospital	Warrenton	100%	53
Henrico Doctors' Hospital	Richmond	100%	165
Inova Fair Oaks Hospital	Fairfax	100%	60
Inova Mount Vernon Hospital	Alexandria	100%	61
John Randolph Medical Center[2]	Hopewell	100%	57
Lewisgale Hospital Alleghany[2]	Low Moor	100%	25
Lewisgale Hospital Montgomery	Blacksburg	100%	33
Lewisgale Hospital Pulaski[2]	Pulaski	100%	30
Lewisgale Medical Center	Salem	100%	177
Martha Jefferson Hospital	Charlottesville	100%	128
Mary Immaculate Hospital	Newport News	100%	37
Mary Washington Hospital	Fredericksburg	100%	269
Medical College of Virginia Hospitals[2]	Richmond	100%	75
Mem Hosp of Martinsville & Henry Co	Martinsville	100%	77
Novant Health Prince William Med Ctr	Manassas	100%	65
Rappahannock General Hospital	Kilmarnock	100%	37
Reston Hospital Center	Reston	100%	124
Riverside Regional Medical Center	Newport News	100%	246
Riverside Shore Memorial Hospital	Nassawadox	100%	44
Riverside Walter Reed Hospital	Gloucester	100%	43
Rockingham Memorial Hospital	Harrisonburg	100%	144
Sentara Careplex Hospital	Hampton	100%	190
Sentara Leigh Hospital	Norfolk	100%	186
Sentara Norfolk General Hospital	Norfolk	100%	238
Sentara Northern Virginia Medical Center	Woodbridge	100%	125
Sentara Princess Anne Hospital	Virginia Beach	100%	109
Sentara Virginia Beach General Hospital	Virginia Beach	100%	176
Sentara Williamsburg Reg Med Ctr	Williamsburg	100%	136
Southside Community Hospital	Farmville	100%	40
Southside Regional Medical Center	Petersburg	100%	149
Stafford Hospital	Stafford	100%	25
Twin County Regional Hospital	Galax	100%	49
Winchester Medical Center	Winchester	100%	287
Bon Secours Depaul Medical Center	Norfolk	99%	97
Inova Alexandria Hospital[2]	Alexandria	99%	120
Inova Loudoun Hospital[2]	Leesburg	99%	108
Johnston Memorial Hospital	Abingdon	99%	69
Sentara Obici Hospital	Suffolk	99%	144
Virginia Hospital Center	Arlington	99%	183
Bon Secours Saint Marys Hospital	Richmond	98%	186
Danville Regional Medical Center[2]	Danville	98%	104
Inova Fairfax Hospital[2]	Falls Church	98%	168
University of Virginia Medical Center[2]	Charlottesville	98%	64
Bon Secours Maryview Medical Center	Portsmouth	97%	147
Halifax Regional Hospital	Halifax	97%	65
Southampton Memorial Hospital	Franklin	97%	29

Discharged on Statin Medication

Hospital Name	City	Rate	Cases
Carilion Roanoke Memorial Hospital	Roanoke	100%	311
Cjw Medical Center[2]	Richmond	100%	216
Community Memorial Healthcenter	South Hill	100%	32
John Randolph Medical Center[2]	Hopewell	100%	46
Lewisgale Medical Center	Salem	100%	135
Mary Immaculate Hospital	Newport News	100%	27
Mem Hosp of Martinsville & Henry Co	Martinsville	100%	62
Novant Health Prince William Med Ctr	Manassas	100%	58
Reston Hospital Center	Reston	100%	101
Sentara Leigh Hospital	Norfolk	100%	141

NOTE: Hospital profiles are in alphabetical order by state, then city, then hospital within the city; Rankings exclude hospitals with less than 25 cases except for patient surveys which excludes hospitals with less than 100 cases; (a) 100-299 cases; (1) The number of cases/patients is too few to report; (2) Data submitted were based on a sample of cases/patients; (3) Results are based on a shorter time period than required; (4) Data suppressed by CMS for one or more quarters; (5) Results are not available for this reporting period; (6) Fewer than 100 patients completed the HCAHPS survey; (7) No cases met the criteria for this measure; (8) The lower limit of the confidence interval cannot be calculated if the number of observed infections equals zero; (9) No data are available from the state/territory for this reporting period; (10) The scores shown reflect fewer than 50 completed surveys; (11) There were discrepancies in the data collection process; (12) This measure does not apply to this hospital for this reporting period; (13) Results cannot be calculated for this reporting period; (14) The results for this state are combined with nearby states to protect confidentiality; Please refer to the User's Guide for a full explanation of data.

Hospital Name	City	Rate	Cases
Sentara Northern Virginia Medical Center	Woodbridge	100%	100
Sentara Obici Hospital	Suffolk	100%	114
Sentara Princess Anne Hospital	Virginia Beach	100%	84
Twin County Regional Hospital	Galax	100%	37
Centra Health[2]	Lynchburg	99%	79
Henrico Doctors' Hospital	Richmond	99%	137
Mary Washington Hospital	Fredericksburg	99%	216
Riverside Regional Medical Center	Newport News	99%	191
Sentara Norfolk General Hospital	Norfolk	99%	175
Sentara Virginia Beach General Hospital	Virginia Beach	99%	134
Sentara Williamsburg Reg Med Ctr	Williamsburg	99%	104
Winchester Medical Center	Winchester	99%	226
Inova Loudoun Hospital[2]	Leesburg	98%	83
Inova Mount Vernon Hospital	Alexandria	98%	45
Rockingham Memorial Hospital	Harrisonburg	98%	117
Southside Regional Medical Center	Petersburg	98%	122
Virginia Hospital Center	Arlington	98%	144
Augusta Health[2]	Fishersville	97%	70
Bon Secours Depaul Medical Center	Norfolk	97%	75
Bon Secours Maryview Medical Center	Portsmouth	97%	103
Inova Alexandria Hospital[2]	Alexandria	97%	97
Martha Jefferson Hospital	Charlottesville	97%	97
Riverside Walter Reed Hospital	Gloucester	97%	35
Sentara Careplex Hospital	Hampton	97%	152
Southside Community Hospital	Farmville	97%	31
Bon Secours Saint Marys Hospital	Richmond	96%	117
Danville Regional Medical Center[2]	Danville	96%	80
Halifax Regional Hospital	Halifax	96%	50
Inova Fair Oaks Hospital	Fairfax	96%	50
Medical College of Virginia Hospitals[2]	Richmond	95%	64
University of Virginia Medical Center[2]	Charlottesville	95%	57
Bon Secours Saint Francis Medical Center	Midlothian	94%	54
Chesapeake General Hospital[2]	Chesapeake	94%	64
Riverside Shore Memorial Hospital	Nassawadox	94%	35
Fauquier Hospital	Warrenton	93%	42
Inova Fairfax Hospital[2]	Falls Church	93%	152
Bon Secours Mem Reg Med Ctr	Mechanicsville	91%	188
Carilion New River Valley Medical Center	Christiansburg	91%	57
Johnston Memorial Hospital	Abingdon	90%	61
Bon Secours Richmond Community Hospital	Richmond	70%	27
Rappahannock General Hospital	Kilmarnock	56%	34

Thrombolytic Therapy Timing

Hospital Name	City	Rate	Cases
Augusta Health[2]	Fishersville	23%	26

Venous Thromboembolism (VTE) Prophylaxis

Hospital Name	City	Rate	Cases
Augusta Health[2]	Fishersville	100%	88
Bon Secours Richmond Community Hospital	Richmond	100%	39
Carilion Roanoke Memorial Hospital	Roanoke	100%	539
Cjw Medical Center[2]	Richmond	100%	296
Clinch Valley Medical Center	Richlands	100%	28
Community Memorial Healthcenter	South Hill	100%	56
Inova Loudoun Hospital[2]	Leesburg	100%	116
John Randolph Medical Center[2]	Hopewell	100%	68
Lewisgale Hospital Alleghany[2]	Low Moor	100%	27
Lewisgale Hospital Montgomery	Blacksburg	100%	40
Lewisgale Hospital Pulaski[2]	Pulaski	100%	32
Lewisgale Medical Center	Salem	100%	198
Mary Washington Hospital	Fredericksburg	100%	282
Norton Community Hospital	Norton	100%	25
Reston Hospital Center	Reston	100%	113
Sentara Careplex Hospital	Hampton	100%	208
Spotsylvania Regional Medical Center[2]	Fredericksburg	100%	29
Riverside Regional Medical Center	Newport News	99%	320
Sentara Leigh Hospital	Norfolk	99%	187
Sentara Norfolk General Hospital	Norfolk	99%	377
University of Virginia Medical Center[2]	Charlottesville	99%	89
Bon Secours Depaul Medical Center	Norfolk	98%	130
Danville Regional Medical Center[2]	Danville	98%	109
Henrico Doctors' Hospital	Richmond	98%	199
Inova Fairfax Hospital[2]	Falls Church	98%	265
Martha Jefferson Hospital	Charlottesville	98%	105
Mary Immaculate Hospital	Newport News	98%	41
Medical College of Virginia Hospitals[2]	Richmond	98%	123
Novant Health Prince William Med Ctr	Manassas	98%	51
Riverside Shore Memorial Hospital	Nassawadox	98%	48
Sentara Northern Virginia Medical Center	Woodbridge	98%	127
Sentara Princess Anne Hospital	Virginia Beach	98%	118
Sentara Williamsburg Reg Med Ctr	Williamsburg	98%	139
Twin County Regional Hospital	Galax	98%	46
Bon Secours Saint Francis Medical Center	Midlothian	97%	72
Carilion New River Valley Medical Center	Christiansburg	97%	69
Mem Hosp of Martinsville & Henry Co	Martinsville	97%	76
Rappahannock General Hospital	Kilmarnock	97%	36
Sentara Virginia Beach General Hospital	Virginia Beach	97%	230
Southside Regional Medical Center	Petersburg	97%	163
Virginia Hospital Center	Arlington	97%	229
Inova Alexandria Hospital[2]	Alexandria	96%	138
Riverside Walter Reed Hospital	Gloucester	96%	47
Winchester Medical Center	Winchester	96%	303
Fauquier Hospital	Warrenton	95%	57
Sentara Obici Hospital	Suffolk	95%	139
Bon Secours Saint Marys Hospital	Richmond	94%	230
Centra Health[2]	Lynchburg	94%	120
Inova Fair Oaks Hospital	Fairfax	94%	69
Johnston Memorial Hospital	Abingdon	93%	72
Rockingham Memorial Hospital	Harrisonburg	93%	121
Bon Secours Mem Reg Med Ctr	Mechanicsville	92%	262
Bon Secours Maryview Medical Center	Portsmouth	91%	167
Inova Mount Vernon Hospital	Alexandria	90%	70
Southside Community Hospital	Farmville	89%	35
Chesapeake General Hospital[2]	Chesapeake	87%	105
Southern Virginia Regional Medical Center	Emporia	85%	27
Southampton Memorial Hospital	Franklin	82%	33
Halifax Regional Hospital	Halifax	80%	66

Written Stroke Educational Materials Given

Hospital Name	City	Rate	Cases
Bon Secours Depaul Medical Center	Norfolk	100%	51
Bon Secours Maryview Medical Center	Portsmouth	100%	91
Fauquier Hospital	Warrenton	100%	35
John Randolph Medical Center[2]	Hopewell	100%	26
Lewisgale Medical Center	Salem	100%	97
Mary Immaculate Hospital	Newport News	100%	31
Mary Washington Hospital	Fredericksburg	100%	170
Novant Health Prince William Med Ctr	Manassas	100%	32
Reston Hospital Center	Reston	100%	93
Rockingham Memorial Hospital	Harrisonburg	100%	84
Cjw Medical Center[2]	Richmond	99%	140
Sentara Obici Hospital	Suffolk	99%	94
Southside Regional Medical Center	Petersburg	99%	80
Henrico Doctors' Hospital	Richmond	98%	105
Inova Loudoun Hospital[2]	Leesburg	98%	65
Inova Mount Vernon Hospital	Alexandria	97%	36
Riverside Regional Medical Center	Newport News	97%	157
Sentara Careplex Hospital	Hampton	97%	117
Sentara Norfolk General Hospital	Norfolk	97%	184
Sentara Northern Virginia Medical Center	Woodbridge	97%	61
Sentara Princess Anne Hospital	Virginia Beach	97%	72
Sentara Williamsburg Reg Med Ctr	Williamsburg	97%	90
Twin County Regional Hospital	Galax	97%	32
Sentara Virginia Beach General Hospital	Virginia Beach	96%	121
Danville Regional Medical Center[2]	Danville	95%	56
Sentara Leigh Hospital	Norfolk	95%	118
Carilion Roanoke Memorial Hospital	Roanoke	94%	234
Inova Fair Oaks Hospital	Fairfax	94%	49
Virginia Hospital Center	Arlington	93%	107
Martha Jefferson Hospital	Charlottesville	92%	83
Inova Alexandria Hospital[2]	Alexandria	89%	75
Inova Fairfax Hospital[2]	Falls Church	89%	118
Bon Secours Saint Francis Medical Center	Midlothian	88%	48
Riverside Shore Memorial Hospital	Nassawadox	88%	32
Winchester Medical Center	Winchester	88%	199
University of Virginia Medical Center[2]	Charlottesville	87%	46
Augusta Health[2]	Fishersville	86%	51
Carilion New River Valley Medical Center	Christiansburg	86%	42
Bon Secours Richmond Community Hospital	Richmond	85%	26
Medical College of Virginia Hospitals[2]	Richmond	85%	74
Bon Secours Mem Reg Med Ctr	Mechanicsville	81%	160
Johnston Memorial Hospital	Abingdon	81%	47
Bon Secours Saint Marys Hospital	Richmond	79%	121
Halifax Regional Hospital	Halifax	79%	42
Centra Health[2]	Lynchburg	76%	58
Mem Hosp of Martinsville & Henry Co	Martinsville	76%	46
Chesapeake General Hospital[2]	Chesapeake	74%	62

Surgical Care Improvement Project

Appropriate Beta Blocker Usage

Hospital Name	City	Rate	Cases
Bon Secours Mem Reg Med Ctr[2]	Mechanicsville	100%	383
Cjw Medical Center[2]	Richmond	100%	328
Clinch Valley Medical Center	Richlands	100%	48
Hampton VA Medical Center[2]	Hampton	100%	25
Henrico Doctors' Hospital[2]	Richmond	100%	240
Inova Mount Vernon Hospital[2]	Alexandria	100%	36
John Randolph Medical Center	Hopewell	100%	42
Lewisgale Hospital Alleghany	Low Moor	100%	47
Lewisgale Hospital Montgomery	Blacksburg	100%	88
Mary Immaculate Hospital[2]	Newport News	100%	426
Reston Hospital Center[2]	Reston	100%	101
Riverside Tappahannock Hospital	Tappahannock	100%	48
Riverside Walter Reed Hospital	Gloucester	100%	53
Sentara Careplex Hospital[2]	Hampton	100%	175
Sentara Leigh Hospital[2]	Norfolk	100%	500
Sentara Norfolk General Hospital[2]	Norfolk	100%	551
Sentara Princess Anne Hospital[2]	Virginia Beach	100%	78
Sentara Virginia Beach General Hospital[2]	Virginia Beach	100%	161
Spotsylvania Regional Medical Center	Fredericksburg	100%	32
University of Virginia Medical Center[2]	Charlottesville	100%	193
Virginia Hospital Center	Arlington	100%	590
Bon Secours Maryview Medical Center[2]	Portsmouth	99%	227
Carilion Roanoke Memorial Hospital[2]	Roanoke	99%	766
Centra Health[2]	Lynchburg	99%	493
Danville Regional Medical Center[2]	Danville	99%	105
Fauquier Hospital	Warrenton	99%	93
Inova Fair Oaks Hospital[2]	Fairfax	99%	95
Lewisgale Medical Center[2]	Salem	99%	176
Medical College of Virginia Hospitals[2]	Richmond	99%	216
Novant Health Prince William Med Ctr[2]	Manassas	99%	158
Rockingham Memorial Hospital[2]	Harrisonburg	99%	197
Sentara Northern Virginia Medical Center[2]	Woodbridge	99%	69
Sentara Williamsburg Reg Med Ctr[2]	Williamsburg	99%	127
Bon Secours Saint Marys Hospital[2]	Richmond	98%	306
Community Memorial Healthcenter[2]	South Hill	98%	53
Inova Alexandria Hospital[2]	Alexandria	98%	112
Mary Washington Hospital[2]	Fredericksburg	98%	343
Richmond VA Medical Center[2]	Richmond	98%	141
Sentara Obici Hospital[2]	Suffolk	98%	151
Augusta Health	Fishersville	97%	319
Bon Secours Saint Francis Medical Center	Midlothian	97%	229
Chesapeake General Hospital[2]	Chesapeake	97%	102
Culpeper Regional Hospital	Culpeper	97%	65
Inova Loudoun Hospital[2]	Leesburg	97%	89
Mem Hosp of Martinsville & Henry Co	Martinsville	97%	62
Riverside Regional Medical Center[2]	Newport News	97%	234
Southampton Memorial Hospital	Franklin	97%	29
Southside Community Hospital	Farmville	97%	31
Twin County Regional Hospital	Galax	97%	30
Winchester Medical Center[2]	Winchester	97%	263
Carilion New River Valley Medical Center	Christiansburg	96%	106
Halifax Regional Hospital	Halifax	96%	46
Inova Fairfax Hospital[2]	Falls Church	96%	246
Johnston Memorial Hospital[2]	Abingdon	96%	90
Martha Jefferson Hospital[2]	Charlottesville	96%	107
Shenandoah Memorial Hospital	Woodstock	96%	55
Wythe County Community Hospital	Wytheville	96%	89
Southside Regional Medical Center	Petersburg	94%	140
Bon Secours Depaul Medical Center[2]	Norfolk	93%	72
Salem VA Medical Center[2]	Salem	92%	59
Stafford Hospital	Stafford	92%	38
Wellmont Lonesome Pine Hospital[2]	Big Stone Gap	88%	25

Appropriate VTP Within 24 Hours

Hospital Name	City	Rate	Cases
Bon Secours Mem Reg Med Ctr[2]	Mechanicsville	100%	842
Carilion Giles Community Hospital	Pearisburg	100%	33
Cjw Medical Center[2]	Richmond	100%	544
Community Memorial Healthcenter[2]	South Hill	100%	125
Hampton VA Medical Center[2]	Hampton	100%	76
Inova Mount Vernon Hospital[2]	Alexandria	100%	235
John Randolph Medical Center	Hopewell	100%	128
Lewisgale Hospital Alleghany	Low Moor	100%	145
Lewisgale Hospital Montgomery	Blacksburg	100%	279
Lewisgale Hospital Pulaski	Pulaski	100%	43
Lewisgale Medical Center[2]	Salem	100%	457
Novant Health Prince William Med Ctr[2]	Manassas	100%	480
Reston Hospital Center[2]	Reston	100%	397
Riverside Tappahannock Hospital	Tappahannock	100%	150
Sentara Careplex Hospital[2]	Hampton	100%	523
Sentara Obici Hospital[2]	Suffolk	100%	416
Sentara Princess Anne Hospital[2]	Virginia Beach	100%	397
Sentara Virginia Beach General Hospital[2]	Virginia Beach	100%	612
Smyth County Community Hospital[2]	Marion	100%	106
Southside Regional Medical Center	Petersburg	100%	474
University of Virginia Medical Center[2]	Charlottesville	100%	401
Warren Memorial Hospital	Front Royal	100%	70
Bon Secours Maryview Medical Center[2]	Portsmouth	99%	575
Bon Secours Saint Francis Medical Center	Midlothian	99%	799
Henrico Doctors' Hospital[2]	Richmond	99%	543
Inova Alexandria Hospital[2]	Alexandria	99%	362
Inova Fair Oaks Hospital[2]	Fairfax	99%	333
Martha Jefferson Hospital[2]	Charlottesville	99%	357
Mary Immaculate Hospital[2]	Newport News	99%	1138
Medical College of Virginia Hospitals[2]	Richmond	99%	476
Riverside Regional Medical Center[2]	Newport News	99%	498
Riverside Walter Reed Hospital	Gloucester	99%	171
Sentara Leigh Hospital[2]	Norfolk	99%	1733
Sentara Northern Virginia Medical Center[2]	Woodbridge	99%	313
Sentara Williamsburg Reg Med Ctr[2]	Williamsburg	99%	375
Virginia Hospital Center	Arlington	99%	1637
Augusta Health	Fishersville	98%	950
Bon Secours Saint Marys Hospital[2]	Richmond	98%	595
Carilion Roanoke Memorial Hospital[2]	Roanoke	98%	1542
Centra Health[2]	Lynchburg	98%	853
Clinch Valley Medical Center	Richlands	98%	172
Danville Regional Medical Center[2]	Danville	98%	237
Fauquier Hospital	Warrenton	98%	361
Mary Washington Hospital[2]	Fredericksburg	98%	644

NOTE: Hospital profiles are in alphabetical order by state, then city, then hospital within the city; Rankings exclude hospitals with less than 25 cases except for patient surveys which excludes hospitals with less than 100 cases; (a) 100-299 cases; (1) The number of cases/patients is too few to report; (2) Data submitted were based on a sample of cases/patients; (3) Results are based on a shorter time period than required; (4) Data suppressed by CMS for one or more quarters; (5) Results are not available for this reporting period; (6) Fewer than 100 patients completed the HCAHPS survey; (7) No cases met the criteria for this measure; (8) The lower limit of the confidence interval cannot be calculated if the number of observed infections equals zero; (9) No data are available from the state/territory for this reporting period; (10) The scores shown reflect fewer than 50 completed surveys; (11) There were discrepancies in the data collection process; (12) This measure does not apply to this hospital for this reporting period; (13) Results cannot be calculated for this reporting period; (14) The results for this state are combined with nearby states to protect confidentiality; Please refer to the User's Guide for a full explanation of data.

Hospital Name	City	Rate	Cases
Mem Hosp of Martinsville & Henry Co	Martinsville	98%	198
Richmond VA Medical Center[2]	Richmond	98%	257
Rockingham Memorial Hospital[2]	Harrisonburg	98%	373
Shenandoah Memorial Hospital	Woodstock	98%	169
Southampton Memorial Hospital	Franklin	98%	118
Southern Virginia Regional Medical Center	Emporia	98%	47
Spotsylvania Regional Medical Center	Fredericksburg	98%	183
Winchester Medical Center[2]	Winchester	98%	496
Bon Secours Depaul Medical Center[2]	Norfolk	97%	204
Chesapeake General Hospital[2]	Chesapeake	97%	376
Inova Fairfax Hospital[2]	Falls Church	97%	440
Sentara Norfolk General Hospital[2]	Norfolk	97%	223
Twin County Regional Hospital	Galax	97%	117
Wythe County Community Hospital	Wytheville	97%	273
Culpeper Regional Hospital	Culpeper	96%	226
Inova Loudoun Hospital[2]	Leesburg	96%	307
Johnston Memorial Hospital[2]	Abingdon	96%	304
Norton Community Hospital[2]	Norton	96%	46
Southside Community Hospital	Farmville	96%	105
Carilion New River Valley Medical Center	Christiansburg	95%	199
Riverside Shore Memorial Hospital	Nassawadox	95%	58
Stafford Hospital	Stafford	95%	149
Rappahannock General Hospital	Kilmarnock	94%	49
Wellmont Lonesome Pine Hospital[2]	Big Stone Gap	91%	90
Salem VA Medical Center[2]	Salem	88%	190
Halifax Regional Hospital	Halifax	87%	177
Carilion Stonewall Jackson Hospital	Lexington	86%	42

Controlled Postoperative Blood Glucose

Hospital Name	City	Rate	Cases
Bon Secours Maryview Medical Center[2]	Portsmouth	100%	65
Bon Secours Mem Reg Med Ctr[2]	Mechanicsville	100%	154
Inova Alexandria Hospital[2]	Alexandria	100%	67
Riverside Regional Medical Center[2]	Newport News	100%	98
Bon Secours Saint Marys Hospital[2]	Richmond	99%	214
Carilion Roanoke Memorial Hospital[2]	Roanoke	99%	346
Henrico Doctors' Hospital[2]	Richmond	99%	141
Inova Fairfax Hospital[2]	Falls Church	99%	155
Winchester Medical Center[2]	Winchester	99%	153
Cjw Medical Center[2]	Richmond	98%	186
Lewisgale Medical Center[2]	Salem	98%	116
Mary Washington Hospital[2]	Fredericksburg	98%	186
Sentara Virginia Beach General Hospital[2]	Virginia Beach	98%	94
Virginia Hospital Center	Arlington	98%	182
Rockingham Memorial Hospital[2]	Harrisonburg	97%	65
Sentara Norfolk General Hospital[2]	Norfolk	97%	541
Centra Health[2]	Lynchburg	96%	250
Medical College of Virginia Hospitals[2]	Richmond	96%	157
University of Virginia Medical Center[2]	Charlottesville	92%	106
Richmond VA Medical Center[2]	Richmond	88%	83
Danville Regional Medical Center[2]	Danville	87%	39

Perioperative Temperature Management

Hospital Name	City	Rate	Cases
Augusta Health	Fishersville	100%	1086
Bon Secours Depaul Medical Center[2]	Norfolk	100%	275
Bon Secours Maryview Medical Center[2]	Portsmouth	100%	703
Bon Secours Mem Reg Med Ctr[2]	Mechanicsville	100%	1035
Bon Secours Saint Francis Medical Center	Midlothian	100%	915
Bon Secours Saint Marys Hospital[2]	Richmond	100%	786
Carilion Franklin Memorial Hospital	Rocky Mount	100%	49
Carilion Roanoke Memorial Hospital[2]	Roanoke	100%	2098
Carilion Stonewall Jackson Hospital	Lexington	100%	45
Centra Health[2]	Lynchburg	100%	1111
Chesapeake General Hospital[2]	Chesapeake	100%	431
Cjw Medical Center[2]	Richmond	100%	681
Community Memorial Healthcenter[2]	South Hill	100%	128
Culpeper Regional Hospital	Culpeper	100%	236
Danville Regional Medical Center[2]	Danville	100%	295
Fauquier Hospital	Warrenton	100%	396
Hampton VA Medical Center[2]	Hampton	100%	108
Henrico Doctors' Hospital[2]	Richmond	100%	677
Inova Alexandria Hospital[2]	Alexandria	100%	416
Inova Fair Oaks Hospital[2]	Fairfax	100%	412
Inova Loudoun Hospital[2]	Leesburg	100%	393
John Randolph Medical Center	Hopewell	100%	151
Lewisgale Hospital Montgomery	Blacksburg	100%	307
Lewisgale Hospital Pulaski	Pulaski	100%	46
Lewisgale Medical Center[2]	Salem	100%	548
Mary Immaculate Hospital[2]	Newport News	100%	1864
Mary Washington Hospital[2]	Fredericksburg	100%	783
Medical College of Virginia Hospitals[2]	Richmond	100%	590
Mem Hosp of Martinsville & Henry Co	Martinsville	100%	215
Novant Health Prince William Med Ctr[2]	Manassas	100%	572
Rappahannock General Hospital	Kilmarnock	100%	52
Reston Hospital Center[2]	Reston	100%	473
Riverside Regional Medical Center[2]	Newport News	100%	650
Riverside Shore Memorial Hospital	Nassawadox	100%	63
Riverside Tappahannock Hospital	Tappahannock	100%	159
Riverside Walter Reed Hospital	Gloucester	100%	176
Rockingham Memorial Hospital[2]	Harrisonburg	100%	478
Sentara Careplex Hospital[2]	Hampton	100%	625
Sentara Leigh Hospital[2]	Norfolk	100%	1802
Sentara Norfolk General Hospital[2]	Norfolk	100%	411
Sentara Northern Virginia Medical Center[2]	Woodbridge	100%	367
Sentara Obici Hospital[2]	Suffolk	100%	501
Sentara Princess Anne Hospital[2]	Virginia Beach	100%	395
Sentara Virginia Beach General Hospital[2]	Virginia Beach	100%	723
Sentara Williamsburg Reg Med Ctr[2]	Williamsburg	100%	436
Smyth County Community Hospital[2]	Marion	100%	111
Southern Virginia Regional Medical Center	Emporia	100%	48
Southside Community Hospital	Farmville	100%	123
Southside Regional Medical Center	Petersburg	100%	522
Spotsylvania Regional Medical Center	Fredericksburg	100%	218
Stafford Hospital	Stafford	100%	155
Twin County Regional Hospital	Galax	100%	129
University of Virginia Medical Center[2]	Charlottesville	100%	523
Virginia Hospital Center	Arlington	100%	1930
Warren Memorial Hospital	Front Royal	100%	81
Winchester Medical Center[2]	Winchester	100%	606
Wythe County Community Hospital	Wytheville	100%	296
Carilion New River Valley Medical Center	Christiansburg	99%	275
Clinch Valley Medical Center	Richlands	99%	186
Halifax Regional Hospital	Halifax	99%	196
Inova Mount Vernon Hospital[2]	Alexandria	99%	347
Johnston Memorial Hospital[2]	Abingdon	99%	332
Lewisgale Hospital Alleghany	Low Moor	99%	166
Martha Jefferson Hospital[2]	Charlottesville	99%	463
Richmond VA Medical Center[2]	Richmond	99%	289
Salem VA Medical Center[2]	Salem	99%	216
Shenandoah Memorial Hospital	Woodstock	99%	178
Southampton Memorial Hospital	Franklin	99%	125
Inova Fairfax Hospital[2]	Falls Church	98%	612
Carilion Giles Community Hospital	Pearisburg	97%	34
Wellmont Lonesome Pine Hospital[2]	Big Stone Gap	97%	105
Norton Community Hospital[2]	Norton	96%	52

Prophylactic Antibiotic Selection

Hospital Name	City	Rate	Cases
Augusta Health	Fishersville	100%	864
Bon Secours Mem Reg Med Ctr[2]	Mechanicsville	100%	851
Centra Health[2]	Lynchburg	100%	925
Cjw Medical Center[2]	Richmond	100%	597
Clinch Valley Medical Center	Richlands	100%	113
Community Memorial Healthcenter[2]	South Hill	100%	93
Inova Alexandria Hospital[2]	Alexandria	100%	323
Inova Mount Vernon Hospital[2]	Alexandria	100%	228
John Randolph Medical Center	Hopewell	100%	91
Lewisgale Hospital Montgomery	Blacksburg	100%	232
Lewisgale Hospital Pulaski	Pulaski	100%	27
Lewisgale Medical Center[2]	Salem	100%	439
Mary Immaculate Hospital[2]	Newport News	100%	1649
Mary Washington Hospital[2]	Fredericksburg	100%	635
Novant Health Prince William Med Ctr[2]	Manassas	100%	429
Rappahannock General Hospital	Kilmarnock	100%	26
Reston Hospital Center[2]	Reston	100%	295
Riverside Tappahannock Hospital	Tappahannock	100%	131
Riverside Walter Reed Hospital	Gloucester	100%	136
Sentara Careplex Hospital[2]	Hampton	100%	442
Sentara Leigh Hospital[2]	Norfolk	100%	1625
Sentara Norfolk General Hospital[2]	Norfolk	100%	681
Sentara Princess Anne Hospital[2]	Virginia Beach	100%	310
Sentara Virginia Beach General Hospital[2]	Virginia Beach	100%	582
Smyth County Community Hospital[2]	Marion	100%	75
Southern Virginia Regional Medical Center	Emporia	100%	29
Southside Community Hospital	Farmville	100%	72
Southside Regional Medical Center	Petersburg	100%	340
Spotsylvania Regional Medical Center	Fredericksburg	100%	148
Twin County Regional Hospital	Galax	100%	88
University of Virginia Medical Center[2]	Charlottesville	100%	372
Virginia Hospital Center	Arlington	100%	1274
Wythe County Community Hospital	Wytheville	100%	239
Bon Secours Maryview Medical Center[2]	Portsmouth	99%	579
Bon Secours Saint Francis Medical Center	Midlothian	99%	585
Carilion New River Valley Medical Center	Christiansburg	99%	184
Carilion Roanoke Memorial Hospital[2]	Roanoke	99%	2087
Chesapeake General Hospital[2]	Chesapeake	99%	285
Danville Regional Medical Center[2]	Danville	99%	231
Fauquier Hospital	Warrenton	99%	289
Hampton VA Medical Center	Hampton	99%	79
Henrico Doctors' Hospital[2]	Richmond	99%	563
Inova Fairfax Hospital[2]	Falls Church	99%	518
Johnston Memorial Hospital[2]	Abingdon	99%	227
Lewisgale Hospital Alleghany	Low Moor	99%	145
Medical College of Virginia Hospitals[2]	Richmond	99%	478
Mem Hosp of Martinsville & Henry Co	Martinsville	99%	124
Richmond VA Medical Center	Richmond	99%	246
Riverside Regional Medical Center[2]	Newport News	99%	454
Rockingham Memorial Hospital[2]	Harrisonburg	99%	409
Salem VA Medical Center	Salem	99%	154
Sentara Northern Virginia Medical Center[2]	Woodbridge	99%	231
Sentara Obici Hospital[2]	Suffolk	99%	363
Sentara Williamsburg Reg Med Ctr[2]	Williamsburg	99%	283
Shenandoah Memorial Hospital	Woodstock	99%	142
Stafford Hospital	Stafford	99%	97
Bon Secours Depaul Medical Center[2]	Norfolk	98%	152
Bon Secours Saint Marys Hospital[2]	Richmond	98%	689
Carilion Franklin Memorial Hospital	Rocky Mount	98%	40
Inova Fair Oaks Hospital[2]	Fairfax	98%	260
Martha Jefferson Hospital[2]	Charlottesville	98%	327
Winchester Medical Center[2]	Winchester	98%	500
Culpeper Regional Hospital	Culpeper	97%	193
Halifax Regional Hospital	Halifax	97%	125
Riverside Shore Memorial Hospital	Nassawadox	97%	39
Carilion Giles Community Hospital	Pearisburg	96%	28
Warren Memorial Hospital	Front Royal	96%	51
Inova Loudoun Hospital[2]	Leesburg	95%	232
Southampton Memorial Hospital	Franklin	94%	105
Wellmont Lonesome Pine Hospital[2]	Big Stone Gap	92%	66

Prophylactic Antibiotic Selection (Outpatient)

Hospital Name	City	Rate	Cases
Cjw Medical Center	Richmond	100%	743
Clinch Valley Medical Center	Richlands	100%	27
Halifax Regional Hospital	Halifax	100%	113
Lewisgale Hospital Montgomery	Blacksburg	100%	57
Novant Health Prince William Med Ctr	Manassas	100%	423
Wellmont Lonesome Pine Hospital	Big Stone Gap	100%	26
Augusta Health	Fishersville	99%	269
Carilion New River Valley Medical Center	Christiansburg	99%	337
Centra Health	Lynchburg	99%	621
Fauquier Hospital	Warrenton	99%	94
Henrico Doctors' Hospital	Richmond	99%	607
Inova Alexandria Hospital	Alexandria	99%	258
Inova Fair Oaks Hospital	Fairfax	99%	548
Inova Fairfax Hospital	Falls Church	99%	941
Lewisgale Medical Center	Salem	99%	555
Mary Washington Hospital	Fredericksburg	99%	779
Medical College of Virginia Hospitals	Richmond	99%	679
Reston Hospital Center	Reston	99%	597
Rockingham Memorial Hospital	Harrisonburg	99%	239
Sentara Norfolk General Hospital	Norfolk	99%	645
Sentara Obici Hospital	Suffolk	99%	196
Southside Regional Medical Center	Petersburg	99%	365
Virginia Hospital Center	Arlington	99%	569
Bon Secours Maryview Medical Center	Portsmouth	98%	393
Chesapeake General Hospital	Chesapeake	98%	511
Inova Loudoun Hospital	Leesburg	98%	374
Inova Mount Vernon Hospital	Alexandria	98%	121
Mary Immaculate Hospital	Newport News	98%	358
Norton Community Hospital	Norton	98%	41
Riverside Regional Medical Center	Newport News	98%	581
Riverside Shore Memorial Hospital	Nassawadox	98%	65
Sentara Princess Anne Hospital	Virginia Beach	98%	174
Southampton Memorial Hospital	Franklin	98%	45
Spotsylvania Regional Medical Center	Fredericksburg	98%	189
Stafford Hospital	Stafford	98%	106
Winchester Medical Center	Winchester	98%	543
Wythe County Community Hospital	Wytheville	98%	60
Bon Secours Mem Reg Med Ctr	Mechanicsville	97%	448
Carilion Roanoke Memorial Hospital	Roanoke	97%	726
Mem Hosp of Martinsville & Henry Co	Martinsville	97%	71
Sentara Careplex Hospital	Hampton	97%	194
Sentara Leigh Hospital	Norfolk	97%	445
Sentara Northern Virginia Medical Center	Woodbridge	97%	153
Sentara Virginia Beach General Hospital	Virginia Beach	97%	298
Southern Virginia Regional Medical Center	Emporia	97%	31
Bon Secours Saint Marys Hospital	Richmond	96%	626
Danville Regional Medical Center	Danville	96%	170
Johnston Memorial Hospital	Abingdon	96%	72
Martha Jefferson Hospital	Charlottesville	95%	283
Bon Secours Depaul Medical Center	Norfolk	94%	429
Riverside Tappahannock Hospital	Tappahannock	93%	45
Culpeper Regional Hospital	Culpeper	91%	32
University of Virginia Medical Center	Charlottesville	90%	366
Sentara Williamsburg Reg Med Ctr	Williamsburg	86%	212
Bon Secours Saint Francis Medical Center	Midlothian	85%	437

Prophylactic Antibiotic Stopped

Hospital Name	City	Rate	Cases
Carilion Franklin Memorial Hospital	Rocky Mount	100%	38
Centra Health[2]	Lynchburg	100%	882
Henrico Doctors' Hospital[2]	Richmond	100%	542
Lewisgale Hospital Alleghany	Low Moor	100%	144
Lewisgale Hospital Montgomery	Blacksburg	100%	224
Lewisgale Hospital Pulaski	Pulaski	100%	27
Lewisgale Medical Center[2]	Salem	100%	419
Reston Hospital Center[2]	Reston	100%	290
Riverside Tappahannock Hospital	Tappahannock	100%	129
Riverside Walter Reed Hospital	Gloucester	100%	135
Sentara Careplex Hospital[2]	Hampton	100%	438

NOTE: Hospital profiles are in alphabetical order by state, then city, then hospital within the city; Rankings exclude hospitals with less than 25 cases except for patient surveys which excludes hospitals with less than 100 cases; (a) 100-299 cases; (1) The number of cases/patients is too few to report; (2) Data submitted were based on a sample of cases/patients; (3) Results are based on a shorter time period than required; (4) Data suppressed by CMS for one or more quarters; (5) Results are not available for this reporting period; (6) Fewer than 100 patients completed the HCAHPS survey; (7) No cases met the criteria for this measure; (8) The lower limit of the confidence interval cannot be calculated if the number of observed infections equals zero; (9) No data are available from the state/territory for this reporting period; (10) The scores shown reflect fewer than 50 completed surveys; (11) There were discrepancies in the data collection process; (12) This measure does not apply to this hospital for this reporting period; (13) Results cannot be calculated for this reporting period; (14) The results for this state are combined with nearby states to protect confidentiality; Please refer to the User's Guide for a full explanation of data.

Hospital Name	City	Rate	Cases
Sentara Princess Anne Hospital[2]	Virginia Beach	100%	310
Sentara Virginia Beach General Hospital[2]	Virginia Beach	100%	579
Smyth County Community Hospital[2]	Marion	100%	71
Stafford Hospital	Stafford	100%	95
Bon Secours Mem Reg Med Ctr[2]	Mechanicsville	99%	843
Carilion Roanoke Memorial Hospital[2]	Roanoke	99%	2046
Cjw Medical Center[2]	Richmond	99%	572
Community Memorial Healthcenter[2]	South Hill	99%	88
Danville Regional Medical Center[2]	Danville	99%	226
Fauquier Hospital	Warrenton	99%	285
Hampton VA Medical Center	Hampton	99%	77
Inova Mount Vernon Hospital[2]	Alexandria	99%	228
John Randolph Medical Center	Hopewell	99%	86
Mary Immaculate Hospital[2]	Newport News	99%	1639
Mary Washington Hospital[2]	Fredericksburg	99%	610
Novant Health Prince William Med Ctr[2]	Manassas	99%	421
Riverside Regional Medical Center[2]	Newport News	99%	436
Sentara Leigh Hospital[2]	Norfolk	99%	1613
Sentara Williamsburg Reg Med Ctr[2]	Williamsburg	99%	279
Southside Regional Medical Center	Petersburg	99%	318
Spotsylvania Regional Medical Center	Fredericksburg	99%	144
Virginia Hospital Center	Arlington	99%	1252
Wythe County Community Hospital	Wytheville	99%	231
Augusta Health	Fishersville	98%	847
Bon Secours Maryview Medical Center[2]	Portsmouth	98%	566
Bon Secours Saint Francis Medical Center	Midlothian	98%	568
Bon Secours Saint Marys Hospital[2]	Richmond	98%	669
Clinch Valley Medical Center	Richlands	98%	105
Inova Alexandria Hospital[2]	Alexandria	98%	320
Inova Loudoun Hospital[2]	Leesburg	98%	229
Martha Jefferson Hospital[2]	Charlottesville	98%	319
Medical College of Virginia Hospitals[2]	Richmond	98%	459
Salem VA Medical Center	Salem	98%	154
Sentara Norfolk General Hospital[2]	Norfolk	98%	646
Sentara Obici Hospital[2]	Suffolk	98%	357
University of Virginia Medical Center[2]	Charlottesville	98%	367
Bon Secours Depaul Medical Center[2]	Norfolk	97%	148
Culpeper Regional Hospital	Culpeper	97%	191
Inova Fairfax Hospital[2]	Falls Church	97%	506
Sentara Northern Virginia Medical Center[2]	Woodbridge	97%	230
Carilion Giles Community Hospital	Pearisburg	96%	27
Carilion New River Valley Medical Center	Christiansburg	96%	180
Chesapeake General Hospital[2]	Chesapeake	96%	280
Inova Fair Oaks Hospital[2]	Fairfax	96%	257
Johnston Memorial Hospital[2]	Abingdon	96%	220
Mem Hosp of Martinsville & Henry Co	Martinsville	96%	108
Southside Community Hospital	Farmville	96%	67
Winchester Medical Center[2]	Winchester	96%	484
Twin County Regional Hospital	Galax	95%	84
Rockingham Memorial Hospital[2]	Harrisonburg	94%	287
Shenandoah Memorial Hospital	Woodstock	94%	140
Warren Memorial Hospital	Front Royal	94%	50
Richmond VA Medical Center	Richmond	93%	242
Southern Virginia Regional Medical Center	Emporia	93%	28
Riverside Shore Memorial Hospital	Nassawadox	92%	37
Southampton Memorial Hospital	Franklin	91%	99
Wellmont Lonesome Pine Hospital[2]	Big Stone Gap	91%	64
Halifax Regional Hospital	Halifax	90%	120

Prophylactic Antibiotic Timing

Hospital Name	City	Rate	Cases
Centra Health[2]	Lynchburg	100%	925
Chesapeake General Hospital[2]	Chesapeake	100%	285
Cjw Medical Center[2]	Richmond	100%	597
Community Memorial Healthcenter[2]	South Hill	100%	93
Culpeper Regional Hospital	Culpeper	100%	197
Danville Regional Medical Center[2]	Danville	100%	231
Hampton VA Medical Center	Hampton	100%	79
Henrico Doctors' Hospital[2]	Richmond	100%	563
Inova Alexandria Hospital[2]	Alexandria	100%	323
Inova Mount Vernon Hospital[2]	Alexandria	100%	230
John Randolph Medical Center	Hopewell	100%	91
Johnston Memorial Hospital[2]	Abingdon	100%	227
Lewisgale Hospital Montgomery	Blacksburg	100%	232
Lewisgale Hospital Pulaski	Pulaski	100%	27
Lewisgale Medical Center[2]	Salem	100%	439
Mary Immaculate Hospital[2]	Newport News	100%	1652
Mary Washington Hospital[2]	Fredericksburg	100%	635
Medical College of Virginia Hospitals[2]	Richmond	100%	479
Novant Health Prince William Med Ctr[2]	Manassas	100%	429
Rappahannock General Hospital	Kilmarnock	100%	26
Reston Hospital Center[2]	Reston	100%	295
Riverside Regional Medical Center[2]	Newport News	100%	455
Riverside Shore Memorial Hospital	Nassawadox	100%	39
Riverside Tappahannock Hospital	Tappahannock	100%	131
Sentara Northern Virginia Medical Center[2]	Woodbridge	100%	235
Sentara Obici Hospital[2]	Suffolk	100%	363
Sentara Virginia Beach General Hospital[2]	Virginia Beach	100%	582
Smyth County Community Hospital[2]	Marion	100%	75
Spotsylvania Regional Medical Center	Fredericksburg	100%	148
Stafford Hospital	Stafford	100%	97
Twin County Regional Hospital	Galax	100%	88
Augusta Health	Fishersville	99%	865
Bon Secours Maryview Medical Center[2]	Portsmouth	99%	579
Bon Secours Saint Marys Hospital[2]	Richmond	99%	689
Carilion New River Valley Medical Center	Christiansburg	99%	184
Clinch Valley Medical Center	Richlands	99%	113
Fauquier Hospital	Warrenton	99%	289
Lewisgale Hospital Alleghany	Low Moor	99%	145
Martha Jefferson Hospital[2]	Charlottesville	99%	327
Riverside Walter Reed Hospital	Gloucester	99%	136
Rockingham Memorial Hospital[2]	Harrisonburg	99%	409
Sentara Careplex Hospital[2]	Hampton	99%	443
Sentara Leigh Hospital[2]	Norfolk	99%	1626
Sentara Norfolk General Hospital[2]	Norfolk	99%	681
Sentara Princess Anne Hospital[2]	Virginia Beach	99%	310
Shenandoah Memorial Hospital	Woodstock	99%	142
Southampton Memorial Hospital	Franklin	99%	105
Southside Regional Medical Center	Petersburg	99%	340
University of Virginia Medical Center[2]	Charlottesville	99%	372
Virginia Hospital Center	Arlington	99%	1274
Wythe County Community Hospital	Wytheville	99%	239
Bon Secours Mem Reg Med Ctr[2]	Mechanicsville	98%	857
Bon Secours Saint Francis Medical Center	Midlothian	98%	585
Carilion Roanoke Memorial Hospital[2]	Roanoke	98%	2103
Inova Fair Oaks Hospital[2]	Fairfax	98%	261
Inova Fairfax Hospital[2]	Falls Church	98%	519
Inova Loudoun Hospital[2]	Leesburg	98%	232
Richmond VA Medical Center	Richmond	98%	247
Bon Secours Depaul Medical Center[2]	Norfolk	97%	154
Halifax Regional Hospital	Halifax	97%	126
Salem VA Medical Center	Salem	97%	154
Sentara Williamsburg Reg Med Ctr[2]	Williamsburg	97%	285
Southern Virginia Regional Medical Center	Emporia	97%	29
Southside Community Hospital	Farmville	97%	72
Warren Memorial Hospital	Front Royal	96%	51
Mem Hosp of Martinsville & Henry Co	Martinsville	95%	124
Winchester Medical Center[2]	Winchester	94%	507
Carilion Giles Community Hospital	Pearisburg	93%	28
Wellmont Lonesome Pine Hospital[2]	Big Stone Gap	91%	67
Carilion Franklin Memorial Hospital	Rocky Mount	90%	41

Prophylactic Antibiotic Timing (Outpatient)

Hospital Name	City	Rate	Cases
Bon Secours Mem Reg Med Ctr	Mechanicsville	100%	445
Clinch Valley Medical Center	Richlands	100%	27
Culpeper Regional Hospital	Culpeper	100%	32
Fauquier Hospital	Warrenton	100%	94
Henrico Doctors' Hospital	Richmond	100%	608
Inova Fair Oaks Hospital	Fairfax	100%	545
Lewisgale Hospital Montgomery	Blacksburg	100%	57
Lewisgale Medical Center	Salem	100%	552
Mary Washington Hospital	Fredericksburg	100%	778
Reston Hospital Center	Reston	100%	597
Riverside Shore Memorial Hospital	Nassawadox	100%	65
Spotsylvania Regional Medical Center	Fredericksburg	100%	189
Stafford Hospital	Stafford	100%	106
Centra Health	Lynchburg	99%	624
Chesapeake General Hospital	Chesapeake	99%	512
Cjw Medical Center	Richmond	99%	742
Inova Alexandria Hospital	Alexandria	99%	261
Inova Mount Vernon Hospital	Alexandria	99%	122
Mary Immaculate Hospital	Newport News	99%	360
Novant Health Prince William Med Ctr	Manassas	99%	420
Rockingham Memorial Hospital	Harrisonburg	99%	241
Sentara Leigh Hospital	Norfolk	99%	448
Sentara Northern Virginia Medical Center	Woodbridge	99%	153
Sentara Obici Hospital	Suffolk	99%	196
Sentara Princess Anne Hospital	Virginia Beach	99%	175
Southside Regional Medical Center	Petersburg	99%	366
Virginia Hospital Center	Arlington	99%	571
Augusta Health	Fishersville	98%	269
Bon Secours Depaul Medical Center	Norfolk	98%	431
Carilion New River Valley Medical Center	Christiansburg	98%	332
Carilion Roanoke Memorial Hospital	Roanoke	98%	727
Inova Fairfax Hospital	Falls Church	98%	949
Inova Loudoun Hospital	Leesburg	98%	358
Medical College of Virginia Hospitals	Richmond	98%	680
Riverside Regional Medical Center	Newport News	98%	587
Sentara Careplex Hospital	Hampton	98%	195
Wythe County Community Hospital	Wytheville	98%	60
Bon Secours Saint Marys Hospital	Richmond	97%	628
Johnston Memorial Hospital	Abingdon	97%	72
Sentara Williamsburg Reg Med Ctr	Williamsburg	97%	217
Bon Secours Maryview Medical Center	Portsmouth	96%	397
Bon Secours Saint Francis Medical Center	Midlothian	96%	439
Mem Hosp of Martinsville & Henry Co	Martinsville	96%	72
Sentara Norfolk General Hospital	Norfolk	96%	666
Sentara Virginia Beach General Hospital	Virginia Beach	96%	301
Danville Regional Medical Center	Danville	95%	172
Martha Jefferson Hospital	Charlottesville	95%	287
Norton Community Hospital	Norton	95%	42
Winchester Medical Center	Winchester	94%	553
University of Virginia Medical Center	Charlottesville	88%	295
Halifax Regional Hospital	Halifax	75%	117

Urinary Catheter Removal

Hospital Name	City	Rate	Cases
Bon Secours Maryview Medical Center[2]	Portsmouth	100%	335
Carilion New River Valley Medical Center	Christiansburg	100%	195
Community Memorial Healthcenter[2]	South Hill	100%	99
Danville Regional Medical Center[2]	Danville	100%	88
Henrico Doctors' Hospital[2]	Richmond	100%	475
Inova Mount Vernon Hospital[2]	Alexandria	100%	232
John Randolph Medical Center	Hopewell	100%	94
Lewisgale Hospital Pulaski	Pulaski	100%	33
Lewisgale Medical Center[2]	Salem	100%	296
Reston Hospital Center[2]	Reston	100%	318
Riverside Tappahannock Hospital	Tappahannock	100%	55
Riverside Walter Reed Hospital	Gloucester	100%	156
Sentara Leigh Hospital[2]	Norfolk	100%	1527
Smyth County Community Hospital[2]	Marion	100%	57
Warren Memorial Hospital	Front Royal	100%	38
Augusta Health	Fishersville	99%	868
Bon Secours Mem Reg Med Ctr[2]	Mechanicsville	99%	884
Clinch Valley Medical Center	Richlands	99%	69
Inova Alexandria Hospital[2]	Alexandria	99%	318
Lewisgale Hospital Montgomery	Blacksburg	99%	181
Novant Health Prince William Med Ctr[2]	Manassas	99%	420
Sentara Norfolk General Hospital[2]	Norfolk	99%	647
Sentara Northern Virginia Medical Center[2]	Woodbridge	99%	151
Sentara Virginia Beach General Hospital[2]	Virginia Beach	99%	551
Spotsylvania Regional Medical Center	Fredericksburg	99%	121
University of Virginia Medical Center[2]	Charlottesville	99%	238
Bon Secours Saint Marys Hospital[2]	Richmond	98%	705
Centra Health[2]	Lynchburg	98%	547
Cjw Medical Center[2]	Richmond	98%	501
Inova Fair Oaks Hospital[2]	Fairfax	98%	250
Inova Loudoun Hospital[2]	Leesburg	98%	121
Medical College of Virginia Hospitals[2]	Richmond	98%	522
Rappahannock General Hospital	Kilmarnock	98%	44
Riverside Regional Medical Center[2]	Newport News	98%	422
Sentara Careplex Hospital[2]	Hampton	98%	157
Sentara Princess Anne Hospital[2]	Virginia Beach	98%	197
Sentara Williamsburg Reg Med Ctr[2]	Williamsburg	98%	259
Twin County Regional Hospital	Galax	98%	63
Virginia Hospital Center	Arlington	98%	851
Wythe County Community Hospital	Wytheville	98%	225
Culpeper Regional Hospital	Culpeper	97%	207
Richmond VA Medical Center[2]	Richmond	97%	191
Southern Virginia Regional Medical Center	Emporia	97%	33
Southside Regional Medical Center	Petersburg	97%	312
Stafford Hospital	Stafford	97%	114
Winchester Medical Center[2]	Winchester	97%	338
Carilion Roanoke Memorial Hospital[2]	Roanoke	96%	1767
Chesapeake General Hospital[2]	Chesapeake	96%	223
Mary Washington Hospital[2]	Fredericksburg	96%	481
Rockingham Memorial Hospital[2]	Harrisonburg	96%	305
Salem VA Medical Center[2]	Salem	96%	110
Sentara Obici Hospital[2]	Suffolk	96%	143
Shenandoah Memorial Hospital	Woodstock	96%	90
Bon Secours Depaul Medical Center[2]	Norfolk	95%	157
Inova Fairfax Hospital[2]	Falls Church	95%	427
Mary Immaculate Hospital[2]	Newport News	95%	78
Mem Hosp of Martinsville & Henry Co	Martinsville	95%	116
Carilion Stonewall Jackson Hospital	Lexington	94%	32
Fauquier Hospital	Warrenton	94%	301
Johnston Memorial Hospital[2]	Abingdon	94%	151
Martha Jefferson Hospital[2]	Charlottesville	94%	188
Carilion Giles Community Hospital	Pearisburg	93%	27
Southside Community Hospital	Farmville	93%	72
Wellmont Lonesome Pine Hospital[2]	Big Stone Gap	92%	61
Bon Secours Saint Francis Medical Center	Midlothian	87%	215
Halifax Regional Hospital	Halifax	78%	94

Survey of Patients' Hospital Experiences

Area Around Room 'Always' Quiet at Night

Hospital Name	City	Rate	Cases
Bon Secours Richmond Community Hospital	Richmond	72%	(a)
Southern Virginia Regional Medical Center	Emporia	71%	300+
Sentara Careplex Hospital	Hampton	70%	300+
Spotsylvania Regional Medical Center	Fredericksburg	69%	300+
Halifax Regional Hospital	Halifax	68%	300+
Wellmont Lonesome Pine Hospital	Big Stone Gap	68%	300+
Carilion Tazewell Community Hospital	Tazewell	67%	(a)
Martha Jefferson Hospital	Charlottesville	67%	300+
Sentara Obici Hospital	Suffolk	67%	300+
Sentara Princess Anne Hospital	Virginia Beach	67%	300+
Bon Secours Maryview Medical Center	Portsmouth	65%	300+
Bon Secours Saint Francis Medical Center	Midlothian	65%	300+
Buchanan General Hospital	Grundy	65%	(a)

NOTE: Hospital profiles are in alphabetical order by state, then city, then hospital within the city; Rankings exclude hospitals with less than 25 cases except for patient surveys which excludes hospitals with less than 100 cases; (a) 100-299 cases; (1) The number of cases/patients is too few to report; (2) Data submitted were based on a sample of cases/patients; (3) Results are based on a shorter time period than required; (4) Data suppressed by CMS for one or more quarters; (5) Results are not available for this reporting period; (6) Fewer than 100 patients completed the HCAHPS survey; (7) No cases met the criteria for this measure; (8) The lower limit of the confidence interval cannot be calculated if the number of observed infections equals zero; (9) No data are available from the state/territory for this reporting period; (10) The scores shown reflect fewer than 50 completed surveys; (11) There were discrepancies in the data collection process; (12) This measure does not apply to this hospital for this reporting period; (13) Results cannot be calculated for this reporting period; (14) The results for this state are combined with nearby states to protect confidentiality; Please refer to the User's Guide for a full explanation of data.

Hospital Name	City	Rate	Cases
Southampton Memorial Hospital	Franklin	65%	300+
Carilion Giles Community Hospital	Pearisburg	64%	(a)
John Randolph Medical Center	Hopewell	64%	300+
Mary Immaculate Hospital	Newport News	63%	300+
Sentara Northern Virginia Medical Center	Woodbridge	63%	300+
Shenandoah Memorial Hospital	Woodstock	63%	300+
Smyth County Community Hospital	Marion	63%	300+
Virginia Hospital Center	Arlington	63%	300+
Bon Secours Depaul Medical Center	Norfolk	62%	300+
Bon Secours Saint Marys Hospital	Richmond	62%	300+
Carilion Franklin Memorial Hospital	Rocky Mount	62%	300+
Centra Health	Lynchburg	62%	300+
Henrico Doctors' Hospital	Richmond	62%	300+
Lewisgale Hospital Montgomery	Blacksburg	62%	300+
Mem Hosp of Martinsville & Henry Co	Martinsville	62%	300+
Page Memorial Hospital	Luray	62%	(a)
Sentara Norfolk General Hospital	Norfolk	62%	300+
Wythe County Community Hospital	Wytheville	62%	300+
Carilion New River Valley Medical Center	Christiansburg	61%	300+
Danville Regional Medical Center	Danville	61%	300+
Fauquier Hospital	Warrenton	61%	300+
Johnston Memorial Hospital	Abingdon	61%	300+
Lewisgale Hospital Pulaski	Pulaski	61%	300+
Carilion Stonewall Jackson Hospital	Lexington	60%	(a)
Clinch Valley Medical Center	Richlands	60%	300+
Community Memorial Healthcenter	South Hill	60%	300+
Riverside Shore Memorial Hospital	Nassawadox	60%	300+
Russell County Medical Center	Lebanon	60%	(a)
Sentara Virginia Beach General Hospital	Virginia Beach	60%	300+
Southside Regional Medical Center	Petersburg	60%	300+
Chesapeake General Hospital	Chesapeake	59%	300+
Lewisgale Hospital Alleghany	Low Moor	59%	300+
Reston Hospital Center	Reston	59%	300+
Riverside Tappahannock Hospital	Tappahannock	59%	300+
Rockingham Memorial Hospital	Harrisonburg	59%	300+
Sentara Williamsburg Reg Med Ctr	Williamsburg	59%	300+
Southside Community Hospital	Farmville	59%	300+
Stafford Hospital	Stafford	59%	300+
Cjw Medical Center	Richmond	58%	300+
Riverside Regional Medical Center	Newport News	58%	300+
Sentara Leigh Hospital	Norfolk	58%	300+
Twin County Regional Hospital	Galax	58%	300+
Bon Secours Mem Reg Med Ctr	Mechanicsville	57%	300+
Medical College of Virginia Hospitals	Richmond	57%	300+
Norton Community Hospital	Norton	57%	300+
Carilion Roanoke Memorial Hospital	Roanoke	56%	300+
Culpeper Regional Hospital	Culpeper	56%	300+
Inova Fair Oaks Hospital	Fairfax	56%	300+
Inova Mount Vernon Hospital	Alexandria	56%	300+
Warren Memorial Hospital	Front Royal	55%	300+
Bedford Memorial Hospital	Bedford	54%	(a)
Inova Alexandria Hospital	Alexandria	54%	300+
Rappahannock General Hospital	Kilmarnock	53%	300+
Lewisgale Medical Center	Salem	52%	300+
Mary Washington Hospital	Fredericksburg	52%	300+
Novant Health Prince William Med Ctr	Manassas	51%	300+
Augusta Health	Fishersville	50%	300+
Inova Fairfax Hospital	Falls Church	50%	300+
Riverside Walter Reed Hospital	Gloucester	50%	300+
Winchester Medical Center	Winchester	48%	300+
Inova Loudoun Hospital	Leesburg	45%	300+
University of Virginia Medical Center	Charlottesville	45%	300+

Doctors 'Always' Communicated Well

Hospital Name	City	Rate	Cases
Carilion Giles Community Hospital	Pearisburg	91%	(a)
Carilion Stonewall Jackson Hospital	Lexington	90%	(a)
Buchanan General Hospital	Grundy	88%	(a)
Bon Secours Richmond Community Hospital	Richmond	87%	(a)
Carilion Tazewell Community Hospital	Tazewell	86%	(a)
Halifax Regional Hospital	Halifax	86%	300+
Clinch Valley Medical Center	Richlands	85%	300+
Martha Jefferson Hospital	Charlottesville	85%	300+
Rappahannock General Hospital	Kilmarnock	85%	300+
Riverside Tappahannock Hospital	Tappahannock	85%	300+
Sentara Obici Hospital	Suffolk	85%	300+
Wythe County Community Hospital	Wytheville	85%	300+
Carilion New River Valley Medical Center	Christiansburg	84%	300+
Page Memorial Hospital	Luray	84%	(a)
Riverside Walter Reed Hospital	Gloucester	84%	300+
Sentara Norfolk General Hospital	Norfolk	84%	300+
Bedford Memorial Hospital	Bedford	83%	(a)
Carilion Franklin Memorial Hospital	Rocky Mount	83%	300+
Centra Health	Lynchburg	83%	300+
Chesapeake General Hospital	Chesapeake	83%	300+
Lewisgale Hospital Alleghany	Low Moor	83%	300+
Lewisgale Hospital Pulaski	Pulaski	83%	300+
Norton Community Hospital	Norton	83%	300+
Russell County Medical Center	Lebanon	83%	(a)
Sentara Careplex Hospital	Hampton	83%	300+
Sentara Princess Anne Hospital	Virginia Beach	83%	300+
Sentara Williamsburg Reg Med Ctr	Williamsburg	83%	300+
Southern Virginia Regional Medical Center	Emporia	83%	300+
Twin County Regional Hospital	Galax	83%	300+
Virginia Hospital Center	Arlington	83%	300+
Wellmont Lonesome Pine Hospital	Big Stone Gap	83%	300+
Augusta Health	Fishersville	82%	300+
Community Memorial Healthcenter	South Hill	82%	300+
Henrico Doctors' Hospital	Richmond	82%	300+
Riverside Shore Memorial Hospital	Nassawadox	82%	300+
Sentara Leigh Hospital	Norfolk	82%	300+
Smyth County Community Hospital	Marion	82%	300+
Bon Secours Maryview Medical Center	Portsmouth	81%	300+
Bon Secours Mem Reg Med Ctr	Mechanicsville	81%	300+
Fauquier Hospital	Warrenton	81%	300+
Lewisgale Hospital Montgomery	Blacksburg	81%	300+
Mary Immaculate Hospital	Newport News	81%	300+
Medical College of Virginia Hospitals	Richmond	81%	300+
Southside Community Hospital	Farmville	81%	300+
Bon Secours Saint Marys Hospital	Richmond	80%	300+
Culpeper Regional Hospital	Culpeper	80%	300+
Inova Mount Vernon Hospital	Alexandria	80%	300+
John Randolph Medical Center	Hopewell	80%	300+
Johnston Memorial Hospital	Abingdon	80%	300+
Sentara Virginia Beach General Hospital	Virginia Beach	80%	300+
Southampton Memorial Hospital	Franklin	80%	300+
Southside Regional Medical Center	Petersburg	80%	300+
Bon Secours Depaul Medical Center	Norfolk	79%	300+
Bon Secours Saint Francis Medical Center	Midlothian	79%	300+
Cjw Medical Center	Richmond	79%	300+
Lewisgale Medical Center	Salem	79%	300+
Riverside Regional Medical Center	Newport News	79%	300+
Rockingham Memorial Hospital	Harrisonburg	79%	300+
Spotsylvania Regional Medical Center	Fredericksburg	79%	300+
University of Virginia Medical Center	Charlottesville	79%	300+
Warren Memorial Hospital	Front Royal	79%	300+
Winchester Medical Center	Winchester	79%	300+
Danville Regional Medical Center	Danville	78%	300+
Inova Fair Oaks Hospital	Fairfax	78%	300+
Inova Loudoun Hospital	Leesburg	78%	300+
Novant Health Prince William Med Ctr	Manassas	78%	300+
Carilion Roanoke Memorial Hospital	Roanoke	77%	300+
Sentara Northern Virginia Medical Center	Woodbridge	77%	300+
Inova Alexandria Hospital	Alexandria	76%	300+
Inova Fairfax Hospital	Falls Church	76%	300+
Mary Washington Hospital	Fredericksburg	76%	300+
Mem Hosp of Martinsville & Henry Co	Martinsville	76%	300+
Shenandoah Memorial Hospital	Woodstock	76%	300+
Reston Hospital Center	Reston	75%	300+
Stafford Hospital	Stafford	74%	300+

Home Recovery Information Given

Hospital Name	City	Rate	Cases
Bon Secours Richmond Community Hospital	Richmond	91%	(a)
Carilion Giles Community Hospital	Pearisburg	91%	(a)
Sentara Leigh Hospital	Norfolk	91%	300+
Sentara Princess Anne Hospital	Virginia Beach	91%	300+
Page Memorial Hospital	Luray	90%	(a)
Rappahannock General Hospital	Kilmarnock	90%	300+
Sentara Careplex Hospital	Hampton	90%	300+
Sentara Virginia Beach General Hospital	Virginia Beach	90%	300+
Martha Jefferson Hospital	Charlottesville	89%	300+
Sentara Norfolk General Hospital	Norfolk	89%	300+
Sentara Williamsburg Reg Med Ctr	Williamsburg	89%	300+
Bon Secours Saint Marys Hospital	Richmond	88%	300+
Carilion Stonewall Jackson Hospital	Lexington	88%	(a)
Centra Health	Lynchburg	88%	300+
Chesapeake General Hospital	Chesapeake	88%	300+
Lewisgale Hospital Montgomery	Blacksburg	88%	300+
Lewisgale Hospital Pulaski	Pulaski	88%	300+
Mary Immaculate Hospital	Newport News	88%	300+
Medical College of Virginia Hospitals	Richmond	88%	300+
Riverside Tappahannock Hospital	Tappahannock	88%	300+
Sentara Obici Hospital	Suffolk	88%	300+
Twin County Regional Hospital	Galax	88%	300+
University of Virginia Medical Center	Charlottesville	88%	300+
Wythe County Community Hospital	Wytheville	88%	300+
Augusta Health	Fishersville	87%	300+
Bon Secours Maryview Medical Center	Portsmouth	87%	300+
Bon Secours Mem Reg Med Ctr	Mechanicsville	87%	300+
Carilion New River Valley Medical Center	Christiansburg	87%	300+
Cjw Medical Center	Richmond	87%	300+
Community Memorial Healthcenter	South Hill	87%	300+
Halifax Regional Hospital	Halifax	87%	300+
Inova Loudoun Hospital	Leesburg	87%	300+
Lewisgale Medical Center	Salem	87%	300+
Southside Community Hospital	Farmville	87%	300+
Virginia Hospital Center	Arlington	87%	300+
Bon Secours Saint Francis Medical Center	Midlothian	86%	300+
Carilion Franklin Memorial Hospital	Rocky Mount	86%	300+
Carilion Roanoke Memorial Hospital	Roanoke	86%	300+
Carilion Tazewell Community Hospital	Tazewell	86%	(a)
Culpeper Regional Hospital	Culpeper	86%	300+
Fauquier Hospital	Warrenton	86%	300+
Henrico Doctors' Hospital	Richmond	86%	300+
Lewisgale Hospital Alleghany	Low Moor	86%	300+
Novant Health Prince William Med Ctr	Manassas	86%	300+
Riverside Walter Reed Hospital	Gloucester	86%	300+
Rockingham Memorial Hospital	Harrisonburg	86%	300+
Southampton Memorial Hospital	Franklin	86%	300+
Spotsylvania Regional Medical Center	Fredericksburg	86%	300+
Bedford Memorial Hospital	Bedford	85%	(a)
Bon Secours Depaul Medical Center	Norfolk	85%	300+
Clinch Valley Medical Center	Richlands	85%	300+
Inova Mount Vernon Hospital	Alexandria	85%	300+
Sentara Northern Virginia Medical Center	Woodbridge	85%	300+
Shenandoah Memorial Hospital	Woodstock	85%	300+
Smyth County Community Hospital	Marion	85%	300+
Inova Fair Oaks Hospital	Fairfax	84%	300+
John Randolph Medical Center	Hopewell	84%	300+
Mary Washington Hospital	Fredericksburg	84%	300+
Mem Hosp of Martinsville & Henry Co	Martinsville	84%	300+
Reston Hospital Center	Reston	84%	300+
Southside Regional Medical Center	Petersburg	84%	300+
Wellmont Lonesome Pine Hospital	Big Stone Gap	84%	300+
Winchester Medical Center	Winchester	84%	300+
Inova Fairfax Hospital	Falls Church	83%	300+
Johnston Memorial Hospital	Abingdon	83%	300+
Riverside Regional Medical Center	Newport News	83%	300+
Riverside Shore Memorial Hospital	Nassawadox	83%	300+
Russell County Medical Center	Lebanon	83%	(a)
Stafford Hospital	Stafford	83%	300+
Danville Regional Medical Center	Danville	82%	300+
Norton Community Hospital	Norton	81%	300+
Warren Memorial Hospital	Front Royal	81%	300+
Buchanan General Hospital	Grundy	80%	(a)
Inova Alexandria Hospital	Alexandria	80%	300+
Southern Virginia Regional Medical Center	Emporia	80%	300+

Hospital Given 9 or 10 on 10 Point Scale

Hospital Name	City	Rate	Cases
Virginia Hospital Center	Arlington	83%	300+
Martha Jefferson Hospital	Charlottesville	80%	300+
Sentara Princess Anne Hospital	Virginia Beach	79%	300+
Carilion New River Valley Medical Center	Christiansburg	78%	300+
Carilion Giles Community Hospital	Pearisburg	77%	(a)
Sentara Norfolk General Hospital	Norfolk	77%	300+
Sentara Obici Hospital	Suffolk	77%	300+
Sentara Williamsburg Reg Med Ctr	Williamsburg	77%	300+
Centra Health	Lynchburg	74%	300+
Sentara Leigh Hospital	Norfolk	74%	300+
Sentara Virginia Beach General Hospital	Virginia Beach	74%	300+
Stafford Hospital	Stafford	74%	300+
Bon Secours Saint Francis Medical Center	Midlothian	73%	300+
Bon Secours Saint Marys Hospital	Richmond	73%	300+
Inova Fair Oaks Hospital	Fairfax	73%	300+
Rockingham Memorial Hospital	Harrisonburg	73%	300+
Fauquier Hospital	Warrenton	72%	300+
Medical College of Virginia Hospitals	Richmond	72%	300+
Rappahannock General Hospital	Kilmarnock	72%	300+
Sentara Careplex Hospital	Hampton	72%	300+
Smyth County Community Hospital	Marion	72%	300+
Bon Secours Mem Reg Med Ctr	Mechanicsville	71%	300+
Henrico Doctors' Hospital	Richmond	71%	300+
Spotsylvania Regional Medical Center	Fredericksburg	71%	300+
Winchester Medical Center	Winchester	71%	300+
Wythe County Community Hospital	Wytheville	71%	300+
Carilion Franklin Memorial Hospital	Rocky Mount	70%	300+
Chesapeake General Hospital	Chesapeake	70%	300+
Halifax Regional Hospital	Halifax	70%	300+
Lewisgale Medical Center	Salem	70%	300+
Bedford Memorial Hospital	Bedford	69%	(a)
Southside Regional Medical Center	Petersburg	69%	300+
Wellmont Lonesome Pine Hospital	Big Stone Gap	69%	300+
Bon Secours Richmond Community Hospital	Richmond	68%	(a)
Carilion Roanoke Memorial Hospital	Roanoke	68%	300+
Lewisgale Hospital Montgomery	Blacksburg	68%	300+
Lewisgale Hospital Pulaski	Pulaski	68%	300+
Riverside Walter Reed Hospital	Gloucester	68%	300+
University of Virginia Medical Center	Charlottesville	68%	300+
Augusta Health	Fishersville	67%	300+
Cjw Medical Center	Richmond	67%	300+
Clinch Valley Medical Center	Richlands	67%	300+
Culpeper Regional Hospital	Culpeper	67%	300+
Inova Mount Vernon Hospital	Alexandria	67%	300+
Norton Community Hospital	Norton	67%	300+
Page Memorial Hospital	Luray	67%	(a)
Reston Hospital Center	Reston	67%	300+
Riverside Regional Medical Center	Newport News	67%	300+
Buchanan General Hospital	Grundy	66%	(a)
Carilion Stonewall Jackson Hospital	Lexington	66%	(a)
Mary Immaculate Hospital	Newport News	66%	300+
Shenandoah Memorial Hospital	Woodstock	66%	300+

NOTE: Hospital profiles are in alphabetical order by state, then city, then hospital within the city; Rankings exclude hospitals with less than 25 cases except for patient surveys which excludes hospitals with less than 100 cases; (a) 100-299 cases; (1) The number of cases/patients is too few to report; (2) Data submitted were based on a sample of cases/patients; (3) Results are based on a shorter time period than required; (4) Data suppressed by CMS for one or more quarters; (5) Results are not available for this reporting period; (6) Fewer than 100 patients completed the HCAHPS survey; (7) No cases met the criteria for this measure; (8) The lower limit of the confidence interval cannot be calculated if the number of observed infections equals zero; (9) No data are available from the state/territory for this reporting period; (10) The scores shown reflect fewer than 50 completed surveys; (11) There were discrepancies in the data collection process; (12) This measure does not apply to this hospital for this reporting period; (13) Results cannot be calculated for this reporting period; (14) The results for this state are combined with nearby states to protect confidentiality; Please refer to the User's Guide for a full explanation of data.

Southampton Memorial Hospital	Franklin	66%	300+
Carilion Tazewell Community Hospital	Tazewell	65%	(a)
Inova Fairfax Hospital	Falls Church	65%	300+
Inova Loudoun Hospital	Leesburg	65%	300+
Riverside Tappahannock Hospital	Tappahannock	65%	300+
Twin County Regional Hospital	Galax	65%	300+
Lewisgale Hospital Alleghany	Low Moor	64%	300+
Mary Washington Hospital	Fredericksburg	64%	300+
Russell County Medical Center	Lebanon	64%	(a)
Bon Secours Depaul Medical Center	Norfolk	63%	300+
Community Memorial Healthcenter	South Hill	63%	300+
Johnston Memorial Hospital	Abingdon	63%	300+
Warren Memorial Hospital	Front Royal	63%	300+
Inova Alexandria Hospital	Alexandria	62%	300+
Bon Secours Maryview Medical Center	Portsmouth	61%	300+
John Randolph Medical Center	Hopewell	61%	300+
Southern Virginia Regional Medical Center	Emporia	60%	300+
Southside Community Hospital	Farmville	60%	300+
Riverside Shore Memorial Hospital	Nassawadox	59%	300+
Novant Health Prince William Med Ctr	Manassas	58%	300+
Sentara Northern Virginia Medical Center	Woodbridge	58%	300+
Danville Regional Medical Center	Danville	54%	300+
Mem Hosp of Martinsville & Henry Co	Martinsville	54%	300+

Meds 'Always' Explained Before Given

Hospital Name	City	Rate	Cases
Carilion Giles Community Hospital	Pearisburg	73%	(a)
Carilion Tazewell Community Hospital	Tazewell	71%	(a)
Carilion Stonewall Jackson Hospital	Lexington	70%	(a)
Virginia Hospital Center	Arlington	70%	300+
Bon Secours Richmond Community Hospital	Richmond	69%	(a)
Carilion New River Valley Medical Center	Christiansburg	68%	300+
Sentara Leigh Hospital	Norfolk	68%	300+
Wellmont Lonesome Pine Hospital	Big Stone Gap	68%	300+
Carilion Franklin Memorial Hospital	Rocky Mount	67%	300+
Halifax Regional Hospital	Halifax	67%	300+
Rappahannock General Hospital	Kilmarnock	67%	300+
Riverside Walter Reed Hospital	Gloucester	67%	300+
Shenandoah Memorial Hospital	Woodstock	67%	300+
Wythe County Community Hospital	Wytheville	67%	300+
Centra Health	Lynchburg	66%	300+
Sentara Williamsburg Reg Med Ctr	Williamsburg	66%	300+
Warren Memorial Hospital	Front Royal	66%	300+
Clinch Valley Medical Center	Richlands	65%	300+
Medical College of Virginia Hospitals	Richmond	65%	300+
Sentara Norfolk General Hospital	Norfolk	65%	300+
Sentara Obici Hospital	Suffolk	65%	300+
Sentara Princess Anne Hospital	Virginia Beach	65%	300+
Chesapeake General Hospital	Chesapeake	64%	300+
Community Memorial Healthcenter	South Hill	64%	300+
Southern Virginia Regional Medical Center	Emporia	64%	300+
Bon Secours Saint Marys Hospital	Richmond	63%	300+
Culpeper Regional Hospital	Culpeper	63%	300+
Fauquier Hospital	Warrenton	63%	300+
Martha Jefferson Hospital	Charlottesville	63%	300+
Page Memorial Hospital	Luray	63%	(a)
Riverside Tappahannock Hospital	Tappahannock	63%	300+
Southampton Memorial Hospital	Franklin	63%	300+
Southside Community Hospital	Farmville	63%	300+
Southside Regional Medical Center	Petersburg	63%	300+
Twin County Regional Hospital	Galax	63%	300+
Bedford Memorial Hospital	Bedford	62%	(a)
Bon Secours Mem Reg Med Ctr	Mechanicsville	62%	300+
Buchanan General Hospital	Grundy	62%	(a)
Norton Community Hospital	Norton	62%	300+
Augusta Health	Fishersville	61%	300+
Inova Fair Oaks Hospital	Fairfax	61%	300+
Lewisgale Hospital Pulaski	Pulaski	61%	300+
Mary Immaculate Hospital	Newport News	61%	300+
Rockingham Memorial Hospital	Harrisonburg	61%	300+
Russell County Medical Center	Lebanon	61%	(a)
Sentara Careplex Hospital	Hampton	61%	300+
Sentara Virginia Beach General Hospital	Virginia Beach	61%	300+
Stafford Hospital	Stafford	61%	300+
University of Virginia Medical Center	Charlottesville	61%	300+
Cjw Medical Center	Richmond	60%	300+
Henrico Doctors' Hospital	Richmond	60%	300+
Inova Alexandria Hospital	Alexandria	60%	300+
Inova Fairfax Hospital	Falls Church	60%	300+
John Randolph Medical Center	Hopewell	60%	300+
Lewisgale Hospital Alleghany	Low Moor	60%	300+
Lewisgale Hospital Montgomery	Blacksburg	60%	300+
Riverside Regional Medical Center	Newport News	60%	300+
Bon Secours Saint Francis Medical Center	Midlothian	59%	300+
Inova Loudoun Hospital	Leesburg	59%	300+
Inova Mount Vernon Hospital	Alexandria	59%	300+
Mary Washington Hospital	Fredericksburg	59%	300+
Spotsylvania Regional Medical Center	Fredericksburg	59%	300+
Winchester Medical Center	Winchester	59%	300+
Bon Secours Maryview Medical Center	Portsmouth	58%	300+
Carilion Roanoke Memorial Hospital	Roanoke	58%	300+
Lewisgale Medical Center	Salem	58%	300+
Novant Health Prince William Med Ctr	Manassas	58%	300+
Reston Hospital Center	Reston	58%	300+
Sentara Northern Virginia Medical Center	Woodbridge	58%	300+
Smyth County Community Hospital	Marion	58%	300+
Danville Regional Medical Center	Danville	57%	300+
Johnston Memorial Hospital	Abingdon	57%	300+
Riverside Shore Memorial Hospital	Nassawadox	57%	300+
Bon Secours Depaul Medical Center	Norfolk	56%	300+
Mem Hosp of Martinsville & Henry Co	Martinsville	56%	300+

Nurses 'Always' Communicated Well

Hospital Name	City	Rate	Cases
Carilion Giles Community Hospital	Pearisburg	86%	(a)
Sentara Obici Hospital	Suffolk	84%	300+
Carilion New River Valley Medical Center	Christiansburg	83%	300+
Rappahannock General Hospital	Kilmarnock	83%	300+
Riverside Tappahannock Hospital	Tappahannock	83%	300+
Virginia Hospital Center	Arlington	83%	300+
Wellmont Lonesome Pine Hospital	Big Stone Gap	83%	300+
Buchanan General Hospital	Grundy	82%	(a)
Centra Health	Lynchburg	82%	300+
Martha Jefferson Hospital	Charlottesville	82%	300+
Page Memorial Hospital	Luray	82%	(a)
Russell County Medical Center	Lebanon	82%	(a)
Sentara Princess Anne Hospital	Virginia Beach	82%	300+
Wythe County Community Hospital	Wytheville	82%	300+
Carilion Franklin Memorial Hospital	Rocky Mount	81%	300+
Carilion Stonewall Jackson Hospital	Lexington	81%	(a)
Community Memorial Healthcenter	South Hill	81%	300+
Halifax Regional Hospital	Halifax	81%	300+
Sentara Careplex Hospital	Hampton	81%	300+
Sentara Norfolk General Hospital	Norfolk	81%	300+
Sentara Virginia Beach General Hospital	Virginia Beach	81%	300+
Sentara Williamsburg Reg Med Ctr	Williamsburg	81%	300+
Bedford Memorial Hospital	Bedford	80%	(a)
Bon Secours Richmond Community Hospital	Richmond	80%	(a)
Carilion Tazewell Community Hospital	Tazewell	80%	(a)
Sentara Leigh Hospital	Norfolk	80%	300+
Smyth County Community Hospital	Marion	80%	300+
Bon Secours Saint Marys Hospital	Richmond	79%	300+
Culpeper Regional Hospital	Culpeper	79%	300+
Fauquier Hospital	Warrenton	79%	300+
Lewisgale Hospital Alleghany	Low Moor	79%	300+
Riverside Walter Reed Hospital	Gloucester	79%	300+
Rockingham Memorial Hospital	Harrisonburg	79%	300+
Shenandoah Memorial Hospital	Woodstock	79%	300+
Southside Regional Medical Center	Petersburg	79%	300+
Warren Memorial Hospital	Front Royal	79%	300+
Carilion Roanoke Memorial Hospital	Roanoke	78%	300+
Clinch Valley Medical Center	Richlands	78%	300+
Medical College of Virginia Hospitals	Richmond	78%	300+
Norton Community Hospital	Norton	78%	300+
Riverside Shore Memorial Hospital	Nassawadox	78%	300+
Southampton Memorial Hospital	Franklin	78%	300+
Stafford Hospital	Stafford	78%	300+
Bon Secours Mem Reg Med Ctr	Mechanicsville	77%	300+
Chesapeake General Hospital	Chesapeake	77%	300+
Henrico Doctors' Hospital	Richmond	77%	300+
Lewisgale Hospital Pulaski	Pulaski	77%	300+
Riverside Regional Medical Center	Newport News	77%	300+
Southside Community Hospital	Farmville	77%	300+
Augusta Health	Fishersville	76%	300+
Cjw Medical Center	Richmond	76%	300+
Inova Fair Oaks Hospital	Fairfax	76%	300+
Inova Loudoun Hospital	Leesburg	76%	300+
Lewisgale Hospital Montgomery	Blacksburg	76%	300+
Mary Washington Hospital	Fredericksburg	76%	300+
Spotsylvania Regional Medical Center	Fredericksburg	76%	300+
Twin County Regional Hospital	Galax	76%	300+
University of Virginia Medical Center	Charlottesville	76%	300+
Winchester Medical Center	Winchester	76%	300+
Bon Secours Saint Francis Medical Center	Midlothian	75%	300+
Danville Regional Medical Center	Danville	74%	300+
John Randolph Medical Center	Hopewell	74%	300+
Lewisgale Medical Center	Salem	74%	300+
Mary Immaculate Hospital	Newport News	74%	300+
Bon Secours Maryview Medical Center	Portsmouth	73%	300+
Inova Alexandria Hospital	Alexandria	73%	300+
Inova Mount Vernon Hospital	Alexandria	73%	300+
Reston Hospital Center	Reston	73%	300+
Sentara Northern Virginia Medical Center	Woodbridge	73%	300+
Inova Fairfax Hospital	Falls Church	72%	300+
Johnston Memorial Hospital	Abingdon	72%	300+
Mem Hosp of Martinsville & Henry Co	Martinsville	72%	300+
Bon Secours Depaul Medical Center	Norfolk	71%	300+
Novant Health Prince William Med Ctr	Manassas	71%	300+
Southern Virginia Regional Medical Center	Emporia	70%	300+

Pain 'Always' Well Controlled

Hospital Name	City	Rate	Cases
Carilion Tazewell Community Hospital	Tazewell	80%	(a)
Sentara Leigh Hospital	Norfolk	76%	300+
Sentara Norfolk General Hospital	Norfolk	76%	300+
Virginia Hospital Center	Arlington	75%	300+
Wellmont Lonesome Pine Hospital	Big Stone Gap	75%	300+
Buchanan General Hospital	Grundy	74%	(a)
Sentara Obici Hospital	Suffolk	74%	300+
Sentara Virginia Beach General Hospital	Virginia Beach	74%	300+
Carilion Roanoke Memorial Hospital	Roanoke	73%	300+
Rappahannock General Hospital	Kilmarnock	73%	300+
Sentara Princess Anne Hospital	Virginia Beach	73%	300+
Bon Secours Saint Marys Hospital	Richmond	72%	300+
Carilion Giles Community Hospital	Pearisburg	72%	(a)
Carilion New River Valley Medical Center	Christiansburg	72%	300+
Carilion Stonewall Jackson Hospital	Lexington	72%	(a)
Centra Health	Lynchburg	72%	300+
Riverside Walter Reed Hospital	Gloucester	72%	300+
Sentara Careplex Hospital	Hampton	72%	300+
Sentara Williamsburg Reg Med Ctr	Williamsburg	72%	300+
Winchester Medical Center	Winchester	72%	300+
Chesapeake General Hospital	Chesapeake	71%	300+
Culpeper Regional Hospital	Culpeper	71%	300+
Halifax Regional Hospital	Halifax	71%	300+
Henrico Doctors' Hospital	Richmond	71%	300+
Lewisgale Hospital Montgomery	Blacksburg	71%	300+
Medical College of Virginia Hospitals	Richmond	71%	300+
Riverside Tappahannock Hospital	Tappahannock	71%	300+
Shenandoah Memorial Hospital	Woodstock	71%	300+
Southampton Memorial Hospital	Franklin	71%	300+
Southside Regional Medical Center	Petersburg	71%	300+
Wythe County Community Hospital	Wytheville	71%	300+
Bon Secours Richmond Community Hospital	Richmond	70%	(a)
Carilion Franklin Memorial Hospital	Rocky Mount	70%	300+
Clinch Valley Medical Center	Richlands	70%	300+
Lewisgale Hospital Pulaski	Pulaski	70%	300+
Martha Jefferson Hospital	Charlottesville	70%	300+
Rockingham Memorial Hospital	Harrisonburg	70%	300+
Sentara Northern Virginia Medical Center	Woodbridge	70%	300+
Smyth County Community Hospital	Marion	70%	300+
Southside Community Hospital	Farmville	70%	300+
Bon Secours Mem Reg Med Ctr	Mechanicsville	69%	300+
Bon Secours Saint Francis Medical Center	Midlothian	69%	300+
Fauquier Hospital	Warrenton	69%	300+
Lewisgale Medical Center	Salem	69%	300+
Mary Washington Hospital	Fredericksburg	69%	300+
Stafford Hospital	Stafford	69%	300+
Warren Memorial Hospital	Front Royal	69%	300+
Augusta Health	Fishersville	68%	300+
Bedford Memorial Hospital	Bedford	68%	(a)
Bon Secours Maryview Medical Center	Portsmouth	68%	300+
Cjw Medical Center	Richmond	68%	300+
Community Memorial Healthcenter	South Hill	68%	300+
Inova Mount Vernon Hospital	Alexandria	68%	300+
Lewisgale Hospital Alleghany	Low Moor	68%	300+
Inova Alexandria Hospital	Alexandria	67%	300+
Inova Fair Oaks Hospital	Fairfax	67%	300+
Inova Loudoun Hospital	Leesburg	67%	300+
John Randolph Medical Center	Hopewell	67%	300+
Page Memorial Hospital	Luray	67%	(a)
Riverside Regional Medical Center	Newport News	67%	300+
Spotsylvania Regional Medical Center	Fredericksburg	67%	300+
Twin County Regional Hospital	Galax	67%	300+
Reston Hospital Center	Reston	66%	300+
Danville Regional Medical Center	Danville	65%	300+
Inova Fairfax Hospital	Falls Church	65%	300+
Mary Immaculate Hospital	Newport News	65%	300+
Riverside Shore Memorial Hospital	Nassawadox	65%	300+
Russell County Medical Center	Lebanon	65%	(a)
University of Virginia Medical Center	Charlottesville	65%	300+
Bon Secours Depaul Medical Center	Norfolk	64%	300+
Johnston Memorial Hospital	Abingdon	64%	300+
Norton Community Hospital	Norton	64%	300+
Novant Health Prince William Med Ctr	Manassas	64%	300+
Southern Virginia Regional Medical Center	Emporia	64%	300+
Mem Hosp of Martinsville & Henry Co	Martinsville	63%	300+

Room and Bathroom 'Always' Clean

Hospital Name	City	Rate	Cases
Shenandoah Memorial Hospital	Woodstock	85%	300+
Carilion Franklin Memorial Hospital	Rocky Mount	83%	300+
Smyth County Community Hospital	Marion	80%	300+
Virginia Hospital Center	Arlington	80%	300+
Wellmont Lonesome Pine Hospital	Big Stone Gap	80%	300+
Carilion Giles Community Hospital	Pearisburg	79%	(a)
Fauquier Hospital	Warrenton	78%	300+
Buchanan General Hospital	Grundy	77%	(a)
Culpeper Regional Hospital	Culpeper	77%	300+
Rockingham Memorial Hospital	Harrisonburg	77%	300+

NOTE: Hospital profiles are in alphabetical order by state, then city, then hospital within the city; Rankings exclude hospitals with less than 25 cases except for patient surveys which excludes hospitals with less than 100 cases; (a) 100-299 cases; (1) The number of cases/patients is too few to report; (2) Data submitted were based on a sample of cases/patients; (3) Results are based on a shorter time period than required; (4) Data suppressed by CMS for one or more quarters; (5) Results are not available for this reporting period; (6) Fewer than 100 patients completed the HCAHPS survey; (7) No cases met the criteria for this measure; (8) The lower limit of the confidence interval cannot be calculated if the number of observed infections equals zero; (9) No data are available from the state/territory for this reporting period; (10) The scores shown reflect fewer than 50 completed surveys; (11) There were discrepancies in the data collection process; (12) This measure does not apply to this hospital for this reporting period; (13) Results cannot be calculated for this reporting period; (14) The results for this state are combined with nearby states to protect confidentiality; Please refer to the User's Guide for a full explanation of data.

Carilion Tazewell Community Hospital	Tazewell	76%	(a)
Sentara Obici Hospital	Suffolk	75%	300+
Southside Community Hospital	Farmville	75%	300+
Bon Secours Richmond Community Hospital	Richmond	74%	(a)
Martha Jefferson Hospital	Charlottesville	74%	300+
Riverside Tappahannock Hospital	Tappahannock	74%	300+
Russell County Medical Center	Lebanon	74%	(a)
Sentara Careplex Hospital	Hampton	74%	300+
Stafford Hospital	Stafford	74%	300+
Twin County Regional Hospital	Galax	74%	300+
Bedford Memorial Hospital	Bedford	73%	(a)
Centra Health	Lynchburg	73%	300+
Halifax Regional Hospital	Halifax	73%	300+
John Randolph Medical Center	Hopewell	73%	300+
Lewisgale Hospital Pulaski	Pulaski	73%	300+
Page Memorial Hospital	Luray	73%	(a)
Rappahannock General Hospital	Kilmarnock	73%	300+
Sentara Williamsburg Reg Med Ctr	Williamsburg	73%	300+
Warren Memorial Hospital	Front Royal	73%	300+
Wythe County Community Hospital	Wytheville	73%	300+
Carilion New River Valley Medical Center	Christiansburg	72%	300+
Clinch Valley Medical Center	Richlands	72%	300+
Lewisgale Hospital Montgomery	Blacksburg	72%	300+
Mary Washington Hospital	Fredericksburg	72%	300+
Norton Community Hospital	Norton	72%	300+
Reston Hospital Center	Reston	72%	300+
Riverside Regional Medical Center	Newport News	72%	300+
Riverside Shore Memorial Hospital	Nassawadox	72%	300+
Southside Regional Medical Center	Petersburg	72%	300+
Riverside Walter Reed Hospital	Gloucester	71%	300+
Sentara Princess Anne Hospital	Virginia Beach	71%	300+
Southampton Memorial Hospital	Franklin	71%	300+
Spotsylvania Regional Medical Center	Fredericksburg	71%	300+
Johnston Memorial Hospital	Abingdon	70%	300+
Medical College of Virginia Hospitals	Richmond	70%	300+
Novant Health Prince William Med Ctr	Manassas	70%	300+
Sentara Northern Virginia Medical Center	Woodbridge	70%	300+
Community Memorial Healthcenter	South Hill	69%	300+
Danville Regional Medical Center	Danville	69%	300+
Winchester Medical Center	Winchester	69%	300+
Augusta Health	Fishersville	68%	300+
Bon Secours Saint Marys Hospital	Richmond	68%	300+
Sentara Norfolk General Hospital	Norfolk	68%	300+
Cjw Medical Center	Richmond	67%	300+
Henrico Doctors' Hospital	Richmond	67%	300+
Inova Mount Vernon Hospital	Alexandria	67%	300+
Sentara Virginia Beach General Hospital	Virginia Beach	67%	300+
Southern Virginia Regional Medical Center	Emporia	67%	300+
University of Virginia Medical Center	Charlottesville	67%	300+
Bon Secours Depaul Medical Center	Norfolk	66%	300+
Bon Secours Saint Francis Medical Center	Midlothian	66%	300+
Inova Fair Oaks Hospital	Fairfax	66%	300+
Bon Secours Mem Reg Med Ctr	Mechanicsville	65%	300+
Mem Hosp of Martinsville & Henry Co	Martinsville	65%	300+
Sentara Leigh Hospital	Norfolk	65%	300+
Carilion Stonewall Jackson Hospital	Lexington	64%	(a)
Inova Fairfax Hospital	Falls Church	64%	300+
Lewisgale Medical Center	Salem	64%	300+
Chesapeake General Hospital	Chesapeake	63%	300+
Inova Alexandria Hospital	Alexandria	63%	300+
Inova Loudoun Hospital	Leesburg	63%	300+
Bon Secours Maryview Medical Center	Portsmouth	62%	300+
Carilion Roanoke Memorial Hospital	Roanoke	61%	300+
Lewisgale Hospital Alleghany	Low Moor	59%	300+
Mary Immaculate Hospital	Newport News	59%	300+

Timely Help 'Always' Received

Hospital Name	City	Rate	Cases
Russell County Medical Center	Lebanon	77%	(a)
Riverside Tappahannock Hospital	Tappahannock	76%	300+
Carilion Giles Community Hospital	Pearisburg	75%	(a)
Rappahannock General Hospital	Kilmarnock	75%	300+
Carilion Franklin Memorial Hospital	Rocky Mount	74%	300+
Carilion Tazewell Community Hospital	Tazewell	74%	(a)
Sentara Obici Hospital	Suffolk	74%	300+
Wellmont Lonesome Pine Hospital	Big Stone Gap	74%	300+
Carilion New River Valley Medical Center	Christiansburg	72%	300+
Virginia Hospital Center	Arlington	72%	300+
Sentara Norfolk General Hospital	Norfolk	71%	300+
Wythe County Community Hospital	Wytheville	71%	300+
Martha Jefferson Hospital	Charlottesville	70%	300+
Buchanan General Hospital	Grundy	69%	(a)
Halifax Regional Hospital	Halifax	69%	300+
Sentara Virginia Beach General Hospital	Virginia Beach	68%	300+
Bon Secours Mem Reg Med Ctr	Mechanicsville	67%	300+
Carilion Stonewall Jackson Hospital	Lexington	67%	(a)
Centra Health	Lynchburg	67%	300+
Sentara Princess Anne Hospital	Virginia Beach	67%	300+
Shenandoah Memorial Hospital	Woodstock	67%	300+
Smyth County Community Hospital	Marion	67%	300+
Carilion Roanoke Memorial Hospital	Roanoke	66%	300+
Clinch Valley Medical Center	Richlands	66%	300+
Community Memorial Healthcenter	South Hill	66%	300+
Riverside Shore Memorial Hospital	Nassawadox	66%	300+
Sentara Careplex Hospital	Hampton	66%	300+
Sentara Leigh Hospital	Norfolk	66%	300+
Southampton Memorial Hospital	Franklin	66%	300+
Southside Regional Medical Center	Petersburg	66%	300+
Stafford Hospital	Stafford	66%	300+
Warren Memorial Hospital	Front Royal	66%	300+
Bon Secours Richmond Community Hospital	Richmond	65%	(a)
Rockingham Memorial Hospital	Harrisonburg	65%	300+
Bedford Memorial Hospital	Bedford	64%	(a)
Bon Secours Saint Marys Hospital	Richmond	64%	300+
Chesapeake General Hospital	Chesapeake	64%	300+
Culpeper Regional Hospital	Culpeper	64%	300+
Fauquier Hospital	Warrenton	64%	300+
Henrico Doctors' Hospital	Richmond	64%	300+
Norton Community Hospital	Norton	64%	300+
Riverside Walter Reed Hospital	Gloucester	64%	300+
Spotsylvania Regional Medical Center	Fredericksburg	64%	300+
Winchester Medical Center	Winchester	64%	300+
Southside Community Hospital	Farmville	62%	300+
Cjw Medical Center	Richmond	61%	300+
Lewisgale Hospital Alleghany	Low Moor	61%	300+
Lewisgale Hospital Montgomery	Blacksburg	61%	300+
Lewisgale Hospital Pulaski	Pulaski	61%	300+
Mary Washington Hospital	Fredericksburg	61%	300+
Medical College of Virginia Hospitals	Richmond	61%	300+
Inova Loudoun Hospital	Leesburg	60%	300+
Page Memorial Hospital	Luray	60%	(a)
Riverside Regional Medical Center	Newport News	60%	300+
Augusta Health	Fishersville	59%	300+
Bon Secours Saint Francis Medical Center	Midlothian	59%	300+
Inova Alexandria Hospital	Alexandria	59%	300+
Inova Fair Oaks Hospital	Fairfax	59%	300+
Mary Immaculate Hospital	Newport News	59%	300+
Sentara Williamsburg Reg Med Ctr	Williamsburg	59%	300+
Twin County Regional Hospital	Galax	59%	300+
Bon Secours Maryview Medical Center	Portsmouth	58%	300+
Inova Mount Vernon Hospital	Alexandria	58%	300+
Johnston Memorial Hospital	Abingdon	58%	300+
Danville Regional Medical Center	Danville	57%	300+
University of Virginia Medical Center	Charlottesville	57%	300+
Bon Secours Depaul Medical Center	Norfolk	56%	300+
John Randolph Medical Center	Hopewell	56%	300+
Lewisgale Medical Center	Salem	56%	300+
Novant Health Prince William Med Ctr	Manassas	56%	300+
Reston Hospital Center	Reston	56%	300+
Sentara Northern Virginia Medical Center	Woodbridge	55%	300+
Inova Fairfax Hospital	Falls Church	54%	300+
Mem Hosp of Martinsville & Henry Co	Martinsville	54%	300+
Southern Virginia Regional Medical Center	Emporia	51%	300+

Would Definitely Recommend Hospital

Hospital Name	City	Rate	Cases
Virginia Hospital Center	Arlington	85%	300+
Martha Jefferson Hospital	Charlottesville	83%	300+
Sentara Princess Anne Hospital	Virginia Beach	83%	300+
Carilion New River Valley Medical Center	Christiansburg	82%	300+
Sentara Williamsburg Reg Med Ctr	Williamsburg	81%	300+
Sentara Norfolk General Hospital	Norfolk	79%	300+
Centra Health	Lynchburg	78%	300+
Inova Fair Oaks Hospital	Fairfax	78%	300+
Sentara Leigh Hospital	Norfolk	78%	300+
Sentara Virginia Beach General Hospital	Virginia Beach	78%	300+
Carilion Giles Community Hospital	Pearisburg	77%	(a)
Winchester Medical Center	Winchester	77%	300+
Bon Secours Saint Francis Medical Center	Midlothian	76%	300+
Bon Secours Saint Marys Hospital	Richmond	76%	300+
Carilion Roanoke Memorial Hospital	Roanoke	76%	300+
Medical College of Virginia Hospitals	Richmond	76%	300+
Sentara Careplex Hospital	Hampton	76%	300+
Bon Secours Mem Reg Med Ctr	Mechanicsville	75%	300+
Henrico Doctors' Hospital	Richmond	75%	300+
Inova Fairfax Hospital	Falls Church	75%	300+
Sentara Obici Hospital	Suffolk	75%	300+
Stafford Hospital	Stafford	75%	300+
University of Virginia Medical Center	Charlottesville	75%	300+
Lewisgale Medical Center	Salem	74%	300+
Fauquier Hospital	Warrenton	73%	300+
Carilion Franklin Memorial Hospital	Rocky Mount	72%	300+
Inova Loudoun Hospital	Leesburg	72%	300+
Spotsylvania Regional Medical Center	Fredericksburg	72%	300+
Chesapeake General Hospital	Chesapeake	71%	300+
Inova Mount Vernon Hospital	Alexandria	71%	300+
Lewisgale Hospital Montgomery	Blacksburg	71%	300+
Reston Hospital Center	Reston	71%	300+
Riverside Regional Medical Center	Newport News	71%	300+
Augusta Health	Fishersville	70%	300+
Bon Secours Richmond Community Hospital	Richmond	70%	(a)
Cjw Medical Center	Richmond	70%	300+
Culpeper Regional Hospital	Culpeper	70%	300+
Lewisgale Hospital Pulaski	Pulaski	70%	300+
Rockingham Memorial Hospital	Harrisonburg	70%	300+
Mary Immaculate Hospital	Newport News	69%	300+
Rappahannock General Hospital	Kilmarnock	69%	300+
Smyth County Community Hospital	Marion	69%	300+
Bedford Memorial Hospital	Bedford	68%	(a)
Clinch Valley Medical Center	Richlands	68%	300+
Wellmont Lonesome Pine Hospital	Big Stone Gap	68%	300+
Carilion Tazewell Community Hospital	Tazewell	67%	(a)
Riverside Walter Reed Hospital	Gloucester	67%	300+
Southside Regional Medical Center	Petersburg	67%	300+
Halifax Regional Hospital	Halifax	66%	300+
Inova Alexandria Hospital	Alexandria	66%	300+
Mary Washington Hospital	Fredericksburg	66%	300+
Riverside Tappahannock Hospital	Tappahannock	66%	300+
Wythe County Community Hospital	Wytheville	65%	300+
Buchanan General Hospital	Grundy	64%	(a)
Page Memorial Hospital	Luray	64%	(a)
Russell County Medical Center	Lebanon	64%	(a)
Sentara Northern Virginia Medical Center	Woodbridge	64%	300+
Shenandoah Memorial Hospital	Woodstock	64%	300+
Bon Secours Depaul Medical Center	Norfolk	63%	300+
Johnston Memorial Hospital	Abingdon	62%	300+
Norton Community Hospital	Norton	62%	300+
Novant Health Prince William Med Ctr	Manassas	62%	300+
Carilion Stonewall Jackson Hospital	Lexington	61%	(a)
Community Memorial Healthcenter	South Hill	61%	300+
Lewisgale Hospital Alleghany	Low Moor	61%	300+
John Randolph Medical Center	Hopewell	60%	300+
Warren Memorial Hospital	Front Royal	60%	300+
Southside Community Hospital	Farmville	58%	300+
Twin County Regional Hospital	Galax	58%	300+
Southampton Memorial Hospital	Franklin	57%	300+
Bon Secours Maryview Medical Center	Portsmouth	56%	300+
Riverside Shore Memorial Hospital	Nassawadox	55%	300+
Danville Regional Medical Center	Danville	50%	300+
Southern Virginia Regional Medical Center	Emporia	50%	300+
Mem Hosp of Martinsville & Henry Co	Martinsville	49%	300+

Use of Medical Imaging

Cardiac Imaging Stress Test before OP Surgery

Hospital Name	City	Rate	Cases
Russell County Medical Center	Lebanon	0.0%	55
Carilion Stonewall Jackson Hospital	Lexington	2.1%	188
Inova Mount Vernon Hospital	Alexandria	2.1%	192
Buchanan General Hospital	Grundy	2.8%	106
Southern Virginia Regional Medical Center	Emporia	2.9%	103
Bon Secours Maryview Medical Center	Portsmouth	3.6%	584
Johnston Memorial Hospital	Abingdon	3.6%	364
Riverside Tappahannock Hospital	Tappahannock	3.6%	249
Southampton Memorial Hospital	Franklin	3.6%	221
Southside Regional Medical Center	Petersburg	3.6%	192
Augusta Health	Fishersville	3.7%	596
Culpeper Regional Hospital	Culpeper	3.8%	79
Wellmont Lonesome Pine Hospital	Big Stone Gap	3.8%	211
Martha Jefferson Hospital	Charlottesville	3.9%	232
Shenandoah Memorial Hospital	Woodstock	3.9%	129
Winchester Medical Center	Winchester	3.9%	558
Page Memorial Hospital	Luray	4.0%	75
Lewisgale Medical Center	Salem	4.1%	712
Southside Community Hospital	Farmville	4.1%	195
Warren Memorial Hospital	Front Royal	4.1%	146
Cjw Medical Center	Richmond	4.2%	357
Lewisgale Hospital Alleghany	Low Moor	4.2%	167
Riverside Regional Medical Center	Newport News	4.2%	1156
Community Memorial Healthcenter	South Hill	4.3%	117
Henrico Doctors' Hospital	Richmond	4.3%	188
Riverside Walter Reed Hospital	Gloucester	4.3%	232
Centra Health	Lynchburg	4.5%	1389
Rockingham Memorial Hospital	Harrisonburg	4.5%	1011
Sentara Princess Anne Hospital	Virginia Beach	4.5%	491
Chesapeake General Hospital	Chesapeake	4.7%	660
Carilion Roanoke Memorial Hospital	Roanoke	4.8%	1351
Medical College of Virginia Hospitals	Richmond	4.8%	921
Reston Hospital Center	Reston	4.8%	63
Sentara Norfolk General Hospital	Norfolk	4.8%	415
Halifax Regional Hospital	Halifax	4.9%	690
Inova Fairfax Hospital	Falls Church	5.1%	256
Sentara Leigh Hospital	Norfolk	5.1%	571
Bon Secours Saint Francis Medical Center	Midlothian	5.2%	96
Riverside Shore Memorial Hospital	Nassawadox	5.3%	320
Sentara Obici Hospital	Suffolk	5.5%	292
Bedford Memorial Hospital	Bedford	5.6%	89
Mem Hosp of Martinsville & Henry Co	Martinsville	5.6%	268
Sentara Virginia Beach General Hospital	Virginia Beach	5.7%	460
Virginia Hospital Center	Arlington	5.7%	123
Bon Secours Saint Marys Hospital	Richmond	5.9%	1213
Fauquier Hospital	Warrenton	5.9%	202

NOTE: Hospital profiles are in alphabetical order by state, then city, then hospital within the city; Rankings exclude hospitals with less than 25 cases except for patient surveys which excludes hospitals with less than 100 cases; (a) 100-299 cases; (1) The number of cases/patients is too few to report; (2) Data submitted were based on a sample of cases/patients; (3) Results are based on a shorter time period than required; (4) Data suppressed by CMS for one or more quarters; (5) Results are not available for this reporting period; (6) Fewer than 100 patients completed the HCAHPS survey; (7) No cases met the criteria for this measure; (8) The lower limit of the confidence interval cannot be calculated if the number of observed infections equals zero; (9) No data are available from the state/territory for this reporting period; (10) The scores shown reflect fewer than 50 completed surveys; (11) There were discrepancies in the data collection process; (12) This measure does not apply to this hospital for this reporting period; (13) Results cannot be calculated for this reporting period; (14) The results for this state are combined with nearby states to protect confidentiality; Please refer to the User's Guide for a full explanation of data.

Hospital Name	City	Rate	Cases
Lewisgale Hospital Montgomery	Blacksburg	5.9%	272
Rappahannock General Hospital	Kilmarnock	6.0%	151
Spotsylvania Regional Medical Center	Fredericksburg	6.0%	83
Sentara Northern Virginia Medical Center	Woodbridge	6.1%	98
Stafford Hospital	Stafford	6.1%	98
Clinch Valley Medical Center	Richlands	6.3%	222
Mary Immaculate Hospital	Newport News	6.3%	383
Mary Washington Hospital	Fredericksburg	6.4%	535
Sentara Williamsburg Reg Med Ctr	Williamsburg	6.4%	409
Danville Regional Medical Center	Danville	6.5%	200
Novant Health Prince William Med Ctr	Manassas	6.6%	76
Smyth County Community Hospital	Marion	6.8%	148
Bon Secours Depaul Medical Center	Norfolk	6.9%	130
Sentara Careplex Hospital	Hampton	7.1%	268
Carilion Franklin Memorial Hospital	Rocky Mount	7.2%	207
Bon Secours Mem Reg Med Ctr	Mechanicsville	7.3%	694
University of Virginia Medical Center	Charlottesville	7.5%	996
Inova Alexandria Hospital	Alexandria	8.2%	110
Norton Community Hospital	Norton	8.2%	194
Carilion New River Valley Medical Center	Christiansburg	8.3%	520
John Randolph Medical Center	Hopewell	12.2%	82

Combination Abdominal CT Scan

Hospital Name	City	Rate	Cases
Dickenson Community Hospital	Clintwood	0.0%	135
Page Memorial Hospital	Luray	0.0%	238
Russell County Medical Center	Lebanon	1.1%	188
Inova Fairfax Hospital	Falls Church	1.3%	1038
Mary Washington Hospital	Fredericksburg	1.3%	906
Bedford Memorial Hospital	Bedford	1.7%	298
Lewisgale Hospital Pulaski	Pulaski	1.8%	394
Stafford Hospital	Stafford	2.1%	236
Warren Memorial Hospital	Front Royal	2.3%	393
Carilion Franklin Memorial Hospital	Rocky Mount	2.6%	418
Culpeper Regional Hospital	Culpeper	2.6%	664
Lewisgale Medical Center	Salem	2.6%	1218
Inova Fair Oaks Hospital	Fairfax	3.2%	665
Fauquier Hospital	Warrenton	3.3%	760
University of Virginia Medical Center	Charlottesville	3.3%	1155
Mary Immaculate Hospital	Newport News	3.5%	347
Novant Health Prince William Med Ctr	Manassas	3.5%	968
Bon Secours Richmond Community Hospital	Richmond	3.6%	84
Riverside Walter Reed Hospital	Gloucester	3.9%	742
Winchester Medical Center	Winchester	4.0%	1563
Spotsylvania Regional Medical Center	Fredericksburg	4.1%	316
Carilion Stonewall Jackson Hospital	Lexington	4.2%	336
Bon Secours Saint Francis Medical Center	Midlothian	4.5%	828
Sentara Obici Hospital	Suffolk	4.5%	1385
Medical College of Virginia Hospitals	Richmond	4.7%	1126
Inova Loudoun Hospital	Leesburg	4.9%	926
Carilion New River Valley Medical Center	Christiansburg	5.3%	1001
Martha Jefferson Hospital	Charlottesville	5.4%	1441
Southside Community Hospital	Farmville	5.4%	627
Sentara Careplex Hospital	Hampton	5.5%	1841
Carilion Roanoke Memorial Hospital	Roanoke	5.6%	1640
Twin County Regional Hospital	Galax	5.7%	777
Lewisgale Hospital Alleghany	Low Moor	5.8%	446
Mem Hosp of Martinsville & Henry Co	Martinsville	5.9%	749
Shenandoah Memorial Hospital	Woodstock	5.9%	543
Sentara Northern Virginia Medical Center	Woodbridge	6.0%	900
Pioneer Health Services of Patrick County	Stuart	6.1%	115
Sentara Princess Anne Hospital	Virginia Beach	6.1%	1308
Norton Community Hospital	Norton	6.4%	503
Bon Secours Mem Reg Med Ctr	Mechanicsville	6.5%	1589
Bon Secours Depaul Medical Center	Norfolk	6.8%	547
Bon Secours Saint Marys Hospital	Richmond	6.8%	1021
Reston Hospital Center	Reston	7.1%	617
Sentara Norfolk General Hospital	Norfolk	7.1%	1231
Riverside Regional Medical Center	Newport News	7.3%	1898
Virginia Hospital Center	Arlington	7.4%	1419
Smyth County Community Hospital	Marion	7.7%	440
Carilion Tazewell Community Hospital	Tazewell	7.8%	193
Danville Regional Medical Center	Danville	7.8%	651
Inova Alexandria Hospital	Alexandria	7.8%	1391
Sentara Williamsburg Reg Med Ctr	Williamsburg	7.9%	1125
Buchanan General Hospital	Grundy	8.0%	324
Chesapeake General Hospital	Chesapeake	8.0%	1354
Centra Health	Lynchburg	8.2%	1880
Sentara Virginia Beach General Hospital	Virginia Beach	8.2%	1794
Johnston Memorial Hospital	Abingdon	8.3%	1115
Rockingham Memorial Hospital	Harrisonburg	8.3%	1386
Rappahannock General Hospital	Kilmarnock	8.4%	514
Sentara Leigh Hospital	Norfolk	8.4%	2074
Henrico Doctors' Hospital	Richmond	8.7%	1304
Bon Secours Maryview Medical Center	Portsmouth	8.9%	1249
Halifax Regional Hospital	Halifax	9.2%	877
Southern Virginia Regional Medical Center	Emporia	9.5%	220
Riverside Tappahannock Hospital	Tappahannock	9.7%	455
Carilion Giles Community Hospital	Pearisburg	10.7%	337
Lewisgale Hospital Montgomery	Blacksburg	11.1%	583
Southampton Memorial Hospital	Franklin	12.1%	371
Augusta Health	Fishersville	13.3%	1775
Riverside Shore Memorial Hospital	Nassawadox	13.7%	445
Inova Mount Vernon Hospital	Alexandria	16.3%	545
Southside Regional Medical Center	Petersburg	17.5%	1025
Community Memorial Healthcenter	South Hill	21.9%	525
Cjw Medical Center	Richmond	30.3%	1966
John Randolph Medical Center	Hopewell	32.4%	544
Wellmont Lonesome Pine Hospital	Big Stone Gap	32.4%	578
Wythe County Community Hospital	Wytheville	36.1%	546
Clinch Valley Medical Center	Richlands	45.3%	545

Combination Brain/Sinus CT Scan

Hospital Name	City	Rate	Cases
Danville Regional Medical Center	Danville	0.2%	1030
Bedford Memorial Hospital	Bedford	0.6%	313
Dickenson Community Hospital	Clintwood	0.6%	178
Russell County Medical Center	Lebanon	0.7%	283
Rappahannock General Hospital	Kilmarnock	0.9%	439
Halifax Regional Hospital	Halifax	1.0%	734
Page Memorial Hospital	Luray	1.0%	287
Sentara Careplex Hospital	Hampton	1.0%	1309
Warren Memorial Hospital	Front Royal	1.0%	398
Bon Secours Saint Marys Hospital	Richmond	1.1%	1134
Medical College of Virginia Hospitals	Richmond	1.1%	527
Stafford Hospital	Stafford	1.1%	273
Chesapeake General Hospital	Chesapeake	1.2%	1126
Mary Washington Hospital	Fredericksburg	1.2%	1065
Southside Community Hospital	Farmville	1.3%	700
Bon Secours Depaul Medical Center	Norfolk	1.5%	602
Culpeper Regional Hospital	Culpeper	1.5%	602
John Randolph Medical Center	Hopewell	1.5%	463
Sentara Norfolk General Hospital	Norfolk	1.5%	739
Sentara Williamsburg Reg Med Ctr	Williamsburg	1.5%	848
Smyth County Community Hospital	Marion	1.5%	392
Winchester Medical Center	Winchester	1.5%	997
Augusta Health	Fishersville	1.6%	1057
Carilion Giles Community Hospital	Pearisburg	1.6%	314
Community Memorial Healthcenter	South Hill	1.6%	502
Norton Community Hospital	Norton	1.6%	376
Riverside Shore Memorial Hospital	Nassawadox	1.6%	432
Riverside Tappahannock Hospital	Tappahannock	1.7%	361
University of Virginia Medical Center	Charlottesville	1.7%	660
Centra Health	Lynchburg	1.8%	1588
Mary Immaculate Hospital	Newport News	1.8%	503
Rockingham Memorial Hospital	Harrisonburg	1.9%	1281
Carilion Franklin Memorial Hospital	Rocky Mount	2.0%	446
Carilion New River Valley Medical Center	Christiansburg	2.0%	587
Riverside Regional Medical Center	Newport News	2.0%	1264
Martha Jefferson Hospital	Charlottesville	2.2%	1070
Virginia Hospital Center	Arlington	2.2%	1073
Bon Secours Saint Francis Medical Center	Midlothian	2.3%	857
Twin County Regional Hospital	Galax	2.3%	660
Wythe County Community Hospital	Wytheville	2.3%	520
Carilion Roanoke Memorial Hospital	Roanoke	2.4%	1227
Novant Health Prince William Med Ctr	Manassas	2.4%	922
Mem Hosp of Martinsville & Henry Co	Martinsville	2.5%	673
Sentara Northern Virginia Medical Center	Woodbridge	2.5%	761
Bon Secours Maryview Medical Center	Portsmouth	2.6%	1125
Johnston Memorial Hospital	Abingdon	2.6%	763
Bon Secours Mem Reg Med Ctr	Mechanicsville	2.7%	1668
Riverside Walter Reed Hospital	Gloucester	2.7%	513
Henrico Doctors' Hospital	Richmond	2.9%	1534
Inova Fairfax Hospital	Falls Church	2.9%	1875
Inova Loudoun Hospital	Leesburg	2.9%	1015
Sentara Leigh Hospital	Norfolk	3.0%	1432
Cjw Medical Center	Richmond	3.1%	1549
Inova Alexandria Hospital	Alexandria	3.1%	1340
Southside Regional Medical Center	Petersburg	3.1%	1087
Lewisgale Medical Center	Salem	3.2%	974
Sentara Princess Anne Hospital	Virginia Beach	3.3%	857
Inova Fair Oaks Hospital	Fairfax	3.4%	787
Fauquier Hospital	Warrenton	3.8%	637
Sentara Obici Hospital	Suffolk	3.8%	1251
Sentara Virginia Beach General Hospital	Virginia Beach	3.8%	1477
Reston Hospital Center	Reston	4.6%	567

Combination Chest CT Scan

Hospital Name	City	Rate	Cases
Bedford Memorial Hospital	Bedford	0.0%	161
Bon Secours Depaul Medical Center	Norfolk	0.0%	440
Carilion Stonewall Jackson Hospital	Lexington	0.0%	126
Culpeper Regional Hospital	Culpeper	0.0%	310
Danville Regional Medical Center	Danville	0.0%	379
Dickenson Community Hospital	Clintwood	0.0%	49
Fauquier Hospital	Warrenton	0.0%	427
Inova Loudoun Hospital	Leesburg	0.0%	554
Lewisgale Hospital Pulaski	Pulaski	0.0%	196
Martha Jefferson Hospital	Charlottesville	0.0%	1166
Mary Immaculate Hospital	Newport News	0.0%	139
Mary Washington Hospital	Fredericksburg	0.0%	135
Riverside Tappahannock Hospital	Tappahannock	0.0%	289
Rockingham Memorial Hospital	Harrisonburg	0.0%	951
Russell County Medical Center	Lebanon	0.0%	76
Sentara Norfolk General Hospital	Norfolk	0.0%	1003
Smyth County Community Hospital	Marion	0.0%	149
Southern Virginia Regional Medical Center	Emporia	0.0%	97
Stafford Hospital	Stafford	0.0%	71
University of Virginia Medical Center	Charlottesville	0.0%	1478
Wythe County Community Hospital	Wytheville	0.0%	224
Medical College of Virginia Hospitals	Richmond	0.1%	1476
Riverside Regional Medical Center	Newport News	0.1%	1499
Sentara Leigh Hospital	Norfolk	0.1%	1796
Virginia Hospital Center	Arlington	0.1%	1186
Inova Fairfax Hospital	Falls Church	0.2%	499
Riverside Walter Reed Hospital	Gloucester	0.2%	525
Halifax Regional Hospital	Halifax	0.3%	367
Novant Health Prince William Med Ctr	Manassas	0.3%	653
Winchester Medical Center	Winchester	0.3%	1054
Augusta Health	Fishersville	0.4%	1317
Chesapeake General Hospital	Chesapeake	0.4%	911
Sentara Careplex Hospital	Hampton	0.4%	1165
Shenandoah Memorial Hospital	Woodstock	0.4%	271
Twin County Regional Hospital	Galax	0.4%	238
Bon Secours Saint Francis Medical Center	Midlothian	0.5%	553
Bon Secours Saint Marys Hospital	Richmond	0.5%	439
Sentara Obici Hospital	Suffolk	0.5%	607
Sentara Princess Anne Hospital	Virginia Beach	0.5%	1106
Warren Memorial Hospital	Front Royal	0.5%	183
Bon Secours Mem Reg Med Ctr	Mechanicsville	0.6%	652
Lewisgale Medical Center	Salem	0.8%	824
Carilion Roanoke Memorial Hospital	Roanoke	0.9%	1294
Sentara Northern Virginia Medical Center	Woodbridge	1.1%	475
Cjw Medical Center	Richmond	1.2%	1241
Rappahannock General Hospital	Kilmarnock	1.2%	335
Spotsylvania Regional Medical Center	Fredericksburg	1.2%	86
Clinch Valley Medical Center	Richlands	1.3%	229
Inova Fair Oaks Hospital	Fairfax	1.3%	310
Sentara Virginia Beach General Hospital	Virginia Beach	1.3%	1333
Page Memorial Hospital	Luray	1.4%	69
Henrico Doctors' Hospital	Richmond	1.5%	816
Lewisgale Hospital Montgomery	Blacksburg	1.6%	316
Reston Hospital Center	Reston	1.7%	460
John Randolph Medical Center	Hopewell	1.8%	392
Centra Health	Lynchburg	1.9%	1193
Sentara Williamsburg Reg Med Ctr	Williamsburg	1.9%	802
Bon Secours Maryview Medical Center	Portsmouth	2.3%	902
Norton Community Hospital	Norton	2.3%	262
Carilion New River Valley Medical Center	Christiansburg	2.4%	736
Southampton Memorial Hospital	Franklin	2.4%	170
Lewisgale Hospital Alleghany	Low Moor	3.1%	320
Inova Alexandria Hospital	Alexandria	3.8%	720
Johnston Memorial Hospital	Abingdon	4.1%	606
Southside Community Hospital	Farmville	4.3%	299
Mem Hosp of Martinsville & Henry Co	Martinsville	4.5%	396
Buchanan General Hospital	Grundy	5.1%	177
Carilion Franklin Memorial Hospital	Rocky Mount	5.1%	177
Riverside Shore Memorial Hospital	Nassawadox	6.6%	212
Community Memorial Healthcenter	South Hill	7.8%	346
Wellmont Lonesome Pine Hospital	Big Stone Gap	14.6%	453
Inova Mount Vernon Hospital	Alexandria	14.8%	284
Carilion Giles Community Hospital	Pearisburg	16.5%	127
Southside Regional Medical Center	Petersburg	16.7%	717

Follow-up Mammogram/Ultrasound

A follow-up rate near zero may indicate missed cancer; a rate higher than 14% may mean there is unnecessary follow up.

Hospital Name	City	Rate	Cases
Riverside Tappahannock Hospital	Tappahannock	2.3%	836
Twin County Regional Hospital	Galax	2.5%	1419
Carilion Stonewall Jackson Hospital	Lexington	3.3%	768
Mem Hosp of Martinsville & Henry Co	Martinsville	3.3%	2116
Johnston Memorial Hospital	Abingdon	3.7%	1795
Russell County Medical Center	Lebanon	3.8%	185
Carilion Franklin Memorial Hospital	Rocky Mount	3.9%	857
Winchester Medical Center	Winchester	3.9%	3749
John Randolph Medical Center	Hopewell	4.1%	752
Smyth County Community Hospital	Marion	4.2%	684
Inova Fairfax Hospital	Falls Church	4.4%	68
Cjw Medical Center	Richmond	4.5%	3092
Carilion Roanoke Memorial Hospital	Roanoke	4.8%	4466
Lewisgale Medical Center	Salem	4.8%	2836
Southern Virginia Regional Medical Center	Emporia	4.9%	467
Medical College of Virginia Hospitals	Richmond	5.1%	2386
Lewisgale Hospital Pulaski	Pulaski	5.2%	365
Carilion New River Valley Medical Center	Christiansburg	5.3%	2025
Community Memorial Healthcenter	South Hill	5.4%	1373
Riverside Shore Memorial Hospital	Nassawadox	5.5%	1108
Southampton Memorial Hospital	Franklin	5.6%	465
Norton Community Hospital	Norton	5.9%	455
Shenandoah Memorial Hospital	Woodstock	5.9%	769
Bon Secours Maryview Medical Center	Portsmouth	6.2%	2151

NOTE: Hospital profiles are in alphabetical order by state, then city, then hospital within the city; Rankings exclude hospitals with less than 25 cases except for patient surveys which excludes hospitals with less than 100 cases; (a) 100-299 cases; (1) The number of cases/patients is too few to report; (2) Data submitted were based on a sample of cases/patients; (3) Results are based on a shorter time period than required; (4) Data suppressed by CMS for one or more quarters; (5) Results are not available for this reporting period; (6) Fewer than 100 patients completed the HCAHPS survey; (7) No cases met the criteria for this measure; (8) The lower limit of the confidence interval cannot be calculated if the number of observed infections equals zero; (9) No data are available from the state/territory for this reporting period; (10) The scores shown reflect fewer than 50 completed surveys; (11) There were discrepancies in the data collection process; (12) This measure does not apply to this hospital for this reporting period; (13) Results cannot be calculated for this reporting period; (14) The results for this state are combined with nearby states to protect confidentiality; Please refer to the User's Guide for a full explanation of data.

Sentara Leigh Hospital	Norfolk	6.4%	4205
Bon Secours Mem Reg Med Ctr	Mechanicsville	6.5%	2010
Carilion Giles Community Hospital	Pearisburg	6.5%	660
Henrico Doctors' Hospital	Richmond	6.5%	2010
Halifax Regional Hospital	Halifax	6.6%	1392
Lewisgale Hospital Alleghany	Low Moor	6.7%	835
Rockingham Memorial Hospital	Harrisonburg	6.9%	3135
Mary Immaculate Hospital	Newport News	7.0%	483
Wellmont Lonesome Pine Hospital	Big Stone Gap	7.0%	561
Bedford Memorial Hospital	Bedford	7.3%	715
Bon Secours Saint Francis Medical Center	Midlothian	7.4%	1484
Riverside Walter Reed Hospital	Gloucester	7.4%	1305
Bon Secours Depaul Medical Center	Norfolk	7.6%	1580
Sentara Virginia Beach General Hospital	Virginia Beach	7.7%	3772
Inova Alexandria Hospital	Alexandria	8.0%	950
Virginia Hospital Center	Arlington	8.0%	2352
Clinch Valley Medical Center	Richlands	8.2%	281
Sentara Norfolk General Hospital	Norfolk	8.2%	2545
Sentara Williamsburg Reg Med Ctr	Williamsburg	8.7%	3670
Inova Mount Vernon Hospital	Alexandria	8.8%	697
Carilion Tazewell Community Hospital	Tazewell	9.0%	178
Sentara Obici Hospital	Suffolk	9.0%	1831
Riverside Regional Medical Center	Newport News	9.1%	3106
Southside Regional Medical Center	Petersburg	9.1%	1620
Bon Secours Richmond Community Hospital	Richmond	9.2%	907
Martha Jefferson Hospital	Charlottesville	9.2%	4321
Sentara Princess Anne Hospital	Virginia Beach	9.2%	1660
Inova Fair Oaks Hospital	Fairfax	9.4%	339
Rappahannock General Hospital	Kilmarnock	9.6%	926
Novant Health Prince William Med Ctr	Manassas	9.7%	1495
Bon Secours Saint Marys Hospital	Richmond	10.0%	2950
Warren Memorial Hospital	Front Royal	10.1%	611
Reston Hospital Center	Reston	10.4%	578
Culpeper Regional Hospital	Culpeper	10.5%	697
Fauquier Hospital	Warrenton	10.6%	1048
Lewisgale Hospital Montgomery	Blacksburg	10.6%	1146
Sentara Careplex Hospital	Hampton	10.7%	3010
Sentara Northern Virginia Medical Center	Woodbridge	11.0%	794
Page Memorial Hospital	Luray	12.0%	367
University of Virginia Medical Center	Charlottesville	12.1%	4028
Wythe County Community Hospital	Wytheville	12.1%	672
Chesapeake General Hospital	Chesapeake	12.2%	2329
Southside Community Hospital	Farmville	12.6%	628
Buchanan General Hospital	Grundy	13.0%	277
Augusta Health	Fishersville	14.0%	3427
Spotsylvania Regional Medical Center	Fredericksburg	14.0%	136
Inova Loudoun Hospital	Leesburg	15.8%	602
Stafford Hospital	Stafford	16.0%	162
Danville Regional Medical Center	Danville	21.4%	103

Lumbar Spine MRI for Low Back Pain

Hospital Name	City	Rate	Cases
Community Memorial Healthcenter	South Hill	25.4%	67
Culpeper Regional Hospital	Culpeper	26.9%	67
Sentara Williamsburg Reg Med Ctr	Williamsburg	27.7%	130
Sentara Careplex Hospital	Hampton	27.8%	115
Chesapeake General Hospital	Chesapeake	28.2%	170
Clinch Valley Medical Center	Richlands	28.7%	87
Cjw Medical Center	Richmond	28.9%	266
Henrico Doctors' Hospital	Richmond	29.1%	141
Bon Secours Mem Reg Med Ctr	Mechanicsville	30.2%	265
Carilion Roanoke Memorial Hospital	Roanoke	30.3%	379
John Randolph Medical Center	Hopewell	30.4%	79
Bon Secours Maryview Medical Center	Portsmouth	31.9%	455
Sentara Virginia Beach General Hospital	Virginia Beach	32.1%	234
Wellmont Lonesome Pine Hospital	Big Stone Gap	32.3%	96
Medical College of Virginia Hospitals	Richmond	32.5%	160
Riverside Regional Medical Center	Newport News	32.6%	239
Inova Loudoun Hospital	Leesburg	33.0%	91
Carilion New River Valley Medical Center	Christiansburg	33.1%	133
Sentara Northern Virginia Medical Center	Woodbridge	33.3%	105
Bon Secours Saint Francis Medical Center	Midlothian	33.4%	293
Virginia Hospital Center	Arlington	33.4%	329
Inova Mount Vernon Hospital	Alexandria	33.6%	125
Sentara Princess Anne Hospital	Virginia Beach	34.2%	146
Southside Regional Medical Center	Petersburg	34.2%	111
Sentara Leigh Hospital	Norfolk	34.3%	169
Lewisgale Hospital Alleghany	Low Moor	34.6%	107
Riverside Walter Reed Hospital	Gloucester	34.6%	104
Inova Fair Oaks Hospital	Fairfax	34.8%	155
Novant Health Prince William Med Ctr	Manassas	34.8%	247
Wythe County Community Hospital	Wytheville	34.8%	89
Sentara Norfolk General Hospital	Norfolk	35.2%	125
Bedford Memorial Hospital	Bedford	35.3%	51
Lewisgale Hospital Pulaski	Pulaski	35.3%	51
Riverside Tappahannock Hospital	Tappahannock	36.2%	47
Sentara Obici Hospital	Suffolk	36.4%	129
Fauquier Hospital	Warrenton	36.6%	191
Inova Alexandria Hospital	Alexandria	36.6%	391
Lewisgale Hospital Montgomery	Blacksburg	36.6%	131
Martha Jefferson Hospital	Charlottesville	37.1%	426
Rockingham Memorial Hospital	Harrisonburg	37.2%	317
Carilion Franklin Memorial Hospital	Rocky Mount	37.7%	61
Southside Community Hospital	Farmville	37.7%	61
Bon Secours Saint Marys Hospital	Richmond	37.8%	294
Winchester Medical Center	Winchester	37.8%	400
Rappahannock General Hospital	Kilmarnock	38.7%	75
Bon Secours Depaul Medical Center	Norfolk	39.0%	82
Twin County Regional Hospital	Galax	39.5%	119
Shenandoah Memorial Hospital	Woodstock	40.0%	50
Augusta Health	Fishersville	40.2%	311
Norton Community Hospital	Norton	40.3%	62
Carilion Stonewall Jackson Hospital	Lexington	40.4%	52
Buchanan General Hospital	Grundy	40.6%	64
Centra Health	Lynchburg	42.8%	152
Lewisgale Medical Center	Salem	43.0%	207
Johnston Memorial Hospital	Abingdon	46.9%	177
Mem Hosp of Martinsville & Henry Co	Martinsville	49.6%	125
Halifax Regional Hospital	Halifax	53.8%	93
Russell County Medical Center	Lebanon	59.1%	44

NOTE: Hospital profiles are in alphabetical order by state, then city, then hospital within the city; Rankings exclude hospitals with less than 25 cases except for patient surveys which excludes hospitals with less than 100 cases; (a) 100-299 cases; (1) The number of cases/patients is too few to report; (2) Data submitted were based on a sample of cases/patients; (3) Results are based on a shorter time period than required; (4) Data suppressed by CMS for one or more quarters; (5) Results are not available for this reporting period; (6) Fewer than 100 patients completed the HCAHPS survey; (7) No cases met the criteria for this measure; (8) The lower limit of the confidence interval cannot be calculated if the number of observed infections equals zero; (9) No data are available from the state/territory for this reporting period; (10) The scores shown reflect fewer than 50 completed surveys; (11) There were discrepancies in the data collection process; (12) This measure does not apply to this hospital for this reporting period; (13) Results cannot be calculated for this reporting period; (14) The results for this state are combined with nearby states to protect confidentiality; Please refer to the User's Guide for a full explanation of data.

Johnston Memorial Hospital

16000 Johnston Memorial Drive
Abingdon, VA 24211
Phone: 276-258-1000
Fax: 276-676-2631
E-mail: info@jmh.org
URL: www.jmh.org
Type: Acute Care Hospitals
Emergency Services: Yes
Ownership: Voluntary non-profit - Private
Beds: 135

Key Personnel:

Chief of Medical Staff.......... Richard Buddington
Radiology.................. Matthew Cobb
CEO/President............... Chuck Elliott
Infection Control............. Sue Greco
Operating Room............. Eleanor E Hess
Pediatric Ambulatory Care...... Donna Hudgens, MD
Pediatric In-Patient Care .... Donna Hudgens, MD
Quality Assurance .... Teresa Tignor, RN

Measure	Cases	This Hosp.	State Avg.	U.S. Avg.
Blood Clot Prevention and Treatment				
Anticoagulation Overlap Therapy[2]	44	98%	95%	93%
ICU Venous Thromboembolism Prophylaxis[2]	69	83%	95%	92%
Incidence of Potentially Preventable VTE[1,2]	-	-	8%	10%
UFH with Dosages/Platelet Monitoring[1,2]	-	-	99%	97%
Venous Thromboembolism Prophylaxis[2]	333	79%	91%	85%
Warfarin Therapy Discharge Instructions[2]	31	52%	78%	75%
Chest Pain/Possible Heart Attack Care				
Aspirin Given Within 24 Hours of Arrival	130	100%	98%	96%
Fibrinolytic Meds Within 30 Min. of Arrival[7]	-	-	68%	58%
Average Time to ECG (minutes)	134	0	7	7
Average Time to Transfer (minutes)	19	34	64	60
Children's Asthma Care				
Received Home Management Plan of Care	-	-	-	88%
Received Reliever Medication	-	-	-	100%
Received Systemic Corticosteroids	-	-	-	100%
Emergency Department				
Admittance Decision Time (minutes)[2]	604	68	96	98
Head CT Results Within 45 Min. of Arrival	13	54%	60%	57%
Patients Who Left ER Before Being Seen	42,676	1%	2%	2%
Time from ER Arrival to Admit. (minutes)[2]	698	210	280	274
Time from ER Arrival to Discharge (minutes)	374	116	167	134
Time in ER Before Being Evaluated (minutes)	407	22	35	26
Time to Pain Meds for Fractures (minutes)	108	46	56	57
Heart Attack Care				
Aspirin Given at Discharge[2]	35	97%	99%	99%
Fibrinolytic Meds Within 30 Min. of Arrival[2,7]	-	-	75%	54%
PCI Within 90 Minutes of Arrival[2,7]	-	-	97%	96%
Statin Prescribed at Discharge[2]	34	94%	99%	98%
Heart Failure Care				
ACE Inhibitor or ARB for LVSD[2]	44	95%	98%	97%
Discharge Instructions Given[2]	132	93%	95%	94%
Evaluation of LVS Function[2]	158	99%	100%	99%
Medicare Spending				
Medicare Spending per Patient (ratio)	-	0.94	0.95	0.98
Pneumonia Care				
Appropriate Initial Antibiotic Given[2]	87	94%	97%	95%
Blood Culture Timing[2]	152	99%	98%	98%
Pregnancy and Delivery Care				
Newborn Deliveries Scheduled Early[2]	17	18%	6%	6%
Preventive Care				
Immunization for Influenza[2]	560	97%	92%	90%
Immunization for Pneumonia[2]	760	94%	93%	92%
Stroke Care				
Anticoagulation Therapy for Atrial Fibrillation[1]	-	-	96%	95%
Antithrombotic Therapy Timing	69	100%	99%	98%
Assessed for Rehabilitation	74	92%	99%	97%
Discharged on Antithrombotic Therapy	69	99%	100%	99%
Discharged on Statin Medication	61	90%	97%	94%
Thrombolytic Therapy Timing[1]	-	-	73%	66%
Venous Thromboembolism Prophylaxis	72	93%	97%	94%
Written Stroke Educational Materials Given	47	81%	92%	88%
Surgical Care Improvement Project				
Appropriate Beta Blocker Usage[2]	90	96%	99%	98%
Appropriate VTP Within 24 Hours[2]	304	96%	99%	98%
Controlled Postoperative Blood Glucose[2,7]	-	-	98%	97%
Perioperative Temperature Management[2]	332	99%	100%	100%
Prophylactic Antibiotic Selection[2]	227	99%	99%	99%
Prophylactic Antibiotic Selection (Outpatient)	72	96%	98%	98%
Prophylactic Antibiotic Stopped[2]	220	96%	98%	98%
Prophylactic Antibiotic Timing[2]	227	100%	99%	99%
Prophylactic Antibiotic Timing (Outpatient)	72	97%	98%	98%
Urinary Catheter Removal[2]	151	94%	98%	97%
Survey of Patients' Hospital Experiences				
Area Around Room 'Always' Quiet at Night	300+	61%	60%	61%
Doctors 'Always' Communicated Well	300+	80%	81%	82%
Home Recovery Information Given	300+	83%	86%	85%
Hospital Given 9 or 10 on 10 Point Scale	300+	63%	68%	71%
Meds 'Always' Explained Before Given	300+	57%	62%	64%
Nurses 'Always' Communicated Well	300+	72%	78%	79%
Pain 'Always' Well Controlled	300+	64%	70%	71%
Room and Bathroom 'Always' Clean	300+	70%	71%	73%
Timely Help 'Always' Received	300+	58%	64%	68%
Would Definitely Recommend Hospital	300+	62%	69%	71%
Use of Medical Imaging				
Cardiac Imaging Stress Test before Surgery	364	3.6%	5.1%	5.3%
Combination Abdominal CT Scan	1,115	8.3%	8.5%	10.5%
Combination Brain/Sinus CT Scan	763	2.6%	2.3%	2.7%
Combination Chest CT Scan	606	4.1%	1.6%	2.7%
Follow-up Mammogram/Ultrasound	1,795	3.7%	7.7%	8.8%
Lumbar Spine MRI for Low Back Pain	177	46.9%	35.3%	37.2%

Inova Alexandria Hospital

4320 Seminary Rd
Alexandria, VA 22304
Phone: 703-504-3167
Fax: 703-504-3700
URL: www.inova.com/inovapublic.srt/iah/index.jsp
Type: Acute Care Hospitals
Emergency Services: Yes
Ownership: Voluntary non-profit - Private
Beds: 320

Key Personnel:

Quality Assurance .... Pam Baker
CEO/President............... Christine Candio
Pediatric In-Patient Care .... Jon Farber, MD
Chief of Medical Staff.......... Loring Flint, MD
Radiology.................. Frank Schert
Operating Room............. Carol Webb

Measure	Cases	This Hosp.	State Avg.	U.S. Avg.
Blood Clot Prevention and Treatment				
Anticoagulation Overlap Therapy[2]	102	96%	95%	93%
ICU Venous Thromboembolism Prophylaxis[2]	60	98%	95%	92%
Incidence of Potentially Preventable VTE[2]	35	6%	8%	10%
UFH with Dosages/Platelet Monitoring[2]	93	100%	99%	97%
Venous Thromboembolism Prophylaxis[2]	354	87%	91%	85%
Warfarin Therapy Discharge Instructions[2]	77	78%	78%	75%
Chest Pain/Possible Heart Attack Care				
Aspirin Given Within 24 Hours of Arrival	33	94%	98%	96%
Fibrinolytic Meds Within 30 Min. of Arrival[3,7]	-	-	68%	58%
Average Time to ECG (minutes)	35	6	7	7
Average Time to Transfer (minutes)[1,3]	-	-	64	60
Children's Asthma Care				
Received Home Management Plan of Care	-	-	-	88%
Received Reliever Medication	-	-	-	100%
Received Systemic Corticosteroids	-	-	-	100%
Emergency Department				
Admittance Decision Time (minutes)[2]	512	111	96	98
Head CT Results Within 45 Min. of Arrival	21	67%	60%	57%
Patients Who Left ER Before Being Seen	>100k	0%	2%	2%
Time from ER Arrival to Admit. (minutes)[2]	514	292	280	274
Time from ER Arrival to Discharge (minutes)	910	123	167	134
Time in ER Before Being Evaluated (minutes)	943	28	35	26
Time to Pain Meds for Fractures (minutes)	246	45	56	57
Heart Attack Care				
Aspirin Given at Discharge	229	100%	99%	99%
Fibrinolytic Meds Within 30 Min. of Arrival[7]	-	-	75%	54%
PCI Within 90 Minutes of Arrival	30	100%	97%	96%
Statin Prescribed at Discharge	226	100%	99%	98%
Heart Failure Care				
ACE Inhibitor or ARB for LVSD[2]	106	100%	98%	97%
Discharge Instructions Given[2]	235	90%	95%	94%
Evaluation of LVS Function[2]	290	99%	100%	99%
Medicare Spending				
Medicare Spending per Patient (ratio)	-	1.01	0.95	0.98
Pneumonia Care				
Appropriate Initial Antibiotic Given[2]	76	99%	97%	95%
Blood Culture Timing[2]	108	98%	98%	98%
Pregnancy and Delivery Care				
Newborn Deliveries Scheduled Early[2]	235	3%	6%	6%
Preventive Care				
Immunization for Influenza[2]	519	93%	92%	90%
Immunization for Pneumonia[2]	510	93%	93%	92%
Stroke Care				
Anticoagulation Therapy for Atrial Fibrillation[2]	16	100%	96%	95%
Antithrombotic Therapy Timing[2]	109	99%	99%	98%
Assessed for Rehabilitation[2]	127	95%	99%	97%
Discharged on Antithrombotic Therapy[2]	120	99%	100%	99%
Discharged on Statin Medication[2]	97	97%	97%	94%
Thrombolytic Therapy Timing[2]	15	93%	73%	66%
Venous Thromboembolism Prophylaxis[2]	138	96%	97%	94%
Written Stroke Educational Materials Given[2]	75	89%	92%	88%
Surgical Care Improvement Project				
Appropriate Beta Blocker Usage[2]	112	98%	99%	98%
Appropriate VTP Within 24 Hours[2]	362	99%	99%	98%
Controlled Postoperative Blood Glucose[2]	67	100%	98%	97%
Perioperative Temperature Management[2]	416	100%	100%	100%
Prophylactic Antibiotic Selection[2]	323	100%	99%	99%
Prophylactic Antibiotic Selection (Outpatient)	258	99%	98%	98%
Prophylactic Antibiotic Stopped[2]	320	98%	98%	98%
Prophylactic Antibiotic Timing[2]	323	100%	99%	99%
Prophylactic Antibiotic Timing (Outpatient)	261	99%	98%	98%
Urinary Catheter Removal[2]	318	99%	98%	97%
Survey of Patients' Hospital Experiences				
Area Around Room 'Always' Quiet at Night	300+	54%	60%	61%
Doctors 'Always' Communicated Well	300+	76%	81%	82%
Home Recovery Information Given	300+	80%	86%	85%
Hospital Given 9 or 10 on 10 Point Scale	300+	62%	68%	71%
Meds 'Always' Explained Before Given	300+	60%	62%	64%
Nurses 'Always' Communicated Well	300+	73%	78%	79%
Pain 'Always' Well Controlled	300+	67%	70%	71%
Room and Bathroom 'Always' Clean	300+	63%	71%	73%
Timely Help 'Always' Received	300+	59%	64%	68%
Would Definitely Recommend Hospital	300+	66%	69%	71%
Use of Medical Imaging				
Cardiac Imaging Stress Test before Surgery	110	8.2%	5.1%	5.3%
Combination Abdominal CT Scan	1,391	7.8%	8.5%	10.5%
Combination Brain/Sinus CT Scan	1,340	3.1%	2.3%	2.7%
Combination Chest CT Scan	720	3.8%	1.6%	2.7%
Follow-up Mammogram/Ultrasound	950	8.0%	7.7%	8.8%
Lumbar Spine MRI for Low Back Pain	391	36.6%	35.3%	37.2%

Inova Mount Vernon Hospital

2501 Parkers Lane
Alexandria, VA 22306
Phone: 703-664-7000
Fax: 703-664-7304
URL: www.inova.com/inovapublic.srt/imvh/index.jsp
Type: Acute Care Hospitals
Emergency Services: Yes
Ownership: Voluntary non-profit - Private
Beds: 232

Key Personnel:

Chief of Medical Staff.......... David M Abbot
Radiology.................. Maria C Alvano, MD
CEO/President............... Barbara Doyle
Pediatric In-Patient Care .... Nancy J Leykan, MD
Quality Assurance .... Judy Perry
Operating Room............. Ann Vandervort

Measure	Cases	This Hosp.	State Avg.	U.S. Avg.
Blood Clot Prevention and Treatment				
Anticoagulation Overlap Therapy[2]	24	96%	95%	93%
ICU Venous Thromboembolism Prophylaxis[2]	38	89%	95%	92%
Incidence of Potentially Preventable VTE[1,2]	-	-	8%	10%
UFH with Dosages/Platelet Monitoring[1,2]	-	-	99%	97%
Venous Thromboembolism Prophylaxis[2]	235	77%	91%	85%
Warfarin Therapy Discharge Instructions[2]	15	73%	78%	75%
Chest Pain/Possible Heart Attack Care				
Aspirin Given Within 24 Hours of Arrival	33	100%	98%	96%
Fibrinolytic Meds Within 30 Min. of Arrival[7]	-	-	68%	58%
Average Time to ECG (minutes)	34	5	7	7
Average Time to Transfer (minutes)[1]	-	-	64	60
Children's Asthma Care				

NOTE: *Hospital profiles are in alphabetical order by state, then city, then hospital within the city; Rankings exclude hospitals with less than 25 cases except for patient surveys which excludes hospitals with less than 100 cases; (a) 100-299 cases; (1) The number of cases/patients is too few to report; (2) Data submitted were based on a sample of cases/patients; (3) Results are based on a shorter time period than required; (4) Data suppressed by CMS for one or more quarters; (5) Results are not available for this reporting period; (6) Fewer than 100 patients completed the HCAHPS survey; (7) No cases met the criteria for this measure; (8) The lower limit of the confidence interval cannot be calculated if the number of observed infections equals zero; (9) No data are available from the state/territory for this reporting period; (10) The scores shown reflect fewer than 50 completed surveys; (11) There were discrepancies in the data collection process; (12) This measure does not apply to this hospital for this reporting period; (13) Results cannot be calculated for this reporting period; (14) The results for this state are combined with nearby states to protect confidentiality; Please refer to the User's Guide for a full explanation of data.*

Received Home Management Plan of Care	-	-	-	88%
Received Reliever Medication	-	-	-	100%
Received Systemic Corticosteroids	-	-	-	100%
Emergency Department				
Admittance Decision Time (minutes)[2]	508	123	96	98
Head CT Results Within 45 Min. of Arrival	15	73%	60%	57%
Patients Who Left ER Before Being Seen	30,461	2%	2%	2%
Time from ER Arrival to Admit. (minutes)[2]	513	292	280	274
Time from ER Arrival to Discharge (minutes)	686	134	167	134
Time in ER Before Being Evaluated (minutes)	735	34	35	26
Time to Pain Meds for Fractures (minutes)	127	55	56	57
Heart Attack Care				
Aspirin Given at Discharge	11	100%	99%	99%
Fibrinolytic Meds Within 30 Min. of Arrival[7]	-	-	75%	54%
PCI Within 90 Minutes of Arrival[7]	-	-	97%	96%
Statin Prescribed at Discharge[1]	-	-	99%	98%
Heart Failure Care				
ACE Inhibitor or ARB for LVSD	58	95%	98%	97%
Discharge Instructions Given	170	92%	95%	94%
Evaluation of LVS Function	193	99%	100%	99%
Medicare Spending				
Medicare Spending per Patient (ratio)	-	0.93	0.95	0.98
Pneumonia Care				
Appropriate Initial Antibiotic Given	67	97%	97%	95%
Blood Culture Timing	91	98%	98%	98%
Pregnancy and Delivery Care				
Newborn Deliveries Scheduled Early[2,7]	-	-	6%	6%
Preventive Care				
Immunization for Influenza[2]	592	93%	92%	90%
Immunization for Pneumonia[2]	752	92%	93%	92%
Stroke Care				
Anticoagulation Therapy for Atrial Fibrillation[1]	-	-	96%	95%
Antithrombotic Therapy Timing	63	100%	99%	98%
Assessed for Rehabilitation	61	98%	99%	97%
Discharged on Antithrombotic Therapy	61	100%	100%	99%
Discharged on Statin Medication	45	98%	97%	94%
Thrombolytic Therapy Timing[1]	-	-	73%	66%
Venous Thromboembolism Prophylaxis	70	90%	97%	94%
Written Stroke Educational Materials Given	36	97%	92%	88%
Surgical Care Improvement Project				
Appropriate Beta Blocker Usage[2]	36	100%	99%	98%
Appropriate VTP Within 24 Hours[2]	235	100%	99%	98%
Controlled Postoperative Blood Glucose[2,7]	-	-	98%	97%
Perioperative Temperature Management[2]	347	99%	100%	100%
Prophylactic Antibiotic Selection[2]	228	100%	99%	99%
Prophylactic Antibiotic Selection (Outpatient)	121	98%	98%	98%
Prophylactic Antibiotic Stopped[2]	228	99%	98%	98%
Prophylactic Antibiotic Timing[2]	230	100%	99%	99%
Prophylactic Antibiotic Timing (Outpatient)	122	99%	98%	98%
Urinary Catheter Removal[2]	232	100%	98%	97%
Survey of Patients' Hospital Experiences				
Area Around Room 'Always' Quiet at Night	300+	56%	60%	61%
Doctors 'Always' Communicated Well	300+	80%	81%	82%
Home Recovery Information Given	300+	85%	86%	85%
Hospital Given 9 or 10 on 10 Point Scale	300+	67%	68%	71%
Meds 'Always' Explained Before Given	300+	59%	62%	64%
Nurses 'Always' Communicated Well	300+	73%	78%	79%
Pain 'Always' Well Controlled	300+	68%	70%	71%
Room and Bathroom 'Always' Clean	300+	67%	71%	73%
Timely Help 'Always' Received	300+	58%	64%	68%
Would Definitely Recommend Hospital	300+	71%	69%	71%
Use of Medical Imaging				
Cardiac Imaging Stress Test before Surgery	192	2.1%	5.1%	5.3%
Combination Abdominal CT Scan	545	16.3%	8.5%	10.5%
Combination Brain/Sinus CT Scan[1]	-	-	2.3%	2.7%
Combination Chest CT Scan	284	14.8%	1.6%	2.7%
Follow-up Mammogram/Ultrasound	697	8.8%	7.7%	8.8%
Lumbar Spine MRI for Low Back Pain	125	33.6%	35.3%	37.2%

Virginia Hospital Center

1701 North George Mason Drive
Arlington, VA 22205
URL: www.virginiahospitalcenter.com
Type: Acute Care Hospitals
Ownership: Voluntary non-profit - Private
Phone: 703-558-5000
Fax: 703-558-6553
Emergency Services: Yes
Beds: 342

Key Personnel:

Emergency Room .... Yorke Allen, MD
Anesthesiology................ David Banks, MD
Operating Room.............. Thomas Butler, MD
CEO/President................ James B Cole
Patient Relations .... Carolyn McCosh
Radiology........................ Russell McWey, MD
Cardiac Laboratory........... Antonio Parente, MD
Pediatric Ambulatory Care ...... David Reese, MD

Measure	Cases	This Hosp.	State Avg.	U.S. Avg.
Blood Clot Prevention and Treatment				
Anticoagulation Overlap Therapy[2]	127	93%	95%	93%
ICU Venous Thromboembolism Prophylaxis[2]	74	100%	95%	92%
Incidence of Potentially Preventable VTE[2]	16	6%	8%	10%
UFH with Dosages/Platelet Monitoring[2]	69	100%	99%	97%
Venous Thromboembolism Prophylaxis[2]	304	96%	91%	85%
Warfarin Therapy Discharge Instructions[2]	102	61%	78%	75%
Chest Pain/Possible Heart Attack Care				
Aspirin Given Within 24 Hours of Arrival[5]	-	-	98%	96%
Fibrinolytic Meds Within 30 Min. of Arrival[5]	-	-	68%	58%
Average Time to ECG (minutes)[5]	-	-	7	7
Average Time to Transfer (minutes)[5]	-	-	64	60
Children's Asthma Care				
Received Home Management Plan of Care	-	-	-	88%
Received Reliever Medication	-	-	-	100%
Received Systemic Corticosteroids	-	-	-	100%
Emergency Department				
Admittance Decision Time (minutes)[2]	398	102	96	98
Head CT Results Within 45 Min. of Arrival[1,3]	-	-	60%	57%
Patients Who Left ER Before Being Seen	65,368	0%	2%	2%
Time from ER Arrival to Admit. (minutes)[2]	404	272	280	274
Time from ER Arrival to Discharge (minutes)	421	152	167	134
Time in ER Before Being Evaluated (minutes)	445	20	35	26
Time to Pain Meds for Fractures (minutes)	203	39	56	57
Heart Attack Care				
Aspirin Given at Discharge	200	100%	99%	99%
Fibrinolytic Meds Within 30 Min. of Arrival[7]	-	-	75%	54%
PCI Within 90 Minutes of Arrival	41	95%	97%	96%
Statin Prescribed at Discharge	190	100%	99%	98%
Heart Failure Care				
ACE Inhibitor or ARB for LVSD	73	97%	98%	97%
Discharge Instructions Given	176	97%	95%	94%
Evaluation of LVS Function	232	100%	100%	99%
Medicare Spending				
Medicare Spending per Patient (ratio)	-	0.95	0.95	0.98
Pneumonia Care				
Appropriate Initial Antibiotic Given[2]	80	99%	97%	95%
Blood Culture Timing[2]	123	99%	98%	98%
Pregnancy and Delivery Care				
Newborn Deliveries Scheduled Early[2]	77	10%	6%	6%
Preventive Care				
Immunization for Influenza[2]	492	97%	92%	90%
Immunization for Pneumonia[2]	548	90%	93%	92%
Stroke Care				
Anticoagulation Therapy for Atrial Fibrillation	30	100%	96%	95%
Antithrombotic Therapy Timing	172	100%	99%	98%
Assessed for Rehabilitation	217	99%	99%	97%
Discharged on Antithrombotic Therapy	183	99%	100%	99%
Discharged on Statin Medication	144	98%	97%	94%
Thrombolytic Therapy Timing[1]	-	-	73%	66%
Venous Thromboembolism Prophylaxis	229	97%	97%	94%
Written Stroke Educational Materials Given	107	93%	92%	88%
Surgical Care Improvement Project				
Appropriate Beta Blocker Usage	590	100%	99%	98%
Appropriate VTP Within 24 Hours	1,637	99%	99%	98%
Controlled Postoperative Blood Glucose	182	98%	98%	97%
Perioperative Temperature Management	1,930	100%	100%	100%
Prophylactic Antibiotic Selection	1,274	100%	99%	99%
Prophylactic Antibiotic Selection (Outpatient)	569	99%	98%	98%
Prophylactic Antibiotic Stopped	1,252	99%	98%	98%
Prophylactic Antibiotic Timing	1,274	99%	99%	99%
Prophylactic Antibiotic Timing (Outpatient)	571	99%	98%	98%
Urinary Catheter Removal	851	98%	98%	97%
Survey of Patients' Hospital Experiences				
Area Around Room 'Always' Quiet at Night	300+	63%	60%	61%
Doctors 'Always' Communicated Well	300+	83%	81%	82%
Home Recovery Information Given	300+	87%	86%	85%
Hospital Given 9 or 10 on 10 Point Scale	300+	83%	68%	71%
Meds 'Always' Explained Before Given	300+	70%	62%	64%
Nurses 'Always' Communicated Well	300+	83%	78%	79%
Pain 'Always' Well Controlled	300+	75%	70%	71%
Room and Bathroom 'Always' Clean	300+	80%	71%	73%
Timely Help 'Always' Received	300+	72%	64%	68%
Would Definitely Recommend Hospital	300+	85%	69%	71%
Use of Medical Imaging				
Cardiac Imaging Stress Test before Surgery	123	5.7%	5.1%	5.3%
Combination Abdominal CT Scan	1,419	7.4%	8.5%	10.5%
Combination Brain/Sinus CT Scan	1,073	2.2%	2.3%	2.7%
Combination Chest CT Scan	1,186	0.1%	1.6%	2.7%
Follow-up Mammogram/Ultrasound	2,352	8.0%	7.7%	8.8%
Lumbar Spine MRI for Low Back Pain	329	33.4%	35.3%	37.2%

Bedford Memorial Hospital

1613 Oakwood Street
Bedford, VA 24523
URL: www.bmhva.com
Type: Acute Care Hospitals
Ownership: Voluntary non-profit - Private
Phone: 540-586-2441
Fax: 540-586-4342
Emergency Services: Yes
Beds: 161

Key Personnel:

Chief of Medical Staff.......... Linda S Beahm, MD
Anesthesiology.................. Martin Dittler
CEO/President.................. William Flattery
Infection Control................ Melisa Hobbs
Administrator .... Patti O. Jurkus
Operating Room................ Eugene W Lowe
Quality Assurance .... Karen McBrite
Emergency Room .... Darrell Vanness

Measure	Cases	This Hosp.	State Avg.	U.S. Avg.
Blood Clot Prevention and Treatment				
Anticoagulation Overlap Therapy[2]	12	92%	95%	93%
ICU Venous Thromboembolism Prophylaxis[2]	90	96%	95%	92%
Incidence of Potentially Preventable VTE[1,2]	-	-	8%	10%
UFH with Dosages/Platelet Monitoring[1,2]	-	-	99%	97%
Venous Thromboembolism Prophylaxis[2]	213	90%	91%	85%
Warfarin Therapy Discharge Instructions[1,2]	-	-	78%	75%
Chest Pain/Possible Heart Attack Care				
Aspirin Given Within 24 Hours of Arrival	53	91%	98%	96%
Fibrinolytic Meds Within 30 Min. of Arrival[1]	-	-	68%	58%
Average Time to ECG (minutes)	54	14	7	7
Average Time to Transfer (minutes)[1]	-	-	64	60
Children's Asthma Care				
Received Home Management Plan of Care	-	-	-	88%
Received Reliever Medication	-	-	-	100%
Received Systemic Corticosteroids	-	-	-	100%
Emergency Department				
Admittance Decision Time (minutes)[2]	576	67	96	98
Head CT Results Within 45 Min. of Arrival[1]	-	-	60%	57%
Patients Who Left ER Before Being Seen	16,626	2%	2%	2%
Time from ER Arrival to Admit. (minutes)[2]	606	260	280	274
Time from ER Arrival to Discharge (minutes)	355	133	167	134
Time in ER Before Being Evaluated (minutes)	289	38	35	26
Time to Pain Meds for Fractures (minutes)	74	90	56	57
Heart Attack Care				
Aspirin Given at Discharge[1]	-	-	99%	99%
Fibrinolytic Meds Within 30 Min. of Arrival[7]	-	-	75%	54%
PCI Within 90 Minutes of Arrival[7]	-	-	97%	96%
Statin Prescribed at Discharge[1]	-	-	99%	98%
Heart Failure Care				
ACE Inhibitor or ARB for LVSD	13	100%	98%	97%
Discharge Instructions Given	41	98%	95%	94%
Evaluation of LVS Function	59	98%	100%	99%
Medicare Spending				

NOTE: Hospital profiles are in alphabetical order by state, then city, then hospital within the city; Rankings exclude hospitals with less than 25 cases except for patient surveys which excludes hospitals with less than 100 cases; (a) 100-299 cases; (1) The number of cases/patients is too few to report; (2) Data submitted were based on a sample of cases/patients; (3) Results are based on a shorter time period than required; (4) Data suppressed by CMS for one or more quarters; (5) Results are not available for this reporting period; (6) Fewer than 100 patients completed the HCAHPS survey; (7) No cases met the criteria for this measure; (8) The lower limit of the confidence interval cannot be calculated if the number of observed infections equals zero; (9) No data are available from the state/territory for this reporting period; (10) The scores shown reflect fewer than 50 completed surveys; (11) There were discrepancies in the data collection process; (12) This measure does not apply to this hospital for this reporting period; (13) Results cannot be calculated for this reporting period; (14) The results for this state are combined with nearby states to protect confidentiality; Please refer to the User's Guide for a full explanation of data.

Measure	Cases	This Hosp.	State Avg.	U.S. Avg.
Medicare Spending per Patient (ratio)	-	0.92	0.95	0.98
Pneumonia Care				
Appropriate Initial Antibiotic Given	66	94%	97%	95%
Blood Culture Timing	111	95%	98%	98%
Pregnancy and Delivery Care				
Newborn Deliveries Scheduled Early[7]	-	-	6%	6%
Preventive Care				
Immunization for Influenza[2]	473	80%	92%	90%
Immunization for Pneumonia[2]	733	88%	93%	92%
Stroke Care				
Anticoagulation Therapy for Atrial Fibrillation[7]	-	-	96%	95%
Antithrombotic Therapy Timing[1]	-	-	99%	98%
Assessed for Rehabilitation[1]	-	-	99%	97%
Discharged on Antithrombotic Therapy[1]	-	-	100%	99%
Discharged on Statin Medication[1]	-	-	97%	94%
Thrombolytic Therapy Timing[1]	-	-	73%	66%
Venous Thromboembolism Prophylaxis[1]	-	-	97%	94%
Written Stroke Educational Materials Given[1]	-	-	92%	88%
Surgical Care Improvement Project				
Appropriate Beta Blocker Usage[1]	-	-	99%	98%
Appropriate VTP Within 24 Hours	14	93%	99%	98%
Controlled Postoperative Blood Glucose[7]	-	-	98%	97%
Perioperative Temperature Management	16	100%	100%	100%
Prophylactic Antibiotic Selection[1]	-	-	99%	99%
Prophylactic Antibiotic Selection (Outpatient)[1,3]	-	-	98%	98%
Prophylactic Antibiotic Stopped[1]	-	-	98%	98%
Prophylactic Antibiotic Timing[1]	-	-	99%	99%
Prophylactic Antibiotic Timing (Outpatient)[1,3]	-	-	98%	98%
Urinary Catheter Removal	11	100%	98%	97%
Survey of Patients' Hospital Experiences				
Area Around Room 'Always' Quiet at Night	(a)	54%	60%	61%
Doctors 'Always' Communicated Well	(a)	83%	81%	82%
Home Recovery Information Given	(a)	85%	86%	85%
Hospital Given 9 or 10 on 10 Point Scale	(a)	69%	68%	71%
Meds 'Always' Explained Before Given	(a)	62%	62%	64%
Nurses 'Always' Communicated Well	(a)	80%	78%	79%
Pain 'Always' Well Controlled	(a)	68%	70%	71%
Room and Bathroom 'Always' Clean	(a)	73%	71%	73%
Timely Help 'Always' Received	(a)	64%	64%	68%
Would Definitely Recommend Hospital	(a)	68%	69%	71%
Use of Medical Imaging				
Cardiac Imaging Stress Test before Surgery	89	5.6%	5.1%	5.3%
Combination Abdominal CT Scan	298	1.7%	8.5%	10.5%
Combination Brain/Sinus CT Scan	313	0.6%	2.3%	2.7%
Combination Chest CT Scan	161	0.0%	1.6%	2.7%
Follow-up Mammogram/Ultrasound	715	7.3%	7.7%	8.8%
Lumbar Spine MRI for Low Back Pain	51	35.3%	35.3%	37.2%

Wellmont Lonesome Pine Hospital

1990 Holton Avenue East
Big Stone Gap, VA 24219
Phone: 276-523-3111
Fax: 423-230-8224
URL: www.wellmont.org
Type: Acute Care Hospitals
Emergency Services: Yes
Ownership: Voluntary non-profit - Other
Beds: 60

Key Personnel:
Emergency Room . . . . Jelly Carter
CEO/President. . . . . Denny DeNarvaez
Chairman/CEO . . . . Ed Roop
Quality Assurance . . . . Paul Trammell

Measure	Cases	This Hosp.	State Avg.	U.S. Avg.
Blood Clot Prevention and Treatment				
Anticoagulation Overlap Therapy[2]	27	81%	95%	93%
ICU Venous Thromboembolism Prophylaxis[2]	115	90%	95%	92%
Incidence of Potentially Preventable VTE[1,2]	-	-	8%	10%
UFH with Dosages/Platelet Monitoring[2]	21	100%	99%	97%
Venous Thromboembolism Prophylaxis[2]	370	83%	91%	85%
Warfarin Therapy Discharge Instructions[2]	17	59%	78%	75%
Chest Pain/Possible Heart Attack Care				
Aspirin Given Within 24 Hours of Arrival	62	95%	98%	96%
Fibrinolytic Meds Within 30 Min. of Arrival[1]	-	-	68%	58%
Average Time to ECG (minutes)	68	6	7	7
Average Time to Transfer (minutes)[1]	-	-	64	60
Children's Asthma Care				
Received Home Management Plan of Care	-	-	-	88%
Received Reliever Medication	-	-	-	100%
Received Systemic Corticosteroids	-	-	-	100%
Emergency Department				
Admittance Decision Time (minutes)[2]	743	53	96	98
Head CT Results Within 45 Min. of Arrival	20	45%	60%	57%
Patients Who Left ER Before Being Seen	28,756	2%	2%	2%
Time from ER Arrival to Admit. (minutes)[2]	743	202	280	274
Time from ER Arrival to Discharge (minutes)	708	125	167	134
Time in ER Before Being Evaluated (minutes)	751	40	35	26
Time to Pain Meds for Fractures (minutes)	67	84	56	57
Heart Attack Care				
Aspirin Given at Discharge	28	100%	99%	99%
Fibrinolytic Meds Within 30 Min. of Arrival[7]	-	-	75%	54%
PCI Within 90 Minutes of Arrival[7]	-	-	97%	96%
Statin Prescribed at Discharge	26	100%	99%	98%
Heart Failure Care				
ACE Inhibitor or ARB for LVSD	31	90%	98%	97%
Discharge Instructions Given	98	91%	95%	94%
Evaluation of LVS Function	121	100%	100%	99%
Medicare Spending				
Medicare Spending per Patient (ratio)	-	0.85	0.95	0.98
Pneumonia Care				
Appropriate Initial Antibiotic Given	98	91%	97%	95%
Blood Culture Timing	149	99%	98%	98%
Pregnancy and Delivery Care				
Newborn Deliveries Scheduled Early	44	2%	6%	6%
Preventive Care				
Immunization for Influenza[2]	516	96%	92%	90%
Immunization for Pneumonia[2]	695	99%	93%	92%
Stroke Care				
Anticoagulation Therapy for Atrial Fibrillation[1]	-	-	96%	95%
Antithrombotic Therapy Timing	17	88%	99%	98%
Assessed for Rehabilitation	18	94%	99%	97%
Discharged on Antithrombotic Therapy	17	88%	100%	99%
Discharged on Statin Medication	17	88%	97%	94%
Thrombolytic Therapy Timing[1]	-	-	73%	66%
Venous Thromboembolism Prophylaxis	18	89%	97%	94%
Written Stroke Educational Materials Given[1]	-	-	92%	88%
Surgical Care Improvement Project				
Appropriate Beta Blocker Usage[2]	25	88%	99%	98%
Appropriate VTP Within 24 Hours[2]	90	91%	99%	98%
Controlled Postoperative Blood Glucose[2,7]	-	-	98%	97%
Perioperative Temperature Management[2]	105	97%	100%	100%
Prophylactic Antibiotic Selection[2]	66	92%	99%	99%
Prophylactic Antibiotic Selection (Outpatient)	26	100%	98%	98%
Prophylactic Antibiotic Stopped[2]	64	91%	98%	98%
Prophylactic Antibiotic Timing[2]	67	91%	99%	99%
Prophylactic Antibiotic Timing (Outpatient)	11	100%	98%	98%
Urinary Catheter Removal[2]	61	92%	98%	97%
Survey of Patients' Hospital Experiences				
Area Around Room 'Always' Quiet at Night	300+	68%	60%	61%
Doctors 'Always' Communicated Well	300+	83%	81%	82%
Home Recovery Information Given	300+	84%	86%	85%
Hospital Given 9 or 10 on 10 Point Scale	300+	69%	68%	71%
Meds 'Always' Explained Before Given	300+	68%	62%	64%
Nurses 'Always' Communicated Well	300+	83%	78%	79%
Pain 'Always' Well Controlled	300+	75%	70%	71%
Room and Bathroom 'Always' Clean	300+	80%	71%	73%
Timely Help 'Always' Received	300+	74%	64%	68%
Would Definitely Recommend Hospital	300+	68%	69%	71%
Use of Medical Imaging				
Cardiac Imaging Stress Test before Surgery	211	3.8%	5.1%	5.3%
Combination Abdominal CT Scan	578	32.4%	8.5%	10.5%
Combination Brain/Sinus CT Scan[1]	-	-	2.3%	2.7%
Combination Chest CT Scan	453	14.6%	1.6%	2.7%
Follow-up Mammogram/Ultrasound	561	7.0%	7.7%	8.8%
Lumbar Spine MRI for Low Back Pain	96	32.3%	35.3%	37.2%

Lewisgale Hospital Montgomery

3700 South Main Street
Blacksburg, VA 24060
Phone: 540-951-1111
Fax: 540-953-5295
URL: www.mrhospital.com
Type: Acute Care Hospitals
Emergency Services: Yes
Ownership: Proprietary
Beds: 146

Key Personnel:
Radiology. . . . . Michael Aronson, MD
Intensive Care Unit. . . . . MJ Bean
Infection Control. . . . . Jennifer Brumfield
CEO/President. . . . . Alan Fabian, FACHE
Operating Room. . . . . Jolene B Henshaw
Chief of Medical Staff . . . . Hing - Har Lo, MD
Quality Assurance . . . . Lori Rakes
Pediatric Ambulatory Care . . . . . . Martha Wunsch, MD

Measure	Cases	This Hosp.	State Avg.	U.S. Avg.
Blood Clot Prevention and Treatment				
Anticoagulation Overlap Therapy[2]	21	95%	95%	93%
ICU Venous Thromboembolism Prophylaxis[2]	48	98%	95%	92%
Incidence of Potentially Preventable VTE[1,2]	-	-	8%	10%
UFH with Dosages/Platelet Monitoring[1,2]	-	-	99%	97%
Venous Thromboembolism Prophylaxis[2]	324	99%	91%	85%
Warfarin Therapy Discharge Instructions[2]	12	100%	78%	75%
Chest Pain/Possible Heart Attack Care				
Aspirin Given Within 24 Hours of Arrival[1,3]	-	-	98%	96%
Fibrinolytic Meds Within 30 Min. of Arrival[3,7]	-	-	68%	58%
Average Time to ECG (minutes)[1,3]	-	-	7	7
Average Time to Transfer (minutes)[1,3]	-	-	64	60
Children's Asthma Care				
Received Home Management Plan of Care	-	-	-	88%
Received Reliever Medication	-	-	-	100%
Received Systemic Corticosteroids	-	-	-	100%
Emergency Department				
Admittance Decision Time (minutes)[2]	472	50	96	98
Head CT Results Within 45 Min. of Arrival[1]	-	-	60%	57%
Patients Who Left ER Before Being Seen	26,490	1%	2%	2%
Time from ER Arrival to Admit. (minutes)[2]	477	211	280	274
Time from ER Arrival to Discharge (minutes)	427	124	167	134
Time in ER Before Being Evaluated (minutes)	474	15	35	26
Time to Pain Meds for Fractures (minutes)	73	29	56	57
Heart Attack Care				
Aspirin Given at Discharge	93	100%	99%	99%
Fibrinolytic Meds Within 30 Min. of Arrival[7]	-	-	75%	54%
PCI Within 90 Minutes of Arrival	12	100%	97%	96%
Statin Prescribed at Discharge	91	100%	99%	98%
Heart Failure Care				
ACE Inhibitor or ARB for LVSD	35	100%	98%	97%
Discharge Instructions Given	62	97%	95%	94%
Evaluation of LVS Function	86	100%	100%	99%
Medicare Spending				
Medicare Spending per Patient (ratio)	-	0.95	0.95	0.98
Pneumonia Care				
Appropriate Initial Antibiotic Given	64	100%	97%	95%
Blood Culture Timing	102	100%	98%	98%
Pregnancy and Delivery Care				
Newborn Deliveries Scheduled Early	33	3%	6%	6%
Preventive Care				
Immunization for Influenza[2]	435	99%	92%	90%
Immunization for Pneumonia[2]	551	99%	93%	92%
Stroke Care				
Anticoagulation Therapy for Atrial Fibrillation[1]	-	-	96%	95%
Antithrombotic Therapy Timing	38	100%	99%	98%
Assessed for Rehabilitation	34	100%	99%	97%
Discharged on Antithrombotic Therapy	33	100%	100%	99%
Discharged on Statin Medication	22	100%	97%	94%
Thrombolytic Therapy Timing[1]	-	-	73%	66%
Venous Thromboembolism Prophylaxis	40	100%	97%	94%
Written Stroke Educational Materials Given	21	100%	92%	88%
Surgical Care Improvement Project				
Appropriate Beta Blocker Usage	88	100%	99%	98%
Appropriate VTP Within 24 Hours	279	100%	99%	98%
Controlled Postoperative Blood Glucose[7]	-	-	98%	97%
Perioperative Temperature Management	307	100%	100%	100%
Prophylactic Antibiotic Selection	232	100%	99%	99%

NOTE: Hospital profiles are in alphabetical order by state, then city, then hospital within the city; Rankings exclude hospitals with less than 25 cases except for patient surveys which excludes hospitals with less than 100 cases; (a) 100-299 cases; (1) The number of cases/patients is too few to report; (2) Data submitted were based on a sample of cases/patients; (3) Results are based on a shorter time period than required; (4) Data suppressed by CMS for one or more quarters; (5) Results are not available for this reporting period; (6) Fewer than 100 patients completed the HCAHPS survey; (7) No cases met the criteria for this measure; (8) The lower limit of the confidence interval cannot be calculated if the number of observed infections equals zero; (9) No data are available from the state/territory for this reporting period; (10) The scores shown reflect fewer than 50 completed surveys; (11) There were discrepancies in the data collection process; (12) This measure does not apply to this hospital for this reporting period; (13) Results cannot be calculated for this reporting period; (14) The results for this state are combined with nearby states to protect confidentiality; Please refer to the User's Guide for a full explanation of data.

Measure	Cases	This Hosp.	State Avg.	U.S. Avg.
Prophylactic Antibiotic Selection (Outpatient)	57	100%	98%	98%
Prophylactic Antibiotic Stopped	224	100%	98%	98%
Prophylactic Antibiotic Timing	232	100%	99%	99%
Prophylactic Antibiotic Timing (Outpatient)	57	100%	98%	98%
Urinary Catheter Removal	181	99%	98%	97%
Survey of Patients' Hospital Experiences				
Area Around Room 'Always' Quiet at Night	300+	62%	60%	61%
Doctors 'Always' Communicated Well	300+	81%	81%	82%
Home Recovery Information Given	300+	88%	86%	85%
Hospital Given 9 or 10 on 10 Point Scale	300+	68%	68%	71%
Meds 'Always' Explained Before Given	300+	60%	62%	64%
Nurses 'Always' Communicated Well	300+	76%	78%	79%
Pain 'Always' Well Controlled	300+	71%	70%	71%
Room and Bathroom 'Always' Clean	300+	72%	71%	73%
Timely Help 'Always' Received	300+	61%	64%	68%
Would Definitely Recommend Hospital	300+	71%	69%	71%
Use of Medical Imaging				
Cardiac Imaging Stress Test before Surgery	272	5.9%	5.1%	5.3%
Combination Abdominal CT Scan	583	11.1%	8.5%	10.5%
Combination Brain/Sinus CT Scan[1]	-	-	2.3%	2.7%
Combination Chest CT Scan	316	1.6%	1.6%	2.7%
Follow-up Mammogram/Ultrasound	1,146	10.6%	7.7%	8.8%
Lumbar Spine MRI for Low Back Pain	131	36.6%	35.3%	37.2%

Piedmont Geriatric Hospital

5001 E Patrick Henry Hwy - Highway 360 & 460
Phone: 434-767-4401
Burkeville, VA 23922 Fax: 434-767-4500
E-mail: mike.wimsatt@pgh.dmhmrsas.virginia.gov
URL: www.pgh.dmhmrsas.virginia.gov
Type: Acute Care Hospitals Emergency Services: No
Ownership: Government - State Beds: 150

Key Personnel:

Chief of Medical Staff . . . . Hugo Falcon
Quality Assurance . . . . H Eugene Overton
CEO/President. . . . . WR Pirece, Jr
Patient Relations . . . . Anne Stiles

Measure	Cases	This Hosp.	State Avg.	U.S. Avg.
Blood Clot Prevention and Treatment				
Anticoagulation Overlap Therapy[2,3]	-	-	95%	93%
ICU Venous Thromboembolism Prophylaxis[2,3]	-	-	95%	92%
Incidence of Potentially Preventable VTE[2,3]	-	-	8%	10%
UFH with Dosages/Platelet Monitoring[2,3]	-	-	99%	97%
Venous Thromboembolism Prophylaxis[2,3]	-	-	91%	85%
Warfarin Therapy Discharge Instructions[2,3]	-	-	78%	75%
Chest Pain/Possible Heart Attack Care				
Aspirin Given Within 24 Hours of Arrival	-	-	98%	96%
Fibrinolytic Meds Within 30 Min. of Arrival	-	-	68%	58%
Average Time to ECG (minutes)	-	-	7	7
Average Time to Transfer (minutes)	-	-	64	60
Children's Asthma Care				
Received Home Management Plan of Care	-	-	-	88%
Received Reliever Medication	-	-	-	100%
Received Systemic Corticosteroids	-	-	-	100%
Emergency Department				
Admittance Decision Time (minutes)[2,3]	-	-	96	98
Head CT Results Within 45 Min. of Arrival	-	-	60%	57%
Patients Who Left ER Before Being Seen	-	-	2%	2%
Time from ER Arrival to Admit. (minutes)[2,3]	-	-	280	274
Time from ER Arrival to Discharge (minutes)	-	-	167	134
Time in ER Before Being Evaluated (minutes)	-	-	35	26
Time to Pain Meds for Fractures (minutes)	-	-	56	57
Heart Attack Care				
Aspirin Given at Discharge[5]	-	-	99%	99%
Fibrinolytic Meds Within 30 Min. of Arrival[5]	-	-	75%	54%
PCI Within 90 Minutes of Arrival[5]	-	-	97%	96%
Statin Prescribed at Discharge[5]	-	-	99%	98%
Heart Failure Care				
ACE Inhibitor or ARB for LVSD[5]	-	-	98%	97%
Discharge Instructions Given[5]	-	-	95%	94%
Evaluation of LVS Function[5]	-	-	100%	99%
Medicare Spending				
Medicare Spending per Patient (ratio)[1]	-	-	0.95	0.98
Pneumonia Care				
Appropriate Initial Antibiotic Given[5]	-	-	97%	95%
Blood Culture Timing[5]	-	-	98%	98%
Pregnancy and Delivery Care				
Newborn Deliveries Scheduled Early[7]	-	-	6%	6%
Preventive Care				
Immunization for Influenza[5]	-	-	92%	90%
Immunization for Pneumonia[1,2]	-	-	93%	92%
Stroke Care				
Anticoagulation Therapy for Atrial Fibrillation[5]	-	-	96%	95%
Antithrombotic Therapy Timing[5]	-	-	99%	98%
Assessed for Rehabilitation[5]	-	-	99%	97%
Discharged on Antithrombotic Therapy[5]	-	-	100%	99%
Discharged on Statin Medication[5]	-	-	97%	94%
Thrombolytic Therapy Timing[5]	-	-	73%	66%
Venous Thromboembolism Prophylaxis[5]	-	-	97%	94%
Written Stroke Educational Materials Given[5]	-	-	92%	88%
Surgical Care Improvement Project				
Appropriate Beta Blocker Usage[5]	-	-	99%	98%
Appropriate VTP Within 24 Hours[5]	-	-	99%	98%
Controlled Postoperative Blood Glucose[5]	-	-	98%	97%
Perioperative Temperature Management[5]	-	-	100%	100%
Prophylactic Antibiotic Selection[5]	-	-	99%	99%
Prophylactic Antibiotic Selection (Outpatient)	-	-	98%	98%
Prophylactic Antibiotic Stopped[5]	-	-	98%	98%
Prophylactic Antibiotic Timing[5]	-	-	99%	99%
Prophylactic Antibiotic Timing (Outpatient)	-	-	98%	98%
Urinary Catheter Removal[5]	-	-	98%	97%
Survey of Patients' Hospital Experiences				
Area Around Room 'Always' Quiet at Night[1]	-	-	60%	61%
Doctors 'Always' Communicated Well[1]	-	-	81%	82%
Home Recovery Information Given[1]	-	-	86%	85%
Hospital Given 9 or 10 on 10 Point Scale[1]	-	-	68%	71%
Meds 'Always' Explained Before Given[1]	-	-	62%	64%
Nurses 'Always' Communicated Well[1]	-	-	78%	79%
Pain 'Always' Well Controlled[1]	-	-	70%	71%
Room and Bathroom 'Always' Clean[1]	-	-	71%	73%
Timely Help 'Always' Received[1]	-	-	64%	68%
Would Definitely Recommend Hospital[1]	-	-	69%	71%
Use of Medical Imaging				
Cardiac Imaging Stress Test before Surgery	-	-	5.1%	5.3%
Combination Abdominal CT Scan	-	-	8.5%	10.5%
Combination Brain/Sinus CT Scan	-	-	2.3%	2.7%
Combination Chest CT Scan	-	-	1.6%	2.7%
Follow-up Mammogram/Ultrasound	-	-	7.7%	8.8%
Lumbar Spine MRI for Low Back Pain	-	-	35.3%	37.2%

Martha Jefferson Hospital

500 Martha Jefferson Drive Phone: 434-654-7000
Charlottesville, VA 22911 Fax: 434-982-7759
URL: www.marthajefferson.org
Type: Acute Care Hospitals Emergency Services: Yes
Ownership: Voluntary non-profit - Private Beds: 176

Key Personnel:

Chief of Medical Staff . . . . K Asao-Ragosta
Operating Room. . . . . Andrew A Bailey
CEO/President. . . . . James E Haden
Pediatric In-Patient Care . . . . Katherine D Mika, MD
Quality Assurance . . . . DD Sandridge
Emergency Room . . . . Sarah White

Measure	Cases	This Hosp.	State Avg.	U.S. Avg.
Blood Clot Prevention and Treatment				
Anticoagulation Overlap Therapy[2]	101	89%	95%	93%
ICU Venous Thromboembolism Prophylaxis[2]	52	88%	95%	92%
Incidence of Potentially Preventable VTE[2]	17	12%	8%	10%
UFH with Dosages/Platelet Monitoring[2]	28	100%	99%	97%
Venous Thromboembolism Prophylaxis[2]	321	82%	91%	85%
Warfarin Therapy Discharge Instructions[2]	74	74%	78%	75%
Chest Pain/Possible Heart Attack Care				
Aspirin Given Within 24 Hours of Arrival[1]	-	-	98%	96%
Fibrinolytic Meds Within 30 Min. of Arrival[3,7]	-	-	68%	58%
Average Time to ECG (minutes)[1]	-	-	7	7
Average Time to Transfer (minutes)[3,7]	-	-	64	60
Children's Asthma Care				
Received Home Management Plan of Care	-	-	-	88%
Received Reliever Medication	-	-	-	100%
Received Systemic Corticosteroids	-	-	-	100%
Emergency Department				
Admittance Decision Time (minutes)[2]	591	141	96	98
Head CT Results Within 45 Min. of Arrival[1]	-	-	60%	57%
Patients Who Left ER Before Being Seen	52,957	1%	2%	2%
Time from ER Arrival to Admit. (minutes)[2]	593	342	280	274
Time from ER Arrival to Discharge (minutes)	386	162	167	134
Time in ER Before Being Evaluated (minutes)	408	18	35	26
Time to Pain Meds for Fractures (minutes)	205	56	56	57
Heart Attack Care				
Aspirin Given at Discharge	170	99%	99%	99%
Fibrinolytic Meds Within 30 Min. of Arrival[7]	-	-	75%	54%
PCI Within 90 Minutes of Arrival	31	97%	97%	96%
Statin Prescribed at Discharge	175	99%	99%	98%
Heart Failure Care				
ACE Inhibitor or ARB for LVSD	78	100%	98%	97%
Discharge Instructions Given	210	90%	95%	94%
Evaluation of LVS Function	257	100%	100%	99%
Medicare Spending				
Medicare Spending per Patient (ratio)	-	0.94	0.95	0.98
Pneumonia Care				
Appropriate Initial Antibiotic Given[2]	90	93%	97%	95%
Blood Culture Timing[2]	181	93%	98%	98%
Pregnancy and Delivery Care				
Newborn Deliveries Scheduled Early[2]	25	20%	6%	6%
Preventive Care				
Immunization for Influenza[2]	542	84%	92%	90%
Immunization for Pneumonia[2]	686	93%	93%	92%
Stroke Care				
Anticoagulation Therapy for Atrial Fibrillation	14	100%	96%	95%
Antithrombotic Therapy Timing	87	97%	99%	98%
Assessed for Rehabilitation	136	99%	99%	97%
Discharged on Antithrombotic Therapy	128	100%	100%	99%
Discharged on Statin Medication	97	97%	97%	94%
Thrombolytic Therapy Timing[1]	-	-	73%	66%
Venous Thromboembolism Prophylaxis	105	98%	97%	94%
Written Stroke Educational Materials Given	83	92%	92%	88%
Surgical Care Improvement Project				
Appropriate Beta Blocker Usage[2]	107	96%	99%	98%
Appropriate VTP Within 24 Hours[2]	357	99%	99%	98%
Controlled Postoperative Blood Glucose[2,7]	-	-	98%	97%
Perioperative Temperature Management[2]	463	99%	100%	100%
Prophylactic Antibiotic Selection[2]	327	98%	99%	99%
Prophylactic Antibiotic Selection (Outpatient)	283	95%	98%	98%
Prophylactic Antibiotic Stopped[2]	319	98%	98%	98%
Prophylactic Antibiotic Timing[2]	327	99%	99%	99%
Prophylactic Antibiotic Timing (Outpatient)	287	95%	98%	98%
Urinary Catheter Removal[2]	188	94%	98%	97%
Survey of Patients' Hospital Experiences				
Area Around Room 'Always' Quiet at Night	300+	67%	60%	61%
Doctors 'Always' Communicated Well	300+	85%	81%	82%
Home Recovery Information Given	300+	89%	86%	85%
Hospital Given 9 or 10 on 10 Point Scale	300+	80%	68%	71%
Meds 'Always' Explained Before Given	300+	63%	62%	64%
Nurses 'Always' Communicated Well	300+	82%	78%	79%
Pain 'Always' Well Controlled	300+	70%	70%	71%
Room and Bathroom 'Always' Clean	300+	74%	71%	73%
Timely Help 'Always' Received	300+	70%	64%	68%
Would Definitely Recommend Hospital	300+	83%	69%	71%
Use of Medical Imaging				
Cardiac Imaging Stress Test before Surgery	232	3.9%	5.1%	5.3%
Combination Abdominal CT Scan	1,441	5.4%	8.5%	10.5%
Combination Brain/Sinus CT Scan	1,070	2.2%	2.3%	2.7%
Combination Chest CT Scan	1,166	0.0%	1.6%	2.7%
Follow-up Mammogram/Ultrasound	4,321	9.2%	7.7%	8.8%
Lumbar Spine MRI for Low Back Pain	426	37.1%	35.3%	37.2%

NOTE: Hospital profiles are in alphabetical order by state, then city, then hospital within the city; Rankings exclude hospitals with less than 25 cases except for patient surveys which excludes hospitals with less than 100 cases; (a) 100-299 cases; (1) The number of cases/patients is too few to report; (2) Data submitted were based on a sample of cases/patients; (3) Results are based on a shorter time period than required; (4) Data suppressed by CMS for one or more quarters; (5) Results are not available for this reporting period; (6) Fewer than 100 patients completed the HCAHPS survey; (7) No cases met the criteria for this measure; (8) The lower limit of the confidence interval cannot be calculated if the number of observed infections equals zero; (9) No data are available from the state/territory for this reporting period; (10) The scores shown reflect fewer than 50 completed surveys; (11) There were discrepancies in the data collection process; (12) This measure does not apply to this hospital for this reporting period; (13) Results cannot be calculated for this reporting period; (14) The results for this state are combined with nearby states to protect confidentiality; Please refer to the User's Guide for a full explanation of data.

University of Virginia Medical Center

Jefferson Park Ave
Charlottesville, VA 22908
Phone: 800-251-3627
URL: www.uvahealth.com
Type: Acute Care Hospitals
Emergency Services: Yes
Ownership: Government - State
Beds: 604

Key Personnel:
Radiology.................. James Carnes
Infection Control.............. Eve Giannetta
CEO/President.............. R Edward Howell
Coronary Care.............. Marian Lawson, RN
Quality Assurance .... Abraham Segres
Pediatric Ambulatory Care ...... Sheila Smith
Pediatric In-Patient Care .... Sheila Smith
Chief of Medical Staff.......... Jonathon D Truwit, MD, MBA

Measure	Cases	This Hosp.	State Avg.	U.S. Avg.
Blood Clot Prevention and Treatment				
Anticoagulation Overlap Therapy[2]	109	92%	95%	93%
ICU Venous Thromboembolism Prophylaxis[2]	111	91%	95%	92%
Incidence of Potentially Preventable VTE[2]	87	8%	8%	10%
UFH with Dosages/Platelet Monitoring[2]	186	88%	99%	97%
Venous Thromboembolism Prophylaxis[2]	281	89%	91%	85%
Warfarin Therapy Discharge Instructions[2]	89	27%	78%	75%
Chest Pain/Possible Heart Attack Care				
Aspirin Given Within 24 Hours of Arrival[5]	-	-	98%	96%
Fibrinolytic Meds Within 30 Min. of Arrival[5]	-	-	68%	58%
Average Time to ECG (minutes)[5]	-	-	7	7
Average Time to Transfer (minutes)[5]	-	-	64	60
Children's Asthma Care				
Received Home Management Plan of Care[2]	39	97%	-	88%
Received Reliever Medication	39	100%	-	100%
Received Systemic Corticosteroids	39	100%	-	100%
Emergency Department				
Admittance Decision Time (minutes)[2]	477	101	96	98
Head CT Results Within 45 Min. of Arrival[1]	-	-	60%	57%
Patients Who Left ER Before Being Seen	61,779	2%	2%	2%
Time from ER Arrival to Admit. (minutes)[2]	477	369	280	274
Time from ER Arrival to Discharge (minutes)	391	190	167	134
Time in ER Before Being Evaluated (minutes)	353	37	35	26
Time to Pain Meds for Fractures (minutes)	117	61	56	57
Heart Attack Care				
Aspirin Given at Discharge[2]	339	99%	99%	99%
Fibrinolytic Meds Within 30 Min. of Arrival[2,7]	-	-	75%	54%
PCI Within 90 Minutes of Arrival[2]	41	93%	97%	96%
Statin Prescribed at Discharge[2]	331	99%	99%	98%
Heart Failure Care				
ACE Inhibitor or ARB for LVSD[2]	99	98%	98%	97%
Discharge Instructions Given[2]	225	97%	95%	94%
Evaluation of LVS Function[2]	277	99%	100%	99%
Medicare Spending				
Medicare Spending per Patient (ratio)	-	1.01	0.95	0.98
Pneumonia Care				
Appropriate Initial Antibiotic Given[2]	47	87%	97%	95%
Blood Culture Timing[2]	134	92%	98%	98%
Pregnancy and Delivery Care				
Newborn Deliveries Scheduled Early[2]	13	0%	6%	6%
Preventive Care				
Immunization for Influenza[2]	533	54%	92%	90%
Immunization for Pneumonia[2]	579	48%	93%	92%
Stroke Care				
Anticoagulation Therapy for Atrial Fibrillation[2]	11	100%	96%	95%
Antithrombotic Therapy Timing[2]	47	98%	99%	98%
Assessed for Rehabilitation[2]	87	100%	99%	97%
Discharged on Antithrombotic Therapy[2]	64	98%	100%	99%
Discharged on Statin Medication[2]	57	95%	97%	94%
Thrombolytic Therapy Timing[1,2]	-	-	73%	66%
Venous Thromboembolism Prophylaxis[2]	89	99%	97%	94%
Written Stroke Educational Materials Given[2]	46	87%	92%	88%
Surgical Care Improvement Project				
Appropriate Beta Blocker Usage[2]	193	100%	99%	98%
Appropriate VTP Within 24 Hours[2]	401	100%	99%	98%
Controlled Postoperative Blood Glucose[2]	106	92%	98%	97%
Perioperative Temperature Management[2]	523	100%	100%	100%
Prophylactic Antibiotic Selection[2]	372	100%	99%	99%
Prophylactic Antibiotic Selection (Outpatient)	366	90%	98%	98%
Prophylactic Antibiotic Stopped[2]	367	98%	98%	98%
Prophylactic Antibiotic Timing[2]	372	99%	99%	99%
Prophylactic Antibiotic Timing (Outpatient)	295	88%	98%	98%
Urinary Catheter Removal[2]	238	99%	98%	97%
Survey of Patients' Hospital Experiences				
Area Around Room 'Always' Quiet at Night	300+	45%	60%	61%
Doctors 'Always' Communicated Well	300+	79%	81%	82%
Home Recovery Information Given	300+	88%	86%	85%
Hospital Given 9 or 10 on 10 Point Scale	300+	68%	68%	71%
Meds 'Always' Explained Before Given	300+	61%	62%	64%
Nurses 'Always' Communicated Well	300+	76%	78%	79%
Pain 'Always' Well Controlled	300+	65%	70%	71%
Room and Bathroom 'Always' Clean	300+	67%	71%	73%
Timely Help 'Always' Received	300+	57%	64%	68%
Would Definitely Recommend Hospital	300+	75%	69%	71%
Use of Medical Imaging				
Cardiac Imaging Stress Test before Surgery	996	7.5%	5.1%	5.3%
Combination Abdominal CT Scan	1,155	3.3%	8.5%	10.5%
Combination Brain/Sinus CT Scan	660	1.7%	2.3%	2.7%
Combination Chest CT Scan	1,478	0.0%	1.6%	2.7%
Follow-up Mammogram/Ultrasound	4,028	12.1%	7.7%	8.8%
Lumbar Spine MRI for Low Back Pain[1]	-	-	35.3%	37.2%

Chesapeake General Hospital

736 Battlefield Blvd, North
Chesapeake, VA 23320
Phone: 757-312-8121
Fax: 757-312-6184
E-mail: info@chealth.org,
URL: www.chesapeakehealth.com
Type: Acute Care Hospitals
Emergency Services: Yes
Ownership: Govt - Hospital Dist/Auth
Beds: 310

Key Personnel:
CEO/President.............. Peter F. Bastone
Chair/CEO.................. Rhonda Bridgeman
Quality Assurance .... Sandra Chellew, RN
Pediatric Ambulatory Care ...... Vernita Peeples, MD
Pediatric In-Patient Care .... Vernita Peeples, MD
Radiology.................. James J Rinaldi, MD
Chief of Medical Staff.......... Francis Watson, MD
Operating Room............. Merle Wilson, RN

Measure	Cases	This Hosp.	State Avg.	U.S. Avg.
Blood Clot Prevention and Treatment				
Anticoagulation Overlap Therapy[2]	138	87%	95%	93%
ICU Venous Thromboembolism Prophylaxis[2]	77	83%	95%	92%
Incidence of Potentially Preventable VTE[2]	21	10%	8%	10%
UFH with Dosages/Platelet Monitoring[2]	83	100%	99%	97%
Venous Thromboembolism Prophylaxis[2]	380	78%	91%	85%
Warfarin Therapy Discharge Instructions[2]	113	65%	78%	75%
Chest Pain/Possible Heart Attack Care				
Aspirin Given Within 24 Hours of Arrival[5]	-	-	98%	96%
Fibrinolytic Meds Within 30 Min. of Arrival[5]	-	-	68%	58%
Average Time to ECG (minutes)[5]	-	-	7	7
Average Time to Transfer (minutes)[5]	-	-	64	60
Children's Asthma Care				
Received Home Management Plan of Care	-	-	-	88%
Received Reliever Medication	-	-	-	100%
Received Systemic Corticosteroids	-	-	-	100%
Emergency Department				
Admittance Decision Time (minutes)[2]	628	121	96	98
Head CT Results Within 45 Min. of Arrival	16	19%	60%	57%
Patients Who Left ER Before Being Seen	72,634	1%	2%	2%
Time from ER Arrival to Admit. (minutes)[2]	661	355	280	274
Time from ER Arrival to Discharge (minutes)	371	159	167	134
Time in ER Before Being Evaluated (minutes)	338	30	35	26
Time to Pain Meds for Fractures (minutes)	186	62	56	57
Heart Attack Care				
Aspirin Given at Discharge	223	99%	99%	99%
Fibrinolytic Meds Within 30 Min. of Arrival[7]	-	-	75%	54%
PCI Within 90 Minutes of Arrival	54	98%	97%	96%
Statin Prescribed at Discharge	220	98%	99%	98%
Heart Failure Care				
ACE Inhibitor or ARB for LVSD[2]	116	97%	98%	97%
Discharge Instructions Given[2]	257	91%	95%	94%
Evaluation of LVS Function[2]	320	100%	100%	99%
Medicare Spending				
Medicare Spending per Patient (ratio)	-	1.00	0.95	0.98
Pneumonia Care				
Appropriate Initial Antibiotic Given[2]	91	97%	97%	95%
Blood Culture Timing[2]	133	95%	98%	98%
Pregnancy and Delivery Care				
Newborn Deliveries Scheduled Early	225	7%	6%	6%
Preventive Care				
Immunization for Influenza[2]	530	96%	92%	90%
Immunization for Pneumonia[2]	618	93%	93%	92%
Stroke Care				
Anticoagulation Therapy for Atrial Fibrillation[2]	13	100%	96%	95%
Antithrombotic Therapy Timing[2]	94	100%	99%	98%
Assessed for Rehabilitation[2]	87	97%	99%	97%
Discharged on Antithrombotic Therapy[2]	81	100%	100%	99%
Discharged on Statin Medication[2]	64	94%	97%	94%
Thrombolytic Therapy Timing[2]	14	7%	73%	66%
Venous Thromboembolism Prophylaxis[2]	105	87%	97%	94%
Written Stroke Educational Materials Given[2]	62	74%	92%	88%
Surgical Care Improvement Project				
Appropriate Beta Blocker Usage[2]	102	97%	99%	98%
Appropriate VTP Within 24 Hours[2]	376	97%	99%	98%
Controlled Postoperative Blood Glucose[2,7]	-	-	98%	97%
Perioperative Temperature Management[2]	431	100%	100%	100%
Prophylactic Antibiotic Selection[2]	285	99%	99%	99%
Prophylactic Antibiotic Selection (Outpatient)	511	98%	98%	98%
Prophylactic Antibiotic Stopped[2]	280	96%	98%	98%
Prophylactic Antibiotic Timing[2]	285	100%	99%	99%
Prophylactic Antibiotic Timing (Outpatient)	512	99%	98%	98%
Urinary Catheter Removal[2]	223	96%	98%	97%
Survey of Patients' Hospital Experiences				
Area Around Room 'Always' Quiet at Night	300+	59%	60%	61%
Doctors 'Always' Communicated Well	300+	83%	81%	82%
Home Recovery Information Given	300+	88%	86%	85%
Hospital Given 9 or 10 on 10 Point Scale	300+	70%	68%	71%
Meds 'Always' Explained Before Given	300+	64%	62%	64%
Nurses 'Always' Communicated Well	300+	77%	78%	79%
Pain 'Always' Well Controlled	300+	71%	70%	71%
Room and Bathroom 'Always' Clean	300+	63%	71%	73%
Timely Help 'Always' Received	300+	64%	64%	68%
Would Definitely Recommend Hospital	300+	71%	69%	71%
Use of Medical Imaging				
Cardiac Imaging Stress Test before Surgery	660	4.7%	5.1%	5.3%
Combination Abdominal CT Scan	1,354	8.0%	8.5%	10.5%
Combination Brain/Sinus CT Scan	1,126	1.2%	2.3%	2.7%
Combination Chest CT Scan	911	0.4%	1.6%	2.7%
Follow-up Mammogram/Ultrasound	2,329	12.2%	7.7%	8.8%
Lumbar Spine MRI for Low Back Pain	170	28.2%	35.3%	37.2%

Carilion New River Valley Medical Center

2900 Lamb Circle
Christiansburg, VA 24073
Phone: 540-731-2000
Fax: 540-731-2850
URL: www.carilion.com
Type: Acute Care Hospitals
Emergency Services: Yes
Ownership: Voluntary non-profit - Other
Beds: 97

Key Personnel:
CEO/President.............. Nancy Howell Agee
Emergency Room .... Gary S Abel
Cardiac Laboratory............ Carlos Fernandez
Chair/CEO.................. James A Hartley
Pediatric Ambulatory Care ...... Joyce Yearout

Measure	Cases	This Hosp.	State Avg.	U.S. Avg.
Blood Clot Prevention and Treatment				
Anticoagulation Overlap Therapy[2]	54	100%	95%	93%
ICU Venous Thromboembolism Prophylaxis[2]	70	81%	95%	92%
Incidence of Potentially Preventable VTE[1,2]	-	-	8%	10%
UFH with Dosages/Platelet Monitoring[2]	28	100%	99%	97%
Venous Thromboembolism Prophylaxis[2]	357	91%	91%	85%
Warfarin Therapy Discharge Instructions[2]	51	100%	78%	75%
Chest Pain/Possible Heart Attack Care				
Aspirin Given Within 24 Hours of Arrival	83	98%	98%	96%
Fibrinolytic Meds Within 30 Min. of Arrival[1]	-	-	68%	58%
Average Time to ECG (minutes)	85	21	7	7

NOTE: Hospital profiles are in alphabetical order by state, then city, then hospital within the city; Rankings exclude hospitals with less than 25 cases except for patient surveys which excludes hospitals with less than 100 cases; (a) 100-299 cases; (1) The number of cases/patients is too few to report; (2) Data submitted were based on a sample of cases/patients; (3) Results are based on a shorter time period than required; (4) Data suppressed by CMS for one or more quarters; (5) Results are not available for this reporting period; (6) Fewer than 100 patients completed the HCAHPS survey; (7) No cases met the criteria for this measure; (8) The lower limit of the confidence interval cannot be calculated if the number of observed infections equals zero; (9) No data are available from the state/territory for this reporting period; (10) The scores shown reflect fewer than 50 completed surveys; (11) There were discrepancies in the data collection process; (12) This measure does not apply to this hospital for this reporting period; (13) Results cannot be calculated for this reporting period; (14) The results for this state are combined with nearby states to protect confidentiality; Please refer to the User's Guide for a full explanation of data.

Measure	Cases	This Hosp.	State Avg.	U.S. Avg.
Average Time to Transfer (minutes)	11	75	64	60
Children's Asthma Care				
Received Home Management Plan of Care	-	-	-	88%
Received Reliever Medication	-	-	-	100%
Received Systemic Corticosteroids	-	-	-	100%
Emergency Department				
Admittance Decision Time (minutes)[2]	567	163	96	98
Head CT Results Within 45 Min. of Arrival[1]	-	-	60%	57%
Patients Who Left ER Before Being Seen	34,278	3%	2%	2%
Time from ER Arrival to Admit. (minutes)[2]	567	372	280	274
Time from ER Arrival to Discharge (minutes)	382	185	167	134
Time in ER Before Being Evaluated (minutes)	399	69	35	26
Time to Pain Meds for Fractures (minutes)	112	64	56	57
Heart Attack Care				
Aspirin Given at Discharge[1]	-	-	99%	99%
Fibrinolytic Meds Within 30 Min. of Arrival[7]	-	-	75%	54%
PCI Within 90 Minutes of Arrival[7]	-	-	97%	96%
Statin Prescribed at Discharge[1]	-	-	99%	98%
Heart Failure Care				
ACE Inhibitor or ARB for LVSD	36	100%	98%	97%
Discharge Instructions Given	162	96%	95%	94%
Evaluation of LVS Function	194	100%	100%	99%
Medicare Spending				
Medicare Spending per Patient (ratio)	-	0.97	0.95	0.98
Pneumonia Care				
Appropriate Initial Antibiotic Given	110	95%	97%	95%
Blood Culture Timing	172	99%	98%	98%
Pregnancy and Delivery Care				
Newborn Deliveries Scheduled Early	94	27%	6%	6%
Preventive Care				
Immunization for Influenza[2]	522	91%	92%	90%
Immunization for Pneumonia[2]	616	96%	93%	92%
Stroke Care				
Anticoagulation Therapy for Atrial Fibrillation[1]	-	-	96%	95%
Antithrombotic Therapy Timing	65	97%	99%	98%
Assessed for Rehabilitation	67	99%	99%	97%
Discharged on Antithrombotic Therapy	66	100%	100%	99%
Discharged on Statin Medication	57	91%	97%	94%
Thrombolytic Therapy Timing[7]	-	-	73%	66%
Venous Thromboembolism Prophylaxis	69	97%	97%	94%
Written Stroke Educational Materials Given	42	86%	92%	88%
Surgical Care Improvement Project				
Appropriate Beta Blocker Usage	106	96%	99%	98%
Appropriate VTP Within 24 Hours	199	95%	99%	98%
Controlled Postoperative Blood Glucose[7]	-	-	98%	97%
Perioperative Temperature Management	275	99%	100%	100%
Prophylactic Antibiotic Selection	184	99%	99%	99%
Prophylactic Antibiotic Selection (Outpatient)	337	99%	98%	98%
Prophylactic Antibiotic Stopped	180	96%	98%	98%
Prophylactic Antibiotic Timing	184	99%	99%	99%
Prophylactic Antibiotic Timing (Outpatient)	332	98%	98%	98%
Urinary Catheter Removal	195	100%	98%	97%
Survey of Patients' Hospital Experiences				
Area Around Room 'Always' Quiet at Night	300+	61%	60%	61%
Doctors 'Always' Communicated Well	300+	84%	81%	82%
Home Recovery Information Given	300+	87%	86%	85%
Hospital Given 9 or 10 on 10 Point Scale	300+	78%	68%	71%
Meds 'Always' Explained Before Given	300+	68%	62%	64%
Nurses 'Always' Communicated Well	300+	83%	78%	79%
Pain 'Always' Well Controlled	300+	72%	70%	71%
Room and Bathroom 'Always' Clean	300+	72%	71%	73%
Timely Help 'Always' Received	300+	72%	64%	68%
Would Definitely Recommend Hospital	300+	82%	69%	71%
Use of Medical Imaging				
Cardiac Imaging Stress Test before Surgery	520	8.3%	5.1%	5.3%
Combination Abdominal CT Scan	1,001	5.3%	8.5%	10.5%
Combination Brain/Sinus CT Scan	587	2.0%	2.3%	2.7%
Combination Chest CT Scan	736	2.4%	1.6%	2.7%
Follow-up Mammogram/Ultrasound	2,025	5.3%	7.7%	8.8%
Lumbar Spine MRI for Low Back Pain	133	33.1%	35.3%	37.2%

Dickenson Community Hospital

312 Hospital Drive
Clintwood, VA 24228
URL: www.dchosp.com
Phone: 276-926-0300
Fax: 276-926-0329
Type: Critical Access Hospitals
Emergency Services: Yes
Ownership: Voluntary non-profit - Private
Beds: 15

Key Personnel:

Operating Room. . . . . Carman Banks, RN
Radiology. . . . . Mark Blair, RT(R)
Quality Assurance . . . . Joan Curry
CEO/President. . . . . Alan Levine

Measure	Cases	This Hosp.	State Avg.	U.S. Avg.
Blood Clot Prevention and Treatment				
Anticoagulation Overlap Therapy[5]	-	-	95%	93%
ICU Venous Thromboembolism Prophylaxis[5]	-	-	95%	92%
Incidence of Potentially Preventable VTE[5]	-	-	8%	10%
UFH with Dosages/Platelet Monitoring[5]	-	-	99%	97%
Venous Thromboembolism Prophylaxis[5]	-	-	91%	85%
Warfarin Therapy Discharge Instructions[5]	-	-	78%	75%
Chest Pain/Possible Heart Attack Care				
Aspirin Given Within 24 Hours of Arrival	98	99%	98%	96%
Fibrinolytic Meds Within 30 Min. of Arrival[1]	-	-	68%	58%
Average Time to ECG (minutes)	100	4	7	7
Average Time to Transfer (minutes)[1]	-	-	64	60
Children's Asthma Care				
Received Home Management Plan of Care	-	-	-	88%
Received Reliever Medication	-	-	-	100%
Received Systemic Corticosteroids	-	-	-	100%
Emergency Department				
Admittance Decision Time (minutes)[5]	-	-	96	98
Head CT Results Within 45 Min. of Arrival[1]	-	-	60%	57%
Patients Who Left ER Before Being Seen	6,949	0%	2%	2%
Time from ER Arrival to Admit. (minutes)[5]	-	-	280	274
Time from ER Arrival to Discharge (minutes)	217	70	167	134
Time in ER Before Being Evaluated (minutes)	228	15	35	26
Time to Pain Meds for Fractures (minutes)	19	39	56	57
Heart Attack Care				
Aspirin Given at Discharge[5]	-	-	99%	99%
Fibrinolytic Meds Within 30 Min. of Arrival[5]	-	-	75%	54%
PCI Within 90 Minutes of Arrival[5]	-	-	97%	96%
Statin Prescribed at Discharge[5]	-	-	99%	98%
Heart Failure Care				
ACE Inhibitor or ARB for LVSD[5]	-	-	98%	97%
Discharge Instructions Given[5]	-	-	95%	94%
Evaluation of LVS Function[5]	-	-	100%	99%
Medicare Spending				
Medicare Spending per Patient (ratio)	-	-	0.95	0.98
Pneumonia Care				
Appropriate Initial Antibiotic Given[5]	-	-	97%	95%
Blood Culture Timing[5]	-	-	98%	98%
Pregnancy and Delivery Care				
Newborn Deliveries Scheduled Early[7]	-	-	6%	6%
Preventive Care				
Immunization for Influenza[5]	-	-	92%	90%
Immunization for Pneumonia[5]	-	-	93%	92%
Stroke Care				
Anticoagulation Therapy for Atrial Fibrillation[5]	-	-	96%	95%
Antithrombotic Therapy Timing[5]	-	-	99%	98%
Assessed for Rehabilitation[5]	-	-	99%	97%
Discharged on Antithrombotic Therapy[5]	-	-	100%	99%
Discharged on Statin Medication[5]	-	-	97%	94%
Thrombolytic Therapy Timing[5]	-	-	73%	66%
Venous Thromboembolism Prophylaxis[5]	-	-	97%	94%
Written Stroke Educational Materials Given[5]	-	-	92%	88%
Surgical Care Improvement Project				
Appropriate Beta Blocker Usage[5]	-	-	99%	98%
Appropriate VTP Within 24 Hours[5]	-	-	99%	98%
Controlled Postoperative Blood Glucose[5]	-	-	98%	97%
Perioperative Temperature Management[5]	-	-	100%	100%
Prophylactic Antibiotic Selection[5]	-	-	99%	99%
Prophylactic Antibiotic Selection (Outpatient)[5]	-	-	98%	98%
Prophylactic Antibiotic Stopped[5]	-	-	98%	98%
Prophylactic Antibiotic Timing[5]	-	-	99%	99%
Prophylactic Antibiotic Timing (Outpatient)[5]	-	-	98%	98%
Urinary Catheter Removal[5]	-	-	98%	97%
Survey of Patients' Hospital Experiences				
Area Around Room 'Always' Quiet at Night[5]	-	-	60%	61%
Doctors 'Always' Communicated Well[5]	-	-	81%	82%
Home Recovery Information Given[5]	-	-	86%	85%
Hospital Given 9 or 10 on 10 Point Scale[5]	-	-	68%	71%
Meds 'Always' Explained Before Given[5]	-	-	62%	64%
Nurses 'Always' Communicated Well[5]	-	-	78%	79%
Pain 'Always' Well Controlled[5]	-	-	70%	71%
Room and Bathroom 'Always' Clean[5]	-	-	71%	73%
Timely Help 'Always' Received[5]	-	-	64%	68%
Would Definitely Recommend Hospital[5]	-	-	69%	71%
Use of Medical Imaging				
Cardiac Imaging Stress Test before Surgery[7]	-	-	5.1%	5.3%
Combination Abdominal CT Scan	135	0.0%	8.5%	10.5%
Combination Brain/Sinus CT Scan	178	0.6%	2.3%	2.7%
Combination Chest CT Scan	49	0.0%	1.6%	2.7%
Follow-up Mammogram/Ultrasound[1]	-	-	7.7%	8.8%
Lumbar Spine MRI for Low Back Pain[7]	-	-	35.3%	37.2%

Culpeper Regional Hospital

501 Sunset Lane
Culpeper, VA 22701
Phone: 540-829-4100
Fax: 540-829-4353
E-mail: webmaster@culpeperhospital.com
URL: www.culpeperhospital.com
Type: Acute Care Hospitals
Emergency Services: Yes
Ownership: Voluntary non-profit - Other
Beds: 70

Key Personnel:

Operating Room. . . . . Tama Auville
Intensive Care Unit. . . . . Janice Beahm, RN
Emergency Room . . . . Michael Bost, MD
CEO/President. . . . . Larry Fitzgerald
Hemotology Center . . . . Vicki Krohn, RN
Quality Assurance . . . . Patricia Mullins, RN
Infection Control. . . . . Lisa Richardson, RN
Chief of Medical Staff . . . . Sok Yi, MD

Measure	Cases	This Hosp.	State Avg.	U.S. Avg.
Blood Clot Prevention and Treatment				
Anticoagulation Overlap Therapy[2]	29	100%	95%	93%
ICU Venous Thromboembolism Prophylaxis[2]	38	87%	95%	92%
Incidence of Potentially Preventable VTE[1,2]	-	-	8%	10%
UFH with Dosages/Platelet Monitoring[1,2]	-	-	99%	97%
Venous Thromboembolism Prophylaxis[2]	246	92%	91%	85%
Warfarin Therapy Discharge Instructions[2]	23	91%	78%	75%
Chest Pain/Possible Heart Attack Care				
Aspirin Given Within 24 Hours of Arrival	147	99%	98%	96%
Fibrinolytic Meds Within 30 Min. of Arrival[7]	-	-	68%	58%
Average Time to ECG (minutes)	150	15	7	7
Average Time to Transfer (minutes)	15	72	64	60
Children's Asthma Care				
Received Home Management Plan of Care	-	-	-	88%
Received Reliever Medication	-	-	-	100%
Received Systemic Corticosteroids	-	-	-	100%
Emergency Department				
Admittance Decision Time (minutes)[2]	455	40	96	98
Head CT Results Within 45 Min. of Arrival	22	68%	60%	57%
Patients Who Left ER Before Being Seen	31,840	1%	2%	2%
Time from ER Arrival to Admit. (minutes)[2]	455	225	280	274
Time from ER Arrival to Discharge (minutes)	335	124	167	134
Time in ER Before Being Evaluated (minutes)	380	30	35	26
Time to Pain Meds for Fractures (minutes)	90	38	56	57
Heart Attack Care				
Aspirin Given at Discharge	22	95%	99%	99%
Fibrinolytic Meds Within 30 Min. of Arrival[7]	-	-	75%	54%
PCI Within 90 Minutes of Arrival[7]	-	-	97%	96%
Statin Prescribed at Discharge	26	88%	99%	98%
Heart Failure Care				
ACE Inhibitor or ARB for LVSD	38	95%	98%	97%
Discharge Instructions Given	124	90%	95%	94%
Evaluation of LVS Function	154	99%	100%	99%
Medicare Spending				
Medicare Spending per Patient (ratio)	-	0.93	0.95	0.98
Pneumonia Care				

NOTE: Hospital profiles are in alphabetical order by state, then city, then hospital within the city; Rankings exclude hospitals with less than 25 cases except for patient surveys which excludes hospitals with less than 100 cases; (a) 100-299 cases; (1) The number of cases/patients is too few to report; (2) Data submitted were based on a sample of cases/patients; (3) Results are based on a shorter time period than required; (4) Data suppressed by CMS for one or more quarters; (5) Results are not available for this reporting period; (6) Fewer than 100 patients completed the HCAHPS survey; (7) No cases met the criteria for this measure; (8) The lower limit of the confidence interval cannot be calculated if the number of observed infections equals zero; (9) No data are available from the state/territory for this reporting period; (10) The scores shown reflect fewer than 50 completed surveys; (11) There were discrepancies in the data collection process; (12) This measure does not apply to this hospital for this reporting period; (13) Results cannot be calculated for this reporting period; (14) The results for this state are combined with nearby states to protect confidentiality; Please refer to the User's Guide for a full explanation of data.

Measure	Cases	This Hosp.	State Avg.	U.S. Avg.
Appropriate Initial Antibiotic Given	87	95%	97%	95%
Blood Culture Timing	194	95%	98%	98%
Pregnancy and Delivery Care				
Newborn Deliveries Scheduled Early	37	11%	6%	6%
Preventive Care				
Immunization for Influenza[2]	300	94%	92%	90%
Immunization for Pneumonia[2]	399	95%	93%	92%
Stroke Care				
Anticoagulation Therapy for Atrial Fibrillation[1]	-	-	96%	95%
Antithrombotic Therapy Timing	21	100%	99%	98%
Assessed for Rehabilitation	22	100%	99%	97%
Discharged on Antithrombotic Therapy	18	100%	100%	99%
Discharged on Statin Medication	17	71%	97%	94%
Thrombolytic Therapy Timing[7]	-	-	73%	66%
Venous Thromboembolism Prophylaxis	23	96%	97%	94%
Written Stroke Educational Materials Given[1]	-	-	92%	88%
Surgical Care Improvement Project				
Appropriate Beta Blocker Usage	65	97%	99%	98%
Appropriate VTP Within 24 Hours	226	96%	99%	98%
Controlled Postoperative Blood Glucose[7]	-	-	98%	97%
Perioperative Temperature Management	236	100%	100%	100%
Prophylactic Antibiotic Selection	193	97%	99%	99%
Prophylactic Antibiotic Selection (Outpatient)	32	91%	98%	98%
Prophylactic Antibiotic Stopped	191	97%	98%	98%
Prophylactic Antibiotic Timing	197	100%	99%	99%
Prophylactic Antibiotic Timing (Outpatient)	32	100%	98%	98%
Urinary Catheter Removal	207	97%	98%	97%
Survey of Patients' Hospital Experiences				
Area Around Room 'Always' Quiet at Night	300+	56%	60%	61%
Doctors 'Always' Communicated Well	300+	80%	81%	82%
Home Recovery Information Given	300+	86%	86%	85%
Hospital Given 9 or 10 on 10 Point Scale	300+	67%	68%	71%
Meds 'Always' Explained Before Given	300+	63%	62%	64%
Nurses 'Always' Communicated Well	300+	79%	78%	79%
Pain 'Always' Well Controlled	300+	71%	70%	71%
Room and Bathroom 'Always' Clean	300+	77%	71%	73%
Timely Help 'Always' Received	300+	64%	64%	68%
Would Definitely Recommend Hospital	300+	70%	69%	71%
Use of Medical Imaging				
Cardiac Imaging Stress Test before Surgery	79	3.8%	5.1%	5.3%
Combination Abdominal CT Scan	664	2.6%	8.5%	10.5%
Combination Brain/Sinus CT Scan	602	1.5%	2.3%	2.7%
Combination Chest CT Scan	310	0.0%	1.6%	2.7%
Follow-up Mammogram/Ultrasound	697	10.5%	7.7%	8.8%
Lumbar Spine MRI for Low Back Pain	67	26.9%	35.3%	37.2%

Danville Regional Medical Center

142 South Main Street
Danville, VA 24541
URL: www.danvilleregional.org
Type: Acute Care Hospitals
Ownership: Proprietary
Phone: 434-799-2100
Fax: 434-799-4449
Emergency Services: Yes
Beds: 350

Key Personnel:
Emergency Room . . . . Mark Brande
Operating Room. . . . . Kathy Dalton
CEO/President. . . . . Eric Deaton
Quality Assurance . . . . Kim Gibson
Radiology. . . . . Gerald Johnson, MD
Anesthesiology. . . . . Richard Pagano, MD
Chief of Medical Staff . . . . Dr. Saria Saccocio, MD, MHA
Intensive Care Unit. . . . . Tari Wyatt

Measure	Cases	This Hosp.	State Avg.	U.S. Avg.
Blood Clot Prevention and Treatment				
Anticoagulation Overlap Therapy[2]	91	95%	95%	93%
ICU Venous Thromboembolism Prophylaxis[2]	85	98%	95%	92%
Incidence of Potentially Preventable VTE[2]	16	6%	8%	10%
UFH with Dosages/Platelet Monitoring[2]	55	100%	99%	97%
Venous Thromboembolism Prophylaxis[2]	371	95%	91%	85%
Warfarin Therapy Discharge Instructions[2]	55	100%	78%	75%
Chest Pain/Possible Heart Attack Care				
Aspirin Given Within 24 Hours of Arrival	19	100%	98%	96%
Fibrinolytic Meds Within 30 Min. of Arrival[1,3]	-	-	68%	58%
Average Time to ECG (minutes)	19	6	7	7
Average Time to Transfer (minutes)[3,7]	-	-	64	60
Children's Asthma Care				
Received Home Management Plan of Care	-	-	-	88%
Received Reliever Medication	-	-	-	100%
Received Systemic Corticosteroids	-	-	-	100%
Emergency Department				
Admittance Decision Time (minutes)[2]	783	85	96	98
Head CT Results Within 45 Min. of Arrival	22	82%	60%	57%
Patients Who Left ER Before Being Seen	43,244	8%	2%	2%
Time from ER Arrival to Admit. (minutes)[2]	807	265	280	274
Time from ER Arrival to Discharge (minutes)	426	199	167	134
Time in ER Before Being Evaluated (minutes)	460	33	35	26
Time to Pain Meds for Fractures (minutes)	164	60	56	57
Heart Attack Care				
Aspirin Given at Discharge	139	100%	99%	99%
Fibrinolytic Meds Within 30 Min. of Arrival[1]	-	-	75%	54%
PCI Within 90 Minutes of Arrival	26	81%	97%	96%
Statin Prescribed at Discharge	134	100%	99%	98%
Heart Failure Care				
ACE Inhibitor or ARB for LVSD[2]	97	99%	98%	97%
Discharge Instructions Given[2]	204	97%	95%	94%
Evaluation of LVS Function[2]	266	100%	100%	99%
Medicare Spending				
Medicare Spending per Patient (ratio)	-	1.00	0.95	0.98
Pneumonia Care				
Appropriate Initial Antibiotic Given[2]	88	98%	97%	95%
Blood Culture Timing[2]	131	96%	98%	98%
Pregnancy and Delivery Care				
Newborn Deliveries Scheduled Early[2]	36	6%	6%	6%
Preventive Care				
Immunization for Influenza[2]	526	90%	92%	90%
Immunization for Pneumonia[2]	711	94%	93%	92%
Stroke Care				
Anticoagulation Therapy for Atrial Fibrillation[2]	16	100%	96%	95%
Antithrombotic Therapy Timing[2]	104	100%	99%	98%
Assessed for Rehabilitation[2]	107	98%	99%	97%
Discharged on Antithrombotic Therapy[2]	104	98%	100%	99%
Discharged on Statin Medication[2]	80	96%	97%	94%
Thrombolytic Therapy Timing[1,2]	-	-	73%	66%
Venous Thromboembolism Prophylaxis[2]	109	98%	97%	94%
Written Stroke Educational Materials Given[2]	56	95%	92%	88%
Surgical Care Improvement Project				
Appropriate Beta Blocker Usage[2]	105	99%	99%	98%
Appropriate VTP Within 24 Hours[2]	237	98%	99%	98%
Controlled Postoperative Blood Glucose[2]	39	87%	98%	97%
Perioperative Temperature Management[2]	295	100%	100%	100%
Prophylactic Antibiotic Selection[2]	231	99%	99%	99%
Prophylactic Antibiotic Selection (Outpatient)	170	96%	98%	98%
Prophylactic Antibiotic Stopped[2]	226	99%	98%	98%
Prophylactic Antibiotic Timing[2]	231	100%	99%	99%
Prophylactic Antibiotic Timing (Outpatient)	172	95%	98%	98%
Urinary Catheter Removal[2]	88	100%	98%	97%
Survey of Patients' Hospital Experiences				
Area Around Room 'Always' Quiet at Night	300+	61%	60%	61%
Doctors 'Always' Communicated Well	300+	78%	81%	82%
Home Recovery Information Given	300+	82%	86%	85%
Hospital Given 9 or 10 on 10 Point Scale	300+	54%	68%	71%
Meds 'Always' Explained Before Given	300+	57%	62%	64%
Nurses 'Always' Communicated Well	300+	74%	78%	79%
Pain 'Always' Well Controlled	300+	65%	70%	71%
Room and Bathroom 'Always' Clean	300+	69%	71%	73%
Timely Help 'Always' Received	300+	57%	64%	68%
Would Definitely Recommend Hospital	300+	50%	69%	71%
Use of Medical Imaging				
Cardiac Imaging Stress Test before Surgery	200	6.5%	5.1%	5.3%
Combination Abdominal CT Scan	651	7.8%	8.5%	10.5%
Combination Brain/Sinus CT Scan	1,030	0.2%	2.3%	2.7%
Combination Chest CT Scan	379	0.0%	1.6%	2.7%
Follow-up Mammogram/Ultrasound	103	21.4%	7.7%	8.8%
Lumbar Spine MRI for Low Back Pain[1]	-	-	35.3%	37.2%

Southern Virginia Regional Medical Center

727 North Main Street
Emporia, VA 23847
URL: www.svrmc.com
Type: Acute Care Hospitals
Ownership: Proprietary
Phone: 434-348-4400
Fax: 434-348-4982
Emergency Services: Yes
Beds: 80

Key Personnel:
Chief of Medical Staff . . . . Michael Anderson
Hemotology Center . . . . Mary Hackney, MD
Anesthesiology. . . . . Manhal Saleeby, MD
Emergency Room . . . . Iqbal Singh, MD
CEO/President. . . . . Robert D Towler

Measure	Cases	This Hosp.	State Avg.	U.S. Avg.
Blood Clot Prevention and Treatment				
Anticoagulation Overlap Therapy[2]	18	100%	95%	93%
ICU Venous Thromboembolism Prophylaxis[2]	53	100%	95%	92%
Incidence of Potentially Preventable VTE[1,2]	-	-	8%	10%
UFH with Dosages/Platelet Monitoring[1,2]	-	-	99%	97%
Venous Thromboembolism Prophylaxis[2]	344	96%	91%	85%
Warfarin Therapy Discharge Instructions[2]	14	100%	78%	75%
Chest Pain/Possible Heart Attack Care				
Aspirin Given Within 24 Hours of Arrival	49	98%	98%	96%
Fibrinolytic Meds Within 30 Min. of Arrival[7]	-	-	68%	58%
Average Time to ECG (minutes)	50	5	7	7
Average Time to Transfer (minutes)	32	42	64	60
Children's Asthma Care				
Received Home Management Plan of Care	-	-	-	88%
Received Reliever Medication	-	-	-	100%
Received Systemic Corticosteroids	-	-	-	100%
Emergency Department				
Admittance Decision Time (minutes)[2]	578	72	96	98
Head CT Results Within 45 Min. of Arrival	16	94%	60%	57%
Patients Who Left ER Before Being Seen	13,483	2%	2%	2%
Time from ER Arrival to Admit. (minutes)[2]	578	210	280	274
Time from ER Arrival to Discharge (minutes)	390	99	167	134
Time in ER Before Being Evaluated (minutes)	422	18	35	26
Time to Pain Meds for Fractures (minutes)	62	44	56	57
Heart Attack Care				
Aspirin Given at Discharge	14	93%	99%	99%
Fibrinolytic Meds Within 30 Min. of Arrival[7]	-	-	75%	54%
PCI Within 90 Minutes of Arrival[7]	-	-	97%	96%
Statin Prescribed at Discharge	14	100%	99%	98%
Heart Failure Care				
ACE Inhibitor or ARB for LVSD	70	97%	98%	97%
Discharge Instructions Given	150	98%	95%	94%
Evaluation of LVS Function	169	100%	100%	99%
Medicare Spending				
Medicare Spending per Patient (ratio)	-	0.91	0.95	0.98
Pneumonia Care				
Appropriate Initial Antibiotic Given	128	92%	97%	95%
Blood Culture Timing	132	98%	98%	98%
Pregnancy and Delivery Care				
Newborn Deliveries Scheduled Early[2,7]	-	-	6%	6%
Preventive Care				
Immunization for Influenza[2]	304	100%	92%	90%
Immunization for Pneumonia[2]	483	99%	93%	92%
Stroke Care				
Anticoagulation Therapy for Atrial Fibrillation[7]	-	-	96%	95%
Antithrombotic Therapy Timing	26	92%	99%	98%
Assessed for Rehabilitation	25	100%	99%	97%
Discharged on Antithrombotic Therapy	23	96%	100%	99%
Discharged on Statin Medication	19	79%	97%	94%
Thrombolytic Therapy Timing[1]	-	-	73%	66%
Venous Thromboembolism Prophylaxis	27	85%	97%	94%
Written Stroke Educational Materials Given	16	88%	92%	88%
Surgical Care Improvement Project				
Appropriate Beta Blocker Usage	18	83%	99%	98%
Appropriate VTP Within 24 Hours	47	98%	99%	98%
Controlled Postoperative Blood Glucose[7]	-	-	98%	97%
Perioperative Temperature Management	48	100%	100%	100%
Prophylactic Antibiotic Selection	29	100%	99%	99%
Prophylactic Antibiotic Selection (Outpatient)	31	97%	98%	98%
Prophylactic Antibiotic Stopped	28	93%	98%	98%

NOTE: Hospital profiles are in alphabetical order by state, then city, then hospital within the city; Rankings exclude hospitals with less than 25 cases except for patient surveys which excludes hospitals with less than 100 cases; (a) 100-299 cases; (1) The number of cases/patients is too few to report; (2) Data submitted were based on a sample of cases/patients; (3) Results are based on a shorter time period than required; (4) Data suppressed by CMS for one or more quarters; (5) Results are not available for this reporting period; (6) Fewer than 100 patients completed the HCAHPS survey; (7) No cases met the criteria for this measure; (8) The lower limit of the confidence interval cannot be calculated if the number of observed infections equals zero; (9) No data are available from the state/territory for this reporting period; (10) The scores shown reflect fewer than 50 completed surveys; (11) There were discrepancies in the data collection process; (12) This measure does not apply to this hospital for this reporting period; (13) Results cannot be calculated for this reporting period; (14) The results for this state are combined with nearby states to protect confidentiality; Please refer to the User's Guide for a full explanation of data.

Prophylactic Antibiotic Timing	29	97%	99%	99%
Prophylactic Antibiotic Timing (Outpatient)[1]	-	-	98%	98%
Urinary Catheter Removal	33	97%	98%	97%
Survey of Patients' Hospital Experiences				
Area Around Room 'Always' Quiet at Night	300+	71%	60%	61%
Doctors 'Always' Communicated Well	300+	83%	81%	82%
Home Recovery Information Given	300+	80%	86%	85%
Hospital Given 9 or 10 on 10 Point Scale	300+	60%	68%	71%
Meds 'Always' Explained Before Given	300+	64%	62%	64%
Nurses 'Always' Communicated Well	300+	70%	78%	79%
Pain 'Always' Well Controlled	300+	64%	70%	71%
Room and Bathroom 'Always' Clean	300+	67%	71%	73%
Timely Help 'Always' Received	300+	51%	64%	68%
Would Definitely Recommend Hospital	300+	50%	69%	71%
Use of Medical Imaging				
Cardiac Imaging Stress Test before Surgery	103	2.9%	5.1%	5.3%
Combination Abdominal CT Scan	220	9.5%	8.5%	10.5%
Combination Brain/Sinus CT Scan[1]	-	-	2.3%	2.7%
Combination Chest CT Scan	97	0.0%	1.6%	2.7%
Follow-up Mammogram/Ultrasound	467	4.9%	7.7%	8.8%
Lumbar Spine MRI for Low Back Pain[1]	-	-	35.3%	37.2%

Inova Fair Oaks Hospital

3600 Joseph Siewick Drive Phone: 703-391-4170
Fairfax, VA 22033 Fax: 703-391-3273
URL: www.inova.org/inovapublic.srt/ifoh/index.jsp
Type: Acute Care Hospitals Emergency Services: Yes
Ownership: Voluntary non-profit - Other Beds: 160

Key Personnel:

Quality Assurance . . . . Robbin Bixler
Anesthesiology. . . . . Ricky Lee Ramsey, MD
Emergency Room . . . . Ellen Ruja
Pediatric Ambulatory Care . . . . . . Alan E Silk, MD
Pediatric In-Patient Care . . . . Alan E Silk, MD
Chair/CEO . . . . J. Knox Singleton
Chief of Medical Staff. . . . . Jay Tyroller, MD
Intensive Care Unit. . . . . Megan Winegarden

Measure	Cases	This Hosp.	State Avg.	U.S. Avg.
Blood Clot Prevention and Treatment				
Anticoagulation Overlap Therapy[2]	77	86%	95%	93%
ICU Venous Thromboembolism Prophylaxis[2]	41	100%	95%	92%
Incidence of Potentially Preventable VTE[2]	17	24%	8%	10%
UFH with Dosages/Platelet Monitoring[2]	18	100%	99%	97%
Venous Thromboembolism Prophylaxis[2]	318	90%	91%	85%
Warfarin Therapy Discharge Instructions[2]	59	66%	78%	75%
Chest Pain/Possible Heart Attack Care				
Aspirin Given Within 24 Hours of Arrival	66	100%	98%	96%
Fibrinolytic Meds Within 30 Min. of Arrival[7]	-	-	68%	58%
Average Time to ECG (minutes)	66	10	7	7
Average Time to Transfer (minutes)[7]	-	-	64	60
Children's Asthma Care				
Received Home Management Plan of Care	-	-	-	88%
Received Reliever Medication	-	-	-	100%
Received Systemic Corticosteroids	-	-	-	100%
Emergency Department				
Admittance Decision Time (minutes)[2]	408	74	96	98
Head CT Results Within 45 Min. of Arrival[1]	-	-	60%	57%
Patients Who Left ER Before Being Seen	55,831	0%	2%	2%
Time from ER Arrival to Admit. (minutes)[2]	408	245	280	274
Time from ER Arrival to Discharge (minutes)	715	137	167	134
Time in ER Before Being Evaluated (minutes)	735	29	35	26
Time to Pain Meds for Fractures (minutes)	245	46	56	57
Heart Attack Care				
Aspirin Given at Discharge	19	95%	99%	99%
Fibrinolytic Meds Within 30 Min. of Arrival[7]	-	-	75%	54%
PCI Within 90 Minutes of Arrival[7]	-	-	97%	96%
Statin Prescribed at Discharge	18	100%	99%	98%
Heart Failure Care				
ACE Inhibitor or ARB for LVSD	22	95%	98%	97%
Discharge Instructions Given	151	92%	95%	94%
Evaluation of LVS Function	177	100%	100%	99%
Medicare Spending				
Medicare Spending per Patient (ratio)	-	0.95	0.95	0.98
Pneumonia Care				
Appropriate Initial Antibiotic Given[2]	109	98%	97%	95%
Blood Culture Timing[2]	154	99%	98%	98%
Pregnancy and Delivery Care				
Newborn Deliveries Scheduled Early[2]	251	7%	6%	6%
Preventive Care				
Immunization for Influenza[2]	462	91%	92%	90%
Immunization for Pneumonia[2]	368	91%	93%	92%
Stroke Care				
Anticoagulation Therapy for Atrial Fibrillation[1]	-	-	96%	95%
Antithrombotic Therapy Timing	62	100%	99%	98%
Assessed for Rehabilitation	68	99%	99%	97%
Discharged on Antithrombotic Therapy	60	100%	100%	99%
Discharged on Statin Medication	50	96%	97%	94%
Thrombolytic Therapy Timing[1]	-	-	73%	66%
Venous Thromboembolism Prophylaxis	69	94%	97%	94%
Written Stroke Educational Materials Given	49	94%	92%	88%
Surgical Care Improvement Project				
Appropriate Beta Blocker Usage[2]	95	99%	99%	98%
Appropriate VTP Within 24 Hours[2]	333	99%	99%	98%
Controlled Postoperative Blood Glucose[2,7]	-	-	98%	97%
Perioperative Temperature Management[2]	412	100%	100%	100%
Prophylactic Antibiotic Selection[2]	260	98%	99%	99%
Prophylactic Antibiotic Selection (Outpatient)	548	99%	98%	98%
Prophylactic Antibiotic Stopped[2]	257	96%	98%	98%
Prophylactic Antibiotic Timing[2]	261	98%	99%	99%
Prophylactic Antibiotic Timing (Outpatient)	545	100%	98%	98%
Urinary Catheter Removal[2]	250	98%	98%	97%
Survey of Patients' Hospital Experiences				
Area Around Room 'Always' Quiet at Night	300+	56%	60%	61%
Doctors 'Always' Communicated Well	300+	78%	81%	82%
Home Recovery Information Given	300+	84%	86%	85%
Hospital Given 9 or 10 on 10 Point Scale	300+	73%	68%	71%
Meds 'Always' Explained Before Given	300+	61%	62%	64%
Nurses 'Always' Communicated Well	300+	76%	78%	79%
Pain 'Always' Well Controlled	300+	67%	70%	71%
Room and Bathroom 'Always' Clean	300+	66%	71%	73%
Timely Help 'Always' Received	300+	59%	64%	68%
Would Definitely Recommend Hospital	300+	78%	69%	71%
Use of Medical Imaging				
Cardiac Imaging Stress Test before Surgery[1]	-	-	5.1%	5.3%
Combination Abdominal CT Scan	665	3.2%	8.5%	10.5%
Combination Brain/Sinus CT Scan	787	3.4%	2.3%	2.7%
Combination Chest CT Scan	310	1.3%	1.6%	2.7%
Follow-up Mammogram/Ultrasound	339	9.4%	7.7%	8.8%
Lumbar Spine MRI for Low Back Pain	155	34.8%	35.3%	37.2%

Inova Fairfax Hospital

8110 Gatehouse Road, 400 West Phone: 703-776-3332
Falls Church, VA 22042 Fax: 703-776-3623
URL: www.inova.org
Type: Acute Care Hospitals Emergency Services: Yes
Ownership: Voluntary non-profit - Other Beds: 833

Key Personnel:

Chairman/CEO . . . . Nicholas Carosi
Emergency Room . . . . Robert Cates, MD
CEO . . . . Patrick Christiansen
Chief of Medical Staff. . . . . F Joseph Hallal
Infection Control. . . . . Allan J Morrison, MD
CEO/President. . . . . Mark Stauder
Quality Assurance . . . . Betty Ann Wilkins

Measure	Cases	This Hosp.	State Avg.	U.S. Avg.
Blood Clot Prevention and Treatment				
Anticoagulation Overlap Therapy[2]	245	99%	95%	93%
ICU Venous Thromboembolism Prophylaxis[2]	85	93%	95%	92%
Incidence of Potentially Preventable VTE[2]	69	19%	8%	10%
UFH with Dosages/Platelet Monitoring[2]	144	100%	99%	97%
Venous Thromboembolism Prophylaxis[2]	322	86%	91%	85%
Warfarin Therapy Discharge Instructions[2]	174	56%	78%	75%
Chest Pain/Possible Heart Attack Care				
Aspirin Given Within 24 Hours of Arrival	29	93%	98%	96%
Fibrinolytic Meds Within 30 Min. of Arrival[5]	-	-	68%	58%
Average Time to ECG (minutes)	29	14	7	7
Average Time to Transfer (minutes)[5]	-	-	64	60
Children's Asthma Care				
Received Home Management Plan of Care[2]	198	95%	-	88%
Received Reliever Medication[2]	199	100%	-	100%
Received Systemic Corticosteroids[2]	199	99%	-	100%
Emergency Department				
Admittance Decision Time (minutes)[2]	443	134	96	98
Head CT Results Within 45 Min. of Arrival[1]	-	-	60%	57%
Patients Who Left ER Before Being Seen	>100k	1%	2%	2%
Time from ER Arrival to Admit. (minutes)[2]	465	342	280	274
Time from ER Arrival to Discharge (minutes)	862	144	167	134
Time in ER Before Being Evaluated (minutes)	934	34	35	26
Time to Pain Meds for Fractures (minutes)	454	54	56	57
Heart Attack Care				
Aspirin Given at Discharge[2]	290	98%	99%	99%
Fibrinolytic Meds Within 30 Min. of Arrival[2,7]	-	-	75%	54%
PCI Within 90 Minutes of Arrival[2]	52	98%	97%	96%
Statin Prescribed at Discharge[2]	286	99%	99%	98%
Heart Failure Care				
ACE Inhibitor or ARB for LVSD[2]	104	93%	98%	97%
Discharge Instructions Given[2]	249	57%	95%	94%
Evaluation of LVS Function[2]	295	98%	100%	99%
Medicare Spending				
Medicare Spending per Patient (ratio)	-	0.98	0.95	0.98
Pneumonia Care				
Appropriate Initial Antibiotic Given[2]	66	95%	97%	95%
Blood Culture Timing[2]	103	94%	98%	98%
Pregnancy and Delivery Care				
Newborn Deliveries Scheduled Early[2]	439	10%	6%	6%
Preventive Care				
Immunization for Influenza[2]	480	88%	92%	90%
Immunization for Pneumonia[2]	401	85%	93%	92%
Stroke Care				
Anticoagulation Therapy for Atrial Fibrillation[2]	24	92%	96%	95%
Antithrombotic Therapy Timing[2]	146	100%	99%	98%
Assessed for Rehabilitation[2]	244	98%	99%	97%
Discharged on Antithrombotic Therapy[2]	168	98%	100%	99%
Discharged on Statin Medication[2]	152	93%	97%	94%
Thrombolytic Therapy Timing[2]	22	55%	73%	66%
Venous Thromboembolism Prophylaxis[2]	265	98%	97%	94%
Written Stroke Educational Materials Given[2]	118	89%	92%	88%
Surgical Care Improvement Project				
Appropriate Beta Blocker Usage[2]	246	96%	99%	98%
Appropriate VTP Within 24 Hours[2]	440	97%	99%	98%
Controlled Postoperative Blood Glucose[2]	155	99%	98%	97%
Perioperative Temperature Management[2]	612	98%	100%	100%
Prophylactic Antibiotic Selection[2]	518	99%	99%	99%
Prophylactic Antibiotic Selection (Outpatient)	941	99%	98%	98%
Prophylactic Antibiotic Stopped[2]	506	97%	98%	98%
Prophylactic Antibiotic Timing[2]	519	98%	99%	99%
Prophylactic Antibiotic Timing (Outpatient)	949	98%	98%	98%
Urinary Catheter Removal[2]	427	95%	98%	97%
Survey of Patients' Hospital Experiences				
Area Around Room 'Always' Quiet at Night	300+	50%	60%	61%
Doctors 'Always' Communicated Well	300+	76%	81%	82%
Home Recovery Information Given	300+	83%	86%	85%
Hospital Given 9 or 10 on 10 Point Scale	300+	65%	68%	71%
Meds 'Always' Explained Before Given	300+	60%	62%	64%
Nurses 'Always' Communicated Well	300+	72%	78%	79%
Pain 'Always' Well Controlled	300+	65%	70%	71%
Room and Bathroom 'Always' Clean	300+	64%	71%	73%
Timely Help 'Always' Received	300+	54%	64%	68%
Would Definitely Recommend Hospital	300+	75%	69%	71%
Use of Medical Imaging				
Cardiac Imaging Stress Test before Surgery	256	5.1%	5.1%	5.3%
Combination Abdominal CT Scan	1,038	1.3%	8.5%	10.5%
Combination Brain/Sinus CT Scan	1,875	2.9%	2.3%	2.7%
Combination Chest CT Scan	499	0.2%	1.6%	2.7%
Follow-up Mammogram/Ultrasound	68	4.4%	7.7%	8.8%
Lumbar Spine MRI for Low Back Pain[1]	-	-	35.3%	37.2%

NOTE: Hospital profiles are in alphabetical order by state, then city, then hospital within the city; Rankings exclude hospitals with less than 25 cases except for patient surveys which excludes hospitals with less than 100 cases; (a) 100-299 cases; (1) The number of cases/patients is too few to report; (2) Data submitted were based on a sample of cases/patients; (3) Results are based on a shorter time period than required; (4) Data suppressed by CMS for one or more quarters; (5) Results are not available for this reporting period; (6) Fewer than 100 patients completed the HCAHPS survey; (7) No cases met the criteria for this measure; (8) The lower limit of the confidence interval cannot be calculated if the number of observed infections equals zero; (9) No data are available from the state/territory for this reporting period; (10) The scores shown reflect fewer than 50 completed surveys; (11) There were discrepancies in the data collection process; (12) This measure does not apply to this hospital for this reporting period; (13) Results cannot be calculated for this reporting period; (14) The results for this state are combined with nearby states to protect confidentiality; Please refer to the User's Guide for a full explanation of data.

Southside Community Hospital

800 Oak Street
Farmville, VA 23901
E-mail: info@sch-farmville.org
URL: www.sch-farmville.org
Type: Acute Care Hospitals
Ownership: Voluntary non-profit - Other

Phone: 434-392-8811
Fax: 434-315-2581

Emergency Services: Yes
Beds: 116

Key Personnel:
Chief of Medical Staff.......... Charles Anderson, MD
CEO/President............... Gwen Eddleman, EdD
Emergency Room .... Kathleen Manis
Quality Assurance .... Judy Neller

Measure	Cases	This Hosp.	State Avg.	U.S. Avg.
Blood Clot Prevention and Treatment				
Anticoagulation Overlap Therapy[2]	26	92%	95%	93%
ICU Venous Thromboembolism Prophylaxis[2]	86	85%	95%	92%
Incidence of Potentially Preventable VTE[1,2]	-	-	8%	10%
UFH with Dosages/Platelet Monitoring[1,2]	-	-	99%	97%
Venous Thromboembolism Prophylaxis[2]	345	76%	91%	85%
Warfarin Therapy Discharge Instructions[2]	21	10%	78%	75%
Chest Pain/Possible Heart Attack Care				
Aspirin Given Within 24 Hours of Arrival	118	96%	98%	96%
Fibrinolytic Meds Within 30 Min. of Arrival[1]	-	-	68%	58%
Average Time to ECG (minutes)	132	5	7	7
Average Time to Transfer (minutes)	15	63	64	60
Children's Asthma Care				
Received Home Management Plan of Care	-	-	-	88%
Received Reliever Medication	-	-	-	100%
Received Systemic Corticosteroids	-	-	-	100%
Emergency Department				
Admittance Decision Time (minutes)[2]	684	73	96	98
Head CT Results Within 45 Min. of Arrival	13	62%	60%	57%
Patients Who Left ER Before Being Seen	33,232	1%	2%	2%
Time from ER Arrival to Admit. (minutes)[2]	695	234	280	274
Time from ER Arrival to Discharge (minutes)	387	130	167	134
Time in ER Before Being Evaluated (minutes)	377	56	35	26
Time to Pain Meds for Fractures (minutes)	78	40	56	57
Heart Attack Care				
Aspirin Given at Discharge	18	100%	99%	99%
Fibrinolytic Meds Within 30 Min. of Arrival[7]	-	-	75%	54%
PCI Within 90 Minutes of Arrival[7]	-	-	97%	96%
Statin Prescribed at Discharge	18	94%	99%	98%
Heart Failure Care				
ACE Inhibitor or ARB for LVSD	78	88%	98%	97%
Discharge Instructions Given	142	70%	95%	94%
Evaluation of LVS Function	187	100%	100%	99%
Medicare Spending				
Medicare Spending per Patient (ratio)	-	1.01	0.95	0.98
Pneumonia Care				
Appropriate Initial Antibiotic Given	96	93%	97%	95%
Blood Culture Timing	169	98%	98%	98%
Pregnancy and Delivery Care				
Newborn Deliveries Scheduled Early	57	7%	6%	6%
Preventive Care				
Immunization for Influenza[2]	469	90%	92%	90%
Immunization for Pneumonia[2]	615	95%	93%	92%
Stroke Care				
Anticoagulation Therapy for Atrial Fibrillation[1]	-	-	96%	95%
Antithrombotic Therapy Timing	35	91%	99%	98%
Assessed for Rehabilitation	40	98%	99%	97%
Discharged on Antithrombotic Therapy	40	100%	100%	99%
Discharged on Statin Medication	31	97%	97%	94%
Thrombolytic Therapy Timing[7]	-	-	73%	66%
Venous Thromboembolism Prophylaxis	35	89%	97%	94%
Written Stroke Educational Materials Given	20	10%	92%	88%
Surgical Care Improvement Project				
Appropriate Beta Blocker Usage	31	97%	99%	98%
Appropriate VTP Within 24 Hours	105	96%	99%	98%
Controlled Postoperative Blood Glucose[7]	-	-	98%	97%
Perioperative Temperature Management	123	100%	100%	100%
Prophylactic Antibiotic Selection	72	100%	99%	99%
Prophylactic Antibiotic Selection (Outpatient)	20	95%	98%	98%
Prophylactic Antibiotic Stopped	67	96%	98%	98%
Prophylactic Antibiotic Timing	72	97%	99%	99%
Prophylactic Antibiotic Timing (Outpatient)	17	82%	98%	98%
Urinary Catheter Removal	72	93%	98%	97%
Survey of Patients' Hospital Experiences				
Area Around Room 'Always' Quiet at Night	300+	59%	60%	61%
Doctors 'Always' Communicated Well	300+	81%	81%	82%
Home Recovery Information Given	300+	87%	86%	85%
Hospital Given 9 or 10 on 10 Point Scale	300+	60%	68%	71%
Meds 'Always' Explained Before Given	300+	63%	62%	64%
Nurses 'Always' Communicated Well	300+	77%	78%	79%
Pain 'Always' Well Controlled	300+	70%	70%	71%
Room and Bathroom 'Always' Clean	300+	75%	71%	73%
Timely Help 'Always' Received	300+	62%	64%	68%
Would Definitely Recommend Hospital	300+	58%	69%	71%
Use of Medical Imaging				
Cardiac Imaging Stress Test before Surgery	195	4.1%	5.1%	5.3%
Combination Abdominal CT Scan	627	5.4%	8.5%	10.5%
Combination Brain/Sinus CT Scan	700	1.3%	2.3%	2.7%
Combination Chest CT Scan	299	4.3%	1.6%	2.7%
Follow-up Mammogram/Ultrasound	628	12.6%	7.7%	8.8%
Lumbar Spine MRI for Low Back Pain	61	37.7%	35.3%	37.2%

Augusta Health

78 Medical Center Drive
Fishersville, VA 22939
URL: www.augustamed.com
Type: Acute Care Hospitals
Ownership: Voluntary non-profit - Private

Phone: 540-932-4000
Fax: 540-332-4809

Emergency Services: Yes
Beds: 255

Key Personnel:
Anesthesiology................ Louis Chaldars, MD
CEO/President............... Richard Graham
Pediatric Ambulatory Care ...... Robert Gunther, MD
Pediatric In-Patient Care .... Robert Gunther, MD
Infection Control.............. Carolyn Palmer, RN
Chief of Medical Staff.......... Joseph Ranzini
Radiology.................. David Tempkin, MD
Emergency Room .... Sally Tucker, MD

Measure	Cases	This Hosp.	State Avg.	U.S. Avg.
Blood Clot Prevention and Treatment				
Anticoagulation Overlap Therapy[2]	80	92%	95%	93%
ICU Venous Thromboembolism Prophylaxis[2]	20	100%	95%	92%
Incidence of Potentially Preventable VTE[2]	12	0%	8%	10%
UFH with Dosages/Platelet Monitoring[2]	39	95%	99%	97%
Venous Thromboembolism Prophylaxis[2]	312	90%	91%	85%
Warfarin Therapy Discharge Instructions[2]	67	73%	78%	75%
Chest Pain/Possible Heart Attack Care				
Aspirin Given Within 24 Hours of Arrival	24	100%	98%	96%
Fibrinolytic Meds Within 30 Min. of Arrival[3,7]	-	-	68%	58%
Average Time to ECG (minutes)	24	8	7	7
Average Time to Transfer (minutes)[3,7]	-	-	64	60
Children's Asthma Care				
Received Home Management Plan of Care	-	-	-	88%
Received Reliever Medication	-	-	-	100%
Received Systemic Corticosteroids	-	-	-	100%
Emergency Department				
Admittance Decision Time (minutes)[2]	603	77	96	98
Head CT Results Within 45 Min. of Arrival	14	43%	60%	57%
Patients Who Left ER Before Being Seen	65,455	3%	2%	2%
Time from ER Arrival to Admit. (minutes)[2]	612	262	280	274
Time from ER Arrival to Discharge (minutes)	439	140	167	134
Time in ER Before Being Evaluated (minutes)	390	22	35	26
Time to Pain Meds for Fractures (minutes)	165	64	56	57
Heart Attack Care				
Aspirin Given at Discharge	222	100%	99%	99%
Fibrinolytic Meds Within 30 Min. of Arrival[7]	-	-	75%	54%
PCI Within 90 Minutes of Arrival	67	100%	97%	96%
Statin Prescribed at Discharge	218	99%	99%	98%
Heart Failure Care				
ACE Inhibitor or ARB for LVSD	96	100%	98%	97%
Discharge Instructions Given	299	96%	95%	94%
Evaluation of LVS Function	394	100%	100%	99%
Medicare Spending				
Medicare Spending per Patient (ratio)	-	0.91	0.95	0.98
Pneumonia Care				
Appropriate Initial Antibiotic Given	170	99%	97%	95%
Blood Culture Timing	330	99%	98%	98%
Pregnancy and Delivery Care				
Newborn Deliveries Scheduled Early[2]	22	9%	6%	6%
Preventive Care				
Immunization for Influenza[2]	543	89%	92%	90%
Immunization for Pneumonia[2]	741	92%	93%	92%
Stroke Care				
Anticoagulation Therapy for Atrial Fibrillation[2]	21	100%	96%	95%
Antithrombotic Therapy Timing[2]	79	99%	99%	98%
Assessed for Rehabilitation[2]	107	97%	99%	97%
Discharged on Antithrombotic Therapy[2]	104	100%	100%	99%
Discharged on Statin Medication[2]	70	97%	97%	94%
Thrombolytic Therapy Timing[2]	26	23%	73%	66%
Venous Thromboembolism Prophylaxis[2]	88	100%	97%	94%
Written Stroke Educational Materials Given[2]	51	86%	92%	88%
Surgical Care Improvement Project				
Appropriate Beta Blocker Usage	319	97%	99%	98%
Appropriate VTP Within 24 Hours	950	98%	99%	98%
Controlled Postoperative Blood Glucose[7]	-	-	98%	97%
Perioperative Temperature Management	1,086	100%	100%	100%
Prophylactic Antibiotic Selection	864	100%	99%	99%
Prophylactic Antibiotic Selection (Outpatient)	269	99%	98%	98%
Prophylactic Antibiotic Stopped	847	98%	98%	98%
Prophylactic Antibiotic Timing	865	99%	99%	99%
Prophylactic Antibiotic Timing (Outpatient)	269	98%	98%	98%
Urinary Catheter Removal	868	99%	98%	97%
Survey of Patients' Hospital Experiences				
Area Around Room 'Always' Quiet at Night	300+	50%	60%	61%
Doctors 'Always' Communicated Well	300+	82%	81%	82%
Home Recovery Information Given	300+	87%	86%	85%
Hospital Given 9 or 10 on 10 Point Scale	300+	67%	68%	71%
Meds 'Always' Explained Before Given	300+	61%	62%	64%
Nurses 'Always' Communicated Well	300+	76%	78%	79%
Pain 'Always' Well Controlled	300+	68%	70%	71%
Room and Bathroom 'Always' Clean	300+	68%	71%	73%
Timely Help 'Always' Received	300+	59%	64%	68%
Would Definitely Recommend Hospital	300+	70%	69%	71%
Use of Medical Imaging				
Cardiac Imaging Stress Test before Surgery	596	3.7%	5.1%	5.3%
Combination Abdominal CT Scan	1,775	13.3%	8.5%	10.5%
Combination Brain/Sinus CT Scan	1,057	1.6%	2.3%	2.7%
Combination Chest CT Scan	1,317	0.4%	1.6%	2.7%
Follow-up Mammogram/Ultrasound	3,427	14.0%	7.7%	8.8%
Lumbar Spine MRI for Low Back Pain	311	40.2%	35.3%	37.2%

Southampton Memorial Hospital

100 Fairview Drive - PO Box 817
Franklin, VA 23851
URL: www.smhfranklin.com
Type: Acute Care Hospitals
Ownership: Proprietary

Phone: 757-569-6100
Fax: 757-569-6390

Emergency Services: Yes
Beds: 221

Key Personnel:
Pediatric Ambulatory Care ...... Mike Cicero
Pediatric In-Patient Care .... Mike Cicero
CEO/President............... Gwen Eddleman
Chief of Medical Staff.......... Rich Holm, MD
Operating Room.............. Gregory Johnson
Emergency Room .... David Sields, RN
Quality Assurance .... Margie Wilson

Measure	Cases	This Hosp.	State Avg.	U.S. Avg.
Blood Clot Prevention and Treatment				
Anticoagulation Overlap Therapy[2]	21	90%	95%	93%
ICU Venous Thromboembolism Prophylaxis[2]	58	100%	95%	92%
Incidence of Potentially Preventable VTE[1,2]	-	-	8%	10%
UFH with Dosages/Platelet Monitoring[1,2]	-	-	99%	97%
Venous Thromboembolism Prophylaxis[2]	218	91%	91%	85%
Warfarin Therapy Discharge Instructions[2]	15	93%	78%	75%
Chest Pain/Possible Heart Attack Care				
Aspirin Given Within 24 Hours of Arrival	50	98%	98%	96%
Fibrinolytic Meds Within 30 Min. of Arrival[1]	-	-	68%	58%
Average Time to ECG (minutes)	52	6	7	7
Average Time to Transfer (minutes)[1]	-	-	64	60
Children's Asthma Care				

NOTE: Hospital profiles are in alphabetical order by state, then city, then hospital within the city; Rankings exclude hospitals with less than 25 cases except for patient surveys which excludes hospitals with less than 100 cases; (a) 100-299 cases; (1) The number of cases/patients is too few to report; (2) Data submitted were based on a sample of cases/patients; (3) Results are based on a shorter time period than required; (4) Data suppressed by CMS for one or more quarters; (5) Results are not available for this reporting period; (6) Fewer than 100 patients completed the HCAHPS survey; (7) No cases met the criteria for this measure; (8) The lower limit of the confidence interval cannot be calculated if the number of observed infections equals zero; (9) No data are available from the state/territory for this reporting period; (10) The scores shown reflect fewer than 50 completed surveys; (11) There were discrepancies in the data collection process; (12) This measure does not apply to this hospital for this reporting period; (13) Results cannot be calculated for this reporting period; (14) The results for this state are combined with nearby states to protect confidentiality; Please refer to the User's Guide for a full explanation of data.

Measure	Cases	This Hosp.	State Avg.	U.S. Avg.
Received Home Management Plan of Care	-	-	-	88%
Received Reliever Medication	-	-	-	100%
Received Systemic Corticosteroids	-	-	-	100%
Emergency Department				
Admittance Decision Time (minutes)[2]	412	70	96	98
Head CT Results Within 45 Min. of Arrival[1]	-	-	60%	57%
Patients Who Left ER Before Being Seen	14,833	1%	2%	2%
Time from ER Arrival to Admit. (minutes)[2]	438	238	280	274
Time from ER Arrival to Discharge (minutes)	396	131	167	134
Time in ER Before Being Evaluated (minutes)	409	26	35	26
Time to Pain Meds for Fractures (minutes)	42	38	56	57
Heart Attack Care				
Aspirin Given at Discharge[1]	-	-	99%	99%
Fibrinolytic Meds Within 30 Min. of Arrival[7]	-	-	75%	54%
PCI Within 90 Minutes of Arrival[7]	-	-	97%	96%
Statin Prescribed at Discharge[1]	-	-	99%	98%
Heart Failure Care				
ACE Inhibitor or ARB for LVSD	40	100%	98%	97%
Discharge Instructions Given	75	92%	95%	94%
Evaluation of LVS Function	90	100%	100%	99%
Medicare Spending				
Medicare Spending per Patient (ratio)	-	0.87	0.95	0.98
Pneumonia Care				
Appropriate Initial Antibiotic Given	37	92%	97%	95%
Blood Culture Timing	75	95%	98%	98%
Pregnancy and Delivery Care				
Newborn Deliveries Scheduled Early[2]	28	0%	6%	6%
Preventive Care				
Immunization for Influenza[2]	312	99%	92%	90%
Immunization for Pneumonia[2]	406	99%	93%	92%
Stroke Care				
Anticoagulation Therapy for Atrial Fibrillation[1]	-	-	96%	95%
Antithrombotic Therapy Timing	30	93%	99%	98%
Assessed for Rehabilitation	31	100%	99%	97%
Discharged on Antithrombotic Therapy	29	97%	100%	99%
Discharged on Statin Medication	24	100%	97%	94%
Thrombolytic Therapy Timing[1]	-	-	73%	66%
Venous Thromboembolism Prophylaxis	33	82%	97%	94%
Written Stroke Educational Materials Given	18	61%	92%	88%
Surgical Care Improvement Project				
Appropriate Beta Blocker Usage	29	97%	99%	98%
Appropriate VTP Within 24 Hours	118	98%	99%	98%
Controlled Postoperative Blood Glucose[7]	-	-	98%	97%
Perioperative Temperature Management	125	99%	100%	100%
Prophylactic Antibiotic Selection	105	94%	99%	99%
Prophylactic Antibiotic Selection (Outpatient)	45	98%	98%	98%
Prophylactic Antibiotic Stopped	99	91%	98%	98%
Prophylactic Antibiotic Timing	105	99%	99%	99%
Prophylactic Antibiotic Timing (Outpatient)[1]	-	-	98%	98%
Urinary Catheter Removal	12	100%	98%	97%
Survey of Patients' Hospital Experiences				
Area Around Room 'Always' Quiet at Night	300+	65%	60%	61%
Doctors 'Always' Communicated Well	300+	80%	81%	82%
Home Recovery Information Given	300+	86%	86%	85%
Hospital Given 9 or 10 on 10 Point Scale	300+	66%	68%	71%
Meds 'Always' Explained Before Given	300+	63%	62%	64%
Nurses 'Always' Communicated Well	300+	78%	78%	79%
Pain 'Always' Well Controlled	300+	71%	70%	71%
Room and Bathroom 'Always' Clean	300+	71%	71%	73%
Timely Help 'Always' Received	300+	66%	64%	68%
Would Definitely Recommend Hospital	300+	57%	69%	71%
Use of Medical Imaging				
Cardiac Imaging Stress Test before Surgery	221	3.6%	5.1%	5.3%
Combination Abdominal CT Scan	371	12.1%	8.5%	10.5%
Combination Brain/Sinus CT Scan[1]	-	-	2.3%	2.7%
Combination Chest CT Scan	170	2.4%	1.6%	2.7%
Follow-up Mammogram/Ultrasound	465	5.6%	7.7%	8.8%
Lumbar Spine MRI for Low Back Pain[1]	-	-	35.3%	37.2%

Mary Washington Hospital

1001 Sam Perry Boulevard
Fredericksburg, VA 22401
Phone: 540-741-1100
Fax: 540-741-2571
URL: www.medicorp.org
Type: Acute Care Hospitals
Emergency Services: Yes
Ownership: Voluntary non-profit - Private
Beds: 412

Key Personnel:
Chief of Medical Staff.......... Rebecca Bigoney, MD
Operating Room.............. Elyse Dorman
Ambulatory Care .... Marie Fredrick
Radiology.................... Michael Hewitt
CEO/President............... Fred M. Rankin, III
Pediatric Ambulatory Care ...... Claudia Sussdorf
Pediatric In-Patient Care .... Claudia Sussdorf
Quality Assurance .... Linda Wallace

Measure	Cases	This Hosp.	State Avg.	U.S. Avg.
Blood Clot Prevention and Treatment				
Anticoagulation Overlap Therapy[2]	154	100%	95%	93%
ICU Venous Thromboembolism Prophylaxis[2]	65	98%	95%	92%
Incidence of Potentially Preventable VTE[2]	33	0%	8%	10%
UFH with Dosages/Platelet Monitoring[2]	53	100%	99%	97%
Venous Thromboembolism Prophylaxis[2]	365	100%	91%	85%
Warfarin Therapy Discharge Instructions[2]	112	11%	78%	75%
Chest Pain/Possible Heart Attack Care				
Aspirin Given Within 24 Hours of Arrival[1,3]	-	-	98%	96%
Fibrinolytic Meds Within 30 Min. of Arrival[3,7]	-	-	68%	58%
Average Time to ECG (minutes)[1,3]	-	-	7	7
Average Time to Transfer (minutes)[3,7]	-	-	64	60
Children's Asthma Care				
Received Home Management Plan of Care	63	70%	-	88%
Received Reliever Medication	69	100%	-	100%
Received Systemic Corticosteroids	69	100%	-	100%
Emergency Department				
Admittance Decision Time (minutes)[2]	647	97	96	98
Head CT Results Within 45 Min. of Arrival	12	42%	60%	57%
Patients Who Left ER Before Being Seen	61,802	3%	2%	2%
Time from ER Arrival to Admit. (minutes)[2]	652	265	280	274
Time from ER Arrival to Discharge (minutes)	391	147	167	134
Time in ER Before Being Evaluated (minutes)	297	32	35	26
Time to Pain Meds for Fractures (minutes)	270	60	56	57
Heart Attack Care				
Aspirin Given at Discharge	420	100%	99%	99%
Fibrinolytic Meds Within 30 Min. of Arrival[7]	-	-	75%	54%
PCI Within 90 Minutes of Arrival	50	98%	97%	96%
Statin Prescribed at Discharge	408	100%	99%	98%
Heart Failure Care				
ACE Inhibitor or ARB for LVSD	147	100%	98%	97%
Discharge Instructions Given	401	99%	95%	94%
Evaluation of LVS Function	486	100%	100%	99%
Medicare Spending				
Medicare Spending per Patient (ratio)	-	1.01	0.95	0.98
Pneumonia Care				
Appropriate Initial Antibiotic Given[2]	236	100%	97%	95%
Blood Culture Timing[2]	323	99%	98%	98%
Pregnancy and Delivery Care				
Newborn Deliveries Scheduled Early	239	9%	6%	6%
Preventive Care				
Immunization for Influenza[2]	544	82%	92%	90%
Immunization for Pneumonia[2]	657	90%	93%	92%
Stroke Care				
Anticoagulation Therapy for Atrial Fibrillation	29	93%	96%	95%
Antithrombotic Therapy Timing	250	98%	99%	98%
Assessed for Rehabilitation	290	95%	99%	97%
Discharged on Antithrombotic Therapy	269	100%	100%	99%
Discharged on Statin Medication	216	99%	97%	94%
Thrombolytic Therapy Timing	24	71%	73%	66%
Venous Thromboembolism Prophylaxis	282	100%	97%	94%
Written Stroke Educational Materials Given	170	100%	92%	88%
Surgical Care Improvement Project				
Appropriate Beta Blocker Usage[2]	343	98%	99%	98%
Appropriate VTP Within 24 Hours[2]	644	98%	99%	98%
Controlled Postoperative Blood Glucose[2]	186	98%	98%	97%
Perioperative Temperature Management[2]	783	100%	100%	100%
Prophylactic Antibiotic Selection[2]	635	100%	99%	99%
Prophylactic Antibiotic Selection (Outpatient)	779	99%	98%	98%
Prophylactic Antibiotic Stopped[2]	610	99%	98%	98%
Prophylactic Antibiotic Timing[2]	635	100%	99%	99%
Prophylactic Antibiotic Timing (Outpatient)	778	100%	98%	98%
Urinary Catheter Removal[2]	481	96%	98%	97%
Survey of Patients' Hospital Experiences				
Area Around Room 'Always' Quiet at Night	300+	52%	60%	61%
Doctors 'Always' Communicated Well	300+	76%	81%	82%
Home Recovery Information Given	300+	84%	86%	85%
Hospital Given 9 or 10 on 10 Point Scale	300+	64%	68%	71%
Meds 'Always' Explained Before Given	300+	59%	62%	64%
Nurses 'Always' Communicated Well	300+	76%	78%	79%
Pain 'Always' Well Controlled	300+	69%	70%	71%
Room and Bathroom 'Always' Clean	300+	72%	71%	73%
Timely Help 'Always' Received	300+	61%	64%	68%
Would Definitely Recommend Hospital	300+	66%	69%	71%
Use of Medical Imaging				
Cardiac Imaging Stress Test before Surgery	535	6.4%	5.1%	5.3%
Combination Abdominal CT Scan	906	1.3%	8.5%	10.5%
Combination Brain/Sinus CT Scan	1,065	1.2%	2.3%	2.7%
Combination Chest CT Scan	135	0.0%	1.6%	2.7%
Follow-up Mammogram/Ultrasound[1]	-	-	7.7%	8.8%
Lumbar Spine MRI for Low Back Pain[1]	-	-	35.3%	37.2%

Spotsylvania Regional Medical Center

4600 Spotsylvania Parkway
Fredericksburg, VA 22408
Phone: 540-498-4000
URL: www.spotsrmc.com
Type: Acute Care Hospitals
Emergency Services: Yes
Ownership: Proprietary

Key Personnel:
CEO .... Greg Madsen

Measure	Cases	This Hosp.	State Avg.	U.S. Avg.
Blood Clot Prevention and Treatment				
Anticoagulation Overlap Therapy[2]	26	100%	95%	93%
ICU Venous Thromboembolism Prophylaxis[2]	51	100%	95%	92%
Incidence of Potentially Preventable VTE[1,2]	-	-	8%	10%
UFH with Dosages/Platelet Monitoring[2]	11	100%	99%	97%
Venous Thromboembolism Prophylaxis[2]	339	99%	91%	85%
Warfarin Therapy Discharge Instructions[2]	20	100%	78%	75%
Chest Pain/Possible Heart Attack Care				
Aspirin Given Within 24 Hours of Arrival[1,3]	-	-	98%	96%
Fibrinolytic Meds Within 30 Min. of Arrival[3,7]	-	-	68%	58%
Average Time to ECG (minutes)[1,3]	-	-	7	7
Average Time to Transfer (minutes)[3,7]	-	-	64	60
Children's Asthma Care				
Received Home Management Plan of Care	-	-	-	88%
Received Reliever Medication	-	-	-	100%
Received Systemic Corticosteroids	-	-	-	100%
Emergency Department				
Admittance Decision Time (minutes)[2]	635	59	96	98
Head CT Results Within 45 Min. of Arrival[1]	-	-	60%	57%
Patients Who Left ER Before Being Seen	36,598	1%	2%	2%
Time from ER Arrival to Admit. (minutes)[2]	635	240	280	274
Time from ER Arrival to Discharge (minutes)	474	123	167	134
Time in ER Before Being Evaluated (minutes)	504	16	35	26
Time to Pain Meds for Fractures (minutes)	103	36	56	57
Heart Attack Care				
Aspirin Given at Discharge	83	100%	99%	99%
Fibrinolytic Meds Within 30 Min. of Arrival[7]	-	-	75%	54%
PCI Within 90 Minutes of Arrival	18	100%	97%	96%
Statin Prescribed at Discharge	79	100%	99%	98%
Heart Failure Care				
ACE Inhibitor or ARB for LVSD	35	100%	98%	97%
Discharge Instructions Given	94	100%	95%	94%
Evaluation of LVS Function	108	100%	100%	99%
Medicare Spending				
Medicare Spending per Patient (ratio)	-	0.93	0.95	0.98
Pneumonia Care				
Appropriate Initial Antibiotic Given	67	100%	97%	95%
Blood Culture Timing	96	100%	98%	98%
Pregnancy and Delivery Care				
Newborn Deliveries Scheduled Early	49	4%	6%	6%

NOTE: Hospital profiles are in alphabetical order by state, then city, then hospital within the city; Rankings exclude hospitals with less than 25 cases except for patient surveys which excludes hospitals with less than 100 cases; (a) 100-299 cases; (1) The number of cases/patients is too few to report; (2) Data submitted were based on a sample of cases/patients; (3) Results are based on a shorter time period than required; (4) Data suppressed by CMS for one or more quarters; (5) Results are not available for this reporting period; (6) Fewer than 100 patients completed the HCAHPS survey; (7) No cases met the criteria for this measure; (8) The lower limit of the confidence interval cannot be calculated if the number of observed infections equals zero; (9) No data are available from the state/territory for this reporting period; (10) The scores shown reflect fewer than 50 completed surveys; (11) There were discrepancies in the data collection process; (12) This measure does not apply to this hospital for this reporting period; (13) Results cannot be calculated for this reporting period; (14) The results for this state are combined with nearby states to protect confidentiality; Please refer to the User's Guide for a full explanation of data.

Preventive Care				
Immunization for Influenza[2]	475	97%	92%	90%
Immunization for Pneumonia[2]	490	99%	93%	92%
Stroke Care				
Anticoagulation Therapy for Atrial Fibrillation[1,2]	-	-	96%	95%
Antithrombotic Therapy Timing[2]	24	100%	99%	98%
Assessed for Rehabilitation[2]	25	100%	99%	97%
Discharged on Antithrombotic Therapy[2]	23	100%	100%	99%
Discharged on Statin Medication[2]	17	94%	97%	94%
Thrombolytic Therapy Timing[2,7]	-	-	73%	66%
Venous Thromboembolism Prophylaxis[2]	29	100%	97%	94%
Written Stroke Educational Materials Given[2]	16	100%	92%	88%
Surgical Care Improvement Project				
Appropriate Beta Blocker Usage	32	100%	99%	98%
Appropriate VTP Within 24 Hours	183	98%	99%	98%
Controlled Postoperative Blood Glucose[7]	-	-	98%	97%
Perioperative Temperature Management	218	100%	100%	100%
Prophylactic Antibiotic Selection	148	100%	99%	99%
Prophylactic Antibiotic Selection (Outpatient)	189	98%	98%	98%
Prophylactic Antibiotic Stopped	144	99%	98%	98%
Prophylactic Antibiotic Timing	148	100%	99%	99%
Prophylactic Antibiotic Timing (Outpatient)	189	100%	98%	98%
Urinary Catheter Removal	121	99%	98%	97%
Survey of Patients' Hospital Experiences				
Area Around Room 'Always' Quiet at Night	300+	69%	60%	61%
Doctors 'Always' Communicated Well	300+	79%	81%	82%
Home Recovery Information Given	300+	86%	86%	85%
Hospital Given 9 or 10 on 10 Point Scale	300+	71%	68%	71%
Meds 'Always' Explained Before Given	300+	59%	62%	64%
Nurses 'Always' Communicated Well	300+	76%	78%	79%
Pain 'Always' Well Controlled	300+	67%	70%	71%
Room and Bathroom 'Always' Clean	300+	71%	71%	73%
Timely Help 'Always' Received	300+	64%	64%	68%
Would Definitely Recommend Hospital	300+	72%	69%	71%
Use of Medical Imaging				
Cardiac Imaging Stress Test before Surgery	83	6.0%	5.1%	5.3%
Combination Abdominal CT Scan	316	4.1%	8.5%	10.5%
Combination Brain/Sinus CT Scan[1]	-	-	2.3%	2.7%
Combination Chest CT Scan	86	1.2%	1.6%	2.7%
Follow-up Mammogram/Ultrasound	136	14.0%	7.7%	8.8%
Lumbar Spine MRI for Low Back Pain[1]	-	-	35.3%	37.2%

Warren Memorial Hospital

1000 North Shenandoah Ave
Front Royal, VA 22630
Phone: 703-636-0300
Fax: 540-636-0258
URL: www.valleyhealthlink.com
Type: Acute Care Hospitals
Emergency Services: Yes
Ownership: Voluntary non-profit - Other
Beds: 196

Key Personnel:
Chief of Medical Staff.......... Floyd Bradd, III, MD
Operating Room.............. Ronnie Duckworth, RN
Radiology.................. Namik Erdag
Intensive Care Unit........... Susan Hawkins, RN
Patient Relations .... Phyllis Himelright
President/CEO.............. Mark H. Merrill
Infection Control............ Trudi Riley, RN
Quality Assurance .... Heather Silvious

Measure	Cases	This Hosp.	State Avg.	U.S. Avg.
Blood Clot Prevention and Treatment				
Anticoagulation Overlap Therapy[2]	12	100%	95%	93%
ICU Venous Thromboembolism Prophylaxis[2]	40	98%	95%	92%
Incidence of Potentially Preventable VTE[1,2]	-	-	8%	10%
UFH with Dosages/Platelet Monitoring[1,2]	-	-	99%	97%
Venous Thromboembolism Prophylaxis[2]	143	97%	91%	85%
Warfarin Therapy Discharge Instructions[2]	11	91%	78%	75%
Chest Pain/Possible Heart Attack Care				
Aspirin Given Within 24 Hours of Arrival[3]	11	100%	98%	96%
Fibrinolytic Meds Within 30 Min. of Arrival[3,7]	-	-	68%	58%
Average Time to ECG (minutes)[1,3]	-	-	7	7
Average Time to Transfer (minutes)[3,7]	-	-	64	60
Children's Asthma Care				
Received Home Management Plan of Care	-	-	-	88%
Received Reliever Medication	-	-	-	100%
Received Systemic Corticosteroids	-	-	-	100%
Emergency Department				
Admittance Decision Time (minutes)[2]	285	87	96	98
Head CT Results Within 45 Min. of Arrival[1]	-	-	60%	57%
Patients Who Left ER Before Being Seen	27,241	1%	2%	2%
Time from ER Arrival to Admit. (minutes)[2]	326	241	280	274
Time from ER Arrival to Discharge (minutes)	334	117	167	134
Time in ER Before Being Evaluated (minutes)	357	25	35	26
Time to Pain Meds for Fractures (minutes)	45	62	56	57
Heart Attack Care				
Aspirin Given at Discharge[1]	-	-	99%	99%
Fibrinolytic Meds Within 30 Min. of Arrival[7]	-	-	75%	54%
PCI Within 90 Minutes of Arrival[7]	-	-	97%	96%
Statin Prescribed at Discharge[1]	-	-	99%	98%
Heart Failure Care				
ACE Inhibitor or ARB for LVSD	21	100%	98%	97%
Discharge Instructions Given	57	95%	95%	94%
Evaluation of LVS Function	72	100%	100%	99%
Medicare Spending				
Medicare Spending per Patient (ratio)	-	0.89	0.95	0.98
Pneumonia Care				
Appropriate Initial Antibiotic Given	64	97%	97%	95%
Blood Culture Timing	114	99%	98%	98%
Pregnancy and Delivery Care				
Newborn Deliveries Scheduled Early	20	0%	6%	6%
Preventive Care				
Immunization for Influenza[2]	258	98%	92%	90%
Immunization for Pneumonia[2]	320	99%	93%	92%
Stroke Care				
Anticoagulation Therapy for Atrial Fibrillation[7]	-	-	96%	95%
Antithrombotic Therapy Timing[1]	-	-	99%	98%
Assessed for Rehabilitation[1]	-	-	99%	97%
Discharged on Antithrombotic Therapy[1]	-	-	100%	99%
Discharged on Statin Medication[1]	-	-	97%	94%
Thrombolytic Therapy Timing[1]	-	-	73%	66%
Venous Thromboembolism Prophylaxis[1]	-	-	97%	94%
Written Stroke Educational Materials Given[1]	-	-	92%	88%
Surgical Care Improvement Project				
Appropriate Beta Blocker Usage	17	100%	99%	98%
Appropriate VTP Within 24 Hours	70	100%	99%	98%
Controlled Postoperative Blood Glucose[7]	-	-	98%	97%
Perioperative Temperature Management	81	100%	100%	100%
Prophylactic Antibiotic Selection	51	96%	99%	99%
Prophylactic Antibiotic Selection (Outpatient)	18	94%	98%	98%
Prophylactic Antibiotic Stopped	50	94%	98%	98%
Prophylactic Antibiotic Timing	51	96%	99%	99%
Prophylactic Antibiotic Timing (Outpatient)	18	94%	98%	98%
Urinary Catheter Removal	38	100%	98%	97%
Survey of Patients' Hospital Experiences				
Area Around Room 'Always' Quiet at Night	300+	55%	60%	61%
Doctors 'Always' Communicated Well	300+	79%	81%	82%
Home Recovery Information Given	300+	81%	86%	85%
Hospital Given 9 or 10 on 10 Point Scale	300+	63%	68%	71%
Meds 'Always' Explained Before Given	300+	66%	62%	64%
Nurses 'Always' Communicated Well	300+	79%	78%	79%
Pain 'Always' Well Controlled	300+	69%	70%	71%
Room and Bathroom 'Always' Clean	300+	73%	71%	73%
Timely Help 'Always' Received	300+	66%	64%	68%
Would Definitely Recommend Hospital	300+	60%	69%	71%
Use of Medical Imaging				
Cardiac Imaging Stress Test before Surgery	146	4.1%	5.1%	5.3%
Combination Abdominal CT Scan	393	2.3%	8.5%	10.5%
Combination Brain/Sinus CT Scan	398	1.0%	2.3%	2.7%
Combination Chest CT Scan	183	0.5%	1.6%	2.7%
Follow-up Mammogram/Ultrasound	611	10.1%	7.7%	8.8%
Lumbar Spine MRI for Low Back Pain[1]	-	-	35.3%	37.2%

Twin County Regional Hospital

200 Hospital Drive
Galax, VA 24333
Phone: 276-236-8181
Fax: 276-236-1718
E-mail: ppeterson@tcrh.hbocvan.com
URL: www.tcrh.org
Type: Acute Care Hospitals
Emergency Services: Yes
Ownership: Voluntary non-profit - Private
Beds: 141

Key Personnel:
Infection Control.............. Julia Banks
Quality Assurance .... Michele Bobbitt
Radiology................. John W Bolen Jr, MD
Anesthesiology.............. James Griffeth, MD
CEO/President............... Marcus Kuhn
Operating Room.............. Shelby Luper, RN
Chief of Medical Staff.......... Julie Williams
Emergency Room .... Scott Wright, MD

Measure	Cases	This Hosp.	State Avg.	U.S. Avg.
Blood Clot Prevention and Treatment				
Anticoagulation Overlap Therapy[2]	27	100%	95%	93%
ICU Venous Thromboembolism Prophylaxis[2]	66	92%	95%	92%
Incidence of Potentially Preventable VTE[2,7]	-	-	8%	10%
UFH with Dosages/Platelet Monitoring[1,2]	-	-	99%	97%
Venous Thromboembolism Prophylaxis[2]	216	80%	91%	85%
Warfarin Therapy Discharge Instructions[2]	14	64%	78%	75%
Chest Pain/Possible Heart Attack Care				
Aspirin Given Within 24 Hours of Arrival	123	97%	98%	96%
Fibrinolytic Meds Within 30 Min. of Arrival[1]	-	-	68%	58%
Average Time to ECG (minutes)	123	7	7	7
Average Time to Transfer (minutes)[1]	-	-	64	60
Children's Asthma Care				
Received Home Management Plan of Care	-	-	-	88%
Received Reliever Medication	-	-	-	100%
Received Systemic Corticosteroids	-	-	-	100%
Emergency Department				
Admittance Decision Time (minutes)[2]	379	61	96	98
Head CT Results Within 45 Min. of Arrival	15	73%	60%	57%
Patients Who Left ER Before Being Seen	24,689	1%	2%	2%
Time from ER Arrival to Admit. (minutes)[2]	380	223	280	274
Time from ER Arrival to Discharge (minutes)	365	113	167	134
Time in ER Before Being Evaluated (minutes)	398	15	35	26
Time to Pain Meds for Fractures (minutes)	82	40	56	57
Heart Attack Care				
Aspirin Given at Discharge	13	100%	99%	99%
Fibrinolytic Meds Within 30 Min. of Arrival[7]	-	-	75%	54%
PCI Within 90 Minutes of Arrival[7]	-	-	97%	96%
Statin Prescribed at Discharge	13	100%	99%	98%
Heart Failure Care				
ACE Inhibitor or ARB for LVSD	22	100%	98%	97%
Discharge Instructions Given	68	90%	95%	94%
Evaluation of LVS Function	105	100%	100%	99%
Medicare Spending				
Medicare Spending per Patient (ratio)	-	1.01	0.95	0.98
Pneumonia Care				
Appropriate Initial Antibiotic Given	97	93%	97%	95%
Blood Culture Timing	204	100%	98%	98%
Pregnancy and Delivery Care				
Newborn Deliveries Scheduled Early	21	0%	6%	6%
Preventive Care				
Immunization for Influenza[2]	315	92%	92%	90%
Immunization for Pneumonia[2]	365	96%	93%	92%
Stroke Care				
Anticoagulation Therapy for Atrial Fibrillation[1]	-	-	96%	95%
Antithrombotic Therapy Timing	43	98%	99%	98%
Assessed for Rehabilitation	50	100%	99%	97%
Discharged on Antithrombotic Therapy	49	100%	100%	99%
Discharged on Statin Medication	37	100%	97%	94%
Thrombolytic Therapy Timing[1]	-	-	73%	66%
Venous Thromboembolism Prophylaxis	46	98%	97%	94%
Written Stroke Educational Materials Given	32	97%	92%	88%
Surgical Care Improvement Project				
Appropriate Beta Blocker Usage	30	97%	99%	98%
Appropriate VTP Within 24 Hours	117	97%	99%	98%
Controlled Postoperative Blood Glucose[7]	-	-	98%	97%
Perioperative Temperature Management	129	100%	100%	100%

NOTE: Hospital profiles are in alphabetical order by state, then city, then hospital within the city; Rankings exclude hospitals with less than 25 cases except for patient surveys which excludes hospitals with less than 100 cases; (a) 100-299 cases; (1) The number of cases/patients is too few to report; (2) Data submitted were based on a sample of cases/patients; (3) Results are based on a shorter time period than required; (4) Data suppressed by CMS for one or more quarters; (5) Results are not available for this reporting period; (6) Fewer than 100 patients completed the HCAHPS survey; (7) No cases met the criteria for this measure; (8) The lower limit of the confidence interval cannot be calculated if the number of observed infections equals zero; (9) No data are available from the state/territory for this reporting period; (10) The scores shown reflect fewer than 50 completed surveys; (11) There were discrepancies in the data collection process; (12) This measure does not apply to this hospital for this reporting period; (13) Results cannot be calculated for this reporting period; (14) The results for this state are combined with nearby states to protect confidentiality; Please refer to the User's Guide for a full explanation of data.

Measure	Cases	This Hosp.	State Avg.	U.S. Avg.
Prophylactic Antibiotic Selection	88	100%	99%	99%
Prophylactic Antibiotic Selection (Outpatient)	14	100%	98%	98%
Prophylactic Antibiotic Stopped	84	95%	98%	98%
Prophylactic Antibiotic Timing	88	100%	99%	99%
Prophylactic Antibiotic Timing (Outpatient)	14	100%	98%	98%
Urinary Catheter Removal	63	98%	98%	97%
Survey of Patients' Hospital Experiences				
Area Around Room 'Always' Quiet at Night	300+	58%	60%	61%
Doctors 'Always' Communicated Well	300+	83%	81%	82%
Home Recovery Information Given	300+	88%	86%	85%
Hospital Given 9 or 10 on 10 Point Scale	300+	65%	68%	71%
Meds 'Always' Explained Before Given	300+	63%	62%	64%
Nurses 'Always' Communicated Well	300+	76%	78%	79%
Pain 'Always' Well Controlled	300+	67%	70%	71%
Room and Bathroom 'Always' Clean	300+	74%	71%	73%
Timely Help 'Always' Received	300+	59%	64%	68%
Would Definitely Recommend Hospital	300+	58%	69%	71%
Use of Medical Imaging				
Cardiac Imaging Stress Test before Surgery[1]	-	-	5.1%	5.3%
Combination Abdominal CT Scan	777	5.7%	8.5%	10.5%
Combination Brain/Sinus CT Scan	660	2.3%	2.3%	2.7%
Combination Chest CT Scan	238	0.4%	1.6%	2.7%
Follow-up Mammogram/Ultrasound	1,419	2.5%	7.7%	8.8%
Lumbar Spine MRI for Low Back Pain	119	39.5%	35.3%	37.2%

Riverside Walter Reed Hospital

7519 Hospital Road
Gloucester, VA 23061
Phone: 804-693-8800
Fax: 804-693-8812
URL: www.riverside-online.com
Type: Acute Care Hospitals
Emergency Services: Yes
Ownership: Voluntary non-profit - Private
Beds: 67

Key Personnel:
Chief of Medical Staff . . . . Robert Cross, MD
Emergency Room . . . . Susan Frishkorn, RN
CEO/President . . . . Richard Pearce
Quality Assurance . . . . David Tate

Measure	Cases	This Hosp.	State Avg.	U.S. Avg.
Blood Clot Prevention and Treatment				
Anticoagulation Overlap Therapy[2]	28	100%	95%	93%
ICU Venous Thromboembolism Prophylaxis[2]	125	96%	95%	92%
Incidence of Potentially Preventable VTE[1,2]	-	-	8%	10%
UFH with Dosages/Platelet Monitoring[1,2]	-	-	99%	97%
Venous Thromboembolism Prophylaxis[2]	291	98%	91%	85%
Warfarin Therapy Discharge Instructions[2]	28	100%	78%	75%
Chest Pain/Possible Heart Attack Care				
Aspirin Given Within 24 Hours of Arrival	51	98%	98%	96%
Fibrinolytic Meds Within 30 Min. of Arrival[7]	-	-	68%	58%
Average Time to ECG (minutes)	52	4	7	7
Average Time to Transfer (minutes)[1]	-	-	64	60
Children's Asthma Care				
Received Home Management Plan of Care	-	-	-	88%
Received Reliever Medication	-	-	-	100%
Received Systemic Corticosteroids	-	-	-	100%
Emergency Department				
Admittance Decision Time (minutes)[2]	546	119	96	98
Head CT Results Within 45 Min. of Arrival	12	75%	60%	57%
Patients Who Left ER Before Being Seen	24,503	1%	2%	2%
Time from ER Arrival to Admit. (minutes)[2]	546	293	280	274
Time from ER Arrival to Discharge (minutes)	353	132	167	134
Time in ER Before Being Evaluated (minutes)	375	52	35	26
Time to Pain Meds for Fractures (minutes)	116	58	56	57
Heart Attack Care				
Aspirin Given at Discharge	28	100%	99%	99%
Fibrinolytic Meds Within 30 Min. of Arrival[1]	-	-	75%	54%
PCI Within 90 Minutes of Arrival[7]	-	-	97%	96%
Statin Prescribed at Discharge	25	100%	99%	98%
Heart Failure Care				
ACE Inhibitor or ARB for LVSD	45	100%	98%	97%
Discharge Instructions Given	101	97%	95%	94%
Evaluation of LVS Function	129	100%	100%	99%
Medicare Spending				
Medicare Spending per Patient (ratio)	-	0.86	0.95	0.98
Pneumonia Care				
Appropriate Initial Antibiotic Given	113	98%	97%	95%
Blood Culture Timing	167	99%	98%	98%
Pregnancy and Delivery Care				
Newborn Deliveries Scheduled Early[7]	-	-	6%	6%
Preventive Care				
Immunization for Influenza[2]	292	94%	92%	90%
Immunization for Pneumonia[2]	470	94%	93%	92%
Stroke Care				
Anticoagulation Therapy for Atrial Fibrillation[1]	-	-	96%	95%
Antithrombotic Therapy Timing	46	98%	99%	98%
Assessed for Rehabilitation	45	100%	99%	97%
Discharged on Antithrombotic Therapy	43	100%	100%	99%
Discharged on Statin Medication	35	97%	97%	94%
Thrombolytic Therapy Timing[7]	-	-	73%	66%
Venous Thromboembolism Prophylaxis	47	96%	97%	94%
Written Stroke Educational Materials Given	22	95%	92%	88%
Surgical Care Improvement Project				
Appropriate Beta Blocker Usage	53	100%	99%	98%
Appropriate VTP Within 24 Hours	171	99%	99%	98%
Controlled Postoperative Blood Glucose[7]	-	-	98%	97%
Perioperative Temperature Management	176	100%	100%	100%
Prophylactic Antibiotic Selection	136	100%	99%	99%
Prophylactic Antibiotic Selection (Outpatient)	15	93%	98%	98%
Prophylactic Antibiotic Stopped	135	100%	98%	98%
Prophylactic Antibiotic Timing	136	99%	99%	99%
Prophylactic Antibiotic Timing (Outpatient)	16	94%	98%	98%
Urinary Catheter Removal	156	100%	98%	97%
Survey of Patients' Hospital Experiences				
Area Around Room 'Always' Quiet at Night	300+	50%	60%	61%
Doctors 'Always' Communicated Well	300+	84%	81%	82%
Home Recovery Information Given	300+	86%	86%	85%
Hospital Given 9 or 10 on 10 Point Scale	300+	68%	68%	71%
Meds 'Always' Explained Before Given	300+	67%	62%	64%
Nurses 'Always' Communicated Well	300+	79%	78%	79%
Pain 'Always' Well Controlled	300+	72%	70%	71%
Room and Bathroom 'Always' Clean	300+	71%	71%	73%
Timely Help 'Always' Received	300+	64%	64%	68%
Would Definitely Recommend Hospital	300+	67%	69%	71%
Use of Medical Imaging				
Cardiac Imaging Stress Test before Surgery	232	4.3%	5.1%	5.3%
Combination Abdominal CT Scan	742	3.9%	8.5%	10.5%
Combination Brain/Sinus CT Scan	513	2.7%	2.3%	2.7%
Combination Chest CT Scan	525	0.2%	1.6%	2.7%
Follow-up Mammogram/Ultrasound	1,305	7.4%	7.7%	8.8%
Lumbar Spine MRI for Low Back Pain	104	34.6%	35.3%	37.2%

Buchanan General Hospital

1535 Slate Creek Road
Grundy, VA 24614
Phone: 276-935-1000
Fax: 276-935-1469
E-mail: roger.cooper@bgh.org
URL: www.bgh.org
Type: Acute Care Hospitals
Emergency Services: Yes
Ownership: Voluntary non-profit - Private
Beds: 134

Key Personnel:
Emergency Room . . . . Dwight Bagano
CEO/President . . . . Roger Cooper
Radiology . . . . Dilip R Patel
Chief of Medical Staff . . . . JG Patel
CEO . . . . Robert D. Ruchti

Measure	Cases	This Hosp.	State Avg.	U.S. Avg.
Blood Clot Prevention and Treatment				
Anticoagulation Overlap Therapy[2]	13	31%	95%	93%
ICU Venous Thromboembolism Prophylaxis[2]	31	94%	95%	92%
Incidence of Potentially Preventable VTE[1,2]	-	-	8%	10%
UFH with Dosages/Platelet Monitoring[1,2]	-	-	99%	97%
Venous Thromboembolism Prophylaxis[2]	108	80%	91%	85%
Warfarin Therapy Discharge Instructions[2]	13	62%	78%	75%
Chest Pain/Possible Heart Attack Care				
Aspirin Given Within 24 Hours of Arrival	108	98%	98%	96%
Fibrinolytic Meds Within 30 Min. of Arrival	12	92%	68%	58%
Average Time to ECG (minutes)	122	4	7	7
Average Time to Transfer (minutes)[7]	-	-	64	60
Children's Asthma Care				
Received Home Management Plan of Care	-	-	-	88%
Received Reliever Medication	-	-	-	100%
Received Systemic Corticosteroids	-	-	-	100%
Emergency Department				
Admittance Decision Time (minutes)[2]	396	50	96	98
Head CT Results Within 45 Min. of Arrival	12	58%	60%	57%
Patients Who Left ER Before Being Seen	10,886	1%	2%	2%
Time from ER Arrival to Admit. (minutes)[2]	396	216	280	274
Time from ER Arrival to Discharge (minutes)	1,104	132	167	134
Time in ER Before Being Evaluated (minutes)	1,325	22	35	26
Time to Pain Meds for Fractures (minutes)	51	40	56	57
Heart Attack Care				
Aspirin Given at Discharge[1]	-	-	99%	99%
Fibrinolytic Meds Within 30 Min. of Arrival[7]	-	-	75%	54%
PCI Within 90 Minutes of Arrival[7]	-	-	97%	96%
Statin Prescribed at Discharge[1]	-	-	99%	98%
Heart Failure Care				
ACE Inhibitor or ARB for LVSD[1]	-	-	98%	97%
Discharge Instructions Given	28	96%	95%	94%
Evaluation of LVS Function	34	100%	100%	99%
Medicare Spending				
Medicare Spending per Patient (ratio)	-	0.95	0.95	0.98
Pneumonia Care				
Appropriate Initial Antibiotic Given	58	100%	97%	95%
Blood Culture Timing	76	100%	98%	98%
Pregnancy and Delivery Care				
Newborn Deliveries Scheduled Early[7]	-	-	6%	6%
Preventive Care				
Immunization for Influenza[2]	283	80%	92%	90%
Immunization for Pneumonia[2]	409	93%	93%	92%
Stroke Care				
Anticoagulation Therapy for Atrial Fibrillation[7]	-	-	96%	95%
Antithrombotic Therapy Timing[1]	-	-	99%	98%
Assessed for Rehabilitation[1]	-	-	99%	97%
Discharged on Antithrombotic Therapy[1]	-	-	100%	99%
Discharged on Statin Medication[1]	-	-	97%	94%
Thrombolytic Therapy Timing[7]	-	-	73%	66%
Venous Thromboembolism Prophylaxis[1]	-	-	97%	94%
Written Stroke Educational Materials Given[7]	-	-	92%	88%
Surgical Care Improvement Project				
Appropriate Beta Blocker Usage[1,3]	-	-	99%	98%
Appropriate VTP Within 24 Hours[1,3]	-	-	99%	98%
Controlled Postoperative Blood Glucose[3,7]	-	-	98%	97%
Perioperative Temperature Management[1,3]	-	-	100%	100%
Prophylactic Antibiotic Selection[1,3]	-	-	99%	99%
Prophylactic Antibiotic Selection (Outpatient)[5]	-	-	98%	98%
Prophylactic Antibiotic Stopped[1,3]	-	-	98%	98%
Prophylactic Antibiotic Timing[1,3]	-	-	99%	99%
Prophylactic Antibiotic Timing (Outpatient)[5]	-	-	98%	98%
Urinary Catheter Removal[1,3]	-	-	98%	97%
Survey of Patients' Hospital Experiences				
Area Around Room 'Always' Quiet at Night	(a)	65%	60%	61%
Doctors 'Always' Communicated Well	(a)	88%	81%	82%
Home Recovery Information Given	(a)	80%	86%	85%
Hospital Given 9 or 10 on 10 Point Scale	(a)	66%	68%	71%
Meds 'Always' Explained Before Given	(a)	62%	62%	64%
Nurses 'Always' Communicated Well	(a)	82%	78%	79%
Pain 'Always' Well Controlled	(a)	74%	70%	71%
Room and Bathroom 'Always' Clean	(a)	77%	71%	73%
Timely Help 'Always' Received	(a)	69%	64%	68%
Would Definitely Recommend Hospital	(a)	64%	69%	71%
Use of Medical Imaging				
Cardiac Imaging Stress Test before Surgery	106	2.8%	5.1%	5.3%
Combination Abdominal CT Scan	324	8.0%	8.5%	10.5%
Combination Brain/Sinus CT Scan[1]	-	-	2.3%	2.7%
Combination Chest CT Scan	177	5.1%	1.6%	2.7%
Follow-up Mammogram/Ultrasound	277	13.0%	7.7%	8.8%
Lumbar Spine MRI for Low Back Pain	64	40.6%	35.3%	37.2%

NOTE: Hospital profiles are in alphabetical order by state, then city, then hospital within the city; Rankings exclude hospitals with less than 25 cases except for patient surveys which excludes hospitals with less than 100 cases; (a) 100-299 cases; (1) The number of cases/patients is too few to report; (2) Data submitted were based on a sample of cases/patients; (3) Results are based on a shorter time period than required; (4) Data suppressed by CMS for one or more quarters; (5) Results are not available for this reporting period; (6) Fewer than 100 patients completed the HCAHPS survey; (7) No cases met the criteria for this measure; (8) The lower limit of the confidence interval cannot be calculated if the number of observed infections equals zero; (9) No data are available from the state/territory for this reporting period; (10) The scores shown reflect fewer than 50 completed surveys; (11) There were discrepancies in the data collection process; (12) This measure does not apply to this hospital for this reporting period; (13) Results cannot be calculated for this reporting period; (14) The results for this state are combined with nearby states to protect confidentiality; Please refer to the User's Guide for a full explanation of data.

Halifax Regional Hospital

2204 Wilborn Avenue
Halifax, VA 24558
Phone: 434-517-3100
Type: Acute Care Hospitals
Emergency Services: Yes
Ownership: Voluntary non-profit - Private

Measure	Cases	This Hosp.	State Avg.	U.S. Avg.
Blood Clot Prevention and Treatment				
Anticoagulation Overlap Therapy[2]	33	85%	95%	93%
ICU Venous Thromboembolism Prophylaxis[2]	110	92%	95%	92%
Incidence of Potentially Preventable VTE[2,7]	-	-	8%	10%
UFH with Dosages/Platelet Monitoring[2]	11	100%	99%	97%
Venous Thromboembolism Prophylaxis[2]	344	83%	91%	85%
Warfarin Therapy Discharge Instructions[2]	23	91%	78%	75%
Chest Pain/Possible Heart Attack Care				
Aspirin Given Within 24 Hours of Arrival	21	95%	98%	96%
Fibrinolytic Meds Within 30 Min. of Arrival	11	91%	68%	58%
Average Time to ECG (minutes)	22	6	7	7
Average Time to Transfer (minutes)[7]	-	-	64	60
Children's Asthma Care				
Received Home Management Plan of Care	-	-	-	88%
Received Reliever Medication	-	-	-	100%
Received Systemic Corticosteroids	-	-	-	100%
Emergency Department				
Admittance Decision Time (minutes)[2]	535	103	96	98
Head CT Results Within 45 Min. of Arrival	15	67%	60%	57%
Patients Who Left ER Before Being Seen	30,553	1%	2%	2%
Time from ER Arrival to Admit. (minutes)[2]	538	285	280	274
Time from ER Arrival to Discharge (minutes)	386	132	167	134
Time in ER Before Being Evaluated (minutes)	399	27	35	26
Time to Pain Meds for Fractures (minutes)	97	77	56	57
Heart Attack Care				
Aspirin Given at Discharge	82	98%	99%	99%
Fibrinolytic Meds Within 30 Min. of Arrival[7]	-	-	75%	54%
PCI Within 90 Minutes of Arrival[1]	-	-	97%	96%
Statin Prescribed at Discharge	73	97%	99%	98%
Heart Failure Care				
ACE Inhibitor or ARB for LVSD	49	98%	98%	97%
Discharge Instructions Given	187	88%	95%	94%
Evaluation of LVS Function	237	100%	100%	99%
Medicare Spending				
Medicare Spending per Patient (ratio)	-	0.89	0.95	0.98
Pneumonia Care				
Appropriate Initial Antibiotic Given	51	92%	97%	95%
Blood Culture Timing	71	94%	98%	98%
Pregnancy and Delivery Care				
Newborn Deliveries Scheduled Early	37	27%	6%	6%
Preventive Care				
Immunization for Influenza[2]	437	86%	92%	90%
Immunization for Pneumonia[2]	582	86%	93%	92%
Stroke Care				
Anticoagulation Therapy for Atrial Fibrillation[1]	-	-	96%	95%
Antithrombotic Therapy Timing	61	100%	99%	98%
Assessed for Rehabilitation	67	90%	99%	97%
Discharged on Antithrombotic Therapy	65	97%	100%	99%
Discharged on Statin Medication	50	96%	97%	94%
Thrombolytic Therapy Timing[1]	-	-	73%	66%
Venous Thromboembolism Prophylaxis	66	80%	97%	94%
Written Stroke Educational Materials Given	42	79%	92%	88%
Surgical Care Improvement Project				
Appropriate Beta Blocker Usage	46	96%	99%	98%
Appropriate VTP Within 24 Hours	177	87%	99%	98%
Controlled Postoperative Blood Glucose[7]	-	-	98%	97%
Perioperative Temperature Management	196	99%	100%	100%
Prophylactic Antibiotic Selection	125	97%	99%	99%
Prophylactic Antibiotic Selection (Outpatient)	113	100%	98%	98%
Prophylactic Antibiotic Stopped	120	90%	98%	98%
Prophylactic Antibiotic Timing	126	97%	99%	99%
Prophylactic Antibiotic Timing (Outpatient)	117	75%	98%	98%
Urinary Catheter Removal	94	78%	98%	97%
Survey of Patients' Hospital Experiences				
Area Around Room 'Always' Quiet at Night	300+	68%	60%	61%
Doctors 'Always' Communicated Well	300+	86%	81%	82%
Home Recovery Information Given	300+	87%	86%	85%
Hospital Given 9 or 10 on 10 Point Scale	300+	70%	68%	71%
Meds 'Always' Explained Before Given	300+	67%	62%	64%
Nurses 'Always' Communicated Well	300+	81%	78%	79%
Pain 'Always' Well Controlled	300+	71%	70%	71%
Room and Bathroom 'Always' Clean	300+	73%	71%	73%
Timely Help 'Always' Received	300+	69%	64%	68%
Would Definitely Recommend Hospital	300+	66%	69%	71%
Use of Medical Imaging				
Cardiac Imaging Stress Test before Surgery	690	4.9%	5.1%	5.3%
Combination Abdominal CT Scan	877	9.2%	8.5%	10.5%
Combination Brain/Sinus CT Scan	734	1.0%	2.3%	2.7%
Combination Chest CT Scan	367	0.3%	1.6%	2.7%
Follow-up Mammogram/Ultrasound	1,392	6.6%	7.7%	8.8%
Lumbar Spine MRI for Low Back Pain	93	53.8%	35.3%	37.2%

Hampton VA Medical Center

100 Emancipation Drive
Hampton, VA 23667
Phone: 757-722-9961
Fax: 757-728-7000
E-mail: sheila.bailey@va.gov
URL: www.va.gov
Type: Acute Care - VA
Emergency Services: No
Ownership: Government Federal
Beds: 516

Key Personnel:

Chief of Medical Staff.......... Gnamani Arul, MD
Radiology.................. Haywood Davis, MD
Infection Control.............. Debra Kerr, RN
CEO/President.............. Wanda Mims, MBA
Operating Room.............. Ida Robinson, RN
Quality Assurance .... Sharon Steinkamp, RN

Measure	Cases	This Hosp.	State Avg.	U.S. Avg.
Blood Clot Prevention and Treatment				
Anticoagulation Overlap Therapy	-	-	95%	93%
ICU Venous Thromboembolism Prophylaxis	-	-	95%	92%
Incidence of Potentially Preventable VTE	-	-	8%	10%
UFH with Dosages/Platelet Monitoring	-	-	99%	97%
Venous Thromboembolism Prophylaxis	-	-	91%	85%
Warfarin Therapy Discharge Instructions	-	-	78%	75%
Chest Pain/Possible Heart Attack Care				
Aspirin Given Within 24 Hours of Arrival	-	-	98%	96%
Fibrinolytic Meds Within 30 Min. of Arrival	-	-	68%	58%
Average Time to ECG (minutes)	-	-	7	7
Average Time to Transfer (minutes)	-	-	64	60
Children's Asthma Care				
Received Home Management Plan of Care	-	-	-	88%
Received Reliever Medication	-	-	-	100%
Received Systemic Corticosteroids	-	-	-	100%
Emergency Department				
Admittance Decision Time (minutes)	-	-	96	98
Head CT Results Within 45 Min. of Arrival	-	-	60%	57%
Patients Who Left ER Before Being Seen	-	-	2%	2%
Time from ER Arrival to Admit. (minutes)	-	-	280	274
Time from ER Arrival to Discharge (minutes)	-	-	167	134
Time in ER Before Being Evaluated (minutes)	-	-	35	26
Time to Pain Meds for Fractures (minutes)	-	-	56	57
Heart Attack Care				
Aspirin Given at Discharge[5]	-	-	99%	99%
Fibrinolytic Meds Within 30 Min. of Arrival[5]	-	-	75%	54%
PCI Within 90 Minutes of Arrival[5]	-	-	97%	96%
Statin Prescribed at Discharge[5]	-	-	99%	98%
Heart Failure Care				
ACE Inhibitor or ARB for LVSD[1]	21	100%	98%	97%
Discharge Instructions Given	76	100%	95%	94%
Evaluation of LVS Function	84	100%	100%	99%
Medicare Spending				
Medicare Spending per Patient (ratio)	-	-	0.95	0.98
Pneumonia Care				
Appropriate Initial Antibiotic Given[1]	23	100%	97%	95%
Blood Culture Timing	34	97%	98%	98%
Pregnancy and Delivery Care				
Newborn Deliveries Scheduled Early	-	-	6%	6%
Preventive Care				
Immunization for Influenza[5]	-	-	92%	90%
Immunization for Pneumonia[5]	-	-	93%	92%
Stroke Care				
Anticoagulation Therapy for Atrial Fibrillation	-	-	96%	95%
Antithrombotic Therapy Timing	-	-	99%	98%
Assessed for Rehabilitation	-	-	99%	97%
Discharged on Antithrombotic Therapy	-	-	100%	99%
Discharged on Statin Medication	-	-	97%	94%
Thrombolytic Therapy Timing	-	-	73%	66%
Venous Thromboembolism Prophylaxis	-	-	97%	94%
Written Stroke Educational Materials Given	-	-	92%	88%
Surgical Care Improvement Project				
Appropriate Beta Blocker Usage[2]	25	100%	99%	98%
Appropriate VTP Within 24 Hours[2]	76	100%	99%	98%
Controlled Postoperative Blood Glucose[5]	-	-	98%	97%
Perioperative Temperature Management[2]	108	100%	100%	100%
Prophylactic Antibiotic Selection	79	99%	99%	99%
Prophylactic Antibiotic Selection (Outpatient)	-	-	98%	98%
Prophylactic Antibiotic Stopped	77	99%	98%	98%
Prophylactic Antibiotic Timing	79	100%	99%	99%
Prophylactic Antibiotic Timing (Outpatient)	-	-	98%	98%
Urinary Catheter Removal[1,2]	12	100%	98%	97%
Survey of Patients' Hospital Experiences				
Area Around Room 'Always' Quiet at Night	-	-	60%	61%
Doctors 'Always' Communicated Well	-	-	81%	82%
Home Recovery Information Given	-	-	86%	85%
Hospital Given 9 or 10 on 10 Point Scale	-	-	68%	71%
Meds 'Always' Explained Before Given	-	-	62%	64%
Nurses 'Always' Communicated Well	-	-	78%	79%
Pain 'Always' Well Controlled	-	-	70%	71%
Room and Bathroom 'Always' Clean	-	-	71%	73%
Timely Help 'Always' Received	-	-	64%	68%
Would Definitely Recommend Hospital	-	-	69%	71%
Use of Medical Imaging				
Cardiac Imaging Stress Test before Surgery	-	-	5.1%	5.3%
Combination Abdominal CT Scan	-	-	8.5%	10.5%
Combination Brain/Sinus CT Scan	-	-	2.3%	2.7%
Combination Chest CT Scan	-	-	1.6%	2.7%
Follow-up Mammogram/Ultrasound	-	-	7.7%	8.8%
Lumbar Spine MRI for Low Back Pain	-	-	35.3%	37.2%

Sentara Careplex Hospital

3000 Coliseum Drive
Hampton, VA 23666
Phone: 757-736-1000
URL: www.sentara.com
Type: Acute Care Hospitals
Emergency Services: Yes
Ownership: Voluntary non-profit - Private
Beds: 224

Measure	Cases	This Hosp.	State Avg.	U.S. Avg.
Blood Clot Prevention and Treatment				
Anticoagulation Overlap Therapy[2]	91	90%	95%	93%
ICU Venous Thromboembolism Prophylaxis[2]	96	97%	95%	92%
Incidence of Potentially Preventable VTE[2]	13	0%	8%	10%
UFH with Dosages/Platelet Monitoring[2]	62	100%	99%	97%
Venous Thromboembolism Prophylaxis[2]	313	92%	91%	85%
Warfarin Therapy Discharge Instructions[2]	64	98%	78%	75%
Chest Pain/Possible Heart Attack Care				
Aspirin Given Within 24 Hours of Arrival	18	100%	98%	96%
Fibrinolytic Meds Within 30 Min. of Arrival[7]	-	-	68%	58%
Average Time to ECG (minutes)	21	2	7	7
Average Time to Transfer (minutes)[1]	-	-	64	60
Children's Asthma Care				
Received Home Management Plan of Care	-	-	-	88%
Received Reliever Medication	-	-	-	100%
Received Systemic Corticosteroids	-	-	-	100%
Emergency Department				
Admittance Decision Time (minutes)[2]	912	126	96	98
Head CT Results Within 45 Min. of Arrival[1]	-	-	60%	57%
Patients Who Left ER Before Being Seen	>100k	1%	2%	2%
Time from ER Arrival to Admit. (minutes)[2]	915	335	280	274
Time from ER Arrival to Discharge (minutes)	8,023	177	167	134
Time in ER Before Being Evaluated (minutes)	8,338	29	35	26
Time to Pain Meds for Fractures (minutes)	146	65	56	57
Heart Attack Care				
Aspirin Given at Discharge	116	100%	99%	99%

NOTE: Hospital profiles are in alphabetical order by state, then city, then hospital within the city; Rankings exclude hospitals with less than 25 cases except for patient surveys which excludes hospitals with less than 100 cases; (a) 100-299 cases; (1) The number of cases/patients is too few to report; (2) Data submitted were based on a sample of cases/patients; (3) Results are based on a shorter time period than required; (4) Data suppressed by CMS for one or more quarters; (5) Results are not available for this reporting period; (6) Fewer than 100 patients completed the HCAHPS survey; (7) No cases met the criteria for this measure; (8) The lower limit of the confidence interval cannot be calculated if the number of observed infections equals zero; (9) No data are available from the state/territory for this reporting period; (10) The scores shown reflect fewer than 50 completed surveys; (11) There were discrepancies in the data collection process; (12) This measure does not apply to this hospital for this reporting period; (13) Results cannot be calculated for this reporting period; (14) The results for this state are combined with nearby states to protect confidentiality; Please refer to the User's Guide for a full explanation of data.

Measure	Cases	This Hosp.	State Avg.	U.S. Avg.
Fibrinolytic Meds Within 30 Min. of Arrival[7]	-	-	75%	54%
PCI Within 90 Minutes of Arrival	43	100%	97%	96%
Statin Prescribed at Discharge	116	100%	99%	98%
Heart Failure Care				
ACE Inhibitor or ARB for LVSD	106	96%	98%	97%
Discharge Instructions Given	321	98%	95%	94%
Evaluation of LVS Function	386	100%	100%	99%
Medicare Spending				
Medicare Spending per Patient (ratio)	-	0.99	0.95	0.98
Pneumonia Care				
Appropriate Initial Antibiotic Given	128	98%	97%	95%
Blood Culture Timing	228	100%	98%	98%
Pregnancy and Delivery Care				
Newborn Deliveries Scheduled Early[7]	-	-	6%	6%
Preventive Care				
Immunization for Influenza[2]	603	98%	92%	90%
Immunization for Pneumonia[2]	891	97%	93%	92%
Stroke Care				
Anticoagulation Therapy for Atrial Fibrillation	16	81%	96%	95%
Antithrombotic Therapy Timing	191	100%	99%	98%
Assessed for Rehabilitation	203	100%	99%	97%
Discharged on Antithrombotic Therapy	190	100%	100%	99%
Discharged on Statin Medication	152	97%	97%	94%
Thrombolytic Therapy Timing[1]	-	-	73%	66%
Venous Thromboembolism Prophylaxis	208	100%	97%	94%
Written Stroke Educational Materials Given	117	97%	92%	88%
Surgical Care Improvement Project				
Appropriate Beta Blocker Usage[2]	175	100%	99%	98%
Appropriate VTP Within 24 Hours[2]	523	100%	99%	98%
Controlled Postoperative Blood Glucose[2,7]	-	-	98%	97%
Perioperative Temperature Management[2]	625	100%	100%	100%
Prophylactic Antibiotic Selection[2]	442	100%	99%	99%
Prophylactic Antibiotic Selection (Outpatient)	194	97%	98%	98%
Prophylactic Antibiotic Stopped[2]	438	100%	98%	98%
Prophylactic Antibiotic Timing[2]	443	99%	99%	99%
Prophylactic Antibiotic Timing (Outpatient)	195	98%	98%	98%
Urinary Catheter Removal[2]	157	98%	98%	97%
Survey of Patients' Hospital Experiences				
Area Around Room 'Always' Quiet at Night	300+	70%	60%	61%
Doctors 'Always' Communicated Well	300+	83%	81%	82%
Home Recovery Information Given	300+	90%	86%	85%
Hospital Given 9 or 10 on 10 Point Scale	300+	72%	68%	71%
Meds 'Always' Explained Before Given	300+	61%	62%	64%
Nurses 'Always' Communicated Well	300+	81%	78%	79%
Pain 'Always' Well Controlled	300+	72%	70%	71%
Room and Bathroom 'Always' Clean	300+	74%	71%	73%
Timely Help 'Always' Received	300+	66%	64%	68%
Would Definitely Recommend Hospital	300+	76%	69%	71%
Use of Medical Imaging				
Cardiac Imaging Stress Test before Surgery	268	7.1%	5.1%	5.3%
Combination Abdominal CT Scan	1,841	5.5%	8.5%	10.5%
Combination Brain/Sinus CT Scan	1,309	1.0%	2.3%	2.7%
Combination Chest CT Scan	1,165	0.4%	1.6%	2.7%
Follow-up Mammogram/Ultrasound	3,010	10.7%	7.7%	8.8%
Lumbar Spine MRI for Low Back Pain	115	27.8%	35.3%	37.2%

Rockingham Memorial Hospital

2010 Health Campus Drive
Harrisonburg, VA 22801
Phone: 540-689-1000
Fax: 540-433-4576
URL: www.rmhonline.com
Type: Acute Care Hospitals
Emergency Services: Yes
Ownership: Voluntary non-profit - Private
Beds: 270

Key Personnel:
Radiology. . . . . Judy Budd
Chief of Medical Staff . . . . Dale Carroll, MD, MPH
CEO/President. . . . . Jim Krauss
Emergency Room . . . . Mary Anne Nolan
Operating Room. . . . . Joan Ridley, RN
Quality Assurance . . . . Helen Youngs

Measure	Cases	This Hosp.	State Avg.	U.S. Avg.
Blood Clot Prevention and Treatment				
Anticoagulation Overlap Therapy[2]	109	100%	95%	93%
ICU Venous Thromboembolism Prophylaxis[2]	30	100%	95%	92%
Incidence of Potentially Preventable VTE[2]	15	13%	8%	10%
UFH with Dosages/Platelet Monitoring[2]	75	100%	99%	97%
Venous Thromboembolism Prophylaxis[2]	314	96%	91%	85%
Warfarin Therapy Discharge Instructions[2]	81	98%	78%	75%
Chest Pain/Possible Heart Attack Care				
Aspirin Given Within 24 Hours of Arrival[1,3]	-	-	98%	96%
Fibrinolytic Meds Within 30 Min. of Arrival[3,7]	-	-	68%	58%
Average Time to ECG (minutes)[1,3]	-	-	7	7
Average Time to Transfer (minutes)[3,7]	-	-	64	60
Children's Asthma Care				
Received Home Management Plan of Care	-	-	-	88%
Received Reliever Medication	-	-	-	100%
Received Systemic Corticosteroids	-	-	-	100%
Emergency Department				
Admittance Decision Time (minutes)[2]	771	137	96	98
Head CT Results Within 45 Min. of Arrival	11	91%	60%	57%
Patients Who Left ER Before Being Seen	75,392	2%	2%	2%
Time from ER Arrival to Admit. (minutes)[2]	772	289	280	274
Time from ER Arrival to Discharge (minutes)	543	130	167	134
Time in ER Before Being Evaluated (minutes)	571	31	35	26
Time to Pain Meds for Fractures (minutes)	202	59	56	57
Heart Attack Care				
Aspirin Given at Discharge[2]	261	100%	99%	99%
Fibrinolytic Meds Within 30 Min. of Arrival[2,7]	-	-	75%	54%
PCI Within 90 Minutes of Arrival[2]	64	100%	97%	96%
Statin Prescribed at Discharge[2]	261	100%	99%	98%
Heart Failure Care				
ACE Inhibitor or ARB for LVSD[2]	78	100%	98%	97%
Discharge Instructions Given[2]	287	96%	95%	94%
Evaluation of LVS Function[2]	355	100%	100%	99%
Medicare Spending				
Medicare Spending per Patient (ratio)	-	0.92	0.95	0.98
Pneumonia Care				
Appropriate Initial Antibiotic Given[2]	143	99%	97%	95%
Blood Culture Timing[2]	286	99%	98%	98%
Pregnancy and Delivery Care				
Newborn Deliveries Scheduled Early[2]	34	3%	6%	6%
Preventive Care				
Immunization for Influenza[2]	591	95%	92%	90%
Immunization for Pneumonia[2]	720	97%	93%	92%
Stroke Care				
Anticoagulation Therapy for Atrial Fibrillation	23	100%	96%	95%
Antithrombotic Therapy Timing	118	99%	99%	98%
Assessed for Rehabilitation	147	99%	99%	97%
Discharged on Antithrombotic Therapy	144	100%	100%	99%
Discharged on Statin Medication	117	98%	97%	94%
Thrombolytic Therapy Timing[1]	-	-	73%	66%
Venous Thromboembolism Prophylaxis	121	93%	97%	94%
Written Stroke Educational Materials Given	84	100%	92%	88%
Surgical Care Improvement Project				
Appropriate Beta Blocker Usage[2]	197	99%	99%	98%
Appropriate VTP Within 24 Hours[2]	373	98%	99%	98%
Controlled Postoperative Blood Glucose[2]	65	97%	98%	97%
Perioperative Temperature Management[2]	478	100%	100%	100%
Prophylactic Antibiotic Selection[2]	409	99%	99%	99%
Prophylactic Antibiotic Selection (Outpatient)	239	99%	98%	98%
Prophylactic Antibiotic Stopped[2]	287	94%	98%	98%
Prophylactic Antibiotic Timing[2]	409	99%	99%	99%
Prophylactic Antibiotic Timing (Outpatient)	241	99%	98%	98%
Urinary Catheter Removal[2]	305	96%	98%	97%
Survey of Patients' Hospital Experiences				
Area Around Room 'Always' Quiet at Night	300+	59%	60%	61%
Doctors 'Always' Communicated Well	300+	79%	81%	82%
Home Recovery Information Given	300+	86%	86%	85%
Hospital Given 9 or 10 on 10 Point Scale	300+	73%	68%	71%
Meds 'Always' Explained Before Given	300+	61%	62%	64%
Nurses 'Always' Communicated Well	300+	79%	78%	79%
Pain 'Always' Well Controlled	300+	70%	70%	71%
Room and Bathroom 'Always' Clean	300+	77%	71%	73%
Timely Help 'Always' Received	300+	65%	64%	68%
Would Definitely Recommend Hospital	300+	70%	69%	71%
Use of Medical Imaging				
Cardiac Imaging Stress Test before Surgery	1,011	4.5%	5.1%	5.3%
Combination Abdominal CT Scan	1,386	8.3%	8.5%	10.5%
Combination Brain/Sinus CT Scan	1,281	1.9%	2.3%	2.7%
Combination Chest CT Scan	951	0.0%	1.6%	2.7%
Follow-up Mammogram/Ultrasound	3,135	6.9%	7.7%	8.8%
Lumbar Spine MRI for Low Back Pain	317	37.2%	35.3%	37.2%

John Randolph Medical Center

411 West Randolph Road
Hopewell, VA 23860
Phone: 804-541-1600
Fax: 804-452-3699
URL: www.johnrandolphmed.com
Type: Acute Care Hospitals
Emergency Services: Yes
Ownership: Proprietary
Beds: 257

Key Personnel:
CEO/President. . . . . E Bernard Boone, III
Operating Room. . . . . Joan Hirsch
Pediatric In-Patient Care . . . . Nancy Lasken, RN
Chief of Medical Staff . . . . Dr Mohammad Mojeebuddin
Radiology. . . . . Rhonda Munson
Quality Assurance . . . . Jeanne Poindexter
Coronary Care . . . . Debbie Young

Measure	Cases	This Hosp.	State Avg.	U.S. Avg.
Blood Clot Prevention and Treatment				
Anticoagulation Overlap Therapy[2]	44	100%	95%	93%
ICU Venous Thromboembolism Prophylaxis[2]	89	100%	95%	92%
Incidence of Potentially Preventable VTE[1,2]	-	-	8%	10%
UFH with Dosages/Platelet Monitoring[2]	33	100%	99%	97%
Venous Thromboembolism Prophylaxis[2]	359	100%	91%	85%
Warfarin Therapy Discharge Instructions[2]	37	100%	78%	75%
Chest Pain/Possible Heart Attack Care				
Aspirin Given Within 24 Hours of Arrival	29	100%	98%	96%
Fibrinolytic Meds Within 30 Min. of Arrival[7]	-	-	68%	58%
Average Time to ECG (minutes)	31	1	7	7
Average Time to Transfer (minutes)	21	33	64	60
Children's Asthma Care				
Received Home Management Plan of Care	-	-	-	88%
Received Reliever Medication	-	-	-	100%
Received Systemic Corticosteroids	-	-	-	100%
Emergency Department				
Admittance Decision Time (minutes)[2]	852	50	96	98
Head CT Results Within 45 Min. of Arrival[1]	-	-	60%	57%
Patients Who Left ER Before Being Seen	36,876	1%	2%	2%
Time from ER Arrival to Admit. (minutes)[2]	852	244	280	274
Time from ER Arrival to Discharge (minutes)	487	110	167	134
Time in ER Before Being Evaluated (minutes)	524	13	35	26
Time to Pain Meds for Fractures (minutes)	92	37	56	57
Heart Attack Care				
Aspirin Given at Discharge	38	100%	99%	99%
Fibrinolytic Meds Within 30 Min. of Arrival[7]	-	-	75%	54%
PCI Within 90 Minutes of Arrival[7]	-	-	97%	96%
Statin Prescribed at Discharge	39	100%	99%	98%
Heart Failure Care				
ACE Inhibitor or ARB for LVSD	68	100%	98%	97%
Discharge Instructions Given	134	100%	95%	94%
Evaluation of LVS Function	173	100%	100%	99%
Medicare Spending				
Medicare Spending per Patient (ratio)	-	1.03	0.95	0.98
Pneumonia Care				
Appropriate Initial Antibiotic Given	85	100%	97%	95%
Blood Culture Timing	133	99%	98%	98%
Pregnancy and Delivery Care				
Newborn Deliveries Scheduled Early[2,7]	-	-	6%	6%
Preventive Care				
Immunization for Influenza[2]	493	100%	92%	90%
Immunization for Pneumonia[2]	717	100%	93%	92%
Stroke Care				
Anticoagulation Therapy for Atrial Fibrillation[1,2]	-	-	96%	95%
Antithrombotic Therapy Timing[2]	66	100%	99%	98%
Assessed for Rehabilitation[2]	59	100%	99%	97%
Discharged on Antithrombotic Therapy[2]	57	100%	100%	99%
Discharged on Statin Medication[2]	46	100%	97%	94%
Thrombolytic Therapy Timing[2,7]	-	-	73%	66%
Venous Thromboembolism Prophylaxis[2]	68	100%	97%	94%
Written Stroke Educational Materials Given[2]	26	100%	92%	88%
Surgical Care Improvement Project				

NOTE: Hospital profiles are in alphabetical order by state, then city, then hospital within the city; Rankings exclude hospitals with less than 25 cases except for patient surveys which excludes hospitals with less than 100 cases; (a) 100-299 cases; (1) The number of cases/patients is too few to report; (2) Data submitted were based on a sample of cases/patients; (3) Results are based on a shorter time period than required; (4) Data suppressed by CMS for one or more quarters; (5) Results are not available for this reporting period; (6) Fewer than 100 patients completed the HCAHPS survey; (7) No cases met the criteria for this measure; (8) The lower limit of the confidence interval cannot be calculated if the number of observed infections equals zero; (9) No data are available from the state/territory for this reporting period; (10) The scores shown reflect fewer than 50 completed surveys; (11) There were discrepancies in the data collection process; (12) This measure does not apply to this hospital for this reporting period; (13) Results cannot be calculated for this reporting period; (14) The results for this state are combined with nearby states to protect confidentiality; Please refer to the User's Guide for a full explanation of data.

Measure	Cases	This Hosp.	State Avg.	U.S. Avg.
Appropriate Beta Blocker Usage	42	100%	99%	98%
Appropriate VTP Within 24 Hours	128	100%	99%	98%
Controlled Postoperative Blood Glucose[7]	-	-	98%	97%
Perioperative Temperature Management	151	100%	100%	100%
Prophylactic Antibiotic Selection	91	100%	99%	99%
Prophylactic Antibiotic Selection (Outpatient)	21	100%	98%	98%
Prophylactic Antibiotic Stopped	86	99%	98%	98%
Prophylactic Antibiotic Timing	91	100%	99%	99%
Prophylactic Antibiotic Timing (Outpatient)	21	100%	98%	98%
Urinary Catheter Removal	94	100%	98%	97%
Survey of Patients' Hospital Experiences				
Area Around Room 'Always' Quiet at Night	300+	64%	60%	61%
Doctors 'Always' Communicated Well	300+	80%	81%	82%
Home Recovery Information Given	300+	84%	86%	85%
Hospital Given 9 or 10 on 10 Point Scale	300+	61%	68%	71%
Meds 'Always' Explained Before Given	300+	60%	62%	64%
Nurses 'Always' Communicated Well	300+	74%	78%	79%
Pain 'Always' Well Controlled	300+	67%	70%	71%
Room and Bathroom 'Always' Clean	300+	73%	71%	73%
Timely Help 'Always' Received	300+	56%	64%	68%
Would Definitely Recommend Hospital	300+	60%	69%	71%
Use of Medical Imaging				
Cardiac Imaging Stress Test before Surgery	82	12.2%	5.1%	5.3%
Combination Abdominal CT Scan	544	32.4%	8.5%	10.5%
Combination Brain/Sinus CT Scan	463	1.5%	2.3%	2.7%
Combination Chest CT Scan	392	1.8%	1.6%	2.7%
Follow-up Mammogram/Ultrasound	752	4.1%	7.7%	8.8%
Lumbar Spine MRI for Low Back Pain	79	30.4%	35.3%	37.2%

Bath Community Hospital

106 Park Drive- PO Drawer Z
Hot Springs, VA 24445
Phone: 540-839-7000
Fax: 540-839-7060
E-mail: dlipes@bcchospital.org
URL: www.bcchospital.org
Type: Critical Access Hospitals
Emergency Services: Yes
Ownership: Voluntary non-profit - Private
Beds: 25

Key Personnel:
Infection Control. . . . . Becky Armstrong
Operating Room. . . . . Mary Ayers
Radiology. . . . . Jo Lamb, MD
CEO/President. . . . . Deborah R Lipes
Chief of Medical Staff. . . . . James Redington, MD
Emergency Room . . . . James Redington, MD
Quality Assurance . . . . Amanda Thornsbury
Cardiology . . . . John Yang, MD

Measure	Cases	This Hosp.	State Avg.	U.S. Avg.
Blood Clot Prevention and Treatment				
Anticoagulation Overlap Therapy[5]	-	-	95%	93%
ICU Venous Thromboembolism Prophylaxis[5]	-	-	95%	92%
Incidence of Potentially Preventable VTE[5]	-	-	8%	10%
UFH with Dosages/Platelet Monitoring[5]	-	-	99%	97%
Venous Thromboembolism Prophylaxis[5]	-	-	91%	85%
Warfarin Therapy Discharge Instructions[5]	-	-	78%	75%
Chest Pain/Possible Heart Attack Care				
Aspirin Given Within 24 Hours of Arrival	-	-	98%	96%
Fibrinolytic Meds Within 30 Min. of Arrival	-	-	68%	58%
Average Time to ECG (minutes)	-	-	7	7
Average Time to Transfer (minutes)	-	-	64	60
Children's Asthma Care				
Received Home Management Plan of Care	-	-	-	88%
Received Reliever Medication	-	-	-	100%
Received Systemic Corticosteroids	-	-	-	100%
Emergency Department				
Admittance Decision Time (minutes)[5]	-	-	96	98
Head CT Results Within 45 Min. of Arrival	-	-	60%	57%
Patients Who Left ER Before Being Seen	-	-	2%	2%
Time from ER Arrival to Admit. (minutes)[5]	-	-	280	274
Time from ER Arrival to Discharge (minutes)	-	-	167	134
Time in ER Before Being Evaluated (minutes)	-	-	35	26
Time to Pain Meds for Fractures (minutes)	-	-	56	57
Heart Attack Care				
Aspirin Given at Discharge[5]	-	-	99%	99%
Fibrinolytic Meds Within 30 Min. of Arrival[5]	-	-	75%	54%
PCI Within 90 Minutes of Arrival[5]	-	-	97%	96%
Statin Prescribed at Discharge[5]	-	-	99%	98%
Heart Failure Care				
ACE Inhibitor or ARB for LVSD[1,3]	-	-	98%	97%
Discharge Instructions Given[3]	19	95%	95%	94%
Evaluation of LVS Function[3]	19	84%	100%	99%
Medicare Spending				
Medicare Spending per Patient (ratio)	-	-	0.95	0.98
Pneumonia Care				
Appropriate Initial Antibiotic Given[1]	-	-	97%	95%
Blood Culture Timing	11	100%	98%	98%
Pregnancy and Delivery Care				
Newborn Deliveries Scheduled Early[5]	-	-	6%	6%
Preventive Care				
Immunization for Influenza[5]	-	-	92%	90%
Immunization for Pneumonia[5]	-	-	93%	92%
Stroke Care				
Anticoagulation Therapy for Atrial Fibrillation[5]	-	-	96%	95%
Antithrombotic Therapy Timing[5]	-	-	99%	98%
Assessed for Rehabilitation[5]	-	-	99%	97%
Discharged on Antithrombotic Therapy[5]	-	-	100%	99%
Discharged on Statin Medication[5]	-	-	97%	94%
Thrombolytic Therapy Timing[5]	-	-	73%	66%
Venous Thromboembolism Prophylaxis[5]	-	-	97%	94%
Written Stroke Educational Materials Given[5]	-	-	92%	88%
Surgical Care Improvement Project				
Appropriate Beta Blocker Usage[5]	-	-	99%	98%
Appropriate VTP Within 24 Hours[5]	-	-	99%	98%
Controlled Postoperative Blood Glucose[5]	-	-	98%	97%
Perioperative Temperature Management[5]	-	-	100%	100%
Prophylactic Antibiotic Selection[5]	-	-	99%	99%
Prophylactic Antibiotic Selection (Outpatient)	-	-	98%	98%
Prophylactic Antibiotic Stopped[5]	-	-	98%	98%
Prophylactic Antibiotic Timing[5]	-	-	99%	99%
Prophylactic Antibiotic Timing (Outpatient)	-	-	98%	98%
Urinary Catheter Removal[5]	-	-	98%	97%
Survey of Patients' Hospital Experiences				
Area Around Room 'Always' Quiet at Night[5]	-	-	60%	61%
Doctors 'Always' Communicated Well[5]	-	-	81%	82%
Home Recovery Information Given[5]	-	-	86%	85%
Hospital Given 9 or 10 on 10 Point Scale[5]	-	-	68%	71%
Meds 'Always' Explained Before Given[5]	-	-	62%	64%
Nurses 'Always' Communicated Well[5]	-	-	78%	79%
Pain 'Always' Well Controlled[5]	-	-	70%	71%
Room and Bathroom 'Always' Clean[5]	-	-	71%	73%
Timely Help 'Always' Received[5]	-	-	64%	68%
Would Definitely Recommend Hospital[5]	-	-	69%	71%
Use of Medical Imaging				
Cardiac Imaging Stress Test before Surgery	-	-	5.1%	5.3%
Combination Abdominal CT Scan	-	-	8.5%	10.5%
Combination Brain/Sinus CT Scan	-	-	2.3%	2.7%
Combination Chest CT Scan	-	-	1.6%	2.7%
Follow-up Mammogram/Ultrasound	-	-	7.7%	8.8%
Lumbar Spine MRI for Low Back Pain	-	-	35.3%	37.2%

Rappahannock General Hospital

101 Harris Road
Kilmarnock, VA 22482
Phone: 804-435-8000
Fax: 804-435-8543
E-mail: egravatt@hotmail.com
URL: www.rgh-hospital.com
Type: Acute Care Hospitals
Emergency Services: Yes
Ownership: Voluntary non-profit - Private
Beds: 76

Key Personnel:
Radiology. . . . . Matthew C Allison, RN
Radiology. . . . . Garrett W Colby
CEO/President. . . . . James M Holmes, Jr
Cardiology . . . . Charles W Nelson
Anesthesiology. . . . . Barbara P Perona, RN
Cardiology . . . . PV Ravindra

Measure	Cases	This Hosp.	State Avg.	U.S. Avg.
Blood Clot Prevention and Treatment				
Anticoagulation Overlap Therapy[1,2]	-	-	95%	93%
ICU Venous Thromboembolism Prophylaxis[2]	43	91%	95%	92%
Incidence of Potentially Preventable VTE[1,2]	-	-	8%	10%
UFH with Dosages/Platelet Monitoring[1,2]	-	-	99%	97%
Venous Thromboembolism Prophylaxis[2]	111	92%	91%	85%
Warfarin Therapy Discharge Instructions[1,2]	-	-	78%	75%
Chest Pain/Possible Heart Attack Care				
Aspirin Given Within 24 Hours of Arrival	86	100%	98%	96%
Fibrinolytic Meds Within 30 Min. of Arrival[1]	-	-	68%	58%
Average Time to ECG (minutes)	92	7	7	7
Average Time to Transfer (minutes)	11	80	64	60
Children's Asthma Care				
Received Home Management Plan of Care	-	-	-	88%
Received Reliever Medication	-	-	-	100%
Received Systemic Corticosteroids	-	-	-	100%
Emergency Department				
Admittance Decision Time (minutes)[2]	606	102	96	98
Head CT Results Within 45 Min. of Arrival	42	24%	60%	57%
Patients Who Left ER Before Being Seen	11,749	3%	2%	2%
Time from ER Arrival to Admit. (minutes)[2]	621	309	280	274
Time from ER Arrival to Discharge (minutes)	331	151	167	134
Time in ER Before Being Evaluated (minutes)	378	35	35	26
Time to Pain Meds for Fractures (minutes)	68	67	56	57
Heart Attack Care				
Aspirin Given at Discharge[1]	-	-	99%	99%
Fibrinolytic Meds Within 30 Min. of Arrival[7]	-	-	75%	54%
PCI Within 90 Minutes of Arrival[7]	-	-	97%	96%
Statin Prescribed at Discharge[1]	-	-	99%	98%
Heart Failure Care				
ACE Inhibitor or ARB for LVSD	23	100%	98%	97%
Discharge Instructions Given	55	98%	95%	94%
Evaluation of LVS Function	66	98%	100%	99%
Medicare Spending				
Medicare Spending per Patient (ratio)	-	0.90	0.95	0.98
Pneumonia Care				
Appropriate Initial Antibiotic Given	47	83%	97%	95%
Blood Culture Timing	63	95%	98%	98%
Pregnancy and Delivery Care				
Newborn Deliveries Scheduled Early[7]	-	-	6%	6%
Preventive Care				
Immunization for Influenza[2]	456	95%	92%	90%
Immunization for Pneumonia[2]	600	97%	93%	92%
Stroke Care				
Anticoagulation Therapy for Atrial Fibrillation[1]	-	-	96%	95%
Antithrombotic Therapy Timing	37	100%	99%	98%
Assessed for Rehabilitation	39	92%	99%	97%
Discharged on Antithrombotic Therapy	37	100%	100%	99%
Discharged on Statin Medication	34	56%	97%	94%
Thrombolytic Therapy Timing[1]	-	-	73%	66%
Venous Thromboembolism Prophylaxis	36	97%	97%	94%
Written Stroke Educational Materials Given	23	74%	92%	88%
Surgical Care Improvement Project				
Appropriate Beta Blocker Usage	15	93%	99%	98%
Appropriate VTP Within 24 Hours	49	94%	99%	98%
Controlled Postoperative Blood Glucose[7]	-	-	98%	97%
Perioperative Temperature Management	52	100%	100%	100%
Prophylactic Antibiotic Selection	26	100%	99%	99%
Prophylactic Antibiotic Selection (Outpatient)	15	100%	98%	98%
Prophylactic Antibiotic Stopped	24	88%	98%	98%
Prophylactic Antibiotic Timing	26	100%	99%	99%
Prophylactic Antibiotic Timing (Outpatient)	15	100%	98%	98%
Urinary Catheter Removal	44	98%	98%	97%
Survey of Patients' Hospital Experiences				
Area Around Room 'Always' Quiet at Night	300+	53%	60%	61%
Doctors 'Always' Communicated Well	300+	85%	81%	82%
Home Recovery Information Given	300+	90%	86%	85%
Hospital Given 9 or 10 on 10 Point Scale	300+	72%	68%	71%
Meds 'Always' Explained Before Given	300+	67%	62%	64%
Nurses 'Always' Communicated Well	300+	83%	78%	79%
Pain 'Always' Well Controlled	300+	73%	70%	71%
Room and Bathroom 'Always' Clean	300+	73%	71%	73%
Timely Help 'Always' Received	300+	75%	64%	68%
Would Definitely Recommend Hospital	300+	69%	69%	71%
Use of Medical Imaging				
Cardiac Imaging Stress Test before Surgery	151	6.0%	5.1%	5.3%
Combination Abdominal CT Scan	514	8.4%	8.5%	10.5%

NOTE: Hospital profiles are in alphabetical order by state, then city, then hospital within the city; Rankings exclude hospitals with less than 25 cases except for patient surveys which excludes hospitals with less than 100 cases; (a) 100-299 cases; (1) The number of cases/patients is too few to report; (2) Data submitted were based on a sample of cases/patients; (3) Results are based on a shorter time period than required; (4) Data suppressed by CMS for one or more quarters; (5) Results are not available for this reporting period; (6) Fewer than 100 patients completed the HCAHPS survey; (7) No cases met the criteria for this measure; (8) The lower limit of the confidence interval cannot be calculated if the number of observed infections equals zero; (9) No data are available from the state/territory for this reporting period; (10) The scores shown reflect fewer than 50 completed surveys; (11) There were discrepancies in the data collection process; (12) This measure does not apply to this hospital for this reporting period; (13) Results cannot be calculated for this reporting period; (14) The results for this state are combined with nearby states to protect confidentiality; Please refer to the User's Guide for a full explanation of data.

Combination Brain/Sinus CT Scan	439	0.9%	2.3%	2.7%
Combination Chest CT Scan	335	1.2%	1.6%	2.7%
Follow-up Mammogram/Ultrasound	926	9.6%	7.7%	8.8%
Lumbar Spine MRI for Low Back Pain	75	38.7%	35.3%	37.2%

Russell County Medical Center

58 Carroll Street
Lebanon, VA 24266
Phone: 276-883-8100
Fax: 276-883-8111
URL: www.msha.com
Type: Acute Care Hospitals
Emergency Services: Yes
Ownership: Voluntary non-profit - Private
Beds: 78

Key Personnel:
Quality Assurance . . . . Brenda Banner
Anesthesiology. . . . . Jennifer Burton, D.O.
Intensive Care Unit. . . . . Karen Chaney, RN
Operating Room. . . . . Debbie Garrett, RN
Chief of Medical Staff . . . . Samuel Milton
CEO/President. . . . . David Parsh
Emergency Room . . . . Norman Rexrode Jr, MD
Infection Control. . . . . William Taylor, RN

Measure	Cases	This Hosp.	State Avg.	U.S. Avg.
Blood Clot Prevention and Treatment				
Anticoagulation Overlap Therapy[2]	12	83%	95%	93%
ICU Venous Thromboembolism Prophylaxis[2]	32	78%	95%	92%
Incidence of Potentially Preventable VTE[1,2]	-	-	8%	10%
UFH with Dosages/Platelet Monitoring[2,7]	-	-	99%	97%
Venous Thromboembolism Prophylaxis[2]	170	71%	91%	85%
Warfarin Therapy Discharge Instructions[2]	11	55%	78%	75%
Chest Pain/Possible Heart Attack Care				
Aspirin Given Within 24 Hours of Arrival	46	98%	98%	96%
Fibrinolytic Meds Within 30 Min. of Arrival[1]	-	-	68%	58%
Average Time to ECG (minutes)	48	5	7	7
Average Time to Transfer (minutes)[7]	-	-	64	60
Children's Asthma Care				
Received Home Management Plan of Care	-	-	-	88%
Received Reliever Medication	-	-	-	100%
Received Systemic Corticosteroids	-	-	-	100%
Emergency Department				
Admittance Decision Time (minutes)[2]	369	47	96	98
Head CT Results Within 45 Min. of Arrival[1]	-	-	60%	57%
Patients Who Left ER Before Being Seen	16,006	1%	2%	2%
Time from ER Arrival to Admit. (minutes)[2]	396	182	280	274
Time from ER Arrival to Discharge (minutes)	349	96	167	134
Time in ER Before Being Evaluated (minutes)	388	20	35	26
Time to Pain Meds for Fractures (minutes)	40	47	56	57
Heart Attack Care				
Aspirin Given at Discharge[1,2]	-	-	99%	99%
Fibrinolytic Meds Within 30 Min. of Arrival[2,3]	-	-	75%	54%
PCI Within 90 Minutes of Arrival[2,3]	-	-	97%	96%
Statin Prescribed at Discharge[1,2]	-	-	99%	98%
Heart Failure Care				
ACE Inhibitor or ARB for LVSD[2]	21	86%	98%	97%
Discharge Instructions Given[2]	60	92%	95%	94%
Evaluation of LVS Function[2]	69	96%	100%	99%
Medicare Spending				
Medicare Spending per Patient (ratio)	-	0.93	0.95	0.98
Pneumonia Care				
Appropriate Initial Antibiotic Given[2]	87	92%	97%	95%
Blood Culture Timing[2]	108	97%	98%	98%
Pregnancy and Delivery Care				
Newborn Deliveries Scheduled Early[7]	-	-	6%	6%
Preventive Care				
Immunization for Influenza[2]	299	97%	92%	90%
Immunization for Pneumonia[2]	468	98%	93%	92%
Stroke Care				
Anticoagulation Therapy for Atrial Fibrillation[3,7]	-	-	96%	95%
Antithrombotic Therapy Timing[1,3]	-	-	99%	98%
Assessed for Rehabilitation[1,3]	-	-	99%	97%
Discharged on Antithrombotic Therapy[1,3]	-	-	100%	99%
Discharged on Statin Medication[1,3]	-	-	97%	94%
Thrombolytic Therapy Timing[3,7]	-	-	73%	66%
Venous Thromboembolism Prophylaxis[1,3]	-	-	97%	94%
Written Stroke Educational Materials Given[1,3]	-	-	92%	88%
Surgical Care Improvement Project				
Appropriate Beta Blocker Usage[5]	-	-	99%	98%
Appropriate VTP Within 24 Hours[5]	-	-	99%	98%
Controlled Postoperative Blood Glucose[5]	-	-	98%	97%
Perioperative Temperature Management[5]	-	-	100%	100%
Prophylactic Antibiotic Selection[5]	-	-	99%	99%
Prophylactic Antibiotic Selection (Outpatient)[5]	-	-	98%	98%
Prophylactic Antibiotic Stopped[5]	-	-	98%	98%
Prophylactic Antibiotic Timing[5]	-	-	99%	99%
Prophylactic Antibiotic Timing (Outpatient)[5]	-	-	98%	98%
Urinary Catheter Removal[5]	-	-	98%	97%
Survey of Patients' Hospital Experiences				
Area Around Room 'Always' Quiet at Night	(a)	60%	60%	61%
Doctors 'Always' Communicated Well	(a)	83%	81%	82%
Home Recovery Information Given	(a)	83%	86%	85%
Hospital Given 9 or 10 on 10 Point Scale	(a)	64%	68%	71%
Meds 'Always' Explained Before Given	(a)	61%	62%	64%
Nurses 'Always' Communicated Well	(a)	82%	78%	79%
Pain 'Always' Well Controlled	(a)	65%	70%	71%
Room and Bathroom 'Always' Clean	(a)	74%	71%	73%
Timely Help 'Always' Received	(a)	77%	64%	68%
Would Definitely Recommend Hospital	(a)	64%	69%	71%
Use of Medical Imaging				
Cardiac Imaging Stress Test before Surgery	55	0.0%	5.1%	5.3%
Combination Abdominal CT Scan	188	1.1%	8.5%	10.5%
Combination Brain/Sinus CT Scan	283	0.7%	2.3%	2.7%
Combination Chest CT Scan	76	0.0%	1.6%	2.7%
Follow-up Mammogram/Ultrasound	185	3.8%	7.7%	8.8%
Lumbar Spine MRI for Low Back Pain	44	59.1%	35.3%	37.2%

Inova Loudoun Hospital

44045 Riverside Parkway
Leesburg, VA 20176
Phone: 703-858-6600
Fax: 703-858-6610
URL: www.loudounhealthcare.org
Type: Acute Care Hospitals
Emergency Services: Yes
Ownership: Voluntary non-profit - Private
Beds: 155

Key Personnel:
Infection Control. . . . . Linda Belomonte
Cardiac Laboratory. . . . . Deidre Cahill
Emergency Room . . . . Lisa Dugan
CEO/President. . . . . Randall Kelley
Operating Room. . . . . Barb McDonnell
Chief of Medical Staff . . . . Kevin O'Connor
CEO . . . . J. Knox Singleton
Quality Assurance . . . . Diane Wilhite

Measure	Cases	This Hosp.	State Avg.	U.S. Avg.
Blood Clot Prevention and Treatment				
Anticoagulation Overlap Therapy[2]	102	97%	95%	93%
ICU Venous Thromboembolism Prophylaxis[2]	57	95%	95%	92%
Incidence of Potentially Preventable VTE[1,2]	-	-	8%	10%
UFH with Dosages/Platelet Monitoring[2]	22	100%	99%	97%
Venous Thromboembolism Prophylaxis[2]	315	84%	91%	85%
Warfarin Therapy Discharge Instructions[2]	86	87%	78%	75%
Chest Pain/Possible Heart Attack Care				
Aspirin Given Within 24 Hours of Arrival	37	97%	98%	96%
Fibrinolytic Meds Within 30 Min. of Arrival[3,7]	-	-	68%	58%
Average Time to ECG (minutes)	41	10	7	7
Average Time to Transfer (minutes)[1,3]	-	-	64	60
Children's Asthma Care				
Received Home Management Plan of Care	-	-	-	88%
Received Reliever Medication	-	-	-	100%
Received Systemic Corticosteroids	-	-	-	100%
Emergency Department				
Admittance Decision Time (minutes)[2]	512	122	96	98
Head CT Results Within 45 Min. of Arrival	14	86%	60%	57%
Patients Who Left ER Before Being Seen	68,033	0%	2%	2%
Time from ER Arrival to Admit. (minutes)[2]	514	305	280	274
Time from ER Arrival to Discharge (minutes)	777	136	167	134
Time in ER Before Being Evaluated (minutes)	821	17	35	26
Time to Pain Meds for Fractures (minutes)	221	50	56	57
Heart Attack Care				
Aspirin Given at Discharge	206	100%	99%	99%
Fibrinolytic Meds Within 30 Min. of Arrival[7]	-	-	75%	54%
PCI Within 90 Minutes of Arrival	42	100%	97%	96%
Statin Prescribed at Discharge	198	99%	99%	98%
Heart Failure Care				
ACE Inhibitor or ARB for LVSD[2]	62	100%	98%	97%
Discharge Instructions Given[2]	219	92%	95%	94%
Evaluation of LVS Function[2]	271	100%	100%	99%
Medicare Spending				
Medicare Spending per Patient (ratio)	-	1.02	0.95	0.98
Pneumonia Care				
Appropriate Initial Antibiotic Given[2]	77	96%	97%	95%
Blood Culture Timing[2]	106	99%	98%	98%
Pregnancy and Delivery Care				
Newborn Deliveries Scheduled Early[2]	135	10%	6%	6%
Preventive Care				
Immunization for Influenza[2]	464	94%	92%	90%
Immunization for Pneumonia[2]	443	93%	93%	92%
Stroke Care				
Anticoagulation Therapy for Atrial Fibrillation[2]	16	100%	96%	95%
Antithrombotic Therapy Timing[2]	105	100%	99%	98%
Assessed for Rehabilitation[2]	110	99%	99%	97%
Discharged on Antithrombotic Therapy[2]	108	99%	100%	99%
Discharged on Statin Medication[2]	83	98%	97%	94%
Thrombolytic Therapy Timing[1,2]	-	-	73%	66%
Venous Thromboembolism Prophylaxis[2]	116	100%	97%	94%
Written Stroke Educational Materials Given[2]	65	98%	92%	88%
Surgical Care Improvement Project				
Appropriate Beta Blocker Usage[2]	89	97%	99%	98%
Appropriate VTP Within 24 Hours[2]	307	96%	99%	98%
Controlled Postoperative Blood Glucose[2,7]	-	-	98%	97%
Perioperative Temperature Management[2]	393	100%	100%	100%
Prophylactic Antibiotic Selection[2]	232	95%	99%	99%
Prophylactic Antibiotic Selection (Outpatient)	374	98%	98%	98%
Prophylactic Antibiotic Stopped[2]	229	98%	98%	98%
Prophylactic Antibiotic Timing[2]	232	98%	99%	99%
Prophylactic Antibiotic Timing (Outpatient)	358	98%	98%	98%
Urinary Catheter Removal[2]	121	98%	98%	97%
Survey of Patients' Hospital Experiences				
Area Around Room 'Always' Quiet at Night	300+	45%	60%	61%
Doctors 'Always' Communicated Well	300+	78%	81%	82%
Home Recovery Information Given	300+	87%	86%	85%
Hospital Given 9 or 10 on 10 Point Scale	300+	65%	68%	71%
Meds 'Always' Explained Before Given	300+	59%	62%	64%
Nurses 'Always' Communicated Well	300+	76%	78%	79%
Pain 'Always' Well Controlled	300+	67%	70%	71%
Room and Bathroom 'Always' Clean	300+	63%	71%	73%
Timely Help 'Always' Received	300+	60%	64%	68%
Would Definitely Recommend Hospital	300+	72%	69%	71%
Use of Medical Imaging				
Cardiac Imaging Stress Test before Surgery[1]	-	-	5.1%	5.3%
Combination Abdominal CT Scan	926	4.9%	8.5%	10.5%
Combination Brain/Sinus CT Scan	1,015	2.9%	2.3%	2.7%
Combination Chest CT Scan	554	0.0%	1.6%	2.7%
Follow-up Mammogram/Ultrasound	602	15.8%	7.7%	8.8%
Lumbar Spine MRI for Low Back Pain	91	33.0%	35.3%	37.2%

Carilion Stonewall Jackson Hospital

1 Health Circle
Lexington, VA 24450
Phone: 540-458-3503
Fax: 540-458-3545
E-mail: crassist@sjhospital.com
URL: www.sjhospital.com
Type: Critical Access Hospitals
Emergency Services: Yes
Ownership: Voluntary non-profit - Other
Beds: 130

Key Personnel:
CEO . . . . Charles E. Carr
Radiology. . . . . Michael Clague
Chair/CEO . . . . H. E. Derrick, Jr.
Chief of Medical Staff . . . . Timothy Harriso, MD
CEO/President. . . . . Thomas McNamara

Measure	Cases	This Hosp.	State Avg.	U.S. Avg.
Blood Clot Prevention and Treatment				
Anticoagulation Overlap Therapy[5]	-	-	95%	93%
ICU Venous Thromboembolism Prophylaxis[5]	-	-	95%	92%
Incidence of Potentially Preventable VTE[5]	-	-	8%	10%
UFH with Dosages/Platelet Monitoring[5]	-	-	99%	97%
Venous Thromboembolism Prophylaxis[5]	-	-	91%	85%
Warfarin Therapy Discharge Instructions[5]	-	-	78%	75%

NOTE: Hospital profiles are in alphabetical order by state, then city, then hospital within the city; Rankings exclude hospitals with less than 25 cases except for patient surveys which excludes hospitals with less than 100 cases; (a) 100-299 cases; (1) The number of cases/patients is too few to report; (2) Data submitted were based on a sample of cases/patients; (3) Results are based on a shorter time period than required; (4) Data suppressed by CMS for one or more quarters; (5) Results are not available for this reporting period; (6) Fewer than 100 patients completed the HCAHPS survey; (7) No cases met the criteria for this measure; (8) The lower limit of the confidence interval cannot be calculated if the number of observed infections equals zero; (9) No data are available from the state/territory for this reporting period; (10) The scores shown reflect fewer than 50 completed surveys; (11) There were discrepancies in the data collection process; (12) This measure does not apply to this hospital for this reporting period; (13) Results cannot be calculated for this reporting period; (14) The results for this state are combined with nearby states to protect confidentiality; Please refer to the User's Guide for a full explanation of data.

Measure	Cases	This Hosp.	State Avg.	U.S. Avg.
Chest Pain/Possible Heart Attack Care				
Aspirin Given Within 24 Hours of Arrival[5]	-	-	98%	96%
Fibrinolytic Meds Within 30 Min. of Arrival[5]	-	-	68%	58%
Average Time to ECG (minutes)[5]	-	-	7	7
Average Time to Transfer (minutes)[5]	-	-	64	60
Children's Asthma Care				
Received Home Management Plan of Care	-	-	-	88%
Received Reliever Medication	-	-	-	100%
Received Systemic Corticosteroids	-	-	-	100%
Emergency Department				
Admittance Decision Time (minutes)[2]	375	107	96	98
Head CT Results Within 45 Min. of Arrival[5]	-	-	60%	57%
Patients Who Left ER Before Being Seen[5]	-	-	2%	2%
Time from ER Arrival to Admit. (minutes)[2]	468	274	280	274
Time from ER Arrival to Discharge (minutes)[5]	-	-	167	134
Time in ER Before Being Evaluated (minutes)[5]	-	-	35	26
Time to Pain Meds for Fractures (minutes)[5]	-	-	56	57
Heart Attack Care				
Aspirin Given at Discharge[1]	-	-	99%	99%
Fibrinolytic Meds Within 30 Min. of Arrival[7]	-	-	75%	54%
PCI Within 90 Minutes of Arrival[7]	-	-	97%	96%
Statin Prescribed at Discharge[1]	-	-	99%	98%
Heart Failure Care				
ACE Inhibitor or ARB for LVSD	21	100%	98%	97%
Discharge Instructions Given	54	98%	95%	94%
Evaluation of LVS Function	86	100%	100%	99%
Medicare Spending				
Medicare Spending per Patient (ratio)	-	-	0.95	0.98
Pneumonia Care				
Appropriate Initial Antibiotic Given	28	96%	97%	95%
Blood Culture Timing	57	95%	98%	98%
Pregnancy and Delivery Care				
Newborn Deliveries Scheduled Early[2,3]	-	-	6%	6%
Preventive Care				
Immunization for Influenza[2]	284	97%	92%	90%
Immunization for Pneumonia[2]	551	97%	93%	92%
Stroke Care				
Anticoagulation Therapy for Atrial Fibrillation[5]	-	-	96%	95%
Antithrombotic Therapy Timing[5]	-	-	99%	98%
Assessed for Rehabilitation[5]	-	-	99%	97%
Discharged on Antithrombotic Therapy[5]	-	-	100%	99%
Discharged on Statin Medication[5]	-	-	97%	94%
Thrombolytic Therapy Timing[5]	-	-	73%	66%
Venous Thromboembolism Prophylaxis[5]	-	-	97%	94%
Written Stroke Educational Materials Given[5]	-	-	92%	88%
Surgical Care Improvement Project				
Appropriate Beta Blocker Usage	13	85%	99%	98%
Appropriate VTP Within 24 Hours	42	86%	99%	98%
Controlled Postoperative Blood Glucose[3,7]	-	-	98%	97%
Perioperative Temperature Management	45	100%	100%	100%
Prophylactic Antibiotic Selection	24	100%	99%	99%
Prophylactic Antibiotic Selection (Outpatient)[5]	-	-	98%	98%
Prophylactic Antibiotic Stopped	24	100%	98%	98%
Prophylactic Antibiotic Timing	24	100%	99%	99%
Prophylactic Antibiotic Timing (Outpatient)[5]	-	-	98%	98%
Urinary Catheter Removal	32	94%	98%	97%
Survey of Patients' Hospital Experiences				
Area Around Room 'Always' Quiet at Night	(a)	60%	60%	61%
Doctors 'Always' Communicated Well	(a)	90%	81%	82%
Home Recovery Information Given	(a)	88%	86%	85%
Hospital Given 9 or 10 on 10 Point Scale	(a)	66%	68%	71%
Meds 'Always' Explained Before Given	(a)	70%	62%	64%
Nurses 'Always' Communicated Well	(a)	81%	78%	79%
Pain 'Always' Well Controlled	(a)	72%	70%	71%
Room and Bathroom 'Always' Clean	(a)	64%	71%	73%
Timely Help 'Always' Received	(a)	67%	64%	68%
Would Definitely Recommend Hospital	(a)	61%	69%	71%
Use of Medical Imaging				
Cardiac Imaging Stress Test before Surgery	188	2.1%	5.1%	5.3%
Combination Abdominal CT Scan	336	4.2%	8.5%	10.5%
Combination Brain/Sinus CT Scan[1]	-	-	2.3%	2.7%
Combination Chest CT Scan	126	0.0%	1.6%	2.7%
Follow-up Mammogram/Ultrasound	768	3.3%	7.7%	8.8%
Lumbar Spine MRI for Low Back Pain	52	40.4%	35.3%	37.2%

Lewisgale Hospital Alleghany

One Arh Lane - PO Box 7
Low Moor, VA 24457
URL: www.alleghanyregional.com
Type: Acute Care Hospitals
Ownership: Proprietary

Phone: 540-862-6011
Fax: 540-862-6472

Emergency Services: Yes
Beds: 156

Key Personnel:

Chief of Medical Staff.......... Michele Ballou, MD
Radiology.................. Bruce C Banning, MD
Quality Assurance .... Debbie Clark, RN
CEO/President............... Greg Madsen
Operating Room............. Gayle Minson, RN
CEO .... Charlotte Tyson, MHA, BSN, FACHE

Measure	Cases	This Hosp.	State Avg.	U.S. Avg.
Blood Clot Prevention and Treatment				
Anticoagulation Overlap Therapy[2]	24	100%	95%	93%
ICU Venous Thromboembolism Prophylaxis[2]	52	100%	95%	92%
Incidence of Potentially Preventable VTE[1,2]	-	-	8%	10%
UFH with Dosages/Platelet Monitoring[1,2]	-	-	99%	97%
Venous Thromboembolism Prophylaxis[2]	222	99%	91%	85%
Warfarin Therapy Discharge Instructions[2]	16	100%	78%	75%
Chest Pain/Possible Heart Attack Care				
Aspirin Given Within 24 Hours of Arrival	67	100%	98%	96%
Fibrinolytic Meds Within 30 Min. of Arrival	12	100%	68%	58%
Average Time to ECG (minutes)	71	7	7	7
Average Time to Transfer (minutes)[1]	-	-	64	60
Children's Asthma Care				
Received Home Management Plan of Care	-	-	-	88%
Received Reliever Medication	-	-	-	100%
Received Systemic Corticosteroids	-	-	-	100%
Emergency Department				
Admittance Decision Time (minutes)[2]	398	50	96	98
Head CT Results Within 45 Min. of Arrival[1]	-	-	60%	57%
Patients Who Left ER Before Being Seen	14,786	2%	2%	2%
Time from ER Arrival to Admit. (minutes)[2]	398	213	280	274
Time from ER Arrival to Discharge (minutes)	409	96	167	134
Time in ER Before Being Evaluated (minutes)	460	21	35	26
Time to Pain Meds for Fractures (minutes)	36	30	56	57
Heart Attack Care				
Aspirin Given at Discharge[1]	-	-	99%	99%
Fibrinolytic Meds Within 30 Min. of Arrival[7]	-	-	75%	54%
PCI Within 90 Minutes of Arrival[7]	-	-	97%	96%
Statin Prescribed at Discharge[1]	-	-	99%	98%
Heart Failure Care				
ACE Inhibitor or ARB for LVSD	15	100%	98%	97%
Discharge Instructions Given	76	92%	95%	94%
Evaluation of LVS Function	100	100%	100%	99%
Medicare Spending				
Medicare Spending per Patient (ratio)	-	0.93	0.95	0.98
Pneumonia Care				
Appropriate Initial Antibiotic Given	77	97%	97%	95%
Blood Culture Timing	107	100%	98%	98%
Pregnancy and Delivery Care				
Newborn Deliveries Scheduled Early[2,7]	-	-	6%	6%
Preventive Care				
Immunization for Influenza[2]	319	98%	92%	90%
Immunization for Pneumonia[2]	523	100%	93%	92%
Stroke Care				
Anticoagulation Therapy for Atrial Fibrillation[1,2]	-	-	96%	95%
Antithrombotic Therapy Timing[2]	25	100%	99%	98%
Assessed for Rehabilitation[2]	26	100%	99%	97%
Discharged on Antithrombotic Therapy[2]	25	100%	100%	99%
Discharged on Statin Medication[2]	18	100%	97%	94%
Thrombolytic Therapy Timing[1,2]	-	-	73%	66%
Venous Thromboembolism Prophylaxis[2]	27	100%	97%	94%
Written Stroke Educational Materials Given[2]	12	100%	92%	88%
Surgical Care Improvement Project				
Appropriate Beta Blocker Usage	47	100%	99%	98%
Appropriate VTP Within 24 Hours	145	100%	99%	98%
Controlled Postoperative Blood Glucose[7]	-	-	98%	97%
Perioperative Temperature Management	166	99%	100%	100%
Prophylactic Antibiotic Selection	145	99%	99%	99%
Prophylactic Antibiotic Selection (Outpatient)	16	100%	98%	98%
Prophylactic Antibiotic Stopped	144	100%	98%	98%
Prophylactic Antibiotic Timing	145	99%	99%	99%
Prophylactic Antibiotic Timing (Outpatient)	16	100%	98%	98%
Urinary Catheter Removal	24	83%	98%	97%
Survey of Patients' Hospital Experiences				
Area Around Room 'Always' Quiet at Night	300+	59%	60%	61%
Doctors 'Always' Communicated Well	300+	83%	81%	82%
Home Recovery Information Given	300+	86%	86%	85%
Hospital Given 9 or 10 on 10 Point Scale	300+	64%	68%	71%
Meds 'Always' Explained Before Given	300+	60%	62%	64%
Nurses 'Always' Communicated Well	300+	79%	78%	79%
Pain 'Always' Well Controlled	300+	68%	70%	71%
Room and Bathroom 'Always' Clean	300+	59%	71%	73%
Timely Help 'Always' Received	300+	61%	64%	68%
Would Definitely Recommend Hospital	300+	61%	69%	71%
Use of Medical Imaging				
Cardiac Imaging Stress Test before Surgery	167	4.2%	5.1%	5.3%
Combination Abdominal CT Scan	446	5.8%	8.5%	10.5%
Combination Brain/Sinus CT Scan[1]	-	-	2.3%	2.7%
Combination Chest CT Scan	320	3.1%	1.6%	2.7%
Follow-up Mammogram/Ultrasound	835	6.7%	7.7%	8.8%
Lumbar Spine MRI for Low Back Pain	107	34.6%	35.3%	37.2%

Page Memorial Hospital

200 Memorial Drive
Luray, VA 22835
E-mail: pmh@shentel.net
URL: www.pagememorialhospital.org
Type: Critical Access Hospitals
Ownership: Voluntary non-profit - Private

Phone: 540-743-4561
Fax: 540-743-9560

Emergency Services: Yes
Beds: 54

Key Personnel:

Quality Assurance .... Clara Layman
CEO/President............... Mark H. Merrill
Emergency Room .... Erin Noser
Radiology.................. Donna M Sefczek
Chairman/CEO .... Joseph F. Silek, JR.
Infection Control.............. John Vollmer

Measure	Cases	This Hosp.	State Avg.	U.S. Avg.
Blood Clot Prevention and Treatment				
Anticoagulation Overlap Therapy[5]	-	-	95%	93%
ICU Venous Thromboembolism Prophylaxis[5]	-	-	95%	92%
Incidence of Potentially Preventable VTE[5]	-	-	8%	10%
UFH with Dosages/Platelet Monitoring[5]	-	-	99%	97%
Venous Thromboembolism Prophylaxis[5]	-	-	91%	85%
Warfarin Therapy Discharge Instructions[5]	-	-	78%	75%
Chest Pain/Possible Heart Attack Care				
Aspirin Given Within 24 Hours of Arrival[5]	-	-	98%	96%
Fibrinolytic Meds Within 30 Min. of Arrival[5]	-	-	68%	58%
Average Time to ECG (minutes)[5]	-	-	7	7
Average Time to Transfer (minutes)[5]	-	-	64	60
Children's Asthma Care				
Received Home Management Plan of Care	-	-	-	88%
Received Reliever Medication	-	-	-	100%
Received Systemic Corticosteroids	-	-	-	100%
Emergency Department				
Admittance Decision Time (minutes)[2]	321	85	96	98
Head CT Results Within 45 Min. of Arrival[5]	-	-	60%	57%
Patients Who Left ER Before Being Seen	14,412	0%	2%	2%
Time from ER Arrival to Admit. (minutes)[2]	333	243	280	274
Time from ER Arrival to Discharge (minutes)[5]	-	-	167	134
Time in ER Before Being Evaluated (minutes)[5]	-	-	35	26
Time to Pain Meds for Fractures (minutes)[5]	-	-	56	57
Heart Attack Care				
Aspirin Given at Discharge[3,7]	-	-	99%	99%
Fibrinolytic Meds Within 30 Min. of Arrival[3,7]	-	-	75%	54%
PCI Within 90 Minutes of Arrival[3,7]	-	-	97%	96%
Statin Prescribed at Discharge[3,7]	-	-	99%	98%
Heart Failure Care				
ACE Inhibitor or ARB for LVSD[1]	-	-	98%	97%
Discharge Instructions Given	22	95%	95%	94%
Evaluation of LVS Function	31	90%	100%	99%

NOTE: Hospital profiles are in alphabetical order by state, then city, then hospital within the city; Rankings exclude hospitals with less than 25 cases except for patient surveys which excludes hospitals with less than 100 cases; (a) 100-299 cases; (1) The number of cases/patients is too few to report; (2) Data submitted were based on a sample of cases/patients; (3) Results are based on a shorter time period than required; (4) Data suppressed by CMS for one or more quarters; (5) Results are not available for this reporting period; (6) Fewer than 100 patients completed the HCAHPS survey; (7) No cases met the criteria for this measure; (8) The lower limit of the confidence interval cannot be calculated if the number of observed infections equals zero; (9) No data are available from the state/territory for this reporting period; (10) The scores shown reflect fewer than 50 completed surveys; (11) There were discrepancies in the data collection process; (12) This measure does not apply to this hospital for this reporting period; (13) Results cannot be calculated for this reporting period; (14) The results for this state are combined with nearby states to protect confidentiality; Please refer to the User's Guide for a full explanation of data.

Measure	Cases	This Hosp.	State Avg.	U.S. Avg.
Medicare Spending				
Medicare Spending per Patient (ratio)	-	-	0.95	0.98
Pneumonia Care				
Appropriate Initial Antibiotic Given	23	100%	97%	95%
Blood Culture Timing	25	100%	98%	98%
Pregnancy and Delivery Care				
Newborn Deliveries Scheduled Early[7]	-	-	6%	6%
Preventive Care				
Immunization for Influenza[2]	288	93%	92%	90%
Immunization for Pneumonia[2]	459	94%	93%	92%
Stroke Care				
Anticoagulation Therapy for Atrial Fibrillation[5]	-	-	96%	95%
Antithrombotic Therapy Timing[5]	-	-	99%	98%
Assessed for Rehabilitation[5]	-	-	99%	97%
Discharged on Antithrombotic Therapy[5]	-	-	100%	99%
Discharged on Statin Medication[5]	-	-	97%	94%
Thrombolytic Therapy Timing[5]	-	-	73%	66%
Venous Thromboembolism Prophylaxis[5]	-	-	97%	94%
Written Stroke Educational Materials Given[5]	-	-	92%	88%
Surgical Care Improvement Project				
Appropriate Beta Blocker Usage[5]	-	-	99%	98%
Appropriate VTP Within 24 Hours[5]	-	-	99%	98%
Controlled Postoperative Blood Glucose[5]	-	-	98%	97%
Perioperative Temperature Management[5]	-	-	100%	100%
Prophylactic Antibiotic Selection[5]	-	-	99%	99%
Prophylactic Antibiotic Selection (Outpatient)[5]	-	-	98%	98%
Prophylactic Antibiotic Stopped[5]	-	-	98%	98%
Prophylactic Antibiotic Timing[5]	-	-	99%	99%
Prophylactic Antibiotic Timing (Outpatient)[5]	-	-	98%	98%
Urinary Catheter Removal[5]	-	-	98%	97%
Survey of Patients' Hospital Experiences				
Area Around Room 'Always' Quiet at Night	(a)	62%	60%	61%
Doctors 'Always' Communicated Well	(a)	84%	81%	82%
Home Recovery Information Given	(a)	90%	86%	85%
Hospital Given 9 or 10 on 10 Point Scale	(a)	67%	68%	71%
Meds 'Always' Explained Before Given	(a)	63%	62%	64%
Nurses 'Always' Communicated Well	(a)	82%	78%	79%
Pain 'Always' Well Controlled	(a)	67%	70%	71%
Room and Bathroom 'Always' Clean	(a)	73%	71%	73%
Timely Help 'Always' Received	(a)	60%	64%	68%
Would Definitely Recommend Hospital	(a)	64%	69%	71%
Use of Medical Imaging				
Cardiac Imaging Stress Test before Surgery	75	4.0%	5.1%	5.3%
Combination Abdominal CT Scan	238	0.0%	8.5%	10.5%
Combination Brain/Sinus CT Scan	287	1.0%	2.3%	2.7%
Combination Chest CT Scan	69	1.4%	1.6%	2.7%
Follow-up Mammogram/Ultrasound	367	12.0%	7.7%	8.8%
Lumbar Spine MRI for Low Back Pain[1]	-	-	35.3%	37.2%

Centra Health

1920 Atherholt Road
Lynchburg, VA 24501
Phone: 434-200-4789
URL: www.centrahealth.com
Type: Acute Care Hospitals
Emergency Services: Yes
Ownership: Voluntary non-profit - Private
Key Personnel:
President/CEO . . . . W Michael Bryant

Measure	Cases	This Hosp.	State Avg.	U.S. Avg.
Blood Clot Prevention and Treatment				
Anticoagulation Overlap Therapy[2]	153	99%	95%	93%
ICU Venous Thromboembolism Prophylaxis[2]	110	84%	95%	92%
Incidence of Potentially Preventable VTE[2]	21	24%	8%	10%
UFH with Dosages/Platelet Monitoring[2]	24	96%	99%	97%
Venous Thromboembolism Prophylaxis[2]	315	82%	91%	85%
Warfarin Therapy Discharge Instructions[2]	115	5%	78%	75%
Chest Pain/Possible Heart Attack Care				
Aspirin Given Within 24 Hours of Arrival[1,3]	-	-	98%	96%
Fibrinolytic Meds Within 30 Min. of Arrival[3,7]	-	-	68%	58%
Average Time to ECG (minutes)[1,3]	-	-	7	7
Average Time to Transfer (minutes)[3,7]	-	-	64	60
Children's Asthma Care				
Received Home Management Plan of Care	97	97%	-	88%
Received Reliever Medication	101	100%	-	100%
Received Systemic Corticosteroids	101	100%	-	100%
Emergency Department				
Admittance Decision Time (minutes)[2]	650	127	96	98
Head CT Results Within 45 Min. of Arrival[1]	-	-	60%	57%
Patients Who Left ER Before Being Seen	99,565	4%	2%	2%
Time from ER Arrival to Admit. (minutes)[2]	665	328	280	274
Time from ER Arrival to Discharge (minutes)	380	211	167	134
Time in ER Before Being Evaluated (minutes)	384	88	35	26
Time to Pain Meds for Fractures (minutes)	164	64	56	57
Heart Attack Care				
Aspirin Given at Discharge	619	100%	99%	99%
Fibrinolytic Meds Within 30 Min. of Arrival[1]	-	-	75%	54%
PCI Within 90 Minutes of Arrival	104	96%	97%	96%
Statin Prescribed at Discharge	615	99%	99%	98%
Heart Failure Care				
ACE Inhibitor or ARB for LVSD[2]	191	98%	98%	97%
Discharge Instructions Given[2]	600	76%	95%	94%
Evaluation of LVS Function[2]	733	100%	100%	99%
Medicare Spending				
Medicare Spending per Patient (ratio)	-	0.96	0.95	0.98
Pneumonia Care				
Appropriate Initial Antibiotic Given[2]	190	97%	97%	95%
Blood Culture Timing[2]	279	99%	98%	98%
Pregnancy and Delivery Care				
Newborn Deliveries Scheduled Early	192	1%	6%	6%
Preventive Care				
Immunization for Influenza[2]	586	90%	92%	90%
Immunization for Pneumonia[2]	733	94%	93%	92%
Stroke Care				
Anticoagulation Therapy for Atrial Fibrillation[2]	23	96%	96%	95%
Antithrombotic Therapy Timing[2]	97	98%	99%	98%
Assessed for Rehabilitation[2]	113	98%	99%	97%
Discharged on Antithrombotic Therapy[2]	100	100%	100%	99%
Discharged on Statin Medication[2]	79	99%	97%	94%
Thrombolytic Therapy Timing[1,2]	-	-	73%	66%
Venous Thromboembolism Prophylaxis[2]	120	94%	97%	94%
Written Stroke Educational Materials Given[2]	58	76%	92%	88%
Surgical Care Improvement Project				
Appropriate Beta Blocker Usage[2]	493	99%	99%	98%
Appropriate VTP Within 24 Hours[2]	853	98%	99%	98%
Controlled Postoperative Blood Glucose[2]	250	96%	98%	97%
Perioperative Temperature Management[2]	1,111	100%	100%	100%
Prophylactic Antibiotic Selection[2]	925	100%	99%	99%
Prophylactic Antibiotic Selection (Outpatient)	621	99%	98%	98%
Prophylactic Antibiotic Stopped[2]	882	100%	98%	98%
Prophylactic Antibiotic Timing[2]	925	100%	99%	99%
Prophylactic Antibiotic Timing (Outpatient)	624	99%	98%	98%
Urinary Catheter Removal[2]	547	98%	98%	97%
Survey of Patients' Hospital Experiences				
Area Around Room 'Always' Quiet at Night	300+	62%	60%	61%
Doctors 'Always' Communicated Well	300+	83%	81%	82%
Home Recovery Information Given	300+	88%	86%	85%
Hospital Given 9 or 10 on 10 Point Scale	300+	74%	68%	71%
Meds 'Always' Explained Before Given	300+	66%	62%	64%
Nurses 'Always' Communicated Well	300+	82%	78%	79%
Pain 'Always' Well Controlled	300+	72%	70%	71%
Room and Bathroom 'Always' Clean	300+	73%	71%	73%
Timely Help 'Always' Received	300+	67%	64%	68%
Would Definitely Recommend Hospital	300+	78%	69%	71%
Use of Medical Imaging				
Cardiac Imaging Stress Test before Surgery	1,389	4.5%	5.1%	5.3%
Combination Abdominal CT Scan	1,880	8.2%	8.5%	10.5%
Combination Brain/Sinus CT Scan	1,588	1.8%	2.3%	2.7%
Combination Chest CT Scan	1,193	1.9%	1.6%	2.7%
Follow-up Mammogram/Ultrasound[1]	-	-	7.7%	8.8%
Lumbar Spine MRI for Low Back Pain	152	42.8%	35.3%	37.2%

Novant Health Prince William Medical Center

8700 Sudley Rd
Manassas, VA 20110
Phone: 703-369-8000
Fax: 703-369-8010
URL: www.pwhs.org
Type: Acute Care Hospitals
Emergency Services: Yes
Ownership: Voluntary non-profit - Private
Beds: 170
Key Personnel:
Emergency Room . . . . Ayan H Ahmed, MD
Quality Assurance . . . . Ginny Blairk
Radiology. . . . . Namik Erdag
Operating Room. . . . . Beatrice Holt, RN
Chief of Medical Staff . . . . Vikram Khot, MD
Pediatric Ambulatory Care . . . . . . Marc Krenytzky
Patient Relations . . . . Sandy Rigsbee
CEO/President. . . . . Michael J Schwartz, MD

Measure	Cases	This Hosp.	State Avg.	U.S. Avg.
Blood Clot Prevention and Treatment				
Anticoagulation Overlap Therapy[2]	55	100%	95%	93%
ICU Venous Thromboembolism Prophylaxis[2]	73	97%	95%	92%
Incidence of Potentially Preventable VTE[1,2]	-	-	8%	10%
UFH with Dosages/Platelet Monitoring[2]	15	100%	99%	97%
Venous Thromboembolism Prophylaxis[2]	230	95%	91%	85%
Warfarin Therapy Discharge Instructions[2]	40	98%	78%	75%
Chest Pain/Possible Heart Attack Care				
Aspirin Given Within 24 Hours of Arrival	14	100%	98%	96%
Fibrinolytic Meds Within 30 Min. of Arrival[7]	-	-	68%	58%
Average Time to ECG (minutes)	16	2	7	7
Average Time to Transfer (minutes)[1]	-	-	64	60
Children's Asthma Care				
Received Home Management Plan of Care	-	-	-	88%
Received Reliever Medication	-	-	-	100%
Received Systemic Corticosteroids	-	-	-	100%
Emergency Department				
Admittance Decision Time (minutes)[2]	454	173	96	98
Head CT Results Within 45 Min. of Arrival	11	64%	60%	57%
Patients Who Left ER Before Being Seen	76,126	1%	2%	2%
Time from ER Arrival to Admit. (minutes)[2]	454	352	280	274
Time from ER Arrival to Discharge (minutes)	487	124	167	134
Time in ER Before Being Evaluated (minutes)	518	19	35	26
Time to Pain Meds for Fractures (minutes)	362	47	56	57
Heart Attack Care				
Aspirin Given at Discharge	167	99%	99%	99%
Fibrinolytic Meds Within 30 Min. of Arrival[7]	-	-	75%	54%
PCI Within 90 Minutes of Arrival	51	96%	97%	96%
Statin Prescribed at Discharge	162	100%	99%	98%
Heart Failure Care				
ACE Inhibitor or ARB for LVSD	59	100%	98%	97%
Discharge Instructions Given	137	91%	95%	94%
Evaluation of LVS Function	156	100%	100%	99%
Medicare Spending				
Medicare Spending per Patient (ratio)	-	1.01	0.95	0.98
Pneumonia Care				
Appropriate Initial Antibiotic Given	92	99%	97%	95%
Blood Culture Timing	179	99%	98%	98%
Pregnancy and Delivery Care				
Newborn Deliveries Scheduled Early[2]	41	0%	6%	6%
Preventive Care				
Immunization for Influenza[2]	628	91%	92%	90%
Immunization for Pneumonia[2]	545	95%	93%	92%
Stroke Care				
Anticoagulation Therapy for Atrial Fibrillation	12	100%	96%	95%
Antithrombotic Therapy Timing	40	98%	99%	98%
Assessed for Rehabilitation	66	98%	99%	97%
Discharged on Antithrombotic Therapy	65	100%	100%	99%
Discharged on Statin Medication	58	100%	97%	94%
Thrombolytic Therapy Timing[1]	-	-	73%	66%
Venous Thromboembolism Prophylaxis	51	98%	97%	94%
Written Stroke Educational Materials Given	32	100%	92%	88%
Surgical Care Improvement Project				
Appropriate Beta Blocker Usage[2]	158	99%	99%	98%
Appropriate VTP Within 24 Hours[2]	480	100%	99%	98%
Controlled Postoperative Blood Glucose[2,7]	-	-	98%	97%
Perioperative Temperature Management[2]	572	100%	100%	100%
Prophylactic Antibiotic Selection[2]	429	100%	99%	99%

NOTE: Hospital profiles are in alphabetical order by state, then city, then hospital within the city; Rankings exclude hospitals with less than 25 cases except for patient surveys which excludes hospitals with less than 100 cases; (a) 100-299 cases; (1) The number of cases/patients is too few to report; (2) Data submitted were based on a sample of cases/patients; (3) Results are based on a shorter time period than required; (4) Data suppressed by CMS for one or more quarters; (5) Results are not available for this reporting period; (6) Fewer than 100 patients completed the HCAHPS survey; (7) No cases met the criteria for this measure; (8) The lower limit of the confidence interval cannot be calculated if the number of observed infections equals zero; (9) No data are available from the state/territory for this reporting period; (10) The scores shown reflect fewer than 50 completed surveys; (11) There were discrepancies in the data collection process; (12) This measure does not apply to this hospital for this reporting period; (13) Results cannot be calculated for this reporting period; (14) The results for this state are combined with nearby states to protect confidentiality; Please refer to the User's Guide for a full explanation of data.

Measure	Cases	This Hosp.	State Avg.	U.S. Avg.
Prophylactic Antibiotic Selection (Outpatient)	423	100%	98%	98%
Prophylactic Antibiotic Stopped[2]	421	99%	98%	98%
Prophylactic Antibiotic Timing[2]	429	100%	99%	99%
Prophylactic Antibiotic Timing (Outpatient)	420	99%	98%	98%
Urinary Catheter Removal[2]	420	99%	98%	97%
Survey of Patients' Hospital Experiences				
Area Around Room 'Always' Quiet at Night	300+	51%	60%	61%
Doctors 'Always' Communicated Well	300+	78%	81%	82%
Home Recovery Information Given	300+	86%	86%	85%
Hospital Given 9 or 10 on 10 Point Scale	300+	58%	68%	71%
Meds 'Always' Explained Before Given	300+	58%	62%	64%
Nurses 'Always' Communicated Well	300+	71%	78%	79%
Pain 'Always' Well Controlled	300+	64%	70%	71%
Room and Bathroom 'Always' Clean	300+	70%	71%	73%
Timely Help 'Always' Received	300+	56%	64%	68%
Would Definitely Recommend Hospital	300+	62%	69%	71%
Use of Medical Imaging				
Cardiac Imaging Stress Test before Surgery	76	6.6%	5.1%	5.3%
Combination Abdominal CT Scan	968	3.5%	8.5%	10.5%
Combination Brain/Sinus CT Scan	922	2.4%	2.3%	2.7%
Combination Chest CT Scan	653	0.3%	1.6%	2.7%
Follow-up Mammogram/Ultrasound	1,495	9.7%	7.7%	8.8%
Lumbar Spine MRI for Low Back Pain	247	34.8%	35.3%	37.2%

Smyth County Community Hospital

245 Medical Park Drive
Marion, VA 24354
Phone: 276-378-1000
Fax: 276-782-1436
URL: www.scchosp.org
Type: Acute Care Hospitals
Emergency Services: Yes
Ownership: Voluntary non-profit - Other
Beds: 50

Key Personnel:

Chair/CEO . . . . Barbara Allen
Quality Assurance . . . . Tim Anderson
Radiology. . . . . Wesley L Asbury Jr
CEO/President. . . . . Houston Bell
Emergency Room . . . . James Paterson

Measure	Cases	This Hosp.	State Avg.	U.S. Avg.
Blood Clot Prevention and Treatment				
Anticoagulation Overlap Therapy[2]	11	100%	95%	93%
ICU Venous Thromboembolism Prophylaxis[2]	19	100%	95%	92%
Incidence of Potentially Preventable VTE[1,2]	-	-	8%	10%
UFH with Dosages/Platelet Monitoring[1,2]	-	-	99%	97%
Venous Thromboembolism Prophylaxis[2]	134	97%	91%	85%
Warfarin Therapy Discharge Instructions[1,2]	-	-	78%	75%
Chest Pain/Possible Heart Attack Care				
Aspirin Given Within 24 Hours of Arrival	107	98%	98%	96%
Fibrinolytic Meds Within 30 Min. of Arrival[1]	-	-	68%	58%
Average Time to ECG (minutes)	111	4	7	7
Average Time to Transfer (minutes)[1]	-	-	64	60
Children's Asthma Care				
Received Home Management Plan of Care	-	-	-	88%
Received Reliever Medication	-	-	-	100%
Received Systemic Corticosteroids	-	-	-	100%
Emergency Department				
Admittance Decision Time (minutes)[2]	323	32	96	98
Head CT Results Within 45 Min. of Arrival[1]	-	-	60%	57%
Patients Who Left ER Before Being Seen	18,053	0%	2%	2%
Time from ER Arrival to Admit. (minutes)[2]	368	168	280	274
Time from ER Arrival to Discharge (minutes)	203	91	167	134
Time in ER Before Being Evaluated (minutes)	383	15	35	26
Time to Pain Meds for Fractures (minutes)	57	46	56	57
Heart Attack Care				
Aspirin Given at Discharge[1,2]	-	-	99%	99%
Fibrinolytic Meds Within 30 Min. of Arrival[2,3]	-	-	75%	54%
PCI Within 90 Minutes of Arrival[2,3]	-	-	97%	96%
Statin Prescribed at Discharge[1,2]	-	-	99%	98%
Heart Failure Care				
ACE Inhibitor or ARB for LVSD[2]	24	100%	98%	97%
Discharge Instructions Given[2]	42	100%	95%	94%
Evaluation of LVS Function[2]	56	100%	100%	99%
Medicare Spending				
Medicare Spending per Patient (ratio)	-	0.94	0.95	0.98
Pneumonia Care				
Appropriate Initial Antibiotic Given[2]	48	98%	97%	95%
Blood Culture Timing[2]	88	100%	98%	98%
Pregnancy and Delivery Care				
Newborn Deliveries Scheduled Early[7]	-	-	6%	6%
Preventive Care				
Immunization for Influenza[2]	304	99%	92%	90%
Immunization for Pneumonia[2]	471	99%	93%	92%
Stroke Care				
Anticoagulation Therapy for Atrial Fibrillation[1]	-	-	96%	95%
Antithrombotic Therapy Timing	22	100%	99%	98%
Assessed for Rehabilitation	21	100%	99%	97%
Discharged on Antithrombotic Therapy	20	100%	100%	99%
Discharged on Statin Medication	16	94%	97%	94%
Thrombolytic Therapy Timing[1]	-	-	73%	66%
Venous Thromboembolism Prophylaxis	18	100%	97%	94%
Written Stroke Educational Materials Given	12	92%	92%	88%
Surgical Care Improvement Project				
Appropriate Beta Blocker Usage[2]	24	96%	99%	98%
Appropriate VTP Within 24 Hours[2]	106	100%	99%	98%
Controlled Postoperative Blood Glucose[2,7]	-	-	98%	97%
Perioperative Temperature Management[2]	111	100%	100%	100%
Prophylactic Antibiotic Selection[2]	75	100%	99%	99%
Prophylactic Antibiotic Selection (Outpatient)[1,3]	-	-	98%	98%
Prophylactic Antibiotic Stopped[2]	71	100%	98%	98%
Prophylactic Antibiotic Timing[2]	75	100%	99%	99%
Prophylactic Antibiotic Timing (Outpatient)[1,3]	-	-	98%	98%
Urinary Catheter Removal[2]	57	100%	98%	97%
Survey of Patients' Hospital Experiences				
Area Around Room 'Always' Quiet at Night	300+	63%	60%	61%
Doctors 'Always' Communicated Well	300+	82%	81%	82%
Home Recovery Information Given	300+	85%	86%	85%
Hospital Given 9 or 10 on 10 Point Scale	300+	72%	68%	71%
Meds 'Always' Explained Before Given	300+	58%	62%	64%
Nurses 'Always' Communicated Well	300+	80%	78%	79%
Pain 'Always' Well Controlled	300+	70%	70%	71%
Room and Bathroom 'Always' Clean	300+	80%	71%	73%
Timely Help 'Always' Received	300+	67%	64%	68%
Would Definitely Recommend Hospital	300+	69%	69%	71%
Use of Medical Imaging				
Cardiac Imaging Stress Test before Surgery	148	6.8%	5.1%	5.3%
Combination Abdominal CT Scan	440	7.7%	8.5%	10.5%
Combination Brain/Sinus CT Scan	392	1.5%	2.3%	2.7%
Combination Chest CT Scan	149	0.0%	1.6%	2.7%
Follow-up Mammogram/Ultrasound	684	4.2%	7.7%	8.8%
Lumbar Spine MRI for Low Back Pain[1]	-	-	35.3%	37.2%

Southwestern Virginia Mental Health Institute

340 Bagley Circle
Marion, VA 24354
Phone: 276-783-1217
Fax: 276-783-9712
URL: www.swvmhi.state.va.us
Type: Acute Care Hospitals
Emergency Services: No
Ownership: Government - State
Beds: 176

Key Personnel:

Quality Assurance . . . . Philip Jones
CEO/President. . . . . Cynthia McLure
Chief of Medical Staff. . . . . Donna Rigolrvo
Infection Control. . . . . Pam Rolen, RN

Measure	Cases	This Hosp.	State Avg.	U.S. Avg.
Blood Clot Prevention and Treatment				
Anticoagulation Overlap Therapy[5]	-	-	95%	93%
ICU Venous Thromboembolism Prophylaxis[5]	-	-	95%	92%
Incidence of Potentially Preventable VTE[5]	-	-	8%	10%
UFH with Dosages/Platelet Monitoring[5]	-	-	99%	97%
Venous Thromboembolism Prophylaxis[5]	-	-	91%	85%
Warfarin Therapy Discharge Instructions[5]	-	-	78%	75%
Chest Pain/Possible Heart Attack Care				
Aspirin Given Within 24 Hours of Arrival	-	-	98%	96%
Fibrinolytic Meds Within 30 Min. of Arrival	-	-	68%	58%
Average Time to ECG (minutes)	-	-	7	7
Average Time to Transfer (minutes)	-	-	64	60
Children's Asthma Care				
Received Home Management Plan of Care	-	-	-	88%
Received Reliever Medication	-	-	-	100%
Received Systemic Corticosteroids	-	-	-	100%
Emergency Department				
Admittance Decision Time (minutes)[5]	-	-	96	98
Head CT Results Within 45 Min. of Arrival	-	-	60%	57%
Patients Who Left ER Before Being Seen	-	-	2%	2%
Time from ER Arrival to Admit. (minutes)[5]	-	-	280	274
Time from ER Arrival to Discharge (minutes)	-	-	167	134
Time in ER Before Being Evaluated (minutes)	-	-	35	26
Time to Pain Meds for Fractures (minutes)	-	-	56	57
Heart Attack Care				
Aspirin Given at Discharge[5]	-	-	99%	99%
Fibrinolytic Meds Within 30 Min. of Arrival[5]	-	-	75%	54%
PCI Within 90 Minutes of Arrival[5]	-	-	97%	96%
Statin Prescribed at Discharge[5]	-	-	99%	98%
Heart Failure Care				
ACE Inhibitor or ARB for LVSD[5]	-	-	98%	97%
Discharge Instructions Given[5]	-	-	95%	94%
Evaluation of LVS Function[5]	-	-	100%	99%
Medicare Spending				
Medicare Spending per Patient (ratio)[1]	-	-	0.95	0.98
Pneumonia Care				
Appropriate Initial Antibiotic Given[5]	-	-	97%	95%
Blood Culture Timing[5]	-	-	98%	98%
Pregnancy and Delivery Care				
Newborn Deliveries Scheduled Early[7]	-	-	6%	6%
Preventive Care				
Immunization for Influenza[5]	-	-	92%	90%
Immunization for Pneumonia[5]	-	-	93%	92%
Stroke Care				
Anticoagulation Therapy for Atrial Fibrillation[5]	-	-	96%	95%
Antithrombotic Therapy Timing[5]	-	-	99%	98%
Assessed for Rehabilitation[5]	-	-	99%	97%
Discharged on Antithrombotic Therapy[5]	-	-	100%	99%
Discharged on Statin Medication[5]	-	-	97%	94%
Thrombolytic Therapy Timing[5]	-	-	73%	66%
Venous Thromboembolism Prophylaxis[5]	-	-	97%	94%
Written Stroke Educational Materials Given[5]	-	-	92%	88%
Surgical Care Improvement Project				
Appropriate Beta Blocker Usage[5]	-	-	99%	98%
Appropriate VTP Within 24 Hours[5]	-	-	99%	98%
Controlled Postoperative Blood Glucose[5]	-	-	98%	97%
Perioperative Temperature Management[5]	-	-	100%	100%
Prophylactic Antibiotic Selection[5]	-	-	99%	99%
Prophylactic Antibiotic Selection (Outpatient)	-	-	98%	98%
Prophylactic Antibiotic Stopped[5]	-	-	98%	98%
Prophylactic Antibiotic Timing[5]	-	-	99%	99%
Prophylactic Antibiotic Timing (Outpatient)	-	-	98%	98%
Urinary Catheter Removal[5]	-	-	98%	97%
Survey of Patients' Hospital Experiences				
Area Around Room 'Always' Quiet at Night[1]	-	-	60%	61%
Doctors 'Always' Communicated Well[1]	-	-	81%	82%
Home Recovery Information Given[1]	-	-	86%	85%
Hospital Given 9 or 10 on 10 Point Scale[1]	-	-	68%	71%
Meds 'Always' Explained Before Given[1]	-	-	62%	64%
Nurses 'Always' Communicated Well[1]	-	-	78%	79%
Pain 'Always' Well Controlled[1]	-	-	70%	71%
Room and Bathroom 'Always' Clean[1]	-	-	71%	73%
Timely Help 'Always' Received[1]	-	-	64%	68%
Would Definitely Recommend Hospital[1]	-	-	69%	71%
Use of Medical Imaging				
Cardiac Imaging Stress Test before Surgery	-	-	5.1%	5.3%
Combination Abdominal CT Scan	-	-	8.5%	10.5%
Combination Brain/Sinus CT Scan	-	-	2.3%	2.7%
Combination Chest CT Scan	-	-	1.6%	2.7%
Follow-up Mammogram/Ultrasound	-	-	7.7%	8.8%
Lumbar Spine MRI for Low Back Pain	-	-	35.3%	37.2%

NOTE: Hospital profiles are in alphabetical order by state, then city, then hospital within the city; Rankings exclude hospitals with less than 25 cases except for patient surveys which excludes hospitals with less than 100 cases; (a) 100-299 cases; (1) The number of cases/patients is too few to report; (2) Data submitted were based on a sample of cases/patients; (3) Results are based on a shorter time period than required; (4) Data suppressed by CMS for one or more quarters; (5) Results are not available for this reporting period; (6) Fewer than 100 patients completed the HCAHPS survey; (7) No cases met the criteria for this measure; (8) The lower limit of the confidence interval cannot be calculated if the number of observed infections equals zero; (9) No data are available from the state/territory for this reporting period; (10) The scores shown reflect fewer than 50 completed surveys; (11) There were discrepancies in the data collection process; (12) This measure does not apply to this hospital for this reporting period; (13) Results cannot be calculated for this reporting period; (14) The results for this state are combined with nearby states to protect confidentiality; Please refer to the User's Guide for a full explanation of data.

Memorial Hospital of Martinsville & Henry County

320 Hospital Drive — Phone: 276-666-7200
Martinsville, VA 24115 — Fax: 276-666-7600
E-mail: info@mhmhc.com
URL: www.martinsvillehospital.com
Type: Acute Care Hospitals — Emergency Services: Yes
Ownership: Proprietary — Beds: 220

Key Personnel:
Operating Room. . . . . Thomas K Berry, RN
Coronary Care . . . . Martha Holland, RN BSN
CEO . . . . Grady W. Phillips
Chief of Medical Staff. . . . . LS Poirer, MD
Radiology. . . . . Leonard S Poirier
Infection Control. . . . . Faye Sedwick, RN MSN
Quality Assurance . . . . Peggy Tunnell, RN

Measure	Cases	This Hosp.	State Avg.	U.S. Avg.
Blood Clot Prevention and Treatment				
Anticoagulation Overlap Therapy[2]	40	90%	95%	93%
ICU Venous Thromboembolism Prophylaxis[2]	128	89%	95%	92%
Incidence of Potentially Preventable VTE[1,2]	-	-	8%	10%
UFH with Dosages/Platelet Monitoring[1,2]	-	-	99%	97%
Venous Thromboembolism Prophylaxis[2]	311	91%	91%	85%
Warfarin Therapy Discharge Instructions[2]	25	92%	78%	75%
Chest Pain/Possible Heart Attack Care				
Aspirin Given Within 24 Hours of Arrival	51	100%	98%	96%
Fibrinolytic Meds Within 30 Min. of Arrival[1]	-	-	68%	58%
Average Time to ECG (minutes)	52	6	7	7
Average Time to Transfer (minutes)[1]	-	-	64	60
Children's Asthma Care				
Received Home Management Plan of Care	-	-	-	88%
Received Reliever Medication	-	-	-	100%
Received Systemic Corticosteroids	-	-	-	100%
Emergency Department				
Admittance Decision Time (minutes)[2]	776	210	96	98
Head CT Results Within 45 Min. of Arrival[1]	-	-	60%	57%
Patients Who Left ER Before Being Seen	43,332	2%	2%	2%
Time from ER Arrival to Admit. (minutes)[2]	777	346	280	274
Time from ER Arrival to Discharge (minutes)	425	146	167	134
Time in ER Before Being Evaluated (minutes)	498	19	35	26
Time to Pain Meds for Fractures (minutes)	145	46	56	57
Heart Attack Care				
Aspirin Given at Discharge	73	100%	99%	99%
Fibrinolytic Meds Within 30 Min. of Arrival[7]	-	-	75%	54%
PCI Within 90 Minutes of Arrival[1]	-	-	97%	96%
Statin Prescribed at Discharge	72	94%	99%	98%
Heart Failure Care				
ACE Inhibitor or ARB for LVSD	66	98%	98%	97%
Discharge Instructions Given	189	80%	95%	94%
Evaluation of LVS Function	274	100%	100%	99%
Medicare Spending				
Medicare Spending per Patient (ratio)	-	1.02	0.95	0.98
Pneumonia Care				
Appropriate Initial Antibiotic Given[2]	87	98%	97%	95%
Blood Culture Timing[2]	161	98%	98%	98%
Pregnancy and Delivery Care				
Newborn Deliveries Scheduled Early[2]	40	8%	6%	6%
Preventive Care				
Immunization for Influenza[2]	521	97%	92%	90%
Immunization for Pneumonia[2]	741	99%	93%	92%
Stroke Care				
Anticoagulation Therapy for Atrial Fibrillation[1]	-	-	96%	95%
Antithrombotic Therapy Timing	78	100%	99%	98%
Assessed for Rehabilitation	77	99%	99%	97%
Discharged on Antithrombotic Therapy	77	100%	100%	99%
Discharged on Statin Medication	62	100%	97%	94%
Thrombolytic Therapy Timing[1]	-	-	73%	66%
Venous Thromboembolism Prophylaxis	76	97%	97%	94%
Written Stroke Educational Materials Given	46	76%	92%	88%
Surgical Care Improvement Project				
Appropriate Beta Blocker Usage	62	97%	99%	98%
Appropriate VTP Within 24 Hours	198	98%	99%	98%
Controlled Postoperative Blood Glucose[7]	-	-	98%	97%
Perioperative Temperature Management	215	100%	100%	100%
Prophylactic Antibiotic Selection	124	99%	99%	99%
Prophylactic Antibiotic Selection (Outpatient)	71	97%	98%	98%
Prophylactic Antibiotic Stopped	108	96%	98%	98%
Prophylactic Antibiotic Timing	124	95%	99%	99%
Prophylactic Antibiotic Timing (Outpatient)	72	96%	98%	98%
Urinary Catheter Removal	116	95%	98%	97%
Survey of Patients' Hospital Experiences				
Area Around Room 'Always' Quiet at Night	300+	62%	60%	61%
Doctors 'Always' Communicated Well	300+	76%	81%	82%
Home Recovery Information Given	300+	84%	86%	85%
Hospital Given 9 or 10 on 10 Point Scale	300+	54%	68%	71%
Meds 'Always' Explained Before Given	300+	56%	62%	64%
Nurses 'Always' Communicated Well	300+	72%	78%	79%
Pain 'Always' Well Controlled	300+	63%	70%	71%
Room and Bathroom 'Always' Clean	300+	65%	71%	73%
Timely Help 'Always' Received	300+	54%	64%	68%
Would Definitely Recommend Hospital	300+	49%	69%	71%
Use of Medical Imaging				
Cardiac Imaging Stress Test before Surgery	268	5.6%	5.1%	5.3%
Combination Abdominal CT Scan	749	5.9%	8.5%	10.5%
Combination Brain/Sinus CT Scan	673	2.5%	2.3%	2.7%
Combination Chest CT Scan	396	4.5%	1.6%	2.7%
Follow-up Mammogram/Ultrasound	2,116	3.3%	7.7%	8.8%
Lumbar Spine MRI for Low Back Pain	125	49.6%	35.3%	37.2%

Bon Secours Memorial Regional Medical Center

8260 Atlee Road — Phone: 804-764-6000
Mechanicsville, VA 23116 — Fax: 804-764-6420
URL: www.bonsecours.com
Type: Acute Care Hospitals — Emergency Services: Yes
Ownership: Voluntary non-profit - Church — Beds: 225

Key Personnel:
Emergency Room . . . . William Azzie
Radiology. . . . . Todd B Baird
Chief of Medical Staff. . . . . John Bowman
Cardiac Laboratory. . . . . Timothy W Hagemann, MD
CEO . . . . Michael C Robinson

Measure	Cases	This Hosp.	State Avg.	U.S. Avg.
Blood Clot Prevention and Treatment				
Anticoagulation Overlap Therapy[2]	90	100%	95%	93%
ICU Venous Thromboembolism Prophylaxis[2]	66	98%	95%	92%
Incidence of Potentially Preventable VTE[1,2]	-	-	8%	10%
UFH with Dosages/Platelet Monitoring[2]	20	100%	99%	97%
Venous Thromboembolism Prophylaxis[2]	369	92%	91%	85%
Warfarin Therapy Discharge Instructions[2]	62	97%	78%	75%
Chest Pain/Possible Heart Attack Care				
Aspirin Given Within 24 Hours of Arrival[5]	-	-	98%	96%
Fibrinolytic Meds Within 30 Min. of Arrival[5]	-	-	68%	58%
Average Time to ECG (minutes)[5]	-	-	7	7
Average Time to Transfer (minutes)[5]	-	-	64	60
Children's Asthma Care				
Received Home Management Plan of Care	-	-	-	88%
Received Reliever Medication	-	-	-	100%
Received Systemic Corticosteroids	-	-	-	100%
Emergency Department				
Admittance Decision Time (minutes)[2]	802	235	96	98
Head CT Results Within 45 Min. of Arrival	15	60%	60%	57%
Patients Who Left ER Before Being Seen	77,623	1%	2%	2%
Time from ER Arrival to Admit. (minutes)[2]	805	423	280	274
Time from ER Arrival to Discharge (minutes)	405	175	167	134
Time in ER Before Being Evaluated (minutes)	414	15	35	26
Time to Pain Meds for Fractures (minutes)	238	73	56	57
Heart Attack Care				
Aspirin Given at Discharge	361	100%	99%	99%
Fibrinolytic Meds Within 30 Min. of Arrival[7]	-	-	75%	54%
PCI Within 90 Minutes of Arrival	52	96%	97%	96%
Statin Prescribed at Discharge	350	99%	99%	98%
Heart Failure Care				
ACE Inhibitor or ARB for LVSD	101	100%	98%	97%
Discharge Instructions Given	334	100%	95%	94%
Evaluation of LVS Function	410	100%	100%	99%
Medicare Spending				
Medicare Spending per Patient (ratio)	-	0.96	0.95	0.98
Pneumonia Care				
Appropriate Initial Antibiotic Given[2]	180	100%	97%	95%
Blood Culture Timing[2]	284	100%	98%	98%
Pregnancy and Delivery Care				
Newborn Deliveries Scheduled Early[2]	29	14%	6%	6%
Preventive Care				
Immunization for Influenza[2]	568	96%	92%	90%
Immunization for Pneumonia[2]	805	96%	93%	92%
Stroke Care				
Anticoagulation Therapy for Atrial Fibrillation	28	100%	96%	95%
Antithrombotic Therapy Timing	237	100%	99%	98%
Assessed for Rehabilitation	267	98%	99%	97%
Discharged on Antithrombotic Therapy	258	100%	100%	99%
Discharged on Statin Medication	188	91%	97%	94%
Thrombolytic Therapy Timing	22	64%	73%	66%
Venous Thromboembolism Prophylaxis	262	92%	97%	94%
Written Stroke Educational Materials Given	160	81%	92%	88%
Surgical Care Improvement Project				
Appropriate Beta Blocker Usage[2]	383	100%	99%	98%
Appropriate VTP Within 24 Hours[2]	842	100%	99%	98%
Controlled Postoperative Blood Glucose[2]	154	100%	98%	97%
Perioperative Temperature Management[2]	1,035	100%	100%	100%
Prophylactic Antibiotic Selection[2]	851	100%	99%	99%
Prophylactic Antibiotic Selection (Outpatient)	448	97%	98%	98%
Prophylactic Antibiotic Stopped[2]	843	99%	98%	98%
Prophylactic Antibiotic Timing[2]	857	98%	99%	99%
Prophylactic Antibiotic Timing (Outpatient)	445	100%	98%	98%
Urinary Catheter Removal[2]	884	99%	98%	97%
Survey of Patients' Hospital Experiences				
Area Around Room 'Always' Quiet at Night	300+	57%	60%	61%
Doctors 'Always' Communicated Well	300+	81%	81%	82%
Home Recovery Information Given	300+	87%	86%	85%
Hospital Given 9 or 10 on 10 Point Scale	300+	71%	68%	71%
Meds 'Always' Explained Before Given	300+	62%	62%	64%
Nurses 'Always' Communicated Well	300+	77%	78%	79%
Pain 'Always' Well Controlled	300+	69%	70%	71%
Room and Bathroom 'Always' Clean	300+	65%	71%	73%
Timely Help 'Always' Received	300+	67%	64%	68%
Would Definitely Recommend Hospital	300+	75%	69%	71%
Use of Medical Imaging				
Cardiac Imaging Stress Test before Surgery	694	7.3%	5.1%	5.3%
Combination Abdominal CT Scan	1,589	6.5%	8.5%	10.5%
Combination Brain/Sinus CT Scan	1,668	2.7%	2.3%	2.7%
Combination Chest CT Scan	652	0.6%	1.6%	2.7%
Follow-up Mammogram/Ultrasound	2,010	6.5%	7.7%	8.8%
Lumbar Spine MRI for Low Back Pain	265	30.2%	35.3%	37.2%

Bon Secours Saint Francis Medical Center

13700 Saint Francis Blvd, Suite 100 — Phone: 804-594-7400
Midlothian, VA 23114
URL: www.richmond.bonsecours.com
Type: Acute Care Hospitals — Emergency Services: Yes
Ownership: Voluntary non-profit - Church

Key Personnel:
CEO/President. . . . . Peter Gallagher

Measure	Cases	This Hosp.	State Avg.	U.S. Avg.
Blood Clot Prevention and Treatment				
Anticoagulation Overlap Therapy[2]	73	97%	95%	93%
ICU Venous Thromboembolism Prophylaxis[2]	53	94%	95%	92%
Incidence of Potentially Preventable VTE[1,2]	-	-	8%	10%
UFH with Dosages/Platelet Monitoring[2]	23	100%	99%	97%
Venous Thromboembolism Prophylaxis[2]	357	94%	91%	85%
Warfarin Therapy Discharge Instructions[2]	53	96%	78%	75%
Chest Pain/Possible Heart Attack Care				
Aspirin Given Within 24 Hours of Arrival	20	90%	98%	96%
Fibrinolytic Meds Within 30 Min. of Arrival[3,7]	-	-	68%	58%
Average Time to ECG (minutes)	21	9	7	7
Average Time to Transfer (minutes)[3,7]	-	-	64	60
Children's Asthma Care				
Received Home Management Plan of Care	-	-	-	88%
Received Reliever Medication	-	-	-	100%
Received Systemic Corticosteroids	-	-	-	100%
Emergency Department				
Admittance Decision Time (minutes)[2]	591	134	96	98

NOTE: Hospital profiles are in alphabetical order by state, then city, then hospital within the city; Rankings exclude hospitals with less than 25 cases except for patient surveys which excludes hospitals with less than 100 cases; (a) 100-299 cases; (1) The number of cases/patients is too few to report; (2) Data submitted were based on a sample of cases/patients; (3) Results are based on a shorter time period than required; (4) Data suppressed by CMS for one or more quarters; (5) Results are not available for this reporting period; (6) Fewer than 100 patients completed the HCAHPS survey; (7) No cases met the criteria for this measure; (8) The lower limit of the confidence interval cannot be calculated if the number of observed infections equals zero; (9) No data are available from the state/territory for this reporting period; (10) The scores shown reflect fewer than 50 completed surveys; (11) There were discrepancies in the data collection process; (12) This measure does not apply to this hospital for this reporting period; (13) Results cannot be calculated for this reporting period; (14) The results for this state are combined with nearby states to protect confidentiality; Please refer to the User's Guide for a full explanation of data.

Measure	Cases	This Hosp.	State Avg.	U.S. Avg.
Head CT Results Within 45 Min. of Arrival[1]	-	-	60%	57%
Patients Who Left ER Before Being Seen	47,167	0%	2%	2%
Time from ER Arrival to Admit. (minutes)[2]	602	291	280	274
Time from ER Arrival to Discharge (minutes)	396	117	167	134
Time in ER Before Being Evaluated (minutes)	421	9	35	26
Time to Pain Meds for Fractures (minutes)	145	49	56	57
Heart Attack Care				
Aspirin Given at Discharge	156	99%	99%	99%
Fibrinolytic Meds Within 30 Min. of Arrival[7]	-	-	75%	54%
PCI Within 90 Minutes of Arrival	40	100%	97%	96%
Statin Prescribed at Discharge	149	100%	99%	98%
Heart Failure Care				
ACE Inhibitor or ARB for LVSD	79	99%	98%	97%
Discharge Instructions Given	195	99%	95%	94%
Evaluation of LVS Function	235	100%	100%	99%
Medicare Spending				
Medicare Spending per Patient (ratio)	-	1.03	0.95	0.98
Pneumonia Care				
Appropriate Initial Antibiotic Given	126	94%	97%	95%
Blood Culture Timing	229	97%	98%	98%
Pregnancy and Delivery Care				
Newborn Deliveries Scheduled Early[2]	35	3%	6%	6%
Preventive Care				
Immunization for Influenza[2]	580	92%	92%	90%
Immunization for Pneumonia[2]	640	89%	93%	92%
Stroke Care				
Anticoagulation Therapy for Atrial Fibrillation[1]	-	-	96%	95%
Antithrombotic Therapy Timing	63	98%	99%	98%
Assessed for Rehabilitation	75	99%	99%	97%
Discharged on Antithrombotic Therapy	72	100%	100%	99%
Discharged on Statin Medication	54	94%	97%	94%
Thrombolytic Therapy Timing[1]	-	-	73%	66%
Venous Thromboembolism Prophylaxis	72	97%	97%	94%
Written Stroke Educational Materials Given	48	88%	92%	88%
Surgical Care Improvement Project				
Appropriate Beta Blocker Usage	229	97%	99%	98%
Appropriate VTP Within 24 Hours	799	99%	99%	98%
Controlled Postoperative Blood Glucose[7]	-	-	98%	97%
Perioperative Temperature Management	915	100%	100%	100%
Prophylactic Antibiotic Selection	585	99%	99%	99%
Prophylactic Antibiotic Selection (Outpatient)	437	85%	98%	98%
Prophylactic Antibiotic Stopped	568	98%	98%	98%
Prophylactic Antibiotic Timing	585	98%	99%	99%
Prophylactic Antibiotic Timing (Outpatient)	439	96%	98%	98%
Urinary Catheter Removal	215	87%	98%	97%
Survey of Patients' Hospital Experiences				
Area Around Room 'Always' Quiet at Night	300+	65%	60%	61%
Doctors 'Always' Communicated Well	300+	79%	81%	82%
Home Recovery Information Given	300+	86%	86%	85%
Hospital Given 9 or 10 on 10 Point Scale	300+	73%	68%	71%
Meds 'Always' Explained Before Given	300+	59%	62%	64%
Nurses 'Always' Communicated Well	300+	75%	78%	79%
Pain 'Always' Well Controlled	300+	69%	70%	71%
Room and Bathroom 'Always' Clean	300+	66%	71%	73%
Timely Help 'Always' Received	300+	59%	64%	68%
Would Definitely Recommend Hospital	300+	76%	69%	71%
Use of Medical Imaging				
Cardiac Imaging Stress Test before Surgery	96	5.2%	5.1%	5.3%
Combination Abdominal CT Scan	828	4.5%	8.5%	10.5%
Combination Brain/Sinus CT Scan	857	2.3%	2.3%	2.7%
Combination Chest CT Scan	553	0.5%	1.6%	2.7%
Follow-up Mammogram/Ultrasound	1,484	7.4%	7.7%	8.8%
Lumbar Spine MRI for Low Back Pain	293	33.4%	35.3%	37.2%

Riverside Shore Memorial Hospital

9507 Hospital Avenue   Phone: 757-414-8000
Nassawadox, VA 23413   Fax: 757-414-8633
E-mail: shorehealth@esva.net
URL: www.shorehealthservices.org
Type: Acute Care Hospitals   Emergency Services: Yes
Ownership: Voluntary non-profit - Private   Beds: 143
Key Personnel:
Infection Control.............. Sharon Angle
Quality Assurance .... Sharon Angle
Radiology.................... Michael J Bigg, MD
Operating Room............... Otis W Doss, MD
CEO/President................ Alan Markowitz
Chief of Medical Staff.......... James L McDaniel, MD
Pediatric Ambulatory Care ...... Cathy Riopel, MD
Pediatric In-Patient Care .... Cathy Riopel, MD

Measure	Cases	This Hosp.	State Avg.	U.S. Avg.
Blood Clot Prevention and Treatment				
Anticoagulation Overlap Therapy[2]	14	79%	95%	93%
ICU Venous Thromboembolism Prophylaxis[2]	102	92%	95%	92%
Incidence of Potentially Preventable VTE[2,7]	-	-	8%	10%
UFH with Dosages/Platelet Monitoring[1,2]	-	-	99%	97%
Venous Thromboembolism Prophylaxis[2]	364	96%	91%	85%
Warfarin Therapy Discharge Instructions[1,2]	-	-	78%	75%
Chest Pain/Possible Heart Attack Care				
Aspirin Given Within 24 Hours of Arrival	26	100%	98%	96%
Fibrinolytic Meds Within 30 Min. of Arrival[1]	-	-	68%	58%
Average Time to ECG (minutes)	27	4	7	7
Average Time to Transfer (minutes)[1]	-	-	64	60
Children's Asthma Care				
Received Home Management Plan of Care	-	-	-	88%
Received Reliever Medication	-	-	-	100%
Received Systemic Corticosteroids	-	-	-	100%
Emergency Department				
Admittance Decision Time (minutes)[2]	495	92	96	98
Head CT Results Within 45 Min. of Arrival	11	82%	60%	57%
Patients Who Left ER Before Being Seen	16,510	2%	2%	2%
Time from ER Arrival to Admit. (minutes)[2]	505	267	280	274
Time from ER Arrival to Discharge (minutes)	359	161	167	134
Time in ER Before Being Evaluated (minutes)	400	30	35	26
Time to Pain Meds for Fractures (minutes)	36	62	56	57
Heart Attack Care				
Aspirin Given at Discharge	20	95%	99%	99%
Fibrinolytic Meds Within 30 Min. of Arrival[7]	-	-	75%	54%
PCI Within 90 Minutes of Arrival[7]	-	-	97%	96%
Statin Prescribed at Discharge	18	89%	99%	98%
Heart Failure Care				
ACE Inhibitor or ARB for LVSD	64	100%	98%	97%
Discharge Instructions Given	107	98%	95%	94%
Evaluation of LVS Function	125	100%	100%	99%
Medicare Spending				
Medicare Spending per Patient (ratio)	-	0.91	0.95	0.98
Pneumonia Care				
Appropriate Initial Antibiotic Given	63	98%	97%	95%
Blood Culture Timing	118	98%	98%	98%
Pregnancy and Delivery Care				
Newborn Deliveries Scheduled Early[2]	28	4%	6%	6%
Preventive Care				
Immunization for Influenza[2]	347	95%	92%	90%
Immunization for Pneumonia[2]	445	97%	93%	92%
Stroke Care				
Anticoagulation Therapy for Atrial Fibrillation[1]	-	-	96%	95%
Antithrombotic Therapy Timing	36	94%	99%	98%
Assessed for Rehabilitation	48	94%	99%	97%
Discharged on Antithrombotic Therapy	44	100%	100%	99%
Discharged on Statin Medication	35	94%	97%	94%
Thrombolytic Therapy Timing[1]	-	-	73%	66%
Venous Thromboembolism Prophylaxis	48	98%	97%	94%
Written Stroke Educational Materials Given	32	88%	92%	88%
Surgical Care Improvement Project				
Appropriate Beta Blocker Usage	18	94%	99%	98%
Appropriate VTP Within 24 Hours	58	95%	99%	98%
Controlled Postoperative Blood Glucose[7]	-	-	98%	97%
Perioperative Temperature Management	63	100%	100%	100%
Prophylactic Antibiotic Selection	39	97%	99%	99%
Prophylactic Antibiotic Selection (Outpatient)	65	98%	98%	98%
Prophylactic Antibiotic Stopped	37	92%	98%	98%
Prophylactic Antibiotic Timing	39	100%	99%	99%
Prophylactic Antibiotic Timing (Outpatient)	65	100%	98%	98%
Urinary Catheter Removal	21	90%	98%	97%
Survey of Patients' Hospital Experiences				
Area Around Room 'Always' Quiet at Night	300+	60%	60%	61%
Doctors 'Always' Communicated Well	300+	82%	81%	82%
Home Recovery Information Given	300+	83%	86%	85%
Hospital Given 9 or 10 on 10 Point Scale	300+	59%	68%	71%
Meds 'Always' Explained Before Given	300+	57%	62%	64%
Nurses 'Always' Communicated Well	300+	78%	78%	79%
Pain 'Always' Well Controlled	300+	65%	70%	71%
Room and Bathroom 'Always' Clean	300+	72%	71%	73%
Timely Help 'Always' Received	300+	66%	64%	68%
Would Definitely Recommend Hospital	300+	55%	69%	71%
Use of Medical Imaging				
Cardiac Imaging Stress Test before Surgery	320	5.3%	5.1%	5.3%
Combination Abdominal CT Scan	445	13.7%	8.5%	10.5%
Combination Brain/Sinus CT Scan	432	1.6%	2.3%	2.7%
Combination Chest CT Scan	212	6.6%	1.6%	2.7%
Follow-up Mammogram/Ultrasound	1,108	5.5%	7.7%	8.8%
Lumbar Spine MRI for Low Back Pain[1]	-	-	35.3%	37.2%

Mary Immaculate Hospital

2 Bernardine Drive   Phone: 757-886-6000
Newport News, VA 23602   Fax: 757-886-6605
URL: www.bonsecourshamptonroad.com
Type: Acute Care Hospitals   Emergency Services: Yes
Ownership: Voluntary non-profit - Church   Beds: 120
Key Personnel:
Radiology.................. Harry Ill
CEO/President............... Pat L Robertson

Measure	Cases	This Hosp.	State Avg.	U.S. Avg.
Blood Clot Prevention and Treatment				
Anticoagulation Overlap Therapy[2]	41	98%	95%	93%
ICU Venous Thromboembolism Prophylaxis[2]	53	100%	95%	92%
Incidence of Potentially Preventable VTE[1,2]	-	-	8%	10%
UFH with Dosages/Platelet Monitoring[2]	24	100%	99%	97%
Venous Thromboembolism Prophylaxis[2]	234	98%	91%	85%
Warfarin Therapy Discharge Instructions[2]	29	100%	78%	75%
Chest Pain/Possible Heart Attack Care				
Aspirin Given Within 24 Hours of Arrival[1,3]	-	-	98%	96%
Fibrinolytic Meds Within 30 Min. of Arrival[3,7]	-	-	68%	58%
Average Time to ECG (minutes)[1,3]	-	-	7	7
Average Time to Transfer (minutes)[3,7]	-	-	64	60
Children's Asthma Care				
Received Home Management Plan of Care	-	-	-	88%
Received Reliever Medication	-	-	-	100%
Received Systemic Corticosteroids	-	-	-	100%
Emergency Department				
Admittance Decision Time (minutes)[2]	458	92	96	98
Head CT Results Within 45 Min. of Arrival[1]	-	-	60%	57%
Patients Who Left ER Before Being Seen	42,518	2%	2%	2%
Time from ER Arrival to Admit. (minutes)[2]	462	286	280	274
Time from ER Arrival to Discharge (minutes)	391	123	167	134
Time in ER Before Being Evaluated (minutes)	376	22	35	26
Time to Pain Meds for Fractures (minutes)	82	56	56	57
Heart Attack Care				
Aspirin Given at Discharge	67	100%	99%	99%
Fibrinolytic Meds Within 30 Min. of Arrival[7]	-	-	75%	54%
PCI Within 90 Minutes of Arrival	16	100%	97%	96%
Statin Prescribed at Discharge	69	99%	99%	98%
Heart Failure Care				
ACE Inhibitor or ARB for LVSD	58	100%	98%	97%
Discharge Instructions Given	173	99%	95%	94%
Evaluation of LVS Function	211	100%	100%	99%
Medicare Spending				
Medicare Spending per Patient (ratio)	-	0.96	0.95	0.98
Pneumonia Care				
Appropriate Initial Antibiotic Given	121	98%	97%	95%
Blood Culture Timing	160	98%	98%	98%
Pregnancy and Delivery Care				
Newborn Deliveries Scheduled Early[2]	38	18%	6%	6%
Preventive Care				
Immunization for Influenza[2]	569	97%	92%	90%
Immunization for Pneumonia[2]	639	96%	93%	92%
Stroke Care				
Anticoagulation Therapy for Atrial Fibrillation[1]	-	-	96%	95%
Antithrombotic Therapy Timing	39	100%	99%	98%
Assessed for Rehabilitation	41	100%	99%	97%

NOTE: Hospital profiles are in alphabetical order by state, then city, then hospital within the city; Rankings exclude hospitals with less than 25 cases except for patient surveys which excludes hospitals with less than 100 cases; (a) 100-299 cases; (1) The number of cases/patients is too few to report; (2) Data submitted were based on a sample of cases/patients; (3) Results are based on a shorter time period than required; (4) Data suppressed by CMS for one or more quarters; (5) Results are not available for this reporting period; (6) Fewer than 100 patients completed the HCAHPS survey; (7) No cases met the criteria for this measure; (8) The lower limit of the confidence interval cannot be calculated if the number of observed infections equals zero; (9) No data are available from the state/territory for this reporting period; (10) The scores shown reflect fewer than 50 completed surveys; (11) There were discrepancies in the data collection process; (12) This measure does not apply to this hospital for this reporting period; (13) Results cannot be calculated for this reporting period; (14) The results for this state are combined with nearby states to protect confidentiality; Please refer to the User's Guide for a full explanation of data.

Measure	Cases	This Hosp.	State Avg.	U.S. Avg.
Discharged on Antithrombotic Therapy	37	100%	100%	99%
Discharged on Statin Medication	27	100%	97%	94%
Thrombolytic Therapy Timing[1]	-	-	73%	66%
Venous Thromboembolism Prophylaxis	41	98%	97%	94%
Written Stroke Educational Materials Given	31	100%	92%	88%
Surgical Care Improvement Project				
Appropriate Beta Blocker Usage[2]	426	100%	99%	98%
Appropriate VTP Within 24 Hours[2]	1,138	99%	99%	98%
Controlled Postoperative Blood Glucose[2,7]	-	-	98%	97%
Perioperative Temperature Management[2]	1,864	100%	100%	100%
Prophylactic Antibiotic Selection[2]	1,649	100%	99%	99%
Prophylactic Antibiotic Selection (Outpatient)	358	98%	98%	98%
Prophylactic Antibiotic Stopped[2]	1,639	99%	98%	98%
Prophylactic Antibiotic Timing[2]	1,652	100%	99%	99%
Prophylactic Antibiotic Timing (Outpatient)	360	99%	98%	98%
Urinary Catheter Removal[2]	78	95%	98%	97%
Survey of Patients' Hospital Experiences				
Area Around Room 'Always' Quiet at Night	300+	63%	60%	61%
Doctors 'Always' Communicated Well	300+	81%	81%	82%
Home Recovery Information Given	300+	88%	86%	85%
Hospital Given 9 or 10 on 10 Point Scale	300+	66%	68%	71%
Meds 'Always' Explained Before Given	300+	61%	62%	64%
Nurses 'Always' Communicated Well	300+	74%	78%	79%
Pain 'Always' Well Controlled	300+	65%	70%	71%
Room and Bathroom 'Always' Clean	300+	59%	71%	73%
Timely Help 'Always' Received	300+	59%	64%	68%
Would Definitely Recommend Hospital	300+	69%	69%	71%
Use of Medical Imaging				
Cardiac Imaging Stress Test before Surgery	383	6.3%	5.1%	5.3%
Combination Abdominal CT Scan	347	3.5%	8.5%	10.5%
Combination Brain/Sinus CT Scan	503	1.8%	2.3%	2.7%
Combination Chest CT Scan	139	0.0%	1.6%	2.7%
Follow-up Mammogram/Ultrasound	483	7.0%	7.7%	8.8%
Lumbar Spine MRI for Low Back Pain[1]	-	-	35.3%	37.2%

Riverside Regional Medical Center

500 J Clyde Morris Blvd
Newport News, VA 23601
Phone: 757-594-2000
Fax: 757-594-3864
URL: www.riversideonline.com
Type: Acute Care Hospitals
Emergency Services: Yes
Ownership: Voluntary non-profit - Private
Beds: 576

Key Personnel:
Radiology. . . . . Paula Burcher
Quality Assurance . . . . Jody Friend
Chief of Medical Staff. . . . . Dr Barry Gross
Coronary Care. . . . . Donna Haughinberry
Intensive Care Unit. . . . . Donna Haughinberry
CEO/President. . . . . Richard J Pearce
Patient Relations . . . . Medford Ramey
Operating Room. . . . . Sheila Rilee

Measure	Cases	This Hosp.	State Avg.	U.S. Avg.
Blood Clot Prevention and Treatment				
Anticoagulation Overlap Therapy[2]	85	99%	95%	93%
ICU Venous Thromboembolism Prophylaxis[2]	155	100%	95%	92%
Incidence of Potentially Preventable VTE[2]	15	0%	8%	10%
UFH with Dosages/Platelet Monitoring[2]	26	100%	99%	97%
Venous Thromboembolism Prophylaxis[2]	427	96%	91%	85%
Warfarin Therapy Discharge Instructions[2]	72	85%	78%	75%
Chest Pain/Possible Heart Attack Care				
Aspirin Given Within 24 Hours of Arrival[5]	-	-	98%	96%
Fibrinolytic Meds Within 30 Min. of Arrival[5]	-	-	68%	58%
Average Time to ECG (minutes)[5]	-	-	7	7
Average Time to Transfer (minutes)[5]	-	-	64	60
Children's Asthma Care				
Received Home Management Plan of Care	-	-	-	88%
Received Reliever Medication	-	-	-	100%
Received Systemic Corticosteroids	-	-	-	100%
Emergency Department				
Admittance Decision Time (minutes)[2]	608	112	96	98
Head CT Results Within 45 Min. of Arrival[1]	-	-	60%	57%
Patients Who Left ER Before Being Seen	65,747	3%	2%	2%
Time from ER Arrival to Admit. (minutes)[2]	609	328	280	274
Time from ER Arrival to Discharge (minutes)	352	192	167	134
Time in ER Before Being Evaluated (minutes)	364	83	35	26
Time to Pain Meds for Fractures (minutes)	170	73	56	57
Heart Attack Care				
Aspirin Given at Discharge	418	100%	99%	99%
Fibrinolytic Meds Within 30 Min. of Arrival[7]	-	-	75%	54%
PCI Within 90 Minutes of Arrival	60	98%	97%	96%
Statin Prescribed at Discharge	412	100%	99%	98%
Heart Failure Care				
ACE Inhibitor or ARB for LVSD	175	100%	98%	97%
Discharge Instructions Given	422	99%	95%	94%
Evaluation of LVS Function	518	100%	100%	99%
Medicare Spending				
Medicare Spending per Patient (ratio)	-	0.98	0.95	0.98
Pneumonia Care				
Appropriate Initial Antibiotic Given	161	97%	97%	95%
Blood Culture Timing	237	98%	98%	98%
Pregnancy and Delivery Care				
Newborn Deliveries Scheduled Early[2]	56	0%	6%	6%
Preventive Care				
Immunization for Influenza[2]	488	95%	92%	90%
Immunization for Pneumonia[2]	611	95%	93%	92%
Stroke Care				
Anticoagulation Therapy for Atrial Fibrillation	31	97%	96%	95%
Antithrombotic Therapy Timing	212	100%	99%	98%
Assessed for Rehabilitation	312	99%	99%	97%
Discharged on Antithrombotic Therapy	246	100%	100%	99%
Discharged on Statin Medication	191	99%	97%	94%
Thrombolytic Therapy Timing	19	100%	73%	66%
Venous Thromboembolism Prophylaxis	320	99%	97%	94%
Written Stroke Educational Materials Given	157	97%	92%	88%
Surgical Care Improvement Project				
Appropriate Beta Blocker Usage[2]	234	97%	99%	98%
Appropriate VTP Within 24 Hours[2]	498	99%	99%	98%
Controlled Postoperative Blood Glucose[2]	98	100%	98%	97%
Perioperative Temperature Management[2]	650	100%	100%	100%
Prophylactic Antibiotic Selection[2]	454	99%	99%	99%
Prophylactic Antibiotic Selection (Outpatient)	581	98%	98%	98%
Prophylactic Antibiotic Stopped[2]	436	99%	98%	98%
Prophylactic Antibiotic Timing[2]	455	100%	99%	99%
Prophylactic Antibiotic Timing (Outpatient)	587	98%	98%	98%
Urinary Catheter Removal[2]	422	98%	98%	97%
Survey of Patients' Hospital Experiences				
Area Around Room 'Always' Quiet at Night	300+	58%	60%	61%
Doctors 'Always' Communicated Well	300+	79%	81%	82%
Home Recovery Information Given	300+	83%	86%	85%
Hospital Given 9 or 10 on 10 Point Scale	300+	67%	68%	71%
Meds 'Always' Explained Before Given	300+	60%	62%	64%
Nurses 'Always' Communicated Well	300+	77%	78%	79%
Pain 'Always' Well Controlled	300+	67%	70%	71%
Room and Bathroom 'Always' Clean	300+	72%	71%	73%
Timely Help 'Always' Received	300+	60%	64%	68%
Would Definitely Recommend Hospital	300+	71%	69%	71%
Use of Medical Imaging				
Cardiac Imaging Stress Test before Surgery	1,156	4.2%	5.1%	5.3%
Combination Abdominal CT Scan	1,898	7.3%	8.5%	10.5%
Combination Brain/Sinus CT Scan	1,264	2.0%	2.3%	2.7%
Combination Chest CT Scan	1,499	0.1%	1.6%	2.7%
Follow-up Mammogram/Ultrasound	3,106	9.1%	7.7%	8.8%
Lumbar Spine MRI for Low Back Pain	239	32.6%	35.3%	37.2%

Bon Secours Depaul Medical Center

150 Kingsley Lane
Norfolk, VA 23505
Phone: 757-889-5000
Fax: 757-489-3450
URL: www.bonsecourshamptonroads.com
Type: Acute Care Hospitals
Emergency Services: Yes
Ownership: Voluntary non-profit - Church
Beds: 189

Key Personnel:
Radiology. . . . . Harry A Allen, III
Operating Room. . . . . L D Britt
Emergency Room . . . . Jane Carty
Infection Control. . . . . Jessica Davis
Quality Assurance . . . . Amy Derion
CEO/President. . . . . Susan Erickson
Chief of Medical Staff. . . . . Judy Meekins-James

Measure	Cases	This Hosp.	State Avg.	U.S. Avg.
Blood Clot Prevention and Treatment				
Anticoagulation Overlap Therapy[2]	19	89%	95%	93%
ICU Venous Thromboembolism Prophylaxis[2]	112	94%	95%	92%
Incidence of Potentially Preventable VTE[1,2]	-	-	8%	10%
UFH with Dosages/Platelet Monitoring[2]	18	100%	99%	97%
Venous Thromboembolism Prophylaxis[2]	313	91%	91%	85%
Warfarin Therapy Discharge Instructions[2]	15	100%	78%	75%
Chest Pain/Possible Heart Attack Care				
Aspirin Given Within 24 Hours of Arrival[1]	-	-	98%	96%
Fibrinolytic Meds Within 30 Min. of Arrival[5]	-	-	68%	58%
Average Time to ECG (minutes)[1]	-	-	7	7
Average Time to Transfer (minutes)[5]	-	-	64	60
Children's Asthma Care				
Received Home Management Plan of Care	-	-	-	88%
Received Reliever Medication	-	-	-	100%
Received Systemic Corticosteroids	-	-	-	100%
Emergency Department				
Admittance Decision Time (minutes)[2]	633	137	96	98
Head CT Results Within 45 Min. of Arrival[3,7]	-	-	60%	57%
Patients Who Left ER Before Being Seen	36,578	3%	2%	2%
Time from ER Arrival to Admit. (minutes)[2]	641	367	280	274
Time from ER Arrival to Discharge (minutes)	372	182	167	134
Time in ER Before Being Evaluated (minutes)	403	41	35	26
Time to Pain Meds for Fractures (minutes)	101	92	56	57
Heart Attack Care				
Aspirin Given at Discharge	94	100%	99%	99%
Fibrinolytic Meds Within 30 Min. of Arrival[7]	-	-	75%	54%
PCI Within 90 Minutes of Arrival	21	100%	97%	96%
Statin Prescribed at Discharge	90	99%	99%	98%
Heart Failure Care				
ACE Inhibitor or ARB for LVSD	68	93%	98%	97%
Discharge Instructions Given	175	97%	95%	94%
Evaluation of LVS Function	211	99%	100%	99%
Medicare Spending				
Medicare Spending per Patient (ratio)	-	1.02	0.95	0.98
Pneumonia Care				
Appropriate Initial Antibiotic Given	106	94%	97%	95%
Blood Culture Timing	179	96%	98%	98%
Pregnancy and Delivery Care				
Newborn Deliveries Scheduled Early[2]	26	8%	6%	6%
Preventive Care				
Immunization for Influenza[2]	556	78%	92%	90%
Immunization for Pneumonia[2]	680	82%	93%	92%
Stroke Care				
Anticoagulation Therapy for Atrial Fibrillation[1]	-	-	96%	95%
Antithrombotic Therapy Timing	83	100%	99%	98%
Assessed for Rehabilitation	124	100%	99%	97%
Discharged on Antithrombotic Therapy	97	99%	100%	99%
Discharged on Statin Medication	75	97%	97%	94%
Thrombolytic Therapy Timing[1]	-	-	73%	66%
Venous Thromboembolism Prophylaxis	130	98%	97%	94%
Written Stroke Educational Materials Given	51	100%	92%	88%
Surgical Care Improvement Project				
Appropriate Beta Blocker Usage[2]	72	93%	99%	98%
Appropriate VTP Within 24 Hours[2]	204	97%	99%	98%
Controlled Postoperative Blood Glucose[2,7]	-	-	98%	97%
Perioperative Temperature Management[2]	275	100%	100%	100%
Prophylactic Antibiotic Selection[2]	152	98%	99%	99%
Prophylactic Antibiotic Selection (Outpatient)	429	94%	98%	98%
Prophylactic Antibiotic Stopped[2]	148	97%	98%	98%
Prophylactic Antibiotic Timing[2]	154	97%	99%	99%
Prophylactic Antibiotic Timing (Outpatient)	431	98%	98%	98%
Urinary Catheter Removal[2]	157	95%	98%	97%
Survey of Patients' Hospital Experiences				
Area Around Room 'Always' Quiet at Night	300+	62%	60%	61%
Doctors 'Always' Communicated Well	300+	79%	81%	82%
Home Recovery Information Given	300+	85%	86%	85%
Hospital Given 9 or 10 on 10 Point Scale	300+	63%	68%	71%
Meds 'Always' Explained Before Given	300+	56%	62%	64%
Nurses 'Always' Communicated Well	300+	71%	78%	79%
Pain 'Always' Well Controlled	300+	64%	70%	71%
Room and Bathroom 'Always' Clean	300+	66%	71%	73%

NOTE: Hospital profiles are in alphabetical order by state, then city, then hospital within the city; Rankings exclude hospitals with less than 25 cases except for patient surveys which excludes hospitals with less than 100 cases; (a) 100-299 cases; (1) The number of cases/patients is too few to report; (2) Data submitted were based on a sample of cases/patients; (3) Results are based on a shorter time period than required; (4) Data suppressed by CMS for one or more quarters; (5) Results are not available for this reporting period; (6) Fewer than 100 patients completed the HCAHPS survey; (7) No cases met the criteria for this measure; (8) The lower limit of the confidence interval cannot be calculated if the number of observed infections equals zero; (9) No data are available from the state/territory for this reporting period; (10) The scores shown reflect fewer than 50 completed surveys; (11) There were discrepancies in the data collection process; (12) This measure does not apply to this hospital for this reporting period; (13) Results cannot be calculated for this reporting period; (14) The results for this state are combined with nearby states to protect confidentiality; Please refer to the User's Guide for a full explanation of data.

Timely Help 'Always' Received	300+	56%	64%	68%
Would Definitely Recommend Hospital	300+	63%	69%	71%
Use of Medical Imaging				
Cardiac Imaging Stress Test before Surgery	130	6.9%	5.1%	5.3%
Combination Abdominal CT Scan	547	6.8%	8.5%	10.5%
Combination Brain/Sinus CT Scan	602	1.5%	2.3%	2.7%
Combination Chest CT Scan	440	0.0%	1.6%	2.7%
Follow-up Mammogram/Ultrasound	1,580	7.6%	7.7%	8.8%
Lumbar Spine MRI for Low Back Pain	82	39.0%	35.3%	37.2%

Sentara Leigh Hospital

830 Kempsville Road
Norfolk, VA 23502
URL: www.sentara.com
Type: Acute Care Hospitals
Ownership: Voluntary non-profit - Other
Phone: 757-261-6601
Fax: 757-455-7164
Emergency Services: Yes
Beds: 250

Key Personnel:
CEO/President. . . . . Darlene Anderson
Quality Assurance . . . . Sam Byrd
Chief of Medical Staff . . . . John Hurre, MD
Operating Room. . . . . Lisa Rogers

Measure	Cases	This Hosp.	State Avg.	U.S. Avg.
Blood Clot Prevention and Treatment				
Anticoagulation Overlap Therapy[2]	103	97%	95%	93%
ICU Venous Thromboembolism Prophylaxis[2]	50	98%	95%	92%
Incidence of Potentially Preventable VTE[2]	24	4%	8%	10%
UFH with Dosages/Platelet Monitoring[2]	71	100%	99%	97%
Venous Thromboembolism Prophylaxis[2]	349	94%	91%	85%
Warfarin Therapy Discharge Instructions[2]	77	97%	78%	75%
Chest Pain/Possible Heart Attack Care				
Aspirin Given Within 24 Hours of Arrival	20	95%	98%	96%
Fibrinolytic Meds Within 30 Min. of Arrival[7]	-	-	68%	58%
Average Time to ECG (minutes)	20	7	7	7
Average Time to Transfer (minutes)[1]	-	-	64	60
Children's Asthma Care				
Received Home Management Plan of Care	-	-	-	88%
Received Reliever Medication	-	-	-	100%
Received Systemic Corticosteroids	-	-	-	100%
Emergency Department				
Admittance Decision Time (minutes)[2]	715	109	96	98
Head CT Results Within 45 Min. of Arrival	23	65%	60%	57%
Patients Who Left ER Before Being Seen	66,722	1%	2%	2%
Time from ER Arrival to Admit. (minutes)[2]	717	355	280	274
Time from ER Arrival to Discharge (minutes)	3,924	226	167	134
Time in ER Before Being Evaluated (minutes)	3,963	71	35	26
Time to Pain Meds for Fractures (minutes)	97	61	56	57
Heart Attack Care				
Aspirin Given at Discharge	111	100%	99%	99%
Fibrinolytic Meds Within 30 Min. of Arrival[7]	-	-	75%	54%
PCI Within 90 Minutes of Arrival	36	97%	97%	96%
Statin Prescribed at Discharge	105	99%	99%	98%
Heart Failure Care				
ACE Inhibitor or ARB for LVSD	158	98%	98%	97%
Discharge Instructions Given	361	100%	95%	94%
Evaluation of LVS Function	428	100%	100%	99%
Medicare Spending				
Medicare Spending per Patient (ratio)	-	0.98	0.95	0.98
Pneumonia Care				
Appropriate Initial Antibiotic Given	157	99%	97%	95%
Blood Culture Timing	278	99%	98%	98%
Pregnancy and Delivery Care				
Newborn Deliveries Scheduled Early	178	0%	6%	6%
Preventive Care				
Immunization for Influenza[2]	554	91%	92%	90%
Immunization for Pneumonia[2]	704	94%	93%	92%
Stroke Care				
Anticoagulation Therapy for Atrial Fibrillation	21	95%	96%	95%
Antithrombotic Therapy Timing	172	100%	99%	98%
Assessed for Rehabilitation	189	99%	99%	97%
Discharged on Antithrombotic Therapy	186	100%	100%	99%
Discharged on Statin Medication	141	100%	97%	94%
Thrombolytic Therapy Timing[1]	-	-	73%	66%
Venous Thromboembolism Prophylaxis	187	99%	97%	94%
Written Stroke Educational Materials Given	118	95%	92%	88%
Surgical Care Improvement Project				
Appropriate Beta Blocker Usage[2]	500	100%	99%	98%
Appropriate VTP Within 24 Hours[2]	1,733	99%	99%	98%
Controlled Postoperative Blood Glucose[2,7]	-	-	98%	97%
Perioperative Temperature Management[2]	1,802	100%	100%	100%
Prophylactic Antibiotic Selection[2]	1,625	100%	99%	99%
Prophylactic Antibiotic Selection (Outpatient)	445	97%	98%	98%
Prophylactic Antibiotic Stopped[2]	1,613	99%	98%	98%
Prophylactic Antibiotic Timing[2]	1,626	99%	99%	99%
Prophylactic Antibiotic Timing (Outpatient)	448	99%	98%	98%
Urinary Catheter Removal[2]	1,527	100%	98%	97%
Survey of Patients' Hospital Experiences				
Area Around Room 'Always' Quiet at Night	300+	58%	60%	61%
Doctors 'Always' Communicated Well	300+	82%	81%	82%
Home Recovery Information Given	300+	91%	86%	85%
Hospital Given 9 or 10 on 10 Point Scale	300+	74%	68%	71%
Meds 'Always' Explained Before Given	300+	68%	62%	64%
Nurses 'Always' Communicated Well	300+	80%	78%	79%
Pain 'Always' Well Controlled	300+	76%	70%	71%
Room and Bathroom 'Always' Clean	300+	65%	71%	73%
Timely Help 'Always' Received	300+	66%	64%	68%
Would Definitely Recommend Hospital	300+	78%	69%	71%
Use of Medical Imaging				
Cardiac Imaging Stress Test before Surgery	571	5.1%	5.1%	5.3%
Combination Abdominal CT Scan	2,074	8.4%	8.5%	10.5%
Combination Brain/Sinus CT Scan	1,432	3.0%	2.3%	2.7%
Combination Chest CT Scan	1,796	0.1%	1.6%	2.7%
Follow-up Mammogram/Ultrasound	4,205	6.4%	7.7%	8.8%
Lumbar Spine MRI for Low Back Pain	169	34.3%	35.3%	37.2%

Sentara Norfolk General Hospital

600 Gresham Dr
Norfolk, VA 23507
URL: www.sentara.com
Type: Acute Care Hospitals
Ownership: Voluntary non-profit - Other
Phone: 757-388-3000
Fax: 757-455-7555
Emergency Services: Yes
Beds: 569

Key Personnel:
Infection Control. . . . . Jackie Butler, RN
Radiology. . . . . Brock Cutchins
Pediatric Ambulatory Care . . . . . . Glen Green, MD
CEO/President. . . . . Howard Kern
Quality Assurance . . . . Jaeque Mitchell
Cardiac Laboratory. . . . . Matt Rheins
Operating Room. . . . . Pam Robertson
Chief of Medical Staff . . . . Leonard Weineter, MD

Measure	Cases	This Hosp.	State Avg.	U.S. Avg.
Blood Clot Prevention and Treatment				
Anticoagulation Overlap Therapy[2]	51	94%	95%	93%
ICU Venous Thromboembolism Prophylaxis[2]	65	98%	95%	92%
Incidence of Potentially Preventable VTE[2]	18	6%	8%	10%
UFH with Dosages/Platelet Monitoring[2]	53	98%	99%	97%
Venous Thromboembolism Prophylaxis[2]	376	92%	91%	85%
Warfarin Therapy Discharge Instructions[2]	41	100%	78%	75%
Chest Pain/Possible Heart Attack Care				
Aspirin Given Within 24 Hours of Arrival[3,7]	-	-	98%	96%
Fibrinolytic Meds Within 30 Min. of Arrival[5]	-	-	68%	58%
Average Time to ECG (minutes)[3,7]	-	-	7	7
Average Time to Transfer (minutes)[5]	-	-	64	60
Children's Asthma Care				
Received Home Management Plan of Care	-	-	-	88%
Received Reliever Medication	-	-	-	100%
Received Systemic Corticosteroids	-	-	-	100%
Emergency Department				
Admittance Decision Time (minutes)[2]	563	137	96	98
Head CT Results Within 45 Min. of Arrival[3,7]	-	-	60%	57%
Patients Who Left ER Before Being Seen	69,401	2%	2%	2%
Time from ER Arrival to Admit. (minutes)[2]	565	378	280	274
Time from ER Arrival to Discharge (minutes)	5,351	229	167	134
Time in ER Before Being Evaluated (minutes)	5,484	51	35	26
Time to Pain Meds for Fractures (minutes)	82	81	56	57
Heart Attack Care				
Aspirin Given at Discharge	643	100%	99%	99%
Fibrinolytic Meds Within 30 Min. of Arrival[7]	-	-	75%	54%
PCI Within 90 Minutes of Arrival	42	100%	97%	96%
Statin Prescribed at Discharge	637	100%	99%	98%
Heart Failure Care				
ACE Inhibitor or ARB for LVSD	408	100%	98%	97%
Discharge Instructions Given	879	100%	95%	94%
Evaluation of LVS Function	971	100%	100%	99%
Medicare Spending				
Medicare Spending per Patient (ratio)	-	0.98	0.95	0.98
Pneumonia Care				
Appropriate Initial Antibiotic Given	120	99%	97%	95%
Blood Culture Timing	259	99%	98%	98%
Pregnancy and Delivery Care				
Newborn Deliveries Scheduled Early	130	0%	6%	6%
Preventive Care				
Immunization for Influenza[2]	527	74%	92%	90%
Immunization for Pneumonia[2]	625	79%	93%	92%
Stroke Care				
Anticoagulation Therapy for Atrial Fibrillation	14	100%	96%	95%
Antithrombotic Therapy Timing	226	100%	99%	98%
Assessed for Rehabilitation	334	100%	99%	97%
Discharged on Antithrombotic Therapy	238	100%	100%	99%
Discharged on Statin Medication	175	99%	97%	94%
Thrombolytic Therapy Timing[1]	-	-	73%	66%
Venous Thromboembolism Prophylaxis	377	99%	97%	94%
Written Stroke Educational Materials Given	184	97%	92%	88%
Surgical Care Improvement Project				
Appropriate Beta Blocker Usage[2]	551	100%	99%	98%
Appropriate VTP Within 24 Hours[2]	223	97%	99%	98%
Controlled Postoperative Blood Glucose[2]	541	97%	98%	97%
Perioperative Temperature Management[2]	411	100%	100%	100%
Prophylactic Antibiotic Selection[2]	681	100%	99%	99%
Prophylactic Antibiotic Selection (Outpatient)	645	99%	98%	98%
Prophylactic Antibiotic Stopped[2]	646	98%	98%	98%
Prophylactic Antibiotic Timing[2]	681	99%	99%	99%
Prophylactic Antibiotic Timing (Outpatient)	666	96%	98%	98%
Urinary Catheter Removal[2]	647	99%	98%	97%
Survey of Patients' Hospital Experiences				
Area Around Room 'Always' Quiet at Night	300+	62%	60%	61%
Doctors 'Always' Communicated Well	300+	84%	81%	82%
Home Recovery Information Given	300+	89%	86%	85%
Hospital Given 9 or 10 on 10 Point Scale	300+	77%	68%	71%
Meds 'Always' Explained Before Given	300+	65%	62%	64%
Nurses 'Always' Communicated Well	300+	81%	78%	79%
Pain 'Always' Well Controlled	300+	76%	70%	71%
Room and Bathroom 'Always' Clean	300+	68%	71%	73%
Timely Help 'Always' Received	300+	71%	64%	68%
Would Definitely Recommend Hospital	300+	79%	69%	71%
Use of Medical Imaging				
Cardiac Imaging Stress Test before Surgery	415	4.8%	5.1%	5.3%
Combination Abdominal CT Scan	1,231	7.1%	8.5%	10.5%
Combination Brain/Sinus CT Scan	739	1.5%	2.3%	2.7%
Combination Chest CT Scan	1,003	0.0%	1.6%	2.7%
Follow-up Mammogram/Ultrasound	2,545	8.2%	7.7%	8.8%
Lumbar Spine MRI for Low Back Pain	125	35.2%	35.3%	37.2%

Norton Community Hospital

100 15th Saint Nw
Norton, VA 24273
URL: www.nchosp.org
Type: Acute Care Hospitals
Ownership: Voluntary non-profit - Other
Phone: 703-679-8865
Fax: 276-679-9003
Emergency Services: Yes
Beds: 129

Key Personnel:
Quality Assurance . . . . Madonna Baker
Chief of Medical Staff . . . . Nicanor Concepcion, MD
Chairman/CEO . . . . Ann Fleming
Operating Room. . . . . Mitch Kennedy, RN
CEO/President. . . . . Alan Levine
Infection Control. . . . . Barbara Mullins, RN
Radiology. . . . . Bryan Mullins
Pediatric Ambulatory Care . . . . . . Nancy Woodward

Measure	Cases	This Hosp.	State Avg.	U.S. Avg.
Blood Clot Prevention and Treatment				
Anticoagulation Overlap Therapy[2]	24	100%	95%	93%
ICU Venous Thromboembolism Prophylaxis[2]	90	98%	95%	92%

NOTE: Hospital profiles are in alphabetical order by state, then city, then hospital within the city; Rankings exclude hospitals with less than 25 cases except for patient surveys which excludes hospitals with less than 100 cases; (a) 100-299 cases; (1) The number of cases/patients is too few to report; (2) Data submitted were based on a sample of cases/patients; (3) Results are based on a shorter time period than required; (4) Data suppressed by CMS for one or more quarters; (5) Results are not available for this reporting period; (6) Fewer than 100 patients completed the HCAHPS survey; (7) No cases met the criteria for this measure; (8) The lower limit of the confidence interval cannot be calculated if the number of observed infections equals zero; (9) No data are available from the state/territory for this reporting period; (10) The scores shown reflect fewer than 50 completed surveys; (11) There were discrepancies in the data collection process; (12) This measure does not apply to this hospital for this reporting period; (13) Results cannot be calculated for this reporting period; (14) The results for this state are combined with nearby states to protect confidentiality; Please refer to the User's Guide for a full explanation of data.

Measure	Cases	This Hosp.	State Avg.	U.S. Avg.
Incidence of Potentially Preventable VTE[1,2]	-	-	8%	10%
UFH with Dosages/Platelet Monitoring[2]	19	100%	99%	97%
Venous Thromboembolism Prophylaxis[2]	215	94%	91%	85%
Warfarin Therapy Discharge Instructions[2]	15	53%	78%	75%
Chest Pain/Possible Heart Attack Care				
Aspirin Given Within 24 Hours of Arrival	215	100%	98%	96%
Fibrinolytic Meds Within 30 Min. of Arrival[1]	-	-	68%	58%
Average Time to ECG (minutes)	227	6	7	7
Average Time to Transfer (minutes)[1]	-	-	64	60
Children's Asthma Care				
Received Home Management Plan of Care	-	-	-	88%
Received Reliever Medication	-	-	-	100%
Received Systemic Corticosteroids	-	-	-	100%
Emergency Department				
Admittance Decision Time (minutes)[2]	209	43	96	98
Head CT Results Within 45 Min. of Arrival[1]	-	-	60%	57%
Patients Who Left ER Before Being Seen	22,143	1%	2%	2%
Time from ER Arrival to Admit. (minutes)[2]	328	242	280	274
Time from ER Arrival to Discharge (minutes)	353	134	167	134
Time in ER Before Being Evaluated (minutes)	360	20	35	26
Time to Pain Meds for Fractures (minutes)	57	50	56	57
Heart Attack Care				
Aspirin Given at Discharge[1,2]	-	-	99%	99%
Fibrinolytic Meds Within 30 Min. of Arrival[2,3]	-	-	75%	54%
PCI Within 90 Minutes of Arrival[2,3]	-	-	97%	96%
Statin Prescribed at Discharge[1,2]	-	-	99%	98%
Heart Failure Care				
ACE Inhibitor or ARB for LVSD[2]	12	100%	98%	97%
Discharge Instructions Given[2]	64	100%	95%	94%
Evaluation of LVS Function[2]	74	100%	100%	99%
Medicare Spending				
Medicare Spending per Patient (ratio)	-	0.94	0.95	0.98
Pneumonia Care				
Appropriate Initial Antibiotic Given[2]	64	97%	97%	95%
Blood Culture Timing[2]	132	91%	98%	98%
Pregnancy and Delivery Care				
Newborn Deliveries Scheduled Early[2]	17	12%	6%	6%
Preventive Care				
Immunization for Influenza[2]	376	88%	92%	90%
Immunization for Pneumonia[2]	393	84%	93%	92%
Stroke Care				
Anticoagulation Therapy for Atrial Fibrillation[7]	-	-	96%	95%
Antithrombotic Therapy Timing	24	100%	99%	98%
Assessed for Rehabilitation	23	100%	99%	97%
Discharged on Antithrombotic Therapy	20	100%	100%	99%
Discharged on Statin Medication	16	88%	97%	94%
Thrombolytic Therapy Timing[1]	-	-	73%	66%
Venous Thromboembolism Prophylaxis	25	100%	97%	94%
Written Stroke Educational Materials Given[1]	-	-	92%	88%
Surgical Care Improvement Project				
Appropriate Beta Blocker Usage[2]	16	100%	99%	98%
Appropriate VTP Within 24 Hours[2]	46	96%	99%	98%
Controlled Postoperative Blood Glucose[2,7]	-	-	98%	97%
Perioperative Temperature Management[2]	52	96%	100%	100%
Prophylactic Antibiotic Selection[2]	20	90%	99%	99%
Prophylactic Antibiotic Selection (Outpatient)	41	98%	98%	98%
Prophylactic Antibiotic Stopped[2]	18	83%	98%	98%
Prophylactic Antibiotic Timing[2]	20	90%	99%	99%
Prophylactic Antibiotic Timing (Outpatient)	42	95%	98%	98%
Urinary Catheter Removal[2]	19	95%	98%	97%
Survey of Patients' Hospital Experiences				
Area Around Room 'Always' Quiet at Night	300+	57%	60%	61%
Doctors 'Always' Communicated Well	300+	83%	81%	82%
Home Recovery Information Given	300+	81%	86%	85%
Hospital Given 9 or 10 on 10 Point Scale	300+	67%	68%	71%
Meds 'Always' Explained Before Given	300+	62%	62%	64%
Nurses 'Always' Communicated Well	300+	78%	78%	79%
Pain 'Always' Well Controlled	300+	64%	70%	71%
Room and Bathroom 'Always' Clean	300+	72%	71%	73%
Timely Help 'Always' Received	300+	64%	64%	68%
Would Definitely Recommend Hospital	300+	62%	69%	71%
Use of Medical Imaging				
Cardiac Imaging Stress Test before Surgery	194	8.2%	5.1%	5.3%
Combination Abdominal CT Scan	503	6.4%	8.5%	10.5%
Combination Brain/Sinus CT Scan	376	1.6%	2.3%	2.7%
Combination Chest CT Scan	262	2.3%	1.6%	2.7%
Follow-up Mammogram/Ultrasound	455	5.9%	7.7%	8.8%
Lumbar Spine MRI for Low Back Pain	62	40.3%	35.3%	37.2%

Carilion Giles Community Hospital

159 Hartley Way
Pearisburg, VA 24134
URL: www.carilion.com/cgmh
Type: Critical Access Hospitals
Ownership: Voluntary non-profit - Private
Phone: 540-921-6000
Fax: 540-921-6858
Emergency Services: Yes
Beds: 65

Key Personnel:
CEO/President. . . . . Morris Reese
Operating Room. . . . . Beverly Rice
Radiology. . . . . John L Tamminen

Measure	Cases	This Hosp.	State Avg.	U.S. Avg.
Blood Clot Prevention and Treatment				
Anticoagulation Overlap Therapy[5]	-	-	95%	93%
ICU Venous Thromboembolism Prophylaxis[5]	-	-	95%	92%
Incidence of Potentially Preventable VTE[5]	-	-	8%	10%
UFH with Dosages/Platelet Monitoring[5]	-	-	99%	97%
Venous Thromboembolism Prophylaxis[5]	-	-	91%	85%
Warfarin Therapy Discharge Instructions[5]	-	-	78%	75%
Chest Pain/Possible Heart Attack Care				
Aspirin Given Within 24 Hours of Arrival	58	95%	98%	96%
Fibrinolytic Meds Within 30 Min. of Arrival[1]	-	-	68%	58%
Average Time to ECG (minutes)	58	10	7	7
Average Time to Transfer (minutes)[1]	-	-	64	60
Children's Asthma Care				
Received Home Management Plan of Care	-	-	-	88%
Received Reliever Medication	-	-	-	100%
Received Systemic Corticosteroids	-	-	-	100%
Emergency Department				
Admittance Decision Time (minutes)[2]	282	112	96	98
Head CT Results Within 45 Min. of Arrival	11	27%	60%	57%
Patients Who Left ER Before Being Seen[5]	-	-	2%	2%
Time from ER Arrival to Admit. (minutes)[2]	350	276	280	274
Time from ER Arrival to Discharge (minutes)	344	160	167	134
Time in ER Before Being Evaluated (minutes)	311	35	35	26
Time to Pain Meds for Fractures (minutes)	68	78	56	57
Heart Attack Care				
Aspirin Given at Discharge[1]	-	-	99%	99%
Fibrinolytic Meds Within 30 Min. of Arrival[7]	-	-	75%	54%
PCI Within 90 Minutes of Arrival[7]	-	-	97%	96%
Statin Prescribed at Discharge[1]	-	-	99%	98%
Heart Failure Care				
ACE Inhibitor or ARB for LVSD	14	93%	98%	97%
Discharge Instructions Given	31	100%	95%	94%
Evaluation of LVS Function	41	100%	100%	99%
Medicare Spending				
Medicare Spending per Patient (ratio)	-	-	0.95	0.98
Pneumonia Care				
Appropriate Initial Antibiotic Given	57	86%	97%	95%
Blood Culture Timing	67	94%	98%	98%
Pregnancy and Delivery Care				
Newborn Deliveries Scheduled Early[2,3]	-	-	6%	6%
Preventive Care				
Immunization for Influenza[2]	277	95%	92%	90%
Immunization for Pneumonia[2]	495	96%	93%	92%
Stroke Care				
Anticoagulation Therapy for Atrial Fibrillation[5]	-	-	96%	95%
Antithrombotic Therapy Timing[5]	-	-	99%	98%
Assessed for Rehabilitation[5]	-	-	99%	97%
Discharged on Antithrombotic Therapy[5]	-	-	100%	99%
Discharged on Statin Medication[5]	-	-	97%	94%
Thrombolytic Therapy Timing[5]	-	-	73%	66%
Venous Thromboembolism Prophylaxis[5]	-	-	97%	94%
Written Stroke Educational Materials Given[5]	-	-	92%	88%
Surgical Care Improvement Project				
Appropriate Beta Blocker Usage	12	100%	99%	98%
Appropriate VTP Within 24 Hours	33	100%	99%	98%
Controlled Postoperative Blood Glucose[7]	-	-	98%	97%
Perioperative Temperature Management	34	97%	100%	100%
Prophylactic Antibiotic Selection	28	96%	99%	99%
Prophylactic Antibiotic Selection (Outpatient)[1,3]	-	-	98%	98%
Prophylactic Antibiotic Stopped	27	96%	98%	98%
Prophylactic Antibiotic Timing	28	93%	99%	99%
Prophylactic Antibiotic Timing (Outpatient)[1,3]	-	-	98%	98%
Urinary Catheter Removal	27	93%	98%	97%
Survey of Patients' Hospital Experiences				
Area Around Room 'Always' Quiet at Night	(a)	64%	60%	61%
Doctors 'Always' Communicated Well	(a)	91%	81%	82%
Home Recovery Information Given	(a)	91%	86%	85%
Hospital Given 9 or 10 on 10 Point Scale	(a)	77%	68%	71%
Meds 'Always' Explained Before Given	(a)	73%	62%	64%
Nurses 'Always' Communicated Well	(a)	86%	78%	79%
Pain 'Always' Well Controlled	(a)	72%	70%	71%
Room and Bathroom 'Always' Clean	(a)	79%	71%	73%
Timely Help 'Always' Received	(a)	75%	64%	68%
Would Definitely Recommend Hospital	(a)	77%	69%	71%
Use of Medical Imaging				
Cardiac Imaging Stress Test before Surgery[7]	-	-	5.1%	5.3%
Combination Abdominal CT Scan	337	10.7%	8.5%	10.5%
Combination Brain/Sinus CT Scan	314	1.6%	2.3%	2.7%
Combination Chest CT Scan	127	16.5%	1.6%	2.7%
Follow-up Mammogram/Ultrasound	660	6.5%	7.7%	8.8%
Lumbar Spine MRI for Low Back Pain[1]	-	-	35.3%	37.2%

Southside Regional Medical Center

200 Medical Park Boulevard
Petersburg, VA 23805
URL: www.srmconline.com
Type: Acute Care Hospitals
Ownership: Proprietary
Phone: 804-765-5000
Fax: 804-957-6000
Emergency Services: Yes
Beds: 408

Key Personnel:
Infection Control. . . . . Linda Atkinson
Radiology. . . . . Rita Baldwin
Pediatric In-Patient Care . . . . Peggy Benton
CEO/President. . . . . David Fikse
Coronary Care . . . . Margaret Greene, RN
Cardiac Laboratory. . . . . Lynn Sule
Operating Room. . . . . Sherry Wilkinson

Measure	Cases	This Hosp.	State Avg.	U.S. Avg.
Blood Clot Prevention and Treatment				
Anticoagulation Overlap Therapy[2]	83	88%	95%	93%
ICU Venous Thromboembolism Prophylaxis[2]	106	93%	95%	92%
Incidence of Potentially Preventable VTE[1,2]	-	-	8%	10%
UFH with Dosages/Platelet Monitoring[2]	64	100%	99%	97%
Venous Thromboembolism Prophylaxis[2]	420	87%	91%	85%
Warfarin Therapy Discharge Instructions[2]	49	88%	78%	75%
Chest Pain/Possible Heart Attack Care				
Aspirin Given Within 24 Hours of Arrival[1]	-	-	98%	96%
Fibrinolytic Meds Within 30 Min. of Arrival[7]	-	-	68%	58%
Average Time to ECG (minutes)[1]	-	-	7	7
Average Time to Transfer (minutes)[7]	-	-	64	60
Children's Asthma Care				
Received Home Management Plan of Care	-	-	-	88%
Received Reliever Medication	-	-	-	100%
Received Systemic Corticosteroids	-	-	-	100%
Emergency Department				
Admittance Decision Time (minutes)[2]	844	125	96	98
Head CT Results Within 45 Min. of Arrival	11	73%	60%	57%
Patients Who Left ER Before Being Seen	60,128	2%	2%	2%
Time from ER Arrival to Admit. (minutes)[2]	863	269	280	274
Time from ER Arrival to Discharge (minutes)	366	138	167	134
Time in ER Before Being Evaluated (minutes)	416	30	35	26
Time to Pain Meds for Fractures (minutes)	155	73	56	57
Heart Attack Care				
Aspirin Given at Discharge	267	99%	99%	99%
Fibrinolytic Meds Within 30 Min. of Arrival[7]	-	-	75%	54%
PCI Within 90 Minutes of Arrival	48	92%	97%	96%
Statin Prescribed at Discharge	255	99%	99%	98%
Heart Failure Care				
ACE Inhibitor or ARB for LVSD	241	99%	98%	97%
Discharge Instructions Given	484	99%	95%	94%

NOTE: Hospital profiles are in alphabetical order by state, then city, then hospital within the city; Rankings exclude hospitals with less than 25 cases except for patient surveys which excludes hospitals with less than 100 cases; (a) 100-299 cases; (1) The number of cases/patients is too few to report; (2) Data submitted were based on a sample of cases/patients; (3) Results are based on a shorter time period than required; (4) Data suppressed by CMS for one or more quarters; (5) Results are not available for this reporting period; (6) Fewer than 100 patients completed the HCAHPS survey; (7) No cases met the criteria for this measure; (8) The lower limit of the confidence interval cannot be calculated if the number of observed infections equals zero; (9) No data are available from the state/territory for this reporting period; (10) The scores shown reflect fewer than 50 completed surveys; (11) There were discrepancies in the data collection process; (12) This measure does not apply to this hospital for this reporting period; (13) Results cannot be calculated for this reporting period; (14) The results for this state are combined with nearby states to protect confidentiality; Please refer to the User's Guide for a full explanation of data.

Evaluation of LVS Function	597	100%	100%	99%
Medicare Spending				
Medicare Spending per Patient (ratio)	-	1.06	0.95	0.98
Pneumonia Care				
Appropriate Initial Antibiotic Given	159	96%	97%	95%
Blood Culture Timing	235	97%	98%	98%
Pregnancy and Delivery Care				
Newborn Deliveries Scheduled Early[2]	72	4%	6%	6%
Preventive Care				
Immunization for Influenza[2]	608	94%	92%	90%
Immunization for Pneumonia[2]	741	96%	93%	92%
Stroke Care				
Anticoagulation Therapy for Atrial Fibrillation	13	92%	96%	95%
Antithrombotic Therapy Timing	147	99%	99%	98%
Assessed for Rehabilitation	155	97%	99%	97%
Discharged on Antithrombotic Therapy	149	100%	100%	99%
Discharged on Statin Medication	122	98%	97%	94%
Thrombolytic Therapy Timing	17	53%	73%	66%
Venous Thromboembolism Prophylaxis	163	97%	97%	94%
Written Stroke Educational Materials Given	80	99%	92%	88%
Surgical Care Improvement Project				
Appropriate Beta Blocker Usage	140	94%	99%	98%
Appropriate VTP Within 24 Hours	474	100%	99%	98%
Controlled Postoperative Blood Glucose[7]	-	-	98%	97%
Perioperative Temperature Management	522	100%	100%	100%
Prophylactic Antibiotic Selection	340	100%	99%	99%
Prophylactic Antibiotic Selection (Outpatient)	365	99%	98%	98%
Prophylactic Antibiotic Stopped	318	99%	98%	98%
Prophylactic Antibiotic Timing	340	99%	99%	99%
Prophylactic Antibiotic Timing (Outpatient)	366	99%	98%	98%
Urinary Catheter Removal	312	97%	98%	97%
Survey of Patients' Hospital Experiences				
Area Around Room 'Always' Quiet at Night	300+	60%	60%	61%
Doctors 'Always' Communicated Well	300+	80%	81%	82%
Home Recovery Information Given	300+	84%	86%	85%
Hospital Given 9 or 10 on 10 Point Scale	300+	69%	68%	71%
Meds 'Always' Explained Before Given	300+	63%	62%	64%
Nurses 'Always' Communicated Well	300+	79%	78%	79%
Pain 'Always' Well Controlled	300+	71%	70%	71%
Room and Bathroom 'Always' Clean	300+	72%	71%	73%
Timely Help 'Always' Received	300+	66%	64%	68%
Would Definitely Recommend Hospital	300+	67%	69%	71%
Use of Medical Imaging				
Cardiac Imaging Stress Test before Surgery	192	3.6%	5.1%	5.3%
Combination Abdominal CT Scan	1,025	17.5%	8.5%	10.5%
Combination Brain/Sinus CT Scan	1,087	3.1%	2.3%	2.7%
Combination Chest CT Scan	717	16.7%	1.6%	2.7%
Follow-up Mammogram/Ultrasound	1,620	9.1%	7.7%	8.8%
Lumbar Spine MRI for Low Back Pain	111	34.2%	35.3%	37.2%

Bon Secours Maryview Medical Center

3636 High Street
Portsmouth, VA 23707
Phone: 757-398-2200
Fax: 757-398-4982
URL: www.bonsecourshamptonroads.com
Type: Acute Care Hospitals
Emergency Services: Yes
Ownership: Voluntary non-profit - Private
Beds: 346

Key Personnel:
Pediatric In-Patient Care .... Sandra Baucom
CEO/President................ Dominick Calgi
Radiology.................. N Devanath
Operating Room............. John Jacobs
Quality Assurance .... Emma Truitt

Measure	Cases	This Hosp.	State Avg.	U.S. Avg.
Blood Clot Prevention and Treatment				
Anticoagulation Overlap Therapy[2]	41	93%	95%	93%
ICU Venous Thromboembolism Prophylaxis[2]	59	85%	95%	92%
Incidence of Potentially Preventable VTE[1,2]	-	-	8%	10%
UFH with Dosages/Platelet Monitoring[2]	36	92%	99%	97%
Venous Thromboembolism Prophylaxis[2]	275	81%	91%	85%
Warfarin Therapy Discharge Instructions[2]	32	97%	78%	75%
Chest Pain/Possible Heart Attack Care				
Aspirin Given Within 24 Hours of Arrival[1,3]	-	-	98%	96%
Fibrinolytic Meds Within 30 Min. of Arrival[3,7]	-	-	68%	58%
Average Time to ECG (minutes)[1,3]	-	-	7	7
Average Time to Transfer (minutes)[3,7]	-	-	64	60
Children's Asthma Care				
Received Home Management Plan of Care	-	-	-	88%
Received Reliever Medication	-	-	-	100%
Received Systemic Corticosteroids	-	-	-	100%
Emergency Department				
Admittance Decision Time (minutes)[2]	466	146	96	98
Head CT Results Within 45 Min. of Arrival	16	56%	60%	57%
Patients Who Left ER Before Being Seen	73,653	5%	2%	2%
Time from ER Arrival to Admit. (minutes)[2]	507	389	280	274
Time from ER Arrival to Discharge (minutes)	378	170	167	134
Time in ER Before Being Evaluated (minutes)	396	31	35	26
Time to Pain Meds for Fractures (minutes)	117	73	56	57
Heart Attack Care				
Aspirin Given at Discharge	210	100%	99%	99%
Fibrinolytic Meds Within 30 Min. of Arrival[7]	-	-	75%	54%
PCI Within 90 Minutes of Arrival	29	97%	97%	96%
Statin Prescribed at Discharge	207	100%	99%	98%
Heart Failure Care				
ACE Inhibitor or ARB for LVSD	83	100%	98%	97%
Discharge Instructions Given	291	100%	95%	94%
Evaluation of LVS Function	330	100%	100%	99%
Medicare Spending				
Medicare Spending per Patient (ratio)	-	0.98	0.95	0.98
Pneumonia Care				
Appropriate Initial Antibiotic Given	113	98%	97%	95%
Blood Culture Timing	243	89%	98%	98%
Pregnancy and Delivery Care				
Newborn Deliveries Scheduled Early[2]	33	6%	6%	6%
Preventive Care				
Immunization for Influenza[2]	593	73%	92%	90%
Immunization for Pneumonia[2]	685	71%	93%	92%
Stroke Care				
Anticoagulation Therapy for Atrial Fibrillation	26	88%	96%	95%
Antithrombotic Therapy Timing	149	97%	99%	98%
Assessed for Rehabilitation	155	100%	99%	97%
Discharged on Antithrombotic Therapy	147	97%	100%	99%
Discharged on Statin Medication	103	97%	97%	94%
Thrombolytic Therapy Timing[1]	-	-	73%	66%
Venous Thromboembolism Prophylaxis	167	91%	97%	94%
Written Stroke Educational Materials Given	91	100%	92%	88%
Surgical Care Improvement Project				
Appropriate Beta Blocker Usage[2]	227	99%	99%	98%
Appropriate VTP Within 24 Hours[2]	575	99%	99%	98%
Controlled Postoperative Blood Glucose[2]	65	100%	98%	97%
Perioperative Temperature Management[2]	703	100%	100%	100%
Prophylactic Antibiotic Selection[2]	579	99%	99%	99%
Prophylactic Antibiotic Selection (Outpatient)	393	98%	98%	98%
Prophylactic Antibiotic Stopped[2]	566	98%	98%	98%
Prophylactic Antibiotic Timing[2]	579	99%	99%	99%
Prophylactic Antibiotic Timing (Outpatient)	397	96%	98%	98%
Urinary Catheter Removal[2]	335	100%	98%	97%
Survey of Patients' Hospital Experiences				
Area Around Room 'Always' Quiet at Night	300+	65%	60%	61%
Doctors 'Always' Communicated Well	300+	81%	81%	82%
Home Recovery Information Given	300+	87%	86%	85%
Hospital Given 9 or 10 on 10 Point Scale	300+	61%	68%	71%
Meds 'Always' Explained Before Given	300+	58%	62%	64%
Nurses 'Always' Communicated Well	300+	73%	78%	79%
Pain 'Always' Well Controlled	300+	68%	70%	71%
Room and Bathroom 'Always' Clean	300+	62%	71%	73%
Timely Help 'Always' Received	300+	58%	64%	68%
Would Definitely Recommend Hospital	300+	56%	69%	71%
Use of Medical Imaging				
Cardiac Imaging Stress Test before Surgery	584	3.6%	5.1%	5.3%
Combination Abdominal CT Scan	1,249	8.9%	8.5%	10.5%
Combination Brain/Sinus CT Scan	1,125	2.6%	2.3%	2.7%
Combination Chest CT Scan	902	2.3%	1.6%	2.7%
Follow-up Mammogram/Ultrasound	2,151	6.2%	7.7%	8.8%
Lumbar Spine MRI for Low Back Pain	455	31.9%	35.3%	37.2%

Lewisgale Hospital Pulaski

2400 Lee Highway
Pulaski, VA 24301
Phone: 540-994-8100
Fax: 540-994-8333
URL: www.lewisgale.com
Type: Acute Care Hospitals
Emergency Services: Yes
Ownership: Proprietary
Beds: 147

Key Personnel:
Pediatric In-Patient Care .... Greg Angle
Operating Room.............. Yung C Chan
Infection Control.............. Lee Cox
Chief of Medical Staff.......... Paul D'Amico, MD
Cardiac Laboratory............ Barbara Farris
Radiology.................. Allen Knull
CEO/President............... Mark Nichols, FACHE
Quality Assurance .... Bob Suddarth

Measure	Cases	This Hosp.	State Avg.	U.S. Avg.
Blood Clot Prevention and Treatment				
Anticoagulation Overlap Therapy[2]	21	100%	95%	93%
ICU Venous Thromboembolism Prophylaxis[2]	61	100%	95%	92%
Incidence of Potentially Preventable VTE[1,2]	-	-	8%	10%
UFH with Dosages/Platelet Monitoring[1,2]	-	-	99%	97%
Venous Thromboembolism Prophylaxis[2]	205	100%	91%	85%
Warfarin Therapy Discharge Instructions[2]	14	100%	78%	75%
Chest Pain/Possible Heart Attack Care				
Aspirin Given Within 24 Hours of Arrival	65	100%	98%	96%
Fibrinolytic Meds Within 30 Min. of Arrival[7]	-	-	68%	58%
Average Time to ECG (minutes)	66	3	7	7
Average Time to Transfer (minutes)	18	40	64	60
Children's Asthma Care				
Received Home Management Plan of Care	-	-	-	88%
Received Reliever Medication	-	-	-	100%
Received Systemic Corticosteroids	-	-	-	100%
Emergency Department				
Admittance Decision Time (minutes)[2]	515	68	96	98
Head CT Results Within 45 Min. of Arrival[1,3]	-	-	60%	57%
Patients Who Left ER Before Being Seen	18,462	1%	2%	2%
Time from ER Arrival to Admit. (minutes)[2]	516	226	280	274
Time from ER Arrival to Discharge (minutes)	478	112	167	134
Time in ER Before Being Evaluated (minutes)	512	14	35	26
Time to Pain Meds for Fractures (minutes)	40	31	56	57
Heart Attack Care				
Aspirin Given at Discharge	16	100%	99%	99%
Fibrinolytic Meds Within 30 Min. of Arrival[7]	-	-	75%	54%
PCI Within 90 Minutes of Arrival[7]	-	-	97%	96%
Statin Prescribed at Discharge	14	93%	99%	98%
Heart Failure Care				
ACE Inhibitor or ARB for LVSD	41	100%	98%	97%
Discharge Instructions Given	64	92%	95%	94%
Evaluation of LVS Function	99	100%	100%	99%
Medicare Spending				
Medicare Spending per Patient (ratio)	-	0.99	0.95	0.98
Pneumonia Care				
Appropriate Initial Antibiotic Given	67	99%	97%	95%
Blood Culture Timing	123	100%	98%	98%
Pregnancy and Delivery Care				
Newborn Deliveries Scheduled Early[2,7]	-	-	6%	6%
Preventive Care				
Immunization for Influenza[2]	303	97%	92%	90%
Immunization for Pneumonia[2]	491	99%	93%	92%
Stroke Care				
Anticoagulation Therapy for Atrial Fibrillation[1,2]	-	-	96%	95%
Antithrombotic Therapy Timing[2]	29	100%	99%	98%
Assessed for Rehabilitation[2]	32	100%	99%	97%
Discharged on Antithrombotic Therapy[2]	30	100%	100%	99%
Discharged on Statin Medication[2]	20	100%	97%	94%
Thrombolytic Therapy Timing[1,2]	-	-	73%	66%
Venous Thromboembolism Prophylaxis[2]	32	100%	97%	94%
Written Stroke Educational Materials Given[2]	15	93%	92%	88%
Surgical Care Improvement Project				
Appropriate Beta Blocker Usage[1]	-	-	99%	98%
Appropriate VTP Within 24 Hours	43	100%	99%	98%
Controlled Postoperative Blood Glucose[7]	-	-	98%	97%
Perioperative Temperature Management	46	100%	100%	100%
Prophylactic Antibiotic Selection	27	100%	99%	99%

NOTE: Hospital profiles are in alphabetical order by state, then city, then hospital within the city; Rankings exclude hospitals with less than 25 cases except for patient surveys which excludes hospitals with less than 100 cases; (a) 100-299 cases; (1) The number of cases/patients is too few to report; (2) Data submitted were based on a sample of cases/patients; (3) Results are based on a shorter time period than required; (4) Data suppressed by CMS for one or more quarters; (5) Results are not available for this reporting period; (6) Fewer than 100 patients completed the HCAHPS survey; (7) No cases met the criteria for this measure; (8) The lower limit of the confidence interval cannot be calculated if the number of observed infections equals zero; (9) No data are available from the state/territory for this reporting period; (10) The scores shown reflect fewer than 50 completed surveys; (11) There were discrepancies in the data collection process; (12) This measure does not apply to this hospital for this reporting period; (13) Results cannot be calculated for this reporting period; (14) The results for this state are combined with nearby states to protect confidentiality; Please refer to the User's Guide for a full explanation of data.

Measure	Cases	This Hosp.	State Avg.	U.S. Avg.
Prophylactic Antibiotic Selection (Outpatient)[3]	12	100%	98%	98%
Prophylactic Antibiotic Stopped	27	100%	98%	98%
Prophylactic Antibiotic Timing	27	100%	99%	99%
Prophylactic Antibiotic Timing (Outpatient)[3]	12	100%	98%	98%
Urinary Catheter Removal	33	100%	98%	97%
Survey of Patients' Hospital Experiences				
Area Around Room 'Always' Quiet at Night	300+	61%	60%	61%
Doctors 'Always' Communicated Well	300+	83%	81%	82%
Home Recovery Information Given	300+	88%	86%	85%
Hospital Given 9 or 10 on 10 Point Scale	300+	68%	68%	71%
Meds 'Always' Explained Before Given	300+	61%	62%	64%
Nurses 'Always' Communicated Well	300+	77%	78%	79%
Pain 'Always' Well Controlled	300+	70%	70%	71%
Room and Bathroom 'Always' Clean	300+	73%	71%	73%
Timely Help 'Always' Received	300+	61%	64%	68%
Would Definitely Recommend Hospital	300+	70%	69%	71%
Use of Medical Imaging				
Cardiac Imaging Stress Test before Surgery[1]	-	-	5.1%	5.3%
Combination Abdominal CT Scan	394	1.8%	8.5%	10.5%
Combination Brain/Sinus CT Scan[1]	-	-	2.3%	2.7%
Combination Chest CT Scan	196	0.0%	1.6%	2.7%
Follow-up Mammogram/Ultrasound	365	5.2%	7.7%	8.8%
Lumbar Spine MRI for Low Back Pain	51	35.3%	35.3%	37.2%

Reston Hospital Center

1850 Town Center Parkway
Reston, VA 20190
Phone: 703-689-9000
Fax: 703-689-0840
E-mail: denise.dancy@hcahealthcare.com
URL: www.restonhospital.com
Type: Acute Care Hospitals
Emergency Services: Yes
Ownership: Proprietary
Beds: 160

Key Personnel:

Operating Room. . . . . Jim Cliett, RN
CEO/President. . . . . John Deardorff, FACHE
Radiology. . . . . David Dubois, MD
Cardiac Laboratory. . . . . Kim Elliotts
Emergency Room . . . . Darren Lisse, MD
Quality Assurance . . . . Judy Riggins
Pediatric In-Patient Care . . . . Carrie Sutara, RN

Measure	Cases	This Hosp.	State Avg.	U.S. Avg.
Blood Clot Prevention and Treatment				
Anticoagulation Overlap Therapy[2]	82	100%	95%	93%
ICU Venous Thromboembolism Prophylaxis[2]	87	98%	95%	92%
Incidence of Potentially Preventable VTE[1,2]	-	-	8%	10%
UFH with Dosages/Platelet Monitoring[2]	28	93%	99%	97%
Venous Thromboembolism Prophylaxis[2]	314	98%	91%	85%
Warfarin Therapy Discharge Instructions[2]	62	100%	78%	75%
Chest Pain/Possible Heart Attack Care				
Aspirin Given Within 24 Hours of Arrival[1]	-	-	98%	96%
Fibrinolytic Meds Within 30 Min. of Arrival[3,7]	-	-	68%	58%
Average Time to ECG (minutes)[1]	-	-	7	7
Average Time to Transfer (minutes)[3,7]	-	-	64	60
Children's Asthma Care				
Received Home Management Plan of Care	-	-	-	88%
Received Reliever Medication	-	-	-	100%
Received Systemic Corticosteroids	-	-	-	100%
Emergency Department				
Admittance Decision Time (minutes)[2]	479	103	96	98
Head CT Results Within 45 Min. of Arrival[1]	-	-	60%	57%
Patients Who Left ER Before Being Seen	44,109	1%	2%	2%
Time from ER Arrival to Admit. (minutes)[2]	479	257	280	274
Time from ER Arrival to Discharge (minutes)	437	125	167	134
Time in ER Before Being Evaluated (minutes)	496	12	35	26
Time to Pain Meds for Fractures (minutes)	288	36	56	57
Heart Attack Care				
Aspirin Given at Discharge	146	100%	99%	99%
Fibrinolytic Meds Within 30 Min. of Arrival[7]	-	-	75%	54%
PCI Within 90 Minutes of Arrival	47	98%	97%	96%
Statin Prescribed at Discharge	136	100%	99%	98%
Heart Failure Care				
ACE Inhibitor or ARB for LVSD	40	100%	98%	97%
Discharge Instructions Given	211	100%	95%	94%
Evaluation of LVS Function	263	100%	100%	99%
Medicare Spending				
Medicare Spending per Patient (ratio)	-	0.99	0.95	0.98
Pneumonia Care				
Appropriate Initial Antibiotic Given	103	100%	97%	95%
Blood Culture Timing	167	99%	98%	98%
Pregnancy and Delivery Care				
Newborn Deliveries Scheduled Early[2]	72	1%	6%	6%
Preventive Care				
Immunization for Influenza[2]	535	99%	92%	90%
Immunization for Pneumonia[2]	494	97%	93%	92%
Stroke Care				
Anticoagulation Therapy for Atrial Fibrillation	20	100%	96%	95%
Antithrombotic Therapy Timing	109	100%	99%	98%
Assessed for Rehabilitation	133	100%	99%	97%
Discharged on Antithrombotic Therapy	124	100%	100%	99%
Discharged on Statin Medication	101	100%	97%	94%
Thrombolytic Therapy Timing	11	100%	73%	66%
Venous Thromboembolism Prophylaxis	113	100%	97%	94%
Written Stroke Educational Materials Given	93	100%	92%	88%
Surgical Care Improvement Project				
Appropriate Beta Blocker Usage[2]	101	100%	99%	98%
Appropriate VTP Within 24 Hours[2]	397	100%	99%	98%
Controlled Postoperative Blood Glucose[2,7]	-	-	98%	97%
Perioperative Temperature Management[2]	473	100%	100%	100%
Prophylactic Antibiotic Selection[2]	295	100%	99%	99%
Prophylactic Antibiotic Selection (Outpatient)	597	99%	98%	98%
Prophylactic Antibiotic Stopped[2]	290	100%	98%	98%
Prophylactic Antibiotic Timing[2]	295	100%	99%	99%
Prophylactic Antibiotic Timing (Outpatient)	597	100%	98%	98%
Urinary Catheter Removal[2]	318	100%	98%	97%
Survey of Patients' Hospital Experiences				
Area Around Room 'Always' Quiet at Night	300+	59%	60%	61%
Doctors 'Always' Communicated Well	300+	75%	81%	82%
Home Recovery Information Given	300+	84%	86%	85%
Hospital Given 9 or 10 on 10 Point Scale	300+	67%	68%	71%
Meds 'Always' Explained Before Given	300+	58%	62%	64%
Nurses 'Always' Communicated Well	300+	73%	78%	79%
Pain 'Always' Well Controlled	300+	66%	70%	71%
Room and Bathroom 'Always' Clean	300+	72%	71%	73%
Timely Help 'Always' Received	300+	56%	64%	68%
Would Definitely Recommend Hospital	300+	71%	69%	71%
Use of Medical Imaging				
Cardiac Imaging Stress Test before Surgery	63	4.8%	5.1%	5.3%
Combination Abdominal CT Scan	617	7.1%	8.5%	10.5%
Combination Brain/Sinus CT Scan	567	4.6%	2.3%	2.7%
Combination Chest CT Scan	460	1.7%	1.6%	2.7%
Follow-up Mammogram/Ultrasound	578	10.4%	7.7%	8.8%
Lumbar Spine MRI for Low Back Pain[1]	-	-	35.3%	37.2%

Clinch Valley Medical Center

2949 West Front Street
Richlands, VA 24641
Phone: 276-596-6000
Fax: 276-596-6009
E-mail: karel.fulton@lpnt.net
URL: www.clinchvalleymedicalcenter.com
Type: Acute Care Hospitals
Emergency Services: Yes
Ownership: Proprietary
Beds: 200

Key Personnel:

Operating Room. . . . . Joseph C Claustro
Chief of Medical Staff. . . . . Glenn Harrison, DDS
Radiology. . . . . Edson L Knapp
Quality Assurance . . . . Jeanna Lambert
CEO . . . . Peter Mulkey
Intensive Care Unit. . . . . Rusty Osborne
Infection Control. . . . . Debi Riffe
Patient Relations . . . . Tracie Rinehardt

Measure	Cases	This Hosp.	State Avg.	U.S. Avg.
Blood Clot Prevention and Treatment				
Anticoagulation Overlap Therapy[2]	35	91%	95%	93%
ICU Venous Thromboembolism Prophylaxis[2]	96	99%	95%	92%
Incidence of Potentially Preventable VTE[1,2]	-	-	8%	10%
UFH with Dosages/Platelet Monitoring[2]	35	100%	99%	97%
Venous Thromboembolism Prophylaxis[2]	380	97%	91%	85%
Warfarin Therapy Discharge Instructions[2]	28	100%	78%	75%
Chest Pain/Possible Heart Attack Care				
Aspirin Given Within 24 Hours of Arrival	55	100%	98%	96%
Fibrinolytic Meds Within 30 Min. of Arrival	12	83%	68%	58%
Average Time to ECG (minutes)	60	8	7	7
Average Time to Transfer (minutes)[7]	-	-	64	60
Children's Asthma Care				
Received Home Management Plan of Care	-	-	-	88%
Received Reliever Medication	-	-	-	100%
Received Systemic Corticosteroids	-	-	-	100%
Emergency Department				
Admittance Decision Time (minutes)[2]	479	54	96	98
Head CT Results Within 45 Min. of Arrival[1]	-	-	60%	57%
Patients Who Left ER Before Being Seen	20,100	1%	2%	2%
Time from ER Arrival to Admit. (minutes)[2]	479	212	280	274
Time from ER Arrival to Discharge (minutes)	383	141	167	134
Time in ER Before Being Evaluated (minutes)	469	14	35	26
Time to Pain Meds for Fractures (minutes)	81	45	56	57
Heart Attack Care				
Aspirin Given at Discharge	37	100%	99%	99%
Fibrinolytic Meds Within 30 Min. of Arrival[7]	-	-	75%	54%
PCI Within 90 Minutes of Arrival[1]	-	-	97%	96%
Statin Prescribed at Discharge	39	100%	99%	98%
Heart Failure Care				
ACE Inhibitor or ARB for LVSD	31	100%	98%	97%
Discharge Instructions Given	134	100%	95%	94%
Evaluation of LVS Function	146	100%	100%	99%
Medicare Spending				
Medicare Spending per Patient (ratio)	-	0.89	0.95	0.98
Pneumonia Care				
Appropriate Initial Antibiotic Given	80	99%	97%	95%
Blood Culture Timing	129	100%	98%	98%
Pregnancy and Delivery Care				
Newborn Deliveries Scheduled Early[2]	28	4%	6%	6%
Preventive Care				
Immunization for Influenza[2]	448	99%	92%	90%
Immunization for Pneumonia[2]	554	99%	93%	92%
Stroke Care				
Anticoagulation Therapy for Atrial Fibrillation[1]	-	-	96%	95%
Antithrombotic Therapy Timing	28	100%	99%	98%
Assessed for Rehabilitation	23	100%	99%	97%
Discharged on Antithrombotic Therapy	23	100%	100%	99%
Discharged on Statin Medication	12	100%	97%	94%
Thrombolytic Therapy Timing[7]	-	-	73%	66%
Venous Thromboembolism Prophylaxis	28	100%	97%	94%
Written Stroke Educational Materials Given	16	81%	92%	88%
Surgical Care Improvement Project				
Appropriate Beta Blocker Usage	48	100%	99%	98%
Appropriate VTP Within 24 Hours	172	98%	99%	98%
Controlled Postoperative Blood Glucose[7]	-	-	98%	97%
Perioperative Temperature Management	186	99%	100%	100%
Prophylactic Antibiotic Selection	113	100%	99%	99%
Prophylactic Antibiotic Selection (Outpatient)	27	100%	98%	98%
Prophylactic Antibiotic Stopped	105	98%	98%	98%
Prophylactic Antibiotic Timing	113	99%	99%	99%
Prophylactic Antibiotic Timing (Outpatient)	27	100%	98%	98%
Urinary Catheter Removal	69	99%	98%	97%
Survey of Patients' Hospital Experiences				
Area Around Room 'Always' Quiet at Night	300+	60%	60%	61%
Doctors 'Always' Communicated Well	300+	85%	81%	82%
Home Recovery Information Given	300+	85%	86%	85%
Hospital Given 9 or 10 on 10 Point Scale	300+	67%	68%	71%
Meds 'Always' Explained Before Given	300+	65%	62%	64%
Nurses 'Always' Communicated Well	300+	78%	78%	79%
Pain 'Always' Well Controlled	300+	70%	70%	71%
Room and Bathroom 'Always' Clean	300+	72%	71%	73%
Timely Help 'Always' Received	300+	66%	64%	68%
Would Definitely Recommend Hospital	300+	68%	69%	71%
Use of Medical Imaging				
Cardiac Imaging Stress Test before Surgery	222	6.3%	5.1%	5.3%
Combination Abdominal CT Scan	545	45.3%	8.5%	10.5%
Combination Brain/Sinus CT Scan[1]	-	-	2.3%	2.7%
Combination Chest CT Scan	229	1.3%	1.6%	2.7%
Follow-up Mammogram/Ultrasound	281	8.2%	7.7%	8.8%
Lumbar Spine MRI for Low Back Pain	87	28.7%	35.3%	37.2%

NOTE: Hospital profiles are in alphabetical order by state, then city, then hospital within the city; Rankings exclude hospitals with less than 25 cases except for patient surveys which excludes hospitals with less than 100 cases; (a) 100-299 cases; (1) The number of cases/patients is too few to report; (2) Data submitted were based on a sample of cases/patients; (3) Results are based on a shorter time period than required; (4) Data suppressed by CMS for one or more quarters; (5) Results are not available for this reporting period; (6) Fewer than 100 patients completed the HCAHPS survey; (7) No cases met the criteria for this measure; (8) The lower limit of the confidence interval cannot be calculated if the number of observed infections equals zero; (9) No data are available from the state/territory for this reporting period; (10) The scores shown reflect fewer than 50 completed surveys; (11) There were discrepancies in the data collection process; (12) This measure does not apply to this hospital for this reporting period; (13) Results cannot be calculated for this reporting period; (14) The results for this state are combined with nearby states to protect confidentiality; Please refer to the User's Guide for a full explanation of data.

Bon Secours Richmond Community Hospital

1500 N. 28th Street | Phone: 804-225-1700
Richmond, VA 23223 | Fax: 804-627-5029
E-mail: webmaster@bshsi.org
URL: www.bonsecours.com
Type: Acute Care Hospitals | Emergency Services: Yes
Ownership: Voluntary non-profit - Private | Beds: 104

Key Personnel:
Radiology. . . . . Todd B Baird
CEO . . . . Peter J. Bernard
Infection Control. . . . . Connie Jones
Anesthesiology. . . . . Mark Kirshner
Operating Room. . . . . Jacqueline Manning
Quality Assurance . . . . Marlene McAnich
Emergency Room . . . . Dean Williams

Measure	Cases	This Hosp.	State Avg.	U.S. Avg.
Blood Clot Prevention and Treatment				
Anticoagulation Overlap Therapy[1,2]	-	-	95%	93%
ICU Venous Thromboembolism Prophylaxis[2]	49	96%	95%	92%
Incidence of Potentially Preventable VTE[2,7]	-	-	8%	10%
UFH with Dosages/Platelet Monitoring[1,2]	-	-	99%	97%
Venous Thromboembolism Prophylaxis[2]	78	96%	91%	85%
Warfarin Therapy Discharge Instructions[1,2]	-	-	78%	75%
Chest Pain/Possible Heart Attack Care				
Aspirin Given Within 24 Hours of Arrival	16	94%	98%	96%
Fibrinolytic Meds Within 30 Min. of Arrival[3,7]	-	-	68%	58%
Average Time to ECG (minutes)	17	10	7	7
Average Time to Transfer (minutes)[1,3]	-	-	64	60
Children's Asthma Care				
Received Home Management Plan of Care	-	-	-	88%
Received Reliever Medication	-	-	-	100%
Received Systemic Corticosteroids	-	-	-	100%
Emergency Department				
Admittance Decision Time (minutes)[2]	234	103	96	98
Head CT Results Within 45 Min. of Arrival[1,3]	-	-	60%	57%
Patients Who Left ER Before Being Seen	33,699	3%	2%	2%
Time from ER Arrival to Admit. (minutes)[2]	234	314	280	274
Time from ER Arrival to Discharge (minutes)	358	121	167	134
Time in ER Before Being Evaluated (minutes)	384	21	35	26
Time to Pain Meds for Fractures (minutes)	37	74	56	57
Heart Attack Care				
Aspirin Given at Discharge[1,3]	-	-	99%	99%
Fibrinolytic Meds Within 30 Min. of Arrival[3,7]	-	-	75%	54%
PCI Within 90 Minutes of Arrival[3,7]	-	-	97%	96%
Statin Prescribed at Discharge[1,3]	-	-	99%	98%
Heart Failure Care				
ACE Inhibitor or ARB for LVSD	25	100%	98%	97%
Discharge Instructions Given	44	100%	95%	94%
Evaluation of LVS Function	56	100%	100%	99%
Medicare Spending				
Medicare Spending per Patient (ratio)	-	0.99	0.95	0.98
Pneumonia Care				
Appropriate Initial Antibiotic Given	46	96%	97%	95%
Blood Culture Timing	66	98%	98%	98%
Pregnancy and Delivery Care				
Newborn Deliveries Scheduled Early[2,7]	-	-	6%	6%
Preventive Care				
Immunization for Influenza[2]	294	96%	92%	90%
Immunization for Pneumonia[2]	300	93%	93%	92%
Stroke Care				
Anticoagulation Therapy for Atrial Fibrillation[7]	-	-	96%	95%
Antithrombotic Therapy Timing	37	100%	99%	98%
Assessed for Rehabilitation	39	97%	99%	97%
Discharged on Antithrombotic Therapy	38	100%	100%	99%
Discharged on Statin Medication	27	70%	97%	94%
Thrombolytic Therapy Timing[1]	-	-	73%	66%
Venous Thromboembolism Prophylaxis	39	100%	97%	94%
Written Stroke Educational Materials Given	26	85%	92%	88%
Surgical Care Improvement Project				
Appropriate Beta Blocker Usage[3,7]	-	-	99%	98%
Appropriate VTP Within 24 Hours[3,7]	-	-	99%	98%
Controlled Postoperative Blood Glucose[3,7]	-	-	98%	97%
Perioperative Temperature Management[3,7]	-	-	100%	100%
Prophylactic Antibiotic Selection[3,7]	-	-	99%	99%
Prophylactic Antibiotic Selection (Outpatient)[3,7]	-	-	98%	98%
Prophylactic Antibiotic Stopped[3,7]	-	-	98%	98%
Prophylactic Antibiotic Timing[3,7]	-	-	99%	99%
Prophylactic Antibiotic Timing (Outpatient)[3,7]	-	-	98%	98%
Urinary Catheter Removal[3,7]	-	-	98%	97%
Survey of Patients' Hospital Experiences				
Area Around Room 'Always' Quiet at Night	(a)	72%	60%	61%
Doctors 'Always' Communicated Well	(a)	87%	81%	82%
Home Recovery Information Given	(a)	91%	86%	85%
Hospital Given 9 or 10 on 10 Point Scale	(a)	68%	68%	71%
Meds 'Always' Explained Before Given	(a)	69%	62%	64%
Nurses 'Always' Communicated Well	(a)	80%	78%	79%
Pain 'Always' Well Controlled	(a)	70%	70%	71%
Room and Bathroom 'Always' Clean	(a)	74%	71%	73%
Timely Help 'Always' Received	(a)	65%	64%	68%
Would Definitely Recommend Hospital	(a)	70%	69%	71%
Use of Medical Imaging				
Cardiac Imaging Stress Test before Surgery[1]	-	-	5.1%	5.3%
Combination Abdominal CT Scan	84	3.6%	8.5%	10.5%
Combination Brain/Sinus CT Scan[1]	-	-	2.3%	2.7%
Combination Chest CT Scan[1]	-	-	1.6%	2.7%
Follow-up Mammogram/Ultrasound	907	9.2%	7.7%	8.8%
Lumbar Spine MRI for Low Back Pain[1]	-	-	35.3%	37.2%

Bon Secours Saint Marys Hospital

5801 Bremo Rd | Phone: 804-285-2011
Richmond, VA 23226 | Fax: 804-285-1338
URL: www.bonsecours.com
Type: Acute Care Hospitals | Emergency Services: Yes
Ownership: Voluntary non-profit - Church | Beds: 391

Key Personnel:
CEO/President. . . . . Toni R. Ardabell
Chief of Medical Staff. . . . . Thomas Davis, MD
Radiology. . . . . David Ekey, MD
Quality Assurance . . . . Marie Kerns
Operating Room. . . . . Khaki Kostetter, RN
Infection Control. . . . . Michael Mandel, MD
Pediatric Ambulatory Care . . . . . . Grover Robinson, MD
Pediatric In-Patient Care . . . . Grover Robinson, MD

Measure	Cases	This Hosp.	State Avg.	U.S. Avg.
Blood Clot Prevention and Treatment				
Anticoagulation Overlap Therapy[2]	98	98%	95%	93%
ICU Venous Thromboembolism Prophylaxis[2]	72	94%	95%	92%
Incidence of Potentially Preventable VTE[2]	15	7%	8%	10%
UFH with Dosages/Platelet Monitoring[2]	31	100%	99%	97%
Venous Thromboembolism Prophylaxis[2]	315	91%	91%	85%
Warfarin Therapy Discharge Instructions[2]	66	100%	78%	75%
Chest Pain/Possible Heart Attack Care				
Aspirin Given Within 24 Hours of Arrival[5]	-	-	98%	96%
Fibrinolytic Meds Within 30 Min. of Arrival[5]	-	-	68%	58%
Average Time to ECG (minutes)[5]	-	-	7	7
Average Time to Transfer (minutes)[5]	-	-	64	60
Children's Asthma Care				
Received Home Management Plan of Care	-	-	-	88%
Received Reliever Medication	-	-	-	100%
Received Systemic Corticosteroids	-	-	-	100%
Emergency Department				
Admittance Decision Time (minutes)[2]	607	124	96	98
Head CT Results Within 45 Min. of Arrival[1]	-	-	60%	57%
Patients Who Left ER Before Being Seen	43,791	1%	2%	2%
Time from ER Arrival to Admit. (minutes)[2]	613	296	280	274
Time from ER Arrival to Discharge (minutes)	431	148	167	134
Time in ER Before Being Evaluated (minutes)	460	18	35	26
Time to Pain Meds for Fractures (minutes)	250	44	56	57
Heart Attack Care				
Aspirin Given at Discharge	206	99%	99%	99%
Fibrinolytic Meds Within 30 Min. of Arrival[7]	-	-	75%	54%
PCI Within 90 Minutes of Arrival	46	96%	97%	96%
Statin Prescribed at Discharge	197	98%	99%	98%
Heart Failure Care				
ACE Inhibitor or ARB for LVSD[2]	97	99%	98%	97%
Discharge Instructions Given[2]	243	100%	95%	94%
Evaluation of LVS Function[2]	323	100%	100%	99%
Medicare Spending				
Medicare Spending per Patient (ratio)	-	1.00	0.95	0.98
Pneumonia Care				
Appropriate Initial Antibiotic Given[2]	81	95%	97%	95%
Blood Culture Timing[2]	154	99%	98%	98%
Pregnancy and Delivery Care				
Newborn Deliveries Scheduled Early[2]	58	24%	6%	6%
Preventive Care				
Immunization for Influenza[2]	578	96%	92%	90%
Immunization for Pneumonia[2]	674	96%	93%	92%
Stroke Care				
Anticoagulation Therapy for Atrial Fibrillation	23	100%	96%	95%
Antithrombotic Therapy Timing	163	99%	99%	98%
Assessed for Rehabilitation	225	99%	99%	97%
Discharged on Antithrombotic Therapy	186	98%	100%	99%
Discharged on Statin Medication	117	96%	97%	94%
Thrombolytic Therapy Timing	17	88%	73%	66%
Venous Thromboembolism Prophylaxis	230	94%	97%	94%
Written Stroke Educational Materials Given	121	79%	92%	88%
Surgical Care Improvement Project				
Appropriate Beta Blocker Usage[2]	306	98%	99%	98%
Appropriate VTP Within 24 Hours[2]	595	98%	99%	98%
Controlled Postoperative Blood Glucose[2]	214	99%	98%	97%
Perioperative Temperature Management[2]	786	100%	100%	100%
Prophylactic Antibiotic Selection[2]	689	98%	99%	99%
Prophylactic Antibiotic Selection (Outpatient)	626	96%	98%	98%
Prophylactic Antibiotic Stopped[2]	669	98%	98%	98%
Prophylactic Antibiotic Timing[2]	689	99%	99%	99%
Prophylactic Antibiotic Timing (Outpatient)	628	97%	98%	98%
Urinary Catheter Removal[2]	705	98%	98%	97%
Survey of Patients' Hospital Experiences				
Area Around Room 'Always' Quiet at Night	300+	62%	60%	61%
Doctors 'Always' Communicated Well	300+	80%	81%	82%
Home Recovery Information Given	300+	88%	86%	85%
Hospital Given 9 or 10 on 10 Point Scale	300+	73%	68%	71%
Meds 'Always' Explained Before Given	300+	63%	62%	64%
Nurses 'Always' Communicated Well	300+	79%	78%	79%
Pain 'Always' Well Controlled	300+	72%	70%	71%
Room and Bathroom 'Always' Clean	300+	68%	71%	73%
Timely Help 'Always' Received	300+	64%	64%	68%
Would Definitely Recommend Hospital	300+	76%	69%	71%
Use of Medical Imaging				
Cardiac Imaging Stress Test before Surgery	1,213	5.9%	5.1%	5.3%
Combination Abdominal CT Scan	1,021	6.8%	8.5%	10.5%
Combination Brain/Sinus CT Scan	1,134	1.1%	2.3%	2.7%
Combination Chest CT Scan	439	0.5%	1.6%	2.7%
Follow-up Mammogram/Ultrasound	2,950	10.0%	7.7%	8.8%
Lumbar Spine MRI for Low Back Pain	294	37.8%	35.3%	37.2%

Cjw Medical Center

7101 Jahnke Road | Phone: 804-330-2001
Richmond, VA 23235
URL: www.hcavirginia.com
Type: Acute Care Hospitals | Emergency Services: Yes
Ownership: Proprietary

Key Personnel:
CEO/President. . . . . Peter Marmerstrin

Measure	Cases	This Hosp.	State Avg.	U.S. Avg.
Blood Clot Prevention and Treatment				
Anticoagulation Overlap Therapy[2]	214	100%	95%	93%
ICU Venous Thromboembolism Prophylaxis[2]	159	97%	95%	92%
Incidence of Potentially Preventable VTE[2]	34	0%	8%	10%
UFH with Dosages/Platelet Monitoring[2]	149	100%	99%	97%
Venous Thromboembolism Prophylaxis[2]	327	98%	91%	85%
Warfarin Therapy Discharge Instructions[2]	167	96%	78%	75%
Chest Pain/Possible Heart Attack Care				
Aspirin Given Within 24 Hours of Arrival[1,3]	-	-	98%	96%
Fibrinolytic Meds Within 30 Min. of Arrival[3,7]	-	-	68%	58%
Average Time to ECG (minutes)[1,3]	-	-	7	7
Average Time to Transfer (minutes)[3,7]	-	-	64	60
Children's Asthma Care				
Received Home Management Plan of Care	-	-	-	88%
Received Reliever Medication	-	-	-	100%
Received Systemic Corticosteroids	-	-	-	100%

NOTE: Hospital profiles are in alphabetical order by state, then city, then hospital within the city; Rankings exclude hospitals with less than 25 cases except for patient surveys which excludes hospitals with less than 100 cases; (a) 100-299 cases; (1) The number of cases/patients is too few to report; (2) Data submitted were based on a sample of cases/patients; (3) Results are based on a shorter time period than required; (4) Data suppressed by CMS for one or more quarters; (5) Results are not available for this reporting period; (6) Fewer than 100 patients completed the HCAHPS survey; (7) No cases met the criteria for this measure; (8) The lower limit of the confidence interval cannot be calculated if the number of observed infections equals zero; (9) No data are available from the state/territory for this reporting period; (10) The scores shown reflect fewer than 50 completed surveys; (11) There were discrepancies in the data collection process; (12) This measure does not apply to this hospital for this reporting period; (13) Results cannot be calculated for this reporting period; (14) The results for this state are combined with nearby states to protect confidentiality; Please refer to the User's Guide for a full explanation of data.

Measure	Cases	This Hosp.	State Avg.	U.S. Avg.
Emergency Department				
Admittance Decision Time (minutes)[2]	848	102	96	98
Head CT Results Within 45 Min. of Arrival[1]	-	-	60%	57%
Patients Who Left ER Before Being Seen	>100k	2%	2%	2%
Time from ER Arrival to Admit. (minutes)[2]	848	253	280	274
Time from ER Arrival to Discharge (minutes)	498	138	167	134
Time in ER Before Being Evaluated (minutes)	548	13	35	26
Time to Pain Meds for Fractures (minutes)	232	34	56	57
Heart Attack Care				
Aspirin Given at Discharge[2]	300	100%	99%	99%
Fibrinolytic Meds Within 30 Min. of Arrival[2,7]	-	-	75%	54%
PCI Within 90 Minutes of Arrival[2]	39	100%	97%	96%
Statin Prescribed at Discharge[2]	284	100%	99%	98%
Heart Failure Care				
ACE Inhibitor or ARB for LVSD[2]	192	100%	98%	97%
Discharge Instructions Given[2]	520	97%	95%	94%
Evaluation of LVS Function[2]	655	100%	100%	99%
Medicare Spending				
Medicare Spending per Patient (ratio)	-	1.02	0.95	0.98
Pneumonia Care				
Appropriate Initial Antibiotic Given[2]	218	98%	97%	95%
Blood Culture Timing[2]	382	100%	98%	98%
Pregnancy and Delivery Care				
Newborn Deliveries Scheduled Early[2]	57	2%	6%	6%
Preventive Care				
Immunization for Influenza[2]	657	98%	92%	90%
Immunization for Pneumonia[2]	788	98%	93%	92%
Stroke Care				
Anticoagulation Therapy for Atrial Fibrillation[2]	36	100%	96%	95%
Antithrombotic Therapy Timing[2]	245	100%	99%	98%
Assessed for Rehabilitation[2]	296	100%	99%	97%
Discharged on Antithrombotic Therapy[2]	260	100%	100%	99%
Discharged on Statin Medication[2]	216	100%	97%	94%
Thrombolytic Therapy Timing[2]	15	100%	73%	66%
Venous Thromboembolism Prophylaxis[2]	296	100%	97%	94%
Written Stroke Educational Materials Given[2]	140	99%	92%	88%
Surgical Care Improvement Project				
Appropriate Beta Blocker Usage[2]	328	100%	99%	98%
Appropriate VTP Within 24 Hours[2]	544	100%	99%	98%
Controlled Postoperative Blood Glucose[2]	186	98%	98%	97%
Perioperative Temperature Management[2]	681	100%	100%	100%
Prophylactic Antibiotic Selection[2]	597	100%	99%	99%
Prophylactic Antibiotic Selection (Outpatient)	743	100%	98%	98%
Prophylactic Antibiotic Stopped[2]	572	99%	98%	98%
Prophylactic Antibiotic Timing[2]	597	100%	99%	99%
Prophylactic Antibiotic Timing (Outpatient)	742	99%	98%	98%
Urinary Catheter Removal[2]	501	98%	98%	97%
Survey of Patients' Hospital Experiences				
Area Around Room 'Always' Quiet at Night	300+	58%	60%	61%
Doctors 'Always' Communicated Well	300+	79%	81%	82%
Home Recovery Information Given	300+	87%	86%	85%
Hospital Given 9 or 10 on 10 Point Scale	300+	67%	68%	71%
Meds 'Always' Explained Before Given	300+	60%	62%	64%
Nurses 'Always' Communicated Well	300+	76%	78%	79%
Pain 'Always' Well Controlled	300+	68%	70%	71%
Room and Bathroom 'Always' Clean	300+	67%	71%	73%
Timely Help 'Always' Received	300+	61%	64%	68%
Would Definitely Recommend Hospital	300+	70%	69%	71%
Use of Medical Imaging				
Cardiac Imaging Stress Test before Surgery	357	4.2%	5.1%	5.3%
Combination Abdominal CT Scan	1,966	30.3%	8.5%	10.5%
Combination Brain/Sinus CT Scan	1,549	3.1%	2.3%	2.7%
Combination Chest CT Scan	1,241	1.2%	1.6%	2.7%
Follow-up Mammogram/Ultrasound	3,092	4.5%	7.7%	8.8%
Lumbar Spine MRI for Low Back Pain	266	28.9%	35.3%	37.2%

Henrico Doctors' Hospital

1602 Skipwith Road
Richmond, VA 23229
Phone: 804-289-4500
Fax: 804-287-4358
URL: www.henricodoctors.com
Type: Acute Care Hospitals
Ownership: Proprietary
Emergency Services: Yes
Beds: 760

Key Personnel:

Infection Control. . . . . Jeanette Daniel
Chief of Medical Staff. . . . . Dr Richard Hamrick
Quality Assurance . . . . Nancy Kindervater
Radiology. . . . . Bob Longley
Pediatric Ambulatory Care . . . . . . Judy Mathews
Pediatric In-Patient Care . . . . Judy Mathews
Coronary Care. . . . . Steve Tarkington
CEO/President. . . . . David Russell Williams

Measure	Cases	This Hosp.	State Avg.	U.S. Avg.
Blood Clot Prevention and Treatment				
Anticoagulation Overlap Therapy[2]	172	99%	95%	93%
ICU Venous Thromboembolism Prophylaxis[2]	97	100%	95%	92%
Incidence of Potentially Preventable VTE[2]	31	0%	8%	10%
UFH with Dosages/Platelet Monitoring[2]	69	100%	99%	97%
Venous Thromboembolism Prophylaxis[2]	382	99%	91%	85%
Warfarin Therapy Discharge Instructions[2]	132	100%	78%	75%
Chest Pain/Possible Heart Attack Care				
Aspirin Given Within 24 Hours of Arrival[1,3]	-	-	98%	96%
Fibrinolytic Meds Within 30 Min. of Arrival[5]	-	-	68%	58%
Average Time to ECG (minutes)[1,3]	-	-	7	7
Average Time to Transfer (minutes)[5]	-	-	64	60
Children's Asthma Care				
Received Home Management Plan of Care	-	-	-	88%
Received Reliever Medication	-	-	-	100%
Received Systemic Corticosteroids	-	-	-	100%
Emergency Department				
Admittance Decision Time (minutes)[2]	683	82	96	98
Head CT Results Within 45 Min. of Arrival[7]	-	-	60%	57%
Patients Who Left ER Before Being Seen	79,496	1%	2%	2%
Time from ER Arrival to Admit. (minutes)[2]	686	243	280	274
Time from ER Arrival to Discharge (minutes)	499	134	167	134
Time in ER Before Being Evaluated (minutes)	530	11	35	26
Time to Pain Meds for Fractures (minutes)	120	33	56	57
Heart Attack Care				
Aspirin Given at Discharge	296	100%	99%	99%
Fibrinolytic Meds Within 30 Min. of Arrival[7]	-	-	75%	54%
PCI Within 90 Minutes of Arrival	54	96%	97%	96%
Statin Prescribed at Discharge	304	100%	99%	98%
Heart Failure Care				
ACE Inhibitor or ARB for LVSD	163	100%	98%	97%
Discharge Instructions Given	417	98%	95%	94%
Evaluation of LVS Function	508	100%	100%	99%
Medicare Spending				
Medicare Spending per Patient (ratio)	-	0.99	0.95	0.98
Pneumonia Care				
Appropriate Initial Antibiotic Given	150	98%	97%	95%
Blood Culture Timing	286	100%	98%	98%
Pregnancy and Delivery Care				
Newborn Deliveries Scheduled Early[2]	76	5%	6%	6%
Preventive Care				
Immunization for Influenza[2]	622	100%	92%	90%
Immunization for Pneumonia[2]	786	99%	93%	92%
Stroke Care				
Anticoagulation Therapy for Atrial Fibrillation	23	100%	96%	95%
Antithrombotic Therapy Timing	151	100%	99%	98%
Assessed for Rehabilitation	191	100%	99%	97%
Discharged on Antithrombotic Therapy	165	100%	100%	99%
Discharged on Statin Medication	137	99%	97%	94%
Thrombolytic Therapy Timing	21	100%	73%	66%
Venous Thromboembolism Prophylaxis	199	98%	97%	94%
Written Stroke Educational Materials Given	105	98%	92%	88%
Surgical Care Improvement Project				
Appropriate Beta Blocker Usage[2]	240	100%	99%	98%
Appropriate VTP Within 24 Hours[2]	543	99%	99%	98%
Controlled Postoperative Blood Glucose[2]	141	99%	98%	97%
Perioperative Temperature Management[2]	677	100%	100%	100%
Prophylactic Antibiotic Selection[2]	563	99%	99%	99%
Prophylactic Antibiotic Selection (Outpatient)	607	99%	98%	98%
Prophylactic Antibiotic Stopped[2]	542	100%	98%	98%
Prophylactic Antibiotic Timing[2]	563	100%	99%	99%
Prophylactic Antibiotic Timing (Outpatient)	608	100%	98%	98%
Urinary Catheter Removal[2]	475	100%	98%	97%
Survey of Patients' Hospital Experiences				
Area Around Room 'Always' Quiet at Night	300+	62%	60%	61%
Doctors 'Always' Communicated Well	300+	82%	81%	82%
Home Recovery Information Given	300+	86%	86%	85%
Hospital Given 9 or 10 on 10 Point Scale	300+	71%	68%	71%
Meds 'Always' Explained Before Given	300+	60%	62%	64%
Nurses 'Always' Communicated Well	300+	77%	78%	79%
Pain 'Always' Well Controlled	300+	71%	70%	71%
Room and Bathroom 'Always' Clean	300+	67%	71%	73%
Timely Help 'Always' Received	300+	64%	64%	68%
Would Definitely Recommend Hospital	300+	75%	69%	71%
Use of Medical Imaging				
Cardiac Imaging Stress Test before Surgery	188	4.3%	5.1%	5.3%
Combination Abdominal CT Scan	1,304	8.7%	8.5%	10.5%
Combination Brain/Sinus CT Scan	1,534	2.9%	2.3%	2.7%
Combination Chest CT Scan	816	1.5%	1.6%	2.7%
Follow-up Mammogram/Ultrasound	2,010	6.5%	7.7%	8.8%
Lumbar Spine MRI for Low Back Pain	141	29.1%	35.3%	37.2%

Medical College of Virginia Hospitals

1250 East Marshall Street - Box 980510
Richmond, VA 23298
Phone: 804-828-0938
Fax: 804-828-1657
E-mail: lcoles@mcvh-vcu.edu
URL: www.vcuhealth.org
Type: Acute Care Hospitals
Ownership: Govt - Hospital Dist/Auth
Emergency Services: Yes
Beds: 779

Key Personnel:

Chief of Medical Staff. . . . . Ralph R Clark, MD
CEO/President. . . . . John F. Duval
Infection Control. . . . . Michael Edmond, MD MPH
Pediatric In-Patient Care . . . . Lauren Goodloe
Pediatric Ambulatory Care . . . . . . Joseph Laver
Radiology. . . . . Ron Miller
Coronary Care. . . . . Wanda Miller
President. . . . . Michael Rao, Ph.D.

Measure	Cases	This Hosp.	State Avg.	U.S. Avg.
Blood Clot Prevention and Treatment				
Anticoagulation Overlap Therapy[2]	167	95%	95%	93%
ICU Venous Thromboembolism Prophylaxis[2]	118	94%	95%	92%
Incidence of Potentially Preventable VTE[2]	70	7%	8%	10%
UFH with Dosages/Platelet Monitoring[2]	144	99%	99%	97%
Venous Thromboembolism Prophylaxis[2]	338	85%	91%	85%
Warfarin Therapy Discharge Instructions[2]	129	60%	78%	75%
Chest Pain/Possible Heart Attack Care				
Aspirin Given Within 24 Hours of Arrival[5]	-	-	98%	96%
Fibrinolytic Meds Within 30 Min. of Arrival[5]	-	-	68%	58%
Average Time to ECG (minutes)[5]	-	-	7	7
Average Time to Transfer (minutes)[5]	-	-	64	60
Children's Asthma Care				
Received Home Management Plan of Care	-	-	-	88%
Received Reliever Medication	-	-	-	100%
Received Systemic Corticosteroids	-	-	-	100%
Emergency Department				
Admittance Decision Time (minutes)[2]	533	164	96	98
Head CT Results Within 45 Min. of Arrival[7]	-	-	60%	57%
Patients Who Left ER Before Being Seen	92,231	7%	2%	2%
Time from ER Arrival to Admit. (minutes)[2]	534	365	280	274
Time from ER Arrival to Discharge (minutes)	399	235	167	134
Time in ER Before Being Evaluated (minutes)	360	74	35	26
Time to Pain Meds for Fractures (minutes)	152	56	56	57
Heart Attack Care				
Aspirin Given at Discharge	385	99%	99%	99%
Fibrinolytic Meds Within 30 Min. of Arrival[7]	-	-	75%	54%
PCI Within 90 Minutes of Arrival	56	100%	97%	96%
Statin Prescribed at Discharge	376	100%	99%	98%
Heart Failure Care				
ACE Inhibitor or ARB for LVSD	337	97%	98%	97%
Discharge Instructions Given	704	99%	95%	94%
Evaluation of LVS Function	761	100%	100%	99%
Medicare Spending				
Medicare Spending per Patient (ratio)	-	0.98	0.95	0.98
Pneumonia Care				
Appropriate Initial Antibiotic Given	109	93%	97%	95%
Blood Culture Timing	202	99%	98%	98%
Pregnancy and Delivery Care				
Newborn Deliveries Scheduled Early[2]	20	5%	6%	6%

NOTE: Hospital profiles are in alphabetical order by state, then city, then hospital within the city; Rankings exclude hospitals with less than 25 cases except for patient surveys which excludes hospitals with less than 100 cases; (a) 100-299 cases; (1) The number of cases/patients is too few to report; (2) Data submitted were based on a sample of cases/patients; (3) Results are based on a shorter time period than required; (4) Data suppressed by CMS for one or more quarters; (5) Results are not available for this reporting period; (6) Fewer than 100 patients completed the HCAHPS survey; (7) No cases met the criteria for this measure; (8) The lower limit of the confidence interval cannot be calculated if the number of observed infections equals zero; (9) No data are available from the state/territory for this reporting period; (10) The scores shown reflect fewer than 50 completed surveys; (11) There were discrepancies in the data collection process; (12) This measure does not apply to this hospital for this reporting period; (13) Results cannot be calculated for this reporting period; (14) The results for this state are combined with nearby states to protect confidentiality; Please refer to the User's Guide for a full explanation of data.

Measure	Cases	This Hosp.	State Avg.	U.S. Avg.
Preventive Care				
Immunization for Influenza[2]	547	98%	92%	90%
Immunization for Pneumonia[2]	562	91%	93%	92%
Stroke Care				
Anticoagulation Therapy for Atrial Fibrillation[1,2]	-	-	96%	95%
Antithrombotic Therapy Timing[2]	61	97%	99%	98%
Assessed for Rehabilitation[2]	121	95%	99%	97%
Discharged on Antithrombotic Therapy[2]	75	100%	100%	99%
Discharged on Statin Medication[2]	64	95%	97%	94%
Thrombolytic Therapy Timing[1,2]	-	-	73%	66%
Venous Thromboembolism Prophylaxis[2]	123	98%	97%	94%
Written Stroke Educational Materials Given[2]	74	85%	92%	88%
Surgical Care Improvement Project				
Appropriate Beta Blocker Usage[2]	216	99%	99%	98%
Appropriate VTP Within 24 Hours[2]	476	99%	99%	98%
Controlled Postoperative Blood Glucose[2]	157	96%	98%	97%
Perioperative Temperature Management[2]	590	100%	100%	100%
Prophylactic Antibiotic Selection[2]	478	99%	99%	99%
Prophylactic Antibiotic Selection (Outpatient)	679	99%	98%	98%
Prophylactic Antibiotic Stopped[2]	459	98%	98%	98%
Prophylactic Antibiotic Timing[2]	479	100%	99%	99%
Prophylactic Antibiotic Timing (Outpatient)	680	98%	98%	98%
Urinary Catheter Removal[2]	522	98%	98%	97%
Survey of Patients' Hospital Experiences				
Area Around Room 'Always' Quiet at Night	300+	57%	60%	61%
Doctors 'Always' Communicated Well	300+	81%	81%	82%
Home Recovery Information Given	300+	88%	86%	85%
Hospital Given 9 or 10 on 10 Point Scale	300+	72%	68%	71%
Meds 'Always' Explained Before Given	300+	65%	62%	64%
Nurses 'Always' Communicated Well	300+	78%	78%	79%
Pain 'Always' Well Controlled	300+	71%	70%	71%
Room and Bathroom 'Always' Clean	300+	70%	71%	73%
Timely Help 'Always' Received	300+	61%	64%	68%
Would Definitely Recommend Hospital	300+	76%	69%	71%
Use of Medical Imaging				
Cardiac Imaging Stress Test before Surgery	921	4.8%	5.1%	5.3%
Combination Abdominal CT Scan	1,126	4.7%	8.5%	10.5%
Combination Brain/Sinus CT Scan	527	1.1%	2.3%	2.7%
Combination Chest CT Scan	1,476	0.1%	1.6%	2.7%
Follow-up Mammogram/Ultrasound	2,386	5.1%	7.7%	8.8%
Lumbar Spine MRI for Low Back Pain	160	32.5%	35.3%	37.2%

Richmond VA Medical Center

1201 Broad Rock Boulevard
Richmond, VA 23249
URL: www.med.va.gov
Type: Acute Care - VA
Ownership: Government Federal

Phone: 804-675-5000
Fax: 804-675-5585

Emergency Services: No
Beds: 427

Key Personnel:
Intensive Care Unit. . . . . Mablene Bailey, RN
Chief of Medical Staff . . . . Julie L. Beales, MD
Operating Room. . . . . Bobbie C Branch, RN
Anesthesiology. . . . . Robert Litwack, MD
Radiology. . . . . Peter Quagliano, MD
Emergency Room . . . . Charles Stuckey, MD
Quality Assurance . . . . Margaret Supensky, RN
Infection Control. . . . . Edward Wong, MD

Measure	Cases	This Hosp.	State Avg.	U.S. Avg.
Blood Clot Prevention and Treatment				
Anticoagulation Overlap Therapy	-	-	95%	93%
ICU Venous Thromboembolism Prophylaxis	-	-	95%	92%
Incidence of Potentially Preventable VTE	-	-	8%	10%
UFH with Dosages/Platelet Monitoring	-	-	99%	97%
Venous Thromboembolism Prophylaxis	-	-	91%	85%
Warfarin Therapy Discharge Instructions	-	-	78%	75%
Chest Pain/Possible Heart Attack Care				
Aspirin Given Within 24 Hours of Arrival	-	-	98%	96%
Fibrinolytic Meds Within 30 Min. of Arrival	-	-	68%	58%
Average Time to ECG (minutes)	-	-	7	7
Average Time to Transfer (minutes)	-	-	64	60
Children's Asthma Care				
Received Home Management Plan of Care	-	-	-	88%
Received Reliever Medication	-	-	-	100%
Received Systemic Corticosteroids	-	-	-	100%
Emergency Department				
Admittance Decision Time (minutes)	-	-	96	98
Head CT Results Within 45 Min. of Arrival	-	-	60%	57%
Patients Who Left ER Before Being Seen	-	-	2%	2%
Time from ER Arrival to Admit. (minutes)	-	-	280	274
Time from ER Arrival to Discharge (minutes)	-	-	167	134
Time in ER Before Being Evaluated (minutes)	-	-	35	26
Time to Pain Meds for Fractures (minutes)	-	-	56	57
Heart Attack Care				
Aspirin Given at Discharge	64	100%	99%	99%
Fibrinolytic Meds Within 30 Min. of Arrival[5]	-	-	75%	54%
PCI Within 90 Minutes of Arrival[1]	-	-	97%	96%
Statin Prescribed at Discharge	60	100%	99%	98%
Heart Failure Care				
ACE Inhibitor or ARB for LVSD	116	97%	98%	97%
Discharge Instructions Given	286	100%	95%	94%
Evaluation of LVS Function	309	100%	100%	99%
Medicare Spending				
Medicare Spending per Patient (ratio)	-	-	0.95	0.98
Pneumonia Care				
Appropriate Initial Antibiotic Given	58	93%	97%	95%
Blood Culture Timing	122	94%	98%	98%
Pregnancy and Delivery Care				
Newborn Deliveries Scheduled Early	-	-	6%	6%
Preventive Care				
Immunization for Influenza[5]	-	-	92%	90%
Immunization for Pneumonia[5]	-	-	93%	92%
Stroke Care				
Anticoagulation Therapy for Atrial Fibrillation	-	-	96%	95%
Antithrombotic Therapy Timing	-	-	99%	98%
Assessed for Rehabilitation	-	-	99%	97%
Discharged on Antithrombotic Therapy	-	-	100%	99%
Discharged on Statin Medication	-	-	97%	94%
Thrombolytic Therapy Timing	-	-	73%	66%
Venous Thromboembolism Prophylaxis	-	-	97%	94%
Written Stroke Educational Materials Given	-	-	92%	88%
Surgical Care Improvement Project				
Appropriate Beta Blocker Usage[2]	141	98%	99%	98%
Appropriate VTP Within 24 Hours[2]	257	98%	99%	98%
Controlled Postoperative Blood Glucose[2]	83	88%	98%	97%
Perioperative Temperature Management[2]	289	99%	100%	100%
Prophylactic Antibiotic Selection	246	99%	99%	99%
Prophylactic Antibiotic Selection (Outpatient)	-	-	98%	98%
Prophylactic Antibiotic Stopped	242	93%	98%	98%
Prophylactic Antibiotic Timing	247	98%	99%	99%
Prophylactic Antibiotic Timing (Outpatient)	-	-	98%	98%
Urinary Catheter Removal[2]	191	97%	98%	97%
Survey of Patients' Hospital Experiences				
Area Around Room 'Always' Quiet at Night	-	-	60%	61%
Doctors 'Always' Communicated Well	-	-	81%	82%
Home Recovery Information Given	-	-	86%	85%
Hospital Given 9 or 10 on 10 Point Scale	-	-	68%	71%
Meds 'Always' Explained Before Given	-	-	62%	64%
Nurses 'Always' Communicated Well	-	-	78%	79%
Pain 'Always' Well Controlled	-	-	70%	71%
Room and Bathroom 'Always' Clean	-	-	71%	73%
Timely Help 'Always' Received	-	-	64%	68%
Would Definitely Recommend Hospital	-	-	69%	71%
Use of Medical Imaging				
Cardiac Imaging Stress Test before Surgery	-	-	5.1%	5.3%
Combination Abdominal CT Scan	-	-	8.5%	10.5%
Combination Brain/Sinus CT Scan	-	-	2.3%	2.7%
Combination Chest CT Scan	-	-	1.6%	2.7%
Follow-up Mammogram/Ultrasound	-	-	7.7%	8.8%
Lumbar Spine MRI for Low Back Pain	-	-	35.3%	37.2%

Carilion Roanoke Memorial Hospital

1906 Belleview Avenue, Se
Roanoke, VA 24014
URL: www.carilion.com/crmh
Type: Acute Care Hospitals
Ownership: Voluntary non-profit - Private

Phone: 540-981-7000
Fax: 540-983-1190

Emergency Services: Yes
Beds: 520

Key Personnel:
Operating Room. . . . . Jeannette Capella
Infection Control. . . . . Debora Demicco, MD
Radiology. . . . . Dana B Fathy, MD
Chief of Medical Staff . . . . Jim Gooding
Emergency Room . . . . Evelyn Menetta
Intensive Care Unit. . . . . Cindy Smith
CEO/President. . . . . Lucas A Snipes
Quality Assurance . . . . Judy Wilson

Measure	Cases	This Hosp.	State Avg.	U.S. Avg.
Blood Clot Prevention and Treatment				
Anticoagulation Overlap Therapy[2]	242	96%	95%	93%
ICU Venous Thromboembolism Prophylaxis[2]	121	93%	95%	92%
Incidence of Potentially Preventable VTE[2]	80	6%	8%	10%
UFH with Dosages/Platelet Monitoring[2]	160	100%	99%	97%
Venous Thromboembolism Prophylaxis[2]	485	87%	91%	85%
Warfarin Therapy Discharge Instructions[2]	164	90%	78%	75%
Chest Pain/Possible Heart Attack Care				
Aspirin Given Within 24 Hours of Arrival[1,3]	-	-	98%	96%
Fibrinolytic Meds Within 30 Min. of Arrival[5]	-	-	68%	58%
Average Time to ECG (minutes)[1,3]	-	-	7	7
Average Time to Transfer (minutes)[5]	-	-	64	60
Children's Asthma Care				
Received Home Management Plan of Care	-	-	-	88%
Received Reliever Medication	-	-	-	100%
Received Systemic Corticosteroids	-	-	-	100%
Emergency Department				
Admittance Decision Time (minutes)[2]	370	173	96	98
Head CT Results Within 45 Min. of Arrival[1]	-	-	60%	57%
Patients Who Left ER Before Being Seen	84,761	5%	2%	2%
Time from ER Arrival to Admit. (minutes)[2]	377	396	280	274
Time from ER Arrival to Discharge (minutes)	352	222	167	134
Time in ER Before Being Evaluated (minutes)	313	60	35	26
Time to Pain Meds for Fractures (minutes)	482	100	56	57
Heart Attack Care				
Aspirin Given at Discharge	1,120	99%	99%	99%
Fibrinolytic Meds Within 30 Min. of Arrival[1]	-	-	75%	54%
PCI Within 90 Minutes of Arrival	127	94%	97%	96%
Statin Prescribed at Discharge	1,060	99%	99%	98%
Heart Failure Care				
ACE Inhibitor or ARB for LVSD	270	95%	98%	97%
Discharge Instructions Given	692	98%	95%	94%
Evaluation of LVS Function	929	99%	100%	99%
Medicare Spending				
Medicare Spending per Patient (ratio)	-	0.97	0.95	0.98
Pneumonia Care				
Appropriate Initial Antibiotic Given	237	95%	97%	95%
Blood Culture Timing	446	98%	98%	98%
Pregnancy and Delivery Care				
Newborn Deliveries Scheduled Early	224	3%	6%	6%
Preventive Care				
Immunization for Influenza[2]	537	90%	92%	90%
Immunization for Pneumonia[2]	662	92%	93%	92%
Stroke Care				
Anticoagulation Therapy for Atrial Fibrillation	43	98%	96%	95%
Antithrombotic Therapy Timing	360	100%	99%	98%
Assessed for Rehabilitation	494	100%	99%	97%
Discharged on Antithrombotic Therapy	390	100%	100%	99%
Discharged on Statin Medication	311	100%	97%	94%
Thrombolytic Therapy Timing	20	100%	73%	66%
Venous Thromboembolism Prophylaxis	539	100%	97%	94%
Written Stroke Educational Materials Given	234	94%	92%	88%
Surgical Care Improvement Project				
Appropriate Beta Blocker Usage[2]	766	99%	99%	98%
Appropriate VTP Within 24 Hours[2]	1,542	98%	99%	98%
Controlled Postoperative Blood Glucose[2]	346	99%	98%	97%
Perioperative Temperature Management[2]	2,098	100%	100%	100%
Prophylactic Antibiotic Selection[2]	2,087	99%	99%	99%
Prophylactic Antibiotic Selection (Outpatient)	726	97%	98%	98%
Prophylactic Antibiotic Stopped[2]	2,046	99%	98%	98%
Prophylactic Antibiotic Timing[2]	2,103	98%	99%	99%
Prophylactic Antibiotic Timing (Outpatient)	727	98%	98%	98%
Urinary Catheter Removal[2]	1,767	96%	98%	97%
Survey of Patients' Hospital Experiences				
Area Around Room 'Always' Quiet at Night	300+	56%	60%	61%

NOTE: Hospital profiles are in alphabetical order by state, then city, then hospital within the city; Rankings exclude hospitals with less than 25 cases except for patient surveys which excludes hospitals with less than 100 cases; (a) 100-299 cases; (1) The number of cases/patients is too few to report; (2) Data submitted were based on a sample of cases/patients; (3) Results are based on a shorter time period than required; (4) Data suppressed by CMS for one or more quarters; (5) Results are not available for this reporting period; (6) Fewer than 100 patients completed the HCAHPS survey; (7) No cases met the criteria for this measure; (8) The lower limit of the confidence interval cannot be calculated if the number of observed infections equals zero; (9) No data are available from the state/territory for this reporting period; (10) The scores shown reflect fewer than 50 completed surveys; (11) There were discrepancies in the data collection process; (12) This measure does not apply to this hospital for this reporting period; (13) Results cannot be calculated for this reporting period; (14) The results for this state are combined with nearby states to protect confidentiality; Please refer to the User's Guide for a full explanation of data.

Doctors 'Always' Communicated Well	300+	77%	81%	82%
Home Recovery Information Given	300+	86%	86%	85%
Hospital Given 9 or 10 on 10 Point Scale	300+	68%	68%	71%
Meds 'Always' Explained Before Given	300+	58%	62%	64%
Nurses 'Always' Communicated Well	300+	78%	78%	79%
Pain 'Always' Well Controlled	300+	73%	70%	71%
Room and Bathroom 'Always' Clean	300+	61%	71%	73%
Timely Help 'Always' Received	300+	66%	64%	68%
Would Definitely Recommend Hospital	300+	76%	69%	71%
Use of Medical Imaging				
Cardiac Imaging Stress Test before Surgery	1,351	4.8%	5.1%	5.3%
Combination Abdominal CT Scan	1,640	5.6%	8.5%	10.5%
Combination Brain/Sinus CT Scan	1,227	2.4%	2.3%	2.7%
Combination Chest CT Scan	1,294	0.9%	1.6%	2.7%
Follow-up Mammogram/Ultrasound	4,466	4.8%	7.7%	8.8%
Lumbar Spine MRI for Low Back Pain	379	30.3%	35.3%	37.2%

Carilion Franklin Memorial Hospital

180 Floyd Avenue
Rocky Mount, VA 24151
Phone: 540-483-5277
Fax: 540-489-6442
URL: www.carilion.com/cfmh
Type: Acute Care Hospitals
Emergency Services: Yes
Ownership: Voluntary non-profit - Other
Beds: 37

Key Personnel:
Chief of Medical Staff. . . . . Christine Barrett, M.D.
Infection Control. . . . . Virginia Crouch
Operating Room. . . . . Charles A Harris
Quality Assurance . . . . Carol Melvin
Emergency Room . . . . Darrell Van Ness

Measure	Cases	This Hosp.	State Avg.	U.S. Avg.
Blood Clot Prevention and Treatment				
Anticoagulation Overlap Therapy[2]	11	100%	95%	93%
ICU Venous Thromboembolism Prophylaxis[2]	55	100%	95%	92%
Incidence of Potentially Preventable VTE[1,2]	-	-	8%	10%
UFH with Dosages/Platelet Monitoring[1,2]	-	-	99%	97%
Venous Thromboembolism Prophylaxis[2]	214	86%	91%	85%
Warfarin Therapy Discharge Instructions[1,2]	-	-	78%	75%
Chest Pain/Possible Heart Attack Care				
Aspirin Given Within 24 Hours of Arrival	97	98%	98%	96%
Fibrinolytic Meds Within 30 Min. of Arrival[7]	-	-	68%	58%
Average Time to ECG (minutes)	107	17	7	7
Average Time to Transfer (minutes)[1]	-	-	64	60
Children's Asthma Care				
Received Home Management Plan of Care	-	-	-	88%
Received Reliever Medication	-	-	-	100%
Received Systemic Corticosteroids	-	-	-	100%
Emergency Department				
Admittance Decision Time (minutes)[2]	447	87	96	98
Head CT Results Within 45 Min. of Arrival	11	64%	60%	57%
Patients Who Left ER Before Being Seen	25,845	3%	2%	2%
Time from ER Arrival to Admit. (minutes)[2]	452	264	280	274
Time from ER Arrival to Discharge (minutes)	332	148	167	134
Time in ER Before Being Evaluated (minutes)	312	45	35	26
Time to Pain Meds for Fractures (minutes)	110	86	56	57
Heart Attack Care				
Aspirin Given at Discharge[1]	-	-	99%	99%
Fibrinolytic Meds Within 30 Min. of Arrival[7]	-	-	75%	54%
PCI Within 90 Minutes of Arrival[7]	-	-	97%	96%
Statin Prescribed at Discharge[1]	-	-	99%	98%
Heart Failure Care				
ACE Inhibitor or ARB for LVSD	20	100%	98%	97%
Discharge Instructions Given	75	100%	95%	94%
Evaluation of LVS Function	93	99%	100%	99%
Medicare Spending				
Medicare Spending per Patient (ratio)	-	0.88	0.95	0.98
Pneumonia Care				
Appropriate Initial Antibiotic Given	88	97%	97%	95%
Blood Culture Timing	133	99%	98%	98%
Pregnancy and Delivery Care				
Newborn Deliveries Scheduled Early[7]	-	-	6%	6%
Preventive Care				
Immunization for Influenza[2]	364	97%	92%	90%
Immunization for Pneumonia[2]	531	98%	93%	92%
Stroke Care				
Anticoagulation Therapy for Atrial Fibrillation[1]	-	-	96%	95%
Antithrombotic Therapy Timing	20	100%	99%	98%
Assessed for Rehabilitation	24	100%	99%	97%
Discharged on Antithrombotic Therapy	24	100%	100%	99%
Discharged on Statin Medication	16	100%	97%	94%
Thrombolytic Therapy Timing[1]	-	-	73%	66%
Venous Thromboembolism Prophylaxis	21	95%	97%	94%
Written Stroke Educational Materials Given	12	33%	92%	88%
Surgical Care Improvement Project				
Appropriate Beta Blocker Usage[1]	-	-	99%	98%
Appropriate VTP Within 24 Hours	16	94%	99%	98%
Controlled Postoperative Blood Glucose[7]	-	-	98%	97%
Perioperative Temperature Management	49	100%	100%	100%
Prophylactic Antibiotic Selection	40	98%	99%	99%
Prophylactic Antibiotic Selection (Outpatient)	13	92%	98%	98%
Prophylactic Antibiotic Stopped	38	100%	98%	98%
Prophylactic Antibiotic Timing	41	90%	99%	99%
Prophylactic Antibiotic Timing (Outpatient)	13	100%	98%	98%
Urinary Catheter Removal[1]	-	-	98%	97%
Survey of Patients' Hospital Experiences				
Area Around Room 'Always' Quiet at Night	300+	62%	60%	61%
Doctors 'Always' Communicated Well	300+	83%	81%	82%
Home Recovery Information Given	300+	86%	86%	85%
Hospital Given 9 or 10 on 10 Point Scale	300+	70%	68%	71%
Meds 'Always' Explained Before Given	300+	67%	62%	64%
Nurses 'Always' Communicated Well	300+	81%	78%	79%
Pain 'Always' Well Controlled	300+	70%	70%	71%
Room and Bathroom 'Always' Clean	300+	83%	71%	73%
Timely Help 'Always' Received	300+	74%	64%	68%
Would Definitely Recommend Hospital	300+	72%	69%	71%
Use of Medical Imaging				
Cardiac Imaging Stress Test before Surgery	207	7.2%	5.1%	5.3%
Combination Abdominal CT Scan	418	2.6%	8.5%	10.5%
Combination Brain/Sinus CT Scan	446	2.0%	2.3%	2.7%
Combination Chest CT Scan	177	5.1%	1.6%	2.7%
Follow-up Mammogram/Ultrasound	857	3.9%	7.7%	8.8%
Lumbar Spine MRI for Low Back Pain	61	37.7%	35.3%	37.2%

Lewisgale Medical Center

1900 Electric Road
Salem, VA 24153
Phone: 540-776-4000
Fax: 540-772-6411
E-mail: james.thweatt@hcahealthcare.com
URL: www.lewis-gale.com
Type: Acute Care Hospitals
Emergency Services: Yes
Ownership: Proprietary
Beds: 521

Key Personnel:
CEO/President. . . . . Jon Bartlett
Pediatric In-Patient Care . . . . Luther A Beazley, MD
Operating Room. . . . . Nancy Boyer, RN
Radiology. . . . . John M Mathis, MD
Chief of Medical Staff. . . . . Rajeev Sharma, MD
Infection Control. . . . . Teresa Stowasser, RN
Quality Assurance . . . . Charlotte Tyson

Measure	Cases	This Hosp.	State Avg.	U.S. Avg.
Blood Clot Prevention and Treatment				
Anticoagulation Overlap Therapy[2]	105	100%	95%	93%
ICU Venous Thromboembolism Prophylaxis[2]	105	100%	95%	92%
Incidence of Potentially Preventable VTE[2]	25	0%	8%	10%
UFH with Dosages/Platelet Monitoring[2]	37	100%	99%	97%
Venous Thromboembolism Prophylaxis[2]	305	99%	91%	85%
Warfarin Therapy Discharge Instructions[2]	64	100%	78%	75%
Chest Pain/Possible Heart Attack Care				
Aspirin Given Within 24 Hours of Arrival[1,3]	-	-	98%	96%
Fibrinolytic Meds Within 30 Min. of Arrival[5]	-	-	68%	58%
Average Time to ECG (minutes)[1,3]	-	-	7	7
Average Time to Transfer (minutes)[5]	-	-	64	60
Children's Asthma Care				
Received Home Management Plan of Care	-	-	-	88%
Received Reliever Medication	-	-	-	100%
Received Systemic Corticosteroids	-	-	-	100%
Emergency Department				
Admittance Decision Time (minutes)[2]	697	61	96	98
Head CT Results Within 45 Min. of Arrival[1]	-	-	60%	57%
Patients Who Left ER Before Being Seen	46,189	2%	2%	2%
Time from ER Arrival to Admit. (minutes)[2]	697	236	280	274
Time from ER Arrival to Discharge (minutes)	457	170	167	134
Time in ER Before Being Evaluated (minutes)	522	14	35	26
Time to Pain Meds for Fractures (minutes)	89	35	56	57
Heart Attack Care				
Aspirin Given at Discharge[2]	303	100%	99%	99%
Fibrinolytic Meds Within 30 Min. of Arrival[2,7]	-	-	75%	54%
PCI Within 90 Minutes of Arrival[2]	35	100%	97%	96%
Statin Prescribed at Discharge[2]	291	100%	99%	98%
Heart Failure Care				
ACE Inhibitor or ARB for LVSD[2]	72	100%	98%	97%
Discharge Instructions Given[2]	244	100%	95%	94%
Evaluation of LVS Function[2]	322	100%	100%	99%
Medicare Spending				
Medicare Spending per Patient (ratio)	-	1.03	0.95	0.98
Pneumonia Care				
Appropriate Initial Antibiotic Given	178	100%	97%	95%
Blood Culture Timing	311	100%	98%	98%
Pregnancy and Delivery Care				
Newborn Deliveries Scheduled Early	81	0%	6%	6%
Preventive Care				
Immunization for Influenza[2]	602	100%	92%	90%
Immunization for Pneumonia[2]	832	100%	93%	92%
Stroke Care				
Anticoagulation Therapy for Atrial Fibrillation	24	100%	96%	95%
Antithrombotic Therapy Timing	176	100%	99%	98%
Assessed for Rehabilitation	191	100%	99%	97%
Discharged on Antithrombotic Therapy	177	100%	100%	99%
Discharged on Statin Medication	135	100%	97%	94%
Thrombolytic Therapy Timing[1]	-	-	73%	66%
Venous Thromboembolism Prophylaxis	198	100%	97%	94%
Written Stroke Educational Materials Given	97	100%	92%	88%
Surgical Care Improvement Project				
Appropriate Beta Blocker Usage[2]	176	99%	99%	98%
Appropriate VTP Within 24 Hours[2]	457	100%	99%	98%
Controlled Postoperative Blood Glucose[2]	116	98%	98%	97%
Perioperative Temperature Management[2]	548	100%	100%	100%
Prophylactic Antibiotic Selection[2]	439	100%	99%	99%
Prophylactic Antibiotic Selection (Outpatient)	555	99%	98%	98%
Prophylactic Antibiotic Stopped[2]	419	100%	98%	98%
Prophylactic Antibiotic Timing[2]	439	100%	99%	99%
Prophylactic Antibiotic Timing (Outpatient)	552	100%	98%	98%
Urinary Catheter Removal[2]	296	100%	98%	97%
Survey of Patients' Hospital Experiences				
Area Around Room 'Always' Quiet at Night	300+	52%	60%	61%
Doctors 'Always' Communicated Well	300+	79%	81%	82%
Home Recovery Information Given	300+	87%	86%	85%
Hospital Given 9 or 10 on 10 Point Scale	300+	70%	68%	71%
Meds 'Always' Explained Before Given	300+	58%	62%	64%
Nurses 'Always' Communicated Well	300+	74%	78%	79%
Pain 'Always' Well Controlled	300+	69%	70%	71%
Room and Bathroom 'Always' Clean	300+	64%	71%	73%
Timely Help 'Always' Received	300+	56%	64%	68%
Would Definitely Recommend Hospital	300+	74%	69%	71%
Use of Medical Imaging				
Cardiac Imaging Stress Test before Surgery	712	4.1%	5.1%	5.3%
Combination Abdominal CT Scan	1,218	2.6%	8.5%	10.5%
Combination Brain/Sinus CT Scan	974	3.2%	2.3%	2.7%
Combination Chest CT Scan	824	0.8%	1.6%	2.7%
Follow-up Mammogram/Ultrasound	2,836	4.8%	7.7%	8.8%
Lumbar Spine MRI for Low Back Pain	207	43.0%	35.3%	37.2%

Salem VA Medical Center

1970 Boulevard
Salem, VA 24153
Phone: 540-982-2463
Fax: 540-983-1096
URL: www.med.va.gov
Type: Acute Care - VA
Emergency Services: No
Ownership: Government Federal
Beds: 282

Key Personnel:
Emergency Room . . . . Matthew T Barnette, RN
Cardiac Laboratory. . . . . Nelson Bernardo, MD
Patient Relations . . . . Debra Burgess
Quality Assurance . . . . Carol Carlson, RN
Chief of Medical Staff. . . . . Anne C. Hutchins, MD
Infection Control. . . . . Charlene McCadden

NOTE: Hospital profiles are in alphabetical order by state, then city, then hospital within the city; Rankings exclude hospitals with less than 25 cases except for patient surveys which excludes hospitals with less than 100 cases; (a) 100-299 cases; (1) The number of cases/patients is too few to report; (2) Data submitted were based on a sample of cases/patients; (3) Results are based on a shorter time period than required; (4) Data suppressed by CMS for one or more quarters; (5) Results are not available for this reporting period; (6) Fewer than 100 patients completed the HCAHPS survey; (7) No cases met the criteria for this measure; (8) The lower limit of the confidence interval cannot be calculated if the number of observed infections equals zero; (9) No data are available from the state/territory for this reporting period; (10) The scores shown reflect fewer than 50 completed surveys; (11) There were discrepancies in the data collection process; (12) This measure does not apply to this hospital for this reporting period; (13) Results cannot be calculated for this reporting period; (14) The results for this state are combined with nearby states to protect confidentiality; Please refer to the User's Guide for a full explanation of data.

Radiology. . . . . Narain Srinivas, MD
Operating Room. . . . . Wayne H Wilson

Measure	Cases	This Hosp.	State Avg.	U.S. Avg.
Blood Clot Prevention and Treatment				
Anticoagulation Overlap Therapy	-	-	95%	93%
ICU Venous Thromboembolism Prophylaxis	-	-	95%	92%
Incidence of Potentially Preventable VTE	-	-	8%	10%
UFH with Dosages/Platelet Monitoring	-	-	99%	97%
Venous Thromboembolism Prophylaxis	-	-	91%	85%
Warfarin Therapy Discharge Instructions	-	-	78%	75%
Chest Pain/Possible Heart Attack Care				
Aspirin Given Within 24 Hours of Arrival	-	-	98%	96%
Fibrinolytic Meds Within 30 Min. of Arrival	-	-	68%	58%
Average Time to ECG (minutes)	-	-	7	7
Average Time to Transfer (minutes)	-	-	64	60
Children's Asthma Care				
Received Home Management Plan of Care	-	-	-	88%
Received Reliever Medication	-	-	-	100%
Received Systemic Corticosteroids	-	-	-	100%
Emergency Department				
Admittance Decision Time (minutes)	-	-	96	98
Head CT Results Within 45 Min. of Arrival	-	-	60%	57%
Patients Who Left ER Before Being Seen	-	-	2%	2%
Time from ER Arrival to Admit. (minutes)	-	-	280	274
Time from ER Arrival to Discharge (minutes)	-	-	167	134
Time in ER Before Being Evaluated (minutes)	-	-	35	26
Time to Pain Meds for Fractures (minutes)	-	-	56	57
Heart Attack Care				
Aspirin Given at Discharge	32	97%	99%	99%
Fibrinolytic Meds Within 30 Min. of Arrival[5]	-	-	75%	54%
PCI Within 90 Minutes of Arrival[1]	-	-	97%	96%
Statin Prescribed at Discharge	30	100%	99%	98%
Heart Failure Care				
ACE Inhibitor or ARB for LVSD	41	100%	98%	97%
Discharge Instructions Given	112	97%	95%	94%
Evaluation of LVS Function	136	100%	100%	99%
Medicare Spending				
Medicare Spending per Patient (ratio)	-	-	0.95	0.98
Pneumonia Care				
Appropriate Initial Antibiotic Given	52	94%	97%	95%
Blood Culture Timing	79	99%	98%	98%
Pregnancy and Delivery Care				
Newborn Deliveries Scheduled Early	-	-	6%	6%
Preventive Care				
Immunization for Influenza[5]	-	-	92%	90%
Immunization for Pneumonia[5]	-	-	93%	92%
Stroke Care				
Anticoagulation Therapy for Atrial Fibrillation	-	-	96%	95%
Antithrombotic Therapy Timing	-	-	99%	98%
Assessed for Rehabilitation	-	-	99%	97%
Discharged on Antithrombotic Therapy	-	-	100%	99%
Discharged on Statin Medication	-	-	97%	94%
Thrombolytic Therapy Timing	-	-	73%	66%
Venous Thromboembolism Prophylaxis	-	-	97%	94%
Written Stroke Educational Materials Given	-	-	92%	88%
Surgical Care Improvement Project				
Appropriate Beta Blocker Usage[2]	59	92%	99%	98%
Appropriate VTP Within 24 Hours[2]	190	88%	99%	98%
Controlled Postoperative Blood Glucose[5]	-	-	98%	97%
Perioperative Temperature Management[2]	216	99%	100%	100%
Prophylactic Antibiotic Selection	154	99%	99%	99%
Prophylactic Antibiotic Selection (Outpatient)	-	-	98%	98%
Prophylactic Antibiotic Stopped	154	98%	98%	98%
Prophylactic Antibiotic Timing	154	97%	99%	99%
Prophylactic Antibiotic Timing (Outpatient)	-	-	98%	98%
Urinary Catheter Removal[2]	110	96%	98%	97%
Survey of Patients' Hospital Experiences				
Area Around Room 'Always' Quiet at Night	-	-	60%	61%
Doctors 'Always' Communicated Well	-	-	81%	82%
Home Recovery Information Given	-	-	86%	85%
Hospital Given 9 or 10 on 10 Point Scale	-	-	68%	71%
Meds 'Always' Explained Before Given	-	-	62%	64%
Nurses 'Always' Communicated Well	-	-	78%	79%
Pain 'Always' Well Controlled	-	-	70%	71%
Room and Bathroom 'Always' Clean	-	-	71%	73%
Timely Help 'Always' Received	-	-	64%	68%
Would Definitely Recommend Hospital	-	-	69%	71%
Use of Medical Imaging				
Cardiac Imaging Stress Test before Surgery	-	-	5.1%	5.3%
Combination Abdominal CT Scan	-	-	8.5%	10.5%
Combination Brain/Sinus CT Scan	-	-	2.3%	2.7%
Combination Chest CT Scan	-	-	1.6%	2.7%
Follow-up Mammogram/Ultrasound	-	-	7.7%	8.8%
Lumbar Spine MRI for Low Back Pain	-	-	35.3%	37.2%

Community Memorial Healthcenter

125 Buena Vista Circle
South Hill, VA 23970
Phone: 434-447-3151
Fax: 434-774-2485
E-mail: ethompson@cmh-sh.org
URL: www.cmh-sh.org
Type: Acute Care Hospitals
Emergency Services: Yes
Ownership: Voluntary non-profit - Private
Beds: 144

Key Personnel:
Quality Assurance . . . . Edward Brandenburg
CEO/President. . . . . W Scott Burnette
Patient Relations . . . . Ursula Butts
Radiology. . . . . Nirpendra Devanath
Emergency Room . . . . Wallace Horne
Operating Room. . . . . Joanne Paynter, TN
Chief of Medical Staff. . . . . David Powers
Infection Control. . . . . Gayle Sutton, RN

Measure	Cases	This Hosp.	State Avg.	U.S. Avg.
Blood Clot Prevention and Treatment				
Anticoagulation Overlap Therapy[2]	34	71%	95%	93%
ICU Venous Thromboembolism Prophylaxis[2]	76	99%	95%	92%
Incidence of Potentially Preventable VTE[1,2]	-	-	8%	10%
UFH with Dosages/Platelet Monitoring[2]	28	100%	99%	97%
Venous Thromboembolism Prophylaxis[2]	322	88%	91%	85%
Warfarin Therapy Discharge Instructions[2]	23	91%	78%	75%
Chest Pain/Possible Heart Attack Care				
Aspirin Given Within 24 Hours of Arrival	132	100%	98%	96%
Fibrinolytic Meds Within 30 Min. of Arrival[1]	-	-	68%	58%
Average Time to ECG (minutes)	136	3	7	7
Average Time to Transfer (minutes)[1]	-	-	64	60
Children's Asthma Care				
Received Home Management Plan of Care	-	-	-	88%
Received Reliever Medication	-	-	-	100%
Received Systemic Corticosteroids	-	-	-	100%
Emergency Department				
Admittance Decision Time (minutes)[2]	549	88	96	98
Head CT Results Within 45 Min. of Arrival[1]	-	-	60%	57%
Patients Who Left ER Before Being Seen	21,372	1%	2%	2%
Time from ER Arrival to Admit. (minutes)[2]	580	267	280	274
Time from ER Arrival to Discharge (minutes)	327	126	167	134
Time in ER Before Being Evaluated (minutes)	382	19	35	26
Time to Pain Meds for Fractures (minutes)	88	48	56	57
Heart Attack Care				
Aspirin Given at Discharge[1]	-	-	99%	99%
Fibrinolytic Meds Within 30 Min. of Arrival[7]	-	-	75%	54%
PCI Within 90 Minutes of Arrival[7]	-	-	97%	96%
Statin Prescribed at Discharge[1]	-	-	99%	98%
Heart Failure Care				
ACE Inhibitor or ARB for LVSD	41	100%	98%	97%
Discharge Instructions Given	160	100%	95%	94%
Evaluation of LVS Function	197	100%	100%	99%
Medicare Spending				
Medicare Spending per Patient (ratio)	-	0.93	0.95	0.98
Pneumonia Care				
Appropriate Initial Antibiotic Given	54	96%	97%	95%
Blood Culture Timing	119	97%	98%	98%
Pregnancy and Delivery Care				
Newborn Deliveries Scheduled Early[7]	-	-	6%	6%
Preventive Care				
Immunization for Influenza[2]	334	93%	92%	90%
Immunization for Pneumonia[2]	515	96%	93%	92%
Stroke Care				
Anticoagulation Therapy for Atrial Fibrillation[1]	-	-	96%	95%
Antithrombotic Therapy Timing	54	100%	99%	98%
Assessed for Rehabilitation	47	100%	99%	97%
Discharged on Antithrombotic Therapy	45	100%	100%	99%
Discharged on Statin Medication	32	100%	97%	94%
Thrombolytic Therapy Timing[7]	-	-	73%	66%
Venous Thromboembolism Prophylaxis	56	100%	97%	94%
Written Stroke Educational Materials Given	19	100%	92%	88%
Surgical Care Improvement Project				
Appropriate Beta Blocker Usage[2]	53	98%	99%	98%
Appropriate VTP Within 24 Hours[2]	125	100%	99%	98%
Controlled Postoperative Blood Glucose[2,7]	-	-	98%	97%
Perioperative Temperature Management[2]	128	100%	100%	100%
Prophylactic Antibiotic Selection[2]	93	100%	99%	99%
Prophylactic Antibiotic Selection (Outpatient)	21	100%	98%	98%
Prophylactic Antibiotic Stopped[2]	88	99%	98%	98%
Prophylactic Antibiotic Timing[2]	93	100%	99%	99%
Prophylactic Antibiotic Timing (Outpatient)	21	95%	98%	98%
Urinary Catheter Removal[2]	99	100%	98%	97%
Survey of Patients' Hospital Experiences				
Area Around Room 'Always' Quiet at Night	300+	60%	60%	61%
Doctors 'Always' Communicated Well	300+	82%	81%	82%
Home Recovery Information Given	300+	87%	86%	85%
Hospital Given 9 or 10 on 10 Point Scale	300+	63%	68%	71%
Meds 'Always' Explained Before Given	300+	64%	62%	64%
Nurses 'Always' Communicated Well	300+	81%	78%	79%
Pain 'Always' Well Controlled	300+	68%	70%	71%
Room and Bathroom 'Always' Clean	300+	69%	71%	73%
Timely Help 'Always' Received	300+	66%	64%	68%
Would Definitely Recommend Hospital	300+	61%	69%	71%
Use of Medical Imaging				
Cardiac Imaging Stress Test before Surgery	117	4.3%	5.1%	5.3%
Combination Abdominal CT Scan	525	21.9%	8.5%	10.5%
Combination Brain/Sinus CT Scan	502	1.6%	2.3%	2.7%
Combination Chest CT Scan	346	7.8%	1.6%	2.7%
Follow-up Mammogram/Ultrasound	1,373	5.4%	7.7%	8.8%
Lumbar Spine MRI for Low Back Pain	67	25.4%	35.3%	37.2%

Stafford Hospital

101 Hospital Center Boulevard, Suite 307
Stafford, VA 22554
Phone: 540-741-9000
URL: www.marywashingtonhealthcare.com
Type: Acute Care Hospitals
Emergency Services: Yes
Ownership: Voluntary non-profit - Private
Beds: 100

Key Personnel:
Chief of Medical Staff. . . . . Rebecca Bigoney
CEO/President. . . . . Fred M. Rankin

Measure	Cases	This Hosp.	State Avg.	U.S. Avg.
Blood Clot Prevention and Treatment				
Anticoagulation Overlap Therapy[2]	59	100%	95%	93%
ICU Venous Thromboembolism Prophylaxis[2]	46	98%	95%	92%
Incidence of Potentially Preventable VTE[1,2]	-	-	8%	10%
UFH with Dosages/Platelet Monitoring[1,2]	-	-	99%	97%
Venous Thromboembolism Prophylaxis[2]	312	100%	91%	85%
Warfarin Therapy Discharge Instructions[2]	48	15%	78%	75%
Chest Pain/Possible Heart Attack Care				
Aspirin Given Within 24 Hours of Arrival	35	94%	98%	96%
Fibrinolytic Meds Within 30 Min. of Arrival[7]	-	-	68%	58%
Average Time to ECG (minutes)	36	9	7	7
Average Time to Transfer (minutes)[1]	-	-	64	60
Children's Asthma Care				
Received Home Management Plan of Care	-	-	-	88%
Received Reliever Medication	-	-	-	100%
Received Systemic Corticosteroids	-	-	-	100%
Emergency Department				
Admittance Decision Time (minutes)[2]	539	85	96	98
Head CT Results Within 45 Min. of Arrival[1]	-	-	60%	57%
Patients Who Left ER Before Being Seen	34,283	1%	2%	2%
Time from ER Arrival to Admit. (minutes)[2]	540	257	280	274
Time from ER Arrival to Discharge (minutes)	395	136	167	134
Time in ER Before Being Evaluated (minutes)	336	24	35	26
Time to Pain Meds for Fractures (minutes)	143	59	56	57
Heart Attack Care				

NOTE: Hospital profiles are in alphabetical order by state, then city, then hospital within the city; Rankings exclude hospitals with less than 25 cases except for patient surveys which excludes hospitals with less than 100 cases; (a) 100-299 cases; (1) The number of cases/patients is too few to report; (2) Data submitted were based on a sample of cases/patients; (3) Results are based on a shorter time period than required; (4) Data suppressed by CMS for one or more quarters; (5) Results are not available for this reporting period; (6) Fewer than 100 patients completed the HCAHPS survey; (7) No cases met the criteria for this measure; (8) The lower limit of the confidence interval cannot be calculated if the number of observed infections equals zero; (9) No data are available from the state/territory for this reporting period; (10) The scores shown reflect fewer than 50 completed surveys; (11) There were discrepancies in the data collection process; (12) This measure does not apply to this hospital for this reporting period; (13) Results cannot be calculated for this reporting period; (14) The results for this state are combined with nearby states to protect confidentiality; Please refer to the User's Guide for a full explanation of data.

Measure	Cases	This Hosp.	State Avg.	U.S. Avg.
Aspirin Given at Discharge	25	100%	99%	99%
Fibrinolytic Meds Within 30 Min. of Arrival[7]	-	-	75%	54%
PCI Within 90 Minutes of Arrival[7]	-	-	97%	96%
Statin Prescribed at Discharge	23	100%	99%	98%
Heart Failure Care				
ACE Inhibitor or ARB for LVSD	31	100%	98%	97%
Discharge Instructions Given	95	97%	95%	94%
Evaluation of LVS Function	102	99%	100%	99%
Medicare Spending				
Medicare Spending per Patient (ratio)	-	0.96	0.95	0.98
Pneumonia Care				
Appropriate Initial Antibiotic Given	86	100%	97%	95%
Blood Culture Timing	104	100%	98%	98%
Pregnancy and Delivery Care				
Newborn Deliveries Scheduled Early	51	10%	6%	6%
Preventive Care				
Immunization for Influenza[2]	360	79%	92%	90%
Immunization for Pneumonia[2]	374	93%	93%	92%
Stroke Care				
Anticoagulation Therapy for Atrial Fibrillation[1]	-	-	96%	95%
Antithrombotic Therapy Timing	25	100%	99%	98%
Assessed for Rehabilitation	26	96%	99%	97%
Discharged on Antithrombotic Therapy	25	100%	100%	99%
Discharged on Statin Medication	21	95%	97%	94%
Thrombolytic Therapy Timing[1]	-	-	73%	66%
Venous Thromboembolism Prophylaxis	23	100%	97%	94%
Written Stroke Educational Materials Given	14	100%	92%	88%
Surgical Care Improvement Project				
Appropriate Beta Blocker Usage	38	92%	99%	98%
Appropriate VTP Within 24 Hours	149	95%	99%	98%
Controlled Postoperative Blood Glucose[7]	-	-	98%	97%
Perioperative Temperature Management	155	100%	100%	100%
Prophylactic Antibiotic Selection	97	99%	99%	99%
Prophylactic Antibiotic Selection (Outpatient)	106	98%	98%	98%
Prophylactic Antibiotic Stopped	95	100%	98%	98%
Prophylactic Antibiotic Timing	97	100%	99%	99%
Prophylactic Antibiotic Timing (Outpatient)	106	100%	98%	98%
Urinary Catheter Removal	114	97%	98%	97%
Survey of Patients' Hospital Experiences				
Area Around Room 'Always' Quiet at Night	300+	59%	60%	61%
Doctors 'Always' Communicated Well	300+	74%	81%	82%
Home Recovery Information Given	300+	83%	86%	85%
Hospital Given 9 or 10 on 10 Point Scale	300+	74%	68%	71%
Meds 'Always' Explained Before Given	300+	61%	62%	64%
Nurses 'Always' Communicated Well	300+	78%	78%	79%
Pain 'Always' Well Controlled	300+	69%	70%	71%
Room and Bathroom 'Always' Clean	300+	74%	71%	73%
Timely Help 'Always' Received	300+	66%	64%	68%
Would Definitely Recommend Hospital	300+	75%	69%	71%
Use of Medical Imaging				
Cardiac Imaging Stress Test before Surgery	98	6.1%	5.1%	5.3%
Combination Abdominal CT Scan	236	2.1%	8.5%	10.5%
Combination Brain/Sinus CT Scan	273	1.1%	2.3%	2.7%
Combination Chest CT Scan	71	0.0%	1.6%	2.7%
Follow-up Mammogram/Ultrasound	162	16.0%	7.7%	8.8%
Lumbar Spine MRI for Low Back Pain[1]	-	-	35.3%	37.2%

Western State Hospital

1301 Richmond Avenue
Staunton, VA 24402
Phone: 703-332-8000
Fax: 540-332-8197
Type: Acute Care Hospitals
Emergency Services: No
Ownership: Government - State
Beds: 517

Key Personnel:

Quality Assurance . . . . Kathy Belcher
Infection Control. . . . . Nancy Davis, RN
Radiology. . . . . Lucy Hanger
Chief of Medical Staff . . . . Marie Claire Smith

Measure	Cases	This Hosp.	State Avg.	U.S. Avg.
Blood Clot Prevention and Treatment				
Anticoagulation Overlap Therapy[2,3]	-	-	95%	93%
ICU Venous Thromboembolism Prophylaxis[2,3]	-	-	95%	92%
Incidence of Potentially Preventable VTE[2,3]	-	-	8%	10%
UFH with Dosages/Platelet Monitoring[2,3]	-	-	99%	97%
Venous Thromboembolism Prophylaxis[1,2]	-	-	91%	85%
Warfarin Therapy Discharge Instructions[2,3]	-	-	78%	75%
Chest Pain/Possible Heart Attack Care				
Aspirin Given Within 24 Hours of Arrival[5]	-	-	98%	96%
Fibrinolytic Meds Within 30 Min. of Arrival[5]	-	-	68%	58%
Average Time to ECG (minutes)[5]	-	-	7	7
Average Time to Transfer (minutes)[5]	-	-	64	60
Children's Asthma Care				
Received Home Management Plan of Care	-	-	-	88%
Received Reliever Medication	-	-	-	100%
Received Systemic Corticosteroids	-	-	-	100%
Emergency Department				
Admittance Decision Time (minutes)[2,3]	-	-	96	98
Head CT Results Within 45 Min. of Arrival[5]	-	-	60%	57%
Patients Who Left ER Before Being Seen[5]	-	-	2%	2%
Time from ER Arrival to Admit. (minutes)[2,3]	-	-	280	274
Time from ER Arrival to Discharge (minutes)[5]	-	-	167	134
Time in ER Before Being Evaluated (minutes)[5]	-	-	35	26
Time to Pain Meds for Fractures (minutes)[5]	-	-	56	57
Heart Attack Care				
Aspirin Given at Discharge[5]	-	-	99%	99%
Fibrinolytic Meds Within 30 Min. of Arrival[5]	-	-	75%	54%
PCI Within 90 Minutes of Arrival[5]	-	-	97%	96%
Statin Prescribed at Discharge[5]	-	-	99%	98%
Heart Failure Care				
ACE Inhibitor or ARB for LVSD[5]	-	-	98%	97%
Discharge Instructions Given[5]	-	-	95%	94%
Evaluation of LVS Function[5]	-	-	100%	99%
Medicare Spending				
Medicare Spending per Patient (ratio)	-	-	0.95	0.98
Pneumonia Care				
Appropriate Initial Antibiotic Given[5]	-	-	97%	95%
Blood Culture Timing[5]	-	-	98%	98%
Pregnancy and Delivery Care				
Newborn Deliveries Scheduled Early[7]	-	-	6%	6%
Preventive Care				
Immunization for Influenza[1,2]	-	-	92%	90%
Immunization for Pneumonia[1,2]	-	-	93%	92%
Stroke Care				
Anticoagulation Therapy for Atrial Fibrillation[5]	-	-	96%	95%
Antithrombotic Therapy Timing[5]	-	-	99%	98%
Assessed for Rehabilitation[5]	-	-	99%	97%
Discharged on Antithrombotic Therapy[5]	-	-	100%	99%
Discharged on Statin Medication[5]	-	-	97%	94%
Thrombolytic Therapy Timing[5]	-	-	73%	66%
Venous Thromboembolism Prophylaxis[5]	-	-	97%	94%
Written Stroke Educational Materials Given[5]	-	-	92%	88%
Surgical Care Improvement Project				
Appropriate Beta Blocker Usage[5]	-	-	99%	98%
Appropriate VTP Within 24 Hours[5]	-	-	99%	98%
Controlled Postoperative Blood Glucose[5]	-	-	98%	97%
Perioperative Temperature Management[5]	-	-	100%	100%
Prophylactic Antibiotic Selection[5]	-	-	99%	99%
Prophylactic Antibiotic Selection (Outpatient)[5]	-	-	98%	98%
Prophylactic Antibiotic Stopped[5]	-	-	98%	98%
Prophylactic Antibiotic Timing[5]	-	-	99%	99%
Prophylactic Antibiotic Timing (Outpatient)[5]	-	-	98%	98%
Urinary Catheter Removal[5]	-	-	98%	97%
Survey of Patients' Hospital Experiences				
Area Around Room 'Always' Quiet at Night[1]	-	-	60%	61%
Doctors 'Always' Communicated Well[1]	-	-	81%	82%
Home Recovery Information Given[1]	-	-	86%	85%
Hospital Given 9 or 10 on 10 Point Scale[1]	-	-	68%	71%
Meds 'Always' Explained Before Given[1]	-	-	62%	64%
Nurses 'Always' Communicated Well[1]	-	-	78%	79%
Pain 'Always' Well Controlled[1]	-	-	70%	71%
Room and Bathroom 'Always' Clean[1]	-	-	71%	73%
Timely Help 'Always' Received[1]	-	-	64%	68%
Would Definitely Recommend Hospital[1]	-	-	69%	71%
Use of Medical Imaging				
Cardiac Imaging Stress Test before Surgery[7]	-	-	5.1%	5.3%
Combination Abdominal CT Scan[7]	-	-	8.5%	10.5%
Combination Brain/Sinus CT Scan[7]	-	-	2.3%	2.7%
Combination Chest CT Scan[7]	-	-	1.6%	2.7%
Follow-up Mammogram/Ultrasound[7]	-	-	7.7%	8.8%
Lumbar Spine MRI for Low Back Pain[7]	-	-	35.3%	37.2%

Pioneer Health Services of Patrick County

18688 Jeb Stuart Highway
Stuart, VA 24171
Phone: 276-694-3151
Fax: 276-694-8655
URL: www.rjrhospital.com
Type: Critical Access Hospitals
Emergency Services: Yes
Ownership: Proprietary
Beds: 50

Key Personnel:

Chief of Medical Staff . . . . Richard Cole
Emergency Room . . . . Cindy Fain
Operating Room. . . . . Sandy Rhodes
CEO/President. . . . . Janice Wilkins, RN, BSN

Measure	Cases	This Hosp.	State Avg.	U.S. Avg.
Blood Clot Prevention and Treatment				
Anticoagulation Overlap Therapy[5]	-	-	95%	93%
ICU Venous Thromboembolism Prophylaxis[5]	-	-	95%	92%
Incidence of Potentially Preventable VTE[5]	-	-	8%	10%
UFH with Dosages/Platelet Monitoring[5]	-	-	99%	97%
Venous Thromboembolism Prophylaxis[5]	-	-	91%	85%
Warfarin Therapy Discharge Instructions[5]	-	-	78%	75%
Chest Pain/Possible Heart Attack Care				
Aspirin Given Within 24 Hours of Arrival[1,3]	-	-	98%	96%
Fibrinolytic Meds Within 30 Min. of Arrival[3,7]	-	-	68%	58%
Average Time to ECG (minutes)[1,3]	-	-	7	7
Average Time to Transfer (minutes)[3,7]	-	-	64	60
Children's Asthma Care				
Received Home Management Plan of Care	-	-	-	88%
Received Reliever Medication	-	-	-	100%
Received Systemic Corticosteroids	-	-	-	100%
Emergency Department				
Admittance Decision Time (minutes)[5]	-	-	96	98
Head CT Results Within 45 Min. of Arrival[3,7]	-	-	60%	57%
Patients Who Left ER Before Being Seen	5,105	1%	2%	2%
Time from ER Arrival to Admit. (minutes)[5]	-	-	280	274
Time from ER Arrival to Discharge (minutes)[5]	-	-	167	134
Time in ER Before Being Evaluated (minutes)[5]	-	-	35	26
Time to Pain Meds for Fractures (minutes)[1,3]	-	-	56	57
Heart Attack Care				
Aspirin Given at Discharge[5]	-	-	99%	99%
Fibrinolytic Meds Within 30 Min. of Arrival[5]	-	-	75%	54%
PCI Within 90 Minutes of Arrival[5]	-	-	97%	96%
Statin Prescribed at Discharge[5]	-	-	99%	98%
Heart Failure Care				
ACE Inhibitor or ARB for LVSD[1]	-	-	98%	97%
Discharge Instructions Given[1]	-	-	95%	94%
Evaluation of LVS Function[1]	-	-	100%	99%
Medicare Spending				
Medicare Spending per Patient (ratio)	-	-	0.95	0.98
Pneumonia Care				
Appropriate Initial Antibiotic Given	38	84%	97%	95%
Blood Culture Timing	45	96%	98%	98%
Pregnancy and Delivery Care				
Newborn Deliveries Scheduled Early[5]	-	-	6%	6%
Preventive Care				
Immunization for Influenza[5]	-	-	92%	90%
Immunization for Pneumonia[5]	-	-	93%	92%
Stroke Care				
Anticoagulation Therapy for Atrial Fibrillation[5]	-	-	96%	95%
Antithrombotic Therapy Timing[5]	-	-	99%	98%
Assessed for Rehabilitation[5]	-	-	99%	97%
Discharged on Antithrombotic Therapy[5]	-	-	100%	99%
Discharged on Statin Medication[5]	-	-	97%	94%
Thrombolytic Therapy Timing[5]	-	-	73%	66%
Venous Thromboembolism Prophylaxis[5]	-	-	97%	94%
Written Stroke Educational Materials Given[5]	-	-	92%	88%
Surgical Care Improvement Project				
Appropriate Beta Blocker Usage[5]	-	-	99%	98%
Appropriate VTP Within 24 Hours[5]	-	-	99%	98%
Controlled Postoperative Blood Glucose[5]	-	-	98%	97%

NOTE: Hospital profiles are in alphabetical order by state, then city, then hospital within the city; Rankings exclude hospitals with less than 25 cases except for patient surveys which excludes hospitals with less than 100 cases; (a) 100-299 cases; (1) The number of cases/patients is too few to report; (2) Data submitted were based on a sample of cases/patients; (3) Results are based on a shorter time period than required; (4) Data suppressed by CMS for one or more quarters; (5) Results are not available for this reporting period; (6) Fewer than 100 patients completed the HCAHPS survey; (7) No cases met the criteria for this measure; (8) The lower limit of the confidence interval cannot be calculated if the number of observed infections equals zero; (9) No data are available from the state/territory for this reporting period; (10) The scores shown reflect fewer than 50 completed surveys; (11) There were discrepancies in the data collection process; (12) This measure does not apply to this hospital for this reporting period; (13) Results cannot be calculated for this reporting period; (14) The results for this state are combined with nearby states to protect confidentiality; Please refer to the User's Guide for a full explanation of data.

Measure	Cases	This Hosp.	State Avg.	U.S. Avg.
Perioperative Temperature Management[5]	-	-	100%	100%
Prophylactic Antibiotic Selection[5]	-	-	99%	99%
Prophylactic Antibiotic Selection (Outpatient)[5]	-	-	98%	98%
Prophylactic Antibiotic Stopped[5]	-	-	98%	98%
Prophylactic Antibiotic Timing[5]	-	-	99%	99%
Prophylactic Antibiotic Timing (Outpatient)[5]	-	-	98%	98%
Urinary Catheter Removal[5]	-	-	98%	97%
Survey of Patients' Hospital Experiences				
Area Around Room 'Always' Quiet at Night[5]	-	-	60%	61%
Doctors 'Always' Communicated Well[5]	-	-	81%	82%
Home Recovery Information Given[5]	-	-	86%	85%
Hospital Given 9 or 10 on 10 Point Scale[5]	-	-	68%	71%
Meds 'Always' Explained Before Given[5]	-	-	62%	64%
Nurses 'Always' Communicated Well[5]	-	-	78%	79%
Pain 'Always' Well Controlled[5]	-	-	70%	71%
Room and Bathroom 'Always' Clean[5]	-	-	71%	73%
Timely Help 'Always' Received[5]	-	-	64%	68%
Would Definitely Recommend Hospital[5]	-	-	69%	71%
Use of Medical Imaging				
Cardiac Imaging Stress Test before Surgery[7]	-	-	5.1%	5.3%
Combination Abdominal CT Scan	115	6.1%	8.5%	10.5%
Combination Brain/Sinus CT Scan[1]	-	-	2.3%	2.7%
Combination Chest CT Scan[1]	-	-	1.6%	2.7%
Follow-up Mammogram/Ultrasound[7]	-	-	7.7%	8.8%
Lumbar Spine MRI for Low Back Pain[7]	-	-	35.3%	37.2%

Sentara Obici Hospital

2800 Godwin Boulevard
Suffolk, VA 23439
URL: www.sentara.com
Type: Acute Care Hospitals
Ownership: Voluntary non-profit - Other
Phone: 757-934-4000
Fax: 757-455-7155
Emergency Services: Yes
Beds: 150

Key Personnel:
Radiology. Gail Byrd
Coronary Care . . . . Theresa Godfrey
Quality Assurance . . . . Amanda Goodwin
Infection Control. . . . . Tammy Irving
CEO/President. . . . . Howard P Kern
Pediatric Ambulatory Care . . . . . . K Sankaran
Pediatric In-Patient Care . . . . K Sankaran
Chief of Medical Staff. . . . . Gary R Yates, MD

Measure	Cases	This Hosp.	State Avg.	U.S. Avg.
Blood Clot Prevention and Treatment				
Anticoagulation Overlap Therapy[2]	56	100%	95%	93%
ICU Venous Thromboembolism Prophylaxis[2]	60	100%	95%	92%
Incidence of Potentially Preventable VTE[2]	17	0%	8%	10%
UFH with Dosages/Platelet Monitoring[2]	63	100%	99%	97%
Venous Thromboembolism Prophylaxis[2]	379	91%	91%	85%
Warfarin Therapy Discharge Instructions[2]	32	97%	78%	75%
Chest Pain/Possible Heart Attack Care				
Aspirin Given Within 24 Hours of Arrival	53	100%	98%	96%
Fibrinolytic Meds Within 30 Min. of Arrival[7]	-	-	68%	58%
Average Time to ECG (minutes)	52	6	7	7
Average Time to Transfer (minutes)[7]	-	-	64	60
Children's Asthma Care				
Received Home Management Plan of Care	-	-	-	88%
Received Reliever Medication	-	-	-	100%
Received Systemic Corticosteroids	-	-	-	100%
Emergency Department				
Admittance Decision Time (minutes)[2]	687	89	96	98
Head CT Results Within 45 Min. of Arrival	14	79%	60%	57%
Patients Who Left ER Before Being Seen	74,968	1%	2%	2%
Time from ER Arrival to Admit. (minutes)[2]	691	294	280	274
Time from ER Arrival to Discharge (minutes)	6,172	163	167	134
Time in ER Before Being Evaluated (minutes)	6,497	35	35	26
Time to Pain Meds for Fractures (minutes)	118	62	56	57
Heart Attack Care				
Aspirin Given at Discharge	55	100%	99%	99%
Fibrinolytic Meds Within 30 Min. of Arrival[7]	-	-	75%	54%
PCI Within 90 Minutes of Arrival[7]	-	-	97%	96%
Statin Prescribed at Discharge	50	98%	99%	98%
Heart Failure Care				
ACE Inhibitor or ARB for LVSD	108	97%	98%	97%
Discharge Instructions Given	303	95%	95%	94%
Evaluation of LVS Function	369	100%	100%	99%
Medicare Spending				
Medicare Spending per Patient (ratio)	-	0.97	0.95	0.98
Pneumonia Care				
Appropriate Initial Antibiotic Given	90	99%	97%	95%
Blood Culture Timing	177	97%	98%	98%
Pregnancy and Delivery Care				
Newborn Deliveries Scheduled Early	128	0%	6%	6%
Preventive Care				
Immunization for Influenza[2]	534	91%	92%	90%
Immunization for Pneumonia[2]	695	95%	93%	92%
Stroke Care				
Anticoagulation Therapy for Atrial Fibrillation	13	100%	96%	95%
Antithrombotic Therapy Timing	136	100%	99%	98%
Assessed for Rehabilitation	146	100%	99%	97%
Discharged on Antithrombotic Therapy	144	99%	100%	99%
Discharged on Statin Medication	114	100%	97%	94%
Thrombolytic Therapy Timing[1]	-	-	73%	66%
Venous Thromboembolism Prophylaxis	139	95%	97%	94%
Written Stroke Educational Materials Given	94	99%	92%	88%
Surgical Care Improvement Project				
Appropriate Beta Blocker Usage[2]	151	98%	99%	98%
Appropriate VTP Within 24 Hours[2]	416	100%	99%	98%
Controlled Postoperative Blood Glucose[2,7]	-	-	98%	97%
Perioperative Temperature Management[2]	501	100%	100%	100%
Prophylactic Antibiotic Selection[2]	363	99%	99%	99%
Prophylactic Antibiotic Selection (Outpatient)	196	99%	98%	98%
Prophylactic Antibiotic Stopped[2]	357	98%	98%	98%
Prophylactic Antibiotic Timing[2]	363	100%	99%	99%
Prophylactic Antibiotic Timing (Outpatient)	196	99%	98%	98%
Urinary Catheter Removal[2]	143	96%	98%	97%
Survey of Patients' Hospital Experiences				
Area Around Room 'Always' Quiet at Night	300+	67%	60%	61%
Doctors 'Always' Communicated Well	300+	85%	81%	82%
Home Recovery Information Given	300+	88%	86%	85%
Hospital Given 9 or 10 on 10 Point Scale	300+	77%	68%	71%
Meds 'Always' Explained Before Given	300+	65%	62%	64%
Nurses 'Always' Communicated Well	300+	84%	78%	79%
Pain 'Always' Well Controlled	300+	74%	70%	71%
Room and Bathroom 'Always' Clean	300+	75%	71%	73%
Timely Help 'Always' Received	300+	74%	64%	68%
Would Definitely Recommend Hospital	300+	75%	69%	71%
Use of Medical Imaging				
Cardiac Imaging Stress Test before Surgery	292	5.5%	5.1%	5.3%
Combination Abdominal CT Scan	1,385	4.5%	8.5%	10.5%
Combination Brain/Sinus CT Scan	1,251	3.8%	2.3%	2.7%
Combination Chest CT Scan	607	0.5%	1.6%	2.7%
Follow-up Mammogram/Ultrasound	1,831	9.0%	7.7%	8.8%
Lumbar Spine MRI for Low Back Pain	129	36.4%	35.3%	37.2%

Riverside Tappahannock Hospital

618 Hospital Road
Tappahannock, VA 22560
Type: Acute Care Hospitals
Ownership: Voluntary non-profit - Private
Phone: 804-443-6189
Fax: 804-443-6004
Emergency Services: Yes
Beds: 92

Key Personnel:
Radiology. . . . . Elizabeth L Abell
Emergency Room . . . . Shafqat H Ashai, ENP
Chief of Medical Staff. . . . . James R Dudley, MD
Quality Assurance . . . . Jodi Friend
CEO/President. . . . . Elizabeth J Martin
Infection Control. . . . . Donna Tigor
Operating Room. . . . . Terri Willaford

Measure	Cases	This Hosp.	State Avg.	U.S. Avg.
Blood Clot Prevention and Treatment				
Anticoagulation Overlap Therapy[1,2]	-	-	95%	93%
ICU Venous Thromboembolism Prophylaxis[2]	92	100%	95%	92%
Incidence of Potentially Preventable VTE[2,7]	-	-	8%	10%
UFH with Dosages/Platelet Monitoring[2,7]	-	-	99%	97%
Venous Thromboembolism Prophylaxis[2]	234	100%	91%	85%
Warfarin Therapy Discharge Instructions[1,2]	-	-	78%	75%
Chest Pain/Possible Heart Attack Care				
Aspirin Given Within 24 Hours of Arrival	44	100%	98%	96%
Fibrinolytic Meds Within 30 Min. of Arrival[7]	-	-	68%	58%
Average Time to ECG (minutes)	44	7	7	7
Average Time to Transfer (minutes)[1]	-	-	64	60
Children's Asthma Care				
Received Home Management Plan of Care	-	-	-	88%
Received Reliever Medication	-	-	-	100%
Received Systemic Corticosteroids	-	-	-	100%
Emergency Department				
Admittance Decision Time (minutes)[2]	532	110	96	98
Head CT Results Within 45 Min. of Arrival[1]	-	-	60%	57%
Patients Who Left ER Before Being Seen	19,508	1%	2%	2%
Time from ER Arrival to Admit. (minutes)[2]	533	298	280	274
Time from ER Arrival to Discharge (minutes)	359	122	167	134
Time in ER Before Being Evaluated (minutes)	382	40	35	26
Time to Pain Meds for Fractures (minutes)	75	52	56	57
Heart Attack Care				
Aspirin Given at Discharge	15	100%	99%	99%
Fibrinolytic Meds Within 30 Min. of Arrival[7]	-	-	75%	54%
PCI Within 90 Minutes of Arrival[7]	-	-	97%	96%
Statin Prescribed at Discharge	14	100%	99%	98%
Heart Failure Care				
ACE Inhibitor or ARB for LVSD	24	100%	98%	97%
Discharge Instructions Given	67	100%	95%	94%
Evaluation of LVS Function	86	100%	100%	99%
Medicare Spending				
Medicare Spending per Patient (ratio)	-	0.89	0.95	0.98
Pneumonia Care				
Appropriate Initial Antibiotic Given	66	100%	97%	95%
Blood Culture Timing	98	99%	98%	98%
Pregnancy and Delivery Care				
Newborn Deliveries Scheduled Early[7]	-	-	6%	6%
Preventive Care				
Immunization for Influenza[2]	290	99%	92%	90%
Immunization for Pneumonia[2]	477	100%	93%	92%
Stroke Care				
Anticoagulation Therapy for Atrial Fibrillation[1]	-	-	96%	95%
Antithrombotic Therapy Timing	17	100%	99%	98%
Assessed for Rehabilitation	20	100%	99%	97%
Discharged on Antithrombotic Therapy	20	100%	100%	99%
Discharged on Statin Medication	18	100%	97%	94%
Thrombolytic Therapy Timing[7]	-	-	73%	66%
Venous Thromboembolism Prophylaxis	17	100%	97%	94%
Written Stroke Educational Materials Given	13	100%	92%	88%
Surgical Care Improvement Project				
Appropriate Beta Blocker Usage	48	100%	99%	98%
Appropriate VTP Within 24 Hours	150	100%	99%	98%
Controlled Postoperative Blood Glucose[7]	-	-	98%	97%
Perioperative Temperature Management	159	100%	100%	100%
Prophylactic Antibiotic Selection	131	100%	99%	99%
Prophylactic Antibiotic Selection (Outpatient)	45	93%	98%	98%
Prophylactic Antibiotic Stopped	129	100%	98%	98%
Prophylactic Antibiotic Timing	131	100%	99%	99%
Prophylactic Antibiotic Timing (Outpatient)	15	87%	98%	98%
Urinary Catheter Removal	55	100%	98%	97%
Survey of Patients' Hospital Experiences				
Area Around Room 'Always' Quiet at Night	300+	59%	60%	61%
Doctors 'Always' Communicated Well	300+	85%	81%	82%
Home Recovery Information Given	300+	88%	86%	85%
Hospital Given 9 or 10 on 10 Point Scale	300+	65%	68%	71%
Meds 'Always' Explained Before Given	300+	63%	62%	64%
Nurses 'Always' Communicated Well	300+	83%	78%	79%
Pain 'Always' Well Controlled	300+	71%	70%	71%
Room and Bathroom 'Always' Clean	300+	74%	71%	73%
Timely Help 'Always' Received	300+	76%	64%	68%
Would Definitely Recommend Hospital	300+	66%	69%	71%
Use of Medical Imaging				
Cardiac Imaging Stress Test before Surgery	249	3.6%	5.1%	5.3%
Combination Abdominal CT Scan	455	9.7%	8.5%	10.5%
Combination Brain/Sinus CT Scan	361	1.7%	2.3%	2.7%
Combination Chest CT Scan	289	0.0%	1.6%	2.7%
Follow-up Mammogram/Ultrasound	836	2.3%	7.7%	8.8%
Lumbar Spine MRI for Low Back Pain	47	36.2%	35.3%	37.2%

NOTE: Hospital profiles are in alphabetical order by state, then city, then hospital within the city; Rankings exclude hospitals with less than 25 cases except for patient surveys which excludes hospitals with less than 100 cases; (a) 100-299 cases; (1) The number of cases/patients is too few to report; (2) Data submitted were based on a sample of cases/patients; (3) Results are based on a shorter time period than required; (4) Data suppressed by CMS for one or more quarters; (5) Results are not available for this reporting period; (6) Fewer than 100 patients completed the HCAHPS survey; (7) No cases met the criteria for this measure; (8) The lower limit of the confidence interval cannot be calculated if the number of observed infections equals zero; (9) No data are available from the state/territory for this reporting period; (10) The scores shown reflect fewer than 50 completed surveys; (11) There were discrepancies in the data collection process; (12) This measure does not apply to this hospital for this reporting period; (13) Results cannot be calculated for this reporting period; (14) The results for this state are combined with nearby states to protect confidentiality; Please refer to the User's Guide for a full explanation of data.

Carilion Tazewell Community Hospital

141 Ben Bolt Avenue Phone: 276-988-8700
Tazewell, VA 24651 Fax: 276-988-8782
URL: www.tazecommhospital.org
Type: Acute Care Hospitals Emergency Services: Yes
Ownership: Voluntary non-profit - Other Beds: 56

Key Personnel:
Anesthesiology. . . . . Alex Fernandez
Intensive Care Unit. . . . . Tanya Hess
CEO/President. . . . . Chris Wearmouth

Measure	Cases	This Hosp.	State Avg.	U.S. Avg.
Blood Clot Prevention and Treatment				
Anticoagulation Overlap Therapy[1,2]	-	-	95%	93%
ICU Venous Thromboembolism Prophylaxis[2,7]	-	-	95%	92%
Incidence of Potentially Preventable VTE[1,2]	-	-	8%	10%
UFH with Dosages/Platelet Monitoring[1,2]	-	-	99%	97%
Venous Thromboembolism Prophylaxis[2]	114	87%	91%	85%
Warfarin Therapy Discharge Instructions[1,2]	-	-	78%	75%
Chest Pain/Possible Heart Attack Care				
Aspirin Given Within 24 Hours of Arrival	70	96%	98%	96%
Fibrinolytic Meds Within 30 Min. of Arrival[1]	-	-	68%	58%
Average Time to ECG (minutes)	62	29	7	7
Average Time to Transfer (minutes)[1]	-	-	64	60
Children's Asthma Care				
Received Home Management Plan of Care	-	-	-	88%
Received Reliever Medication	-	-	-	100%
Received Systemic Corticosteroids	-	-	-	100%
Emergency Department				
Admittance Decision Time (minutes)[2]	476	44	96	98
Head CT Results Within 45 Min. of Arrival[1]	-	-	60%	57%
Patients Who Left ER Before Being Seen	11,661	4%	2%	2%
Time from ER Arrival to Admit. (minutes)[2]	488	259	280	274
Time from ER Arrival to Discharge (minutes)	323	158	167	134
Time in ER Before Being Evaluated (minutes)	342	42	35	26
Time to Pain Meds for Fractures (minutes)	43	69	56	57
Heart Attack Care				
Aspirin Given at Discharge[5]	-	-	99%	99%
Fibrinolytic Meds Within 30 Min. of Arrival[5]	-	-	75%	54%
PCI Within 90 Minutes of Arrival[5]	-	-	97%	96%
Statin Prescribed at Discharge[5]	-	-	99%	98%
Heart Failure Care				
ACE Inhibitor or ARB for LVSD[1]	-	-	98%	97%
Discharge Instructions Given	24	100%	95%	94%
Evaluation of LVS Function	33	100%	100%	99%
Medicare Spending				
Medicare Spending per Patient (ratio)	-	1.08	0.95	0.98
Pneumonia Care				
Appropriate Initial Antibiotic Given	39	97%	97%	95%
Blood Culture Timing	72	97%	98%	98%
Pregnancy and Delivery Care				
Newborn Deliveries Scheduled Early[7]	-	-	6%	6%
Preventive Care				
Immunization for Influenza[2]	270	91%	92%	90%
Immunization for Pneumonia[2]	405	95%	93%	92%
Stroke Care				
Anticoagulation Therapy for Atrial Fibrillation[7]	-	-	96%	95%
Antithrombotic Therapy Timing[1]	-	-	99%	98%
Assessed for Rehabilitation[1]	-	-	99%	97%
Discharged on Antithrombotic Therapy[1]	-	-	100%	99%
Discharged on Statin Medication[1]	-	-	97%	94%
Thrombolytic Therapy Timing[7]	-	-	73%	66%
Venous Thromboembolism Prophylaxis[1]	-	-	97%	94%
Written Stroke Educational Materials Given[1]	-	-	92%	88%
Surgical Care Improvement Project				
Appropriate Beta Blocker Usage[5]	-	-	99%	98%
Appropriate VTP Within 24 Hours[5]	-	-	99%	98%
Controlled Postoperative Blood Glucose[5]	-	-	98%	97%
Perioperative Temperature Management[5]	-	-	100%	100%
Prophylactic Antibiotic Selection[5]	-	-	99%	99%
Prophylactic Antibiotic Selection (Outpatient)[5]	-	-	98%	98%
Prophylactic Antibiotic Stopped[5]	-	-	98%	98%
Prophylactic Antibiotic Timing[5]	-	-	99%	99%
Prophylactic Antibiotic Timing (Outpatient)[5]	-	-	98%	98%
Urinary Catheter Removal[5]	-	-	98%	97%
Survey of Patients' Hospital Experiences				
Area Around Room 'Always' Quiet at Night	(a)	67%	60%	61%
Doctors 'Always' Communicated Well	(a)	86%	81%	82%
Home Recovery Information Given	(a)	86%	86%	85%
Hospital Given 9 or 10 on 10 Point Scale	(a)	65%	68%	71%
Meds 'Always' Explained Before Given	(a)	71%	62%	64%
Nurses 'Always' Communicated Well	(a)	80%	78%	79%
Pain 'Always' Well Controlled	(a)	80%	70%	71%
Room and Bathroom 'Always' Clean	(a)	76%	71%	73%
Timely Help 'Always' Received	(a)	74%	64%	68%
Would Definitely Recommend Hospital	(a)	67%	69%	71%
Use of Medical Imaging				
Cardiac Imaging Stress Test before Surgery[7]	-	-	5.1%	5.3%
Combination Abdominal CT Scan	193	7.8%	8.5%	10.5%
Combination Brain/Sinus CT Scan[1]	-	-	2.3%	2.7%
Combination Chest CT Scan[1]	-	-	1.6%	2.7%
Follow-up Mammogram/Ultrasound	178	9.0%	7.7%	8.8%
Lumbar Spine MRI for Low Back Pain[1]	-	-	35.3%	37.2%

Sentara Princess Anne Hospital

2025 Glenn Mitchell Drive Phone: 757-507-1520
Virginia Beach, VA 23456 Fax: 757-363-6650
URL: www.sentara.com
Type: Acute Care Hospitals Emergency Services: Yes
Ownership: Voluntary non-profit - Other Beds: 158

Key Personnel:
Quality Assurance . . . . Sam Byrd
Operating Room. . . . . Thomas G Clifford Jr
CEO/President. . . . . Mark Gaven
Emergency Room . . . . Su Harvell

Measure	Cases	This Hosp.	State Avg.	U.S. Avg.
Blood Clot Prevention and Treatment				
Anticoagulation Overlap Therapy[2]	88	100%	95%	93%
ICU Venous Thromboembolism Prophylaxis[2]	85	96%	95%	92%
Incidence of Potentially Preventable VTE[2]	22	5%	8%	10%
UFH with Dosages/Platelet Monitoring[2]	81	99%	99%	97%
Venous Thromboembolism Prophylaxis[2]	386	94%	91%	85%
Warfarin Therapy Discharge Instructions[2]	71	93%	78%	75%
Chest Pain/Possible Heart Attack Care				
Aspirin Given Within 24 Hours of Arrival	35	100%	98%	96%
Fibrinolytic Meds Within 30 Min. of Arrival[7]	-	-	68%	58%
Average Time to ECG (minutes)	36	5	7	7
Average Time to Transfer (minutes)	19	59	64	60
Children's Asthma Care				
Received Home Management Plan of Care	-	-	-	88%
Received Reliever Medication	-	-	-	100%
Received Systemic Corticosteroids	-	-	-	100%
Emergency Department				
Admittance Decision Time (minutes)[2]	649	95	96	98
Head CT Results Within 45 Min. of Arrival[1]	-	-	60%	57%
Patients Who Left ER Before Being Seen	74,620	1%	2%	2%
Time from ER Arrival to Admit. (minutes)[2]	657	314	280	274
Time from ER Arrival to Discharge (minutes)	5,914	195	167	134
Time in ER Before Being Evaluated (minutes)	6,184	58	35	26
Time to Pain Meds for Fractures (minutes)	173	56	56	57
Heart Attack Care				
Aspirin Given at Discharge	57	100%	99%	99%
Fibrinolytic Meds Within 30 Min. of Arrival[7]	-	-	75%	54%
PCI Within 90 Minutes of Arrival	12	100%	97%	96%
Statin Prescribed at Discharge	48	96%	99%	98%
Heart Failure Care				
ACE Inhibitor or ARB for LVSD	99	100%	98%	97%
Discharge Instructions Given	298	98%	95%	94%
Evaluation of LVS Function	340	100%	100%	99%
Medicare Spending				
Medicare Spending per Patient (ratio)	-	0.95	0.95	0.98
Pneumonia Care				
Appropriate Initial Antibiotic Given	162	100%	97%	95%
Blood Culture Timing	312	97%	98%	98%
Pregnancy and Delivery Care				
Newborn Deliveries Scheduled Early	178	0%	6%	6%
Preventive Care				
Immunization for Influenza[2]	489	90%	92%	90%
Immunization for Pneumonia[2]	557	93%	93%	92%
Stroke Care				
Anticoagulation Therapy for Atrial Fibrillation	11	100%	96%	95%
Antithrombotic Therapy Timing	104	100%	99%	98%
Assessed for Rehabilitation	114	100%	99%	97%
Discharged on Antithrombotic Therapy	109	100%	100%	99%
Discharged on Statin Medication	84	100%	97%	94%
Thrombolytic Therapy Timing[7]	-	-	73%	66%
Venous Thromboembolism Prophylaxis	118	98%	97%	94%
Written Stroke Educational Materials Given	72	97%	92%	88%
Surgical Care Improvement Project				
Appropriate Beta Blocker Usage[2]	78	100%	99%	98%
Appropriate VTP Within 24 Hours[2]	397	100%	99%	98%
Controlled Postoperative Blood Glucose[2,7]	-	-	98%	97%
Perioperative Temperature Management[2]	395	100%	100%	100%
Prophylactic Antibiotic Selection[2]	310	100%	99%	99%
Prophylactic Antibiotic Selection (Outpatient)	174	98%	98%	98%
Prophylactic Antibiotic Stopped[2]	310	100%	98%	98%
Prophylactic Antibiotic Timing[2]	310	99%	99%	99%
Prophylactic Antibiotic Timing (Outpatient)	175	99%	98%	98%
Urinary Catheter Removal[2]	197	98%	98%	97%
Survey of Patients' Hospital Experiences				
Area Around Room 'Always' Quiet at Night	300+	67%	60%	61%
Doctors 'Always' Communicated Well	300+	83%	81%	82%
Home Recovery Information Given	300+	91%	86%	85%
Hospital Given 9 or 10 on 10 Point Scale	300+	79%	68%	71%
Meds 'Always' Explained Before Given	300+	65%	62%	64%
Nurses 'Always' Communicated Well	300+	82%	78%	79%
Pain 'Always' Well Controlled	300+	73%	70%	71%
Room and Bathroom 'Always' Clean	300+	71%	71%	73%
Timely Help 'Always' Received	300+	67%	64%	68%
Would Definitely Recommend Hospital	300+	83%	69%	71%
Use of Medical Imaging				
Cardiac Imaging Stress Test before Surgery	491	4.5%	5.1%	5.3%
Combination Abdominal CT Scan	1,308	6.1%	8.5%	10.5%
Combination Brain/Sinus CT Scan	857	3.3%	2.3%	2.7%
Combination Chest CT Scan	1,106	0.5%	1.6%	2.7%
Follow-up Mammogram/Ultrasound	1,660	9.2%	7.7%	8.8%
Lumbar Spine MRI for Low Back Pain	146	34.2%	35.3%	37.2%

Sentara Virginia Beach General Hospital

1060 First Colonial Road Phone: 757-395-8000
Virginia Beach, VA 23454 Fax: 757-455-7964
URL: www.sentara.com
Type: Acute Care Hospitals Emergency Services: Yes
Ownership: Voluntary non-profit - Other Beds: 274

Key Personnel:
Radiology. . . . . John Arvny, MD
Emergency Room . . . . Linda Baker
CEO/President. . . . . Robert Graves
Chief of Medical Staff . . . . HC Harrison
Operating Room. . . . . R William Hoefer
Quality Assurance . . . . Deborah Pelech
Pediatric Ambulatory Care . . . . . . Glenn Snyders, MD
Pediatric In-Patient Care . . . . Glenn Snyders, MD

Measure	Cases	This Hosp.	State Avg.	U.S. Avg.
Blood Clot Prevention and Treatment				
Anticoagulation Overlap Therapy[2]	103	93%	95%	93%
ICU Venous Thromboembolism Prophylaxis[2]	56	93%	95%	92%
Incidence of Potentially Preventable VTE[2]	29	0%	8%	10%
UFH with Dosages/Platelet Monitoring[2]	129	100%	99%	97%
Venous Thromboembolism Prophylaxis[2]	386	82%	91%	85%
Warfarin Therapy Discharge Instructions[2]	64	94%	78%	75%
Chest Pain/Possible Heart Attack Care				
Aspirin Given Within 24 Hours of Arrival	37	100%	98%	96%
Fibrinolytic Meds Within 30 Min. of Arrival[3,7]	-	-	68%	58%
Average Time to ECG (minutes)	36	6	7	7
Average Time to Transfer (minutes)[1,3]	-	-	64	60
Children's Asthma Care				
Received Home Management Plan of Care	-	-	-	88%
Received Reliever Medication	-	-	-	100%
Received Systemic Corticosteroids	-	-	-	100%
Emergency Department				

NOTE: Hospital profiles are in alphabetical order by state, then city, then hospital within the city; Rankings exclude hospitals with less than 25 cases except for patient surveys which excludes hospitals with less than 100 cases; (a) 100-299 cases; (1) The number of cases/patients is too few to report; (2) Data submitted were based on a sample of cases/patients; (3) Results are based on a shorter time period than required; (4) Data suppressed by CMS for one or more quarters; (5) Results are not available for this reporting period; (6) Fewer than 100 patients completed the HCAHPS survey; (7) No cases met the criteria for this measure; (8) The lower limit of the confidence interval cannot be calculated if the number of observed infections equals zero; (9) No data are available from the state/territory for this reporting period; (10) The scores shown reflect fewer than 50 completed surveys; (11) There were discrepancies in the data collection process; (12) This measure does not apply to this hospital for this reporting period; (13) Results cannot be calculated for this reporting period; (14) The results for this state are combined with nearby states to protect confidentiality; Please refer to the User's Guide for a full explanation of data.

Measure	Cases	This Hosp.	State Avg.	U.S. Avg.
Admittance Decision Time (minutes)[2]	918	103	96	98
Head CT Results Within 45 Min. of Arrival[1]	-	-	60%	57%
Patients Who Left ER Before Being Seen	82,555	1%	2%	2%
Time from ER Arrival to Admit. (minutes)[2]	918	312	280	274
Time from ER Arrival to Discharge (minutes)	6,423	173	167	134
Time in ER Before Being Evaluated (minutes)	6,844	43	35	26
Time to Pain Meds for Fractures (minutes)	192	56	56	57
Heart Attack Care				
Aspirin Given at Discharge	291	99%	99%	99%
Fibrinolytic Meds Within 30 Min. of Arrival[1]	-	-	75%	54%
PCI Within 90 Minutes of Arrival	41	100%	97%	96%
Statin Prescribed at Discharge	288	100%	99%	98%
Heart Failure Care				
ACE Inhibitor or ARB for LVSD	129	100%	98%	97%
Discharge Instructions Given	399	99%	95%	94%
Evaluation of LVS Function	484	100%	100%	99%
Medicare Spending				
Medicare Spending per Patient (ratio)	-	0.97	0.95	0.98
Pneumonia Care				
Appropriate Initial Antibiotic Given	180	100%	97%	95%
Blood Culture Timing	404	99%	98%	98%
Pregnancy and Delivery Care				
Newborn Deliveries Scheduled Early[7]	-	-	6%	6%
Preventive Care				
Immunization for Influenza[2]	594	95%	92%	90%
Immunization for Pneumonia[2]	883	92%	93%	92%
Stroke Care				
Anticoagulation Therapy for Atrial Fibrillation	28	96%	96%	95%
Antithrombotic Therapy Timing	174	99%	99%	98%
Assessed for Rehabilitation	206	100%	99%	97%
Discharged on Antithrombotic Therapy	176	100%	100%	99%
Discharged on Statin Medication	134	99%	97%	94%
Thrombolytic Therapy Timing[1]	-	-	73%	66%
Venous Thromboembolism Prophylaxis	230	97%	97%	94%
Written Stroke Educational Materials Given	121	96%	92%	88%
Surgical Care Improvement Project				
Appropriate Beta Blocker Usage[2]	161	100%	99%	98%
Appropriate VTP Within 24 Hours[2]	612	100%	99%	98%
Controlled Postoperative Blood Glucose[2]	94	98%	98%	97%
Perioperative Temperature Management[2]	723	100%	100%	100%
Prophylactic Antibiotic Selection[2]	582	100%	99%	99%
Prophylactic Antibiotic Selection (Outpatient)	298	97%	98%	98%
Prophylactic Antibiotic Stopped[2]	579	100%	98%	98%
Prophylactic Antibiotic Timing[2]	582	100%	99%	99%
Prophylactic Antibiotic Timing (Outpatient)	301	96%	98%	98%
Urinary Catheter Removal[2]	551	99%	98%	97%
Survey of Patients' Hospital Experiences				
Area Around Room 'Always' Quiet at Night	300+	60%	60%	61%
Doctors 'Always' Communicated Well	300+	80%	81%	82%
Home Recovery Information Given	300+	90%	86%	85%
Hospital Given 9 or 10 on 10 Point Scale	300+	74%	68%	71%
Meds 'Always' Explained Before Given	300+	61%	62%	64%
Nurses 'Always' Communicated Well	300+	81%	78%	79%
Pain 'Always' Well Controlled	300+	74%	70%	71%
Room and Bathroom 'Always' Clean	300+	67%	71%	73%
Timely Help 'Always' Received	300+	68%	64%	68%
Would Definitely Recommend Hospital	300+	78%	69%	71%
Use of Medical Imaging				
Cardiac Imaging Stress Test before Surgery	460	5.7%	5.1%	5.3%
Combination Abdominal CT Scan	1,794	8.2%	8.5%	10.5%
Combination Brain/Sinus CT Scan	1,477	3.8%	2.3%	2.7%
Combination Chest CT Scan	1,333	1.3%	1.6%	2.7%
Follow-up Mammogram/Ultrasound	3,772	7.7%	7.7%	8.8%
Lumbar Spine MRI for Low Back Pain	234	32.1%	35.3%	37.2%

Fauquier Hospital

500 Hospital Drive
Warrenton, VA 20186
E-mail: referral@fauquierhospital.org
URL: www.fauquierhospital.org
Type: Acute Care Hospitals
Ownership: Voluntary non-profit - Private

Phone: 540-316-5000
Fax: 540-341-0823
Emergency Services: No
Beds: 86

Key Personnel:
CEO/President . . . . Rodger H Baker
Cardiology . . . . Keith Chu, MD
Radiology. . . . . Hasan Huq, MD
Quality Assurance . . . . Lee Laughter
Operating Room. . . . . Angela Schob
Infection Control. . . . . Dorothy Siebert, RN
Pulmonology . . . . Richard Swift
Anesthesiology. . . . . Beejal Taylor

Measure	Cases	This Hosp.	State Avg.	U.S. Avg.
Blood Clot Prevention and Treatment				
Anticoagulation Overlap Therapy[2]	62	97%	95%	93%
ICU Venous Thromboembolism Prophylaxis[2]	67	99%	95%	92%
Incidence of Potentially Preventable VTE[1,2]	-	-	8%	10%
UFH with Dosages/Platelet Monitoring[1,2]	-	-	99%	97%
Venous Thromboembolism Prophylaxis[2]	354	88%	91%	85%
Warfarin Therapy Discharge Instructions[2]	53	94%	78%	75%
Chest Pain/Possible Heart Attack Care				
Aspirin Given Within 24 Hours of Arrival	62	97%	98%	96%
Fibrinolytic Meds Within 30 Min. of Arrival[1]	-	-	68%	58%
Average Time to ECG (minutes)	65	7	7	7
Average Time to Transfer (minutes)[1]	-	-	64	60
Children's Asthma Care				
Received Home Management Plan of Care	-	-	-	88%
Received Reliever Medication	-	-	-	100%
Received Systemic Corticosteroids	-	-	-	100%
Emergency Department				
Admittance Decision Time (minutes)[2]	662	116	96	98
Head CT Results Within 45 Min. of Arrival	11	73%	60%	57%
Patients Who Left ER Before Being Seen	35,278	1%	2%	2%
Time from ER Arrival to Admit. (minutes)[2]	761	302	280	274
Time from ER Arrival to Discharge (minutes)	380	169	167	134
Time in ER Before Being Evaluated (minutes)	406	32	35	26
Time to Pain Meds for Fractures (minutes)	153	63	56	57
Heart Attack Care				
Aspirin Given at Discharge	19	100%	99%	99%
Fibrinolytic Meds Within 30 Min. of Arrival[7]	-	-	75%	54%
PCI Within 90 Minutes of Arrival[7]	-	-	97%	96%
Statin Prescribed at Discharge	18	94%	99%	98%
Heart Failure Care				
ACE Inhibitor or ARB for LVSD	34	91%	98%	97%
Discharge Instructions Given	104	92%	95%	94%
Evaluation of LVS Function	127	100%	100%	99%
Medicare Spending				
Medicare Spending per Patient (ratio)	-	0.99	0.95	0.98
Pneumonia Care				
Appropriate Initial Antibiotic Given	118	96%	97%	95%
Blood Culture Timing	213	97%	98%	98%
Pregnancy and Delivery Care				
Newborn Deliveries Scheduled Early	70	4%	6%	6%
Preventive Care				
Immunization for Influenza[2]	536	98%	92%	90%
Immunization for Pneumonia[2]	659	98%	93%	92%
Stroke Care				
Anticoagulation Therapy for Atrial Fibrillation[1]	-	-	96%	95%
Antithrombotic Therapy Timing	52	94%	99%	98%
Assessed for Rehabilitation	54	98%	99%	97%
Discharged on Antithrombotic Therapy	53	100%	100%	99%
Discharged on Statin Medication	42	93%	97%	94%
Thrombolytic Therapy Timing[1]	-	-	73%	66%
Venous Thromboembolism Prophylaxis	57	95%	97%	94%
Written Stroke Educational Materials Given	35	100%	92%	88%
Surgical Care Improvement Project				
Appropriate Beta Blocker Usage	93	99%	99%	98%
Appropriate VTP Within 24 Hours	361	98%	99%	98%
Controlled Postoperative Blood Glucose[7]	-	-	98%	97%
Perioperative Temperature Management	396	100%	100%	100%
Prophylactic Antibiotic Selection	289	99%	99%	99%
Prophylactic Antibiotic Selection (Outpatient)	94	99%	98%	98%
Prophylactic Antibiotic Stopped	285	99%	98%	98%
Prophylactic Antibiotic Timing	289	99%	99%	99%
Prophylactic Antibiotic Timing (Outpatient)	94	100%	98%	98%
Urinary Catheter Removal	301	94%	98%	97%
Survey of Patients' Hospital Experiences				
Area Around Room 'Always' Quiet at Night	300+	61%	60%	61%
Doctors 'Always' Communicated Well	300+	81%	81%	82%
Home Recovery Information Given	300+	86%	86%	85%
Hospital Given 9 or 10 on 10 Point Scale	300+	72%	68%	71%
Meds 'Always' Explained Before Given	300+	63%	62%	64%
Nurses 'Always' Communicated Well	300+	79%	78%	79%
Pain 'Always' Well Controlled	300+	69%	70%	71%
Room and Bathroom 'Always' Clean	300+	78%	71%	73%
Timely Help 'Always' Received	300+	64%	64%	68%
Would Definitely Recommend Hospital	300+	73%	69%	71%
Use of Medical Imaging				
Cardiac Imaging Stress Test before Surgery	202	5.9%	5.1%	5.3%
Combination Abdominal CT Scan	760	3.3%	8.5%	10.5%
Combination Brain/Sinus CT Scan	637	3.8%	2.3%	2.7%
Combination Chest CT Scan	427	0.0%	1.6%	2.7%
Follow-up Mammogram/Ultrasound	1,048	10.6%	7.7%	8.8%
Lumbar Spine MRI for Low Back Pain	191	36.6%	35.3%	37.2%

Eastern State Hospital

4601 Ironbound Road
Williamsburg, VA 23188
URL: www.ehs.dmhmrsas.virginia.gov
Type: Acute Care Hospitals
Ownership: Government - State

Phone: 757-253-5161
Fax: 757-253-5065
Emergency Services: No
Beds: 362

Key Personnel:
Patient Relations . . . . Willie Barnes
Infection Control. . . . . Karol Curtis, RN
CEO/President. . . . . John M Favret NHA
Quality Assurance . . . . Barbara Lambert, RN
Chief of Medical Staff . . . . Guillermo Schrader, MD
Radiology. . . . . Mary Wilson, MT

Measure	Cases	This Hosp.	State Avg.	U.S. Avg.
Blood Clot Prevention and Treatment				
Anticoagulation Overlap Therapy[2,7]	-	-	95%	93%
ICU Venous Thromboembolism Prophylaxis[2,7]	-	-	95%	92%
Incidence of Potentially Preventable VTE[2,7]	-	-	8%	10%
UFH with Dosages/Platelet Monitoring[2,7]	-	-	99%	97%
Venous Thromboembolism Prophylaxis[2]	38	11%	91%	85%
Warfarin Therapy Discharge Instructions[2,7]	-	-	78%	75%
Chest Pain/Possible Heart Attack Care				
Aspirin Given Within 24 Hours of Arrival[5]	-	-	98%	96%
Fibrinolytic Meds Within 30 Min. of Arrival[5]	-	-	68%	58%
Average Time to ECG (minutes)[5]	-	-	7	7
Average Time to Transfer (minutes)[5]	-	-	64	60
Children's Asthma Care				
Received Home Management Plan of Care	-	-	-	88%
Received Reliever Medication	-	-	-	100%
Received Systemic Corticosteroids	-	-	-	100%
Emergency Department				
Admittance Decision Time (minutes)[2,7]	-	-	96	98
Head CT Results Within 45 Min. of Arrival[5]	-	-	60%	57%
Patients Who Left ER Before Being Seen[5]	-	-	2%	2%
Time from ER Arrival to Admit. (minutes)[2,7]	-	-	280	274
Time from ER Arrival to Discharge (minutes)[5]	-	-	167	134
Time in ER Before Being Evaluated (minutes)[5]	-	-	35	26
Time to Pain Meds for Fractures (minutes)[5]	-	-	56	57
Heart Attack Care				
Aspirin Given at Discharge[5]	-	-	99%	99%
Fibrinolytic Meds Within 30 Min. of Arrival[5]	-	-	75%	54%
PCI Within 90 Minutes of Arrival[5]	-	-	97%	96%
Statin Prescribed at Discharge[5]	-	-	99%	98%
Heart Failure Care				
ACE Inhibitor or ARB for LVSD[2,3]	-	-	98%	97%
Discharge Instructions Given[2,3]	-	-	95%	94%
Evaluation of LVS Function[2,3]	-	-	100%	99%
Medicare Spending				
Medicare Spending per Patient (ratio)	-	0.66	0.95	0.98
Pneumonia Care				
Appropriate Initial Antibiotic Given[1,2]	-	-	97%	95%
Blood Culture Timing[2,7]	-	-	98%	98%
Pregnancy and Delivery Care				
Newborn Deliveries Scheduled Early[7]	-	-	6%	6%
Preventive Care				
Immunization for Influenza[2]	33	76%	92%	90%
Immunization for Pneumonia[2]	53	89%	93%	92%

NOTE: Hospital profiles are in alphabetical order by state, then city, then hospital within the city; Rankings exclude hospitals with less than 25 cases except for patient surveys which excludes hospitals with less than 100 cases; (a) 100-299 cases; (1) The number of cases/patients is too few to report; (2) Data submitted were based on a sample of cases/patients; (3) Results are based on a shorter time period than required; (4) Data suppressed by CMS for one or more quarters; (5) Results are not available for this reporting period; (6) Fewer than 100 patients completed the HCAHPS survey; (7) No cases met the criteria for this measure; (8) The lower limit of the confidence interval cannot be calculated if the number of observed infections equals zero; (9) No data are available from the state/territory for this reporting period; (10) The scores shown reflect fewer than 50 completed surveys; (11) There were discrepancies in the data collection process; (12) This measure does not apply to this hospital for this reporting period; (13) Results cannot be calculated for this reporting period; (14) The results for this state are combined with nearby states to protect confidentiality; Please refer to the User's Guide for a full explanation of data.

Stroke Care				
Anticoagulation Therapy for Atrial Fibrillation[5]	-	-	96%	95%
Antithrombotic Therapy Timing[5]	-	-	99%	98%
Assessed for Rehabilitation[5]	-	-	99%	97%
Discharged on Antithrombotic Therapy[5]	-	-	100%	99%
Discharged on Statin Medication[5]	-	-	97%	94%
Thrombolytic Therapy Timing[5]	-	-	73%	66%
Venous Thromboembolism Prophylaxis[5]	-	-	97%	94%
Written Stroke Educational Materials Given[5]	-	-	92%	88%
Surgical Care Improvement Project				
Appropriate Beta Blocker Usage[5]	-	-	99%	98%
Appropriate VTP Within 24 Hours[5]	-	-	99%	98%
Controlled Postoperative Blood Glucose[5]	-	-	98%	97%
Perioperative Temperature Management[5]	-	-	100%	100%
Prophylactic Antibiotic Selection[5]	-	-	99%	99%
Prophylactic Antibiotic Selection (Outpatient)[5]	-	-	98%	98%
Prophylactic Antibiotic Stopped[5]	-	-	98%	98%
Prophylactic Antibiotic Timing[5]	-	-	99%	99%
Prophylactic Antibiotic Timing (Outpatient)[5]	-	-	98%	98%
Urinary Catheter Removal[5]	-	-	98%	97%
Survey of Patients' Hospital Experiences				
Area Around Room 'Always' Quiet at Night[1]	-	-	60%	61%
Doctors 'Always' Communicated Well[1]	-	-	81%	82%
Home Recovery Information Given[1]	-	-	86%	85%
Hospital Given 9 or 10 on 10 Point Scale[1]	-	-	68%	71%
Meds 'Always' Explained Before Given[1]	-	-	62%	64%
Nurses 'Always' Communicated Well[1]	-	-	78%	79%
Pain 'Always' Well Controlled[1]	-	-	70%	71%
Room and Bathroom 'Always' Clean[1]	-	-	71%	73%
Timely Help 'Always' Received[1]	-	-	64%	68%
Would Definitely Recommend Hospital[1]	-	-	69%	71%
Use of Medical Imaging				
Cardiac Imaging Stress Test before Surgery[7]	-	-	5.1%	5.3%
Combination Abdominal CT Scan[7]	-	-	8.5%	10.5%
Combination Brain/Sinus CT Scan[7]	-	-	2.3%	2.7%
Combination Chest CT Scan[7]	-	-	1.6%	2.7%
Follow-up Mammogram/Ultrasound[7]	-	-	7.7%	8.8%
Lumbar Spine MRI for Low Back Pain[7]	-	-	35.3%	37.2%

Riverside Doctors' Hospital of Williamsburg

1500 Commonwealth Avenue
Williamsburg, VA 23185
Phone: 757-345-3000
Type: Acute Care Hospitals
Emergency Services: Yes
Ownership: Voluntary non-profit - Private

Measure	Cases	This Hosp.	State Avg.	U.S. Avg.
Blood Clot Prevention and Treatment				
Anticoagulation Overlap Therapy[5]	-	-	95%	93%
ICU Venous Thromboembolism Prophylaxis[5]	-	-	95%	92%
Incidence of Potentially Preventable VTE[5]	-	-	8%	10%
UFH with Dosages/Platelet Monitoring[5]	-	-	99%	97%
Venous Thromboembolism Prophylaxis[5]	-	-	91%	85%
Warfarin Therapy Discharge Instructions[5]	-	-	78%	75%
Chest Pain/Possible Heart Attack Care				
Aspirin Given Within 24 Hours of Arrival[5]	-	-	98%	96%
Fibrinolytic Meds Within 30 Min. of Arrival[5]	-	-	68%	58%
Average Time to ECG (minutes)[5]	-	-	7	7
Average Time to Transfer (minutes)[5]	-	-	64	60
Children's Asthma Care				
Received Home Management Plan of Care	-	-	-	88%
Received Reliever Medication	-	-	-	100%
Received Systemic Corticosteroids	-	-	-	100%
Emergency Department				
Admittance Decision Time (minutes)[5]	-	-	96	98
Head CT Results Within 45 Min. of Arrival[5]	-	-	60%	57%
Patients Who Left ER Before Being Seen[5]	-	-	2%	2%
Time from ER Arrival to Admit. (minutes)[5]	-	-	280	274
Time from ER Arrival to Discharge (minutes)[5]	-	-	167	134
Time in ER Before Being Evaluated (minutes)[5]	-	-	35	26
Time to Pain Meds for Fractures (minutes)[5]	-	-	56	57
Heart Attack Care				
Aspirin Given at Discharge[5]	-	-	99%	99%
Fibrinolytic Meds Within 30 Min. of Arrival[5]	-	-	75%	54%
PCI Within 90 Minutes of Arrival[5]	-	-	97%	96%
Statin Prescribed at Discharge[5]	-	-	99%	98%
Heart Failure Care				
ACE Inhibitor or ARB for LVSD[5]	-	-	98%	97%
Discharge Instructions Given[5]	-	-	95%	94%
Evaluation of LVS Function[5]	-	-	100%	99%
Medicare Spending				
Medicare Spending per Patient (ratio)	-	-	0.95	0.98
Pneumonia Care				
Appropriate Initial Antibiotic Given[5]	-	-	97%	95%
Blood Culture Timing[5]	-	-	98%	98%
Pregnancy and Delivery Care				
Newborn Deliveries Scheduled Early[5]	-	-	6%	6%
Preventive Care				
Immunization for Influenza[5]	-	-	92%	90%
Immunization for Pneumonia[5]	-	-	93%	92%
Stroke Care				
Anticoagulation Therapy for Atrial Fibrillation[5]	-	-	96%	95%
Antithrombotic Therapy Timing[5]	-	-	99%	98%
Assessed for Rehabilitation[5]	-	-	99%	97%
Discharged on Antithrombotic Therapy[5]	-	-	100%	99%
Discharged on Statin Medication[5]	-	-	97%	94%
Thrombolytic Therapy Timing[5]	-	-	73%	66%
Venous Thromboembolism Prophylaxis[5]	-	-	97%	94%
Written Stroke Educational Materials Given[5]	-	-	92%	88%
Surgical Care Improvement Project				
Appropriate Beta Blocker Usage[5]	-	-	99%	98%
Appropriate VTP Within 24 Hours[5]	-	-	99%	98%
Controlled Postoperative Blood Glucose[5]	-	-	98%	97%
Perioperative Temperature Management[5]	-	-	100%	100%
Prophylactic Antibiotic Selection[5]	-	-	99%	99%
Prophylactic Antibiotic Selection (Outpatient)[5]	-	-	98%	98%
Prophylactic Antibiotic Stopped[5]	-	-	98%	98%
Prophylactic Antibiotic Timing[5]	-	-	99%	99%
Prophylactic Antibiotic Timing (Outpatient)[5]	-	-	98%	98%
Urinary Catheter Removal[5]	-	-	98%	97%
Survey of Patients' Hospital Experiences				
Area Around Room 'Always' Quiet at Night[5]	-	-	60%	61%
Doctors 'Always' Communicated Well[5]	-	-	81%	82%
Home Recovery Information Given[5]	-	-	86%	85%
Hospital Given 9 or 10 on 10 Point Scale[5]	-	-	68%	71%
Meds 'Always' Explained Before Given[5]	-	-	62%	64%
Nurses 'Always' Communicated Well[5]	-	-	78%	79%
Pain 'Always' Well Controlled[5]	-	-	70%	71%
Room and Bathroom 'Always' Clean[5]	-	-	71%	73%
Timely Help 'Always' Received[5]	-	-	64%	68%
Would Definitely Recommend Hospital[5]	-	-	69%	71%
Use of Medical Imaging				
Cardiac Imaging Stress Test before Surgery[7]	-	-	5.1%	5.3%
Combination Abdominal CT Scan[1]	-	-	8.5%	10.5%
Combination Brain/Sinus CT Scan[1]	-	-	2.3%	2.7%
Combination Chest CT Scan[1]	-	-	1.6%	2.7%
Follow-up Mammogram/Ultrasound[7]	-	-	7.7%	8.8%
Lumbar Spine MRI for Low Back Pain[7]	-	-	35.3%	37.2%

Sentara Williamsburg Regional Medical Center

100 Sentara Circle
Williamsburg, VA 23188
Phone: 757-984-6000
Fax: 757-984-7421
URL: www.sentara.com
Type: Acute Care Hospitals
Emergency Services: Yes
Ownership: Voluntary non-profit - Private
Beds: 139
Key Personnel:
Operating Room. . . . . Linda Silver

Measure	Cases	This Hosp.	State Avg.	U.S. Avg.
Blood Clot Prevention and Treatment				
Anticoagulation Overlap Therapy[2]	95	91%	95%	93%
ICU Venous Thromboembolism Prophylaxis[2]	74	96%	95%	92%
Incidence of Potentially Preventable VTE[1,2]	-	-	8%	10%
UFH with Dosages/Platelet Monitoring[2]	50	96%	99%	97%
Venous Thromboembolism Prophylaxis[2]	354	90%	91%	85%
Warfarin Therapy Discharge Instructions[2]	75	96%	78%	75%
Chest Pain/Possible Heart Attack Care				
Aspirin Given Within 24 Hours of Arrival[1,3]	-	-	98%	96%
Fibrinolytic Meds Within 30 Min. of Arrival[3,7]	-	-	68%	58%
Average Time to ECG (minutes)[1,3]	-	-	7	7
Average Time to Transfer (minutes)[3,7]	-	-	64	60
Children's Asthma Care				
Received Home Management Plan of Care	-	-	-	88%
Received Reliever Medication	-	-	-	100%
Received Systemic Corticosteroids	-	-	-	100%
Emergency Department				
Admittance Decision Time (minutes)[2]	777	107	96	98
Head CT Results Within 45 Min. of Arrival[1]	-	-	60%	57%
Patients Who Left ER Before Being Seen	44,104	1%	2%	2%
Time from ER Arrival to Admit. (minutes)[2]	777	283	280	274
Time from ER Arrival to Discharge (minutes)	3,348	197	167	134
Time in ER Before Being Evaluated (minutes)	3,850	38	35	26
Time to Pain Meds for Fractures (minutes)	107	83	56	57
Heart Attack Care				
Aspirin Given at Discharge	103	100%	99%	99%
Fibrinolytic Meds Within 30 Min. of Arrival[7]	-	-	75%	54%
PCI Within 90 Minutes of Arrival	35	100%	97%	96%
Statin Prescribed at Discharge	101	99%	99%	98%
Heart Failure Care				
ACE Inhibitor or ARB for LVSD	78	100%	98%	97%
Discharge Instructions Given	251	99%	95%	94%
Evaluation of LVS Function	306	100%	100%	99%
Medicare Spending				
Medicare Spending per Patient (ratio)	-	0.95	0.95	0.98
Pneumonia Care				
Appropriate Initial Antibiotic Given	135	90%	97%	95%
Blood Culture Timing	181	99%	98%	98%
Pregnancy and Delivery Care				
Newborn Deliveries Scheduled Early	76	0%	6%	6%
Preventive Care				
Immunization for Influenza[2]	542	94%	92%	90%
Immunization for Pneumonia[2]	752	96%	93%	92%
Stroke Care				
Anticoagulation Therapy for Atrial Fibrillation	22	100%	96%	95%
Antithrombotic Therapy Timing	133	100%	99%	98%
Assessed for Rehabilitation	139	100%	99%	97%
Discharged on Antithrombotic Therapy	136	100%	100%	99%
Discharged on Statin Medication	104	99%	97%	94%
Thrombolytic Therapy Timing	11	100%	73%	66%
Venous Thromboembolism Prophylaxis	139	98%	97%	94%
Written Stroke Educational Materials Given	90	97%	92%	88%
Surgical Care Improvement Project				
Appropriate Beta Blocker Usage[2]	127	99%	99%	98%
Appropriate VTP Within 24 Hours[2]	375	99%	99%	98%
Controlled Postoperative Blood Glucose[2,7]	-	-	98%	97%
Perioperative Temperature Management[2]	436	100%	100%	100%
Prophylactic Antibiotic Selection[2]	283	99%	99%	99%
Prophylactic Antibiotic Selection (Outpatient)	212	86%	98%	98%
Prophylactic Antibiotic Stopped[2]	279	99%	98%	98%
Prophylactic Antibiotic Timing[2]	285	97%	99%	99%
Prophylactic Antibiotic Timing (Outpatient)	217	97%	98%	98%
Urinary Catheter Removal[2]	259	98%	98%	97%
Survey of Patients' Hospital Experiences				
Area Around Room 'Always' Quiet at Night	300+	59%	60%	61%
Doctors 'Always' Communicated Well	300+	83%	81%	82%
Home Recovery Information Given	300+	89%	86%	85%
Hospital Given 9 or 10 on 10 Point Scale	300+	77%	68%	71%
Meds 'Always' Explained Before Given	300+	66%	62%	64%
Nurses 'Always' Communicated Well	300+	81%	78%	79%
Pain 'Always' Well Controlled	300+	72%	70%	71%
Room and Bathroom 'Always' Clean	300+	73%	71%	73%
Timely Help 'Always' Received	300+	59%	64%	68%
Would Definitely Recommend Hospital	300+	81%	69%	71%
Use of Medical Imaging				
Cardiac Imaging Stress Test before Surgery	409	6.4%	5.1%	5.3%
Combination Abdominal CT Scan	1,125	7.9%	8.5%	10.5%
Combination Brain/Sinus CT Scan	848	1.5%	2.3%	2.7%
Combination Chest CT Scan	802	1.9%	1.6%	2.7%
Follow-up Mammogram/Ultrasound	3,670	8.7%	7.7%	8.8%
Lumbar Spine MRI for Low Back Pain	130	27.7%	35.3%	37.2%

NOTE: Hospital profiles are in alphabetical order by state, then city, then hospital within the city; Rankings exclude hospitals with less than 25 cases except for patient surveys which excludes hospitals with less than 100 cases; (a) 100-299 cases; (1) The number of cases/patients is too few to report; (2) Data submitted were based on a sample of cases/patients; (3) Results are based on a shorter time period than required; (4) Data suppressed by CMS for one or more quarters; (5) Results are not available for this reporting period; (6) Fewer than 100 patients completed the HCAHPS survey; (7) No cases met the criteria for this measure; (8) The lower limit of the confidence interval cannot be calculated if the number of observed infections equals zero; (9) No data are available from the state/territory for this reporting period; (10) The scores shown reflect fewer than 50 completed surveys; (11) There were discrepancies in the data collection process; (12) This measure does not apply to this hospital for this reporting period; (13) Results cannot be calculated for this reporting period; (14) The results for this state are combined with nearby states to protect confidentiality; Please refer to the User's Guide for a full explanation of data.

Winchester Medical Center

220 Campus Blvd Suite 210
Winchester, VA 22601
Phone: 540-536-8000
Fax: 540-536-8606
URL: www.valleyhealthlink.com
Type: Acute Care Hospitals
Emergency Services: Yes
Ownership: Voluntary non-profit - Private
Beds: 445

Key Personnel:
Infection Control. . . . . Jack Armstrong, MD
Emergency Room . . . . Ahmad Baray
Radiology. . . . . Namik Erdag
Chairman/CEO . . . . Thomas T. Gilpin
Operating Room. . . . . Kathleen Johnson
CEO/President. . . . . Mark H. Merrill
Chief of Medical Staff. . . . . Nicolas C. Restrepo, MD
Cardiac Laboratory. . . . . James Warner, MD

Measure	Cases	This Hosp.	State Avg.	U.S. Avg.
Blood Clot Prevention and Treatment				
Anticoagulation Overlap Therapy[2]	155	88%	95%	93%
ICU Venous Thromboembolism Prophylaxis[2]	69	88%	95%	92%
Incidence of Potentially Preventable VTE[2]	29	24%	8%	10%
UFH with Dosages/Platelet Monitoring[2]	126	100%	99%	97%
Venous Thromboembolism Prophylaxis[2]	319	89%	91%	85%
Warfarin Therapy Discharge Instructions[2]	138	78%	78%	75%
Chest Pain/Possible Heart Attack Care				
Aspirin Given Within 24 Hours of Arrival[5]	-	-	98%	96%
Fibrinolytic Meds Within 30 Min. of Arrival[5]	-	-	68%	58%
Average Time to ECG (minutes)[5]	-	-	7	7
Average Time to Transfer (minutes)[5]	-	-	64	60
Children's Asthma Care				
Received Home Management Plan of Care	-	-	-	88%
Received Reliever Medication	-	-	-	100%
Received Systemic Corticosteroids	-	-	-	100%
Emergency Department				
Admittance Decision Time (minutes)[2]	428	124	96	98
Head CT Results Within 45 Min. of Arrival[1]	-	-	60%	57%
Patients Who Left ER Before Being Seen	70,046	1%	2%	2%
Time from ER Arrival to Admit. (minutes)[2]	467	377	280	274
Time from ER Arrival to Discharge (minutes)	330	196	167	134
Time in ER Before Being Evaluated (minutes)	342	63	35	26
Time to Pain Meds for Fractures (minutes)	143	96	56	57
Heart Attack Care				
Aspirin Given at Discharge[2]	298	100%	99%	99%
Fibrinolytic Meds Within 30 Min. of Arrival[2,7]	-	-	75%	54%
PCI Within 90 Minutes of Arrival[2]	28	100%	97%	96%
Statin Prescribed at Discharge[2]	283	100%	99%	98%
Heart Failure Care				
ACE Inhibitor or ARB for LVSD[2]	103	100%	98%	97%
Discharge Instructions Given[2]	315	94%	95%	94%
Evaluation of LVS Function[2]	360	100%	100%	99%
Medicare Spending				
Medicare Spending per Patient (ratio)	-	0.95	0.95	0.98
Pneumonia Care				
Appropriate Initial Antibiotic Given[2]	98	96%	97%	95%
Blood Culture Timing[2]	154	94%	98%	98%
Pregnancy and Delivery Care				
Newborn Deliveries Scheduled Early[2]	26	4%	6%	6%
Preventive Care				
Immunization for Influenza[2]	515	90%	92%	90%
Immunization for Pneumonia[2]	691	90%	93%	92%
Stroke Care				
Anticoagulation Therapy for Atrial Fibrillation	55	93%	96%	95%
Antithrombotic Therapy Timing	251	99%	99%	98%
Assessed for Rehabilitation	308	100%	99%	97%
Discharged on Antithrombotic Therapy	287	100%	100%	99%
Discharged on Statin Medication	226	99%	97%	94%
Thrombolytic Therapy Timing	19	84%	73%	66%
Venous Thromboembolism Prophylaxis	303	96%	97%	94%
Written Stroke Educational Materials Given	199	88%	92%	88%
Surgical Care Improvement Project				
Appropriate Beta Blocker Usage[2]	263	97%	99%	98%
Appropriate VTP Within 24 Hours[2]	496	98%	99%	98%
Controlled Postoperative Blood Glucose[2]	153	99%	98%	97%
Perioperative Temperature Management[2]	606	100%	100%	100%
Prophylactic Antibiotic Selection[2]	500	98%	99%	99%
Prophylactic Antibiotic Selection (Outpatient)	543	98%	98%	98%
Prophylactic Antibiotic Stopped[2]	484	96%	98%	98%
Prophylactic Antibiotic Timing[2]	507	94%	99%	99%
Prophylactic Antibiotic Timing (Outpatient)	553	94%	98%	98%
Urinary Catheter Removal[2]	338	97%	98%	97%
Survey of Patients' Hospital Experiences				
Area Around Room 'Always' Quiet at Night	300+	48%	60%	61%
Doctors 'Always' Communicated Well	300+	79%	81%	82%
Home Recovery Information Given	300+	84%	86%	85%
Hospital Given 9 or 10 on 10 Point Scale	300+	71%	68%	71%
Meds 'Always' Explained Before Given	300+	59%	62%	64%
Nurses 'Always' Communicated Well	300+	76%	78%	79%
Pain 'Always' Well Controlled	300+	72%	70%	71%
Room and Bathroom 'Always' Clean	300+	69%	71%	73%
Timely Help 'Always' Received	300+	64%	64%	68%
Would Definitely Recommend Hospital	300+	77%	69%	71%
Use of Medical Imaging				
Cardiac Imaging Stress Test before Surgery	558	3.9%	5.1%	5.3%
Combination Abdominal CT Scan	1,563	4.0%	8.5%	10.5%
Combination Brain/Sinus CT Scan	997	1.5%	2.3%	2.7%
Combination Chest CT Scan	1,054	0.3%	1.6%	2.7%
Follow-up Mammogram/Ultrasound	3,749	3.9%	7.7%	8.8%
Lumbar Spine MRI for Low Back Pain	400	37.8%	35.3%	37.2%

Sentara Northern Virginia Medical Center

2300 Opitz Boulevard
Woodbridge, VA 22191
Phone: 703-523-1000
Fax: 703-670-7643
E-mail: email@potomachospital.com
URL: www.potomachospital.com
Type: Acute Care Hospitals
Emergency Services: Yes
Ownership: Voluntary non-profit - Private
Beds: 153

Key Personnel:
Radiology. . . . . Norbertina Bans, MD
Pediatric Ambulatory Care . . . . . . William Carr, MD
Pediatric In-Patient Care . . . . William Carr, MD
Infection Control. . . . . Suzanne Davis
Operating Room. . . . . Todd Henderson
Quality Assurance . . . . Valerie Keane
CEO/President. . . . . William M Moss
Chief of Medical Staff. . . . . Bill Reha

Measure	Cases	This Hosp.	State Avg.	U.S. Avg.
Blood Clot Prevention and Treatment				
Anticoagulation Overlap Therapy[2]	64	92%	95%	93%
ICU Venous Thromboembolism Prophylaxis[2]	91	95%	95%	92%
Incidence of Potentially Preventable VTE[2]	13	0%	8%	10%
UFH with Dosages/Platelet Monitoring[2]	38	100%	99%	97%
Venous Thromboembolism Prophylaxis[2]	354	91%	91%	85%
Warfarin Therapy Discharge Instructions[2]	44	95%	78%	75%
Chest Pain/Possible Heart Attack Care				
Aspirin Given Within 24 Hours of Arrival[1,3]	-	-	98%	96%
Fibrinolytic Meds Within 30 Min. of Arrival[3,7]	-	-	68%	58%
Average Time to ECG (minutes)[1,3]	-	-	7	7
Average Time to Transfer (minutes)[1,3]	-	-	64	60
Children's Asthma Care				
Received Home Management Plan of Care	-	-	-	88%
Received Reliever Medication	-	-	-	100%
Received Systemic Corticosteroids	-	-	-	100%
Emergency Department				
Admittance Decision Time (minutes)[2]	598	149	96	98
Head CT Results Within 45 Min. of Arrival	15	60%	60%	57%
Patients Who Left ER Before Being Seen	74,293	2%	2%	2%
Time from ER Arrival to Admit. (minutes)[2]	601	344	280	274
Time from ER Arrival to Discharge (minutes)	5,753	170	167	134
Time in ER Before Being Evaluated (minutes)	6,828	40	35	26
Time to Pain Meds for Fractures (minutes)	241	55	56	57
Heart Attack Care				
Aspirin Given at Discharge	106	98%	99%	99%
Fibrinolytic Meds Within 30 Min. of Arrival[7]	-	-	75%	54%
PCI Within 90 Minutes of Arrival	18	94%	97%	96%
Statin Prescribed at Discharge	103	98%	99%	98%
Heart Failure Care				
ACE Inhibitor or ARB for LVSD	92	100%	98%	97%
Discharge Instructions Given	305	99%	95%	94%
Evaluation of LVS Function	355	100%	100%	99%
Medicare Spending				
Medicare Spending per Patient (ratio)	-	1.04	0.95	0.98
Pneumonia Care				
Appropriate Initial Antibiotic Given	137	100%	97%	95%
Blood Culture Timing	233	99%	98%	98%
Pregnancy and Delivery Care				
Newborn Deliveries Scheduled Early	149	0%	6%	6%
Preventive Care				
Immunization for Influenza[2]	516	79%	92%	90%
Immunization for Pneumonia[2]	542	80%	93%	92%
Stroke Care				
Anticoagulation Therapy for Atrial Fibrillation	17	100%	96%	95%
Antithrombotic Therapy Timing	108	100%	99%	98%
Assessed for Rehabilitation	127	100%	99%	97%
Discharged on Antithrombotic Therapy	125	100%	100%	99%
Discharged on Statin Medication	100	100%	97%	94%
Thrombolytic Therapy Timing	17	88%	73%	66%
Venous Thromboembolism Prophylaxis	127	98%	97%	94%
Written Stroke Educational Materials Given	61	97%	92%	88%
Surgical Care Improvement Project				
Appropriate Beta Blocker Usage[2]	69	99%	99%	98%
Appropriate VTP Within 24 Hours[2]	313	99%	99%	98%
Controlled Postoperative Blood Glucose[2,7]	-	-	98%	97%
Perioperative Temperature Management[2]	367	100%	100%	100%
Prophylactic Antibiotic Selection[2]	231	99%	99%	99%
Prophylactic Antibiotic Selection (Outpatient)	153	97%	98%	98%
Prophylactic Antibiotic Stopped[2]	230	97%	98%	98%
Prophylactic Antibiotic Timing[2]	235	100%	99%	99%
Prophylactic Antibiotic Timing (Outpatient)	153	99%	98%	98%
Urinary Catheter Removal[2]	151	99%	98%	97%
Survey of Patients' Hospital Experiences				
Area Around Room 'Always' Quiet at Night	300+	63%	60%	61%
Doctors 'Always' Communicated Well	300+	77%	81%	82%
Home Recovery Information Given	300+	85%	86%	85%
Hospital Given 9 or 10 on 10 Point Scale	300+	58%	68%	71%
Meds 'Always' Explained Before Given	300+	58%	62%	64%
Nurses 'Always' Communicated Well	300+	73%	78%	79%
Pain 'Always' Well Controlled	300+	70%	70%	71%
Room and Bathroom 'Always' Clean	300+	70%	71%	73%
Timely Help 'Always' Received	300+	55%	64%	68%
Would Definitely Recommend Hospital	300+	64%	69%	71%
Use of Medical Imaging				
Cardiac Imaging Stress Test before Surgery	98	6.1%	5.1%	5.3%
Combination Abdominal CT Scan	900	6.0%	8.5%	10.5%
Combination Brain/Sinus CT Scan	761	2.5%	2.3%	2.7%
Combination Chest CT Scan	475	1.1%	1.6%	2.7%
Follow-up Mammogram/Ultrasound	794	11.0%	7.7%	8.8%
Lumbar Spine MRI for Low Back Pain	105	33.3%	35.3%	37.2%

Shenandoah Memorial Hospital

759 South Main Street
Woodstock, VA 22664
Phone: 540-459-1100
Fax: 540-459-1136
E-mail: marketingmail@valleyhealthlink.com
URL: www.valleyhealthlink.com
Type: Critical Access Hospitals
Emergency Services: Yes
Ownership: Voluntary non-profit - Private
Beds: 25

Key Personnel:
CEO/President. . . . . Floyd Heater

Measure	Cases	This Hosp.	State Avg.	U.S. Avg.
Blood Clot Prevention and Treatment				
Anticoagulation Overlap Therapy[5]	-	-	95%	93%
ICU Venous Thromboembolism Prophylaxis[5]	-	-	95%	92%
Incidence of Potentially Preventable VTE[5]	-	-	8%	10%
UFH with Dosages/Platelet Monitoring[5]	-	-	99%	97%
Venous Thromboembolism Prophylaxis[5]	-	-	91%	85%
Warfarin Therapy Discharge Instructions[5]	-	-	78%	75%
Chest Pain/Possible Heart Attack Care				
Aspirin Given Within 24 Hours of Arrival[5]	-	-	98%	96%
Fibrinolytic Meds Within 30 Min. of Arrival[5]	-	-	68%	58%
Average Time to ECG (minutes)[5]	-	-	7	7
Average Time to Transfer (minutes)[5]	-	-	64	60
Children's Asthma Care				
Received Home Management Plan of Care	-	-	-	88%

NOTE: Hospital profiles are in alphabetical order by state, then city, then hospital within the city; Rankings exclude hospitals with less than 25 cases except for patient surveys which excludes hospitals with less than 100 cases; (a) 100-299 cases; (1) The number of cases/patients is too few to report; (2) Data submitted were based on a sample of cases/patients; (3) Results are based on a shorter time period than required; (4) Data suppressed by CMS for one or more quarters; (5) Results are not available for this reporting period; (6) Fewer than 100 patients completed the HCAHPS survey; (7) No cases met the criteria for this measure; (8) The lower limit of the confidence interval cannot be calculated if the number of observed infections equals zero; (9) No data are available from the state/territory for this reporting period; (10) The scores shown reflect fewer than 50 completed surveys; (11) There were discrepancies in the data collection process; (12) This measure does not apply to this hospital for this reporting period; (13) Results cannot be calculated for this reporting period; (14) The results for this state are combined with nearby states to protect confidentiality; Please refer to the User's Guide for a full explanation of data.

Measure	Cases	This Hosp.	State Avg.	U.S. Avg.
Received Reliever Medication	-	-	-	100%
Received Systemic Corticosteroids	-	-	-	100%
Emergency Department				
Admittance Decision Time (minutes)[5]	-	-	96	98
Head CT Results Within 45 Min. of Arrival[5]	-	-	60%	57%
Patients Who Left ER Before Being Seen	18,622	1%	2%	2%
Time from ER Arrival to Admit. (minutes)[5]	-	-	280	274
Time from ER Arrival to Discharge (minutes)[5]	-	-	167	134
Time in ER Before Being Evaluated (minutes)[5]	-	-	35	26
Time to Pain Meds for Fractures (minutes)[5]	-	-	56	57
Heart Attack Care				
Aspirin Given at Discharge[3,7]	-	-	99%	99%
Fibrinolytic Meds Within 30 Min. of Arrival[3,7]	-	-	75%	54%
PCI Within 90 Minutes of Arrival[3,7]	-	-	97%	96%
Statin Prescribed at Discharge[3,7]	-	-	99%	98%
Heart Failure Care				
ACE Inhibitor or ARB for LVSD[1]	-	-	98%	97%
Discharge Instructions Given	32	81%	95%	94%
Evaluation of LVS Function	44	100%	100%	99%
Medicare Spending				
Medicare Spending per Patient (ratio)	-	-	0.95	0.98
Pneumonia Care				
Appropriate Initial Antibiotic Given	96	95%	97%	95%
Blood Culture Timing	153	96%	98%	98%
Pregnancy and Delivery Care				
Newborn Deliveries Scheduled Early[5]	-	-	6%	6%
Preventive Care				
Immunization for Influenza[2,3]	140	96%	92%	90%
Immunization for Pneumonia[2,3]	335	94%	93%	92%
Stroke Care				
Anticoagulation Therapy for Atrial Fibrillation[5]	-	-	96%	95%
Antithrombotic Therapy Timing[5]	-	-	99%	98%
Assessed for Rehabilitation[5]	-	-	99%	97%
Discharged on Antithrombotic Therapy[5]	-	-	100%	99%
Discharged on Statin Medication[5]	-	-	97%	94%
Thrombolytic Therapy Timing[5]	-	-	73%	66%
Venous Thromboembolism Prophylaxis[5]	-	-	97%	94%
Written Stroke Educational Materials Given[5]	-	-	92%	88%
Surgical Care Improvement Project				
Appropriate Beta Blocker Usage	55	96%	99%	98%
Appropriate VTP Within 24 Hours	169	98%	99%	98%
Controlled Postoperative Blood Glucose[7]	-	-	98%	97%
Perioperative Temperature Management	178	99%	100%	100%
Prophylactic Antibiotic Selection	142	99%	99%	99%
Prophylactic Antibiotic Selection (Outpatient)[5]	-	-	98%	98%
Prophylactic Antibiotic Stopped	140	94%	98%	98%
Prophylactic Antibiotic Timing	142	99%	99%	99%
Prophylactic Antibiotic Timing (Outpatient)[5]	-	-	98%	98%
Urinary Catheter Removal	90	96%	98%	97%
Survey of Patients' Hospital Experiences				
Area Around Room 'Always' Quiet at Night	300+	63%	60%	61%
Doctors 'Always' Communicated Well	300+	76%	81%	82%
Home Recovery Information Given	300+	85%	86%	85%
Hospital Given 9 or 10 on 10 Point Scale	300+	66%	68%	71%
Meds 'Always' Explained Before Given	300+	67%	62%	64%
Nurses 'Always' Communicated Well	300+	79%	78%	79%
Pain 'Always' Well Controlled	300+	71%	70%	71%
Room and Bathroom 'Always' Clean	300+	85%	71%	73%
Timely Help 'Always' Received	300+	67%	64%	68%
Would Definitely Recommend Hospital	300+	64%	69%	71%
Use of Medical Imaging				
Cardiac Imaging Stress Test before Surgery	129	3.9%	5.1%	5.3%
Combination Abdominal CT Scan	543	5.9%	8.5%	10.5%
Combination Brain/Sinus CT Scan[1]	-	-	2.3%	2.7%
Combination Chest CT Scan	271	0.4%	1.6%	2.7%
Follow-up Mammogram/Ultrasound	769	5.9%	7.7%	8.8%
Lumbar Spine MRI for Low Back Pain	50	40.0%	35.3%	37.2%

Wythe County Community Hospital

600 West Ridge Road
Wytheville, VA 24382
URL: www.wcch.org
Phone: 276-228-0200
Fax: 276-228-0397
Type: Acute Care Hospitals
Emergency Services: Yes
Ownership: Voluntary non-profit - Private
Beds: 104

Key Personnel:
CEO . . . . Timothy A. Bess
Coronary Care . . . . Marsha Jones
Infection Control . . . . Becky McDonald, RN
Operating Room. . . . . Paul Morin
Radiology. . . . . Karl Ritch
Quality Assurance . . . . Carolyn Rudzinski
Chief of Medical Staff . . . . Michael Stoker, MD

Measure	Cases	This Hosp.	State Avg.	U.S. Avg.
Blood Clot Prevention and Treatment				
Anticoagulation Overlap Therapy[2]	12	92%	95%	93%
ICU Venous Thromboembolism Prophylaxis[2]	44	100%	95%	92%
Incidence of Potentially Preventable VTE[2,7]	-	-	8%	10%
UFH with Dosages/Platelet Monitoring[2,7]	-	-	99%	97%
Venous Thromboembolism Prophylaxis[2]	140	94%	91%	85%
Warfarin Therapy Discharge Instructions[2]	12	100%	78%	75%
Chest Pain/Possible Heart Attack Care				
Aspirin Given Within 24 Hours of Arrival	100	97%	98%	96%
Fibrinolytic Meds Within 30 Min. of Arrival	13	100%	68%	58%
Average Time to ECG (minutes)	102	8	7	7
Average Time to Transfer (minutes)[1]	-	-	64	60
Children's Asthma Care				
Received Home Management Plan of Care	-	-	-	88%
Received Reliever Medication	-	-	-	100%
Received Systemic Corticosteroids	-	-	-	100%
Emergency Department				
Admittance Decision Time (minutes)[2]	374	42	96	98
Head CT Results Within 45 Min. of Arrival	11	64%	60%	57%
Patients Who Left ER Before Being Seen	18,356	1%	2%	2%
Time from ER Arrival to Admit. (minutes)[2]	375	204	280	274
Time from ER Arrival to Discharge (minutes)	470	127	167	134
Time in ER Before Being Evaluated (minutes)	512	24	35	26
Time to Pain Meds for Fractures (minutes)	114	46	56	57
Heart Attack Care				
Aspirin Given at Discharge	12	100%	99%	99%
Fibrinolytic Meds Within 30 Min. of Arrival[7]	-	-	75%	54%
PCI Within 90 Minutes of Arrival[7]	-	-	97%	96%
Statin Prescribed at Discharge	12	100%	99%	98%
Heart Failure Care				
ACE Inhibitor or ARB for LVSD	22	95%	98%	97%
Discharge Instructions Given	48	98%	95%	94%
Evaluation of LVS Function	75	100%	100%	99%
Medicare Spending				
Medicare Spending per Patient (ratio)	-	0.97	0.95	0.98
Pneumonia Care				
Appropriate Initial Antibiotic Given	115	100%	97%	95%
Blood Culture Timing	168	98%	98%	98%
Pregnancy and Delivery Care				
Newborn Deliveries Scheduled Early[2]	21	0%	6%	6%
Preventive Care				
Immunization for Influenza[2]	294	99%	92%	90%
Immunization for Pneumonia[2]	364	98%	93%	92%
Stroke Care				
Anticoagulation Therapy for Atrial Fibrillation[1]	-	-	96%	95%
Antithrombotic Therapy Timing	22	100%	99%	98%
Assessed for Rehabilitation	24	100%	99%	97%
Discharged on Antithrombotic Therapy	23	100%	100%	99%
Discharged on Statin Medication	22	86%	97%	94%
Thrombolytic Therapy Timing[1]	-	-	73%	66%
Venous Thromboembolism Prophylaxis	22	91%	97%	94%
Written Stroke Educational Materials Given	11	91%	92%	88%
Surgical Care Improvement Project				
Appropriate Beta Blocker Usage	89	96%	99%	98%
Appropriate VTP Within 24 Hours	273	97%	99%	98%
Controlled Postoperative Blood Glucose[7]	-	-	98%	97%
Perioperative Temperature Management	296	100%	100%	100%
Prophylactic Antibiotic Selection	239	100%	99%	99%
Prophylactic Antibiotic Selection (Outpatient)	60	98%	98%	98%
Prophylactic Antibiotic Stopped	231	99%	98%	98%
Prophylactic Antibiotic Timing	239	99%	99%	99%
Prophylactic Antibiotic Timing (Outpatient)	60	98%	98%	98%
Urinary Catheter Removal	225	98%	98%	97%
Survey of Patients' Hospital Experiences				
Area Around Room 'Always' Quiet at Night	300+	62%	60%	61%
Doctors 'Always' Communicated Well	300+	85%	81%	82%
Home Recovery Information Given	300+	88%	86%	85%
Hospital Given 9 or 10 on 10 Point Scale	300+	71%	68%	71%
Meds 'Always' Explained Before Given	300+	67%	62%	64%
Nurses 'Always' Communicated Well	300+	82%	78%	79%
Pain 'Always' Well Controlled	300+	71%	70%	71%
Room and Bathroom 'Always' Clean	300+	73%	71%	73%
Timely Help 'Always' Received	300+	71%	64%	68%
Would Definitely Recommend Hospital	300+	65%	69%	71%
Use of Medical Imaging				
Cardiac Imaging Stress Test before Surgery[1]	-	-	5.1%	5.3%
Combination Abdominal CT Scan	546	36.1%	8.5%	10.5%
Combination Brain/Sinus CT Scan	520	2.3%	2.3%	2.7%
Combination Chest CT Scan	224	0.0%	1.6%	2.7%
Follow-up Mammogram/Ultrasound	672	12.1%	7.7%	8.8%
Lumbar Spine MRI for Low Back Pain	89	34.8%	35.3%	37.2%

NOTE: Hospital profiles are in alphabetical order by state, then city, then hospital within the city; Rankings exclude hospitals with less than 25 cases except for patient surveys which excludes hospitals with less than 100 cases; (a) 100-299 cases; (1) The number of cases/patients is too few to report; (2) Data submitted were based on a sample of cases/patients; (3) Results are based on a shorter time period than required; (4) Data suppressed by CMS for one or more quarters; (5) Results are not available for this reporting period; (6) Fewer than 100 patients completed the HCAHPS survey; (7) No cases met the criteria for this measure; (8) The lower limit of the confidence interval cannot be calculated if the number of observed infections equals zero; (9) No data are available from the state/territory for this reporting period; (10) The scores shown reflect fewer than 50 completed surveys; (11) There were discrepancies in the data collection process; (12) This measure does not apply to this hospital for this reporting period; (13) Results cannot be calculated for this reporting period; (14) The results for this state are combined with nearby states to protect confidentiality; Please refer to the User's Guide for a full explanation of data.

Blood Clot Prevention and Treatment

Anticoagulation Overlap Therapy

Hospital Name	City	Rate	Cases
Berkeley Medical Center[2]	Martinsburg	100%	60
United Hospital Center[2]	Bridgeport	100%	91
West Virginia University Hospitals[2]	Morgantown	100%	135
Bluefield Regional Medical Center[2]	Bluefield	98%	47
Raleigh General Hospital[2]	Beckley	97%	118
Saint Mary's Medical Center[2]	Huntington	97%	146
Greenbrier Valley Medical Center[2]	Ronceverte	96%	46
Charleston Area Medical Center[2]	Charleston	95%	219
Cabell Huntington Hospital[2]	Huntington	94%	105
Thomas Memorial Hospital[2]	S Charleston	92%	52
Wheeling Hospital[2]	Wheeling	90%	92
Beckley ARH Hospital[2]	Beckley	85%	40
Monongalia County General Hospital[2]	Morgantown	83%	77
Princeton Community Hospital[2]	Princeton	82%	57
Camden Clark Medical Center[2]	Parkersburg	76%	76
Logan Regional Medical Center[2]	Logan	76%	45
Weirton Medical Center[2]	Weirton	63%	60
Ohio Valley Medical Center[2]	Wheeling	54%	35

ICU Venous Thromboembolism Prophylaxis

Hospital Name	City	Rate	Cases
United Hospital Center[2]	Bridgeport	100%	52
West Virginia University Hospitals[2]	Morgantown	100%	99
Williamson Memorial Hospital[2]	Williamson	100%	32
Berkeley Medical Center[2]	Martinsburg	99%	108
Bluefield Regional Medical Center[2]	Bluefield	99%	107
Greenbrier Valley Medical Center[2]	Ronceverte	99%	142
Plateau Medical Center[2]	Oak Hill	98%	64
Logan Regional Medical Center[2]	Logan	96%	101
Ohio Valley Medical Center[2]	Wheeling	95%	92
Raleigh General Hospital[2]	Beckley	95%	94
Cabell Huntington Hospital[2]	Huntington	94%	101
Camden Clark Medical Center[2]	Parkersburg	94%	78
Saint Mary's Medical Center[2]	Huntington	94%	129
Beckley ARH Hospital[2]	Beckley	93%	96
Stonewall Jackson Memorial Hospital[2]	Weston	92%	38
Saint Francis Hospital[2]	Charleston	91%	45
Davis Memorial Hospital[2]	Elkins	90%	67
Monongalia County General Hospital[2]	Morgantown	84%	115
Thomas Memorial Hospital[2]	S Charleston	84%	51
Charleston Area Medical Center[2]	Charleston	82%	129
Fairmont General Hospital[2]	Fairmont	80%	56
Wheeling Hospital[2]	Wheeling	78%	82
Camc Teays Valley Hospital[2]	Hurricane	77%	125
Summersville Regional Medical Center[2]	Summersville	73%	44
Princeton Community Hospital[2]	Princeton	68%	100
Welch Community Hospital[2]	Welch	68%	34
Weirton Medical Center[2]	Weirton	63%	84
Reynolds Memorial Hospital[2]	Glen Dale	61%	56

Incidence of Potentially Preventable VTE

Hospital Name	City	Rate	Cases
West Virginia University Hospitals[2]	Morgantown	0%	33
Charleston Area Medical Center[2]	Charleston	5%	74
Raleigh General Hospital[2]	Beckley	17%	29

UFH with Dosages/Platelet Count Monitoring

Hospital Name	City	Rate	Cases
Berkeley Medical Center[2]	Martinsburg	100%	49
Bluefield Regional Medical Center[2]	Bluefield	100%	28
Cabell Huntington Hospital[2]	Huntington	100%	86
Logan Regional Medical Center[2]	Logan	100%	40
Saint Mary's Medical Center[2]	Huntington	100%	151
United Hospital Center[2]	Bridgeport	100%	58
West Virginia University Hospitals[2]	Morgantown	100%	129
Weirton Medical Center[2]	Weirton	98%	48
Camden Clark Medical Center[2]	Parkersburg	97%	39
Monongalia County General Hospital[2]	Morgantown	97%	64
Wheeling Hospital[2]	Wheeling	97%	59
Charleston Area Medical Center[2]	Charleston	96%	167

Venous Thromboembolism Prophylaxis

Hospital Name	City	Rate	Cases
Greenbrier Valley Medical Center[2]	Ronceverte	100%	261
United Hospital Center[2]	Bridgeport	100%	345
West Virginia University Hospitals[2]	Morgantown	100%	288
Williamson Memorial Hospital[2]	Williamson	100%	154
Berkeley Medical Center[2]	Martinsburg	98%	333
Jackson General Hospital[2]	Ripley	98%	128
Bluefield Regional Medical Center[2]	Bluefield	96%	326
Plateau Medical Center[2]	Oak Hill	96%	351
Beckley ARH Hospital[2]	Beckley	92%	413
Cabell Huntington Hospital[2]	Huntington	91%	275
Davis Memorial Hospital[2]	Elkins	91%	320
Preston Memorial Hospital[2,3]	Kingwood	91%	53
Saint Mary's Medical Center[2]	Huntington	90%	571
Saint Joseph Hospital[2]	Buckhannon	87%	76
Camden Clark Medical Center[2]	Parkersburg	86%	333
Pleasant Valley Hospital[2]	Point Pleasant	86%	97
Logan Regional Medical Center[2]	Logan	83%	377
Stonewall Jackson Memorial Hospital[2]	Weston	83%	206
Wetzel County Hospital[2]	New Martinsville	82%	107
Saint Francis Hospital[2]	Charleston	81%	240
Raleigh General Hospital[2]	Beckley	79%	422
Charleston Area Medical Center[2]	Charleston	73%	353
Thomas Memorial Hospital[2]	S Charleston	71%	344
Summersville Regional Medical Center[2]	Summersville	68%	128
Fairmont General Hospital[2]	Fairmont	66%	227
Ohio Valley Medical Center[2]	Wheeling	65%	231
Monongalia County General Hospital[2]	Morgantown	63%	301
Wheeling Hospital[2]	Wheeling	60%	400
Camc Teays Valley Hospital[2]	Hurricane	56%	499
Welch Community Hospital[2]	Welch	52%	54
Princeton Community Hospital[2]	Princeton	50%	316
Reynolds Memorial Hospital[2]	Glen Dale	45%	197
Weirton Medical Center[2]	Weirton	44%	369

Warfarin Therapy Discharge Instructions

Hospital Name	City	Rate	Cases
Greenbrier Valley Medical Center[2]	Ronceverte	100%	43
Raleigh General Hospital[2]	Beckley	100%	93
West Virginia University Hospitals[2]	Morgantown	100%	93
United Hospital Center[2]	Bridgeport	99%	74
Cabell Huntington Hospital[2]	Huntington	97%	79
Berkeley Medical Center[2]	Martinsburg	96%	47
Bluefield Regional Medical Center[2]	Bluefield	96%	27
Beckley ARH Hospital[2]	Beckley	94%	31
Logan Regional Medical Center[2]	Logan	94%	32
Wheeling Hospital[2]	Wheeling	92%	61
Monongalia County General Hospital[2]	Morgantown	89%	64
Saint Mary's Medical Center[2]	Huntington	86%	107
Princeton Community Hospital[2]	Princeton	83%	47
Weirton Medical Center[2]	Weirton	51%	39
Charleston Area Medical Center[2]	Charleston	48%	159
Thomas Memorial Hospital[2]	S Charleston	47%	34
Ohio Valley Medical Center[2]	Wheeling	33%	27
Camden Clark Medical Center[2]	Parkersburg	20%	59

Chest Pain/Possible Heart Attack Care

Aspirin Given Within 24 Hours of Arrival

Hospital Name	City	Rate	Cases
Fairmont General Hospital	Fairmont	100%	83
Greenbrier Valley Medical Center	Ronceverte	100%	178
Ohio Valley Medical Center	Wheeling	100%	33
Plateau Medical Center	Oak Hill	100%	89
Pleasant Valley Hospital	Point Pleasant	100%	28
Preston Memorial Hospital[3]	Kingwood	100%	32
Saint Joseph Hospital	Buckhannon	100%	71
Davis Memorial Hospital	Elkins	99%	105
Logan Regional Medical Center	Logan	99%	84
Princeton Community Hospital	Princeton	99%	171
Stonewall Jackson Memorial Hospital	Weston	98%	65
Beckley ARH Hospital	Beckley	97%	31
Williamson Memorial Hospital	Williamson	97%	33
Jackson General Hospital	Ripley	96%	50
Jefferson Medical Center	Ranson	94%	48
Roane General Hospital	Spencer	94%	35
Summersville Regional Medical Center	Summersville	94%	127
Raleigh General Hospital	Beckley	93%	27
Wetzel County Hospital	New Martinsville	86%	58

Average Time to ECG (minutes)

Hospital Name	City	Min.	Cases
Greenbrier Valley Medical Center	Ronceverte	1	181
Williamson Memorial Hospital	Williamson	1	37
Stonewall Jackson Memorial Hospital	Weston	2	64
Roane General Hospital	Spencer	3	35
Jefferson Medical Center	Ranson	4	47
Plateau Medical Center	Oak Hill	4	90
Pleasant Valley Hospital	Point Pleasant	5	34
Beckley ARH Hospital	Beckley	7	31
Logan Regional Medical Center	Logan	7	87
Ohio Valley Medical Center	Wheeling	7	33
Wetzel County Hospital	New Martinsville	7	59
Davis Memorial Hospital	Elkins	8	112
Saint Joseph Hospital	Buckhannon	9	74
Summersville Regional Medical Center	Summersville	9	134
Fairmont General Hospital	Fairmont	10	83
Preston Memorial Hospital[3]	Kingwood	10	36
Princeton Community Hospital	Princeton	11	176
Jackson General Hospital	Ripley	14	54
Raleigh General Hospital	Beckley	14	30

Children's Asthma Care

No hospitals met the 25 case threshold.

Emergency Department

Admittance Decision Time (minutes)

Hospital Name	City	Min.	Cases
Pocahontas Memorial Hospital[2]	Buckeye	24	76
United Hospital Center[2]	Bridgeport	35	564
Grant Memorial Hospital[3]	Petersburg	36	226
Wetzel County Hospital[2]	New Martinsville	50	355
Stonewall Jackson Memorial Hospital[2]	Weston	51	342
Fairmont General Hospital[2]	Fairmont	58	300
Jackson General Hospital[2]	Ripley	58	345
Potomac Valley Hospital	Keyser	60	194
Saint Joseph Hospital[2]	Buckhannon	60	117
Weirton Medical Center[2]	Weirton	60	528
Ohio Valley Medical Center[2]	Wheeling	63	479
Raleigh General Hospital[2]	Beckley	65	706
Reynolds Memorial Hospital[2]	Glen Dale	66	146
Plateau Medical Center[2]	Oak Hill	68	473
Davis Memorial Hospital[2]	Elkins	69	482
West Virginia University Hospitals[2]	Morgantown	70	468
Williamson Memorial Hospital[2]	Williamson	71	376
Boone Memorial Hospital	Madison	72	340
Pleasant Valley Hospital[2]	Point Pleasant	72	265
Logan Regional Medical Center[2]	Logan	74	780
Minnie Hamilton Health Care Center[2]	Grantsville	75	138
Roane General Hospital	Spencer	75	158
Welch Community Hospital[2]	Welch	75	260
Wheeling Hospital[2]	Wheeling	75	515
Camden Clark Medical Center[2]	Parkersburg	76	486
Monongalia County General Hospital[2]	Morgantown	82	395
Cabell Huntington Hospital[2]	Huntington	84	465
Berkeley Medical Center[2]	Martinsburg	86	738
Bluefield Regional Medical Center[2]	Bluefield	89	476
Princeton Community Hospital[2]	Princeton	94	630
Camc Teays Valley Hospital[2]	Hurricane	97	260
Summersville Regional Medical Center[2]	Summersville	100	271
Greenbrier Valley Medical Center[2]	Ronceverte	117	535
Saint Francis Hospital[2]	Charleston	117	243
Beckley ARH Hospital[2]	Beckley	126	510
Saint Mary's Medical Center[2]	Huntington	129	231
Thomas Memorial Hospital[2]	S Charleston	143	666
Charleston Area Medical Center[2]	Charleston	145	631

Patients Who Left ER Before Being Seen

Hospital Name	City	Rate	Cases
Fairmont General Hospital	Fairmont	0%	31941
Pleasant Valley Hospital	Point Pleasant	0%	19885
Weirton Medical Center	Weirton	0%	37638
Berkeley Medical Center	Martinsburg	1%	50838
Cabell Huntington Hospital	Huntington	1%	57100
Grant Memorial Hospital	Petersburg	1%	12428
Greenbrier Valley Medical Center	Ronceverte	1%	24070
Monongalia County General Hospital	Morgantown	1%	31199
Preston Memorial Hospital	Kingwood	1%	9530
Roane General Hospital	Spencer	1%	8344
Saint Mary's Medical Center	Huntington	1%	69957
Sistersville General Hospital	Sistersville	1%	7311
Stonewall Jackson Memorial Hospital	Weston	1%	15863
Wetzel County Hospital	New Martinsville	1%	13853
Beckley ARH Hospital	Beckley	2%	24171
Bluefield Regional Medical Center	Bluefield	2%	30672
Charleston Area Medical Center	Charleston	2%	101795
Raleigh General Hospital	Beckley	2%	51064
Saint Joseph Hospital	Buckhannon	2%	14469
Summersville Regional Medical Center	Summersville	2%	24070
United Hospital Center	Bridgeport	2%	56181
Welch Community Hospital	Welch	2%	9615
West Virginia University Hospitals	Morgantown	2%	46697
Wheeling Hospital	Wheeling	2%	49320
Williamson Memorial Hospital	Williamson	2%	13736
Ohio Valley Medical Center	Wheeling	3%	31790
Plateau Medical Center	Oak Hill	3%	14419
Princeton Community Hospital	Princeton	3%	48663
Saint Francis Hospital	Charleston	3%	15872
Camc Teays Valley Hospital	Hurricane	4%	20181
Davis Memorial Hospital	Elkins	4%	28506
Reynolds Memorial Hospital	Glen Dale	4%	12028
Jackson General Hospital	Ripley	5%	12133
Logan Regional Medical Center	Logan	5%	33299
Thomas Memorial Hospital	S Charleston	5%	35328
Camden Clark Medical Center	Parkersburg	9%	55798

Time from ER Arrival to Being Admitted (minutes)

Hospital Name	City	Min.	Cases
Pocahontas Memorial Hospital[2]	Buckeye	130	78
Stonewall Jackson Memorial Hospital[2]	Weston	152	359

NOTE: Hospital profiles are in alphabetical order by state, then city, then hospital within the city; Rankings exclude hospitals with less than 25 cases except for patient surveys which excludes hospitals with less than 100 cases; (a) 100-299 cases; (1) The number of cases/patients is too few to report; (2) Data submitted were based on a sample of cases/patients; (3) Results are based on a shorter time period than required; (4) Data suppressed by CMS for one or more quarters; (5) Results are not available for this reporting period; (6) Fewer than 100 patients completed the HCAHPS survey; (7) No cases met the criteria for this measure; (8) The lower limit of the confidence interval cannot be calculated if the number of observed infections equals zero; (9) No data are available from the state/territory for this reporting period; (10) The scores shown reflect fewer than 50 completed surveys; (11) There were discrepancies in the data collection process; (12) This measure does not apply to this hospital for this reporting period; (13) Results cannot be calculated for this reporting period; (14) The results for this state are combined with nearby states to protect confidentiality; Please refer to the User's Guide for a full explanation of data.

Hospital Name	City	Min.	Cases
Saint Joseph Hospital[2]	Buckhannon	182	150
Grant Memorial Hospital[3]	Petersburg	184	226
Fairmont General Hospital[2]	Fairmont	187	300
Weirton Medical Center[2]	Weirton	199	642
United Hospital Center[2]	Bridgeport	204	564
Jackson General Hospital[2]	Ripley	206	351
Roane General Hospital	Spencer	208	211
Raleigh General Hospital[2]	Beckley	211	733
Plateau Medical Center[2]	Oak Hill	214	475
Minnie Hamilton Health Care Center[2]	Grantsville	215	151
Wetzel County Hospital[2]	New Martinsville	228	375
Ohio Valley Medical Center[2]	Wheeling	230	479
Pleasant Valley Hospital[2]	Point Pleasant	238	297
Williamson Memorial Hospital[2]	Williamson	240	376
Davis Memorial Hospital[2]	Elkins	245	517
Monongalia County General Hospital[2]	Morgantown	245	404
Wheeling Hospital[2]	Wheeling	249	564
Reynolds Memorial Hospital[2]	Glen Dale	250	154
Cabell Huntington Hospital[2]	Huntington	261	475
Greenbrier Valley Medical Center[2]	Ronceverte	263	543
Bluefield Regional Medical Center[2]	Bluefield	274	478
Potomac Valley Hospital	Keyser	274	414
Summersville Regional Medical Center[2]	Summersville	275	275
West Virginia University Hospitals[2]	Morgantown	275	457
Logan Regional Medical Center[2]	Logan	276	780
Berkeley Medical Center[2]	Martinsburg	280	738
Saint Francis Hospital[2]	Charleston	293	243
Camden Clark Medical Center[2]	Parkersburg	298	547
Princeton Community Hospital[2]	Princeton	302	634
Welch Community Hospital[2]	Welch	308	290
Boone Memorial Hospital	Madison	312	352
Beckley ARH Hospital[2]	Beckley	320	511
Saint Mary's Medical Center[2]	Huntington	325	301
Charleston Area Medical Center[2]	Charleston	333	699
Camc Teays Valley Hospital[2]	Hurricane	335	317
Thomas Memorial Hospital[2]	S Charleston	395	680

Time from ER Arrival to Discharge (minutes)

Hospital Name	City	Min.	Cases
Stonewall Jackson Memorial Hospital	Weston	76	393
Fairmont General Hospital	Fairmont	82	370
Weirton Medical Center	Weirton	104	369
Saint Joseph Hospital	Buckhannon	105	283
Raleigh General Hospital	Beckley	108	403
Plateau Medical Center	Oak Hill	110	374
Sistersville General Hospital[3]	Sistersville	110	211
Jackson General Hospital	Ripley	113	375
Wetzel County Hospital	New Martinsville	113	361
Jefferson Medical Center	Ranson	114	349
Pleasant Valley Hospital	Point Pleasant	118	378
Grant Memorial Hospital[3]	Petersburg	121	337
Ohio Valley Medical Center	Wheeling	122	363
Berkeley Medical Center	Martinsburg	128	383
Reynolds Memorial Hospital	Glen Dale	130	359
Greenbrier Valley Medical Center	Ronceverte	133	363
Davis Memorial Hospital	Elkins	136	366
United Hospital Center	Bridgeport	137	346
Saint Francis Hospital	Charleston	142	338
Cabell Huntington Hospital	Huntington	144	484
Summersville Regional Medical Center	Summersville	150	371
Saint Mary's Medical Center	Huntington	153	736
Williamson Memorial Hospital	Williamson	153	1149
Monongalia County General Hospital	Morgantown	158	369
Princeton Community Hospital	Princeton	161	377
Wheeling Hospital	Wheeling	170	423
Bluefield Regional Medical Center	Bluefield	172	364
Welch Community Hospital	Welch	175	327
Beckley ARH Hospital	Beckley	180	354
Camc Teays Valley Hospital	Hurricane	182	365
Logan Regional Medical Center	Logan	185	458
Charleston Area Medical Center	Charleston	190	844
West Virginia University Hospitals	Morgantown	200	346
Camden Clark Medical Center	Parkersburg	216	339
Thomas Memorial Hospital	S Charleston	249	349

Time in ER Before Being Evaluated (minutes)

Hospital Name	City	Min.	Cases
Fairmont General Hospital	Fairmont	11	415
Stonewall Jackson Memorial Hospital	Weston	13	414
Saint Joseph Hospital	Buckhannon	15	366
Plateau Medical Center	Oak Hill	16	418
Jefferson Medical Center	Ranson	17	384
Ohio Valley Medical Center	Wheeling	19	423
Greenbrier Valley Medical Center	Ronceverte	20	420
Logan Regional Medical Center	Logan	21	567
Raleigh General Hospital	Beckley	21	443
Saint Francis Hospital	Charleston	22	384
West Virginia University Hospitals	Morgantown	22	379
Monongalia County General Hospital	Morgantown	23	467
Sistersville General Hospital[3]	Sistersville	25	252
Davis Memorial Hospital	Elkins	26	393
Pleasant Valley Hospital	Point Pleasant	27	398
Jackson General Hospital	Ripley	29	405
Princeton Community Hospital	Princeton	29	403
Beckley ARH Hospital	Beckley	31	440
Weirton Medical Center	Weirton	31	378
Wheeling Hospital	Wheeling	31	433
Grant Memorial Hospital[3]	Petersburg	32	378
Reynolds Memorial Hospital	Glen Dale	32	122
Wetzel County Hospital	New Martinsville	32	322
Berkeley Medical Center	Martinsburg	33	411
Welch Community Hospital	Welch	34	434
Bluefield Regional Medical Center	Bluefield	36	408
Summersville Regional Medical Center	Summersville	36	404
Cabell Huntington Hospital	Huntington	41	504
Camc Teays Valley Hospital	Hurricane	46	408
Charleston Area Medical Center	Charleston	46	875
Williamson Memorial Hospital	Williamson	52	1313
United Hospital Center	Bridgeport	61	384
Camden Clark Medical Center	Parkersburg	62	328
Saint Mary's Medical Center	Huntington	62	656
Thomas Memorial Hospital	S Charleston	76	364

Time to Pain Meds for Bone Fractures (minutes)

Hospital Name	City	Min.	Cases
Ohio Valley Medical Center	Wheeling	43	99
Saint Joseph Hospital	Buckhannon	48	41
Fairmont General Hospital	Fairmont	49	69
Greenbrier Valley Medical Center	Ronceverte	50	77
Weirton Medical Center	Weirton	52	94
Stonewall Jackson Memorial Hospital	Weston	53	44
Reynolds Memorial Hospital	Glen Dale	54	34
Saint Francis Hospital	Charleston	55	31
Davis Memorial Hospital	Elkins	57	67
Jefferson Medical Center	Ranson	58	110
Plateau Medical Center	Oak Hill	60	86
Pleasant Valley Hospital	Point Pleasant	60	41
Raleigh General Hospital	Beckley	61	153
Princeton Community Hospital	Princeton	63	136
Summersville Regional Medical Center	Summersville	64	114
Bluefield Regional Medical Center	Bluefield	65	100
Charleston Area Medical Center	Charleston	65	225
Saint Mary's Medical Center	Huntington	65	187
Berkeley Medical Center	Martinsburg	67	181
Wetzel County Hospital	New Martinsville	67	65
Monongalia County General Hospital	Morgantown	68	70
Jackson General Hospital	Ripley	73	29
Cabell Huntington Hospital	Huntington	74	200
United Hospital Center	Bridgeport	74	151
Welch Community Hospital	Welch	74	49
Williamson Memorial Hospital	Williamson	78	56
Logan Regional Medical Center	Logan	83	112
West Virginia University Hospitals	Morgantown	85	35
Camden Clark Medical Center	Parkersburg	86	102
Wheeling Hospital	Wheeling	86	85
Camc Teays Valley Hospital	Hurricane	94	56
Beckley ARH Hospital	Beckley	95	81
Thomas Memorial Hospital	S Charleston	108	84

Heart Attack Care

Aspirin Given at Discharge

Hospital Name	City	Rate	Cases
Berkeley Medical Center	Martinsburg	100%	164
Bluefield Regional Medical Center	Bluefield	100%	86
Cabell Huntington Hospital	Huntington	100%	40
Fairmont General Hospital	Fairmont	100%	43
Monongalia County General Hospital	Morgantown	100%	342
Saint Francis Hospital	Charleston	100%	31
United Hospital Center	Bridgeport	100%	331
West Virginia University Hospitals	Morgantown	100%	502
Wheeling Hospital	Wheeling	100%	462
Camden Clark Medical Center	Parkersburg	99%	395
Charleston Area Medical Center[2]	Charleston	99%	578
Raleigh General Hospital	Beckley	99%	310
Saint Mary's Medical Center[2]	Huntington	99%	338
Thomas Memorial Hospital	S Charleston	97%	115
Weirton Medical Center	Weirton	95%	59
Ohio Valley Medical Center	Wheeling	91%	33

PCI Within 90 Minutes of Arrival

Hospital Name	City	Rate	Cases
United Hospital Center	Bridgeport	100%	27
West Virginia University Hospitals	Morgantown	100%	37
Berkeley Medical Center	Martinsburg	97%	33
Wheeling Hospital	Wheeling	97%	60
Saint Mary's Medical Center[2]	Huntington	94%	36
Camden Clark Medical Center	Parkersburg	88%	43
Monongalia County General Hospital	Morgantown	88%	49
Raleigh General Hospital	Beckley	88%	52
Charleston Area Medical Center[2]	Charleston	84%	45

Statin Prescribed at Discharge

Hospital Name	City	Rate	Cases
Berkeley Medical Center	Martinsburg	100%	157
Cabell Huntington Hospital	Huntington	100%	41
Fairmont General Hospital	Fairmont	100%	37
Raleigh General Hospital	Beckley	100%	297
United Hospital Center	Bridgeport	100%	310
West Virginia University Hospitals	Morgantown	100%	485
Wheeling Hospital	Wheeling	100%	425
Camden Clark Medical Center	Parkersburg	98%	367
Monongalia County General Hospital	Morgantown	98%	304
Saint Mary's Medical Center[2]	Huntington	98%	328
Charleston Area Medical Center[2]	Charleston	97%	574
Bluefield Regional Medical Center	Bluefield	96%	84
Saint Francis Hospital	Charleston	96%	28
Weirton Medical Center	Weirton	91%	56
Thomas Memorial Hospital	S Charleston	90%	114
Ohio Valley Medical Center	Wheeling	83%	29

Heart Failure Care

ACE Inhibitor or ARB for LVSD

Hospital Name	City	Rate	Cases
Beckley VA Medical Center	Beckley	100%	28
Berkeley Medical Center	Martinsburg	100%	63
Cabell Huntington Hospital	Huntington	100%	49
Fairmont General Hospital	Fairmont	100%	46
Logan Regional Medical Center	Logan	100%	45
Princeton Community Hospital	Princeton	100%	32
Stonewall Jackson Memorial Hospital	Weston	100%	34
United Hospital Center	Bridgeport	100%	99
Weirton Medical Center	Weirton	100%	37
West Virginia University Hospitals	Morgantown	100%	119
Wheeling Hospital	Wheeling	100%	71
Monongalia County General Hospital	Morgantown	98%	42
Raleigh General Hospital	Beckley	98%	93
Bluefield Regional Medical Center	Bluefield	97%	37
Camden Clark Medical Center	Parkersburg	96%	131
Huntington VA Medical Center	Huntington	96%	70
Saint Mary's Medical Center[2]	Huntington	95%	88
Thomas Memorial Hospital	S Charleston	95%	88
Martinsburg VA Medical Center	Martinsburg	94%	50
Charleston Area Medical Center[2]	Charleston	92%	195
Greenbrier Valley Medical Center	Ronceverte	92%	52
Davis Memorial Hospital	Elkins	91%	34
Saint Francis Hospital	Charleston	88%	26
Reynolds Memorial Hospital	Glen Dale	86%	28
Ohio Valley Medical Center	Wheeling	85%	26
Beckley ARH Hospital	Beckley	77%	35

Discharge Instructions Given

Hospital Name	City	Rate	Cases
Beckley VA Medical Center	Beckley	100%	51
Huntington VA Medical Center	Huntington	100%	154
Jefferson Medical Center	Ranson	100%	27
Pleasant Valley Hospital	Point Pleasant	100%	90
Thomas Memorial Hospital	S Charleston	100%	231
West Virginia University Hospitals	Morgantown	100%	305
Logan Regional Medical Center	Logan	99%	199
Saint Mary's Medical Center[2]	Huntington	99%	280
Cabell Huntington Hospital	Huntington	98%	113
Princeton Community Hospital	Princeton	98%	126
United Hospital Center	Bridgeport	98%	268
Wheeling Hospital	Wheeling	98%	206
Berkeley Medical Center	Martinsburg	97%	201
Martinsburg VA Medical Center	Martinsburg	97%	96
Clarksburg VA Medical Center	Clarksburg	96%	67
Monongalia County General Hospital	Morgantown	96%	167
Davis Memorial Hospital	Elkins	95%	115
Greenbrier Valley Medical Center	Ronceverte	95%	103
Weirton Medical Center	Weirton	95%	129
Stonewall Jackson Memorial Hospital	Weston	94%	78
Summersville Regional Medical Center	Summersville	94%	35
Williamson Memorial Hospital	Williamson	94%	64
Camden Clark Medical Center	Parkersburg	93%	440
Saint Francis Hospital	Charleston	93%	88
Saint Joseph Hospital[2]	Buckhannon	93%	30
Bluefield Regional Medical Center	Bluefield	92%	122
Fairmont General Hospital	Fairmont	92%	142
Summers County ARH Hospital	Hinton	92%	25
Charleston Area Medical Center[2]	Charleston	91%	416
Ohio Valley Medical Center	Wheeling	91%	99
Grant Memorial Hospital	Petersburg	90%	30
Plateau Medical Center	Oak Hill	90%	61
Jackson General Hospital	Ripley	89%	37
Beckley ARH Hospital	Beckley	88%	108

NOTE: Hospital profiles are in alphabetical order by state, then city, then hospital within the city; Rankings exclude hospitals with less than 25 cases except for patient surveys which excludes hospitals with less than 100 cases; (a) 100-299 cases; (1) The number of cases/patients is too few to report; (2) Data submitted were based on a sample of cases/patients; (3) Results are based on a shorter time period than required; (4) Data suppressed by CMS for one or more quarters; (5) Results are not available for this reporting period; (6) Fewer than 100 patients completed the HCAHPS survey; (7) No cases met the criteria for this measure; (8) The lower limit of the confidence interval cannot be calculated if the number of observed infections equals zero; (9) No data are available from the state/territory for this reporting period; (10) The scores shown reflect fewer than 50 completed surveys; (11) There were discrepancies in the data collection process; (12) This measure does not apply to this hospital for this reporting period; (13) Results cannot be calculated for this reporting period; (14) The results for this state are combined with nearby states to protect confidentiality; Please refer to the User's Guide for a full explanation of data.

Hospital Name	City	Rate	Cases
Raleigh General Hospital	Beckley	83%	269
Reynolds Memorial Hospital	Glen Dale	82%	71
Camc Teays Valley Hospital	Hurricane	78%	37

Evaluation of LVS Function

Hospital Name	City	Rate	Cases
Beckley VA Medical Center	Beckley	100%	55
Berkeley Medical Center	Martinsburg	100%	223
Bluefield Regional Medical Center	Bluefield	100%	155
Cabell Huntington Hospital	Huntington	100%	144
Davis Memorial Hospital	Elkins	100%	122
Fairmont General Hospital	Fairmont	100%	179
Greenbrier Valley Medical Center	Ronceverte	100%	118
Huntington VA Medical Center	Huntington	100%	174
Jefferson Medical Center	Ranson	100%	39
Logan Regional Medical Center	Logan	100%	213
Martinsburg VA Medical Center	Martinsburg	100%	109
Monongalia County General Hospital	Morgantown	100%	197
Plateau Medical Center	Oak Hill	100%	83
Pleasant Valley Hospital	Point Pleasant	100%	118
Raleigh General Hospital	Beckley	100%	315
Saint Joseph Hospital[2]	Buckhannon	100%	41
Saint Mary's Medical Center[2]	Huntington	100%	324
Stonewall Jackson Memorial Hospital	Weston	100%	88
Thomas Memorial Hospital	S Charleston	100%	269
United Hospital Center	Bridgeport	100%	324
West Virginia University Hospitals	Morgantown	100%	363
Wetzel County Hospital	New Martinsville	100%	30
Wheeling Hospital	Wheeling	100%	274
Camden Clark Medical Center	Parkersburg	99%	560
Charleston Area Medical Center[2]	Charleston	99%	465
Clarksburg VA Medical Center	Clarksburg	99%	72
Princeton Community Hospital	Princeton	99%	158
Saint Francis Hospital	Charleston	99%	104
Weirton Medical Center	Weirton	99%	181
Williamson Memorial Hospital	Williamson	99%	70
Jackson General Hospital	Ripley	98%	47
Beckley ARH Hospital	Beckley	97%	138
Ohio Valley Medical Center	Wheeling	97%	123
Potomac Valley Hospital	Keyser	97%	35
Camc Teays Valley Hospital	Hurricane	95%	44
Reynolds Memorial Hospital	Glen Dale	94%	123
Summers County ARH Hospital	Hinton	94%	33
Preston Memorial Hospital[2]	Kingwood	90%	30
Summersville Regional Medical Center	Summersville	90%	40
Grant Memorial Hospital	Petersburg	78%	36

Medicare Spending

Medicare Spending per Patient (ratio)

Hospital Name	City	Ratio	Cases
Davis Memorial Hospital	Elkins	0.85	-
Greenbrier Valley Medical Center	Ronceverte	0.89	-
Stonewall Jackson Memorial Hospital	Weston	0.90	-
Saint Francis Hospital	Charleston	0.92	-
Summersville Regional Medical Center	Summersville	0.92	-
Welch Community Hospital	Welch	0.92	-
Logan Regional Medical Center	Logan	0.93	-
Saint Joseph Hospital	Buckhannon	0.93	-
Cabell Huntington Hospital	Huntington	0.94	-
United Hospital Center	Bridgeport	0.94	-
Berkeley Medical Center	Martinsburg	0.95	-
Thomas Memorial Hospital	S Charleston	0.95	-
Pleasant Valley Hospital	Point Pleasant	0.96	-
Princeton Community Hospital	Princeton	0.96	-
Williamson Memorial Hospital	Williamson	0.96	-
Charleston Area Medical Center	Charleston	0.97	-
Saint Mary's Medical Center	Huntington	0.98	-
Beckley ARH Hospital	Beckley	0.99	-
Ohio Valley Medical Center	Wheeling	0.99	-
Raleigh General Hospital	Beckley	0.99	-
Wetzel County Hospital	New Martinsville	0.99	-
Wheeling Hospital	Wheeling	0.99	-
Reynolds Memorial Hospital	Glen Dale	1.00	-
West Virginia University Hospitals	Morgantown	1.00	-
Bluefield Regional Medical Center	Bluefield	1.01	-
Fairmont General Hospital	Fairmont	1.01	-
Weirton Medical Center	Weirton	1.01	-
Camc Teays Valley Hospital	Hurricane	1.02	-
Monongalia County General Hospital	Morgantown	1.02	-
Camden Clark Medical Center	Parkersburg	1.04	-

Pneumonia Care

Appropriate Initial Antibiotic Given

Hospital Name	City	Rate	Cases
Cabell Huntington Hospital	Huntington	100%	72
Jefferson Medical Center	Ranson	100%	25
Plateau Medical Center	Oak Hill	100%	64
Pleasant Valley Hospital[2]	Point Pleasant	100%	68
Huntington VA Medical Center	Huntington	99%	72
Jackson General Hospital	Ripley	99%	67
Raleigh General Hospital	Beckley	99%	228
West Virginia University Hospitals	Morgantown	99%	90
Wetzel County Hospital	New Martinsville	99%	75
Logan Regional Medical Center	Logan	98%	196
Williamson Memorial Hospital	Williamson	98%	49
Berkeley Medical Center	Martinsburg	97%	172
Bluefield Regional Medical Center	Bluefield	97%	69
Clarksburg VA Medical Center	Clarksburg	97%	74
Davis Memorial Hospital	Elkins	97%	116
Ohio Valley Medical Center	Wheeling	97%	77
Saint Francis Hospital	Charleston	97%	75
Stonewall Jackson Memorial Hospital	Weston	97%	75
Wheeling Hospital	Wheeling	97%	197
Beckley ARH Hospital	Beckley	96%	105
Camc Teays Valley Hospital	Hurricane	96%	89
Greenbrier Valley Medical Center	Ronceverte	96%	137
United Hospital Center	Bridgeport	96%	255
Weirton Medical Center	Weirton	96%	202
Fairmont General Hospital	Fairmont	95%	103
Saint Mary's Medical Center[2]	Huntington	95%	152
Princeton Community Hospital	Princeton	94%	232
Thomas Memorial Hospital	S Charleston	94%	245
Beckley VA Medical Center	Beckley	93%	70
Charleston Area Medical Center[2]	Charleston	92%	118
Martinsburg VA Medical Center	Martinsburg	92%	75
Camden Clark Medical Center	Parkersburg	91%	212
Monongalia County General Hospital	Morgantown	91%	91
Reynolds Memorial Hospital	Glen Dale	90%	61
Welch Community Hospital[2]	Welch	90%	40
Montgomery General Hospital	Montgomery	86%	58
Summers County ARH Hospital	Hinton	86%	29
Potomac Valley Hospital	Keyser	85%	39
Grant Memorial Hospital	Petersburg	81%	27
Saint Joseph Hospital[2]	Buckhannon	79%	39
Webster County Memorial Hospital[3]	Webster Springs	64%	28
Pocahontas Memorial Hospital[2]	Buckeye	60%	30
Boone Memorial Hospital	Madison	56%	39

Blood Culture Timing

Hospital Name	City	Rate	Cases
Beckley VA Medical Center	Beckley	100%	112
Davis Memorial Hospital	Elkins	100%	171
Jefferson Medical Center	Ranson	100%	41
Monongalia County General Hospital	Morgantown	100%	124
Plateau Medical Center	Oak Hill	100%	87
Pleasant Valley Hospital[2]	Point Pleasant	100%	101
Summers County ARH Hospital	Hinton	100%	33
Weirton Medical Center	Weirton	100%	292
West Virginia University Hospitals	Morgantown	100%	240
Berkeley Medical Center	Martinsburg	99%	330
Greenbrier Valley Medical Center	Ronceverte	99%	249
Logan Regional Medical Center	Logan	99%	304
Princeton Community Hospital	Princeton	99%	392
Stonewall Jackson Memorial Hospital	Weston	99%	103
Thomas Memorial Hospital	S Charleston	99%	433
Wheeling Hospital	Wheeling	99%	353
Cabell Huntington Hospital	Huntington	98%	135
Camc Teays Valley Hospital	Hurricane	98%	121
Clarksburg VA Medical Center	Clarksburg	98%	139
Fairmont General Hospital	Fairmont	98%	127
Jackson General Hospital	Ripley	98%	105
Martinsburg VA Medical Center	Martinsburg	98%	116
Ohio Valley Medical Center	Wheeling	98%	130
Raleigh General Hospital	Beckley	98%	333
Reynolds Memorial Hospital	Glen Dale	98%	65
United Hospital Center	Bridgeport	98%	328
Wetzel County Hospital	New Martinsville	98%	86
Bluefield Regional Medical Center	Bluefield	97%	133
Braxton County Memorial Hospital	Gassaway	97%	33
Camden Clark Medical Center	Parkersburg	97%	325
Preston Memorial Hospital[2]	Kingwood	97%	30
Huntington VA Medical Center	Huntington	96%	125
Saint Mary's Medical Center[2]	Huntington	96%	319
Saint Francis Hospital	Charleston	95%	146
Summersville Regional Medical Center	Summersville	95%	117
Beckley ARH Hospital	Beckley	93%	171
Charleston Area Medical Center[2]	Charleston	93%	283
Boone Memorial Hospital	Madison	92%	59
Williamson Memorial Hospital	Williamson	92%	76
Potomac Valley Hospital	Keyser	88%	51
Saint Joseph Hospital[2]	Buckhannon	88%	48
Webster County Memorial Hospital[3]	Webster Springs	88%	25
Montgomery General Hospital	Montgomery	86%	83
Sistersville General Hospital[2]	Sistersville	84%	25
Grant Memorial Hospital	Petersburg	76%	34
Welch Community Hospital[2]	Welch	73%	52

Pregnancy and Delivery Care

Newborns whose Deliveries were Scheduled Early

Hospital Name	City	Rate	Cases
Saint Joseph Hospital	Buckhannon	0%	46
Stonewall Jackson Memorial Hospital[2]	Weston	0%	28
United Hospital Center	Bridgeport	0%	50
Logan Regional Medical Center[2]	Logan	2%	45
Davis Memorial Hospital	Elkins	3%	29
Pleasant Valley Hospital[2]	Point Pleasant	4%	47
Princeton Community Hospital[2]	Princeton	5%	65
Raleigh General Hospital[2]	Beckley	6%	33
Charleston Area Medical Center[2]	Charleston	7%	60
Summersville Regional Medical Center[2]	Summersville	7%	27
Ohio Valley Medical Center[2]	Wheeling	10%	41
Wheeling Hospital	Wheeling	10%	137
Cabell Huntington Hospital[2]	Huntington	12%	40
Thomas Memorial Hospital[2]	S Charleston	18%	28
Camden Clark Medical Center[2]	Parkersburg	20%	40
Saint Mary's Medical Center	Huntington	34%	53
Weirton Medical Center[2]	Weirton	80%	25

Preventive Care

Immunization for Influenza

Hospital Name	City	Rate	Cases
Greenbrier Valley Medical Center[2]	Ronceverte	100%	406
Logan Regional Medical Center[2]	Logan	100%	509
West Virginia University Hospitals[2]	Morgantown	100%	534
Cabell Huntington Hospital[2]	Huntington	99%	501
Fairmont General Hospital[2]	Fairmont	99%	436
Monongalia County General Hospital[2]	Morgantown	99%	557
Plateau Medical Center[2]	Oak Hill	99%	428
Princeton Community Hospital[2]	Princeton	99%	546
Williamson Memorial Hospital[2]	Williamson	99%	267
Pleasant Valley Hospital[2]	Point Pleasant	98%	295
Raleigh General Hospital[2]	Beckley	98%	523
Saint Francis Hospital[2]	Charleston	98%	336
Wheeling Hospital[2]	Wheeling	98%	598
Preston Memorial Hospital[2]	Kingwood	97%	147
Stonewall Jackson Memorial Hospital[2]	Weston	97%	274
Beckley VA Medical Center[2,3]	Beckley	96%	144
Berkeley Medical Center[2]	Martinsburg	96%	564
Camc Teays Valley Hospital[2]	Hurricane	96%	316
Jackson General Hospital[2]	Ripley	96%	295
Wetzel County Hospital[2]	New Martinsville	96%	238
Beckley ARH Hospital[2]	Beckley	95%	412
Bluefield Regional Medical Center[2]	Bluefield	95%	507
Pocahontas Memorial Hospital	Buckeye	95%	55
Thomas Memorial Hospital[2]	S Charleston	94%	519
Camden Clark Medical Center[2]	Parkersburg	92%	542
Davis Memorial Hospital[2]	Elkins	92%	420
Weirton Medical Center[2]	Weirton	92%	545
Charleston Area Medical Center[2]	Charleston	91%	569
Clarksburg VA Medical Center[2,3]	Clarksburg	91%	139
Minnie Hamilton Health Care Center	Grantsville	91%	94
United Hospital Center[2]	Bridgeport	91%	540
Ohio Valley Medical Center[2]	Wheeling	90%	575
Saint Mary's Medical Center[2]	Huntington	89%	615
Reynolds Memorial Hospital[2]	Glen Dale	88%	288
Saint Joseph Hospital[2]	Buckhannon	87%	242
Roane General Hospital	Spencer	86%	132
Summersville Regional Medical Center[2]	Summersville	85%	252
Welch Community Hospital[2]	Welch	79%	271
Boone Memorial Hospital	Madison	70%	181

Immunization for Pneumonia

Hospital Name	City	Rate	Cases
Cabell Huntington Hospital[2]	Huntington	100%	448
Greenbrier Valley Medical Center[2]	Ronceverte	100%	525
Logan Regional Medical Center[2]	Logan	100%	729
Stonewall Jackson Memorial Hospital[2]	Weston	100%	370
West Virginia University Hospitals[2]	Morgantown	100%	580
Williamson Memorial Hospital[2]	Williamson	100%	328
Bluefield Regional Medical Center[2]	Bluefield	99%	631
Fairmont General Hospital[2]	Fairmont	99%	534
Jackson General Hospital[2]	Ripley	99%	508
Monongalia County General Hospital[2]	Morgantown	99%	709
Plateau Medical Center[2]	Oak Hill	99%	696
Pleasant Valley Hospital[2]	Point Pleasant	99%	403
Saint Francis Hospital[2]	Charleston	99%	496
Wetzel County Hospital[2]	New Martinsville	99%	372
Princeton Community Hospital[2]	Princeton	98%	744
Raleigh General Hospital[2]	Beckley	98%	739
Wheeling Hospital[2]	Wheeling	98%	763
Thomas Memorial Hospital[2]	S Charleston	97%	682
Beckley ARH Hospital[2]	Beckley	96%	673
Davis Memorial Hospital[2]	Elkins	96%	513
Camc Teays Valley Hospital[2]	Hurricane	95%	485
Ohio Valley Medical Center[2]	Wheeling	95%	582

NOTE: Hospital profiles are in alphabetical order by state, then city, then hospital within the city; Rankings exclude hospitals with less than 25 cases except for patient surveys which excludes hospitals with less than 100 cases; (a) 100-299 cases; (1) The number of cases/patients is too few to report; (2) Data submitted were based on a sample of cases/patients; (3) Results are based on a shorter time period than required; (4) Data suppressed by CMS for one or more quarters; (5) Results are not available for this reporting period; (6) Fewer than 100 patients completed the HCAHPS survey; (7) No cases met the criteria for this measure; (8) The lower limit of the confidence interval cannot be calculated if the number of observed infections equals zero; (9) No data are available from the state/territory for this reporting period; (10) The scores shown reflect fewer than 50 completed surveys; (11) There were discrepancies in the data collection process; (12) This measure does not apply to this hospital for this reporting period; (13) Results cannot be calculated for this reporting period; (14) The results for this state are combined with nearby states to protect confidentiality; Please refer to the User's Guide for a full explanation of data.

Hospital Name	City	Rate	Cases
Preston Memorial Hospital[2]	Kingwood	95%	248
United Hospital Center[2]	Bridgeport	95%	732
Beckley VA Medical Center[2,3]	Beckley	94%	360
Berkeley Medical Center[2]	Martinsburg	94%	653
Camden Clark Medical Center[2]	Parkersburg	93%	738
Saint Mary's Medical Center[2]	Huntington	92%	886
Clarksburg VA Medical Center[2,3]	Clarksburg	90%	315
Minnie Hamilton Health Care Center	Grantsville	90%	139
Pocahontas Memorial Hospital	Buckeye	90%	59
Weirton Medical Center[2]	Weirton	90%	802
Roane General Hospital	Spencer	89%	226
Reynolds Memorial Hospital[2]	Glen Dale	88%	463
Summersville Regional Medical Center[2]	Summersville	88%	301
Charleston Area Medical Center[2]	Charleston	86%	782
Welch Community Hospital[2]	Welch	86%	290
Saint Joseph Hospital[2]	Buckhannon	84%	254
Boone Memorial Hospital	Madison	77%	288

Stroke Care

Anticoagulation Therapy for Atrial Fibrillation

Hospital Name	City	Rate	Cases
Charleston Area Medical Center	Charleston	100%	60
Saint Mary's Medical Center	Huntington	100%	37
West Virginia University Hospitals	Morgantown	100%	40

Antithrombotic Therapy Timing

Hospital Name	City	Rate	Cases
Berkeley Medical Center	Martinsburg	100%	78
Bluefield Regional Medical Center	Bluefield	100%	37
Cabell Huntington Hospital	Huntington	100%	85
Camden Clark Medical Center[2]	Parkersburg	100%	77
Greenbrier Valley Medical Center	Ronceverte	100%	32
Logan Regional Medical Center	Logan	100%	30
Saint Mary's Medical Center	Huntington	100%	274
United Hospital Center	Bridgeport	100%	57
Raleigh General Hospital	Beckley	99%	100
West Virginia University Hospitals	Morgantown	99%	329
Charleston Area Medical Center	Charleston	98%	396
Ohio Valley Medical Center	Wheeling	98%	44
Thomas Memorial Hospital	S Charleston	96%	94
Weirton Medical Center[2]	Weirton	96%	48
Wheeling Hospital	Wheeling	95%	96
Princeton Community Hospital	Princeton	89%	46

Assessed for Rehabilitation

Hospital Name	City	Rate	Cases
Berkeley Medical Center	Martinsburg	100%	75
Cabell Huntington Hospital	Huntington	100%	123
Greenbrier Valley Medical Center	Ronceverte	100%	30
Logan Regional Medical Center	Logan	100%	29
Saint Mary's Medical Center	Huntington	100%	347
United Hospital Center	Bridgeport	100%	62
Raleigh General Hospital	Beckley	99%	105
West Virginia University Hospitals	Morgantown	99%	504
Camden Clark Medical Center[2]	Parkersburg	98%	84
Bluefield Regional Medical Center	Bluefield	97%	38
Ohio Valley Medical Center	Wheeling	96%	52
Charleston Area Medical Center	Charleston	93%	462
Princeton Community Hospital	Princeton	93%	60
Thomas Memorial Hospital	S Charleston	93%	88
Wheeling Hospital	Wheeling	92%	104
Weirton Medical Center[2]	Weirton	69%	48

Discharged on Antithrombotic Therapy

Hospital Name	City	Rate	Cases
Berkeley Medical Center	Martinsburg	100%	70
Bluefield Regional Medical Center	Bluefield	100%	35
Cabell Huntington Hospital	Huntington	100%	98
Camden Clark Medical Center[2]	Parkersburg	100%	79
Logan Regional Medical Center	Logan	100%	28
United Hospital Center	Bridgeport	100%	53
Charleston Area Medical Center	Charleston	99%	408
Raleigh General Hospital	Beckley	99%	100
Saint Mary's Medical Center	Huntington	99%	297
West Virginia University Hospitals	Morgantown	99%	393
Ohio Valley Medical Center	Wheeling	98%	40
Greenbrier Valley Medical Center	Ronceverte	97%	30
Wheeling Hospital	Wheeling	96%	95
Thomas Memorial Hospital	S Charleston	94%	86
Weirton Medical Center[2]	Weirton	93%	45
Princeton Community Hospital	Princeton	92%	52

Discharged on Statin Medication

Hospital Name	City	Rate	Cases
Cabell Huntington Hospital	Huntington	100%	80
United Hospital Center	Bridgeport	100%	47
Charleston Area Medical Center	Charleston	98%	313
Raleigh General Hospital	Beckley	98%	86
Saint Mary's Medical Center	Huntington	98%	224
West Virginia University Hospitals	Morgantown	95%	308
Berkeley Medical Center	Martinsburg	93%	60
Thomas Memorial Hospital	S Charleston	92%	63
Camden Clark Medical Center[2]	Parkersburg	89%	64
Ohio Valley Medical Center	Wheeling	84%	37
Princeton Community Hospital	Princeton	80%	49
Weirton Medical Center[2]	Weirton	55%	40
Wheeling Hospital	Wheeling	54%	72

Thrombolytic Therapy Timing

Hospital Name	City	Rate	Cases
West Virginia University Hospitals	Morgantown	100%	35

Venous Thromboembolism (VTE) Prophylaxis

Hospital Name	City	Rate	Cases
Cabell Huntington Hospital	Huntington	100%	124
Greenbrier Valley Medical Center	Ronceverte	100%	35
Saint Mary's Medical Center	Huntington	99%	354
Berkeley Medical Center	Martinsburg	98%	88
Raleigh General Hospital	Beckley	98%	112
West Virginia University Hospitals	Morgantown	98%	535
Logan Regional Medical Center	Logan	97%	31
United Hospital Center	Bridgeport	97%	64
Bluefield Regional Medical Center	Bluefield	95%	39
Charleston Area Medical Center	Charleston	93%	492
Camden Clark Medical Center[2]	Parkersburg	90%	80
Thomas Memorial Hospital	S Charleston	77%	93
Ohio Valley Medical Center	Wheeling	70%	61
Wheeling Hospital	Wheeling	63%	111
Princeton Community Hospital	Princeton	57%	49
Weirton Medical Center[2]	Weirton	30%	50

Written Stroke Educational Materials Given

Hospital Name	City	Rate	Cases
Cabell Huntington Hospital	Huntington	99%	86
West Virginia University Hospitals	Morgantown	97%	297
Saint Mary's Medical Center	Huntington	94%	196
Charleston Area Medical Center	Charleston	92%	314
Berkeley Medical Center	Martinsburg	90%	49
Princeton Community Hospital	Princeton	85%	41
United Hospital Center	Bridgeport	82%	39
Raleigh General Hospital	Beckley	73%	64
Camden Clark Medical Center[2]	Parkersburg	72%	54
Wheeling Hospital	Wheeling	71%	62
Thomas Memorial Hospital	S Charleston	69%	64
Weirton Medical Center[2]	Weirton	0%	34

Surgical Care Improvement Project

Appropriate Beta Blocker Usage

Hospital Name	City	Rate	Cases
Beckley ARH Hospital	Beckley	100%	45
Fairmont General Hospital	Fairmont	100%	40
Huntington VA Medical Center[2]	Huntington	100%	72
Monongalia County General Hospital[2]	Morgantown	100%	512
Plateau Medical Center	Oak Hill	100%	58
Pleasant Valley Hospital	Point Pleasant	100%	27
Princeton Community Hospital	Princeton	100%	207
United Hospital Center[2]	Bridgeport	100%	213
Berkeley Medical Center	Martinsburg	99%	126
Charleston Area Medical Center[2]	Charleston	99%	652
Saint Mary's Medical Center[2]	Huntington	99%	538
West Virginia University Hospitals[2]	Morgantown	99%	217
Cabell Huntington Hospital[2]	Huntington	98%	195
Camden Clark Medical Center[2]	Parkersburg	98%	377
Ohio Valley Medical Center	Wheeling	98%	155
Stonewall Jackson Memorial Hospital	Weston	98%	43
Thomas Memorial Hospital	S Charleston	98%	221
Weirton Medical Center	Weirton	98%	90
Wheeling Hospital	Wheeling	98%	310
Raleigh General Hospital	Beckley	97%	114
Davis Memorial Hospital	Elkins	96%	89
Martinsburg VA Medical Center[2]	Martinsburg	96%	75
Saint Francis Hospital	Charleston	96%	325
Camc Teays Valley Hospital	Hurricane	94%	53
Reynolds Memorial Hospital	Glen Dale	90%	31
Bluefield Regional Medical Center	Bluefield	89%	111
Summersville Regional Medical Center	Summersville	82%	28

Appropriate VTP Within 24 Hours

Hospital Name	City	Rate	Cases
Berkeley Medical Center	Martinsburg	100%	387
Jefferson Medical Center	Ranson	100%	35
Logan Regional Medical Center	Logan	100%	89
Plateau Medical Center	Oak Hill	100%	194
Stonewall Jackson Memorial Hospital	Weston	100%	134
United Hospital Center[2]	Bridgeport	100%	630
Williamson Memorial Hospital	Williamson	100%	36
Bluefield Regional Medical Center	Bluefield	99%	174
Cabell Huntington Hospital[2]	Huntington	99%	548
Camden Clark Medical Center[2]	Parkersburg	99%	784
Fairmont General Hospital	Fairmont	99%	95
Monongalia County General Hospital[2]	Morgantown	99%	796
Raleigh General Hospital	Beckley	99%	272
West Virginia University Hospitals[2]	Morgantown	99%	433
Wheeling Hospital	Wheeling	99%	515
Huntington VA Medical Center[2]	Huntington	98%	124
Princeton Community Hospital	Princeton	98%	531
Saint Mary's Medical Center[2]	Huntington	98%	739
Davis Memorial Hospital	Elkins	97%	240
Grant Memorial Hospital	Petersburg	97%	65
Greenbrier Valley Medical Center	Ronceverte	97%	69
Martinsburg VA Medical Center[2]	Martinsburg	97%	147
Pleasant Valley Hospital	Point Pleasant	97%	72
Saint Francis Hospital	Charleston	97%	806
Beckley ARH Hospital	Beckley	96%	111
Charleston Area Medical Center[2]	Charleston	96%	526
Ohio Valley Medical Center	Wheeling	96%	451
Weirton Medical Center	Weirton	96%	226
Camc Teays Valley Hospital	Hurricane	95%	130
Summersville Regional Medical Center	Summersville	94%	70
Saint Joseph Hospital[2]	Buckhannon	93%	74
Thomas Memorial Hospital	S Charleston	92%	499
Reynolds Memorial Hospital	Glen Dale	87%	63
Welch Community Hospital	Welch	74%	31

Controlled Postoperative Blood Glucose

Hospital Name	City	Rate	Cases
West Virginia University Hospitals[2]	Morgantown	99%	169
Monongalia County General Hospital[2]	Morgantown	97%	277
Saint Mary's Medical Center[2]	Huntington	97%	377
Camden Clark Medical Center[2]	Parkersburg	96%	131
Charleston Area Medical Center[2]	Charleston	93%	558
Wheeling Hospital	Wheeling	89%	203

Perioperative Temperature Management

Hospital Name	City	Rate	Cases
Beckley ARH Hospital	Beckley	100%	130
Berkeley Medical Center	Martinsburg	100%	475
Bluefield Regional Medical Center	Bluefield	100%	313
Cabell Huntington Hospital[2]	Huntington	100%	668
Charleston Area Medical Center[2]	Charleston	100%	711
Davis Memorial Hospital	Elkins	100%	262
Fairmont General Hospital	Fairmont	100%	136
Greenbrier Valley Medical Center	Ronceverte	100%	93
Huntington VA Medical Center[2]	Huntington	100%	137
Jefferson Medical Center	Ranson	100%	36
Logan Regional Medical Center	Logan	100%	96
Monongalia County General Hospital[2]	Morgantown	100%	941
Ohio Valley Medical Center	Wheeling	100%	510
Plateau Medical Center	Oak Hill	100%	201
Raleigh General Hospital	Beckley	100%	338
Reynolds Memorial Hospital	Glen Dale	100%	86
Saint Francis Hospital	Charleston	100%	874
Saint Joseph Hospital[2]	Buckhannon	100%	92
Saint Mary's Medical Center[2]	Huntington	100%	862
Stonewall Jackson Memorial Hospital	Weston	100%	140
Thomas Memorial Hospital	S Charleston	100%	615
United Hospital Center[2]	Bridgeport	100%	749
Weirton Medical Center	Weirton	100%	270
West Virginia University Hospitals[2]	Morgantown	100%	595
Williamson Memorial Hospital	Williamson	100%	38
Camden Clark Medical Center[2]	Parkersburg	99%	975
Martinsburg VA Medical Center[2]	Martinsburg	99%	160
Pleasant Valley Hospital	Point Pleasant	99%	76
Princeton Community Hospital	Princeton	99%	595
Summersville Regional Medical Center	Summersville	99%	74
Camc Teays Valley Hospital	Hurricane	98%	149
Grant Memorial Hospital	Petersburg	97%	66
Wheeling Hospital	Wheeling	97%	724
Jackson General Hospital	Ripley	92%	25
Welch Community Hospital	Welch	85%	34

Prophylactic Antibiotic Selection

Hospital Name	City	Rate	Cases
Berkeley Medical Center	Martinsburg	100%	324
Cabell Huntington Hospital[2]	Huntington	100%	362
Charleston Area Medical Center[2]	Charleston	100%	896
Davis Memorial Hospital	Elkins	100%	182
Fairmont General Hospital	Fairmont	100%	87
Greenbrier Valley Medical Center	Ronceverte	100%	61
Huntington VA Medical Center	Huntington	100%	92
Monongalia County General Hospital[2]	Morgantown	100%	1070
Pleasant Valley Hospital	Point Pleasant	100%	35
Saint Joseph Hospital[2]	Buckhannon	100%	28
Stonewall Jackson Memorial Hospital	Weston	100%	110

NOTE: Hospital profiles are in alphabetical order by state, then city, then hospital within the city; Rankings exclude hospitals with less than 25 cases except for patient surveys which excludes hospitals with less than 100 cases; (a) 100-299 cases; (1) The number of cases/patients is too few to report; (2) Data submitted were based on a sample of cases/patients; (3) Results are based on a shorter time period than required; (4) Data suppressed by CMS for one or more quarters; (5) Results are not available for this reporting period; (6) Fewer than 100 patients completed the HCAHPS survey; (7) No cases met the criteria for this measure; (8) The lower limit of the confidence interval cannot be calculated if the number of observed infections equals zero; (9) No data are available from the state/territory for this reporting period; (10) The scores shown reflect fewer than 50 completed surveys; (11) There were discrepancies in the data collection process; (12) This measure does not apply to this hospital for this reporting period; (13) Results cannot be calculated for this reporting period; (14) The results for this state are combined with nearby states to protect confidentiality; Please refer to the User's Guide for a full explanation of data.

Hospital Name	City	Rate	Cases
United Hospital Center[2]	Bridgeport	100%	585
West Virginia University Hospitals[2]	Morgantown	100%	565
Wheeling Hospital	Wheeling	100%	604
Camden Clark Medical Center[2]	Parkersburg	99%	811
Martinsburg VA Medical Center	Martinsburg	99%	112
Ohio Valley Medical Center	Wheeling	99%	406
Plateau Medical Center	Oak Hill	99%	169
Princeton Community Hospital	Princeton	99%	476
Raleigh General Hospital	Beckley	99%	150
Saint Francis Hospital	Charleston	99%	725
Saint Mary's Medical Center[2]	Huntington	99%	1013
Thomas Memorial Hospital	S Charleston	99%	399
Bluefield Regional Medical Center	Bluefield	98%	248
Camc Teays Valley Hospital	Hurricane	98%	95
Weirton Medical Center	Weirton	98%	178
Beckley ARH Hospital	Beckley	97%	75
Logan Regional Medical Center	Logan	97%	65
Summersville Regional Medical Center	Summersville	95%	43
Grant Memorial Hospital	Petersburg	92%	62
Reynolds Memorial Hospital	Glen Dale	91%	54

Prophylactic Antibiotic Selection (Outpatient)

Hospital Name	City	Rate	Cases
Camc Teays Valley Hospital	Hurricane	100%	64
Davis Memorial Hospital	Elkins	100%	75
Reynolds Memorial Hospital	Glen Dale	100%	25
Stonewall Jackson Memorial Hospital	Weston	100%	67
Cabell Huntington Hospital	Huntington	99%	294
Monongalia County General Hospital	Morgantown	99%	558
West Virginia University Hospitals	Morgantown	99%	260
Wheeling Hospital	Wheeling	99%	353
Berkeley Medical Center	Martinsburg	98%	115
Bluefield Regional Medical Center	Bluefield	98%	109
Camden Clark Medical Center	Parkersburg	98%	217
Charleston Area Medical Center	Charleston	98%	942
Greenbrier Valley Medical Center	Ronceverte	98%	109
Saint Mary's Medical Center	Huntington	98%	635
Beckley ARH Hospital	Beckley	97%	77
Fairmont General Hospital	Fairmont	97%	73
Raleigh General Hospital	Beckley	97%	394
United Hospital Center	Bridgeport	97%	175
Ohio Valley Medical Center	Wheeling	96%	75
Thomas Memorial Hospital	S Charleston	96%	313
Pleasant Valley Hospital	Point Pleasant	95%	43
Weirton Medical Center	Weirton	95%	104
Logan Regional Medical Center	Logan	93%	82
Princeton Community Hospital	Princeton	93%	81
Saint Francis Hospital	Charleston	92%	189

Prophylactic Antibiotic Stopped

Hospital Name	City	Rate	Cases
Berkeley Medical Center	Martinsburg	100%	321
Cabell Huntington Hospital[2]	Huntington	100%	355
Fairmont General Hospital	Fairmont	100%	84
Huntington VA Medical Center	Huntington	100%	92
Plateau Medical Center	Oak Hill	100%	167
Pleasant Valley Hospital	Point Pleasant	100%	35
Summersville Regional Medical Center	Summersville	100%	43
Monongalia County General Hospital[2]	Morgantown	99%	1051
Stonewall Jackson Memorial Hospital	Weston	99%	105
Thomas Memorial Hospital	S Charleston	99%	390
United Hospital Center[2]	Bridgeport	99%	557
Camden Clark Medical Center[2]	Parkersburg	98%	796
Charleston Area Medical Center[2]	Charleston	98%	813
Princeton Community Hospital	Princeton	98%	467
Raleigh General Hospital	Beckley	98%	142
Saint Mary's Medical Center[2]	Huntington	98%	972
Bluefield Regional Medical Center	Bluefield	97%	245
Greenbrier Valley Medical Center	Ronceverte	97%	60
Logan Regional Medical Center	Logan	97%	38
Ohio Valley Medical Center	Wheeling	97%	402
Saint Francis Hospital	Charleston	97%	719
West Virginia University Hospitals[2]	Morgantown	97%	541
Davis Memorial Hospital	Elkins	96%	179
Martinsburg VA Medical Center	Martinsburg	96%	110
Saint Joseph Hospital[2]	Buckhannon	96%	28
Wheeling Hospital	Wheeling	96%	572
Beckley ARH Hospital	Beckley	95%	66
Camc Teays Valley Hospital	Hurricane	92%	89
Reynolds Memorial Hospital	Glen Dale	90%	48
Weirton Medical Center	Weirton	89%	174
Grant Memorial Hospital	Petersburg	85%	61

Prophylactic Antibiotic Timing

Hospital Name	City	Rate	Cases
Beckley ARH Hospital	Beckley	100%	75
Berkeley Medical Center	Martinsburg	100%	325
Cabell Huntington Hospital[2]	Huntington	100%	362
Davis Memorial Hospital	Elkins	100%	183
Fairmont General Hospital	Fairmont	100%	87
Greenbrier Valley Medical Center	Ronceverte	100%	61
Huntington VA Medical Center	Huntington	100%	92
Logan Regional Medical Center	Logan	100%	65
Monongalia County General Hospital[2]	Morgantown	100%	1071
Plateau Medical Center	Oak Hill	100%	171
Pleasant Valley Hospital	Point Pleasant	100%	35
Saint Joseph Hospital[2]	Buckhannon	100%	28
Stonewall Jackson Memorial Hospital	Weston	100%	110
West Virginia University Hospitals[2]	Morgantown	100%	568
Bluefield Regional Medical Center	Bluefield	99%	248
Camden Clark Medical Center[2]	Parkersburg	99%	812
Charleston Area Medical Center[2]	Charleston	99%	899
Princeton Community Hospital	Princeton	99%	477
Raleigh General Hospital	Beckley	99%	150
Saint Francis Hospital	Charleston	99%	727
Saint Mary's Medical Center[2]	Huntington	99%	1014
Thomas Memorial Hospital	S Charleston	99%	399
United Hospital Center[2]	Bridgeport	99%	591
Weirton Medical Center	Weirton	99%	178
Ohio Valley Medical Center	Wheeling	98%	407
Reynolds Memorial Hospital	Glen Dale	98%	54
Summersville Regional Medical Center	Summersville	98%	43
Camc Teays Valley Hospital	Hurricane	97%	95
Grant Memorial Hospital	Petersburg	97%	62
Wheeling Hospital	Wheeling	97%	606
Martinsburg VA Medical Center	Martinsburg	94%	112

Prophylactic Antibiotic Timing (Outpatient)

Hospital Name	City	Rate	Cases
Beckley ARH Hospital	Beckley	100%	76
Berkeley Medical Center	Martinsburg	100%	115
Greenbrier Valley Medical Center	Ronceverte	100%	109
Pleasant Valley Hospital	Point Pleasant	100%	43
Reynolds Memorial Hospital	Glen Dale	100%	25
Stonewall Jackson Memorial Hospital	Weston	100%	41
Charleston Area Medical Center	Charleston	99%	942
Fairmont General Hospital	Fairmont	99%	74
Logan Regional Medical Center	Logan	99%	83
United Hospital Center	Bridgeport	99%	145
Cabell Huntington Hospital	Huntington	98%	173
Monongalia County General Hospital	Morgantown	98%	562
Raleigh General Hospital	Beckley	98%	396
West Virginia University Hospitals	Morgantown	98%	252
Bluefield Regional Medical Center	Bluefield	97%	109
Saint Mary's Medical Center	Huntington	97%	638
Wheeling Hospital	Wheeling	97%	327
Camc Teays Valley Hospital	Hurricane	96%	67
Camden Clark Medical Center	Parkersburg	95%	222
Thomas Memorial Hospital	S Charleston	95%	319
Davis Memorial Hospital	Elkins	94%	78
Princeton Community Hospital	Princeton	94%	77
Weirton Medical Center	Weirton	93%	108
Ohio Valley Medical Center	Wheeling	92%	78
Saint Francis Hospital	Charleston	90%	189
Jefferson Medical Center[3]	Ranson	88%	26
Summersville Regional Medical Center	Summersville	79%	28

Urinary Catheter Removal

Hospital Name	City	Rate	Cases
Berkeley Medical Center	Martinsburg	100%	278
Fairmont General Hospital	Fairmont	100%	77
Huntington VA Medical Center[2]	Huntington	100%	117
Martinsburg VA Medical Center[2]	Martinsburg	100%	128
Plateau Medical Center	Oak Hill	100%	150
Pleasant Valley Hospital	Point Pleasant	100%	39
Saint Joseph Hospital[2]	Buckhannon	100%	38
Stonewall Jackson Memorial Hospital	Weston	100%	107
United Hospital Center[2]	Bridgeport	100%	501
West Virginia University Hospitals[2]	Morgantown	100%	444
Cabell Huntington Hospital[2]	Huntington	99%	353
Raleigh General Hospital	Beckley	99%	160
Saint Mary's Medical Center[2]	Huntington	99%	788
Bluefield Regional Medical Center	Bluefield	98%	48
Camden Clark Medical Center[2]	Parkersburg	98%	684
Ohio Valley Medical Center	Wheeling	98%	404
Saint Francis Hospital	Charleston	98%	490
Wheeling Hospital	Wheeling	98%	460
Charleston Area Medical Center[2]	Charleston	97%	710
Grant Memorial Hospital	Petersburg	97%	33
Greenbrier Valley Medical Center	Ronceverte	97%	37
Monongalia County General Hospital[2]	Morgantown	97%	283
Thomas Memorial Hospital	S Charleston	97%	183
Logan Regional Medical Center	Logan	96%	46
Beckley ARH Hospital	Beckley	95%	65
Camc Teays Valley Hospital	Hurricane	94%	105
Weirton Medical Center	Weirton	94%	145
Princeton Community Hospital	Princeton	93%	45
Reynolds Memorial Hospital	Glen Dale	90%	29
Davis Memorial Hospital	Elkins	82%	38
Summersville Regional Medical Center	Summersville	82%	51

Survey of Patients' Hospital Experiences

Area Around Room 'Always' Quiet at Night

Hospital Name	City	Rate	Cases
Hampshire Memorial Hospital	Romney	72%	(a)
Summers County ARH Hospital	Hinton	72%	(a)
Pleasant Valley Hospital	Point Pleasant	68%	300+
War Memorial Hospital	Berkeley Springs	68%	(a)
Plateau Medical Center	Oak Hill	66%	300+
Cabell Huntington Hospital	Huntington	65%	300+
Saint Francis Hospital	Charleston	65%	300+
Saint Joseph Hospital	Buckhannon	64%	300+
Ohio Valley Medical Center	Wheeling	63%	300+
Welch Community Hospital	Welch	63%	(a)
Monongalia County General Hospital	Morgantown	62%	300+
Jefferson Medical Center	Ranson	61%	(a)
Wetzel County Hospital	New Martinsville	61%	(a)
Bluefield Regional Medical Center	Bluefield	60%	300+
Princeton Community Hospital	Princeton	60%	300+
Saint Mary's Medical Center	Huntington	60%	300+
United Hospital Center	Bridgeport	60%	300+
Wheeling Hospital	Wheeling	60%	300+
Beckley ARH Hospital	Beckley	59%	300+
Davis Memorial Hospital	Elkins	59%	300+
Thomas Memorial Hospital	S Charleston	59%	300+
Fairmont General Hospital	Fairmont	58%	300+
Greenbrier Valley Medical Center	Ronceverte	58%	300+
Stonewall Jackson Memorial Hospital	Weston	55%	300+
Jackson General Hospital	Ripley	54%	(a)
Logan Regional Medical Center	Logan	54%	300+
Raleigh General Hospital	Beckley	51%	300+
Reynolds Memorial Hospital	Glen Dale	50%	300+
Williamson Memorial Hospital	Williamson	50%	(a)
Summersville Regional Medical Center	Summersville	49%	300+
Charleston Area Medical Center	Charleston	48%	300+
West Virginia University Hospitals	Morgantown	48%	300+
Camden Clark Medical Center	Parkersburg	46%	300+
Grant Memorial Hospital	Petersburg	46%	300+
Berkeley Medical Center	Martinsburg	45%	300+
Weirton Medical Center	Weirton	42%	300+
Camc Teays Valley Hospital	Hurricane	39%	300+

Doctors 'Always' Communicated Well

Hospital Name	City	Rate	Cases
Summers County ARH Hospital	Hinton	90%	(a)
Plateau Medical Center	Oak Hill	89%	300+
Jackson General Hospital	Ripley	88%	(a)
Williamson Memorial Hospital	Williamson	88%	(a)
Pleasant Valley Hospital	Point Pleasant	87%	300+
Princeton Community Hospital	Princeton	86%	300+
Grant Memorial Hospital	Petersburg	85%	300+
Jefferson Medical Center	Ranson	85%	(a)
Stonewall Jackson Memorial Hospital	Weston	84%	300+
Fairmont General Hospital	Fairmont	83%	300+
Logan Regional Medical Center	Logan	83%	300+
War Memorial Hospital	Berkeley Springs	83%	(a)
Welch Community Hospital	Welch	83%	(a)
Greenbrier Valley Medical Center	Ronceverte	82%	300+
Monongalia County General Hospital	Morgantown	82%	300+
Saint Joseph Hospital	Buckhannon	82%	300+
Summersville Regional Medical Center	Summersville	82%	300+
Wetzel County Hospital	New Martinsville	82%	(a)
Bluefield Regional Medical Center	Bluefield	81%	300+
Davis Memorial Hospital	Elkins	81%	300+
Reynolds Memorial Hospital	Glen Dale	81%	300+
Saint Mary's Medical Center	Huntington	81%	300+
United Hospital Center	Bridgeport	81%	300+
Cabell Huntington Hospital	Huntington	80%	300+
Thomas Memorial Hospital	S Charleston	80%	300+
Wheeling Hospital	Wheeling	80%	300+
Charleston Area Medical Center	Charleston	79%	300+
Saint Francis Hospital	Charleston	79%	300+
Beckley ARH Hospital	Beckley	78%	300+
Camc Teays Valley Hospital	Hurricane	78%	300+
Camden Clark Medical Center	Parkersburg	78%	300+
West Virginia University Hospitals	Morgantown	78%	300+
Berkeley Medical Center	Martinsburg	77%	300+
Hampshire Memorial Hospital	Romney	77%	(a)
Weirton Medical Center	Weirton	76%	300+
Raleigh General Hospital	Beckley	75%	300+
Ohio Valley Medical Center	Wheeling	74%	300+

Home Recovery Information Given

Hospital Name	City	Rate	Cases
Grant Memorial Hospital	Petersburg	90%	300+
Plateau Medical Center	Oak Hill	90%	300+
Wheeling Hospital	Wheeling	90%	300+
Summers County ARH Hospital	Hinton	89%	(a)
Welch Community Hospital	Welch	89%	(a)
Cabell Huntington Hospital	Huntington	88%	300+

NOTE: Hospital profiles are in alphabetical order by state, then city, then hospital within the city; Rankings exclude hospitals with less than 25 cases except for patient surveys which excludes hospitals with less than 100 cases; (a) 100-299 cases; (1) The number of cases/patients is too few to report; (2) Data submitted were based on a sample of cases/patients; (3) Results are based on a shorter time period than required; (4) Data suppressed by CMS for one or more quarters; (5) Results are not available for this reporting period; (6) Fewer than 100 patients completed the HCAHPS survey; (7) No cases met the criteria for this measure; (8) The lower limit of the confidence interval cannot be calculated if the number of observed infections equals zero; (9) No data are available from the state/territory for this reporting period; (10) The scores shown reflect fewer than 50 completed surveys; (11) There were discrepancies in the data collection process; (12) This measure does not apply to this hospital for this reporting period; (13) Results cannot be calculated for this reporting period; (14) The results for this state are combined with nearby states to protect confidentiality; Please refer to the User's Guide for a full explanation of data.

Hospital Name	City	Rate	Cases
Pleasant Valley Hospital	Point Pleasant	88%	300+
Saint Mary's Medical Center	Huntington	88%	300+
Jackson General Hospital	Ripley	87%	(a)
Monongalia County General Hospital	Morgantown	87%	300+
Saint Francis Hospital	Charleston	87%	300+
Stonewall Jackson Memorial Hospital	Weston	87%	300+
Wetzel County Hospital	New Martinsville	87%	(a)
Greenbrier Valley Medical Center	Ronceverte	86%	300+
Princeton Community Hospital	Princeton	86%	300+
Saint Joseph Hospital	Buckhannon	86%	300+
Beckley ARH Hospital	Beckley	85%	300+
Davis Memorial Hospital	Elkins	85%	300+
Jefferson Medical Center	Ranson	85%	(a)
Bluefield Regional Medical Center	Bluefield	84%	300+
Camden Clark Medical Center	Parkersburg	84%	300+
Reynolds Memorial Hospital	Glen Dale	84%	300+
War Memorial Hospital	Berkeley Springs	84%	(a)
West Virginia University Hospitals	Morgantown	84%	300+
Charleston Area Medical Center	Charleston	83%	300+
Fairmont General Hospital	Fairmont	83%	300+
Logan Regional Medical Center	Logan	83%	300+
Thomas Memorial Hospital	S Charleston	83%	300+
United Hospital Center	Bridgeport	83%	300+
Weirton Medical Center	Weirton	83%	300+
Williamson Memorial Hospital	Williamson	82%	(a)
Berkeley Medical Center	Martinsburg	81%	300+
Ohio Valley Medical Center	Wheeling	81%	300+
Raleigh General Hospital	Beckley	81%	300+
Camc Teays Valley Hospital	Hurricane	80%	300+
Summersville Regional Medical Center	Summersville	80%	300+
Hampshire Memorial Hospital	Romney	79%	(a)

Hospital Given 9 or 10 on 10 Point Scale

Hospital Name	City	Rate	Cases
Monongalia County General Hospital	Morgantown	78%	300+
Saint Mary's Medical Center	Huntington	77%	300+
Cabell Huntington Hospital	Huntington	76%	300+
Plateau Medical Center	Oak Hill	75%	300+
War Memorial Hospital	Berkeley Springs	75%	(a)
West Virginia University Hospitals	Morgantown	75%	300+
Jefferson Medical Center	Ranson	74%	(a)
Pleasant Valley Hospital	Point Pleasant	74%	300+
Princeton Community Hospital	Princeton	74%	300+
Jackson General Hospital	Ripley	72%	(a)
Wheeling Hospital	Wheeling	71%	300+
Saint Francis Hospital	Charleston	70%	300+
Beckley ARH Hospital	Beckley	69%	300+
Charleston Area Medical Center	Charleston	68%	300+
Greenbrier Valley Medical Center	Ronceverte	68%	300+
Saint Joseph Hospital	Buckhannon	68%	300+
Stonewall Jackson Memorial Hospital	Weston	67%	300+
Summers County ARH Hospital	Hinton	67%	(a)
Thomas Memorial Hospital	S Charleston	67%	300+
United Hospital Center	Bridgeport	67%	300+
Welch Community Hospital	Welch	67%	(a)
Hampshire Memorial Hospital	Romney	66%	(a)
Ohio Valley Medical Center	Wheeling	65%	300+
Wetzel County Hospital	New Martinsville	65%	(a)
Grant Memorial Hospital	Petersburg	62%	300+
Reynolds Memorial Hospital	Glen Dale	62%	300+
Bluefield Regional Medical Center	Bluefield	61%	300+
Williamson Memorial Hospital	Williamson	61%	(a)
Davis Memorial Hospital	Elkins	60%	300+
Berkeley Medical Center	Martinsburg	58%	300+
Logan Regional Medical Center	Logan	58%	300+
Fairmont General Hospital	Fairmont	57%	300+
Raleigh General Hospital	Beckley	57%	300+
Camden Clark Medical Center	Parkersburg	56%	300+
Summersville Regional Medical Center	Summersville	55%	300+
Camc Teays Valley Hospital	Hurricane	54%	300+
Weirton Medical Center	Weirton	49%	300+

Meds 'Always' Explained Before Given

Hospital Name	City	Rate	Cases
Summers County ARH Hospital	Hinton	74%	(a)
Stonewall Jackson Memorial Hospital	Weston	71%	300+
Hampshire Memorial Hospital	Romney	69%	(a)
Plateau Medical Center	Oak Hill	69%	300+
Grant Memorial Hospital	Petersburg	67%	300+
Jackson General Hospital	Ripley	67%	(a)
Pleasant Valley Hospital	Point Pleasant	67%	300+
Welch Community Hospital	Welch	66%	(a)
West Virginia University Hospitals	Morgantown	66%	300+
Cabell Huntington Hospital	Huntington	65%	300+
Fairmont General Hospital	Fairmont	65%	300+
Greenbrier Valley Medical Center	Ronceverte	65%	300+
Monongalia County General Hospital	Morgantown	65%	300+
Saint Joseph Hospital	Buckhannon	65%	300+
Summersville Regional Medical Center	Summersville	65%	300+
Wetzel County Hospital	New Martinsville	65%	(a)
Davis Memorial Hospital	Elkins	64%	300+
Jefferson Medical Center	Ranson	64%	(a)
United Hospital Center	Bridgeport	64%	300+
War Memorial Hospital	Berkeley Springs	64%	(a)
Saint Mary's Medical Center	Huntington	63%	300+
Berkeley Medical Center	Martinsburg	62%	300+
Bluefield Regional Medical Center	Bluefield	62%	300+
Beckley ARH Hospital	Beckley	61%	300+
Charleston Area Medical Center	Charleston	61%	300+
Wheeling Hospital	Wheeling	61%	300+
Princeton Community Hospital	Princeton	60%	300+
Camden Clark Medical Center	Parkersburg	59%	300+
Ohio Valley Medical Center	Wheeling	59%	300+
Reynolds Memorial Hospital	Glen Dale	59%	300+
Williamson Memorial Hospital	Williamson	59%	(a)
Logan Regional Medical Center	Logan	57%	300+
Saint Francis Hospital	Charleston	57%	300+
Camc Teays Valley Hospital	Hurricane	56%	300+
Raleigh General Hospital	Beckley	56%	300+
Weirton Medical Center	Weirton	56%	300+
Thomas Memorial Hospital	S Charleston	55%	300+

Nurses 'Always' Communicated Well

Hospital Name	City	Rate	Cases
Jefferson Medical Center	Ranson	85%	(a)
Plateau Medical Center	Oak Hill	85%	300+
Hampshire Memorial Hospital	Romney	84%	(a)
Summers County ARH Hospital	Hinton	84%	(a)
War Memorial Hospital	Berkeley Springs	84%	(a)
Pleasant Valley Hospital	Point Pleasant	81%	300+
Saint Mary's Medical Center	Huntington	81%	300+
West Virginia University Hospitals	Morgantown	81%	300+
Grant Memorial Hospital	Petersburg	80%	300+
Monongalia County General Hospital	Morgantown	80%	300+
Stonewall Jackson Memorial Hospital	Weston	80%	300+
Greenbrier Valley Medical Center	Ronceverte	79%	300+
Jackson General Hospital	Ripley	79%	(a)
Princeton Community Hospital	Princeton	79%	300+
Saint Joseph Hospital	Buckhannon	79%	300+
Welch Community Hospital	Welch	79%	(a)
Wheeling Hospital	Wheeling	79%	300+
Cabell Huntington Hospital	Huntington	78%	300+
Saint Francis Hospital	Charleston	78%	300+
Davis Memorial Hospital	Elkins	77%	300+
Fairmont General Hospital	Fairmont	77%	300+
United Hospital Center	Bridgeport	76%	300+
Beckley ARH Hospital	Beckley	75%	300+
Berkeley Medical Center	Martinsburg	75%	300+
Bluefield Regional Medical Center	Bluefield	75%	300+
Camden Clark Medical Center	Parkersburg	75%	300+
Charleston Area Medical Center	Charleston	75%	300+
Ohio Valley Medical Center	Wheeling	75%	300+
Summersville Regional Medical Center	Summersville	75%	300+
Wetzel County Hospital	New Martinsville	75%	(a)
Logan Regional Medical Center	Logan	73%	300+
Reynolds Memorial Hospital	Glen Dale	73%	300+
Weirton Medical Center	Weirton	73%	300+
Williamson Memorial Hospital	Williamson	73%	(a)
Raleigh General Hospital	Beckley	71%	300+
Thomas Memorial Hospital	S Charleston	71%	300+
Camc Teays Valley Hospital	Hurricane	69%	300+

Pain 'Always' Well Controlled

Hospital Name	City	Rate	Cases
Plateau Medical Center	Oak Hill	75%	300+
Saint Mary's Medical Center	Huntington	75%	300+
Summers County ARH Hospital	Hinton	75%	(a)
Jackson General Hospital	Ripley	74%	(a)
Pleasant Valley Hospital	Point Pleasant	74%	300+
Monongalia County General Hospital	Morgantown	73%	300+
Wheeling Hospital	Wheeling	73%	300+
Greenbrier Valley Medical Center	Ronceverte	72%	300+
Hampshire Memorial Hospital	Romney	72%	(a)
Princeton Community Hospital	Princeton	72%	300+
Saint Francis Hospital	Charleston	72%	300+
Stonewall Jackson Memorial Hospital	Weston	72%	300+
Beckley ARH Hospital	Beckley	71%	300+
Cabell Huntington Hospital	Huntington	71%	300+
Fairmont General Hospital	Fairmont	71%	300+
Saint Joseph Hospital	Buckhannon	71%	300+
Welch Community Hospital	Welch	71%	(a)
Grant Memorial Hospital	Petersburg	70%	300+
Jefferson Medical Center	Ranson	70%	(a)
Ohio Valley Medical Center	Wheeling	70%	300+
War Memorial Hospital	Berkeley Springs	70%	(a)
West Virginia University Hospitals	Morgantown	69%	300+
Davis Memorial Hospital	Elkins	68%	300+
Reynolds Memorial Hospital	Glen Dale	68%	300+
United Hospital Center	Bridgeport	68%	300+
Wetzel County Hospital	New Martinsville	68%	(a)
Berkeley Medical Center	Martinsburg	67%	300+
Bluefield Regional Medical Center	Bluefield	67%	300+
Camc Teays Valley Hospital	Hurricane	67%	300+
Charleston Area Medical Center	Charleston	67%	300+
Thomas Memorial Hospital	S Charleston	67%	300+
Camden Clark Medical Center	Parkersburg	66%	300+
Summersville Regional Medical Center	Summersville	66%	300+
Logan Regional Medical Center	Logan	65%	300+
Weirton Medical Center	Weirton	65%	300+
Raleigh General Hospital	Beckley	64%	300+
Williamson Memorial Hospital	Williamson	64%	(a)

Room and Bathroom 'Always' Clean

Hospital Name	City	Rate	Cases
Jefferson Medical Center	Ranson	85%	(a)
War Memorial Hospital	Berkeley Springs	85%	(a)
Welch Community Hospital	Welch	84%	(a)
Grant Memorial Hospital	Petersburg	83%	300+
Hampshire Memorial Hospital	Romney	82%	(a)
Stonewall Jackson Memorial Hospital	Weston	81%	300+
Summers County ARH Hospital	Hinton	81%	(a)
Pleasant Valley Hospital	Point Pleasant	80%	300+
Wetzel County Hospital	New Martinsville	80%	(a)
Jackson General Hospital	Ripley	79%	(a)
Saint Mary's Medical Center	Huntington	78%	300+
Berkeley Medical Center	Martinsburg	77%	300+
United Hospital Center	Bridgeport	77%	300+
Davis Memorial Hospital	Elkins	76%	300+
Greenbrier Valley Medical Center	Ronceverte	76%	300+
Plateau Medical Center	Oak Hill	76%	300+
Ohio Valley Medical Center	Wheeling	74%	300+
Cabell Huntington Hospital	Huntington	73%	300+
Monongalia County General Hospital	Morgantown	73%	300+
Wheeling Hospital	Wheeling	73%	300+
Logan Regional Medical Center	Logan	72%	300+
Bluefield Regional Medical Center	Bluefield	71%	300+
Princeton Community Hospital	Princeton	71%	300+
Summersville Regional Medical Center	Summersville	71%	300+
Reynolds Memorial Hospital	Glen Dale	68%	300+
Saint Francis Hospital	Charleston	68%	300+
West Virginia University Hospitals	Morgantown	68%	300+
Beckley ARH Hospital	Beckley	67%	300+
Camc Teays Valley Hospital	Hurricane	67%	300+
Fairmont General Hospital	Fairmont	67%	300+
Raleigh General Hospital	Beckley	67%	300+
Williamson Memorial Hospital	Williamson	67%	(a)
Weirton Medical Center	Weirton	66%	300+
Charleston Area Medical Center	Charleston	65%	300+
Thomas Memorial Hospital	S Charleston	65%	300+
Camden Clark Medical Center	Parkersburg	64%	300+
Saint Joseph Hospital	Buckhannon	62%	300+

Timely Help 'Always' Received

Hospital Name	City	Rate	Cases
Summers County ARH Hospital	Hinton	79%	(a)
Grant Memorial Hospital	Petersburg	75%	300+
Jefferson Medical Center	Ranson	75%	(a)
Plateau Medical Center	Oak Hill	75%	300+
Hampshire Memorial Hospital	Romney	74%	(a)
Saint Joseph Hospital	Buckhannon	73%	300+
Stonewall Jackson Memorial Hospital	Weston	73%	300+
Pleasant Valley Hospital	Point Pleasant	72%	300+
Welch Community Hospital	Welch	72%	(a)
Saint Mary's Medical Center	Huntington	71%	300+
Jackson General Hospital	Ripley	69%	(a)
Saint Francis Hospital	Charleston	69%	300+
Wetzel County Hospital	New Martinsville	69%	(a)
Cabell Huntington Hospital	Huntington	68%	300+
Davis Memorial Hospital	Elkins	68%	300+
Monongalia County General Hospital	Morgantown	68%	300+
Princeton Community Hospital	Princeton	67%	300+
West Virginia University Hospitals	Morgantown	67%	300+
Greenbrier Valley Medical Center	Ronceverte	66%	300+
Wheeling Hospital	Wheeling	66%	300+
Berkeley Medical Center	Martinsburg	65%	300+
Camden Clark Medical Center	Parkersburg	65%	300+
Beckley ARH Hospital	Beckley	64%	300+
Reynolds Memorial Hospital	Glen Dale	64%	300+
Charleston Area Medical Center	Charleston	63%	300+
Thomas Memorial Hospital	S Charleston	63%	300+
Fairmont General Hospital	Fairmont	62%	300+
War Memorial Hospital	Berkeley Springs	61%	(a)
Bluefield Regional Medical Center	Bluefield	59%	300+
Ohio Valley Medical Center	Wheeling	59%	300+
Summersville Regional Medical Center	Summersville	59%	300+
United Hospital Center	Bridgeport	59%	300+
Logan Regional Medical Center	Logan	58%	300+
Weirton Medical Center	Weirton	58%	300+
Camc Teays Valley Hospital	Hurricane	57%	300+
Williamson Memorial Hospital	Williamson	51%	(a)

NOTE: Hospital profiles are in alphabetical order by state, then city, then hospital within the city; Rankings exclude hospitals with less than 25 cases except for patient surveys which excludes hospitals with less than 100 cases; (a) 100-299 cases; (1) The number of cases/patients is too few to report; (2) Data submitted were based on a sample of cases/patients; (3) Results are based on a shorter time period than required; (4) Data suppressed by CMS for one or more quarters; (5) Results are not available for this reporting period; (6) Fewer than 100 patients completed the HCAHPS survey; (7) No cases met the criteria for this measure; (8) The lower limit of the confidence interval cannot be calculated if the number of observed infections equals zero; (9) No data are available from the state/territory for this reporting period; (10) The scores shown reflect fewer than 50 completed surveys; (11) There were discrepancies in the data collection process; (12) This measure does not apply to this hospital for this reporting period; (13) Results cannot be calculated for this reporting period; (14) The results for this state are combined with nearby states to protect confidentiality; Please refer to the User's Guide for a full explanation of data.

Raleigh General Hospital	Beckley	50%	300+

Would Definitely Recommend Hospital

Hospital Name	City	Rate	Cases
Monongalia County General Hospital	Morgantown	83%	300+
Saint Mary's Medical Center	Huntington	82%	300+
Cabell Huntington Hospital	Huntington	78%	300+
West Virginia University Hospitals	Morgantown	78%	300+
Saint Francis Hospital	Charleston	76%	300+
Pleasant Valley Hospital	Point Pleasant	75%	300+
Beckley ARH Hospital	Beckley	73%	300+
Plateau Medical Center	Oak Hill	73%	300+
Wheeling Hospital	Wheeling	73%	300+
Charleston Area Medical Center	Charleston	72%	300+
Jefferson Medical Center	Ranson	72%	(a)
Princeton Community Hospital	Princeton	72%	300+
Thomas Memorial Hospital	S Charleston	72%	300+
Ohio Valley Medical Center	Wheeling	71%	300+
Summers County ARH Hospital	Hinton	70%	(a)
Wetzel County Hospital	New Martinsville	68%	(a)
War Memorial Hospital	Berkeley Springs	67%	(a)
Jackson General Hospital	Ripley	66%	(a)
Saint Joseph Hospital	Buckhannon	66%	300+
United Hospital Center	Bridgeport	65%	300+
Stonewall Jackson Memorial Hospital	Weston	64%	300+
Greenbrier Valley Medical Center	Ronceverte	63%	300+
Bluefield Regional Medical Center	Bluefield	62%	300+
Hampshire Memorial Hospital	Romney	62%	(a)
Reynolds Memorial Hospital	Glen Dale	60%	300+
Welch Community Hospital	Welch	59%	(a)
Camden Clark Medical Center	Parkersburg	58%	300+
Berkeley Medical Center	Martinsburg	57%	300+
Grant Memorial Hospital	Petersburg	57%	300+
Raleigh General Hospital	Beckley	57%	300+
Williamson Memorial Hospital	Williamson	57%	(a)
Summersville Regional Medical Center	Summersville	56%	300+
Davis Memorial Hospital	Elkins	55%	300+
Logan Regional Medical Center	Logan	55%	300+
Camc Teays Valley Hospital	Hurricane	54%	300+
Fairmont General Hospital	Fairmont	54%	300+
Weirton Medical Center	Weirton	51%	300+

Use of Medical Imaging

Cardiac Imaging Stress Test before OP Surgery

Hospital Name	City	Rate	Cases
Jefferson Medical Center	Ranson	0.0%	45
Preston Memorial Hospital	Kingwood	2.0%	49
Beckley ARH Hospital	Beckley	3.0%	199
Saint Mary's Medical Center	Huntington	3.0%	302
United Hospital Center	Bridgeport	3.1%	360
Camden Clark Medical Center	Parkersburg	3.2%	94
Berkeley Medical Center	Martinsburg	3.6%	393
Wheeling Hospital	Wheeling	3.8%	133
Davis Memorial Hospital	Elkins	4.1%	363
West Virginia University Hospitals	Morgantown	4.1%	542
Weirton Medical Center	Weirton	4.2%	261
Pleasant Valley Hospital	Point Pleasant	4.4%	180
Summersville Regional Medical Center	Summersville	4.4%	91
Stonewall Jackson Memorial Hospital	Weston	4.5%	177
Camc Teays Valley Hospital	Hurricane	4.7%	64
Greenbrier Valley Medical Center	Ronceverte	4.8%	248
Fairmont General Hospital	Fairmont	5.0%	400
Logan Regional Medical Center	Logan	5.1%	297
Raleigh General Hospital	Beckley	5.1%	257
Bluefield Regional Medical Center	Bluefield	5.2%	231
Charleston Area Medical Center	Charleston	5.3%	1619
Thomas Memorial Hospital	S Charleston	5.9%	204
Monongalia County General Hospital	Morgantown	6.3%	366
Williamson Memorial Hospital	Williamson	6.5%	77
Princeton Community Hospital	Princeton	6.7%	417
Saint Joseph Hospital	Buckhannon	7.0%	115
Cabell Huntington Hospital	Huntington	8.9%	135
Jackson General Hospital	Ripley	9.2%	152
Boone Memorial Hospital	Madison	11.9%	67

Combination Abdominal CT Scan

Hospital Name	City	Rate	Cases
Jefferson Medical Center	Ranson	1.2%	333
Logan Regional Medical Center	Logan	1.8%	682
Welch Community Hospital	Welch	1.8%	163
Boone Memorial Hospital	Madison	2.3%	311
Plateau Medical Center	Oak Hill	2.4%	379
Saint Francis Hospital	Charleston	3.1%	225
Camc Teays Valley Hospital	Hurricane	3.3%	491
Saint Mary's Medical Center	Huntington	3.4%	1538
Grant Memorial Hospital	Petersburg	3.5%	287
Williamson Memorial Hospital	Williamson	4.2%	287
Bluefield Regional Medical Center	Bluefield	5.5%	531
Pleasant Valley Hospital	Point Pleasant	5.5%	328
Berkeley Medical Center	Martinsburg	5.6%	1221
Cabell Huntington Hospital	Huntington	5.9%	1073
Wetzel County Hospital	New Martinsville	7.3%	259
Wheeling Hospital	Wheeling	8.0%	916
War Memorial Hospital	Berkeley Springs	8.8%	148
Charleston Area Medical Center	Charleston	9.1%	1876
West Virginia University Hospitals	Morgantown	9.2%	731
Weirton Medical Center	Weirton	9.3%	603
Greenbrier Valley Medical Center	Ronceverte	9.9%	957
Raleigh General Hospital	Beckley	9.9%	657
Summersville Regional Medical Center	Summersville	10.1%	483
Preston Memorial Hospital	Kingwood	11.2%	143
Jackson General Hospital	Ripley	12.6%	269
Camden Clark Medical Center	Parkersburg	13.5%	1861
Thomas Memorial Hospital	S Charleston	13.6%	1004
Reynolds Memorial Hospital	Glen Dale	15.2%	204
Monongalia County General Hospital	Morgantown	18.3%	885
Davis Memorial Hospital	Elkins	21.2%	820
Beckley ARH Hospital	Beckley	21.4%	463
United Hospital Center	Bridgeport	29.8%	1270
Fairmont General Hospital	Fairmont	30.5%	581
Broaddus Hospital Association	Philippi	32.2%	118
Roane General Hospital	Spencer	34.7%	190
Stonewall Jackson Memorial Hospital	Weston	37.4%	227
Saint Joseph Hospital	Buckhannon	37.9%	240
Sistersville General Hospital	Sistersville	39.8%	83
Ohio Valley Medical Center	Wheeling	53.7%	406
Princeton Community Hospital	Princeton	60.2%	962

Combination Brain/Sinus CT Scan

Hospital Name	City	Rate	Cases
Camc Teays Valley Hospital	Hurricane	0.6%	321
Roane General Hospital	Spencer	0.6%	181
Broaddus Hospital Association	Philippi	0.7%	135
Charleston Area Medical Center	Charleston	0.8%	1192
West Virginia University Hospitals	Morgantown	0.8%	722
Jefferson Medical Center	Ranson	1.5%	532
Berkeley Medical Center	Martinsburg	1.8%	609
Plateau Medical Center	Oak Hill	1.9%	516
Raleigh General Hospital	Beckley	2.0%	664
Camden Clark Medical Center	Parkersburg	2.1%	1362
Princeton Community Hospital	Princeton	2.1%	986
United Hospital Center	Bridgeport	2.4%	914
Fairmont General Hospital	Fairmont	2.5%	568
Monongalia County General Hospital	Morgantown	2.5%	600
Summersville Regional Medical Center	Summersville	2.7%	566
Thomas Memorial Hospital	S Charleston	2.8%	709
Wheeling Hospital	Wheeling	2.9%	799
Davis Memorial Hospital	Elkins	4.0%	598
Logan Regional Medical Center	Logan	4.4%	661
Beckley ARH Hospital	Beckley	4.5%	513
Greenbrier Valley Medical Center	Ronceverte	4.7%	749
Saint Mary's Medical Center	Huntington	4.9%	1662
Bluefield Regional Medical Center	Bluefield	5.2%	572
Ohio Valley Medical Center	Wheeling	5.2%	327
Preston Memorial Hospital	Kingwood	6.8%	220
Saint Francis Hospital	Charleston	7.3%	274
Williamson Memorial Hospital	Williamson	8.2%	306

Combination Chest CT Scan

Hospital Name	City	Rate	Cases
Camc Teays Valley Hospital	Hurricane	0.0%	232
Plateau Medical Center	Oak Hill	0.0%	128
Roane General Hospital	Spencer	0.0%	85
Saint Francis Hospital	Charleston	0.0%	48
Saint Joseph Hospital	Buckhannon	0.0%	123
Saint Mary's Medical Center	Huntington	0.0%	1034
United Hospital Center	Bridgeport	0.0%	698
Welch Community Hospital	Welch	0.0%	78
Wetzel County Hospital	New Martinsville	0.0%	150
Monongalia County General Hospital	Morgantown	0.1%	742
Logan Regional Medical Center	Logan	0.2%	555
Wheeling Hospital	Wheeling	0.3%	682
Cabell Huntington Hospital	Huntington	0.4%	906
Charleston Area Medical Center	Charleston	0.4%	1616
Ohio Valley Medical Center	Wheeling	0.6%	311
Stonewall Jackson Memorial Hospital	Weston	0.6%	166
Greenbrier Valley Medical Center	Ronceverte	0.7%	540
Grant Memorial Hospital	Petersburg	1.0%	96
Princeton Community Hospital	Princeton	1.0%	727
Reynolds Memorial Hospital	Glen Dale	1.1%	91
Fairmont General Hospital	Fairmont	1.2%	340
Boone Memorial Hospital	Madison	1.6%	188
Jefferson Medical Center	Ranson	2.0%	102
Weirton Medical Center	Weirton	2.1%	241
Camden Clark Medical Center	Parkersburg	2.5%	933
West Virginia University Hospitals	Morgantown	2.7%	813
Thomas Memorial Hospital	S Charleston	3.0%	670
Williamson Memorial Hospital	Williamson	4.7%	85
Berkeley Medical Center	Martinsburg	5.4%	541
Pleasant Valley Hospital	Point Pleasant	5.4%	129
Bluefield Regional Medical Center	Bluefield	6.0%	235
Davis Memorial Hospital	Elkins	6.3%	458
Raleigh General Hospital	Beckley	6.6%	454
Jackson General Hospital	Ripley	8.3%	180
Broaddus Hospital Association	Philippi	9.3%	97
Preston Memorial Hospital	Kingwood	11.8%	68
Summersville Regional Medical Center	Summersville	19.3%	187
Beckley ARH Hospital	Beckley	29.3%	157

Follow-up Mammogram/Ultrasound

A follow-up rate near zero may indicate missed cancer; a rate higher than 14% may mean there is unnecessary follow up.

Hospital Name	City	Rate	Cases
Jefferson Medical Center	Ranson	1.9%	363
Sistersville General Hospital	Sistersville	1.9%	107
Bluefield Regional Medical Center	Bluefield	3.8%	652
Roane General Hospital	Spencer	4.4%	226
Stonewall Jackson Memorial Hospital	Weston	4.8%	230
Berkeley Medical Center	Martinsburg	5.5%	1173
Camden Clark Medical Center	Parkersburg	5.8%	3132
Davis Memorial Hospital	Elkins	6.0%	906
Pleasant Valley Hospital	Point Pleasant	6.7%	419
Saint Joseph Hospital	Buckhannon	6.7%	401
Princeton Community Hospital	Princeton	6.8%	1193
United Hospital Center	Bridgeport	6.9%	1698
Welch Community Hospital	Welch	6.9%	87
Charleston Area Medical Center	Charleston	7.4%	3184
Camc Teays Valley Hospital	Hurricane	7.6%	370
Monongalia County General Hospital	Morgantown	7.7%	1185
Fairmont General Hospital	Fairmont	7.9%	595
Plateau Medical Center	Oak Hill	8.2%	97
Summersville Regional Medical Center	Summersville	8.4%	249
Wheeling Hospital	Wheeling	8.8%	1455
Saint Mary's Medical Center	Huntington	9.4%	1106
Cabell Huntington Hospital	Huntington	9.6%	1876
Preston Memorial Hospital	Kingwood	9.6%	198
Beckley ARH Hospital	Beckley	9.8%	255
Jackson General Hospital	Ripley	9.8%	256
Thomas Memorial Hospital	S Charleston	10.0%	1304
Raleigh General Hospital	Beckley	10.7%	122
Wetzel County Hospital	New Martinsville	11.1%	396
Boone Memorial Hospital	Madison	11.2%	187
Broaddus Hospital Association	Philippi	11.3%	142
Saint Francis Hospital	Charleston	11.5%	918
Weirton Medical Center	Weirton	11.7%	626
West Virginia University Hospitals	Morgantown	11.9%	2029
Logan Regional Medical Center	Logan	14.3%	505
Grant Memorial Hospital	Petersburg	14.5%	346
Williamson Memorial Hospital	Williamson	14.6%	82
Reynolds Memorial Hospital	Glen Dale	15.5%	304
Greenbrier Valley Medical Center	Ronceverte	17.1%	432
Ohio Valley Medical Center	Wheeling	17.8%	597
War Memorial Hospital	Berkeley Springs	21.8%	220

Lumbar Spine MRI for Low Back Pain

Hospital Name	City	Rate	Cases
Beckley ARH Hospital	Beckley	17.1%	70
Jackson General Hospital	Ripley	30.9%	55
United Hospital Center	Bridgeport	31.3%	387
Pleasant Valley Hospital	Point Pleasant	34.3%	67
Cabell Huntington Hospital	Huntington	34.6%	208
Wheeling Hospital	Wheeling	35.4%	113
Saint Francis Hospital	Charleston	35.7%	70
Greenbrier Valley Medical Center	Ronceverte	36.1%	166
Fairmont General Hospital	Fairmont	36.9%	122
Saint Mary's Medical Center	Huntington	37.2%	304
Logan Regional Medical Center	Logan	37.5%	72
Raleigh General Hospital	Beckley	37.5%	277
Camden Clark Medical Center	Parkersburg	38.1%	244
Davis Memorial Hospital	Elkins	38.5%	78
Berkeley Medical Center	Martinsburg	39.3%	122
Summersville Regional Medical Center	Summersville	39.5%	81
Princeton Community Hospital	Princeton	40.1%	207
Monongalia County General Hospital	Morgantown	41.2%	119
Charleston Area Medical Center	Charleston	41.4%	222
Bluefield Regional Medical Center	Bluefield	42.2%	83
Thomas Memorial Hospital	S Charleston	42.9%	275
Weirton Medical Center	Weirton	43.9%	82
Camc Teays Valley Hospital	Hurricane	44.3%	70
Wetzel County Hospital	New Martinsville	45.0%	40
Plateau Medical Center	Oak Hill	46.7%	45
Reynolds Memorial Hospital	Glen Dale	47.3%	55
Grant Memorial Hospital	Petersburg	47.7%	44

NOTE: Hospital profiles are in alphabetical order by state, then city, then hospital within the city; Rankings exclude hospitals with less than 25 cases except for patient surveys which excludes hospitals with less than 100 cases; (a) 100-299 cases; (1) The number of cases/patients is too few to report; (2) Data submitted were based on a sample of cases/patients; (3) Results are based on a shorter time period than required; (4) Data suppressed by CMS for one or more quarters; (5) Results are not available for this reporting period; (6) Fewer than 100 patients completed the HCAHPS survey; (7) No cases met the criteria for this measure; (8) The lower limit of the confidence interval cannot be calculated if the number of observed infections equals zero; (9) No data are available from the state/territory for this reporting period; (10) The scores shown reflect fewer than 50 completed surveys; (11) There were discrepancies in the data collection process; (12) This measure does not apply to this hospital for this reporting period; (13) Results cannot be calculated for this reporting period; (14) The results for this state are combined with nearby states to protect confidentiality; Please refer to the User's Guide for a full explanation of data.

Beckley ARH Hospital

306 Stanaford Road
Beckley, WV 25801
E-mail: beckleyarh@arh.org
URL: www.arh.org/beckley
Type: Acute Care Hospitals
Ownership: Voluntary non-profit - Private
Phone: 304-255-3456
Fax: 304-255-3544
Emergency Services: Yes
Beds: 173

Key Personnel:
CEO/President.............. Stephen C Hanson
Operating Room.............. Elias Isaac
Chief of Medical Staff.......... Rajiv Khanna, MD
Infection Control.............. Kathy Martin
Radiology.................. Daniel D Maxwell
Intensive Care Unit............ Brenda Ward
Quality Assurance............ Robert Wayne
Emergency Room............ Rob Williams, MD

Measure	Cases	This Hosp.	State Avg.	U.S. Avg.
Blood Clot Prevention and Treatment				
Anticoagulation Overlap Therapy[2]	40	85%	90%	93%
ICU Venous Thromboembolism Prophylaxis[2]	96	93%	88%	92%
Incidence of Potentially Preventable VTE[1,2]	-	-	12%	10%
UFH with Dosages/Platelet Monitoring[2]	11	100%	98%	97%
Venous Thromboembolism Prophylaxis[2]	413	92%	79%	85%
Warfarin Therapy Discharge Instructions[2]	31	94%	80%	75%
Chest Pain/Possible Heart Attack Care				
Aspirin Given Within 24 Hours of Arrival	31	97%	96%	96%
Fibrinolytic Meds Within 30 Min. of Arrival[7]	-	-	74%	58%
Average Time to ECG (minutes)	31	7	8	7
Average Time to Transfer (minutes)[1]	-	-	109	60
Children's Asthma Care				
Received Home Management Plan of Care	-	-	-	88%
Received Reliever Medication	-	-	-	100%
Received Systemic Corticosteroids	-	-	-	100%
Emergency Department				
Admittance Decision Time (minutes)[2]	510	126	76	98
Head CT Results Within 45 Min. of Arrival[1]	-	-	43%	57%
Patients Who Left ER Before Being Seen	24,171	2%	2%	2%
Time from ER Arrival to Admit. (minutes)[2]	511	320	257	274
Time from ER Arrival to Discharge (minutes)	354	180	142	134
Time in ER Before Being Evaluated (minutes)	440	31	30	26
Time to Pain Meds for Fractures (minutes)	81	95	67	57
Heart Attack Care				
Aspirin Given at Discharge[1]	-	-	99%	99%
Fibrinolytic Meds Within 30 Min. of Arrival[7]	-	-	50%	54%
PCI Within 90 Minutes of Arrival[7]	-	-	93%	96%
Statin Prescribed at Discharge[1]	-	-	98%	98%
Heart Failure Care				
ACE Inhibitor or ARB for LVSD	35	77%	96%	97%
Discharge Instructions Given	108	88%	94%	94%
Evaluation of LVS Function	138	97%	98%	99%
Medicare Spending				
Medicare Spending per Patient (ratio)	-	0.99	0.96	0.98
Pneumonia Care				
Appropriate Initial Antibiotic Given	105	96%	94%	95%
Blood Culture Timing	171	93%	97%	98%
Pregnancy and Delivery Care				
Newborn Deliveries Scheduled Early[7]	-	-	10%	6%
Preventive Care				
Immunization for Influenza[2]	412	95%	94%	90%
Immunization for Pneumonia[2]	673	96%	95%	92%
Stroke Care				
Anticoagulation Therapy for Atrial Fibrillation[1]	-	-	94%	95%
Antithrombotic Therapy Timing	11	91%	98%	98%
Assessed for Rehabilitation	12	92%	96%	97%
Discharged on Antithrombotic Therapy[1]	-	-	98%	99%
Discharged on Statin Medication[1]	-	-	91%	94%
Thrombolytic Therapy Timing[7]	-	-	67%	66%
Venous Thromboembolism Prophylaxis	15	73%	91%	94%
Written Stroke Educational Materials Given[1]	-	-	84%	88%
Surgical Care Improvement Project				
Appropriate Beta Blocker Usage	45	100%	98%	98%
Appropriate VTP Within 24 Hours	111	96%	98%	98%
Controlled Postoperative Blood Glucose[7]	-	-	95%	97%
Perioperative Temperature Management	130	100%	100%	100%
Prophylactic Antibiotic Selection	75	97%	99%	99%
Prophylactic Antibiotic Selection (Outpatient)	77	97%	97%	98%
Prophylactic Antibiotic Stopped	66	95%	98%	98%
Prophylactic Antibiotic Timing	75	100%	99%	99%
Prophylactic Antibiotic Timing (Outpatient)	76	100%	97%	98%
Urinary Catheter Removal	65	95%	98%	97%
Survey of Patients' Hospital Experiences				
Area Around Room 'Always' Quiet at Night	300+	59%	58%	61%
Doctors 'Always' Communicated Well	300+	78%	82%	82%
Home Recovery Information Given	300+	85%	85%	85%
Hospital Given 9 or 10 on 10 Point Scale	300+	69%	66%	71%
Meds 'Always' Explained Before Given	300+	61%	64%	64%
Nurses 'Always' Communicated Well	300+	75%	78%	79%
Pain 'Always' Well Controlled	300+	71%	70%	71%
Room and Bathroom 'Always' Clean	300+	67%	75%	73%
Timely Help 'Always' Received	300+	64%	68%	68%
Would Definitely Recommend Hospital	300+	73%	66%	71%
Use of Medical Imaging				
Cardiac Imaging Stress Test before Surgery	199	3.0%	4.9%	5.3%
Combination Abdominal CT Scan	463	21.4%	14.4%	10.5%
Combination Brain/Sinus CT Scan	513	4.5%	3%	2.7%
Combination Chest CT Scan	157	29.3%	2.8%	2.7%
Follow-up Mammogram/Ultrasound	255	9.8%	8.8%	8.8%
Lumbar Spine MRI for Low Back Pain	70	17.1%	38.4%	37.2%

Beckley VA Medical Center

200 Veterans Avenue
Beckley, WV 25801
URL: www.beckley.va.gov
Type: Acute Care - VA
Ownership: Government Federal
Phone: 304-255-2121
Fax: 304-255-2431
Emergency Services: No
Beds: 111

Key Personnel:
Quality Assurance............ Sandra Mane
Emergency Room............ James Pawell
Chief of Medical Staff.......... Edward Shooler

Measure	Cases	This Hosp.	State Avg.	U.S. Avg.
Blood Clot Prevention and Treatment				
Anticoagulation Overlap Therapy	-	-	90%	93%
ICU Venous Thromboembolism Prophylaxis	-	-	88%	92%
Incidence of Potentially Preventable VTE	-	-	12%	10%
UFH with Dosages/Platelet Monitoring	-	-	98%	97%
Venous Thromboembolism Prophylaxis	-	-	79%	85%
Warfarin Therapy Discharge Instructions	-	-	80%	75%
Chest Pain/Possible Heart Attack Care				
Aspirin Given Within 24 Hours of Arrival	-	-	96%	96%
Fibrinolytic Meds Within 30 Min. of Arrival	-	-	74%	58%
Average Time to ECG (minutes)	-	-	8	7
Average Time to Transfer (minutes)	-	-	109	60
Children's Asthma Care				
Received Home Management Plan of Care	-	-	-	88%
Received Reliever Medication	-	-	-	100%
Received Systemic Corticosteroids	-	-	-	100%
Emergency Department				
Admittance Decision Time (minutes)	-	-	76	98
Head CT Results Within 45 Min. of Arrival	-	-	43%	57%
Patients Who Left ER Before Being Seen	-	-	2%	2%
Time from ER Arrival to Admit. (minutes)	-	-	257	274
Time from ER Arrival to Discharge (minutes)	-	-	142	134
Time in ER Before Being Evaluated (minutes)	-	-	30	26
Time to Pain Meds for Fractures (minutes)	-	-	67	57
Heart Attack Care				
Aspirin Given at Discharge[5]	-	-	99%	99%
Fibrinolytic Meds Within 30 Min. of Arrival[5]	-	-	50%	54%
PCI Within 90 Minutes of Arrival[5]	-	-	93%	96%
Statin Prescribed at Discharge[5]	-	-	98%	98%
Heart Failure Care				
ACE Inhibitor or ARB for LVSD	28	100%	96%	97%
Discharge Instructions Given	51	100%	94%	94%
Evaluation of LVS Function	55	100%	98%	99%
Medicare Spending				
Medicare Spending per Patient (ratio)	-	-	0.96	0.98
Pneumonia Care				
Appropriate Initial Antibiotic Given	70	93%	94%	95%
Blood Culture Timing	112	100%	97%	98%
Pregnancy and Delivery Care				
Newborn Deliveries Scheduled Early	-	-	10%	6%
Preventive Care				
Immunization for Influenza[2,3]	144	96%	94%	90%
Immunization for Pneumonia[2,3]	360	94%	95%	92%
Stroke Care				
Anticoagulation Therapy for Atrial Fibrillation	-	-	94%	95%
Antithrombotic Therapy Timing	-	-	98%	98%
Assessed for Rehabilitation	-	-	96%	97%
Discharged on Antithrombotic Therapy	-	-	98%	99%
Discharged on Statin Medication	-	-	91%	94%
Thrombolytic Therapy Timing	-	-	67%	66%
Venous Thromboembolism Prophylaxis	-	-	91%	94%
Written Stroke Educational Materials Given	-	-	84%	88%
Surgical Care Improvement Project				
Appropriate Beta Blocker Usage[5]	-	-	98%	98%
Appropriate VTP Within 24 Hours[5]	-	-	98%	98%
Controlled Postoperative Blood Glucose[5]	-	-	95%	97%
Perioperative Temperature Management[5]	-	-	100%	100%
Prophylactic Antibiotic Selection[5]	-	-	99%	99%
Prophylactic Antibiotic Selection (Outpatient)	-	-	97%	98%
Prophylactic Antibiotic Stopped[5]	-	-	98%	98%
Prophylactic Antibiotic Timing[5]	-	-	99%	99%
Prophylactic Antibiotic Timing (Outpatient)	-	-	97%	98%
Urinary Catheter Removal[5]	-	-	98%	97%
Survey of Patients' Hospital Experiences				
Area Around Room 'Always' Quiet at Night	-	-	58%	61%
Doctors 'Always' Communicated Well	-	-	82%	82%
Home Recovery Information Given	-	-	85%	85%
Hospital Given 9 or 10 on 10 Point Scale	-	-	66%	71%
Meds 'Always' Explained Before Given	-	-	64%	64%
Nurses 'Always' Communicated Well	-	-	78%	79%
Pain 'Always' Well Controlled	-	-	70%	71%
Room and Bathroom 'Always' Clean	-	-	75%	73%
Timely Help 'Always' Received	-	-	68%	68%
Would Definitely Recommend Hospital	-	-	66%	71%
Use of Medical Imaging				
Cardiac Imaging Stress Test before Surgery	-	-	4.9%	5.3%
Combination Abdominal CT Scan	-	-	14.4%	10.5%
Combination Brain/Sinus CT Scan	-	-	3%	2.7%
Combination Chest CT Scan	-	-	2.8%	2.7%
Follow-up Mammogram/Ultrasound	-	-	8.8%	8.8%
Lumbar Spine MRI for Low Back Pain	-	-	38.4%	37.2%

Raleigh General Hospital

1710 Harper Road
Beckley, WV 25801
URL: www.raleighgeneral.com
Type: Acute Care Hospitals
Ownership: Proprietary
Phone: 304-256-4100
Fax: 304-256-4009
Emergency Services: Yes
Beds: 392

Key Personnel:
CEO/President.............. David Darden
Chief of Medical Staff.......... Anthony Dinh
Quality Assurance............ Shievonna Shamblin
Pediatric Ambulatory Care...... Ted Solari, MD
Pediatric In-Patient Care....... Ted Solari, MD
Infection Control.............. Nancy Ward
Operating Room.............. Doug Wyandt

Measure	Cases	This Hosp.	State Avg.	U.S. Avg.
Blood Clot Prevention and Treatment				
Anticoagulation Overlap Therapy[2]	118	97%	90%	93%
ICU Venous Thromboembolism Prophylaxis[2]	94	95%	88%	92%
Incidence of Potentially Preventable VTE[2]	29	17%	12%	10%
UFH with Dosages/Platelet Monitoring[2]	22	95%	98%	97%
Venous Thromboembolism Prophylaxis[2]	422	79%	79%	85%
Warfarin Therapy Discharge Instructions[2]	93	100%	80%	75%
Chest Pain/Possible Heart Attack Care				
Aspirin Given Within 24 Hours of Arrival	27	93%	96%	96%
Fibrinolytic Meds Within 30 Min. of Arrival[1,3]	-	-	74%	58%
Average Time to ECG (minutes)	30	14	8	7
Average Time to Transfer (minutes)[3,7]	-	-	109	60
Children's Asthma Care				
Received Home Management Plan of Care	13	85%	-	88%

NOTE: *Hospital profiles are in alphabetical order by state, then city, then hospital within the city; Rankings exclude hospitals with less than 25 cases except for patient surveys which excludes hospitals with less than 100 cases; (a) 100-299 cases; (1) The number of cases/patients is too few to report; (2) Data submitted were based on a sample of cases/patients; (3) Results are based on a shorter time period than required; (4) Data suppressed by CMS for one or more quarters; (5) Results are not available for this reporting period; (6) Fewer than 100 patients completed the HCAHPS survey; (7) No cases met the criteria for this measure; (8) The lower limit of the confidence interval cannot be calculated if the number of observed infections equals zero; (9) No data are available from the state/territory for this reporting period; (10) The scores shown reflect fewer than 50 completed surveys; (11) There were discrepancies in the data collection process; (12) This measure does not apply to this hospital for this reporting period; (13) Results cannot be calculated for this reporting period; (14) The results for this state are combined with nearby states to protect confidentiality; Please refer to the User's Guide for a full explanation of data.*

Measure	Cases	This Hosp.	State Avg.	U.S. Avg.
Received Reliever Medication	13	100%	-	100%
Received Systemic Corticosteroids	13	100%	-	100%
Emergency Department				
Admittance Decision Time (minutes)[2]	706	65	76	98
Head CT Results Within 45 Min. of Arrival[1]	-	-	43%	57%
Patients Who Left ER Before Being Seen	51,064	2%	2%	2%
Time from ER Arrival to Admit. (minutes)[2]	733	211	257	274
Time from ER Arrival to Discharge (minutes)	403	108	142	134
Time in ER Before Being Evaluated (minutes)	443	21	30	26
Time to Pain Meds for Fractures (minutes)	153	61	67	57
Heart Attack Care				
Aspirin Given at Discharge	310	99%	99%	99%
Fibrinolytic Meds Within 30 Min. of Arrival[7]	-	-	50%	54%
PCI Within 90 Minutes of Arrival	52	88%	93%	96%
Statin Prescribed at Discharge	297	100%	98%	98%
Heart Failure Care				
ACE Inhibitor or ARB for LVSD	93	98%	96%	97%
Discharge Instructions Given	269	83%	94%	94%
Evaluation of LVS Function	315	100%	98%	99%
Medicare Spending				
Medicare Spending per Patient (ratio)	-	0.99	0.96	0.98
Pneumonia Care				
Appropriate Initial Antibiotic Given	228	99%	94%	95%
Blood Culture Timing	333	98%	97%	98%
Pregnancy and Delivery Care				
Newborn Deliveries Scheduled Early[2]	33	6%	10%	6%
Preventive Care				
Immunization for Influenza[2]	523	98%	94%	90%
Immunization for Pneumonia[2]	739	98%	95%	92%
Stroke Care				
Anticoagulation Therapy for Atrial Fibrillation	13	85%	94%	95%
Antithrombotic Therapy Timing	100	99%	98%	98%
Assessed for Rehabilitation	105	99%	96%	97%
Discharged on Antithrombotic Therapy	100	99%	98%	99%
Discharged on Statin Medication	86	98%	91%	94%
Thrombolytic Therapy Timing[1]	-	-	67%	66%
Venous Thromboembolism Prophylaxis	112	98%	91%	94%
Written Stroke Educational Materials Given	64	73%	84%	88%
Surgical Care Improvement Project				
Appropriate Beta Blocker Usage	114	97%	98%	98%
Appropriate VTP Within 24 Hours	272	99%	98%	98%
Controlled Postoperative Blood Glucose[7]	-	-	95%	97%
Perioperative Temperature Management	338	100%	100%	100%
Prophylactic Antibiotic Selection	150	99%	99%	99%
Prophylactic Antibiotic Selection (Outpatient)	394	97%	97%	98%
Prophylactic Antibiotic Stopped	142	98%	98%	98%
Prophylactic Antibiotic Timing	150	99%	99%	99%
Prophylactic Antibiotic Timing (Outpatient)	396	98%	97%	98%
Urinary Catheter Removal	160	99%	98%	97%
Survey of Patients' Hospital Experiences				
Area Around Room 'Always' Quiet at Night	300+	51%	58%	61%
Doctors 'Always' Communicated Well	300+	75%	82%	82%
Home Recovery Information Given	300+	81%	85%	85%
Hospital Given 9 or 10 on 10 Point Scale	300+	57%	66%	71%
Meds 'Always' Explained Before Given	300+	56%	64%	64%
Nurses 'Always' Communicated Well	300+	71%	78%	79%
Pain 'Always' Well Controlled	300+	64%	70%	71%
Room and Bathroom 'Always' Clean	300+	67%	75%	73%
Timely Help 'Always' Received	300+	50%	68%	68%
Would Definitely Recommend Hospital	300+	57%	66%	71%
Use of Medical Imaging				
Cardiac Imaging Stress Test before Surgery	257	5.1%	4.9%	5.3%
Combination Abdominal CT Scan	657	9.9%	14.4%	10.5%
Combination Brain/Sinus CT Scan	664	2.0%	3%	2.7%
Combination Chest CT Scan	454	6.6%	2.8%	2.7%
Follow-up Mammogram/Ultrasound	122	10.7%	8.8%	8.8%
Lumbar Spine MRI for Low Back Pain	277	37.5%	38.4%	37.2%

War Memorial Hospital

1 Healthy Way
Berkeley Springs, WV 25411
Type: Critical Access Hospitals
Ownership: Voluntary non-profit - Private
Phone: 304-258-1234
Fax: 304-258-5618
Emergency Services: Yes
Beds: 60

Key Personnel:
Quality Assurance . . . . Evelyn Clonch, RN
Chairman/CEO . . . . Bradley Close
Radiology. . . . . Stephen B Eigles
Chief of Medical Staff. . . . . Joseph Hashem
CEO/President. . . . . Neil R. McLaughlin

Measure	Cases	This Hosp.	State Avg.	U.S. Avg.
Blood Clot Prevention and Treatment				
Anticoagulation Overlap Therapy[5]	-	-	90%	93%
ICU Venous Thromboembolism Prophylaxis[5]	-	-	88%	92%
Incidence of Potentially Preventable VTE[5]	-	-	12%	10%
UFH with Dosages/Platelet Monitoring[5]	-	-	98%	97%
Venous Thromboembolism Prophylaxis[5]	-	-	79%	85%
Warfarin Therapy Discharge Instructions[5]	-	-	80%	75%
Chest Pain/Possible Heart Attack Care				
Aspirin Given Within 24 Hours of Arrival[5]	-	-	96%	96%
Fibrinolytic Meds Within 30 Min. of Arrival[5]	-	-	74%	58%
Average Time to ECG (minutes)[5]	-	-	8	7
Average Time to Transfer (minutes)[5]	-	-	109	60
Children's Asthma Care				
Received Home Management Plan of Care	-	-	-	88%
Received Reliever Medication	-	-	-	100%
Received Systemic Corticosteroids	-	-	-	100%
Emergency Department				
Admittance Decision Time (minutes)[5]	-	-	76	98
Head CT Results Within 45 Min. of Arrival[5]	-	-	43%	57%
Patients Who Left ER Before Being Seen[5]	-	-	2%	2%
Time from ER Arrival to Admit. (minutes)[5]	-	-	257	274
Time from ER Arrival to Discharge (minutes)[5]	-	-	142	134
Time in ER Before Being Evaluated (minutes)[5]	-	-	30	26
Time to Pain Meds for Fractures (minutes)[5]	-	-	67	57
Heart Attack Care				
Aspirin Given at Discharge[1,3]	-	-	99%	99%
Fibrinolytic Meds Within 30 Min. of Arrival[3,7]	-	-	50%	54%
PCI Within 90 Minutes of Arrival[3,7]	-	-	93%	96%
Statin Prescribed at Discharge[1,3]	-	-	98%	98%
Heart Failure Care				
ACE Inhibitor or ARB for LVSD[1,3]	-	-	96%	97%
Discharge Instructions Given[1,3]	-	-	94%	94%
Evaluation of LVS Function[1,3]	-	-	98%	99%
Medicare Spending				
Medicare Spending per Patient (ratio)	-	-	0.96	0.98
Pneumonia Care				
Appropriate Initial Antibiotic Given[3]	12	67%	94%	95%
Blood Culture Timing[3]	13	85%	97%	98%
Pregnancy and Delivery Care				
Newborn Deliveries Scheduled Early[5]	-	-	10%	6%
Preventive Care				
Immunization for Influenza[5]	-	-	94%	90%
Immunization for Pneumonia[5]	-	-	95%	92%
Stroke Care				
Anticoagulation Therapy for Atrial Fibrillation[5]	-	-	94%	95%
Antithrombotic Therapy Timing[5]	-	-	98%	98%
Assessed for Rehabilitation[5]	-	-	96%	97%
Discharged on Antithrombotic Therapy[5]	-	-	98%	99%
Discharged on Statin Medication[5]	-	-	91%	94%
Thrombolytic Therapy Timing[5]	-	-	67%	66%
Venous Thromboembolism Prophylaxis[5]	-	-	91%	94%
Written Stroke Educational Materials Given[5]	-	-	84%	88%
Surgical Care Improvement Project				
Appropriate Beta Blocker Usage[5]	-	-	98%	98%
Appropriate VTP Within 24 Hours[5]	-	-	98%	98%
Controlled Postoperative Blood Glucose[5]	-	-	95%	97%
Perioperative Temperature Management[5]	-	-	100%	100%
Prophylactic Antibiotic Selection[5]	-	-	99%	99%
Prophylactic Antibiotic Selection (Outpatient)[5]	-	-	97%	98%
Prophylactic Antibiotic Stopped[5]	-	-	98%	98%
Prophylactic Antibiotic Timing[5]	-	-	99%	99%
Prophylactic Antibiotic Timing (Outpatient)[5]	-	-	97%	98%
Urinary Catheter Removal[5]	-	-	98%	97%
Survey of Patients' Hospital Experiences				
Area Around Room 'Always' Quiet at Night	(a)	68%	58%	61%
Doctors 'Always' Communicated Well	(a)	83%	82%	82%
Home Recovery Information Given	(a)	84%	85%	85%
Hospital Given 9 or 10 on 10 Point Scale	(a)	75%	66%	71%
Meds 'Always' Explained Before Given	(a)	64%	64%	64%
Nurses 'Always' Communicated Well	(a)	84%	78%	79%
Pain 'Always' Well Controlled	(a)	70%	70%	71%
Room and Bathroom 'Always' Clean	(a)	85%	75%	73%
Timely Help 'Always' Received	(a)	61%	68%	68%
Would Definitely Recommend Hospital	(a)	67%	66%	71%
Use of Medical Imaging				
Cardiac Imaging Stress Test before Surgery[7]		-	4.9%	5.3%
Combination Abdominal CT Scan	148	8.8%	14.4%	10.5%
Combination Brain/Sinus CT Scan[1]		-	3%	2.7%
Combination Chest CT Scan[1]	-	-	2.8%	2.7%
Follow-up Mammogram/Ultrasound	220	21.8%	8.8%	8.8%
Lumbar Spine MRI for Low Back Pain[1]	-	-	38.4%	37.2%

Bluefield Regional Medical Center

500 Cherry St
Bluefield, WV 24701
URL: www.bluefield.org
Type: Acute Care Hospitals
Ownership: Proprietary
Phone: 304-327-1100
Fax: 304-327-1896
Emergency Services: Yes
Beds: 210

Key Personnel:
Chief of Medical Staff. . . . . Donald Asbury, MD
Emergency Room . . . . Gary Butt
Intensive Care Unit. . . . . Gary Butt
Radiology. . . . . Kay Cooper
CEO/President. . . . . Leland Farnell
Pediatric In-Patient Care . . . . Kathy Glover
Operating Room. . . . . Martha Plant
Pediatric Ambulatory Care . . . . . . Thomas E Richardon, MD

Measure	Cases	This Hosp.	State Avg.	U.S. Avg.
Blood Clot Prevention and Treatment				
Anticoagulation Overlap Therapy[2]	47	98%	90%	93%
ICU Venous Thromboembolism Prophylaxis[2]	107	99%	88%	92%
Incidence of Potentially Preventable VTE[2]	14	14%	12%	10%
UFH with Dosages/Platelet Monitoring[2]	28	100%	98%	97%
Venous Thromboembolism Prophylaxis[2]	326	96%	79%	85%
Warfarin Therapy Discharge Instructions[2]	27	96%	80%	75%
Chest Pain/Possible Heart Attack Care				
Aspirin Given Within 24 Hours of Arrival	11	100%	96%	96%
Fibrinolytic Meds Within 30 Min. of Arrival[1,3]	-	-	74%	58%
Average Time to ECG (minutes)	12	0	8	7
Average Time to Transfer (minutes)[1,3]	-	-	109	60
Children's Asthma Care				
Received Home Management Plan of Care	-	-	-	88%
Received Reliever Medication	-	-	-	100%
Received Systemic Corticosteroids	-	-	-	100%
Emergency Department				
Admittance Decision Time (minutes)[2]	476	89	76	98
Head CT Results Within 45 Min. of Arrival[1]	-	-	43%	57%
Patients Who Left ER Before Being Seen	30,672	2%	2%	2%
Time from ER Arrival to Admit. (minutes)[2]	478	274	257	274
Time from ER Arrival to Discharge (minutes)	364	172	142	134
Time in ER Before Being Evaluated (minutes)	408	36	30	26
Time to Pain Meds for Fractures (minutes)	100	65	67	57
Heart Attack Care				
Aspirin Given at Discharge	86	100%	99%	99%
Fibrinolytic Meds Within 30 Min. of Arrival[1]	-	-	50%	54%
PCI Within 90 Minutes of Arrival[1]	-	-	93%	96%
Statin Prescribed at Discharge	84	96%	98%	98%
Heart Failure Care				
ACE Inhibitor or ARB for LVSD	37	97%	96%	97%
Discharge Instructions Given	122	92%	94%	94%
Evaluation of LVS Function	155	100%	98%	99%
Medicare Spending				
Medicare Spending per Patient (ratio)	-	1.01	0.96	0.98
Pneumonia Care				
Appropriate Initial Antibiotic Given	69	97%	94%	95%

NOTE: Hospital profiles are in alphabetical order by state, then city, then hospital within the city; Rankings exclude hospitals with less than 25 cases except for patient surveys which excludes hospitals with less than 100 cases; (a) 100-299 cases; (1) The number of cases/patients is too few to report; (2) Data submitted were based on a sample of cases/patients; (3) Results are based on a shorter time period than required; (4) Data suppressed by CMS for one or more quarters; (5) Results are not available for this reporting period; (6) Fewer than 100 patients completed the HCAHPS survey; (7) No cases met the criteria for this measure; (8) The lower limit of the confidence interval cannot be calculated if the number of observed infections equals zero; (9) No data are available from the state/territory for this reporting period; (10) The scores shown reflect fewer than 50 completed surveys; (11) There were discrepancies in the data collection process; (12) This measure does not apply to this hospital for this reporting period; (13) Results cannot be calculated for this reporting period; (14) The results for this state are combined with nearby states to protect confidentiality; Please refer to the User's Guide for a full explanation of data.

Measure	Cases	This Hosp.	State Avg.	U.S. Avg.
Blood Culture Timing	133	97%	97%	98%
Pregnancy and Delivery Care				
Newborn Deliveries Scheduled Early[2]	22	5%	10%	6%
Preventive Care				
Immunization for Influenza[2]	507	95%	94%	90%
Immunization for Pneumonia[2]	631	99%	95%	92%
Stroke Care				
Anticoagulation Therapy for Atrial Fibrillation[1]	-	-	94%	95%
Antithrombotic Therapy Timing	37	100%	98%	98%
Assessed for Rehabilitation	38	97%	96%	97%
Discharged on Antithrombotic Therapy	35	100%	98%	99%
Discharged on Statin Medication	23	91%	91%	94%
Thrombolytic Therapy Timing[7]		-	67%	66%
Venous Thromboembolism Prophylaxis	39	95%	91%	94%
Written Stroke Educational Materials Given	23	87%	84%	88%
Surgical Care Improvement Project				
Appropriate Beta Blocker Usage	111	89%	98%	98%
Appropriate VTP Within 24 Hours	174	99%	98%	98%
Controlled Postoperative Blood Glucose[7]		-	95%	97%
Perioperative Temperature Management	313	100%	100%	100%
Prophylactic Antibiotic Selection	248	98%	99%	99%
Prophylactic Antibiotic Selection (Outpatient)	109	98%	97%	98%
Prophylactic Antibiotic Stopped	245	97%	98%	98%
Prophylactic Antibiotic Timing	248	99%	99%	99%
Prophylactic Antibiotic Timing (Outpatient)	109	97%	97%	98%
Urinary Catheter Removal	48	98%	98%	97%
Survey of Patients' Hospital Experiences				
Area Around Room 'Always' Quiet at Night	300+	60%	58%	61%
Doctors 'Always' Communicated Well	300+	81%	82%	82%
Home Recovery Information Given	300+	84%	85%	85%
Hospital Given 9 or 10 on 10 Point Scale	300+	61%	66%	71%
Meds 'Always' Explained Before Given	300+	62%	64%	64%
Nurses 'Always' Communicated Well	300+	75%	78%	79%
Pain 'Always' Well Controlled	300+	67%	70%	71%
Room and Bathroom 'Always' Clean	300+	71%	75%	73%
Timely Help 'Always' Received	300+	59%	68%	68%
Would Definitely Recommend Hospital	300+	62%	66%	71%
Use of Medical Imaging				
Cardiac Imaging Stress Test before Surgery	231	5.2%	4.9%	5.3%
Combination Abdominal CT Scan	531	5.5%	14.4%	10.5%
Combination Brain/Sinus CT Scan	572	5.2%	3%	2.7%
Combination Chest CT Scan	235	6.0%	2.8%	2.7%
Follow-up Mammogram/Ultrasound	652	3.8%	8.8%	8.8%
Lumbar Spine MRI for Low Back Pain	83	42.2%	38.4%	37.2%

United Hospital Center

327 Medical Park Drive
Bridgeport, WV 26330
Phone: 681-342-1000
URL: www.uhcwv.org
Type: Acute Care Hospitals
Emergency Services: Yes
Ownership: Voluntary non-profit - Private
Beds: 292
Key Personnel:
Radiology. . . . . Parke Thrush

Measure	Cases	This Hosp.	State Avg.	U.S. Avg.
Blood Clot Prevention and Treatment				
Anticoagulation Overlap Therapy[2]	91	100%	90%	93%
ICU Venous Thromboembolism Prophylaxis[2]	52	100%	88%	92%
Incidence of Potentially Preventable VTE[2]	15	0%	12%	10%
UFH with Dosages/Platelet Monitoring[2]	58	100%	98%	97%
Venous Thromboembolism Prophylaxis[2]	345	100%	79%	85%
Warfarin Therapy Discharge Instructions[2]	74	99%	80%	75%
Chest Pain/Possible Heart Attack Care				
Aspirin Given Within 24 Hours of Arrival	19	100%	96%	96%
Fibrinolytic Meds Within 30 Min. of Arrival[3,7]	-	-	74%	58%
Average Time to ECG (minutes)	19	8	8	7
Average Time to Transfer (minutes)[3,7]	-	-	109	60
Children's Asthma Care				
Received Home Management Plan of Care	-	-	-	88%
Received Reliever Medication	-	-	-	100%
Received Systemic Corticosteroids	-	-	-	100%
Emergency Department				
Admittance Decision Time (minutes)[2]	564	35	76	98
Head CT Results Within 45 Min. of Arrival	22	36%	43%	57%
Patients Who Left ER Before Being Seen	56,181	2%	2%	2%
Time from ER Arrival to Admit. (minutes)[2]	564	204	257	274
Time from ER Arrival to Discharge (minutes)	346	137	142	134
Time in ER Before Being Evaluated (minutes)	384	61	30	26
Time to Pain Meds for Fractures (minutes)	151	74	67	57
Heart Attack Care				
Aspirin Given at Discharge	331	100%	99%	99%
Fibrinolytic Meds Within 30 Min. of Arrival[7]	-	-	50%	54%
PCI Within 90 Minutes of Arrival	27	100%	93%	96%
Statin Prescribed at Discharge	310	100%	98%	98%
Heart Failure Care				
ACE Inhibitor or ARB for LVSD	99	100%	96%	97%
Discharge Instructions Given	268	98%	94%	94%
Evaluation of LVS Function	324	100%	98%	99%
Medicare Spending				
Medicare Spending per Patient (ratio)	-	0.94	0.96	0.98
Pneumonia Care				
Appropriate Initial Antibiotic Given	255	96%	94%	95%
Blood Culture Timing	328	98%	97%	98%
Pregnancy and Delivery Care				
Newborn Deliveries Scheduled Early	50	0%	10%	6%
Preventive Care				
Immunization for Influenza[2]	540	91%	94%	90%
Immunization for Pneumonia[2]	732	95%	95%	92%
Stroke Care				
Anticoagulation Therapy for Atrial Fibrillation[1]	-	-	94%	95%
Antithrombotic Therapy Timing	57	100%	98%	98%
Assessed for Rehabilitation	62	100%	96%	97%
Discharged on Antithrombotic Therapy	53	100%	98%	99%
Discharged on Statin Medication	47	100%	91%	94%
Thrombolytic Therapy Timing[1]	-	-	67%	66%
Venous Thromboembolism Prophylaxis	64	97%	91%	94%
Written Stroke Educational Materials Given	39	82%	84%	88%
Surgical Care Improvement Project				
Appropriate Beta Blocker Usage[2]	213	100%	98%	98%
Appropriate VTP Within 24 Hours[2]	630	100%	98%	98%
Controlled Postoperative Blood Glucose[2,7]	-	-	95%	97%
Perioperative Temperature Management[2]	749	100%	100%	100%
Prophylactic Antibiotic Selection[2]	585	100%	99%	99%
Prophylactic Antibiotic Selection (Outpatient)	175	97%	97%	98%
Prophylactic Antibiotic Stopped[2]	557	99%	98%	98%
Prophylactic Antibiotic Timing[2]	591	99%	99%	99%
Prophylactic Antibiotic Timing (Outpatient)	145	99%	97%	98%
Urinary Catheter Removal[2]	501	100%	98%	97%
Survey of Patients' Hospital Experiences				
Area Around Room 'Always' Quiet at Night	300+	60%	58%	61%
Doctors 'Always' Communicated Well	300+	81%	82%	82%
Home Recovery Information Given	300+	83%	85%	85%
Hospital Given 9 or 10 on 10 Point Scale	300+	67%	66%	71%
Meds 'Always' Explained Before Given	300+	64%	64%	64%
Nurses 'Always' Communicated Well	300+	76%	78%	79%
Pain 'Always' Well Controlled	300+	68%	70%	71%
Room and Bathroom 'Always' Clean	300+	77%	75%	73%
Timely Help 'Always' Received	300+	59%	68%	68%
Would Definitely Recommend Hospital	300+	65%	66%	71%
Use of Medical Imaging				
Cardiac Imaging Stress Test before Surgery	360	3.1%	4.9%	5.3%
Combination Abdominal CT Scan	1,270	29.8%	14.4%	10.5%
Combination Brain/Sinus CT Scan	914	2.4%	3%	2.7%
Combination Chest CT Scan	698	0.0%	2.8%	2.7%
Follow-up Mammogram/Ultrasound	1,698	6.9%	8.8%	8.8%
Lumbar Spine MRI for Low Back Pain	387	31.3%	38.4%	37.2%

Pocahontas Memorial Hospital

Rr Box 52 West
Buckeye, WV 24924
Phone: 304-799-7400
Fax: 304-799-6636
Type: Critical Access Hospitals
Emergency Services: Yes
Ownership: Government - Local
Beds: 27
Key Personnel:
Chief of Medical Staff. . . . . Luis Soriano
Emergency Room . . . . Luis Soriano, MD
Quality Assurance . . . . Amy Wade

Measure	Cases	This Hosp.	State Avg.	U.S. Avg.
Blood Clot Prevention and Treatment				
Anticoagulation Overlap Therapy[5]	-	-	90%	93%
ICU Venous Thromboembolism Prophylaxis[5]	-	-	88%	92%
Incidence of Potentially Preventable VTE[5]	-	-	12%	10%
UFH with Dosages/Platelet Monitoring[5]	-	-	98%	97%
Venous Thromboembolism Prophylaxis[5]	-	-	79%	85%
Warfarin Therapy Discharge Instructions[5]	-	-	80%	75%
Chest Pain/Possible Heart Attack Care				
Aspirin Given Within 24 Hours of Arrival	-	-	96%	96%
Fibrinolytic Meds Within 30 Min. of Arrival	-	-	74%	58%
Average Time to ECG (minutes)	-	-	8	7
Average Time to Transfer (minutes)	-	-	109	60
Children's Asthma Care				
Received Home Management Plan of Care	-	-	-	88%
Received Reliever Medication	-	-	-	100%
Received Systemic Corticosteroids	-	-	-	100%
Emergency Department				
Admittance Decision Time (minutes)[2]	76	24	76	98
Head CT Results Within 45 Min. of Arrival	-	-	43%	57%
Patients Who Left ER Before Being Seen	-	-	2%	2%
Time from ER Arrival to Admit. (minutes)[2]	78	130	257	274
Time from ER Arrival to Discharge (minutes)	-	-	142	134
Time in ER Before Being Evaluated (minutes)	-	-	30	26
Time to Pain Meds for Fractures (minutes)	-	-	67	57
Heart Attack Care				
Aspirin Given at Discharge[1,3]	-	-	99%	99%
Fibrinolytic Meds Within 30 Min. of Arrival[3,7]	-	-	50%	54%
PCI Within 90 Minutes of Arrival[3,7]	-	-	93%	96%
Statin Prescribed at Discharge[1,3]	-	-	98%	98%
Heart Failure Care				
ACE Inhibitor or ARB for LVSD[1]	-	-	96%	97%
Discharge Instructions Given[1]	-	-	94%	94%
Evaluation of LVS Function	14	86%	98%	99%
Medicare Spending				
Medicare Spending per Patient (ratio)	-	-	0.96	0.98
Pneumonia Care				
Appropriate Initial Antibiotic Given[2]	30	60%	94%	95%
Blood Culture Timing[2]	20	95%	97%	98%
Pregnancy and Delivery Care				
Newborn Deliveries Scheduled Early[5]	-	-	10%	6%
Preventive Care				
Immunization for Influenza	55	95%	94%	90%
Immunization for Pneumonia	59	90%	95%	92%
Stroke Care				
Anticoagulation Therapy for Atrial Fibrillation[5]	-	-	94%	95%
Antithrombotic Therapy Timing[5]	-	-	98%	98%
Assessed for Rehabilitation[5]	-	-	96%	97%
Discharged on Antithrombotic Therapy[5]	-	-	98%	99%
Discharged on Statin Medication[5]	-	-	91%	94%
Thrombolytic Therapy Timing[5]	-	-	67%	66%
Venous Thromboembolism Prophylaxis[5]	-	-	91%	94%
Written Stroke Educational Materials Given[5]	-	-	84%	88%
Surgical Care Improvement Project				
Appropriate Beta Blocker Usage[5]	-	-	98%	98%
Appropriate VTP Within 24 Hours[5]	-	-	98%	98%
Controlled Postoperative Blood Glucose[5]	-	-	95%	97%
Perioperative Temperature Management[5]	-	-	100%	100%
Prophylactic Antibiotic Selection[5]	-	-	99%	99%
Prophylactic Antibiotic Selection (Outpatient)	-	-	97%	98%
Prophylactic Antibiotic Stopped[5]	-	-	98%	98%
Prophylactic Antibiotic Timing[5]	-	-	99%	99%
Prophylactic Antibiotic Timing (Outpatient)	-	-	97%	98%
Urinary Catheter Removal[5]	-	-	98%	97%
Survey of Patients' Hospital Experiences				
Area Around Room 'Always' Quiet at Night[6]	<100	64%	58%	61%
Doctors 'Always' Communicated Well[6]	<100	71%	82%	82%
Home Recovery Information Given[6]	<100	81%	85%	85%
Hospital Given 9 or 10 on 10 Point Scale[6]	<100	65%	66%	71%
Meds 'Always' Explained Before Given[6]	<100	74%	64%	64%
Nurses 'Always' Communicated Well[6]	<100	82%	78%	79%
Pain 'Always' Well Controlled[6]	<100	80%	70%	71%
Room and Bathroom 'Always' Clean[6]	<100	90%	75%	73%

NOTE: Hospital profiles are in alphabetical order by state, then city, then hospital within the city; Rankings exclude hospitals with less than 25 cases except for patient surveys which excludes hospitals with less than 100 cases; (a) 100-299 cases; (1) The number of cases/patients is too few to report; (2) Data submitted were based on a sample of cases/patients; (3) Results are based on a shorter time period than required; (4) Data suppressed by CMS for one or more quarters; (5) Results are not available for this reporting period; (6) Fewer than 100 patients completed the HCAHPS survey; (7) No cases met the criteria for this measure; (8) The lower limit of the confidence interval cannot be calculated if the number of observed infections equals zero; (9) No data are available from the state/territory for this reporting period; (10) The scores shown reflect fewer than 50 completed surveys; (11) There were discrepancies in the data collection process; (12) This measure does not apply to this hospital for this reporting period; (13) Results cannot be calculated for this reporting period; (14) The results for this state are combined with nearby states to protect confidentiality; Please refer to the User's Guide for a full explanation of data.

Measure	Cases	This Hosp.	State Avg.	U.S. Avg.
Timely Help 'Always' Received[6]	<100	85%	68%	68%
Would Definitely Recommend Hospital[6]	<100	63%	66%	71%
Use of Medical Imaging				
Cardiac Imaging Stress Test before Surgery	-	-	4.9%	5.3%
Combination Abdominal CT Scan	-	-	14.4%	10.5%
Combination Brain/Sinus CT Scan	-	-	3%	2.7%
Combination Chest CT Scan	-	-	2.8%	2.7%
Follow-up Mammogram/Ultrasound	-	-	8.8%	8.8%
Lumbar Spine MRI for Low Back Pain	-	-	38.4%	37.2%

Saint Joseph Hospital

1 Amalia Drive
Buckhannon, WV 26201
Phone: 304-472-2000
Fax: 304-472-6620
E-mail: webmaster@stj.net
URL: www.stj.net
Type: Acute Care Hospitals
Emergency Services: Yes
Ownership: Voluntary non-profit - Church
Beds: 95

Key Personnel:
Emergency Room . . . . John Freed, MD
CEO/President. . . . . Wayne B Griffith
Quality Assurance . . . . Elly Mick

Measure	Cases	This Hosp.	State Avg.	U.S. Avg.
Blood Clot Prevention and Treatment				
Anticoagulation Overlap Therapy[1,2]	-	-	90%	93%
ICU Venous Thromboembolism Prophylaxis[2]	24	96%	88%	92%
Incidence of Potentially Preventable VTE[2,7]	-	-	12%	10%
UFH with Dosages/Platelet Monitoring[2,7]	-	-	98%	97%
Venous Thromboembolism Prophylaxis[2]	76	87%	79%	85%
Warfarin Therapy Discharge Instructions[1,2]	-	-	80%	75%
Chest Pain/Possible Heart Attack Care				
Aspirin Given Within 24 Hours of Arrival	71	100%	96%	96%
Fibrinolytic Meds Within 30 Min. of Arrival[1]	-	-	74%	58%
Average Time to ECG (minutes)	74	9	8	7
Average Time to Transfer (minutes)[7]	-	-	109	60
Children's Asthma Care				
Received Home Management Plan of Care	-	-	-	88%
Received Reliever Medication	-	-	-	100%
Received Systemic Corticosteroids	-	-	-	100%
Emergency Department				
Admittance Decision Time (minutes)[2]	117	60	76	98
Head CT Results Within 45 Min. of Arrival	16	19%	43%	57%
Patients Who Left ER Before Being Seen	14,469	2%	2%	2%
Time from ER Arrival to Admit. (minutes)[2]	150	182	257	274
Time from ER Arrival to Discharge (minutes)	283	105	142	134
Time in ER Before Being Evaluated (minutes)	366	15	30	26
Time to Pain Meds for Fractures (minutes)	41	48	67	57
Heart Attack Care				
Aspirin Given at Discharge[1,2]	-	-	99%	99%
Fibrinolytic Meds Within 30 Min. of Arrival[2,7]	-	-	50%	54%
PCI Within 90 Minutes of Arrival[2,7]	-	-	93%	96%
Statin Prescribed at Discharge[2,7]	-	-	98%	98%
Heart Failure Care				
ACE Inhibitor or ARB for LVSD[1,2]	-	-	96%	97%
Discharge Instructions Given[2]	30	93%	94%	94%
Evaluation of LVS Function[2]	41	100%	98%	99%
Medicare Spending				
Medicare Spending per Patient (ratio)	-	0.93	0.96	0.98
Pneumonia Care				
Appropriate Initial Antibiotic Given[2]	39	79%	94%	95%
Blood Culture Timing[2]	48	88%	97%	98%
Pregnancy and Delivery Care				
Newborn Deliveries Scheduled Early	46	0%	10%	6%
Preventive Care				
Immunization for Influenza[2]	242	87%	94%	90%
Immunization for Pneumonia[2]	254	84%	95%	92%
Stroke Care				
Anticoagulation Therapy for Atrial Fibrillation[2,7]	-	-	94%	95%
Antithrombotic Therapy Timing[1,2]	-	-	98%	98%
Assessed for Rehabilitation[1,2]	-	-	96%	97%
Discharged on Antithrombotic Therapy[1,2]	-	-	98%	99%
Discharged on Statin Medication[2,7]	-	-	91%	94%
Thrombolytic Therapy Timing[2,7]	-	-	67%	66%
Venous Thromboembolism Prophylaxis[1,2]	-	-	91%	94%
Written Stroke Educational Materials Given[1,2]	-	-	84%	88%
Surgical Care Improvement Project				
Appropriate Beta Blocker Usage[2]	24	100%	98%	98%
Appropriate VTP Within 24 Hours[2]	74	93%	98%	98%
Controlled Postoperative Blood Glucose[2,7]	-	-	95%	97%
Perioperative Temperature Management[2]	92	100%	100%	100%
Prophylactic Antibiotic Selection[2]	28	100%	99%	99%
Prophylactic Antibiotic Selection (Outpatient)[1]	-	-	97%	98%
Prophylactic Antibiotic Stopped[2]	28	96%	98%	98%
Prophylactic Antibiotic Timing[2]	28	100%	99%	99%
Prophylactic Antibiotic Timing (Outpatient)[1]	-	-	97%	98%
Urinary Catheter Removal[2]	38	100%	98%	97%
Survey of Patients' Hospital Experiences				
Area Around Room 'Always' Quiet at Night	300+	64%	58%	61%
Doctors 'Always' Communicated Well	300+	82%	82%	82%
Home Recovery Information Given	300+	86%	85%	85%
Hospital Given 9 or 10 on 10 Point Scale	300+	68%	66%	71%
Meds 'Always' Explained Before Given	300+	65%	64%	64%
Nurses 'Always' Communicated Well	300+	79%	78%	79%
Pain 'Always' Well Controlled	300+	71%	70%	71%
Room and Bathroom 'Always' Clean	300+	62%	75%	73%
Timely Help 'Always' Received	300+	73%	68%	68%
Would Definitely Recommend Hospital	300+	66%	66%	71%
Use of Medical Imaging				
Cardiac Imaging Stress Test before Surgery	115	7.0%	4.9%	5.3%
Combination Abdominal CT Scan	240	37.9%	14.4%	10.5%
Combination Brain/Sinus CT Scan[1]	-	-	3%	2.7%
Combination Chest CT Scan	123	0.0%	2.8%	2.7%
Follow-up Mammogram/Ultrasound	401	6.7%	8.8%	8.8%
Lumbar Spine MRI for Low Back Pain[1]	-	-	38.4%	37.2%

Charleston Area Medical Center

501 Morris Street
Charleston, WV 25301
Phone: 304-388-6203
Fax: 304-388-6314
URL: www.camc.org
Type: Acute Care Hospitals
Emergency Services: Yes
Ownership: Voluntary non-profit - Private
Beds: 400

Key Personnel:
Cardiac Laboratory. . . . . Jamal Kahken
Infection Control. . . . . Terrie Lee
Pediatric Ambulatory Care . . . . . . Stefan Maxwell, MD
Quality Assurance . . . . Jean Morgan
CEO/President. . . . . David Ramsey
Emergency Room . . . . David Seidler, MD
Radiology. . . . . Joseph Skeens, MD
Operating Room. . . . . Susan Taber, RN

Measure	Cases	This Hosp.	State Avg.	U.S. Avg.
Blood Clot Prevention and Treatment				
Anticoagulation Overlap Therapy[2]	219	95%	90%	93%
ICU Venous Thromboembolism Prophylaxis[2]	129	82%	88%	92%
Incidence of Potentially Preventable VTE[2]	74	5%	12%	10%
UFH with Dosages/Platelet Monitoring[2]	167	96%	98%	97%
Venous Thromboembolism Prophylaxis[2]	353	73%	79%	85%
Warfarin Therapy Discharge Instructions[2]	159	48%	80%	75%
Chest Pain/Possible Heart Attack Care				
Aspirin Given Within 24 Hours of Arrival[1,3]	-	-	96%	96%
Fibrinolytic Meds Within 30 Min. of Arrival[5]	-	-	74%	58%
Average Time to ECG (minutes)[1,3]	-	-	8	7
Average Time to Transfer (minutes)[5]	-	-	109	60
Children's Asthma Care				
Received Home Management Plan of Care	-	-	-	88%
Received Reliever Medication	-	-	-	100%
Received Systemic Corticosteroids	-	-	-	100%
Emergency Department				
Admittance Decision Time (minutes)[2]	631	145	76	98
Head CT Results Within 45 Min. of Arrival[1,3]	-	-	43%	57%
Patients Who Left ER Before Being Seen	>100k	2%	2%	2%
Time from ER Arrival to Admit. (minutes)[2]	699	333	257	274
Time from ER Arrival to Discharge (minutes)	844	190	142	134
Time in ER Before Being Evaluated (minutes)	875	46	30	26
Time to Pain Meds for Fractures (minutes)	225	65	67	57
Heart Attack Care				
Aspirin Given at Discharge[2]	578	99%	99%	99%
Fibrinolytic Meds Within 30 Min. of Arrival[2,7]	-	-	50%	54%
PCI Within 90 Minutes of Arrival[2]	45	84%	93%	96%
Statin Prescribed at Discharge[2]	574	97%	98%	98%
Heart Failure Care				
ACE Inhibitor or ARB for LVSD[2]	195	92%	96%	97%
Discharge Instructions Given[2]	416	91%	94%	94%
Evaluation of LVS Function[2]	465	99%	98%	99%
Medicare Spending				
Medicare Spending per Patient (ratio)	-	0.97	0.96	0.98
Pneumonia Care				
Appropriate Initial Antibiotic Given[2]	118	92%	94%	95%
Blood Culture Timing[2]	283	93%	97%	98%
Pregnancy and Delivery Care				
Newborn Deliveries Scheduled Early[2]	60	7%	10%	6%
Preventive Care				
Immunization for Influenza[2]	569	91%	94%	90%
Immunization for Pneumonia[2]	782	86%	95%	92%
Stroke Care				
Anticoagulation Therapy for Atrial Fibrillation	60	100%	94%	95%
Antithrombotic Therapy Timing	396	98%	98%	98%
Assessed for Rehabilitation	462	93%	96%	97%
Discharged on Antithrombotic Therapy	408	99%	98%	99%
Discharged on Statin Medication	313	98%	91%	94%
Thrombolytic Therapy Timing	17	76%	67%	66%
Venous Thromboembolism Prophylaxis	492	93%	91%	94%
Written Stroke Educational Materials Given	314	92%	84%	88%
Surgical Care Improvement Project				
Appropriate Beta Blocker Usage[2]	652	99%	98%	98%
Appropriate VTP Within 24 Hours[2]	526	96%	98%	98%
Controlled Postoperative Blood Glucose[2]	558	93%	95%	97%
Perioperative Temperature Management[2]	711	100%	100%	100%
Prophylactic Antibiotic Selection[2]	896	100%	99%	99%
Prophylactic Antibiotic Selection (Outpatient)	942	98%	97%	98%
Prophylactic Antibiotic Stopped[2]	813	98%	98%	98%
Prophylactic Antibiotic Timing[2]	899	99%	99%	99%
Prophylactic Antibiotic Timing (Outpatient)	942	99%	97%	98%
Urinary Catheter Removal[2]	710	97%	98%	97%
Survey of Patients' Hospital Experiences				
Area Around Room 'Always' Quiet at Night	300+	48%	58%	61%
Doctors 'Always' Communicated Well	300+	79%	82%	82%
Home Recovery Information Given	300+	83%	85%	85%
Hospital Given 9 or 10 on 10 Point Scale	300+	68%	66%	71%
Meds 'Always' Explained Before Given	300+	61%	64%	64%
Nurses 'Always' Communicated Well	300+	75%	78%	79%
Pain 'Always' Well Controlled	300+	67%	70%	71%
Room and Bathroom 'Always' Clean	300+	65%	75%	73%
Timely Help 'Always' Received	300+	63%	68%	68%
Would Definitely Recommend Hospital	300+	72%	66%	71%
Use of Medical Imaging				
Cardiac Imaging Stress Test before Surgery	1,619	5.3%	4.9%	5.3%
Combination Abdominal CT Scan	1,876	9.1%	14.4%	10.5%
Combination Brain/Sinus CT Scan	1,192	0.8%	3%	2.7%
Combination Chest CT Scan	1,616	0.4%	2.8%	2.7%
Follow-up Mammogram/Ultrasound	3,184	7.4%	8.8%	8.8%
Lumbar Spine MRI for Low Back Pain	222	41.4%	38.4%	37.2%

Charleston Surgical Hospital

1306 Kanawha Bl E
Charleston, WV 25301
Phone: 304-343-4371
Fax: 304-353-0215
E-mail: ashelton@citynet.net
URL: www.eyeandearclinicwv.com
Type: Acute Care Hospitals
Emergency Services: No
Ownership: Physician
Beds: 35

Key Personnel:
Anesthesiology. . . . . Phillip Casingal, MD
Operating Room. . . . . Carmen Palmer, RN
Chief of Medical Staff. . . . . Robert E Pollard, MD
CEO/President. . . . . W Allen Shelton

Measure	Cases	This Hosp.	State Avg.	U.S. Avg.
Blood Clot Prevention and Treatment				
Anticoagulation Overlap Therapy[5]	-	-	90%	93%
ICU Venous Thromboembolism Prophylaxis[5]	-	-	88%	92%
Incidence of Potentially Preventable VTE[5]	-	-	12%	10%
UFH with Dosages/Platelet Monitoring[5]	-	-	98%	97%

NOTE: Hospital profiles are in alphabetical order by state, then city, then hospital within the city; Rankings exclude hospitals with less than 25 cases except for patient surveys which excludes hospitals with less than 100 cases; (a) 100-299 cases; (1) The number of cases/patients is too few to report; (2) Data submitted were based on a sample of cases/patients; (3) Results are based on a shorter time period than required; (4) Data suppressed by CMS for one or more quarters; (5) Results are not available for this reporting period; (6) Fewer than 100 patients completed the HCAHPS survey; (7) No cases met the criteria for this measure; (8) The lower limit of the confidence interval cannot be calculated if the number of observed infections equals zero; (9) No data are available from the state/territory for this reporting period; (10) The scores shown reflect fewer than 50 completed surveys; (11) There were discrepancies in the data collection process; (12) This measure does not apply to this hospital for this reporting period; (13) Results cannot be calculated for this reporting period; (14) The results for this state are combined with nearby states to protect confidentiality; Please refer to the User's Guide for a full explanation of data.

Measure	Cases	This Hosp.	State Avg.	U.S. Avg.
Venous Thromboembolism Prophylaxis[5]	-	-	79%	85%
Warfarin Therapy Discharge Instructions[5]	-	-	80%	75%
Chest Pain/Possible Heart Attack Care				
Aspirin Given Within 24 Hours of Arrival[5]	-	-	96%	96%
Fibrinolytic Meds Within 30 Min. of Arrival[5]	-	-	74%	58%
Average Time to ECG (minutes)[5]	-	-	8	7
Average Time to Transfer (minutes)[5]	-	-	109	60
Children's Asthma Care				
Received Home Management Plan of Care	-	-	-	88%
Received Reliever Medication	-	-	-	100%
Received Systemic Corticosteroids	-	-	-	100%
Emergency Department				
Admittance Decision Time (minutes)[5]	-	-	76	98
Head CT Results Within 45 Min. of Arrival[5]	-	-	43%	57%
Patients Who Left ER Before Being Seen[5]	-	-	2%	2%
Time from ER Arrival to Admit. (minutes)[5]	-	-	257	274
Time from ER Arrival to Discharge (minutes)[5]	-	-	142	134
Time in ER Before Being Evaluated (minutes)[5]	-	-	30	26
Time to Pain Meds for Fractures (minutes)[5]	-	-	67	57
Heart Attack Care				
Aspirin Given at Discharge[5]	-	-	99%	99%
Fibrinolytic Meds Within 30 Min. of Arrival[5]	-	-	50%	54%
PCI Within 90 Minutes of Arrival[5]	-	-	93%	96%
Statin Prescribed at Discharge[5]	-	-	98%	98%
Heart Failure Care				
ACE Inhibitor or ARB for LVSD[5]	-	-	96%	97%
Discharge Instructions Given[5]	-	-	94%	94%
Evaluation of LVS Function[5]	-	-	98%	99%
Medicare Spending				
Medicare Spending per Patient (ratio)	-	-	0.96	0.98
Pneumonia Care				
Appropriate Initial Antibiotic Given[5]	-	-	94%	95%
Blood Culture Timing[5]	-	-	97%	98%
Pregnancy and Delivery Care				
Newborn Deliveries Scheduled Early[7]	-	-	10%	6%
Preventive Care				
Immunization for Influenza[5]	-	-	94%	90%
Immunization for Pneumonia[5]	-	-	95%	92%
Stroke Care				
Anticoagulation Therapy for Atrial Fibrillation[5]	-	-	94%	95%
Antithrombotic Therapy Timing[5]	-	-	98%	98%
Assessed for Rehabilitation[5]	-	-	96%	97%
Discharged on Antithrombotic Therapy[5]	-	-	98%	99%
Discharged on Statin Medication[5]	-	-	91%	94%
Thrombolytic Therapy Timing[5]	-	-	67%	66%
Venous Thromboembolism Prophylaxis[5]	-	-	91%	94%
Written Stroke Educational Materials Given[5]	-	-	84%	88%
Surgical Care Improvement Project				
Appropriate Beta Blocker Usage[5]	-	-	98%	98%
Appropriate VTP Within 24 Hours[5]	-	-	98%	98%
Controlled Postoperative Blood Glucose[5]	-	-	95%	97%
Perioperative Temperature Management[5]	-	-	100%	100%
Prophylactic Antibiotic Selection[5]	-	-	99%	99%
Prophylactic Antibiotic Selection (Outpatient)[5]	-	-	97%	98%
Prophylactic Antibiotic Stopped[5]	-	-	98%	98%
Prophylactic Antibiotic Timing[5]	-	-	99%	99%
Prophylactic Antibiotic Timing (Outpatient)[5]	-	-	97%	98%
Urinary Catheter Removal[5]	-	-	98%	97%
Survey of Patients' Hospital Experiences				
Area Around Room 'Always' Quiet at Night[1]	-	-	58%	61%
Doctors 'Always' Communicated Well[1]	-	-	82%	82%
Home Recovery Information Given[1]	-	-	85%	85%
Hospital Given 9 or 10 on 10 Point Scale[1]	-	-	66%	71%
Meds 'Always' Explained Before Given[1]	-	-	64%	64%
Nurses 'Always' Communicated Well[1]	-	-	78%	79%
Pain 'Always' Well Controlled[1]	-	-	70%	71%
Room and Bathroom 'Always' Clean[1]	-	-	75%	73%
Timely Help 'Always' Received[1]	-	-	68%	68%
Would Definitely Recommend Hospital[1]	-	-	66%	71%
Use of Medical Imaging				
Cardiac Imaging Stress Test before Surgery[7]	-	-	4.9%	5.3%
Combination Abdominal CT Scan[7]	-	-	14.4%	10.5%
Combination Brain/Sinus CT Scan[7]	-	-	3%	2.7%
Combination Chest CT Scan[7]	-	-	2.8%	2.7%
Follow-up Mammogram/Ultrasound[7]	-	-	8.8%	8.8%
Lumbar Spine MRI for Low Back Pain[1]	-	-	38.4%	37.2%

Saint Francis Hospital

333 Laidley St
Charleston, WV 25301
Type: Acute Care Hospitals
Ownership: Proprietary
Phone: 304-347-6500
Fax: 304-347-6885
Emergency Services: Yes
Beds: 155

Key Personnel:
Emergency Room . . . . Ed Bowdifh
CEO/President. . . . . Alan D. Guerci, MD
Administrator . . . . Ruth E. Hennessey
Chair/CEO . . . . Richard J. J. Sullivan, Jr.
Chief of Medical Staff . . . . Mallinath Kay, MD
Operating Room. . . . . Cindy Kranz
Cardiac Laboratory. . . . . Brian Lilly
Quality Assurance . . . . Patty Skaff

Measure	Cases	This Hosp.	State Avg.	U.S. Avg.
Blood Clot Prevention and Treatment				
Anticoagulation Overlap Therapy[2]	12	100%	90%	93%
ICU Venous Thromboembolism Prophylaxis[2]	45	91%	88%	92%
Incidence of Potentially Preventable VTE[1,2]	-	-	12%	10%
UFH with Dosages/Platelet Monitoring[1,2]	-	-	98%	97%
Venous Thromboembolism Prophylaxis[2]	240	81%	79%	85%
Warfarin Therapy Discharge Instructions[1,2]	-	-	80%	75%
Chest Pain/Possible Heart Attack Care				
Aspirin Given Within 24 Hours of Arrival[5]	-	-	96%	96%
Fibrinolytic Meds Within 30 Min. of Arrival[5]	-	-	74%	58%
Average Time to ECG (minutes)[5]	-	-	8	7
Average Time to Transfer (minutes)[5]	-	-	109	60
Children's Asthma Care				
Received Home Management Plan of Care	-	-	-	88%
Received Reliever Medication	-	-	-	100%
Received Systemic Corticosteroids	-	-	-	100%
Emergency Department				
Admittance Decision Time (minutes)[2]	243	117	76	98
Head CT Results Within 45 Min. of Arrival[1]	-	-	43%	57%
Patients Who Left ER Before Being Seen	15,872	3%	2%	2%
Time from ER Arrival to Admit. (minutes)[2]	243	293	257	274
Time from ER Arrival to Discharge (minutes)	338	142	142	134
Time in ER Before Being Evaluated (minutes)	384	22	30	26
Time to Pain Meds for Fractures (minutes)	31	55	67	57
Heart Attack Care				
Aspirin Given at Discharge	31	100%	99%	99%
Fibrinolytic Meds Within 30 Min. of Arrival[7]	-	-	50%	54%
PCI Within 90 Minutes of Arrival[1]	-	-	93%	96%
Statin Prescribed at Discharge	28	96%	98%	98%
Heart Failure Care				
ACE Inhibitor or ARB for LVSD	26	88%	96%	97%
Discharge Instructions Given	88	93%	94%	94%
Evaluation of LVS Function	104	99%	98%	99%
Medicare Spending				
Medicare Spending per Patient (ratio)	-	0.92	0.96	0.98
Pneumonia Care				
Appropriate Initial Antibiotic Given	75	97%	94%	95%
Blood Culture Timing	146	95%	97%	98%
Pregnancy and Delivery Care				
Newborn Deliveries Scheduled Early[7]	-	-	10%	6%
Preventive Care				
Immunization for Influenza[2]	336	98%	94%	90%
Immunization for Pneumonia[2]	496	99%	95%	92%
Stroke Care				
Anticoagulation Therapy for Atrial Fibrillation[1]	-	-	94%	95%
Antithrombotic Therapy Timing	18	83%	98%	98%
Assessed for Rehabilitation	19	95%	96%	97%
Discharged on Antithrombotic Therapy	18	94%	98%	99%
Discharged on Statin Medication	12	75%	91%	94%
Thrombolytic Therapy Timing[1]	-	-	67%	66%
Venous Thromboembolism Prophylaxis	16	81%	91%	94%
Written Stroke Educational Materials Given	12	17%	84%	88%
Surgical Care Improvement Project				
Appropriate Beta Blocker Usage	325	96%	98%	98%
Appropriate VTP Within 24 Hours	806	97%	98%	98%
Controlled Postoperative Blood Glucose[7]	-	-	95%	97%
Perioperative Temperature Management	874	100%	100%	100%
Prophylactic Antibiotic Selection	725	99%	99%	99%
Prophylactic Antibiotic Selection (Outpatient)	189	92%	97%	98%
Prophylactic Antibiotic Stopped	719	97%	98%	98%
Prophylactic Antibiotic Timing	727	99%	99%	99%
Prophylactic Antibiotic Timing (Outpatient)	189	90%	97%	98%
Urinary Catheter Removal	490	98%	98%	97%
Survey of Patients' Hospital Experiences				
Area Around Room 'Always' Quiet at Night	300+	65%	58%	61%
Doctors 'Always' Communicated Well	300+	79%	82%	82%
Home Recovery Information Given	300+	87%	85%	85%
Hospital Given 9 or 10 on 10 Point Scale	300+	70%	66%	71%
Meds 'Always' Explained Before Given	300+	57%	64%	64%
Nurses 'Always' Communicated Well	300+	78%	78%	79%
Pain 'Always' Well Controlled	300+	72%	70%	71%
Room and Bathroom 'Always' Clean	300+	68%	75%	73%
Timely Help 'Always' Received	300+	69%	68%	68%
Would Definitely Recommend Hospital	300+	76%	66%	71%
Use of Medical Imaging				
Cardiac Imaging Stress Test before Surgery[7]	-	-	4.9%	5.3%
Combination Abdominal CT Scan	225	3.1%	14.4%	10.5%
Combination Brain/Sinus CT Scan	274	7.3%	3%	2.7%
Combination Chest CT Scan	48	0.0%	2.8%	2.7%
Follow-up Mammogram/Ultrasound	918	11.5%	8.8%	8.8%
Lumbar Spine MRI for Low Back Pain	70	35.7%	38.4%	37.2%

Clarksburg VA Medical Center

1 Medical Center Drive
Clarksburg, WV 26301
URL: www.clarksburg.va.gov
Type: Acute Care - VA
Ownership: Government Federal
Phone: 304-623-3461
Emergency Services: No

Measure	Cases	This Hosp.	State Avg.	U.S. Avg.
Blood Clot Prevention and Treatment				
Anticoagulation Overlap Therapy	-	-	90%	93%
ICU Venous Thromboembolism Prophylaxis	-	-	88%	92%
Incidence of Potentially Preventable VTE	-	-	12%	10%
UFH with Dosages/Platelet Monitoring	-	-	98%	97%
Venous Thromboembolism Prophylaxis	-	-	79%	85%
Warfarin Therapy Discharge Instructions	-	-	80%	75%
Chest Pain/Possible Heart Attack Care				
Aspirin Given Within 24 Hours of Arrival	-	-	96%	96%
Fibrinolytic Meds Within 30 Min. of Arrival	-	-	74%	58%
Average Time to ECG (minutes)	-	-	8	7
Average Time to Transfer (minutes)	-	-	109	60
Children's Asthma Care				
Received Home Management Plan of Care	-	-	-	88%
Received Reliever Medication	-	-	-	100%
Received Systemic Corticosteroids	-	-	-	100%
Emergency Department				
Admittance Decision Time (minutes)	-	-	76	98
Head CT Results Within 45 Min. of Arrival	-	-	43%	57%
Patients Who Left ER Before Being Seen	-	-	2%	2%
Time from ER Arrival to Admit. (minutes)	-	-	257	274
Time from ER Arrival to Discharge (minutes)	-	-	142	134
Time in ER Before Being Evaluated (minutes)	-	-	30	26
Time to Pain Meds for Fractures (minutes)	-	-	67	57
Heart Attack Care				
Aspirin Given at Discharge[1]	-	-	99%	99%
Fibrinolytic Meds Within 30 Min. of Arrival[5]	-	-	50%	54%
PCI Within 90 Minutes of Arrival[5]	-	-	93%	96%
Statin Prescribed at Discharge[1]	-	-	98%	98%
Heart Failure Care				
ACE Inhibitor or ARB for LVSD[1]	21	95%	96%	97%
Discharge Instructions Given	67	96%	94%	94%
Evaluation of LVS Function	72	99%	98%	99%
Medicare Spending				
Medicare Spending per Patient (ratio)	-	-	0.96	0.98
Pneumonia Care				
Appropriate Initial Antibiotic Given	74	97%	94%	95%

NOTE: Hospital profiles are in alphabetical order by state, then city, then hospital within the city; Rankings exclude hospitals with less than 25 cases except for patient surveys which excludes hospitals with less than 100 cases; (a) 100-299 cases; (1) The number of cases/patients is too few to report; (2) Data submitted were based on a sample of cases/patients; (3) Results are based on a shorter time period than required; (4) Data suppressed by CMS for one or more quarters; (5) Results are not available for this reporting period; (6) Fewer than 100 patients completed the HCAHPS survey; (7) No cases met the criteria for this measure; (8) The lower limit of the confidence interval cannot be calculated if the number of observed infections equals zero; (9) No data are available from the state/territory for this reporting period; (10) The scores shown reflect fewer than 50 completed surveys; (11) There were discrepancies in the data collection process; (12) This measure does not apply to this hospital for this reporting period; (13) Results cannot be calculated for this reporting period; (14) The results for this state are combined with nearby states to protect confidentiality; Please refer to the User's Guide for a full explanation of data.

Measure	Cases	This Hosp.	State Avg.	U.S. Avg.
Blood Culture Timing	139	98%	97%	98%
Pregnancy and Delivery Care				
Newborn Deliveries Scheduled Early	-	-	10%	6%
Preventive Care				
Immunization for Influenza[2,3]	139	91%	94%	90%
Immunization for Pneumonia[2,3]	315	90%	95%	92%
Stroke Care				
Anticoagulation Therapy for Atrial Fibrillation	-	-	94%	95%
Antithrombotic Therapy Timing	-	-	98%	98%
Assessed for Rehabilitation	-	-	96%	97%
Discharged on Antithrombotic Therapy	-	-	98%	99%
Discharged on Statin Medication	-	-	91%	94%
Thrombolytic Therapy Timing	-	-	67%	66%
Venous Thromboembolism Prophylaxis	-	-	91%	94%
Written Stroke Educational Materials Given	-	-	84%	88%
Surgical Care Improvement Project				
Appropriate Beta Blocker Usage[5]	-	-	98%	98%
Appropriate VTP Within 24 Hours[5]	-	-	98%	98%
Controlled Postoperative Blood Glucose[5]	-	-	95%	97%
Perioperative Temperature Management[5]	-	-	100%	100%
Prophylactic Antibiotic Selection[5]	-	-	99%	99%
Prophylactic Antibiotic Selection (Outpatient)	-	-	97%	98%
Prophylactic Antibiotic Stopped[5]	-	-	98%	98%
Prophylactic Antibiotic Timing[5]	-	-	99%	99%
Prophylactic Antibiotic Timing (Outpatient)	-	-	97%	98%
Urinary Catheter Removal[5]	-	-	98%	97%
Survey of Patients' Hospital Experiences				
Area Around Room 'Always' Quiet at Night	-	-	58%	61%
Doctors 'Always' Communicated Well	-	-	82%	82%
Home Recovery Information Given	-	-	85%	85%
Hospital Given 9 or 10 on 10 Point Scale	-	-	66%	71%
Meds 'Always' Explained Before Given	-	-	64%	64%
Nurses 'Always' Communicated Well	-	-	78%	79%
Pain 'Always' Well Controlled	-	-	70%	71%
Room and Bathroom 'Always' Clean	-	-	75%	73%
Timely Help 'Always' Received	-	-	68%	68%
Would Definitely Recommend Hospital	-	-	66%	71%
Use of Medical Imaging				
Cardiac Imaging Stress Test before Surgery	-	-	4.9%	5.3%
Combination Abdominal CT Scan	-	-	14.4%	10.5%
Combination Brain/Sinus CT Scan	-	-	3%	2.7%
Combination Chest CT Scan	-	-	2.8%	2.7%
Follow-up Mammogram/Ultrasound	-	-	8.8%	8.8%
Lumbar Spine MRI for Low Back Pain	-	-	38.4%	37.2%

Davis Memorial Hospital

PO Box 1484
Elkins, WV 26241
Phone: 304-636-3300
Fax: 304-637-3384
URL: www.davishealthcare.org
Type: Acute Care Hospitals
Emergency Services: Yes
Ownership: Voluntary non-profit - Private
Beds: 90

Key Personnel:
Radiology. . . . . Steven M Barnett
Emergency Room . . . . Susan E Bobes, MD
CEO/President. . . . . Mark Doak
Infection Control. . . . . Margaret Emma, RN
Quality Assurance . . . . Sandra Phillips

Measure	Cases	This Hosp.	State Avg.	U.S. Avg.
Blood Clot Prevention and Treatment				
Anticoagulation Overlap Therapy[2]	23	74%	90%	93%
ICU Venous Thromboembolism Prophylaxis[2]	67	90%	88%	92%
Incidence of Potentially Preventable VTE[1,2]	-	-	12%	10%
UFH with Dosages/Platelet Monitoring[1,2]	-	-	98%	97%
Venous Thromboembolism Prophylaxis[2]	320	91%	79%	85%
Warfarin Therapy Discharge Instructions[2]	17	82%	80%	75%
Chest Pain/Possible Heart Attack Care				
Aspirin Given Within 24 Hours of Arrival	105	99%	96%	96%
Fibrinolytic Meds Within 30 Min. of Arrival	11	73%	74%	58%
Average Time to ECG (minutes)	112	8	8	7
Average Time to Transfer (minutes)[1]	-	-	109	60
Children's Asthma Care				
Received Home Management Plan of Care	-	-	-	88%
Received Reliever Medication	-	-	-	100%
Received Systemic Corticosteroids	-	-	-	100%
Emergency Department				
Admittance Decision Time (minutes)[2]	482	69	76	98
Head CT Results Within 45 Min. of Arrival	13	38%	43%	57%
Patients Who Left ER Before Being Seen	28,506	4%	2%	2%
Time from ER Arrival to Admit. (minutes)[2]	517	245	257	274
Time from ER Arrival to Discharge (minutes)	366	136	142	134
Time in ER Before Being Evaluated (minutes)	393	26	30	26
Time to Pain Meds for Fractures (minutes)	67	57	67	57
Heart Attack Care				
Aspirin Given at Discharge	13	100%	99%	99%
Fibrinolytic Meds Within 30 Min. of Arrival[7]	-	-	50%	54%
PCI Within 90 Minutes of Arrival[7]	-	-	93%	96%
Statin Prescribed at Discharge	11	91%	98%	98%
Heart Failure Care				
ACE Inhibitor or ARB for LVSD	34	91%	96%	97%
Discharge Instructions Given	115	95%	94%	94%
Evaluation of LVS Function	122	100%	98%	99%
Medicare Spending				
Medicare Spending per Patient (ratio)	-	0.85	0.96	0.98
Pneumonia Care				
Appropriate Initial Antibiotic Given	116	97%	94%	95%
Blood Culture Timing	171	100%	97%	98%
Pregnancy and Delivery Care				
Newborn Deliveries Scheduled Early	29	3%	10%	6%
Preventive Care				
Immunization for Influenza[2]	420	92%	94%	90%
Immunization for Pneumonia[2]	513	96%	95%	92%
Stroke Care				
Anticoagulation Therapy for Atrial Fibrillation[1]	-	-	94%	95%
Antithrombotic Therapy Timing	22	95%	98%	98%
Assessed for Rehabilitation	18	100%	96%	97%
Discharged on Antithrombotic Therapy	16	100%	98%	99%
Discharged on Statin Medication	15	87%	91%	94%
Thrombolytic Therapy Timing[1]	-	-	67%	66%
Venous Thromboembolism Prophylaxis	24	92%	91%	94%
Written Stroke Educational Materials Given	11	82%	84%	88%
Surgical Care Improvement Project				
Appropriate Beta Blocker Usage	89	96%	98%	98%
Appropriate VTP Within 24 Hours	240	97%	98%	98%
Controlled Postoperative Blood Glucose[7]	-	-	95%	97%
Perioperative Temperature Management	262	100%	100%	100%
Prophylactic Antibiotic Selection	182	100%	99%	99%
Prophylactic Antibiotic Selection (Outpatient)	75	100%	97%	98%
Prophylactic Antibiotic Stopped	179	96%	98%	98%
Prophylactic Antibiotic Timing	183	100%	99%	99%
Prophylactic Antibiotic Timing (Outpatient)	78	94%	97%	98%
Urinary Catheter Removal	38	82%	98%	97%
Survey of Patients' Hospital Experiences				
Area Around Room 'Always' Quiet at Night	300+	59%	58%	61%
Doctors 'Always' Communicated Well	300+	81%	82%	82%
Home Recovery Information Given	300+	85%	85%	85%
Hospital Given 9 or 10 on 10 Point Scale	300+	60%	66%	71%
Meds 'Always' Explained Before Given	300+	64%	64%	64%
Nurses 'Always' Communicated Well	300+	77%	78%	79%
Pain 'Always' Well Controlled	300+	68%	70%	71%
Room and Bathroom 'Always' Clean	300+	76%	75%	73%
Timely Help 'Always' Received	300+	68%	68%	68%
Would Definitely Recommend Hospital	300+	55%	66%	71%
Use of Medical Imaging				
Cardiac Imaging Stress Test before Surgery	363	4.1%	4.9%	5.3%
Combination Abdominal CT Scan	820	21.2%	14.4%	10.5%
Combination Brain/Sinus CT Scan	598	4.0%	3%	2.7%
Combination Chest CT Scan	458	6.3%	2.8%	2.7%
Follow-up Mammogram/Ultrasound	906	6.0%	8.8%	8.8%
Lumbar Spine MRI for Low Back Pain	78	38.5%	38.4%	37.2%

Fairmont General Hospital

1325 Locust Avenue
Fairmont, WV 26554
Phone: 304-367-7100
Fax: 304-367-7167
E-mail: info@fghi.com
URL: www.fghi.com
Type: Acute Care Hospitals
Emergency Services: Yes
Ownership: Voluntary non-profit - Private
Beds: 268

Key Personnel:
Cardiac Laboratory. . . . . Paul Alappha
CEO/President. . . . . Peggy Coster, RN, MSN, CEO
Infection Control. . . . . Janet Crigler
Chief of Medical Staff. . . . . Joedy Daristotle, MD
Chairman/CEO . . . . Toni Nesselrotte
Emergency Room . . . . Tina Straight

Measure	Cases	This Hosp.	State Avg.	U.S. Avg.
Blood Clot Prevention and Treatment				
Anticoagulation Overlap Therapy[2]	23	96%	90%	93%
ICU Venous Thromboembolism Prophylaxis[2]	56	80%	88%	92%
Incidence of Potentially Preventable VTE[1,2]	-	-	12%	10%
UFH with Dosages/Platelet Monitoring[2]	15	93%	98%	97%
Venous Thromboembolism Prophylaxis[2]	227	66%	79%	85%
Warfarin Therapy Discharge Instructions[2]	14	100%	80%	75%
Chest Pain/Possible Heart Attack Care				
Aspirin Given Within 24 Hours of Arrival	83	100%	96%	96%
Fibrinolytic Meds Within 30 Min. of Arrival[1]	-	-	74%	58%
Average Time to ECG (minutes)	83	10	8	7
Average Time to Transfer (minutes)[1]	-	-	109	60
Children's Asthma Care				
Received Home Management Plan of Care	-	-	-	88%
Received Reliever Medication	-	-	-	100%
Received Systemic Corticosteroids	-	-	-	100%
Emergency Department				
Admittance Decision Time (minutes)[2]	300	58	76	98
Head CT Results Within 45 Min. of Arrival	20	60%	43%	57%
Patients Who Left ER Before Being Seen	31,941	0%	2%	2%
Time from ER Arrival to Admit. (minutes)[2]	300	187	257	274
Time from ER Arrival to Discharge (minutes)	370	82	142	134
Time in ER Before Being Evaluated (minutes)	415	11	30	26
Time to Pain Meds for Fractures (minutes)	69	49	67	57
Heart Attack Care				
Aspirin Given at Discharge	43	100%	99%	99%
Fibrinolytic Meds Within 30 Min. of Arrival[1]	-	-	50%	54%
PCI Within 90 Minutes of Arrival[7]	-	-	93%	96%
Statin Prescribed at Discharge	37	100%	98%	98%
Heart Failure Care				
ACE Inhibitor or ARB for LVSD	46	100%	96%	97%
Discharge Instructions Given	142	92%	94%	94%
Evaluation of LVS Function	179	100%	98%	99%
Medicare Spending				
Medicare Spending per Patient (ratio)	-	1.01	0.96	0.98
Pneumonia Care				
Appropriate Initial Antibiotic Given	103	95%	94%	95%
Blood Culture Timing	127	98%	97%	98%
Pregnancy and Delivery Care				
Newborn Deliveries Scheduled Early[2]	21	0%	10%	6%
Preventive Care				
Immunization for Influenza[2]	436	99%	94%	90%
Immunization for Pneumonia[2]	534	99%	95%	92%
Stroke Care				
Anticoagulation Therapy for Atrial Fibrillation[1]	-	-	94%	95%
Antithrombotic Therapy Timing[1]	-	-	98%	98%
Assessed for Rehabilitation[1]	-	-	96%	97%
Discharged on Antithrombotic Therapy[1]	-	-	98%	99%
Discharged on Statin Medication[1]	-	-	91%	94%
Thrombolytic Therapy Timing[7]	-	-	67%	66%
Venous Thromboembolism Prophylaxis[1]	-	-	91%	94%
Written Stroke Educational Materials Given[1]	-	-	84%	88%
Surgical Care Improvement Project				
Appropriate Beta Blocker Usage	40	100%	98%	98%
Appropriate VTP Within 24 Hours	95	99%	98%	98%
Controlled Postoperative Blood Glucose[7]	-	-	95%	97%
Perioperative Temperature Management	136	100%	100%	100%
Prophylactic Antibiotic Selection	87	100%	99%	99%
Prophylactic Antibiotic Selection (Outpatient)	73	97%	97%	98%

NOTE: Hospital profiles are in alphabetical order by state, then city, then hospital within the city; Rankings exclude hospitals with less than 25 cases except for patient surveys which excludes hospitals with less than 100 cases; (a) 100-299 cases; (1) The number of cases/patients is too few to report; (2) Data submitted were based on a sample of cases/patients; (3) Results are based on a shorter time period than required; (4) Data suppressed by CMS for one or more quarters; (5) Results are not available for this reporting period; (6) Fewer than 100 patients completed the HCAHPS survey; (7) No cases met the criteria for this measure; (8) The lower limit of the confidence interval cannot be calculated if the number of observed infections equals zero; (9) No data are available from the state/territory for this reporting period; (10) The scores shown reflect fewer than 50 completed surveys; (11) There were discrepancies in the data collection process; (12) This measure does not apply to this hospital for this reporting period; (13) Results cannot be calculated for this reporting period; (14) The results for this state are combined with nearby states to protect confidentiality; Please refer to the User's Guide for a full explanation of data.

Prophylactic Antibiotic Stopped	84	100%	98%	98%
Prophylactic Antibiotic Timing	87	100%	99%	99%
Prophylactic Antibiotic Timing (Outpatient)	74	99%	97%	98%
Urinary Catheter Removal	77	100%	98%	97%
Survey of Patients' Hospital Experiences				
Area Around Room 'Always' Quiet at Night	300+	58%	58%	61%
Doctors 'Always' Communicated Well	300+	83%	82%	82%
Home Recovery Information Given	300+	83%	85%	85%
Hospital Given 9 or 10 on 10 Point Scale	300+	57%	66%	71%
Meds 'Always' Explained Before Given	300+	65%	64%	64%
Nurses 'Always' Communicated Well	300+	77%	78%	79%
Pain 'Always' Well Controlled	300+	71%	70%	71%
Room and Bathroom 'Always' Clean	300+	67%	75%	73%
Timely Help 'Always' Received	300+	62%	68%	68%
Would Definitely Recommend Hospital	300+	54%	66%	71%
Use of Medical Imaging				
Cardiac Imaging Stress Test before Surgery	400	5.0%	4.9%	5.3%
Combination Abdominal CT Scan	581	30.5%	14.4%	10.5%
Combination Brain/Sinus CT Scan	568	2.5%	3%	2.7%
Combination Chest CT Scan	340	1.2%	2.8%	2.7%
Follow-up Mammogram/Ultrasound	595	7.9%	8.8%	8.8%
Lumbar Spine MRI for Low Back Pain	122	36.9%	38.4%	37.2%

Braxton County Memorial Hospital

100 Hoylman Drive Phone: 304-364-5156
Gassaway, WV 26624 Fax: 304-364-1154
URL: www.braxtonmemorial.org
Type: Critical Access Hospitals Emergency Services: Yes
Ownership: Voluntary non-profit - Private Beds: 25

Key Personnel:
CEO/President. . . . . Barbara Adams
Anesthesiology. . . . . Pam Bender, RN
Operating Room. . . . . Pam Bender, RN
Emergency Room . . . . Jill Cotrill, RN
Infection Control. . . . . Sharon Gaston, RN
Quality Assurance . . . . Sharon Gaston, RN
Chief of Medical Staff. . . . . Russell Stewart, MD

Measure	Cases	This Hosp.	State Avg.	U.S. Avg.
Blood Clot Prevention and Treatment				
Anticoagulation Overlap Therapy[5]	-	-	90%	93%
ICU Venous Thromboembolism Prophylaxis[5]	-	-	88%	92%
Incidence of Potentially Preventable VTE[5]	-	-	12%	10%
UFH with Dosages/Platelet Monitoring[5]	-	-	98%	97%
Venous Thromboembolism Prophylaxis[5]	-	-	79%	85%
Warfarin Therapy Discharge Instructions[5]	-	-	80%	75%
Chest Pain/Possible Heart Attack Care				
Aspirin Given Within 24 Hours of Arrival	-	-	96%	96%
Fibrinolytic Meds Within 30 Min. of Arrival	-	-	74%	58%
Average Time to ECG (minutes)	-	-	8	7
Average Time to Transfer (minutes)	-	-	109	60
Children's Asthma Care				
Received Home Management Plan of Care	-	-	-	88%
Received Reliever Medication	-	-	-	100%
Received Systemic Corticosteroids	-	-	-	100%
Emergency Department				
Admittance Decision Time (minutes)[5]	-	-	76	98
Head CT Results Within 45 Min. of Arrival	-	-	43%	57%
Patients Who Left ER Before Being Seen	-	-	2%	2%
Time from ER Arrival to Admit. (minutes)[5]	-	-	257	274
Time from ER Arrival to Discharge (minutes)	-	-	142	134
Time in ER Before Being Evaluated (minutes)	-	-	30	26
Time to Pain Meds for Fractures (minutes)	-	-	67	57
Heart Attack Care				
Aspirin Given at Discharge[5]	-	-	99%	99%
Fibrinolytic Meds Within 30 Min. of Arrival[5]	-	-	50%	54%
PCI Within 90 Minutes of Arrival[5]	-	-	93%	96%
Statin Prescribed at Discharge[5]	-	-	98%	98%
Heart Failure Care				
ACE Inhibitor or ARB for LVSD[1,3]	-	-	96%	97%
Discharge Instructions Given[1,3]	-	-	94%	94%
Evaluation of LVS Function[1,3]	-	-	98%	99%
Medicare Spending				
Medicare Spending per Patient (ratio)	-	-	0.96	0.98
Pneumonia Care				
Appropriate Initial Antibiotic Given	18	67%	94%	95%
Blood Culture Timing	33	97%	97%	98%
Pregnancy and Delivery Care				
Newborn Deliveries Scheduled Early[5]	-	-	10%	6%
Preventive Care				
Immunization for Influenza[5]	-	-	94%	90%
Immunization for Pneumonia[5]	-	-	95%	92%
Stroke Care				
Anticoagulation Therapy for Atrial Fibrillation[5]	-	-	94%	95%
Antithrombotic Therapy Timing[5]	-	-	98%	98%
Assessed for Rehabilitation[5]	-	-	96%	97%
Discharged on Antithrombotic Therapy[5]	-	-	98%	99%
Discharged on Statin Medication[5]	-	-	91%	94%
Thrombolytic Therapy Timing[5]	-	-	67%	66%
Venous Thromboembolism Prophylaxis[5]	-	-	91%	94%
Written Stroke Educational Materials Given[5]	-	-	84%	88%
Surgical Care Improvement Project				
Appropriate Beta Blocker Usage[1,3]	-	-	98%	98%
Appropriate VTP Within 24 Hours[1,3]	-	-	98%	98%
Controlled Postoperative Blood Glucose[3,7]	-	-	95%	97%
Perioperative Temperature Management[1,3]	-	-	100%	100%
Prophylactic Antibiotic Selection[1,3]	-	-	99%	99%
Prophylactic Antibiotic Selection (Outpatient)	-	-	97%	98%
Prophylactic Antibiotic Stopped[1,3]	-	-	98%	98%
Prophylactic Antibiotic Timing[1,3]	-	-	99%	99%
Prophylactic Antibiotic Timing (Outpatient)	-	-	97%	98%
Urinary Catheter Removal[1,3]	-	-	98%	97%
Survey of Patients' Hospital Experiences				
Area Around Room 'Always' Quiet at Night[6]	<100	67%	58%	61%
Doctors 'Always' Communicated Well[6]	<100	85%	82%	82%
Home Recovery Information Given[6]	<100	76%	85%	85%
Hospital Given 9 or 10 on 10 Point Scale[6]	<100	72%	66%	71%
Meds 'Always' Explained Before Given[6]	<100	64%	64%	64%
Nurses 'Always' Communicated Well[6]	<100	82%	78%	79%
Pain 'Always' Well Controlled[6]	<100	67%	70%	71%
Room and Bathroom 'Always' Clean[6]	<100	76%	75%	73%
Timely Help 'Always' Received[6]	<100	79%	68%	68%
Would Definitely Recommend Hospital[6]	<100	71%	66%	71%
Use of Medical Imaging				
Cardiac Imaging Stress Test before Surgery	-	-	4.9%	5.3%
Combination Abdominal CT Scan	-	-	14.4%	10.5%
Combination Brain/Sinus CT Scan	-	-	3%	2.7%
Combination Chest CT Scan	-	-	2.8%	2.7%
Follow-up Mammogram/Ultrasound	-	-	8.8%	8.8%
Lumbar Spine MRI for Low Back Pain	-	-	38.4%	37.2%

Reynolds Memorial Hospital

800 Wheeling Ave Phone: 304-843-3230
Glen Dale, WV 26038 Fax: 304-843-3202
URL: www.reynoldsmemorial.com
Type: Acute Care Hospitals Emergency Services: Yes
Ownership: Voluntary non-profit - Private Beds: 233

Key Personnel:
Radiology. . . . . Frank D Diettinger
Quality Assurance . . . . Patricia Downey
Emergency Room . . . . Debra L Henry, MD
Infection Control. . . . . Patti Kimpel, RN
Coronary Care . . . . Patti Kimple, RN
CEO/President. . . . . John A Sicurella
Chief of Medical Staff. . . . . Robert B Wade, MD

Measure	Cases	This Hosp.	State Avg.	U.S. Avg.
Blood Clot Prevention and Treatment				
Anticoagulation Overlap Therapy[1,2]	-	-	90%	93%
ICU Venous Thromboembolism Prophylaxis[2]	56	61%	88%	92%
Incidence of Potentially Preventable VTE[1,2]	-	-	12%	10%
UFH with Dosages/Platelet Monitoring[1,2]	-	-	98%	97%
Venous Thromboembolism Prophylaxis[2]	197	45%	79%	85%
Warfarin Therapy Discharge Instructions[1,2]	-	-	80%	75%
Chest Pain/Possible Heart Attack Care				
Aspirin Given Within 24 Hours of Arrival	22	86%	96%	96%
Fibrinolytic Meds Within 30 Min. of Arrival[7]	-	-	74%	58%
Average Time to ECG (minutes)	22	9	8	7
Average Time to Transfer (minutes)	11	63	109	60
Children's Asthma Care				
Received Home Management Plan of Care	-	-	-	88%
Received Reliever Medication	-	-	-	100%
Received Systemic Corticosteroids	-	-	-	100%
Emergency Department				
Admittance Decision Time (minutes)[2]	146	66	76	98
Head CT Results Within 45 Min. of Arrival[1,3]	-	-	43%	57%
Patients Who Left ER Before Being Seen	12,028	4%	2%	2%
Time from ER Arrival to Admit. (minutes)[2]	154	250	257	274
Time from ER Arrival to Discharge (minutes)	359	130	142	134
Time in ER Before Being Evaluated (minutes)	122	32	30	26
Time to Pain Meds for Fractures (minutes)	34	54	67	57
Heart Attack Care				
Aspirin Given at Discharge	17	100%	99%	99%
Fibrinolytic Meds Within 30 Min. of Arrival[7]	-	-	50%	54%
PCI Within 90 Minutes of Arrival[7]	-	-	93%	96%
Statin Prescribed at Discharge	13	54%	98%	98%
Heart Failure Care				
ACE Inhibitor or ARB for LVSD	28	86%	96%	97%
Discharge Instructions Given	71	82%	94%	94%
Evaluation of LVS Function	123	94%	98%	99%
Medicare Spending				
Medicare Spending per Patient (ratio)	-	1.00	0.96	0.98
Pneumonia Care				
Appropriate Initial Antibiotic Given	61	90%	94%	95%
Blood Culture Timing	65	98%	97%	98%
Pregnancy and Delivery Care				
Newborn Deliveries Scheduled Early[1]	-	-	10%	6%
Preventive Care				
Immunization for Influenza[2]	288	88%	94%	90%
Immunization for Pneumonia[2]	463	88%	95%	92%
Stroke Care				
Anticoagulation Therapy for Atrial Fibrillation[1]	-	-	94%	95%
Antithrombotic Therapy Timing	20	95%	98%	98%
Assessed for Rehabilitation	19	89%	96%	97%
Discharged on Antithrombotic Therapy	19	100%	98%	99%
Discharged on Statin Medication	16	62%	91%	94%
Thrombolytic Therapy Timing[1]	-	-	67%	66%
Venous Thromboembolism Prophylaxis	20	45%	91%	94%
Written Stroke Educational Materials Given[1]	-	-	84%	88%
Surgical Care Improvement Project				
Appropriate Beta Blocker Usage	31	90%	98%	98%
Appropriate VTP Within 24 Hours	63	87%	98%	98%
Controlled Postoperative Blood Glucose[7]	-	-	95%	97%
Perioperative Temperature Management	86	100%	100%	100%
Prophylactic Antibiotic Selection	54	91%	99%	99%
Prophylactic Antibiotic Selection (Outpatient)	25	100%	97%	98%
Prophylactic Antibiotic Stopped	48	90%	98%	98%
Prophylactic Antibiotic Timing	54	98%	99%	99%
Prophylactic Antibiotic Timing (Outpatient)	25	100%	97%	98%
Urinary Catheter Removal	29	90%	98%	97%
Survey of Patients' Hospital Experiences				
Area Around Room 'Always' Quiet at Night	300+	50%	58%	61%
Doctors 'Always' Communicated Well	300+	81%	82%	82%
Home Recovery Information Given	300+	84%	85%	85%
Hospital Given 9 or 10 on 10 Point Scale	300+	62%	66%	71%
Meds 'Always' Explained Before Given	300+	59%	64%	64%
Nurses 'Always' Communicated Well	300+	73%	78%	79%
Pain 'Always' Well Controlled	300+	68%	70%	71%
Room and Bathroom 'Always' Clean	300+	68%	75%	73%
Timely Help 'Always' Received	300+	64%	68%	68%
Would Definitely Recommend Hospital	300+	60%	66%	71%
Use of Medical Imaging				
Cardiac Imaging Stress Test before Surgery[1]	-	-	4.9%	5.3%
Combination Abdominal CT Scan	204	15.2%	14.4%	10.5%
Combination Brain/Sinus CT Scan[1]	-	-	3%	2.7%
Combination Chest CT Scan	91	1.1%	2.8%	2.7%
Follow-up Mammogram/Ultrasound	304	15.5%	8.8%	8.8%
Lumbar Spine MRI for Low Back Pain	55	47.3%	38.4%	37.2%

NOTE: Hospital profiles are in alphabetical order by state, then city, then hospital within the city; Rankings exclude hospitals with less than 25 cases except for patient surveys which excludes hospitals with less than 100 cases; (a) 100-299 cases; (1) The number of cases/patients is too few to report; (2) Data submitted were based on a sample of cases/patients; (3) Results are based on a shorter time period than required; (4) Data suppressed by CMS for one or more quarters; (5) Results are not available for this reporting period; (6) Fewer than 100 patients completed the HCAHPS survey; (7) No cases met the criteria for this measure; (8) The lower limit of the confidence interval cannot be calculated if the number of observed infections equals zero; (9) No data are available from the state/territory for this reporting period; (10) The scores shown reflect fewer than 50 completed surveys; (11) There were discrepancies in the data collection process; (12) This measure does not apply to this hospital for this reporting period; (13) Results cannot be calculated for this reporting period; (14) The results for this state are combined with nearby states to protect confidentiality; Please refer to the User's Guide for a full explanation of data.

Grafton City Hospital

1 Hospital Plaza
Grafton, WV 26354
URL: www.graftonhospital.com
Phone: 304-265-0400
Fax: 304-265-3926
Type: Critical Access Hospitals
Emergency Services: Yes
Ownership: Government - Local
Beds: 136

Key Personnel:
Anesthesiology. . . . . Mona Grandstaff CRNA
Infection Control. . . . . Diana Knight
Emergency Room . . . . Thomas Lauderman
Operating Room. . . . . Debbie Lemasters
CEO/President. . . . . Jeff Lilley
Patient Relations . . . . Kathy Matheney
Quality Assurance . . . . Dan Swiger
Chief of Medical Staff. . . . . Christopher Z Villaraza, II

Measure	Cases	This Hosp.	State Avg.	U.S. Avg.
Blood Clot Prevention and Treatment				
Anticoagulation Overlap Therapy[5]	-	-	90%	93%
ICU Venous Thromboembolism Prophylaxis[5]	-	-	88%	92%
Incidence of Potentially Preventable VTE[5]	-	-	12%	10%
UFH with Dosages/Platelet Monitoring[5]	-	-	98%	97%
Venous Thromboembolism Prophylaxis[5]	-	-	79%	85%
Warfarin Therapy Discharge Instructions[5]	-	-	80%	75%
Chest Pain/Possible Heart Attack Care				
Aspirin Given Within 24 Hours of Arrival	-	-	96%	96%
Fibrinolytic Meds Within 30 Min. of Arrival	-	-	74%	58%
Average Time to ECG (minutes)	-	-	8	7
Average Time to Transfer (minutes)	-	-	109	60
Children's Asthma Care				
Received Home Management Plan of Care	-	-	-	88%
Received Reliever Medication	-	-	-	100%
Received Systemic Corticosteroids	-	-	-	100%
Emergency Department				
Admittance Decision Time (minutes)[5]	-	-	76	98
Head CT Results Within 45 Min. of Arrival	-	-	43%	57%
Patients Who Left ER Before Being Seen	-	-	2%	2%
Time from ER Arrival to Admit. (minutes)[5]	-	-	257	274
Time from ER Arrival to Discharge (minutes)	-	-	142	134
Time in ER Before Being Evaluated (minutes)	-	-	30	26
Time to Pain Meds for Fractures (minutes)	-	-	67	57
Heart Attack Care				
Aspirin Given at Discharge[5]	-	-	99%	99%
Fibrinolytic Meds Within 30 Min. of Arrival[5]	-	-	50%	54%
PCI Within 90 Minutes of Arrival[5]	-	-	93%	96%
Statin Prescribed at Discharge[5]	-	-	98%	98%
Heart Failure Care				
ACE Inhibitor or ARB for LVSD[1]	-	-	96%	97%
Discharge Instructions Given[1]	-	-	94%	94%
Evaluation of LVS Function[1]	-	-	98%	99%
Medicare Spending				
Medicare Spending per Patient (ratio)	-	-	0.96	0.98
Pneumonia Care				
Appropriate Initial Antibiotic Given[2]	15	73%	94%	95%
Blood Culture Timing[2]	11	82%	97%	98%
Pregnancy and Delivery Care				
Newborn Deliveries Scheduled Early[5]	-	-	10%	6%
Preventive Care				
Immunization for Influenza[5]	-	-	94%	90%
Immunization for Pneumonia[5]	-	-	95%	92%
Stroke Care				
Anticoagulation Therapy for Atrial Fibrillation[5]	-	-	94%	95%
Antithrombotic Therapy Timing[5]	-	-	98%	98%
Assessed for Rehabilitation[5]	-	-	96%	97%
Discharged on Antithrombotic Therapy[5]	-	-	98%	99%
Discharged on Statin Medication[5]	-	-	91%	94%
Thrombolytic Therapy Timing[5]	-	-	67%	66%
Venous Thromboembolism Prophylaxis[5]	-	-	91%	94%
Written Stroke Educational Materials Given[5]	-	-	84%	88%
Surgical Care Improvement Project				
Appropriate Beta Blocker Usage[5]	-	-	98%	98%
Appropriate VTP Within 24 Hours[5]	-	-	98%	98%
Controlled Postoperative Blood Glucose[5]	-	-	95%	97%
Perioperative Temperature Management[5]	-	-	100%	100%
Prophylactic Antibiotic Selection[5]	-	-	99%	99%
Prophylactic Antibiotic Selection (Outpatient)	-	-	97%	98%
Prophylactic Antibiotic Stopped[5]	-	-	98%	98%
Prophylactic Antibiotic Timing[5]	-	-	99%	99%
Prophylactic Antibiotic Timing (Outpatient)	-	-	97%	98%
Urinary Catheter Removal[5]	-	-	98%	97%
Survey of Patients' Hospital Experiences				
Area Around Room 'Always' Quiet at Night[5]	-	-	58%	61%
Doctors 'Always' Communicated Well[5]	-	-	82%	82%
Home Recovery Information Given[5]	-	-	85%	85%
Hospital Given 9 or 10 on 10 Point Scale[5]	-	-	66%	71%
Meds 'Always' Explained Before Given[5]	-	-	64%	64%
Nurses 'Always' Communicated Well[5]	-	-	78%	79%
Pain 'Always' Well Controlled[5]	-	-	70%	71%
Room and Bathroom 'Always' Clean[5]	-	-	75%	73%
Timely Help 'Always' Received[5]	-	-	68%	68%
Would Definitely Recommend Hospital[5]	-	-	66%	71%
Use of Medical Imaging				
Cardiac Imaging Stress Test before Surgery	-	-	4.9%	5.3%
Combination Abdominal CT Scan	-	-	14.4%	10.5%
Combination Brain/Sinus CT Scan	-	-	3%	2.7%
Combination Chest CT Scan	-	-	2.8%	2.7%
Follow-up Mammogram/Ultrasound	-	-	8.8%	8.8%
Lumbar Spine MRI for Low Back Pain	-	-	38.4%	37.2%

Minnie Hamilton Health Care Center

186 Hospital Drive
Grantsville, WV 26147
Phone: 304-354-9244
Type: Critical Access Hospitals
Emergency Services: Yes
Ownership: Voluntary non-profit - Private

Key Personnel:
Emergency Room . . . . Trudy Anderson, RN
Radiology. . . . . Cheryl Balisciano
Quality Assurance . . . . Sandra Ellis
Chief of Medical Staff. . . . . Vishwanath Hande, MD
CEO/President. . . . . Barbara Lay

Measure	Cases	This Hosp.	State Avg.	U.S. Avg.
Blood Clot Prevention and Treatment				
Anticoagulation Overlap Therapy[5]	-	-	90%	93%
ICU Venous Thromboembolism Prophylaxis[5]	-	-	88%	92%
Incidence of Potentially Preventable VTE[5]	-	-	12%	10%
UFH with Dosages/Platelet Monitoring[5]	-	-	98%	97%
Venous Thromboembolism Prophylaxis[5]	-	-	79%	85%
Warfarin Therapy Discharge Instructions[5]	-	-	80%	75%
Chest Pain/Possible Heart Attack Care				
Aspirin Given Within 24 Hours of Arrival	-	-	96%	96%
Fibrinolytic Meds Within 30 Min. of Arrival	-	-	74%	58%
Average Time to ECG (minutes)	-	-	8	7
Average Time to Transfer (minutes)	-	-	109	60
Children's Asthma Care				
Received Home Management Plan of Care	-	-	-	88%
Received Reliever Medication	-	-	-	100%
Received Systemic Corticosteroids	-	-	-	100%
Emergency Department				
Admittance Decision Time (minutes)[2]	138	75	76	98
Head CT Results Within 45 Min. of Arrival	-	-	43%	57%
Patients Who Left ER Before Being Seen	-	-	2%	2%
Time from ER Arrival to Admit. (minutes)[2]	151	215	257	274
Time from ER Arrival to Discharge (minutes)	-	-	142	134
Time in ER Before Being Evaluated (minutes)	-	-	30	26
Time to Pain Meds for Fractures (minutes)	-	-	67	57
Heart Attack Care				
Aspirin Given at Discharge[1,3]	-	-	99%	99%
Fibrinolytic Meds Within 30 Min. of Arrival[3,7]	-	-	50%	54%
PCI Within 90 Minutes of Arrival[3,7]	-	-	93%	96%
Statin Prescribed at Discharge[1,3]	-	-	98%	98%
Heart Failure Care				
ACE Inhibitor or ARB for LVSD[1]	-	-	96%	97%
Discharge Instructions Given[1]	-	-	94%	94%
Evaluation of LVS Function	14	64%	98%	99%
Medicare Spending				
Medicare Spending per Patient (ratio)	-	-	0.96	0.98
Pneumonia Care				
Appropriate Initial Antibiotic Given	14	50%	94%	95%
Blood Culture Timing	22	82%	97%	98%
Pregnancy and Delivery Care				
Newborn Deliveries Scheduled Early[5]	-	-	10%	6%
Preventive Care				
Immunization for Influenza	94	91%	94%	90%
Immunization for Pneumonia	139	90%	95%	92%
Stroke Care				
Anticoagulation Therapy for Atrial Fibrillation[5]	-	-	94%	95%
Antithrombotic Therapy Timing[5]	-	-	98%	98%
Assessed for Rehabilitation[5]	-	-	96%	97%
Discharged on Antithrombotic Therapy[5]	-	-	98%	99%
Discharged on Statin Medication[5]	-	-	91%	94%
Thrombolytic Therapy Timing[5]	-	-	67%	66%
Venous Thromboembolism Prophylaxis[5]	-	-	91%	94%
Written Stroke Educational Materials Given[5]	-	-	84%	88%
Surgical Care Improvement Project				
Appropriate Beta Blocker Usage[5]	-	-	98%	98%
Appropriate VTP Within 24 Hours[5]	-	-	98%	98%
Controlled Postoperative Blood Glucose[5]	-	-	95%	97%
Perioperative Temperature Management[5]	-	-	100%	100%
Prophylactic Antibiotic Selection[5]	-	-	99%	99%
Prophylactic Antibiotic Selection (Outpatient)	-	-	97%	98%
Prophylactic Antibiotic Stopped[5]	-	-	98%	98%
Prophylactic Antibiotic Timing[5]	-	-	99%	99%
Prophylactic Antibiotic Timing (Outpatient)	-	-	97%	98%
Urinary Catheter Removal[5]	-	-	98%	97%
Survey of Patients' Hospital Experiences				
Area Around Room 'Always' Quiet at Night[6]	<100	50%	58%	61%
Doctors 'Always' Communicated Well[6]	<100	84%	82%	82%
Home Recovery Information Given[6]	<100	86%	85%	85%
Hospital Given 9 or 10 on 10 Point Scale[6]	<100	62%	66%	71%
Meds 'Always' Explained Before Given[6]	<100	67%	64%	64%
Nurses 'Always' Communicated Well[6]	<100	79%	78%	79%
Pain 'Always' Well Controlled[6]	<100	82%	70%	71%
Room and Bathroom 'Always' Clean[6]	<100	72%	75%	73%
Timely Help 'Always' Received[6]	<100	75%	68%	68%
Would Definitely Recommend Hospital[6]	<100	61%	66%	71%
Use of Medical Imaging				
Cardiac Imaging Stress Test before Surgery	-	-	4.9%	5.3%
Combination Abdominal CT Scan	-	-	14.4%	10.5%
Combination Brain/Sinus CT Scan	-	-	3%	2.7%
Combination Chest CT Scan	-	-	2.8%	2.7%
Follow-up Mammogram/Ultrasound	-	-	8.8%	8.8%
Lumbar Spine MRI for Low Back Pain	-	-	38.4%	37.2%

Summers County ARH Hospital

Terrace Street, PO Box 940
Hinton, WV 25951
E-mail: nwhitleck@arh.org
URL: www.arh.org/summers%20county
Phone: 304-466-1000
Fax: 304-466-1690
Type: Critical Access Hospitals
Emergency Services: Yes
Ownership: Voluntary non-profit - Private
Beds: 89

Key Personnel:
Cardiac Laboratory. . . . . Ajay Anand, MD
Emergency Room . . . . Amarinder S Chhabra, MD
Radiology. . . . . Daniel D Maxwell
CEO/President. . . . . Chris Vaught

Measure	Cases	This Hosp.	State Avg.	U.S. Avg.
Blood Clot Prevention and Treatment				
Anticoagulation Overlap Therapy[5]	-	-	90%	93%
ICU Venous Thromboembolism Prophylaxis[5]	-	-	88%	92%
Incidence of Potentially Preventable VTE[5]	-	-	12%	10%
UFH with Dosages/Platelet Monitoring[5]	-	-	98%	97%
Venous Thromboembolism Prophylaxis[5]	-	-	79%	85%
Warfarin Therapy Discharge Instructions[5]	-	-	80%	75%
Chest Pain/Possible Heart Attack Care				
Aspirin Given Within 24 Hours of Arrival	-	-	96%	96%
Fibrinolytic Meds Within 30 Min. of Arrival	-	-	74%	58%
Average Time to ECG (minutes)	-	-	8	7
Average Time to Transfer (minutes)	-	-	109	60
Children's Asthma Care				
Received Home Management Plan of Care	-	-	-	88%
Received Reliever Medication	-	-	-	100%

NOTE: Hospital profiles are in alphabetical order by state, then city, then hospital within the city; Rankings exclude hospitals with less than 25 cases except for patient surveys which excludes hospitals with less than 100 cases; (a) 100-299 cases; (1) The number of cases/patients is too few to report; (2) Data submitted were based on a sample of cases/patients; (3) Results are based on a shorter time period than required; (4) Data suppressed by CMS for one or more quarters; (5) Results are not available for this reporting period; (6) Fewer than 100 patients completed the HCAHPS survey; (7) No cases met the criteria for this measure; (8) The lower limit of the confidence interval cannot be calculated if the number of observed infections equals zero; (9) No data are available from the state/territory for this reporting period; (10) The scores shown reflect fewer than 50 completed surveys; (11) There were discrepancies in the data collection process; (12) This measure does not apply to this hospital for this reporting period; (13) Results cannot be calculated for this reporting period; (14) The results for this state are combined with nearby states to protect confidentiality; Please refer to the User's Guide for a full explanation of data.

Measure	Cases	This Hosp.	State Avg.	U.S. Avg.
Received Systemic Corticosteroids	-	-	-	100%
Emergency Department				
Admittance Decision Time (minutes)[5]	-	-	76	98
Head CT Results Within 45 Min. of Arrival	-	-	43%	57%
Patients Who Left ER Before Being Seen	-	-	2%	2%
Time from ER Arrival to Admit. (minutes)[5]	-	-	257	274
Time from ER Arrival to Discharge (minutes)	-	-	142	134
Time in ER Before Being Evaluated (minutes)	-	-	30	26
Time to Pain Meds for Fractures (minutes)	-	-	67	57
Heart Attack Care				
Aspirin Given at Discharge[7]	-	-	99%	99%
Fibrinolytic Meds Within 30 Min. of Arrival[3,7]	-	-	50%	54%
PCI Within 90 Minutes of Arrival[3,7]	-	-	93%	96%
Statin Prescribed at Discharge[7]	-	-	98%	98%
Heart Failure Care				
ACE Inhibitor or ARB for LVSD	14	100%	96%	97%
Discharge Instructions Given	25	92%	94%	94%
Evaluation of LVS Function	33	94%	98%	99%
Medicare Spending				
Medicare Spending per Patient (ratio)	-	-	0.96	0.98
Pneumonia Care				
Appropriate Initial Antibiotic Given	29	86%	94%	95%
Blood Culture Timing	33	100%	97%	98%
Pregnancy and Delivery Care				
Newborn Deliveries Scheduled Early[5]	-	-	10%	6%
Preventive Care				
Immunization for Influenza[5]	-	-	94%	90%
Immunization for Pneumonia[5]	-	-	95%	92%
Stroke Care				
Anticoagulation Therapy for Atrial Fibrillation[5]	-	-	94%	95%
Antithrombotic Therapy Timing[5]	-	-	98%	98%
Assessed for Rehabilitation[5]	-	-	96%	97%
Discharged on Antithrombotic Therapy[5]	-	-	98%	99%
Discharged on Statin Medication[5]	-	-	91%	94%
Thrombolytic Therapy Timing[5]	-	-	67%	66%
Venous Thromboembolism Prophylaxis[5]	-	-	91%	94%
Written Stroke Educational Materials Given[5]	-	-	84%	88%
Surgical Care Improvement Project				
Appropriate Beta Blocker Usage[5]	-	-	98%	98%
Appropriate VTP Within 24 Hours[5]	-	-	98%	98%
Controlled Postoperative Blood Glucose[5]	-	-	95%	97%
Perioperative Temperature Management[5]	-	-	100%	100%
Prophylactic Antibiotic Selection[5]	-	-	99%	99%
Prophylactic Antibiotic Selection (Outpatient)	-	-	97%	98%
Prophylactic Antibiotic Stopped[5]	-	-	98%	98%
Prophylactic Antibiotic Timing[5]	-	-	99%	99%
Prophylactic Antibiotic Timing (Outpatient)	-	-	97%	98%
Urinary Catheter Removal[5]	-	-	98%	97%
Survey of Patients' Hospital Experiences				
Area Around Room 'Always' Quiet at Night	(a)	72%	58%	61%
Doctors 'Always' Communicated Well	(a)	90%	82%	82%
Home Recovery Information Given	(a)	89%	85%	85%
Hospital Given 9 or 10 on 10 Point Scale	(a)	67%	66%	71%
Meds 'Always' Explained Before Given	(a)	74%	64%	64%
Nurses 'Always' Communicated Well	(a)	84%	78%	79%
Pain 'Always' Well Controlled	(a)	75%	70%	71%
Room and Bathroom 'Always' Clean	(a)	81%	75%	73%
Timely Help 'Always' Received	(a)	79%	68%	68%
Would Definitely Recommend Hospital	(a)	70%	66%	71%
Use of Medical Imaging				
Cardiac Imaging Stress Test before Surgery	-	-	4.9%	5.3%
Combination Abdominal CT Scan	-	-	14.4%	10.5%
Combination Brain/Sinus CT Scan	-	-	3%	2.7%
Combination Chest CT Scan	-	-	2.8%	2.7%
Follow-up Mammogram/Ultrasound	-	-	8.8%	8.8%
Lumbar Spine MRI for Low Back Pain	-	-	38.4%	37.2%

Cabell Huntington Hospital

1340 Hal Greer Boulevard
Huntington, WV 25701
E-mail: info@cabellhuntington.org
URL: www.cabellhuntington.org
Type: Acute Care Hospitals
Ownership: Voluntary non-profit - Private
Phone: 304-526-2000
Fax: 304-526-6077
Emergency Services: Yes
Beds: 303

Key Personnel:
Operating Room. . . . . Debbie Ball, RN
Chief of Medical Staff. . . . . Hoyt Burdick
Radiology. . . . . John Duncan
CEO/President. . . . . Brent A Marsteller
Quality Assurance . . . . Deanna Parsons
Pediatric In-Patient Care . . . . Gilbert Ratcliff

Measure	Cases	This Hosp.	State Avg.	U.S. Avg.
Blood Clot Prevention and Treatment				
Anticoagulation Overlap Therapy[2]	105	94%	90%	93%
ICU Venous Thromboembolism Prophylaxis[2]	101	94%	88%	92%
Incidence of Potentially Preventable VTE[2]	17	6%	12%	10%
UFH with Dosages/Platelet Monitoring[2]	86	100%	98%	97%
Venous Thromboembolism Prophylaxis[2]	275	91%	79%	85%
Warfarin Therapy Discharge Instructions[2]	79	97%	80%	75%
Chest Pain/Possible Heart Attack Care				
Aspirin Given Within 24 Hours of Arrival	11	91%	96%	96%
Fibrinolytic Meds Within 30 Min. of Arrival[7]	-	-	74%	58%
Average Time to ECG (minutes)	11	10	8	7
Average Time to Transfer (minutes)[1]	-	-	109	60
Children's Asthma Care				
Received Home Management Plan of Care	-	-	-	88%
Received Reliever Medication	-	-	-	100%
Received Systemic Corticosteroids	-	-	-	100%
Emergency Department				
Admittance Decision Time (minutes)[2]	465	84	76	98
Head CT Results Within 45 Min. of Arrival[3,7]	-	-	43%	57%
Patients Who Left ER Before Being Seen	57,100	1%	2%	2%
Time from ER Arrival to Admit. (minutes)[2]	475	261	257	274
Time from ER Arrival to Discharge (minutes)	484	144	142	134
Time in ER Before Being Evaluated (minutes)	504	41	30	26
Time to Pain Meds for Fractures (minutes)	200	74	67	57
Heart Attack Care				
Aspirin Given at Discharge	40	100%	99%	99%
Fibrinolytic Meds Within 30 Min. of Arrival[7]	-	-	50%	54%
PCI Within 90 Minutes of Arrival[1]	-	-	93%	96%
Statin Prescribed at Discharge	41	100%	98%	98%
Heart Failure Care				
ACE Inhibitor or ARB for LVSD	49	100%	96%	97%
Discharge Instructions Given	113	98%	94%	94%
Evaluation of LVS Function	144	100%	98%	99%
Medicare Spending				
Medicare Spending per Patient (ratio)	-	0.94	0.96	0.98
Pneumonia Care				
Appropriate Initial Antibiotic Given	72	100%	94%	95%
Blood Culture Timing	135	98%	97%	98%
Pregnancy and Delivery Care				
Newborn Deliveries Scheduled Early[2]	40	12%	10%	6%
Preventive Care				
Immunization for Influenza[2]	501	99%	94%	90%
Immunization for Pneumonia[2]	448	100%	95%	92%
Stroke Care				
Anticoagulation Therapy for Atrial Fibrillation[1]	-	-	94%	95%
Antithrombotic Therapy Timing	85	100%	98%	98%
Assessed for Rehabilitation	123	100%	96%	97%
Discharged on Antithrombotic Therapy	98	100%	98%	99%
Discharged on Statin Medication	80	100%	91%	94%
Thrombolytic Therapy Timing[1]	-	-	67%	66%
Venous Thromboembolism Prophylaxis	124	100%	91%	94%
Written Stroke Educational Materials Given	86	99%	84%	88%
Surgical Care Improvement Project				
Appropriate Beta Blocker Usage[2]	195	98%	98%	98%
Appropriate VTP Within 24 Hours[2]	548	99%	98%	98%
Controlled Postoperative Blood Glucose[2,7]	-	-	95%	97%
Perioperative Temperature Management[2]	668	100%	100%	100%
Prophylactic Antibiotic Selection[2]	362	100%	99%	99%
Prophylactic Antibiotic Selection (Outpatient)	294	99%	97%	98%
Prophylactic Antibiotic Stopped[2]	355	100%	98%	98%
Prophylactic Antibiotic Timing[2]	362	100%	99%	99%
Prophylactic Antibiotic Timing (Outpatient)	173	98%	97%	98%
Urinary Catheter Removal[2]	353	99%	98%	97%
Survey of Patients' Hospital Experiences				
Area Around Room 'Always' Quiet at Night	300+	65%	58%	61%
Doctors 'Always' Communicated Well	300+	80%	82%	82%
Home Recovery Information Given	300+	88%	85%	85%
Hospital Given 9 or 10 on 10 Point Scale	300+	76%	66%	71%
Meds 'Always' Explained Before Given	300+	65%	64%	64%
Nurses 'Always' Communicated Well	300+	78%	78%	79%
Pain 'Always' Well Controlled	300+	71%	70%	71%
Room and Bathroom 'Always' Clean	300+	73%	75%	73%
Timely Help 'Always' Received	300+	68%	68%	68%
Would Definitely Recommend Hospital	300+	78%	66%	71%
Use of Medical Imaging				
Cardiac Imaging Stress Test before Surgery	135	8.9%	4.9%	5.3%
Combination Abdominal CT Scan	1,073	5.9%	14.4%	10.5%
Combination Brain/Sinus CT Scan[1]	-	-	3%	2.7%
Combination Chest CT Scan	906	0.4%	2.8%	2.7%
Follow-up Mammogram/Ultrasound	1,876	9.6%	8.8%	8.8%
Lumbar Spine MRI for Low Back Pain	208	34.6%	38.4%	37.2%

Huntington VA Medical Center

1540 Spring Valley Road
Huntington, WV 25704
E-mail: jerrishaffer@med.va.gov
URL: www.huntington.med.gov
Type: Acute Care - VA
Ownership: Government Federal
Phone: 304-429-0241
Fax: 304-429-6713
Emergency Services: No
Beds: 80

Key Personnel:
Quality Assurance . . . . Carole Bachtel, RN
CEO/President. . . . . Gale Beamen
Operating Room. . . . . Nancy Hutchinson, RN
Infection Control. . . . . Roberta Messner, RN
Chief of Medical Staff. . . . . Joseph A Pellecchia, MD
Cardiac Laboratory. . . . . Richard Stevenson, MD

Measure	Cases	This Hosp.	State Avg.	U.S. Avg.
Blood Clot Prevention and Treatment				
Anticoagulation Overlap Therapy	-	-	90%	93%
ICU Venous Thromboembolism Prophylaxis	-	-	88%	92%
Incidence of Potentially Preventable VTE	-	-	12%	10%
UFH with Dosages/Platelet Monitoring	-	-	98%	97%
Venous Thromboembolism Prophylaxis	-	-	79%	85%
Warfarin Therapy Discharge Instructions	-	-	80%	75%
Chest Pain/Possible Heart Attack Care				
Aspirin Given Within 24 Hours of Arrival	-	-	96%	96%
Fibrinolytic Meds Within 30 Min. of Arrival	-	-	74%	58%
Average Time to ECG (minutes)	-	-	8	7
Average Time to Transfer (minutes)	-	-	109	60
Children's Asthma Care				
Received Home Management Plan of Care	-	-	-	88%
Received Reliever Medication	-	-	-	100%
Received Systemic Corticosteroids	-	-	-	100%
Emergency Department				
Admittance Decision Time (minutes)	-	-	76	98
Head CT Results Within 45 Min. of Arrival	-	-	43%	57%
Patients Who Left ER Before Being Seen	-	-	2%	2%
Time from ER Arrival to Admit. (minutes)	-	-	257	274
Time from ER Arrival to Discharge (minutes)	-	-	142	134
Time in ER Before Being Evaluated (minutes)	-	-	30	26
Time to Pain Meds for Fractures (minutes)	-	-	67	57
Heart Attack Care				
Aspirin Given at Discharge[1]	-	-	99%	99%
Fibrinolytic Meds Within 30 Min. of Arrival[5]	-	-	50%	54%
PCI Within 90 Minutes of Arrival[5]	-	-	93%	96%
Statin Prescribed at Discharge[1]	-	-	98%	98%
Heart Failure Care				
ACE Inhibitor or ARB for LVSD	70	96%	96%	97%
Discharge Instructions Given	154	100%	94%	94%
Evaluation of LVS Function	174	100%	98%	99%
Medicare Spending				
Medicare Spending per Patient (ratio)	-	-	0.96	0.98
Pneumonia Care				

NOTE: Hospital profiles are in alphabetical order by state, then city, then hospital within the city; Rankings exclude hospitals with less than 25 cases except for patient surveys which excludes hospitals with less than 100 cases; (a) 100-299 cases; (1) The number of cases/patients is too few to report; (2) Data submitted were based on a sample of cases/patients; (3) Results are based on a shorter time period than required; (4) Data suppressed by CMS for one or more quarters; (5) Results are not available for this reporting period; (6) Fewer than 100 patients completed the HCAHPS survey; (7) No cases met the criteria for this measure; (8) The lower limit of the confidence interval cannot be calculated if the number of observed infections equals zero; (9) No data are available from the state/territory for this reporting period; (10) The scores shown reflect fewer than 50 completed surveys; (11) There were discrepancies in the data collection process; (12) This measure does not apply to this hospital for this reporting period; (13) Results cannot be calculated for this reporting period; (14) The results for this state are combined with nearby states to protect confidentiality; Please refer to the User's Guide for a full explanation of data.

Measure	Cases	This Hosp.	State Avg.	U.S. Avg.
Appropriate Initial Antibiotic Given	72	99%	94%	95%
Blood Culture Timing	125	96%	97%	98%
Pregnancy and Delivery Care				
Newborn Deliveries Scheduled Early	-	-	10%	6%
Preventive Care				
Immunization for Influenza[5]	-	-	94%	90%
Immunization for Pneumonia[5]	-	-	95%	92%
Stroke Care				
Anticoagulation Therapy for Atrial Fibrillation	-	-	94%	95%
Antithrombotic Therapy Timing	-	-	98%	98%
Assessed for Rehabilitation	-	-	96%	97%
Discharged on Antithrombotic Therapy	-	-	98%	99%
Discharged on Statin Medication	-	-	91%	94%
Thrombolytic Therapy Timing	-	-	67%	66%
Venous Thromboembolism Prophylaxis	-	-	91%	94%
Written Stroke Educational Materials Given	-	-	84%	88%
Surgical Care Improvement Project				
Appropriate Beta Blocker Usage[2]	72	100%	98%	98%
Appropriate VTP Within 24 Hours[2]	124	98%	98%	98%
Controlled Postoperative Blood Glucose[5]	-	-	95%	97%
Perioperative Temperature Management[2]	137	100%	100%	100%
Prophylactic Antibiotic Selection	92	100%	99%	99%
Prophylactic Antibiotic Selection (Outpatient)	-	-	97%	98%
Prophylactic Antibiotic Stopped	92	100%	98%	98%
Prophylactic Antibiotic Timing	92	100%	99%	99%
Prophylactic Antibiotic Timing (Outpatient)	-	-	97%	98%
Urinary Catheter Removal[2]	117	100%	98%	97%
Survey of Patients' Hospital Experiences				
Area Around Room 'Always' Quiet at Night	-	-	58%	61%
Doctors 'Always' Communicated Well	-	-	82%	82%
Home Recovery Information Given	-	-	85%	85%
Hospital Given 9 or 10 on 10 Point Scale	-	-	66%	71%
Meds 'Always' Explained Before Given	-	-	64%	64%
Nurses 'Always' Communicated Well	-	-	78%	79%
Pain 'Always' Well Controlled	-	-	70%	71%
Room and Bathroom 'Always' Clean	-	-	75%	73%
Timely Help 'Always' Received	-	-	68%	68%
Would Definitely Recommend Hospital	-	-	66%	71%
Use of Medical Imaging				
Cardiac Imaging Stress Test before Surgery	-	-	4.9%	5.3%
Combination Abdominal CT Scan	-	-	14.4%	10.5%
Combination Brain/Sinus CT Scan	-	-	3%	2.7%
Combination Chest CT Scan	-	-	2.8%	2.7%
Follow-up Mammogram/Ultrasound	-	-	8.8%	8.8%
Lumbar Spine MRI for Low Back Pain	-	-	38.4%	37.2%

Saint Mary's Medical Center

2900 1st Avenue
Huntington, WV 25701
URL: www.st-marys.org
Type: Acute Care Hospitals
Ownership: Voluntary non-profit - Church
Phone: 304-526-1234
Fax: 304-526-8996
Emergency Services: Yes
Beds: 393

Key Personnel:
Radiology. Paul Akers
Infection Control. . . . . Anita Fahirety
Pediatric Ambulatory Care . . . . . . James Lewis
Pediatric In-Patient Care . . . . James Lewis
Operating Room. . . . . Tammy Nimmo
CEO/President. . . . . Michael G Sellards
Quality Assurance . . . . Pat Stultz
Chief of Medical Staff. . . . . Dr. Lee Taylor

Measure	Cases	This Hosp.	State Avg.	U.S. Avg.
Blood Clot Prevention and Treatment				
Anticoagulation Overlap Therapy[2]	146	97%	90%	93%
ICU Venous Thromboembolism Prophylaxis[2]	129	94%	88%	92%
Incidence of Potentially Preventable VTE[1,2]	-	-	12%	10%
UFH with Dosages/Platelet Monitoring[2]	151	100%	98%	97%
Venous Thromboembolism Prophylaxis[2]	571	90%	79%	85%
Warfarin Therapy Discharge Instructions[2]	107	86%	80%	75%
Chest Pain/Possible Heart Attack Care				
Aspirin Given Within 24 Hours of Arrival	21	86%	96%	96%
Fibrinolytic Meds Within 30 Min. of Arrival[3,7]	-	-	74%	58%
Average Time to ECG (minutes)	21	9	8	7
Average Time to Transfer (minutes)[3,7]	-	-	109	60
Children's Asthma Care				
Received Home Management Plan of Care	-	-	-	88%
Received Reliever Medication	-	-	-	100%
Received Systemic Corticosteroids	-	-	-	100%
Emergency Department				
Admittance Decision Time (minutes)[2]	231	129	76	98
Head CT Results Within 45 Min. of Arrival[1]	-	-	43%	57%
Patients Who Left ER Before Being Seen	69,957	1%	2%	2%
Time from ER Arrival to Admit. (minutes)[2]	301	325	257	274
Time from ER Arrival to Discharge (minutes)	736	153	142	134
Time in ER Before Being Evaluated (minutes)	656	62	30	26
Time to Pain Meds for Fractures (minutes)	187	65	67	57
Heart Attack Care				
Aspirin Given at Discharge[2]	338	99%	99%	99%
Fibrinolytic Meds Within 30 Min. of Arrival[2,7]	-	-	50%	54%
PCI Within 90 Minutes of Arrival[2]	36	94%	93%	96%
Statin Prescribed at Discharge[2]	328	98%	98%	98%
Heart Failure Care				
ACE Inhibitor or ARB for LVSD[2]	88	95%	96%	97%
Discharge Instructions Given[2]	280	99%	94%	94%
Evaluation of LVS Function[2]	324	100%	98%	99%
Medicare Spending				
Medicare Spending per Patient (ratio)	-	0.98	0.96	0.98
Pneumonia Care				
Appropriate Initial Antibiotic Given[2]	152	95%	94%	95%
Blood Culture Timing[2]	319	96%	97%	98%
Pregnancy and Delivery Care				
Newborn Deliveries Scheduled Early	53	34%	10%	6%
Preventive Care				
Immunization for Influenza[2]	615	89%	94%	90%
Immunization for Pneumonia[2]	886	92%	95%	92%
Stroke Care				
Anticoagulation Therapy for Atrial Fibrillation	37	100%	94%	95%
Antithrombotic Therapy Timing	274	100%	98%	98%
Assessed for Rehabilitation	347	100%	96%	97%
Discharged on Antithrombotic Therapy	297	99%	98%	99%
Discharged on Statin Medication	224	98%	91%	94%
Thrombolytic Therapy Timing	15	100%	67%	66%
Venous Thromboembolism Prophylaxis	354	99%	91%	94%
Written Stroke Educational Materials Given	196	94%	84%	88%
Surgical Care Improvement Project				
Appropriate Beta Blocker Usage[2]	538	99%	98%	98%
Appropriate VTP Within 24 Hours[2]	739	98%	98%	98%
Controlled Postoperative Blood Glucose[2]	377	97%	95%	97%
Perioperative Temperature Management[2]	862	100%	100%	100%
Prophylactic Antibiotic Selection[2]	1,013	99%	99%	99%
Prophylactic Antibiotic Selection (Outpatient)	635	98%	97%	98%
Prophylactic Antibiotic Stopped[2]	972	98%	98%	98%
Prophylactic Antibiotic Timing[2]	1,014	99%	99%	99%
Prophylactic Antibiotic Timing (Outpatient)	638	97%	97%	98%
Urinary Catheter Removal[2]	788	99%	98%	97%
Survey of Patients' Hospital Experiences				
Area Around Room 'Always' Quiet at Night	300+	60%	58%	61%
Doctors 'Always' Communicated Well	300+	81%	82%	82%
Home Recovery Information Given	300+	88%	85%	85%
Hospital Given 9 or 10 on 10 Point Scale	300+	77%	66%	71%
Meds 'Always' Explained Before Given	300+	63%	64%	64%
Nurses 'Always' Communicated Well	300+	81%	78%	79%
Pain 'Always' Well Controlled	300+	75%	70%	71%
Room and Bathroom 'Always' Clean	300+	78%	75%	73%
Timely Help 'Always' Received	300+	71%	68%	68%
Would Definitely Recommend Hospital	300+	82%	66%	71%
Use of Medical Imaging				
Cardiac Imaging Stress Test before Surgery	302	3.0%	4.9%	5.3%
Combination Abdominal CT Scan	1,538	3.4%	14.4%	10.5%
Combination Brain/Sinus CT Scan	1,662	4.9%	3%	2.7%
Combination Chest CT Scan	1,034	0.0%	2.8%	2.7%
Follow-up Mammogram/Ultrasound	1,106	9.4%	8.8%	8.8%
Lumbar Spine MRI for Low Back Pain	304	37.2%	38.4%	37.2%

Camc Teays Valley Hospital

1400 Hospital Drive
Hurricane, WV 25526
Type: Acute Care Hospitals
Ownership: Voluntary non-profit - Private
Phone: 304-757-1700
Fax: 304-757-1732
Emergency Services: Yes
Beds: 68

Key Personnel:
Infection Control. . . . . Sue Ellis, RN
Quality Assurance . . . . Sue Ellis
Operating Room. . . . . Jeff Fleck, RN
CEO/President. . . . . Patsy Hardy
Intensive Care Unit. . . . . Tammie Hiles, RN
Chief of Medical Staff. . . . . Rick Houdersheldt, DO
Emergency Room . . . . Gregory Kelly, DO
Anesthesiology. . . . . David Maxson, MD

Measure	Cases	This Hosp.	State Avg.	U.S. Avg.
Blood Clot Prevention and Treatment				
Anticoagulation Overlap Therapy[2]	20	75%	90%	93%
ICU Venous Thromboembolism Prophylaxis[2]	125	77%	88%	92%
Incidence of Potentially Preventable VTE[1,2]	-	-	12%	10%
UFH with Dosages/Platelet Monitoring[2]	11	100%	98%	97%
Venous Thromboembolism Prophylaxis[2]	499	56%	79%	85%
Warfarin Therapy Discharge Instructions[2]	11	73%	80%	75%
Chest Pain/Possible Heart Attack Care				
Aspirin Given Within 24 Hours of Arrival	15	73%	96%	96%
Fibrinolytic Meds Within 30 Min. of Arrival[3,7]	-	-	74%	58%
Average Time to ECG (minutes)	16	33	8	7
Average Time to Transfer (minutes)[1,3]	-	-	109	60
Children's Asthma Care				
Received Home Management Plan of Care	-	-	-	88%
Received Reliever Medication	-	-	-	100%
Received Systemic Corticosteroids	-	-	-	100%
Emergency Department				
Admittance Decision Time (minutes)[2]	260	97	76	98
Head CT Results Within 45 Min. of Arrival[1]	-	-	43%	57%
Patients Who Left ER Before Being Seen	20,181	4%	2%	2%
Time from ER Arrival to Admit. (minutes)[2]	317	335	257	274
Time from ER Arrival to Discharge (minutes)	365	182	142	134
Time in ER Before Being Evaluated (minutes)	408	46	30	26
Time to Pain Meds for Fractures (minutes)	56	94	67	57
Heart Attack Care				
Aspirin Given at Discharge[1]	-	-	99%	99%
Fibrinolytic Meds Within 30 Min. of Arrival[7]	-	-	50%	54%
PCI Within 90 Minutes of Arrival[7]	-	-	93%	96%
Statin Prescribed at Discharge[1]	-	-	98%	98%
Heart Failure Care				
ACE Inhibitor or ARB for LVSD[1]	-	-	96%	97%
Discharge Instructions Given	37	78%	94%	94%
Evaluation of LVS Function	44	95%	98%	99%
Medicare Spending				
Medicare Spending per Patient (ratio)	-	1.02	0.96	0.98
Pneumonia Care				
Appropriate Initial Antibiotic Given	89	96%	94%	95%
Blood Culture Timing	121	98%	97%	98%
Pregnancy and Delivery Care				
Newborn Deliveries Scheduled Early[7]	-	-	10%	6%
Preventive Care				
Immunization for Influenza[2]	316	96%	94%	90%
Immunization for Pneumonia[2]	485	95%	95%	92%
Stroke Care				
Anticoagulation Therapy for Atrial Fibrillation[1]	-	-	94%	95%
Antithrombotic Therapy Timing[1]	-	-	98%	98%
Assessed for Rehabilitation[1]	-	-	96%	97%
Discharged on Antithrombotic Therapy[1]	-	-	98%	99%
Discharged on Statin Medication[1]	-	-	91%	94%
Thrombolytic Therapy Timing[7]	-	-	67%	66%
Venous Thromboembolism Prophylaxis[1]	-	-	91%	94%
Written Stroke Educational Materials Given[1]	-	-	84%	88%
Surgical Care Improvement Project				
Appropriate Beta Blocker Usage	53	94%	98%	98%
Appropriate VTP Within 24 Hours	130	95%	98%	98%
Controlled Postoperative Blood Glucose[7]	-	-	95%	97%
Perioperative Temperature Management	149	98%	100%	100%
Prophylactic Antibiotic Selection	95	98%	99%	99%
Prophylactic Antibiotic Selection (Outpatient)	64	100%	97%	98%

NOTE: Hospital profiles are in alphabetical order by state, then city, then hospital within the city; Rankings exclude hospitals with less than 25 cases except for patient surveys which excludes hospitals with less than 100 cases; (a) 100-299 cases; (1) The number of cases/patients is too few to report; (2) Data submitted were based on a sample of cases/patients; (3) Results are based on a shorter time period than required; (4) Data suppressed by CMS for one or more quarters; (5) Results are not available for this reporting period; (6) Fewer than 100 patients completed the HCAHPS survey; (7) No cases met the criteria for this measure; (8) The lower limit of the confidence interval cannot be calculated if the number of observed infections equals zero; (9) No data are available from the state/territory for this reporting period; (10) The scores shown reflect fewer than 50 completed surveys; (11) There were discrepancies in the data collection process; (12) This measure does not apply to this hospital for this reporting period; (13) Results cannot be calculated for this reporting period; (14) The results for this state are combined with nearby states to protect confidentiality; Please refer to the User's Guide for a full explanation of data.

Prophylactic Antibiotic Stopped	89	92%	98%	98%
Prophylactic Antibiotic Timing	95	97%	99%	99%
Prophylactic Antibiotic Timing (Outpatient)	67	96%	97%	98%
Urinary Catheter Removal	105	94%	98%	97%
Survey of Patients' Hospital Experiences				
Area Around Room 'Always' Quiet at Night	300+	39%	58%	61%
Doctors 'Always' Communicated Well	300+	78%	82%	82%
Home Recovery Information Given	300+	80%	85%	85%
Hospital Given 9 or 10 on 10 Point Scale	300+	54%	66%	71%
Meds 'Always' Explained Before Given	300+	56%	64%	64%
Nurses 'Always' Communicated Well	300+	69%	78%	79%
Pain 'Always' Well Controlled	300+	67%	70%	71%
Room and Bathroom 'Always' Clean	300+	67%	75%	73%
Timely Help 'Always' Received	300+	57%	68%	68%
Would Definitely Recommend Hospital	300+	54%	66%	71%
Use of Medical Imaging				
Cardiac Imaging Stress Test before Surgery	64	4.7%	4.9%	5.3%
Combination Abdominal CT Scan	491	3.3%	14.4%	10.5%
Combination Brain/Sinus CT Scan	321	0.6%	3%	2.7%
Combination Chest CT Scan	232	0.0%	2.8%	2.7%
Follow-up Mammogram/Ultrasound	370	7.6%	8.8%	8.8%
Lumbar Spine MRI for Low Back Pain	70	44.3%	38.4%	37.2%

Potomac Valley Hospital

100 Pin Oak Lane
Keyser, WV 26726
Phone: 304-597-3500
Fax: 304-597-1118
Type: Critical Access Hospitals
Emergency Services: Yes
Ownership: Voluntary non-profit - Private
Beds: 25

Measure	Cases	This Hosp.	State Avg.	U.S. Avg.
Blood Clot Prevention and Treatment				
Anticoagulation Overlap Therapy[5]	-	-	90%	93%
ICU Venous Thromboembolism Prophylaxis[5]	-	-	88%	92%
Incidence of Potentially Preventable VTE[5]	-	-	12%	10%
UFH with Dosages/Platelet Monitoring[5]	-	-	98%	97%
Venous Thromboembolism Prophylaxis[5]	-	-	79%	85%
Warfarin Therapy Discharge Instructions[5]	-	-	80%	75%
Chest Pain/Possible Heart Attack Care				
Aspirin Given Within 24 Hours of Arrival	-	-	96%	96%
Fibrinolytic Meds Within 30 Min. of Arrival	-	-	74%	58%
Average Time to ECG (minutes)	-	-	8	7
Average Time to Transfer (minutes)	-	-	109	60
Children's Asthma Care				
Received Home Management Plan of Care	-	-	-	88%
Received Reliever Medication	-	-	-	100%
Received Systemic Corticosteroids	-	-	-	100%
Emergency Department				
Admittance Decision Time (minutes)	194	60	76	98
Head CT Results Within 45 Min. of Arrival	-	-	43%	57%
Patients Who Left ER Before Being Seen	-	-	2%	2%
Time from ER Arrival to Admit. (minutes)	414	274	257	274
Time from ER Arrival to Discharge (minutes)	-	-	142	134
Time in ER Before Being Evaluated (minutes)	-	-	30	26
Time to Pain Meds for Fractures (minutes)	-	-	67	57
Heart Attack Care				
Aspirin Given at Discharge[1,3]	-	-	99%	99%
Fibrinolytic Meds Within 30 Min. of Arrival[3,7]	-	-	50%	54%
PCI Within 90 Minutes of Arrival[3,7]	-	-	93%	96%
Statin Prescribed at Discharge[1,3]	-	-	98%	98%
Heart Failure Care				
ACE Inhibitor or ARB for LVSD[1]	-	-	96%	97%
Discharge Instructions Given	23	57%	94%	94%
Evaluation of LVS Function	35	97%	98%	99%
Medicare Spending				
Medicare Spending per Patient (ratio)	-	-	0.96	0.98
Pneumonia Care				
Appropriate Initial Antibiotic Given	39	85%	94%	95%
Blood Culture Timing	51	88%	97%	98%
Pregnancy and Delivery Care				
Newborn Deliveries Scheduled Early[5]	-	-	10%	6%
Preventive Care				
Immunization for Influenza[5]	-	-	94%	90%
Immunization for Pneumonia[5]	-	-	95%	92%
Stroke Care				
Anticoagulation Therapy for Atrial Fibrillation[1]	-	-	94%	95%
Antithrombotic Therapy Timing[1]	-	-	98%	98%
Assessed for Rehabilitation[1]	-	-	96%	97%
Discharged on Antithrombotic Therapy[1]	-	-	98%	99%
Discharged on Statin Medication[1]	-	-	91%	94%
Thrombolytic Therapy Timing[1]	-	-	67%	66%
Venous Thromboembolism Prophylaxis[1]	-	-	91%	94%
Written Stroke Educational Materials Given[7]	-	-	84%	88%
Surgical Care Improvement Project				
Appropriate Beta Blocker Usage[1]	-	-	98%	98%
Appropriate VTP Within 24 Hours[1]	-	-	98%	98%
Controlled Postoperative Blood Glucose[7]	-	-	95%	97%
Perioperative Temperature Management	13	100%	100%	100%
Prophylactic Antibiotic Selection[7]	-	-	99%	99%
Prophylactic Antibiotic Selection (Outpatient)	-	-	97%	98%
Prophylactic Antibiotic Stopped[7]	-	-	98%	98%
Prophylactic Antibiotic Timing[7]	-	-	99%	99%
Prophylactic Antibiotic Timing (Outpatient)	-	-	97%	98%
Urinary Catheter Removal	13	100%	98%	97%
Survey of Patients' Hospital Experiences				
Area Around Room 'Always' Quiet at Night[5]	-	-	58%	61%
Doctors 'Always' Communicated Well[5]	-	-	82%	82%
Home Recovery Information Given[5]	-	-	85%	85%
Hospital Given 9 or 10 on 10 Point Scale[5]	-	-	66%	71%
Meds 'Always' Explained Before Given[5]	-	-	64%	64%
Nurses 'Always' Communicated Well[5]	-	-	78%	79%
Pain 'Always' Well Controlled[5]	-	-	70%	71%
Room and Bathroom 'Always' Clean[5]	-	-	75%	73%
Timely Help 'Always' Received[5]	-	-	68%	68%
Would Definitely Recommend Hospital[5]	-	-	66%	71%
Use of Medical Imaging				
Cardiac Imaging Stress Test before Surgery	-	-	4.9%	5.3%
Combination Abdominal CT Scan	-	-	14.4%	10.5%
Combination Brain/Sinus CT Scan	-	-	3%	2.7%
Combination Chest CT Scan	-	-	2.8%	2.7%
Follow-up Mammogram/Ultrasound	-	-	8.8%	8.8%
Lumbar Spine MRI for Low Back Pain	-	-	38.4%	37.2%

Preston Memorial Hospital

300 S Price Street
Kingwood, WV 26537
Phone: 304-329-1400
Fax: 304-329-1175
URL: www.prestonmemorial.com
Type: Critical Access Hospitals
Emergency Services: Yes
Ownership: Voluntary non-profit - Private
Beds: 76

Key Personnel:

Pediatrics. . . . . Bernice Schwarzenberg
Emergency Room . . . . Fred Conley, MD
Pediatrics. . . . . Jennifer Pumphrey
Cardiology . . . . Richard Smith
Radiology. . . . . Leisa Stalnaker
CEO/President. . . . . Michael Thompson

Measure	Cases	This Hosp.	State Avg.	U.S. Avg.
Blood Clot Prevention and Treatment				
Anticoagulation Overlap Therapy[2,3]	-	-	90%	93%
ICU Venous Thromboembolism Prophylaxis[1,2]	-	-	88%	92%
Incidence of Potentially Preventable VTE[2,3]	-	-	12%	10%
UFH with Dosages/Platelet Monitoring[2,3]	-	-	98%	97%
Venous Thromboembolism Prophylaxis[2,3]	53	91%	79%	85%
Warfarin Therapy Discharge Instructions[2,3]	-	-	80%	75%
Chest Pain/Possible Heart Attack Care				
Aspirin Given Within 24 Hours of Arrival[3]	32	100%	96%	96%
Fibrinolytic Meds Within 30 Min. of Arrival[1,3]	-	-	74%	58%
Average Time to ECG (minutes)[3]	36	10	8	7
Average Time to Transfer (minutes)[1,3]	-	-	109	60
Children's Asthma Care				
Received Home Management Plan of Care	-	-	-	88%
Received Reliever Medication	-	-	-	100%
Received Systemic Corticosteroids	-	-	-	100%
Emergency Department				
Admittance Decision Time (minutes)[5]	-	-	76	98
Head CT Results Within 45 Min. of Arrival[5]	-	-	43%	57%
Patients Who Left ER Before Being Seen	9,530	1%	2%	2%
Time from ER Arrival to Admit. (minutes)[5]	-	-	257	274
Time from ER Arrival to Discharge (minutes)[5]	-	-	142	134
Time in ER Before Being Evaluated (minutes)[5]	-	-	30	26
Time to Pain Meds for Fractures (minutes)[5]	-	-	67	57
Heart Attack Care				
Aspirin Given at Discharge[1]	-	-	99%	99%
Fibrinolytic Meds Within 30 Min. of Arrival[7]	-	-	50%	54%
PCI Within 90 Minutes of Arrival[7]	-	-	93%	96%
Statin Prescribed at Discharge[1]	-	-	98%	98%
Heart Failure Care				
ACE Inhibitor or ARB for LVSD[1,2]	-	-	96%	97%
Discharge Instructions Given[2]	24	88%	94%	94%
Evaluation of LVS Function[2]	30	90%	98%	99%
Medicare Spending				
Medicare Spending per Patient (ratio)	-	-	0.96	0.98
Pneumonia Care				
Appropriate Initial Antibiotic Given[2]	21	95%	94%	95%
Blood Culture Timing[2]	30	97%	97%	98%
Pregnancy and Delivery Care				
Newborn Deliveries Scheduled Early[3,7]	-	-	10%	6%
Preventive Care				
Immunization for Influenza[2]	147	97%	94%	90%
Immunization for Pneumonia[2]	248	95%	95%	92%
Stroke Care				
Anticoagulation Therapy for Atrial Fibrillation[5]	-	-	94%	95%
Antithrombotic Therapy Timing[5]	-	-	98%	98%
Assessed for Rehabilitation[5]	-	-	96%	97%
Discharged on Antithrombotic Therapy[5]	-	-	98%	99%
Discharged on Statin Medication[5]	-	-	91%	94%
Thrombolytic Therapy Timing[5]	-	-	67%	66%
Venous Thromboembolism Prophylaxis[5]	-	-	91%	94%
Written Stroke Educational Materials Given[5]	-	-	84%	88%
Surgical Care Improvement Project				
Appropriate Beta Blocker Usage[1,3]	-	-	98%	98%
Appropriate VTP Within 24 Hours[3]	13	100%	98%	98%
Controlled Postoperative Blood Glucose[5]	-	-	95%	97%
Perioperative Temperature Management[3]	15	100%	100%	100%
Prophylactic Antibiotic Selection[1,3]	-	-	99%	99%
Prophylactic Antibiotic Selection (Outpatient)[1,3]	-	-	97%	98%
Prophylactic Antibiotic Stopped[1,3]	-	-	98%	98%
Prophylactic Antibiotic Timing[1,3]	-	-	99%	99%
Prophylactic Antibiotic Timing (Outpatient)[1,3]	-	-	97%	98%
Urinary Catheter Removal[3]	12	100%	98%	97%
Survey of Patients' Hospital Experiences				
Area Around Room 'Always' Quiet at Night[6]	<100	55%	58%	61%
Doctors 'Always' Communicated Well[6]	<100	92%	82%	82%
Home Recovery Information Given[6]	<100	87%	85%	85%
Hospital Given 9 or 10 on 10 Point Scale[6]	<100	61%	66%	71%
Meds 'Always' Explained Before Given[6]	<100	67%	64%	64%
Nurses 'Always' Communicated Well[6]	<100	80%	78%	79%
Pain 'Always' Well Controlled[6]	<100	66%	70%	71%
Room and Bathroom 'Always' Clean[6]	<100	76%	75%	73%
Timely Help 'Always' Received[6]	<100	70%	68%	68%
Would Definitely Recommend Hospital[6]	<100	71%	66%	71%
Use of Medical Imaging				
Cardiac Imaging Stress Test before Surgery	49	2.0%	4.9%	5.3%
Combination Abdominal CT Scan	143	11.2%	14.4%	10.5%
Combination Brain/Sinus CT Scan	220	6.8%	3%	2.7%
Combination Chest CT Scan	68	11.8%	2.8%	2.7%
Follow-up Mammogram/Ultrasound	198	9.6%	8.8%	8.8%
Lumbar Spine MRI for Low Back Pain[1]	-	-	38.4%	37.2%

Logan Regional Medical Center

20 Hospital Drive
Logan, WV 25601
Phone: 304-831-1350
Fax: 304-831-1871
URL: www.loganregionalmedicalcenter.com
Type: Acute Care Hospitals
Emergency Services: Yes
Ownership: Proprietary
Beds: 140

Key Personnel:

Intensive Care Unit. . . . . Jenny Baxter
Quality Assurance . . . . Alisa Bently
Chief of Medical Staff . . . . S Chevy, MD
CEO . . . . Jerry Dooley
CEO/President. . . . . Kevin Fowler
Anesthesiology. . . . . Billy Mullen, DO
Operating Room. . . . . Richard Skibo

NOTE: Hospital profiles are in alphabetical order by state, then city, then hospital within the city; Rankings exclude hospitals with less than 25 cases except for patient surveys which excludes hospitals with less than 100 cases; (a) 100-299 cases; (1) The number of cases/patients is too few to report; (2) Data submitted were based on a sample of cases/patients; (3) Results are based on a shorter time period than required; (4) Data suppressed by CMS for one or more quarters; (5) Results are not available for this reporting period; (6) Fewer than 100 patients completed the HCAHPS survey; (7) No cases met the criteria for this measure; (8) The lower limit of the confidence interval cannot be calculated if the number of observed infections equals zero; (9) No data are available from the state/territory for this reporting period; (10) The scores shown reflect fewer than 50 completed surveys; (11) There were discrepancies in the data collection process; (12) This measure does not apply to this hospital for this reporting period; (13) Results cannot be calculated for this reporting period; (14) The results for this state are combined with nearby states to protect confidentiality; Please refer to the User's Guide for a full explanation of data.

Measure	Cases	This Hosp.	State Avg.	U.S. Avg.
Blood Clot Prevention and Treatment				
Anticoagulation Overlap Therapy[2]	45	76%	90%	93%
ICU Venous Thromboembolism Prophylaxis[2]	101	96%	88%	92%
Incidence of Potentially Preventable VTE[1,2]	-	-	12%	10%
UFH with Dosages/Platelet Monitoring[2]	40	100%	98%	97%
Venous Thromboembolism Prophylaxis[2]	377	83%	79%	85%
Warfarin Therapy Discharge Instructions[2]	32	94%	80%	75%
Chest Pain/Possible Heart Attack Care				
Aspirin Given Within 24 Hours of Arrival	84	99%	96%	96%
Fibrinolytic Meds Within 30 Min. of Arrival[1,3]	-	-	74%	58%
Average Time to ECG (minutes)	87	7	8	7
Average Time to Transfer (minutes)[1,3]	-	-	109	60
Children's Asthma Care				
Received Home Management Plan of Care	-	-	-	88%
Received Reliever Medication	-	-	-	100%
Received Systemic Corticosteroids	-	-	-	100%
Emergency Department				
Admittance Decision Time (minutes)[2]	780	74	76	98
Head CT Results Within 45 Min. of Arrival[1]	-	-	43%	57%
Patients Who Left ER Before Being Seen	33,299	5%	2%	2%
Time from ER Arrival to Admit. (minutes)[2]	780	276	257	274
Time from ER Arrival to Discharge (minutes)	458	185	142	134
Time in ER Before Being Evaluated (minutes)	567	21	30	26
Time to Pain Meds for Fractures (minutes)	112	83	67	57
Heart Attack Care				
Aspirin Given at Discharge	15	93%	99%	99%
Fibrinolytic Meds Within 30 Min. of Arrival[7]	-	-	50%	54%
PCI Within 90 Minutes of Arrival[7]	-	-	93%	96%
Statin Prescribed at Discharge	12	100%	98%	98%
Heart Failure Care				
ACE Inhibitor or ARB for LVSD	45	100%	96%	97%
Discharge Instructions Given	199	99%	94%	94%
Evaluation of LVS Function	213	100%	98%	99%
Medicare Spending				
Medicare Spending per Patient (ratio)	-	0.93	0.96	0.98
Pneumonia Care				
Appropriate Initial Antibiotic Given	196	98%	94%	95%
Blood Culture Timing	304	99%	97%	98%
Pregnancy and Delivery Care				
Newborn Deliveries Scheduled Early[2]	45	2%	10%	6%
Preventive Care				
Immunization for Influenza[2]	509	100%	94%	90%
Immunization for Pneumonia[2]	729	100%	95%	92%
Stroke Care				
Anticoagulation Therapy for Atrial Fibrillation[1]	-	-	94%	95%
Antithrombotic Therapy Timing	30	100%	98%	98%
Assessed for Rehabilitation	29	100%	96%	97%
Discharged on Antithrombotic Therapy	28	100%	98%	99%
Discharged on Statin Medication	21	100%	91%	94%
Thrombolytic Therapy Timing[7]	-	-	67%	66%
Venous Thromboembolism Prophylaxis	31	97%	91%	94%
Written Stroke Educational Materials Given	19	100%	84%	88%
Surgical Care Improvement Project				
Appropriate Beta Blocker Usage	23	100%	98%	98%
Appropriate VTP Within 24 Hours	89	100%	98%	98%
Controlled Postoperative Blood Glucose[7]	-	-	95%	97%
Perioperative Temperature Management	96	100%	100%	100%
Prophylactic Antibiotic Selection	65	97%	99%	99%
Prophylactic Antibiotic Selection (Outpatient)	82	93%	97%	98%
Prophylactic Antibiotic Stopped	38	97%	98%	98%
Prophylactic Antibiotic Timing	65	100%	99%	99%
Prophylactic Antibiotic Timing (Outpatient)	83	99%	97%	98%
Urinary Catheter Removal	46	96%	98%	97%
Survey of Patients' Hospital Experiences				
Area Around Room 'Always' Quiet at Night	300+	54%	58%	61%
Doctors 'Always' Communicated Well	300+	83%	82%	82%
Home Recovery Information Given	300+	83%	85%	85%
Hospital Given 9 or 10 on 10 Point Scale	300+	58%	66%	71%
Meds 'Always' Explained Before Given	300+	57%	64%	64%
Nurses 'Always' Communicated Well	300+	73%	78%	79%
Pain 'Always' Well Controlled	300+	65%	70%	71%
Room and Bathroom 'Always' Clean	300+	72%	75%	73%
Timely Help 'Always' Received	300+	58%	68%	68%
Would Definitely Recommend Hospital	300+	55%	66%	71%
Use of Medical Imaging				
Cardiac Imaging Stress Test before Surgery	297	5.1%	4.9%	5.3%
Combination Abdominal CT Scan	682	1.8%	14.4%	10.5%
Combination Brain/Sinus CT Scan	661	4.4%	3%	2.7%
Combination Chest CT Scan	555	0.2%	2.8%	2.7%
Follow-up Mammogram/Ultrasound	505	14.3%	8.8%	8.8%
Lumbar Spine MRI for Low Back Pain	72	37.5%	38.4%	37.2%

Boone Memorial Hospital

701 Madison Avenue
Madison, WV 25130
E-mail: mlinville@bmh.org
URL: www.bmh.org
Type: Critical Access Hospitals
Ownership: Government - Local

Phone: 304-369-1230
Fax: 304-369-1525
Emergency Services: Yes
Beds: 25

Key Personnel:
Chief of Medical Staff.......... Robert B Atkins
Cardiac Laboratory............ Matt Downey
Infection Control.............. Teresa Meade
Administrator .... Tommy Mullins
CEO/President................ Tommy H Mullins
Radiology.................... Greg Zornes

Measure	Cases	This Hosp.	State Avg.	U.S. Avg.
Blood Clot Prevention and Treatment				
Anticoagulation Overlap Therapy[5]	-	-	90%	93%
ICU Venous Thromboembolism Prophylaxis[5]	-	-	88%	92%
Incidence of Potentially Preventable VTE[5]	-	-	12%	10%
UFH with Dosages/Platelet Monitoring[5]	-	-	98%	97%
Venous Thromboembolism Prophylaxis[5]	-	-	79%	85%
Warfarin Therapy Discharge Instructions[5]	-	-	80%	75%
Chest Pain/Possible Heart Attack Care				
Aspirin Given Within 24 Hours of Arrival[5]	-	-	96%	96%
Fibrinolytic Meds Within 30 Min. of Arrival[5]	-	-	74%	58%
Average Time to ECG (minutes)[5]	-	-	8	7
Average Time to Transfer (minutes)[5]	-	-	109	60
Children's Asthma Care				
Received Home Management Plan of Care	-	-	-	88%
Received Reliever Medication	-	-	-	100%
Received Systemic Corticosteroids	-	-	-	100%
Emergency Department				
Admittance Decision Time (minutes)	340	72	76	98
Head CT Results Within 45 Min. of Arrival[5]	-	-	43%	57%
Patients Who Left ER Before Being Seen[5]	-	-	2%	2%
Time from ER Arrival to Admit. (minutes)	352	312	257	274
Time from ER Arrival to Discharge (minutes)[5]	-	-	142	134
Time in ER Before Being Evaluated (minutes)[5]	-	-	30	26
Time to Pain Meds for Fractures (minutes)[5]	-	-	67	57
Heart Attack Care				
Aspirin Given at Discharge[5]	-	-	99%	99%
Fibrinolytic Meds Within 30 Min. of Arrival[5]	-	-	50%	54%
PCI Within 90 Minutes of Arrival[5]	-	-	93%	96%
Statin Prescribed at Discharge[5]	-	-	98%	98%
Heart Failure Care				
ACE Inhibitor or ARB for LVSD[1]	-	-	96%	97%
Discharge Instructions Given	12	42%	94%	94%
Evaluation of LVS Function	20	60%	98%	99%
Medicare Spending				
Medicare Spending per Patient (ratio)	-	-	0.96	0.98
Pneumonia Care				
Appropriate Initial Antibiotic Given	39	56%	94%	95%
Blood Culture Timing	59	92%	97%	98%
Pregnancy and Delivery Care				
Newborn Deliveries Scheduled Early[5]	-	-	10%	6%
Preventive Care				
Immunization for Influenza	181	70%	94%	90%
Immunization for Pneumonia	288	77%	95%	92%
Stroke Care				
Anticoagulation Therapy for Atrial Fibrillation[5]	-	-	94%	95%
Antithrombotic Therapy Timing[5]	-	-	98%	98%
Assessed for Rehabilitation[5]	-	-	96%	97%
Discharged on Antithrombotic Therapy[5]	-	-	98%	99%
Discharged on Statin Medication[5]	-	-	91%	94%
Thrombolytic Therapy Timing[5]	-	-	67%	66%
Venous Thromboembolism Prophylaxis[5]	-	-	91%	94%
Written Stroke Educational Materials Given[5]	-	-	84%	88%
Surgical Care Improvement Project				
Appropriate Beta Blocker Usage[5]	-	-	98%	98%
Appropriate VTP Within 24 Hours[5]	-	-	98%	98%
Controlled Postoperative Blood Glucose[5]	-	-	95%	97%
Perioperative Temperature Management[5]	-	-	100%	100%
Prophylactic Antibiotic Selection[5]	-	-	99%	99%
Prophylactic Antibiotic Selection (Outpatient)[5]	-	-	97%	98%
Prophylactic Antibiotic Stopped[5]	-	-	98%	98%
Prophylactic Antibiotic Timing[5]	-	-	99%	99%
Prophylactic Antibiotic Timing (Outpatient)[5]	-	-	97%	98%
Urinary Catheter Removal[5]	-	-	98%	97%
Survey of Patients' Hospital Experiences				
Area Around Room 'Always' Quiet at Night[6]	<100	53%	58%	61%
Doctors 'Always' Communicated Well[6]	<100	88%	82%	82%
Home Recovery Information Given[6]	<100	84%	85%	85%
Hospital Given 9 or 10 on 10 Point Scale[6]	<100	67%	66%	71%
Meds 'Always' Explained Before Given[6]	<100	73%	64%	64%
Nurses 'Always' Communicated Well[6]	<100	79%	78%	79%
Pain 'Always' Well Controlled[6]	<100	71%	70%	71%
Room and Bathroom 'Always' Clean[6]	<100	81%	75%	73%
Timely Help 'Always' Received[6]	<100	74%	68%	68%
Would Definitely Recommend Hospital[6]	<100	63%	66%	71%
Use of Medical Imaging				
Cardiac Imaging Stress Test before Surgery	67	11.9%	4.9%	5.3%
Combination Abdominal CT Scan	311	2.3%	14.4%	10.5%
Combination Brain/Sinus CT Scan[1]	-	-	3%	2.7%
Combination Chest CT Scan	188	1.6%	2.8%	2.7%
Follow-up Mammogram/Ultrasound	187	11.2%	8.8%	8.8%
Lumbar Spine MRI for Low Back Pain[1]	-	-	38.4%	37.2%

Berkeley Medical Center

2500 Hospital Drive
Martinsburg, WV 25401
URL: www.cityhospital.org
Type: Acute Care Hospitals
Ownership: Voluntary non-profit - Other

Phone: 304-264-1000
Fax: 304-264-1255
Emergency Services: Yes
Beds: 144

Key Personnel:
Radiology.................. Frederick Ammer
CEO/President.............. Jon Applebaum
Chief of Medical Staff.......... C Joseph Cincinnati, DO
Intensive Care Unit........... Mary Ellen Clark, RN
Infection Control............. Paula Donahue, RN
Pediatric In-Patient Care .... Mary Jo Ostrowski, RN
Hemotology Center .... Bernie Raney, RN
Quality Assurance .... Barbara Sherman

Measure	Cases	This Hosp.	State Avg.	U.S. Avg.
Blood Clot Prevention and Treatment				
Anticoagulation Overlap Therapy[2]	60	100%	90%	93%
ICU Venous Thromboembolism Prophylaxis[2]	108	99%	88%	92%
Incidence of Potentially Preventable VTE[1,2]	-	-	12%	10%
UFH with Dosages/Platelet Monitoring[2]	49	100%	98%	97%
Venous Thromboembolism Prophylaxis[2]	333	98%	79%	85%
Warfarin Therapy Discharge Instructions[2]	47	96%	80%	75%
Chest Pain/Possible Heart Attack Care				
Aspirin Given Within 24 Hours of Arrival	18	100%	96%	96%
Fibrinolytic Meds Within 30 Min. of Arrival[1]	-	-	74%	58%
Average Time to ECG (minutes)	18	10	8	7
Average Time to Transfer (minutes)[7]	-	-	109	60
Children's Asthma Care				
Received Home Management Plan of Care	-	-	-	88%
Received Reliever Medication	-	-	-	100%
Received Systemic Corticosteroids	-	-	-	100%
Emergency Department				
Admittance Decision Time (minutes)[2]	738	86	76	98
Head CT Results Within 45 Min. of Arrival[1]	-	-	43%	57%
Patients Who Left ER Before Being Seen	50,838	1%	2%	2%
Time from ER Arrival to Admit. (minutes)[2]	738	280	257	274
Time from ER Arrival to Discharge (minutes)	383	128	142	134
Time in ER Before Being Evaluated (minutes)	411	33	30	26
Time to Pain Meds for Fractures (minutes)	181	67	67	57

NOTE: Hospital profiles are in alphabetical order by state, then city, then hospital within the city; Rankings exclude hospitals with less than 25 cases except for patient surveys which excludes hospitals with less than 100 cases; (a) 100-299 cases; (1) The number of cases/patients is too few to report; (2) Data submitted were based on a sample of cases/patients; (3) Results are based on a shorter time period than required; (4) Data suppressed by CMS for one or more quarters; (5) Results are not available for this reporting period; (6) Fewer than 100 patients completed the HCAHPS survey; (7) No cases met the criteria for this measure; (8) The lower limit of the confidence interval cannot be calculated if the number of observed infections equals zero; (9) No data are available from the state/territory for this reporting period; (10) The scores shown reflect fewer than 50 completed surveys; (11) There were discrepancies in the data collection process; (12) This measure does not apply to this hospital for this reporting period; (13) Results cannot be calculated for this reporting period; (14) The results for this state are combined with nearby states to protect confidentiality; Please refer to the User's Guide for a full explanation of data.

Measure	Cases	This Hosp.	State Avg.	U.S. Avg.
Heart Attack Care				
Aspirin Given at Discharge	164	100%	99%	99%
Fibrinolytic Meds Within 30 Min. of Arrival[7]	-	-	50%	54%
PCI Within 90 Minutes of Arrival	33	97%	93%	96%
Statin Prescribed at Discharge	157	100%	98%	98%
Heart Failure Care				
ACE Inhibitor or ARB for LVSD	63	100%	96%	97%
Discharge Instructions Given	201	97%	94%	94%
Evaluation of LVS Function	223	100%	98%	99%
Medicare Spending				
Medicare Spending per Patient (ratio)	-	0.95	0.96	0.98
Pneumonia Care				
Appropriate Initial Antibiotic Given	172	97%	94%	95%
Blood Culture Timing	330	99%	97%	98%
Pregnancy and Delivery Care				
Newborn Deliveries Scheduled Early[2]	20	0%	10%	6%
Preventive Care				
Immunization for Influenza[2]	564	96%	94%	90%
Immunization for Pneumonia[2]	653	94%	95%	92%
Stroke Care				
Anticoagulation Therapy for Atrial Fibrillation[1]	-	-	94%	95%
Antithrombotic Therapy Timing	78	100%	98%	98%
Assessed for Rehabilitation	75	100%	96%	97%
Discharged on Antithrombotic Therapy	70	100%	98%	99%
Discharged on Statin Medication	60	93%	91%	94%
Thrombolytic Therapy Timing[1]	-	-	67%	66%
Venous Thromboembolism Prophylaxis	88	98%	91%	94%
Written Stroke Educational Materials Given	49	90%	84%	88%
Surgical Care Improvement Project				
Appropriate Beta Blocker Usage	126	99%	98%	98%
Appropriate VTP Within 24 Hours	387	100%	98%	98%
Controlled Postoperative Blood Glucose[7]	-	-	95%	97%
Perioperative Temperature Management	475	100%	100%	100%
Prophylactic Antibiotic Selection	324	100%	99%	99%
Prophylactic Antibiotic Selection (Outpatient)	115	98%	97%	98%
Prophylactic Antibiotic Stopped	321	100%	98%	98%
Prophylactic Antibiotic Timing	325	100%	99%	99%
Prophylactic Antibiotic Timing (Outpatient)	115	100%	97%	98%
Urinary Catheter Removal	278	100%	98%	97%
Survey of Patients' Hospital Experiences				
Area Around Room 'Always' Quiet at Night	300+	45%	58%	61%
Doctors 'Always' Communicated Well	300+	77%	82%	82%
Home Recovery Information Given	300+	81%	85%	85%
Hospital Given 9 or 10 on 10 Point Scale	300+	58%	66%	71%
Meds 'Always' Explained Before Given	300+	62%	64%	64%
Nurses 'Always' Communicated Well	300+	75%	78%	79%
Pain 'Always' Well Controlled	300+	67%	70%	71%
Room and Bathroom 'Always' Clean	300+	77%	75%	73%
Timely Help 'Always' Received	300+	65%	68%	68%
Would Definitely Recommend Hospital	300+	57%	66%	71%
Use of Medical Imaging				
Cardiac Imaging Stress Test before Surgery	393	3.6%	4.9%	5.3%
Combination Abdominal CT Scan	1,221	5.6%	14.4%	10.5%
Combination Brain/Sinus CT Scan	609	1.8%	3%	2.7%
Combination Chest CT Scan	541	5.4%	2.8%	2.7%
Follow-up Mammogram/Ultrasound	1,173	5.5%	8.8%	8.8%
Lumbar Spine MRI for Low Back Pain	122	39.3%	38.4%	37.2%

Martinsburg VA Medical Center

510 Butler Ave.
Martinsburg, WV 25401
Phone: 304-263-0811
Fax: 304-262-7433
URL: www.martinsburg.va.gov
Type: Acute Care - VA
Emergency Services: No
Ownership: Government Federal
Beds: 566

Key Personnel:
Operating Room. . . . . Kati Jo Brown, RN
Infection Control. . . . . Linda Coffman, RN
Chief of Medical Staff . . . . Timothy J. Cooke, MD
Radiology. . . . . Satinder Gill, MD
Coronary Care . . . . Sonya Racey, RN
CEO/President. . . . . Fernando O Rivera
Quality Assurance . . . . Debra Rogers

Measure	Cases	This Hosp.	State Avg.	U.S. Avg.
Blood Clot Prevention and Treatment				
Anticoagulation Overlap Therapy	-	-	90%	93%
ICU Venous Thromboembolism Prophylaxis	-	-	88%	92%
Incidence of Potentially Preventable VTE	-	-	12%	10%
UFH with Dosages/Platelet Monitoring	-	-	98%	97%
Venous Thromboembolism Prophylaxis	-	-	79%	85%
Warfarin Therapy Discharge Instructions	-	-	80%	75%
Chest Pain/Possible Heart Attack Care				
Aspirin Given Within 24 Hours of Arrival	-	-	96%	96%
Fibrinolytic Meds Within 30 Min. of Arrival	-	-	74%	58%
Average Time to ECG (minutes)	-	-	8	7
Average Time to Transfer (minutes)	-	-	109	60
Children's Asthma Care				
Received Home Management Plan of Care	-	-	-	88%
Received Reliever Medication	-	-	-	100%
Received Systemic Corticosteroids	-	-	-	100%
Emergency Department				
Admittance Decision Time (minutes)	-	-	76	98
Head CT Results Within 45 Min. of Arrival	-	-	43%	57%
Patients Who Left ER Before Being Seen	-	-	2%	2%
Time from ER Arrival to Admit. (minutes)	-	-	257	274
Time from ER Arrival to Discharge (minutes)	-	-	142	134
Time in ER Before Being Evaluated (minutes)	-	-	30	26
Time to Pain Meds for Fractures (minutes)	-	-	67	57
Heart Attack Care				
Aspirin Given at Discharge[1]	-	-	99%	99%
Fibrinolytic Meds Within 30 Min. of Arrival[5]	-	-	50%	54%
PCI Within 90 Minutes of Arrival[5]	-	-	93%	96%
Statin Prescribed at Discharge[1]	-	-	98%	98%
Heart Failure Care				
ACE Inhibitor or ARB for LVSD	50	94%	96%	97%
Discharge Instructions Given	96	97%	94%	94%
Evaluation of LVS Function	109	100%	98%	99%
Medicare Spending				
Medicare Spending per Patient (ratio)	-	-	0.96	0.98
Pneumonia Care				
Appropriate Initial Antibiotic Given	75	92%	94%	95%
Blood Culture Timing	116	98%	97%	98%
Pregnancy and Delivery Care				
Newborn Deliveries Scheduled Early	-	-	10%	6%
Preventive Care				
Immunization for Influenza[5]	-	-	94%	90%
Immunization for Pneumonia[5]	-	-	95%	92%
Stroke Care				
Anticoagulation Therapy for Atrial Fibrillation	-	-	94%	95%
Antithrombotic Therapy Timing	-	-	98%	98%
Assessed for Rehabilitation	-	-	96%	97%
Discharged on Antithrombotic Therapy	-	-	98%	99%
Discharged on Statin Medication	-	-	91%	94%
Thrombolytic Therapy Timing	-	-	67%	66%
Venous Thromboembolism Prophylaxis	-	-	91%	94%
Written Stroke Educational Materials Given	-	-	84%	88%
Surgical Care Improvement Project				
Appropriate Beta Blocker Usage[2]	75	96%	98%	98%
Appropriate VTP Within 24 Hours[2]	147	97%	98%	98%
Controlled Postoperative Blood Glucose[5]	-	-	95%	97%
Perioperative Temperature Management[2]	160	99%	100%	100%
Prophylactic Antibiotic Selection	112	99%	99%	99%
Prophylactic Antibiotic Selection (Outpatient)	-	-	97%	98%
Prophylactic Antibiotic Stopped	110	96%	98%	98%
Prophylactic Antibiotic Timing	112	94%	99%	99%
Prophylactic Antibiotic Timing (Outpatient)	-	-	97%	98%
Urinary Catheter Removal[2]	128	100%	98%	97%
Survey of Patients' Hospital Experiences				
Area Around Room 'Always' Quiet at Night	-	-	58%	61%
Doctors 'Always' Communicated Well	-	-	82%	82%
Home Recovery Information Given	-	-	85%	85%
Hospital Given 9 or 10 on 10 Point Scale	-	-	66%	71%
Meds 'Always' Explained Before Given	-	-	64%	64%
Nurses 'Always' Communicated Well	-	-	78%	79%
Pain 'Always' Well Controlled	-	-	70%	71%
Room and Bathroom 'Always' Clean	-	-	75%	73%
Timely Help 'Always' Received	-	-	68%	68%
Would Definitely Recommend Hospital	-	-	66%	71%
Use of Medical Imaging				
Cardiac Imaging Stress Test before Surgery	-	-	4.9%	5.3%
Combination Abdominal CT Scan	-	-	14.4%	10.5%
Combination Brain/Sinus CT Scan	-	-	3%	2.7%
Combination Chest CT Scan	-	-	2.8%	2.7%
Follow-up Mammogram/Ultrasound	-	-	8.8%	8.8%
Lumbar Spine MRI for Low Back Pain	-	-	38.4%	37.2%

Montgomery General Hospital

401 Sixth Avenue, Fayette County
Montgomery, WV 25136
Phone: 304-442-5151
Fax: 304-442-7494
URL: www.montgomerygeneral.com
Type: Critical Access Hospitals
Emergency Services: Yes
Ownership: Voluntary non-profit - Private
Beds: 191

Key Personnel:
Chief of Medical Staff. . . . . John D Maylath
President/CEO. . . . . Peter W Monge, FACHE
Patient Relations . . . . Marylou Watson, MS, RN

Measure	Cases	This Hosp.	State Avg.	U.S. Avg.
Blood Clot Prevention and Treatment				
Anticoagulation Overlap Therapy[5]	-	-	90%	93%
ICU Venous Thromboembolism Prophylaxis[5]	-	-	88%	92%
Incidence of Potentially Preventable VTE[5]	-	-	12%	10%
UFH with Dosages/Platelet Monitoring[5]	-	-	98%	97%
Venous Thromboembolism Prophylaxis[5]	-	-	79%	85%
Warfarin Therapy Discharge Instructions[5]	-	-	80%	75%
Chest Pain/Possible Heart Attack Care				
Aspirin Given Within 24 Hours of Arrival	-	-	96%	96%
Fibrinolytic Meds Within 30 Min. of Arrival	-	-	74%	58%
Average Time to ECG (minutes)	-	-	8	7
Average Time to Transfer (minutes)	-	-	109	60
Children's Asthma Care				
Received Home Management Plan of Care	-	-	-	88%
Received Reliever Medication	-	-	-	100%
Received Systemic Corticosteroids	-	-	-	100%
Emergency Department				
Admittance Decision Time (minutes)[5]	-	-	76	98
Head CT Results Within 45 Min. of Arrival	-	-	43%	57%
Patients Who Left ER Before Being Seen	-	-	2%	2%
Time from ER Arrival to Admit. (minutes)[5]	-	-	257	274
Time from ER Arrival to Discharge (minutes)	-	-	142	134
Time in ER Before Being Evaluated (minutes)	-	-	30	26
Time to Pain Meds for Fractures (minutes)	-	-	67	57
Heart Attack Care				
Aspirin Given at Discharge[1]	-	-	99%	99%
Fibrinolytic Meds Within 30 Min. of Arrival[7]	-	-	50%	54%
PCI Within 90 Minutes of Arrival[7]	-	-	93%	96%
Statin Prescribed at Discharge[1]	-	-	98%	98%
Heart Failure Care				
ACE Inhibitor or ARB for LVSD[1]	-	-	96%	97%
Discharge Instructions Given[1]	-	-	94%	94%
Evaluation of LVS Function	14	93%	98%	99%
Medicare Spending				
Medicare Spending per Patient (ratio)	-	-	0.96	0.98
Pneumonia Care				
Appropriate Initial Antibiotic Given	58	86%	94%	95%
Blood Culture Timing	83	86%	97%	98%
Pregnancy and Delivery Care				
Newborn Deliveries Scheduled Early[5]	-	-	10%	6%
Preventive Care				
Immunization for Influenza[5]	-	-	94%	90%
Immunization for Pneumonia[5]	-	-	95%	92%
Stroke Care				
Anticoagulation Therapy for Atrial Fibrillation[5]	-	-	94%	95%
Antithrombotic Therapy Timing[5]	-	-	98%	98%
Assessed for Rehabilitation[5]	-	-	96%	97%
Discharged on Antithrombotic Therapy[5]	-	-	98%	99%
Discharged on Statin Medication[5]	-	-	91%	94%
Thrombolytic Therapy Timing[5]	-	-	67%	66%
Venous Thromboembolism Prophylaxis[5]	-	-	91%	94%
Written Stroke Educational Materials Given[5]	-	-	84%	88%
Surgical Care Improvement Project				

NOTE: Hospital profiles are in alphabetical order by state, then city, then hospital within the city; Rankings exclude hospitals with less than 25 cases except for patient surveys which excludes hospitals with less than 100 cases; (a) 100-299 cases; (1) The number of cases/patients is too few to report; (2) Data submitted were based on a sample of cases/patients; (3) Results are based on a shorter time period than required; (4) Data suppressed by CMS for one or more quarters; (5) Results are not available for this reporting period; (6) Fewer than 100 patients completed the HCAHPS survey; (7) No cases met the criteria for this measure; (8) The lower limit of the confidence interval cannot be calculated if the number of observed infections equals zero; (9) No data are available from the state/territory for this reporting period; (10) The scores shown reflect fewer than 50 completed surveys; (11) There were discrepancies in the data collection process; (12) This measure does not apply to this hospital for this reporting period; (13) Results cannot be calculated for this reporting period; (14) The results for this state are combined with nearby states to protect confidentiality; Please refer to the User's Guide for a full explanation of data.

Measure	Cases	This Hosp.	State Avg.	U.S. Avg.
Appropriate Beta Blocker Usage[5]	-	-	98%	98%
Appropriate VTP Within 24 Hours[5]	-	-	98%	98%
Controlled Postoperative Blood Glucose[5]	-	-	95%	97%
Perioperative Temperature Management[5]	-	-	100%	100%
Prophylactic Antibiotic Selection[5]	-	-	99%	99%
Prophylactic Antibiotic Selection (Outpatient)	-	-	97%	98%
Prophylactic Antibiotic Stopped[5]	-	-	98%	98%
Prophylactic Antibiotic Timing[5]	-	-	99%	99%
Prophylactic Antibiotic Timing (Outpatient)	-	-	97%	98%
Urinary Catheter Removal[5]	-	-	98%	97%
Survey of Patients' Hospital Experiences				
Area Around Room 'Always' Quiet at Night[6]	<100	57%	58%	61%
Doctors 'Always' Communicated Well[6]	<100	75%	82%	82%
Home Recovery Information Given[6]	<100	84%	85%	85%
Hospital Given 9 or 10 on 10 Point Scale[6]	<100	59%	66%	71%
Meds 'Always' Explained Before Given[6]	<100	61%	64%	64%
Nurses 'Always' Communicated Well[6]	<100	74%	78%	79%
Pain 'Always' Well Controlled[6]	<100	66%	70%	71%
Room and Bathroom 'Always' Clean[6]	<100	71%	75%	73%
Timely Help 'Always' Received[6]	<100	68%	68%	68%
Would Definitely Recommend Hospital[6]	<100	48%	66%	71%
Use of Medical Imaging				
Cardiac Imaging Stress Test before Surgery	-	-	4.9%	5.3%
Combination Abdominal CT Scan	-	-	14.4%	10.5%
Combination Brain/Sinus CT Scan	-	-	3%	2.7%
Combination Chest CT Scan	-	-	2.8%	2.7%
Follow-up Mammogram/Ultrasound	-	-	8.8%	8.8%
Lumbar Spine MRI for Low Back Pain	-	-	38.4%	37.2%

Monongalia County General Hospital

1200 Jd Anderson Dr Phone: 304-598-1200
Morgantown, WV 26505 Fax: 304-599-8382
URL: www.mongeneral.com
Type: Acute Care Hospitals Emergency Services: Yes
Ownership: Voluntary non-profit - Private Beds: 199

Key Personnel:

Operating Room. . . . . Roberto H Burns, RN
Emergency Room . . . . Jo Anne Liptock
Radiology. . . . . Surendra V Pawar
CEO/President. . . . . Dave Robertson
Chief of Medical Staff. . . . . Todd Tallman, MD

Measure	Cases	This Hosp.	State Avg.	U.S. Avg.
Blood Clot Prevention and Treatment				
Anticoagulation Overlap Therapy[2]	77	83%	90%	93%
ICU Venous Thromboembolism Prophylaxis[2]	115	84%	88%	92%
Incidence of Potentially Preventable VTE[2]	16	12%	12%	10%
UFH with Dosages/Platelet Monitoring[2]	64	97%	98%	97%
Venous Thromboembolism Prophylaxis[2]	301	63%	79%	85%
Warfarin Therapy Discharge Instructions[2]	64	89%	80%	75%
Chest Pain/Possible Heart Attack Care				
Aspirin Given Within 24 Hours of Arrival	17	88%	96%	96%
Fibrinolytic Meds Within 30 Min. of Arrival[5]	-	-	74%	58%
Average Time to ECG (minutes)	17	18	8	7
Average Time to Transfer (minutes)[5]	-	-	109	60
Children's Asthma Care				
Received Home Management Plan of Care	-	-	-	88%
Received Reliever Medication	-	-	-	100%
Received Systemic Corticosteroids	-	-	-	100%
Emergency Department				
Admittance Decision Time (minutes)[2]	395	82	76	98
Head CT Results Within 45 Min. of Arrival[7]	-	-	43%	57%
Patients Who Left ER Before Being Seen	31,199	1%	2%	2%
Time from ER Arrival to Admit. (minutes)[2]	404	245	257	274
Time from ER Arrival to Discharge (minutes)	369	158	142	134
Time in ER Before Being Evaluated (minutes)	467	23	30	26
Time to Pain Meds for Fractures (minutes)	70	68	67	57
Heart Attack Care				
Aspirin Given at Discharge	342	100%	99%	99%
Fibrinolytic Meds Within 30 Min. of Arrival[7]	-	-	50%	54%
PCI Within 90 Minutes of Arrival	49	88%	93%	96%
Statin Prescribed at Discharge	304	98%	98%	98%
Heart Failure Care				
ACE Inhibitor or ARB for LVSD	42	98%	96%	97%
Discharge Instructions Given	167	96%	94%	94%
Evaluation of LVS Function	197	100%	98%	99%
Medicare Spending				
Medicare Spending per Patient (ratio)	-	1.02	0.96	0.98
Pneumonia Care				
Appropriate Initial Antibiotic Given	91	91%	94%	95%
Blood Culture Timing	124	100%	97%	98%
Pregnancy and Delivery Care				
Newborn Deliveries Scheduled Early[2]	24	21%	10%	6%
Preventive Care				
Immunization for Influenza[2]	557	99%	94%	90%
Immunization for Pneumonia[2]	709	99%	95%	92%
Stroke Care				
Anticoagulation Therapy for Atrial Fibrillation[1]	-	-	94%	95%
Antithrombotic Therapy Timing	16	100%	98%	98%
Assessed for Rehabilitation	17	88%	96%	97%
Discharged on Antithrombotic Therapy	16	100%	98%	99%
Discharged on Statin Medication	12	92%	91%	94%
Thrombolytic Therapy Timing[7]	-	-	67%	66%
Venous Thromboembolism Prophylaxis	15	73%	91%	94%
Written Stroke Educational Materials Given[1]	-	-	84%	88%
Surgical Care Improvement Project				
Appropriate Beta Blocker Usage[2]	512	100%	98%	98%
Appropriate VTP Within 24 Hours[2]	796	99%	98%	98%
Controlled Postoperative Blood Glucose[2]	277	97%	95%	97%
Perioperative Temperature Management[2]	941	100%	100%	100%
Prophylactic Antibiotic Selection[2]	1,070	100%	99%	99%
Prophylactic Antibiotic Selection (Outpatient)	558	99%	97%	98%
Prophylactic Antibiotic Stopped[2]	1,051	99%	98%	98%
Prophylactic Antibiotic Timing[2]	1,071	100%	99%	99%
Prophylactic Antibiotic Timing (Outpatient)	562	98%	97%	98%
Urinary Catheter Removal[2]	283	97%	98%	97%
Survey of Patients' Hospital Experiences				
Area Around Room 'Always' Quiet at Night	300+	62%	58%	61%
Doctors 'Always' Communicated Well	300+	82%	82%	82%
Home Recovery Information Given	300+	87%	85%	85%
Hospital Given 9 or 10 on 10 Point Scale	300+	78%	66%	71%
Meds 'Always' Explained Before Given	300+	65%	64%	64%
Nurses 'Always' Communicated Well	300+	80%	78%	79%
Pain 'Always' Well Controlled	300+	73%	70%	71%
Room and Bathroom 'Always' Clean	300+	73%	75%	73%
Timely Help 'Always' Received	300+	68%	68%	68%
Would Definitely Recommend Hospital	300+	83%	66%	71%
Use of Medical Imaging				
Cardiac Imaging Stress Test before Surgery	366	6.3%	4.9%	5.3%
Combination Abdominal CT Scan	885	18.3%	14.4%	10.5%
Combination Brain/Sinus CT Scan	600	2.5%	3%	2.7%
Combination Chest CT Scan	742	0.1%	2.8%	2.7%
Follow-up Mammogram/Ultrasound	1,185	7.7%	8.8%	8.8%
Lumbar Spine MRI for Low Back Pain	119	41.2%	38.4%	37.2%

West Virginia University Hospitals

Medical Center Drive Phone: 304-598-4000
Morgantown, WV 26506 Fax: 304-598-4124
URL: www.wvuh.com
Type: Acute Care Hospitals Emergency Services: Yes
Ownership: Voluntary non-profit - Private Beds: 440

Key Personnel:

Operating Room. . . . . Ehab Akkary
Radiology. . . . . Mary Cannon, MD
Emergency Room . . . . Ann Chinnis, MD
Chief of Medical Staff. . . . . Kevin Halbritter
Anesthesiology. . . . . Robert Johnstone, MD
Infection Control. . . . . Rashida Khakoo, MD
CEO/President. . . . . Bruce McClymounds

Measure	Cases	This Hosp.	State Avg.	U.S. Avg.
Blood Clot Prevention and Treatment				
Anticoagulation Overlap Therapy[2]	135	100%	90%	93%
ICU Venous Thromboembolism Prophylaxis[2]	99	100%	88%	92%
Incidence of Potentially Preventable VTE[2]	33	0%	12%	10%
UFH with Dosages/Platelet Monitoring[2]	129	100%	98%	97%
Venous Thromboembolism Prophylaxis[2]	288	100%	79%	85%
Warfarin Therapy Discharge Instructions[2]	93	100%	80%	75%
Chest Pain/Possible Heart Attack Care				
Aspirin Given Within 24 Hours of Arrival[5]	-	-	96%	96%
Fibrinolytic Meds Within 30 Min. of Arrival[5]	-	-	74%	58%
Average Time to ECG (minutes)[5]	-	-	8	7
Average Time to Transfer (minutes)[5]	-	-	109	60
Children's Asthma Care				
Received Home Management Plan of Care	-	-	-	88%
Received Reliever Medication	-	-	-	100%
Received Systemic Corticosteroids	-	-	-	100%
Emergency Department				
Admittance Decision Time (minutes)[2]	468	70	76	98
Head CT Results Within 45 Min. of Arrival[1,3]	-	-	43%	57%
Patients Who Left ER Before Being Seen	46,697	2%	2%	2%
Time from ER Arrival to Admit. (minutes)[2]	457	275	257	274
Time from ER Arrival to Discharge (minutes)	346	200	142	134
Time in ER Before Being Evaluated (minutes)	379	22	30	26
Time to Pain Meds for Fractures (minutes)	35	85	67	57
Heart Attack Care				
Aspirin Given at Discharge	502	100%	99%	99%
Fibrinolytic Meds Within 30 Min. of Arrival[1]	-	-	50%	54%
PCI Within 90 Minutes of Arrival	37	100%	93%	96%
Statin Prescribed at Discharge	485	100%	98%	98%
Heart Failure Care				
ACE Inhibitor or ARB for LVSD	119	100%	96%	97%
Discharge Instructions Given	305	100%	94%	94%
Evaluation of LVS Function	363	100%	98%	99%
Medicare Spending				
Medicare Spending per Patient (ratio)	-	1.00	0.96	0.98
Pneumonia Care				
Appropriate Initial Antibiotic Given	90	99%	94%	95%
Blood Culture Timing	240	100%	97%	98%
Pregnancy and Delivery Care				
Newborn Deliveries Scheduled Early[2]	11	0%	10%	6%
Preventive Care				
Immunization for Influenza[2]	534	100%	94%	90%
Immunization for Pneumonia[2]	580	100%	95%	92%
Stroke Care				
Anticoagulation Therapy for Atrial Fibrillation	40	100%	94%	95%
Antithrombotic Therapy Timing	329	99%	98%	98%
Assessed for Rehabilitation	504	99%	96%	97%
Discharged on Antithrombotic Therapy	393	99%	98%	99%
Discharged on Statin Medication	308	95%	91%	94%
Thrombolytic Therapy Timing	35	100%	67%	66%
Venous Thromboembolism Prophylaxis	535	98%	91%	94%
Written Stroke Educational Materials Given	297	97%	84%	88%
Surgical Care Improvement Project				
Appropriate Beta Blocker Usage[2]	217	99%	98%	98%
Appropriate VTP Within 24 Hours[2]	433	99%	98%	98%
Controlled Postoperative Blood Glucose[2]	169	99%	95%	97%
Perioperative Temperature Management[2]	595	100%	100%	100%
Prophylactic Antibiotic Selection[2]	565	100%	99%	99%
Prophylactic Antibiotic Selection (Outpatient)	260	99%	97%	98%
Prophylactic Antibiotic Stopped[2]	541	97%	98%	98%
Prophylactic Antibiotic Timing[2]	568	100%	99%	99%
Prophylactic Antibiotic Timing (Outpatient)	252	98%	97%	98%
Urinary Catheter Removal[2]	444	100%	98%	97%
Survey of Patients' Hospital Experiences				
Area Around Room 'Always' Quiet at Night	300+	48%	58%	61%
Doctors 'Always' Communicated Well	300+	78%	82%	82%
Home Recovery Information Given	300+	84%	85%	85%
Hospital Given 9 or 10 on 10 Point Scale	300+	75%	66%	71%
Meds 'Always' Explained Before Given	300+	66%	64%	64%
Nurses 'Always' Communicated Well	300+	81%	78%	79%
Pain 'Always' Well Controlled	300+	69%	70%	71%
Room and Bathroom 'Always' Clean	300+	68%	75%	73%
Timely Help 'Always' Received	300+	67%	68%	68%
Would Definitely Recommend Hospital	300+	78%	66%	71%
Use of Medical Imaging				
Cardiac Imaging Stress Test before Surgery	542	4.1%	4.9%	5.3%
Combination Abdominal CT Scan	731	9.2%	14.4%	10.5%
Combination Brain/Sinus CT Scan	722	0.8%	3%	2.7%
Combination Chest CT Scan	813	2.7%	2.8%	2.7%
Follow-up Mammogram/Ultrasound	2,029	11.9%	8.8%	8.8%

NOTE: Hospital profiles are in alphabetical order by state, then city, then hospital within the city; Rankings exclude hospitals with less than 25 cases except for patient surveys which excludes hospitals with less than 100 cases; (a) 100-299 cases; (1) The number of cases/patients is too few to report; (2) Data submitted were based on a sample of cases/patients; (3) Results are based on a shorter time period than required; (4) Data suppressed by CMS for one or more quarters; (5) Results are not available for this reporting period; (6) Fewer than 100 patients completed the HCAHPS survey; (7) No cases met the criteria for this measure; (8) The lower limit of the confidence interval cannot be calculated if the number of observed infections equals zero; (9) No data are available from the state/territory for this reporting period; (10) The scores shown reflect fewer than 50 completed surveys; (11) There were discrepancies in the data collection process; (12) This measure does not apply to this hospital for this reporting period; (13) Results cannot be calculated for this reporting period; (14) The results for this state are combined with nearby states to protect confidentiality; Please refer to the User's Guide for a full explanation of data.

Measure	Cases	This Hosp.	State Avg.	U.S. Avg.
Lumbar Spine MRI for Low Back Pain[7]	-	-	38.4%	37.2%

Wetzel County Hospital

#3 East Benjamin Drive
New Martinsville, WV 26155
Type: Acute Care Hospitals
Ownership: Government - Local

Phone: 304-455-8000
Fax: 304-455-4259
Emergency Services: Yes
Beds: 68

Key Personnel:
Infection Control. . . . . Jenny Abbott, RN
Chief of Medical Staff. . . . . Donald Blum
CEO/President. . . . . George Couch
Quality Assurance . . . . Jane Flor, RN
Emergency Room . . . . John King, MD
Cardiac Laboratory. . . . . Bradley Miller
Anesthesiology. . . . . Santwara Souani, MD
Operating Room. . . . . Debbie Starchen, RN

Measure	Cases	This Hosp.	State Avg.	U.S. Avg.
Blood Clot Prevention and Treatment				
Anticoagulation Overlap Therapy[1,2]	-	-	90%	93%
ICU Venous Thromboembolism Prophylaxis[2]	19	79%	88%	92%
Incidence of Potentially Preventable VTE[2,7]	-	-	12%	10%
UFH with Dosages/Platelet Monitoring[1,2]	-	-	98%	97%
Venous Thromboembolism Prophylaxis[2]	107	82%	79%	85%
Warfarin Therapy Discharge Instructions[1,2]	-	-	80%	75%
Chest Pain/Possible Heart Attack Care				
Aspirin Given Within 24 Hours of Arrival	58	86%	96%	96%
Fibrinolytic Meds Within 30 Min. of Arrival[7]	-	-	74%	58%
Average Time to ECG (minutes)	59	7	8	7
Average Time to Transfer (minutes)[1]	-	-	109	60
Children's Asthma Care				
Received Home Management Plan of Care	-	-	-	88%
Received Reliever Medication	-	-	-	100%
Received Systemic Corticosteroids	-	-	-	100%
Emergency Department				
Admittance Decision Time (minutes)[2]	355	50	76	98
Head CT Results Within 45 Min. of Arrival[1]	-	-	43%	57%
Patients Who Left ER Before Being Seen	13,853	1%	2%	2%
Time from ER Arrival to Admit. (minutes)[2]	375	228	257	274
Time from ER Arrival to Discharge (minutes)	361	113	142	134
Time in ER Before Being Evaluated (minutes)	322	32	30	26
Time to Pain Meds for Fractures (minutes)	65	67	67	57
Heart Attack Care				
Aspirin Given at Discharge[1]	-	-	99%	99%
Fibrinolytic Meds Within 30 Min. of Arrival[7]	-	-	50%	54%
PCI Within 90 Minutes of Arrival[7]	-	-	93%	96%
Statin Prescribed at Discharge[1]	-	-	98%	98%
Heart Failure Care				
ACE Inhibitor or ARB for LVSD[1]	-	-	96%	97%
Discharge Instructions Given	21	100%	94%	94%
Evaluation of LVS Function	30	100%	98%	99%
Medicare Spending				
Medicare Spending per Patient (ratio)	-	0.99	0.96	0.98
Pneumonia Care				
Appropriate Initial Antibiotic Given	75	99%	94%	95%
Blood Culture Timing	86	98%	97%	98%
Pregnancy and Delivery Care				
Newborn Deliveries Scheduled Early[7]	-	-	10%	6%
Preventive Care				
Immunization for Influenza[2]	238	96%	94%	90%
Immunization for Pneumonia[2]	372	99%	95%	92%
Stroke Care				
Anticoagulation Therapy for Atrial Fibrillation[7]	-	-	94%	95%
Antithrombotic Therapy Timing[1]	-	-	98%	98%
Assessed for Rehabilitation[1]	-	-	96%	97%
Discharged on Antithrombotic Therapy[1]	-	-	98%	99%
Discharged on Statin Medication[1]	-	-	91%	94%
Thrombolytic Therapy Timing[1]	-	-	67%	66%
Venous Thromboembolism Prophylaxis[1]	-	-	91%	94%
Written Stroke Educational Materials Given[7]	-	-	84%	88%
Surgical Care Improvement Project				
Appropriate Beta Blocker Usage[1,3]	-	-	98%	98%
Appropriate VTP Within 24 Hours[3,7]	-	-	98%	98%
Controlled Postoperative Blood Glucose[3,7]	-	-	95%	97%
Perioperative Temperature Management[1,3]	-	-	100%	100%
Prophylactic Antibiotic Selection[1,3]	-	-	99%	99%
Prophylactic Antibiotic Selection (Outpatient)[1,3]	-	-	97%	98%
Prophylactic Antibiotic Stopped[1,3]	-	-	98%	98%
Prophylactic Antibiotic Timing[1,3]	-	-	99%	99%
Prophylactic Antibiotic Timing (Outpatient)[1,3]	-	-	97%	98%
Urinary Catheter Removal[3,7]	-	-	98%	97%
Survey of Patients' Hospital Experiences				
Area Around Room 'Always' Quiet at Night	(a)	61%	58%	61%
Doctors 'Always' Communicated Well	(a)	82%	82%	82%
Home Recovery Information Given	(a)	87%	85%	85%
Hospital Given 9 or 10 on 10 Point Scale	(a)	65%	66%	71%
Meds 'Always' Explained Before Given	(a)	65%	64%	64%
Nurses 'Always' Communicated Well	(a)	75%	78%	79%
Pain 'Always' Well Controlled	(a)	68%	70%	71%
Room and Bathroom 'Always' Clean	(a)	80%	75%	73%
Timely Help 'Always' Received	(a)	69%	68%	68%
Would Definitely Recommend Hospital	(a)	68%	66%	71%
Use of Medical Imaging				
Cardiac Imaging Stress Test before Surgery[1]	-	-	4.9%	5.3%
Combination Abdominal CT Scan	259	7.3%	14.4%	10.5%
Combination Brain/Sinus CT Scan[1]	-	-	3%	2.7%
Combination Chest CT Scan	150	0.0%	2.8%	2.7%
Follow-up Mammogram/Ultrasound	396	11.1%	8.8%	8.8%
Lumbar Spine MRI for Low Back Pain	40	45.0%	38.4%	37.2%

Plateau Medical Center

430 Main Street
Oak Hill, WV 25901
URL: www.plateaumedicalcenter.com
Type: Critical Access Hospitals
Ownership: Proprietary

Phone: 304-469-8600
Fax: 304-469-8605
Emergency Services: Yes
Beds: 90

Key Personnel:
CEO/President. . . . . David Bunch
Chief of Medical Staff. . . . . Clint Curtis
Intensive Care Unit. . . . . Linda DeBord
Quality Assurance . . . . Lynn Legg
Anesthesiology. . . . . Jessie Loot, MD
Infection Control. . . . . Linda Roach
Emergency Room . . . . Burnon Stanly
Operating Room. . . . . Joyce Stover, RN

Measure	Cases	This Hosp.	State Avg.	U.S. Avg.
Blood Clot Prevention and Treatment				
Anticoagulation Overlap Therapy[1,2]	-	-	90%	93%
ICU Venous Thromboembolism Prophylaxis[2]	64	98%	88%	92%
Incidence of Potentially Preventable VTE[2,7]	-	-	12%	10%
UFH with Dosages/Platelet Monitoring[1,2]	-	-	98%	97%
Venous Thromboembolism Prophylaxis[2]	351	96%	79%	85%
Warfarin Therapy Discharge Instructions[1,2]	-	-	80%	75%
Chest Pain/Possible Heart Attack Care				
Aspirin Given Within 24 Hours of Arrival	89	100%	96%	96%
Fibrinolytic Meds Within 30 Min. of Arrival[1]	-	-	74%	58%
Average Time to ECG (minutes)	90	4	8	7
Average Time to Transfer (minutes)[1]	-	-	109	60
Children's Asthma Care				
Received Home Management Plan of Care	-	-	-	88%
Received Reliever Medication	-	-	-	100%
Received Systemic Corticosteroids	-	-	-	100%
Emergency Department				
Admittance Decision Time (minutes)[2]	473	68	76	98
Head CT Results Within 45 Min. of Arrival	14	86%	43%	57%
Patients Who Left ER Before Being Seen	14,419	3%	2%	2%
Time from ER Arrival to Admit. (minutes)[2]	475	214	257	274
Time from ER Arrival to Discharge (minutes)	374	110	142	134
Time in ER Before Being Evaluated (minutes)	418	16	30	26
Time to Pain Meds for Fractures (minutes)	86	60	67	57
Heart Attack Care				
Aspirin Given at Discharge[1]	-	-	99%	99%
Fibrinolytic Meds Within 30 Min. of Arrival[7]	-	-	50%	54%
PCI Within 90 Minutes of Arrival[7]	-	-	93%	96%
Statin Prescribed at Discharge[1]	-	-	98%	98%
Heart Failure Care				
ACE Inhibitor or ARB for LVSD	19	100%	96%	97%
Discharge Instructions Given	61	90%	94%	94%
Evaluation of LVS Function	83	100%	98%	99%
Medicare Spending				
Medicare Spending per Patient (ratio)	-	-	0.96	0.98
Pneumonia Care				
Appropriate Initial Antibiotic Given	64	100%	94%	95%
Blood Culture Timing	87	100%	97%	98%
Pregnancy and Delivery Care				
Newborn Deliveries Scheduled Early[5]	-	-	10%	6%
Preventive Care				
Immunization for Influenza[2]	428	99%	94%	90%
Immunization for Pneumonia[2]	696	99%	95%	92%
Stroke Care				
Anticoagulation Therapy for Atrial Fibrillation[1]	-	-	94%	95%
Antithrombotic Therapy Timing[1]	-	-	98%	98%
Assessed for Rehabilitation[1]	-	-	96%	97%
Discharged on Antithrombotic Therapy[1]	-	-	98%	99%
Discharged on Statin Medication[1]	-	-	91%	94%
Thrombolytic Therapy Timing[7]	-	-	67%	66%
Venous Thromboembolism Prophylaxis	13	100%	91%	94%
Written Stroke Educational Materials Given[1]	-	-	84%	88%
Surgical Care Improvement Project				
Appropriate Beta Blocker Usage	58	100%	98%	98%
Appropriate VTP Within 24 Hours	194	100%	98%	98%
Controlled Postoperative Blood Glucose[7]	-	-	95%	97%
Perioperative Temperature Management	201	100%	100%	100%
Prophylactic Antibiotic Selection	169	99%	99%	99%
Prophylactic Antibiotic Selection (Outpatient)[1,3]	-	-	97%	98%
Prophylactic Antibiotic Stopped	167	100%	98%	98%
Prophylactic Antibiotic Timing	171	100%	99%	99%
Prophylactic Antibiotic Timing (Outpatient)[1,3]	-	-	97%	98%
Urinary Catheter Removal	150	100%	98%	97%
Survey of Patients' Hospital Experiences				
Area Around Room 'Always' Quiet at Night	300+	66%	58%	61%
Doctors 'Always' Communicated Well	300+	89%	82%	82%
Home Recovery Information Given	300+	90%	85%	85%
Hospital Given 9 or 10 on 10 Point Scale	300+	75%	66%	71%
Meds 'Always' Explained Before Given	300+	69%	64%	64%
Nurses 'Always' Communicated Well	300+	85%	78%	79%
Pain 'Always' Well Controlled	300+	75%	70%	71%
Room and Bathroom 'Always' Clean	300+	76%	75%	73%
Timely Help 'Always' Received	300+	75%	68%	68%
Would Definitely Recommend Hospital	300+	73%	66%	71%
Use of Medical Imaging				
Cardiac Imaging Stress Test before Surgery[1]	-	-	4.9%	5.3%
Combination Abdominal CT Scan	379	2.4%	14.4%	10.5%
Combination Brain/Sinus CT Scan	516	1.9%	3%	2.7%
Combination Chest CT Scan	128	0.0%	2.8%	2.7%
Follow-up Mammogram/Ultrasound	97	8.2%	8.8%	8.8%
Lumbar Spine MRI for Low Back Pain	45	46.7%	38.4%	37.2%

Camden Clark Medical Center

800 Garfield Ave
Parkersburg, WV 26101
E-mail: prccmh@ccmh.org
URL: www.ccmh.org
Type: Acute Care Hospitals
Ownership: Voluntary non-profit - Private

Phone: 304-424-2111
Fax: 304-424-2688
Emergency Services: Yes
Beds: 269

Key Personnel:
Radiology. . . . . Robert Al-Aly, MD
Emergency Room . . . . Dominic Bagnoli, MD
Intensive Care Unit. . . . . Patty Blanchard
Patient Relations . . . . Nancy Brooks
CEO/President. . . . . Thomas Corder
Infection Control. . . . . Susan Dearman
Quality Assurance . . . . Sherry Johnston
Chief of Medical Staff. . . . . Judy Kemp, MD

Measure	Cases	This Hosp.	State Avg.	U.S. Avg.
Blood Clot Prevention and Treatment				
Anticoagulation Overlap Therapy[2]	76	76%	90%	93%
ICU Venous Thromboembolism Prophylaxis[2]	78	94%	88%	92%
Incidence of Potentially Preventable VTE[1,2]	-	-	12%	10%
UFH with Dosages/Platelet Monitoring[2]	39	97%	98%	97%
Venous Thromboembolism Prophylaxis[2]	333	86%	79%	85%
Warfarin Therapy Discharge Instructions[2]	59	20%	80%	75%
Chest Pain/Possible Heart Attack Care				

NOTE: Hospital profiles are in alphabetical order by state, then city, then hospital within the city; Rankings exclude hospitals with less than 25 cases except for patient surveys which excludes hospitals with less than 100 cases; (a) 100-299 cases; (1) The number of cases/patients is too few to report; (2) Data submitted were based on a sample of cases/patients; (3) Results are based on a shorter time period than required; (4) Data suppressed by CMS for one or more quarters; (5) Results are not available for this reporting period; (6) Fewer than 100 patients completed the HCAHPS survey; (7) No cases met the criteria for this measure; (8) The lower limit of the confidence interval cannot be calculated if the number of observed infections equals zero; (9) No data are available from the state/territory for this reporting period; (10) The scores shown reflect fewer than 50 completed surveys; (11) There were discrepancies in the data collection process; (12) This measure does not apply to this hospital for this reporting period; (13) Results cannot be calculated for this reporting period; (14) The results for this state are combined with nearby states to protect confidentiality; Please refer to the User's Guide for a full explanation of data.

Measure	Cases	This Hosp.	State Avg.	U.S. Avg.
Aspirin Given Within 24 Hours of Arrival[1]	-	-	96%	96%
Fibrinolytic Meds Within 30 Min. of Arrival[3,7]	-	-	74%	58%
Average Time to ECG (minutes)[1]	-	-	8	7
Average Time to Transfer (minutes)[3,7]	-	-	109	60
Children's Asthma Care				
Received Home Management Plan of Care	-	-	-	88%
Received Reliever Medication	-	-	-	100%
Received Systemic Corticosteroids	-	-	-	100%
Emergency Department				
Admittance Decision Time (minutes)[2]	486	76	76	98
Head CT Results Within 45 Min. of Arrival	11	27%	43%	57%
Patients Who Left ER Before Being Seen	55,798	9%	2%	2%
Time from ER Arrival to Admit. (minutes)[2]	547	298	257	274
Time from ER Arrival to Discharge (minutes)	339	216	142	134
Time in ER Before Being Evaluated (minutes)	328	62	30	26
Time to Pain Meds for Fractures (minutes)	102	86	67	57
Heart Attack Care				
Aspirin Given at Discharge	395	99%	99%	99%
Fibrinolytic Meds Within 30 Min. of Arrival[7]	-	-	50%	54%
PCI Within 90 Minutes of Arrival	43	88%	93%	96%
Statin Prescribed at Discharge	367	98%	98%	98%
Heart Failure Care				
ACE Inhibitor or ARB for LVSD	131	96%	96%	97%
Discharge Instructions Given	440	93%	94%	94%
Evaluation of LVS Function	560	99%	98%	99%
Medicare Spending				
Medicare Spending per Patient (ratio)	-	1.04	0.96	0.98
Pneumonia Care				
Appropriate Initial Antibiotic Given	212	91%	94%	95%
Blood Culture Timing	325	97%	97%	98%
Pregnancy and Delivery Care				
Newborn Deliveries Scheduled Early[2]	40	20%	10%	6%
Preventive Care				
Immunization for Influenza[2]	542	92%	94%	90%
Immunization for Pneumonia[2]	738	93%	95%	92%
Stroke Care				
Anticoagulation Therapy for Atrial Fibrillation[2]	14	71%	94%	95%
Antithrombotic Therapy Timing[2]	77	100%	98%	98%
Assessed for Rehabilitation[2]	84	98%	96%	97%
Discharged on Antithrombotic Therapy[2]	79	100%	98%	99%
Discharged on Statin Medication[2]	64	89%	91%	94%
Thrombolytic Therapy Timing[1,2]	-	-	67%	66%
Venous Thromboembolism Prophylaxis[2]	80	90%	91%	94%
Written Stroke Educational Materials Given[2]	54	72%	84%	88%
Surgical Care Improvement Project				
Appropriate Beta Blocker Usage[2]	377	98%	98%	98%
Appropriate VTP Within 24 Hours[2]	784	99%	98%	98%
Controlled Postoperative Blood Glucose[2]	131	96%	95%	97%
Perioperative Temperature Management[2]	975	99%	100%	100%
Prophylactic Antibiotic Selection[2]	811	99%	99%	99%
Prophylactic Antibiotic Selection (Outpatient)	217	98%	97%	98%
Prophylactic Antibiotic Stopped[2]	796	98%	98%	98%
Prophylactic Antibiotic Timing[2]	812	99%	99%	99%
Prophylactic Antibiotic Timing (Outpatient)	222	95%	97%	98%
Urinary Catheter Removal[2]	684	98%	98%	97%
Survey of Patients' Hospital Experiences				
Area Around Room 'Always' Quiet at Night	300+	46%	58%	61%
Doctors 'Always' Communicated Well	300+	78%	82%	82%
Home Recovery Information Given	300+	84%	85%	85%
Hospital Given 9 or 10 on 10 Point Scale	300+	56%	66%	71%
Meds 'Always' Explained Before Given	300+	59%	64%	64%
Nurses 'Always' Communicated Well	300+	75%	78%	79%
Pain 'Always' Well Controlled	300+	66%	70%	71%
Room and Bathroom 'Always' Clean	300+	64%	75%	73%
Timely Help 'Always' Received	300+	65%	68%	68%
Would Definitely Recommend Hospital	300+	58%	66%	71%
Use of Medical Imaging				
Cardiac Imaging Stress Test before Surgery	94	3.2%	4.9%	5.3%
Combination Abdominal CT Scan	1,861	13.5%	14.4%	10.5%
Combination Brain/Sinus CT Scan	1,362	2.1%	3%	2.7%
Combination Chest CT Scan	933	2.5%	2.8%	2.7%
Follow-up Mammogram/Ultrasound	3,132	5.8%	8.8%	8.8%
Lumbar Spine MRI for Low Back Pain	244	38.1%	38.4%	37.2%

Grant Memorial Hospital

PO Box 1019
Petersburg, WV 26847
Phone: 304-257-1026
Fax: 304-257-2537
Type: Critical Access Hospitals
Emergency Services: Yes
Ownership: Voluntary non-profit - Other
Beds: 61

Key Personnel:
Emergency Room . . . . Mark Geary II, DO
CEO/President. . . . . Robert Harman
Surgery . . . . Anil K. Makani, M.D., FACS FRCS
Anesthesiology. . . . . L. Ray McKinney, CRNA,APRN,MHS,D
Radiology. . . . . J. Tim, MD
Pediatrics. . . . . Anish Trehun, MD

Measure	Cases	This Hosp.	State Avg.	U.S. Avg.
Blood Clot Prevention and Treatment				
Anticoagulation Overlap Therapy[5]	-	-	90%	93%
ICU Venous Thromboembolism Prophylaxis[5]	-	-	88%	92%
Incidence of Potentially Preventable VTE[5]	-	-	12%	10%
UFH with Dosages/Platelet Monitoring[5]	-	-	98%	97%
Venous Thromboembolism Prophylaxis[5]	-	-	79%	85%
Warfarin Therapy Discharge Instructions[5]	-	-	80%	75%
Chest Pain/Possible Heart Attack Care				
Aspirin Given Within 24 Hours of Arrival[1,3]	-	-	96%	96%
Fibrinolytic Meds Within 30 Min. of Arrival[3,7]	-	-	74%	58%
Average Time to ECG (minutes)[1,3]	-	-	8	7
Average Time to Transfer (minutes)[3,7]	-	-	109	60
Children's Asthma Care				
Received Home Management Plan of Care	-	-	-	88%
Received Reliever Medication	-	-	-	100%
Received Systemic Corticosteroids	-	-	-	100%
Emergency Department				
Admittance Decision Time (minutes)[3]	226	36	76	98
Head CT Results Within 45 Min. of Arrival[1,3]	-	-	43%	57%
Patients Who Left ER Before Being Seen	12,428	1%	2%	2%
Time from ER Arrival to Admit. (minutes)[3]	226	184	257	274
Time from ER Arrival to Discharge (minutes)[3]	337	121	142	134
Time in ER Before Being Evaluated (minutes)[3]	378	32	30	26
Time to Pain Meds for Fractures (minutes)[5]	-	-	67	57
Heart Attack Care				
Aspirin Given at Discharge[1,3]	-	-	99%	99%
Fibrinolytic Meds Within 30 Min. of Arrival[3,7]	-	-	50%	54%
PCI Within 90 Minutes of Arrival[3,7]	-	-	93%	96%
Statin Prescribed at Discharge[1,3]	-	-	98%	98%
Heart Failure Care				
ACE Inhibitor or ARB for LVSD[1]	-	-	96%	97%
Discharge Instructions Given	30	90%	94%	94%
Evaluation of LVS Function	36	78%	98%	99%
Medicare Spending				
Medicare Spending per Patient (ratio)	-	-	0.96	0.98
Pneumonia Care				
Appropriate Initial Antibiotic Given	27	81%	94%	95%
Blood Culture Timing	34	76%	97%	98%
Pregnancy and Delivery Care				
Newborn Deliveries Scheduled Early[5]	-	-	10%	6%
Preventive Care				
Immunization for Influenza[5]	-	-	94%	90%
Immunization for Pneumonia[5]	-	-	95%	92%
Stroke Care				
Anticoagulation Therapy for Atrial Fibrillation[5]	-	-	94%	95%
Antithrombotic Therapy Timing[5]	-	-	98%	98%
Assessed for Rehabilitation[5]	-	-	96%	97%
Discharged on Antithrombotic Therapy[5]	-	-	98%	99%
Discharged on Statin Medication[5]	-	-	91%	94%
Thrombolytic Therapy Timing[5]	-	-	67%	66%
Venous Thromboembolism Prophylaxis[5]	-	-	91%	94%
Written Stroke Educational Materials Given[5]	-	-	84%	88%
Surgical Care Improvement Project				
Appropriate Beta Blocker Usage[1]	-	-	98%	98%
Appropriate VTP Within 24 Hours	65	97%	98%	98%
Controlled Postoperative Blood Glucose[3,7]	-	-	95%	97%
Perioperative Temperature Management	66	97%	100%	100%
Prophylactic Antibiotic Selection	62	92%	99%	99%
Prophylactic Antibiotic Selection (Outpatient)[1,3]	-	-	97%	98%
Prophylactic Antibiotic Stopped	61	85%	98%	98%
Prophylactic Antibiotic Timing	62	97%	99%	99%
Prophylactic Antibiotic Timing (Outpatient)[1,3]	-	-	97%	98%
Urinary Catheter Removal	33	97%	98%	97%
Survey of Patients' Hospital Experiences				
Area Around Room 'Always' Quiet at Night	300+	46%	58%	61%
Doctors 'Always' Communicated Well	300+	85%	82%	82%
Home Recovery Information Given	300+	90%	85%	85%
Hospital Given 9 or 10 on 10 Point Scale	300+	62%	66%	71%
Meds 'Always' Explained Before Given	300+	67%	64%	64%
Nurses 'Always' Communicated Well	300+	80%	78%	79%
Pain 'Always' Well Controlled	300+	70%	70%	71%
Room and Bathroom 'Always' Clean	300+	83%	75%	73%
Timely Help 'Always' Received	300+	75%	68%	68%
Would Definitely Recommend Hospital	300+	57%	66%	71%
Use of Medical Imaging				
Cardiac Imaging Stress Test before Surgery[1]	-	-	4.9%	5.3%
Combination Abdominal CT Scan	287	3.5%	14.4%	10.5%
Combination Brain/Sinus CT Scan[1]	-	-	3%	2.7%
Combination Chest CT Scan	96	1.0%	2.8%	2.7%
Follow-up Mammogram/Ultrasound	346	14.5%	8.8%	8.8%
Lumbar Spine MRI for Low Back Pain	44	47.7%	38.4%	37.2%

Broaddus Hospital Association

Mansfield Hill PO Box 930
Philippi, WV 26416
Phone: 304-457-1760
Fax: 304-457-1516
E-mail: higginss@davishealthsystem.org
URL: www.davishealthcare.com
Type: Critical Access Hospitals
Emergency Services: Yes
Ownership: Voluntary non-profit - Private
Beds: 72

Key Personnel:
Radiology. . . . . Steven M Barnett
Chief of Medical Staff . . . . Pecel Hollbert
Emergency Room . . . . Sharon Mots, RN
CEO/President. . . . . Jeff Powpofon

Measure	Cases	This Hosp.	State Avg.	U.S. Avg.
Blood Clot Prevention and Treatment				
Anticoagulation Overlap Therapy[5]	-	-	90%	93%
ICU Venous Thromboembolism Prophylaxis[5]	-	-	88%	92%
Incidence of Potentially Preventable VTE[5]	-	-	12%	10%
UFH with Dosages/Platelet Monitoring[5]	-	-	98%	97%
Venous Thromboembolism Prophylaxis[5]	-	-	79%	85%
Warfarin Therapy Discharge Instructions[5]	-	-	80%	75%
Chest Pain/Possible Heart Attack Care				
Aspirin Given Within 24 Hours of Arrival[5]	-	-	96%	96%
Fibrinolytic Meds Within 30 Min. of Arrival[5]	-	-	74%	58%
Average Time to ECG (minutes)[5]	-	-	8	7
Average Time to Transfer (minutes)[5]	-	-	109	60
Children's Asthma Care				
Received Home Management Plan of Care	-	-	-	88%
Received Reliever Medication	-	-	-	100%
Received Systemic Corticosteroids	-	-	-	100%
Emergency Department				
Admittance Decision Time (minutes)[5]	-	-	76	98
Head CT Results Within 45 Min. of Arrival[5]	-	-	43%	57%
Patients Who Left ER Before Being Seen[5]	-	-	2%	2%
Time from ER Arrival to Admit. (minutes)[5]	-	-	257	274
Time from ER Arrival to Discharge (minutes)[5]	-	-	142	134
Time in ER Before Being Evaluated (minutes)[5]	-	-	30	26
Time to Pain Meds for Fractures (minutes)[5]	-	-	67	57
Heart Attack Care				
Aspirin Given at Discharge[5]	-	-	99%	99%
Fibrinolytic Meds Within 30 Min. of Arrival[5]	-	-	50%	54%
PCI Within 90 Minutes of Arrival[5]	-	-	93%	96%
Statin Prescribed at Discharge[5]	-	-	98%	98%
Heart Failure Care				
ACE Inhibitor or ARB for LVSD[5]	-	-	96%	97%
Discharge Instructions Given[5]	-	-	94%	94%
Evaluation of LVS Function[5]	-	-	98%	99%
Medicare Spending				
Medicare Spending per Patient (ratio)	-	-	0.96	0.98
Pneumonia Care				

NOTE: Hospital profiles are in alphabetical order by state, then city, then hospital within the city; Rankings exclude hospitals with less than 25 cases except for patient surveys which excludes hospitals with less than 100 cases; (a) 100-299 cases; (1) The number of cases/patients is too few to report; (2) Data submitted were based on a sample of cases/patients; (3) Results are based on a shorter time period than required; (4) Data suppressed by CMS for one or more quarters; (5) Results are not available for this reporting period; (6) Fewer than 100 patients completed the HCAHPS survey; (7) No cases met the criteria for this measure; (8) The lower limit of the confidence interval cannot be calculated if the number of observed infections equals zero; (9) No data are available from the state/territory for this reporting period; (10) The scores shown reflect fewer than 50 completed surveys; (11) There were discrepancies in the data collection process; (12) This measure does not apply to this hospital for this reporting period; (13) Results cannot be calculated for this reporting period; (14) The results for this state are combined with nearby states to protect confidentiality; Please refer to the User's Guide for a full explanation of data.

Appropriate Initial Antibiotic Given[1,3]	-	-	94%	95%
Blood Culture Timing[1,3]	-	-	97%	98%
Pregnancy and Delivery Care				
Newborn Deliveries Scheduled Early[5]	-	-	10%	6%
Preventive Care				
Immunization for Influenza[5]	-	-	94%	90%
Immunization for Pneumonia[5]	-	-	95%	92%
Stroke Care				
Anticoagulation Therapy for Atrial Fibrillation[5]	-	-	94%	95%
Antithrombotic Therapy Timing[5]	-	-	98%	98%
Assessed for Rehabilitation[5]	-	-	96%	97%
Discharged on Antithrombotic Therapy[5]	-	-	98%	99%
Discharged on Statin Medication[5]	-	-	91%	94%
Thrombolytic Therapy Timing[5]	-	-	67%	66%
Venous Thromboembolism Prophylaxis[5]	-	-	91%	94%
Written Stroke Educational Materials Given[5]	-	-	84%	88%
Surgical Care Improvement Project				
Appropriate Beta Blocker Usage[5]	-	-	98%	98%
Appropriate VTP Within 24 Hours[5]	-	-	98%	98%
Controlled Postoperative Blood Glucose[5]	-	-	95%	97%
Perioperative Temperature Management[5]	-	-	100%	100%
Prophylactic Antibiotic Selection[5]	-	-	99%	99%
Prophylactic Antibiotic Selection (Outpatient)[5]	-	-	97%	98%
Prophylactic Antibiotic Stopped[5]	-	-	98%	98%
Prophylactic Antibiotic Timing[5]	-	-	99%	99%
Prophylactic Antibiotic Timing (Outpatient)[5]	-	-	97%	98%
Urinary Catheter Removal[5]	-	-	98%	97%
Survey of Patients' Hospital Experiences				
Area Around Room 'Always' Quiet at Night[6]	<100	70%	58%	61%
Doctors 'Always' Communicated Well[6]	<100	92%	82%	82%
Home Recovery Information Given[6]	<100	87%	85%	85%
Hospital Given 9 or 10 on 10 Point Scale[6]	<100	88%	66%	71%
Meds 'Always' Explained Before Given[6]	<100	78%	64%	64%
Nurses 'Always' Communicated Well[6]	<100	87%	78%	79%
Pain 'Always' Well Controlled[6]	<100	82%	70%	71%
Room and Bathroom 'Always' Clean[6]	<100	89%	75%	73%
Timely Help 'Always' Received[6]	<100	83%	68%	68%
Would Definitely Recommend Hospital[6]	<100	78%	66%	71%
Use of Medical Imaging				
Cardiac Imaging Stress Test before Surgery[7]	-	-	4.9%	5.3%
Combination Abdominal CT Scan	118	32.2%	14.4%	10.5%
Combination Brain/Sinus CT Scan	135	0.7%	3%	2.7%
Combination Chest CT Scan	97	9.3%	2.8%	2.7%
Follow-up Mammogram/Ultrasound	142	11.3%	8.8%	8.8%
Lumbar Spine MRI for Low Back Pain[1]	-	-	38.4%	37.2%

Pleasant Valley Hospital

2520 Valley Drive
Point Pleasant, WV 25550
Phone: 304-675-4340
Fax: 304-675-5243
E-mail: ssprouse@pvalley.org
URL: www.pvalley.org
Type: Acute Care Hospitals
Emergency Services: Yes
Ownership: Voluntary non-profit - Private
Beds: 201

Key Personnel:

Radiology. . . . . Suresh K Agrawal
Intensive Care Unit. . . . . Doug Eades
Operating Room. . . . . Doug Eades
Infection Control. . . . . Susan Garten
Patient Relations . . . . Sue Hussel
Cardiac Laboratory. . . . . Israel Jamora
CEO/President. . . . . Alvin R Lawson, JD
Chief of Medical Staff. . . . . Shrikant Vaidya, MD

Measure	Cases	This Hosp.	State Avg.	U.S. Avg.
Blood Clot Prevention and Treatment				
Anticoagulation Overlap Therapy[2]	22	95%	90%	93%
ICU Venous Thromboembolism Prophylaxis[2]	24	79%	88%	92%
Incidence of Potentially Preventable VTE[2,7]	-	-	12%	10%
UFH with Dosages/Platelet Monitoring[1,2]	-	-	98%	97%
Venous Thromboembolism Prophylaxis[2]	97	86%	79%	85%
Warfarin Therapy Discharge Instructions[2]	18	94%	80%	75%
Chest Pain/Possible Heart Attack Care				
Aspirin Given Within 24 Hours of Arrival	28	100%	96%	96%
Fibrinolytic Meds Within 30 Min. of Arrival[7]	-	-	74%	58%
Average Time to ECG (minutes)	34	5	8	7
Average Time to Transfer (minutes)	15	68	109	60
Children's Asthma Care				
Received Home Management Plan of Care	-	-	-	88%
Received Reliever Medication	-	-	-	100%
Received Systemic Corticosteroids	-	-	-	100%
Emergency Department				
Admittance Decision Time (minutes)[2]	265	72	76	98
Head CT Results Within 45 Min. of Arrival[1]	-	-	43%	57%
Patients Who Left ER Before Being Seen	19,885	0%	2%	2%
Time from ER Arrival to Admit. (minutes)[2]	297	238	257	274
Time from ER Arrival to Discharge (minutes)	378	118	142	134
Time in ER Before Being Evaluated (minutes)	398	27	30	26
Time to Pain Meds for Fractures (minutes)	41	60	67	57
Heart Attack Care				
Aspirin Given at Discharge[1]	-	-	99%	99%
Fibrinolytic Meds Within 30 Min. of Arrival[7]	-	-	50%	54%
PCI Within 90 Minutes of Arrival[7]	-	-	93%	96%
Statin Prescribed at Discharge[1]	-	-	98%	98%
Heart Failure Care				
ACE Inhibitor or ARB for LVSD	15	100%	96%	97%
Discharge Instructions Given	90	100%	94%	94%
Evaluation of LVS Function	118	100%	98%	99%
Medicare Spending				
Medicare Spending per Patient (ratio)	-	0.96	0.96	0.98
Pneumonia Care				
Appropriate Initial Antibiotic Given[2]	68	100%	94%	95%
Blood Culture Timing[2]	101	100%	97%	98%
Pregnancy and Delivery Care				
Newborn Deliveries Scheduled Early[2]	47	4%	10%	6%
Preventive Care				
Immunization for Influenza[2]	295	98%	94%	90%
Immunization for Pneumonia[2]	403	99%	95%	92%
Stroke Care				
Anticoagulation Therapy for Atrial Fibrillation[7]	-	-	94%	95%
Antithrombotic Therapy Timing[1]	-	-	98%	98%
Assessed for Rehabilitation	14	79%	96%	97%
Discharged on Antithrombotic Therapy[1]	-	-	98%	99%
Discharged on Statin Medication[1]	-	-	91%	94%
Thrombolytic Therapy Timing[1]	-	-	67%	66%
Venous Thromboembolism Prophylaxis	11	82%	91%	94%
Written Stroke Educational Materials Given[1]	-	-	84%	88%
Surgical Care Improvement Project				
Appropriate Beta Blocker Usage	27	100%	98%	98%
Appropriate VTP Within 24 Hours	72	97%	98%	98%
Controlled Postoperative Blood Glucose[7]	-	-	95%	97%
Perioperative Temperature Management	76	99%	100%	100%
Prophylactic Antibiotic Selection	35	100%	99%	99%
Prophylactic Antibiotic Selection (Outpatient)	43	95%	97%	98%
Prophylactic Antibiotic Stopped	35	100%	98%	98%
Prophylactic Antibiotic Timing	35	100%	99%	99%
Prophylactic Antibiotic Timing (Outpatient)	43	100%	97%	98%
Urinary Catheter Removal	39	100%	98%	97%
Survey of Patients' Hospital Experiences				
Area Around Room 'Always' Quiet at Night	300+	68%	58%	61%
Doctors 'Always' Communicated Well	300+	87%	82%	82%
Home Recovery Information Given	300+	88%	85%	85%
Hospital Given 9 or 10 on 10 Point Scale	300+	74%	66%	71%
Meds 'Always' Explained Before Given	300+	67%	64%	64%
Nurses 'Always' Communicated Well	300+	81%	78%	79%
Pain 'Always' Well Controlled	300+	74%	70%	71%
Room and Bathroom 'Always' Clean	300+	80%	75%	73%
Timely Help 'Always' Received	300+	72%	68%	68%
Would Definitely Recommend Hospital	300+	75%	66%	71%
Use of Medical Imaging				
Cardiac Imaging Stress Test before Surgery	180	4.4%	4.9%	5.3%
Combination Abdominal CT Scan	328	5.5%	14.4%	10.5%
Combination Brain/Sinus CT Scan[1]	-	-	3%	2.7%
Combination Chest CT Scan	129	5.4%	2.8%	2.7%
Follow-up Mammogram/Ultrasound	419	6.7%	8.8%	8.8%
Lumbar Spine MRI for Low Back Pain	67	34.3%	38.4%	37.2%

Princeton Community Hospital

122 12th Street
Princeton, WV 24740
Phone: 304-487-7260
Fax: 304-487-2161
URL: www.pchonline.org
Type: Acute Care Hospitals
Emergency Services: Yes
Ownership: Government - Local
Beds: 267

Key Personnel:

Infection Control. . . . . Cindy Belcher
Chief of Medical Staff . . . . Philip Branson, MD
CEO/President. . . . . Wayne Griffith
Operating Room. . . . . Larry Perdue
Quality Assurance . . . . Rick Puckett

Measure	Cases	This Hosp.	State Avg.	U.S. Avg.
Blood Clot Prevention and Treatment				
Anticoagulation Overlap Therapy[2]	57	82%	90%	93%
ICU Venous Thromboembolism Prophylaxis[2]	100	68%	88%	92%
Incidence of Potentially Preventable VTE[2]	15	27%	12%	10%
UFH with Dosages/Platelet Monitoring[1,2]	-	-	98%	97%
Venous Thromboembolism Prophylaxis[2]	316	50%	79%	85%
Warfarin Therapy Discharge Instructions[2]	47	83%	80%	75%
Chest Pain/Possible Heart Attack Care				
Aspirin Given Within 24 Hours of Arrival	171	99%	96%	96%
Fibrinolytic Meds Within 30 Min. of Arrival	17	71%	74%	58%
Average Time to ECG (minutes)	176	11	8	7
Average Time to Transfer (minutes)[1]	-	-	109	60
Children's Asthma Care				
Received Home Management Plan of Care	-	-	-	88%
Received Reliever Medication	-	-	-	100%
Received Systemic Corticosteroids	-	-	-	100%
Emergency Department				
Admittance Decision Time (minutes)[2]	630	94	76	98
Head CT Results Within 45 Min. of Arrival	19	53%	43%	57%
Patients Who Left ER Before Being Seen	48,663	3%	2%	2%
Time from ER Arrival to Admit. (minutes)[2]	634	302	257	274
Time from ER Arrival to Discharge (minutes)	377	161	142	134
Time in ER Before Being Evaluated (minutes)	403	29	30	26
Time to Pain Meds for Fractures (minutes)	136	63	67	57
Heart Attack Care				
Aspirin Given at Discharge	16	100%	99%	99%
Fibrinolytic Meds Within 30 Min. of Arrival[7]	-	-	50%	54%
PCI Within 90 Minutes of Arrival[7]	-	-	93%	96%
Statin Prescribed at Discharge	17	94%	98%	98%
Heart Failure Care				
ACE Inhibitor or ARB for LVSD	32	100%	96%	97%
Discharge Instructions Given	126	98%	94%	94%
Evaluation of LVS Function	158	99%	98%	99%
Medicare Spending				
Medicare Spending per Patient (ratio)	-	0.96	0.96	0.98
Pneumonia Care				
Appropriate Initial Antibiotic Given	232	94%	94%	95%
Blood Culture Timing	392	99%	97%	98%
Pregnancy and Delivery Care				
Newborn Deliveries Scheduled Early[2]	65	5%	10%	6%
Preventive Care				
Immunization for Influenza[2]	546	99%	94%	90%
Immunization for Pneumonia[2]	744	98%	95%	92%
Stroke Care				
Anticoagulation Therapy for Atrial Fibrillation[1]	-	-	94%	95%
Antithrombotic Therapy Timing	46	89%	98%	98%
Assessed for Rehabilitation	60	93%	96%	97%
Discharged on Antithrombotic Therapy	52	92%	98%	99%
Discharged on Statin Medication	49	80%	91%	94%
Thrombolytic Therapy Timing[1]	-	-	67%	66%
Venous Thromboembolism Prophylaxis	49	57%	91%	94%
Written Stroke Educational Materials Given	41	85%	84%	88%
Surgical Care Improvement Project				
Appropriate Beta Blocker Usage	207	100%	98%	98%
Appropriate VTP Within 24 Hours	531	98%	98%	98%
Controlled Postoperative Blood Glucose[7]	-	-	95%	97%
Perioperative Temperature Management	595	99%	100%	100%
Prophylactic Antibiotic Selection	476	99%	99%	99%
Prophylactic Antibiotic Selection (Outpatient)	81	93%	97%	98%
Prophylactic Antibiotic Stopped	467	98%	98%	98%

NOTE: Hospital profiles are in alphabetical order by state, then city, then hospital within the city; Rankings exclude hospitals with less than 25 cases except for patient surveys which excludes hospitals with less than 100 cases; (a) 100-299 cases; (1) The number of cases/patients is too few to report; (2) Data submitted were based on a sample of cases/patients; (3) Results are based on a shorter time period than required; (4) Data suppressed by CMS for one or more quarters; (5) Results are not available for this reporting period; (6) Fewer than 100 patients completed the HCAHPS survey; (7) No cases met the criteria for this measure; (8) The lower limit of the confidence interval cannot be calculated if the number of observed infections equals zero; (9) No data are available from the state/territory for this reporting period; (10) The scores shown reflect fewer than 50 completed surveys; (11) There were discrepancies in the data collection process; (12) This measure does not apply to this hospital for this reporting period; (13) Results cannot be calculated for this reporting period; (14) The results for this state are combined with nearby states to protect confidentiality; Please refer to the User's Guide for a full explanation of data.

Measure	Cases	This Hosp.	State Avg.	U.S. Avg.
Prophylactic Antibiotic Timing	477	99%	99%	99%
Prophylactic Antibiotic Timing (Outpatient)	77	94%	97%	98%
Urinary Catheter Removal	45	93%	98%	97%
Survey of Patients' Hospital Experiences				
Area Around Room 'Always' Quiet at Night	300+	60%	58%	61%
Doctors 'Always' Communicated Well	300+	86%	82%	82%
Home Recovery Information Given	300+	86%	85%	85%
Hospital Given 9 or 10 on 10 Point Scale	300+	74%	66%	71%
Meds 'Always' Explained Before Given	300+	60%	64%	64%
Nurses 'Always' Communicated Well	300+	79%	78%	79%
Pain 'Always' Well Controlled	300+	72%	70%	71%
Room and Bathroom 'Always' Clean	300+	71%	75%	73%
Timely Help 'Always' Received	300+	67%	68%	68%
Would Definitely Recommend Hospital	300+	72%	66%	71%
Use of Medical Imaging				
Cardiac Imaging Stress Test before Surgery	417	6.7%	4.9%	5.3%
Combination Abdominal CT Scan	962	60.2%	14.4%	10.5%
Combination Brain/Sinus CT Scan	986	2.1%	3%	2.7%
Combination Chest CT Scan	727	1.0%	2.8%	2.7%
Follow-up Mammogram/Ultrasound	1,193	6.8%	8.8%	8.8%
Lumbar Spine MRI for Low Back Pain	207	40.1%	38.4%	37.2%

Jefferson Medical Center

300 South Preston Street
Ranson, WV 25438
Phone: 304-728-1600
Fax: 304-725-9492
E-mail: tstover@jeffmem.com
URL: www.jeffmem.com
Type: Critical Access Hospitals
Emergency Services: Yes
Ownership: Voluntary non-profit - Private
Beds: 114

Key Personnel:
Infection Control.............. Robin Akin, RN
Pediatric In-Patient Care .... Linda Blanc
Chief of Medical Staff.......... Vikram Dayal, MD
Intensive Care Unit............ Tammy Fitch
Quality Assurance .... Sarah Johnson
Pediatric Ambulatory Care ...... Sarah Moerschel, MD
Patient Relations .... Suzanne Shackelford
CEO/President................ John M Sherwood

Measure	Cases	This Hosp.	State Avg.	U.S. Avg.
Blood Clot Prevention and Treatment				
Anticoagulation Overlap Therapy[5]	-	-	90%	93%
ICU Venous Thromboembolism Prophylaxis[5]	-	-	88%	92%
Incidence of Potentially Preventable VTE[5]	-	-	12%	10%
UFH with Dosages/Platelet Monitoring[5]	-	-	98%	97%
Venous Thromboembolism Prophylaxis[5]	-	-	79%	85%
Warfarin Therapy Discharge Instructions[5]	-	-	80%	75%
Chest Pain/Possible Heart Attack Care				
Aspirin Given Within 24 Hours of Arrival	48	94%	96%	96%
Fibrinolytic Meds Within 30 Min. of Arrival[7]	-	-	74%	58%
Average Time to ECG (minutes)	47	4	8	7
Average Time to Transfer (minutes)[7]	-	-	109	60
Children's Asthma Care				
Received Home Management Plan of Care	-	-	-	88%
Received Reliever Medication	-	-	-	100%
Received Systemic Corticosteroids	-	-	-	100%
Emergency Department				
Admittance Decision Time (minutes)[5]	-	-	76	98
Head CT Results Within 45 Min. of Arrival	11	64%	43%	57%
Patients Who Left ER Before Being Seen[5]	-	-	2%	2%
Time from ER Arrival to Admit. (minutes)[5]	-	-	257	274
Time from ER Arrival to Discharge (minutes)	349	114	142	134
Time in ER Before Being Evaluated (minutes)	384	17	30	26
Time to Pain Meds for Fractures (minutes)	110	58	67	57
Heart Attack Care				
Aspirin Given at Discharge[1]	-	-	99%	99%
Fibrinolytic Meds Within 30 Min. of Arrival[7]	-	-	50%	54%
PCI Within 90 Minutes of Arrival[3,7]	-	-	93%	96%
Statin Prescribed at Discharge[1]	-	-	98%	98%
Heart Failure Care				
ACE Inhibitor or ARB for LVSD	13	100%	96%	97%
Discharge Instructions Given	27	100%	94%	94%
Evaluation of LVS Function	39	100%	98%	99%
Medicare Spending				
Medicare Spending per Patient (ratio)	-	-	0.96	0.98
Pneumonia Care				
Appropriate Initial Antibiotic Given	25	100%	94%	95%
Blood Culture Timing	41	100%	97%	98%
Pregnancy and Delivery Care				
Newborn Deliveries Scheduled Early[5]	-	-	10%	6%
Preventive Care				
Immunization for Influenza[5]	-	-	94%	90%
Immunization for Pneumonia[5]	-	-	95%	92%
Stroke Care				
Anticoagulation Therapy for Atrial Fibrillation[5]	-	-	94%	95%
Antithrombotic Therapy Timing[5]	-	-	98%	98%
Assessed for Rehabilitation[5]	-	-	96%	97%
Discharged on Antithrombotic Therapy[5]	-	-	98%	99%
Discharged on Statin Medication[5]	-	-	91%	94%
Thrombolytic Therapy Timing[5]	-	-	67%	66%
Venous Thromboembolism Prophylaxis[5]	-	-	91%	94%
Written Stroke Educational Materials Given[5]	-	-	84%	88%
Surgical Care Improvement Project				
Appropriate Beta Blocker Usage[1]	-	-	98%	98%
Appropriate VTP Within 24 Hours	35	100%	98%	98%
Controlled Postoperative Blood Glucose[7]	-	-	95%	97%
Perioperative Temperature Management	36	100%	100%	100%
Prophylactic Antibiotic Selection	15	93%	99%	99%
Prophylactic Antibiotic Selection (Outpatient)[3]	23	87%	97%	98%
Prophylactic Antibiotic Stopped[1]	-	-	98%	98%
Prophylactic Antibiotic Timing	15	100%	99%	99%
Prophylactic Antibiotic Timing (Outpatient)[3]	26	88%	97%	98%
Urinary Catheter Removal	16	94%	98%	97%
Survey of Patients' Hospital Experiences				
Area Around Room 'Always' Quiet at Night	(a)	61%	58%	61%
Doctors 'Always' Communicated Well	(a)	85%	82%	82%
Home Recovery Information Given	(a)	85%	85%	85%
Hospital Given 9 or 10 on 10 Point Scale	(a)	74%	66%	71%
Meds 'Always' Explained Before Given	(a)	64%	64%	64%
Nurses 'Always' Communicated Well	(a)	85%	78%	79%
Pain 'Always' Well Controlled	(a)	70%	70%	71%
Room and Bathroom 'Always' Clean	(a)	85%	75%	73%
Timely Help 'Always' Received	(a)	75%	68%	68%
Would Definitely Recommend Hospital	(a)	72%	66%	71%
Use of Medical Imaging				
Cardiac Imaging Stress Test before Surgery	45	0.0%	4.9%	5.3%
Combination Abdominal CT Scan	333	1.2%	14.4%	10.5%
Combination Brain/Sinus CT Scan	532	1.5%	3%	2.7%
Combination Chest CT Scan	102	2.0%	2.8%	2.7%
Follow-up Mammogram/Ultrasound	363	1.9%	8.8%	8.8%
Lumbar Spine MRI for Low Back Pain[1]	-	-	38.4%	37.2%

Jackson General Hospital

122 Pinnell St
Ripley, WV 25271
Phone: 304-372-2731
Type: Critical Access Hospitals
Emergency Services: Yes
Ownership: Voluntary non-profit - Other

Measure	Cases	This Hosp.	State Avg.	U.S. Avg.
Blood Clot Prevention and Treatment				
Anticoagulation Overlap Therapy[2]	15	67%	90%	93%
ICU Venous Thromboembolism Prophylaxis[2]	22	95%	88%	92%
Incidence of Potentially Preventable VTE[2,7]	-	-	12%	10%
UFH with Dosages/Platelet Monitoring[1,2]	-	-	98%	97%
Venous Thromboembolism Prophylaxis[2]	128	98%	79%	85%
Warfarin Therapy Discharge Instructions[2]	14	93%	80%	75%
Chest Pain/Possible Heart Attack Care				
Aspirin Given Within 24 Hours of Arrival	50	96%	96%	96%
Fibrinolytic Meds Within 30 Min. of Arrival[1]	-	-	74%	58%
Average Time to ECG (minutes)	54	14	8	7
Average Time to Transfer (minutes)[1]	-	-	109	60
Children's Asthma Care				
Received Home Management Plan of Care	-	-	-	88%
Received Reliever Medication	-	-	-	100%
Received Systemic Corticosteroids	-	-	-	100%
Emergency Department				
Admittance Decision Time (minutes)[2]	345	58	76	98
Head CT Results Within 45 Min. of Arrival[1]	-	-	43%	57%
Patients Who Left ER Before Being Seen	12,133	5%	2%	2%
Time from ER Arrival to Admit. (minutes)[2]	351	206	257	274
Time from ER Arrival to Discharge (minutes)	375	113	142	134
Time in ER Before Being Evaluated (minutes)	405	29	30	26
Time to Pain Meds for Fractures (minutes)	29	73	67	57
Heart Attack Care				
Aspirin Given at Discharge[2,3]	-	-	99%	99%
Fibrinolytic Meds Within 30 Min. of Arrival[2,3]	-	-	50%	54%
PCI Within 90 Minutes of Arrival[2,3]	-	-	93%	96%
Statin Prescribed at Discharge[2,3]	-	-	98%	98%
Heart Failure Care				
ACE Inhibitor or ARB for LVSD	12	100%	96%	97%
Discharge Instructions Given	37	89%	94%	94%
Evaluation of LVS Function	47	98%	98%	99%
Medicare Spending				
Medicare Spending per Patient (ratio)	-	-	0.96	0.98
Pneumonia Care				
Appropriate Initial Antibiotic Given	67	99%	94%	95%
Blood Culture Timing	105	98%	97%	98%
Pregnancy and Delivery Care				
Newborn Deliveries Scheduled Early[5]	-	-	10%	6%
Preventive Care				
Immunization for Influenza[2]	295	96%	94%	90%
Immunization for Pneumonia[2]	508	99%	95%	92%
Stroke Care				
Anticoagulation Therapy for Atrial Fibrillation[5]	-	-	94%	95%
Antithrombotic Therapy Timing[5]	-	-	98%	98%
Assessed for Rehabilitation[5]	-	-	96%	97%
Discharged on Antithrombotic Therapy[5]	-	-	98%	99%
Discharged on Statin Medication[5]	-	-	91%	94%
Thrombolytic Therapy Timing[5]	-	-	67%	66%
Venous Thromboembolism Prophylaxis[5]	-	-	91%	94%
Written Stroke Educational Materials Given[5]	-	-	84%	88%
Surgical Care Improvement Project				
Appropriate Beta Blocker Usage[1]	-	-	98%	98%
Appropriate VTP Within 24 Hours	24	92%	98%	98%
Controlled Postoperative Blood Glucose[7]	-	-	95%	97%
Perioperative Temperature Management	25	92%	100%	100%
Prophylactic Antibiotic Selection[1]	-	-	99%	99%
Prophylactic Antibiotic Selection (Outpatient)[1,3]	-	-	97%	98%
Prophylactic Antibiotic Stopped[1]	-	-	98%	98%
Prophylactic Antibiotic Timing[1]	-	-	99%	99%
Prophylactic Antibiotic Timing (Outpatient)[1,3]	-	-	97%	98%
Urinary Catheter Removal[1]	-	-	98%	97%
Survey of Patients' Hospital Experiences				
Area Around Room 'Always' Quiet at Night	(a)	54%	58%	61%
Doctors 'Always' Communicated Well	(a)	88%	82%	82%
Home Recovery Information Given	(a)	87%	85%	85%
Hospital Given 9 or 10 on 10 Point Scale	(a)	72%	66%	71%
Meds 'Always' Explained Before Given	(a)	67%	64%	64%
Nurses 'Always' Communicated Well	(a)	79%	78%	79%
Pain 'Always' Well Controlled	(a)	74%	70%	71%
Room and Bathroom 'Always' Clean	(a)	79%	75%	73%
Timely Help 'Always' Received	(a)	69%	68%	68%
Would Definitely Recommend Hospital	(a)	66%	66%	71%
Use of Medical Imaging				
Cardiac Imaging Stress Test before Surgery	152	9.2%	4.9%	5.3%
Combination Abdominal CT Scan	269	12.6%	14.4%	10.5%
Combination Brain/Sinus CT Scan[1]	-	-	3%	2.7%
Combination Chest CT Scan	180	8.3%	2.8%	2.7%
Follow-up Mammogram/Ultrasound	256	9.8%	8.8%	8.8%
Lumbar Spine MRI for Low Back Pain	55	30.9%	38.4%	37.2%

Hampshire Memorial Hospital

363 Sunrise Boulevard
Romney, WV 26757
Phone: 304-822-4561
Fax: 304-822-7809
E-mail: hmhi@access.mountain.net
Type: Critical Access Hospitals
Emergency Services: Yes
Ownership: Voluntary non-profit - Private
Beds: 47

Key Personnel:
Chief of Medical Staff.......... Vijay K Chowdhary, MD
Emergency Room .... Anthony K Haywood, DO
CEO/President............... Mark H. Merrill, Sr
Quality Assurance .... Julia A Sites, RN
Operating Room.............. Carlotte Staudt

NOTE: Hospital profiles are in alphabetical order by state, then city, then hospital within the city; Rankings exclude hospitals with less than 25 cases except for patient surveys which excludes hospitals with less than 100 cases; (a) 100-299 cases; (1) The number of cases/patients is too few to report; (2) Data submitted were based on a sample of cases/patients; (3) Results are based on a shorter time period than required; (4) Data suppressed by CMS for one or more quarters; (5) Results are not available for this reporting period; (6) Fewer than 100 patients completed the HCAHPS survey; (7) No cases met the criteria for this measure; (8) The lower limit of the confidence interval cannot be calculated if the number of observed infections equals zero; (9) No data are available from the state/territory for this reporting period; (10) The scores shown reflect fewer than 50 completed surveys; (11) There were discrepancies in the data collection process; (12) This measure does not apply to this hospital for this reporting period; (13) Results cannot be calculated for this reporting period; (14) The results for this state are combined with nearby states to protect confidentiality; Please refer to the User's Guide for a full explanation of data.

Infection Control. . . . . Jonathan R Walburn, MD

Measure	Cases	This Hosp.	State Avg.	U.S. Avg.
Blood Clot Prevention and Treatment				
Anticoagulation Overlap Therapy[5]	-	-	90%	93%
ICU Venous Thromboembolism Prophylaxis[5]	-	-	88%	92%
Incidence of Potentially Preventable VTE[5]	-	-	12%	10%
UFH with Dosages/Platelet Monitoring[5]	-	-	98%	97%
Venous Thromboembolism Prophylaxis[5]	-	-	79%	85%
Warfarin Therapy Discharge Instructions[5]	-	-	80%	75%
Chest Pain/Possible Heart Attack Care				
Aspirin Given Within 24 Hours of Arrival	-	-	96%	96%
Fibrinolytic Meds Within 30 Min. of Arrival	-	-	74%	58%
Average Time to ECG (minutes)	-	-	8	7
Average Time to Transfer (minutes)	-	-	109	60
Children's Asthma Care				
Received Home Management Plan of Care	-	-	-	88%
Received Reliever Medication	-	-	-	100%
Received Systemic Corticosteroids	-	-	-	100%
Emergency Department				
Admittance Decision Time (minutes)[5]	-	-	76	98
Head CT Results Within 45 Min. of Arrival	-	-	43%	57%
Patients Who Left ER Before Being Seen	-	-	2%	2%
Time from ER Arrival to Admit. (minutes)[5]	-	-	257	274
Time from ER Arrival to Discharge (minutes)	-	-	142	134
Time in ER Before Being Evaluated (minutes)	-	-	30	26
Time to Pain Meds for Fractures (minutes)	-	-	67	57
Heart Attack Care				
Aspirin Given at Discharge[5]	-	-	99%	99%
Fibrinolytic Meds Within 30 Min. of Arrival[5]	-	-	50%	54%
PCI Within 90 Minutes of Arrival[5]	-	-	93%	96%
Statin Prescribed at Discharge[5]	-	-	98%	98%
Heart Failure Care				
ACE Inhibitor or ARB for LVSD[3,7]	-	-	96%	97%
Discharge Instructions Given[1,3]	-	-	94%	94%
Evaluation of LVS Function[1,3]	-	-	98%	99%
Medicare Spending				
Medicare Spending per Patient (ratio)	-	-	0.96	0.98
Pneumonia Care				
Appropriate Initial Antibiotic Given[1,3]	-	-	94%	95%
Blood Culture Timing[3]	15	100%	97%	98%
Pregnancy and Delivery Care				
Newborn Deliveries Scheduled Early[5]	-	-	10%	6%
Preventive Care				
Immunization for Influenza[5]	-	-	94%	90%
Immunization for Pneumonia[5]	-	-	95%	92%
Stroke Care				
Anticoagulation Therapy for Atrial Fibrillation[5]	-	-	94%	95%
Antithrombotic Therapy Timing[5]	-	-	98%	98%
Assessed for Rehabilitation[5]	-	-	96%	97%
Discharged on Antithrombotic Therapy[5]	-	-	98%	99%
Discharged on Statin Medication[5]	-	-	91%	94%
Thrombolytic Therapy Timing[5]	-	-	67%	66%
Venous Thromboembolism Prophylaxis[5]	-	-	91%	94%
Written Stroke Educational Materials Given[5]	-	-	84%	88%
Surgical Care Improvement Project				
Appropriate Beta Blocker Usage[5]	-	-	98%	98%
Appropriate VTP Within 24 Hours[5]	-	-	98%	98%
Controlled Postoperative Blood Glucose[5]	-	-	95%	97%
Perioperative Temperature Management[5]	-	-	100%	100%
Prophylactic Antibiotic Selection[5]	-	-	99%	99%
Prophylactic Antibiotic Selection (Outpatient)	-	-	97%	98%
Prophylactic Antibiotic Stopped[5]	-	-	98%	98%
Prophylactic Antibiotic Timing[5]	-	-	99%	99%
Prophylactic Antibiotic Timing (Outpatient)	-	-	97%	98%
Urinary Catheter Removal[5]	-	-	98%	97%
Survey of Patients' Hospital Experiences				
Area Around Room 'Always' Quiet at Night	(a)	72%	58%	61%
Doctors 'Always' Communicated Well	(a)	77%	82%	82%
Home Recovery Information Given	(a)	79%	85%	85%
Hospital Given 9 or 10 on 10 Point Scale	(a)	66%	66%	71%
Meds 'Always' Explained Before Given	(a)	69%	64%	64%
Nurses 'Always' Communicated Well	(a)	84%	78%	79%
Pain 'Always' Well Controlled	(a)	72%	70%	71%
Room and Bathroom 'Always' Clean	(a)	82%	75%	73%
Timely Help 'Always' Received	(a)	74%	68%	68%
Would Definitely Recommend Hospital	(a)	62%	66%	71%
Use of Medical Imaging				
Cardiac Imaging Stress Test before Surgery	-	-	4.9%	5.3%
Combination Abdominal CT Scan	-	-	14.4%	10.5%
Combination Brain/Sinus CT Scan	-	-	3%	2.7%
Combination Chest CT Scan	-	-	2.8%	2.7%
Follow-up Mammogram/Ultrasound	-	-	8.8%	8.8%
Lumbar Spine MRI for Low Back Pain	-	-	38.4%	37.2%

Greenbrier Valley Medical Center

202 Maplewood Avenue PO Box 497
Ronceverte, WV 24970
Phone: 304-647-4411
Fax: 304-647-6010
URL: www.gvmc.com
Type: Acute Care Hospitals
Ownership: Proprietary
Emergency Services: Yes
Beds: 122

Key Personnel:

Anesthesiology. . . . . Glenn Avidon, MD
Operating Room. . . . . Paula Bishop, RN
Radiology. . . . . David Maki
Intensive Care Unit. . . . . Tammy Murphy
CEO/President. . . . . Mark Nosacka
Chief of Medical Staff. . . . . Oshfaq Ohsannidin, MD
Emergency Room . . . . Jon Stout, DO
Infection Control. . . . . Barbara Walker

Measure	Cases	This Hosp.	State Avg.	U.S. Avg.
Blood Clot Prevention and Treatment				
Anticoagulation Overlap Therapy[2]	46	96%	90%	93%
ICU Venous Thromboembolism Prophylaxis[2]	142	99%	88%	92%
Incidence of Potentially Preventable VTE[1,2]	-	-	12%	10%
UFH with Dosages/Platelet Monitoring[2]	15	100%	98%	97%
Venous Thromboembolism Prophylaxis[2]	261	100%	79%	85%
Warfarin Therapy Discharge Instructions[2]	43	100%	80%	75%
Chest Pain/Possible Heart Attack Care				
Aspirin Given Within 24 Hours of Arrival	178	100%	96%	96%
Fibrinolytic Meds Within 30 Min. of Arrival	20	100%	74%	58%
Average Time to ECG (minutes)	181	1	8	7
Average Time to Transfer (minutes)[1]	-	-	109	60
Children's Asthma Care				
Received Home Management Plan of Care	-	-	-	88%
Received Reliever Medication	-	-	-	100%
Received Systemic Corticosteroids	-	-	-	100%
Emergency Department				
Admittance Decision Time (minutes)[2]	535	117	76	98
Head CT Results Within 45 Min. of Arrival[1]	-	-	43%	57%
Patients Who Left ER Before Being Seen	24,070	1%	2%	2%
Time from ER Arrival to Admit. (minutes)[2]	543	263	257	274
Time from ER Arrival to Discharge (minutes)	363	133	142	134
Time in ER Before Being Evaluated (minutes)	420	20	30	26
Time to Pain Meds for Fractures (minutes)	77	50	67	57
Heart Attack Care				
Aspirin Given at Discharge	18	94%	99%	99%
Fibrinolytic Meds Within 30 Min. of Arrival[7]	-	-	50%	54%
PCI Within 90 Minutes of Arrival[7]	-	-	93%	96%
Statin Prescribed at Discharge	15	73%	98%	98%
Heart Failure Care				
ACE Inhibitor or ARB for LVSD	52	92%	96%	97%
Discharge Instructions Given	103	95%	94%	94%
Evaluation of LVS Function	118	100%	98%	99%
Medicare Spending				
Medicare Spending per Patient (ratio)	-	0.89	0.96	0.98
Pneumonia Care				
Appropriate Initial Antibiotic Given	137	96%	94%	95%
Blood Culture Timing	249	99%	97%	98%
Pregnancy and Delivery Care				
Newborn Deliveries Scheduled Early[2]	24	0%	10%	6%
Preventive Care				
Immunization for Influenza[2]	406	100%	94%	90%
Immunization for Pneumonia[2]	525	100%	95%	92%
Stroke Care				
Anticoagulation Therapy for Atrial Fibrillation[1]	-	-	94%	95%
Antithrombotic Therapy Timing	32	100%	98%	98%
Assessed for Rehabilitation	30	100%	96%	97%
Discharged on Antithrombotic Therapy	30	97%	98%	99%
Discharged on Statin Medication	22	82%	91%	94%
Thrombolytic Therapy Timing[7]	-	-	67%	66%
Venous Thromboembolism Prophylaxis	35	100%	91%	94%
Written Stroke Educational Materials Given	17	82%	84%	88%
Surgical Care Improvement Project				
Appropriate Beta Blocker Usage	24	100%	98%	98%
Appropriate VTP Within 24 Hours	69	97%	98%	98%
Controlled Postoperative Blood Glucose[7]	-	-	95%	97%
Perioperative Temperature Management	93	100%	100%	100%
Prophylactic Antibiotic Selection	61	100%	99%	99%
Prophylactic Antibiotic Selection (Outpatient)	109	98%	97%	98%
Prophylactic Antibiotic Stopped	60	97%	98%	98%
Prophylactic Antibiotic Timing	61	100%	99%	99%
Prophylactic Antibiotic Timing (Outpatient)	109	100%	97%	98%
Urinary Catheter Removal	37	97%	98%	97%
Survey of Patients' Hospital Experiences				
Area Around Room 'Always' Quiet at Night	300+	58%	58%	61%
Doctors 'Always' Communicated Well	300+	82%	82%	82%
Home Recovery Information Given	300+	86%	85%	85%
Hospital Given 9 or 10 on 10 Point Scale	300+	68%	66%	71%
Meds 'Always' Explained Before Given	300+	65%	64%	64%
Nurses 'Always' Communicated Well	300+	79%	78%	79%
Pain 'Always' Well Controlled	300+	72%	70%	71%
Room and Bathroom 'Always' Clean	300+	76%	75%	73%
Timely Help 'Always' Received	300+	66%	68%	68%
Would Definitely Recommend Hospital	300+	63%	66%	71%
Use of Medical Imaging				
Cardiac Imaging Stress Test before Surgery	248	4.8%	4.9%	5.3%
Combination Abdominal CT Scan	957	9.9%	14.4%	10.5%
Combination Brain/Sinus CT Scan	749	4.7%	3%	2.7%
Combination Chest CT Scan	540	0.7%	2.8%	2.7%
Follow-up Mammogram/Ultrasound	432	17.1%	8.8%	8.8%
Lumbar Spine MRI for Low Back Pain	166	36.1%	38.4%	37.2%

Sistersville General Hospital

314 South Wells Street
Sistersville, WV 26175
Phone: 304-652-2611
Fax: 304-652-1448
E-mail: sisgen@ovis.net
URL: www.sistersvillegeneral.com
Type: Critical Access Hospitals
Ownership: Voluntary non-profit - Private
Emergency Services: Yes
Beds: 12

Key Personnel:

Radiology. . . . . Anna Carson
Cardiology . . . . Jack Casas, MD
Emergency Room . . . . Jason Enoch
Chief of Medical Staff. . . . . Ramon Fagundo
CEO/President. . . . . Brian Lowther
Pulmonology . . . . Melvin Saludes, MD

Measure	Cases	This Hosp.	State Avg.	U.S. Avg.
Blood Clot Prevention and Treatment				
Anticoagulation Overlap Therapy[5]	-	-	90%	93%
ICU Venous Thromboembolism Prophylaxis[5]	-	-	88%	92%
Incidence of Potentially Preventable VTE[5]	-	-	12%	10%
UFH with Dosages/Platelet Monitoring[5]	-	-	98%	97%
Venous Thromboembolism Prophylaxis[5]	-	-	79%	85%
Warfarin Therapy Discharge Instructions[5]	-	-	80%	75%
Chest Pain/Possible Heart Attack Care				
Aspirin Given Within 24 Hours of Arrival[1,3]	-	-	96%	96%
Fibrinolytic Meds Within 30 Min. of Arrival[3,7]	-	-	74%	58%
Average Time to ECG (minutes)[1,3]	-	-	8	7
Average Time to Transfer (minutes)[1,3]	-	-	109	60
Children's Asthma Care				
Received Home Management Plan of Care	-	-	-	88%
Received Reliever Medication	-	-	-	100%
Received Systemic Corticosteroids	-	-	-	100%
Emergency Department				
Admittance Decision Time (minutes)[5]	-	-	76	98
Head CT Results Within 45 Min. of Arrival[3,7]	-	-	43%	57%
Patients Who Left ER Before Being Seen	7,311	1%	2%	2%
Time from ER Arrival to Admit. (minutes)[5]	-	-	257	274
Time from ER Arrival to Discharge (minutes)[3]	211	110	142	134

NOTE: Hospital profiles are in alphabetical order by state, then city, then hospital within the city; Rankings exclude hospitals with less than 25 cases except for patient surveys which excludes hospitals with less than 100 cases; (a) 100-299 cases; (1) The number of cases/patients is too few to report; (2) Data submitted were based on a sample of cases/patients; (3) Results are based on a shorter time period than required; (4) Data suppressed by CMS for one or more quarters; (5) Results are not available for this reporting period; (6) Fewer than 100 patients completed the HCAHPS survey; (7) No cases met the criteria for this measure; (8) The lower limit of the confidence interval cannot be calculated if the number of observed infections equals zero; (9) No data are available from the state/territory for this reporting period; (10) The scores shown reflect fewer than 50 completed surveys; (11) There were discrepancies in the data collection process; (12) This measure does not apply to this hospital for this reporting period; (13) Results cannot be calculated for this reporting period; (14) The results for this state are combined with nearby states to protect confidentiality; Please refer to the User's Guide for a full explanation of data.

Time in ER Before Being Evaluated (minutes)[3]	252	25	30	26
Time to Pain Meds for Fractures (minutes)[1,3]	-	-	67	57
Heart Attack Care				
Aspirin Given at Discharge[2,3]	-	-	99%	99%
Fibrinolytic Meds Within 30 Min. of Arrival[2,3]	-	-	50%	54%
PCI Within 90 Minutes of Arrival[2,3]	-	-	93%	96%
Statin Prescribed at Discharge[2,3]	-	-	98%	98%
Heart Failure Care				
ACE Inhibitor or ARB for LVSD[1,2]	-	-	96%	97%
Discharge Instructions Given[2,3]	11	91%	94%	94%
Evaluation of LVS Function[2,3]	17	76%	98%	99%
Medicare Spending				
Medicare Spending per Patient (ratio)	-	-	0.96	0.98
Pneumonia Care				
Appropriate Initial Antibiotic Given[2]	13	92%	94%	95%
Blood Culture Timing[2]	25	84%	97%	98%
Pregnancy and Delivery Care				
Newborn Deliveries Scheduled Early[5]	-	-	10%	6%
Preventive Care				
Immunization for Influenza[5]	-	-	94%	90%
Immunization for Pneumonia[5]	-	-	95%	92%
Stroke Care				
Anticoagulation Therapy for Atrial Fibrillation[5]	-	-	94%	95%
Antithrombotic Therapy Timing[5]	-	-	98%	98%
Assessed for Rehabilitation[5]	-	-	96%	97%
Discharged on Antithrombotic Therapy[5]	-	-	98%	99%
Discharged on Statin Medication[5]	-	-	91%	94%
Thrombolytic Therapy Timing[5]	-	-	67%	66%
Venous Thromboembolism Prophylaxis[5]	-	-	91%	94%
Written Stroke Educational Materials Given[5]	-	-	84%	88%
Surgical Care Improvement Project				
Appropriate Beta Blocker Usage[5]	-	-	98%	98%
Appropriate VTP Within 24 Hours[5]	-	-	98%	98%
Controlled Postoperative Blood Glucose[5]	-	-	95%	97%
Perioperative Temperature Management[5]	-	-	100%	100%
Prophylactic Antibiotic Selection[5]	-	-	99%	99%
Prophylactic Antibiotic Selection (Outpatient)[5]	-	-	97%	98%
Prophylactic Antibiotic Stopped[5]	-	-	98%	98%
Prophylactic Antibiotic Timing[5]	-	-	99%	99%
Prophylactic Antibiotic Timing (Outpatient)[5]	-	-	97%	98%
Urinary Catheter Removal[5]	-	-	98%	97%
Survey of Patients' Hospital Experiences				
Area Around Room 'Always' Quiet at Night[5]	-	-	58%	61%
Doctors 'Always' Communicated Well[5]	-	-	82%	82%
Home Recovery Information Given[5]	-	-	85%	85%
Hospital Given 9 or 10 on 10 Point Scale[5]	-	-	66%	71%
Meds 'Always' Explained Before Given[5]	-	-	64%	64%
Nurses 'Always' Communicated Well[5]	-	-	78%	79%
Pain 'Always' Well Controlled[5]	-	-	70%	71%
Room and Bathroom 'Always' Clean[5]	-	-	75%	73%
Timely Help 'Always' Received[5]	-	-	68%	68%
Would Definitely Recommend Hospital[5]	-	-	66%	71%
Use of Medical Imaging				
Cardiac Imaging Stress Test before Surgery[7]	-	-	4.9%	5.3%
Combination Abdominal CT Scan	83	39.8%	14.4%	10.5%
Combination Brain/Sinus CT Scan[1]	-	-	3%	2.7%
Combination Chest CT Scan[1]	-	-	2.8%	2.7%
Follow-up Mammogram/Ultrasound	107	1.9%	8.8%	8.8%
Lumbar Spine MRI for Low Back Pain[1]	-	-	38.4%	37.2%

Thomas Memorial Hospital

4605 Maccorkle Ave Sw
South Charleston, WV 25309
Phone: 304-766-3600
Fax: 304-766-3477
URL: www.thomaswv.org
Type: Acute Care Hospitals
Emergency Services: Yes
Ownership: Voluntary non-profit - Private
Beds: 296

Key Personnel:

Quality Assurance . . . . Renee Amend
CEO/President. . . . . Stephen P Dexter
Operating Room. . . . . Rudy Mancuso
Chief of Medical Staff. . . . . James Mears, MD
Infection Control. . . . . Sara K Spencer
Coronary Care . . . . Lynn Storrick
Radiology. . . . . Mark Wilcox
Pediatric Ambulatory Care . . . . . . Sandy Young

Measure	Cases	This Hosp.	State Avg.	U.S. Avg.
Blood Clot Prevention and Treatment				
Anticoagulation Overlap Therapy[2]	52	92%	90%	93%
ICU Venous Thromboembolism Prophylaxis[2]	51	84%	88%	92%
Incidence of Potentially Preventable VTE[2]	12	8%	12%	10%
UFH with Dosages/Platelet Monitoring[2]	19	95%	98%	97%
Venous Thromboembolism Prophylaxis[2]	344	71%	79%	85%
Warfarin Therapy Discharge Instructions[2]	34	47%	80%	75%
Chest Pain/Possible Heart Attack Care				
Aspirin Given Within 24 Hours of Arrival[3]	14	93%	96%	96%
Fibrinolytic Meds Within 30 Min. of Arrival[3,7]	-	-	74%	58%
Average Time to ECG (minutes)[3]	16	26	8	7
Average Time to Transfer (minutes)[1,3]	-	-	109	60
Children's Asthma Care				
Received Home Management Plan of Care	-	-	-	88%
Received Reliever Medication	-	-	-	100%
Received Systemic Corticosteroids	-	-	-	100%
Emergency Department				
Admittance Decision Time (minutes)[2]	666	143	76	98
Head CT Results Within 45 Min. of Arrival[1]	-	-	43%	57%
Patients Who Left ER Before Being Seen	35,328	5%	2%	2%
Time from ER Arrival to Admit. (minutes)[2]	680	395	257	274
Time from ER Arrival to Discharge (minutes)	349	249	142	134
Time in ER Before Being Evaluated (minutes)	364	76	30	26
Time to Pain Meds for Fractures (minutes)	84	108	67	57
Heart Attack Care				
Aspirin Given at Discharge	115	97%	99%	99%
Fibrinolytic Meds Within 30 Min. of Arrival[7]	-	-	50%	54%
PCI Within 90 Minutes of Arrival	17	88%	93%	96%
Statin Prescribed at Discharge	114	90%	98%	98%
Heart Failure Care				
ACE Inhibitor or ARB for LVSD	88	95%	96%	97%
Discharge Instructions Given	231	100%	94%	94%
Evaluation of LVS Function	269	100%	98%	99%
Medicare Spending				
Medicare Spending per Patient (ratio)	-	0.95	0.96	0.98
Pneumonia Care				
Appropriate Initial Antibiotic Given	245	94%	94%	95%
Blood Culture Timing	433	99%	97%	98%
Pregnancy and Delivery Care				
Newborn Deliveries Scheduled Early[2]	28	18%	10%	6%
Preventive Care				
Immunization for Influenza[2]	519	94%	94%	90%
Immunization for Pneumonia[2]	682	97%	95%	92%
Stroke Care				
Anticoagulation Therapy for Atrial Fibrillation	12	100%	94%	95%
Antithrombotic Therapy Timing	94	96%	98%	98%
Assessed for Rehabilitation	88	93%	96%	97%
Discharged on Antithrombotic Therapy	86	94%	98%	99%
Discharged on Statin Medication	63	92%	91%	94%
Thrombolytic Therapy Timing[1]	-	-	67%	66%
Venous Thromboembolism Prophylaxis	93	77%	91%	94%
Written Stroke Educational Materials Given	64	69%	84%	88%
Surgical Care Improvement Project				
Appropriate Beta Blocker Usage	221	98%	98%	98%
Appropriate VTP Within 24 Hours	499	92%	98%	98%
Controlled Postoperative Blood Glucose[7]	-	-	95%	97%
Perioperative Temperature Management	615	100%	100%	100%
Prophylactic Antibiotic Selection	399	99%	99%	99%
Prophylactic Antibiotic Selection (Outpatient)	313	96%	97%	98%
Prophylactic Antibiotic Stopped	390	99%	98%	98%
Prophylactic Antibiotic Timing	399	99%	99%	99%
Prophylactic Antibiotic Timing (Outpatient)	319	95%	97%	98%
Urinary Catheter Removal	183	97%	98%	97%
Survey of Patients' Hospital Experiences				
Area Around Room 'Always' Quiet at Night	300+	59%	58%	61%
Doctors 'Always' Communicated Well	300+	80%	82%	82%
Home Recovery Information Given	300+	83%	85%	85%
Hospital Given 9 or 10 on 10 Point Scale	300+	67%	66%	71%
Meds 'Always' Explained Before Given	300+	55%	64%	64%
Nurses 'Always' Communicated Well	300+	71%	78%	79%
Pain 'Always' Well Controlled	300+	67%	70%	71%
Room and Bathroom 'Always' Clean	300+	65%	75%	73%
Timely Help 'Always' Received	300+	63%	68%	68%
Would Definitely Recommend Hospital	300+	72%	66%	71%
Use of Medical Imaging				
Cardiac Imaging Stress Test before Surgery	204	5.9%	4.9%	5.3%
Combination Abdominal CT Scan	1,004	13.6%	14.4%	10.5%
Combination Brain/Sinus CT Scan	709	2.8%	3%	2.7%
Combination Chest CT Scan	670	3.0%	2.8%	2.7%
Follow-up Mammogram/Ultrasound	1,304	10.0%	8.8%	8.8%
Lumbar Spine MRI for Low Back Pain	275	42.9%	38.4%	37.2%

Roane General Hospital

200 Hospital Drive
Spencer, WV 25276
Phone: 304-927-4444
Fax: 304-927-6390
URL: www.roanegeneralhospital.com
Type: Critical Access Hospitals
Emergency Services: Yes
Ownership: Voluntary non-profit - Private
Beds: 60

Key Personnel:

CEO/President. . . . . Douglas E. Bentz
Emergency Room . . . . Julie Carr
Quality Assurance . . . . Martha Hardman
Operating Room. . . . . Robin Miller, RN
Anesthesiology. . . . . Gerald Princesa, MD
Patient Relations . . . . Louise Ward
Chief of Medical Staff . . . . Brent Watson, MD
Radiology. . . . . George Wilson

Measure	Cases	This Hosp.	State Avg.	U.S. Avg.
Blood Clot Prevention and Treatment				
Anticoagulation Overlap Therapy[5]	-	-	90%	93%
ICU Venous Thromboembolism Prophylaxis[5]	-	-	88%	92%
Incidence of Potentially Preventable VTE[5]	-	-	12%	10%
UFH with Dosages/Platelet Monitoring[5]	-	-	98%	97%
Venous Thromboembolism Prophylaxis[5]	-	-	79%	85%
Warfarin Therapy Discharge Instructions[5]	-	-	80%	75%
Chest Pain/Possible Heart Attack Care				
Aspirin Given Within 24 Hours of Arrival	35	94%	96%	96%
Fibrinolytic Meds Within 30 Min. of Arrival[1]	-	-	74%	58%
Average Time to ECG (minutes)	35	3	8	7
Average Time to Transfer (minutes)[7]	-	-	109	60
Children's Asthma Care				
Received Home Management Plan of Care	-	-	-	88%
Received Reliever Medication	-	-	-	100%
Received Systemic Corticosteroids	-	-	-	100%
Emergency Department				
Admittance Decision Time (minutes)	158	75	76	98
Head CT Results Within 45 Min. of Arrival[1]	-	-	43%	57%
Patients Who Left ER Before Being Seen	8,344	1%	2%	2%
Time from ER Arrival to Admit. (minutes)	211	208	257	274
Time from ER Arrival to Discharge (minutes)[5]	-	-	142	134
Time in ER Before Being Evaluated (minutes)[5]	-	-	30	26
Time to Pain Meds for Fractures (minutes)	24	53	67	57
Heart Attack Care				
Aspirin Given at Discharge[1,3]	-	-	99%	99%
Fibrinolytic Meds Within 30 Min. of Arrival[3,7]	-	-	50%	54%
PCI Within 90 Minutes of Arrival[3,7]	-	-	93%	96%
Statin Prescribed at Discharge[1,3]	-	-	98%	98%
Heart Failure Care				
ACE Inhibitor or ARB for LVSD[1,3]	-	-	96%	97%
Discharge Instructions Given[1,3]	-	-	94%	94%
Evaluation of LVS Function[1,3]	-	-	98%	99%
Medicare Spending				
Medicare Spending per Patient (ratio)	-	-	0.96	0.98
Pneumonia Care				
Appropriate Initial Antibiotic Given	15	87%	94%	95%
Blood Culture Timing	21	95%	97%	98%
Pregnancy and Delivery Care				
Newborn Deliveries Scheduled Early[5]	-	-	10%	6%
Preventive Care				
Immunization for Influenza	132	86%	94%	90%
Immunization for Pneumonia	226	89%	95%	92%
Stroke Care				
Anticoagulation Therapy for Atrial Fibrillation[5]	-	-	94%	95%
Antithrombotic Therapy Timing[5]	-	-	98%	98%
Assessed for Rehabilitation[5]	-	-	96%	97%

NOTE: Hospital profiles are in alphabetical order by state, then city, then hospital within the city; Rankings exclude hospitals with less than 25 cases except for patient surveys which excludes hospitals with less than 100 cases; (a) 100-299 cases; (1) The number of cases/patients is too few to report; (2) Data submitted were based on a sample of cases/patients; (3) Results are based on a shorter time period than required; (4) Data suppressed by CMS for one or more quarters; (5) Results are not available for this reporting period; (6) Fewer than 100 patients completed the HCAHPS survey; (7) No cases met the criteria for this measure; (8) The lower limit of the confidence interval cannot be calculated if the number of observed infections equals zero; (9) No data are available from the state/territory for this reporting period; (10) The scores shown reflect fewer than 50 completed surveys; (11) There were discrepancies in the data collection process; (12) This measure does not apply to this hospital for this reporting period; (13) Results cannot be calculated for this reporting period; (14) The results for this state are combined with nearby states to protect confidentiality; Please refer to the User's Guide for a full explanation of data.

Discharged on Antithrombotic Therapy[5]	-	-	98%	99%
Discharged on Statin Medication[5]	-	-	91%	94%
Thrombolytic Therapy Timing[5]	-	-	67%	66%
Venous Thromboembolism Prophylaxis[5]	-	-	91%	94%
Written Stroke Educational Materials Given[5]	-	-	84%	88%
Surgical Care Improvement Project				
Appropriate Beta Blocker Usage[3,7]	-	-	98%	98%
Appropriate VTP Within 24 Hours[1,3]	-	-	98%	98%
Controlled Postoperative Blood Glucose[3,7]	-	-	95%	97%
Perioperative Temperature Management[1,3]	-	-	100%	100%
Prophylactic Antibiotic Selection[1,3]	-	-	99%	99%
Prophylactic Antibiotic Selection (Outpatient)[5]	-	-	97%	98%
Prophylactic Antibiotic Stopped[1,3]	-	-	98%	98%
Prophylactic Antibiotic Timing[1,3]	-	-	99%	99%
Prophylactic Antibiotic Timing (Outpatient)[5]	-	-	97%	98%
Urinary Catheter Removal[1,3]	-	-	98%	97%
Survey of Patients' Hospital Experiences				
Area Around Room 'Always' Quiet at Night[6]	<100	56%	58%	61%
Doctors 'Always' Communicated Well[6]	<100	89%	82%	82%
Home Recovery Information Given[6]	<100	91%	85%	85%
Hospital Given 9 or 10 on 10 Point Scale[6]	<100	70%	66%	71%
Meds 'Always' Explained Before Given[6]	<100	71%	64%	64%
Nurses 'Always' Communicated Well[6]	<100	79%	78%	79%
Pain 'Always' Well Controlled[6]	<100	64%	70%	71%
Room and Bathroom 'Always' Clean[6]	<100	81%	75%	73%
Timely Help 'Always' Received[6]	<100	75%	68%	68%
Would Definitely Recommend Hospital[6]	<100	64%	66%	71%
Use of Medical Imaging				
Cardiac Imaging Stress Test before Surgery[1]			4.9%	5.3%
Combination Abdominal CT Scan	190	34.7%	14.4%	10.5%
Combination Brain/Sinus CT Scan	181	0.6%	3%	2.7%
Combination Chest CT Scan	85	0.0%	2.8%	2.7%
Follow-up Mammogram/Ultrasound	226	4.4%	8.8%	8.8%
Lumbar Spine MRI for Low Back Pain[1]	-	-	38.4%	37.2%

Summersville Regional Medical Center

400 Fairview Heights Road
Summersville, WV 26651
Phone: 304-872-2891
Fax: 304-872-4546
E-mail: susies@wirefire.com
URL: www.summersvillememorial.org
Type: Acute Care Hospitals
Emergency Services: Yes
Ownership: Government - Local
Beds: 109

Key Personnel:
Infection Control.............. Paula Fields, RN
Emergency Room .... Robert Fleer, MD
Anesthesiology................ Cecil Graham, MD
CEO/President................ Debra Hill
Quality Assurance .... Susie Keaton, RN
Operating Room.............. Betty O'Neil, RN
Chief of Medical Staff.......... Mark Wanez

Measure	Cases	This Hosp.	State Avg.	U.S. Avg.
Blood Clot Prevention and Treatment				
Anticoagulation Overlap Therapy[2]	12	67%	90%	93%
ICU Venous Thromboembolism Prophylaxis[2]	44	73%	88%	92%
Incidence of Potentially Preventable VTE[1,2]	-	-	12%	10%
UFH with Dosages/Platelet Monitoring[1,2]	-	-	98%	97%
Venous Thromboembolism Prophylaxis[2]	128	68%	79%	85%
Warfarin Therapy Discharge Instructions[2]	11	91%	80%	75%
Chest Pain/Possible Heart Attack Care				
Aspirin Given Within 24 Hours of Arrival	127	94%	96%	96%
Fibrinolytic Meds Within 30 Min. of Arrival	14	86%	74%	58%
Average Time to ECG (minutes)	134	9	8	7
Average Time to Transfer (minutes)[1]	-	-	109	60
Children's Asthma Care				
Received Home Management Plan of Care	-	-	-	88%
Received Reliever Medication	-	-	-	100%
Received Systemic Corticosteroids	-	-	-	100%
Emergency Department				
Admittance Decision Time (minutes)[2]	271	100	76	98
Head CT Results Within 45 Min. of Arrival	14	57%	43%	57%
Patients Who Left ER Before Being Seen	24,070	2%	2%	2%
Time from ER Arrival to Admit. (minutes)[2]	275	275	257	274
Time from ER Arrival to Discharge (minutes)	371	150	142	134
Time in ER Before Being Evaluated (minutes)	404	36	30	26
Time to Pain Meds for Fractures (minutes)	114	64	67	57
Heart Attack Care				
Aspirin Given at Discharge[1,3]	-	-	99%	99%
Fibrinolytic Meds Within 30 Min. of Arrival[3,7]	-	-	50%	54%
PCI Within 90 Minutes of Arrival[3,7]	-	-	93%	96%
Statin Prescribed at Discharge[1,3]	-	-	98%	98%
Heart Failure Care				
ACE Inhibitor or ARB for LVSD	20	70%	96%	97%
Discharge Instructions Given	35	94%	94%	94%
Evaluation of LVS Function	40	90%	98%	99%
Medicare Spending				
Medicare Spending per Patient (ratio)	-	0.92	0.96	0.98
Pneumonia Care				
Appropriate Initial Antibiotic Given[1]	-	-	94%	95%
Blood Culture Timing	117	95%	97%	98%
Pregnancy and Delivery Care				
Newborn Deliveries Scheduled Early[2]	27	7%	10%	6%
Preventive Care				
Immunization for Influenza[2]	252	85%	94%	90%
Immunization for Pneumonia[2]	301	88%	95%	92%
Stroke Care				
Anticoagulation Therapy for Atrial Fibrillation[1]	-	-	94%	95%
Antithrombotic Therapy Timing	18	89%	98%	98%
Assessed for Rehabilitation	17	100%	96%	97%
Discharged on Antithrombotic Therapy	16	94%	98%	99%
Discharged on Statin Medication	13	54%	91%	94%
Thrombolytic Therapy Timing[1]	-	-	67%	66%
Venous Thromboembolism Prophylaxis	19	89%	91%	94%
Written Stroke Educational Materials Given[1]	-	-	84%	88%
Surgical Care Improvement Project				
Appropriate Beta Blocker Usage	28	82%	98%	98%
Appropriate VTP Within 24 Hours	70	94%	98%	98%
Controlled Postoperative Blood Glucose[7]	-	-	95%	97%
Perioperative Temperature Management	74	99%	100%	100%
Prophylactic Antibiotic Selection	43	95%	99%	99%
Prophylactic Antibiotic Selection (Outpatient)	23	96%	97%	98%
Prophylactic Antibiotic Stopped	43	100%	98%	98%
Prophylactic Antibiotic Timing	43	98%	99%	99%
Prophylactic Antibiotic Timing (Outpatient)	28	79%	97%	98%
Urinary Catheter Removal	51	82%	98%	97%
Survey of Patients' Hospital Experiences				
Area Around Room 'Always' Quiet at Night	300+	49%	58%	61%
Doctors 'Always' Communicated Well	300+	82%	82%	82%
Home Recovery Information Given	300+	80%	85%	85%
Hospital Given 9 or 10 on 10 Point Scale	300+	55%	66%	71%
Meds 'Always' Explained Before Given	300+	65%	64%	64%
Nurses 'Always' Communicated Well	300+	75%	78%	79%
Pain 'Always' Well Controlled	300+	66%	70%	71%
Room and Bathroom 'Always' Clean	300+	71%	75%	73%
Timely Help 'Always' Received	300+	59%	68%	68%
Would Definitely Recommend Hospital	300+	56%	66%	71%
Use of Medical Imaging				
Cardiac Imaging Stress Test before Surgery	91	4.4%	4.9%	5.3%
Combination Abdominal CT Scan	483	10.1%	14.4%	10.5%
Combination Brain/Sinus CT Scan	566	2.7%	3%	2.7%
Combination Chest CT Scan	187	19.3%	2.8%	2.7%
Follow-up Mammogram/Ultrasound	249	8.4%	8.8%	8.8%
Lumbar Spine MRI for Low Back Pain	81	39.5%	38.4%	37.2%

Webster County Memorial Hospital

PO Box 312 (miller Mountain Drive)
Webster Springs, WV 26288
Phone: 304-847-5682
Fax: 304-847-7660
E-mail: admin@wcmhwv.com
URL: www.wcmhwv.com
Type: Critical Access Hospitals
Emergency Services: Yes
Ownership: Voluntary non-profit - Private
Beds: 25

Key Personnel:
Emergency Room .... Larry Clevenger, MD
Pediatric Ambulatory Care ...... Mark Hardway, MD
Infection Control.............. Mary Leonard
Chief of Medical Staff.......... Robert Mace, MD
Patient Relations .... Betty Skidmore
Quality Assurance .... Betty Skidmore

Measure	Cases	This Hosp.	State Avg.	U.S. Avg.
Blood Clot Prevention and Treatment				
Anticoagulation Overlap Therapy[5]	-	-	90%	93%
ICU Venous Thromboembolism Prophylaxis[5]	-	-	88%	92%
Incidence of Potentially Preventable VTE[5]	-	-	12%	10%
UFH with Dosages/Platelet Monitoring[5]	-	-	98%	97%
Venous Thromboembolism Prophylaxis[5]	-	-	79%	85%
Warfarin Therapy Discharge Instructions[5]	-	-	80%	75%
Chest Pain/Possible Heart Attack Care				
Aspirin Given Within 24 Hours of Arrival	-	-	96%	96%
Fibrinolytic Meds Within 30 Min. of Arrival	-	-	74%	58%
Average Time to ECG (minutes)	-	-	8	7
Average Time to Transfer (minutes)	-	-	109	60
Children's Asthma Care				
Received Home Management Plan of Care	-	-	-	88%
Received Reliever Medication	-	-	-	100%
Received Systemic Corticosteroids	-	-	-	100%
Emergency Department				
Admittance Decision Time (minutes)[5]	-	-	76	98
Head CT Results Within 45 Min. of Arrival	-	-	43%	57%
Patients Who Left ER Before Being Seen	-	-	2%	2%
Time from ER Arrival to Admit. (minutes)[5]	-	-	257	274
Time from ER Arrival to Discharge (minutes)	-	-	142	134
Time in ER Before Being Evaluated (minutes)	-	-	30	26
Time to Pain Meds for Fractures (minutes)	-	-	67	57
Heart Attack Care				
Aspirin Given at Discharge[5]	-	-	99%	99%
Fibrinolytic Meds Within 30 Min. of Arrival[5]	-	-	50%	54%
PCI Within 90 Minutes of Arrival[5]	-	-	93%	96%
Statin Prescribed at Discharge[5]	-	-	98%	98%
Heart Failure Care				
ACE Inhibitor or ARB for LVSD[3,7]	-	-	96%	97%
Discharge Instructions Given[1,3]	-	-	94%	94%
Evaluation of LVS Function[1,3]	-	-	98%	99%
Medicare Spending				
Medicare Spending per Patient (ratio)	-	-	0.96	0.98
Pneumonia Care				
Appropriate Initial Antibiotic Given[3]	28	64%	94%	95%
Blood Culture Timing[3]	25	88%	97%	98%
Pregnancy and Delivery Care				
Newborn Deliveries Scheduled Early[5]	-	-	10%	6%
Preventive Care				
Immunization for Influenza[5]	-	-	94%	90%
Immunization for Pneumonia[5]	-	-	95%	92%
Stroke Care				
Anticoagulation Therapy for Atrial Fibrillation[5]	-	-	94%	95%
Antithrombotic Therapy Timing[5]	-	-	98%	98%
Assessed for Rehabilitation[5]	-	-	96%	97%
Discharged on Antithrombotic Therapy[5]	-	-	98%	99%
Discharged on Statin Medication[5]	-	-	91%	94%
Thrombolytic Therapy Timing[5]	-	-	67%	66%
Venous Thromboembolism Prophylaxis[5]	-	-	91%	94%
Written Stroke Educational Materials Given[5]	-	-	84%	88%
Surgical Care Improvement Project				
Appropriate Beta Blocker Usage[5]	-	-	98%	98%
Appropriate VTP Within 24 Hours[5]	-	-	98%	98%
Controlled Postoperative Blood Glucose[5]	-	-	95%	97%
Perioperative Temperature Management[5]	-	-	100%	100%
Prophylactic Antibiotic Selection[5]	-	-	99%	99%
Prophylactic Antibiotic Selection (Outpatient)	-	-	97%	98%
Prophylactic Antibiotic Stopped[5]	-	-	98%	98%
Prophylactic Antibiotic Timing[5]	-	-	99%	99%
Prophylactic Antibiotic Timing (Outpatient)	-	-	97%	98%
Urinary Catheter Removal[5]	-	-	98%	97%
Survey of Patients' Hospital Experiences				
Area Around Room 'Always' Quiet at Night[5]	-	-	58%	61%
Doctors 'Always' Communicated Well[5]	-	-	82%	82%
Home Recovery Information Given[5]	-	-	85%	85%
Hospital Given 9 or 10 on 10 Point Scale[5]	-	-	66%	71%
Meds 'Always' Explained Before Given[5]	-	-	64%	64%
Nurses 'Always' Communicated Well[5]	-	-	78%	79%
Pain 'Always' Well Controlled[5]	-	-	70%	71%
Room and Bathroom 'Always' Clean[5]	-	-	75%	73%

NOTE: Hospital profiles are in alphabetical order by state, then city, then hospital within the city; Rankings exclude hospitals with less than 25 cases except for patient surveys which excludes hospitals with less than 100 cases; (a) 100-299 cases; (1) The number of cases/patients is too few to report; (2) Data submitted were based on a sample of cases/patients; (3) Results are based on a shorter time period than required; (4) Data suppressed by CMS for one or more quarters; (5) Results are not available for this reporting period; (6) Fewer than 100 patients completed the HCAHPS survey; (7) No cases met the criteria for this measure; (8) The lower limit of the confidence interval cannot be calculated if the number of observed infections equals zero; (9) No data are available from the state/territory for this reporting period; (10) The scores shown reflect fewer than 50 completed surveys; (11) There were discrepancies in the data collection process; (12) This measure does not apply to this hospital for this reporting period; (13) Results cannot be calculated for this reporting period; (14) The results for this state are combined with nearby states to protect confidentiality; Please refer to the User's Guide for a full explanation of data.

Measure	Cases	This Hosp.	State Avg.	U.S. Avg.
Timely Help 'Always' Received[5]	-	-	68%	68%
Would Definitely Recommend Hospital[5]	-	-	66%	71%
Use of Medical Imaging				
Cardiac Imaging Stress Test before Surgery	-	-	4.9%	5.3%
Combination Abdominal CT Scan	-	-	14.4%	10.5%
Combination Brain/Sinus CT Scan	-	-	3%	2.7%
Combination Chest CT Scan	-	-	2.8%	2.7%
Follow-up Mammogram/Ultrasound	-	-	8.8%	8.8%
Lumbar Spine MRI for Low Back Pain	-	-	38.4%	37.2%

Weirton Medical Center

601 Colliers Way
Weirton, WV 26062
Phone: 304-797-6000
Fax: 304-797-6449
URL: www.weirtonmedical.com
Type: Acute Care Hospitals
Emergency Services: Yes
Ownership: Government - Local
Beds: 240

Key Personnel:
Operating Room.............. Adnan Abla, RN
Radiology................... Peter Aragones
Emergency Room .... Neal Aulick
CEO/President............... Joseph P Endrich, MD
Chief of Medical Staff.......... Garry Hanson
Quality Assurance .... R Nolan
Cardiac Laboratory............ Carletta Williams

Measure	Cases	This Hosp.	State Avg.	U.S. Avg.
Blood Clot Prevention and Treatment				
Anticoagulation Overlap Therapy[2]	60	63%	90%	93%
ICU Venous Thromboembolism Prophylaxis[2]	84	63%	88%	92%
Incidence of Potentially Preventable VTE[1,2]	-	-	12%	10%
UFH with Dosages/Platelet Monitoring[2]	48	98%	98%	97%
Venous Thromboembolism Prophylaxis[2]	369	44%	79%	85%
Warfarin Therapy Discharge Instructions[2]	39	51%	80%	75%
Chest Pain/Possible Heart Attack Care				
Aspirin Given Within 24 Hours of Arrival[1,3]	-	-	96%	96%
Fibrinolytic Meds Within 30 Min. of Arrival[3,7]	-	-	74%	58%
Average Time to ECG (minutes)[1,3]	-	-	8	7
Average Time to Transfer (minutes)[3,7]	-	-	109	60
Children's Asthma Care				
Received Home Management Plan of Care	-	-	-	88%
Received Reliever Medication	-	-	-	100%
Received Systemic Corticosteroids	-	-	-	100%
Emergency Department				
Admittance Decision Time (minutes)[2]	528	60	76	98
Head CT Results Within 45 Min. of Arrival[1]	-	-	43%	57%
Patients Who Left ER Before Being Seen	37,638	0%	2%	2%
Time from ER Arrival to Admit. (minutes)[2]	642	199	257	274
Time from ER Arrival to Discharge (minutes)	369	104	142	134
Time in ER Before Being Evaluated (minutes)	378	31	30	26
Time to Pain Meds for Fractures (minutes)	94	52	67	57
Heart Attack Care				
Aspirin Given at Discharge	59	95%	99%	99%
Fibrinolytic Meds Within 30 Min. of Arrival[7]	-	-	50%	54%
PCI Within 90 Minutes of Arrival[1]	-	-	93%	96%
Statin Prescribed at Discharge	56	91%	98%	98%
Heart Failure Care				
ACE Inhibitor or ARB for LVSD	37	100%	96%	97%
Discharge Instructions Given	129	95%	94%	94%
Evaluation of LVS Function	181	99%	98%	99%
Medicare Spending				
Medicare Spending per Patient (ratio)	-	1.01	0.96	0.98
Pneumonia Care				
Appropriate Initial Antibiotic Given	202	96%	94%	95%
Blood Culture Timing	292	100%	97%	98%
Pregnancy and Delivery Care				
Newborn Deliveries Scheduled Early[2]	25	80%	10%	6%
Preventive Care				
Immunization for Influenza[2]	545	92%	94%	90%
Immunization for Pneumonia[2]	802	90%	95%	92%
Stroke Care				
Anticoagulation Therapy for Atrial Fibrillation[1,2]	-	-	94%	95%
Antithrombotic Therapy Timing[2]	48	96%	98%	98%
Assessed for Rehabilitation[2]	48	69%	96%	97%
Discharged on Antithrombotic Therapy[2]	45	93%	98%	99%
Discharged on Statin Medication[2]	40	55%	91%	94%
Thrombolytic Therapy Timing[1,2]	-	-	67%	66%
Venous Thromboembolism Prophylaxis[2]	50	30%	91%	94%
Written Stroke Educational Materials Given[2]	34	0%	84%	88%
Surgical Care Improvement Project				
Appropriate Beta Blocker Usage	90	98%	98%	98%
Appropriate VTP Within 24 Hours	226	96%	98%	98%
Controlled Postoperative Blood Glucose[7]	-	-	95%	97%
Perioperative Temperature Management	270	100%	100%	100%
Prophylactic Antibiotic Selection	178	98%	99%	99%
Prophylactic Antibiotic Selection (Outpatient)	104	95%	97%	98%
Prophylactic Antibiotic Stopped	174	89%	98%	98%
Prophylactic Antibiotic Timing	178	99%	99%	99%
Prophylactic Antibiotic Timing (Outpatient)	108	93%	97%	98%
Urinary Catheter Removal	145	94%	98%	97%
Survey of Patients' Hospital Experiences				
Area Around Room 'Always' Quiet at Night	300+	42%	58%	61%
Doctors 'Always' Communicated Well	300+	76%	82%	82%
Home Recovery Information Given	300+	83%	85%	85%
Hospital Given 9 or 10 on 10 Point Scale	300+	49%	66%	71%
Meds 'Always' Explained Before Given	300+	56%	64%	64%
Nurses 'Always' Communicated Well	300+	73%	78%	79%
Pain 'Always' Well Controlled	300+	65%	70%	71%
Room and Bathroom 'Always' Clean	300+	66%	75%	73%
Timely Help 'Always' Received	300+	58%	68%	68%
Would Definitely Recommend Hospital	300+	51%	66%	71%
Use of Medical Imaging				
Cardiac Imaging Stress Test before Surgery	261	4.2%	4.9%	5.3%
Combination Abdominal CT Scan	603	9.3%	14.4%	10.5%
Combination Brain/Sinus CT Scan[1]	-	-	3%	2.7%
Combination Chest CT Scan	241	2.1%	2.8%	2.7%
Follow-up Mammogram/Ultrasound	626	11.7%	8.8%	8.8%
Lumbar Spine MRI for Low Back Pain	82	43.9%	38.4%	37.2%

Welch Community Hospital

454 Mcdowell Street
Welch, WV 24801
Phone: 304-436-8461
Fax: 304-436-6380
Type: Acute Care Hospitals
Emergency Services: Yes
Ownership: Government - State
Beds: 124

Key Personnel:
Emergency Room .... Barbara Dalton, RN
CEO/President.............. Walter J Garrett
Administrator .... Walter J. Garrett
Intensive Care Unit........... Janice Hagy, RN
Infection Control............. Peggy Miller, RN
Operating Room.............. Debbie Myers, RN
Chief of Medical Staff......... Chandra P. Sharma, MD
Anesthesiology............... Bill Shrewsberry

Measure	Cases	This Hosp.	State Avg.	U.S. Avg.
Blood Clot Prevention and Treatment				
Anticoagulation Overlap Therapy[1,2]	-	-	90%	93%
ICU Venous Thromboembolism Prophylaxis[2]	34	68%	88%	92%
Incidence of Potentially Preventable VTE[2,7]	-	-	12%	10%
UFH with Dosages/Platelet Monitoring[2,7]	-	-	98%	97%
Venous Thromboembolism Prophylaxis[2]	54	52%	79%	85%
Warfarin Therapy Discharge Instructions[1,2]	-	-	80%	75%
Chest Pain/Possible Heart Attack Care				
Aspirin Given Within 24 Hours of Arrival[5]	-	-	96%	96%
Fibrinolytic Meds Within 30 Min. of Arrival[5]	-	-	74%	58%
Average Time to ECG (minutes)[5]	-	-	8	7
Average Time to Transfer (minutes)[5]	-	-	109	60
Children's Asthma Care				
Received Home Management Plan of Care	-	-	-	88%
Received Reliever Medication	-	-	-	100%
Received Systemic Corticosteroids	-	-	-	100%
Emergency Department				
Admittance Decision Time (minutes)[2]	260	75	76	98
Head CT Results Within 45 Min. of Arrival[1]	-	-	43%	57%
Patients Who Left ER Before Being Seen	9,615	2%	2%	2%
Time from ER Arrival to Admit. (minutes)[2]	290	308	257	274
Time from ER Arrival to Discharge (minutes)	327	175	142	134
Time in ER Before Being Evaluated (minutes)	434	34	30	26
Time to Pain Meds for Fractures (minutes)	49	74	67	57
Heart Attack Care				
Aspirin Given at Discharge[5]	-	-	99%	99%
Fibrinolytic Meds Within 30 Min. of Arrival[5]	-	-	50%	54%
PCI Within 90 Minutes of Arrival[5]	-	-	93%	96%
Statin Prescribed at Discharge[5]	-	-	98%	98%
Heart Failure Care				
ACE Inhibitor or ARB for LVSD[3,7]	-	-	96%	97%
Discharge Instructions Given[1,3]	-	-	94%	94%
Evaluation of LVS Function[1,3]	-	-	98%	99%
Medicare Spending				
Medicare Spending per Patient (ratio)	-	0.92	0.96	0.98
Pneumonia Care				
Appropriate Initial Antibiotic Given[2]	40	90%	94%	95%
Blood Culture Timing[2]	52	73%	97%	98%
Pregnancy and Delivery Care				
Newborn Deliveries Scheduled Early[2]	12	25%	10%	6%
Preventive Care				
Immunization for Influenza[2]	271	79%	94%	90%
Immunization for Pneumonia[2]	290	86%	95%	92%
Stroke Care				
Anticoagulation Therapy for Atrial Fibrillation[5]	-	-	94%	95%
Antithrombotic Therapy Timing[5]	-	-	98%	98%
Assessed for Rehabilitation[5]	-	-	96%	97%
Discharged on Antithrombotic Therapy[5]	-	-	98%	99%
Discharged on Statin Medication[5]	-	-	91%	94%
Thrombolytic Therapy Timing[5]	-	-	67%	66%
Venous Thromboembolism Prophylaxis[5]	-	-	91%	94%
Written Stroke Educational Materials Given[5]	-	-	84%	88%
Surgical Care Improvement Project				
Appropriate Beta Blocker Usage[1]	-	-	98%	98%
Appropriate VTP Within 24 Hours	31	74%	98%	98%
Controlled Postoperative Blood Glucose[7]	-	-	95%	97%
Perioperative Temperature Management	34	85%	100%	100%
Prophylactic Antibiotic Selection	17	88%	99%	99%
Prophylactic Antibiotic Selection (Outpatient)[5]	-	-	97%	98%
Prophylactic Antibiotic Stopped	16	62%	98%	98%
Prophylactic Antibiotic Timing	17	100%	99%	99%
Prophylactic Antibiotic Timing (Outpatient)[5]	-	-	97%	98%
Urinary Catheter Removal[1]	-	-	98%	97%
Survey of Patients' Hospital Experiences				
Area Around Room 'Always' Quiet at Night	(a)	63%	58%	61%
Doctors 'Always' Communicated Well	(a)	83%	82%	82%
Home Recovery Information Given	(a)	89%	85%	85%
Hospital Given 9 or 10 on 10 Point Scale	(a)	67%	66%	71%
Meds 'Always' Explained Before Given	(a)	66%	64%	64%
Nurses 'Always' Communicated Well	(a)	79%	78%	79%
Pain 'Always' Well Controlled	(a)	71%	70%	71%
Room and Bathroom 'Always' Clean	(a)	84%	75%	73%
Timely Help 'Always' Received	(a)	72%	68%	68%
Would Definitely Recommend Hospital	(a)	59%	66%	71%
Use of Medical Imaging				
Cardiac Imaging Stress Test before Surgery[7]	-	-	4.9%	5.3%
Combination Abdominal CT Scan	163	1.8%	14.4%	10.5%
Combination Brain/Sinus CT Scan[1]	-	-	3%	2.7%
Combination Chest CT Scan	78	0.0%	2.8%	2.7%
Follow-up Mammogram/Ultrasound	87	6.9%	8.8%	8.8%
Lumbar Spine MRI for Low Back Pain[7]	-	-	38.4%	37.2%

Stonewall Jackson Memorial Hospital

230 Hospital Plaza
Weston, WV 26452
Phone: 304-269-8080
Fax: 304-269-8090
E-mail: hospital@stonewallhospital.com
URL: www.stonewallhospital.com
Type: Acute Care Hospitals
Emergency Services: Yes
Ownership: Voluntary non-profit - Private
Beds: 70

Key Personnel:
Infection Control.............. Diane Bennett, RN
Operating Room.............. Mark Casto, RN
Quality Assurance .... Debbie Corder
Emergency Room .... Carla Hamner, RN
Intensive Care Unit........... Lisa Henry, RN
Chief of Medical Staff.......... K Mahmoud, MD
CEO/President............... David D Shaffer
Patient Relations .... Julia Spelsburg

Measure	Cases	This Hosp.	State Avg.	U.S. Avg.
Blood Clot Prevention and Treatment				

NOTE: Hospital profiles are in alphabetical order by state, then city, then hospital within the city; Rankings exclude hospitals with less than 25 cases except for patient surveys which excludes hospitals with less than 100 cases; (a) 100-299 cases; (1) The number of cases/patients is too few to report; (2) Data submitted were based on a sample of cases/patients; (3) Results are based on a shorter time period than required; (4) Data suppressed by CMS for one or more quarters; (5) Results are not available for this reporting period; (6) Fewer than 100 patients completed the HCAHPS survey; (7) No cases met the criteria for this measure; (8) The lower limit of the confidence interval cannot be calculated if the number of observed infections equals zero; (9) No data are available from the state/territory for this reporting period; (10) The scores shown reflect fewer than 50 completed surveys; (11) There were discrepancies in the data collection process; (12) This measure does not apply to this hospital for this reporting period; (13) Results cannot be calculated for this reporting period; (14) The results for this state are combined with nearby states to protect confidentiality; Please refer to the User's Guide for a full explanation of data.

Measure	Cases	This Hosp.	State Avg.	U.S. Avg.
Anticoagulation Overlap Therapy[2]	18	100%	90%	93%
ICU Venous Thromboembolism Prophylaxis[2]	38	92%	88%	92%
Incidence of Potentially Preventable VTE[1,2]	-	-	12%	10%
UFH with Dosages/Platelet Monitoring[1,2]	-	-	98%	97%
Venous Thromboembolism Prophylaxis[2]	206	83%	79%	85%
Warfarin Therapy Discharge Instructions[2]	16	94%	80%	75%
Chest Pain/Possible Heart Attack Care				
Aspirin Given Within 24 Hours of Arrival	65	98%	96%	96%
Fibrinolytic Meds Within 30 Min. of Arrival[1]	-	-	74%	58%
Average Time to ECG (minutes)	64	2	8	7
Average Time to Transfer (minutes)[1]	-	-	109	60
Children's Asthma Care				
Received Home Management Plan of Care	-	-	-	88%
Received Reliever Medication	-	-	-	100%
Received Systemic Corticosteroids	-	-	-	100%
Emergency Department				
Admittance Decision Time (minutes)[2]	342	51	76	98
Head CT Results Within 45 Min. of Arrival[1]	-	-	43%	57%
Patients Who Left ER Before Being Seen	15,863	1%	2%	2%
Time from ER Arrival to Admit. (minutes)[2]	359	152	257	274
Time from ER Arrival to Discharge (minutes)	393	76	142	134
Time in ER Before Being Evaluated (minutes)	414	13	30	26
Time to Pain Meds for Fractures (minutes)	44	53	67	57
Heart Attack Care				
Aspirin Given at Discharge	12	100%	99%	99%
Fibrinolytic Meds Within 30 Min. of Arrival[7]	-	-	50%	54%
PCI Within 90 Minutes of Arrival[7]	-	-	93%	96%
Statin Prescribed at Discharge	14	100%	98%	98%
Heart Failure Care				
ACE Inhibitor or ARB for LVSD	34	100%	96%	97%
Discharge Instructions Given	78	94%	94%	94%
Evaluation of LVS Function	88	100%	98%	99%
Medicare Spending				
Medicare Spending per Patient (ratio)	-	0.90	0.96	0.98
Pneumonia Care				
Appropriate Initial Antibiotic Given	75	97%	94%	95%
Blood Culture Timing	103	99%	97%	98%
Pregnancy and Delivery Care				
Newborn Deliveries Scheduled Early[2]	28	0%	10%	6%
Preventive Care				
Immunization for Influenza[2]	274	97%	94%	90%
Immunization for Pneumonia[2]	370	100%	95%	92%
Stroke Care				
Anticoagulation Therapy for Atrial Fibrillation[1]	-	-	94%	95%
Antithrombotic Therapy Timing[1]	-	-	98%	98%
Assessed for Rehabilitation[1]	-	-	96%	97%
Discharged on Antithrombotic Therapy[1]	-	-	98%	99%
Discharged on Statin Medication[1]	-	-	91%	94%
Thrombolytic Therapy Timing[7]	-	-	67%	66%
Venous Thromboembolism Prophylaxis[1]	-	-	91%	94%
Written Stroke Educational Materials Given[1]	-	-	84%	88%
Surgical Care Improvement Project				
Appropriate Beta Blocker Usage	43	98%	98%	98%
Appropriate VTP Within 24 Hours	134	100%	98%	98%
Controlled Postoperative Blood Glucose[7]	-	-	95%	97%
Perioperative Temperature Management	140	100%	100%	100%
Prophylactic Antibiotic Selection	110	100%	99%	99%
Prophylactic Antibiotic Selection (Outpatient)	67	100%	97%	98%
Prophylactic Antibiotic Stopped	105	99%	98%	98%
Prophylactic Antibiotic Timing	110	100%	99%	99%
Prophylactic Antibiotic Timing (Outpatient)	41	100%	97%	98%
Urinary Catheter Removal	107	100%	98%	97%
Survey of Patients' Hospital Experiences				
Area Around Room 'Always' Quiet at Night	300+	55%	58%	61%
Doctors 'Always' Communicated Well	300+	84%	82%	82%
Home Recovery Information Given	300+	87%	85%	85%
Hospital Given 9 or 10 on 10 Point Scale	300+	67%	66%	71%
Meds 'Always' Explained Before Given	300+	71%	64%	64%
Nurses 'Always' Communicated Well	300+	80%	78%	79%
Pain 'Always' Well Controlled	300+	72%	70%	71%
Room and Bathroom 'Always' Clean	300+	81%	75%	73%
Timely Help 'Always' Received	300+	73%	68%	68%
Would Definitely Recommend Hospital	300+	64%	66%	71%
Use of Medical Imaging				
Cardiac Imaging Stress Test before Surgery	177	4.5%	4.9%	5.3%
Combination Abdominal CT Scan	227	37.4%	14.4%	10.5%
Combination Brain/Sinus CT Scan[1]	-	-	3%	2.7%
Combination Chest CT Scan	166	0.6%	2.8%	2.7%
Follow-up Mammogram/Ultrasound	230	4.8%	8.8%	8.8%
Lumbar Spine MRI for Low Back Pain[1]	-	-	38.4%	37.2%

Ohio Valley Medical Center

2000 Eoff Street
Wheeling, WV 26003
Phone: 304-234-0123
Fax: 304-234-1830
URL: www.ohiovalleymedicalcenter.com
Type: Acute Care Hospitals
Emergency Services: Yes
Ownership: Voluntary non-profit - Private
Beds: 200

Key Personnel:
Radiology. . . . . Vicente P Almario
Administrator . . . . Kelly Bettem, FACHE
Chief of Medical Staff. . . . . Satinder Bhullar
President/CEO. . . . . Michael J. Caruso
Quality Assurance . . . . Staci L. Turdo, BSN, RN, CCRN,

Measure	Cases	This Hosp.	State Avg.	U.S. Avg.
Blood Clot Prevention and Treatment				
Anticoagulation Overlap Therapy[2]	35	54%	90%	93%
ICU Venous Thromboembolism Prophylaxis[2]	92	95%	88%	92%
Incidence of Potentially Preventable VTE[1,2]	-	-	12%	10%
UFH with Dosages/Platelet Monitoring[2]	23	100%	98%	97%
Venous Thromboembolism Prophylaxis[2]	231	65%	79%	85%
Warfarin Therapy Discharge Instructions[2]	27	33%	80%	75%
Chest Pain/Possible Heart Attack Care				
Aspirin Given Within 24 Hours of Arrival	33	100%	96%	96%
Fibrinolytic Meds Within 30 Min. of Arrival[7]	-	-	74%	58%
Average Time to ECG (minutes)	33	7	8	7
Average Time to Transfer (minutes)	14	67	109	60
Children's Asthma Care				
Received Home Management Plan of Care	-	-	-	88%
Received Reliever Medication	-	-	-	100%
Received Systemic Corticosteroids	-	-	-	100%
Emergency Department				
Admittance Decision Time (minutes)[2]	479	63	76	98
Head CT Results Within 45 Min. of Arrival[1]	-	-	43%	57%
Patients Who Left ER Before Being Seen	31,790	3%	2%	2%
Time from ER Arrival to Admit. (minutes)[2]	479	230	257	274
Time from ER Arrival to Discharge (minutes)	363	122	142	134
Time in ER Before Being Evaluated (minutes)	423	19	30	26
Time to Pain Meds for Fractures (minutes)	99	43	67	57
Heart Attack Care				
Aspirin Given at Discharge	33	91%	99%	99%
Fibrinolytic Meds Within 30 Min. of Arrival[7]	-	-	50%	54%
PCI Within 90 Minutes of Arrival[7]	-	-	93%	96%
Statin Prescribed at Discharge	29	83%	98%	98%
Heart Failure Care				
ACE Inhibitor or ARB for LVSD	26	85%	96%	97%
Discharge Instructions Given	99	91%	94%	94%
Evaluation of LVS Function	123	97%	98%	99%
Medicare Spending				
Medicare Spending per Patient (ratio)	-	0.99	0.96	0.98
Pneumonia Care				
Appropriate Initial Antibiotic Given	77	97%	94%	95%
Blood Culture Timing	130	98%	97%	98%
Pregnancy and Delivery Care				
Newborn Deliveries Scheduled Early[2]	41	10%	10%	6%
Preventive Care				
Immunization for Influenza[2]	575	90%	94%	90%
Immunization for Pneumonia[2]	582	95%	95%	92%
Stroke Care				
Anticoagulation Therapy for Atrial Fibrillation[1]	-	-	94%	95%
Antithrombotic Therapy Timing	44	98%	98%	98%
Assessed for Rehabilitation	52	96%	96%	97%
Discharged on Antithrombotic Therapy	40	98%	98%	99%
Discharged on Statin Medication	37	84%	91%	94%
Thrombolytic Therapy Timing[1]	-	-	67%	66%
Venous Thromboembolism Prophylaxis	61	70%	91%	94%
Written Stroke Educational Materials Given	24	12%	84%	88%
Surgical Care Improvement Project				
Appropriate Beta Blocker Usage	155	98%	98%	98%
Appropriate VTP Within 24 Hours	451	96%	98%	98%
Controlled Postoperative Blood Glucose[7]	-	-	95%	97%
Perioperative Temperature Management	510	100%	100%	100%
Prophylactic Antibiotic Selection	406	99%	99%	99%
Prophylactic Antibiotic Selection (Outpatient)	75	96%	97%	98%
Prophylactic Antibiotic Stopped	402	97%	98%	98%
Prophylactic Antibiotic Timing	407	98%	99%	99%
Prophylactic Antibiotic Timing (Outpatient)	78	92%	97%	98%
Urinary Catheter Removal	404	98%	98%	97%
Survey of Patients' Hospital Experiences				
Area Around Room 'Always' Quiet at Night	300+	63%	58%	61%
Doctors 'Always' Communicated Well	300+	74%	82%	82%
Home Recovery Information Given	300+	81%	85%	85%
Hospital Given 9 or 10 on 10 Point Scale	300+	65%	66%	71%
Meds 'Always' Explained Before Given	300+	59%	64%	64%
Nurses 'Always' Communicated Well	300+	75%	78%	79%
Pain 'Always' Well Controlled	300+	70%	70%	71%
Room and Bathroom 'Always' Clean	300+	74%	75%	73%
Timely Help 'Always' Received	300+	59%	68%	68%
Would Definitely Recommend Hospital	300+	71%	66%	71%
Use of Medical Imaging				
Cardiac Imaging Stress Test before Surgery[1]	-	-	4.9%	5.3%
Combination Abdominal CT Scan	406	53.7%	14.4%	10.5%
Combination Brain/Sinus CT Scan	327	5.2%	3%	2.7%
Combination Chest CT Scan	311	0.6%	2.8%	2.7%
Follow-up Mammogram/Ultrasound	597	17.8%	8.8%	8.8%
Lumbar Spine MRI for Low Back Pain[1]	-	-	38.4%	37.2%

Wheeling Hospital

1 Medical Park
Wheeling, WV 26003
Phone: 304-243-3000
Fax: 304-243-3060
E-mail: webmaster@wheelinghospital.com
URL: www.wheelinghospital.com
Type: Acute Care Hospitals
Emergency Services: Yes
Ownership: Voluntary non-profit - Church
Beds: 277

Key Personnel:
CEO/President. . . . . Donald H Hofreuter, MD

Measure	Cases	This Hosp.	State Avg.	U.S. Avg.
Blood Clot Prevention and Treatment				
Anticoagulation Overlap Therapy[2]	92	90%	90%	93%
ICU Venous Thromboembolism Prophylaxis[2]	82	78%	88%	92%
Incidence of Potentially Preventable VTE[2]	12	8%	12%	10%
UFH with Dosages/Platelet Monitoring[2]	59	97%	98%	97%
Venous Thromboembolism Prophylaxis[2]	400	60%	79%	85%
Warfarin Therapy Discharge Instructions[2]	61	92%	80%	75%
Chest Pain/Possible Heart Attack Care				
Aspirin Given Within 24 Hours of Arrival[1]	-	-	96%	96%
Fibrinolytic Meds Within 30 Min. of Arrival[3,7]	-	-	74%	58%
Average Time to ECG (minutes)[1]	-	-	8	7
Average Time to Transfer (minutes)[3,7]	-	-	109	60
Children's Asthma Care				
Received Home Management Plan of Care	-	-	-	88%
Received Reliever Medication	-	-	-	100%
Received Systemic Corticosteroids	-	-	-	100%
Emergency Department				
Admittance Decision Time (minutes)[2]	515	75	76	98
Head CT Results Within 45 Min. of Arrival[1]	-	-	43%	57%
Patients Who Left ER Before Being Seen	49,320	2%	2%	2%
Time from ER Arrival to Admit. (minutes)[2]	564	249	257	274
Time from ER Arrival to Discharge (minutes)	423	170	142	134
Time in ER Before Being Evaluated (minutes)	433	31	30	26
Time to Pain Meds for Fractures (minutes)	85	86	67	57
Heart Attack Care				
Aspirin Given at Discharge	462	100%	99%	99%
Fibrinolytic Meds Within 30 Min. of Arrival[7]	-	-	50%	54%
PCI Within 90 Minutes of Arrival	60	97%	93%	96%
Statin Prescribed at Discharge	425	100%	98%	98%
Heart Failure Care				
ACE Inhibitor or ARB for LVSD	71	100%	96%	97%
Discharge Instructions Given	206	98%	94%	94%
Evaluation of LVS Function	274	100%	98%	99%

NOTE: Hospital profiles are in alphabetical order by state, then city, then hospital within the city; Rankings exclude hospitals with less than 25 cases except for patient surveys which excludes hospitals with less than 100 cases; (a) 100-299 cases; (1) The number of cases/patients is too few to report; (2) Data submitted were based on a sample of cases/patients; (3) Results are based on a shorter time period than required; (4) Data suppressed by CMS for one or more quarters; (5) Results are not available for this reporting period; (6) Fewer than 100 patients completed the HCAHPS survey; (7) No cases met the criteria for this measure; (8) The lower limit of the confidence interval cannot be calculated if the number of observed infections equals zero; (9) No data are available from the state/territory for this reporting period; (10) The scores shown reflect fewer than 50 completed surveys; (11) There were discrepancies in the data collection process; (12) This measure does not apply to this hospital for this reporting period; (13) Results cannot be calculated for this reporting period; (14) The results for this state are combined with nearby states to protect confidentiality; Please refer to the User's Guide for a full explanation of data.

Medicare Spending				
Medicare Spending per Patient (ratio)	-	0.99	0.96	0.98
Pneumonia Care				
Appropriate Initial Antibiotic Given	197	97%	94%	95%
Blood Culture Timing	353	99%	97%	98%
Pregnancy and Delivery Care				
Newborn Deliveries Scheduled Early	137	10%	10%	6%
Preventive Care				
Immunization for Influenza[2]	598	98%	94%	90%
Immunization for Pneumonia[2]	763	98%	95%	92%
Stroke Care				
Anticoagulation Therapy for Atrial Fibrillation	19	79%	94%	95%
Antithrombotic Therapy Timing	96	95%	98%	98%
Assessed for Rehabilitation	104	92%	96%	97%
Discharged on Antithrombotic Therapy	95	96%	98%	99%
Discharged on Statin Medication	72	54%	91%	94%
Thrombolytic Therapy Timing	12	42%	67%	66%
Venous Thromboembolism Prophylaxis	111	63%	91%	94%
Written Stroke Educational Materials Given	62	71%	84%	88%
Surgical Care Improvement Project				
Appropriate Beta Blocker Usage	310	98%	98%	98%
Appropriate VTP Within 24 Hours	515	99%	98%	98%
Controlled Postoperative Blood Glucose	203	89%	95%	97%
Perioperative Temperature Management	724	97%	100%	100%
Prophylactic Antibiotic Selection	604	100%	99%	99%
Prophylactic Antibiotic Selection (Outpatient)	353	99%	97%	98%
Prophylactic Antibiotic Stopped	572	96%	98%	98%
Prophylactic Antibiotic Timing	606	97%	99%	99%
Prophylactic Antibiotic Timing (Outpatient)	327	97%	97%	98%
Urinary Catheter Removal	460	98%	98%	97%
Survey of Patients' Hospital Experiences				
Area Around Room 'Always' Quiet at Night	300+	60%	58%	61%
Doctors 'Always' Communicated Well	300+	80%	82%	82%
Home Recovery Information Given	300+	90%	85%	85%
Hospital Given 9 or 10 on 10 Point Scale	300+	71%	66%	71%
Meds 'Always' Explained Before Given	300+	61%	64%	64%
Nurses 'Always' Communicated Well	300+	79%	78%	79%
Pain 'Always' Well Controlled	300+	73%	70%	71%
Room and Bathroom 'Always' Clean	300+	73%	75%	73%
Timely Help 'Always' Received	300+	66%	68%	68%
Would Definitely Recommend Hospital	300+	73%	66%	71%
Use of Medical Imaging				
Cardiac Imaging Stress Test before Surgery	133	3.8%	4.9%	5.3%
Combination Abdominal CT Scan	916	8.0%	14.4%	10.5%
Combination Brain/Sinus CT Scan	799	2.9%	3%	2.7%
Combination Chest CT Scan	682	0.3%	2.8%	2.7%
Follow-up Mammogram/Ultrasound	1,455	8.8%	8.8%	8.8%
Lumbar Spine MRI for Low Back Pain	113	35.4%	38.4%	37.2%

Williamson Memorial Hospital

859 Alderson Street
Williamson, WV 25661
Phone: 304-235-2500
Fax: 304-235-0538
URL: www.hmawmh.com
Type: Acute Care Hospitals
Emergency Services: Yes
Ownership: Voluntary non-profit - Private
Beds: 76

Key Personnel:

Chief of Medical Staff.......... Manuel Angco, MD
Operating Room.............. Nyoka Farley
Anesthesiology............... Jhansi Rani Lanka, MD
Infection Control.............. Sandy Loew
Cardiac Laboratory............ Ashik Patnaik, MD
CEO/President............... Stephen Young

Measure	Cases	This Hosp.	State Avg.	U.S. Avg.
Blood Clot Prevention and Treatment				
Anticoagulation Overlap Therapy[2]	11	100%	90%	93%
ICU Venous Thromboembolism Prophylaxis[2]	32	100%	88%	92%
Incidence of Potentially Preventable VTE[2,7]	-	-	12%	10%
UFH with Dosages/Platelet Monitoring[2,7]	-	-	98%	97%
Venous Thromboembolism Prophylaxis[2]	154	100%	79%	85%
Warfarin Therapy Discharge Instructions[1,2]	-	-	80%	75%
Chest Pain/Possible Heart Attack Care				
Aspirin Given Within 24 Hours of Arrival	33	97%	96%	96%
Fibrinolytic Meds Within 30 Min. of Arrival[7]	-	-	74%	58%
Average Time to ECG (minutes)	37	1	8	7
Average Time to Transfer (minutes)	17	197	109	60
Children's Asthma Care				
Received Home Management Plan of Care	-	-	-	88%
Received Reliever Medication	-	-	-	100%
Received Systemic Corticosteroids	-	-	-	100%
Emergency Department				
Admittance Decision Time (minutes)[2]	376	71	76	98
Head CT Results Within 45 Min. of Arrival[1]	-	-	43%	57%
Patients Who Left ER Before Being Seen	13,736	2%	2%	2%
Time from ER Arrival to Admit. (minutes)[2]	376	240	257	274
Time from ER Arrival to Discharge (minutes)	1,149	153	142	134
Time in ER Before Being Evaluated (minutes)	1,313	52	30	26
Time to Pain Meds for Fractures (minutes)	56	78	67	57
Heart Attack Care				
Aspirin Given at Discharge[1]	-	-	99%	99%
Fibrinolytic Meds Within 30 Min. of Arrival[7]	-	-	50%	54%
PCI Within 90 Minutes of Arrival[7]	-	-	93%	96%
Statin Prescribed at Discharge[1]	-	-	98%	98%
Heart Failure Care				
ACE Inhibitor or ARB for LVSD	12	100%	96%	97%
Discharge Instructions Given	64	94%	94%	94%
Evaluation of LVS Function	70	99%	98%	99%
Medicare Spending				
Medicare Spending per Patient (ratio)	-	0.96	0.96	0.98
Pneumonia Care				
Appropriate Initial Antibiotic Given	49	98%	94%	95%
Blood Culture Timing	76	92%	97%	98%
Pregnancy and Delivery Care				
Newborn Deliveries Scheduled Early[1]	-	-	10%	6%
Preventive Care				
Immunization for Influenza[2]	267	99%	94%	90%
Immunization for Pneumonia[2]	328	100%	95%	92%
Stroke Care				
Anticoagulation Therapy for Atrial Fibrillation[1]	-	-	94%	95%
Antithrombotic Therapy Timing[1]	-	-	98%	98%
Assessed for Rehabilitation[1]	-	-	96%	97%
Discharged on Antithrombotic Therapy[1]	-	-	98%	99%
Discharged on Statin Medication[1]	-	-	91%	94%
Thrombolytic Therapy Timing[7]	-	-	67%	66%
Venous Thromboembolism Prophylaxis[1]	-	-	91%	94%
Written Stroke Educational Materials Given[1]	-	-	84%	88%
Surgical Care Improvement Project				
Appropriate Beta Blocker Usage[1]	-	-	98%	98%
Appropriate VTP Within 24 Hours	36	100%	98%	98%
Controlled Postoperative Blood Glucose[7]	-	-	95%	97%
Perioperative Temperature Management	38	100%	100%	100%
Prophylactic Antibiotic Selection	12	100%	99%	99%
Prophylactic Antibiotic Selection (Outpatient)	15	100%	97%	98%
Prophylactic Antibiotic Stopped	13	92%	98%	98%
Prophylactic Antibiotic Timing	13	69%	99%	99%
Prophylactic Antibiotic Timing (Outpatient)	15	87%	97%	98%
Urinary Catheter Removal[1]	-	-	98%	97%
Survey of Patients' Hospital Experiences				
Area Around Room 'Always' Quiet at Night	(a)	50%	58%	61%
Doctors 'Always' Communicated Well	(a)	88%	82%	82%
Home Recovery Information Given	(a)	82%	85%	85%
Hospital Given 9 or 10 on 10 Point Scale	(a)	61%	66%	71%
Meds 'Always' Explained Before Given	(a)	59%	64%	64%
Nurses 'Always' Communicated Well	(a)	73%	78%	79%
Pain 'Always' Well Controlled	(a)	64%	70%	71%
Room and Bathroom 'Always' Clean	(a)	67%	75%	73%
Timely Help 'Always' Received	(a)	51%	68%	68%
Would Definitely Recommend Hospital	(a)	57%	66%	71%
Use of Medical Imaging				
Cardiac Imaging Stress Test before Surgery	77	6.5%	4.9%	5.3%
Combination Abdominal CT Scan	287	4.2%	14.4%	10.5%
Combination Brain/Sinus CT Scan	306	8.2%	3%	2.7%
Combination Chest CT Scan	85	4.7%	2.8%	2.7%
Follow-up Mammogram/Ultrasound	82	14.6%	8.8%	8.8%
Lumbar Spine MRI for Low Back Pain[1]	-	-	38.4%	37.2%

NOTE: Hospital profiles are in alphabetical order by state, then city, then hospital within the city; Rankings exclude hospitals with less than 25 cases except for patient surveys which excludes hospitals with less than 100 cases; (a) 100-299 cases; (1) The number of cases/patients is too few to report; (2) Data submitted were based on a sample of cases/patients; (3) Results are based on a shorter time period than required; (4) Data suppressed by CMS for one or more quarters; (5) Results are not available for this reporting period; (6) Fewer than 100 patients completed the HCAHPS survey; (7) No cases met the criteria for this measure; (8) The lower limit of the confidence interval cannot be calculated if the number of observed infections equals zero; (9) No data are available from the state/territory for this reporting period; (10) The scores shown reflect fewer than 50 completed surveys; (11) There were discrepancies in the data collection process; (12) This measure does not apply to this hospital for this reporting period; (13) Results cannot be calculated for this reporting period; (14) The results for this state are combined with nearby states to protect confidentiality; Please refer to the User's Guide for a full explanation of data.

Appendix A: 30-Day Death (Mortality) Rates

What Do These Mortality Categories Show?

These categories show how hospitals' risk-adjusted 30-day death (mortality) rates for heart attack, heart failure, and pneumonia compare to the rate across the U.S., after making adjustments for how sick patients were before they were admitted to the hospital and taking into account differences in death rates that might be due to chance.

This first part of this appendix shows hospitals with 30-day risk-adjusted death (mortality) rates that are lower (better) or higher (worse) than the national rate for all three categories. Hospitals are shown to be better or worse than the U.S. national rate only if the data shows with 95% certainty, that the difference between their surgical complication rates and the U.S. national rate is not due to chance.

The second part of this appendix contains state and national summaries with the following column headers:

- **Better Than U.S. National Rate.** Hospitals in the Better Than U.S. National Rate category have risk-adjusted 30-day death (mortality) rates that are lower than the U.S. National Rate, with 95% certainty that this difference is not due to chance.
- **Worse Than U.S. National Rate.** Hospitals in the Worse Than U.S. National Rate category have risk-adjusted 30-day death (mortality) rates that are higher than the U.S. National Rate, with 95% certainty that this difference is not due to chance.
- **No Different Than U.S. National Rate.** Many hospitals in the No Different Than U.S. National Rate category have risk-adjusted 30-day death (mortality) rates that are about the same as the U.S. National Rate. Other hospitals in this category have rates that are higher or lower than the U.S. National Rate, without 95% certainty that these differences are not due to chance.
- **Number of Cases Too Small.** The number of cases is too small to classify the hospital.

Why are Death Rates for Individual Hospitals Not Shown?

Comparisons based on estimated death (mortality) rates alone can be misleading. Risk-adjusted death (mortality) rates are estimated for individual hospitals based on information taken from a particular time period. If a slightly different time period had been chosen, chances are that each hospital's results would have been somewhat different.

A range ("confidence interval" or in this case an "interval estimate") around estimates show how much variation might be due to this kind of chance. In this case, researchers are 95% confident that a hospital's death (mortality) rate fell somewhere within this specified range. The smaller the range, the more precise the estimate.

When hospitals treat a very large number of patients, chance differences will not have much effect on the overall rates. The range will be small, and the estimated death (mortality) rates will be more precise. In hospitals that treat smaller numbers of patients, however, even small chance differences could have a big impact on death (mortality) rates. The 95% confidence interval, or range, will be large, and the estimated death (mortality) rates will be less precise.

Because the number of patients treated at U.S. hospitals varies widely, the precision of hospitals' estimated death (mortality) rates also varies.

Calculation of 30-Day Risk-Standardized Mortality Rates

The 30-day death (mortality) measures are estimates of deaths from any cause within 30 days of a hospital admission, for patients hospitalized with one of several primary diagnoses. Deaths can be counted in the measures regardless of whether the patient dies while still in the hospital or after discharge. Using deaths within 30 days instead of inpatient deaths show a more consistent measurement time window because length of hospital stay varies across patients and hospitals. Also, mortality over longer time periods (such as 90 days) may have less to do with the care received in the hospital and more to do with other complicating illnesses, patients' own behavior, or care provided to patients after hospital discharge. *The Comparative Guide to American Hospitals* reports on the following 30-day mortality measures:

- 30-day death rate for heart attack (acute myocardial infarction [AMI]) patients
- 30-day death rate for heart failure (HF) patients
- 30-day death rate for pneumonia patients

Which Patients are Included

The 30-day death (mortality) measures include hospitalizations for Medicare beneficiaries aged 65 or older who were enrolled in Original Medicare (traditional fee-for-service Medicare) for the entire 12 months prior to their hospital admission. The AMI, heart failure, and pneumonia (death) mortality measures also include patients aged 65 or older who were admitted to Veteran's Health Administration (VA) hospitals. Beneficiaries enrolled in Medicare managed care plans are not included.

Where the Information Comes From

The Centers for Medicare & Medicaid Services (CMS) calculates hospital-specific 30-day mortality rates using Medicare claims and eligibility information. The AMI, HF, and pneumonia mortality measures are also calculated using VA administrative data. Using administrative data makes it possible to calculate mortality rates without having to do medical chart reviews or requiring hospitals to report additional information to CMS. Research conducted during development of the AMI, HF, and pneumonia death (mortality) measures showed that statistical models based on claims data performed well in estimating hospital mortality rates compared to models that are based on information from medical chart reviews.

Risk Adjustment

To make comparison of hospital performance equitable, the 30-day (death) mortality measures adjust for patient characteristics that may make death more likely, even if the hospital provided higher quality of care. These characteristics include the patient's age, past medical history, and other diseases or conditions (comorbidities) the patient had when admitted that are known to increase the patient's risk of dying.

Significance Testing

The statistical model used to calculate 30-day (death) mortality measures also determines how precise the estimates are, and provides the upper and lower bounds of the 95% interval estimates for each hospital's risk-adjusted mortality rates. Interval estimates, which are like confidence intervals, describe the level of uncertainty around the estimated mortality rates.

Comparing Individual Hospital Rates to the U.S. National Rate

To assign hospitals to performance categories, the hospital's interval estimate is compared to the U.S. national 30-day observed (death) mortality rate. If the 95% interval estimate includes the national observed rate for that measure, the hospital's performance is in the "No Different than U.S. National Rate" category. If the entire 95% interval estimate is below the national observed rate for that measure, then the hospital is performing "Better Than U.S. National Rate." If the entire 95% interval estimate is above the national observed rate for that measure, its performance is "WorseThan U.S. National Rate." Hospitals with fewer than 25 eligible cases are placed into a separate category that indicates that the hospital did not have enough cases to reliably tell how well the hospital is performing.

Additional Information

For more detail on how the 30-day (death) mortality rates are calculated, visit QualityNet—Mortality Measures at www.qualitynet.org.

Hospitals whose Acute Myocardial Infarction (Heart Attack) 30-Day Mortality Rate is Better (Lower) than the U.S. National Rate

Hospital	City	State	Phone	Web Site
Advocate Lutheran General Hospital	Park Ridge	Illinois	847-723-2210	www.advocatehealth.com
Alexian Brothers Medical Center	Elk Grove Village	Illinois	847-437-5500	www.alexian.org
Arkansas Heart Hospital	Little Rock	Arkansas	501-219-7000	www.arheart.com
The Aroostook Medical Center	Presque Isle	Maine	207-768-4000	www.tamc.org
Avera Heart Hospital of South Dakota	Sioux Falls	South Dakota	605-977-7000	www.avera.org/heart-hospital
Baptist Memorial Hospital	Memphis	Tennessee	901-226-5000	www.bmhcc.org
Baptist Saint Anthony's Hospital	Amarillo	Texas	806-212-2000	www.bsahs.com
Beebe Medical Center	Lewes	Delaware	302-645-3300	www.beebemed.org
Beth Israel Deaconess Medical Center	Boston	Massachusetts	617-667-7000	www.bidmc.harvard.edu
Boca Raton Regional Hospital	Boca Raton	Florida	561-362-5002	www.brrh.com
Boone Hospital Center	Columbia	Missouri	573-815-8000	www.boone.org
Catholic Medical Center	Manchester	New Hampshire	603-668-3545	www.catholicmedicalcenter.org
Cedars - Sinai Medical Center	Los Angeles	California	310-423-5000	www.cedars-sinai.edu
Centegra Health System - Woodstock Hospital	Woodstock	Illinois	815-788-5823	www.centegra.org
Centinela Hospital Medical Center	Inglewood	California	310-673-4660	www.centinelafreeman.com
Chambersburg Hospital	Chambersburg	Pennsylvania	717-267-3000	www.summithealth.org
Champlain Valley Physicians Hospital Medical Center	Plattsburgh	New York	518-561-2000	www.cvph.org
Cypress Fairbanks Medical Center	Houston	Texas	281-897-3100	www.cyfairhospital.com
Doylestown Hospital	Doylestown	Pennsylvania	215-345-2200	www.dh.org
East Orange General Hospital	East Orange	New Jersey	973-266-4401	www.evh.org
Englewood Hospital & Medical Center	Englewood	New Jersey	201-894-3000	www.englewoodhospital.com
Evangelical Community Hospital	Lewisburg	Pennsylvania	570-522-2200	www.evanhospital.com
Firsthealth Moore Regional Hospital	Pinehurst	North Carolina	910-715-1000	www.firsthealth.org
French Hospital Medical Center	San Luis Obispo	California	805-543-5353	www.frenchmedicalcenter.org
Glendale Adventist Medical Center	Glendale	California	818-409-8202	www.glendaleadventist.com
Good Samaritan Hospital	Dayton	Ohio	937-278-2612	www.goodsamdayton.org
Hackensack University Medical Center	Hackensack	New Jersey	201-996-2000	www.humed.com
Hays Medical Center	Hays	Kansas	785-623-5000	www.haysmed.com
Henry Ford Hospital	Detroit	Michigan	313-916-2600	www.henryfordhospital.com
Holy Cross Hospital	Silver Spring	Maryland	301-754-7000	www.holycrosshealth.org
Holy Name Medical Center	Teaneck	New Jersey	201-833-3000	www.holyname.org
John T Mather Memorial Hospital of Port Jefferson	Port Jefferson	New York	631-473-1320	www.matherhospital.com
Lawrence Hospital Center	Bronxville	New York	914-787-1000	www.lawrencehealth.org
Lehigh Valley Hospital	Allentown	Pennsylvania	610-402-2273	www.lvhhn.org
Lehigh Valley Hospital - Hazleton	Hazleton	Pennsylvania	570-501-4000	www.ghha.org
Loyola Gottlieb Memorial Hospital	Melrose Park	Illinois	708-450-4924	www.gottliebhospital.org
Maimonides Medical Center	Brooklyn	New York	718-283-6000	www.maimonidesmed.org
Massachusetts General Hospital	Boston	Massachusetts	617-726-2000	www.massgeneral.org
Minneapolis VA Medical Center	Minneapolis	Minnesota	612-725-2000	www1.va.gov/minneapolis
Miriam Hospital	Providence	Rhode Island	401-793-2500	www.lifespan.org/partners/tmh
Missouri Baptist Medical Center	Town & Country	Missouri	314-996-5000	www.missouribaptistmedicalcenter.org
Montefiore Medical Center	Bronx	New York	718-920-4321	www.montefiore.org
Morristown Medical Center	Morristown	New Jersey	973-971-5450	www.morristownmemorialhospital.org
Mount Sinai Medical Center	Miami Beach	Florida	305-674-2121	www.msmc.com
Munson Medical Center	Traverse City	Michigan	231-935-5000	www.munsonhealthcare.org
New York - Presbyterian Hospital	New York	New York	212-746-4189	www.nyp.org
North Shore University Hospital	Manhasset	New York	516-562-0100	www.northshorelij.com
Northwestern Memorial Hospital	Chicago	Illinois	312-926-2000	www.nmh.org
NYU Hospitals Center	New York	New York	212-263-7300	www.med.nyu.edu
Oakwood Hospital - Dearborn	Dearborn	Michigan	313-593-7125	www.oakwood.org
Olympia Medical Center	Los Angeles	California	310-657-5900	www.olympiamc.com
Overlook Medical Center	Summit	New Jersey	908-522-2000	www.atlantichealth.org
Palisades Medical Center	North Bergen	New Jersey	201-854-5000	www.palisadesmedical.org
Presence Saint Joseph Hospital - Chicago	Chicago	Illinois	773-665-3000	www.res-health.org
Presence Saint Joseph Medical Center	Joliet	Illinois	815-725-7133	www.provena.org/stjoes
Providence Hospital & Medical Centers	Southfield	Michigan	248-849-3011	www.stjohn.org/providence
Rhode Island Hospital	Providence	Rhode Island	401-444-4000	www.rhodeislandhospital.org
Sarasota Memorial Hospital	Sarasota	Florida	941-917-9000	www.smh.com
Sherman Oaks Hospital	Sherman Oaks	California	818-981-7111	www.shermanoakshospital.com
Southcoast Hospital Group	Fall River	Massachusetts	508-679-3131	www.southcoast.org/charlton
Southside Hospital	Bay Shore	New York	631-968-3000	www.northshorelij.com
Saint Francis Hospital - Roslyn	Roslyn	New York	516-562-6000	www.stfrancisheartcenter.com
Saint Joseph Mercy Hospital	Ann Arbor	Michigan	734-712-3791	www.stjoesannarbor.or
Saint Luke's Hospital Bethlehem	Bethlehem	Pennsylvania	610-954-4000	www.slhn-lehighvalley.org
Saint Luke's Hospital	Chesterfield	Missouri	314-434-1500	www.goodhealthmatters.com

Hospital	City	State	Phone	Web Site
Saint Luke's Hospital of Kansas City	Kansas City	Missouri	816-932-2000	www.staintlukeshealthsystem.org
Saint Mary's Medical Center	Huntington	West Virginia	304-526-1234	www.st-marys.org
Saint Vincent Heart Center of Indiana	Indianapolis	Indiana	317-583-5000	www.theheartcenter.com
Trinity Rock Island	Rock Island	Illinois	309-779-5000	www.trinityqc.com
University of California Davis Medical Center	Sacramento	California	916-734-2011	www.ucdmc.ucdavis.edu
Valley Hospital	Ridgewood	New Jersey	201-447-8000	www.valleyhealth.com
Wakemed - Cary Hospital	Cary	North Carolina	919-350-2550	www.wakemed.org
Waterbury Hospital	Waterbury	Connecticut	203-573-6000	www.waterburyhospital.org
William Beaumont Hospital - Troy	Troy	Michigan	248-964-8800	www.beaumonthospitals.com
Winchester Hospital	Winchester	Massachusetts	781-729-9000	www.winchesterhospital.org
Yale-New Haven Hospital	New Haven	Connecticut	203-688-4242	www.ynhh.org
Yuma Regional Medical Center	Yuma	Arizona	928-336-7275	www.yumaregional.org

Note: Table shows hospitals nationwide whose acute myocardial infarction 30-day risk-adjusted mortality rate is better (lower) than U.S. rate of 15.2%

Hospitals whose Acute Myocardial Infarction (Heart Attack) 30-Day Mortality Rate is Worse (Higher) than the U.S. National Rate

Hospital	City	State	Phone	Web Site
Altru Hospital	Grand Forks	North Dakota	701-780-5000	www.altru.org
Baptist Health Corbin	Corbin	Kentucky	606-528-1212	www.baptistregional.com
Bronson Battle Creek Hospital	Battle Creek	Michigan	269-966-8000	www.bchealth.com
Dallas Regional Medical Center	Mesquite	Texas	214-320-7000	www.dallasregionalmedicalcenter.com
Desert Springs Hospital	Las Vegas	Nevada	702-369-7600	www.desertspringshospital.net/p12.html
Hurley Medical Center	Flint	Michigan	810-257-9000	www.hurleymc.com
Kaweah Delta Medical Center	Visalia	California	559-624-2000	www.kaweahdelta.org
Lafayette General Medical Center	Lafayette	Louisiana	337-289-7991	www.lafayettegeneral.org
Lakes Region General Hospital	Laconia	New Hampshire	603-524-3211	www.lrgh.org
Laredo Medical Center	Laredo	Texas	956-796-5000	www.laredomedical.com
Mclaren Bay Region	Bay City	Michigan	989-894-3000	www.baymed.org
National Park Medical Center	Hot Springs	Arkansas	501-321-1000	www.nationalparkmedical.com
North Hills Hospital	North Richland Hills	Texas	817-255-1000	www.northhillshospital.com
Penobscot Valley Hospital	Lincoln	Maine	207-794-3321	www.pvhhealthcare.org
Robert Wood Johnson University Hospital at Rahway	Rahway	New Jersey	732-381-4200	www.rwjuhr.com/about/history.html
Schuylkill Medical Center - East Norwegian Street	Pottsville	Pennsylvania	570-621-4000	www.schuylkillhealth.com
Saint Marys Regional Medical Center	Russellville	Arkansas	479-968-2841	www.saintmarysregional.com
University Hospital SUNY Health Science Center	Syracuse	New York	315-473-4240	www.upstate.edu
Winter Haven Hospital	Winter Haven	Florida	863-293-1121	www.winterhavenhospital.com

Note: Table shows hospitals nationwide whose acute myocardial infarction 30-day risk-adjusted mortality rate is worse (higher) than U.S. rate of 15.2%

Hospitals whose Heart Failure 30-Day Mortality Rate is Better (Lower) than the U.S. National Rate

Hospital	City	State	Phone	Web Site
Abbott Northwestern Hospital	Minneapolis	Minnesota	612-863-4509	www.abbottnorthwestern.com
Advocate Trinity Hospital	Chicago	Illinois	773-967-2000	www.advocatehealth.com/trin
Alexian Brothers Medical Center	Elk Grove Village	Illinois	847-437-5500	www.alexian.org
Atlanticare Regional Medical Center	Atlantic City	New Jersey	609-441-8020	www.atlanticare.org/acmc/index.html
Aurora Saint Lukes Medical Center	Milwaukee	Wisconsin	414-649-6000	www.aurorahealthcare.org
Banner Thunderbird Medical Center	Glendale	Arizona	602-588-5555	www.bannerhealth.com
Baptist Medical Center	San Antonio	Texas	210-297-1020	www.baptisthealthsystem.org
Bay Medical Center Sacred Heart Health System	Panama City	Florida	850-769-1511	www.baymedical.org
Bayhealth - Kent General Hospital	Dover	Delaware	302-744-7001	www.bayhealth.org/about/kent.asp
Beaumont Health System	Royal Oak	Michigan	248-898-5000	www.beaumonthospitals.com
Beth Israel Deaconess Medical Center	Boston	Massachusetts	617-667-7000	www.bidmc.harvard.edu
Beverly Hospital	Montebello	California	323-726-1222	www.beverly.org
Birmingham VA Medical Center	Birmingham	Alabama	205-933-4515	www.birmingham.va.gov
Boston Medical Center Corporation	Boston	Massachusetts	617-638-8000	www.bmc.org
Brigham & Women's Hospital	Boston	Massachusetts	617-732-5500	www.brighamandwomens.org
California Hospital Medical Center Los Angeles	Los Angeles	California	213-748-2411	www.chmcla.org
Cedars - Sinai Medical Center	Los Angeles	California	310-423-5000	www.cedars-sinai.edu
Centinela Hospital Medical Center	Inglewood	California	310-673-4660	www.centinelafreeman.com
Centrastate Medical Center	Freehold	New Jersey	732-431-2000	www.centrastate.com
Champlain Valley Physicians Hospital Medical Center	Plattsburgh	New York	518-561-2000	www.cvph.org
Charleston Area Medical Center	Charleston	West Virginia	304-388-6203	www.camc.org
Clara Maass Medical Center	Belleville	New Jersey	973-450-2002	www.sbhcs.com/hospitals
Cleveland - Wade Park VA Medical Center	Cleveland	Ohio	216-791-3800	www.cleveland.va.gov
Community Hospital	Munster	Indiana	219-836-1600	www.comhs.org/community
Conemaugh Valley Memorial Hospital	Johnstown	Pennsylvania	814-534-9000	www.conemaugh.org
Desert Valley Hospital	Victorville	California	760-241-8000	www.dvmc.com
East Orange General Hospital	East Orange	New Jersey	973-266-4401	www.evh.org
Edward Hospital	Naperville	Illinois	630-527-3000	www.edward.org
Emory University Hospital Midtown	Atlanta	Georgia	404-686-4411	www.emoryhealthcare.org
Essentia Health Saint Joseph's Medical Center	Brainerd	Minnesota	218-829-2861	www.sjmcmn.org
Excela Health Frick Hospital	Mount Pleasant	Pennsylvania	724-547-1500	www.excelahealth.org
Fairview Hospital	Cleveland	Ohio	216-476-7000	www.fairviewhospital.org
Falmouth Hospital	Falmouth	Massachusetts	508-548-5300	www.capecodhealth.com
Fawcett Memorial Hospital	Port Charlotte	Florida	941-629-1181	www.fawcetthospital.com
Firsthealth Moore Regional Hospital	Pinehurst	North Carolina	910-715-1000	www.firsthealth.org
Flagler Hospital	Saint Augustine	Florida	904-819-4426	www.flaglerhospital.com
Florida Hospital Heartland Medical Center	Sebring	Florida	863-314-4466	www.fhhd.org
Forbes Regional Hospital	Monroeville	Pennsylvania	412-858-2000	www.wpahs.org
Fort Duncan Medical Center	Eagle Pass	Texas	830-773-5321	www.fortduncanmedicalcenter.com
Fountain Valley Regional Hospital & Medical Center	Fountain Valley	California	714-966-7200	www.fountainvalleyhospital.com
Franciscan Saint James Health	Olympia Fields	Illinois	708-747-4000	www.franciscanalliance.org
Franciscan Saint Margaret Health - Hammond	Hammond	Indiana	219-932-2300	www.smmhc.com
Frederick Memorial Hospital	Frederick	Maryland	240-566-3300	www.fmh.org
Genesys Regional Medical Center - Health Park	Grand Blanc	Michigan	810-606-5000	www.genesys.org
Glendale Adventist Medical Center	Glendale	California	818-409-8202	www.glendaleadventist.com
Glendale Memorial Hospital & Health Center	Glendale	California	818-502-1900	www.glendalememorialhospital.org
Good Samaritan Hospital	Los Angeles	California	213-977-2121	www.goodsam.org
Good Shepherd Medical Center	Longview	Texas	903-315-2000	www.goodshepherdhealth.org
Grand View Hospital	Sellersville	Pennsylvania	215-453-4615	www.gvh.org
Hahnemann University Hospital	Philadelphia	Pennsylvania	215-762-7000	www.hahnemannhospital.com
Harper University Hospital	Detroit	Michigan	313-745-6211	www.harperhospital.org
Henry Ford Hospital	Detroit	Michigan	313-916-2600	www.henryfordhospital.com
Henry Ford Wyandotte Hospital	Wyandotte	Michigan	734-246-6000	www.henryfordwyandotte.com
Hillcrest Hospital	Mayfield Heights	Ohio	440-312-4500	www.hillcresthospital.org
Hollywood Presbyterian Medical Center	Los Angeles	California	213-413-3000	www.qahpmc.com
Holy Name Medical Center	Teaneck	New Jersey	201-833-3000	www.holyname.org
Houston VA Medical Center	Houston	Texas	713-794-7100	www.houston.med.va.gov
Howard County General Hospital	Columbia	Maryland	410-740-7890	www.hcgh.org
Huntington Beach Hospital	Huntington Beach	California	714-843-5000	www.hbhospital.com
Huron Valley - Sinai Hospital	Commerce Township	Michigan	248-937-3370	www.hvsh.org
Ingalls Memorial Hospital	Harvey	Illinois	708-333-2300	www.ingalls.org
Inova Fairfax Hospital	Falls Church	Virginia	703-776-3332	www.inova.org
Jersey Shore University Medical Center	Neptune	New Jersey	732-776-4900	www.meridianhealth.com
Jesse Brown VA Medical Center - VA Chicago	Chicago	Illinois	312-569-8387	www.va.gov
Kingsbrook Jewish Medical Center	Brooklyn	New York	718-604-5789	www.kingsbrook.org

Hospital	City	State	Phone	Web Site
Lawrence General Hospital	Lawrence	Massachusetts	978-683-4000	www.lawrencegeneral.org
Lehigh Valley Hospital	Allentown	Pennsylvania	610-402-2273	www.lvhhn.org
Lehigh Valley Hospital - Hazleton	Hazleton	Pennsylvania	570-501-4000	www.ghha.org
Lenox Hill Hospital	New York	New York	212-439-2345	www.lenoxhillhospital.org
Libertyhealth - Jersey City Medical Center Campus	Jersey City	New Jersey	201-915-2000	www.libertyhcs.org
Long Beach Memorial Medical Center	Long Beach	California	562-933-2000	www.memorialcare.com/long_beach
Louis A Weiss Memorial Hospital	Chicago	Illinois	773-878-8700	www.weisshospital.org
Maimonides Medical Center	Brooklyn	New York	718-283-6000	www.maimonidesmed.org
Main Line Hospital Bryn Mawr Campus	Bryn Mawr	Pennsylvania	610-526-3000	www.mainlinehealth.org
Main Line Hospital Lankenau	Wynnewood	Pennsylvania	610-645-2000	www.mainlinehealth.org/lh
Marymount Hospital	Garfield Heights	Ohio	216-581-0500	www.marymount.org
Mclaren Flint	Flint	Michigan	810-342-2000	www.mclaren.org
Medical Center of Southeastern Oklahoma	Durant	Oklahoma	405-924-3080	www.mcsohealth.com
Medstar Franklin Square Medical Center	Baltimore	Maryland	443-777-7850	www.franklinsquare.org
Medstar Good Samaritan Hospital	Baltimore	Maryland	443-444-3902	www.goodsam-md.org
Medstar Washington Hospital Center	Washington	District of Columbia	202-877-7000	www.whcenter.org
Mercy Fitzgerald Hospital	Darby	Pennsylvania	215-237-4000	www.mercyhealth.org
Mercy Hospital & Medical Center	Chicago	Illinois	312-567-2000	www.mercy-chicago.org
Mercy Medical Center	Springfield	Massachusetts	413-748-9000	www.mercycares.com
Mercy Saint Vincent Medical Center	Toledo	Ohio	419-251-3232	www.mhsnr.org
The Methodist Hospital	Houston	Texas	713-790-2221	www.methodisthealth.com
Mission Hospital Regional Medical Center	Mission Viejo	California	949-364-1400	www.mission4health.com
Missouri Baptist Medical Center	Town & Country	Missouri	314-996-5000	www.missouribaptistmedicalcenter.org
Montefiore Medical Center	Bronx	New York	718-920-4321	www.montefiore.org
Morristown Medical Center	Morristown	New Jersey	973-971-5450	www.morristownmemorialhospital.org
Mount Sinai Hospital	New York	New York	212-241-7981	www.mountsinai.org
Mountainview Hospital	Las Vegas	Nevada	702-255-5065	www.mountainview-hospital.com
New York Hospital Medical Center of Queens	Flushing	New York	718-670-1231	www.nyhq.org
New York - Presbyterian Hospital	New York	New York	212-746-4189	www.nyp.org
Newark Beth Israel Medical Center	Newark	New Jersey	973-926-7850	www.sbhcs.com
Newton - Wellesley Hospital	Newton	Massachusetts	617-243-6000	www.nwh.org
North Florida Regional Medical Center	Gainesville	Florida	352-333-4100	www.nfrmc.com
North Shore Medical Center	Salem	Massachusetts	978-741-1215	www.nsmc.partners.org
Northridge Hospital Medical Center	Northridge	California	818-885-8500	www.northridgehospital.org
Northwestern Memorial Hospital	Chicago	Illinois	312-926-2000	www.nmh.org
NYU Hospitals Center	New York	New York	212-263-7300	www.med.nyu.edu
Oakwood Hospital - Dearborn	Dearborn	Michigan	313-593-7125	www.oakwood.org
Oklahoma Heart Hospital South	Oklahoma City	Oklahoma	405-628-6000	www.okheart.com/south-campus
Olympia Medical Center	Los Angeles	California	310-657-5900	www.olympiamc.com
Oroville Hospital	Oroville	California	530-533-8500	www.orovillehospital.com
Palm Beach Gardens Medical Center	Palm Beach Gardens	Florida	561-622-1411	www.pbgmc.com
Palmetto Health Richland	Columbia	South Carolina	803-296-5678	www.palmettohealth.org
Paradise Valley Hospital	National City	California	619-470-4321	www.paradisevalleyhospital.org
Penn Presbyterian Medical Center	Philadelphia	Pennsylvania	215-662-8000	www.pennhealth.com
Pennsylvania Hospital of the Univ of PA Health Sys	Philadelphia	Pennsylvania	215-829-3000	www.pennmedicine.org/pahosp
Philadelphia VA Medical Center	Philadelphia	Pennsylvania	215-823-5857	www.philadelphia.va.gov
Portland VA Medical Center	Portland	Oregon	503-220-8262	www.va.gov/portland/index.asp
Presence Saint Joseph Hospital - Chicago	Chicago	Illinois	773-665-3000	www.res-health.org
Presence Saint Joseph Medical Center	Joliet	Illinois	815-725-7133	www.provena.org/stjoes
Presence Saints Mary & Elizabeth Medical Center	Chicago	Illinois	312-770-2000	www.reshealth.org
Providence Holy Cross Medical Center	Mission Hills	California	818-365-8051	www.providence.org
Providence Hospital	Washington	District of Columbia	202-269-7000	www.provhosp.org
Providence Hospital & Medical Centers	Southfield	Michigan	248-849-3011	www.stjohn.org/providence
Providence Little Co of Mary Medical Center Torrance	Torrance	California	310-540-7676	www.lcmhs.org
Providence Tarzana Medical Center	Tarzana	California	818-881-0800	www.encino-tarzana.com
Raritan Bay Medical Center	Perth Amboy	New Jersey	732-442-3700	www.rbmc.org
Regional Medical Center of San Jose	San Jose	California	408-259-5000	www.regionalmedicalsanjose.com
Rex Hospital	Raleigh	North Carolina	919-784-3100	www.rexhealth.com
Rio Grande Regional Hospital	Mcallen	Texas	956-632-6000	www.riohealth.com
Ronald Reagan UCLA Medical Center	Los Angeles	California	310-825-6301	www.uclahealth.org
Rush Oak Park Hospital	Oak Park	Illinois	708-383-9300	www.oakparkhospital.org
Rush University Medical Center	Chicago	Illinois	312-942-5000	www.ruch.edu
Saint Agnes Hospital	Baltimore	Maryland	410-368-2101	www.stagnes.org
Saint Francis Medical Center	Lynwood	California	310-900-8900	www.stfrancis.dochs.org
Saint Michael's Medical Center	Newark	New Jersey	973-877-5350	www.cathedralhealth.org
Saint Vincent Medical Center	Los Angeles	California	213-484-7111	www.stvincent.dochs.org
Santa Monica - UCLA Medical Center & Orthopaedic Hospital	Santa Monica	California	310-319-4000	www.healthcare.ucla.edu

Hospital	City	State	Phone	Web Site
Scottsdale Healthcare - Shea Medical Center	Scottsdale	Arizona	480-323-3009	www.shc.org
Scripps Green Hospital	La Jolla	California	858-554-3600	www.scrippshealth.org
Scripps Mercy Hospital	San Diego	California	619-294-8111	www.scrippshealth.org
Shore Medical Center	Somers Point	New Jersey	609-653-3545	www.shorememorial.org
Sinai Hospital of Baltimore	Baltimore	Maryland	410-601-5131	www.sinai-balt.com
Sinai - Grace Hospital	Detroit	Michigan	313-966-3300	www.sinaigrace.org
South Pointe Hospital	Warrensville Heights	Ohio	216-491-6000	www.southpointehospital.org
South Texas Health System	Edinburg	Texas	956-632-4000	www.edinburgregional.com
Southcoast Hospital Group	Fall River	Massachusetts	508-679-3131	www.southcoast.org/charlton
Southeastern Regional Medical Center	Lumberton	North Carolina	910-671-5000	www.srmc.org
SSM Saint Marys Health Center	Richmond Heights	Missouri	314-768-8000	www.ssmhealth.com/stmarys
Saint Alexius Medical Center	Hoffman Estates	Illinois	847-843-2000	www.alexianbrothershealth.org
Saint Catherine Hospital	East Chicago	Indiana	219-392-7004	www.comhs.org/stcatherine
Saint Elizabeth's Medical Center	Brighton	Massachusetts	617-789-3000	www.semc.org
Saint Francis Hospital & Medical Center	Hartford	Connecticut	860-714-4000	www.saintfranciscare.com
Saint Francis Hospital - Roslyn	Roslyn	New York	516-562-6000	www.stfrancisheartcenter.com
Saint John Hospital & Medical Center	Detroit	Michigan	313-343-4000	www.stjohnprovidence.org
Saint Luke's Hospital	Chesterfield	Missouri	314-434-1500	www.goodhealthmatters.com
Saint Luke's Hospital of Kansas City	Kansas City	Missouri	816-932-2000	www.staintlukeshealthsystem.org
Saint Vincent's Medical Center Southside	Jacksonville	Florida	904-296-3700	www.jaxhealth.com
Thomas Jefferson University Hospital	Philadelphia	Pennsylvania	215-955-6000	www.jeffersonhospital.org
Touro Infirmary	New Orleans	Louisiana	504-897-7011	www.touro.com
Tufts Medical Center	Boston	Massachusetts	617-636-5000	www.tuftsmedicalcenter.org
University Hospital of Brooklyn - Downstate Medical Center	Brooklyn	New York	718-270-1000	www.downstate.edu
University of Maryland Charles Regional Medical Center	La Plata	Maryland	301-609-4265	www.civista.org
University of Miami Hospital	Miami	Florida	305-325-5511	www.cedarsmedicalcenter.com
UPMC Mckeesport	Mc Keesport	Pennsylvania	412-664-2000	www.selectmedicalcorp.com
UPMC Passavant	Pittsburgh	Pennsylvania	412-367-6700	www.passavant.upmc.com
UT Southwestern University Hospital	Dallas	Texas	214-879-3758	www.utsouthwestern.edu
VA Boston Healthcare System - Jamaica Plain	Jamaica Plain	Massachusetts	617-232-9500	www.vaww.visn1.med.va.gov/boston
VA Greater Los Angeles Healthcare System	West Los Angeles	California	310-478-3711	www1.va.gov
VA New York Harbor Healthcare System	New York	New York	212-686-7500	www.nyharbor.va.gov
Valley Hospital	Ridgewood	New Jersey	201-447-8000	www.valleyhealth.com
Valley Presbyterian Hospital	Van Nuys	California	818-902-3906	www.valleypres.org
Wakemed - Raleigh Campus	Raleigh	North Carolina	919-350-8000	www.wakemed.org
Washington Adventist Hospital	Takoma Park	Maryland	301-891-5651	www.adventisthealthcare.com/wah
Waukesha Memorial Hospital	Waukesha	Wisconsin	262-928-1000	www.waukeshamemorial.org
West Haven VA Medical Center	West Haven	Connecticut	203-932-5711	www.visn1.med.va.gov/vact
Wheaton Franciscan Healthcare Saint Francis	Milwaukee	Wisconsin	414-647-5000	www.mywheaton.org
White Memorial Medical Center	Los Angeles	California	323-268-5000	www.whitememorial.com
William Beaumont Hospital - Troy	Troy	Michigan	248-964-8800	www.beaumonthospitals.com
Willis Knighton Medical Center	Shreveport	Louisiana	318-212-4000	www.wkhs.com//locations/medicalcenter.aspx
Winchester Hospital	Winchester	Massachusetts	781-729-9000	www.winchesterhospital.org
Wing Memorial Hospital & Medical Center	Palmer	Massachusetts	413-283-7651	www.winghealth.org
Yale-New Haven Hospital	New Haven	Connecticut	203-688-4242	www.ynhh.org

Note: Table shows hospitals nationwide whose heart failure 30-day risk-adjusted mortality rate is better (lower) than U.S. rate of 11.7%

Hospitals whose Heart Failure 30-Day Mortality Rate is Worse (Higher) than the U.S. National Rate

Hospital	City	State	Phone	Web Site
Abbeville General Hospital	Abbeville	Louisiana	337-893-5466	www.abgen.net
Abrom Kaplan Memorial Hospital	Kaplan	Louisiana	337-643-8300	www.compasshealthcare.com/site78.php
Albany Memorial Hospital	Albany	New York	518-471-3221	www.nehealth.com
Alegent Creighton Health Immanuel Medical Center	Omaha	Nebraska	402-572-2121	www.alegent.com
Anne Arundel Medical Center	Annapolis	Maryland	443-481-1307	www.aahs.org
Appleton Medical Center	Appleton	Wisconsin	920-731-4101	www.thedacare.org
Arkansas Methodist Medical Center	Paragould	Arkansas	870-239-7000	www.arkansasmethodist.org
Baptist Health Medical Center - North Little Rock	North Little Rock	Arkansas	501-202-3000	www.baptist-health.org
Baptist Memorial Hospital/Golden Triangle	Columbus	Mississippi	662-244-1500	www.bmhcc.org/facilities/goldentriangle
Baxter Regional Medical Center	Mountain Home	Arkansas	870-508-1000	www.baxterregional.org
Blanchard Valley Hospital	Findlay	Ohio	419-423-4500	www.bvha.org
Bolivar Medical Center	Cleveland	Mississippi	662-846-2551	www.bolivarmedical.com
Brattleboro Memorial Hospital	Brattleboro	Vermont	802-257-0341	www.bmhvt.org
Bronson Methodist Hospital	Kalamazoo	Michigan	269-341-6000	www.bronsonhealth.com
Capital Region Medical Center	Jefferson City	Missouri	573-632-5000	www.crmc.org
Carilion Roanoke Memorial Hospital	Roanoke	Virginia	540-981-7000	www.carilion.com/crmh
Carolinas Medical Center/Behaviorial Health	Charlotte	North Carolina	704-355-2000	www.carolinasmedicalcenter.org
Carroll Hospital Center	Westminster	Maryland	410-848-3000	www.carrollhospitalcenter.org
Carson Tahoe Regional Medical Center	Carson City	Nevada	775-445-8000	www.carsontahoehospital.com
Cayuga Medical Center at Ithaca	Ithaca	New York	607-274-4401	www.cayugamed.org
Central Maine Medical Center	Lewiston	Maine	207-795-0111	www.cmmc.org
Central Washington Hospital	Wenatchee	Washington	509-662-1511	www.cwhs.com
Cherokee Regional Medical Center	Cherokee	Iowa	712-225-5101	www.cherokeermc.org
Chicot Memorial Medical Center	Lake Village	Arkansas	870-265-5351	www.chicotmemorial.com
Christus Hospital	Beaumont	Texas	409-892-7171	www.christushealth.org
Citizens Baptist Medical Center	Talladega	Alabama	256-761-4542	www.bhsala.com
Citrus Memorial Hospital	Inverness	Florida	352-726-1551	www.citrusmh.com
Clarion Hospital	Clarion	Pennsylvania	814-226-9500	www.clarionhospital.org
Clovis Community Medical Center	Clovis	California	559-324-4000	www.communitymedical.org
Columbia Saint Marys Hospital Ozaukee	Mequon	Wisconsin	262-243-7300	www.columbia-stmarys.org
Community Hospital North	Indianapolis	Indiana	317-621-5335	www.ecommunity.com/north
Conway Regional Medical Center	Conway	Arkansas	501-329-3831	www.conwayregional.org
Copley Memorial Hospital	Aurora	Illinois	630-978-6200	www.rushcopley.com
Coshocton County Memorial Hospital	Coshocton	Ohio	740-622-6411	www.ccmh.com
Dekalb Regional Medical Center	Fort Payne	Alabama	256-845-3150	www.baptistmedical.org
Dominican Hospital	Santa Cruz	California	831-462-7700	www.dominicanhospital.org
Edward W Sparrow Hospital	Lansing	Michigan	517-364-1000	www.sparrow.org
Emerson Hospital	W Concord	Massachusetts	978-369-1400	www.emersonhospital.org
Fletcher Allen Hospital of Vermont	Burlington	Vermont	802-847-0000	www.fletcherallen.org
Floyd Medical Center	Rome	Georgia	706-509-6900	www.floydmed.org
Geisinger Medical Center	Danville	Pennsylvania	570-271-6211	www.geisinger.org
Geneva General Hospital	Geneva	New York	315-787-4175	www.flhealth.org
GHS Greenville Memorial Medical Center	Greenville	South Carolina	864-455-7000	www.ghs.org
Good Samaritan Hospital	Lebanon	Pennsylvania	717-270-7500	www.gshleb.org
Grossmont Hospital	La Mesa	California	619-465-0711	www.sharp.com
Hendrick Medical Center	Abilene	Texas	325-670-2000	www.ehendrick.org
Highland Hospital	Rochester	New York	585-473-2200	www.urmc.rochester.edu
Hilton Head Regional Medical Center	Hilton Head Island	South Carolina	843-681-6122	www.hiltonheadmedctr.com
Hopkins County Memorial Hospital	Sulphur Springs	Texas	903-885-7671	www.hcmh.com
Hutchinson Regional Medical Center	Hutchinson	Kansas	620-665-2001	www.hutchinsonhospital.com
Iberia General Hospital & Medical Center	New Iberia	Louisiana	337-364-0441	www.iberiamedicalcenter.com
Indiana University Health La Porte Hospital	La Porte	Indiana	219-326-1234	www.laportehealth.org
Integris Grove Hospital	Grove	Oklahoma	918-786-2243	www.integris-health.com
IU Health Goshen Hospital	Goshen	Indiana	574-364-1000	www.goshenhosp.com
Jane Phillips Medical Center	Bartlesville	Oklahoma	918-333-7200	www.jpmc.org
JFK Medical Center - A M Yelencsics Comm Hospital	Edison	New Jersey	732-321-7000	www.jfkmc.org
Johnson Memorial Hospital	Franklin	Indiana	317-736-3300	www.johnsonmemorial.org
Kadlec Regional Medical Center	Richland	Washington	509-946-4611	www.kadlecmed.org
Kootenai Medical Center	Coeur D'alene	Idaho	208-625-4001	www.kootenaihealth.org
Lake Cumberland Regional Hospital	Somerset	Kentucky	606-679-7441	www.lakecumberlandhospital.com
Lake Granbury Medical Center	Granbury	Texas	817-573-2683	www.lakegranburymedicalcenter.com
Lawrence & Memorial Hospital	New London	Connecticut	860-442-0711	www.lmhospital.org
Los Alamitos Medical Center	Los Alamitos	California	562-799-3220	www.losalamitosmedctr.com
Manatee Memorial Hospital	Bradenton	Florida	941-746-5111	www.manateememorial.com
Manchester Memorial Hospital	Manchester	Connecticut	860-647-4780	www.echn.org

Hospital	City	State	Phone	Web Site
Maury Regional Hospital	Columbia	Tennessee	931-381-1111	www.maurgregional.com
Mclaren - Greater Lansing	Lansing	Michigan	517-975-6000	www.mclaren.org
Meadville Medical Center	Meadville	Pennsylvania	814-333-5000	www.mmchs.org
Medcentral Health System Mansfield Hospital	Mansfield	Ohio	419-526-8000	www.medcentral.org
Memorial Hospital of South Bend	South Bend	Indiana	574-647-1000	www.qualityoflife.org
Mercy Health System Corp	Janesville	Wisconsin	608-756-6080	www.mercyhealthsystem.org
Mercy Hospital Springfield	Springfield	Missouri	417-820-2000	www.stjohns.com
Mercy Medical Center - Redding	Redding	California	530-225-6102	www.redding.mercy.org
Mercy Medical Center - North Iowa	Mason City	Iowa	641-428-7000	www.mercynorthiowa.com
Mountain View Regional Medical Center	Las Cruces	New Mexico	575-556-7600	www.mountainviewregional.com
Nathan Littauer Hospital	Gloversville	New York	518-725-8621	www.nlh.org
Nea Baptist Memorial Hospital	Jonesboro	Arkansas	870-972-7000	www.baptistonline.com
New Hanover Regional Medical Center	Wilmington	North Carolina	910-343-7000	www.nhrmc.org
New Milford Hospital	New Milford	Connecticut	860-355-2611	www.newmilfordhospital.org
Norman Regional Health System	Norman	Oklahoma	405-321-1700	www.normanregional.com
North Mississippi Medical Center	Tupelo	Mississippi	662-377-3000	www.nmhs.net/nmmc
North Shore University Hospital	Manhasset	New York	516-562-0100	www.northshorelij.com
Northwest Community Hospital	Arlington Heights	Illinois	847-618-1000	www.nch.org
Northwest Hospital	Seattle	Washington	206-364-0500	www.nwhospital.org
O'Connor Hospital	San Jose	California	408-947-2500	www.oconnorhospital.org
Olympic Medical Center	Port Angeles	Washington	360-417-7000	www.olympicmedical.org
Our Lady of the Lake Regional Medical Center	Baton Rouge	Louisiana	225-765-6565	www.ololrmc.com
Overton Brooks VA Medical Center - Shreveport	Shreveport	Louisiana	318-424-6037	www.va.gov/sta/guide/home.asp
Pinnacle Health Hospitals	Harrisburg	Pennsylvania	717-782-5181	www.pinnaclehealth.org
Poplar Bluff Regional Medical Center	Poplar Bluff	Missouri	573-785-7721	www.poplarbluffregional.com
Porter Regional Hospital	Valparaiso	Indiana	219-983-8300	www.portermemorial.org
Providence Alaska Medical Center	Anchorage	Alaska	907-261-3675	www.providence.org
Providence Sacred Heart Medical Center	Spokane	Washington	509-474-3040	www.shmc.org
Rideout Memorial Hospital	Marysville	California	530-749-4300	www.frhg.org
Riverview Hospital Assoc	Wisconsin Rapids	Wisconsin	715-423-6060	www.riverviewhospital.net
Sacred Heart Medical Center - Riverbend	Springfield	Oregon	541-222-7300	www.peacehealth.org/sacred-heart-riverbend
Saint Anthony Medical Center	Rockford	Illinois	815-226-2000	www.osfhealth.com
Saint Francis Medical Center	Peoria	Illinois	309-655-2000	www.osfsaintfrancis.org
Salem Hospital	Salem	Oregon	503-561-5200	www.salemhospital.org
Saline Memorial Hospital	Benton	Arkansas	501-776-6000	www.salinememorial.org
San Juan Regional Medical Center	Farmington	New Mexico	505-609-2000	www.sanjuanregional.com
Sanford Usd Medical Center	Sioux Falls	South Dakota	605-333-1000	www.sanfordhealth.org
Santa Rosa Memorial Hospital	Santa Rosa	California	707-525-5300	www.stjosephhealth.org
Sarasota Memorial Hospital	Sarasota	Florida	941-917-9000	www.smh.com
Scenic Mountain Medical Center	Big Spring	Texas	432-263-1211	www.smmccares.com
Sentara Obici Hospital	Suffolk	Virginia	757-934-4000	www.sentara.com
Saint Anthony's Hospital	Saint Petersburg	Florida	727-825-1100	www.stanthonys.com
Saint Bernards Medical Center	Jonesboro	Arkansas	870-972-4100	www.sbrmc.com
Saint Francis - Downtown	Greenville	South Carolina	864-255-1000	www.stfrancishealth.org
Saint Johns Hospital	Springfield	Illinois	217-544-6464	www.st-johns.org
Saint Joseph Regional Health Center	Bryan	Texas	979-776-3912	www.st-joseph.org/sjrhc
Saint Joseph's Mercy Health Center	Hot Springs	Arkansas	501-622-1000	www.saintjosephs.com
Saint Lucie Medical Center	Port Saint Lucie	Florida	772-335-4000	www.stluciemed.com
Saint Marys Hospital Medical Center	Green Bay	Wisconsin	920-498-4200	www.stmgb.org
Saint Marys Regional Medical Center	Russellville	Arkansas	479-968-2841	www.saintmarysregional.com
Saint Nicholas Hospital	Sheboygan	Wisconsin	920-459-8300	www.stnicholashospital.org
Saint Rose Dominican Hospitals - Rose De Lima Campus	Henderson	Nevada	702-616-5000	www.dignityhealth.org/las-vegas
Starr Regional Medical Center Athens	Athens	Tennessee	423-745-1411	www.athensrmc.com
Swedish Edmonds Hospital	Edmonds	Washington	425-640-4000	www.stevenshealthcare.org
Texas Health Harris Methodist Fort Worth	Fort Worth	Texas	817-250-2100	www.texashealth.org
The Nebraska Medical Center	Omaha	Nebraska	402-552-2040	www.nebraskamed.com
Theda Clark Medical Center	Neenah	Wisconsin	920-729-3100	www.thedacare.org
Thibodaux Regional Medical Center	Thibodaux	Louisiana	985-447-5500	www.thibodaux.com
Tulare Regional Medical Center	Tulare	California	559-688-0821	www.tdhs.org
Ukiah Valley Medical Center	Ukiah	California	707-462-3111	www.uvmc.org
Union General Hospital	Blairsville	Georgia	706-745-2111	www.uniongeneralhospital.com
United Health Services Hospitals	Johnson City	New York	607-763-6000	www.vhs.ent
United Regional Health Care System	Wichita Falls	Texas	940-764-3055	www.urhcs.org
University of Missouri Health Care	Columbia	Missouri	573-882-4141	www.missouri.edu
Utah Valley Regional Medical Center	Provo	Utah	801-373-7850	www.intermountainhealthcare.org/hospitals/uvrmc
VA Southern Arizona Healthcare System	Tucson	Arizona	520-629-1821	www.va.gov/sta/guide/home.asp
Valley Hospital	Spokane	Washington	509-924-6650	www.valleyhospital.org

Hospital	City	State	Phone	Web Site
Western Missouri Medical Center	Warrensburg	Missouri	660-747-2500	www.wmmc.com
White County Medical Center	Searcy	Arkansas	501-278-3100	www.centralarkhospital.com
Wilkes-Barre General Hospital	Wilkes-Barre	Pennsylvania	570-829-8111	www.wvhcs.org
Wyoming Medical Center	Casper	Wyoming	307-577-7201	www.wyomingmedicalcenter.com

Note: Table shows hospitals nationwide whose heart failure 30-day risk-adjusted mortality rate is worse (higher) than U.S. rate of 11.7%

Hospitals whose Pneumonia 30-Day Mortality Rate is Better (Lower) than the U.S. National Rate

Hospital	City	State	Phone	Web Site
Adventist La Grange Memorial Hospital	La Grange	Illinois	708-352-1200	www.keepingyouwell.com
Ahmc Anaheim Regional Medical Center	Anaheim	California	714-774-1450	www.memorialcare.org/anaheim
Akron General Medical Center	Akron	Ohio	330-344-6000	www.akrongeneral.org
Alhambra Hospital Medical Center	Alhambra	California	626-570-1606	www.alhambrahospital.com
Arnot Ogden Medical Center	Elmira	New York	607-737-4100	www.arnothealth.org
Augusta Health	Fishersville	Virginia	540-932-4000	www.augustamed.com
Aurora Saint Lukes Medical Center	Milwaukee	Wisconsin	414-649-6000	www.aurorahealthcare.org
Aventura Hospital & Medical Center	Aventura	Florida	305-682-7000	www.aventurahospital.com
Banner Thunderbird Medical Center	Glendale	Arizona	602-588-5555	www.bannerhealth.com
Baptist Hospital of Miami	Miami	Florida	786-596-1960	www.baptisthealth.net
Barnes-Jewish Saint Peters Hospital	Saint Peters	Missouri	636-916-9000	www.bjsph.org
Bay Medical Center Sacred Heart Health System	Panama City	Florida	850-769-1511	www.baymedical.org
Baylor Regional Medical Center at Grapevine	Grapevine	Texas	817-481-1588	www.baylorhealth.com
Beaumont Health System	Grosse Pointe	Michigan	313-343-1000	www.beaumonthospitals.com
Beaumont Health System	Royal Oak	Michigan	248-898-5000	www.beaumonthospitals.com
Benefis Hospitals	Great Falls	Montana	406-455-5000	www.benefis.org
Berkshire Medical Center	Pittsfield	Massachusetts	413-447-2000	www.berkshirehealthsystems.org
Beth Israel Deaconess Medical Center	Boston	Massachusetts	617-667-7000	www.bidmc.harvard.edu
Betsy Johnson Regional Hospital	Dunn	North Carolina	910-892-7161	www.bjrh.org
Cape Cod Hospital	Hyannis	Massachusetts	508-771-1800	www.capecodhealth.org
Casey County Hospital	Liberty	Kentucky	606-787-6275	
Cedars - Sinai Medical Center	Los Angeles	California	310-423-5000	www.cedars-sinai.edu
Centinela Hospital Medical Center	Inglewood	California	310-673-4660	www.centinelafreeman.com
Centura Health - Littleton Adventist Hospital	Littleton	Colorado	303-730-5888	www.littletonhosp.org
Christ Hospital	Cincinnati	Ohio	513-585-2000	www.thechristhospital.com
Cobre Valley Regional Medical Center	Globe	Arizona	928-425-3261	www.cvchospital.com
Community Medical Center	Toms River	New Jersey	732-557-8000	www.sbhcs.com
Corning Hospital	Corning	New York	607-937-7200	www.corninghospital.org
Cox Medical Center Branson	Branson	Missouri	417-335-7000	www.skaggs.net
Delray Medical Center	Delray Beach	Florida	561-498-4440	www.delraymedicalctr.com
Desert Valley Hospital	Victorville	California	760-241-8000	www.dvmc.com
Doctors Hospital at Renaissance	Edinburg	Texas	956-362-8677	www.dhr-rgv.com
Duke University Hospital	Durham	North Carolina	919-684-8111	www.dukehealth.org
East Valley Hospital Medical Center	Glendora	California	626-335-0231	www.eastvalleyhospital.org
Edward Hospital	Naperville	Illinois	630-527-3000	www.edward.org
Eisenhower Medical Center	Rancho Mirage	California	760-340-3911	www.emc.org
Elmhurst Memorial Hospital	Elmhurst	Illinois	630-833-1400	www.emhc.org
Englewood Hospital & Medical Center	Englewood	New Jersey	201-894-3000	www.englewoodhospital.com
Evanston Hospital	Evanston	Illinois	847-432-8000	www.enh.org
Evergreen Hospital Medical Center	Kirkland	Washington	425-899-1000	www.evergreenhospital.org
Exempla Lutheran Medical Center	Wheat Ridge	Colorado	303-425-4500	www.exemlpa.org
Falmouth Hospital	Falmouth	Massachusetts	508-548-5300	www.capecodhealth.com
Firsthealth Moore Regional Hospital	Pinehurst	North Carolina	910-715-1000	www.firsthealth.org
Flagler Hospital	Saint Augustine	Florida	904-819-4426	www.flaglerhospital.com
Forbes Regional Hospital	Monroeville	Pennsylvania	412-858-2000	www.wpahs.org
Fountain Valley Regional Hospital & Medical Center	Fountain Valley	California	714-966-7200	www.fountainvalleyhospital.com
Franklin Woods Community Hospital	Johnson City	Tennessee	423-302-1120	www.msha.com
Frederick Memorial Hospital	Frederick	Maryland	240-566-3300	www.fmh.org
Frisbie Memorial Hospital	Rochester	New Hampshire	603-332-5211	www.frisbiehospital.com
Garden Grove Hospital & Medical Center	Garden Grove	California	714-537-5160	www.gardengrovehospital.com
Garfield Medical Center	Monterey Park	California	626-573-2222	www.garfieldmedicalcenter.com
Geisinger - Bloomsburg Hospital	Bloomsburg	Pennsylvania	570-387-2100	www.tbhonline.org
Genesis Healthcare System	Zanesville	Ohio	740-454-5000	www.genesishcs.org
Genesys Regional Medical Center - Health Park	Grand Blanc	Michigan	810-606-5000	www.genesys.org
Glendale Adventist Medical Center	Glendale	California	818-409-8202	www.glendaleadventist.com
Grandview Hospital & Medical Center	Dayton	Ohio	937-723-3312	www.kmcnetwork.org
Greater Baltimore Medical Center	Baltimore	Maryland	443-849-2000	www.gbmc.org
Harper University Hospital	Detroit	Michigan	313-745-6211	www.harperhospital.org
Heartland Regional Medical Center	Saint Joseph	Missouri	816-271-6000	www.heartland-health.com
Henry Ford Macomb Hospital	Clinton Township	Michigan	586-263-2300	www.stjoe-macomb.com
Hillcrest Hospital	Mayfield Heights	Ohio	440-312-4500	www.hillcresthospital.org
Hinsdale Hospital	Hinsdale	Illinois	630-856-9000	www.keepingyouwell.com
Hollywood Presbyterian Medical Center	Los Angeles	California	213-413-3000	www.qahpmc.com
Holy Name Medical Center	Teaneck	New Jersey	201-833-3000	www.holyname.org
The Hospital of Central Connecticut	New Britain	Connecticut	860-224-5011	www.thocc.org

Hospital	City	State	Phone	Web Site
Huntington Beach Hospital	Huntington Beach	California	714-843-5000	www.hbhospital.com
Huntington Memorial Hospital	Pasadena	California	626-397-5000	www.huntingtonhospital.com
Indiana University Health	Indianapolis	Indiana	317-962-5900	www.iuhealth.org
Ingalls Memorial Hospital	Harvey	Illinois	708-333-2300	www.ingalls.org
Inova Loudoun Hospital	Leesburg	Virginia	703-858-6600	www.loudounhealthcare.org
Jersey Shore University Medical Center	Neptune	New Jersey	732-776-4900	www.meridianhealth.com
Jupiter Medical Center	Jupiter	Florida	561-747-2234	www.jupitermed.com
Kane Community Hospital	Kane	Pennsylvania	814-837-8585	www.kanehosp.com
Kingsbrook Jewish Medical Center	Brooklyn	New York	718-604-5789	www.kingsbrook.org
Lehigh Valley Hospital	Allentown	Pennsylvania	610-402-2273	www.lvhhn.org
Lehigh Valley Hospital - Hazleton	Hazleton	Pennsylvania	570-501-4000	www.ghha.org
Lehigh Valley Hospital - Muhlenberg	Bethlehem	Pennsylvania	610-402-2273	www.lvhn.org
Liberty Hospital	Liberty	Missouri	816-781-7200	www.libertyhospital.org
Los Angeles Community Hospital	Los Angeles	California	323-267-0477	www.altacorp.com
Los Robles Hospital & Medical Center	Thousand Oaks	California	805-497-2727	www.losrobleshospital.com
Maimonides Medical Center	Brooklyn	New York	718-283-6000	www.maimonidesmed.org
Mary Greeley Medical Center	Ames	Iowa	515-239-2011	www.mgmc.org
Mayo Clinic Hospital	Phoenix	Arizona	480-342-2000	www.mayoclinic.org
Medical Center of Southeastern Oklahoma	Durant	Oklahoma	405-924-3080	www.mcsohealth.com
Medical City Dallas Hospital	Dallas	Texas	972-566-6222	www.medicalcityhospital.com
Medstar Franklin Square Medical Center	Baltimore	Maryland	443-777-7850	www.franklinsquare.org
Medstar Good Samaritan Hospital	Baltimore	Maryland	443-444-3902	www.goodsam-md.org
Medstar Harbor Hospital	Baltimore	Maryland	410-350-3201	www.harborhospital.org
Memorial Mission Hospital & Asheville Surgery Center	Asheville	North Carolina	828-213-1111	www.missionhospitals.org
Mercy Memorial Hospital System	Monroe	Michigan	734-240-8400	www.mercymemorial.org
The Methodist Hospital	Houston	Texas	713-790-2221	www.methodisthealth.com
Methodist Sugar Land Hospital	Sugar Land	Texas	281-274-8000	www.methodisthealth.com/sugarland
Milford Regional Medical Center	Milford	Massachusetts	508-473-1190	www.milfordregional.org
Missouri Baptist Medical Center	Town & Country	Missouri	314-996-5000	www.missouribaptistmedicalcenter.org
Monmouth Medical Center - Southern Campus	Lakewood	New Jersey	732-363-1900	www.sbhcs.com
Montefiore Medical Center	Bronx	New York	718-920-4321	www.montefiore.org
Morristown Medical Center	Morristown	New Jersey	973-971-5450	www.morristownmemorialhospital.org
Mount Auburn Hospital	Cambridge	Massachusetts	617-492-3500	www.mountauburnhospital.org
Mount Sinai Hospital	New York	New York	212-241-7981	www.mountsinai.org
Mount Sinai Medical Center	Miami Beach	Florida	305-674-2121	www.msmc.com
New York - Presbyterian Hospital	New York	New York	212-746-4189	www.nyp.org
Newton Memorial Hospital	Newton	New Jersey	973-383-2121	www.itsyourlife.com
North Shore Medical Center	Salem	Massachusetts	978-741-1215	www.nsmc.partners.org
North Shore University Hospital	Manhasset	New York	516-562-0100	www.northshorelij.com
Northern Westchester Hospital	Mount Kisco	New York	914-666-1200	www.nwhc.net
Northwestern Memorial Hospital	Chicago	Illinois	312-926-2000	www.nmh.org
Norton Community Hospital	Norton	Virginia	703-679-8865	www.nchosp.org
NYU Hospitals Center	New York	New York	212-263-7300	www.med.nyu.edu
Oakwood Hospital - Dearborn	Dearborn	Michigan	313-593-7125	www.oakwood.org
Olympia Medical Center	Los Angeles	California	310-657-5900	www.olympiamc.com
Oroville Hospital	Oroville	California	530-533-8500	www.orovillehospital.com
Our Lady of Lourdes Medical Center	Camden	New Jersey	856-757-3500	www.lourdesnet.org
Overlook Medical Center	Summit	New Jersey	908-522-2000	www.atlantichealth.org
Owensboro Health Regional Hospital	Owensboro	Kentucky	270-688-2000	www.omhs.org
Palos Community Hospital	Palos Heights	Illinois	708-923-4000	www.paloshospital.org
Paradise Valley Hospital	National City	California	619-470-4321	www.paradisevalleyhospital.org
Park Plaza Hospital	Houston	Texas	713-527-5019	www.parkplazahospital.com
Parkland Health Center	Farmington	Missouri	573-431-6005	www.bjc.org
Piedmont Hospital	Atlanta	Georgia	404-605-5000	www.piedmonthospital.org
Portland VA Medical Center	Portland	Oregon	503-220-8262	www.va.gov/portland/index.asp
Presbyterian Intercommunity Hospital	Whittier	California	526-698-0811	www.whittierpres.com
Presence Resurrection Medical Center	Chicago	Illinois	773-774-8000	www.reshealthcare.org
Presence Saint Joseph Hospital - Chicago	Chicago	Illinois	773-665-3000	www.res-health.org
Presence Saint Joseph Medical Center	Joliet	Illinois	815-725-7133	www.provena.org/stjoes
Presence Saint Marys Hospital	Kankakee	Illinois	815-937-2490	www.provenastmarys.com
Providence Hospital & Medical Centers	Southfield	Michigan	248-849-3011	www.stjohn.org/providence
Providence Little Co of Mary Medical Center Torrance	Torrance	California	310-540-7676	www.lcmhs.org
Providence Saint Joseph Medical Center	Burbank	California	818-843-5111	www.providence.org/losangeles
Providence Tarzana Medical Center	Tarzana	California	818-881-0800	www.encino-tarzana.com
Randolph Hospital	Asheboro	North Carolina	336-625-5151	www.randolphhospital.org
Raritan Bay Medical Center	Perth Amboy	New Jersey	732-442-3700	www.rbmc.org
Reading Hospital	Reading	Pennsylvania	610-988-8000	www.readinghospital.org

Hospital	City	State	Phone	Web Site
Rex Hospital	Raleigh	North Carolina	919-784-3100	www.rexhealth.com
Rhode Island Hospital	Providence	Rhode Island	401-444-4000	www.rhodeislandhospital.org
Rio Grande Regional Hospital	Mcallen	Texas	956-632-6000	www.riohealth.com
Riverside Medical Center	Kankakee	Illinois	815-933-1671	www.riversidehealthcare.org
Riverview Medical Center	Red Bank	New Jersey	732-741-2700	www.meridianhealth.com
Robert Wood Johnson University Hospital	New Brunswick	New Jersey	732-937-8900	www.rwjuh.edu
Rockingham Memorial Hospital	Harrisonburg	Virginia	540-689-1000	www.rmhonline.com
Ronald Reagan UCLA Medical Center	Los Angeles	California	310-825-6301	www.uclahealth.org
Saint Clare's Hospital	Denville	New Jersey	973-625-6000	www.saintclares.org
Saint Francis Hospital	Tulsa	Oklahoma	918-494-2200	www.saintfrancis.com
Saint Vincent Medical Center	Los Angeles	California	213-484-7111	www.stvincent.dochs.org
San Francisco VA Medical Center	San Francisco	California	415-221-4810	www.sanfrancisco.va.gov
San Gabriel Valley Medical Center	San Gabriel	California	626-289-5454	www.sangabrielvalleymedctr.org
Santa Monica - UCLA Medical Center & Orthopaedic Hospital	Santa Monica	California	310-319-4000	www.healthcare.ucla.edu
Scott & White Hospital - Round Rock	Round Rock	Texas	512-509-0100	www.sw.org
Scott & White Memorial Hospital	Temple	Texas	254-724-2111	www.sw.org
Scripps Memorial Hospital La Jolla	La Jolla	California	858-626-4123	www.scrippshealth.org
Scripps Mercy Hospital	San Diego	California	619-294-8111	www.scrippshealth.org
Sharon Regional Health System	Sharon	Pennsylvania	724-983-3800	www.sharonregional.com
Sinai Hospital of Baltimore	Baltimore	Maryland	410-601-5131	www.sinai-balt.com
South Pointe Hospital	Warrensville Heights	Ohio	216-491-6000	www.southpointehospital.org
Southampton Hospital	Southampton	New York	516-726-8200	www.southamptonhospital.org
Southcoast Hospital Group	Fall River	Massachusetts	508-679-3131	www.southcoast.org/charlton
Southwest General Health Center	Middleburg Heights	Ohio	440-816-8000	www.swgeneral.com
Spartanburg Regional Medical Center	Spartanburg	South Carolina	864-560-6000	www.srhs.com
Spring Valley Hospital Medical Center	Las Vegas	Nevada	702-853-3000	www.springvalleyhospital.com
Saint Alexius Medical Center	Hoffman Estates	Illinois	847-843-2000	www.alexianbrothershealth.org
Saint Anthony Community Hospital	Warwick	New York	845-986-2276	www.stanthonycommunityhosp.org
Saint Luke's Hospital Bethlehem	Bethlehem	Pennsylvania	610-954-4000	www.slhn-lehighvalley.org
Saint Luke's Roosevelt Hospital	New York	New York	212-523-4000	www.wehealny.org
Saint Luke's Episcopal Hospital	Houston	Texas	832-355-1000	www.sleh.com
Saint Luke's Hospital	Cedar Rapids	Iowa	319-369-7211	www.crstlukes.com
Saint Luke's Hospital	Chesterfield	Missouri	314-434-1500	www.goodhealthmatters.com
Saint Marys Hospital	Madison	Wisconsin	608-251-6100	www.stmarysmadison.com
Saint Peter's Hospital	Albany	New York	518-525-1550	www.stpetershealthcare.org
Stafford Hospital	Stafford	Virginia	540-741-9000	www.marywashingtonhealthcare.com
Swedish Covenant Hospital	Chicago	Illinois	773-878-8200	www.swedishcovenant.org
Tomball Regional Medical Center	Tomball	Texas	281-351-1623	www.tomballhospital.org
Tri Valley Health System	Cambridge	Nebraska	308-697-3329	www.trivalleyhealth.com
Tri - City Regional Medical Center	Hawaiian Gardens	California	562-860-0401	www.tri-cityrmc.org
Trumbull Memorial Hospital	Warren	Ohio	330-841-9011	www.trumhosp.org
Tufts Medical Center	Boston	Massachusetts	617-636-5000	www.tuftsmedicalcenter.org
United Regional Medical Center	Manchester	Tennessee	931-728-3586	www.urmchealthcare.com
University Medical Center of Princeton at Plainsboro	Plainsboro	New Jersey	866-460-4776	www.princetonhcs.org
University Hospitals - Elyria Medical Center	Elyria	Ohio	440-329-7500	www.emh-healthcare.org
University of California San Diego Medical Center	San Diego	California	619-543-6222	www.health.ucsd.edu
University of Maryland Shore Medical Center at Easton	Easton	Maryland	410-822-1000	www.shorehealth.org
University of Michigan Health System	Ann Arbor	Michigan	734-764-1505	www.med.umich.edu
University of Texas Health Science Center at Tyler	Tyler	Texas	903-877-7777	www.uthct.edu
UPMC Mckeesport	Mc Keesport	Pennsylvania	412-664-2000	www.selectmedicalcorp.com
VA Boston Healthcare System - Jamaica Plain	Jamaica Plain	Massachusetts	617-232-9500	www.vaww.visn1.med.va.gov/boston
VA North Florida/South Georgia Healthcare System	Gainesville	Florida	352-376-1611	www.northflorida.va.gov
VA Sierra Nevada Healthcare System	Reno	Nevada	775-328-1263	www.reno.va.gov
Valley Hospital	Ridgewood	New Jersey	201-447-8000	www.valleyhealth.com
VHS Harlingen Hospital Company	Harlingen	Texas	956-389-1100	www.vbmc.org
Virginia Mason Medical Center	Seattle	Washington	206-223-6600	www.vmmc.org
W Palm Beach VA Medical Center	West Palm Beach	Florida	561-422-8600	www.va.gov
Waukesha Memorial Hospital	Waukesha	Wisconsin	262-928-1000	www.waukeshamemorial.org
Weirton Medical Center	Weirton	West Virginia	304-797-6000	www.weirtonmedical.com
West Anaheim Medical Center	Anaheim	California	714-827-3000	www.wamc.phcs.us
West Haven VA Medical Center	West Haven	Connecticut	203-932-5711	www.visn1.med.va.gov/vact
Wheaton Franciscan Healthcare Saint Francis	Milwaukee	Wisconsin	414-647-5000	www.mywheaton.org
White Memorial Medical Center	Los Angeles	California	323-268-5000	www.whitememorial.com
William Beaumont Hospital - Troy	Troy	Michigan	248-964-8800	www.beaumonthospitals.com
Willis Knighton Medical Center	Shreveport	Louisiana	318-212-4000	www.wkhs.com//locations/medicalcenter.aspx
Yale-New Haven Hospital	New Haven	Connecticut	203-688-4242	www.ynhh.org

Note: Table shows hospitals nationwide whose pneumonia 30-day risk-adjusted mortality rate is better (lower) than U.S. rate of 11.9%

Hospitals whose Pneumonia 30-Day Mortality Rate is Worse (Higher) than the U.S. National Rate

Hospital	City	State	Phone	Web Site
Abilene Regional Medical Center	Abilene	Texas	325-428-1000	www.abileneregional.com
Acmh Hospital	Kittanning	Pennsylvania	724-543-8404	www.acmh.org
Albemarle Hospital Authority	Elizabeth City	North Carolina	252-335-0531	www.albemarlehealth.org
Antelope Valley Hospital	Lancaster	California	661-949-5000	www.avhospital.org
Aspirus Grand View Hospital	Ironwood	Michigan	906-932-2525	www.gvhs.org
Augusta VA Medical Center	Augusta	Georgia	706-823-2201	www.va.gov
Auxilio Mutuo Hospital	Hato Rey	Puerto Rico	787-758-2000	www.auxiliopr.com
Avera Sacred Heart Hospital	Yankton	South Dakota	605-668-8000	www.avera.org/sacred-heart
Bacon County Hospital	Alma	Georgia	912-632-8961	www.baconcountyhospital.com
Baptist Memorial Hospital/Golden Triangle	Columbus	Mississippi	662-244-1500	www.bmhcc.org/facilities/goldentriangle
Baptist Memorial Hospital Union City	Union City	Tennessee	731-885-2410	www.bmhcc.org
Baxter Regional Medical Center	Mountain Home	Arkansas	870-508-1000	www.baxterregional.org
Bay Area Hospital	Coos Bay	Oregon	541-269-8111	www.bayareahospital.org
Bolivar Medical Center	Cleveland	Mississippi	662-846-2551	www.bolivarmedical.com
Bon Secours Maryview Medical Center	Portsmouth	Virginia	757-398-2200	www.bonsecourshamptonroads.com
Caldwell Medical Center	Princeton	Kentucky	270-365-0300	www.caldwellhosp.org
Cameron Regional Medical Center	Cameron	Missouri	816-632-2101	www.cameronregional.org
Carilion Roanoke Memorial Hospital	Roanoke	Virginia	540-981-7000	www.carilion.com/crmh
Carondelet Saint Joseph's Hospital	Tucson	Arizona	520-873-3000	www.carondelet.org
Carson Tahoe Regional Medical Center	Carson City	Nevada	775-445-8000	www.carsontahoehospital.com
Catawba Valley Medical Center	Hickory	North Carolina	828-326-3809	www.catawbavalleymc.org
Central Carolina Hospital	Sanford	North Carolina	919-774-2100	www.centralcarolinahosp.com
Citizens Memorial Hospital	Bolivar	Missouri	417-326-6000	www.citizensmemorial.com
Cleveland Regional Medical Center	Shelby	North Carolina	704-487-3000	www.clevelandregional.org
Community Hospital East	Indianapolis	Indiana	317-355-5411	www.ecommunity.com
Conway Regional Medical Center	Conway	Arkansas	501-329-3831	www.conwayregional.org
Coshocton County Memorial Hospital	Coshocton	Ohio	740-622-6411	www.ccmh.com
Dallas County Medical Center	Fordyce	Arkansas	870-352-6300	www.dallascountymedicalcenter.com
Dekalb Regional Medical Center	Fort Payne	Alabama	256-845-3150	www.baptistmedical.org
Delano Regional Medical Center	Delano	California	661-725-4800	www.drmc.com
Desert Springs Hospital	Las Vegas	Nevada	702-369-7600	www.desertspringshospital.net/p12.html
Doctors Medical Center	Modesto	California	209-578-1211	www.dmc-modesto.com
East Georgia Regional Medical Center	Statesboro	Georgia	912-486-1500	www.egrmc.com
East Liverpool City Hospital	East Liverpool	Ohio	330-385-7200	www.elch.org
Eastern Niagara Hospital	Lockport	New York	716-514-5700	www.enhs.org
El Centro Regional Medical Center	El Centro	California	760-339-7100	www.ecrmc.org
Eliza Coffee Memorial Hospital	Florence	Alabama	256-768-8400	www.chgroup.org
Erlanger Medical Center	Chattanooga	Tennessee	423-778-7000	www.erlanger.org
Essentia Health Saint Mary's Medical Center	Duluth	Minnesota	218-786-4000	www.smdc.org
Florida Hospital Deland	Deland	Florida	386-943-4772	www.fhdeland.org
Floyd County Memorial Hospital	Charles City	Iowa	641-228-6830	www.fcmc.us.com
Franklin General Hospital	Hampton	Iowa	641-456-5000	www.franklingeneral.com
Franklin Medical Center	Winnsboro	Louisiana	318-435-9411	www.fmc-cares.com
Fremont Area Medical Center	Fremont	Nebraska	402-721-1610	www.famc.org
Frye Regional Medical Center	Hickory	North Carolina	828-322-6070	www.fryemedctr.com
Fulton County Hospital	Salem	Arkansas	870-895-2691	www.fultoncountyhospital.org
GV (Sonny) Montgomery VA Medical Center Jackson	Jackson	Mississippi	601-362-4471	www.visn16.med.va.gov
Gadsden Regional Medical Center	Gadsden	Alabama	256-494-4000	www.gadsdenregional.com
Galesburg Cottage Hospital	Galesburg	Illinois	309-345-4555	www.cottagehospital.com
Gateway Medical Center	Clarksville	Tennessee	931-502-1000	www.todaysgateway.com
GHS Laurens County Memorial Hospital	Clinton	South Carolina	864-833-9100	www.lchcs.org
Glenwood Regional Medical Center	West Monroe	Louisiana	318-329-4600	www.grmc.com
Good Samaritan Hospital	Kearney	Nebraska	308-865-7100	www.gshs.org
Good Samaritan Hospital	Lebanon	Pennsylvania	717-270-7500	www.gshleb.org
Greenview Regional Hospital	Bowling Green	Kentucky	270-793-1000	www.greenviewhospital.com
Grossmont Hospital	La Mesa	California	619-465-0711	www.sharp.com
Halifax Health Medical Center	Daytona Beach	Florida	386-254-4000	www.halifax.org
Hammond Henry Hospital	Geneseo	Illinois	309-944-6431	www.hammondhenry.com
Harrison County Hospital	Corydon	Indiana	812-738-4251	www.hchin.org
Harrison Memorial Hospital	Cynthiana	Kentucky	859-234-2300	www.harrisonmemhosp.com
Harton Regional Medical Center	Tullahoma	Tennessee	931-393-3000	www.hartonmedicalcenter.com
Helen Keller Memorial Hospital	Sheffield	Alabama	256-386-4556	www.helenkeller.com
Helena Regional Medical Center	Helena	Arkansas	870-338-5800	www.helenaregionalmedicalcenter.com
Hemet Valley Medical Center	Hemet	California	951-652-2811	www.valleyhealthsystem.com/hemmain
Highland Hospital	Rochester	New York	585-473-2200	www.urmc.rochester.edu

Hospital	City	State	Phone	Web Site
Highlands Regional Medical Center	Sebring	Florida	863-385-6101	www.highlandsregional.com
Highline Medical Center	Burien	Washington	206-244-9970	www.hchnet.org
Hospital Pavia Santurce	Fernandez Juncos	Puerto Rico	787-727-6060	www.paviahospitalsanturce.com
Howard Memorial Hospital	Nashville	Arkansas	870-845-4400	www.howardmemorial.com
Hutchinson Regional Medical Center	Hutchinson	Kansas	620-665-2001	www.hutchinsonhospital.com
Iberia General Hospital & Medical Center	New Iberia	Louisiana	337-364-0441	www.iberiamedicalcenter.com
Indiana University Health Bloomington Hospital	Bloomington	Indiana	812-353-9555	www.bloomingtonhospital.org
Indiana University Health La Porte Hospital	La Porte	Indiana	219-326-1234	www.laportehealth.org
Inspira Medical Center Vineland	Vineland	New Jersey	856-641-6610	www.sjhs.com
Integris Grove Hospital	Grove	Oklahoma	918-786-2243	www.integris-health.com
IU Health Goshen Hospital	Goshen	Indiana	574-364-1000	www.goshenhosp.com
Jackson Hospital & Clinic	Montgomery	Alabama	334-293-8000	www.jackson.org
Jackson Memorial Hospital	Miami	Florida	305-585-1111	www.jhsmiami.org
Jacksonville Medical Center	Jacksonville	Alabama	256-782-4538	www.jmchealth.com
Jane Phillips Medical Center	Bartlesville	Oklahoma	918-333-7200	www.jpmc.org
Jeff Davis Hospital	Hazlehurst	Georgia	912-375-7781	www.jeffdavishospital.org
Jennie Stuart Medical Center	Hopkinsville	Kentucky	270-887-0100	www.jsmc.org
JFK Medical Center - A M Yelencsics Comm Hospital	Edison	New Jersey	732-321-7000	www.jfkmc.org
Keokuk Area Hospital	Keokuk	Iowa	319-524-7150	www.keokukhealthsystems.org
Lafayette General Medical Center	Lafayette	Louisiana	337-289-7991	www.lafayettegeneral.org
Lake Charles Memorial Hospital	Lake Charles	Louisiana	337-494-3200	www.lcmh.com
Lake Cumberland Regional Hospital	Somerset	Kentucky	606-679-7441	www.lakecumberlandhospital.com
Lake Granbury Medical Center	Granbury	Texas	817-573-2683	www.lakegranburymedicalcenter.com
Lexington Medical Center	West Columbia	South Carolina	803-791-2000	www.lexmed.com
Lexington VA Medical Center	Lexington	Kentucky	859-233-4511	www.lexington.va.gov
Livingston Regional Hospital	Livingston	Tennessee	931-823-5611	www.livingstonregionalhospital.com
Lompoc Valley Medical Center	Lompoc	California	805-737-3300	www.lompochospital.org
Louisville VA Medical Center	Louisville	Kentucky	502-287-4000	www.va.gov/603louisville
Madera Community Hospital	Madera	California	559-675-5555	www.maderahospital.org
Mahaska Health Partnership	Oskaloosa	Iowa	641-672-3100	www.mahaskahospital.com
Margaret Mary Community Hospital	Batesville	Indiana	812-934-6624	www.mmch.org
Marion General Hospital	Columbia	Mississippi	601-736-6303	
Marshall Medical Center South	Boaz	Alabama	256-593-8310	www.mmcenters.com/mmcsouth.php
McGehee Hospital	Mcgehee	Arkansas	870-222-5600	
Medical Center Hospital	Odessa	Texas	432-640-4000	www.mchodessa.com
Memorial Medical Center	Modesto	California	209-526-4500	www.memorialmedicalcenter.org
Memorial Healthcare	Owosso	Michigan	989-723-5211	www.memorialhealthcare.org
Memorial Hospital & Manor	Bainbridge	Georgia	229-246-3500	www.mh-m.org
Memorial Hospital of Martinsville & Henry County	Martinsville	Virginia	276-666-7200	www.martinsvillehospital.com
Memorial Hospital of South Bend	South Bend	Indiana	574-647-1000	www.qualityoflife.org
Memorial Medical Center of East Texas	Lufkin	Texas	936-634-8111	www.mymemorialhealth.org
Mercy Health - West Hospital	Cincinnati	Ohio	513-215-5000	www.e-mercy.com/west-hospital.aspx
Mercy Hospital Oklahoma City	Oklahoma City	Oklahoma	405-752-3754	www.mercyok.net/mhc
Mercy Hospital Springfield	Springfield	Missouri	417-820-2000	www.stjohns.com
Mercy Medical Center	Merced	California	209-564-5000	www.mercymercedcares.org
Mercy Medical Center	Rockville Centre	New York	516-705-2525	www.mercymedicalcenter.info
Mercy Medical Center - Mount Shasta	Mount Shasta	California	530-926-6111	www.mercymtshasta.org
Mercy Memorial Health Center	Ardmore	Oklahoma	405-223-5400	www.mercyok.com/mmhc
Methodist Healthcare Memphis Hospitals	Memphis	Tennessee	901-516-8274	www.methodisthealth.org
Mid Coast Hospital	Brunswick	Maine	207-729-0181	www.midcoasthealth.com
Midtown Medical Center	Columbus	Georgia	706-571-1000	www.columbusregional.com
Milford Hospital	Milford	Connecticut	203-876-4000	www.milfordhospital.org
Mississippi Baptist Medical Center	Jackson	Mississippi	601-968-1000	www.mbmc.org
Mizell Memorial Hospital	Opp	Alabama	334-493-3541	www.mizellmh.com
Mobile Infirmary	Mobile	Alabama	251-435-4700	www.mimc.com
Morris Hospital & Healthcare Centers	Morris	Illinois	815-942-2932	www.morrishospital.org
Mount Carmel West	Columbus	Ohio	614-234-5000	www.mountcarmelhealth.com
Multicare Good Samaritan Hospital	Puyallup	Washington	253-697-2102	www.multicare.org/goodsam
Neshoba County General Hospital	Philadelphia	Mississippi	601-663-1200	www.neshobageneral.com
New London Family Medical Center	New London	Wisconsin	920-531-2000	www.thedacare.org
North Mississippi Medical Center	Tupelo	Mississippi	662-377-3000	www.nmhs.net/nmmc
North Valley Hospital	Whitefish	Montana	406-863-3550	www.nvhosp.org
Northern Louisiana Medical Center	Ruston	Louisiana	318-254-2100	www.lincolnhealth.com
Novant Health Rowan Medical Center	Salisbury	North Carolina	704-210-5000	www.rowan.org
Novant Health Thomasville Medical Center	Thomasville	North Carolina	336-472-2000	www.thomasvillemedicalcenter.org
Och Regional Medical Center	Starkville	Mississippi	662-323-4320	www.och.org
Ohio Valley General Hospital	Mckees Rocks	Pennsylvania	412-777-6161	www.ohiovalleyhospital.org

Hospital	City	State	Phone	Web Site
Olympic Medical Center	Port Angeles	Washington	360-417-7000	www.olympicmedical.org
Orange Park Medical Center	Orange Park	Florida	904-276-8500	www.opmedical.com
Paris Regional Medical Center	Paris	Texas	903-785-4521	www.parisregional.com
Passavant Area Hospital	Jacksonville	Illinois	217-245-9551	www.passavanthospital.com
Petaluma Valley Hospital	Petaluma	California	707-778-1111	www.stjosephhealth.org
Peterson Regional Medical Center	Kerrville	Texas	830-896-4200	www.petersonrmc.com
Piedmont Medical Center	Rock Hill	South Carolina	803-329-1234	www.piedmontmedicalcenter.com
Pike Community Hospital	Waverly	Ohio	740-947-2186	www.adena.org
Pinnacle Health Hospitals	Harrisburg	Pennsylvania	717-782-5181	www.pinnaclehealth.org
Pottstown Memorial Medical Center	Pottstown	Pennsylvania	610-327-7000	www.pmmctr.org
Rappahannock General Hospital	Kilmarnock	Virginia	804-435-8000	www.rgh-hospital.com
Redlands Community Hospital	Redlands	California	909-335-5500	www.redlandshospital.com
River Parishes Hospital	Laplace	Louisiana	985-652-7000	www.riverparisheshospital.com
River Valley Medical Center	Dardanelle	Arkansas	479-229-4677	
Rockcastle County Hospital	Mount Vernon	Kentucky	606-256-2195	www.rockcastlehospital.com
Rush Foundation Hospital	Meridian	Mississippi	601-483-0011	www.rushhealthsystems.org
Rush Memorial Hospital	Rushville	Indiana	765-932-7513	www.rushmemorial.com
Russell Hospital	Alexander City	Alabama	256-329-7100	www.russellmedcenter.com
Saint Joseph Mount Sterling	Mount Sterling	Kentucky	859-498-1220	www.marychiles.org
San Gorgonio Memorial Hospital	Banning	California	951-769-2101	www.sgmh.org
San Juan VA Medical Center	San Juan	Puerto Rico	800-449-8729	www.visn8.med.va.gov/caribbean
Sentara Careplex Hospital	Hampton	Virginia	757-736-1000	www.sentara.com
Sentara Leigh Hospital	Norfolk	Virginia	757-261-6601	www.sentara.com
Sentara Obici Hospital	Suffolk	Virginia	757-934-4000	www.sentara.com
Seven Rivers Regional Medical Center	Crystal River	Florida	352-795-6560	www.srrmc.com
Shands Live Oak Regional Medical Center	Live Oak	Florida	904-362-1413	www.shands.org
Sierra View District Hospital	Porterville	California	559-784-1110	www.sierra-view.com
Skyridge Medical Center	Cleveland	Tennessee	423-339-4132	www.skyridgemedcenter.com
Somerset Medical Center	Somerville	New Jersey	908-685-2200	www.somersetmedicalcenter.com
South Central Regional Medical Center	Laurel	Mississippi	601-649-4000	www.scrmc.com
South Shore Hospital	South Weymouth	Massachusetts	781-340-8000	www.southshorehospital.org
Southampton Memorial Hospital	Franklin	Virginia	757-569-6100	www.smhfranklin.com
Southern Virginia Regional Medical Center	Emporia	Virginia	434-348-4400	www.svrmc.com
Spectrum Health - Reed City Campus	Reed City	Michigan	231-832-3271	www.spectrum-health.org
Spencer Municipal Hospital	Spencer	Iowa	712-264-8300	www.spencerhospital.org
Springfield Regional Medical Center	Springfield	Ohio	937-523-1000	www.communityhospital.com
Springs Memorial Hospital	Lancaster	South Carolina	803-286-1481	www.springsmemorial.com
Saint Anthony Regional Hospital & Nursing Home	Carroll	Iowa	712-792-3581	www.stanthonyhospital.org
Saint Anthony Shawnee Hospital	Shawnee	Oklahoma	405-273-2270	www.unityhealthcenter.com
Saint Catherine Hospital	Garden City	Kansas	620-272-2561	www.stcath-hosp.org
Saint Francis Community Hospital	Federal Way	Washington	253-944-8100	www.fhshealth.org
Saint Francis Hospital	Litchfield	Illinois	217-324-2191	www.stfrancis-litchfield.org
Saint Francis Hospital	Memphis	Tennessee	901-765-1000	www.saintfrancishosp.com
Saint Francis Hospital	Columbus	Georgia	706-596-4020	www.wecareforlife.com
Saint Francis - Downtown	Greenville	South Carolina	864-255-1000	www.stfrancishealth.org
Saint Joseph Hospital	Orange	California	714-633-9111	www.sjo.org
Saint Joseph Hospital & Health Center	Kokomo	Indiana	765-456-5300	www.stvincent.org
Saint Joseph's Hospital - Savannah	Savannah	Georgia	912-819-4100	www.sjchs.org
Saint Joseph's Medical Center of Stockton	Stockton	California	209-943-2000	www.stjospehscares.org
Saint Peter's Hospital	Helena	Montana	406-442-2480	www.stpetes.org
Saint Vincent Dunn Hospital	Bedford	Indiana	812-275-3331	www.stvincent.org/St-Vincent-Dunn
Saint Vincent's East	Birmingham	Alabama	205-838-3122	www.nolandhealth.com
Starr Regional Medical Center Athens	Athens	Tennessee	423-745-1411	www.athensrmc.com
Sumner Regional Medical Center	Gallatin	Tennessee	615-452-4210	www.mysumnermedical.com
Sunbury Community Hospital	Sunbury	Pennsylvania	570-286-3333	www.schopc.org
Sunrise Hospital & Medical Center	Las Vegas	Nevada	702-731-8000	www.sunrisehospital.com
Teche Regional Medical Center	Morgan City	Louisiana	985-384-2200	www.techeregional.com
Terrebonne General Medical Center	Houma	Louisiana	985-873-4141	www.tgmc.com
Texoma Medical Center	Denison	Texas	903-416-4000	www.texomamedicalcenter.net
Thibodaux Regional Medical Center	Thibodaux	Louisiana	985-447-5500	www.thibodaux.com
Thomas Memorial Hospital	South Charleston	West Virginia	304-766-3600	www.thomaswv.org
Trinity Medical Center	Birmingham	Alabama	205-592-1000	www.bhsala.com/montclair
Trinity Rock Island	Rock Island	Illinois	309-779-5000	www.trinityqc.com
Tuality Community Hospital	Hillsboro	Oregon	503-681-1111	www.tuality.com
Twin County Regional Hospital	Galax	Virginia	276-236-8181	www.tcrh.org
Union General Hospital	Farmerville	Louisiana	318-368-9751	www.uniongen.org
United Health Services Hospitals	Johnson City	New York	607-763-6000	www.vhs.ent

Hospital	City	State	Phone	Web Site
University Mcduffie County Regional Medical Center	Thomson	Georgia	706-595-1411	www.mrmc.org
University of Missouri Health Care	Columbia	Missouri	573-882-4141	www.missouri.edu
Upson Regional Medical Center	Thomaston	Georgia	706-647-8111	www.urmc.org
Upstate New York VA Healthcare System - Western NY	Buffalo	New York	716-862-3611	www.buffalo.va.gov
Utah Valley Regional Medical Center	Provo	Utah	801-373-7850	www.intermountainhealthcare.org/hospitals/uvrmc
VA Middle Tennessee Healthcare System	Nashville	Tennessee	615-327-5332	www.tennesseevalley.va.gov
VA Salt Lake City Healthcare - George E. Wahlen VA	Salt Lake City	Utah	801-584-1211	www1.va.gov/directory/guide/facility.asp?
Vidant Edgecombe Hospital	Tarboro	North Carolina	252-641-7700	www.vidanthealth.com/edgecombe
Vista Medical Center East	Waukegan	Illinois	847-360-4000	www.vistahealth.com
Western Plains Medical Complex	Dodge City	Kansas	620-225-8400	www.westernplainsmc.com
Wilkes-Barre General Hospital	Wilkes-Barre	Pennsylvania	570-829-8111	www.wvhcs.org
Wilson Medical Center	Wilson	North Carolina	252-399-8040	www.wilmed.org/contact.asp
Wise Regional Health System	Decatur	Texas	940-627-5921	www.wiseregional.com
Woodland Heights Medical Center	Lufkin	Texas	936-634-8311	www.woodlandheights.net
Woodland Memorial Hospital	Woodland	California	530-662-3961	www.woodlandhealthcare.org
Yakima Valley Memorial Hospital	Yakima	Washington	509-575-8000	www.yakimamemorialhospital.org
Yuma Regional Medical Center	Yuma	Arizona	928-336-7275	www.yumaregional.org

Note: Table shows hospitals nationwide whose pneumonia 30-day risk-adjusted mortality rate is worse (higher) than U.S. rate of 11.9%

Hospital Mortality from Heart Attack: State and National Summary

Area	Number of Hospitals			
	Better than U.S. National Rate[1]	Worse than U.S. National Rate[2]	No Different than U.S. National Rate[3]	Number of Cases Too Small[4]
U.S. and Territories	77	19	2579	1889
Alabama	0	0	50	50
Alaska	0	0	5	15
American Samoa	0	0	0	1
Arizona	1	0	49	19
Arkansas	1	2	30	40
California	7	1	219	103
Colorado	0	0	33	35
Connecticut	2	0	28	1
Delaware	1	0	5	1
District of Columbia	0	0	6	2
Florida	3	1	157	22
Georgia	0	0	74	65
Guam	0	0	1	0
Hawaii	0	0	12	4
Idaho	0	0	10	23
Illinois	8	0	112	61
Indiana	1	0	68	49
Iowa	0	0	35	81
Kansas	1	0	29	91
Kentucky	0	1	51	43
Louisiana	0	1	49	52
Maine	1	1	30	5
Maryland	1	0	40	6
Massachusetts	4	0	54	6
Michigan	6	3	72	49
Minnesota	1	0	36	85
Mississippi	0	0	34	50
Missouri	4	0	57	54
Montana	0	0	8	39
N. Mariana Islands	0	0	0	1
Nebraska	0	0	20	56
Nevada	0	1	18	13
New Hampshire	1	1	17	6
New Jersey	8	1	54	3
New Mexico	0	0	13	26
New York	10	1	141	31
North Carolina	2	0	83	24
North Dakota	0	1	8	32
Ohio	1	0	112	47
Oklahoma	0	0	35	71
Oregon	0	0	29	31
Pennsylvania	6	1	122	33
Puerto Rico	0	0	21	24
Rhode Island	2	0	9	0
South Carolina	0	0	42	20
South Dakota	1	0	10	40
Tennessee	1	0	66	46
Texas	2	3	189	149
Utah	0	0	16	19
Vermont	0	0	10	5
Virgin Islands	0	0	1	1
Virginia	0	0	73	9
Washington	0	0	44	40
West Virginia	1	0	29	24
Wisconsin	0	0	60	62
Wyoming	0	0	3	24

Note: (1) 30-day risk-adjusted mortality rate is better (lower) than U.S. rate of 15.2%; (2) 30-day risk-adjusted mortality rate is worse (higher) than U.S. rate of 15.2%; (3) 30-day risk-adjusted mortality rate is about the same as U.S. rate of 15.2%; (4) The number of cases is too small to classify the hospital

Hospital Mortality from Heart Failure: State and National Summary

Area	Number of Hospitals			
	Better than U.S. National Rate[1]	Worse than U.S. National Rate[2]	No Different than U.S. National Rate[3]	Number of Cases Too Small[4]
U.S. and Territories	181	139	3732	725
Alabama	1	2	89	8
Alaska	0	1	9	12
American Samoa	0	0	0	1
Arizona	2	1	57	17
Arkansas	0	11	59	7
California	30	10	246	51
Colorado	0	0	55	19
Connecticut	4	3	24	1
Delaware	1	0	6	0
District of Columbia	2	0	6	0
Florida	8	5	166	8
Georgia	1	2	126	15
Guam	0	0	1	0
Hawaii	0	0	14	5
Idaho	0	1	21	15
Illinois	16	5	156	7
Indiana	3	7	108	2
Iowa	0	2	95	21
Kansas	0	1	83	49
Kentucky	0	1	92	3
Louisiana	2	6	82	19
Maine	0	1	34	2
Maryland	9	2	35	1
Massachusetts	14	1	47	2
Michigan	12	3	106	14
Minnesota	2	0	81	48
Mississippi	0	3	77	18
Missouri	4	5	96	11
Montana	0	0	26	35
N. Mariana Islands	0	0	0	1
Nebraska	0	2	48	35
Nevada	1	2	27	5
New Hampshire	0	0	25	1
New Jersey	13	1	52	0
New Mexico	0	2	30	9
New York	13	7	156	7
North Carolina	4	3	97	8
North Dakota	0	0	24	20
Ohio	6	3	144	13
Oklahoma	2	3	84	29
Oregon	1	2	49	8
Pennsylvania	16	6	136	6
Puerto Rico	0	0	28	21
Rhode Island	0	0	11	1
South Carolina	1	3	57	2
South Dakota	0	1	26	26
Tennessee	0	2	107	7
Texas	8	8	294	62
Utah	0	1	24	17
Vermont	0	2	12	1
Virgin Islands	0	0	2	0
Virginia	1	2	79	2
Washington	0	7	58	24
West Virginia	1	0	47	6
Wisconsin	3	8	101	12
Wyoming	0	1	17	11

Note: (1) 30-day risk-adjusted mortality rate is better (lower) than U.S. rate of 11.7%; (2) 30-day risk-adjusted mortality rate is worse (higher) than U.S. rate of 11.7%; (3) 30-day risk-adjusted mortality rate is about the same as U.S. rate of 11.7%; (4) The number of cases is too small to classify the hospital

Hospital Mortality from Pneumonia: State and National Summary

Area	Number of Hospitals			
	Better than U.S. National Rate[1]	Worse than U.S. National Rate[2]	No Different than U.S. National Rate[3]	Number of Cases Too Small[4]
U.S. and Territories	203	223	4014	377
Alabama	0	13	84	4
Alaska	0	0	15	7
American Samoa	0	0	1	0
Arizona	3	2	66	10
Arkansas	0	8	66	3
California	34	19	244	45
Colorado	2	0	60	13
Connecticut	4	1	27	0
Delaware	0	0	7	0
District of Columbia	0	0	8	0
Florida	9	7	167	5
Georgia	1	11	128	3
Guam	0	0	1	0
Hawaii	0	0	14	8
Idaho	0	0	33	6
Illinois	16	7	157	4
Indiana	1	10	107	2
Iowa	2	6	105	5
Kansas	0	3	116	13
Kentucky	2	9	85	0
Louisiana	1	11	86	14
Maine	0	1	35	1
Maryland	8	0	37	1
Massachusetts	10	1	51	3
Michigan	10	3	116	6
Minnesota	1	1	112	17
Mississippi	0	10	78	10
Missouri	7	4	101	5
Montana	1	2	39	20
N. Mariana Islands	0	0	1	0
Nebraska	1	2	70	13
Nevada	3	3	24	6
New Hampshire	1	0	25	0
New Jersey	15	3	48	0
New Mexico	0	0	38	4
New York	14	6	161	4
North Carolina	6	9	94	4
North Dakota	0	0	39	5
Ohio	9	6	146	4
Oklahoma	2	5	101	11
Oregon	1	2	54	3
Pennsylvania	10	7	143	5
Puerto Rico	0	3	26	21
Rhode Island	1	0	10	1
South Carolina	1	5	55	2
South Dakota	0	1	49	6
Tennessee	2	13	96	5
Texas	13	10	306	48
Utah	0	2	33	7
Vermont	0	0	15	0
Virgin Islands	0	0	2	0
Virginia	5	10	67	5
Washington	2	5	73	9
West Virginia	1	1	51	1
Wisconsin	4	1	115	5
Wyoming	0	0	26	3

Note: (1) 30-day risk-adjusted mortality rate is better (lower) than U.S. rate of 11.9%; (2) 30-day risk-adjusted mortality rate is worse (higher) than U.S. rate of 11.9%; (3) 30-day risk-adjusted mortality rate is about the same as U.S. rate of 11.9%; (4) The number of cases is too small to classify the hospital

Appendix B: 30-Day Readmission Rates

What Do These Readmission Categories Show?

"Readmission" is when patients who have had a recent stay in the hospital go back into a hospital again. The information shows how often patients are readmitted within 30 days of discharge from a previous hospital stay for heart attack, heart failure, or pneumonia. Patients may have been readmitted back to the same hospital or to a different hospital or acute care facility. They may have been readmitted for the same condition as their recent hospital stay, or for a different reason.

This first part of this appendix shows hospitals with risk-adjusted 30-day unplanned readmission rates that are lower (better) or higher (worse) than the national rate for all three categories. Hospitals are shown to be better or worse than the U.S. national rate only if the data shows with 95% certainty, that the difference between their surgical complication rates and the U.S. national rate is not due to chance.

The second part of this appendix contains state and national summaries with the following column headers:

- **Better Than U.S. National Rate.** Hospitals in the Better Than U.S. National Rate category have risk-adjusted 30-day unplanned readmission rates that are lower than the U.S. National Rate, and with 95% certainty that this difference is not due to chance.
- **Worse Than U.S. National Rate.** Hospitals in the Worse Than U.S. National Rate category have risk-adjusted 30-day unplanned readmission rates that are higher than the U.S. National Rate, and with 95% certainty that this difference is not due to chance.
- **No Different Than U.S. National Rate.** Many hospitals in the No Different Than U.S. National Rate category have risk-adjusted 30-day unplanned readmission rates that are about the same as the U.S. National Rate. Other hospitals in this category have rates that are higher or lower than the U.S. National Rate, but without 95% certainty that these differences are not due to chance.
- **Number of Cases Too Small.** The number of cases is too small to classify the hospital..

Why are Readmission Rates for Individual Hospitals Not Shown?

Comparisons based on estimated readmission rates alone can be misleading. Risk-adjusted readmission rates are estimated for individual hospitals based on information taken from a particular time period. If a slightly different time period had been chosen, chances are that each hospital's results would have been somewhat different.

A range ("confidence interval" or in this case an "interval estimate") around estimates show how much variation might be due to this kind of chance. In this case, researchers are 95% confident that a hospital's readmission rate fell somewhere within this specified range. The smaller the range, the more precise the estimate.

When hospitals treat a very large number of patients, chance differences will not have much effect on the overall rates. The range will be small, and the estimated readmission rates will be more precise. In hospitals that treat smaller numbers of patients, however, even small chance differences could have a big impact on readmission rates. The 95% confidence interval, or range, will be large, and the estimated readmission rates will be less precise.

Because the number of patients treated at U.S. hospitals varies widely, the precision of hospitals' estimated readmission rates also varies.

Calculation of 30-Day Risk-Standardized Rates of Readmission

The 30-day readmission measures are estimates of unplanned readmission for any cause to any acute care hospital within 30 days of discharge from a hospitalization. Using unplanned readmissions within 30 days instead of over longer time periods (such as 90 days) eliminate factors outside hospitals' control such as other complicating illnesses, patients' own behavior, or care provided to patients after discharge. *The Comparative Guide to American Hospitals* reports the following 30-day readmission measures:

- 30-day unplanned readmission for heart attack (AMI) patients
- 30-day unplanned readmission for heart failure (HF) patients
- 30-day unplanned readmission for pneumonia patients
- 30-day unplanned readmission for hip/knee replacement patients
- 30-day overall rate of unplanned readmission after discharge from the hospital (hospital-wide readmission). Note: This measure includes patients admitted for internal medicine, surgery/gynecology, cardiorespiratory, cardiovascular, and neurology services. It is not a composite measure.

Which Patients are Included

The 30-day unplanned readmission measures include hospitalizations for Medicare beneficiaries aged 65 or older who were enrolled in Original Medicare (traditional fee-for-service Medicare) for the entire 12 months prior to their hospital admission (and for readmissions, for 30 days after their original admission). The AMI, heart failure, and pneumonia unplanned readmission measures also include patients aged 65 or older who were admitted to Veteran's Health Administration (VA) hospitals. Beneficiaries enrolled in Medicare managed care plans are not included. The unplanned readmission measures do not include patients who died during the index admission, or who left the hospital against medical advice.

Where the Information Comes From

The Centers for Medicare & Medicaid Services (CMS) calculates hospital-specific 30-day readmission rates using Medicare claims and eligibility information. The AMI, HF, and pneumonia readmission measures are also calculated using VA administrative data. Using administrative data makes it possible to calculate readmission rates without having to do medical chart reviews or requiring hospitals to report additional information to CMS.

Risk Adjustment

To make comparison of hospital performance equitable, the 30-day unplanned readmission measures adjust for patient characteristics that may make unplanned readmission more likely, even if the hospital provided higher quality of care. These characteristics include the patient's age, past medical history, and other diseases or conditions (comorbidities) the patient had when admitted that are known to increase the patient's risk of having an unplanned readmission.

Significance Testing

The statistical model used to calculate 30-day unplanned readmission measures also determines how precise the estimates are, and provides the upper and lower bounds of the 95% interval estimates for each hospital's readmission rates. Interval estimates, which are like confidence intervals, describe the level of uncertainty around the estimated readmission rates.

Comparing Individual Hospital Rates to the U.S. National Rate

To assign hospitals to performance categories, the hospital's interval estimate is compared to the U.S. national 30-day observed unplanned readmission rate. If the 95% interval estimate includes the national observed rate for that measure, the hospital's performance is in the "No Different than U.S. National Rate" category. If the entire 95% interval estimate is below the national observed rate for that measure, then the hospital is performing "Better Than U.S. National Rate." If the entire 95% interval estimate is above the national observed rate for that measure, its performance is "Worse Than U.S. National Rate." Hospitals with fewer than 25 eligible cases are placed into a separate category that indicates that the hospital did not have enough cases to reliably tell how well the hospital is performing.

Additional information

For more detail on how the 30-day unplanned readmission rates are calculated, please visit QualityNet—Readmission Measures at www.qualitynet.org.

Hospitals whose Acute Myocardial Infarction (Heart Attack) 30-Day Readmission Rate is Better (Lower) than the U.S. National Rate

Hospital	City	State	Phone	Web Site
Asante Rogue Regional Medical Center	Medford	Oregon	541-789-7000	www.asante.org
Aspirus Wausau Hospital	Wausau	Wisconsin	715-847-2121	www.aspirus.org
Aurora Saint Lukes Medical Center	Milwaukee	Wisconsin	414-649-6000	www.aurorahealthcare.org
Baylor Heart & Vascular Hospital	Dallas	Texas	214-820-0670	www.baylorhearthospital.com
Bellin Memorial Hospital	Green Bay	Wisconsin	920-433-3500	www.bellin.org
Central Washington Hospital	Wenatchee	Washington	509-662-1511	www.cwhs.com
Frye Regional Medical Center	Hickory	North Carolina	828-322-6070	www.fryemedctr.com
GHS Greenville Memorial Medical Center	Greenville	South Carolina	864-455-7000	www.ghs.org
Lancaster General Hospital	Lancaster	Pennsylvania	717-299-5511	www.lancastergeneral.org
Lovelace Medical Center	Albuquerque	New Mexico	505-727-8000	www.lovelace.com
Maine Medical Center	Portland	Maine	207-662-0111	www.mmc.org
Mercy Health Partners - Mercy Campus	Muskegon	Michigan	231-672-3901	www.mghp.com
Munroe Regional Medical Center	Ocala	Florida	352-351-7200	www.munroeregional.com
Parkview Regional Medical Center	Fort Wayne	Indiana	260-266-1000	www.parkview.com
Providence Sacred Heart Medical Center	Spokane	Washington	509-474-3040	www.shmc.org
Saint Joseph's Hospital of Atlanta	Atlanta	Georgia	678-843-5720	www.stjosephsatlanta.org
Sanford Medical Center Fargo	Fargo	North Dakota	701-234-2000	www.meritcare.com
Sarasota Memorial Hospital	Sarasota	Florida	941-917-9000	www.smh.com
Saint Luke's Episcopal Hospital	Houston	Texas	832-355-1000	www.sleh.com
Saint Vincent Heart Center of Indiana	Indianapolis	Indiana	317-583-5000	www.theheartcenter.com
Sutter Roseville Medical Center	Roseville	California	916-781-1000	www.sutterroseville.org
University Colo Health Memorial Hospital Central	Colorado Springs	Colorado	719-365-5000	www.memorialhospital.com
Venice Regional Medical Center - Bayfront Health	Venice	Florida	941-485-7711	www.veniceregional.com

Note: Table shows hospitals nationwide whose acute myocardial infarction 30-day readmission rate is better (lower) than U.S. rate of 18.3%

Hospitals whose Acute Myocardial Infarction (Heart Attack) 30-Day Readmission Rate is Worse (Higher) than the U.S. National Rate

Hospital	City	State	Phone	Web Site
Baxter Regional Medical Center	Mountain Home	Arkansas	870-508-1000	www.baxterregional.org
Boston Medical Center Corporation	Boston	Massachusetts	617-638-8000	www.bmc.org
Carolinas Hospital System	Florence	South Carolina	843-674-2500	www.carolinashospital.com
Centra Health	Lynchburg	Virginia	434-200-4789	www.centrahealth.com
Community Medical Center	Toms River	New Jersey	732-557-8000	www.sbhcs.com
Florida Hospital	Orlando	Florida	407-303-1976	www.floridahospital.com
Good Samaritan Regional Health Center	Mount Vernon	Illinois	618-899-1469	www.smgsi.com
Hillcrest Medical Center	Tulsa	Oklahoma	918-579-1000	www.hillcrest.com
Ingalls Memorial Hospital	Harvey	Illinois	708-333-2300	www.ingalls.org
Johnson City Medical Center	Johnson City	Tennessee	423-431-6111	www.msha.com
Kaleida Health	Buffalo	New York	716-859-8620	www.kaleidahealth.org
Lewisgale Medical Center	Salem	Virginia	540-776-4000	www.lewis-gale.com
Mercy Hospital & Medical Center	Chicago	Illinois	312-567-2000	www.mercy-chicago.org
Montefiore Medical Center	Bronx	New York	718-920-4321	www.montefiore.org
Newark Beth Israel Medical Center	Newark	New Jersey	973-926-7850	www.sbhcs.com
North Shore University Hospital	Manhasset	New York	516-562-0100	www.northshorelij.com
Northside Hospital	Saint Petersburg	Florida	813-521-5000	www.northsidehospital.com
Northwest Community Hospital	Arlington Heights	Illinois	847-618-1000	www.nch.org
Olympia Medical Center	Los Angeles	California	310-657-5900	www.olympiamc.com
Presence Saint Joseph Medical Center	Joliet	Illinois	815-725-7133	www.provena.org/stjoes
Raleigh General Hospital	Beckley	West Virginia	304-256-4100	www.raleighgeneral.com
Saint Clare's Hospital	Denville	New Jersey	973-625-6000	www.saintclares.org
Saint Michael's Medical Center	Newark	New Jersey	973-877-5350	www.cathedralhealth.org
San Juan VA Medical Center	San Juan	Puerto Rico	800-449-8729	www.visn8.med.va.gov/caribbean
Saint Joseph's Regional Medical Center	Paterson	New Jersey	973-754-2010	www.sjhmc.org
Saint Vincent's Medical Center	Bridgeport	Connecticut	203-576-5551	www.stvincents.org
Tampa VA Medical Center	Tampa	Florida	813-972-2000	www.tampa.va.gov
University Hospital - Stony Brook	Stony Brook	New York	631-444-4000	www.stonybrookmedicalcenter.org
Vidant Medical Center	Greenville	North Carolina	252-847-4100	www.uhseast.com

Note: Table shows hospitals nationwide whose acute myocardial infarction 30-day readmission rate is worse (higher) than U.S. rate of 18.3%

Hospitals whose Heart Failure 30-Day Readmission Rate is Better (Lower) than the U.S. National Rate

Hospital	City	State	Phone	Web Site
Abilene Regional Medical Center	Abilene	Texas	325-428-1000	www.abileneregional.com
Alegent Creighton Health Bergan Mercy Medical Center	Omaha	Nebraska	402-398-6060	www.alegent.com
Alpena Regional Medical Center	Alpena	Michigan	989-356-7390	www.agh.org
Asante Rogue Regional Medical Center	Medford	Oregon	541-789-7000	www.asante.org
Audrain Medical Center	Mexico	Missouri	573-582-5000	www.audrainmedicalcenter.com
Aurora Sheboygan Memorial Medical Center	Sheboygan	Wisconsin	920-451-5000	www.aurorahealthcare.org/facilities
Banner Boswell Medical Center	Sun City	Arizona	623-977-7211	www.bannerhealth.com
Banner Good Samaritan Medical Center	Phoenix	Arizona	602-239-2000	www.bannerhealth.com
Baptist Memorial Hospital	Memphis	Tennessee	901-226-5000	www.bmhcc.org
Baptist Saint Anthony's Hospital	Amarillo	Texas	806-212-2000	www.bsahs.com
Bay Medical Center Sacred Heart Health System	Panama City	Florida	850-769-1511	www.baymedical.org
Baylor All Saints Medical Center at FW	Fort Worth	Texas	817-926-2544	www.baylorhealth.com/locations/allsaints
Baylor Medical Center at Garland	Garland	Texas	972-487-5000	www.baylorhealth.com
Baylor University Medical Center	Dallas	Texas	214-820-0111	www.baylorhealth.com
Bellin Memorial Hospital	Green Bay	Wisconsin	920-433-3500	www.bellin.org
Billings Clinic Hospital	Billings	Montana	406-657-4000	www.billngsclinic.com
Boca Raton Regional Hospital	Boca Raton	Florida	561-362-5002	www.brrh.com
Boone Hospital Center	Columbia	Missouri	573-815-8000	www.boone.org
Boulder Community Hospital	Boulder	Colorado	303-440-2273	www.bch.org
Bronson Methodist Hospital	Kalamazoo	Michigan	269-341-6000	www.bronsonhealth.com
Bryan Medical Center	Lincoln	Nebraska	402-481-1111	www.bryan.org
Carolinas Medical Center/Behaviorial Health	Charlotte	North Carolina	704-355-2000	www.carolinasmedicalcenter.org
Carondelet Saint Marys Hospital	Tucson	Arizona	520-872-3000	www.carondelet.org
Catawba Valley Medical Center	Hickory	North Carolina	828-326-3809	www.catawbavalleymc.org
Cedars - Sinai Medical Center	Los Angeles	California	310-423-5000	www.cedars-sinai.edu
Central Maine Medical Center	Lewiston	Maine	207-795-0111	www.cmmc.org
Central Washington Hospital	Wenatchee	Washington	509-662-1511	www.cwhs.com
Chester County Hospital	West Chester	Pennsylvania	610-431-5000	www.cchosp.com
Christus Santa Rosa Hospital	San Antonio	Texas	210-704-2011	www.christussantarosa.org
Citrus Memorial Hospital	Inverness	Florida	352-726-1551	www.citrusmh.com
Columbia Saint Marys Hospital Ozaukee	Mequon	Wisconsin	262-243-7300	www.columbia-stmarys.org
Columbus Regional Hospital	Columbus	Indiana	812-379-4441	www.crh.org
Community Hospital of the Monterey Peninsula	Monterey	California	831-624-5311	www.chomp.org
Cox Medical Center	Springfield	Missouri	417-269-6000	www.coxhealth.com
Decatur Morgan Hospital - Decatur Campus	Decatur	Alabama	256-341-2000	www.decaturgeneral.org
Dixie Regional Medical Center	Saint George	Utah	435-251-2100	www.intermountainhealthcare.org
Dominican Hospital	Santa Cruz	California	831-462-7700	www.dominicanhospital.org
East Jefferson General Hospital	Metairie	Louisiana	504-454-4000	www.eastjeffhospital.org
Eisenhower Medical Center	Rancho Mirage	California	760-340-3911	www.emc.org
Eliza Coffee Memorial Hospital	Florence	Alabama	256-768-8400	www.chgroup.org
Elmhurst Memorial Hospital	Elmhurst	Illinois	630-833-1400	www.emhc.org
Emory University Hospital	Atlanta	Georgia	404-686-8500	www.emoryhealthcare.org
Exempla Lutheran Medical Center	Wheat Ridge	Colorado	303-425-4500	www.exemlpa.org
Fargo VA Medical Center	Fargo	North Dakota	701-232-3241	www.fargo.va.gov
Fremont Area Medical Center	Fremont	Nebraska	402-721-1610	www.famc.org
Frye Regional Medical Center	Hickory	North Carolina	828-322-6070	www.fryemedctr.com
Genesis Medical Center - Davenport	Davenport	Iowa	563-421-1000	www.genesishealth.com
GHS Greenville Memorial Medical Center	Greenville	South Carolina	864-455-7000	www.ghs.org
Hartford Hospital	Hartford	Connecticut	860-545-5000	www.harthosp.org
Hutchinson Regional Medical Center	Hutchinson	Kansas	620-665-2001	www.hutchinsonhospital.com
Integris Baptist Medical Center	Oklahoma City	Oklahoma	405-951-8110	www.integris-health.com
Intermountain Medical Center	Murray	Utah	801-507-7000	www.intermountainhealthcare.org
Iowa Methodist Medical Center	Des Moines	Iowa	515-241-6212	www.iowahealth.org
John D Archbold Memorial Hospital	Thomasville	Georgia	229-228-2880	www.archbold.org
John Muir Medical Center - Concord Campus	Concord	California	925-674-2002	www.johnmuirhealth.com
John Muir Medical Center - Walnut Creek Campus	Walnut Creek	California	925-939-3000	www.jmmdhs.com
Lancaster General Hospital	Lancaster	Pennsylvania	717-299-5511	www.lancastergeneral.org
Licking Memorial Hospital	Newark	Ohio	740-348-4000	www.lmhealth.org
Lima Memorial Health System	Lima	Ohio	419-998-4731	www.limamemorial.org
Maine Medical Center	Portland	Maine	207-662-0111	www.mmc.org
Marshalltown Medical & Surgical Center	Marshalltown	Iowa	641-754-5151	www.everydaychampions.org
Mary Hitchcock Memorial Hospital	Lebanon	New Hampshire	603-650-5000	www.dhmc.org
Mayo Clinic Health System - Eau Claire Hospital	Eau Claire	Wisconsin	715-838-3311	www.luthermidelfort.org
McKay Dee Hospital	Ogden	Utah	801-387-2800	www.intermountainhealthcare.org
Mclaren Bay Region	Bay City	Michigan	989-894-3000	www.baymed.org

Hospital	City	State	Phone	Web Site
Memorial Healthcare System	Chattanooga	Tennessee	423-495-2525	www.memorial.org
Memorial Hermann Hospital System	Houston	Texas	713-448-6796	www.memorialhermann.org
Memorial Hermann Memorial City Medical Center	Houston	Texas	713-242-3000	www.mhhs.org
Memorial Hospital of South Bend	South Bend	Indiana	574-647-1000	www.qualityoflife.org
Memorial Mission Hospital & Asheville Surgery Center	Asheville	North Carolina	828-213-1111	www.missionhospitals.org
Mercy Health Partners - Mercy Campus	Muskegon	Michigan	231-672-3901	www.mghp.com
Mercy Hospital Springfield	Springfield	Missouri	417-820-2000	www.stjohns.com
Mercy Medical Center - Redding	Redding	California	530-225-6102	www.redding.mercy.org
Methodist Charlton Medical Center	Dallas	Texas	214-947-7777	www.methodisthealthsystem.org
Methodist Hospital	San Antonio	Texas	210-575-4000	www.mh.sahealth.com
The Methodist Hospital	Houston	Texas	713-790-2221	www.methodisthealth.com
Morristown Medical Center	Morristown	New Jersey	973-971-5450	www.morristownmemorialhospital.org
Morton Plant Hospital	Clearwater	Florida	727-462-7000	www.measehospitals.com
Munson Medical Center	Traverse City	Michigan	231-935-5000	www.munsonhealthcare.org
Naples Community Hospital	Naples	Florida	239-436-5000	www.nchmd.org
New Hanover Regional Medical Center	Wilmington	North Carolina	910-343-7000	www.nhrmc.org
North Shore Medical Center	Salem	Massachusetts	978-741-1215	www.nsmc.partners.org
Northeast Georgia Medical Center	Gainesville	Georgia	770-535-3553	www.nghs.com
Oklahoma Heart Hospital	Oklahoma City	Oklahoma	405-608-3200	www.okheart.com
Owensboro Health Regional Hospital	Owensboro	Kentucky	270-688-2000	www.omhs.org
Parkview Regional Medical Center	Fort Wayne	Indiana	260-266-1000	www.parkview.com
Penn Highlands Dubois	Dubois	Pennsylvania	814-371-2200	www.drmc.org
Penn Presbyterian Medical Center	Philadelphia	Pennsylvania	215-662-8000	www.pennhealth.com
Pocono Medical Center	East Stroudsburg	Pennsylvania	570-476-3348	www.poconohealthsystem.org
Portneuf Medical Center	Pocatello	Idaho	208-239-1000	www.portmed.org
Providence Saint Peter Hospital	Olympia	Washington	360-491-9480	www.providence.org/swsa
Providence Saint Vincent Medical Center	Portland	Oregon	503-216-1234	www.providence.org
Reading Hospital	Reading	Pennsylvania	610-988-8000	www.readinghospital.org
Rex Hospital	Raleigh	North Carolina	919-784-3100	www.rexhealth.com
Roper Hospital	Charleston	South Carolina	843-724-2800	www.ropersaintfrancis.com
Sacred Heart Medical Center - Riverbend	Springfield	Oregon	541-222-7300	www.peacehealth.org/sacred-heart-riverbend
Saint Vincent Hospital	Erie	Pennsylvania	814-452-5000	www.svhs.org
Santa Rosa Memorial Hospital	Santa Rosa	California	707-525-5300	www.stjosephhealth.org
Sarasota Memorial Hospital	Sarasota	Florida	941-917-9000	www.smh.com
Scripps Green Hospital	La Jolla	California	858-554-3600	www.scrippshealth.org
Sisters of Charity Providence Hospitals	Columbia	South Carolina	803-256-5300	www.providencehospitals.com
Spartanburg Regional Medical Center	Spartanburg	South Carolina	864-560-6000	www.srhs.com
Spectrum Health - Butterworth Campus	Grand Rapids	Michigan	616-391-1774	www.spectrum-health.org
Saint Charles Medical Center - Bend	Bend	Oregon	541-382-4321	www.scmc.org
Saint Francis - Downtown	Greenville	South Carolina	864-255-1000	www.stfrancishealth.org
Saint Joseph's Hospital	Saint Paul	Minnesota	651-232-7707	www.stjosephs-stpaul.org
Saint Luke's Regional Medical Center	Boise	Idaho	208-381-2222	www.slrmc.org
Saint Vincent Hospital	Santa Fe	New Mexico	505-913-5201	www.stvin.org
Sutter Roseville Medical Center	Roseville	California	916-781-1000	www.sutterroseville.org
Tallahassee Memorial Hospital	Tallahassee	Florida	850-431-1155	www.tmh.org
Tennova Healthcare	Knoxville	Tennessee	865-545-8000	www.stmaryshealth.com
The Queens Medical Center	Honolulu	Hawaii	808-538-9011	www.queens.org
Trident Medical Center	Charleston	South Carolina	843-797-8800	www.tridenthealthsystem.com
University Colo Health Memorial Hospital Central	Colorado Springs	Colorado	719-365-5000	www.memorialhospital.com
UPMC Hamot	Erie	Pennsylvania	814-877-6000	www.hamot.org
Venice Regional Medical Center - Bayfront Health	Venice	Florida	941-485-7711	www.veniceregional.com
Virginia Hospital Center	Arlington	Virginia	703-558-5000	www.virginiahospitalcenter.com
Wesley Medical Center	Wichita	Kansas	316-962-2000	www.wesleymc.com
Williamsport Regional Medical Center	Williamsport	Pennsylvania	570-321-1000	www.susquehannahealth.org
Willis Knighton Medical Center	Shreveport	Louisiana	318-212-4000	www.wkhs.com//locations/medicalcenter.aspx

Note: Table shows hospitals nationwide whose heart failure 30-day readmission rate is better (lower) than U.S. rate of 23.0%

Hospitals whose Heart Failure 30-Day Readmission Rate is Worse (Higher) than the U.S. National Rate

Hospital	City	State	Phone	Web Site
Abbeville General Hospital	Abbeville	Louisiana	337-893-5466	www.abgen.net
Advocate Trinity Hospital	Chicago	Illinois	773-967-2000	www.advocatehealth.com/trin
Banner Baywood Medical Center	Mesa	Arizona	480-321-2000	www.bannerhealth.com
Baptist Health Medical Center - North Little Rock	North Little Rock	Arkansas	501-202-3000	www.baptist-health.org
Barnes-Jewish Hospital	Saint Louis	Missouri	314-747-3000	www.barnesjewish.org
Beaumont Health System	Royal Oak	Michigan	248-898-5000	www.beaumonthospitals.com
Beckley ARH Hospital	Beckley	West Virginia	304-255-3456	www.arh.org/beckley
Beth Israel Medical Center	New York	New York	212-420-2000	www.wehealny.org
Bolivar Medical Center	Cleveland	Mississippi	662-846-2551	www.bolivarmedical.com
Brookhaven Memorial Hospital Medical Center	Patchogue	New York	631-654-7100	www.brookhavenhospitalorg
Camden Clark Medical Center	Parkersburg	West Virginia	304-424-2111	www.ccmh.org
Capital Health System - Fuld Campus	Trenton	New Jersey	609-394-6000	www.capitalhealth.org
Capital Regional Medical Center	Tallahassee	Florida	850-656-5000	www.capitalregionalmedicalcenter.com
Carepoint Health - Bayonne Hospital Center	Bayonne	New Jersey	201-858-5000	www.bayonnemedicalcenter.org
Carepoint Health - Christ Hospital	Jersey City	New Jersey	201-795-8200	www.christhospital.org
Carepoint Health - Hoboken UMC	Hoboken	New Jersey	201-418-1004	www.bonsecoursnj.com
Carolinas Hospital System	Florence	South Carolina	843-674-2500	www.carolinashospital.com
Centegra Health System - Mc Henry Hospital	Mchenry	Illinois	815-344-5000	www.centegra.org
Chicot Memorial Medical Center	Lake Village	Arkansas	870-265-5351	www.chicotmemorial.com
Cincinnati VA Medical Center	Cincinnati	Ohio	513-861-3100	www.cincinnati.va.gov
Clinch Valley Medical Center	Richlands	Virginia	276-596-6000	www.clinchvalleymedicalcenter.com
Community Medical Center	Toms River	New Jersey	732-557-8000	www.sbhcs.com
Coney Island Hospital	Brooklyn	New York	718-616-3000	www.coneyislandhospital.com
Covenant Medical Center	Saginaw	Michigan	989-583-4000	www.covenanthealthcare.com
Crozer Chester Medical Center	Upland	Pennsylvania	610-447-2000	www.crozer.org
Culpeper Regional Hospital	Culpeper	Virginia	540-829-4100	www.culpeperhospital.com
Dallas VA Medical Center - VA North Texas	Dallas	Texas	214-742-8387	www.north-texas.med.va.gov
Danville Regional Medical Center	Danville	Virginia	434-799-2100	www.danvilleregional.org
Davis Memorial Hospital	Elkins	West Virginia	304-636-3300	www.davishealthcare.org
Detroit Receiving Hospital & University Health Center	Detroit	Michigan	313-745-3104	www.drhuhc.org
Doctors Hospital of Manteca	Manteca	California	209-823-3111	www.doctorsmanteca.com
East Georgia Regional Medical Center	Statesboro	Georgia	912-486-1500	www.egrmc.com
East Orange General Hospital	East Orange	New Jersey	973-266-4401	www.evh.org
Etmc Henderson	Henderson	Texas	903-657-7541	www.hmhtx.org
Florida Hospital	Orlando	Florida	407-303-1976	www.floridahospital.com
Flushing Hospital Medical Center	Flushing	New York	718-670-5000	www.flushinghospital.org
Forrest General Hospital	Hattiesburg	Mississippi	601-288-7000	www.forrestgeneral.com
Fountain Valley Regional Hospital & Medical Center	Fountain Valley	California	714-966-7200	www.fountainvalleyhospital.com
Franciscan Saint James Health	Olympia Fields	Illinois	708-747-4000	www.franciscanalliance.org
GV (Sonny) Montgomery VA Medical Center Jackson	Jackson	Mississippi	601-362-4471	www.visn16.med.va.gov
Georgetown Memorial Hospital	Georgetown	South Carolina	843-527-7000	www.gmhsc.com
Glenwood Regional Medical Center	West Monroe	Louisiana	318-329-4600	www.grmc.com
Griffin Hospital	Derby	Connecticut	203-732-7500	www.griffinhealth.org
Harlan Appalachian Regional Healthcare Hospital	Harlan	Kentucky	606-573-8100	www.arh.org
Harmon Memorial Hospital	Hollis	Oklahoma	580-688-3363	
Hazard ARH Regional Medical Center	Hazard	Kentucky	606-439-6600	www.arh.org/hazard
Henry Ford Hospital	Detroit	Michigan	313-916-2600	www.henryfordhospital.com
Hialeah Hospital	Hialeah	Florida	305-693-6100	www.hialeahhosp.com
Highlands Regional Medical Center	Prestonsburg	Kentucky	606-886-8511	www.hrmc.org
Hines VA Medical Center	Hines	Illinois	708-202-8387	www.visn12.med.va.gov/hines
Holy Name Medical Center	Teaneck	New Jersey	201-833-3000	www.holyname.org
Holzer Medical Center	Gallipolis	Ohio	740-446-5000	www.holzer.org
Howard University Hospital	Washington	District of Columbia	202-745-6100	www.huhosp.org
Huntington VA Medical Center	Huntington	West Virginia	304-429-0241	www.huntington.med.gov
Inspira Medical Center Woodbury	Woodbury	New Jersey	856-845-0100	www.umhospital.org
Interfaith Medical Center	Brooklyn	New York	718-613-4000	www.interfaithmedical.com
Jackson Memorial Hospital	Miami	Florida	305-585-1111	www.jhsmiami.org
Jamestown Regional Medical Center	Jamestown	Tennessee	931-879-3352	www.jamestownregional.org
Jefferson Regional Medical Center	Pittsburgh	Pennsylvania	412-469-5000	www.jeffersonregional.com
Jennings American Legion Hospital	Jennings	Louisiana	337-616-7000	www.jalh.com
Jesse Brown VA Medical Center - VA Chicago	Chicago	Illinois	312-569-8387	www.va.gov
JFK Medical Center	Atlantis	Florida	561-965-7300	www.jfkmc.com
Johns Hopkins Bayview Medical Center	Baltimore	Maryland	410-550-0123	www.hopkinsbayview.org
Jordan Hospital	Plymouth	Massachusetts	508-746-2000	www.jordanhospital.org
Kennedy University Hospital - Stratford Div	Stratford	New Jersey	856-346-6000	www.kennedyhealth.org

Hospital	City	State	Phone	Web Site
King's Daughters' Medical Center	Ashland	Kentucky	606-408-4000	www.kdmc.com
Leesburg Regional Medical Center	Leesburg	Florida	352-323-5762	www.leesburgregional.org
Lewisgale Hospital Pulaski	Pulaski	Virginia	540-994-8100	www.lewisgale.com
Libertyhealth - Jersey City Medical Center Campus	Jersey City	New Jersey	201-915-2000	www.libertyhcs.org
Lutheran Medical Center	Brooklyn	New York	718-630-8000	www.lmcmc.com
Madison River Oaks Medical Center	Canton	Mississippi	601-855-5323	www.madisonriveroaks.com
Mayo Clinic Health System - Fairmont	Fairmont	Minnesota	507-238-8101	www.fairmontmedicalcenter.org
Medical Center of Southeastern Oklahoma	Durant	Oklahoma	405-924-3080	www.mcsohealth.com
Medical Center of Trinity	Trinity	Florida	727-848-1733	www.communityhospitalnpr.com
Medstar Harbor Hospital	Baltimore	Maryland	410-350-3201	www.harborhospital.org
Memorial Hospital of Rhode Island	Pawtucket	Rhode Island	401-729-2000	www.mhriweb.org
Memorial Regional Hospital	Hollywood	Florida	954-987-2000	www.memorialregional.com
Mercy Fitzgerald Hospital	Darby	Pennsylvania	215-237-4000	www.mercyhealth.org
Mercy Hospital Saint Louis	Saint Louis	Missouri	314-569-6000	www.stjohnsmercy.org
Methodist Healthcare Memphis Hospitals	Memphis	Tennessee	901-516-8274	www.methodisthealth.org
Methodist Hospitals	Gary	Indiana	219-886-4642	www.methodisthospital.org
Metrosouth Medical Center	Blue Island	Illinois	708-597-2000	www.stfrancisblueisland.com
Midwest Regional Medical Center	Midwest City	Oklahoma	405-610-8530	www.midwestregional.com
Monmouth Medical Center - Southern Campus	Lakewood	New Jersey	732-363-1900	www.sbhcs.com
Montefiore Medical Center	Bronx	New York	718-920-4321	www.montefiore.org
Montefiore New Rochelle Hospital	New Rochelle	New York	914-632-5000	www.ssmc.org
Morton Hospital	Taunton	Massachusetts	508-828-7000	www.mortonhospital.org
Multicare Auburn Medical Center	Auburn	Washington	253-833-7711	www.armcuhs.com/p1.html
Nassau University Medical Center	East Meadow	New York	516-572-0123	www.numc.edu
New York Community Hospital of Brooklyn	Brooklyn	New York	718-692-5302	www.nych.com
New York Methodist Hospital	Brooklyn	New York	718-780-3000	www.nym.org
New York - Presbyterian Hospital	New York	New York	212-746-4189	www.nyp.org
North Carolina Baptist Hospital	Winston-Salem	North Carolina	336-716-2011	www.wfubmc.edu
North Shore Medical Center	Miami	Florida	305-835-6000	www.northshoremedical.com
North Shore University Hospital	Manhasset	New York	516-562-0100	www.northshorelij.com
Northwest Hospital Center	Randallstown	Maryland	410-521-5995	www.lifebridgehealth.org
Northwest Mississippi Regional Medical Center	Clarksdale	Mississippi	662-627-3211	www.nwmsregionalmedcenter.com
Oakwood Hospital - Dearborn	Dearborn	Michigan	313-593-7125	www.oakwood.org
Ochsner Medical Center	New Orleans	Louisiana	504-842-3000	www.ochsner.org
Olympia Medical Center	Los Angeles	California	310-657-5900	www.olympiamc.com
Orange Regional Medical Center	Middletown	New York	845-343-2424	www.ormc.org
Palisades Medical Center	North Bergen	New Jersey	201-854-5000	www.palisadesmedical.org
Palm Springs General Hospital	Hialeah	Florida	305-558-2500	www.psghosp.com
Pineville Community Hospital	Pineville	Kentucky	606-337-3051	www.pinevillehospital.com
Poplar Bluff VA Medical Center	Poplar Bluff	Missouri	573-686-4151	www.poplarbluff.va.gov
Port Huron Hospital	Port Huron	Michigan	810-987-5000	www.porthuronhospital.org
Presence Saint Joseph Medical Center	Joliet	Illinois	815-725-7133	www.provena.org/stjoes
Presence United Samaritans Medical Center	Danville	Illinois	217-443-5000	www.provena.org/usmc
Prince Georges Hospital Center	Cheverly	Maryland	301-618-2000	www.princegeorgeshospital.org
Providence VA Medical Center	Providence	Rhode Island	401-457-3042	www.visn1.med.va.gov/providence
Raritan Bay Medical Center	Perth Amboy	New Jersey	732-442-3700	www.rbmc.org
Riverview Regional Medical Center	Gadsden	Alabama	256-543-5200	www.riverviewregional.com
San Antonio VA Medical Center	San Antonio	Texas	210-617-5300	www.vasthcs.med.va.gov
San Juan VA Medical Center	San Juan	Puerto Rico	800-449-8729	www.visn8.med.va.gov/caribbean
Schuylkill Medical Center - East Norwegian Street	Pottsville	Pennsylvania	570-621-4000	www.schuylkillhealth.com
Sinai - Grace Hospital	Detroit	Michigan	313-966-3300	www.sinaigrace.org
Singing River Hospital	Pascagoula	Mississippi	228-809-5000	www.srhshealth.com
Skyridge Medical Center	Cleveland	Tennessee	423-339-4132	www.skyridgemedcenter.com
Somerset Medical Center	Somerville	New Jersey	908-685-2200	www.somersetmedicalcenter.com
South Nassau Communities Hospital	Oceanside	New York	516-632-3000	www.southnassau.org
Southcoast Hospital Group	Fall River	Massachusetts	508-679-3131	www.southcoast.org/charlton
Southeastern Regional Medical Center	Lumberton	North Carolina	910-671-5000	www.srmc.org
Southern Tennessee Medical Center	Winchester	Tennessee	931-967-8295	www.southerntennessee.com
Southside Regional Medical Center	Petersburg	Virginia	804-765-5000	www.srmconline.com
SSM Depaul Health Center	Bridgeton	Missouri	314-344-6000	www.ssmdepaul.com
SSM Saint Marys Health Center	Richmond Heights	Missouri	314-768-8000	www.ssmhealth.com/stmarys
Saint Catherine of Siena Hospital	Smithtown	New York	631-862-3000	www.stcatherines.chsli.org
Saint Francis Medical Center	Monroe	Louisiana	318-966-4000	www.stfran.com
Saint John Hospital & Medical Center	Detroit	Michigan	313-343-4000	www.stjohnprovidence.org
Saint John's Episcopal Hospital at South Shore	Far Rockaway	New York	718-869-7000	www.ehs.org
Saint John's Riverside Hospital	Yonkers	New York	914-964-4444	www.riversidehealth.org
Saint Joseph's Hospital	Tampa	Florida	813-870-4398	www.stjosephstampa.org

Hospital	City	State	Phone	Web Site
Saint Joseph's Regional Medical Center	Paterson	New Jersey	973-754-2010	www.sjhmc.org
Saint Louis - John Cochran VA Medical Center	Saint Louis	Missouri	314-652-4100	www.stlouis.va.gov
Saint Luke's Hospital Bethlehem	Bethlehem	Pennsylvania	610-954-4000	www.slhn-lehighvalley.org
Saint Luke's Roosevelt Hospital	New York	New York	212-523-4000	www.wehealny.org
Saint Mary Mercy Hospital	Livonia	Michigan	734-655-4800	www.stmarymercy.org
Saint Marys Hospital	Centralia	Illinois	618-436-6519	www.stmarys-goodsamaritan.com
Swedish Covenant Hospital	Chicago	Illinois	773-878-8200	www.swedishcovenant.org
Tampa VA Medical Center	Tampa	Florida	813-972-2000	www.tampa.va.gov
Univerity of MD Balto Washington Medical Center	Glen Burnie	Maryland	410-595-1967	www.bwmc.umms.org
University Hospital of Brooklyn - Downstate Medical Center	Brooklyn	New York	718-270-1000	www.downstate.edu
University of Miami Hospital	Miami	Florida	305-325-5511	www.cedarsmedicalcenter.com
VA Middle Tennessee Healthcare System	Nashville	Tennessee	615-327-5332	www.tennesseevalley.va.gov
VA New York Harbor Healthcare System	New York	New York	212-686-7500	www.nyharbor.va.gov
VA North Florida/South Georgia Healthcare System	Gainesville	Florida	352-376-1611	www.northflorida.va.gov
Valley Hospital	Ridgewood	New Jersey	201-447-8000	www.valleyhealth.com
W Palm Beach VA Medical Center	West Palm Beach	Florida	561-422-8600	www.va.gov
Wellmont Bristol Regional Medical Center	Bristol	Tennessee	423-844-1121	www.wellmont.org
Western Maryland Regional Medical Center	Cumberland	Maryland	240-964-8001	www.wmhs.com
Westlake Regional Hospital	Columbia	Kentucky	270-384-4753	www.westlake-healthcare.org
Whitesburg ARH Hospital	Whitesburg	Kentucky	606-633-3500	www.arh.org/whitesburg
William Beaumont Hospital - Troy	Troy	Michigan	248-964-8800	www.beaumonthospitals.com
Williamson ARH Hospital	South Williamson	Kentucky	606-237-1700	www.arh.org
Wuesthoff Medical Center Rockledge	Rockledge	Florida	321-637-2603	www.wuesthoff.org
Wyckoff Heights Medical Center	Brooklyn	New York	718-963-7272	www.wyckoffhospital.org

Note: Table shows hospitals nationwide whose heart failure 30-day readmission rate is worse (higher) than U.S. rate of 23.0%

Hospitals whose Pneumonia 30-Day Readmission Rate is Better (Lower) than the U.S. National Rate

Hospital	City	State	Phone	Web Site
Bay Medical Center Sacred Heart Health System	Panama City	Florida	850-769-1511	www.baymedical.org
Boca Raton Regional Hospital	Boca Raton	Florida	561-362-5002	www.brrh.com
Bronson Methodist Hospital	Kalamazoo	Michigan	269-341-6000	www.bronsonhealth.com
Cayuga Medical Center at Ithaca	Ithaca	New York	607-274-4401	www.cayugamed.org
Citrus Memorial Hospital	Inverness	Florida	352-726-1551	www.citrusmh.com
Eisenhower Medical Center	Rancho Mirage	California	760-340-3911	www.emc.org
Evergreen Hospital Medical Center	Kirkland	Washington	425-899-1000	www.evergreenhospital.org
Florida Hospital Waterman	Tavares	Florida	352-253-3300	www.fhwat.org
Freeman Health System - Freeman West	Joplin	Missouri	417-347-1111	www.freemanhealth.com
Kalispell Regional Medical Center	Kalispell	Montana	406-752-5111	www.krmc.org
Lake Regional Health System	Osage Beach	Missouri	573-348-8000	www.lakeregional.com
Memorial Healthcare System	Chattanooga	Tennessee	423-495-2525	www.memorial.org
Memorial Hermann Hospital System	Houston	Texas	713-448-6796	www.memorialhermann.org
Memorial Hermann Memorial City Medical Center	Houston	Texas	713-242-3000	www.mhhs.org
Memorial Medical Center of West Michigan	Ludington	Michigan	231-843-2591	www.mmcwm.com
Mercy Medical Center - Redding	Redding	California	530-225-6102	www.redding.mercy.org
Owensboro Health Regional Hospital	Owensboro	Kentucky	270-688-2000	www.omhs.org
Parkview Medical Center	Pueblo	Colorado	719-584-4000	www.parkviewmc.com
Parkview Regional Medical Center	Fort Wayne	Indiana	260-266-1000	www.parkview.com
Providence Saint Vincent Medical Center	Portland	Oregon	503-216-1234	www.providence.org
Rex Hospital	Raleigh	North Carolina	919-784-3100	www.rexhealth.com
Saint Joseph Regional Medical Center	Mishawaka	Indiana	574-335-5000	www.sjmed.com
Saint Joseph's Hospital of Atlanta	Atlanta	Georgia	678-843-5720	www.stjosephsatlanta.org
Salem Regional Medical Center	Salem	Ohio	330-332-1551	www.salemhosp.com
San Antonio Community Hospital	Upland	California	714-985-2811	www.sach.org
Sarasota Memorial Hospital	Sarasota	Florida	941-917-9000	www.smh.com
South Texas Health System	Edinburg	Texas	956-632-4000	www.edinburgregional.com
Spartanburg Regional Medical Center	Spartanburg	South Carolina	864-560-6000	www.srhs.com
Saint Edward Mercy Medical Center	Fort Smith	Arkansas	479-314-6000	www.stedwardmercy.com
Saint Francis Hospital - Roslyn	Roslyn	New York	516-562-6000	www.stfrancisheartcenter.com
Saint Francis - Downtown	Greenville	South Carolina	864-255-1000	www.stfrancishealth.org
Saint Mary's Regional Medical Center	Enid	Oklahoma	580-233-6100	www.stmarysregional.com
Saint Patrick Hospital	Missoula	Montana	406-543-7271	www.saintpatrick.org
Stormont - Vail Healthcare	Topeka	Kansas	785-354-6121	www.stormontvail.org
Virtua Memorial Hospital of Burlington County	Mount Holly	New Jersey	609-914-6200	www.virtua.org
Williamsport Regional Medical Center	Williamsport	Pennsylvania	570-321-1000	www.susquehannahealth.org
Willis Knighton Medical Center	Shreveport	Louisiana	318-212-4000	www.wkhs.com//locations/medicalcenter.aspx

Note: Table shows hospitals nationwide whose pneumonia 30-day readmission rate is better (lower) than U.S. rate of 17.6%

Hospitals whose Pneumonia 30-Day Readmission Rate is Worse (Higher) than the U.S. National Rate

Hospital	City	State	Phone	Web Site
Adena Regional Medical Center	Chillicothe	Ohio	740-779-7500	www.adena.org
Advocate Lutheran General Hospital	Park Ridge	Illinois	847-723-2210	www.advocatehealth.com
Advocate South Suburban Hospital	Hazel Crest	Illinois	708-799-8000	www.advocatehealth.com
Arnot Ogden Medical Center	Elmira	New York	607-737-4100	www.arnothealth.org
Baptist Memorial Hospital Desoto	Southaven	Mississippi	662-772-4000	www.bmhcc.org/facilities/desoto
Barnes-Jewish Hospital	Saint Louis	Missouri	314-747-3000	www.barnesjewish.org
Baxter Regional Medical Center	Mountain Home	Arkansas	870-508-1000	www.baxterregional.org
Bay Area Hospital	Coos Bay	Oregon	541-269-8111	www.bayareahospital.org
Bay Pines VA Medical Center	Bay Pines	Florida	727-398-6661	www.baypines.va.gov
Bayfront Health Punta Gorda	Punta Gorda	Florida	941-639-3131	www.charlotteregional.com
Beaumont Health System	Royal Oak	Michigan	248-898-5000	www.beaumonthospitals.com
Beckley VA Medical Center	Beckley	West Virginia	304-255-2121	www.beckley.va.gov
Beth Israel Medical Center	New York	New York	212-420-2000	www.wehealny.org
Blount Memorial Hospital	Maryville	Tennessee	865-983-7211	www.blountmemorial.org
Brandon Regional Hospital	Brandon	Florida	813-681-5551	www.brandonregionalhospital.com
Bronx VA Medical Center	Bronx	New York	718-584-9000	www.med.va.gov
Bronx - Lebanon Hospital Center	Bronx	New York	212-588-7000	www.bronx-leb.org
Brookhaven Memorial Hospital Medical Center	Patchogue	New York	631-654-7100	www.brookhavenhospitalorg
Cape Fear Valley Medical Center	Fayetteville	North Carolina	910-609-4000	www.capefearvalley.com
Casey County Hospital	Liberty	Kentucky	606-787-6275	
Chambers Memorial Hospital	Danville	Arkansas	479-495-2241	www.chambershospital.com
Cleveland Clinic	Cleveland	Ohio	216-444-2200	www.clevelandclinic.org
Cleveland - Wade Park VA Medical Center	Cleveland	Ohio	216-791-3800	www.cleveland.va.gov
Columbia MO VA Medical Center	Columbia	Missouri	573-814-6000	www.columbiamo.vc.gov
Community Hospital	Munster	Indiana	219-836-1600	www.comhs.org/community
Dallas VA Medical Center - VA North Texas	Dallas	Texas	214-742-8387	www.north-texas.med.va.gov
Davis Regional Medical Center	Statesville	North Carolina	704-873-0281	www.davisregional.com
Doctors' Community Hospital	Lanham	Maryland	301-552-8085	www.dchweb.org
East Orange General Hospital	East Orange	New Jersey	973-266-4401	www.evh.org
Florida Hospital	Orlando	Florida	407-303-1976	www.floridahospital.com
Florida Hospital Tampa	Tampa	Florida	813-615-7200	www.uch.org
Forest Hills Hospital	Forest Hills	New York	718-830-4000	www.northshorelij.com
Franklin Medical Center	Winnsboro	Louisiana	318-435-9411	www.fmc-cares.com
Garden City Hospital	Garden City	Michigan	734-421-3300	www.gchosp.org
Great River Medical Center	Blytheville	Arkansas	870-838-7300	www.greatrivermc.com
Harlan Appalachian Regional Healthcare Hospital	Harlan	Kentucky	606-573-8100	www.arh.org
Hazard ARH Regional Medical Center	Hazard	Kentucky	606-439-6600	www.arh.org/hazard
Heartland Regional Medical Center	Marion	Illinois	618-998-7000	www.heartlandregional.com
Henry Ford Hospital	Detroit	Michigan	313-916-2600	www.henryfordhospital.com
Highlands Regional Medical Center	Sebring	Florida	863-385-6101	www.highlandsregional.com
Hillcrest Hospital	Mayfield Heights	Ohio	440-312-4500	www.hillcresthospital.org
Hines VA Medical Center	Hines	Illinois	708-202-8387	www.visn12.med.va.gov/hines
Holzer Medical Center	Gallipolis	Ohio	740-446-5000	www.holzer.org
Houston VA Medical Center	Houston	Texas	713-794-7100	www.houston.med.va.gov
Howard County General Hospital	Columbia	Maryland	410-740-7890	www.hcgh.org
Huntington Hospital	Huntington	New York	631-351-2000	www.hunthosp.org
Huntington VA Medical Center	Huntington	West Virginia	304-429-0241	www.huntington.med.gov
Jackson Parish Hospital	Jonesboro	Louisiana	318-259-4435	www.jacksonparishhospital.com
Jewish Hospital & Saint Mary's Healthcare	Louisville	Kentucky	502-587-4011	www.jhhs.org
Johns Hopkins Bayview Medical Center	Baltimore	Maryland	410-550-0123	www.hopkinsbayview.org
Kennedy University Hospital - Stratford Div	Stratford	New Jersey	856-346-6000	www.kennedyhealth.org
King's Daughters' Medical Center	Ashland	Kentucky	606-408-4000	www.kdmc.com
Lake City Medical Center	Lake City	Florida	386-719-9000	www.lakecitymedical.com
Lake Health	Concord	Ohio	440-953-9600	www.lakehealth.org
Lehigh Valley Hospital - Hazleton	Hazleton	Pennsylvania	570-501-4000	www.ghha.org
Lenox Hill Hospital	New York	New York	212-439-2345	www.lenoxhillhospital.org
Little Company of Mary Hospital	Evergreen Park	Illinois	708-422-6200	www.lcmh.org
Livingston Regional Hospital	Livingston	Tennessee	931-823-5611	www.livingstonregionalhospital.com
Logan Regional Medical Center	Logan	West Virginia	304-831-1350	www.loganregionalmedicalcenter.com
Marymount Hospital	Garfield Heights	Ohio	216-581-0500	www.marymount.org
Medical Center of Southeastern Oklahoma	Durant	Oklahoma	405-924-3080	www.mcsohealth.com
Medstar Good Samaritan Hospital	Baltimore	Maryland	443-444-3902	www.goodsam-md.org
Memorial Hospital	Manchester	Kentucky	606-598-5104	www.manchestermemorial.com
Mercy Memorial Health Center	Ardmore	Oklahoma	405-223-5400	www.mercyok.com/mmhc
Metrosouth Medical Center	Blue Island	Illinois	708-597-2000	www.stfrancisblueisland.com

Hospital	City	State	Phone	Web Site
Mississippi Baptist Medical Center	Jackson	Mississippi	601-968-1000	www.mbmc.org
Monroe County Medical Center	Tompkinsville	Kentucky	270-487-9231	www.mcmccares.com
Mount Sinai Hospital	New York	New York	212-241-7981	www.mountsinai.org
Muskogee VA Medical Center	Muskogee	Oklahoma	918-577-3000	www.visn16.med.va.gov/muskogee.asp
Nassau University Medical Center	East Meadow	New York	516-572-0123	www.numc.edu
New York Hospital Medical Center of Queens	Flushing	New York	718-670-1231	www.nyhq.org
New York Methodist Hospital	Brooklyn	New York	718-780-3000	www.nym.org
North Carolina Baptist Hospital	Winston-Salem	North Carolina	336-716-2011	www.wfubmc.edu
North Oaks Medical Center	Hammond	Louisiana	985-345-2700	www.northoaks.org
Northern Westchester Hospital	Mount Kisco	New York	914-666-1200	www.nwhc.net
Northwest Hospital Center	Randallstown	Maryland	410-521-5995	www.lifebridgehealth.org
Northwestern Memorial Hospital	Chicago	Illinois	312-926-2000	www.nmh.org
Oakwood Hospital - Wayne	Wayne	Michigan	734-467-4175	www.oakwood.org
Orange Regional Medical Center	Middletown	New York	845-343-2424	www.ormc.org
Oroville Hospital	Oroville	California	530-533-8500	www.orovillehospital.com
Palos Community Hospital	Palos Heights	Illinois	708-923-4000	www.paloshospital.org
Piedmont Medical Center	Rock Hill	South Carolina	803-329-1234	www.piedmontmedicalcenter.com
Pineville Community Hospital	Pineville	Kentucky	606-337-3051	www.pinevillehospital.com
Presence United Samaritans Medical Center	Danville	Illinois	217-443-5000	www.provena.org/usmc
Princeton Community Hospital	Princeton	West Virginia	304-487-7260	www.pchonline.org
Raleigh General Hospital	Beckley	West Virginia	304-256-4100	www.raleighgeneral.com
Richmond VA Medical Center	Richmond	Virginia	804-675-5000	www.med.va.gov
Robert Packer Hospital	Sayre	Pennsylvania	570-888-6666	www.guthrie.org
Russell County Medical Center	Lebanon	Virginia	276-883-8100	www.msha.com
Saint Anne's Hospital	Fall River	Massachusetts	508-674-5600	www.saintanneshospital.org
Saint Thomas Rutherford Hospital	Murfreesboro	Tennessee	615-396-4100	www.mtmc.org
San Gabriel Valley Medical Center	San Gabriel	California	626-289-5454	www.sangabrielvalleymedctr.org
San Juan VA Medical Center	San Juan	Puerto Rico	800-449-8729	www.visn8.med.va.gov/caribbean
Santa Monica - UCLA Medical Center & Orthopaedic Hospital	Santa Monica	California	310-319-4000	www.healthcare.ucla.edu
Sentara Careplex Hospital	Hampton	Virginia	757-736-1000	www.sentara.com
Silver Cross Hospital & Medical Centers	New Lenox	Illinois	815-300-1100	www.silvercross.org
Sinai Hospital of Baltimore	Baltimore	Maryland	410-601-5131	www.sinai-balt.com
Singing River Hospital	Pascagoula	Mississippi	228-809-5000	www.srhshealth.com
Springfield Regional Medical Center	Springfield	Ohio	937-523-1000	www.communityhospital.com
Saint Anthony's Medical Center	Saint Louis	Missouri	314-525-1000	www.samcstl.org
Saint Bernard Hospital	Chicago	Illinois	773-962-3900	www.stbernardhospital.com
Saint Catherine of Siena Hospital	Smithtown	New York	631-862-3000	www.stcatherines.chsli.org
Saint Francis Hospital	Poughkeepsie	New York	845-483-5000	www.sfhhc.org
Saint Joseph's Hospital Health Center	Syracuse	New York	315-448-5111	www.sjhsyr.org
Saint Luke's Roosevelt Hospital	New York	New York	212-523-4000	www.wehealny.org
Saint Rose Dominican Hospitals - Rose De Lima Campus	Henderson	Nevada	702-616-5000	www.dignityhealth.org/las-vegas
Sumner Regional Medical Center	Gallatin	Tennessee	615-452-4210	www.mysumnermedical.com
Syracuse VA Medical Center	Syracuse	New York	315-425-4400	www1.va.gov/visns/visn02
Tampa VA Medical Center	Tampa	Florida	813-972-2000	www.tampa.va.gov
Univerity of MD Balto Washington Medical Center	Glen Burnie	Maryland	410-595-1967	www.bwmc.umms.org
University Hospital - Stony Brook	Stony Brook	New York	631-444-4000	www.stonybrookmedicalcenter.org
University Hospitals - Elyria Medical Center	Elyria	Ohio	440-329-7500	www.emh-healthcare.org
University of Alabama Hospital	Birmingham	Alabama	205-934-4011	www.health.uab.edu
University of Maryland Medical Center	Baltimore	Maryland	410-328-8667	www.umm.edu
University of Maryland Charles Regional Medical Center	La Plata	Maryland	301-609-4265	www.civista.org
Upper Valley Medical Center	Troy	Ohio	937-440-7853	www.uvmc.com
Upstate New York VA Healthcare System - Western NY	Buffalo	New York	716-862-3611	www.buffalo.va.gov
VA Central Arkansas Veterans Healthcare System	Little Rock	Arkansas	501-257-1000	www.visn16.med.va.gov
VA Maryland Healthcare System - Baltimore	Baltimore	Maryland	410-605-7016	www.maryland.va.gov
VA Middle Tennessee Healthcare System	Nashville	Tennessee	615-327-5332	www.tennesseevalley.va.gov
VA Pittsburgh Healthcare System	Pittsburgh	Pennsylvania	412-688-6100	www.pittsburg.va.gov
Vassar Brothers Medical Center	Poughkeepsie	New York	845-454-8500	www.vasserbrothers.org
Wadley Regional Medical Center	Texarkana	Texas	903-798-8000	www.wadleyhealth.com
Washington Hospital	Fremont	California	510-797-1111	www.whhs.com
Wayne Memorial Hospital	Goldsboro	North Carolina	919-736-1110	www.waynehealth.org
White County Medical Center	Searcy	Arkansas	501-278-3100	www.centralarkhospital.com
White Plains Hospital Center	White Plains	New York	914-681-0600	www.wphospital.org
William Beaumont Hospital - Troy	Troy	Michigan	248-964-8800	www.beaumonthospitals.com
Wing Memorial Hospital & Medical Center	Palmer	Massachusetts	413-283-7651	www.winghealth.org
Wyckoff Heights Medical Center	Brooklyn	New York	718-963-7272	www.wyckoffhospital.org

Note: Table shows hospitals nationwide whose pneumonia 30-day readmission rate is worse (higher) than U.S. rate of 17.6%

Hospitals whose Rate of Readmission After Hip/Knee Surgery is Better (Lower) than the U.S. National Rate

Hospital	City	State	Phone	Web Site
Arkansas Surgical Hospital	No Little Rock	Arkansas	501-748-8000	www.arksurgicalhospital.com
Blake Medical Center	Bradenton	Florida	941-792-6611	www.blakemedicalcenter.com
Boca Raton Regional Hospital	Boca Raton	Florida	561-362-5002	www.brrh.com
Christus Santa Rosa Hospital	San Antonio	Texas	210-704-2011	www.christussantarosa.org
Community Memorial Hospital	Hamilton	New York	315-824-1100	www.communitymemorial.org
Eisenhower Medical Center	Rancho Mirage	California	760-340-3911	www.emc.org
Elkhart General Hospital	Elkhart	Indiana	574-294-2621	www.egh.org
Emory University Hospital	Atlanta	Georgia	404-686-8500	www.emoryhealthcare.org
Evanston Hospital	Evanston	Illinois	847-432-8000	www.enh.org
Grace Medical Center	Lubbock	Texas	806-788-4100	www.highlandcommunityhospital.com
Heart of Florida Regional Medical Center	Davenport	Florida	863-422-4971	www.heartofflorida.com
Heartland Regional Medical Center	Saint Joseph	Missouri	816-271-6000	www.heartland-health.com
Hoag Orthopedic Institute	Irvine	California	949-727-5000	www.orthopedichospital.com
Holy Cross Hospital	Fort Lauderdale	Florida	954-771-8000	www.holy-cross.com
Hospital For Special Surgery	New York	New York	212-606-1000	www.hss.edu
Inova Mount Vernon Hospital	Alexandria	Virginia	703-664-7000	www.inova.com/inovapublic.srt/imvh/index.jsp
Kalispell Regional Medical Center	Kalispell	Montana	406-752-5111	www.krmc.org
Kansas Medical Center	Andover	Kansas	316-300-4000	www.ksmedcenter.com
Kettering Medical Center	Kettering	Ohio	937-298-4331	www.khnetwork.org
Maine Medical Center	Portland	Maine	207-662-0111	www.mmc.org
Meadville Medical Center	Meadville	Pennsylvania	814-333-5000	www.mmchs.org
Memorial Healthcare System	Chattanooga	Tennessee	423-495-2525	www.memorial.org
Memorial Mission Hospital & Asheville Surgery Center	Asheville	North Carolina	828-213-1111	www.missionhospitals.org
Mercy Medical Center - Cedar Rapids	Cedar Rapids	Iowa	319-398-6011	www.mercycare.org
Mercy Medical Center - Redding	Redding	California	530-225-6102	www.redding.mercy.org
New England Baptist Hospital	Boston	Massachusetts	617-754-5800	www.nebh.caregroup.org
Ocala Regional Medical Center	Ocala	Florida	352-401-1000	www.ocalaregional.com
Oklahoma Surgical Hospital	Tulsa	Oklahoma	918-477-5000	www.oklahomasurgicalhospital.com
Orthopaedic Hospital at Parkview North	Fort Wayne	Indiana	260-672-4050	www.parkview.com
Orthopaedic Hospital of Wisconsin	Glendale	Wisconsin	414-961-6800	www.ohow.org
Poudre Valley Hospital	Fort Collins	Colorado	970-495-7000	www.pvhs.org
Presbyterian Hospital	Albuquerque	New Mexico	505-724-8386	www.phs.org
Providence Saint John's Health Center	Santa Monica	California	310-829-5511	www.stjohns.org
Reading Hospital	Reading	Pennsylvania	610-988-8000	www.readinghospital.org
Sacred Heart Medical Center - Riverbend	Springfield	Oregon	541-222-7300	www.peacehealth.org/sacred-heart-riverbend
Saint Elizabeth Regional Medical Center	Lincoln	Nebraska	402-219-7700	www.stelizabethonline.com
Saint Joseph's Hospital of Atlanta	Atlanta	Georgia	678-843-5720	www.stjosephsatlanta.org
Saint Thomas West Hospital	Nashville	Tennessee	615-222-2111	www.stthomas.org
Salinas Valley Memorial Hospital	Salinas	California	831-757-4333	www.svmh.com
Samaritan Regional Health System	Ashland	Ohio	419-289-0491	www.samho.org
Sanford Medical Center Fargo	Fargo	North Dakota	701-234-2000	www.meritcare.com
Scottsdale Healthcare - Shea Medical Center	Scottsdale	Arizona	480-323-3009	www.shc.org
Sentara Leigh Hospital	Norfolk	Virginia	757-261-6601	www.sentara.com
Saint Joseph Hospital	Orange	California	714-633-9111	www.sjo.org
Saint Joseph Mercy Oakland	Pontiac	Michigan	248-858-3000	www.stjoesoakland.org
Sutter General Hospital	Sacramento	California	916-733-8999	www.suttermedicalcenter.org
The Orthopaedic Hospital of Lutheran Health Network	Fort Wayne	Indiana	260-435-2999	www.lutheranhealth.net
United Health Services Hospitals	Johnson City	New York	607-763-6000	www.vhs.ent
VHS Harlingen Hospital Company	Harlingen	Texas	956-389-1100	www.vbmc.org
Washington Hospital	Fremont	California	510-797-1111	www.whhs.com
Wythe County Community Hospital	Wytheville	Virginia	276-228-0200	www.wcch.org

Note: Table shows hospitals nationwide whose rate of readmission after hip/knee surgery is better (lower) than U.S. rate of 5.4%

Hospitals whose Rate of Readmission After Hip/Knee Surgery is Worse (Higher) than the U.S. National Rate

Hospital	City	State	Phone	Web Site
Abington Memorial Hospital	Abington	Pennsylvania	215-481-2000	www.amh.org
Advocate Christ Hospital & Medical Center	Oak Lawn	Illinois	708-684-8000	www.advocatehealth.com
Advocate Good Samaritan Hospital	Downers Grove	Illinois	630-275-5900	www.advocatehealth.com/gsam
Bayfront Health - Saint Petersburg	Saint Petersburg	Florida	727-823-1234	www.bayfront.org
Beaufort County Memorial Hospital	Beaufort	South Carolina	843-522-5200	www.bmhsc.org
Beaumont Health System	Royal Oak	Michigan	248-898-5000	www.beaumonthospitals.com
Centrastate Medical Center	Freehold	New Jersey	732-431-2000	www.centrastate.com
Christus Saint Michael Health System	Texarkana	Texas	903-614-1000	www.christusstmichael.org
Des Peres Hospital	Saint Louis	Missouri	314-966-9100	www.despereshospital.com
Doctors' Community Hospital	Lanham	Maryland	301-552-8085	www.dchweb.org
Enloe Medical Center	Chico	California	530-332-7300	www.enloe.org
Froedtert Memorial Lutheran Hospital	Milwaukee	Wisconsin	414-805-3000	www.froedtert.com
Galesburg Cottage Hospital	Galesburg	Illinois	309-345-4555	www.cottagehospital.com
Grant Medical Center	Columbus	Ohio	614-566-9978	www.ohiohealth.com
Jackson County Memorial Hospital	Altus	Oklahoma	580-379-5000	www.jcmh.com
Leesburg Regional Medical Center	Leesburg	Florida	352-323-5762	www.leesburgregional.org
Mercy Hospital Saint Louis	Saint Louis	Missouri	314-569-6000	www.stjohnsmercy.org
Mercy Saint Anne Hospital	Toledo	Ohio	419-407-2663	www.mercyweb.org
Minden Medical Center	Minden	Louisiana	318-377-2321	www.mindenmedicalcenter.com
Northwestern Memorial Hospital	Chicago	Illinois	312-926-2000	www.nmh.org
Orlando Health	Orlando	Florida	321-841-5111	www.orlandoregionalmedicalcenter.org
Parkwest Medical Center	Knoxville	Tennessee	865-970-9800	www.yesparkwest.com
Penn Presbyterian Medical Center	Philadelphia	Pennsylvania	215-662-8000	www.pennhealth.com
Pennsylvania Hospital of the Univ of PA Health Sys	Philadelphia	Pennsylvania	215-829-3000	www.pennmedicine.org/pahosp
Peterson Regional Medical Center	Kerrville	Texas	830-896-4200	www.petersonrmc.com
Providence Hospital	Washington	District of Columbia	202-269-7000	www.provhosp.org
Reston Hospital Center	Reston	Virginia	703-689-9000	www.restonhospital.com
Saint Agnes Hospital	Baltimore	Maryland	410-368-2101	www.stagnes.org
Saline Memorial Hospital	Benton	Arkansas	501-776-6000	www.salinememorial.org
Shannon Medical Center	San Angelo	Texas	325-653-6741	www.shannonhealth.com
Sinai Hospital of Baltimore	Baltimore	Maryland	410-601-5131	www.sinai-balt.com
Southside Regional Medical Center	Petersburg	Virginia	804-765-5000	www.srmconline.com
Saint Joseph Regional Health Center	Bryan	Texas	979-776-3912	www.st-joseph.org/sjrhc
Saint Joseph's Hospital	Tampa	Florida	813-870-4398	www.stjosephstampa.org
Thomas Jefferson University Hospital	Philadelphia	Pennsylvania	215-955-6000	www.jeffersonhospital.org
Wellmont Holston Valley Medical Center	Kingsport	Tennessee	423-224-4000	www.wellmont.org
Woodland Heights Medical Center	Lufkin	Texas	936-634-8311	www.woodlandheights.net

Note: Table shows hospitals nationwide whose rate of readmission after hip/knee surgery is better (lower) than U.S. rate of 5.4%

Hospitals whose Rate of Readmission After Discharge From Hospital (Hospital-wide) is Better (Lower) than the U.S. National Rate

Hospital	City	State	Phone	Web Site
Abbott Northwestern Hospital	Minneapolis	Minnesota	612-863-4509	www.abbottnorthwestern.com
Alegent Creighton Health Bergan Mercy Medical Center	Omaha	Nebraska	402-398-6060	www.alegent.com
Alexian Brothers Medical Center	Elk Grove Village	Illinois	847-437-5500	www.alexian.org
Alpena Regional Medical Center	Alpena	Michigan	989-356-7390	www.agh.org
Alta Bates Summit Medical Center	Oakland	California	510-655-4000	www.altabates.com
American Fork Hospital	American Fork	Utah	801-855-3305	www.ihc.com/facility/facilityresults.jsp
Anderson Regional Medical Center	Meridian	Mississippi	601-553-6000	www.jarmc.org
Appleton Medical Center	Appleton	Wisconsin	920-731-4101	www.thedacare.org
Arkansas Surgical Hospital	No Little Rock	Arkansas	501-748-8000	www.arksurgicalhospital.com
Asante Rogue Regional Medical Center	Medford	Oregon	541-789-7000	www.asante.org
Aspirus Wausau Hospital	Wausau	Wisconsin	715-847-2121	www.aspirus.org
Athens Regional Medical Center	Athens	Georgia	706-475-7000	www.armc.org
Augusta Health	Fishersville	Virginia	540-932-4000	www.augustamed.com
Aurora Lakeland Medical Center	Elkhorn	Wisconsin	262-741-2000	www.aurorahealthcare.org/facilities
Aurora Medical Center Manitowoc County	Two Rivers	Wisconsin	920-794-5000	www.aurorahealthcare.org
Aurora Medical Center Washington County	Hartford	Wisconsin	262-673-2300	www.aurorahealthcare.org
Aurora Saint Lukes Medical Center	Milwaukee	Wisconsin	414-649-6000	www.aurorahealthcare.org
Aurora West Allis Medical Center	West Allis	Wisconsin	414-328-6000	www.aurorahealthcare.org
Avera Mckennan Hospital & University Health Center	Sioux Falls	South Dakota	605-322-8000	www.mckennan.org
Avera Queen of Peace	Mitchell	South Dakota	605-995-2000	www.averaqueenofpeace.org
Avera Saint Lukes	Aberdeen	South Dakota	605-622-5000	www.averastlukes.org
Banner Good Samaritan Medical Center	Phoenix	Arizona	602-239-2000	www.bannerhealth.com
Baptist Health Louisville	Louisville	Kentucky	502-897-8100	www.baptisteast.com
Baptist Medical Center	San Antonio	Texas	210-297-1020	www.baptisthealthsystem.org
Baptist Memorial Hospital	Memphis	Tennessee	901-226-5000	www.bmhcc.org
Baptist Saint Anthony's Hospital	Amarillo	Texas	806-212-2000	www.bsahs.com
Baylor All Saints Medical Center at FW	Fort Worth	Texas	817-926-2544	www.baylorhealth.com/locations/allsaints
Baylor Medical Center at Garland	Garland	Texas	972-487-5000	www.baylorhealth.com
Baylor Medical Center at Irving	Irving	Texas	972-579-8100	www.baylorhealth.com
Baylor Regional Medical Center at Grapevine	Grapevine	Texas	817-481-1588	www.baylorhealth.com
Baylor University Medical Center	Dallas	Texas	214-820-0111	www.baylorhealth.com
Baystate Medical Center	Springfield	Massachusetts	413-794-0000	www.baystatehealth.com
Bellin Memorial Hospital	Green Bay	Wisconsin	920-433-3500	www.bellin.org
Billings Clinic Hospital	Billings	Montana	406-657-4000	www.billingsclinic.com
Blanchard Valley Hospital	Findlay	Ohio	419-423-4500	www.bvha.org
Bon Secours Maryview Medical Center	Portsmouth	Virginia	757-398-2200	www.bonsecourshamptonroads.com
Boone Hospital Center	Columbia	Missouri	573-815-8000	www.boone.org
Borgess Medical Center	Kalamazoo	Michigan	269-226-7000	www.borgess.com
Boulder Community Hospital	Boulder	Colorado	303-440-2273	www.bch.org
Bronson Methodist Hospital	Kalamazoo	Michigan	269-341-6000	www.bronsonhealth.com
Bryan Medical Center	Lincoln	Nebraska	402-481-1111	www.bryan.org
Caldwell Memorial Hospital	Lenoir	North Carolina	828-757-5100	www.caldwellmemorial.org
California Pacific Medical Center - Pacific Campus Hospital	San Francisco	California	415-600-6000	www.cpmc.org
Cape Cod Hospital	Hyannis	Massachusetts	508-771-1800	www.capecodhealth.org
Carolinas Medical Center - Pineville	Charlotte	North Carolina	704-379-5000	www.carolinashealthcare.org
Carondelet Saint Marys Hospital	Tucson	Arizona	520-872-3000	www.carondelet.org
Carondelet Saint Joseph's Hospital	Tucson	Arizona	520-873-3000	www.carondelet.org
Carteret General Hospital	Morehead City	North Carolina	252-808-6000	www.ccgh.org
Catawba Valley Medical Center	Hickory	North Carolina	828-326-3809	www.catawbavalleymc.org
Central Dupage Hospital	Winfield	Illinois	630-682-1600	www.cdh.org
Central Vermont Medical Center	Barre	Vermont	802-371-4100	www.cvmc.hitchcock.org
Central Washington Hospital	Wenatchee	Washington	509-662-1511	www.cwhs.com
Centura Health - Penrose Saint Francis Health Services	Colorado Springs	Colorado	719-776-5000	www.centurahealth.com
Centura Health - Saint Mary Corwin Medical Center	Pueblo	Colorado	719-557-4000	www.stmarycorwin.org
Chandler Regional Medical Center	Chandler	Arizona	480-963-4561	www.chandlerregional.com
Charlotte Hungerford Hospital	Torrington	Connecticut	860-496-6666	www.charlottesweb.hungerford.org
Cheyenne Regional Medical Center	Cheyenne	Wyoming	307-634-2273	www.crmcwy.org
Christus Health Shreveport - Bossier	Shreveport	Louisiana	318-681-5000	www.christusschumpert.org
Citizens Medical Center	Victoria	Texas	361-572-5113	www.citizensmedicalcenter.org
Citrus Memorial Hospital	Inverness	Florida	352-726-1551	www.citrusmh.com
CMC - Blue Ridge	Morganton	North Carolina	828-580-5000	www.gracehcs.org
Comanche County Memorial Hospital	Lawton	Oklahoma	580-355-8620	www.memorialhealthsource.org
Community Hospital of the Monterey Peninsula	Monterey	California	831-624-5311	www.chomp.org
Community Memorial Hospital San Buenaventura	Ventura	California	805-652-5011	www.cmhhospital.org
The Corpus Christi Medical Center	Corpus Christi	Texas	361-761-1501	www.ccmedicalcenter.com

Hospital	City	State	Phone	Web Site
Covenant Medical Center	Lubbock	Texas	806-725-6000	www.covenanthealth.org
Deaconess Hospital	Oklahoma City	Oklahoma	405-604-6109	www.deaconessokc.com
Dixie Regional Medical Center	Saint George	Utah	435-251-2100	www.intermountainhealthcare.org
Doctors Hospital of Sarasota	Sarasota	Florida	941-342-1100	www.doctorsofsarasota.com
Dominican Hospital	Santa Cruz	California	831-462-7700	www.dominicanhospital.org
East Jefferson General Hospital	Metairie	Louisiana	504-454-4000	www.eastjeffhospital.org
Eastern Idaho Regional Medical Center	Idaho Falls	Idaho	208-529-6111	www.eirmc.org
Eisenhower Medical Center	Rancho Mirage	California	760-340-3911	www.emc.org
Englewood Community Hospital	Englewood	Florida	941-475-6571	www.englewoodcommunityhospital.com
Ephrata Community Hospital	Ephrata	Pennsylvania	717-733-0311	www.ephratahospital.org
Evergreen Hospital Medical Center	Kirkland	Washington	425-899-1000	www.evergreenhospital.org
Exempla Lutheran Medical Center	Wheat Ridge	Colorado	303-425-4500	www.exemlpa.org
Fairview Southdale Hospital	Edina	Minnesota	952-924-5000	www.fairview.org
Falmouth Hospital	Falmouth	Massachusetts	508-548-5300	www.capecodhealth.com
Flagler Hospital	Saint Augustine	Florida	904-819-4426	www.flaglerhospital.com
Flagstaff Medical Center	Flagstaff	Arizona	928-773-2009	www.nahealth.com
Franciscan Saint Elizabeth Health - Lafayette East	Lafayette	Indiana	765-502-4334	www.ste.org
Freeman Health System - Freeman West	Joplin	Missouri	417-347-1111	www.freemanhealth.com
Genesis Medical Center - Davenport	Davenport	Iowa	563-421-1000	www.genesishealth.com
GHS Greenville Memorial Medical Center	Greenville	South Carolina	864-455-7000	www.ghs.org
Grand View Hospital	Sellersville	Pennsylvania	215-453-4615	www.gvh.org
Greater Baltimore Medical Center	Baltimore	Maryland	443-849-2000	www.gbmc.org
Gundersen Lutheran Medical Center	La Crosse	Wisconsin	608-782-7300	www.gundluth.org
Gwinnett Medical Center	Lawrenceville	Georgia	678-312-1000	www.gwinnettmedicalcenter.org
Harlingen Medical Center	Harlingen	Texas	956-365-1000	www.harlingenmedicalcenter.com
Harrison Memorial Center	Bremerton	Washington	360-377-3911	www.harrisonmedical.org
Hill Country Memorial Hospital	Fredericksburg	Texas	830-997-4353	www.hcmbs.org
Hinsdale Hospital	Hinsdale	Illinois	630-856-9000	www.keepingyouwell.com
Hoag Memorial Hospital Presbyterian	Newport Beach	California	949-645-8600	www.hoaghospital.org
Hoag Orthopedic Institute	Irvine	California	949-727-5000	www.orthopedichospital.com
Hospital For Special Surgery	New York	New York	212-606-1000	www.hss.edu
Huguley Memorial Medical Center	Burleson	Texas	817-568-5317	www.huguley.org
Huntington Memorial Hospital	Pasadena	California	626-397-5000	www.huntingtonhospital.com
Hutchinson Regional Medical Center	Hutchinson	Kansas	620-665-2001	www.hutchinsonhospital.com
Indian River Medical Center	Vero Beach	Florida	772-567-4311	www.irmh.com
Indiana University Health Ball Memorial Hospital	Muncie	Indiana	765-747-3111	www.accesschs.org/baal-memorial-l
Indiana University Health North Hospital	Carmel	Indiana	317-688-2000	www.iuhealth.org/north
Integris Baptist Medical Center	Oklahoma City	Oklahoma	405-951-8110	www.integris-health.com
Intermountain Medical Center	Murray	Utah	801-507-7000	www.intermountainhealthcare.org
Iowa Lutheran Hospital	Des Moines	Iowa	515-263-5612	www.ihsdesmoines.org
Iowa Methodist Medical Center	Des Moines	Iowa	515-241-6212	www.iowahealth.org
IU Health West Hospital	Avon	Indiana	317-217-3000	www.iuhealth.org/west
Jane Phillips Medical Center	Bartlesville	Oklahoma	918-333-7200	www.jpmc.org
John Muir Medical Center - Walnut Creek Campus	Walnut Creek	California	925-939-3000	www.jmmdhs.com
Kalispell Regional Medical Center	Kalispell	Montana	406-752-5111	www.krmc.org
Kaweah Delta Medical Center	Visalia	California	559-624-2000	www.kaweahdelta.org
Kenmore Mercy Hospital	Kenmore	New York	716-447-6100	www.chsbuffalo.org
Kettering Medical Center	Kettering	Ohio	937-298-4331	www.khnetwork.org
Kootenai Medical Center	Coeur D'alene	Idaho	208-625-4001	www.kootenaihealth.org
Lakeview Memorial Hospital	Stillwater	Minnesota	651-439-5330	www.lakeview.org
Lancaster General Hospital	Lancaster	Pennsylvania	717-299-5511	www.lancastergeneral.org
Lawrence & Memorial Hospital	New London	Connecticut	860-442-0711	www.lmhospital.org
Lawrence Memorial Hospital	Lawrence	Kansas	785-505-6100	www.lmh.org
Lehigh Valley Hospital	Allentown	Pennsylvania	610-402-2273	www.lvhhn.org
Lexington Medical Center	West Columbia	South Carolina	803-791-2000	www.lexmed.com
Lovelace Medical Center	Albuquerque	New Mexico	505-727-8000	www.lovelace.com
Mainegeneral Medical Center	Augusta	Maine	207-872-1000	www.mainegeneral.org
Margaret R Pardee Memorial Hospital	Hendersonville	North Carolina	828-696-1000	www.pardeehospital.org
Marian Regional Medical Center	Santa Maria	California	805-739-3000	www.marinmedicalcenter.org
Marion General Hospital	Marion	Indiana	765-660-6000	www.mgh.net
Marquette General Hospital	Marquette	Michigan	906-228-9440	www.mgh.org
Marshalltown Medical & Surgical Center	Marshalltown	Iowa	641-754-5151	www.everydaychampions.org
Mary Lanning Healthcare	Hastings	Nebraska	402-463-4521	www.marylanning.org
Maui Memorial Medical Center	Wailuku	Hawaii	808-442-5101	www.mauimemorialmedical.org
Mayo Clinic Health System - Eau Claire Hospital	Eau Claire	Wisconsin	715-838-3311	www.luthermidelfort.org
Mayo Clinic Hospital	Phoenix	Arizona	480-342-2000	www.mayoclinic.org
McBride Clinic Orthopedic Hospital	Oklahoma City	Oklahoma	405-478-1717	www.mcbrideclinic.com

Hospital	City	State	Phone	Web Site
McKay Dee Hospital	Ogden	Utah	801-387-2800	www.intermountainhealthcare.org
Mclaren - Northern Michigan	Petoskey	Michigan	231-487-4000	www.northernhealth.org
The Medical Center of Aurora	Aurora	Colorado	303-695-2600	www.auroramed.com
Medical City Dallas Hospital	Dallas	Texas	972-566-6222	www.medicalcityhospital.com
Medwest Haywood	Clyde	North Carolina	828-456-7311	www.haymed.org
Memorial Healthcare System	Chattanooga	Tennessee	423-495-2525	www.memorial.org
Memorial Hermann Hospital System	Houston	Texas	713-448-6796	www.memorialhermann.org
Memorial Hermann Memorial City Medical Center	Houston	Texas	713-242-3000	www.mhhs.org
Memorial Hospital & Health Care Center	Jasper	Indiana	812-996-2345	www.mhhcc.org
Memorial Hospital of South Bend	South Bend	Indiana	574-647-1000	www.qualityoflife.org
Memorial Medical Center of West Michigan	Ludington	Michigan	231-843-2591	www.mmcwm.com
Memorial Mission Hospital & Asheville Surgery Center	Asheville	North Carolina	828-213-1111	www.missionhospitals.org
Mercy General Hospital	Sacramento	California	916-453-4545	www.mercygeneral.org
Mercy Health Partners - Mercy Campus	Muskegon	Michigan	231-672-3901	www.mghp.com
Mercy Hospital	Iowa City	Iowa	319-339-0300	www.mercyiowacity.org
Mercy Hospital	Portland	Maine	207-879-3000	www.mercyhospital.com
Mercy Hospital	Buffalo	New York	716-826-7000	www.chsbuffalo.org
Mercy Hospital - Grayling	Grayling	Michigan	989-348-5461	www.mercygrayling.munsonhealthcare.org
Mercy Hospital Northwest Arkansas	Rogers	Arkansas	479-338-8000	www.mercy4u.com
Mercy Hospital Springfield	Springfield	Missouri	417-820-2000	www.stjohns.com
Mercy Medical Center	Canton	Ohio	330-489-1001	www.thequalityhospital.com
Mercy Medical Center	Roseburg	Oregon	541-673-0611	www.mercyrose.org
Mercy Medical Center - Redding	Redding	California	530-225-6102	www.redding.mercy.org
Mercy Medical Center - Des Moines	Des Moines	Iowa	515-247-3121	www.mercydesmoines.org
Meriter Hospital	Madison	Wisconsin	608-417-6000	www.meriter.com
Methodist Hospital	San Antonio	Texas	210-575-4000	www.mh.sahealth.com
Methodist Stone Oak Hospital	San Antonio	Texas	210-638-2100	www.stoneoakhealth.com
Methodist Sugar Land Hospital	Sugar Land	Texas	281-274-8000	www.methodisthealth.com/sugarland
Midland Memorial Hospital	Midland	Texas	432-685-1111	www.midland-memorial.com
Mills - Peninsula Medical Center	Burlingame	California	650-696-5270	www.mills-peninsula.org
Morristown Medical Center	Morristown	New Jersey	973-971-5450	www.morristownmemorialhospital.org
Morton Plant Hospital	Clearwater	Florida	727-462-7000	www.measehospitals.com
The Moses H Cone Memorial Hospital	Greensboro	North Carolina	336-832-7000	www.mosescone.com
Mother Frances Hospital	Tyler	Texas	903-593-8441	www.tmfhs.org
Munroe Regional Medical Center	Ocala	Florida	352-351-7200	www.munroeregional.com
Munson Medical Center	Traverse City	Michigan	231-935-5000	www.munsonhealthcare.org
Naples Community Hospital	Naples	Florida	239-436-5000	www.nchmd.org
Nebraska Heart Hospital	Lincoln	Nebraska	402-328-3000	www.neheart.com
New England Baptist Hospital	Boston	Massachusetts	617-754-5800	www.nebh.caregroup.org
New Hanover Regional Medical Center	Wilmington	North Carolina	910-343-7000	www.nhrmc.org
Newton Medical Center	Newton	Kansas	316-804-6001	www.newtonmedicalcenter.com
Norman Regional Health System	Norman	Oklahoma	405-321-1700	www.normanregional.com
North Memorial Medical Center	Robbinsdale	Minnesota	763-520-5200	www.northmemorial.com
North Shore Medical Center	Salem	Massachusetts	978-741-1215	www.nsmc.partners.org
Northside Hospital	Atlanta	Georgia	404-851-8000	www.northside.com
Northwest Community Hospital	Arlington Heights	Illinois	847-618-1000	www.nch.org
Northwest Hospital	Seattle	Washington	206-364-0500	www.nwhospital.org
Northwest Texas Hospital	Amarillo	Texas	806-354-1110	www.nxtexashealthcare.com
Novant Health Huntersville Medical Center	Huntersville	North Carolina	704-316-4000	www.presbyterian.org
Oklahoma Heart Hospital	Oklahoma City	Oklahoma	405-608-3200	www.okheart.com
Oklahoma Surgical Hospital	Tulsa	Oklahoma	918-477-5000	www.oklahomasurgicalhospital.com
Olympic Medical Center	Port Angeles	Washington	360-417-7000	www.olympicmedical.org
Our Lady of the Lake Regional Medical Center	Baton Rouge	Louisiana	225-765-6565	www.ololrmc.com
Overlake Hospital Medical Center	Bellevue	Washington	425-688-5000	www.overlakehospital.org
Owensboro Health Regional Hospital	Owensboro	Kentucky	270-688-2000	www.omhs.org
Palmetto Health Baptist	Columbia	South Carolina	803-296-5678	www.palmettohealth.org
Palmetto Health Richland	Columbia	South Carolina	803-296-5678	www.palmettohealth.org
Park Nicollet Methodist Hospital	Saint Louis Park	Minnesota	952-993-5000	www.parknicollet.com/methodist
Parkview Medical Center	Pueblo	Colorado	719-584-4000	www.parkviewmc.com
Parkview Regional Medical Center	Fort Wayne	Indiana	260-266-1000	www.parkview.com
Peacehealth Saint Joseph Medical Center	Bellingham	Washington	360-734-5400	www.peacehealth.org
Peninsula Regional Medical Center	Salisbury	Maryland	410-543-7111	www.peninsula.org
Penn Highlands Dubois	Dubois	Pennsylvania	814-371-2200	www.drmc.org
Petaluma Valley Hospital	Petaluma	California	707-778-1111	www.stjosephhealth.org
Phelps County Regional Medical Center	Rolla	Missouri	573-458-8899	www.rollanet.org/~pcrmc
Piedmont Fayette Hospital	Fayetteville	Georgia	770-719-7071	www.fayettehospital.org
Piedmont Hospital	Atlanta	Georgia	404-605-5000	www.piedmonthospital.org

Hospital	City	State	Phone	Web Site
Plaza Medical Center of Fort Worth	Fort Worth	Texas	817-336-2100	www.plazamedicalcenter.com
Porter Regional Hospital	Valparaiso	Indiana	219-983-8300	www.portermemorial.org
Portneuf Medical Center	Pocatello	Idaho	208-239-1000	www.portmed.org
Presbyterian Hospital	Albuquerque	New Mexico	505-724-8386	www.phs.org
Presbyterian Hospital Matthews	Matthews	North Carolina	704-384-6500	www.presbyterian.org
Providence Alaska Medical Center	Anchorage	Alaska	907-261-3675	www.providence.org
Providence Holy Family Hospital	Spokane	Washington	509-482-2450	www.holy-family.org
Providence Hospital	Mobile	Alabama	251-633-1000	www.providencehospital.org
Providence Regional Medical Center Everett	Everett	Washington	425-261-2000	www.providence.org
Providence Sacred Heart Medical Center	Spokane	Washington	509-474-3040	www.shmc.org
Providence Saint John's Health Center	Santa Monica	California	310-829-5511	www.stjohns.org
Providence Saint Mary Medical Center	Walla Walla	Washington	509-522-5900	www.smmc.com
Providence Saint Peter Hospital	Olympia	Washington	360-491-9480	www.providence.org/swsa
Providence Saint Vincent Medical Center	Portland	Oregon	503-216-1234	www.providence.org
Rapid City Regional Hospital	Rapid City	South Dakota	605-719-1000	www.rcrh.org
Reading Hospital	Reading	Pennsylvania	610-988-8000	www.readinghospital.org
Reid Hospital & Health Care Services	Richmond	Indiana	765-983-3000	www.reidhosp.com
Rex Hospital	Raleigh	North Carolina	919-784-3100	www.rexhealth.com
Roper Hospital	Charleston	South Carolina	843-724-2800	www.ropersaintfrancis.com
Sacred Heart Medical Center - Riverbend	Springfield	Oregon	541-222-7300	www.peacehealth.org/sacred-heart-riverbend
Saddleback Memorial Medical Center	Laguna Hills	California	949-837-4500	www.memorialcare.org/saddleback
Saint Barnabas Medical Center	Livingston	New Jersey	973-322-5000	www.saintbarnabas.com
Saint Elizabeth Regional Medical Center	Lincoln	Nebraska	402-219-7700	www.stelizabethonline.com
Saint Joseph Regional Medical Center	Mishawaka	Indiana	574-335-5000	www.sjmed.com
Saint Joseph's Hospital of Atlanta	Atlanta	Georgia	678-843-5720	www.stjosephsatlanta.org
Saint Mary's Health Care	Grand Rapids	Michigan	616-685-5000	www.smhealthcare.org
Saint Thomas West Hospital	Nashville	Tennessee	615-222-2111	www.stthomas.org
Saint Vincent Hospital	Erie	Pennsylvania	814-452-5000	www.svhs.org
Salem Hospital	Salem	Oregon	503-561-5200	www.salemhospital.org
Salem Regional Medical Center	Salem	Ohio	330-332-1551	www.salemhosp.com
Salina Regional Health Center	Salina	Kansas	785-452-7000	www.srhc.com
Salinas Valley Memorial Hospital	Salinas	California	831-757-4333	www.svmh.com
Samaritan Albany General Hospital	Albany	Oregon	541-812-4000	www.samhealth.org/shs_facilities
Sampson Regional Medical Center	Clinton	North Carolina	910-592-8511	www.sampsonrmc.org
San Jacinto Methodist Hospital	Baytown	Texas	281-420-8600	www.methodisthealth.com/sanjacinto
Sanford Bemidji Medical Center	Bemidji	Minnesota	218-751-5430	www.nchs.com
Sanford Medical Center Fargo	Fargo	North Dakota	701-234-2000	www.meritcare.com
Sanford Usd Medical Center	Sioux Falls	South Dakota	605-333-1000	www.sanfordhealth.org
Santa Barbara Cottage Hospital	Santa Barbara	California	805-682-7111	www.cottagehealthsystem.org
Santa Rosa Memorial Hospital	Santa Rosa	California	707-525-5300	www.stjosephhealth.org
Sarasota Memorial Hospital	Sarasota	Florida	941-917-9000	www.smh.com
Saratoga Hospital	Saratoga Springs	New York	518-587-3222	www.saratogacare.org
Scottsdale Healthcare Osborn Medical Center	Scottsdale	Arizona	480-882-4000	www.shc.org
Scottsdale Healthcare - Shea Medical Center	Scottsdale	Arizona	480-323-3009	www.shc.org
Scottsdale Healthcare - Thompson Peak Hospital	Scottsdale	Arizona	480-324-7004	www.shc.org
Scripps Memorial Hospital - Encinitas	Encinitas	California	760-753-6501	www.scripps.org
Sentara Williamsburg Regional Medical Center	Williamsburg	Virginia	757-984-6000	www.sentara.com
Sequoia Hospital	Redwood City	California	650-367-5551	www.sequoiahospital.org
Seven Rivers Regional Medical Center	Crystal River	Florida	352-795-6560	www.srrmc.com
Sisters of Charity Providence Hospitals	Columbia	South Carolina	803-256-5300	www.providencehospitals.com
Sky Lakes Medical Center	Klamath Falls	Oregon	541-274-6150	www.skylakes.org
Sky Ridge Medical Center	Lone Tree	Colorado	720-225-1000	www.skyridgemedcenter.com
Sonoma Valley Hospital	Sonoma	California	707-935-5000	www.svh.com
Sonora Regional Medical Center	Sonora	California	209-532-3161	www.sonorahospital.org
South Lake Hospital	Clermont	Florida	352-394-4071	www.southlakehospital.com
Spartanburg Regional Medical Center	Spartanburg	South Carolina	864-560-6000	www.srhs.com
Spectrum Health - Butterworth Campus	Grand Rapids	Michigan	616-391-1774	www.spectrum-health.org
Saint Agnes Hospital	Fond Du Lac	Wisconsin	920-929-2300	www.agnesian.com
Saint Alexius Medical Center	Bismarck	North Dakota	701-530-7000	www.st.alexius.org
Saint Alphonsus Regional Medical Center	Boise	Idaho	208-367-2121	www.saintalphonsus.org
Saint Bernardine Medical Center	San Bernardino	California	909-881-4440	www.stbernardinemedicalcenter.com
Saint Charles Medical Center - Bend	Bend	Oregon	541-382-4321	www.scmc.org
Saint David's Medical Center	Austin	Texas	512-476-7111	www.stdavidsrehab.com
Saint Edward Mercy Medical Center	Fort Smith	Arkansas	479-314-6000	www.stedwardmercy.com
Saint Francis Hospital	Columbus	Georgia	706-596-4020	www.wecareforlife.com
Saint Francis Hospital - Roslyn	Roslyn	New York	516-562-6000	www.stfrancisheartcenter.com
Saint Francis Medical Center	Grand Island	Nebraska	308-384-4600	www.saintfrancisgi.org

Hospital	City	State	Phone	Web Site
Saint Francis - Downtown	Greenville	South Carolina	864-255-1000	www.stfrancishealth.org
Saint Joseph Hospital	Eureka	California	707-445-8121	www.stjosepheureka.org
Saint Joseph Hospital & Health Center	Kokomo	Indiana	765-456-5300	www.stvincent.org
Saint Joseph Medical Center	Reading	Pennsylvania	610-378-2300	www.sjmcberks.org
Saint Joseph Regional Medical Center	Lewiston	Idaho	208-743-2511	www.sjrmc.org
Saint Luke's Regional Medical Center	Boise	Idaho	208-381-2222	www.slrmc.org
Saint Luke's Hospital	Cedar Rapids	Iowa	319-369-7211	www.crstlukes.com
Saint Luke's Hospital	Duluth	Minnesota	218-249-5555	www.slhduluth.com
Saint Marks Hospital	Salt Lake City	Utah	801-268-7700	www.stmarkshospital.com
Saint Mary's Regional Medical Center	Enid	Oklahoma	580-233-6100	www.stmarysregional.com
Saint Marys Hospital	Madison	Wisconsin	608-251-6100	www.stmarysmadison.com
Saint Marys Hospital & Medical Center	Grand Junction	Colorado	970-298-1950	www.stmarygj.org
Saint Marys Regional Medical Center	Lewiston	Maine	207-777-8100	www.stmarysmaine.com
Saint Patrick Hospital	Missoula	Montana	406-543-7271	www.saintpatrick.org
Saint Peter's Hospital	Albany	New York	518-525-1550	www.stpetershealthcare.org
Saint Rose Dominican Hospitals - Siena Campus	Henderson	Nevada	702-616-5000	www.strosehospitals.org
Saint Vincent Heart Center of Indiana	Indianapolis	Indiana	317-583-5000	www.theheartcenter.com
Saint Vincent Hospital	Green Bay	Wisconsin	920-433-0111	www.stvincenthospital.org
Saint Vincent Hospital & Health Services	Indianapolis	Indiana	317-338-7000	www.indianapolis.stvincent.org
Sutter Auburn Faith Hospital	Auburn	California	530-888-4500	www.sutterauburnfaith.org
Sutter Roseville Medical Center	Roseville	California	916-781-1000	www.sutterroseville.org
Tallahassee Memorial Hospital	Tallahassee	Florida	850-431-1155	www.tmh.org
Tennova Healthcare	Knoxville	Tennessee	865-545-8000	www.stmaryshealth.com
Texas Health Harris Methodist Fort Worth	Fort Worth	Texas	817-250-2100	www.texashealth.org
Texas Health Presbyterian Hospital Plano	Plano	Texas	972-981-8000	www.presbyplano.org
Texas Health Presbyterian Hospital - WNJ	Sherman	Texas	903-870-4611	www.wnj.org
Texas Orthopedic Hospital	Houston	Texas	713-799-8600	www.texasorthopedic.com
The Queens Medical Center	Honolulu	Hawaii	808-538-9011	www.queens.org
The Toledo Hospital	Toledo	Ohio	419-291-7463	www.promedica.org
Touro Infirmary	New Orleans	Louisiana	504-897-7011	www.touro.com
United Hospital	Saint Paul	Minnesota	651-241-8802	www.allinahealth.org/ahs/united.nsf
University Colo Health Memorial Hospital Central	Colorado Springs	Colorado	719-365-5000	www.memorialhospital.com
University of Wisconsin Hospitals & Clinics Authority	Madison	Wisconsin	608-263-8991	www.uwhealth.org
UPMC Altoona	Altoona	Pennsylvania	814-889-2011	www.altoonaregional.org
UPMC Hamot	Erie	Pennsylvania	814-877-6000	www.hamot.org
Utah Valley Regional Medical Center	Provo	Utah	801-373-7850	www.intermountainhealthcare.org/hospitals/uvrmc
Venice Regional Medical Center - Bayfront Health	Venice	Florida	941-485-7711	www.veniceregional.com
VHS Harlingen Hospital Company	Harlingen	Texas	956-389-1100	www.vbmc.org
Via Christi Hospital Pittsburg	Pittsburg	Kansas	620-231-6100	www.via-christi.org
Via Christi Hospitals Wichita	Wichita	Kansas	316-268-5000	www.via-christi.org
Wakemed - Raleigh Campus	Raleigh	North Carolina	919-350-8000	www.wakemed.org
Wentworth - Douglass Hospital	Dover	New Hampshire	603-740-2580	www.wdhospital.com
Wesley Medical Center	Wichita	Kansas	316-962-2000	www.wesleymc.com
West Calcasieu Cameron Hospital	Sulphur	Louisiana	337-527-7034	www.wcch.com
West Shore Medical Center	Manistee	Michigan	231-398-1000	www.westshoremedcenter.org
Williamsport Regional Medical Center	Williamsport	Pennsylvania	570-321-1000	www.susquehannahealth.org
Willis Knighton Medical Center	Shreveport	Louisiana	318-212-4000	www.wkhs.com//locations/medicalcenter.aspx
Woodland Heights Medical Center	Lufkin	Texas	936-634-8311	www.woodlandheights.net
Wooster Community Hospital	Wooster	Ohio	330-263-8100	www.woosterhospital.org

Note: Table shows hospitals nationwide whose rate of readmission after discharge from hospital (hospital-wide) is better (lower) than U.S. rate of 16.0%

Hospitals whose Rate of Readmission After Discharge From Hospital (Hospital-wide) is Worse (Higher) than the U.S. National Rate

Hospital	City	State	Phone	Web Site
Adena Regional Medical Center	Chillicothe	Ohio	740-779-7500	www.adena.org
Advocate Christ Hospital & Medical Center	Oak Lawn	Illinois	708-684-8000	www.advocatehealth.com
Advocate Illinois Masonic Medical Center	Chicago	Illinois	773-975-1600	www.advocatehealth.com/immc
Advocate Trinity Hospital	Chicago	Illinois	773-967-2000	www.advocatehealth.com/trin
Albert Einstein Medical Center	Philadelphia	Pennsylvania	215-456-6090	www.einstein.edu
Anne Arundel Medical Center	Annapolis	Maryland	443-481-1307	www.aahs.org
Aria Health	Philadelphia	Pennsylvania	215-612-4129	www.ariahealth.com
Arkansas Methodist Medical Center	Paragould	Arkansas	870-239-7000	www.arkansasmethodist.org
Atlanticare Regional Medical Center	Atlantic City	New Jersey	609-441-8020	www.atlanticare.org/acmc/index.html
Aventura Hospital & Medical Center	Aventura	Florida	305-682-7000	www.aventurahospital.com
B R F Hospital Holdings	Shreveport	Louisiana	318-675-5000	www.lsumc.edu
Banner Desert Medical Center	Mesa	Arizona	480-412-3000	www.bannerhealth.com
Baptist Beaumont Hospital	Beaumont	Texas	409-212-5012	www.mhbh.org
Baptist Memorial Hospital Desoto	Southaven	Mississippi	662-772-4000	www.bmhcc.org/facilities/desoto
Barnes-Jewish Hospital	Saint Louis	Missouri	314-747-3000	www.barnesjewish.org
Baxter Regional Medical Center	Mountain Home	Arkansas	870-508-1000	www.baxterregional.org
Beaumont Health System	Grosse Pointe	Michigan	313-343-1000	www.beaumonthospitals.com
Beaumont Health System	Royal Oak	Michigan	248-898-5000	www.beaumonthospitals.com
Beckley ARH Hospital	Beckley	West Virginia	304-255-3456	www.arh.org/beckley
Bellevue Hospital Center	New York	New York	212-561-4132	www.nyc.gov/html/hhc/html/facilities/bellevue.shtml
Beth Israel Deaconess Hospital - Milton	Milton	Massachusetts	617-696-4600	www.miltonhosital.org
Beth Israel Deaconess Medical Center	Boston	Massachusetts	617-667-7000	www.bidmc.harvard.edu
Beth Israel Medical Center	New York	New York	212-420-2000	www.wehealny.org
Bluefield Regional Medical Center	Bluefield	West Virginia	304-327-1100	www.bluefield.org
Bolivar Medical Center	Cleveland	Mississippi	662-846-2551	www.bolivarmedical.com
Boston Medical Center Corporation	Boston	Massachusetts	617-638-8000	www.bmc.org
Botsford Hospital	Farmington Hills	Michigan	248-471-8000	www.botsfordsystem.org
Bridgeport Hospital	Bridgeport	Connecticut	203-384-3000	www.bridgeporthospital.com
Brigham & Women's Faulkner Hospital	Boston	Massachusetts	617-983-7000	www.brighamandwomensfaulkner.org
Brigham & Women's Hospital	Boston	Massachusetts	617-732-5500	www.brighamandwomens.org
Bronx - Lebanon Hospital Center	Bronx	New York	212-588-7000	www.bronx-leb.org
Brookdale Hospital Medical Center	Brooklyn	New York	718-240-5966	www.brookdalehospital.org
Brookhaven Memorial Hospital Medical Center	Patchogue	New York	631-654-7100	www.brookhavenhospitalorg
Brooklyn Hospital Center at Downtown Campus	Brooklyn	New York	718-250-8000	www.tbh.org
Byrd Regional Hospital	Leesville	Louisiana	337-239-9041	www.chs.net
California Hospital Medical Center Los Angeles	Los Angeles	California	213-748-2411	www.chmcla.org
Camden Clark Medical Center	Parkersburg	West Virginia	304-424-2111	www.ccmh.org
Capital Health System - Fuld Campus	Trenton	New Jersey	609-394-6000	www.capitalhealth.org
Capital Regional Medical Center	Tallahassee	Florida	850-656-5000	www.capitalregionalmedicalcenter.com
Carepoint Health - Christ Hospital	Jersey City	New Jersey	201-795-8200	www.christhospital.org
Carepoint Health - Hoboken UMC	Hoboken	New Jersey	201-418-1004	www.bonsecoursnj.com
Carolinas Hospital System	Florence	South Carolina	843-674-2500	www.carolinashospital.com
Casey County Hospital	Liberty	Kentucky	606-787-6275	
Catskill Regional Medical Center	Harris	New York	845-794-3300	www.crmcny.org
Chambers Memorial Hospital	Danville	Arkansas	479-495-2241	www.chambershospital.com
Chesapeake General Hospital	Chesapeake	Virginia	757-312-8121	www.chesapeakehealth.com
Clay County Hospital	Flora	Illinois	618-662-2131	www.claycountyhospital.org
Cleveland Clinic	Cleveland	Ohio	216-444-2200	www.clevelandclinic.org
Cleveland Clinic Hospital	Weston	Florida	954-689-5000	www.clevelandclinic.org
Clinch Valley Medical Center	Richlands	Virginia	276-596-6000	www.clinchvalleymedicalcenter.com
Coffee Regional Medical Center	Douglas	Georgia	229-384-1900	www.coffeeregional.org
Coliseum Medical Center	Macon	Georgia	478-765-4100	www.coliseumhealthsystem.com
Community Regional Medical Center	Fresno	California	559-459-6000	www.communitymedical.org
Conemaugh Valley Memorial Hospital	Johnstown	Pennsylvania	814-534-9000	www.conemaugh.org
Coney Island Hospital	Brooklyn	New York	718-616-3000	www.coneyislandhospital.com
Cooper University Hospital	Camden	New Jersey	856-342-2000	www.cooperhealth.org
Covenant Medical Center	Saginaw	Michigan	989-583-4000	www.covenanthealthcare.com
Crittenden Health System	Marion	Kentucky	270-965-5281	www.crittenden-health.org
Danville Regional Medical Center	Danville	Virginia	434-799-2100	www.danvilleregional.org
Davis Memorial Hospital	Elkins	West Virginia	304-636-3300	www.davishealthcare.org
Desert Valley Hospital	Victorville	California	760-241-8000	www.dvmc.com
Desoto Memorial Hospital	Arcadia	Florida	863-494-3535	www.dmh.org
Detroit Receiving Hospital & University Health Center	Detroit	Michigan	313-745-3104	www.drhuhc.org
Doctors Hospital	Columbus	Ohio	614-544-1000	www.columbusregional.com
Doctors Hospital of Manteca	Manteca	California	209-823-3111	www.doctorsmanteca.com

Hospital	City	State	Phone	Web Site
Drew Memorial Hospital	Monticello	Arkansas	870-367-2411	www.drewmemorial.org
Duke University Hospital	Durham	North Carolina	919-684-8111	www.dukehealth.org
Dyersburg Regional Medical Center	Dyersburg	Tennessee	731-285-2410	www.dyersburgregionalmc.com
East Georgia Regional Medical Center	Statesboro	Georgia	912-486-1500	www.egrmc.com
East Ohio Regional Hospital	Martins Ferry	Ohio	740-633-4151	www.eastohioregionalhospital.com
East Orange General Hospital	East Orange	New Jersey	973-266-4401	www.evh.org
Eastern Niagara Hospital	Lockport	New York	716-514-5700	www.enhs.org
Eastern State Hospital	Williamsburg	Virginia	757-253-5161	www.ehs.dmhmrsas.virginia.gov
Easton Hospital	Easton	Pennsylvania	610-250-4076	www.easton-hospital.com
Elmhurst Hospital Center	Elmhurst	New York	718-334-1141	www.nyc.gov
Emanuel Medical Center	Turlock	California	209-667-4200	www.emanuelmedicalcenter.org
Excela Health Frick Hospital	Mount Pleasant	Pennsylvania	724-547-1500	www.excelahealth.org
Fauquier Hospital	Warrenton	Virginia	540-316-5000	www.fauquierhospital.org
Fayette County Hospital	Vandalia	Illinois	618-283-1231	www.fayettecountyhospital.org
Fitzgibbon Hospital	Marshall	Missouri	660-886-7431	www.fitzgibbon.org
Florida Hospital	Orlando	Florida	407-303-1976	www.floridahospital.com
Flushing Hospital Medical Center	Flushing	New York	718-670-5000	www.flushinghospital.org
Forest Hills Hospital	Forest Hills	New York	718-830-4000	www.northshorelij.com
Franciscan Saint James Health	Olympia Fields	Illinois	708-747-4000	www.franciscanalliance.org
Franciscan Saint Margaret Health - Hammond	Hammond	Indiana	219-932-2300	www.smmhc.com
Franklin Hospital	Valley Stream	New York	516-256-6000	www.northshorelij.com
Frederick Memorial Hospital	Frederick	Maryland	240-566-3300	www.fmh.org
Garden City Hospital	Garden City	Michigan	734-421-3300	www.gchosp.org
Gateway Medical Center	Clarksville	Tennessee	931-502-1000	www.todaysgateway.com
Genesis Healthcare System	Zanesville	Ohio	740-454-5000	www.genesishcs.org
George Washington Univ Hospital	Washington	District of Columbia	202-716-4605	www.gwhospital.com
Glenwood Regional Medical Center	West Monroe	Louisiana	318-329-4600	www.grmc.com
Good Samaritan Hospital of Suffern	Suffern	New York	914-368-5000	www.goodsamhosp.org
Grant Medical Center	Columbus	Ohio	614-566-9978	www.ohiohealth.com
Great River Medical Center	Blytheville	Arkansas	870-838-7300	www.greatrivermc.com
Harlan Appalachian Regional Healthcare Hospital	Harlan	Kentucky	606-573-8100	www.arh.org
Harlem Hospital Center	New York	New York	212-491-8400	www.nyc.gov/hhc
Harper University Hospital	Detroit	Michigan	313-745-6211	www.harperhospital.org
Harris Hospital	Newport	Arkansas	870-523-8911	www.harrishospital.com
Harton Regional Medical Center	Tullahoma	Tennessee	931-393-3000	www.hartonmedicalcenter.com
Hazard ARH Regional Medical Center	Hazard	Kentucky	606-439-6600	www.arh.org/hazard
Health Alliance Hospital Broadway Campus	Kingston	New York	914-331-3131	www.kingstonregionalhealth.org
Henry Ford Hospital	Detroit	Michigan	313-916-2600	www.henryfordhospital.com
Hialeah Hospital	Hialeah	Florida	305-693-6100	www.hialeahhosp.com
Highlands Regional Medical Center	Prestonsburg	Kentucky	606-886-8511	www.hrmc.org
Hollywood Presbyterian Medical Center	Los Angeles	California	213-413-3000	www.qahpmc.com
Holy Cross Hospital	Chicago	Illinois	773-471-8000	www.holycrosshospital.org
Holzer Medical Center	Gallipolis	Ohio	740-446-5000	www.holzer.org
Hospital of Univ of Pennsylvania	Philadelphia	Pennsylvania	215-662-3227	www.upenn.edu
Howard University Hospital	Washington	District of Columbia	202-745-6100	www.huhosp.org
Hudson Valley Hospital Center	Cortlandt Manor	New York	914-734-3611	www.hvhc.org
Illinois Valley Community Hospital	Peru	Illinois	815-223-3300	www.ivch.org
Ingalls Memorial Hospital	Harvey	Illinois	708-333-2300	www.ingalls.org
Jackson Memorial Hospital	Miami	Florida	305-585-1111	www.jhsmiami.org
Jackson Parish Hospital	Jonesboro	Louisiana	318-259-4435	www.jacksonparishhospital.com
Jackson Park Hospital	Chicago	Illinois	773-947-7500	www.jacksonparkhospital.org
Jacobi Medical Center	Bronx	New York	718-918-5000	www.ci.nyc.ny.us/html/hhc
Jamaica Hospital Medical Center	Jamaica	New York	718-262-6000	www.jamaicahospital.org
Jane Todd Crawford Hospital	Greensburg	Kentucky	270-932-4211	
Jeanes Hospital	Philadelphia	Pennsylvania	215-728-2000	www.jeanes.com
Jennie Stuart Medical Center	Hopkinsville	Kentucky	270-887-0100	www.jsmc.org
Jennings American Legion Hospital	Jennings	Louisiana	337-616-7000	www.jalh.com
JFK Medical Center	Atlantis	Florida	561-965-7300	www.jfkmc.com
JFK Medical Center - A M Yelencsics Comm Hospital	Edison	New Jersey	732-321-7000	www.jfkmc.org
John H Stroger Jr Hospital	Chicago	Illinois	312-864-6000	www.cookcountygov.com
Johns Hopkins Bayview Medical Center	Baltimore	Maryland	410-550-0123	www.hopkinsbayview.org
The Johns Hopkins Hospital	Baltimore	Maryland	410-955-9540	www.jhmi.edu
Johnson City Medical Center	Johnson City	Tennessee	423-431-6111	www.msha.com
Kendall Regional Medical Center	Miami	Florida	305-223-3000	www.kendallmed.com
Kennedy University Hospital - Stratford Div	Stratford	New Jersey	856-346-6000	www.kennedyhealth.org
Kent County Memorial Hospital	Warwick	Rhode Island	401-737-7000	www.kentri.org
Kentucky River Medical Center	Jackson	Kentucky	606-666-6000	www.kentuckyrivermc.com

Hospital	City	State	Phone	Web Site
King's Daughters' Medical Center	Ashland	Kentucky	606-408-4000	www.kdmc.com
Kings County Hospital Center	Brooklyn	New York	718-245-3901	www.nyc.gov/html/hhc/html/facilities/kings.shtml
Kingsbrook Jewish Medical Center	Brooklyn	New York	718-604-5789	www.kingsbrook.org
Knox County Hospital	Barbourville	Kentucky	606-546-4175	www.knoxcohospital.com
Lahey Hospital & Medical Center - Burlington	Burlington	Massachusetts	781-744-5100	www.lahey.org
Lake Pointe Medical Center	Rowlett	Texas	972-412-2273	www.lakepointemedical.com
Lake Wales Medical Center	Lake Wales	Florida	863-676-1433	www.lakewalesmedicalcenter.com
Larkin Community Hospital	South Miami	Florida	305-284-7500	www.larkinhospital.com
Laurel Regional Medical Center	Laurel	Maryland	301-725-4300	www.laurelregionalhospital.org
Lawrence Hospital Center	Bronxville	New York	914-787-1000	www.lawrencehealth.org
Leesburg Regional Medical Center	Leesburg	Florida	352-323-5762	www.leesburgregional.org
Lenox Hill Hospital	New York	New York	212-439-2345	www.lenoxhillhospital.org
Lewisgale Hospital Pulaski	Pulaski	Virginia	540-994-8100	www.lewisgale.com
Libertyhealth - Jersey City Medical Center Campus	Jersey City	New Jersey	201-915-2000	www.libertyhcs.org
Lincoln Medical & Mental Health Center	Bronx	New York	718-579-5000	www.nyc.gov/html/hhc/lincoln
Little Company of Mary Hospital	Evergreen Park	Illinois	708-422-6200	www.lcmh.org
Long Island Jewish Medical Center	New Hyde Park	New York	718-470-7000	www.northshorelij.com
Lowell General Hospital	Lowell	Massachusetts	978-937-6000	www.lowellgeneral.org
Loyola University Medical Center	Maywood	Illinois	708-216-9000	www.lumc.edu
Lutheran Medical Center	Brooklyn	New York	718-630-8000	www.lmcmc.com
Maimonides Medical Center	Brooklyn	New York	718-283-6000	www.maimonidesmed.org
Mary Immaculate Hospital	Newport News	Virginia	757-886-6000	www.bonsecourshamptonroad.com
Medical Center of Southeastern Oklahoma	Durant	Oklahoma	405-924-3080	www.mcsohealth.com
Medical College of Georgia Hospitals & Clinics	Augusta	Georgia	706-721-6569	www.mcghealth.org
Medical College of Virginia Hospitals	Richmond	Virginia	804-828-0938	www.vcuhealth.org
Medstar Good Samaritan Hospital	Baltimore	Maryland	443-444-3902	www.goodsam-md.org
Medstar Montgomery Medical Center	Olney	Maryland	301-774-8882	www.montgomerygeneral.com
Memorial Hospital	Manchester	Kentucky	606-598-5104	www.manchestermemorial.com
Memorial Hospital	Nacogdoches	Texas	936-564-4611	www.nacmem.org
Memorial Hospital of Gardena	Gardena	California	310-532-4200	www.avantihospitals.com
Memorial Hospital of Salem County	Salem	New Jersey	856-935-1000	www.mhshealth.com
Memorial Hospital of Stilwell	Stilwell	Oklahoma	918-696-3101	www.stilwellmemorialhospital.com
Memorial Regional Hospital	Hollywood	Florida	954-987-2000	www.memorialregional.com
Mercy Fitzgerald Hospital	Darby	Pennsylvania	215-237-4000	www.mercyhealth.org
Mercy Hospital & Medical Center	Chicago	Illinois	312-567-2000	www.mercy-chicago.org
Mercy Hospital Anderson	Cincinnati	Ohio	513-624-4006	www.e-mercy.com/mercy-hospital-anderson.aspx
Mercy Hospital Fairfield	Fairfield	Ohio	513-870-7197	www.e-mercy.com/mercy-hospital-fairfield.aspx
Mercy Hospital Jefferson	Crystal City	Missouri	636-933-1000	www.jeffersonmemorial.org
Mercy Medical Center	Baltimore	Maryland	410-332-9237	www.mdmercy.com
Mercy Regional Medical Center	Ville Platte	Louisiana	337-363-5684	www.vpmc.com
Methodist Hospital	Henderson	Kentucky	270-827-7700	www.methodisthospital.net
Methodist Hospitals	Gary	Indiana	219-886-4642	www.methodisthospital.org
Metrosouth Medical Center	Blue Island	Illinois	708-597-2000	www.stfrancisblueisland.com
Middlesboro Appalachian Regional Healthcare Hospital	Middlesboro	Kentucky	606-242-1101	www.arh.org/middlesboro
Midwest Regional Medical Center	Midwest City	Oklahoma	405-610-8530	www.midwestregional.com
Milford Regional Medical Center	Milford	Massachusetts	508-473-1190	www.milfordregional.org
Miriam Hospital	Providence	Rhode Island	401-793-2500	www.lifespan.org/partners/tmh
Mission Regional Medical Center	Mission	Texas	956-323-9000	www.missionhospital.org
Monmouth Medical Center - Southern Campus	Lakewood	New Jersey	732-363-1900	www.sbhcs.com
Monroe County Medical Center	Tompkinsville	Kentucky	270-487-9231	www.mcmccares.com
Montefiore Medical Center	Bronx	New York	718-920-4321	www.montefiore.org
Montefiore New Rochelle Hospital	New Rochelle	New York	914-632-5000	www.ssmc.org
Morgan County ARH Hospital	West Liberty	Kentucky	606-743-3186	www.arh.org/morgan
Morton Hospital	Taunton	Massachusetts	508-828-7000	www.mortonhospital.org
Mountainview Hospital	Las Vegas	Nevada	702-255-5065	www.mountainview-hospital.com
Musc Medical Center	Charleston	South Carolina	843-792-2300	www.musc.edu
Nacogdoches Medical Center	Nacogdoches	Texas	936-569-9481	www.nacmedicalcenter.com
Nassau University Medical Center	East Meadow	New York	516-572-0123	www.numc.edu
Natchez Community Hospital	Natchez	Mississippi	601-445-6205	www.natchezcommunityhospital.com
Nazareth Hospital	Philadelphia	Pennsylvania	215-335-6000	www.nazarethhospital.org
New York Community Hospital of Brooklyn	Brooklyn	New York	718-692-5302	www.nych.com
New York Hospital Medical Center of Queens	Flushing	New York	718-670-1231	www.nyhq.org
New York Methodist Hospital	Brooklyn	New York	718-780-3000	www.nym.org
New York - Presbyterian Hospital	New York	New York	212-746-4189	www.nyp.org
Newark Beth Israel Medical Center	Newark	New Jersey	973-926-7850	www.sbhcs.com
North Oaks Medical Center	Hammond	Louisiana	985-345-2700	www.northoaks.org
North Shore University Hospital	Manhasset	New York	516-562-0100	www.northshorelij.com

Hospital	City	State	Phone	Web Site
Northside Hospital	Saint Petersburg	Florida	813-521-5000	www.northsidehospital.com
Northwest Hospital Center	Randallstown	Maryland	410-521-5995	www.lifebridgehealth.org
Northwest Mississippi Regional Medical Center	Clarksdale	Mississippi	662-627-3211	www.nwmsregionalmedcenter.com
Northwestern Memorial Hospital	Chicago	Illinois	312-926-2000	www.nmh.org
Norwegian - American Hospital	Chicago	Illinois	773-292-8200	www.nahospital.org
Nyack Hospital	Nyack	New York	845-348-2000	www.nyackhospital.org
NYU Hospitals Center	New York	New York	212-263-7300	www.med.nyu.edu
Oakwood Hospital - Dearborn	Dearborn	Michigan	313-593-7125	www.oakwood.org
Oakwood Hospital - Taylor	Taylor	Michigan	313-295-5253	www.oakwod.org
Oakwood Hospital - Wayne	Wayne	Michigan	734-467-4175	www.oakwood.org
Ohio State University Hospitals	Columbus	Ohio	614-293-9700	www.jamesline.com
Olympia Medical Center	Los Angeles	California	310-657-5900	www.olympiamc.com
Orange Regional Medical Center	Middletown	New York	845-343-2424	www.ormc.org
Oroville Hospital	Oroville	California	530-533-8500	www.orovillehospital.com
Osceola Regional Medical Center	Kissimmee	Florida	407-846-2266	www.osceolaregional.com
Pacifica Hospital of the Valley	Sun Valley	California	818-767-3310	www.pacificahospital.com
Palisades Medical Center	North Bergen	New Jersey	201-854-5000	www.palisadesmedical.org
Palm Springs General Hospital	Hialeah	Florida	305-558-2500	www.psghosp.com
Palmetto General Hospital	Hialeah	Florida	305-823-5000	www.palmettogeneral.com
Palms West Hospital	Loxahatchee	Florida	561-753-4245	www.palmswesthospital.com
Peacehealth Southwest Medical Center	Vancouver	Washington	360-256-2000	www.swmedicalcenter.org
Peconic Bay Medical Center	Riverhead	New York	631-548-6000	www.pbmedicalcenter.org
Pekin Memorial Hospital	Pekin	Illinois	309-347-1151	www.pekinhospital.org
Pennsylvania Hospital of the Univ of PA Health Sys	Philadelphia	Pennsylvania	215-829-3000	www.pennmedicine.org/pahosp
Perry Community Hospital	Linden	Tennessee	931-589-2121	
Pineville Community Hospital	Pineville	Kentucky	606-337-3051	www.pinevillehospital.com
Poplar Bluff Regional Medical Center	Poplar Bluff	Missouri	573-785-7721	www.poplarbluffregional.com
Pottstown Memorial Medical Center	Pottstown	Pennsylvania	610-327-7000	www.pmmctr.org
Presence Saint Francis Hospital	Evanston	Illinois	847-316-4000	www.reshealth.org
Presence Saint Joseph Hospital - Chicago	Chicago	Illinois	773-665-3000	www.res-health.org
Presence Saint Joseph Medical Center	Joliet	Illinois	815-725-7133	www.provena.org/stjoes
Presence Saints Mary & Elizabeth Medical Center	Chicago	Illinois	312-770-2000	www.reshealth.org
Presence Saint Marys Hospital	Kankakee	Illinois	815-937-2490	www.provenastmarys.com
Presence United Samaritans Medical Center	Danville	Illinois	217-443-5000	www.provena.org/usmc
Providence Hospital	Washington	District of Columbia	202-269-7000	www.provhosp.org
Providence Hospital & Medical Centers	Southfield	Michigan	248-849-3011	www.stjohn.org/providence
Queens Hospital Center	Jamaica	New York	718-883-3000	www.nyc.gov/html/hhc/qhn/home.html
Raleigh General Hospital	Beckley	West Virginia	304-256-4100	www.raleighgeneral.com
Raritan Bay Medical Center	Perth Amboy	New Jersey	732-442-3700	www.rbmc.org
Reston Hospital Center	Reston	Virginia	703-689-9000	www.restonhospital.com
Rhode Island Hospital	Providence	Rhode Island	401-444-4000	www.rhodeislandhospital.org
Richmond University Medical Center	Staten Island	New York	718-818-1234	www.rumcsi.org
Riverside Methodist Hospital	Columbus	Ohio	614-566-5000	www.ohiohealth.com
Robert Packer Hospital	Sayre	Pennsylvania	570-888-6666	www.guthrie.org
Robert Wood Johnson University Hospital	New Brunswick	New Jersey	732-937-8900	www.rwjuh.edu
Ronald Reagan UCLA Medical Center	Los Angeles	California	310-825-6301	www.uclahealth.org
Roseland Community Hospital	Chicago	Illinois	773-995-3000	www.roselandhospital.org
Roxborough Memorial Hospital	Philadelphia	Pennsylvania	215-483-9900	www.roxboroughmemorial.com
Rush University Medical Center	Chicago	Illinois	312-942-5000	www.ruch.edu
Saint Francis Hospital	Tulsa	Oklahoma	918-494-2200	www.saintfrancis.com
Saint Francis Medical Center	Peoria	Illinois	309-655-2000	www.osfsaintfrancis.org
Saint Michael's Medical Center	Newark	New Jersey	973-877-5350	www.cathedralhealth.org
Saint Peter's University Hospital	New Brunswick	New Jersey	732-745-8600	www.saintpetersuh.com
Saint Thomas Rutherford Hospital	Murfreesboro	Tennessee	615-396-4100	www.mtmc.org
Saline Memorial Hospital	Benton	Arkansas	501-776-6000	www.salinememorial.org
San Joaquin Community Hospital	Bakersfield	California	661-395-3000	www.sanjoaquinhospital.org
San Luke's Memorial Hospital	Ponce	Puerto Rico	787-844-2080	www.ssepr.com/hospital_sanlucas.html
Sandhills Regional Medical Center	Hamlet	North Carolina	910-958-2361	www.hma-corp.com
Santa Monica - UCLA Medical Center & Orthopaedic Hospital	Santa Monica	California	310-319-4000	www.healthcare.ucla.edu
Scotland Memorial Hospital	Laurinburg	North Carolina	910-291-7000	www.scotlandhealth.org
Silver Cross Hospital & Medical Centers	New Lenox	Illinois	815-300-1100	www.silvercross.org
Sinai Hospital of Baltimore	Baltimore	Maryland	410-601-5131	www.sinai-balt.com
Sinai - Grace Hospital	Detroit	Michigan	313-966-3300	www.sinaigrace.org
Singing River Hospital	Pascagoula	Mississippi	228-809-5000	www.srhshealth.com
South Nassau Communities Hospital	Oceanside	New York	516-632-3000	www.southnassau.org
South Shore Hospital	Chicago	Illinois	773-768-0810	www.southshorehospital.com
Southern Tennessee Medical Center	Winchester	Tennessee	931-967-8295	www.southerntennessee.com

Hospital	City	State	Phone	Web Site
Southern Virginia Regional Medical Center	Emporia	Virginia	434-348-4400	www.svrmc.com
Southwest Healthcare System	Murrieta	California	951-696-6000	www.ivrmc-rsmc.com
Saint Anthony's Medical Center	Saint Louis	Missouri	314-525-1000	www.samcstl.org
Saint Barnabas Hospital	Bronx	New York	212-960-9000	www.stbarnabashospital.org
Saint Bernard Hospital	Chicago	Illinois	773-962-3900	www.stbernardhospital.com
Saint Catherine of Siena Hospital	Smithtown	New York	631-862-3000	www.stcatherines.chsli.org
Saint Claire Regional Medical Center	Morehead	Kentucky	606-783-6500	www.st-claire.org
Saint Elizabeth Hospital	Belleville	Illinois	618-234-2120	www.steliz.org
Saint Elizabeth's Medical Center	Brighton	Massachusetts	617-789-3000	www.semc.org
Saint Francis Hospital	Poughkeepsie	New York	845-483-5000	www.sfhhc.org
Saint John Hospital & Medical Center	Detroit	Michigan	313-343-4000	www.stjohnprovidence.org
Saint John Macomb - Oakland Hospital - Macomb Center	Warren	Michigan	586-573-5000	www.stjohn.org
Saint John's Episcopal Hospital at South Shore	Far Rockaway	New York	718-869-7000	www.ehs.org
Saint John's Riverside Hospital	Yonkers	New York	914-964-4444	www.riversidehealth.org
Saint Joseph Health Services of RI	North Providence	Rhode Island	401-456-3000	www.fatimahospital.com
Saint Joseph Mercy Oakland	Pontiac	Michigan	248-858-3000	www.stjoesoakland.org
Saint Joseph Regional Health Center	Bryan	Texas	979-776-3912	www.st-joseph.org/sjrhc
Saint Joseph's Hospital	Philadelphia	Pennsylvania	215-787-2000	www.nphs.com
Saint Joseph's Medical Center	Yonkers	New York	914-378-7000	www.saintjosephs.org
Saint Joseph's Regional Medical Center	Paterson	New Jersey	973-754-2010	www.sjhmc.org
Saint Louis University Hospital	Saint Louis	Missouri	314-577-8000	www.slucare.edu/clinical
Saint Luke's Roosevelt Hospital	New York	New York	212-523-4000	www.wehealny.org
Saint Luke's Episcopal Hospital	Houston	Texas	832-355-1000	www.sleh.com
Saint Mary Medical Center	Hobart	Indiana	219-942-0551	www.comhs.org/stmary
Saint Mary Mercy Hospital	Livonia	Michigan	734-655-4800	www.stmarymercy.org
Saint Mary's of Michigan Medical Center	Saginaw	Michigan	989-776-8000	www.stmarysofmichigan.org
Saint Marys Hospital	Centralia	Illinois	618-436-6519	www.stmarys-goodsamaritan.com
Saint Rose Hospital	Hayward	California	510-782-6200	www.strosehospital.org
Saint Vincent Hospital	Worcester	Massachusetts	508-363-5000	www.stvincenthospital.com
Saint Vincent's Medical Center	Bridgeport	Connecticut	203-576-5551	www.stvincents.org
Saint Vincent's Medical Center	Jacksonville	Florida	904-308-7300	www.jaxhealth.com
Staten Island University Hospital	Staten Island	New York	718-226-9000	www.siuh.edu
Stephens County Hospital	Toccoa	Georgia	706-282-4250	www.stephenscountyhospital.com
Strong Memorial Hospital	Rochester	New York	585-275-2121	www.urmc.rochester.edu
Summa Health System Barberton Hospital	Barberton	Ohio	330-615-3000	www.barbhosp.com
Sumner Regional Medical Center	Gallatin	Tennessee	615-452-4210	www.mysumnermedical.com
Sunrise Hospital & Medical Center	Las Vegas	Nevada	702-731-8000	www.sunrisehospital.com
Swedish Covenant Hospital	Chicago	Illinois	773-878-8200	www.swedishcovenant.org
Temple University Hospital	Philadelphia	Pennsylvania	215-707-2000	www.tuh.templehealth.org
The University of Chicago Medical Center	Chicago	Illinois	773-702-1000	www.uchospitals.edu
Thomas Jefferson University Hospital	Philadelphia	Pennsylvania	215-955-6000	www.jeffersonhospital.org
Thorek Memorial Hospital	Chicago	Illinois	312-525-6780	www.thorek.org
Trinitas Regional Medical Center	Elizabeth	New Jersey	908-994-5000	www.trinitashospital.org
Tristar Summit Medical Center	Hermitage	Tennessee	615-316-3000	www.summitmedctr.com
Tufts Medical Center	Boston	Massachusetts	617-636-5000	www.tuftsmedicalcenter.org
Tulane Medical Center	New Orleans	Louisiana	504-988-1900	www.tuhc.com
UAMS Medical Center	Little Rock	Arkansas	501-686-5000	www.uams.edu/medcenter
UF Health Shands Hospital	Gainesville	Florida	352-265-8000	www.shands.org
Umass Memorial Medical Center	Worcester	Massachusetts	508-334-1000	www.umassmemorial.org
Union Hospital	Terre Haute	Indiana	812-238-7606	www.uhhg.org
University Health Care/University Hospitals & Clinics	Salt Lake City	Utah	801-581-2121	www.healthcare.utah.edu
University Hospital	Newark	New Jersey	973-972-5658	www.theuniversityhospital.com
University Hospital - Stony Brook	Stony Brook	New York	631-444-4000	www.stonybrookmedicalcenter.org
University Hospital of Brooklyn - Downstate Medical Center	Brooklyn	New York	718-270-1000	www.downstate.edu
University Hospitals - Elyria Medical Center	Elyria	Ohio	440-329-7500	www.emh-healthcare.org
University Hospitals Ahuja Medical Center	Beachwood	Ohio	216-767-8793	www.uhhospitals.org/ahuja
University Hospitals Case Medical Center	Cleveland	Ohio	216-844-1000	www.uhhs.com
University of Alabama Hospital	Birmingham	Alabama	205-934-4011	www.health.uab.edu
University of Arizona Medical Center	Tucson	Arizona	520-694-0111	www.azumc.com
University of Cincinnati Medical Center	Cincinnati	Ohio	513-584-1000	www.universityhospitalcincinnati.com
University of Illinois Hospital	Chicago	Illinois	312-996-3900	www.uic.edu
University of Iowa Hospital & Clinics	Iowa City	Iowa	319-356-1616	www.uihealthcare.com
University of Kentucky Hospital	Lexington	Kentucky	859-323-5000	www.uhealthcare.uky.edu
University of Louisville Hospital	Louisville	Kentucky	502-562-3000	www.uoflhealthcare.org
University of Maryland Medical Center	Baltimore	Maryland	410-328-8667	www.umm.edu
University of Maryland Medical Center Midtown Campus	Baltimore	Maryland	410-225-8996	www.marylandgeneral.org
University of Miami Hospital	Miami	Florida	305-325-5511	www.cedarsmedicalcenter.com

Hospital	City	State	Phone	Web Site
University of Michigan Health System	Ann Arbor	Michigan	734-764-1505	www.med.umich.edu
University of North Carolina Hospital	Chapel Hill	North Carolina	919-966-4131	www.unchealthcare.org
University of Texas Medical Branch Galveston	Galveston	Texas	409-772-1011	www.utmb.edu
University of Virginia Medical Center	Charlottesville	Virginia	800-251-3627	www.uvahealth.com
UPMC Presbyterian Shadyside	Pittsburgh	Pennsylvania	412-647-8788	www.upmc.edu
Valley Hospital	Ridgewood	New Jersey	201-447-8000	www.valleyhealth.com
Valley Hospital Medical Center	Las Vegas	Nevada	702-388-4000	www.valleyhealthsystem.org
Vanderbilt University Hospital	Nashville	Tennessee	615-322-3454	www.mc.vanderbilt.edu
Vassar Brothers Medical Center	Poughkeepsie	New York	845-454-8500	www.vasserbrothers.org
Vidant Medical Center	Greenville	North Carolina	252-847-4100	www.uhseast.com
Vidant Roanoke Chowan Hospital	Ahoskie	North Carolina	252-209-3000	www.uhseast.com
Washington Hospital	Fremont	California	510-797-1111	www.whhs.com
Wellmont Bristol Regional Medical Center	Bristol	Tennessee	423-844-1121	www.wellmont.org
Wellmont Holston Valley Medical Center	Kingsport	Tennessee	423-224-4000	www.wellmont.org
Wesley Medical Center	Hattiesburg	Mississippi	601-268-8000	www.wesley.com
West Chester Hospital	West Chester	Ohio	513-298-3000	www.westchesterhospital.uchealth.com
West River Regional Medical Center	Hettinger	North Dakota	701-567-4561	www.wrhs.com
West Virginia University Hospitals	Morgantown	West Virginia	304-598-4000	www.wvuh.com
Westchester General Hospital	Miami	Florida	305-263-9270	www.westchestergeneralhospital.com
Westchester Medical Center	Valhalla	New York	914-285-7017	www.wcmc.com
Western Arizona Regional Medical Center	Bullhead City	Arizona	928-763-2273	www.warmc.com
Western Maryland Regional Medical Center	Cumberland	Maryland	240-964-8001	www.wmhs.com
White County Medical Center	Searcy	Arkansas	501-278-3100	www.centralarkhospital.com
White River Medical Center	Batesville	Arkansas	870-262-1200	www.wrmc.com
William Beaumont Hospital - Troy	Troy	Michigan	248-964-8800	www.beaumonthospitals.com
Williamson ARH Hospital	South Williamson	Kentucky	606-237-1700	www.arh.org
Williamson Memorial Hospital	Williamson	West Virginia	304-235-2500	www.hmawmh.com
Winter Haven Hospital	Winter Haven	Florida	863-293-1121	www.winterhavenhospital.com
Wyckoff Heights Medical Center	Brooklyn	New York	718-963-7272	www.wyckoffhospital.org
Yale-New Haven Hospital	New Haven	Connecticut	203-688-4242	www.ynhh.org

Note: Table shows hospitals nationwide whose rate of readmission after discharge from hospital (hospital-wide) is better (lower) than U.S. rate of 16.0%

Hospital Heart Attack Readmission Rates: State and National Summary

Area	Number of Hospitals			
	Better than U.S. National Rate[1]	Worse than U.S. National Rate[2]	No Different than U.S. National Rate[3]	Number of Cases Too Small[4]
U.S. and Territories	23	29	2327	2085
Alabama	0	0	39	58
Alaska	0	0	5	14
American Samoa	0	0	0	1
Arizona	0	0	47	21
Arkansas	0	1	27	46
California	1	1	201	122
Colorado	1	0	32	33
Connecticut	0	1	27	3
Delaware	0	0	6	1
District of Columbia	0	0	6	2
Florida	3	3	144	32
Georgia	1	0	64	72
Guam	0	0	1	0
Hawaii	0	0	11	5
Idaho	0	0	9	23
Illinois	0	5	103	71
Indiana	2	0	61	54
Iowa	0	0	27	82
Kansas	0	0	27	82
Kentucky	0	0	40	55
Louisiana	0	0	44	56
Maine	1	0	21	15
Maryland	0	0	39	7
Massachusetts	0	1	52	10
Michigan	1	0	76	51
Minnesota	0	0	31	89
Mississippi	0	0	30	49
Missouri	0	0	53	59
Montana	0	0	8	35
N. Mariana Islands	0	0	1	0
Nebraska	0	0	19	53
Nevada	0	0	18	14
New Hampshire	0	0	15	10
New Jersey	0	5	55	6
New Mexico	1	0	11	26
New York	0	4	132	45
North Carolina	1	1	67	40
North Dakota	1	0	7	33
Ohio	0	0	96	61
Oklahoma	0	1	31	67
Oregon	1	0	23	36
Pennsylvania	1	0	120	41
Puerto Rico	0	1	12	32
Rhode Island	0	0	11	0
South Carolina	1	1	36	22
South Dakota	0	0	9	38
Tennessee	0	1	56	55
Texas	2	0	176	153
Utah	0	0	14	20
Vermont	0	0	8	7
Virgin Islands	0	0	1	1
Virginia	0	2	62	17
Washington	2	0	40	40
West Virginia	0	1	24	28
Wisconsin	3	0	50	68
Wyoming	0	0	2	24

Note: (1) 30-day readmission rate is better (lower) than U.S. rate of 18.3%; (2) 30-day readmission rate is worse (higher) than U.S. rate of 18.3%; (3) 30-day readmission rate is about the same as U.S. rate of 18.3%; (4) The number of cases is too small to classify the hospital

Hospital Heart Failure Readmission Rates: State and National Summary

Area	Number of Hospitals			
	Better than U.S. National Rate[1]	Worse than U.S. National Rate[2]	No Different than U.S. National Rate[3]	Number of Cases Too Small[4]
U.S. and Territories	120	159	3876	631
Alabama	2	1	92	6
Alaska	0	0	12	10
American Samoa	0	0	0	1
Arizona	3	1	60	14
Arkansas	0	3	71	3
California	10	3	280	46
Colorado	3	0	54	17
Connecticut	1	2	29	0
Delaware	0	0	7	0
District of Columbia	0	1	7	0
Florida	8	16	157	6
Georgia	3	1	129	11
Guam	0	0	1	0
Hawaii	1	0	13	5
Idaho	2	0	20	16
Illinois	1	10	168	5
Indiana	3	1	113	3
Iowa	3	0	97	18
Kansas	2	0	85	46
Kentucky	1	8	86	1
Louisiana	2	5	86	16
Maine	2	0	33	2
Maryland	0	6	40	1
Massachusetts	1	3	59	1
Michigan	6	10	108	11
Minnesota	1	1	86	43
Mississippi	0	6	77	13
Missouri	4	6	101	6
Montana	1	0	30	29
N. Mariana Islands	0	0	0	1
Nebraska	3	0	47	35
Nevada	0	0	30	5
New Hampshire	1	0	24	1
New Jersey	1	16	49	1
New Mexico	1	0	32	9
New York	0	22	156	5
North Carolina	6	2	97	8
North Dakota	1	0	24	19
Ohio	2	2	153	10
Oklahoma	2	3	87	25
Oregon	4	0	51	5
Pennsylvania	9	5	144	6
Puerto Rico	0	1	28	20
Rhode Island	0	2	9	1
South Carolina	6	2	53	2
South Dakota	0	0	29	26
Tennessee	3	6	102	4
Texas	11	3	308	52
Utah	3	0	22	17
Vermont	0	0	14	1
Virgin Islands	0	0	2	0
Virginia	1	5	76	2
Washington	2	1	64	21
West Virginia	0	5	45	4
Wisconsin	4	0	111	10
Wyoming	0	0	18	11

Note: (1) 30-day readmission rate is better (lower) than U.S. rate of 23.0%; (2) 30-day readmission rate is worse (higher) than U.S. rate of 23.0%; (3) 30-day readmission rate is about the same as U.S. rate of 23.0%; (4) The number of cases is too small to classify the hospital

Hospital Pneumonia Readmission Rates: State and National Summary

Area	Number of Hospitals			
	Better than U.S. National Rate[1]	Worse than U.S. National Rate[2]	No Different than U.S. National Rate[3]	Number of Cases Too Small[4]
U.S. and Territories	37	135	4285	376
Alabama	0	1	96	5
Alaska	0	0	15	6
American Samoa	0	0	1	0
Arizona	0	0	72	9
Arkansas	1	5	68	3
California	3	5	290	46
Colorado	1	0	62	12
Connecticut	0	1	31	0
Delaware	0	0	7	0
District of Columbia	0	0	8	0
Florida	5	8	170	5
Georgia	1	0	138	4
Guam	0	0	1	0
Hawaii	0	0	14	8
Idaho	0	0	33	7
Illinois	0	11	169	5
Indiana	2	1	115	2
Iowa	0	0	113	5
Kansas	1	0	118	13
Kentucky	1	8	87	0
Louisiana	1	3	95	13
Maine	0	0	36	1
Maryland	0	11	34	1
Massachusetts	0	2	62	1
Michigan	2	5	122	6
Minnesota	0	0	112	19
Mississippi	0	3	87	8
Missouri	2	3	107	6
Montana	2	0	40	20
N. Mariana Islands	0	0	1	0
Nebraska	0	0	77	9
Nevada	0	1	29	6
New Hampshire	0	0	26	0
New Jersey	1	2	63	2
New Mexico	0	0	39	3
New York	2	24	154	5
North Carolina	1	4	104	5
North Dakota	0	0	40	4
Ohio	1	11	149	6
Oklahoma	1	3	103	12
Oregon	1	1	55	3
Pennsylvania	1	3	157	4
Puerto Rico	0	1	26	23
Rhode Island	0	0	11	1
South Carolina	2	1	58	2
South Dakota	0	0	51	5
Tennessee	1	5	105	5
Texas	3	4	325	49
Utah	0	0	37	5
Vermont	0	0	15	0
Virgin Islands	0	0	2	0
Virginia	0	3	79	7
Washington	1	0	81	7
West Virginia	0	5	48	1
Wisconsin	0	0	120	5
Wyoming	0	0	27	2

Note: (1) 30-day readmission rate is better (lower) than U.S. rate of 17.6%; (2) 30-day readmission rate is worse (higher) than U.S. rate of 17.6%; (3) 30-day readmission rate is about the same as U.S. rate of 17.6%; (4) The number of cases is too small to classify the hospital

Hospital Readmission Rate After Hip/Knee Surgery: State and National Summary

Area	Number of Hospitals			
	Better than U.S. National Rate[1]	Worse than U.S. National Rate[2]	No Different than U.S. National Rate[3]	Number of Cases Too Small[4]
U.S. and Territories	51	38	2738	665
Alabama	0	0	52	9
Alaska	0	0	8	0
American Samoa	0	0	0	0
Arizona	1	0	48	7
Arkansas	1	1	28	7
California	8	1	199	90
Colorado	1	0	49	6
Connecticut	0	1	28	0
Delaware	0	0	5	1
District of Columbia	0	1	4	2
Florida	5	4	138	15
Georgia	2	0	77	15
Guam	0	0	0	0
Hawaii	0	0	8	6
Idaho	0	0	23	5
Illinois	1	4	110	24
Indiana	3	0	78	29
Iowa	1	0	47	17
Kansas	1	0	42	12
Kentucky	0	0	42	19
Louisiana	0	1	59	15
Maine	1	0	25	6
Maryland	0	3	40	2
Massachusetts	1	0	55	5
Michigan	1	1	96	18
Minnesota	0	0	67	16
Mississippi	0	0	29	7
Missouri	1	2	64	13
Montana	1	0	19	6
N. Mariana Islands	0	0	0	0
Nebraska	1	0	31	13
Nevada	0	0	23	2
New Hampshire	0	0	22	4
New Jersey	0	1	54	7
New Mexico	1	0	21	3
New York	3	0	119	30
North Carolina	1	0	82	6
North Dakota	1	0	7	1
Ohio	2	2	133	20
Oklahoma	1	1	45	19
Oregon	1	0	39	10
Pennsylvania	2	4	123	29
Puerto Rico	0	0	8	28
Rhode Island	0	0	9	1
South Carolina	0	1	40	13
South Dakota	0	0	17	1
Tennessee	2	2	53	19
Texas	3	5	204	51
Utah	0	0	26	6
Vermont	0	0	12	1
Virgin Islands	0	0	1	0
Virginia	3	2	55	9
Washington	0	0	53	9
West Virginia	0	0	26	6
Wisconsin	1	1	82	21
Wyoming	0	0	13	4

Note: (1) 30-day readmission rate is better (lower) than U.S. rate of 5.4%; (2) 30-day readmission rate is worse (higher) than U.S. rate of 5.4%; (3) 30-day readmission rate is about the same as U.S. rate of 5.4%; (4) The number of cases is too small to classify the hospital

Hospital Readmission Rate After Discharge From Hospital (Hospital-wide): State and National Summary

Area	Number of Hospitals			
	Better than U.S. National Rate[1]	Worse than U.S. National Rate[2]	No Different than U.S. National Rate[3]	Number of Cases Too Small[4]
U.S. and Territories	316	369	3966	158
Alabama	1	1	92	3
Alaska	1	0	20	1
American Samoa	0	0	1	0
Arizona	9	3	64	5
Arkansas	3	11	60	0
California	29	17	283	10
Colorado	9	0	63	3
Connecticut	2	4	25	0
Delaware	0	0	6	0
District of Columbia	0	3	4	0
Florida	13	23	143	2
Georgia	7	5	129	1
Guam	0	0	1	0
Hawaii	2	0	13	6
Idaho	6	0	32	2
Illinois	4	37	137	1
Indiana	14	4	104	2
Iowa	7	1	106	2
Kansas	7	0	125	6
Kentucky	2	20	72	0
Louisiana	6	8	102	9
Maine	3	0	32	1
Maryland	3	14	28	0
Massachusetts	5	13	46	0
Michigan	12	20	93	6
Minnesota	8	0	119	4
Mississippi	1	6	86	5
Missouri	4	6	100	2
Montana	3	0	50	8
N. Mariana Islands	0	0	0	1
Nebraska	6	0	79	4
Nevada	1	3	28	3
New Hampshire	1	0	25	0
New Jersey	2	21	41	0
New Mexico	2	0	38	2
New York	6	57	110	4
North Carolina	15	6	88	2
North Dakota	2	1	38	2
Ohio	6	17	141	7
Oklahoma	9	4	106	6
Oregon	8	0	48	2
Pennsylvania	11	17	134	7
Puerto Rico	0	1	47	4
Rhode Island	0	4	7	0
South Carolina	8	2	52	0
South Dakota	5	0	52	2
Tennessee	4	12	96	1
Texas	31	8	341	20
Utah	6	1	34	2
Vermont	1	0	13	0
Virgin Islands	0	0	2	0
Virginia	3	11	66	4
Washington	12	1	71	2
West Virginia	0	7	42	1
Wisconsin	15	0	107	1
Wyoming	1	0	24	2

Note: (1) 30-day readmission rate is better (lower) than U.S. rate of 16.0%; (2) 30-day readmission rate is worse (higher) than U.S. rate of 16.0%; (3) 30-day readmission rate is about the same as U.S. rate of 16.0%; (4) The number of cases is too small to classify the hospital

Appendix C: Surgical Complication Rates

What Do These Surgical Complication Measures Show?

This appendix shows how hospitals' surgical complication rates compare to the rate across the U.S. The categories are:

- A Wound That Splits Open After Surgery on the Abdomen or Pelvis
- Accidental Cuts and Tears From Medical Treatment
- Collapsed Lung Due to Medical Treatment
- Deaths Among Patients With Serious Treatable Complications After Surgery
- Rate of Complications for Hip/Knee Replacement Patients
- Serious Blood Clots After Surgery
- Serious Complications (see below for details)

This first part of this appendix shows hospitals with surgical complication rates that are lower (better) or higher (worse) than the national rate for all categories. Hospitals are shown to be better or worse than the U.S. national rate only if the data shows with 95% certainty, the difference between their surgical complication rates and the U.S. national rate is not due to chance.

The second part of this appendix contains state and national summaries with the following column headers:

- **Better Than U.S. National Rate.** Hospitals in the Better Than U.S. National Rate category have surgical complication rates that are lower than the U.S. National Rate, with 95% certainty that this difference is not due to chance.
- **Worse Than U.S. National Rate.** Hospitals in the Worse Than U.S. National Rate category have surgical complication rates that are higher than the U.S. National Rate, with 95% certainty that this difference is not due to chance.
- **No Different Than U.S. National Rate.** Many hospitals in the No Different Than U.S. National Rate category have surgical complication rates that are about the same as the U.S. National Rate. Other hospitals in this category have rates that are higher or lower than the U.S. National Rate, without 95% certainty that these differences are not due to chance.
- **Number of Cases Too Small.** The number of cases is too small to classify the hospital.

Serious Complications

Measures of serious complications are drawn from the Agency for Healthcare Research and Quality (AHRQ) Patient Safety Indicators (PSIs). The overall score for serious complications is based on how often adult patients had certain serious, but potentially preventable, complications related to medical or surgical inpatient hospital care. This composite or summary measure is based on the following measures:

- Collapsed lung that results from medical treatment (Iatrogenic pneumothorax, adult)
- Blood clots, in the lung or a large vein, after surgery (Postoperative Pulmonary Embolism or Deep Vein Thrombosis Rate)
- A wound that splits open after surgery (Postoperative wound dehiscence)
- Accidental cuts and tears (Accidental puncture or laceration)
- Pressure sores (Pressure ulcers)
- Infections from a large venous catheters (Central venous catheter-related blood stream infection rate)
- Broken hip from a fall after surgery (Postoperative hip fracture rate)
- Blood stream infection after surgery (Postoperative sepsis)

Which Patients are Included

The Serious Complications measure applies only to Medicare beneficiaries enrolled in Original Medicare (traditional fee-for-service (FFS) Medicare) who were discharged from a hospital that was paid through the inpatient prospective payment system (IPPS) after the beneficiary had an inpatient stay. Non-Medicare patients and beneficiaries enrolled in Medicare managed care plans are also excluded from the data.

Where the Information Comes From

The Centers for Medicare & Medicaid Services (CMS) calculates the indicators of patient safety data from the claims hospitals submit for Medicare beneficiaries enrolled in Original Medicare(traditional FFS Medicare). The rate for each PSI is calculated by dividing the actual number of outcomes at each hospital by the number of eligible discharges for that measure at each hospital, multiplied by 1,000. The composite value reported on Hospital Compare is the weighted averages of the component indicators. PSI data are only calculated for hospitals that are paid through the IPPS, which excludes Critical Access hospitals (CAHs), long-term care hospitals (LTCHs), Maryland waiver hospitals, cancer hospitals, children's inpatient facilities, rural health clinics, federally qualified health centers, inpatient psychiatric hospitals, inpatient rehabilitation facilities, Veterans Administration/ Department of Defense hospitals, and religious, non-medical health care institutions.

Risk Adjustment

The measures of serious complications reported are risk adjusted to account for differences in hospital patients' characteristics. In addition, the rates reported are "smoothed" to reflect the fact that measures for small hospitals are measured less accurately (i.e., are less reliable) than for larger hospitals.

Comparing Individual Hospital Rates to Benchmarks

For the composite measure, CMS assigns comparative performance categories. If the interval estimate includes and/or overlaps with the national composite value, the hospital's performance is in the "no different than U.S. national rate" category. If the entire interval estimate is below the national composite value, then the hospital is performing "better than U.S. national rate." If the entire interval estimate is above the national composite value, it is "worse than U.S. national rate."

Additional Information

For more detail on Serious Complications measures (AHRQ Patient Safety Indicators) visit the Agency for Healthcare Research and Quality (AHRQ) Patient Safety Indicator Resources Web site at www.qualityindicators.ahrq.gov.

Hospitals whose Surgical Complication Rate is Better (Lower) than the U.S. National Rate

Measure: A Wound That Splits Open After Surgery on the Abdomen or Pelvis

Hospital	City	State	Phone	Web Site
No hospitals met this criteria.				

Note: Table shows hospitals nationwide whose surgical complication rate is better (lower) than U.S. rate of 0.92%

Hospitals whose Surgical Complication Rate is Worse (Higher) than the U.S. National Rate

Measure: A Wound That Splits Open After Surgery on the Abdomen or Pelvis

Hospital	City	State	Phone	Web Site
Aurora Lakeland Medical Center	Elkhorn	Wisconsin	262-741-2000	www.aurorahealthcare.org/facilities
Banner Thunderbird Medical Center	Glendale	Arizona	602-588-5555	www.bannerhealth.com
Beaumont Health System	Royal Oak	Michigan	248-898-5000	www.beaumonthospitals.com
Bronson Methodist Hospital	Kalamazoo	Michigan	269-341-6000	www.bronsonhealth.com
Central Carolina Hospital	Sanford	North Carolina	919-774-2100	www.centralcarolinahosp.com
Cjw Medical Center	Richmond	Virginia	804-330-2001	www.hcavirginia.com
Eastern Idaho Regional Medical Center	Idaho Falls	Idaho	208-529-6111	www.eirmc.org
Erlanger Medical Center	Chattanooga	Tennessee	423-778-7000	www.erlanger.org
Exeter Hospital	Exeter	New Hampshire	603-778-7311	www.exeterhospital.com
Fairfield Medical Center	Lancaster	Ohio	740-687-8009	www.fmchealth.org
Florida Hospital Deland	Deland	Florida	386-943-4772	www.fhdeland.org
Florida Hospital Fish Memorial	Orange City	Florida	386-917-5000	www.fhfishmemorial.org
Frye Regional Medical Center	Hickory	North Carolina	828-322-6070	www.fryemedctr.com
Genesys Regional Medical Center - Health Park	Grand Blanc	Michigan	810-606-5000	www.genesys.org
Good Samaritan Hospital	San Jose	California	408-559-2011	www.goodsamsj.org
Health Alliance Hospital Broadway Campus	Kingston	New York	914-331-3131	www.kingstonregionalhealth.org
Inspira Medical Center Woodbury	Woodbury	New Jersey	856-845-0100	www.umhospital.org
Lake Cumberland Regional Hospital	Somerset	Kentucky	606-679-7441	www.lakecumberlandhospital.com
Lake Regional Health System	Osage Beach	Missouri	573-348-8000	www.lakeregional.com
Lakeland Hospital - Saint Joseph	Saint Joseph	Michigan	269-983-8300	www.lakelandhealth.org
Longmont United Hospital	Longmont	Colorado	303-651-5111	www.luhcares.org
Maine Medical Center	Portland	Maine	207-662-0111	www.mmc.org
Mayo Clinic Hospital Rochester	Rochester	Minnesota	507-255-5123	www.mayoclinic.org/saintmaryshospital
The Medical Center of Aurora	Aurora	Colorado	303-695-2600	www.auroramed.com
Medstar Washington Hospital Center	Washington	District of Columbia	202-877-7000	www.whcenter.org
Memorial Health Univ Medical Center	Savannah	Georgia	912-350-8000	www.memorialhealth.com
Mercy Saint Anne Hospital	Toledo	Ohio	419-407-2663	www.mercyweb.org
Miami Valley Hospital	Dayton	Ohio	937-208-8000	www.miamivalleyhospital.com
Mountainview Hospital	Las Vegas	Nevada	702-255-5065	www.mountainview-hospital.com
Norton Hospitals	Louisville	Kentucky	502-629-6560	www.nortonhealthcare.com
Pali Momi Medical Center	Aiea	Hawaii	808-486-6000	www.kapiolani.org
Pottstown Memorial Medical Center	Pottstown	Pennsylvania	610-327-7000	www.pmmctr.org
Robert Wood Johnson University Hospital at Rahway	Rahway	New Jersey	732-381-4200	www.rwjuhr.com/about/history.html
Southeast Georgia Health System - Brunswick Campus	Brunswick	Georgia	912-466-7000	www.sghs.org
Spring Valley Hospital Medical Center	Las Vegas	Nevada	702-853-3000	www.springvalleyhospital.com
Saint Joseph Regional Health Center	Bryan	Texas	979-776-3912	www.st-joseph.org/sjrhc
Saint Luke's Episcopal Hospital	Houston	Texas	832-355-1000	www.sleh.com
Touro Infirmary	New Orleans	Louisiana	504-897-7011	www.touro.com
University of Wisconsin Hospitals & Clinics Authority	Madison	Wisconsin	608-263-8991	www.uwhealth.org
UNM Hospital	Albuquerque	New Mexico	505-272-2111	www.hospitals.unm.edu/unmh
Wayne Memorial Hospital	Honesdale	Pennsylvania	570-253-8100	www.wmh.org

Note: Table shows hospitals nationwide whose surgical complication rate is worse (higher) than U.S. rate of 0.92%

Hospitals whose Surgical Complication Rate is Better (Lower) than the U.S. National Rate

Measure: Accidental Cuts and Tears From Medical Treatment

Hospital	City	State	Phone	Web Site
Advocate Christ Hospital & Medical Center	Oak Lawn	Illinois	708-684-8000	www.advocatehealth.com
Advocate Good Samaritan Hospital	Downers Grove	Illinois	630-275-5900	www.advocatehealth.com/gsam
Advocate Lutheran General Hospital	Park Ridge	Illinois	847-723-2210	www.advocatehealth.com
Arkansas Heart Hospital	Little Rock	Arkansas	501-219-7000	www.arheart.com
Asante Rogue Regional Medical Center	Medford	Oregon	541-789-7000	www.asante.org
Atlanticare Regional Medical Center	Atlantic City	New Jersey	609-441-8020	www.atlanticare.org/acmc/index.html
Aventura Hospital & Medical Center	Aventura	Florida	305-682-7000	www.aventurahospital.com
Baptist Beaumont Hospital	Beaumont	Texas	409-212-5012	www.mhbh.org
Baystate Medical Center	Springfield	Massachusetts	413-794-0000	www.baystatehealth.com
Bethesda Hospital East	Boynton Beach	Florida	561-737-7733	www.bethesdahealthcare.com
Cape Regional Medical Center	Cape May Ct House	New Jersey	609-463-2000	www.caperegional.com
Cedars - Sinai Medical Center	Los Angeles	California	310-423-5000	www.cedars-sinai.edu
Central Dupage Hospital	Winfield	Illinois	630-682-1600	www.cdh.org
Christiana Care Health Services	Newark	Delaware	302-733-1000	www.christianacare.org
Christus Spohn Hospital Corpus Christi	Corpus Christi	Texas	361-902-4103	www.christusspohn.org
Clear Lake Regional Medical Center	Webster	Texas	281-332-2511	www.clearlakermc.com
Community Medical Center	Toms River	New Jersey	732-557-8000	www.sbhcs.com
Delray Medical Center	Delray Beach	Florida	561-498-4440	www.delraymedicalctr.com
Duke University Hospital	Durham	North Carolina	919-684-8111	www.dukehealth.org
Englewood Hospital & Medical Center	Englewood	New Jersey	201-894-3000	www.englewoodhospital.com
Florida Hospital	Orlando	Florida	407-303-1976	www.floridahospital.com
Floyd Medical Center	Rome	Georgia	706-509-6900	www.floydmed.org
Glendale Adventist Medical Center	Glendale	California	818-409-8202	www.glendaleadventist.com
Good Samaritan Hospital Medical Center	West Islip	New York	631-376-3000	www.good-samaritan-hospital.org
Good Samaritan Medical Center	Brockton	Massachusetts	508-427-3000	www.goodsamaritanmedical.org
Indiana University Health	Indianapolis	Indiana	317-962-5900	www.iuhealth.org
Integris Baptist Medical Center	Oklahoma City	Oklahoma	405-951-8110	www.integris-health.com
Integris Southwest Medical Center	Oklahoma City	Oklahoma	405-636-7000	www.integris-health.com
Jackson - Madison County General Hospital	Jackson	Tennessee	731-541-5000	www.wth.org
Lakeland Regional Medical Center	Lakeland	Florida	863-687-1100	www.lrmc.com
Laredo Medical Center	Laredo	Texas	956-796-5000	www.laredomedical.com
Lovelace Medical Center	Albuquerque	New Mexico	505-727-8000	www.lovelace.com
Marietta Memorial Hospital	Marietta	Ohio	740-374-1400	www.mmhospital.org
Marion General Hospital	Marion	Ohio	740-383-8400	www.mariongeneral.com
Mayo Clinic	Jacksonville	Florida	904-953-2000	www.mayoclinic.org/jacksonville
Mayo Clinic Hospital	Phoenix	Arizona	480-342-2000	www.mayoclinic.org
Mayo Clinic Hospital Rochester	Rochester	Minnesota	507-255-5123	www.mayoclinic.org/saintmaryshospital
Mayo Clinic Methodist- Hospital	Rochester	Minnesota	507-266-7890	www.mayoclinic.org/methodisthospital
Mclaren Bay Region	Bay City	Michigan	989-894-3000	www.baymed.org
Memorial Healthcare System	Chattanooga	Tennessee	423-495-2525	www.memorial.org
Memorial Hermann Hospital System	Houston	Texas	713-448-6796	www.memorialhermann.org
Memorial Hermann Memorial City Medical Center	Houston	Texas	713-242-3000	www.mhhs.org
Memorial Hermann Texas Medical Center	Houston	Texas	713-704-3700	www.mhhs.org
Memorial Hospital	Belleville	Illinois	618-233-7750	www.memhosp.com
Memorial Regional Hospital	Hollywood	Florida	954-987-2000	www.memorialregional.com
Mercy Hospital Fairfield	Fairfield	Ohio	513-870-7197	www.e-mercy.com/mercy-hospital-fairfield.aspx
Methodist Hospital	San Antonio	Texas	210-575-4000	www.mh.sahealth.com
The Methodist Hospital	Houston	Texas	713-790-2221	www.methodisthealth.com
Methodist Willowbrook Hospital	Houston	Texas	281-477-1000	www.houstonmethodist.org/willowbrook-hospital
Mississippi Baptist Medical Center	Jackson	Mississippi	601-968-1000	www.mbmc.org
Munroe Regional Medical Center	Ocala	Florida	352-351-7200	www.munroeregional.com
North Florida Regional Medical Center	Gainesville	Florida	352-333-4100	www.nfrmc.com
Northwestern Memorial Hospital	Chicago	Illinois	312-926-2000	www.nmh.org
Ocala Regional Medical Center	Ocala	Florida	352-401-1000	www.ocalaregional.com
Our Lady of Lourdes Medical Center	Camden	New Jersey	856-757-3500	www.lourdesnet.org
Overlook Medical Center	Summit	New Jersey	908-522-2000	www.atlantichealth.org
Palos Community Hospital	Palos Heights	Illinois	708-923-4000	www.paloshospital.org
Presence Resurrection Medical Center	Chicago	Illinois	773-774-8000	www.reshealthcare.org
Presence Saint Joseph Medical Center	Joliet	Illinois	815-725-7133	www.provena.org/stjoes
Providence Little Co of Mary Medical Center Torrance	Torrance	California	310-540-7676	www.lcmhs.org
Providence Tarzana Medical Center	Tarzana	California	818-881-0800	www.encino-tarzana.com
Roper Hospital	Charleston	South Carolina	843-724-2800	www.ropersaintfrancis.com
Saint Thomas West Hospital	Nashville	Tennessee	615-222-2111	www.stthomas.org
Scripps Memorial Hospital La Jolla	La Jolla	California	858-626-4123	www.scrippshealth.org

Hospital	City	State	Phone	Web Site
Sentara Careplex Hospital	Hampton	Virginia	757-736-1000	www.sentara.com
Sentara Leigh Hospital	Norfolk	Virginia	757-261-6601	www.sentara.com
Sentara Norfolk General Hospital	Norfolk	Virginia	757-388-3000	www.sentara.com
Sentara Virginia Beach General Hospital	Virginia Beach	Virginia	757-395-8000	www.sentara.com
Shasta Regional Medical Center	Redding	California	530-244-5454	www.shastaregional.com
South Shore Hospital	South Weymouth	Massachusetts	781-340-8000	www.southshorehospital.org
Saint Francis Hospital	Columbus	Georgia	706-596-4020	www.wecareforlife.com
Saint Francis Hospital - Roslyn	Roslyn	New York	516-562-6000	www.stfrancisheartcenter.com
Saint John Medical Center	Tulsa	Oklahoma	918-744-3606	www.sjmc.org
Saint John's Riverside Hospital	Yonkers	New York	914-964-4444	www.riversidehealth.org
Saint Luke's Episcopal Hospital	Houston	Texas	832-355-1000	www.sleh.com
Saint Mary Medical Center	Langhorne	Pennsylvania	215-750-2003	www.stmaryhealthcare.org
Saint Mary Mercy Hospital	Livonia	Michigan	734-655-4800	www.stmarymercy.org
Saint Vincent Heart Center of Indiana	Indianapolis	Indiana	317-583-5000	www.theheartcenter.com
Staten Island University Hospital	Staten Island	New York	718-226-9000	www.siuh.edu
Sutter General Hospital	Sacramento	California	916-733-8999	www.suttermedicalcenter.org
Swedish Covenant Hospital	Chicago	Illinois	773-878-8200	www.swedishcovenant.org
Tennova Healthcare	Knoxville	Tennessee	865-545-8000	www.stmaryshealth.com
The Nebraska Medical Center	Omaha	Nebraska	402-552-2040	www.nebraskamed.com
Tuomey Healthcare System	Sumter	South Carolina	803-774-8900	www.tuomey.com
UF Health Shands Hospital	Gainesville	Florida	352-265-8000	www.shands.org
United Hospital Center	Bridgeport	West Virginia	681-342-1000	www.uhcwv.org
University of Kentucky Hospital	Lexington	Kentucky	859-323-5000	www.uhealthcare.uky.edu
University of Michigan Health System	Ann Arbor	Michigan	734-764-1505	www.med.umich.edu
Valley Hospital	Ridgewood	New Jersey	201-447-8000	www.valleyhealth.com
Vanderbilt University Hospital	Nashville	Tennessee	615-322-3454	www.mc.vanderbilt.edu
Virtua West Jersey Hospitals Berlin	Berlin	New Jersey	856-322-3200	www.virtua.org
Williamsport Regional Medical Center	Williamsport	Pennsylvania	570-321-1000	www.susquehannahealth.org
Winchester Medical Center	Winchester	Virginia	540-536-8000	www.valleyhealthlink.com
Winthrop - University Hospital	Mineola	New York	516-663-0333	www.winthrop.org

Note: Table shows hospitals nationwide whose surgical complication rate is better (lower) than U.S. rate of 1.83%

Hospitals whose Surgical Complication Rate is Worse (Higher) than the U.S. National Rate

Measure: Accidental Cuts and Tears From Medical Treatment

Hospital	City	State	Phone	Web Site
Adena Regional Medical Center	Chillicothe	Ohio	740-779-7500	www.adena.org
Adirondack Medical Center	Saranac Lake	New York	518-891-4141	www.amccares.org
Aiken Regional Medical Center	Aiken	South Carolina	803-641-5900	www.aikenregional.com
Alaska Native Medical Center	Anchorage	Alaska	907-563-2662	www.anmc.org
Appleton Medical Center	Appleton	Wisconsin	920-731-4101	www.thedacare.org
Atlanta Medical Center	Atlanta	Georgia	404-265-4000	www.atlantamedcenter.com
B R F Hospital Holdings	Shreveport	Louisiana	318-675-5000	www.lsumc.edu
Baptist Saint Anthony's Hospital	Amarillo	Texas	806-212-2000	www.bsahs.com
Barnes-Jewish Hospital	Saint Louis	Missouri	314-747-3000	www.barnesjewish.org
Baylor University Medical Center	Dallas	Texas	214-820-0111	www.baylorhealth.com
Beth Israel Deaconess Medical Center	Boston	Massachusetts	617-667-7000	www.bidmc.harvard.edu
Blessing Hospital	Quincy	Illinois	217-223-5811	www.blessinghealthsystem.org
Borgess Medical Center	Kalamazoo	Michigan	269-226-7000	www.borgess.com
Boston Medical Center Corporation	Boston	Massachusetts	617-638-8000	www.bmc.org
Bridgeport Hospital	Bridgeport	Connecticut	203-384-3000	www.bridgeporthospital.com
Carney Hospital	Boston	Massachusetts	617-506-2000	www.caritascarney.org
Caromont Regional Medical Center	Gastonia	North Carolina	704-834-4891	www.caromont.org
Catholic Medical Center	Manchester	New Hampshire	603-668-3545	www.catholicmedicalcenter.org
Centra Health	Lynchburg	Virginia	434-200-4789	www.centrahealth.com
Central Texas Medical Center	San Marcos	Texas	512-753-3690	www.ctmc.org
Centrastate Medical Center	Freehold	New Jersey	732-431-2000	www.centrastate.com
Cheshire Medical Center	Keene	New Hampshire	603-354-5400	www.cheshire-med.com
Chilton Medical Center	Pompton Plains	New Jersey	973-831-5000	www.chiltonmemorial.org
Clearview Regional Medical Center	Monroe	Georgia	770-267-1792	www.clearviewregionalmedicalcenter.com
Cleveland Clinic	Cleveland	Ohio	216-444-2200	www.clevelandclinic.org
Clovis Community Medical Center	Clovis	California	559-324-4000	www.communitymedical.org
Community Regional Medical Center	Fresno	California	559-459-6000	www.communitymedical.org
Covenant Hospital Plainview	Plainview	Texas	806-296-5531	www.covenantplainview.org
Crestwood Medical Center	Huntsville	Alabama	256-882-3100	www.crestwoodmedcenter.com
Crossgates River Oaks Hospital	Brandon	Mississippi	601-825-2811	www.rankinmedcenter.com
Crouse Hospital	Syracuse	New York	315-470-7449	www.crouse.org
Dameron Hospital	Stockton	California	209-944-5550	www.dameronhospital.org
Deaconess Hospital	Spokane	Washington	509-473-5800	www.deaconessmedicalcenter.org
Deaconess Hospital	Evansville	Indiana	812-450-5000	www.deaconess.com
Desert Regional Medical Center	Palm Springs	California	760-323-6511	www.desertmedctr.com
Eisenhower Medical Center	Rancho Mirage	California	760-340-3911	www.emc.org
El Camino Hospital	Mountain View	California	650-940-7000	www.elcaminohospital.org
Eliza Coffee Memorial Hospital	Florence	Alabama	256-768-8400	www.chgroup.org
Emory University Hospital Midtown	Atlanta	Georgia	404-686-4411	www.emoryhealthcare.org
Faith Regional Health Services	Norfolk	Nebraska	402-371-4880	www.frhs.org
Firsthealth Moore Regional Hospital	Pinehurst	North Carolina	910-715-1000	www.firsthealth.org
Geisinger Medical Center	Danville	Pennsylvania	570-271-6211	www.geisinger.org
Geisinger Wyoming Valley Medical Center	Wilkes Barre	Pennsylvania	570-826-7300	www.geisinger.org
Gila Regional Medical Center	Silver City	New Mexico	575-538-4000	www.grmc.org
Good Samaritan Hospital	San Jose	California	408-559-2011	www.goodsamsj.org
Good Samaritan Hospital	Dayton	Ohio	937-278-2612	www.goodsamdayton.org
Good Shepherd Medical Center Marshall	Marshall	Texas	903-927-6712	www.marshallregional.org
Grady Memorial Hospital	Atlanta	Georgia	404-616-4252	www.gradyhealthsystem.org
Grinnell Regional Medical Center	Grinnell	Iowa	641-236-7511	www.grmc.us
Grossmont Hospital	La Mesa	California	619-465-0711	www.sharp.com
Harborview Medical Center	Seattle	Washington	206-731-3000	www.harborview.org
Hennepin County Medical Center	Minneapolis	Minnesota	612-873-3000	www.hcmc.org
Henrico Doctors' Hospital	Richmond	Virginia	804-289-4500	www.henricodoctors.com
Heritage Valley Beaver	Beaver	Pennsylvania	412-728-7000	www.heritagevalley.org
The Indiana Heart Hospital	Indianapolis	Indiana	317-621-8063	www.hearthospital.com
Inspira Medical Center Vineland	Vineland	New Jersey	856-641-6610	www.sjhs.com
Intermountain Medical Center	Murray	Utah	801-507-7000	www.intermountainhealthcare.org
Jewish Hospital & Saint Mary's Healthcare	Louisville	Kentucky	502-587-4011	www.jhhs.org
John Dempsey Hospital	Farmington	Connecticut	860-679-1145	www.uconnhealth.orgorwww.uchc.edu
JPS Health Network	Fort Worth	Texas	817-921-3431	www.jpshealthnet.org
Jupiter Medical Center	Jupiter	Florida	561-747-2234	www.jupitermed.com
Kadlec Regional Medical Center	Richland	Washington	509-946-4611	www.kadlecmed.org
Kaiser Foundation Hospital - Fontana	Fontana	California	909-427-5500	www.kaiserpermanente.com
Kaweah Delta Medical Center	Visalia	California	559-624-2000	www.kaweahdelta.org

Hospital	City	State	Phone	Web Site
Keck Hospital of USC	Los Angeles	California	323-442-8656	www.uscuh.com
Kingman Regional Medical Center	Kingman	Arizona	928-757-2101	www.azkrmc.com
Kuakini Medical Center	Honolulu	Hawaii	808-536-2236	www.kuakini.org
LDS Hospital	Salt Lake City	Utah	801-408-1100	www.intermountainhealthcare.org
Lourdes Hospital	Paducah	Kentucky	270-444-2444	www.ehealthconnection.com
Magee Womens Hospital of UPMC Health System	Pittsburgh	Pennsylvania	412-641-4010	www.magee.edu
Maine Medical Center	Portland	Maine	207-662-0111	www.mmc.org
Manchester Memorial Hospital	Manchester	Connecticut	860-647-4780	www.echn.org
Marin General Hospital	Greenbrae	California	415-925-7900	www.maringeneral.com
Mary Hitchcock Memorial Hospital	Lebanon	New Hampshire	603-650-5000	www.dhmc.org
Mat-Su Regional Medical Center	Palmer	Alaska	907-746-8600	www.matsuregional.com
Mayo Clinic Health System - Mankato	Mankato	Minnesota	507-625-4031	www.isj-mhs.org
Mayo Clinic Health System - Eau Claire Hospital	Eau Claire	Wisconsin	715-838-3311	www.luthermidelfort.org
McKay Dee Hospital	Ogden	Utah	801-387-2800	www.intermountainhealthcare.org
Medical College of Virginia Hospitals	Richmond	Virginia	804-828-0938	www.vcuhealth.org
Medical West	Bessemer	Alabama	205-481-7000	www.uab.edu
Medstar Washington Hospital Center	Washington	District of Columbia	202-877-7000	www.whcenter.org
Memorial Medical Center	Modesto	California	209-526-4500	www.memorialmedicalcenter.org
Memorial Health Univ Medical Center	Savannah	Georgia	912-350-8000	www.memorialhealth.com
Memorial Hospital	York	Pennsylvania	717-843-8623	www.mhyork.org
Memorial Hospital & Health Care Center	Jasper	Indiana	812-996-2345	www.mhhcc.org
Memorial Hospital of Carbondale	Carbondale	Illinois	618-549-0721	www.sih.net
Memorial Medical Center	Springfield	Illinois	217-788-3000	www.memorialmedical.com
Mercy General Hospital	Sacramento	California	916-453-4545	www.mercygeneral.org
Mercy Health Hackley Campus	Muskegon	Michigan	231-726-3511	www.hackley.org
Mercy Hospital - Cadillac	Cadillac	Michigan	231-876-7200	www.mercycadillac.munsonhealthcare.org
Mercy Medical Center - Des Moines	Des Moines	Iowa	515-247-3121	www.mercydesmoines.org
Mercy Memorial Health Center	Ardmore	Oklahoma	405-223-5400	www.mercyok.com/mmhc
Methodist Hospital of Sacramento	Sacramento	California	916-423-6010	www.methodistsacramento.org
Methodist Jennie Edmundson	Council Bluffs	Iowa	712-396-6000	www.bestcare.org
Metro Health Hospital	Wyoming	Michigan	616-252-7200	www.metrohealth.net
Metrohealth System	Cleveland	Ohio	216-778-7089	www.metrohealth.org
Miami Valley Hospital	Dayton	Ohio	937-208-8000	www.miamivalleyhospital.com
Milton S Hershey Medical Center	Hershey	Pennsylvania	717-531-8521	www.hmc.psu.edu
Montrose Memorial Hospital	Montrose	Colorado	970-249-2211	www.montrosehospital.com
Morton Plant Hospital	Clearwater	Florida	727-462-7000	www.measehospitals.com
Mount Sinai Hospital	New York	New York	212-241-7981	www.mountsinai.org
Muhlenberg Community Hospital	Greenville	Kentucky	270-338-8000	www.mchky.org
Multicare Good Samaritan Hospital	Puyallup	Washington	253-697-2102	www.multicare.org/goodsam
Musc Medical Center	Charleston	South Carolina	843-792-2300	www.musc.edu
Nash General Hospital	Rocky Mount	North Carolina	252-443-8000	www.nhcs.org
New Hanover Regional Medical Center	Wilmington	North Carolina	910-343-7000	www.nhrmc.org
Newport Hospital	Newport	Rhode Island	401-846-6400	www.newporthospital.org
Northwest Medical Center	Tucson	Arizona	520-742-9000	www.northwestmedicalcenter.com
Novant Health Presbyterian Medical Center	Charlotte	North Carolina	704-384-4000	www.presbyterian.org
O U Medical Center	Oklahoma City	Oklahoma	405-271-5911	www.oumedcenter.com
OHSU Hospital & Clinics	Portland	Oregon	503-494-4036	www.ohsu.edu
Oklahoma State University Medical Center	Tulsa	Oklahoma	918-587-2561	www.tulsaregional.com
Our Lady of the Lake Regional Medical Center	Baton Rouge	Louisiana	225-765-6565	www.ololrmc.com
Overland Park Regional Medical Center	Overland Park	Kansas	913-541-5301	www.oprmc.com
Parkview Medical Center	Pueblo	Colorado	719-584-4000	www.parkviewmc.com
Peacehealth Saint Joseph Medical Center	Bellingham	Washington	360-734-5400	www.peacehealth.org
Phelps County Regional Medical Center	Rolla	Missouri	573-458-8899	www.rollanet.org/~pcrmc
Physicians Regional Medical Center - Pine Ridge	Naples	Florida	239-348-4000	www.physiciansregional.com
Pinnacle Health Hospitals	Harrisburg	Pennsylvania	717-782-5181	www.pinnaclehealth.org
Providence Holy Cross Medical Center	Mission Hills	California	818-365-8051	www.providence.org
Providence Sacred Heart Medical Center	Spokane	Washington	509-474-3040	www.shmc.org
Rhode Island Hospital	Providence	Rhode Island	401-444-4000	www.rhodeislandhospital.org
Ridgeview Medical Center	Waconia	Minnesota	952-442-2191	www.ridgeviewmedical.org
Riverview Hospital Assoc	Wisconsin Rapids	Wisconsin	715-423-6060	www.riverviewhospital.net
Ronald Reagan UCLA Medical Center	Los Angeles	California	310-825-6301	www.uclahealth.org
Rush University Medical Center	Chicago	Illinois	312-942-5000	www.ruch.edu
Russellville Hospital	Russellville	Alabama	256-332-1611	www.russellvillehospital.com
Sacred Heart Hospital	Eau Claire	Wisconsin	715-717-4121	www.sacredhearteauclaire.org
Saint Anthony Medical Center	Rockford	Illinois	815-226-2000	www.osfhealth.com
Saint Francis Medical Center	Peoria	Illinois	309-655-2000	www.osfsaintfrancis.org
Saint Joseph's Hospital of Atlanta	Atlanta	Georgia	678-843-5720	www.stjosephsatlanta.org

Hospital	City	State	Phone	Web Site
Saint Mary's Health Care	Grand Rapids	Michigan	616-685-5000	www.smhealthcare.org
Saint Mary's Regional Medical Center	Reno	Nevada	775-770-3000	www.saintmarysreno.com
Salem Hospital	Salem	Oregon	503-561-5200	www.salemhospital.org
Salina Regional Health Center	Salina	Kansas	785-452-7000	www.srhc.com
Sanford Usd Medical Center	Sioux Falls	South Dakota	605-333-1000	www.sanfordhealth.org
Santiam Memorial Hospital	Stayton	Oregon	503-769-2175	www.santiamhospital.com
Sarasota Memorial Hospital	Sarasota	Florida	941-917-9000	www.smh.com
Seton Medical Center Austin	Austin	Texas	512-324-1000	www.seton.net
Sharp Memorial Hospital	San Diego	California	858-939-3400	www.sharp.com/memorial
Sky Ridge Medical Center	Lone Tree	Colorado	720-225-1000	www.skyridgemedcenter.com
Slidell Memorial Hospital	Slidell	Louisiana	985-643-2200	www.sliddelmemorial.org
Southeast Alabama Medical Center	Dothan	Alabama	334-793-8701	www.samc.org
Southwestern Vermont Medical Center	Bennington	Vermont	802-442-6361	www.svhealthcare.org
Spectrum Health - Butterworth Campus	Grand Rapids	Michigan	616-391-1774	www.spectrum-health.org
Springhill Medical Center	Mobile	Alabama	251-344-9630	www.springhillmedicalcenter.com
Saint Elizabeth Health Center	Youngstown	Ohio	330-746-7211	www.hmhs.org
Saint Elizabeth Medical Center	Utica	New York	315-798-8100	www.stemc.org
Saint Francis Health Center	Topeka	Kansas	785-295-8000	www.stfrancistopeka.org
Saint Francis - Downtown	Greenville	South Carolina	864-255-1000	www.stfrancishealth.org
Saint Helena Hospital	Saint Helena	California	707-963-3611	www.sthelenahospital.org
Saint Joseph Medical Center	Tacoma	Washington	253-627-4101	www.fhshealth.org
Saint Joseph Mercy Hospital	Ann Arbor	Michigan	734-712-3791	www.stjoesannarbor.or
Saint Joseph's Hospital & Medical Center	Phoenix	Arizona	602-406-3000	www.stjosephs-phx.org
Saint Louis University Hospital	Saint Louis	Missouri	314-577-8000	www.slucare.edu/clinical
Saint Luke's Hospital Bethlehem	Bethlehem	Pennsylvania	610-954-4000	www.slhn-lehighvalley.org
Saint Luke's Hospital	Chesterfield	Missouri	314-434-1500	www.goodhealthmatters.com
Saint Luke's Hospital of Kansas City	Kansas City	Missouri	816-932-2000	www.staintlukeshealthsystem.org
Saint Marys Hospital	Madison	Wisconsin	608-251-6100	www.stmarysmadison.com
Stanford Hospital	Stanford	California	650-723-5708	www.stanfordhospital.com
Swedish Medical Center	Seattle	Washington	206-386-6000	www.swedish.org
Swedish Medical Center - Cherry Hill	Seattle	Washington	206-320-2000	www.swedish.org
Tacoma General Allenmore Hospital	Tacoma	Washington	253-403-1000	www.multicare.org
Tampa General Hospital	Tampa	Florida	813-844-7000	www.tgh.org
Heart Hospital Baylor Plano	Plano	Texas	469-814-3278	www.thehearthospitalbaylor.com
Theda Clark Medical Center	Neenah	Wisconsin	920-729-3100	www.thedacare.org
Thomas Hospital	Fairhope	Alabama	251-928-2375	www.thomashospital.com
Town & Country Hospital	Tampa	Florida	813-882-7159	www.townandcountryhospital.com
Trinity Hospitals	Minot	North Dakota	701-857-5000	www.trinityhealth.org
Trinity Medical Center	Birmingham	Alabama	205-592-1000	www.bhsala.com/montclair
Trinity Rock Island	Rock Island	Illinois	309-779-5000	www.trinityqc.com
Trumbull Memorial Hospital	Warren	Ohio	330-841-9011	www.trumhosp.org
Tulane Medical Center	New Orleans	Louisiana	504-988-1900	www.tuhc.com
UF Health Jacksonville	Jacksonville	Florida	904-244-0411	www.shandsjacksonville.org
UMC of Southern Nevada	Las Vegas	Nevada	702-383-2000	www.umc-cares.org
University Colo Health Memorial Hospital Central	Colorado Springs	Colorado	719-365-5000	www.memorialhospital.com
University Health Care/University Hospitals & Clinics	Salt Lake City	Utah	801-581-2121	www.healthcare.utah.edu
University Health System	San Antonio	Texas	210-358-4000	www.universityhealthsystem.com
University of California Davis Medical Center	Sacramento	California	916-734-2011	www.ucdmc.ucdavis.edu
University of Cincinnati Medical Center	Cincinnati	Ohio	513-584-1000	www.universityhospitalcincinnati.com
University of Colorado Hospital	Aurora	Colorado	720-848-0000	www.uch.edu
University of Kansas Hospital	Kansas City	Kansas	913-588-7332	www.kumc.edu
University of Miami Hospital	Miami	Florida	305-325-5511	www.cedarsmedicalcenter.com
University of Minnesota Medical Center - Fairview	Minneapolis	Minnesota	612-273-3000	www.uofmmedicalcenter.org
University of Toledo Medical Center	Toledo	Ohio	419-383-3407	www.utmc.utoledo.edu
University of Wisconsin Hospitals & Clinics Authority	Madison	Wisconsin	608-263-8991	www.uwhealth.org
UPMC Hamot	Erie	Pennsylvania	814-877-6000	www.hamot.org
UPMC Passavant	Pittsburgh	Pennsylvania	412-367-6700	www.passavant.upmc.com
UPMC Presbyterian Shadyside	Pittsburgh	Pennsylvania	412-647-8788	www.upmc.edu
UT Southwestern University Hospital	Dallas	Texas	214-879-3758	www.utsouthwestern.edu
Utah Valley Regional Medical Center	Provo	Utah	801-373-7850	www.intermountainhealthcare.org/hospitals/uvrmc
Ventura County Medical Center	Ventura	California	805-652-6075	www.vchca.org
Vidant Medical Center	Greenville	North Carolina	252-847-4100	www.uhseast.com
Virginia Mason Medical Center	Seattle	Washington	206-223-6600	www.vmmc.org
Waukesha Memorial Hospital	Waukesha	Wisconsin	262-928-1000	www.waukeshamemorial.org
Wesley Medical Center	Hattiesburg	Mississippi	601-268-8000	www.wesley.com
West Virginia University Hospitals	Morgantown	West Virginia	304-598-4000	www.wvuh.com
Wheaton Franciscan Saint Joseph	Milwaukee	Wisconsin	414-447-2000	www.wfhealthcare.org

Hospital	City	State	Phone	Web Site
Winchester Hospital	Winchester	Massachusetts	781-729-9000	www.winchesterhospital.org
Women & Infants Hospital of Rhode Island	Providence	Rhode Island	401-274-1100	www.womenandinfants.com
The Women's Hospital	Newburgh	Indiana	812-842-4200	www.deaconess.com
Yavapai Regional Medical Center	Prescott	Arizona	928-771-5676	www.yrmc.org

Note: Table shows hospitals nationwide whose surgical complication rate is worse (higher) than U.S. rate of 1.83%

Hospitals whose Surgical Complication Rate is Better (Lower) than the U.S. National Rate

Measure: Collapsed Lung Due to Medical Treatment

Hospital	City	State	Phone	Web Site
Centinela Hospital Medical Center	Inglewood	California	310-673-4660	www.centinelafreeman.com
Centra Health	Lynchburg	Virginia	434-200-4789	www.centrahealth.com
Community Medical Center	Toms River	New Jersey	732-557-8000	www.sbhcs.com
Evanston Hospital	Evanston	Illinois	847-432-8000	www.enh.org
New York - Presbyterian Hospital	New York	New York	212-746-4189	www.nyp.org
Norton Hospitals	Louisville	Kentucky	502-629-6560	www.nortonhealthcare.com
Spectrum Health - Butterworth Campus	Grand Rapids	Michigan	616-391-1774	www.spectrum-health.org
Virtua West Jersey Hospitals Berlin	Berlin	New Jersey	856-322-3200	www.virtua.org
Willis Knighton Medical Center	Shreveport	Louisiana	318-212-4000	www.wkhs.com//locations/medicalcenter.aspx

Note: Table shows hospitals nationwide whose surgical complication rate is better (lower) than U.S. rate of 0.32%

Hospitals whose Surgical Complication Rate is Worse (Higher) than the U.S. National Rate

Measure: Collapsed Lung Due to Medical Treatment

Hospital	City	State	Phone	Web Site
Abilene Regional Medical Center	Abilene	Texas	325-428-1000	www.abileneregional.com
Banner Heart Hospital	Mesa	Arizona	480-854-5050	www.bannerhealth.com
Baylor Medical Center at Garland	Garland	Texas	972-487-5000	www.baylorhealth.com
Baylor Regional Medical Center at Grapevine	Grapevine	Texas	817-481-1588	www.baylorhealth.com
Bert Fish Medical Center	New Smyrna Beach	Florida	386-424-5000	www.bertfish.com
Beth Israel Deaconess Medical Center	Boston	Massachusetts	617-667-7000	www.bidmc.harvard.edu
Bryan Medical Center	Lincoln	Nebraska	402-481-1111	www.bryan.org
Capital Region Medical Center	Jefferson City	Missouri	573-632-5000	www.crmc.org
Carolinas Medical Center - Union	Monroe	North Carolina	704-283-3100	www.carolinashealthcare.org/cmc-union
Champlain Valley Physicians Hospital Medical Center	Plattsburgh	New York	518-561-2000	www.cvph.org
Community Regional Medical Center	Fresno	California	559-459-6000	www.communitymedical.org
Des Peres Hospital	Saint Louis	Missouri	314-966-9100	www.desperes hospital.com
Feather River Hospital	Paradise	California	530-877-9361	www.frhosp.org
Florida Hospital	Orlando	Florida	407-303-1976	www.floridahospital.com
Hays Medical Center	Hays	Kansas	785-623-5000	www.haysmed.com
Inova Fairfax Hospital	Falls Church	Virginia	703-776-3332	www.inova.org
Kansas Medical Center	Andover	Kansas	316-300-4000	www.ksmedcenter.com
Largo Medical Center	Largo	Florida	727-588-5200	www.largomedical.com
Lawrence Memorial Hospital	Lawrence	Kansas	785-505-6100	www.lmh.org
Loma Linda University Medical Center	Loma Linda	California	909-558-4000	www.llumc.edu
Madera Community Hospital	Madera	California	559-675-5555	www.maderahospital.org
Maine Medical Center	Portland	Maine	207-662-0111	www.mmc.org
Massachusetts General Hospital	Boston	Massachusetts	617-726-2000	www.massgeneral.org
Mclaren - Northern Michigan	Petoskey	Michigan	231-487-4000	www.northernhealth.org
Medical West	Bessemer	Alabama	205-481-7000	www.uab.edu
Midmichigan Medical Center - Midland	Midland	Michigan	989-839-3000	www.midmichigan.org
Mills - Peninsula Medical Center	Burlingame	California	650-696-5270	www.mills-peninsula.org
Norman Regional Health System	Norman	Oklahoma	405-321-1700	www.normanregional.com
Northwest Texas Hospital	Amarillo	Texas	806-354-1110	www.nxtexashealthcare.com
NYU Hospitals Center	New York	New York	212-263-7300	www.med.nyu.edu
Orange Regional Medical Center	Middletown	New York	845-343-2424	www.ormc.org
Orlando Health	Orlando	Florida	321-841-5111	www.orlandoregionalmedicalcenter.org
Parkridge Medical Center	Chattanooga	Tennessee	423-894-4220	www.tristarhealth.com
Piedmont Hospital	Atlanta	Georgia	404-605-5000	www.piedmonthospital.org
Pikeville Medical Center	Pikeville	Kentucky	606-218-3500	www.pikevillehospital.org
Providence Health Center	Waco	Texas	254-751-4000	www.providence.net
Providence Saint Vincent Medical Center	Portland	Oregon	503-216-1234	www.providence.org
Ronald Reagan UCLA Medical Center	Los Angeles	California	310-825-6301	www.uclahealth.org
Saint Francis Medical Center	Peoria	Illinois	309-655-2000	www.osfsaintfrancis.org
Saint Joseph Hospital	Lexington	Kentucky	859-313-1000	www.sjhlex.org
Saint Joseph's Hospital of Atlanta	Atlanta	Georgia	678-843-5720	www.stjosephsatlanta.org
Sanford Medical Center Fargo	Fargo	North Dakota	701-234-2000	www.meritcare.com
Self Regional Healthcare	Greenwood	South Carolina	864-227-4111	www.selfregional.org
Sentara Norfolk General Hospital	Norfolk	Virginia	757-388-3000	www.sentara.com
Sharp Memorial Hospital	San Diego	California	858-939-3400	www.sharp.com/memorial
Silver Cross Hospital & Medical Centers	New Lenox	Illinois	815-300-1100	www.silvercross.org
SSM Depaul Health Center	Bridgeton	Missouri	314-344-6000	www.ssmdepaul.com
Saint Bernards Medical Center	Jonesboro	Arkansas	870-972-4100	www.sbrmc.com
Saint John Medical Center	Tulsa	Oklahoma	918-744-3606	www.sjmc.org
Saint John's Episcopal Hospital at South Shore	Far Rockaway	New York	718-869-7000	www.ehs.org
Saint Luke's Hospital of Kansas City	Kansas City	Missouri	816-932-2000	www.staintlukeshealthsystem.org
Saint Tammany Parish Hospital	Covington	Louisiana	985-898-4000	www.stph.org
Sturdy Memorial Hospital	Attleboro	Massachusetts	508-222-5200	www.sturdymemorial.org
Theda Clark Medical Center	Neenah	Wisconsin	920-729-3100	www.thedacare.org
UMC of Southern Nevada	Las Vegas	Nevada	702-383-2000	www.umc-cares.org
University Medical Center of El Paso	El Paso	Texas	915-521-7602	www.thomasoncares.org
University of Alabama Hospital	Birmingham	Alabama	205-934-4011	www.health.uab.edu
University of Toledo Medical Center	Toledo	Ohio	419-383-3407	www.utmc.utoledo.edu
UPMC Presbyterian Shadyside	Pittsburgh	Pennsylvania	412-647-8788	www.upmc.edu
Williamsport Regional Medical Center	Williamsport	Pennsylvania	570-321-1000	www.susquehannahealth.org

Note: Table shows hospitals nationwide whose surgical complication rate is worse (higher) than U.S. rate of 0.32%

Hospitals whose Surgical Complication Rate is Better (Lower) than the U.S. National Rate

Measure: Deaths Among Patients With Serious Treatable Complications After Surgery

Hospital	City	State	Phone	Web Site
Advocate Lutheran General Hospital	Park Ridge	Illinois	847-723-2210	www.advocatehealth.com
Alexian Brothers Medical Center	Elk Grove Village	Illinois	847-437-5500	www.alexian.org
Aurora West Allis Medical Center	West Allis	Wisconsin	414-328-6000	www.aurorahealthcare.org
Banner Thunderbird Medical Center	Glendale	Arizona	602-588-5555	www.bannerhealth.com
Baptist Saint Anthony's Hospital	Amarillo	Texas	806-212-2000	www.bsahs.com
Bayfront Health Punta Gorda	Punta Gorda	Florida	941-639-3131	www.charlotteregional.com
Delray Medical Center	Delray Beach	Florida	561-498-4440	www.delraymedicalctr.com
Emory University Hospital	Atlanta	Georgia	404-686-8500	www.emoryhealthcare.org
Evanston Hospital	Evanston	Illinois	847-432-8000	www.enh.org
Fawcett Memorial Hospital	Port Charlotte	Florida	941-629-1181	www.fawcetthospital.com
Franciscan Saint Francis Health - Indianapolis	Indianapolis	Indiana	317-865-5001	www.stfrancishospitals.org
Gwinnett Medical Center	Lawrenceville	Georgia	678-312-1000	www.gwinnettmedicalcenter.org
Hackensack University Medical Center	Hackensack	New Jersey	201-996-2000	www.humed.com
Henry Ford Wyandotte Hospital	Wyandotte	Michigan	734-246-6000	www.henryfordwyandotte.com
Hinsdale Hospital	Hinsdale	Illinois	630-856-9000	www.keepingyouwell.com
Hospital For Special Surgery	New York	New York	212-606-1000	www.hss.edu
JFK Medical Center	Atlantis	Florida	561-965-7300	www.jfkmc.com
JFK Medical Center - A M Yelencsics Comm Hospital	Edison	New Jersey	732-321-7000	www.jfkmc.org
Los Robles Hospital & Medical Center	Thousand Oaks	California	805-497-2727	www.losrobleshospital.com
Martin Medical Center	Stuart	Florida	772-287-5200	www.mmhs.com
Mayo Clinic Hospital	Phoenix	Arizona	480-342-2000	www.mayoclinic.org
Mayo Clinic Methodist- Hospital	Rochester	Minnesota	507-266-7890	www.mayoclinic.org/methodisthospital
Mclaren Flint	Flint	Michigan	810-342-2000	www.mclaren.org
Memorial Hermann Memorial City Medical Center	Houston	Texas	713-242-3000	www.mhhs.org
Missouri Baptist Medical Center	Town & Country	Missouri	314-996-5000	www.missouribaptistmedicalcenter.org
Mother Frances Hospital	Tyler	Texas	903-593-8441	www.tmfhs.org
North Colorado Medical Center	Greeley	Colorado	970-352-4121	www.bannerhealth.com
North Kansas City Hospital	North Kansas City	Missouri	816-691-2000	www.nkch.org
Northwestern Memorial Hospital	Chicago	Illinois	312-926-2000	www.nmh.org
NYU Hospitals Center	New York	New York	212-263-7300	www.med.nyu.edu
OHSU Hospital & Clinics	Portland	Oregon	503-494-4036	www.ohsu.edu
Palm Beach Gardens Medical Center	Palm Beach Gardens	Florida	561-622-1411	www.pbgmc.com
Palos Community Hospital	Palos Heights	Illinois	708-923-4000	www.paloshospital.org
Providence Hospital & Medical Centers	Southfield	Michigan	248-849-3011	www.stjohn.org/providence
Saint Alexius Medical Center	Hoffman Estates	Illinois	847-843-2000	www.alexianbrothershealth.org
Saint Alexius Medical Center	Bismarck	North Dakota	701-530-7000	www.st.alexius.org
Saint David's Medical Center	Austin	Texas	512-476-7111	www.stdavidsrehab.com
Saint Elizabeth Health Center	Youngstown	Ohio	330-746-7211	www.hmhs.org
Saint John Macomb - Oakland Hospital - Macomb Center	Warren	Michigan	586-573-5000	www.stjohn.org
Saint Joseph's Hospital & Medical Center	Phoenix	Arizona	602-406-3000	www.stjosephs-phx.org
Saint Luke's Hospital	Cedar Rapids	Iowa	319-369-7211	www.crstlukes.com
Heart Hospital Baylor Plano	Plano	Texas	469-814-3278	www.thehearthospitalbaylor.com
University of Wisconsin Hospitals & Clinics Authority	Madison	Wisconsin	608-263-8991	www.uwhealth.org

Note: Table shows hospitals nationwide whose surgical complication rate is better (lower) than U.S. rate of 110.25%

Hospitals whose Surgical Complication Rate is Worse (Higher) than the U.S. National Rate

Measure: Deaths Among Patients With Serious Treatable Complications After Surgery

Hospital	City	State	Phone	Web Site
Baptist Health Medical Center - Little Rock	Little Rock	Arkansas	501-202-2000	www.baptist-health.com
Baptist Medical Center	San Antonio	Texas	210-297-1020	www.baptisthealthsystem.org
Carolinas Hospital System	Florence	South Carolina	843-674-2500	www.carolinashospital.com
Carolinas Medical Center/Behaviorial Health	Charlotte	North Carolina	704-355-2000	www.carolinasmedicalcenter.org
Christian Hospital Northeast - Northwest	Saint Louis	Missouri	314-653-5000	www.christianhospital.org
Christiana Care Health Services	Newark	Delaware	302-733-1000	www.christianacare.org
Community Regional Medical Center	Fresno	California	559-459-6000	www.communitymedical.org
Conway Medical Center	Conway	South Carolina	843-347-8037	www.conwayhospital.com
Cooper University Hospital	Camden	New Jersey	856-342-2000	www.cooperhealth.org
Cullman Regional Medical Center	Cullman	Alabama	256-737-2000	www.crmchospital.com
Doctors Hospital	Augusta	Georgia	706-651-6008	www.doctors-hospital.net
Doctors Medical Center	Modesto	California	209-578-1211	www.dmc-modesto.com
Duke University Hospital	Durham	North Carolina	919-684-8111	www.dukehealth.org
East Texas Medical Center	Tyler	Texas	903-597-0351	www.etmc.org
Erlanger Medical Center	Chattanooga	Tennessee	423-778-7000	www.erlanger.org
Fairbanks Memorial Hospital	Fairbanks	Alaska	907-452-8181	www.bannerhealth.com
Fletcher Allen Hospital of Vermont	Burlington	Vermont	802-847-0000	www.fletcherallen.org
Florida Hospital Tampa	Tampa	Florida	813-615-7200	www.uch.org
Good Samaritan Hospital Medical Center	West Islip	New York	631-376-3000	www.good-samaritan-hospital.org
Halifax Health Medical Center	Daytona Beach	Florida	386-254-4000	www.halifax.org
Health Alliance Hospital Broadway Campus	Kingston	New York	914-331-3131	www.kingstonregionalhealth.org
Hillcrest Medical Center	Tulsa	Oklahoma	918-579-1000	www.hillcrest.com
Integris Baptist Medical Center	Oklahoma City	Oklahoma	405-951-8110	www.integris-health.com
Jewish Hospital & Saint Mary's Healthcare	Louisville	Kentucky	502-587-4011	www.jhhs.org
Kaleida Health	Buffalo	New York	716-859-8620	www.kaleidahealth.org
Lake Cumberland Regional Hospital	Somerset	Kentucky	606-679-7441	www.lakecumberlandhospital.com
Lakeland Regional Medical Center	Lakeland	Florida	863-687-1100	www.lrmc.com
Magnolia Regional Health Center	Corinth	Mississippi	662-293-7660	www.mrhc.org
Marian Regional Medical Center	Santa Maria	California	805-739-3000	www.marinmedicalcenter.org
Mary Hitchcock Memorial Hospital	Lebanon	New Hampshire	603-650-5000	www.dhmc.org
Medical Center of Central Georgia	Macon	Georgia	478-633-6805	www.mccg.org
Medical Center of Plano	Plano	Texas	972-596-6800	www.medicalcenterofplano.com
Medical College of Georgia Hospitals & Clinics	Augusta	Georgia	706-721-6569	www.mcghealth.org
Methodist Healthcare Memphis Hospitals	Memphis	Tennessee	901-516-8274	www.methodisthealth.org
Milton S Hershey Medical Center	Hershey	Pennsylvania	717-531-8521	www.hmc.psu.edu
Mobile Infirmary	Mobile	Alabama	251-435-4700	www.mimc.com
Nazareth Hospital	Philadelphia	Pennsylvania	215-335-6000	www.nazarethhospital.org
North Carolina Baptist Hospital	Winston-Salem	North Carolina	336-716-2011	www.wfubmc.edu
North Mississippi Medical Center	Tupelo	Mississippi	662-377-3000	www.nmhs.net/nmmc
Northeast Alabama Regional Medical Center	Anniston	Alabama	256-235-5121	www.rmccares.org
Oklahoma State University Medical Center	Tulsa	Oklahoma	918-587-2561	www.tulsaregional.com
Phoebe Putney Memorial Hospital	Albany	Georgia	229-312-4068	www.phoebeputney.com
Renown Regional Medical Center	Reno	Nevada	775-982-4100	www.renown.org
Riverside Methodist Hospital	Columbus	Ohio	614-566-5000	www.ohiohealth.com
Robert Wood Johnson University Hospital	New Brunswick	New Jersey	732-937-8900	www.rwjuh.edu
Robert Wood Johnson University Hospital - Hamilton	Hamilton	New Jersey	609-586-7900	www.rwjhamilton.org
Saint Francis Medical Center	Peoria	Illinois	309-655-2000	www.osfsaintfrancis.org
Sentara Norfolk General Hospital	Norfolk	Virginia	757-388-3000	www.sentara.com
Saint John Medical Center	Tulsa	Oklahoma	918-744-3606	www.sjmc.org
Saint Joseph's Hospital - Savannah	Savannah	Georgia	912-819-4100	www.sjchs.org
Saint Luke's Episcopal Hospital	Houston	Texas	832-355-1000	www.sleh.com
Saint Mary's Medical Center	Huntington	West Virginia	304-526-1234	www.st-marys.org
Saint Vincent's East	Birmingham	Alabama	205-838-3122	www.nolandhealth.com
Strong Memorial Hospital	Rochester	New York	585-275-2121	www.urmc.rochester.edu
Sunrise Hospital & Medical Center	Las Vegas	Nevada	702-731-8000	www.sunrisehospital.com
Tampa General Hospital	Tampa	Florida	813-844-7000	www.tgh.org
Trident Medical Center	Charleston	South Carolina	843-797-8800	www.tridenthealthsystem.com
UF Health Shands Hospital	Gainesville	Florida	352-265-8000	www.shands.org
Umass Memorial Medical Center	Worcester	Massachusetts	508-334-1000	www.umassmemorial.org
University Hospital	Newark	New Jersey	973-972-5658	www.theuniversityhospital.com
University Medical Center	Lubbock	Texas	806-775-8200	www.teamumc.org
University of Alabama Hospital	Birmingham	Alabama	205-934-4011	www.health.uab.edu
University of Kentucky Hospital	Lexington	Kentucky	859-323-5000	www.uhealthcare.uky.edu
University of Mississippi Medical Center	Jackson	Mississippi	601-984-4100	www.umc.edu

Hospital	City	State	Phone	Web Site
University of South Alabama Medical Center	Mobile	Alabama	251-471-7110	www.southalabama.edu/usamc
Vidant Medical Center	Greenville	North Carolina	252-847-4100	www.uhseast.com
Virtua West Jersey Hospitals Berlin	Berlin	New Jersey	856-322-3200	www.virtua.org

Note: Table shows hospitals nationwide whose surgical complication rate is worse (higher) than U.S. rate of 110.25%

Hospitals whose Surgical Complication Rate is Better (Lower) than the U.S. National Rate

Measure: Rate of Complications for Hip/Knee Replacement Patients

Hospital	City	State	Phone	Web Site
Arkansas Surgical Hospital	No Little Rock	Arkansas	501-748-8000	www.arksurgicalhospital.com
Baptist Health Louisville	Louisville	Kentucky	502-897-8100	www.baptisteast.com
Barnes-Jewish Hospital	Saint Louis	Missouri	314-747-3000	www.barnesjewish.org
Beaumont Health System	Royal Oak	Michigan	248-898-5000	www.beaumonthospitals.com
Boone Hospital Center	Columbia	Missouri	573-815-8000	www.boone.org
Bronson Methodist Hospital	Kalamazoo	Michigan	269-341-6000	www.bronsonhealth.com
Cape Cod Hospital	Hyannis	Massachusetts	508-771-1800	www.capecodhealth.org
Carilion Roanoke Memorial Hospital	Roanoke	Virginia	540-981-7000	www.carilion.com/crmh
Covenant Medical Center	Lubbock	Texas	806-725-6000	www.covenanthealth.org
Crittenton Hospital Medical Center	Rochester	Michigan	248-652-5000	www.crittenton.com
Delray Medical Center	Delray Beach	Florida	561-498-4440	www.delraymedicalctr.com
Doctors Hospital at Renaissance	Edinburg	Texas	956-362-8677	www.dhr-rgv.com
Florida Hospital Memorial Medical Center	Daytona Beach	Florida	386-676-6000	www.fhmd.com
Franciscan Saint Elizabeth Health - Lafayette East	Lafayette	Indiana	765-502-4334	www.ste.org
Heart of Florida Regional Medical Center	Davenport	Florida	863-422-4971	www.heartofflorida.com
Heartland Regional Medical Center	Saint Joseph	Missouri	816-271-6000	www.heartland-health.com
Hoag Orthopedic Institute	Irvine	California	949-727-5000	www.orthopedichospital.com
Holy Cross Hospital	Fort Lauderdale	Florida	954-771-8000	www.holy-cross.com
Hospital For Special Surgery	New York	New York	212-606-1000	www.hss.edu
Indian River Medical Center	Vero Beach	Florida	772-567-4311	www.irmh.com
Indiana Orthopaedic Hospital	Indianapolis	Indiana	317-956-1000	www.indianaorthopaedichospital.com
Jupiter Medical Center	Jupiter	Florida	561-747-2234	www.jupitermed.com
Kansas Medical Center	Andover	Kansas	316-300-4000	www.ksmedcenter.com
Kansas Surgery & Recovery Center	Wichita	Kansas	316-634-0090	www.ksrc.org
Maine Medical Center	Portland	Maine	207-662-0111	www.mmc.org
Mayo Clinic Methodist- Hospital	Rochester	Minnesota	507-266-7890	www.mayoclinic.org/methodisthospital
Mclaren - Greater Lansing	Lansing	Michigan	517-975-6000	www.mclaren.org
Memorial Healthcare System	Chattanooga	Tennessee	423-495-2525	www.memorial.org
Memorial Mission Hospital & Asheville Surgery Center	Asheville	North Carolina	828-213-1111	www.missionhospitals.org
Mississippi Baptist Medical Center	Jackson	Mississippi	601-968-1000	www.mbmc.org
Nebraska Orthopaedic Hospital	Omaha	Nebraska	402-609-1600	www.neorthohospital.com
New England Baptist Hospital	Boston	Massachusetts	617-754-5800	www.nebh.caregroup.org
North Mississippi Medical Center	Tupelo	Mississippi	662-377-3000	www.nmhs.net/nmmc
Ocala Regional Medical Center	Ocala	Florida	352-401-1000	www.ocalaregional.com
Oklahoma Surgical Hospital	Tulsa	Oklahoma	918-477-5000	www.oklahomasurgicalhospital.com
Olathe Medical Center	Olathe	Kansas	913-791-4200	www.ohsi.com
Orthopaedic Hospital at Parkview North	Fort Wayne	Indiana	260-672-4050	www.parkview.com
Plaza Medical Center of Fort Worth	Fort Worth	Texas	817-336-2100	www.plazamedicalcenter.com
Poudre Valley Hospital	Fort Collins	Colorado	970-495-7000	www.pvhs.org
Proctor Hospital	Peoria	Illinois	309-691-1000	www.proctor.org
Providence Saint John's Health Center	Santa Monica	California	310-829-5511	www.stjohns.org
Quail Creek Surgical Hospital	Amarillo	Texas	806-354-6100	www.physurg.com
Riverside Medical Center	Kankakee	Illinois	815-933-1671	www.riversidehealthcare.org
Roper Hospital	Charleston	South Carolina	843-724-2800	www.ropersaintfrancis.com
Sacred Heart Hospital	Pensacola	Florida	850-416-7000	www.sacred-heart.org
Saint Elizabeth Regional Medical Center	Lincoln	Nebraska	402-219-7700	www.stelizabethonline.com
Saint Joseph Regional Medical Center	Mishawaka	Indiana	574-335-5000	www.sjmed.com
Saint Joseph's Hospital of Atlanta	Atlanta	Georgia	678-843-5720	www.stjosephsatlanta.org
Saint Thomas Midtown Hospital	Nashville	Tennessee	615-284-5555	www.baptisthospital.com
Samaritan Regional Health System	Ashland	Ohio	419-289-0491	www.samho.org
Sanford Medical Center Bismarck	Bismarck	North Dakota	701-323-6000	www.medcenterone.com
Sentara Leigh Hospital	Norfolk	Virginia	757-261-6601	www.sentara.com
Seton Medical Center Austin	Austin	Texas	512-324-1000	www.seton.net
South Nassau Communities Hospital	Oceanside	New York	516-632-3000	www.southnassau.org
Southside Hospital	Bay Shore	New York	631-968-3000	www.northshorelij.com
Southwest General Health Center	Middleburg Heights	Ohio	440-816-8000	www.swgeneral.com
Saint Francis Hospital & Medical Center	Hartford	Connecticut	860-714-4000	www.saintfranciscare.com
Saint Helena Hospital	Saint Helena	California	707-963-3611	www.sthelenahospital.org
Saint Joseph Hospital	Orange	California	714-633-9111	www.sjo.org
Saint Joseph Mercy Oakland	Pontiac	Michigan	248-858-3000	www.stjoesoakland.org
Saint Joseph's Hospital - Savannah	Savannah	Georgia	912-819-4100	www.sjchs.org
Saint Peter's Hospital	Albany	New York	518-525-1550	www.stpetershealthcare.org
Saint Vincent's Medical Center	Jacksonville	Florida	904-308-7300	www.jaxhealth.com
Sutter General Hospital	Sacramento	California	916-733-8999	www.suttermedicalcenter.org

Hospital	City	State	Phone	Web Site
Tampa General Hospital	Tampa	Florida	813-844-7000	www.tgh.org
Texas Health Presbyterian Hospital Dallas	Dallas	Texas	214-345-6789	www.texashealth.org
Torrance Memorial Medical Center	Torrance	California	310-325-9110	www.torrancememorial.org
Valley Medical Center	Renton	Washington	425-228-3450	www.valleymed.org
VHS Harlingen Hospital Company	Harlingen	Texas	956-389-1100	www.vbmc.org
Washington Hospital	Fremont	California	510-797-1111	www.whhs.com
Western Maryland Regional Medical Center	Cumberland	Maryland	240-964-8001	www.wmhs.com
William Beaumont Hospital - Troy	Troy	Michigan	248-964-8800	www.beaumonthospitals.com
Yavapai Regional Medical Center	Prescott	Arizona	928-771-5676	www.yrmc.org

Note: Table shows hospitals nationwide whose surgical complication rate is better (lower) than U.S. rate of 3.4%

Hospitals whose Surgical Complication Rate is Worse (Higher) than the U.S. National Rate

Measure: Rate of Complications for Hip/Knee Replacement Patients

Hospital	City	State	Phone	Web Site
Alegent Health Mercy Hospital	Council Bluffs	Iowa	712-328-5000	www.alegent.com/mercy
Atrium Medical Center	Franklin	Ohio	513-420-5102	www.atriummedcenter.org
Baptist Memorial Hospital	Memphis	Tennessee	901-226-5000	www.bmhcc.org
Baptist Saint Anthony's Hospital	Amarillo	Texas	806-212-2000	www.bsahs.com
Beaumont Health System	Grosse Pointe	Michigan	313-343-1000	www.beaumonthospitals.com
Bridgeport Hospital	Bridgeport	Connecticut	203-384-3000	www.bridgeporthospital.com
Carolinas Medical Center - Northeast	Concord	North Carolina	704-783-3000	www.northeastmedical.org
Central Maine Medical Center	Lewiston	Maine	207-795-0111	www.cmmc.org
Community Memorial Hospital San Buenaventura	Ventura	California	805-652-5011	www.cmhhospital.org
D C H Regional Medical Center	Tuscaloosa	Alabama	205-759-7111	www.dchsystem.com
Decatur Morgan Hospital - Decatur Campus	Decatur	Alabama	256-341-2000	www.decaturgeneral.org
Defiance Regional Medical Center	Defiance	Ohio	419-783-6955	www.promedica.org/defiance
Doctors Medical Center	Modesto	California	209-578-1211	www.dmc-modesto.com
East Ohio Regional Hospital	Martins Ferry	Ohio	740-633-4151	www.eastohioregionalhospital.com
Floyd Medical Center	Rome	Georgia	706-509-6900	www.floydmed.org
Froedtert Memorial Lutheran Hospital	Milwaukee	Wisconsin	414-805-3000	www.froedtert.com
Gadsden Regional Medical Center	Gadsden	Alabama	256-494-4000	www.gadsdenregional.com
Genesis Medical Center - Davenport	Davenport	Iowa	563-421-1000	www.genesishealth.com
Genesys Regional Medical Center - Health Park	Grand Blanc	Michigan	810-606-5000	www.genesys.org
Grant Medical Center	Columbus	Ohio	614-566-9978	www.ohiohealth.com
Henry County Medical Center	Paris	Tennessee	731-642-1220	www.hcmc-tn.org
Houston Orthopedic & Spine Hospital	Bellaire	Texas	713-622-2262	www.foundationsurgicalhospital.com
Johnson City Medical Center	Johnson City	Tennessee	423-431-6111	www.msha.com
Lancaster General Hospital	Lancaster	Pennsylvania	717-299-5511	www.lancastergeneral.org
Louis A Weiss Memorial Hospital	Chicago	Illinois	773-878-8700	www.weisshospital.org
The Medical Center of Aurora	Aurora	Colorado	303-695-2600	www.auroramed.com
Mercy Health System Corp	Janesville	Wisconsin	608-756-6080	www.mercyhealthsystem.org
Mercy Saint Anne Hospital	Toledo	Ohio	419-407-2663	www.mercyweb.org
Mountain View Hospital	Payson	Utah	801-465-7100	www.mvhpayson.com
North Colorado Medical Center	Greeley	Colorado	970-352-4121	www.bannerhealth.com
North Kansas City Hospital	North Kansas City	Missouri	816-691-2000	www.nkch.org
Northwestern Memorial Hospital	Chicago	Illinois	312-926-2000	www.nmh.org
Novant Health Rowan Medical Center	Salisbury	North Carolina	704-210-5000	www.rowan.org
NYU Hospitals Center	New York	New York	212-263-7300	www.med.nyu.edu
Onslow Memorial Hospital	Jacksonville	North Carolina	910-577-2345	www.onslowmemorial.org
Overland Park Regional Medical Center	Overland Park	Kansas	913-541-5301	www.oprmc.com
Park Ridge Health	Hendersonville	North Carolina	828-684-8501	www.parkridgehospital.org
Pennsylvania Hospital of the Univ of PA Health Sys	Philadelphia	Pennsylvania	215-829-3000	www.pennmedicine.org/pahosp
Peterson Regional Medical Center	Kerrville	Texas	830-896-4200	www.petersonrmc.com
Pinnacle Health Hospitals	Harrisburg	Pennsylvania	717-782-5181	www.pinnaclehealth.org
Poplar Bluff Regional Medical Center	Poplar Bluff	Missouri	573-785-7721	www.poplarbluffregional.com
Reston Hospital Center	Reston	Virginia	703-689-9000	www.restonhospital.com
Riddle Memorial Hospital	Media	Pennsylvania	610-566-9400	www.riddlehospital.org
Saint Michael's Medical Center	Newark	New Jersey	973-877-5350	www.cathedralhealth.org
Shady Grove Adventist Hospital	Rockville	Maryland	240-826-6517	www.adventisthealthcare.com/sgah
Shannon Medical Center	San Angelo	Texas	325-653-6741	www.shannonhealth.com
South Central Regional Medical Center	Laurel	Mississippi	601-649-4000	www.scrmc.com
South Lake Hospital	Clermont	Florida	352-394-4071	www.southlakehospital.com
Southside Regional Medical Center	Petersburg	Virginia	804-765-5000	www.srmconline.com
Spring Valley Hospital Medical Center	Las Vegas	Nevada	702-853-3000	www.springvalleyhospital.com
Saint Alexius Medical Center	Hoffman Estates	Illinois	847-843-2000	www.alexianbrothershealth.org
Saint Anthony Hospital	Oklahoma City	Oklahoma	405-272-7000	www.saintsok.com
Saint Catherine of Siena Hospital	Smithtown	New York	631-862-3000	www.stcatherines.chsli.org
Saint Clair Memorial Hospital	Pittsburgh	Pennsylvania	412-942-6209	www.stclair.org
Saint Elizabeth Hospital	Appleton	Wisconsin	920-738-2000	www.affinityhealth.org
Saint Luke's Hospital Bethlehem	Bethlehem	Pennsylvania	610-954-4000	www.slhn-lehighvalley.org
Saint Marys Hospital	Madison	Wisconsin	608-251-6100	www.stmarysmadison.com
Saint Vincent Anderson Regional Hospital	Anderson	Indiana	765-646-8373	www.stjohnshealthsystem.org
Saint Vincent Healthcare	Billings	Montana	406-657-7000	www.svh-mt.org
Saint Vincent's Medical Center	Bridgeport	Connecticut	203-576-5551	www.stvincents.org
Sutter Auburn Faith Hospital	Auburn	California	530-888-4500	www.sutterauburnfaith.org
Sutter Solano Medical Center	Vallejo	California	707-554-5280	www.suttersolano.org
Swedish Medical Center	Englewood	Colorado	303-788-5000	www.swedishhospital.com/default.asp
Trinity Medical Center	Birmingham	Alabama	205-592-1000	www.bhsala.com/montclair

Hospital	City	State	Phone	Web Site
University of Kansas Hospital	Kansas City	Kansas	913-588-7332	www.kumc.edu
University of Toledo Medical Center	Toledo	Ohio	419-383-3407	www.utmc.utoledo.edu
Wentworth - Douglass Hospital	Dover	New Hampshire	603-740-2580	www.wdhospital.com
White River Medical Center	Batesville	Arkansas	870-262-1200	www.wrmc.com

Note: Table shows hospitals nationwide whose surgical complication rate is worse (higher) than U.S. rate of 3.4%

Hospitals whose Surgical Complication Rate is Better (Lower) than the U.S. National Rate

Measure: Serious Blood Clots After Surgery

Hospital	City	State	Phone	Web Site
Abbott Northwestern Hospital	Minneapolis	Minnesota	612-863-4509	www.abbottnorthwestern.com
Advocate Condell Medical Center	Libertyville	Illinois	847-990-5200	www.condell.org
Allegiance Health	Jackson	Michigan	517-788-4800	www.footehealth.org
Arkansas Heart Hospital	Little Rock	Arkansas	501-219-7000	www.arheart.com
Asante Rogue Regional Medical Center	Medford	Oregon	541-789-7000	www.asante.org
Aurora Saint Lukes Medical Center	Milwaukee	Wisconsin	414-649-6000	www.aurorahealthcare.org
Avera Mckennan Hospital & University Health Center	Sioux Falls	South Dakota	605-322-8000	www.mckennan.org
Avera Saint Lukes	Aberdeen	South Dakota	605-622-5000	www.averastlukes.org
Bakersfield Memorial Hospital	Bakersfield	California	661-327-1792	www.bakersfieldmemorial.org
Banner Baywood Medical Center	Mesa	Arizona	480-321-2000	www.bannerhealth.com
Banner Good Samaritan Medical Center	Phoenix	Arizona	602-239-2000	www.bannerhealth.com
Baptist Beaumont Hospital	Beaumont	Texas	409-212-5012	www.mhbh.org
Baptist Health Lexington	Lexington	Kentucky	859-260-6104	www.centralbap.com
Baptist Health Louisville	Louisville	Kentucky	502-897-8100	www.baptisteast.com
Baptist Health Medical Center - Little Rock	Little Rock	Arkansas	501-202-2000	www.baptist-health.com
Baystate Medical Center	Springfield	Massachusetts	413-794-0000	www.baystatehealth.com
Benefis Hospitals	Great Falls	Montana	406-455-5000	www.benefis.org
Berkshire Medical Center	Pittsfield	Massachusetts	413-447-2000	www.berkshirehealthsystems.org
Billings Clinic Hospital	Billings	Montana	406-657-4000	www.billngsclinic.com
Camden Clark Medical Center	Parkersburg	West Virginia	304-424-2111	www.ccmh.org
Cape Cod Hospital	Hyannis	Massachusetts	508-771-1800	www.capecodhealth.org
Carilion New River Valley Medical Center	Christiansburg	Virginia	540-731-2000	www.carilion.com
Carolinas Medical Center/Behaviorial Health	Charlotte	North Carolina	704-355-2000	www.carolinasmedicalcenter.org
Caromont Regional Medical Center	Gastonia	North Carolina	704-834-4891	www.caromont.org
Carson Tahoe Regional Medical Center	Carson City	Nevada	775-445-8000	www.carsontahoehospital.com
Centra Health	Lynchburg	Virginia	434-200-4789	www.centrahealth.com
Central Maine Medical Center	Lewiston	Maine	207-795-0111	www.cmmc.org
Charlotte Hungerford Hospital	Torrington	Connecticut	860-496-6666	www.charlottesweb.hungerford.org
Comanche County Memorial Hospital	Lawton	Oklahoma	580-355-8620	www.memorialhealthsource.org
Community Hospital North	Indianapolis	Indiana	317-621-5335	www.ecommunity.com/north
Community Medical Center	Toms River	New Jersey	732-557-8000	www.sbhcs.com
Cox Medical Center	Springfield	Missouri	417-269-6000	www.coxhealth.com
Doctors Hospital of Sarasota	Sarasota	Florida	941-342-1100	www.doctorsofsarasota.com
Duke University Hospital	Durham	North Carolina	919-684-8111	www.dukehealth.org
Eastern Idaho Regional Medical Center	Idaho Falls	Idaho	208-529-6111	www.eirmc.org
Eisenhower Medical Center	Rancho Mirage	California	760-340-3911	www.emc.org
El Camino Hospital	Mountain View	California	650-940-7000	www.elcaminohospital.org
Elkhart General Hospital	Elkhart	Indiana	574-294-2621	www.egh.org
Essentia Health - Fargo	Fargo	North Dakota	701-364-8000	www.dakotaclinic.com
Exeter Hospital	Exeter	New Hampshire	603-778-7311	www.exeterhospital.com
Flagstaff Medical Center	Flagstaff	Arizona	928-773-2009	www.nahealth.com
Fort Sanders Regional Medical Center	Knoxville	Tennessee	865-541-1101	www.fsregional.com
Franciscan Saint Elizabeth Health - Lafayette East	Lafayette	Indiana	765-502-4334	www.ste.org
Geisinger - Community Medical Center	Scranton	Pennsylvania	570-969-8240	www.cmchealthsys.org
Genesis Medical Center - Davenport	Davenport	Iowa	563-421-1000	www.genesishealth.com
Glens Falls Hospital	Glens Falls	New York	518-926-1000	www.glensfallshospital.org
Good Samaritan Regional Medical Center	Corvallis	Oregon	541-768-5111	www.samhealth.org/shs_facilities
Gundersen Lutheran Medical Center	La Crosse	Wisconsin	608-782-7300	www.gundluth.org
Harrison Memorial Center	Bremerton	Washington	360-377-3911	www.harrisonmedical.org
Hays Medical Center	Hays	Kansas	785-623-5000	www.haysmed.com
Heartland Regional Medical Center	Saint Joseph	Missouri	816-271-6000	www.heartland-health.com
Hendrick Medical Center	Abilene	Texas	325-670-2000	www.ehendrick.org
Holy Cross Hospital	Fort Lauderdale	Florida	954-771-8000	www.holy-cross.com
Indiana University Health Bloomington Hospital	Bloomington	Indiana	812-353-9555	www.bloomingtonhospital.org
Indiana University Health North Hospital	Carmel	Indiana	317-688-2000	www.iuhealth.org/north
Inova Mount Vernon Hospital	Alexandria	Virginia	703-664-7000	www.inova.com/inovapublic.srt/imvh/index.jsp
Integris Baptist Medical Center	Oklahoma City	Oklahoma	405-951-8110	www.integris-health.com
Jackson Hospital & Clinic	Montgomery	Alabama	334-293-8000	www.jackson.org
Jackson - Madison County General Hospital	Jackson	Tennessee	731-541-5000	www.wth.org
John Muir Medical Center - Concord Campus	Concord	California	925-674-2002	www.johnmuirhealth.com
John Muir Medical Center - Walnut Creek Campus	Walnut Creek	California	925-939-3000	www.jmmdhs.com
Kalispell Regional Medical Center	Kalispell	Montana	406-752-5111	www.krmc.org
Kootenai Medical Center	Coeur D'alene	Idaho	208-625-4001	www.kootenaihealth.org
Lakeland Hospital - Saint Joseph	Saint Joseph	Michigan	269-983-8300	www.lakelandhealth.org

Hospital	City	State	Phone	Web Site
Marian Regional Medical Center	Santa Maria	California	805-739-3000	www.marinmedicalcenter.org
Mary Washington Hospital	Fredericksburg	Virginia	540-741-1100	www.medicorp.org
Maury Regional Hospital	Columbia	Tennessee	931-381-1111	www.maurgregional.com
Mayo Clinic Methodist- Hospital	Rochester	Minnesota	507-266-7890	www.mayoclinic.org/methodisthospital
Mcleod Regional Medical Center - Pee Dee	Florence	South Carolina	843-777-2900	www.mcleodhealth.org
Medical Center of Central Georgia	Macon	Georgia	478-633-6805	www.mccg.org
Memorial Healthcare System	Chattanooga	Tennessee	423-495-2525	www.memorial.org
Memorial Hospital at Gulfport	Gulfport	Mississippi	228-867-4000	www.gulfportmemorial.com
Memorial Hospital of Carbondale	Carbondale	Illinois	618-549-0721	www.sih.net
Memorial Mission Hospital & Asheville Surgery Center	Asheville	North Carolina	828-213-1111	www.missionhospitals.org
Mercy Hospital	Coon Rapids	Minnesota	763-236-8205	www.allinamercy.org
Mercy Medical Center - Cedar Rapids	Cedar Rapids	Iowa	319-398-6011	www.mercycare.org
Mercy Medical Center - Redding	Redding	California	530-225-6102	www.redding.mercy.org
Mercy Medical Center - North Iowa	Mason City	Iowa	641-428-7000	www.mercynorthiowa.com
Methodist Hospital	San Antonio	Texas	210-575-4000	www.mh.sahealth.com
Methodist Medical Center of Oak Ridge	Oak Ridge	Tennessee	865-835-1000	www.mmcoakridge.com
Mother Frances Hospital	Tyler	Texas	903-593-8441	www.tmfhs.org
Munson Medical Center	Traverse City	Michigan	231-935-5000	www.munsonhealthcare.org
New England Baptist Hospital	Boston	Massachusetts	617-754-5800	www.nebh.caregroup.org
Novant Health Charlotte Orthopedic Hospital	Charlotte	North Carolina	704-316-2000	www.presbyterian.org
NW Arkansas Hospitals	Springdale	Arkansas	479-751-5711	www.northwesthealth.org
Ochsner Medical Center	New Orleans	Louisiana	504-842-3000	www.ochsner.org
Oklahoma Heart Hospital	Oklahoma City	Oklahoma	405-608-3200	www.okheart.com
Olathe Medical Center	Olathe	Kansas	913-791-4200	www.ohsi.com
Parker Adventist Hospital	Parker	Colorado	303-269-4000	www.parkerhospital.org
Parkview Medical Center	Pueblo	Colorado	719-584-4000	www.parkviewmc.com
Parkview Regional Medical Center	Fort Wayne	Indiana	260-266-1000	www.parkview.com
Parkwest Medical Center	Knoxville	Tennessee	865-970-9800	www.yesparkwest.com
Peacehealth Saint Joseph Medical Center	Bellingham	Washington	360-734-5400	www.peacehealth.org
Peconic Bay Medical Center	Riverhead	New York	631-548-6000	www.pbmedicalcenter.org
Presence Covenant Medical Center	Urbana	Illinois	217-337-2000	www.provena.org/covenant
Providence Sacred Heart Medical Center	Spokane	Washington	509-474-3040	www.shmc.org
Providence Saint John's Health Center	Santa Monica	California	310-829-5511	www.stjohns.org
Providence Saint Joseph Medical Center	Burbank	California	818-843-5111	www.providence.org/losangeles
Regional Medical Center Bayonet Point	Hudson	Florida	727-819-2929	www.mchealth.comorwww.heartoftampa.com
Riverview Medical Center	Red Bank	New Jersey	732-741-2700	www.meridianhealth.com
Sacred Heart Medical Center - Riverbend	Springfield	Oregon	541-222-7300	www.peacehealth.org/sacred-heart-riverbend
Saint Francis Medical Center	Cape Girardeau	Missouri	573-331-3000	www.sfmc.net
Saint Joseph Hospital	Lexington	Kentucky	859-313-1000	www.sjhlex.org
Saint Joseph Regional Medical Center	Mishawaka	Indiana	574-335-5000	www.sjmed.com
Saint Mary's Health Care	Grand Rapids	Michigan	616-685-5000	www.smhealthcare.org
Saint Thomas West Hospital	Nashville	Tennessee	615-222-2111	www.stthomas.org
Salinas Valley Memorial Hospital	Salinas	California	831-757-4333	www.svmh.com
San Jacinto Methodist Hospital	Baytown	Texas	281-420-8600	www.methodisthealth.com/sanjacinto
Sanford Medical Center Fargo	Fargo	North Dakota	701-234-2000	www.meritcare.com
Sanford Usd Medical Center	Sioux Falls	South Dakota	605-333-1000	www.sanfordhealth.org
Sarasota Memorial Hospital	Sarasota	Florida	941-917-9000	www.smh.com
Scott & White Memorial Hospital	Temple	Texas	254-724-2111	www.sw.org
Seton Medical Center Austin	Austin	Texas	512-324-1000	www.seton.net
Shannon Medical Center	San Angelo	Texas	325-653-6741	www.shannonhealth.com
Shasta Regional Medical Center	Redding	California	530-244-5454	www.shastaregional.com
South Georgia Medical Center	Valdosta	Georgia	229-333-1020	www.sgmc.org
Saint Charles Medical Center - Bend	Bend	Oregon	541-382-4321	www.scmc.org
Saint Cloud Hospital	Saint Cloud	Minnesota	320-251-2700	www.centracare.com
Saint David's Medical Center	Austin	Texas	512-476-7111	www.stdavidsrehab.com
Saint Elizabeth Medical Center	Lakeside Park	Kentucky	859-292-2000	www.stelizabeth.com
Saint Helena Hospital	Saint Helena	California	707-963-3611	www.sthelenahospital.org
Saint Joseph Hospital	Orange	California	714-633-9111	www.sjo.org
Saint Joseph Mercy Oakland	Pontiac	Michigan	248-858-3000	www.stjoesoakland.org
Saint Joseph's Hospital Health Center	Syracuse	New York	315-448-5111	www.sjhsyr.org
Saint Joseph's Medical Center of Stockton	Stockton	California	209-943-2000	www.stjospehscares.org
Saint Luke's Hospital	Cedar Rapids	Iowa	319-369-7211	www.crstlukes.com
Saint Mary's Regional Medical Center	Enid	Oklahoma	580-233-6100	www.stmarysregional.com
Saint Marys Hospital	Madison	Wisconsin	608-251-6100	www.stmarysmadison.com
Saint Patrick Hospital	Missoula	Montana	406-543-7271	www.saintpatrick.org
Saint Vincent Healthcare	Billings	Montana	406-657-7000	www.svh-mt.org
Saint Vincent Hospital	Santa Fe	New Mexico	505-913-5201	www.stvin.org

Hospital	City	State	Phone	Web Site
Saint Vincent Hospital & Health Services	Indianapolis	Indiana	317-338-7000	www.indianapolis.stvincent.org
Saint Vincent's Medical Center	Jacksonville	Florida	904-308-7300	www.jaxhealth.com
Sutter General Hospital	Sacramento	California	916-733-8999	www.suttermedicalcenter.org
Swedish American Hospital	Rockford	Illinois	815-968-4400	www.swedishamerican.org
Swedish Medical Center	Seattle	Washington	206-386-6000	www.swedish.org
Tallahassee Memorial Hospital	Tallahassee	Florida	850-431-1155	www.tmh.org
Texas Health Harris Methodist Hurst - Euless - Bedford	Bedford	Texas	817-848-4000	www.texashealth.org
Thibodaux Regional Medical Center	Thibodaux	Louisiana	985-447-5500	www.thibodaux.com
Trinity Rock Island	Rock Island	Illinois	309-779-5000	www.trinityqc.com
United Regional Health Care System	Wichita Falls	Texas	940-764-3055	www.urhcs.org
University Health Care/University Hospitals & Clinics	Salt Lake City	Utah	801-581-2121	www.healthcare.utah.edu
University Medical Center	Lubbock	Texas	806-775-8200	www.teamumc.org
University of Washington Medical Center	Seattle	Washington	206-598-3300	www.washington.edu/medical/uwmc
Vanderbilt University Hospital	Nashville	Tennessee	615-322-3454	www.mc.vanderbilt.edu
VHS Harlingen Hospital Company	Harlingen	Texas	956-389-1100	www.vbmc.org
Via Christi Hospitals Wichita	Wichita	Kansas	316-268-5000	www.via-christi.org
Virginia Mason Medical Center	Seattle	Washington	206-223-6600	www.vmmc.org
Wakemed - Raleigh Campus	Raleigh	North Carolina	919-350-8000	www.wakemed.org
Washington Hospital	Fremont	California	510-797-1111	www.whhs.com
Wesley Medical Center	Wichita	Kansas	316-962-2000	www.wesleymc.com
Winchester Medical Center	Winchester	Virginia	540-536-8000	www.valleyhealthlink.com
Winter Haven Hospital	Winter Haven	Florida	863-293-1121	www.winterhavenhospital.com
Wyoming Medical Center	Casper	Wyoming	307-577-7201	www.wyomingmedicalcenter.com
Yakima Valley Memorial Hospital	Yakima	Washington	509-575-8000	www.yakimamemorialhospital.org

Note: Table shows hospitals nationwide whose surgical complication rate is better (lower) than U.S. rate of 4.14%

Hospitals whose Surgical Complication Rate is Worse (Higher) than the U.S. National Rate

Measure: Serious Blood Clots After Surgery

Hospital	City	State	Phone	Web Site
Advocate Good Samaritan Hospital	Downers Grove	Illinois	630-275-5900	www.advocatehealth.com/gsam
Advocate Illinois Masonic Medical Center	Chicago	Illinois	773-975-1600	www.advocatehealth.com/immc
Advocate Lutheran General Hospital	Park Ridge	Illinois	847-723-2210	www.advocatehealth.com
Albert Einstein Medical Center	Philadelphia	Pennsylvania	215-456-6090	www.einstein.edu
Alegent Health Mercy Hospital	Council Bluffs	Iowa	712-328-5000	www.alegent.com/mercy
Alexian Brothers Medical Center	Elk Grove Village	Illinois	847-437-5500	www.alexian.org
Aultman Hospital	Canton	Ohio	330-452-9911	www.aultman.com
B R F Hospital Holdings	Shreveport	Louisiana	318-675-5000	www.lsumc.edu
Baptist Memorial Hospital Desoto	Southaven	Mississippi	662-772-4000	www.bmhcc.org/facilities/desoto
Barnes-Jewish Hospital	Saint Louis	Missouri	314-747-3000	www.barnesjewish.org
Beaumont Health System	Grosse Pointe	Michigan	313-343-1000	www.beaumonthospitals.com
Beaumont Health System	Royal Oak	Michigan	248-898-5000	www.beaumonthospitals.com
Bon Secours Saint Francis Medical Center	Midlothian	Virginia	804-594-7400	www.richmond.bonsecours.com
Bridgeport Hospital	Bridgeport	Connecticut	203-384-3000	www.bridgeporthospital.com
Brigham & Women's Hospital	Boston	Massachusetts	617-732-5500	www.brighamandwomens.org
Brookdale Hospital Medical Center	Brooklyn	New York	718-240-5966	www.brookdalehospital.org
Brookwood Medical Center	Birmingham	Alabama	205-877-1000	www.bwmc.com
Cape Coral Hospital	Cape Coral	Florida	239-574-2323	www.leememorial.org
Carilion Roanoke Memorial Hospital	Roanoke	Virginia	540-981-7000	www.carilion.com/crmh
Cedars - Sinai Medical Center	Los Angeles	California	310-423-5000	www.cedars-sinai.edu
Centennial Medical Center	Frisco	Texas	972-963-3333	www.centennialmedcenter.com
Charleston Area Medical Center	Charleston	West Virginia	304-388-6203	www.camc.org
Christian Hospital Northeast - Northwest	Saint Louis	Missouri	314-653-5000	www.christianhospital.org
Christiana Care Health Services	Newark	Delaware	302-733-1000	www.christianacare.org
Christus Saint Frances Cabrini Hospital	Alexandria	Louisiana	318-487-1122	www.cabrini.org
Christus Saint Michael Health System	Texarkana	Texas	903-614-1000	www.christusstmichael.org
Cleveland Clinic	Cleveland	Ohio	216-444-2200	www.clevelandclinic.org
Conemaugh Valley Memorial Hospital	Johnstown	Pennsylvania	814-534-9000	www.conemaugh.org
Coney Island Hospital	Brooklyn	New York	718-616-3000	www.coneyislandhospital.com
Cooper University Hospital	Camden	New Jersey	856-342-2000	www.cooperhealth.org
Crouse Hospital	Syracuse	New York	315-470-7449	www.crouse.org
D C H Regional Medical Center	Tuscaloosa	Alabama	205-759-7111	www.dchsystem.com
Danbury Hospital	Danbury	Connecticut	203-797-7000	www.danburyhospital.com
Delnor Community Hospital	Geneva	Illinois	630-208-3000	www.delnor.com
Doctors Hospital	Augusta	Georgia	706-651-6008	www.doctors-hospital.net
Doctors Hospital	Coral Gables	Florida	305-666-2111	www.baptisthealth.net
Edward Hospital	Naperville	Illinois	630-527-3000	www.edward.org
El Paso Specialty Hospital	El Paso	Texas	915-544-3636	www.elpasospecialtyhospital.com
Emory University Hospital Midtown	Atlanta	Georgia	404-686-4411	www.emoryhealthcare.org
Evanston Hospital	Evanston	Illinois	847-432-8000	www.enh.org
Flagler Hospital	Saint Augustine	Florida	904-819-4426	www.flaglerhospital.com
Florida Hospital	Orlando	Florida	407-303-1976	www.floridahospital.com
Franciscan Saint Margaret Health - Hammond	Hammond	Indiana	219-932-2300	www.smmhc.com
Geisinger Medical Center	Danville	Pennsylvania	570-271-6211	www.geisinger.org
Genesys Regional Medical Center - Health Park	Grand Blanc	Michigan	810-606-5000	www.genesys.org
Glen Cove Hospital	Glen Cove	New York	516-674-7300	www.northshorelij.com
Grady Memorial Hospital	Atlanta	Georgia	404-616-4252	www.gradyhealthsystem.org
Grand View Hospital	Sellersville	Pennsylvania	215-453-4615	www.gvh.org
Gulf Coast Medical Center Lee Memorial Health System	Fort Myers	Florida	239-768-5000	www.leememorial.org
Hackensack University Medical Center	Hackensack	New Jersey	201-996-2000	www.humed.com
Hackettstown Regional Medical Center	Hackettstown	New Jersey	908-852-5100	www.hrmcnj.org
Hahnemann University Hospital	Philadelphia	Pennsylvania	215-762-7000	www.hahnemannhospital.com
Harris Health System	Houston	Texas	713-566-6417	www.hchdonline.com
Hartford Hospital	Hartford	Connecticut	860-545-5000	www.harthosp.org
Henry Ford Hospital	Detroit	Michigan	313-916-2600	www.henryfordhospital.com
Henry Ford West Bloomfield Hospital	W Bloomfield	Michigan	248-325-1000	www.henryford.com
Henry Ford Wyandotte Hospital	Wyandotte	Michigan	734-246-6000	www.henryfordwyandotte.com
Heritage Valley Beaver	Beaver	Pennsylvania	412-728-7000	www.heritagevalley.org
Heritage Valley Sewickley	Sewickley	Pennsylvania	412-741-6600	www.heritagevalley.org
Hillcrest Hospital	Mayfield Heights	Ohio	440-312-4500	www.hillcresthospital.org
Holmes Regional Medical Center	Melbourne	Florida	321-434-7000	www.healthfirst.org
Holy Name Medical Center	Teaneck	New Jersey	201-833-3000	www.holyname.org
Hospital of Univ of Pennsylvania	Philadelphia	Pennsylvania	215-662-3227	www.upenn.edu
Huntington Memorial Hospital	Pasadena	California	626-397-5000	www.huntingtonhospital.com

Hospital	City	State	Phone	Web Site
Hurley Medical Center	Flint	Michigan	810-257-9000	www.hurleymc.com
Ingalls Memorial Hospital	Harvey	Illinois	708-333-2300	www.ingalls.org
Intermountain Medical Center	Murray	Utah	801-507-7000	www.intermountainhealthcare.org
Jackson Memorial Hospital	Miami	Florida	305-585-1111	www.jhsmiami.org
Jeanes Hospital	Philadelphia	Pennsylvania	215-728-2000	www.jeanes.com
JFK Medical Center	Atlantis	Florida	561-965-7300	www.jfkmc.com
JFK Medical Center - A M Yelencsics Comm Hospital	Edison	New Jersey	732-321-7000	www.jfkmc.org
John H Stroger Jr Hospital	Chicago	Illinois	312-864-6000	www.cookcountygov.com
JPS Health Network	Fort Worth	Texas	817-921-3431	www.jpshealthnet.org
Jupiter Medical Center	Jupiter	Florida	561-747-2234	www.jupitermed.com
Lancaster General Hospital	Lancaster	Pennsylvania	717-299-5511	www.lancastergeneral.org
Lee Memorial Hospital	Fort Myers	Florida	239-332-1111	www.leememorial.org
Legacy Emanuel Medical Center	Portland	Oregon	503-413-2200	www.legacyhealth.org
Lehigh Valley Hospital	Allentown	Pennsylvania	610-402-2273	www.lvhhn.org
Lehigh Valley Hospital - Muhlenberg	Bethlehem	Pennsylvania	610-402-2273	www.lvhn.org
Lenox Hill Hospital	New York	New York	212-439-2345	www.lenoxhillhospital.org
Little Company of Mary Hospital	Evergreen Park	Illinois	708-422-6200	www.lcmh.org
Louis A Weiss Memorial Hospital	Chicago	Illinois	773-878-8700	www.weisshospital.org
Lourdes Hospital	Paducah	Kentucky	270-444-2444	www.ehealthconnection.com
Lovelace Medical Center	Albuquerque	New Mexico	505-727-8000	www.lovelace.com
Loyola University Medical Center	Maywood	Illinois	708-216-9000	www.lumc.edu
Magee Womens Hospital of UPMC Health System	Pittsburgh	Pennsylvania	412-641-4010	www.magee.edu
Maimonides Medical Center	Brooklyn	New York	718-283-6000	www.maimonidesmed.org
Marin General Hospital	Greenbrae	California	415-925-7900	www.maringeneral.com
Mary Hitchcock Memorial Hospital	Lebanon	New Hampshire	603-650-5000	www.dhmc.org
Marymount Hospital	Garfield Heights	Ohio	216-581-0500	www.marymount.org
Mclaren Flint	Flint	Michigan	810-342-2000	www.mclaren.org
The Medical Center of Aurora	Aurora	Colorado	303-695-2600	www.auroramed.com
Medical Center of Mckinney	Mckinney	Texas	972-547-8000	www.medicalcenterofmckinney.com
Medical Center of Plano	Plano	Texas	972-596-6800	www.medicalcenterofplano.com
Medstar Georgetown University Hospital	Washington	District of Columbia	202-784-3000	www.georgetownuniversityhospital.org
Memorial Healthcare	Owosso	Michigan	989-723-5211	www.memorialhealthcare.org
Memorial Hermann Texas Medical Center	Houston	Texas	713-704-3700	www.mhhs.org
Memorial Hospital Jacksonville	Jacksonville	Florida	904-399-6111	www.memorialhospitaljax.com
Memorial Medical Center	Las Cruces	New Mexico	575-522-8641	www.mmclc.org
Menorah Medical Center	Overland Park	Kansas	913-498-6773	www.menorahmedicalcenter.com
Mercy Fitzgerald Hospital	Darby	Pennsylvania	215-237-4000	www.mercyhealth.org
Mercy Hospital Springfield	Springfield	Missouri	417-820-2000	www.stjohns.com
Mercy Saint Vincent Medical Center	Toledo	Ohio	419-251-3232	www.mhsnr.org
Miami Valley Hospital	Dayton	Ohio	937-208-8000	www.miamivalleyhospital.com
Midwest Orthopedic Specialty Hospital	Franklin	Wisconsin	414-817-5800	www.mymosh.com
Milton S Hershey Medical Center	Hershey	Pennsylvania	717-531-8521	www.hmc.psu.edu
Ministry Saint Josephs Hospital	Marshfield	Wisconsin	715-387-7850	www.stjosephs-marshfield.org
Mobile Infirmary	Mobile	Alabama	251-435-4700	www.mimc.com
Montefiore Medical Center	Bronx	New York	718-920-4321	www.montefiore.org
Morristown Medical Center	Morristown	New Jersey	973-971-5450	www.morristownmemorialhospital.org
Naples Community Hospital	Naples	Florida	239-436-5000	www.nchmd.org
Nason Hospital	Roaring Spring	Pennsylvania	814-224-2141	www.nasonhospital.com
Nathan Littauer Hospital	Gloversville	New York	518-725-8621	www.nlh.org
Newark Beth Israel Medical Center	Newark	New Jersey	973-926-7850	www.sbhcs.com
North Shore University Hospital	Manhasset	New York	516-562-0100	www.northshorelij.com
North Suburban Medical Center	Thornton	Colorado	303-451-7800	www.northsuburban.com
Northside Hospital	Atlanta	Georgia	404-851-8000	www.northside.com
Northwestern Memorial Hospital	Chicago	Illinois	312-926-2000	www.nmh.org
Novant Health Rowan Medical Center	Salisbury	North Carolina	704-210-5000	www.rowan.org
NYU Hospitals Center	New York	New York	212-263-7300	www.med.nyu.edu
O U Medical Center	Oklahoma City	Oklahoma	405-271-5911	www.oumedcenter.com
Oakwood Hospital - Southshore	Trenton	Michigan	734-671-3800	www.oakwood.org/oakwood-hospital-southshore
Och Regional Medical Center	Starkville	Mississippi	662-323-4320	www.och.org
OHSU Hospital & Clinics	Portland	Oregon	503-494-4036	www.ohsu.edu
Orlando Health	Orlando	Florida	321-841-5111	www.orlandoregionalmedicalcenter.org
Our Lady of the Lake Regional Medical Center	Baton Rouge	Louisiana	225-765-6565	www.ololrmc.com
Overlook Medical Center	Summit	New Jersey	908-522-2000	www.atlantichealth.org
Owensboro Health Regional Hospital	Owensboro	Kentucky	270-688-2000	www.omhs.org
Palmetto General Hospital	Hialeah	Florida	305-823-5000	www.palmettogeneral.com
Parkland Health & Hospital System	Dallas	Texas	214-590-8000	www.parklandhospital.com
Pennsylvania Hospital of the Univ of PA Health Sys	Philadelphia	Pennsylvania	215-829-3000	www.pennmedicine.org/pahosp
Piedmont Hospital	Atlanta	Georgia	404-605-5000	www.piedmonthospital.org

Hospital	City	State	Phone	Web Site
Pinnacle Health Hospitals	Harrisburg	Pennsylvania	717-782-5181	www.pinnaclehealth.org
Plainview Hospital	Plainview	New York	516-719-3000	www.nslij.com
Pratt Regional Medical Center	Pratt	Kansas	620-450-1160	www.prmc.org
Proctor Hospital	Peoria	Illinois	309-691-1000	www.proctor.org
Providence Hospital & Medical Centers	Southfield	Michigan	248-849-3011	www.stjohn.org/providence
Providence Memorial Hospital	El Paso	Texas	915-577-6011	www.sphn.com
Raleigh General Hospital	Beckley	West Virginia	304-256-4100	www.raleighgeneral.com
Regional Medical Center at Memphis	Memphis	Tennessee	901-545-7928	www.the-med.org
Riddle Memorial Hospital	Media	Pennsylvania	610-566-9400	www.riddlehospital.org
Robert Wood Johnson University Hospital	New Brunswick	New Jersey	732-937-8900	www.rwjuh.edu
Rose Medical Center	Denver	Colorado	303-320-2121	www.rosemed.com
Saint Barnabas Medical Center	Livingston	New Jersey	973-322-5000	www.saintbarnabas.com
Saint Peter's University Hospital	New Brunswick	New Jersey	732-745-8600	www.saintpetersuh.com
Saratoga Hospital	Saratoga Springs	New York	518-587-3222	www.saratogacare.org
Scripps Memorial Hospital La Jolla	La Jolla	California	858-626-4123	www.scrippshealth.org
Scripps Mercy Hospital	San Diego	California	619-294-8111	www.scrippshealth.org
Sentara Norfolk General Hospital	Norfolk	Virginia	757-388-3000	www.sentara.com
Sharp Memorial Hospital	San Diego	California	858-939-3400	www.sharp.com/memorial
Sierra Medical Center	El Paso	Texas	915-747-4000	www.sphn.com
Sinai - Grace Hospital	Detroit	Michigan	313-966-3300	www.sinaigrace.org
Somerset Medical Center	Somerville	New Jersey	908-685-2200	www.somersetmedicalcenter.com
South Lake Hospital	Clermont	Florida	352-394-4071	www.southlakehospital.com
Saint Alphonsus Regional Medical Center	Boise	Idaho	208-367-2121	www.saintalphonsus.org
Saint Anthonys Memorial Hospital	Effingham	Illinois	217-342-2121	www.stanthonyshospital.org
Saint Catherine of Siena Hospital	Smithtown	New York	631-862-3000	www.stcatherines.chsli.org
Saint Clare Hospital	Lakewood	Washington	253-588-1711	www.fhshealth.org
Saint Elizabeth Hospital	Belleville	Illinois	618-234-2120	www.steliz.org
Saint John's Episcopal Hospital at South Shore	Far Rockaway	New York	718-869-7000	www.ehs.org
Saint Joseph Hospital	Nashua	New Hampshire	603-882-3000	www.stjosephhospital.com
Saint Joseph Medical Center	Tacoma	Washington	253-627-4101	www.fhshealth.org
Saint Louis University Hospital	Saint Louis	Missouri	314-577-8000	www.slucare.edu/clinical
Saint Luke's Hospital Bethlehem	Bethlehem	Pennsylvania	610-954-4000	www.slhn-lehighvalley.org
Saint Luke's Roosevelt Hospital	New York	New York	212-523-4000	www.wehealny.org
Saint Luke's Warren Hospital	Phillipsburg	New Jersey	908-859-6700	www.warrenhospital.org
Saint Luke's Episcopal Hospital	Houston	Texas	832-355-1000	www.sleh.com
Saint Luke's Hospital	Chesterfield	Missouri	314-434-1500	www.goodhealthmatters.com
Saint Mary's Medical Center	West Palm Beach	Florida	561-840-6202	www.stmarysmc.com
Saint Mary's of Michigan Medical Center	Saginaw	Michigan	989-776-8000	www.stmarysofmichigan.org
Saint Vincent Hospital	Worcester	Massachusetts	508-363-5000	www.stvincenthospital.com
Staten Island University Hospital	Staten Island	New York	718-226-9000	www.siuh.edu
Summa Health Systems Hospitals	Akron	Ohio	330-375-3000	www.summahealth.org
Swedish Medical Center	Englewood	Colorado	303-788-5000	www.swedishhospital.com/default.asp
Tampa General Hospital	Tampa	Florida	813-844-7000	www.tgh.org
Temple University Hospital	Philadelphia	Pennsylvania	215-707-2000	www.tuh.templehealth.org
Carle Foundation Hospital	Urbana	Illinois	217-383-3311	www.carle.com
The University of Chicago Medical Center	Chicago	Illinois	773-702-1000	www.uchospitals.edu
Thomas Jefferson University Hospital	Philadelphia	Pennsylvania	215-955-6000	www.jeffersonhospital.org
Tri - City Medical Center	Oceanside	California	760-724-8411	www.tricitymed.org
Tucson Medical Center	Tucson	Arizona	520-327-5461	www.tmcaz.com
University Hospital	Augusta	Georgia	706-722-9011	www.universityhealth.org
University Hospital	Newark	New Jersey	973-972-5658	www.theuniversityhospital.com
University Hospital - Stony Brook	Stony Brook	New York	631-444-4000	www.stonybrookmedicalcenter.org
University Hospital SUNY Health Science Center	Syracuse	New York	315-473-4240	www.upstate.edu
University of California Davis Medical Center	Sacramento	California	916-734-2011	www.ucdmc.ucdavis.edu
University of Cincinnati Medical Center	Cincinnati	Ohio	513-584-1000	www.universityhospitalcincinnati.com
University of Illinois Hospital	Chicago	Illinois	312-996-3900	www.uic.edu
University of Miami Hospital	Miami	Florida	305-325-5511	www.cedarsmedicalcenter.com
University of Mississippi Medical Center	Jackson	Mississippi	601-984-4100	www.umc.edu
University of North Carolina Hospital	Chapel Hill	North Carolina	919-966-4131	www.unchealthcare.org
University of Tn Memorial Hospital	Knoxville	Tennessee	865-544-9000	www.utmedicalcenter.org
University of Toledo Medical Center	Toledo	Ohio	419-383-3407	www.utmc.utoledo.edu
University of Virginia Medical Center	Charlottesville	Virginia	800-251-3627	www.uvahealth.com
UPMC Presbyterian Shadyside	Pittsburgh	Pennsylvania	412-647-8788	www.upmc.edu
Valley Hospital	Ridgewood	New Jersey	201-447-8000	www.valleyhealth.com
Westchester Medical Center	Valhalla	New York	914-285-7017	www.wcmc.com
Wyckoff Heights Medical Center	Brooklyn	New York	718-963-7272	www.wyckoffhospital.org
Yale-New Haven Hospital	New Haven	Connecticut	203-688-4242	www.ynhh.org

Note: Table shows hospitals nationwide whose surgical complication rate is worse (higher) than U.S. rate of 4.14%

Hospitals whose Surgical Complication Rate is Better (Lower) than the U.S. National Rate

Measure: Serious Complications

Hospital	City	State	Phone	Web Site
Advocate Christ Hospital & Medical Center	Oak Lawn	Illinois	708-684-8000	www.advocatehealth.com
Allegiance Health	Jackson	Michigan	517-788-4800	www.footehealth.org
Anmed Health	Anderson	South Carolina	864-261-1109	www.anmed.com
Arkansas Heart Hospital	Little Rock	Arkansas	501-219-7000	www.arheart.com
Asante Rogue Regional Medical Center	Medford	Oregon	541-789-7000	www.asante.org
Atlanticare Regional Medical Center	Atlantic City	New Jersey	609-441-8020	www.atlanticare.org/acmc/index.html
Avera Mckennan Hospital & University Health Center	Sioux Falls	South Dakota	605-322-8000	www.mckennan.org
Baptist Beaumont Hospital	Beaumont	Texas	409-212-5012	www.mhbh.org
Baptist Health Lexington	Lexington	Kentucky	859-260-6104	www.centralbap.com
Baptist Health Louisville	Louisville	Kentucky	502-897-8100	www.baptisteast.com
Baystate Medical Center	Springfield	Massachusetts	413-794-0000	www.baystatehealth.com
Bethesda Hospital East	Boynton Beach	Florida	561-737-7733	www.bethesdahealthcare.com
Bethesda North	Cincinnati	Ohio	513-865-1241	www.trihealth.com
Billings Clinic Hospital	Billings	Montana	406-657-4000	www.billingsclinic.com
Carolina East Medical Center	New Bern	North Carolina	252-633-8640	www.cravenhealthcare.org
Carson Tahoe Regional Medical Center	Carson City	Nevada	775-445-8000	www.carsontahoehospital.com
Centinela Hospital Medical Center	Inglewood	California	310-673-4660	www.centinelafreeman.com
Central Dupage Hospital	Winfield	Illinois	630-682-1600	www.cdh.org
Christus Hospital	Beaumont	Texas	409-892-7171	www.christushealth.org
Christus Spohn Hospital Corpus Christi	Corpus Christi	Texas	361-902-4103	www.christusspohn.org
Community Hospital	Munster	Indiana	219-836-1600	www.comhs.org/community
Community Medical Center	Toms River	New Jersey	732-557-8000	www.sbhcs.com
Conway Regional Medical Center	Conway	Arkansas	501-329-3831	www.conwayregional.org
Cox Medical Center	Springfield	Missouri	417-269-6000	www.coxhealth.com
Delray Medical Center	Delray Beach	Florida	561-498-4440	www.delraymedicalctr.com
Duke University Hospital	Durham	North Carolina	919-684-8111	www.dukehealth.org
East Texas Medical Center	Tyler	Texas	903-597-0351	www.etmc.org
Englewood Hospital & Medical Center	Englewood	New Jersey	201-894-3000	www.englewoodhospital.com
Exeter Hospital	Exeter	New Hampshire	603-778-7311	www.exeterhospital.com
Floyd Medical Center	Rome	Georgia	706-509-6900	www.floydmed.org
Floyd Memorial Hospital & Health Services	New Albany	Indiana	812-949-5500	www.floydmedical.org
Genesis Medical Center - Davenport	Davenport	Iowa	563-421-1000	www.genesishealth.com
Glens Falls Hospital	Glens Falls	New York	518-926-1000	www.glensfallshospital.org
Heartland Regional Medical Center	Saint Joseph	Missouri	816-271-6000	www.heartland-health.com
Holy Cross Hospital	Fort Lauderdale	Florida	954-771-8000	www.holy-cross.com
Indiana University Health	Indianapolis	Indiana	317-962-5900	www.iuhealth.org
Indiana University Health Arnett Hospital	Lafayette	Indiana	765-448-8000	www.iuhealth.org/arnett
Integris Baptist Medical Center	Oklahoma City	Oklahoma	405-951-8110	www.integris-health.com
Integris Southwest Medical Center	Oklahoma City	Oklahoma	405-636-7000	www.integris-health.com
Jackson - Madison County General Hospital	Jackson	Tennessee	731-541-5000	www.wth.org
John Muir Medical Center - Concord Campus	Concord	California	925-674-2002	www.johnmuirhealth.com
Lakeland Hospital - Saint Joseph	Saint Joseph	Michigan	269-983-8300	www.lakelandhealth.org
Laredo Medical Center	Laredo	Texas	956-796-5000	www.laredomedical.com
Lehigh Valley Hospital - Hazleton	Hazleton	Pennsylvania	570-501-4000	www.ghha.org
Marietta Memorial Hospital	Marietta	Ohio	740-374-1400	www.mmhospital.org
Mary Washington Hospital	Fredericksburg	Virginia	540-741-1100	www.medicorp.org
Mayo Clinic	Jacksonville	Florida	904-953-2000	www.mayoclinic.org/jacksonville
Mayo Clinic Hospital	Phoenix	Arizona	480-342-2000	www.mayoclinic.org
Mayo Clinic Methodist- Hospital	Rochester	Minnesota	507-266-7890	www.mayoclinic.org/methodisthospital
Mclaren Bay Region	Bay City	Michigan	989-894-3000	www.baymed.org
Mcleod Regional Medical Center - Pee Dee	Florence	South Carolina	843-777-2900	www.mcleodhealth.org
Medcentral Health System Mansfield Hospital	Mansfield	Ohio	419-526-8000	www.medcentral.org
Memorial Healthcare System	Chattanooga	Tennessee	423-495-2525	www.memorial.org
Memorial Hermann Hospital System	Houston	Texas	713-448-6796	www.memorialhermann.org
Memorial Mission Hospital & Asheville Surgery Center	Asheville	North Carolina	828-213-1111	www.missionhospitals.org
Mercy Medical Center - Cedar Rapids	Cedar Rapids	Iowa	319-398-6011	www.mercycare.org
Methodist Hospital	San Antonio	Texas	210-575-4000	www.mh.sahealth.com
Methodist Medical Center of Illinois	Peoria	Illinois	309-672-5522	www.mmci.org
Methodist Willowbrook Hospital	Houston	Texas	281-477-1000	www.houstonmethodist.org/willowbrook-hospital
Metrowest Medical Center	Framingham	Massachusetts	508-383-1000	www.mwmc.com
Mississippi Baptist Medical Center	Jackson	Mississippi	601-968-1000	www.mbmc.org
Monongalia County General Hospital	Morgantown	West Virginia	304-598-1200	www.mongeneral.com
Mother Frances Hospital	Tyler	Texas	903-593-8441	www.tmfhs.org
Munroe Regional Medical Center	Ocala	Florida	352-351-7200	www.munroeregional.com

Hospital	City	State	Phone	Web Site
Munson Medical Center	Traverse City	Michigan	231-935-5000	www.munsonhealthcare.org
Nebraska Heart Hospital	Lincoln	Nebraska	402-328-3000	www.neheart.com
New York Community Hospital of Brooklyn	Brooklyn	New York	718-692-5302	www.nych.com
North Mississippi Medical Center	Tupelo	Mississippi	662-377-3000	www.nmhs.net/nmmc
Oklahoma Heart Hospital	Oklahoma City	Oklahoma	405-608-3200	www.okheart.com
Our Lady of Lourdes Medical Center	Camden	New Jersey	856-757-3500	www.lourdesnet.org
Palos Community Hospital	Palos Heights	Illinois	708-923-4000	www.paloshospital.org
Parkview Regional Medical Center	Fort Wayne	Indiana	260-266-1000	www.parkview.com
Parkwest Medical Center	Knoxville	Tennessee	865-970-9800	www.yesparkwest.com
Pomona Valley Hospital Medical Center	Pomona	California	909-865-9500	www.pvhmc.com
Presence Saint Joseph Medical Center	Joliet	Illinois	815-725-7133	www.provena.org/stjoes
Providence Little Co of Mary Medical Center Torrance	Torrance	California	310-540-7676	www.lcmhs.org
Providence Saint Joseph Medical Center	Burbank	California	818-843-5111	www.providence.org/losangeles
Redmond Regional Medical Center	Rome	Georgia	706-802-3012	www.redmondregional.com
Regional Medical Center Bayonet Point	Hudson	Florida	727-819-2929	www.mchealth.comorwww.heartoftampa.com
Roper Hospital	Charleston	South Carolina	843-724-2800	www.ropersaintfrancis.com
Saint Thomas West Hospital	Nashville	Tennessee	615-222-2111	www.stthomas.org
Sentara Careplex Hospital	Hampton	Virginia	757-736-1000	www.sentara.com
Sentara Leigh Hospital	Norfolk	Virginia	757-261-6601	www.sentara.com
Shasta Regional Medical Center	Redding	California	530-244-5454	www.shastaregional.com
Southcoast Hospital Group	Fall River	Massachusetts	508-679-3131	www.southcoast.org/charlton
Saint Elizabeth Medical Center	Lakeside Park	Kentucky	859-292-2000	www.stelizabeth.com
Saint Francis Hospital	Columbus	Georgia	706-596-4020	www.wecareforlife.com
Saint Francis Hospital - Roslyn	Roslyn	New York	516-562-6000	www.stfrancisheartcenter.com
Saint Luke's Hospital	Cedar Rapids	Iowa	319-369-7211	www.crstlukes.com
Saint Mary Medical Center	Langhorne	Pennsylvania	215-750-2003	www.stmaryhealthcare.org
Saint Mary Mercy Hospital	Livonia	Michigan	734-655-4800	www.stmarymercy.org
Saint Vincent Heart Center of Indiana	Indianapolis	Indiana	317-583-5000	www.theheartcenter.com
Saint Vincent Hospital & Health Services	Indianapolis	Indiana	317-338-7000	www.indianapolis.stvincent.org
Saint Vincent's Medical Center	Jacksonville	Florida	904-308-7300	www.jaxhealth.com
Sutter General Hospital	Sacramento	California	916-733-8999	www.suttermedicalcenter.org
Texas Health Harris Methodist Hurst - Euless - Bedford	Bedford	Texas	817-848-4000	www.texashealth.org
Thibodaux Regional Medical Center	Thibodaux	Louisiana	985-447-5500	www.thibodaux.com
Tuomey Healthcare System	Sumter	South Carolina	803-774-8900	www.tuomey.com
United Hospital Center	Bridgeport	West Virginia	681-342-1000	www.uhcwv.org
University Hospitals - Elyria Medical Center	Elyria	Ohio	440-329-7500	www.emh-healthcare.org
University of Michigan Health System	Ann Arbor	Michigan	734-764-1505	www.med.umich.edu
UPMC Altoona	Altoona	Pennsylvania	814-889-2011	www.altoonaregional.org
Vanderbilt University Hospital	Nashville	Tennessee	615-322-3454	www.mc.vanderbilt.edu
Virtua West Jersey Hospitals Berlin	Berlin	New Jersey	856-322-3200	www.virtua.org
Washington Hospital	Fremont	California	510-797-1111	www.whhs.com
Williamsport Regional Medical Center	Williamsport	Pennsylvania	570-321-1000	www.susquehannahealth.org
Willis Knighton Bossier Health Center	Bossier City	Louisiana	318-212-7000	www.wkhs.com/locations/bossier.aspx
Winchester Medical Center	Winchester	Virginia	540-536-8000	www.valleyhealthlink.com

Note: Table shows hospitals nationwide whose surgical complication rate is better (lower) than U.S. rate of 0.61%

Hospitals whose Surgical Complication Rate is Worse (Higher) than the U.S. National Rate

Measure: Serious Complications

Hospital	City	State	Phone	Web Site
Adirondack Medical Center	Saranac Lake	New York	518-891-4141	www.amccares.org
Appleton Medical Center	Appleton	Wisconsin	920-731-4101	www.thedacare.org
Aurora Medical Center Kenosha	Kenosha	Wisconsin	262-948-5600	www.aurorahealthcare.org
B R F Hospital Holdings	Shreveport	Louisiana	318-675-5000	www.lsumc.edu
Baptist Memorial Hospital Desoto	Southaven	Mississippi	662-772-4000	www.bmhcc.org/facilities/desoto
Baptist Saint Anthony's Hospital	Amarillo	Texas	806-212-2000	www.bsahs.com
Barnes-Jewish Hospital	Saint Louis	Missouri	314-747-3000	www.barnesjewish.org
Baylor University Medical Center	Dallas	Texas	214-820-0111	www.baylorhealth.com
Beaumont Health System	Royal Oak	Michigan	248-898-5000	www.beaumonthospitals.com
Beth Israel Deaconess Medical Center	Boston	Massachusetts	617-667-7000	www.bidmc.harvard.edu
Blessing Hospital	Quincy	Illinois	217-223-5811	www.blessinghealthsystem.org
Boston Medical Center Corporation	Boston	Massachusetts	617-638-8000	www.bmc.org
Bridgeport Hospital	Bridgeport	Connecticut	203-384-3000	www.bridgeporthospital.com
Brigham & Women's Hospital	Boston	Massachusetts	617-732-5500	www.brighamandwomens.org
Cape Coral Hospital	Cape Coral	Florida	239-574-2323	www.leememorial.org
Carilion Roanoke Memorial Hospital	Roanoke	Virginia	540-981-7000	www.carilion.com/crmh
Centennial Medical Center	Frisco	Texas	972-963-3333	www.centennialmedcenter.com
Central Texas Medical Center	San Marcos	Texas	512-753-3690	www.ctmc.org
Charleston Area Medical Center	Charleston	West Virginia	304-388-6203	www.camc.org
Chilton Medical Center	Pompton Plains	New Jersey	973-831-5000	www.chiltonmemorial.org
Christus Saint Frances Cabrini Hospital	Alexandria	Louisiana	318-487-1122	www.cabrini.org
Clearview Regional Medical Center	Monroe	Georgia	770-267-1792	www.clearviewregionalmedicalcenter.com
Cleveland Clinic	Cleveland	Ohio	216-444-2200	www.clevelandclinic.org
Clovis Community Medical Center	Clovis	California	559-324-4000	www.communitymedical.org
Community Regional Medical Center	Fresno	California	559-459-6000	www.communitymedical.org
Conemaugh Valley Memorial Hospital	Johnstown	Pennsylvania	814-534-9000	www.conemaugh.org
Cooper University Hospital	Camden	New Jersey	856-342-2000	www.cooperhealth.org
Crouse Hospital	Syracuse	New York	315-470-7449	www.crouse.org
Dameron Hospital	Stockton	California	209-944-5550	www.dameronhospital.org
Deaconess Hospital	Spokane	Washington	509-473-5800	www.deaconessmedicalcenter.org
Emory University Hospital Midtown	Atlanta	Georgia	404-686-4411	www.emoryhealthcare.org
Evanston Hospital	Evanston	Illinois	847-432-8000	www.enh.org
Firsthealth Moore Regional Hospital	Pinehurst	North Carolina	910-715-1000	www.firsthealth.org
Geisinger Medical Center	Danville	Pennsylvania	570-271-6211	www.geisinger.org
Geisinger Wyoming Valley Medical Center	Wilkes Barre	Pennsylvania	570-826-7300	www.geisinger.org
Genesys Regional Medical Center - Health Park	Grand Blanc	Michigan	810-606-5000	www.genesys.org
Gila Regional Medical Center	Silver City	New Mexico	575-538-4000	www.grmc.org
Good Samaritan Hospital	San Jose	California	408-559-2011	www.goodsamsj.org
Good Shepherd Medical Center Marshall	Marshall	Texas	903-927-6712	www.marshallregional.org
Grady Memorial Hospital	Atlanta	Georgia	404-616-4252	www.gradyhealthsystem.org
Grand View Hospital	Sellersville	Pennsylvania	215-453-4615	www.gvh.org
Grossmont Hospital	La Mesa	California	619-465-0711	www.sharp.com
Gulf Coast Medical Center Lee Memorial Health System	Fort Myers	Florida	239-768-5000	www.leememorial.org
Hackettstown Regional Medical Center	Hackettstown	New Jersey	908-852-5100	www.hrmcnj.org
Hahnemann University Hospital	Philadelphia	Pennsylvania	215-762-7000	www.hahnemannhospital.com
Harborview Medical Center	Seattle	Washington	206-731-3000	www.harborview.org
Hartford Hospital	Hartford	Connecticut	860-545-5000	www.harthosp.org
Hennepin County Medical Center	Minneapolis	Minnesota	612-873-3000	www.hcmc.org
Henry Ford Hospital	Detroit	Michigan	313-916-2600	www.henryfordhospital.com
Henry Ford West Bloomfield Hospital	W Bloomfield	Michigan	248-325-1000	www.henryford.com
Heritage Valley Beaver	Beaver	Pennsylvania	412-728-7000	www.heritagevalley.org
Holy Cross Hospital	Taos	New Mexico	575-758-8883	www.taoshospital.org
Hospital of Univ of Pennsylvania	Philadelphia	Pennsylvania	215-662-3227	www.upenn.edu
Huntington Memorial Hospital	Pasadena	California	626-397-5000	www.huntingtonhospital.com
Inova Fairfax Hospital	Falls Church	Virginia	703-776-3332	www.inova.org
Inspira Medical Center Vineland	Vineland	New Jersey	856-641-6610	www.sjhs.com
Intermountain Medical Center	Murray	Utah	801-507-7000	www.intermountainhealthcare.org
Jackson Memorial Hospital	Miami	Florida	305-585-1111	www.jhsmiami.org
JFK Medical Center - A M Yelencsics Comm Hospital	Edison	New Jersey	732-321-7000	www.jfkmc.org
John Dempsey Hospital	Farmington	Connecticut	860-679-1145	www.uconnhealth.orgorwww.uchc.edu
JPS Health Network	Fort Worth	Texas	817-921-3431	www.jpshealthnet.org
Kaweah Delta Medical Center	Visalia	California	559-624-2000	www.kaweahdelta.org
Keck Hospital of USC	Los Angeles	California	323-442-8656	www.uscuh.com
Lancaster General Hospital	Lancaster	Pennsylvania	717-299-5511	www.lancastergeneral.org

Hospital	City	State	Phone	Web Site
LDS Hospital	Salt Lake City	Utah	801-408-1100	www.intermountainhealthcare.org
Lee Memorial Hospital	Fort Myers	Florida	239-332-1111	www.leememorial.org
Lenox Hill Hospital	New York	New York	212-439-2345	www.lenoxhillhospital.org
Lourdes Hospital	Paducah	Kentucky	270-444-2444	www.ehealthconnection.com
Lower Keys Medical Center	Key West	Florida	305-294-5531	www.lkmc.com
Loyola University Medical Center	Maywood	Illinois	708-216-9000	www.lumc.edu
Magee Womens Hospital of UPMC Health System	Pittsburgh	Pennsylvania	412-641-4010	www.magee.edu
Maine Medical Center	Portland	Maine	207-662-0111	www.mmc.org
Marin General Hospital	Greenbrae	California	415-925-7900	www.maringeneral.com
Mary Hitchcock Memorial Hospital	Lebanon	New Hampshire	603-650-5000	www.dhmc.org
Mayo Clinic Health System - Mankato	Mankato	Minnesota	507-625-4031	www.isj-mhs.org
McKay Dee Hospital	Ogden	Utah	801-387-2800	www.intermountainhealthcare.org
The Medical Center of Aurora	Aurora	Colorado	303-695-2600	www.auroramed.com
Medical Center of Plano	Plano	Texas	972-596-6800	www.medicalcenterofplano.com
Medical College of Virginia Hospitals	Richmond	Virginia	804-828-0938	www.vcuhealth.org
Medical West	Bessemer	Alabama	205-481-7000	www.uab.edu
Medstar Georgetown University Hospital	Washington	District of Columbia	202-784-3000	www.georgetownuniversityhospital.org
Medstar Washington Hospital Center	Washington	District of Columbia	202-877-7000	www.whcenter.org
Memorial Medical Center	Modesto	California	209-526-4500	www.memorialmedicalcenter.org
Memorial Hospital Jacksonville	Jacksonville	Florida	904-399-6111	www.memorialhospitaljax.com
Memorial Medical Center	Springfield	Illinois	217-788-3000	www.memorialmedical.com
Menorah Medical Center	Overland Park	Kansas	913-498-6773	www.menorahmedicalcenter.com
Mercy Hospital - Cadillac	Cadillac	Michigan	231-876-7200	www.mercycadillac.munsonhealthcare.org
Mercy Memorial Health Center	Ardmore	Oklahoma	405-223-5400	www.mercyok.com/mmhc
Mercy Saint Vincent Medical Center	Toledo	Ohio	419-251-3232	www.mhsnr.org
Metrohealth System	Cleveland	Ohio	216-778-7089	www.metrohealth.org
Miami Valley Hospital	Dayton	Ohio	937-208-8000	www.miamivalleyhospital.com
Milton S Hershey Medical Center	Hershey	Pennsylvania	717-531-8521	www.hmc.psu.edu
Ministry Saint Josephs Hospital	Marshfield	Wisconsin	715-387-7850	www.stjosephs-marshfield.org
Montefiore Medical Center	Bronx	New York	718-920-4321	www.montefiore.org
Newark Beth Israel Medical Center	Newark	New Jersey	973-926-7850	www.sbhcs.com
North Shore University Hospital	Manhasset	New York	516-562-0100	www.northshorelij.com
North Suburban Medical Center	Thornton	Colorado	303-451-7800	www.northsuburban.com
Novant Health Presbyterian Medical Center	Charlotte	North Carolina	704-384-4000	www.presbyterian.org
NYU Hospitals Center	New York	New York	212-263-7300	www.med.nyu.edu
O U Medical Center	Oklahoma City	Oklahoma	405-271-5911	www.oumedcenter.com
OHSU Hospital & Clinics	Portland	Oregon	503-494-4036	www.ohsu.edu
Our Lady of the Lake Regional Medical Center	Baton Rouge	Louisiana	225-765-6565	www.ololrmc.com
Overland Park Regional Medical Center	Overland Park	Kansas	913-541-5301	www.oprmc.com
Parkland Health & Hospital System	Dallas	Texas	214-590-8000	www.parklandhospital.com
Parkview Medical Center	Pueblo	Colorado	719-584-4000	www.parkviewmc.com
Piedmont Hospital	Atlanta	Georgia	404-605-5000	www.piedmonthospital.org
Pinnacle Health Hospitals	Harrisburg	Pennsylvania	717-782-5181	www.pinnaclehealth.org
Plainview Hospital	Plainview	New York	516-719-3000	www.nslij.com
Providence Holy Cross Medical Center	Mission Hills	California	818-365-8051	www.providence.org
Providence Sacred Heart Medical Center	Spokane	Washington	509-474-3040	www.shmc.org
Rhode Island Hospital	Providence	Rhode Island	401-444-4000	www.rhodeislandhospital.org
Ridgeview Medical Center	Waconia	Minnesota	952-442-2191	www.ridgeviewmedical.org
Robert Wood Johnson University Hospital	New Brunswick	New Jersey	732-937-8900	www.rwjuh.edu
Ronald Reagan UCLA Medical Center	Los Angeles	California	310-825-6301	www.uclahealth.org
Rose Medical Center	Denver	Colorado	303-320-2121	www.rosemed.com
Rush University Medical Center	Chicago	Illinois	312-942-5000	www.ruch.edu
Sacred Heart Hospital	Eau Claire	Wisconsin	715-717-4121	www.sacredhearteauclaire.org
Saint Anthony Medical Center	Rockford	Illinois	815-226-2000	www.osfhealth.com
Saint Barnabas Medical Center	Livingston	New Jersey	973-322-5000	www.saintbarnabas.com
Saint Francis Medical Center	Peoria	Illinois	309-655-2000	www.osfsaintfrancis.org
Saint Mary's Health Care	Grand Rapids	Michigan	616-685-5000	www.smhealthcare.org
Santa Clara Valley Medical Center	San Jose	California	408-885-5000	www.sccgov.org
Saratoga Hospital	Saratoga Springs	New York	518-587-3222	www.saratogacare.org
Sentara Norfolk General Hospital	Norfolk	Virginia	757-388-3000	www.sentara.com
Sharp Memorial Hospital	San Diego	California	858-939-3400	www.sharp.com/memorial
Sierra Medical Center	El Paso	Texas	915-747-4000	www.sphn.com
Sinai - Grace Hospital	Detroit	Michigan	313-966-3300	www.sinaigrace.org
Somerset Medical Center	Somerville	New Jersey	908-685-2200	www.somersetmedicalcenter.com
Springhill Medical Center	Mobile	Alabama	251-344-9630	www.springhillmedicalcenter.com
Saint Alphonsus Regional Medical Center	Boise	Idaho	208-367-2121	www.saintalphonsus.org
Saint Clare Hospital	Lakewood	Washington	253-588-1711	www.fhshealth.org

Hospital	City	State	Phone	Web Site
Saint Elizabeth Health Center	Youngstown	Ohio	330-746-7211	www.hmhs.org
Saint Joseph Medical Center	Tacoma	Washington	253-627-4101	www.fhshealth.org
Saint Joseph Mercy Hospital	Ann Arbor	Michigan	734-712-3791	www.stjoesannarbor.or
Saint Joseph's Hospital & Medical Center	Phoenix	Arizona	602-406-3000	www.stjosephs-phx.org
Saint Louis University Hospital	Saint Louis	Missouri	314-577-8000	www.slucare.edu/clinical
Saint Luke's Hospital Bethlehem	Bethlehem	Pennsylvania	610-954-4000	www.slhn-lehighvalley.org
Saint Luke's Episcopal Hospital	Houston	Texas	832-355-1000	www.sleh.com
Saint Luke's Hospital	Chesterfield	Missouri	314-434-1500	www.goodhealthmatters.com
Saint Luke's Hospital of Kansas City	Kansas City	Missouri	816-932-2000	www.staintlukeshealthsystem.org
Stamford Hospital	Stamford	Connecticut	203-276-1000	www.stamhealth.org
Summa Health Systems Hospitals	Akron	Ohio	330-375-3000	www.summahealth.org
Sunrise Hospital & Medical Center	Las Vegas	Nevada	702-731-8000	www.sunrisehospital.com
Swedish Medical Center	Englewood	Colorado	303-788-5000	www.swedishhospital.com/default.asp
Swedish Medical Center - Cherry Hill	Seattle	Washington	206-320-2000	www.swedish.org
Tampa General Hospital	Tampa	Florida	813-844-7000	www.tgh.org
The University of Chicago Medical Center	Chicago	Illinois	773-702-1000	www.uchospitals.edu
Theda Clark Medical Center	Neenah	Wisconsin	920-729-3100	www.thedacare.org
Thomas Hospital	Fairhope	Alabama	251-928-2375	www.thomashospital.com
Thomas Jefferson University Hospital	Philadelphia	Pennsylvania	215-955-6000	www.jeffersonhospital.org
Trinity Hospitals	Minot	North Dakota	701-857-5000	www.trinityhealth.org
Trinity Medical Center	Birmingham	Alabama	205-592-1000	www.bhsala.com/montclair
Tucson Medical Center	Tucson	Arizona	520-327-5461	www.tmcaz.com
Tulane Medical Center	New Orleans	Louisiana	504-988-1900	www.tuhc.com
UF Health Jacksonville	Jacksonville	Florida	904-244-0411	www.shandsjacksonville.org
UMC of Southern Nevada	Las Vegas	Nevada	702-383-2000	www.umc-cares.org
University Colo Health Memorial Hospital Central	Colorado Springs	Colorado	719-365-5000	www.memorialhospital.com
University Health System	San Antonio	Texas	210-358-4000	www.universityhealthsystem.com
University Hospital - Stony Brook	Stony Brook	New York	631-444-4000	www.stonybrookmedicalcenter.org
University Hospital SUNY Health Science Center	Syracuse	New York	315-473-4240	www.upstate.edu
University Medical Center of El Paso	El Paso	Texas	915-521-7602	www.thomasoncares.org
University of Alabama Hospital	Birmingham	Alabama	205-934-4011	www.health.uab.edu
University of California Davis Medical Center	Sacramento	California	916-734-2011	www.ucdmc.ucdavis.edu
University of Cincinnati Medical Center	Cincinnati	Ohio	513-584-1000	www.universityhospitalcincinnati.com
University of Illinois Hospital	Chicago	Illinois	312-996-3900	www.uic.edu
University of Kansas Hospital	Kansas City	Kansas	913-588-7332	www.kumc.edu
University of Miami Hospital	Miami	Florida	305-325-5511	www.cedarsmedicalcenter.com
University of Mississippi Medical Center	Jackson	Mississippi	601-984-4100	www.umc.edu
University of Toledo Medical Center	Toledo	Ohio	419-383-3407	www.utmc.utoledo.edu
UPMC Hamot	Erie	Pennsylvania	814-877-6000	www.hamot.org
UPMC Passavant	Pittsburgh	Pennsylvania	412-367-6700	www.passavant.upmc.com
UPMC Presbyterian Shadyside	Pittsburgh	Pennsylvania	412-647-8788	www.upmc.edu
UT Southwestern University Hospital	Dallas	Texas	214-879-3758	www.utsouthwestern.edu
Utah Valley Regional Medical Center	Provo	Utah	801-373-7850	www.intermountainhealthcare.org/hospitals/uvrmc
Valley Hospital	Ridgewood	New Jersey	201-447-8000	www.valleyhealth.com
Vidant Medical Center	Greenville	North Carolina	252-847-4100	www.uhseast.com
Waukesha Memorial Hospital	Waukesha	Wisconsin	262-928-1000	www.waukeshamemorial.org
Wesley Medical Center	Hattiesburg	Mississippi	601-268-8000	www.wesley.com
West Virginia University Hospitals	Morgantown	West Virginia	304-598-4000	www.wvuh.com
Wheaton Franciscan Saint Joseph	Milwaukee	Wisconsin	414-447-2000	www.wfhealthcare.org
Yale-New Haven Hospital	New Haven	Connecticut	203-688-4242	www.ynhh.org

Note: Table shows hospitals nationwide whose surgical complication rate is worse (higher) than U.S. rate of 0.61%

Surgical Complication Rate: State and National Summary

Measure: A Wound That Splits Open After Surgery on the Abdomen or Pelvis

Area	Number of Hospitals			
	Better than U.S. National Rate[1]	Worse than U.S. National Rate[2]	No Different than U.S. National Rate[3]	Number of Cases Too Small[4]
U.S. and Territories	0	42	2703	391
Alabama	0	0	58	18
Alaska	0	0	8	0
American Samoa	n/a	n/a	n/a	n/a
Arizona	0	1	49	9
Arkansas	0	0	35	9
California	0	2	245	49
Colorado	0	2	37	4
Connecticut	0	0	29	0
Delaware	0	0	6	0
District of Columbia	0	1	6	0
Florida	0	2	157	3
Georgia	0	2	83	15
Guam	n/a	n/a	n/a	n/a
Hawaii	0	1	11	2
Idaho	0	1	10	1
Illinois	0	0	122	3
Indiana	0	0	72	11
Iowa	0	0	30	4
Kansas	0	0	39	11
Kentucky	0	2	51	10
Louisiana	0	1	62	17
Maine	0	1	18	1
Maryland	n/a	n/a	n/a	n/a
Massachusetts	0	0	57	1
Michigan	0	4	80	6
Minnesota	0	1	40	9
Mississippi	0	0	37	7
Missouri	0	1	61	10
Montana	0	0	11	1
N. Mariana Islands	n/a	n/a	n/a	n/a
Nebraska	0	0	19	0
Nevada	0	2	19	0
New Hampshire	0	1	12	0
New Jersey	0	2	59	3
New Mexico	0	1	22	3
New York	0	1	146	9
North Carolina	0	2	79	4
North Dakota	0	0	6	0
Ohio	0	3	117	7
Oklahoma	0	0	47	21
Oregon	0	0	32	0
Pennsylvania	0	2	128	14
Puerto Rico	n/a	n/a	n/a	n/a
Rhode Island	0	0	11	0
South Carolina	0	0	49	4
South Dakota	0	0	10	7
Tennessee	0	1	66	22
Texas	0	2	205	55
Utah	0	0	23	4
Vermont	0	0	6	0
Virgin Islands	n/a	n/a	n/a	n/a
Virginia	0	1	64	7
Washington	0	0	46	2
West Virginia	0	0	28	3
Wisconsin	0	2	58	4
Wyoming	0	0	9	2

Note: (1) Surgical complication rate is better (lower) than U.S. rate of 0.92%; (2) Surgical complication rate is worse (higher) than U.S. rate of 0.92%; (3) Surgical complication rate is about the same as U.S. rate of 0.92%; (4) The number of cases is too small to classify the hospital; n/a not available

Surgical Complication Rate: State and National Summary

Measure: Accidental Cuts and Tears From Medical Treatment

Area	Number of Hospitals			
	Better than U.S. National Rate[1]	Worse than U.S. National Rate[2]	No Different than U.S. National Rate[3]	Number of Cases Too Small[4]
U.S. and Territories	95	203	3133	42
Alabama	0	8	89	0
Alaska	0	2	7	0
American Samoa	n/a	n/a	n/a	n/a
Arizona	1	4	61	1
Arkansas	1	0	45	0
California	7	22	280	1
Colorado	0	5	40	1
Connecticut	0	4	27	1
Delaware	1	0	5	0
District of Columbia	0	1	6	0
Florida	11	8	151	1
Georgia	2	6	100	0
Guam	n/a	n/a	n/a	n/a
Hawaii	0	1	13	0
Idaho	0	0	13	1
Illinois	10	7	111	1
Indiana	2	4	83	1
Iowa	0	3	31	0
Kansas	0	4	52	0
Kentucky	1	3	61	0
Louisiana	0	4	88	6
Maine	0	1	19	0
Maryland	n/a	n/a	n/a	n/a
Massachusetts	3	4	54	0
Michigan	3	7	85	0
Minnesota	2	4	46	0
Mississippi	1	2	61	3
Missouri	0	5	71	2
Montana	0	0	13	0
N. Mariana Islands	n/a	n/a	n/a	n/a
Nebraska	1	1	21	1
Nevada	0	2	22	0
New Hampshire	0	3	10	0
New Jersey	8	3	54	1
New Mexico	1	1	31	0
New York	5	4	158	2
North Carolina	1	6	82	0
North Dakota	0	1	6	0
Ohio	3	9	126	3
Oklahoma	3	3	83	2
Oregon	1	3	29	0
Pennsylvania	2	11	140	3
Puerto Rico	n/a	n/a	n/a	n/a
Rhode Island	0	3	8	0
South Carolina	2	3	52	0
South Dakota	0	1	20	0
Tennessee	5	0	92	0
Texas	11	10	301	7
Utah	0	5	26	1
Vermont	0	1	5	0
Virgin Islands	n/a	n/a	n/a	n/a
Virginia	5	3	70	2
Washington	0	11	37	0
West Virginia	1	1	29	0
Wisconsin	0	9	57	0
Wyoming	0	0	11	0

Note: (1) Surgical complication rate is better (lower) than U.S. rate of 1.83%; (2) Surgical complication rate is worse (higher) than U.S. rate of 1.83%; (3) Surgical complication rate is about the same as U.S. rate of 1.83%; (4) The number of cases is too small to classify the hospital; n/a not available

Surgical Complication Rate: State and National Summary

Measure: Collapsed Lung Due to Medical Treatment

Area	Number of Hospitals			
	Better than U.S. National Rate[1]	Worse than U.S. National Rate[2]	No Different than U.S. National Rate[3]	Number of Cases Too Small[4]
U.S. and Territories	9	60	3366	38
Alabama	0	2	95	0
Alaska	0	0	9	0
American Samoa	n/a	n/a	n/a	n/a
Arizona	0	1	65	1
Arkansas	0	1	45	0
California	1	7	302	0
Colorado	0	0	45	1
Connecticut	0	0	31	1
Delaware	0	0	6	0
District of Columbia	0	0	7	0
Florida	0	4	166	1
Georgia	0	2	106	0
Guam	n/a	n/a	n/a	n/a
Hawaii	0	0	14	0
Idaho	0	0	13	1
Illinois	1	2	125	1
Indiana	0	0	89	1
Iowa	0	0	34	0
Kansas	0	3	52	1
Kentucky	1	2	62	0
Louisiana	1	1	92	4
Maine	0	1	19	0
Maryland	n/a	n/a	n/a	n/a
Massachusetts	0	3	58	0
Michigan	1	2	92	0
Minnesota	0	0	52	0
Mississippi	0	0	64	3
Missouri	0	4	72	2
Montana	0	0	13	0
N. Mariana Islands	n/a	n/a	n/a	n/a
Nebraska	0	1	23	0
Nevada	0	1	23	0
New Hampshire	0	0	13	0
New Jersey	2	0	63	1
New Mexico	0	0	33	0
New York	1	4	162	2
North Carolina	0	1	88	0
North Dakota	0	1	6	0
Ohio	0	1	136	4
Oklahoma	0	2	88	1
Oregon	0	1	32	0
Pennsylvania	0	2	152	2
Puerto Rico	n/a	n/a	n/a	n/a
Rhode Island	0	0	11	0
South Carolina	0	1	56	0
South Dakota	0	0	21	0
Tennessee	0	1	96	0
Texas	0	6	316	7
Utah	0	0	31	1
Vermont	0	0	6	0
Virgin Islands	n/a	n/a	n/a	n/a
Virginia	1	2	75	2
Washington	0	0	48	0
West Virginia	0	0	31	0
Wisconsin	0	1	65	0
Wyoming	0	0	11	0

Note: (1) Surgical complication rate is better (lower) than U.S. rate of 0.32%; (2) Surgical complication rate is worse (higher) than U.S. rate of 0.32%; (3) Surgical complication rate is about the same as U.S. rate of 0.32%; (4) The number of cases is too small to classify the hospital; n/a not available

Surgical Complication Rate: State and National Summary

Measure: Deaths Among Patients With Serious Treatable Complications After Surgery

Area	Number of Hospitals			
	Better than U.S. National Rate[1]	Worse than U.S. National Rate[2]	No Different than U.S. National Rate[3]	Number of Cases Too Small[4]
U.S. and Territories	43	70	1831	1058
Alabama	0	6	33	29
Alaska	0	1	4	3
American Samoa	n/a	n/a	n/a	n/a
Arizona	3	0	39	15
Arkansas	0	1	20	17
California	1	3	164	116
Colorado	1	0	27	14
Connecticut	0	0	22	7
Delaware	0	1	4	1
District of Columbia	0	0	6	1
Florida	6	5	124	26
Georgia	2	5	50	41
Guam	n/a	n/a	n/a	n/a
Hawaii	0	0	5	9
Idaho	0	0	8	4
Illinois	7	1	87	29
Indiana	1	0	54	29
Iowa	1	0	22	10
Kansas	0	0	25	23
Kentucky	0	3	31	25
Louisiana	0	0	38	28
Maine	0	0	9	11
Maryland	n/a	n/a	n/a	n/a
Massachusetts	0	1	42	15
Michigan	4	0	56	28
Minnesota	1	0	23	24
Mississippi	0	3	20	16
Missouri	2	1	44	23
Montana	0	0	9	2
N. Mariana Islands	n/a	n/a	n/a	n/a
Nebraska	0	0	17	5
Nevada	0	2	14	5
New Hampshire	0	1	10	2
New Jersey	2	5	50	7
New Mexico	0	0	10	14
New York	2	4	91	58
North Carolina	0	4	57	25
North Dakota	1	0	5	0
Ohio	1	1	84	37
Oklahoma	0	4	27	27
Oregon	1	0	17	14
Pennsylvania	0	2	80	60
Puerto Rico	n/a	n/a	n/a	n/a
Rhode Island	0	0	7	4
South Carolina	0	3	29	21
South Dakota	0	0	6	9
Tennessee	0	2	45	30
Texas	5	5	147	81
Utah	0	0	16	11
Vermont	0	1	3	2
Virgin Islands	n/a	n/a	n/a	n/a
Virginia	0	1	46	21
Washington	0	0	40	6
West Virginia	0	1	19	8
Wisconsin	2	0	39	25
Wyoming	0	0	2	9

Note: (1) Surgical complication rate is better (lower) than U.S. rate of 110.25%; (2) Surgical complication rate is worse (higher) than U.S. rate of 110.25%; (3) Surgical complication rate is about the same as U.S. rate of 110.25%; (4) The number of cases is too small to classify the hospital; n/a not available

Surgical Complication Rate: State and National Summary

Measure: Rate of Complications for Hip/Knee Replacement Patients

Area	Number of Hospitals			
	Better than U.S. National Rate[1]	Worse than U.S. National Rate[2]	No Different than U.S. National Rate[3]	Number of Cases Too Small[4]
U.S. and Territories	75	68	2655	687
Alabama	0	4	46	11
Alaska	0	0	7	1
American Samoa	0	0	0	0
Arizona	1	0	48	6
Arkansas	1	1	28	7
California	7	4	196	89
Colorado	1	3	46	6
Connecticut	1	2	26	0
Delaware	0	0	5	1
District of Columbia	0	0	5	2
Florida	11	1	134	16
Georgia	2	1	76	15
Guam	0	0	0	0
Hawaii	0	0	8	6
Idaho	0	0	23	5
Illinois	2	3	108	25
Indiana	4	1	73	32
Iowa	0	2	46	17
Kansas	3	2	37	13
Kentucky	1	0	41	19
Louisiana	0	0	59	16
Maine	1	1	24	5
Maryland	2	1	41	1
Massachusetts	2	0	54	5
Michigan	6	2	88	20
Minnesota	1	0	65	17
Mississippi	2	1	24	9
Missouri	3	2	61	14
Montana	0	1	19	6
N. Mariana Islands	0	0	0	0
Nebraska	2	0	30	13
Nevada	0	1	22	2
New Hampshire	0	1	21	4
New Jersey	0	1	53	9
New Mexico	0	0	22	2
New York	4	2	116	30
North Carolina	1	4	77	8
North Dakota	1	0	7	1
Ohio	2	6	128	21
Oklahoma	1	1	46	18
Oregon	0	0	40	10
Pennsylvania	0	6	123	27
Puerto Rico	0	0	8	27
Rhode Island	0	0	9	1
South Carolina	1	0	39	14
South Dakota	0	0	16	2
Tennessee	2	3	50	21
Texas	7	4	198	54
Utah	0	1	25	6
Vermont	0	0	12	1
Virgin Islands	0	0	1	0
Virginia	2	2	54	11
Washington	1	0	52	9
West Virginia	0	0	26	6
Wisconsin	0	4	79	22
Wyoming	0	0	13	4

Note: (1) Surgical complication rate is better (lower) than U.S. rate of 3.4%; (2) Surgical complication rate is worse (higher) than U.S. rate of 3.4%; (3) Surgical complication rate is about the same as U.S. rate of 3.4%; (4) The number of cases is too small to classify the hospital; n/a not available

Surgical Complication Rate: State and National Summary

Measure: Serious Blood Clots After Surgery

Area	Number of Hospitals			
	Better than U.S. National Rate[1]	Worse than U.S. National Rate[2]	No Different than U.S. National Rate[3]	Number of Cases Too Small[4]
U.S. and Territories	155	203	2846	114
Alabama	1	3	72	5
Alaska	0	0	8	1
American Samoa	n/a	n/a	n/a	n/a
Arizona	3	1	58	1
Arkansas	3	0	41	2
California	16	8	274	5
Colorado	2	4	38	0
Connecticut	1	5	23	0
Delaware	0	1	5	0
District of Columbia	0	1	6	0
Florida	7	18	138	2
Georgia	2	6	92	4
Guam	n/a	n/a	n/a	n/a
Hawaii	0	0	14	0
Idaho	2	1	10	1
Illinois	5	20	100	2
Indiana	8	1	79	1
Iowa	4	1	29	0
Kansas	4	2	46	3
Kentucky	4	2	57	2
Louisiana	2	3	80	7
Maine	1	0	19	0
Maryland	n/a	n/a	n/a	n/a
Massachusetts	4	2	52	2
Michigan	5	13	74	0
Minnesota	4	0	47	0
Mississippi	1	3	39	9
Missouri	3	5	62	5
Montana	5	0	7	1
N. Mariana Islands	n/a	n/a	n/a	n/a
Nebraska	0	0	23	0
Nevada	1	0	20	0
New Hampshire	1	2	10	0
New Jersey	2	15	47	1
New Mexico	1	2	23	3
New York	3	21	133	5
North Carolina	6	2	79	0
North Dakota	2	0	4	0
Ohio	0	9	122	4
Oklahoma	4	1	68	11
Oregon	4	2	26	1
Pennsylvania	1	23	127	2
Puerto Rico	n/a	n/a	n/a	n/a
Rhode Island	0	0	11	0
South Carolina	1	0	54	2
South Dakota	3	0	15	1
Tennessee	8	2	77	5
Texas	13	12	257	23
Utah	1	1	27	1
Vermont	0	0	6	0
Virgin Islands	n/a	n/a	n/a	n/a
Virginia	5	4	62	1
Washington	7	2	39	0
West Virginia	1	2	28	0
Wisconsin	3	2	61	0
Wyoming	1	0	10	0

Note: (1) Surgical complication rate is better (lower) than U.S. rate of 4.14%; (2) Surgical complication rate is worse (higher) than U.S. rate of 4.14%; (3) Surgical complication rate is about the same as U.S. rate of 4.14%; (4) The number of cases is too small to classify the hospital; n/a not available

Surgical Complication Rate: State and National Summary

Measure: Serious Complications

Area	Number of Hospitals			
	Better than U.S. National Rate[1]	Worse than U.S. National Rate[2]	No Different than U.S. National Rate[3]	Number of Cases Too Small[4]
U.S. and Territories	108	182	3184	0
Alabama	0	5	92	0
Alaska	0	0	9	0
American Samoa	n/a	n/a	n/a	n/a
Arizona	1	2	64	0
Arkansas	2	0	44	0
California	8	15	287	0
Colorado	0	6	40	0
Connecticut	0	6	26	0
Delaware	0	0	6	0
District of Columbia	0	2	5	0
Florida	7	9	155	0
Georgia	3	4	101	0
Guam	n/a	n/a	n/a	n/a
Hawaii	0	0	14	0
Idaho	0	1	13	0
Illinois	5	9	115	0
Indiana	7	0	83	0
Iowa	3	0	31	0
Kansas	0	3	53	0
Kentucky	3	1	61	0
Louisiana	2	4	92	0
Maine	0	1	19	0
Maryland	n/a	n/a	n/a	n/a
Massachusetts	3	3	55	0
Michigan	6	8	81	0
Minnesota	1	3	48	0
Mississippi	2	3	62	0
Missouri	2	4	72	0
Montana	1	0	12	0
N. Mariana Islands	n/a	n/a	n/a	n/a
Nebraska	1	0	23	0
Nevada	1	2	21	0
New Hampshire	1	1	11	0
New Jersey	5	10	51	0
New Mexico	0	2	31	0
New York	3	10	157	0
North Carolina	3	3	83	0
North Dakota	0	1	6	0
Ohio	4	8	129	0
Oklahoma	3	2	86	0
Oregon	1	1	31	0
Pennsylvania	4	16	136	0
Puerto Rico	n/a	n/a	n/a	n/a
Rhode Island	0	1	10	0
South Carolina	4	0	53	0
South Dakota	1	0	20	0
Tennessee	5	0	92	0
Texas	10	13	306	0
Utah	0	4	28	0
Vermont	0	0	6	0
Virgin Islands	n/a	n/a	n/a	n/a
Virginia	4	4	72	0
Washington	0	6	42	0
West Virginia	2	2	27	0
Wisconsin	0	7	59	0
Wyoming	0	0	11	0

Note: (1) Surgical complication rate is better (lower) than U.S. rate of 0.61%; (2) Surgical complication rate is worse (higher) than U.S. rate of 0.61%; (3) Surgical complication rate is about the same as U.S. rate of 0.61%; (4) The number of cases is too small to classify the hospital; n/a not available

Appendix D: Best Hospitals by Selected Category

What Do These Tables Show?

This appendix shows the best hospitals nationwide based on their average scores in 11 categories. The categories are:

- Blood Clot Prevention and Treatment
- Children's Asthma Care
- Emergency Department Care
- Heart Care
- Pneumonia Care
- Preventative Care
- Stroke Care
- Surgical Care
- Patient's Hospital Experiences
- Use of Medical Imaging
- Lowest Medicare Spending per Beneficiary

How Were the Hospitals Selected?

Hospitals were selected for inclusion in three ways:

- Hospitals that achieved a perfect 100% average score in all qualified measures in a given category.
- Hospitals that were in the top 5% of hospitals based on their average score in a given category.
- Hospitals whose Medicare spending ratios fell below a certain threshold.

How Were Average Scores Calculated?

The average score for any given category was calculated by averaging the scores of the individual measures that made up that category. In some instances, not all measures were included in the average score calculation. A meaure was omitted if: 1) data was not available 2) the measure did not meet the 25 case threshold for inclusion (except Patient's Hospital Experiences in which the threshold was 100 or more completed surveys). Note that the Pregnancy Care category did not have enough information available to calculate an average score.

Best Hospitals for Blood Clot Prevention and Treatment

Hospital	City	State	Phone	Web Site
Baptist Hospital of Miami	Miami	Florida	786-596-1960	www.baptisthealth.net
Berkshire Medical Center	Pittsfield	Massachusetts	413-447-2000	www.berkshirehealthsystems.org
Blanchard Valley Hospital	Findlay	Ohio	419-423-4500	www.bvha.org
Boca Raton Regional Hospital	Boca Raton	Florida	561-362-5002	www.brrh.com
Brandon Regional Hospital	Brandon	Florida	813-681-5551	www.brandonregionalhospital.com
Capital Regional Medical Center	Tallahassee	Florida	850-656-5000	www.capitalregionalmedicalcenter.com
Centerpoint Medical Center	Independence	Missouri	816-698-7000	www.centerpointmedical.com
Community Hospital of the Monterey Peninsula	Monterey	California	831-624-5311	www.chomp.org
Delray Medical Center	Delray Beach	Florida	561-498-4440	www.delraymedicalctr.com
Doctors' Community Hospital	Lanham	Maryland	301-552-8085	www.dchweb.org
Fairview Southdale Hospital	Edina	Minnesota	952-924-5000	www.fairview.org
Flushing Hospital Medical Center	Flushing	New York	718-670-5000	www.flushinghospital.org
Fort Sanders Regional Medical Center	Knoxville	Tennessee	865-541-1101	www.fsregional.com
Henrico Doctors' Hospital	Richmond	Virginia	804-289-4500	www.henricodoctors.com
Heritage Valley Beaver	Beaver	Pennsylvania	412-728-7000	www.heritagevalley.org
Heritage Valley Sewickley	Sewickley	Pennsylvania	412-741-6600	www.heritagevalley.org
John Randolph Medical Center	Hopewell	Virginia	804-541-1600	www.johnrandolphmed.com
Kaiser Foundation Hospital - Roseville	Roseville	California	916-784-4000	www.kaiserpermanente.org/roseville
Kendall Regional Medical Center	Miami	Florida	305-223-3000	www.kendallmed.com
Lewisgale Medical Center	Salem	Virginia	540-776-4000	www.lewis-gale.com
Lovelace Medical Center	Albuquerque	New Mexico	505-727-8000	www.lovelace.com
Mclaren Lapeer Region	Lapeer	Michigan	810-667-5500	www.lapeerregional.org
The Medical Center of Aurora	Aurora	Colorado	303-695-2600	www.auroramed.com
Medical Center of Plano	Plano	Texas	972-596-6800	www.medicalcenterofplano.com
Memorial Hospital Pembroke	Pembroke Pines	Florida	954-962-9650	www.memorialpembroke.com\
Memorial Hospital West	Pembroke Pines	Florida	954-436-5000	www.memorialwest.com
Memorial Regional Hospital	Hollywood	Florida	954-987-2000	www.memorialregional.com
Mercy Hospital of Folsom	Folsom	California	916-983-7400	www.mercyfolsom.org
Mercy Memorial Hospital System	Monroe	Michigan	734-240-8400	www.mercymemorial.org
Methodist Dallas Medical Center	Dallas	Texas	214-947-2879	www.mhd.com
Mountain View Regional Medical Center	Las Cruces	New Mexico	575-556-7600	www.mountainviewregional.com
Nazareth Hospital	Philadelphia	Pennsylvania	215-335-6000	www.nazarethhospital.org
North Florida Regional Medical Center	Gainesville	Florida	352-333-4100	www.nfrmc.com
Northside Hospital	Atlanta	Georgia	404-851-8000	www.northside.com
Northside Hospital Cherokee	Canton	Georgia	770-720-5298	www.northside.com/cherokee
Northside Hospital Forsyth	Cumming	Georgia	404-851-8700	www.gbhcs.org
Novant Health Forsyth Medical Center	Winston-Salem	North Carolina	336-718-5000	www.forsythmedicalcenter.org
Oak Hill Hospital	Brooksville	Florida	352-596-6632	www.oakhillhospital.com
Orange Park Medical Center	Orange Park	Florida	904-276-8500	www.opmedical.com
Overland Park Regional Medical Center	Overland Park	Kansas	913-541-5301	www.oprmc.com
Rapides Regional Medical Center	Alexandria	Louisiana	318-769-3000	www.rapidesregional.com
Regional Medical Center Bayonet Point	Hudson	Florida	727-819-2929	www.mchealth.comorwww.heartoftampa.com
Riverside Medical Center	Kankakee	Illinois	815-933-1671	www.riversidehealthcare.org
Rockdale Medical Center	Conyers	Georgia	770-918-3000	www.rockdalehospital.org
Rose Medical Center	Denver	Colorado	303-320-2121	www.rosemed.com
Saint Clares Hospital of Weston	Weston	Wisconsin	715-393-3000	www.ministryhealth.org
Saint Lucie Medical Center	Port Saint Lucie	Florida	772-335-4000	www.stluciemed.com
Saint Mary Medical Center	Hobart	Indiana	219-942-0551	www.comhs.org/stmary
Saint Mary's Medical Center	West Palm Beach	Florida	561-840-6202	www.stmarysmc.com
Saint Mary's Medical Center	Blue Springs	Missouri	816-228-5900	www.stmaryskc.com
Saint Vincent's Medical Center Southside	Jacksonville	Florida	904-296-3700	www.jaxhealth.com
Sisters of Charity Hospital	Buffalo	New York	716-862-1000	www.chsbuffalo.org
South Miami Hospital	South Miami	Florida	786-662-4000	www.baptisthealth.net
Southern Hills Hospital & Medical Center	Las Vegas	Nevada	702-880-2100	www.southernhillshospital.com
Springs Memorial Hospital	Lancaster	South Carolina	803-286-1481	www.springsmemorial.com
Summa Western Reserve Hospital	Cuyahoga Falls	Ohio	330-971-7000	www.westernreservehospital.org
Texoma Medical Center	Denison	Texas	903-416-4000	www.texomamedicalcenter.net
Trinity Medical Center	Birmingham	Alabama	205-592-1000	www.bhsala.com/montclair
Tulane Medical Center	New Orleans	Louisiana	504-988-1900	www.tuhc.com
United Hospital Center	Bridgeport	West Virginia	681-342-1000	www.uhcwv.org
University Medical Center of El Paso	El Paso	Texas	915-521-7602	www.thomasoncares.org
UPMC Horizon	Greenville	Pennsylvania	724-588-2100	www.upmc.com
UPMC Mckeesport	Mc Keesport	Pennsylvania	412-664-2000	www.selectmedicalcorp.com
Venice Regional Medical Center - Bayfront Health	Venice	Florida	941-485-7711	www.veniceregional.com
Vista Medical Center East	Waukegan	Illinois	847-360-4000	www.vistahealth.com

Hospital	City	State	Phone	Web Site
Wesley Medical Center	Wichita	Kansas	316-962-2000	www.wesleymc.com
West Georgia Medical Center	Lagrange	Georgia	706-882-1411	www.wghealth.org
West Virginia University Hospitals	Morgantown	West Virginia	304-598-4000	www.wvuh.com

Note: The hospitals shown above represent the top 5% of the 1,268 hospitals nationwide for which an average score was calculated. Average scores were calculated for hospitals with qualifying data (25 cases or more) in at least 5 of 6 measures in the Blood Clot Prevention and Treatment category.

Best Hospitals for Children's Asthma Care

Hospital	City	State	Phone	Web Site
Carroll Hospital Center	Westminster	Maryland	410-848-3000	www.carrollhospitalcenter.org
Cleveland Clinic	Cleveland	Ohio	216-444-2200	www.clevelandclinic.org
Lawnwood Regional Medical Center & Heart Institute	Fort Pierce	Florida	772-461-4000	www.lawnwoodmed.com
Memorial Regional Hospital	Hollywood	Florida	954-987-2000	www.memorialregional.com
Renown Regional Medical Center	Reno	Nevada	775-982-4100	www.renown.org

Note: The hospitals shown above represent the top 5% of the 90 hospitals nationwide for which an average score was calculated. Average scores were calculated for hospitals with qualifying data (25 cases or more) in all three measures in the Children's Asthma category.

Best Hospitals for Emergency Department Care

Hospital	City	State	Phone	Web Site
Abraham Lincoln Memorial Hospital	Lincoln	Illinois	217-732-2161	www.almh.org
Albemarle Hospital Authority	Elizabeth City	North Carolina	252-335-0531	www.albemarlehealth.org
Alliance Community Hospital	Alliance	Ohio	330-596-7527	www.achosp.org
Ashtabula County Medical Center	Ashtabula	Ohio	440-997-2262	www.acmchealth.org
Aspirus Wausau Hospital	Wausau	Wisconsin	715-847-2121	www.aspirus.org
Aurora Medical Center	Summit	Wisconsin	262-434-1000	www.aurorahealthcare.org
Avera Sacred Heart Hospital	Yankton	South Dakota	605-668-8000	www.avera.org/sacred-heart
Avera Saint Mary's Hospital	Pierre	South Dakota	605-224-3100	www.st-marys.com
Avoyelles Hospital	Marksville	Louisiana	318-253-8611	www.avoyelleshospital.com
Bates County Memorial Hospital	Butler	Missouri	660-200-7000	www.bcmhospital.com
Bear River Valley Hospital	Tremonton	Utah	435-207-4708	www.intermountainhealthcare.org
Bellevue Hospital	Bellevue	Ohio	419-483-4040	www.bellevuehospital.com
Bluffton Hospital	Bluffton	Ohio	419-358-9010	www.bvhealthsystem.org
Bourbon Community Hospital	Paris	Kentucky	859-987-3600	www.bourbonhospital.com
Brigham City Community Hospital	Brigham City	Utah	435-734-9471	www.brighamcityhospital.com
Brookings Hospital	Brookings	South Dakota	605-696-7701	www.brookingshospital.org
Cache Valley Speciality Hospital	North Logan	Utah	435-713-9700	www.cachevalleyhospital.com
Cameron Regional Medical Center	Cameron	Missouri	816-632-2101	www.cameronregional.org
Carson City Hospital	Carson City	Michigan	989-584-3131	www.carsoncityhospital.com
Cogdell Memorial Hospital	Snyder	Texas	325-574-7437	www.cogdellhospital.com
Colorado Plains Medical Center	Fort Morgan	Colorado	970-867-3391	www.coloradoplainsmedicalcenter.com
Crossroads Community Hospital	Mount Vernon	Illinois	618-244-5500	www.crossroadscommnityhospital.com
Custer Regional Hospital	Custer	South Dakota	605-673-2229	www.rcrh.org/facilities
Dauterive Hospital	New Iberia	Louisiana	337-365-7311	www.dauterivehospital.com
Daviess Community Hospital	Washington	Indiana	812-254-2760	www.dchosp.org
Decatur County Memorial Hospital	Greensburg	Indiana	812-663-4331	www.dcmh.net
Detroit Receiving Hospital & University Health Center	Detroit	Michigan	313-745-3104	www.drhuhc.org
Dupont Hospital	Fort Wayne	Indiana	260-416-3000	www.theduponthospital.com
East Cooper Medical Center	Mount Pleasant	South Carolina	843-881-0100	www.eastcoopermedctr.com
El Paso Specialty Hospital	El Paso	Texas	915-544-3636	www.elpasospecialtyhospital.com
Encino Hospital Medical Center	Encino	California	818-995-5000	www.encino-tarzana.com
Englewood Community Hospital	Englewood	Florida	941-475-6571	www.englewoodcommunityhospital.com
Evanston Regional Hospital	Evanston	Wyoming	307-789-3636	www.evanstonregionalhospital.com
Excela Health Frick Hospital	Mount Pleasant	Pennsylvania	724-547-1500	www.excelahealth.org
Fairmont General Hospital	Fairmont	West Virginia	304-367-7100	www.fghi.com
Fort Hamilton Hughes Memorial Hospital	Hamilton	Ohio	513-867-2000	www.forthamiltonhospital.com
Fremont Area Medical Center	Fremont	Nebraska	402-721-1610	www.famc.org
Genesis Medical Center - Dewitt	Dewitt	Iowa	563-659-4200	www.genesishealth.com
Good Samaritan Health Center	Merrill	Wisconsin	715-536-5511	www.ministryhealth.org/GSHC/home.nws
Good Samaritan Hospital	Kearney	Nebraska	308-865-7100	www.gshs.org
Graham Hospital Association	Canton	Illinois	309-647-5240	www.grahamhospital.org
Great Bend Regional Hospital	Great Bend	Kansas	620-792-8833	www.greatbendsurgical.com
Grove City Medical Center	Grove City	Pennsylvania	724-450-7000	www.uchpa.org
Hamilton General Hospital	Hamilton	Texas	254-386-3151	www.hamiltonhospital.org
Harrington Memorial Hospital	Southbridge	Massachusetts	508-765-9771	www.harringtonhospital.org
Harris Hospital	Newport	Arkansas	870-523-8911	www.harrishospital.com
Heber Valley Medical Center	Heber City	Utah	435-654-2500	www.intermountainhealthcare.org
Henderson County Community Hospital	Lexington	Tennessee	731-968-1801	www.hendersoncchospital.com
Hill Regional Hospital	Hillsboro	Texas	254-580-8500	www.hillregionalhospital.com
Hillside Hospital	Pulaski	Tennessee	931-363-7531	www.hillsidehospital.com
Holdenville Hospital Authority	Holdenville	Oklahoma	405-379-4200	
The Hospital at Westlake Medical Center	Austin	Texas	512-327-0000	www.westlakemedical.com
Hutchinson Health	Hutchinson	Minnesota	320-234-5000	www.hahc-hmc.com
Illinois Valley Community Hospital	Peru	Illinois	815-223-3300	www.ivch.org
Integris Blackwell Regional Hospital	Blackwell	Oklahoma	580-363-2311	www.integrisblackwell.com
Integris Health Edmond	Edmond	Oklahoma	405-657-3000	www.integrisok.com/integris-health-edmond-ok
Integris Marshall County Medical Center	Madill	Oklahoma	580-795-3384	www.integris-health.com/integris
Iroquois Memorial Hospital	Watseka	Illinois	815-432-5201	www.iroquoismemorial.com
Kansas Medical Center	Andover	Kansas	316-300-4000	www.ksmedcenter.com
Lafayette Regional Health Center	Lexington	Missouri	660-259-2203	www.lafayetteregionalhealthcenter.com
Lake Region Healthcare Corporation	Fergus Falls	Minnesota	218-736-8000	www.lrhc.org
Lakeland Community Hospital	Haleyville	Alabama	205-485-7117	www.lifepointhospitals.com
Lakeland Regional Medical Center	Lakeland	Florida	863-687-1100	www.lrmc.com
Lander Regional Hospital	Lander	Wyoming	307-332-4420	www.landerhospital.com
Lawrence Medical Center	Moulton	Alabama	256-974-2200	www.lawrencemedicalcenter.com

Hospital	City	State	Phone	Web Site
Livingston Regional Hospital	Livingston	Tennessee	931-823-5611	www.livingstonregionalhospital.com
Madison Memorial Hospital	Rexburg	Idaho	208-359-6900	www.madisonhospital.org
Maple Grove Hospital	Maple Grove	Minnesota	763-581-1000	www.maplegrove.org
Mary Greeley Medical Center	Ames	Iowa	515-239-2011	www.mgmc.org
Mary Lanning Healthcare	Hastings	Nebraska	402-463-4521	www.marylanning.org
Mayo Clinic Health System - Fairmont	Fairmont	Minnesota	507-238-8101	www.fairmontmedicalcenter.org
McBride Clinic Orthopedic Hospital	Oklahoma City	Oklahoma	405-478-1717	www.mcbrideclinic.com
McCullough - Hyde Memorial Hospital	Oxford	Ohio	513-523-2111	www.mhmh.org
McDonough District Hospital	Macomb	Illinois	309-833-4101	www.mdh.org
Mercer County Joint Township Community Hospital	Coldwater	Ohio	419-678-4843	www.mercer-health.com
Mercy Health System Corp	Janesville	Wisconsin	608-756-6080	www.mercyhealthsystem.org
Mercy Medical Center	Roseburg	Oregon	541-673-0611	www.mercyrose.org
Mercy Medical Center - Dubuque	Dubuque	Iowa	563-589-8000	www.mercydubuque.com
Mercy Regional Medical Center	Ville Platte	Louisiana	337-363-5684	www.vpmc.com
Meriter Hospital	Madison	Wisconsin	608-417-6000	www.meriter.com
Mesa View Regional Hospital	Mesquite	Nevada	702-346-8040	www.mesaviewhospital.com
Minden Medical Center	Minden	Louisiana	318-377-2321	www.mindenmedicalcenter.com
Ministry Saint Michaels Hospital of Stevens Point	Stevens Point	Wisconsin	715-346-5000	www.saintmichaelshospital.org
Moore County Hospital District	Dumas	Texas	806-935-7171	www.mchd.net
Mount Pleasant Hospital	Mount Pleasant	South Carolina	843-724-2954	www.rsfh.com
Mountain View Hospital	Payson	Utah	801-465-7100	www.mvhpayson.com
Neshoba County General Hospital	Philadelphia	Mississippi	601-663-1200	www.neshobageneral.com
Nevada Regional Medical Center	Nevada	Missouri	417-667-3355	www.nrmchealth.com
Ottawa Regional Hospital & Healthcare Center	Ottawa	Illinois	815-433-3100	www.community-hospital.org
Park City Medical Center	Park City	Utah	435-658-7000	www.intermountainhealthcare.org
Parkview Lagrange Hospital	Lagrange	Indiana	260-463-9000	www.parkview.com
Ponca City Medical Center	Ponca City	Oklahoma	580-765-3321	www.poncamedcenter.com
Portage Health	Hancock	Michigan	906-483-1000	www.portagehealth.org
Prairie Lakes Hospital	Watertown	South Dakota	605-882-7000	www.prairielakes.com
Presbyterian Saint Lukes Medical Center	Denver	Colorado	303-839-6000	www.pslmc.com
Proctor Hospital	Peoria	Illinois	309-691-1000	www.proctor.org
Providence Seaside Hospital	Seaside	Oregon	503-717-7000	www.providence.org/northcoast
Pushmataha County - Town of Antlers Hospital Authority	Antlers	Oklahoma	580-298-3341	www.pushhospital.com
Riverview Regional Medical Center	Carthage	Tennessee	615-735-9815	www.sumner.org
Rockcastle County Hospital	Mount Vernon	Kentucky	606-256-2195	www.rockcastlehospital.com
Sagewest Health Care	Riverton	Wyoming	307-856-4161	www.riverton-hospital.com
Saint Charles Parish Hospital	Luling	Louisiana	985-785-6242	www.stch.net
Saint Clare Hospital Health Services	Baraboo	Wisconsin	608-356-1400	www.stclare.com
Saint Elizabeth Grant	Williamstown	Kentucky	859-824-8240	www.stelizabeth.com
Saint Elizabeth Hospital	Appleton	Wisconsin	920-738-2000	www.affinityhealth.org
Saint James Healthcare	Butte	Montana	406-723-2500	www.stjameshealthcare.org
Saint James Hospital	Pontiac	Illinois	815-842-2828	www.osfsaintjames.org
Saint John Hospital	Leavenworth	Kansas	913-596-3930	www.providence-health.org
Saint Johns Medical Center	Jackson	Wyoming	307-733-3636	www.tetonhospital.org
Saint Margarets Hospital	Spring Valley	Illinois	815-664-1176	www.aboutsmh.org
Saint Marys Hospital	Madison	Wisconsin	608-251-6100	www.stmarysmadison.com
Saint Marys Hospital Superior	Superior	Wisconsin	715-817-7000	www.smdc.org
Saint Marys Janesville Hospital	Janesville	Wisconsin	608-373-8000	www.stmarysjanesville.com
Samaritan Albany General Hospital	Albany	Oregon	541-812-4000	www.samhealth.org/shs_facilities
Sanford Medical Center Bismarck	Bismarck	North Dakota	701-323-6000	www.medcenterone.com
Sanford Worthington Medical Center	Worthington	Minnesota	507-372-2941	www.worthingtonhospital.com
Santa Ynez Valley Cottage Hospital	Solvang	California	805-688-6431	www.cottagehealthsystem.org
Seton Smithville Regional Hospital	Smithville	Texas	512-237-3214	www.srhnet.com
Share Memorial Hospital	Alva	Oklahoma	580-327-2800	www.smcok.com
Shelby Memorial Hospital	Shelbyville	Illinois	217-774-3961	www.mysmh.org
Silverton Hospital	Silverton	Oregon	503-873-1500	www.silvertonhospital.org
Smyth County Community Hospital	Marion	Virginia	276-378-1000	www.scchosp.org
South Central Kansas Medical Center	Arkansas City	Kansas	620-442-2500	www.sckrmc.com
Spearfish Regional Hospital	Spearfish	South Dakota	605-644-4000	www.rcrh.org
Spencer Municipal Hospital	Spencer	Iowa	712-264-8300	www.spencerhospital.org
Springhill Medical Center	Springhill	Louisiana	318-539-1000	www.smccare.com
Stephens Memorial Hospital	Breckenridge	Texas	254-559-2241	www.smhtx.com
Stonewall Jackson Memorial Hospital	Weston	West Virginia	304-269-8080	www.stonewallhospital.com
Swedish Issaquah	Issaquah	Washington	425-313-4000	www.swedish.org/locations/issaquah-campus
Swedish Medical Center	Seattle	Washington	206-386-6000	www.swedish.org
Taylorville Memorial Hospital	Taylorville	Illinois	217-824-3331	www.svmh.org
Toppenish Community Hospital	Toppenish	Washington	509-865-1520	www.hma-corp.com

Hospital	City	State	Phone	Web Site
Tristar Ashland City Medical Center	Ashland City	Tennessee	615-792-3030	www.centennialashlandcity.com
UPMC Bedford Memorial	Everett	Pennsylvania	814-623-6161	www.upmc.com
UPMC Northwest	Seneca	Pennsylvania	814-676-7600	www.northwest.upmc.com
Valley West Community Hospital	Sandwich	Illinois	815-786-8484	www.snd.softfarm.com/sandhosp
Via Christi Hospital Wichita Saint Teresa	Wichita	Kansas	316-796-7800	www.via-christi.org
Walla Walla General Hospital	Walla Walla	Washington	509-525-0480	www.wwgh.com
Winn Parish Medical Center	Winnfield	Louisiana	318-648-3000	www.winnparishmedical.com
Winona Health Services	Winona	Minnesota	507-454-3650	www.winonahealth.org
Woodward Regional Hospital	Woodward	Oklahoma	580-254-8492	www.woodwardhospital.com
Yampa Valley Medical Center	Steamboat Springs	Colorado	970-879-1322	www.yvmc.org
York Hospital	York	Maine	207-363-4321	www.yorkhospital.com

Note: The hospitals shown above represent the top 5% of the 2,872 hospitals nationwide for which an average score was calculated. Average scores were calculated for hospitals with qualifying data (25 cases or more) in at least 6 of 7 measures in the Emergency Department Care category.

Best Hospitals for Heart Care

Hospital	City	State	Phone	Web Site
Advocate Good Shepherd Hospital	Barrington	Illinois	847-381-9600	www.advocatehealth.com
Advocate Illinois Masonic Medical Center	Chicago	Illinois	773-975-1600	www.advocatehealth.com/immc
Alegent Creighton Health Immanuel Medical Center	Omaha	Nebraska	402-572-2121	www.alegent.com
Arkansas Heart Hospital	Little Rock	Arkansas	501-219-7000	www.arheart.com
Baptist Hospital of Miami	Miami	Florida	786-596-1960	www.baptisthealth.net
Baylor Heart & Vascular Hospital	Dallas	Texas	214-820-0670	www.baylorhearthospital.com
Beaumont Health System	Grosse Pointe	Michigan	313-343-1000	www.beaumonthospitals.com
Blanchard Valley Hospital	Findlay	Ohio	419-423-4500	www.bvha.org
Boca Raton Regional Hospital	Boca Raton	Florida	561-362-5002	www.brrh.com
Brooklyn Hospital Center at Downtown Campus	Brooklyn	New York	718-250-8000	www.tbh.org
Broward Health North	Pompano Beach	Florida	954-786-6950	www.browardhealth.org
Calvert Memorial Hospital	Prince Frederick	Maryland	410-535-8239	www.calverthospital.com
Carepoint Health - Bayonne Hospital Center	Bayonne	New Jersey	201-858-5000	www.bayonnemedicalcenter.org
Cedars - Sinai Medical Center	Los Angeles	California	310-423-5000	www.cedars-sinai.edu
Centinela Hospital Medical Center	Inglewood	California	310-673-4660	www.centinelafreeman.com
Decatur Memorial Hospital	Decatur	Illinois	217-877-8121	www.dmhcares.org
Dekalb Regional Medical Center	Fort Payne	Alabama	256-845-3150	www.baptistmedical.org
Delray Medical Center	Delray Beach	Florida	561-498-4440	www.delraymedicalctr.com
Doctors Hospital	Augusta	Georgia	706-651-6008	www.doctors-hospital.net
Doctors Hospital	Columbus	Ohio	614-544-1000	www.columbusregional.com
Eastern Idaho Regional Medical Center	Idaho Falls	Idaho	208-529-6111	www.eirmc.org
Fairview Southdale Hospital	Edina	Minnesota	952-924-5000	www.fairview.org
Florida Hospital North Pinellas	Tarpon Springs	Florida	727-942-5000	www.hemh.com
Fort Sanders Regional Medical Center	Knoxville	Tennessee	865-541-1101	www.fsregional.com
Gateway Regional Medical Center	Granite City	Illinois	618-798-3175	www.sehs.com
Good Samaritan Hospital Medical Center	West Islip	New York	631-376-3000	www.good-samaritan-hospital.org
Good Samaritan Hospital of Suffern	Suffern	New York	914-368-5000	www.goodsamhosp.org
Hackettstown Regional Medical Center	Hackettstown	New Jersey	908-852-5100	www.hrmcnj.org
Health Central	Ocoee	Florida	407-296-1820	www.health-central.org
High Point Regional Hospital	High Point	North Carolina	336-878-6000	www.highpointregional.com
Holy Name Medical Center	Teaneck	New Jersey	201-833-3000	www.holyname.org
Homestead Hospital	Homestead	Florida	786-243-8000	www.baptisthealth.net
Hospital De La Concepcion	San German	Puerto Rico	787-892-1860	www.hospitalconcepcion.org
Hospital of Univ of Pennsylvania	Philadelphia	Pennsylvania	215-662-3227	www.upenn.edu
Hudson Valley Hospital Center	Cortlandt Manor	New York	914-734-3611	www.hvhc.org
Indiana University Health Bloomington Hospital	Bloomington	Indiana	812-353-9555	www.bloomingtonhospital.org
Ingalls Memorial Hospital	Harvey	Illinois	708-333-2300	www.ingalls.org
Jamaica Hospital Medical Center	Jamaica	New York	718-262-6000	www.jamaicahospital.org
JFK Medical Center	Atlantis	Florida	561-965-7300	www.jfkmc.com
John Dempsey Hospital	Farmington	Connecticut	860-679-1145	www.uconnhealth.orgorwww.uchc.edu
Kaiser Foundation Hospital	Honolulu	Hawaii	808-432-0000	www.kaiserpermanente.com
Kaiser Foundation Hospital - Fremont/Hayward	Hayward	California	510-784-4000	www.kaiserpermanente.org
Kaiser Foundation Hospital - Manteca	Manteca	California	209-825-3700	www.healthy.kaiserpermanente.org
Kaiser Foundation Hospital - Orange Co-Anaheim	Anaheim	California	714-644-2000	www.healthy.kaiserpermanente.org
Kaiser Foundation Hospital - Redwood City	Redwood City	California	650-299-2000	www.seiu-uhw.org/aboutuhw
Kaiser Foundation Hospital - Sacramento	Sacramento	California	916-973-5000	www.kaiserpermanente.org
Kaiser Foundation Hospital - Santa Clara	Santa Clara	California	408-236-6400	www.members.kaiserpermanente.org
Kaiser Foundation Hospital - South Bay	Harbor City	California	310-517-6441	www.kaiserpermanente.org
Kaiser Foundation Hospital - South San Francisco	South San Francisco	California	650-742-3200	www.healthy.kaiserpermanente.org
Kaiser Foundation Hospital South Sacramento	Sacramento	California	916-688-2000	www.mydoctor.kaiserpermanente.org
Kansas Medical Center	Andover	Kansas	316-300-4000	www.ksmedcenter.com
Keck Hospital of USC	Los Angeles	California	323-442-8656	www.uscuh.com
La Palma Intercommunity Hospital	La Palma	California	714-670-7400	www.lapalmaintercommunityhospital.com
Lakeview Hospital	Bountiful	Utah	801-299-2211	www.lakeviewhospital.com
Lakeview Regional Medical Center	Covington	Louisiana	985-867-4443	www.lakeviewregional.com
Laredo Medical Center	Laredo	Texas	956-796-5000	www.laredomedical.com
Las Colinas Medical Center	Irving	Texas	972-969-2000	www.lascolinas.com
Lawnwood Regional Medical Center & Heart Institute	Fort Pierce	Florida	772-461-4000	www.lawnwoodmed.com
Lawrence Memorial Hospital	Lawrence	Kansas	785-505-6100	www.lmh.org
Lewisgale Medical Center	Salem	Virginia	540-776-4000	www.lewis-gale.com
Loyola University Medical Center	Maywood	Illinois	708-216-9000	www.lumc.edu
Manatee Memorial Hospital	Bradenton	Florida	941-746-5111	www.manateememorial.com
Mary Greeley Medical Center	Ames	Iowa	515-239-2011	www.mgmc.org
Medical Center of Arlington	Arlington	Texas	817-465-3241	www.medicalcenterarlington.com
Medical Center of Trinity	Trinity	Florida	727-848-1733	www.communityhospitalnpr.com

Hospital	City	State	Phone	Web Site
Memorial Regional Hospital	Hollywood	Florida	954-987-2000	www.memorialregional.com
Mercy Fitzgerald Hospital	Darby	Pennsylvania	215-237-4000	www.mercyhealth.org
Methodist Mansfield Medical Center	Mansfield	Texas	682-622-2059	www.methodisthealthsystem.com
Methodist Sugar Land Hospital	Sugar Land	Texas	281-274-8000	www.methodisthealth.com/sugarland
Metropolitan Hospital of Miami	Miami	Florida	305-264-1000	www.pahnet.org
Mid Coast Hospital	Brunswick	Maine	207-729-0181	www.midcoasthealth.com
Newark Beth Israel Medical Center	Newark	New Jersey	973-926-7850	www.sbhcs.com
North Florida Regional Medical Center	Gainesville	Florida	352-333-4100	www.nfrmc.com
North Hills Hospital	North Richland Hills	Texas	817-255-1000	www.northhillshospital.com
North Okaloosa Medical Center	Crestview	Florida	850-689-8100	www.northokaloosa.com
North Suburban Medical Center	Thornton	Colorado	303-451-7800	www.northsuburban.com
Novant Health Forsyth Medical Center	Winston-Salem	North Carolina	336-718-5000	www.forsythmedicalcenter.org
NYU Hospitals Center	New York	New York	212-263-7300	www.med.nyu.edu
Ocala Regional Medical Center	Ocala	Florida	352-401-1000	www.ocalaregional.com
Orange Park Medical Center	Orange Park	Florida	904-276-8500	www.opmedical.com
Palms West Hospital	Loxahatchee	Florida	561-753-4245	www.palmswesthospital.com
Paradise Valley Hospital	Phoenix	Arizona	602-923-5000	www.paradisevalleyhospital.com
Paradise Valley Hospital	National City	California	619-470-4321	www.paradisevalleyhospital.org
Parma Community General Hospital	Parma	Ohio	440-743-3000	www.parmahopsital.org
Penn Presbyterian Medical Center	Philadelphia	Pennsylvania	215-662-8000	www.pennhealth.com
Phelps Memorial Hospital Assn	Sleepy Hollow	New York	914-366-3000	www.phelpshospital.org
Pikeville Medical Center	Pikeville	Kentucky	606-218-3500	www.pikevillehospital.org
Plaza Medical Center of Fort Worth	Fort Worth	Texas	817-336-2100	www.plazamedicalcenter.com
Porter Regional Hospital	Valparaiso	Indiana	219-983-8300	www.portermemorial.org
Portsmouth Regional Hospital	Portsmouth	New Hampshire	603-436-5110	www.portsmouthhospital.com
Presbyterian Community Hospital	San Juan	Puerto Rico	787-721-2160	www.presbypr.com
Providence Memorial Hospital	El Paso	Texas	915-577-6011	www.sphn.com
Riverside Community Hospital	Riverside	California	951-788-3000	www.rchc.org
Riverside Methodist Hospital	Columbus	Ohio	614-566-5000	www.ohiohealth.com
Riverview Regional Medical Center	Gadsden	Alabama	256-543-5200	www.riverviewregional.com
Roper Hospital	Charleston	South Carolina	843-724-2800	www.ropersaintfrancis.com
Rose Medical Center	Denver	Colorado	303-320-2121	www.rosemed.com
Round Rock Medical Center	Round Rock	Texas	512-341-1000	www.roundrockmedicalcenter.com
Saint Anthony Hospital	Oklahoma City	Oklahoma	405-272-7000	www.saintsok.com
Saint John's Riverside Hospital	Yonkers	New York	914-964-4444	www.riversidehealth.org
Saint Luke's Magic Valley Rmc	Twin Falls	Idaho	208-814-1000	www.stlukesonline.org/magic_valley
Saint Mary Medical Center	Hobart	Indiana	219-942-0551	www.comhs.org/stmary
Saint Mary Medical Center	Langhorne	Pennsylvania	215-750-2003	www.stmaryhealthcare.org
Saint Mary's Health Center	Jefferson City	Missouri	573-761-7000	www.stmarys-jeffcity.com
Saint Mary's Hospital - Passaic	Passaic	New Jersey	973-365-4300	www.smh-nj.com
Sanford Medical Center Bismarck	Bismarck	North Dakota	701-323-6000	www.medcenterone.com
Scripps Green Hospital	La Jolla	California	858-554-3600	www.scrippshealth.org
Scripps Memorial Hospital La Jolla	La Jolla	California	858-626-4123	www.scrippshealth.org
Sebastian River Medical Center	Sebastian	Florida	772-589-3187	www.srmcenter.com
Sentara Norfolk General Hospital	Norfolk	Virginia	757-388-3000	www.sentara.com
Shady Grove Adventist Hospital	Rockville	Maryland	240-826-6517	www.adventisthealthcare.com/sgah
Sistema Integrados De Salud Del Sur Oeste	Mayaguez	Puerto Rico	787-652-9200	
Southern Hills Hospital & Medical Center	Las Vegas	Nevada	702-880-2100	www.southernhillshospital.com
Spotsylvania Regional Medical Center	Fredericksburg	Virginia	540-498-4000	www.spotsrmc.com
SSM Depaul Health Center	Bridgeton	Missouri	314-344-6000	www.ssmdepaul.com
SSM Saint Marys Health Center	Richmond Heights	Missouri	314-768-8000	www.ssmhealth.com/stmarys
Sutter Medical Center of Santa Rosa	Santa Rosa	California	707-576-4000	www.suttersantarosa.org
University Hospital	Newark	New Jersey	973-972-5658	www.theuniversityhospital.com
University of South Alabama Medical Center	Mobile	Alabama	251-471-7110	www.southalabama.edu/usamc
Venice Regional Medical Center - Bayfront Health	Venice	Florida	941-485-7711	www.veniceregional.com
Vista Medical Center East	Waukegan	Illinois	847-360-4000	www.vistahealth.com
Walker Baptist Medical Center	Jasper	Alabama	205-387-4000	www.bhsala.com/walker
Wellmont Bristol Regional Medical Center	Bristol	Tennessee	423-844-1121	www.wellmont.org
Wesley Medical Center	Wichita	Kansas	316-962-2000	www.wesleymc.com
West Florida Hospital	Pensacola	Florida	850-494-4000	www.westfloridahospital.com
West Virginia University Hospitals	Morgantown	West Virginia	304-598-4000	www.wvuh.com
Wichita VA Medical Center	Wichita	Kansas	316-685-2221	www.wichita.va.gov

Note: The 127 hospitals shown above all achieved a perfect 100% average score. Average scores were calculated for hospitals with qualifying data (25 cases or more) in at least 5 of 11 measures in the following categories: Chest Pain/Possible Heart Attack; Heart Attack; Heart Failure. A total of 2,234 hospitals nationwide were considered.

Best Hospitals for Pneumonia Care

Hospital	City	State	Phone	Web Site
Abilene Regional Medical Center	Abilene	Texas	325-428-1000	www.abileneregional.com
Advocate Christ Hospital & Medical Center	Oak Lawn	Illinois	708-684-8000	www.advocatehealth.com
Advocate Illinois Masonic Medical Center	Chicago	Illinois	773-975-1600	www.advocatehealth.com/immc
Alaska Regional Hospital	Anchorage	Alaska	907-276-1131	www.alaskaregional.com
Alegent Creighton Health Creighton University Med	Omaha	Nebraska	402-449-4000	www.creightonhospital.com
Alegent Creighton Health Midlands Hospital	Papillion	Nebraska	402-593-3000	www.alegent.com
Allegheny General Hospital	Pittsburgh	Pennsylvania	412-359-3131	www.allhealth.edu
Asante Ashland Community Hospital	Ashland	Oregon	541-201-4001	www.ashlandhospital.org
Asante Rogue Regional Medical Center	Medford	Oregon	541-789-7000	www.asante.org
Ashtabula County Medical Center	Ashtabula	Ohio	440-997-2262	www.acmchealth.org
Aurora Baycare Medical Center	Green Bay	Wisconsin	920-288-8000	www.aurorabaycare.com
Aurora West Allis Medical Center	West Allis	Wisconsin	414-328-6000	www.aurorahealthcare.org
Aventura Hospital & Medical Center	Aventura	Florida	305-682-7000	www.aventurahospital.com
Avera Marshall Regional Medical Center	Marshall	Minnesota	507-537-9661	www.averamarshall.org
Baptist Hospital of Miami	Miami	Florida	786-596-1960	www.baptisthealth.net
Baptist Memorial Hospital Huntingdon	Huntingdon	Tennessee	731-986-4461	www.bmhcc.org
Baptist Memorial Hospital North Mississippi	Oxford	Mississippi	662-232-8100	www.baptistonline.org/facilities/oxford
Baptist Memorial Hospital Union City	Union City	Tennessee	731-885-2410	www.bmhcc.org
Beaumont Health System	Grosse Pointe	Michigan	313-343-1000	www.beaumonthospitals.com
Bellevue Medical Center	Bellevue	Nebraska	402-763-3600	www.bellevuemed.com
Berkshire Medical Center	Pittsfield	Massachusetts	413-447-2000	www.berkshirehealthsystems.org
Big Bend Regional Medical Center	Alpine	Texas	432-837-3447	www.bigbendhealthcare.com
Bolivar Medical Center	Cleveland	Mississippi	662-846-2551	www.bolivarmedical.com
Bon Secours Memorial Regional Medical Center	Mechanicsville	Virginia	804-764-6000	www.bonsecours.com
Bonner General Hospital	Sandpoint	Idaho	208-263-1441	www.bonnergeneral.org
Brigham & Women's Faulkner Hospital	Boston	Massachusetts	617-983-7000	www.brighamandwomensfaulkner.org
Broadlawns Medical Center	Des Moines	Iowa	515-282-2200	www.broadlawns.org
Brookings Hospital	Brookings	South Dakota	605-696-7701	www.brookingshospital.org
Broward Health North	Pompano Beach	Florida	954-786-6950	www.browardhealth.org
Buchanan General Hospital	Grundy	Virginia	276-935-1000	www.bgh.org
Bucyrus Community Hospital	Bucyrus	Ohio	419-562-4677	www.bchonline.org
California Pacific Medical Center - Pacific Campus Hospital	San Francisco	California	415-600-6000	www.cpmc.org
California Pacific Medical Center - Saint Luke's Campus	San Francisco	California	415-641-6562	www.stlukes.sf.org
Carepoint Health - Bayonne Hospital Center	Bayonne	New Jersey	201-858-5000	www.bayonnemedicalcenter.org
Carney Hospital	Boston	Massachusetts	617-506-2000	www.caritascarney.org
Carolinas Hospital System	Florence	South Carolina	843-674-2500	www.carolinashospital.com
Centinela Hospital Medical Center	Inglewood	California	310-673-4660	www.centinelafreeman.com
Central Peninsula General Hospital	Soldotna	Alaska	907-262-4404	www.cpgh.org
Chatuge Regional Hospital	Hiawassee	Georgia	706-896-2222	www.chatugeregionalhospital.org
Coffee Regional Medical Center	Douglas	Georgia	229-384-1900	www.coffeeregional.org
Conroe Regional Medical Center	Conroe	Texas	936-539-1111	www.conroeregional.com
Coosa Valley Medical Center	Sylacauga	Alabama	256-249-5000	www.cvhealth.net
Coral Gables Hospital	Coral Gables	Florida	305-445-8461	www.coralgableshospital.com
The Corpus Christi Medical Center	Corpus Christi	Texas	361-761-1501	www.ccmedicalcenter.com
Davis Hospital & Medical Center	Layton	Utah	801-807-1000	www.davishospital.com
Delray Medical Center	Delray Beach	Florida	561-498-4440	www.delraymedicalctr.com
Detar Hospital Navarro	Victoria	Texas	361-575-7441	www.detar.com
Detroit (John D. Dingell) VA Medical Center	Detroit	Michigan	313-576-1000	www.detroit.va.gov
Doctors Hospital	Augusta	Georgia	706-651-6008	www.doctors-hospital.net
Dominican Hospital	Santa Cruz	California	831-462-7700	www.dominicanhospital.org
Down East Community Hospital	Machias	Maine	207-255-3356	www.dech.org
Dupont Hospital	Fort Wayne	Indiana	260-416-3000	www.theduponthospital.com
East Texas Medical Center - Gilmer	Gilmer	Texas	903-841-7100	www.etmc.org
Eastern Idaho Regional Medical Center	Idaho Falls	Idaho	208-529-6111	www.eirmc.org
El Camino Hospital	Mountain View	California	650-940-7000	www.elcaminohospital.org
Encino Hospital Medical Center	Encino	California	818-995-5000	www.encino-tarzana.com
Englewood Community Hospital	Englewood	Florida	941-475-6571	www.englewoodcommunityhospital.com
Excela Health Latrobe Hospital	Latrobe	Pennsylvania	724-537-1000	www.excelahealth.org
Faith Regional Health Services	Norfolk	Nebraska	402-371-4880	www.frhs.org
Falmouth Hospital	Falmouth	Massachusetts	508-548-5300	www.capecodhealth.com
Fannin Regional Hospital	Blue Ridge	Georgia	706-632-3711	www.fanninregionalhospital.com
Fawcett Memorial Hospital	Port Charlotte	Florida	941-629-1181	www.fawcetthospital.com
Florida Hospital North Pinellas	Tarpon Springs	Florida	727-942-5000	www.hemh.com
Flowers Hospital	Dothan	Alabama	334-793-5000	www.flowershospital.com
Forest Hills Hospital	Forest Hills	New York	718-830-4000	www.northshorelij.com

Hospital	City	State	Phone	Web Site
Fostoria Community Hospital	Fostoria	Ohio	419-435-7734	www.promedica.org
Franciscan Saint Anthony Health - Michigan City	Michigan City	Indiana	219-879-8511	www.samhc.org
Franciscan Saint Elizabeth Health - Lafayette East	Lafayette	Indiana	765-502-4334	www.ste.org
Frankfort Regional Medical Center	Frankfort	Kentucky	502-875-5240	www.frankfortregional.com
Garden Grove Hospital & Medical Center	Garden Grove	California	714-537-5160	www.gardengrovehospital.com
Garden Park Medical Center	Gulfport	Mississippi	228-575-7000	www.gardenparkmedical.com
Genesis Medical Center - Davenport	Davenport	Iowa	563-421-1000	www.genesishealth.com
Georgetown Memorial Hospital	Georgetown	South Carolina	843-527-7000	www.gmhsc.com
Good Samaritan Hospital Medical Center	West Islip	New York	631-376-3000	www.good-samaritan-hospital.org
Greene Memorial Hospital	Xenia	Ohio	937-352-2000	www.ketteringhealth.org/greene
Hackensack - Umc Mountainside	Montclair	New Jersey	973-429-6000	www.mountainsidenow.org
Hackettstown Regional Medical Center	Hackettstown	New Jersey	908-852-5100	www.hrmcnj.org
Hammond Henry Hospital	Geneseo	Illinois	309-944-6431	www.hammondhenry.com
Hardin Memorial Hospital	Kenton	Ohio	419-673-0761	www.hardinmemorial.org
Harlingen Medical Center	Harlingen	Texas	956-365-1000	www.harlingenmedicalcenter.com
Heart of Lancaster Regional Medical Center	Lititz	Pennsylvania	717-625-5000	www.heartoflancaster.com
Helena Regional Medical Center	Helena	Arkansas	870-338-5800	www.helenaregionalmedicalcenter.com
Henderson County Community Hospital	Lexington	Tennessee	731-968-1801	www.hendersoncchospital.com
Holy Family Memorial	Manitowoc	Wisconsin	920-320-2011	www.hfmhealth.org
Hospital Pavia Santurce	Fernandez Juncos	Puerto Rico	787-727-6060	www.paviahospitalsanturce.com
Howard Memorial Hospital	Nashville	Arkansas	870-845-4400	www.howardmemorial.com
Huntington Beach Hospital	Huntington Beach	California	714-843-5000	www.hbhospital.com
Hutchinson Health	Hutchinson	Minnesota	320-234-5000	www.hahc-hmc.com
Ingalls Memorial Hospital	Harvey	Illinois	708-333-2300	www.ingalls.org
Intermountain Medical Center	Murray	Utah	801-507-7000	www.intermountainhealthcare.org
Jackson Hospital & Clinic	Montgomery	Alabama	334-293-8000	www.jackson.org
Jamaica Hospital Medical Center	Jamaica	New York	718-262-6000	www.jamaicahospital.org
Jay Hospital	Jay	Florida	850-675-4532	www.bhcpns.org
Jefferson Medical Center	Ranson	West Virginia	304-728-1600	www.jeffmem.com
Jennings American Legion Hospital	Jennings	Louisiana	337-616-7000	www.jalh.com
JFK Medical Center	Atlantis	Florida	561-965-7300	www.jfkmc.com
The Johns Hopkins Hospital	Baltimore	Maryland	410-955-9540	www.jhmi.edu
Kaiser Foundation Hospital - Orange Co-Anaheim	Anaheim	California	714-644-2000	www.healthy.kaiserpermanente.org
Kaiser Foundation Hospital - San Jose	San Jose	California	408-972-7000	www.mydoctor.kaiserpermanente.org
Kaiser Foundation Hospital - Santa Clara	Santa Clara	California	408-236-6400	www.members.kaiserpermanente.org
Kendall Regional Medical Center	Miami	Florida	305-223-3000	www.kendallmed.com
Kenmore Mercy Hospital	Kenmore	New York	716-447-6100	www.chsbuffalo.org
Kennewick General Hospital	Kennewick	Washington	509-586-6111	www.kennewickgeneral.com
Lake City Medical Center	Lake City	Florida	386-719-9000	www.lakecitymedical.com
Lake Forest Hospital	Lake Forest	Illinois	847-234-5600	www.lakeforesthospital.com
Lake Wales Medical Center	Lake Wales	Florida	863-676-1433	www.lakewalesmedicalcenter.com
Lakeview Medical Center	Rice Lake	Wisconsin	715-234-1515	www.lakeviewmedical.com
Lakeview Regional Medical Center	Covington	Louisiana	985-867-4443	www.lakeviewregional.com
Lancaster Regional Medical Center	Lancaster	Pennsylvania	717-291-8123	www.lancasterregional.com
Laredo Medical Center	Laredo	Texas	956-796-5000	www.laredomedical.com
Largo Medical Center	Largo	Florida	727-588-5200	www.largomedical.com
Las Colinas Medical Center	Irving	Texas	972-969-2000	www.lascolinas.com
Lawnwood Regional Medical Center & Heart Institute	Fort Pierce	Florida	772-461-4000	www.lawnwoodmed.com
Lawrence Memorial Hospital	Walnut Ridge	Arkansas	870-886-1200	www.lawrencehealth.net
Lee's Summit Medical Center	Lees Summit	Missouri	816-282-5000	www.leessummithospital.com
Lehigh Regional Medical Center	Lehigh Acres	Florida	239-369-2101	www.lehighregional.com
Lewisgale Hospital Montgomery	Blacksburg	Virginia	540-951-1111	www.mrhospital.com
Lewisgale Medical Center	Salem	Virginia	540-776-4000	www.lewis-gale.com
Libertyhealth - Jersey City Medical Center Campus	Jersey City	New Jersey	201-915-2000	www.libertyhcs.org
Little Company of Mary Hospital	Evergreen Park	Illinois	708-422-6200	www.lcmh.org
Littleton Regional Healthcare	Littleton	New Hampshire	603-444-9000	www.littletonhospital.org
Lock Haven Hospital	Lock Haven	Pennsylvania	570-893-5000	www.lockhavenhospital.com
Lucas County Health Center	Chariton	Iowa	641-774-3000	www.lchcia.com
Marin General Hospital	Greenbrae	California	415-925-7900	www.maringeneral.com
Mary Greeley Medical Center	Ames	Iowa	515-239-2011	www.mgmc.org
Maryvale Hospital	Phoenix	Arizona	623-848-5000	www.maryvalehospital.com
Mat-Su Regional Medical Center	Palmer	Alaska	907-746-8600	www.matsuregional.com
Mayo Clinic Health System - Fairmont	Fairmont	Minnesota	507-238-8101	www.fairmontmedicalcenter.org
Mayo Clinic Health System - Northland	Barron	Wisconsin	715-537-3186	www.luthermidelfortnorthland.org
McKenzie Regional Hospital	Mc Kenzie	Tennessee	731-352-5344	www.mckenzieregionalhospital.com
Mease Hospital Dunedin	Dunedin	Florida	727-733-1111	www.measehospitals.com
Medical Center of Arlington	Arlington	Texas	817-465-3241	www.medicalcenterarlington.com

Hospital	City	State	Phone	Web Site
Medical Center of Trinity	Trinity	Florida	727-848-1733	www.communityhospitalnpr.com
Medical City Dallas Hospital	Dallas	Texas	972-566-6222	www.medicalcityhospital.com
Medwest Swain	Bryson City	North Carolina	828-488-2155	www.westcarehealth.org
Memorial Healthcare System	Chattanooga	Tennessee	423-495-2525	www.memorial.org
Memorial Hospital Los Banos	Los Banos	California	209-826-0591	www.memoriallosbanos.org
Memorial Hospital Pembroke	Pembroke Pines	Florida	954-962-9650	www.memorialpembroke.com\
Memorial Hospital West	Pembroke Pines	Florida	954-436-5000	www.memorialwest.com
Memorial Regional Hospital	Hollywood	Florida	954-987-2000	www.memorialregional.com
Menorah Medical Center	Overland Park	Kansas	913-498-6773	www.menorahmedicalcenter.com
Mercy General Hospital	Sacramento	California	916-453-4545	www.mercygeneral.org
Mercy Hospital - Fort Scott	Fort Scott	Kansas	620-223-7057	www.mercy.net
Mercy Hospital of Defiance	Defiance	Ohio	419-782-8444	www.mercyweb.org/mercy_defiance.aspx
Mercy Medical Center	Springfield	Massachusetts	413-748-9000	www.mercycares.com
Mercy Regional Health Center	Manhattan	Kansas	785-776-2831	www.mercyregional.org
Methodist Medical Center of Oak Ridge	Oak Ridge	Tennessee	865-835-1000	www.mmcoakridge.com
Methodist Richardson Medical Center	Richardson	Texas	972-498-4000	www.richardsonregional.com
Metroplex Hospital	Killeen	Texas	254-526-7523	www.mplex.org
Minden Medical Center	Minden	Louisiana	318-377-2321	www.mindenmedicalcenter.com
Ministry Sacred Heart Hospital	Tomahawk	Wisconsin	715-453-7700	www.ministryhealth.org
Ministry Saint Marys Hospital	Rhinelander	Wisconsin	715-361-2000	www.ministryhealth.org
Ministry Saint Michaels Hospital of Stevens Point	Stevens Point	Wisconsin	715-346-5000	www.saintmichaelshospital.org
Moberly Regional Medical Center	Moberly	Missouri	660-263-8400	www.moberlyhospital.com
Monmouth Medical Center - Southern Campus	Lakewood	New Jersey	732-363-1900	www.sbhcs.com
Mount Pleasant Hospital	Mount Pleasant	South Carolina	843-724-2954	www.rsfh.com
Mountain Home VA Medical Center	Mountain Home	Tennessee	423-926-1171	www.mountainhome.va.gov
Mountain View Hospital	Payson	Utah	801-465-7100	www.mvhpayson.com
Mountain View Regional Medical Center	Las Cruces	New Mexico	575-556-7600	www.mountainviewregional.com
Myrtue Medical Center	Harlan	Iowa	712-755-5161	www.shelbycohealth.com
New Ulm Medical Center	New Ulm	Minnesota	507-233-1000	www.newulmmedicalcenter.com
New York Community Hospital of Brooklyn	Brooklyn	New York	718-692-5302	www.nych.com
Noble Hospital	Westfield	Massachusetts	413-568-2811	www.noblehospital.org
North Austin Medical Center	Austin	Texas	512-901-1000	www.cornerstonehealthcaregroup.com
North Florida Regional Medical Center	Gainesville	Florida	352-333-4100	www.nfrmc.com
North Shore Medical Center	Miami	Florida	305-835-6000	www.northshoremedical.com
North Suburban Medical Center	Thornton	Colorado	303-451-7800	www.northsuburban.com
Northeast Regional Medical Center	Kirksville	Missouri	660-785-1000	www.nermc.com
Northern Westchester Hospital	Mount Kisco	New York	914-666-1200	www.nwhc.net
Northside Hospital	Saint Petersburg	Florida	813-521-5000	www.northsidehospital.com
Northside Hospital	Atlanta	Georgia	404-851-8000	www.northside.com
Northside Hospital Cherokee	Canton	Georgia	770-720-5298	www.northside.com/cherokee
Norwalk Hospital Association	Norwalk	Connecticut	203-852-2000	www.norwalkhosp.org
Novant Health Forsyth Medical Center	Winston-Salem	North Carolina	336-718-5000	www.forsythmedicalcenter.org
Novant Health Franklin Medical Center	Louisburg	North Carolina	919-496-5131	www.franklinregionalmedicalctr.com
Novant Health Huntersville Medical Center	Huntersville	North Carolina	704-316-4000	www.presbyterian.org
Novant Health Thomasville Medical Center	Thomasville	North Carolina	336-472-2000	www.thomasvillemedicalcenter.org
Oak Hill Hospital	Brooksville	Florida	352-596-6632	www.oakhillhospital.com
Oaklawn Hospital	Marshall	Michigan	269-781-4271	www.oaklawnhospital.org
OHSU Hospital & Clinics	Portland	Oregon	503-494-4036	www.ohsu.edu
Oklahoma State University Medical Center	Tulsa	Oklahoma	918-587-2561	www.tulsaregional.com
Orange Park Medical Center	Orange Park	Florida	904-276-8500	www.opmedical.com
Overton Brooks VA Medical Center - Shreveport	Shreveport	Louisiana	318-424-6037	www.va.gov/sta/guide/home.asp
Palm Bay Hospital	Palm Bay	Florida	321-434-8000	www.health-first.org
Parkway Regional Hospital	Fulton	Kentucky	270-472-2522	www.parkwayregionalhospital.com
Piggott Community Hospital	Piggott	Arkansas	870-598-3881	www.piggottcommunityhospital.com
Plateau Medical Center	Oak Hill	West Virginia	304-469-8600	www.plateaumedicalcenter.com
Pleasant Valley Hospital	Point Pleasant	West Virginia	304-675-4340	www.pvalley.org
Pomerene Hospital	Millersburg	Ohio	330-674-1015	www.pomerenehospital.org
Portsmouth Regional Hospital	Portsmouth	New Hampshire	603-436-5110	www.portsmouthhospital.com
Promedica Herrick Hospital	Tecumseh	Michigan	517-424-3000	www.promedica.org/herrick
Putnam General Hospital	Eatonton	Georgia	706-485-2711	www.putnamgeneral.com
Rapides Regional Medical Center	Alexandria	Louisiana	318-769-3000	www.rapidesregional.com
Raulerson Hospital	Okeechobee	Florida	863-763-2151	www.raulersonhospital.com
Regional Hospital of Jackson	Jackson	Tennessee	731-661-2000	www.regionalhospitaljackson.com
Regional Medical Center of San Jose	San Jose	California	408-259-5000	www.regionalmedicalsanjose.com
Renown South Meadows Medical Center	Reno	Nevada	775-982-7000	www.renown.org
River Parishes Hospital	Laplace	Louisiana	985-652-7000	www.riverparisheshospital.com
Riverview Medical Center	Red Bank	New Jersey	732-741-2700	www.meridianhealth.com

Hospital	City	State	Phone	Web Site
Rockford Memorial Hospital	Rockford	Illinois	815-968-6861	www.rhsnet.org
Roper Hospital	Charleston	South Carolina	843-724-2800	www.ropersaintfrancis.com
Rose Medical Center	Denver	Colorado	303-320-2121	www.rosemed.com
Roxborough Memorial Hospital	Philadelphia	Pennsylvania	215-483-9900	www.roxboroughmemorial.com
Saint Anthony Hospital	Chicago	Illinois	773-521-1710	www.cath-health.org
Saint Anthony Shawnee Hospital	Shawnee	Oklahoma	405-273-2270	www.unityhealthcenter.com
Saint Anthony's Health Center	Alton	Illinois	618-465-2571	www.sahc.org
Saint Barnabas Medical Center	Livingston	New Jersey	973-322-5000	www.saintbarnabas.com
Saint Catherine Hospital	East Chicago	Indiana	219-392-7004	www.comhs.org/stcatherine
Saint Clare Hospital Health Services	Baraboo	Wisconsin	608-356-1400	www.stclare.com
Saint Clares Hospital of Weston	Weston	Wisconsin	715-393-3000	www.ministryhealth.org
Saint Francis Hospital	Escanaba	Michigan	906-786-3311	www.osfstfrancis.or
Saint Francis Medical Center	Trenton	New Jersey	609-599-5000	www.stfrancismedical.com
Saint James Hospital	Pontiac	Illinois	815-842-2828	www.osfsaintjames.org
Saint Joseph Hospital	Fort Wayne	Indiana	260-425-3000	www.stjoehospital.com
Saint Joseph Hospital & Health Center	Kokomo	Indiana	765-456-5300	www.stvincent.org
Saint Joseph Mercy Port Huron	Port Huron	Michigan	810-985-1510	www.mercyporthuron.com
Saint Joseph Regional Medical Center - Plymouth	Plymouth	Indiana	574-948-4000	www.sjmed.com
Saint Joseph's Hospital	Breese	Illinois	618-526-4511	www.stjoebreese.com
Saint Joseph's Mercy Health Center	Hot Springs	Arkansas	501-622-1000	www.saintjosephs.com
Saint Louise Regional Hospital	Gilroy	California	408-848-2000	www.saintlouiseregionalhospital.org
Saint Lucie Medical Center	Port Saint Lucie	Florida	772-335-4000	www.stluciemed.com
Saint Luke's Magic Valley Rmc	Twin Falls	Idaho	208-814-1000	www.stlukesonline.org/magic_valley
Saint Luke's Quakertown Hospital	Quakertown	Pennsylvania	215-538-4500	www.slhn-lehighvalley.com
Saint Margarets Hospital	Spring Valley	Illinois	815-664-1176	www.aboutsmh.org
Saint Mary Medical Center	Hobart	Indiana	219-942-0551	www.comhs.org/stmary
Saint Mary's Good Samaritan Hospital	Greensboro	Georgia	706-453-7331	www.stmarysgoodsam.org
Saint Vincent Anderson Regional Hospital	Anderson	Indiana	765-646-8373	www.stjohnshealthsystem.org
Saint Vincent's Birmingham	Birmingham	Alabama	205-939-7000	www.stv.org
Saint Vincent's East	Birmingham	Alabama	205-838-3122	www.nolandhealth.com
Saint Vincent's Medical Center Southside	Jacksonville	Florida	904-296-3700	www.jaxhealth.com
Samaritan Hospital	Moses Lake	Washington	509-765-5606	www.samaritanhealthcare.com
San Angelo Community Medical Center	San Angelo	Texas	325-949-9511	www.sacmc.com
Scripps Mercy Hospital	San Diego	California	619-294-8111	www.scrippshealth.org
Sebastian River Medical Center	Sebastian	Florida	772-589-3187	www.srmcenter.com
Seton Highland Lakes	Burnet	Texas	512-715-3000	www.seton.net
Shands Lake Shore Regional Medical Center	Lake City	Florida	386-292-8000	www.shands.org
Sharp Coronado Hospital & Healthcare Center	Coronado	California	619-435-6251	www.sharp.com/coronado
Shasta Regional Medical Center	Redding	California	530-244-5454	www.shastaregional.com
Sibley Memorial Hospital	Washington	District of Columbia	202-537-4680	www.sibley.org
Signature Healthcare Brockton Hospital	Brockton	Massachusetts	508-941-7000	www.brocktonhospital.com
Silverton Hospital	Silverton	Oregon	503-873-1500	www.silvertonhospital.org
Singing River Hospital	Pascagoula	Mississippi	228-809-5000	www.srhshealth.com
Sisters of Charity Hospital	Buffalo	New York	716-862-1000	www.chsbuffalo.org
South Miami Hospital	South Miami	Florida	786-662-4000	www.baptisthealth.net
Southern Nh Medical Center	Nashua	New Hampshire	603-577-2000	www.snhmc.org
Sparks Regional Medical Center	Fort Smith	Arkansas	501-441-4000	www.sparks.org
Spokane VA Medical Center	Spokane	Washington	509-434-7000	www.spokane.med.va.gov
Spotsylvania Regional Medical Center	Fredericksburg	Virginia	540-498-4000	www.spotsrmc.com
Stafford Hospital	Stafford	Virginia	540-741-9000	www.marywashingtonhealthcare.com
Staten Island University Hospital	Staten Island	New York	718-226-9000	www.siuh.edu
Summit Medical Center	Van Buren	Arkansas	479-471-4300	www.summitmc.net
Sutter Medical Center of Santa Rosa	Santa Rosa	California	707-576-4000	www.suttersantarosa.org
Sycamore Medical Center	Miamisburg	Ohio	937-384-8776	www.khnetwork.org/sycamore
Takoma Regional Hospital	Greeneville	Tennessee	423-639-3151	www.takoma.org
Texas Health Arlington Memorial Hospital	Arlington	Texas	817-548-6100	www.texashealth.org
Texas Health Harris Methodist Hospital Alliance	Fort Worth	Texas	682-212-2004	www.texashealth.org/alliance
Texoma Medical Center	Denison	Texas	903-416-4000	www.texomamedicalcenter.net
Thorek Memorial Hospital	Chicago	Illinois	312-525-6780	www.thorek.org
Three Rivers Medical Center	Louisa	Kentucky	606-638-9451	www.threeriversmedicalcenter.com
Togus VA Medical Center	Augusta	Maine	207-623-8411	www.maine.va.gov
Transylvania Regional Hospital	Brevard	North Carolina	828-883-5302	www.tchospital.org
Trinity Medical Center	Birmingham	Alabama	205-592-1000	www.bhsala.com/montclair
Tristar Hendersonville Medical Center	Hendersonville	Tennessee	615-338-1000	www.hendersonvillemedicalcenter.com
Tristar Southern Hills Medical Center	Nashville	Tennessee	615-781-4000	www.southernhills.com
Tristar Stonecrest Medical Center	Smyrna	Tennessee	615-768-2000	www.stonecrestmedical.com
Tucson Medical Center	Tucson	Arizona	520-327-5461	www.tmcaz.com

Hospital	City	State	Phone	Web Site
Twin Cities Hospital	Niceville	Florida	850-678-4131	www.tchealthcare.com
UH Geauga Medical Center	Chardon	Ohio	440-269-6000	www.uhgeauga.org
UHHS Memorial Hospital of Geneva	Geneva	Ohio	440-466-1141	www.uhhospitals.org/geneva
University of Maryland Medical Center	Baltimore	Maryland	410-328-8667	www.umm.edu
University of Miami Hospital	Miami	Florida	305-325-5511	www.cedarsmedicalcenter.com
UPMC Mckeesport	Mc Keesport	Pennsylvania	412-664-2000	www.selectmedicalcorp.com
VA Pittsburgh Healthcare System	Pittsburgh	Pennsylvania	412-688-6100	www.pittsburg.va.gov
Valley West Community Hospital	Sandwich	Illinois	815-786-8484	www.snd.softfarm.com/sandhosp
Venice Regional Medical Center - Bayfront Health	Venice	Florida	941-485-7711	www.veniceregional.com
Viera Hospital	Melbourne	Florida	321-434-9000	www.health-first.org
Waupun Memorial Hospital	Waupun	Wisconsin	920-324-6530	www.agnesian.com
Wayne County Hospital	Monticello	Kentucky	606-348-9343	www.waynehospital.org
Weatherford Regional Medical Center	Weatherford	Texas	817-599-1190	www.campbellhealth.com
Wesley Medical Center	Wichita	Kansas	316-962-2000	www.wesleymc.com
West Palm Hospital	West Palm Beach	Florida	561-844-6141	www.columbiahospital.com
Western Pennsylvania Hospital	Pittsburgh	Pennsylvania	412-578-5000	www.wpahs.org/wph/contact/index.html
White County Medical Center	Searcy	Arkansas	501-278-3100	www.centralarkhospital.com
Wichita VA Medical Center	Wichita	Kansas	316-685-2221	www.wichita.va.gov
Wilcox Memorial Hospital	Lihue	Hawaii	808-245-1103	www.wilcoxhealth.org
William Beaumont Hospital - Troy	Troy	Michigan	248-964-8800	www.beaumonthospitals.com
Williamsport Regional Medical Center	Williamsport	Pennsylvania	570-321-1000	www.susquehannahealth.org
Woodward Regional Hospital	Woodward	Oklahoma	580-254-8492	www.woodwardhospital.com

Note: The 288 hospitals shown above all achieved a perfect 100% average score. Average scores were calculated for hospitals with qualifying data (25 cases or more) in both measures in the Pneumonia Care category. A total of 3,347 hospitals nationwide were considered.

Best Hospitals for Preventative Care

Hospital	City	State	Phone	Web Site
Abilene Regional Medical Center	Abilene	Texas	325-428-1000	www.abileneregional.com
Adena Regional Medical Center	Chillicothe	Ohio	740-779-7500	www.adena.org
Alton Memorial Hospital	Alton	Illinois	618-463-7300	www.altonmemorialhospital.org
Arizona Spine & Joint Hospital	Mesa	Arizona	480-832-4770	www.azspineandjoint.com
Atrium Medical Center	Franklin	Ohio	513-420-5102	www.atriummedcenter.org
Avera Heart Hospital of South Dakota	Sioux Falls	South Dakota	605-977-7000	www.avera.org/heart-hospital
Bailey Medical Center	Owasso	Oklahoma	918-376-8000	www.baileymedicalcenter.com
Baptist Hospital of Miami	Miami	Florida	786-596-1960	www.baptisthealth.net
Baptist Memorial Hospital Huntingdon	Huntingdon	Tennessee	731-986-4461	www.bmhcc.org
Barstow Community Hospital	Barstow	California	760-256-1761	www.barstowhospital.com
Belton Regional Medical Center	Belton	Missouri	816-348-1236	www.beltonregionalmedicalcenter.com
Biloxi Regional Medical Center	Biloxi	Mississippi	228-436-1104	www.hmabrmc.com
Broward Health North	Pompano Beach	Florida	954-786-6950	www.browardhealth.org
Byrd Regional Hospital	Leesville	Louisiana	337-239-9041	www.chs.net
Calhoun Health Services	Calhoun City	Mississippi	662-628-6611	www.nmhs.net
Carepoint Health - Bayonne Hospital Center	Bayonne	New Jersey	201-858-5000	www.bayonnemedicalcenter.org
Carrington Health Center	Carrington	North Dakota	701-652-3141	www.carringtonhealthcenter.net
Centerpoint Medical Center	Independence	Missouri	816-698-7000	www.centerpointmedical.com
Centinela Hospital Medical Center	Inglewood	California	310-673-4660	www.centinelafreeman.com
Central Mississippi Medical Center	Jackson	Mississippi	601-376-1000	www.centralmississippimedicalcenter.com
Chesterfield General Hospital	Cheraw	South Carolina	843-537-7881	www.chesterfieldgeneral.com
Clay County Hospital	Flora	Illinois	618-662-2131	www.claycountyhospital.org
Coosa Valley Medical Center	Sylacauga	Alabama	256-249-5000	www.cvhealth.net
Coral Gables Hospital	Coral Gables	Florida	305-445-8461	www.coralgableshospital.com
The Corpus Christi Medical Center	Corpus Christi	Texas	361-761-1501	www.ccmedicalcenter.com
Cypress Pointe Hospital East	Slidell	Louisiana	504-690-8200	
Delray Medical Center	Delray Beach	Florida	561-498-4440	www.delraymedicalctr.com
Detar Hospital Navarro	Victoria	Texas	361-575-7441	www.detar.com
Dyersburg Regional Medical Center	Dyersburg	Tennessee	731-285-2410	www.dyersburgregionalmc.com
Encino Hospital Medical Center	Encino	California	818-995-5000	www.encino-tarzana.com
Fannin Regional Hospital	Blue Ridge	Georgia	706-632-3711	www.fanninregionalhospital.com
Flowers Hospital	Dothan	Alabama	334-793-5000	www.flowershospital.com
Garden Grove Hospital & Medical Center	Garden Grove	California	714-537-5160	www.gardengrovehospital.com
Garden Park Medical Center	Gulfport	Mississippi	228-575-7000	www.gardenparkmedical.com
Greenbrier Valley Medical Center	Ronceverte	West Virginia	304-647-4411	www.gvmc.com
Hedrick Medical Center	Chillicothe	Missouri	660-646-1480	www.saintlukeshealthsystem.org
Helena Regional Medical Center	Helena	Arkansas	870-338-5800	www.helenaregionalmedicalcenter.com
Henderson County Community Hospital	Lexington	Tennessee	731-968-1801	www.hendersoncchospital.com
Henry County Memorial Hospital	New Castle	Indiana	765-521-0890	www.hcmhcares.org
Heritage Medical Center	Shelbyville	Tennessee	931-685-5433	www.heritagemedicalcenter.com
Highlands Regional Medical Center	Sebring	Florida	863-385-6101	www.highlandsregional.com
Holy Name Medical Center	Teaneck	New Jersey	201-833-3000	www.holyname.org
The Hospital at Westlake Medical Center	Austin	Texas	512-327-0000	www.westlakemedical.com
Huntington Beach Hospital	Huntington Beach	California	714-843-5000	www.hbhospital.com
Indiana University Health Blackford Hospital	Hartford City	Indiana	765-348-0300	www.accesschs.org
Ingalls Memorial Hospital	Harvey	Illinois	708-333-2300	www.ingalls.org
Integris Mayes County Medical Center	Pryor	Oklahoma	918-825-1600	www.integris-health.com
Jeff Davis Hospital	Hazlehurst	Georgia	912-375-7781	www.jeffdavishospital.org
JFK Medical Center	Atlantis	Florida	561-965-7300	www.jfkmc.com
John Randolph Medical Center	Hopewell	Virginia	804-541-1600	www.johnrandolphmed.com
Kansas Medical Center	Andover	Kansas	316-300-4000	www.ksmedcenter.com
Kentucky River Medical Center	Jackson	Kentucky	606-666-6000	www.kentuckyrivermc.com
L V Stabler Memorial Hospital	Greenville	Alabama	334-382-2200	www.lvstabler.com
Lafayette Regional Health Center	Lexington	Missouri	660-259-2203	www.lafayetteregionalhealthcenter.com
Lakeview Regional Medical Center	Covington	Louisiana	985-867-4443	www.lakeviewregional.com
Laredo Medical Center	Laredo	Texas	956-796-5000	www.laredomedical.com
Lawnwood Regional Medical Center & Heart Institute	Fort Pierce	Florida	772-461-4000	www.lawnwoodmed.com
Lehigh Regional Medical Center	Lehigh Acres	Florida	239-369-2101	www.lehighregional.com
Lehigh Valley Hospital - Hazleton	Hazleton	Pennsylvania	570-501-4000	www.ghha.org
Lewisgale Medical Center	Salem	Virginia	540-776-4000	www.lewis-gale.com
Livingston Regional Hospital	Livingston	Tennessee	931-823-5611	www.livingstonregionalhospital.com
Logan Regional Medical Center	Logan	West Virginia	304-831-1350	www.loganregionalmedicalcenter.com
McNairy Regional Hospital	Selmer	Tennessee	731-645-3221	www.mcnairyregionalhospital.com
Medical Center of Plano	Plano	Texas	972-596-6800	www.medicalcenterofplano.com
Medical Center of Southeastern Oklahoma	Durant	Oklahoma	405-924-3080	www.mcsohealth.com

Hospital	City	State	Phone	Web Site
Medical Center South Arkansas	El Dorado	Arkansas	870-863-2000	www.themedcenter.net
Memorial Hospital Los Banos	Los Banos	California	209-826-0591	www.memoriallosbanos.org
Memorial Hospital Pembroke	Pembroke Pines	Florida	954-962-9650	www.memorialpembroke.com\
Memorial Hospital West	Pembroke Pines	Florida	954-436-5000	www.memorialwest.com
Menorah Medical Center	Overland Park	Kansas	913-498-6773	www.menorahmedicalcenter.com
Methodist Stone Oak Hospital	San Antonio	Texas	210-638-2100	www.stoneoakhealth.com
Mills - Peninsula Medical Center	Burlingame	California	650-696-5270	www.mills-peninsula.org
Mimbres Memorial Hospital	Deming	New Mexico	575-546-5803	www.mimbresmemorial.com
Minden Medical Center	Minden	Louisiana	318-377-2321	www.mindenmedicalcenter.com
Moberly Regional Medical Center	Moberly	Missouri	660-263-8400	www.moberlyhospital.com
Mount Desert Island Hospital	Bar Harbor	Maine	207-288-5081	www.mdihospital.com
Mountain View Hospital	Idaho Falls	Idaho	208-557-2899	www.mountainviewhospital.org
Mountain View Regional Medical Center	Las Cruces	New Mexico	575-556-7600	www.mountainviewregional.com
Newberry County Memorial Hospital	Newberry	South Carolina	803-405-7145	www.newberryhospital.org
North Carolina Specialty Hospital	Durham	North Carolina	919-956-9300	www.ncspecialty.com
Northeast Regional Medical Center	Kirksville	Missouri	660-785-1000	www.nermc.com
Northern Louisiana Medical Center	Ruston	Louisiana	318-254-2100	www.lincolnhealth.com
Northern Maine Medical Center	Fort Kent	Maine	207-834-3195	www.nmmc.org
Ocala Regional Medical Center	Ocala	Florida	352-401-1000	www.ocalaregional.com
Oconee Regional Medical Center	Milledgeville	Georgia	478-454-3550	www.oconeeregional.com
Oklahoma Heart Hospital South	Oklahoma City	Oklahoma	405-628-6000	www.okheart.com/south-campus
Oklahoma Surgical Hospital	Tulsa	Oklahoma	918-477-5000	www.oklahomasurgicalhospital.com
Orange Park Medical Center	Orange Park	Florida	904-276-8500	www.opmedical.com
Palm Springs General Hospital	Hialeah	Florida	305-558-2500	www.psghosp.com
Pampa Regional Medical Center	Pampa	Texas	806-665-3721	www.prmctx.com
Parkway Regional Hospital	Fulton	Kentucky	270-472-2522	www.parkwayregionalhospital.com
Person Memorial Hospital	Roxboro	North Carolina	336-599-2121	www.personhospital.com
Ponca City Medical Center	Ponca City	Oklahoma	580-765-3321	www.poncamedcenter.com
Rapides Regional Medical Center	Alexandria	Louisiana	318-769-3000	www.rapidesregional.com
Raulerson Hospital	Okeechobee	Florida	863-763-2151	www.raulersonhospital.com
Regional Hospital of Jackson	Jackson	Tennessee	731-661-2000	www.regionalhospitaljackson.com
Regional Medical Center Bayonet Point	Hudson	Florida	727-819-2929	www.mchealth.comorwww.heartoftampa.com
The Regional Medical Center of Acadiana	Lafayette	Louisiana	337-981-2949	www.medicalcentersw.com
Renown South Meadows Medical Center	Reno	Nevada	775-982-7000	www.renown.org
Research Medical Center	Kansas City	Missouri	816-276-4000	www.researchmedicalcenter.com
Riverview Medical Center	Red Bank	New Jersey	732-741-2700	www.meridianhealth.com
Riverview Regional Medical Center	Gadsden	Alabama	256-543-5200	www.riverviewregional.com
Rolling Plains Memorial Hospital	Sweetwater	Texas	325-235-1701	www.rpmh.net
Rush University Medical Center	Chicago	Illinois	312-942-5000	www.ruch.edu
Russellville Hospital	Russellville	Alabama	256-332-1611	www.russellvillehospital.com
Saint Elizabeth Florence	Florence	Kentucky	859-212-5220	www.stlukehospitals.com
Saint Elizabeth Ft Thomas	Fort Thomas	Kentucky	859-572-3100	www.cardinalhill.org
Saint Elizabeth Grant	Williamstown	Kentucky	859-824-8240	www.stelizabeth.com
Saint Elizabeth Medical Center	Lakeside Park	Kentucky	859-292-2000	www.stelizabeth.com
Saint James Mercy Hospital	Hornell	New York	607-324-8000	www.stjamesmercy.org
Saint Joseph Hospital & Health Center	Kokomo	Indiana	765-456-5300	www.stvincent.org
Saint Luke's Miners Memorial Hospital	Coaldale	Pennsylvania	570-645-2131	www.slhn-lehighvalley.org
Saint Mary's Health Center	Jefferson City	Missouri	573-761-7000	www.stmarys-jeffcity.com
Sebastian River Medical Center	Sebastian	Florida	772-589-3187	www.srmcenter.com
Sherman Oaks Hospital	Sherman Oaks	California	818-981-7111	www.shermanoakshospital.com
Skagit Valley Hospital	Mount Vernon	Washington	360-424-4111	www.skagitvalleyhospital.org
Sonoma Developmental Center	Eldridge	California	707-938-6393	www.dds.ca.gov/sonoma/index.cfm
South Baldwin Regional Medical Center	Foley	Alabama	251-949-3400	www.southbaldwinrmc.com
South Bay Hospital	Sun City Center	Florida	813-634-3301	www.southbayhospital.com
Southwest General Hospital	San Antonio	Texas	210-921-2000	www.swgeneralhospital.com
Stones River Hospital & Dekalb Community Hospital	Smithville	Tennessee	615-215-5000	www.dekalb-hospital.com
Stormont - Vail Healthcare	Topeka	Kansas	785-354-6121	www.stormontvail.org
Temple Community Hospital	Los Angeles	California	213-382-7252	www.templecommunityhospital.com
Terre Haute Regional Hospital	Terre Haute	Indiana	812-232-0021	www.regionalhospital.com
Texas Health Harris Methodist Hospital Azle	Azle	Texas	817-444-8700	www.hmhs.org
Tomah Memorial Hospital	Tomah	Wisconsin	608-372-2181	www.tomahhospital.org
Trinity Hospital of Augusta	Augusta	Georgia	706-481-7000	www.trinityofaugusta.com
Trinity Medical Center	Birmingham	Alabama	205-592-1000	www.bhsala.com/montclair
Twin Cities Hospital	Niceville	Florida	850-678-4131	www.tchealthcare.com
Tyrone Hospital	Tyrone	Pennsylvania	814-684-1255	www.tyronehospital.org
UPMC East	Monroeville	Pennsylvania	412-357-3000	www.upmc.com
Valley West Community Hospital	Sandwich	Illinois	815-786-8484	www.snd.softfarm.com/sandhosp

Hospital	City	State	Phone	Web Site
Vaughan Regional Medical Center Parkway Campus	Selma	Alabama	334-418-4100	www.vaughanregional.com
Vista Medical Center East	Waukegan	Illinois	847-360-4000	www.vistahealth.com
Walker Baptist Medical Center	Jasper	Alabama	205-387-4000	www.bhsala.com/walker
Weatherford Regional Medical Center	Weatherford	Texas	817-599-1190	www.campbellhealth.com
West Anaheim Medical Center	Anaheim	California	714-827-3000	www.wamc.phcs.us
West Kendall Baptist Hospital	Miami	Florida	786-467-2011	www.baptisthealth.net
West Palm Hospital	West Palm Beach	Florida	561-844-6141	www.columbiahospital.com
West Virginia University Hospitals	Morgantown	West Virginia	304-598-4000	www.wvuh.com
Western Arizona Regional Medical Center	Bullhead City	Arizona	928-763-2273	www.warmc.com
Westside Regional Medical Center	Plantation	Florida	954-473-6600	www.westsidehospital.com
Woodland Heights Medical Center	Lufkin	Texas	936-634-8311	www.woodlandheights.net
Woodward Regional Hospital	Woodward	Oklahoma	580-254-8492	www.woodwardhospital.com

Note: The 144 hospitals shown above all achieved a perfect 100% average score. Average scores were calculated for hospitals with qualifying data (25 cases or more) in both measures in the Preventative Care category. A total of 3,674 hospitals nationwide were considered.

Best Hospitals for Stroke Care

Hospital	City	State	Phone	Web Site
Baptist Hospital of Miami	Miami	Florida	786-596-1960	www.baptisthealth.net
Bellevue Medical Center	Bellevue	Nebraska	402-763-3600	www.bellevuemed.com
Blanchard Valley Hospital	Findlay	Ohio	419-423-4500	www.bvha.org
Boca Raton Regional Hospital	Boca Raton	Florida	561-362-5002	www.brrh.com
Bronx - Lebanon Hospital Center	Bronx	New York	212-588-7000	www.bronx-leb.org
Brookdale Hospital Medical Center	Brooklyn	New York	718-240-5966	www.brookdalehospital.org
Cabell Huntington Hospital	Huntington	West Virginia	304-526-2000	www.cabellhuntington.org
Capital Health Medical Center - Hopewell	Pennington	New Jersey	609-303-4000	www.capitalhealth.org
Capital Regional Medical Center	Tallahassee	Florida	850-656-5000	www.capitalregionalmedicalcenter.com
Caromont Regional Medical Center	Gastonia	North Carolina	704-834-4891	www.caromont.org
Catawba Valley Medical Center	Hickory	North Carolina	828-326-3809	www.catawbavalleymc.org
Central Carolina Hospital	Sanford	North Carolina	919-774-2100	www.centralcarolinahosp.com
Cjw Medical Center	Richmond	Virginia	804-330-2001	www.hcavirginia.com
Cleveland Clinic Hospital	Weston	Florida	954-689-5000	www.clevelandclinic.org
Cox Medical Center Branson	Branson	Missouri	417-335-7000	www.skaggs.net
Delray Medical Center	Delray Beach	Florida	561-498-4440	www.delraymedicalctr.com
Detar Hospital Navarro	Victoria	Texas	361-575-7441	www.detar.com
Doctors Hospital	Augusta	Georgia	706-651-6008	www.doctors-hospital.net
Falmouth Hospital	Falmouth	Massachusetts	508-548-5300	www.capecodhealth.com
Fawcett Memorial Hospital	Port Charlotte	Florida	941-629-1181	www.fawcetthospital.com
Forest Hills Hospital	Forest Hills	New York	718-830-4000	www.northshorelij.com
Fort Walton Beach Medical Center	Fort Walton Beach	Florida	850-862-1111	www.fwbmedicalcenter.com
Good Samaritan Hospital Medical Center	West Islip	New York	631-376-3000	www.good-samaritan-hospital.org
Grant Medical Center	Columbus	Ohio	614-566-9978	www.ohiohealth.com
Heartland Regional Medical Center	Saint Joseph	Missouri	816-271-6000	www.heartland-health.com
Holland Community Hospital	Holland	Michigan	616-392-5141	www.hoho.org
Homestead Hospital	Homestead	Florida	786-243-8000	www.baptisthealth.net
John Randolph Medical Center	Hopewell	Virginia	804-541-1600	www.johnrandolphmed.com
Kaiser Foundation Hospital - Redwood City	Redwood City	California	650-299-2000	www.seiu-uhw.org/aboutuhw
Kaiser Foundation Hospital - San Diego	San Diego	California	619-528-5000	www.members.kaiserpermanente.org
Kaiser Foundation Hospital - South Bay	Harbor City	California	310-517-6441	www.kaiserpermanente.org
Kaiser Foundation Hospital - South San Francisco	South San Francisco	California	650-742-3200	www.healthy.kaiserpermanente.org
Lake Pointe Medical Center	Rowlett	Texas	972-412-2273	www.lakepointemedical.com
Lakeview Regional Medical Center	Covington	Louisiana	985-867-4443	www.lakeviewregional.com
Lawnwood Regional Medical Center & Heart Institute	Fort Pierce	Florida	772-461-4000	www.lawnwoodmed.com
Lewisgale Medical Center	Salem	Virginia	540-776-4000	www.lewis-gale.com
Libertyhealth - Jersey City Medical Center Campus	Jersey City	New Jersey	201-915-2000	www.libertyhcs.org
Los Alamitos Medical Center	Los Alamitos	California	562-799-3220	www.losalamitosmedctr.com
Lovelace Medical Center	Albuquerque	New Mexico	505-727-8000	www.lovelace.com
Main Line Hospital Paoli	Paoli	Pennsylvania	610-648-1000	www.mainlinehealth.org
Marshall Medical Center	Placerville	California	530-622-1441	www.marshallmedical.org
Mary Immaculate Hospital	Newport News	Virginia	757-886-6000	www.bonsecourshamptonroad.com
Maui Memorial Medical Center	Wailuku	Hawaii	808-442-5101	www.mauimemorialmedical.org
Memorial Hospital Pembroke	Pembroke Pines	Florida	954-962-9650	www.memorialpembroke.com\
Memorial Hospital West	Pembroke Pines	Florida	954-436-5000	www.memorialwest.com
Mercy Hospital	Bakersfield	California	661-632-5000	www.mercybakersfield.org
Methodist Dallas Medical Center	Dallas	Texas	214-947-2879	www.mhd.com
Methodist Hospital of Southern California	Arcadia	California	626-445-4441	www.methodisthospital.org
Methodist Mansfield Medical Center	Mansfield	Texas	682-622-2059	www.methodisthealthsystem.com
Methodist Medical Center of Oak Ridge	Oak Ridge	Tennessee	865-835-1000	www.mmcoakridge.com
Methodist Richardson Medical Center	Richardson	Texas	972-498-4000	www.richardsonregional.com
Methodist Stone Oak Hospital	San Antonio	Texas	210-638-2100	www.stoneoakhealth.com
Metroplex Hospital	Killeen	Texas	254-526-7523	www.mplex.org
Mills - Peninsula Medical Center	Burlingame	California	650-696-5270	www.mills-peninsula.org
Monmouth Medical Center - Southern Campus	Lakewood	New Jersey	732-363-1900	www.sbhcs.com
Morristown Hamblen Hospital Association	Morristown	Tennessee	423-586-4231	www.mhhs1.org
Newton - Wellesley Hospital	Newton	Massachusetts	617-243-6000	www.nwh.org
North Austin Medical Center	Austin	Texas	512-901-1000	www.cornerstonehealthcaregroup.com
North Cypress Medical Center	Cypress	Texas	281-890-0203	www.ncmc-hospital.com
North Hills Hospital	North Richland Hills	Texas	817-255-1000	www.northhillshospital.com
Northside Hospital	Saint Petersburg	Florida	813-521-5000	www.northsidehospital.com
Northwest Community Hospital	Arlington Heights	Illinois	847-618-1000	www.nch.org
Novant Health Forsyth Medical Center	Winston-Salem	North Carolina	336-718-5000	www.forsythmedicalcenter.org
Novant Health Thomasville Medical Center	Thomasville	North Carolina	336-472-2000	www.thomasvillemedicalcenter.org
Oak Hill Hospital	Brooksville	Florida	352-596-6632	www.oakhillhospital.com

Hospital	City	State	Phone	Web Site
Pali Momi Medical Center	Aiea	Hawaii	808-486-6000	www.kapiolani.org
Palms of Pasadena Hospital	Saint Petersburg	Florida	727-381-1000	www.palmspasadena.com
Pikeville Medical Center	Pikeville	Kentucky	606-218-3500	www.pikevillehospital.org
Portsmouth Regional Hospital	Portsmouth	New Hampshire	603-436-5110	www.portsmouthhospital.com
Presence Saints Mary & Elizabeth Medical Center	Chicago	Illinois	312-770-2000	www.reshealth.org
Reston Hospital Center	Reston	Virginia	703-689-9000	www.restonhospital.com
Richmond University Medical Center	Staten Island	New York	718-818-1234	www.rumcsi.org
Saint Catherine of Siena Hospital	Smithtown	New York	631-862-3000	www.stcatherines.chsli.org
Saint Clair Memorial Hospital	Pittsburgh	Pennsylvania	412-942-6209	www.stclair.org
Saint Joseph Medical Center	Kansas City	Missouri	816-942-4000	www.stjosehkc.com
Saint Mary's Medical Center	San Francisco	California	415-668-1000	www.stmarysmedicalcenter.org
Salinas Valley Memorial Hospital	Salinas	California	831-757-4333	www.svmh.com
San Gabriel Valley Medical Center	San Gabriel	California	626-289-5454	www.sangabrielvalleymedctr.org
San Ramon Regional Medical Center	San Ramon	California	925-275-9200	www.sanramonmedctr.com
Scripps Memorial Hospital La Jolla	La Jolla	California	858-626-4123	www.scrippshealth.org
Sebastian River Medical Center	Sebastian	Florida	772-589-3187	www.srmcenter.com
Shasta Regional Medical Center	Redding	California	530-244-5454	www.shastaregional.com
Sherman Hospital	Elgin	Illinois	847-742-9800	www.shermanhealth.com
Sierra Nevada Memorial Hospital	Grass Valley	California	530-274-6000	www.snmh.org
South Baldwin Regional Medical Center	Foley	Alabama	251-949-3400	www.southbaldwinrmc.com
South Bay Hospital	Sun City Center	Florida	813-634-3301	www.southbayhospital.com
South Miami Hospital	South Miami	Florida	786-662-4000	www.baptisthealth.net
South Pointe Hospital	Warrensville Heights	Ohio	216-491-6000	www.southpointehospital.org
Southern Nh Medical Center	Nashua	New Hampshire	603-577-2000	www.snhmc.org
Sparks Regional Medical Center	Fort Smith	Arkansas	501-441-4000	www.sparks.org
Springs Memorial Hospital	Lancaster	South Carolina	803-286-1481	www.springsmemorial.com
Sunrise Hospital & Medical Center	Las Vegas	Nevada	702-731-8000	www.sunrisehospital.com
Sutter Auburn Faith Hospital	Auburn	California	530-888-4500	www.sutterauburnfaith.org
Temple Community Hospital	Los Angeles	California	213-382-7252	www.templecommunityhospital.com
Texas Health Harris Methodist Hurst - Euless - Bedford	Bedford	Texas	817-848-4000	www.texashealth.org
Texas Health Presbyterian Hospital Plano	Plano	Texas	972-981-8000	www.presbyplano.org
Texoma Medical Center	Denison	Texas	903-416-4000	www.texomamedicalcenter.net
Thibodaux Regional Medical Center	Thibodaux	Louisiana	985-447-5500	www.thibodaux.com
Trinity Medical Center	Birmingham	Alabama	205-592-1000	www.bhsala.com/montclair
University Hospitals Case Medical Center	Cleveland	Ohio	216-844-1000	www.uhhs.com
University of Kentucky Hospital	Lexington	Kentucky	859-323-5000	www.uhealthcare.uky.edu
UPMC East	Monroeville	Pennsylvania	412-357-3000	www.upmc.com
Vaughan Regional Medical Center Parkway Campus	Selma	Alabama	334-418-4100	www.vaughanregional.com
Vista Medical Center East	Waukegan	Illinois	847-360-4000	www.vistahealth.com
Wellmont Bristol Regional Medical Center	Bristol	Tennessee	423-844-1121	www.wellmont.org
Wesley Medical Center	Wichita	Kansas	316-962-2000	www.wesleymc.com
West Florida Hospital	Pensacola	Florida	850-494-4000	www.westfloridahospital.com
West Houston Medical Center	Houston	Texas	281-588-8080	www.westhoustonmedical.com
Wilcox Memorial Hospital	Lihue	Hawaii	808-245-1103	www.wilcoxhealth.org

Note: The hospitals shown above represent the top 5% of the 1,762 hospitals nationwide for which an average score was calculated. Average scores were calculated for hospitals with qualifying data (25 cases or more) in at least 6 of 11 measures in the Stroke Care category.

Best Hospitals for Surgical Care

Hospital	City	State	Phone	Web Site
Arizona Orthopedic & Surgical Speciality Hospital	Chandler	Arizona	480-603-9000	www.azosh.com
Avera Queen of Peace	Mitchell	South Dakota	605-995-2000	www.averaqueenofpeace.org
Baptist Health Corbin	Corbin	Kentucky	606-528-1212	www.baptistregional.com
Baptist Memorial Hospital Union City	Union City	Tennessee	731-885-2410	www.bmhcc.org
Baptist Memorial Hospital Union County	New Albany	Mississippi	662-538-7631	www.baptistonline.org
Baylor Medical Center at Uptown	Dallas	Texas	214-443-3000	www.bmcuptown.com
Baylor Regional Medical Center at Plano	Plano	Texas	469-814-2000	www.baylorhealth.com
Belton Regional Medical Center	Belton	Missouri	816-348-1236	www.beltonregionalmedicalcenter.com
Boca Raton Regional Hospital	Boca Raton	Florida	561-362-5002	www.brrh.com
Broward Health Coral Springs	Coral Springs	Florida	954-344-3000	www.coralspringsmedicalcenter.org
Broward Health Imperial Point	Fort Lauderdale	Florida	954-776-8500	www.nbhd.org
Broward Health Medical Center	Fort Lauderdale	Florida	954-355-4400	www.browardhealth.org
Carolinas Medical Center - Pineville	Charlotte	North Carolina	704-379-5000	www.carolinashealthcare.org
Caromont Regional Medical Center	Gastonia	North Carolina	704-834-4891	www.caromont.org
Dauterive Hospital	New Iberia	Louisiana	337-365-7311	www.dauterivehospital.com
Doctors Hospital	Augusta	Georgia	706-651-6008	www.doctors-hospital.net
Dupont Hospital	Fort Wayne	Indiana	260-416-3000	www.theduponthospital.com
East Alabama Medical Center	Opelika	Alabama	334-749-3411	www.eamc.org
Englewood Community Hospital	Englewood	Florida	941-475-6571	www.englewoodcommunityhospital.com
Exempla Good Samaritan Medical Center	Lafayette	Colorado	303-689-4000	www.exempla.org
Fairview Park Hospital	Dublin	Georgia	478-274-3100	www.fairviewparkhospital.com
Fannin Regional Hospital	Blue Ridge	Georgia	706-632-3711	www.fanninregionalhospital.com
Flowers Hospital	Dothan	Alabama	334-793-5000	www.flowershospital.com
Fort Walton Beach Medical Center	Fort Walton Beach	Florida	850-862-1111	www.fwbmedicalcenter.com
Garden Park Medical Center	Gulfport	Mississippi	228-575-7000	www.gardenparkmedical.com
GHS Patewood Memorial Hospital	Greenville	South Carolina	864-797-1000	www.ghs.org
Holland Community Hospital	Holland	Michigan	616-392-5141	www.hoho.org
Ingalls Memorial Hospital	Harvey	Illinois	708-333-2300	www.ingalls.org
Institute For Orthopaedic Surgery	Lima	Ohio	419-224-7586	www.ioshospital.com
Jefferson Regional Medical Center	Pine Bluff	Arkansas	870-541-7100	www.jrmc.org
JFK Medical Center	Atlantis	Florida	561-965-7300	www.jfkmc.com
Jupiter Medical Center	Jupiter	Florida	561-747-2234	www.jupitermed.com
Kansas Medical Center	Andover	Kansas	316-300-4000	www.ksmedcenter.com
Lake City Medical Center	Lake City	Florida	386-719-9000	www.lakecitymedical.com
Lawnwood Regional Medical Center & Heart Institute	Fort Pierce	Florida	772-461-4000	www.lawnwoodmed.com
Lee's Summit Medical Center	Lees Summit	Missouri	816-282-5000	www.leessummithospital.com
Lewisgale Hospital Montgomery	Blacksburg	Virginia	540-951-1111	www.mrhospital.com
Magee Womens Hospital of UPMC Health System	Pittsburgh	Pennsylvania	412-641-4010	www.magee.edu
Margaret R Pardee Memorial Hospital	Hendersonville	North Carolina	828-696-1000	www.pardeehospital.org
Marion General Hospital	Marion	Ohio	740-383-8400	www.mariongeneral.com
Mary Greeley Medical Center	Ames	Iowa	515-239-2011	www.mgmc.org
McKenzie - Willamette Medical Center	Springfield	Oregon	541-726-4400	www.mckweb.com
Medical Center Enterprise	Enterprise	Alabama	334-347-0584	www.mcehospital.com
Memorial Hospital Pembroke	Pembroke Pines	Florida	954-962-9650	www.memorialpembroke.com\
Memorial Hospital West	Pembroke Pines	Florida	954-436-5000	www.memorialwest.com
Memorial Regional Hospital	Hollywood	Florida	954-987-2000	www.memorialregional.com
Mercy Medical Center	Roseburg	Oregon	541-673-0611	www.mercyrose.org
Methodist Dallas Medical Center	Dallas	Texas	214-947-2879	www.mhd.com
Methodist Mansfield Medical Center	Mansfield	Texas	682-622-2059	www.methodisthealthsystem.com
Mountain View Regional Medical Center	Las Cruces	New Mexico	575-556-7600	www.mountainviewregional.com
Mountainview Hospital	Las Vegas	Nevada	702-255-5065	www.mountainview-hospital.com
North Carolina Specialty Hospital	Durham	North Carolina	919-956-9300	www.ncspecialty.com
North Central Surgical Center	Dallas	Texas	214-265-2810	www.northcentral-sc.com
North Florida Regional Medical Center	Gainesville	Florida	352-333-4100	www.nfrmc.com
North Mississippi Medical Center	Tupelo	Mississippi	662-377-3000	www.nmhs.net/nmmc
North Suburban Medical Center	Thornton	Colorado	303-451-7800	www.northsuburban.com
Northern Westchester Hospital	Mount Kisco	New York	914-666-1200	www.nwhc.net
Northside Hospital	Atlanta	Georgia	404-851-8000	www.northside.com
Northside Hospital Cherokee	Canton	Georgia	770-720-5298	www.northside.com/cherokee
Northside Hospital Forsyth	Cumming	Georgia	404-851-8700	www.gbhcs.org
Northwest Medical Center	Margate	Florida	954-974-0400	www.northwestmed.com
Novant Health Charlotte Orthopedic Hospital	Charlotte	North Carolina	704-316-2000	www.presbyterian.org
Novant Health Forsyth Medical Center	Winston-Salem	North Carolina	336-718-5000	www.forsythmedicalcenter.org
Novant Health Park Hospital	Winston-Salem	North Carolina	336-718-0600	www.novanthealth.org
Novant Health Rowan Medical Center	Salisbury	North Carolina	704-210-5000	www.rowan.org

Hospital	City	State	Phone	Web Site
Ocala Regional Medical Center	Ocala	Florida	352-401-1000	www.ocalaregional.com
Oklahoma Surgical Hospital	Tulsa	Oklahoma	918-477-5000	www.oklahomasurgicalhospital.com
Orange Park Medical Center	Orange Park	Florida	904-276-8500	www.opmedical.com
The Orthopaedic Hospital of Lutheran Health Network	Fort Wayne	Indiana	260-435-2999	www.lutheranhealth.net
Orthopaedic Hospital of Wisconsin	Glendale	Wisconsin	414-961-6800	www.ohow.org
Oss Orthopaedic Hospital	York	Pennsylvania	717-718-2000	www.osshealth.com
Pinnacle Health Hospitals	Harrisburg	Pennsylvania	717-782-5181	www.pinnaclehealth.org
Portsmouth Regional Hospital	Portsmouth	New Hampshire	603-436-5110	www.portsmouthhospital.com
Quail Creek Surgical Hospital	Amarillo	Texas	806-354-6100	www.physurg.com
Rapides Regional Medical Center	Alexandria	Louisiana	318-769-3000	www.rapidesregional.com
Raulerson Hospital	Okeechobee	Florida	863-763-2151	www.raulersonhospital.com
Regional Hospital of Jackson	Jackson	Tennessee	731-661-2000	www.regionalhospitaljackson.com
The Regional Medical Center of Acadiana	Lafayette	Louisiana	337-981-2949	www.medicalcentersw.com
Renown South Meadows Medical Center	Reno	Nevada	775-982-7000	www.renown.org
Reston Hospital Center	Reston	Virginia	703-689-9000	www.restonhospital.com
River Oaks Hospital	Flowood	Mississippi	601-936-2390	www.riveroakshospital.org
Rose Medical Center	Denver	Colorado	303-320-2121	www.rosemed.com
Saint Anthony's Health Center	Alton	Illinois	618-465-2571	www.sahc.org
Saint Charles Hospital	Port Jefferson	New York	631-474-6000	www.stcharles.org
Saint Elizabeth Florence	Florence	Kentucky	859-212-5220	www.stlukehospitals.com
Saint Elizabeth Medical Center	Lakeside Park	Kentucky	859-292-2000	www.stelizabeth.com
Saint Francis Regional Medical Center	Shakopee	Minnesota	952-403-3000	www.stfrancis-shakopee.com
Saint Lucie Medical Center	Port Saint Lucie	Florida	772-335-4000	www.stluciemed.com
Saint Luke's Lakeside Hospital	The Woodlands	Texas	936-266-4055	www.stlukeslakeside.com
Saint Luke's South Hospital	Overland Park	Kansas	913-317-7904	www.saintlukeshealthsystem.org
Saint Mary Medical Center	Hobart	Indiana	219-942-0551	www.comhs.org/stmary
Saint Vincent Healthcare	Billings	Montana	406-657-7000	www.svh-mt.org
Saint Vincent's Medical Center Southside	Jacksonville	Florida	904-296-3700	www.jaxhealth.com
San Angelo Community Medical Center	San Angelo	Texas	325-949-9511	www.sacmc.com
Scripps Green Hospital	La Jolla	California	858-554-3600	www.scrippshealth.org
Scripps Memorial Hospital - Encinitas	Encinitas	California	760-753-6501	www.scripps.org
Sebastian River Medical Center	Sebastian	Florida	772-589-3187	www.srmcenter.com
South Baldwin Regional Medical Center	Foley	Alabama	251-949-3400	www.southbaldwinrmc.com
South Miami Hospital	South Miami	Florida	786-662-4000	www.baptisthealth.net
South Nassau Communities Hospital	Oceanside	New York	516-632-3000	www.southnassau.org
Sparks Regional Medical Center	Fort Smith	Arkansas	501-441-4000	www.sparks.org
Springs Memorial Hospital	Lancaster	South Carolina	803-286-1481	www.springsmemorial.com
Strong Memorial Hospital	Rochester	New York	585-275-2121	www.urmc.rochester.edu
Tanner Medical Center - Carrollton	Carrollton	Georgia	770-836-9580	www.tanner.org
Texas Health Harris Methodist Hospital Southlake	Southlake	Texas	817-748-8700	www.texashealthsouthlake.com
Texas Orthopedic Hospital	Houston	Texas	713-799-8600	www.texasorthopedic.com
Trinity Medical Center	Birmingham	Alabama	205-592-1000	www.bhsala.com/montclair
Twin Cities Hospital	Niceville	Florida	850-678-4131	www.tchealthcare.com
UH Geauga Medical Center	Chardon	Ohio	440-269-6000	www.uhgeauga.org
UPMC East	Monroeville	Pennsylvania	412-357-3000	www.upmc.com
Venice Regional Medical Center - Bayfront Health	Venice	Florida	941-485-7711	www.veniceregional.com
Walker Baptist Medical Center	Jasper	Alabama	205-387-4000	www.bhsala.com/walker
West Florida Hospital	Pensacola	Florida	850-494-4000	www.westfloridahospital.com
West Georgia Medical Center	Lagrange	Georgia	706-882-1411	www.wghealth.org
West Kendall Baptist Hospital	Miami	Florida	786-467-2011	www.baptisthealth.net
West Palm Hospital	West Palm Beach	Florida	561-844-6141	www.columbiahospital.com

Note: The hospitals shown above represent the top 5% of the 2,338 hospitals nationwide for which an average score was calculated. Average scores were calculated for hospitals with qualifying data (25 cases or more) in at least 9 of 10 measures in the Surgical Care Improvment Project category.

Best Hospitals in Terms of Patient's Hospital Experiences

Hospital	City	State	Phone	Web Site
Abbeville Area Medical Center	Abbeville	South Carolina	864-366-5011	www.abbevilleareamc.com
Advanced Surgical Hospital	Washington	Pennsylvania	724-884-0710	www.ashospital.net
Animas Surgical Hospital	Durango	Colorado	970-247-3537	www.animassorgical.com
Arizona Orthopedic & Surgical Speciality Hospital	Chandler	Arizona	480-603-9000	www.azosh.com
Arkansas Heart Hospital	Little Rock	Arkansas	501-219-7000	www.arheart.com
Arkansas Surgical Hospital	No Little Rock	Arkansas	501-748-8000	www.arksurgicalhospital.com
Avera Heart Hospital of South Dakota	Sioux Falls	South Dakota	605-977-7000	www.avera.org/heart-hospital
Avera Saint Anthony's Hospital	O' Neill	Nebraska	402-336-2611	www.avera-sta.org
Baptist Emergency Hospital	San Antonio	Texas	210-402-4092	www.baptistemergencyhospital.com
Barton County Memorial Hospital	Lamar	Missouri	417-682-6081	www.bcmh.net
Baylor Heart & Vascular Hospital	Dallas	Texas	214-820-0670	www.baylorhearthospital.com
Baylor Medical Center at Frisco	Frisco	Texas	214-618-2000	www.bmcf.com
Baylor Medical Center at Trophy Club	Trophy Club	Texas	817-837-4600	www.tc-mc.com
Baylor Medical Center at Uptown	Dallas	Texas	214-443-3000	www.bmcuptown.com
Baylor Orthopedic & Spine Hospital at Arlington	Arlington	Texas	817-549-2364	www.baylorarlington.com
Baylor Surgical Hospital at Las Colinas	Irving	Texas	972-868-4000	www.ic-sh.com
Bear River Valley Hospital	Tremonton	Utah	435-207-4708	www.intermountainhealthcare.org
Bigfork Valley Hospital	Bigfork	Minnesota	218-743-3177	www.bigforkvalley.org
Black Hills Surgical Hospital	Rapid City	South Dakota	605-721-4700	www.bhsh.com
Black River Memorial Hospital	Black River Falls	Wisconsin	715-284-5361	www.brmh.net
Blue Hill Memorial Hospital	Blue Hill	Maine	207-374-2836	www.bhmh.org/default.html
Bluffton Hospital	Bluffton	Ohio	419-358-9010	www.bvhealthsystem.org
Boone County Health Center	Albion	Nebraska	402-395-2191	www.boonecohealth.org
Brodstone Memorial Hospital	Superior	Nebraska	402-879-3281	www.brodstonehospital.org
Bucks County Specialty Hospital	Bensalem	Pennsylvania	215-244-7400	www.bcshospital.com
Caldwell Memorial Hospital	Columbia	Louisiana	318-649-6111	
Central Louisiana Surgical Hospital	Alexandria	Louisiana	318-449-6400	www.clshospital.com
Chickasaw Nation Medical Center	Ada	Oklahoma	580-436-3980	www.chickasaw.net
Choctaw Nation Healthcare	Talihina	Oklahoma	918-567-7000	www.choctawnationhealth.com
Citizens Medical Center	Columbia	Louisiana	318-649-6106	www.citizensmedcenter.com
Clinton County Hospital	Albany	Kentucky	606-387-6421	www.clintoncountyhospital.com
Columbia Center	Mequon	Wisconsin	262-243-7408	www.columbiacenter.org
Community Hospital	Torrington	Wyoming	307-532-4181	www.bannerhealth.com
Community Medical Center	Falls City	Nebraska	402-245-2428	www.hhs.state.ne.us/index.htm
Community Memorial Hospital	Hicksville	Ohio	419-542-6692	www.cmhosp.com
Coordinated Health Orthopedic Hospital	Bethlehem	Pennsylvania	610-691-4300	www.coordinatedhealth.com
Cypress Pointe Surgical Hospital	Hammond	Louisiana	985-510-6200	www.cpsh.org
Dakota Plains Surgical Center	Aberdeen	South Dakota	605-225-3300	www.orthopediccenterofthedakotas.com
Doctors Hospital at Deer Creek	Leesville	Louisiana	337-392-5088	www.dhdc.md
East Texas Medical Center - Gilmer	Gilmer	Texas	903-841-7100	www.etmc.org
East Texas Medical Center Pittsburg	Pittsburg	Texas	903-856-4520	www.etmc.org
Electra Memorial Hospital	Electra	Texas	940-495-3981	www.electrahospital.com
Fairview Hospital	Great Barrington	Massachusetts	413-528-0790	www.berkshirehealthsystems.com
Fairway Medical Center	Covington	Louisiana	985-801-3010	www.fairwaymedical.com
Fayette Medical Center	Fayette	Alabama	205-932-5966	www.dchsystem.com
First Care Health Center	Park River	North Dakota	701-284-7500	www.firstcarehc.com
Floyd County Memorial Hospital	Charles City	Iowa	641-228-6830	www.fcmc.us.com
Fostoria Community Hospital	Fostoria	Ohio	419-435-7734	www.promedica.org
Foundation Surgical Hospital of San Antonio	San Antonio	Texas	210-478-5400	www.fshsanantonio.com
Fresno Surgical Hospital	Fresno	California	559-431-8000	www.fresnosurgerycenter.com
GHS Patewood Memorial Hospital	Greenville	South Carolina	864-797-1000	www.ghs.org
Glacial Ridge Hospital	Glenwood	Minnesota	320-634-2208	www.glacialridge.org
Grant Regional Health Center	Lancaster	Wisconsin	608-723-2143	www.grantregional.com
Great Falls Clinic Medical Center	Great Falls	Montana	406-216-8000	www.gfclinic.com
Green Clinic Surgical Hospital	Ruston	Louisiana	318-232-7700	www.green-clinic.com
Grundy County Memorial Hospital	Grundy Center	Iowa	319-824-5421	www.grundyhospital.com
H B Magruder Memorial Hospital	Port Clinton	Ohio	419-734-3131	www.magruderhospital.com
Heart Hospital Baylor Plano	Plano	Texas	469-814-3278	www.thehearthospitalbaylor.com
Heart Hospital of Lafayette	Lafayette	Louisiana	337-521-1000	www.hearthospitaloflafayette.com
Heritage Park Surgical Hospital	Sherman	Texas	903-813-3728	www.heritageparksurgicalhospital.com
Hill Country Memorial Hospital	Fredericksburg	Texas	830-997-4353	www.hcmbs.org
Hillsboro Area Hospital	Hillsboro	Illinois	217-532-6111	www.hillsboroareahospital.org
Hoag Orthopedic Institute	Irvine	California	949-727-5000	www.orthopedichospital.com
Houston Orthopedic & Spine Hospital	Bellaire	Texas	713-622-2262	www.foundationsurgicalhospital.com
Houston Physicians' Hospital	Webster	Texas	281-335-1700	www.houstonphysicianshospital.com

Hospital	City	State	Phone	Web Site
Indiana Orthopaedic Hospital	Indianapolis	Indiana	317-956-1000	www.indianaorthopaedichospital.com
Institute For Orthopaedic Surgery	Lima	Ohio	419-224-7586	www.ioshospital.com
Integris Health Edmond	Edmond	Oklahoma	405-657-3000	www.integrisok.com/integris-health-edmond-ok
Jefferson County Health Center	Fairfield	Iowa	641-472-4111	www.jchospital.org
Kansas City Orthopaedic Institute	Leawood	Kansas	913-319-7633	www.kcoi.com
Kentuckiana Medical Center	Clarksville	Indiana	812-280-3300	www.kentuckianamedcen.com
King's Daughters Medical Center - Brookhaven	Brookhaven	Mississippi	601-833-6011	www.kdmc.org
Lady of the Sea General Hospital	Cut Off	Louisiana	985-632-6401	www.losgh.org
Lafayette Surgical Specialty Hospital	Lafayette	Louisiana	337-769-4100	www.lafayettesurgical.com
Lakeview Memorial Hospital	Stillwater	Minnesota	651-439-5330	www.lakeview.org
Lawrence County Hospital	Monticello	Mississippi	601-587-4051	www.smrmc.com/index.php
Lincoln Surgical Hospital	Lincoln	Nebraska	402-484-9090	www.lincolnsurgery.com
Mackinac Straits Hospital & Health Center	Saint Ignace	Michigan	906-643-8585	www.mackinacstraitshealth.org
Manhattan Surgical Hospital	Manhattan	Kansas	785-776-5100	www.manhattansurgical.com
Mariners Hospital	Tavernier	Florida	305-434-3000	www.baptisthealth.net
Marion Regional Medical Center	Hamilton	Alabama	205-921-6200	www.nmhs.net
Mayo Clinic Hospital	Phoenix	Arizona	480-342-2000	www.mayoclinic.org
McBride Clinic Orthopedic Hospital	Oklahoma City	Oklahoma	405-478-1717	www.mcbrideclinic.com
Menlo Park Surgical Hospital	Menlo Park	California	650-324-8500	www.pamf.org/mpsh
Mercy Willard Hospital	Willard	Ohio	419-964-5000	www.mercyweb.org/mercy_willard.aspx
Miami County Medical Center	Paola	Kansas	913-557-4385	www.olathehealth.org
Mid - Valley Hospital	Peckville	Pennsylvania	570-383-5000	
Midwest Orthopedic Specialty Hospital	Franklin	Wisconsin	414-817-5800	www.mymosh.com
Midwest Surgical Hospital	Omaha	Nebraska	402-399-1900	www.mwsurgicalhospital.com
Millinocket Regional Hospital	Millinocket	Maine	207-723-5161	www.mrhme.org
Ministry Door County Medical Center	Sturgeon Bay	Wisconsin	920-743-5566	www.doorcountymemorial.org
Mount Carmel New Albany Surgical Hospital	New Albany	Ohio	614-775-6600	www.mountcarmelhealth.com
Mount Desert Island Hospital	Bar Harbor	Maine	207-288-5081	www.mdihospital.com
Mountain View Regional Hospital	Casper	Wyoming	307-995-8100	www.monroehospital.com
Nebraska Orthopaedic Hospital	Omaha	Nebraska	402-609-1600	www.neorthohospital.com
The Neuromedical Center Hospital	Baton Rouge	Louisiana	225-763-9900	www.theneuromedicalcenter.com
North Carolina Specialty Hospital	Durham	North Carolina	919-956-9300	www.ncspecialty.com
North Central Surgical Center	Dallas	Texas	214-265-2810	www.northcentral-sc.com
Northside Medical Center	Columbus	Georgia	706-494-2100	www.hughstonsports.com
Northwest Hills Surgical Hospital	Austin	Texas	512-346-1994	www.scasurgery.com
Northwest Specialty Hospital	Post Falls	Idaho	208-262-2300	www.northwestspecialtyhospital.com
Northwest Surgical Hospital	Oklahoma City	Oklahoma	404-848-1918	www.nwsurgicalokc.com
Oak Leaf Surgical Hospital	Eau Claire	Wisconsin	715-831-8130	www.oakleafsurgical.com
Ogallala Community Hospital	Ogallala	Nebraska	308-284-4011	www.bannerhealth.com
Oklahoma Center for Orthopaedic & Multi-Spec	Oklahoma City	Oklahoma	405-602-6500	www.ocomhospital.com
Oklahoma Heart Hospital	Oklahoma City	Oklahoma	405-608-3200	www.okheart.com
Oklahoma Heart Hospital South	Oklahoma City	Oklahoma	405-628-6000	www.okheart.com/south-campus
Oklahoma Spine Hospital	Oklahoma City	Oklahoma	405-749-2700	www.oklahomaspine.com
Oklahoma Surgical Hospital	Tulsa	Oklahoma	918-477-5000	www.oklahomasurgicalhospital.com
Orange City Area Health System	Orange City	Iowa	712-737-4984	www.ochealthsystem.org
Orthopaedic Hospital of Wisconsin	Glendale	Wisconsin	414-961-6800	www.ohow.org
OSF Holy Family Medical Center	Monmouth	Illinois	309-734-3141	www.cmchospital.com
Oss Orthopaedic Hospital	York	Pennsylvania	717-718-2000	www.osshealth.com
Ouachita Community Hospital	West Monroe	Louisiana	318-322-1339	www.ouachitahospital.com
P & S Surgical Hospital	Monroe	Louisiana	318-388-4040	www.pssurgery.com
Patients' Hospital of Redding	Redding	California	530-225-8700	www.patientshospital.com
Pella Regional Health Center	Pella	Iowa	641-628-3150	www.pellahealth.org
Pender Community Hospital	Pender	Nebraska	402-385-3083	www.pendercommunityhospital.com
Physician's Care Surgical Hospital	Royersford	Pennsylvania	610-495-4793	www.phycarehospital.com
The Physicians Centre	Bryan	Texas	979-731-3100	www.thephysicianscentre.com
Physicians Medical Center	Houma	Louisiana	985-853-1390	www.physicianshouma.com
Physicians' Medical Center	New Albany	Indiana	812-206-7660	www.pmcdev.interactivemedialab.com
Physicians' Specialty Hospital	Fayetteville	Arkansas	479-571-7002	www.pshfay.com
Quail Creek Surgical Hospital	Amarillo	Texas	806-354-6100	www.physurg.com
Richland Parish Hospital - Delhi	Delhi	Louisiana	318-878-5171	www.delhihospital.com
River Falls Area Hospital	River Falls	Wisconsin	715-307-6000	www.allina.com
Rochelle Community Hospital	Rochelle	Illinois	815-562-2181	www.rcha.net
Rockcastle County Hospital	Mount Vernon	Kentucky	606-256-2195	www.rockcastlehospital.com
Rollins Brook Community Hospital	Lampasas	Texas	512-556-3682	www.mplex.org
Sacred Heart Hospital on the Gulf	Port Saint Joe	Florida	850-229-5600	www.sacred-heart.org/gulf
Saint Joseph Memorial Hospital	Murphysboro	Illinois	618-684-3156	www.sih.net
Saint Joseph's Hospital	Breese	Illinois	618-526-4511	www.stjoebreese.com

Hospital	City	State	Phone	Web Site
Saint Luke's Lakeside Hospital	The Woodlands	Texas	936-266-4055	www.stlukeslakeside.com
Saint Luke's Wood River Medical Center	Ketchum	Idaho	208-727-8800	www.stlukesonline.org/wood_river
Saint Thomas Hospital for Spinal Surgery	Nashville	Tennessee	615-515-8200	www.hospitalforspinalsurgery.com
Salina Surgical Hospital	Salina	Kansas	785-827-0610	www.salinasurgical.com
Sanford Luverne Medical Center	Luverne	Minnesota	507-283-2321	www.sanfordluverne.org
Sauk Prairie Hospital	Prairie Du Sac	Wisconsin	608-643-3311	www.spmh.org
Sharp Coronado Hospital & Healthcare Center	Coronado	California	619-435-6251	www.sharp.com/coronado
Sioux Falls Specialty Hospital	Sioux Falls	South Dakota	605-334-6730	www.sfsurgical.com
Siouxland Surgery Center	Dakota Dunes	South Dakota	605-232-3332	www.siouxlandsurg.com
South Texas Spine & Surgical Hospital	San Antonio	Texas	210-404-0800	www.southtexassurgical.com
South Texas Surgical Hospital	Corpus Christi	Texas	361-993-2000	www.nshinc.com
Southern Surgical Hospital	Slidell	Louisiana	985-641-0600	www.sshla.com
Southwestern Regional Medical Center	Tulsa	Oklahoma	918-496-5000	www.cancercenter.com/southwestern
Specialists Hospital Shreveport	Shreveport	Louisiana	318-213-3800	www.specialistshospitalshreveport.com
Stanislaus Surgical Hospital	Modesto	California	209-572-2700	www.stanislaussurgical.com
Stewart Memorial Community Hospital	Lake City	Iowa	712-464-3171	www.stewartmemorial.org
Stoughton Hospital	Stoughton	Wisconsin	608-873-6611	www.stoughtonhospital.com
Sugar Land Surgical Hospital	Sugar Land	Texas	281-243-1000	www.sugarlandsurgicalhospital.com
Surgical Hospital at Southwoods	Youngstown	Ohio	330-758-1954	www.surgeryatsouthwoods.com
Surgical Institute of Reading	Wyomissing	Pennsylvania	717-999-9999	www.sireading.com
Surgical Specialty Center at Coordinated Health	Allentown	Pennsylvania	610-871-9110	www.coordinatedhealth.com
Surgical Specialty Center of Baton Rouge	Baton Rouge	Louisiana	225-408-5730	www.sscbr.com
Sutter Surgical Hospital - North Valley	Yuba City	California	530-749-5700	www.suttersurgicalhospitalnorthvalley.org
Texas Health Center for Diagnostics & Surgery	Plano	Texas	972-403-2700	www.ppcds.com
Texas Health Harris Methodist Hospital Southlake	Southlake	Texas	817-748-8700	www.texashealthsouthlake.com
Texas Institute for Surgery at Presbyterian Hospital	Dallas	Texas	214-647-5300	www.texasinstituteforsurgery.org
Texas Spine & Joint Hospital	Tyler	Texas	903-525-3300	www.tsjh.org
Tishomingo Health Services	Iuka	Mississippi	662-423-6051	www.nmhs.net/iuka
Tops Surgical Specialty Hospital	Houston	Texas	281-539-2900	www.tops-hospital.com
Treasure Valley Hospital	Boise	Idaho	208-373-5000	www.treasurevalleyhospital.com
Tulsa Spine & Specialty Hospital	Tulsa	Oklahoma	918-388-5701	www.tulsaspinehospital.com
United Regional Medical Center	Manchester	Tennessee	931-728-3586	www.urmchealthcare.com
University Hospitals Conneaut Medical Center	Conneaut	Ohio	440-593-1131	www.uhhospitals.org/conneaut
Upland Hills Health	Dodgeville	Wisconsin	608-930-8000	www.uplandhillshealth.org
USMD Hospital at Arlington	Arlington	Texas	817-472-3400	www.usmdhospital.com
USMD Hospital at Fort Worth	Fort Worth	Texas	817-433-9100	www.usmdfortworth.com
Vernon Memorial Hospital	Viroqua	Wisconsin	608-637-2101	www.vmh.org
Vidant Bertie Hospital	Windsor	North Carolina	252-794-6600	www.vidanthealth.com/bertie
W J Mangold Memorial Hospital	Lockney	Texas	806-652-3373	www.mangoldmemorial.org
Wellspan Surgery & Rehabilitation Hospital	York	Pennsylvania	717-812-6100	www.wellspan.org
West Kendall Baptist Hospital	Miami	Florida	786-467-2011	www.baptisthealth.net
Westlake Regional Hospital	Columbia	Kentucky	270-384-4753	www.westlake-healthcare.org
Whitman Hospital & Medical Center	Colfax	Washington	509-397-3435	www.whitmanhospital.com
Wright Memorial Hospital	Trenton	Missouri	660-359-5621	www.saintlukeshealthsystem.org
York Hospital	York	Maine	207-363-4321	www.yorkhospital.com

Note: The hospitals shown above represent the top 5% of the 3,591 hospitals nationwide for which an average score was calculated. Average scores were calculated for hospitals with qualifying data (100 completed surveys or more) in all ten measures in the Survey of Patient's Hospital Experiences category.

Best Hospitals in Terms of Use of Medical Imaging

Hospital	City	State	Phone	Web Site
Alameda Hospital	Alameda	California	510-522-3700	www.alamedahospital.org
Bartlett Regional Hospital	Juneau	Alaska	907-796-8900	www.bartletthospital.org
Caldwell Memorial Hospital	Lenoir	North Carolina	828-757-5100	www.caldwellmemorial.org
Capital Regional Medical Center	Tallahassee	Florida	850-656-5000	www.capitalregionalmedicalcenter.com
Carroll County Memorial Hospital	Carrollton	Kentucky	502-732-4321	www.ccmhosp.com
Centrastate Medical Center	Freehold	New Jersey	732-431-2000	www.centrastate.com
Chandler Regional Medical Center	Chandler	Arizona	480-963-4561	www.chandlerregional.com
Chinese Hospital	San Francisco	California	415-982-2400	www.chinesehospital-sf.org
Community Regional Medical Center	Fresno	California	559-459-6000	www.communitymedical.org
Conemaugh Valley Memorial Hospital	Johnstown	Pennsylvania	814-534-9000	www.conemaugh.org
Deaconess Hospital	Spokane	Washington	509-473-5800	www.deaconessmedicalcenter.org
Doctors Medical Center	Modesto	California	209-578-1211	www.dmc-modesto.com
Doctors Medical Center - San Pablo	San Pablo	California	510-970-5000	www.doctorsmedicalcenter.org
Dominican Hospital	Santa Cruz	California	831-462-7700	www.dominicanhospital.org
Emanuel Medical Center	Turlock	California	209-667-4200	www.emanuelmedicalcenter.org
Enloe Medical Center	Chico	California	530-332-7300	www.enloe.org
Evergreen Hospital Medical Center	Kirkland	Washington	425-899-1000	www.evergreenhospital.org
Exempla Saint Joseph Hospital	Denver	Colorado	303-837-7111	www.exempla.org
Fairview Hospital	Cleveland	Ohio	216-476-7000	www.fairviewhospital.org
Fairview Park Hospital	Dublin	Georgia	478-274-3100	www.fairviewparkhospital.com
Glens Falls Hospital	Glens Falls	New York	518-926-1000	www.glensfallshospital.org
Good Samaritan Hospital	San Jose	California	408-559-2011	www.goodsamsj.org
Halifax Health Medical Center	Daytona Beach	Florida	386-254-4000	www.halifax.org
Harrison Memorial Center	Bremerton	Washington	360-377-3911	www.harrisonmedical.org
Hartford Hospital	Hartford	Connecticut	860-545-5000	www.harthosp.org
Healthalliance Hospitals	Leominster	Massachusetts	978-466-2000	www.healthalliance.com
Heart Hospital Baylor Plano	Plano	Texas	469-814-3278	www.thehearthospitalbaylor.com
Holy Redeemer Hospital & Medical Center	Meadowbrook	Pennsylvania	215-947-3000	www.holyredeemer.com
Huntington Hospital	Huntington	New York	631-351-2000	www.hunthosp.org
Huntington Memorial Hospital	Pasadena	California	626-397-5000	www.huntingtonhospital.com
Indiana University Health White Memorial Hospital	Monticello	Indiana	574-583-7111	www.whitecmh.org
Inova Fairfax Hospital	Falls Church	Virginia	703-776-3332	www.inova.org
Jefferson Medical Center	Ranson	West Virginia	304-728-1600	www.jeffmem.com
Johnson Memorial Hospital	Stafford Springs	Connecticut	860-684-4251	www.johnsonhealthnetwork.com
Lake City Medical Center	Lake City	Florida	386-719-9000	www.lakecitymedical.com
Lake Regional Health System	Osage Beach	Missouri	573-348-8000	www.lakeregional.com
Lakewood Regional Medical Center	Lakewood	California	562-602-6751	www.lakewoodregional.com
Lasalle General Hospital	Jena	Louisiana	318-992-9200	www.lasallegeneralhospital.com
Little Falls Hospital	Little Falls	New York	315-823-5261	www.lfhny.org
Long Island Jewish Medical Center	New Hyde Park	New York	718-470-7000	www.northshorelij.com
Lourdes Medical Center of Burlington County	Willingboro	New Jersey	609-835-2900	www.lourdesnet.org/lourdes
Lovelace Medical Center	Albuquerque	New Mexico	505-727-8000	www.lovelace.com
Lowell General Hospital	Lowell	Massachusetts	978-937-6000	www.lowellgeneral.org
Mainegeneral Medical Center	Augusta	Maine	207-872-1000	www.mainegeneral.org
Maria Parham Medical Center	Henderson	North Carolina	252-438-4143	www.mphosp.org
Marin General Hospital	Greenbrae	California	415-925-7900	www.maringeneral.com
Mary Greeley Medical Center	Ames	Iowa	515-239-2011	www.mgmc.org
Mary Washington Hospital	Fredericksburg	Virginia	540-741-1100	www.medicorp.org
Maui Memorial Medical Center	Wailuku	Hawaii	808-442-5101	www.mauimemorialmedical.org
Mayo Clinic Health System - Albert Lea	Albert Lea	Minnesota	507-373-2384	www.mayoclinichealthsystem.org
McKenzie - Willamette Medical Center	Springfield	Oregon	541-726-4400	www.mckweb.com
Medstar Franklin Square Medical Center	Baltimore	Maryland	443-777-7850	www.franklinsquare.org
Medstar Southern Maryland Hospital Center	Clinton	Maryland	301-868-8000	www.medstarhealth.org
Memorial Medical Center	Modesto	California	209-526-4500	www.memorialmedicalcenter.org
Mercy General Hospital	Sacramento	California	916-453-4545	www.mercygeneral.org
Mercy Gilbert Medical Center	Gilbert	Arizona	480-728-8327	www.dignityhealth.org/mercygilbert
Mercy Hospital	Coon Rapids	Minnesota	763-236-8205	www.allinamercy.org
Mercy Medical Center - Clinton	Clinton	Iowa	563-244-5555	www.mercyclinton.com
Mercy Medical Center - Redding	Redding	California	530-225-6102	www.redding.mercy.org
Mercy San Juan Medical Center	Carmichael	California	916-537-5000	www.mercysanjuan.org
Mercy Willard Hospital	Willard	Ohio	419-964-5000	www.mercyweb.org/mercy_willard.aspx
Methodist Hospital of Sacramento	Sacramento	California	916-423-6010	www.methodistsacramento.org
Methodist Hospital of Southern California	Arcadia	California	626-445-4441	www.methodisthospital.org
Metrosouth Medical Center	Blue Island	Illinois	708-597-2000	www.stfrancisblueisland.com
Miriam Hospital	Providence	Rhode Island	401-793-2500	www.lifespan.org/partners/tmh

Hospital	City	State	Phone	Web Site
Nashoba Valley Medical Center	Ayer	Massachusetts	978-784-9000	www.nashobamed.com
Newton Memorial Hospital	Newton	New Jersey	973-383-2121	www.itsyourlife.com
North Florida Regional Medical Center	Gainesville	Florida	352-333-4100	www.nfrmc.com
Northbay Medical Center	Fairfield	California	707-646-5000	www.northbay.org
Ocala Regional Medical Center	Ocala	Florida	352-401-1000	www.ocalaregional.com
Page Memorial Hospital	Luray	Virginia	540-743-4561	www.pagememorialhospital.org
Palomar Health Downtown Campus	Escondido	California	760-739-3000	www.pph.org
Paris Regional Medical Center	Paris	Texas	903-785-4521	www.parisregional.com
Peacehealth Saint Joseph Medical Center	Bellingham	Washington	360-734-5400	www.peacehealth.org
Penobscot Bay Medical Center	Rockport	Maine	207-596-8000	www.nehealth.org
PIH Hospital - Downey	Downey	California	526-904-5000	www.drmci.org
Pomerado Hospital	Poway	California	858-485-6511	www.pph.org
Providence Sacred Heart Medical Center	Spokane	Washington	509-474-3040	www.shmc.org
Regional Medical Center of San Jose	San Jose	California	408-259-5000	www.regionalmedicalsanjose.com
Riverview Hospital Assoc	Wisconsin Rapids	Wisconsin	715-423-6060	www.riverviewhospital.net
Robert Wood Johnson University Hospital	New Brunswick	New Jersey	732-937-8900	www.rwjuh.edu
Saint Alphonsus Medical Center - Ontario	Ontario	Oregon	541-881-7000	www.holyrosary-ontario.org
Saint Alphonsus Regional Medical Center	Boise	Idaho	208-367-2121	www.saintalphonsus.org
Saint David's Medical Center	Austin	Texas	512-476-7111	www.stdavidsrehab.com
Saint Joseph Mercy Port Huron	Port Huron	Michigan	810-985-1510	www.mercyporthuron.com
Saint Joseph's Hospital Health Center	Syracuse	New York	315-448-5111	www.sjhsyr.org
Saint Mary's Hospital - Troy	Troy	New York	518-272-5000	www.setonhealth.org
Saint Marys Hospital	Waterbury	Connecticut	203-574-6000	www.stmh.org
Saint Thomas Rutherford Hospital	Murfreesboro	Tennessee	615-396-4100	www.mtmc.org
Salinas Valley Memorial Hospital	Salinas	California	831-757-4333	www.svmh.com
Santa Rosa Memorial Hospital	Santa Rosa	California	707-525-5300	www.stjosephhealth.org
Santiam Memorial Hospital	Stayton	Oregon	503-769-2175	www.santiamhospital.com
Scottsdale Healthcare - Thompson Peak Hospital	Scottsdale	Arizona	480-324-7004	www.shc.org
Scottsdale Healthcare Osborn Medical Center	Scottsdale	Arizona	480-882-4000	www.shc.org
Shady Grove Adventist Hospital	Rockville	Maryland	240-826-6517	www.adventisthealthcare.com/sgah
Sharp Chula Vista Medical Center	Chula Vista	California	619-502-5800	www.sharp.com
Southwest Regional Medical Center	Georgetown	Ohio	513-378-7800	www.browncountygeneralhospital.com
Stafford Hospital	Stafford	Virginia	540-741-9000	www.marywashingtonhealthcare.com
Sutter Delta Medical Center	Antioch	California	925-779-7200	www.sutterdelta.org
Sutter General Hospital	Sacramento	California	916-733-8999	www.suttermedicalcenter.org
Sutter Roseville Medical Center	Roseville	California	916-781-1000	www.sutterroseville.org
Swedish Edmonds Hospital	Edmonds	Washington	425-640-4000	www.stevenshealthcare.org
Tallahassee Memorial Hospital	Tallahassee	Florida	850-431-1155	www.tmh.org
Texas Health Presbyterian Hospital Dallas	Dallas	Texas	214-345-6789	www.texashealth.org
Trinity Rock Island	Rock Island	Illinois	309-779-5000	www.trinityqc.com
Union Hospital Clinton	Clinton	Indiana	765-832-1234	www.unionhospitalhealthgroup.org/wcch
University Medical Center at Brackenridge	Austin	Texas	512-324-7000	www.seton.net/locations/brackenridge
University Medical Center of Princeton at Plainsboro	Plainsboro	New Jersey	866-460-4776	www.princetonhcs.org
Valley Hospital	Spokane	Washington	509-924-6650	www.valleyhospital.org
Vidant Duplin Hospital	Kenansville	North Carolina	910-296-0941	www.dgh.org
Virtua Memorial Hospital of Burlington County	Mount Holly	New Jersey	609-914-6200	www.virtua.org
Warren Memorial Hospital	Front Royal	Virginia	703-636-0300	www.valleyhealthlink.com
Waterbury Hospital	Waterbury	Connecticut	203-573-6000	www.waterburyhospital.org
Watsonville Community Hospital	Watsonville	California	831-724-4741	www.watsonvillehospital.com
West Hills Hospital & Medical Center	West Hills	California	818-676-4100	www.westhillshospital.com
West Valley Medical Center	Caldwell	Idaho	208-459-4641	www.westvalleymedctr.com
Wooster Community Hospital	Wooster	Ohio	330-263-8100	www.woosterhospital.org

Note: The hospitals shown above represent the top 5% of the 2,308 hospitals nationwide for which an average score was calculated. Average scores were calculated for hospitals with qualifying data (25 cases or more) in at least 4 of 5 measures in the Use of Medical Imaging category. The measure, Follow-up Mammogram/Ultrasound, was not included in the average score.

Hospitals with the Lowest Medicare Spending per Beneficiary

Hospital	City	State	Phone	Web Site
Basin Healthcare Center	Odessa	Texas	432-425-9510	www.bhcodessa.com
Beaver Valley Hospital	Beaver	Utah	435-438-7102	
Bob Wilson Memorial Grant County Hospital	Ulysses	Kansas	620-356-1266	www.bwmgch.com
Brighton Hospital	Brighton	Michigan	810-227-1211	www.stjohn.org/brighton
Cherokee Indian Hospital Authority	Cherokee	North Carolina	704-497-9163	
Chinle Comprehensive Health Care Facility	Chinle	Arizona	928-674-7001	
Crownpoint Healthcare Facility	Crownpoint	New Mexico	505-786-5291	www.ihs.gov
Dhhs Usphs Indian Health Services	San Fidel	New Mexico	505-552-5300	www.ihs.gov
Eastern State Hospital	Williamsburg	Virginia	757-253-5161	www.ehs.dmhmrsas.virginia.gov
Epic Medical Center	Eufaula	Oklahoma	918-689-2535	
Fort Defiance Indian Hospital	Fort Defiance	Arizona	928-729-8000	www.home.navajo.his.gov
Gallup Indian Medical Center	Gallup	New Mexico	505-722-1000	www.ihs.gov/facilitiesservices
Guadalupe County Hospital	Santa Rosa	New Mexico	575-472-3417	
Harmon Memorial Hospital	Hollis	Oklahoma	580-688-3363	
Ira Davenport Memorial Hospital	Bath	New York	607-776-8500	www.davenportandtaylor.org
Kaiser Foundation Hospital - Antioch	Antioch	California	925-813-6500	www.kaiserpermanente.org
Kaiser Foundation Hospital - Fresno	Fresno	California	559-448-4500	www.kaiserpermanente.org
Kaiser Foundation Hospital - San Diego	San Diego	California	619-528-5000	www.members.kaiserpermanente.org
Kaiser Foundation Hospital - San Francisco	San Francisco	California	415-833-2646	www.permanente.net
Kaiser Foundation Hospital - South San Francisco	South San Francisco	California	650-742-3200	www.healthy.kaiserpermanente.org
Kaiser Foundation Hospital - Vacaville	Vacaville	California	707-624-4000	www.kaiserpermanente.org
Kaiser Sunnyside Medical Center	Clackamas	Oregon	503-571-2880	www.members.kaiserpermanente.org
Keefe Memorial Hospital	Cheyenne Wells	Colorado	719-767-5661	
Laguna Honda Hospital & Rehabilitation Center	San Francisco	California	415-759-2300	www.dph.sf.ca.us/chn/lagunahondahosp
Lewis County General Hospital	Lowville	New York	315-376-5200	www.lcgh.net
Memorial Hospital of Texas County	Guymon	Oklahoma	580-338-6515	www.mhtcguymon.org
Morton County Hospital	Elkhart	Kansas	620-697-2141	www.mchswecare.com
Mount Edgecumbe Hospital	Sitka	Alaska	907-966-2411	www.searhc.org
Newman Memorial Hospital	Shattuck	Oklahoma	580-938-2551	
P H S Indian Hospital at Belcourt - Quentin N Burdick	Belcourt	North Dakota	701-477-6111	
P H S Indian Hospital at Browning - Blackfeet	Browning	Montana	406-338-6157	www.ihs.gov
Phoenix Indian Medical Center	Phoenix	Arizona	602-263-1200	www.ihs.gov
PHS Indian Hospital at Pine Ridge	Pine Ridge	South Dakota	605-867-5131	www.ihs.gov
PHS Indian Hospital at Rosebud	Rosebud	South Dakota	605-747-2231	www.ihs.gov
Provident Hospital of Chicago	Chicago	Illinois	312-572-2000	www.providentfoundation.org
Red Lake Hospital	Redlake	Minnesota	218-679-3912	
Sacred Heart University District	Eugene	Oregon	541-686-7300	www.peacehealth.org
Sonoma Developmental Center	Eldridge	California	707-938-6393	www.dds.ca.gov/sonoma/index.cfm
South Lyon Medical Center	Yerington	Nevada	775-781-3761	
Tuba City Regional Health Care Corporation	Tuba City	Arizona	928-283-2501	www.tcrhcc.org
USPHS Lawton Indian Hospital	Lawton	Oklahoma	580-354-5000	
Valley Forge Medical Center & Hospital	Norristown	Pennsylvania	215-539-8500	www.vfmc.net
Wayne Medical Center	Waynesboro	Tennessee	931-722-5411	
Whiteriver PHS Indian Hospital	Whiteriver	Arizona	928-338-4911	
Whitfield Medical Surgical Hospital	Whitfield	Mississippi	601-351-8001	
Yalobusha General Hospital	Water Valley	Mississippi	662-473-1411	
Yukon Kuskokwim Delta Regional Hospital	Bethel	Alaska	907-543-6300	www.ykhc.org
Zuni Comprehensive Community Health Center	Zuni	New Mexico	505-782-4431	www.ihs.gov

Note: These 48 hospitals had an average ratio of 0.75 or less in the Medicare Spending per Beneficiary category. A total of 3,229 hospitals had medicare spending data available.

Appendix E: Glossary

Accreditation
An evaluative process in which a healthcare organization undergoes an examination of its policies, procedures and performance by an external private sector organization ("accrediting body") to ensure that it is meeting predetermined criteria. It usually involves both on- and off-site surveys. Also see the terms American Osteopathic Association, The Joint Commission, and Medicare-Certified Hospitals.

Acute Care—VA Medical Center
The Veterans Health Administration (VA) Medical Centers deliver inpatient hospital care and related services for surgery and short-term health conditions, as well as comprehensive primary, specialty and long-term care. The VA's medical benefits package is available to Veterans (including Reservists and National Guard) who served on active duty and meet eligibility requirements. Other groups can also be eligible. For more information, visit the U.S. Department of Veterans Affairs.

Acute care hospital
A hospital that provides inpatient medical care and other related services for surgery, acute medical conditions or injuries (usually for a short-term illness or condition).

Acute myocardial infarction (AMI)
See Heart Attack.

American Hospital Association (AHA)
The national organization that represents and serves all types of hospitals, health care networks, and their patients and communities. AHA takes part in national health policy development, legislative and regulatory debates, and legal matters. It also provides education for health care leaders and is a source of information on health care issues and trends.

American Osteopathic Association (AOA)
A member association representing approximately 52,000 osteopathic physicians (D.O.s). The AOA serves as the primary certifying body for D.O.s, and is the accrediting agency for all osteopathic medical colleges and health care facilities. The AOA writes a performance report on each hospital that it checks. You can call or write to AOA to find out a hospital's level of accreditation.

Angioplasty
In angioplasty, a catheter is used to insert a balloon that is inflated to open a blocked blood vessel. Percutaneous transluminal coronary angioplasty (PTCA) is one of several procedures used to open a blocked blood vessel, known collectively as a percutaneous coronary intervention (PCI).

Angiotensin converting enzyme (ACE) inhibitor
A drug used to treat heart attacks, heart failure, or a decreased function of the left heart. It stops production of a hormone that can narrow blood vessels, which helps reduce the pressure in the heart and lower blood pressure.

Angiotensin receptor blocker (ARB)
A drug used to treat patients with heart failure and a decreased function of the left heart. ARBs block the action of a hormone that can narrow blood vessels. This helps reduce the pressure in the heart and lower blood pressure.

Antibiotic
Drugs used to fight bacteria in the body.

ASA Physical Status Classification
Assessment by the anesthesiologist of the patient's preoperative physical condition using the American Society of Anesthesiologists' (ASA) Classification of Physical Status.

Asthma
A chronic lung condition that causes problems getting air in and out of the lungs. Children with asthma may experience wheezing, coughing, chest tightness and trouble breathing.

Atherectomy
A procedure where a blade or laser on a catheter cuts through and removes blockages in blood vessels. It is one of several procedures used to open a blocked blood vessel (known as a Percutaneous Coronary Intervention or PCI).

Beta blocker
A type of drug that is used to lower blood pressure, treat chest pain (angina) and heart failure, and to help prevent a heart attack. Beta blockers relieve the stress on the heart by slowing the heart rate and reducing the force with which the heart muscles contract to pump blood. They also help keep blood vessels from constricting in the heart, brain, and body.

Blood clot
Blood clots are clumps that occur when blood hardens from a liquid to a solid. A blood clot can partly or completely block the flow of blood in a blood vessel.

Blood culture
A blood test that shows if there are bacteria in the blood and what type of bacteria exist. It helps your doctor decide which antibiotic to use to treat a bacterial infection.

Blood thinners
Blood thinners reduce the risk of heart attack and stroke by reducing the formation of blood clots in arteries and veins. There are two main types of blood thinners-anticoagulants, such as heparin or warfarin (also called Coumadin) and antiplatelet drugs, such as aspirin.

Cardiac surgery registry
A registry collects and analyzes information on certain medical topics, conditions, or procedures for hospitals or other providers. The registry then provides the hospitals or providers with information to help them improve the care they provide. A cardiac surgery registry is one example of a registry in which hospitals or providers that perform cardiac surgery can participate.

Centers for Medicare & Medicaid Services (CMS)
The federal agency that runs the Medicare program for the elderly aged and disabled. In addition, CMS works with the states to run the Medicaid program for low-income individuals. CMS works to make sure that the people in these programs are able to get high quality health care.

Centers for Medicare & Medicaid Services (CMS) National Surgical Quality Pilot
In September of 2011, CMS engaged the American College of Surgeons (ACS) to publicly report surgical outcome measures on the Hospital Compare website. Hospitals volunteering in this multispecialty surgical registry are provided with nationally validated, risk-adjusted, outcomes-based surgical quality measures. Hospitals report for one or any combination of three surgical measures—elderly surgical outcomes, colectomy outcomes, and lower-extremity bypass outcomes—collected through participation in the American College of Surgeons National Surgical Quality Improvement Program (ACS NSQIP®), a nationally validated, risk-adjusted, outcomes-based program to measure and improve the quality of surgical care in the private sector.

Certification (Medicare-certified)
State government agencies inspect health care providers, including hospitals, nursing homes, dialysis facilities and home health agencies, as well as other health care providers. These providers are certified if they pass inspection. Being certified is not the same as being accredited. Medicare or Medicaid only pays for care provided by certified or accredited providers.

Cesarean section (C-section)
A cesarean section (C-section) is the delivery of a baby through a surgical opening in the mother's lower belly area. A C-section delivery is done when it is not possible or safe for the mother to deliver the baby through the vagina.

Children's hospital
A hospital with a majority of its inpatients under the age of 18, which participates and is paid in the Medicare program as a children's hospital.

Chronic illness
An illness that persists over a long period of time.

Comorbidities
Two or more diseases that are present at the same time.

Critical access hospital (CAH)
A small facility that provides outpatient services, as well as inpatient services on a limited basis, to people in rural areas.

Computerized tomography (CT) scan
An imaging test that uses multiple x-rays to produce detailed pictures of the inside of the body (bones, organs, and other body parts).

Department of Health And Human Services (DHHS)
A federal agency that administers programs for protecting the health of all Americans, including Medicare, Medicaid, and the Children's Health Insurance Program (CHIP).

Diastolic pressure
The lowest pressure in the artery, occurring when the heart is filling with blood. In a blood pressure reading, the diastolic pressure is the second number recorded.

Elective delivery
An elective delivery is a delivery performed for a nonmedical reason. Some nonmedical reasons include wanting to schedule the birth of the baby on a specific date, living far away from the hospital, or discomfort in the last weeks of pregnancy.

Fibrinolysis, fibrinolytic drugs
Fibrinolytic drugs are "clot-busting" drugs that can help dissolve blood clots in blood vessels and improve blood flow to your heart. They are important for treating heart attacks. If you have a heart attack, your doctor may give you a fibrinolytic drug, perform a percutaneous coronary intervention (PCI), or both.

Heart attack
A heart attack, also called an acute myocardial infarction (AMI), happens when one of the heart's arteries becomes blocked and the supply of blood and oxygen to part of the heart muscle is slowed or stopped. When the heart muscle doesn't get the oxygen and nutrients it needs, the affected heart tissue may die.

Heart failure
In heart failure, the heart cannot pump enough blood through the body. The heart cannot fill with enough blood or pump with enough force, or both. Heart failure develops over time as the pumping action of the heart gets weaker. It can affect the right, the left, or both sides of the heart. Heart failure does not mean that the heart has stopped working or is about to stop working.

Hemorrhagic stroke
A hemorrhagic stroke occurs when a blood vessel in part of the brain becomes weak and bursts open, causing blood to leak into the brain. Some people have defects in the blood vessels of the brain that make this more likely.

Heparin injection
Heparin is a type of anticoagulant or "blood thinner," and is used to prevent blood clots from forming in people who have certain medical conditions or who are undergoing certain medical procedures that increase the chance that clots will form. Heparin is also used to stop the growth of clots that have already formed in the blood vessels.

Index admission
An index admission is the admission with a principal diagnosis of a specified condition that meets the inclusion and exclusion criteria for the measure.

Influenza
A serious and sometimes deadly lung infection that can spread quickly in a community. Symptoms include fever-often a high temperature of more than 102° Fahrenheit (38.9° Celsius), headache, muscle aches and pains, chills, cough and chest pain when you take a breath ("pleuritic chest pain"). Although most people recover from the illness, the Centers for Disease Control and Prevention (the CDC) estimates that in the United States more than 200,000 people are hospitalized and about 36,000 people die from the flu and its complications every year.

Influenza vaccination ("Flu Shot")
The main way to keep from getting flu is to get a yearly flu vaccination. Learn more about the flu from the Centers for Disease Control and Prevention (CDC). Hospitals should check to make sure that pneumonia patients get a flu shot during flu season to protect them from another lung infection and to help prevent the spread of influenza in the community.

Inpatient hospital services
Services you get when you're admitted to a hospital, including bed and board, nursing services, diagnostic or therapeutic services, and medical or surgical services.

International Classification of Diseases, Ninth Revision, Clinical Modification (ICD-9-CM)
The classification used to code and classify mortality data from death certificates.

Ischemic stroke
Ischemic stroke occurs when a blood vessel that supplies blood to the brain is blocked by a blood clot. Ischemic strokes may be caused by clogged arteries. Fat, cholesterol, and other substances collect on the artery walls, forming a sticky substance called plaque.

Left ventricular function assessment
A test to check how well the heart is pumping.

Long-term care hospital
Acute care hospitals that provide treatment for patients who stay, on average, more than 25 days. Most patients are transferred from an intensive or critical care unit. These hospitals provide services like comprehensive rehabilitation, respiratory therapy, head trauma treatment, and pain management.

Magnetic resonance imaging (MRI)
An imaging test that uses powerful magnets and radio waves to create pictures of the body. It does not use radiation (x-rays).

Measurement
The process of collecting data to assess performance conducted at a single point in time or repeated over time.

Medicaid
A joint federal and state program that helps with medical costs for some people with low incomes and limited resources. Medicaid programs vary from state to state, but most health care costs are covered if you qualify for both Medicare and Medicaid.

Medical imaging
Tests that create images of various parts of the body to screen for or diagnose medical conditions. Examples of medical imaging include CT Scans, MRIs, and mammograms.

Medicare Advantage Plan (Part C)
A type of Medicare health plan offered by a private company that contracts with Medicare to provide you with all your Part A and Part B benefits. Medicare Advantage Plans include Health Maintenance Organizations (HMOs), Preferred Provider Organizations (PPOs), Private Fee-for-Service Plans, Special Needs Plans, and Medicare Medical Savings Account Plans. If you're enrolled in a Medicare Advantage Plan, Medicare services are covered through the plan and aren't paid for under Original Medicare. Most Medicare Advantage Plans offer prescription drug coverage.

Medicare health plan
A plan offered by a private company that contracts with Medicare to provide Part A and Part B benefits to people with Medicare who enroll in the plan. Medicare health plans include all Medicare Advantage Plans, Medicare Cost Plans, Demonstration/Pilot Programs, and Programs of All-inclusive Care for the Elderly (PACE).

Medicare Severity-Diagnosis Related Group (MS-DRG)
The Medicare Severity - Diagnosis Related Groups (MS-DRGs) are payment groups designed for the Medicare population. Patients who have similar clinical characteristics and similar costs are assigned to an MS-DRG. The MS-DRG will be linked to a fixed payment amount based on the average cost of patients in the group. Patients can be assigned to an MS-DRG based on their diagnosis, surgical procedures, age and other information. Hospitals provide this information on their bills and Medicare uses this information to decide how much the hospitals should be paid. There may be some groups of MS-DRGs that are based on complications or comorbidities (CCs) or major complications or comorbidities (MCCs). Complications are new problems that are the result of a procedure, treatment, or illness.

Medicare-certified hospital
In order to receive any payment from either the Medicare or Medicaid programs, a hospital must meet a set of basic standards for quality of care, called "conditions of participation." Medicare-certified hospitals are reviewed periodically (every three years), either by their State Survey Agency or a CMS-approved national accreditation organization, to assure that they are continuing to provide services of acceptable quality. Accreditation is optional, but most short-term acute hospitals in the United States choose to be Medicare-certified based on accreditation by a CMS approved national accreditation organization. There are currently three CMS-approved national hospital accreditation organizations: the American Osteopathic Association/health care Facilities Accreditation Program (AOA/HFAP), Det Norske Veritas Healthcare (DNV Healthcare), and The Joint Commission (TJC).

Number of completed surveys
The "number of completed surveys" is the total number of patients who completed a survey. When at least 300 patients have completed the survey for a hospital, we can be more confident that the survey results are fully representative of patients' experiences at that hospital and are reliable for assessing the hospital's performance. However, smaller hospitals could sample all of their HCAHPS-eligible discharges but, because of their small size, still have fewer than 300 completed surveys.

Original Medicare
Original Medicare is fee-for-service coverage under which the government pays your health care providers directly for your Part A and/or Part B benefits.

Osteopathic doctor
A licensed physician who can do surgery and prescribe drugs who has training in manipulative therapy. Also called a Doctor of Osteopathy (DO).

Outpatient hospital care
Medical or surgical care you get from a hospital when your doctor hasn't written an order to admit you to the hospital as an inpatient. Outpatient hospital care may include emergency department services, observation services, outpatient surgery, lab tests, or X-rays. Your care may be considered outpatient hospital care even if you spend the night at the hospital.

Outpatient Prospective Payment System (OPPS)
Under the Outpatient Prospective Payment System (OPPS), hospitals are paid a set amount of money (called the payment rate) to provide certain outpatient services to people with Medicare.

Oxygenation assessment
Test that measures the amount of oxygen in your blood to see if you need oxygen therapy.

Patient discharge
Patients are considered "discharged" from a hospital when they are released to go home or to another health care setting, or when they die during the hospital stay.

Percutaneous coronary interventions (PCI)
The procedures called percutaneous coronary interventions (PCI), such as angioplasty and atherectomy are among those that are the most effective for opening blocked blood vessels that cause heart attacks. Doctors may perform a PCI, or give certain drugs to open the blockage, and in some cases, they may do both.

Plan of care
A written plan of care created with your physician and hospital staff. It tells what services you will get to reach and keep your best physical, mental, and social wellbeing. The hospital staff keeps your doctor up-to-date on how you are doing and updates your care plan as needed.

Pneumonia
An inflammation of the lungs caused by a viral or bacterial infection. This fills your lungs with mucus and lowers the oxygen level in your blood. Symptoms can include fever, fatigue, difficulty breathing, chills, a "wet" cough, and chest pain. For more on pneumonia, visit MedlinePlus

Pneumonia (pneumococcal) vaccination
Vaccine given to prevent pneumonia, estimated to protect against 80% of bacteria causing pneumonia.

Provider
A doctor, hospital, health care professional or health care facility.

Psychiatric hospital
A facility that provides inpatient psychiatric services for the diagnosis and treatment of mental illness on a 24-hour basis, by or under the supervision of a physician.

Quality
Quality health care is how well a doctor, hospital, health plan, or other provider of health care, keeps its patients healthy or treats them when they are sick. Good quality health care means doing the right thing at the right time, in the right way, for the right person and getting the best possible results.

Quality assurance
The process of looking at how well a medical service is provided. The process may include formally reviewing health care given to a person, or group of persons, locating the problem, correcting the problem, and then checking to see if what was done worked.

Quality Improvement Organizations (QIOs)
A group of practicing doctors and other health care experts paid by the federal government to check and improve the care given to people with Medicare.

Ratio
The amount of one thing compared to the amount of another, such as the number of combination CT scans done compared to the number of all CT scans done.

Readmissions
Patients who are admitted to the hospital for treatment of medical problems sometimes get other serious injuries, complications, or conditions, and may even die. Some patients may experience problems soon after they are discharged and need to be admitted to the hospital again. These events can often be prevented if hospitals follow best practices for treating patients.

Registry
A registry collects and analyzes information on certain medical topics, conditions, or procedures for hospitals or other providers. The registry then provides the hospitals or providers with information to help them improve the care they provide. Examples of registries in which hospitals can participate include: a multispecialty surgical registry , a nursing care registry, and a stroke care registry.

Rehabilitation hospital
A hospital that specializes in improving or restoring a patient's functional ability through therapies. Sometimes called a post-acute hospital.

Reliever medications
Relievers are medications that relax the bands of muscle surrounding the airways and are used to quickly make breathing easier.

Risk-adjusted
"Risk-adjusted" means that the measure calculations take into account how sick patients were when they went in for their initial hospital stay. When rates are risk-adjusted, it means that hospitals that usually take care of sicker patients won't have a worse rate just because their patients were sicker when they arrived at the hospital. When rates are risk-adjusted, it helps make comparisons fair and meaningful.

Risk-adjusted 30-day death (mortality) rates
The 30-day Risk-Adjusted Death (Mortality) Rates are produced using a complex statistical model, that relies on Medicare claims and enrollment information. The model predicts patient deaths for any cause within 30 days of hospital admission for heart attack or heart failure, whether the patients die while still in the hospital or after discharge. Thirty-day mortality is used because this is the time period when deaths are most likely to be related to the care patients received in the hospital. Deaths that occur outside the hospital within 30 days are included along with deaths that occur in the hospital, because some hospitals discharge patients sooner than others.

Screening mammogram
A medical procedure to check for breast cancer before you or a doctor may be able to find it manually.

Stent
A small wire tube inserted in a blood vessel by a catheter to hold open a blocked blood vessel. This is one of several procedures called a percutaneous coronary intervention (PCI) that are used to open a blocked blood vessel.

Structural measures
A structural measure reflects the environment in which providers care for patients, such as whether or not a hospital uses an electronic health record.

Survey of patients' experiences
A national, standardized survey of hospital patients about their experiences during a recent inpatient hospital stay. This is also referred to as HCAHPS (Hospital Consumer Assessment of Healthcare Providers and Systems).

Survey response rate
Tells what percentage of patients who were asked to complete the survey actually did complete it. In general, the higher this response rate percentage, the more confident we can be that the survey results for a hospital are representative of patients' experiences at that hospital and are reliable for assessing the hospital's performance.

Systemic corticosteroid
Inflammation-reducing, anti-allergic medications that affect the body as a whole.

Teaching hospital
Hospitals that train residents in approved medical, osteopathic, dental or podiatry residency programs.

The Joint Commission (JC)
An independent, not-for-profit organization that accredits and certifies a large number of health care organizations and programs in the United States. The Joint Commission's hospital accreditation program has held deeming authority since the inception of the Medicare program in 1965. The Joint Commission's mission is to continuously improve health care for the public, in collaboration with other stakeholders, by evaluating health care organizations and inspiring them to excel in providing safe and effective care of the highest quality and value.

Thrombolytic therapy
Thrombolytic therapy is the use of drugs to break up or dissolve blood clots, which are the main cause of both heart attacks and stroke.

Treatment
Something done to help with a health problem. For example, giving certain drugs and performing surgery are treatments.

Treatment options
The choices you have when there is more than one way to treat your health problem.

Venous thromboembolism (VTE)
Venous thromboembolism (VTE) is a term that includes both deep vein thrombosis and pulmonary embolism. A deep vein thrombosis (DVT) is a blood clot that forms in a vein deep in the body. A pulmonary embolism (PE) is a loose blood clot that travels to an artery in the lungs and can block blood flow.

Warfarin
A medication used to prevent blood clots from forming or growing larger in your blood and blood vessels.

Source: Medicare.gov

Regional Hospital Profile Index

2014 Title List

Visit **www.GreyHouse.com** for Product Information, Table of Contents and Sample Pages

General Reference

America's College Museums
American Environmental Leaders: From Colonial Times to the Present
An African Biographical Dictionary
An Encyclopedia of Human Rights in the United States
Constitutional Amendments
Encyclopedia of African-American Writing
Encyclopedia of the Continental Congress
Encyclopedia of Gun Control & Gun Rights
Encyclopedia of Invasions & Conquests
Encyclopedia of Prisoners of War & Internment
Encyclopedia of Religion & Law in America
Encyclopedia of Rural America
Encyclopedia of the United States Cabinet, 1789-2010
Encyclopedia of War Journalism
Encyclopedia of Warrior Peoples & Fighting Groups
From Suffrage to the Senate: America's Political Women
Nations of the World
Political Corruption in America
Speakers of the House of Representatives, 1789-2009
The Environmental Debate: A Documentary History
The Evolution Wars: A Guide to the Debates
The Religious Right: A Reference Handbook
The Value of a Dollar: 1860-2009
The Value of a Dollar: Colonial Era
This is Who We Were: A Companion to the 1940 Census
This is Who We Were: The 1920s
This is Who We Were: The 1950s
This is Who We Were: The 1960s
US Land & Natural Resource Policy
Working Americans 1770-1869 Vol. IX: Revolutionary War to the Civil War
Working Americans 1880-1999 Vol. I: The Working Class
Working Americans 1880-1999 Vol. II: The Middle Class
Working Americans 1880-1999 Vol. III: The Upper Class
Working Americans 1880-1999 Vol. IV: Their Children
Working Americans 1880-2003 Vol. V: At War
Working Americans 1880-2005 Vol. VI: Women at Work
Working Americans 1880-2006 Vol. VII: Social Movements
Working Americans 1880-2007 Vol. VIII: Immigrants
Working Americans 1880-2009 Vol. X: Sports & Recreation
Working Americans 1880-2010 Vol. XI: Inventors & Entrepreneurs
Working Americans 1880-2011 Vol. XII: Our History through Music
Working Americans 1880-2012 Vol. XIII: Education & Educators
World Cultural Leaders of the 20th & 21st Centuries

Business Information

Complete Television, Radio & Cable Industry Directory
Directory of Business Information Resources
Directory of Mail Order Catalogs
Directory of Venture Capital & Private Equity Firms
Environmental Resource Handbook
Food & Beverage Market Place
Grey House Homeland Security Directory
Grey House Performing Arts Directory
Hudson's Washington News Media Contacts Directory
New York State Directory
Sports Market Place Directory

Education Information

Charter School Movement
Comparative Guide to American Elementary & Secondary Schools
Complete Learning Disabilities Directory
Educators Resource Directory
Special Education

Health Information

Comparative Guide to American Hospitals
Complete Directory for Pediatric Disorders
Complete Directory for People with Chronic Illness
Complete Directory for People with Disabilities
Complete Mental Health Directory
Diabetes in America: A Geographic & Demographic Analysis
Directory of Health Care Group Purchasing Organizations
Directory of Hospital Personnel
HMO/PPO Directory
Medical Device Register
Older Americans Information Directory

Statistics & Demographics

America's Top-Rated Cities
America's Top-Rated Small Towns & Cities
America's Top-Rated Smaller Cities
American Tally
Ancestry & Ethnicity in America
Comparative Guide to American Hospitals
Comparative Guide to American Suburbs
Profiles of America
Profiles of... Series – State Handbooks
The Hispanic Databook
Weather America

Financial Ratings Series

TheStreet.com Ratings Guide to Bond & Money Market Mutual Funds
TheStreet.com Ratings Guide to Common Stocks
TheStreet.com Ratings Guide to Exchange-Traded Funds
TheStreet.com Ratings Guide to Stock Mutual Funds
TheStreet.com Ratings Ultimate Guided Tour of Stock Investing
Weiss Ratings Consumer Guides
Weiss Ratings Guide to Banks & Thrifts
Weiss Ratings Guide to Credit Unions
Weiss Ratings Guide to Health Insurers
Weiss Ratings Guide to Life & Annuity Insurers
Weiss Ratings Guide to Property & Casualty Insurers

Bowker's Books In Print® Titles

Books In Print®
Books In Print® Supplement
American Book Publishing Record® Annual
American Book Publishing Record® Monthly
Books Out Loud™
Bowker's Complete Video Directory™
Children's Books In Print®
El-Hi Textbooks & Serials In Print®
Forthcoming Books®
Law Books & Serials In Print™
Medical & Health Care Books In Print™
Publishers, Distributors & Wholesalers of the US™
Subject Guide to Books In Print®
Subject Guide to Children's Books In Print®

Canadian General Reference

Associations Canada
Canadian Almanac & Directory
Canadian Environmental Resource Guide
Canadian Parliamentary Guide
Financial Services Canada
Governments Canada
Health Services Canada
Libraries Canada
Major Canadian Cities
The History of Canada

Grey House Publishing | Salem Press | H.W. Wilson
4919 Route, 22 PO Box 56, Amenia NY 12501-0056

2014 Title List

Visit **www.SalemPress.com** for Product Information, Table of Contents and Sample Pages

Literature

American Ethnic Writers
Critical Insights: Authors
Critical Insights: New Literary Collection Bundles
Critical Insights: Themes
Critical Insights: Works
Critical Survey of Drama
Critical Survey of Graphic Novels: Heroes & Super Heroes
Critical Survey of Graphic Novels: History, Theme & Technique
Critical Survey of Graphic Novels: Independents & Underground Classics
Critical Survey of Graphic Novels: Manga
Critical Survey of Long Fiction
Critical Survey of Mystery & Detective Fiction
Critical Survey of Mythology and Folklore: Heroes and Heroines
Critical Survey of Mythology and Folklore: Love, Sexuality & Desire
Critical Survey of Mythology and Folklore: World Mythology
Critical Survey of Poetry
Critical Survey of Poetry: American Poetry
Critical Survey of Poetry: British, Irish & Commonwealth Poets
Critical Survey of Poetry: European Poets
Critical Survey of Poetry: European Poets
Critical Survey of Poetry: Topical Essays
Critical Survey of Poetry: World Poets
Critical Survey of Science Fiction & Fantasy Literature
Critical Survey of Shakespeare's Sonnets
Critical Survey of Short Fiction
Critical Survey of Short Fiction: American Writers
Critical Survey of Short Fiction: British, Irish & Commonwealth Poets
Critical Survey of Short Fiction: European Writers
Critical Survey of Short Fiction: Topical Essays
Critical Survey of Short Fiction: World Writers
Cyclopedia of Literary Characters
Introduction to Literary Context: American Post-Modernist Novels
Introduction to Literary Context: American Short Fiction
Introduction to Literary Context: English Literature
Introduction to Literary Context: World Literature
Magill's Literary Annual 2014
Magill's Survey of American Literature
Magill's Survey of World Literature
Masterplots
Masterplots II: African American Literature
Masterplots II: Christian Literature
Masterplots II: Drama Series
Masterplots II: Short Story Series
Notable African American Writers
Notable American Novelists
Notable Playwrights
Short Story Writers

Science, Careers & Mathematics

Applied Science
Applied Science: Engineering & Mathematics
Applied Science: Science & Medicine
Applied Science: Technology
Biomes and Ecosystems
Careers in Chemistry
Careers in Communications & Media
Careers in Healthcare
Careers in Hospitality & Tourism
Careers in Law & Criminology
Careers in Physics
Computer Technology Inventors
Contemporary Biographies in Chemistry
Contemporary Biographies in Communications & Media
Contemporary Biographies in Healthcare
Contemporary Biographies in Hospitality & Tourism
Contemporary Biographies in Law & Criminology
Contemporary Biographies in Physics
Earth Science
Earth Science: Earth Materials & Resources
Earth Science: Earth's Surface and History
Earth Science: Physics & Chemistry of the Earth
Earth Science: Weather, Water & Atmosphere
Encyclopedia of Energy
Encyclopedia of Environmental Issues
Encyclopedia of Global Resources
Encyclopedia of Global Warming
Encyclopedia of Mathematics and Society
Encyclopedia of the Ancient World
Forensic Science
Internet Innovators
Introduction to Chemistry
Magill's Encyclopedia of Science: Animal Life
Magill's Encyclopedia of Science: Plant life
Magill's Medical Guide
Notable Natural Disasters
Solar System

Health

Addictions & Substance Abuse
Cancer
Complementary & Alternative Medicine
Genetics & Inherited Conditions
Infectious Diseases & Conditions
Magill's Medical Guide
Psychology & Mental Health
Psychology Basics

Grey House Publishing | Salem Press | H.W. Wilson
4919 Route, 22 PO Box 56, Amenia NY 12501-0056

 SALEM PRESS

2014 Title List

Visit **www.SalemPress.com** for Product Information, Table of Contents and Sample Pages

History and Social Science

A 2000s in America
50 States
African American History
Agriculture in History (check)
American First Ladies
American Heroes
American Indian Tribes
American Presidents
American Villains
Ancient Greece
Bill of Rights, The
Cold War, The
Defining Documents: American Revolution 1754-1805
Defining Documents: Civil War 1860-1865
Defining Documents: Emergence of Modern America, 1868-1918
Defining Documents: Exploration & Colonial America 1492-1755
Defining Documents: Manifest Destiny 1803-1860
Defining Documents: Reconstruction, 1865-1880
Defining Documents: The 1920s
Defining Documents: The 1930s
Defining Documents: World War I
Eighties in America
Encyclopedia of American Immigration
Fifties in America
Forties in America
Great Athletes
Great Events from History: 17th Century
Great Events from History: 18th Century
Great Events from History: 19th Century
Great Events from History: 20th Century, 1901-1940
Great Events from History: 20th Century, 1941-1970
Great Events from History: 20th Century, 1971-200
Great Events from History: Ancient World
Great Events from History: Middle Ages
Great Events from History: Modern Scandals
Great Events from History: Renaissance & Early Modern Era
Great Lives from History: 17th Century
Great Lives from History: 18th Century
Great Lives from History: 19th Century
Great Lives from History: 20th Century
Great Lives from History: African Americans
Great Lives from History: Ancient World
Great Lives from History: Asian & Pacific Islander Americans
Great Lives from History: Incredibly Wealthy
Great Lives from History: Inventors & Inventions
Great Lives from History: Jewish Americans
Great Lives from History: Latinos
Great Lives from History: Middle Ages
Great Lives from History: Notorious Lives
Great Lives from History: Renaissance & Early Modern Era
Great Lives from History: Scientists & Science
Historical Encyclopedia of American Business
Immigration in U.S. History
Magill's Guide to Military History
Milestone Documents in African American History
Milestone Documents in American History
Milestone Documents in World History
Milestone Documents of American Leaders
Milestone Documents of World Religions
Musicians & Composers 20th Century
Nineties in America
Seventies in America
Sixties in America
Survey of American Industry and Careers
Thirties in America
Twenties in America
U.S. Court Cases
U.S. Laws, Acts, and Treaties
U.S. Legal System
U.S. Supreme Court
United States at War
USA in Space
Weapons and Warfare
World Conflicts: Asia and the Middle East

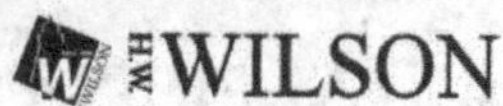
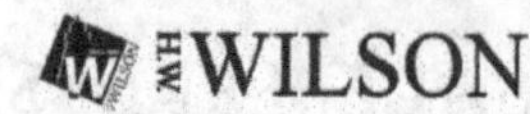

2014 Title List

Visit **www.HwWilsonInPrint.com** for Product Information, Table of Contents and Sample Pages

Current Biography
Current Biography Cumulative Index 1946-2013
Current Biography Magazine
Current Biography Yearbook-2004
Current Biography Yearbook-2005
Current Biography Yearbook-2006
Current Biography Yearbook-2007
Current Biography Yearbook-2008
Current Biography Yearbook-2009
Current Biography Yearbook-2010
Current Biography Yearbook-2011
Current Biography Yearbook-2012
Current Biography Yearbook-2013
Current Biography Yearbook-2014

Core Collections
Senior High Core Collection
Middle & Junior High School Core
Children's Core Collection
Fiction Core Collection
Public Library Core Collection: Nonfiction

Sears List
Sears List of Subject Headings
Sears: Lista de Encabezamientos de Materia

The Reference Shelf
Aging in America
Revisiting Gender
The U.S. National Debate Topic, 2014/2015
Embracing New Paradigms in education
Marijuana Reform
Representative American Speeches 2013-2014
Reality Television
The Business of Food
The Future of U.S. Economic Relations: Mexico, Cuba, and Venezuela
Sports in America
Global Climate Change
Representative American Speeches, 2012-2013
Conspiracy Theories
The Arab Spring
U.S. National Debate Topic: Transportation Infrastructure
Families: Traditional and New Structures
Faith & Science
Representative American Speeches 2011-2012
Social Networking
Dinosaurs
Space Exploration & Development
U.S. Infrastructure
Politics of the Ocean
Representative American Speeches 2010-2011
Robotics
The News and its Future
American Military Presence Overseas
Russia
Graphic Novels and Comic Books
Representative American Speeches 2009-2010

Readers' Guide
Readers Guide to Periodicals Literature
Abridged Readers' Guide to Periodical Literature
Short Story Index

Indexes
Short Story Index
Index to Legal Periodicals & Books

Facts About Series
Facts About the Presidents, Eighth Edition
Facts About China
Facts About the 20th Century
Facts About American Immigration
Facts About World's Languages

Nobel Prize Winners
Nobel Prize Winners, 2002-2013

World Authors
World Authors 2000-2005
World Authors 2006-2013

Famous First Facts
Famous First Facts, Seventh Edition
Famous First Facts About American Politics
Famous First Facts About Sports
Famous First Facts About the Environment
Famous First Facts, International Edition

American Book of Days
The American Book of Days, Fifth Edition
The International Book of Days

Junior Authors & Illustrators
Tenth Book of Junior Authors & Illustrations

Monographs
The Barnhart Dictionary of Etymology
Celebrate the World
Indexing from A to Z
Radical Change: Books for Youth in a Digital Age
The Poetry Break
Guide to the Ancient World

Wilson Chronology
Wilson Chronology of Asia and the Pacific
Wilson Chronology of Human Rights
Wilson Chronology of Ideas
Wilson Chronology of the Arts
Wilson Chronology of the World's Religions
Wilson Chronology of Women's Achievements

Book Review Digest
Book Review Digest, 2014

Grey House Publishing | Salem Press | H.W. Wilson
4919 Route, 22 PO Box 56, Amenia NY 12501-0056

LINDENHURST MEMORIAL LIBRARY